SABISTON
TEXTBOOK
of SURGERY

SABISTON
TEXTBOOK
of SURGERY

The Biological Basis of Modern Surgical Practice

17*th*
EDITION

COURTNEY M. TOWNSEND, JR., M.D.
Professor and John Woods Harris Distinguished Chairman
Department of Surgery
The University of Texas Medical Branch
Galveston, Texas

R. DANIEL BEAUCHAMP, M.D.
J. C. Foshee Distinguished Professor of Surgery
Chairman, Section of Surgical Sciences
Vanderbilt University School of Medicine
Surgeon-in-Chief
Vanderbilt University Hospital
Nashville, Tennessee

B. MARK EVERS, M.D.
Professor and Robertson-Poth Distinguished Chair in
General Surgery
Department of Surgery
The University of Texas Medical Branch
Galveston, Texas

KENNETH L. MATTOX, M.D.
Professor and Vice Chairman
Department of Surgery
Baylor College of Medicine
Chief of Staff and Chief of Surgery
Ben Taub General Hospital
Houston, Texas

ELSEVIER
SAUNDERS

**ELSEVIER
SAUNDERS**

The Curtis Center
170 S Independence Mall W 300E
Philadelphia, Pennsylvania 19106

SABISTON TEXTBOOK OF SURGERY

ISBN 0-7216-0409-9
International Edition ISBN 0-8089-2295-5
e-dition ISBN 0-7216-5368-5

NOTICE

Surgery is an ever-changing field. Standard safety precautions must be followed, but as new research and clinical experience broaden our knowledge, changes in treatment and drug therapy may become necessary or appropriate. Readers are advised to check the most current product information provided by the manufacturer of each drug to be administered to verify the recommended dose, the method and duration of administration, and contraindications. It is the responsibility of the licensed prescriber, relying on experience and knowledge of the patient, to determine dosages and the best treatment for each individual patient. Neither the publisher nor the author assumes any liability for any injury and/or damage to persons or property arising from this publication.

Library of Congress Cataloging-in-Publication Data

Sabiston textbook of surgery: the biological basis of modern surgical practice.—17th ed.
  Courtney M. Townsend Jr. ... [et al.].
    p.; cm.
  Includes bibliographical references and index.
  ISBN 0-7216-0409-9
    1. Surgery.   I. Title: Textbook of surgery.   II. Townsend, Courtney M.   III. Sabiston, David C.,
  [DNLM: 1. Surgical Procedures, Operative.   2. Perioperative Care.   3. Surgery. WO 100 T3552
2004]
RD31.S234 2004
617–dc22

2004046677

Vice President Global Surgery: Richard H. Lampert
Acquisitions Editor: Joe Rusko
Developmental Editor: Kim J. Davis
Publishing Services Manager: Tina Rebane
Project Manager: Norm Stellander
Design Coordinator: Gene Harris

Printed in the United States of America

Last digit is the print number: 9   8   7   6   5   4   3   2   1

DEDICATION

*To our patients who grant us the privilege of practicing our craft;
to our students, residents, and colleagues from whom we learn;
and to our wives—Mary, Shannon, Karen, and June—without
their support, this would not have been possible.*

REVIEWERS

The Publisher wishes to acknowledge the following individuals, who previewed advance materials from *Sabiston Textbook of Medicine*, 17th edition.

MOHAMED BAGUNEID, M.B.Ch.B., FRCS(Ed)
Executive officer, Association of Surgeons in Training, London; Specialist Registrar in General Surgery, Manchester Royal Infirmary, Manchester, UK

MICHAEL J. LAMPARELLI, FRCS(GenSurg)
Dorset County Hospital, Dorchester, Dorset, UK

John Sebastian Knight, B.Sc.(Hons), M.B.B.S.(Lon), MRCS(Eng)
Specialist Registrar in General Surgery, Dorset County Hospital, Dorchester, Dorset, UK

Guy Nash, M.D., FRCS
Resident Surgical Officer, St. Mark's Hospital, Harrow, Middlesex, UK

Andrew Renwick, M.D., FRCS
Colorectal Fellow, Concord Repatriation General Hospital, Sydney, New South Wales, Australia

CONTRIBUTORS

STEVEN A. AHRENDT, M.D.
Associate Professor of Surgery, Oncology, and Pathology, University of Rochester; Attending Surgeon and Director of Gastrointestinal Malignancy Program, Strong Memorial Hospital, Rochester, New York
Biliary Tract

FRANK G. ALBERTA, M.D.
Active Orthopaedics and Sports Medicine, Westwood, New Jersey
Emergent Care of Musculoskeletal Injuries

E. FRANCOIS ALDRICH, M.D.
Associate Professor, Department of Neurosurgery, University of Maryland Medical Center, Baltimore, Maryland
Neurosurgery

DANIEL A. ANAYA, M.D.
Resident in Surgery, University of Washington School of Medicine, Seattle, Washington
Surgical Infections and Choice of Antibiotics

RICHARD J. ANDRASSY, M.D. FACS, FAAP
Denton A. Cooley Professor and Chairman, Department of Surgery, and Executive Vice-President for Clinical Affairs, The University of Texas Health Science Center, Houston, Texas
Appendix

NIREN ANGLE, M.D.
Assistant Professor of Surgery, Section of Vascular Surgery, University of California, San Diego; Attending Surgeon, University of California San Diego Medical Center, San Diego, California
Venous Disease

PAUL S. AUERBACH, M.D., M.S.
Clinical Professor of Surgery, Division of Emergency Medicine, Department of Surgery, Stanford University School of Medicine; Attending Physician, Emergency Medicine, Stanford University Hospital, Stanford, California
Bites and Stings

CLYDE F. BARKER, M.D.
Donald Guthrie Professor of Surgery, University of Pennsylvania, School of Medicine; Attending Surgeon, Hospital of the University of Pennsylvania, Philadelphia, Pennsylvania
Transplantation of Abdominal Organs

BARBARA LEE BASS, M.D.
Professor of Surgery and Associate Chair for Research and Academic Affairs, University of Maryland School of Medicine, Baltimore, Maryland
Acute Gastrointestinal Hemorrhage

B. TIMOTHY BAXTER, M.D.
Professor of Surgery, University of Nebraska Medical Center; Staff Surgeon, Methodist Hospital, Omaha, Nebraska
The Lymphatics

R. DANIEL BEAUCHAMP, M.D.
J. C. Foshee Distinguished Professor of Surgery and Chairman, Section of Surgical Sciences, Vanderbilt University School of Medicine; Surgeon-in-Chief, Vanderbilt University Hospital, Nashville, Tennessee
Spleen

PAUL R. BEERY II, M.D.
Surgical Resident and Critical Care Fellow, Department of Surgery, The Ohio State University, Columbus, Ohio
Surgery in the Pregnant Patient

MICHAEL BELKIN, M.D.
Associate Professor, Department of Surgery, Harvard Medical School; Chief of Vascular Surgery, Brigham and Women's Hospital, Boston, Massachusetts
Peripheral Arterial Occlusive Disease

MANOOP S. BHUTANI, M.D.
Co-Director, Center for Endoscopic Research, Training and Innovation; Director, Center for Endoscopic Ultrasound; Professor of Medicine, Department of Internal Medicine—Gastroenterology, The University of Texas Medical Branch, Galveston, Texas
Esophagus

WALTER L. BIFFL, M.D., FACS
Associate Professor of Surgery and Chief, Division of Trauma and Surgical Critical Care, Brown University Medical School; Chief, Division of Trauma and Surgical Critical Care, Rhode Island Hospital, Providence, Rhode Island
Surgical Critical Care

JOHN D. BIRKMEYER, M.D.
Professor of Surgery, University of Michigan; Staff Surgeon, University of Michigan Medical Center, Ann Arbor, Michigan
Critical Assessment of Surgical Outcomes

STEVEN J. BLACKWELL, M.D.
Stephen R. Lewis, M.D., Professor of Plastic Surgery, Division of Plastic Surgery, Department of Surgery, The University of Texas Medical Branch, Galveston, Texas
Plastic Surgery

KENNETH L. BRAYMAN, M.D.
Professor of Surgery, Department of Surgery, and Director, Renal, Pancreas and Islet Transplant Program, University of Virginia Health System, Chanlottesville, Virginia
Transplantation of Abdominal Organs

MURRAY F. BRENNAN, M.D.
Professor of Surgery, Cornell University, Weill Medical College; Chairman, Department of Surgery, Memorial Sloan-Kettering Cancer Center, New York, New York
Soft Tissue Sarcomas

PHILIP M. BROWN, JR., M.D.
Assistant Professor of Surgery, East Carolina University School of Medicine; Attending, Pitt County Memorial Hospital, Greenville, North Carolina
Access and Ports

BRUCE D. BROWNER, M.D.
Chairman and Residency Program Director, Department of Orthopaedic Surgery, University of Connecticut Health Center, Farmington; Director, Department of Orthopaedics, Hartford Hospital, Hartford, Connecticut
Emergent Care of Musculoskeletal Injuries

L. MICHAEL BRUNT, M.D.
Associate Professor of Surgery, Section of Endocrine and Oncologic Surgery, Department of Surgery, Washington University School of Medicine, Barnes-Jewish Hospital, St. Louis, Missouri
The Pituitary and Adrenal Glands

BRIAN B. BURKEY, M.D., FACS
Vice Chairman for Clinical Affairs and Education, Associate Professor of Otolaryngology, and Residency Program Director, Vanderbilt University Medical Center, Nashville, Tennessee
Head and Neck

JOHN L. BURNS, M.D.
Clinical Instructor, Department of Plastic Surgery, University of Texas Southwestern Medical Center; Associate, Dallas Plastic Surgery Institute, Tom Landry Center at Baylor University Medical Center, Dallas, Texas
Plastic Surgery

PHILLIP C. CAMP, JR., M.D.
Assistant Professor, University of Kentucky; Assistant Professor, University of Kentucky Cardiothoracic Surgery, Lexington, Kentucky
Surgical Treatment of Coronary Artery Disease

RONALD A. CARSON, Ph.D.
Harris L. Kempner Distinguished Professor, The University of Texas Medical Branch; Director, Institute for the Medical Humanities, Galveston, Texas
Ethics in Surgery

ELLIOT L. CHAIKOF, M.D.
Professor, Emory University School of Medicine; Professor, Chief of Vascular Surgery Division, Emory University Hospital, Atlanta, Georgia
Endovascular Surgery

CRAIG CHANG, M.D.
Fellow in Minimally Invasive Surgery and Bariatrics, The University of Texas Southwestern Medical Center, Dallas, Texas
Minimally Invasive Surgery

LAWRENCE S. CHIN, M.D.
Associate Professor, Department of Neurosurgery, University of Maryland Medical Center, Baltimore, Maryland
Neurosurgery

WILLIAM G. CIOFFI, M.D.
J. Murray Beardsley Professor and Chairman, Department of Surgery, Brown Medical School; Surgeon-in-Chief, Rhode Island Hospital, Providence, Rhode Island
Surgical Critical Care

G. PATRICK CLAGETT, M.D.
Professor of Surgery and Chairman, Division of Vascular Surgery, University of Texas Southwestern Medical Center Dallas, Texas
Cerebrovascular Disease

JEFFREY A. CLARIDGE, M.D.
Chief Resident in Surgery, University of Virginia Health System, Charlottesville, Virginia
Acute Abdomen

RAUL COIMBRA, M.D., Ph.D.
Associate Professor of Surgery, University of California, San Diego; Associate Director of Trauma, University of California San Diego Medical Center, San Diego, California
Management of Acute Trauma

MICHAEL S. CONTE, M.D.
Associate Professor of Surgery, Department of Surgery, Harvard Medical School; Associate Surgeon, Vascular Surgery, Brigham and Women's Hospital, Boston, Massachusetts
Peripheral Arterial Occlusive Disease

CHARLES S. COX, JR., M.D.
The Children's Fund Distinguished Associate Professor of Surgery and Pediatrics, The University of Texas—Houston Medical School; Attending Surgeon, Memorial Hermann Children's Hospital, Houston, Texas
Appendix

MICHAEL D'ANGELICA, M.D.
Assistant Professor of Surgery, Cornell University Medical College; Assistant Attending, Memorial Sloan-Kettering Cancer Center, New York, New York
The Liver

R. DUANE DAVIS, JR., M.D.
Professor of Surgery, and Chief of Cardiothoracic Transplantation, Division of Cardiovascular and Thoracic Surgery, Department of Surgery, Duke University Medical Center, Durham, North Carolina
The Mediastinum

MERRIL T. DAYTON, M.D.
Professor and Chairman, Department of Surgery, State University of New York-Buffalo; Chief of Surgery, Kaleida Health, Buffalo, New York
Surgical Complications

E. PATCHEN DELLINGER, M.D.
Professor of Surgery, Department of Surgery, and Chair, Division of General Surgery, University of Washington, Seattle, Washington
Surgical Infections and Choice of Antibiotics

CHRISTOPHER J. DENTE, M.D.
Assistant Professor of Surgery, Emory University School of Medicine; Surgeon, Grady Memorial Hospital, Atlanta, Georgia
Ultrasound for Surgeons

ARTHUR J. DIPATRI, M.D.
Assistant Professor, Department of Neurosurgery, University of Maryland Medical Center, Baltimore, Maryland
Neurosurgery

GERARD M. DOHERTY, M.D.
Norman W. Thompson Professor of Surgery, Division of Endocrine Surgery, Department of Surgery, University of Michigan, Ann Arbor, Michigan
Parathyroid Glands

MICHELE A. DOMENICK, M.D.
Staff Surgeon, Kent General Hospital, Dover, Delaware
Transplantation Immunology and Immunosuppression

MAGRUDER C. DONALDSON, M.D.
Associate Professor of Surgery, Harvard Medical School; Attending, Brigham and Women's Hospital, Boston, Massachusetts
Peripheral Arterial Occlusive Disease

JAY DOUCET, M.D.
Assistant Professor of Surgery, Keck School of Medicine, University of Southern California; Attending Surgeon, Division of Trauma, Navy Trauma Training Center, LAC + USC Medical Center, Los Angeles, California
The Surgeon's Role in Unconventional Civilian Disasters

JONATHAN J. DRUMMOND-WEBB, M.B., B.Ch., FCS (SA)
Associate Professor, Department of Surgery, University of Arkansas for Medical Sciences; Chief, Pediatric Cardiac Surgery, Arkansas Children's Hospital, Little Rock, Arkansas
Congenital Heart Disease

TIMOTHY J. EBERLEIN, M.D.
Professor and Chairman, Department of Surgery, and Director, Alvin J. Siteman Cancer Center, Washington University School of Medicine; Surgeon-in-Chief, Barnes-Jewish Hospital, St. Louis, Missouri
Tumor Biology and Tumor Markers

HOWARD M. EISENBERG, M.D.
R. K. Thompson Professor and Chairman, Department of Neurosurgery, University of Maryland Medical Center, Baltimore, Maryland
Neurosurgery

E. CHRISTOPHER ELLISON, M.D.
Professor and Robert M. Zollinger Chair, Department of Surgery, The Ohio State University, Columbus, Ohio
Surgery in the Pregnant Patient

STEPHEN S. ENTMAN, M.D.
Professor, Obstetrics and Gynecology, and Chairman, Department of Obstetrics and Gynecology, Vanderbilt University School of Medicine, Nashville, Tennessee
Gynecologic Surgery

ANTHONY L. ESTRERA, M.D.
Assistant Professor, University of Texas Medical School; Attending Surgeon, Memorial Hermann Hospital, Houston, Texas
Thoracic Vasculature (with Emphasis on the Thoracic Aorta)

THOMAS R. EUBANKS, D.O.
Portland Surgical Specialists, Portland, Oregon
Hiatal Hernia and Gastroesophageal Reflux Disease

B. MARK EVERS, M.D.
Professor and Robertson-Poth Distinguished Chair in General Surgery, Department of Surgery, and Interim Director, Sealy Center for Cancer Cell Biology, The University of Texas Medical Branch, Galveston, Texas
Small Intestine; Molecular and Cell Biology

TIMOTHY C. FABIAN, M.D.
Harwell Wilson Alumni Professor and Chairman, Department of Surgery, University of Tennessee Health Science Center, Memphis, Tennessee
Spleen

SAMIR M. FAKHRY, M.D.
Chief, Trauma and Surgical Critical Care, Department of Surgery, Inova Fairfax Hospital, Falls Church, Virginia
Hematologic Principles in Surgery

MITCHELL P. FINK, M.D.
Professor, University of Pittsburgh, School of Medicine; Chair, Department of Critical Care Medicine, University of Pittsburgh Medical Center, Pittsburgh, Pennsylvania
The Role of Cytokines as Mediators of the Inflammatory Response

SAMUEL R. G. FINLAYSON, M.D., M.P.H.
Assistant Professor of Surgery and of Community and Family Medicine, Dartmouth Medical School, Hanover; Staff Surgeon, Dartmouth-Hitchcock Medical Center, Lebanon, New Hampshire
Critical Assessment of Surgical Outcomes

JOSEF E. FISCHER, M.D.
Mallinckrodt Professor of Surgery, Harvard Medical School; Surgeon-in-Chief, Beth Israel Deaconess Medical Center, Boston, Massachusetts
Metabolism in Surgical Patients

YUMAN FONG, M.D.
Professor of Surgery, Cornell University Medical College; Chief, GMT Service, and Murray F. Brennan Chair in Surgery, Memorial Sloan-Kettering Cancer Center, New York, New York
The Liver

JULIE A. FREISCHLAG, M.D.
William Stewart Halsted Professor of Surgery, Chair, Department of Surgery, and Surgeon-in Chief, Johns Hopkins Medical Center, Baltimore, Maryland
Venous Disease

DONALD E. FRY, M.D.
Professor and Chairman, Department of Surgery, University of New Mexico School of Medicine; Chief of Surgery, University of New Mexico Hospital, Albuquerque, New Mexico
Surgical Problems in the Immunosuppressed Patient; The Surgeon's Role in Unconventional Civilian Disasters

ROBERT D. FRY, M.D.
Professor of Surgery and Chief of Division of Colon and Rectal Surgery, University of Pennsylvania; Attending Surgeon, Hospital of the University of Pennsylvania, Philadelphia, Pennsylvania
Colon and Rectum

DAVID A. FULLERTON, M.D.
Professor of Surgery and Chief, Division of Cardiothoracic Surgery, Department of Surgery, University of Colorado Health Sciences Center, Denver, Colorado
Acquired Heart Disease: Valvular

PATRICIA C. FUREY, M.D.
The Orthopaedic Center, Manchester, New Hampshire
Emergent Care of Musculoskeletal Injuries

RAYMOND J. GAGLIARDI, M.D.
Assistant Professor of Surgery, Case Western Reserve University; Faculty, MetroHealth Medical Center, Cleveland, Ohio
Hernias

PAUL G. GAUGER, M.D.
Assistant Professor of Surgery, Division of Endocrine Surgery, Department of Surgery, University of Michigan, Ann Arbor, Michigan
Parathyroid Glands

PETER S. GEODEGEBUURE, Ph.D.
Research Assistant Professor of Surgery, Department of Surgery, Washington University, School of Medicine, St. Louis, Missouri
Tumor Biology and Tumor Markers

GUILLERMO GOMEZ, M.D.
Granville T. Hall Chair and Associate Professor, Department of Surgery, The University of Texas Medical Branch, Galveston, Texas
Emerging Technology in Surgery: Informatics, Electronics, Robotics

DOUGLAS GOUMAS, M.D.
The Orthopaedic Center, Manchester, New Hampshire
Emergent Care of Musculoskeletal Injuries

DARLA K. GRANGER, M.D.
Associate Professor, Department of Surgery, Wayne State University, Detroit, Michigan
Transplantation Immunology and Immunosuppression

EDWIN GRAVEREAUX, M.D.
Instructor of Surgery, Division of Vascular Surgery, Harvard Medical School; Director, Endovascular Surgery and Vascular Intervention, Brigham and Women's Hospital, Boston, Massachusetts
Peripheral Arterial Occlusive Disease

CORNELIA R. GRAVES, M.D.
Associate Professor, Department of Obstetrics and Gynecology, Division of Maternal/Fetal Medicine, and Section Chief, Maternal/Fetal Medicine, Vanderbilt University School of Medicine, Nashville, Tennessee
Gynecologic Surgery

CARL E. HAISCH, M.D.
Professor of Surgery, East Carolina University School of Medicine; Attending and Director of Surgical Immunology and Transplantation, Pitt County Memorial Hospital, Greenville, North Carolina
Access and Ports

JOHN B. HANKS, M.D.
C. Bruce Morton Professor and Chief, Division of General Surgery, Department of Surgery, University of Virginia Health Sciences Center, Charlottesville, Virginia
Thyroid

ALDEN H. HARKEN, M.D.
Professor and Chairman, Department of Surgery, University of California, San Francisco-East Bay, Oakland, California
Acquired Heart Disease: Valvular

JOHN H. HEALEY, M.D.
Professor, Orthopaedic Surgery, Weill Medical College of Cornell University; Chief, Orthopaedic Surgery, Memorial Sloan-Kettering Cancer Center, New York, New York
Primary Bone Tumors

MAARIT A. HEIKKINEN, M.D., Ph.D.
Postdoctoral Fellow, Stanford University, Stanford, California
Aneurysmal Vascular Disease

DAVID N. HERNDON, M.D.
Jesse H. Jones Distinguished Chair in Burn Surgery and Professor of Surgery, Department of Surgery, The University of Texas Medical Branch; Chief of Staff, Shriners Hospital for Children, Galveston, Texas
Burns

BRADLEY B. HILL, M.D.
Assistant Professor of Surgery, Stanford University; Vascular Surgeon, Stanford University Medical Center, Stanford, California
Aneurysmal Vascular Disease

ASHER HIRSHBERG, M.D.
Associate Professor, Department of Surgery, Baylor College of Medicine; Director of Vascular Surgery, Ben Taub General Hospital, Houston, Texas
Vascular Trauma

MICHAEL D. HOLZMAN, M.D., M.P.H.
Associate Professor, General Surgery Division, Vanderbilt University Medical Center, Nashville, Tennessee
Spleen

DAVID B. HOYT, M.D.
The Monroe E. Trout Professor of Surgery, Department of Surgery, University of California, San Diego; Interim Chairman, Department of Surgery, and Director, Trauma, Burns, and Critical Care, University of California, San Diego, Medical Center, San Diego, California
Management of Acute Trauma; The Surgeon's Role in Unconventional Civilian Disasters

JOHN P. HUNT, M.D., M.P.H.
Associate Professor of Surgery and Section Chief, Trauma/Critical Care/General Surgery, Louisiana State University Health Sciences Center; Assistant Director of Trauma, Charity Hospital, Medical Center of Louisiana, New Orleans, Louisiana
Principles of Preoperative and Operative Surgery

TAM T. T. HUYNH, M.D.
Assistant Professor, University of Texas Medical School; Attending Surgeon, Memorial Hermann Hospital, Houston, Texas
Thoracic Vasculature (With Emphasis on the Thoracic Aorta)

J. DIRK IGLEHART, M.D.
Anne E. Dyson Professor of Women's Cancers at the Harvard Medical School, Harvard Medical School; Chief of Surgical Oncology, Brigham and Women's Hospital, Boston, Massachusetts
Diseases of the Breast

SUZANNE T. ILDSTAD, M.D.
Director, Institute for Cellular Therapeutics, Jewish Hospital Distinguished Professor of Transplantation, and Professor of Surgery, University of Louisville and University of Louisville Hospital, Louisville, Kentucky
Transplantation Immunology and Immunosuppression

BARRY K. JARNAGIN, M.D.
Assistant Professor, Department of Obstetrics and Gynecology, Division of Urogynecology, Vanderbilt University School of Medicine, Nashville, Tennessee
Gynecologic Surgery

SANDEEP S. JEJURIKAR, M.D.
Suburban Plastic Surgery Associates, and Attending Surgeon, Plastic and Reconstructive Surgery, Good Samaritan Hospital, Downers Grove, Illinois
Hand Surgery

R. SCOTT JONES, M.D.
Professor of Surgery, University of Virginia School of Medicine, Charlottesville, Virginia
Acute Abdomen

CAROLYN M. KAELIN, M.D., M.P.H.
Assistant Professor of Surgery, Department of Surgery, Harvard Medical School; Director, Comprehensive Breast Health Center, Brigham and Women's Hospital, Boston, Massachusetts
Diseases of the Breast

HAROLD E. KLEINERT, M.D.
Clinical Professor of Surgery, University of Louisville School of Medicine, Louisville, Kentucky; Clinical Professor of Surgery, Indiana University-Purdue University School of Medicine, Indianapolis, Indiana
Hand Surgery

TIEN C. KO, M.D.
Chela and Jimmy Storm Distinguished Associate Professor of Surgery, Department of Surgery, and Associate Professor, Department of Human Biological Chemistry and Genetics, The University of Texas Medical Branch, Galveston, Texas
Molecular and Cell Biology

TERRY C. LAIRMORE, M.D.
Associate Professor, Endocrine and Oncologic Surgery, Washington University School of Medicine; Attending Surgeon, Barnes-Jewish Hospital, St. Louis, Missouri
The Multiple Endocrine Neoplasia Syndromes

KEVIN P. LALLY, M.D.
A. G. McNeese Professor of Surgery, The University of Texas—Houston Medical School; Attending Surgeon, Memorial Hermann Children's Hospital, Houston, Texas
Appendix

CHRISTINE L. LAU, M.D.
Cardiothoracic Surgery Fellow, Division of Cardiothoracic Surgery, Department of Surgery, Washington University School of Medicine, Barnes-Jewish Hospital, St. Louis, Missouri
The Mediastinum

MIMI LEONG, M.D.
Resident, Division of Plastic and Reconstructive Surgery, Department of Surgery, University of Texas at Houston, Houston, Texas
Wound Healing

BENJAMIN D. L. LI, M.D.
Professor of Surgery, Chief, Division of Surgical Oncology, and Co-Director, Breast and Solid Organ Cancer Program, Feist-Weiller Cancer Center, Louisiana State University Health Sciences Center-Shreveport, Shreveport, Louisiana
Abdominal Wall, Umbilicus, Peritoneum, Mesenteries, Omentum, and Retroperitoneum

UDAYA K. LIYANAGE, M.D.
Resident in General Surgery, Barnes-Jewish Hospital/Washington University School of Medicine, St. Louis, Missouri
Tumor Biology and Tumor Markers

ROBERT R. LORENZ, M.D.
Staff Physician, Section of Head and Neck Surgery, Department of Otolaryngology, Cleveland Clinic Foundation, Cleveland, Ohio
Head and Neck

JEANNE M. LUKANICH, M.D.
Instructor in Surgery, Division of Thoracic Surgery, Harvard
Medical School; Staff Surgeon, Division of Thoracic Surgery,
Brigham and Women's Hospital, Boston, Massachusetts
Chest Wall and Pleura

NAJJIA MAHMOUD, M.D.
Assistant Professor of Surgery, University of Pennsylvania;
Attending Surgeon, Hospital of the University of Pennsylvania,
Philadelphia, Pennsylvania
Colon and Rectum

MARK A. MALANGONI, M.D.
Professor of Surgery, Case Western Reserve University; Chair-
person, Department of Surgery, MetroHealth Medical Center,
Cleveland, Ohio
Hernias

JAMES F. MARKMANN, M.D., Ph.D.
Associate Professor of Surgery, University of Pennsylvania
School of Medicine; Associate Professor of Surgery, Director of
Pancreas Transplant Program, and Attending Surgeon, Hospital
of the University of Pennsylvania, Philadelphia, Pennsylvania
Transplantation of Abdominal Organs

KENNETH L. MATTOX, M.D.
Professor and Vice Chairman, Michael E. DeBakey Department
of Surgery, Baylor College of Medicine; Chief of Staff/Chief of
Surgery, Ben Taub General Hospital, Houston, Texas
Vascular Trauma

JUSTIN A. MAYKEL, M.D.
Clinical Fellow in Surgery, Harvard Medical School; Chief Resi-
dent in Surgery, Beth Israel Deaconess Medical Center, Boston,
Massachusetts
Metabolism in Surgical Patients

JOHN C. McDONALD, M.D.
Professor of Surgery, and Chancellor and Dean, Louisiana State
University Health Sciences Center-Shreveport, Shreveport,
Louisiana
*Abdominal Wall, Umbilicus, Peritoneum, Mesenteries,
Omentum, and Retroperitoneum*

ROGER B. B. MEE, M.B., CH.B., F.R.A.C.S.
Chairman, Department of Pediatric and Congenital Heart
Surgery, Cleveland Clinic Foundation, Cleveland, Ohio
Congenital Heart Disease

ROBERT M. MENTZER, JR., M.D.
Professor of Surgery, University of Kentucky; Chairman,
Department of Surgery, A. B. Chandler Medical Center,
Lexington, Kentucky
Surgical Treatment of Coronary Artery Disease

DAVID W. MERCER, M.D.
Professor of Surgery, The University of Texas Health Science
Center—Houston; Chief of Surgery, Lyndon Baines Johnson
General Hospital, Houston, Texas
Stomach

CHARLES C. MILLER, III, Ph.D.
University of Texas Medical School, Houston, Texas
*Thoracic Vasculature (With Emphasis on
the Thoracic Aorta)*

JOHN H. MILLER, M.D.
Gulfport, Mississippi
Hand Surgery

ROSS MILNER, M.D.
Assistant Professor, Emory University School of Medicine;
Assistant Professor of Surgery, Emory University Hospital,
Atlanta, Georgia
Endovascular Surgery

JEFFREY F. MOLEY, M.D.
Professor of Surgery and Chief, Endocrine and Oncologic
Surgery, Washington University School of Medicine; Associate
Director, Alvin J. Siteman Cancer Center; Attending Surgeon,
Barnes Jewish Hospital, St. Louis, Missouri
*The Pituitary and Adrenal Glands; The Multiple Endocrine
Neoplasia Syndromes*

RICHARD J. MULLINS, M.D.
Chief, Trauma/Critical Care Section; Surgeon, Division of
General Surgery; and Professor, Department of Surgery,
Oregon Health and Science University, Portland, Oregon
Shock, Electrolytes, and Fluid

ALI NAJI, M.D., Ph.D.
Professor of Surgery, University of Pennsylvania School of
Medicine; Professor of Surgery, University of Pennsylvania
Medical Center, Philadelphia, Pennsylvania
Transplantation of Abdominal Organs

ELAINE E. NELSON, M.D.
Vice Chair and Section Chief of Emergency Medicine, San Jose
Medical Center, San Jose, California
Bites and Stings

HEIDI NELSON, M.D.
Professor of Surgery, Mayo Medical School; Chair, Division of
Colon and Rectal Surgery, Mayo Clinic and Foundation,
Rochester, Minnesota
Anus

JAMES L. NETTERVILLE, M.D.
Professor and Director of Head and Neck Surgery,
Department of Otolaryngology, Vanderbilt Medical Center,
Nashville, Tennessee
Head and Neck

ROBERT L. NORRIS, M.D.
Associate Professor of Surgery/Emergency Medicine, Stanford
University; Chief, Emergency Medicine, Stanford University
Hospital, Stanford, California
Bites and Stings

BRANT K. OELSCHLAGER, M.D.
Assistant Professor of Surgery, Co-Director of Swallowing
Center, and Director of Laparoscopic Fellowship, University of
Washington, Seattle, Washington
Hiatal Hernia and Gastroesophageal Reflux Disease

TOMOMI OKA, M.D.

Resident, Brown Medical School, Providence, Rhode Island
Surgical Critical Care

J. PATRICK O'LEARY, M.D.

The Isidore Cohn, Jr. Professor and Chairman of Surgery, Louisiana State University Health Sciences Center, New Orleans, Louisiana
Principles of Preoperative and Operative Surgery

KIM M. OLTHOFF, M.D.

Associate Professor of Surgery, University of Pennsylvania School of Medicine, Philadelphia, Pennsylvania
Transplantation of Abdominal Organs

ARIA F. OLUMI, M.D.

Assistant Professor of Surgery, Harvard Medical School; Medical Director of Urologic Research, Division of Urology, Beth Israel Deaconess Medical Center, Boston, Massachusetts
Urologic Surgery

FRANK M. PARKER, JR., D.O.

Assistant Professor for Surgery, East Carolina University School of Medicine; Attending, Pitt County Memorial Hospital, Greenville, North Carolina
Access and Ports

LYNN P. PARKER, M.D.

Assistant Professor, Department of Obstetrics and Gynecology, Division of Gynecologic Oncology, Vanderbilt University School of Medicine, Nashville, Tennessee
Gynecologic Surgery

NEIL G. PARRY, M.D., FRCSC

Assistant Professor of Surgery, University of Western Ontario; General and Trauma Surgery, Critical Care, Victoria Campus, London Health Sciences Centre, London, Ontario, Canada
Ultrasound for Surgeons

CARLOS A. PELLEGRINI, M.D.

The Henry N. Harkins Professor and Chairman, Department of Surgery, University of Washington Medical Center, Seattle, Washington
Hiatal Hernia and Gastroesophageal Reflux

LINDA G. PHILLIPS, M.D.

Truman G. Blocker, Jr., M.D. Distinguished Professor and Chief, Division of Plastic Surgery, Department of Surgery, The University of Texas Medical Branch, Galveston, Texas
Breast Reconstruction; Wound Healing

IRAKLIS I. PIPINOS, M.D.

Assistant Professor, Vascular Surgery, University of Nebraska Medical Center, Omaha, Nebraska
The Lymphatics

HENRY A. PITT, M.D.

Professor of Surgery, Medical College of Wisconsin; Attending Surgeon, Froedtert Memorial Hospital, Milwaukee, Wisconsin
Biliary Tract

BRUCE M. POTENZA, M.D.

Assistant Professor of Surgery, University of California, San Diego; Assistant Professor of Surgery, University of California, San Diego, Medical Center, San Diego, California
Management of Acute Trauma

DONALD S. PROUGH, M.D.

Professor of Anesthesiology, Neurology, and Pathology and Rebecca Terry White Distinguished Chair, Department of Anesthesiology, The University of Texas Medical Branch, Galveston, Texas
Anesthesiology Principles, Pain Management, and Conscious Sedation

JOE B. PUTNAM, JR., M.D.

Professor and Chairman, Department of Thoracic Surgery, Vanderbilt University Medical Center, Nashville, Tennessee
Lung (Including Pulmonary Embolism and Thoracic Outlet Syndrome)

ROBERT V. REGE, M.D.

Professor and Chairman, Department of Surgery, The University of Texas Southwestern Medical Center, Dallas, Texas
Minimally Invasive Surgery

JEROME P. RICHIE, M.D.

Elliott C. Cutler Professor of Urological Surgery and Chairman, Harvard Program in Urology, Harvard Medical School; Chief of Urology, Brigham and Women's Hospital, Boston, Massachusetts
Urologic Surgery

LAYTON F. RIKKERS, M.D.

A. R. Curreri Professor of Surgery and Chairman, Department of Surgery, University of Wisconsin-Madison, Madison, Wisconsin
Surgical Complications of Cirrhosis and Portal Hypertension

EMILY K. ROBINSON, M.D.

Assistant Professor of Surgery, The University of Texas Health Science Center—Houston; Attending, Lyndon Baines Johnson General Hospital, Houston, Texas
Stomach

JOHN ROMBEAU, M.D.

Professor of Surgery, University of Pennsylvania; Attending Surgeon, Hospital of the University of Pennsylvania, Philadelphia, Pennsylvania
Colon and Rectum

RONNIE A. ROSENTHAL, M.S., M.D.

Associate Professor of Surgery, Yale University School of Medicine, New Haven; Chief, Surgical Service, VA Connecticut Healthcare System, West Haven, Connecticut
Surgery in the Elderly

HOWARD M. ROSS, M.D.

Assistant Professor of Surgery, University of Pennsylvania; Attending Surgeon, Hospital of the University of Pennsylvania, Presbyterian Campus, Philadelphia, Pennsylvania
Colon and Rectum

GRACE S. ROZYCKI, M.D.

Professor of Surgery, Emory University School of Medicine; Director, Trauma/Surgical Critical Care, Emory University School of Medicine, Grady Memorial Hospital, Atlanta, Georgia
Ultrasound for Surgeons

EDMUND J. RUTHERFORD, M.D.
Associate Professor of Surgery, University of North Carolina, Chapel Hill, North Carolina
Hematologic Principles in Surgery

IRA M. RUTKOW, M.D., M.P.H., Dr.P.H.
Clinical Professor of Surgery, University of Medicine and Dentistry of New Jersey-Newark, Newark; Surgical Director, The Hernia Center, Freehold, New Jersey
History of Surgery

HAZIM J. SAFI, M.D.
Professor and Chairman, University of Texas Medical School; Attending Surgeon, Memorial Hermann Hospital, Houston, Texas
Thoracic Vasculature (With Emphasis on the Thoracic Aorta)

CLARE SAVAGE, M.D.
Radiology Resident, University of Texas-Houston, Houston, Texas
Esophagus

BRUCE DAVID SCHIRMER, M.D.
Stephen H. Watts Professor of Surgery, Department of Surgery, University of Virginia Health System, Charlottesville, Virginia
Morbid Obesity

WESLEY G. SCHOOLER, M.D.
Resident Physician, Division of Plastic and Reconstructive Surgery, Department of Surgery, University of California, San Francisco, San Francisco, California
Hematologic Principles in Surgery

ABRAHAM SHAKED, M.D., Ph.D.
Professor of Surgery, University of Pennsylvania School of Medicine, Hospital of the University of Pennsylvania, Liver Transplant Program, Philadelphia, Pennsylvania
Transplantation of Abdominal Organs

EDWARD SHERWOOD, M.D., Ph.D.
Associate Professor and James F. Arens Endowed Chair, Department of Anesthesiology, University of Texas Medical Branch, Galveston, Texas
Anesthesiology Principles, Pain Management, and Conscious Sedation

SAMUEL SINGER, M.D.
Associate Professor of Surgery, Weill Medical College of Cornell University; Associate Attending, Memorial Sloan-Kettering Cancer Center, New York, New York
Soft Tissue Sarcomas

DIONNE SKEETE, M.D.
Assistant Professor of Surgery, University of Iowa, Iowa City, Iowa
Hematologic Principles in Surgery

SENG-JAW SOONG, Ph.D.
Professor of Medicine and Biostatistics, and Director of Biostatistics and Bioinformatics Unit, University of Alabama at Birmingham, Birmingham, Alabama
Melanoma and Cutaneous Malignancies

MICHAEL L. STEER, M.D.
Professor of Surgery, Anatomy, and Cellular Biology, Tufts University School of Medicine; Professor of Surgery Emeritus, Harvard Medical School; Chief of General Surgery and Vice Chairman of Surgery, Tufts-New England Medical Center, Boston, Massachusetts
Exocrine Pancreas

DAVID J. SUGARBAKER, M.D.
Richard E. Wilson Professor of Surgery, Division of Thoracic Surgery, Harvard Medical School; Chief, Division of Thoracic Surgery, Brigham and Women's Hospital; Chief, Department of Surgical Services, and Philip L. Lowe Senior Surgeon, Dana-Farber Cancer Institute, Boston, Massachusetts
Chest Wall and Pleura

T.M. SUNIL, M.S. ORTH., D.N.B. ORTH.
Christine Kleinert Fellow in Hand Surgery, Department of Surgery, University of Louisville School of Medicine, Louisville, Kentucky
Hand Surgery

NICHOLAS E. TAWA, JR., M.D., Ph.D.
Assistant Professor of Surgery (Cell Biology), Harvard Medical School; Associate in Surgery, Beth Israel Deaconess Medical Center, Boston, Massachusetts
Metabolism in Surgical Patients

JAMES C. THOMPSON, M.D.
Ashbel Smith Professor of Surgery, Department of Surgery, The University of Texas Medical Branch, Galveston, Texas
Endocrine Pancreas

COURTNEY M. TOWNSEND, JR., M.D.
Professor and John Woods Harris Distinguished Chairman, Department of Surgery, The University of Texas Medical Branch, Galveston, Texas
Endocrine Pancreas

RICHARD H. TURNAGE, M.D.
Professor of Surgery, and Chairman, Department of Surgery, Louisiana State University Health Sciences Center-Shreveport, Shreveport, Louisiana
Abdominal Wall, Umbilicus, Peritoneum, Mesenteries, Omentum, and Retroperitoneum

DOUGLAS J. TURNER, M.D.
Assistant Professor of Surgery, Division of General Surgery, Department of Surgery, University of Maryland School of Medicine, Baltimore, Maryland
Acute Gastrointestinal Hemorrhage

MARSHALL M. URIST, M.D.
Professor of Surgery and Program Co-Director, General Surgery Residency Program, University of Alabama at Birmingham, Birmingham, Alabama
Melanoma and Cutaneous Malignancies

VIKAS VARMA, M.D.
Orthopaedic Surgery Resident, The University of Connecticut Health Center, Farmington, Connecticut
Emergent Care of Musculoskeletal Injuries

YI-ZARN WANG, D.D.S., M.D.

Associate Professor of Surgery, Louisiana State University Health Sciences Center; Chief of General Surgery, Medical Center of Louisiana, New Orleans, Louisiana
Principles of Preoperative and Operative Surgery

BRAD W. WARNER, M.D.

Professor, University of Cincinnati College of Medicine; Attending Surgeon, Cincinnati Children's Hospital Medical Center, Cincinnati, Ohio
Pediatric Surgery

SHARON L. WEINTRAUB, M.D.

Assistant Professor of Clinical Surgery, Louisiana State University Health Sciences Center; Staff Surgeon, Medical Center of Louisiana, New Orleans, Louisiana
Principles of Preoperative and Operative Surgery

ANTHONY D. WHITTEMORE, M.D.

Professor of Surgery, Harvard Medical School, Chief Medical Officer, Brigham and Women's Hospital, Boston, Massachusetts
Peripheral Arterial Occlusive Disease

BRADON J. WILHELMI, M.D.

Assistant Professor, Division of Plastic Surgery, Department of Surgery, Southern Illinois University School of Medicine, Springfield, Illinois
Breast Reconstruction

COURTNEY G. WILLIAMS, M.D.

Associate Professor of Anesthesiology and Director of Pain Management, Department of Anesthesiology, University of Texas Medical Branch, Galveston, Texas
Anesthesiology Principles, Pain Management, and Conscious Sedation

STEVEN E. WOLF, M.D.

Associate Professor, Department of Surgery, and Director, Blocker Burn Unit, The University of Texas Medical Branch; Assistant Chief of Staff, Shriners Hospital for Children, Galveston, Texas
Burns

CHRISTOPHER K. ZARINS, M.D.

Chidester Professor of Surgery, Stanford University; Chief, Division of Vascular Surgery, Stanford University Medical Center, Stanford, California
Aneurysmal Vascular Disease

MICHAEL E. ZENILMAN, M.D.

Clarence and Mary Dennis Professor and Chairman, Department of Surgery, SUNY Downstate Medical Center, Brooklyn, New York
Surgery in the Elderly

JOSEPH B. ZWISCHENBERGER, M.D.

Professor of Surgery, Medicine and Radiology; Director, General Thoracic Surgery and ECMO Programs, Division of Cardiothoracic Surgery, Department of Surgery, The University of Texas Medical Branch, Galveston, Texas
Esophagus

FOREWORD

"Once you start studying medicine, you never get through with it"

Charles H. Mayo (1865–1939)

The 17th edition of *Sabiston Textbook of Surgery*, edited by Courtney Townsend, represents an historical landmark. It is the oldest continuously published surgery textbook in the English language. The long list of distinguished authors has included Christopher, Davis, Sabiston, and now Townsend. The editor-in-chief is joined by three distinguished members of the surgical community, that is, R. Daniel Beauchamp, B. Mark Evers, and Kenneth L. Mattox. They have assembled an outstanding group of diverse contributors that cross national boundaries, disciplines, age, and gender. All are well-informed and known major contributors to the fields for which they have written chapters.

The editors have employed several innovative concepts in this design. The opinions and suggestions of general surgery residents from a variety of institutions were solicited anonymously to evaluate the quality, accuracy, and relevance of the previous edition of this historical document. This novel, aggressive, and productive exercise to improve the relevance and practicality of the current edition has met with success. The editors and publisher have adopted an attitude of "customer satisfaction guaranteed," a long-established successful business concept made workable for their readership.

The co-editors have brought to this bold departure from previous editions significant clinical and research experience and important elements of balanced functionality. The 76 chapters are well focused and represent information that is useful to the practitioner, resident, and student. To keep abreast of this exploding knowledge base, the 17th edition has included expanded chapters on Critical Assessment of Outcomes, Ultrasound for Surgeons, Surgery in the Elderly, Emerging Technology, Informatics, and The Surgeon's Role in Unconventional Civilian Disasters.

Bound into each copy is a useful CD-ROM, which includes all of the figures and illustrations, all of which can be downloaded into PowerPoint™ presentations. The 17th edition of Townsend: *Sabiston Textbook of Surgery* has a website with all references linked to PubMed. This publication is a reasoned departure from the previous genre of textbooks. Theodore Billroth was correct: "It is a most gratifying sign of the rapid progress of our time that our best textbooks become antiquated so quickly."

CLAUDE ORGAN, M.D.

PREFACE

Surgery continues to evolve as new technology, techniques, and knowledge are incorporated into the care of surgical patients. Surgeons, traditional leaders in mass casualty situations, face new problems and challenges in the era of bioterrorism. Distant surgery, employing robotic and telementoring technology, has become a reality. Minimally invasive techniques are being used in almost all invasive procedures. Increased understanding of molecular genetic abnormalities has expanded the application of preemptive surgical operations to prevent cancer.

The 17th edition of the *Sabiston Textbook of Surgery* reflects these exciting changes and new knowledge; it has been extensively revised and updated to ensure that the most current information is presented. We have recruited 31 new authors for chapters that appeared in previous editions and have added 6 new chapters. The goal of this new edition is to remain the most thorough, useful, readable, and understandable textbook presenting the principles and techniques of surgery. It is designed to be equally useful to students, trainees, and experts in the field. We are committed to maintaining this tradition of excellence begun in 1936. Surgery, after all, remains a discipline in which the knowledge and skill of a surgeon combine for the welfare of our patients.

COURTNEY M. TOWNSEND, JR., M.D.

ACKNOWLEDGMENTS

We would like to recognize the invaluable contributions of Liz Cook, Kelly Lee, Karen Martin, and Steve Schuenke. Their dedicated professionalism, indefatigable efforts, and cheerful cooperation are without parallel. They did whatever was required, often on short or instantaneous deadlines, and were vital for the successful completion of the endeavor.

Our authors, respected authorities in their fields, and busy physicians and surgeons all, did an outstanding job in sharing their wealth of knowledge.

We would also like to acknowledge the professionalism of our colleagues at Elsevier: developmental editor Kim Davis, production services manager Tina Rebane, and designer Paul Fry. We would particularly thank our editor, Joe Rusko, who provided leadership and support throughout.

CONTENTS

SECTION XI
CHEST

SECTION XII
VASCULAR

SECTION XIII
SPECIALTIES IN GENERAL SURGERY

INDEX

SURGICAL BASIC PRINCIPLES

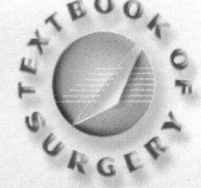

CHAPTER 1

HISTORY OF SURGERY

Ira M. Rutkow, M.D., M.P.H., Dr.P.H.

IMPORTANCE OF UNDERSTANDING SURGICAL HISTORY

It remains a rhetorical question whether an understanding of surgical history is important to the maturation and continued education and training of a surgeon. Conversely, it is hardly necessary to dwell on the heuristic value that an appreciation of history provides in developing adjunctive humanistic, literary, and philosophic tastes. Clearly, the study of medicine is a lifelong learning process that should be an enjoyable and rewarding experience. For a surgeon, the study of surgical history can contribute toward making this educational effort more pleasurable and can provide constant invigoration. Tracing the evolution of what one does on a daily basis and understanding it from a historical perspective become enviable goals. In reality, there is no way to separate present-day surgery and one's own clinical practice from the experiences of all surgeons and all the years that have gone before. For the budding surgeon, it is a magnificent adventure to appreciate what he or she is currently learning within the context of past and present cultural, economic, political, and social institutions. The active practitioner will find that the study of the profession—dealing, as it rightly must, with all aspects of the human condition—affords an excellent opportunity to approach current clinical concepts in ways not previously appreciated.

In studying our profession's past, it is certainly easier to relate to the history of "modern" surgery of the past 100 or so years than to the seemingly "primitive" practices of prior periods because the closer to the present, the more likely it is that surgical practices resemble those of nowadays. Yet, writing the history of modern surgery is in many respects more difficult than describing the development of surgery before the late 19th century. One significant reason for this is the ever-increasing pace of scientific development coapted with unrelenting fragmentation (i.e., specialization and subspecialization) within the profession. The craft of surgery is in constant flux, and the more rapid the change, the more difficult it is to obtain a satisfactory historical perspective. Only the lengthy passage of time permits a truly valid historical analysis.

HISTORICAL RELATIONSHIP BETWEEN SURGERY AND MEDICINE

Despite outward appearances, it was actually not until the latter decades of the 19th century that the surgeon truly emerged as a specialist within the whole of medicine to become a recognized and respected clinical practitioner. Similarly, it was not until the first decades of the 20th century that surgery could be considered to have achieved the status of a bona fide profession. Before this time, the scope of surgery remained quite limited. Surgeons, or at least those medical men who used the sobriquet "surgeon," whether university educated or trained in private apprenticeships, at best treated only simple fractures, dislocations, and abscesses and occasionally performed amputations with dexterity but also with high mortality rates. They managed to ligate major arteries for common and accessible aneurysms and made heroic attempts to excise external tumors. Some individuals focused on the treatment of anal fistulas, hernias, cataracts, and bladder stones. Inept attempts at reduction of incarcerated and strangulated hernias were made, and, hesitatingly, rather rudimentary colostomies or ileostomies were created by simply incising the skin over an expanding intra-abdominal mass, representing the end stage of a long-standing intestinal obstruction. Compound fractures of the limbs with attendant sepsis remained mostly unmanageable, with staggering morbidity a likely surgical outcome. Although a few bold surgeons endeavored to incise the abdomen, hoping to divide obstructing bands and adhesions, abdominal and other intrabody surgeries were virtually unknown.

Despite it all, including an ignorance of anesthesia and antisepsis tempered with the not uncommon result of the patient suffering from and/or succumbing to the effects of a surgical operation, surgery was long considered an important and medically valid therapy. This seeming paradox, in view of the terrifying nature of surgical intervention, its limited technical scope, and its damning consequences before the development of modern conditions, is explained by the simple fact that surgical procedures were usually performed only for external difficulties that required an "objective" anatomic diagnosis. Surgeons or followers of the surgical cause saw what needed to be fixed (e.g., abscesses, broken bones, bulging tumors, cataracts, hernias) and would treat the problem in as rational a manner as the times permitted. Conversely, the physician was forced to render "subjective" care for disease processes that were neither visible nor understood. After all, it is a difficult task to treat the symptoms of illnesses such as arthritis, asthma, heart failure, and diabetes, to name but a few, if there is no scientific understanding or "internal" knowledge of what constitutes their basic pathologic and physiologic underpinnings.

With the breathtaking advances made in pathologic anatomy and experimental physiology during the 18th and the first part of the 19th centuries, physicians would soon adopt a therapeutic viewpoint that had long been prevalent among surgeons. It was no longer a question of just treating symptoms; the actual pathologic problem could ultimately be understood. Internal disease processes that manifested themselves through difficult-to-treat external signs and symptoms were finally described via physiology-based experimentation or viewed pathologically through the lens of a microscope. Because this reorientation of internal medicine occurred within a relatively short time and brought about such dramatic results in the classification, diagnosis, and treatment of disease, the rapid ascent of mid-19th century "internal" medicine might seem more impressive than the agonizingly slow but steady advance of surgery. In a seeming contradiction of mid-19th century scientific and social reality, medicine appeared as the more progressive branch, with surgery lagging behind. The art and craft of surgery, for all its practical possibilities, would be severely restricted until the discovery of anesthesia in 1846 and an understanding and acceptance of the need for surgical antisepsis and asepsis during the 1870s and 1880s. Still, surgeons never needed a diagnostic and pathologic revolution in the manner of the physician. Despite the imperfection of their scientific knowledge, the pre–modern era surgeon did cure with some technical confidence.

That the gradual evolution of surgery was superseded in the 1880s and 1890s by a rapid introduction of startling new technical advances was based on a simple culminating axiom—the four fundamental clinical prerequisites that were required before a surgical operation could ever be considered a truly viable therapeutic procedure had finally been identified and understood: (1) knowledge of human anatomy; (2) a method for controlling hemorrhage and maintaining intraoperative hemostasis; (3) anesthesia to permit the performance of pain-free procedures; and (4) an explanation of the nature of infection along with the elaboration of methods necessary to achieve an antiseptic and aseptic operating room environment. The first two prerequisites were essentially solved in the 16th century, but the latter two would not be fully resolved until those ending decades of the 19th century. In turn, the ascent of 20th century scientific surgery would unify the profession and allow what had always been an art and craft to become a learned vocation. Standardized postgraduate surgical education and training programs could be established to help produce a cadre of scientifically knowledgeable practitioners. And in a final snub to an unscientific past, newly established basic surgical research laboratories offered the means of proving or disproving the latest theories while providing a testing ground for bold and exciting clinical breakthroughs.

KNOWLEDGE OF HUMAN ANATOMY

Few individuals have had an influence on the history of surgery as overwhelming as that of the Brussels-born Andreas Vesalius (1514-1564) (Fig. 1-1). As professor of anatomy and surgery at Padua, Italy, Vesalius taught that human anatomy could be learned only through the study of structures revealed by human dissection. In particular, his great anatomic treatise, *De Humani Corporis Fabrica Libri Septem* (1543), provided a fuller and more detailed description of the human anatomy than any of his illustrious predecessors. Most importantly, Vesalius corrected errors in traditional anatomic teachings propagated 13 centuries earlier by Greek and Roman authorities, whose findings were based on animal rather than human dissection. Even more radical was Vesalius' blunt assertion that anatomic dissection must be completed by physician/surgeons themselves—a direct renunciation of the long-standing doctrine that dissection was a grisly and loathsome task to be performed by a diener-like individ-

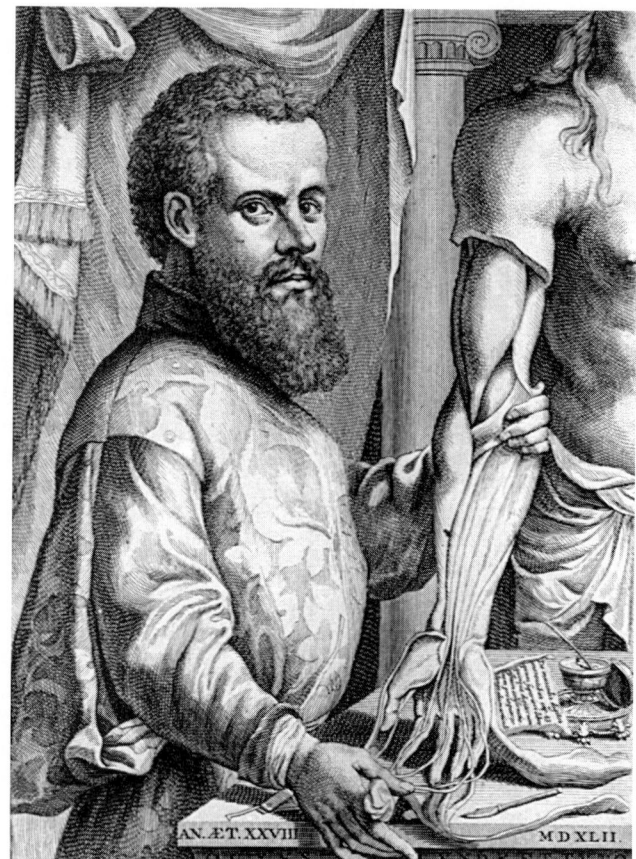

FIGURE 1-1. Andreas Vesalius (1514-1564).

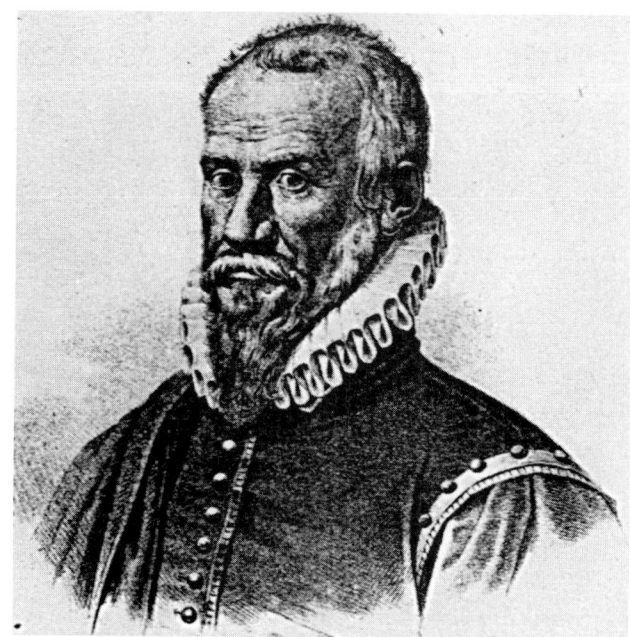

FIGURE 1-2. Ambroise Paré (1510-1590).

ual, while from on high the perched physician/surgeon lectured by reading from an orthodox anatomic text. This principle of hands-on education would remain Vesalius' most important and long-lasting contribution to the teaching of anatomy. Vesalius' Latin *literae scriptae* assured its accessibility to the most well-known physicians and scientists of the day. Latin was the language of the intelligentsia and the *Fabrica* became instantly popular, so it was only natural that over the next two centuries the work would go through numerous adaptations, editions, and revisions, although always remaining an authoritative anatomic text.

METHOD FOR CONTROLLING HEMORRHAGE

Ambroise Paré's (1510-1590) (Fig. 1-2) position in the evolution of surgery remains of supreme importance. He played the major role in reinvigorating and updating Renaissance surgery and represents the severing of the final link between surgical thought and techniques of the ancients and the push toward more modern eras. From 1536 until just before his death, Paré was either engaged as an army surgeon, accompanying different French armies on their military expeditions, or performing surgery in civilian practice in Paris. Although other surgeons made similar observations about the difficulties and

nonsensical aspects of using boiling oil as a means of cauterizing fresh gunshot wounds, Paré's employment of a less irritating emollient of egg yolk, rose oil, and turpentine brought him lasting fame and glory. His ability to articulate such a finding in multiple textbooks, all written in the vernacular, allowed his writings to reach more than just the educated elite. Among Paré's important corollary observations was that in performing an amputation, it was more efficacious to ligate individual blood vessels than to attempt to control hemorrhage by means of mass ligation of tissue or with hot oleum. Described in his *Dix Livres de la Chirurgie avec le Magasin des Instruments Necessaires à Icelle* (1564), the free or cut end of a blood vessel was doubly ligated and the ligature was allowed to remain undisturbed in situ until, as the result of local suppuration, it was cast off. Paré humbly attributed his success with patients to God, as noted in his famous motto, "Je le pansay. Dieu le guérit," that is, "I treated him. God cured him."

PATHOPHYSIOLOGIC BASIS OF SURGICAL DISEASES

Although it would be another three centuries before the third desideratum, that of anesthesia, was discovered, much of the scientific understanding concerning efforts to relieve discomfort secondary to surgical operations was based on the 18th century work of England's premier surgical scientist, John Hunter (1728-1793) (Fig. 1-3). Considered one of the most influential surgeons of all time, his endeavors stand out because of the prolificacy of his written word and the quality of his research, especially in using experimental animal surgery as a way to understand the pathophysiologic basis of surgical diseases. Most impressively, Hunter relied little on the theories of past

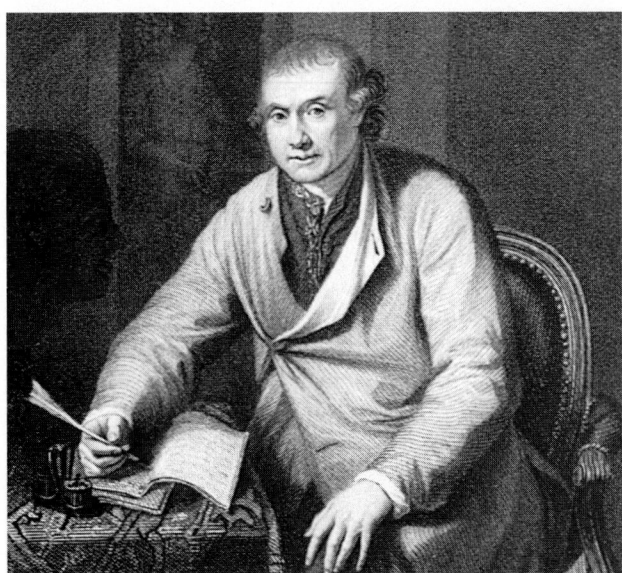

FIGURE 1-3.   John Hunter (1728-1793).

authorities but rather on personal observations, with his fundamental pathologic studies first described in the renowned textbook *A Treatise on the Blood, Inflammation, and Gun-Shot Wounds* (1794). Ultimately, his voluminous research and clinical work resulted in a collection of more than 13,000 specimens, which became one of his most important legacies to the world of surgery. It represented a unique warehousing of separate organ systems, with comparisons of these systems, from the simplest animal or plant to humans, demonstrating the interaction of structure and function. For decades, Hunter's collection, housed in England's Royal College of Surgeons, remained the outstanding museum of comparative anatomy and pathology in the world. That was until a World War II Nazi bombing attack of London created a conflagration that destroyed most of Hunter's assemblage.

ANESTHESIA

Since time immemorial, the inability of surgeons to complete pain-free operations had been among the most terrifying of medical problems. In the preanesthetic era, surgeons were forced to be more concerned about the speed with which an operation was completed than with the clinical efficacy of their dissection. In a similar vein, patients refused or delayed surgical procedures for as long as possible to avoid the personal horror of experiencing the surgeon's knife. Analgesic, narcotic, and soporific agents such as hashish, mandrake, and opium had been put to use for thousands of years. However, the systematic operative invasion of body cavities and the inevitable progression of surgical history could not occur until an effective means of rendering a patient insensitive to pain was developed.

As anatomic knowledge and surgical techniques improved, the search for safe methods to prevent pain became more pressing. By the early 1830s, chloroform,

ether, and nitrous oxide had been discovered and "laughing gas parties" and "ether frolics" were in vogue, especially in America. Young people were amusing themselves with the pleasant side effects of these compounds as itinerant "professors" of chemistry traveled to hamlets, towns, and cities, lecturing on and demonstrating the exhilarating effects of these new gases. It soon became evident to various physicians and dentists that the "pain-relieving" qualities of ether and nitrous oxide could be applicable to surgical operations and tooth extraction. On October 16, 1846, William T. G. Morton (1819-1868), a Boston dentist, persuaded John Collins Warren (1778-1856), professor of surgery at the Massachusetts General Hospital, to let him administer sulfuric ether to a surgical patient from whom Warren went on to painlessly remove a small, congenital vascular tumor of the neck. After the operation, Warren, greatly impressed with the new discovery, uttered his famous words: "Gentlemen, this is no humbug."

Few medical discoveries have been so readily accepted as inhalation anesthesia. News of the momentous event spread rapidly throughout the United States and Europe: A new era in the history of surgery had begun. Within a few months after the first public demonstration in Boston, ether was used in hospitals throughout the world. Yet, no matter how much it contributed to the relief of pain during surgical operations and decreased the surgeon's angst, the discovery did not immediately further the scope of elective surgery. Such technical triumphs awaited the recognition and acceptance of antisepsis and asepsis. Anesthesia helped make the illusion of surgical cures more seductive, but it could not bring forth the final prerequisite: all-important hygienic reforms.

Still, by the mid-19th century, both doctors and patients were coming to hold surgery in relatively high regard for its pragmatic appeal, technologic virtuosity, and unambiguously measurable results. After all, surgery appeared to some a mystical craft. To be allowed to consensually cut into another human's body, to gaze at the depth of that person's suffering, and to excise the demon of disease seemed an awesome responsibility. Yet, it was this very mysticism, long associated with religious overtones, that so fascinated the public and their own feared but inevitable date with a surgeon's knife. Surgeons had finally begun to view themselves as combining art and nature, essentially assisting nature in its continual process of destruction and rebuilding. This regard for the natural would spring from the eventual, although preternaturally slow, understanding and use of Joseph Lister's (1827-1912) techniques (Fig. 1-4).

ANTISEPSIS, ASEPSIS, AND UNDERSTANDING THE NATURE OF INFECTION

In many respects, the recognition of antisepsis and asepsis was a more important event in the evolution of surgical history than was the advent of inhalation anesthesia. There was no arguing that the deadening of pain permitted a surgical operation to be conducted in a more efficacious manner. Haste was no longer of prime concern.

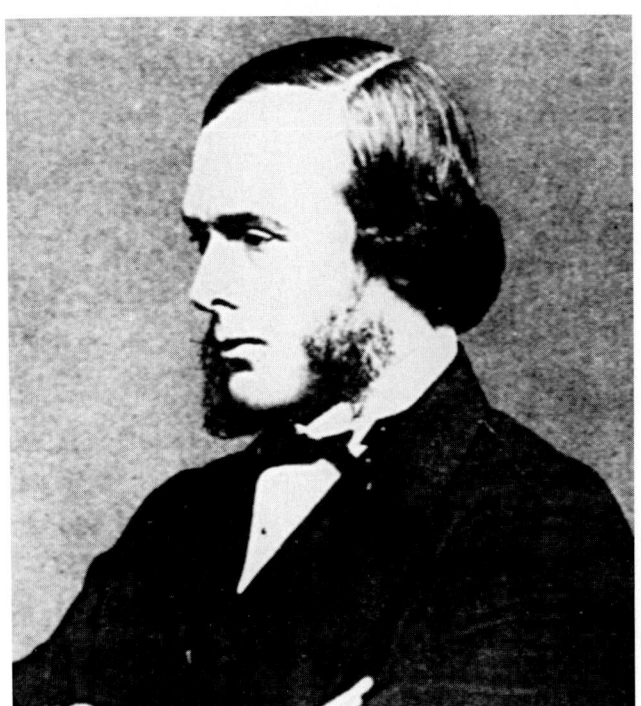

FIGURE 1-4. Joseph Lister (1827-1912).

He did not emphasize hand scrubbing but merely dipped his fingers into a solution of phenol and corrosive sublimate. Lister was incorrectly convinced that scrubbing created crevices in the palms of the hands where bacteria would proliferate. A second important advance by Lister was the development of sterile absorbable sutures. He believed that much of the deep suppuration found in wounds was created by previously contaminated silk ligatures. Lister evolved a carbolized catgut suture that was better than any previously produced. He was able to cut short the ends of the ligature, thereby closing the wound tightly, and eliminate the necessity of bringing the ends of the suture out through the incision, a surgical practice that had persisted since the days of Paré.

The acceptance of listerism was an uneven and distinctly slow process. There were many reasons for this. First, the various procedural changes Lister made during the evolution of his methodology created confusion. Second, listerism, as a technical exercise, was complicated with the use of carbolic acid, an unpleasant and time-consuming nuisance. Third, various early attempts to use antisepsis in surgery had proved abject failures, with many leading surgeons unable to replicate Lister's generally good results. Finally, and most important, the acceptance of listerism depended entirely on an understanding and ultimate recognition of the veracity of the germ theory, a hypothesis that many practical-minded surgeons were loath to accept.

As a professional group, German-speaking surgeons would be the first to grasp the importance of bacteriology and the germ theory. Consequently, they were among the earliest to expand on Lister's message of antisepsis, with his spray being discarded in favor of boiling and use of the autoclave. The availability of heat sterilization engendered sterile aprons, drapes, instruments, and sutures. Similarly, the use of face masks, gloves, hats, and operating gowns also naturally evolved. By the mid 1890s, less clumsy aseptic techniques had found their way into most European surgical amphitheaters and were coming near to total acceptance by American surgeons. Any lingering doubts about the validity and significance of the momentous concepts Lister had put forth were eliminated on the battlefields of World War I. There the importance of just plain antisepsis became an invaluable lesson for scalpel bearers, whereas the exigencies of the battlefield helped bring about the final maturation and equitable standing of surgery and surgeons within the worldwide medical community.

However, if anesthesia had never been conceived, a surgical procedure could still be performed, albeit with much difficulty. Such was not the case with listerism. Without antisepsis and asepsis, major surgical operations more than likely ended in death rather than just pain. Clearly, surgery needed both anesthesia and antisepsis, but in terms of overall importance, antisepsis proved of greater singular impact.

In the long evolution of world surgery, the contributions of several individuals stand out as being preeminent. Lister, an English surgeon, can be placed on such a select list because of his monumental efforts to introduce systematic, scientifically based antisepsis in the treatment of wounds and the performance of surgical operations. He pragmatically applied others' research into fermentation and microorganisms to the world of surgery by devising a means of preventing surgical infection and securing its adoption by a skeptical profession.

It was evident to Lister that a method of destroying bacteria by excessive heat could not be applied to a surgical patient. He turned, instead, to chemical antisepsis and, after experimenting with zinc chloride and the sulfites, decided on carbolic acid. By 1865, Lister was instilling pure carbolic acid into wounds and onto dressings. He would eventually make numerous modifications in the technique of the dressings, the manner of applying and retaining them, and the choice of antiseptic solutions of varying concentrations. Although the carbolic acid spray remains the best remembered of his many contributions, it was eventually abandoned in favor of other germicidal substances. Lister not only used carbolic acid in the wound and on dressings but also went so far as to spray it in the atmosphere around the operative field and table.

X-RAYS

Especially prominent among other late 19th century discoveries that had an enormous impact on the evolution of surgery was research conducted by Wilhelm Roentgen (1845-1923), leading to his 1895 elucidation of x-rays. Having grown interested in the phosphorescence from metallic salts that were exposed to lights, Roentgen made a chance observation when passing a current through a vacuum tube, noticing a greenish glow coming from a screen on a shelf 9 feet away. This strange effect continued after the current was turned off. He found that the screen had been painted with a phosphorescent substance. Proceeding with full experimental vigor, Roentgen soon realized that there were "invisible" rays capable of passing through solid objects made of wood, metal, and other materials. Most significant, these rays also penetrated the soft parts of the body in such a manner that the more dense bones of his hand were able to be revealed on a specially treated photographic plate. In a short time, numerous applications were developed as surgeons rapidly applied the new discovery to the diagnosis and location of fractures and dislocations and the removal of foreign bodies.

TURN OF THE 20TH CENTURY

By the late 1890s, the interactions of political, scientific, socioeconomic, and technical factors set the stage for what would become a spectacular showcasing of surgery's newfound prestige and accomplishments. Surgeons were finally wearing antiseptic-looking white coats. Patients and tables were draped in white, and basins for bathing instruments in bichloride solution abounded. Suddenly all was clean and tidy, with the conduct of the surgical operation no longer a haphazard affair. This reformation would be successful not because surgeons had fundamentally changed but because medicine and its relationship to scientific inquiry had been irrevocably altered. Sectarianism and quackery, the consequences of earlier medical dogmatism, would no longer be tenable within the confines of scientific truth.

With all four fundamental clinical prerequisites in place by the turn of the century and highlighted with the emerging clinical triumphs of various English surgeons including Robert Tait (1845-1899), William Macewen (1848-1924), and Frederick Treves (1853-1923); German-speaking surgeons, among whom were Theodor Billroth (1829-1894) (Fig. 1-5), Theodor Kocher (1841-1917) (Fig. 1-6), Friedrich Trendelenburg (1844-1924), and Johann von Mikulicz-Radecki (1850-1905); French surgeons, including Jules Peán (1830-1898), Just Lucas-Championière (1843-1913), and Marin-Theodore Tuffiér (1857-1929); the Italians, most notably Eduardo Bassini (1844-1924) and Antonio Ceci (1852-1920); and several American surgeons, exemplified by William Williams Keen (1837-1932), Nicholas Senn (1844-1908), and John Benjamin Murphy (1857-1916), scalpel wielders had essentially explored all cavities of the human body. Nonetheless, surgeons retained a lingering sense of professional and social discomfort and continued to be pejoratively described by nouveau "scientific" physicians as "nonthinkers" who worked in little more than an inferior and crude manual craft.

It was becoming increasingly evident that research models, theoretical concepts, and valid clinical applications would be necessary to demonstrate the scientific basis of surgery to a wary public. The effort to devise new operative methods called for an even greater reliance on experimental surgery and an absolute encouragement of it by all concerned parties. Most importantly, a scientific

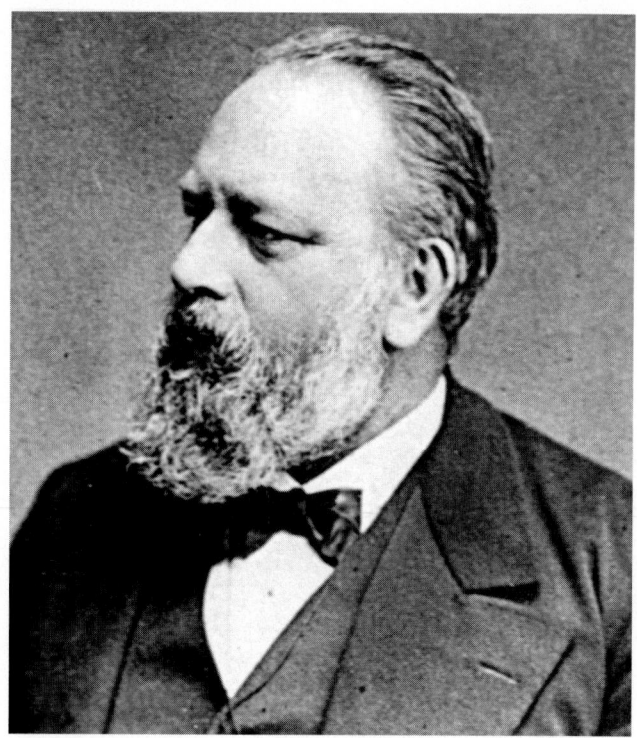

FIGURE 1-5. Theodor Billroth (1829-1894).

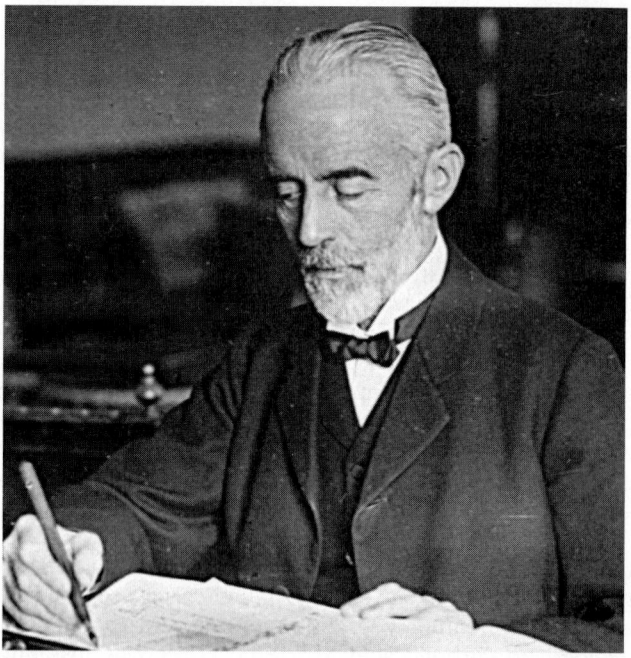

FIGURE 1-6. Theodor Kocher (1841-1917).

basis for therapeutic surgical recommendations—consisting of empirical data, collected and analyzed according to nationally and internationally accepted rules and set apart from individual authoritative assumptions—would have to be developed. In contrast with previously unexplainable doctrines, scientific research would triumph as the final arbiter between valid and invalid surgical therapies.

In turn, surgeons had no choice but to allay society's fear of the surgical unknown by presenting surgery as an accepted part of a newly established medical armamentarium. This would not be an easy task. The immediate consequences of surgical operations, such as discomfort and associated complications, were often of more concern to patients than was the positive knowledge that an operation could eliminate potentially devastating disease processes. Accordingly, the most consequential achievement by surgeons during the early 20th century was assuring the social acceptability of surgery as a legitimate scientific endeavor and the surgical operation as a therapeutic necessity.

ASCENT OF SCIENTIFIC SURGERY

William Stewart Halsted (1852-1922) (Fig. 1-7), more than any other surgeon, set the scientific tone for this most important period in surgical history. He moved surgery from the melodramatics of the 19th century operating "theater" to the starkness and sterility of the modern operating "room," commingled with the privacy and soberness of the research laboratory. As professor of surgery at the newly opened Johns Hopkins Hospital and School of Medicine, Halsted proved a complex personality, but the impact of this aloof and reticent man would become widespread. He introduced a "new" surgery, showing that research based on anatomic, pathologic, and physiologic principles and employing animal experimentation made it possible to develop sophisticated operative procedures and perform them clinically with outstanding results.

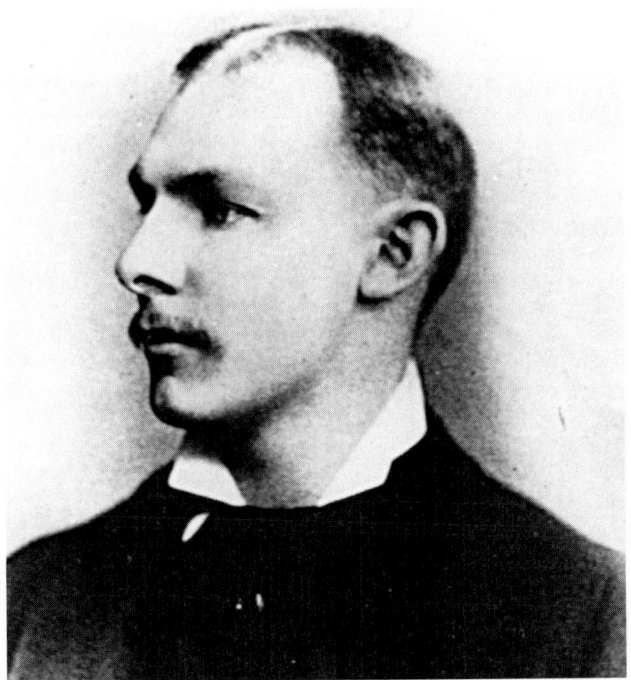

FIGURE 1-7. William Halsted (1852-1922).

Halsted proved, to an often leery profession and public, that an unambiguous sequence could be constructed from the laboratory of basic surgical research to the clinical operating room. Most importantly, for surgery's own self-respect, he demonstrated during this turn-of-the-century renaissance in medical education that departments of surgery could command a faculty whose stature was equal in importance and prestige to that of other more academic or research-oriented fields such as anatomy, bacteriology, biochemistry, internal medicine, pathology, and physiology.

As a single individual, Halsted developed and disseminated a different system of surgery so characteristic that it was referred to as a *school of surgery.* More to the point, Halsted's methods revolutionized the world of surgery and earned his work the epithet *halstedian principles,* which remains a widely acknowledged and accepted scientific imprimatur. Halsted subordinated technical brilliance and speed of dissection to a meticulous and safe, albeit sometimes slow, performance. As a direct result, Halsted's effort did much to bring about surgery's self-sustaining transformation from therapeutic subservience to clinical necessity.

Despite his demeanor as a professional recluse, Halsted's clinical and research achievements were overwhelming in number and scope. His residency system of training surgeons was not merely the first such program of its kind; it was unique in its primary purpose. Above all other concerns, Halsted desired to establish a school of surgery that would eventually disseminate throughout the surgical world the principles and attributes he considered sound and proper. His aim was to train able surgical teachers, not merely competent operating surgeons. There is little doubt that Halsted achieved his stated goal of producing "not only surgeons but surgeons of the highest type, men who will stimulate the first youth of our country to study surgery and to devote their energies and their lives to raising the standards of surgical science." So fundamental were his contributions that without them, surgery might never have fully developed and could have remained mired in a quasi-professional state.

The heroic and dangerous nature of surgery seemed appealing in less scientifically sophisticated times. But now, surgeons were courted for personal attributes beyond their unmitigated technical boldness. A trend toward hospital-based surgery was increasingly evident, owing in equal parts to new, technically demanding operations and to modern hospital physical structures within which surgeons could work more effectively. The increasing complexity and effectiveness of aseptic surgery, the diagnostic necessity of the x-ray and clinical laboratory, the convenience of 24-hour nursing, and the availability of capable surgical residents living within a hospital were making the hospital operating room the most plausible and convenient place for a surgical operation to be completed.

It was obvious to both hospital superintendents and the whole of medicine that acute-care institutions were becoming a necessity more for the surgeon than for the physician. As a consequence, increasing numbers of hospitals went to great lengths to supply their surgical staffs with the finest facilities in which to complete operations. For centuries, surgical operations had been performed under the illumination of sunlight and/or candles. Now, however, electric lights installed in operating rooms offered a far more reliable and unwavering source of illumination. Surgery became a more proficient craft because surgical operations could be completed on stormy summer mornings as well as wet winter afternoons.

INTERNATIONALIZATION, SURGICAL SOCIETIES, AND JOURNALS

As the sophistication of surgery grew, internationalization became one of its underlying themes, with surgeons crossing the great oceans to visit and learn from one another. Halsted and Hermann Küttner (1870-1932), director of the surgical clinic in Breslau, Germany (now known as Wroclaw and located in southwestern Poland), instituted the first known official exchange of surgical residents in 1914. This experiment in surgical education was meant to underscore the true international spirit that had engulfed surgery. Halsted firmly believed that young surgeons achieved greater clinical maturity by observing the practice of surgery in other countries as well as in their own.

An inevitable formation of national and international surgical societies and the emergence and development of periodicals devoted to surgical subjects proved important adjuncts to the professionalization process of surgery. For the most part, professional societies began as a method of providing mutual improvement via personal interaction with surgical peers and the publication of presented papers. Unlike surgeons of earlier centuries, who were known to closely guard "trade secrets," members of these new organizations were emphatic about publishing transactions of their meetings. In this way, not only would their surgical peers read of their clinical accomplishments but also a written record was established to be circulated throughout the world of medicine.

The first of these surgical societies was the Académie Royale de Chirurgie in Paris, with its *Mémoires* appearing sporadically from 1743 through 1838. Of 19th century associations, the most prominent published proceedings were the *Mémoires* and *Bulletins* of the Société de Chirurgie of Paris (1847), the *Verhandlungen* of the Deutsche Gesellschaft für Chirurgie (1872), and the *Transactions* of the American Surgical Association (1883). No surgical association that published professional reports existed in 19th century Great Britain, and the Royal Colleges of Surgeons of England, Ireland, and Scotland never undertook such projects. Although textbooks, monographs, and treatises had always been the mainstay of medical writing, the introduction of monthly journals, including August Richter's (1742-1812) *Chirurgische Bibliothek* (1771), Joseph Malgaigne's (1806-1865) *Journal de Chirurgie* (1843), Bernard Langenbeck's (1810-1887) *Archiv für Klinische Chirurgie* (1860), and Lewis Pilcher's (1844-1917) *Annals of Surgery* (1885), had a tremendous impact on the updating and continuing education of surgeons.

WORLD WAR I

Austria-Hungary and Germany continued as the dominating forces in world surgery until World War I. However, results of the conflict proved disastrous to the central powers (Austria-Hungary, Bulgaria, Germany, and the Ottoman Empire) and especially German-speaking surgeons. Europe took on a new social and political look, with the demise of Germany's status as the world leader in surgery a sad but foregone conclusion. As with most armed conflicts, because of the massive human toll, especially battlefield injuries, tremendous strides were made in multiple areas of surgery. Undoubtedly, the greatest surgical achievement was in the treatment of wound infection. Trench warfare in soil contaminated by decades of cultivation and animal manure made every wounded soldier a potential carrier of any number of pathogenic bacilli. On the battlefront, sepsis was inevitable. Most attempts to maintain aseptic technique proved inadequate, but the treatment of infected wounds by antisepsis was becoming a pragmatic reality.

Surgeons experimented with numerous antiseptic solutions and various types of surgical dressing. A principle of wound treatment applied by means of débridement and irrigation eventually evolved. Henry Dakin (1880-1952), an English chemist, and Alexis Carrel (1873-1944) (Fig. 1-8), the Nobel prize-winning French American surgeon, were the principal protagonists in the development of this extensive system of wound management. In addition to successes with wound sterility, surgical advances were made in the use of x-rays in the diagnosis of battlefield injuries, and remarkable operative ingenuity was evident in reconstructive facial surgery and the treatment of fractures resulting from gunshot wounds.

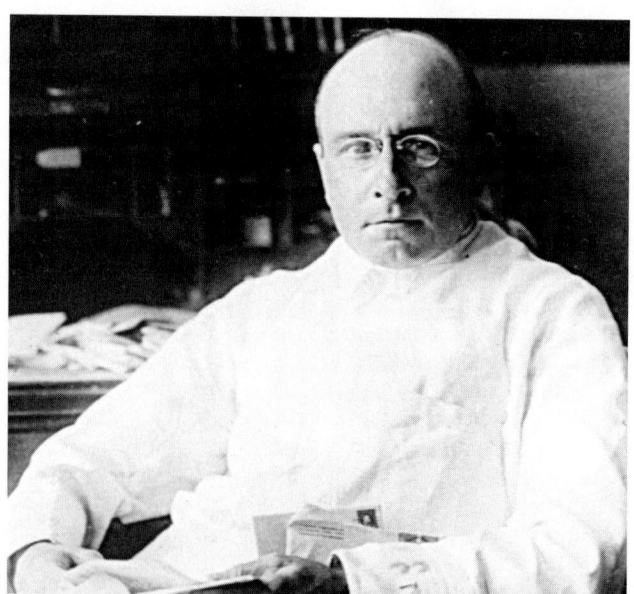

FIGURE 1-8. Alexis Carrel (1873-1944).

AMERICAN COLLEGE OF SURGEONS

For American surgeons, the years just before World War I were a time of active coalescence into various social and educational organizations. The most important and influential of these societies was the American College of Surgeons, founded by Franklin Martin (1857-1935), a Chicago-based gynecologist, in 1913. Patterned after the Royal Colleges of Surgeons of England, Ireland, and Scotland, the American College of Surgeons established professional, ethical, and moral standards for every graduate in medicine who practiced in surgery and conferred the designation *Fellow of the American College of Surgeons* (FACS) on its members. From the outset, its primary aim was the continuing education of surgical practitioners. Accordingly, the requirements for fellowship were always related to the educational opportunities of the period. In 1914, an applicant had to be a licensed graduate of medicine, receive the backing of three fellows, and be endorsed by his local credentials committee.

In view of the stipulated peer recommendations, many practitioners, realistically or not, viewed the American College of Surgeons as an elitist organization. With an obvious "blackball" system built into the membership requirements, there was a difficult-to-deny belief that many surgeons, who were immigrants, females, or members of particular religious and racial minorities, were granted fellowships sparingly. Such inherent bias, in addition to questionable accusations of fee-splitting along with unbridled contempt of certain surgeons' business practices, resulted in some very prominent American surgeons never being permitted the "privilege" of membership.

The 1920s and beyond proved a prosperous time for American society and its surgeons. After all, the history of world surgery in the 20th century is more a tale of American triumphs than it ever was in the 18th or 19th centuries. Physicians' incomes dramatically increased and surgeons' prestige, aided by the ever-mounting successes of medical science, became securely established in American culture. Still, a noticeable lack of standards and regulations in surgical specialty practice became a serious concern to leaders in the profession. The difficulties of World War I had greatly accentuated this realistic need for specialty standards when many of the physicians who were self-proclaimed surgical specialists were found to be unqualified by military examining boards. In ophthalmology, for example, over 50% of tested individuals were deemed unfit to treat diseases of the eye.

There was an unmistakable reality that there were no established criteria with which to distinguish the well-qualified ophthalmologist from the "upstart" optometrist or to clarify the differences in clinical expertise between the well-trained, full-time ophthalmologic specialist and the inadequately trained, part-time "general practitioner/ophthalmologist." In recognition of the gravity of the situation, the self-patrolling concept of a professional examining board, sponsored by leading voluntary ophthalmologic organizations, was proposed as a mechanism for certifying competency. In 1916, uniform standards and regulations were set forth in the form of minimal educational requirements and written and oral examinations, and the American Board for Ophthalmic Examinations, the country's first, was formally incorporated. By 1940, six additional surgical specialty boards were established, including orthopaedic (1934), colon and rectal (1934), urology (1935), plastic (1937), surgery (1937), and neurologic (1940).

As order was introduced into surgical specialty training and the process of certification matured, it was apparent that the continued growth of residency programs carried important implications for the future structure of medical practice and the social relations of medicine to overall society. Professional power had been consolidated, and specialization, which had been evolving since the time of the Civil War, was now recognized as an essential if not integral part of modern medicine. Although the creation of surgical specialty boards was justified under the broad imprimatur of raising the educational status and evaluating the clinical competency of specialists, board certification undeniably began to restrict entry into the specialties.

As the specialties evolved, the political influence and cultural authority enjoyed by the profession of surgery were growing. This socioeconomic strength was most prominently expressed in reform efforts directed toward the modernization and standardization of America's hospital system. Any vestiges of "kitchen surgery" had essentially disappeared, and other than numerous small private hospitals predominantly constructed by surgeons for their personal use, the only facilities where major surgery could be adequately conducted and postoperative patients appropriately cared for were the well-equipped and physically impressive modern hospitals. For this reason, the American College of Surgeons and its expanding list of fellows had a strong motive to ensure that America's hospital system was as up to date and efficient as possible.

On an international level, surgeons were confronted with the lack of any formal organizational body. Not until the International College of Surgeons was founded in 1935 in Geneva would such a society exist. At its inception, the International College was intended to serve as a liaison to the existing colleges and surgical societies in the various countries of the world. However, its goals of elevating the art and science of surgery, creating greater understanding among the surgeons of the world, and affording a means of international postgraduate study never came to full fruition, in part because the American College of Surgeons adamantly opposed the establishment, and continues to do so, of a viable American chapter of the International College of Surgeons.

WOMEN SURGEONS

One of the many overlooked areas of surgical history concerns the involvement of women. Until recent times, women's options for obtaining advanced surgical training were severely restricted. The major reason was that through the mid-20th century, only a handful of women had performed enough surgery to become skilled mentors. Without role models and with limited access to hospital positions, the ability of the few practicing female physicians to specialize in surgery seemed an impossibility. Consequently, women surgeons were forced to utilize different career strategies than men and to have more divergent goals of personal success to achieve professional satisfaction. Despite these difficulties and through the determination and aid of several enlightened male surgeons, most notably William Byford (1817-1890) of Chicago and William Keen of Philadelphia, a small cadre of female surgeons did exist in late 19th century America. Mary Dixon Jones (1828-1908), Emmeline Horton Cleveland (1829-1878), Mary Harris Thompson (1829-1895), Anna Elizabeth Broomall (1847-1931), and Marie Mergler (1851-1901) would act as a nidus toward greater equality of the genders in 20th century surgery.

AFRICAN AMERICAN SURGEONS

There is little disputing the fact that both gender and racial bias have affected the evolution of surgery. Every aspect of society is affected by such discrimination, and African Americans, like women, were innocent victims of injustices that forced them into never-ending struggles to attain competency in surgery. As early as 1868, a department of surgery was established at Howard University. However, the first three chairmen were all white Anglo-Saxon Protestants. Not until Austin Curtis was appointed professor of surgery in 1928 did the department have its first African American head. Like all black physicians of his era, he was forced to train at "Negro" hospitals, in Curtis' case Provident Hospital in Chicago, where he came under the tutelage of Daniel Hale Williams (1858-1931), the most influential and highly regarded of early African American surgeons. In 1897, Williams received considerable notoriety when he reported a successful suturing of the pericardium for a stab wound of the heart.

With little likelihood of obtaining membership in the American Medical Association or its related societies, in 1895, African American physicians joined together to form the National Medical Association. Black surgeons identified an even more specific need when the Surgical Section of the National Medical Association was opened in 1906. These National Medical Association surgical clinics, which preceded the Clinical Congress of Surgeons of North America, the forerunner to the annual congress of the American College of Surgeons, by almost half a decade, represented the earliest instances of organized "show-me" surgical education in the United States.

Admittance to surgical societies and attainment of specialty certification were important social and psychological accomplishments for early African American surgeons. When Daniel Williams was named a Fellow of the American College of Surgeons in 1913, the news spread rapidly throughout the African American surgical community. Still, African American surgeons' fellowship applications were often acted on rather slowly, which suggested that denials based on race were clandestinely conducted throughout much of the country. As late as the mid 1940s, Charles Drew (1904-1950) (Fig. 1-9), chairman of the department of surgery at Howard University School

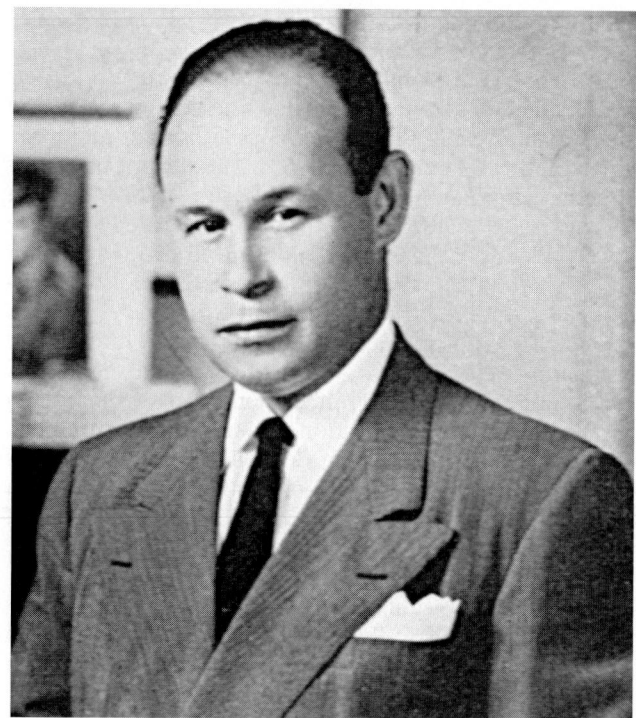

FIGURE 1-9.   Charles Drew (1904-1950).

of Medicine, acknowledged that he refused to accept membership in the American College of Surgeons because this "nationally representative" surgical society had, in his opinion, not yet begun to freely accept capable and well-qualified African American surgeons.

MODERN ERA

Despite World War I's aftermath of a global economic depression, the 1920s and 1930s signaled the ascent of American surgery to its current position of international leadership. Highlighted by educational reforms in its medical schools, Halsted's redefinition of surgical residency programs, and the growth of surgical specialties, the stage was set for the blossoming of scientific surgery. Basic surgical research became an established reality as George Crile (1864-1943), Alfred Blalock (1899-1964) (Fig. 1-10), Dallas Phemister (1882-1951), and Charles Huggins (1901-1997) became world-renowned "surgeon-scientists."

Much as the ascendancy of the surgeon-scientist brought about changes in the way in which the public and the profession viewed surgical research, the introduction of increasingly sophisticated technologies had an enormous impact on the practice of surgery. Throughout the evolution of surgery, the practice of surgery—the art, the craft, and finally, the science of working with one's hands—had been largely defined by its tools. From crude flint instruments of ancient peoples, through the simple tonsillotomes and lithotrites of the 19th century, up to the increasingly complex surgical instruments developed in

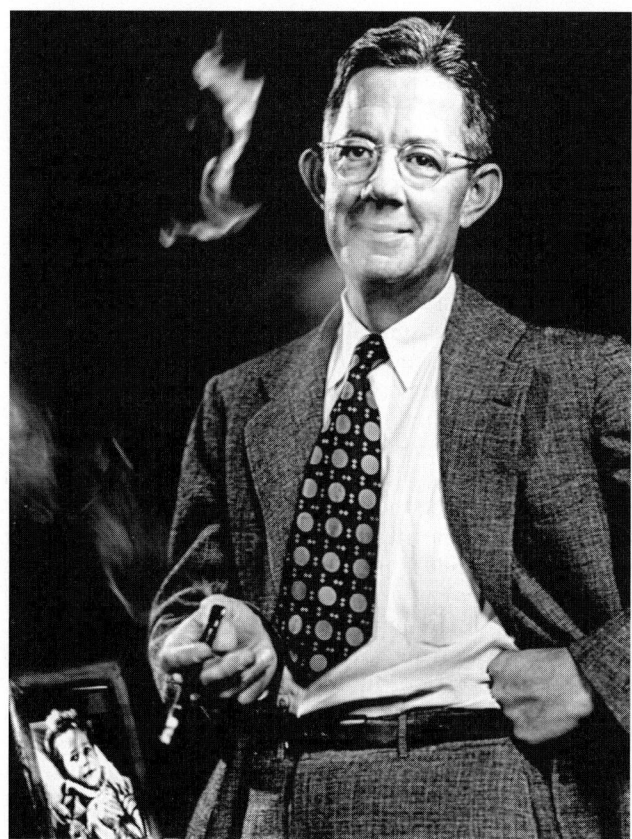

FIGURE 1-10. Alfred Blalock (1899-1964).

the 20th century, new and improved instruments usually led to a better surgical result. Progress in surgical instrumentation and surgical techniques went hand in hand.

Surgical techniques would, of course, become more sophisticated with the passage of time, but by the conclusion of World War II, essentially all organs and areas of the body had been fully explored. Essentially, within a short half-century the domain of surgery had become so well established that the profession's foundation of basic operative procedures was already completed. As a consequence, there were few technical surgical mysteries left. What surgery now needed to sustain its continued growth was the ability to diagnose surgical diseases at earlier stages, to locate malignant growths while they remained small, and to have more effective postoperative treatment so that patients could survive ever more technically complex operations. Such thinking was exemplified by the introduction in 1924 of cholecystography by Evarts Graham (1883-1957) and Warren Cole (1898-1990). In this case, an emerging scientific technology introduced new possibilities into surgical practice that were not necessarily related solely to improvements in technique. To the surgeon, the discovery and application of cholecystography proved most important not only because it brought about more accurate diagnoses of cholecystitis but also because it created an influx of surgical patients where few had previously existed. If surgery was to grow, then large numbers of individuals with surgical diseases were needed.

It was an exciting era for surgeons, with important clinical advances being made both in the operating room and in the basic science laboratory. Among the most notable highlights were the introduction in 1935 of pancreatico-duodenectomy for cancer of the pancreas by Allen Oldfather Whipple (1881-1963) and a report in 1943 on vagotomy for operative therapy for peptic ulcer by Lester Dragstedt (1893-1976). Frank Lahey (1880-1953) stressed the importance of identifying the recurrent laryngeal nerve during the course of thyroid surgery; Owen Wangensteen (1898-1981) successfully decompressed mechanical bowel obstructions using a newly devised suction apparatus in 1932; George Vaughan (1859-1948) completed a successful ligation of the abdominal aorta for aneurysmal disease in 1921; Max Peet (1885-1949) presented his splanchnic resection for hypertension in 1935; Walter Dandy (1886-1946) performed intracranial section of various cranial nerves in the 1920s; Walter Freeman (1895-1972) described prefrontal lobotomy as a means of treatment for various mental illnesses in 1936; Harvey Cushing (1869-1939) introduced electrocoagulation in neurosurgery in 1928; Marius Smith-Petersen (1886-1953) described a flanged nail for pinning a fracture of the neck of the femur in 1931 and introduced Vitallium cup arthroplasty in 1939; Vilray Blair (1871-1955) and James Brown (1899-1971) popularized the use of split-skin grafts to cover large areas of granulating wounds; Earl Padgett (1893-1946) devised an operative dermatome, which allowed calibration of the thickness of skin grafts, in 1939; Elliott Cutler (1888-1947) performed a successful section of the mitral valve for relief of mitral stenosis in 1923; Evarts Graham completed the first successful removal of an entire lung for cancer in 1933; Claude Beck (1894-1971) implanted pectoral muscle into the pericardium and attached a pedicled omental graft to the surface of the heart, thus providing collateral circulation to that organ, in 1935; Robert Gross (1905-1988) reported the first successful ligation of a patent arterial duct in 1939 and a resection for coarctation of the aorta with direct anastomosis of the remaining ends in 1945; and John Alexander (1891-1954) resected a saccular aneurysm of the thoracic aorta in 1944.

With such a wide variety of technically complex surgical operations now possible, it had clearly become impossible for any single surgeon to master all the manual skills combined with the pathophysiologic knowledge necessary to perform such cases. Therefore, by mid century, a consolidation of professional power inherent in the movement toward specialization, with numerous individuals restricting their surgical practice to one highly structured field, had become among the most significant and dominating events in 20th century surgery. Ironically, the United States, which had been much slower than European countries to recognize surgeons as a distinct group of clinicians separate from physicians, would now spearhead this move toward surgical specialization with great alacrity. Clearly, the course of surgical fragmentation into specialties and subspecialties was gathering tremendous speed as the dark clouds of World War II settled over the globe. The socioeconomic and political ramifications of this war would bring about a fundamental change in the way surgeons viewed themselves and their interactions with the society in which they lived and worked.

LAST HALF OF THE 20TH CENTURY

The decades of economic expansion after World War II had a dramatic impact on surgery's scale, particularly in the United States. It was as if being victorious in battle permitted medicine to become big business overnight, with the single-minded pursuit of health care rapidly transformed into society's largest growth industry. Spacious hospital complexes were built that not only represented the scientific advancement of the healing arts but also vividly demonstrated the strength of American's postwar socioeconomic boom. Society was willing to give surgical science unprecedented recognition as a prized national asset.

The overwhelming impact of World War II on surgery was the sudden expansion of the profession and the beginnings of an extensive distribution of surgeons throughout the country. Many of these individuals, newly baptized to the rigors of technically complex trauma operations, became leaders in the construction and improvement of hospitals, multispecialty clinics, and surgical facilities in their hometowns. Large urban and community hospitals established surgical education and training programs, finding it a relatively easy matter to attract interns and residents. For the first time, residency programs in general surgery were rivaled in growth and educational sophistication by those in all the special fields of surgery. These changes served as fodder for further increases in the number of students entering surgery. Not only would surgeons command the highest salaries, but society was also enamored of the drama of the operating room. Television series, movies, novels, and the more-than-occasional live performance of a heart operation on network broadcast beckoned the lay individual.

Despite lay approval, success and acceptability in the biomedical sciences are sometimes difficult to determine, but one measure of both in recent times has been the awarding of the Nobel Prize in medicine and physiology. Society's continued approbation of surgery's accomplishments is seen in the naming of nine surgeons as Nobel laureates (Table 1-1).

CARDIAC SURGERY AND ORGAN TRANSPLANTATION

Two clinical developments truly epitomized the magnificence of post–World War II surgery and concurrently fascinated the public: the maturation of cardiac surgery as a "new" surgical specialty and the emergence of organ transplantation. Together they would stand as signposts along the new surgical highway. Fascination with the heart goes far beyond that of clinical medicine. From the historical perspective of art, customs, literature, philosophy, religion, and science, the heart has represented the seat of the soul and the wellspring of life itself. Such reverence also meant that this noble organ was long considered a surgical untouchable. Whereas the late 19th and 20th centuries witnessed a steady march of surgical triumphs for opening successive cavities of the body, the final achievement awaited the perfection of methods for surgical operations in the thoracic space.

Such a scientific and technologic accomplishment can be traced back to the repair of cardiac stab wounds by direct suture and the earliest attempts at fixing faulty heart valves. As triumphant as Luther Hill's (1862-1946) first known successful suture of a wound that penetrated a cardiac chamber was in 1902, it would not be until the 1940s that the development of safe intrapleural surgery could be counted on as something other than an occasional event. During World War II, Dwight Harken (1910-1993) gained extensive battlefield experience in removing bullets and shrapnel in or in relation to the heart and great vessels without a single fatality. Building on his wartime experience, Harken and other pioneering surgeons, including Charles Bailey (1910-1993) of Philadelphia and Russell Brock (1903-1980) of London, proceeded to expand intracardiac surgery by developing operations for the relief of mitral valve stenosis. The procedure was

TABLE 1-1.   Surgeons Named Nobel Laureates in Medicine and Physiology

Surgeon (Dates)	Country	Field (Year of Award)
Theodor Kocher (1841-1917)	Switzerland	Thyroid disease (1909)
Allvar Gullstrand (1862-1930)	Sweden	Ocular dioptrics (1911)
Alexis Carrel (1873-1944)	France and United States	Vascular surgery (1912)
Robert Bárány (1876-1936)	Austria	Vestibular disease (1914)
Frederick Banting (1891-1941)	Canada	Insulin (1922)
Walter Hess (1881-1973)	Switzerland	Midbrain physiology (1949)
Werner Forssmann (1904-1979)	Germany	Cardiac catheterization (1956)
Charles Huggins (1901-1997)	United States	Oncology (1966)
Joseph Murray (1919-	United States	Organ transplantation (1990)

progressively refined, evolving into the open commissurotomy repair used today.

Despite mounting clinical successes, surgeons who operated on the heart had to contend not only with the quagmire of blood flowing through the area where a difficult dissection was taking place but also with the unrelenting to-and-fro movement of a beating heart. Technically complex cardiac repair procedures could not be developed further until these problems were solved. John Gibbon (1903-1973) (Fig. 1-11) addressed this enigma by devising a machine that would take on the work of the heart and lungs while the patient was under anesthesia, in essence pumping oxygen-rich blood through the circulatory system while bypassing the heart so that the organ could be operated on at leisure. The first successful open-heart operation in 1953, using a heart-lung machine, was a momentous surgical contribution. Through single-mindedness of purpose, Gibbon's research paved the way for all future cardiac surgery, including procedures for correction of congenital heart defects, repair of heart valves, and transplantation of the heart.

Since time immemorial, the focus of surgery was mostly on excision and repair. However, beginning in the 20th century, the opposite end of the surgical spectrum—reconstruction and transplantation—became realities. Nineteenth century experience had shown that skin and bone tissues could be "autotransplanted" from one site to another in the same patient. It would take the horrendous and mutilating injuries of World War I to decisively advance skin transplants and legitimize the concept of surgery as a method of reconstruction. With Harold Gillies (1882-1960) of England and America's Vilray Blair establishing military-based "plastic surgery" units to deal with complex maxillofacial injuries, a turning point in the way in which society viewed surgery's raison d'être occurred. Now, not only would surgeons enhance nature's healing powers but they could also dramatically alter what had previously been little more than one's physical foregone conclusion. For example, Hippolyte Morestin (1869-1919) described a method of mammaplasty in 1902. John Staige Davis (1872-1946) of Baltimore popularized a manner of splinting skin grafts and later wrote the first comprehensive textbook on this new specialty, *Plastic Surgery: Its Principles and Practice* (1919). Immediately after the war, Blair would go on to establish the first separate plastic surgery service in a civilian institution at Barnes Hospital in St. Louis. Vladimir Filatov (1875-1956) of Odessa, Russia, used a tubed pedicle flap in 1916; and, in the following year, Gillies introduced a similar technique.

What about the replacement of damaged or diseased organs? After all, even at mid century, the very thought of successfully transplanting worn-out or unhealthy body parts verged on scientific fantasy. At the beginning of the 20th century, Alexis Carrel developed revolutionary new suturing techniques to anastomose the smallest of blood vessels. Using his surgical élan on experimental animals, Carrel began to "transplant" kidneys, hearts, and spleens. Technically, his research was a success, but some unknown biologic process always led to the rejection of the transplanted organ and death of the animal. By mid century, medical researchers had begun to clarify the presence of underlying "defensive" immune reactions and the necessity of creating "immunosuppression" as a method to allow the host to "accept" the foreign transplant. Using high-powered immunosuppressant drugs and other modern modalities, kidney transplantation soon blazed the way, and it was not long before a slew of organs and even whole hands were being replaced.

POLITICAL AND SOCIOECONOMIC INFLUENCES

Despite the 1950s and 1960s witnessing some of the most magnificent advances in the history of surgery, by the 1970s, political and socioeconomic influences were starting to overshadow many of the clinical triumphs. It was the beginning of a schizophrenic existence for surgeons: Complex and dramatic lifesaving operations were completed to innumerable accolades, while concurrently, public criticism of the economics of medicine, in particular high-priced surgical practice, portrayed the scalpel holder as an acquisitive, financially driven, selfish individual. This was in stark contrast to the relatively selfless and sanctified image of the surgeon before the growth of specialty work and the introduction of government involvement in health care delivery.

Although they are philosophically inconsistent, the dramatic and theatrical features of surgery that make surgeons heroes from one perspective and symbols of corruption, mendacity, and greed from the opposite point

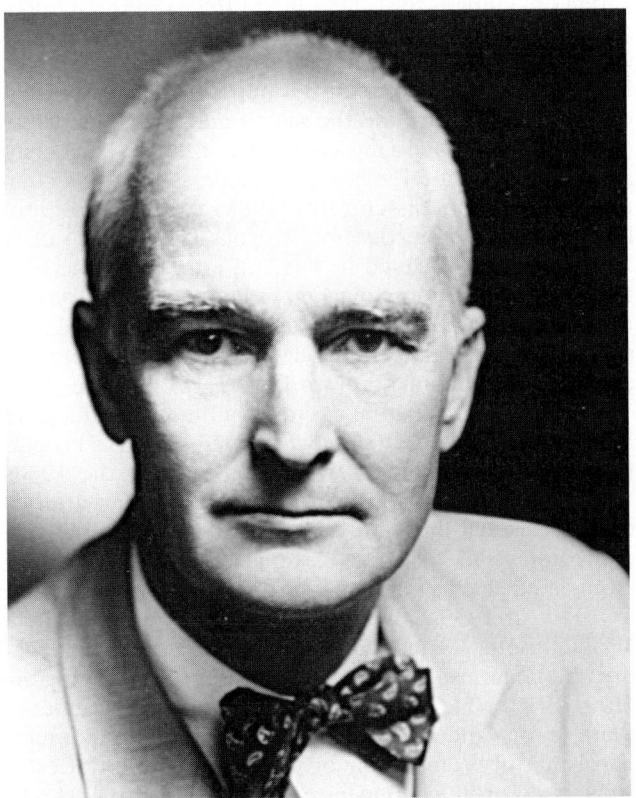

FIGURE 1-11. John Gibbon (1903-1973).

of view are the very reasons why society demands so much of its surgeons. There is the precise and definitive nature of surgical intervention, the expectation of success that surrounds an operation, the short time frame in which outcomes are realized, the high income levels of most surgeons, and the almost insatiable inquisitiveness of lay individuals concerning all aspects of the act of consensually cutting into another human's flesh. These phenomena, ever more sensitized in an age of mass media and instantaneous telecommunication, make the surgeon seem more accountable than his or her medical colleague and, simultaneously, symbolic of the best and the worst in medicine. In ways previously unimaginable, this vast social transformation of surgery controls the fate of the individual practitioner in the present era to a much greater extent than surgeons as a collective force are able to control it by their attempts to direct their own profession.

20TH CENTURY SURGICAL HIGHLIGHTS

Among the difficulties in studying 20th century surgery is the abundance of famous names and important written contributions. So much so that it becomes a difficult and invidious task to attempt any rational selection of representative personalities along with their significant journal or book-length writings. Although many justly famous names might be missing, the following description of surgical advances is intended to chronologically highlight some of the stunning clinical achievements of the past century.

In 1900, the German surgeon Hermann Pfannenstiel (1862-1909) described his technique for a suprapubic surgical incision. That same year, William Mayo (1861-1939) presented his results concerning partial gastrectomy before the American Surgical Association. The treatment of breast cancer was radically altered when George Beatson (1848-1933), professor of surgery in Glasgow, Scotland, proposed oophorectomy and the administration of thyroid extract as a possible cure (1901). John Finney (1863-1942) of The Johns Hopkins Hospital authored a paper on a new method of gastroduodenostomy, or widened pyloroplasty (1903). In Germany, Fedor Krause (1856-1937) was writing about total cystectomy and bilateral ureterosigmoidostomy. In 1905, Hugh Hampton Young (1870-1945) of Baltimore was presenting early studies of his radical prostatectomy for carcinoma. William Handley (1872-1962) was surgeon to the Middlesex Hospital in London when he authored *Cancer of the Breast and its Treatment* (1906). In that work, he advanced the theory that in breast cancer metastasis is due to extension along lymphatic vessels and not to dissemination via the bloodstream. That same year, José Goyanes (1876-1964) of Madrid used vein grafts to restore arterial flow. William Miles (1869-1947) of England first wrote about his operation of abdominoperineal resection in 1908, the same year that Friedrich Trendelenburg (1844-1924) attempted pulmonary embolectomy. Three years later, Martin Kirschner (1879-1942) of Germany described a wire for skeletal traction and for stabilization of bone fragments or joint immobilization. Donald Balfour (1882-

1963) of the Mayo Clinic provided the initial account of his important operation for resection of the sigmoid colon, as did William Mayo for his radical operation for carcinoma of the rectum in 1910.

In 1911, Fred Albee (1876-1945) of New York City began to employ living bone grafts as internal splints. Wilhelm Ramstedt (1867-1963), a German surgeon, described a pyloromyotomy (1912) at the same time that Pierre Fredet (1870-1946) was reporting a similar operation. In 1913, Henry Janeway (1873-1921) of New York City developed a technique for gastrostomy in which he wrapped the anterior wall of the stomach around a catheter and sutured it in place, establishing a permanent fistula. Hans Finsterer (1877-1955), professor of surgery in Vienna, improved on Franz von Hofmeister's (1867-1926) description of a partial gastrectomy with closure of a portion of the lesser curvature and retrocolic anastomosis of the remainder of the stomach to the jejunum (1918). Thomas Dunhill (1876-1957) of London was a pioneer in thyroid surgery, especially in his operation for exophthalmic goiter (1919). William Gallie (1882-1959) of Canada used sutures fashioned from the fascia lata in herniorrhaphy (1923). Barney Brooks (1884-1952), professor of surgery at Vanderbilt University in Nashville, Tennessee, initially introduced clinical angiography and femoral arteriography in 1924. Five years later, Reynaldo dos Santos (1880-1970), a Portuguese urologist, reported the first translumbar aortogram. Cecil Joll (1885-1945), professor of surgery in London, fully described the treatment of thyrotoxicosis by means of a subtotal thyroidectomy in the 1930s.

In 1931, George Cheatle (1865-1951), professor of surgery in London, and Max Cutler (1899-1984), a surgeon from New York City, published their important treatise *Tumours of the Breast.* In that same year, Cutler detailed his systemic use of ovarian hormone in the treatment of chronic mastitis. Around the same time, Ernst Sauerbruch (1875-1951) of Germany completed the first successful surgical intervention for cardiac aneurysm, and his countrymate Rudolph Nissen (1896-1981) removed an entire bronchiectatic lung. Geoffrey Keynes (1887-1982) of St. Bartholomew's Hospital in England articulated the basis for the opposition to radical mastectomy and his favoring of radium treatment in breast cancer (1932). The Irish surgeon Arnold Henry (1886-1962) devised an operative approach for femoral hernia in 1936. Earl Shouldice (1891-1965) of Toronto first began to experiment with a groin hernia repair based on overlapping layers brought together by a continuous wire suture during the 1930s. René Leriche (1879-1955) proposed in 1937 an arteriectomy in arterial thrombosis and, later, a periarterial sympathectomy to improve arterial flow. Leriche also enunciated a syndrome of aortoiliac occlusive disease in 1940. In 1939, Edward Churchill (1895-1972) of the Massachusetts General Hospital performed a segmental pneumonectomy for bronchiectasis. Charles Huggins (1901-1997) (Fig. 1-12), a pioneer in the endocrine therapy for cancer, found that antiandrogenic treatment consisting of orchiectomy or the administration of estrogens could produce long-term regression in patients with advanced prostatic cancer. These observations formed the

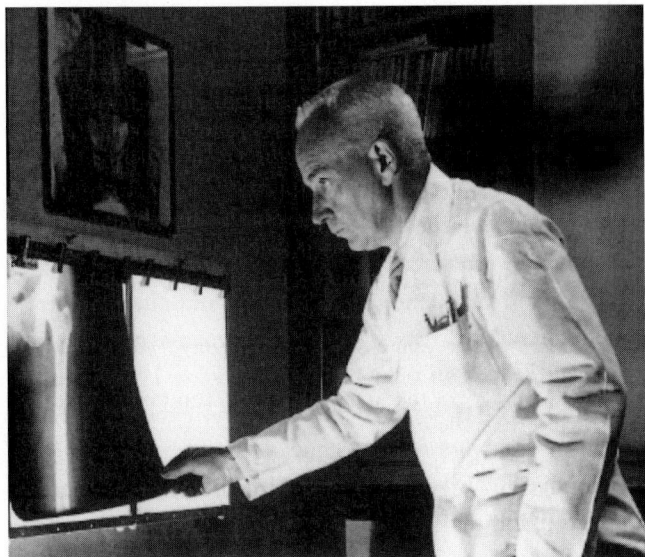

FIGURE 1-12. Charles Huggins (1901-1997). (Used with permission from the University of Chicago Hospitals.)

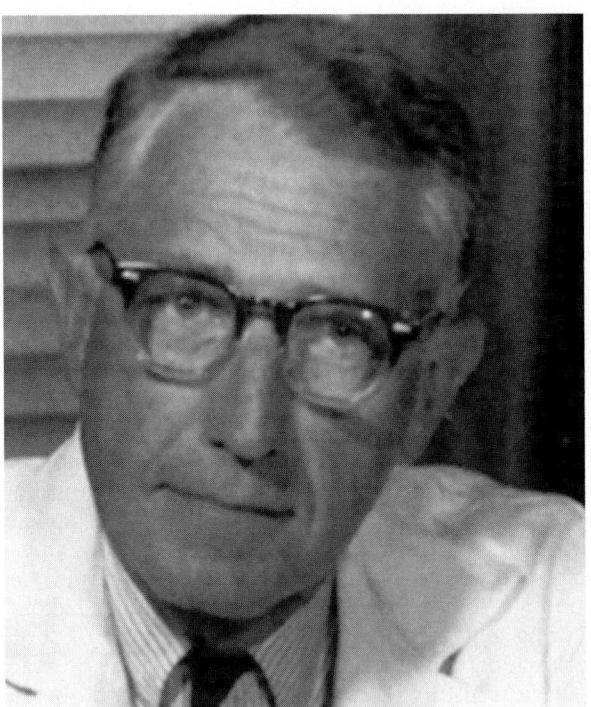

FIGURE 1-13. Francis D. Moore (1913-2001).

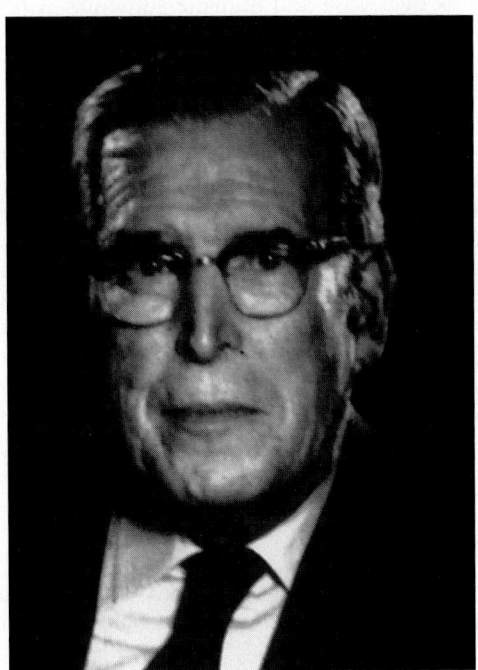

FIGURE 1-14. Jonathan Rhoads (1907-2002). (Photograph courtesy of James C. Thompson, M.D.)

basis for the current treatment of prostate and breast cancers by hormonal manipulation; Dr. Huggins was awarded the Nobel Prize in 1966 for these monumental discoveries. Clarence Crafoord (1899-1984) pioneered his surgical treatment of coarctation of the aorta in 1945. The following year, Willis Potts (1895-1968) completed an anastomosis of the aorta to a pulmonary vein for certain types of congenital heart disease. Chester McVay (1911-1987) popularized a repair of groin hernias based on the pectineal ligament in 1948. Working at Georgetown University Medical Center in Washington, DC, Charles Hufnagel (1916-1989) designed and inserted the first workable prosthetic heart valve in a man (1951). That same year, Charles Dubost (1914-1991) of Paris performed the first successful resection of an abdominal aortic aneurysm and insertion of a homologous graft. Robert Zollinger (1903-1994) and Edwin Ellison (1918-1970) first described their eponymic polyendocrine adenomatosis in 1955. The following year, Donald Murray (1894-1976) completed the first successful aortic valve homograft. At the same time, John Merrill (1917-1986) was performing the world's first successful homotransplantation of the human kidney between identical twin brothers. Francis D. Moore (1913-2001) (Fig. 1-13) defined objectives of metabolism in surgical patients and in 1959 published his widely quoted book *Metabolic Care of the Surgical Patient.* Moore was also a driving force in the field of transplantation and pioneered the technique of using radioactive isotopes to locate abscesses and tumors. In the 1960s, Jonathan E. Rhoads (1907-2002) (Fig. 1-14), in collaboration with colleagues Harry Vars and Stan Dudrick, described the technique of total parenteral nutrition, which has become an important and lifesaving treatment in the management of the critically ill patient who cannot tolerate standard enteral feedings. James D. Hardy (1918-2003), at the University of Mississippi, performed the first lung (1963) and heart (1964) transplants in a human.

FUTURE TRENDS

Throughout most of its evolution, the practice of surgery has been largely defined by its tools and the manual aspects of the craft. The last decades of the 20th century saw unprecedented progress in the development of new

instrumentation and imaging techniques. These refinements have not come without noticeable social and
economic cost. Advancement will assuredly continue,
because if the study of surgical history offers any lesson,
it is that progress can always be expected, at least relative
to technology. There will be more sophisticated surgical
operations with better results. Eventually, automation may
even robotize the surgeon's hand for certain procedures.
Still, the surgical sciences will always retain their historical roots as fundamentally a manual-based art and craft.

In many respects, the surgeon's most difficult future
challenges are not in the clinical realm but instead in
better understanding the socioeconomic forces that affect
the practice of surgery and in learning how to effectively
manage them. Many splendid schools of surgery now exist
in virtually every major industrialized city, but none can
lay claim to dominance in all the disciplines that make up
surgery. Likewise, the presence of authoritative individual
personalities who help guide surgery is more unusual
today than in previous times. National aims and socioeconomic status have become overwhelming factors in
securing and shepherding the future growth of surgery
worldwide. In light of an understanding of the intricacies
of surgical history, it seems an unenviable and obviously
impossible task to predict what will happen in the future.
In 1874, John Erichsen (1818-1896) of London wrote that
"the abdomen, chest, and brain will forever be closed to
operations by a wise and humane surgeon." A few years
later Theodor Billroth remarked, "A surgeon who tries to
suture a heart wound deserves to lose the esteem of his
colleagues." Obviously, the surgical crystal ball is a cloudy
one at best.

To study the fascinating history of our profession, with
its many magnificent personalities and outstanding scientific and social achievements, may not necessarily help us
predict the future of surgery. However, it does shed much
light on the clinical practices of our own time. To a certain
extent, if surgeons in the future wish to be regarded as
more than mere technicians, the profession needs to better
appreciate the value of its past experiences. Surgery has a
distinguished heritage that is in danger of being forgotten.
Although the future of the art, craft, and science of surgery
remains unknown, it assuredly rests on a glorious past.

Selected References

Allbutt TC: The Historical Relations of Medicine and Surgery to
the End of the Sixteenth Century. London, Macmillan, 1905.

An incisive and provocative address by the Regius Professor of Physic in the University of Cambridge concerning
the sometimes strained relations between early medical
and surgical practitioners.

Billings JS: The history and literature of surgery. In Dennis FS
(ed): System of Surgery, vol 1. Philadelphia, Lea Brothers,
1895, pp 17-144.

Surgeon, hospital architect, originator of the Index
Medicus, and director of the New York Public Library,
Billings' chapter is a comprehensive review of surgery,
albeit based on a hagiographic theme.

Bishop WJ: The Early History of Surgery. London, Robert Hale,
1960.

A distinguished medical bibliophile, Bishop's text is best
for its description of surgery in the Middle Ages, Renaissance, and 17th and 18th centuries.

Cartwright FF: The Development of Modern Surgery from 1830.
London, Arthur Barker, 1967.

An anesthetist at King's College Hospital in London,
Cartwright's work is rich in detail and interpretation.

Cope Z: Pioneers in Acute Abdominal Surgery. London, Oxford
University Press, 1939.
Cope Z: A History of the Acute Abdomen. London, Oxford Uni-
versity Press, 1965.

These two works by the highly regarded English surgeon
provide overall reviews of the evolution of surgical intervention for intra-abdominal pathology.

Gurlt EJ: Geschichte der Chirurgie und ihrer Ausübung (3 vols).
Berlin, A Hirschwald, 1898.

A monumentally detailed history of surgery from the
beginnings of recorded history to the end of the 16th
century. Gurlt, a German surgeon, includes innumerable
translations from ancient manuscripts. Unfortunately, this
work has not been translated into English.

Hurwitz A, Degenshein GA: Milestones in Modern Surgery. New
York, Hoeber-Harper, 1958.

Surgical attendings at Maimonides Hospital in Brooklyn,
their numerous chapters contain prefatory information,
including a short biography of each surgeon (with por-
trait) and a reprinted or translated excerpt of each one's
most important surgical contribution.

Leonardo RA: History of Surgery. New York, Froben, 1943.
Leonardo RA: Lives of Master Surgeons. New York, Froben,
1948 [plus Lives of Master Surgeons, Supplement 1, Froben,
1949].

These texts, by the eminent Rochester, New York, surgeon
and historian, together provide an in-depth description
of the whole of surgery from ancient times to the mid-
20th century. Especially valuable are the countless
biographies of both famous and near-famous scalpel
bearers.

Malgaigne JF: Histoire de la Chirurgie en Occident depuis de VIe
Jusqu'au XVIe Siècle, et Histoire de la Vie et des Travaux
d'Ambroise Paré. In Malgaigne JF (ed): Ambroise Paré,
Oeuvres Complètes, Vol 1, Introduction. Paris, JB Baillière,
1840-1841.

Considered among the most brilliant French surgeons
of the 19th century, Malgaigne's history is particularly
noteworthy for its study of 15th and 16th century
European surgery. This entire work was admirably
translated into English by Wallace Hamby, an American
neurosurgeon, in Surgery and Ambrose Paré by J. F.
Malgaigne (Norman, University of Oklahoma Press,
1965).

Meade RH: An Introduction to the History of General Surgery.
Philadelphia, WB Saunders, 1968.

Meade RH: A History of Thoracic Surgery. Springfield, IL, Charles C Thomas, 1961.

Meade, an indefatigable researcher of historical topics, practiced surgery in Grand Rapids, Michigan. With extensive bibliographies, his two books are among the most ambitious of such systematic works.

Porter R: The Greatest Benefit to Mankind, a Medical History of Humanity. New York, WW Norton, 1997.

A wonderful literary tour de force by one of the most erudite and entertaining of modern medical historians. Although more a history of the whole of medicine than of surgery specifically, this text has become an instantaneous classic and should be required reading for all physicians and surgeons.

Rutkow IM: Surgery, An Illustrated History. St. Louis, Mosby–Year Book, 1993.

Rutkow IM: American Surgery, An Illustrated History. Philadelphia, Lippincott-Raven, 1998.

Combining both a detailed text and numerous colored illustrations, these books explore the evolution of surgery, worldwide and in the United States.

Thompson CJS: The History and Evolution of Surgical Instruments. New York, Schuman's, 1942.

Surgeons are often defined by their surgical armamentarium, and this text provides detailed discussions on the evolution of instruments such as the scalpel, amputation knife, headsaws, tourniquets, trocars, and even operating tables.

Thorwald J: The Century of the Surgeon. New York, Pantheon, 1956.

Thorwald J: The Triumph of Surgery. New York, Pantheon, 1960.

In a most dramatic literary fashion, Thorwald uses a fictional eyewitness narrator to create a continuity in the story of the development of surgery during its most important decades of growth, the late 19th and early 20th centuries. Imbued with a myriad of true historical facts, these books are among the most enjoyable to be found within the genre of surgical history.

Wangensteen OH, Wangensteen SD: The Rise of Surgery, from Empiric Craft to Scientific Discipline. Minneapolis, University of Minnesota Press, 1978.

Not a systematic history but an assessment of various operative techniques (e.g., gastric surgery, tracheostomy, ovariotomy, vascular surgery) and technical factors (e.g., débridement, phlebotomy, surgical amphitheater, preparations for operation) that contributed to or retarded the evolution of surgery. Wangensteen was a noted teacher of experimental and clinical surgery at the University of Minnesota and his wife, an accomplished medical historian.

Zimmerman LM, Veith I: Great Ideas in the History of Surgery. Baltimore, Williams & Wilkins, 1961.

Zimmerman, late professor of surgery at the Chicago Medical School, and Veith, a masterful medical historian, provide well-written biographic narratives to accompany numerous readings and translations from the works of almost 50 renowned surgeons of varying eras.

CHAPTER 2

ETHICS IN SURGERY

Ronald A. Carson, Ph.D.

Renewed public attention is being paid to ethics today. There are governmental ethics commissions, research ethics boards, and corporate ethics committees. Some of these institutional entities are little more than "window dressing," whereas others are investigative bodies called into being, for example, on suspicion that financial records have been altered or data have been presented in a deceptive manner. But many of these groups do important work, and the fact that they have been established at all suggests that we are not as certain as we once were, or thought we were, about where the moral boundaries are and how we would know if we overstepped them. In search of insight and guidance, we turn to ethics. In the professions, which are largely self-regulating, and especially in the medical profession, whose primary purpose is to be responsive to people in need, ethics is at the heart of the enterprise.

It is important to be clear at the outset about what ethics is and is not. Although physicians are expected to uphold such standards of professionalism as reporting impaired colleagues, medical ethics is not primarily about keeping transgressors in line. That is the domain of laws, courts, and boards of medical examiners. Ethics has to do with discerning where the lines should be drawn in the first place and to what we should aspire. It is about thinking through what we believe is good or bad or right or wrong and why we think that way. The emphasis is on reflecting and deliberating. Ethical reflection is especially useful in a social and cultural environment such as ours in which values often conflict.

The ethical precepts of the medical profession have traditionally been summarized in various oaths and codes. For example, it is still customary for students to repeat the Hippocratic Oath, or some contemporary adaptation of it, on graduation from medical school. The American College of Surgeons' Statements on Principles contains a fellowship pledge that includes a promise to maintain the college's historical commitment to "the ethical practice of medicine."[1] The American College of Obstetricians and Gynecologists (ACOG) subscribes to a code of ethics that governs the patient-physician relationship, physician conduct and practice, conflicts of interest, professional relations, and societal responsibilities.[2] Moreover, ACOG's publication *Ethics in Obstetrics and Gynecology* is exemplary in its comprehensiveness and specificity in discussing ethical issues ranging from reproductive choice to end-of-life care.[3] Several other surgical subspecialties, as well as anesthesiology, have also given careful thought to ethical issues that arise in practice, research, education, and the introduction of innovative surgical technologies and techniques.[4-13]

For more than a century and a half, the American Medical Association has promulgated a statement of ethical principles. Although this code has evolved over time to accommodate changes in society and in medicine, it has always enunciated the ethical principles on which the profession perceives itself to be grounded. The most recent version of this statement of principles is more patient centered than ever before. It asserts that "a physician must recognize responsibility to patients first and foremost" and spells out this responsibility as the provision of "competent medical care, with compassion and respect for human dignity and rights." Principle VIII states, "A physician shall, while caring for a patient, regard responsibility to the patient as paramount."[14]

Responsibility to the patient in contemporary clinical ethics entails maximal patient participation, permitted by the patient's condition, in decisions regarding the course of care. For the surgeon, this means arriving at an accurate diagnosis of the patient's presenting problem, making a treatment recommendation based on the best knowledge available, and then talking with the patient about the merits and drawbacks of the recommended course in light of the patient's life values. For the patient, maximal participation in decision making means having a conversation with the surgeon about the recommendation, why it seems reasonable and desirable, what the alternatives are, if any, and what the likely risks are of accepting the recommendation or pursuing an alternate course.

This view of ethically sound clinical care has evolved over the past half century from a doctor-knows-best ethic that worked reasonably well for both patients and physicians at a time when medical knowledge was limited and most of what medicine could do for patients could be carried in the doctor's black bag or handled in a small, uncluttered office or operating room.

The subsequent explosion of biomedical knowledge and the resulting proliferation of treatment options, many of them involving new technologic apparatus and interventions, were accompanied by a growing dissatisfaction with medical paternalism. As medicine grew more complex, and doctors became more reliant on specialty knowledge and instrumentation, physicians and patients became less familiar with each other. Patients could no longer assume that they and their physicians shared a common set of personal values sufficient to guide physicians in judging what was best for their patients. For example, faced with a variety of treatment options, women diagnosed with breast cancer and men diagnosed with prostate cancer want to participate personally in decisions that will affect not only their bodies but also their lives.

In response to these new complexities, and following on the various rights movements of the 1960s, some bioethicists began to advocate giving pride of place to patient autonomy (respecting the patient's right to decide by seeking his or her consent to treatment) over physician beneficence (doing that which, in the physician's judgment, is in the patient's best interest) in the hierarchy of principles governing ethical medicine (autonomy, nonmaleficence, beneficence, and justice).[15]

Consent is permission, granted by the patient to the surgeon, to make a diagnostic or therapeutic intervention on the patient's behalf. For consent to be valid, it must be informed. The patient must be provided all relevant information. To be valid, it must also be voluntary, that is, as free from coercion as possible, recognizing that in extremis the patient's condition itself may be inherently coercive. The surgeon's ethical objective is to judiciously provide the patient sufficient information on which to decide what course to follow. This entails selectively presenting all information pertinent to the patient's condition regarding benefits, risks, and alternatives while avoiding overwhelming the patient with extraneous data. To walk the line between what is pertinent and what is extraneous requires prudent judgment.

Informed consent has become a baseline best-practice ethical standard in modern medical care. It is a necessary but insufficient condition for ethically sound patient care. More moral work remains to be done if the physician-patient relationship is to be more than a contractual arrangement for rendering services. The ultimate goal is to achieve the best outcome, not only in terms of adherence to ethical principles of practice but also in keeping with patients' moral values, with what matters most to patients in their relationships and their lives. Achieving this goal certainly entails the provision of information and the granting of consent, but this exchange must take place in the context of a conversation about how the proposed intervention will affect a particular patient's life.

Twenty years ago Jay Katz foresaw the moral work that would be required to construct a contemporary medical ethic capable of overcoming what he termed a prevailing "silence" between doctors and patients. Katz was referring to the practice of physicians deciding what was best for patients and of patients abiding by the decision. He proposed that this silence be supplanted by "meaningful conversation" based on "the humaneness of mutual understanding."[16]

Meaningful conversation requires conversation partners jointly committed to treating the patient's ailment in a context of mutual respect and understanding. In addition to enhancing mutuality and promoting understanding, meaningful conversation contributes to better health outcomes and to patients' satisfaction with their care. It stands to reason that patients whose doctors are responsive to their questions are likely to feel better. Is such attentiveness a luxury in today's time-conscious, monitored, and managed environment? On the contrary, studies show that when doctors miss clues to emotional and social matters that their patients cannot broach explicitly, visits tend to be prolonged as the patient continues to try to elicit an acknowledgment from the physician of concerns that may not seem immediately relevant to the patient's chief complaint.[17]

Anticipating the need for physicians to cultivate the ability to engage patients in meaningful conversation, the Accreditation Council for Graduate Medical Education (ACGME) has included ethical and professional skills and behaviors among the general clinical competencies on which residency training programs are evaluated. Accreditation criteria for programs include adherence to accepted ethical principles of patient care as well as respectful personal interactions with diverse patients, families, and other professionals.[18] Nowhere are such qualities of physicians more in demand than in the care of patients near the end of life.

In 1998 the American College of Surgeons adopted a "Statement on Principles Guiding Care at the End of Life,"[19] which includes the following principles:

- Respect the dignity of both patient and caregivers.
- Be sensitive to and respectful of the patient's and family's wishes.
- Use the most appropriate measures that are consistent with the choices of the patient or the patient's legal surrogate.
- Ensure alleviation of pain and management of other physical symptoms.
- Recognize, assess, and address psychological, social, and spiritual problems.
- Ensure appropriate continuity of care by the patient's primary and/or specialist physician.
- Provide access to therapies that may realistically be expected to improve the patient's quality of life.
- Provide access to appropriate palliative care and hospice care.
- Respect the patient's right to refuse treatment.
- Recognize the physician's responsibility to forgo treatments that are futile.

A Surgeons Palliative Care Workgroup was convened in 2001 to put these principles into operation and to introduce the precepts and techniques of palliative care into surgical practice and education by means of symposia, a palliative care website, and focused contributions to the surgical literature.

In a paper introducing a monthly series from members of the workgroup written for and by surgeons, Geoffrey P. Dunn and Robert A. Milch observe that caring for patients near the end of life offers surgeons an "opportunity to rebalance decisiveness with introspection, detachment with empathy," and thereby "restore the integrity of our relationships with our patients."[20] Other contributions to this series provide expert discussions of such ethically difficult issues as decision making in palliative surgery[21]; chronic pain management and opioid tolerance[22,23]; withdrawing life support, including tube feeding and hydration and total parenteral nutrition[24,25]; management of dyspnea,[26] depression, and anxiety[27]; and attending to dying patients' spiritual needs.[28] Two themes thread their way through these discussions. Patients in a surgeon's care near the end of life stand not only to gain from the surgeon's cognitive and technical expertise as long as rescue is an option but also to benefit from the surgeon's attentiveness and guidance when what ails the patient cannot be remedied or reversed.[29] Moreover, surgeons themselves can derive satisfaction from staying the course with dying patients and their families, responding to their trust, seeing them through difficult times, and caring for them even when curative options are no longer indicated or available.[30]

Among other responsibilities articulated in the American Medical Association's Principles of Medical Ethics, two suggest a growing sense within the profession of medicine's role as a public-spirited profession: (1) contributing to the betterment of the health of the community and (2) supporting access to medical care for everyone. Additional evidence of public-spiritedness is to be found in the association's Declaration of Professional Responsibility, which was forged in response to the terrorist attacks on New York and Washington in September 2001. Subtitled "Medicine's Social Contract with Humanity," this unprecedented oath contains the following declaration[31]:

We, the members of the world community of physicians, solemnly commit ourselves to:

  I. Respect human life and the dignity of every individual.
 II. Refrain from supporting or committing crimes against humanity and condemn all such acts.
III. Treat the sick and injured with competence and compassion and without prejudice.
 IV. Apply our knowledge and skill when needed, though doing so may put us at risk.
  V. Protect the privacy and confidentiality of those for whom we care and breach that confidence only when keeping it would seriously threaten their health and safety and that of others.

 VI. Work freely with colleagues to discover, develop, and promote advances in medicine and public health that ameliorate suffering and contribute to human well-being.
VII. Educate the public and polity about present and future threats to the health of humanity.
VIII. Advocate for social, economic, educational, and political changes that ameliorate suffering and contribute to human well-being.
 IX. Teach and mentor those who follow us for they are the future of our caring profession.

We make these promises solemnly, freely, and upon our personal and professional honor.

Recognizing the social value of volunteerism, the Governors' Committee on Socioeconomic Issues of the American College of Surgeons created the "Giving Back" project in the year 2000. Based on survey data from 500 Fellows, the committee recommended that the College "Promote surgeon volunteerism as 'The right thing to do' and 'Part of being a physician'."[32]

Taken together, these three documents, along with the emphasis on professional values in the medical ethics literature and the ACGME *General Competencies,* indicate a renewed commitment on the part of clinicians to competent, respectful, compassionate patient care and a growing awareness within the profession of the ethical obligations of physicians in their various roles as clinicians, researchers, educators, and citizens that arise from and extend beyond the traditional patient-physician relationship.[33-35]

Contemporary clinical ethics is evolving toward a relational understanding of interactions between doctors and patients. In the parlance of ethics, this means that ethical principles are being supplemented by moral virtues. Adherence to principles leads one to ask: what should I do? Attention to virtues prompts the question: what kind of person or doctor should I be? How to conduct oneself with patients in an economic and social environment that rewards haste, encourages narrow self-interest and inattention to the patient as a person, and is increasingly inhospitable to underserved populations is motivating a re-evaluation of medical professionalism not only at the bedside but in society as well.

Selected References

Barnard D, Boston P, Towers A, Lambrinidou Y: Crossing Over: Narratives of Palliative Care. New York, Oxford University Press, 2000.

> **Accounts of patients, families and health care professionals working together to maintain hope in the face of incurable illness.**

Cassell EJ: The Nature of Suffering and the Goals of Medicine. New York, Oxford University Press, 1991.

> **Experienced internist's reflections on suffering and the relationship between patient and doctor.**

Gawande A: Complications: A Surgeon's Notes on an Imperfect Science. New York, Metropolitan Books, 2002.

A young surgeon's thoughts on fallibility, mystery, and uncertainty in surgical practice.

Jonsen AR, Siegler M, Winslade WJ: Clinical Ethics. New York, McGraw-Hill, 2002.

The standard physician's pocket guide to clinical-ethical decision making.

Lynn J, Lynch Schuster J, Kabcenell A: Improving Care for the End of Life. New York, Oxford University Press, 2000.

A source book for improving health care practices and systems, with appendices containing helpful instruments for assessing pain, survival time, comfort, and grief.

May WF: The Physician's Covenant: Images of the Healer in Medical Ethics. Philadelphia, Westminster Press, 1983.

Reflections on the physician as parent, fighter, technician, and teacher.

McCullough LB, Jones JW, Brody BA: Surgical Ethics. New York, Oxford University Press, 1998.

Nineteen chapters on surgical ethics, varying from principles and practice through research and innovation to finances and institutional relations.

Nuland SB: How We Die: Reflections on Life's Final Chapter. New York, Alfred A. Knopf, 1994.

A national bestseller by a senior surgeon, writer, and historian of medicine.

Selzer R: Letters to a Young Doctor. New York, Simon & Schuster, 1982.

Sage advice for young surgeons from a seasoned surgeon-writer.

References

1. American College of Surgeons Statements on Principles. These statements were collated, approved by the Board of Regents, and initially published in 1974. They were last revised in October 1997. (Electronic version) Retrieved April 30, 2003 from http://www.facs.org
2. Code of Professional Ethics of the American College of Obstetricians and Gynecologists. Approved by the Executive Board of the American College of Obstetricians and Gynecologists. (Electronic version) Retrieved April 28, 2003 from http://www.acog.org/
3. American College of Obstetricians and Gynecologists: Ethics in Obstetrics and Gynecology. (2002). (Electronic version) Retrieved April 30, 2003 from http://www.acog.org/
4. Gates E: Ethical considerations in the incorporation of new technologies into gynecologic practice. Clin Obstet Gynecol 43:540-550, 2000.
5. Shaw A: Historical review of pediatric surgical ethics. Semin Pediatr Surg 10:171-178, 2001.
6. Boudreaux AM, Tilden SJ: Ethical dilemmas for pediatric surgical patients. Anesthesiol Clin North Am 20:227-240, 2002.
7. Frader JE, Flanagan-Klygis E: Innovation and research in pediatric surgery. Semin Pediatr Surg 10:198-203, 2001.
8. Levin AV: IOLs, innovation, and ethics in pediatric ophthalmology: Let's be honest. J AAPOS 6:133-135, 2002.
9. Day SH: Teaching ethics: A structured curriculum on ethics for ophthalmology residents is valuable. Arch Ophthalmol 120:963-964, 2002.
10. Wenger NS, Liu H, Lieberman JR: Teaching medical ethics to orthopaedic surgery residents. J Bone Joint Surg Am 80A:1125-1131, 1998.
11. Capozzi JD, Rhodes R, Springfield DS: Ethical considerations in orthopaedic surgery. Am Acad Orthop Surg Instruct Course Lect 49:633-637, 2000.
12. Committee on Ethics of the American Society of Anesthesiologists: Syllabus on Ethics: Informed Consent (1997). (Electronic version) Retrieved October 10, 2002 from http://www.asahq.org/wlm/Ethics.html
13. ABIM Foundation, American Board of Internal Medicine, ACP-ASIM Foundation, American College of Physicians-American Society of Internal Medicine, European Federation of Internal Medicine: Medical professionalism in the new millennium: A physician charter. Ann Intern Med 136:243-246, 2002.
14. American Medical Association: E-Principles of Medical Ethics. Current Opinions of the Council on Ethical and Judicial Affairs (2001). (Electronic version) Retrieved April 30, 2003 from http://www.ama-assn.org/ama/pub/category/8289.html
15. Beauchamp TL, Childress JF: Principles of Biomedical Ethics, 5th ed. New York, Oxford University Press, 2001.
16. Katz J: The Silent World of Doctor and Patient. New York, The Free Press, 1984.
17. Levinson W, Gorawara-Phat R, Lamb J: A study of patient clues and physician responses in primary care and surgical settings. JAMA 284:1021-1027, 2000.
18. Accreditation Council for Graduate Medical Education: General Competencies (Electronic version) http://www.acgme.org/Outcome/
19. American College of Surgeons' Committee on Ethics: Statement on Principles Guiding Care at the End of Life. Bull Am Coll Surg 83:46, 1998.
20. Dunn GP, Milch RA: Introduction and historical background of palliative care: Where does the surgeon fit in? J Am Coll Surg 193:325-328, 2001.
21. McCahill LE, Krouse RS, Chu DZJ, et al: Decision making in palliative surgery. J Am Coll Surg 195:411-422, 2002.
22. Lee KF, James B, Ray JB, Dunn GP: Chronic pain management and the surgeon: Barriers and opportunities. J Am Coll Surg 193:689-701, 2001.
23. Thompson AR, Ray JB: The importance of opioid tolerance: A therapeutic paradox. J Am Coll Surg 196:321-324, 2003.
24. Easson AM, Hinshaw DB, Johnson DL: The role of tube feeding and total parenteral nutrition in advanced illness. J Am Coll Surg 194:225-228, 2002.
25. Huffman JL, Dunn GP: The paradox of hydration in advanced terminal illness. J Am Coll Surg 194:835-839, 2002.
26. Mosenthal AC, Lees KF: Management of dyspnea at the end of life: Relief for patients and surgeons. J Am Coll Surg 194:377-386, 2002.
27. Hinshaw DB, Carnahan JM, Johnson DL: Depression, anxiety, and asthenia in advanced illness. J Am Coll Surg 195:271-277, 2002.
28. Hinshaw DB: The spiritual needs of the dying patient. J Am Coll Surg 195:565-568, 2002.
29. Little M: Invited commentary: Is there a distinctively surgical ethics? Surgery 129:668-671, 2001.
30. The Kaiser Family Foundation: 2001 National Survey of Physicians (Electronic version). Retrieved from http://www.kff.org/content/2003/3223/National_Survey_Physicians_Toplines_Revised.pdf

31. American Medical Association: Declaration of Professional Responsibility (Electronic version). Retrieved April 30, 2003 from http://www.ama-assn.org/ama/pub/category/7491.html

32. The American College of Surgeons: Volunteerism and Giving Back to Society Among Surgeons Project: Phase Three—Survey of ACS Fellows (Electronic version). Retrieved April 30, 2003 from http://www.facs.org/about/governors/phase3givingback.pdf

33. Mechanic D: Managed care and the imperative for a new professional ethic. Health Affairs 19:100-111, 2000.

34. Bloche MG: Clinical loyalties and the social purpose of medicine. JAMA 281:268-274, 1999.

35. Little M: Ethonomics: The ethics of the unaffordable. Arch Surg 135:17-21, 2000.

CHAPTER 3

MOLECULAR AND CELL BIOLOGY

Tien C. Ko, M.D. and B. Mark Evers, M.D.

Human Genome	**Apoptosis**
Recombinant DNA Technology	**Human Genome Project**
Cell Signaling	**Novel Treatment Strategies**
Cell Division Cycle	**Ethical, Psychological, and Legal Implications**

Since the 1980s, there has been an explosion in knowledge regarding molecular and cell biology. These advances will transform the practice of surgery to one that is based on molecular techniques for prevention, diagnosis, and treatment of many surgical diseases. This is made possible by the achievements of the Human Genome Project, which intends to reveal the complete genetic instruction of humans. The core knowledge of molecular and cell biology has been presented in detail in several textbooks.[1,2] An overview of the field is presented here, with emphasis on basic concepts and techniques.

HUMAN GENOME

Mendel first defined genes as information-containing elements that are distributed from parents to offspring. Genes contain the design that is essential for the development of each human. The field of molecular biology began in 1944 when Avery demonstrated that DNA was the hereditary material that made up genes. This genetic information is translated into RNA and then protein, leading to the expression of specific biologic characteristics or phenotypes. Major advances made in the field of molecular biology are listed in Table 3-1. In this section, the structures of genes and DNA are reviewed, as are the processes by which genetic information is translated into biologic characteristics.

Structure of Genes and DNA

DNA is composed of two antiparallel strands of unbranched polymer wrapped around each other to form a right-handed double helix (Fig. 3-1).[3] Each strand is composed of four types of deoxyribonucleotides containing the bases adenine (A), cytosine (C), guanine (G), and thymine (T). The nucleotides are joined together by phosphodiester bonds that join the 5′ carbon of one deoxyribose group to the 3′ carbon of the next. Although the sugar-phosphate backbone remains constant, the attached bases can vary to encode different genetic information. The nucleotide sequences of the opposing strands of DNA are complementary to each other, allowing formation of hydrogen bonds that stabilize the double-helix structure. Complementary base pairs require that A always pairs with T and C always pairs with G. For example, if the sense strand (5′-to-3′ direction) of DNA has the nucleotide sequence of GAATTC, then the complementary antisense strand (3′-to-5′ direction) has the sequence CTTAAG.

The entire human genetic information, or human genome, contains 3×10^9 nucleotide pairs. However, less than 10% of DNA sequences are copied into either messenger RNA (mRNA) molecules that encode proteins or structural RNA, such as transfer RNA (tRNA) or ribosomal RNA (rRNA) molecules. Each nucleotide sequence in a DNA molecule that directs the synthesis of a functional RNA molecule is called a *gene* (Fig. 3-2). Those DNA sequences that do not encode genetic information may have structural or other unknown functions. Human genes commonly contain more than 100,000 nucleotide pairs in length, yet most mRNA molecule-encoding proteins consist of only 1000 nucleotide pairs. Most of the extra nucleotides consist of long stretches of noncoding sequences called *introns* that interrupt the relatively short segments of coding sequences called *exons*. For example, the thyroglobulin gene has 300,000 nucleotide bases and 36 introns, while its mRNA has only 8700 nucleotide bases. The processes by which genetic information encoded in DNA is transferred to RNA and protein molecules are discussed later.

TABLE 3-1.	Major Events in Molecular Biology
Year	**Event**
1941	Genes are found to encode proteins
1944	DNA is determined to carry the genetic information
1953	DNA structure is determined
1962	Restriction endonucleases are discovered
1966	Genetic code is deciphered
1973	DNA cloning technique is established
1976	First oncogene is discovered
1977	Human growth hormone is produced in bacteria
1978	Human insulin gene is cloned
1981	First transgenic animal is produced
1985	Polymerase chain reaction is invented First tumor suppressor gene is discovered
1990	Human Genome Project is created
1998	First mammal is cloned

The human genome contains 24 different DNA molecules; each DNA has 10^8 bases and is packaged in a separate chromosome. Thus, the human genome is organized into 22 different autosomes and two different sex chromosomes. Since humans are diploid organisms, each somatic cell contains two copies of each different autosome and two sex chromosomes for a total of 46 chromosomes. One copy of chromosomes is inherited from the mother and one is inherited from the father. Germ cells contain only 22 autosomes and one sex chromosome. Each chromosome contains three types of specialized DNA sequences that are important in the replication or segregation of chromosomes during cell division (Fig. 3-3). To replicate, each chromosome contains many short, specific DNA sequences that act as *replication origins*.[4] A second sequence element, called a *centromere*, attaches DNA to the mitotic spindle during cell division.[5] The third sequence element is a *telomere*, which contains G-rich repeats located at each end of the chromosome.[6] During DNA replication, one strand of DNA becomes a few bases shorter at its 3′ end due to limitation in the replication machinery. If this is not remedied, DNA molecules will become progressively shorter in their telomere segments with each cell division. This problem is solved by an

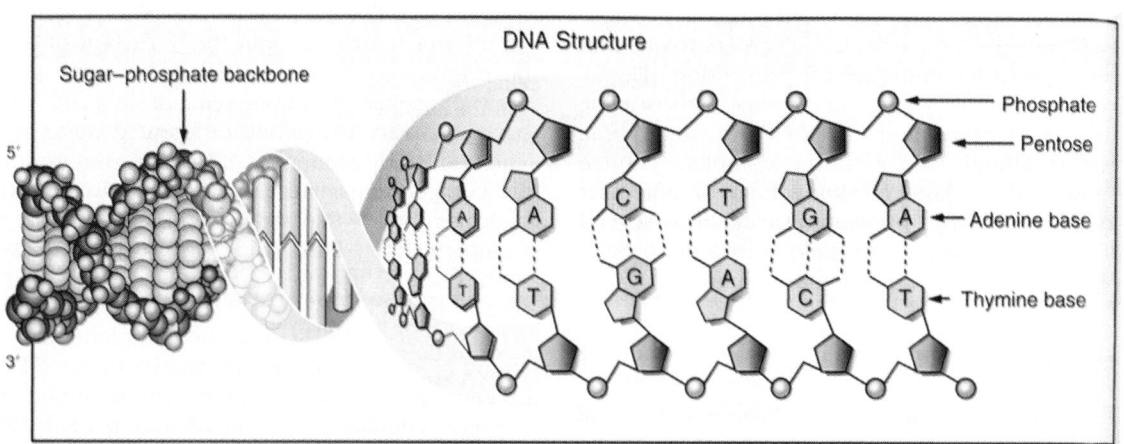

FIGURE 3-1.   DNA double-helix structure. Sequence of four bases (guanine, adenine, thymine, and cytosine), which determines the specificity of genetic information. The bases face inward from the sugar-phosphate backbone and form pairs (*dashed lines*) with complementary bases on the opposing strand. (Adapted from Rosenthal N: DNA and the genetic code. N Engl J Med 331:39, 1994. Copyright © 1994 Massachusetts Medical Society. All rights reserved.)

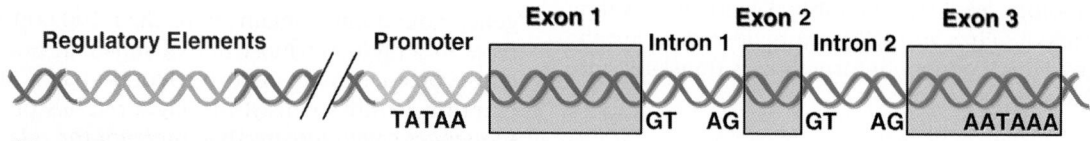

FIGURE 3-2.   Gene structure. The DNA sequences that are transcribed as RNA are collectively called the *gene* and include exons (expressed sequences) and introns (intervening sequences). Introns invariably begin with the nucleotide sequence GT and end with AG. An AT-rich sequence in the last exon forms a signal for processing the end of the RNA transcript. Regulatory sequences that make up the promoter and include the TATA box occur close to the site where transcription starts. Additional regulatory elements are located at variable distances from the gene. (Adapted from Rosenthal N: Regulation of gene expression. N Engl J Med 331:932, 1994. Copyright © 1994 Massachusetts Medical Society. All rights reserved.)

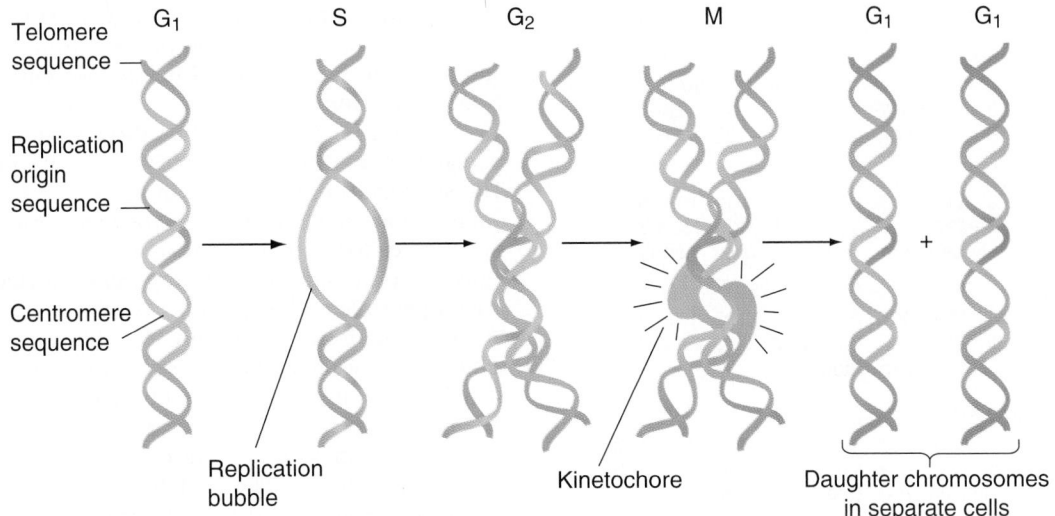

FIGURE 3-3. Chromosome structure. Each chromosome has three types of specific sequences that facilitate its replication during the cell cycle. Origins of replication are located throughout each chromosome to facilitate DNA synthesis. The centromere holds the duplicated chromosome together and is attached to the mitotic spindle through a protein complex called a *kinetochore*. Telomere sequences are located at each end of the chromosome and are replicated in a special way to preserve chromosome integrity.

enzyme called *telomerase*, which periodically extends the telomerase sequence by several bases.

Each chromosome, when stretched out, would span the cell nucleus thousands of times. To facilitate DNA replication and segregation, each chromosome is packaged into a compact structure with the aid of special proteins including histones.[7] DNA and histones form a repeated array of particles called *nucleosomes*; each consists of an octomeric core of histone proteins around which the DNA is wrapped twice. The condensed complex of DNA and proteins is known as *chromatin*. Not only does chromosome packaging facilitate DNA replication and segregation, it also influences the activity of genes, which is discussed later.

DNA Replication and Repair

Prior to cell division, DNA must be precisely duplicated, such that a complete set of chromosomes can be passed to each progeny. DNA replication must occur rapidly, yet with extremely high accuracy.[8] In humans, DNA is replicated at the rate of approximately 50 nucleotides per second with an error rate of 1 in every 10^9 base pair replications. This efficient replication of genetic material requires an elaborate replication machinery consisting of several enzymes. Since each strand of DNA double helix encodes nucleotide sequences complementary to its partner strand, both strands contain identical genetic information and serve as templates for the formation of an entirely new strand. DNA replication occurs in the 5′-to-3′ direction along each strand by the sequential addition of complementary deoxyribonucleoside triphosphates. Eventually, two complete DNA double helices are formed containing identical genetic information. The fidelity of

DNA replication is of critical importance since any mistake, called a *mutation*, will result in wrong DNA sequences being copied to daughter cells. Change in a single base pair is called a *point mutation*, which can result in one of two types of mutations (Fig. 3-4). A single amino acid change as the consequence of the point mutation is called a *missense mutation*. Missense mutations may cause changes in the structure of the protein, leading to altered biologic activity. If the point mutation results in the replacement of an amino acid codon with a stop codon, it is called a *nonsense mutation*. Nonsense mutations lead to premature termination of translation and often results in the loss of the encoded protein. If there is an addition or deletion of a few base pairs, it is called *frameshift mutation*, which leads to the introduction of unrelated amino acids or a stop codon (see Fig. 3-4). Some mutations are silent and do not affect the function of the organisms. Several proofreading mechanisms are used to eliminate mistakes during DNA replication.

RNA and Protein Synthesis

In the early 1940s, geneticists demonstrated that genes specify the structure of individual proteins. The transfer of information from DNA to protein proceeds through the synthesis of an intermediate molecule known as *RNA*. RNA, like DNA, is made up of a linear sequence of nucleotides composed of four complementary bases. RNA differs from DNA in two respects: (1) its sugar-phosphate backbone contains ribose instead of deoxyribose sugar and (2) thymine (T) is replaced by uracil (U), a closely related base that pairs with adenine (A). RNA molecules are synthesized from DNA by a process known as *DNA transcription*, which uses one strand of DNA as a

Wild-type sequences

Amino acid	N-Phe	Arg	Trp	Ile	Ala	Asn-C
mRNA	5'–UUU	CGA	UGG	AUA	GCC	AAU–3'
DNA	3'–AAA	GCT	ACC	TAT	CGG	TTA–5'
	5'–TTT	CGA	TGG	ATA	GCC	AAT–3'

Missense

	3'–AA[T]	GCT	ACC	TAT	CGG	TTA–5'
	5'–TT[A]	CGA	TGG	ATA	GCC	AAT–3'
	N-[Leu]	Arg	Trp	Ile	Ala	Asn-C

Nonsense

	3'–AAA	GCT	A[T]C	TAT	CGG	TTA–5'
	5'–TTT	CGA	T[A]G	ATA	GCC	AAT–3'
	N-Phe	Arg	[Stop]			

Frameshift by addition

	3'–AAA	GCT	ACC	[A]TA	TCG	GTT	A–5'
	5'–TTT	CGA	TGG	[T]AT	AGC	CAA	T–3'
	N-Phe	Arg	Trp	[Tyr]	[Ser]	[Gln]	

Frameshift by deletion

GCTA
CGAT

	3'–AAA ◢ CCT	ATC	GGT	TA–5'
	5'–TTT GGA	TAG	CCA	AT–3'
	N-Phe [Gly]	[Stop]		

FIGURE 3-4. Different types of mutations. Point mutations involve alteration in a single base pair. Small additions or deletions of several base pairs directly affect the sequence of only one gene. A wild-type peptide sequence and the messenger RNA and DNA encoding it are shown at the top. Altered nucleotides and amino acid residues are enclosed in a box. Missense mutations lead to a change in a single amino acid in the encoding protein. In a nonsense mutation, a nucleotide base change leads to the formation of a stop codon. This results in premature termination of translation, thereby generating a truncated protein. Frameshift mutations involve the addition or deletion of any number of nucleotides that is not a multiple of three, causing a change in the reading frame. (From Lodish HF, Baltimore D, Berk A, et al [eds]: Molecular Cell Biology, 3rd ed. New York, Scientific American, 1998, p 267.)

template. DNA transcription differs from DNA replication in that RNA is synthesized as single-stranded molecule and is relatively short compared to DNA. Several classes of RNA transcripts are made, including mRNA, tRNA, and rRNA. Although all of these RNA molecules are involved in the translation of information from RNA to protein, only mRNA serves as the template. RNA synthesis is a highly selective process, with only about 1% of the entire human DNA nucleotide sequence transcribed into functional RNA sequences. Those DNA nucleotide sequences that code for proteins are called *exons* and are separated by noncoding sequences called *introns* (see Fig. 3-2). After RNA transcription, intron sequences are removed by RNA-processing enzymes (Fig. 3-5). This RNA-processing step, called *RNA splicing*, occurs in the nucleus. Although each cell contains the same genetic material, only specific genes are transcribed. RNA transcription is controlled by regulatory proteins that bind to specific sites on DNA

close to the coding sequence of a gene. The complex regulation of gene transcription occurs during development and tissue differentiation, allowing differential patterns of gene expression.

Once in the cytoplasm, RNA directs synthesis of a particular protein through a process called *RNA translation*. The sequences of nucleotide in mRNA are translated into amino acid sequences of a protein. Each triplet of nucleotides forms a codon that specifies one amino acid. Since RNA is composed of four types of nucleotides, there are 64 possible codon triplets ($4 \times 4 \times 4$). However, only 20 amino acids are commonly found in proteins, so most amino acids are specified by several codons. The rule by which different codons are translated into amino acids is called the genetic code (Table 3-2).

Protein translation requires ribosomes, which are composed of more than 50 different proteins and several rRNAs. Ribosomes bind a mRNA molecule at the initiation codon (AUG) and begin translation in the 5'-to-3' direction. Protein synthesis ceases once one of the three termination codons is encountered. The rate of protein synthesis is controlled by initiation factors that respond to the external environment, such as growth factor and nutrients. These regulatory factors help coordinate cell growth and proliferation.

Control of Gene Expression

The human body is made up of millions of specialized cells, each performing predetermined functions. This is characteristic of all multicellular organisms. In general, different human cell types contain the same genetic material (i.e., DNA), yet they synthesize and accumulate different sets of RNA and protein molecules. This difference in gene expression determines whether a cell is a hepatocyte or a cholangiocyte. Gene expression can be controlled at six major steps in the synthetic pathway from DNA to RNA to protein.[9] The first and most important control of gene expression is at the level of gene transcription, which determines when and how often a given gene is transcribed into RNA molecules. The next step is RNA processing control, which regulates how many mature mRNA molecules are produced in the nucleus. The third step is RNA transport control that determines which mature mRNAs are exported into the cytoplasm where protein synthesis occurs. The fourth step involves mRNA stability control, which determines the rate of mRNA degradation. These steps involve translational control, which determines how often mRNA is translated by ribosomes into proteins. The final step is protein activity control, which regulates the function of protein molecules.

Control of gene transcription is the most important step of regulation for most genes. RNA synthesis begins with the binding and assembly of the *general transcription machinery* to the *promoter* region of a gene (see Fig. 3-5). The promoter is located upstream of the transcription initiation site at the 5' end of the gene and consists of a stretch of DNA sequence primarily composed of T and A nucleotides (i.e., the TATA box). The general transcription

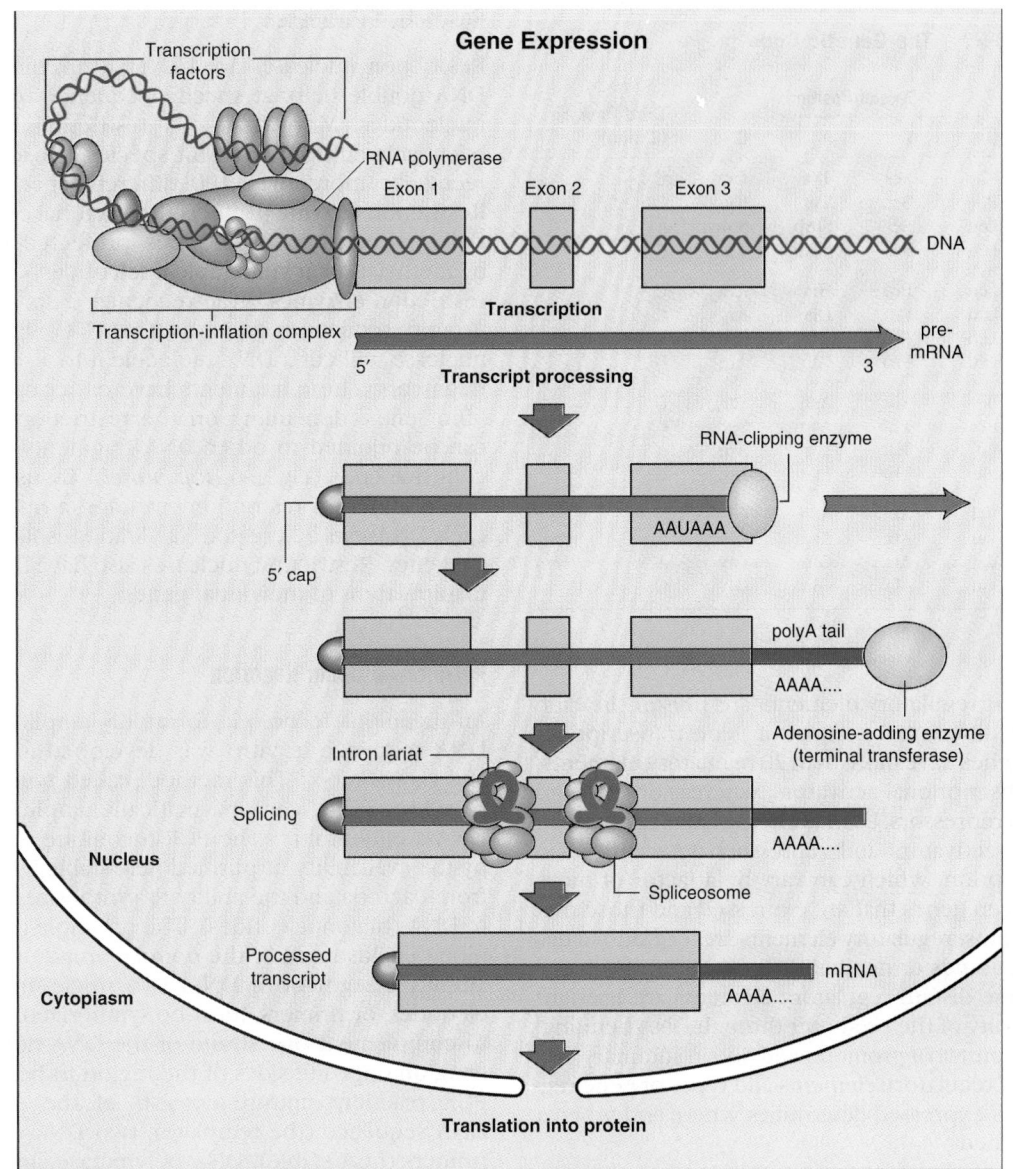

Gene Expression

Transcription factors

RNA polymerase

Exon 1 Exon 2 Exon 3

DNA

Transcription

Transcription-inflation complex

5' 3'

pre-mRNA

Transcript processing

RNA-clipping enzyme

5' cap

AAUAAA

polyA tail

AAAA....

Adenosine-adding enzyme (terminal transferase)

Intron lariat

Splicing

AAAA....

Nucleus

Spliceosome

Processed transcript

mRNA

AAAA....

Cytopiasm

Translation into protein

FIGURE 3-5. Process of gene transcription. Gene expression begins with the binding of multiple protein factors to enhancer sequences and promoter sequences. These factors help form the transcription-initiation complex, which includes the enzyme RNA polymerase and multiple polymerase-associated proteins. The primary transcript (pre-messenger RNA [pre-mRNA]) includes both exon and intron sequences. Post-transcriptional processing begins with changes at both ends of the RNA transcript. At the 5' end, enzymes add a special nucleotide cap; at the 3' end, an enzyme clips the pre-mRNA approximately 30 base pairs after the AAUAAA sequence in the last exon. Another enzyme adds a polyA tail, which consists of as many as 200 adenine nucleotides. Next, spliceosomes remove the introns by cutting the RNA at the boundaries between exons and introns. The process of excision forms lariats of the intron sequences. The spliced mRNA is then mature and can leave the nucleus for protein translation in the cytoplasm. (Adapted from Rosenthal N: Regulation of gene expression. N Engl J Med 331:932, 1994. Copyright © 1994 Massachusetts Medical Society. All rights reserved.)

machinery is composed of several proteins, including RNA polymerase II and general transcription proteins. These general transcription factors are abundantly expressed in all cells and are required for transcription of most mammalian genes. The rate of assembly of the general transcription machinery to the promoter determines the rate of transcription, which is regulated by *gene regulatory* *proteins*. In contrast to the small number of general transcription proteins, there are thousands of different gene regulatory proteins. Most bind to specific DNA sequences, called *regulatory elements*, to either activate or repress transcription. Gene regulatory proteins are expressed in small amounts in a cell and different selections of proteins are expressed in different cell types. Similarly, different

TABLE 3-2. The Genetic Code

First Position (5' end)	Second Position				Third Position (3' end)
	U	**C**	**A**	**G**	
U	Phe	Ser	Tyr	Cys	U
	Phe	Ser	Tyr	Cys	C
	Leu	Ser	Stop	Stop	A
	Leu	Ser	Stop	Trp	G
C	Leu	Pro	His	Arg	U
	Leu	Pro	His	Arg	C
	Leu	Pro	Gln	Arg	A
	Leu	Pro	Gln	Arg	G
A	Ile	Thr	Asn	Ser	U
	Ile	Thr	Asn	Ser	C
	Ile	Thr	Lys	Arg	A
	Met	Thr	Lys	Arg	G
G	Val	Ala	Asp	Gly	U
	Val	Ala	Asp	Gly	C
	Val	Ala	Glu	Gly	A
	Val	Ala	Glu	Gly	G

combinations of regulatory elements are present in each gene to allow differential control of gene transcription. Many human genes have more than 20 regulatory elements; some bind transcriptional activators, whereas others bind transcriptional repressors. Ultimately, the balance between transcriptional activators and repressors determines the rate of transcription, which can vary by a factor of more than 10^6 between genes that are expressed and those that are repressed. Most regulatory elements are located at a distance (i.e., thousands of nucleotide bases) away from the promoter. These distant regulatory elements are brought into the proximity of the promoter through DNA bending, thus enabling control of promoter activity. In summary, the combination of regulatory elements and types of gene regulatory proteins expressed determines where and when a gene is transcribed.

Although controls of gene transcription are the predominant form of regulation of gene expression for most genes, post-transcriptional controls are also crucial for many genes.

RECOMBINANT DNA TECHNOLOGY

Advances in recombinant DNA technology, beginning in the 1970s, have greatly facilitated the study of the human genome. It is now routine practice in molecular laboratories to excise a specific region of DNA, to produce unlimited copies of it, and to determine its nucleotide sequences. Furthermore, isolated genes can be altered (engineered) and transferred back into cells in culture or into a germline of an animal or plant, so that the altered gene is inherited as part of the organism's genome. The most important recombinant DNA technology includes the ability to cut DNA at specific sites by restriction nucleases, to rapidly amplify DNA sequences, to rapidly determine the nucleotide sequences, to clone a DNA fragment, and to create a DNA sequence.[10]

Restriction Nucleases

Restriction nucleases are bacterial enzymes that cut the DNA double helix at specific sequences of four to eight nucleotides. More than 400 restriction nucleases have been isolated from different species of bacteria, and they recognize more than 100 different specific sequences. Restriction enzyme protects the bacterial cell from foreign DNA, whereas native DNA is protected from cleavage by methylation at vulnerable nucleotides. Commonly used restriction enzymes often recognize a six-base pair palindromic sequence, such as GAATTC. Each restriction nuclease will cut a DNA molecule into a series of specific fragments. These fragments have either cohesive ends or blunt ends, depending on the restriction nuclease, and can be rejoined to other DNA fragments with the same cohesive ends (Fig. 3-6, *top panel*). By using a combination of different restriction enzymes, a restriction map of each DNA can be created, facilitating isolation of individual genes. Restriction nucleases also have been used in the manipulation of individual genes.

Polymerase Chain Reaction

An ingenious technique to rapidly amplify a segment of DNA sequence in vitro was developed in 1985 by Saiki and coworkers.[11] This method, called *polymerase chain reaction* (PCR), can enzymatically amplify a segment of DNA a billionfold.[12] The PCR technique is made possible by the availability of purified heat-stable DNA polymerase from bacteria and the ability to synthesize small segments of DNA (oligonucleotides). The principle of the PCR technique is illustrated in the *bottom panel* of Figure 3-6. To amplify a segment of DNA, two single-stranded oligonucleotides, or primers, must be synthesized, each designed to complement one strand of the DNA double helix and lying on opposite sides of the region to be amplified. The PCR reaction mixture consists of the double-stranded DNA sequence (the template), two DNA oligonucleotide primers (heat stable), DNA polymerase, and four types of deoxynucleotide triphosphate. Each round of amplification involves three thermal-controlled steps. First, the reaction mixture is briefly heated to 94°C to separate the double helix structure of the DNA template into two single strands. Next, the reaction mixture is cooled to below 55°C, resulting in hybridization of the two DNA primers to complementary sequences on each strand of the DNA template. Finally, the reaction is heated to 72°C to allow DNA synthesis downstream of each primer. Each round of PCR reaction requires only about 5 minutes and results in a doubling of the double-stranded DNA molecules, which serve as templates for subsequent reactions. After only 32 cycles, more than 1 billion copies of the desired DNA segment are produced. Not only is the PCR technique extremely powerful, it is also the most sensitive technique to detect a single copy of a DNA or RNA molecule in a sample. To detect RNA molecules, they must be first transcribed into complementary DNA sequences using the enzyme reverse transcriptase. The number of research and clinical applications for PCR continues to grow. In molecular laboratories, PCR has been

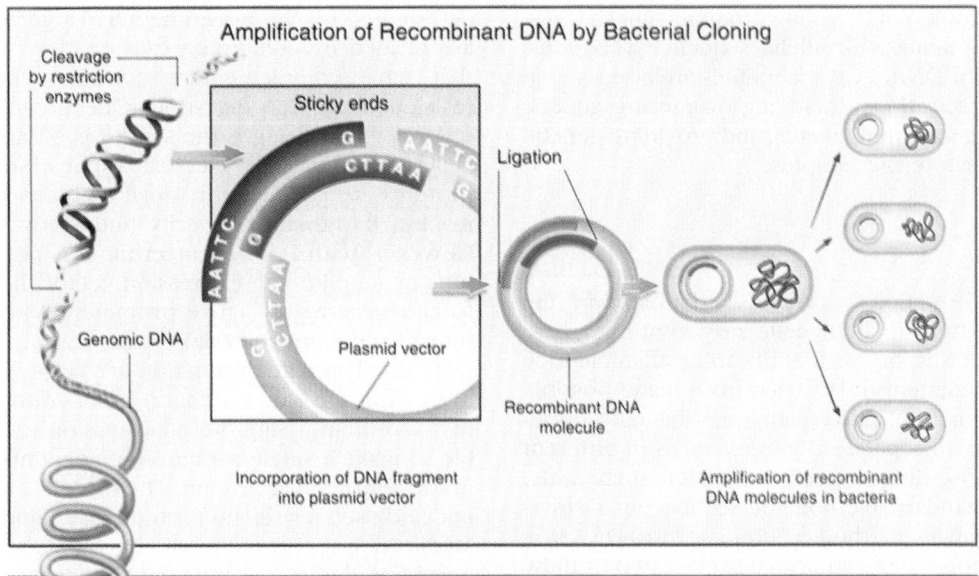

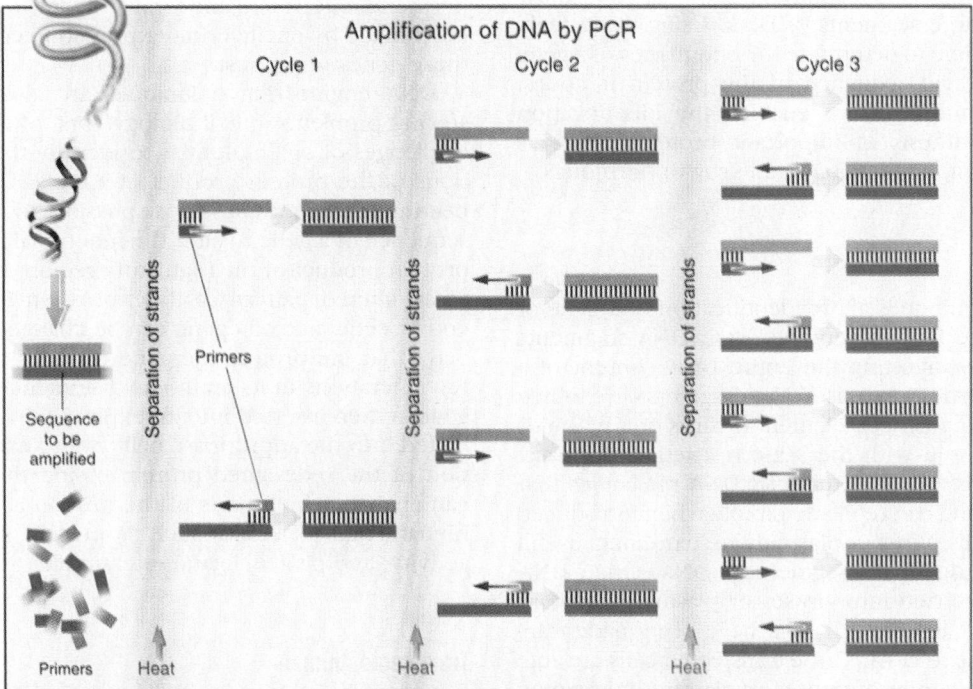

■ FIGURE 3-6.   Amplification of recombinant DNA and amplification by polymerase chain reaction. At the top, the DNA segment to be amplified is separated from surrounding genomic DNA by cleavage with a restriction enzyme. The enzymatic cuts often produce staggered or "sticky" ends. In the example shown, the restriction enzyme *Eco*RI recognizes the sequence GAATTC and cuts each strand between G (guanine) and A (adenine); the two strands of the genomic DNA are shown as black (C denotes cytosine and T denotes thymine). The same restriction enzyme cuts the circular plasmid DNA (gray) at a single site, generating sticky ends that are complementary to the sticky ends of the genomic DNA fragment. The cut genomic DNA and the remainder of the plasmid, when mixed together in the presence of a ligase enzyme, form smooth joints on each side of the plasmid-genomic DNA junction. This new molecule—recombinant DNA—is carried into bacteria, which replicate the plasmid as they grow in culture. At the bottom, the DNA sequence to be amplified is selected by primers, which are short, synthetic oligonucleotides that correspond to sequences flanking the DNA to be amplified. After an excess of primers is added to the DNA, together with a heat-stable DNA polymerase, the strands of both the genomic DNA and the primers are separated by heating and allowed to cool. A heat-stable polymerase elongates the primers on either strand, thus generating two new, identical double-stranded DNA molecules and doubling the number of DNA fragments. Each cycle takes just a few minutes and doubles the number of copies of the original DNA fragment. (From Rosenthal N: Tools of the trade—recombinant DNA. N Engl J Med 331:316, 1994. Copyright © 1994 Massachusetts Medical Society. All rights reserved.)

used for direct cloning of DNA, in vitro mutagenesis, engineering of DNA, analysis of allelic sequence variations, and sequencing of DNA. PCR techniques are also used in many clinical applications, including diagnosing genetic diseases, assaying infectious agents, and providing genetic fingerprinting for forensic samples.

DNA Sequencing

DNA encodes information for proteins and, ultimately, the phenotype of a human. Each gene may continue more than 3000 nucleotide bases. Identification of nucleotide sequences of a fragment of DNA has been made possible through development of rapid techniques that take advantage of the ability to separate DNA molecules of different lengths, even those differing only by a single nucleotide. Currently, the standard method for sequencing DNA is based on an enzymatic method requiring in vitro DNA synthesis. This method is rapid and can be automated to allow sequencing of large segments of DNA. Using these techniques, it is possible to determine the boundaries of a gene and the amino acid sequence of the protein it codes. Sequencing techniques have enabled the identification and in vitro synthesis of important proteins, such as insulin, interferon, hemoglobin, and growth hormones.

DNA Cloning

DNA cloning techniques allow identification of a gene of interest from the human genome. First, DNA fragments are generated by digesting the entire DNA content of a cell with a restriction nuclease. DNA fragments are joined to a self-replicating genetic element (a virus or a plasmid) that is also digested with the same restriction nuclease. Virus or plasmids are small, circular DNA molecules that occur naturally and can replicate rapidly when introduced into bacterial cells. Virus or plasmids are extremely useful vectors for propagating a segment of DNA. Once DNA fragments are inserted into viruses or plasmids, they are introduced into bacterial cells that have been made transiently permeable to DNA. These transfected cells are able to produce large copies of viruses or plasmids containing the DNA fragment. Using this method, a collection of bacteria plasmids containing the entire human genome can be created. This human DNA library can then be used to identify genes of interest.

DNA Engineering

One of the most important outcomes of recombinant DNA technologies is the ability to generate new DNA molecules of any sequence through DNA engineering. New DNA molecules can be synthesized either by the PCR method or by using automated oligonucleotide synthesizers. PCR can be used to amplify any known segment of human genome and to redesign its two ends. Automated oligonucleotide synthesizers enable the rapid production of DNA molecules up to about 100 nucleotides in length. The sequence of such synthetic DNA molecules is entirely determined by the experimenter. Larger DNA molecules are formed by combining two or more DNA molecules that have complementary cohesive ends created by restriction enzyme digestion. One powerful application of DNA engineering is the synthesis of large quantities of cellular proteins for medical application. Most cellular proteins are produced in small amounts in human cells, making it difficult to purify and study these proteins. However, with DNA engineering, it is possible to place a human gene into an expression vector that is engineered to contain a highly active promoter. When the vector is transfected into bacterial, yeast, insect, or mammalian cells, it will initiate production of a large amount of mRNA of the human gene, leading to production of a large quantity of protein. Using these expression vectors, it is possible to make a single protein that accounts for 1% to 10% of the total cellular protein. The protein can easily be purified and used for scientific studies or clinical applications. Medically useful proteins, such as human insulin, growth hormone, interferon, and viral antigens for vaccines, have been made by engineering expression vectors containing these genes of interest.

DNA engineering techniques are also important for solving problems in cell biology. One of the fundamental challenges of cell biology is to identify the biologic functions of the protein product of a gene. Using DNA engineering techniques, it is now possible to alter the coding sequence of a gene to alter the functional properties of its protein product or the regulatory region of a gene leading to an altered pattern of its expression in the cell. The coding sequence of a gene can be changed in such subtle ways that the protein the gene encodes has only one or few alterations in its amino acid sequence. The modified gene is then inserted into an expression vector and transfected into the appropriate cell type to examine the function of the redesigned protein. Using this strategy, one can analyze which parts of the protein are important for fundamental processes such as protein folding, enzyme activity, and protein-ligand interactions.

Transgenic Animals

The ultimate test of the function of a gene is to either overexpress the gene in an organism and see what effect it has or to delete it from the genome and evaluate the consequences. It is much easier to overexpress a gene of interest than to delete it from the genome of an organism.[13] To overexpress a gene, the DNA fragment encoding the gene of interest, or the *transgene,* must be constructed using recombinant DNA techniques.[12,14] The DNA fragment must contain all the components necessary for efficient expression of the gene, including a promoter and a regulatory region that drives transcription. The type of promoter used can determine whether the transgene is expressed in many tissues of the transgenic animal or in a specific tissue. For example, selective expression in the acinar pancreas can be achieved by placing the amylase promoter 5′ upstream of the coding sequence of the transgene. The transgene DNA fragments are then introduced into the male pronucleus of a fertilized egg using microinjection techniques. Typically, 2% to 6% of injected embryos have the transgene integrated into their germline DNA. Animals are then screened for the presence of the transgene. Analyzing these animals has provided important insights into the functions of many human genes and has provided animal models of human diseases. For example, transgenic animals engineered to overexpress a mutant form of the gene for β-amyloid protein precursor (the *APP* gene) have neuropathologic changes similar to patients with Alzheimer's disease. This transgenic model not only supports the role of the APP gene in the development of Alzheimer's disease but is also a model for testing methods of prevention or treatment of Alzheimer's disease.

A major disadvantage of using transgenic animals is that they reveal only dominant effects of the transgene, since these animals still retain two normal copies of the gene in its genome. Therefore, it is extremely useful to produce animals that do not express both copies of the gene of interest.[15] These knockout animals are much more difficult to develop than transgenic animals and require gene targeting techniques. To knock out a gene, it is important to modify the gene of interest by DNA engineering to create a nonfunctioning gene. This altered gene is inserted into a vector and inserted into germ cell lines. Although most mutated genes are inserted randomly into one of the chromosomes, rarely a mutated gene will replace one of the two copies of the normal gene by *homologous recombination*. Germ cells with one copy of normal gene and one copy of mutated gene give rise to heterozygous animals. Heterozygous males and females are generated and can then be bred to produce animals that are homozygous for the mutated gene. These knockout animals can be studied to determine which cellular functions are altered compared to normal animals, thereby identifying the biologic function of the gene of interest. The ability to produce knockout animals that lack a known normal gene has greatly facilitated studies of the functions of specific mammalian genes.

RNA Interference

Since the majority of the approximately 30,000 to 40,000 human genes encoding potential proteins has unknown function, uncovering their biologic activities has been an area of intense investigation. The most effective way to assess the function of a gene is using reverse genetics, that is, target deletion of the expression of a specific gene, and examine the biologic consequences. Until recently, only a few reverse genetic approaches have been available, such as homologous recombination and antisense oligonucleotide strategies. Each of these technologies has significant limitations, making reverse genetic studies both slow and costly. However, a new powerful tool was developed in 1998 by Andrew Fire and Craig Mello that is based on the silencing of specific genes by double-stranded RNA (dsRNA).[16] This technology, termed *RNA interference* (RNAi), requires the synthesis of a dsRNA that is homologous to the target gene.[17] Once taken up by the cells, the dsRNA is cleaved into 21 to 23 nucleotide long RNAs

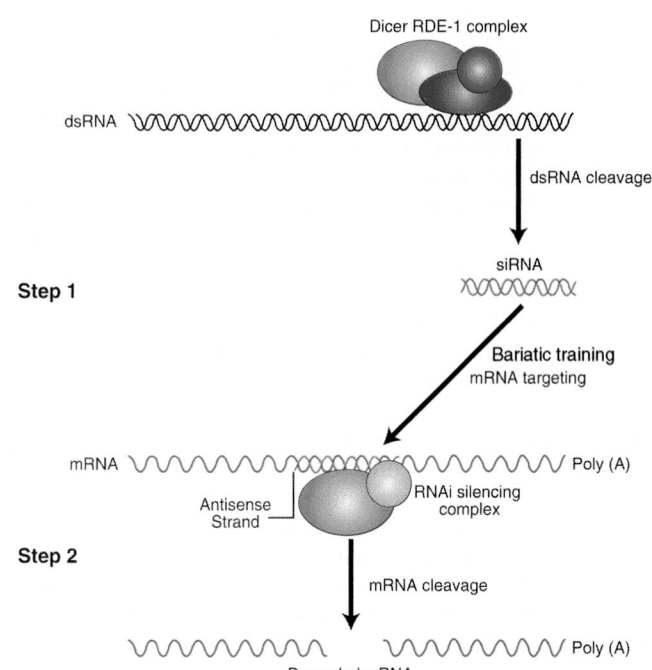

FIGURE 3-7. RNA interference. Long double-stranded RNA (dsRNA) is processed by the Dicer-RDE-1 complex to form short interfering RNA (siRNA). The antisense strand of siRNA is used by an RNA interference (RNAi) silencing complex to guide specific messenger RNA (mRNA) cleavage, so promoting mRNA degradation. RDE-1, RNAi-deficient-1.

called *short interfering RNAs* (siRNAs) by an enzyme complex (Dicer-RDE-1) (Fig. 3-7).[18,19] The antisense strand of the siRNA binds to the target mRNA, leading to its degradation by an RNAi silencing complex. Recent advancement has allowed for the direct design and synthesis of siRNAs as well as placing these siRNAs in viral vectors. This technology not only will transform future studies in the analysis of gene function but, potentially, siRNAs may be used as gene therapy to silence the function of specific genes.

CELL SIGNALING

The human body is composed of billions of cells that must be coordinated to form specific tissues. Both neighboring and distant cells influence behavior of cells through intercellular signaling mechanisms. Whereas normal cell signaling ensures the health of the human, abnormal cell signaling can lead to diseases, such as cancer. Through powerful molecular techniques, the sophisticated signaling mechanisms used by mammalian cells are becoming better understood. This section reviews the general principles of intercellular signaling and examines the signaling mechanisms of two main families of cell surface receptor proteins.[20]

Ligands and Receptors

Cells communicate with one another by means of multiple signaling molecules, including proteins, small peptides, amino acids, nucleotides, steroids, fatty acid derivatives, and even dissolved gases such as nitric oxide and carbon monoxide. Once these signaling molecules are synthesized and released by a cell, they may act on the signaling cell (autocrine signaling), affect adjacent cells (paracrine signaling), or enter the systemic circulation to act on distant target cells (endocrine signaling). These signaling molecules, also called *ligands*, bind to specific proteins, called *receptors*, expressed either in the plasma membrane or the cytoplasm of the target cells. On ligand binding, the receptor becomes activated and generates a cascade of intracellular signals that alter the behavior of the cell. Each human cell is exposed to hundreds of different signals from its environment, but it is genetically programmed to respond to only specific sets of signals. Cells may respond to one set of signals by proliferating, to another set by differentiating, and to another by achieving cell death. Furthermore, different cells may respond to the same set of signals with different biologic activities.

Most extracellular signals are mediated by hydrophilic molecules that bind to receptors on the cell surface of the target cells. These cell surface receptors are divided into three classes based on the transduction mechanism used to propagate signals intracellularly. *Ion channel–coupled receptors* are involved in rapid synaptic signaling between electrically excitable cells. These receptors form gated ion channels that open or close rapidly in response to neurotransmitters. *G-protein-coupled receptors* regulate the activity of other membrane proteins through a guanosine triphosphate–binding regulatory protein called *G protein*.[21] *Enzyme-coupled receptors* act either directly as enzymes or are associated with enzymes.[22,23] Most of these receptors are protein kinases or are associated with protein kinases that phosphorylate specific proteins in the cell.

Some extracellular signals are small hydrophobic molecules, such as steroid hormones, thyroid hormones, retinoids, and vitamin D. They communicate with the target cells by diffusing across the plasma membrane and binding to intracellular receptor proteins. These cytoplasmic receptors are structurally related and constitute the intracellular receptor superfamily. On ligand activation, the intracellular receptors enter the nucleus, bind specific DNA sequences, and regulate transcription of the adjacent gene.

Some dissolved gases, such as nitric oxide and carbon monoxide, act as local signals by diffusing across the plasma membrane and activating intracellular enzymes in the target cells. In the case of nitric oxide, it binds and activates the enzyme guanylyl cyclase, leading to production of the intracellular mediator cyclic guanosine monophosphate (cGMP).

G-Protein-Coupled Receptors

G-protein-coupled receptors are the largest family of cell surface receptors and mediate cellular responses to a broad range of signaling molecules, including hormones, neurotransmitters, and local mediators.[24,25] These receptors include β-adrenergic receptors, α₂-adrenergic recep-

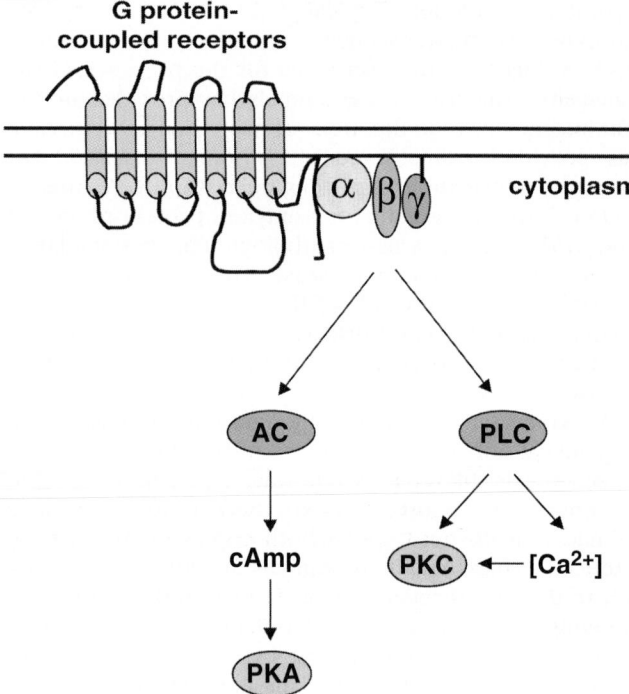

FIGURE 3-8.   G-protein–coupled receptors signaling pathway. G-protein–coupled receptors are seven transmembrane domain proteins that are activated by the binding of ligands. Activated receptors initiate a cascade of events leading to the amplification of the original signal. First, the receptor activates a trimer G protein, consisting of α, β, and γ subunits. G proteins can activate adenylyl cyclase (AC) to generate cyclic adenosine monophosphate (cAMP) or phospholipase C (PLC) to release intracellular calcium. cAMP can activate protein kinase A (PKA), whereas PLC or intracellular calcium can activate protein kinase C (PKC).

tors, and glucagon receptors. They share a similar structure with an extracellular domain that binds ligand and an intracellular domain that binds to a specific trimeric G protein.[26] There are at least six distinct trimeric G proteins based on their intracellular signaling mechanisms; each is composed of three different polypeptide chains, called α, β, and γ.[21,27] On ligand binding, the G-protein–coupled receptor activates its trimeric G protein (Fig. 3-8). Activated trimeric G protein alters the concentrations of one or more small intracellular signaling molecules, referred to as *second messengers*. Two major second messengers regulated by G-protein-coupled receptors are cyclic adenosine monophosphate (cAMP) and calcium. cAMP is synthesized by the enzyme adenylyl cyclase and can be rapidly degraded by cAMP phosphodiesterase.[28] Intracellular calcium is stored in the endoplasmic reticulum and released into the cytoplasm on proper signaling. Some trimeric G proteins can activate adenylyl cyclase, whereas others inhibit its activity. Trimeric G protein can also activate the enzyme phospholipase C, which produces the necessary signal molecules to activate calcium release from the endoplasmic reticulum. Activation of phospholipase C can also lead to activation of protein kinase C, which initiates a cascade of kinases. Changes in cAMP or calcium concentrations in the cell directly affect the activities of specific kinases that phosphorylate target proteins.

The end result is altered biologic activity of these target proteins, leading to a specific biologic response to the initial signal molecule. Despite the differences in signaling details, all G-protein–coupled receptors use a complex cascade of intracellular mediators to greatly amplify the biologic response to the initial extracellular signals.

Enzyme-Coupled Receptors

Enzyme-coupled receptors are a diverse family of transmembrane proteins with similar structure. Each receptor has an extracellular ligand-binding domain and a cytosolic domain that either has intrinsic enzyme activity or is associated directly with an enzyme. Enzyme-coupled receptors are classified based on the type of enzymatic activity used for their intracellular signal transduction. Some receptors have guanylyl cyclase activity and generate cGMP as an intracellular mediator. Others have tyrosine kinase activity or are associated with tyrosine kinase proteins, which phosphorylate specific tyrosine residues on intracellular proteins to propagate intracellular signals. Finally, some enzyme-coupled receptors have serine/threonine kinase activities and can phosphorylate specific serine or threonine residues to transduce intracellular signals.

The receptors for most known growth factors belong to the tyrosine kinase receptor family.[22,23] These include receptors for epidermal growth factor, platelet-derived growth factor, fibroblast growth factor, hepatocyte growth factor, insulin, insulin-like growth factor-1, vascular endothelial growth factor, and macrophage-colony stimulating factor. These growth factor receptors play crucial roles during normal development and tissue homeostasis. Furthermore, many of the genes that encode the proteins in the intracellular signaling cascades that are activated by receptor tyrosine kinases were first identified as oncogenes in cancer cells. Their inappropriate activation causes a cell to proliferate excessively. Similar to G-protein–coupled receptors, tyrosine kinase receptors use a complex cascade of intracellular mediators to propagate and amplify the initial signals (Fig. 3-9). On ligand binding, the tyrosine kinase receptor dimerizes, which activates the kinase activity. Activated receptor kinase initiates an intracellular relay system, first by cross-phosphorylation of tyrosine residues of the cytoplasmic domain of the receptor. Next, small intracellular signaling proteins bind to phosphotyrosine residues on the receptor, forming a multiprotein signaling complex from which the signal propagates to the nucleus. The Ras proteins serve as crucial links in the signaling cascade.[29] On activation, Ras proteins initiate a cascade of serine/threonine phosphorylation that converges on mitogen-activated protein (MAP) kinases. Activated MAP kinases relay signals downstream by phosphorylating transcription factors, leading to regulation of gene expression.

As mentioned previously, human cells integrate many different extracellular signals and respond with biologic behaviors such as proliferation, differentiation, and programmed cell death. In the following sections, we review the mechanisms governing these important biologic processes.

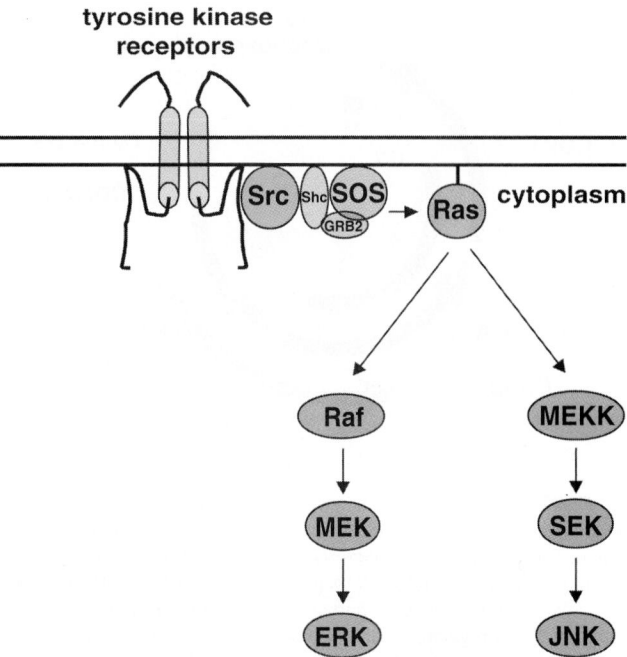

FIGURE 3-9. Tyrosine kinase receptors signaling pathway. Tyrosine kinase receptors are single transmembrane proteins that form a dimer on ligand binding. The activated receptors bind to several proteins (Src, shc, SOS, GRB2) to form a multiprotein signal complex. This protein complex can activate RAS, which can initiate several kinase cascades. One kinase cascade includes the Raf, MEK, and ERK members, whereas another includes the MEKK, SEK, and JNK proteins.

CELL DIVISION CYCLE

Cell division cycle is the fundamental means by which organisms propagate and by which normal tissue homeostasis is maintained. The cell division cycle is an organized sequence of complex biologic processes that is traditionally divided into four distinct phases (Fig. 3-10). Replication of DNA occurs in the S phase (S = synthesis), whereas nuclear division and cell fission occur in the mitotic, or M, phase. The intervals between these two phases are called the G_1 and G_2 phases (G = gap). After cell division, cells enter the G_1 phase, where they are able to receive extracellular signals, and a determination is made whether to proceed with DNA replication or to exit the cell cycle. In this section, we review the proteins that regulate the progression through each phase of the cell cycle and how they control key checkpoints of the cell cycle. Then, we discuss how many cell cycle proteins are mutated or deleted in human cancers.

Cyclin, CDK, and CKI Regulate Cell Division Cycle

The progression of the mammalian cell cycle through these specific phases is governed by the sequential activation and inactivation of a highly conserved family of regulatory proteins, cyclin-dependent kinases (Cdks).[30-32] Cdk activation requires the binding of a regulatory protein (cyclin) and is controlled by both positive and negative phosphorylation.[33,34] Cdk activities are inhibited by Cdk

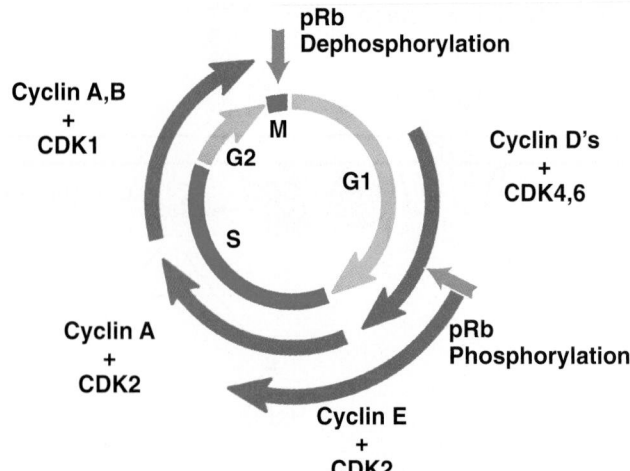

FIGURE 3-10. Mechanisms regulating mammalian cell cycle progression. The cell cycle consists of four phases: G_1 (first gap) phase, S (DNA synthetic) phase, G_2 (second gap) phase, and M (mitotic) phase. Progression through the cell cycle is regulated by a highly conserved family of serine/threonine protein kinases that are composed of a regulatory subunit (the cyclins) and a catalytic subunit (the cyclin-dependent kinases [CDKs]). Cell-cycle progression can be inhibited by a class of regulators called the *cyclin kinase inhibitors* and by phosphorylation of the retinoblastoma (pRb) protein.

inhibitory proteins (CKIs).[35,36] The active cyclin/Cdk complex is involved in the phosphorylation of other cell cycle regulatory proteins. Cyclin proteins are classified based on their structural similarities. Each cyclin exhibits a cell cycle/phase–specific pattern of expression. In contrast, Cdk proteins are expressed throughout the cell cycle. The cyclins, Cdks, and CKIs form the fundamental regulatory units of the cell cycle machinery.

Cell Cycle Check Points

In proliferating cells, cell cycle progression is regulated at two key checkpoints: the G_1/S and the G_2/M transitions. Progression through early-to-mid G_1 is dependent on Cdk4 and Cdk6, which are activated by association with one of the D-type cyclins, D1, D2, or D3.[37] Progression through late G_1 and into the S phase requires activation of Cdk2, which is sequentially regulated by cyclins E and A, respectively. The subsequent activation of Cdk1 (cdc2) by cyclin B is essential for the transition from G_2 into the M phase. There are two families of Cdk inhibitory proteins: the CIP/KIP family and the INK family. The four known INK proteins (p15[INK4B], p16[INK4A], p18[INK4C], and p19[INK4D]) selectively bind and inhibit Cdk4 and Cdk6 and are expressed in a tissue-specific pattern. The three members of the CIP/KIP family (p21[CIP1], p27[KIP1] and p57[KIP2]) share a conserved amino-terminal domain that is sufficient for both binding to cyclin/Cdk complexes and inhibition of Cdk-associated kinase activity. Each CIP/KIP protein can inhibit all known Cdks. One of the key targets of the G_1 Cdks is the retinoblastoma tumor suppressor protein (pRb), which belongs to the Rb family of pocket proteins (pRb, p107, p130).[38] In their hypophosphorylated form, pocket proteins can sequester cell cycle regulatory

transcription factors, including heterodimers of E2F and DP families of proteins.[39] Phosphorylation of pRb, first by cyclin D–dependent kinases followed by cyclin E/Cdk2 during late G_1, leads to release of E2F/DP and subsequent activation of genes that participate in S phase entry.

Oncogenes and Tumor Suppressor Genes

The genes encoding cell cycle regulatory proteins are often targets of mutations during neoplastic transformations. If the mutated gene is cancer causing, it is referred to as an *oncogene* and its normal counterpart is called a *protooncogene*. Many protooncogenes have been identified, and they are typically involved in relay stimulatory signals from the growth factor receptors to the nucleus. They include the intracellular signaling protein Ras, as well as the cell cycle regulatory protein cyclin D1. Mutation of a single copy of a protooncogene is sufficient to bring about increased cellular proliferation, one of the hallmarks of cancer. Several antiproliferative gene-encoding proteins such as pRb, p15, and p16 also negatively control the cell division cycle. These genes are often referred to as *tumor suppressor genes* because they prevent excess and uncontrolled cellular proliferation. These genes are inactivated in some forms of cancer to bring about the loss of proliferation control. However, unlike protooncogenes, both copies of a tumor suppressor gene must be deleted or inactivated during malignant transformation.

APOPTOSIS

Cell proliferation must be balanced by an appropriate process of cell elimination to maintain tissue homeostasis. Physiologic cell death is a genetic program pathway and is called *apoptosis*. Apoptosis has been implicated in various physiologic functions, including the remodeling of tissues during development, removal of senescent cells and cells with genetic damage beyond repair, and the maintenance of tissue homeostasis. In this section we review the biologic and morphologic features of apoptosis and the molecular machinery that controls apoptosis.

Biochemical and Morphologic Features of Apoptosis

Apoptosis is a physiologic process of cell elimination in contrast to another form of cell death called *necrosis*. Necrosis is a passive, adenosine triphosphate–independent form of cell death requiring an acute nonphysiologic injury (i.e., ischemia, mechanical injury, and toxins) that results in destruction of the cytoplasmic and organellar membranes with subsequent cellular swelling and lysis.[37,38] The lysis of necrotic cells releases cytoplasmic and organelle contents into the extracellular milieu, resulting in inflammation with surrounding tissue necrosis and destruction. In contrast, apoptosis is a highly regulated energy-requiring form of cell death that is genetically programmed. Apoptotic cells undergo the following sequence of morphologic and biochemical events:

1. In the early phase of apoptosis, cells exhibit a shrunken cytoplasm and detach from neighboring cells. One of the earliest biochemical features of apoptotic cells is

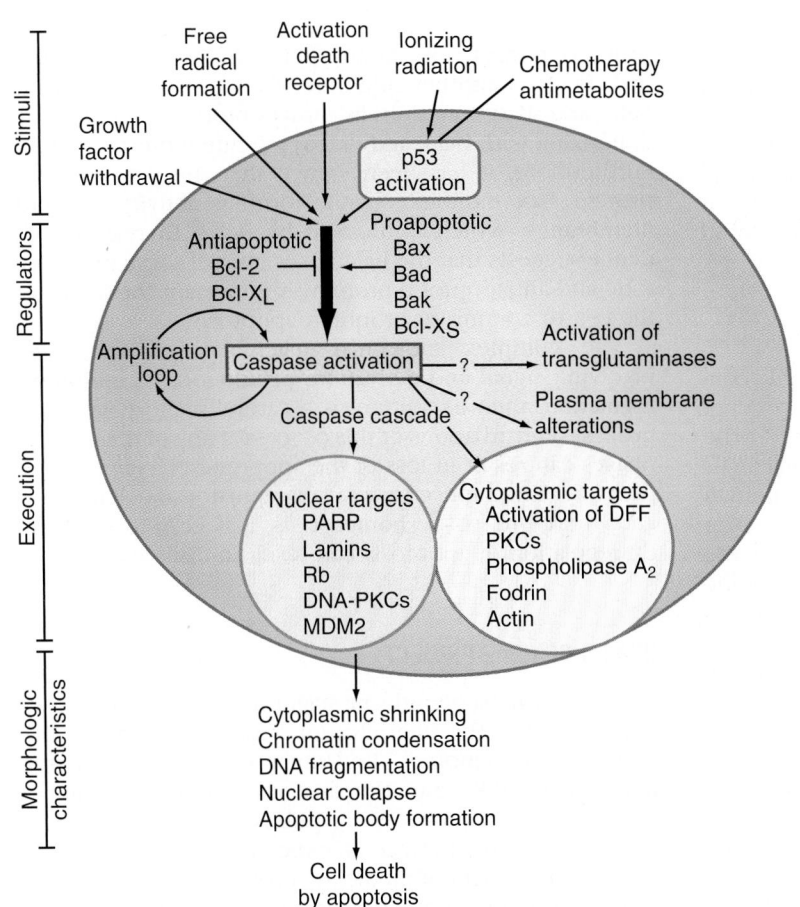

FIGURE 3-11. The apoptotic pathway of cell death. The molecular mechanisms involved in apoptosis are divided into three parts. First, stimuli of the apoptotic pathway include DNA damage through ionizing radiation or chemotherapeutic agents (p53 activation), activation of death receptors such as Fas and tumor necrosis factor (TNF)-α, free radical formation, or loss of growth factor signaling. Second, the progression of these stimuli to the central execution pathway is either positively or negatively regulated by expression of the Bcl-2 family of proteins. Third, the execution phase of apoptosis involves the activation of a family of evolutionarily conserved proteases called caspases. Caspase activation targets various nuclear and cytoplasmic proteins for activation or destruction, leading to the morphologic and biochemical characteristics of apoptosis. (From Papaconstantinou HT, Ko TC: Cell cycle and apoptosis regulation in GI cancers. *In* Evers BM [ed]: Molecular Mechanisms in Gastrointestinal Cancer. Austin, TX, Landes Bioscience, 1999, p 59.)

the externalization of phosphatidyl serine residues on the plasma membrane. It has been proposed that these signaling intermediates may be involved in alerting surrounding cells when apoptosis occurs.

2. Middle events include chromatin condensation with resultant crescent-shaped nuclei and subsequent nuclear fragmentation. During this phase, endonuclease activation results in the fragmentation of DNA into 180 to 200 base pair (bp) internucleosomal sized fragments.

3. Late in apoptosis, the cells begin to fragment into discrete plasma membrane–bound vesicles termed *apoptotic bodies*, which are then phagocytized by neighboring cells and macrophages without inducing an inflammatory response.

The molecular machinery that governs apoptosis can be divided into three parts (Fig. 3-11): (1) signaling of apoptosis by a stimulus, (2) regulation by proapoptotic and antiapoptotic factors, and (3) the execution machinery. These molecular events result in the morphologic and biochemical characteristics of the apoptotic cell.

Apoptotic Stimuli

Many stimuli activate the process of apoptosis (see Fig. 3-11). These include DNA damage through ionizing radiation, growth factor and nutritional deprivation, activation of certain death receptors (e.g., Fas receptor [FasR] and tumor necrosis factor receptor [TNF-R1]), metabolic or cell cycle perturbations, oxidative stress, and many chemotherapeutic agents.[40-43] Signal sensors proximal in the apoptotic pathway recognize these stimuli and include cell surface receptors requiring ligand binding or intracellular sensors detecting the loss of an advantageous environment for survival or irreparable damage. The nerve growth factor/tumor necrosis factor (NGF/TNF) receptor family is the typical example of membrane receptor signal sensors and includes the FasR and TNF-R1 receptors.[44,45] FasR is a 45-kD protein expressed at the surface of activated T cells, hepatocytes, and enterocytes and can be found expressed in tissues including the liver, heart, lung, kidney, and small intestine. Extensive studies with the T-cell model have revealed the downstream events of receptor activation. The binding of a death-promoting ligand to the receptor triggers the death signal, resulting in a conformational change in the intracellular region of the receptor. This protein structure change allows binding of cytoplasmic adapter proteins. These receptor-adapter protein complexes, such as the Fas-activated death domain (FADD), catalyze the activation of downstream proteases involved in the execution phase of apoptosis. Intracellular signal sensors include the *p53* tumor suppressor gene. The identification of DNA damage activates *p53* functional activity and results in G_1 phase cell cycle arrest to allow DNA repair; however, irreparable damage commits the cell to death by apoptosis.[46,47] This differential function may be a result of intracellular expression levels of *p53*. Finally, the lack of certain survival factors results in decreased cytoplasmic signals from cell surface receptors, such as interleukin (IL)-2 receptors, on activated T cells. This loss of exogenous survival signals results in the activation of the endogenous death program. Similar results have been seen with serum withdrawal or growth factor receptor blockade, both of which induce apoptosis. Regardless of the many different signals and signal sensors involved in the activation of apoptosis, each of these pathways converge to activate a common central execution process, the caspase cascade.

Caspases

Caspases, or *cysteine aspartate proteases*, are highly conserved proteins first recognized as the *ced-3* gene product from the nematode *Caenorhabditis elegans*.[48,49] The sequence of Ced-3 exhibits homology to the mammalian IL-1β–converting enzyme (ICE), which is now known as *caspase-1*. To date there are 14 known mammalian caspases, each of which is intimately involved in the conserved biochemical pathway that mediates apoptotic cell death. These proteolytic enzymes are synthesized as inactive proenzymes requiring cleavage for activation. Each activated caspase has specific functions, which may overlap with other caspases. This overlap in function shows the evolutionary significance of apoptosis. The protein substrates cleaved by activated caspases play a functional role in the morphologic and biochemical features seen in apoptotic cells. As indicated in Figure 3-11, activated caspases result in the destruction of cytoskeletal and structural proteins (α-fodrin and actin), nuclear structural components (NuMA and lamins), and cell adhesion factors (FAK). They induce cell cycle arrest through Rb cleavage, cytoplasmic release of p53 by cleavage of the regulatory double-minute 2 (MDM2) protein with subsequent nuclear translocation, and PKC-δ activation. DNA repair enzymes, such as poly (ADP-ribose) polymerase and the 140-kD component of DNA replication complex C, are inactivated by caspase proteolysis. Finally, DNA fragmentation is induced by the activation and nuclear translocation of a 45-kD cytoplasmic protein called *DNA fragmentation factor*. Although there is no known caspase involved in the redistribution of phosphatidyl serine residues on the plasma membrane, caspase inhibitors have been shown to block this event. Overall, the net effect of caspase activation is to halt cell cycle progression, disable homeostatic and repair mechanisms, initiate the detachment of the cell from its surrounding tissue structures, disassemble structural components, and mark the dying cell for engulfment by surrounding cells and macrophages.

Bcl-2 Family

The process of apoptosis is regulated by the expression of certain intracellular proteins belonging to the *Bcl-2* family of genes (see Fig. 3-11).[50-52] Bcl-2 is a potent inhibitor of apoptosis and is predominantly expressed in cholangiocytes, colonic epithelial cells, and pancreatic duct cells. The precise mechanism of apoptotic inhibition by Bcl-2 is not known, but this protein is found on organelle membranes and may function as an antioxidant, protease inhibitor, or gate keeper, preventing the apop-

totic machinery from entering a target organelle. Other proteins in this family include Bcl-x$_L$, Bcl- x$_s$, Bax, Bak, and Bad. Bcl-x$_L$ is another inhibitor of apoptosis. Bcl-x$_s$, Bax, Bak, and Bad function as proapoptotic regulators by dimerizing with Bcl-2 and Bcl-x$_L$, inhibiting their function. Furthermore, it has been shown that the proapoptotic protein Bax exhibits channel-forming activity in lipid membranes, which is blocked by Bcl-2. Increasing evidence suggests that the balance or ratio of these proapoptotic and antiapoptotic proteins is important for signaling the cell to commit to or inhibit apoptosis.

The complex molecular machinery of apoptosis, involving signal and activation, promotion, or inhibition regulation, then execution, is a carefully choreographed process. Perturbations of this process at any of these three phases can result in loss of the apoptotic cell elimination pathway. Since apoptosis is a key regulator of cell number and, therefore, tissue homeostasis, it is easy to see how dysregulation of apoptosis can result in diseases.

HUMAN GENOME PROJECT

One of the most significant scientific undertakings of all times involves the identification and sequencing of the entire human genome. The Human Genome Project was initiated in 1990, and the first versions of the human genome DNA sequence were published in 2001.[53,54] The Human Genome Project is expected to have a major impact on the field of medicine, providing clinicians with an unprecedented arsenal of genetic information that will hopefully lead to a better understanding and treatment of a variety of genetic diseases. As an example, the Human Genome Project is providing new information on the genetic variations in the human population by identifying DNA variants such as single nucleotide polymorphisms (SNPs) that occur about once every 300 to 500 bases along the 3 billion-base human genome.[55] SNPs are thought to serve as genetic markers for identifying diseased genes by linkage studies in families or from the discovery of genes involved in human diseases. These findings may lead to a better screening and help implement preventive medical therapy in the hope of reducing the development of certain diseases in patients found to have predisposing conditions. It is anticipated that knowing the sequence of human DNA will allow scientists to better understand a host of diseases. With new information and techniques to unravel the mysteries of human biology, this knowledge will dramatically accelerate the development of new strategies for the diagnosis, prevention, and treatment of disease, not just for single-gene disorders but for the more common complex diseases, such as diabetes, heart disease, and cancer, for which genetic differences may contribute to the risk of contracting the disease and the response to particular therapies.

The transition from genetics to genomics marks the evolution from an understanding of single genes and their individual functions to a more global understanding of the actions of multiple genes and their control of biologic systems. Technology emanating from the Human Genome Project is currently available to assess an array of genes that may change (either increase or decrease) over time or with treatment. This technology using DNA "chips" provides for one of the most promising approaches to large-scale studies of genetic variations, detection of heterogenous gene mutations, and gene expression. DNA chips, which are also called *microarrays*, generally consist of a thin slice of glass or silicone about the size of a postage stamp on which threads of synthetic nucleic acids are arrayed.[56,57] Literally thousands of genes can be assessed on a single DNA chip. A clinical example of the use of microarrays includes the detection of human immunodeficiency virus (HIV) sequence variations, *p53* gene mutations in breast tissue, and expression of cytochrome p450 genes. In addition, microarray technology has been applied to genomic comparisons across species, genetic recombination, and large-scale analysis of gene copy number and expression, as well as protein expression in cancers.

As genome technology moves from the laboratory to the clinical setting, new methods will make it possible to read the instructions contained in an individual person's DNA. Such knowledge may predict future disease and alert patients and their health care providers to initiate preventive strategies. Individual DNA profile as well as DNA profiles of tumors may provide better stratification of patients for cancer therapies. The Human Genome Project is certain to have an important impact on all areas of clinical medicine. All surgical disciplines will be directly affected by this information. We focus on some specific examples where we foresee major developments occurring that will greatly influence our clinical management.

Transplantation

Despite the remarkable advances made in transplantation, organ procurement, and immunosuppression, a significant impediment remains the availability of suitable organs. The level of organ and tissue demand cannot be met by organ donation alone. Xenotransplantation has been proposed as a possible solution to the problem of organ availability and suitability for transplantation. A number of investigators have examined the possibility of using xenotransplanted organs. However, whereas short-term successes have been reported, there have been no long-term survivors using these techniques. Data obtained from the Human Genome Project may enable transplant investigators to genetically engineer animals to potentially have more specific combinations of human antigens. It is anticipated that, in the future, animals can be developed whose immune systems have been engineered to more closely resemble that of humans, thus eliminating dependence on organ donors.

Another possibility to address the organ donation problem is the potential for organ cloning. With the recent cloning of sheep and cattle, this has received a considerable amount of attention. Although the issue of whole animal cloning is fascinating, the area that offers the greatest hope for transplant patients is the growing field of stem cell biology. By identifying stem cells of interest, the information gathered from the Human Genome Project could enable scientists to develop organ-cloning techniques that will revolutionize the field of transplantation. These pluripotent stem cells have the ability to divide without limit and to give rise to many types of differentiated and specialized tissues with a specific purpose. It is anticipated that the identification of stem cells and the potential modification of these cells by gene therapy may allow investigators to genetically engineer tissues of interest.

Oncology

The results of the Human Genome Project will have far-reaching effects on diagnostic studies, treatment, and counseling of cancer patients and family members.[57] Genetic testing is currently available for many disorders including Tay-Sachs disease and cystic fibrosis. New tests have been developed to detect predispositions to Alzheimer's disease, colon cancer, breast cancer, and other conditions. The identification of the entire human genome will provide for an unprecedented and powerful modality to increase our ability to screen high-risk groups and the general population.

With identification of certain high-risk groups for the development of cancer, surgeons will play an ever-increasing role in both the genetic assessment and ultimate therapy. Prophylactic surgery may soon become more prevalent as a first-line treatment in the fight against cancer. For example, the discovery of the association between mutations of the *ret* protooncogene and hereditary medullary thyroid carcinoma has allowed surgeons to identify patients who will eventually develop medullary thyroid cancer. Genetic screening for mutations of the *ret* protooncogene in patients with the multiple endocrine neoplasia type 2 (MEN 2) syndrome allows prophylactic thyroidectomy to be performed at an earlier stage of the disease process than does traditional biochemical screening. Other areas of active interest include the testing of patients with familial adenomatous polyposis in which the timing and extent of therapy may be based on exact location of the APC mutations. Furthermore, additional testing will allow investigators to better determine other genes that may contribute to this syndrome. Another area of controversy is in the treatment of patients with mutations of the breast cancer susceptibility genes, *BRCA-1* and *BRCA-2*. As more information becomes known regarding mutations of these genes and the clinical implications of these mutations, cancer treatment protocols will be altered accordingly.

Pediatric and Fetal Surgery

Identification of the human genome will further aid in prenatal diagnostic testing and screening. With the identification of fetuses at risk for a number of identifiable genetic diseases, the Human Genome Project will increase research and activity in the field of fetal surgery by expanding the current knowledge of genetic diseases and the rate of fetal surgical interventions using not only the current techniques but also the combination or use of somatic gene therapy. In utero manipulation of identifiable genetic defects may, in the future, become a common intervention.

NOVEL TREATMENT STRATEGIES

Gene Therapy

The ability to alter specific genes of interest represents an exciting and powerful tool in the potential treatment of a wide array of diseases.[58-60] Instead of giving a patient a drug to treat or control the symptoms of a genetic disorder, physicians may be capable of treating the basic problem by altering the genetic makeup of the patient's cells. Several methods are currently available to introduce new genetic material into mammalian cells. Typically, two strategies have been considered: germline and somatic cell gene therapy. In the germline strategy, foreign DNA is introduced into the zygote or early embryo with the expectation that the newly introduced material will contribute to the germline of the recipient and, therefore, it will be passed on to the next generation. In contrast, somatic cell gene therapy models represent the introduction of genetic material into somatic cells, which cannot be transmitted to the germ cells.

A wide array of somatic cell gene therapy protocols designed to treat single-gene diseases, a variety of cancers, or HIV is currently under development with some gene therapy protocols in clinical trials. The goals of human somatic gene therapy are usually one of the following: to repair or compensate for a defective gene, to enhance the immune response directed at a tumor or pathogen, to protect vulnerable cell populations against treatments such as chemotherapy, or to kill tumor cells directly.[61,62]

Several single-gene disorders are candidates for gene therapy, and a number of protocols have been developed. In addition, current thinking has expanded from the treatment of single-cell gene disorders to include treatment of acquired immunodeficiency syndrome and atherosclerosis using gene therapy techniques. Also, many protocols for the treatment of cancer are under evaluation, particularly for otherwise untreatable conditions. Strategies include alteration of cancer cells or other host cells to produce cytokines or other molecules to alter the host response to the malignancy, expression of antigens on cancer cells to induce a host immune response, insertion of tumor suppressor genes or the sequences to slow cell growth, and introduction of drug-resistant genes into normal cells to facilitate more aggressive chemotherapy.

Although a number of in vitro experiments have shown great promise, the current in vivo trials have failed to match the in vitro results, owing partly to the vehicles used for transfecting the DNA into cells. A repertoire of viral-based vectors has been analyzed, with each generation showing more promise than the previous modification.[63] Initially, retroviruses were used as vectors and are still used in certain instances. However, other potential vectors include adenovirus, herpesvirus, vaccinia, and other viruses. Nonviral systems, such as liposomes, DNA-protein conjugates, and DNA-protein-defective virus conjugates, also appear promising.[64] Safety issues, improvement of in vivo gene delivery, efficiency, and gene regulation after cellular transduction are the difficult issues that must be resolved in vector design. However exciting and appealing the prospects of gene therapy may appear, this technique is still in the experimental stages.

Drug Design

Based on information from the fields of genomics and structural biology, rational drug design can be devised to treat a host of diseases.[65] This technique has been used to generate potent drugs, many of which are currently in use or under study. For example, a rational design based on crystallographic data has led to the development of new classes of anti-HIV agents targeted against the HIV protease. Once the critical proteins accounting for a disease are identified and their abnormal function understood, drugs can be designed to stimulate, inhibit, or substitute function.

The identification of human genetic variations will eventually allow clinicians to subclassify diseases and adapt therapies that are appropriate to the individual patient.[66] There may be differences in the effectiveness of medicines from one patient to the next. Also, toxic reactions can occur that may be a consequence of genetically encoded host factors. These observations have spawned the field of pharmacogenomics, which attempts to use information regarding genetic variations in patients to predict responses to drug therapies. In addition to genetic tests, which will predict responsiveness to therapies currently available, these genetic approaches to disease prevention and treatment should provide an expanding array of gene products that will be used in developing future drug therapies.

Genetic Engineering of Antibodies

Monoclonal antibodies, directed against specific antigens, have been generated using hybridoma techniques and are widely used in a number of fields of medicine, including oncology and transplantation. However, a major drawback is the fact that repeated treatment using murine antibodies results in an immune response directed against the antibody. Genetic engineering techniques have allowed for the modification of mouse monoclonal antibodies so as to reduce the immune response directed against them by human recipients and to provide nonhuman resources of human antibodies.[67] This modification involves cloning either the variable or the hypervariable regions of the antibody from the mRNA of a hybridoma and fusing them with a human constant region, thus resulting in clones that can be expressed in human cell lines to produce large amounts of modified antibody. It is anticipated that techniques such as this will become more commonplace in the future and provide a ready source of antibodies directed against a wide array of antigens.

ETHICAL, PSYCHOLOGICAL, AND LEGAL IMPLICATIONS

The possibilities of genetic-based medicine are endless and one can predict that, in the next decade, our lives will be greatly altered due to these rapid advances.[53,68] A number of ethical, psychological, and legal implications can be envisioned and will need to be addressed.[69,70] Such issues include the ownership of the genetic information and who should have access to this information.[71] Another issue is how to correctly counsel both the patient and other family members based on information obtained from genetic testing. The surgeon of the future will need to actively participate and be knowledgeable in these emerging technologies since our management of specific problems will be greatly altered by the new knowledge gained from the analysis of the human genome.[68,72,73] Most assuredly, these rapid advances will continue to alter current treatment strategies and challenge existing dogmas. Surgeons have the opportunity to be active participants and leaders in the research and complex decision-making process that will affect our treatment of patients with surgical diseases. Surgeons, as well as all physicians, must rise to the occasion or otherwise we will be relegated to a bystander status with these complex clinical and ethical decisions made by nonclinicians.

Selected References

Alberts B, Johnson A, Lewis J, et al (eds): Molecular Biology of the Cell, 4th ed. New York, Garland, 2002.

> This textbook provides an excellent primer for the reader to better understand the fundamental concepts of molecular biology.

Collins FS: Shattuck Lecture: Medical and societal consequences of the Human Genome Project. N Engl J Med 341:28-37, 1999.

> This paper by the leader of the Human Genome Project provides an assessment of the progress toward completing this project, as well as future implications for human disease prevention and treatment.

McManus MT, Sharp PA: Gene silencing in mammals by small interfering RNAs. Nat Rev Genet 3:737-747, 2002.

> This paper provides a review of RNA interference technology as a tool to silence genes.

Papaconstantinou HT, Ko TC: Cell cycle and apoptosis regulation in GI cancers. *In* Evers BM (ed): Molecular Mechanisms of Gastrointestinal Cancers. Austin, TX, Landes Bioscience, 1999, pp 49-78.

> This chapter provides an excellent review for the reader to better understand regulation of the cell cycle and apoptosis.

Sambrook J, Russell D (eds): Molecular Cloning: A Laboratory Manual, 3rd ed. Plainview, NY, Cold Spring Harbor Laboratory Press, 2001.

> This manual is a collection of laboratory protocols, including detailed discussion of DNA recombinant technology.

The Chipping Forecast. Nat Genet 21:Supplement, 1999.

> This entire supplement provides an excellent primer for the reader to better understand and appreciate the vast scientific potential and utility of microarray (i.e., gene chip) technology. A basic description of these techniques and possible limitations is presented.

References

1. Alberts B, Johnson A, Lewis J, et al: Molecular Biology of the Cell. New York, Garland, 2002.
2. Lodish HF, Baltimore D, Berk A, et al: Molecular Cell Biology. New York, Scientific American Books, 1998.
3. Rosenthal N: DNA and the genetic code. N Engl J Med 331:39-41, 1994.
4. Donaldson AD, Blow JJ: The regulation of replication origin activation. Curr Opin Genet Dev 9:62-68, 1999.
5. Craig JM, Earnshaw WC, Vagnarelli P: Mammalian centromeres: DNA sequence, protein composition, and role in cell cycle progression. Exp Cell Res 246:249-262, 1999.
6. Urquidi V, Tarin D, Goodison S: Telomerase in cancer: Clinical applications. Ann Med 30:419-430, 1998.
7. Benbow RM: Chromosome structures. Sci Prog 76:425-450, 1992.
8. Malkas LH: DNA replication machinery of the mammalian cell. J Cell Biochem Suppl 30-31:18-29, 1998.
9. Rosenthal N: Regulation of gene expression. N Engl J Med 331:931-933, 1994.
10. Rosenthal N: Tools of the trade—recombinant DNA. N Engl J Med 331:315-317, 1994.
11. Saiki RK, Scharf S, Faloona F, et al: Enzymatic amplification of beta-globin genomic sequences and restriction site analysis for diagnosis of sickle cell anemia. Science 230:1350-1354, 1985.
12. Templeton NS: The polymerase chain reaction: History, methods, and applications. Diagn Mol Pathol 1:58-72, 1992.
13. Yamamura K: Overview of transgenic and gene knockout mice. Prog Exp Tumor Res 35:13-24, 1999.
14. Hofker MH, Breuer M: Generation of transgenic mice. Methods Mol Biol 110:63-78, 1998.
15. Majzoub JA, Muglia LJ: Knockout mice. N Engl J Med 334:904-907, 1996.
16. Fire A, Xu S, Montgomery MK, et al: Potent and specific genetic interference by double-stranded RNA in *Caenorhabditis elegans*. Nature 391:806-811, 1998.
17. McManus MT, Sharp PA: Gene silencing in mammals by small interfering RNAs. Nat Rev Genet 3:737-747, 2002.
18. Grishok A, Pasquinelli AE, Conte D, et al: Genes and mechanisms related to RNA interference regulate expression of the small temporal RNAs that control *C. elegans* developmental timing. Cell 106:23-34, 2001.
19. Ketting RF, Fischer SE, Bernstein E, et al: Dicer functions in RNA interference and in synthesis of small RNA involved in developmental timing in *C. elegans*. Genes Dev 15:2654-2659, 2001.
20. Nishizuka Y: Signal transduction: Crosstalk. Trends Biochem Sci 17:367-443, 1992.
21. Offermanns S: G-proteins as transducers in transmembrane signalling. Prog Biophys Mol Biol 83:101-130, 2003.
22. Heldin CH: Protein tyrosine kinase receptors. Cancer Surv 27:7-24, 1996.
23. Parsons JT, Parsons SJ: Src family protein tyrosine kinases: Cooperating with growth factor and adhesion signaling pathways. Curr Opin Cell Biol 9:187-192, 1997.

24. Ji TH, Grossmann M, Ji I: G protein–coupled receptors: I. Diversity of receptor-ligand interactions. J Biol Chem 273:17299-17302, 1998.

25. Marinissen MJ, Gutkind JS: G-protein–coupled receptors and signaling networks: Emerging paradigms. Trends Pharmacol Sci 22:368-376, 2001.

26. Strader CD, Fong TM, Tota MR, et al: Structure and function of G protein–coupled receptors. Annu Rev Biochem 63:101-132, 1994.

27. Birnbaumer L: Receptor-to-effector signaling through G proteins: Roles for beta-gamma dimers as well as alpha subunits. Cell 71:1069-1072, 1992.

28. Hurley JH: Structure, mechanism, and regulation of mammalian adenylyl cyclase. J Biol Chem 274:7599-7602, 1999.

29. Campbell SL, Khosravi-Far R, Rossman KL, et al: Increasing complexity of Ras signaling. Oncogene 17:1395-1413, 1998.

30. Nigg EA: Cyclin-dependent protein kinases: Key regulators of the eukaryotic cell cycle. Bioessays 17:471-480, 1995.

31. Pavletich NP: Mechanisms of cyclin-dependent kinase regulation: Structures of Cdks, their cyclin activators, and Cip and INK4 inhibitors. J Mol Biol 287:821-828, 1999.

32. Morgan DO: Cyclin-dependent kinases: Engines, clocks, and microprocessors. Annu Rev Cell Dev Biol 13:261-291, 1997.

33. Olashaw N, Pledger WJ: Paradigms of growth control: Relation to Cdk activation. Sci STKE 2002:RE7, 2002.

34. Yang J, Kornbluth S: All aboard the cyclin train: Subcellular trafficking of cyclins and their CDK partners. Trends Cell Biol 9:207-210, 1999.

35. Vidal A, Koff A: Cell-cycle inhibitors: Three families united by a common cause. Gene 247:1-15, 2000.

36. Sherr CJ, Roberts JM: CDK inhibitors: Positive and negative regulators of G_1-phase progression. Genes Dev 13:1501-1512, 1999.

37. Ekholm SV, Reed SI: Regulation of G_1 cyclin-dependent kinases in the mammalian cell cycle. Curr Opin Cell Biol 12:676-684, 2000.

38. Tonini T, Hillson C, Claudio PP: Interview with the retinoblastoma family members: Do they help each other? J Cell Physiol 192:138-150, 2002.

39. DeGregori J: The genetics of the E2F family of transcription factors: Shared functions and unique roles. Biochim Biophys Acta 1602:131-150, 2002.

40. Abastado JP: Apoptosis: Function and regulation of cell death. Res Immunol 147:443-456, 1996.

41. Konopleva M, Zhao S, Xie Z, et al: Apoptosis: Molecules and mechanisms. Adv Exp Med Biol 457:217-236, 1999.

42. Kaufmann SH, Earnshaw WC: Induction of apoptosis by cancer chemotherapy. Exp Cell Res 256:42-49, 2000.

43. Ashkenazi A, Dixit VM: Death receptors: Signaling and modulation. Science 281:1305-1308, 1998.

44. Rath PC, Aggarwal BB: TNF-induced signaling in apoptosis. J Clin Immunol 19:350-364, 1999.

45. Sharma K, Wang RX, Zhang LY, et al: Death the Fas way: Regulation and pathophysiology of CD95 and its ligand. Pharmacol Ther 88:333-347, 2000.

46. Sheikh MS, Fornace AJ Jr: Role of *p53* family members in apoptosis. J Cell Physiol 182:171-181, 2000.

47. Vousden KH, Lu X: Live or let die: The cell's response to *p53*. Nat Rev Cancer 2:594-604, 2002.

48. Creagh EM, Martin SJ: Caspases: Cellular demolition experts. Biochem Soc Trans 29:696-702, 2001.

49. Denault JB, Salvesen GS: Caspases: Keys in the ignition of cell death. Chem Rev 102:4489-4500, 2002.

50. Adams JM, Cory S: The Bcl-2 protein family: Arbiters of cell survival. Science 281:1322-1326, 1998.

51. Antonsson B, Martinou JC: The Bcl-2 protein family. Exp Cell Res 256:50-57, 2000.

52. Tsujimoto Y, Shimizu S: Bcl-2 family: Life-or-death switch. FEBS Lett 466:6-10, 2000.

53. Lander ES, Linton LM, Birren B, et al: Initial sequencing and analysis of the human genome. Nature 409:860-921, 2001.

54. Venter JC, Adams MD, Myers EW, et al: The sequence of the human genome. Science 291:1304-1351, 2001.

55. Wang DG, Fan JB, Siao CJ, et al: Large-scale identification, mapping, and genotyping of single-nucleotide polymorphisms in the human genome. Science 280:1077-1082, 1998.

56. The Chipping Forecast. Nature Genet Suppl 21, 1999.

57. Khan J, Bittner ML, Chen Y, et al: DNA microarray technology: The anticipated impact on the study of human disease. Biochim Biophys Acta 1423:M17-M28, 1999.

58. Prieto J, Herraiz M, Sangro B, et al: The promise of gene therapy in gastrointestinal and liver diseases. Gut 52(Suppl 2):49-54, 2003.

59. Meyerson SL, Schwartz LB: Gene therapy as a therapeutic intervention for vascular disease. J Cardiovasc Nurs 13:91-109, 1999.

60. Petrie NC, Yao F, Eriksson E: Gene therapy in wound healing. Surg Clin North Am 83:597-616, 2003.

61. Lee JH, Klein HG: Cellular gene therapy. Hematol Oncol Clin North Am 9:91-113, 1995.

62. Crystal RG: In vivo and ex vivo gene therapy strategies to treat tumors using adenovirus gene transfer vectors. Cancer Chemother Pharmacol 43(Suppl):S90-S99, 1999.

63. Mah C, Byrne BJ, Flotte TR: Virus-based gene delivery systems. Clin Pharmacokinet 41:901-911, 2002.

64. Niidome T, Huang L: Gene therapy progress and prospects: Nonviral vectors. Gene Ther 9:1647-1652, 2002.

65. Bailey DS, Bondar A, Furness LM: Pharmacogenomics—it's not just pharmacogenetics. Curr Opin Biotechnol 9:595-601, 1998.

66. Evans WE, McLeod HL: Pharmacogenomics—drug disposition, drug targets, and side effects. N Engl J Med 348:538-549, 2003.

67. Brekke OH, Sandlie I: Therapeutic antibodies for human diseases at the dawn of the twenty-first century. Nat Rev Drug Discov 2:52-62, 2003.

68. Hernandez A, Evers BM: Functional genomics: Clinical effect and the evolving role of the surgeon. Arch Surg 134:1209-1215, 1999.

69. Vineis P: Ethical issues in genetic screening for cancer. Ann Oncol 8:945-949, 1997.

70. Grady C: Ethics and genetic testing. Adv Intern Med 44:389-411, 1999.

71. Nowlan W: Human genetics: A rational view of insurance and genetic discrimination. Science 297:195-196, 2002.

72. Vogelstein B: Genetic testings for cancer—the surgeon's critical role: Familial colon cancer. J Am Coll Surg 188:74-79, 1999.

73. Moulton G: Surgeons have critical role in genetic testing decisions, medical, legal experts say. J Natl Cancer Inst 90:804-805, 1998.

CHAPTER 4

THE ROLE OF CYTOKINES AS MEDIATORS OF THE INFLAMMATORY RESPONSE

Mitchell P. Fink, M.D.

Basic Definitions and Classification Systems
Interferon-γ
Interleukin-1 and Tumor Necrosis Factor
Interleukin-6 and Interleukin-11
Interleukin-8 and Other Chemokines
Interleukin-12

Interleukin-18
Interleukin-4, Interleukin-10, and Interleukin-13
High Mobility Group B1
Inducible Nitric Oxide Synthase and
    Cyclooxygenase-2

Classically, the term *inflammation* was used to denote the pathologic reaction whereby fluid and circulating leukocytes accumulate in extravascular tissues in response to injury or infection. As it is currently used, the term connotes not only localized effects, such as edema, hyperemia, and leukocytic infiltration, but also systemic phenomena, such as fever and increased synthesis of certain acute-phase proteins. The inflammatory response is closely interrelated with the processes of healing and repair. Indeed, healing is impossible in the absence of inflammation. Accordingly, inflammation is involved in virtually every aspect of surgery because the proper healing of traumatic wounds, surgical incisions, and various kinds of anastomoses is entirely dependent on the expression of a tightly orchestrated and well-controlled inflammatory process.

Inflammation is fundamentally a protective response that has evolved to permit higher forms of life to rid themselves of injurious agents, to remove necrotic cells and cellular debris, and to repair damage to tissues and organs. However, the mechanisms used to kill invading microorganisms and/or to ingest and destroy devitalized cells as part of the inflammatory response can also be injurious to normal tissues. Thus, inflammation is a major pathogenic mechanism underlying numerous diseases and syndromes. Many of these pathologic conditions, such as inflammatory bowel disease, sepsis, and the adult respiratory distress syndrome (ARDS), are of importance in the practice of surgery.

The initiation, maintenance, and termination of the inflammatory response are extremely complex processes involving numerous different cell types as well as hundreds of different humoral mediators. A thorough account of the cellular and humoral mediators of inflammation would fill volumes and is obviously beyond the scope of a single chapter in a text covering many other topics. Accordingly, the primary objective of this chapter is to provide an overview of the properties and interrelationships of one the most important classes of humoral inflammatory mediators, namely, the diverse group of proteins called *cytokines*. In addition, this chapter provides brief accounts of the roles of several small molecules (e.g., the prostaglandins and nitric oxide) as mediators and modulators of the inflammatory response.

In an effort to avoid presenting an overly dry scientific treatise divorced from the day-to-day practice of surgery, this overview uses a single, albeit complicated, clinical entity—septic shock—as a paradigm of the inflammatory response. *Septic shock* is the clinical manifestation of a systemic inflammatory response run amok. Sepsis is the most common cause of mortality among patients requiring care in an intensive care unit. Severe sepsis, which occurs in about 750,000 people in the United States every year, carries a mortality rate close to 30%.[1] It is generally believed that the incidence of sepsis and septic shock is increasing, probably as a result of advances in many fields of medicine that have extended the use of complex invasive procedures and potent immunosuppressive agents. Given the importance of sepsis as a public health problem, efforts have been made to translate improvements in our understanding of inflammation and inflammatory mediators into the development of useful therapeutic agents. Some of these therapeutic agents are mentioned in the context of the overall discussion of inflammation.

BASIC DEFINITIONS AND CLASSIFICATION SYSTEMS

Cytokines are small proteins or glycoproteins secreted for the purpose of altering the function of target cells in an endocrine (uncommon), paracrine, or autocrine fashion. In contrast to classic hormones like insulin or thyroxine, cytokines are not secreted by specialized glands but, instead, are produced by cells acting individually (e.g., lymphocytes or macrophages) or as components of a tissue (e.g., the intestinal epithelium). Many cytokines are pleiotropic; these cytokines are capable of inducing many different biologic effects, depending on the target cell types involved and the presence or absence of other modulating factors. Redundancy is another characteristic feature of cytokines; that is, several different cytokines can exert very similar biologic effects.

Cytokines can be classified according to several different schemes, all of which are somewhat arbitrary and not completely satisfactory. In an older nomenclature, cytokines were classified according to the type of cell responsible for their synthesis; cytokines produced by lymphocytes were called *lymphokines,* whereas cytokines secreted by macrophages or monocytes were called *monokines.* However, cytokines can be produced by more than one type of cell. Thus, the terms lymphokine and monokine are rarely used in the current literature.

Another way cytokines can be categorized is on the basis of structure. Thus, *type I* cytokines are a large group of proteins that share a characteristic tertiary structure, consisting of a bundle of four α helices. The receptors for the type I cytokines also share structural similarities and are referred to as *type I cytokine receptors.* Type I cytokines include the following proteins: interleukin (IL)-2, IL-3, IL-4, IL-5, IL-6, IL-7, IL-9, IL-11, IL-13, IL-15 and granulocyte colony-stimulating factor (G-CSF). The *type II* cytokines, including interferon (IFN)-α, IFN-β, IFN-γ, and IL-10, are a second structurally related group of proteins. The *type II cytokine receptors* are also structurally related.

Yet another way of grouping cytokines is based on the recognition that naive CD4$^+$ T cells (T$_H$0 cells) can differentiate into either of two T helper (T$_H$) subsets, called T$_H$1 and T$_H$2. T$_H$1 cells, responsible for directing the cell-mediated immune responses necessary for the eradication of intracellular pathogens, favor macrophage activation. T$_H$2 cells have been implicated in the pathogenesis of atopy and allergic inflammation and favor B-cell growth and differentiation. T$_H$1 cells produce IL-2 as well as the potent proinflammatory cytokines, IFN-γ and lymphotoxin (LT)-α. T$_H$2 cells produce IL-4, IL-5, IL-6, IL-9, IL-10, and IL-13.

The actions of IL-4, IL-10, IL-13 and, to some extent, IL-6 are largely anti-inflammatory. Thus, T$_H$1 cytokines are often viewed as being proinflammatory, whereas T$_H$2 cytokines are thought of as being anti-inflammatory. The cytokine IL-12 drives T$_H$1 differentiation, whereas IL-4 induces T$_H$2 differentiation.[2]

A special family of cytokines, the *chemokines,* comprises small proteins with molecular weights in the range of 8 to 11 kD. The chemokines have as their primary biologic activity the ability to act as chemoattractants for leukocytes or fibroblasts. Another cytokine subclass is a group of proteins that act primarily to stimulate the growth and/or differentiation of hematopoietic progenitor cells; these mediators are collectively referred to as *colony-stimulating factors.* Other growth and differentiation factors, including the various platelet-derived growth factors, epidermal growth factor, and keratinocyte growth factor, also fit into the broad category of cytokines.

Overall, hundreds of soluble proteins involved in cell-to-cell signaling, variously called cytokines, chemokines, interleukins, colony-stimulating factors, and growth factors, have been identified and characterized. An exhaustive account of each and every one of these mediators is beyond the scope of this chapter and would be a futile exercise in any event, given the rapid pace of discovery in this broad field of research. Some pertinent facts about some of the most important cytokines are provided in Table 4-1. Some of these mediators are discussed in greater detail in the paragraphs that follow.

INTERFERON-γ

The immune response to infection has two broad components. The *innate* responses, which occur early and are not antigen specific, depend largely on the proper functioning of natural killer (NK) cells and phagocytic cells, such as monocytes, macrophages, and neutrophils. The *acquired* responses, which develop later after antigen processing and the clonal expansion of T- and B-cell subsets, are antigen specific. A number of cytokines, including transforming growth factor-β (TGF-β), tumor necrosis factor (TNF), IL-1, IL-6, IL-10, IL-12, and IL-18, are synthesized by cells of the innate immune system and contribute to the ability of the host to mount an early, innate immune response to an infectious challenge. Another group of cytokines, the interferons, are also key components of the innate immune system.

The *interferons,* named for their ability to interfere with viral infection, were initially discovered in the 1950s as soluble factors secreted by leukocytes.[3,4] The type 1 interferons, IFN-α and IFN-β, are primarily involved as mediators of innate (and acquired) immune responses to viral infection.[5] IFN-γ, although also important in the immune response to viral infection, has much broader activity as a proinflammatory mediator.

For the most part, IFN-γ is produced by three types of cells: CD4$^+$ T$_H$1 cells, CD8$^+$ T$_H$1 cells, and NK cells. IFN-γ, along with two other cytokines, IL-12 and IL-18, plays a critical role in promoting the differentiation of CD4$^+$ T cells to the T$_H$1 phenotype. Because T$_H$1 cells also produce IFN-γ,

TABLE 4-1. Cellular Sources and Important Biologic Effects of Selected Cytokines

Cytokine	Abbreviation	Main Source(s)	Important Biologic Effect(s)
Tumor necrosis factor	TNF	Mφ*, others	See Table 4-3
Lymphotoxin-α	LT-α	$T_H1^†$, NK‡	Same as TNF
Interferon-α	IFN-α	Leukocytes	Increases expression of cell-surface class I major histocompatibility complex (MHC) molecules; inhibits viral replication
Interferon-β	IFN-β	Fibroblasts	Same as IFN-α
Interferon-γ	IFN-γ	T_H1	Activates Mφ; promotes differentiation of CD4$^+$ T cells into T_H1 cells; inhibits differentiation of CD4$^+$ T cells into T_H2 cells
Interleukin-1α	IL-1α	Keratinocytes, others	See Table 4-3
Interleukin-1β	IL-1β	Mφ, NK, PMN§, others	See Table 4-3
Interleukin-2	IL-2	T_H1	In combination with other stimuli, promotes proliferation of T cells; promotes proliferation of activated B cells; stimulates secretion of cytokines by T cells; increases cytotoxicity of NK cells
Interleukin-3	IL-3	T cells	Stimulates pluripotent bone marrow stem cells, increasing production of leukocytes, erythrocytes, and platelets
Interleukin-4	IL-4	T_H2	Promotes growth and differentiation of B cells; promotes differentiation of CD4$^+$ T cells into T_H2 cells; inhibits secretion of proinflammatory cytokines by Mφ
Interleukin-5	IL-5	T cells, mast cells	Induces production of eosinophils from myeloid precursor cells
Interleukin-6	IL-6	Mφ, T_H2, enterocytes, others	Induces fever; promotes B-cell maturation and differentiation; stimulates hypothalamic-pituitary-adrenal axis; induces hepatic synthesis of acute-phase proteins
Interleukin-8	IL-8	Mφ, endothelial cells, others	Stimulates chemotaxis by PMN; stimulates oxidative burst by PMN
Interleukin-9	IL-9	T_H2	Promotes proliferation of activated T cells; promotes immunoglobulin secretion by B cells
Interleukin-10	IL-10	T_H2, Mφ	Inhibits secretion of proinflammatory cytokines by Mφ
Interleukin-11	IL-11	Neurons, fibroblasts, others	Increases production of platelets; inhibits proliferation of enterocytes
Interleukin-12	IL-12	Mφ	Promotes differentiation of CD4$^+$ T cells into T_H1 cells; enhances IFN-γ secretion by T_H1 cells and NK cells
Interleukin-13	IL-13	T_H2, others	Inhibits secretion of proinflammatory cytokines by Mφ
Interleukin-18	IL-18	Mφ, others	Co-stimulation with IL-12 of IFN-γ secretion by T_H1 cells and NK cells
Monocyte chemotactic protein-1	MCP-1	Mφ, endothelial cells, others	Stimulates chemotaxis by monocytes; stimulates oxidative burst by macrophages
Granulocyte-macrophage colony-stimulating factor	GM-CSF	T cells, Mφ, endothelial cells, others	Enhances production by the bone marrow of granulocytes and monocytes; primes Mφ to produce proinflammatory mediators after activation by another stimulus
Granulocyte colony-stimulating factor	G-CSF	Mφ fibroblasts	Enhances production by the bone marrow of granulocytes
Erythropoietin	EPO	Kidney cells	Enhances production by the bone marrow of erythrocytes
Transforming growth factor-β	TGF-β	T cells, Mφ, platelets, others	Stimulates chemotaxis by monocytes and fibroblasts; induces synthesis of extracellular matrix proteins by fibroblasts; inhibits secretion of cytokines by T cells; inhibits immunoglobulin secretion by B cells; downregulates activation of NK cells

*Cells of the monocyte-macrophage lineage.

$^†T_H1$ subset of differentiated CD4$^+$ T helper cells.

‡Natural killer cells.

§Polymorphonuclear neutrophils.

$^¶T_H2$ subset of differentiated CD4$^+$ T helper cells.

the potential exists for a positive-feedback loop. IL-12 and IL-18 produced by monocytes and macrophages stimulate the production of IFN-γ, by T_H1 and NK cells (Fig. 4-1). In turn, IFN-γ further activates monocytes and macrophages, thereby creating another positive-feedback loop.

In addition to promoting the differentiation of uncommitted $CD4^+$ T cells into T_H1 cells, IFN-γ also inhibits the differentiation of lymphocytes into cells with the T_H2 phenotype. Because T_H2 cells secrete the anti-inflammatory cytokines IL-4 and IL-10, the effect of IFN-γ, to downregulate production of these cytokines by T_H2 cells, further promotes development of an inflammatory response to an invading pathogen. In target cells, such as macrophages or enterocytes, IFN-γ induces expression or activation of a number of key proteins involved in the innate immune response to microbes. Among these proteins are other cytokines, such as TNF and IL-1, and enzymes, such as inducible nitric oxide synthase (iNOS) and the nicotinamide adenine dinucleotide phosphate, reduced form

(NADPH) oxidase complex. Thus, IFN-γ stimulates the release of a number of other proinflammatory mediators, including cytokines, like TNF, and small molecules, like superoxide radical anion ($O_2 \cdot^-$), an oxidant produced by NADPH oxidase, and nitric oxide (NO·), produced by iNOS. The secretion of these inflammatory mediators by activated macrophages and other cell types is inhibited by IL-4 and IL-10. Accordingly, IFN-γ–mediated downregulation of the T_H2 phenotype, and thereby production of IL-4 and IL-10, further promotes development of an inflammatory response.

The crucial role of IFN-γ in the host's innate immune response to microbial invasion, particularly by intracellular pathogens, has been emphasized by experiments using transgenic mice with targeted disruptions of the genes coding for IFN-γ[6] or the ligand-binding subunit of the IFN-γ receptor (IFN-γR).[7] These knock-out mice manifest increased susceptibility to infections caused by *Listeria monocytogenes,*[7] *Mycobacterium tuberculosis,*[7] or bacille Calmette-Guérin.[8]

When responsive target cells are exposed to IFN-γ, a number of genes are activated within minutes and without the synthesis of new copies of intermediate signaling proteins. IFN-γ–induced signal transduction occurs via activation of a protein tyrosine phosphorylation cascade known as the *JAK-STAT pathway.*[9] JAK initially stood for "*j*ust *a*nother *k*inase," because the biologic role of these proteins was not established when they were initially discovered.[10] Because these receptor-associated kinases look both outside and inside the cell, JAK has now come to stand for *Janus kinases,* after the two-faced Roman god.[9] The moniker, STAT, an acronym for "signal *t*ransducers and *a*ctivators of *t*ranscription," was appropriately chosen because, in medical parlance, an action to be carried out immediately is a *stat* order and signaling involving these proteins similarly occurs without delay. In addition to IFN-γ, a large number of other cytokines, including IL-6 and IL-11 (see later), also utilize versions of the JAK-STAT signaling mechanism. In mammals, there are four JAK proteins (JAK1, JAK2, JAK3, and TYK2) and seven STAT proteins (STAT1, STAT2, STAT3, STAT4, STAT5A, STAT5B, and STAT6).[11]

The IFN-γR is a heterodimer, consisting of a 90-kD glycoprotein, the α chain, that is required for binding of the ligand and a transmembrane protein, the β chain, that is required for signaling. Associated with the receptor are two members of the JAK family of kinases, JAK1 and JAK2.[11,12] Interaction of IFN-γ with its receptor leads to dimerization of IFN-γR, bringing JAK1 and JAK2 into close association, resulting in mutual phosphorylation and activation (Fig. 4-2). The activated JAK kinases then catalyze phosphorylation of tyrosine residues on the α chains of IFN-γR, leading to docking to the receptor complex by the transcription factor STAT1. After tyrosine phosphorylation, two copies of STAT1 form a homodimer (the IFN-γ–activated factor, or GAF), which subsequently dissociates from the receptor complex and translocates to the nucleus, where binding to the regulatory regions of target genes, containing the IFN-γ activation site (GAS) nucleotide sequence, leads to transcriptional activation.[11,12]

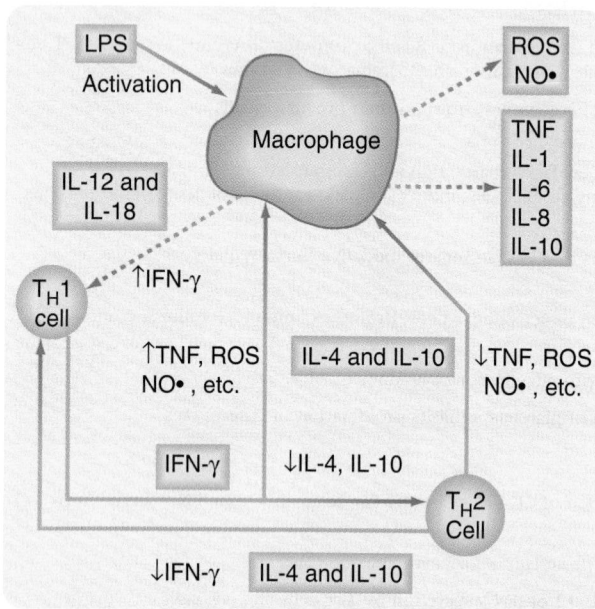

FIGURE 4-1. Simplified representation of the responses of three important cell types (macrophages, T helper cells with a T_H1 phenotype, and T helper cells with a T_H2 phenotype) involved in the inflammatory response to an archetypical proinflammatory stimulus, namely, exposure to lipopolysaccharide (LPS), a component of the outer cell wall of gram-negative bacteria. In response to stimulation by LPS, macrophages secrete the cytokines IL-12 and IL-18. IL-12 promotes the differentiation of naive $CD4^+$ T cells (T_H0 cells) into T_H1 cells capable of producing IFN-γ after activation, and together IL-12 and IL-18 stimulate secretion of IFN-γ by T_H1 cells. IFN-γ, in turn, further upregulates the production of proinflammatory cytokines (e.g., TNF, IL-1, IL-6, and IL-8) and other proinflammatory mediators (e.g., reactive oxygen species [ROS] and nitric oxide [NO·]) by LPS-stimulated macrophages. IFN-γ also downregulates production of anti-inflammatory cytokines (IL-4 and IL-10) by T_H2 cells. IL-4 and IL-10 act to downregulate production of IFN-γ by T_H1 cells and production of proinflammatory cytokines and other proinflammatory mediators by macrophages. IL-10 is not only produced by T_H2 cells but is also secreted by stimulated macrophages as well, creating an autocrine negative feedback loop.

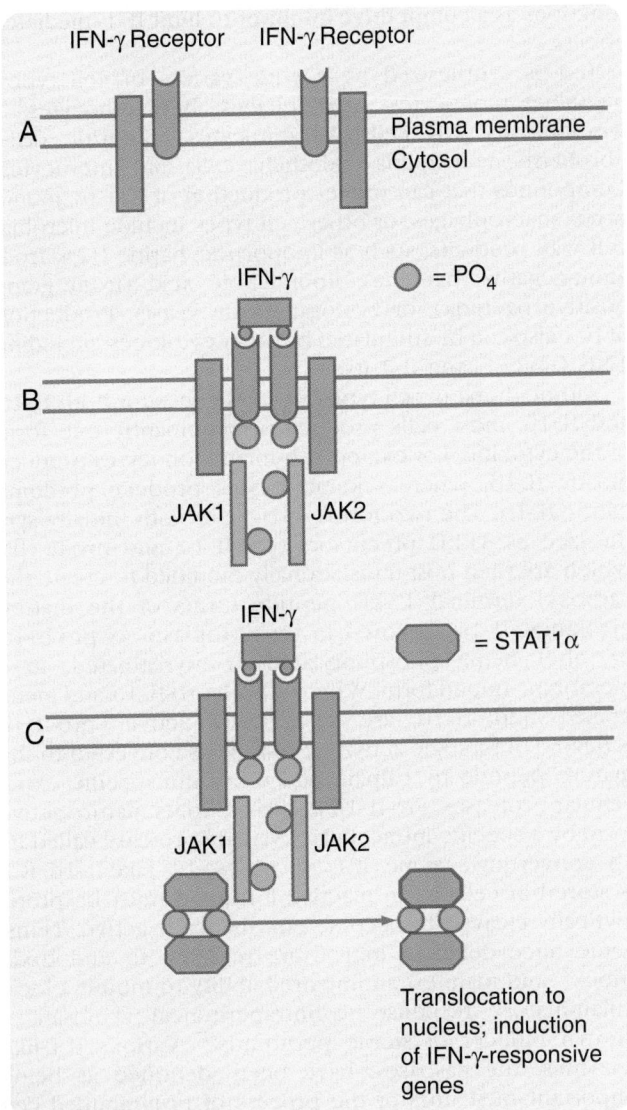

FIGURE 4-2. Simplified representation of intracellular signaling mediated by binding of IFN-γ to its receptor (IFN-γR). **A,** The IFN-γ receptor is a dimer, consisting of a ligand-binding α chain and a transmembrane signaling β chain. **B,** Binding of IFN-γ leads to dimerization of IFN-γR and brings two signaling proteins, JAK1 and JAK2, into association with the receptor complex. **C,** The association of JAK1 and JAK2 with the receptor leads to mutual tyrosine phosphorylation of these proteins, as well as phosphorylation of tyrosine residues on the ligand-binding chains of IFN-γR and docking to the receptor complex of two copies of the preformed transcription factor STAT1α. After tyrosine phosphorylation, STAT1α forms a homodimer. The homodimer dissociates from the receptor complex and translocates to the nucleus, where binding to the promoter regions of various IFN-γ–responsive genes leads to transcriptional activation.

Prompted by the pivotal role played by IFN-γ in the regulation and expression of innate immunity to microbial pathogens, investigators have been interested in using this cytokine as a therapeutic agent to increase host resistance to infection, particularly for patients with congenital or acquired immunosuppression. For example, prophylactic treatment with recombinant IFN-γ has been shown to markedly reduce the frequency of infections in patients with chronic granulomatous disease,[13] a life-threatening condition caused by an inherited defect in NADPH oxidase, the enzyme complex responsible for generating reactive oxygen metabolites in phagocytes. IFN-γ has been approved for this indication by the U.S. Food and Drug Administration (FDA). Severe trauma and burns are associated with defects in host antibacterial and antifungal defenses[14,15]; and in animal models of these conditions, treatment with IFN-γ has been found to increase resistance to infection.[16,17] Based on these encouraging results, three major clinical trials of prophylactic treatment with IFN-γ have been conducted in patients with multiple trauma[18,19] or major thermal injury.[20] Unfortunately, in all three studies, the incidence of infections and mortality was similar in cytokine- and placebo-treated patients.

It is unclear why treatment with IFN-γ failed to improve outcome in these trials. However, treatment with IFN-γ was not individualized based on immunologic phenotype; thus, some of the deleterious effects of inflammation might have been fostered in certain subjects by administration of this potent proinflammatory cytokine. This notion is supported by results from an uncontrolled trial wherein patients with sepsis *and* laboratory findings indicative of excessive immunosuppression (downregulation of human leukocyte antigen [HLA]-DR expression on circulating monocytes) were treated with IFN-γ.[21] In this small study, administration of IFN-γ resulted in resolution of sepsis in eight of nine patients. Prompted by this reasoning, a small pilot study evaluated the use of prophylactic perioperative therapy with IFN-γ to decrease the risk of infection in anergic high-risk patients undergoing major operations.[22] Another approach may be to substitute granulocyte-macrophage colony stimulating factor (GM-CSF) for IFN-γ. GM-CSF, a hematopoietic growth factor that promotes an increase in the number of circulating polymorphonuclear neutrophils, has a number of IFN-γ–like features, including use of JAK-STAT signaling pathways. A randomized trial of adjuvant treatment with GM-CSF in neonates with sepsis and neutropenia showed that survival was significantly improved in the group treated with the cytokine/growth factor.[23]

INTERLEUKIN-1 AND TUMOR NECROSIS FACTOR

IL-1 and TNF are structurally dissimilar pluripotent cytokines. Although these compounds bind to different cellular receptors, their multiple biologic activities overlap considerably, as can be appreciated by inspecting Tables 4-2 and 4-3. Table 4-2 summarizes some of the biologic effects observed when humans are injected with recombinant IL-1 or TNF. Table 4-3 summarizes some important effects observed when certain representative cell types are incubated in the presence of IL-1 or TNF in vitro. Through their ability to potentiate the activation of helper T cells, IL-1 and TNF can promote nearly all types of humoral and cellular immune responses. Furthermore, both of these cytokines are capable of activating neutrophils and macrophages and of inducing the expression of many other cytokines and inflammatory mediators.

TABLE 4-2. Partial List of the Physiologic Effects Induced by Infusing Human Subjects IL-1 or TNF

Effect	IL-1	TNF
Fever	+	+
Headache	+	+
Anorexia	+	+
Increased plasma ACTH level	+	+
Hypercortisolemia	+	+
Increased plasma nitrite/nitrate levels	+	+
Systemic arterial hypotension	+	+
Neutrophilia	+	+
Transient neutropenia	+	+
Increased plasma acute-phase protein levels	+	+
Hypoferremia	+	+
Hypozincemia		+
Increased plasma level of IL-1RA	+	+
Increased plasma level of TNF-R1 and TNF-R2	+	+
Increased plasma level of IL-6	+	+
Increased plasma level of IL-8	+	+
Activation of coagulation cascades	–	+
Increased platelet count	+	–
Pulmonary edema		+
Hepatocellular injury	–	+

Many of the biologic effects of either IL-1 or TNF are greatly potentiated by the presence of the other cytokine. The molecular basis for these synergistic actions remains poorly understood because many of the signal transduction pathways that are activated by the two cytokines are the same.

Interleukin-1 and the IL-1R/TLR Superfamily of Receptors

IL-1 was first described as a *lymphocyte-activating factor* produced by stimulated macrophages.[24] IL-1 is not a single compound but rather a family of three distinct proteins, IL-1α, IL-1β, and IL-1 receptor antagonist (IL-1RA), which are products of different genes located close to one another on the long arm of human chromosome 2. The genes for the two receptors for IL-1, IL-1RI and IL-1RII, are also located on chromosome 2. IL-1α and IL-1β are peptides composed of 159 and 153 amino acids, respectively. Although IL-1α and IL-1β are structurally distinct—only 26% of their amino acid sequences are homologous—the two compounds are virtually identical from a functional standpoint. IL-1RA, the third member of the IL-1 family of proteins, is biologically inactive but competes with IL-1α and IL-1β for binding to IL-1 receptors on cells and thereby

functions as a competitive inhibitor to limit IL-1–mediated effects.

IL-1 is synthesized by a wide variety of cell types, including monocytes, macrophages, B lymphocytes, T lymphocytes, NK cells, keratinocytes, dendritic cells, fibroblasts, neutrophils, endothelial cells, and enterocytes. Compounds that can trigger production of IL-1 by monocytes, macrophages, or other cell types include microbial cell wall products, such as lipopolysaccharide (LPS; from gram-negative bacteria), lipoteichoic acid (from gram-positive bacteria), or zymosan (from yeast). Production of IL-1 also can be stimulated by other cytokines, including TNF, GM-CSF, and IL-1 itself.

Although many cell types express genes for both IL-1α and IL-1β, most cells produce predominantly one form of the cytokine. For example, human monocytes produce mostly IL-1β, whereas keratinocytes produce predominantly IL-1α. The two forms of IL-1 are both initially synthesized as 31-kD precursors (pro-IL-1α and pro-IL-1β), which are then post-translationally modified to create the carboxyl terminal 17-kD peptide forms of the mature cytokines. IL-1α is stored in the cytoplasm as pro-IL-1α or, after being phosphorylated or myristolated, in a membrane-bound form. Whereas both pro-IL-1α and membrane-bound IL-1α are biologically active, pro-IL-1β is devoid of biologic activity. Pro-IL-1β is converted to the mature peptide by calpain and other nonspecific extracellular proteases. Pro-IL-1β is cleaved to its mature active form by a specific intracellular cysteine protease called IL-1β–converting enzyme (ICE) or caspase-1.[25] Like IL-1β, ICE is stored in cells in an inactive form and must be proteolytically cleaved to become enzymatically active. Transgenic mice deficient in ICE are resistant to endotoxic shock[26] and manifest an impaired ability to mount a local inflammatory response to intraperitoneal zymosan, a known inducer of sterile peritonitis.[27] Various ICE-like enzymes, the caspases, have been identified as being important mediators of the process of programmed cell death or apoptosis.[28]

Because it lacks a secretory signal peptide, the mature 17-kD form of IL-1β is not targeted to the endoplasmic reticulum and is not secreted via the classical exocytic pathway used for the secretion of most proteins (including other cytokines) from cells. ICE-dependent processing of pro-IL-1β and the secretory step appear to occur at the same time. Secretion of the leaderless mature peptide apparently occurs through the action of a specific transporter called ABC1, which can be inhibited by the oral hypoglycemic agent glyburide.[29]

Similar to the other members of the IL-1 family, IL-1RA can be produced by a variety of cell types. However, unlike IL-1α and IL-1β , IL-RA is synthesized with a leader peptide that allows for normal secretion of the protein. A specialized form of IL-1RA, intracellular IL-1RA, is synthesized without a leader peptide sequence and, therefore, accumulates intracellularly in certain cell types. In some tissues, such as the intestinal epithelium, formation of intracellular IL-1RA may serve a counter-regulatory function to limit inflammation and thereby confer mucosal protection. Moreover, an imbalance between the production of IL-1 and of IL-1RA may promote the development of

TABLE 4-3.   Partial List of the Effects of IL-1 and TNF on Various Target Cells

Cell Type	Important Effects	IL-1	TNF
T cell	IL-2 synthesis	↑	↑
	IL-2R expression	↑	↑
Monocyte/macrophage	IL-1 synthesis	↑	
	TNF synthesis	↑	
	IL-6 synthesis	↑	↑
	IL-10 synthesis	↑	
	GM-CSF synthesis	↑	→
	G-CSF synthesis	↑	↑
	Prostaglandin synthesis	↑	→
	Tissue factor expression	↑	↑
Neutrophils	Complement receptor 3 expression	→	↑
	IL-8 synthesis	↑	↑
	Priming for increased oxidant production	↑	↑
Endothelial cells	GM-CSF synthesis	↑	↑
	G-CSF synthesis	↑	↑
	Prostacyclin synthesis	↑	↑
	E-selectin expression	↑	↑
	VCAM-1 expression	↑	↑
	ICAM-1 expression	↑	↑
	Tissue factor expression	↑	↑
Hepatocytes	Albumin synthesis	↓	↓
	C-reactive protein synthesis	↑	↑
	Insulin-like growth factor-1 synthesis	↓	↓
	Complement component 3	↑	↑
	Inducible nitric oxide synthase expression	↑	→
Fibroblasts	Hepatocyte growth factor synthesis	↑	↑
	Vascular endothelial growth factor	↑	→

chronic inflammation in certain pathologic conditions, such as Crohn's disease.[30] Production by cells of IL-1 and IL-1RA is differentially regulated. Certain cytokines, notably IL-4, IL-10, and IL-13, which function in many ways as counter-regulatory cytokines, serve as anti-inflammatory mediators in part by promoting the synthesis of IL-1RA. IL-6, although not usually thought of as an anti-inflammatory cytokine, is also capable of triggering production of IL-1RA.

The importance of IL-1β as a proinflammatory cytokine and of IL-1RA as an anti-inflammatory cytokine is emphasized by experiments using transgenic mouse strains deficient in IL-1RA, IL-1α or IL-1β, or both IL-1α and IL-1β (double *knock-out* mice).[31] In these studies, IL-1α knock-out mice were able to mount a normal inflammatory response, whereas the IL-1β knock-out animals manifested an impaired ability to mount a normal inflammatory response. In contrast, mice functionally deficient in IL-RA manifested an exaggerated response to a systemic proinflammatory stimulus (intraperitoneal injection of turpentine).

There are two distinct IL-1 receptors, called *IL-1RI* and *IL-1RII*. IL-1RI is an 80-kD transmembrane protein with a long cytoplasmic tail. In contrast, IL-1RII, a 60-kD protein, has only a very short cytoplasmic tail and is incapable of signaling. As a consequence, IL-1RII is actually a *decoy receptor,* which serves a counter-regulatory role by competing with IL-1RI, the fully functional IL-1 receptor, for IL-1 in the extracellular space. IL-1RI is present on a wide variety of cell types, including T cells, endothelial cells, hepatocytes, and fibroblasts. IL-1RII is the predominant IL-1 receptor found on B cells, monocytes, and neutrophils. The extracellular domains of IL-1RI and IL-1RII are shed by activated neutrophils and monocytes. The shed receptors can act as a sink for secreted IL-1 and, thus, along with IL-1RA, represent an important counter-regulatory component of the inflammatory response.

In 1991, Gay and Keith noted that the cytosolic region of IL-1RI is homologous to a protein, Toll, found in the fruit fly, *Drosophila melanogaster*.[32] In the fruit fly, Toll plays a role in both development and host defense against infection. In mammalian cells, a large family of Toll homologues—the IL-1R/Toll-like receptor (TLR) superfamily—is involved in the recognition of microbial components as well as endogenous ligands induced during the inflammatory response.[2,33] Whereas the cytoplasmic portions of all the members of this superfamily of transmembrane proteins are homologous, the extracellular domains fall into two main subdivisions. In one subdivision, the extracellular portion of the molecule contains three immunoglobulin-like domains and is homologous to the structure of IL-1RI. In the other subdivision, which includes 10 different TLRs (i.e., TLR1-10), the extracellular domain contains leucine-rich repeats.

One of the members of the TLR family, TLR4, has been shown to be important for the activation of inflammatory cells by lipopolysaccharide (LPS; endotoxin), a proinflammatory component of the cell wall of gram-negative bacteria. LPS is a complex glycolipid composed of a polysaccharide tail attached to a lipophilic domain called lipid A. The polysaccharide portion of the molecule tends to be structurally different among different species and strains of gram-negative bacteria, whereas the structure of lipid A (as well as a few neighboring sugar residues) is highly conserved across different species and strains of gram-negative microorganisms. A complex of LPS and a serum protein, LPS-binding protein (LBP), initiates the activation of monocytes and macrophages by binding to a surface protein, CD14. Being a glycophosphatidylinositol-anchored membrane protein, CD14 lacks a cytosolic domain and is unable to directly initiate intracellular signaling. Accordingly, investigators sought to identify another protein that presumably participates with CD14 to initiate cellular response to LPS. The putative LPS co-receptor ultimately was identified as TLR4 by studying an inbred strain of mice, C3H/HeJ, that is congenitally hyporesponsive to endotoxin.[34] Subsequently, TLR4 knock-out mice were generated and shown to be as hyporesponsive to LPS as are C3H/HeJ mice, confirming the concept that expression of functional TLR4 is necessary for activation of macrophages and monocytes by endotoxin.[35] TLR4 mutations are also associated with endotoxin hyporesponsiveness in humans.[36] MD-2, another protein that is associated with the extracellular domain of TLR4, is required for LPS responsiveness.[37,38]

In addition to LPS, other microbial products are recognized by various TLRs. For example, TLR2 recognizes various bacterial lipoproteins as well as peptidoglycan derived from gram-positive bacteria.[2] TLR5 recognizes flagellin, a 55-kD protein found in the flagella of certain bacteria.[2] TLR9 recognizes certain oligonucleotides containing unmethylated CpG motifs that are more common in bacterial DNA than in mammalian DNA.[2]

Because the cytoplasmic domains of all of these TLRs are homologous to the cytoplasmic region of IL-1RI, it is not surprising that shared mechanisms are responsible for downstream signaling (Fig. 4-3). In all cases, an adapter protein, MyD88, links the receptor to another protein, called *IL-1 receptor-associated kinase* (IRAK). On binding of the ligand to the TLR (or IL-1RI), IRAK is phosphorylated and dissociates from the receptor complex, allowing it to interact with another signaling protein, *tumor necrosis factor receptor–activated factor 6* (TRAF6). This process results in the activation of the key proinflammatory transcription factor, nuclear factor kappa B (NF-κB), as well as the phosphorylation signaling cascades involving *mitogen activated protein kinases* (MAPKs).[2]

In the case of activation of this signaling pathway by the binding of IL-1β to IL-1RI, the ligand-receptor interaction does not initiate signal transduction without the association of another transcytoplasmic protein, called *IL-1 receptor accessory protein* (IL-1RAcP).[33] Interestingly, the interaction of IL-18 (structurally related to IL-1) with IL-18R (another member of the IL-1R/TLR superfamily) does not trigger downstream signal transduction without the cooperation of a similar accessory protein called IL-18RAcP (or AcPL).

TLRs also may be involved in the activation of the innate immune response secondary to tissue injury even

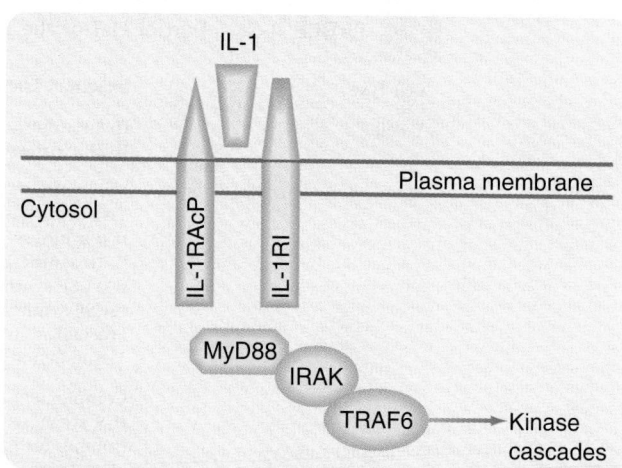

FIGURE 4-3. Simplified representation of intracellular signal transduction initiated by binding of IL-1 to its receptor. There are two IL-1 receptors called IL-1RI and IL-1RII. Only IL-1RI participates in signal transduction, and signaling via this receptor requires the participation of another transcytoplasmic protein called IL-1 receptor accessory protein (IL-1RAcP). The interaction of IL-1 with IL-1RI and IL-1RAcP leads to formation of a trimolecular complex, which, in turn, leads to the docking of yet another protein, MyD88. This molecule then binds another protein, called IL-1 receptor–associated kinase (IRAK). As a result of its interaction with MyD88, IRAK is phosphorylated and activates another signaling protein, TRAF6. The IRAK/TRAF6 complex activates various downstream kinase cascades, ultimately leading to activation of key transcription factors, such as nuclear factor kappa B (NF-κB), and transcriptional activation of various IL-1-responsive genes.

in the absence of infection. Two likely candidates for triggering this pathway for immune cell activation are the proteins called *heat shock protein 60* (HSP60) and *heat shock protein 70* (HSP70).[39-41] Like other members of this family of proteins, HSP60 and HSP70 normally play an important role as chaperones to promote the proper folding of newly translated polypeptides. However, when cells undergo necrosis, these intracellular proteins are released into the extracellular milieu where they can bind to TLRs on macrophages thereby inducing an inflammatory response. This pathway or others like it may help explain how the immune system can respond to danger (e.g., tissue injury) even in the absence of a "foreign" antigen.[42]

IL-1 is an extremely potent mediator. Injecting healthy humans with as little as 1 ng/kg of recombinant IL-1β induces symptoms.[43] Many IL-1–induced physiologic effects occur as a result of enhanced biosynthesis of other inflammatory mediators, including prostaglandin E_2 (PGE$_2$) and NO·. Thus, IL-1 increases expression of the enzyme cyclooxygenase-2 (COX-2) in many cell types, leading to increased production of PGE$_2$. IL-1–induced hyperthermia is mediated by enhanced biosynthesis of PGE$_2$ within the central nervous system and can be blocked by the administration of cyclooxygenase inhibitors. IL-1 induces the enzyme iNOS in vascular smooth muscle cells as well as in other cell types. Induction of iNOS, leading to increased production of the potent vasodilator NO· in the vascular wall, probably plays a key role in mediating hypotension triggered by the production of IL-1 and other cytokines released in response to LPS or other bacterial products.

Elevated circulating concentrations of IL-1β have been detected in normal human volunteers injected with tiny doses of LPS and patients with septic shock.[44] However, in subjects with acute endotoxemia or septic shock, circulating concentrations of IL-1β are relatively low compared with levels of other cytokines such as IL-6, IL-8, and TNF. In contrast, in normal subjects injected with LPS and in patients with sepsis or septic shock, circulating levels of IL-1RA increase substantially and, in some studies, have been shown to correlate with the severity of disease.[45-47] Plasma levels of IL-1RII also increase dramatically in patients with serious infections, leading to systemic inflammatory response syndrome.[47] Although circulating concentrations of IL-1β tend to be relatively low in patients with sepsis, local concentrations of the cytokine can be quite elevated in patients with sepsis or related conditions, such as ARDS.[48]

Tumor Necrosis Factor

TNF was initially obtained from LPS-challenged animals and identified as a serum factor that was capable of killing tumor cells in vitro and causing necrosis of transplantable tumors in mice.[49] The gene coding for the protein was sequenced and cloned shortly thereafter.[50] At about the same time, another protein, named *cachectin,* was identified in supernatants from LPS-stimulated macrophages on the basis of its ability to suppress the expression of lipoprotein lipase and other anabolic hormones in adipocytes.[51,52] TNF and cachectin were later shown to be the same protein.[53] Administration of a large dose of TNF/cachectin to mice was shown to induce a lethal shocklike state remarkably similar to that induced by the injection of LPS,[54] and passive immunization with antibodies to TNF/cachectin was shown to protect mice from endotoxin-induced mortality.[55] Thus, a modern version of Koch's postulates was satisfied, and TNF/cachectin was identified as a pivotal mediator of endotoxic shock in animals. Gradually, the term *cachectin* was abandoned; the name TNF has survived. TNF is sometimes called TNF-α because it is structurally related to another cytokine that was originally called TNF-β but is now generally referred to as lymphotoxin-α (LT-α). TNF and LT-α are both members of a large family of ligands that activate a corresponding family of structurally similar receptors. Other members of the TNF family include Fas ligand (FasL), receptor activator of NF-κB ligand (RANKL), CD40 ligand (CD40L), and TNF-related apoptosis-inducing ligand (TRAIL).[56] Although cells of the monocyte/macrophage lineage are the major sources of TNF, other cell types, including mast cells, keratinocytes, T cells, and B cells, are also capable of releasing the cytokine. A wide variety of endogenous and exogenous stimuli can trigger induction of TNF expression (Box 4-1). LT-α is produced by lymphocytes and NK cells.

TNF is initially synthesized as a 26-kD cell surface–associated molecule that is anchored by an amino-terminal hydrophobic domain. This membrane-bound

Box 4-1. Partial List of Stimuli Known to Initiate Release of Tumor Necrosis Factor

Endogenous Factors

Cytokines (TNF-α, IL-1, IFN-γ, GM-CSF, IL-2)
Platelet-activating factor
Myelin P2 protein
HMGB1
HSP70
HSP60

Microbe-Derived Factors

Lipopolysaccharide
Zymosan
Peptidoglycan
Streptococcal pyrogenic exotoxin A
Streptolysin O
Lipoteichoic acid
Staphylococcal enterotoxin B
Staphylococcal toxic shock syndrome toxin-1
Lipoarabinomannan
Bacterial (CpG) DNA
Flagellin

form of TNF possesses biologic activity. The membrane-bound form of TNF is cleaved to form a soluble 17-kD form by a specific TNF-converting enzyme that is a member of the matrix metalloproteinase family of proteins. Like most of the other members of the TNF family of ligands, the soluble form of TNF exists as a homotrimer, a feature that is important for the cross-linking and activation of TNF receptors.

TNF and LT-α are both capable of binding to two different receptors, TNFR1 (p55) and TNFR2 (p75). Both of these receptors, like other receptors in the TNF-receptor family, are transmembrane proteins that consist of two identical subunits. The extracellular domains of TNFR1 and TNFR2 are relatively homologous and manifest similar affinity for TNF, but the cytoplasmic regions of the two receptors are distinct. Accordingly, TNFR1 and TNFR2 signal through different pathways. Both receptors are present on most cell types except erythrocytes, but TNFR1 tends to be quantitatively dominant on cells of nonhematopoietic lineage.

The precise functions of the two TNF receptors remain to be elucidated. Nevertheless, considerable information about the roles of TNFR1 and TNFR2 has already been gleaned from experiments using genetically engineered strains of mice lacking one or the other or both of the TNF receptors. TNFR1 knock-out mice are relatively resistant to LPS-induced lethality but manifest increased susceptibility to mortality caused by infection with the intracellular pathogens *L. monocytogenes*[57] and *Salmonella typhimurium.*[58] TNFR2 knock-out mice are relatively resistant to lethality induced by large doses of recombinant TNF[59] but have an exaggerated circulating TNF response and manifest exacerbated pulmonary inflammation after intravenous challenge with LPS.[60] Double knock-out mice deficient in both TNFR1 and TNFR2 are phenotypically similar to mice lacking only TNFR1.[60]

Most of the members of the TNF family of ligands are primarily involved with the regulation of cellular proliferation or the converse process, programmed cell death (apoptosis). For example, interaction of the Fas ligand (FasL) with the Fas receptor is essential for the normal process of apoptosis in T lymphocytes. TNF itself is somewhat different from other members of the TNF family of ligands because it is both an initiator of apoptosis and a potent proinflammatory mediator. Activation of inflammation by TNF depends, at least in part, on activation of the transcription factor NF-κB. Because activation of NF-κB tends to suppress apoptosis, it is generally necessary to suppress synthesis of new proteins to observe TNF-mediated induction of apoptosis.[56]

TNF-mediated signaling is initiated by trimerization of receptor subunits. The subsequent downstream events involved in TNF-mediated signaling are different for the two TNF receptors because the cytoplasmic domains for TNFR1 and TNFR2 are distinct. After ligand-induced trimerization of TNFR1, the first protein recruited to receptor complex is *TNFR1-associated death domain protein* (TRADD).[56] Subsequently, three more proteins are recruited to the receptor complex: *receptor-interacting protein 1* (RIP1), *Fas-associated death domain protein* (FADD), and *TNF-receptor associated factor 2* (TRAF2). When TNFR2 is trimerized after association of the ligand with the receptor, TRAF2 is recruited directly. *TNF-receptor associated factor 1* (TRAF1) then associates with TRAF2. The cytoplasmic domains of Fas, TNFR1, FADD, and TRADD all share a highly conserved sequence of about 80 amino acids called the *death domain,* which seems to serve as a mediator of critical protein-protein interactions involved in Fas- and TNFR1-mediated signaling.

The downstream events leading to caspase activation (i.e., apoptosis) or gene transcription (i.e., inflammation) after recruitment of TRADD and/or TRAF2 are exceedingly complex. A deliberately oversimplified model is depicted in Figure 4-4. In the pro-apoptotic pathway, TRADD interacts with FADD, which in turn interacts with a protein called caspase-8 (also known *as Fas-associated death domain–like interleukin-1β converting enzyme* [FLICE]), the proximal element in the caspase cascade leading to programmed cell death (apoptosis). In the proinflammatory pathway induced by activation of TNFR1 or TNFR2, TRAF2 plays a central role in the early events that lead to activation of NF-κB and two important MAPK pathways: namely, those involving the proteins p38 MAPK and *c-Jun N-terminal kinase* (JNK). Overexpression of TRAF2 in engineered cells is sufficient to activate signaling pathways leading to activation of NF-κB as well as another proinflammatory transcription factor, *activator protein-1* (AP-1).[56] By triggering the association of FADD with the receptor complex, the interaction of FasL with Fas directly leads to the induction of apoptosis, whereas the recruitment of FADD to the TNF/TNFR1 receptor

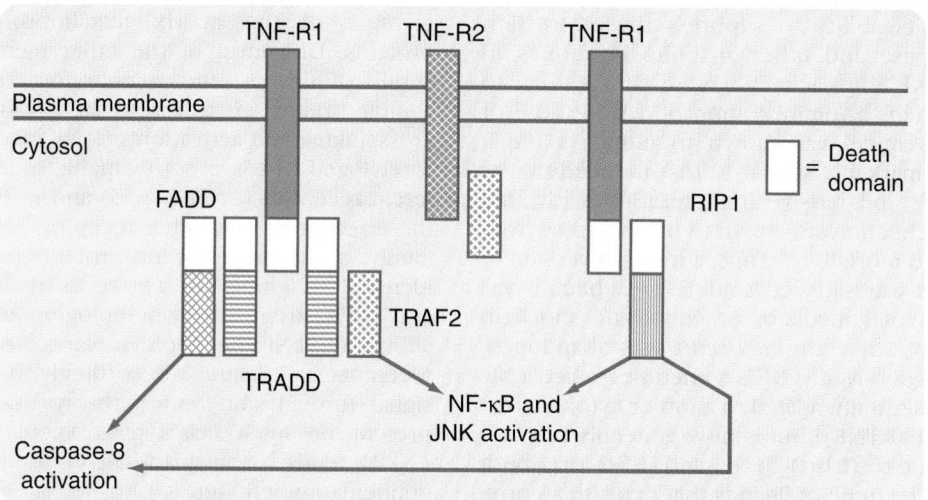

FIGURE 4-4. Simplified view of intracellular signal transduction events initiated by binding of TNF to its cellular receptors. There are two TNF receptors, called TNF-R1 and TNF-R2. Both receptors are homodimeric transmembrane proteins. Although both TNF-R1 and TNF-R2 are capable of initiating signal transduction, different pathways are involved. After TNF binds to TNF-R1, a number of proteins, including receptor interacting protein 1 (RIP1), Fas-associated death domain (FADD), and TNF-receptor-associated death domain (TRADD), associate with the receptor. The intracytoplasmic tail of TNF-R1 and portions of these other signaling molecules share a highly conserved sequence of about 80 amino acids, which is called the "death domain." Homotypic interactions among the death domains of these various proteins are essential for formation of the functional signaling complex. After docking to the receptor complex, TRADD recruits other proteins (e.g., TRAF2 and MADD), which, in turn, initiate protein kinase pathways, leading to activation of the transcription factor NF-κB and the protein kinase c-JUN N-terminal kinase (JNK). TRAF2 also can interact with TNF-R2. Association of FADD with the TNF-R1 receptor complex leads to activation of the proteolytic enzyme caspase-8, which is the proximal element in a signaling cascade leading to apoptosis ("programmed cell death").

complex requires an adapter protein, TRADD, and thus initiates apoptotic processes less directly. Furthermore, the FasL/Fas interaction does not lead to activation of NF-κB, whereas signaling through NF-κB apparently can be initiated by TNF through more than one pathway (TRAF2 and RIP1).[56]

The extracellular domains of TNFR1 and TNFR2 are constitutively released by monocytes, and the release of these soluble receptors is increased when the cells are activated by LPS or phorbol ester. Both soluble (s) TNFR1 and sTNFR2 are present at low concentrations in the circulation of normal subjects.[61] In patients with sepsis or septic shock, circulating levels of both sTNF-R1 and sTNF-R2 increase significantly. Moreover, higher concentrations portend a worse prognosis.[62-64] When present in great molar excess, sTNF receptors can inhibit the biologic effects of TNF. However, when present at lower concentrations, sTNF receptors can stabilize the cytokine and potentially augment some of its actions.

The amount of TNF produced in response to a proinflammatory stimulus, such as exposure of cells to LPS, is determined, in part, by inherited differences (polymorphisms) in noncoding regions of the TNF gene. For example, if the base at position −308 in the TNF promoter is adenine (A), then in vitro spontaneous and stimulated TNF production by monocytes is greater than if the base at this position is guanine (G). The more common allelic form of the TNF gene (TNF1) has guanine at position −308, whereas the less common allele (TNF2) has adenine at this position. Some studies suggest that presence of the TNF2 allele markedly increases the risk of mortality in patients with septic shock,[65,66] although other data dispute this notion.[67] A G to A substitution at position +250 in the LT-α gene is also associated with increased production of TNF by stimulated mononuclear cells, and patients carrying this allele are also at higher risk for mortality due to septic shock.[68] Among patients with community-acquired pneumonia (a relatively homogeneous population of patients with infection), the risk of developing septic shock is greatest for those who are homozygous for the "high TNF secretor" genotype (i.e., AA) at position +250 in the LT-α gene.[69] Data like these suggest that genotyping of patients may prove to be very valuable in the coming years for tailoring anticytokine and other forms of adjuvant therapy for critically ill patients.

Interleukin-1 and/or Tumor Necrosis Factor as Targets for Anti-inflammatory Therapeutic Agents

In view of the central importance of IL-1 and TNF as mediators of the inflammatory response, investigators have regarded blocking the production or the actions of these cytokines as a reasonable strategy for treating a variety of conditions associated with excessive or poorly controlled inflammation. Although clearly different in many respects from sepsis in humans, the shocklike syndrome induced in rodents by injecting LPS intravenously or intraperitoneally has served as a useful paradigm for evaluating various anti-inflammatory strategies.[70] In this model system, survival is improved when animals are treated with any one of a variety of different pharmacologic, immunologic, or genetic strategies that either block the release of TNF or prevent this cytokine from interacting with its receptor(s) after it is released. To a lesser extent, the same statement also applies to IL-1.

Clinicians and scientists have recognized for decades that glucocorticoids, such as hydrocortisone and dexamethasone, are potent anti-inflammatory agents. Additionally, it is now well established that corticosteroids inhibit the release of TNF and IL-1 from activated monocytes and other cell types. These anti-inflammatory actions of hydrocortisone and related compounds are mediated by more than one mechanism. One important action of glucocorticoids is to downregulate signaling mediated by a key transcription factor, NF-κB, known to activate many genes (including those coding for TNF and IL-1) associated with the inflammatory response.[71] Glucocorticoid-induced downregulation of NF-κB activation is a result of augmented expression of a protein, IκB, that is an inhibitory component of the NF-κB complex.[71] Another anti-inflammatory action of glucocorticoids is to inhibit activation of another signaling pathway, the JNK/SAPK cascade, leading to decreased translation of TNF mRNA and, thus, decreased production of TNF.[72] Still another mechanism whereby glucocorticoids inhibit inflammation is through decreased expression of the enzyme ICE required for post-translational processing of pro-IL-1β and, thus, decreased secretion of mature IL-1β.[73]

In experimental models of sepsis, early treatment with high doses of a potent synthetic glucocorticoid, such as methylprednisolone or dexamethasone, improves survival.[74] Unfortunately, several large clinical trials have failed to confirm the benefit of high-dose glucocorticoid therapy for the adjuvant treatment of patients with septic shock or the related condition ARDS.[75-79] As a result, the notion of using glucocorticoids for these indications seemed to be a dead issue. However, in the past few years, the concept of using glucocorticoids as anti-inflammatory agents in the management of ARDS or septic shock has been resurrected. Several small studies showed that prolonged therapy with relatively low doses of hydrocortisone or methylprednisolone can improve systemic hemodynamics and/or pulmonary function in patients with ARDS or septic shock.[80-83] These tantalizing findings were confirmed by the results obtained in a 300-patient multicentric randomized clinical trial carried out in a single country (France).[84] Although somewhat controversial, the results of this study support the view that administration of a relatively low dose of hydrocortisone (50 mg IV every 6 hours for 7 days) improves survival in patients with volume-unresponsive pressor-dependent septic shock. At present, it is not clear whether hydrocortisone is effective in this setting because many patients with septic shock are functionally adrenally insufficient (i.e., hydrocortisone is functioning as replacement therapy) or because administration of the glucocorticoid modulates the inflammatory response. Of course, these two potential mechanisms are not mutually exclusive.

Glucocorticoids are an old-fashioned and not very selective way to block IL-1– or TNF-mediated proinflammatory effects. As our understanding of the role of cytokines as mediators of inflammation has progressed, newer and more specific pharmacologic anti-inflammatory strategies have been developed and evaluated as adjunctive agents for the treatment of sepsis in placebo-controlled prospective clinical trials. Unfortunately, results in these trials have been disappointing. Positive results have been obtained in only a single study, an open-label trial of recombinant IL-1RA that enrolled a relatively small number of patients.[85] With the exception of this study, none of the agents tested has been shown to significantly improve survival. Indeed, in one trial, treatment of septic patients with a "fusion protein" incorporating the extracellular domain of TNFR2 resulted in increased mortality, particularly in patients with gram-positive infections.[86]

Despite the negative results obtained in sepsis trials, at least two agents designed to neutralize the effects of secreted TNF have been shown to have significant clinical efficacy in other important inflammatory conditions, such as Crohn's disease[87,88] and rheumatoid arthritis.[89,90] Infliximab, a monoclonal anti-TNF antibody, has been approved by the FDA for administration to patients to provide long-term remission-level control of the debilitating symptoms of Crohn's disease. Infliximab also has been approved for use, in combination with methotrexate, to reduce the signs and symptoms, inhibit the progression of structural damage, and improve physical function in patients with moderately to severely active rheumatoid arthritis who have had an inadequate response to methotrexate. Etanercept, the TNFR2 fusion protein evaluated unsuccessfully for the treatment of sepsis, has been approved by the FDA for the management of psoriatic arthritis, for reducing the signs and symptoms and inhibiting the progression of structural damage in patients with moderately to severely active rheumatoid arthritis, and for reducing signs and symptoms in patients 4 years of age and older with moderately to severely active polyarticular-course juvenile rheumatoid arthritis. Thus, cytokine-specific approaches toward managing inflammatory conditions have moved from the research bench to the clinic and now occupy an important role in the clinical management of common clinical conditions, even though this approach has not panned out for the treatment of sepsis and septic shock.

The network of cytokines that is associated with the inflammatory response interacts at multiple points with another component of the host's defense against injury and infection, namely, the coagulation system. TNF and IL-1 (as well as some other pro-inflammatory cytokines) can activate the extrinsic pathway of coagulation, in part by promoting expression of tissue factor (TF) on endothelial cells and monocytes. In addition, these cytokines also downregulate the expression of an important endogenous inhibitor of coagulation, thrombomodulin, on the surface of endothelial cells. Thus, TNF and IL-1 promote activation of the coagulation cascade.[91] Numerous studies have documented that the extrinsic coagulation pathway is activated in patients with sepsis, even in the absence of frank, clinically evident disseminated intravascular coagulation (DIC). Of note, circulating levels of a natural inhibitor of coagulation, protein C, tend to decrease in patients with severe sepsis or septic shock, and a marked deficiency of protein C in these patients is a prognostic indicator for an unfavorable outcome.[92] Prompted by these concepts, various strategies to inhibit excessive activation of the coagulation system have been extensively evaluated in both animal models of endotoxemia and sepsis as well as in clinical trials. Recently, one of these approaches, namely, administration of recombinant human activated protein C, also called drotrecogin alfa (activated), was shown in a large multicentric randomized clinical trial to significantly improve survival in patients with severe sepsis.[93] Drotrecogin alfa (activated) has been approved for this indication by the FDA.

INTERLEUKIN-6 AND INTERLEUKIN-11

IL-6 and IL-11 warrant consideration together because, along with several other proteins (e.g., oncostatin M), both of these cytokines utilize a specific transmembrane protein, gp130, for receptor function. IL-6 consists of 184 amino acids plus a 28-amino acid hydrophobic signal sequence. The protein is variably phosphorylated and glycosylated before secretion. IL-11 is translated as a precursor protein containing 199 amino acids, including a 21-amino acid leader sequence.

Like IL-1 and TNF, IL-6 is a pluripotent cytokine, intimately associated with the inflammatory response to injury or infection. IL-6 can be produced not only by immunocytes (e.g., monocytes, macrophages, and lymphocytes) but also by many other cell types, including endothelial cells and intestinal epithelial cells. Factors known to induce expression of IL-6 include IL-1, TNF, platelet activating factor, LPS, and reactive oxygen metabolites. The promoter region of the IL-6 gene contains functional elements capable of binding NF-κB as well as another important transcription factor, *CCAAT/enhancer binding protein* (C/EBP), previously called NF-IL-6. The cellular and physiologic effects of IL-6 are diverse and include induction of fever, promotion of B-cell maturation and differentiation, stimulation of T-cell proliferation and differentiation, promotion of differentiation of nerve cells, stimulation of the hypothalamic-pituitary-adrenal axis, and induction of synthesis of acute-phase proteins (e.g., C-reactive protein) by hepatocytes. Transgenic mice that overexpress IL-6 develop plasmacytosis and hypergammaglobulinemia.[94] Conversely, transgenic IL-6 knock-out mice have an impaired acute-phase response to inflammatory stimuli, abnormal B-cell maturation, deficient mucosal immunoglobulin (Ig) A production, and impaired host resistance to the intracellular pathogen *L. monocytogenes*.[95,96] In other murine models of inflammation, the effects of genetic IL-6 deficiency are highly variable. For example, in a murine model of acute pancreatitis induced by repetitive injections of cerulein, inflammation is exacerbated in IL-6 knock-out mice as compared with wild-type controls, a finding that emphasizes the anti-inflammatory effects of IL-6.[97] In contrast, in a murine model of hemorrhagic shock and resuscitation, IL-6 knock-out mice develop less pulmonary inflammation and lung injury than do wild-type controls, an observation that emphasizes the proinflammatory effects of IL-6.[98] Although IL-6 knock-out mice are not protected from the lethal effects of sepsis, treatment of septic wild-type mice with a carefully calibrated dose of an anti-IL-6 antibody improves survival.[99] Whether modulation of IL-6 activity by administration of a neutralizing anti-IL-6 monoclonal antibody will prove to be beneficial in the management of disease in humans remains to be seen.

IL-11 is expressed in a variety of cell types, including neurons, fibroblasts, and epithelial cells. Although constitutive expression of IL-11 can be detected in a range of normal adult tissues, expression of IL-11 can also be upregulated by IL-1, TGF-β, and other cytokines or growth factors. Regulation of IL-11 expression is under both transcriptional and translational control. From a functional standpoint, IL-11 is a hematopoietic growth factor, having particular activity as a stimulator of megakaryocytopoiesis and thrombopoiesis. IL-11 also can interact with epithelial cells in the gastrointestinal tract and inhibit proliferation of enterocytic cell lines in vitro.

The mechanisms whereby IL-6- or IL-11-induced signals are transduced in target cells have been studied extensively. Activation of target cells via the IL-6 or IL-11 receptor complexes requires the cooperation of two distinct proteins. In the case of IL-6, the ligand-binding subunit is called IL-6R, whereas in the case of IL-11 the ligand-binding subunit is called IL-11R. For both receptors, a distinct protein, called gp130, is required for signal transduction. Intracellular signal transduction involves the association of the IL-6/IL-6R complex or the IL-11/IL-11R complex with gp130. Dimerization of gp130 leads to downstream signaling via members of the JAK family of protein tyrosine kinases. JAK kinase activation leads, in turn, to phosphorylation and activation of STAT3, a member of the STAT family of signaling proteins. Phosphorylation of STAT proteins leads to dimerization, translocation to the nucleus, binding to DNA, and transcriptional activation.

Circulating concentrations of IL-6 increase dramatically after tissue injury, such as occurs as a consequence of elective surgical procedures,[100,101] accidental trauma,[102] or burns.[103,104] Elevated plasma levels of IL-6 are consistently observed in patients with sepsis or septic shock.[105,106] The degree to which circulating IL-6 levels are elevated after tissue trauma or during sepsis has been shown to correlate with the risk of postinjury complications[102] or death.[105] Although it remains to be established whether high circulating IL-6 levels are directly or indirectly injurious to patients with sepsis or are simply a marker of severity of illness, the observation that immunoneutralization of IL-6 improves outcome in experimental bacterial peritonitis suggests that elevated concentrations of this cytokine are deleterious.[99]

Circulating levels of IL-11 increase in patients with disseminated intravascular coagulation and sepsis. Intravenous or oral administration of recombinant IL-11 improves survival in neutropenic rodents with sepsis, possibly by preserving the integrity of the intestinal mucosal barrier.[107,108]

INTERLEUKIN-8 AND OTHER CHEMOKINES

Chemotaxis is the term used to denote the directed migration of cells toward increasing concentrations of an activating substance (chemotaxin). The ability to recruit leukocytes to an inflammatory focus by promoting chemotaxis is the primary biologic activity of a special group of cytokines that are called *chemokines.* More than 40 of these small proteins have been identified. Each contains 70 to 80 amino acids, including three or four conserved cysteine residues. Four chemokine subgroups have been described: CXC, CC, C, and CX$_3$C. The subgroups are defined by the degree of separation of the first two NH$_2$-terminal cysteine residues. In the CXC or α-chemokines, the first two cysteine moieties are separated by a single nonconserved amino acid residue, whereas in the CC or β-chemokines, the NH$_2$-terminal cysteines are directly adjacent to each other. The C chemokine subgroup is characterized by the presence of only a single NH$_2$-terminal cysteine moiety. The CX$_3$C subgroup has only one member (fractalkine); in this chemokine, the NH$_2$-terminal cysteine residues are separated by three intervening amino acids. A subclass of the CXC chemokines, exemplified by IL-8, contains a characteristic amino acid sequence (glu-tamate-leucine-arginine) near the NH$_2$-terminal end of the protein; these chemokines act primarily on polymorphonuclear neutrophils. Other chemokines, including the CC chemokines and members of CXC subgroup not containing the glutamate-leucine-arginine sequence, act, for the most part, on monocytes, macrophages, lymphocytes, or eosinophils. Many different cell types are capable of secreting chemokines; cells of monocyte/macrophage lineage and endothelial cells are particularly important in this regard. Numerous proinflammatory stimuli, including cytokines, such as TNF and IL-1, and bacterial products, such as LPS, can stimulate the production of chemokines.

IL-8, the prototypical CXC chemokine, was first identified as a chemotactic protein by Yoshimura and associates in 1987.[109] IL-8 is translated as a 99-amino acid precursor and is secreted after cleavage of a 20-amino acid leader sequence. In addition to attracting neutrophils along a chemotactic gradient, IL-8 also activates these cells, triggering degranulation, increased expression of surface adhesion molecules, and the production of reactive oxygen metabolites. At least two distinct IL-8 receptors have been identified; these receptors are called CXCR1 (IL-8R1) and CXCR2 (IL-8R2). CXCR1 is predominantly expressed on neutrophils. Like other chemokine receptors, CXCR1 and CXCR2 are coupled to G proteins, and binding of ligand to these receptors leads to intracellular signal transduction through generation of inositol triphosphate, activation of protein kinase C, and perturbations in intracellular ionized calcium concentration.

Increased circulating concentrations of IL-8 have been detected in experimental animal models of infection or endotoxemia[110,111] and in patients with sepsis.[112,113] High circulating levels of IL-8 have been associated with a fatal outcome in patients with sepsis.[112,113] Treatment of experimental animals with antibodies against IL-8 has been shown to improve survival or prevent pulmonary injury in models of sepsis or ischemia/reperfusion injury.[114] These observations support the view that IL-8-mediated activation of neutrophils plays an important role in the pathogenesis of organ system damage in these syndromes.

Monocyte chemotactic protein (MCP)-1, the prototypical CC chemokine, was identified in the same year by two groups of investigators.[115,116] MCP-1 is a chemotaxin for monocytes (but not neutrophils) and also activates monocytes, triggering the production of reactive oxygen metabolites and the expression of β_2-integrins (cell-surface adhesion molecules). Elevated circulating concentrations of MCP-1 have been detected in endotoxemic mice[117] and patients with sepsis.[118,119] Pretreatment of mice with a polyclonal anti-MIP-1 antiserum ameliorates LPS-induced lung injury, suggesting an important role for this chemokine in the pathogenesis of sepsis-induced ARDS.[117]

INTERLEUKIN-12

IL-12, a cytokine produced primarily by antigen-presenting cells, is a heterodimeric protein composed of two disulfide-linked peptides (p35 and p40) that are encoded by distinct genes. Both subunits are required for biologic activity. The IL-12 receptor (IL-12R) is expressed on T cells and NK cells. The most important biologic activity associated with IL-12 is to promote T_H1 responses by T helper cells. In this regard, IL-12 promotes the differentiation of naive T cells into T_H1 cells capable of producing IFN-γ after activation and serves to augment IFN-γ secretion by T_H1 cells responding to an antigenic stimulus. Stimulation of IFN-γ production of IL-12 by T or NK cells can be synergistically enhanced by the presence of other proinflammatory cytokines, notably TNF, IL-1, and IL-2. Conversely, counter-regulatory cytokines, such as IL-4 and IL-10, are capable of inhibiting IL-12–induced IFN-γ secretion.

The immunologic responses governed by T_H1 cells are central to the development of cell-mediated immunity necessary for appropriate host resistance to intracellular pathogens. It is not surprising, therefore, that transgenic mice deficient in IL-12 manifest markedly increased susceptibility to infections caused by a number of intracellular pathogens, including *Mycobacterium avium*[120] and *Cryptococcus neoformans*.[121]

IL-12 may be a key factor in some of the deleterious inflammatory responses to LPS and gram-negative bacteria. Elevated circulating levels of IL-12 have been measured in endotoxemic mice[122,123] and baboons infused with viable *Escherichia coli*.[110] Elevated plasma levels of IL-12 also have been detected in children with meningococcal septic shock and have been shown to correlate with outcome.[124] However, in patients with postoperative sepsis, circulating IL-12 levels tend to be less than those in control subjects without sepsis and do not correlate with outcome.[125] Defective production of IL-12 by peripheral blood mononuclear cells after stimulation with IFN-γ and LPS is associated with an increased risk for the development of postoperative sepsis in preoperative patients.[126]

IL-12 also has been implicated in the pathogenesis of inflammatory bowel disease. T cells eluted from the lamina propria of intestinal resection specimens from patients with Crohn's disease secrete cytokines consistent with a T_H1-like profile.[127] In addition, IL-12–secreting macrophages are present in large numbers in tissue specimens from patients with Crohn's disease but are rare in histologic sections from appropriate control subjects.[10] Treatment with anti–IL-12 antibodies ameliorates the severity of disease in certain murine models of inflammatory bowel disease.[128] Treatment of patients with refractory inflammatory bowel disease with thalidomide, a potent anti-inflammatory agent, decreases production of both TNF and IL-12 by mononuclear cells isolated from the lamina propria of gut mucosal biopsies and decreases disease activity.[129]

Although excessive production of IL-12 has been implicated in the pathogenesis of acute inflammatory conditions such as septic shock and chronic inflammatory states such as Crohn's disease, adequate production of IL-12 appears to be essential for orchestration of the normal host response to infection. When antibodies to IL-12 are administered to mice with fecal peritonitis induced by cecal ligation and perforation, mortality is increased and clearance of the bacterial load is impaired.[130] Conversely, pre- or even post-treatment with recombinant IL-12 has been shown to improve survival in a murine model of bacterial peritonitis.[131]

INTERLEUKIN-18

IL-18 is structurally related to IL-1β and functionally is a member of the T_H1-inducing family of cytokines.[132] Like IL-1β, IL-18 is translated in the form of a precursor protein (pro-IL-18). This precursor molecule requires cleavage by the same converting enzyme that activates IL-1β (i.e., ICE) to form biologically active IL-18. The two cytokines, IL-1β and IL-18, are also similar with respect to the way that intracellular signaling occurs after association of the cytokine with its receptor on target cells. Binding of IL-18 to its receptor (IL-18R) initiates a cascade of events that involves participation by a number of the same accessory proteins required for IL-1β–induced signaling, including IRAK, TRAF6, and MyD88.

IL-18 is expressed constitutively by human peripheral blood mononuclear cells and murine intestinal epithelial cells, but IL-18 production also can be stimulated by a variety of proinflammatory microbial products. The main biologic activity of IL-18 is to induce production of IFN-γ by T cells and NK cells. In this regard, IL-18 acts most potently as a co-stimulant in combination with IL-12. Indeed, IL-12–induced IFN-γ expression appears to depend on the presence of IL-18, because transgenic mice (or cells from mice) deficient in IL-18 or ICE produce little IFN-γ in response to appropriate stimulation even in the presence of ample IL-12.[133,134] In addition to stimulating IFN-γ production, IL-18 also has been shown to induce production of CC and CXC chemokines from human mononuclear cells. IL-18 also activates neutrophils, an effect that may contribute to organ injury and dysfunction in conditions such as sepsis and ARDS.[135] Circulating concentrations of IL-18 increased in patients with sepsis as compared with those with just injuries, and high levels of this cytokine are associated with a fatal outcome in patients with postoperative sepsis.[125,136]

INTERLEUKIN-4, INTERLEUKIN-10, and INTERLEUKIN-13

IL-4, IL-10, and IL-13 can be regarded as inhibitory, anti-inflammatory, or *counter-regulatory* cytokines. All three of these cytokines are produced by T_H2 cells and, among other roles, serve to modulate the production and effects of proinflammatory cytokines, such as TNF and IL-1.

IL-4, originally described as a B-cell growth factor, is a 15- to 20-kD glycoprotein that is synthesized by T_H2 cells, mast cells, basophils, and eosinophils. IL-4 has many biologic actions that promote expression of the T_H2 phenotype, characterized by downregulation of proinflammatory and cell-mediated immune responses and upregulation of humoral (B-cell–mediated) immune responses. IL-4 induces differentiation of CD4+ T cells into T_H2 cells and, conversely, downregulates differentiation of CD4+ T cells into T_H1 cells. IL-4 inhibits the production of TNF, IL-1, IL-8, and PGE_2 by stimulated monocytes or macrophages and downregulates endothelial cell activation induced by TNF. IL-4 acts as a co-mitogen for B cells and promotes the expression of the class II major histocompatibility complex on B cells.

IL-10, originally called *cytokine synthesis inhibitory factor,* was first isolated from supernatants of cultures of activated T cells.[137] This cytokine is an 18-kD protein that is produced primarily by T_H2 cells but also is released by activated monocytes and other cell types. IL-10 acts to downregulate the inflammatory response through numerous mechanisms. For example, IL-10 inhibits production of numerous proinflammatory cytokines, including IL-1, TNF, IL-6, IL-8, 1L-12, and GM-CSF, by monocytes and macrophages and, conversely, increases synthesis of the counter-regulatory cytokine IL-1RA by activated monocytes. In addition, IL-10 downregulates the proliferation and secretion of IFN-γ and IL-2 by activated T_H1 cells, primarily by inhibiting the production of IL-12 by macrophages or other *accessory* cells. Conversely, IFN-γ downregulates IL-10 production by monocytes. At least some of the inhibitory effects of IL-10 are mediated by blocking IFN-γ–induced tyrosine phosphorylation of STAT1α, a key protein in the signal transduction pathway for IFN-γ.

The importance of IL-10 as a regulatory cytokine has been illustrated by experiments using transgenic mice deficient in IL-10. Such animals manifest markedly increased resistance to the intracellular bacterial pathogen *L. monocytogenes,* suggesting that IL-10–mediated suppression of the T_H1-type phenotype can impair the host's ability to eradicate certain types of infections.[43] In contrast to these results, IL-10 knock-out mice succumb to the lethal effects of excessive inflammation when infected with another intracellular pathogen, the protozoan parasite *Toxoplasma gondii.*[138] Results have been variable in mice with severe sepsis, but a genetic deficiency of IL-10 production most likely alters the kinetics of the inflammatory process without affecting long-term survival.[139] IL-10–deficient mice spontaneously develop a form of enterocolitis that is reminiscent of inflammatory bowel disease in humans.[140] Because the inflammatory bowel disease–like syndrome in these animals can be suppressed by treating the animals with either exogenous IL-10 or a neutralizing anti-IFN-γ antibody, the enterocolitis associated with IL-10 deficiency is thought to be caused by excessive expression of the T_H1-type phenotype.[140]

Production of IL-10 by peripheral blood mononuclear cells and CD4+ T cells is increased in trauma victims,[14] and elevated circulating concentrations of this cytokine have been measured in patients with trauma[141,142] or sepsis.[143-145] Moreover, in trauma and burn patients, increased production of IL-10 has been associated with a greater risk of serious infection[141,142] and, in patients with sepsis, a greater risk of mortality[143,145] or shock.[144] These findings support the view that whereas excessive production of proinflammatory mediators may be deleterious in trauma and sepsis, the development of the T_H2 phenotype, characterized by markedly increased production of IL-10 and IL-4 and decreased expression on monocytes of the major histocompatibility complex type II (MHC II) antigen HLA-DR, may lead to excessive immunosuppression and deleteriously affect outcome on this basis. Evidence has been presented supporting the view that HLA-DR expression on monocytes is post-translationally downregulated by IL-10 in patients with sepsis.[146] Prompted by this view, some investigators have begun investigating the notion of using an agent like IFN-γ to restore immunocompetence (i.e., shift the balance toward the T_H1 phenotype) in patients with sepsis and evidence of impaired cell-mediated immunity.[21] Whether this strategy ultimately will prove to be successful remains to be seen.

Administering exogenous IL-10 in an effort to blunt excessive inflammation has led to mixed results in experimental models of sepsis or septic shock. In models, wherein experimental animals are challenged with intravenous LPS, treatment with recombinant IL-10 has been shown to ameliorate fever[147] and improve survival.[148] In models such as cecal ligation and perforation, wherein the sepsis syndrome is induced by infection with viable bacteria, administration of exogenous IL-10 has been shown to be either beneficial[149,150] or without effect.[151] However, in mice with pneumonia caused by *Pseudomonas aeruginosa,* survival is improved when animals are treated with an anti–IL-10 antibody to neutralize endogenous IL-10.[152] Thus, whereas the use of recombinant IL-10 as an adjuvant treatment for sepsis is appealing, caution will need to be exercised in the design and conduct of clinical trials, because excessive immunosuppression could adversely affect antibacterial defense mechanisms.

IL-13 is a 12-kD protein closely related to IL-4. The two proteins have about 25% homology and share many structural characteristics. IL-13 is produced by T_H2 cells and also undifferentiated CD4+ T cells and CD8+ T cells. The IL-13 receptor (IL-13R) consists of two chains, one of which binds IL-4 but not IL-13 and another that binds IL-13 with high affinity. Binding of either IL-4 or IL-13 to their respective receptors induces signaling by activating the same JAK kinases, JAK1 and Tyk2. IL-4, but not IL-13, also activates JAK3. The biologic activities of IL-13 are very similar to those of IL-4 with respect to B-cell functions, although, unlike IL-4, IL-13 does not have any direct effect on T cells. IL-13 downregulates production of proinflammatory cytokines (e.g., IL-1, TNF, IL-6, IL-8, 1L-12, G-CSF, GM-CSF, and MIP-1α) and PGE_2 by activated monocytes and macrophages and, by the same token, increases production of anti-inflammatory proteins, including IL-1RA and IL-1RII, from these cells. Additional anti-inflammatory properties of IL-13 include inhibition of the induction of the enzyme COX-2 required for the production of prostaglandins and induction of the enzyme 15-lipoxygenase that catalyzes the formation of a lipid mediator (lipoxin A4) with anti-inflammatory properties. Treatment of mice with recombinant IL-13 has been shown to prevent LPS-induced lethality and to decrease circulating levels of TNF and other proinflammatory cytokines.[153] Conversely, treatment of septic mice with an anti–IL-13 antibody has been shown to increase mortality.[154]

HIGH MOBILITY GROUP B1

When mice are injected with a lethal bolus dose of LPS, circulating levels of TNF peak 60 to 90 minutes later and are virtually undetectable within 4 hours. Although the animals show clinical signs of endotoxemia (e.g., decreased activity and ruffled fur) within a few hours after the injection of LPS, mortality typically does not occur until more than 24 hours later, that is, long after circulating levels of the "alarm phase" cytokines (TNF and IL-1β) have returned to normal. These observations suggested the possibility to Tracey and colleagues that LPS-induced lethality might be mediated by a previously unidentified factor that is released much later than TNF or IL-1β.[155] They identified high mobility group B1 (HMGB1, formerly called HMG-1) as a novel mediator of LPS-induced lethality.

HMGB1 was originally identified in 1973 as a non-histone nuclear protein with high electrophoretic mobility.[156] A characteristic feature of the protein is the presence of two folded DNA-binding motifs that are termed the *A domain* and the *B domain*.[157] Both of these domains contain a characteristic grouping of aromatic and basic amino acids within a block of 75 residues termed the *HMGB1 box*.[158] HMGB1 has several functions within the nucleus, including facilitating DNA repair[159] and supporting the transcriptional regulation of genes.[160]

Although HMGB1 is normally not secreted by cells and levels of this protein are normally undetectable in plasma or serum, high circulating concentrations of HMGB1 can be detected in mice 16 to 32 hours after the onset of endotoxemia.[161] Remarkably, delayed passive immunization of mice with antibodies against HMGB1 confers significant protection against LPS-induced mortality.[161] Furthermore, administration of highly purified recombinant HMGB1 to mice is lethal.[161] Thus, HMGB1 fulfills (a modified version of) Koch's criteria for being a mediator of LPS-induced lethality in mice. Subsequent studies have shown that direct application of HMGB1 into the airways of mice initiates an acute inflammatory response and lung injury reminiscent of ARDS in humans.[162] Furthermore, HMGB1 (or a truncated form of the protein including only the B box domain) increases the permeability of human enterocyte-like monolayers in culture and promotes intestinal

barrier dysfunction when injected into mice.[163] Thus, it seems plausible that HMGB1 contributes to the development of organ dysfunction in human sepsis, a notion that is supported by the observation that circulating HMGB1 concentrations are significantly higher in patients with ultimately fatal sepsis as compared with patients with a less severe form of the syndrome.[161] Ethyl pyruvate, a compound that blocks the release of HMGB1 from LPS-stimulated murine macrophage-like cells and inhibits release of the mediator in vivo, improves survival in mice with bacterial peritonitis, even when treatment with the compound is delayed for 24 hours after the onset of infection.[164]

INDUCIBLE NITRIC OXIDE SYNTHASE AND CYCLOOXYGENASE-2

Many of the downstream actions of the proinflammatory cytokines occur as a result of increased expression of two key enzymes: iNOS (NOS-2) and COX-2. Because these two enzymes share some common features and are both centrally involved in many aspects of the inflammatory response, they are discussed together briefly here.

iNOS is one of three isoforms of an enzyme, nitric oxide synthase (NOS), that catalyzes to conversion of the amino acid L-arginine to the free radical gas NO·. One of the simplest stable molecules in nature, NO· is produced by many different types of cells and serves as both a signaling and an effector molecule in mammalian biology. Whereas NOS-1 (also called neuronal NOS or nNOS) and NOS-3 (also called endothelial or eNOS) tend to be expressed constitutively in various cell types, iNOS is expressed for the most part only after stimulation of cells by proinflammatory cytokines (particularly IFN-γ, TNF, and IL-1) or LPS. NOS-1 and NOS-2 produce small "puffs" of NO· in response to transient changes in intracellular ionized calcium concentration. In contrast, iNOS, once induced, produces large quantities of NO· for a prolonged period of time.

All three NOS isoforms require L-arginine as a substrate and in a complex five-electron redox reaction, convert one of the guanidino nitrogens of the amino acid into NO·. In addition to L-arginine, the redox reaction catalyzed by the various NOS isoforms requires the presence of molecular oxygen and a number of cofactors, including flavin mononucleotide, flavin adenine dinucleotide, iron-protoporphyrin IX, and tetrahydrobiopterin (BH_4). The rate-limiting step in the biosynthesis of BH_4 is the reaction catalyzed by guanosine triphosphate (GTP) cyclohydrolase I, an enzyme that, like iNOS, is induced in certain cell types by cytokines and/or LPS.

Many of the biologic actions of NO·, including vasodilatation, induction of vascular hyperpermeability, and inhibition of platelet aggregation, are mediated through activation of the enzyme, soluble guanylyl cyclase (sGC). Binding of NO· to the heme moiety of sGC activates the enzyme, enabling it to catalyze the conversion of GTP to cyclic guanosine monophosphate (GMP). NO· is not the only ligand that is capable of activating sGC; carbon monoxide (CO), another small gaseous molecule produced by mammalian cells, has also been shown to activate this enzyme. Signal transduction via the NO·-sGC (or the CO-sGC) pathway entails activation of various cyclic GMP–dependent protein kinase (PKG) isoforms. In vascular smooth muscle cells, NO·-induced vasodilatation occurs as a result of PKG-mediated opening of high-conductance calcium and voltage-activated potassium channels. Excessive production of NO· as a result of iNOS induction in vascular smooth muscle cells is thought to be a major factor contributing to the loss of vasomotor tone and the loss of responsiveness to vasopressor agents ("vasoplegia") in patients with septic shock. Treatment with a drug, such as N^G-monomethyl-L-arginine (L-NMMA)], that blocks production of NO· ameliorates hypotension in patients with septic shock.[165] Unfortunately, treatment of septic patients with L-NMMA actually worsens survival, possibly because the drug does not selectively inhibit iNOS but also inhibits NOS-3 as well and therefore interferes with the normal regulation of microcirculatory perfusion. Some,[166,167] but not all,[168,169] studies suggest that iNOS knock-out mice are partially resistant to the lethal effects of acute endotoxemia. In contrast, one study showed that iNOS knock-out mice are more susceptible than wild-type controls to lethality induced by bacterial peritonitis,[170] possibly because enhanced NO· production is important for the host's defense against infection. On the other hand, iNOS knock-out mice are protected from sepsis-induced acute lung injury.[171]

Signaling via the sGC-PKG pathway is not the only way that NO· functions as an inflammatory mediator. In addition, NO· reacts rapidly with another free radical, superoxide anion ($O_2^{·-}$), to form peroxynitrite anion ($ONOO^-$), the conjugate base of the weak acid peroxynitrous acid (ONOOH). Being a potent oxidizing and nitrosating agent, $ONOO^-$/ONOOH is thought to be responsible for many of the toxic effects of NO·. For example, $ONOO^-$/ONOOH is capable of oxidizing sulfhydryl groups on various proteins at a rapid rate, peroxidizing membrane lipids, and inactivating mitochondrial aconitase. $ONOO^-$/ONOOH is also capable of damaging nuclear DNA, setting up a chain of events that ultimately leads to activation of the enzyme polyadenosine ribose diphosphate polymerase-1 (PARP-1). On activation, PARP-1 catalyzes the polyadenosine diphosphate (ADP) ribosylation of proteins, a reaction that consumes nicotine adenine dinucleotide (oxidized form) (NAD^+), leading to energetic failure in cells.[172,173] Treatment using pharmacologic agents that scavenge $ONOO^-$/ONOOH,[13] selectively block iNOS[162] (without blocking the NOS-1 or NOS-3), or block the activity of PARP-1[2] has been shown to improve organ system function and/or survival in certain experimental models of inflammation, such as acute endotoxemia, mesenteric ischemia and reperfusion, hemorrhagic shock and resuscitation, and stroke.

The prostaglandins, including PGE_2 and PGI_2 (prostacyclin) and thromboxane A_2 (TxA_2), are lipid mediators derived from the unstable intermediate compound PGG_2. The formation of PGG_2 depends on the activity of two families of enzymes. First, isoforms of the enzyme, phospholipase A_2, liberate the polyunsaturated fatty acid arachidonate from membrane phospholipids. Second, the

two cyclooxygenase isoforms, COX-1 and COX-2, catalyze the stereospecific oxidation of arachidonate to form the cyclic endoperoxide PGG_2. Both of these reactions are major regulatory steps in the formation of prostaglandins and TxA_2.

COX-1 is expressed constitutively in many tissues, and mediators produced by this isoform are thought to be important in a variety of homeostatic processes, such as regulating renal perfusion and salt and water handling, maintaining hemostasis by modulating platelet aggregation, and preserving gastrointestinal mucosal integrity. COX-2, however, is an inducible enzyme like iNOS. COX-2 expression is induced by a number of stimuli, including various growth factors and proinflammatory cytokines. In cells subjected to inflammatory stimuli, activation of COX-2 is thought to be mediated by the powerful oxidant $ONOO^-$, thereby providing a tight functional linkage between the NO· and prostaglandin mediator systems.[174]

Once expressed and activated, COX-2 promotes the formation of PGG_2 and PGH_2 and, ultimately, various prostaglandins and TxA_2. These mediators, in turn, interact with cell surface receptors belonging to the G-protein–coupled receptor superfamily. These receptors interact with cytosolic signaling pathways, leading to rapid alterations in cell physiology, which are manifested as physiologic or pathophysiologic phenomena, such as vasodilation and increased microvascular permeability. Pharmacologic inhibition of cyclooxygenase activity is the basis for the anti-inflammatory actions of the class of compounds called nonsteroidal anti-inflammatory drugs (NSAIDs). Whereas the beneficial effects of the NSAIDs are thought to be mediated by blocking the enzymatic activity of COX-2, some of the adverse side effects of these agents (e.g., gastric mucosal ulceration) are thought to be mediated by inhibition of COX-1. Accordingly, the identification of COX-2 as the "inflammatory" isoform of cyclooxygenase led to intense efforts to develop drugs selective for the inducible enzyme.

Selected References

Angus DC, Linde-Zwirble WT, Lidicker J, et al: Epidemiology of severe sepsis in the United States: Analysis of incidence, outcome, and associated costs of care. Crit Care Med 29:1303-1310, 2001.

> This study used data from all hospitalized patients during a single year from seven states to draw inferences about the incidence and outcome of severe sepsis. The authors showed that about 750,000 cases of severe sepsis occur annually in the United States and the overall mortality rate is about 30%.

Bernard GR, Luce JM, Sprung CL, et al: High-dose corticosteroids in patients with the adult respiratory distress syndrome. N Engl J Med 317:1565-1570, 1987.

> This study was the first large multicentric randomized double-blind clinical trial to demonstrate efficacy for a novel adjuvant treatment for patients with severe sepsis or septic shock. The study demonstrated that treatment with drotrecogin alfa (activated) significantly improves survival in selected patients with severe sepsis.

Beutler B, Milsark IW, Cerami A: Passive immunization against cachectin/tumor necrosis factor protects mice from lethal effect of endotoxin. Science 229:869-871, 1985.

> **This paper was one of series of landmark publications from the Rockefeller University during the 1980s that identified TNF as a crucial mediator of the lethal effects of lipopolysaccharide (endotoxin) from gram-negative bacteria.**

Poltorak A, He X, Smirnova I, et al: Defective LPS signaling in C3H/HeJ and C57BL/10ScCr mice: Mutations in *Tlr4* gene. Science 282:2085-2088, 1998.

> **This paper showed that mice with a mutation in the gene encoding TLR4 are unable to respond to lipopolysaccharide (endotoxin) from gram-negative bacteria and thereby established that the receptor, TLR4, is a key element in the signaling pathway involved in cellular responses to this proinflammatory bacterial substance.**

Sappington PL, Yang R, Yang H, et al: HMGB1 B box increases the permeability of Caco-2 enterocytic monolayers and impairs intestinal barrier function in mice. Gastroenterology 23:790-802, 2002.

> **This study showed that HMGB1, a novel late-acting cytokine-like molecule, is capable of causing marked alterations in intestinal epithelial barrier function.**

Wang H, Bloom O, Zhang M, et al: HMG-1 as a late mediator of endotoxin lethality in mice. Science 285:248-251, 1999.

> **This landmark study showed that HMGB1, already well-known as a nuclear protein involved in the regulation of gene transcription, is also a late-acting proinflammatory cytokine-like mediator that is at least partly responsible for lipopolysaccharide-induced lethality in mice.**

References

1. Angus DC, Linde-Zwirble WT, Lidicker J, et al: Epidemiology of severe sepsis in the United States: Analysis of incidence, outcome, and associated costs of care. Crit Care Med 29:1303-1310, 2001.
2. Akira S, Takeda K, Kaisho T: Toll-like receptors: Critical proteins linking innate and acquired immunity. Nat Immunol 2:675-680, 2001.
3. Issacs A, Lindemann J: Virus interference: I: The interferons. Proc R Soc Lond (Biol) 147:258-267, 1957.
4. Nagano Y, Kojima Y: Pouvoir immunisant du virus vaccinal inactive par des rayons ultraviolets. C R Soc Biol (Paris) 148:1700-1702, 1954.
5. Biron CA: Role of early cytokines, including alpha and beta interferons (IFN-alpha/beta), in innate and adaptive immune responses to viral infections. Semin Immunol 10:383-390, 1998.
6. Dalton DK, Pitts-Meek S, Keshav S, et al: Multiple defects of immune cell function in mice with disrupted interferon-gamma genes. Science 259:1739-1742, 1993.
7. Huang S, Hendriks W, Althage A, et al: Immune response in mice that lack the interferon-gamma receptor. Science 259:1742-1745, 1993.
8. Kamijo R, Le J, Shapiro D, et al: Mice that lack the interferon-gamma receptor have profoundly altered responses to infection with bacillus Calmette-Guérin and subsequent challenge with lipopolysaccharide. J Exp Med 178:1435-1440, 1993.
9. Ransohoff RM: Cellular responses to interferons and other cytokines: The JAK-STAT paradigm. N Engl J Med 338:616-618, 1998.
10. Parronchi P, Romagnani P, Annunziato F, et al: Type 1 T-helper cell predominance and interleukin-12 expression in the gut of patients with Crohn's disease. Am J Pathol 150:823-832, 1997.
11. Aaronson DS, Horvath CM: A road map for those who know JAK-STAT. Science 296:1653-1655, 2002.
12. Gallin JI, Farber JM, Holland SM, et al: Interferon-gamma in the management of infectious diseases. Ann Intern Med 123:216-224, 1995.
13. A controlled trial of interferon gamma to prevent infection in chronic granulomatous disease. The International Chronic Granulomatous Disease Cooperative Study Group. N Engl J Med 324:509-516, 1991.
14. Lyons A, Kelly JL, Rodrick ML, et al: Major injury induces increased production of interleukin-10 by cells of the immune system with a negative impact on resistance to infection. Ann Surg 226:450-460, 1997.
15. O'Sullivan ST, Lederer JA, Horgan AF, et al: Major injury leads to predominance of the T helper-2 lymphocyte phenotype and diminished interleukin-12 production associated with decreased resistance to infection. Ann Surg 222:482-492, 1995.
16. Hershman MJ, Polk HC Jr, Pietsch JD, et al: Modulation of infection by gamma interferon treatment following trauma. Infect Immun 56:2412-2416, 1988.
17. Hershman MJ, Sonnenfeld G, Logan WA, et al: Effect of interferon-gamma treatment on the course of a burn wound infection. J Interferon Res 8:367-373, 1988.
18. Dries DJ, Jurkovich GJ, Maier RV, et al: Effect of interferon gamma on infection-related death in patients with severe injuries: A randomized, double-blind, placebo-controlled trial. Arch Surg 129:1031-1042, 1994.
19. Polk HC Jr, Cheadle WG, Livingston DH, et al: A randomized prospective clinical trial to determine the efficacy of interferon-gamma in severely injured patients. Am J Surg 163:191-196, 1992.
20. Wasserman D, Ioannovich JD, Hinzmann RD, et al: Interferon-gamma in the prevention of severe burn-related infections: A European phase III multicenter trial. The Severe Burns Study Group. Crit Care Med 26:434-439, 1998.
21. Docke WD, Randow F, Syrbe U, et al: Monocyte deactivation in septic patients: Restoration by IFN-gamma treatment. Nat Med 3:678-681, 1997.
22. Schinkel C, Licht K, Zedler S, et al: Perioperative treatment with human recombinant interferon-gamma: A randomized double-blind clinical trial. Shock 16:329-333, 2001.
23. Bilgin K, Yaramis A, Haspolat K, et al: A randomized trial of granulocyte-macrophage colony-stimulating factor in neonates with sepsis and neutropenia. Pediatrics 107:36-41, 2001.
24. Gery I, Gershon RK, Waksman BH: Potentiation of the T-lymphocyte response to mitogens. I. The responding cell. J Exp Med 136:128-142, 1972.
25. Thornberry NA, Bull HG, Calaycay JR, et al: A novel heterodimeric cysteine protease is required for interleukin-1 beta processing in monocytes. Nature 356:768-774, 1992.
26. Li P, Allen H, Banerjee S, et al: Mice deficient in IL-1 beta-converting enzyme are defective in production of mature IL-1 beta and resistant to endotoxic shock. Cell 80:401-411, 1995.
27. Fantuzzi G, Ku G, Harding MW, et al: Response to local inflammation of IL-1 beta-converting enzyme-deficient mice. J Immunol 158:1818-1824, 1997.

28. Thornberry NA, Lazebnik Y: Caspases: Enemies within. Science 281:1312-1316, 1998.

29. Hamon Y, Luciani MF, Becq F, et al: Interleukin-1beta secretion is impaired by inhibitors of the Atp binding cassette transporter, ABC1. Blood 90:2911-2915, 1997.

30. Andus T, Daig R, Vogl D, et al: Imbalance of the interleukin 1 system in colonic mucosa—association with intestinal inflammation and interleukin 1 receptor antagonist [corrected] genotype 2. Gut 41:651-657, 1997.

31. Horai R, Asano M, Sudo K, et al: Production of mice deficient in genes for interleukin (IL)-1alpha, IL-1beta, IL-1alpha/beta, and IL-1 receptor antagonist shows that IL-1beta is crucial in turpentine-induced fever development and glucocorticoid secretion. J Exp Med 187:1463-1475, 1998.

32. Gay NJ, Keith FJ: *Drosophila* Toll and IL-1 receptor. Nature 351:355-356, 1991.

33. Bowie A, O'Neill LA: The interleukin-1 receptor/Toll-like receptor superfamily: Signal generators for pro-inflammatory interleukins and microbial products. J Leukoc Biol 67:508-514, 2000.

34. Poltorak A, He X, Smirnova I, et al: Defective LPS signaling in C3H/HeJ and C57BL/10ScCr mice: Mutations in *Tlr4* gene. Science 282:2085-2088, 1998.

35. Hoshino K, Takeuchi O, Kawai T, et al: Cutting edge: Toll-like receptor 4 (TLR4)-deficient mice are hyporesponsive to lipopolysaccharide: Evidence for TLR4 as the Lps gene product. J Immunol 162:3749-3752, 1999.

36. Arbour NC, Lorenz E, Schutte BC, et al: *TLR4* mutations are associated with endotoxin hyporesponsiveness in humans. Nat Genet 25:187-191, 2000.

37. Nagai Y, Akashi S, Nagafuku M, et al: Essential role of MD-2 in LPS responsiveness and TLR4 distribution. Nat Immunol 3:667-672, 2002.

38. Shimazu R, Akashi S, Ogata H, et al: MD-2, a molecule that confers lipopolysaccharide responsiveness on Toll-like receptor 4. J Exp Med 189:1777-1782, 1999.

39. Asea A, Rehli M, Kabingu E, et al: Novel signal transduction pathway utilized by extracellular HSP70: Role of toll-like receptor (TLR) 2 and TLR4. J Biol Chem 277:15028-15034, 2002.

40. Ohashi K, Burkart V, Flohe S, et al: Cutting edge: Heat shock protein 60 is a putative endogenous ligand of the toll-like receptor-4 complex. J Immunol 164:558-561, 2000.

41. Vabulas RM, Ahmad-Nejad P, Ghose S, et al: HSP70 as endogenous stimulus of the Toll/interleukin-1 receptor signal pathway. J Biol Chem 277:15107-15112, 2002.

42. Matzinger P: The danger model: A renewed sense of self. Science 296:301-305, 2002.

43. Dai WJ, Kohler G, Brombacher F: Both innate and acquired immunity to *Listeria monocytogenes* infection are increased in IL-10–deficient mice. J Immunol 158:2259-2267, 1997.

44. Cannon JG, Tompkins RG, Gelfand JA, et al: Circulating interleukin-1 and tumor necrosis factor in septic shock and experimental endotoxin fever. J Infect Dis 161:79-84, 1990.

45. Fischer E, Van Zee KJ, Marano MA, et al: Interleukin-1 receptor antagonist circulates in experimental inflammation and in human disease. Blood 79:2196-2200, 1992.

46. Goldie AS, Fearon KC, Ross JA, et al: Natural cytokine antagonists and endogenous antiendotoxin core antibodies in sepsis syndrome. The Sepsis Intervention Group. JAMA 274:172-177, 1995.

47. van Deuren M, van der Ven-Jongekrijg J, Vannier E, et al: The pattern of interleukin-1beta (IL-1beta) and its modulating agents IL-1 receptor antagonist and IL-1 soluble receptor type II in acute meningococcal infections. Blood 90:1101-1108, 1997.

48. Donnelly SC, Strieter RM, Reid PT, et al: The association between mortality rates and decreased concentrations of interleukin-10 and interleukin-1 receptor antagonist in the lung fluids of patients with the adult respiratory distress syndrome. Ann Intern Med 125:191-196, 1996.

49. Carswell EA, Old LJ, Kassel RL, et al: An endotoxin-induced serum factor that causes necrosis of tumors. Proc Natl Acad Sci U S A 72:3666-3670, 1975.

50. Pennica D, Nedwin GE, Hayflick JS, et al: Human tumour necrosis factor: Precursor structure, expression and homology to lymphotoxin. Nature 312:724-729, 1984.

51. Beutler B, Mahoney J, Le Trang N, et al: Purification of cachectin, a lipoprotein lipase-suppressing hormone secreted by endotoxin-induced RAW 264.7 cells. J Exp Med 161:984-995, 1985.

52. Torti FM, Dieckmann B, Beutler B, et al: A macrophage factor inhibits adipocyte gene expression: An in vitro model of cachexia. Science 229:867-869, 1985.

53. Beutler B, Greenwald D, Hulmes JD, et al: Identity of tumour necrosis factor and the macrophage-secreted factor cachectin. Nature 316:552-554, 1985.

54. Tracey KJ, Beutler B, Lowry SF, et al: Shock and tissue injury induced by recombinant human cachectin. Science 234:470-474, 1986.

55. Beutler B, Milsark IW, Cerami AC: Passive immunization against cachectin/tumor necrosis factor protects mice from lethal effect of endotoxin. Science 229:869-871, 1985.

56. Baud V, Karin M: Signal transduction by tumor necrosis factor and its relatives. Trends Cell Biol 11:372-377, 2001.

57. Pfeffer K, Matsuyama T, Kundig TM, et al: Mice deficient for the 55 kd tumor necrosis factor receptor are resistant to endotoxic shock, yet succumb to *L. monocytogenes* infection. Cell 73:457-467, 1993.

58. Everest P, Roberts M, Dougan G: Susceptibility to *Salmonella typhimurium* infection and effectiveness of vaccination in mice deficient in the tumor necrosis factor alpha p55 receptor. Infect Immun 66:3355-3364, 1998.

59. Erickson SL, de Sauvage FJ, Kikly K, et al: Decreased sensitivity to tumour-necrosis factor but normal T-cell development in TNF receptor-2-deficient mice. Nature 372:560-563, 1994.

60. Peschon JJ, Torrance DS, Stocking KL, et al: TNF receptor-deficient mice reveal divergent roles for p55 and p75 in several models of inflammation. J Immunol 160:943-952, 1998.

61. Dinarello CA: Proinflammatory and anti-inflammatory cytokines as mediators in the pathogenesis of septic shock. Chest 112:321S-329S, 1997.

62. Ertel W, Scholl FA, Gallati H, et al: Increased release of soluble tumor necrosis factor receptors into blood during clinical sepsis. Arch Surg 129:1330-1337, 1994.

63. Froon AH, Bemelmans MH, Greve JW, et al: Increased plasma concentrations of soluble tumor necrosis factor receptors in sepsis syndrome: Correlation with plasma creatinine values. Crit Care Med 22:803-809, 1994.

64. Gogos CA, Drosou E, Bassaris HP, et al: Pro- versus anti-inflammatory cytokine profile in patients with severe sepsis: A marker for prognosis and future therapeutic options. J Infect Dis 181:176-180, 2000.

65. Mira JP, Cariou A, Grall F, et al: Association of TNF2, a TNF-alpha promoter polymorphism, with septic shock susceptibility and mortality: A multicenter study. JAMA 282:561-568, 1999.

66. Tang GJ, Huang SL, Yien HW, et al: Tumor necrosis factor gene polymorphism and septic shock in surgical infection. Crit Care Med 28:2733-2736, 2000.

67. Stuber F, Udalova IA, Book M, et al: −308 tumor necrosis factor (TNF) polymorphism is not associated with survival in severe sepsis and is unrelated to lipopolysaccharide inducibility of the human TNF promoter. J Inflamm 46:42-50, 1995.

68. Stuber F, Petersen M, Bokelmann F, et al: A genomic polymorphism within the tumor necrosis factor locus influences plasma tumor necrosis factor-alpha concentrations and outcome of patients with severe sepsis. Crit Care Med 24:381-384, 1996.

69. Waterer GW, Quasney MW, Cantor RM, et al: Septic shock and respiratory failure in community-acquired pneumonia have different TNF polymorphism associations. Am J Respir Crit Care Med 163:1599-1604, 2001.

70. Fink MP, Heard SO: Laboratory models of sepsis and septic shock. J Surg Res 49:186-196, 1990.

71. Auphan N, DiDonato JA, Rosette C, et al: Immunosuppression by glucocorticoids: Inhibition of NF-kappa B activity through induction of I kappa B synthesis. Science 270:286-290, 1995.

72. Swantek JL, Cobb MH, Geppert TD: Jun N-terminal kinase/stress-activated protein kinase (JNK/SAPK) is required for lipopolysaccharide stimulation of tumor necrosis factor alpha (TNF-alpha) translation: Glucocorticoids inhibit TNF-alpha translation by blocking JNK/SAPK. Mol Cell Biol 17:6274-6282, 1997.

73. Yao J, Johnson RW: Induction of interleukin-1 beta-converting enzyme (ICE) in murine microglia by lipopolysaccharide. Brain Res Mol Brain Res 51:170-178, 1997.

74. Hinshaw LB, Beller-Todd BK, Archer LT, et al: Effectiveness of steroid/antibiotic treatment in primates administered LD100 Escherichia coli. Ann Surg 194:51-56, 1981.

75. Bernard GR, Luce JM, Sprung CL, et al: High-dose corticosteroids in patients with the adult respiratory distress syndrome. N Engl J Med 317:1565-1570, 1987.

76. Bone RC, Fisher CJ, Jr, Clemmer TP, et al: A controlled clinical trial of high-dose methylprednisolone in the treatment of severe sepsis and septic shock. N Engl J Med 317:653-658, 1987.

77. Luce JM, Montgomery AB, Marks JD, et al: Ineffectiveness of high-dose methylprednisolone in preventing parenchymal lung injury and improving mortality in patients with septic shock. Am Rev Respir Dis 138:62-68, 1988.

78. Sprung CL, Caralis PV, Marcial EH, et al: The effects of high-dose corticosteroids in patients with septic shock: A prospective, controlled study. N Engl J Med 311:1137-1143, 1984.

79. The Veterans Administration Systemic Sepsis Cooperative Study Group. Effect of high-dose glucocorticoid therapy on mortality in patients with clinical signs of systemic sepsis. N Engl J Med 317:659-665, 1987.

80. Bollaert PE, Charpentier C, Levy B, et al: Reversal of late septic shock with supraphysiologic doses of hydrocortisone. Crit Care Med 26:645-650, 1998.

81. Briegel J, Forst H, Haller M, et al: Stress doses of hydrocortisone reverse hyperdynamic septic shock: A prospective, randomized, double-blind, single-center study. Crit Care Med 27:723-732, 1999.

82. Meduri GU, Headley AS, Golden E, et al: Effect of prolonged methylprednisolone therapy in unresolving acute respiratory distress syndrome: A randomized controlled trial. JAMA 280:159-165, 1998.

83. Meduri GU, Headley S, Tolley E, et al: Plasma and BAL cytokine response to corticosteroid rescue treatment in late ARDS. Chest 108:1315-1325, 1995.

84. Annane D, Sebille V, Charpentier C, et al: Effect of treatment with low doses of hydrocortisone and fludrocortisone on mortality in patients with septic shock. JAMA 288:862-871, 2002.

85. Fisher CJ Jr, Slotman GJ, Opal SM, et al: Initial evaluation of human recombinant interleukin-1 receptor antagonist in the treatment of sepsis syndrome: A randomized, open-label, placebo-controlled multicenter trial. The IL-1RA Sepsis Syndrome Study Group. Crit Care Med 22:12-21, 1994.

86. Fisher CJ Jr, Agosti JM, Opal SM, et al: Treatment of septic shock with the tumor necrosis factor receptor:Fc fusion protein. The Soluble TNF Receptor Sepsis Study Group. N Engl J Med 334:1697-1702, 1996.

87. Baert FJ, D'Haens GR, Peeters M, et al: Tumor necrosis factor alpha antibody (infliximab) therapy profoundly down-regulates the inflammation in Crohn's ileocolitis. Gastroenterology 116:22-28, 1999.

88. Present DH, Rutgeerts P, Targan S, et al: Infliximab for the treatment of fistulas in patients with Crohn's disease. N Engl J Med 340:1398-1405, 1999.

89. Moreland LW, Baumgartner SW, Schiff MH, et al: Treatment of rheumatoid arthritis with a recombinant human tumor necrosis factor receptor (p75)-Fc fusion protein. N Engl J Med 337:141-147, 1997.

90. Moreland LW, Schiff MH, Baumgartner SW, et al: Etanercept therapy in rheumatoid arthritis: A randomized, controlled trial. Ann Intern Med 130:478-486, 1999.

91. Hack CE: Tissue factor pathway of coagulation in sepsis. Crit Care Med 28:S25-30, 2000.

92. Fisher CJ Jr, Yan SB: Protein C levels as a prognostic indicator of outcome in sepsis and related diseases. Crit Care Med 28:S49-56, 2000.

93. Bernard GR, Vincent JL, Laterre PF, et al: Efficacy and safety of recombinant human activated protein C for severe sepsis. N Engl J Med 344:699-709, 2001.

94. Suematsu S, Matsuda T, Aozasa K, et al: IgG1 plasmacytosis in interleukin 6 transgenic mice. Proc Natl Acad Sci U S A 86:7547-7551, 1989.

95. Dalrymple SA, Lucian LA, Slattery R, et al: Interleukin-6-deficient mice are highly susceptible to Listeria monocytogenes infection: Correlation with inefficient neutrophilia. Infect Immun 63:2262-2268, 1995.

96. Kopf M, Baumann H, Freer G, et al: Impaired immune and acute-phase responses in interleukin-6-deficient mice. Nature 368:339-342, 1994.

97. Cuzzocrea S, Mazzon E, Dugo L, et al: Absence of endogenous interleukin-6 enhances the inflammatory response during acute pancreatitis induced by cerulein in mice. Cytokine 18:274-285, 2002.

98. Hierholzer C, Kalff JC, Omert L, et al: Interleukin-6 production in hemorrhagic shock is accompanied by neutrophil recruitment and lung injury. Am J Physiol 275:L611-621, 1998.

99. Riedemann NC, Neff TA, Guo RF, et al: Protective effects of IL-6 blockade in sepsis are linked to reduced C5a receptor expression. J Immunol 170:503-507, 2003.

100. Cruickshank AM, Fraser WD, Burns HJ, et al: Response of serum interleukin-6 in patients undergoing elective surgery of varying severity. Clin Sci (Lond) 79:161-165, 1990.

101. Shenkin A, Fraser WD, Series J, et al: The serum interleukin 6 response to elective surgery. Lymphokine Res 8:123-127, 1989.

102. Ertel W, Faist E, Nestle C, et al: Kinetics of interleukin-2 and interleukin-6 synthesis following major mechanical trauma. J Surg Res 48:622-628, 1990.

103. Guo Y, Dickerson C, Chrest FJ, et al: Increased levels of circulating interleukin 6 in burn patients. Clin Immunol Immunopathol 54:361-371, 1990.

104. Nijsten MW, Hack CE, Helle M, et al: Interleukin-6 and its relation to the humoral immune response and clinical parameters in burned patients. Surgery 109:761-767, 1991.

105. Calandra T, Gerain J, Heumann D, et al: High circulating levels of interleukin-6 in patients with septic shock: Evolution during sepsis, prognostic value, and interplay with other cytokines. The Swiss-Dutch J5 Immunoglobulin Study Group. Am J Med 91:23-29, 1991.

106. Presterl E, Staudinger T, Pettermann M, et al: Cytokine profile and correlation to the APACHE III and MPM II scores in patients with sepsis. Am J Respir Crit Care Med 156:825-832, 1997.

107. Opal SM, Jhung JW, Keith JC Jr, et al: Recombinant human interleukin-11 in experimental *Pseudomonas aeruginosa* sepsis in immunocompromised animals. J Infect Dis 178:1205-1208, 1998.

108. Opal SM, Keith JC Jr, Jhung J, et al: Orally administered recombinant human interleukin-11 is protective in experimental neutropenic sepsis. J Infect Dis 187:70-76, 2003.

109. Yoshimura T, Matsushima K, Tanaka S, et al: Purification of a human monocyte-derived neutrophil chemotactic factor that has peptide sequence similarity to other host defense cytokines. Proc Natl Acad Sci U S A 84:9233-9237, 1987.

110. Jansen PM, van der Pouw Kraan TC, de Jong IW, et al: Release of interleukin-12 in experimental *Escherichia coli* septic shock in baboons: Relation to plasma levels of interleukin-10 and interferon-gamma. Blood 87:5144-5151, 1996.

111. Van Zee KJ, DeForge LE, Fischer E, et al: IL-8 in septic shock, endotoxemia, and after IL-1 administration. J Immunol 146:3478-3482, 1991.

112. Hack CE, Hart M, van Schijndel RJ, et al: Interleukin-8 in sepsis: Relation to shock and inflammatory mediators. Infect Immun 60:2835-2842, 1992.

113. Marty C, Misset B, Tamion F, et al: Circulating interleukin-8 concentrations in patients with multiple organ failure of septic and nonseptic origin. Crit Care Med 22:673-679, 1994.

114. Carvalho GL, Wakabayashi G, Shimazu M, et al: Anti-interleukin-8 monoclonal antibody reduces free radical production and improves hemodynamics and survival rate in endotoxic shock in rabbits. Surgery 122:60-68, 1997.

115. Black RA, Rauch CT, Kozlosky CJ, et al: A metalloproteinase disintegrin that releases tumour-necrosis factor-alpha from cells. Nature 385:729-733, 1997.

116. Yoshimura T, Robinson EA, Tanaka S, et al: Purification and amino acid analysis of two human monocyte chemoattractants produced by phytohemagglutinin-stimulated human blood mononuclear leukocytes. J Immunol 142:1956-1962, 1989.

117. Standiford TJ, Kunkel SL, Lukacs NW, et al: Macrophage inflammatory protein-1 alpha mediates lung leukocyte recruitment, lung capillary leak, and early mortality in murine endotoxemia. J Immunol 155:1515-1524, 1995.

118. Bossink AW, Paemen L, Jansen PM, et al: Plasma levels of the chemokines monocyte chemotactic proteins-1 and -2 are elevated in human sepsis. Blood 86:3841-3847, 1995.

119. O'Grady NP, Tropea M, Preas HL II, et al: Detection of macrophage inflammatory protein (MIP)-1alpha and MIP-1beta during experimental endotoxemia and human sepsis. J Infect Dis 179:136-141, 1999.

120. Cooper AM, Magram J, Ferrante J, et al: Interleukin 12 (IL-12) is crucial to the development of protective immunity in mice intravenously infected with *Mycobacterium tuberculosis*. J Exp Med 186:39-45, 1997.

121. Decken K, Kohler G, Palmer-Lehmann K, et al: Interleukin-12 is essential for a protective Th1 response in mice infected with *Cryptococcus neoformans*. Infect Immun 66:4994-5000, 1998.

122. Heinzel FP, Rerko RM, Ling P, et al: Interleukin 12 is produced in vivo during endotoxemia and stimulates synthesis of gamma interferon. Infect Immun 62:4244-4249, 1994.

123. Wysocka M, Kubin M, Vieira LQ, et al: Interleukin-12 is required for interferon-gamma production and lethality in lipopolysaccharide-induced shock in mice. Eur J Immunol 25:672-676, 1995.

124. Hazelzet JA, Kornelisse RF, van der Pouw Kraan TC, et al: Interleukin 12 levels during the initial phase of septic shock with purpura in children: Relation to severity of disease. Cytokine 9:711-716, 1997.

125. Emmanuilidis K, Weighardt H, Matevossian E, et al: Differential regulation of systemic IL-18 and IL-12 release during postoperative sepsis: High serum IL-18 as an early predictive indicator of lethal outcome. Shock 18:301-305, 2002.

126. Weighardt H, Heidecke CD, Westerholt A, et al: Impaired monocyte IL-12 production before surgery as a predictive factor for the lethal outcome of postoperative sepsis. Ann Surg 235:560-567, 2002.

127. Fuss IJ, Neurath M, Boirivant M, et al: Disparate CD4$^+$ lamina propria (LP) lymphokine secretion profiles in inflammatory bowel disease: Crohn's disease LP cells manifest increased secretion of IFN-gamma, whereas ulcerative colitis LP cells manifest increased secretion of IL-5. J Immunol 157:1261-1270, 1996.

128. Neurath MF, Fuss I, Kelsall BL, et al: Antibodies to interleukin 12 abrogate established experimental colitis in mice. J Exp Med 182:1281-1290, 1995.

129. Bauditz J, Wedel S, Lochs H: Thalidomide reduces tumour necrosis factor alpha and interleukin 12 production in patients with chronic active Crohn's disease. Gut 50:196-200, 2002.

130. Steinhauser ML, Hogaboam CM, Lukacs NW, et al: Multiple roles for IL-12 in a model of acute septic peritonitis. J Immunol 162:5437-5443, 1999.

131. Ono S, Ueno C, Aosasa S, et al: Severe sepsis induces deficient interferon-gamma and interleukin-12 production, but interleukin-12 therapy improves survival in peritonitis. Am J Surg 182:491-497, 2001.

132. Dinarello CA: IL-18: A TH1-inducing, proinflammatory cytokine and new member of the IL-1 family. J Allergy Clin Immunol 103:11-24, 1999.

133. Fantuzzi G, Puren AJ, Harding MW, et al: Interleukin-18 regulation of interferon gamma production and cell proliferation as shown in interleukin-1beta-converting enzyme (caspase-1)-deficient mice. Blood 91:2118-2125, 1998.

134. Ghayur T, Banerjee S, Hugunin M, et al: Caspase-1 processes IFN-gamma-inducing factor and regulates LPS-induced IFN-gamma production. Nature 386:619-623, 1997.

135. Wyman TH, Dinarello CA, Banerjee A, et al: Physiological levels of interleukin-18 stimulate multiple neutrophil functions through p38 MAP kinase activation. J Leukoc Biol 72:401-409, 2002.

136. Oberholzer A, Steckholzer U, Kurimoto M, et al: Interleukin-18 plasma levels are increased in patients with sepsis compared to severely injured patients. Shock 16:411-414, 2001.

137. Fiorentino DF, Bond MW, Mosmann TR: Two types of mouse T helper cell: IV. Th2 clones secrete a factor that inhibits cytokine production by Th1 clones. J Exp Med 170:2081-2095, 1989.

138. Gazzinelli RT, Wysocka M, Hieny S, et al: In the absence of endogenous IL-10, mice acutely infected with *Toxoplasma gondii* succumb to a lethal immune response dependent on CD4[+] T cells and accompanied by overproduction of IL-12, IFN-gamma and TNF-alpha. J Immunol 157:798-805, 1996.

139. Latifi SQ, O'Riordan MA, Levine AD: Interleukin-10 controls the onset of irreversible septic shock. Infect Immun 70:4441-4446, 2002.

140. Berg DJ, Davidson N, Kuhn R, et al: Enterocolitis and colon cancer in interleukin-10-deficient mice are associated with aberrant cytokine production and CD4(+) T_H1-like responses. J Clin Invest 98:1010-1020, 1996.

141. Neidhardt R, Keel M, Steckholzer U, et al: Relationship of interleukin-10 plasma levels to severity of injury and clinical outcome in injured patients. J Trauma 42:863-871, 1997.

142. Sherry RM, Cue JI, Goddard JK, et al: Interleukin-10 is associated with the development of sepsis in trauma patients. J Trauma 40:613-617, 1996.

143. Lehmann AK, Halstensen A, Sornes S, et al: High levels of interleukin 10 in serum are associated with fatality in meningococcal disease. Infect Immun 63:2109-2112, 1995.

144. Marchant A, Deviere J, Byl B, et al: Interleukin-10 production during septicaemia. Lancet 343:707-708, 1994.

145. van Dissel JT, van Langevelde P, Westendorp RG, et al: Anti-inflammatory cytokine profile and mortality in febrile patients. Lancet 351:950-953, 1998.

146. Fumeaux T, Pugin J: Role of interleukin-10 in the intracellular sequestration of human leukocyte antigen-DR in monocytes during septic shock. Am J Respir Crit Care Med 166:1475-1482, 2002.

147. Leon LR, Kozak W, Rudolph K, et al: An antipyretic role for interleukin-10 in LPS fever in mice. Am J Physiol 276:R81-89, 1999.

148. Gerard C, Bruyns C, Marchant A, et al: Interleukin 10 reduces the release of tumor necrosis factor and prevents lethality in experimental endotoxemia. J Exp Med 177:547-550, 1993.

149. Kato T, Murata A, Ishida H, et al: Interleukin 10 reduces mortality from severe peritonitis in mice. Antimicrob Agents Chemother 39:1336-1340, 1995.

150. Matsumoto T, Tateda K, Miyazaki S, et al: Effect of interleukin-10 on gut-derived sepsis caused by *Pseudomonas aeruginosa* in mice. Antimicrob Agents Chemother 42:2853-2857, 1998.

151. Remick DG, Garg SJ, Newcomb DE, et al: Exogenous interleukin-10 fails to decrease the mortality or morbidity of sepsis. Crit Care Med 26:895-904, 1998.

152. Steinhauser ML, Hogaboam CM, Kunkel SL, et al: IL-10 is a major mediator of sepsis-induced impairment in lung antibacterial host defense. J Immunol 162:392-399, 1999.

153. Muchamuel T, Menon S, Pisacane P, et al: IL-13 protects mice from lipopolysaccharide-induced lethal endotoxemia: Correlation with down-modulation of TNF-alpha, IFN-gamma, and IL-12 production. J Immunol 158:2898-2903, 1997.

154. Matsukawa A, Hogaboam CM, Lukacs NW, et al: Expression and contribution of endogenous IL-13 in an experimental model of sepsis. J Immunol 164:2738-2744, 2000.

155. Yang H, Wang H, Tracey KJ: HMG-1 rediscovered as a cytokine. Shock 15:247-253, 2001.

156. Goodwin GH, Sanders C, Johns EW: A new group of chromatin-associated proteins with a high content of acidic and basic amino acids. Eur J Biochem 38:14-19, 1973.

157. Baxevanis AD, Landsman D: The HMG-1 box protein family: Classification and functional relationships. Nucleic Acids Res 23:1604-1613, 1995.

158. Jantzen HM, Admon A, Bell SP, et al: Nucleolar transcription factor hUBF contains a DNA-binding motif with homology to HMG proteins. Nature 344:830-836, 1990.

159. Imamura T, Izumi H, Nagatani G, et al: Interaction with p53 enhances binding of cisplatin-modified DNA by high mobility group 1 protein. J Biol Chem 276:7534-7540, 2001.

160. Zappavigna V, Falciola L, Helmer-Citterich M, et al: HMG1 interacts with HOX proteins and enhances their DNA binding and transcriptional activation. Embo J 15:4981-4991, 1996.

161. Wang H, Bloom O, Zhang M, et al: HMG-1 as a late mediator of endotoxin lethality in mice. Science 285:248-251, 1999.

162. Abraham E, Arcaroli J, Carmody A, et al: HMG-1 as a mediator of acute lung inflammation. J Immunol 165:2950-2954, 2000.

163. Sappington PL, Yang R, Yang H, et al: HMGB1 B box increases the permeability of Caco-2 enterocytic monolayers and impairs intestinal barrier function in mice. Gastroenterology 123:790-802, 2002.

164. Ulloa L, Ochani M, Yang H, et al: Ethyl pyruvate prevents lethality in mice with established lethal sepsis and systemic inflammation. Proc Natl Acad Sci U S A 99:12351-12356, 2002.

165. Grover R, Zaccardelli D, Colice G, et al: An open-label dose escalation study of the nitric oxide synthase inhibitor, N(G)-methyl-L-arginine hydrochloride (546C88), in patients with septic shock. Glaxo Wellcome International Septic Shock Study Group. Crit Care Med 27:913-922, 1999.

166. MacMicking JD, Nathan C, Hom G, et al: Altered responses to bacterial infection and endotoxic shock in mice lacking inducible nitric oxide synthase. Cell 81:641-650, 1995.

167. Wei XQ, Charles IG, Smith A, et al: Altered immune responses in mice lacking inducible nitric oxide synthase. Nature 375:408-411, 1995.

168. Laubach VE, Shesely EG, Smithies O, et al: Mice lacking inducible nitric oxide synthase are not resistant to lipopolysaccharide-induced death. Proc Natl Acad Sci U S A 92:10688-10692, 1995.

169. Nicholson SC, Grobmyer SR, Shiloh MU, et al: Lethality of endotoxin in mice genetically deficient in the respiratory burst oxidase, inducible nitric oxide synthase, or both. Shock 11:253-258, 1999.

170. Cobb JP, Hotchkiss RS, Swanson PE, et al: Inducible nitric oxide synthase (iNOS) gene deficiency increases the mortality of sepsis in mice. Surgery 126:438-442, 1999.

171. Wang LF, Patel M, Razavi HM, et al: Role of inducible nitric oxide synthase in pulmonary microvascular protein leak in murine sepsis. Am J Respir Crit Care Med 165:1634-1639, 2002.

172. Fink MP: Cytopathic hypoxia: Mitochondrial dysfunction as mechanism contributing to organ dysfunction in sepsis. Crit Care Clin 17:219-237, 2001.

173. Khan AU, Delude RL, Han YY, et al: Liposomal NAD[+] prevents diminished O_2 consumption by immunostimulated Caco-2 cells. Am J Physiol Lung Cell Mol Physiol 282:L1082-1091, 2002.

174. Marnett LJ, Rowlinson SW, Goodwin DC, et al: Arachidonic acid oxygenation by COX-1 and COX-2: Mechanisms of catalysis and inhibition. J Biol Chem 274:22903-22906, 1999.

CHAPTER 5

SHOCK, ELECTROLYTES, AND FLUID

Richard J. Mullins, M.D.

Body Water and Solute Composition
Extracellular Water and Electrolytes
Biochemistry and Physiology of Acid-Base
   Regulation
Hyponatremia and Hypotonicity
Hypernatremia and Syndromes of Hypertonicity
Pathophysiology of Potassium
Calcium and Magnesium

Control of Plasma Volume and the Circulation of
   Interstitial Fluid
Cellular Aerobic Function and Dysfunction
Hypovolemic Shock
Shock from Sepsis
Shock from Cardiac Disease
Shock from Adrenal Insufficiency

In health, an individual maintains physiologic balance termed *homeostasis*. The body is divided into compartments separated by membranes of variable permeability characteristics. Each compartment has a different composition, and within each is a directed flow of fluid and movement of solutes. The physiologic balance of homeostasis controls the exchange of water and solutes between these compartments. In a healthy individual a wide range of physiologic systems are coordinated and in equipoise. For example, coordinated function of normal circulatory, pulmonary, and renal organ function maintains delivery of energy to cells throughout the body despite fluctuations in the external environment. Most physiologic systems have the capacity to accelerate and decelerate and are modulated by feedback mechanisms; homeostasis is intricately regulated with interactions between physiologic systems. Claude Bernard was a 19th century French physician whose studies of function led him to propose the concept of *milieu interieur:* physiologic function is adjusted for the purpose of maintaining the optimal internal environment within cells. Homeostasis is maintained only if there is adequate delivery of energy, that is, fuels and oxygen to cells.

Shock is a circumstance in which homeostasis is disrupted. A universal physiologic threat to the patient in shock is deficient oxygen delivery to the mitochondria of cells. As a consequence, aerobic metabolism cannot be sustained at the rate needed to maintain cell function. The cell cannot recover from sustained interruption of aerobic metabolism. As cells die, organ failure ensues. A wide range of mechanisms cause shock. Surgeons treat many of these patients by focusing therapy on restoring cardiovascular function, by treating either impaired cardiac contractility, a decline in systemic vascular resistance, or depleted intravascular volume. But an emphasis on therapy that measurably influences whole-organ function should not deflect the appreciation that patient survival will ultimately be determined by events within cells. Profound hemorrhage leads to a rapidly lethal form of shock; a sustained period of a modestly reduced oxygen delivery leading to irreversible intracellular dysfunction is just as lethal.

In this chapter priority is given to information with a clinical basis. Information on normal human structure and function is reviewed, as well as pathologic conditions encountered in clinical practice. The mechanisms by which homeostasis are maintained are described, and the role that shock plays in disruption of these normal balances is defined. Therapy is described in the context of restoring the capacity of the body's physiologic systems to maintain the normal *milieu interieur*. Focus is on the challenge of diagnosis and treatment of shock. In other chapters in the textbook, details are presented regarding blood transfusion, nutritional support, and management of specific diseases.

BODY WATER AND SOLUTE COMPOSITION

Total Body Water

In most adults, water accounts for 45% to 60% of the total body weight. In a young adult 70-kg male, total body water (TBW) therefore approximates 40 kg, corresponding to 40 L. Female subjects have smaller measured TBWs compared with male subjects of the same height and weight. The proportion of the body weight made up of fat is associated with the variance of TBW per kilogram of body weight in both genders.

Investigators have measured TBW in humans using indicator dilution methods with deuterium oxide (D$_2$O, an isotope of water), tritium,[1] and nonradioactive water enriched with the heavy isotope ^{18}O.[2] In practice, the subject ingests a known mass of D$_2$O and, based on the steady-state plasma concentration of the isotope achieved in 3 hours, the distribution volume of the tracer isotope is calculated as a measure of the TBW.[3] Chumlea and colleagues reported TBW using serial D$_2$O measurements made on a selected cohort of United States adults with long-term follow-up.[4] TBW was measured as 56% of the body weight in young men and 46% of body weight in 60-year-old men. Women had a smaller proportion of TBW than men. The TBW measured in young women was 47% of their body weight, whereas in women older than age 60 TBW was measured as 43% of their body weight. Predicting for an individual patient body composition should be done with models that include, as independent predictor variables, age, gender, and race, as well as the standard measures of stature such as height and weight (Table 5-1).[5] In their longitudinal study, these investigators observed that healthy adults had relatively little decline in TBW from age 20 to age 60. The lower proportion of TBW in older subjects was principally related to fat being a larger proportion of the body weight in the geriatric age group.[4] Chumlea and colleagues also reported that blacks had a larger TBW than whites. Thus, predicting the ideal TBW requires consideration of age, gender, and race, as well as the standard measures of stature such as height and weight.

Compartments of Total Body Water

TBW largely distributes in two compartments, the intracellular water (ICW) and extracellular water (ECW) spaces. Cell membranes are permeable to water but selectively permeable to solutes. ICW averages 66% of TBW; therefore, 40% of a lean adult male's body weight is composed solely of water in cells, chiefly skeletal muscle cells. ECW accounts for 20% of the total body weight.

Movement of solutes (particularly sodium and potassium) across the cell membrane is both tightly controlled and energy dependent. In contrast, water moves passively and quickly across the cell membranes separating the ECW and ICW. Water moves to establish osmotic equilibrium between these two compartments (Fig. 5-1).[6] Surgeons should interpret measured changes in the osmolality of plasma samples in terms of the predictable influence on the distribution of TBW between the ICW and ECW.

Several methods can be used to measure the size of ECW and ICW in humans. As previously described, TBW can be measured via indicator dilution methods, most commonly with deuterium oxide (D$_2$O). Similarly, ECW can be measured as the distribution volume of bromide (administered as NaBr) or sulfate (^{35}SO$_4$), although new methods using heavy isotopes of sulfate have been reported that have the advantage of avoiding patient exposure to radioactive isotopes.[7] Sulfate provides a 20% smaller measurement of ECW volume than bromide.[8] Using these methods, TBW and ECW can be measured simultaneously and ICW is calculated as TBW minus ECW. Such indicator dilution methods are laborious, require meticulous technique, and are expensive; therefore these techniques are limited to research applications.

When measuring TBW one must also consider the relative size of "transcellular" water, defined as body water not readily exchangeable with either the ECW or ICW. This water is fixed in synovial, cerebrospinal, and intraocular fluids. In addition, patients may have a highly variable volume of water within the lumen of the bowel or bladder that contributes to the plus or minus 5% daily variance in body weight that can be recorded in patients. It is important to realize that indicator dilution measurements of body water compartments are best achieved in patients in a steady state and without pathologic conditions such as ascites, pleural effusions, or subcutaneous edema.

Bioimpedance spectroscopy has been reported as a useful and clinically practical method of measuring ECW and ICW.[7,8] These studies found that wrist-to-ankle bioimpedance spectroscopy, which measures total body

TABLE 5-1.   Body Composition* Estimated in Younger and Older Women of Similar Height and Weight, Separated by Race as Percent of Body Weight

Compartment	Age 20		Age 70	
	Black	White	Black	White
ICW	30.3	30.7	26.3	25.1
ECW	19.9	19.0	13.4	12.8
TBW	50.2	49.7	39.7	37.9
Protein	15.1	14.8	13.4	12.8
Fat	29.6	30.7	36.2	37.5
Mineral	5.0	4.7	3.9	3.6

*Total body water (TBW) is measured as the dilution volume of ingested dose of tritiated water. Extracellular water (ECW) was measured as the delayed gamma neutron activation for total body chloride. Intracellular water (ICW) was the difference TBW − ECW. Total body protein was calculated from total body nitrogen using gamma neutron activation. Total body fat was calculated from total body carbon, measured in vivo by neutron inelastic scattering and total body nitrogen.
From Aloia JF, Vaswani A, Flaster E, Ma R: Relationship of body water compartments to age, race, and fat-free mass. J Lab Clin Med 132:483-490, 1998.

DISTRIBUTION OF SOLUTES

EXTRACELLULAR		INTRACELLULAR	
Na$^+$	142	Na$^+$	10
K$^+$	4	K$^+$	140
CL$^-$	110	CL$^-$	3
HCO$_3^-$	24	HCO$_3^-$	10
Inorganic$^-$	12	Organic$^-$	137
Glucose	3	Glucose	2.5
OSM	300 ⟷	300	
Urea	⟷	UREA	
(ETOH)	⟷	(ETOH)	

Units: mmole/kg of water, except organic$^-$
*Units: mEq/kg of water

■ FIGURE 5-1.   The cell membrane forms a selective barrier to electrolyte solutes. The osmolality (mmol/kg of water) of intracellular and extracellular water is equivalent because water can freely cross the cell membrane. Organic anions in intracellular water are macromolecules with multiple sites per molecule of phosphate ester charge. These organic anions include DNA, RNA, creatinine phosphate, adenosine triphosphate, and phospholipids. Urea and ethanol can, like water, equilibrate rapidly by diffusion across the cell membrane. (From Halperin ML, Goldstein M: Fluid, Electrolyte, and Acid-Base Physiology: A Problem-based Approach, 3rd ed. Philadelphia, WB Saunders, 1999.)

impedance over a range of electrical impulse frequencies, when analyzed with appropriate biophysical models provided acceptably accurate measures of ECW and ICW in normal men and women. Bioimpedance spectroscopy has also been demonstrated by Finn and colleagues to be reliable in seriously injured and ill patients.[1] O'Brien and coworkers evaluated the utility of bioimpedance spectroscopy for assessment of TBW in normal humans with induced dehydration by two methods: sweating associated with exercise and a diuretic-induced water loss.[9] Using D$_2$O as the standard, these authors concluded that the bioimpedance assessment of dehydration was reliable.

The majority of potassium in the human body is found within the cells, and measures of the total body potassium content can be used to indicate ICW. The mass of total body potassium-40 (K-40), a naturally occurring isotope, can be measured using a scintillation counter composed of an array of ^{32}NaI detectors in a heavily shielded room.[1] To calculate the ICW, two measures are needed: the size of the ECW and the concentration of K-40 in a serum sample. These two values multiplied together provide the mass of K-40 in ECW; this mass is then subtracted from the total body K-40 value (as measured with a scintillation counter) to provide the mass of K-40 in cells. It is assumed that the concentration of K-40 in cells is essentially unchanged over a wide range of conditions, and thus an increase or decrease in calculated K-40 mass reflects either an increase or decrease in cell volume.

Two studies demonstrate the utility of K-40 and other measures of body composition. Finn and associates found that over a period of 3 weeks, severe stress from injury or sepsis leads to cell shrinkage in patients in an intensive care unit (ICU). In this study, TBW was measured with tritium dilution and ECW was measured with both bromide tracers and bioimpedance spectroscopy. The authors observed that, despite total body overhydration, patients still experienced cellular dehydration (Figs. 5-2 and 5-3). In meticulous investigation of metabolic response to injury, Herndon and coworkers reported that administration of β blockers to catabolic children with serious burns was beneficial. β Blockers reduced the accelerated proteolysis that depletes intracellular protein in these children despite aggressive nutritional support. In summary, a patient with a smaller intracellular space compared with normal controls is a patient with a measurable deficit in lean body mass and functional reserve.

Filtered Plasma Forms Interstitial Fluid

The ECW is subdivided into the plasma and interstitial compartments. Fluid and solutes circulate from the plasma

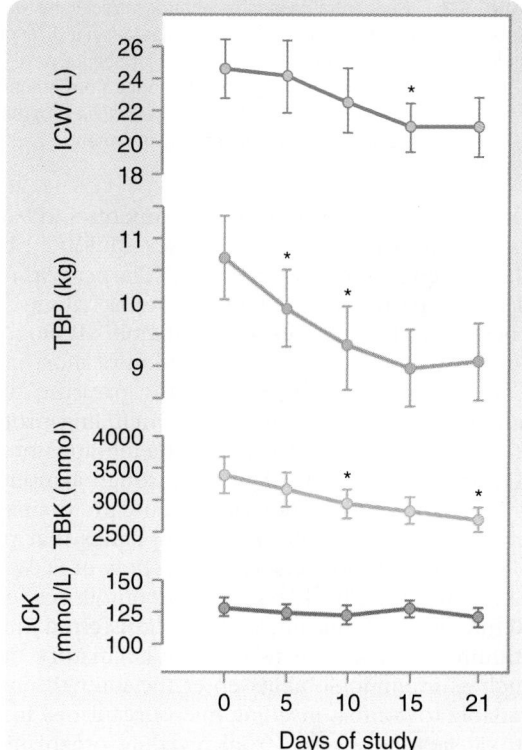

■ FIGURE 5-2.   Sequential measurements of intracellular water (ICW), total body protein (TBP), total body potassium (TBK), and intracellular potassium (ICK) concentration in nine multiply injured patients. *Asterisk* indicates significant change from preceding measurement. (From Finn PJ, Plank LD, Clark MA, et al: Progressive cellular dehydration and proteolysis in critically ill patients. Lancet 347:654-656, 1996.)

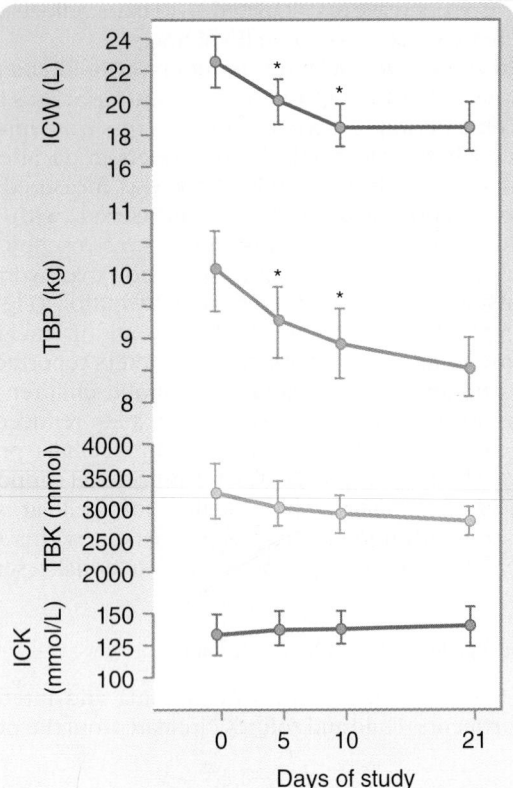

FIGURE 5-3. Sequential measurements of intracellular water (ICW), total body protein (TBP), total body potassium (TBK), and intracellular potassium (ICK) concentration in 11 patients with severe sepsis. *Asterisk* indicates significant change from preceding measurement. (From Finn PJ, Plank LD, Clark MA, et al: Progressive cellular dehydration and proteolysis in critically ill patients. Lancet 347:654-656, 1996.)

compartment to the interstitial compartments and back to the plasma compartment via lymphatics. Multiple physiologic factors control the flow of ECW. Plasma within the vascular compartment contains proteins along with erythrocytes and other cellular elements of blood. As blood flows through the microcirculation of most organs (the brain is an exception), hydrostatic pressure within the lumen drives a filtrate of plasma, including proteins, across the semipermeable capillary membrane into the interstitium. Interstitial fluid flows through lymphatics, passes through lymph nodes, and eventually drains into the thoracic duct and other large lymphatics that pump lymph into the superior vena cava. The flow of ECW from plasma to lymph and back to plasma accomplishes several critical functions. Plasma nutrients are transferred into the interstitium and delivered to cells. Inflammatory mediators such as immunoglobulins enter the interstitium and are available to combat invading microorganisms. In addition, toxic factors released from invading organisms are cleared through lymph nodes, where an immune response is escalated, and then returned to the plasma for transport to the reticuloendothelial system. The flow of fluid and protein across the microvascular membrane is an important method for control of the intravascular volume.

The plasma volume is measured by indicator dilution methods that depend on intravenous injection of a large molecule that can be easily assayed. Considerable experience has been reported using radioactively labeled albumin. Labeled albumin is injected, and several plasma samples are drawn for the subsequent hour. The concentration, measured as specific activity, of albumin isotope in plasma is determined from these samples and should demonstrate a decline. The decline in albumin concentration results from the constant shift of albumin across capillary membranes. Logarithms of plasma albumin concentrations are extrapolated over the hour, and the intercept with time zero is estimated; this intercept is accepted as the plasma concentration if there had been complete mixing of the intravenously injected isotope. This estimated time zero concentration is divided by the mass of albumin isotope injected to provide an estimate of plasma volume. Clinical investigators have also used Evans Blue dye (which preferentially binds albumin) or indocyanine green dye as alternatives to radioactive labeled albumin.[10] Measurement of transient changes in plasma volume in response to intravenous infusion of therapeutic fluids indicates that renal function, lymph flow, and ECW fluid shifts govern the restoration of homeostasis after an expansion in blood volume.[11]

EXTRACELLULAR WATER AND ELECTROLYTES

Control of Extracellular Sodium

Sodium is the predominant cation in ECW and associates with the anions chloride and bicarbonate. These three electrolytes constitute over 90% of the active osmoles in the ECW. The predominant cation in ICW is potassium, which is electrochemically balanced primarily by organic phosphates. In addition, DNA, RNA, adenosine triphosphate (ATP), adenosine diphosphate (ADP), and creatine phosphate provide a negative charge to balance the positive charge of potassium in ICW. The difference in electrolyte composition between ICW and ECW is sustained because the normally functioning cell membrane, predominantly composed of lipids, acts as a barrier to sodium. Large enzyme molecules structurally embedded in the cell membrane form pores capable of actively transporting sodium from the ICW to ECW. The ubiquitous enzyme Na^+/K^+-ATPase, for example, plays a key role in sustaining the difference in electrolyte composition of the ECW and ICW.[12] Na^+/K^+-ATPase, also known as the "sodium pump," moves sodium across the cell membrane by undergoing molecular conformational changes that consume energy (Fig. 5-4). The pump binds three sodium ions in the ICW, and then energy provided by hydrolysis of ATP to ADP changes the conformation within the Na^+/K^+-ATPase. The bonded intracellular sodium is then moved across the membrane and released into the extracellular fluid. Two potassium ions enter the cell in association with the three sodium ions leaving the cell in active transport by Na^+/K^+-ATPase. With three cations out and two cations into the cell, the electrochemical consequence is a net negative intracellular charge termed the *resting membrane potential*. The majority of anionic

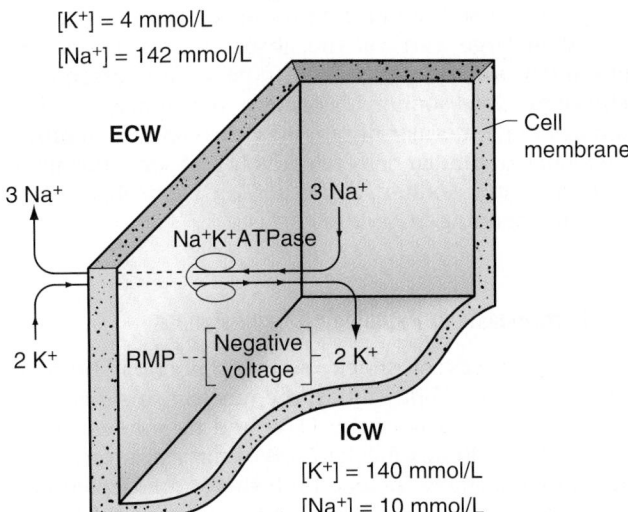

[K⁺] = 4 mmol/L

[Na⁺] = 142 mmol/L

ECW

Cell membrane

3 Na⁺

3 Na⁺

Na⁺K⁺ATPase

2 K⁺   RMP   Negative voltage   2 K⁺

ICW

[K⁺] = 140 mmol/L

[Na⁺] = 10 mmol/L

FIGURE 5-4. The resting membrane potential within cells of a negative charge is established by the cell membrane enzyme Na⁺/K⁺-ATPase using energy to pump three sodium molecules out of the cell for every two potassium molecules transported into the cell. ECW, extracellular water; ICW, intracellular water.

centration is 10 mmol/L and the potassium concentration is 150 mmol/L. Conversely, in the ECW, the sodium concentration is 140 mmol/L and the potassium concentration averages 4 mmol/L. Because small amounts of sodium continuously regain access to ICW, the sodium pump is constantly active and converts the energy in ATP to restore the resting membrane potential. In circumstances in which insufficient oxygen is available to sustain aerobic metabolism and, consequently, cellular ATP levels fall, the sodium pump cannot function. Cell death becomes imminent as intracellular sodium concentration increases and resting membrane potential declines.

Total Body Sodium Mass Determines the Size of the ECW and Is Regulated by Renal Function

The nephron is the basic functional unit of renal function (Fig. 5-5). Patients with normal renal function have glomerular filtration rates in excess of 100 mL/min. Over 6 L of ECW filtrate enters Bowman's capsule every hour in a healthy adult. At this rate of filtration, every 4 hours the sodium load filtered into the nephron exceeds the total mass of sodium in the body. The size of ECW and total body sodium mass is regulated through multiple

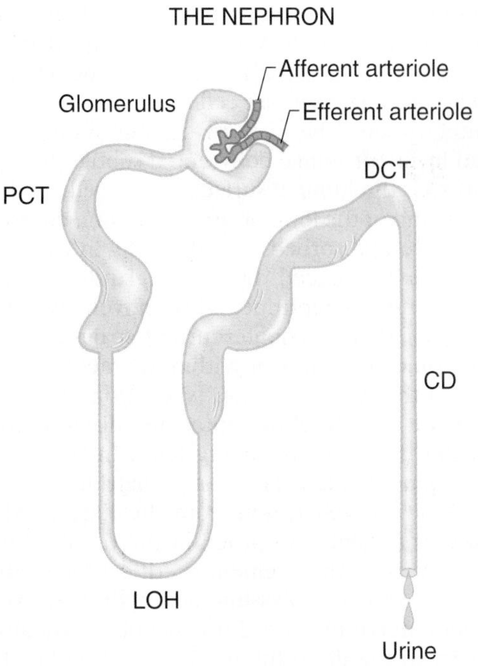

molecules in the cell are large and cannot diffuse across the cell membrane; thus restricted to ICW, these negatively charged macromolecules contribute to resting membrane potential. Voltage of the resting membrane potential is essential for cell function and is the basis for nerve cell conduction and muscle cell contraction.

The control of Na⁺/K⁺-ATPase involves multiple factors. An increase in ICW sodium concentration occurs during an action potential, when a sodium pore opens in the cell membrane, allowing sodium to transiently shift along its concentration gradient into the cell. In response to greater ICW sodium concentration, the activity of Na⁺/K⁺-ATPase increases. Circulating extracellular hormones can attach to the cell membrane and increase ATP synthesis, which accelerates the ion transport of Na⁺/K⁺-ATPase. β₂-Adrenergic agonists and insulin can similarly lead to more sodium and potassium exchange. When patients deficient in the mineralocorticoid hormone aldosterone receive doses of the hormone, serum potassium concentration abruptly falls. Aldosterone achieves this effect by directly binding to Na⁺/K⁺-ATPase and accelerating cation exchange across the cell membrane. The regulation of electrolyte concentration is a critical function for survival and is accomplished within cells via local feedback mechanisms along with circulating hormones.

The substantial difference between potassium concentration in ICW and ECW favors diffusion of potassium along a concentration gradient to the ECW. The transport of potassium along this gradient is passive, meaning no energy is required. However, the negative charge of the resting membrane potential powerfully favors potassium to remain intracellular. As potassium moves through pores into the ECW unaccompanied by an anion, the intracellular negative charge increases, which attracts more K⁺ ions back into the cell. In normal cells, the ICW sodium con-

THE NEPHRON

Afferent arteriole

Efferent arteriole

Glomerulus

DCT

PCT

CD

LOH

Urine

FIGURE 5-5. The major components of the nephron are the glomerulus, where plasma delivered in afferent arterioles is filtered; the proximal convoluted tubule (PCT); the loop of Henle (LOH); the distal convoluted tubule (DCT); and the collecting duct (CD). Different components of renal function occur along the nephron. A normal glomerular filtration rate of 125 mL/min would generate 180 L/day of filtrate containing 27,000 mmol of sodium. Approximately two thirds of the filtered sodium is absorbed in the PCT, 20% in the LOH, 7% in the DCT, and 3% in the CD; and the net excretion of urinary sodium, as a fraction of the total sodium filtered load, per day is less than 1%.

mechanisms that influence nephron tubular function. Tubule cells absorb over 95% of the enormous volume of daily glomerular filtrate. Selective reabsorption is the process by which solutes are separated into those excreted in urine and those returned to ECW. Excess dietary sodium and consumed water loads are eliminated in urine, and patients remain in sodium and water balance becoming neither edematous nor dehydrated. Renal tubular function varies along the path of the nephron, and four regions of distinct function have been defined: the proximal convoluted tubule, the thin descending and thick ascending limbs of the loop of Henle, and the distal convoluted tubule and the medullary collecting duct that transverses the renal medulla and drains urine into the renal pelvis. Endocrine mechanisms and internal renal regulatory functions adjust the properties of sodium resorption in each segment, although specific cellular events vary among the four segments. Urinary excretion of water and electrolytes reflects the result of complex homeostatic processes intended to preserve the composition and size of the ECW.

At the luminal surface of cells in the proximal convoluted tubules, 60% to 70% of the filtered sodium and water is absorbed into cells.[13] The tubular cells depend on Na^+/K^+-ATPase to remove sodium at the basilar side of the cell where sodium diffuses into postglomerular capillaries and is cleared from the kidney. This sodium pump activity creates an environment within the tubule cell that favors filtrate electrolytes, particularly sodium and chloride, to move into the ICW of tubular cells. Sympathetic nerves, angiotensin, parathyroid hormone (PTH), and endothelin modulate tubular cell function in the proximal convoluted tubule. The majority of filtered bicarbonate is absorbed in the proximal convoluted tubule through specific pores on the luminal surface of the cell. In the thick ascending limb of the loop of Henle, sodium, chloride, and potassium are reabsorbed. Tubular cells in this nephron segment are influenced by prostaglandins, glucagon, calcitonin, and epinephrine. This movement of solute in the loop of Henle's countercurrent structure produces the hypertonic environment within the medullary section essential for the reabsorption of water from the collecting ducts. Dilute filtrate flows into the distal convoluted tubule from the thick ascending limb. In the distal convoluted segment, aldosterone and natriuretic peptides influence sodium absorption from the filtrate. Although the amount of sodium absorbed in the distal convoluted tubule is not large, this segment is critical for establishing the extent of urinary potassium and hydrogen excretion. Sympathetic nerve fibers and the macula densa also regulate activity in the distal tubule. The final segment of the nephron is the collecting duct, which passes through the hypertonic interstitial fluid of the medullary portion of the kidney. Water absorption from the filtrate, which enables the production of concentrated urine and thus, when the individual is threatened by dehydrations, preserves TBW, is accomplished in the collecting duct under the control of the hormone arginine vasopressin. The normal function of the renal nephron enables reabsorption of between 97% and 99.1% of glomerular filtrate water and sodium.

Absorption of sodium in the proximal nephron is accomplished in large part via the absorption of anions, but substantial urinary excretion of potassium is essential to achieve maximal sodium absorption. In summary, as huge volumes of glomerular filtrate flow through the nephron, a sequence of tubular cells selectively reabsorbs the majority of the water, sodium, and other key electrolytes essential to maintaining ECW homeostasis.

ECW Homeostasis in Pathologic Circumstances

In circumstances of shock, serious infection, burn, or pathologic loss of body fluids, the mechanisms that maintain the homeostasis of the ECW and its solutes can be overwhelmed. Reflex mechanisms of survival advantage in these circumstances include both short-term depletion of ICW to preserve ECW size and shifts of interstitial fluid to the plasma volume. These mechanisms preserve blood volume and especially the flow of blood to vital organs. Surgeons effectively resuscitate patients with these life-threatening conditions by intravenously infusing replacement fluids and medications. The results of successful resuscitation typically involve a major expansion of the ECW and a restoration of oxygen delivery to a disturbed intracellular environment.[14] After an episode of shock and resuscitation, patients have a substantial perturbation in composition, including an expanded ECW space and excess sodium. Multiple homeostatic mechanisms lead to a restoration of normal ECW size and composition. These include intrinsic renal function.

Natriuretic peptides are a family of at least three molecules named atrial natriuretic peptide (ANP), brain natriuretic peptide (BNP), and C-type natriuretic peptide.[15] ANP is released from cells located in the cardiac atrial walls. Humans principally secrete BNP from cells in the ventricular wall. Both ANP and BNP levels are elevated in patients with hypertension, expanded blood volume, congestive heart failure, and other forms of heart disease.[16] Controlled physiologic experiments have demonstrated that these peptides are released into plasma and circulate at higher levels in circumstances of overdistention of the heart. The physiologic effects of these peptides are proposed to compensate for an overdistended blood volume. Compensatory cardiovascular actions of ANP and BNP include arterial smooth muscle relaxation and vasodilation and increased microvascular membrane permeability. These latter actions result in a shift of plasma fluid and proteins into the interstitium that combined with venous capacitance vessel dilation reduces cardiac preload.[16] The additional volume-reducing effect of natriuretic peptides occurs through direct action on renal function. These peptides are antagonists to the antidiuretic effect of aldosterone in the renal tubules.

C-type natriuretic peptides have been identified in vascular smooth muscle cells as well as endothelial cells and are hypothesized to act locally to produce paracrine or autocrine vasodilation. All natriuretic peptides work by binding to receptors on the cell surface, resulting in increased intracellular cyclic guanosine monophosphate, which acts as the intracellular mediator of natriuretic peptide effects.

Control of the ECW size is influenced by a second major physiologic mechanism that influences the ECW osmolality. Arginine vasopressin (AVP) is a peptide synthesized in the hypothalamus and is released when ECW osmolality exceeds 280 mOsm/L. This molecule increases the absorption of water from the distal tubule in the nephron. As more water is absorbed and urine osmolality exceeds ECW osmolality, the net result is gain in ECW. Because water distributes in ECW and ICW to achieve osmolar equilibrium, retention of water by the nephron usually expands both the ECW and ICW compartments. Additionally, thirst—a compelling drive to drink generated when central nervous system sensors determine osmolality has increased beyond a certain threshold—acts to expand the volume of body water.

In summary, the body has two parallel but separate groups of physiologic mechanisms for control of ECW. Sodium balance is determined by renal function, which is regulated by hormones. In circumstances where sodium balance is positive, an increase in ECW osmolality occurs. As osmolality exceeds its threshold, a second and independent mechanism dependent on AVP becomes activated, resulting in a net gain of body water. In circumstances in which the ECW volume exceeds normal, renal function accomplishes diuresis along with a net loss of sodium and water, thereby reducing ECW. In normal conditions, osmolality and sodium balance are modulated within a narrow range. In shock caused by acute depletion of ECW through hemorrhage, these compensatory mechanisms are stressed to produce a rapid correction. Hypotension is a strong stimulant for AVP release, and patients will produce concentrated urine and retain excess water to the extent that serum sodium concentration is diluted below normal. Thus, in shock, restoring ECW has precedence over maintaining a normal ECW osmolality of 280 mOsm/L.

BIOCHEMISTRY AND PHYSIOLOGY OF ACID-BASE REGULATION

With its single positive charge and the lowest elemental molecular weight, the ubiquitous proton influences all vital biochemical reactions. The molar concentration of protons in ECW, H^+, is normally 40 ± 2 nmol/L. Proton concentration is maintained in a narrow range by multiple regulatory pathways. The concentrations of other solutes (Na^+, K^+, Cl^-, HCO_3^-) in ECW and ICW are 10^6 fold greater than H^+. Despite these differences in magnitude of concentration, the tolerable range of H^+ fluctuation is narrow compared with other electrolytes. In clinical practice, H^+ is measured as pH, the logarithm to the base 10 of $1/H^+$ in nanomoles per liter. The normal plasma pH value is 7.40. Patients with excess protons in arterial blood have an acidemia. Patients with an arterial pH above 7.40 have an alkalemia. Patients with acid-base disorders that produce a pH less than 7.00 or a pH greater than 7.70 have low rates of survival, and therefore homeostasis of pH is

critical. Acidemia is the more serious clinical perturbation in acid-base status. Fuels and proteins are consumed and metabolized, with the consequence of a daily positive proton balance. Plasma pH is maintained at 7.40 because urinary proton excretion equals the gain in protons from diet. An adult consuming a standard Western diet generates 50 to 100 mEq of protons daily from absorbed nutrients. Renal function principally eliminates the excess protons as the urinary solutes NH_4^+ and $H_2PO_4^-$. In contrast to slow accumulation of excess protons through diet, rapid increases in H^+ concentration in ICW and ECW that occur in shock can threaten life. Whereas normal renal function provides the capacity to excrete a large number of protons, hours are required to fully excrete large excesses, and renal function cannot compensate for sudden increases in H^+. Two physiologic functions protect the body against substantial falls in pH after the sudden release of a large number of protons: the neutralizing capacity of buffers and the exhalation of CO_2 by the lungs.

Buffers are anions that bind protons and dampen changes in pH. As mentioned, most patients with a serious clinical acid-base condition suffer acidemia. However, patients can also develop life-threatening alkalemia, and ICW and ECW buffering capacities can also resist increases in pH when a sudden decline in available protons occurs. Bicarbonate is the predominant buffer in ICW and ECW (Table 5-2).[6] Protons and a bicarbonate reversibly combine to form carbonic acid (H_2CO_3). Carbonic acid can further disassociate into water and the gas CO_2. In pulmonary capillaries, the CO_2 in blood readily diffuses into alveoli. This loss of CO_2 drives the conversion of more carbonic acid into CO_2 to be exhaled as a respiratory gas. As CO_2 is exhaled, the body achieves a net proton loss. The physiologic capacity to rapidly rid the body of excess protons through increased alveolar ventilation is a critical response to sudden increases in H^+. In addition, arterial pH regulation is achieved by alterations in pulmonary function that increase and decrease alveolar ventilation and the amount of carbon dioxide exhaled.

TABLE 5-2. **Buffers as Total Percent of Buffer Capacity Active in Intracellular and Extracellular Water***

	HCO_3^-	$H_2PO_4^{2-}$	Imidazole on Proteins
ECW	95%	4%	1%
ICW	42%	6%	52%

*It is estimated that a 70-kg person has 400 mmol of buffer in ECW and 800 mmol of buffer in ICW.

Adapted from Halperin ML, Goldstein M: Fluid, Electrolyte, and Acid-Base Physiology: A Problem-based Approach, 3rd ed. Philadelphia, WB Saunders, 1999.

Bicarbonate acts as a major buffer in ICW and ECW but proteins are important buffers only in ICW. Hydrogen ions can bind the imidazole site in the amino acid histidine present in cell proteins; however, as a consequence, bound protons can adversely alter the protein's charge and function. The third major system for intracellular buffering involves inorganic phosphates. Dibasic phosphate converts to a monobasic phosphate with the addition of a proton. Two thirds of ICW inorganic phosphate is normally present as monovalent HPO_4^{2-} and can readily assist in blunting the fall in pH associated with an acid load. The inorganic phosphate buffer system accounts for less than 10% of intracellular buffer capacity and makes only a minimal contribution to control of extracellular pH.

Correction of a suddenly imposed acid-base abnormality depends on an interaction between the ICW and ECW, which have substantially different solute compositions and are separated by a cell membrane not readily permeable to protons. The ICW pH is 7.10, substantially lower than the normal ECW pH of 7.40. Normal metabolism generates protons in ICW. As H^+ increases, bicarbonate is buffered and more CO_2 is generated. While the transport of ions across the cell membrane is restricted, the neutral gas CO_2 readily crosses cell membranes. As CO_2 builds in the ECW, the bicarbonate buffer system shifts toward protons. The enzyme carbonic anhydrase accelerates the kinetics of carbonic acid hydrolysis to carbon dioxide and water and vice versa. Excess carbonic acid is transported to the pulmonary microcirculation, where carbonic anhydrase facilitates its rapid conversion into gaseous CO_2 that diffuses into alveolar gas. Carbon dioxide exchange across the cell membrane can occur in either direction, however, and if P_{CO_2} builds in the ECW owing to reduced pulmonary function, carbonic acid will instead shift into the cell and lower ICW H^+.

Cells contain complex biochemical machines that integrate into enormous physiologic mechanisms to accomplish the work of the body. Cells principally depend on the high-energy terminal phosphate bond in ATP to do this work. In multiple reactions, cell machinery hydrolyzes ATP to ADP in a reaction that releases the inorganic phosphate and a proton. Using oxygen and fuels, oxidative phosphorylation occurs in cells, and in the mitochondria in particular, to convert ADP back to ATP. In oxidative phosphorylation, the high-energy phosphate bond and proton are recaptured. Thus, in steady-state conditions within cells in the presence of adequate fuel and oxygen delivery, pH does not change. However, in the circumstance of impaired oxygen delivery to the extent that oxidative phosphorylation cannot proceed at the rate needed to restore ATP, H^+ increases. Buffers are essential to human physiology in the clinical circumstances of depressed oxidative phosphorylation. A rapid rise in H^+ can be partially buffered by proteins in ICW as well as bicarbonate, but transport of CO_2 from ICW to ECW is essential to preventing a lethal depression in pH. Whereas buffer mechanisms can temporarily reduce the risk of acidosis, if the primary problem of energy production by oxidative phosphorylation is not resolved, cell death will occur within minutes.

Renal Function and Control of pH

The kidney plays an essential role in control of the body acid-base balance, because the excess protons produced through daily dietary intake are eliminated through the urine in a tightly regulated manner. The distal convoluted tubule segment is critical to the control of acid-base balance; here protons are secreted into the filtrate to produce an acidic urine, while bicarbonate and sodium are transported into the ECW. To achieve proton excretion, glutamine is converted into ammonium, which is transported into the filtrate. As protons are added to the filtrate, ammonium buffers the protons and forms NH_4^+. Inorganic phosphate acts as another important urine buffer that facilitates acid clearance from the body. While a normal adult daily generates 4500 mEq of bicarbonate in glomerular filtrate, the nephron reabsorbs the bicarbonate and achieves a net urinary excretion of 50 to 100 mEq of protons each day. In circumstances of sustained alkalemia or acidemia, the tightly regulated renal mechanisms of hydrogen excretion and bicarbonate absorption are adjusted in a manner that restores the extracellular pH to 7.40.

Several factors determine the capacity of renal function to achieve adequate H^+ excretion. Patients in renal failure with low glomerular filtration rate cannot clear sufficient amounts of protons to compensate for dietary intake, and thus they develop acidemia. Aldosterone released from the adrenal gland in response to the renin-angiotensin-aldosterone axis increases tubular absorption of filtered sodium in the distal convoluted tubule by increasing its exchange for protons; as a result, more bicarbonate is released by the tubule cells into ECW even if the pH is greater than 7.40. Patients suffering malnutrition and glutamine deficiency cannot provide sufficient substrate to generate the NH_3 needed to achieve the required proton excretion. Thus, renal function is pivotal in the control of acid-base status; depending on arterial pH, either an acid or alkaline urine can be produced to achieve a net loss or gain in extracellular protons.

Clinical Practice and Measurement of Acid-Base Status

Clinicians depend on analysis of arterial blood composition to assess total body acid-base balance. Three components of the arterial blood gas are used: the pH, the Pa_{CO_2}, and the bicarbonate concentration. The pH is a measure of H^+ concentration in ECW and indicates whether the ICW is acidotic or alkalotic. Pa_{CO_2} provides the clinician a measure of pulmonary alveolar ventilation. Electrodes in blood gas machines enable immediate measure of the pH and Pa_{CO_2}, and these values can help define the patient's acid-base status using the Henderson-Hasselbalch equation. In 1909, Henderson used physical chemistry terminology to present a fixed (incorporated in the formula as the constant "K") relationship of proton concentration and the bicarbonate buffer system. Hasselbalch added the concept that by taking the base 10 log of an inverted form of Henderson's formula, the resulting Henderson-Hasselbalch equation can calculate pH in a linear relationship to bicarbonate:

$$pH = pK + \log[HCO_3^-/(0.03\ H\ PaCO_2)]$$

The variable ($0.03\ H\ PaCO_2$) reflects the fixed relationship of carbonic acid concentration and partial pressure of CO_2 at body temperature. In physiologic homeostasis, the molar ratio of 20 bicarbonate ions to 1 carbonic acid molecule gives the ECW a normal pH of 7.40. The Henderson-Hasselbalch equation implies the concept that two factors, bicarbonate and $PaCO_2$, are principal determinants of a patient's acid-base status. Assuming the blood sample temperature is 37°C, the Henderson-Hasselbalch equation describes normal arterial blood gas as:

$$pH = 7.40 = 6.1 + \log_{10}(24/1.33)$$

The Henderson-Hasselbalch–based blood gas analysis carries the advantage that a change in proton concentration is linearly proportional to changes in the two most important extracellular buffers: the bicarbonate concentration, which is influenced by renal function, and the $PaCO_2$, which is influenced by alveolar ventilation. One disadvantage of this formula for some clinicians is the difficulty of thinking intuitively in terms of logarithms; as proton concentration increases, pH declines.

Whereas arterial $PvCO_2$ reflects alveolar ventilation, mixed venous $PvCO_2$ indicates the "average" partial pressure of this oxidative phosphorylation gas product. Patients in shock, defined as a low cardiac output, not only have impaired oxygen delivery to tissues but also suffer slowed clearance of carbon dioxide. These patients may have a markedly elevated mixed venous $PaCO_2$. Alternatively, acid-base status can be measured by the total carbon dioxide value reported by venous serum electrolyte analysis. The total carbon dioxide corresponds to the combination of bicarbonate and carbonic acid and includes dissolved carbon dioxide. The total carbon dioxide in a venous blood sample should be greater than the bicarbonate reported in arterial blood gas analysis. Venous total carbon dioxide can be greater or less than normal, and although this can be useful as an indicator of trends in change in bicarbonate concentration, it is unreliable as an indicator of whether the patient has acidemia or alkalemia.

Acidosis and Alkalosis

The four paradigms of acid-base disorder are metabolic acidosis, metabolic alkalosis, respiratory acidosis, and respiratory alkalosis. These disorders are described based on the assumption that a patient with normal acid-base status has an acutely imposed perturbation in acid-base status. However, in clinical reality, altered acid-base status is often due to the complex influence of a primary insult and compensatory physiologic changes to correct pH to normal. The clinician who comprehends the biochemistry of theoretical disorder based on an isolated change has a basis for interpreting the causes and treatment of more complex acid-base disorders in patients. In this discussion, the premise of the Henderson-Hasselbalch equation will be adopted such that acid-base disorders can be defined with an arterial blood sample in terms of changes in bicarbonate base or partial pressure of carbon dioxide (Box 5-1).[17] Acidemia is an increase in H^+ concentration in ECW. The pH in arterial blood of patients with acidemia falls from the normal value of 7.40. Protons are produced in these patients at a rate faster than renal excretion or pulmonary exhalation can clear them. Patients who develop metabolic acidemia experience a decrease in bicarbonate concentration from the normal 24 mEq/L in proportion to the molar load of excess protons. Metabolic acidemia is

---

Box 5-1. Four Paradigms of Acid-Base Disorder Interpreted with the Henderson-Hasselbalch Equation

Normal Components of the Henderson-Hasselbalch Equation

$pH = 6.1 + \log\ [(HCO_3^-)/(0.03 \times PaCO_2)]$
pH is log to base 10 of proton concentration in nmol/L
HCO_3^- is bicarbonate concentration in mEq/L
$PaCO_2$ is partial pressure in mm Hg of carbon dioxide in arterial blood sample. The partial pressure multiplied by 0.03 predicts the carbonic acid concentration

Normal Arterial Blood Gas

$pH = 7.40 = 6.1 + \log(24/1.33)$

Acidemia

Metabolic acidemia: An abrupt addition of sufficient protons to reduce bicarbonate buffer 50%.

$pH = 7.10 = 6.1 + \log(12/1.33)$

Respiratory acidemia: A sudden reduction in alveolar ventilation causes an increase in $PaCO_2$ to 50 torr.

$pH = 7.30 = 6.1 + \log(24/1.5)$

Alkalemia

Metabolic alkalemia: An abrupt addition of sufficient bicarbonate to increase the buffer concentration to 30 mEq/L.

$pH = 7.45 = 6.1 + \log(30/1.33)$

Respiratory alkalemia: A sudden increase in alveolar ventilation causes a decrease in $PaCO_2$ to 20 torr.

$pH = 7.70 = 6.1 + \log(24/0.6)$

presented in the Henderson-Hasselbalch equation as a decline in bicarbonate buffer, the numerator in the right side of the equation. Impaired alveolar ventilation causes increased partial pressure of carbon dioxide and a respiratory acidemia that is demonstrated in the Henderson-Hasselbalch equation as an increase in the denominator. A decrease in H^+ concentration in an arterial blood sample—an increased pH, or alkalemia—occurs as a result of added bicarbonate buffer, or because the $PaCO_2$ is decreased by hyperventilation.

In summary, the four paradigms of acid-base dysfunction can be linked to consequences of increases or decreases in the physiologic function of the renal or pulmonary organ systems. Clinicians can interpret a patient's arterial blood gas sample in terms of these four ideal and simplistic categories of acid-base disorder. These interpretations then indicate appropriate therapy to correct pH to normal.

The four paradigms of acid-base abnormality were described as abrupt directional changes in bicarbonate concentration or $PaCO_2$ that produce quantifiable alterations in pH. Thus, the arterial blood gas analysis is essential in understanding a patient's acid-base status. In most clinical situations, physiologic compensatory adjustments have already taken place in response to the sudden pathologic change in acid-base status. For example, the arterial pH of an inadequately ventilating patient decreases as $PaCO_2$ increases. Over several hours, this patient with respiratory acidosis would experience increased renal bicarbonate production as the excess protons were excreted in an acidic urine. The arterial pH would consequently shift back toward 7.40 as bicarbonate concentration increased above 24 mEq/L. A clinician must interpret an arterial blood gas finding in the context of the patient's medical history and physical examination to acquire a comprehensive understanding of the acid-base status.

A calculated base deficit using information reported in the arterial blood gas provides a method to assess a patient's status. Calculation of base deficit is based on the mass balance implicit in the Henderson-Hasselbalch equation. The pH and $PaCO_2$ are used to predict what the bicarbonate would be if that same sample of arterial blood had a normal pH of 7.40 and a normal $PaCO_2$ of 40 mm Hg. If the predicted bicarbonate is less than the normal value of 24 mEq/L, this indicates a base deficit and the patient has a component of metabolic acidosis. If a patient's arterial blood gas sample has a predicted bicarbonate that exceeds 24 mEq/L, this indicates a negative base deficit, or "metabolic alkalosis." Clinicians who prefer semantics that avoid the double negative designate a patient with the excess bicarbonate of metabolic alkalosis as having a "base excess."

Clinicians can evaluate a patient's acid-base status in a six-step process based on the Henderson-Hasselbalch equation (Table 5-3). First, the clinician interprets the pH of the arterial blood gas and categorizes the patient as acidemic, normal, or alkalemic and assigns a severity of acid-base disorder. Next, one must reason if the increase or decrease in $PaCO_2$ contributes to the abnormality or compensates for the pH status. Furthermore, the clinician can conclude whether a therapeutic change in $PaCO_2$—usually accomplished by some form of assisted ventilation—would restore a normal pH. At this point it is possible to conclude whether the primary problem is metabolic or respiratory dysfunction. In the fourth step of the analysis, the base deficit status is interpreted to determine whether

TABLE 5-3. A Six-Step Sequential Approach to Interpretation of Arterial Blood Gas with Supplemental Information from Serum Sodium, Potassium, and Chloride Concentrations*

Observation	Interpretation	Intervention
Is the pH other than 7.40?	Acidosis if < 7.35 Alkalosis if > 7.45	Clinical evaluation for what causal disease
Is the pH < 7.20 or > 7.55?	Severe disorder	Prompt correction required
Is the $PaCO_2$ other than 40 mm Hg?	Ventilation compensates or contributes to disorder	Change ventilation so $PaCO_2$ compensates
Is the base deficit other than zero?	Bicarbonate loss/gain compensates or contributes to disorder	Infuse $NaHCO_3$/HCl to correct proton concentration
Does the urine pH reflect acidosis/alkalosis?	Acid/alkaline urine indicates renal function compensates or contributes	Renal active drugs or electrolyte replacement so nephron contributes
Is the anion gap† 12 mmol/L?	Under 12 mmol/L suggests lactic or ketoacidosis	Correct primary metabolic problem

*The goal is to achieve a normal pH of 7.40.
†Anion gap = $[Na^+] + [K^+] - [Cl^-]$

there are too many protons (a base deficit) or an excess in bicarbonate anions. After this fourth step, the clinician can conclude whether infusion of bicarbonate or some chemical form of protons, such as HCl, will increase or decrease the available buffer in ECW to achieve a favorable influence on pH. Urine pH indicates whether renal function contributes or is attempting to compensate for the acid-base disorder. Calculation of the anion gap informs the clinician if the acidotic patient is likely to have lactic or keto acids. Using this six-step method, clinicians can identify the magnitude of the acid-base disorder as well as which interventions that could be therapeutic. Critics of the Henderson-Hasselbalch method of acid-base status analysis argue that specific information necessary to establish the root clinical diagnosis is missing.

Stewart proposed an alternative approach to the interpretation of laboratory data regarding acid-base status. In contrast to the Henderson-Hasselbalch approach, the Stewart method is based quantitatively on buffer and acid concentrations[18,19]; data from serum chemistry and arterial blood gas are combined, and three groups of variables are identified to determine the pH status of a patient. The strong ion difference is the sum of sodium, potassium, calcium, and magnesium concentrations minus lactate and chloride concentrations. The concentration of weak acids (proteins and phosphates—also called the nonvolatile buffers to contrast these with bicarbonate) is a defining aspect of the Stewart approach. The third variable is the $PaCO_2$. Several authors believe the Stewart approach offers advantages over the more traditional Henderson-Hasselbalch method not only because it accounts for the influence of weak acids but also because it enables exact diagnosis of the cause of excess or deficient protons. For example, after shock the Stewart method readily enables a metabolic acidemia to be differentiated into acidemia caused by either hypoxia-related lactic acid production or dilution of the ECW after volume-restoring treatments.[20] Whether the clinician depends on the Stewart method or the Henderson-Hasselbalch bicarbonate method of determining acid-base status, it is essential to comprehend both the differential diagnosis of the clinical problems that cause these disorders and proper therapeutic decisions.

The Henderson-Hasselbalch equation indicates the pH status of the extracellular fluid environment where the bicarbonate buffer system dominates. This equation does not reliably inform the clinician regarding the acid-base status of the intracellular environment, where pH is lower and buffer systems other than bicarbonate influence pH. Alterations in extracellular pH that occur over hours usually directly reflect similar pH trends within the cytosol. In circumstances of a rapid change in proton concentration, however, the pH of the ECW and ICW may not change in parallel. For example, hypoxia can cause a rapid and possibly fatal accumulation of acid load in the ICW with only a modest change evident in arterial pH. Therapy for patients with profound acidemia may involve intravenous injection of sodium bicarbonate as a buffer. A patient treated for a metabolic acidemia generates large amounts of carbonic acid in ECW after rapid injection of bicarbonate. In circumstances in which the rate of increase in ECW carbonic acid concentration exceeds the

capacity of alveolar ventilation to exhale carbon dioxide, the excess carbon dioxide shifts into the cell and causes ICW pH decreases. To avoid this paradoxical ICW acidosis, intravenous bicarbonate therapy should be infused slowly in patients with profound metabolic acidemia.

Clinical Patterns of Acid-Base Disorders

Metabolic Acidosis

Lactic acidosis is a common problem in seriously ill and injured patients who suffer impaired delivery of oxygen. In mitochondria, oxidative phosphorylation uses chemical energy derived from oxygen and fuels to transform ADP to ATP. In hypoxic circumstances, as oxidative phosphorylation slows, intracellular ADP, inorganic phosphate, and proton concentrations increase. In a normal adult, mitochondria consume approximately 12 mmol of O_2 per minute to support oxidative phosphorylation. Glucose is a six-carbon primary fuel that is hydrolyzed to a pair of three-carbon pyruvate molecules during the glycolysis process. The enzyme pyruvate dehydrogenase accelerates conversion of pyruvate into a series of intermediate molecules that generate the electrons required to support oxidative phosphorylation. Anaerobic glycolysis occurs when pyruvate molecules are diverted to an alternative biochemical pathway that produces l-lactic acid. For patients in shock, the rate of lactic acid production is proportional to the severity of the oxygen deficiency. People who briefly and strenuously exercise may experience a transient period of lactic acidemia that quickly resolves during the recovery phase. Drowning victims suffer acute anoxia that within moments leads to profound intracellular ATP deficiency and severe lactic acidemia that quickly becomes irreversible and lethal. The concept that lactic acidemia associated with shock is entirely related to hypoxia has been challenged. Luchette and associates proposed that lactic acidosis during shock is in part a catecholamine-mediated accelerated anaerobic glycolysis. They have provided experimental evidence that elevations in circulating epinephrine associated with shock induce increased cell membrane enzyme activity, which in turn drives glycolysis and excess pyruvate production. As pyruvate concentration increases in the cytosol it is diverted into lactic acid.[21]

The arterial blood gas analysis of a patient with lactic acidosis from shock typically demonstrates a base deficit and a decrease in pH that, in patients who are spontaneously breathing, is usually associated with compensatory hyperventilation to reduce $PaCO_2$. Clinical circumstances that cause lactic acidemia include hemorrhage, impaired cardiac function due to a large myocardial infarction, and vasodilatory shock associated with sepsis. Serum lactate levels can be measured to confirm the lactic acidosis contribution to metabolic acidemia. Calculating the anion gap is an alternative but less specific method to determine the presence of lactic acidosis. The anion gap equals the plasma sodium concentration minus the chloride and bicarbonate anion concentrations. Normally, the anion gap is 12 mEq/L. Acidemic patients with clinical evidence of shock whose anion gap exceeds this value likely have lactic acidosis. From another perspective, acidemia associated with an increased anion gap should prompt the clinician to determine the cause of underperfusion.

To successfully treat lactic acidemia, the clinician must correct the primary cause. For patients in shock, effective treatments vary depending on the pathophysiologic process involved. In brief, patients in hemorrhagic shock need restoration of intravascular volume; patients in cardiogenic shock may require drugs to improve cardiac contractility. After resuscitation, the rate at which plasma lactate concentration corrects to normal indicates prognosis. Patients with delayed resolution of lactic acidemia are at substantially higher risk for death.[22] Abramson and colleagues reported that among severely compromised patients with elevated serum lactate levels, a good predictor of outcome was not the maximum level of lactate elevation but rather whether the lactate level had returned to normal within 24 hours of initiating resuscitation.[23] These authors emphasized that patients whose elevated lactic acid levels do not resolve promptly should be evaluated for missed injuries, ischemic bowel, or untreated causes of continued shock. Carbon monoxide poisoning is another, rare cause of profound lactic acidemia. Carbon monoxide binds hemoglobin, blocks oxygen uptake, and substantially reduces oxygen transport in blood. The patient with carbon monoxide poisoning may have a transiently elevated cardiac output but deliver very little oxygen to mitochondria. Patients with this disease process quickly develop a profound intracellular energy deficit and deteriorate into coma and irreversible lactic acidemia. Successful treatment of a patient with lactic acidemia of any cause is determined more by the capacity of the clinician to correct the primary clinical problem than by infusion of buffer to reverse acidemia.

The indications for intravenous infusion of bicarbonate in patients with lactic acidemia are debated, but most authors conclude that patients with a pH less than 7.20 benefit from slow sodium bicarbonate infusions. Clinicians must understand that bicarbonate infusion accomplishes only a temporary reduction in proton concentration and is incomplete therapy because it does not resolve the life-threatening problem of impaired oxidative phosphorylation and ATP deficiency. Furthermore, rapid intravenous infusion of sodium bicarbonate may produce a paradoxical further decline in ICW pH. Alternative chemical forms of buffer are available; for example, the organic buffer tris(hydroxymethyl)aminomethane (THAM) will increase pH without producing carbonic acid.[24]

Patients with severe sepsis and septic shock who require treatment with catecholamine infusions to sustain perfusion pressure have been noted to develop profound lactic acidemia despite hyperdynamic circulation and high rates of oxygen delivery. Levy and coworkers proposed that lactic acidosis in septic patients is a multifactorial process consistent with reduced mitochondrial oxygen availability and dysfunction of normal biochemical processes in the cytosol.[25] These authors reported that more than 12 hours of septic shock and lactic acidemia

indicated a global and irreversible failure in cell functions with subsequent organ failure and death. However, the surgeon should always consider the possibility that a septic patient with persistent lactic acidosis may have a focal area of persistent ischemia (e.g., dead bowel or necrotic tissue) that would require surgical intervention.

In contrast, Hotchkiss and Karl observed that serial plasma lactate levels were unreliable indicators of cellular bioenergetic failure in patients with septic shock.[26] A specific pathophysiologic mechanism for lactic acidosis is thiamine deficiency, a clinical problem commonly seen in alcoholics who consume a diet deficient in vegetables. Thiamine deficiency leads to lactic acidosis because pyruvate dehydrogenase requires thiamine as a critical cofactor. Without thiamine, pyruvate levels build up and are unable to be oxidatively metabolized; consequently, more pyruvate is converted to lactic acid.

Normally, lactic acid is released in small amounts from cells, circulates to the liver, and is cleared. Hepatic cells take up the lactate and a proton and convert these back into glucose in an enzymatic process termed *gluconeogenesis*. Therefore, lactic acidosis can occur due to impaired clearance as well as overproduction. Type A lactic acidosis encompasses any mechanism resulting in excessive production of lactate from pyruvate. Type B lactic acidosis occurs in patients with impaired hepatic clearance of lactate. Patients can develop type B lactic acidosis when hepatocytes fail to function owing to infection or alcoholic hepatitis. Similarly, the drug metformin is one of several that can cause hepatic cellular dysfunction and lead to profound lactic acidosis.

Not all patients resuscitated from shock have acidemia due to lactic acid. Dilution metabolic acidemia occurs in situations in which large volumes of isotonic sodium chloride solutions have been rapidly infused. The rapid repletion by isotonic sodium chloride restores the ECW but dilutes the bicarbonate concentration. Patients with this form of acidemia have a depressed bicarbonate concentration, an elevated chloride level, and a normal or decreased anion gap. Patients with this form of postresuscitation hyperchloremic acidemia correct their pH to normal by renal tubular generation of bicarbonate while urinary excretion of $NH_4^+Cl^-$ produces a net loss of protons and chloride. Clinicians have recommended avoiding this form of hyperchloremic acidemia by using a balanced electrolyte solution (e.g., lactated Ringer's) for resuscitation fluid.[27]

Patients with gastrointestinal fistula drainage or diarrhea exceeding 4 L/day can experience enough bicarbonate loss to induce acidemia. Duodenal, proximal small bowel, and pancreatic fistulas can produce large volumes of fluid rich in sodium bicarbonate. Diarrhea contains sodium, potassium, and bicarbonate, and patients who report multiple watery stools may have a substantial reduction in ECW and low concentrations of sodium and potassium as well as being acidotic. Treatment should include normal saline infusion to restore ECW and potassium supplements as indicated; these interventions enable renal function to restore the bicarbonate deficit. Intravenous sodium bicarbonate is indicated only if the patient has severe acidemia. Patients who develop a small bowel obstruction and have fluid-filled loops may also develop a severe bicarbonate deficiency owing to fluid and sodium bicarbonate sequestration in loops of small bowel and thus have an occult gastrointestinal loss that accounts for acidemia.

In patients with diabetes mellitus, insulin deficiency leads to dysfunction of two major biochemical pathways, and diabetic ketoacidosis may result. Depressed insulin levels trigger lipolysis, in which triglycerides are converted into glycerol and free fatty acids. These free fatty acids are released to the circulation and are taken up by the liver, where they are converted into two-carbon ketoacids: β-hydroxybutyric acid and acetoacetic acid. These ketoacid fuels can support oxidative phosphorylation in brain and kidney cells. However, oxidative phosphorylation of ketoacids in mitochondria is slowed in patients without sufficient insulin to maintain glucose transport across cell membranes. In the cytosol, depressed glycolysis leads to an inability to metabolize ketones in the citric acid cycle. Serum and urine ketone levels become markedly elevated in this disease process, and acetone can often be easily detected on the breath of these patients.

Acidemia develops in ketoacidosis as protons are generated during hepatic ketone production and as ADP and protons accumulate owing to impaired oxidative phosphorylation. The arterial blood gas level of a patient with diabetic ketoacidosis shows a low pH and a depressed bicarbonate concentration; these patients also exhibit an increased anion gap corresponding to the excess ketones. Kussmaul respirations (in which the patient ventilates with rapid, large tidal volumes) are common in these patients, and they usually have a $PaCO_2$ of less than 20 mm Hg in an attempt to correct their arterial blood pH to normal.

Proper treatment of diabetic ketoacidosis involves insulin infusion, which repletes the intracellular supply of glucose and enables the excess ketones to be used as fuels. Clinicians can monitor the success of the initial response to insulin therapy in patients with ketoacidosis by measuring a decrease in serum or urine ketones in the first few hours. In contrast to the precipitous onset of lactic acidosis from shock, diabetics experience a slow onset of ketoacidosis over hours. During these hours, a hyperglycemic osmotic diuresis depletes the ECW and sodium and potassium concentrations. Therefore, in addition to ordering sufficient insulin to lower blood glucose levels, the clinician must anticipate a need to infuse several liters of balanced electrolyte and substantial amounts of supplemental potassium chloride to avoid precipitous hypokalemia.

Patients with diabetes mellitus who suddenly cease taking their insulin develop ketoacidosis within days. However, a diabetic with stress related to an injury or illness can rapidly develop ketoacidosis owing to an increase in epinephrine and glucocorticoids, which block insulin actions and accelerate the onset of diabetic ketoacidosis. Patients with diabetic ketoacidosis can develop profound acidemia, and some clinicians have advocated correction of a plasma pH of less than 7.10 by intravenous infusion of sodium bicarbonate. Several series

indicate that in patients with uncomplicated ketoacidosis, bicarbonate therapy is *not* indicated. Equivalent clinical outcome is achieved by aggressive insulin therapy, correction of hypokalemia, and fluid resuscitation; with resuscitation, renal function restores pH to normal.[28]

Alcoholics develop a ketoacidosis syndrome, but the pathophysiologic mechanism is not insulin deficiency. Alcoholics who binge drink large amounts of ethanol over days and fail to consume a normal diet experience a fall in insulin due to starvation and consequently undergo lipolysis and hepatic conversion of free fatty acids to ketones. At the same time, these heavily intoxicated individuals experience a diuresis and do not replete their intravascular volume by consuming sufficient water and electrolytes. The contracted ECW produces an increased sympathetic tone and higher levels of circulating epinephrine. Insulin effectiveness is consequently reduced in the presence of exaggerated α-adrenergic tone. This constellation of biochemical events leads to ketoacidosis. Surgeons encounter ketoacidosis in alcoholic patients when injury or an acute surgical emergency such as pancreatitis or invasive infection suddenly interrupts a period of sustained heavy ethanol ingestion. Ketoacidosis should be suspected in alcoholic patients with acidemia if they exhibit an increased anion gap. These patients will correct their acid-base disorder if they are treated with glucose and infused with balanced electrolyte solutions to restore ECW. In addition, many of these patients have poor diets and may be thiamine deficient.

Acidemia is a hallmark of renal failure. Patients with low glomerular filtration rates develop acidemia because they cannot clear protons at a rate equal to the production of protons through normal metabolism. Patients with uremia have an increased anion gap and elevated concentrations of anions such as phosphate and sulfate in serum. Renal replacement therapies provide definitive clearance of these excess anions, but bicarbonate replacement therapy at a dose of 50 to 100 mmol ingested daily can be useful in the management of acidemia in chronic renal failure.

Renal tubular acidosis syndromes are rare causes of mild to moderate acidemia. The acidosis is caused by impaired tubular cell capacity to excrete protons and synthesize bicarbonate. Specifically, these cells are unable to generate and secrete sufficient NH_3 to the filtrate to bind protons. Another mechanism of renal tubular acidosis involves the inability to generate a high proton gradient across the abluminal membrane of tubular cells; most of these patients suffer a mild acidemia.

Metabolic Alkalosis

Metabolic alkalosis develops as excess bicarbonate accumulates in the ECW. Clinicians can produce this problem by infusing large amounts of bicarbonate to treat patients with acute lactic acidosis, especially when the acidosis is successfully and promptly cleared. Similarly, mechanical ventilation of patients with chronic hypoventilation syndromes (as occurs in restrictive lung disease or morbid obesity) can also produce a metabolic alkalemia. As these patients gradually developed increased $PaCO_2$, their renal function compensated by retaining bicarbonate. If these patients are intubated for surgery or to treat acute respiratory failure, and with mechanical ventilation a normal $PaCO_2$ is rapidly achieved, the excess bicarbonate causes a metabolic alkalosis. This complication can be avoided if mechanical ventilation is modulated to achieve a slow return to normal $PaCO_2$. A sudden correction of hypercapnia can precipitate severe alkalemia, arrhythmias, and death.[29]

Hypokalemic, hypochloremic metabolic alkalosis is a pattern of acid-base disorder that occurs in patients with prolonged vomiting or sustained high gastric fluid drainage. Gastric fluid has a high hydrochloric acid concentration because gastric mucosal cells secrete protons into the gastric lumen. With each proton secreted, the stomach adds a bicarbonate molecule to the ECW. Sustained loss of gastric fluid by tube suctioning or vomiting results in a net loss of water, HCl, and potassium. This dehydration results in elevated aldosterone, which stimulates sodium exchange for K^+ and H^+ in the nephron's distal convoluted tubule. Also, the depletion of chloride leads to impaired sodium absorption in the proximal tubule, and more filtered sodium is delivered to the distal nephron segments, where it can be exchanged for K^+ and H^+. To compound the problem, these patients are hypokalemic, owing to KCl losses in the gastric fluid, so less potassium is available for exchange. As an end result, alkalotic patients with low chloride and potassium concentrations actually produce an acidic urine. This situation is best corrected by the intravenous infusion of isotonic fluids with sufficient KCl to replete deficits of these ions. As ECW expands and KCl levels correct, aldosterone levels decline and the nephron produces an alkaline urine to correct the alkalemia.

Diuretic therapy can also produce a metabolic alkalemia. Loop diuretics that alter tubule cell function in the loop of Henle increase urinary excretion of sodium chloride and can reduce plasma volume in patients with heart failure or hepatic cirrhosis, even in the presence of an increased ECW caused by edema or ascites. Hypokalemia develops because elevated aldosterone promotes high losses of potassium in the distal nephron. Administration of a potassium-sparing diuretic (e.g., spironolactone) inhibits sodium absorption in the distal nephron and dampens the loss of protons and potassium in urine. A rare clinical form of metabolic alkalosis occurs in patients who ingest huge amounts of calcium carbonate to control peptic acid–related symptoms. Patients with severe alkalemia (pH > 7.60) may require infusion of hydrochloric acid to correct the elevated bicarbonate concentration by converting it to carbonic acid and exhaling carbon dioxide.[17]

Respiratory Alkalosis

Normal rates of oxidative phosphorylation in mitochondria maintain the biochemical energy in ATP necessary to sustain life; this is achieved by daily consumption of a predictable molecular mass of oxygen and synthesis of carbon dioxide. If carbohydrates are the only source of fuels to sustain oxidative phosphorylation, the molar ratio of CO_2 produced to O_2 consumed, termed the *respiratory quotient,* equals 1. As fats become a larger proportion of the fuels that support oxidative phosphorylation, the respiratory quotient declines toward 0.7. The $PaCO_2$ in venous blood reflects the rate of carbon dioxide production. Regulatory centers in the brain normally respond to fluctuations in $PaCO_2$ levels by either increasing or decreasing minute ventilation to keep $PaCO_2$ in the range of 40 ± 2 mm Hg. In circumstances of fear, stress, sepsis, fever, or pain, patients can experience an abrupt increase in alveolar ventilation that results in a decline in $PaCO_2$ and an associated alkalemia.[30] Maintaining normal oxygen tension takes precedence over normal pH, and acutely hypoxic patients will also hyperventilate and cause alkalemia. Respiratory alkalemia, also *termed hypocapnia,* can be a serious complication of mechanical ventilation when a patient with pharmacologic paralysis is inadvertently overventilated. The ventilator settings for respiratory rate and tidal volume that achieve a normal arterial $PaCO_2$ vary depending on multiple factors. Respiratory alkalosis can be therapeutic. Brief periods of induced hypocapnia are utilized in mechanically ventilated patients with brain injuries who demonstrate sudden elevations in intracranial pressure. In alkalemia, cerebral blood vessels constrict, cerebral blood flow and blood volume decline, and an increase in intracranial pressure can be temporarily relieved. Evidence does not support sustained use of hypocapnia in patients with brain injury.[31]

Respiratory Acidosis

Acute onset of respiratory acidosis is most commonly the consequence of an abrupt decline in alveolar ventilation. A patient who has a normal result of arterial blood gas analysis and suddenly stops ventilating will double his or her $PaCO_2$ from 40 to 80 mm Hg within minutes. With this magnitude of hypercarbia, arterial blood gas demonstrates a decrease in pH from 7.40 to 7.25 as protons accumulate and an increase in bicarbonate from 24 to 26.5 mEq/L as a consequence of carbonic acid accumulation. Acute lethal hypoventilation may be a consequence of suppression of the respiratory control center by narcotic or sedative drugs; sudden damage to the respiratory drive centers in the brain stem can have similar results.

The acidemia of acute hypercarbia can be compensated in a few hours by increased renal excretion of NH_4^+ and concurrent bicarbonate release into the ECW. As the plasma concentration of bicarbonate increases, the pH returns toward 7.40 despite elevated $PaCO_2$. Under normal circumstances two reflex mechanisms provide feedback stimulation to ventilation centers. Central chemoreceptors in the brain stem provide primary control over ventilation and respond to higher proton concentrations by stimulating increased respiratory rates. However, in situations of chronic hypercarbia, renal compensation blunts the capacity of chemoreceptors to respond to further increases in $PaCO_2$ by increasing bicarbonate concentration in ECW. Therefore, these patients depend on the second reflex mechanism to stimulate ventilatory drive: chemoreceptors in the carotid bodies that are stimulated by decreased arterial oxygen saturation. Patients with chronic hypercarbia who are given supplemental oxygen to maintain high oxygen saturations are at high risk for sudden death from a hypoventilation-induced critical increase in $PaCO_2$; such an increase may induce carbon dioxide narcosis that suppresses even chemoreflex-driven ventilation.

Obese patients are encountered with increasing frequency on surgical services as more and more bariatric procedures are performed to control the lethal complications of morbid obesity. Obesity-associated hypoventilation syndromes incorporate a spectrum of conditions in which obstructed airways, reduced pulmonary compliance, and central hypoventilation lead to chronic hypercarbia. Clinical trials have demonstrated that patients with sleep apnea can be successfully managed with noninvasive nocturnal ventilation support and avoid metabolic alkalosis.[32]

HYPONATREMIA AND HYPOTONICITY

Sodium, with the corresponding anions chloride and bicarbonate, normally determines over 95% of the osmolality of ECW. Thus, the diagnosis and management of disorders in sodium concentration and ECW osmolality are linked. The normal serum Na^+ should range between 138 and 145 mEq/L. Hyponatremia, or low Na^+, can be classified as mild, moderate, or severe. Mild hyponatremia exists when serum Na^+ lies between 130 and 138 mEq/L. Whereas patients have few signs or symptoms caused by mild hyponatremia, a falling serum Na^+ should prompt the surgeon to consider reversible causes for the decline, and corrective therapy should be instituted. Moderate hyponatremia exists when serum Na^+ measures between 120 and 130 mEq/L. Rapid onset of moderate hyponatremia produces a sudden decline in osmolality that corresponds to an expansion of ICW. Swelling of intracranial cells leads to the acute onset of moderate hyponatremia and the development of headaches or lethargy. Patients with coexisting brain injury, infection, or tumor who develop moderate hyponatremia are at risk for deteriorated neurologic function. Severe hyponatremia is defined as a serum Na^+ concentration less than 120 mEq/L. As the serum Na^+ level declines, risk of seizure increases and patients become comatose. Patients are at risk for death from cerebral swelling if the serum Na^+ value drops below 110 mEq/L.

Acute hyponatremia evolves over a few hours and poses a risk of cerebral swelling as TBW osmolality declines. Chronic hyponatremia develops over days, allowing solute transport out of cells and decreasing the amount of cell swelling. It is clinically important to differentiate acute from chronic hyponatremia because rates of correction should differ substantially.

Acute Hyponatremia Syndromes

Acute hyponatremia can occur when a patient is rapidly depleted of sodium and water and then either drinks water or is intravenously infused with a hypo-osmotic fluid. Surgeons encounter dilutional hyponatremia in a variety of patients. For example, hyponatremia can develop after infusion of D_5W into a patient who has hemorrhaged, suffered an acute bout of diarrhea, or has had fluid shifts into an inflamed pancreas or burn wound. The hyponatremia problem is exacerbated in these hypovolemic patients by elevated levels of AVP. As AVP increases urine osmolality above the osmolality of ECW, a further increase in ECW free water follows. To avoid hyponatremia, clinicians should resuscitate hypovolemic or dehydrated patients with iso-osmotic sodium-containing electrolyte solutions. Hypovolemic patients complaining of thirst should have limited access to drinking water. These patients typically produce small volumes of concentrated urine with urinary sodium concentrations less than 20 mEq/L, indicating the acute hyponatremia is principally caused by renal free-water retention.

Postoperative Hyponatremia

While the serum sodium drops below 130 mEq/L in up to 4% of patients after surgery, a rare but treacherous syndrome of acute hyponatremia occurs in predominantly female patients who have undergone routine surgery without significant blood loss. Arieff described 15 women who developed a decline in serum Na^+ concentration from a mean of 138 mEq/L to 108 mEq/L by the second postoperative day.[33] Signs of neurologic dysfunction, decreased responsiveness, and seizures were the first indication of hyponatremia. Arieff measured an average urine Na^+ level of 68 mEq/L and an average urine osmolality of 501 mOsm/L at the time when the serum Na^+ level was at its nadir. The special risk to menstruating women for the development of postoperative hyponatremia was reported by Ayus and colleagues.[34] The authors observed that menstruating women with hyponatremia had more symptoms than men with equivalent suppressions in serum Na^+. Surgeons can reduce the risk of postoperative hyponatremia by always ordering isotonic intravenous fluids. Furthermore, patients (particularly small-statured women) who develop lethargy, headache, and altered mental status in the postoperative period should have serum sodium concentrations checked.

Steele and coworkers proposed the concept of desalination to account for hyponatremia in postoperative patients. They noted that selected patients developed modest hyponatremia despite normal saline infusions.[35] During the first 24 hours after surgery they measured urine osmolality as more than twice serum osmolality. Elevated AVP levels were associated with the increase in urine osmolality. These authors concluded that pain, apprehension, or stresses related to surgery can cause a sustained release of AVP during the first 1 to 2 days after surgery. Because of the production of a large amount of concentrated urine, desalination led to acute hyponatremia.

Acute hyponatremia can complicate a diuretic-induced, forced diuresis. In addition to loop diuretics, infusion of mannitol causes an osmotic diuresis that includes an obligatory loss of sodium. Diabetics with sustained hyperglycemia can induce an osmotic diuresis that depletes liters of water from the body. Furthermore, the ketonuria of a patient with diabetic ketoacidosis exacerbates renal sodium losses. A large osmotic diuresis can also occur in patients receiving total parental nutritional fluids who develop sustained and marked elevations in serum glucose concentration. In each of these situations, the ECW space becomes dehydrated; and if replacement fluids in the form of intravenous solutions, enteral tube feedings, or a liquid diet are hypotonic fluids, hyponatremia will result.

Cerebral salt wasting is a cause of hyponatremia most commonly reported in neurosurgical patients. Patients with a brain lesion develop hyponatremia associated with sustained, elevated urine sodium concentrations in the setting of a normal creatinine clearance. Berendes and colleagues studied a group of patients with aneurysmal subarachnoid hemorrhage whom they aggressively infused with sodium to maintain a normal serum Na^+.[36] They noted high urine outputs of 4 to 6 L/day and fractional urine sodium levels twice normal. They correlated markedly elevated brain natriuretic peptide levels that persisted for 8 days with salt wasting in these patients and hypothesized that this peptide, rather than elevated AVP, accounted for the onset of low serum sodium concentrations. Treatment of patients with cerebral salt wasting requires administration of sufficient daily sodium to sustain normal total body sodium balance. Thus, sodium replacement therapy can be guided by determination of 24-hour urinary sodium excretion. Some patients with severe cerebral salt wasting require intravenous infusion of 3% hypertonic saline solutions.

Acute water intoxication is a rare cause of hyponatremia. Water intoxication can develop in patients undergoing transcervical endometrial resection or transurethral resection of the prostrate, endoscopic procedures performed with hypo-osmotic irrigation fluids. These patients can suffer the abrupt onset of severe hyponatremia with potentially lethal neurologic complications. Treatment includes discontinuation of water irrigations and intravenous infusion of hypertonic saline.[37]

Chronic Hyponatremia

The syndrome of inappropriate release of antidiuretic hormone (SIADH) has been a carefully studied cause of chronic hyponatremia. The diagnosis of SIADH can only be made in euvolemic patients. Patients with SIADH have serum osmolalities less than 270 mOsm/kg H_2O along with an inappropriately concentrated urine osmolality, defined as a urine osmolality greater than 300 mOsm/kg H_2O. Establishing euvolemia is key to the diagnosis of SIADH, as demonstrated by normal systolic and orthostatic blood pressures. Endocrine diseases (hypothyroidism or adrenal insufficiency) and renal dysfunction must also be ruled out. Patients with indisputable SIADH are those with an AVP-secreting tumor, usually a carcinoid or small cell carcinoma of the lung. AVP can also be inappropriately released from the hypothalamus because of cerebral injury, infection, or tumor. Up to 35% of AIDS patients admitted with an active infection have hyponatremia and meet the criteria of SIADH.[38] Many patients with SIADH are asymptomatic and live with lower serum sodium concentrations.

Patients with chronic renal disease may develop an impaired capacity to retain sodium and subsequently develop hyponatremia. Renal diagnoses associated with obligatory sodium losses include medullary cystic disease, polycystic kidney disease, analgesic nephropathy, chronic pyelonephritis, and obstructive uropathy post-decompression syndromes. These patients require supplemental sodium as well as fluid to compensate for daily fixed losses in sodium and water. A rare cause of hyponatremia is decreased adrenal production of mineralocorticoids due to adrenal infarction, hemorrhage, tumor infiltration, or autoimmune adrenalitis.

Treatment of Hyponatremia

Surgeons must differentiate between patients with acute and chronic hyponatremia. Patients who suffer the acute onset of serum Na^+ levels below 110 mEq/L and develop neurologic symptoms should be corrected to a serum Na^+ value of about 120 mEq/L over the first 24 hours of therapy. In contrast, patients who present with a chronically reduced serum Na^+ concentration of less than 110 mEq/L will not commonly exhibit neurologic symptoms. Rapid correction in patients with chronic hyponatremia can lead to central pontine myelinolysis, a severe, permanent neurologic disorder characterized by spastic quadriparesis, pseudobulbar palsy, and depressed levels of consciousness.[39] This condition can be definitively diagnosed by demonstrating a characteristic intense central pontine lesion on T2-weighted magnetic resonance images.

Safe corrective treatment requires the surgeon to monitor the patient's physical examination, as well as serial checks of serum Na^+ concentration over the first 48 hours of treatment. Patients with profound acute hyponatremia who manifest signs of severe encephalopathy (lethargy, seizures, or coma) should undergo prompt therapy that accomplishes a slow increase in the ECW Na^+. To avoid the complications of central pontine myelinolysis, the maximal rate of sodium correction should not exceed 0.25 mEq/L/hr. Thus, the rate of increase in serum Na^+ concentration should not exceed 8 mOsm/kg H_2O per day. Correction rates should remain slow when the serum Na^+ level exceeds 120 mEq/L, and prescribed treatments accomplish over several days the goal of restoring serum Na^+ to the normal range of 135 to 140 mEq/L.

Patients with chronic hyponatremia are less likely to have encephalopathy or other neurologic symptoms, and thus there is less urgency to bring about a correction of the serum Na^+ level. Several additional factors should be kept in mind during correction of chronic hyponatremia. The compensatory depletion of intracellular K^+ during prolonged hyponatremia requires that as ECW sodium is repleted, large amounts of supplemental potassium must also be administered to restore ICW deficits. In practical terms, this means correction must be accomplished in a closely monitored environment that enables frequent assessment of water balance and serum electrolyte composition.

HYPERNATREMIA AND SYNDROMES OF HYPERTONICITY

Hypernatremia is the most common cause of hypertonicity. Patients have moderate hypernatremia if serum Na^+ lies between 146 and 159 mEq/L, and they have severe, life-threatening hypernatremia if serum Na^+ exceeds 160 mEq/L.[38] As serum Na^+ increases in response to dehydration, a corresponding reduction in the volume of both ECW and ICW occurs. The danger of hypernatremia is brain shrinkage and, consequently, neurologic dysfunction. Brain cell dehydration manifests clinically as altered levels of consciousness, seizures, and coma. Sudden contraction in cerebral ICW can lead to intracerebral hemorrhage.[40] Although severe hypernatremia may not be associated with hypotension in the supine patient, postural hypotension, dry mucous membranes, and decreased skin turgor are useful indicators of a significant contraction in ECW.

As a normal response to increased serum Na^+ concentration and osmolality, the kidney produces a concentrated urine. As urine osmolality exceeds serum osmolality, the kidneys achieve a net gain for TBW of solute-free water. Nephrons accomplish antidiuresis by responding to AVP, which the hypothalamus releases in amounts proportional to the extent the serum osmolality exceeds a threshold of approximately 280 mOsm/kg H_2O. However, renal corrections of hypernatremia depend on patient access to water. Ethanol suppresses AVP release. Intoxicated patients with hypernatremia may produce large volumes of hypo-osmolar urine, and, consequently, renal water losses inappropriately further increase serum Na^+ levels. Severe hypernatremia rarely occurs in conscious patients because relentless thirst compels the individual to drink water. Hospitalized hypovolemic intoxicated patients pharmacologically sedated can rapidly experience a dangerous increase in serum Na^+ level unless they are given intravenous fluids. Typically, as blood ETOH levels fall, urine outputs decline and urine specific gravity approaches 1.030, leading to a renal correction of hypernatremia.

Causes of Hypernatremia

Diabetes insipidus is a syndrome of excessive excretion of greater than 500 mL hr of hypotonic urine and results in TBW contraction and hypernatremia if the patient does not drink water at rates that exceed urine flow rates. There are two main types of diabetes insipidus: central and nephrogenic. Patients present with the complaint of onset of continuous polyuria and polydipsia that interrupts their sleep. Continual production of a dilute urine (osmolality less than 200 mOsm/kg H_2O) by a patient whose serum Osm exceeds 300 mOsm/L is a pathognomonic finding of diabetes insipidus.

Central diabetes insipidus is characterized by a decline or loss in the ability of the hypothalamus to produce and excrete AVP. The acute onset of diabetes insipidus occurs in patients with brain injury, intracerebral hemorrhage, skull base or pituitary surgery, or cerebral infection. Suddenly without AVP, the patient may have the abrupt onset of hourly hypotonic (1.010 specific gravity) urine flows in excess of 1 L. In most published series of central diabetes insipidus, 50% of patients have no pathologic reason to account for the onset of central diabetes insipidus; evidence suggests that idiopathic diabetes insipidus is caused by autoimmune mechanisms. One subset of patients with central diabetes insipidus has adjusted the osmolality threshold to a higher value. As serum osmolality exceeds 280 mOsm/L, AVP levels in serum remain undetectable until the new threshold is reached and blood levels of AVP increase in proportion to serum osmolality.

Nephrogenic diabetes insipidus is defined as an impaired capacity of renal tubules to respond to AVP and concentrate urine. Patients with nephrogenic diabetes insipidus have elevated levels of circulating AVP and polyuria and can develop moderate hypernatremia. These patients produce a dilute urine unchanged by the intravenous administration of exogenous AVP. Several pathologic conditions have been identified as causes of nephrogenic diabetes insipidus. Renal tubular cells may be poorly responsive to AVP after decompression of chronically obstructed ureters. Patients with sickle cell nephropathy and medullary cystic disease may also develop nephrogenic diabetes insipidus. Lithium, glyburide, demeclocycline, and amphotericin B can all induce nephrogenic diabetes insipidus through direct effects on tubular cells. Hypercalcemia and severe hypokalemia can also cause renal tubular cell dysfunction. Patients with end-stage renal dysfunction and low glomerular filtration rates may produce a fixed volume of 2 to 4 L/day of urine that is always iso-osmolar. These patients, in hot and arid environments, are susceptible to dehydration and the development of hypernatremia.

Hypernatremia can also emerge rapidly in patients owing to excessive and uncontrollable losses of hypotonic fluids. In most patients, acute-onset hypernatremia is due to the loss of several liters of ECW. A water deficit of 3 L in a 70-kg young man represents a 7% reduction in TBW. This magnitude of dehydration would increase the serum Na^+ concentration by 11 mEq/L. In 24 hours, a patient can lose liters of water due to copious sweating in a hot environment. The gastrointestinal tract can be the source of hypotonic fluid losses as well, owing to vomiting, enteric tube suctioning, enterocutaneous fistula drainage, or diarrhea. Patients with large body surface area burns or dermatitis conditions may experience large volumes of transcutaneous water evaporation owing to an impaired dermal barrier. Patients with a sustained osmotic diuresis, whether from hyperglycemia or after mannitol infusion, may develop elevated serum Na^+ levels as solute diuresis leads to irretrievable urinary water losses. Without oral or intravenous water replacement, the dehydrated patient with hypernatremia cannot produce sufficient amounts of concentrated urine to restore TBW and reduce serum Na^+ values. Hospitalized patients who are sedated or have impaired neurologic function are at higher risk for developing hypernatremia because they cannot respond to thirst and drink fluids to rehydrate. Hypernatremia is rarely caused by ingestion or intravenous infusion of a large sodium load.

Two populations at particular risk for dehydration and hypernatremia are very young children and the infirm elderly. Symptoms of hypernatremia are nonspecific in children and include muscle weakness, restlessness, and lethargy. Palevsky and colleagues noted that geriatric patients who develop serious infections were at a higher risk for presenting to a hospital with hypernatremia. On the other hand, these authors observed that hypernatremia was a problem in all age groups of hospitalized patients. They concluded that in many cases, hypernatremia developed because physicians ordered inadequate hydration or inappropriate fluids.[41]

Treatment of Hypernatremia

Treatment of patients with hypernatremia due to dehydration involves intravenous or oral administration of water. Hypernatremic patients typically have significantly reduced blood volumes. These patients are usually hypotensive, and initial resuscitation with balanced electrolyte solution or blood product infusion may be indicated. Physical examination can indicate the magnitude of ECW depletion. Postural hypotension, low central venous pressure, and poor skin turgor are signs of significant dehydration. Evaluation may also involve measurement of urine characteristics to categorize the problem as either a nonrenal water loss or diabetes insipidus. Patients produce small volumes of maximally hyperosmolar urine if their hypernatremia is a consequence of nonrenal water loss. In contrast, urine osmolality is inappropriately less than serum osmolality in patients with diabetes insipidus. Hypernatremic patients with either mechanism of hypernatremia require rehydration; the key difference is that patients with central diabetes insipidus should be given AVP or a synthetic analogue, desmopressin.

To correct an elevated serum Na^+ concentration the surgeon orders either an intravenous infusion or enteral intake of sufficient solute-free water to achieve a positive water balance. Correction of a sustained hypernatremia should be cautious because a rapid decline in ECW osmolality can lead to cerebral injury due to rapid cytosol swelling. Serum Na^+ should be corrected at a rate of no more than 10 mEq/day, unless the patient is symptomatic

from severe acute hypernatremia. Adrogue and Madias provided a formula that, adjusting for the sodium content of the infusate, predicts a patient's change in serum Na^+ content in response to intravenous infusion of 1 L of fluid; such formulas are useful guidelines (Table 5-4).[40] Patients with hypernatremia may also have deficits in total body potassium related to the shrinkage of the ICW. KCl may need to be added as ECW and ICW return to normal, and therefore serial serum chemistry studies are indicated during correction. Finally, in addition to the administration of water to rehydrate the ECW and ICW, the surgeon must either stop the excessive water loss that caused the hypernatremia or, if that is not possible, devise a fluid replacement protocol that offsets the ongoing fluid losses.

Patients with hypernatremia due to central diabetes insipidus should be treated with antidiuretic hormone. AVP may be continuously infused in patients and adjusted to achieve desired urine flow rates. Unfortunately, AVP is a potent vascular smooth muscle constrictor, and it may cause ischemia, including coronary artery constriction that precipitates angina. Desmopressin (1-desamino-8-D-arginine vasopressin [DDAVP]) is a synthetic analogue of AVP that has a half-life of several hours after intravenous injection. Desmopressin is the agent of choice for treating patients with central diabetes insipidus because it effectively induces renal tubular water reabsorption without acting as a vasopressor. Patients with a partial AVP deficiency typically have mild diabetes insipidus and are successfully managed with intranasal desmopressin and copious water intake. Patients with central diabetes insipidus treated with drugs as outpatients risk rapid development of hypernatremia in the event of a surgical emergency and discontinuation of desmopressin.

Rarely has a gain in total body sodium been identified as the cause of hypernatremia. Intravenous infusions of hypertonic sodium bicarbonate during aggressive treatment of severe acidemia and infusion of hypertonic saline during resuscitation of hypovolemic patients can increase serum Na^+ levels. Hypernatremic patients with peripheral edema constitute a particular challenge. Correction of this problem depends on achieving a net loss of sodium and water. Administration of the loop diuretic furosemide

TABLE 5-4.　Given a Patient with Hypernatremia (Serum $[Na^+]$ = 160 mEq/L), the Estimated Change in $[Na^+]$ after Infusion of 1 Liter

$$\frac{\text{Change in } [Na^+]}{L} = \frac{(\text{Infusate } [Na^+] - \text{Serum } [Na^+])_{[CN1]}}{TBW + 1}$$

Infusate	Woman, Age 70 50 kg × 0.45 = 22.5 L TBW	Man, Age 20 80 kg × 0.60 = 48.0 L TBW
D_5W	$\frac{(0-160)}{22.5+1} = -6.8$	$\frac{(0-160)}{48+1} = -3.3$
D_5 0.2% NaCl	$\frac{(34-160)}{22.5+1} = -5.3$	$\frac{(34-160)}{48+1} = -2.6$
D_5 0.45% NaCl	$\frac{(77-160)}{22.5+1} = -3.5$	$\frac{(77-160)}{48+1} = -1.7$

produces increased urine flow and sodium excretion, but unless the patient is given electrolyte-free water, the serum Na^+ level may increase as a diuresis occurs.

PATHOPHYSIOLOGY OF POTASSIUM

An increase or decrease of potassium concentration greater than 3 mmol/L can lead to death. Thus, control of the amount of extracellular potassium is essential. The kidney controls the concentration of potassium in the ECW by adjusting potassium excretion in urine. An individual consuming a typical Western diet absorbs from the gut lumen approximately 1 mmol/kg of body weight of potassium. A normal ECW K^+ level is maintained at 4 mmol/L largely because renal function in the distal convoluted tubule (DCT) segment of the nephron excretes excess potassium (Fig. 5-5). A patient with a normal glomerular filtration rate has approximately 20 L of tubule fluid flow daily into the DCT. This filtrate fluid has a K^+ equivalent to plasma, and if additional potassium is not excreted urinary potassium excretion would approximate 80 mmol/day. Enzymes in the luminal membrane of DCT cells enable electrogenic reabsorption of sodium, which, without cotransport of chloride, produces a net negative charge in the tubule. Potassium and protons in the tubule cell cytosol are pulled by this charge difference into the tubule fluid. The more negative charge produced in the tubule by the electrogenic reabsorption of sodium, the more moles of potassium enter the tubule fluid. The urinary concentration of potassium is a function of both the moles of potassium that shift into the tubule fluid and the volume of water eventually excreted as urine. The hormone aldosterone controls potassium excretion by increasing the activity of the enzyme responsible for electrogenic reabsorption of sodium. More aldosterone means greater amounts of sodium are transported into the cell and more potassium is excreted in urine.

The excretion of potassium in the DCT is also influenced by the availability of bicarbonate ions in filtrate fluid. Greater amounts of $NaHCO_3$ in filtrate fluid and lesser amounts of NaCl produce electrogenic forces favorable for potassium diffusion into lumen of the DCT. Thus, an alkaline diuresis facilitates the loss of potassium. The renal response to an abnormal potassium concentration can be best judged by examination of its 24-hour excretion. Patients on a normal diet with an elevated serum K^+ concentration are capable of excreting over 400 mmol of potassium per day. Patients with a depressed serum K^+ concentration should produce less than 20 mmol of potassium per day.

Hyperkalemia

Hyperkalemia is defined as a K^+ value greater than 5.0 mmol/L. As extracellular K^+ concentration exceeds 6 mmol/L, alterations occur in the resting cell membrane potential that impair normal depolarization and repolarization. Cardiac arrhythmias caused by the rapid onset of hyperkalemia resist standard pharmacologic therapy and often prove lethal. ECG changes may provide the first clin-

ical indication of hyperkalemia. Hyperkalemia in the range of 6 to 7 mmol/L may be associated with tall T waves. Symmetrically peaked T waves indicate dangerous hyperkalemia, particularly if T waves are higher than the R wave in more than one lead (Fig. 5-6). As K^+ exceeds 7 mmol/L, P-wave amplitudes decrease, PR segments increase, and the QRS complex widens. As the K^+ level exceeds 8 mmol/L, suddenly lethal arrhythmias ensue, such as asystole, ventricular fibrillation, or a wide pulseless idioventricular rhythm. Severely hyperkalemic patients who develop these arrhythmias rarely respond to treatment.

Rapid-onset hyperkalemia is most commonly due to renal dysfunction or failure. Patients with significant renal dysfunction may not require dialysis because they have an adequate fixed volume of urine output that enables clearance of their daily ingested potassium load. However, patients with renal dysfunction are at risk for hyperkalemia because they can suddenly release a large amount of intercellular potassium if they develop injury or sepsis. Patients whose number of functional nephrons has declined to less than 20% of normal cannot respond to aldosterone to achieve greater urinary potassium excretion. Patients who do not release aldosterone in response to hyperkalemia may develop a modest elevation in serum potassium concentration. Alternatively, hyperkalemia is a consequence of an excessive dose of an angiotensin-converting enzyme inhibitor that suppresses the renin-angiotensin-aldosterone axis. Drugs with a direct effect on renal tubule cells that increase serum potassium concentration include the diuretics spironolactone and triamterene, β blockers, cyclosporine, and tacrolimus (FK506); in most patients with hyperkalemia, these drugs are one of several contributing factors.

Precipitous hyperkalemia should be anticipated in patients who experience sudden reperfusion of a vascular bed that had been ischemic for hours. At the completion of a repair of an arterial injury, hyperkalemia follows release of a vascular clamp. Intravenous bicarbonate infusion before clamp release may help reduce the risk of

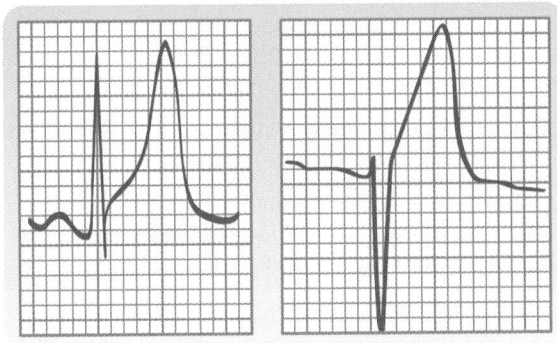

FIGURE 5-6. **A,** ECG changes indicating hyperkalemia. The T wave is tall, narrow, and symmetrical. **B,** ECG changes indicating acute myocardial infarction. The T wave is tall but broad-based and asymmetrical. (From Somers MP, Brady WJ, Perron AD, Mattu A: The prominent T wave: Electrocardiographic differential diagnosis. Am J Emerg Med 20:243-251, 2002.)

arrhythmia. Precipitous hyperkalemia can be a complication of intravenous injection of succinylcholine, a depolarizing paralytic agent, when used in patients who have muscle atrophy from disuse, neurologic denervation syndromes, severe burns, direct muscle trauma, or rhabdomyolysis syndromes or who have required prolonged bed rest. Succinylcholine induces a sustained reduction of resting membrane potential in myocytes, and without a negative charge in the cell there is accelerated movement of K^+ from skeletal muscle cells into the ECW.[42]

Treatment of Acute Hyperkalemia

Several interventions are useful in patients at risk from cardiac arrhythmias from hyperkalemia. Intravenous calcium can immediately reduce the risk of arrhythmia in hyperkalemic patients with characteristic ECG changes (Box 5-2). Calcium antagonizes the depolarization effect of elevated extracellular K^+. Sodium bicarbonate infusion buffers ECW protons and allows net transfer of cytosol protons across the cell membrane via carbonic acid. The shift of protons out of the cell is associated with a shift of potassium into the cell. This treatment is most effective in hyperkalemic patients with metabolic acidemia related to deficient bicarbonate. Insulin and glucose infusions prompt increased Na^+/K^+-ATPase activity and a decline in ECW potassium concentration as the ECW potassium is pumped into the ICW. Patients who suffer aldosterone deficiency as well as hyperkalemia will increase renal excretion of potassium if treated with a mineralocorticoid drug such as 9α-fludrocortisone. In the patient with acute renal failure, definitive reduction of K^+ can only be accomplished by renal replacement therapy; hemodialysis can be used to achieve a negative potassium balance in minutes, whereas continuous filtration methods clear potassium at a much slower rate. Chronic hyperkalemia associated with renal dysfunction can be managed by oral or rectal administration of sodium polystyrene sulfonate, a cation-exchange resin that binds potassium in the gut lumen. Rectally administered binding resins are particularly effective because the colonic mucosa can excrete mucus with large amounts of potassium.

Hypokalemia

Patients with hypokalemia have a serum K^+ concentration less than 3.5 mmol/L. Generalized symptoms commonly associated with depressed serum K^+ levels include fatigue, weakness, and ileus. Rarely, rhabdomyolysis may occur in patients whose ECW K^+ level drops below 2.5 mmol/L. Flaccid paralysis with respiratory compromise can occur at K^+ levels less than 2 mmol/L. Patients treated with digoxin are at high risk for cardiac arrhythmias if they develop hypokalemia. Hepatic encephalopathy may be due to elevated ammonium levels.

Hypokalemia is a common problem among hospitalized patients and can usually be attributed to gastrointestinal or renal losses.[12] Patients with persistent vomiting or who drain large volumes from gastric tubes, diarrhea, or high-output enteric or pancreatic fistulas can lose large amounts of potassium. Patients with normal renal function should be able to reduce daily urinary losses of potassium to less than 20 mmol/day. If daily urinary losses exceed that amount in a hypokalemic patient, then an element of renal dysfunction or marked elevations in aldosterone are contributing to the hypokalemia.

Hypokalemia is a common problem in patients with congestive heart failure managed with multiple drugs, including diuretics.[43] In these patients, renal dysfunction and neurohormonal activation of the renin-angiotensin-aldosterone axis can lead to hypokalemia. Contracted intravascular volume enhances sympathetic nervous tone and elevates plasma levels of catecholamines. The combination of catecholamines and aldosterone alters function in the DCT segment of the nephron, and the consequence is greater renal excretion of potassium.

Sustained renal losses of potassium deplete intracellular K^+ stores. The Nernst equation defines the resting membrane potential of myocardial cells as related to the intracellular and extracellular concentrations of potassium:

$$RMP = -61.5 \times \log (ICW\ [K^+]/ECW\ [K^+])$$

Long-term diuretic therapy can reduce ICW K^+ levels, with the consequence of impaired conduction and electrical automaticity leading to arrhythmias. In this situation, the electrocardiogram will show depressed T waves and

---

Box 5-2. Guidelines for Treatment of Adult Patients With Hyperkalemia

FIRST: Stop all infusion of potassium

ELECTROCARDIOGRAPHIC EVIDENCE OF PENDING ARREST: Loss of P wave and broad slurring of QRS; immediate effective therapy indicated

1. Intravenous infusion of calcium salts
   a. 10 mL of 10% calcium chloride over 10 minutes

   or

   b. 10 mL of 10% calcium gluconate over 3-5 minutes

2. Intravenous infusion of sodium bicarbonate
   a. 50-100 mEq over 10-20 minutes; benefit proportional to extent of pretherapy acidemia

ELECTROCARDIOGRAPHIC EVIDENCE OF POTASSIUM EFFECT: Peaked T waves; prompt therapy needed

1. Glucose and insulin infusion
   a. Intravenously infused 50 mL of $D_{50}W$ and 10 units of regular insulin; monitor glucose

2. Immediate hemodialysis

BIOCHEMICAL EVIDENCE OF HYPERKALEMIA AND NO ECG CHANGES: Effective therapy needed within hours

1. Potassium-binding resins into GI tract, with 20% sorbitol
2. Promotion of renal kaliuresis by loop diuretic

the onset of U waves. Hypokalemia leads to cardiac arrhythmias, particularly atrial tachycardia with or without block, atrioventricular dissociation, ventricular tachycardia, and ventricular fibrillation. The risk of hypokalemia-associated arrhythmia is higher in patients treated with digoxin, even when potassium concentrations are in the "low normal" range.

Clinical Syndromes of Acute Hypokalemia

Most patients with hypokalemia develop the problem while excreting more than 20 mmol of urinary potassium each day, which indicates that renal losses contribute to hypokalemia. Diuretic administration is a common iatrogenic mechanism of reducing serum K^+ levels. Thiazide and loop diuretics, as well as osmotic diuresis produced by mannitol infusion, increase delivery of sodium to the DCT segment of the nephron. In the presence of elevated aldosterone, sodium is absorbed while potassium enters the filtrate and is lost in urine. Patients with congestive heart failure are particularly sensitive to aggressive diuretic therapy that is often necessary to relieve pulmonary or peripheral edema. Diuresis reduces effective blood volume and activates the renin-angiotensin-aldosterone axis.

Patients with vomiting or diarrhea suffer losses of sodium, potassium, protons, and chloride. In addition, they become dehydrated and have elevated aldosterone levels. Excessive losses of urinary potassium occur in these patients because preservation of ECW by optimal sodium reabsorption takes precedence over maintaining a normal serum K^+ concentration.

Transient changes in serum K^+ can occur due to K^+ shifts into the cells. Intravenous infusions of epinephrine or isoproterenol can activate β_2-adrenergic receptors and activate Na^+/K^+-ATPase. Even inhalation of nebulized β agonists for asthma has been demonstrated to transiently reduce serum K^+ concentration. Alcoholic patients who present after a sustained period of drinking and associated vomiting often have profound electrolyte imbalances, including hypokalemia and hypophosphatemia. In the alcoholic population, hypomagnesemia also frequently contributes to hypokalemia. Onset of delirium tremens with epinephrine surges can further exacerbate hypokalemia in alcoholic patients. Primary aldosteronism is caused by aldosterone-producing hyperplasia or adenoma in the adrenal gland; and in the rare patient with this endocrine abnormality, hypokalemia with mild alkalosis is a common presenting finding.

Treatment of Hypokalemia

Hypokalemic patients require potassium replacement. Because being serum K^+ poor reflects ICW deficits, patients should be closely monitored during replacement therapy. Administered either intravenously or enterally, KCl is preferred because chloride deficits and alkalosis are common in patients with a contracted ECW. Potassium in foods is linked to phosphate. Potassium phosphate salts may need to be given intravenously, particularly when an expansion of the ICW is anticipated. To reduce the risk of serious cardiac arrhythmias in patients with cardiac disease or postoperative cardiac surgery who have a serum K^+ value less than 3.5 mmol/L, patients should be promptly corrected to a serum K^+ concentration of over 4.0 mmol/L.[44] Potassium infusion should not exceed a rate of 0.3 mmol/kg/hr to avoid overcorrection. High concentrations of potassium in intravenous fluids can be irritating to peripheral small veins, and infusions may require a central venous catheter. Patients rarely require more than 200 mmol of potassium in 1 day. The exception is patients with substantial losses who may require extraordinary potassium replacement.

Hypokalemic patients with concurrent acidemia should have delayed correction of ECW pH. These patients should receive potassium before bicarbonate. Rapid reduction in ECW H^+ leads to an H^+ for K^+ exchange across the cell membrane. As extracellular K^+ concentration decreases, there occurs a further disruption of normal resting membrane potential.

Diabetics in ketoacidosis may present with normal serum K^+ but rapidly develop hypokalemia as insulin is administered and glucose shifts into cells. Potassium supplements should be added to resuscitation fluid of the diabetic in ketoacidosis once the physician is confident the patient has adequate renal function.

Treatment of hypokalemia should include interventions to reduce potassium loss. If the patient is on a diuretic that wastes potassium, he or she should either receive supplemental potassium or be given an additional drug that spares potassium, such as triamterene or spironolactone. Hypokalemic patients may also need magnesium, which is an important cofactor for potassium uptake and maintenance of intracellular K^+ levels. Supplemental magnesium also reduces the risk of arrhythmia. The hypokalemic patient not on diuretic therapy can have a rare endocrine disorder including primary hyperaldosteronism and renin-secreting tumors. Amphotericin B therapy may have a toxic effect on renal tubule function, and drug-induced potassium losses can be substantial.[45]

CALCIUM AND MAGNESIUM

Calcium, a divalent cation, is a critical component of many extracellular and intracellular reactions. It is an essential cofactor in the coagulation cascade, and intracellular ionized calcium participates in regulation of neuronal, myocardial, and renal tubular functions. Calcium is assayed in a serum sample as total serum calcium concentration (normally, 8.5 to 10.5 mg/dL). Total calcium assays encompass the three molecular forms of calcium in serum: protein-bound calcium, diffusible calcium complexed to anions (bicarbonate, phosphate, and acetate), and freely diffusible. Ionized calcium Ca^{2+}_i is the biochemically active species that constitutes approximately 45% of the total serum calcium. Over 80% of protein-bound calcium is attached to an albumin. Acidemia decreases calcium binding to albumin; and as pH falls, the ionized proportion increases; conversely, alkalemia reduces Ca^{2+}_i. Thus, in patients with diluted albumin concentrations or fluctuating acid-base status, the total serum calcium concentration inadequately indicates the concentration of Ca^{2+}_i available to support biochemical reactions. Electrodes are used to measure Ca^{2+}_i in anaerobic samples of blood or plasma and normally range between 1.1 and 1.4 mmol/L.

The serum calcium concentration is controlled by the interaction of PTH, calcitonin, and vitamin D. Vitamin D is not one molecule but a mixture of sterols with antirachitic activity. The ICW Ca^{2+}_i is substantially lower than the ECW Ca^{2+}_i. Calcium functions in the cytosol as a second messenger, and Ca^{2+}_i concentrations are narrowly controlled by enzymes in the cell membrane that transport the ions out of the cell. In muscle cells, ionized calcium is stored in the sarcoplasmic reticulum from which it can be quickly released into ICW. Muscle contraction occurs during a molecular interaction of actin and myosin molecules that depends on calcium. Tight control of Ca^{2+}_i in ICW and ECW is essential. Shock leads to a depletion of intracellular energy, which in turn leads to impaired active transport of calcium out of the cell. As ICW Ca^{2+}_i increases in patients in shock, biochemical reactions are altered; if prolonged or substantial elevations in ICW Ca^{2+}_i occur, the cells die.[46] Similarly, an increase or decrease in ECW Ca^{2+}_i can occur rapidly, and severe perturbations can lead to organ dysfunction and death. The multiple regulatory mechanisms that modulate Ca^{2+}_i reflect the critical importance of this divalent cation.[47]

Bone is an enormous reservoir of calcium. Turnover of calcium salts in bone is constant and integral to maintaining a stable $Ca^{2+}i$ in ECW. Receptors in the membranes of parathyroid cells can identify low or falling Ca^{2+}_i, which rapidly stimulates the release of PTH. PTH has several target tissues. It activates osteoclasts, which release calcium from the structural matrix of bone. PTH stimulates tubule cells in the proximal nephron to both absorb calcium in the filtrate and excrete phosphates. The hormone also works with vitamin D to enhance absorption of calcium from the lumen of the gut. Increased extracellular Ca^{2+}_i suppresses the release of PTH, and, as hormone levels fall, osteoblasts use calcium to synthesize new bone. Vitamin D also assists in the control of calcium homeostasis. The potency of dietary vitamin D is increased by conversion to 1,25-dihydroxycholecalciferol in the kidneys, the most active form of the vitamin; PTH also stimulates this conversion. In turn, 1,25-dihydroxycholecalciferol promotes production of more mRNA for the peptide PTH in parathyroid cells. In summary, multiple mechanisms produce a balance of forces that increase and decrease Ca^{2+}_i and thus modulate the availability of this critical cation to support metabolic activity.

Magnesium is an essential cation in the enzymatic activity that enables ATP conversion to ADP and energy release. Less than 1% of the total body magnesium content is found in the extracellular fluid. The normal concentration of magnesium Mg^{2+} in plasma ranges between 1.4 and 2.0 mEq/L, and approximately 20% is bound to proteins. Mg^{2+} can be assayed in the hydrolysate of erythrocytes, and this measurement indicates intracellular magnesium stores. Patients with ICW Mg^{2+} measures of less than 4.4 to 6.0 mEq/L have a substantial total body magnesium deficiency. Several diseases that deplete magnesium have parallel effects on calcium. Furthermore, these two divalent cations have similar effects on biochemical reactions. Thus, hypomagnesemic patients exhibit central nervous, muscular, and cardiovascular signs and symptoms similar to those of depressed ECW calcium concentration; in actuality, symptoms are often the net result of deficiencies in both cations.

Hypercalcemia

Hypercalcemia can be suspected when serum calcium levels exceed the normal range (9 to 11 mg/dL, 2.2 to 2.7 mmol/L). Confirmation of the diagnosis of hypercalcemia requires that Ca^{2+}_i exceeds 1.4 mmol/L. Patients with transient modest elevations in serum calcium levels are generally asymptomatic, whereas those with sustained elevations in renal calcium excretion may develop renal lithiasis. Calcium levels greater than 15 mg/dL produce symptoms of weakness, stupor, and other central nervous system dysfunction. A renal concentrating defect also occurs in hypercalcemic patients, which leads to polyuria and a loss of sodium; indeed, many hypercalcemic patients present with dehydration. Hypercalcemic crisis is a syndrome in which the total serum calcium levels exceed 17 mg/dL. These patients suffer life-threatening cardiac tachyarrhythmias, coma, acute renal failure, and an ileus with abdominal distention.

Several clinical syndromes or circumstances account for the majority of hypercalcemia cases. Hyperparathyroidism, or unregulated PTH secretion, is a common cause of significant hypercalcemia.[48] Continual PTH stimulation causes accelerated osteoclastic activity, which releases large amounts of calcium from bone and produces a sustained elevation in Ca^{2+}_i.[47] Bone demineralization is found in patients with severe and prolonged hyperparathyroidism. Eighty-five percent of patients with this syndrome are found to have a solitary hyperfunctioning adenoma in one parathyroid gland, and the remainder have excessive PTH release from all four glands. PTH induces phosphaturia and depresses serum phosphate concentrations, and these laboratory findings corroborate the diagnosis of primary hyperparathyroidism.

Patients with chronic renal failure develop secondary hyperparathyroidism, an endocrine disease characterized by hyperplasia of the parathyroid glands. A period of hypocalcemia due to either decreased renal production of 1,25-dihydroxycholecalciferol or hyperphosphatemia leads to hypertrophy of the parathyroid glands. Hypercalcemia is the eventual complication of an unregulated elevation in PTH.

Patients with malignancies can develop hypercalcemia independent of the hormone PTH. Selected tumors have been demonstrated to produce a PTH-related peptide that shares 8 of its first 13 amino acids with PTH, which induces calcium release from bone and reduces calcium loss in urine.[49] Multiple myeloma and other hematologic malignancies and tumors metastatic to bone (particularly breast, lung, and prostate cancers) cause hypercalcemia by excessive osteoclastic activity. Selected tumors that directly invade bone increase Ca^{2+}_i by nonhormonal mechanisms involving cytokines (IL-1, TNF, IL-6) that activate osteo-clasts. Drugs can also cause hypercalcemia, including thiazide diuretics and extraordinary doses of vitamins A and D. Young, normally active patients with high bone turnover rates can develop hypercalcemia when suddenly forced into immobility, as may occur during forced bed rest after injury or major illness. This hypercalcemia of immobilization resolves with return to normal activity.[50]

Definitive management of hypercalcemia depends on correction of the primary problem. Thus, patients with hyperparathyroidism due to a parathyroid adenoma or hyperplasia are cured of hypercalcemia by excision of the diseased parathyroid tissue. Hypercalcemic patients on thiazide drugs should be converted to alternative therapies. Patients with a malignancy and hypercalcemia may respond to surgical excision, radiation therapy, or chemotherapy. Symptomatic patients with malignancy-related severe hypercalcemia can be quickly and effectively treated by saline infusion to expand the ECW followed by loop diuretic administration (i.e., furosemide) to induce a saline diuresis with associated urinary calcium clearance. In fact, patients with severe hypercalcemia frequently suffer a contracted ECW volume and thus isotonic saline infusion is essential. Hypercalcemic patients in renal failure who cannot benefit from a drug-induced diuresis can be managed by hemodialysis.

Severe hypercalcemia related to release of calcium from bone can be successfully managed by bisphospho-nate treatment. These drugs have a potent capacity to reduce osteoclast-mediated release of calcium from bone.[51] Several formulations of bisphosphonates are available (in order of preference, zolendronic acid, pamidronate disodium, etidronate disodium), all of which produce a slow decline in plasma Ca^{2+} over several days.[48] Bisphosphonates given as long-term prophylactic agents to patients with metastatic breast cancer, and administered at a regular dosage, have been proven to effectively prevent hypercalcemia.[52]

Calcitonin is the calcium-lowering hormone produced by parafollicular cells of the thyroid gland. Administration of exogenous calcitonin effectively induces renal excretion of calcium and suppresses osteoclast bone reabsorption. While calcitonin therapy for hypercalcemia is often initially effective, long-term therapy frequently leads to tachyphylaxis, possibly related to the development of antibodies to the exogenous calcitonin.[48] Chelating agents (EDTA or phosphate salts) that bind and neutralize ionized calcium are rarely indicated, owing to their associations with complications of metastatic calcifications, acute renal failure, and the risk that Ca^{2+}_i may be depressed to hypocalcemic levels.

Hypocalcemia

Acute hypocalcemia can be a life-threatening event. This condition impairs transmembrane depolarization, and Ca^{2+}_i below 0.8 mEq/L can lead to CNS dysfunction. Hypocalcemic patients complain of paresthesias and muscle spasms (including tetany) and develop seizures. The consequences of a rapid decline in Ca^{2+}_i can be clearly demonstrated in patients after parathyroid surgery that becomes complicated by a precipitous decline in PTH. Within hours, these patients develop hypocalcemia and complain of numbness, paresthesias of the distal extremities and circumoral region, and painful muscle spasms. Patients may exacerbate the condition if they hyperventilate and induce a respiratory alkalosis, which further reduces ionized calcium concentrations. The Chvostek sign is a twitch of facial muscles elicited by tapping gently on the facial nerve. Trousseau's sign is a carpopedal spasm induced by 3 minutes of inflation of a sphygmomanometer cuff above the brachial artery. These provocative tests, though neither sensitive nor specific for hypocalcemia, can readily indicate in a clinical setting a potential problem.

Cardiac dysfunction also occurs in patients with hypocalcemia. Low plasma Ca^{2+}_i is associated with impaired cardiac contractility, and intravenous infusion of calcium can improve cardiac output in these patients. Electrocardiograms show a prolonged QT interval that may progress to complete heart block or ventricular fibrillation.

The tumor lysis syndrome is a constellation of electrolyte abnormalities including hypocalcemia, hyperphosphatemia, hyperuricemia, and hyperkalemia. These electrolyte aberrations occur when antineoplastic therapy causes a sudden surge in tumor cell death and release of cytosol contents. Solid tumors and lymphomas have been associated with this problem. Acute renal failure occurs in patients suffering from the tumor lysis syndrome and prevents spontaneous correction of the electrolyte abnormalities; emergency dialysis may be the only therapy providing comprehensive correction of the problems.[53]

Acute hypocalcemia can also be a complication of severe pancreatitis and is speculated to be the consequence of ionized extracellular calcium becoming linked to fats in the peripancreatic inflammatory phlegmon. Rapid infusion of a citrate load during transfusion of blood products (particularly platelet concentrates and fresh frozen plasma) may also lead to acute severe hypocalcemia (Ca^{2+}_i < 0.62 mmol/L) and hypotension[54]; clinicians have advocated routine administration of supplemental calcium linked to units of blood products during massive transfusion protocols to prevent hypocalcemia. Rapid increases in serum phosphate can occur after improper administration or excessive dosing of phosphate-containing cathartics and can cause severe hypocalcemia.

Chronic hypocalcemia is usually secondary to parathyroid dysfunction after thyroid or parathyroid surgery.[47] Patients with diets deficient in vitamin D, or in whom the conversion of vitamin D to a 1,25-dihydroxycholecalciferol is impaired owing to liver or renal disease, can become hypocalcemic. Vitamin D deficiency can also develop in patients with short gut syndrome or if the gastrointestinal mucosa malabsorbs fat-soluble vitamins owing to biliary, pancreatic, or mucosa dysfunction. A decrease in total serum calcium concentration may not represent a reduction in the functionally important and diffusible Ca^{2+}_i. Therapy must correct both the magnesium and calcium defects, which may be substantial in the ICW. For more chronic forms of hypocalcemia, treatment with supplemental calcium and vitamin D in the diet are often sufficient measures to maintain an adequate calcium level and avoid the symptoms of muscle spasms, paresthesias, and weakness.

In the ICU, where multiple blood tests are continuously monitored, mild hypocalcemia is common. While replacement therapy is appropriate in the symptomatic hypocalcemic patient, it is controversial whether correcting to a normal ionized calcium value of 0.8 to 1.1 mmol/L is beneficial. Patients with severe hypocalcemia (Ca^{2+}_i < 0.62 mmol/L) at risk for impending cardiac failure or a fatal arrhythmia are treated with intravenous calcium salt infusions. Infusion of 10 mL of a 10% $CaCl_2$ solution provides 272 mg of calcium (equivalent to 13.6 mmol of ionized calcium), whereas the same volume of 10% calcium gluconate contains only 90 mg of calcium (equivalent to 4.5 mmol of ionized calcium). Intravenous calcium infusion should be performed with caution because rapid shifts in ECW Ca^{2+}_i concentration can cause cardiac arrhythmias, particularly in patients treated with digoxin. Also in patients with low Ca^{2+}_i but elevated serum phosphate, rapid calcium infusion can result in the widespread precipitation of calcium. Furthermore, intravenous calcium preparations are caustic and infiltration in a peripheral vein leads to necrosis of skin and is best administered rapidly through central venous catheters.

Hypermagnesemia and Hypomagnesemia

Hypermagnesemia is an electrolyte abnormality most often seen in patients with renal failure. It can be exacerbated by ingestion of magnesium-containing drugs, particularly antacids, and such agents should be avoided. Magnesium blocks the shift of calcium into myocardial cells, and patients with severe hypermagnesemia show evidence of heart failure.

Intracellular magnesium stores can become substantially depleted in patients afflicted with chronic diarrhea or who undergo prolonged aggressive diuretic therapy.[55] Magnesium deficiency is also common in patients with heavy ethanol intakes. Diabetic patients with persistent osmotic diuresis from glucosuria commonly have hypomagnesemia. These categories of patients often benefit by adding magnesium salts to resuscitation fluids. Correction of hypomagnesemia is accomplished by the intravenous infusion of magnesium sulfate ($MgSO_4$). Severe hypomagnesemia (<1.0 mEq/L) requires sustained therapy owing to the slow equilibration of extracellular magnesium with intracellular stores. Correction of hypomagnesemia can also reduce the risk of cardiac arrhythmias. Often, the magnitude of magnesium deficiency parallels the magnitude of hypocalcemia. Hypocalcemia in patients with magnesium deficiency is resistant to calcium replacement alone, and these patients should receive magnesium concurrently.

CONTROL OF PLASMA VOLUME AND THE CIRCULATION OF INTERSTITIAL FLUID

Blood flow delivers oxygen to the arterioles, capillaries, and venules, which together form the microcirculation. As oxygen diffuses into the tissues, carbon dioxide released from cells enters the blood and is transported to the lungs for excretion. The flow of lymph, a filtrate of plasma, is a second circulation of fluid and solutes that also plays a vital role in sustaining a viable cell environment. Fluid in the plasma compartment crosses the endothelial cell barrier in the microcirculation, enters the interstitial compartment, and is returned to the plasma compartment through lymphatic channels.

Several factors are critical to the control of the second circulation. Driving forces in the capillary move water and solute across the microvascular membrane. The permeability characteristics of the microvascular membrane determine the proportion of plasma proteins blocked from entry into the interstitium. The compliance of the interstitial matrix modulates to an extent which pressures change as the matrix contracts or swells and the interstitial pressure drives fluid into lymphatics. The driving forces within the capillaries are modulated by local factors or systemic neuroendocrine function. The permeability characteristics of the microvascular membrane can be adjusted by mediators of inflammation or altered with drugs. The interstitium fluctuates in size and composition and forms a reservoir that can restore or decompress the plasma volume. The lymphatic flow mechanism controls the size of interstitial volume and marshals an immune response.

An important function of the second circulation is the unidirectional flux of soluble proteins from plasma to the interstitium and through lymphatics back to the venous circulation. Renkin estimated that the total circulating protein mass (primarily albumin, immunoglobulins, and fibrinogen) could be 450 g in a 65-kg man (Fig. 5-7).[56] Of this protein, 210 g reside within the 3 L of plasma volume and 240 g are found in the 12 L of ECW, which principally constitutes interstitial fluid. In the daily filtration of fluid from the plasma to the interstitium, Renkin estimates that approximately one half of the interstitial protein mass drains into lymphatics, which is eventually delivered as 4 L of thoracic duct lymph into the venous circulation each day. Each organ has unique lymph characteristics that correspond to the function of the organ. There is negligible interstitial fluid and no lymph flow from the brain. Skin and skeletal muscle, which contain the largest proportion of the interstitial volume, have relatively impermeable microvascular membranes, a rich network of lymphatics, and a compliant interstitial volume. Hepatic microvascular membranes are highly permeable, and lymph flow from the liver is high. Furthermore, lymphatics act as conduits to deliver proteins synthesized in hepatocytes to blood. The circulation of interstitial fluid as lymph flow clears the interstitial fluid that bathes the cells as new plasma filtrate enters the interstitium.

The microvascular walls are composed of endothelial cells attached to a basement membrane. These cells lie in a continuous monolayer, and adjacent cells are connected with cell-cell junctions. The basement membrane consists of thin, multilayered molecules that form a barrier, particularly for highly charged molecules. The endothelial cell layer and the basement membrane constitute a semipermeable barrier that separates the plasma compartment from the interstitium. Plasma water and solutes can cross

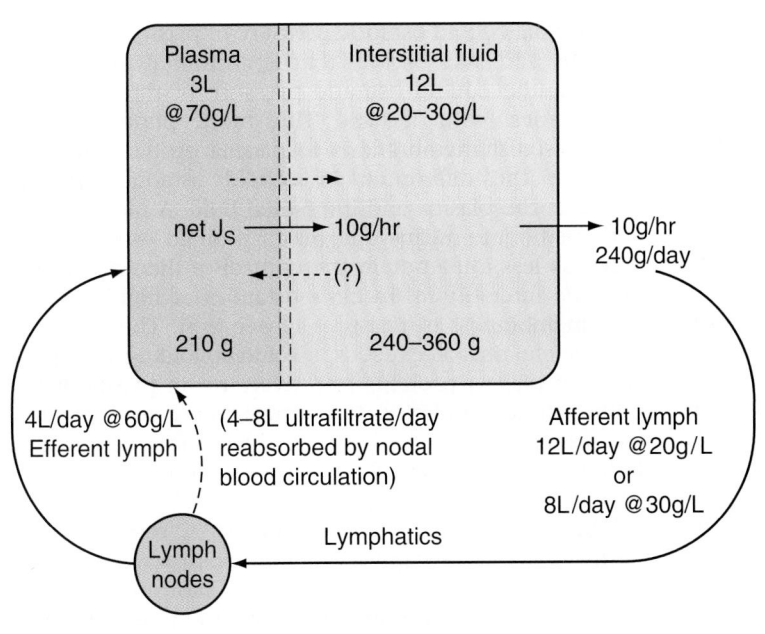

FIGURE 5-7. Magnitudes of lymphatic turnover of fluid and plasma protein. (From Renkin EM: Some consequences of capillary permeability to macromolecules: Starling's hypothesis reconsidered. Am J Physiol 250:H706, 1986.)

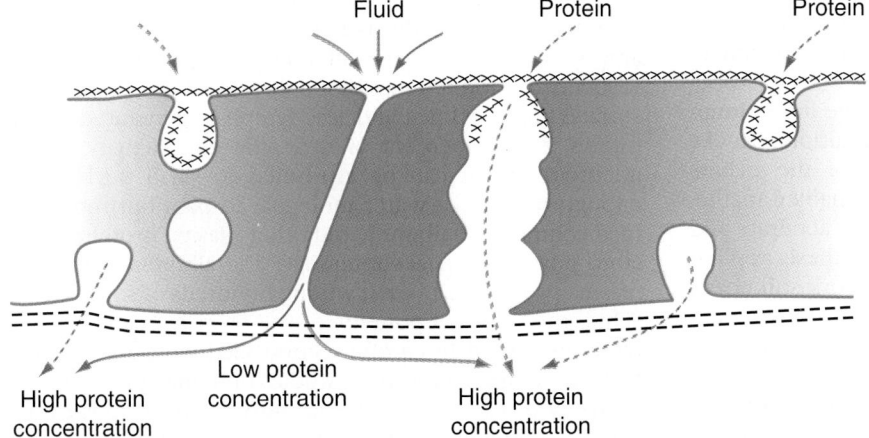

FIGURE 5-8. Diagrammatic representation of microvascular endothelium barrier, which shows separate pathways for fluid and protein to cross from the plasma space to the interstitium. (From Michel CC, Curry FE: Microvascular permeability. Physiol Rev 79:703-761, 1999.)

the microvascular membranes by passing through intercellular gaps and pores in the capillary and venular segments. In addition, fluid transport from the plasma to the interstitium occurs through vesicles. These small spheres form as the cell membrane invaginates, trapping an aliquot of extracellular fluid. They then appear to migrate from the luminal to the abluminal side of the endothelial cell, where the vesicles fuse with the cell membrane and release their contents to the interstitium. A group of vesicles are hypothesized to be able to coalesce within the endothelial cell to transiently form large channels through the cell and connect the plasma and interstitial fluid (Fig. 5-8).[57]

The microvascular membrane is nearly as permeable to small solutes (e.g., electrolytes, glucose, and urea) as it is water, and the concentration of these solutes in plasma and interstitial fluid are essentially equivalent. In contrast to small molecules, large solutes in plasma, the plasma proteins, are too large to cross the microvascular membrane through the pores that accommodate water and small solutes. Plasma proteins pass into the interstitium through large pores that may contain an extracellular glycocalyx, a network of fibers permeable to water but which sieves plasma proteins. Fluid entering the interstitium contains plasma protein with a diluted concentration compared with that within the capillary lumen. The lymph concentration over plasma concentration ratios (L/P) for small molecules, such as glucose, equals 1. For proteins circulating in the blood, the L/P is less than 1. Furthermore, the larger the size of a plasma protein, the lower the L/P ratio; the L/P for albumin may be 0.6, whereas the L/P for IgG is 0.3. Investigators attribute the semi-permeable characteristics of the microvascular membrane to two groups of pores. Small pores enable transmembrane movement of water and electrolytes but cannot accommodate molecules the size of proteins. Larger pores are able to accommodate albumin and other large proteins. The pore theory asserts that the number of small pores substantially exceeds the number of large pores; thus, more water than protein enters the interstitium.

Control of Fluid Movement and Solute Flux Across the Microvascular Membrane

In 1896, Ernst Starling hypothesized that a balance of forces across the microvascular membrane is responsible for controlling the distribution of fluid and proteins between the intravascular and interstitial spaces. Starling's hypothesis proposed that an oncotic pressure from plasma proteins exists across the capillary wall that favors the retention of water in the vascular compartment and counterbalances the intraluminal hydrostatic pressure that forces fluid into the interstitium. Research in the subsequent 100 years has elaborated many details of Starling's hypothesis, but the basic concept that initiating events for lymph flow occurs across the capillary wall is still accepted.[57] Proteins in a solution generate an oncotic pressure proportional to the concentration of the proteins. Oncotic pressure moves water across a membrane effectively only if that membrane is more permeable to water than to proteins. While changes in oncotic pressure occur relatively slowly, physiologic mechanisms can rapidly adjust arteriolar vascular tone and thus hydrostatic pressure in the capillary. In addition, vascular tone controls the distribution of cardiac output to the organs. Each organ has different microvascular membrane permeability characteristics, and the influence on total body distribution of ECW between plasma volume and the interstitium is a summation of Starling forces across multiple circulations in parallel. Considerable research of the events occurring across individual capillaries has enabled mathematical models to evolve and provide a more accurate and complete description than the Starling hypothesis applied to a single-vessel exchange. Considerable work still needs to be done before clinicians can, with comparable confidence, define the application of Starling's hypothesis to total body exchange of fluid and protein.

The following equation describes a contemporary mathematical model of Starling's hypothesis as applied to a single vessel such as a capillary or venule.[57]

$$J_v = L_p S \left[(P_c - P_i) - \sigma(COP_c - COP_i) \right]$$

In steady-state conditions, the J_v for a defined mass of tissue is equivalent to the lymph flow for that tissue, and as a consequence, interstitial size remains stable. The driving forces responsible for water flow, presented in the equation as P and COP, correspond to hydrostatic and colloid oncotic pressure. A key component of the model is that four pressures exist, two on each side of the microvascular membrane, to define the net balance of forces. The subscripts i and c designate locations, in the interstitium or in the capillary. The component $(P_c - P_i)$ in the equation indicates what the driving pressures in millimeters of mercury are for plasma fluid to flow across the microvascular membrane into the interstitium. The component $(COP_c - COP_i)$ represents the force attributed to osmotic pressure of proteins in a solution in millimeters of mercury, which favors water retention on the plasma side of the membrane. Sigma, σ, has a value between 0 and 1 and corresponds to the effectiveness of the microvascular membrane as a barrier to plasma proteins.

The normal colloid osmotic pressure of plasma is 25 to 30 mm Hg, and over 50% of that is attributed to albumin, whereas the colloid osmotic pressure of the interstitial fluid varies with tissues. The more permeable the microvascular membrane is to plasma proteins, the less effective the difference in colloid osmotic pressure between the plasma and interstitial fluid. A more permeable membrane means that plasma colloid osmotic pressure has less influence in the control of fluid movement into the interstitium. In circumstances of highly permeable membranes, σ measures closer to 0. The σ in skin and skeletal muscle exceeds 0.9, and colloid osmotic pressures of plasma proteins effectively retain plasma water within these capillaries. In contrast, the σ in liver capillaries approaches zero, and colloid pressures have limited influence. High lymph flow and a tightly restrictive liver capsule prevent liver edema.

The term $L_p S$ has two components. L_p represents the permeability of the capillary membrane to water, also designated as hydraulic conductivity. S indicates capillary membrane surface area available for water to move across. Thus, tissues with many capillaries have large surface areas. Arteriolar vasomotor tone is a physiologic mechanism that not only adjusts P_c but also controls the surface area within the microcirculation of a specific tissue. As vasoconstriction reduces blood flow to a capillary bed, the surface area declines and less lymph is generated by filtration. Ninety percent of hydraulic conductivity in the microcirculation can be attributed to small pores large enough to allow a water molecule to pass but too small to accommodate albumin and other plasma proteins. One large pore able to accommodate the albumin and other plasma proteins may exist among hundreds of small pores. While the two components of the term $L_p S$ can be separately measured in carefully controlled experiments performed on single vessels, in studies of human permeability these two factors are fused into a single term, the capillary filtration coefficient (CFC). The CFC measures the combined influence of microvascular hydraulic conductivity (water permeability) and the number of capillaries being perfused at a given point in time per 100 g of tissue. This has been measured in the human forearm with strain-gauge plethysmography, which precisely measures the rate of arm swelling when venous pressure is increased. Groban and colleagues reported that infusion of atrial natriuretic peptide (ANP) increased CFC between 37% and 63%. These authors reasoned that release of ANP from the heart in response to increased atrial distention led to increased CFC in skin and skeletal muscle; they further proposed this phenomenon as a rapidly acting mechanism to reduce intravascular volume.[58] In summary, based on decades of research, a mathematical model of microvascular membrane permeability has been refined. Multiple interacting forces are in balance and govern the net movement of fluid into the interstitium.

Fluid and solutes cross from the plasma compartment and enter the interstitium. Fluid flows through the interstitium and enters terminal lymphatics. The interstitium comprises cells, macromolecules, and a free-fluid phase of the ECW. In skeletal muscles, at most 10% of interstitial water is ECW and the majority of mass is made up by myocyte ICW. In skin, 50% of interstitial water is ECW and cells components include primarily fibroblasts, endothelium, and inflammatory cells. Macromolecules constitute a hydrated gel matrix and a major acellular component of the interstitium. The third component is the free-fluid phase of ECW in direct continuity with lymphatics; prenodal lymph and interstitial free fluid are similar in composition. Edema is the pathologic condition of increased interstitial volume. A variety of conditions that increase microvascular membrane permeability or change the Starling forces across the membrane can cause edema. Evidence indicates that edema fluid characteristics vary depending on the mechanism of edema formation. Furthermore, increasing evidence suggests that the interstitium is a modulated environment, and signals or actions from interstitial cells can modify the matrix and increase compliance; therefore, edema may be the consequence of a pathologic change in the interstitial gel matrix.

Collagen molecules are composed of three long polypeptide chains that coil into a helix. Collagen is secreted by fibroblasts into the interstitial fluid as precursors that coalesce into chains. Multiple collagen molecules cross-link and assemble into fibers. The collagen fibers form a framework that supports the interstitium structure. Glycosaminoglycans, which are polyanionic polysaccharide chains composed of repeated carbohydrate units, are also synthesized by fibroblasts; several forms have been identified, and most are linked to proteins to form entangled coils that intertwine with collagen fibers to form the gel phase of the interstitium.

The gel matrix of collagen and glycosaminoglycans endows the interstitium with several properties. It provides a structure of fibers that, attached to fibroblasts, resist hydration. Its properties have been speculated to determine the interstitial hydrostatic pressure; experimental evidence indicates that a net pressure to imbibe water and swell exists under normal conditions. The matrix also influences interstitial colloid osmotic pressure. Whereas small water molecules can hydrate the interstices of the tightly interwoven glycosaminoglycans, large protein solutes such as albumin cannot gain access. This produces an excluded water volume, which can be altered by hydration of the gel matrix, and thus can amplify interstitial fluid protein concentration dilution and reduce COP$_i$.

Lymphatics are endothelial-lined tubes that connect the interstitium to lymph nodes and eventually to major veins in the chest. Lymphatics are thought to be impermeable, with the exception of the terminal lymphatics where lymph flow begins. The interstitial fluid concentrations of solutes, including albumin and other proteins, are equivalent to the concentration of these solutes in prenodal lymph. Interstitial fluid pressure drives lymph flow and increases with movement; one-way valves in the lymphatics enable only anterograde flow. Prenodal lymphatics drain into the cortical surface of a lymph node. The fluid percolates through the lymphoid tissue, where its composition may be altered and then drains into a lymphatic vessel that exits from the node's hilum. Centripetal flow propels postnodal lymph toward the chest, where it drains into the main thoracic right thoracic ducts. These vessels have smooth muscle that generates peristaltic contractions. Lymph is finally pumped into the superior vena cava or its major tributaries. It is estimated that a normal adult drains 2 to 4 L of thoracic duct lymph into the plasma compartment per day. The flow of lymph clears metabolites from the interstitium and toxins from the pericellular environment. Lymph flow is also a critical component of the mechanisms the body utilizes to respond to infection.

Pathologic Changes in Interstitial Volume; Dehydration and Edema

The size of the plasma volume is regulated by multiple physiologic factors that influence the distribution of fluid and proteins between the plasma and interstitium. Dehydrated patients preserve plasma volume and contract interstitial volume, whereas overhydrated patients proportionally increase the interstitial volume more than the plasma volume. Control of the size and composition of the interstitial volume is influenced by multiple factors.

The interstitium can serve to restore blood volume after hemorrhage. Acute hemorrhage reduces intravascular volume, and capillary perfusion pressures decline. Decreased capillary hydrostatic pressure leads to reduced plasma fluid transport across the microvascular membrane. Thoracic duct flow is sustained; and for a transient period of time, return of interstitial fluid and proteins exceeds filtration of plasma, with the consequence that plasma volume is restored. Small volumes of hypertonic saline have been successfully utilized to resuscitate patients in hemorrhagic shock by osmotically shifting ICW into the interstitium, which sustains fluid return to the plasma compartment through the thoracic duct.

Edema is defined as an excessive increase in interstitial fluid. Several mechanisms that cause edema have been carefully defined. Infusion of a balanced electrolyte solution normally prompts a compensatory renal response and diuresis. In patients with a depleted blood volume after hemorrhage, rapid infusion of isotonic saline expands the blood volume; however, a great proportion of the fluid shifts into the interstitium. The plasma oncotic pressure becomes diluted by infusion of isotonic fluid with the result of a net fluid transport increase. While lymph flow increases to compensate, interstitial edema develops, along with associated dilution of the interstitial protein concentration. After resuscitation from hypovolemic shock, transient edema is apparent in the largest ECW reservoirs, particularly the skin. When hemorrhage is controlled, edema resolves, in part owing to synthesis of new plasma proteins that restore the plasma oncotic pressure to normal. Also, fibroblasts restore depleted hyaluronan and interstitial matrix gel characteristics return to normal, with subsequent extrusion of excess interstitial fluid.

Congestive heart failure commonly precipitates peripheral edema. Elevated venous pressures shift retrograde into the capillaries, and increased hydrostatic pressure results in higher transmicrovascular fluid shift and edema. These patients classically have edema in the lower extremities or the dependent tissues of the back if supine. Resolution of this form of edema depends on reducing the elevated venous pressure; this is often achieved with diuretics to reduce the plasma volume, which is replaced with lymph drainage from the interstitium.

High-permeability edema occurs when the number or size of large pores in the endothelial membrane increases. Two endogenously produced molecules, histamine and the polypeptide bradykinin, cause gaps to develop between venular endothelial cells; other inflammatory agents can also cause these changes. These large gaps enable greater amounts of fluid with a protein concentration equal to plasma to enter the interstitium. High-permeability edema is characterized by an interstitial fluid high in protein concentration. Studies of the interstitial matrix properties after bradykinin-induced edema indicate the swelling is principally protein-enriched fluid.

Control of Blood Pressure in Response to Shock

The two types of adrenergic receptors of the autonomic nervous system are pivotal in the hemodynamic response to shock. Receptors are located throughout the cardiovascular system and the myocardium. The α receptors are subdivided into α_1 and α_2 types. The β receptors are subdivided into β_1 and β_2 types. When the receptors are occupied by agonists, variable effects are induced. In general, α-adrenergic agonists stimulate vasoconstriction via smooth muscle contraction, whereas β-adrenergic agonists induce smooth muscle relaxation while increasing heart contractility and rate.

The central nervous system regulates reflexes that sustain a normal blood pressure despite fluctuations in the intravascular volume. Baroreceptors located in the aortic arch and other major vessels respond to perfusion pressure changes that are measures of vessel wall stretch during systole. Increases and decreases in systolic pressure prompt reflex signals to centers in the brain stem that control the catecholamines norepinephrine (NE) and epinephrine (EPI). In response to a fall in blood pressure, sympathetic postganglionic neurons release NE into synaptic junctions where NE binds α- and β-adrenergic receptors. Receptors in the myocardium and vascular smooth muscle in response to NE induce increased cardiac function and vasoconstriction to counter the hypotension. Furthermore, during hypotension baroreceptors through the central nervous system direct adrenal release of EPI that circulates in blood and can bind adrenergic receptors throughout the body. Baroreceptors also augment release of arginine vasopressin from the supraoptic and paraventricular nuclei of the hypothalamus, which act to constrict arterioles and increase renal water absorption. In contrast, during episodes of hypertension, baroreceptors detect greater stretch in the vessel wall. Through the central nervous system, release of catecholamines by the autonomic nervous system is suppressed.

The kidney is both an endocrine organ and an effector organ that acts to physiologically adjust total body sodium and water balance and, thus, control blood pressure. The juxtaglomerular apparatus is located in the nephron at the site where the DCT segment comes close to the glomerulus. The endocrine cells of the apparatus control the renin-angiotensin-aldosterone endocrine reflex. Decreased systolic pressure reduces afferent arteriolar perfusion pressure, and less filtered sodium is reabsorbed. The juxtaglomerular apparatus response to hypotension is release of renin, an enzyme that cleaves angiotensinogen in plasma to produce angiotensin I, a peptide of limited physiologic effectiveness. Angiotensin-converting enzyme (ACE) is located on the pulmonary endothelium. ACE converts angiotensin I to angiotensin II, and this second molecule is a potent hormonal vasoconstrictor. Angiotensin II also stimulates secretion of aldosterone by the adrenal glomerulosa. As plasma aldosterone levels increase, more sodium is reabsorbed in the DCT segment of the nephron. Patients in shock activate the renin-angiotensin-aldosterone system with the benefit of an expanded plasma volume, owing to less renal losses of sodium and water. Higher angiotensin II levels also enhance AVP release in a process that links these two endocrine pathways, both of which depend on renal function for an effect.

Renal function adjusts to restore intravascular volume in the circumstance of hypovolemia. Renal blood flow shifts during shock to the juxtamedullary nephrons. With longer loops of Henle than the outer cortical nephrons, these nephrons create the hyperosmolality of the medullary interstitium essential for AVP to produce a small amount of maximally concentrated urine.

Severe hypotension induces a baroreceptor-mediated surge in sympathetic nervous system activity that redistributes blood flow. The increase in vasoconstriction is greatest in the vessels that deliver blood to skin, muscle, and bowel. Available blood flow is diverted to the brain and coronary circulations. Increased renal sympathetic tone constricts efferent arterioles with a range of effects. Modest increases in sympathetic tone preserve glomerular filtration rates and increase water and sodium reabsorption. Maximum sympathetic tone reduces glomerular filtration and may initiate a vasomotor nephropathy that, once established, causes acute renal failure.

CELLULAR AEROBIC FUNCTION AND DYSFUNCTION

Shock in patients is ultimately a problem of dysfunction of intracellular energy metabolism. Patients in shock develop energy deficits in cells that impair cell function. At some threshold, cell energy deficits become irreversible. Widespread energy failure kills cells and consequently the individual dies. In the past century investigators have defined the pathophysiology of shock in terms of organ system dysfunction. Successful therapies for patients in shock have focused on restoring organ function. The discovery of new therapies effective for the problem of irreversible shock may depend on interventions that directly reverse cellular energy deficit and restore normal metabolism to cells.

Cellular Energy Metabolism

Cellular metabolism depends primarily on hydrolysis of the high-energy bond in ATP.[59] The phosphoanhydride bond between the terminal phosphate and ADP is the source of chemical energy for most cellular work. Cellular work performed with ATP includes the contraction of actin and myosin, transport of electrolytes across cell membranes, synthesis of constitutive molecules, and generation of heat. ATP is hydrolyzed to ADP, and, with cleavage of the terminal phosphate bond, energy is released.

$$ATP^{4-} + H_2O \rightarrow ADP^{3-} + P_i^{2-} + H^+ + energy$$

P_i^{2-} is an inorganic phosphate, and *energy* may be up to 12,000 calories for each mole of ATP hydrolyzed. ATP must be constantly replenished. Respiration is a process of biochemical reactions in cells that synthesize ATP from ADP. The final steps in the process of the respiration reaction synthesize high-energy phosphate bonds in ATP and reclaim protons, thereby increasing the pH in ICW. In respiration, the energy in fuels, primarily glucose and fatty acids, is used for ATP synthesis. The energy in carbon-carbon bonds and carbon-hydrogen bonds in fuels is transferred to oxygen in a sequence of chemical reactions that first occur in the cytosol. Six-carbon glucose is degraded to a pair of three-carbon pyruvate molecules through a chain of reactions designated the glycolytic pathway. Without consuming oxygen, the glycolytic pathway can produce 2 moles of ATP for each mole of glucose that is catabolized. This reaction is critical to temporarily sustain minimal amounts of ATP in a cell suddenly deprived of oxygen. Complete oxidation of 1 mole of glucose generates 38 moles of ATP. The process of respiration is continued in the cytosol by pyruvate being directed, with the enzyme pyruvate dehydrogenase, into acetyl-CoA, which then enters the citric acid cycle. Electrons released from the breakage in the chemical bonds of fuels are transported by coenzymes into the mitochondria where oxidative phosphorylation occurs, and oxygen is reduced and converted into carbon dioxide and water.

Clinical Syndromes of Cellular Energy Failure

Several clinical problems demonstrate the consequences for the entire body if the failure of intracellular aerobic metabolism occurs. Ketoacidosis develops in insulin-dependent diabetics because without insulin glucose concentrations decline in the ICW of cells, chiefly in skeletal muscle and adipose cells, and an ATP deficiency ensues. Insulin facilitates the transport of glucose across the cell membrane, so if insulin is not present, glucose cannot enter cells. The cellular H^+ increases in patients with diabetic ketoacidosis because without glucose in the cell, glycolysis and the subsequent cascade of biochemical events needed to support oxidative phosphorylation do not occur. ATP levels fall in the cell while ADP, phosphate, and protons increase. Treatment of these patients with insulin corrects the profound acidemia. As glucose is transported into the cells, aerobic metabolism will rapidly reduce ICW H^+. Patients with diabetic ketoacidosis can develop profound acidemia, and some have advocated

correction of plasma pH less than 7.10 by intravenous infusion of sodium bicarbonate. Several series indicate that in patients with uncomplicated ketoacidosis, bicarbonate therapy is not indicated and equivalent clinical outcome is achieved by aggressive insulin therapy.[28]

Pyruvate dehydrogenase requires the cofactor thiamine (vitamin B_1) to convert pyruvate into acetyl-CoA. Patients must ingest thiamine in their diet, which is available in vegetables. Patients with malabsorption syndromes may fail to deliver the dietary thiamine to their cells. Alcoholic patients who are continually intoxicated can be indifferent to their diet and present with a thiamine deficiency. A specific clinical scenario is that the alcoholic has an acute surgical condition and during treatment develops, owing to thiamine deficiency, lactic acidosis and brain damage because pyruvate dehydrogenase cannot function and support synthesis of ATP by oxidative phosphorylation. This serious metabolic failure can be readily corrected by administration of thiamine.

Patients with acute anoxia experience profound neurocellular dysfunction and death within minutes. The rapidly lethal consequences of anoxia are demonstrated by carbon monoxide poisoning. The carbon monoxide binds to hemoglobin preferentially, and the supply of oxygen in tissues plummets. Patients present unconscious, and death occurs quickly from shock.

In the circumstances of impaired blood flow, the delivery of oxygen to tissues is insufficient to sustain oxidative phosphorylation in the mitochondria at a rate that matches the turnover of ATP to ADP. Patients in shock have an increase in lactate that is coupled with an increase in H^+. In hypoxic conditions, conversion rates of pyruvate into acetyl CoA are low, and lactate dehydrogenase converts the accumulating pyruvate into lactate. Liver and renal cells can extract lactate circulating in blood and metabolize lactate. However, definitive correction of lactic acidosis caused by hypoxia usually depends on restoring adequate blood flow. Patients in shock with lactic acidosis respond to resuscitation with a fall in serum lactate concentration. Abramson and associates reported that among severely compromised patients with elevated serum lactate levels, a good predictor of outcome was not the maximum level of lactate elevation but rather whether the lactate level had returned to normal within 24 hours of initiating resuscitation.[23] One clinical utility of their observation was that patients whose elevated lactic acid levels do not resolve should be carefully examined for missed injuries or untreated causes of continued shock, such as ischemic bowel.

Induced Superoxygen Endpoints of Resuscitation

A hypothesis regarding treatment of shock that has been debated for decades has asserted that the outcome of seriously ill patients resuscitated from shock was optimal if the resuscitation achieved a supernormal oxygen delivery. The hypothesis's core concept was that during shock cells without sufficient oxygen delivery developed an energy debt. The rationale for supernormal oxygen delivery after shock was that the additional oxygen was consumed in higher rates of oxidative phosphorylation to restore the deficit in ATP. Randomized controlled trials intended to test this hypothesis have been conducted. The specific protocols varied, but in general each advocated that seriously injured patients who required resuscitation from shock should have three sequential interventions in the ICU. First, sufficient blood should be transfused to exceed hemoglobin of 10 g/dL. In addition, fluid should be intravenously infused to raise the pulmonary artery wedge pressure to the range of 15 to 20 mm Hg. Second, if cardiac output fails to reach a threshold level after appropriate volume loading, the patient was infused with an inotropic agent such as dopamine or dobutamine. Third, adjustments were made in fluid and drug therapy to achieve a goal of a calculated oxygen delivery. Oxygen delivery is determined using the cardiac output and oxygen content of blood. Randomized clinical trials have been reported that tested the hypothesis that achieving supernormal delivery of oxygen is beneficial. The results have been inconclusive. Boyd and coworkers reported in a randomized control trial of high-risk surgery patients that survival was improved when infusion of inotropes was used to increase oxygen delivery.[60] Gattinoni and colleagues, in large populations of a diverse group of patients requiring resuscitation in an ICU, were unable to demonstrate a benefit to achieving a supernormal oxygen delivery.[61] Hayes and associates reported more deaths in the group pushed to higher oxygen delivery.[101] These clinical trials vary in details, such as the timing of when the supernormal oxygen delivery was achieved and the heterogeneous profile of patients included. Clinical investigators continue to study the concept of tailoring resuscitation after an anaerobic stress to optimize the recovery of cells from an ATP deficit.[62] In reporting on such a protocol, McKinley and coworkers advocated that the goal for oxygen delivery index (DO_2I) should be over 500 mL/min/m², rather than the value of 600 that others have advocated.[63] They demonstrated that among a group of seriously injured patients with hemorrhagic shock, resuscitation of patients to either threshold had equivalent outcome. Specifically, acidemia, measured as a base excess, resolved within 18 hours, and lactate levels had declined to 2.6 mmol/L, both indicating that the hypoxic insult to cells during shock had resolved. One criticism of earlier randomized studies was that there was a delay in achieving the goal of supernormal oxygen delivery. Velmahos and colleagues addressed this criticism in their protocol applied to trauma patients resuscitated from hemorrhagic shock.[64] They used as their DO_2I a threshold of 600 mL/min/m². They relied on thoracic bioimpedance methods to determine early in resuscitation if the patients needed additional therapy to achieve a hyperdynamic status. The authors used blood transfusion and inotropes to achieve the supernormal oxygen delivery goal in the treatment group. The results were that survival was the same in the two groups, and the conclusion was that there was no advantage to their treatment protocol. What did emerge in this study and others is that there exists a group of patients who fail to achieve supernormal oxygen delivery and that among these nonresponders death rates are high. One explanation for this observation is that in non-

responders shock had quickly led to an irreversible oxygen debt in cells. Thus, death is inevitable even if the patients are aggressively resuscitated. Improved outcome for these moribund patients may depend on the discovery of therapies that can restore the aerobic metabolism in profoundly dysfunctional cells.

HYPOVOLEMIC SHOCK

Hypovolemic shock is defined as insufficient delivery of oxygen to tissues caused by a reduced intravascular volume. Surgeons routinely encounter hypovolemic shock, and hemorrhage is the most common specific cause. Hemorrhagic shock follows sudden bleeding from gastrointestinal ulcerations, wounds, or fractures. Intravascular volume deficits are sufficient that venous blood return to the heart is critically reduced. Three forms of hemorrhagic shock have been defined: compensated, uncompensated, and lethal exsanguination.

Compensated shock occurs with hemorrhage of less than 20% of the blood volume. While perfusion is suboptimal, physiologic mechanisms act to adjust systemic vascular resistance and sustain mean systemic pressure. In compensated shock, brain and heart perfusions remain near normal while other less critical organ systems are, in proportion to the blood volume deficit, stressed by ischemia. Patients who develop uncompensated shock become hypotensive because the intravascular volume deficit exceeds the capacity of vasoconstrictive mechanisms to maintain systemic perfusion pressure. Patients in uncompensated shock are at risk for death owing to deficient delivery of oxygen to vital organs and impaired mitochondrial aerobic energy production. These patients must have cellular perfusion restored before irreversible damage to cell biochemical pathways occurs. The third form of hemorrhagic shock is exsanguinating hemorrhage. Patients who lose over 40% of their blood volume develop profound hypotension; without blood flow to the brain, syncope occurs, followed within minutes by cardiopulmonary arrest. The concept of three levels of hemorrhagic shock has been used to design, analyze, and interpret in vivo laboratory studies to test treatments for hemorrhagic shock.

Physiologic and biochemical characteristics of animals in acute hemorrhagic shock have been studied for over a century.[65] However, for a surgeon treating hemorrhagic shock, the patient's survival depends less on a single intervention and more on a series of treatments. The patient's intravascular volume often fluctuates during a sequence of therapeutic interventions. Blood loss is treated with first asanguineous fluid and then, if still hypotensive, blood product infusions that expand the intravascular volume and restore perfusion. However, if the site of bleeding has not been controlled, bleeding continues and hypovolemia recurs. Furthermore, the patient's plasma protein losses are exacerbated by hemodilution. Successful treatment of hypovolemic shock is linked to timely and effective interventions that control sites of active hemorrhage. Therefore, the problem of shock is dynamic. Experimentally defined consequences of severe hemorrhage as an isolated insult not linked to resuscitation may fall short of describing clinically relevant interactions between patient physiology and therapies. Patients survive hemorrhagic shock as a consequence of timely hemostasis and infusions that replete blood volume and support physiologic mechanisms that restore normal cell and organ function.

Causes of hypovolemic shock other than hemorrhage exist. Severe dehydration—a substantial reduction in ECW space and total body sodium—can occur over a few hours and result in hypovolemic shock. For example, patients who suffer the acute onset of *Clostridium difficile* colitis diarrhea can defecate liters of isotonic fluid over a few hours. Diabetics who sustain hours of hyperglycemia can deplete their total body water via osmotic diuresis. The intravascular volume can also be depleted by shifts of fluid within the ECW space; large body surface area burns or fluid sequestration in the intestinal lumen due to a small bowel obstruction can lead to hypovolemic shock. Patients who experience anaphylactic shock shift a large proportion of their plasma into the interstitium due to histamine-induced increase in microvascular membrane permeability. An increase in hematocrit is associated with the hypovolemic shock that occurs in patients with ECW fluid shifts; in these circumstances, increased blood viscosity exacerbates the low perfusion related to hypotension.

The clinical findings of patients in hemorrhagic shock vary depending on several factors, including the capacity to increase sympathetic tone.[66] Patients in hypovolemic shock have diaphoresis and pallor of vasoconstricted digits due to increased α-adrenergic function. Healthy patients whose baroreceptor-mediated reflexes are robust can sustain large losses of blood before precipitously developing profound hypotension. In contrast, patients with marginal cardiac function or on sympatholytic drugs for cardiovascular disease may develop shock after a modest hemorrhage.[67] Decreased mental status or agitation in a hemorrhaging patient indicates impaired cerebral blood flow and impending cardiovascular collapse. Normal volunteers experimentally subjected to hemorrhage of prescribed volumes have enabled investigators to describe the quantitative relationship between blood volume deficit and decline in systolic pressure.[66] Burri and coworkers reported a correlation between the magnitude of blood loss and systolic blood pressure. Most patients who lost less than 25% of blood volume had systolic pressures greater than 110 mm Hg. Subjects with estimated blood losses of 25% to 33% had systolic pressures approximating 100 mm Hg. When losses exceeded 33% of blood volume, most patients had systolic pressures under 100 mm Hg; however, there was considerable variance in this population.[68] Tachycardia is not a reliable indication of significant hemorrhage.[69,70] Demetriades and colleagues reviewed patients in hemorrhagic shock who presented to a level 1 trauma center with systolic blood pressures less than 90 mm Hg and pulse rates less than 90 beats/min. In a multivariate analysis, these investigators could not determine that patients with bradycardia had a different risk of death compared with patients without bradycardia.[71] The widespread use of β blockers further undermines reliance on pulse rate as an indication of shock severity in hemorrhagic patients.

Pathophysiology of Hypovolemic Shock

Baroreceptor-mediated vasoconstriction can readily compensate for a sudden hemorrhage of 15% or less of the blood volume. Vasoconstriction of arterial vessels is the consequence of increased sympathetic tone (measurable as elevated plasma norepinephrine levels), increased blood levels of angiotensin II generated in response to activation of the renin-angiotensin system, higher levels of circulating epinephrine released from the adrenal medulla, and a surge in pituitary release of arginine vasopressin.[72] Vasoconstriction also occurs in the venous circulation. Venoconstriction reduces the compliance of the venous reservoirs, and pressure in the superior and inferior venae cavae is sustained despite reduced intravascular volume. Arterial vasoconstriction maintains mean arterial pressure and perfusion to the heart and brain at the expense of reduced blood flow to skin and skeletal muscles. The vascular tone of patients in hemorrhagic shock can abruptly increase the response to sudden hypotension. Miyagatani and colleagues noted that vascular tone returns to normal in the 4 to 12 hours after an episode of shock reversed by resuscitation.[73]

Patients who hemorrhage 15% to 40% of blood volume experience a decrease in mean arterial pressure. As venous return declines and end-diastolic ventricular filling pressures fall, there is a decrease in left ventricular stroke volume. Patients with substantial vasoconstriction after sudden hemorrhage present with low mean arterial pressure and signs of marked adrenergic vasoconstriction, including pale peripheral capillary beds, agitation, and diaphoresis. Interstitial fluid and proteins can shift to the plasma compartment. Riddez and associates studied normal adults with controlled hemorrhage of 900 mL of blood. Based on hematocrit dilution they estimated up to 50% refill of depleted intravascular volume due to fluid shifts from interstitial reservoirs to the blood volume.[74] Hypotensive baroreceptor stimulation increases adrenergic activity and one consequence may be an accelerated heart rate. However, injured patients without hypovolemia but experiencing pain or fear release epinephrine from their adrenals and also develop tachycardia. Patients with hypovolemia may, in addition to adrenergic activity, have markedly increased parasympathetic tone, and consequently a vagal-mediated decrease in heart rate. These opposing neuroendocrine influences on heart rate explain why pulse rate is neither a sensitive nor a specific indication of the patient's severity of hemorrhagic shock.

Acidemia has been used as a clinical measure of the severity of shock. The metabolic acidemia of hemorrhagic shock is attributed to impaired delivery of oxygen to cells, resulting in a reduced capacity to conduct aerobic metabolism. As the ratio of ADP/ATP increases, protons accumulate. Furthermore, lack of mitochondrial fuel consumption leads to a back-up of molecules synthesized from pyruvate and consequently more pyruvate becomes available for lactate synthesis. Davis and colleagues reported that the severity of hemorrhagic shock relates to the patient's base deficit.[75] Patients whose initial base deficit exceeded 6 mmol/L and whose acidemia did not correct by 24 hours had death rates exceeding 60%. Other investigators have reported the base deficit measurement superior to pH as an indicator of high-risk patients in need of additional resuscitation from hemorrhagic shock.[76,77]

Treatment of Patients in Hemorrhagic Shock

The successful resuscitation of patients in hemorrhagic shock depends on two events: restoration of blood volume and therapeutic interventions to stop hemorrhage.[78] Adults who present in hemorrhagic shock initially receive 2 L of isotonic fluid. Children are resuscitated with up to 20 mL/kg. The surgeon should assess the hemodynamic response to initial intravenous fluids. Patients who remain hypotensive may be severely hypovolemic or have ongoing hemorrhage and in either case will probably require blood transfusion to restore intravascular volume. In addition to systolic blood pressure, resuscitation can be guided by measures of right or left ventricular filling pressure. Pulmonary artery catheters determine central venous pressure (CVP) and pulmonary artery wedge pressure (PCWP). In addition, pulmonary artery catheters enable the clinician to follow cardiac index and systemic vascular resistance, as well as calculate more complex measures of resuscitation such as oxygen delivery or consumption. There is considerable debate in the medical literature regarding the merits of routine use of drugs and intravenous infusions to achieve a prescribed level of resuscitation as oxygen delivery and oxygen consumption.[61,63] Clearly in patients with complex comorbidities who develop hemorrhagic shock, pulmonary artery catheter data provide more precise measurements of response to therapeutic interventions.

Controversy surrounds the timing of resuscitation in actively hemorrhaging patients. Bickell and associates studied the merits of delayed resuscitation in patients with penetrating torso trauma and shock[79]; patients had superior outcomes when resuscitation fluids were not administered until the incision to control hemorrhage was being made in the operating room. In contrast, patients whose intravenous fluid infusions were begun on arrival in the emergency department had inferior survival rates and more complications. In another randomized controlled trial that included a broader group of patients but excluded those with brain injury, Dutton and colleagues reported no adverse effects to what they termed "hypotensive resuscitation."[80] These studies all demonstrated that attempts to restore blood volume during active hemorrhage from large vessels were futile and possibly detrimental. The surgeon's most effective intervention for a hypotensive patient in hemorrhagic shock is to achieve hemostasis.

Debate continues regarding the composition of the ideal resuscitation fluid to treat patients in hemorrhagic shock.[78] Isotonic saline solutions have been effective in the resuscitation of injured and burned patients in hemorrhagic shock as reported in the surgical literature for 40 years.[81] The successful use of balanced electrolyte solutions for resuscitation does require administration of 3 to 4 mL of fluid for each milliliter of shed blood. After resuscitation, metabolic acidosis with an elevated chloride con-

centration is often noted. This form of acidemia should be differentiated from lactic acidemia. To avoid hyperchloremic acidosis, clinical investigators advocate using isotonic saline solutions that include alternative anions to chloride, such as lactated Ringer's.[82] Massive blood transfusions may be required in patients with severe hemorrhage. Coagulopathy may develop as a complication of massive transfusion, and selected blood components (i.e., coagulation factors, fresh frozen plasma, cryoprecipitate, and platelet concentrates) may be necessary to replenish coagulation factors as well as to restore blood volume.[83] Several authors have concluded colloid-containing solutions are superior to isotonic saline for resuscitation from hemorrhagic shock. Schierhout and Roberts reported a systematic review of 26 randomized controlled trials that compared crystalloid with colloid fluid use in critically ill patients, including those with hemorrhagic shock.[84] The authors' analysis calculated that colloid infusion was associated with a 4% increased risk of death. They concluded that no evidence supported the use of colloid fluids.

The Three Phases of Hemorrhagic Shock

Clinicians treating patients in shock must understand that restoration of fluid deficit does not restore the patient to normal. Instead, recovering patients require time to resolve base deficits, normalize lactate levels, and dissipate sympathetic tone, all of which indicate improved delivery of oxygen to tissues. Furthermore, patients who have suffered profound or sustained periods of shock initiate inflammatory responses during reperfusion of ischemic organs. Specific changes during this reperfusion period can include sustained vasodilation leading to a hyperdynamic circulation and rapid onset of edema.

Events After Resuscitation From Shock

Three phases have been described in the human response to acute hemorrhagic shock.[14] In *phase I* (beginning with injury and ending with surgery or a procedure to control active hemorrhage), the patient is hypovolemic, is usually vasoconstricted, and has impaired organ perfusion. It is during this phase that cellular bioenergetics deteriorate and patients develop progressive acidemia, measurable as reduced bicarbonate in arterial blood gases. Therapy is infusion of balanced electrolyte solution given in volume ratios of three to four volumes of isotonic saline for every volume of shed blood. Transfusion is essential when patients have sustained a hemorrhage of more than 30% blood volume. During phase I, severely injured patients with active hemorrhage may require liters of blood during the operation or procedure to control hemorrhage yet experience minimal shock.

Phase II starts at the completion of hemostasis and is a period of fluid sequestration. Both intracellular and interstitial expansions occur during this period of fluid uptake.[59] The duration and magnitude of fluid gain during phase II are proportional to the severity of shock. In the period after severe shock, patients gain weight in excess fluid equivalent to 10% of body weight. Respiratory failure

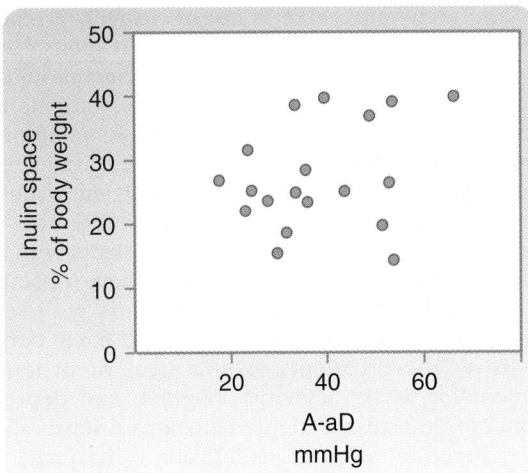

FIGURE 5-9. Expansion in extracellular water during phase II does not consistently correlate with pulmonary dysfunction. Note random relationship of alveolar-arterial P_{O_2} difference (A-aD). (From Rosenburg IK, Gupta SL, Lucas CE, et al: Renal insufficiency after trauma and sepsis: A prospective functional and ultrastructural analysis. Arch Surg 103:175-183, 1971. Copyright 1971, American Medical Association.)

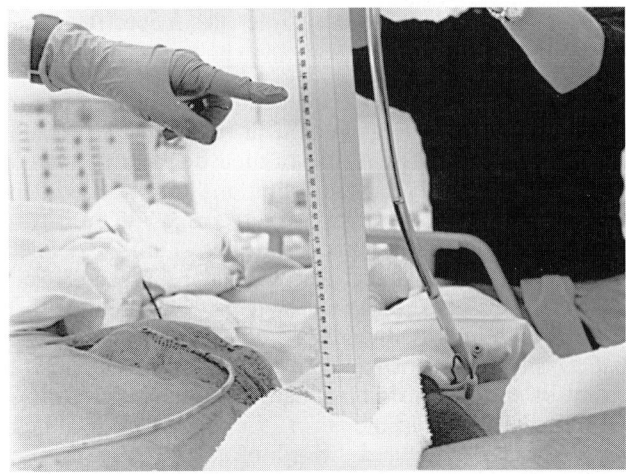

FIGURE 5-10. Measurement of the abdominal compartment pressure is easily accomplished by determining the height of the meniscus of a urine column above the pubic symphysis. A fluid height above 30 cm should prompt consideration of interventions that decompress the abdominal pressure. In this case, insertion of prosthesis material, polyglycolic acid mesh, in the abdominal wound reduced abdominal pressure to less than 20 cm and reversed shock.

is rarely a direct result of the excess fluid retained during phase II (Fig. 5-9). However, abdominal viscera edema can be enormous, particularly in patients with peritonitis. During phase II, patients can develop an abdominal compartment hypertension syndrome, prompting many surgeons to avoid tight closure of the abdomen by inserting a prosthesis (Fig. 5-10).[85] Lucas[14] attributed the expansion of interstitial volume during phase II to an alteration in the interstitial matrix. Shires and coworkers[78] attributed the events after shock to impaired sodium pump activity at the cell membrane and subsequent cell swelling. Other investigators have suggested the increases in microvascular membrane permeability may contribute to widespread fluid gain during phase II. During phase II, occult hypoperfusion may jeopardize the recovery of a patient. Claridge and associates[22] reported that delayed correction of an elevated lactic acid level indicates occult hypoperfusion.

The final recovery phase after hemorrhagic shock begins with negative fluid balance. *Phase III* involves a diuretic period when the excess fluid gained during phase II is mobilized and excreted by the kidneys. The onset of phase III should occur within 2 to 4 days of phase I, and failure of phase III onset may indicate that the patient either has developed a complication (usually sepsis) or, in the case of patients with preexisting heart disease, may have limited cardiac reserve and would benefit from diuretic therapy or inotropic drugs.

In summary, the treatment of hypovolemic shock has two components: repleting blood volume and interventions that terminate the pathologic events that incited the hypovolemia. Patients should follow a sequence of events after an episode of shock, and clinicians should investigate for complications in those patients who deviate from the expected pattern of recovery from hemorrhagic shock.

SHOCK FROM SEPSIS

Shock associated with the sepsis syndrome is a common cause of death in surgical intensive care units. In 1995, Rangel-Frausto estimated that over 500,000 patients with serious sepsis and shock are treated annually in hospitals in the United States.[86] Angus and associates, in 2001, projected that, because of the aging United States population, over 1 million patients will be threatened each year by shock associated with sepsis by the year 2010.[87] The hospital mortality rate from hypotension associated with sepsis is over 35%, and the long-term death rate for patients who had sustained septic shock exceeds 45%.[88]

Surgeons treating patients with septic shock must consider several issues. First, the patient must be resuscitated from shock. Second, the source of infection and pathogens must either be identified or predicted pending culture results. Patients in septic shock should receive antibiotics effective against the documented or suspected invading organisms. The surgeon's third problem is to decide whether the sepsis is caused by a condition requiring surgical intervention. To have an optimal probability of survival, patients with an abscess and shock commonly require resuscitation of intravascular volume deficits, antibiotics, and drainage or extirpation of the site of infection. Patients in shock from sepsis are at risk for subsequent multiple organ failure. Research over the past 30 years has supported the hypothesis that multiple organ failure can be caused by an exaggerated endogenous inflammatory response to invasive infection.[89] Ultimate survival of the infected patient in shock may depend on therapies that ameliorate the immune response while the patient retains the capacity to kill invading microorganisms.

Systemic Inflammatory Response Syndrome: A Spectrum of Clinical Disease

Bone and colleagues convened a consensus conference to define criteria for categorization of sepsis-related inflammatory response.[30] The results of their deliberations were published in 1992, and these definitions have been widely used in subsequent studies to categorize inflammatory responses to infection (Box 5-3). These authors defined four categories of clinical disease that represented successive levels of escalating severity of inflammatory response. The core concept of Bone and colleagues was that as the burden of bacterial toxins increases and the extent of endogenous inflammatory response intensifies, the clinical manifestations of the severity of illness become exaggerated and the risk of death increases.

The consensus conference described the response to infection as beginning with a systemic inflammatory response syndrome (SIRS) characterized by fever, tachycardia, and tachypnea. SIRS is not exclusively a reaction to infection but can also be observed in response to the sterile insults of pancreatitis, aspiration pneumonitis, or burn injury. To meet the criteria of SIRS, patients must have two or more of the clinical conditions identified in the consensus conference and subsequently validated in clinical studies. Patients with clinical sepsis meet the SIRS criteria and also have a documented infection. This category reflects the observation that some patients with clear clinical evidence of being infected never have a bacterial, fungal, or viral pathogen cultured. Patients with severe sepsis meet the criteria of sepsis and have become hypotensive; these patients exhibit signs of hypoperfusion, including lactic acidemia, oliguria, and depressed level of consciousness. Patients with severe sepsis should be resuscitated by intravenous infusion of balanced electrolyte solution. Many respond with improved perfusion and restored organ function. Patients who remain hypotensive despite adequate intravenous fluid infusion have the most lethal of the four categories: septic shock. Patients in septic shock have organ dysfunction that may progress to organ failure. Although hypotension may respond to resuscitation with inotropic and vasoactive drugs, these patients are at immediate risk for death from shock.

Patients with an exaggerated inflammatory response to uncontrolled infection risk progression from the mild SIRS to the lethal problem of septic shock. Rangel-Frausto and associates reported a prospective study of a large cohort of patients treated in tertiary care hospitals. Sixty-eight percent of patients treated in the ICUs developed one or more of the SIRS criteria.[86] These authors determined the natural histories of SIRS patients with 1-month follow-up: 61% progressed and met the criteria of sepsis, 18% developed severe sepsis, and 4% developed septic shock. Patients had a greater risk for death if they progressed into successive categories (Table 5-5). Other factors in SIRS patients associated with an increased risk of death include the number of failed organs (pulmonary, renal, cardiac, and coagulopathy) and hypothermia. Arons and coworkers reported that while the prevalence of hypothermia was only 10% among a group of patients with severe sepsis, the mortality of hypothermic patients was twice that of hyperthermic patients.[90]

Clinical Observations; Patterns of Infection and Organisms

The majority of SIRS patients have a clinically suspected or culture-positive proven site of infection. Sands and associates reported that the four most prevalent sites of infection at university medical centers were, in order of prevalence, pulmonary, bloodstream, genitourinary tract, and intra-abdominal wounds.[88] Among patients with sepsis or severe sepsis, Rangel-Frausto and associates reported bloodstream infections in 17% of patients with sepsis, in 25% of patients with severe sepsis, and in 69% of patients with septic shock.[86]

Hadley and colleagues, who studied a placebo group of 930 patients in the North American Septic Shock Trial,

---

Box 5-3. Criteria for Four Categories of Systemic Inflammatory Response Syndrome

Systemic Inflammatory Response Syndrome (SIRS)

Two or more of the following:

- Temperature (core) above 38° or below 36°
- Heart rate over 90 beats/min
- Respiratory rate of over 20 breaths/min for patients spontaneously ventilating, of $Paco_2$ <32 torr
- WBC count >12,000 cells/mm^3, or <4000 cells/mm^3, or >10% immature (band) cells in peripheral blood smear

Sepsis

Same criteria as SIRS with clearly established focus of infection

Severe Sepsis

Sepsis associated with organ dysfunction and hypoperfusion

Indicators of hypoperfusion:

- Systolic blood pressure <90 torr
- >40 torr fall from normal systolic blood pressure
- Lactic acidemia
- Oliguria
- Acute mental status changes

Septic Shock

Patients with severe sepsis who:

- Are not responsive to intravenous fluid infusion for resuscitation
- Require inotropic or vasopressor agents to maintain systolic blood pressure

TABLE 5-5. Categories of Systemic Inflammatory Response Syndromes among 857 Patients Treated in Surgical Intensive Care Settings

	Culture Positive*	Culture Negative†	Death Prevalence(%)†
Sepsis	305	165	16-10
Severe sepsis	260	130	20-16
Septic shock	40	22	46

* Indicates incidence density as episodes per 1000 patient-days.
† Death rates for culture-positive and culture-negative subgroups.
Adapted from Rangel-Frausto MS, Pitter D, Costigan M, et al: The natural history of the systemic inflammatory response syndrome. JAMA 273:117, 1995.

summarized the bacteria responsible for septic shock.[91] Among 392 patients with positive blood cultures, 44% had gram-positive species, 44% had gram-negative species, and 3% had fungemia (only *Candida* species). The remaining patients were infected by mixed species of organisms. The top three gram-positive organisms included *Staphylococcus aureus*, *Enterococcus* species, and coagulase-negative *Staphylococcus* species. The three most prevalent gram-negative species were *Escherichia coli*, *Klebsiella* species, and *Pseudomonas aeruginosa*. These findings indicate that clinicians managing patients with a new diagnosis of SIRS should obtain blood cultures, as well as cultures from suspected sites of infection before instituting empirical therapy with antibiotics. Given the diversity in bacteria associated with SIRS, surgeons treating a patient with serious infection may need to initially order broad-spectrum antibiotics with the understanding that effective antibiotic therapy may prevent the progression to septic shock.

Empirical antifungal therapy should not be routinely given unless the patient is immunosuppressed. Pelz and coworkers tested the value of prophylactic antifungal therapy (fluconazole, 800-mg loading dose with 400-mg daily dose) given to high-risk patients in a surgical ICU. The therapy was well tolerated and may have reduced the prevalence of serious fungal infection by 55%; however, these researchers were unable to demonstrate an improved survival rate by routinely adding antifungal therapy to antibacterial therapy.[92] Finally, although invading microorganisms are the most common cause of severe sepsis and septic shock, 20% to 40% of patients with these syndromes do not have culture-positive sites of infection. This indicates that toxins released by bacteria killed by antibiotics are capable of provoking the inflammatory response. Duration and choice of antibiotics in these patients is determined by clinical response.

SIRS as an Exaggerated Inflammatory Response

The normal response to microbial invasion encompasses a complex immune response that involves circulating immune cells (e.g., neutrophils, macrophages, and lymphocytes), the activation of coagulation and complement cascades, and biochemical alterations within constitutive cells (e.g., endothelial cells and fibroblasts). The bene-

cial consequence of the inflammatory response is destruction or at least containment of invading microorganisms. On the other hand, a major hypothesis regarding severe sepsis and septic shock holds that damage to organs remote from those infected is caused by an excessive and unmitigated inflammatory response of endogenous immune mechanisms (Fig. 5-11).[93,94]

Cytokines are protein molecules produced by activated inflammatory cells that function as messengers and incite production of intermediate metabolites. Proinflammatory cytokines include TNF-α, IL-1, and IL-8, which induce endothelial cell production of proteases, nitric oxide release, coagulation pathway activation, vasoactive arachidonic acid metabolite production, and increased microvascular membrane permeability, which leads to edema. Cytokines also activate neutrophils, the cells that engulf and destroy invading pathogens with oxygen radicals and proteases. Mediators of bacterial destruction can be released by activated neutrophils that adhere to endothelium in organs remote from the site of infection (e.g., the pulmonary circulation) where the mediators damage the endothelial cells and structural components of the interstitium. Neutrophil-mediated injury is thought to be a major source of organ damage and dysfunction in patients with severe sepsis and septic shock.[89] In circumstances of increased numbers of activated neutrophils, proinflammatory cytokine release can overwhelmingly activate the entire inflammatory cascade and cause profound hypotension. Therapies that reduce neutrophil capacity may reduce the risk of remote organ damage in patients with septic shock but introduce the risk of impaired immunocompetency.[95] Anti-inflammatory cytokines suppress the immune response to infection, injury, and shock. There is evidence that in selected patients overwhelming sepsis and death may be caused by failure to provide a robust resistance to bacterial toxins.[93] In summary, successful treatment of a patient at risk from severe sepsis and septic shock requires careful assessment of the individual. The source of infection must be treated promptly by appropriate antibiotics in therapeutic doses, and effective, appropriate surgical intervention should be performed. In immunosuppressed patients, immune-enhancing treatments such as granulocyte-stimulating factor are indicated. The treatment of shock due to sepsis must be individualized.

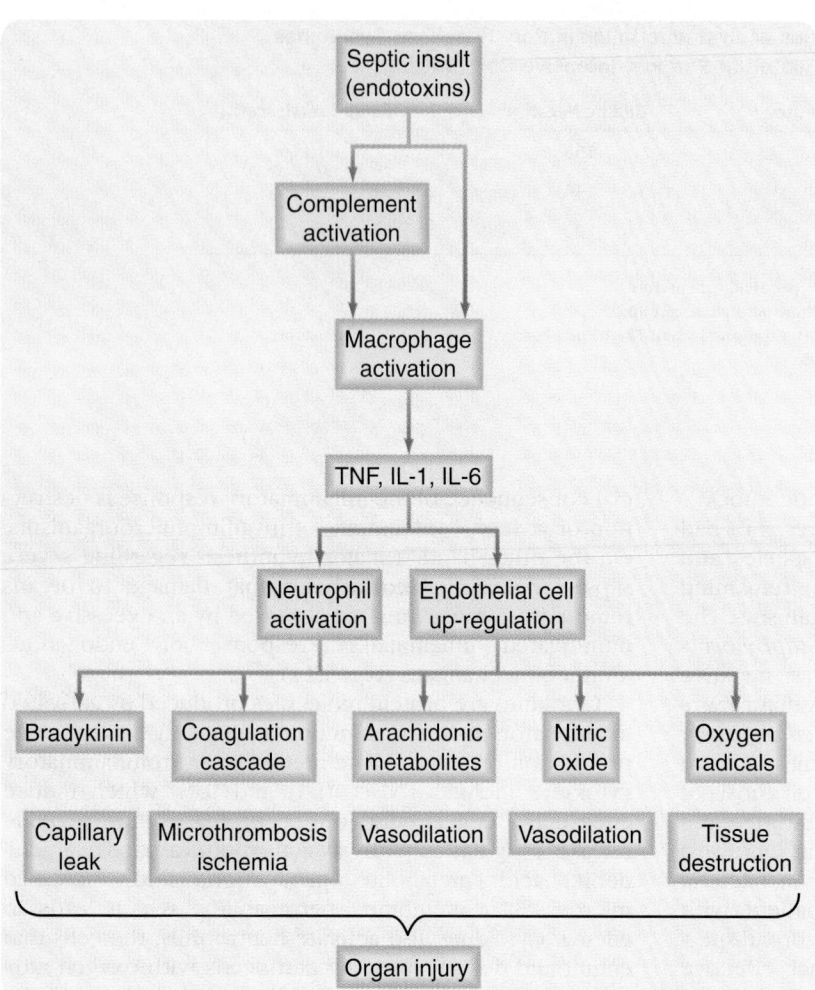

FIGURE 5-11.   Septic shock-mediated inflammatory cascade.

Pathogenetic Mechanisms of Shock in Patients With Sepsis

Patients with severe sepsis or septic shock commonly suffer hypotension due to arteriolar vasodilation. Hyperdynamic patterns in patients with septic shock have been measured with pulmonary artery catheters. Typically, these patients have cardiac outputs twice normal, and their hypotension corresponds to marked reductions in systemic vascular resistance attributed to uncontrolled vasodilation in organs with high capillary densities, such as skeletal muscle. Patients in septic shock have markedly elevated cardiac outputs; however, owing to hypotension, effective perfusion is deficient to the critical organs such as the heart, liver, and brain. Patients in septic shock can die within a few hours resistant to interventions intended to increase systemic vascular resistance and, thus, mean arterial pressure. Although most patients in refractory septic shock have profound vasodilation, a minority of patients are severely hypovolemic and have marked vasoconstriction and low-flow shock (Table 5-6).

Impaired function of the smooth muscle cells that surround arterioles has been identified as one mechanism

TABLE 5-6.   Hemodynamic Characteristics of Patients in Septic Shock*

Characteristic	Mean	Minimum	Maximum
Heart rate (beats/min)	121	47	142
MAP (mm Hg)	60	48	66
PCWP (mm Hg)	14	8	20
CI (L/min/m²)	4.2	3.0	5.6
SVRI (dynes cm⁻⁵ sec/m²)	868	675	1110
O_2 delivery (mL/min/m²)	498	344	573
O_2 consumption (mL/min/m²)	141	101	183

*Average of mean values reported in 11 manuscripts describing findings in patients with severe sepsis or septic shock.
MAP, mean arterial pressure; PCWP, pulmonary capillary wedge pressure; CI, cardiac index; SVRI, systemic vascular resistance index calculated as the mean systemic arterial pressure minus right atrial pressure divided by cardiac index; O_2 delivery, cardiac index multiplied by arterial oxygen content; O_2 consumption, cardiac index multiplied by arterial oxygen content minus venous oxygen content.

for vasodilatory shock.[96] Patients in septic shock release inflammatory mediators from endothelial cells and activated phagocytes, which impairs the capacity of vascular smooth muscle cells to constrict in response to catecholamines and angiotensin II, two vasoconstrictors normally generated in response to hypotension. In a normal response, these vascular smooth muscle cells bind norepinephrine and angiotensin II with cell surface receptors, which triggers an increase in intracellular Ca^{2+}. Nitric oxide is a potent but effervescent vasodilator synthesized and released into adjacent interstitial fluid by endothelial cells. In response to hypoxia and inflammation caused by invasive infection, an upregulation of enzymes that generate nitric oxide occurs, and nitric oxide release is increased. In addition to elevated levels of nitric oxide, patients in septic shock exhibit depressed plasma levels of arginine vasopressin, perhaps owing to impaired neurohypophyseal function in response to the infection.[96] Treatment of humans in vasodilatory shock with administration of nonselective nitric oxide synthetase inhibitors has been unsuccessful, perhaps because of the multiple effects of nitric oxide on tissues other than smooth muscle.[97]

Myocardial dysfunction is a second major factor contributing to hypotension in patients with septic shock. Despite the high cardiac output of patients in septic shock, cardiac function becomes impaired. Parrillo summarized the clinical evidence in support of myocardial dysfunction and proposed that a pathogenetic sequence of events led to shock in infected patients.[98] Endotoxins and exotoxins release endogenous mediators of inflammation that, when circulating in the blood, impair cardiac myocytes. Right and left ventricular end-systolic dilation was demonstrated in the hearts of septic, hypotensive patients. Using radionuclide gated blood-pool scanning, Parrillo and colleagues measured cardiac dysfunction in

patients in septic shock and demonstrated that despite adequate pulmonary artery wedge pressures, ejection fraction averaged only 33%, compared with an ejection fraction of 50% in control patients.[98] Among patients who recovered from septic shock, cardiac function returned to normal with an improvement in ejection fraction to 60%. Parrillo and colleagues provided convincing evidence that a substance circulating in the blood accounts for the suppression in myocardial function in patients in septic shock (Fig. 5-12).[99] Kumar and associates proposed that TNF-α and IL-1 (elevated during sepsis) had direct toxic effects on contracting cardiac muscle[100] and speculated that effective therapy that neutralizes these mediators of myocardial depression will eventually be devised.

Resuscitation of Impaired Hemodynamics in Patients With Septic Shock

Persistently hypotensive patients who meet the definition of septic shock should be managed with the assistance of invasive hemodynamic monitoring, including pulmonary artery catheters. The first step in resuscitation involves intravenous infusion of fluid to restore intravascular volume deficits; in most patients, full restoration is achieved when pulmonary artery wedge pressures stabilize between 15 and 20 mm Hg. Successful resuscitation is demonstrated by preservation of normal renal function and resolution of metabolic (often lactic) acidosis.[89] Patients in septic shock may require large volumes of fluid to achieve full resuscitation. Crystalloid fluids equal in volume to 10% of the body weight have been reported as necessary to restore central venous pressure. Balanced electrolyte solutions are the preferred resuscitation fluids for patients with severe sepsis and septic shock.[84] However, investigators have shown that infusions of

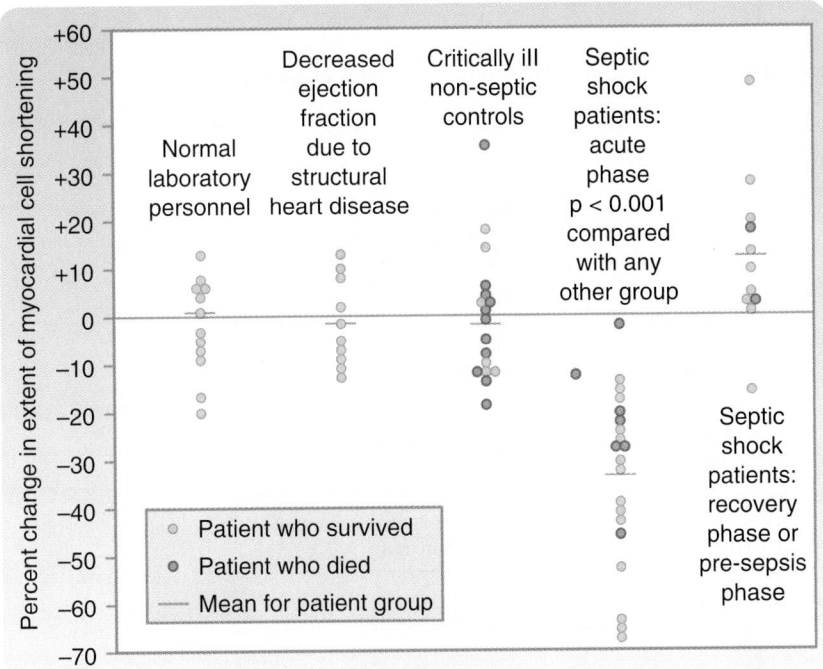

FIGURE 5-12. Suppression of myocardial cell function specifically by serum of patients in septic shock. (From Parrillo JE, Burch C, Shelhamer JH, et al: A circulating myocardial depressant substance in humans with septic shock: Septic shock patients with a reduced ejection fraction have a circulating factor that depresses in vitro myocardial cell performance. J Clin Invest 76:1539-1553, 1985. Copyright 1985, Journal of Clinical Investigation. Reproduced with permission in the format Textbook via Copyright Clearance Center.)

colloid solutions can achieve greater cardiac filling pressures for each milliliter of infused fluid than can crystalloid solutions. A more complex method to determine optimal volume expansion requires plotting the increase in left ventricular stroke work index (LVSWI) in response to volume loading. When the LVSWI plateaus despite further fluid infusions, the surgeon should conclude that the intravascular volume has been fully restored.[101] Patients who remain hypotensive despite increased pulmonary artery wedge pressure should be infused with inotropic agents.

Patients with restored intravascular volume who remain in septic shock should be given drugs to improve cardiac function, namely, dopamine, dobutamine, and epinephrine (Table 5-7). These three inotropic agents have different pharmacologic modes of action. Epinephrine and dobutamine increase cardiac contractility through β-adrenergic mechanisms; epinephrine also carries an α-adrenergic effect. Dopamine at lower doses has an inotropic effect through dopaminergic receptors.[102]

Dopamine binds to dopamine receptors and β-adrenergic receptors at doses of 2 to 20 μg/kg/min but provides a greater α-adrenergic effect at higher doses. In 1994, Marik and coworkers reported that dopamine infusion into patients with septic shock, despite an expanded intravascular volume, effectively increased mean arterial blood pressure.[103] This increase in pressure was due to an inotropic influence on the myocardium. These authors observed that, by all criteria of hemodynamic performance, dopamine infusion rates of 2 to 20 μg/kg/min improved patient status. However, the authors expressed the concern that dopamine caused an uncompensated increase in splanchnic oxygen consumption. In a subsequent study, Marik and Iglesias examined the influence of dopamine infusions on patients with septic shock and oliguria and found no evidence of benefit as determined by the criteria of improved renal function. These studies support the conclusion that dopamine may have a favorable influence on hemodynamic parameters, but surgeons must remain open to the possibility that drugs that alter one parameter may have unintended consequences on another.

Dobutamine is a β-adrenergic agonist that not only increases contractility of the myocardium but also may have a vasodilatory effect at doses of 5 to 15 μg/kg/min. Hayes and coworkers reported dobutamine infusion increased cardiac index and oxygen delivery in patients in septic shock but that dobutamine treatment did not have a survival advantage.[101] The authors divided patients into two categories: those who increased oxygen consumption when delivery increased, and those who did not. The authors concluded that for an inotropic drug infusion to save patients at risk for death from septic shock, the cellular apparatus necessary for aerobic metabolism must be intact; in other words, increasing the oxygen delivery to dysfunctional cells is futile in septic patients. This conclusion implies that early resuscitation is critical to avoid the onset of an irreversible defect in cellular biochemical function. The authors of this study also raised the concern that infusion of very large doses of dobutamine can be stressful to cardiac function and detrimental.

Epinephrine infused usually in doses of 1 to 20 μg/min acts as a powerful α- and β-adrenergic agonist. Epinephrine was compared with dobutamine-plus-norepinephrine infusion in a randomized controlled trial that studied patients in septic shock.[104] Patients infused with epinephrine experienced similar improvements in hemodynamic status as the patients infused with the two-drug regimen. Both treatment groups increased mean arterial pressure and cardiac index and showed reduced oxygen extraction ratios with increased oxygen delivery; a reduced extraction ratio corresponds to improved intra-

TABLE 5-7.   Vasoactive Drugs Reported as Therapeutic in Shock in Adults*

Drug	Range of Dose	Principal Mechanism[†]
INOTROPIC AGENTS (MAY BE CHRONOTROPIC)		
Dobutamine	2-20 μg/kg/min	β_1-adrenergic
Dopamine (low dose)	5-10 μg/kg/min	β_1-adrenergic: dopaminergic
Epinephrine (low dose)	0.06-0.20 μg/kg/min	β_1 and β_2-adrenergic: less α
VASOCONSTRICTOR AND INOTROPIC AGENT		
Dopamine (high dose)	>10 μg/kg/min	α-adrenergic: less dopaminergic
Epinephrine (high dose)	0.21-0.42 μg/kg/min	α-adrenergic: less β_1 and β_2
Norepinephrine	0.02-0.25 μg/kg/min	α-adrenergic: less β_1 and β_2
VASOCONSTRICTOR		
Phenylephrine	0.2-2.5 μg/kg/min	α-adrenergic
Vasopressin	0.4-0.10 units/min	V1 receptor
VASODILATOR		
Milrinone	0.4-0.6 μg/kg/min	Phosphodiesterase inhibitor[‡]
Dopamine (very low dose)	1-4 μg/kg/min	Dopaminergic

*An individual patient's response to a given drug or dose is variable

[†]α and β refer to adrenergic agonists. β_1-adrenergic effects are inotropic and increase contractility. β_2-adrenergic effects are chronotropic.

[‡]After loading dose of 50 μg/kg/min over 10 minutes.

cellular oxygen tensions. The key difference between these two groups was that epinephrine-treated patients had higher gastric mucosal blood flows. The authors hypothesized that higher rates of mesenteric circulation reduced the risk of gut-induced multiple organ dysfunctions. They concluded that adrenergic effective pharmacologic therapy for septic shock depends jointly on the drug and the dose. Clinicians treating patients should monitor the individual's hemodynamic response to select the optimal drug and dose.

Patients in septic shock commonly have profound vasodilatation and often appear flushed and have pink, well-perfused digits with brisk capillary refill despite being hypotensive. Vasodilatory shock can be clinically demonstrated by a pulmonary artery catheter measurement of high cardiac output and a low calculated systemic vascular resistance (Table 5-6). These patients will increase their mean arterial pressures if given vasoconstrictors. Improved systolic blood pressure can be accomplished in these patients by infusing a vasoconstrictor agent; the two most commonly used drugs are α-adrenergic agents and vasopressin.

α-Adrenergic agents used effectively in patients with vasodilatory shock include norepinephrine and phenylephrine. Infusion of norepinephrine is most beneficial when attempting to selectively vasoconstrict noncritical vascular beds (e.g., skin and skeletal muscle) with the consequence of increasing mean aortic pressure and improving the perfusion of renal, cerebral, and cardiac circulations. As an alternative, phenylephrine which has a pure α_1 effect, may be used in vasodilatory shock. In several studies reporting multiple drug therapy for the treatment of hemodynamic consequences of septic shock, norepinephrine has been used as a second drug to control systemic vascular resistance, whereas another drug was used to influence contractility.[101,104]

Vasopressin infusion has been reported as an effective treatment of vasodilatory shock.[105] This peptide is an antidiuretic hormone synthesized in the hypothalamus and released from the posterior pituitary in response to several stimuli, including increased ECW osmolality, hypoxia, pain, and baroreceptor-detected hypotension. V1 receptors on the surface of smooth muscle cells that surround blood vessels bind circulating vasopressin. Vascular smooth muscles contract, causing constriction of the arteriole vascular lumen. Skin, skeletal muscle, and fat are three tissues that contain arterioles responsive to vasopressin. Evidence indicates that patients with sustained septic shock (over hours) deplete endogenous vasopressin stores. These observations explain why vasopressin infused into patients with catecholamine-resistant septic shock can reverse vasodilation. Arginine vasopressin (AVP) is an alternative vasoconstrictor agent in patients with refractory hypotension from vasodilatory shock.[105]

Many reports regarding the range of medications used to provide hemodynamic support to patients in septic shock have been published (see Table 5-7). Whereas randomized controlled trials suggest a specific drug or combination of drugs as more effective, an individual's response may vary. Thus, the surgeon resuscitating a patient must monitor hemodynamic responses and adjust therapies as indicated. One may resuscitate these patients by following a protocol specific to the selected intervention. Rivers and colleagues reported that patients in septic shock who presented to an emergency department benefited from the successful implementation of a protocol intended to rapidly achieve a balance of oxygen delivery and demand.[106] Patients in the protocol were resuscitated within 6 hours of arrival in the emergency department and compared with patients whose resuscitation began when admitted to the ICU. The death rate for protocol patients was 30%, compared with 45% in the control group. Patients in shock from sepsis resuscitated according to an efficient protocol are protected from a prolonged insult and avoid irreversible cellular damage. Guiding principles in the resuscitation of any patient in septic shock must include the adjustment of fluid infusions, selection of vasoactive drugs, and modulation of drug doses based on the individual patient's response. Thus, invasive hemodynamic monitoring is essential in complex patients to determine the effectiveness of interventions intended to restore delivery of oxygen to tissues. As a final consideration in the treatment of any patient in septic shock, resuscitation often is futile without amelioration of the source of sepsis (Box 5-4).

Anti-inflammatory Treatment for Severe Sepsis and Septic Shock

As sepsis progresses to severe sepsis and septic shock, the risk for organ failure increases in proportion to excessive activation of the inflammatory cascade. Over the past 10

Box 5-4. A Protocol for Resuscitation of the Adult Patient in Septic Shock

Hypotensive and suspected sepsis?
  Culture relevant body fluids including blood.
  Infuse balanced electrolyte solution of 500 cc/15 minutes. Monitor systolic blood pressure response.
  Insert central venous or pulmonary artery catheter.
  If, after bolus 500 cc of saline, patient remains hypotensive, and CVP less than 8-12 mm Hg or PAWP less than 8-12 mm Hg, then infuse another 500 cc bolus of fluid; repeat as needed.
  If CVP is over 15 or PAWP 15-20 and patient remains hypotensive (less than 65), start infusion of the inotropes, dobutamine or dopamine. Goal is mean systemic pressure over 65 and pulse rate less than 120 beats/min.
  Determine cardiac index and systemic vascular resistance.
  If, after fluid and infusion and inotropes, the SVR is under 600 then infuse vasopressor—either norepinephrine or vasopressin to increase SVR.
  Monitor mixed venous oxygen saturation and urine output as an indication that therapeutic interventions have improved perfusion.

TABLE 5-8.　Hemodynamic Characteristics of Patients in Cardiogenic Shock

Anterior myocardial infarction	60.5%
Median time from myocardial infarction to shock	5.6 hr
Lowest systolic blood pressure	88 mm Hg
Lowest diastolic blood pressure	54 mm Hg
Heart rate	102 beats/min
Pulmonary-capillary wedge pressure	24 mm Hg
Cardiac index	1.75 L/min/m²
Left ventricular ejection fraction	31%
Number of diseased coronary vessels	
1	13%
2	23%
3	64%
Left main coronary artery disease	20%

Adapted from Hochman JS, Sleeper LA, Webb JG, et al: Early revascularization in acute myocardial infarction complicated by cardiogenic shock. SHOCK Investigators. Should we emergently revascularize occluded coronaries for cardiogenic shock? N Engl J Med 341:625-634, 1999.

years, multiple clinical investigators have reported several large randomized controlled trials intended to evaluate the safety and effectiveness of a variety of agents designed to modulate inflammation. Until a report in 2001 by Bernard and colleagues, results of multicenter trials have been disappointing. These investigators compared the 28-day survival of patients in severe sepsis who received either placebo or recombinant human activated protein C (APC).[107] This anticoagulant agent inhibits thrombosis and accelerates fibrinolysis. Furthermore, this protein blocks tissue factor monocyte activation and cytokine release. The trial showed a significant reduction in mortality rates from 31% to 25% with APC treatment. Although recombinant human APC increased the prevalence of bleeding complications from 2% to 3.5%, this genetically engineered protein did favorably alter the capacity to survive overwhelming infection.

Previous trials of anti-inflammatory therapies had failed to show improved survival. For example, therapies intended to neutralize TNF-α failed to enhance survival rates, although a trend toward improved survival was observed in the subset of patients with markedly elevated IL-6 levels.[108,109] Similar studies using drugs to neutralize inflammatory mediators such as IL-1, platelet-activating factor, and bradykinin have been undertaken; disappointingly, large randomized controlled trials did not show improved survival rates of treated patients over those who received placebo. Large doses of ibuprofen, which inhibits cyclooxygenase, infused into septic patients did substantially reduce prostacyclin and thromboxane synthesis. While fever, tachycardia, and lactic acidosis all improved, no improvement in 28-day survival was observed, and both groups had 38% mortality rates.[110] Multiple trials of a range of anti-inflammatory therapies have demonstrated that therapies targeted to influence specific components of the immune response and inflammatory

cascade can have the intended focal impact. However, these interventions may not improve survival because the machinery of exaggerated inflammation is complex and multiple parallel events interact. Thus, altering one component fails to achieve overall change and durable benefit. Future treatments may be more effective if these therapies (e.g., recombinant human APC) influence several components of the inflammatory response at multiple sites.

Severe sepsis has been demonstrated to cause relative adrenal insufficiency, defined as impaired glucocorticoid response to adrenal cortex stimulation. Annane and colleagues reported that treatment of patients in septic shock with low doses of hydrocortisone and fludrocortisone reduced risk of death at 28 days.[111] Specifically benefiting were those patients who required catecholamines to support hemodynamic function and were classified as "nonresponders" to corticotropin stimulation tests. Nonresponders included those patients whose serum cortisol levels increased less than 9 μg/dL; these patients were considered to have a sepsis-related dysfunction in the hypothalamic-pituitary-adrenal axis. Among treated patients, death rates were 53% compared with 63% in the placebo group. The authors emphasized that the benefit of adrenal steroid therapy in their protocol was related to reversal of adrenal insufficiency and that this therapeutic goal contrasted to other studies in which immunosuppressive doses of glucocorticoids failed to improve survival rates of patients in septic shock.[112]

SHOCK FROM CARDIAC DISEASE

Surgical patients develop acute hypotension as a consequence of several cardiac diseases that share the general problem that cardiac output from the left ventricle is inadequate. The conditions that cause cardiogenic shock have variable pathophysiologic characteristics, but all are highly lethal. Successful treatment must be directed to correct the specific cause. To identify the correct treatment, patients in cardiogenic shock need a systematic diagnostic work-up that is accomplished rapidly. The patient's history regarding the current illness and previous cardiac diseases, a physical examination, an electrocardiogram, and a few laboratory tests can lead the surgeon to the specific diagnosis. In selected patients, cardiac echocardiography or coronary artery angiography is required to establish the anatomic cause for shock and the precise nature of cardiac pump dysfunction.

Shock From Acute Myocardial Infarction

Seven to 10 percent of patients with an acute myocardial infarction develop cardiogenic shock, and 70% of patients die who develop cardiogenic shock.[113] Sudden occlusion of a coronary artery leads to myocardial ischemia, and typically patients complain of chest pain, unless the patient is sedated or under general anesthesia, in which case the indication of myocardial ischemia may be hypotension, arrhythmia, or ECG changes. Blood flow through coronary arteries stops, and myocardial infarction will occur owing to vessel occlusion and secondary hemorrhage beneath an atherosclerotic plaque that displaces the plaque and obstructs the vessel's lumen. Troponins are contractile proteins in myocytes that are released when infarction occurs. The ECG evidence that a patient has ischemic myocardium includes ST segment depression, which is ischemic. Patients with myocardial infarction have new onset of left bundle branch block and develop Q waves. An elevation in serum concentration of troponin within 8 hours of the initial symptoms or signs is a sensitive indicator of myocardial damage. Cardiogenic shock occurs in patients with acute occlusion of the left main or right main coronary artery or multiple occlusions.

Patients who develop cardiogenic shock after a myocardial infarction typically have onset of symptoms 6 to 12 hours after initial angina symptoms. Poor contractility of the left ventricular wall results in impaired development of pressures within the ventricular chamber and a decline in cardiac ejection fraction. Other causes of severe cardiac dysfunction associated with myocardial infarction are acute mitral regurgitation, rupture of the interventricular septum, or, rarely, right ventricular dysfunction. Patients in cardiogenic shock typically have a systolic blood pressure less than 90 mm Hg, distended neck veins, and dyspnea associated with audible rales. These patients look desperately ill and typically have a gray or cyanotic face, diaphoresis, vasoconstricted extremities, weakly palpable pulses, and decreased level of consciousness.[114] In addition to hemodynamic deterioration, patients with cardiogenic shock are at risk for lethal arrhythmias.

Cardiogenic shock can be confirmed by echocardiography, which demonstrates poorly contractile left ventricle, or passing a pulmonary artery catheter, which reveals pulmonary artery wedge pressure over 20 mm Hg and cardiac index under 2.0 L/min/m². Initial therapy in patients with myocardial ischemia should include oxygen, nitroglycerin, aspirin, and adequate intravenous morphine to provide pain relief and reduce anxiety.[115] Patients in cardiogenic shock may need an intra-aortic balloon pump to sustain perfusion while more definitive therapies are planned.

Multiple studies have confirmed that fibrinolytic therapy (i.e., tissue plasminogen activator) improves the survival of patients having acute myocardial ischemia. Fibrinolytic therapy is not effective in patients in established cardiogenic shock.[114] The best hope for long-term survival of patients is having a cardiologist or surgeon achieve coronary artery revascularization. Immediate cardiac catheterization and angioplasty, performed by experts, are able to restore perfusion in over 70% of occluded coronary arteries. Percutaneous transluminal coronary angiography with balloon dilatation and stent insertion across the plaque can avert cardiogenic shock. Antiplatelet therapy with the glycoprotein IIb/IIIa has been demonstrated to improve patency of coronary stent grafts. These revascularization procedures, as well as emergency coronary artery bypass surgery, are less effective in patients once cardiogenic shock has developed.[113] The key to successful definitive management of patients in cardiogenic shock is immediate revascularization by endovascular techniques or coronary artery bypass surgery. Cardiogenic shock can develop in patients who may develop a cardiac arrhythmia, and prompt conversion of the patient to normal sinus rhythm can correct the shock. Selected patients are best treated immediately with cardioversion. Correction of hypokalemia and hypomagnesemia may also improve probability of restoring a sinus rhythm that improves perfusion. A common problem in postoperative patients with acute coronary artery occlusion is that anticoagulation or fibrinolytic therapy increases the risk of postoperative hemorrhage. Coronary artery dilation and stent placement should be performed with the patient heparinized. In addition, infusion of fibrinolytic agents is associated with a substantial risk of serious wound bleeding. Thus, choosing a therapeutic intervention in a postoperative patient with an acute myocardial infarction is a complicated balance of risk and benefits.

Shock From Cardiac Tamponade and Cardiac Contusion

Injury to the heart can lead to rapid death from cardiogenic causes. A blow to the anterior chest that transmits substantial energy to the myocardium can cause myocardial hemorrhage and tissue edema. Cardiac contusion may be a common cause of immediate death to patients who sustain chest trauma in such high-energy circumstances as a motor vehicle crash. However, cardiac contusion is rarely the cause of shock in a blunt trauma patient who is hypotensive on arrival at a hospital's emergency department. Although several blood tests have been advocated for making the diagnosis of acute cardiac contusion, the cardiac echocardiogram is most specific.[116] Hypotensive patients who sustained chest trauma and have, by echocardiography, a dilated ventricular chamber associated with poor contractility of the wall have either a cardiac contusion to the ventricle or a proximal main coronary artery occlusion and an acute myocardial infarction in association with their episode of injury. Infusion of dobutamine, epinephrine, or dopamine may improve myocardial contraction in the patient with cardiac contusion and profound pump dysfunction. Intra-aortic balloon pump may provide temporary support while the contused cardiac muscle recovers.

Cardiac tamponade is a readily reversible cause of shock. Tamponade occurs when fluid or blood accumulates between the pericardium and heart. If pericardial fluid develops under significant pressure, filling of the heart cannot occur during diastole, and thus there is little blood within the ventricle available for ejection. Cardiac tamponade is principally a clinical problem in patients who have sustained penetrating chest trauma in proximity to the sternum. Knife or gunshot wounds that perforate the heart wall bleed; and as blood accumulates under pressure between the tough pericardium and the beating heart, heart size is compressed. Tamponade can occur after perforation of the heart during passage of a right-sided cardiac catheter. The physical findings in patients with cardiac tamponade are hypotension, distended neck veins, and pulsus paradoxus, defined as more than 10 mm Hg decline in systolic pressure at the end of the inspiratory phase of respiration. Echocardiography is an excellent diagnostic tool for identification of fluid or blood in the pericardium.[116] Patients with hemodynamically significant cardiac tamponade have compression of the atrium. Passage of a pulmonary artery catheter from the superior vena cava to the pulmonary artery through the right atrium and ventricle that shows equalization of pressures is an indication of hemodynamically significant cardiac tamponade. Aspiration of fluid or blood in the pericardial space can temporarily relieve the cardiac compression and improve systolic pressure. In most cases of trauma-related cardiac tamponade, patients need surgical exploration to relieve the tamponade and repair the heart wound that caused it.[117]

Shock From Massive Pulmonary Embolism

A massive pulmonary embolism can cause the acute onset of shock. A large clot that becomes impacted at the bifurcation, a central "saddle" pulmonary embolus, obstructs the flow of blood into the pulmonary artery. With the embolism there is insufficient delivery of blood to the left side of the heart, and systemic hypotension occurs as well as hypoxia. Right-sided heart failure has been identified as the usual cause of death. Echocardiogram shows an enlarged right ventricle. Clinical examination reveals distended neck veins and a tricuspid regurgitation murmur. The ECG findings indicate right ventricular strain with an $S_1Q_3T_3$ pattern, which means a prominent S wave in lead I and Q wave and T-wave inversion in lead III. Patients who are hypotensive with acute heart failure after an acute pulmonary embolus may benefit from infusion of inotropic agents that sustain cardiac output pending dissolution or removal of the emboli.

Intravenous heparin should be given to most patients in whom a diagnosis of acute pulmonary embolism has been established. Vena cava filters inserted into patients can trap additional emboli from residual lower extremity clots and avert the catastrophe of additional emboli. The effectiveness of thrombolytic therapy for massive pulmonary embolism has been established, but there is debate regarding the value of thrombolytic therapy for small pulmonary embolism not associated with shock.[118,119] Most recent thrombolytic studies have been conducted using as the thrombolytic agent, recombinant tissue-type plasminogen activator. For patients with recent wounds or incisions, bleeding complications are a risk after thrombolytic therapy. Embolectomy is an alternative to thrombolysis. Embolectomy can be performed through a sternotomy with the patient on cardiopulmonary bypass or by endovascular techniques.[120]

SHOCK FROM ADRENAL INSUFFICIENCY

Control of Adrenal Function

The two adrenal glands release hormones essential for life, and individuals with sudden stress depend on accelerated adrenal hormone release. For patients in shock, three adrenal hormones secreted into the blood have been defined as needed if the patient is to survive. Cortisol is released from the zona fasciculata of the adrenal cortex. Cortisol supports accelerated intracellular synthesis of proteins in response to stress and is crucial in the energy metabolism essential for maintenance of cell homeostasis. Cortisol release from the adrenal cortex can increase 5- to 10-fold under conditions of severe stress. The zona glomerulosa layer in the adrenal cortex secretes aldosterone, a mineralocorticoid essential in sustaining homeostasis of body sodium and potassium content and ECW volume. The adrenal medulla secretes epinephrine, a powerful α- and β-adrenergic agonist, which accelerates cardiac function and sustains vasomotor tone. Other organs control release of adrenal hormones. The hypothalamic-pituitary-adrenal axis enables the brain to direct the release of cortisol. Corticotropin-releasing hormone produced in the hypothalamus stimulates the release of corticotropin (ACTH) from the anterior pituitary. ACTH circulates in the blood to the adrenals and stimulates release of cortisol. The renin-angiotensin-aldosterone axis starts with cells of the juxtaglomerular apparatus of the kidney capable of responding to alterations in perfusion pressure. Cells in the juxtaglomerular apparatus release renin, which generates angiotensin, modified by pulmonary artery endothelial cells into angiotensin II. As the concentration of angiotensin II increases, more aldosterone is released from the adrenal cortex. Cardiovascular control centers in the brain stem through sympathetic nerves modulate release of epinephrine, which adjusts perfusion.

Primary and Secondary Adrenal Insufficiency

Primary adrenal insufficiency is a pathologic process of the adrenal gland. The critical nature of adrenal function is dramatically demonstrated by the rapid clinical deterioration of patients who have a sudden loss of adrenal function.[121] Patients have abrupt termination of adrenal hormone release after bilateral adrenalectomy, after acute infarction of both adrenal glands as occurs in meningococcal or other forms of overwhelming sepsis, or as a consequence of bilateral adrenal hemorrhage in an anticoagulated patient. Sudden hemorrhage of adrenal glands after idiopathic thrombosis of the adrenal veins causes acute hemorrhage into the two glands. Patients who suddenly have declining levels in blood of adrenal hormones experience the rapid onset of an abdominal pain syndrome, vomiting, and tender abdomen and rapidly deteriorate into irreversible hypotension. Two conditions associated with adrenal infarction in the postoperative patient are antiphospholipid antibody syndrome and heparin-associated thrombocytopenia.[122]

Secondary adrenal insufficiency occurs when there is injury or disease of the pituitary or hypothalamus.[121] Brain injury involving the skull base or pituitary surgery can suddenly terminate release of ACTH from the pituitary. A confounding event in these patients may be the onset of diabetes insipidus because AVP is neither synthesized in the hypothalamus nor released from the pituitary. A rare manifestation of this problem is the postpartum pituitary necrosis.

The clinical finding of patients who have sudden acute adrenal insufficiency can be nonspecific. Acute onset of hypocortisolemia leads to malaise, hyponatremia with hyperkalemia, and hypotension unresponsive to catecholamine infusion. Patients with this syndrome can die within hours unless they receive glucocorticoid replacement therapy. Treatment of glucocorticoid deficiency in the adult is intravenous infusion of 100 mg of hydrocortisone, which has an onset of action within 1 to 2 hours and a duration of action of 8 hours. Thus the commonly recommended replacement dose used in acute severe stress would be 100 mg intravenously every 8 hours with a rapid taper over the subsequent days as the patient's condition stabilizes. Other glucocorticoids used for intravenous replacement therapy include methylprednisolone and dexamethasone, which have been determined to have an anti-inflammatory milligram-per-milligram potency (relative to hydrocortisone of 1.0) of 5 and 25, respectively. Treatment of mineralocorticoid insufficiency in patients with primary adrenal failure can be accomplished by administration of 0.05 to 0.2 mg/day of 9α-fluorhydrocortisone.

Relative Adrenal Glucocorticoid Insufficiency

Adrenal glucocorticoid insufficiency, but not complete failure, occurs in patients with impaired function of their hypothalamic-pituitary-adrenal axis. These patients produce limited amounts of corticosteroids and develop clinical problems when stressed by hypovolemia from hemorrhage, onset of an infection, fear, or hypothermia. Thus the patient with chronic adrenal insufficiency may be initially diagnosed when he or she presents with intractable hypotension with a surgical emergency. The pathologic causes of chronic adrenal insufficiency include an autoimmune destruction of the adrenal gland, adrenalitis, in which cytotoxic lymphocytes gradually destroy the cortisol-synthesizing cells in the adrenal cortex. Patients with adrenalitis gradually develop fatigue, inanition, weight loss, and postural dizziness symptoms. These patients may have as a chief complaint vague crampy abdominal pain, nausea, and a change in bowel habits. Laboratory tests suggesting adrenal insufficiency are hyperkalemia, acidemia, hyponatremia, and an elevation in serum creatinine level. These laboratory findings are an indication of total body sodium deficit and a contracted ECW volume. To establish the diagnosis of adrenal insufficiency owing to end-organ failure requires the patient have a disproportionate elevation in ACTH in comparison to cortisol levels. In countries in which tuberculosis is still endemic, tuberculosis destruction of the adrenals is another pathologic condition that can cause the gradual onset of first adrenal insufficiency and then adrenal failure.

Adrenal insufficiency occurs in patients who have received long-term therapy with glucocorticoids.[123] Patients are given these drugs as immunosuppression after transplantation or to treat inflammatory conditions, including autoimmune diseases, inflammatory bowel disease, reactive airway disease, and arthritis. Because patients on these drugs have sustained elevations of circulating corticosteroids, corticotropin-releasing hormone synthesis by the hypothalamus is suppressed and ACTH release by the pituitary is impaired; with no stimulation delivered to cells in the adrenal cortex, the zona fasciculata cells atrophy. In circumstances of stress these patients may be unable to respond by an increased release of glucocorticoids required to meet the stress. Patients on glucocorticoids who have elective surgical procedures have been studied, and there is a variance in the extent of suppression in glucocorticoids. The recommended dosages of supplemental corticosteroids are adjusted to the severity of the surgical stress and remain debated.[123] Indicators that the dosage of corticosteroid is adequate are stable and adequate systolic blood pressure and a sustained normal serum sodium level.

Critical Adrenal Insufficiency in Sepsis

Annane and associates have reported evidence that severe sepsis and septic shock are associated with a relative adrenal insufficiency.[111] These investigators observed a cohort of patients with septic shock and could predict 28-day mortality rates based on the measure of response to intravenous corticotropin. Specifically, failure of the serum cortisol to increase more than 9 μg/dL at 30 or 60 minutes after corticotropin injection was associated with increased odds of death. In a randomized, prospective, placebo-controlled trial to evaluate the effectiveness of replacement therapy, these investigators administered low doses of hydrocortisone and fludrocortisone, a synthetic mineralocorticoid, to the treatment group for 7 days. This therapy improved survival of patients, specifically those with occult adrenal insufficiency. This study suggests that other patient groups besides those in septic shock may have relative adrenal insufficiency and that the use of provocative tests may be beneficial to determine who would benefit from adrenal hormone replacement.

Selected References

Lucas CE: Resuscitation through the three phases of hemorrhagic shock. Can J Surg 33:451, 1990.

> The author presents a description of the three phases that patients resuscitated from hemorrhagic shock with balanced electrolyte solution can be expected to follow. A pathophysiologic rationale to account for the temporal sequence is provided.

Parrillo JE: Pathogenic mechanisms of septic shock. N Engl J Med 328:1473, 1993.

> In this detailed and extensively referenced review, the author summarizes the physiologic characteristics of patients in shock with infection. The hyperdynamic pattern of perfusion and impaired cardiac function is described.

Renkin EM: Some consequences of capillary permeability to macromolecules: Starling's hypothesis reconsidered. Am J Physiol 250:H706, 1986.

> In this summary the physiologic and biochemical factors are defined that determine the balance of fluid and plasma protein solutes between the intervascular and interstitial spaces.

Shires T, Coln CD, Carrico CJ, Lightfoot S: Fluid therapy in hemorrhagic shock. Arch Surg 88:688, 1964.

> **This landmark article discusses the pathophysiologic influence of anaerobic insult associated with the hemorrhagic shock on sodium and water balance across the cell membrane, which is hypothesized to account for the need of a period of fluid and sodium gain after the reversal of hemorrhagic shock.**

Velanovich V: Crystalloid versus colloid fluid resuscitation: A meta-analysis of mortality. Surgery 105:65, 1989.

> **A meta-analysis provides a summary of published evidence reporting the effectiveness of crystalloid versus colloid fluid resuscitation in the management of patients in shock.**

References

1. Finn PJ, Plank LD, Clark MA, et al: Progressive cellular dehydration and proteolysis in critically ill patients. Lancet 347:654-656, 1996.
2. Chambrier C, Normand S, Ecochard R, et al: Total-body-water measurement with (18)O-labeled water in short-bowel patients with an ileostomy. Nutrition 17:287-291, 2001.
3. Forbes GB: Body composition: Overview. J Nutr 129(1S Suppl):270S-272S, 1999.
4. Chumlea WC, Guo SS, Zeller CM, et al: Total body water reference values and prediction equations for adults. Kidney Int 59:2250-2258, 2001.
5. Aloia JF, Vaswani A, Flaster E, Ma R: Relationship of body water compartments to age, race, and fat-free mass. J Lab Clin Med 132:483-490, 1998.
6. Halperin ML, Goldstein M: Fluid, Electrolyte, and Acid-Base Physiology: A Problem-based Approach, 3rd ed. Philadelphia, WB Saunders, 1999.
7. Hamadeh MJ, Robitaille L, Boismenu D, et al: Human extracellular water volume can be measured using the stable isotope Na234SO4. J Nutr 129:722-727, 1999.
8. De Lorenzo A, Andreoli A, Matthie J, Withers P: Predicting body cell mass with bioimpedance by using theoretical methods: A technological review. J App Physiol 82:1542-1558, 1997.
9. O'Brien C, Baker-Fulco CJ, Young AJ, Sawka MN: Bioimpedance assessment of hypohydration. Med Sci Sports Exerc 31:1466-1471, 1999.
10. Ishihara H, Matsui A, Muraoka M, et al: Detection of capillary protein leakage by indocyanine green and glucose dilutions in septic patients. Crit Care Med 28:620-626, 2000.
11. Svensen C, Hahn RG: Volume kinetics of Ringer solution, dextran 70, and hypertonic saline in male volunteers. Anesthesiology 87:204-212, 1997.
12. Gennari FJ: Hypokalemia. N Engl J Med 339:451-458, 1998.
13. Greger R: Physiology of renal sodium transport. Am J Med Sci 319:51-62, 2000.
14. Lucas CE: The water of life: A century of confusion. J Am Coll Surg 192:86-93, 2001.
15. Berendes E, Van Aken H, Raufhake C, et al: Differential secretion of atrial and brain natriuretic peptide in critically ill patients. Anesth Anal 93:676-682, 2001.
16. Levin ER, Gardner DG, Samson WK: Natriuretic peptides. N Engl J Med 339:321-328, 1998.
17. Adrogue HJ, Madias NE: Management of life-threatening acid-base disorders: Second of two parts. N Engl J Med 338:107-111, 1998.
18. Fencl V, Leith DE: Stewart's quantitative acid-base chemistry: Applications in biology and medicine. Respir Physiol 91(1):1-16, 1993.
19. Sirker AA, Rhodes A, Grounds RM, Bennett ED: Acid-base physiology: The "traditional" and the "modern" approaches. Anaesthesia 57:348-356, 2002.
20. Story DA, Poustie S, Bellomo R: Quantitative physical chemistry analysis of acid-base disorders in critically ill patients. Anaesthesia 56:530-533, 2001.
21. Luchette FA, Jenkins WA, Friend LA, et al: Hypoxia is not the sole cause of lactate production during shock. J Trauma 52:415-419, 2002.
22. Claridge JA, Crabtree TD, Pelletier SJ, et al: Persistent occult hypoperfusion is associated with a significant increase in infection rate and mortality in major trauma patients. J Trauma 48:8-14; discussion 14-15, 2000.
23. Abramson D, Scalea TM, Hitchcock R, et al: Lactate clearance and survival following injury. J Trauma 35:584-588; discussion 588-589, 1993.
24. Bjerneroth G: Tribonat—a comprehensive summary of its properties. Crit Care Med 27:1009-1013, 1999.
25. Levy B, Sadoune LO, Gelot AM, et al: Evolution of lactate/pyruvate and arterial ketone body ratios in the early course of catecholamine-treated septic shock. Crit Care Med 28:114-119, 2000.
26. Hotchkiss RS, Karl IE: Reevaluation of the role of cellular hypoxia and bioenergetic failure in sepsis. JAMA 267:1503-1510, 1992.
27. Prough DS, White RT: Acidosis associated with perioperative saline administration: Dilution or delusion? Anesthesiology 93:1167-1169, 2000.
28. Viallon A, Zeni F, Lafond P, et al: Does bicarbonate therapy improve the management of severe diabetic ketoacidosis? Crit Care Med 27:2690-2693, 1999.
29. Miller F, Brown E, Buckley J: Respiratory acidosis: Its relationship to cardiac function and other physiologic mechanisms. Surgery 32:171, 1952.
30. Bone R, Balk R, Cerra F, et al: Definitions for sepsis and organ failure and guidelines for the use of innovative therapies in sepsis. The ACCP/SCCM Consensus Conference Committee. American College of Chest Physicians/Society of Critical Care Medicine. Chest 101:1644-1655, 1992.
31. Laffey JG, Kavanagh BP: Hypocapnia. N Engl J Med Online 347:43-53, 2002.
32. Berger KI, Ayappa I, Chatr-Amontri B, et al: Obesity hypoventilation syndrome as a spectrum of respiratory disturbances during sleep. Chest 120:1231-1238, 2001.
33. Arieff AI: Hyponatremia, convulsions, respiratory arrest, and permanent brain damage after elective surgery in healthy women. N Engl J Med 314:1529-1535, 1986.
34. Ayus JC, Wheeler JM, Arieff AI: Postoperative hyponatremic encephalopathy in menstruant women. Ann Intern Med 117:891-897, 1992.
35. Steele A, Gowrishankar M, Abrahamson S, et al: Postoperative hyponatremia despite near-isotonic saline infusion: A phenomenon of desalination. Ann Intern Med 126:20-25, 1997.
36. Berendes E, Walter M, Cullen P, et al: Secretion of brain natriuretic peptide in patients with aneurysmal subarachnoid haemorrhage. Lancet 349:245-249, 1997.
37. Ayus JC, Arieff AI: Glycine-induced hypo-osmolar hyponatremia. Arch Intern Med 157:223-226, 1997.
38. Kumar S, Berl T: Sodium. Lancet 352:220-228, 1998.
39. Laureno R, Karp BI: Myelinolysis after correction of hyponatremia. Ann Intern Med 126:57-62, 1997.
40. Adrogue HJ, Madias NE: Hypernatremia. N Engl J Med 342:1493-1499, 2000.

41. Palevsky PM, Bhagrath R, Greenberg A: Hypernatremia in hospitalized patients. Ann Intern Med 124:197-203, 1996.
42. Gronert GA: Cardiac arrest after succinylcholine: Mortality greater with rhabdomyolysis than receptor upregulation. Anesthesiology 94:523-529, 2001.
43. Schulman M, Narins RG: Hypokalemia and cardiovascular disease. Am J Cardiol 65:4E-9E; discussion 22E-23E, 1990.
44. Johnson RG, Shafique T, Sirois C, et al: Potassium concentrations and ventricular ectopy: A prospective, observational study in post-cardiac surgery patients. Crit Care Med 27:2430-2434, 1999.
45. Halperin ML, Kamel KS: Potassium. Lancet 352:135-140, 1998.
46. Zaloga GP: Hypocalcemia in critically ill patients. Crit Care Med 20:251-262, 1992.
47. Marx SJ: Hyperparathyroid and hypoparathyroid disorders [erratum appears in N Engl J Med 2001 Jan 18;344(3):240]. N Engl J Med 343:1863-1875, 2000.
48. Bushinsky DA, Monk RD: Calcium. Lancet 352:306-311, 1998.
49. Martin TJ, Moseley JM, Gillespie MT: Parathyroid hormone-related protein: Biochemistry and molecular biology. Crit Rev Biochem Mol Biol 26:377-395, 1991.
50. Kedlaya D, Brandstater M, Lee J: Immobilization hypercalcemia in incomplete paraplegia: Successful treatment with pamidronate. Arch Phys Med Rehabil 79:222, 1998.
51. Bloomfield D: Should bisphosphonates be part of the standard therapy of patients with multiple myeloma or bone metastases from other cancers? An evidence-based review. J Clin Oncol 16:1218, 1998.
52. Hortobagyi G, Theriault R, Porter L: Efficacy of pamidronate in reducing skeletal complications in patients with breast cancer and lytic bone metastases. N Engl J Med 335:1785, 1996.
53. Kalemkerian G, Darwish B, Varterasian M: Tumor lysis syndrome in small cell carcinoma and other solid tumors. Am J Med 103:363, 1997.
54. Denlinger J, Nahrwold M, Gibbs P: Hypocalcemia during rapid blood transfusion in anaesthetized man. Br J Anaesth 48:995, 1976.
55. Gascon A, Cobeta-Garcia J, Iglesias E: Hypomagnesemia and chondrocalcinosis in Gitelman syndrome. Am J Med 107:301, 1999.
56. Renkin EM: Some consequences of capillary permeability to macromolecules: Starling's hypothesis reconsidered. Am J Physiol 250(5 Pt 2):H706-710, 1986.
57. Michel CC, Curry FE: Microvascular permeability. Physiol Rev 79:703-761, 1999.
58. Groban L, Cowley AW Jr, Ebert TJ: Atrial natriuretic peptide augments forearm capillary filtration in humans. Am J Physiol Heart Circ Physiol 259:H258-263, 1990.
59. Shires GT, Coln CD, Carrico CJ, Lightfoot S: Fluid therapy in hemorrhagic shock. Arch Surg 88:688, 1964.
60. Boyd O, Grounds RM, Bennett ED: A randomized clinical trial of the effect of deliberate perioperative increase of oxygen delivery on mortality in high-risk surgical patients. JAMA 270:2699-2707, 1993.
61. Gattinoni L, Brazzi L, Pelosi P, et al: A trial of goal-oriented hemodynamic therapy in critically ill patients. SvO2 Collaborative Group. N Engl J Med 333:1025-1032, 1995.
62. Porter JM, Ivatury RR: In search of the optimal end points of resuscitation in trauma patients: A review. J Trauma 44:908-914, 1998.
63. McKinley BAP, Kozar RAMDP, Cocanour CSMD, et al: Normal versus supranormal oxygen delivery goals in shock resuscitation: The response is the same. J Trauma 53:825-832, 2002.
64. Velmahos GCMDP, Demetriades DMDP, Shoemaker WCMD, et al: Endpoints of resuscitation of critically injured patients: Normal or supranormal?: A prospective randomized trial. Ann Surg 232:409-418, 2000.
65. Shoemaker WC, Peitzman AB, Bellamy R, et al: Resuscitation from severe hemorrhage. Crit Care Med 24(2 Suppl):S12-23, 1996.
66. McGee S, Abernethy WB III, Simel DL: The rational clinical examination: Is this patient hypovolemic? JAMA 281:1022-1029, 1999.
67. Auerbach AD, Goldman L: Beta-blockers and reduction of cardiac events in noncardiac surgery: scientific review [comment]. JAMA 287:1435-1444, 2002.
68. Burri C, Henkemeyer H, Passler HH, Allgower M: Evaluation of acute blood loss by means of simple hemodynamic parameters. Prog Surg 11:108-131, 1973.
69. Hanson JM, Van Hoeyweghen R, Kirkman E, et al: Use of stroke distance in the early detection of simulated blood loss. J Trauma 44:128-134, 1998.
70. Thompson D, Adams SL, Barrett J: Relative bradycardia in patients with isolated penetrating abdominal trauma and isolated extremity trauma. Ann Emerg Med 19:268-275, 1990.
71. Demetriades D, Chan LS, Bhasin P, et al: Relative bradycardia in patients with traumatic hypotension. J Trauma 45:534-539, 1998.
72. Velasquez MT, Menitove JE, Skelton MM, Cowley AW Jr: Hormonal responses and blood pressure maintenance in normal and hypertensive subjects during acute blood loss. Hypertension 9:423-428, 1987.
73. Miyagatani Y, Yukioka T, Ohta S, et al: Vascular tone in patients with hemorrhagic shock. J Trauma 47:282-287, 1999.
74. Riddez L, Hahn RG, Brismar B, et al: Central and regional hemodynamics during acute hypovolemia and volume substitution in volunteers. Crit Care Med 25:635-640, 1997.
75. Davis JW, Kaups KL, Parks SN: Base deficit is superior to pH in evaluating clearance of acidosis after traumatic shock. J Trauma 44:114-118, 1998.
76. Rutherford EJ, Morris JA Jr, Reed GW, Hall KS: Base deficit stratifies mortality and determines therapy. J Trauma 33:417-423, 1992.
77. Tremblay LN, Feliciano DV, Rozycki GS: Assessment of initial base deficit as a predictor of outcome: Mechanism of injury does make a difference. Am Surg 68:689-693; discussion 693-694, 2002.
78. Shires GT, Barber AE, Illner HP: Current status of resuscitation: Solutions including hypertonic saline. Adv Surg 28:133-170, 1995.
79. Bickell WH, Wall MJ Jr, Pepe PE, et al: Immediate versus delayed fluid resuscitation for hypotensive patients with penetrating torso injuries. N Engl J Med 331:1105-1109, 1994.
80. Dutton RP, Mackenzie CF, Scalea TM: Hypotensive resuscitation during active hemorrhage: Impact on in-hospital mortality. J Trauma 52:1141-1146, 2002.
81. McClelland RN, Shires GT, Baxter CR, et al: Balanced salt solution in the treatment of hemorrhagic shock: Studies in dogs. JAMA 199:830-834, 1967.
82. Brill SA, Tuel RJ, Mass DP: Rescue of reapproximated flexor profundus tendons in vitro following segmental irradiation. J Surg Res 57:487-494, 1994.
83. Faringer PD, Mullins RJ, Johnson RL, Trunkey DD: Blood component supplementation during massive transfusion of AS-1 red cells in trauma patients. J Trauma 34:481-485; discussion 485-487, 1993.

84. Schierhout G, Roberts I: Fluid resuscitation with colloid or crystalloid solutions in critically ill patients: A systematic review of randomised trials. BMJ 316:961-964, 1998.

85. Mayberry JC, Mullins RJ, Crass RA, Trunkey DD: Prevention of abdominal compartment syndrome by absorbable mesh prosthesis closure. Arch Surg 132(9):957-961; discussion 961-962, 1997.

86. Rangel-Frausto MS, Pittet D, Costigan M, et al: The natural history of the systemic inflammatory response syndrome (SIRS): A prospective study. JAMA 273:117-123, 1995.

87. Angus DC, Linde-Zwirble WT, Lidicker J, et al: Epidemiology of severe sepsis in the United States: Analysis of incidence, outcome, and associated costs of care. Crit Care Med 29:1303-1310, 2001.

88. Sands KE, Bates DW, Lanken PN, et al: Epidemiology of sepsis syndrome in 8 academic medical centers. JAMA 278:234-240, 1997.

89. Wheeler A, Bernard G: Treating patients with severe sepsis. N Engl J Med 340:207-214, 1999.

90. Arons MM, Wheeler AP, Bernard GR, et al: Effects of ibuprofen on the physiology and survival of hypothermic sepsis. Ibuprofen in Sepsis Study Group. Crit Care Med 27:699-707, 1999.

91. Hadley S, Lee WW, Ruthazer R, Nasraway SA Jr: Candidemia as a cause of septic shock and multiple organ failure in nonimmunocompromised patients. Crit Care Med 30:1808-1814, 2002.

92. Pelz RK, Hendrix CW, Swoboda SM, et al: Double-blind placebo-controlled trial of fluconazole to prevent candidal infections in critically ill surgical patients. Ann Surg 233:542-548, 2001.

93. Hotchkiss RS, Karl IE: The pathophysiology and treatment of sepsis. N Engl J Med 348:138-150, 2003.

94. Fink MP, Evans TW: Mechanisms of organ dysfunction in critical illness: Report from a Round Table Conference held in Brussels. Intensive Care Med 28:369-375, 2002.

95. Heller AR, Groth G, Heller SC, et al: N-Acetylcysteine reduces respiratory burst but augments neutrophil phagocytosis in intensive care unit patients. Crit Care Med 29:272-276, 2001.

96. Landry DW, Oliver JA: The pathogenesis of vasodilatory shock. N Engl J Med 345:588-595, 2001.

97. Cobb JP: Use of nitric oxide synthase inhibitors to treat septic shock: The light has changed from yellow to red. Crit Care Med 27:855-856, 1999.

98. Parrillo JE: Pathogenetic mechanisms of septic shock. N Engl J Med 328(20):1471-1477, 1993.

99. Parrillo JE, Burch C, Shelhamer JH, et al: A circulating myocardial depressant substance in humans with septic shock: Septic shock patients with a reduced ejection fraction have a circulating factor that depresses in vitro myocardial cell performance. J Clin Invest 76:1539-1553, 1985.

100. Kumar A, Haery C, Parrillo JE: Myocardial dysfunction in septic shock. Crit Care Clin 16:251-287, 2001.

101. Hayes MA, Timmins AC, Yau EH, et al: Elevation of systemic oxygen delivery in the treatment of critically ill patients. N Engl J Med 330:1717-1722, 1994.

102. Schremmer B, Dhainaut JF: Heart failure in septic shock: Effects of inotropic support. Crit Care Med 18(1 Pt 2):S49-55, 1990.

103. Marik PE, Mohedin M: The contrasting effects of dopamine and norepinephrine on systemic and splanchnic oxygen utilization in hyperdynamic sepsis. JAMA 272:1354-1357, 1994.

104. Seguin P, Bellissant E, Le Tulzo Y, et al: Effects of epinephrine compared with the combination of dobutamine and norepinephrine on gastric perfusion in septic shock. Clin Pharmacol Ther 71:381-388, 2001.

105. Holmes CL, Patel BM, Russell JA, Walley KR: Physiology of vasopressin relevant to management of septic shock. Chest 120:989-1002, 2001.

106. Rivers E, Nguyen B, Havstad S, et al: Early goal-directed therapy in the treatment of severe sepsis and septic shock. N Engl J Med 345:1368-1377, 2001.

107. Bernard GR, Vincent JL, Laterre PF, et al: Efficacy and safety of recombinant human activated protein C for severe sepsis. N Engl J Med 344:699-709, 2001.

108. Abraham E, Laterre PF, Garbino J, et al: Lenercept (p55 tumor necrosis factor receptor fusion protein) in severe sepsis and early septic shock: A randomized, double-blind, placebo-controlled, multicenter phase III trial with 1,342 patients. Crit Care Med 29:503-510, 2001.

109. Reinhart K, Menges T, Gardlund B, et al: Randomized, placebo-controlled trial of the anti-tumor necrosis factor antibody fragment afelimomab in hyperinflammatory response during severe sepsis: The RAMSES Study. Crit Care Med 29:765-769, 2001.

110. Bernard GR, Wheeler AP, Russell JA, et al: The effects of ibuprofen on the physiology and survival of patients with sepsis. The Ibuprofen in Sepsis Study Group. N Engl J Med 336:912-918, 1997.

111. Annane D, Sebille V, Charpentier C, et al: Effect of treatment with low doses of hydrocortisone and fludrocortisone on mortality in patients with septic shock. JAMA 288:862-871, 2002.

112. Lefering R, Neugebauer EA: Steroid controversy in sepsis and septic shock: A meta-analysis [comment]. Crit Care Med 23:1294-1303, 1995.

113. Hochman JS, Sleeper LA, Webb JG, et al: Early revascularization in acute myocardial infarction complicated by cardiogenic shock. SHOCK Investigators. Should we emergently revascularize occluded coronaries for cardiogenic shock? N Engl J Med 341:625-634, 1999.

114. Hollenberg SM, Kavinsky CJ, Parrillo JE: Cardiogenic shock. Ann Intern Med 131:47-59, 1999.

115. Collins R, Peto R, Baigent C, Sleight P: Aspirin, heparin, and fibrinolytic therapy in suspected acute myocardial infarction. N Engl J Med 336:847-860, 1997.

116. Karalis DG, Victor MF, Davis GA, et al: The role of echocardiography in blunt chest trauma: A transthoracic and transesophageal echocardiographic study. J Trauma 36:53-58, 1994.

117. Asensio JA, Murray J, Demetriades D, et al: Penetrating cardiac injuries: A prospective study of variables predicting outcomes. J Am Coll Surg 186:24-34, 1998.

118. Dalen JE, Alpert JS, Hirsch J: Thrombolytic therapy for pulmonary embolism: Is it effective? Is it safe? When is it indicated? Arch Intern Med 157:2550-2556, 1997.

119. Konstantinides S, Geibel A, Kasper W: Submassive and massive pulmonary embolism: A target for thrombolytic therapy? Thromb Haemost 82(Suppl 1):104-108, 1999.

120. Tai NR, Atwal AS, Hamilton G: Modern management of pulmonary embolism. Br J Surg 86:853-868, 1999.

121. Oelkers W: Adrenal insufficiency. N Engl J Med 335:1206-1212, 1996.

122. Vella A, Nippoldt TB, Morris JC III: Adrenal hemorrhage: A 25-year experience at the Mayo Clinic. Mayo Clin Proc 76:161-168, 2001.

123. Coursin DB, Wood KE: Corticosteroid supplementation for adrenal insufficiency. JAMA 287:236-240, 2002.

CHAPTER 6

HEMATOLOGIC PRINCIPLES IN SURGERY

Edmund J. Rutherford, M.D., Dionne Skeete, M.D., Wesley G. Schooler, M.D., and Samir M. Fakhry, M.D.

Background

Hemostasis and Coagulation

Evaluation of Disorders of Hemostasis and Coagulation

Congenital Bleeding Disorders

Acquired Bleeding Disorders

Disseminated Intravascular Coagulation

Preparation of Blood Components

Clinical Indications and Use of Blood Components

Risks of Blood Transfusion

Massive Transfusion

Blood Substitutes and Alternatives to Transfusion

The management of bleeding disorders and administration of blood products are important therapeutic modalities used by surgeons caring for patients with acute and chronic problems. When used with a thorough understanding of appropriate indications, risks, and benefits, blood transfusion is safe and effective. Surgeons encounter congenital and acquired bleeding disorders in many clinical settings. Congenital conditions such as hemophilia present challenges for both elective and emergent operations. Acquired bleeding disorders are associated with conditions such as inflammatory states, massive transfusion, hypothermia, malnutrition, liver dysfunction, and drugs. Knowledge of the fundamentals of normal and deranged hemostasis is critical to successful operative procedures and complete care of surgical patients.

In this chapter, normal hemostatic mechanisms are discussed and appropriate diagnostic and therapeutic measures for disorders of surgical bleeding are reviewed. The indications and use of blood components, potential risks of blood products, and alternatives to blood transfusion are reviewed. Because blood products are a limited resource with potential serious adverse effects, knowledge of appropriate indications, potential risks, and available alternatives should allow clinicians to exercise judgment in using this important resource.

BACKGROUND

Although now routine, the ability to transfuse blood successfully is relatively recent. Accounts of bloodletting and phlebotomy appear in many early historical references and were recommended for many ailments. Jean-Baptiste Denis in France and Richard Lower in England recorded the first known successful transfusion to humans in 1667.[1] Denis gave 3 pints of sheep blood to a patient with no apparent ill effects. Subsequent attempts to give blood to a young man "to mollify his fiery nature" failed, and the patient died shortly after the transfusion. A lawsuit resulted, and Denis went to trial but was ultimately exonerated. The Paris medical faculty subsequently forbade blood transfusions, which led to bans on transfusion throughout France and Italy that lasted until modern times. In 1795, Dr. Philip Syng Physick of Philadelphia performed the first successful transfusion of human blood.

The discovery of the A, B, and O blood types by Karl Landsteiner in 1900 and the AB blood type by Alfred Decastello and Adriano Sturli in 1902 began the era of modern blood transfusion. The first blood bank was established in the United States in 1937, and the introduction of plastic storage containers and plasmapheresis instruments made component therapy possible. By the 1940s, techniques of crossmatching, anticoagulation, and storage of blood and the establishment of blood banks made routine blood transfusion possible.

Replacing blood intraoperatively is an important prerequisite in modern surgical practice. A majority of blood products are transfused at or near operation. Blood component therapy has made successful operation possible in patients with symptomatic anemia, thrombocytopenia, or coagulopathy. Approximately 10 million units of packed red blood cells (RBCs) were transfused in the United States in 1980. The number peaked at 12.2 million in 1986 and then declined to 11.4 million units in 1997.[2] This decrease is notable given the growth and increasing age of the U.S. population. The use of other components, especially platelets, has increased. Because only 4% to 5% of eligible donors ever donate blood, future increases may exacerbate shortages.

HEMOSTASIS AND COAGULATION

Traditional concepts of coagulation held that two pathways exist by which coagulation could occur: the intrinsic pathway and the extrinsic pathway (Fig. 6-1). In this cascade model, the two pathways converge to a common pathway.[3] In the intrinsic pathway, interaction of circulating factors already within the blood initiates coagulation. This begins with the binding of factor XII to

negatively charged surfaces, whereby it undergoes a conformational change. Partial activation results, and factor XII interacts with prekallikrein and high-molecular-weight kininogen. More complete activation of factor XII (factor XIIa) occurs. In the process, factor XIIa activates prekallikrein to kallikrein, which itself becomes a potent activator of factor XII. Factor XIIa activates factor XI (factor XIa). Factor XIa activates factor IX (factor IXa) in the presence of calcium. Factor IXa forms a complex with activated factor VIII (factor VIIIa), calcium ion, and phospholipids to activate factor X (factor Xa). Factor Xa is able to convert prothrombin to thrombin, changing fibrinogen into fibrin. Factor XIII converts the fibrin monomers into a cross-linked fibrin clot in the presence of calcium. The clinical relevance of the intrinsic pathway is not associated with clinically significant bleeding in vivo, although it does produce aberrations in tests of coagulation. In particular, deficiencies of factor XII or prekallikrein are not associated with a bleeding tendency in humans, whereas patients with deficiencies of factor VIII or factor IX exhibit pronounced bleeding disorders (hemophilia A and B, respectively).

The interaction of factor VII with tissue factor (TF), its high-affinity receptor and cofactor, initiates the extrinsic cascade. In the presence of calcium, the factor VII/TF complex activates factor X (factor Xa). Factor Xa converts prothrombin to thrombin and fibrin monomers from fibrinogen. A thrombus is formed from fibrin, entrapped platelets, and other blood elements and is stabilized by cross-linking of the fibrin monomers. Ultimately, clot retraction follows the interaction of platelets and the fibrin strands. Under normal circumstances, local blood flow, vasodilatory substances, and regulatory feedback mechanisms limit the clotting process to the area of injury. The thrombus is ultimately dissolved by fibrinolysis, which involves the formation of plasmin from plasminogen. These processes are highly interrelated and interdependent in vivo and are involved in regulatory feedback loops that maintain a fine balance between procoagulant hemostatic mechanisms and normal anticoagulant functions.

Deficiencies in the cascade model and recent discoveries have prompted a model of cell-based coagulation,[3] with TF-bearing cells and platelets at the center (Fig. 6-2). When the integrity of the blood vessel wall is disrupted, the exposure of cells expressing TF to plasma activates the coagulation system. The distribution of TF is highly cell specific and includes adventitial cells, outer layers of the epidermis, other squamous epithelial cells, and myoepithelial cells. This corresponds to a hemostatic envelope surrounding blood vessels and organs.[4] Endothelial cells also express TF. Monroe and associates describe three phases of the cell-based coagulation: initiation, priming, and propagation.[3] In the first phase, factor VII binds to TF and is rapidly activated. The TF/VIIa complex catalyzes the activation of factor IX. In addition, the TF/VIIa complex can directly activate factor X. The TF/VIIa/Xa complex binds activated factor V (factor Va) and converts prothrombin to thrombin. The relatively small amount of thrombin formed serves to further enhance platelet activation and accelerate the coagulation

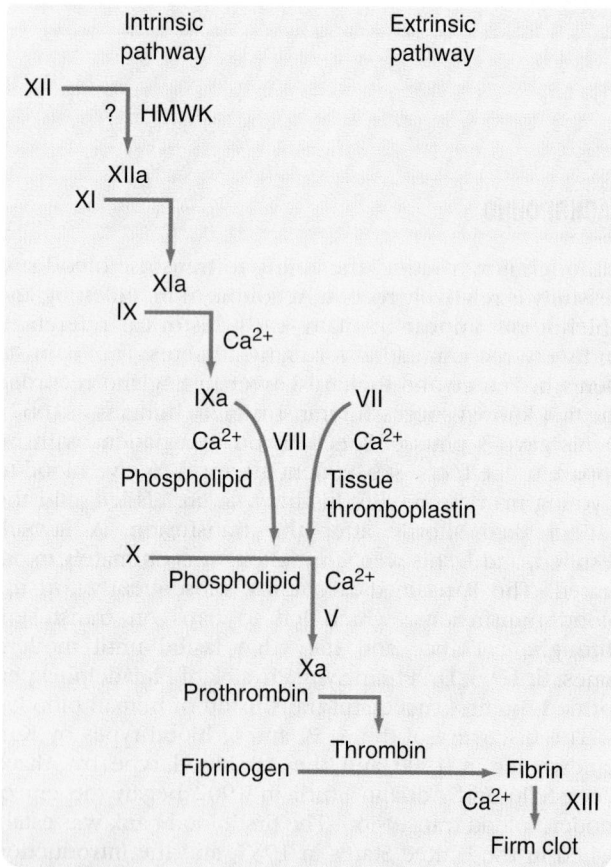

FIGURE 6-1. Traditional schematic version of the coagulation system. HMWK, high-molecular-weight kininogen.

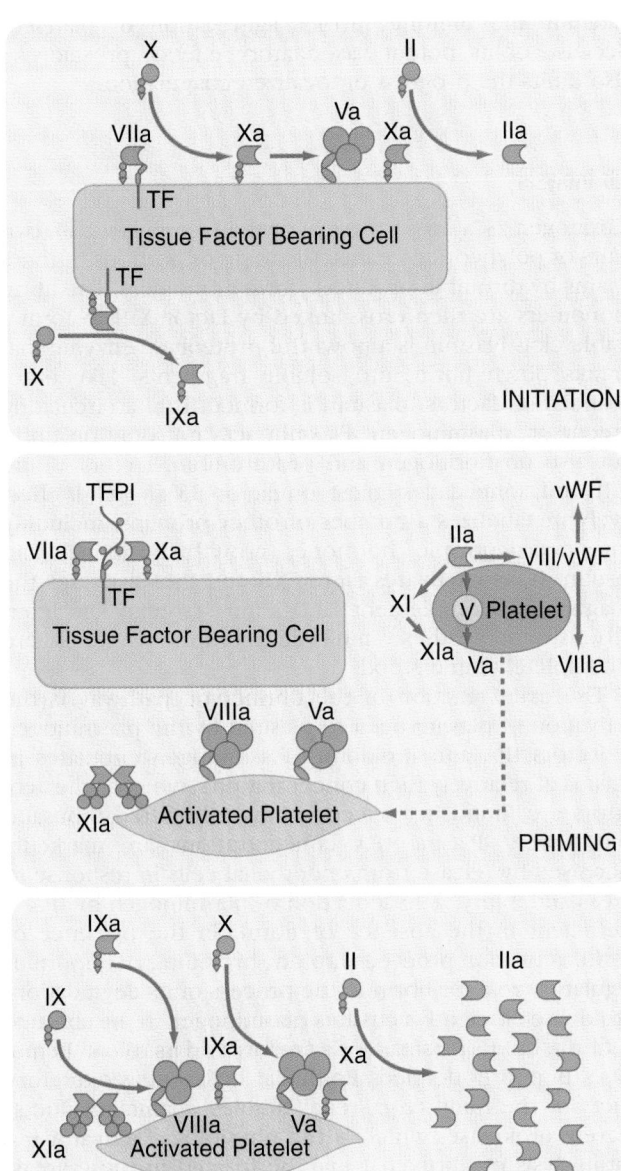

FIGURE 6-2. Cell-based model of coagulation. (From Monroe DM, Hoffman M, Roberts HR: Platelets and thrombin generation. Arterioscler Thromb Vasc Biol 22:1381-1389, 2002.)

response. Platelets, already primed by the exposure to collagen, are synergistically primed by the addition of thrombin. In the second priming phase, platelets release granules containing factor V, which is cleaved to factor Va. Thrombin cleaves factor VIII′ from von Willebrand factor (factor VIIIR) converting it to factor VIII′. In the propagation phase, the activated primed platelets are now able to rapidly bind factors Va, VIIIa, and IXa. On the platelet membrane, factor VIII′/IXa complex is formed. This complex is the major activator of factor X and is estimated to be 50 times more efficient than the TF/VIIa complex. Factor Xa binds with factor Va to form the major converter of prothrombin to thrombin. It is believed that the complexes formed on the platelet surface are more efficient because they are protected from blood-borne

inhibitors.[3] The significant amount of thrombin formed serves to form a stable fibrin clot. This revised scheme of blood coagulation explains the observed clinical syndromes of deficiency of various factors and clarifies the relatively limited role that factor XII plays in coagulation in vivo.

Coagulation is strictly regulated at different steps through the process. Tissue factor pathway inhibitor (TFPI) blocks the TF/VIIa/Va/Xa complex by binding to factor Xa.[5] TFPI is present in small amounts usually, but more is released in the presence of heparin.[5] Antithrombin III (AT-III) is a member of the serine protease inhibitor superfamily and is a weak inhibitor of the TF/VIIa complex. AT-III more effectively neutralizes the coagulation system enzymes like factors IXa, Xa, and XIa, affecting thrombin production. Heparin accelerates these inhibitory reactions by causing a conformational change in AT-III. Thrombin is inactivated by AT-III in the presence of heparin. Heparin cofactor 2 is similar to AT-III as a naturally occurring anticoagulant. Heparin cofactor 2, however, inhibits only thrombin. Its activity is enhanced by both heparin and dermatan sulfate. Deficiency of AT-III is also associated with a tendency to venous thrombosis. Thrombin binds thrombomodulin on the cell surface of endothelial cells. The thrombin-thrombomodulin complex activates protein C in the presence of its cofactor protein S. Activated protein C competitively binds factors Va and VIIIa, limiting the production of factor Xa and thrombin. As a clinically important anticoagulant pathway in humans, either protein C or protein S deficiency is known to cause a significant tendency toward thrombosis. Activated protein C has also been used to treat patients with significant systemic inflammatory response syndrome, who appear to have a procoagulant state with decreased expression of thrombomodulin and decreased levels of protein C.[6]

Blood Vessels and Endothelial Cells

Hemostasis is the physiologic cessation of bleeding. Under normal circumstances, blood maintains its fluidity because of the balance of procoagulant and anticoagulant influences, including interactions at the blood-endothelium interface and many circulating factors.[3] When injury to a vessel occurs, TF and collagen are exposed. Platelets adhere to the site of injury and undergo a release phenomenon with further platelet aggregation and a platelet plug forms.

Vasoconstriction occurs in response to the release of vasoactive substances from platelets (e.g., thromboxane A_2 and serotonin) and endothelin from endothelial cells. Thromboxane A_2 is produced locally at the site of injury and is a very potent constrictor of smooth muscle, especially in smaller and medium-sized vessels. Larger vessels constrict in response to innervation and circulating constrictive factors, such as norepinephrine.

Endothelial cells are highly active cells with many important products and effects, including both procoagulant and antithrombotic effects.[4] Under normal conditions, endothelial cells are crucial in the maintenance of a nonthrombogenic interface between vessels and the circulating blood. Among the contributory mechanisms identified thus far are the elaboration of prostacyclin (a potent inhibitor of platelet aggregation), nitric oxide, thrombomodulin, and tissue plasminogen activator (tPA) and binding of the anticoagulant AT-III to heparin sulfate on the endothelial cell surface. Endothelial cell injury exposes subendothelial TF and collagen, reduces thrombomodulin availability, increases phospholipid sites for coagulation protein binding, and expresses TF on the cell surface. These changes promote the procoagulant effect of injury. During inflammatory states, agents such as endotoxin, interleukin-1, and tumor necrosis factor promote the expression of tissue factor on the endothelial cell surface and the downregulation of thrombomodulin, which leads to procoagulant effects.[4]

Platelets

Platelets participate in hemostasis through a sequence of adherence to the site of injury, release of the contents of their alpha and dense granules, aggregation to form a platelet plug, and promotion of coagulation by providing a procoagulant surface on their phospholipid membranes.[3] Platelets rapidly adhere to exposed subendothelial collagen and other basement membrane proteins. The presence of fibrinogen and factor VIIIR is important for the successful adherence of platelets. Factor VIIIR is a large protein that produces several important effects in hemostasis and coagulation. In addition to its role in the adhesion of platelets to injured vessel walls, it is a carrier for factor VIII in plasma, thus protecting it from degradation.

Factor VIIIR binds to collagen, undergoes a conformational change, and binds the platelet surface receptor glycoprotein Ib/IX. After adhering to the subendothelium, platelets develop pseudopods. Platelets are activated with release of the contents of their alpha granules (platelet factor 4, β-thromboglobulin, thrombospondin, platelet-derived growth factor, fibrinogen, factor VIIIR) and dense granules (adenosine diphosphate, serotonin). With the release of platelet granule contents, particularly adenosine diphosphate, further platelet aggregation at the site of injury occurs. The glycoprotein IIb/IIIa receptors on adjacent platelets are joined by fibrinogen. Platelet activation also produces platelet procoagulant activity through surface coagulation factors, as discussed previously. These events lead to the formation of a platelet plug within 1 to 3 minutes of vessel injury. Ionized calcium and thromboxane A_2, a potent platelet aggregator, are important in many steps of this process. Thrombin production causes further platelet degranulation and aggregation with incorporation of more platelets into the clot. As fibrin is deposited, the clot is stabilized. Retraction of the clot occurs with a reduction in clot size within 10 minutes of the initial injury.

The production of prostacyclin by the endothelial cell serves to counterbalance the local hemostatic process. In particular, prostacyclin elevates levels of adenyl cyclase with an increase in cyclic adenosine monophosphate levels within platelets, decreasing available ionized calcium and limiting further aggregation of platelets. Because of its potent vasodilatory effects, prostacyclin also limits the progress of localized coagulation.

Fibrinolysis

Fibrinogen is a large plasma protein composed of two pairs of polypeptide chains. Cleavage of portions of these chains by thrombin produces fibrin monomers. The fibrin monomers are then cross-linked by factor XIII to form a stable clot. Plasmin is a powerful proteolytic enzyme that breaks down fibrin into soluble fragments. Like other coagulation factors, plasmin is formed from a circulating precursor, plasminogen. Plasmin acts not only on fibrin but also on fibrinogen and prothrombin, factors V and VIII, and, some data suggest, on factors IX and XI. It effectively metabolizes a number of other proteins, including adrenocorticotropic hormone, growth hormone, and insulin. It also activates factor XII and thus activates the coagulation, complement, and kinin systems. The interactions among these multiple, complex systems are incompletely understood.

The main reaction of the fibrinolytic pathway is the activation of plasminogen to plasmin by the plasminogen activators tPA and urokinase. Plasminogen circulates in plasma at relatively high concentrations, whereas the activators are found in concentrations a hundred thousand fold lower.[7] Plasma tPA concentrations are markedly increased by release from endothelial cells in response to stress and injury. The activation of plasminogen by tPA is inefficient in the absence of fibrin. In the presence of fibrin, activation proceeds rapidly, providing an important regulatory role for fibrin in the process of its degradation. Urokinase efficiently activates plasminogen in the absence of fibrin, but its plasma levels are low and its role in hemostasis is poorly defined. Epithelial cells lining excretory ducts of the body (e.g., renal tubules, mammary ducts) secrete urokinase, which is the physiologic activator initiating lysis of fibrin that may be formed in these areas. Streptokinase, a bacterial product, is a potent activator of plasminogen and has been used to induce fibrinolysis therapeutically.

The reactions of the fibrinolytic cascade are catalyzed by serine proteases in a manner analogous to the coagulation cascade. These reactions are believed to occur on the surface of endothelial cells. The serine proteases are regulated by inhibitors from the serine protease inhibitors superfamily, which act as pseudosubstrates for the proteases. Fibrin helps regulate fibrinolysis in addition to serving as its major substrate. Physiologic fibrinolysis is a reparative process that occurs in response to hemostatic plug or formation of thrombus. The final enzymatic step, fibrin proteolysis, results from a coordinated interaction of enzymes and inhibitors, which produces effective action at the site of the process and spares the proteins of the blood or uninvolved parts of the vascular system.

The major inhibitor of plasminogen activation is plasminogen activator inhibitor (PAI-1), which is found in low concentration in plasma but at higher concentration within platelets. Plasma PAI-1 is probably synthesized in endothelial cells and/or hepatocytes. This inhibitor of the fibrinolytic system increases after trauma and operation. The synthesis of PAI-1 is affected by many compounds, including endotoxin, thrombin, transforming growth factor-β, interleukin-1, and tumor necrosis factor-α. The major inhibitor of plasmin, α_2-antiplasmin or plasmin inhibitor, circulates in plasma at relatively high concentrations and can neutralize large amounts of plasmin. Plasmin inhibitor binds fibrin during the process of fibrin cross-linking by activated factor XIII and protects the thrombus from fibrinolysis.[8] Plasmin inhibitor also interferes with plasminogen and inhibits the effect of plasminogen activators.[8] Another recent discovery has been thrombin activatable fibrinolysis inhibitor (TAFI). This proenzyme is activated by thrombin, providing a link between coagulation and fibrinolysis. Its main mechanism of action involves interference of plasminogen binding to degrading fibrin, but interference of plasmin binding and direct plasmin inhibition has also been demonstrated.[7]

Degradation of cross-linked fibrin creates distinctive products characterized by cross-linked (factor XIIIa-induced) derivatives such as D-dimer. Disease states occurring after abnormalities in the fibrinolytic system include both hemorrhagic disorders, resulting from excessive fibrinolysis, and thrombotic disorders, resulting from deficient fibrinolysis. Hyperfibrinolysis can result from pharmacologic administration of activators such as streptokinase, urokinase, and tPA or from defective inhibition produced by α_2-antiplasmin deficiency. Thrombosis can result from hereditary defects of plasminogen or from pharmacologic inhibition of fibrinolysis, such as with ϵ-aminocaproic acid. Laboratory evaluation of fibrinolysis can aid assessment of thrombotic disorders, including specific measurements of plasminogen activators, plasminogen, plasmin inhibitors, and circulating fibrinogen and products of cross-linked fibrin degradation.

EVALUATION OF DISORDERS OF HEMOSTASIS AND COAGULATION

The surgeon may encounter disorders of hemostasis and coagulation either in the preoperative evaluation of the patients for elective surgery or in the perioperative care of patients with acute bleeding disorders. Diagnosis of the specific disorder involved requires a detailed evaluation of the patient's history, review of medical records related to risk factors for bleeding or previously obtained laboratory data, physical examination, and appropriate laboratory tests.[9]

An accurate history and physical examination of a patient scheduled to undergo elective operation offers the most valuable source of information regarding the risk of bleeding. A patient with a history of bleeding, easy bruising (either spontaneous or traumatic), frequent or unusual mucosal bleeding, metromenorrhagia (irregular, prolonged, and excessive menstrual flow), hematuria, epistaxis, prior history of significant or life-threatening hemorrhage associated with invasive procedures, or a family history may be at risk. The intake of medications should always be elicited. Especially important are drugs

such as aspirin and nonsteroidal anti-inflammatory drugs (NSAIDs); patients may not consider their intake as being important to mention when interviewed unless specifically asked. In addition, a history of liver dysfunction, renal dysfunction, or major metabolic or endocrine disorder is useful in directing preoperative screening. Evidence of excessive bruising, joint deformities, petechiae or ecchymosis, adenopathy, hepatosplenomegaly, excessive mobility of joints, or increased elasticity of the skin are symptoms of disorders associated with excessive perioperative bleeding. Evidence of amyloidosis (e.g., thickening of the skin or tongue), multiple myeloma, or other hematologic malignancies can also affect hemostasis and coagulation.

Screening Tests for Bleeding Disorders

The extent of laboratory testing needed for patients with a normal history and physical examination has been debated. For most patients undergoing either minor operations or procedures that do not involve extensive dissection, laboratory testing is unlikely to provide additional information over a properly performed history and physical examination. Preoperative laboratory screening may be useful for patients undergoing major procedures, especially involving body cavities or operations with significant dissection and the creation of raw surfaces, or patients with an abnormal history or physical examination. Patients with infection, systemic inflammatory response syndrome, sepsis syndrome, malnutrition, organ failure, and other major systemic disorders also warrant preoperative screening. The commonly obtained tests include the prothrombin time (PT), the activated partial thromboplastin time (aPTT), a complete blood cell count with platelet count, and, occasionally, a bleeding time. The PT measures the function of factor VII and the *extrinsic pathway* as well as the *common pathway* factors (factor X, prothrombin/thrombin, fibrinogen, and fibrin). Prolongation of the PT occurs when levels of factors V, VII, or X fall below 50% of normal. A prothrombin level less than 30% of normal also prolongs the PT. Warfarin therapy and vitamin K deficiency deplete the vitamin K–dependent proteins (prothrombin, factors VII, IX, X, protein C and S) and prolong the PT.

The aPTT detects decreased levels of the intrinsic pathway factors (high-molecular-weight kininogen, prekallikrein, factors XII, XI, IX, and VIII) and the common pathway factors (fibrinogen, prothrombin, factors V and X). Factor levels of 30% or less are usually required to affect the aPTT. The anticoagulant heparin is a commonly employed drug that causes prolongation of the aPTT without significantly prolonging the PT by depleting the intrinsic pathway factors.

The PT and aPTT can be used together in an attempt to localize coagulation defects. A normal PT with an abnormal aPTT suggests deficiency of the proximal intrinsic pathway factors. A prolonged PT with a normal aPTT suggests abnormalities of the vitamin K–dependent factors such as factor VII. An abnormal PT or aPTT may indicate the presence of an inhibitor (e.g., lupus anticoagulant, heparin, or an inhibitor of a specific factor). To differentiate an inhibitor from a factor deficiency, the patient's plasma is mixed in a 1:1 ratio with normal plasma and the PT or aPTT is repeated. If the abnormal value corrects to the normal range, the presence of a coagulation factor deficiency in the patient's plasma is indicated. If the abnormality does not correct, an inhibitor is presumed to exist.

The platelet count identifies numbers of platelets, whereas the bleeding time estimates qualitative platelet function. None of the commonly recommended screening tests measures fibrinolytic function. Additional screening tests that may be used include a fibrinogen level and the thrombin time (TT). The TT detects abnormalities of globulin, fibrinogen, excess fibrinolysis, and heparin-like substances. In patients suspected of having platelet dysfunction, additional assessments include platelet function tests (aggregation with epinephrine, adenosine diphosphate, collagen, and ristocetin). If a deficiency or specific factor is suspected, as in patients with a family history of hemophilia, specific factor assays should be obtained.

The bleeding time is a crude screening test for platelet function that also reflects endothelial cell function. This test is performed by placing a standardized cut in the skin of either the forearm (Ivy method) or the earlobe (Duke method). Because the bleeding time is affected by many variables, including the manner in which the cut is placed, the location of the cut, endothelial cell function, platelet counts, and overall platelet function, it is a difficult test to standardize. Data suggest that although the bleeding time may be useful in evaluating patients with bleeding disorders, it has no role in the preoperative evaluation of a normal patient.[9]

Patients with familial thrombocytopenia (May-Hegglin anomaly) have an autosomal dominant disorder associated with petechiae and hyperpigmentation of the distal lower extremities. These patients may have abnormal bleeding owing to decreased platelet numbers. Patients with Marfan's syndrome, Ehlers-Danlos syndrome, or osteogenesis imperfecta may have abnormal bleeding and poor wound healing despite normal screening tests. Other bleeding disorders often missed by routine coagulation testing include mild von Willebrand's disease, platelet function defect, factor XIII deficiency, hyperglobulinemic states, α_2-antiplasmin deficiency, and amyloidosis.

If a patient scheduled for an elective procedure has a history of significant risk for bleeding, abnormal findings on physical examination, or deranged screening laboratory tests, the procedure should be postponed pending a more complete evaluation and treatment. Patients about to undergo emergency operative procedures may require urgent correction of their hemostatic abnormalities before and during operation (see guidelines in Clinical Indications and Use of Blood Components).

Thromboelastography

Thromboelastography (TEG) was first described by Hartnet in 1948.[10] Although it is not widely used, this tech-

nique has reliability and validity and is in current clinical use in liver transplant and cardiovascular specialties.[11] It can be performed at the bedside and uses only 0.36 mL of whole blood, and initial results are available in less than 20 minutes if an activator is used. A pin suspended from a torsion wire is lowered into a heated cup. The cup rotates beneath the pin and, as the fibrin forms, it couples the pin to the cup. The rotational motion is transferred and recorded through an electromagnetic transducer and displayed graphically (Fig. 6-3). The computer-generated tracings give information on platelet function, enzyme activity, and overall coagulation properties.

Enzyme inhibition is manifested as a slowing of clotting on TEG and is measured by the reaction time (R), the time first clotting is noted, the angle (α), and the rate of clot growth. A prolonged R time or a decreased α is indicative of factor deficiencies and/or enzyme inhibition. The time to 20 mm of firmness (K-time) and the maximal amplitude (MA) measure platelet alteration, both measures of the strength of the clot. A strong clot depends on the interaction of platelets and fibrin. A prolonged K or decreased MA indicates that there is fibrin formation but insufficient platelet function to form an adequate clot. A mathematical algorithm calculates the coagulation index from R, K, MA, and α and measures overall clotting.

The advantage of TEG is to provide both a numerical and a graphic representation of coagulation and detect both hypocoagulability and hypercoagulability with a single sample. TEG provides two measures each for enzyme activity—platelet function and fibrinolysis—as well as a single overall coagulation index. Disadvantages include operator error and inability for hematology laboratories to perform multiple-batch analyses.

CONGENITAL BLEEDING DISORDERS

Congenital disorders of coagulation usually involve a single coagulation protein. Diagnosis depends on the history, physical examination, PT and aPTT determinations, and assay of factor levels. If available, a history of bleeding problems before presentation usually suggests the presence of the disease. Careful management should include specific factor replacement, meticulous intraoperative hemostasis, and careful monitoring of blood coagulation in the perioperative period. Early consultation with a coagulation specialist is important.

Hemophilia

Hemophilia A (classic hemophilia) is a congenital coagulation disorder that results from a deficiency or abnormality of factor VIII. It is transmitted as an X-linked recessive disorder, with males being affected almost exclusively. A female patient with laboratory abnormalities consistent with hemophilia A is unusual but may represent a carrier state, an unusual chromosomal aberration, or other rare disorder. A large number of different mutations accounting for the genetic abnormality have been identified, with up to 30% of cases representing spontaneous mutations. The severity of the disease can be cate-

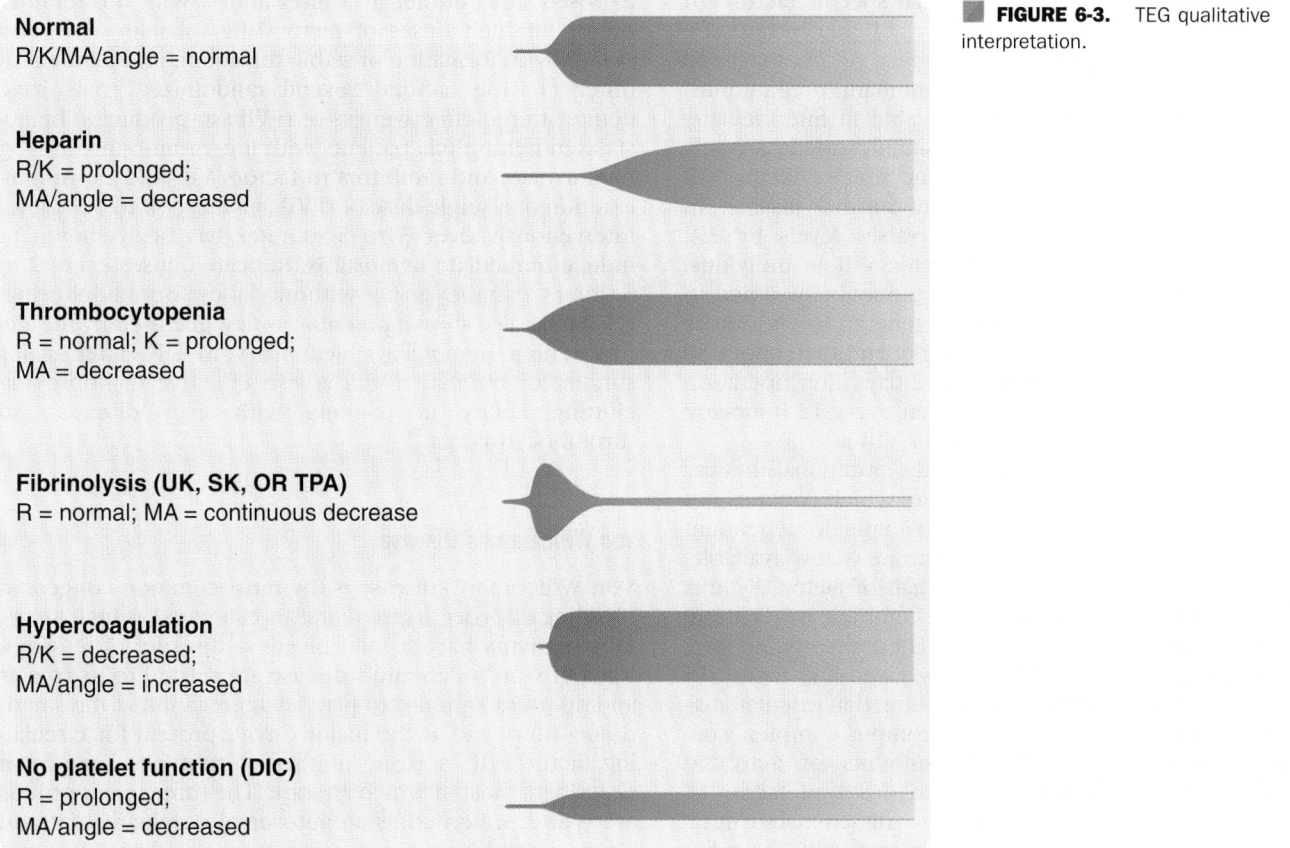

Normal
R/K/MA/angle = normal

Heparin
R/K = prolonged;
MA/angle = decreased

Thrombocytopenia
R = normal; K = prolonged;
MA = decreased

Fibrinolysis (UK, SK, OR TPA)
R = normal; MA = continuous decrease

Hypercoagulation
R/K = decreased;
MA/angle = increased

No platelet function (DIC)
R = prolonged;
MA/angle = decreased

FIGURE 6-3. TEG qualitative interpretation.

gorized based on the functional levels of factor VIII (factor VIII:C) in contradistinction to factor VIII:Ag, which refers to the antigenic level. Patients generally have severe bleeding with factor levels less than 2%, moderate bleeding with levels between 2% and 5%, and mild disease in the range of 5% to 30%. The patient with hemophilia A generally presents with large hematomas and hemarthroses as opposed to mucosal bleeding commonly seen with platelet disorders. Bleeding is often delayed by hours or days after injury, because the platelet plug is the first line of defense against bleeding, followed later by formation of thrombus.

The laboratory evaluation of patients with hemophilia A reveals a prolonged aPTT with decreased factor VIII:C with normal PT, bleeding time, and normal factor VIIIR antigen levels, which excludes the diagnosis of von Willebrand's disease. A small proportion of patients with hemophilia A (10% to 20%) develop inhibitors or IgG antibodies to factor VIII:C. Inhibitors can be detected with a mixing study.

Hemophilia B, also known as Christmas disease, is an inherited X-linked bleeding disorder that reflects a deficiency or defect in factor IX. Patients present with deep bleeding and hemarthroses. Severity of symptoms correlates directly with the level of circulating factor IX. The laboratory diagnosis of hemophilia B consists of the detection of an abnormal aPTT with decreased factor IX levels in a male patient with a normal PT, bleeding time, platelet count, and factor VIII and VIIIR antigen levels. Because factor IX is a vitamin K–dependent factor, vitamin K deficiency may produce depressed levels; however, the PT is prolonged and levels correct with the administration of exogenous vitamin K. As with hemophilia A, inhibitors can develop to factor IX and are diagnosed in similar fashion.

Desmopressin (DDAVP) may temporarily raise factor VIII levels in the patient with mild hemophilia A (basal factor VIII levels of 5% to 10%). Its administration to such patients after minor trauma or before elective dental surgery may obviate or reduce the need for replacement therapy. An intravenous dose of 0.3 µg/kg raises factor VIII levels 2- to 10-fold. Intranasal desmopressin is also effective and raises factor VIII levels 2- to 3-fold. Desmopressin is ineffective in severe hemophilia A. Antifibrinolytic therapy with ε-aminocaproic acid or tranexamic acid has also been effective in combination with desmopressin to decrease bleeding, particularly after dental procedures and in pediatric patients. Both ε-aminocaproic acid and tranexamic acid can be administered intravenously or orally and can be given in combination with factor replacement. They are contraindicated when prothrombin-complex concentrates are used, owing to increased risk of thrombosis.[12] Although fresh frozen plasma (FFP) contains factors VIII and IX, sufficient whole plasma cannot be given to patients with severe hemophilia, unless plasma exchange is done, to raise factors VIII or IX concentrations to levels that effectively prevent or control bleeding episodes. Cryoprecipitate is a good source of factor VIII but is rarely used now that specific factor VIII concentrates are available. Two types of concentrates are available for treatment of hemophilia A: plasma-based factor VIII preparations and recombinant preparations. Plasma-based preparations are available in intermediate- and high-purity strengths and are significantly less costly than recombinant preparations. One unit of factor VIII activity is the amount in 1 mL of normal plasma. In general, 1 unit/kg of factor VIII raises levels by 2%. Although the concentration of factor VIII in individual bags of cryoprecipitate varies, a bag may be assumed to contain 80 units of factor VIII. In general, levels can be achieved by administering 50 units/kg and then about 30 units/kg every 8 hours for the first 2 days after operation or injury. Subsequent infusions given every 12 hours are adjusted, depending on serum factor VIII assays.

For treatment of hemophilia B, the traditional therapy is prothrombin complex concentrate, which contains not only factor IX but also all of the vitamin K–dependent factors. High-purity factor IX concentrate is now available. For unknown reasons, only about half of factor IX units listed on a bottle of prothrombin complex concentrate can be recovered after infusion. Therefore, when prothrombin complex concentrate is given for factor IX replacement therapy, an amount double that calculated as necessary is given. Because prothrombin complex concentrate may contain variable amounts of activated factors, patients receiving repeated doses of factor IX concentrate are at increased risk for disseminated intravascular coagulation (DIC) and, paradoxically, thrombosis. For this reason, heparin (5 to 10 units) is often added to each milliliter of reconstituted prothrombin complex concentrate.

The levels of factors VIII or IX should be raised transiently to about 30% to protect against bleeding after dental extraction or to abort a beginning joint hemorrhage, to 50% if major joint or intramuscular bleeding is already evident, and to 100% in life-threatening bleeding or before major operation. The transmission of human immunodeficiency virus (HIV) to the hemophiliac population through replacement blood products was a major complication of transfusion therapy, with 55% of hemophiliacs infected with HIV-1 by the mid 1980s; this complication has been eliminated by viral inactivation procedures, mandatory blood donor screening for HIV blood screening, and the use of recombinant products.[13]

In hemophiliacs with a factor VIII inhibitor who are bleeding, treatment with factor VIII will stimulate further production of antibodies; therefore, consultation of a coagulation specialist is necessary. Special preparations of prothrombin complex concentrates that bypass the role of factor VIII in coagulation are available but expensive. Recombinant factor VIII preparations are also often effective in patients with inhibitors.

Recombinant factor VIIa (rFVIIa) has been used successfully to stop active bleeding in hemophilia patients and nonhemophilia patients with antibodies to factor VIII. Although the exact mechanism of action has not been elucidated, there appears to be a TF-independent activation of platelets. Normally 1% of total-body factor VII is circulating in activated form, which forms a complex with exposed subendothelial TF after injury. With the administration of high doses of factor VIIa, platelet activation occurs with formation of stable thrombin, independent of other clotting factors. Several randomized trials have demonstrated effectiveness of rFVIIa in producing hemostasis in hemophilia patients with life- or limb-threatening hemorrhage and inhibitors to factors VIII and IX. Administration of a single dose of rFVIIa given at 90 to 120 µg/kg intravenously over 3 to 5 minutes has been shown to induce immediate hemostasis. Repeated doses every 2 to 3 hours can be given without laboratory monitoring. rFVIIa has also shown potential as first-line therapy for life-threatening hemorrhage secondary to DIC after major surgery or trauma. rFVIIa is also effective in improving clotting ability in patients with liver disease and thrombocytopenia.[14]

Von Willebrand's Disease

Von Willebrand's disease is the most common congenital bleeding disorder; its frequency is estimated as high as 1%. Most patients have a mild bleeding disorder. The symptoms of von Willebrand's disease are related to its role as an important stimulus to platelet aggregation at the site of tissue injury and as the major carrier protein for circulating factor VIII. A large number of subtypes have been described, most of which are rare. The three major groups are type I, inherited as an autosomal dominant trait and characterized by a quantitative decrease of an otherwise normally functioning factor VIIIR; type II, which is variably inherited and characterized by qualitative defects in factor VIIIR; and type III, an autosomal recessive severe bleeding disorder with essentially absent levels of factor VIIIR. Bleeding encountered in patients with von Willebrand's disease is similar to that of patients with bleeding from platelet dysfunction with mucosal bleeding, petechiae, epistaxis, and menorrhagia.

The laboratory diagnosis of von Willebrand's disease varies by subtype. Type I von Willebrand's disease is characterized by a normal PT, a mildly prolonged aPTT, an abnormal bleeding time, a normal platelet count, and a mild reduction in factors VIII:C and VIII:Ag. The reduction in factor VIII:C occurs because factor VIIIR is the serum carrier for factor VIII. Patients with blood type O have lower normal levels of factors VIII:C and VIII:Ag and may be erroneously thought to have mild type I von Willebrand's disease. The diagnosis of type II von Willebrand's disease is complicated by many subgroups. In general, decreased functional activity of factor VIIIR produces a depressed ristocetin cofactor assay (factor VIIIR:Cof), which measures the effectiveness of factor VIIIR in agglutinating platelets when stimulated with the antibiotic ristocetin. A further subtype of type II von Willebrand's disease, called *pseudo-von Willebrand's disease,* is a platelet disorder characterized by the presence of very large platelets that aggregate in the presence of cryoprecipitate. Near-complete absence of factors VIII:C, VIII:Ag, and VIIIR:C characterize type III von Willebrand's disease. These patients have prolonged aPTT levels, abnormal bleeding times, and low platelet counts. The help of a coagulation specialist is important in determining the subtype and treatment.

The administration of desmopressin, 0.3 µg/kg, causes significant shortening in the bleeding time and normalization of factors VIII and VIIIR activities. It is effective in reducing blood loss in the perioperative setting.[15] About 48 hours must elapse for new endothelial stores of factor VIIIR to accumulate and so permit a second injection of desmopressin to be as effective as an initial dose. Replacement of factor VIIIR by infusing cryoprecipitate is effective in the control or prevention of bleeding in von Willebrand's disease. Dosage is often selected empirically (e.g., 1 bag/10 kg every 8 to 12 hours for several days to prevent excessive bleeding after major operation). The choice of treatment is based on the subtype of disease.[16]

Other Congenital Deficiencies

Other congenital deficiencies may rarely be encountered, including deficiencies of factors XI and XII, prekallikrein, and high-molecular-weight kininogen, also called the *contact factors.* Deficiencies of factors VII, V, and prothrombin have been described but are extremely rare. Disorders of fibrinogen, including afibrinogenemia, hypofibrinogenemia, and dysfibrinogenemia may occur. Bleeding disorders in these patients range from mild to severe, depending on the level and function of factor in circulation. Factor XIII deficiency creates abnormalities of the cross-linking of fibrin monomers. This is a rare autosomal recessive disorder characterized by poor wound healing and delayed bleeding. Standard laboratory testing is not diagnostic, and determination of factor XIII levels is necessary for the diagnosis.

ACQUIRED BLEEDING DISORDERS

Many coagulation abnormalities may be present in the surgical patient. Acquired defects are more common than congenital defects.

Vitamin K Deficiency

Vitamin K is necessary for the reaction that attaches a carboxyl group to glutamic acid, and the proteins containing carboxyglutamic acid residues are therefore called *vitamin K–dependent clotting factors* (including prothrombin, factors VII, IX, and X, and proteins C and S). When synthesized in the absence of vitamin K, these proteins, lacking carboxyglutamic acid residues, cannot bind calcium normally. This is also the site of action of warfarin. The causes of vitamin K deficiency may be inadequate dietary intake, malabsorption, lack of bile salts, obstructive jaundice, biliary fistula, oral administration of antibiotics, or parenteral alimentation. A number of broad-spectrum antibiotics can cause a vitamin K–dependent coagulopathy, including cephalosporins, quinolones, doxycycline, and trimethoprim-sulfamethoxazole.

Vitamin K may be administered parenterally and produces a correction in clotting times within 6 to 12 hours.

Up to 5 mg intravenously is given slowly as an initial dose. Older preparations of vitamin K were less purified than those used at present, and anaphylaxis and death were reported with intravenous administration of these older agents. The more purified forms are less likely to cause complications, but intravenous vitamin K should be given cautiously. Intramuscular or subcutaneous vitamin K may be given in doses of 10 to 25 mg/day. Repeated doses of intramuscular or subcutaneous vitamin K allow total body repletion (10 to 25 mg/day for 3 days). Administration of FFP rapidly corrects the coagulation deficit and should be given with vitamin K to patients with ongoing bleeding.

Anticoagulant Drugs

Warfarin acts by blocking the synthesis of vitamin K–dependent factors, prolongs the PT, and causes a slight elevation of the aPTT by reducing the levels of prothrombin and factors VII, IX, and X. Warfarin has a half-life of 40 hours, and treatment of major bleeding caused by warfarin consists of either administration of vitamin K or infusion of FFP for life-threatening bleeding.

Unfractionated heparin (UFH) blocks the activation of factor X by binding with AT-III and thrombin. All coagulation tests can be affected by UFH, including the PT, but the aPTT is most sensitive. A dose of UFH is cleared from the blood in approximately 6 hours but varies depending on other factors such as hepatic function, body temperature, and shock. UFH can be neutralized with intravenous protamine sulfate (100 units of UFH is equal to 1 mg of protamine). UFH can cause thrombocytopenia in up to 5% of patients owing to the formation of IgG antibodies to heparin-platelet factor 4 complexes. In most patients this leads to a reversible drop in circulating platelets, but it also rarely causes a profound thrombocytopenia with secondary arterial and venous thrombosis.[17] In any patient who has a decrease in platelet count, all heparin should be withdrawn immediately and another anticoagulant such as lepirudin or argatroban initiated if necessary.

Low-molecular-weight heparins (LMWH) derived from UFH have more selective anti-Xa activity than UFH. LMWH have been associated with less bleeding complications and have become the first-line therapy for deep venous thrombosis prophylaxis and treatment and acute coronary syndromes. The PT is not usually affected by LMWH, and anti-Xa activity should be measured if dose efficacy is questioned. Thrombocytopenia can also occur with LMWH.

Hepatic Failure

Liver diseases including major hepatic trauma, cirrhosis, and biliary obstruction can impair coagulation. The liver is the major site of synthesis of all the coagulation factors except factor VIII. Hemostasis may be further impaired by an associated thrombocytopenia or platelet dysfunction, which also occurs frequently with liver disease. Thrombocytopenia has been attributed to decreased production, splenic sequestration, circulating antiplatelet antibodies, and viral hepatitis infection (particularly hepatitis C). The prolonged bleeding times frequently seen in cirrhotic patients can be improved by administration of desmopressin.[18] Desmopressin is often ineffective with thrombocytopenia or congenital platelet dysfunction. Hyperfibrinolysis in cirrhosis also contributes to coagulopathy. The liver is important in clearing blood of the activated metabolites of both fibrinolysis and coagulation, and the coagulation system may be pushed either toward coagulation or bleeding in patients with liver dysfunction.

Liver disease is commonly associated with a low level of serum fibrinogen, a prolonged PT,[19] and a normal to slightly increased aPTT. An elevated TT usually indicates abnormal or decreased fibrinogen. In patients with severe liver dysfunction, large volumes of FFP may be required to maintain normal factor levels. Up to 2 units of FFP may be needed every 2 hours in patients with complete liver failure to maintain adequate coagulation factor levels.

Renal Failure

Renal disease and uremia cause a reversible bleeding disorder related to platelet dysfunction. There is a decrease in aggregation and adhesiveness of platelets and levels of platelet factor II, resulting in a prolonged bleeding time. The nature of the lesion caused by renal insufficiency is not known. The administration of desmopressin helps decrease bleeding problems after procedures in these patients.[15] Intravenous desmopressin, 0.3 μg/kg, decreases bleeding time, increases platelet retention on glass beads, and increases activity of factor VIII. Cryoprecipitate and conjugated estrogens can also shorten the bleeding time.

Thrombocytopenia

Normal platelet counts range from 150,000 to 400,000/mm³. A platelet count of less than 100,000/mm³ generally constitutes thrombocytopenia. With platelet counts between 40,000 and 100,000/mm³, bleeding may occur after injury or operation but spontaneous bleeding is uncommon. Spontaneous bleeding may occur with platelet counts between 10,000 and 20,000/mm³; with counts below 10,000/mm³, spontaneous bleeding is frequent and often severe.

Thrombocytopenia may be secondary to failure of production of platelets, splenic sequestration, increased destruction of platelets, increased use of platelets, or dilution. Defects in platelets often cause spontaneous bleeding into the skin, manifested by petechiae, purpura, or confluent ecchymoses. Thrombocytopenia also causes mucosal bleeding and excessive bleeding after operation. Heavy gastrointestinal bleeding and bleeding into the central nervous system may be life-threatening manifestations of thrombocytopenia. Thrombocytopenia does not generally cause massive bleeding into tissues or hemarthroses.

Drugs (e.g., quinidine, sulfa preparations, H₂ blockers, oral antidiabetic agents, gold salts, rifampin, and heparin) can cause thrombocytopenia. Contributing factors include a recent blood transfusion with post-transfusion purpura,

heavy consumption of alcohol (alcohol-induced thrombocytopenia), and underlying immunologic disease (e.g., arthralgia, Raynaud's phenomenon, unexplained fever). The presence or absence of fever is an important point of differential diagnosis. It is usually present in thrombocytopenia secondary to infection or active systemic lupus erythematosus and in thrombotic thrombocytopenic purpura but absent in idiopathic thrombocytopenic purpura and in drug-related thrombocytopenias. Size of the spleen on physical examination is a second important diagnostic point. The spleen is not palpably enlarged in most thrombocytopenias caused by increased destruction of platelets (e.g., idiopathic thrombocytopenic purpura, drug-related immune thrombocytopenias), whereas it is usually palpably enlarged in thrombocytopenia secondary to splenic sequestration of platelets and often in patients with thrombocytopenia secondary to lymphoma or a myeloproliferative disorder.

The peripheral blood cell count provides clues to the diagnosis and severity of thrombocytopenia. An increased proportion of large platelets suggests compensatory increased production of platelets and is often found in thrombocytopenias secondary to increased destruction or utilization of platelets. The bleeding time is prolonged in severe thrombocytopenia of any cause. Bone marrow aspiration is useful.

Management of thrombocytopenia secondary to decreased production is directed toward correcting its cause. Platelet concentrates can raise the platelet count temporarily; however, repeated use reduces their effectiveness, owing to development of platelet alloantibodies. If rapid correction of bone marrow failure is not expected, transfusions of platelets are often reserved to treat an active bleeding episode. Corticosteroids have not proved beneficial in the management of patients with thrombocytopenia secondary to bone marrow failure.

Thrombocytopathy

Platelet dysfunction can occur secondary to drugs, congenital disorders, and metabolic derangement. Drugs to consider with important effects on platelets include chemotherapeutic agents, thiazide diuretics, alcohol, estrogen, antibiotics such as the sulfa agents, quinidine and quinine, methyldopa, and gold salts. The most common drugs that block platelet function are prostaglandin inhibitors, particularly aspirin, indomethacin, and other NSAIDs. Aspirin and other NSAIDs act to block prostaglandin metabolism in the platelet. Aspirin permanently acetylates cyclooxygenase, and affected platelets remain dysfunctional throughout their 7-day life span after exposure to aspirin. NSAIDs cause a reversible defect that lasts 3 to 4 days. Desmopressin may be effective in normalizing the prolonged bleeding time caused by aspirin.[20] A normal platelet count with dysfunctional platelets can occur with congenital disorders such as Glanzmann's thrombasthenia (glycoprotein IIb/IIIa dysfunction) and Bernard-Soulier syndrome (platelet glycoprotein Ib/IX/V receptor deficiency) and with metabolic derangement.

Hypothermia

Hypothermia is one of the most common and least well-recognized causes of altered coagulation in surgical patients, especially those receiving massive transfusion.[21] This is exacerbated in patients who have an open thoracic or abdominal cavity, which accelerates heat loss. The coagulation system is a series of proteolytic enzymes, activity of which decreases with decreasing temperature. Hypothermia is characterized by a marked increase in fibrinolytic activity, thrombocytopenia, impaired platelet function,[22] decrease in collagen-induced platelet aggregation, and increased affinity of hemoglobin for oxygen. Hypothermia has been associated with hepatic dysfunction and increased levels of blood citrate and hypocalcemia with transfusion, an effect exacerbated by shock. If blood is being rapidly infused through a central line with its tip near the sinoatrial node, fatal dysrhythmias can result.

Hypothermia and bleeding usually occur in a patient who receives large-volume resuscitation during an extensive surgical procedure or in the perioperative period. Temperatures as low as 30°C to 34°C can be associated with coagulopathy even if levels of factors and platelets are normal. Nonmechanical bleeding can occur and be uncontrollable and lethal. The best course is to terminate the surgical procedure as expeditiously as possible, pack bleeding areas as needed, close the surgical incision, and attempt to rewarm the patient as rapidly as possible in the intensive care unit. Damage control celiotomy for trauma, which includes an abbreviated celiotomy with control of gross bleeding, overt enteric contamination, packing and staged delayed definitive repair of injuries, and abdominal closure has become key in preventing the triangle of death: hypothermia, acidosis, and coagulopathy. Continued administration of FFP, platelets, and other blood products can worsen hypothermia with continued bleeding. Warming intravenous fluids before they are given can ameliorate hypothermia. Care must be taken not to heat RBCs above 40°C because shortened survival or acute hemolysis can result. Hemorrhage accounts for 90% of deaths after abdominal injury, and half of these deaths are secondary to a recalcitrant coagulopathy.[23]

DISSEMINATED INTRAVASCULAR COAGULATION

DIC is a syndrome rather than a specific disease. Much confusion and controversy surround the diagnosis and treatment. Although DIC is generally considered a hemorrhagic disorder because of the obvious bleeding problems encountered, it is important to recognize the very serious sequelae resulting from microvascular (and sometimes large vessel) thrombosis that always accompanies true DIC and leads to end-organ failure and death. DIC is a systemic thrombohemorrhagic disorder seen in association with many clinical situations with laboratory evidence of coagulant activation, fibrinolytic activation, inhibitor consumption, and end-organ dysfunction.[24] The disorder may have a spectrum of presentations, from *low-grade* DIC, with minimal symptoms and minor laboratory abnormalities, to *fulminant DIC,* presenting with life-threatening bleeding and coagulation abnormalities producing end-organ dysfunction and death. Disorders associated with DIC include hemolysis, massive transfusion, amniotic fluid embolism, placental abruption, retained fetus, gram-negative and gram-positive sepsis, viremia, burns, crush injury and tissue destruction, leukemia, malignancy (especially metastatic), liver disease, and miscellaneous inflammatory and autoimmune conditions, including vasculitis. Although the diagnosis of DIC is often attached to patients who are receiving massive transfusion, platelet dysfunction due to hypothermia or a specific factor deficiency should be excluded before making a diagnosis of DIC. In most cases, such patients will respond to rewarming and replenishment of coagulation factors and platelets (see Massive Transfusion).

With the activation of the coagulation and fibrinolytic systems, both thrombin and plasmin are in circulation. Thrombin cleaves fibrinopeptides A and B from fibrinogen, converting it to fibrin monomers. These monomers form soluble fibrin clots, causing microvascular thrombosis with entrapment and depletion of platelets. Simultaneous degradation of these factors by plasmin occurs. Depressed levels of fibrinogen and elevated levels of fibrinogen degradation products (fibrin-split products) result. These degradation products inhibit the normal coagulation of blood by delaying polymerization of fibrin. Fibrin degradation products may also interpose themselves between fibrin and polymers, forming a weak fibrin clot. The fibrin degradation products include X, Y, D, and E fragments; platelet dysfunction is attributable to the latter two fragments. Plasmin also degrades factors V, VIII, IX, and XI and activates the complement system. These changes produce the clinically observed changes characteristic of DIC.

Laboratory abnormalities in DIC are variable and related to the many diseases that are associated with this condition. Common abnormalities include abnormal PT and aPTT levels with depressed fibrinogen levels and abnormal platelet counts. Levels of fibrin degradation products and D-dimer are elevated. The peripheral smear reveals fragmented RBCs, but this finding is not specific. Because of the continued activation of coagulation, thrombin/antithrombin complexes will be formed. Levels of thrombin/antithrombin and AT-III are depressed. Fragments of coagulation factor degradation are elevated, including F1.2 and FpA. Because of the activation of the fibrinolytic system, plasminogen and α_2-antiplasmin inhibitor levels are decreased.

Low-grade DIC generally responds to management of the underlying disorder, with some patients requiring heparin therapy. The appropriate therapy for fulminant DIC remains controversial, compounded by the lack of objective studies and many underlying causes. The help of a physician experienced in managing DIC is valuable. The treatment of the underlying condition is critical to the successful management of DIC. Also important is the treatment of the thrombotic intravascular process that causes end-organ failure. Therapy with heparin is begun if treatment of the underlying pathology does not ameliorate DIC after 6 to 8 hours. Intravenous heparin is administered in doses of 80 to 100 units/kg every 4 to 6 hours.[24] Higher doses of heparin may be needed if the patient does not respond. Antithrombin concentrates administered to attain a serum level of 125% of normal have been useful in some patients. Continued bleeding may be related to depletion of components, but random administration of blood products, especially those containing fibrinogen, may exacerbate the syndrome. Washed RBCs, platelets, AT-III concentrate, and crystalloid and colloid volume expanders may be used. If other therapeutic measures are unsuccessful, inhibition of fibrinolysis may be employed. ε-Aminocaproic acid may be given along with heparin. Despite improved diagnostic and therapeutic modalities, mortality from DIC remains high and closely related to the underlying disorder.

PREPARATION OF BLOOD COMPONENTS

Component therapy is the accepted standard for the optimal management of the blood supply. Blood is separated into its individual components (packed RBCs, plasma, platelets) to optimize therapeutic potency. This strategy maximizes the benefit derived from each individual unit while minimizing the risk to each recipient. Blood is withdrawn from the donor and mixed with a citrate solution to prevent coagulation by binding calcium. The solutions used commonly are citrate phosphate dextrose (CPD), citrate phosphate double dextrose (CP2D), and citrate phosphate dextrose adenine (CPDA-1). Solutions containing some combination of dextrose, adenine, sodium chloride, and either phosphate (AS-3) or mannitol (AS-1 and AS-5) extend the storage life of cells. The unit is gently centrifuged (Fig. 6-4) to pack the RBCs and leave

about 70% of the platelets suspended in plasma. The platelet-rich plasma is removed and centrifuged again at a faster speed to precipitate the platelets. All but 50 mL of supernatant plasma is removed and rapidly frozen at less than −30°C. The platelets are resuspended to yield platelet concentrate. Frozen plasma that is stored at less than −18°C is termed *fresh frozen plasma.* If the frozen plasma is allowed to thaw at 4°C, the precipitate that remains can be collected to yield cryoprecipitate. Proteins, such as albumin, can be isolated from the remaining supernatant plasma by ethanol fractionation (Table 6-1).

Manual or mechanical apheresis can be employed to collect leukocytes, platelets, or plasma. In manual apheresis, a unit of whole blood is drawn from the donor and centrifuged; plasma, platelets, or both are removed, and the remaining blood is returned to the donor. In mechanical apheresis, blood is withdrawn continuously from the donor. The blood is separated by centrifuge, and the desired component is removed. The remaining blood is then returned to the donor in a continuous loop. Large numbers of units of leukocytes or platelets can be removed in a relatively short period.

The storage and refrigeration of packed RBCs create progressive changes, known as *storage lesions,* which include altered affinity of hemoglobin for oxygen; decrease in pH; changes in RBC deformability; hemolysis; an increase in the concentration of potassium, phosphate, and ammonia; development of microaggregates; release of vasoactive substances; and denaturation of proteins. The survival of RBCs is shorter the longer cells are stored. This is associated with a decrease in intracellular 2,3-diphosphoglycerate (2,3-DPG). The transfusion of cold blood may also contribute to the development of hypothermia, especially in patients receiving large volumes of banked blood rapidly. Many of the changes

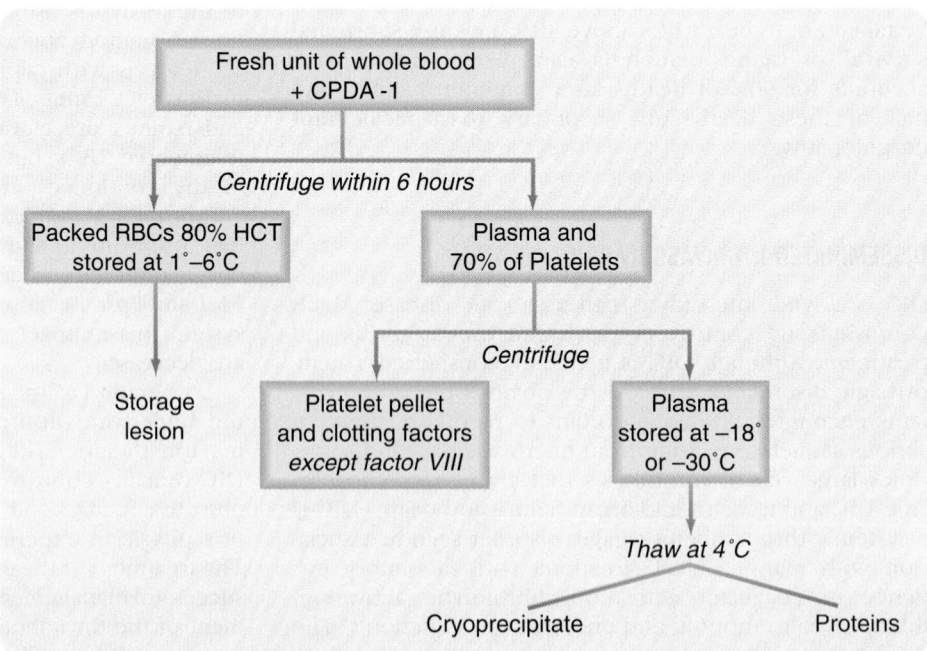

FIGURE 6-4.   Preparation of blood components. CPDA-1, citrate phosphate dextrose adenine; HCT, hematocrit; RBC, red blood cell.

TABLE 6-1. Summary of Available Blood Components

Component	Composition	Shelf Life
Whole blood	RBCs; nonfunctional WBCs and platelets; plasma (450 mL total volume contains 200 mL of RBCs)	CPDA-1: 35 days (1° to 6°C)
Packed RBCs	RBCs; some plasma; nonfunctional WBCs and platelets (250 to 350 mL total volume contains 200 mL of RBCs)	AS-1: 42 days
Leukocyte-reduced RBCs	RBCs; minimum plasma and nonfunctional WBCs and platelets (200 mL total volume contains 170 to 190 mL of RBCs)	24 hr (1° to 6°C)
Platelets (single unit from whole blood donation)	Platelets; some nonfunctional WBCs; few RBCs; plasma (50 to 70 mL total volume contains 5.5 (10^{10} platelets); levels of labile clotting factors depend on storage time	5 days (20° to 24°C)
Platelets (apheresis from random donor)	As above; usually contains as many platelets as 6 to 10 single units (>30 (10^{10})	Usually 24 hr; up to 5 days (20° to 24°C)
Leukocyte concentrate	WBCs; may contain large numbers of platelets, some RBCs (600 mL total volume contains 5 to 30 (10^9 granulocytes)	24 hr (20° to 24°C)
Fresh frozen plasma	Plasma, all coagulation factors (180 to 250 mL contains 0.7 to 1 unit/mL of prothrombin; factors V, VII, VIII, IX, XII, and XIII; and 500 mg of fibrinogen)	Frozen: 1 yr (<−30°C) Thawed: 24 hr (1° to 6°C)
Cryoprecipitate	Fibrinogen, factors VIII, VIIIR, XIII, fibronectin (10 to 20 mL contains 80 units/mL factor VIII, 200 mg fibrinogen)	Frozen: 1 yr (<−30°C) Thawed: 4 hr if pooled (20° to 24°C)
Albumin	Albumin (12.5 g albumin in 50 or 250 mL)	3 yr (room temperature)

RBCs, red blood cells; WBCs, white blood cells; CPDA-1, citrate phosphate dextrose adenine; AS-1, Adsol.

described may be reversed within a short time after transfusion and may cause metabolic patterns different from those predicted.

CLINICAL INDICATIONS AND USE OF BLOOD COMPONENTS

Transfusion based on sound physiologic principles and an understanding of relative risks and benefits should give maximal benefit to the patient, with efficient use of a valuable and finite resource. A consensus conference reviewed the existing literature and developed 11 policies for surgical blood management and proposed interventions.[25] The standards, guidelines, and options are summarized in Table 6-2. The specific needs of some patients may require consultation with specialists in transfusion medicine.

Whole Blood

Storage of whole blood precludes the production of components and is highly inefficient. Whole blood is thus unavailable in most blood banks in the United States because oxygen-carrying capacity and replacement of volume can be achieved with packed RBCs and crystalloid solutions. There are currently few indications for whole blood, and many U.S. blood banks do not routinely store this product.

Red Blood Cells

Packed RBCs can be stored in AS-1 solution with a shelf life of 42 days. With longer storage, fewer than 70% of the RBCs remain viable in circulation 24 hours after transfusion, which is the current U.S. Food and Drug Administration (FDA) definition of an outdated unit. Platelets degenerate at refrigerator temperatures, so banked packed RBCs contain essentially no functioning platelets. The levels of factors V and VIII decrease significantly over 24 hours at 1°C to 6°C, although the levels of other factors remain essentially unchanged.

Packed RBCs provide oxygen-carrying capacity and maintain oxygen delivery provided intravascular volume and cardiac function are adequate. The decision to transfuse and the amount to transfuse depend on the clinical situation. The use of a hematocrit of 30% (or a hemoglobin of 10 g/dL) as a *transfusion trigger* is no longer acceptable. Oxygen delivery is maintained by a series of complex interactions and compensatory mechanisms when red cell mass (measured by hemoglobin or hematocrit) falls. This includes increased cardiac output,

TABLE 6-2. Blood Management Policies* and Interventions

Policies/Interventions	Settings		
	Preop	**Intraop**	**Postop**
Transfusion need should be assessed on a case-by-case basis	X	X	X
Blood should be transfused 1 U at a time, followed by an assessment of benefit and further need	X	X	X
Exposure to allogeneic blood should be limited to appropriate need	X	X	X
Modify the "transfusion trigger" based on hemoglobin/hematocrit level (option)	X	X	X
Consider the use of directed-donor blood (option)	X	X	X
Perioperative blood loss should be prevented or controlled	X	X	X
Consider stopping aspirin, nonsteroidal anti-inflammatory drugs, warfarin, heparin, similar anticoagulant drugs, and thrombolytic agents before surgery (standard)	X		
Identify and address any existing coagulopathy (standard)	X	X	X
Restrict perioperative phlebotomy to necessary tests (standard)	X	X	X
Consider use of regional anesthesia (option)		X	
Consider use of hypotensive anesthesia (option)		X	
Maintain careful surgical hemostasis (standard)		X	
Modify surgical approach (option)		X	
Employ locally acting agents that encourage clotting, such as fibrin glue, collagen, and topical thrombin (option)		X	
Employ fibrinolytic drugs such as aprotinin, aminocaproic acid, desmopressin acetate, and tranexamic acid (option)	X	X	X
Employ drugs designed specifically to reduce or stop bleeding in gynecologic conditions (option)	X	X	X
Before resorting to surgery, consider tumor embolization using angiographic techniques (option)	X		
Autologous blood should be considered for use as an alternative to allogeneic transfusion	X	X	X
Consider preoperative autologous blood procurement (option/guideline)	X		
Consider intraoperative acute normovolemic hemodiluion (option/guideline)		X	
Consider intraoperative autologous blood salvage and autotransfusion (option/guideline)		X	
Consider postoperative autologous blood salvage and autotransfusion (option)			X
Efforts should be made to maximize oxygen delivery in the surgical patient	X	X	X
Treat underlying cardiopulmonary disease (standard)	X	X	X
Red blood cell mass should be increased or restored by means other than red blood cell transfusion	X		X
Replace iron stores in patients with documented iron deficiency (standard)	X		X
Consider the use of epoetin alfa to increase or restore red blood cell mass (guideline)	X		X
The patient should be involved in the transfusion decision	X		X
The reasons for and results of the transfusion decision should be documented contemporaneously in the patient's record	X	X	X
Hospital transfusion policies and procedures should be developed as a cooperative effort that includes input from all those involved in the transfusion decision	X		X
Transfusion practices, both individual and institutional, should be reassessed yearly or more often	X		X

Abbreviations: Preop, preoperative; Intraop, intraoperative; Postop, postoperative.
*Boldface rows are practice policies.
(Reprinted from American Journal of Surgery, Vol. 170, No. 6A, supplement, Spence RK, Surgical red blood cell transfusion practice policies. pp. 3S–15S. Copyright 1995, with permission from Excerpta Medica Inc.)

increased extraction ratio, rightward shift of the oxyhemoglobin curve, and expansion of volume. Many chronically anemic patients tolerate hemoglobin levels of 7 to 8 g/dL or less, as has been demonstrated in chronic renal failure and Jehovah's Witnesses. The cardiac output does not increase until hemoglobin falls below approximately 7 g/dL. Young healthy patients tolerate acute anemia to hemoglobin levels of 7 g/dL or less, provided they have a normal intravascular volume and high arterial oxygen saturation. The primary compensation in this setting is an increased cardiac output (heart rate and stroke volume). The response to the lowered RBC mass and the need for RBC transfusion can be assessed by clinical criteria, such as ongoing blood loss, increased heart rate, dizziness, decreased urinary output, base deficit, lactic acidosis, mixed venous oxygen saturation, and oxygen delivery, and then weighed against potential untoward effects.

A retrospective, multicenter, cohort study of 8787 patients older than age 60 undergoing surgical repair of hip fracture was conducted to determine the effect of perioperative transfusion on 30- and 90-day mortality. No differences were demonstrated in outcome of patients transfused at a transfusion trigger of 8 g/dL of hemoglobin compared with those receiving blood for a hemoglobin level of 10 g/dL.[26] In a multicenter, randomized, controlled study of transfusion in 838 patients in the critical care setting, a liberal transfusion strategy (transfusion for hemoglobin <10 g/dL) was compared with a restrictive strategy (transfusion for hemoglobin <7 g/dL). The restrictive strategy was found to be at least as effective as the liberal strategy, with the possible exception of patients with acute myocardial infarction and unstable angina.[27]

In patients with significant cardiopulmonary disease, transfusion may be considered because increases in cardiac output may cause myocardial ischemia. Stable, asymptomatic patients should not receive packed RBCs solely for a hematocrit below 30% (Box 6-1). Each unit of packed RBCs usually raises the hematocrit 2% to 3% in a 70-kg adult, although this varies depending on the donor, the recipient's fluid status, the method of storage, and its duration.

Leukocyte-Reduced RBCs

An association between immunosuppression and allogeneic transfusion has been noted and subsequently challenged. This effect is thought to be related to exposure to leukocytes and may be decreased or prevented with leukocyte-reduced components. Despite significant cost and the lack of a definitive conclusion, the Blood Products Advisory Committee of the U.S. FDA has recommended "the benefit-to-risk ratio associated with leukoreduction is sufficiently great to justify requiring the universal leukoreduction of all non-leukocyte cellular transfusion blood components."[28] A University HealthSystem Consortium Expert Panel reviewed the literature and identified four indications for WBC-reduced blood components[29]: (1) to decrease the incidence of subsequent refractoriness to platelet transfusion caused by HLA alloimmunization in patients requiring long-term platelet support; (2) to provide blood components with reduced risk for CMV transmission; (3) to prevent subsequent febrile non-

---

Box 6-1. Suggested Transfusion Guidelines for Red Blood Cells

Hemoglobin <8 g/dL or acute blood loss in an otherwise healthy patient with signs and symptoms of decreased oxygen delivery with two or more of the following:
  Estimated or anticipated acute blood loss of >15% of total blood volume (750 mL in 70-kg male)
  Diastolic blood pressure <60 mm Hg
  Systolic blood pressure drop >30 mm Hg from baseline
  Tachycardia (>100 beats/min)
  Oliguria/anuria
  Mental status changes

Hemoglobin <10 g/dL in patients with known increased risk of coronary artery disease or pulmonary insufficiency who have sustained or are expected to sustain significant blood loss
  Symptomatic anemia with any of the following:
  Tachycardia (>100 beats/min)
  Mental status changes
  Evidence of myocardial ischemia including angina
  Shortness of breath or dizziness with mild exertion
  Orthostatic hypotension

Unfounded/questionable indications:
  To increase wound healing
  To improve the patient's sense of well-being
  7 g/dL < hemoglobin <10 g/dL (or 21% < hematocrit <30%) in otherwise stable, asymptomatic patient
  Mere availability of pre-donated autologous blood without medical indication

---

hemolytic transfusion reaction (FNHTR) in patients who have had one documented FNHTR; and (4) to decrease the incidence of HLA alloimmunization in nonhepatic solid-organ transplant candidates. Other indications lack evidence for benefit and may increase risk secondary to increased financial burden.

Platelets

Platelet transfusions are indicated for patients suffering from or at significant risk of bleeding owing to thrombocytopenia and/or platelet dysfunction. Three types of platelet concentrate are available. A single, random-donor unit of platelets is prepared from a single donation of whole blood from one donor (Fig. 6-4). Multiple-unit, single-donor platelets are harvested from one donor by apheresis. This yields as many platelets as 6 to 10 single random-donor units. Multiple-unit, single-donor platelets can be obtained by apheresis from donors who are selected by human leukocyte antigen (HLA) type to yield HLA-matched platelets. Besides monitoring the patient for evidence of improved hemostasis, follow-up platelet counts at 1 hour and 12 or 24 hours can provide an esti-

Box 6-2. Suggested Transfusion Guidelines for Platelets

Recent (within 24 hours) platelet count <10,000/mm^3 (for prophylaxis)

   Recent (within 24 hours) platelet count <50,000/mm^3 with demonstrated microvascular bleeding ("oozing") or a planned surgical/invasive procedure

   Demonstrated microvascular bleeding and a precipitous fall in platelet count

   Adult patients in the operating room who have had complicated procedures or have required more than 10 units of blood **AND** have microvascular bleeding. Giving platelets assumes adequate surgical hemostasis has been achieved.

   Documented platelet dysfunction (e.g., prolonged bleeding time greater than 15 minutes, abnormal platelet function tests) with petechiae, purpura, microvascular bleeding ("oozing"), or surgical/invasive procedure

   Unwarranted indications:

      Empirical use with massive transfusion when patient is not having clinically evident microvascular bleeding ("oozing")

   Prophylaxis in thrombotic thrombocytopenic purpura/ hemolytic-uremic syndrome or idiopathic thrombocytopenic purpura

   Extrinsic platelet dysfunction (e.g., renal failure, von Willebrand's disease)

Box 6-3. Suggested Transfusion Guidelines for Fresh Frozen Plasma

Treatment of multiple or specific coagulation factor deficiency with abnormal prothrombin time and/or activated partial thromboplastin time

   Abnormal specific factor deficiency in the presence of one of the following:

      Congenital deficiency of AT-III; prothrombin, factors V, VII, IX, X, and XI; protein C or S; plasminogen or antiplasmin

      Acquired deficiency related to warfarin therapy, vitamin K deficiency, liver disease, massive transfusion, or disseminated intravascular coagulation

   Also indicated as prophylaxis for the above if a surgical/invasive procedure is planned

   Unwarranted indications:

      Empirical use during massive transfusion if patient does not exhibit clinical coagulopathy

      Volume replacement

      Nutritional supplement

      Hypoalbuminemia

mate of platelet survival. After platelet transfusion, the platelet count obtained at 1 hour should increase at least 5000 platelets/mm^3 for each unit of platelets transfused. Patients may experience a lesser response, especially after repeated transfusion and the development of alloimmunization or because of fever, sepsis, splenomegaly, drug effects, or uremia. When alloimmunization causes the poor response, single-donor units may provide an adequate response. Platelets from a donor of HLA type similar to that of the patient may also be needed.

Platelets should not be transfused prophylactically in the absence of microvascular bleeding, a low platelet count in a patient undergoing a surgical procedure, or a platelet count that has fallen below 10,000/mm^3 (Box 6-2). A threshold of 10,000/mm^3 causes no added bleeding while significantly reducing use of the resource. Patients receiving massive transfusion should not automatically receive prophylactic platelets in the absence of microvascular bleeding.[30] Hypothermia depresses platelet function, and platelet transfusion is generally ineffective.[22] Restoration of a normal temperature returns platelet function to normal and ameliorates microvascular bleeding.

Leukocyte Concentrate

Leukocyte transfusions are indicated in profound granulocytopenia (<500/mm^3) with evidence of infection (e.g., positive blood culture, persistent temperature above

38.5°C) unresponsive to antibiotic therapy. Daily transfusions are given until the infection is under control or the granulocyte count is greater than 1000/mm^3. Because leukocyte concentrate is usually prepared by mechanical apheresis from donors typically premedicated with corticosteroids to increase the number of circulating granulocytes, using hydroxyethyl starch to enhance the separation of cells, there is more risk to the donor than with a routine blood donation. Consultation with specialists in infectious disease is recommended.

Fresh Frozen Plasma

FFP is used to replace labile factors in patients with coagulopathy and documented factor deficiency. This condition may derive from liver dysfunction, congenital absence of factors, or transfusion of factor-deficient blood products. A unit of FFP contains near-normal levels of all factors, including about 400 mg of fibrinogen, and increases factor levels by about 3%. Adequate clotting is usually achieved with factor levels above 30%, although higher levels are advisable in patients undergoing operative or invasive procedures. The PT and the aPTT can be used to assess patients for FFP transfusion and to follow the efficacy of administered FFP.

Documentation of factor deficiency or abnormal PT or aPTT in a patient with clinical bleeding minimizes unnecessary use of FFP (Box 6-3). FFP should not be used routinely by preset formula after RBC transfusion (e.g., 2 units of FFP for every 5 units of packed RBCs) or *prophylactically* after cardiac bypass or other procedures. With equally effective but safer and less expensive crystalloids, FFP should not be used as a volume expander.[31]

Solvent detergent (SD) treated plasma was approved by the U.S. FDA to inactivate enveloped viruses, particularly HIV, hepatitis B (HBV), and hepatitis C (HCV). Because of reports of deaths from thromboembolic complications or severe bleeding, SD plasma should not be used in patients with severe liver disease with a known coagulopathy or in patients undergoing liver transplant. The American Red Cross has discontinued supplying the product, and SD plasma is no longer available in the United States.

Cryoprecipitate

Cryoprecipitate is useful in treating factor deficiency (hemophilia A), von Willebrand's disease, and hypofibrinogenemia and may help treat uremic bleeding. Each 5- to 15-mL unit contains 80 units of factor VIII, about 200 mg of fibrinogen, and fibronectin. Because the proteins mentioned previously are in relatively high concentration, a smaller volume may be given than would be required if FFP were used. Cryoprecipitate is usually administered as a transfusion of 10 single units.

Perioperative Transfusion

The decision to transfuse a patient before operation should address several factors. No specific hematocrit is an indication for preoperative transfusion in a stable patient. A symptomatic patient with anemia who is about to undergo a procedure that involves significant blood loss may benefit from perioperative transfusion. If the patient is anemic with a low (or normal) reticulocyte count, transfusion may be the only way to raise the hemoglobin level before operation. Patients with chronic anemia whose condition is otherwise stable should not be transfused based on a hematocrit of 30%. The goal of transfusion of a symptomatic patient is the relief of symptoms. Previously a single-unit transfusion was condemned; but if one unit is sufficient to alleviate symptoms, no additional transfusion should be given because each unit adds to the risk.

The maximal surgical blood order schedule was designed to minimize the use of perioperative RBC-containing products and is usually based on the institution's or physician's record of transfusion for certain operative procedures. When a surgeon requests blood preoperatively, a *type-and-screen* procedure is performed to determine the patient's ABO and D types and to detect preformed antibodies to RBC antigens. If the antibody screen is negative and the probability that the patient will require blood in the operating room is less than 10%, RBCs are not crossmatched unless the patient needs blood during the procedure. An abbreviated crossmatch is then performed within a few minutes. If the probability of transfusion is greater than 10%, blood is crossmatched preoperatively. The number of units prepared is a function of the number of units transfused during the procedure in the past. In operations in which blood is frequently used, such as open heart or vascular procedures, the minimal number of units is crossmatched and additional units are made available if they are needed. When a procedure is completed, blood is held for 24 to 48 hours and then automatically released for other patients. This process allows the most efficient use of blood products and avoids the full, three-phase crossmatch.

Transfusion of the Patient in Shock

During World War I, it was believed that toxins caused vascular collapse in injured patients. Experiments in the 1930s by Dallas B. Phemister and Alfred Blalock showed that fluid was lost from the circulation into damaged tissues—the concept of a *third space*. In World War II, plasma was the resuscitation solution of choice. Although solutions containing electrolytes were used for children with diarrhea and advances had increased the understanding of metabolic and endocrine changes seen with injury, the use of plasma solutions prevailed until the Korean conflict. Subsequent experimental work indicated that extracellular fluids shifted into the intracellular space after significant hemorrhage with shock.[32] Providing volume resuscitation in excess of shed blood became standard practice to maintain adequate circulation.

During World War II, acute tubular necrosis was a common consequence of hypovolemic shock. As fluid resuscitation became more prevalent during the Korean and Vietnam conflicts, the incidence of acute tubular necrosis decreased. Although acute tubular necrosis after hypovolemic shock became less common with better fluid resuscitation, adult respiratory distress syndrome became increasingly common. The lung injury in adult respiratory distress syndrome, however, is a function of the shock state rather than the resuscitation solution used.

The goal of resuscitation from shock is prompt restoration of adequate perfusion and transport of oxygen. The American College of Surgeons Committee on Trauma developed a classification of shock that permits useful guidelines for resuscitation. Crystalloid is infused at a 3:1 ratio for every unit of RBCs administered, and therapy is monitored by hemodynamic response. Because crystalloid solutions are universally available and some delay is required to prepare blood products, crystalloid is the proper initial resuscitation fluid. Resuscitation proceeds with the use of blood products depending on the patient's response. The choice of a colloid solution (e.g., albumin, plasma) or a crystalloid solution (e.g., lactated Ringer's solution) has been controversial. Both can expand the extracellular space and provide effective resuscitation. Crystalloid solutions are favored because they are less expensive, need not be crossmatched, do not transmit disease, and probably create less fluid accumulation in the lung. No experimental data indicate that using colloid rather than crystalloid solutions can prevent pulmonary edema. A review of randomized controlled trials of albumin suggested an increased mortality in critically ill patients with hypovolemia, burns, or hypoalbuminemia.[33]

Several crystalloid solutions are available for resuscitation, but isotonic solutions should be used to avoid overload of free water. Lactated Ringer's solution is recommended as initial therapy. Metabolic alkalosis is common after successful resuscitation with lactated Ringer's solution and blood products because the lactate in Ringer's solution and citrate in banked blood are both converted to bicarbonate in the liver. Lactated Ringer's solution contains calcium; and if it is mixed with a blood product, the blood may clot in the bag. Normal saline solution is an acceptable alternative to lactated Ringer's solution, but large volumes can produce a hyperchloremic metabolic acidosis, which may complicate the use of base deficit in resuscitation.

RISKS OF BLOOD TRANSFUSION

Physicians should exercise judgment when prescribing a blood transfusion; a transfusion that is not clearly indicated is contraindicated. A transfusion of incompatible RBCs is potentially fatal, but other significant concerns exist when a patient receives blood products, including infectious hazards and immunologic effects. With the introduction of predonation screening for risk factors of hepatitis and HIV infection as well as donor blood testing, the risk of viral transmission has fallen dramatically since the early 1980s. Administrative error leading to ABO incompatibility, bacterial contamination, and transfusion-related lung injury are the three leading causes for fatalities after blood transfusion.[34] To the public though, HIV and viral hepatitis remain the major risks of transfusion. Other transfusion risks include nonhemolytic reactions, graft-versus-host disease, volume overload, and immunomodulation. Physicians prescribing transfusions should recognize these transfusion-related complications and be prepared to discuss these risks with patients and their families.

Transfusion Reactions

Transfusion reactions can be categorized broadly into hemolytic and nonhemolytic reactions, with febrile and allergic nonhemolytic subtypes. Hemolytic reactions are caused by complement-mediated destruction of transfused RBCs secondary to preexisting antibodies, and the severity of the reaction is determined by the degree of complement activation and cytokine release.[35] Severe acute hemolytic reactions generally involve the transfusion of ABO-incompatible blood, with fatalities occurring in 1 in 600,000 units.[36] As the RBCs are rapidly destroyed, peptides derived from complement are released and produce hypotension, compromise renal blood flow, activate coagulation, and lead to DIC. Signs and symptoms include pain and redness along the infused vein, chest tightness and pain, a feeling of doom, hypotension, oozing from intravenous sites, oliguria, chills, fever, hemoglobinemia, and hemoglobinuria. In the unconscious patient, hypotension, hemoglobinuria, and diffuse oozing may be the only clues.

When a transfusion reaction is suspected, the infusion should be stopped immediately and the label on the unit checked against the recipient's wristband. The unit, with all attached intravenous solutions and tubing, should be sent to the blood bank with blood samples drawn from a remote site. The blood should be tested for hemoglobinemia, and the urine should be tested for free hemoglobin. The blood bank should check all samples and

records and perform a direct antiglobulin test. The patient should receive aggressive fluid resuscitation to correct hypotension and maintain renal blood flow. A brisk diuresis may be initiated with mannitol or furosemide, and agents that increase renal blood flow should be considered. Patients who develop hypotension and DIC early are at greatest risk of death.

Delayed hemolytic reactions tend to present 5 to 10 days after transfusion[35] with approximately 1 in 260,000 patients developing a significant hemolytic reaction.[2] The degree of hemolysis may be significant in the patient whose total RBC mass has been replaced by massive transfusion. A transfused patient who develops an unexplained fall in hematocrit, fever, or jaundice should be evaluated for the possibility of a hemolytic reaction. The work-up is similar to that for acute hemolytic reactions, and the need for clinical intervention is less likely.

Allergic nonhemolytic reactions are generally believed to be caused by recipient antibodies to infusing donor plasma proteins. The manifestations vary from a slight rash or urticaria to hemodynamic instability with bronchospasm and anaphylaxis. Allergic reactions may be prevented by premedication with diphenhydramine. Recipient antibodies against antigens on donor leukocytes or platelets cause febrile nonhemolytic reactions. Fevers and chills characterize these reactions shortly after the transfusion has started. An acute hemolytic reaction and bacterial contamination of the unit should be excluded. Treatment consists of antipyretics and transfusion of leukocyte-depleted blood components when pharmacotherapy fails.

Transmission of Infection

Viral and bacterial diseases may be transmitted by blood transfusion, including Epstein-Barr virus, cytomegalovirus (CMV), hepatitis viruses, HIV and human T-cell leukemia virus (HTLV) types I and II, parvovirus B19, human herpesvirus 8, and TT (transfusion transmitted) virus. There are current investigations as to the possibility of transfusion transmission of the new variant Creutzfeldt-Jacob disease and West Nile virus. Since March 1999, pooled nucleic acid amplification testing (NAT) has been used to test for HIV and hepatitis C virus (HCV), which involves pooling of 16 to 24 individual blood samples and polymerase chain reaction or amplification techniques to test for HIV and HCV nucleic sequences. Bacterial and protozoal diseases include syphilis, malaria, and infection with *Babesia microti, Trypanosoma cruzi, Yersinia enterocolitica, Serratia marcescens, Staphylococcus aureus, Staphylococcus epidermidis,* or *Klebsiella pneumoniae.*[2] *Trypanosoma cruzi* causes Chagas' disease, but transmission of this infection is very rare in the United States.

Bacterial Contamination

Bacterial contamination of blood is the most frequent cause of transfusion-transmitted infectious disease.[37] After hemolytic reactions, it is the most frequently reported cause of transfusion-related fatalities to the U.S. FDA.[38] A recent study from the Centers for Disease Control and Prevention found the rates of transfusion-transmitted bacteremia to be 1/100,000 units for single donor and pooled platelets and 1 in 5 million units for packed red cells.[38] The agents implicated in packed RBC bacteremia were *Serratia* and *Yersinia*. For platelets, *Staphylococcus aureus, Escherichia coli, Enterobacter,* and *Serratia* species were more frequently identified. Fever, chills, hypotension, tachycardia, and shock after transfusion should raise the suspicion of bacterial contamination, and blood cultures of the patient and unit should be obtained.

Transfusion-Related Acute Lung Injury

Fatal pulmonary edema associated with transfusion was first described in 1951 by Barnard and the term transfusion-related acute lung injury (TRALI) was first coined in 1983 by Popovsky.[39] The incidence is estimated to be 1 case per 5000 units transfused,[2] but the syndrome is often underdiagnosed. It is believed to be the third most common cause of fatal transfusion reactions.[39] TRALI is a clinical syndrome associated with the transfusion of all blood components, but especially whole blood, packed red cells, and FFP. TRALI is characterized by the onset of dyspnea, hypotension, hypoxemia, fever, and bilateral noncardiogenic pulmonary edema within 4 hours of transfusion. The diagnosis is one of exclusion after volume overload, cardiogenic pulmonary edema, or acute respiratory distress syndrome has been ruled out. The pathophysiology is thought to be due to the transfusion of donor leukocyte antibodies or biologically active lipids from donor blood cell membranes into recipients.[2] Some recipients are more susceptible to developing the syndrome, such as those with infection, cytokine administration, recent surgery, and massive transfusion.[39] The donor antibodies attack the recipient leukocytes that localize to the pulmonary microvasculature and release cytokines that lead to an increase in vascular permeability and fluid exudation. Biologically active lipids serve to prime the recipient's neutrophils, leading to similar effects on the pulmonary microcirculation.[39] The treatment of TRALI is mainly supportive and consists of hemodynamic and respiratory support. Overall mortality is 5% to 10%.[39] The blood bank should be notified so the donated blood can be tested for anti-HLA and/or antigranulocyte antibodies. Blood donations from multiparous women have been implicated as a contributor to the disease.[39]

Hepatitis

Transmission of the infectious agents for hepatitis is among the most serious risks of blood transfusion. Past estimates of post-transfusion hepatitis were approximately 10%. Current data suggest that the infectious risk of hepatitis is 1% or less per unit transfused.[2] All blood is screened for the hepatitis B virus (HBV) surface antigen. In addition, blood is screened for surrogate markers for non-A, non-B hepatitis and for HCV. The risk of transfusion-associated HBV infection is approximately 1:30,000 to 1:250,000 per unit.[35] With the development of pooled NAT tests for HCV, the window period has decreased, and the risk of HCV transmission is now as low as 1 in 1 million.[34]

Approximately half of the blood recipients who contract HBV infection develop symptoms. A much smaller percentage requires hospitalization. Approximately half of patients who contract post-transfusion HCV infection develop a chronic form of the disease. Many of those patients eventually develop significant liver dysfunction, including cirrhosis.

Human Immunodeficiency Virus

The risk of HIV transmission from blood transfusion has decreased dramatically since the early 1980s despite an increasing incidence of HIV infection in the general population. The window period from initial infection to the development of antibody to the virus poses a problem with the ability to detect all seropositive donors. With pooled NAT, the window period for detection of HIV has been reduced by 30% to 50%,[33] and the risk of HIV transmission is estimated to be as low as 1 in 2 million units.[34]

Human T-cell Leukemia Virus

In addition to the transmission of CMV, hepatitis infection, and HIV, blood transfusion carries the risk of transmission of HTLV I and II infection. Transmission of the virus, especially to immunocompromised patients, may cause illnesses such as T-cell leukemia, spastic paraparesis, and myelopathy and has prompted routine screening of donors in the United States since 1989. The risk of HTLV I and II transmission is estimated to be 1 in 641,000 units.

Herpesviruses

CMV infection is endemic so routine screening is not performed in the United States. About 20% of blood donors are infected with CMV by 20 years of age, and approximately 70% are infected by 70 years of age. The infection is carried in WBCs. Most patients who encounter problems with CMV are immunocompromised, especially transplant recipients on immunosuppressive drugs. Such patients require transfusion with CMV-negative blood products to avoid the transmission of this viral infection. Human herpesvirus 8 causes Kaposi's sarcoma and lymphoma in patients with AIDS and other immunosuppressed states, such as transplantation.

Graft-Versus-Host Reaction

Blood transfusion exposes the recipient to many cells and proteins from the donor. When immunologically competent lymphocytes are introduced into an immunocompromised patient, a graft-versus-host reaction can occur.[35] The functional donor lymphocytes attack recipient tissues, notably the bone marrow, causing aplasia. Patients present with fever, rash, nausea, vomiting, diarrhea, liver function test abnormalities, and depressed cell counts.

This complication is fatal in as many as 90% of the cases. The prevalence of this complication in the U.S. is not known but is thought to be rare. Gamma irradiation of blood products may decrease this risk.

Immunomodulation

Allogeneic blood transfusion alters the immune response in individuals and susceptibility to infection, tumor recurrence, and reactivation of latent viruses.[40] It has been known since 1973 that the transfusion of packed RBCs depresses the immune response in patients undergoing renal transplantation[40]; however, it is unclear to what extent these immunosuppressive effects exist in other recipients. A study of critically ill patients showed that transfusing patients to maintain a higher hemoglobin level resulted in an increase in mortality,[26] but the reasons for this increase are undefined. Contradictory evidence exists about increased infections in patients given allogeneic blood transfusions. One recent study showed increased infections in trauma patients given older banked blood.[41] Other studies have had contradictory results.[40] Similar controversy also exists regarding the exact relationship of blood transfusions to increased recurrence of tumor and poor prognosis.[40] Early studies on colorectal cancer showed decreased survival and increased tumor recurrence in patients who were heavily transfused. Since then, studies on many tumors have been performed that have not yielded a decisive answer. The possibility exists that blood transfusion may represent a covariable because very ill patients and those undergoing more difficult procedures for more extensive disease are more likely to receive blood transfusion. In light of the immunomodulating effects of allogeneic blood transfusion, leukocyte-depleted transfusions have been suggested as an alternative. Recent studies have shown significant reductions in mortality and incidence of postoperative infections.[40] In view of the data on immunosuppression from blood transfusion, it would seem reasonable to adopt a policy of blood conservation in the perioperative period in the absence of clear indications and acute symptoms.

MASSIVE TRANSFUSION

Massive transfusion is defined as replacement of the patient's blood volume with packed RBCs in 24 hours or transfusion of more than 10 units of blood over a few hours. Massive transfusion can create significant changes in the patient's metabolic status because of the infusion of large volumes of cold citrate-containing blood that has undergone changes during storage. When blood is stored at 1°C to 6°C, changes occur over time, including leakage of intracellular potassium, decrease in pH, reduced levels of intracellular adenosine triphosphate and 2,3-DPG in the RBCs with increased affinity of hemoglobin for oxygen, degeneration of functional granulocytes and platelets, and deterioration of factors V and VIII. If a large volume of stored blood is infused rapidly, significant effects may be seen in the recipient. Many of the expected changes can

be reversed after transfusion or may produce metabolic patterns different from those predicted. Consequently, the use of standard formulas for the infusion of FFP, platelets, calcium, bicarbonate, and other substances for a specific number of units of packed RBCs transfused is unwarranted and may add risk for the patient.

Acid-Base Changes

Even though stored RBCs and whole blood have an acid pH (about 6.3), alkalosis is the usual result of massive transfusion. Sodium citrate, the anticoagulant in blood products, is converted to sodium bicarbonate in the liver. The alkalosis increases the oxygen affinity of hemoglobin. Because alkalosis stimulates enzymes in the Embden-Meyerhof pathway of glycolysis, the net effect is to increase intracellular 2,3-DPG and restore RBC transport of oxygen. The post-transfusion pH may range from 7.48 to 7.50 and is associated with an increased excretion of potassium. The routine administration of bicarbonate with large transfusion volumes is contraindicated because it causes more severe alkalosis, with undesirable effects on myocardial contractility and greater affinity of hemoglobin for oxygen.

Changes in 2,3-Diphosphoglycerate

Because 2,3-DPG is greatly reduced in RBCs after about 3 weeks of storage, massive transfusion of a patient with blood near the end of its storage life may decrease oxygen off-loading. Rapid correction occurs in most cases after the RBCs are transfused and rewarmed. If the patient's hematocrit is low with depressed cardiac function, as in elderly persons with atherosclerosis, the reduced level of 2,3-DPG may be detrimental.

Changes in Potassium

Hyperkalemia is theoretically possible with massive blood transfusion because stored blood has elevated potassium concentrations, as high as 30 to 40 mEq/L by 3 weeks of storage. Unless the transfusion rate exceeds 100 to 150 mL/min, clinical problems associated with potassium are rare. Most patients requiring rapid transfusion are in shock and have an increase in aldosterone, antidiuretic hormone, and permissive steroid hormones, causing hypokalemia unless renal function ceases. Hyperkalemia may cause peaked T waves on the electrocardiogram. Hyperkalemia, especially if associated with hypocalcemia, may significantly alter cardiac function. Immediate treatment of hyperkalemia is aimed at depressing the membrane threshold potential with calcium, 5 mmol, given intravenously over 5 minutes.

Hypocalcemia

Massive transfusion of citrated blood products can lead to transiently decreased levels of ionized calcium. The effects of hypocalcemia include hypotension, narrowed pulse pressure, and elevated left ventricular end-diastolic pulmonary artery and central venous pressures. Electrocardiographic abnormalities (e.g., prolonged QT intervals) also occur. Most normothermic adults who are not in shock can withstand the infusion of 1 unit of RBCs every 5 minutes without requiring calcium supplementation. Indiscriminate administration of calcium can produce transient hypercalcemia and should be avoided.

Hemostasis

Dilutional thrombocytopenia may occur in a patient who is massively transfused because the number of viable platelets is almost nil in blood stored for 24 hours at 1°C to 6°C. The decrease is often less than expected on the basis of simple dilution. This effect is not completely understood. Release of platelets from the spleen and the bone marrow may account for part of the difference. Despite the fact that platelet counts may fall with massive transfusion, dilutional thrombocytopenia alone usually does not account for microvascular bleeding. Prophylactic use of platelet concentrate in the massively transfused patient is not justified without evidence of microvascular bleeding. Platelet concentrate contains significant amounts of all factors except factor VIII, which is often increased in shock victims. Patients receiving large-volume blood transfusion who experience microvascular bleeding unrelated to hypothermia are best treated with platelet concentrate, which provides factors in addition to platelets. The PT and aPTT provide a reliable indicator for the need for FFP and factor replacement. The prophylactic use of FFP along with transfusion of RBCs is no longer acceptable in light of convincing data and the added risk of transfusion. In patients who develop DIC, large doses of platelet concentrate, FFP, and cryoprecipitate may be required.

Some major changes in the massively transfused patient are opposite to what might be expected based on the changes that occur during the storage of RBCs. In patients requiring massive transfusion, packed RBCs should be transfused to provide oxygen-carrying capacity, platelets given for microvascular bleeding in a normothermic patient, and crystalloid solution infused to restore intravascular volume. In most instances, addition of bicarbonate or calcium and prophylactic transfusion of FFP are not warranted.

BLOOD SUBSTITUTES AND ALTERNATIVES TO TRANSFUSION

Autologous Blood

Patients scheduled for elective procedures in which significant blood loss, requiring transfusion, is expected may be considered for autologous blood donation. Autologous blood transfusion has many advantages, including compatibility and the lack of viral transfusion risk. If the patient is free of infection and has severe cardiac disease and a hematocrit of at least 30%, he or she should be able to pre-donate. Usually 2 to 3 units can be obtained. Disadvantages of autologous blood donation are the increased costs as compared with allogeneic blood transfusion, postoperative anemia, increased risk for allogeneic blood transfusion,[2] and a discard rate of 20% to 73% of the units.[42] Because acute normovolemic hemodilution (ANH) is effective and is less costly than preoperative donation, ANH is more likely to be used in future blood-conserving strategies.[43]

Acute Normovolemic Hemodilution

ANH involves the removal of 1 to 3 units of the patient's blood and replaces it with crystalloid and/or colloid to restore the intravascular volume. Done after induction of anesthesia but before commencement of the operative procedure, ANH is tolerated well in most patient populations. The withdrawn blood is anticoagulated and maintained at room temperature for up to 4 hours. It is reinfused into the patient as needed during the surgical procedure. If ANH is combined with autologous predonation, 6 or more units of blood can be available for a procedure in which significant blood loss is expected. Studies comparing ANH with preoperative autologous blood donation show equal rates of allogeneic blood transfusion, but ANH costs are lower.[42,43] There is no role for this technique in acute hemorrhage.

Autologous Cell Salvage

The salvage of intraoperative blood loss can minimize the need for blood transfusion. This technique has had successful applications in many operative procedures, including cardiac surgery, spine surgery, liver transplantation, trauma, and vascular surgery. Blood is suctioned from the field, washed and/or filtered, and returned to the patient. Relative contraindications include fields with gross bacterial contamination, ascitic or amniotic fluid, and free tumor tissue.[2] Filtering and irradiation has been proposed to further eliminate tumor cells.[42] Risks of intraoperative cell salvage include air embolism, dilutional coagulopathy, and hemolysis. The procedure is cost effective when at least two shed units are able to be salvaged.[2]

Iron Supplementation

Oral iron supplementation with either ferrous gluconate or ferrous sulfate is indicated for iron-deficiency anemia. It is inexpensive and generally well tolerated. It can cause constipation or diarrhea and may also cause a false-positive reaction on occult fecal blood testing.

Erythropoietin

Erythropoietin is a glycoprotein that acts on the bone marrow to selectively increase erythropoiesis. It is produced predominantly in the kidney in response to hypoxia, but extrarenal production sites such as the liver have been identified. Recombinant human erythropoietin (rHuEPO) is commercially available and commonly used to treat anemia associated with renal insufficiency, cancer-related anemia, and anemia in the critically ill.[36]

Preoperative rHuEPO has been shown to decrease the need for allogeneic blood transfusion in orthopedic and urologic procedures.[36] Monk and colleagues[44] compared ANH, preoperative rHuEPO plus ANH, and preoperative autologous blood donation plus ANH in radical prostatectomies. They found similar rates of allogeneic transfusion in all three, but ANH was the least costly. The preoperative rHuEPO plus ANH regimen, however, resulted in less postoperative anemia.

Adverse effects, including hypertension, seizures, and thrombotic events, are few. The major disadvantages of erythropoietin are cost and the interval required for effect, which limits its usefulness in acute hemorrhagic conditions.

Red Blood Cell Substitutes

Concerns over the short supply of donated blood and risk of infection transmission had driven the development of RBC substitutes. At this time, RBC transfusion is the only available clinical method for increasing oxygen-carrying capacity. Several substances that have been considered as RBC substitutes can be divided into two general groups: (1) synthetic molecules, such as the porphyrins and the perfluorocarbon compounds and (2) molecules that incorporate hemoglobin in their structure, such as the conjugated and polymerized stroma-free hemoglobin solutions. Acceptable RBC substitutes must be able to carry at least as much oxygen as hemoglobin normally carries (1.34 mL of oxygen/g of hemoglobin). In addition, these molecules should be stable and have an acceptable half-life. The RBC substitute should have properties that allow it to be completely saturated with oxygen at a normal fraction of inspired oxygen, while unloading substantial portions of its transported oxygen at tissue partial pressure of oxygen levels. Solutions prepared must be highly purified and free of contaminants and endotoxins.

Perfluorocarbons efficiently transport significant quantities of oxygen and carbon dioxide and have the potential to be an effective RBC substitute. Perfluorocarbons can transport 40 to 50 mL of oxygen/100 mL of solution, which is greater than twice the quantity of oxygen that completely saturated hemoglobin carries in the normal adult. Unfortunately, the loading and unloading of oxygen is linear and not sigmoid as the native hemoglobin. Several perfluorocarbon molecules have been tested in humans but at present are not approved in the context of acute hemorrhage. At present, Oxygent (Alliance Pharmaceutical Cooperation) is undergoing clinical trial testing as an adjunct to acute intraoperative normovolemic hemodilution.

Early attempts to prepare hemoglobin solutions consisted of pooling outdated blood, breaking the RBCs open, and extracting the hemoglobin molecules. This solution is termed *stroma-free hemoglobin*. Limitations to the use of stroma-free hemoglobin included its very short half-life in

the circulation, its relatively low oxygen-carrying capacity, and its clearance through the kidneys, with vasoconstriction and direct toxic effects to the kidney. To circumvent these problems, the hemoglobin tetramer was stabilized, polymerized, or pyridoxylated. The resultant hemoglobin-based oxygen carriers (HBOC) have the same oxygen-carrying capacity as normal blood and stay in circulation 4 to 5 days without being cleared through the kidneys. Subsequent trials in healthy volunteers demonstrated the safety of the solution in humans. Clinical trials are being performed to determine the efficacy of the HBOCs for acute blood loss and perioperative applications.[45]

Most HBOCs have been found in trials to have a clinical hypertensive or pressor effect,[45] the mechanisms of which are not entirely understood. Some postulate that HBOCs bind available nitric oxide, leading to a surplus of vasoconstrictive agents.[45] Others point to the lower viscosity of the HBOCs, which decreases flow velocity and shear stress on the endothelial lining, resulting in a decrease in endothelial relaxation factors.[46] Another theory names the decreased oxygen affinity of HBOCs as the source, which leads to lower oxygen concentration at the tissue level. Autoregulatory mechanisms lead to subsequent vasoconstriction,[46] causing a decrease in cardiac output. A major advantage of most HBOCs is the lack of ability to prime neutrophils as compared with allogeneic blood, resulting in fewer immunomodulatory effects.[45]

Hemoglobin-based oxygen carriers have been produced from bovine hemoglobin, human hemoglobin, and recombinant hemoglobin (Table 6-3).[47] They have been tested in animals and humans, but so far only one product (Hemopure) has been licensed for human use in South Africa. Hemopure, produced by Biopure, is a bovine HBOC that has been tested in animals and humans and found to enhance oxygen utilization and erythropoiesis. At present this product is in phase III trial in the United States. Polyethylene glycol (PEG)-modified hemoglobin (Enzon) is also a bovine HBOC that is being studied as a sensitizer in radiation therapy.

Human HBOCs have been produced and tested by Baxter and Northfield. The Baxter product, HemAssist or diaspirin cross-linked hemoglobin, has been studied in multiple animal models and limited human studies. In both animals and humans, diaspirin cross-linked hemoglobin demonstrates a potent vasopressor effect. A phase I study demonstrated the product to be well tolerated, but a phase III trial with diaspirin cross-linked hemoglobin in trauma patients was closed owing to an increased mortality in the study group. The Northfield product, Polyheme, has not been associated with vasoactive or toxic side effects. In trauma patients, Polyheme demonstrated effective oxygen transport and safety and a decreased requirement for allogeneic blood transfusions.[48] Polyheme has been submitted for approval as a human RBC substitute to the U.S. FDA.[49]

Optro (Somatogen Baxter) is a recombinant HBOC that was produced using *Escherichia coli*.[50] The product has been tested in phase I and II trials, but its development has been halted by the parent company Baxter.

TABLE 6-3   Alternatives to Allogeneic Transfusion

Technique	Product	Disadvantages/Status
Autologous blood		Requires donation days to weeks before planned blood loss Potential for clerical error Cost
Acute normovolemic hemodilution		No role in acute hemorrhage Increased logistic requirements
Autologous cell salvage	Cell Saver Chest tube Drains	Potential for contamination Cost
Iron supplementation	Ferrous gluconate Ferrous sulfate	Constipation/diarrhea False-positive fecal occult blood test Requires days to weeks for effect
Epoetin alfa (recombinant human erythropoietin)	Epogen (Amgen) Procrit (Ortho Biotech)	Hypertension, seizures, thrombotic events Cost
Perflubron (perfluorocarbon) Hemoglobin-based substitutes (bovine)	Oxygent HT (Alliance Pharmaceutical) Hemopure (Biopure) PEG-hemoglobin (Enzon)	FDA approval pending Hypertension Approved in South Africa, FDA approval pending Early phase trials as radiosensitizer
Hemoglobin-based substitutes (human)	Diaspirin cross-linked hemoglobin/ HemAssist (Baxter) PolyHeme (Northfield) Hemolink (Hemosol) PHP (Apex Bioscience) Hemospan (Sangart)	Increased mortality in phase III trials Trials closed Phase III trials FDA approval pending Phase III trials in cardiac surgery Phase II trials in acute normovolemic hemodilution Phase III trials Preclinical testing phase
Hemoglobin-based substitutes (recombinant)	Optro (Somatogen/Baxter)	All phase II trials terminated

Selected References

Carson JL, Duff A, Berlin JA, et al: Perioperative blood transfusion and postoperative mortality. JAMA 279:199-205, 1998.

> **This study was a retrospective review of 8787 consecutive hip fracture patients, examining the lowest hemoglobin before transfusion. Transfusion for hemoglobin levels 8.0 g/dL or higher did not influence 30- or 90-day mortality.**

Goodnough LT, Brecher ME, Kanter MH, AuBuchon JP: Blood transfusion. N Engl J Med 340:438-447 and 525-533, 1999.

> **This is a review article in two parts covering blood transfusion and blood conservation. Risks of transfusion, indications for transfusion, alternatives to transfusion, and emerging developments in transfusion medicine are discussed.**

Herbert PC, Wells G, Blajchman MA, et al: A multicenter, randomized, controlled clinical trial of transfusion requirements in critical care. N Engl J Med 340:409-417, 1999.

> **A prospective, randomized study comparing a restrictive strategy of transfusion (transfusion for hemoglobin <7.0 g/dL) versus a liberal strategy (transfusion for hemoglobin <10.0 g/dL). Overall, there was no difference in 30-day mortality; however, the rates were significantly lower for those with Acute Physiology and Chronic Health Evaluation (APACHE) II score of 20 or less and those younger than 55 years old but not those with clinically significant cardiac disease.**

Monroe DM, Hoffman M, Roberts HR: Platelets and thrombin generation. Arterioscler Thromb Vasc Biol 22:1381-1389, 2002.

> **This article reviews the major role of platelets in thrombin generation and presents a cell-based model of coagulation.**

Moore EE: Blood substitutes: The future is now. J Am Coll Surg 196:1-17, 2003.

> **The Scudder Oration on Trauma presented at the American College of Surgeons 88th Annual Clinical Congress, San Francisco, CA, October 8, 2002. This is an excellent review of the background leading up to, and the latest clinical experience with, blood substitutes.**

References

1. American Association of Blood Banks website, www.aabb.org/ Accessed February 5, 2003.
2. Goodnough LT, Brecher ME, Kanter MH, AuBuchon JP: Blood transfusion. N Engl J Med 340:438-447 and 525-533, 1999.
3. Monroe DM, Hoffman M, Roberts HR: Platelets and thrombin generation. Arterioscler Thromb Vasc Biol 22:1381-1389, 2002.
4. Levi M, ten Cate H, van der Poll T: Endothelium: Interface between coagulation and inflammation. Crit Care Med 30:S220-S224, 2002.

5. Mann KG, Butenas S, Brummel K: The dynamics of thrombin formation. Arterioscler Thromb Vasc Biol 23:17-25, 2003.

6. Bernard GR, Vincent JL, Laterre PF, et al: Recombinant human protein C: Efficacy and safety of recombinant human activated protein C for severe sepsis. Worldwide Evaluation in Severe Sepsis (PROWESS) study group. N Engl J Med 344:699-709, 2001.

7. Rijken DC, Sakharov DV: Basic principles of thrombolysis: Regulatory role of plasminogen. Thromb Res 103:S41-S49, 2001.

8. Sidelmann JJ, Gram J, Jespersen J, Kluft C: Fibrin clot formation and lysis: Basic mechanisms. Semin Thromb Hemost 26:605-618, 2000.

9. Cobas M: Preoperative assessment of coagulation disorders. Int Anesthesiol Clin 39:1-15, 2001.

10. Haemoscope Corporation: Thromboelastograph Coagulation Analyzer: The Global Coagulation Test for Functional Analysis of Haemostasis Using Whole Blood. Skokie, IL, Haemoscope Corporation, 1991.

11. Salooja N, Perry DJ: Thromboelastography. Blood Coagul Fibrinolysis 12:327-337, 2001.

12. Triplett DA: Coagulation and bleeding disorders: Review and update. Clin Chem 46:1260-1269, 2000.

13. DiMichele D, Neufeld E: Hemophilia: A new approach to an old disease. Hematol Oncol Clin North Am 12:1315-1344, 1998.

14. Hedner U, Erhardtsen E: Potential role for rFVIIa in transfusion medicine. Transfusion 42:114-124, 2002.

15. Lethagen S: Desmopressin (DDAVP) and hemostasis. Ann Hematol 69:173-180, 1994.

16. Mannucci PM: Treatment of Von Willebrand disease. Thromb Haemost 86:149-153, 2001.

17. Walenga JM, Frenkel EP, Bick RL: Heparin-induced thrombocytopenia, paradoxical thromboembolism, and other adverse effects of heparin-type therapy: Hematol Oncol Clin N Am 17:259, 2003.

18. Rao AK: Congenital disorders of platelet function: Disorders of signal transduction and secretion. Am J Med Sci 316:69-76, 1998.

19. Amitrano L, Guardascione MA, Brancaccio V, et al: Coagulation disorders in liver disease. Semin Liver Dis 22:83-96, 2002.

20. Kottke-Marchant K, Corcoran G: The laboratory diagnosis of platelet disorders. Arch Pathol Lab Med 126:133-146, 2002.

21. Peng RY, Bongard FS: Hypothermia in trauma patients. J Am Coll Surg 188:685-696, 1999.

22. Valeri CR, Feingold H, Cassidy G, et al: Hypothermia induced reversible platelet dysfunction. Ann Surg 205:175-181, 1987.

23. Eddy VA, Morris JA: Early issues in the intensive care unit: The second golden hour. Surg Clin North Am 80:845-854, 2000.

24. Levi M, Ten Cate H: Disseminated intravascular coagulation. N Engl J Med 341:586-592, 1999.

25. Spence RK: Surgical red blood cell transfusion practice policies. Am J Surg 170:3S-15S, 1995.

26. Carson JL, Duff A, Berlin JA, et al: Perioperative blood transfusion and postoperative mortality. JAMA 279:199-205, 1998.

27. Hebert PC, Wells G, Blajchman MA, et al: A multicenter, randomized, controlled clinical trial of transfusion requirements in critical care. N Engl J Med 340:409-417, 1999.

28. American Association of Blood Banks: Blood Products Advisory Committee recommends universal leukoreduction. AABB News Briefs 20:16, 1998.

29. Ratko TA, Cummings JP, Oberman HA, et al: Evidence-based recommendations for the use of WBC-reduced cellular blood components. Transfusion 41:1310-1319, 2001.

30. Reed RL II, Ciavarella D, Heimbach DM, et al: Prophylactic platelet transfusion during massive transfusion: A prospective double-blind clinical study. Ann Surg 203:40-48, 1986.

31. Consensus conference: Fresh-frozen plasma: Indications and risks. JAMA 253:551-553, 1985.

32. Shires T, Coln D, Carrico J, et al: Fluid therapy in hemorrhagic shock. Arch Surg 88:688-693, 1964.

33. Cochrane Injuries Group Albumin Reviewers: Human albumin administration in critically ill patients: Systematic review of randomized controlled trials. BMJ 317:235-240, 1998.

34. Strong DM: Infectious risks of blood transfusions. America's Blood Centers Blood Bulletin 4(2): 2001.

35. Snyder E: Transfusion reactions. In Hoffman R, Benz EJ, Shattil SJ, et al (eds): Hematology: Basic Principles and Practice, 3rd ed. Churchill Livingstone, 2000.

36. Goodnough LT: Erythropoietin therapy versus red cell transfusion. Curr Opin Hematol 8:405-410, 2001.

37. Reading FC, Brecher ME: Transfusion-related bacterial sepsis. Curr Opin Hematol 8:380-386, 2001.

38. Kuehnert MJ, Roth VR, Haley NR, et al: Transfusion-transmitted bacterial infection in the United States, 1998 through 2000. Transfusion 41:1493-1499, 2001.

39. Kopko PM, Holland PV: Transfusion related lung injury. Br J Haematol 105:322-329,1999.

40. Klein HG: Immunomodulatory aspects of transfusion: A once and future risk? Anesthesiology 91:861-865, 1999.

41. Offner PJ, Moore EE, Biffl WL, et al: Increased rate of infection associated with transfusion of old blood after severe injury: Arch Surg 137:711-717, 2002.

42. Spahn DR, Casutt M: Eliminating blood transfusions: New aspects and perspectives. Anesthesiology 93:242-255, 2000.

43. Goodnough LT, Monk TG, Brecher ME: Acute normovolemic hemodilution should replace the preoperative donation of autologous blood as a method of autologous-blood procurement. Transfusion 38:473-476, 1998.

44. Monk TG, Goodnough LT, Brecher ME, et al: A prospectively randomized comparison of three blood conservation strategies for radical prostatectomy: Anesthesiology 91:24-33, 1999.

45. Stowell CP: Hemoglobin based oxygen carriers. Curr Opin Hematol 9:537-543, 2002.

46. Winslow RM: Blood substitutes: Curr Opin Hematol 9:146-151, 2002.

47. Cohn SM: Blood substitutes. N Horiz 7:54-60, 1999.

48. Gould SA, Moore EE, Hoyt DB, et al: The first randomized trial of human polymerized hemoglobin as a blood substitute in acute trauma and emergency surgery. J Am Coll Surg 187:113-122, 1998.

49. Moore EE: Blood substitutes: The future is now. J Am Coll Surg 196:1-17, 2003.

50. Siegel JH, Fabian M, Smith JA, Costantino D: Use of recombinant hemoglobin solution in reversing lethal hemorrhagic hypovolemic oxygen debt shock. J Trauma 42:199-212, 1997.

CHAPTER 7

METABOLISM IN SURGICAL PATIENTS

Nicholas E. Tawa, Jr., M.D., Ph.D.,   Justin A. Maykel, M.D.

and   Josef E. Fischer, M.D.

OVERVIEW

Artificial Nutrition: Importance and History

Nutritional support, along with antibiotics, blood transfusion, critical care monitoring, advances in anesthesia, organ transplantation, and cardiopulmonary bypass, ranks high among advances in surgery achieved in the 20th century. Dudrick and associates in 1968 first demonstrated that intravenous nutrition would support normal growth rates in puppies, and parenteral alimentation began to be widely applied in the United States. Parenteral nutrition has evolved from initial enthusiastic acceptance to more critical review, with demands for efficacy. In the 1960s and 1970s, it was standard practice to feed patients 3000 to 5000 kcal/day ("hyperalimentation") in an effort to attain an anabolic state. It was not appreciated at that time that such overfeeding practices were potentially dangerous and that, with excessive carbohydrate and lipid infusion, the body's ability to metabolize these nutrients was exceeded, thus predisposing patients to iatrogenic immune and hepatic dysfunction. Today, nutrition is provided in more moderate amounts, while nutritional needs in specific disease states have been explored. Some investigators have also proposed the use of specific nutrient components as drugs (termed *nutritional pharmacology*), an approach that will be validated only when pathophysiologic mechanisms are better defined. Although modern practice is to make aggressive use of the gut for nutritional support, intravenous nutrition remains a critical therapy in instances in which enteral support cannot be achieved, either because the gut cannot be used or because caloric requirements cannot be met by the gut alone and must be supplemented parenterally. Studies of body composition in critical illness show, however, that even current approaches to intravenous nutrition remain unsatisfactory. Thus, in a normal individual, body tissue is compartmentalized as approximately 30% adipose, 30% lean body mass (protein), and 30% extracellular fluid (water). In catabolic illness extracellular fluid increases secondary to sodium retention to 50% to 60% of total body mass, whereas fat and lean body tissue decrease to approximately 20% each. Although intravenous nutrition can clearly retard the loss of lean body mass under such conditions, it has proven difficult to induce a net accumulation of body protein in a nongrowing adult host without strenuous exercise. Increasing the amount of intravenous nutrition beyond basal requirements—without exercise, insulin, or other hormonal alterations—in an effort to enhance lean body mass, only increases total body water and fat content further, with no beneficial effect on body protein.[1]

Clinical Sequelae of Impaired Nutrition

Numerous studies have clearly shown an increased incidence of nosocomial infection, longer hospital stay, and increased mortality in patients with significant unintentional weight loss (>10%) prior to their acute illness. Even in an individual with initially normal nutritional status, after 7 to 10 days of inanition, the body's ability to heal wounds and to support normal immune function begins to be impaired. Such deficits include diminished complement and immunoglobulin production, poor cellular immunity, as well as impairment of various aspects of leukocyte action including chemotaxis, phagocytosis, and oxidative burst. Other consequences of inadequate nutrition in the postoperative period include poor tissue repair and wound healing and loss of muscle function and strength due to progressive muscle wasting, which may contribute to reduced ventilatory performance and prolonged ventilator dependence. Overall, malnutrition will be limiting to all aggressive surgical and medical therapies.

Incidence of Malnutrition in Hospitalized Patients

In the early 1970s, the widespread prevalence of malnutrition in hospitalized medical and surgical patients was recognized and suggested to have a major influence on clinical outcome.[2] Today, it is estimated that as many as 50% of hospitalized patients may be malnourished. In the usual U.S. hospital setting, starvation is usually the result of either anorexia, such as occurs in cancer, sepsis, or liver disease, or poor intake caused by esophageal or gastrointestinal obstruction. Other conditions, such as scleroderma, motility disorders or pseudo-obstruction, major gastric resection, inflammatory bowel disease, or short bowel syndrome, may result in inadequate absorption of nutrients. Inadequate nutrition may also be due to excessive losses, as in patients with gastrointestinal fistulas or protein-losing enteropathies. However, the most common cause of in-hospital malnutrition is poor food served without assistance to frail individuals and timed for the benefit of personnel rather than of the patients. Patients are also given nothing by mouth for the most trivial reasons (e.g., radiologic studies) and diets are often not advanced rapidly even after minor operations.

METABOLIC ADAPTATIONS IN CATABOLIC STATES AND REGULATION OF NITROGEN BALANCE

Amino Acid Metabolism and Transport

Roles of Specific Amino Acids

Amino acids have a core configuration of an amino and a carboxyl group adjacent to a carbon atom from which a side chain extends and are thus zwitterions. Amino acids are grouped based on electrical charge and the side chain. The neutral amino acid group comprises the following 12 amino acids: glycine and alanine; the hydroxyamino acids serine and threonine; the branched-chain amino acids valine, leucine, and isoleucine; the aromatic amino acids phenylalanine, tyrosine, and tryptophan; and the sulfur-containing amino acids methionine and cysteine. Aspartate and glutamate are diacidic amino acids, while arginine, lysine, and histidine are dibasic. These features largely determine transport across membranes. The essential or indispensable amino acids are those whose carbon skeleton cannot be synthesized by the body and include valine, leucine, isoleucine, lysine, methionine, phenylala-

nine, threonine, and tryptophan. Cysteine and tyrosine may be essential in that they are synthesized from the essential amino acids methionine and phenylalanine, respectively. The remaining 10 amino acids alanine, arginine, aspartate, asparagine, glutamate, glutamine, glycine, histidine, proline, and serine are not essential. Although not classically essential, histidine, proline, glutamine, and arginine may become conditionally essential under catabolic conditions, when needs are increased and synthetic rates fall short of increased requirements. This concept of conditionally essential amino acids remains controversial and is discussed later in this chapter. Three major fates of amino acids are (1) protein synthesis; (2) oxidation by the tricarboxylic acid cycle, either for energy production or ultimately leading to storage as carbohydrate or fat, with the production of urea and carbon dioxide; or (3) the synthesis of nonessential amino acids and other small molecules, such as purines and pyrimidines.

The plasma amino acid pool is regulated by exchange of amino acids among skeletal muscle, the liver, and other viscera (kidney and lung). Of the essential amino acids, 7 of the 10 are degraded by the liver, the exceptions being the branched-chain amino acids, for which skeletal muscle plays a major role in catabolism. Two amino acids, alanine and glutamine, are carriers for organ exchanges of nitrogen, in a complex process discussed later (Fig. 7-1).

Amino Acid Transport

The transport of free amino acids across cell membranes has been studied in only a few types of cells; it is probably universal. Christensen[3] proposed several transport systems:

1. The A system is an energy- and sodium-dependent system with a high affinity for alanine and other neutral amino acids, including the synthetic amino acid α-aminoisobutyric acid. It is concentrative against a gradient and is stimulated by insulin. Insulin stimulates amino acid transport into muscle via the A system, by recruiting specific sodium-dependent amino acid transporters to the plasma membrane (see later).[4]
2. The L system is sodium independent and transports the branched-chain amino acids (leucine, isoleucine, and valine) and the aromatic amino acids (phenylalanine, tyrosine, and tryptophan) and probably methionine and histidine as well. It operates by exchange for intracellular amino acids and is competitive.
3. Two transport systems are available for the basic amino acids. The carriers for transport of dibasic amino acids and the L system may be linked in some as yet unknown way.
4. Dicarboxylic amino acids have their own transport system.

Current knowledge about amino acid transport in muscle is summarized in Table 7-1.

Amino Acid Metabolism in Liver and Viscera

The liver is the major site in the body for the degradation and synthesis of amino acids and is the most important organ regulating plasma amino acid levels. The liver processes and stores ingested nutrients delivered by the portal venous system and releases them in response to neural and hormonal signals. The liver may extract between 75% and 100% of all portal vein nutrients in one

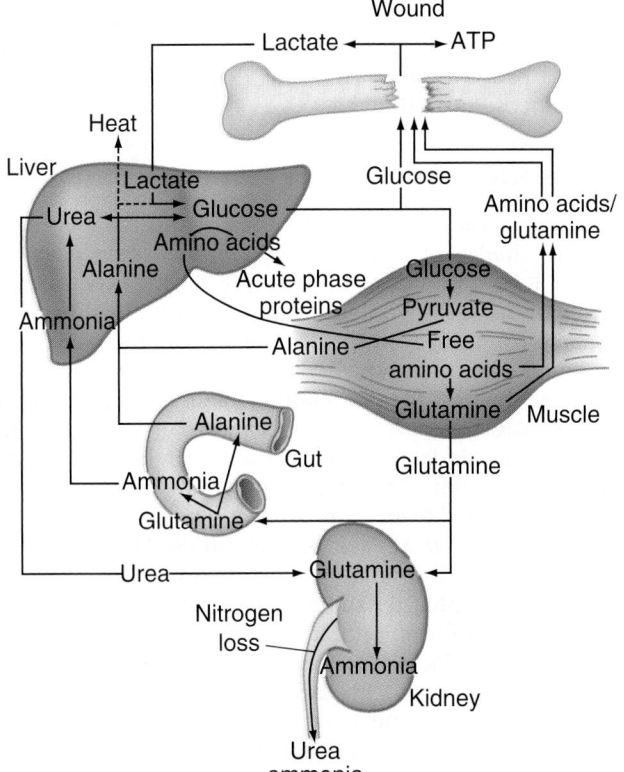

FIGURE 7-1. Overall scheme of the metabolic response to illness. This scheme includes the metabolic relationship among organs. This feature has heretofore not been prominently addressed but is now receiving increased attention. One of the articles of faith is that such responses occur in response to injury and are teleologically correct and beneficial. Thus, the wound requires glucose, probably glutamine, and certainly arginine with respect to certain cellular elements. The movement of amino acids from the periphery (muscle) to the liver presumably results in the secretion of acute-phase protein, the purpose of which, in turn, is to fight infection. The muscle-gut-liver-alanine-glutamine-glucose cycle is prominently displayed. ATP, adenosine triphosphate. (Adapted from Bessey PQ: Metabolic response to critical illness. *In* Wilmore DW, Cheung LY, Harken AH, et al (eds): Scientific American Surgery, Sect. II, Subsect. 11. New York, Healtheon/WebMD, 2000.)

pass, and only 25% of ingested protein reaches the general (nonportal) circulation as free amino acids. Most (~60%) is converted to urea, a small amount (6%) is synthesized to plasma protein, and 14% becomes liver protein. Although the affinity constants for hepatic amino acid degradation are high, and those for synthesis are low, favoring net synthesis, excessive postprandial accumulation of plasma amino acids is prevented, helping for example to prevent rapid and possibly disruptive increases in amino acid brain neurotransmitter precursors. It is not clear whether the large postprandial urea production from absorbed amino acids is wasteful or is somehow required for hepatic functional integrity. During starvation, the liver metabolizes amino acids released by proteolysis in muscle to form glucose, in the process of gluconeogenesis (see later). In parenteral nutrition, nutrients are first supplied to the systemic, rather than the portal, circulation and thus override the liver. Furthermore, as the normal postprandial production of gut hormones (which may have a role in anabolic signaling) is bypassed by parenteral feeding, overall nutrient disposal is probably less efficient, and this phenomenon may contribute to the difficulty in achieving positive nitrogen balance discussed earlier.

The role of the kidney in amino acid homeostasis has not been as well studied as that of muscle or liver but is probably more important than heretofore supposed. Amino acids in the kidney can have several fates, including (1) the production of urea (with the liver) from ammonia by means of the argininosuccinate cycle; (2) the production of ammonia (from glutamine) for urinary acid-base balance; (3) metabolism of other amino acids, such as the branched-chain amino acids; and (4) participation with the liver in gluconeogenesis from muscle-derived glutamine (see later). The lung may also have a greater role in regulation of amino acid levels than has been appreciated, especially when the liver is bypassed or diseased and thus is incapable of modifying portal flow. For example, in sepsis, the lung, in addition to skeletal muscle, can become a major source for glutamine production.

Amino Acid Metabolism in Muscle

Skeletal and cardiac muscle are the major site in the body for the catabolism of several amino acids, most notably leucine, isoleucine, and valine, and for the

TABLE 7-1. Amino Acid Transporters in Muscle

Transporter	Na$^+$ Coupling	Typical Substrates	Comments
X–A,G	Yes	Glutamate, aspartate	Insulin insensitive
y$^+$	No	Lysine, cystine, arginine, ornithine	Insulin insensitive
L	No	Neutral amino acids	Insulin insensitive
A	Yes	Short-chain neutral amino acids	Insulin sensitive, reduced by starvation
ASC	Yes	Alanine, cysteine, serine, threonine	Insulin insensitive
N^m	Yes	Glutamine, histidine, asparagine	Insulin sensitive

synthesis of others, specifically alanine and glutamine.[5] By contrast, muscle does not degrade to any significant extent the carbon skeletons of other amino acids found in plasma.

Branched-Chain Amino Acid Oxidation

The rate of degradation of the branched-chain amino acids in muscle is greater than in the liver, and given that muscle comprises up to 40% of body mass, it is probably the major site for degradation of branched-chain amino acids. Unlike most ingested amino acids, the branched-chain amino acids are not efficiently extracted from the portal circulation by the liver and pass directly into the systemic circulation, to be taken up by peripheral tissues. Though leucine is readily oxidized by muscle, it is also degraded by the kidney, adipose tissue, and brain. The physiologic significance of branched-chain amino acid metabolism in these tissues is probably distinct from that in skeletal muscle. For example, in adipose tissue, leucine degradation serves an anabolic function by providing precursors for triglyceride synthesis, whereas in muscle, leucine is degraded to acetyl-CoA moieties, which are then oxidized in the tricarboxylic acid cycle to provide energy.

In certain catabolic states, including fasting, diabetes, and following traumatic injury, the rates of degradation of the branched-chain amino acids increase markedly in skeletal and cardiac muscle and in the kidney, whereas liver and brain show no such effects. This increased oxidation in muscle is regulated by glucocorticoids and other stimuli.[6] Since leucine can serve as an alternative energy source for muscle during fasting, it can also reduce glucose utilization in this tissue. Therefore, during fasting, when leucine rises in blood and muscle, its degradation in muscle increases, and gluconeogenic precursor molecules such as pyruvate are preserved.[7]

Production and Release of Alanine

The breakdown of branched-chain amino acids in muscle generates amino groups whose accumulation could be toxic. Unlike liver, muscle lacks the enzymes necessary to dispose of ammonia as urea. Instead, alanine and glutamine are released in much greater amounts than would be expected simply by the net breakdown of muscle proteins. Amino groups generated by degradation of branched-chain amino acids and aspartate contribute to the de novo synthesis of alanine and glutamine in muscle.[5] Alanine production by this tissue seems to play an important role in the maintenance of blood glucose in the fasted state. The liver is very active in extracting alanine from the blood, and in the liver, alanine is the most important amino acid utilized for gluconeogenesis. Felig in the mid-1970s proposed the existence of a "glucose-alanine cycle," in which alanine derived from amino acid metabolism in muscle is carried in the circulation to the liver for conversion into urea and glucose. The glucose synthesized by the liver can then be taken up again by muscle and be con-

verted back to alanine. This flux of alanine between muscle and liver is similar to that of lactate in the Cori (glucose-lactate) cycle, but in addition alanine helps ferry potentially toxic amino groups to the liver for disposal as urea. Since alanine is derived from preexistent glucose, this cycle does not allow the generation of new carbohydrate from muscle proteins, and overall, as an amino group is ultimately lost, the glucose-alanine cycle is not a "true" metabolic cycle. However, the oxidation of leucine and the prevention of pyruvate degradation in muscle spare glucose in fasting.

Glutamine Production by Muscle and Interorgan Relationships

Skeletal and cardiac muscle synthesize and release glutamine in similar or even greater amounts than alanine. Studies in isolated muscles[5] and more recent experiments in humans have shown that the carbon atoms in glutamine originate primarily from protein-derived amino acids that can enter the tricarboxylic acid (TCA) cycle and are mainly converted to glutamine, which is then released from muscle. This process is an important initial step in gluconeogenesis from muscle protein. It has been estimated that about 87% of the glutamine released from muscle is derived from de novo synthesis rather than glutamine liberated as a result of proteolysis. The glutamine released by muscle is an important energy source by many cells. For example, glutamine is extensively oxidized by leukocytes and fibroblasts. It is taken up from the blood primarily by the kidney, where it serves as a precursor for urinary ammonia, and its carbon skeleton may be used either for gluconeogenesis, or energy production, or some of the carbons are released into the blood as alanine. In addition, as originally described by Windmueller and Spaeth,[8] the small intestine takes up and metabolizes large amounts of glutamine; it in turn releases appreciable amounts of alanine. The liver then uses the released alanine for glucose production. This complex multiorgan process appears to play an important role in net gluconeogenesis from the five amino acids originating in proteins and converted to glutamine in muscle.

The level of glutamine within different tissues is determined by the relative activities of glutamine synthase and glutaminase. The transcription of glutamine synthase is strongly activated by corticosteroids in lung and muscle tissue. This leads to enhanced glutamine production and underlies the increased production and release of glutamine from muscle in starvation and disease states such as sepsis, or other critical illness, where glucocorticoid levels are high.[9] As indicated earlier, the lung also has a high capacity for synthesizing glutamine, and this process rises in sepsis. For example, after induction of a sepsis-like state with lipopolysaccharide in experimental animals, and in studies with pulmonary artery catheters measuring lung flux in human patients with sepsis, lung release of glutamine at least doubles, presumably as the result of increased levels of glutamine synthase. Under these conditions, glutamine uptake by the small intestine decreases, and glutamine uptake by the liver increases dramatically. The benefit of these changes is not clear (see later section on controversies in artificial nutrition).

Regulation of Intracellular Protein Synthesis and Degradation

Physiologic Significance of Protein Turnover

Classic experiments by Schoenheimer in the 1940s with ^{15}N-labeled amino acids demonstrated that cellular proteins are synthesized and degraded continuously. Net mobilization of muscle protein can provide amino acids for metabolism by other tissues, for example during fasting, whereas net uptake of amino acids by muscle and their incorporation into protein is a form of energy storage. However, there is no generic protein store; muscle may serve that purpose, but not perfectly.

A major technical factor limiting the study of protein metabolism in muscle and other tissues has been problems involving measurement of degradative rates. A variety of in vivo methods are available, but all are subject to a number of potential artifacts. Urinary urea or total nitrogen excretion are often regarded as an index of muscle protein breakdown, but these measurements actually represent processes of amino acid catabolism and will be influenced by amino acids released from nonmuscle tissues and from the diet. One useful method for estimating rates of degradation of certain muscle proteins in vivo is the measurement of urinary N-methylhistidine excretion. This amino acid is formed by a post-translational modification of histidine residues in actin and myosin. When generated by proteolysis, it cannot be reincorporated into protein or significantly metabolized and therefore its release in urine must reflect breakdown of these contractile proteins. However, actin and myosin also exist in other tissues, and skin, gastrointestinal tract, and possibly other organs, besides muscle, may contribute significantly to urinary N-methylhistidine excretion. To analyze rates of protein degradation under controlled conditions, in vitro techniques that employ thin rodent muscles offer many advantages. Similar techniques have been applied for measuring rates of protein synthesis and degradation in human muscle biopsies. Rates of protein synthesis are determined by measuring rates of incorporation of [14C]-tyrosine or phenylalanine into muscle protein, whereas rates of protein degradation are measured by following the release of tyrosine from the muscle.

Biochemical Pathways for Intracellular Protein Breakdown

Several pathways for intracellular proteolysis have been identified, and each pathway uses a unique complement of proteases. These include the acid-dependent proteases (cathepsins) in lysosomes and proteases active at neutral pH and found in the cytosol. This latter group includes the calcium-dependent calpains, the caspases, and the adenosine triphosphate (ATP)-dependent ubiquitin-proteasome pathway. It is now well established that the proteasome is responsible for the majority of protein degradation in mammalian cells including skeletal muscle.[10] There is now also considerable evidence that the ubiquitin-proteasome pathway is responsible for the majority of accelerated proteolysis in many different catabolic conditions characterized by muscle wasting. However, calpains may have a complementary role, as explored by Williams and associates[11] in rats wasting due to sepsis. A calcium-dependent release of myofibrils, and disintegration of the Z-band, along with increased messenger RNA (mRNA) levels for calpains 1, 2, and 3, was noted. This suggests that, in sepsis, calpains might be important in releasing myofibrils from the contractile apparatus, and these then, presumably, serve as substrate for ubiquitination and degradation by the proteasome (Fig. 7-2).[11]

The importance of the ATP-ubiquitin-proteasome pathway in muscle atrophy is now well established.[12] The majority of the acceleration in proteolysis induced by a variety of catabolic conditions, including diabetes, acidosis, sepsis, thyroid hormone treatment, and denervation atrophy, can be blocked by proteasome inhibitors.[13] These muscles also show dramatic increases in ubiquitin-protein conjugates, which are intermediates in proteolysis via this

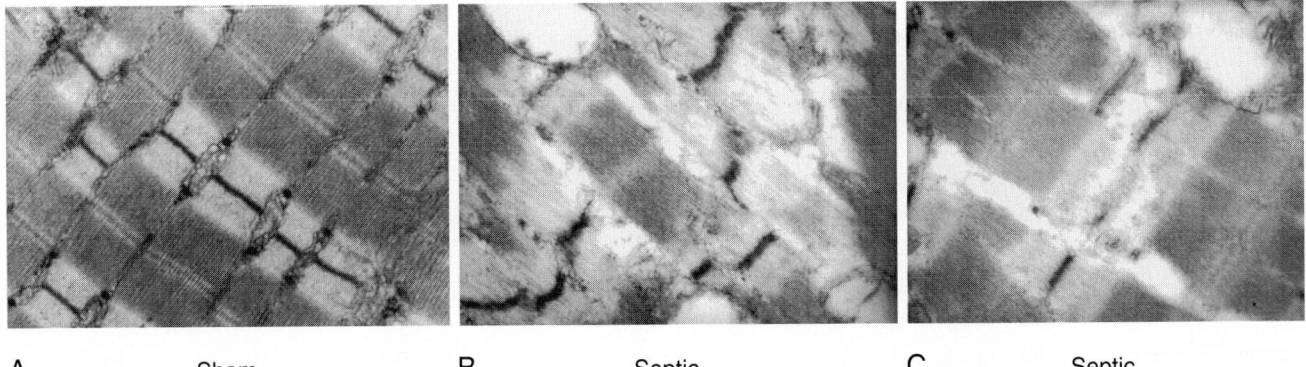

FIGURE 7-2. Electron micrographs of extensor digitorum longus (EDL) muscles from sham-operated (**A**) and septic (**B** and **C**) rats. Note the loss of registry between adjacent sarcomeres in septic muscles. Z disks were thickened, fragmented, or completely lost in septic muscles. Magnification × 33,200. (**A** and **B**, From Williams AB, deCourten-Myers GM, Fischer JE, et al: Sepsis stimulates release of myofilaments in skeletal muscle by a calcium-dependent mechanism. FASEB J 13:1435, 1999.)

pathway, as well as increases in mRNAs encoding components of the ubiquitin-proteasome pathway.[12,14] Degradation of proteins via the ubiquitin-proteasome pathway is a multistep process that requires the hydrolysis of ATP, in addition to the 8-kD protein cofactor ubiquitin and the 26S proteasome.[10] The 26S proteasome is a very large (2-MD) complex made up of at least 50 subunits. Unlike typical proteases, the proteasome requires ATP for the degradation of proteins; in particular, ATP hydrolysis is thought to be needed to drive the unfolding and translocation of globular proteins into the proteolytic compartment. The majority of protein substrates are marked for degradation by covalent linkage of a chain of ubiquitin molecules to an internal lysine of the protein substrate. This process requires at least three enzymes, the so-called E1, E2, and E3s. The E3 ubiquitin-protein ligase can bind only specific protein substrates and ubiquitinates these proteins with the aid of a specific E2. However, which E2s and E3s are involved in the accelerated proteolysis during muscle wasting is still incompletely understood.[14] Recently, genomic approaches have been used to identify genes regulated during muscle atrophy. These exciting studies have revealed E3s that appear to be directly involved in accelerated proteolysis under a number of different conditions. For example, mRNA levels for one new E3 increase severalfold in fasting, diabetes, cancer, or uremia[15] and during immobilization or denervation.[16] The importance of this E3 in muscle wasting was highlighted by studies showing that when muscles from transgenic knockout mice lacking the functional E3 gene were denervated, they lost half as much mass than muscles from wild-type mice.[16]

Nutrients and Hormones Regulating Nitrogen Balance

The hormonal milieu of the body provides for either a storage state or a breakdown state. Insulin, the dominant anabolic signal, inhibits lipolysis and increases nitrogen accrual in muscle, liver, and other tissues. In addition to

hormonal and nutrient factors, a lack of tension or disuse is a major signal activating muscle proteolysis, a phenomenon of great relevance clinically. Great advances have been made in understanding the signaling mechanisms mediating the effects of various nutrients and anabolic hormones (Table 7-2). In particular, two protein kinases, Akt and mTOR (the latter inhibited by the immunosuppressive drug rapamycin), appear particularly important in regulating mRNA translation and thus protein synthesis in response to various growth factors and nutrients.

It has been known for some time that leucine has regulatory effects on muscle protein balance. Studies from several laboratories have shown that branched-chain amino acids stimulate protein synthesis and reduce protein breakdown in isolated skeletal and cardiac muscle. Leucine appears to stimulate protein synthesis and mRNA translation principally via the pathway that involves mTOR, although the inhibitory effects of leucine on protein degradation have been less extensively investigated. However, this action of leucine is not related to its role as a metabolic fuel, because other carbon sources such as alanine and pyruvate fail to have the same anabolic effects, despite being consumed by cells.

Insulin stimulates amino acid transport into muscle (see earlier),[4] increases rates of protein synthesis, and inhibits muscle protein breakdown. Thus, the rise in insulin after meals promotes net protein accumulation in muscle, whereas in the postabsorptive state, when insulin is low, there is a net loss of protein and a release of amino acids from muscle. Binding of insulin to its receptor on the plasma membrane leads to activation of phophatidylinositol-3 kinase (PI-3 kinase), followed by Akt and S6 kinase, and ultimately enhanced translation initiation. Insulin can have a limited role in promoting protein synthesis in some catabolic conditions such as after burns. In addition to its effects on protein synthesis, insulin inhibits protein degradation in many tissues.[17] Insulin's direct inhibition of protein breakdown in liver and muscle results largely from an inhibition of lysosomal proteolysis. However, the sys-

---

TABLE 7-2. **Hormones Influencing Energy Utilization and Nitrogen Balance**

Hormone	Muscle Protein Degradation	Muscle Protein Synthesis	Glucose Utilization	Effect on Growth
Insulin	Decrease	Increase	Increase	Anabolic
Glucocorticoids	Increase	Decrease	Decrease	Catabolic
Cytokines	Increase	Decrease	Decrease	Catabolic
IGF-1	Decrease	Increase	Increase	Anabolic
Growth hormone	No change	Increase	Decrease	Anabolic
Thyroid hormone	Increase	Increase	Increase	Anabolic
Leucine	Decrease	Increase	Decrease	Anabolic
Fasting	Increase	Decrease	Decrease	Catabolic
Long-term fasting	Decrease	Decrease	Decrease	Catabolic
Protein deficiency	Decrease	Decrease	Unknown	Catabolic

IGF, insulin growth factor.

temic effects of low insulin states such as fasting or diabetes include muscle wasting due to accelerated proteolysis via the ATP-ubiquitin-proteasome pathway, a process that appears insensitive to insulin. Under these conditions, glucocorticoids clearly contribute to the activation of the ubiquitin-proteasome pathway and are required for muscle wasting. Possibly insulin somehow inhibits this catabolic response to glucocorticoids.

Glucose by itself can inhibit protein degradation in isolated muscles and in liver without affecting overall protein synthesis. This effect of glucose in muscle is not simply due to supplying energy to the tissue, since fatty acids or ketone bodies do not reduce proteolysis despite their rapid oxidation. Therefore, elevated plasma levels of insulin and glucose following food intake together promote the accumulation of amino acids in muscle.

Hypophysectomy of young animals prevents growth, including that of skeletal muscle. When hypophysectomized animals are treated with growth hormone, overall body growth is reinitiated and rates of protein synthesis in muscle increase. Growth hormone does not appear to suppress proteolysis directly. Rather, the polypeptide insulin-like growth factors, IGF-I and IGF-II, synthesized in part under the stimulation of growth hormone, mediate the reduction in proteolysis. IGF-I has well-documented insulin-like effects, enhancing protein synthesis by activating the PI3 kinase/Akt/mTOR pathway that accelerates translation initiation. In addition to enhancing protein synthesis, IGF-I and IGF-II inhibit protein breakdown in muscle. For example, the increase in protein degradation in isolated muscles following burn injury can be reversed by IGF-I, but this effect was not seen in muscles from septic animals, where IGF-I increased protein synthesis but had no effect on protein degradation rates.[18] The inhibition of protein breakdown by IGF-I is thought to involve a suppression of the lysosomal process, as shown previously for insulin. However, recent evidence suggests that IGF-I, but not growth hormone, can reduce mRNA levels for components of the ubiquitin-proteasome pathway, and this might be an additional mechanism to reduce proteolysis.

Glucocorticoids are another class of hormones that influence muscle size. For example, the overproduction of adrenal steroids in Cushing's syndrome or the high levels used clinically lead to marked muscle weakness and wasting. Glucocorticoids act in several complex ways to retard growth and to promote the release of amino acids from muscle. These include decreasing DNA and protein synthesis and reducing amino acid uptake by muscle. In the fasted state, glucocorticoids play an important physiologic role in promoting the net breakdown of muscle protein, and this response appears important in the regulation of blood glucose. This action of glucocorticoids thus complements the other "permissive actions" of cortisol in enhancing gluconeogenesis in liver and kidney. It is now clear that the accelerated proteolysis due to glucocorticoids in experimental animals is largely due to activation of the ubiquitin-proteasome pathway in muscle, and in general, pale (glycolytic) muscle fibers appear more sensitive to these catabolic effects than dark (oxidative) fibers. In addition to fasting, glucocorticoids are also

important for the increase in proteolysis seen in other physiologic or pathologic states. Thus, the increased ATP-dependent protein breakdown occurring in the muscles of rats with metabolic acidosis, diabetes, and sepsis[19] is dependent on this class of hormone. However, it should be noted that in human studies, no increase in transcripts for proteolytic pathway components has been demonstrated, whether after short exposure to high-dose prednisolone, which induced proteolysis,[20] or in those with untreated Cushing's disease. Recent experiments to define the effects of glucocorticoids on protein synthesis have shown these hormones appear to antagonize the stimulatory effects of insulin and leucine on the PI3 kinase/Akt/mTOR pathway described earlier.

Physiologic Adaptations to Food Deprivation

Short-Term Fasting

Complete food deprivation leads to a mobilization of body protein to support energy needs. Although the normal turnover of protein is 2.5% to 3% of lean body mass per day (Fig. 7-3), in starvation as much as 300 g of protein per day may be lost initially in humans. Early in fasting, amino acid release from skeletal muscle increases, which results from a decrease in protein synthesis and from a marked rise in protein degradation. These adaptive changes in muscle protein metabolism seem to result from the low level of circulating insulin, although glucocorticoids also play an essential permissive role (see earlier). Early in fasting, under the influence of decreased insulin and elevated glucagon, hepatic glycogenolysis provides a limited store (≤100 g) for maintenance of systemic glucose.

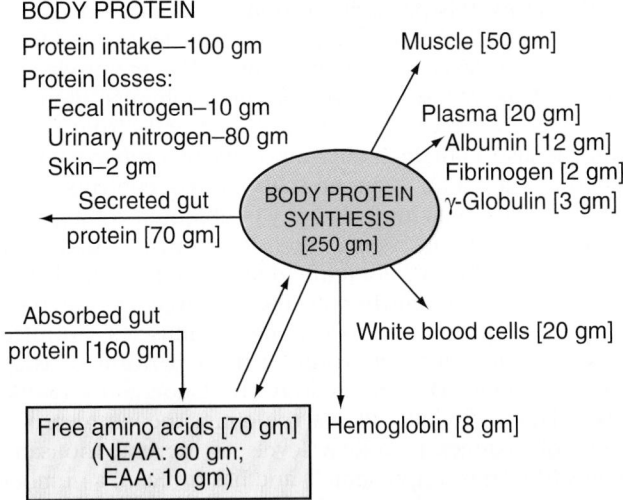

FIGURE 7-3. Diagram shows the daily flux of amino acids in the body of a 70-kg man. Total-body protein synthesis is 250 g per 24 hours, of which 50 g is muscle; proteolysis contributes approximately the same. Thus, with adequate amounts of energy, nitrogen equilibrium is the result. NEAA, nonessential amino acid; EAA, essential amino acid. (Data from Munro HN: Parenteral nutrition: Metabolic consequences of bypassing the gut and liver. *In* Clinical Nutrition Update: Amino Acids. Chicago, American Medical Association, 1977, p 141.)

TABLE 7-3.   Normal Stores of Available Energy and Rates of Utilization in a Man Weighing 65 kg

	Total Body Content (g)	Available Store			Daily Utilization* (g)	Exhaustion Time (days)
		g	mJ	kcal		
Carbohydrate	500	150	2.5	600	All used in first 24 hr	<1
Protein	11,000	2,400	40	9,600	60	About 40[†]
Fat	9,000	6,500	235	58,500	150	About 40[†]

*Assuming an energy expenditure of about 6.7 mJ (1600 kcal)/day.
[†]Experience in voluntary starvation suggests that the limit of resting starvation in young men in excellent physical condition may be as much as 60 to 70 days (Maize Prison, Northern Ireland).
From Passmore R, Robson JS: A Companion to Medical Studies, Vol. 3. Oxford, Blackwell Scientific, 1974.

However, fat constitutes the bulk of calories available (Table 7-3), and lipolysis and release of free fatty acids occur in response to the low insulin levels. For example, the average adult fat reserve is approximately 10 kg, or 100,000 kcal, 60 times hepatic glycogen stores. In peripheral tissues during fasting, free fatty acid and ketone body utilization for ATP production increase, whereas glucose oxidation is inhibited. As discussed earlier, branched-chain amino acid oxidation in muscle rises, thus sparing glucose. Most important, gluconeogenesis in the liver and kidney is activated, using muscle-derived glutamine and alanine, lactate, and glycerol released from lipid oxidation, with increased urea production. This process, in addition to metabolic cycles such as the glucose-alanine or glucose-lactate cycle (see earlier), maintains blood glucose for tissues that initially are highly dependent on glucose for energy (e.g., brain, erythrocytes, and kidney).

In the liver, the accelerated proteolysis induced by fasting occurs largely in lysosomes. However, in muscle tissue, activation of the ATP-ubiquitin–dependent proteolytic pathway is primarily responsible for the increased protein degradation in fasting. In rodents deprived of food for 48 hours, levels of total ubiquitin mRNA in muscle and the mRNAs for several proteasome subunits increase coordinately threefold to sixfold.[12,14] Muscles from fasted animals also contain higher amounts of proteins conjugated to ubiquitin than muscles of fed controls. This finding suggests an increased rate of ubiquitin conjugation in muscle during fasting, and it correlates with the activation of the ATP-ubiquitin–dependent pathway in the isolated muscles. Further detailed analysis of the transcriptional adaptations occurring in muscles of mice fasted for 48 hours has recently been performed using complementary DNA microarrays by Jagoe and coworkers.[21] This technique allows the simultaneous measurement of changes in mRNA levels for several thousand genes (the "transcriptosome") and has revealed a number of important new changes of gene expression that had not been noted before. One new gene is markedly induced, which has subsequently proved to be the new ubiquitin-ligase or E3, named *atrogin-1*[15,16] and discussed earlier. Other features in fasting include reduced transcripts for many of the enzymes involved in later stages of glycolysis and coordinated changes in mRNAs encoding translation initiation factors that might favor translation of a subset of stress-related proteins.

Long-Term Fasting and Dietary Protein Deficiency

In prolonged fasting, gluconeogenesis from body proteins and loss of muscle mass is gradually reduced. The most important factor reducing glucose needs during fasting is a decrease in the brain's requirement for glucose, because this organ comes to utilize ketone bodies for a large part of its ATP production. As the use of alternative fuels to glucose increases, muscle proteolysis falls below levels seen early in starvation, and eventually proteolysis is lower than in the fed state. In humans, 1 week of fasting is necessary for this adaptation, as indicated by a diminished forearm arteriovenous difference of amino acids and by decreased urinary N-methylhistidine excretion. Both the lysosomal and nonlysosomal ATP-dependent pathways are suppressed in muscle of rats fasted for prolonged periods, and very similar reductions in muscle proteolysis occur in animals fed a protein-deficient diet.[22] It remains likely that these nutritional states share common signals and mechanisms for reducing proteolysis, for example, through reduced thyroid status, although additional mechanisms may also be important for these adaptations.

Physiology of Inflammation and Sepsis

Changes in Energy Metabolism and Protein Turnover

Sepsis is the major cause of surgical mortality. The metabolic tragedy of sepsis is that the suppression of proteolysis seen in prolonged starvation does not occur and breakdown of protein continues. In fact, lean tissue losses can approximate 900 g/day in patients with severe sepsis, traumatic injuries, closed head injury, or major burns, with generalized muscle wasting. In humans and animals with sepsis, there is clear evidence of increased proteolysis and net release of amino acids from muscle, and furthermore, most of the increased proteolysis results from activation of the ubiquitin-proteasome pathway. Pale glycolytic muscles appear far more sensitive to sepsis than dark oxidative ones. For example, ubiquitin mRNA increased by several times in pale extensor digitorum longus muscles, whereas ATP-dependent proteolysis rose, but did not change, in dark soleus muscles, in which ATP-dependent proteolytic activity was unchanged.[23] The mRNAs for many other components of the ubiquitin-proteasome pathway increase in muscle in experimental

INTEGRATED CONCEPT OF SEPSIS

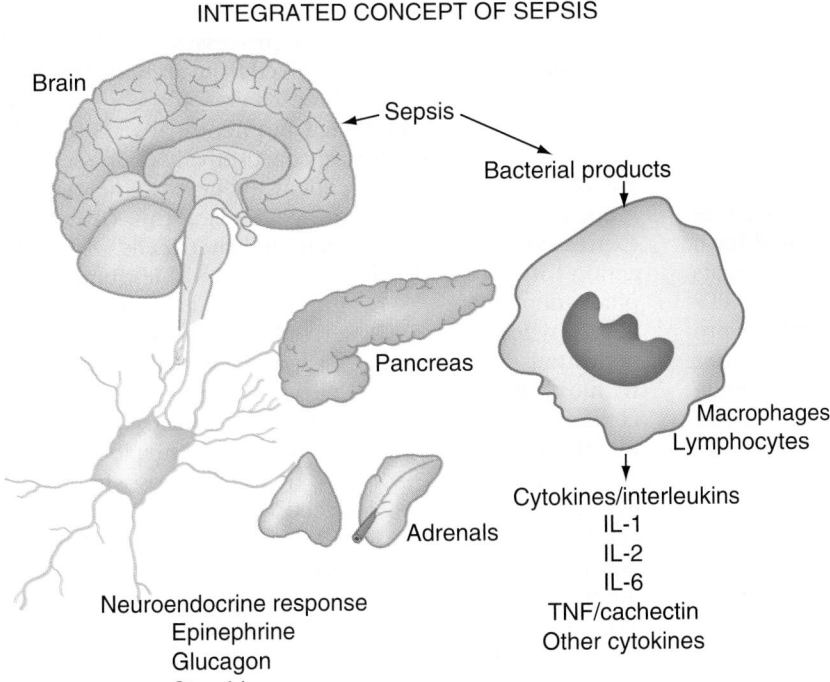

FIGURE 7-4. An emerging concept of the response to stress and sepsis. In previous years, the neurosympathetic response to sepsis was emphasized, with the secretion of epinephrine, glucagon, and corticosteroids—the so-called counter-regulatory hormones. It is now clear that this is but one half of the efferent limb and that cytokines are extremely important. IL, interleukin; TNF, tumor necrosis factor.

models of sepsis[19,24] and in septic patients. Sepsis increases rates of ubiquitination of muscle proteins,[14] and inhibitors of the proteasome dramatically reduce total and myofibrillar proteolysis in muscle from septic animals.[13] Though they contribute little to overall proteolysis, other pathways, in addition to the ubiquitin-proteasome pathway, may also have a role in muscle wasting in sepsis. For example, increased mRNA levels for cathepsin B and calpain have been found in muscle during sepsis, and the calpains also appear to play a role (see earlier).

Sepsis leads to reduced protein synthesis, especially in fast-twitch muscles, owing to reduced rates of translation initiation. Furthermore, the response to stimuli that normally promote increased protein synthesis, such as the branched-chain amino acids or insulin, is diminished. In contrast, hepatic protein synthesis, largely of acute-phase-reactant proteins found in plasma, is increased in the septic state.

As discussed earlier, insulin normally inhibits gluconeogenesis. However, in sepsis and other inflammatory states, gluconeogenesis continues despite the administration of either fat or carbohydrate, and peripheral insulin resistance with impaired skeletal muscle uptake of glucose occurs. For these reasons, hyperglycemia in response to intravenous feeding during sepsis is common, particularly in patients predisposed to diabetes. This insulin resistance or stress-induced hyperglycemia is caused by multiple factors, including elevated counter-regulatory hormones (catecholamines, glucagon, and glucocorticoids) and cytokines (primarily tumor necrosis factor [TNF]) (see later) (Fig. 7-4). Numerous strategies have been proposed to counter hyperglycemia while providing intravenous nutrition to patients with sepsis or severe inflammation, such as that due to burn injury. One approach is by lipid supplementation. However, whether lipid metabolism continues normally in sepsis is controversial. Perhaps in moderate sepsis, fat continues to be used, whereas in severe sepsis, fat is inefficiently utilized. To truly understand why these metabolic profiles are altered will require a better understanding of the effect of the various mediators released during severe inflammation and sepsis on the pancreatic beta cell and peripheral tissues.

Role of Cytokines and Other Mediators in the Response to Sepsis

Many of the systemic manifestations of sepsis are mediated by cytokines, levels of which rise in the blood in infection and in other inflammatory states such as burn injury (see Fig. 7-4) (for a complete discussion of the biology of cytokines and inflammation, the reader is directed to Chapter 4). Clowes, a general surgeon, in 1983 proposed for the first time that a "proteolysis-inducing factor" (most likely an interleukin [IL] split product), was responsible for increased muscle proteolysis and hepatic protein synthesis in sepsis, and this proposal stimulated broad interest in the cytokines as mediators of these processes. Although probably more than 100 products of macrophages exist, attention has focused largely on only a few, primarily IL-1, IL-6, TNF, and interferon (IFN)-γ. Enterocytes, in addition to inflammatory cells, may also serve as a source of these cytokines. In muscle, the activation of proteolysis by TNF and other cytokines appears to depend, at least in part, on activation of a nuclear transcription factor that serves as a common signaling pathway for inflammation, termed *NF-κB*. An increasingly commonly held view is that cytokine release is an appropriate response to a modest-sized insult, but sustained enormous cytokine release is deleterious and may contribute to the so-called multiple organ failure syndrome, the end-stage physiologic state accompanying sepsis.

Elucidating the roles of particular cytokines in the activation of muscle proteolysis during sepsis has proved difficult. Although many of the cytokines mentioned have, when administered in recombinant form to intact animals, been shown singly or in combination to activate the ATP-ubiquitin-proteasome dependent pathway of muscle proteolysis,[25] in isolated muscle preparations their actions are less clear. Unlike IL-1, TNF, or IFN-γ, IL-6 does not induce changes in muscle mRNA for ubiquitin,[25] and this is consistent with the observation in Dr. Fischer's laboratory that in an IL-6–deficient mouse, the sepsis-related acceleration in proteolysis still occurs. One important factor present in the intact animal but perhaps lacking during in vitro experiments are the corticosteroids. Studies from Dr. Fischer and Dr. Hasselgren's laboratory strongly suggest that in septic animals, glucocorticoids are required for full activation of the ubiquitin-proteasome pathway in muscle and thus appear to be a permissive factor for the response to cytokines.[19] Inhibition of TNF production in sepsis and other conditions may be of benefit in inhibiting muscle wasting. For example, recent experiments with a xanthine derivative, torbafylline, demonstrated inhibition of proteolysis via the ubiquitin-proteasome pathway and prevented muscle wasting in animal models of cancer cachexia and sepsis.[26]

Both IL-1 and TNF elicit the release of prostaglandin E_2 from muscle. Although prostaglandin E_2 had been proposed to be critical for increased muscle proteolysis in septic models, no decrease in ATP-dependent proteolysis or in ubiquitin mRNA levels occurred in muscles from endotoxin-treated rats that received naproxen, a potent inhibitor of prostaglandin E_2 production. To summarize both in vivo and in vitro studies, prostaglandins appear unnecessary for the rise in muscle proteolysis during infection.[12]

Another signal for increased proteolysis in muscle during systemic infection is fever. Studies by V. Baracos and A. Goldberg in 1984 of the influence of temperature on protein degradation and synthesis in isolated muscles demonstrated a linear increase in the rate of proteolysis, whereas protein synthesis was relatively unchanged. Therefore, in febrile animals, the rise in body temperature induced by cytokines and their direct catabolic effects on skeletal muscle appear to act synergistically to induce amino acid release and to promote muscle wasting.

The effects of cytokines on the liver are complex. IL-1 is associated with increased hepatic protein synthesis of some of the complement intermediates, whereas synthesis of transferrin is steroid dependent. IL-6 appears to increase synthesis of certain α-glycoproteins, but undoubtedly other cytokines are involved as well.

Role of Oxidizing Agents

Oxidizing agents such as nitric oxide and hydroxyl radicals are generated in a variety of tissues and play impor-

tant roles in metabolic regulation. Nitric oxide (NO), a mediator of diverse physiologic processes, is a short-lived free radical gas and oxidant derived from arginine by nitric oxide synthase (NOS).[27] Three NOS isoforms have been identified in cells. Endothelial and neuronal NOS (ecNOS and ncNOS, respectively) are constitutively expressed and are Ca^{2+}calmodulin dependent, whereas the largely inducible Ca^{2+}independent NOS isoform (iNOS) is expressed in immunologically activated cells. A classic action of ecNOS is the cyclic guanosine monophosphate–dependent vasodilation mediated by the endothelium, whereas ncNOS-derived NO functions as a neurotransmitter in numerous pathways. NO reacts avidly with oxygen-derived free radicals, thiols, and active metal centers of proteins, and a complex chemistry governs its functions in cell signaling and in altering metabolic activity. Of the three isoforms, iNOS is most important because, once it is induced by lipopolysaccharide, cytokines, or other factors, large and sustained amounts of nitric oxide may be produced. The increase in NO production in sepsis has been proposed to mediate increased hepatic protein synthesis, killing of pathogens, and programmed cell death (apoptosis).[28] Various studies have also shown that skeletal muscle produces NO and that NOS activity in this tissue is influenced by contraction[29] and cytokines. In fact, our recent studies in incubated muscles have shown that NO donors or hydroxyl radicals activate proteolysis by up to 80%.[30] These mediators may therefore be important for accelerated muscle proteolysis during strenuous exercise, ischemia, after muscle injury, and in inflammatory states.

Cachexia of Cancer

Patients with neoplastic disease may suffer profound weight loss and generalized cachexia. There are probably many contributing factors to this response, including reduced food intake, altered metabolic rate, endocrine abnormalities, and the effects of anticancer treatments, but various cytokines and other circulating factors have been identified that undoubtedly play a role, including TNF, IL-1, IL-6, and IFN-γ.[31] Anorexia is common, even when the tumor is small, a finding suggesting deranged central nervous system satiety mechanisms (see later). Marked muscle wasting is a debilitating feature of advanced cancer. In rats bearing tumors, severe muscle wasting occurs, apparently mediated by TNF and resulting primarily from an increased rate of ATP-dependent proteolysis, with increased levels of mRNAs for ubiquitin and subunits of the proteasome, especially in the pale muscle fibers that atrophy most profoundly. However, additional proteolytic pathways may also be activated, and different cytokines or other circulating factors are frequently implicated in the genesis of cachexia.[31] One other factor implicated in some types of cancer cachexia is proteolysis-inducing factor (PIF). This was identified first in tumor-bearing mice and when injected into healthy mice produced profound weight loss. Purified PIF induces catabolism in muscle cells and activates the ubiquitin-proteasome pathway in muscle.[32] PIF has also been found in urine of a large proportion of patients with weight loss due to pancreatic cancer, and treatment with eicosapentaenoic acid, which blocks formation of 15-hydroxyeicosatetraenoic acid by PIF in muscle cells, inhibits weight loss even in those with advanced disease.[33] However, whether these mechanisms have broad applicability in cancer remains unclear.

New Concepts in the Regulation of Body Energy Expenditure

In the past decade, exciting insights have been achieved in inter-related areas of mechanisms regulating body size and resting energy expenditure, satiety, and the metabolic phenomena thought relevant to aging. These findings have relevance to diverse disease entities, including the etiology of insulin resistance (e.g., in sepsis), type II diabetes mellitus, and morbid obesity. One surprising realization has been that adipose tissue is not only a storage depot for calories but, in a complex network of hormonal and neuronal signals, this tissue also plays an important role in endocrine regulation. Beginning with the discovery by J. Friedman in 1994 of the adipocyte-derived circulating hormone leptin, adipose tissue is now known to be an important source of endocrine mediators, including TNF, angiotensinogen, resistin, and adiponectin. In conjunction with gut hormones such as ghrelin, CCK, PYY, and insulin, the adipocyte-derived hormones interact in the brain, in particular at the arcuate nucleus, to control food intake and energy expenditure. In the arcuate nucleus, two sets of neurons appear to interact with opposing effects. Activation of agouti-related peptide (AgRP)/ neuropeptide Y (NPY) neurons increases appetite and metabolism, whereas activation of POMC/CART neurons has the opposing effect to inhibit eating, in part by causing the release of α-melanocyte–stimulating hormone, a satiety signal. Such mechanisms are clearly relevant to understanding the inanition accompanying advanced cancer, and there is some evidence to suggest that appetite-promoting agents such as ghrelin may find clinical use in this regard. How these newly described regulatory pathways influence the metabolism of particular nutrients or nitrogen balance remains poorly understood.

Although under ongoing and intense investigation, recent discoveries in aging research appear connected, if indirectly, to the metabolic signaling pathways described earlier. It is now well accepted that dietary caloric restriction enhances longevity and may have other desirable effects, such as a reduction in primary tumors, in experimental animals and lower organisms. Similar genetic mechanisms may underlie such responses, beginning with the discovery by L. Guarente and coworkers of the *Sir2* gene in yeast, and by G. Ruvkun and colleagues of the daf-2 genetic pathway in *Caenorhabditis elegans*. These mechanisms appear to involve changes in nicotinamide adenine dinucleotide–dependent functions such as histone acetylation, in insulin signaling, and in cellular responses to reactive oxygen species generated in the mitochondria. These exciting studies will undoubtedly contribute to our future understanding of overall metabolism, carcinogenesis, and free radical–induced injury.

FUNDAMENTALS OF ARTIFICIAL NUTRITION

General Indications for Nutrition Support and Choice of Route of Administration

Indications for nutritional support should consider the following:

1. The premorbid state (healthy or otherwise)
2. Poor nutritional status (the current oral intake meets <50% of total energy needs)
3. Significant weight loss (initial body weight less than the usual body weight by ≥10%, or a decrease in inpatient weight by >10% of the admission weight)
4. The duration of starvation (>7 days' inanition)
5. An anticipated duration of artificial nutrition (particularly for total parenteral nutrition [TPN]) of more than 7 days
6. The degree of the anticipated insult, surgical or otherwise
7. A serum albumin value less than 3.0 g/100 mL measured in the absence of an inflammatory state

Each practitioner must choose the criteria in a given patient. Obviously, in critically ill patients, nutritional supplementation should be undertaken more readily than in patients who are less severely stressed. Finally, when patients are either malnourished or in the postinjury stressed state, there is no obvious harm and there may be a clinical benefit to the initiation of immediate enteral feeding, particularly in the more critically ill patient (see later).

Two routes of administration are possible: the enteral route, using stomach or preferably small intestine, and the parenteral route. The enteral route is considered to be more physiologic in that the liver is not bypassed, allowing this organ to efficiently process and store various portally supplied nutrients, and the release of gut hormones and insulin is facilitated, presumably leading to more efficient nutrient disposal in the periphery. However, despite these and other putative advantages, the relative benefits of enteral versus parenteral nutrition in humans remain unclear (see the sections on controversies in artificial nutrition).

Nutritional Assessment

Nutritional assessment is a process by which changes in body nutritional composition are estimated, in part to predict risk for surgery or other stressful therapeutic activity. Ideally, valid methods of assessment should facilitate patient selection for instituting artificial nutrition and for determining the efficacy of nutritional interventions. Although functional measures of lean body mass, such as skeletal muscle strength, respiratory and cardiac performance, hepatic synthetic function, renal status, and immunologic reactivity seem most desirable, in practice such approaches have proven difficult (see later). Acceptable studies of nutritional assessment techniques should be randomized, prospective, and blinded. However, most published studies are retrospective for selected patients, usually those judged to be severely at risk. Studies that emphasize hepatic synthesis of short-lived or immunologically active proteins, and those which measure neutrophil function, may be more successful in identifying patients at risk of infection. The University of Pennsylvania group suggested a prognostic nutritional index, but the patients were nonconsecutive and were studied retrospectively. When the same index was studied prospectively, it failed to reveal a group at risk. In several studies, a careful history and physical examination by a seasoned clinician yield the same accuracy as extensive testing for the estimation of nutritional risk, particularly when functionality is assessed.

Clinical History

Weight loss, anorexia, weakness, inability to carry out normal functions, or a disease process that interferes with intake, such as esophageal carcinoma, should alert the examiner to the possibility of malnutrition. Certain disorders such as burns, sepsis, head injury, or pancreatitis are particularly catabolic and must be anticipated to raise caloric requirements significantly. The clinical criteria described earlier for the degree of acceptable body weight loss and duration of inanition must be calculated. Finally, on physical examination, muscle wasting, loose or otherwise abnormal skin, the edema of hypoproteinemia, weakness, loss of body fat, and pallor should suggest the diagnosis of malnutrition.

Body Composition Analysis

Accumulation of lean body mass is the principal objective of nutritional support; thus, determination of lean body mass is the most appropriate means of nutritional assessment. Such determinations are usually available only on a research basis.

Bioelectrical Impedance. This method estimates total body water and lean muscle mass by measuring electrical resistance at various surface locations. Although simple to perform, the values derived are often inaccurate and poorly reproducible.

Displacement. Probably the most sensitive determination of lean body mass is displacement. Various body components are estimated by displacement of water volume.

Exchange of Labeled Ions. Total-body water may be determined by administration of tritiated water. Lean body mass is estimated by exchangeable potassium (^{42}K) and extracellular water by total exchangeable sodium (^{22}Na) Shizgal suggested that a ratio of exchangeable sodium to exchangeable potassium greater than 1.2 indicates the increased extracellular water and decreased body mass accompanying malnutrition. Shizgal also proposed derivative ratios to estimate total-body fat, but because of compounded error, these ratios are probably inaccurate.

Neutron Activation Analysis. This technique is accurate but requires sophisticated apparatus in which the body is bombarded with activated neutrons. Nitrogen, indicative of lean body mass, is then measured. Other ions may also be determined.

Total-Body Counters. These large devices measure spontaneous decay of naturally occurring isotopes, such as ^{40}K, which reflects lean body mass. However, these measurements are not suitable for patients who are ill, because subjects must remain stationary within the counter for prolonged periods.

Magnetic Resonance Imaging. Magnetic resonance imaging may accurately measure lean body mass, although most current work has focused on energy metabolism and the relationships among high-energy phosphate stores in starvation and refeeding. For example, in rats, phosphocreatine is decreased after 6 to 8 days of starvation. Other studies suggest a possible decrease in ATP synthetic efficiency in the starved muscle, presumably secondary to insufficient stores of phosphocreatine to maintain ATP.

Computed Tomography. Computed tomography (CT) with three-dimensional reconstruction can yield accurate values for organ size and volume. Radiographic tissue density can also be used to monitor the response to therapy. For example, the studies of Buchman and associates have shown that the hepatic steatosis which commonly occurs during long-term TPN administration can be at least partially reversed by supplementation of the TPN solution with carnitine or choline, as shown by a reduction in hepatic fat content (with increased radiographic density) on serial CT scanning.[34]

Indirect Calorimetry

Indirect calorimetry, performed using a bedside metabolic cart, is used increasingly to measure energy balance and to estimate caloric requirements. The measurement is carried out with the patient in the resting state, and in general 15% should be added for activity. Oxygen consumption can be determined directly and caloric expenditure calculated. In addition, if carbon dioxide production is measured simultaneously, the respiratory quotient (RQ) can be estimated for an assessment of overfeeding. An alternative method for the determination of oxygen consumption involves placement of a pulmonary artery catheter. If cardiac output is measured by thermodilution and the oxygen content in arterial and mixed venous blood is measured, the Fick equation can then be used to calculate Vo_2. In certain patient populations, particularly following severe burn injury, direct measurement of Vo_2 has proven useful in estimating caloric needs, as in these patients, standard formulas such as the Harris-Benedict equation (see the later section on practical approaches to artificial nutrition) often prove particularly inaccurate.

Metabolic carts can also determine which fuel is being consumed in a clinical setting. An RQ of 1 indicates pure carbohydrate utilization, 0.8 indicates pure protein oxidation, and 0.7 is consistent with pure fat utilization. Theoretically, the RQ with lipogenesis can be as high as 9. Although an RQ of greater than 1 is rarely seen, such data are indicative of overfeeding of glucose and/or fat, whereas an RQ of less than 0.7 indicates ketogenesis. Without such measurements, when fat is administered indirect measures of utilization, such as the absence of plasma lipemia and the presence of ketone bodies, are necessary to confirm efficient metabolism. Although indirect calorimetry is an attractive approach, a recent multicenter study of RQs derived by this method suggests that, in practice, low sensitivity and specificity may limit its efficacy as an indicator of overfeeding or underfeeding.[35]

Anthropomorphic Measurements

These parameters are controversial with regard to normative values and their relevance to nitrogen depletion. Characteristic measurements include the creatinine-height index, triceps skinfold thickness, and the measurement of arm muscle circumference. Although these values may be proportional to muscle or fat stores, they do not reflect function. A more practical anthropomorphic approach is the calculation of "ideal body weight" (IBW), particularly when the usual body weight (UBW) (i.e., the weight of the patient prior to the onset of illness) is unknown. The IBW can be found from standardized tables developed by the insurance industry that relate height to expected weight, or IBW can be estimated by the following formulas:

- For males: 106 lb for the first 5 feet and 6 lb for each inch thereafter
- For females: 100 lb for the first 5 feet and 5 lb for each inch thereafter

As these tables were derived from population norms in the 1950s, prior to the current trend toward obesity in Americans, they tend to underestimate weight. However, in keeping with the general principle of avoiding excessive provision of calories during artificial feeding, use of the IBW in calculating caloric needs is not harmful and is commonly used (see the later section on practical approaches to artificial nutrition).

Functional Studies of Muscle Function

Because many of the tests described earlier are not readily available, muscle strength, either as evaluated by hand-grip dynamometry, as force-frequency characteristics, or as the rate of recovery from fatigue after electrical stimulation of the ulnar nerve, has been evaluated. When properly conducted, such studies provide a functional counterpart of severe protein-calorie malnutrition, and they may be used to assess for a beneficial response to nutritional or other anabolic interventions. For example, an ongoing study at Beth Israel Deaconess Medical Center suggests that hand grip strength may improve in elderly patients administered growth hormone. In most studies, however, patients with deficits in hand dynamometry are easily identifiable by other means such as a simple functional history, physical examination, or global nutritional assessment. The importance of functional studies was recently emphasized by the work of Herridge and colleagues (and see accompanying editorial), who demonstrated residual muscle wasting and weakness for up to 1 year following discharge from the intensive care unit (ICU) and treatment of the acute respiratory distress syndrome.[36]

Biochemical Measurements

A variety of biochemical approaches have been described for determining malnutrition. Although useful, such methods are often inaccurate and usually do not give added value when compared to a clinical approach to nutritional assessment.

Serum Proteins. The measurement of serum proteins, in particular albumin, is often used as an index of malnutrition, with a concentration of less than 3.0 g/dL of albumin the usual indicator. The half-life of albumin is as long as 14 to 18 days, and for this reason other more short-lived proteins, such as prealbumin (half-life, 3 to 5 days) or transferrin (<200 mg/dL; half-life, 7 days), have been proposed as more sensitive indicators of rapid changes in nutritional status. However, the meaning of the lowered serum albumin concentration in patients who are malnourished and at risk has always been controversial. Some investigators have attributed the low serum albumin to decreased synthesis, possibly due to low-grade sepsis or stress, and others have attributed it to increased degradation. In a model of long-term sepsis, von Allmen and associates[37] found that whereas albumin synthesis was decreased for the first 24 hours, after 4 days synthesis of this protein actually rose to normal levels. These results suggest that decreased albumin synthesis because of downregulation may not be tenable in long-term malnutrition. In malnutrition one usually expects an increase in extravascular volume. With greater extravascular volume, a greater amount of albumin is likely to be present in the extravascular space, where it appears to be degraded more rapidly. Thus, increased albumin in the extravascular space with an increased rate of degradation may well explain the lowered serum albumin level in patients who are at risk.

Nitrogen Balance. The measurement of nitrogen balance is a tedious technique that requires the collection of all integumentary, wound, and excretory losses. Overall, such measurements tend to be inaccurate and will often favor the erroneous conclusion that positive nitrogen balance has been achieved. In the clinical setting, nitrogen balance is determined by measuring 24-hour urinary and gastrointestinal losses. Because most patients receiving parenteral nutrition do not eat, stool nitrogen can be assumed to be 1 g/day, or it can be disregarded altogether. The 24-hour urine collection must be accurate, as monitored by measuring urinary creatinine. The value for the rate of nitrogen loss is compared with nitrogen intake, and nitrogen balance is thus obtained.

Therefore, nitrogen balance
= intake − loss [urine 90%, stool 5%, integument 5%]

or

= [protein intake (g)/6.25] − urinary urea (g)
 − 2 (for stool and skin) − 2 (for non-urea nitrogen)

Measurement of Protein Breakdown. Nitrogen turnover, particularly that of lean body mass, can be estimated by urinary excretion of 3-methylhistidine, as described earlier. However, 3-methylhistidine measures breakdown of not only muscle but also of a more rapidly turning over protein pool derived from the gut and skin, invalidating it as a measurement of turnover of skeletal muscle protein alone. Short of actual in vitro measurement in isolated muscle tissue (see earlier), common in vivo approaches for the measurement of protein breakdown include pulse-chase and other isotopic methods, which involve infusion of ^{15}N-labeled amino acids and other metabolites. All of these methods, unfortunately, are highly derivative and are subject to a variety of artifacts.

Measurements of Immunologic Function. Delayed cutaneous hypersensitivity or anergy, most commonly tested by delayed reaction to skin recall antigens, was widely used in early studies of nutritional assessment and is a manifestation of cell-mediated immunity. Although most studies showed a statistical relationship between anergy and mortality, investigators have concluded that delayed cutaneous hypersensitivity is without value for measuring specific nutritional or operative risk. On the other hand, more recent data suggest that when skin testing is carefully performed by trained personnel and done at defined times (e.g., on admission rather than at random throughout the hospital course), skin reactivity may have some value. For example, in patients admitted after trauma or with infection, anergy to cutaneous recall antigens is associated with high mortality and morbidity. These patients are likely those with severe malnutrition. However, not all malnourished patients are at risk and the defect is immunologic, not nutritional. Furthermore, delayed cutaneous hypersensitivity is complicated by extraneous factors such as operation, which is followed by immediate anergy in many patients. Patients with cancer are also anergic, and this condition may be reversed after resection. Thus, the significance of delayed cutaneous hypersensitivity must be assessed in concert with other tests. Another method for determining immunologic function in the clinical setting is neutrophil function, but this approach appears even less relevant to nutritional status than are assays of cell-mediated immunity

Specific Fuels

The sources of calories in a normal diet and during artificial feeding are carbohydrate, lipid, and protein. We discuss each of these fuels, with particular emphasis on their relative roles during intravenous feeding and required adjustments for concurrent illness such as diabetes and liver or renal failure.

Carbohydrate

Glucose is the preferred carbohydrate source in traditional TPN. Glucose administration during fasting or stress appears to decrease urinary urea production, the so-called protein-sparing effect, with a minimum of 100 g of glucose per 24 hours required for this response based on Gamble's classic work of the 1940s. It was not until the late 1970s that the metabolism of exogenously supplied carbohydrate was evaluated in detail. The nitrogen-sparing effect of infused glucose was found to occur via two mechanisms. First, hepatic gluconeogenesis is suppressed, so

protein need not be broken down to generate gluconeogenic precursors. Second, glucose itself is used as an energy substrate, so fewer amino acids need be oxidized for energy. Wolfe and coworkers showed that maximum suppression of gluconeogenesis is achieved at infusion rates of 4 mg/kg/min (~400 g/day for a 70-kg man) and that glucose infusion beyond this level had minimal effects in further suppressing glucose production during TPN administration in postoperative surgical patients.[38] In this work, although any additional nitrogen-sparing effects of glucose would be expected to be derived from its direct oxidation, at infusion rates higher than 9 mg/kg/min all glucose was degraded by nonoxidative pathways, that is, those leading to net synthesis of lipid.

Toxicity of Hyperglycemia and Excessive Calorie Administration. When provided in excess, carbohydrate is converted to fat in the liver, a consequence referred to as *de novo lipogenesis*, and which likely contributes to TPN-related liver dysfunction (see later). In addition, the accompanying increase in V_{CO_2}, as reflected in an elevated RQ (see earlier), may lead to impaired ventilatory function in patients with already compromised pulmonary status. Finally, the resultant hyperglycemic state, most pronounced with blood glucose greater than 300 mg/dL, leads to immunosuppression and increased nosocomial infections. Hyperglycemia is a prevalent metabolic disorder that can be particularly pronounced in the ICU setting and postinjury state and is clearly exacerbated by the excessive administration of dextrose.

The immunosuppressive effects of hyperglycemia have been well studied. In vitro data suggest that hyperglycemia leads to immune cell dysfunction owing to impaired chemotaxis, adherence, phagocytosis, and bactericidal function. In prospective studies, tight postoperative glycemic control has been shown to significantly decrease nosocomial infections in diabetic patients. In the ICU setting, fastidious glycemic control achieved through intensive insulin therapy has been shown to dramatically improve patient outcomes. In the recent prospective, randomized study of Van den Berghe and coworkers,[39] 1548 ICU patients were randomized to either standard glycemic control (to maintain blood glucose at 180 to 200 mg/dL) or to "tight" glycemic control (insulin infusion to maintain glucose 80 to 110 mg/dL). All patents were fed 25 kcal/kg by either enteral or parenteral routes. By maintaining blood glucose in the 80- to 110-mg/dL range, these investigators demonstrated significant improvement in various clinical outcomes and a decrease in overall mortality by 42%. This landmark study highlights the importance of maintaining normoglycemia during feeding, because the benefits of nutritional intervention may be negated by the detrimental consequences associated with the hyperglycemic state.

In an effort to avoid the potential complications of overfeeding, one reasonable short-term option is the practice of hypocaloric feeding. The clinician must often balance the optimal administration of nutrition with a patient's overall clinical status. One could easily envision the desire to limit the volume of TPN received by a diabetic patient with difficult-to-control blood sugars, for the patient in renal failure who is not dialyzed but massively volume overloaded, or for the patient with poor oxygenation on high ventilatory support. In this setting it appears reasonable to provide goal protein (1.5 g/kg/day, see later) while limiting total calories to approximately 1000 kcal/day. This practice will decrease net protein catabolism while still allowing the mobilization of endogenous fat stores to close the expected caloric gap and will limit excessive volume administration. This approach is particularly acceptable when applied over a limited time course such as 1 to 2 weeks and in the obese patient population, when there is an abundance of lipid available for mobilization, but it is not a viable option for standard nutrition support.

Additional Sources of Dextrose. One must be careful to recognize all sources of exogenous dextrose administration, in addition to the patient's feeding solution, because significant amounts of dextrose can be found in

- Intravenous fluids containing 5% dextrose (50 g/L)
- Medications mixed in 5% dextrose instead of normal saline
- Patients on continuous venovenous dialysis, who often have 5% solutions as return fluid
- Patients on peritoneal dialysis with dextrose in the dialysate

Alternative Carbohydrate Sources. Carbohydrate sources other than glucose have not achieved popularity in the United States. Fructose, which some investigators have proposed for use in glucose resistance, may cause fatal lactic acidosis. The polyalcohols xylitol and sorbitol also undergo transformation to glucose, but xylitol may be hepatotoxic and has likely contributed to several deaths in the literature. Glycerol, another potential source of glucose, is potentially advantageous in that it may be sterilized in solution with amino acids, without caramelization, and its osmolality is low. The safety and efficacy of glycerol were studied in patients recovering from major trauma or surgery.[40] In one group, nitrogen equilibrium was achieved with combined lipid and glycerol administration. However, glycerol in large doses may cause renal failure in experimental animals and caution is appropriate.

Lipid

In starvation, fat provides the bulk of calories, in the form of free fatty acids and as ketone bodies manufactured by the liver from long-chain fatty acids. Net lipolysis during fasting or stress is promoted by steroids, catechols, glucagon, and some cytokines and is extremely sensitive to inhibition by insulin. Under normal circumstances or in moderate stress, fat and carbohydrate are indistinguishable with respect to their positive effects on nitrogen balance, with 25% of nonprotein calories as fat seemingly optimal for hepatic protein synthesis. What is not clear is at which point in stress or during sepsis fat utilization becomes impaired. Most investigators agree that whereas hepatic manufacture of ketone bodies is reduced early in sepsis, fat clearance remains relatively normal until comparatively late, even though fat oxidation is clearly impaired at a prior stage. Many sources of lipid are available for intravenous use.

Long-Chain Triglycerides. The safe administration of intravenous lipid became a reality in the late 1970s when an emulsion (Intralipid) composed of soybean oil and egg lecithin and containing predominantly long-chain triglycerides (LCTs) became commercially available in the United States. Although initially administered as a source of essential fatty acids (linoleic acid and α-linolenic acid) these n-3 and n-6 LCT emulsions now serve as a valuable caloric source in parenteral alimentation. Lipid emulsions are particularly versatile because they are calorically dense (9 kcal/g) and can be safely infused via a peripheral vein. Their role as a supplemental caloric source is particularly valuable when blood sugars are difficult to control or when carbohydrate administration reaches safe limits.

Medium-Chain Triglycerides. Because of the potential adverse effect of LCT emulsions (see later), alternative lipid fuels have been considered. In comparison to LCTs, medium-chain triglycerides (MCTs), containing only 8 to 10 carbons, are cleared more rapidly from plasma, are oxidized more rapidly, do not require a carnitine-dependent transport system to enter liver mitochondria, and are more soluble in TPN solutions. MCTs may also have a favorable effect on protein metabolism, leading to improved nitrogen balance. However, MCTs can be neurotoxic in patients with cirrhosis who cannot adequately clear them, and overall, mixed MCT-LCT emulsions are thought to be most desirable. Such mixed emulsions may be of particular benefit in patients with inflammatory disorders, because they contain approximately 50% less n-6 LCTs than the traditional Intralipid. Such LCTs may serve as precursors of potentially deleterious prostaglandins.

Structured Lipids. Structured lipids are a synthetic triglyceride molecule where medium-chain and long-chain fatty acids are esterified to the same glycerol backbone. The composition of the three fatty acid side chains can vary randomly or can be chemically defined by a specific enzymatic re-esterification process. Studies have proven structured lipids to be safe and to carry the metabolic advantages seen with MCT-LCT physical mixtures. Future studies will determine their role in the routine clinical setting.

Essential or Unsaturated Fatty Acids. Unsaturated fatty acids can be classified as monounsaturated (MUFA) or polyunsaturated (PUFA) depending on the location of their double bond. The three families of PUFAs (n-3, n-6, and n-9) start as the "essential" 18-carbon unsaturated fatty acids linoleic acid (C18:2Δ6) and α-linolenic acid (C18:3Δ3), and as the nonessential oleic acid (C18:2Δ9). Via sequential steps of elongation and desaturation, linoleic acid (LA) is converted to arachidonic acid (AA), while α-linolenic acid (ALA) is converted to eicosapentaenoic acid (EPA) and docosahexaenoic acid (DHA). These desaturase and elongase enzymes are found predominantly in the liver and have as their order of preferred substrate n-3 > n-6 > n-9. This process is under tight control, and the enzymes δ-5-desaturase and δ-6-desaturase appear to be key regulatory points. EPA and DHA can be derived only from direct ingestion or by synthesis from dietary ALA.

AA and EPA are the precursors of the eicosanoids, namely prostaglandins, thromboxanes, and leukotrienes. More specifically, AA is the precursor of the 2-series of prostaglandins and thromboxanes and the 4-series of the leukotrienes. EPA and DHA are the precursors of the 3-series of prostaglandins and thromboxanes and the 5-series of leukotrienes. Therefore, at the level of the cyclooxygenase and lipoxygenase enzymes critical for eicosanoid synthesis, there exists competition between AA and EPA. With the ingestion of fish or fish oil, the primary dietary source of omega-3 fatty acids (see later), EPA and DHA levels rise and these lipids can displace arachidonic acid in the membranes of cells active in eicosanoid synthesis, namely platelets, erythrocytes, neutrophils, monocytes, and liver cells. As a result, with omega-3 fatty acid administration there is (1) decreased production of prostaglandin E_2 and its metabolites; (2) a decrease in the production of thromboxane A_2, a potent platelet aggregator and vasoconstrictor; (3) a decrease in leukotriene B_4, an inducer of inflammation and potent inducer of leukocyte chemotaxis and adherence; (4) an increase in thromboxane A_3, a weak platelet aggregator and weak vasoconstrictor; (5) an increase in prostacyclin PGI_3, an active vasodilator and inhibitor of platelet aggregation; and (6) an increase in leukotriene B_5, a weak inducer of inflammation and weak chemotactic agent.[41] Accordingly, the administration of the omega-3 fatty acids (ALA or its products EPA and DHA) may produce an environment where the inflammatory response, if not halted, is modulated or downregulated to a less profound provasoconstrictive and prothrombotic state.

Recognition of Essential Fatty Acid Deficiency. The deficiency of essential fatty acids may be prevented by administration of between 2% and 5% of daily calories as either soybean or safflower oil fat emulsion, or a minimum of 30 to 50 g of lipid emulsion weekly. Plasma alterations, which occur within 1 week of administration of fat-free parenteral nutrition, include decreases in linoleic and arachidonic acids and increases in 5,8,11-eicosatrienoic acid and in the "triene-to-tetraene" ratio. The triene-to-tetraene ratio is normally less than 0.2%, and if greater than this value, essential fatty acid deficiency may be suspected. A common clinical sign is dry, flaky skin with small reddish papules and alopecia. Patients with essential fatty acid deficiency absorb essential fatty acids through the skin, but this approach is not practical except in infants. Patients who have excess adipose tissue can live for months without exogenous essential fatty acid administration because they maintain a mobilizable depot of linolenic acid in their adipose tissue.

Omega-3 Fatty Acids in the Clinical Setting. Omega-3 and omega-6 polyunsaturated fatty acids are important components of human cell membranes. Their composition within the cell membrane is primarily determined by dietary intake, because the omega-3/omega-6 ratio changes with changes in dietary consumption. As indicated earlier, the omega-3 fatty acids EPA and DHA play important roles in prostaglandin metabolism, thrombosis and atherosclerosis, immunology and inflammation, and membrane function. Once epidemiologists recognized that the paucity of heart disease in the Greenland Inuits was due to a diet high in long-chain n-3 fatty acids, subsequent human studies examining n-3 supplementation have documented their important role in the prevention and treatment of coronary artery disease, hypertension, arthritis, inflammatory and autoimmune disorders, and cancer.

In the clinical setting, the benefits of omega-3 fatty acid administration in surgical patients has been realized when administered as a key component of "immune-modulating" enteral feeding formulas. This topic is discussed in more detail elsewhere in this chapter. The use of intravenous n-3 lipid emulsions to modulate the immune system is only now being studied in clinical trials in the United States. Because lipid emulsions containing n-3 fatty acids inhibit triglyceride hydrolysis by lipoprotein lipase, fish oil cannot be infused alone or in combination only with LCTs. Instead, n-3 fatty acids must be combined with MCTs and LCTs in a solution composed of 50% MCT, 40% soybean (LCT), and 10% fish oil. Clinical studies that have administered this combined lipid solution have confirmed an increase in the ratio of 5-series leukotrienes compared to the 4-series in peripheral leukocytes, an improvement in inflammatory disorders such as atopic dermatitis, and an attenuated inflammatory response in experimental models of both pancreatic injury and acute colitis.

Omega-3 supplementation may be particularly advantageous in cirrhosis and liver dysfunction. For example, it is well accepted that patients with end-stage liver disease (ESLD) have very low serum and possibly tissue levels of the polyunsaturated fatty acids. Several investigators have demonstrated low levels of the long-chain PUFAs, namely AA, EPA, and DHA in patients with advanced cirrhosis, and these deficiencies appear to serve as independent predictors of mortality. Patients with ESLD cannot mount an appropriate inflammatory response when facing a severe insult or injury, and cirrhotic patients have a well-documented defect in T-cell-mediated immune function. These phenomena may in part be due to a deficiency in second messengers important in the inflammatory cascade, that is, low levels of long-chain PUFA and of derived eicosanoids. In fact, one of the principal consequences of essential fatty acid deficiency in animals and humans is a reduced resistance to infection.

Potential Toxicities of Lipid Administration. Recent reviews of the literature reveal that no adverse effects related to LCT lipid administration have been observed when intravenous lipids are administered in modest amounts, as long as infusion rates are less than 0.1 g/kg/hour or 1 kcal/kg/hour. Before this critical level was determined, many adverse effects ensued when LCT solutions were infused at excessive rates and quantities. Lipid accumulating in the liver may inhibit the reticuloendothelial system, the major site of RES function, by overloading and impairing Kupffer cell phagocytosis with lipid micelles. The phospholipid-emulsifying agent used in lipid solutions can also interfere with the action of lipoprotein lipase, potentially leading to a clinically relevant hypertriglyceridemic state. Therefore, lipid emulsions are not administered when serum triglyceride levels are greater than 400 mg/dL. The possibility of hypertriglyceride-related pancreatitis also arises when serum triglyceride levels reach the 800- to 1000-mg/dL range. Excessive lipid may also have deleterious effects in patients with severe pulmonary disease such as adult respiratory distress syndrome (ARDS). The downstream prostaglandin products of lipid emulsion precursors, such as thromboxane A_2 or prostaglandin E_2, can suppress lymphocyte proliferation and natural killer cell activity while reversing hypoxic vasoconstriction in patients with ARDS, thus further worsening pulmonary gas diffusion, oxygenation, and resistance to infection. Impaired plasma clearance of lipids can result in "fat overload syndrome," a particularly significant problem in children manifested by fever, back pain, chills, pulmonary insufficiency, and blocking of the reticuloendothelial system. Fat overload syndrome can result from the administration of a stable fat emulsion over a brief interval or from more modest doses of lipid that might be physicochemically unstable, and is avoided when fat is administered at a limit of 2 g/kg/day. In infants, up to 4 g/kg/day of fat is tolerated.

Protein

A 70-kg man has between 10 and 11 kg of protein, otherwise referred to as *lean body mass*. In the fed state, daily protein turnover is between 250 and 300 g, or 3%. The gut is the largest component of this turnover, the source of nitrogen loss being shed enterocytes and secreted digestive enzymes. After digestion of food, all amino acids are absorbed, save 1 g of nitrogen excreted in the stool. Although intracellular proteolysis accounts for 50 to 70 g of amino acids added to the amino acid pool daily, if adequate energy is present, most of these amino acids are reincorporated into protein. The nonessential amino acids can be synthesized from carbon skeletons and sources of nitrogen such as glutamine, through transamination. Twenty grams of plasma protein, 8 g of hemoglobin, 20 g of white blood cells, and a few grams of skin constitute the remainder of total body protein synthesis (see Fig. 7-3). Protein turnover decreases markedly with age. Thus, turnover in a neonate approximates 25 g/kg of protein per 24 hours, decreases to 7 g/kg per 24 hours at 1 year, and in adults, turnover falls to 3 g/kg per 24 hours.

Determining Protein Requirements. The minimal intake of protein required for neutral nitrogen balance can be determined empirically by two approaches. The first method involves measuring all nitrogen losses while the human or animal subject is fed a calorically adequate, but protein-free diet. In general, this approach will underestimate the true protein requirement, particularly when a superimposed stressor is present. For example, after several days of a protein-free diet in humans, 37 mg/kg of nitrogen is excreted into the urine, whereas 12 mg/kg of nitrogen is lost in the feces. Integumentary losses account for another 5 mg/kg, with another 2 to 3 mg/kg of nitrogen by evaporation, for a total of 56 to 57 mg/kg of nitrogen, or in terms of whole protein, 0.34 g/kg of protein per day is lost. This latter value is well below commonly accepted norms for the daily protein requirement in humans. A second approach that appears more relevant to clinical practice is to determine the minimal quantity of ingested protein necessary to maintain nitrogen equilibrium. When derived in this manner, with various corrections, the average normal requirement is 0.8 g/kg of protein or between 56 and 60 g of protein per day. Trauma, infection, and other catabolic conditions increase this requirement. In addi-

tion, in the postinjury state, the increased rate of whole-body protein catabolism appears unusually resistant to exogenous supplementation with amino acids. However, this obligate protein loss, driven by the overexpression of catecholamines and cytokines during the systemic inflammatory response, can be offset to some degree by protein administration, decreasing the rate of net protein catabolism to about one fourth the rate seen in the absence of TPN. The extensive studies of Graham Hill and Robert Wolfe of whole-body protein turnover during the 1980s documented that exogenous protein administration of 1.5 g/kg/day achieves maximal protein sparing and that when amounts exceeding that are administered, no further incorporation of nitrogen into protein is possible, with the excess protein converted to urea and excreted, at least in relatively normal patients. Accordingly, it is most common to administer protein during artificial nutrition, whether enteral or parenteral, at a value of 1.5 g/kg/day. It is not clear in patients with severe protein losses, such as after major burns, whether limiting protein intake to this level is efficacious, and many centers have attempted to administer even greater amounts of protein (e.g., 2 g/day) to correct measured deficits.

Alterations for Liver and Renal Failure. Patients who are intolerant of nitrogen in the surgical setting usually manifest renal or hepatic impairment, and patients with advanced hepatic failure may have both hepatic and renal insufficiency, the so-called hepatorenal syndrome. Both groups of patients tend to be hypercatabolic, and sepsis is a common accompaniment. For some patients, for example following an episode of hypotension, a crush injury involving muscle, or dye toxicity in radiologic procedures, renal failure will hopefully be self-limited. In this latter instance, the goal is to decrease the rise in blood urea nitrogen (BUN) level, thus avoiding dialysis, which in turn may add to the mortality of an accompanying surgical condition. There are good data in the literature suggesting that essential amino acids are a useful treatment in acute renal failure. In the case of hepatic failure, a branched-chain amino acid–enriched, aromatic amino acid–deficient solution, given in an effort to avoid encephalopathy but to administer enough protein to these particularly hypercatabolic patients, is the approach that is also supported by much experimental and clinical data.

Renal Failure. The practice of administering essential amino acids and hypertonic dextrose in a restricted volume, usually in the surgical setting with superimposed acute tubular necrosis, is based on studies published independently in the early 1950s by Giordano and Giovannetti. This work attempted to decrease the frequency of dialysis in chronic renal failure patients. Substantial protein equivalents are lost during dialysis, but in the surgical setting, dialysis is usually thought to be necessary when the BUN approaches 90 or 100 (at which point coagulopathy and other azotemic complications may occur). In addition, encephalopathy may be seen, which may or may not be correlated with the rise in BUN in a given patient. Giordano and Giovannetti found that patients with chronic renal failure given high-biologic-value protein, such as egg albumin, with adequate calories, required less frequent dialysis. Whether this approach might also decrease damage to the few remaining functioning nephrons by decreasing their filtered load, a concept promoted by Brenner, currently lacks scientific support. According to the Giordano and Giovannetti hypothesis, urea was not an end product, as had been commonly supposed, but diffused into the gastrointestinal tract and was converted to ammonia by urease-producing bacteria. If one supplied essential amino acids with high-biologic-value protein and adequate calories, the hypothesis continued, the ammonia could be re-incorporated into nonessential amino acids. Accordingly, a full complement of amino acids would result, thus supporting protein synthesis and adequate nutrition. This hypothesis, however, ultimately proved incorrect. In retrospect, most of the effect of the essential amino acids on BUN appears to be the result of decreased urea generation resulting from their administration.

Although essential amino acids seemed helpful in the chronic setting, the question was, Would they work in the surgical patient with acute renal failure? A series of studies by Wilmore, Dudrick, Abel, Abbot, Fischer, and coworkers in the late 1960s and early 1970s demonstrated conclusively that when such patients were treated with essential amino acids and hypotonic dextrose, a number of beneficial effects could be demonstrated, as follows:

1. Hyperkalemia was improved.
2. Dialysis was averted in patients treated with essential amino acids and hypertonic dextrose, as opposed to hypertonic dextrose alone.
3. Survival was improved, especially in patients with some urine production.
4. There was a lower incidence of pneumonia, gastrointestinal bleeding and other complications, contributing to the improvement in survival.
5. There was a decreased incidence of encephalopathy.

In patients with major procedures, such as following repair of a ruptured abdominal aortic aneurysm in which the peritoneum has not sealed, essential amino acids and hypertonic dextrose may also be sufficient to tide the patient over until hemodialysis can be tolerated hemodynamically, or if desired, peritoneal dialysis initiated.

Other investigators, without satisfactory studies, have advocated increasing the complexity of amino acids from the essential eight (namely, the branched-chain amino acids isoleucine, leucine, and valine, the aromatic amino acids phenylalanine, tyrosine, and tryptophan, and the sulfur-containing amino acids methionine and cysteine), to include histidine and arginine, "semi-essential" amino acids for which rates of synthesis may be insufficient to support the patient during acute stress. However, by adding these additional amino acids, the ability of the solution to hold down the rise in BUN is diminished. Other practices, such as giving branched-chain amino acids in large amounts with standard solutions, have little support in the literature. Utilizing much reduced amounts of standard amino acid solutions, as advocated by some, resulted in considerably worsened survival than in patients treated with essential amino acids, in one study. Other studies failed to show any difference between patients given dilute standard solutions or essential amino acids, but the numbers of subjects were small.

One should be alert to the possibility of hyperammonemia in patients receiving only essential amino acids for a prolonged period, that is, heralded by mental status changes. In infants, an arginine deficiency may develop, or the enzymes for conversion of arginine to ornithine may be insufficiently mature. The amino acids histidine, isoleucine, and leucine, if abundant, may suppress arginosuccinate synthetase, which is necessary for the conversion of arginine to ornithine. Whatever the mechanism, when ornithine stores are depleted, it can no longer serve its role as a carrier amino acid in the urea cycle, and as a result, ammonia is no longer detoxified in the liver and hyperammonemia may ensue. Therefore, it is important that when essential amino acid solutions are administered, particularly over prolonged periods, sufficient quantities of ornithine should be included and serum ammonia levels monitored. Since this ordinarily does not happen, there is little reason to fear.

When used, the average duration of therapy with essential amino acids in hypertonic (35%) dextrose is usually 10 to 14 days. Once the patient is on dialysis, a more complete amino acid solution is appropriate. In the outpatient setting, protein intakes of 0.5 to 0.6 g/kg have been shown to slow the progression of chronic renal insufficiency. However, in renal failure patients with an acute superimposed illness or for those on hemodialysis, protein intakes of up to 1.2 g/kg are recommended, because most recent studies support improved patient outcome when adequate nutrition is administered, even if it requires more frequent or even daily hemodialysis to clear the accumulated urea.

Hepatic Insufficiency. These patients are protein intolerant as well, but here the result of excessive protein administration is potentially severe encephalopathy. In the surgical setting, most such patients manifest sudden hepatic insufficiency, such as that resulting from cirrhosis with acute decompensation secondary to gastrointestinal bleeding, from sepsis, from hepatic resection or transplantation, or from portal venous diversion with resulting encephalopathy. The situation is doubly difficult because these patients are hypercatabolic, with a protein requirement of 1.1 g/kg/day, approximately double the minimal 0.55 g/kg/day adequate for a patient with well-compensated cirrhosis. Although it is generally acknowledged that patients with hepatic failure receiving intravenous amino acid solutions tolerate these better than oral protein, most patients with significant liver disease do not tolerate 1.5 or even 1.1 g/kg of amino acids per day, when efforts are made to achieve nitrogen equilibrium. Many practitioners confronted with these patients believe that an aromatic amino acid–deficient, but branched-chain amino acid–enriched solution is efficacious, and it is not unusual with such an approach to achieve levels of up to 120 g of amino acids per day, for example, and be rewarded not only with adequate nutrition but also by the absence of hepatic encephalopathy.

The basis for using enriched branched-chain and deficient aromatic amino acid solutions is the so-called false neurotransmitter hypothesis, in which hepatic encephalopathy is not a nonspecific toxic phenomenon as heretofore had been thought but instead results from abnormalities in brain synaptic function. The basis for this phenomenon is an abnormal plasma amino acid profile, as demonstrated by James, Fischer, and coworkers in the 1970s. In patients with hepatic failure, decreased circulating levels of branched-chain amino acids and increased aromatic amino acids, including phenylalanine, tyrosine, methionine, and tryptophan, appear to result in abnormal amine neurotransmitter products, in which norepinephrine and dopamine are replaced by compounds such as octopamine and phenylethanolamine. These false neurotransmitters are postulated to be responsible for the disturbances in consciousness known as *hepatic encephalopathy*. Accordingly, if the deranged plasma amino acid pattern can be normalized, increasing the branched-chain amino acids and decreasing aromatic amino acids, the system L transport pathway of the blood-brain barrier will be presented with an improved amino acid pattern, with a more functional brain amino acid profile resulting. Glutamine also may play some role, as levels of glutamine in the brain reflect the availability of ammonia ion, and glutamine is used for exchange of ammonia across the blood-brain barrier. The "unified hypothesis" for hepatic encephalopathy proposes that the deranged levels of plasma amino acids, resulting from decreased hepatic function or anatomic shunting of blood flow, coupled with increased ammonia (glutamine) within the central nervous system, are synergistic in altering transport of amino acids across the blood-brain barrier.

Other workers have suggested the use of increased branched-chain amino acids alone in standard amino acid solutions, instead of the modified amino acid solution described earlier. However, there is no evidence to support efficacy. Addition of branched-chain amino acids to standard solutions also creates a solution containing excessive concentrations of many aromatic amino acids, which with the decreased albumin present in most of these patients, results in increased free plasma and brain tryptophan. Thus, the only formula for which there is adequate data is a hepatamine type of solution, consisting of 35% branched-chain amino acids and decreased aromatic amino acids. Numerous randomized, prospective trials clearly show that encephalopathy is well treated by such formulas. Although some trials, particularly one in which glucose was used as the primary calorie source, resulted in increased survival in the group receiving these special solutions when compared to neomycin alone, other trials have not. Furthermore, a large meta-analysis did not support increased overall survival as a beneficial effect of such practices, although encephalopathy was improved. This topic is further discussed in following sections (see "Controversies in Artificial Nutrition").

Plasma Electrolytes

Abnormalities in plasma electrolytes are minimized by careful monitoring. At least 50 mEq of sodium and 20 to 40 mEq of potassium should be administered daily to most patients receiving parenteral nutrition. The daily mainte-nance requirement for calcium is 0.2 to 0.3 mEq/kg/day, for magnesium 0.35 to 0.45 mEq/kg/day, and for phosphate 30 to 40 mmol/day. Patients who are rapidly anabolic, such as extremely cachectic patients during the initiation of TPN, may require additional potassium, magnesium, and phosphorus (the so-called phosphate steal or refeeding syndrome). One must also be careful to limit sodium and volume administration because these patients are sodium avid and can easily develop volume overload and congestive heart failure. Acid-base imbalance is prevented by adding acetate to TPN solutions when acidosis or hyperchloremia is present, or conversely, solutions are supplemented with potassium chloride when gastric or other gastrointestinal losses are significant. If potassium chloride is insufficient to prevent metabolic alkalosis, as in patients with gastric outlet obstruction, administration of dilute hydrochloric acid or arginine hydrochloride may also be necessary. In general, in the face of changing fluid and electrolyte requirements, it is usually possible to use the TPN solution to address such needs, unless instability is volatile. However, frequent changes in volume or electrolyte requirements are best dealt with by an alternative route of intravenous administration, minimizing wastage of TPN solutions.

Vitamins and Micronutrients

In the modern era, micronutrient deficiencies in parenteral nutrition are rarely seen but result from inadequate provision of essential fatty acids (see earlier), trace elements, or vitamins (Table 7-4). Such mineral deficiencies

TABLE 7-4. Suggested Dosage of Vitamins and Trace Metals During Severe Illness

Vitamins and Trace Metals	Suggested Daily Dosage
VITAMIN	
Water soluble	
Thiamine	25 mg
Riboflavin	25 mg
Niacin	200 mg
Pantothenic acid	50 mg
Pyridoxine	50 mg
Folic acid[*]	2.5 mg
B_{12}[†]	5 mg
Fat soluble	
A[†]	5000 µg
D[†]	400 µg
E[†]	100 µg
K[*]	10 mg
TRACE METAL	
Zinc	10–20 mg
Copper	0.5–2.0 mg
Chromium	20 µg
Selenium	70–150 µg
Manganese	2–2.5 mg
Iron	25 mg

[*]Inactivated (oxidized) by addition to hypertonic glucose amino acid solutions.
[†]Sufficient stores of these vitamins exist, so deficiency states are unlikely during short-term (2- to 4-week) parenteral nutrition. In practice, however, it is wise to provide them.

are avoided with modern additives, and available assays for deficiency are often unreliable and not too useful. Therefore, routine testing is not indicated. Some agents require portal passage for metabolic conversion or activation, which is potentially bypassed during parenteral infusion. Furthermore, in short bowel syndrome or following extensive ileal resection, substances that normally require the enterohepatic circulation for maximal absorption and utilization, such as zinc, copper, manganese, selenium, and many vitamins (cobalamin, folate, and the fat-soluble vitamins A, D, E, and K), are particularly vulnerable. Fat malabsorption, as induced by pancreatic insufficiency for example, can also lead to inadequate uptake of fat-soluble micronutrients.

Thiamine. Severe thiamine deficiency leads to the classic nutritional disease beri-beri, characterized by a refractory lactic acidosis that results from thiamine's role to facilitate entry of glucose into the TCA cycle. The clinical syndrome consists of disturbed mentation, diabetes insipidus, hyperbilirubinemia, thrombocytopenia, and lactic acidosis mimicking sepsis. The plasma amino acid pattern is distorted, with high levels of proline and hydroxyproline. Thiamine deficiency in patients receiving normal amounts of thiamine has occasionally been seen, usually in a depleted patient given a sudden carbohydrate load. Once this condition is recognized, thiamine deficiency is easily treated with 100 mg of thiamine per day. One of the authors (JEF) observed such a case when the U.S. Food and Drug Administration withheld the source of multivitamins for several months.

Biotin. Because biotin is ubiquitous, deficiency hardly ever occurs in patients taking anything by mouth, although biotin deficiency has been reported in patients entirely dependent on TPN.

Vitamin D. Deficiency of vitamin D is primarily an issue during long-term TPN administration or in the face of concurrent metabolic bone disease, such as severe osteoporosis (see "Complications of TPN Administration"). Most standard multivitamin solutions used routinely in TPN contain 200 units of vitamin D. When assayed, aberrations in vitamin D levels (25-OH-vitamin D in normal subjects or 1,25-OH-vitamin D in chronic renal failure) should be evaluated with knowledge of levels of parathyroid hormone measured concurrently. If vitamin D is to be repleted, oral administration is best (50,000 units per week for 6 to 8 weeks), because intravenous replacement can be dangerous, with vitamin D overload and osteomalacia likely.

Vitamin K. In patients who maintain some oral intake in addition to TPN, vitamin K deficiency is unlikely. However, for patients who are entirely dependent on TPN, supplementation weekly with 10 mg of intravenous vitamin K is necessary. In addition, if chronic warfarin (Coumadin) therapy is required, such as for a history of catheter-related superior vena caval syndrome, having a baseline amount of vitamin K in the TPN solution is probably helpful in "buffering" the inhibitory effect of warfarin on post-translation carboxylation of the coagulation proteins. In this way, large variations in the warfarin requirement can be avoided. Conversely, other practitioners avoid vitamin K entirely under such circumstances.

Zinc. Patients who are extremely catabolic or who have excessive diarrhea may develop zinc deficiency. Massive diarrhea and malabsorption may increase losses to as great as 10 mEq of zinc per liter of stool. Neither plasma zinc nor hair zinc is an accurate reflection of total-body stores, which may be markedly depleted even when blood levels appear normal. Three to 6 mg of elemental zinc per day is required in patients with normal stool losses and between 12 and 20 mg is required in patients with short bowel syndrome or excessive diarrhea. Zinc deficiency has numerous manifestations, including alopecia, poor wound healing, immunosuppression, night blindness or photophobia, impaired taste or smell (anosmia), neuritis, and a variety of skin disorders (generalized eruptions, a perioral pustular rash, darkening of the skin creases), and is similar to the syndrome of zinc deficiency seen in sheep (acrodermatitis enteropathica).

Copper. Copper deficiency has been observed in a few patients receiving long-term parenteral nutrition, manifesting as microcytic anemia, pancytopenia, depigmentation, and osteopenia. The microcytic anemia may be mistaken for pyridoxine deficiency. In standard mineral solutions used for TPN, up to 2 mg of copper per day is given as the sulfate.

Chromium. This deficiency is also likely to occur only in patients receiving long-term TPN with minimal or no oral intake. Chromium is necessary for the adequate utilization of glucose, and deficiency is often manifest as a sudden diabetic state in which blood sugar is difficult to control, along with peripheral neuropathy and encephalopathy. Fifteen to 20 μg per day of chromium is adequate to meet daily requirements. To treat chromium deficiency, 150 μg of chromium per day is given for several days.

Molybdenum. This metal is a cofactor for the enzymes superoxide dismutase and xanthine oxidase. The rare deficiency state is characterized by the toxic accumulation of sulfur-containing amino acids and encephalopathy.

Selenium. Selenium deficiency has not been clearly established and is clearly rare. Selenium deficiency may result in diffuse skeletal and cardiomyopathy (with abnormalities in basement and plasma membranes on muscle biopsy), loss of pigmentation, and erythrocyte macrocytosis.

Iron. Calcium, iron, and other metals are absorbed in the duodenum. Consequently, duodenal bypass (as after Billroth II gastrectomy) or resection (as after a Whipple procedure) often results in long-term deficiencies of these ions. Iron deficiency can be classified as early (no anemia, serum iron and ferritin decreased, transferrin increased), intermediate (no anemia, transferrin saturation <15%, ferritin <12 μg/L), or late (hypochromic microcytic anemia). The daily requirement for oral iron is 15 mg/day, of which 5% to 10% is absorbed. Therefore, the parenteral requirement is 1 to 2 mg/day. Although there are obligate iron losses from desquamation of skin and gut mucosa, overall there is limited ability to excrete parenteral iron when administered in excess, and a significant number of patients given iron routinely will develop iron overload. Patients most likely to manifest iron deficiency are premenopausal women (menstruation may increase iron loss by an additional 1 mg/day), patients receiving more than

50% of their total caloric needs from TPN, patients with chronic gastrointestinal bleeding (e.g., Crohn's disease in women), and patients on hemodialysis (especially with concurrent erythropoietin therapy). Iron replacement should be avoided in the face of a concurrent inflammatory state or with active infection, because in these conditions iron utilization is poor and such supplementation may have immunosuppressant activity or may promote bacterial growth. In addition, in short gut syndrome, some patients appear to carry out iron absorption in the intact duodenum and proximal jejunum "too" avidly and may be at risk for iron overload. Finally, concurrent inherited hemochromatosis must be recognized because 0.2% to 0.7% of the population are homozygotic and 8% to 14% are heterozygotes. Even heterozygotic subjects appear predisposed to atherosclerosis, the possible mechanism being iron excess and increased free radical generation. A full discussion of iron deficiency and strategies for iron repletion in TPN is found elsewhere.[42]

PRACTICAL APPROACH TO ARTIFICIAL NUTRITION

A major change in nutritional support over the past decade is the realization that the gut may be more efficacious, particularly in patients with burns or other trauma, than parenteral nutrition. This topic is explored more thoroughly later in this chapter (see "Controversies in Artificial Nutrition"), and was discussed briefly earlier as well (see "Fundamentals of Artificial Nutrition"). Historically, enteral nutrition has not been emphasized as much as parenteral nutrition, because it has been assumed that in many disease states the gut will not function to allow adequate nutrient absorption. In contrast, it is now clear that enteral feeding is often well tolerated even in severe illness, even though it may not provide total nutritional support in all cases. Nonetheless, use of the gut for partial nutritional support probably has significant benefit in areas of immunologic and hepatic function and should be encouraged. As little as 20% of overall nutrient calories administered to the gut may be sufficient to show benefit versus TPN alone in certain studies. Therefore, one should approach nutritional support with two goals in mind: (1) to use the gut if possible, and (2) if total nutritional supplementation cannot be provided by the gastrointestinal tract, to administer at least 20% of the caloric and protein requirements enterally while reaching goal support with TPN until the gastrointestinal tract returns to full functionality.

Principles of Enteral Feeding

The stomach is the principal defense against an enteral osmotic load. After bolus administration of hyperosmotic fluid, gastric motility is inhibited and gastric secretion proceeds until the gastric contents are isosmotic, at which point transfer across the pylorus begins. The small bowel is less able to dilute and tolerate large osmotic loads when they are administered directly. The small intestine is the principal area for nutrient absorption, with the products of protein digestion, such as dipeptides, oligopeptides,

and single amino acids completely absorbed in the first 120 cm of jejunum. With short or diseased bowel, dipeptides may have an absorptive advantage. Carbohydrate is also absorbed high in the jejunum, with simple sugars preferred. Complex sugars, such as disaccharides, require additional enzymatic cleavage. A common difficulty for patients who are ill is acquired lactase deficiency, which often corrects itself in time, although in the early recovery phase lactose-containing foods may cause diarrhea. Fat is most difficult to absorb because it depends on proper release and mixing of bile and pancreatic enzymes. After gastrectomy, pancreatic resection, or complex upper abdominal operations, such relationships are disturbed, and proper mixing of bile and pancreatic enzymes does not occur. Thus, fat absorption after gastrectomy is diminished after Billroth II, and less so after Billroth I, procedures. Aside from mechanical issues related to the feeding tube (see later), the most common complications of enteral feedings result from solute overload. Inappropriately rapid administration of hyperosmolar solutions may result in diarrhea, dehydration, electrolyte imbalance, and hyperglycemia, as well as loss of potassium, magnesium, and other ions through diarrhea. If aggressive administration of hyperosmolar solute continues, pneumatosis intestinalis with bowel necrosis, perforation, and potentially death will result. Hyperosmolar, nonketotic coma can also occur with enteral feedings as with parenteral nutrition.

Routes for Administration of Enteral Feeding

Patients with a functioning gastrointestinal tract who cannot achieve adequate nutritional intake orally and are malnourished or at risk for developing malnutrition are candidates for feeding tube placement. The choice of access route and device must be tailored to the individual, considering the disease process and how long nutritional support will likely be required.

Nasoenteric and Postpyloric Feeding

Nasoenteric feeding (gastric, duodenal, or jejunal) is the least expensive and most widely used modality of enteral nutrition. Most commonly, postsurgical patients have nasogastric tubes in place. These are reasonable tubes for the short term because they are typically large bored, do not clog easily, and allow for gastric residuals to be checked in assessing gastrointestinal tolerance. However, the traditional 16- or 18-French nasogastric tube (intended for gastric drainage) is uncomfortable and may promote relatively greater gastroesophageal reflux by holding the lower esophageal sphincter (LES) open more than a narrower tube. Such smaller-caliber feeding tubes (e.g., the Dobhoff tube, 8 to 10 French) are more comfortable and less erosive to the nasopharynx and esophagus but can clog when not carefully maintained and also collapse easily, making it difficult to follow gastric residuals. Although generally considered to be relatively innocuous, nasoenteric feeding tubes are associated with multiple adverse consequences including tube migration, esophageal and gastric mucosal erosions, pulmonary aspiration, sinusitis, pneumothorax, esophageal stricture, esophageal perforation, and fatal arrhythmias. In particular, feeding tubes with an indwelling removable metal stylet to aid their passage, although often used, appear particularly dangerous. In ventilated patients with indwelling endotracheal tubes, malposition in the bronchus with perforation into the pleural cavity seems to be associated most commonly with such styleted tubes. A more promising design, although not widely available, is the use of a rigid plastic "overtube" from which a narrower, soft feeding tube may be deployed after satisfactory gastric positioning. Many of these complications are avoidable with care. For example, aspiration may be minimized by positioning the patient head-up and by monitoring of gastric residuals, which should generally be less than 150 mL, although some authors have advocated a more aggressive approach, such as tolerance of residuals as great as 300 to 400 mL.

Many enteral feeding studies are handicapped by the high prevalence of gastrointestinal intolerance leading to inadequate protein and calorie administration. Such intolerance, in particular attributable to elevated gastric residual volumes, can affect up to 60% of patients. A variety of approaches have been tried to address poor gastric emptying in critically ill patients, including the use of promotility agents such as metoclopramide or erythromycin. Another strategy proposed as a means of bypassing the region of gastroduodenal ileus is postpyloric feeding. Nasoenteric feeding tubes can be placed with their tip positioned in the duodenum or jejunum, either under fluoroscopic guidance or by endoscopic manipulation and visualization. The hypothesis is that the jejunum may be more tolerant of continuous feeds and that by administering feeds beyond the ligament of Treitz, the risk of aspiration is lessened. However, when these putative advantages have been studied in prospective, randomized trials, there does not appear to be any difference when compared to intragastric feeding practices. In fact, when patients receiving radiolabeled feeds were studied,[43] regurgitation of postpylorically delivered feeds and the incidence of actual aspiration or of clinically definable pneumonia were no different than in patients fed gastrically. It seems reasonable to assume that in most instances, whether the tube tip terminates prepylorically or postpylorically, because all tubes are introduced nasally the LES is held open regardless, and this is probably the most important mechanism to allow aspiration.

As for feeding tolerance, there also does not appear to be any clear benefit attributable to postpyloric feeding. When aggressive advancement protocols are followed, nasogastrically fed patients, despite having higher gastric residual volumes, receive equivalent amounts of enteral nutrition to those fed nasojejunally. This finding has been confirmed in two separate prospective, randomized trials including 180 patients.[44,45] On the other hand, in postoperative trauma patients, Montecalvo and associates[46] showed that patients who received jejunal feeds did reach a significantly higher percentage of their daily caloric goal when compared to patients fed intragastrically. In conclusion, although the concept of postpyloric feeding remains controversial, it appears reasonable to obtain postpyloric access in patients with specific indications such as those suffering from significant gastroparesis or with severe pancreatitis (see later). Such access can easily be obtained at the time of surgery directed toward the primary disease process, when a well-carried-out feeding jejunostomy obviates most risks of aspiration and will anticipate a gastric ileus if sepsis ensues.

Gastrostomy

If long-term access to the stomach will be needed, a permanent gastrostomy can be placed. This goal can be achieved either by the open approach or by percutaneous techniques, the latter using endoscopic, radiologic, or laparoscopic methods. The Stamm gastrostomy is the most widely used open technique for gastric tube insertion, which requires a small laparotomy incision. Either inhalational, or in many cases awake intravenous sedation with local anesthesia, are acceptable anesthetic approaches for this procedure. In more recent years, the percutaneous endoscopic gastrostomy (PEG) technique has become the procedure of choice for many patients because it is generally considered less expensive and less morbid, although some studies indicate open gastrostomy and PEG carry equivalent perioperative risk. Necrosis of the gastric wall, attributable to excessive tension, is a recognized but avoidable complication of percutaneous gastrostomy. Percutaneous gastric tubes can also be placed by the interventional radiologist, which, although seemingly "less invasive" than other procedures for gastrostomy insertion and utilized with increasing frequency, actually appears to have a slightly higher incidence of complications and need for open revision than do surgical or endoscopic approaches. On the other hand, for moribund patients or patients requiring gastric drainage with no attractive operative approach (e.g., in the face of intestinal obstruction due to terminal carcinomatosis), the radiologic technique can be an ideal solution. An important factor limiting any percutaneous gastrostomy insertion is a history of prior upper abdominal surgery, with the potential for adhesions and structures such as the colon superimposed between the stomach and the abdominal wall. Perforation of the colon, which may go unrecognized for many days, is a well-described complication of all percutaneous techniques. Under such circumstances, a Stamm gastrostomy performed via a left upper quadrant incision can usually be carried out. Another drawback of gastrostomy tubes of all types is that they generally do not lie in a dependent position, so it is difficult to aspirate and follow gastric residual volumes.

Jejunostomy

Jejunal or small bowel feeding tube access can be obtained via open jejunostomy (either at the time of laparotomy or as a separate procedure), percutaneously via an extension through an existing gastrostomy tube (often termed a *G-J tube*), by a laparoscopic approach, or rarely as a percutaneous jejunostomy placed under fluoroscopic or CT guidance by the interventional radiologist.

This latter procedure has an undefined but presumably high frequency of complications and is of dubious value. True percutaneous jejunostomies (as opposed to G-J tubes), although often life-saving, are complicated more frequently than desired by dislodgment, occlusion, bowel obstruction, and small bowel ischemia. Furthermore, because the small bowel does not accommodate bolus feeding, feeds delivered to the jejunum must be delivered in a continuous fashion, carefully watching for signs of intolerance such as abdominal distention, abdominal pain or tenderness, diarrhea, or constipation. In the critically ill patient, usually hypo-osmolar, or at most iso-osmolar, solutions should be used. Hyper-osmolar solutions in critical illness are often not tolerated, because the bowel is stressed to begin with, and are much more likely to result in pneumatosis, necrosis, perforation, and death.

Management of Tube Tract Infections

A complication common to any percutaneous feeding tube is chronic infection or erosion of the tube tract as it traverses the abdominal wall. As indicated earlier, excessive traction, particularly in the case of a PEG, may induce frank gastric wall necrosis and free perforation of the stomach. More commonly, patients may experience chronic drainage, erythema, or excessive build-up of granulation tissue with intermittent bleeding. Factors contributing to such phenomena appear to involve excessive tube motion, the choice of catheter material (latex being less desirable than silicone), and chronic bacterial colonization. Simple hygiene and antibacterial ointment daily usually suffice.

Enteral Formulas and Approach to Feed Advancement

Mortality from enteral feeding is largely the result of aspiration, or as indicated earlier, occasionally from hyperosmolar feeding. Patients should be infused constantly, with the bolus technique reserved for special situations. To prevent reflux and aspiration, patients should be kept at a 30-degree angle. In general, there is no commonly agreed-on protocol for advancing enteral feeds. For gastric feeding, first osmolality and then volume are increased, usually beginning with solutions that are slightly hyposmolar. Most commonly, feeds are started at 10 to 20 mL/hour and gastric residual volumes followed every 4 to 6 hours. As long as gastric residual volumes remain less than 100 to 150 mL, feeds are advanced in 10- to 20-mL increments until the goal rate is attained. Unfortunately, this conservative protocol often results in unnecessary cessation of feeding, leading to slow or inadequate provision of nutrition. Several investigators have had better success when feeds are advanced more aggressively and when standardized protocols that outline rules for feed advancement and cessation are followed. Such practices, which tolerate gastric residual volumes as high as 250 to 300 mL and increase infusion rates in increments of 20 mL every 2 to 4 hours, have not resulted in increased complication rates or adverse outcomes. If administration is into the small bowel, volume is increased first, then osmo-

lality. Most patients do not tolerate small bowel administration of tube feeds containing greater than 300 to 400 mOsm, especially when critically ill. Dehydration is prevented by carefully increasing osmolality and using kaolin-pectin (Kaopectate) and opioids to slow diarrhea, as well as by the addition of free water.

Enteral Formulas

Many different enteral products are available, and almost all are hyper-osmolar (Table 7-5). Most formulas provide 1 kcal/mL, although some higher-calorie formulas (1.5 to 2 cal/mL) are also available, allowing smaller volumes of administration. These high-density formulas tend to have greater proportions of fat and relatively less protein (e.g., Nepro, a formula optimized for renal failure). For patients with normal gut function, an inexpensive tube feed analogous to a blenderized meal, such as a hydrolysate, is well tolerated. Some products have various degrees of complexity, ranging from oligopeptides to individual amino acids. The carbohydrate source varies from dextrose to complex starches, the latter solving a major problem in gut feeding—hyperosmolality. Modular diets are those in which the protein, fat, and carbohydrate components can be individually supplied. In patients with reasonably normal gut function, elemental diets (e.g., Vivonex) appear to have no advantage over hydrolysates. Elemental formulations may be more efficiently absorbed in patients suffering from short gut syndrome or in those with chronic diarrhea, although this idea is unproved. Finally, a recent development is the formulation of tube feeding solutions with potential immune-enhancing properties (e.g., Impact), which is discussed subsequently (see "Controversies in Artificial Nutrition").

Parenteral Feeding

When enteral feeding is poorly tolerated or impossible to deliver, parenteral nutrition administered safely is the only alternative (Box 7-1). If the parenteral route is chosen, concentrated TPN (>900 mOsm/L) delivered to a large central vein (termed *central TPN*), with the line tip in the superior vena cava, is the preferred method. The potential sources of calories (e.g., carbohydrate, lipid, and protein) have been discussed in detail earlier. In the absence of central access, a less concentrated formula (dextrose not to exceed 5%) may be delivered via a peripheral vein (termed *peripheral TPN*). This latter method is usually for a short term only (4 to 7 days) and provides less than optimal calories, although nitrogen loss may be retarded. If lipid is included (250 to 500 mL of 20% fat emulsion daily) and up to 3 L of dilute solution can be tolerated, peripheral TPN can satisfy the daily caloric requirement. However, the needs of sick patients are rarely satisfied by this approach, and no clinical trials have yet attributed any benefit to the routine use of peripheral intravenous alimentation. As discussed earlier, there is some experimental evidence to support the provision of (hypocaloric) amino acids and 5% dextrose or glycerol in an attempt to minimize nitrogen breakdown for limited

TABLE 7-5. Enteral Nutrition Products

Descriptor	Product							
	Criticare HN	Vivonex TEN	Peptamen VHP	Impact w/fiber	Impact	Respalor	Nepro	Promod (100 g)
Calories (kcal/mL)	1.06	1.00	1.0	1.00	1.00	1.52	2.00	424
Protein (g/L)	38 (14.4%)	38.2 (15%)	62.5 (25%)	56 (22%)	56 (22%)	75 (20%)	70 (14%)	76 (72%)
Carbohydrate (g/L)	220 (81%)	206 (82%)	104.5 (42%)	133 (53%)	130 (53%)	146 (40%)	215 (43%)	10 (10%)
Fat (g/L)	5.3 (4.5%)	2.8 (3%)	39 (33%)	28 (25%)	28 (25%)	68 (40%)	96 (43%)	9 (19%)
Fat as MCT (%)	0	0	70%	27%	27%	30%	0%	0
Osmolality (mOsm/L)	650	630	300 unflav/ 430 flav	375	375	400	665	—
Free water (ml/L)	850	853	840	868	853	770	699	—
Sodium (mEq/L)	27	20	24	48	48	55	37	10
Potassium (mEq/L)	34	20	38	33	36	38	27	25
Calcium (mg/L)	530	500	800	800	800	1000	1370	607
Phosphorus (mg/L)	530	500	700	800	800	1000	695	500
Magnesium (mg/L)	210	200	300	270	270	400	215	—
Vitamin K (mg/L)	131	22	50	67	67	84	85	—
Dietary fiber (g/L)	0	0	0	10	0	0	0	—
Vol for 100% DRI (mL)	1890	2000	1500	1500	1500	1000	947	NA
Comments	Elemental amino acids and peptides, ready to feed, gluten and lactose free	Elemental amino acids and peptides, oral or tube feeding, 4.9 g/L glutamine, requires mixing, gluten and lactose free	Semi-elemental high-protein oral or tube feeding, 4.6 g/L glutamine, gluten and lactose free	Immune-enhancing tube feeding for critical care, with fiber, high protein, fish oil, RNA, arginine, gluten and lactose free	See Impact no fiber.	For respiratory failure (low carbohydrate, volume restrict), oral or tube feeding, gluten and lactose free	For renal failure (low electrolyte, Mg, Pi, volume restricted), oral or tube feeding gluten and lactose free	Protein supplement, gluten free, low residue; 4.5 g/100 g lactose
Flavors	Unflavored	+ Flavor packets	+ Flavor packets	Unflavored	Unflavored	Vanilla	Vanilla, Pecan	NA
Cost per 1500 kcal	$13.50	$13.80	$23.50	$27.00	$25.50	$3.16	$4.90	—

Descriptor	Product						
	Boost	Boost Plus	Boost High Protein	Ultracal	Promote	Promote w/fiber	Probalance	Deliver 2.0
Calories (kcal/mL)	1.01	1.52	1.01	1.06	1.0	1.0	1.20	2.00
Protein (g/L)	43 (17%)	61 (16%)	61 (24%)	44 (17%)	62.5 (25%)	62.5 (25%)	54 (18%)	75 (15%)
Carbohydrate (g/L)	170 (67%)	190 (50%)	139 (55%)	123 (46%)	130 (52%)	138 (50%)	156 (52%)	200 (40%)
Fat (g/L)	18 (16%)	57 (34%)	23 (21%)	45 (37%)	26 (23%)	28 (25%)	40.8 (30%)	102 (45%)

TABLE 7-5. Cont'd

Descriptor	Product							
	Boost	Boost Plus	Boost High Protein	Ultracal	Promote	Promote w/fiber	Probalance	Deliver 2.0
Fat as MCT (%)	0	0	0	40	19	19	20	30
Osmolality (mOsm/L)	590	630–670	650	310	340	380	450	640
Free water (mL/L)	840	780	850	850	830	830	810	710
Sodium (mEq/L)	24	37	40	40	43	57	33	35
Potassium (mEq/L)	43	38	54	41	51	51	40	43
Calcium (mg/L)	1270	850	1010	850	1200	1200	1250	1010
Phosphorus (mg/L)	1060	850	930	850	1200	1200	1000	1010
Magnesium (mg/L)	420	340	380	340	400	400	400	400
Vitamin K (mg/L)	127	68	240	68	80	80	80	250
Dietary fiber (g/L)	0	<4	0	14	0	14	10	0
Vol for 100% DRI (mL)	1590	1180	1060	1250	1000	1000	1000	1000
Comments	Oral supplement only, gluten and lactose free	Oral, nutrient dense, may be used as tube feeding, gluten and lactose free	Standard high-protein oral or tube feeding, gluten and lactose free	Standard tube feeding with fiber, gluten and lactose free	Standard high-protein oral or tube feeding, lactose and gluten free, low residue	See Promote, with fiber	Higher calorie (1.2 cal/mL) oral or tube feeding with fiber, gluten and lactose free	Volume restricted oral or tube feeding, gluten and lactose free
Flavors	Vanilla, chocolate, strawberry	Vanilla, chocolate, strawberry	Vanilla, chocolate	Unflavored	Vanilla	Vanilla	Many	Vanilla
Cost per 1500 kcal	$1.20	$0.80	$1.20	$3.50	$3.40	$3.40	$2.60	$2.10

MCT, medium-chain triglyceride; DRI, daily recommended intake.

periods. However, in a European trial by Culebras and coworkers, a limited 14-hour infusion of amino acids and 5% dextrose after operations of modest severity did not show improved nitrogen balance.

Practical Approach to Calculation of the Ideal Parenteral Formula

Physicochemical Considerations

Today, most TPN solutions are administered as a total nutrient admixture (TNA or "3-in-1" solution), with lipid emulsions incorporated into the final solution, as opposed to the older method of a separate "piggyback" infusion of lipid. The TNA protocol is clinically advantageous because it (1) limits the number of central venous catheter violations and chance for contamination; (2) produces a hyperosmolar environment in the TNA solution that protects against bacterial growth; and (3) allows a continuous infusion, assuring lipid administration at a safe rate (<0.11 g/kg per hour). TPN is generally compounded in the pharmacy using concentrated stock solutions, which can in turn limit the range of individual solute concentrations achievable. These factors often lead to a requirement for greater volumes of solution to be delivered than initially might seem apparent. For example, common stock solutions of dextrose are 70%, amino acids 10% to 20%, and lipid 20%.

Box 7-1. Indications for Parenteral Nutrition

Primary Therapy

Efficacy shown*
  Gastrointestinal cutaneous fistulas
  Renal failure (acute tubular necrosis)
  Short bowel syndrome
  Acute burns
  Hepatic failure (acute decompensation superimposed on cirrhosis)
Efficacy not shown
  Crohn's disease
  Anorexia nervosa

Supportive Therapy

Efficacy shown*
  Acute radiation enteritis
  Acute chemotherapy toxicity
  Prolonged ileus
  Weight loss preliminary to major surgery
Efficacy not shown
  Before cardiac surgery
  Prolonged respiratory support
  Large wound losses

Areas Under Intensive Study

Patients with cancer
Patients with sepsis

*This indicates that randomized, prospective trials or similar investigations have suggested that such nutritional intervention results in changed (improved) outcome.

Therefore, for 1 L of solution in the absence of fat, the maximal achievable concentrations are 7% amino acids (70 g/L) and 21% dextrose (210 g/L). These amounts become even lower when fat is added to a 3-in-1 mixture. In addition, the pharmacist must take into account the physicochemical stability of the 3-in-1 solution with respect to the effect of mineral additives and of the relative proportions of caloric sources on the stability of the lipid emulsion and on overall solubility (Table 7-6).

Estimation of Energy Needs

In an earlier section (see "Nutritional Assessment" earlier), a variety of approaches were described to estimate energy needs, including indirect calorimetry, use of the ideal body weight, and calculation by standard methods such as the Harris-Benedict equation. The resting energy expenditure or basal metabolic rate (BMR) determined by the Harris-Benedict equation relies on the following formulas:

$$\text{Male BMR} = 66 + (13.7 \times \text{weight in kg}) + (5 \times \text{ht in cm}) - (6.8 \times \text{age in yr})$$

$$\text{Female BMR} = 65.5 + (9.6 \times \text{weight}) + (1.7 \times \text{ht in cm}) - (4.7 \times \text{age in yr})$$

The weight used for this calculation should be the subject's actual body weight. The value obtained for BMR must then be corrected for normal activity, such as ambulation and the work of breathing (+ 15%), and for stress. The added caloric expenditure, or relevant "stress factor" for an uncomplicated postoperative patient is 10%; for peritonitis, 10% to 30%; for sepsis, respiratory failure, or trauma, 30% to 50%; and in burns, caloric requirements may be 50% to 100% greater than normal. Additional stress factors include fever (hyperthermia), for which each 1°C increment of increased body temperature causes a 5% to 8% increase in BMR, and conditions of uncontrolled heat loss, pain, sleep deprivation, and anxiety (Fig. 7-5).

Caloric requirements for TPN administration can also be estimated using normative values, consisting of body weight and the accepted parameter of 25 to 35 kcal/kg/day for the rate of caloric infusion. This latter approach is safe and easy and is the most commonly used in clinical practice. However, as patients can be at, below, or above their IBW (as defined in "Nutritional Assessment" earlier), one must have a method of choosing an appropriate weight that will be used to calculate nutritional goals. This weight is called the "feeding weight" and is calculated by first determining the IBW, as found in standardized tables or estimated by the equations given earlier. Second, the IBW is compared to the actual body weight (ABW). In comparing the IBW and ABW:

■ If the patient is underweight, use the IBW as the feeding weight.
■ If the patient is obese (ABW is >120% of IBW), then add 25% of the difference between the ABW and IBW to the IBW as the feeding weight.
■ If no reliable weight is available, use the IBW alone.

Formulation of the TPN Solution

For the calculation of caloric content in TPN, glucose contains 3.4 kcal/g, protein 4 kcal/g, and fat 9 kcal/g. In general, minimal fluid requirements in the absence of gastrointestinal or other losses are 25 to 25 mL/kg/day. Using the example of a 70-kg person as the feeding weight, one first calculates the overall caloric goal and the proportion contributed by protein, usually

Total kilocalories (25–35 kcal/kg/day):
  $30 \times 70 = 2100\,\text{kcal}$

Protein (1.5 g/kg/day): $1.5 \times 70 = 105\,\text{g}$ amino acids

For TPN formulated without lipid ("2-in-1 solution"):

Total kilocalories = 2100 kcal

Calories from amino acids = $105\,\text{g} \times 4\,\text{kcal/g} = 420\,\text{kcal}$

Remaining calories = $2100 - 420 = 1680\,\text{kcal}$

Then make up the difference with dextrose:

$1680\,\text{kcal} \div 3.4\,\text{kcal/g} = 494\,\text{g}$ dextrose

For TPN formulated with lipid ("3-in-1 solution"):

Total kilocalories = 2100 kcal

TABLE 7-6. Allowable Additive Supplementation (at University of Cincinnati Hospital, Cincinnati, Ohio)*

Additives	Available Products (Injection)	Maximal Allowable Total per Liter
Calcium	Calcium gluconate Calcium chloride	9 mEq
Magnesium	Magnesium sulfate	12 mEq
Phosphate	Sodium phosphate Potassium phosphate	15 mmol
Potassium	Potassium chloride Potassium acetate	80 mEq
Sodium	Sodium chloride Sodium acetate	Patient tolerance and/or need
Chloride	Sodium chloride Calcium chloride Potassium chloride	Limited by amount of cation
Acetate	Sodium acetate Potassium acetate	Limited by amount of cation
Insulin	Regular insulin	100 units (in conjunction with fingerstick blood sugars)

*Some points to remember: (1) Bicarbonate salts must not be added to parenteral nutrition formulations because they create certain incompatibilities and are ineffective given in this manner; (2) Medicinal agents not mentioned must not be admixed or administered with parenteral nutrition formulations unless compatibility data are available; and (3) Phosphate supplementation must be ordered in terms of millimoles (mmol) of phosphate. Phosphate is available only as the sodium or potassium salt, and when the potassium salt is used for "added" phosphate, it must not exceed the maximum allowable concentration of potassium (i.e., 80 mEq).

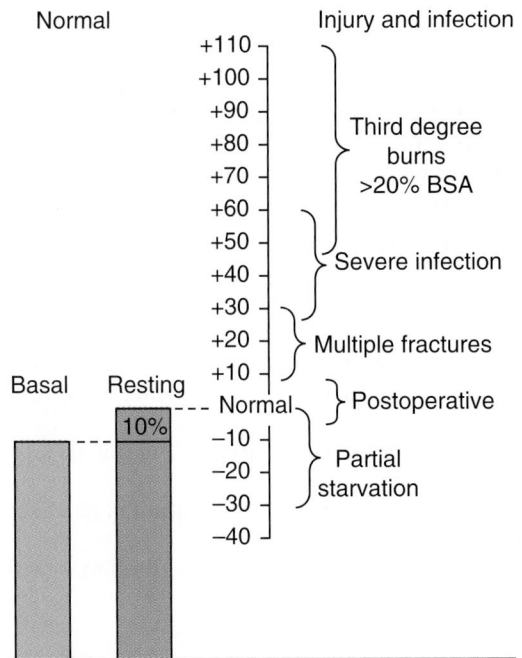

FIGURE 7-5. The increases in resting energy expenditure that have been shown to occur during the acute catabolic phase of injury or infection, when compared with the decreases that develop during partial starvation. BSA, body surface area. (From Kinney JM: The application of indirect calorimetry to clinical studies. *In* Kinney JM [ed]: Assessment of Energy Metabolism in Health and Disease. Columbus, OH, Ross Laboratories, 1980.)

Provide 20% of the total calories as

$$\text{Lipid} = 2100 \times 0.2 = 420 \, \text{kcal}$$

Then

$$420 \, \text{kcal} \div 9 \, \text{kcal/g} = 47 \, \text{g lipid}$$

••

Calories from amino acids = $105 \, \text{g} \times 4 \, \text{kcal/g} = 420 \, \text{kcal}$

Remaining calories = $2100 - 420 - 420 = 1260 \, \text{kcal}$

Then make up the difference with dextrose:

$$1260 \, \text{kcal} \div 3.4 \, \text{kcal/g} = 370 \, \text{g dextrose}$$

••

Final volume (for "3-in-1" maximally concentrated):

Amino acids (10% stock solution): 105 g = 1050 mL

Dextrose (70% stock solution): 370 g = 528 mL

Lipids (20% stock solution): 47 g = 235 mL

Total volume = 1813 mL/day

Final concentrations (wt/vol):

Amino acids 5.8%

Dextrose 20.4%

Lipid 2.6%

For critically ill patients who may have unusually high caloric requirements or who require fine adjustment of the glucose or amino acid content in the TPN solution, it is important to facilitate the clinician's writing of the "custom" TPN order as just described, if necessary. On the other hand, in the hospital setting, most providers have minimal experience managing TPN. For this reason, and to avoid the inefficiencies and waste caused by inappropriately formulated TPN, our institution has implemented a weight-based standard TPN ordering process (Fig. 7-6). Values of 25 kcal/kg/day for total kilocalories and of 1.5 g/kg/day for amino acids are assumed, and either a nonlipid 2-in-1 formula or a lipid-containing 3-in-1 formula (2% lipid, or 18% total calories from lipid) are provided, in 10-kg ranges for weight. The order form also provides a suggested schedule for caloric advancement (see later), and the entire process has now been computerized in a web/HTML-based format. For individuals who desire higher calories, the orders can and should be adjusted upward. In many institutions a very similar, but somewhat different approach to standardized TPN ordering is taken. A uniform, maximally concentrated solution is provided (e.g., for 2-in-1 formulas, 7% amino acids/21% dextrose, with caloric intake individualized by continuously varying the rate of infusion vs. the step-wise increments described earlier). This latter approach may best minimize wastage of solutions (Fig. 7-7).

Schedule for Advancement

The most important aspect of TPN administration is to ensure that it is delivered in a safe manner, one that prevents the development of hyperglycemia and metabolic derangements. At our institution, on the first day TPN is initiated as a "starter solution" providing 70 g of amino acids and 150 g of dextrose in 1000 mL. Tolerance of the infusion is carefully monitored by assessing blood glucose every 6 hours, daily electrolytes, and monitoring for signs of volume overload. If well tolerated, the solution is advanced to the "Day 2" formula comprised of 70 g of amino acids and 210 g of dextrose. On the third day, protein is advanced to goal levels, lipids are added if desired, and dextrose is advanced gradually toward goal amounts, by increments of 50 to 100 g per day. If blood sugars rise to levels higher than 150 mg/dL, the dextrose content of the TPN is not increased until glycemic control is secured. In those institutions that use a single standard solution, the initial infusion may start at 40 mL/hour and advance in 20 mL/hour daily increments until the desired level of caloric intake is reached.

Management of Insulin

All patients who are started on TPN must be provided a subcutaneous sliding scale regimen for regular insulin administration, or in some cases, an intravenous regular insulin infusion. The choice depends on the patient's baseline insulin requirement (e.g., concurrent diabetes mellitus) and the presence of factors leading to insulin resistance (steroids, stress), along with the available level of nursing care. In general, it is safe to add an initial 10 units of regular insulin to every bag of TPN because this dose is below the basal rate of insulin production by the pancreatic beta cells and some insulin will be lost due to unavoidable binding to the plastic components of the infusion equipment. The keys to maintaining blood sugars in the normal range lie in the following maneuvers:

1. Never increase the amount of dextrose in the TPN solution until blood sugars are well controlled (i.e., <150 mg/dL).
2. Determine the amount of sliding scale insulin administered over the previous 24 hours and add $1/2$ to $2/3$ of that amount to the new TPN solution for the ensuing 24 hours.
3. When advancing the dextrose content of the TPN solution, advance the insulin concentration proportionally. For example, if a TPN solution contains 200 g of dextrose and 10 units of insulin, and the dextrose will be advanced to 300 g, add 15 units of insulin to the solution. Be quick to convert to a constant insulin infusion if it is difficult to gain control using subcutaneous insulin, especially in the setting of critical illness.

The insulin added to the TPN solution should cover only the dextrose in the TPN. This insulin should not be used to treat elevated blood sugars due to additional sources of dextrose, such as that contributed by an enteral feeding formula administered concurrently. For instance, if the enteral feed was stopped for any reason, the patient would be at risk for developing hypoglycemia from the excessive insulin in the TPN solution.

Mandatory Monitoring During Intravenous Nutrition

It is important to monitor a variety of parameters in the patient receiving intravenous feeding, both to ensure tolerance and to potentially witness a beneficial response (e.g., appropriate weight gain). These include clinical observations and blood analyses, as follows:

Clinical—daily fluid balance, body weight, evidence of infection
Laboratory—baseline: electrolytes, BUN, creatinine, glucose, calcium, magnesium, Pi, liver function (bilirubin, alanine aminotransferase, aspartate aminotransferase, alkaline phosphatase), triglyceride, albumin, prothrombin time
　Every 6 to 12 hours: glucose, usually for initial 3 to 5 days or until stable
　Daily until stable: electrolytes, BUN, creatinine, glucose, calcium, magnesium, phosphate
　Weekly: liver function, triglyceride, albumin, prothrombin time

Catheter Issues in Parenteral Nutrition

Many different types of venous catheters are available for central infusion, and which is most appropriate for a given patient depends on many factors. In a later chapter (see Chapter 69), the subject of venous access devices is covered in depth, and for this reason we focus here on aspects particularly relevant to the TPN patient. The most important issue is patient safety. Therefore, the avoidance

1954-0711-0279

Beth Israel Deaconess Medical Center
Adult Central Parenteral Nutrition (TPN) Order

Orders must be faxed to Pharmacy daily by 1300   Fax #: 2-8950
PN order has a 24 hr automatic stop time

☐ **DAY 1–2 / STARTER TPN**
A standard parenteral nutrition formulation that can be used
initially while assessing glucose and volume tolerance

Amino acid	70 g
Dextrose	150 g
Total volume	1000 ml (providing 800 Kcal)

☐ **DAY 2 AND/OR THEREAFTER: INTERMEDIATE TPN**
An advanced TPN formulation for patients who have demonstrated glucose
tolerance to Day 1 TPN. If the patient demonstrates tolerance to this TPN, the
patient can be advanced to goal with a Central Standard formula or continued
with this formulation for up to 10 days without adverse clinical consequence.

Amino acid	70 g
Dextrose	210 g
Total volume	1000 ml (providing 1000 Kcal)

DAY 3 AND/OR THEREAFTER: CENTRAL STANDARD FORMULAS:
The Central Standard TPNs are weight-based parenteral nutrition formulas providing protein 1.5g/kg/day and 25 kcal/kg/d. Select either the **2-in-1** formula (amino acid/ dextrose) or the **3-in-1** "mixed fuel" formula (amino acid/ dextrose/ lipid) based on the calculated feeding weight. *(See reverse side for calculation. Round to nearest 10 kg.)* For patients with a calculated feeding weight greater than 80 kg or for obese patients (greater than 130% IBW) consult the Nutrition Support Team for patient-specific recommendations.

CENTRAL STANDARD 2-in-1 TPN

	Feeding Weight	TPN Volume	Amino Acid (g/d)	Dextrose (g/d)	Kcal/day
☐	40 kg	1000	60	223	1000
☐	50 kg	1250	75	279	1250
☐	60 kg	1500	90	335	1500
☐	70 kg	1750	105	390	1750
☐	80 kg (or greater)	2000	120	446	2000

CENTRAL STANDARD 3-in-1 TPN

	Feeding Weight	TPN Volume	Amino Acid (g/d)	Dextrose (g/d)	Fat (g/d)	Kcal/day
☐	40 kg	1000	60	170	20	1000
☐	50 kg	1250	75	213	25	1250
☐	60 kg	1500	90	255	30	1500
☐	70 kg	1750	105	298	35	1750
☐	80 kg (or greater)	2000	120	340	40	2000

NON-STANDARD TPN: **Nutrition Support consult recommended.** *See reverse side for general recommendations.*
For patients with liver and/or kidney failure, protein and volume restriction may be required.

☐ Volume _____ ml/d   Amino Acid _____ g/d   50% Branched-chain AA _____ g/d   Dextrose _____ g/d   Fat _____ g/d

ADDITIVE OPTIONS

Vitamin / Trace Element Additives:

Parenteral Multivitamins will be added daily

Trace Elements will be added daily unless specified:

☐ No

Vitamin K 10 mg will be added each Monday unless specified:

☐ No

☐ Standard electrolytes
Total amount below will be added per day.

Na	70 mEq
K	40 mEq
Ca	9 mEq
Mg	10 mEq
Cl	40 mEq
Ac	30 mEq
PO_4	30 mM

☐ Non-standard electrolytes
Designate amount to be added **per day.**

NaCl _____ mEq (60–150 mEq/day)
NaAc _____ mEq (as required)
$NaPO_4$ _____ mEq (30–60 mEq/day)
KCl _____ mEq (60–100 mEq/day)
KAc _____ mEq (as required)
KPO_4 _____ mEq (as required)
$MgSO_4$ _____ mEq (10–20 mEq/day)
CaGluc _____ mEq (10–20 mEq/day)

☐ Other Additives
See reverse side for general recommendations.

Heparin _____ units
(usual range: 3000-6000 units/day)

Rantidine _____ mg

Insulin _____ units
(Regular Human)

Zinc _____ mg

Other _____

RATE OPTION:
☐ Total volume of solution per 24 hours. Rate of continuous infusion determined by pharmacy-SEE TPN label.
☐ Cycle over _____ hrs. Start at: _ _ _ _
Decrease rate to _____ ml/h at: _ _ _ _ Stop at: _ _ _ _ Plug and flush line with _____ units heparin.

Date: _____ Physician Signature _____ MD   Beeper: _____
Time Posted: _____ by _____ RN

White - MEDICAL RECORDS   Yellow - PHARMACY

(FACE)

FIGURE 7-6. Order form for parenteral formulation used at the Beth Israel Deaconess Medical Center, Boston, MA.

UNIVERSITY OF CINCINNATI HOSPITAL

**PARENTERAL NUTRITION
ORDER FORM**
Dealine for orders at 9:30 A.M.

Date: _____   Time: _____

UMC-375, 8/92

STEP 1:   SELECT BASE FORMULA:
Total Nutrient Admixture (TNA) contains: Fat emulsion, Dextrose, and Amino acids.
Non-TNA contains: Dextrose and Amino acids.

Standard Formula:			**High Dextrose Formula:**		
	❑TNA ❑ NON-TNA			❑TNA ❑ NON-TNA	
Each liter contains:			Each liter contains:		
Non-protein Calorie: N	119	67	Non-protein Calorie: N	141	89
Total kcal/ml	1.1	0.71	Total kcal/ml	1.3	0.88
Dextrose (15%)	150 gm		Dextrose (20%)	200 gm	
Amino Acids (5%)	50 gm		Amino Acids (5%)	50 gm	
Fat Emulsion (4%)	40 gm (as TNA)		Fat Emulsion (4%)	40 gm (as TNA)	

MVI-12 (10 ml) and Trace elements-5 (3 ml) daily   MVI-12 (10 ml) and Trace elements-5 (3 ml) daily
Vit K   5 mg weekly   Vit K   5 mg weekly

Standard Electrolytes (mEq/L)   Standard Electrolytes (mEq/L)

Na	K	Ca	Mg	P(mM)	Cl	Acetate		Na	K	Ca	Mg	P(mM)	Cl	Acetate
30	18	4.5	5	10	37	55		30	18	4.5	5	10	37	55

STEP 2:   ORDER <u>TOTAL</u> ADDITIVES IF DIFFERENT FROM ABOVE:

Total Na _____ mEq/L   Other per Liter:
Total K _____ mEq/L   _____
Total Ca _____ mEq/L   _____
Total Mg _____ mEq/L   _____
Total Phos _____ mM/L   _____
Reg. Insulin _____ units/L   _____

MAXIMUM TOTAL CONC/LITER		**DAILY TRACE ELEMENTS**	
K+	80 mEq	Zn	3.0 mg
Ca	9.4 mEq	Cu	1.2 mg
Mg	12 mEq	Cr	12 mcg
Phos	15 mM	Mn	0.3 mg
Ac	80 mEq	Se	60 mcg

STEP 3:   SELECT INFUSION RATE:
       INFUSE AT _____ ml/hr or Cycle: _____ ml Total Volume

PHYSICIAN SIGNATURE _____   PAGER #: _____

White–CHART   Yellow–PHARMACY

FIGURE 7-7.   Order form for parenteral formulation used at the University of Cincinnati Medical Center, Cincinnati, OH. The variety of solutions minimizes the chance of error and enables one to handle almost any metabolic situation. The various possible contents of each solution are given.

of surgical complications related to catheter placement, avoidance of infection, and preventing late complications (e.g., thrombosis) are paramount.

Catheter Choice and Rationale

In choosing a catheter for TPN administration, the first consideration should be the anticipated duration of therapy. In the inpatient setting, the traditional percutaneous "central line," introduced via the subclavian or internal jugular vein and often containing multiple lumina (e.g., the so-called triple-lumen catheter), is most common. As the number of lumina increases, infection rates will rise proportionally, arguing in favor of single-lumen catheters when the device is intended solely for TPN administration. A more recent trend is to use peripherally inserted central catheters ("PICCs"), introduced via the basilic vein, both in the inpatient setting and also for longer-term outpatient therapy. When evaluated in controlled trials, PICC lines show similar rates of line sepsis to traditional central catheters but have an increased incidence of local complications such as leakage, thrombophlebitis, and malpositioning. At best, a PICC line in the outpatient setting has a lifetime of 4 to 6 weeks before malfunctioning or becoming infected. Therefore, for long-term TPN administration, a more permanent solution is needed. The devices available consist of either subcutaneously tunneled central catheters (Hickman, Broviac, Groshong) or self-contained implantable chambers that connect to the central venous system (Port-A-Cath). The catheter of these devices can be inserted into the vein percutaneously (e.g., the subclavian, internal jugular, or femoral) and then tunneled to the final skin exit site (or to connect to the Port-A-Cath chamber). Alternatively, access may be obtained by venous cut-down, for example the cephalic vein within the deltopectoral groove, the external or internal jugular vein, the saphenous vein, or a branch of the subclavian vein within the axilla.

The principal underlying tunneled catheters is that the subcutaneous tract forms a barrier to bacterial encroachment and colonization, thus discouraging a so-called tunnel or tract infection, although a competing mode of infection for these or any other catheters, with resultant bacteremia, is by an intraluminal route. Tunneled catheters are desirable when frequent access is required, or perhaps if a high incidence of infection is anticipated, because they are easily removed. However, these devices are disfiguring, and proper care of the exit site usually implies an inability to fully bathe or swim. Port-A-Caths are completely subcutaneous and thus obviate some of the limitations of the Hickman design (improved appearance, ability to immerse the body totally). However, when accessed, these devices require a special low-profile needle (Hubner needle) to be inserted percutaneously, which then passes through the self-sealing diaphragm of the device into the chamber. Particularly if accessed frequently, Port-A-Caths may have a higher rate of infection and overall rate of failure than tunneled catheters in the setting of TPN, as opposed to other common scenarios, such as when used for chemotherapy.

Catheter Sepsis

Catheter sepsis is potentially the most lethal complication in patients receiving TPN. This problem is directly related to catheter care and to the incidence of hyperglycemia attributable to TPN and can be reduced to an acceptable minimum of less than 1% per year by attention to detail, the avoidance of multiuse catheters, and careful metabolic management. Organisms causing line infections are generally 80% Staphylococcus (50:50 aureus vs. epidermidis), 15% yeast, and 5% gram-negative bacteria. Additional factors influencing the incidence of line sepsis include the presence of a percutaneous stoma, such as a colostomy or tracheostomy, pre-existent malnutrition with an increased susceptibility to infection, corticosteroid administration, recent broad-spectrum antibiotic

therapy, concurrent chemotherapy, or severe neutropenia (e.g., in acute leukemia). The absence of a protocol for inpatient line care is also important, because in the ideal circumstance of a hyperalimentation team and a rigid protocol, sepsis rates may be as low as 0.6%.

If a patient on TPN develops a fever or signs suggestive of bacteremia, the TPN bottle should be taken down. Blood cultures, both from the central catheter and peripherally, should be performed, and a thorough search should be made of other possible sources of fever, such as pneumonia, an intra-abdominal abscess, the urinary tract, or a wound infection. If the fever persists or blood cultures suggest an infected catheter, the catheter should be removed and the tip cultured quantitatively by rolling it on an agar plate. Such "tip cultures" are considered positive if more than 15 colonies of organisms appear. Whether a percutaneous central line is simply removed under these circumstances or exchanged over a wire depends on many factors, as does the decision to treat such an incident with antibiotics and for what duration. Fungemia constitutes the most serious type of line infection, with the entry site of Candida, the most common fungal pathogen, most probably the gastrointestinal tract. It is important to treat colonization with yeast (defined as two positive site cultures, e.g., urine and skin) in the critically ill patient aggressively, with either fluconazole or amphotericin, to avoid further complications such as line sepsis.

In the instance of a permanent catheter (Hickman, Port-A-Cath), these devices can often be salvaged in the setting of confirmed bacteremia with prolonged antibiotic therapy, usually of 2 weeks' duration. For patients on long-term TPN who may have limited access options remaining due to multiple previous lines, line salvage becomes even more attractive. For S. epidermidis or gram-negative cultures, antibiotic therapy is effective in 60% to 70% of patients. At times a fibrin sheath at the catheter tip may be a nidus, and dissolution with tissue plasminogen activator or urokinase may be useful. Line tract infections can be more difficult to eradicate. In general, if S. aureus or yeast is documented on blood culture, the line should simply be removed with subsequent intravenous antimicrobial therapy, because these organisms are too virulent and dangerous to treat in lesser fashion. Although beyond the scope of this chapter, additional approaches to the avoidance of line infection are the use of impregnated catheters (e.g., with silver or bonded antibiotics) or the so-called antibiotic lock. The latter consists of antibiotics in high concentration, such as rifampicin, instilled into the catheter at the time it is disconnected from the infusion, either as prophylaxis, or in some centers, as definitive therapy for line colonization.

Catheter Thrombosis and Other Complications

Catheter failure due to intraluminal thrombus or a fibrin tip sheath, leading to clogging and lack of function, is quite common. This problem can often be corrected by instillation of tissue plasminogen activator or urokinase and can be avoided by administering long-term prophylactic low-dose heparin (usually 6000 units/bag) or by use of low-dose warfarin (1 to 2 mg/day), as shown effective in randomized trials.[47] Thrombosis of the great veins (subclavian, superior vena cava) occurs much less frequently, although some series report an incidence as high as 5% to 10% of patients. Signs include upper arm or facial swelling and/or pain. When thrombosis of the great veins is suspected, the catheter should be removed, and, after confirmation of the diagnosis, thrombolytic therapy should be begun. Heparin should then be continued, followed by warfarin therapy for 6 months or indefinitely. Other catheter complications include pneumothorax, vascular injuries (arterial or venous lacerations, delayed arteriovenous fistulas), brachial plexus injury, chronic pain, thoracic duct injury after left-sided cannulation, air embolism, and catheter embolism. Erosion of the catheter may occur into the bronchus, right atrium, or other structures. Septic venous thrombosis is a life-threatening complication, and if antibiotics and anticoagulation are not successful, excision of the involved vein or Fogarty catheter embolectomy may occasionally be successful. Hydrothorax results from catheter malposition and fluid administration into the thoracic cavity. This is particularly common with the more rigid percutaneous triple-lumen temporary central venous catheters, especially when introduced via the left subclavian vein. Such catheters should be 20 cm long, versus the 16-cm catheter manufactured for placement in the right chest or neck. If the catheter is too short, thus allowing the line tip to terminate or rub against the wall of the superior vena cava, erosion of the catheter tip into the left pleural cavity can result. Additional information concerning techniques for central venous catheter insertion is presented in Chapter 69.

Home Parenteral Nutrition

A major contribution of parenteral nutrition has been the ability to maintain patients in a functional state for decades with minimal oral intake. Unlike the continuous infusion approach appropriate for a hospitalized patient, home parenteral alimentation is generally "cycled" and performed overnight over an 8- to 14-hour period.

Common Indications for Long-Term Parenteral Nutrition

The most appropriate patients receiving home parenteral nutrition suffer from short gut syndrome, having lost a large portion of the gastrointestinal tract either by repeated resections for Crohn's disease or by massive small bowel resection after midgut volvulus and/or mesenteric thrombosis. Additional indications may include gastrointestinal motility disorders (chronic pseudo-obstruction, sprue, scleroderma), management of a high-output enterocutaneous fistula, intractable chylous ascites, active Crohn's disease, cystic fibrosis, and chronic pancreatitis. Although home TPN for patients with cancer seems rarely indicated (see "Controversies in Artificial Nutrition"), Medicare data indicate an increasing proportion of patients receiving home TPN carry this diagnosis (18% in 1984, 39% in 1988). The best candidates appear to be those with either (1) a curable malignancy requiring aggressive treatment resulting in anorexia, ileus, or intolerance to gastrointestinal feeds or (2) a cured patient with residual bowel dysfunction secondary to radiation enteritis or short gut syndrome. For these patients, survival rates and TPN-related complications appear similar to non-cancer TPN patients. On the other hand, if an incurable cancer is present or the overall prognosis is poor, only 15% of patients placed on TPN will survive 1 year. Human immunodeficiency virus (HIV) infection is rarely an indication for TPN, usually in the presence of intractable diarrhea or treatment-related pancreatitis. However, although a prospective, randomized trial showed improvements in nutritional global assessment, subjective health feelings, and Karnofsky performance index in HIV patients receiving TPN for 2 months, there was no difference in survival.[48]

Economic Aspects and Outcome Measures in Home Parenteral Nutrition

A variety of statistical sources, including the OASIS (Oley-ASPEN Information System) database, Medicare, and the Mayo Clinic, suggest that the primary disease process of patients on home TPN, rather than complications of TPN administration alone, has the strongest influence on survival and rehabilitation. Most are deaths related to the primary disease, with only 8% TPN-related (e.g., superior vena cava thrombosis, sepsis, or liver failure). For the most favorable candidates, there is an average rehospitalization rate of 1 per patient per year, of which 50% are for sepsis, and at least 1 in 6 patients will eventually discontinue TPN. Advanced age alone does not appear to be a reason to deny TPN. Overall, the predicted quality of survival at home for several months, rather than a specific diagnosis, seems the best justification for prolonged TPN. In view of the profound impact of such therapies on lifestyle, quality of life measures are reduced in patients on chronic TPN and are comparable to those reported for patients with chronic renal failure treated by dialysis.[49] Home hyperalimentation is a costly proposition. Depending on the area of the United States and the technique used, such costs may run from $30,000 to $60,000 per year for home therapy, with an annual cost of hospitalization of up to $140,000. Clearly, patient function, rehabilitation, quality of life, and other considerations enter the cost-to-benefit ratio. Patients on home TPN and without concurrent or chronic illness are usually extremely well motivated, and many work and/or have returned to their premorbid situation.

Metabolic Complications of Long-Term Parenteral Nutrition Administration

A variety of problems can arise when TPN is administered over prolonged periods, particularly in patients who have little if any oral intake and are therefore completely dependent on the solution for the provision of essential vitamins, minerals, and fatty acids. The rare deficiency states involving these nutrients, and mechanical and infectious disease considerations relevant to the TPN catheter and common in the outpatient population, have been discussed earlier.

Liver Disease

Hepatic dysfunction is commonly observed in patients receiving TPN, and these disorders occupy a spectrum ranging from simple LFT elevations to cirrhosis. Most often, if hyperbilirubinemia occurs acutely in a patient receiving TPN, the cause is generally sepsis. The factors responsible for liver disease attributable primarily to TPN administration, as opposed to other causes, remain unclear and are a source of controversy. Hepatic steatosis, cholestasis (presumably due to a lack of enteral stimulation and reduced cholecystokinin release), and the presence of chronic inflammation all have been implicated as relevant mechanisms. Predisposing factors include short gut syndrome (ileal disease or resection), a history of bacterial overgrowth, and recurrent sepsis or a chronic inflammatory state. For example, in a study of patients with severe short gut syndrome requiring duodenocolostomy, the risk of TPN-induced liver disease appeared higher than if some jejunum or ileum remained.[50] However, short bowel syndrome alone seemed an insufficient risk factor unless combined with a chronic inflammatory state, such as Crohn's disease. TPN-specific factors include excessive glucose or insulin administration (with increased hepatic lipogenesis), excessive lipid administration (sequestration in hepatocytes), and alterations in fatty acid metabolism leading to the release of arachidonate-derived inflammatory leukotrienes.[51] In home TPN patients, a recent study at our institution has also suggested that levels of inflammatory mediators such as TNF and C-reactive protein are chronically elevated when compared to normal subjects.[52] Nussbaum and coworkers proposed an altered insulin-to-glucagon ratio in chronic TPN patients and were able to ameliorate hepatic steatosis in rats maintained on TPN by administering glucagon. Deficiencies in particular nutrients, such as carnitine, choline, taurine, cysteine, and S-adenosyl methionine, have also been implicated in TPN-related liver disease. However, although the studies of Buchman (see "Fundamentals of Artificial Nutrition" earlier) have shown that hepatic steatosis can be improved by supplementation of TPN solutions with carnitine or choline,[34] these workers have not shown histologic or other evidence for reversal of TPN-induced liver damage.

In infants dependent on TPN, hepatic dysfunction is a more serious and potentially lethal disease, and it may have a different pathophysiology than that seen in adults. It is frequently associated with cholestasis. Even when enteral feeding is begun and TPN is discontinued, hepatic dysfunction may persist and may progress to cirrhosis and death. Whether translocation of gut bacteria or their products across the immature gut, immaturity of other enzyme systems, or other factors may play a role is not clear. The ultimate solution to TPN-induced liver failure, if other maneuvers are unsuccessful (e.g., reduced caloric intake, avoidance of inflammation, carnitine supplementation), is combined liver and small bowel transplantation, an extreme intervention with disappointing outcomes at present. Our group is currently testing whether dietary supplementation with omega-3 fatty acids may be effective in improving the deleterious pattern of inflammatory mediators, and potentially liver dysfunction, recognized in patients on long-term TPN (also see "Fundamentals of Artificial Nutrition" earlier).

Metabolic Bone Disease

In various studies, from 40% to nearly 100% of patients administered TPN over prolonged periods have decreased bone mineral density (BMD) or histologic evidence of bone disease. Some individuals can be shown to have increased urinary calcium or phosphate excretion, decreased parathyroid hormone levels, or vitamin D deficiency as possible mechanisms, but even in these patients there is a poor correlation with BMD.[53] Patients at greatest risk are postmenopausal women, patients with longstanding malnutrition or malabsorption (e.g., Crohn's disease), those with preexisting liver disease, or patients receiving steroids. Some TPN-specific mechanisms postulated to contribute to bone loss are TPN-induced hypercalciuria, in which fixed acids generated by metabolism are buffered by bone calcium carbonate, and calcium diuresis induced by hyperglycemia or excessive sodium. TPN-associated deficiency states, such as calcium or magnesium (magnesium deficiency may decrease parathyroid hormone release and vitamin D formation), copper (a cofactor for lysyl oxidase and collagen synthesis), boron, or silicon have also been suggested to play a role. Given that reduced BMD is so common in long-term TPN patients, routine evaluation is probably unnecessary. However, in the patient population at greatest risk, annual assessment of BMD by neutron activation, possibly with measurement of urinary N-telopeptides (a marker of bone resorption), is a valid approach. If BMD is markedly decreased (e.g., >2 SD from average), a search for easily corrected problems (vitamin D deficiency, parathyroid hormone excess or deficiency) is carried out. A relatively new, but unproven, intervention in such patients is the use of bisphosphonates, synthetic nonbiodegradable analogues of pyrophosphate that decrease osteoclast-mediated bone resorption. Pamidronate, a second-generation agent shown effective in randomized trials in inhibiting postmenopausal osteoporosis, can be administered intravenously to TPN patients in the outpatient setting (30 mg/200 mL 5% dextrose in water over 2 hours) every 3 months, with minimal toxicity.

ARTIFICIAL NUTRITION IN SPECIFIC DISEASE STATES

Pediatrics

Requirements for pediatric patients differ from those for adults. Growth is more rapid, and the distribution of visceral versus lean body mass is considerably different in an infant, which has little muscle compared to an adult.

Enzyme systems are incompletely developed, and excessive administration of certain amino acids may result in abnormally high concentrations of potentially toxic amino acids in the brain and perhaps in other viscera. The requirement for protein is far in excess of that for adults and decreases progressively with age. Energy requirements are also greater than for adults but may be decreased by providing a thermoneutral environment. The amount of lipid that can safely be administered is approximately 4 g/kg in the infant, whereas the upper limit of normal in the adult is thought to be 2 g/kg. Whether this difference results from proportionally larger amounts of viscera in the neonate, the caloric requirements of which are largely met by fat, is unclear. Vitamins and trace metals must be carefully administered because the ability to store these substances is limited and the opportunity for toxicity is greater. Venous access is a problem; the use of the umbilical artery or vein is mentioned only to be condemned, because catheter sepsis at this site is a disaster. In certain catastrophes, such as meconium ileus, gastroschisis, and neonatal enterocolitis, the increased survival now seen is almost certainly the result of aggressive nutritional support as well as improved perioperative care. However, the contribution of nutritional support to the survival of low-birth-weight babies, although suggestive, remains unproven. Requirements for nutritional support in infants are given in Table 7-7.

Pancreatitis

Severe pancreatitis has traditionally been treated with bowel rest and intravenous feeding, on the assumption that gut-derived hormones released with enteral feeding (secretin, cholecystokinin) would have the deleterious effect of stimulating pancreatic secretion, thus worsening pancreatic inflammation. In addition, there is an unfounded belief that lipid-containing TPN may aggravate pancreatitis in some way, whereas a 2-in-1 solution will not. Aside from avoiding severe hypertriglyceridemia, a known precipitant of pancreatitis, there is no evidence to support a negative effect of intravenous lipid on the course of this disease. Furthermore, pancreatitis is often accompanied by glucose intolerance, particularly when sepsis is concurrent, and in this regard the substitution of fat for dextrose in the TPN can be useful. McClave and coworkers[54] have championed the use of early postpyloric enteral feeding in acute pancreatitis. These workers have provided evidence that decreasing degrees of stimulation of the pancreas occur as the site of feeding descends in the gastrointestinal tract, and results of randomized trials in acute pancreatitis suggest that jejunal feeding is at least as safe and well tolerated as TPN. Whether early gut feeding in this setting is beneficial in any other way, for example by decreasing the incidence of nosocomial infections (see later), is unproven. However, one of the authors (JEF), in two separate studies in two different institutions, both with rigorous catheter care protocols, found an increased incidence of catheter infection in patients with pancreatitis.

TABLE 7-7. Nutritional Requirements in Infants

Protein (g/kg/day)	
Newborn to 6 mo	2.5–3
6–12 mo	2.0–2.5
School age	1.75
Adolescent	1.2
kcal/nitrogen	150:1
Calories (kcal/kg/day)	
Newborn or premature infant	120
Infant ≤10 kg	100
Infant 10–20 kg	100 + 50
Infant >20 kg	100 + 50 + 20
Fat	? 35% of calories (≤3.5 g/kg/day)
Electrolytes (mEq/kg/day)	
Na^+	24
K^+	1–2
Urine Na^+:K^+	>1.0 adequate
Trace elements (per day)	
Term infants	
Ca^{2+}	500–600 mg/L
Mg^{2+}	50–70 mg/L
P	400–450 mg/L
Zn	800 µg/L
Cu	100 µg/L
Children >1 year	
Ca^{2+}	200–400 mg/L
Mg^{2+}	20–40 mg/L
P	150–300 mg/L
Vitamins (per day)	
A	2000 IU
C	80 mg
D	400 IU
B_1	1.2 mg
B_2	1.4 mg
B_6	1.0 mg
E	7 IU
Niacin	17 mg
Dexpanthenol	5 mg
Folic acid	40 µg
B_{12}	50 µg
K	200 µg

CONTROVERSIES IN ARTIFICIAL NUTRITION

Advantages of Enteral Compared with Parenteral Feeding

It is increasingly accepted that enteral feeding is associated with improved clinical outcomes when compared to parenteral feeding alone, and furthermore, that early enteral feeding (i.e., following surgery or traumatic injury) is more efficacious than when such feeding is delayed. In addition, enteral feeding solutions for critically ill patients are now commonly formulated with "conditional" nutrients thought to have special properties for enhancing immune function, reducing inflammation, and improving nitrogen balance. However, this area of inquiry is confused by a lack of clarity in proposed mechanisms and by potentially overlapping or unrelated explanations for the benefit of a given intervention. For example, in studies proposing a benefit to arginine supplementation (see later), does this agent improve immune function directly, or does it promote anabolism by enhancing growth hormone or insulin release, with a nonspecific secondary improvement in immune and other physiologic functions? Furthermore, when "immune function" appears improved by a nutritional intervention (the most common claim), does this mean a specific molecular effect was documented, or as in most studies, was simply the overall incidence of infection or another clinical parameter such as length of stay in the ICU studied? Finally, if infection is lessened by enteral feeding, is this because of some laudatory effect on the permeability of the intestine to bacteria, or are the relevant mechanisms more poorly defined?

Translocation Hypothesis and Role of Gut Mucosa

Translocation is a process by which live bacteria or their byproducts (e.g., lipopolysaccharide) gain access to the lymphatic system or portal circulation by passing across the intestinal mucosa. This phenomenon is now fairly well accepted to occur in animal studies following burns and perhaps in hemorrhagic shock but not in other catabolic states such as starvation alone. Whereas the translocated bacteria are normally cleared by the lymph nodes, bacterial products persisting in the portal or systemic circulation under pathologic conditions are postulated to contribute to hepatic dysfunction, nosocomial infection, and multiple organ system failure.[55] One problem with the translocation hypothesis as a whole is that any beneficial result of enteral feeding or of dietary supplementation with particular nutrients (e.g., glutamine) is automatically attributed to an improvement in gut mucosal integrity, often with little or no evidence. Conversely, increased substrate supply to the liver and improved hepatic acute phase protein synthesis may be another mechanism by which outcome is improved by enteral feeding. Alexander and coworkers[56] provided initial evidence that gut feeding early in burn injury in guinea pigs and subsequently in human patients could ameliorate the usual catabolic response. The working hypothesis was that gut feeding prevented bacterial translocation, with a resultant decrease in the release of catecholamines and other negative stimuli, and thus prevented catabolism. In trauma patients, several prospective and randomized studies suggest that early gut feeding lowers mortality and septic complications (see later).[57] Kudsk and colleagues,[58] in a series of studies in traumatized patients, concluded that early jejunal feeding results in a lower rate of sepsis than in patients receiving parenteral nutrition, but their results remain controversial due to differences in nutrient administration and glycemic control (see later). These authors promoted the concept of total mucosal immunity, that is, improved barrier function of gut, respiratory, and nasal mucosa, and provided some evidence that this is mediated through immunoglobulin A.

Although it is likely true that in patients close to death, or in those with defined ischemic colitis, a breakdown of gut mucosal integrity leading to bacteremia can occur, clinically significant loss of gut mucosal integrity has been demonstrated only in patients with burns, trauma, and perhaps hemorrhagic shock. In addition, although bacterial translocation probably does occur in humans, there is little evidence that it is either reduced by the use of enteral nutrition or increased in patients given parenteral nutrition (as suggested by some). In addition, in humans supported with parenteral nutrition, remaining without enteral feeding has no substantial effect on mucosal architecture or permeability,[59] whereas chronic starvation and malnutrition do. Furthermore, when illness results in increased intestinal permeability, there remains no clear association between changes in permeability and actual bacterial translocation.[60]

Benefit of Early Enteral Feeding Versus Parenteral Nutrition

It is often said that enteral nutrition is safer and more efficacious than the parenteral route. However, a preliminary note of caution is raised from observations in experimental animals, which concluded that outcomes of enteral and parenteral nutrition were equivalent when animals with catheter sepsis were eliminated. Numerous studies have shown that it is safe to feed the gut in the immediate postoperative period and that this practice does not place the integrity of intestinal anastomoses at risk. Early feeding has been studied primarily in two patient populations: those who have undergone gastrointestinal surgery and in traumatically injured or critically ill persons. A recent meta-analysis reviewed 11 prospective, randomized, controlled trials that compared the practice of early enteral feeding to maintaining patients NPO after elective gastrointestinal surgery.[61] This analysis of 837 patients concluded that there is no clear advantage to keeping patients NPO postoperatively and that early feeding may be of benefit in decreasing infections and shortening postoperative length of stay. However, a closer evaluation of this data reveals that the length of stay was reduced only by 0.84 day, and although there was an increase in "any type of infection" in the NPO group, when considered individually, there was no difference in the incidence of anastomotic dehiscence, wound infections, pneumonia, intra-abdominal abscess, or mortality. In 2001 Marik and Zaloga performed a meta-analysis of 15 randomized, controlled trials involving 753 subjects that compared early with delayed enteral nutrition in critically ill surgical patients.[62] Early enteral nutrition was associated with a significantly lower incidence of infection (relative risk reduction of 0.45) and reduced length of hospital stay (2.2 days less). There were no differences in noninfectious complications or in mortality. The authors concluded that early initiation of enteral feeding was beneficial, but this result must be interpreted with caution because of substantial heterogeneity between studies.

The studies that compared enteral and parenteral nutrition in the trauma population,[57,58] as discussed earlier, concluded that enteral nutrition was superior because of an attenuated inflammatory response and a decrease in septic morbidity. When these studies are examined more closely, it is clear that patients who were fed enterally usually received significantly less calories than those fed parenterally. This discrepancy of "relative overfeeding" in the TPN groups in many instances led to hyperglycemia, presumably predisposing patients to immune dysfunction and nosocomial infection. Thus, poor glucose control alone may account for the observed differences in outcome. In more contemporary studies where feeds are carefully advanced in a manner that avoids hyperglycemia and groups are fed equivalent protein and calories, there appears to be little difference in clinical outcome between enteral and parenteral routes of feeding.[63] Enteral nutrition also can endanger patient safety in unique ways. Deaths in persons receiving enteral nutrition are often due to aspiration, for example when gastric motility suddenly is impaired with the onset of sepsis. One death from aspiration is equivalent to the mortality over 2 to 3 years of a well-operated parenteral nutrition program, despite the danger of catheter sepsis, which in well-operated units is now less than 1% to 3%.

In conclusion, when possible the gut should be used preferentially for the following reasons:

1. Enteral feeding is much less expensive, costing as little as $25 to $50 per day, compared with up to $200 per day for parenteral nutrition.
2. It likely improves hepatic function and mimics the normal ingress of nutrients to the liver.
3. Gut mucosal integrity is probably maintained, particularly in patients with burns and hemorrhagic shock.
4. Enteral nutrition may have beneficial effects on nonintestinal mucosa, possibly mediated by IgA secretion by the liver.

It seems fair to say that when delivered appropriately, both forms of nutritional support can be expected to improve organ function, immune competence, and wound healing equally in appropriately selected patients. The two forms of nutrition should be considered complementary, feeding both enterally and parenterally to ensure the adequate delivery of protein and calories, with a goal of progressively converting to full enteral feeds when safely tolerated by the patient.

Modulation of the Immune Response by Diet, or "Immunonutrition"

Major injury, whether traumatic or surgery induced, results in significant suppression of immune function, which may influence patient recovery. Specific nutrients, such as arginine and nucleotides (discussed later) and omega-3 fatty acids (see "Fundamentals of Artificial Nutrition") have been shown to modulate the host response in experimental animals, with potential improvements in immune function. The working hypothesis is that clinical use of a solution containing increased amounts of arginine stimulates T lymphocytes and provides a substrate for nitric oxide generation, whereas including omega-3 fatty acids promotes the synthesis of more favorable prostaglandins, and inclusion of RNA nonspecifically enhances immune competence. A variety of clinical trials have evaluated the efficacy of enteral formulas supplemented with such "immune-modulating" substances.

In 1992 Daly and coworkers[64,65] were the first to study the clinical effects of immune-enhancing diets, by prospectively randomizing 85 patients undergoing surgery for upper gastrointestinal malignancies to either a standard (Osmolite) or experimental (Impact) enteral formula. Postoperative nutrition was delivered via a jejunostomy tube, starting on day 1 and continuing until the 7th postoperative day. Patients administered the immune-modulating diet experienced a significant improvement in both postoperative wound healing and infectious complications, along with a shorter length of hospital stay. A potential flaw in this study is that although patients were fed isocalorically, the diets were not isonitrogenous (15.6 vs. 9.0 g of nitrogen per day), leaving it possible that the findings may be partially explained by greater protein administration in the subjects given Impact. A prospective, randomized, double-blinded, multicenter study was conducted by Bower and associates[66] in 1995 of 296 critically ill ICU patients. Subjects stratified as having either sepsis or the systemic inflammatory response syndrome were administered enteral feeding within 48 hours of the precipitating study entry event (trauma, operation, new onset of infection), consisting of Impact or a control diet (Osmolite HN). Feeding formulas were not equivalent, because the patients given Impact received more nitrogen and fewer calories. There were no statistically significant differences noted overall. However, patients stratified as septic and receiving the immune-modulating formula experienced a significant reduction in hospital length of stay (by 10 days) and a reduction in acquired infections. On subgroup analysis, the patients who received a minimum of 821 mL/day for at least 7 days experienced the greatest decrease in hospital stay.

Braga and colleagues[67] in 1999 showed fairly convincingly that the administration of an immune-enhancing diet perioperatively yields significant clinical benefit. These workers randomized 206 candidates undergoing elective surgery for malignancies of the colon, rectum, stomach, or pancreas to receive either an immune-enhancing formula (Impact) or a control formula that was isonitrogenous and isocaloric. Patients were administered 1 L/day for 7 days preoperatively followed by jejunal infusions of the same formula postoperatively, starting 6 hours after operation and continuing until postoperative day 7. The "immunonutrition" group experienced significantly fewer postoperative infections (14% vs. 30%) and a shorter hospital length of stay (11.1 vs. 12.9 days). These findings did not appear influenced by the baseline nutritional status of the patient. The authors concluded that attaining adequate intake before the surgical insult gives perioperative immunonutrition metabolic and immunologic advantages compared with less aggressive approaches to feeding. Despite this positive finding, subsequent studies were less consistent, and therefore several meta-analyses were performed between 1999 and 2001 to further delineate the efficacy of immune-enhancing diets in clinical practice.[68] Common to these meta-analyses was the universal finding of shorter hospital length of stay and an overall reduction in numbers of infectious complications. Although there were positive conclusions overall in each of these more recent meta-analyses, the heterogeneity of the data makes broad recommendations about the use of immune-enhancing diets tentative. What does appear clear is that if it is possible to give immune-modifying nutrition support early in the course of illness, and to give it in rather large amounts, its benefits are more easily detected.

Nutritional Pharmacology: Conditionally Essential and Other "Special" Metabolites in Critical Illness

Nutritional pharmacology is a poorly defined but often used term that emphasizes the role of particular nutrients to change the pathophysiology of a disease process, presumably by distinct molecular mechanisms. Early examples include administering essential amino acids to patients in acute renal failure and using modified amino acid mixtures for the treatment of patients with hepatic failure. As just discussed, one major area of potential advance in nutritional pharmacology has been the use of immunity-enhancing enteral formulas. However, many other proposed approaches in this area remain unproven. In some instances, "nutritional pharmacology" appears to refer to agents that, although not metabolically limiting, may be useful if given in supranormal amounts (e.g., the beneficial changes in lipid metabolism induced by omega-3 fatty acids). Another interpretation is the use of substances that may be metabolized with improved efficiency under conditions of stress (e.g., branched-chain amino acids). Yet another definition of nutritional pharmacology involves the concept of "conditionally essential" amino acids, nucleosides, or other substances, which presumably become rate limiting for protein or nucleic acid synthesis during stress but are sufficiently abundant under normal conditions. The classic example of the latter is glutamine, an amino acid easily synthesized in many cells and normally present in high levels in the circulation. However, despite some literature supporting a relative deficiency of glutamine during stress (see later), even under such conditions, the circulating and intracellular levels of glutamine remain well above the low-affinity constants for glutamyl transfer RNA and other relevant enzymes.

Glutamine

Within 24 hours of operation or trauma, levels of free intracellular glutamine fall in many tissues and do not return to normal until as long as 8 weeks later. The significance of this glutamine export is not clear. Glutamine as a fuel for enterocytes has received much attention. It has been proposed that in pathologic conditions, such as following traumatic injury or during infection, energy production from glutamine released from muscle is critical for maintaining the function of gastrointestinal and immune cells.[1] Furthermore, it has also been suggested that under these conditions, a state of glutamine "deficiency" may exist, and that the administration of supplemental glutamine under such circumstances is beneficial.[1] Glutamine's effects in either preventing or healing chemotherapeutic or radiation toxicity, and in promoting mucosal regrowth after massive small bowel resection, are most impressive when it is given enterally. In severe stress, such as following bone marrow transplantation, beneficial effects of glutamine in decreasing hospital stay, improving nitrogen balance, and decreasing infection have been demonstrated.[69] These effects have been attributed to improved gut barrier function, but improved gut protein and hepatic protein synthesis are equally possible. Although most studies of gut histology with supplemental glutamine have involved enteral delivery, some investigators have proposed that the addition of glutamine to parenteral solutions may prevent the gut atrophy that often accompanies intravenous feeding. In certain animal studies, the addition of glutamine to parenteral nutrition solutions showed maintenance of small intestinal mucosal thickness, protein content, and DNA when compared to glutamine-free solutions, but other investigators failed to show any difference in gut protein, RNA, or wall thickness.[70] These inconclusive experimental results may explain the lack of enthusiasm for glutamine-supplemented parenteral nutrition in clinical practice. Glutamine is also highly unstable when added to TPN solutions, thus limiting its practical use. Another potential concern in neoplastic disease is the observation that glutamine is preferentially metabolized by many tumors, with the potential for augmented tumor growth.

Another putative beneficial effect of glutamine is improved nitrogen balance, particularly in muscle. Attempts to prevent depletion of free glutamine pools in muscle by glutamine supplementation in parenteral nutrition solutions have shown some glutamine sparing. Glutamine supplementation can also raise levels of TCA cycle intermediates, and though this response does not appear to increase energy production or endurance in healthy skeletal muscle, there is some evidence to suggest improved functioning of ischemic heart muscle.[71] Administration of high amounts of glutamine with parenteral nutrition has been reported to promote protein accretion in skeletal muscle.[1] However, although the marginal improvements in nitrogen balance are statistically significant, they seem unlikely to improve clinical outcome.

Arginine

A deficiency of arginine and the dibasic amino acids in the plasma of patients with overwhelming sepsis was observed as early as 1978. Although arginine was thought to be a nonessential amino acid, investigators now recognize that the ability to synthesize arginine in the presence of increased requirements may be exceeded, and it probably is semi-essential. Aside from its metabolic functions, arginine supplementation in critical illness may be beneficial by at least two potential mechanisms: (1) improving immune function and (2) stimulating growth hormone and insulin secretion, a recognized action of this amino acid. Arginine is also known to enhance the responsiveness of T lymphocytes to mitogenic stimulation in vitro. In the study by Daly and colleagues discussed earlier[65] of immune-enhancing enteral diets, T-cell proliferation in response to concanavalin A or phytohemagglutinin was improved in the arginine-supplemented patients, although nitrogen balance was no different between the two groups. Such clinical studies are difficult to interpret with respect to effects attributable to arginine alone, because additional substances (e.g., fish oil) are usually present in the experimental formulas.

Ketone Bodies

The ketone bodies acetoacetate, propionate, and butyrate have been considerably investigated in experimental studies, with respect to their beneficial effect on the gut and especially the effect of butyrate on the ileum and colon. No clinical studies involving exogenous administration of ketone bodies or other short-chain fatty acids are available, however. Acetoacetate, propionate, and butyrate are produced by the fermentation of soluble pectin by colonic bacteria. Because the short-chain fatty acids are not synthesized endogenously, the colonic mucosa can obtain these metabolites only from bacterial fermentation. As compared with other fuels, butyrate appears to be the principal energy source for the colonic mucosa, with acetoacetate, glutamine, and glucose following in order of importance. Diminished short-chain fatty acid oxidation may therefore disrupt the colonic mucosal barrier and presumably, although certainly not proven in human patients, its immune function. In experimental studies, intravenous butyrate results in wall thickening and increased protein content of both the colon and the ileum, and short-chain fatty acids derived from soluble pectin prevent and heal chemotherapy-related gut mucosal damage in animals, as well as improving diversion colitis. Some investigators have proposed a deficiency of short-chain fatty acids in colonocytes as a precursor to ulcerative colitis, but evidence to support this concept is lacking.[72]

Branched-Chain Amino Acids

For many years, the experimental observations that branched-chain amino acids promote positive nitrogen balance in muscle and are preferentially oxidized by this tissue (see "Metabolic Adaptations in Catabolic States and Regulation of Nitrogen Balance") have stimulated broad interest in using branched-chain amino acids as nutritional supplements in critical illness, particularly for the management of hepatic encephalopathy and uremia. However, despite many attempts, little proof of clinical efficacy for branched-chain amino acids is available. As discussed elsewhere in this chapter, branched-chain amino acids do appear helpful in improving severe hepatic encephalopathy, but only in patients to whom a solution deficient in aromatic amino acids is given. However, in incubated muscles from septic animals or humans, branched-chain amino acids do not decrease protein breakdown even when present in pharmacologic quantities (5 mM). Intravenous feeding with solutions enriched in branched-chain amino acids appears to reduce proteolysis in experimental animals with sepsis, but in septic patients, prospective, randomized trials using solutions high in branched-chain amino acids (≤50% of total amino acids) or containing leucine show marginal efficacy in preventing breakdown of lean body mass, perhaps increasing hepatic protein synthesis slightly, and only in severely ill patients. No difference in outcome was seen. Similar results have been obtained in patients undergoing bone marrow transplantation.

Essential Amino Acids

Most amino acids can be recycled, provided energy is adequate. Thus, small amounts of essential amino acids with adequate energy are sufficient for nitrogen equilibrium. In infants, 40% to 50% of the protein intake should be essential amino acids, whereas in an adult in nitrogen equilibrium without stress, sepsis, or trauma, 19% to 20% is sufficient. The percentage of essential amino acids should increase with injury or depletion. The use of essential amino acids in the management of renal failure is discussed elsewhere in this chapter.

Purines and Pyrimidines

These nucleic acid precursors have been proposed to be conditionally essential under conditions of stress, potentially limiting cell division and the generation of new immune or other cells. For example, immune-enhancing enteral formulas such as Impact contain mRNA for this reason. However, as in the case of glutamine, it seems extremely unlikely that these nucleotides would ever be rate limiting, given the numerous salvage pathways available in the cell to regenerate them.

WHO BENEFITS FROM PARENTERAL NUTRITION?

Indications for parenteral nutrition may be organized into three categories, depending on the desired outcome: (1) primary therapy, in which parenteral nutrition is thought to influence the disease process beneficially; (2) supportive therapy, in which nutritional support is important but does not alter the primary disease process; and (3) controversial indications or those under ongoing study. In many cases, the efficacy of intravenous feeding remains controversial because of the limited availability of prospective, randomized trials capable of answering such questions.

Primary Therapy: Efficacy Shown

Gastrointestinal-Cutaneous Fistulas. Patients with gastrointestinal-cutaneous fistulas represent the classic indication for TPN. Increased oral intake increases fistula output. Two longitudinal reviews of fistulas concluded the following:

1. TPN increases spontaneous closure of fistulas.
2. TPN has not resulted in decreased mortality in centers experienced in the treatment of fistulas. The major decrease in mortality in the series at Massachusetts General Hospital and the University of California at San Francisco occurred in the 1960s, probably the result of improved intensive care, including monitoring, respiratory care, and better fluid and electrolyte balance.
3. TPN probably has contributed to decreased mortality in patients with fistulas in most other institutions.
4. The treatment of patients with fistulas has been altered by nutritional support. If spontaneous closure does not occur, patients are in better condition for operation after being supported by TPN.

Respectable rates of fistula closure are also achieved with enteral nutrition, although these rates are slightly lower than with TPN. Initially, fistula drainage increases and then decreases toward closure. A useful compromise, if total caloric replacement is not possible enterally, is to give 20% to 30% of calories enterally, a method that is likely to give all the benefits of enteral feeding, and to give the remainder parenterally.

Renal Failure. TPN results in decreased mortality in patients with acute renal failure, but controversy persists concerning the amino acid solution to use. In 1973, Abel and coworkers, using a mixture of essential amino acids with hypertonic dextrose largely in patients with surgically related renal failure, described decreased urea appearance, earlier diuresis, and a statistically significant improvement in survival in treated patients as compared with those receiving dextrose alone. Other investigators have argued for a more complete amino acid formula and for dealing with the rise in blood urea nitrogen by dialysis. Whereas a few studies have attempted to compare the two formulas, no study with adequate patients concurrently studied is available. A useful compromise is to use essential amino acids early on, in an effort to avoid dialysis, but once dialysis is required, a complete formulation is used (see earlier discussion in "Fundamentals of Artificial Nutrition").

Short Bowel Syndrome. Repeated small bowel resections for Crohn's disease and major enterectomy after mesenteric thrombosis or volvulus are the major causes of short bowel syndrome. No randomized, prospective trials have been undertaken, but patients with short bowel syndrome have no alternative to long-term home TPN. Patients receiving home TPN who would otherwise almost certainly have died commonly survive for 10 to 20 years or even longer. Some patients undergo sufficient hypertrophy of the remaining small bowel to ultimately decrease or obviate the need for home TPN. If a patient is left with 1.5 feet of small bowel anastomosed to the left colon, hypertrophy in 1 or 2 years will, in most cases, enable survival without daily parenteral nutritional support, although twice-weekly supplementation may be necessary. Efforts to promote more rapid hypertrophy of small bowel using gut-specific hormones, fuels, and isotonic solutions have been reported.

Burns. The sharp decrease in mortality from 1965 to 1970 in patients with burns was likely the result of aggressive nutritional support. Early aggressive nutritional support in patients with major burns is associated with improved survival,[56] and aggressive enteral feeding within 3 hours of burn injury is increasingly practiced. Parenteral nutritional support is reserved for those few patients in whom enteral nutrition cannot meet the patient's caloric needs. Moreover, as discussed earlier, nutritional pharmacology is increasingly used in enteral diets specifically designed for burned patients, most likely contributing to lower rates of sepsis, fewer days of bacteremia, lower mortality, and shorter hospital stay.[66]

Hepatic Failure. Improved survival is also seen in patients with hepatic failure who are given aggressive nutritional support. Patients with liver disease are often malnour-ished secondary to excessive alcohol ingestion and decreased food intake and have decreased tolerance to stress. Protein is the important nutritional component they require, but these patients are specifically protein intolerant if hepatic encephalopathy is present (see earlier discussion in "Fundamentals of Artificial Nutrition"). Of the seven randomized, prospective trials thus far reported, in the five in which hypertonic dextrose was used as the caloric source, branched-chain–enriched amino acid solutions were at least as effective as lactulose or neomycin in the treatment of hepatic encephalopathy. In two studies, improved survival was seen. For reasons that are unclear, in studies in which the major caloric source was fat, efficacy for branched-chain amino acids was not seen.[73]

Fan and associates[55] randomized 124 patients undergoing hepatic resection for hepatocellular carcinoma. Half the patients received only oral nutrition, whereas the other half received perioperative intravenous nutritional support using a branched-chain–enriched solution. Dextrose and lipid were the caloric sources, with MCTs comprising 50% of the lipids. A statistically significant reduction occurred in the overall postoperative morbidity rate in the perioperative nutrition group as compared with the control group (34% vs. 55%), predominantly because of fewer septic complications (17% vs. 37%). In addition, there was a reduced need for diuretic agents to control ascites (25% vs. 50%), less weight loss (0 kg vs. 1.4 kg), and less deterioration of liver function as measured by indocyanine green clearance (2.8% vs. 4.8%). However, the difference in mortality (5 of 64 in the perioperative nutrition group and 9 of 60 in the control group) did not reach statistical significance. Thus, during hepatectomy, outcome can be considerably improved by perioperative parenteral nutrition.

Primary Therapy: Efficacy Not Shown

Inflammatory Bowel Disease. In patients with inflammatory bowel disease, oral intake often provokes diarrhea, protein-losing enteropathy, bleeding, and abdominal pain. Although TPN and bowel rest are useful in the treatment of Crohn's disease (particularly disease limited to the small bowel, in which a remission rate of 75% can be expected), such therapy has not been subjected to a randomized, prospective trial. The mean duration of remission is approximately 11 months. Patients with colonic involvement do less well; their rates of initial remission and duration are considerably lower than those of patients with small bowel disease alone. Patients with extensive, severe, and chronically recurrent Crohn's disease are suitable for home hyperalimentation, particularly when surgical therapy would leave the patient almost anenteric. Patients with ulcerative colitis should not receive long-term TPN to induce remission, because definitive resection with a sphincter-saving operation (e.g., an ileoanal pouch or Soave procedure) produces a long-term cure. On the other hand, TPN for usually less than 2 weeks, in conjunction with intravenous antibiotics, may allow the rectal mucosa to heal and thus facilitates rectal mucosal stripping.

Anorexia Nervosa. Patients with anorexia nervosa starve to a moribund state, with enormous losses of lean body mass, tissue, and protein. Anorectic patients are difficult to treat; they are self-destructive by disconnecting their intravenous lines and thus inviting air embolism. A prospective trial has not been carried out in patients with anorexia nervosa.

Supportive Therapy: Efficacy Shown

Acute Radiation Enteritis or Chemotherapy Toxicity. Acute radiation enteritis and/or gastrointestinal complications of chemotherapy may prevent oral intake. Experimental studies of soluble pectin in rats receiving 5-fluorouracil chemotherapy showed reduced toxicity and improved mucosal healing, but no clinical trials in patients have been conducted. TPN administered until the gut mucosa heals enables the patient to survive. Chronic radiation enteritis with multiple strictures may render the patient a candidate for home parenteral nutrition or, rarely, enteral feeding with minimal-residue diets, provided the original neoplasm has been cured.

Prolonged Ileus. Prolonged ileus after an abdominal procedure may necessitate a course of TPN until the ileus subsides. Obviously, this therapy is only supportive.

Supportive Therapy: Efficacy Probably Present

Weight Loss Preliminary to Major Surgery (Perioperative Parenteral Nutrition). Four important questions concern the use of parenteral nutrition in patients experiencing weight loss prior to major surgical procedures: (1) Are operative complications of surgery increased in patients who have lost weight? (2) If so, can these patients be identified? (3) If these patients are identified, does short-term parenteral nutrition change the outcome? (4) If all these conditions are met, what mode of nutritional repletion should be used and for how long?

1. Are surgical complications of major operative procedures increased in patients who have lost weight? In an older review analyzing 18 randomized and nonrandomized studies, Detsky and colleagues[74] concluded that the case had not yet been made for the use of TPN before major operation. Yet a critical Veterans Affairs study, one of the best randomized, controlled, prospective studies available in the entire field of parenteral nutrition, appears to identify a group at risk, namely patients who lost more than 15% of their body weight prior to surgery.[75] In this group, the incidence of surgical complications was greater and was ameliorated by TPN.

2. Can this group be identified? Observations as early as those of Studley in 1936 suggested that patients with profound (20%) weight loss and low serum albumin level experienced increased complications and mortality after gastrectomy. Thus, identifying the group at risk includes a careful history and global assessment. A history of greater than 10% or certainly 15% weight loss and an albumin value of less than 3 g/100 mL would place these patients in a high-risk group. Delayed cutaneous hypersensitivity testing by injected antigens,

hand dynamometry, and serum transferrin is confirmatory and optional.

3. Does short-term nutritional intervention change the outcome? Yes, provided nutritional intervention is limited to the group with severe malnutrition and immunologic dysfunction. In the Veterans Affairs multicenter trial,[75] in patients who were judged severely malnourished and who had lost more than 15% of their body weight, preoperative nutritional intervention for 7 to 10 days decreased operative septic complications. However, in the group stratified as having mild to moderate malnutrition, the decrease in surgical complications was more than offset by the increase in catheter-related infectious complications. The total energy intake of the TPN group was 46 kcal/kg (2944 kcal/day), whereas the ad libitum group consumed 20 kcal/kg (1280 kcal/day). With this degree of TPN-induced hyperglycemia, the immunosuppressive effects would be great enough to negate any potential benefit to preoperative feeding, with the exception of the subgroup that was severely malnourished. Thus, improperly administered TPN increased the risk of catheter-related and non–catheter-related infection. Whether fewer calories or a shorter period or preoperative repletion would have resulted in greater benefit to the minimally or moderately malnourished group is not clear.

4. How long should preoperative repletion last? In previous studies, with 3 days of parenteral nutritional support before operation, the trend was toward decreased sepsis, but statistical significance was not achieved because of the small number of patients. With preoperative repletion, patients begin to feel better at approximately 5 days, a point that generally coincides with an increase in the shortest-turnover proteins, that is, retinol-binding protein and thyroxin-binding prealbumin. In the Veterans Affairs cooperative study[75] the duration of preoperative parenteral nutrition was between 7 and 10 days, and efficacy was seen. Thus, a period of 5 to 7 days should be used for preoperative nutritional repletion.

Cancer. In the 1980s, the initial enthusiasm for nutritional support in patients with cancer waned as evidence suggested that tumor growth is stimulated by such intervention and that nutritional supplementation of patients undergoing chemotherapy and/or radiation therapy might decrease survival and/or the remission-free interval. This important area is plagued by a lack of uniformity in studies, by the inclusion of both malnourished and normally nourished patients in studies, and by the finding that responses to nutritional support may differ depending on whether the treatment modality is to be radiation therapy, chemotherapy, or resection. The sources of calories supplied in standard feeding regimens may also be inappropriate in the patient with cancer, because glucose rather than fat may be used preferentially by many tumors. Randomized, prospective trials in patients with cancer have shown efficacy for preoperative intravenous nutritional support only in severely malnourished patients with upper gastrointestinal tumors. For example, in the Veterans Affairs study discussed earlier, patients with carcinoma of the esophagus or the gastric cardia benefited from perioperative nutritional support and had decreased mortality and morbidity without apparent stimulation of the tumor.[75] In addition, several studies in patients with cancer have suggested that postoperative nutritional support using an "immunologically active" tube feeding may improve postoperative outcome in general (see "Immunonutrition").

Cardiac Surgery. Patients with cardiac cachexia are at increased risk of complications and mortality after cardiac surgery. The conventional wisdom is based on Starling's pronouncement in 1912 that the heart is spared the ravages of starvation. This is not true. Protein depletion in experimental animals results in decreased myocardial contractility, with distortion of cardiac histology manifested as edema and necrosis of myofibrils, conditions that are not totally reversed even after prolonged nutritional repletion. In the single prospective randomized trial in which nutritional supplementation was begun on the day of operation (and thus unlikely to show efficacy), no improvement in outcome was seen. A study in which patients with cardiac cachexia about to undergo surgical treatment are subjected to prolonged nutritional repletion has yet to be done. Anecdotal clinical evidence suggests that patients with cardiac cachexia require nutritional supplementation for at least 2 to 3 weeks, and perhaps as long as 6 weeks before operation, a finding supported by experimental evidence. Fluid limitations in such patients require more concentrated solutions.

Respiratory Failure and Requirements for Prolonged Respiratory Support. No evidence indicates that pulmonary function itself, rather than muscles of respiration, is improved by nutritional support. Although some information is available concerning the metabolic needs of the alveolar cells responsible for surfactant production and gas exchange, a tailored intravenous solution has not appeared. Whereas weaning from ventilators may improve with nutritional support, a potential, deleterious effect of hypertonic dextrose is overproduction of carbon dioxide. Although this phenomenon is extensively discussed in the ICU setting, it is not common; occasionally, in patients with marginal pulmonary function, carbon dioxide overproduction may require replacing glucose with fat to promote weaning from the ventilator. Carbon dioxide production and RQ can be measured in most ICU settings, as described earlier.

Large Wounds and Other Sources of Nitrogen Loss. Many patients with large wounds such as decubitus ulcers are unable to eat. Provision of nutritional support to improve wound healing is logical, but no randomized studies exist.

HIV Infection. The place of TPN in the treatment of patients with acquired immunodeficiency syndrome is controversial[48] and was discussed in an earlier section in the context of home TPN.

FUTURE DIRECTIONS IN ARTIFICIAL NUTRITION: NOVEL APPROACHES FOR REDUCING CACHEXIA

Besides the primarily nutritional approaches described earlier and designed to promote positive nitrogen balance and improved overall outcome in critically ill patients,

additional strategies are available and are a focus of present and future research. Certain initially promising approaches, such as growth hormone administration, have not been clearly shown to be of clinical benefit, whereas others, such as the pharmacologic inhibition of protein breakdown, are in their infancy.

Inhibition of the Stress Response

A variety of approaches have been used to inhibit the actions of inflammatory mediators and catabolic hormones that are released under conditions of stress and are presumably responsible for protein loss and cachexia. Included in this category are the omega-3 fatty acids, which have been amply discussed in earlier sections and which continue to show promise as therapeutic agents. Unfortunately, alternative strategies (e.g., the use of neutralizing antibodies to TNF or to endotoxin during sepsis) have either been shown to be ineffective, or in some cases, actually seem to cause increased mortality in clinical trials. An attractive drug is the glucocorticoid receptor antagonist RU-486, but no data are available for this agent in cachectic patients, perhaps in part because of societal unease with RU-486's identity as an abortifacient. An important issue for all such approaches is whether the signals commonly thought of as harmful in conditions of stress (e.g., the cytokines) should be interpreted in such a simple manner, or alternatively, these mediators serve critical and useful functions during the stress response as well.

Administration of Anabolic Factors

Gut-Derived Hormones

Studies have suggested that glucagon-like peptide-2 (GLP-2) has a robust effect on stimulating gut hypertrophy, DNA, and wall thickness in animals receiving parenteral nutrition. In one of the authors' (JEF) preliminary studies, the effects of GLP-2 have been impressive in the sense that continued administration of GLP-2 in rats receiving TPN results in gut hypertrophy exceeding that seen in orally fed animals. It is hoped that clinical trials will take place within several years.

Growth Hormone and Insulin-Like Growth Factors

In experimental studies discussed earlier, growth hormone and IGFs promoted positive nitrogen balance in muscle. Furthermore, the IGFs inhibit muscle proteolysis and stimulate protein synthesis directly (unlike growth hormone), and during systemic administration the IGFs may be less diabetogenic than growth hormone. These agents may also have beneficial effects on lipolysis. These anabolic effects have led to the clinical use of cloned human growth hormone. Pharmacologic levels of this hormone, when given with hypocaloric TPN to humans, can promote positive nitrogen balance in sepsis and following major injury.[1] The increase in protein degradation in isolated muscles following burn injury can also be reversed by IGF-I in a dose-dependent manner,[76] but this effect was not seen in muscles from septic animals, where IGF-I increased protein synthesis but had no effect on protein degradation rates.[18,76] Although the role of growth hormone in clinical practice remains poorly defined, a cautionary note is raised by a recent clinical trial of growth hormone administration to ventilated ICU patients,[77] in which mortality, the duration of ventilator dependence, and length of stay were seemingly worsened, not improved, by the hormone.

Anabolic Steroids

The increased secretion of testosterone in males at puberty is thought to determine the increased skeletal muscle mass that occurs at this stage in development and is maintained into adult life. Accordingly, suppressing testosterone in healthy young men reduces fat-free mass and fractional muscle protein synthesis, and androgen supplementation to normal physiologic levels in androgen-deficient men leads to increased muscle mass and strength.[78] The potential therapeutic use of testosterone has also been explored in a number of studies. There is some evidence for the use of testosterone to reverse the loss of muscle mass and strength that occurs in normal aging in men.[78] In HIV-infected men with weight loss and low testosterone levels, testosterone supplements led to improved strength, and injections of testosterone after severe burn injury reduced muscle loss by improving protein synthetic efficiency and reducing muscle protein degradation rates.

Catecholamines

Catecholamines appear to exert an anabolic effect on muscle principally by reducing calcium-dependent proteolysis and by increasing protein synthesis. The anabolic effect of catecholamines can also be mimicked by the adrenergic β_2 agonist, clenbuterol. Numerous studies in animals have shown that clenbuterol treatment increases carcass and muscle weights, and furthermore, clenbuterol can inhibit wasting due to hind-limb suspension or denervation in rats and can also attenuate cachexia after scald injury. Clenbuterol also improved lean body mass and muscle size in animals with experimental tumors while increasing the utilization of lipid.[79] The exact mechanism by which drugs such as clenbuterol promote positive nitrogen balance in vivo remains unclear. For example, a pure β-antagonist, propranolol, was shown by Herndon and coworkers to improve protein balance and reduce energy expenditure in children with severe burns randomized to 2 weeks of oral therapy.[80]

Inhibition of Proteolysis

Pharmacologic Inhibition

An extremely attractive approach to the treatment of muscle wasting is the direct inhibition of intracellular proteolysis. As knowledge grows concerning the biochemical pathways for protein breakdown in muscle and other tissues, the potential for such intervention increases. Low-molecular-weight active site inhibitors of the proteasome are now available,[13,14] and newer generation inhibitors have been shown to be fairly safe in humans during initial trials of their use as antineoplastic agents, for example in treating multiple myeloma. More recently, specific E3s induced in muscle under catabolic conditions have been identified,[15,16] and these proteins may offer tissue-specific targets for inhibition of ubiquitination and proteolysis during future drug development. Such specificity will likely prove important to avoid toxicity, because intracellular protein breakdown has fundamental and pleiotropic functions, including regulation of the cell cycle, antigen presentation, and preventing the accumulation of abnormal proteins in cells.

Lessons From Nature

Muscle proteolysis is suppressed in certain physiologic conditions, including following dietary protein deficiency and prolonged fasting.[22] Muscles from such animals are also resistant to many catabolic signals, such as the proteolysis induced by denervation. An improved understanding of the intracellular mechanisms and endocrine signals responsible for these adaptations should suggest new strategies relevant to clinical practice and useful for reducing muscle wasting in ill patients.

SUMMARY

Nutritional support has been available since the mid 1960s and has proved its value as one of the most important therapeutic modalities of the 20th century. As investigators who are equally familiar with the operating room and with molecular biology are trained, the basic mechanisms and pathophysiology of disease states relevant to surgical patients are being elucidated increasingly at the molecular level. As knowledge of nutrition and metabolism becomes more sophisticated, our ability to intervene in disease states that cause significant mortality in patients today will continue to improve markedly.

Selected References

Articles

Abel RM, Beck CH Jr, Abbott WM, et al: Improved survival from acute renal failure after treatment with intravenous essential L-amino acids and glucose: Results of a prospective, double-blind study. N Engl J Med 288:695, 1973.

> An early, randomized, double-blinded trial showed improved survival after the application of techniques of parenteral nutrition and administration of a specialized solution to patients with renal failure. The eight essential L-amino acids in hypertonic dextrose were administered to patients with renal failure, and these patients were compared with a group receiving isocaloric hypertonic dextrose alone. Improved survival and perhaps early healing of the renal lesion were seen.

Clowes GHA, George BC, Villee CA, Saravis CA: Muscle proteolysis induced by a circulating peptide in patients with sepsis or trauma. N Engl J Med 308:545, 1983.

> Few articles have inspired as much interest and excitement as this description of a 4200-dalton protein isolated in the plasma of patients with sepsis. This hypothetical cytokine, PIF, increased hepatic protein synthesis and muscle breakdown. Subsequent experiments revealed that the particular conditions used in these experiments may have contributed to these findings. Nonetheless, this article probably contributed more to the research in surgery of cytokines than any other and inspired a great deal of work over subsequent years.

Cuthbertson DP: Observations on the disturbance of metabolism produced by injury to the limbs. Q J Med 1:233, 1932.

> This study may well have begun contemporary nutritional support. This classic description of loss of nitrogen and breakdown of lean body mass after injury is a careful study in a classic tradition.

Dominioni L, Trocki O, Mochizuki H, et al: Prevention of severe postburn hypermetabolism and catabolism by immediate intragastric feeding. J Burn Care Rehabil 5:106, 1984.

> The first demonstration that changes in gut flora and the translocation of bacteria or absorption of bacterial products after thinning of mucosa in burns contribute to hypermetabolism is presented. With the confirmation of similar results in patients with burns, it is clear that this hypothesis with respect to gut products is operant in other patients as well.

Dudrick SJ, Wilmore DW, Vars HM, Rhoads JE: Long-term total parenteral nutrition with growth, development, and positive nitrogen balance. Surgery 64:134, 1968.

> This is one of the classic articles originally describing high-glucose central TPN from which stems the current popularity of parenteral nutrition in the United States. In this ambitious project, the biochemical requirements for growth in puppies were investigated with astounding results: Normal growth comparable with that seen in puppies who were eating freely could be achieved without any oral intake, provided one infused the necessary nutrients by vein.

Fischer JE, Rosen HM, Ebeid AM, et al: The effect of normalization of plasma amino acids on hepatic encephalopathy in man. Surgery 80:77, 1976.

> An approach to liver disease and the intolerance to protein in patients with hepatic encephalopathy is described. This study represents the culmination of a hypothesis of hepatic encephalopathy, depending on altered plasma amino acid patterns, changes subsequently discovered to be amplified by changes in the blood-brain barrier secondary to disturbed metabolism in liver disease. It represents an early anecdotal attempt to enable patients with severe hepatic deficiency to receive adequate nutrition at the same time as awakening from hepatic encephalopathy while they received increased protein equivalent in the form of a branched-chain–enriched (to 36%) amino acid solution now commercially available as HepatAmine.

Ryan JA Jr, Abel RM, Abbott WM, et al: Catheter complications in total parenteral nutrition: A prospective study of 200 consecutive patients. N Engl J Med 290:757, 1974.

> A study of the complications of parenteral nutrition was done in a large hospital with one of the first centralized nutritional support teams. This study confirmed that rigid asepsis in the care of catheters and minimizing catheter manipulation were the most important factors in preventing line catheter sepsis.

Wilmore DW, Dudrick SJ: Treatment of acute renal failure with intravenous essential L-amino acids. Arch Surg 99:669, 1969.

> This study represents the earliest approach to disease-specific parenteral nutrition. The principle of attempting to define the metabolic abnormalities in a given patient and infusing an appropriate nutritional substrate was first proposed in this study. The intravenous equivalent of a Giordano-Giovanetti diet, containing only the eight L-essential amino acids (an oral diet of high biologic value), was used.

Van den Berghe G, Wouters P, Weekers F, et al: Intensive insulin therapy in the surgical intensive care unit. N Engl J Med 345:1359-1367, 2001.

> This carefully conducted study emphasizes the importance of stringent control of blood glucose for the prevention of sepsis and other complications in critically ill patients.

Books

Fischer JE (ed): Total Parenteral Nutrition, 2nd ed. Boston, Little, Brown, 1991.

> This book represents an attempt to standardize the practical approach to TPN.

Fischer JE (ed): Nutrition and Metabolism in Surgical Patients. Boston, Little, Brown, 1996.

> The basic science and practical knowledge relevant to surgical nutrition are presented in one volume. The various chapters also address the efficacy of parenteral nutrition.

Grant JP (ed): Handbook of Total Parenteral Nutrition, 2nd ed. Philadelphia, WB Saunders, 1992.

> This short version is an attempt to detail knowledge in the area of parenteral nutrition. The bibliography is particularly exhaustive and useful.

Rombeau JL, Caldwell MD (eds): Clinical Nutrition, 2nd ed. Vol. 1, Enteral and Tube Nutrition; Vol. 2, Parenteral Nutrition. Philadelphia, WB Saunders, 1990 (Vol. 1) and 1993 (Vol. 2).

> This is the most recent large textbook on enteral and parenteral nutrition. It is well done and has been updated, with many specialized chapters.

References

1. Wilmore DW: Catabolic illness: Strategies for enhancing recovery. N Engl J Med 325:695-702, 1991.
2. Bistrian BR, Blackburn GL, Vitale J, et al: Incidence of malnutrition in general medical patients. JAMA 235:1567-1570, 1976.
3. Christensen HN: Role of amino acid transport and counter transport in nutrition and metabolism. Physiol Rev 70:43, 1990.
4. Hyde R, Peyrollier K, Hundal HS: Insulin promotes the cell surface recruitment of the SAT2/ATA2 system A amino acid

transporter from an endosomal compartment in skeletal muscle cells. J Biol Chem 277:13628-13634, 2002.

5. Goldberg AL, Chang TW: Regulation and significance of amino acid metabolism in skeletal muscle. Fed Proc 37:2301-2307, 1978.

6. Price SR, Wang X, Bailey JL: Tissue-specific responses of branched-chain α-ketoacid dehydrogenase activity in metabolic acidosis. J Am Soc Nephrol 9:1892-1898, 1998.

7. Goldberg AL, Tischler ME: Regulatory effects of leucine on carbohydrate and protein metabolism. In Walser M, Williamson JR (eds): Metabolism and Clinical Implications of Branched-Chain Amino and Ketoacids. New York, Elsevier/North-Holland, 1981, pp 205-216.

8. Windmueller HG, Spaeth AE: Respiratory fuels and nitrogen metabolism in vivo in small intestine of fed rats: Quantitative importance of glutamine, glutamate, and aspartate. J Biol Chem 255:107-112, 1980.

9. Karinch AM, Pan M, Lin CM, et al: Glutamine metabolism in sepsis and infection. J Nutr 131:2535S-2538S, 2001.

10. Schwartz AL, Ciechanover A: The ubiquitin-proteasome pathway and pathogenesis of human diseases. Annu Rev Med 50:57-74, 1999.

11. Williams AB, DeCourten-Myers GM, Fischer JE, et al: Sepsis stimulates release of myofilaments in skeletal muscle by a calcium-dependent mechanism. FASEB J 13:1435-1443, 1999.

12. Mitch WE, Goldberg AL: Mechanisms of muscle wasting: The role of the ubiquitin-proteasome pathway. N Engl J Med 335:1897-1905, 1996.

13. Tawa NE, Jr., Odessey R, Goldberg AL: Inhibitors of the proteasome reduce the accelerated proteolysis in atrophying rat skeletal muscles. J Clin Invest 100:197-203, 1997.

14. Jagoe RT, Goldberg AL: What do we really know about the ubiquitin-proteasome pathway in muscle atrophy? Curr Opin Clin Nutr Metab Care 4:183-190, 2001.

15. Gomes MD, Lecker SH, Jagoe RT, et al: Atrogin-1, a muscle-specific F-box protein highly expressed during muscle atrophy. Proc Natl Acad Sci U S A 98:14440-14445, 2001.

16. Bodine SC, Latres E, Baumhueter S: Identification of ubiquitin ligases required for skeletal muscle atrophy. Science 294:1704-1708, 2001.

17. Larbaud D, Balage M, Taillandier D, et al: Differential regulation of the lysosomal, Ca^{2+}-dependent and ubiquitin/proteasome-dependent proteolytic pathways in fast-twitch and slow-twitch rat muscle following hyperinsulinaemia. Clin Sci (Lond) 101:551-558, 2001.

18. Hobler SC, Williams AB, Fischer JE, et al: IGF-I stimulates protein synthesis but does not inhibit protein breakdown in muscle from septic rats. Am J Physiol 274:R571-R576, 1998.

19. Tiao G, Fagan J, Roegner V, et al: Energy-ubiquitin–dependent muscle proteolysis during sepsis in rats is regulated by glucocorticoids. J Clin Invest 97:339-348, 1996.

20. Lofberg E, Gutierrez A, Wernerman J, et al: Effects of high doses of glucocorticoids on free amino acids, ribosomes, and protein turnover in human muscle. Eur J Clin Invest 32:345-353, 2002.

21. Jagoe RT, Lecker SH, Gomes MD, et al: Patterns of gene expression in atrophying skeletal muscles: Response to food deprivation. FASEB J 16:1697-1712, 2002.

22. Tawa NE Jr, Kettelhut IC, Goldberg AL: Dietary protein deficiency reduces lysosomal and nonlysosomal ATP-dependent proteolysis in muscle. Am J Physiol 263:E326-E334, 1992.

23. Attaix D, Taillandier D, Temparis S, et al: Regulation of ATP-ubiquitin–dependent proteolysis in muscle wasting. Reprod Nutr Dev 34:583-597, 1994.

24. Hobler SC, Williams AB, Fischer D, et al: Activity and expression of the 20S proteasome are increased in skeletal muscle during sepsis. Am J Physiol 277:R434-R440, 1999.

25. Llovera M, Carbo N, Lopez-Soriano J, et al: Different cytokines modulate ubiquitin gene expression in rat skeletal muscle. Cancer Lett 133:83-87, 1998.

26. Combaret L, Tilignac T, Claustre A, et al: Torbafylline (HWA 448) inhibits enhanced skeletal muscle ubiquitin-proteasome–dependent proteolysis in cancer and septic rats. Biochem J 361:185-192, 2002.

27. Nathan C, Xie QW: Nitric oxide synthases: Roles, tolls, and controls. Cell 78:915-918, 1994.

28. Billiar TR, Simmons RL: Arginine and nitric oxide. In Fischer JE (ed): Surgical Nutrition, 2nd ed. Boston, Little, Brown, 1996.

29. Kobzik L, Reid MB, Bredt DS, et al: Nitric oxide in skeletal muscle [see comments]. Nature 372:546-548, 1994.

30. Tawa NE Jr, Warren MS: Activation of intracellular protein breakdown in skeletal muscle by nitric oxide and oxygen free radicals. Surg Forum 48:30-32, 1997.

31. Baracos VE: Regulation of skeletal-muscle-protein turnover in cancer-associated cachexia. Nutrition 16:1015, 2000.

32. Lorite MJ, Smith HJ, Arnold JA, et al: Activation of ATP-ubiquitin–dependent proteolysis in skeletal muscle in vivo and murine myoblasts in vitro by a proteolysis-inducing factor (PIF). Br J Cancer 85:297-302, 2001.

33. Wigmore SJ, Barber MD, Ross JA, et al: Effect of oral eicosapentaenoic acid on weight loss in patients with pancreatic cancer. Nutr Cancer 36:177-184, 2000.

34. Buchman AL, Ament ME, Sohel M, et al: Choline deficiency causes reversible hepatic abnormalities in patients receiving parenteral nutrition—proof of a human choline requirement: A placebo controlled trial. JPEN J Parenter Enteral Nutr 25:260-268, 2001.

35. McClave SA, Lowen CC, Kleber MJ, et al: Clinical use of the respiratory quotient obtained from indirect calorimetry. JPEN J Parenter Enteral Nutr 27:21-26, 2003.

36. Herridge MS, Cheung AM, Tansey CM, et al: One-year outcomes in survivors of the adult respiratory distress syndrome. N Engl J Med 348:683-693, 2003.

37. Von Allmen D, Hasselgren PO, Fischer JE: Hepatic protein synthesis in a modified septic rat model. J Surg Res 48:476, 1990.

38. Wolfe RR, O'Donnell TF, Stone MD, et al: Investigation of factors determining the optimal glucose infusion rate in total parenteral nutrition. Metabolism 9:892-900, 1980.

39. Van den Berghe G, Wouters P, Weekers F, et al: Intensive insulin therapy in critically ill patients. N Engl J Med 345:1359-1367, 2001.

40. Waxman K, Day AT, Stellin GP, et al: Safety and efficacy of glycerol and amino acids in combination with lipid emulsion for peripheral parenteral nutrition support. JPEN J Parenter Enteral Nutr 16:374, 1992.

41. Simopoulos AP: Omega-3 fatty acids in health and disease and in growth and development. Am J Clin Nutr 54:438-463, 1991.

42. Khaodhiar L, Keane-Ellison M, Tawa NE, et al: Iron deficiency anemia in patients receiving home total parenteral nutrition. JPEN J Parenter Enteral Nutr 26:114-119, 2002.

43. Esparza J, Boivin MA, Hartshorne MF, et al: Equal aspiration rates in gastrically and transpylorically fed critically ill patients. Intensive Care Med 27:660-664, 2001.

44. Davies AR, Froomes PR, French CJ, et al: A randomized comparison of nasojejunal and nasogastric feeding in critically ill patients. Crit Care Med 30:586-590, 2001.

45. Montejo JC, Grau T, Acosta J, et al: Multicenter, prospective, randomized, single-blind study comparing the efficacy and gastrointestinal complications of early jejunal feeding with

early gastric feeding in critically ill patients. Crit Care Med 30:796-800, 2002.

46. Montecalvo MA, Steger KA, Farber HW, et al: Nutritional outcome and pneumonia in critical care patients randomized to gastric versus jejunal tube feedings. Crit Care Med 20:1377-1387, 1992.

47. Bern MM, Lokich JJ, Wallach SR, et al: Very low doses of warfarin can prevent thrombosis in central venous catheters: A randomized prospective trial. Ann Intern Med 112:423-428, 1990.

48. Melchior JC, Chastang C, Gelas P, et al: Efficacy of 2-month total parenteral nutrition in AIDS patients: A controlled randomized prospective trial. The French Multicenter Total Parenteral Nutrition Cooperative Group Study. AIDS 10:379-384, 1996.

49. Jeppesen PB, Langholz E, Mortensen PB: Quality of life in patients receiving home parenteral nutrition. Gut 44:844-852, 1999.

50. Chan S, McCowen KC, Bistrian BR, et al: Incidence, prognosis, and etiology of end-stage liver disease in patients receiving home total parenteral nutrition. Surgery 126:28-34, 1999.

51. Ling PR, Ollero M, Khaodhiar L, et al: Disturbances in essential fatty acid metabolism in patients receiving long-term home parenteral nutrition. Dig Dis Sci 47:1679-1685, 2002.

52. Ling PR, Khaodhiar L, Bistrian BR, et al: Inflammatory mediators in patients receiving long-term home parenteral nutrition. Dig Dis Sci 46:2484-2489, 2001.

53. Saitta JC, Ott SM, Sherrard DJ, et al: Metabolic bone disease in adults receiving long-term parenteral nutrition: Longitudinal study with regional densitometry and bone biopsy. JPEN J Parenter Enteral Nutr 17:214-219, 1993.

54. McClave SA, Spain DA, Snider HL: Nutritional management in acute and chronic pancreatitis. Gastroenterol Clin North Am 27:421-434, 1998.

55. Fan ST, Lo CM, Lai ECS, et al: Perioperative nutritional support in patients undergoing hepatectomy for hepatocellular carcinoma. N Engl J Med 331:547, 1994.

56. Jenkins M, Gottschlich M, Alexander JW, et al: Effect of immediate enteral feeding on the hypermetabolic response following severe burn injury. JPEN J Parenter Enteral Nutr 13:12S, 1989.

57. Moore FA, Feliciano DV, Andrassy RJ, et al: Early enteral feeding, compared with parenteral, reduces postoperative septic complications: The results of a meta-analysis. Ann Surg 216:172, 1992.

58. Kudsk KA, Croce MA, Fabian TC, et al: Enteral versus parenteral feeding: Effects on septic morbidity after blunt and penetrating abdominal trauma. Ann Surg 215:503, 1992.

59. Reynolds JV, Kanwar S, Welsh FK, et al: Does the route of feeding modify gut barrier function and clinical outcome in patients after major upper gastrointestinal surgery? JPEN J Parenter Enteral Nutr 21:196-201, 1997.

60. Gennari R, Alexander JW, Gianotti L, et al: Granulocyte macrophage colony-stimulating factor improves survival in two models of gut-derived sepsis by improving gut barrier function and modulating bacterial clearance. Ann Surg 56:530, 1994.

61. Lewis SJ, Egger M, Sylvester PA, et al: Early enteral feeding versus "nil by mouth" after gastrointestinal surgery: Systematic review and meta-analysis of controlled trials. BMJ 323:1-5, 2001.

62. Marik PE, Zaloga GP: Early enteral nutrition in acutely ill patients: A systematic review. Crit Care Med 29:2264-2270, 2001.

63. Pacelli F, Bossola M, Papa V, et al: Enteral versus parenteral nutrition after major abdominal surgery: An even match. Arch Surg 136:933-936, 2001.

64. Daly JM, Lieberman MD, Goldfine J, et al: Enteral nutrition with supplemental arginine, RNA, and omega-3 fatty acids in patients after operation: Immunologic, metabolic, and clinical outcome. Surgery 112:56-67, 1992.

65. Daly JM, Reynolds J, Thom A, et al: Immune and metabolic effects of arginine in the surgical patient. Ann Surg 208:512, 1988.

66. Bower RH, Cerra FB, Bershadsky B, et al: Early enteral administration of a formula (Impact) supplemented with arginine, nucleotides, and fish oil in intensive care unit patients: Results of a randomized prospective clinical trial. Crit Care Med 23:436, 1995.

67. Braga M, Gianotti L, Radaelli G, et al: Perioperative immunonutrition in patients undergoing cancer surgery: Results of a randomized double-blind phase III trial. Arch Surg 134:428-433, 1999.

68. Heyland DK, Novak F, Drover JW, et al: Should immunonutrition become routine in critically ill patients? A systematic review of the evidence. JAMA 286:944-953, 2001.

69. Ziegler TR, Young LS, Benfall K, et al: Clinical and metabolic efficacy of glutamine-supplemented parenteral nutrition after bone marrow transplantation: A randomized, double-blind, controlled study. Ann Intern Med 116:821, 1992.

70. Li S, Nussbaum MS, McFadden DW, et al: Addition of L-glutamine to total parenteral nutrition (TPN) and its effects on portal insulin and glucagon and the development of hepatic steatosis in rats. J Surg Res 48:421, 1990.

71. Rennie MJ, Bowtell JL, Bruce M, et al: Interaction between glutamine availability and metabolism of glycogen, tricarboxylic acid cycle intermediates, and glutathione. J Nutr 131:2488S-2490S, 2001.

72. Roediger WEW: The place of SCFAs in colonocyte metabolism in health and ulcerative colitis: The impaired colonocyte barrier. In Cummings JH, Sakata T, Rombeau JL (eds): Physiologic and Clinical Aspects of Short-Chain Fatty Acids. Cambridge, Cambridge University Press, 1993.

73. Naylor CD, O'Rourke K, Detsky AS, et al: Parenteral nutrition with branched-chain amino acids in hepatic encephalopathy: A meta-analysis. Gastroenterology 97:1033, 1989.

74. Detsky AS, Baker JP, O'Rourke K, et al: Perioperative parenteral nutrition: A meta-analysis. Ann Intern Med 107:195, 1987.

75. Buzby GP: Perioperative total parenteral nutrition in surgical patients. The Veterans Affairs Total Parenteral Nutrition Cooperative Study Group. N Engl J Med 325:525-532, 1991.

76. Fang CH, Li BG, Wang JJ, et al: Insulin-like growth factor 1 stimulates protein synthesis and inhibits protein breakdown in muscle from burned rats. JPEN J Parenter Enteral Nutr 21:245-251, 1997.

77. Takala J, Ruokonen E, Webster NR, et al: Increased mortality associated with growth hormone treatment in critically ill adults. N Engl J Med 341:785-792, 1999.

78. Bhasin S, Woodhouse L, Storer TW: Proof of the effect of testosterone on skeletal muscle. J Endocrinol 170:27-38, 2001.

79. Chance WT, Cao L, Zhang FS, et al: Clenbuterol treatment increases muscle mass and protein content of tumor-bearing rats maintained on total parenteral nutrition. JPEN J Parenter Enteral Nutr 15:530, 1991.

80. Herndon DN, Hart DW, Wolf SE, et al: Reversal of catabolism by β blockade after severe burns. N Engl J Med 345:1223-1229, 2001.

CHAPTER 8

WOUND HEALING

Mimi Leong, M.D. and **Linda G. Phillips, M.D.**

Tissue Injury and Response	Hypertrophic Scars and Keloids
Wound Healing Phases	Fetal Wound Healing
Abnormal Wound Healing	New Horizons

The treatment and healing of wounds are some of the oldest subjects discussed in the medical literature. The same events, in the same order, occur in every healing process regardless of the tissue type or the inciting injury. Duodenal ulcers, myocardial infarctions, cerebrovascular accidents, cellulitis, long bone fractures, surgical incisions, and traumatic wounds all undergo the same reparative processes. Knowledge of wound healing allows physicians to manipulate wounds to achieve optimal results in a short period. The surgical and anesthetic advances of the 18th and 19th centuries resulted in improved surgical outcomes. The basic science discoveries of the 1980s and 1990s demonstrated that physicians could manipulate the wound with cellular and molecular biology techniques and accelerate healing. Yet, despite the advances in the last 2 decades in elucidating the pathobiology of wound healing, complications, such as nonhealing wounds, excessively healing wounds, and wounds with uncontrolled growth, such as tumors, are still incompletely understood.

TISSUE INJURY AND RESPONSE

Wound repair is the effort of tissues to restore normal function and structure after injury. To reform barriers to fluid loss and infection, limit further entry of foreign organisms and material, re-establish normal blood and lymphatic flow patterns, and restore the mechanical integrity of the injured system, perfect reorganization is sacrificed for the sake of urgent return to function. *Regeneration*, in contrast, is the perfect restoration of the preexisting tissue architecture in the absence of scar information. Although regeneration is the ideal in the world of wound healing, it is only found in embryonic development, in lower organisms, such as the stone crab and the salamander, or in certain tissue compartments, such as bone and liver. In wound healing in the adult human, however, the accuracy of regeneration is traded for the speed of repair. All tissues proceed through the same series of events, and for ease of understanding, these are divided into specific stages. However, these phases overlap in both time and activity.

All wounds undergo the same basic steps of repair. Acute wounds proceed in an orderly and timely reparative process to achieve sustained restoration of structure and function. The chronic wound, however, does not proceed to a restoration of functional integrity. It is stalled in the inflammatory phase owing to a variety of etiologies and does not proceed to closure.

Wound closure types are divided into *primary, secondary,* and *tertiary* repair (Fig. 8-1). *Primary,* or first-intention, closures are those wounds that are immediately sealed with simple suturing, skin graft placement, or flap closure, such as the closure of the wound at the end of a surgical procedure. Closure by *secondary,* or spontaneous, intention involves no active intent to seal the wound. Generally, this type of closure is represented by the highly contaminated wound, which will close by reepithelialization and contraction of the wound. Wound closure by *tertiary* intention is also referred to as *delayed primary closure.* A contaminated wound is initially treated with repeated débridement and perhaps systemic or topical antibiotics for several days to control infection. Once it is assessed as ready for closure, surgical intervention, such as suturing, skin graft placement, or flap design, is performed.

WOUND HEALING PHASES

The immediate response to injury is the *inflammatory* (also called *reactive*) *phase.* The body's defenses are aimed at limiting the amount of damage and preventing

Primary healing

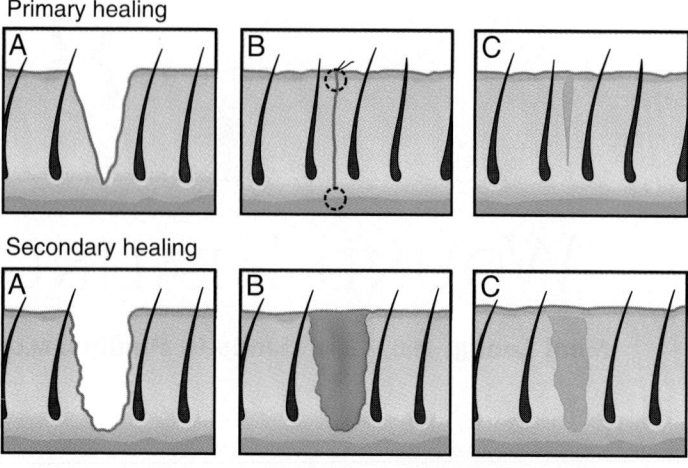

■ **FIGURE 8-1.**   Wound closure types. *Top,* Primary or first-intention closure: a clean incision is made in the tissue (**A**) and the wound edges are reapproximated (**B**) with sutures, staples, or adhesive strips. **C,** Minimal scarring is the end result. *Bottom,* Secondary intention healing: the wound is left open to heal (**A** and **B**) by a combination of contraction, granulation, and epithelialization. **C,** A large scar results.

Secondary healing

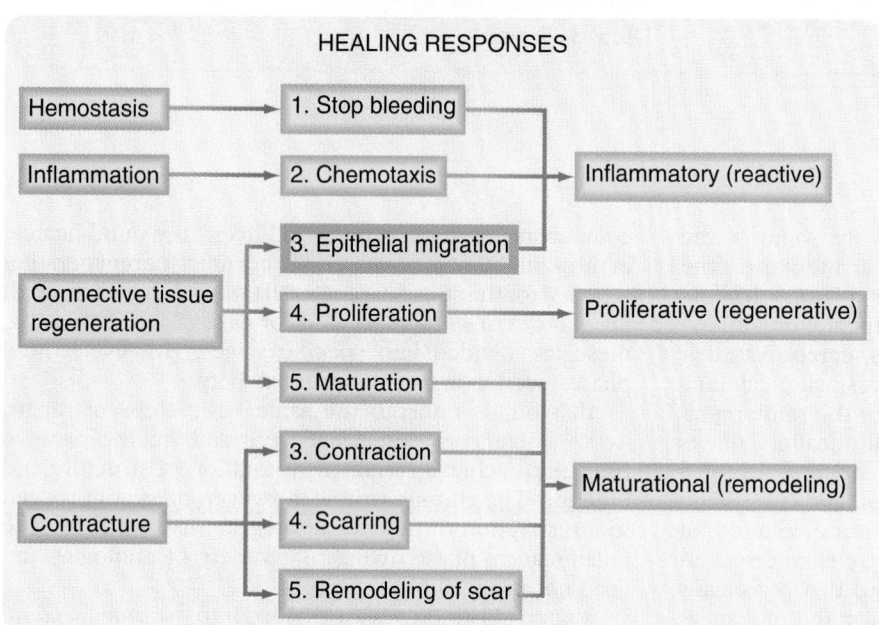

■ **FIGURE 8-2.**   Schematic diagram of the wound healing continuum.

further injury. The *proliferative* (also called *regenerative* or *reparative*) *phase* is the reparative process with reepithelialization, matrix synthesis, and neovascularization to relieve the ischemia of the trauma itself. The final *maturational* (or *remodeling*) *phase* is the period of scar contraction with collagen cross-linking, shrinking, and a loss of edema. In a large wound such as a pressure sore, the eschar or fibrinous exudate reflects the inflammatory phase; the granulation tissue is part of the proliferative phase; the contracting or advancing edge is part of the maturational phase. All three phases may occur simultaneously, and the phases with their individual processes may overlap (Fig. 8-2).

Inflammatory Phase

During the immediate reaction of the tissue to injury, hemostasis and inflammation occur. This phase represents the tissue's attempt to limit damage by stopping the bleeding, sealing the surface of the wound, and removing any necrotic tissue, foreign debris, or bacteria present. This phase is characterized by increased vascular permeability, migration of cells into the wound by chemotaxis, secretion of cytokines and growth factors into the wound, and activation of the migrating cells (Fig. 8-3).

Hemostasis and Inflammation

During tissue injury, blood vessel damage results in exposure of subendothelial collagen to platelets, leading to platelet aggregation and activation of the coagulation pathway. Initial intense local vasoconstriction of arterioles and capillaries is followed by vasodilation and increased vascular permeability. Cessation of hemorrhage is aided by plugging of capillaries with erythrocytes and platelets, which adhere to the damaged capillary endothelium. Exposure of types IV and V collagen promotes platelet

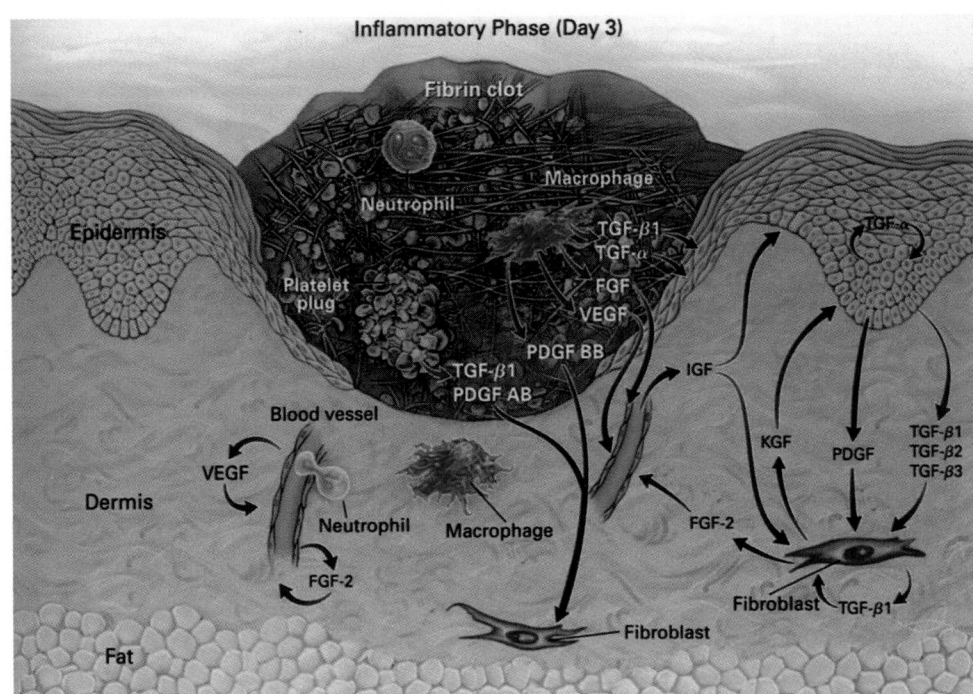

Inflammatory Phase (Day 3)

FIGURE 8-3. A cutaneous wound 3 days after injury. The cells and growth factors necessary to facilitate cell migration into the wound are shown. TGF, transforming growth factor; FGF, fibroblast growth factor; VEGF, vascular endothelial growth factor; PDGF, platelet-derived growth factor; IGF, insulin-like growth factor; KGF, keratinocyte growth factor. (From Singer AJ, Clark RAF: Mechanisms of disease: Cutaneous wound healing. N Engl J Med 341:738, 1999.)

aggregation as platelets bind to these proteins and become activated. The initial contact between platelets and collagen requires the von Willebrand factor (vWF) VIII, a heterodimeric protein synthesized by megakaryocytes and endothelial cells. Platelet adhesion to the endothelium is principally mediated through the interaction between high-affinity glycoprotein receptors and the integrin receptor GPIIb-IIIa ($\alpha_{IIb}\beta_3$). In addition, platelets express other integrin receptors that mediate direct binding of collagen ($\alpha_2\beta_1$), laminin ($\alpha_6\beta_1$), or indirectly by attaching to subendothelial matrix-bound fibronectin ($\alpha_5\beta_1$), vitronectin ($\alpha_v\beta_3$), and other ligands.[1]

Increased Vascular Permeability

Binding results in changes in platelet conformation, triggering intracellular signal transduction pathways that result in platelet activation and the release of biologically active proteins. Platelet α granules are storage organelles that contain platelet-derived growth factor (PDGF), transforming growth factor (TGF)-β, insulin-like growth factor (IGF)-1, fibronectin, fibrinogen, thrombospondin, and vWF. The dense bodies contain the vasoactive amines, such as serotonin, which cause vasodilation and increased vascular permeability. Mast cells adherent to the endothelial surface release histamine and serotonin, affecting the permeability of the endothelial cells and causing leakage of plasma from the intravascular space to the extracellular compartment. The clotting cascade is initiated through both the intrinsic and the extrinsic pathways. As the platelets become activated, the membrane phospholipids bind clotting factor V, allowing interaction with clotting factor X. Membrane-bound prothrombinase activity is generated, potentiating thrombin production exponentially. The thrombin itself activates platelets and catalyzes the formation of fibrinogen into fibrin. The

fibrin strands trap red blood cells, forming the clot, and seal the wound. The lattice framework that results will be the scaffold for endothelial cells, inflammatory cells, and fibroblasts. Thromboxane A_2 and prostaglandin $F_{2\alpha}$, formed from degradation of cell membranes in the arachidonic acid cascade, also assist with platelet aggregation and vasoconstriction. Although these activities serve to limit the amount of injury, they can also cause localized ischemia, resulting in further damage to cell membranes and release of more prostaglandin $F_{2\alpha}$ and thromboxane A_2.

Polymorphonuclear Cells (Fig. 8-4)

The release of histamine and serotonin causes vascular permeability of the capillary bed. Complement factors such as C5a and leukotriene B_4 promote neutrophil adherence and chemoattraction. In the presence of thrombin, endothelial cells exposed to leukotriene C_4 and D_4 release platelet-aggregating factor, further enhancing neutrophil adhesion. Monocytes and endothelial cells produce the inflammatory mediators interleukin (IL)-1 and tumor necrosis factor (TNF)-α, which further promote endothelial-neutrophil adherence. The increased capillary permeability and the various chemotactic factors facilitate diapedesis of neutrophils into the inflammatory site. As the neutrophils begin their migration, they release the contents of their lysosomes and enzymes such as elastase and other proteases into the extracellular matrix (ECM), facilitating the migration of the neutrophils. The combination of intense vasodilation and increased vascular permeability leads to clinical findings of inflammation, *rubor* (redness), *tumor* (swelling), *calor* (heat), and *dolor* (pain). Local tissue swelling is further promoted by the deposition of fibrin, a protein end product of coagulation, which becomes entrapped in lymphatic vessels.

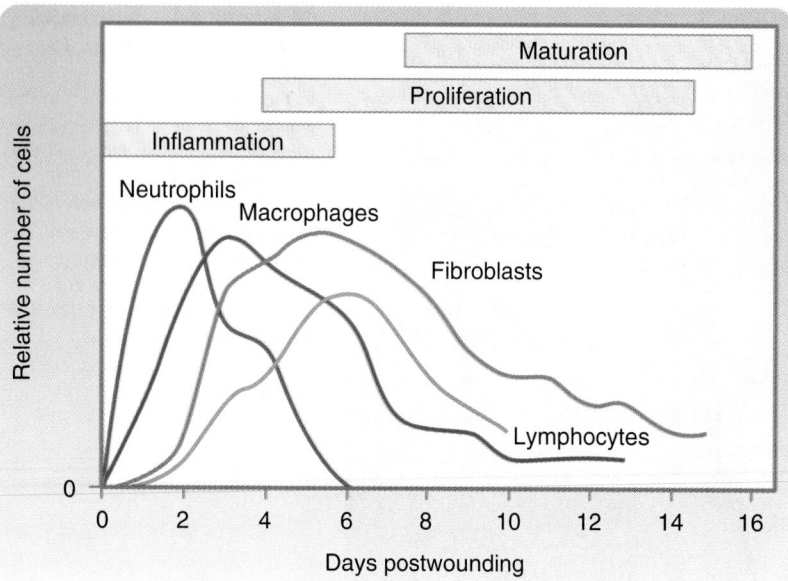

FIGURE 8-4. Time course of the appearance of the different cells in the wound during healing. Macrophages and neutrophils are predominant during the inflammatory phase (peaks at days 2 and 3, respectively). Lymphocytes appear later and peak at day 7. Fibroblasts are the predominant cells during the proliferative phase. (Modified from Witte MB, Barbul A: General principles of wound healing. Surg Clin North Am 77:512, 1997.)

There is evidence to suggest that polymorphonuclear cell (PMN) migration requires sequential adhesive and de-adhesive interactions between β_1 and β_2 integrins and ECM components.[2] *Integrin* molecules are a family of cell surface receptors that are closely coupled with the cell's cytoskeleton. These molecules serve two major functions: (1) to interact with components of the ECM, such as fibronectin, to provide adhesion and (2) to provide signal transduction to the cell interior. Integrins are crucial for cell motility and are required in inflammation and normal wound healing, as well as in embryonic development and tumor metastases. Following extravasation, PMNs, attracted by chemotaxins, migrate through the ECM by means of transient interactions between integrin receptors and their ligands. Four phases of integrin-mediated cell motility have been described: adhesion, spreading, contractility or traction, and retraction. Activation of specific integrins though ligand binding has been shown to increase cell adhesion and activate reorganization of the cell's actin cytoskeleton.[2] Spreading is characterized by the development of lamellipodia and filopodia. Traction at the leading edge of the cell develops through binding of the integrin, followed by translocation of the cell over the adherent segment of the plasma membrane. The integrin is shifted to the rear of the cell and releases its substrate, permitting cell advancement (Fig. 8-5).[2,3] Regulation of integrin function by adhesive substrates offers a mechanism for local control of migrant cells. Within the assembled framework of the ECM, binding sites for integrins have been identified on collagen, laminin, and fibronectin.[2,4]

The chemotactic agent mediates the PMN response through signal transduction, as the chemotaxin binds to receptors on the cell surface. Bacterial products such as N-formyl-methionyl-leucyl-phenylalanine bind to induce cyclic adenosine monophosphate (cAMP), but if there is maximal receptor occupancy, superoxide is produced at peak rates. Neutrophils also possess receptors for immunoglobulin G and the complement proteins C3b and

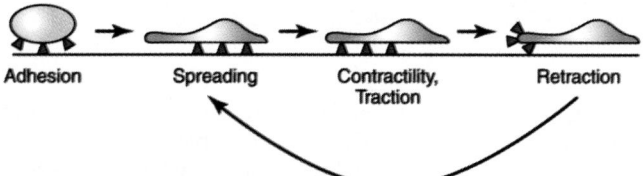

FIGURE 8-5. Schematic of a cycle of integrin-mediated cell migration. Migration is a cyclic process involving integrins at each step. Entry into the migration cycle can take place at either of the first two steps. For example, nonadherent cell types such as lymphomas and circulating carcinomas begin at the first step of attachment, whereas adherent cells such as fibroblasts and solid tumors may begin the migration cycle at the spreading step. Regardless of cell type, however, cells must maintain an attachment to the extracellular matrix once the cycle has begun. (Modified from Holly SP, Larson MK, Parise LV: Multiple roles of integrins in cell motility. Exp Cell Res 261:72, 2000.)

C3bi. As the complement cascade is released and bacteria are opsonized, these proteins bind to cell receptors on the neutrophils, allowing neutrophil recognition and phagocytosis of these bacteria. When neutrophils are stimulated, they express more of the CR1 and CR3 receptors, allowing more efficient binding and phagocytosis of these bacteria.

Functional activation occurs following migration of the PMNs into the wound site, which may induce new cell surface antigen expression, increased cytotoxicity, or increased production and release of cytokines. These activated neutrophils scavenge necrotic debris, foreign material, and bacteria. Stimulated neutrophils generate free oxygen radicals with electrons donated by the reduced form of nicotinamide adenine dinucleotide phosphate, (NADPH). The electrons are transported across the membrane into lysosomes where superoxide anion (O_2^-) is formed. Superoxide dismutase catalyzes formation of hydrogen peroxide (H_2O_2), which is then degraded by myeloperoxidase in the azurophilic

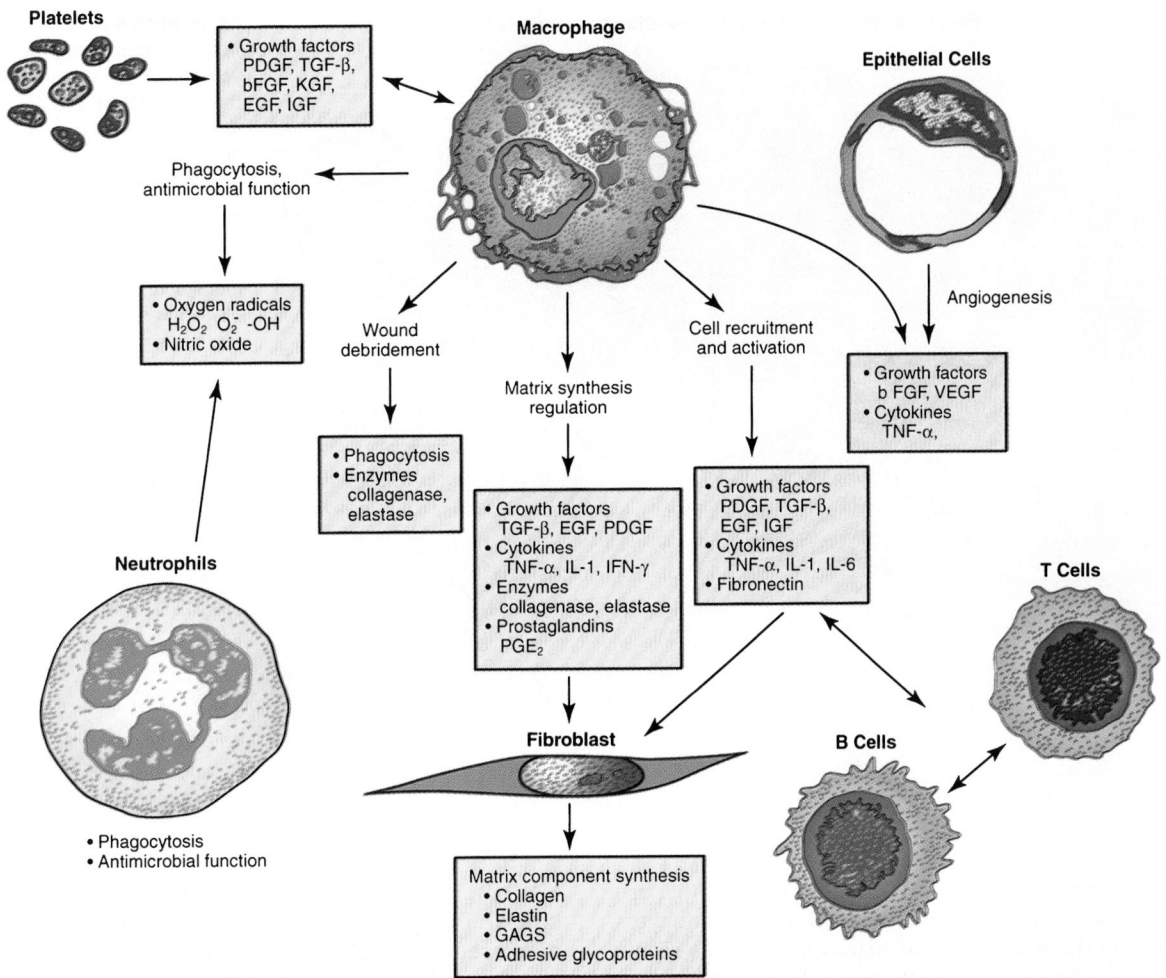

FIGURE 8-6. Interaction of cellular and humoral factors in wound healing. Note the key role of the macrophage. bFGF, basic fibroblast growth factor; EGF, epidermal growth factor; GAGs, glycosaminoglycans; IGF-1, insulin-like growth factor-1; KGF, keratinocyte growth factor; PDGF, platelet-derived growth factor; TGF-β, transforming growth factor-beta; TNF-α, tumor necrosis factor-alpha; KGF, keratinocyte growth factor; H_2O_2, hydrogen peroxide; O_2^-, superoxide; IL, interleukin; IFN-γ, interferon-gamma; PGE_2, prostaglandin E_2; VEGF, vascular endothelial growth factor. (Modified from Witte MB, Barbul A: General principles of wound healing. Surg Clin North Am 77:513, 1997.)

granules of neutrophils. This interaction oxidizes halides, forming by-products such as hypochlorous acid. The iron catalyzed reaction between H_2O_2 and O_2^- forms hydroxyl radicals (O•H). This very potent free radical is bactericidal, but it is also toxic to neutrophils and surrounding viable tissues.

Migration of PMNs stops when wound contamination has been controlled, usually within the first few days after injury. PMNs do not survive longer than 24 hours. After 24 to 48 hours, the predominance of cells in the wound cleft shifts to mononuclear cells. If wound contamination persists or secondary infection occurs, continuous activation of the complement system and other pathways provides a steady supply of chemotactic factors, resulting in a sustained influx of PMNs into the wound. Beyond delay in healing, prolonged inflammation can be deleterious in terms of destruction of normal tissue, progressing to tissue necrosis, abscess formation, and possibly systemic infection. PMNs are not essential to wound healing because their role in phagocytosis and

antimicrobial defense may be taken over by macrophages. Sterile incisions will heal normally without the presence of PMNs.

Macrophages

The macrophage is the one cell that is truly central to wound healing, serving to orchestrate the release of cytokines and stimulate many of the subsequent processes of wound healing (Fig. 8-6). Macrophages in the wound appear at the same time that neutrophils disappear. Macrophages induce PMN apoptosis. Chemotaxis of migrating blood monocytes occurs within 24 to 48 hours. Chemotactic factors specific for monocytes include bacterial products, complement degradation products (C5a), thrombin, fibronectin, collagen, TGF-β, and PGDF-BB. Monocyte chemotaxis is also facilitated by the interaction of the integrin receptors on the monocyte surface with ECM proteins, such as fibrin and fibronectin. The β integrin receptor also transduces the signal for macrophage

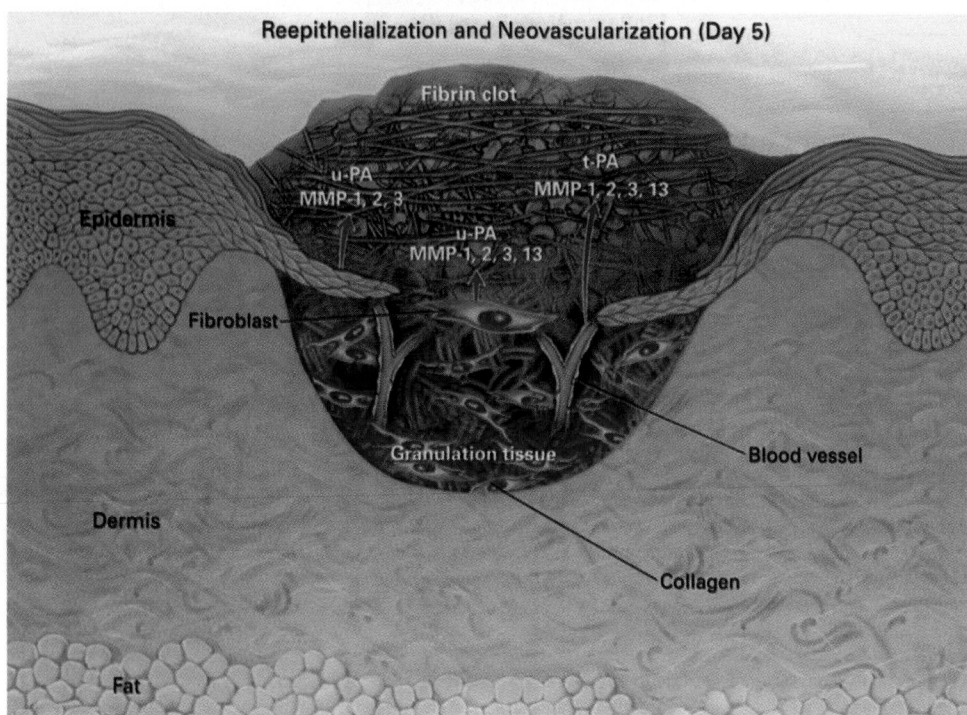

Reepithelialization and Neovascularization (Day 5)

Fibrin clot

u-PA
MMP-1, 2, 3

t-PA
MMP-1, 2, 3, 13

u-PA
MMP-1, 2, 3, 13

Epidermis

Fibroblast

Granulation tissue

Blood vessel

Dermis

Collagen

Fat

FIGURE 8-7. A cutaneous wound 5 days after injury. Blood vessels are seen sprouting into the fibrin clot as epidermal cells resurface the wound. Some of the proteinases involved in cell movement at this time point are shown. u-PA, urokinase-type plasminogen activator; MMP-1, 2, 3, and 13, matrix metalloproteinases 1, 2, 3, and 13 (collagenase 1, gelatinase A, stromelysin 1, and collagenase 3, respectively); t-PA tissue plasminogen activator. (Adapted from Singer AJ, Clark RAF: Mechanisms of disease: Cutaneous wound healing. N Engl J Med 341:738, 1999.)

phagocytic activity. Activated integrin expression promotes adhesion-mediated gene induction in monocytes, transforming them into wound macrophages; this results in increased phagocytic activity and selective messenger RNA (mRNA) expression of cytokines and signal transduction elements, including the early growth response genes *EGR2* and c-*fos*.[5] Macrophages have specific receptors for IgG (Fc-receptor), C3b (CR1 and CR3), and fibronectin (integrin receptors), which permit surface recognition of opsonized pathogens and facilitate phagocytosis.[5]

Bacterial debris, such as lipopolysaccharide, can activate the monocyte to release free radicals and cytokines that mediate angiogenesis and fibroplasia.[6] In the presence of IL-2, there is an increased release of free radicals and bactericidal activity with IL-2 potentiation of the activity of the free radicals. The free radicals cause bacterial debris that potentiates the activation of the monocyte. Activated wound macrophages also produce nitric oxide, which has been demonstrated to have many functions other than antimicrobial properties.

As the monocyte or macrophage is activated, phospholipase is induced, causing enzymatic degradation of the cell membrane phospholipids, releasing thromboxane A_2 and prostaglandin $F_{2\alpha}$. The macrophage also releases leukotrienes B_4 and C_4 and 15- and 5-hydroxyeicosatetraenoic acid. Leukotriene B_4 is a potent chemotaxin for neutrophils and increases their adherence to endothelial cells.

Wound macrophages release proteinases, including matrix metalloproteinases (MMP-1, MMP-2, MMP-3, and

MMP-9) (Fig. 8-7),[5] which degrade the ECM and are crucial for removing foreign material, promoting cell movement through tissue spaces, and regulating ECM turnover. For example, macrophages secrete collagenase when activated by bacterial degradation byproducts such as lipopolysaccharide or activated lymphocytes. This activity is dependent on the cAMP pathway and thus can be blocked by nonsteroidal anti-inflammatory or glucocorticoid drugs. Colchicine and retinoic acid appear to decrease collagenase production as well.

Macrophages secrete numerous cytokines and growth factors (Tables 8-1 and 8-2). IL-1, a proinflammatory cytokine, is an acute-phase-response cytokine. In experimental wound models, IL-1 levels become detectable within the first 24 hours, peak between 72 hours, and then rapidly decline throughout the first week. This endogenous pyrogen causes lymphocyte activation and stimulation of the hypothalamus, inducing the febrile response. It also directly affects hemostasis by causing release of vasodilators and stimulating coagulation. IL-1's effect is further amplified as the endothelial cells produce it in the presence of TNF-α and endotoxin. IL-1 has numerous effects: enhancement of collagenase production, stimulation of cartilage degradation and bone reabsorption, neutrophil activation, adhesion molecule regulation, and promotion of chemotaxis. It promotes other cells to secrete proinflammatory cytokines. IL-1's effects also extend into the proliferative phase, increasing fibroblast and keratinocyte growth and collagen synthesis.

TABLE 8-1. Cytokine Activity in Wound Healing

Cytokine	Cell Source	Biological Activity
Proinflammatory Cytokines		
TNF-α	Macrophages	PMN margination and cytotoxicity, $\pm$ collagen synthesis; provides metabolic substrate
IL-1	Macrophages Keratinocytes	Fibroblast and keratinocyte chemotaxis, collagen synthesis
IL-2	T lymphocytes	Increases fibroblast infiltration and metabolism
IL-6	Macrophages PMNs Fibroblasts	Fibroblast proliferation, hepatic acute-phase protein synthesis
IL-8	Macrophages Fibroblasts	Macrophage and PMN chemotaxis, keratinocyte maturation
IFN-γ	T lymphocytes Macrophages	Macrophage and PMN activation; retards collagen synthesis and cross-linking; stimulates collagenase activity
Anti-inflammatory Cytokines		
IL-4	T lymphocytes Basophils Mast cells	Inhibition of TNF, IL-1, IL-6 production; fibroblast proliferation, collagen synthesis
IL-10	T lymphocytes Macrophages Keratinocytes	Inhibition of TNF, IL-1, IL-6 production; inhibits macrophage and PMN activation

TNF, tumor necrosis factor; IL, interleukin; IFN-γ, interferon-γ; PMNs, polymorphonuclear leukocytes.
From Rumalla VK, Borah GL: Cytokines, growth factors, and plastic surgery. Plast Reconstr Surg 108:719-733, 2001.

TABLE 8-2. Cytokines that Affect Wound Healing

Cytokine	Abbreviation	Source	Functions
Platelet-derived growth factor	PDGF	Platelets, macrophages, endothelial cells, keratinocytes	Chemotactic for PMNs, macrophages, fibroblasts, and smooth muscle cells; activates PMNs, macrophages, and fibroblasts; mitogenic for fibroblasts, endothelial cells; stimulates production of MMPs, fibronectin, and HA; stimulates angiogenesis and wound contraction; remodeling
Transforming growth factor-beta (including isoforms β_1, β_2, and β_3)	TGF-β	Platelets, T lymphocytes, macrophages, endothelial cells, keratinocytes, fibroblasts	Chemotactic for PMNs, macrophages, lymphocytes, fibroblasts; stimulates TIMP synthesis, keratinocyte migration, angiogenesis, and fibroplasia; inhibits production of MMPs and keratinocyte proliferation; induces TGF-β production
Epidermal growth factor	EGF	Platelets, macrophages	Mitogenic for keratinocytes and fibroblasts; stimulates keratinocyte migration
Transforming growth factor-alpha	TGF-α	Macrophages, T lymphocytes, keratinocytes	Similar to EGF
Fibroblast growth factor-1 and -2 family	FGF	Macrophages, mast cells, T lymphocytes, endothelial cells, fibroblasts	Chemotactic for fibroblasts; mitogenic for fibroblasts and keratinocytes; stimulates keratinocyte migration, angiogenesis, wound contraction, and matrix deposition
Keratinocyte growth factor (also called FGF-7)	KGF	Fibroblasts	Stimulates keratinocyte migration, proliferation, and differentiation
Insulin-like growth factor	IGF-1	Macrophages, fibroblasts	Stimulates synthesis of sulfated proteoglycans, collagen, keratinocyte migration, and fibroblast proliferation; endocrine effects similar to those of growth hormone
Vascular endothelial cell growth factor	VEGF	Keratinocytes	Increases vasopermeability; mitogenic for endothelial cells

HA, hyaluronic acid; MMPs, matrix metalloproteinases; PMNs, polymorphonuclear leukocytes; TIMP, tissue inhibitor of matrix metalloproteinase.
Modified from Schwartz SI (ed): Principles of Surgery, 7th ed. New York, McGraw-Hill, 1999, p 269.

Studies have demonstrated increased levels of IL-1 in chronic nonhealing wounds, suggesting its role in the pathogenesis of poor wound healing.[7,8] The early beneficial responses of IL-1 in wound healing appear to be maladaptive if elevated levels last beyond the first week after injury.

Microbial by-products induce macrophages to release TNF (previously called *cachectin*). TNF-α is crucial in initiating the response to injury or bacteria. TNF is chemotactic for the cellular components of inflammation. It upregulates cell surface adhesion molecules that promote the interaction of immune cells and endothelium. TNF-α is detected in the wound within 12 hours after wounding and peaks after 72 hours.[9] Its effects include hemostasis, increased vascular permeability, and increased endothelial proliferation. Like IL-1, TNF-α induces fever, increased collagenase production, cartilage and bone reabsorption, and release of PDGF, as well as the production of more IL-1. Excessive production of TNF-α, however, has been associated with multisystem organ failure and increased morbidity and mortality in inflammatory disease states, partly through its effects on activating macrophages and neutrophils. Recent studies have observed elevated levels of TNF-α in nonhealing versus healing chronic venous ulcers.[7,10] Thus, as in the case of IL-1, TNF-α appears to be essential in the early inflammatory response required for wound healing, but its local and systemic persistence may lead to impaired wound maturation.

IL-6, which is produced by monocytes and macrophages, is involved in stem cell growth, activation of B and T cells, and hepatic acute-phase protein synthesis regulation. Within acute wounds, IL-6 is also secreted by PMNs and fibroblasts, and its rise parallels the increase in PMN count locally.[11] IL-6 is detectable within 12 hours of experimental wounding and may persist at high concentrations for longer than a week.[12] It also works synergistically with IL-1, TNF-α, and endotoxins. It is a potent stimulator of fibroblast proliferation that is decreased in aging fibroblasts and fetal wounds.[13]

Another important proinflammatory cytokine following injury is IL-8. IL-8 is secreted primarily by macrophages and fibroblasts in the acute wound with peak expression within the first 24 hours.[14,15] Its major effects include increased PMN and monocyte chemotaxis, PMN degranulation, and expression of endothelial cell adhesion molecules. In vitro experiments on the effect of recombinant human (rh) IL-8 revealed increased keratinocyte proliferation with an increased number of cells in S phase and the overexpression of the integrin subunit α_6.[16] In vivo, topically applied IL-8 on human skin grafts in a chimeric mouse model enhanced re-epithelialization over controls due to elevated numbers of mitotic keratinocytes.[16] In contrast, other investigators found that IL-8 levels were elevated in delayed human burn wound healing and appeared to inhibit keratinocyte replication.[17] These findings suggest that IL-8 may have a role in keratinocyte maturation but that excess levels may be detrimental.

Interferon (IFN)-γ, another proinflammatory cytokine, is secreted by T lymphocytes and macrophages. Its major effects are macrophage and PMN activation and increased cytotoxicity. It has also been shown to reduce local

wound contraction and aid in tissue remodeling. IFN-γ has been used in the treatment of hypertrophic and keloid scars, possibly by its effect in slowing collagen production and cross-linking while collagenase (MMP-1) production increases.[18] Experimentally, however, it has been shown to impair re-epithelialization and wound strength in a dose-dependent manner when applied either locally or systemically. These findings suggest that IFN-γ administration may improve scar hypertrophy by decreasing the strength of the wound.

Macrophages also release growth factors that stimulate fibroblast, endothelial cell, and keratinocyte proliferation and are important in the proliferative phase (see Table 8-2). Macrophage-secreted PDGF stimulates collagen and proteoglycan synthesis. PDGF exists as three isomers—PDGF-AA, PDGF-AB, and PDGF-BB; however, the PDGF-BB isomer is the only U.S. Food and Drug Administration (FDA)-approved growth factor preparation and is the most widely studied clinically. Topical application of recombinant PDGF improved wound breaking strength and healing time in both human and murine models of acute wounding.[19,20] The administration of PDGF-BB improved wound closure in chronic and diabetic nonhealing ulcers in both humans and rodents but did not have the same effect in steroid-treated animals.[21]

TGF-α and TGF-β are both released by activated monocytes. TGF-α stimulates epidermal growth and angiogenesis. TGF-β itself stimulates the monocytes to express other peptides such as TGF-α, IL-1, and PDGF. TGF-β, which is also released by platelets and fibroblasts within wounds, exists as at least three isomers—$\beta1$, $\beta2$, and $\beta3$—and its effects include fibroblast migration, maturation, and ECM synthesis. TGF-$\beta1$ has been shown to play an important role in collagen metabolism and healing of gastrointestinal injuries and anastomoses.[22] In experimental models, TGF-$\beta1$ accelerated wound healing in normal, steroid-impaired, and irradiated animals. TGF-β is the most potent stimulant of fibroplasia, and its potent fibroblast mitogenic effects have been implicated in the fibrogenesis seen in disease states such as scleroderma and interstitial pulmonary fibrosis. Enhanced expression of TGF-$\beta1$ mRNA is found in both keloid and hypertrophic scars.[18] In contrast, fetal wounds have been demonstrated to have a paucity of TGF-β, suggesting that the scarless repair seen in utero occurs because of low or absent amounts of TGF-β.[23] Studies of the three isomers suggest that although TGF-$\beta1$ and TGF-$\beta2$ play an important role in tissue fibrosis and post-injury scarring, TGF-$\beta3$ may limit scarring.[24] As the concentration of TGF-β rises in the inflammatory site, the fibroblasts are directly stimulated to produce collagen and fibronectin, thus leading into the proliferative phase.

Lymphocytes

T lymphocytes appear in significant numbers in the wound at around the 5th day, with a peak occurring at around the 7th day. B lymphocytes do not appear to play a significant role in wound healing but appear to be involved in downregulating healing as the wound closes.[25] Lymphocytes exert most of their effects on fibroblasts by producing stimulatory cytokines, such as IL-2 and fibroblast activating factor, and inhibitory ones, such as TGF-β, TNF-α, and IFN-γ.[26] Initially, lymphocytes were thought to play a minimal role in acute wound healing, particularly in the absence of excessive inflammation. The macrophage processes foreign debris such as bacteria or enzymatically degraded host proteins and serves as an antigen-presenting cell to the lymphocytes. This interaction stimulates lymphocyte proliferation and cytokine release. T cells produce IFN-γ, which stimulates the macrophage to release a cascade of cytokines including TNF-α and IL-1. IFN-γ also causes decreased synthesis of prostaglandins, which enhances the effect of inflammatory mediators. In addition, IFN-γ also suppresses collagen synthesis and inhibits macrophages from leaving the site of injury. Thus, IFN-γ appears to be an important mediator of the chronic nonhealing wound and its presence suggests that T lymphocytes are primarily involved in chronic wound healing.

Recent studies, however, question the belief that lymphocytes are not essential for acute wound healing. Drugs that suppress T-lymphocyte function and proliferation, such as steroids and immunosuppressive agents (cyclosporine and tacrolimus), have been found to result in impaired wound healing in experimental wound models, possibly through decreased nitric oxide synthesis. In vivo lymphocyte depletion suggests the existence of an incompletely characterized T-cell lymphocyte population that is neither CD4+ nor CD8+ and that it is this subset that seems to be responsible for the promotion of wound healing.[27]

Proliferative Phase

As the acute responses of hemostasis and inflammation begin to resolve, the scaffolding is laid for repair of the wound with angiogenesis, fibroplasia, and epithelialization. This stage is characterized by the formation of granulation tissue, consisting of a capillary bed, fibroblasts, macrophages, a loose arrangement of collagen, fibronectin, and hyaluronic acid.

Multiple studies have used growth factors to modify granulation tissue, particularly fibroplasia. Adenoviral transfer, topical application, or subcutaneous injection of PDGF, TGF-β, keratinocyte growth factor (KGF), vascular endothelial growth factor (VEGF), and epidermal growth factor (EGF) have been tested to increase granulation tissue proliferation.[28-30]

Angiogenesis

Angiogenesis is the process of new blood vessel formation and is necessary to support a healing wound environment. Following injury, activated endothelial cells degrade the basement membrane of postcapillary venules, allowing migration of cells through this gap. Division of these migrating endothelial cells results in tubule or lumen formation. Eventually, deposition of the basement membrane occurs, resulting in capillary maturation.

Following injury, the endothelium is exposed to numerous soluble factors and comes in contact with adhering blood cells. These interactions result in the upregulation of the expression of cell surface adhesion molecules, such as vascular cell surface adhesion molecule (VCAM)-1. Matrix-degrading enzymes, such as plasmin and the metalloproteinases, are released and activated, degrading the endothelial basement membrane. Fragmentation of the basement membrane allows endothelial cell migration into the wound, promoted by fibroblast growth factor (FGF), PDGF, and TGF-β. Injured endothelial cells express adhesion molecules, such as the integrin $\alpha_v\beta_3$, which facilitates attachment to fibrin, fibronectin, and fibrinogen and thus facilitates endothelial cell migration along the provisional matrix scaffold. Platelet endothelial cell adhesion molecule (PECAM)-1, also found on endothelial cells, modulates their interaction with each other as they migrate into the wound.[5]

Capillary tube formation is a complex process involving cell-cell and cell-matrix interactions, modulated by adhesion molecules on endothelial cell surfaces. PECAM-1 has been observed to mediate cell-cell contact, whereas β_1 integrin receptors may aid in stabilizing these contacts and forming tight junctions between endothelial cells. Some of the new capillaries differentiate into arterioles and venules, whereas others undergo involution and apoptosis, with ingestion by macrophages.[5] The regulation of endothelial apoptosis is not well understood.[31,32]

Angiogenesis appears to be stimulated and manipulated by a variety of cytokines, predominantly produced by macrophages and platelets. As the macrophage produces TNF-α, it orchestrates angiogenesis during the inflammatory phase. Heparin, which can stimulate the migration of capillary endothelial cells, binds with high affinity to a group of angiogenic factors. VEGF, a membrane of the PDGF family of growth factors, has potent angiogenic activity. It is produced in large amounts by keratinocytes, macrophages, and fibroblasts during wound healing. Cell disruption and hypoxia, hallmarks of tissue injury, appear to be strong initial inducers of potent angiogenic factors at the wound site, such as VEGF and its receptor.

Both acidic and basic FGFs, or FGF-1 and -2, released from disrupted parenchymal cells, are early stimulants of angiogenesis. FGF-2 provides the initial angiogenic stimulus within the first 3 days of wound repair, followed by a subsequent prolonged stimulus mediated by VEGF from days 4 through 7.[33] There is a dose-dependent effect of VEGF and FGF-2 on angiogenesis.[33,34] Recent investigations to develop collateral circulation by introduction of VEGF and FGF-2 or their genes have shown promise in preclinical models and even in clinical trials. Both TGF-α and EGF stimulate endothelial cell proliferation. TNF-α is chemotactic for endothelial cells and promotes formation of the capillary tube. Recent work suggests that TNF may mediate angiogenesis through its induction of hypoxia-inducible factor (HIF)-1.[35] It regulates the expression of other hypoxia-responsive genes, including inducible nitric oxide (NO) synthase, and VEGF. HIF-1α mRNA is prominently present in wound inflammatory cells during the initial 24 hours and HIF-1α protein is present in wound cells isolated from the wound 1 and 5 days after injury in vitro.[35] Data also suggest that there is a positive interaction between endogenous NO and VEGF with endogenous

NO-enhancing VEGF synthesis.[36] Similarly, VEGF has been shown to promote NO synthesis in angiogenesis, suggesting that NO mediates aspects of VEGF signaling required for endothelial cell proliferation and organization. An in vivo study of NO on wound healing examining the effect of the NO synthase inhibitor aminoguanidine in murine burn wounds demonstrated that epithelial proliferation, collagen formation, and granulation tissue with rich capillaries were greater in the control group compared to the group that received aminoguanidine intraperitoneally.[37]

TGF-β is a chemoattractant for fibroblasts and probably assists angiogenesis by signaling the fibroblast to produce the FGFs. Other factors that have been shown to induce angiogenesis include angiogenin, IL-8, and lactic acid.[38,39] Several of the matrix materials, such as fibronectin and hyaluronic acid from the wound site, are angiogenic. Fibronectin and fibrin are produced by macrophages and damaged endothelial cells. Collagen appears to interact by causing tubular formation of endothelial cells in vitro. The complex interaction of ECM material and cytokines causes angiogenesis.

Fibroplasia

Fibroblasts are specialized cells that differentiate from resting mesenchymal cells in connective tissue; they do not arrive in the wound cleft by diapedesis from circulating cells. After injury, the normally quiescent and sparse fibroblasts are chemoattracted to the inflammatory site, where they divide and produce the components of the ECM. After stimulation by macrophage and platelet-derived cytokines and growth factors, the fibroblast, which is normally arrested in the G_0 phase, undergoes replication and proliferation. Platelet-derived TGF-β stimulates fibroblast proliferation indirectly, by releasing PDGF. The fibroblast can also stimulate replication in an autocrine manner by releasing FGF-2. To continue proliferating, fibroblasts require further stimulation by factors such as EGF or IGF-1.[40] Although fibroblasts require growth factors for proliferation, they do not need growth factors to survive. Fibroblasts can live quiescently in growth factor–free media in either monolayers or three-dimensional cultures.[41]

The primary function of fibroblasts is to synthesize collagen that they begin to produce during the cellular phase of inflammation. The time required for undifferentiated mesenchymal cells to differentiate into highly specialized fibroblasts accounts for the delay between injury and the appearance of collagen in a healing wound. This period, generally 3 to 5 days depending on the type of tissue injured, is called the *lag phase* of wound healing. Fibroblasts begin to migrate in response to chemotactic substances, such as growth factors (PDGF, TGF-β), C5 fragments, thrombin, TNF-α, eicosanoids, elastin fragments, leukotriene B₄, and fragments of collagen and fibronectin.[5]

Collagen synthesis rates decline after 4 weeks, eventually balancing the rate of collagen destruction by collagenase (MMP-1). At this point, the wound enters a phase of collagen maturation. The maturation phase continues for months or even years. Glycoproteins and mucopolysaccharide levels decrease during the maturation phase, and new capillaries regress and disappear. These changes alter the appearance of the wound and increase its strength.

Epithelialization

The epidermis serves as a physical barrier to prevent fluid loss and bacterial invasion. Tight cell junctions within the epithelium contribute to its impermeability while the basement membrane zone gives structural support and attachment between the epidermis and the dermis. The basement membrane zone consists of several layers: (1) the lamina lucida (electron clear), consisting of laminin and heparan sulfate; (2) lamina densa (electron dense), containing type IV collagen; and (3) anchoring fibrils, consisting of type IV collagen, that secure the epidermodermal interface and connect from the lamina densa into the dermis. The basal layer of the epidermis attaches to the basement membrane zone by hemidesmosomes. Re-epithelialization of wounds begins within hours after injury. Initially, the wound is rapidly sealed by clot formation and then by epithelial (epidermal) cell migration across the defect. Keratinocytes located at the basal layer of the residual epidermis or in the depths of epithelium-lined dermal appendages migrate to resurface the wound. Epithelialization involves a sequence of changes in wound keratinocytes: detachment, migration, proliferation, differentiation, and stratification. If the basement membrane zone is intact, epithelialization proceeds more rapidly. The cells are stimulated to migrate. Attachments to neighboring and adjoining cells and to the dermis are loosened as demonstrated by intracellular tonofilament retraction, dissolution of intercellular desmosomes and hemidesmosomes linking the epidermis to the basement membrane, and formation of cytoplasmic actin filaments.[5] Epidermal cells express integrin receptors that allow them to interact with ECM proteins, such as fibronectin. The migrating cells dissect the wound, separating the desiccated eschar from the viable tissue. This path of dissection is determined by the integrins that the epidermal cells express on their cell membranes.[42] Degradation of the ECM, which is required if the epidermal cells are to migrate between the collagenous dermis and fibrin eschar, is driven by epidermal cell production of collagenase (MMP-1) and plasminogen activator,[43] which activates collagenase and plasmin. The migrating cells are also phagocytic, removing debris in their path. Cells behind the leading edge of migrating cells begin to proliferate. The epithelial cells move in a leapfrog and tumbling fashion[5] until the edges establish contact. If the basement membrane zone is not intact, it will be repaired first. The absence of neighbor cells at the wound margin may be a signal for the migration and proliferation of epidermal cells. Local release of EGF, TGF-α, and KGF and increased expression of their receptors may also stimulate these processes.[40] Topical application of KGF-2 in both young and aged animals accelerated re-epithelialization.[29] Basement membrane proteins, such as laminin, reappear in a highly ordered sequence from the margin of the wound inward. After the wound is completely re-epithelialized, the cells become

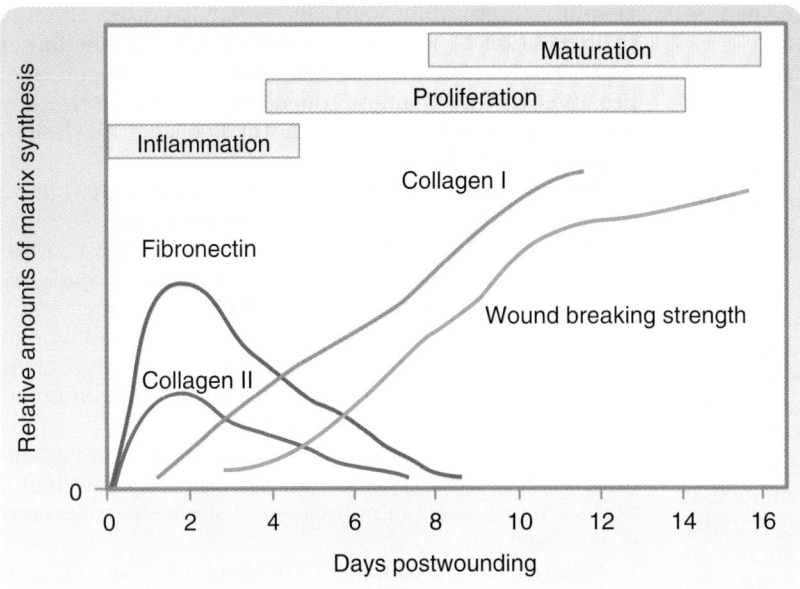

FIGURE 8-8. Wound matrix deposition over time. Fibronectin and type III collagen constitute the early matrix. Type I collagen accumulates later and corresponds to the increase in wound-breaking strength. (Adapted from Witte MB, Barbul A: General principles of wound healing. Surg Clin North Am 77:515, 1997.)

columnar and stratified again, while firmly attaching to the re-established basement membrane and underlying dermis.

Extracellular Matrix (Fig. 8-8)

The ECM exists as a scaffold to stabilize the physical structure of tissues but also plays an active and complex role by regulating the behavior of the cells that contact it. Cells within it produce the macromolecular constituents, including (1) glycosaminoglycans (GAGs), polysaccharide chains, usually found covalently linked to protein in the form of proteoglycans; and (2) fibrous proteins, such as collagen, elastin, fibronectin, and laminin.[44]

In connective tissue, proteoglycan molecules form a gel-like "ground substance." This highly hydrated gel allows the matrix to withstand compressive forces while permitting the rapid diffusion of nutrients, metabolites, and hormones between the blood and the tissue cells. Collagen fibers within the matrix serve to organize and strengthen it, whereas elastin fibers give it resilience and matrix proteins have adhesive functions.[44]

The wound matrix accumulates, changing in composition as healing progresses, balanced between new deposition and degradation. The provisional matrix is a scaffold for cellular migration composed of fibrin, fibrinogen, fibronectin, and vitronectin. GAGs and proteoglycans are synthesized next, supporting further matrix deposition and remodeling. Collagens, which are the predominant scar proteins, are the end result.[6] Attachment proteins, such as fibrin and fibronectin, provide linkage to the ECM through binding to cell surface integrin receptors.

Stimulation of fibroblasts by growth factors induces upregulated expression of the integrin receptors, facilitating cell-matrix interactions. Ligand binding induces integrin clustering into "focal adhesion sites."[45] The regulation of integrin-mediated cell signaling by the extracellular divalent cations Mg^{2+}, Mn^{2+}, and Ca^{2+} is

perhaps due to induction of conformational changes in the integrins.[4]

A dynamic and reciprocal relationship exists between the fibroblasts and the ECM. Cytokine regulation of fibroblast responses is altered by variations in the composition of the ECM. For example, the expression of matrix-degrading enzymes, such as the MMPs, is upregulated after cytokine stimulation of fibroblasts. Collagenolytic MMP-1 is induced by IL-1 and downregulated by TGF-β.[5] Plasminogen activator activates plasminogen to plasmin; plasmin activates procollagenase into collagenase. This results in matrix degradation and facilitates cell migration. Modulation of these processes provides additional mechanisms by which cell-matrix interaction can be regulated during wound healing. Matrix modulation is also seen in tumor metastasis. Neoplastic cells lose anchorage dependence, which is mediated mainly by integrins and is probably due to the decreased production of fibronectin and the subsequent decreased adhesion, allowing these cells to break away from the primary tumor and metastasize.

An example of the necessary dynamic interactions occurring in the provisional matrix during wound healing is the effect of TGF-β on incisional wounds sealed with fibrin sealant. Fibrin sealant is a derivative of plasma components that mimics the last step in the coagulation cascade. Commercially available fibrin sealant has an approximately 10-fold greater concentration of fibrin than in plasma and as a result provides a more airtight, waterproof seal. Fibrin sealant may serve as a mechanical barrier to the early cell-mediated events occurring in wound healing. Supplementation of fibrin sealant with TGF-β has been demonstrated to reverse the inhibitory effects of fibrin sealant on wound healing and increases tensile strength compared to sutured wounds.[46] The increased tensile strength may be a result of improved cell migration into the wound site, more rapid clearance of fibrin sealant, suppression of gelatinase (MMP-9), and enhancement of ECM synthesis in the TGF-β-supplemented wounds.

Collagen Structure

Collagens are found in all multicellular animals and are secreted by a variety of cell types. They are a major component of skin and bone and constitute 25% of the total protein mass in mammals. The proline and glycine-rich collagen molecule is a long, stiff, triple-stranded helical structure, and comprises three collagen polypeptide α chains wound around one another in a ropelike superhelix. With its ringlike structure, proline provides stability to the helical conformation in each α chain, whereas glycine, because of its small size, allows tight packing of the three alpha chains to form the final superhelix. There are at least 20 types of collagen; the main constituents of connective tissue are types I, II, II, V, and XI. Type I is the principal collagen of skin and bone and is the most common.[44] In the adult, the skin is approximately 80% type I and 20% type III. In newborns, the content of type III collagen is greater than that found in the adult. In early wound healing, there is also an increased expression of type III collagen.[47] Type I collagens are the fibrillar collagens, or the fibril-forming collagens. They are secreted into the extracellular space where they assemble into collagen fibrils (10 to 300 nm in diameter), which then aggregate into larger, cablelike bundles called collagen fibers (several micrometers in diameter).

Other types of collagens include types IX and XII (fibril-associated collagens) and types IV and VII (network-forming collagens). Types IX and XII are found on the surface of the collagen fibrils and serve to link the fibrils to one another and to other components in the ECM. Type IV molecules assemble into a meshlike pattern and are a major part of the mature basal lamina. Dimers of type VII form anchoring fibrils, which help attach the basal lamina to the underlying connective tissue and are especially abundant in the skin.

Type XVII and XVIII collagens are two of a number of "collagen-like" proteins. Type XVII has a transmembrane domain and is found in hemidesmosomes. Type XVIII is located in the basal laminae of blood vessels. The peptide endostatin, which inhibits angiogenesis and shows promise as an anticancer drug, is formed by the cleavage of the C-terminal domain of type XVIII collagen.[48]

Collagen Synthesis (Figs. 8-9 and 8-10)

Collagen polypeptide chains are synthesized on membrane-bound ribosomes and enter the endoplasmic reticulum (ER) lumen as proalpha chains. These precursors have amino-terminal signal peptides to direct them to the ER as well as propeptides at both N- and C-terminal ends. Within the lumen of the ER, some of the prolines and lysines undergo hydroxylation, forming hydroxyproline and hydroxylysine. Hydroxylation results in the stable triple-stranded helix through the formation of interchain hydrogen bonds. The proalpha chain then combines with two others to form procollagen that is a hydrogen-bonded, triple-stranded helical molecule. In conditions such as

vitamin C (ascorbic acid) deficiency (scurvy), proline hydroxylation is prevented, resulting in the formation of unstable triple helices secondary to synthesis of defective proalpha chains. Vitamin C deficiency is characterized by the gradual loss of preexisting normal collagen, leading to fragile blood vessels and loose teeth.

After secretion into the ECM, specific proteases cleave the propeptides of the procollagen molecules, forming collagen monomers. These monomers assemble to form collagen fibrils in the ECM, driven by collagen's tendency to self-assemble. Covalent cross-linking of the lysine residues provides tensile strength. The extent and type of cross-linking varies from tissue to tissue. In tissues such as tendons where tensile strength is crucial, collagen cross-linking is extremely high. In mammalian skin, the fibrils are organized in a basket-weave pattern to resist multidirectional tensile stress. In tendons, on the other hand, fibrils are in parallel bundles aligned along the major axis of tension.[6,44,47]

Multiple factors can affect collagen synthesis. Vitamin C (ascorbic acid), TGF-β, IGF-1, and IGF-2 increase collagen synthesis.[40] IFN-γ decreases type I procollagen mRNA synthesis, and glucocorticoids inhibit procollagen gene transcription, leading to decreased collagen synthesis.[49,50]

Several genetic disorders are caused by abnormalities in collagen fibril formation. In *osteogenesis imperfecta*, deletion of one procollagen α_1 allele results in weak and easily fractured bones. Ehlers-Danlos syndrome is a result of mutations affecting type III collagen and is characterized by fragile skin and blood vessels and hypermobile joints.

Elastic Fibers

Tissues such as skin, blood vessels, and lungs require strength and elasticity to function. Elastic fibers in the ECM of these tissues provide the resilience to allow for recoil after transient stretch.

Elastic fibers are predominantly composed of elastin, a highly hydrophobic protein (about 750 amino acids long). Soluble tropoelastin is secreted into the extracellular space where it forms lysine cross-links to other tropoelastin molecules to generate a large network of elastin fibers and sheets. Elastin is composed of hydrophobic and alanine- and lysine-rich α-helical segments that alternate along the polypeptide chain. The hydrophobic segments are responsible for the molecule's elastic properties. The alanine- and lysine-rich α-helical segments form cross-links between adjacent molecules. Although the proposed conformation of elastin molecules is controversial, the predominant theory is that the elastin polypeptide chain adopts a "random coil" conformation that allows the network to stretch and recoil like a rubber band.[51] Elastic fibers consist of an elastin core covered with a sheath of microfibrils, which are composed of several distinct glycoproteins, such as fibrillin. Elastin-binding fibrillin is essential for the integrity of the elastic fibers.

Microfibrils appear before elastin in developing tissues and seem to form a scaffold on which the secreted elastin molecules are deposited. Elastin is produced early in life, stabilizes, and does not undergo much further synthesis

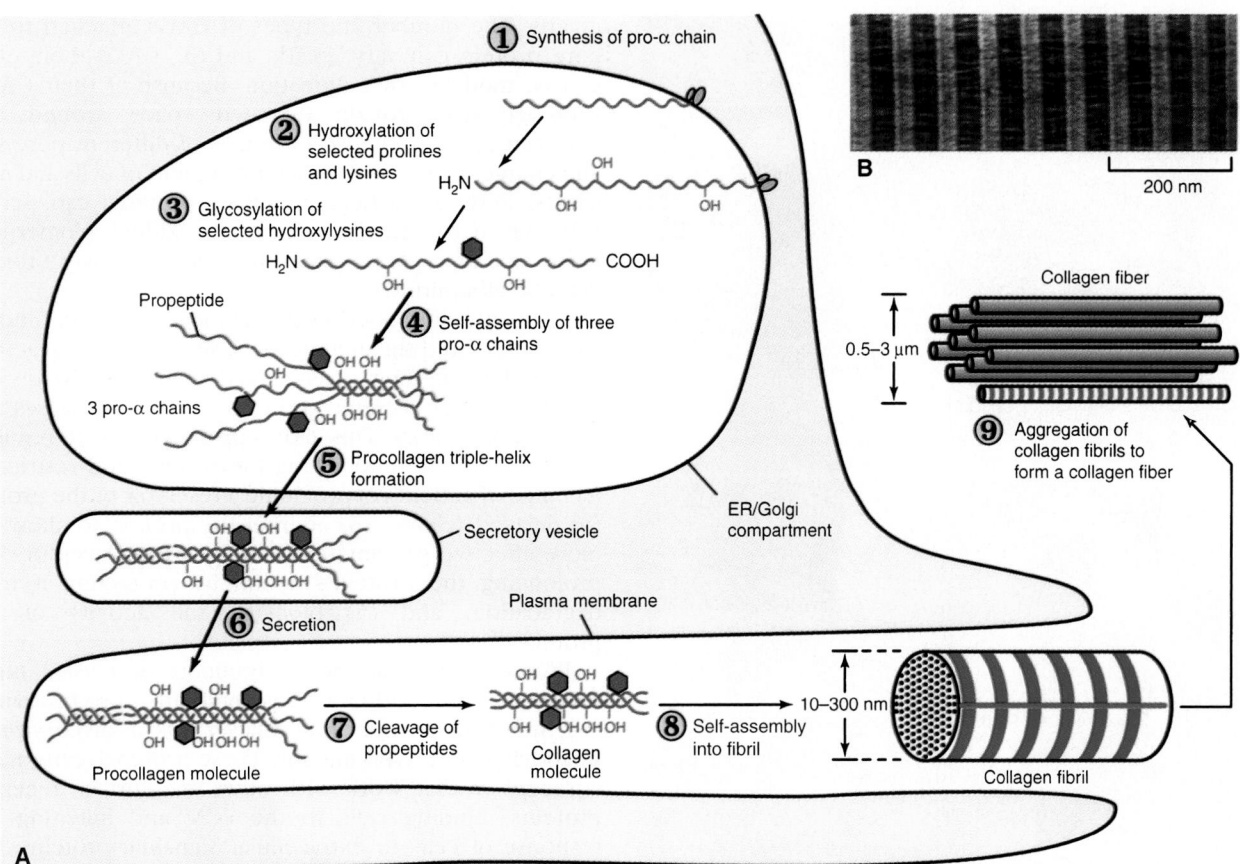

① Synthesis of pro-α chain

② Hydroxylation of selected prolines and lysines

③ Glycosylation of selected hydroxylysines

Propeptide

3 pro-α chains

④ Self-assembly of three pro-α chains

⑤ Procollagen triple-helix formation

Secretory vesicle

⑥ Secretion

Procollagen molecule

⑦ Cleavage of propeptides

Collagen molecule

⑧ Self-assembly into fibril

ER/Golgi compartment

Plasma membrane

10–300 nm

Collagen fibril

B   200 nm

Collagen fiber

0.5–3 μm

⑨ Aggregation of collagen fibrils to form a collagen fiber

A

FIGURE 8-9.   The intracellular and extracellular events in the formation of a collagen fibril. **A,** Note that collagen fibrils are shown assembling in the extracellular space contained within a large infolding in the plasma membrane. As one example of how collagen fibrils can form ordered arrays in the extracellular space, they are shown further assembling into large collagen fibers, which are visible in the light microscope. The covalent cross-links that stabilize the extracellular assemblies are not shown. **B,** Electron micrograph of a negatively stained collagen fibril reveals its typical striated appearance. (**A,** From Alberts B, Johnson A, Lewis J, et al [eds]: Molecular Biology of the Cell, 4th ed. New York, Garland, 2002, p 1100; **B,** Courtesy of Robert Horne.)

or degradation, with a turnover that approaches the life span.[52] Age-related modification is a result of progressive degradation as elastic fibers gradually become tortuous, frayed, and porous. Scanning electron microscopy shows that, in humans, the elastic meshwork grows largely undistorted during postnatal growth, where fibers seem to enlarge in synchrony with the growth of the tissue. In nonwounded circumstances, there is very little elastin degradation. This is probably due to elastin's extremely hydrophobic nature making the interior of this highly folded protein inaccessible. Because of this high degree of three-dimensionality and extensive cross-linking, cleavage must be considerable before there is much loss of elasticity. Both IGF-1 and TGF-β stimulate production of elastin. Glucocorticoids and basic FGF reduce adult skin cell production of elastin.

Mutations causing elastin protein deficiency results in excessive smooth muscle cell proliferation in the arterial wall (intimal hyperplasia), leading to arterial narrowing. These findings suggest that the normal elasticity of an artery is needed to prevent proliferation of these cells. Fibrillin gene mutations result in Marfan's syndrome; severely affected individuals are prone to aortic rupture.[53]

Glycosaminoglycans and Proteoglycans

GAGs are unbranched polysaccharide chains composed of repeating disaccharide units: a sulfated amino sugar (N-acetylglucosamine or N-acetylgalactosamine), and uronic acid (glucuronic or iduronic). The GAGs are highly negatively charged because of the sulfate or carboxyl groups on most of their sugars. Four types of GAGS exist: (1) hyaluronan (HA), (2) chondroitin sulfate and dermatan sulfate, (3) heparan sulfate, and (4) keratan sulfate.[44,54]

The GAGs in connective tissue usually constitute less than 10% of the weight of the fibrous proteins. Their highly negative charge attracts osmotically active cations, such as Na^+, causing large amounts of water to be incorporated into the matrix. This results in porous hydrated gels and is responsible for the turgor that enables the matrix to withstand compressive forces.[44]

HA is the simplest of the GAGs.[54] It is composed of repeating nonsulfated disaccharide units and is found in adult tissues, but is especially prevalent in fetal tissues. Its abundance in fetal wounds is believed to be a factor in the scarless wound healing seen in fetal tissues.[55] Unlike the other GAGs, it is not covalently attached to any protein

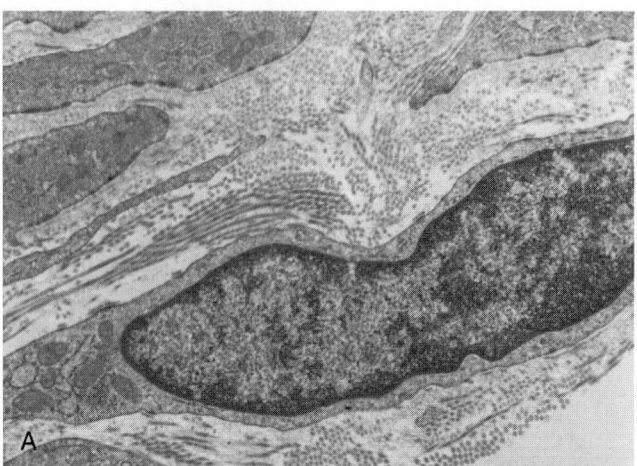

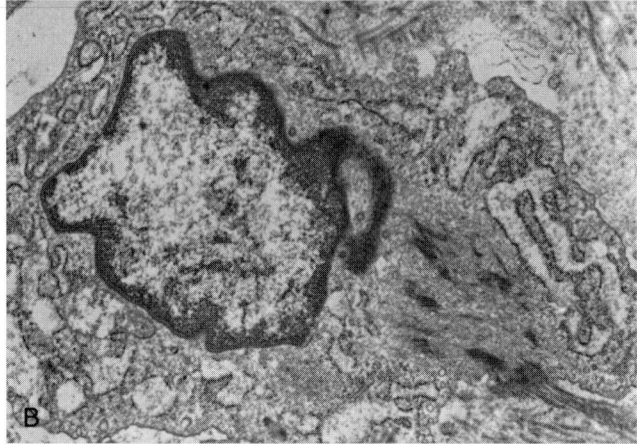

FIGURE 8-10. **A,** Normal resting fibroblast from human connective tissue. Note the large, smooth, oval nucleus; normal mitochondria; and a small amount of rough endoplasmic reticulum. The cell is surrounded by collagen fibrils cut in longitudinal and cross section. The cell fragments seen in the upper left are typical smooth muscle cells. Electron micrograph, ×22,000. **B,** Myofibroblast from a patient with plantar fasciitis. Compared with the fibroblast, note the highly irregular nucleus, the large amount of rough endoplasmic reticulum, and the dense collection of myofilaments. There are numerous dense bodies adjacent to and intermingled with the myofilaments. No basal lamina is seen, and the cell is surrounded by numerous collagen fibrils. This cell has ultrastructural features typical of both a fibroblast and a smooth muscle cell. Electron micrograph, ×25,000. (**A** and **B**, Courtesy of Edward C. Carlson, PhD.)

and is synthesized directly from the cell surface by an enzyme complex embedded in the plasma membrane.

HA serves several different roles because of its large hydration shell. HA is produced in large quantities during wound healing where it facilitates cell migration by physically expanding the ECM, allowing cells additional space for migration and reducing the strength of adhesion of migrating cells to matrix fibers. HA synthesized from the basal side of an epithelium creates a cell-free space for cell migration, as in during embryogenesis and formation of the heart and other organs. When cell migration finishes, the excess HA is degraded by hyaluronidase.[54]

Proteoglycans are a diverse group of glycoproteins with functions mediated by both their core proteins and GAG chains. The number and types of GAGs attached to the core protein can vary greatly and the GAGs themselves can be modified by sulfonation. Because of their GAGs, proteoglycans provide hydrated space around and between cells. They also form gels of different pore size and charge density to regulate movement of cells and molecules. Perlecan, a heparan sulfate proteoglycan, serves this role in the basal lamina of the kidney glomerulus. Decreased levels of perlecan are believed to play a role in diabetic albuminuria.

Proteoglycans function in chemical signaling, binding various secreted signal molecules, such as growth factors, and modulating their signaling activity. Proteoglycans can also bind other secreted proteins, such as proteases and protease inhibitors. This allows proteoglycans to regulate proteins by (1) immobilizing the protein and restricting its range of action; (2) providing a reservoir of the protein for delayed release; (3) altering the protein to allow for more effective presentation to cell surface receptors; (4) prolonging the protein's action by protecting it from degradation; and (5) blocking the activity of the protein.[54,56]

Proteoglycans can be components of plasma membranes and have either a transmembrane core protein or are attached to the lipid bilayer by a glycosylphosphatidylinositol (GPI) anchor. These proteoglycans act as coreceptors that work with other cell surface receptor proteins, binding cells to the ECM and initiating the response of cells to extracellular signaling proteins. For example, the syndecans are transmembrane proteoglycans that are located on the surface of many cells, including fibroblasts and epithelial cells. In fibroblasts, syndecans are found in focal adhesions, where they interact with fibronectin on the cell surface and with cytoskeletal and signaling proteins inside the cell. Severe developmental defects are a result of mutations leading to the inactivation of these coreceptor proteoglycans.[44]

The ECM has other noncollagen proteins, such as the fibronectins, that have multiple domains and can bind to other matrix macromolecules and cell surface receptors. These interactions help organize the matrix and facilitate cell attachment. Fibronectin is important in animal embryogenesis.

Fibronectin exists as soluble and fibrillar isoforms. Soluble plasma fibronectin circulates in various body fluids, enhancing blood clotting, wound healing, and phagocytosis. The highly insoluble fibrillar forms assemble on cell surfaces and are deposited in the ECM. The fibronectin fibrils that form on the surface of fibroblasts are usually coupled with neighboring intracellular actin stress fibers. The actin filaments promote the fibronectin fibril assembly and influence fibril orientation. Integrin transmembrane adhesion proteins mediate these interactions. The contractile actin and myosin cytoskeleton pulls on the fibronectin matrix, generating tension.[44]

Basal Lamina

Basal laminae are flexible, thin (40- to 120-nm thick) mats of specialized ECM that separate cells and epithelia from the underlying or surrounding connective tissue. In the skin, the basal lamina is tethered to the underlying connective tissue by specialized anchoring fibrils. This composite of basal lamina and collagen is the basement membrane.

The basal lamina serves numerous functions; it acts (1) as a molecular filter, preventing passage of macromolecules (i.e., in kidney glomerulus); (2) as a selective barrier to certain cells (i.e., the lamina beneath the epithelium prevents fibroblasts from contacting epithelial cells, but does not stop macrophages or lymphocytes); (3) as a scaffold for regenerating cells to migrate; and (4) is important in tissue regeneration where the basal lamina survives.

Though its composition may vary from tissue to tissue, most mature basal laminae contain type IV collagen, perlecan, and the glycoproteins laminin and nidogen. Type IV collagen has a more flexible structure than the fibrillar collagens; their triple-stranded helix is interrupted, allowing multiple bends.

Laminins, in general, consist of three long polypeptide chains (α, β, and γ). Mice lacking the laminin-γ_1 chain die during embryogenesis because they cannot make a basal lamina.[57] The laminin in basement membranes consists of several domains that bind to perlecan, nidogen, and laminin receptor proteins found on cell surfaces. The type IV collagen and laminin networks are connected by nidogen and perlecan, which act as stabilizing bridges. Many of the cell surface receptors for type IV collagen and laminin are members of the integrin family. Another important type of laminin receptor is dystroglycan, a transmembrane protein, which, together with integrins, may organize the assembly of the basal lamina.[58]

Degradation of the ECM

The regulated turnover of the ECM is crucial to many biologic processes. ECM degradation occurs during metastasis when neoplastic cells migrate from their site of origin to distant organs via the bloodstream or lymphatics. In injury or infection, a localized degradation of the ECM occurs so that cells can migrate across the basal lamina to reach the site of injury or infection. Locally secreted cellular proteases, such as MMPs or serine proteases, degrade the ECM components. Matrix proteolysis helps the cell migrate by (1) clearing a path through the matrix; (2) exposing binding sites, promoting cell binding or migration; (3) facilitating cell detachment so that a cell can move forward; or (4) releasing signal proteins that promote cell migration.

Proteolysis is tightly regulated. Many are secreted as inactive precursors that are activated when required. In addition, cell surface receptors bind these proteases, ensuring that these enzymes act only on sites where they are needed. Finally, protease inhibitors, such as the tissue inhibitors of metalloproteinase (TIMP), can bind these enzymes and block their activity.

Maturational Phase

Wound *contraction* is the centripetal movement of the whole thickness of the surrounding skin, reducing the amount of disorganized scar. Wound *contracture*, in contrast, is a physical constriction or limitation of function and is the result of the process of wound contraction. Contractures occur when excessive scar exceeds normal wound contraction and results in a functional disability. Scars that traverse joints and prevent extension or scars that involve the eyelid or mouth and cause ectropions are examples of contractures.

Wound contraction appears to occur by a complex interaction of the extracellular materials and the fibroblast, which is not completely understood. Using a fibroblast-populated collagen lattice, Ehrlich demonstrated that aborted cell locomotion appears to cause bunching and contraction of the collagen fibers.[59] In this in vitro model, trypsinized collagen is populated by fibroblasts that adhere to it in culture. If normal dermal fibroblasts are cultured, they attempt to move but are trapped by the collagen fibers. The tractional forces cause the lattice to bunch and contract.

Numerous studies have shown that fibroblasts in a contracting wound undergo change to stimulated cells, referred to as *myofibroblasts*. These cells have both function and structure in common with fibroblasts and smooth muscle cells and express alpha smooth muscle actin in bundles called *stress fibers*. The actin appears at day 6 after wounding and persists at high levels for 15 days and is gone by 4 weeks when the cell undergoes apoptosis.[6] It appears that the stimulated fibroblast develops a contractile ability related to formation of cytoplasmic actin-myosin complexes. When this stimulated cell is placed in the fibroblast-populated collagen lattice, contraction occurs even faster. The tension that is exerted by the fibroblasts' attempt at contraction appears to stimulate the actin-myosin structures in their cytoplasm. If colchicine, which inhibits microtubules, or cytochalasin D, which inhibits microfilaments, is added to the tissue culture, the result is minimal contraction of the collagen gels. Fibroblasts develop a linear arrangement in the line of tension that, when removed, causes the cells to round up.

Stimulated fibroblasts or myofibroblasts are found to be a constant feature present in abundance in diseases of excessive fibrosis. These include hepatic cirrhosis, renal and pulmonary fibrosis, Dupuytren's contracture, and desmoplastic reactions induced by neoplasia. The actin microfilaments are arranged linearly along the long axis of the fibroblast. They are associated with dense bodies that allow attachment to the surrounding ECM. Fibronexus is the attachment entity that connects the cytoskeleton to the ECM and spans the cell membrane in doing so.

MMPs also appear to be important for wound contraction. It has been demonstrated that stromelysin-1 (MMP-3) strongly affects wound contraction.[60] MMPs may be necessary to allow cleavage of the attachment between the fibroblast and the collagen so that the lattice can be made to contract. Different populations of fibroblasts, from different organs, respond to the contraction stimulus in a heterogeneous fashion. It is likely that the stromelysin-1 allows modification of attachment sites between the fibroblast and the collagen fibrils involving the β_1 integrins. Similarly, cytokines, such as TGF-β_1, affect contraction by increasing β_1 integrin expression.

Remodeling

The fibroblast population decreases and the dense capillary network regresses. Wound strength increases rapidly within 1 to 6 weeks and then appears to plateau up to 1 year after the injury (see Fig. 8-8). Compared with unwounded skin, the tensile strength is only 30% in the scar. There is an increase in breaking strength after approximately 21 days, which is mostly a result of cross-linking. Although collagen cross-linking causes further wound contraction and increase in strength, it also results in a scar that is more brittle and less elastic than normal skin. Unlike normal skin the epidermodermal interface in the healed wound is devoid of rete pegs, the undulating projections of epidermis that penetrate into the papillary dermis. Loss of this anchorage results in increased fragility and predisposes the neoepidermis to avulsion after minor trauma.

ABNORMAL WOUND HEALING (Box 8-1)

In such a complex series of interweaving events as wound healing, multiple factors can impede the outcome. The amount of tissue lost or damaged, the amount of foreign material or bacterial inoculation, and the length of time of exposure to the toxic factors will affect the period of time to recovery. The greater the insult, the longer the reparative process, and the greater the amount of residual scar. Intrinsic factors such as chemotherapeutic agents, atherosclerosis, cardiac or renal failure, and location on the body all affect wound healing. Blood supply in the lower extremity is the worst in the body; blood supply on the face and hands is the best. The older the patient, the slower the healing.

Ultimately, the type of scar—whether it is adequate, inadequate, or proliferative—is dictated by the amount of collagen deposition and balanced by the amount of collagen degradation. If the balance is tipped in either direction, the result is poor.

Box 8-1. Factors that Inhibit Wound Healing

Infection	Vitamin deficiencies
Ischemia	Vitamin C
Circulation	Vitamin A
Respiration	Mineral deficiencies
Local tension	Zinc
Diabetes mellitus	Iron
Ionizing radiation	Exogenous drugs
Advanced age	Doxorubicin (Adriamycin)
Malnutrition	Glucocorticosteroids

HYPERTROPHIC SCARS AND KELOIDS
(Figs. 8-11 and 8-12)

An example of proliferative scar is the hypertrophic scar or keloid. Pathologic scarring in other areas of the body can cause hepatic cirrhosis, pulmonary fibrosis, scleroderma, retrolental fibroplasia, diabetic retinopathy, or osteoarthritis, among others. Both keloids and hypertrophic scars are characterized by excessive collagen deposition versus collagen degradation. *Keloids* are defined as scars that grow beyond the borders of the original wounds, and these scars rarely regress with time. Keloid formation is more prevalent among patients with darker pigmented skin, occurring in 15% to 20% of African Americans, Asians, and Hispanics.[61] It appears to have a genetic predisposition. The keloid scar tends to occur above the clavicles on the trunk, in the upper extremities, and on the face. Keloids cannot be prevented at this time and are refractory to medical and surgical intervention. Hyper-

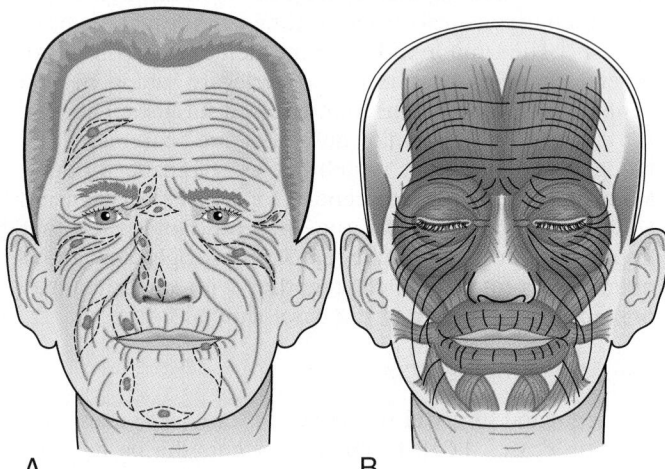

A   B

FIGURE 8-11. Preferred orientation for elective skin incisions (**A**) is parallel to lines of facial expression (**B**) (*A* and *B*, From Kraissl CJ: The selection of appropriate lines for elective surgical incisions. Plast Reconstr Surg 8:1-28, 1951.)

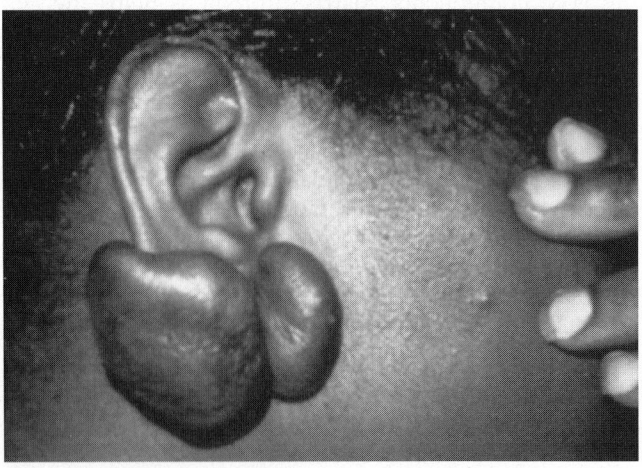

FIGURE 8-12. Keloids caused by ear piercing.

trophic scars, in contrast, are raised scars that remain within the confines of the original wound and frequently regress spontaneously. The hypertrophic scar can occur anywhere on the body. These scars also differ histologically from normal scars. Keloids and hypertrophic scars have stretched collagen bundles aligned in the same plane as the epidermis as opposed to normal scar tissue, where the collagen bundles are randomly arrayed and relaxed. Keloid scars also have thicker, more abundant collagen bundles that form acellular nodelike structures in the deep dermal portion of the keloid lesion. The center of keloid lesions also contains a paucity of cells compared to that of the hypertrophic scar that has islands composed of aggregates of fibroblasts, small vessels, and collagen fibers throughout the dermis.

The hypertrophic scar is in many cases preventable. Prolonged inflammation and insufficient resurfacing, such as can occur with a burn wound, lead to hypertrophic scar. It appears that the tension that signals formation of activated fibroblasts also causes deposition of excessive collagen. Scar that is perpendicular to the underlying muscle fibers tends to be flatter, narrower, with less collagen formation than that which is parallel to the underlying muscle fibers. The position of an elective scar can be chosen in such a way to make a narrower and less obvious scar in the distant future. As muscle fibers contract, they reapproximate the wound edges if they are perpendicular to the underlying muscle. If, however, the scar is parallel to the underlying muscle, then contraction of that muscle will tend to cause gaping of the wound edges and lead to more tension and scar formation.

At this time, there is some indication of biochemical differences between the proliferative scars and normal wound scars. Hypertrophic scars represent a hyperproliferative phenotype following multiple stimulatory effects. This phenotype can be reversed, once the stimulation, such as excessive skin tension or growth factors, is removed. Keloids, however, are a unique phenotype that appears to be genetically predisposed to changes in ECM production and is switched on irreversibly by factors such as TGF-β.[62] The isoforms TGF-β1 and β2 are increased in expression from human keloid cells compared with normal human dermal fibroblasts.[63] Hypertrophic scar fibroblasts produce more TGF-β1.[64] The addition of exogenous TGF-β2 activates proliferative scar fibroblasts from both keloids and burn hypertrophic scars.[57,63] In contrast to the elevated collagen synthesis seen in these scars, collagen degradation is low. Both MMP-1 (collagenase) and MMP-9 (gelatinase involved in early tissue repair) are decreased in hypertrophic scars and keloids.[65,66] MMP-2 (gelatinase in late tissue remodeling) is significantly elevated in hypertrophic scars and keloids.[65,66] Studies being done with antibody to TGF-β show that its activity can be blocked and fibrosis decreased.[67] Recently, studies examining the genetic susceptibility of certain individuals to keloid and hypertrophic scar formation have been reported, yet the findings failed to demonstrate an association between TGF-β1 plasma levels and the common polymorphisms with increased keloid and hypertrophic scars.[68] Growth factors have also been implicated in fibrosis and are being studied as targets for the blockade of fibrosis.[69] IFN-γ, which suppresses collagen synthesis, has been tested clinically in keloid scars and has shown an average of 30% reduction in scar thickness (Fig. 8-13).

Chronic Nonhealing Wounds

Chronic wounds, like other abnormal wounds, appear to have derangements in various stages of wound healing and unusually elevated or depressed levels of cytokines, growth factors, or proteinases. Chronic wound fluid, unlike acute wound fluid, has been demonstrated to have greater levels of IL-1, IL-6, and TNF-α; levels of these proinflammatory cytokines decreased as the wound healed.[7] In addition, an inverse relationship between TNF-α and essential growth factors such as EGF and PDGF has been demonstrated.[7]

The amount of normal wound ECM is determined by a dynamic balance between overall matrix synthesis, deposition, and degradation. Proteolytic degradation of ECM is an essential feature of repair and remodeling during cutaneous repair. Current evidence suggests that proteolytic degradation in the wound environment is a major cause of failure to heal. MMPs are a family of structurally related enzymes that have the ability to degrade ECM components and are differentiated by their substrate specificity and inhibited by TIMPs. TNF-α has been shown to increase the production of MMPs, while inhibiting the production of TIMPs. Conversely, inhibition of MMPs results in decreased levels of TNF-α in wound fluid and decreased inflammatory cell numbers, while increasing wound tensile strength and levels of TGF-β.[70]

Studies in chronic wounds such as pressure ulcers in both human and animal models have demonstrated elevations of MMPs, particularly MMP-1, -2, -8, and -9, and decreased levels of TIMPs.[71,72] This has led many investigators to conclude that the chronic wound is a result of persistently elevated levels of MMPs and depressed levels of their inhibitors. These MMPs have been shown to degrade the adhesive substrates for cell migration and signaling molecules, such as growth factors and cytokines. In addition, excessive proteolysis may cause a release of high levels of breakdown products of connective tissue that will inappropriately activate inflammatory cell processes. With increased inflammation of the wound, there is less likelihood that the wound will progress to healing. The balance is slanted in favor of collagen degradation rather than collagen synthesis.

Wounds that are chronically inflamed and do not proceed to closure can develop squamous cell carcinoma (Fig. 8-14). Originally reported in chronic burn scars by Marjolin,[73] other conditions have been associated with this problem, including osteomyelitis, pressure sores, venous stasis ulcers, and hidradenitis. The wound appears irregular, raised above the surface, with a white, pearly discoloration. The premalignant state is pseudoepitheliomatous hyperplasia. If this report is obtained on biopsy, the biopsy should be repeated because there may be squamous cell carcinoma present in other areas.

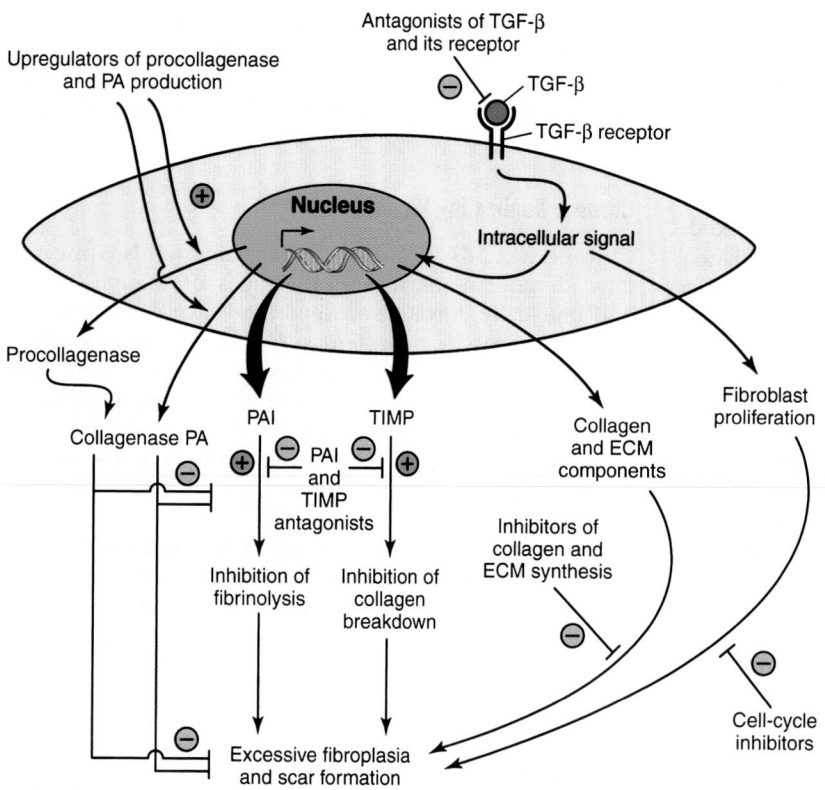

FIGURE 8-13. Pathways in causing excessive fibroplasia by transforming growth factor-β (TGF-β) and means for therapeutic intervention. TGF-β increases the cellular production of extracellular matrix (ECM) proteins, such as fibronectin and collagen, and also increases the cellular expression of integrins (not shown). Furthermore, the synthesis of inhibitors of degrading enzymes of plasminogen activator inhibitor (PAI) and tissue inhibitor of matrix metalloproteinases (TIMP) are also increased by TGF-β, whereas the expression of collagenase and plasminogen activator (PA) are decreased. This upregulation of inhibitor synthesis and downregulation of protease synthesis further augments the accumulation of ECM proteins induced by TGF-β and is the basis for fibrotic tissue formation due to excessive action of TGF-β. Possible means of therapeutic intervention are highlighted. Antagonists of TGF-β and its receptor would shift the ECM equilibrium toward degradation, as would upregulators of PA production and PAI antagonists. Inhibitors of collagen and ECM synthesis would prevent excessive ECM deposition. Cell-cycle inhibitors would prevent the proliferation of fibroblasts. (From Tuan TL, Nichter LS: The molecular basis of keloid and hypertrophic scar formation. Mol Med Today 41:21, 1998.)

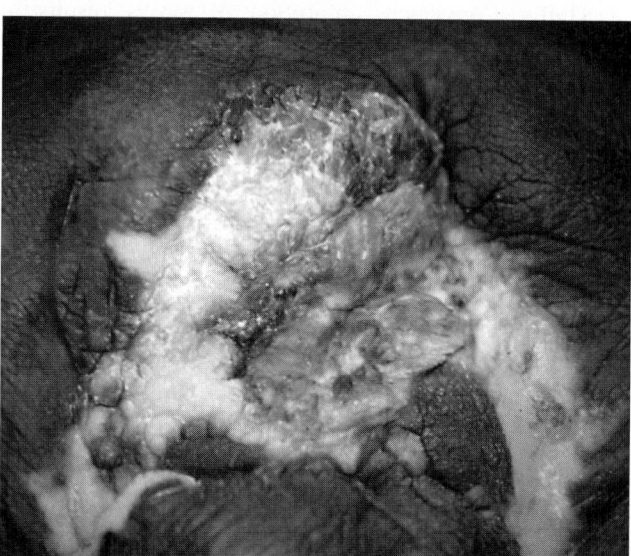

FIGURE 8-14. Squamous cell carcinoma in chronic pressure sore.

Infection

Probably the most common cause of healing delays is wound infection. If the bacterial count in the wound exceeds 10^5 organisms per gram of tissue, or if any β-hemolytic streptococci are present, the wound will not heal by any means including flap closure, skin graft placement, or primary sutures.[74] Bacteria prolong the inflammatory phase and interfere with epithelialization, contraction, and collagen deposition. The endotoxins themselves stimulate phagocytosis and release of collagenase that contribute to collagen degradation and destruction of surrounding previously normal tissue. Treatment to decrease the bacterial count, either mechanically or with the use of systemic antibiotics, therefore limits the amount of inflammation and allows closure of the wound.

Bacteria may accelerate expression or increase concentrations of MMPs, growth factors, and cytokines in chronic-type wounds; their role, as yet, has not been clearly defined. Neutrophils release pro-MMP-8 and fibroblasts and macrophages express pro-MMP-1 and pro-MMP-9. These inactive precursors are activated by bacterial proteinases of the thermolysin family (*Pseudomonas, Vibrio,* and *Serratia*), supporting the role of bacteria in remodeling the ECM.[75] Bacterial phospholipase C can disrupt normal reepithelialization by decreasing cell-cell contact and increasing cell migration, possibly by altering integrin expression and by upregulating MMP-9.[76] However, some studies refute the importance of bacterial induction of MMPs in chronic wounds. Trengove and associates[7] performed quantitative bacteriology on tissue biopsies from 10 nonhealing and healing leg ulcers and found that there was no significant difference in the number of bacteria present in the two groups of wounds.

Hypoxia

Molecular oxygen is essential for collagen formation. Ischemia can be caused by atherosclerosis, cardiac failure, or simple wound tension preventing localized perfusion.

Under hypoxic conditions, energy derived from glycolysis may be sufficient to initiate collagen synthesis, but the presence of molecular oxygen is critical for the post-translational hydroxylation of prolyl and lysyl residues required for triple-helix formation and cross-linking of collagen fibrils. Although hypoxia will stimulate angiogenesis, this essential step in collagen fibril assembly proceeds poorly when PO_2 falls below 40 mm Hg. An optimal PO_2 for collagen synthesis is present at the periphery of the wound while the center remains hypoxic.

The role of anemia in wound healing has long been attributed to be predominantly secondary to hypoperfusion. However, recent work evaluating colonic anastomoses in a crystalloid-resuscitated hemorrhagic shock model demonstrated altered histologic parameters (decreased white blood cell infiltration, angiogenesis, fibroblast production, and collagen production).[77] Use of tobacco products has a similar impact on wound healing due to both the vasoconstriction that occurs with smoking and the elevated carbon monoxide serum levels that can limit the oxygen-carrying capacity of the blood.[78]

Diabetes

Diabetes mellitus impairs wound healing at all stages of the process. The diabetic patient with associated neuropathy and atherosclerosis is prone to tissue ischemia, repetitive trauma, and infection. Tissue hypoxia, as indicated by reduced dorsal foot transcutaneous oxygen tension, is a consequence of vascular disease and has been well demonstrated in the diabetic patient. In addition to large-vessel disease, many diabetic patients have abnormalities at the microvascular level. The basement membrane of the capillaries is thickened, causing decreased perfusion in the microenvironment, and there is increased perivascular localization of albumin, suggesting that these capillaries are leaky. Diabetic patients are prone to repeated trauma as a result of the diabetic neuropathy that affects both sensory and motor functions both in somatic and autonomic pathways. Furthermore, diabetics are susceptible to infection because of an attenuated inflammatory response, impaired chemotaxis, and inefficient bacterial killing. Infection also increases local tissue metabolism, further imposing a burden on an already tenuous blood supply and thereby amplifying the risk for tissue necrosis. Lymphocyte and leukocyte function is impaired, and there is increased collagen degradation and decreased collagen deposition. The collagen that is formed is more brittle than normal collagen, probably owing to glycosylation from the increased levels of glucose present in the ECM.

Ionizing Radiation

Ionizing radiation causes endothelial cell injury with endarteritis resulting in atrophy, fibrosis, and delayed tissue repair. Unlike most hypoxic wound beds, angiogenesis is not initiated. As its greatest effect is on cells in the G_2 through M phase, rapidly dividing cell populations are most sensitive to radiation. This would include the keratinocytes and fibroblasts during wound healing, impairing epithelialization and granulation tissue formation.

Aging

Elderly patients are more likely to have surgical wound ruptures and delayed healing, compared with younger patients. The same patient as he or she ages will heal more slowly. With aging, collagen undergoes qualitative and quantitative changes. Dermal collagen content decreases with aging and aging collagen fibers show distorted architecture and organization. Upregulation of MMP-2 and -9 was elevated in elderly healthy subjects following experimental wounding when compared to young controls.[79] Studies in aged animals have also demonstrated decreased re-epithelialization, depressed collagen synthesis, and impaired angiogenesis with decreased levels of multiple growth factors, including proangiogenic factors FGF-2 and VEGF.[80] Other studies have suggested that the early inflammatory period of wound healing is altered in the elderly, including impaired macrophage activity, with reduced phagocytosis and delayed infiltration of macrophages and B lymphocytes into wounds.[79] In addition, with aging, there is a decrease in response to hypoxia, as demonstrated by decreased MMP activation and decreased TGF-β_1 receptor expression by keratinocytes isolated from aged donors.[81]

Malnutrition

Malnutrition impacts wound healing. Protein catabolism can result in a delay in wound healing. The hypoalbuminemic patient can experience wound healing delay or even dehiscence, although the albumin must be below 2.0 g/dL to have an effect on wound healing.[82] Protein supplements can reverse this deficiency.

Vitamin deficiencies affect wound healing primarily owing to their effect as cofactors. Delayed healing can occur in as few as 3 months of vitamin C deprivation. This deficiency can be reversed by administration of 100 to 1000 g/day. Deficiency of vitamin A impedes monocyte activation, fibronectin deposition that further affects cellular adhesion, and impairment of the TGF-β receptors. Vitamin A contributes to lysosomal membrane destabilization and directly counteracts the effect of glucocorticoids. The main effect of vitamin K deficiency is to limit the synthesis of prothrombin and factors VII, IX, and X. Vitamin K metabolism is impeded by antibiotics. Those patients who have chronic or recurrent infections should have their clotting parameters checked before surgical procedures.

A few minerals, if deficient in the diet, adversely affect wound healing. Zinc deficiency is rare, except in cases such as large burns, severe multiple trauma, and hepatic cirrhosis. Zinc is a necessary cofactor for RNA polymerase and DNA polymerase. Zinc deficiency results in early wound healing delays.[83] Iron deficiency anemia is a debatable cause of wound healing delay. Although the ferrous ion is a cofactor necessary to convert hydroxyproline to proline, there are conflicting reports as to the effects that acute and chronic anemia have on wound healing. In general, the patient is most benefited by a well-rounded diet of adequate protein intake and caloric value with vitamin and mineral supplementation.

Drugs

Some exogenous drugs directly inhibit wound healing. Doxorubicin (Adriamycin) is a potent inhibitor, particularly if it is administered preoperatively. Although clinical studies have shown little impairment, experimental models have indicated that nitrogen mustard, cyclophosphamide, methotrexate, bis-chloroethyl-nitrosourea (BCNU), and doxorubicin are the most potent wound inhibitors. These chemotherapeutic agents reduce mesenchymal cell proliferation and reduce the number of platelets, inflammatory cells, and growth factors available, especially if given preoperatively. Tamoxifen, an anti-estrogen, is known to decrease cellular proliferation. In addition, there appears to be a dose-dependent decrease in wound breaking strength associated with tamoxifen. This may be due to decreased TGF-β production. Glucocorticosteroid impairs fibroblast proliferation and collagen synthesis. The amount of granulation tissue formed is also decreased. Steroids stabilize the lysosomal membranes. This particular effect can be reversed by the administration of vitamin A. The decrease in breaking strength caused by the administration of exogenous steroids appears to be both time and dose related. High doses of nonsteroidal anti-inflammatory drugs have been reported to delay healing, but doses in the therapeutic range are unlikely to have an effect.[84]

FETAL WOUND HEALING (Fig. 8-15)

Fetal skin wounds heal rapidly and without the scarring and inflammation that are characteristic of adult skin wounds. As a result, in the early 1990s a great deal of wound healing research focused on fetal wounds. It was thought that fetal wound healing represented ideal tissue repair and that understanding fetal wound healing would provide surgeons with the tools to regulate and control the different steps in adult wound healing. In adult cutaneous healing as opposed to fetal healing, there is a failure of regeneration of dermal appendages, such as hair follicles, sweat glands, and sebaceous glands. Furthermore, in adult wounds, there are changes in collagen, with the healed wound demonstrating densely packed collagen bundles oriented perpendicularly to the wound surface, unlike that of normal uninjured skin and fetal skin, both of which have a reticular pattern.

Fetal wounds re-epithelialize faster with less neovascularization and faster increase in strength. Fetal wound research has demonstrated that fetal wounds differ from adults in inflammatory responses, ECM components, and in growth factor expression and responses.

Fetal repair is both gestational-age and wound-size dependent. There may be a wound size threshold (the diameter of excised skin at which 50% of the wounds heal scarlessly at a given gestational age). The wound size

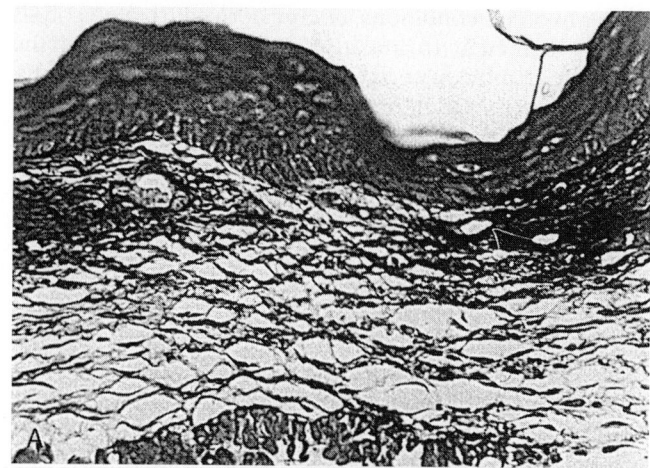

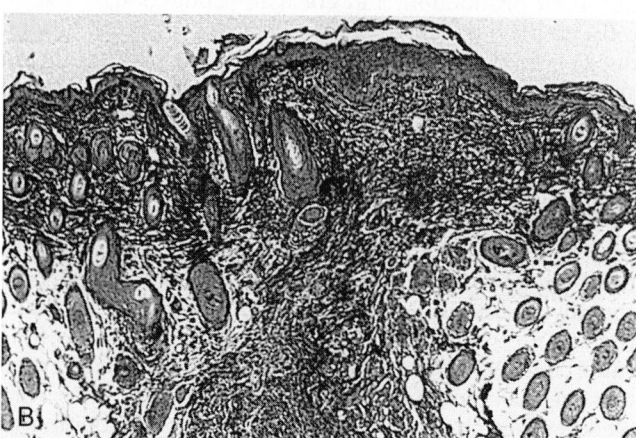

FIGURE 8-15. Comparison of scar-free repair and healing with scar using Mallory trichrome staining. **A,** Healed skin wound in a 2-day-old opossum pouch young, 2 days after wounding, illustrates the absence of scar formation in the dermis and the very rapid repair process. There is epithelial thickening at the wound site and a fine reticular collagen pattern in the healed dermis. **B,** Day 28 pouch young wound, 7 days postoperatively, demonstrates extensive scarring in the dermis as well as abnormal orientation of the collagen fibers perpendicular to the dermis.

thresholds for 60- and 70-day gestation animals is 6 to 10 mm and 4 to 6 mm for 80- and 90-day gestation animals. It has been suggested that larger wounds may extend the time of the healing response and expose wound tissue to a different ECM and growth factor profile. The larger excisional wounds may also stimulate the formation of myofibroblasts in the wound, resulting in scar formation. The transition from scarless to scarring repair occurs near the end of the second trimester and the beginning of the third. Wounds heal faster in the fetus than in the neonate and wounds heal slowest in adults. Normal development of skin appendages occurs when fibroblasts of the dermis induce the epithelium to form hair follicles or glands. Wounds created early in gestation heal scarlessly and with dermal appendages, suggesting tissue regeneration versus repair. Late-gestation wounds, on the other hand, heal with scar and without dermal appendages. The transition from scarless healing to healing without dermal appendages suggests that the fetal fibroblast loses its ability to induce the epithelium to form dermal appendages with advancing gestational age.[85]

Investigators have cited intrinsic (i.e., oxygen tension of the human fetus) and extrinsic (environment-amniotic fluid) differences between fetal and adult wound healing, with most stating that the intrinsic differences are the key determinants in whether or not wounds will heal with scars.[86] Intrinsic differences include fetal oxygen tension, which is markedly decreased (fetal sheep, mean PaO_2 of 20 mm Hg) when compared to adult animals (adult sheep, mean PaO_2 of 116 mm Hg).[87] This decrease in fetal oxygenation is partially compensated by the relative affinity of fetal hemoglobin for oxygen.

The fetal environment, an extrinsic difference between fetal and adult wounds, is characterized by a hyaluronic acid–rich amniotic fluid. Studies suggest that the increased number of hyaluronic acid receptors and increased amount of hyaluronic acid may create a permissive environment in which fibroblast movement is facilitated and results in the increased rate and efficiency of fetal healing.[86]

Much of fetal wound healing research has focused on the role of the fibroblasts. The fetal fibroblast appears to have quite different characteristics from that of the adult fibroblast. Proline hydroxylation is a rate-limiting step in collagen synthesis by dermal cells; early-gestation fetal human fibroblasts have increased prolyl hydroxylase activity, which gradually falls off to adult levels after 20 weeks of gestation. Collagens I, III, V, and VI appear earlier in fetal wounds and the ratio of type III to type I is greater in fetal wounds, which is consistent with the higher prevalence of type III collagen in normal fetal tissue. Fetal fibroblasts in vitro have higher collagen production than adult counterparts. This may be secondary to the unique regulatory mechanism for prolyl hydroxylase and may explain why there is a higher fibroblast activity in fetuses less than 20 weeks' gestation.

Collagen synthesis falls to adult levels after 20 weeks' gestation. There appears to be an increase in collagen degradation as a function of gestational age. Recent work found that there were marked increases in gene expression of MMP-1, MMP-3, and MMP-9 that correlated with the onset of scar formation in nonwounded fetal skin.[88] These findings suggest that late-gestational-age fetal rat skin undergoes an adult-type of tissue remodeling post-wounding, leading to the scarring seen in adult skin.

There are also differences in the components of the ECM of fetal and adult wounds. After injury, fibronectin levels are similar in adults and fetuses, but tenascin, an inhibitor of fibronectin, rises earlier and returns to normal more rapidly in the fetus. Larger amounts of fibronectin in fetal wounds stimulate immediate cell attachment, whereas the more rapid deposition of tenascin in the fetus allows cells to migrate and fully epithelialize the wound more rapidly and decrease wound healing time.

There are persistently elevated hyaluronic acid levels found in fetal wounds. During gestation, levels of hyaluronic acid decrease, correlating with increasing scarring potential. The unique ECM composition of fetal tissues may influence collagen fibril deposition by facilitating cell mobility, cell migration, leading to the loose collagen pattern seen in healed fetal wounds as opposed to the dense collagenous pattern seen in the adult scar. There are, however, few studies examining the effect of modifying the ECM components.

Differences in fetal wound healing also occur in the inflammatory phase. In the fetus, there is a reduced inflammatory response with a lack of neutrophil infiltration and decreased infiltration of endogenous immunoglobulins. The paucity of macrophages and a difference in the temporal appearance of macrophages in the fetal wound may explain why there are differences in the growth factor profiles between adult and fetal wounds and why there is a reduced inflammatory response.[89] These studies cite a direct correlation between increased macrophage recruitment in older fetuses and development of increased scarring.

Fetal wounds have been demonstrated to have minimal levels of TGF-β and FGF-2 by immunohistochemistry. Furthermore, PDGF in fetal wounds disappears more rapidly than in adult wounds. This lack of growth factors may be explained by the decreased inflammatory cell recruitment. The normal inflammatory (adult-type) wound healing may have evolved to reduce the risk of infection at the expense of the healing quality.

TGF-β is the growth factor that has been most extensively studied in fetal wound repair. TGF-β1 has been shown to induce rapid healing and scar formation when added to adult rat wounds and inflammation and fibrosis when added to fetal rabbit wounds. TGF-β production may be blunted in hypoxemic conditions, and this has led to the theory that the decreased oxygen tension in the fetal environment inhibits TGF-β production and results in decreased scar formation. More recent work has suggested that the differential expression of the different TGF-β isoforms, rather than the mere presence of TGF-β, may be important in explaining differences in repair.[90]

Growth factor manipulation to make wounds more fetal-like with less angiogenesis, less fibrosis, and improved ECM migratibility has not resulted in completely scarless healing and there is still a failure of regeneration of dermal appendages. These findings suggest that the mechanisms of scarless fetal wound healing have yet to be completely elucidated. There are some inconsistencies of fetal wound healing that are not clearly understood. It has been shown that there are differences in species in regard to scarless fetal wound healing and that not all fetal tissues are capable of scarless healing. For example, fetal lamb diaphragm and gastric wounds scar whereas concurrent skin wounds heal scarlessly.

Studies have demonstrated the correlation between the presence of myofibroblasts and scar formation; this suggests that a transition in fibroblast phenotype may contribute to the onset of scarring. Excisional wounds in 75-day gestation fetal lambs show an absence of scar formation and alpha smooth muscle actin expression. Alpha smooth muscle actin appears after 100 days of gestation along with scar formation.[91] Although attempts to make wounds more fetal-like has failed to reproduce scarless healing, the differences in fetal and adult wounds have not yet been completely elucidated.

NEW HORIZONS

In the mid-1990s, research targeted the concept of wound manipulation. Prospective, randomized studies were published showing a more rapid closure of venous stasis ulcers, pressure sores, and diabetic foot wounds using a variety of cytokines such as TGF-β, basic FGF-2, and PDGF. Although the patients healed more rapidly on this treatment, drug therapy cost at least $80,000 alone for each patient. Furthermore, until the precise cytokine deficit is known for each wound type, application of growth factor remains an educated guess. In addition, some of these clinical studies have been launched with multiple dosing and administration regimens, making proof of statistical significance difficult to achieve.

Genetic intervention also allows for manipulation of the wound. Application of the gene responsible for these growth factors, performed less frequently, holds promise of being more cost effective and possibly more targeted. Safety factors with viral vectors, such as the adenovirus or the herpes simplex virus, continue to limit this research to animal and in vitro models.

Further advances in understanding the molecular mechanisms regulating wound healing are still progressing, largely aided by innovative techniques to identify novel genes. The development of technologies such as microarrays and differential-display polymerase chain reaction (DD-PCR) have provided new techniques to analyze gene expression.[92,93] Microarray-based technologies allow for rapid and easy large-scale gene expression analysis in a single experiment,[92] while DD-PCR has been reported to be extremely useful as a genetic screening tool for complicated dynamic processes, such as wound healing. Proponents for DD-PCR claim that it is particularly powerful when multiple, small-sized samples are involved.[93]

Tissue engineering allows manipulation of the injured tissue, whether it is a cutaneous wound or infarcted myocardium or even a cirrhotic liver. Tissue engineering represents the merger of clinical surgery, engineering, and biology to restore, sustain, or enhance tissues or organs.[94] Engineered living-skin products, which are FDA approved, are already in use for the treatment of diabetic and venous stasis ulcers. One of these products consists of cultured dermal fibroblasts grown onto a scaffold composed of the water-soluble polymer polylactide coglycolide. Another is composed of dermal fibroblasts in a collagen solution coated with several layers of keratinocytes. After transfer to the patient, the host skin cells replace the skin product as healing occurs. The dermal fibroblasts in these skin products secrete ECM proteins and are able to respond to the patient's own growth factors.[95]

Three principal strategies exist in creating new tissue: (1) implantation of isolated or cultured cells either by direct injection, or combined in vitro with a biodegradable implantable scaffold; (2) implantation of a complete three-dimensional tissue that was grown in vitro using a composite of the patient's cells and a biodegradable scaffold; and (3) in situ tissue regeneration—a scaffold is placed directly into the injured tissue and stimulates the patient's cells to undergo repair. The greatest challenges in tissue engineering are the development of capillary networks to support these implanted cells and the development of scaffolds made of biomaterials that will degrade slowly after placement in the patient and be replaced by the patient's own tissue. These implanted cells and scaffolds will also need to acquire the appropriate tissue architecture in vivo. Finally, the greatest obstacle may be in enlarging these in vitro engineered tissues for clinical use.[95]

The interest in embryonic stem cells is understandable, given that these cells can be expanded in vitro in an undifferentiated state and then induced to form many different cell types, allowing treatment of damaged tissue where the source of cells for repair is either limited or unavailable.

Tissue engineering has the potential to dramatically change the practice of surgery. It offers new tools to modify tissues at the cellular and molecular level. It also offers the promise to replace tissue with living tissue that is designed and built to meet the needs of each individual patient. Cells can be isolated from healthy sites, expanded in vitro or modified by gene therapy, and then reimplanted to correct the functional defect. Surgeons, using minimally invasive surgical skills, can potentially adapt tissue engineering techniques, treating disease by replacement with nearly identical tissue.

Selected References

Alberts B, Johnson A, Lewis J, et al (eds): Cell junctions, cell adhesion, and the extracellular matrix. *In* The Molecular Biology of the Cell, 4th ed. New York, Garland, 2002, pp 1091-1114.

> **This chapter gives a comprehensive review of matrix and integrin biology and their critical role in biologic processes, including tissue repair.**

Cohen IK, Diegelmann RF, Lindblad WJ: Wound Healing: Biochemical and Clinical Aspects. Philadelphia, WB Saunders, 1992.

> **This textbook remains one of the most comprehensive works available on wound healing.**

Dang C, Ting K, Soo C, et al: Fetal wound healing: Current perspectives. Clin Plast Surg 30:13-23, 2003.

> **This review article discusses the morphologic, cellular, and molecular aspects of scarless fetal wound healing.**

Rumalla VK, Borah GL: Cytokines, growth factors, and plastic surgery. Plast Reconstr Surg 108:719-733, 2001.

> **The authors review the critical role of cytokines and growth factors in wound healing.**

Schultz GS, Sibbald RG, Falanga V, et al: Wound bed preparation: A systematic approach to wound management. Wound Rep Reg 11(2 Suppl):S1-S28, 2003.

> **This monograph reviews the current status, role, and key elements in wound bed preparation. It gives an analysis of acute and chronic wound environments and how healing can take place in these settings.**

Singer AJ, Clark, RAF: Mechanisms of disease: Cutaneous wound healing. N Engl J Med 341:738-746, 1999.

This journal article provides a comprehensive review of the cellular and molecular aspects of wound healing.

References

1. Clemetson KJ, Clemetson JM: Platelet collagen receptors. Thromb Haemost 86:189-197, 2001.
2. Harler MB, Wakshull E, Filardo EJ, et al: Promotion of neutrophil chemotaxis through differential regulation of β_1 and β_2 integrins. J Immunol 162:6792-6799, 1999.
3. Holly SP, Larson MK, Parise LV: Multiple roles of integrins in cell motility. Exp Cell Res 261:69-74, 2000.
4. Plow EF, Haas TA, Zhang L, et al: Ligand binding to integrins. J Biol Chem 275:21785-21788, 2000.
5. Nwometh BC, Olutoye OO, Diegelmann RF, et al: The basic biology of wound healing. J Surg Pathol 2:143-162, 1997.
6. Witte MB, Barbul A: General principles of wound healing. Surg Clin North Am 77:509-528, 1997.
7. Trengove NJ, Bielefeldt-Ohmann H, Stacey MC: Mitogenic activity and cytokine levels in non-healing and healing chronic leg ulcers. Wound Repair Regen 8:13-25, 2000.
8. Barone EJ, Yager DR, Pozez AL, et al: Interleukin-1-α and collagenase activity are elevated in chronic wounds. Plast Reconstr Surg 102:1023-1029, 1998.
9. Feiken E, Romer J, Eriksen J, et al: Neutrophils express tumor necrosis factor-α during mouse skin wound healing. J Invest Dermatol 105:120-123, 1995.
10. Wallace HJ, Stacey MC: Levels of tumor necrosis factor-α (TNF-α) and soluble TNF receptors in chronic venous leg ulcers—correlations to healing status. J Invest Dermatol 110:292-296, 1998.
11. Pajulo OT, Pulkki KJ, Alanen MS, et al: Correlation between interleukin-6 and matrix metalloproteinase-9 in early wound healing in children. Wound Repair Regen 7:453-457, 1999.
12. Goretsky MJ, Harriger MD, Supp AP, et al: Expression of interleukin-1-α, interleukin-6, and basic fibroblast growth factor by cultured skin substitutes before and after grafting to full-thickness wounds in athymic mice. J Trauma 40:894-900, 1996.
13. Liechty KW, Adzick NS, Crombleholme TM: Diminished interleukin-6 (IL-6) production during scarless human fetal wound repair. Cytokine 12:671-676, 2000.
14. Liechty KW, Crombleholme TM, Cass DL, et al: Diminished interleukin-8 (IL-8) production in the fetal wound healing response. J Surg Res 77:80-84, 1998.
15. Engelhardt E, Toksoy A, Goebeler M, et al: Chemokines IL-8, GRO-α, MCP-1, IP-10, and Mig are sequentially and differentially expressed during phase-specific infiltration of leukocyte subsets in human wound healing. Am J Pathol 153:1849-1860, 1998.
16. Rennekampff HO, Hansbrough JF, Kiessig V, et al: Bioactive interleukin-8 is expressed in wounds and enhances wound healing. J Surg Res 93:41-54, 2000.
17. Iocono JA, Colleran KR, Remick DG, et al: Interleukin-8 levels and activity in delayed-healing human thermal wounds. Wound Repair Regen 8:216-225, 2000.
18. Tredget EE, Wang R, Shen Q, et al: Transforming growth factor-β mRNA and protein in hypertrophic scar tissues and fibroblasts: Antagonism by IFN-α and IFN-γ in vitro and in vivo. J Interferon Cytokine Res 20:143-151, 2000.
19. Desai H, Dyson M, Hart J: The effect of pretreatment with platelet-derived growth factor-AB (PDGF-AB) on acute wound repair. Wound Repair Regen 5:A110, 1997.
20. Smith PD, Kuhn MA, Franz MG, et al: Initiating the inflammatory phase of incisional healing prior to tissue injury. J Surg Res 92:11-17, 2000.
21. Karr BP, Bubak PJ, Sprugel KH, et al: Platelet-derived growth factor and wound contraction in the rat. J Surg Res 59:739-742, 1995.
22. Buckmire MA, Parquet G, Greenway S, et al: Temporal expression of TGF-β_1, EGF, and PDGF-BB in a model of colonic wound healing. J Surg Res 80:52-57, 1998.
23. Sullivan KM, Lorenz HP, Meuli M, et al: A model of scarless human fetal wound repair is deficient in transforming growth factor-β. J Pediatr Surg 30:198-203, 1995.
24. Shah M, Foreman DM, Ferguson MW: Neutralisation of TGF-β_1 and TGF-β_2 or exogenous addition of TGF-β_3 to cutaneous rat wounds reduces scarring. J Cell Sci 108:985-1002, 1995.
25. Boyce DE, Jones WD, Ruge F, et al: The role of lymphocytes in human dermal wound healing. Br J Dermatol 143:59-65, 2000.
26. Schaffer M, Barbul A: Lymphocyte function in wound healing and following injury. Br J Surg 85:444-460, 1998.
27. Barbul A, Regan MC: Immune involvement in wound healing. Otolaryngol Clin North Am 28:955-968, 1995.
28. Liechty KW, Nesbit M, Herlyn M, et al: Adenoviral-mediated overexpression of platelet-derived growth factor-B corrects ischemic impaired wound healing. J Invest Dermatol 113:375-383, 1999.
29. Xia YP, Zhao Y, Marcus J, et al: Effects of keratinocyte growth factor-2 (KGF-2) on wound healing in an ischaemia-impaired rabbit ear model and on scar formation. J Pathol 188:431-438, 1999.
30. Deodato B, Arsic N, Zentilin L, et al: Recombinant AAV vector encoding human VEGF165 enhances wound healing. Gene Ther 9:777-785, 2002.
31. O'Reilly MS, Holmgren L, Chen C, et al: Angiostatin induces and sustains dormancy of human primary tumors in mice. Nat Med 2:689-692, 1996.
32. O'Reilly MS, Boehm T, Shing Y, et al: Endostatin: An endogenous inhibitor of angiogenesis and tumor growth. Cell 88:277-285, 1997.
33. Nissen NN, Polverini PJ, Koch AE, et al: Vascular endothelial growth factor mediates angiogenic activity during the proliferative phase of wound healing. Am J Pathol 152:1445-1452, 1998.
34. Nissen NN, Polverini PJ, Gamelli RL, et al: Basic fibroblast growth factor mediates angiogenic activity in early surgical wounds. Surgery 119:457-465, 1996.
35. Albina JE, Mastrofrancesco B, Vessella JA, et al: HIF-1 expression in healing wounds: HIF-1α induction in primary inflammatory cells by TNF-α. Am J Physiol Cell Physiol 281:C1971-1977, 2001.
36. Dulak J, Jozkowicz A, Dembinska-Kiec A, et al: Nitric oxide induces the synthesis of vascular endothelial growth factor by rat vascular smooth muscle cells. Arterioscler Thromb Vasc Biol 20:659-666, 2000.
37. Akcay MN, Ozcan O, Gundogdu C, et al: Effect of nitric oxide synthase inhibitor on experimentally induced burn wounds. J Trauma 49:327-330, 2000.
38. Liu S, Yu D, Xu ZP, et al: Angiogenin activates Erk1/2 in human umbilical vein endothelial cells. Biochem Biophys Res Commun 287:305-310, 2001.
39. Constant JS, Feng JJ, Zabel DD, et al: Lactate elicits vascular endothelial growth factor from macrophages: A possible alternative to hypoxia. Wound Repair Regen 8:353-360, 2000.
40. Rumalla VK, Borah GL: Cytokines, growth factors, and plastic surgery. Plast Reconstr Surg 108:719-733, 2001.

41. Ilic D, Almeida EA, Schlaepfer DD, et al: Extracellular matrix survival signals transduced by focal adhesion kinase suppress p53-mediated apoptosis. J Cell Biol 143:547-560, 1998.

42. Decline F, Rousselle P: Keratinocyte migration requires $\alpha_2\beta_1$ integrin-mediated interaction with the laminin-5γ_2 chain. J Cell Sci 114:811-823, 2001.

43. Pilcher BK, Dumin JA, Sudbeck BD, et al: The activity of collagenase-1 is required for keratinocyte migration on a type I collagen matrix. J Cell Biol 137:1445-1457, 1997.

44. Alberts B, Johnson A, Lewis J, et al (eds): Cell junctions, cell adhesion, and the extracellular matrix. *In* The Molecular Biology of the Cell, 4th ed. New York, Garland, 2002, pp 1091-1114.

45. Giancotti FG, Ruoslahti E: Integrin signaling. Science 285:1028-1032, 1999.

46. Petratos PB, Felsen D, Trierweiler G, et al: Transforming growth factor-β_2 (TGF-β_2) reverses the inhibitory effects of fibrin sealant on cutaneous wound repair in the pig. Wound Repair Regen 10:252-258, 2002.

47. Diegelmann RF: Collagen metabolism. Wounds 13:177, 2001.

48. Cattaneo MG, Pola S, Francescato P, et al: Human endostatin–derived synthetic peptides possess potent antiangiogenic properties in vitro and in vivo. Exp Cell Res 283:230-236, 2003.

49. Laato M, Heino J, Gerdin B, et al: Interferon-γ–induced inhibition of wound healing in vivo and in vitro. Ann Chir Gynaecol 90(Suppl 215):19-23, 2001.

50. Shukla A, Meisler N, Cutroneo KR: Transforming growth factor-β: Crossroad of glucocorticoid and bleomycin regulation of collagen synthesis in lung fibroblasts. Wound Repair Regen 7:133-140, 1999.

51. Debelle L, Tamburro AM: Elastin: Molecular description and function. Int J Biochem Cell Biol 31:261-272, 1999.

52. Bailey AJ: Molecular mechanisms of ageing in connective tissues. Mech Ageing Dev 122:735-755, 2001.

53. Nollen GJ, Groenink M, van der Wall EE, et al: Current insights in diagnosis and management of the cardiovascular complications of Marfan's syndrome. Cardiol Young 12:320-327, 2002.

54. Gallo RL: Proteoglycans and cutaneous vascular defense and repair. J Invest Dermatol Symp Proc 5:55-60, 2000.

55. Kennedy CI, Diegelmann RF, Haynes JH, et al: Proinflammatory cytokines differentially regulate hyaluronan synthase isoforms in fetal and adult fibroblasts. J Pediatr Surg 35:874-879, 2000.

56. Iozzo RV: Matrix proteoglycans: From molecular design to cellular function. Annu Rev Biochem 67:609-652, 1998.

57. Smith P, Mosiello G, Deluca L, et al: TGF-β_2 activates proliferative scar fibroblasts. J Surg Res 82:319-323, 1999.

58. Ghohestani RF, Li K, Rousselle P, et al: Molecular organization of the cutaneous basement membrane zone. Clin Dermatol 19:551-562, 2001.

59. Ehrlich HP: Wound closure: Evidence of cooperation between fibroblasts and collagen matrix. Eye 2:149-157, 1988.

60. Bullard KM, Mudgett J, Scheuenstuhl H, et al: Stromelysin-1–deficient fibroblasts display impaired contraction in vitro. J Surg Res 84:31-34, 1999.

61. Tuan TL, Nichter LS: The molecular basis of keloid and hypertrophic scar formation. Mol Med Today 4:19-24, 1998.

62. Tuan TL, Zhu JY, Sun B, et al: Elevated levels of plasminogen activator inhibitor-1 may account for the altered fibrinolysis by keloid fibroblasts. J Invest Dermatol 106:1007-1011, 1996.

63. Lee TY, Chin GS, Kim WJ, et al: Expression of transforming growth factor-β_1, β_2, and β_3 proteins in keloids. Ann Plast Surg 43:179-184, 1999.

64. Wang R, Ghahary A, Shen Q, et al: Hypertrophic scar tissues and fibroblasts produce more transforming growth factor-β_1 mRNA and protein than normal skin and cells. Wound Repair Regen 8:128-137, 2000.

65. Arakawa M, Hatamochi A, Mori Y, et al: Reduced collagenase gene expression in fibroblasts from hypertrophic scar tissue. Br J Dermatol 134:863-868, 1996.

66. Neely AN, Clendening CE, Gardner J, et al: Gelatinase activity in keloids and hypertrophic scars. Wound Repair Regen 7:166-171, 1999.

67. Brahmatewari J, Serafini A, Serralta V, et al: The effects of topical transforming growth factor-β_2 and anti-transforming growth factor-$\beta_{2,3}$ on scarring in pigs. J Cutan Med Surg 4:126-131, 2000.

68. Bayat A, Bock O, Mrowietz U, et al: Genetic susceptibility to keloid disease and hypertrophic scarring: Transforming growth factor-β_1 common polymorphisms and plasma levels. Plast Reconstr Surg 111:535-546, 2003.

69. Blom IE, Goldschmeding R, Leask A: Gene regulation of connective tissue growth factor: new targets for antifibrotic therapy? Matrix Biol 21:473-482, 2002.

70. Witte MB, Thornton FJ, Kiyama T, et al: Metalloproteinase inhibitors and wound healing: A novel enhancer of wound strength. Surgery 124:464-470, 1998.

71. Nwomeh BC, Liang HX, Cohen IK, et al: MMP-8 is the predominant collagenase in healing wounds and nonhealing ulcers. J Surg Res 81:189-195, 1999.

72. Chen C, Schultz GS, Bloch M, et al: Molecular and mechanistic validation of delayed healing rat wounds as a model for human chronic wounds. Wound Repair Regen 7:486-494, 1999.

73. Marjolin J-N: Ulcère. Dictionnaire de Medecine, Vol 21, Pratique, 1828.

74. Robson MC, Heggers JP: Surgical infection: II. The β-hemolytic streptococcus. J Surg Res 9:289-292, 1969.

75. Okamoto T, Akaike T, Suga M, et al: Activation of human matrix metalloproteinases by various bacterial proteinases. J Biol Chem 272:6059-6066, 1997.

76. Firth JD, Putnins EE, Larjava H, et al: Exogenous phospholipase C stimulates epithelial cell migration and integrin expression in vitro. Wound Repair Regen 9:86-94, 2001.

77. Buchmiller-Crair TL, Kim CS, Won NH, et al: Effect of acute anemia on the healing of intestinal anastomoses in the rabbit. J Trauma 51:363-368, 2001.

78. Smith JB, Fenske NA: Cutaneous manifestations and consequences of smoking. J Am Acad Dermatol 34:717-732; quiz 733-741, 1996.

79. Ashcroft GS, Horan MA, Ferguson MW: Aging is associated with reduced deposition of specific extracellular matrix components, an upregulation of angiogenesis, and an altered inflammatory response in a murine incisional wound healing model. J Invest Dermatol 108:430-437, 1997.

80. Swift ME, Kleinman HK, DiPietro LA: Impaired wound repair and delayed angiogenesis in aged mice. Lab Invest 79:1479-1487, 1999.

81. Xia YP, Zhao Y, Tyrone JW, et al: Differential activation of migration by hypoxia in keratinocytes isolated from donors of increasing age: Implication for chronic wounds in the elderly. J Invest Dermatol 116:50-56, 2001.

82. Hill DP Jr, Cooper DM, Robson MC: Serum albumin is a poor prognostic factor for pressure ulcer healing in controlled clinical trials. Wounds 6:174-178, 1994.

83. Lansdown AB, Sampson B, Rowe A: Sequential changes in trace metal, metallothionein, and calmodulin con-

centrations in healing skin wounds. J Anat 195:375-386, 1999.

84. Thomas DR: Specific nutritional factors in wound healing. Adv Wound Care 10:40-43, 1997.

85. Mackool RJ, Gittes GK, Longaker MT: Scarless healing: The fetal wound. Clin Plast Surg 25:357-365, 1998.

86. Dang C, Ting K, Soo C, et al: Fetal wound healing: Current perspectives. Clin Plast Surg 30:13-23, 2003.

87. Scheid A, Wenger RH, Christina H, et al: Hypoxia-regulated gene expression in fetal wound regeneration and adult wound repair. Pediatr Surg Int 16:232-236, 2000.

88. Peled ZM, Phelps ED, Updike DL, et al: Matrix metalloproteinases and the ontogeny of scarless repair: The other side of the wound healing balance. Plast Reconstr Surg 110:801-811, 2002.

89. Cowin AJ, Brosnan MP, Holmes TM, et al: Endogenous inflammatory response to dermal wound healing in the fetal and adult mouse. Dev Dyn 212:385-393, 1998.

90. Cowin AJ, Holmes TM, Brosnan P, et al: Expression of TGF-β and its receptors in murine fetal and adult dermal wounds. Eur J Dermatol 11:424-431, 2001.

91. Estes JM, Vande Berg JS, Adzick NS, et al: Phenotypic and functional features of myofibroblasts in sheep fetal wounds. Differentiation 56:173-181, 1994.

92. Duggan DJ, Bittner M, Chen Y, et al: Expression profiling using cDNA microarrays. Nat Genet 21:10-14, 1999.

93. Soo C, Sayah DN, Zhang X, et al: The identification of novel wound-healing genes through differential display. Plast Reconstr Surg 110:787-800, 2002.

94. Miller MJ, Patrick CW Jr: Tissue engineering. Clin Plast Surg 30:91-103, vii, 2003.

95. Griffith LG, Naughton G: Tissue engineering: Current challenges and expanding opportunities. Science 295:1009-1014, 2002.

CHAPTER 9

CRITICAL ASSESSMENT OF SURGICAL OUTCOMES

John D. Birkmeyer, M.D., and **Samuel R. G. Finlayson**, M.D., M.P.H.

Two Main Applications of Outcomes Research

Data Sources

Is the Study Valid?

Is the Study Focusing on the Right Outcome Measure?

Is the Intervention Cost-Effective?

Studies assessing surgical outcomes have become ubiquitous in the medical literature, employing a wide range of research tools and methodologies collectively known as "outcomes research."[1] Outcome studies take many forms, from prospective clinical studies to population-based studies using administrative data. They apply an ever-broadening range of quality of life measures and economic endpoints. Some focus on evaluating the effectiveness of a clinical intervention, whereas others focus on quality of care or broader policy issues.

Despite the increasing popularity of outcome studies, the quality of this research is highly variable. Many studies have limited validity because they fail to account adequately for the role of chance, bias, or confounding or because their findings cannot be generalized to other settings. Other surgical outcome studies fail to use the most appropriate outcome measures or fail to consider clinical benefits in the context of cost-effectiveness. To judge the usefulness of published studies, surgeons must consider these basic issues.

In this chapter, we provide a framework for critical assessment of surgical outcome studies. In the process, we describe many of the common methodologies and data sources employed by outcomes researchers, illustrating, where appropriate, their strengths and weaknesses.

TWO MAIN APPLICATIONS OF OUTCOMES RESEARCH

There is no perfect taxonomy for categorizing the very heterogeneous field of outcomes research. Instead, we consider the field according to its two main applications:

(1) to study the effectiveness of a clinical intervention and (2) to assess quality of care across providers.

Studies Assessing the Effectiveness of a Clinical Intervention

The most prevalent surgical outcome studies are aimed at making inferences about the effectiveness of a clinical intervention. In this context, evaluation of a clinical intervention may imply assessment of an existing procedure (e.g., surgery vs. medical therapy in patients with carotid stenosis), modification of an existing procedure (e.g., open vs. laparoscopic appendectomy), or adjunctive surgical care (e.g., prophylactic perioperative antibiotics vs. no antibiotics). Each case, however, involves an explicit (or sometimes implicit) comparison between two or more interventions.

A variety of different study designs are employed in making such comparisons (Table 9-1). Many consider the "gold standard" to be the randomized controlled trial (RCT), in which patients are assigned in prospective, random fashion to treatment and control groups. By ensuring that patients are as similar as possible between comparison groups, RCTs minimize the risk that observed differences in outcomes are attributable to other factors (confounding). Cohort studies, which are observational, are much more common, however. These may be either prospective (study and research questions established before data are collected and analyzed) or retrospective. With cohort studies, investigators use a variety of control groups for their comparisons. These may include patients

TABLE 9-1. Common Types of Studies Used to Assess the Effectiveness of Interventions

Study Type	Description	Strengths	Weaknesses	Example: Does fundoplication surgery prevent Barrett's esophagus in patients with GERD?
Case series	Measure outcomes of an intervention in a single case or in a series of cases	Simple; inexpensive	No comparison group	Perform surgery on GERD patients, measure the proportion progressing to Barrett's esophagus
Case-control study	Identify subjects with and without the outcome of interest, then look back in time to find factors that might predict the difference in outcome	Useful for studying rare outcomes; relatively inexpensive; retrospective, therefore no prolonged follow-up	Potential sampling bias, as well as bias measuring predictors; limited to one outcome variable	Identify a group of GERD patients with Barrett's and a group without Barrett's; compare the proportion in each group who have previously undergone surgery
Cohort study				
Retrospective	Select population to study, then measure predictor variables and outcomes by looking back in time	Inexpensive, events already happened and just need to be analyzed	Less control over selection of subjects and measurement of variables; limited to using existing data	Select population of GERD patients, look back over time to discover if those who underwent surgery are less likely to have Barrett's
Prospective	Select population to study, then measure predictor variables and outcomes by following the subjects over time	More control over selection of subjects and measurement of variables	Expensive, requires prolonged follow-up	Select a population of GERD patients without Barrett's esophagus, follow them through time to discover if those who undergo surgery are less likely to progress to Barrett's esophagus
Randomized controlled trial	Randomly assign patients to different interventions, then compare outcomes	Avoids confounding; strongest evidence for cause and effect	Patients may not be willing to be randomized; relatively expensive; difficult to study rare outcomes	Randomize GERD patients to surgical or nonsurgical treatment, compare proportions in each group who progress to Barrett's esophagus

GERD, gastroesophageal reflux disease.

with the same clinical condition not undergoing the treatment of interest during the study period (concurrent controls) or similar patients from an earlier period (historical controls). Many studies (i.e., case series) lack explicit control groups and instead make inferences based on contrasts between their findings and results of previously published studies.

Studies Assessing Quality of Care

An increasing number of surgical outcome studies focus on assessing the quality of surgical care. Such studies are inherently observational. They often involve direct comparisons across individual hospitals or surgeons (e.g., variation in coronary artery bypass grafting mortality rates across New York State hospitals[2]). Others involve comparisons in which providers are aggregated according to specific characteristics. Common examples include studies examining the effects of procedure volume or surgeon specialty on patient outcomes.[3,4]

DATA SOURCES

A variety of data sources are used in outcome studies assessing the effectiveness of a clinical intervention. Many studies rely exclusively on clinical data from a single insti-

tution or a small number of selected institutions. For studies assessing quality of care, however, big datasets involving large numbers of patients and providers are required. These are typically either large clinical registries or administrative datasets. Understanding the advantages and disadvantages of these data sources is crucial for critically assessing a surgical outcome study.

Clinical Registries

Large clinical registries contain medical information collected for purposes of research and/or quality improvement. Clinical registries are occasionally population based (capture all patients in a defined geographic region), such as cardiac surgery registries maintained by state departments of health in New York or California. In other instances, clinical registries capture all patients within a defined health care system or consortium (e.g., the National Surgical Quality Improvement Program of the Department of Veterans Affairs[5]). Some clinical registries are voluntary, capturing data from participating members of professional societies or other groups. For example, in the outcomes initiative managed by the Society of American Gastrointestinal and Endoscopic Surgeons (SAGES), participating surgeons submit data on outcomes of their laparoscopic cases. The level of clinical detail captured in various clinical registries varies widely.

Administrative Data

A large number of studies focusing on the quality of surgical care rely on administrative data—clinical and non-clinical information collected for purposes other than research (most often billing). Large, administrative databases are produced and maintained by the federal and state government, as well as many private health payers and providers (Box 9-1).

Most studies using administrative data to examine surgical outcomes rely on hospital discharge abstract files. These include the national Medicare files or samples of state-level files (e.g., Nationwide Inpatient Sample). Within each of these databases, a uniform set of informa-

tion is collected for every patient experiencing an acute care hospitalization. Because hospitalization is required for inclusion, these files are generally only useful for studying surgical procedures with (at least) overnight hospital stays. Data collected for each hospital discharge abstract include demographic information: age, sex, race/ethnicity, and patient residence. Administrative data include admission and discharge dates, total charges and amount reimbursed, expected payment source, admission type (elective, urgent, emergent), and discharge disposition (including vital status). Based on their unique physician identification numbers (UPINs), attending physicians and operating physicians are also identified. Hospital discharge abstracts contain codes and dates for at least nine diagnoses, which reflect the reason for admission or surgery (principal diagnosis), preexisting conditions (secondary diagnoses), and complications occurring during hospitalization. They also contain fields for the principal and other procedures (at least 5). Both diagnoses and procedures are classified by codes from the *International Classification of Diseases* (ICD).

There are distinct tradeoffs associated with using administrative data for clinical research.[6-10] Among the advantages, administrative databases contain large amounts of longitudinal data already collected for other purposes, which makes these data relatively inexpensive to obtain. They tend to be very accurate for identifying patients undergoing surgical interventions and for assessing "hard" endpoints (e.g., mortality). Many administrative databases are very large (which ensures that studies have adequate power) and contain information about a wide range of surgical conditions and interventions. Patient-level files can be linked to databases containing information about characteristics of hospitals and surgeons and are ideal for studying issues related to health care delivery and quality. Because they are generally population based and often national in scope, administrative databases are often the only way to study surgical outcomes in the "real world" (i.e., effectiveness rather than efficacy).

However, there are several pitfalls associated with using administrative data for clinical research. Most are related to the relative lack of specificity of clinical information contained in these files. ICD codes can be very imprecise, often aggregating heterogeneous clinical conditions (or procedures) under a single code. They do not adequately account for severity (e.g., mild stable angina or end-stage ischemic heart disease). There is wide variability in coding practices across hospitals, and a general tendency to undercode clinical diagnoses, particularly preexisting conditions. Such problems in coding and coding accuracy create obvious limitations in the ability to perform risk adjustment, particularly relevant in studies focusing on quality of care (discussed later).

Finally, administrative data lack specificity about the timing of clinical events and thus are limited in their ability to distinguish between preexisting conditions and surgical complications. Thus, administrative data are not well suited to assessing nonfatal outcomes of surgical interventions.

Box 9-1. Administrative Databases Commonly Used for Surgical Outcomes Research

National Level

Medicare population (Center for Medicare and Medicaid Services files)
   MEDPAR and Inpatient files (hospital discharge abstracts for acute care hospitalizations)
   Part B file (contains claims for all physicians' services based on CPT codes)
   Provider files (information about characteristics of physicians participating in Medicare program)
Health Care Utilization Project (Agency for Healthcare Quality and Research)
   Nationwide Inpatient Sample (all-payer database containing hospital discharge abstracts from large number of states)
   Analogous files pertaining to ambulatory surgery, emergency care, and pediatrics
Department of Veterans Affairs
   Patient Treatment File (use and outcomes of inpatient services)
   Outpatient File
Vital and Health Statistics Databases
   National Death Index (collates death certificate information from all 50 states)

State Level

   Medicaid management system
   State discharge databases (all-payer hospital discharge abstract databases maintained by most but not all states)
   Birth and death certificate data

Private/Proprietary Databases

   Large insurer databases (e.g., Blue Cross/Blue Shield)
   Provider network, managed care organization databases (content and availability varies widely)

TABLE 9-2. Critical Assessment of Surgical Outcome Studies

Questions to Ask	Things to Watch for
Are the conclusions valid? Chance—could the findings be simply "luck of the draw"?	Use of appropriate statistical tests for studies reporting "significant" effects (i.e., to avoid Type I errors) Adequate sample sizes for studies reporting no effect (i.e., to rule out Type II errors)
Bias—were there systematic errors in how study subjects were selected or assessed?	Process of selecting study subjects which does not distort treatment outcomes across comparison groups (i.e., selection bias) Process of collecting outcomes information or other data that does not favor one of the comparison groups (i.e., information bias)
Confounding—could findings be explained by other differences in patient groups?	Comparison groups similar in their baseline risks and likelihood of experiencing outcomes (independent of intervention) Risk factors adequately measured and accounted for with appropriate risk adjustment techniques Observed differences in outcomes large enough to rule out important confounding by unmeasured risk factors
Generalizability (external validity)—can the findings be extrapolated to general clinical practice?	Study population or providers that are representative enough to reflect outcomes in the "real world"
Is the study focusing on the right outcome measure?	Use of primary outcome measure that reflects most important outcome from clinical and/or patient perspective Appropriate instruments used to capture general health status, disease-specific quality of life, or patient preferences
Is the intervention cost-effective?	Benefits of the intervention sufficiently large to justify its costs (relative to other commonly accepted clinical practices)

IS THE STUDY VALID?

Despite the heterogeneity of published studies, critical readers must consider several basic questions as they make inferences from studies assessing the effectiveness of a clinical intervention or quality of care (Table 9-2). The first question is most fundamental to clinical research: Is the study valid? Validity reflects the degree to which an observed association (e.g., between a given intervention and outcome) cannot be attributed to alternative explanations. Factors that can lead to erroneous inferences include *chance* ("luck of the draw"), *bias* (there is a systematic error in how study subjects were selected or assessed), and *confounding* (the findings are due to other differences in patient groups). These three potential sources of error are generally considered criteria for internal validity. External validity refers to *generalizability*—the extent to which findings from a given study can be generalized to other patient populations and settings.

Chance

In clinical research, inference involves making a generalization about a larger group (or universe) of patients based on observations from a smaller subset or sample. Whenever inferences are based on samples, there is always the possibility that results could be inaccurate due to chance alone. For studies comparing outcomes across groups, there are two types of chance-related errors: type I and type II. Each is best defined relative to the *null hypothesis*—the assumption that there is no difference in outcomes between comparison groups. With type I errors,

the null hypothesis is erroneously rejected, that is, outcomes are asserted to differ by group when in reality they are equivalent. With type II errors, the null hypothesis is erroneously accepted, that is, outcomes are asserted to be equivalent, when they are really different.

Type I Errors

Although type I errors (also called α errors) can occur with any study, they are particularly prevalent for those involving multiple comparisons, such as studies comparing operative mortality rates across a very large number of hospitals or surgeons. In such cases, it is virtually certain that some providers will be outliers (good or bad) by chance alone.

The likelihood of a type I error is quantified by statistical testing. A "p value" reflects the probability that observed differences between groups would be observed by chance alone, under the assumption that the comparison groups are truly equivalent (the null hypothesis). Thus, a p value of .05, the conventional threshold for "statistical significance," signifies that the likelihood of observing differences of at least that magnitude by chance alone is 5 of 100. Confidence intervals (e.g., 95% CIs), an alternative to p values, reflect the degree of statistical imprecision by bracketing the observed difference between groups in a range of values that might be expected if the same study were repeated an infinite number of times.

There are a variety of statistical tests for calculating both p values and confidence intervals. Tests are generally selected according to (1) how many groups are being compared, (2) whether one group is being compared with

TABLE 9-3. Simple Overview of Statistical Tests for Evaluating the Role of Chance in Studies Comparing Outcome Data of Different Types

Type of Outcome Data Being Compared	Common Statistical Approach/Test	Example
Proportions		
Unadjusted	Chi-square test (Fisher's exact test if small number of observations)	Compare proportions of smokers and nonsmokers who develop lung cancer
Risk-adjusted	Logistic regression	Compare proportions of smokers and nonsmokers who develop lung cancer, adjusting for age, race, and gender
Means		
Within individuals	Paired t-test	Compare mean hemoglobin A1C levels in diabetic patients before and after pancreas transplantation
Between groups	Unpaired t-test	Compare mean hemoglobin A1C levels between diabetic patients with a transplanted pancreas and diabetic patients without a transplanted pancreas
Risk-adjusted	Linear regression	Compare hemoglobin A1C levels as above, adjusting for age, race, and gender
Survival time		
Unadjusted	Life table analysis or Kaplan-Meier plots	Compare 3 year survival with cryosurgery versus radiofrequency ablation for hepatoma
Risk-adjusted	Cox Proportional Hazards	Compare 3 year survival as above, adjusting for age, race, and gender

different groups or a single group is being compared with itself after an intervention or event, (3) whether risk adjustment is required, and (4) what kind of numerical data are being analyzed (e.g., continuous vs. categorical) (Table 9-3). Although a detailed discussion about choosing the appropriate test is beyond the scope of this chapter, Glantz's *Primer on Biostatistics* is useful.[11]

Type II Errors

Type II errors occur when studies erroneously conclude no difference in outcomes between comparison groups when such a difference really does exist. A large proportion of surgical studies lack sufficient sample size to detect small but clinically important benefits of a clinical intervention.[12] When the sample size in a study is too small to detect a meaningful difference in outcomes, the study can be said to lack sufficient statistical power. Type II errors are also prevalent in studies assessing quality of care. Detecting small but clinically meaningful differences in outcomes (e.g., a 1% vs. 2% stroke rate with carotid endarterectomy) requires thousands of patients, which are sample sizes often available only with administrative data. Type II errors are best avoided by assessing statistical power before conducting the study to ensure that a sufficient number of patients are enrolled in the study. Type II errors cannot be addressed in any way by statistical testing after the study is complete.

Bias

Bias refers to any systematic error in a clinical study that results in an incorrect estimate of differences in outcomes between comparison groups. Bias reflects problems with the design and conduct of the study, not with how the analysis is performed once data are collected. There are two general categories of bias: (1) *selection bias* (errors arising from the process of choosing study populations) and (2) *information bias* (errors related to the process of ascertaining outcomes and other pertinent data).

Selection Bias

Selection bias can occur whenever the manner in which study subjects are identified influences the likelihood of the outcome of interest (independent of the treatment being studied). For example, consider a hypothetical cohort study at a single academic center assessing the effectiveness of antireflux surgery by comparing long-term quality of life in medical and surgical patients with gastroesophageal reflux disease. If the medical arm consisted of patients identified from a gastroenterology clinic, the study might be preferentially including patients most bothered by their reflux (enough to seek care by a specialist).

Selection bias, usually at the provider level, can also occur in studies focusing on quality of care. This is a particular problem for databases that do not include outcomes for all patients and providers from a defined population (i.e., are not population based). For example, with clinical registries based on voluntary participation, surgeons with better than average outcomes may be more predisposed to share their data than other surgeons.

Information Bias

Information bias refers to a broad category of problems that arise from the process by which information about outcomes is collected. For example, bias can be introduced by the technique used to ascertain outcomes. Consider the same study (described earlier) of outcomes with medical and surgical therapy for gastroesophageal reflux.

A patient might respond one way to his or her surgeon about satisfaction with surgery but another way to an anonymous survey. For studies assessing the effectiveness of a clinical intervention, information bias is best avoided by prospective studies with standardized outcomes definitions and, when possible, by blinded assessment of treatment outcomes.

Information bias can occur even with "hard" endpoints. For example, consider a study comparing hospital mortality rates with a given procedure, using in-hospital death to reflect operative mortality. In this case, in-hospital mortality rates would be biased with regard to length of stay, which varies widely by hospital. Hospitals with relatively short lengths of stay would be predisposed to fewer in-hospital deaths; those with longer lengths of stay would be biased toward higher observed mortality. This type of information bias would be avoided by use of a uniform outcome measure (e.g., 30-day mortality).

Confounding

Confounding occurs when outcomes differ because of differences in the baseline risks of the comparison groups (often as a result of selection bias). Consider a hypothetical study comparing mortality rates between open and laparoscopic cholecystectomy. While laparoscopy may have an independent (protective) effect on mortality, it is also true that patients undergoing open cholecystectomy are more likely to have acute cholecystitis and, independent of the surgical approach, are more likely to die after surgery than patients without this condition. Thus, disease severity (acute cholecystitis) confounds the observed relationship between treatment choice and outcome. Of course, confounding can also occur in studies assessing quality of care: some hospitals may have higher mortality rates because their patients are "sicker" at the outset.

Confounding is optimally addressed by randomized controlled clinical trials—randomization ensures that potentially confounding patient characteristics are equally distributed between the study groups. Restricting patient eligibility criteria is another study design option (e.g., restricting the study sample (see earlier) to patients with acute cholecystitis). While randomization or restriction may be feasible for prospective studies assessing the effectiveness of an intervention, these approaches are rarely feasible for studies focusing on quality of care, which are inherently observational in nature.

For these reasons, outcome studies most commonly deal with potential confounding using analytical techniques, collectively known as *risk adjustment*. Risk adjustment refers to a variety of statistical approaches used to control for patient case mix. Typically, potentially confounding patient characteristics are entered as independent variables into multivariable regression equations that best predict the outcome of interest. For studies focusing on quality of care (e.g., mortality), these equations adjust observed mortality rates according to the average baseline risk of patients treated by each provider: downward for providers caring for sicker than average patients, upward for providers with healthier patients. There is a large body of literature addressing various issues related to risk adjustment in studies addressing quality of care.[13-15] In general, the statistical approach is less important than the completeness and quality of data used for risk adjustment.

Critical readers must be able to assess the adequacy of risk adjustment and, equally important, whether risk adjustment is important in the first place. To address these issues, surgeons should ask the follow questions:

How Reliably Are the Important Risk Factors Measured?

In studies based on clinical data, information collected about patient characteristics (potential confounders) is generally accurate. Thus, the main question about clinical registries is their completeness. Administrative databases reliably capture some important predictors of surgical outcomes (e.g., patient age, procedure type). However, such data are particularly limited in their ability to reflect surgical indication and procedure acuity (elective vs. emergent). In addition, preexisting comorbidities (e.g., diabetes, coronary artery disease) tend to be underreported, frequently misclassified, and often difficult to distinguish from postoperative complications.[16-18]

Do Important Risk Factors Vary Between Comparison Groups?

Regardless of the strength of its relationship with the outcome measure or how well it is measured, a variable can only be an important confounder if it varies across comparison groups. For measured risk factors, this question can be addressed directly by comparing the distribution of patient characteristics (or predicted mortality rates) across providers. For unmeasured variables, surgeons must consider the *a priori* likelihood that case mix varies between comparison groups.

How Large Are the Observed Outcome Differences?

Finally, in judging the likelihood of confounding, surgeons should consider the magnitude of reported differences in outcomes across comparison groups. In practice, differences in case mix can readily explain small differences in outcomes (e.g., 4% vs. 5% mortality rates with lower extremity bypass between high- and low-volume hospitals).[19] However, confounding would be a very implausible explanation for large differences (e.g., 4% vs. 16% mortality rates with pancreatic resection between high- and low-volume hospitals).

Generalizability

In any surgical outcome study, observations from a specific study population are used to make broader inferences about effectiveness or quality in the broader population of patients or providers. Thus, it is important to judge the extent to which a study's findings can be safely generalized to other settings.

In assessing generalizability, critical readers should first focus on the patients. In many studies, the study subjects do not adequately represent patients from the general population. Patients who "volunteer" for clinical trials are often more motivated and thus tend to have better outcomes than other patients. Study populations may also do better for more obvious reasons. In the Asymptomatic Carotid Artery Stenosis (ACAS) trial,[20] for example, study patients were substantially younger and healthier than most patients undergoing carotid endarterectomy. As a result, their risks of perioperative mortality (0.1%) were considerably lower than those observed in other patients at the same centers and in the general population.[21] Because net benefit of carotid endarterectomy was ultimately relatively small in this trial, even small differences in procedure-related risks could dramatically alter conclusions about the effectiveness of this procedure.

In considering generalizability, it is also important to focus on the providers and the care that patients are receiving, particularly in studies focusing on quality of care. Clinical trials generally imply careful, standardized protocols for patient selection, operative and perioperative care, and follow-up, often very different than the variable care that patients receive in real-world clinical practice. For obvious reasons, many surgical outcome studies are conducted at large academic centers. Outcomes at these centers tend to be systematically better than those achieved in the "real world." For example, hospitals participating in the ACAS trial had markedly lower mortality rates than other U.S. hospitals.[21] Although some of this difference was attributable to hospital procedure volume, ACAS hospitals also had lower mortality rates than other high-volume hospitals. Thus, the special attributes of study populations or providers can sometimes make it unsafe to extrapolate the findings of a study to the general population.

IS THE STUDY FOCUSING ON THE RIGHT OUTCOME MEASURE?

Clinical research in surgery has traditionally focused on intermediate outcomes (biologic or physiologic measures) and clinical endpoints (mortality or specific complications). Physiologic measures are useful for exploring mechanisms underlying an intervention's effectiveness and for improving the precision and statistical power of a study. For example, in assessing the effectiveness of peripheral arterial stenting, a study focusing on ankle-brachial indices, a continuous measure obtained on all patients, would have much more power than one centered on limb amputations, which occur much less commonly. Clinical endpoints also have the advantage of being discrete and generally simple to measure.

Despite these strengths, however, intermediate outcomes and clinical endpoints may not always correlate with what matters to patients. Thus, these measures may not reflect the relative success of interventions aimed at improving quality of life. For example, 24-hour pH probe results and mortality rates will provide a very incomplete picture of the effectiveness of laparoscopic fundoplication in patients with gastroesophageal reflux.

For this reason, surgical outcome studies rely on a heterogeneous collection of instruments and techniques for assessing outcomes important to patients, so-called patient-centered outcomes. These surgical outcomes measures can be grouped according to five different aspects of health-related quality of life: (1) general health status, (2) disease-specific symptom scores, (3) pain, (4) utilities, and (5) satisfaction (Table 9-4).

General Health Status

General health status, which is most commonly assessed using survey instruments, is the broadest measure of

TABLE 9-4. Common Measures of Health Status and Health-Related Quality of Life

Measure	Definition	Most Common Assessment Tools
General health status	Overall health status, assessed as composite of broad domains of physical and mental health	Previously developed and validated survey instruments (e.g., MOS SF-36, Activities of Daily Living Scale)
Disease-specific symptoms	Effect of specific condition on health and quality of life	Symptom scores using either off-the-shelf or project-specific survey instruments
Pain	Component of health status particularly relevant in assessing outcomes of surgery	Visual Analogue Scale
Utilities	Quantitative expressions of patient preferences for a particular state of health, important for decision analysis and cost-effectiveness analysis	Visual Analogue Scale, time trade-off, standard gamble
Satisfaction	What patients think about the health care or intervention itself	Survey with Likert style questions

MOS SF-36, 36-question Medical Outcomes Study Short-Form survey.

health-related quality of life. Several well-tested and well-known health status surveys are used widely in clinical research. Although beyond the scope of this chapter, detailed summaries and critiques of these instruments are available elsewhere.[22]

Among the best known general health surveys is the Medical Outcomes Study Short-Form survey, which comprises 36 questions (SF-36) or, in its abridged version, 12 questions.[23,24] We describe it here in more detail because it has become a standard tool for assessing baseline health status and/or outcomes in clinical trials involving surgical interventions. The 36 questions are distributed across eight health domains: physical functioning (10 questions), role limitations (4), bodily pain (2), general health (5), emotional functioning (4), social functioning (2), role limitations due to emotional problems (3), mental health (5), and a single item on perceptions of health changes over the past 12 months. Typical questions take the form: "In general, would you say your health is: excellent, very good, good, fair, or poor?" In scoring the SF-36, "subscale" scores are calculated for each of the eight domains and rolled up to create separate summary scores for physical and mental function. Scores are transformed to a linear,100-point scale using population-based weights (mean score: 50).

Many surgical outcome studies focus on patient disability, a component of general health status. The most widely used scale to measure activities of daily living is the Activities of Daily Living (ADL) Scale developed by Katz and colleagues.[25] Designed primarily for elderly or institutionalized patients, it summarizes the degree of independence in bathing, dressing, using the toilet, moving around the house, continence, and eating. Each function is scaled on a three-point scale ranging from complete dependence to independence. The survey is scored according to the number of functions associated with dependence.

Disease-Specific Symptom Scores

Although general health status surveys have the advantage of generalizability and capture broadly the implications of a given disease for overall health, they often lack the sensitivity and precision necessary to assess clinically meaningful changes in how patients experience a single clinical condition. For example, in a trial of therapy for gastroesophageal reflux disease, heartburn symptoms that are very bothersome to patients may not be sufficient to produce large effects on overall health-related quality of life as measured by the SF-36.

For this reason, many surgical outcome studies apply instruments that measure symptoms and quality of life specific to the clinical condition under study. A large number of symptom classification scores have been developed and widely tested for various clinical conditions.[22]

Pain

Pain, whether disease or procedure related, is an essential outcome measure in many surgical studies. Most studies rely on instruments that assess pain in a summary (or global) sense. Among the most commonly used methods for measuring pain is the Visual Analogue Scale, in which patients mark a continuous 10-cm line with "no pain" on one end and "worst pain" on the other. Some survey instruments assess pain in multiple dimensions.[26]

Utilities

Utilities—quantitative expressions of patient preferences for a particular state of health—are most commonly used in the context of decision analysis and cost-effectiveness analysis (described later in this chapter). Although both reflect "quality of life," utilities should be distinguished from measures of health status described earlier in this chapter, which generally describe how patients are affected by a given clinical condition, what they can and cannot do, and so on. Instead, utilities reflect how patients feel about or value living in a specific state of health.[27] Techniques for assessing utilities, which are usually measured on a scale from 0 (death or worst health imaginable) to 10 (best health), include Visual Analogue Scale, the time trade-off, and standard gamble methods.

Satisfaction

Patient satisfaction surveys assess what patients think about the health care or intervention itself, not their effects on an underlying disease process. In general terms, patient satisfaction surveys ask patients to judge their actual care against their underlying expectations. Most surgical outcome studies rely on relatively simple instruments, often based on Likert-style questions (e.g., How satisfied were you with your surgical procedure: not at all, somewhat satisfied, satisfied, or very satisfied?). Studies focusing on patient satisfaction as a primary outcome often employ surveys that assess satisfaction in multiple dimensions.[28,29]

IS THE INTERVENTION COST-EFFECTIVE?

As resources available for health care become increasingly constrained, accepting a new intervention as standard practice requires more than scientific evidence of its effectiveness. Unless the intervention is "cost-effective," limited health care dollars may be better spent elsewhere.

Cost-effectiveness analysis is a systematic approach to assessing whether an intervention provides sufficient "bang for the buck." It is only appropriate for assessing interventions that produce benefit at some additional cost. It is not useful for interventions that are (1) not effective (which should not be adopted regardless of cost) or (2) both effective and cost-saving (which should always be adopted).

The cost-effectiveness of a medical intervention is determined as the ratio of its net costs to its net benefits. Net costs are determined by comparing the direct and indirect costs associated with the intervention versus those associated with treating the same condition without

TABLE 9-5. League Table of Selected Cost-Effectiveness Analyses of Interest to Surgeons

Intervention	Cost-Effectiveness (dollars per QALY)
Primary closure of contaminated appendectomy wound vs. delayed primary or secondary closure in perforated or gangrenous appendicitis	Cost-saving
Endoscopic surveillance with esophagectomy for high-grade dysplasia vs. endoscopic surveillance with esophagectomy for cancer in Barrett's esophagus	Cost-saving
Total hip arthroplasty vs. no surgery for osteoarthritis	Cost-saving
Carotid endarterectomy vs. medical management for asymptomatic patients with > 60% internal carotid stenosis	$8,300
Coronary artery bypass grafting vs. medical therapy for 3-vessel-disease male with normal ventricular function	$13,000
Breast-conserving surgery vs. modified radical mastectomy in women with stages I & II breast cancer	$21,000
Elective surgical repair of asymptomatic, unruptured intracranial aneurysms vs. expectant management	$26,000
Heart transplantation vs. optimal conventional treatment	$46,000
Biennial breast cancer screening from age 40 vs. biennial screening from age 50	$70,000
Ursodiol vs. elective cholecystectomy for symptomatic gallstones	$77,000
Lithotripsy vs. cholecystectomy for symptomatic gallstones	$84,000
Simultaneous pancreas-kidney transplantation vs. kidney transplantation alone in type I diabetics with end-stage renal disease	$280,000
Prostate biopsy vs. no biopsy in men with abnormally high prostate-specific antigen levels but low cancer probabilities	Dominated
Shunt surgery vs. propranolol in cirrhotic patients with non-bleeding esophageal varices	Dominated

"Cost-saving" indicates that the intervention costs less and is more effective than the alternative. "Dominated" indicates that the intervention costs more and is less effective.

From Chapman RH, Stone PW, Sandberg EA, et al: A comprehensive league table of cost-utility ratios and a sub-table of 'panel-worthy' studies. Med Decis Making 20:451-467, 2000.

it (i.e., current practice). Net benefits, which are assessed in similar fashion, are usually expressed in terms of quality-adjusted life years (QALYs) A QALY is a composite measure reflecting both quality and quantity of life and is obtained by multiplying the length of time spent in a given health state by its associated utility. For example, 15 years of life with a stroke (average utility, hypothetically, 0.5) would be equivalent to 7.5 QALYs. Although cost-effectiveness analyses are becoming increasingly common components of prospective clinical trials, cost-effectiveness analysis is most frequently conducted using decision analysis models that simulate costs and benefits in hypothetical cohorts of patients.[30]

Cost-effectiveness ratios are only interpretable in relative terms. Although there is considerable disagreement about where to "set the bar," interventions that cost less than $50,000 to $100,000 per QALY saved are generally considered cost-effective. For comparative purposes, Table 9-5 lists estimates of cost-effectiveness for several common surgical procedures.[31]

Selected References

Birkmeyer JD: Using administrative data for clinical research. *In* Souba WW, Wilmore DW (eds): Surgical Research. San Diego, Academic Press, 2002, pp 127-136.

This chapter provides a broad overview of administrative databases used for clinical research, as well as a description of the potential pitfalls associated with their use.

Glantz SA: Primer of Biostatistics. New York, McGraw-Hill, 2002.

This popular primer introduces the fundamentals of biostatistics, uses many examples from medical literature, and is written in a manner that is both enjoyable and accessible to the uninitiated.

Gold M, Siegel JE, Russell LB, Weinstein MC: Cost-effectiveness in Health and Medicine. New York, Oxford University Press, 1996.

This concise and highly readable book was written by a panel of experts charged by the U.S. Public Health Service with the task of creating guidelines for the appropriate conduct of cost-effectiveness analysis.

Iezzoni LI: The risks of risk adjustment. JAMA 278:1600-1607, 1997.

This paper examines the history and current practices of risk adjustment with particular reference to the implications for quality assessment across hospitals.

McDowell I, Newell C: Measuring Health: A Guide to Rating Scales and Questionnaires. New York, Oxford University Press, 1996.

> **This book describes in detail a wide variety of patient-based surveys and other health measurement instruments that are commonly used in clinical outcomes research.**

Torrance G: Utility approach to measure health-related quality of life. J Chron Dis 40:593-600, 1987.

> **This landmark article describes the rationale and use of utility assessment, a technique that measures the "bottom line" of health from the patients' perspective: how patients feel about or value living in a specific health state.**

Ware JE Jr, Snow KK, Kosinski M, et al: SF-36 Health Survey: Manual and Interpretation Guide. Boston, The Health Institute, New England Medical Center, 1993.

> **This publication describes in detail the most ubiquitous and widely accepted general health assessment tool—the Medical Outcome Study SF-36—along with an overview of health dimension scores and their interpretation.**

References

1. Birkmeyer JD: Outcomes research and surgeons. Surgery 124:477-483, 1998.
2. Hannan EL, Kilburn H Jr, O'Donnell JF, et al: Adult open heart surgery in New York State: An analysis of risk factors and hospital mortality rates. JAMA 264:2768-2774, 1990.
3. Begg CB, Cramer LD, Hoskins WJ, Brennan MF: Impact of hospital volume on operative mortality for major cancer surgery. JAMA 280:1747-1751, 1998.
4. Porter GA, Soskolne CL, Yakimets WW, Newman SC: Surgeon-related factors and outcome in rectal cancer. Ann Surg 227:157-167, 1998.
5. Khuri SF, Daley J, Henderson W: The Department of Veterans Affairs' NSQIP: The first national, validated, outcome-based, risk-adjusted, and peer-controlled program for the measurement and enhancement of the quality of surgical care. National VA Surgical Quality Improvement Program. Ann Surg 228:491-507, 1998.
6. Birkmeyer JD: Using administrative data for clinical research. *In* Souba WW, Wilmore DW (eds): Surgical Research. San Diego, Academic Press, 2002, pp 127-136.
7. Iezzoni LI: Assessing quality using administrative data. Ann Intern Med 127:666-674, 1997.
8. Paul JE, Weis K, Epstein RA: Databases for variations research. Med Care 31:S96-S102, 1993.
9. Mitchell JB, Bubolz T, Paul JE, et al: Using Medicare claims for outcomes research. Med Care 32:S38-S51, 1994.
10. Epstein MH: Guest alliance: Uses of state-level hospital discharge databases. J Am Health Inform Manage Assoc 63:32-39, 1992.
11. Glantz SA: Primer of Biostatistics. New York, McGraw-Hill, 2002.
12. Dimick JB, Diener-West M, Lipsett PA: Negative results of randomized clinical trials published in the surgical literature: Equivalency or error? Arch Surg 136:796-800, 2001.
13. Iezzoni LI, Ash AS, Shwartz M, et al: Predicting who dies depends on how severity is measured: Implications for evaluating patient outcomes. Ann Intern Med 123:763-770, 1995.
14. Iezzoni LI: An introduction to risk adjustment. Am J Med Quality 11:S8-S11, 1996.
15. Iezzoni LI: The risks of risk adjustment. JAMA 278:1600-1607, 1997.
16. Concato J, Horwitz RI, Feinstein AR, et al: Problems of comorbidity in mortality after prostatectomy. JAMA 267:1077-1082, 1992.
17. Fisher ES, Whaley FS, Krushat WM, et al: The accuracy of Medicare's hospital claims data: Progress has been made, but problems remain. Am J Public Health 82:243-248, 1992.
18. Roos LL, Stranc L, James RC, Li J: Complications, comorbidities, and mortality: Improving classification and prediction. Health Serv Res 32:229-242, 1997.
19. Birkmeyer JD, Siewers AE, Finlayson EVA, et al: Hospital volume and surgical mortality in the United States. N Engl J Med 346:1128-1137, 2002.
20. Executive Committee for the Asymptomatic Carotid Atherosclerosis Study: Endarterectomy for asymptomatic carotid artery stenosis. JAMA 273:1421-1428, 1995.
21. Wennberg DE, Lucas FL, Birkmeyer JD, et al: Variation in carotid endarterectomy mortality in the Medicare population: Trial hospitals, volume, and patient characteristics. JAMA 279:1278-1281, 1998.
22. McDowell I, Newell C: Measuring Health: A Guide to Rating Scales and Questionnaires. New York, Oxford University Press, 1996.
23. Ware JE Jr, Snow KK, Kosinski M, et al: SF-36 Health Survey: Manual and Interpretation Guide. Boston, The Health Institute, New England Medical Center, 1993.
24. Ware JE Jr, Kosinski M, Keller SD: A 12-item short-form health survey construction of scales and preliminary tests of reliability and validity. Med Care 34:220-233, 1996.
25. Katz S, Ford AB, Moskowitz RW, et al: Studies of illness in the aged: The index of ADL—a standardized measure of biological and psychosocial function. JAMA 185:914-919, 1963.
26. Melzack R, Casey K: Sensory, motivational, and central control determinants of pain: A new conceptual model. *In* Kenshalo D (ed): The Skin Senses. Springfield, IL, Charles C Thomas, 1968, pp 423-443.
27. Torrance G: Utility approach to measure health-related quality of life. J Chron Dis 40:593-600, 1987.
28. Pascoe G: Patient satisfaction in primary health care: A literature review and analysis. Eval Program Plan 6:185-210, 1983.
29. Ware JE Jr, Snyder MK, Wright WR, et al: Defining and measuring patient satisfaction with medical care. Eval Program Plan 6:247-263, 1983.
30. Gold M, Siegel JE, Russell LB, Weinstein MC: Cost-effectiveness in Health and Medicine. New York, Oxford University Press, 1996.
31. Chapman RH, Stone PW, Sandberg EA, et al: A comprehensive league table of cost-utility ratios and a sub-table of "panel-worthy" studies. Med Decis Making 20:451-467, 2000.

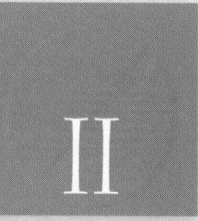

PERIOPERATIVE MANAGEMENT

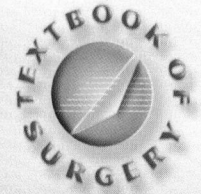

CHAPTER 10

PRINCIPLES OF PREOPERATIVE AND OPERATIVE SURGERY

Sharon L. Weintraub, M.D.,   Yi-Zarn Wang, D.D.S., M.D.,

John P. Hunt, M.D., M.P.H.,   and   J. Patrick O'Leary, M.D.

Preoperative Preparation of the Patient	**Potential Causes of Intraoperative Instability**
Systems Approach to Preoperative Evaluation	**Principles of Operative Surgery**
Additional Preoperative Considerations	**The Operating Room**
Preoperative Checklist	**Surgical Devices and Energy Sources**

PREOPERATIVE PREPARATION OF THE PATIENT

The modern preparation of a patient for operation characterizes the convergence of the art and science of the surgical discipline. The context in which preoperative preparation is conducted ranges from outpatient office visit to hospital inpatient consultation to the emergency department evaluation of a patient. The approaches to preoperative evaluation differ significantly, depending on the nature of the complaint and proposed surgical intervention, patient health and assessment of risk factors, and the results of directed investigation and intervention to optimize the patient's overall status and readiness for operation. This chapter reviews the components of risk assessment applicable to the evaluation of any patient for surgery and attempts to provide some basic algorithms to aid in the preparation of patients for surgery.

Determining the Need for Operation

Patients are often referred to the surgeon with a suspected surgical diagnosis and the results of supporting investigations in hand. In this context, the surgeon's initial encounter with the patient may be largely directed toward confirmation of relevant physical findings and review of clinical history and laboratory and investigative tests that support the diagnosis. A recommendation regarding the need for operative intervention can then be made by the surgeon and discussed with the patient's family members. A decision for further investigative tests, or consideration

of alternative therapeutic options, may postpone the decision for surgical intervention from this initial encounter to a later time. It is important for the surgeon to explain the context of the illness and the benefit of different surgical interventions, further investigation, and possible nonsurgical alternatives, when appropriate.

The surgeon's approach to the patient and the family during the initial encounter should be one that fosters a bond of trust and opens a line of communication among all participants. A professional and unhurried approach is mandatory, with time taken to listen to concerns and answer questions posed by the patient and his or her family members. The surgeon's initial encounter with a patient should result in the patient being able to express a basic understanding of the disease process and the need for further investigation and possible surgical management. A well-articulated follow-up plan is essential.

Perioperative Decision Making

Once the decision has been made to proceed with operative management, a number of considerations must be addressed regarding the timing, site of operation, anesthesia type, and preoperative preparation necessary to understand patient risk and optimize patient outcome. These components of risk assessment take into account both the perioperative (intraoperative through 48 hours postoperative) and later postoperative (up to 30 day) periods and seek to identify factors that may contribute to patient morbidity during these periods.

Preoperative Evaluation

The aim of preoperative evaluation is not to screen broadly for undiagnosed disease but rather to identify and quantify comorbidity that may impact operative outcome. This evaluation is driven by findings on history and physical examination suggestive of organ system dysfunction or by epidemiologic data suggesting the benefit of evaluation based on age, gender, or patterns of disease progression. The goal is to uncover problems areas that may require further investigation or be amenable to preoperative optimization (Table 10-1).[1,2]

If preoperative evaluation uncovers significant comorbidity or evidence of poor control of an underlying disease process, consultation with an internist or medical subspecialist may be required to facilitate the work-up and direct management. In this process, communication between the surgeon and consultants is essential to define realistic goals for this optimization process and to expedite surgical management.

SYSTEMS APPROACH TO PREOPERATIVE EVALUATION

Cardiovascular

Cardiovascular disease is the leading cause of death in the industrialized world, and its contribution to perioperative mortality for noncardiac surgery is significant. Of the 27 million patients undergoing surgery in the United States every year, 8 million, nearly 30%, have significant coronary artery disease or other cardiac comorbidities. One million of those patients will go on to have perioperative cardiac complications, with substantial morbidity, mortality, and cost.[3] As such, much of the preoperative risk assessment and patient preparation centers on the cardiovascular system.

Early risk-stratification schemes for surgery requiring general or spinal anesthesia were based on consensus panel recommendations, poorly defined criteria, and cross-sectional statistics. One of the first anesthesia risk categorization systems was the American Society of

---

TABLE 10-1.   Consensus Recommendations for Preoperative Screening Tests

Test	Age	Procedure Type	Disease or Condition
ECG	Male > 40–45 yr Female > 50–55 yr	Cardiovascular	Cardiovascular disease Hypertension Diabetes
Chest radiograph	>60–65 yr	Thoracic	Respiratory disease Cardiovascular disease Heavy smoker (relative)
Hemoglobin	***	Procedure for which > 500 mL blood loss is expected	Cardiovascular disease Renal disease Malignancy Diabetes Aspirin use NSAID use Full-dose anticoagulation
Creatinine	>50–65 yr	Procedure with high risk for postoperative renal failure	Use of drugs with renal excretion Renal disease Cardiovascular disease Hypertension Diabetes NSAID use
Glucose	>45 yr Possibly younger with risk factors	***	Diabetes Steroid use
Urinalysis	***	Genitourinary Use of a bladder catheter or other infection risk and orthopedic implant or valve replacement	Use of drugs with renal excretion Renal disease (relative) Cardiovascular disease (relative) Hypertension (relative) Diabetes
Pregnancy (qualitative HCG)	***	***	Women of childbearing age for whom pregnancy status is uncertain
Coagulation studies	***	***	Bleeding risk by history Plan full-dose anticoagulation

ECG, electrocardiogram; NSAID, nonsteroidal anti-inflammatory drug; HCG, human chorionic gonadotropin.
From Nierman E, Zakrzewski K: Recognition and management of preoperative risk. Rheum Dis Clin North Am 25:587, 1999.

Anesthesiologists (ASA) classification. This had five stratifications:

I—normal healthy patient
II—patient with mild systemic disease
III—patient with severe systemic disease that limits activity, but is not incapacitating
IV—patient that has incapacitating disease that is a constant threat to life
V—moribund patient not expected to survive 24 hours with or without an operation

The respective anesthetic-related mortalities were 0%, 0.17%, 0.6%, 4.3%, and 10.0%, respectively.[4] The ASA classification lacks accuracy for predicting risk and is not easily reproducible among physicians.[5]

Later assessment tools for anesthetic risk stratification revolved around more easily defined and measured parameters and were enhanced by multivariate statistical methodology. The premiere example is Goldman's criteria (Table 10-2).[6] This strategy, designed using multivariate analysis, assigns points to easily reproducible characteristics. These points are then added to yield a total, which has been correlated with perioperative cardiac risk, as follows:

Class I (0 to 5 points) has a 0.9% risk of serious cardiac event or death
Class II (6 to 12 points) has a 7.1% risk
Class III (13 to 25 points) has a 16.0% risk
Class IV (>26 points) has a 63.6% risk

TABLE 10-2. Computation of the Cardiac Risk Index

Criteria	Points
History	
Age > 70 yr	5
Myocardial infarction < 6 mo	10
Physical examination	
S_3 gallop or jugular venous distention	11
Aortic valvular stenosis	3
ECG	
Rhythm other than sinus or PACs	7
> 5 PVCs/min	7
General status	
Po_2 < 60 or Pco_2 > 50	
K < 3.0 or HCO_3 < 20 mEq/L	
BUN > 50 or creatinine > 3.0 mg/dL	3
Abnormal SGOT or chronic liver disease	
Bedridden	
Operation	
Intraperitoneal, intrathoracic, or aortic operation	3
Emergency operation	4
Total	Possible 53 points

ECG, electrocardiogram; PAC, premature atrial contraction; PVC, premature ventricular contraction; BUN, blood urea nitrogen; SGOT, serum glutamic-oxaloacetic transaminase.

From Goldman L, Caldera DL, Nussbaum SR, et al: Multifactorial index of cardiac risk in noncardiac surgical procedures. N Engl J Med 297:26, 1977.

One of the more important contributions of this work was the inclusion of patient's functional capacity, clinical signs and symptoms, and operative risk assessment to estimate overall risk and plan preoperative intervention. This concept has been further built on in the Revised Cardiac Risk Index, which uses six predictors of complications to estimate cardiac risk in noncardiac surgical patients. The factors include (1) high-risk type of surgery, (2) history of ischemic heart disease, (3) history of congestive heart failure, (4) history of cerebrovascular disease, (5) preoperative treatment with insulin, and (6) preoperative serum creatinine higher than 2.0 mg/dL. Major complications occurred in association with 0, 1, 2, or 3 or more of these factors in 0.5%, 1.3%, 4%, and 9%, respectively, in a cohort of patients from which these factors were originally derived.[7]

Further, in an attempt to best assess and optimize the cardiac status of patients undergoing noncardiac surgery, a joint committee of the American College of Cardiology and the American Heart Association has developed an easily used tool (Fig. 10-1).[8] This methodology takes into account previous coronary revascularization and evaluation and clinical risk assessment, which are divided into major, intermediate, and minor clinical predictors. The next factor taken into account is the patient's functional capacity, which is estimated by obtaining a history of the patient's daily activities. The next step involves using the earlier-mentioned variables and the surgery type to determine whether pretest probability can be altered via noninvasive testing. The standard exercise stress test with or without thallium for perfusion imaging can be limited by the functional capacity of the patient. Patients not able to exercise to an acceptable stress level may require pharmacologic stress testing with dipyridamole; thereafter, perfusion defects can be assessed via thallium or a dobutamine-induced stress followed by functional evaluation with echocardiography. Angiography can then be used to exactly define anatomic abnormalities contributing to ischemia.[9]

Once these data have been obtained, the surgeon and consultants need to weigh the benefits of surgery versus the risk and determine whether perioperative intervention will reduce the probability of a cardiac event. This intervention usually centers on coronary revascularization using coronary artery bypass or percutaneous transluminal coronary angioplasty but may include modification of anesthetic choice or the use of invasive intraoperative monitoring.

The optimal timing of a surgical procedure after myocardial infarction (MI) is dependent on the duration of time since the event and assessment of ischemic risk, either by clinical symptoms or noninvasive study. Any patient can be evaluated as a surgical candidate after an acute MI (within 7 days of evaluation), or a recent MI (between 7 and 30 days of evaluation). The infarction event is considered a major clinical predictor in the context of ongoing ischemic risk. Risk of reinfarction is generally considered low in the absence of such demonstrated risk. General recommendations are to wait 4 to 6 weeks after MI to perform elective surgery.[10]

Improvements in postoperative care have centered on decreasing the adrenergic surge associated with surgery

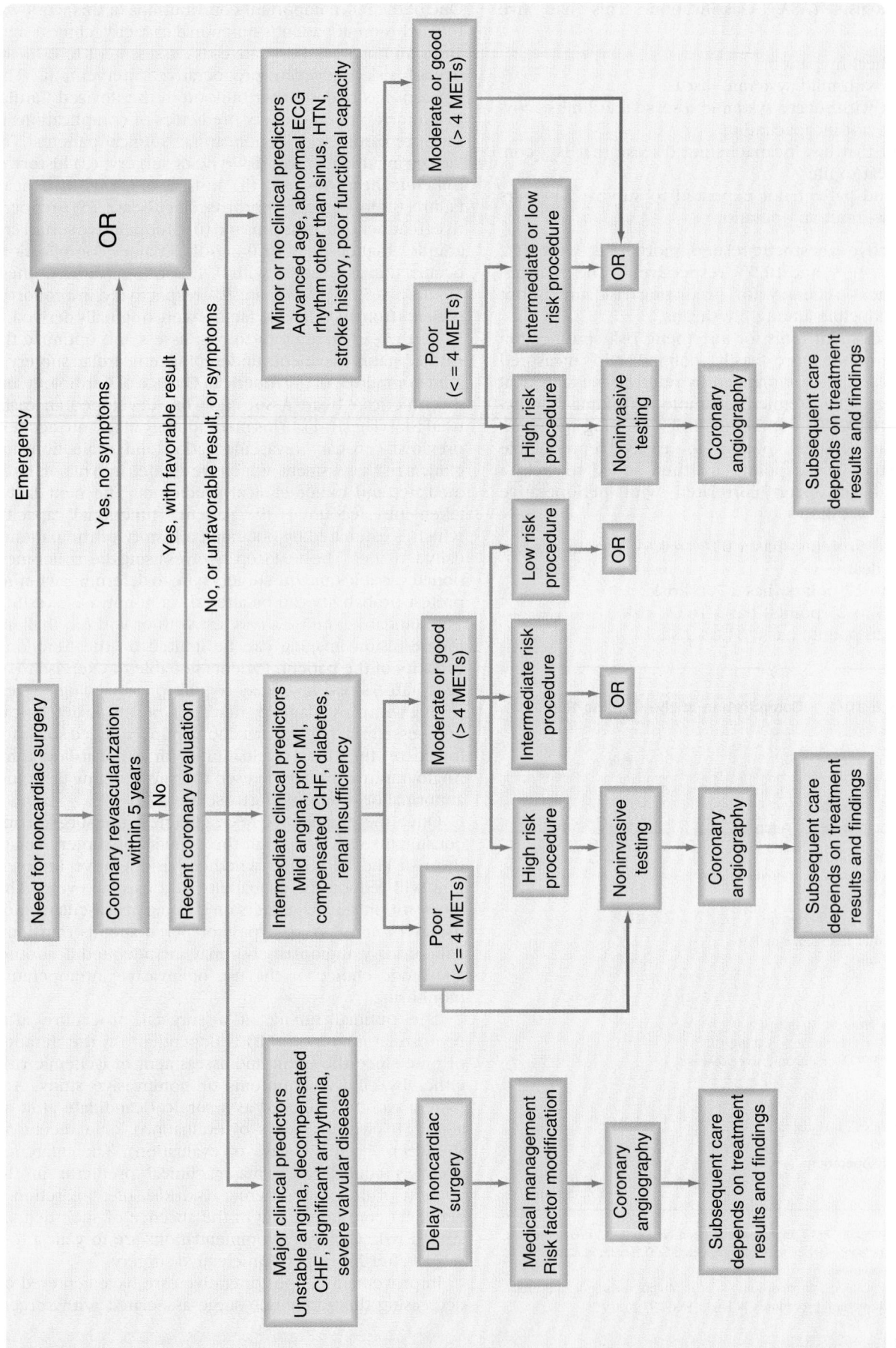

FIGURE 10-1.   Stepwise approach to preoperative cardiac assessment. An abbreviated list of metabolic equivalents (METs) includes the following: *1*—Take care of yourself, eat, dress, and so forth; *4*—Light housework; *5*—Climb a flight of stairs or walk up a hill; *10*—Strenuous sports. "Procedure risks" are defined as the following: *High*—emergent major operations, aortic surgery, other vascular surgery, large blood loss; *Intermediate*—carotid, head and neck, intraperitoneal, intrathoracic, orthopedic, or prostate surgery; *Low*—all others. OR, operating room; CHF, congestive heart failure; MI, myocardial infarction; ECG, electrocardiogram.

and halting platelet activation and microvascular thrombosis. Perioperative risk for cardiovascular morbidity and mortality was decreased by 67% and 55%, respectively, in patients receiving β blockade in the perioperative period versus those receiving placebo. Although the benefit was most noticeable in the 6 months following surgery, the event-free survival difference between the two groups was significantly better in the group that received β blockade up to 2 years after surgery.[11] There is also significant evidence to show that use of aspirin in the immediate postoperative period decreases morbidity and mortality in the cardiac surgery population.[12] Whether this benefit will extend to the noncardiac surgery population remains to be seen.

Pulmonary

Preoperative evaluation of pulmonary function may be necessary for either thoracic or general surgical procedures. Whereas extremity, neurosurgical, and lower abdominal surgical procedures have little effect on pulmonary function and do not routinely require pulmonary function studies, thoracic and upper abdominal procedures can decrease pulmonary function and predispose to pulmonary complications. As such, it is wise to consider assessing pulmonary function for all lung resection cases, for thoracic procedures requiring single-lung ventilation, and for major abdominal and thoracic cases in patients who are older than 60 years of age, have significant underlying medical disease, smoke, or have overt pulmonary symptomatology. Necessary tests include the forced expiratory volume at 1 second (FEV_1), the forced vital capacity, and the diffusing capacity of carbon monoxide.[13] Adults with an FEV_1 of less than 0.8 L/second, or 30% of predicted, have a high risk of complications and postoperative pulmonary insufficiency; nonsurgical solutions should be sought. Pulmonary resections should be planned so that the postoperative FEV_1 is greater than 0.8 L/second or 30% of predicted. This planning can be done with the aid of quantitative lung scans, which can indicate which segments of the lung are functional. The formula is as follows[14]:

> Anticipated loss of function = (preoperative FEV_1) × (% of function of the affected lung from scan) × (number of segments resected/total number of segments)

Conventional wisdom is employed with regard to intervention that may decrease postoperative pulmonary complications, including smoking cessation, bronchodilator therapy, antibiotic therapy for preexisting infection, and pretreatment of asthmatic patients with steroids. Perioperative strategies include the use of epidural anesthesia, vigorous pulmonary toilet and rehabilitation, and continued bronchodilator therapy.[15]

Renal

Approximately 5% of the adult population have some degree of renal dysfunction, which can affect the physiology of multiorgan systems and cause additional morbidity in the perioperative period. The identification of cardiovascular, circulatory, hematologic, and metabolic derangements secondary to renal dysfunction should be the goal of preoperative evaluation of these patients.

The patient with known renal insufficiency should have a thorough history and physical examination. The patient should be questioned about prior MI and symptoms consistent with ischemic heart disease. Cardiovascular examination should seek to document signs of fluid overload. The patient's functional status and exercise tolerance should be carefully elicited. Diagnostic testing for patients with renal dysfunction should include electrocardiogram (ECG), serum chemistry panel, and complete blood count (CBC). If physical examination findings are suggestive of heart failure, a chest radiograph may be helpful. Urinalysis and urinary electrolyte studies are not often helpful in the setting of established renal insufficiency, though they may be diagnostic in the setting of new-onset renal dysfunction.

Laboratory abnormalities are often seen in the patient with advanced renal insufficiency. Some metabolic derangements in the patient with advanced renal failure may be mild and asymptomatic and are uncovered with electrolyte or blood gas determination. Anemia, when present in these patients, may range from mild and asymptomatic to that associated with fatigue, low exercise tolerance, and exertional angina. Such anemia, if not treated with erythropoietin, will often require preoperative transfusion in the setting of acute operative blood loss. History of coagulation dysfunction should trigger evaluation of prothrombin time (PT) and partial thromboplastin time in these patients. As the platelet dysfunction of uremia is often a qualitative one, the bleeding time should be evaluated as well. The patient with end-stage renal disease often requires additional attention in the perioperative period. Pharmacologic manipulation of hyperkalemia, replacement of calcium for symptomatic hypocalcemia, and the use of phosphate-binding antacids for hyperphosphatemia are often required. Sodium bicarbonate is used in the setting of metabolic acidosis when serum bicarbonate levels are below 15 mEq/L. This can be administered in intravenous (IV) fluid as 1 to 2 ampules in 5% dextrose solution. Hyponatremia is treated with volume restriction, although dialysis is often required within the perioperative period for control of volume and electrolyte abnormalities.

Patients with chronic end-stage renal disease should undergo dialysis prior to surgery, to optimize their volume status and control the potassium level. Intraoperative hyperkalemia can result from surgical manipulation of tissue or the transfusion of blood. Such patients are often dialyzed on the day after surgery as well. In the acute setting, patients who have a stable volume status can undergo surgery without preoperative dialysis, provided that no other indication exists for emergent dialysis.[16] The prevention of secondary renal insult in the perioperative period must be the focus of the anesthesia and surgical teams. This includes the avoidance of nephrotoxic agents and maintenance of adequate intravascular volume throughout this period. In the postoperative period, the pharmacokinetics of many drugs may be unpredictable, and adjustments of dosages should be made according to pharmacy recommendation. Notably, narcotics used for postoperative pain control may have prolonged effects, despite hepatic clearance.

Hepatobiliary

Hepatic dysfunction may reflect the common pathway of a number of insults to the liver, including viral-, drug-, and toxin-mediated disease. The patient with liver dysfunction requires careful assessment of the degree of functional impairment as well a coordinated effort to avoid additional insult in the perioperative period.

Evidence of hepatic dysfunction may be seen on physical examination. Jaundice and scleral icterus may be evident with serum bilirubin levels higher than 3 mg/dL. Skin changes include spider angiomas, caput medusae, palmar erythema, and clubbing of the fingertips. Abdominal examination may reveal distention, evidence of fluid shift, and hepatomegaly. Encephalopathy or asterixis may be evident. Muscle wasting or cachexia can be prominent. The patient with liver dysfunction should have standard hepatocellular enzyme determinations, including aspartate aminotransferase (AST), alanine aminotransferase (ALT), lactate dehydrogenase, bilirubin, alkaline phosphatase, and albumin levels. Coagulation profile should also be done. Elevations in hepatocellular enzymes may suggest a diagnosis of acute or chronic hepatitis, which can be investigated with serologic testing for hepatitis A, B, and C. Alcoholic hepatitis is suggested by lower transaminase levels and an AST/ALT ratio greater than 2. Laboratory evidence of chronic hepatitis or clinical findings consistent with cirrhosis should be investigated with tests of hepatic synthetic function, notably serum albumin, prothrombin, and fibrinogen. Patients with evidence of impaired hepatic synthetic function should also have a CBC and serum electrolytes. Type and crossmatch usually is required for all but minor procedures. Platelet transfusion may be required for thrombocytopenia in the setting of acute operative intervention.

Preoperative liver function tests reveal asymptomatic abnormalities in some patients, without history or physical findings supportive of liver disease. In the preoperative setting, liver function tests should be further investigated to exclude a diagnosis of acute hepatitis and to clarify the degree of hepatic dysfunction prior to operation (Fig. 10-2).[17] In the event of an emergent situation requiring operation, such an investigation may not be possible. The patient with acute hepatitis with elevated transaminases should be managed nonoperatively, when feasible, until several weeks beyond normalization of laboratory values. Urgent or emergent procedures in these patients are associated with increased morbidity and mortality. The patient with evidence of chronic hepatitis may often safely undergo operation. The patient with cirrhosis may be assessed using the Child-Pugh classification, which stratifies operative risk according to a score based on abnormal albumin and bilirubin levels, prolongation of the PT, and degree of ascites and encephalopathy (Table 10-

3). This scoring system was initially applied to predict mortality in cirrhotic patients undergoing portacaval shunt procedures, though it has been shown to correlate with mortality in cirrhotic patients undergoing a wider spectrum of procedures as well. Data generated 20 years ago showed patients with Child's classes A, B, and C cirrhosis had mortality rates of 10%, 31%, and 76%, respectively during abdominal operations[18]; these figures have been more recently validated.[19] Although the figures may not represent current risk for all types of abdominal operations, little doubt exists that the presence of cirrhosis confers additional risk for abdominal surgery and that this risk is proportional to the severity of disease. Other factors that impact outcome in these patients are the emergent nature of a procedure, prolongation of the PT beyond 3 seconds and refractory to correction with vitamin K, and the presence of infection.

Two common problems requiring surgical evaluation in the cirrhotic patient are hernia (umbilical and groin) and cholecystitis. The presence of umbilical hernia is strongly associated with the presence of ascites, and failure to operate can lead to spontaneous rupture, with an associated mortality of 50%. Elective repair with perioperative control of ascites is the preferred approach in these cases, though still associated with mortality rates as high as 14%.[20] Groin hernias are less strongly associated with the presence of ascites; their repair is associated with far less risk of recurrence than umbilical hernias.[21]

Several recent reports have shown decreased rates of complication with laparoscopic procedures performed in cirrhotic patients. Among the best-described procedures is the laparoscopic cholecystectomy, performed in patients with Child's classes A through C. When compared to open cholecystectomy, less morbidity in terms of blood loss and wound infection has been observed.[22]

Malnutrition is common in the cirrhotic patient and is associated with a reduction in hepatic glycogen stores and reduced hepatic protein synthesis. Patients with advanced liver disease often have poor appetites, tense ascites, and abdominal pain. Attention must be given to appropriate enteral supplementation, as is done for all patients at significant nutritional risk.

Endocrine

The patient with an endocrine condition such as diabetes mellitus, hyperthyroidism or hypothyroidism, or adrenal insufficiency is subject to additional physiologic stress during surgery. The preoperative evaluation should identify the type and degree of endocrine dysfunction to allow for preoperative optimization. Careful monitoring should identify signs of metabolic stress related to inadequate endocrine control during operation and throughout the postoperative course.

The evaluation of a diabetic patient for operation should assess adequacy of glycemic control and identify the presence of diabetic complications, which may impact the patient's perioperative course. The patient's history and physical examination should document evidence of diabetic complications, including cardiac disease; circula-

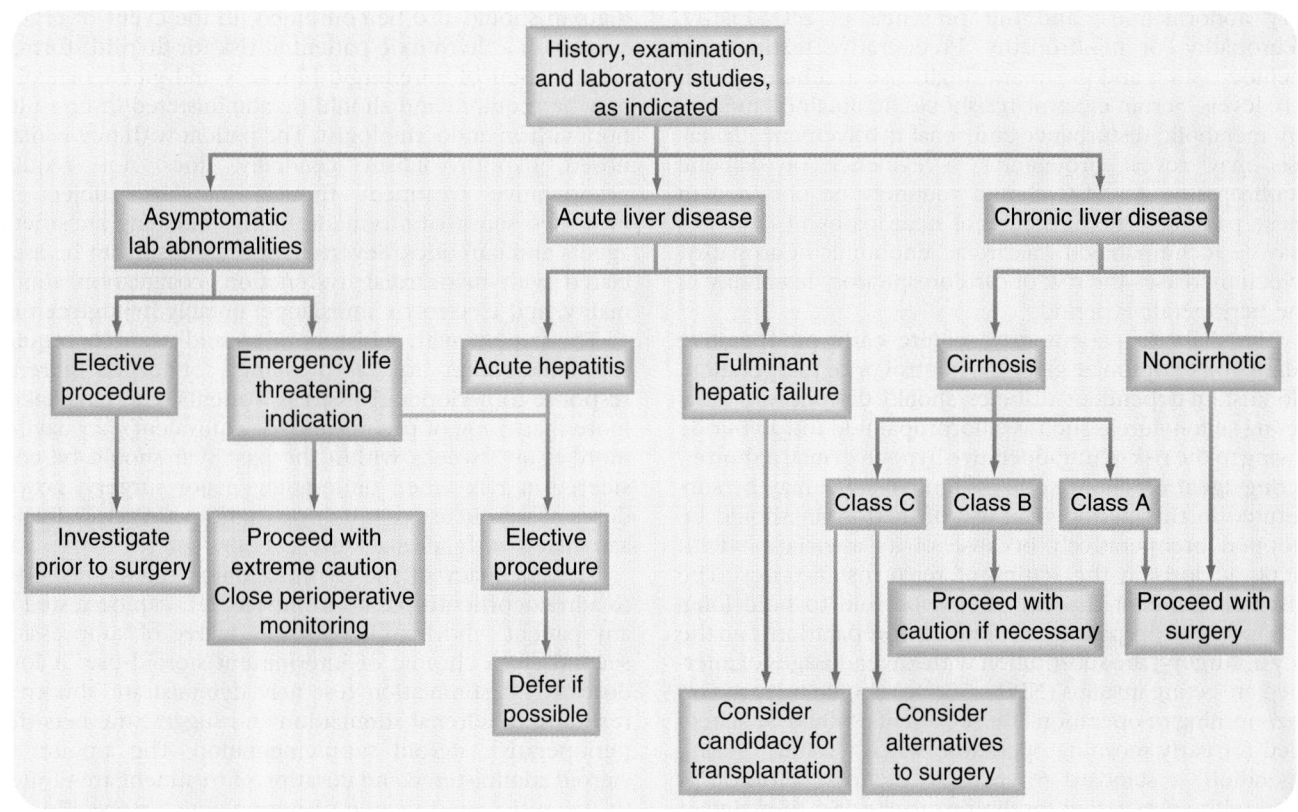

FIGURE 10-2. Approach to the patient with liver disease. (Adapted from Patel T: Surgery in the patient with liver disease. Mayo Clin Proc 74:593-599, 1999.)

TABLE 10-3. Child-Pugh Scoring System

	Points		
	1	**2**	**3**
Encephalopathy	None	Stage I or II	Stage III or IV
Ascites	Absent	Slight (controlled with diuretics)	Moderate despite diuretic treatment
Bilirubin (mg/dL)	<2	2-3	>3
Albumin (g/L)	>3.5	2.8-3.5	<2.8
PT (prolonged seconds)	<4	4-6	>6
INR	<1.7	1.7-2.3	>2.3

PT, prothrombin time; INR, International Normalized Ratio.
Class A = 5-6 points; Class B = 7-9 points; Class C = 10-15 points.

tory abnormalities; and the presence of retinopathy, neuropathy, or nephropathy. Preoperative testing may include fasting and postprandial glucose and hemoglobin A1c levels. Serum electrolytes should be obtained to identify metabolic disturbance and renal involvement. Urinalysis may reveal proteinuria as evidence of diabetic nephropathy. An ECG should routinely be obtained in these patients. The existence of neuropathy in diabetics may be accompanied by a cardiac autonomic neuropathy, which increases the risk of cardiorespiratory instability in the perioperative period.

The diabetic patient may require early preoperative admission to optimize glycemic control prior to operation. Noninsulin-dependent diabetes should discontinue long-acting sulfonylureas such as chlorpropamide and glyburide owing to the risk of intraoperative hypoglycemia; a shorter-acting agent or sliding-scale insulin coverage may be substituted in this period. The use of metformin should be stopped preoperatively because of its association with lactic acidosis in the setting of renal insufficiency. The insulin-dependent diabetic should be told to hold long-acting insulin preparations (Ultralente preparations) on the day of surgery; the substitution with lower dosages of intermediate-acting insulins (NPH or Lente) should be made on the morning of operation. These patients should be scheduled for early morning operation, when feasible. During operation, a standard 5% or 10% dextrose infusion is used with short-acting insulin or insulin drip to maintain glycemic control. The patient with diabetes mellitus that is well controlled by diet or oral medication may not require insulin perioperatively, but those with poorer control or on insulin therapy may require preoperative dosing and both glucose and insulin infusion during surgery.[23] Frequent assessment of glucose levels should be continued through the postoperative period. Adequate hydration must be maintained with avoidance of hypovolemia.

Postoperative orders should include frequent (2- to 4-hour) fingerstick glucose checks, with use of short-acting insulin in the form of sliding-scale coverage. Twice-daily doses of intermediate-acting insulin can be supplemented with sliding-scale coverage until the patient is eating and can resume his or her usual regimen. These patients may require postoperative ECGs to detect perioperative MI, which can be silent. Serum electrolyte levels should be followed daily, and adequate deep venous thrombosis (DVT) prophylaxis is essential due to increased risk of thrombosis. The adequacy of perioperative glycemic control impacts wound healing and the risk of surgical site infection.

The patient with known or suspected thyroid disease should be evaluated with a thyroid function panel. Evidence of hyperthyroidism should be addressed preoperatively and operation deferred until a euthyroid state is achieved, when feasible. These patients should have electrolyte levels and ECGs as part of their preoperative evaluation. In addition, if physical examination suggests signs of airway compromise, further imaging may be warranted. The patient with hyperthyroidism who takes antithyroid medication such as propylthiouracil or methimazole should be instructed to continue this regimen on the day of surgery. The patient's usual doses of β blockers or digoxin should also be continued. In the event of urgent surgery in a thyrotoxic patient at risk for thyroid storm, a combination of adrenergic blockers and glucocorticoids may be required and should be administered in consultation with an endocrinologist. The patient with newly diagnosed hypothyroidism generally does not require preoperative treatment though may be subject to increased sensitivity to medications, including anesthetic agents and narcotics. Severe hypothyroidism can be associated with myocardial dysfunction, coagulation abnormality, and electrolyte imbalance, notably hypoglycemia.

The patient with a history of steroid use may require supplementation for a presumed abnormal adrenal response to perioperative stress. Patients who have taken more than 5 mg of prednisone (or equivalent) per day for more than 2 weeks within the past year should be considered at risk when undergoing major surgery. Lower doses of steroid use or minor procedures are generally not associated with adrenal suppression.

The adequacy of the hypothalamic-pituitary response to adrenocorticotropic hormone (ACTH) can be tested in any patient who may have some degree of suppression secondary to chronic or intermittent steroid use. A low-dose ACTH stimulation test may demonstrate abnormal response to adrenal stimulation and suggest the need for perioperative steroid supplementation. The amount of steroid administered and duration of treatment are titrated to the anticipated degree of perioperative stress. Recent guidelines suggest titrating the dosage of glucocorticoid replacement to the degree of surgical stress. Minor operations such as hernia repair require approximately 25 mg of hydrocortisone equivalent. Moderate operations such as open cholecystectomy or lower extremity revascularization require 50 to 75 mg of hydrocortisone equivalent for 1 or 2 days. Major operations such as colectomy or cardiac surgery should be covered with 100 to 150 mg of hydrocortisone equivalent for 2 to 3 days.[24] Inadequacy of the hypothalamic-pituitary-adrenal axis in the perioperative period can lead to unexplained hypotension.

Patients with pheochromocytoma require preoperative pharmacologic management to prevent intraoperative hypertensive crises or hypotension leading to cardiovascular collapse. The state of catecholamine excess associated with pheochromocytoma should be controlled by a combination of α-adrenergic and β-adrenergic blockade prior to surgery. One to two weeks is usually required to achieve adequate therapeutic effect by α blockade; this can be accomplished with either a nonselective agent such as phenoxybenzamine, or selective α_1 agents such as prazosin. β Blockade is initiated several days after the α agent is begun and serves to inhibit the tachycardia that accompanies nonselective α blockade, as well as to control arrhythmia. Patients with pheochromocytoma may undergo surgery when pharmacologic blood pressure control is achieved.

Immunologic

The approach to a patient with suspected immunosuppression is the same, regardless of whether this state results from antineoplastic drugs in a cancer patient or immunosuppressive therapy in a transplant patient or is the result of advanced disease in patients with acquired immunodeficiency syndrome. The goal is to optimize immunologic function prior to operation and to minimize the risks of infection and wound breakdown.

Preoperative assessment should include a thorough history of the patient's underlying disease and current functional status; history of immunosuppressive treatment, including names of medications and duration of treatment; and history of recent changes in weight. Physical examination should seek to document signs of organ dysfunction, which may underlie the progression of disease or be related to its treatment. Laboratory assessment should include CBC with differential and electrolytes and liver function tests, and an ECG and chest radiograph should be obtained when age or physical findings suggest risk. Possible sites of infection should be investigated, including examination of any indwelling catheters, and may warrant complete work-up of any suspected infectious focus. Additional studies of T-cell, B-cell, polymorphonuclear, or complement function may be helpful to delineate the degree of immunocompromise. Neutropenia, anemia, or thrombocytopenia may accompany the underlying disease process or result from its treatment with immunosuppressive medication. Decisions regarding red blood cell transfusion or the use of synthetic erythropoietin or colony-stimulating factors are often based on the degree of dysfunction and other patient risk factors. Careful attention is given to nutritional deficiency in this patient population, with supplementation indicated in the perioperative period. Appropriate antibiotic prophylaxis is critical.

Patients who are immunocompromised may be at risk of wound complications, especially if on exogenous steroid therapy. When taken within 3 days of surgery, steroids reduce the degree of wound inflammation, epithelialization, and collagen synthesis. This can lead to wound breakdown and infection.

Hematologic

Hematologic assessment may lead to the identification of disorders such as anemia, inherited or acquired coagulopathy, or the hypercoagulable state. Substantial morbidity may derive from failure to identify these abnormalities preoperatively. The need for perioperative anticoagulation must be carefully reviewed for every surgical patient.

Anemia is the most common laboratory abnormality encountered in preoperative patients. It is often asymptomatic and can require further investigation to understand its cause. History and physical examination may uncover subjective complaints of energy loss, dyspnea, or palpitations, and pallor or cyanosis may be evident. Physical examination for lymphadenopathy, hepatomegaly, or splenomegaly should be made, and pelvic and rectal examinations should be performed. CBC, reticulocyte count, and serum iron, total iron-binding capacity, ferritin, vitamin B_{12}, and folate levels should be obtained to inves-

tigate the cause of anemia. Preoperative treatment and optimization are appropriate for the anemic patient. The decision to transfuse a patient perioperatively is made in consideration of the patient's underlying risk factors for ischemic heart disease and the magnitude of blood loss estimated during surgery. Generally, patients with normovolemic anemia without significant cardiac risk or anticipated blood loss can be managed safely without transfusion, with many healthy patients tolerating hemoglobin levels of 6 or 7 g/dL (Box 10-1).[25]

All patients undergoing surgery should be questioned to assess bleeding risk. Coagulopathy may result from inherited or acquired platelet or factor disorders or may be associated with organ dysfunction or medications. The inquiry begins with direct questioning about personal or family history of abnormal bleeding. Supporting information includes history of easy bruising or abnormal bleeding associated with minor procedures or injury. History of liver or kidney dysfunction should be elicited, as well as an assessment of nutritional status. Medications should be carefully reviewed, and the use of anticoagulants, salicylates, nonsteroidal anti-inflammatory agents (NSAIDs), and antiplatelet drugs should be noted. Physical examination may reveal bruising, petechiae, or signs of liver dysfunction. Patients with thrombocytopenia may have qualitative or quantitative defects, due to immune-related disease, infection, drugs, or liver or kidney dysfunction. Qualitative defects may respond to medical management of the underlying disease process, whereas quantitative defects may require platelet transfusion when counts are less than 50,000 in a patient at risk for bleeding. Although coagulation studies should not be routinely ordered, patients with a history suggestive of coagulopathy should undergo coagulation studies prior to operation. Patients with

---

Box 10-1. Guidelines for Red Blood Cell Transfusion for Acute Blood Loss

- Evaluate risk of ischemia.
- Estimate/anticipate degree of blood loss. Less than 30% rapid volume loss probably does not require transfusion in a previously healthy individual.
- Measure hemoglobin concentration: < 6 g/dL, transfusion usually required; 6–10 g/dL, transfusion dictated by clinical circumstance; >10 g/dL, transfusion rarely required.
- Measure vital signs/tissue oxygenation when hemoglobin is 6 to 10 g/dL and extent of blood loss is unknown. Tachycardia and hypotension refractory to volume suggest the need for transfusion; O_2 extraction ratio > 50%, V_{O_2} decreased, suggest that transfusion usually is needed.

From Simon TL, Alverson DC, AuBuchon J, et al: Practice parameters for the use of red blood cell transfusions: Developed by the Red Blood Cell Administration Practice Guideline Development Task Force of the College of American Pathologists. Arch Pathol Lab Med 122:130-138, 1998.

documented disorders of coagulation may require perioperative management of factor deficiencies, often in consultation with a hematologist.

Patients who receive anticoagulation therapy can require preoperative reversal of the anticoagulant effect. In patients taking warfarin, the drug can be held for several days preoperatively to allow the International Normalized Ratio (INR) to fall to the range of 1.5 or less. Patients with a recent history of venous thromboembolism or acute arterial embolism often require perioperative IV heparinization due to increased risk of recurrent events in the perioperative period. Systemic heparinization can often be stopped within 6 hours of surgery and restarted within 12 hours postoperatively. When possible, surgery should be postponed in the first month after an episode of venous or arterial thromboembolism. Patients on anticoagulation for less than 2 weeks for pulmonary embolism or proximal DVT should be considered for inferior vena cava filter placement prior to operation (Table 10-4).[26]

All surgical patients should be assessed for risk of venous thromboembolism and receive adequate prophylaxis according to current guidelines (Table 10-5).[27] Patients should be questioned to elicit personal or family history suggestive of a hypercoagulable state. Laboratory levels of protein C, protein S, antithrombin III, and antiphospholipid antibody panel can be obtained. Risk factor stratification is consideration of multiple factors including age, type of surgical procedure, previous thromboembolism, cancer, obesity, varicose veins, cardiac dysfunction, indwelling central venous catheters, inflammatory bowel disease, nephrotic syndrome, and pregnancy or estrogen use. A number of regimens may be appropriate for venous thromboembolism prophylaxis, depending on assessed risk (see Table 10-5). These include the use of unfractionated heparin, low-molecular-weight heparin, intermittent compression devices or elastic stockings, and early ambulation. Initial prophylactic doses of heparin can be given preoperatively, within 2 hours of operation, and compression devices should be in place prior to induction of anesthesia.

ADDITIONAL PREOPERATIVE CONSIDERATIONS

Age

Older adults comprise a disproportionate percentage of surgical patients. Risk assessment in this population must carefully consider the effect of comorbid illness in this population. Although age has been reported as an inde-

TABLE 10-4.   Recommendations for Perioperative Anticoagulation in Patients Taking Oral Anticoagulants

Indication	Preoperative	Postoperative
Acute venous thromboembolism		
Month 1	IV heparin	IV heparin
Months 2 and 3	No change	IV heparin
Recurrent venous thromboembolism Acute arterial embolism	No change	SC heparin
Month 1	IV heparin	IV heparin
Mechanical heart valve	No change	SC heparin
Nonvalvular atrial fibrillation	No change	SC heparin

IV, intravenous; SC, subcutaneous.
From Kearon C, Hirsh J: Management of anticoagulation before and after elective surgery. N Engl J Med 336:1506, 1997.

TABLE 10-5.   Levels of Thromboembolism Risk in Surgical Patients Without Prophylaxis and Successful Prevention Strategies

Level of Risk	Definition of Risk Level	Calf DVT (%)	Proximal DVT (%)	Clinical PE (%)	Fatal PE (%)	Prevention Strategy
Low	Minor surgery in patients < 40 yr with no additional risk factors	2	0.4	0.2	0.002	No specific measures Aggressive mobilization
Moderate	Minor surgery in patients with additional risk factors: nonmajor surgery in patients aged 40-60 yr with no additional risk factors; major surgery in patients < 40 yr with no additional risk factors	10-20	2-4	1-2	0.1-0.4	LDUH q 12 hr, LMWH, ES or IPC
High	Nonmajor surgery in patients > 60 yr or with additional risk factors; major surgery in patients > 40 yr or with additional risk factors	20-40	4-8	2-4	0.4-1.0	LDUH q 8 hr, LMWH or IPC
Highest	Major surgery in patients > 40 yr plus prior VTE, cancer, or molecular hypercoagulable state; hip or knee arthroplasty, hip fracture surgery; major trauma; spinal cord injury	40-80	10-20	4-10	0.2-5	LMWH, oral anticoagulants, IPC/ES + LDUH/LMWH or ADH

DVT, deep venous thrombosis; PE, pulmonary embolus; VTE, venous thromboembolism; LDUH, low-dose unfractionated heparin; LMWH, low-molecular-weight heparin; ES, elastic stockings; IPC, intermittent pneumatic compression; ADH, adjusted dose heparin.
From Geerts WH, Heit JA, Clagett GP, et al: Prevention of venous thromboembolism. Chest 119:132S-175S, 2001.

pendent risk factor for postoperative mortality, this observation may represent the more relevant issues of comorbid disease, severity of illness, and functional status.[28] Age alone should not be an exclusionary criterion for surgery.

The older adult patient should have a preoperative evaluation that seeks to identify and quantify the magnitude of comorbid disease and to optimize the patient's condition prior to surgery, where possible. Preoperative testing should be based on findings suggested in the history and physical examination of the patient. Generally, elderly patients should undergo ECG, chest radiograph, CBC, and glucose, blood urea nitrogen, and albumin levels. Appropriate preoperative studies should be based on the criteria discussed earlier for estimation of cardiac risk.

Nutritional Status

Evaluation of the patient's nutritional status should be a part of the preoperative evaluation. History of weight loss greater than 10% of body weight over 6 months or 5% over a month is significant. Albumin or prealbumin levels and immune competence (as assessed by delayed hypersensitivity reaction) may help identify patients with some degree of malnutrition, and physical findings of temporal wasting, cachexia, poor dentition, ascites, or peripheral edema may corroborate. The degree of malnutrition is estimated on the basis of weight loss, physical findings, and plasma protein assessment. The adequacy of a nutritional regimen can be followed with a number of serum markers. Albumin (half-life, 21 days), transferrin (half-life, 8 days), and prealbumin (half-life, 2 to 3 days) can be obtained on a regular basis in hospitalized patients. These proteins are responsive to stress conditions, however, and their synthesis may be inhibited in the immediate perioperative period. Once a patient is on a stable regimen and in an anabolic phase of recovery, these markers should reflect the adequacy of nutritional efforts.

The effect of perioperative nutritional support on outcomes has been studied in a number of trials. Patients with severe malnutrition (as defined by a combination of weight loss, visceral protein indicators, or prognostic indices) appear to benefit most from preoperative parenteral nutrition, as demonstrated in study groups treated with total parenteral nutrition for 7 to 10 days before surgery for gastrointestinal malignancy. The majority of studies show a reduction in the rate of postoperative complications from approximately 40% to 30%. The use of total parenteral nutrition postoperatively in similar groups of patients is associated with an increase in complication rates of approximately 10%.[29] Well-nourished patients undergoing surgery appear not to benefit from aggressive perioperative nutritional support, with parenteral nutrition further associated with increased septic complications. Generally, nutritional support should begin within 5 to 10 days of surgery for all patients unable to resume their normal diet. This may take the form of nasoenteric feeding, parenteral nutrition, or a combination of the two.

PREOPERATIVE CHECKLIST

The preoperative evaluation concludes with a review of all pertinent studies and information obtained from investigative tests. Documentation should be made in the chart of this review, which represents an opportunity to ensure that all necessary and pertinent data have been obtained and appropriately interpreted. Informed consent should be documented in the chart, which represents the result of discussion(s) with the patient and family members regarding the indication for the anticipated surgical procedure, as well as its risks and proposed benefits.

Preoperative orders should be written and reviewed as well. The patient should receive written instructions regarding time of surgery and management of special perioperative issues such as bowel preparation or medication usage.

Antibiotic Prophylaxis

Appropriate antibiotics for prophylaxis in surgery depends on the most likely pathogens encountered during the surgical procedure. The type of operative wound encountered[30] (Table 10-6) is helpful in deciding the

---

TABLE 10-6.   National Research Council Classification of Operative Wounds

Clean (class I)	Nontraumatic No inflammation No break in technique Respiratory, alimentary, or genitourinary tract not entered
Clean-contaminated (class II)	Gastrointestinal or respiratory tract entered without significant spillage
Contaminated (class III)	Major break in technique Gross spillage from gastrointestinal tract Traumatic wound, fresh Entrance of genitourinary or biliary tracts in presence of infected urine or bile
Dirty and infected (class IV)	Acute bacterial inflammation encountered, without pus Transection of "clean" tissue for the purpose of surgical access to a collection of pus Traumatic wound with retained devitalized tissue, foreign bodies, fecal contamination, or delayed treatment, or all of these; or from dirty source

Adapted from Cruse PJE: Wound infections: Epidemiology and clinical characteristics. *In* Howard RJ, Simmons RL (eds): Surgical Infectious Disease, 2nd ed. Norwalk, CT, Appleton & Lange, 1988.

appropriate antibiotic spectrum and should be considered prior to ordering or administering any preoperative medication. Prophylactic antibiotics are not generally required for clean (class I) cases, except in the setting of indwelling prosthesis placement, or in patients who have higher risk. This includes patients with three or more concomitant diagnoses and those whose operations are abdominal or longer than 2 hours.[31] Patients who undergo class II procedures benefit from a single dose of appropriate antibiotic administered prior to skin incision. For abdominal (hepatobiliary, pancreatic, gastroduodenal) cases, cefazolin is generally used. Contaminated (class III) cases require mechanical preparation or parenteral antibiotics with both aerobic and anaerobic activity. Such an approach should be taken in the setting of emergency abdominal surgery, as for suspected appendicitis, and in trauma cases. Dirty or infected cases often require the same antibiotic spectrum, which can be continued into the postoperative period in the setting of ongoing infection or delayed treatment.

The appropriate antibiotic should be chosen prior to surgery and administered before the skin incision is made. Repeat dosing should occur at an appropriate interval, generally 3 hours for abdominal cases or twice the half-life of the antibiotic. Perioperative antibiotic prophylaxis should generally not be continued beyond the day of operation. With the advent of minimal access surgery, the use of antibiotics seems less justified because the risk of wound infection is extremely low. For example, routine antibiotic prophylaxis in laparoscopic cholecystectomy for symptomatic cholelithiasis is of questionable value. It may have a role, however, in those cases that result in prosthetic graft (i.e., mesh) placement, such as laparoscopic hernia repair.

Review of Medications

A careful review of the patient's home medications should be a part of the preoperative evaluation prior to any operation; the goal is to appropriately use the medications that control the patient's medical illnesses, while minimizing the risk due to anesthetic-drug interactions or hematologic or metabolic effects of some commonly used medications and therapies. The patient should be asked to name all medications, including psychiatric drugs, hormones, and alternative/herbal medications, and to provide dosages and frequency.

In general, patients taking cardiac drugs, including β blockers and antiarrhythmics; pulmonary drugs such as inhaled or nebulized medications; or anticonvulsants, antihypertensives, or psychiatric drugs, should be advised to take their medications with a sip of water on the morning of surgery. Parenteral forms or substitutions are available for many drugs and may be employed if the patient remains NPO for any significant period postoperatively. It is important to return patients to their normal medication regimen as soon as possible. Two notable examples are the additional cardiovascular morbidity associated with the perioperative discontinuation of β blockers and rebound hypertension with abrupt cessation of the antihypertensive clonidine. Medications such as lipid-lowering agents or vitamins can be omitted on the day of surgery.

Some drugs are associated with increased risk of perioperative bleeding and should be held prior to operation. Drugs that affect platelet function should be held for variable periods: aspirin and clopidogrel (Plavix) should be held for 7 to 10 days, whereas NSAIDs should be held between 1 day (ibuprofen and indomethacin) and 3 days (naproxen and sulindac), depending on the drug's half-life. Estrogen use has been associated with an increased risk of thromboembolism and should probably be withheld for a period of 4 weeks preoperatively.[32]

The widespread use of herbal medications has prompted review of the effects of some commonly used preparations and their potential adverse outcomes in the perioperative period. These substances may fail to be recorded in the preoperative evaluation, although important metabolic and hematologic effects can result from their regular usage (Table 10-7).[33] Generally, the use of herbal medications should be stopped preoperatively. This may be done with caution in patients who report the use of valerian, which may be associated with a benzodiazepine-like withdrawal syndrome.

POTENTIAL CAUSES OF INTRAOPERATIVE INSTABILITY

Anaphylaxis/Latex Allergy

Intraoperative anaphylactic reactions may occur as frequently as one in every 4500 surgical procedures and carry a risk of mortality of 3% to 6%.[34] Causative agents are most often muscle relaxants, latex, induction agents such as etomidate and propofol, and narcotic drugs. Additional agents administered while patients are under anesthesia and that may be associated with anaphylaxis include colloid solutions, antibiotics, blood products, protamine, and mannitol.

The manifestations of anaphylactic reactions occurring under anesthesia may range from mild cutaneous eruptions to hypotension, cardiovascular collapse, bronchospasm, and death. When suspected, the offending agent should be discontinued and the patient given epinephrine 0.3 to 0.5 mL of 1:1000 subcutaneously; in severe anaphylaxis, this is given IV and repeated at 5- to 10-minute intervals, as needed. Histamine-1 (H_1) blockade with diphenhydramine 50 mg IV or intramuscularly and H_2 blockade with ranitidine 50 mg IV as well as hydrocortisone 100 to 250 mg IV every 6 hours are usually required. Additional supportive measures in the setting of hemodynamic or respiratory collapse may require fluid boluses, pressors, orotracheal intubation, and nebulized $β_2$ agonists or racemic epinephrine. Postoperative monitoring in the intensive care unit usually is required for a patient who has had an intraoperative anaphylactic reaction.

Latex sensitivity is the second-most common cause of anaphylactic reactions (after muscle relaxants) and should be screened for in the medical history. Although the incidence of such sensitivity may be less than 5% in the

TABLE 10-7. Perioperative Concerns and Recommendations for Eight Herbal Medicines

Common Name of Herb	Perioperative Concerns	Preoperative Recommendations
Echinacea	Allergic reactions; decreased effectiveness of immunosuppressants; potential for immunosuppression with long-term use	No data
Ephedra	Risk of myocardial ischemia and stroke from tachycardia and hypertension; ventricular arrhythmias with halothane; long-term use depletes endogenous catecholamines and may cause intraoperative hemodynamic instability; life-threatening interaction with monoamine oxidase inhibitors	At least 24 hr before surgery
Garlic	Potential to increase risk of bleeding, especially when combined with other medications that inhibit platelet aggregation	At least 7 days before surgery
Ginkgo	Potential to increase risk of bleeding, especially when combined with other medications that inhibit platelet aggregation	At least 36 hours before surgery
Ginseng	Hypoglycemia; potential to increase risk of bleeding; potential to decrease anticoagulation effect of warfarin	At least 7 days before surgery
Kava	Potential to increase sedative effect of anesthetics; potential for addiction, tolerance, and withdrawal after abstinence unstudied	At least 24 hr before surgery
St. John's wort	Induction of cytochrome P450 enzymes, affecting cyclosporine, warfarin, steroids, protease inhibitors, and possibly benzodiazepines, calcium-channel blockers, and many other drugs; decreased serum digoxin levels	At least 5 days before surgery
Valerian	Potential to increase sedative effect of anesthetics; benzodiazepine-like acute withdrawal; potential to increase anesthetic requirements with long-term use	No data

From Ang-Lee MK, Moss J, Yuan C-S: Herbal medicines and perioperative care. JAMA 286:208-216, 2001.

general population, higher-risk groups including those with genetic predisposition (atopic conditions) or chronic exposure to latex may have rates as high as 72%.[35] Those who give a history consistent with possible latex sensitivity should undergo skin testing prior to anticipated operative procedures. Appropriate intraoperative measures to ensure a "latex-free" environment should obviate most perioperative risks to the patient with latex allergy.

Malignant Hyperthermia

The incidence of malignant hyperthermia (MH) is higher in children and young adults than in adults; a rate of 1:15,000 is approximate in the group at highest risk, boys younger than 15 years of age.[36] MH represents an acute episode of hypermetabolism and muscle injury related to the administration of halogenated anesthetic agents or succinylcholine. MH susceptibility is inherited according to an autosomal dominant pattern, with apparent incomplete penetrance. The patient may therefore fail to reveal familial knowledge of the trait, and personal history of muscle disorder may not be evident.

An acute episode of MH may be recognized by increased sympathetic nervous system activity, muscle rigidity, and high fevers. Associated derangements include hypercarbia, arrhythmia, acidosis, hypoxemia, and rhabdomyolysis. When suspected, MH should be treated by discontinuation of inhalational anesthetic agents and succinylcholine, and with the administration of dantrolene sodium, in doses of 2 to 3 mg/kg IV. This may be titrated to the abatement of symptoms. Additional supportive measures include active or passive cooling and pharmacologic treatment of arrhythmia, hyperkalemia, and acidosis.

PRINCIPLES OF OPERATIVE SURGERY

Proper operative technique is of paramount importance in optimizing outcome and enhancing the wound healing process. There is no substitute for a well-planned and conducted operation to provide the best possible surgical outcome. One of the most reliable ways of ensuring that surgeons provide quality care in the operating room is through participation in high-quality surgical training programs, which provide the opportunities of repetitive observation and performance of surgical procedures in a well-structured environment. With their participation, young surgeons-in-training can progressively develop the technical skills necessary to perform the most demanding and complex operative procedures.

THE OPERATING ROOM

The operating room should be an extension of the classroom for surgical trainees and practicing surgeons. Each should understand the pathophysiology of surgical disease, as well as the treatment options available and their relative risks, benefits, and outcomes. Once surgical intervention is decided on, the choice of procedure and approach should follow. The surgeon should be familiar with the anatomy, sequence of a procedure, and possible complications related to the procedure. Alternative procedures should be considered if circumstances require it. The surgeon should be familiar with any new equipment that might be called on during the procedure.

To run an operating room efficiently requires well-trained surgeons, anesthesia, and operating room staff, and an operating room equipped with an easily maneuverable operating table, good lighting, and ample space for personnel and equipment. The room should be cleaned and the table checked for malfunction before and after each case. It is extremely costly and stressful to replace the operating table or other equipment with the patient already in the operating room. For more complex and unusual procedures, preoperative communication among surgeons, anesthesiologists, and operating room staff is vitally important. This helps save time, prevents confusion and undue frustration in the management of equipment usage, accounts for patient needs and personnel requirements, and makes planned procedures progress in a safe and efficient manner. The modern operating room for a trauma service, in particular, should have a temperature control panel that allows room temperature to be modified rapidly when dealing with a hypothermic patient. Patients should be appropriately positioned and secured on the table. Position-related neuromuscular or orthopedic injury should be prevented. Barriers should be established between the surgeon, patient, and other operating room staff with sterile drapes and gowns. The barriers should be impermeable to water and other body fluids. Finally, the intercom system must be functioning in the room. This facilitates communication between surgeons and pathologists, radiologists, blood bank, pharmacy, and the patient's family members. Most important, should an unexpected situation arise, help can be summoned immediately.

Hemostasis

Minimizing blood loss is an important technical aspect of surgery. Increased blood loss exacerbates the stress of surgery; less blood loss and resuscitation allow for the performance of a technically superior operation. In the presence of adequate hemostasis, one can conduct a more precise dissection and shorten both the operating time and the recovery time of the patient. Avoidance of blood transfusion obviates the risk of transfusion-related complications and blood-borne disease transmission. The negative impact of transfusion, which has been described in both oncologic and critical care populations, is similarly avoided.[37]

Essential operative technique dictates that larger vessels (about ≥1 mm) be tied, clipped, or sealed with monopolar or bipolar electrocautery or high-frequency ultrasonic devices. Major named vessels, in particular, should not only be tied but also undergo suture ligation. Hemoclip application is acceptable, especially in an operating field with an extremely confined space or when dealing with delicate vessels, such as portal vein branches. With limited-access procedures such as those performed with minimal access techniques, clip application seems to be a better choice than knot tying. At times it is necessary to use hemoclips, for example while performing an oncologic procedure in which outlining of margins provides a radiopaque marker for postoperative radiation.

In cases of catastrophic bleeding, such as when confronted by an unexpected intraoperative major vessel injury, intraperitoneal rupture of an aortic aneurysm, or bleeding resulting from major intra-abdominal trauma, temporary occlusion of the aorta at the esophageal hiatus with a compression device such as a T-bar or vascular clamp or manual compression should be considered. Such a maneuver may be lifesaving, by allowing anesthesia staff to catch up with blood loss by aggressive resuscitation. It also allows for the surgeon to remove intraperitoneal blood and clots with lap sponges or suction devices until the exact bleeding site can be identified, controlled, and repaired primarily or with an interposition graft. Occasionally, a partial vascular injury may need to be extended or converted to a complete transection to allow for better repair. This approach is particularly applicable to injury of the aorta and vena cava. Bleeding that occurs from multiple sites in a trauma patient, such as liver laceration or splenic injury, especially in a hypothermic patient, may best be treated with packing alone or in conjunction with angiographic embolization to achieve temporary control followed by a second-look operation. This maneuver of damage control is of paramount importance. It may represent the only way that a patient's life can be saved. Other adjuncts that may be helpful in dealing with wide areas of surface tissue oozing include microwave coagulation, laser coagulation, and application of topical hemostatic agents (i.e., Surgicel, thrombin, Gelfoam, and fibrin glue).

Wound Closure

Wound closure can be temporary or permanent; the latter can be primary or secondary. Critical factors in making this decision are the patient's condition, the clinical setting, the area of the body involved, the condition of the wound itself, and the disease process that led to surgical intervention.

Various methods can be chosen to close wounds in different part of the body, depending on clinical circumstance. In general, clean, noncontaminated wounds with healthy local tissue conditions are best closed by primary permanent closure. In a patient with a condition requiring re-exploration or one suffering from abdominal compartment syndrome, temporary closure is preferable. Heavily contaminated extremity or trunk wounds should be left open with packing. Heavily contaminated abdominal wounds are best served by fascial closure alone, with skin left open and packed. The principle of eliminating dead space to reduce the risk of seroma and hematoma formation is important and can be achieved internally with sutures or suction device or externally with a compression appliance.

Permanent closure can be achieved with either running or interrupted sutures. Suture can be monofilament or multifilament, braided or nonbraided, and dissolvable or nondissolvable (Tables 10-8 and 10-9). In general, when proven infection or contamination is a concern, monofilament, nonbraided suture is preferred. For abdominal wall closure in a debilitated, malnourished cancer patient, permanent closure with nondissolvable suture seems prudent. In a cirrhotic patient with established ascites or a patient who has the potential to develop post-

TABLE 10-8.   Comparison of Absorbable Sutures

Name	Material	Configuration	Absorption (days)
Surgical gut (chromic)	Animal collagen	Twisted	Unpredictable (14–80)
Monocryl	Poliglecaprone	Monofilament	Predictable (90)
Coated Vicryl	Polyglactin	Braided	Predictable (80)
Dexon	Polyglycolic acid	Braided	Predictable (90)
PDS	Polydioxanone	Monofilament	Predictable (180)
Maxon	Polyglyconate	Monofilament	Predictable (180)

Adapted from Ethicon Wound Closure Manual. Sommerville, NJ, Ethicon, Inc., 1999.

TABLE 10-9.   Comparison of Nonabsorbable Sutures

Name	Material	Configuration	Comments
Silk	Silk	Braided	Good handling and knotting characteristics; low durability of tensile strength
Ethilon	Polyamide (nylon)	Monofilament	Tissue reactivity minimal; good tensile strength over time
Dermalon	Polyamide (nylon)	Braided	Less tissue cutting in braided form
Prolene	Polyolefin (polypropylene)	Monofilament	Low reactivity, excellent retained tensile strength
Dacron	Polyester	Braided	Superior strength and durability; poor choice in contaminated field
Tevdek	Polyester (coated with Teflon—heavy)	Braided	Coating minimizes tendency to cut tissue

Adapted from Ethicon Wound Closure Manual. Sommerville, NJ, Ethicon, Inc., 1999.

operative ascites, the abdomen should be closed with running suture, and a multilayer watertight closure must be achieved. In this setting, our practice is to use a tunneled drain that enters the anterior and posterior fascia in different spots. Intermittent drainage helps reduce the tensile stress on the midline abdominal wound closure in the immediate postoperative period.

Temporary closure of the abdominal wall may be appropriate in the setting of a multiply injured patient or in the setting of intra-abdominal hypertension. This can be achieved with a vacuum suction device or via a prosthesis bridging technique using either a sterile IV bag or polypropylene mesh. The vacuum suction technique ("vac pack") uses a two-sided temporary closing material made of a biodrape over a blue towel. The biodrape faces the intestine and prevents adhesion to the blue towel. The membrane is tucked beneath the abdominal wall with the blue towel side facing up to provide retention and prevent potential loss of domain. The central portion of the drape is fenestrated prior to placement. Suction catheters and gauze dressings are placed beneath a second biodrape, which covers the entire abdominal wall and seals the closure. This technique has a number of advantages: it is quick and easy to employ, with materials that are readily available in the operating room; it requires no suturing and therefore maintains the integrity of the abdominal fascia for later permanent closure; and the applied suction prohibits fluid from accumulating in the abdominal cavity.

Disadvantages include inability to inspect the intestine (as with an IV bag) at the bedside, and the increased complexity of fluid and electrolyte balance due to potentially large fluid losses.

Two other new ideas in abdominal surgery include the use of adhesion reduction barriers and synthetic biomembranes for abdominal wall closure. There are two types of adhesion reduction barriers available: hyaluronic acid/carboxymethylcellulose and oxidized regenerated cellulose. Both of these materials are applied to the raw surface of bowel prior to abdominal closure, and within an hour they turn to a gelatinous substance.[38] Although the use of these membranes does not totally obviate adhesions, they have been demonstrated in clinical trials to decrease their severity.[39]

The second innovation is that of engineered tissue matrices that can be used for abdominal wall closure. These materials are constructed from donor integumentary tissue and processed to remove the epidermal and dermal cellular portions and thus antigenic component of the allograft. The resulting product is the collagen-based matrix with its native tensile strength intact but its capacity to generate an immune response abrogated. The interstices of the allograft are then colonized by cellular populations from the recipient.[40] This material promises to yield an adjunct to complex abdominal wall defect closures that has good strength and is more resistant to infection than synthetic materials such as polypropylene mesh (Table 10-10).

TABLE 10-10. Types of Synthetic Mesh and Their Uses

Type of Mesh	Trade Name	Type	Comments
NONABSORBABLE			
Polypropylene	Marlex, Prolene, Atrium	Monofilament	Highly elastic, withstands infection well; widely used for abdominal wall reconstruction, hernia repair
Polytetrafluoroethylene (PTFE)	Teflon	Multifilament	"Nonexpanded" mesh; associated with a large number of complications; limited utility
Expanded PTFE	Gore-Tex	Multifilament	Greatest elongation compared to other nonabsorbable meshes; minimal tissue incorporation; multiple uses in abdominal, vascular reconstruction
Polyethylene terephthalate	Mersilene, Dacron	Multifilament	Polyester fiber mesh with broad utility in abdominal wall, hernia repair; less extensively used than polypropylene
ABSORBABLE			
Polyglycolic acid	Dexon	Multifilament	Useful for temporary abdominal closure; resists infection
Polyglactin 910	Vicryl	Multifilament	Useful for temporary abdominal closure; resists infection

Adapted from Fenner DE: New surgical mesh. Clin Obstet Gynecol 43:650-658, 2000.

Staplers

Surgical staplers have changed the practice of surgery in a profound way, most notably within the field of minimally invasive technology. There are several different devices available for stapling: (1) skin staplers; (2) ligating and dividing staplers (LDSs); (3) gastrointestinal anastomosis (GIA) staplers; (4) thoracoabdominal (TA) staplers; (5) end-to-end anastomosis (EEA) staplers; (6) laparoscopic hernia mesh tackers; (7) open hernia mesh staplers; and (8) endo-GIA.

A modification of the GIA stapler for laparoscopic use, the endo-GIA, has particularly broad utility. It can facilitate the ligation and transection of major vascular pedicles in laparoscopy, as in splenectomy, nephrectomy, or hepatectomy, or facilitate gastrointestinal anastomosis or transection of solid organs such as pancreas. In the video-assisted thoracoscopic surgery procedure, it can aid in wedge resection of injured or diseased lung. The GIA (endo- or standard version) may aid in the transection of thick or indurated mesentery during intestinal resection for patients with inflammatory bowel disease.

Surgical Adhesives

Surgical adhesives have been widely used in modern surgery. Their application can be to a simple task such as skin closure or to more complex wound problems. Many agents are clinically available and are used for a variety of purposes. Fibrin seal adhesive has been used to close fistulae, prevent lymphatic leakage after a complete lymphadenectomy in the axilla or groin, and prevent leakage from tissue surfaces which have been newly transected, such as stapler lines of lung or pancreatic resection. It also has been adapted to seal the terminal bronchus via bronchoscopy as a noninvasive way to treat a small subset of patients with pneumothorax. It has become the preferred way to treat pseudoaneurysms in the groin or axilla that result from arterial puncture. The success of ultrasound-guided direct injection into such lesions has been reported with low complication rates.[41,42] Adhesives can also be used as an adjunct to reinforce and provide a watertight seal to a delicate gastrointestinal anastomosis, such as one of the biliary tract or pancreas.[43] This technique may have special relevance for anastomoses performed via the minimal access approach.

Surgical adhesives work by admixing a two-component agent derived from whole blood; each is secured in separate containers for shipping and storage. When mixed, the components form viscous semi-liquid tissue glue that can be applied onto a suture line, fistula tract or cavity, or other raw tissue surface or potential small dead space. When set, it becomes a solid adhesive biomembrane, sealant, or plug that will be self-retained. The major obstacles to its widespread use are the cost and the potential for complication related to disease transmission with the use of blood products. Two other commonly used agents are 2-octylcyanoacrylate (Dermabond) and butyl-2-cyanoacrylate (Histoacryl). Cyanoacrylate has been used for repair of organs and as an adhesive in many orthopedic procedures. Dermabond has been demonstrated as an adequate replacement for the traditional suture closure of simple skin lacerations.

SURGICAL DEVICES AND ENERGY SOURCES

Electrosurgery and Electrocautery

In 1928, Cushing first published a series of 500 neurosurgical procedures performed using an electrocautery device that was developed by Bovie. Since that time, electrocautery and electrosurgery have become the most important and basic surgical tools in the operating room.

High-frequency alternating current can be delivered in either a unipolar or a bipolar fashion. The unipolar (or monopolar) device is composed of a generator, an electrode of application and an electrode for the returning current to complete the circuit. The patient's body becomes part of the circuit when the system is activated. Since the effectiveness of energy conversion into heat is inversely related to the area of contact, the application electrode is designed to be small to generate heat efficiently, and the returning electrode is designed to be large to disperse energy and prevent burn injury to the patient. The heat generated is dependent on three other factors in addition to the size of contact area: the power setting/frequency of the current; the length of activation time; and whether the waveform released from the generator is continuous or intermittent. Unipolar devices can be used to incise tissue when activated with a constant waveform, and to coagulate when activated with an intermittent waveform. In the cutting mode, much heat is generated relatively quickly over the target with minimum lateral thermal spread. As a result, the device cuts through tissue without coagulating underlying vessels. In contrast, with the coagulation mode, the electrocautery generates less heat on a slower frequency, with potential for large lateral thermal spread. This results in tissue dehydration and vessel thrombosis. A blind waveform can be chosen that will be able to take the advantages of both cutting and coagulation mode. A large grounding pad must be placed securely on the patient for the unipolar electrosurgery/electrocautery device to function properly, and to prevent thermal burn injury to the patient at the current re-entry electrode site.

Bipolar electrocautery establishes a short circuit between the tips of the instrument, whether a tissue grasper or forceps, without the requirement of grounding pad. The tissue grasped between the tips of the instrument completes the circuit. In generating heat that only affects the tissue within the short circuit, it provides precise thermal coagulation. Bipolar electrocautery is more effective than the monopolar instrument in coagulating vessels because it adds the mechanical advantage of compression of tissue between the tips of the instrument to the thermal coagulation. Bipolar electrocautery is particularly useful in conducting a procedure in which lateral thermal injury or arcing phenomenon need to be avoided.

Lasers

Lasers use photons to excite the chromophore molecules within target tissue, generating kinetic energy that is released as heat, causing protein denaturation and coagulation necrosis. This occurs without much collateral damage to surrounding tissue. It can be applied onto the surface of target tissue or interstitially with a fiberoptic probe placed with precision image guidance. The energy generated and the depth of tissue penetration can be varied based on the power setting selected and the photon chosen for the particular task. Laser effect can be enhanced by photosensitizing agents. The most common types of laser in use today are the argon, carbon dioxide, and neodymium-yttrium aluminum garnet (Nd-YAG) lasers. The depth of energy penetration within the target organ is least with the argon laser, moderate with the carbon dioxide laser, and deepest with the Nd-YAG laser.

Interstitial laser photocoagulation is a recently adopted laser treatment technology. With a precisely placed optic fiber (or fibers) inside target tissue, laser light is delivered and absorbed by the surrounding structure and tissue. The degree of absorption within and around the target tissue depends on the wavelength of the laser chosen and the specific optical properties of the tissue. The optical properties of different tumors or tissues are markedly different based on their tissue composition and density, degree of parenchymal fibrosis, vascularity, and presence or absence of necrosis. This technology was initially used in the treatment of hepatic parenchymal tumors. Recently, its use has been reported in the treatment of lesions in the breast, thyroid, kidney, prostate, and even bone.[44-47]

Photodynamic Therapy

Photodynamic therapy is a new treatment that allows destruction of cancer cells and has recently been expanded to the eradication of metaplastic cells. It begins with the administration of a target-specific photosensitizer that is eventually concentrated in the target tissue. The photosensitizing agent is then activated with a wavelength-specific light energy source leading to the generation of free radicals cytotoxic to the target tissue. Photodynamic therapy has been used to treat different types of late-stage cancers, mainly in a palliative setting, but has also been used in the treatment of some chemoresistant tumors. Applications reported in the literature include treating early radiographically detected non-small cell lung cancer, pancreatic cancer, squamous cell and basal cell carcinoma of skin, recurrent superficial bladder cancer, chest wall involvement from breast cancer, and even a chest wall recurrence of breast cancer.[48,49] Its utility has recently expanded to include the treatment of noncancer conditions such as Barrett's esophagus and psoriasis.[50,51]

Argon Beam Coagulator

The argon beam coagulator creates a monopolar electric circuit between a handheld probe and target tissue by establishing a steady flow of electrons through a channel of electrically activated and ionized argon gas. This high-flow argon gas conducts electrical current to the target tissue and generates thermal coagulation on the target tissue. The depth of the thermal penetration of tissue varies from fractions of a millimeter to a maximum of 6 mm, depending on three factors: (1) the power setting; (2) the distance between the probe and the target; and (3) the length of its application. The handheld control is usually combined with the regular Bovie, which can provide much more focused tissue coagulation for any such vessels. Since the argon gas blows blood away from the surface or parenchyma of the target organ, coagulation is more effective in this setting. Visibility is also improved by the same mechanism. It is most commonly used to treat organ parenchymal hemorrhage, particularly the liver, but it can be used on spleen, kidney, or any other solid organs with surface oozing.

High-Frequency Sound Wave Techniques

Ultrasound has had a strong impact on the practice of modern medicine. It has different functions depending on the frequency of ultrasound generated by the machine. At low-power level, it causes no tissue damage and it is mainly used for diagnostic purposes. With a high-frequency setting, ultrasound can be used to dissect, cut, and coagulate. There are several high-frequency ultrasonic devices available for surgical practice.

Another beneficial manipulation of acoustic wave technology is that of extracorporeal shock-wave lithotripsy. It has been used in treating cholelithiasis and nephrolithiasis. In this modality, the patient is placed in a water bath and a high-energy acoustic shock wave is generated by piezoelectric or electromagnetic technology and focused. The water-tissue interface allows the wave to pass through normal tissue without injuring it. The energy of the shock wave is focused on the offending stone by ultrasound and causes disruption and fragmentation of the calculus, which is then passed via the ureter or biliary tree. Its use has been validated as a useful way to deal with renal calculi, but its value for cholelithiasis is still in question.[52,53]

Harmonic Scalpel

The harmonic scalpel is an instrument that uses ultrasound technology to dissect tissue in a bipolar fashion with only minimal collateral tissue damage. The device vibrates at a high frequency, usually around 55,000 times per second, to cut tissue. The high-frequency vibration of tissue molecules generates stress and friction in the tissue, which in turn generate heat and protein denaturation. Because of this unique capability to dissect tissue and coagulate small blood vessels all at once with minimal energy transfer to surrounding tissue, the device has gained recognition among surgeons. It has been used in many different types of minimally invasive surgery, and its application has recently been extended to many open procedures as well.

Ultrasonic Tissue Ablation Device—High-Intensity Focused Ultrasound

High-intensity focused ultrasound (HIFU) is a new ultrasonic device that has been applied to tissue ablation. The major advantage of this technique is that it can be applied extracorporeally and without any surrounding tissue damage. It delivers intense ultrasound energy from multiple ultrasonic beams activated simultaneously. Target lesions are ablated by this intensely focused ultrasonic energy that can heat target tissue to more than 60°C in less than a second, causing thermal coagulation necrosis. Liver, breast, kidney, spleen, prostate, and bladder all are conceivable targets for its application. The major disadvantage of this technique is that it needs a direct ultrasonic pathway without interference of air and bone and currently can deal only with lesions that are extremely small (~1 mm^3).[54]

Ultrasonic Cavitation Devices

The Cavitron ultrasonic surgical aspirator is an ultrasonic instrument that uses lower frequency ultrasound energy to fragment and dissect tissue of low fiber content. It is basically an ultrasound probe combined with an aspirator, so it functions as an acoustic vibrator and suction device at the same time. Cavitron ultrasonic surgical aspirator has a variety of applications. Because the instrument fragments and aspirates tissue of low collagen and high water content, it can be an effective surgical instrument for liver and pancreas procedures without causing damage to the surrounding tissue. Compared to the dissection technique using other instruments such as scalpel or cautery, the advantages of using this device are less blood loss, improved visibility, and reduced collateral tissue injury. The device has been used for resecting lesions in a noncirrhotic liver and pancreatic tumors, especially those small endocrine tumors within a soft normal pancreas without fibrosis. It has also been used for partial nephrectomy, salvaging splenectomy, head and neck procedures, and treatment of many gynecologic tumors as well.

Radiofrequency Ablation

Radiofrequency energy can be used for tissue ablation either in a curative or palliative attempt to treat different cancers. It is also effective in treating benign conditions such as neuralgia, bone pain, and cardiac arrhythmias (e.g., atrial fibrillation). It has recently been adapted to treat gastroesophageal reflux disease by an endoscopic approach.[55] The basic mechanism for the radiofrequency application is placing an electrode(s) into or over the target tissue to transmit a high-frequency alternating current at the range of 350 to 500 kHz to the tissue. Rapid alternating directional movements of ions result in the release of kinetic energy. It can raise the temperature of target tissue to higher than 100°C and cause protein denaturation, desiccation, and coagulation necrosis, with a built-in sensor terminating the transmission of the current automatically at a particular set point, preventing overheating and unwanted collateral damage. The main use of this modality is for tumors in the liver parenchyma. Its applications have been expanded to tumors in the lung, kidney, adrenal gland, breast, thyroid, pancreas, and bone. The indications for radiofrequency use will continue to grow in the future because it is inexpensive and can reliably be used to destroy a larger tumor mass.[43,56-62]

Cryoablation

Cryotherapy can be applied topically to treat skin conditions or tumors or interstitially in the ablation of liver lesions. It destroys cells by the processes of freezing and thawing. With liquid nitrogen or argon circulating through a probe placed over or within the target lesion, the tissue can be frozen to a temperature of −35°C or lower. Cell damage occurs due to the disruption of subcellular structures with ice crystal formation in the freezing phase and degradation during the thawing process. Ischemia of the tissue from focal disruption of circulation, shifting of water and electrolyte content in situ, and protein denaturation also contribute to the tissue damage induced by cryotherapy. Lesions that contact major vessels can be difficult to treat with this modality, due to the heat-sink effect introduced by circulating blood. Despite this, it has been reported effective in treating both primary and secondary lesions of the liver that are unresectable. The major disadvantage of interstitial cryotherapy is the cost. Patients usually need general anesthesia for the procedure, the equipment is more expensive compared to radiofrequency system, and the process itself is time consuming. Complications such as hemorrhage due to tissue fracture are a concern. With the availability of multiple alternative image-guided tissue ablation techniques, cryotherapy will have limited application in the future.[56,63-65]

Microwave Ablation and Radiosurgery

Microwave coagulation is achieved using a generator to transmit microwave energy at a frequency of 2450 MHz via a probe placed under image guidance within target organs or tissue. A rapidly alternating electrical field is created within the target tissue, which in turn induces motion of polar molecules in the tissue, such as water. Kinetic energy is dissipated as heat, causing coagulation necrosis. Its usage was initially for lesions in the liver; however, its application has been expanded into treatment of cardiac rhythm disturbances of the heart, prostatic hyperplasia, endometrial bleeding, sterilization of bony margins, and partial nephrectomy. The major limiting factor is that the area that can be ablated with current equipment is very small, necessitating multiple insertions of the microwave probe to treat a single lesion.[43,61]

The premiere tool in radiosurgery is the gamma knife, and its principal area of use is in neurosurgery. This tool allows more than 200 separate sources of high-energy gamma radiation, arranged in a circular fashion, to be stereotactically focused to a minute area within the brain. Essential to avoiding injury to normal brain tissue is that the head be held motionless by an external fixation device. This ability to destroy finite areas within the brain has been applied to the treatment of benign and malignant brain neoplasms, arteriovenous malformations, and epilepsy.[66-68]

Selected References

Cohn SL (ed): Preoperative Medical Consultation. *In* Medical Clinics of North America, Vol 87. Philadelphia, WB Saunders, January 2003.

   An overview of the components of risk assessment and organized approach to medical consultation for preoperative evaluation.

Eagle KA, Berger PB, Calkins H, et al: ACC/AHA guideline update on perioperative cardiovascular evaluation for noncardiac surgery: A report of the American College of Cardiology/American Heart Association Task Force on Practice Guidelines (Committee to Update the 1996 Guidelines on Perioperative Cardiovascular Evaluation for Noncardiac Surgery). Circulation 105:1257-1267, 2002.

   Evidence-based guidelines for perioperative cardiovascular evaluation for noncardiac surgery, updated in 2002 by the American College of Cardiology/American Heart Association Task Force on Practice Guidelines.

Geerts WH, Heit JA, Clagett GP, et al: Prevention of venous thromboembolism. Chest 119:132S-175S, 2001.

   Evidence-based guidelines for the prevention of venous thromboembolism among patients of varying risk groups. Published by the American College of Chest Physicians, 2001.

Gulec SA, Wang YZ, Reinbold RB, et al: Selected technologies in general surgery. *In* The Physiologic Basis of Surgery, 3rd ed. Philadelphia, Lippincott Williams & Wilkins, 2002.

   An overview of the basic principles behind technology commonly used in the operating room and for diagnostic purposes.

Klein S, Kinney J, Jeejeebhoy K, et al: Nutrition support in clinical practice: Review of published data and recommendations for future research directions. JPEN J Parenter Enteral Nutr 21:133-156, 1997.

   A summary of nutritional support data, relevant to the treatment of patients requiring all levels of nutritional support.

Litaker D: Preoperative screening. Med Clin North Am 83:6, 1999.

   A discussion of how to understand risk in the preoperative patient and a review of effective screening tools to highlight sources of risk. From the IMPACT (Internal Medicine Preoperative Assessment, Consultation, and Treatment) Center and Department of General Internal Medicine, The Cleveland Clinic.

Mack MJ: Minimally invasive and robotic surgery. JAMA 285:568-572, 2001.

   An overview of emerging technologies relevant to practitioners-in-training in the surgical fields.

References

1. Barnard NA, Williams RW, Spencer EM: Preoperative patient assessment: A review of the literature and recommendations. Ann R Coll Surg Engl 76:293-297, 1994.
2. Nierman E, Zakrzewski K: Recognition and management of preoperative risk. Rheum Dis Clin North Am 25:585-622, 1999.
3. Mangano DT, Goldman L: Preoperative assessment of patients with known or suspected coronary disease. N Engl J Med 333:1750-1756, 1995.
4. Dripps RD, Lamont A, Eckenhoff JE: The role of anesthesia in surgical mortality. JAMA 178:261-267, 1961.
5. Goldman L, Caldera DL, Nussbaum SR, et al: Multifactorial index of cardiac risk in noncardiac surgical procedures. N Engl J Med 297:845-850, 1977.

6. Haynes SR, Lawler PG: An assessment of the consistency of ASA physical status classification allocation. Anaesthesia 50:195-199, 1995.

7. Lee TH, Marcantonio ER, Mangione CM, et al: Derivation and prospective validation of a simple index for prediction of cardiac risk of major noncardiac surgery. Circulation 100:1043-1049, 1999.

8. Fleischer LA, Froelich JB, Gusberg RJ, et al: American College of Cardiology/American Heart Association (ACC/AHA) guideline update on perioperative cardiovascular evaluation for noncardiac surgery: A report. Circulation 105:1257-1267, 2002.

9. Paul SD, Eagle KA: A stepwise strategy for coronary risk assessment for noncardiac surgery. Med Clin North Am 79:1241-1262, 1995.

10. Eagle KA, Berger PB, Calkins H, et al: ACC/AHA guideline update for perioperative cardiovascular evaluation for noncardiac surgery: A report of the American College of Cardiology/American Heart Association Task Force on Practice Guidelines (Committee to Update the 1996 Guidelines on Perioperative Cardiovascular Evaluation for Noncardiac Surgery). Circulation 105:1257-1267, 2002.

11. Mangano DT, Layug EL, Wallace A, et al: Effect of atenolol on mortality and cardiovascular morbidity after noncardiac surgery. Multicenter Study of Perioperative Ischemia Research Group. N Engl J Med 335:1713-1720, 1996.

12. Mangano DT: Aspirin and mortality from coronary bypass surgery. N Engl J Med 347:1309-1317, 2002.

13. Tisi GM: Preoperative evaluation of pulmonary function: Validity, indications, and benefits. Am Rev Respir Dis 119:293-310, 1979.

14. Wait J: Southwestern Internal Medicine Conference: Preoperative pulmonary evaluation. Am J Med Sci 310:118-125, 1995.

15. Reilly JJ Jr, Mentzer SJ, Sugarbaker DJ: Preoperative assessment of patients undergoing pulmonary resection. Chest 103:342S-345S, 1993.

16. Joseph AJ, Cohn SL: Perioperative care of the patient with renal failure. Med Clin North Am 87:193-210, 2003.

17. Patel T: Surgery in the patient with liver disease. Mayo Clin Proc 74:593-599, 1999.

18. Garrison RN, Cryer HM, Howard DA, et al: Clarification of risk factors for abdominal operations in patients with hepatic cirrhosis. Ann Surg 199:648-655, 1984.

19. Mansour A, Watson W, Shayani V, et al: Abdominal operations in patients with cirrhosis: Still a major surgical challenge. Surgery 122:730-736, 1997.

20. Maniatis AG, Hunt CM: Therapy for spontaneous umbilical hernia rupture. Am J Gastroenterol 90:310-312, 1995.

21. Hurst RD, Butler BN, Soybel DI, et al: Management of groin hernias in patients with ascites. Ann Surg 216:696-700, 1992.

22. Yerdel MA, Koksoy C, Aras N, et al: Laparoscopic versus open cholecystectomy in cirrhotic patients: A prospective study. Surg Laparosc Endosc 7:483-486, 1997.

23. Schiff RL, Welsh GA: Perioperative evaluation and management of the patient with endocrine dysfunction. Med Clin North Am 87:175-192, 2003.

24. Salem M, Tainsh RE Jr, Bromberg J, et al: Perioperative glucocorticoid coverage: A reassessment 42 years after emergence of a problem. Ann Surg 219:416-425, 1994.

25. Simon TL, Alverson DC, AuBuchon J, et al: Practice parameter for the use of red blood cell transfusions: Developed by the Red Blood Cell Administration Practice Guideline Development Task Force of the College of American Pathologists. Arch Pathol Lab Med 122:130-138, 1998.

26. Kearon C, Hirsh J: Management of anticoagulation before and after elective surgery. N Engl J Med 336:1506-1511, 1997.

27. Geerts WH, Heit JA, Clagett GP, et al: Prevention of venous thromboembolism. Chest 119:132S-175S, 2001.

28. Cruse PJE: Wound infections: Epidemiology and clinical characteristics. In Howard RJ, Simmons RL (eds): Surgical Infectious Disease, 2nd ed. Norwalk, CT, Appleton & Lange, 1988, pp 319-329.

29. Klein S, Kinney J, Jeejeebhoy K, et al: Nutrition support in clinical practice: Review of published data and recommendations for future research directions. National Institutes of Health, American Society for Parenteral and Enteral Nutrition, and American Society for Clinical Nutrition. JPEN J Parenter Enteral Nutr 21:133-156, 1997.

30. Haley RW, Culver DH, Morgan WM, et al: Identifying patients at high risk of surgical wound infection: A simple multivariate index of patient susceptibility and wound contamination. Am J Epidemiol 121:206-215, 1985.

31. Thomas DR, Ritchie CS: Preoperative assessment of older adults. J Am Geriatr Soc 43:811-821, 1995.

32. Mercado DL, Petty BG: Perioperative medication management. Med Clin North Am 87:41-57, 2003.

33. Ang-Lee MK, Moss J, Yuan CS: Herbal medicines and perioperative care. JAMA 286:208-216, 2001.

34. Lieberman P: Anaphylactic reactions during surgical and medical procedures. J Allergy Clin Immunol 110:S64-S69, 2002.

35. Ricci G, Gentili A, Di Lorenzo F, et al: Latex allergy in subjects who had undergone multiple surgical procedures for bladder exstrophy: Relationship with clinical intervention and atopic diseases. BJU Int 84:1058-1062, 1999.

36. Rosenbaum HK, Miller JD: Malignant hyperthermia and myotonic disorders. Anesthesiol Clin North Am 20:385-426, 2002.

37. Hebert PC, Wells G, Tweeddale M, et al: Does transfusion practice affect mortality in critically ill patients? Transfusion Requirements in Critical Care (TRICC) Investigators and the Canadian Critical Care Trials Group. Am J Respir Crit Care Med 155:1618-1623, 1997.

38. DeCherney AH, diZerega GS: Clinical problem of intraperitoneal postsurgical adhesion formation following general surgery and the use of adhesion prevention barriers. Surg Clin North Am 77:671-688, 1997.

39. Vrijland WW, Tseng LN, Eijkman HJ, et al: Fewer intraperitoneal adhesions with use of hyaluronic acid–carboxymethylcellulose membrane: A randomized clinical trial. Ann Surg 235:193-199, 2002.

40. Mizuno H, Takeda A, Uchinuma E: Creation of an acellular dermal matrix from frozen skin. Aesthetic Plast Surg 23:316-322, 1999.

41. Loose HW, Haslam PJ: The management of peripheral arterial aneurysms using percutaneous injection of fibrin adhesive. Br J Radiol 71:1255-1259, 1998.

42. Friedman SG, Pellerito JS, Scher L, et al: Ultrasound-guided thrombin injection is the treatment of choice for femoral pseudoaneurysms. Arch Surg 137:462-464, 2002.

43. Izumi N, Asahina Y, Noguchi O, et al: Risk factors for distant recurrence of hepatocellular carcinoma in the liver after complete coagulation by microwave or radiofrequency ablation. Cancer 91:949-956, 2001.

44. Shankar A, Lees WR, Gillams AR, et al: Treatment of recurrent colorectal liver metastases by interstitial laser photocoagulation. Br J Surg 87:298-300, 2000.

45. Milne PJ, Parel JM, Manns F, et al: Development of stereotactically guided laser interstitial thermotherapy of breast cancer: In situ measurement and analysis of the temperature field in ex vivo and in vivo adipose tissue. Lasers Surg Med 26:67-75, 2000.

46. Basu S, Ravi B, Kant R: Interstitial laser hyperthermia—a new method in the management of fibroadenoma of the breast: A pilot study. Lasers Surg Med 25:148-152, 1999.

47. Tanaka H, Hashimoto K, Yamada I, et al: Interstitial photodynamic therapy with rotating and reciprocating optical fibers. Cancer 91:1791-1796, 2001.

48. Taber SW, Fingar VH, Wieman TJ: Photodynamic therapy for palliation of chest wall recurrence in patients with breast cancer. J Surg Oncol 68:209-214, 1998.

49. Allison R, Mang T, Hewson G, et al: Photodynamic therapy for chest wall progression from breast carcinoma is an underutilized treatment modality. Cancer 91:1-8, 2001.

50. Lim KN, Waring PJ, Saidi R: Therapeutic options in patients with Barrett's esophagus. Dig Dis 17:145-152, 1999.

51. Salo JA, Salminen JT, Kiviluoto TA, et al: Treatment of Barrett's esophagus by endoscopic laser ablation and antireflux surgery. Ann Surg 227:40-44, 1998.

52. Nahrwold DL: Gallstone lithotripsy. Am J Surg 165:431-434, 1993.

53. Strasberg SM, Clavien PA: Overview of therapeutic modalities for the treatment of gallstone diseases. Am J Surg 165:420-426, 1993.

54. Hill CR, ter Haar GR: High-intensity focused ultrasound: Potential for cancer treatment. Br J Radiol 68:1296-1303, 1995.

55. Triadafilopoulos G, DiBaise JK, Nostrant TT, et al: The Stretta procedure for the treatment of GERD: 6 and 12 month follow-up of the U.S. open label trial. Gastrointest Endosc 55:149-156, 2002.

56. Pearson AS, Izzo F, Fleming RY, et al: Intraoperative radiofrequency ablation or cryoablation for hepatic malignancies. Am J Surg 178:592-599, 1999.

57. Wood BJ, Abraham J, Hvizda JL, et al: Radiofrequency ablation of adrenal tumors and adrenocortical carcinoma metastases. Cancer 97:554-560, 2003.

58. Benussi S, Nascimbene S, Agricola E, et al: Surgical ablation of atrial fibrillation using the epicardial radiofrequency approach: Mid-term results and risk analysis. Ann Thorac Surg 74:1050-1057, 2002.

59. Dupuy DE, Monchik JM, Decrea C, et al: Radiofrequency ablation of regional recurrence from well-differentiated thyroid malignancy. Surgery 130:971-977, 2001.

60. Izzo F, Thomas R, Delrio P, et al: Radiofrequency ablation in patients with primary breast carcinoma: A pilot study in 26 patients. Cancer 92:2036-2044, 2001.

61. Maessen JG, Nijs JF, Smeets JL, et al: Beating-heart surgical treatment of atrial fibrillation with microwave ablation. Ann Thorac Surg 74:S1307-S1311, 2002.

62. Mathur PN, Edell E, Sutedja T, et al: Treatment of early-stage non-small cell lung cancer. Chest 123:176S-180S, 2003.

63. Adam R, Majno P, Castaing D, et al: Treatment of irresectable liver tumours by percutaneous cryosurgery. Br J Surg 85:1493-1494, 1998.

64. Bilchik AJ, Wood TF, Allegra D, et al: Cryosurgical ablation and radiofrequency ablation for unresectable hepatic malignant neoplasms: A proposed algorithm. Arch Surg 135:657-664, 2000.

65. Adam R, Akpinar E, Johann M, et al: Place of cryosurgery in the treatment of malignant liver tumors. Ann Surg 225:39-50, 1997.

66. Weil MD: Stereotactic radiosurgery for brain tumors. Hematol Oncol Clin North Am 15:1017-1026, 2001.

67. Hartford AC, Loeffler JS: Radiosurgery for benign tumors and arteriovenous malformations of the central nervous system. Front Radiat Ther Oncol 35:30-47, 2001.

68. McKhann GM II, Bourgeois BF, Goodman RR: Epilepsy surgery: Indications, approaches, and results. Semin Neurol 22:269-278, 2002.

CHAPTER 11

ULTRASOUND FOR SURGEONS

Neil G. Parry, M.D.,   Christopher J. Dente, M.D.,

and   Grace S. Rozycki, M.D., R.D.M.S., F.A.C.S.

Physics and Instrumentation	**Education of Surgeons in Ultrasound**
Clinical Uses of Ultrasound	**Summary**

Although the scientific principles underlying ultrasonography first began to be elucidated in the 19th century, it was not until the second half of the 20th century that this technology could be effectively applied to medicine. Surgeons, first in Europe, and more recently in the United States, have now embraced ultrasonography as a key diagnostic tool in many areas of clinical practice.[1-4] Because ultrasonography is noninvasive, portable, rapid, and easily repeatable, it is especially well suited to surgical practice. The use of this diagnostic tool as an extension of the physical examination allows the surgeon to receive immediate information about the patient's disease process and thus allows for expedited patient management. In addition, computer-enhanced high-resolution imaging and multifrequency specialized transducers have made ultrasonography increasingly user friendly, enhancing its applicability to a variety of surgical settings.

The objectives of this chapter include an introduction to some of the basic principles of ultrasound technology, with a discussion of the physics of ultrasound as well as definitions of the common terminology used. This chapter also describes the current use for ultrasound in various clinical settings, including the office, the operating room, the trauma resuscitation room, and the intensive care unit (ICU).

PHYSICS AND INSTRUMENTATION

Nowhere in diagnostic imaging is the understanding of wave physics more important than in ultrasound, because ultrasonography is highly operator dependent. To perform an ultrasound examination correctly, a surgeon must be able to interpret echo patterns, determine artifacts, and adjust the machine appropriately to obtain the best images.

In diagnostic ultrasonography, the transducer or probe interconverts electrical and acoustic energy (Fig. 11-1).[5] To accomplish this interconversion, the transducer contains the following essential components:

1. An *active element:* Electrical energy is applied to the piezoelectric crystals within the transducer, and an ultrasound pulse is thereby generated via the piezoelectric effect. The pulse distorts the crystals, and an electrical signal is produced. This signal causes an ultrasound image to form on the screen via the reverse-piezoelectric effect.
2. *Damping* or *backing material:* An epoxy resin absorbs the vibrations and reduces the number of cycles in a pulse, thereby improving the resolution of the ultrasound image.
3. A *matching layer:* This substance reduces the reflection that occurs at the transducer-tissue interface. The great difference in density (i.e., the impedance mismatch) between the soft tissue and the transducer results in reflection of the ultrasound waves. The matching material decreases this reflection and facilitates the transit of the ultrasound waves through the body and into the target organ.

Transducers are classified according to (1) the arrangement of the active elements (array) contained within the transducer and (2) the frequency of the ultrasound wave produced. Transducer arrays contain closely packed piezoelectric elements, each with its own electrical con-

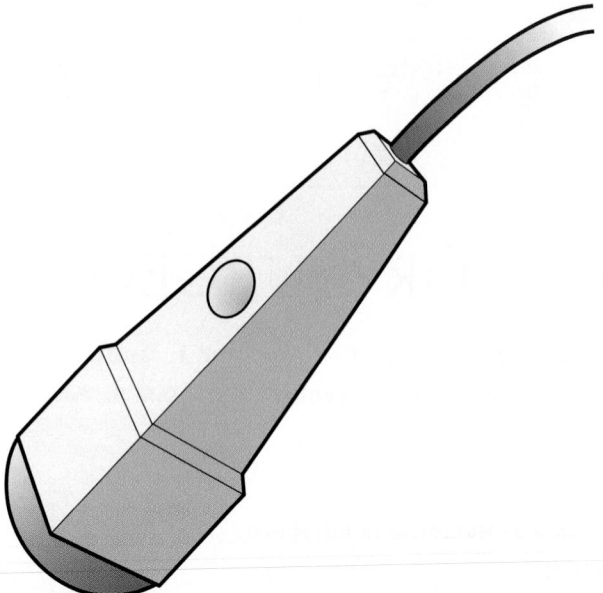

FIGURE 11-1.   A standard curved-array ultrasound probe.

TABLE 11-1. Commonly Used Transducer Frequencies

Frequency (MHz)	Clinical Application
2.5–3.5	Abdominal, aorta, renal, FAST
5.0	Transvaginal, pediatric abdominal, testicular
7.5	Vascular, superficial soft tissue, thyroid, breast
10.0	Endorectal

FAST, focused assessment for sonography in trauma.

nection to the ultrasound instrument. These elements can be excited individually or in groups to produce the ultrasound beam. There are four main transducer arrays: (1) the rectangular linear array, which yields a rectangular image; (2) the curved array, which yields a trapezoidal image; (3) the phased array, a small transducer in which the sound pulses are generated by activating all of the elements in the array; and (4) the annular array, in which the elements are arranged in a circular fashion. Transducer arrays allow the ultrasound beam to be electronically steered without any moving mechanical parts (except for the annular array) and focused.[6] In the clinical setting, this arrangement allows the operator to adjust the focal zone to accurately image a large organ (e.g., the liver) while still being able to obtain fine details of a lesion.

The frequency of the transducer is determined by the thickness of the piezoelectric elements within the transducer: the thinner the piezoelectric elements, the higher the frequency. Although diagnostic ultrasonography makes use of transducer frequencies ranging from 1 to 20 MHz, the most commonly used frequencies for medical diagnostic imaging are those between 2.5 and 10 MHz (Table 11-1). Ultrasound beams of different fre-

quencies have different characteristics: higher frequencies penetrate tissue poorly but yield excellent resolution, whereas lower frequencies penetrate well but at the cost of compromised resolution. Accordingly, transducers are generally chosen on the basis of the depth of the structure to be imaged.[6] For example, a 7.5-MHz transducer is a suitable choice for imaging a superficial organ such as the thyroid, but a 3.5-MHz transducer would be preferable for imaging a deep structure such as the abdominal aorta.

Ultrasound machines vary in complexity, but each has the following essential components:

1. A *transmitter* to control electrical signals sent to the transducer
2. A *receiver* or *image processor* that admits the electrical signal
3. A *transducer* to interconvert electrical and acoustic energy
4. A *monitor* to display the ultrasound image
5. An *image recorder* to produce copies of the ultrasound images

Finally, there are three scanning modes, A, B, and M; these modes evolved over several years.[7] "A" mode (amplitude modulation), the most basic form of diagnostic ultrasonography, yields a one-dimensional image that displays the amplitude or strength of the wave along the vertical axis and the time along the horizontal axis. Therefore, the greater the signal returning to the transducer, the higher the "spike." B mode (brightness modulation), the mode most commonly used today, relates the brightness of the image to the amplitude of the ultrasound wave. Thus, denser structures appear brighter (i.e., whiter, more echogenic) on the image because they reflect the ultrasound waves better. M mode relates the amplitude of the ultrasound wave to the imaging of moving structures, such as cardiac muscle. Before real-time imaging became available, M-mode scanning formed the basis for echocardiography.[7,8]

A summary of technical terms used commonly in ultrasound physics and their definitions is found in Table 11-2. Essential ultrasound principles are listed in Table 11-3 and clinical terminology is found in Table 11-4.

CLINICAL USES OF ULTRASOUND

As an extension of the physical examination, ultrasonography is a valuable adjunct to surgical practice in the office, the operating room, the emergency department, and the surgical ICU. Once surgeons have learned the essential principles of ultrasonography, they can readily build on this experience and extend the use of this technology to various specific aspects of surgery. What follows is a list and description of several clinical areas in which surgeon-performed ultrasonography has proven to be an effective diagnostic and interventional tool.

Outpatient Use of Ultrasound

Breast

Ultrasound-directed biopsy of breast lesions is now a common office procedure for general surgeons. The

TABLE 11-2. Ultrasound Physics Terminology

Term	Definition	Clinical Application
Frequency	Number of cycles/sec (10^6 cycles/sec = 1 MHz)	Increasing frequency improves resolution Diagnostic ultrasound: 1–20 MHz
Wavelength	Distance traveled by wave/cycle (as frequency increases, wavelength decreases)	Shorter wavelengths yield better resolution but poorer penetration
Amplitude	Strength or height of wave	—
Attenuation	Decrease in amplitude and intensity of wave as it travels	Time-gain compensation circuit compensates for attenuation through a medium
Absorption	Conversion of sound energy to heat	Method of attenuation
Scatter	Redirection of wave as it strikes a rough boundary	Method of attenuation
Reflection	Return of wave toward the transducer	Method of attenuation
Propagation speed	Speed with which wave passes through soft tissue (1540 m/sec)	Speed is greater in solids than in liquids and greater in liquids than in gases

TABLE 11-3. Principles of Ultrasound

Principle	Explanation
Piezoelectric effect	Piezoelectric crystals expand and contract to interconvert electrical and mechanical energy.
Pulse-echo principle	When ultrasound waves contact tissue, some of the signal is reflected and some is transmitted. The waves that are reflected back to the crystals generate an electrical impulse comparable to the strength of the returning wave.
Acoustic impedance	Defined as density of tissue × speed of sound in tissue. The strength of the returning echo depends on the difference in density between structures imaged. Structures with significant differences in acoustic impedance are easy to distinguish from one another (e.g., bile and gallstone).

TABLE 11-4. Ultrasound Clinical Terminology

Term	Definition
Echogenicity	Degree to which a tissue reflects ultrasound waves (reflected in images as degree of brightness)
Anechoic	No internal echoes, appearing dark or black
Isoechoic	Having similar appearance to surrounding tissue
Hypoechoic	Less echoic (darker) than surrounding tissue
Hyperechoic	More echoic (whiter) than surrounding tissue
Resolution	Ability to distinguish between two adjacent structures; may be lateral (width of structure) or axial (depth of structure)

increase in the number of screening mammograms performed since the late 1970s has led to the detection of more nonpalpable breast lesions. The traditional choice for further evaluation of such masses has been open surgical excision, but the yield of malignancies with this approach has been only about 20%.[9] Advances in ultrasound technology, including automated biopsy needles, high-resolution transducers,[10] and computer-aided diagnosis programs,[11] have prompted a surge of interest in fine-needle and core biopsy tissue sampling as an alternative to open biopsy. Such procedures are appealing because they are minimally invasive, are about as accurate as open biopsy,[12] and can be performed by the surgeon in the office setting.[13] Surgeons use ultrasound to evaluate the breast for a solid or cystic lesion and also to identify characteristics of the lesion that suggest whether it is benign or malignant.

Current indications for breast ultrasonography include (1) evaluation of a nonpalpable, new, growing mass, or microcalcifications detected on mammography; (2) evaluation of duct size in the presence of nipple discharge; (3) assessment of a dense breast or a vaguely palpable mass; (4) differentiation between a solid palpable mass and a cystic one; and (5) guidance of percutaneous drainage of an abscess.[14] Additional uses include postoperative follow-up for hematomas, seromas, and prostheses. Ultrasound-guided interventions can be used for cyst aspirations, biopsy of solid lesions, preoperative needle localization, axillary lymph node fine-needle aspiration, and peritumoral injection for sentinel lymph node biopsy. Recent reports suggest that high-resolution ultrasonography can demonstrate the intraductal spread of tumors and their multiple foci. Because of new technologies and contrast agents, perfusional studies show enhanced contrast resolution that increases the sensitivity of ultrasound for small nodal metastases. Therefore, the use of breast ultrasound in the office practice has become more sophisticated and sensitive, allowing more patients to be screened for microdisease.[13]

Gastrointestinal Tract

Endoscopic and endorectal ultrasonography have added a new dimension to the preoperative assessment and treatment of many gastrointestinal (GI) lesions. Endoscopic ultrasonography (EUS) involves the visualization of the GI tract via a high-frequency (12- to 20-MHz) ultrasound transducer placed through an endoscope. With the transducer near the target organ, images of the gut wall and the surrounding parenchymal organs can be obtained that are detailed enough to define the depth of tumor penetration with precision and to detect the presence of involved lymph nodes as small as 2 mm. When done preoperatively, EUS is 80% to 90% accurate at predicting the stage of the upper GI tumor; if an endoscopically directed biopsy attachment is used, the diagnostic potential is even higher.[15]

Indications for EUS include (1) preoperative staging of esophageal malignancies; (2) preoperative localization of pancreatic endocrine tumors, particularly insulinomas; (3) evaluation of submucosal lesions of the GI tract; and (4) guidance of imaging during interventional procedures (e.g., tissue sampling and drainage of a pancreatic pseudocyst).[16] Recently, endoscopic ultrasound has been used to direct fine-needle aspiration biopsy of submucosal lesions in the GI tract as well as lesions in the pancreas. Especially in the latter, endoscopic ultrasound-guided fine-needle aspiration accurately detects neoplastic pancreatic cysts and, therefore, may assist in the decision making for either the medical or surgical approach in these patients.[17,18]

Endorectal ultrasonography, used in the evaluation of patients with benign and malignant rectal conditions,[19] is commonly performed with an axial 7.0- or 10.0-MHz rotating transducer that produces a 360-degree horizontal cross-sectional view of the rectal wall. This special transducer is 24 cm long and is covered with a water-filled latex balloon. After the transducer is advanced above the rectal lesion, the balloon that surrounds the transducer is filled with degassed water to create an acoustic window for ultrasound imaging. The transducer is gradually withdrawn while the examiner views the layers of the rectal wall by means of real-time imaging (Fig. 11-2).[20] These layers are important landmarks in ultrasonographic staging, just as they are in postoperative pathologic staging. For example, if the middle white line (i.e., the submucosa) is intact, a benign lesion may be removed via a submucosal resection. A classification of preoperative tumor staging called uTNM has been proposed that is analogous to the TNM classification for tumor staging.[21] This classification is based on ultrasonographic determination of the infiltrative tumor depth (the prefix "u" stands for ultrasonography).

The sensitivity of ultrasonography in determining the depth of tumor invasion is about 85% to 90%; however, it can sometimes overestimate the extent of invasion due to the presence of tissue inflammation and edema.[22] Errors

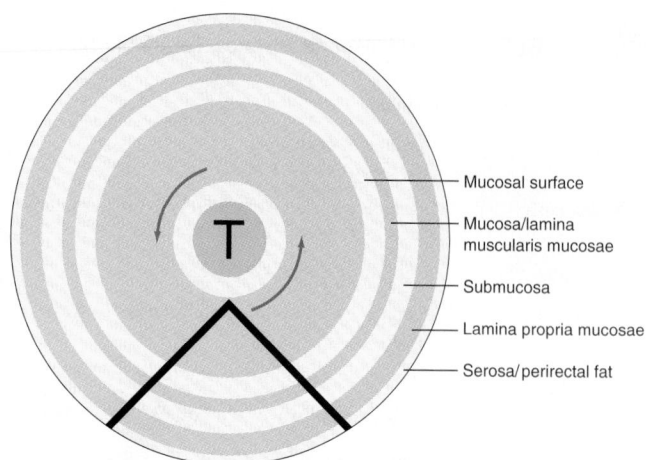

FIGURE 11-2.   Five-layer rectal wall anatomy as delineated by endorectal ultrasonography. (From Wong WK: Endorectral ultrasonography for benign disease. *In* Staren ED, Arregui ME [eds]: Ultrasound for the Surgeon. Philadelphia, Lippincott-Raven, 1997, p 66.)

Labels in figure: Mucosal surface; Mucosa/lamina muscularis mucosae; Submucosa; Lamina propria mucosae; Serosa/perirectal fat

in staging are likely to occur with tumors that invade the lamina muscularis mucosae or are associated with inflammation of the lamina propria mucosae.[23] In addition, lesions characterized by ultramicroscopic invasion of the submucosa may be mis-staged because the technology currently available cannot provide the fine resolution necessary to assess such invasion.[22] With recent advances in technology, a flexible 360-degree rotating transducer is now being used to evaluate rectal lesions. Steele and colleagues from Madigan Army Medical Center found that although the rigid endoscopic transducers were slightly more sensitive for the detection of lesions, the flexible devices showed a high accuracy (77%) for the staging of rectal cancers, and learning curves were similar for both types of transducers.[24]

Finally, endoanal ultrasonography is an important part of the evaluation of anal incontinence because it is capable of detecting defects in the internal and external sphincters.[25] It is done in much the same way as endorectal ultrasonography, except that the 10-MHz transducer is covered with a sonolucent hard plastic cone instead of a water-filled balloon. Although endoanal ultrasonography does not measure sphincter function, ultrasound-detected sphincter disruption correlates well with pressure measurements and operative findings.[26] Additional indications for endoanal ultrasonography include evaluation of patients with an exophytic distal rectal tumor (e.g., a villous adenoma) and assessment of patients who have a perianal abscess, a fistula in ano, a presacral cyst, or a rectal ulcer.

Vascular System

Color-flow duplex imaging and endoluminal ultrasonography have significantly expanded the diagnostic and therapeutic aspects of vascular imaging. Vascular diagnostic imaging is commonly used for evaluation of arterial disease or deep vein thrombosis (DVT) and other disorders such as Raynaud's disease and thoracic outlet syndrome. In the office setting, surgeons use ultrasonography to screen for abdominal aortic aneurysm or to follow patients with an aneurysm, because it is capable of detecting change in aortic diameter as small as a few millimeters.[27] In patients who have undergone repair of an abdominal aortic aneurysm, color-flow duplex imaging is highly specific for the diagnosis of anastomotic false aneurysms. In one study, this modality was compared with B-mode ultrasonography, computed tomography (CT), digital subtraction arteriography, and magnetic resonance imaging and emerged as the diagnostic test of choice when the accuracy, cost, safety, and availability of each method were assessed.[28]

Color-flow duplex scanning is also used to examine the patency and size of the portal vein and the hepatic artery in patients who have undergone liver transplantation, to assess the resectability of pancreatic tumors, to detect superior mesenteric artery occlusion, and for diagnosis of pseudoaneurysm or an arteriovenous fistula after percutaneous arterial catheterization.

Duplex imaging of the lower extremity is used to assess the patency of the deep venous system and is capable of detecting DVT reliably. The addition of color-flow imaging facilitates the examination by making the artery and its associated vein easier to identify. By performing serial duplex venous ultrasound imaging to detect DVT, one group of investigators was able to identify a subgroup of injured patients who were at highest risk for pulmonary embolism; they suggested that these patients be given DVT prophylaxis and undergo close surveillance with duplex imaging.[29]

Intraoperative Use of Ultrasound

Gastrointestinal Tract

Examination with intraoperative or laparoscopic ultrasonography is an integral part of many hepatic, biliary, and pancreatic surgical procedures. With this tool, surgeons can detect previously undiagnosed lesions or bile duct stones,[30] avoid unnecessary dissection of vessels or ducts, clarify tumor margins, and perform biopsy and cryoablation procedures.[31] Compared with preoperative imaging modalities, intraoperative ultrasonography is much more sensitive in detecting malignant or benign lesions.[32] The precision with which intraoperative ultrasonography can delineate small lesions (5 mm) and define their relationship to other structures facilitates resection, reduces operative time, and frequently alters the surgeon's operative strategy.

Intraoperative ultrasonography makes use of both contact scanning and so-called standoff scanning for imaging.[33] In contact scanning, the transducer is directly applied to the organ so that the deepest part of the organ is accurately depicted. This technique is most often used for imaging large organs (e.g., the liver). In standoff scanning, the transducer is placed about 1 to 2 cm away from the structure in a pool of sterile saline solution that permits the transmission of ultrasound waves. This technique is often used to image blood vessels, bile ducts, or the spinal cord; it allows good visualization of the structure without compression by the transducer. The size, shape, and type of ultrasound transducer used for intraoperative scanning depend on the anatomic structure to be examined. For example, a pencil-like 7.5-MHz transducer is used for scanning the common bile duct, whereas a side-viewing T-shaped 5-MHz transducer is preferable for imaging a cirrhotic liver. Intraoperative ultrasound examinations are conducted systematically to ensure that no subtle pathology is missed and that the examination is reproducible. For example, the liver is imaged sequentially according to a system based on Couinaud's anatomic segments.

Similar principles apply to laparoscopic ultrasonography, except that the transducers are made to adapt to the laparoscopic equipment. Indications for this modality include detection of common bile duct stones, staging of pancreatic cancer to prevent unnecessary celiotomy, and resection or cryoablation of hepatic metastases.

Vascular System

Intraoperative duplex imaging can be used to detect technical errors in vascular anastomoses as well as abnormalities in flow. Arteriography assesses the patency of an anastomosis and measures distal arterial runoff, but it is invasive. Intraoperative duplex imaging, on the other hand, permits rapid visualization of the anatomic and hemodynamic aspects of a vascular reconstruction, and it is noninvasive, easily repeatable, and less time consuming than arteriography.

Use of Ultrasound in Acute Settings and Trauma Resuscitation

FAST Examination in Trauma Resuscitation

The focused assessment for sonography in trauma (FAST) is a rapid diagnostic examination to assess patients with potential thoracoabdominal injuries. The test sequentially surveys for the presence or absence of blood in the pericardial sac and dependent abdominal regions, including the right upper quadrant (RUQ), left upper quadrant (LUQ), and pelvis. Surgeons perform the FAST during the American College of Surgeons Advanced Trauma Life Support (ATLS) secondary survey,[34] and although minimal patient preparation is needed, a full urinary bladder is necessary to provide an acoustic window for visualization of blood in the pelvis.

The FAST is designed to assess blood accumulation in dependent areas of the pericardial sac and abdomen while the patient is in the supine position, and the FAST examination is performed in a specific sequence. The pericardial area is visualized first so that blood within the heart can be used as a standard to set the gain. Most modern ultrasound machines have presets so that the gain does not need to be reset each time the machine is turned on. Occasionally, if multiple types of examinations are performed with different transducers, the gain should be checked to ensure that intracardiac blood appears anechoic. This maneuver ensures that hemoperitoneum will also appear anechoic and therefore will be readily detected on the ultrasound image. The abdominal part of the FAST should begin with a survey of the RUQ, which is the location within the peritoneal cavity where blood most often accumulates and is, therefore, readily detected with the FAST. Investigators from four Level I trauma centers examined true positive ultrasound images of 275 patients who sustained either blunt (220 patients) or penetrating (55 patients) injuries.[35] They found that regardless of the injured organ (with the exception of those patients who had an isolated perforated viscus), blood was most often identified on the RUQ image of the FAST. This can be a time-saving measure because when hemoperitoneum is identified on the FAST examination of a hemodynamically unstable patient, then that image alone, in combination with the patient's clinical picture, is sufficient to justify an immediate abdominal exploration.[35]

Technique. Ultrasound transmission gel is applied on four areas of the thorax and abdomen, and the examination is conducted in the following sequence: the pericardial area, RUQ, LUQ, and the pelvis (Fig. 11-3). A 3.5-MHz convex array transducer is oriented for sagittal or longitudinal views and positioned in the subxiphoid region to identify the heart and to examine for blood in the pericardial sac. The normal and abnormal views of the pericardial area are shown in Figure 11-4. The subcostal image usually is not difficult to obtain, but a severe chest wall injury, a very narrow subcostal area, subcutaneous emphysema, or morbid obesity can prevent a satisfactory examination. Both of the latter conditions are associated with poor imaging because air and fat reflect the wave too strongly and prevent penetration into the target organ. If the subcostal pericardial image cannot be obtained or is suboptimal, a parasternal ultrasound view of the heart should be performed (Fig. 11-5).

Next, the transducer is placed in the right midaxillary line between the 11th and 12th ribs to identify in the sagittal section the liver, kidney, and diaphragm (Fig. 11-6). The presence or absence of blood is sought in Morison's pouch and in the subphrenic space. With the transducer positioned in the left posterior axillary line between the 10th and 11th ribs, the spleen and kidney are visualized and blood is sought in between the two organs and in the subphrenic space (Fig. 11-7).

Finally, the transducer is directed for a transverse view and placed about 4 cm superior to the symphysis pubis. It is swept inferiorly to obtain a coronal view of the full bladder and the pelvis searching for blood (Fig. 11-8).

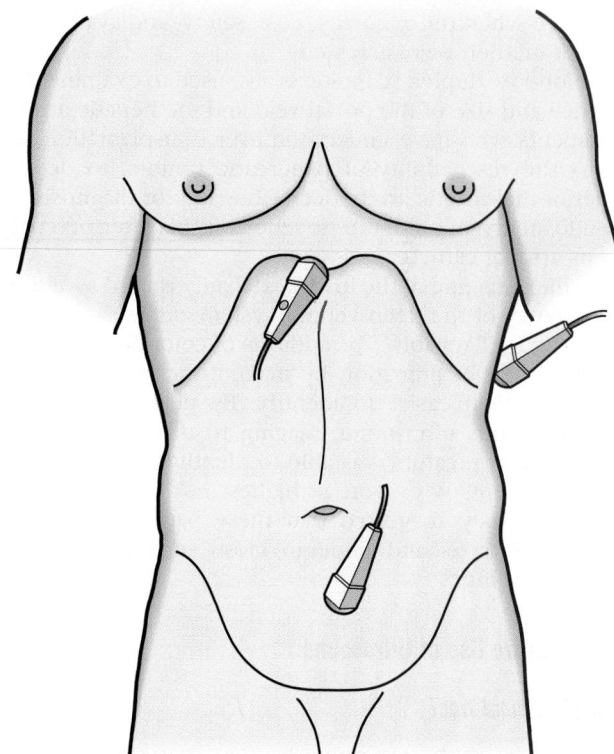

FIGURE 11-3. Transducer positions for FAST: pericardial, right upper quadrant, left upper quadrant, and pelvis.

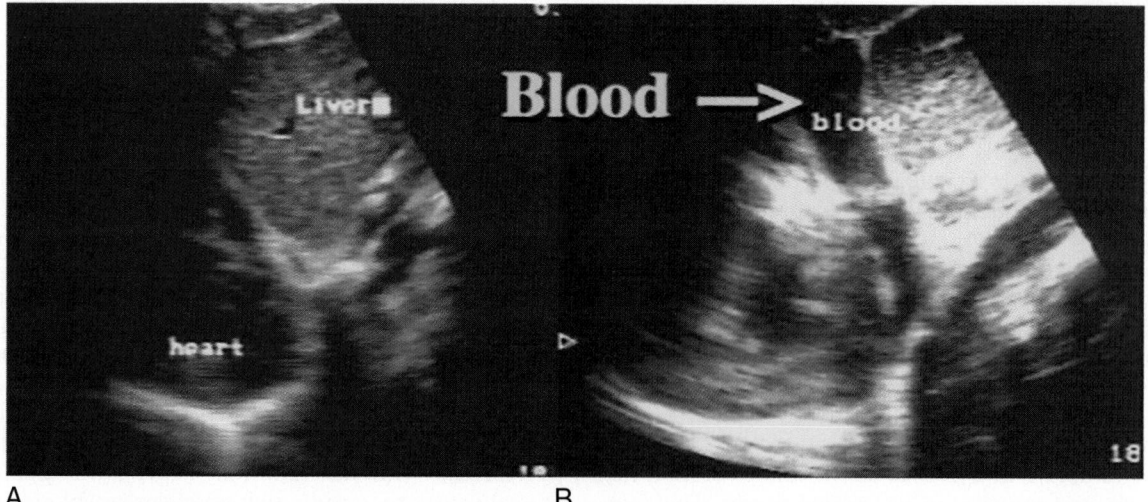

A   B

FIGURE 11-4. **A,** Normal pericardial window in FAST examination. **B,** Pericardial window showing blood in FAST examination.

Accuracy of the FAST. Improper technique, inexperience of the examiner, and inappropriate use of ultrasound are known to adversely impact ultrasound imaging, but the etiology of injury, the presence of hypotension on admission, and select associated injuries have also been shown to influence the accuracy of this modality.[36] Failure to consider these factors has led to inaccurate assessments of the accuracy of the FAST by inappropriately comparing it to a CT scan and not recognizing its role in the evaluation of patients with penetrating torso trauma.[37] Both false-positive and false-negative pericardial ultrasound examinations have been reported to occur in the presence of a massive hemothorax or mediastinal blood.[1,36] Repeating the FAST after the insertion of a tube thoracostomy improves the visualization of the pericardial area, thereby decreasing the number of false-positive and false-negative studies. Notwithstanding these circumstances in which false studies may occur, a rapid-focused ultrasound survey of the subcostal pericardial area is a highly accurate method to detect hemopericardium in most patients with penetrating wounds in the "cardiac box."[1] In a recent large study of patients who sustained either blunt or penetrating injuries, the FAST was 100% sensitive and 99.3% specific for detecting hemopericardium in patients with precordial or transthoracic wounds.[1] Furthermore, the use of pericardial ultrasound has been shown to be especially helpful in the evaluation of patients who have no overt signs of pericardial tamponade. This was highlighted in a study in which 10 of 22 patients with precordial wounds and hemopericardium on the ultrasound examinations had admission systolic blood pressures higher than 110 mm Hg and were relatively asymptomatic. Based on these signs and the lack of symptoms, it is unlikely that the presence of cardiac wounds would have been strongly suspected in these patients and, therefore, this rapid ultrasound examination provided an early diagnosis of hemopericardium before the patients underwent physiologic deterioration.

The FAST is accurate when it is used to evaluate hypotensive patients who present with blunt abdominal trauma. In this scenario, ultrasound is so accurate that when the FAST is positive, an immediate operation is justified.[1,36] However, because the FAST is a focused examination for the detection of blood in dependent areas of the abdomen, its results should not be compared to those of a CT scan because the FAST does not readily identify intraparenchymal or retroperitoneal injuries. Therefore, select patients considered to be at high risk for occult intra-abdominal injury should undergo a CT scan of the abdomen regardless of the results of the FAST examination. These patients include those with fractures of the pelvis or thoracolumbar spine, major thoracic trauma (pulmonary contusion, lower rib fractures), and hematuria. These recommendations are based on the results of

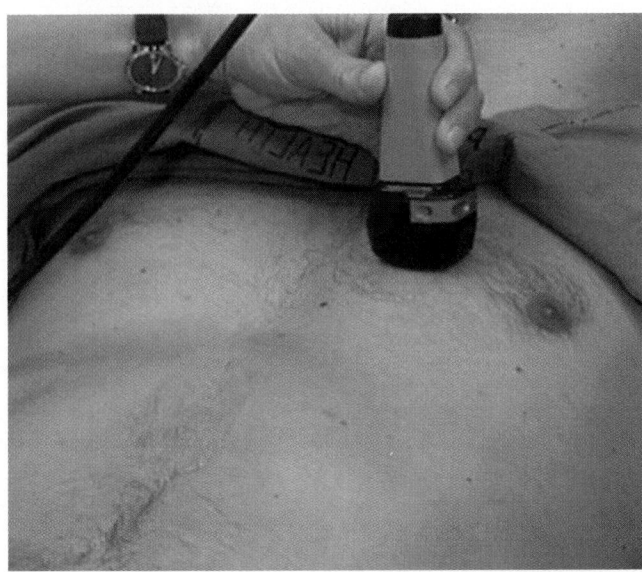

FIGURE 11-5. Transducer position for parasternal view of pericardial area.

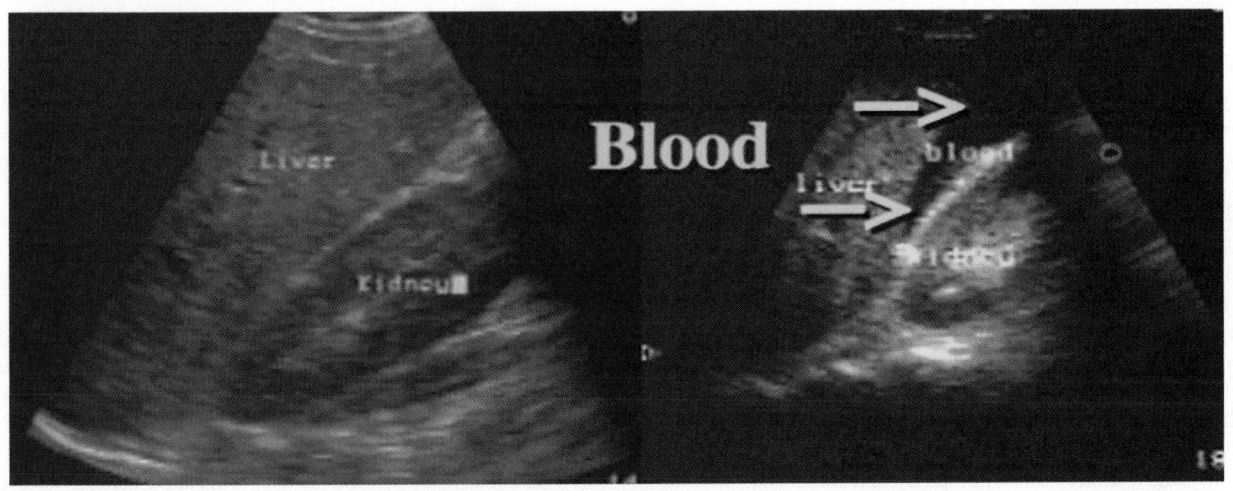

A   B

FIGURE 11-6. **A,** Normal sagittal view of liver, kidney, and diaphragm. **B,** Sagittal view of liver, kidney, and diaphragm with blood in Morison's pouch.

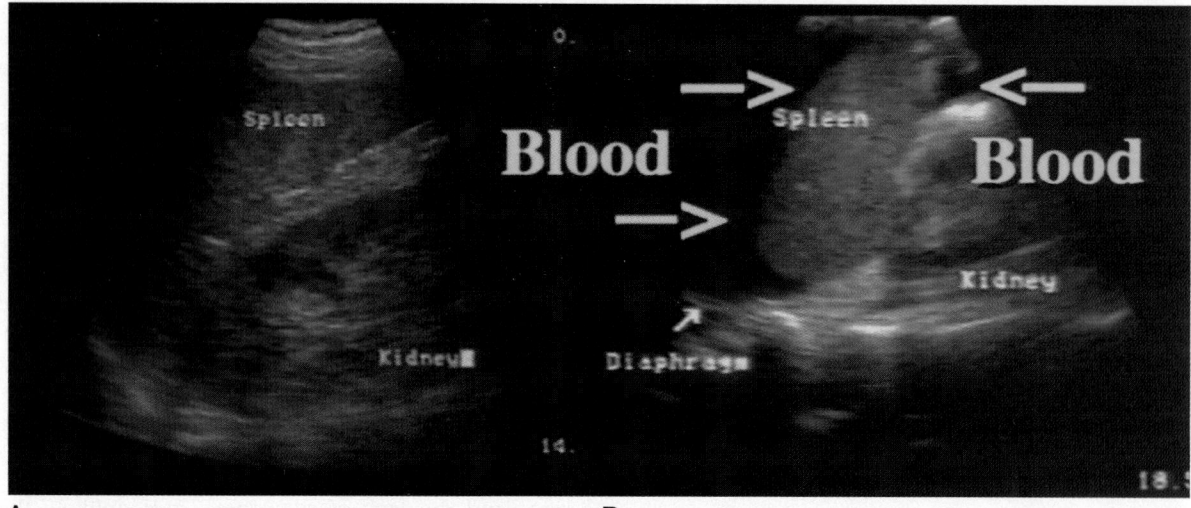

FIGURE 11-7.   A, Normal sagittal view of spleen, kidney, and diaphragm. **B,** Sagittal view of spleen, kidney, and diaphragm with blood between spleen and diaphragm and in the splenorenal recess.

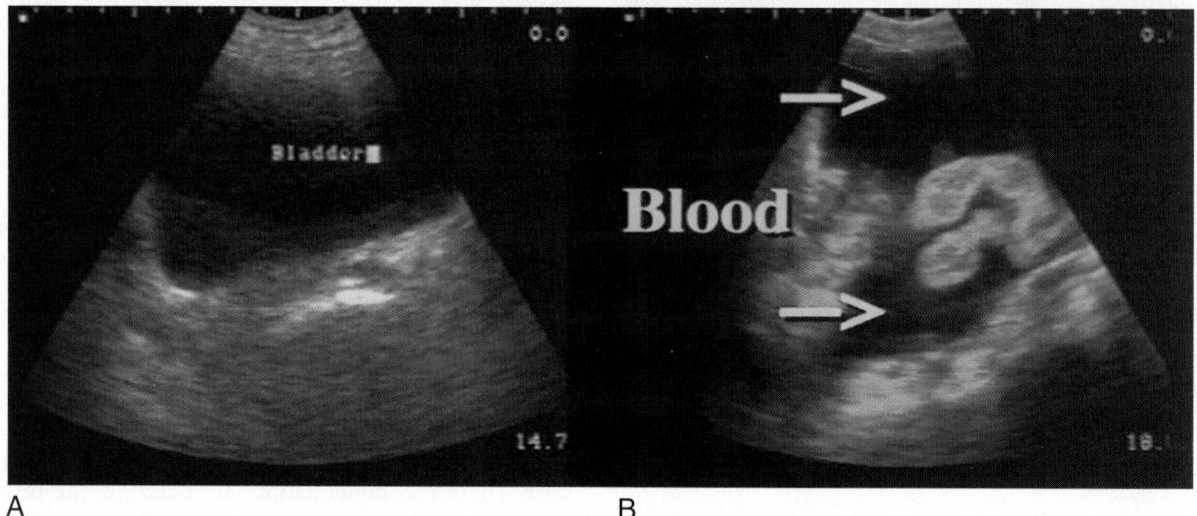

FIGURE 11-8.   A, Normal coronal view of full urinary bladder. **B,** Coronal view of full bladder with fluid in pelvis. Note floating bowel loops.

two studies, from Chiu and associates in 1997[38] and Rozycki and colleagues in 1998.[36] Chiu and associates reviewed their data on 772 patients who underwent FAST examinations after sustaining blunt torso injury. Of the 772 patients, 52 had intra-abdominal injury, but 15 (29%) of them had no hemoperitoneum on the admitting FAST examination or on the CT scan of the abdomen. In the study by Rozycki and colleagues at Grady Memorial Hospital, an algorithm was developed and tested over a 3.5-year period to identify patients who were at high risk for occult intra-abdominal injuries after sustaining blunt thoracoabdominal trauma. Of the 1490 patients admitted with severe blunt trauma, there were 102 (70 with pelvic fractures, 32 with spine injuries) who were considered to be at high risk for occult intra-abdominal injuries. Although there was only one false-negative FAST examination in the 32 patients who had spine injuries, there were 13 false-negative examinations in those with pelvic

fractures. Based on these data, the authors concluded that patients with pelvic fractures should have a CT scan of the abdomen regardless of the result of the FAST examination. Both studies provide guidelines to decrease the number of false-negative FAST studies, but as with the use of any diagnostic modality, it is important to correlate the results of the test with the patient's clinical picture. Suggested algorithms for the use of FAST are depicted in Figure 11-9.

Quantification of Blood. The amount of blood detected on the abdominal CT scan or in the diagnostic peritoneal lavage aspirate (or effluent) has been shown to predict the need for operative intervention.[34] Similarly, the quantity of blood that is detected with ultrasound may be predictive of a therapeutic operation.[39,40] Huang and coworkers[39] developed a scoring system based on the identification of hemoperitoneum in specific areas, such as Morison's pouch or the perisplenic space, with each abdominal area

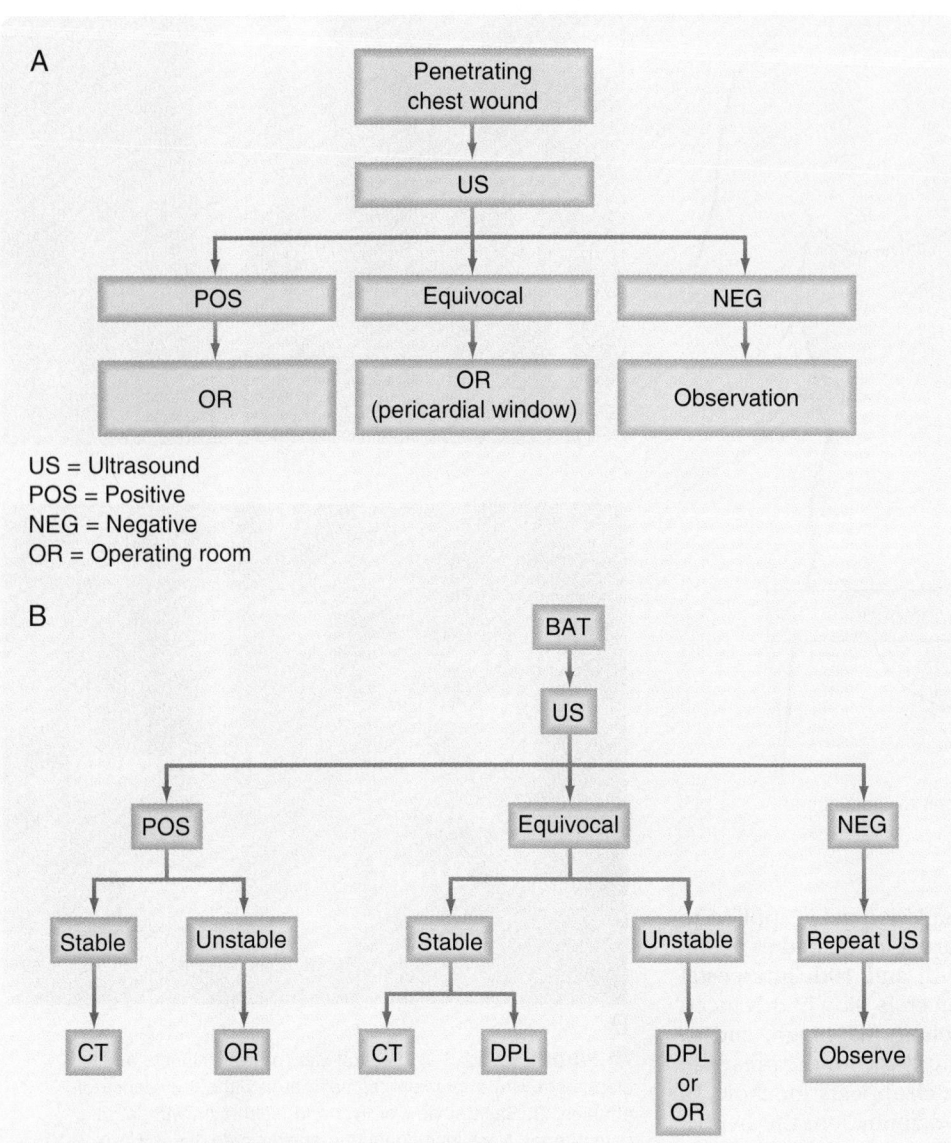

A

US = Ultrasound
POS = Positive
NEG = Negative
OR = Operating room

B

FIGURE 11-9. Algorithms for the use of ultrasound in penetrating chest wounds (**A**) and in blunt abdominal trauma (BAT) (**B**).

being assigned a score from 1 to 3. The authors found that a total score of 3 or higher corresponded to more than 1 L of hemoperitoneum, and it had a sensitivity of 84% for determining the need for an immediate abdominal operation. Another scoring system, developed and prospectively validated by McKenney and colleagues,[40] examined the patient's admission blood pressure, base deficit, and the amount of hemoperitoneum present on the ultrasound examination of 100 patients. The hemoperitoneum was categorized by its measurement and its distribution in the peritoneal cavity, so that a score of 1 was considered a minimal amount of hemoperitoneum, but a score higher than 3 was a large hemoperitoneum. Forty-six of the 100 patients had a score higher than 3, and 40 (87%) of them underwent a therapeutic abdominal operation. Their scoring system had a sensitivity, specificity, and accuracy of 83%, 87%, and 85%, respectively. The authors concluded that an ultrasound score higher than 3 is statistically more accurate than a combination of the initial systolic blood pressure and base deficit for determining which patients will undergo a therapeutic abdominal operation. Although the quantification of hemoperitoneum is not exact and not uniformly accepted, it can provide valuable information about the need for an abdominal operation and its potential to be therapeutic.

Hemothorax in Trauma Resuscitation

A focused thoracic ultrasound examination was developed by surgeons to rapidly detect the presence or absence of a traumatic hemothorax in patients during the ATLS secondary survey.[41] A test that promptly detects a traumatic effusion or hemothorax is worthwhile because it dramatically shortens the interval from diagnosis of a hemothorax to tube thoracostomy insertion, and this facilitates patient management.

Technique. The technique for this examination is similar to that used to interrogate the upper quadrants of the abdomen in the FAST, uses the same type and frequency transducers, and is performed with the patient in the

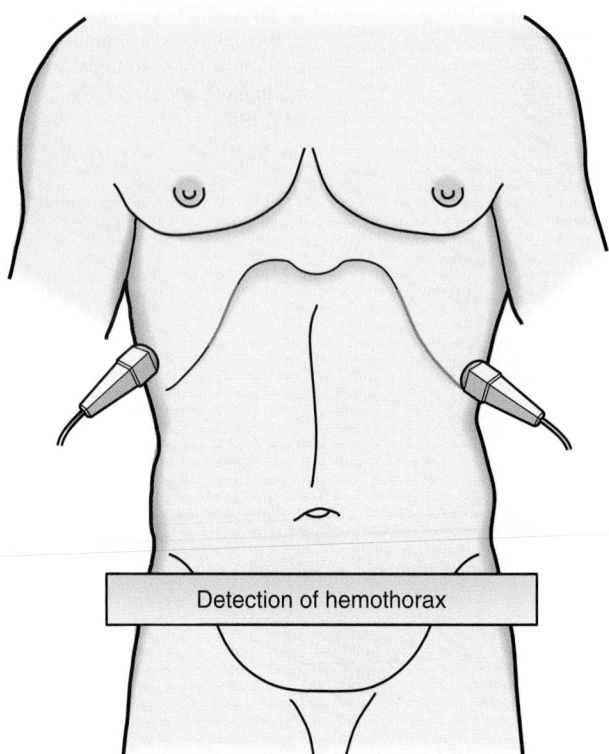

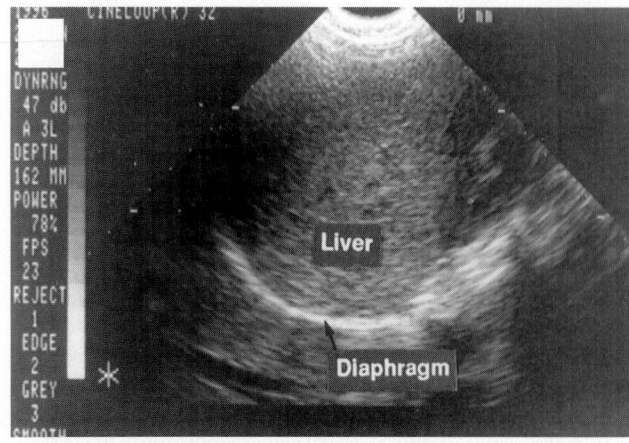

A

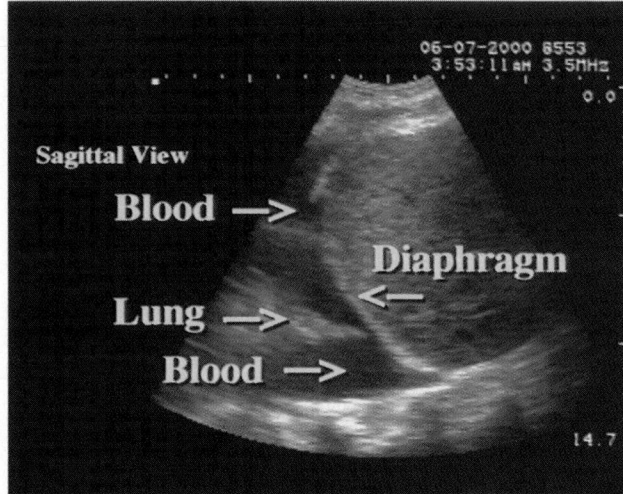

B

FIGURE 11-10.   Transducer positions for hemothorax evaluation.

FIGURE 11-11.   **A,** Sagittal view of liver, kidney, and diaphragm with supradiaphragmatic area without evidence of effusion. **B,** Sagittal view of liver and diaphragm with large hemothorax. Note lung floating in anechoic fluid.

supine position. Ultrasound transmission gel is applied to the right and left lower thoracic areas in the mid to posterior axillary lines between the 9th and 10th intercostal spaces (Fig. 11-10). The transducer is slowly advanced cephalad to identify the hyperechoic diaphragm and to interrogate the supradiaphragmatic space for the presence or absence of fluid (Fig. 11-11) which appears anechoic. In the positive thoracic ultrasound examination, the hypoechoic lung can be seen "floating" amidst the fluid. The same technique can be used to evaluate a critically ill patient for a pleural effusion, as discussed later in this chapter.

Accuracy. Surgeons have examined the accuracy of this examination in 360 patients with blunt and penetrating torso injuries.[41] They compared the time and accuracy of ultrasound with those of the supine portable chest radiograph and found both to be very similar, 97.4% sensitivity and 99.7% specificity observed for thoracic ultrasound versus 92.5% sensitivity and 99.7% specificity for the portable chest radiograph. Performance times, however, for the thoracic ultrasound examinations were statistically much faster ($P < 0.0001$) than those for the portable chest radiograph. Although it is not recommended that the thoracic ultrasound examination replace the chest radiograph, its use can expedite treatment in many patients and decrease the number of chest radiographs obtained.

Pneumothorax in Trauma Resuscitation

The use of ultrasound for the detection of a pneumothorax is not a new concept, having been reported by several authors, most recently Wernecke and associates.[42] This examination is useful to the surgeon to evaluate a patient for a potential pneumothorax if (1) radiographic equipment is not readily available; (2) inordinate delays for obtaining a chest radiograph are anticipated; or (3) numerous injured patients (mass casualty situation) must be rapidly assessed and triaged.[42] Although useful in the trauma resuscitation area, surgeons may also find this examination helpful to detect a pneumothorax in a critically ill patient who is on a ventilator, after a thoracentesis procedure, or after discontinuing the suction on a Pleur-Evac.

Technique. A 5.0- to 7.5-MHz linear array transducer is used to evaluate a patient for the presence of a pneumothorax. The examination may be performed while the patient is in the erect or the supine position. Ultrasound transmission gel is applied to the right and left upper thoracic areas at about the 3rd to 4th intercostal space in the mid-clavicular line, and the presumed unaffected thoracic cavity is examined first. The transducer, oriented for transverse imaging, is placed parallel to the ribs and is slowly advanced medially toward the sternum, then laterally

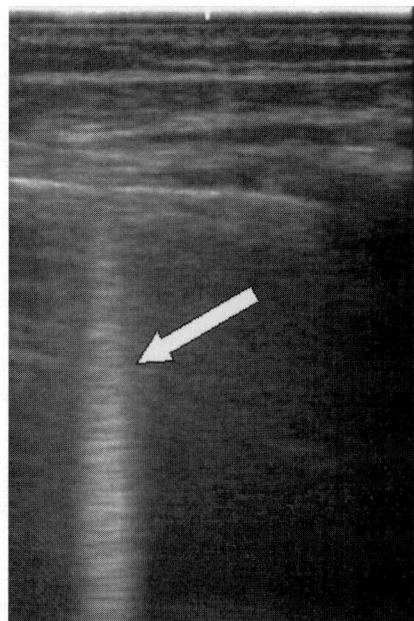

FIGURE 11-12. Comet-tail artifact during pleural examination for pneumothorax *(arrow)*.

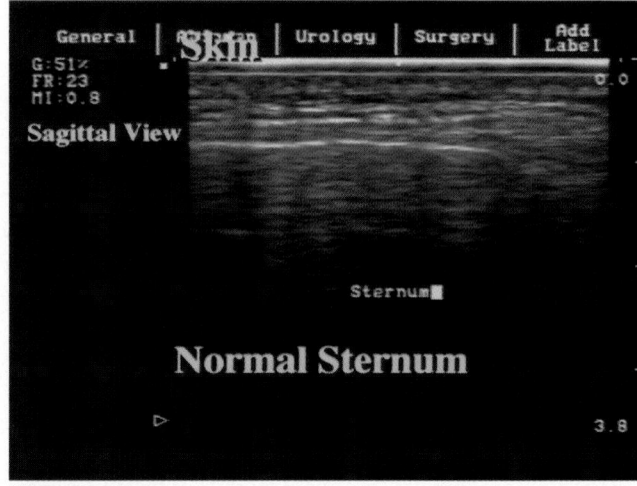

FIGURE 11-13. Sagittal view of normal sternum.

toward the anterior axillary line. The normal examination of the thoracic cavity identifies the rib (seen as black on the ultrasound image because it is a refraction artifact), pleural sliding, and a comet-tail artifact. Pleural sliding is the identification of the visceral and parietal layers of the lung seen as hyperechoic pleural lines. When a pneumothorax is present, air becomes trapped beyond the parietal pleura and does not allow for the transmission of the ultrasound waves. Therefore, the visceral pleura is not imaged and pleural sliding is not observed. The comet-tail artifact is generated because of the interaction of two highly reflective opposing interfaces, such as air and pleura (Fig. 11-12). When air separates the visceral and parietal pleura, the comet-tail artifact is not visualized. Lack of pleural sliding, however, is a more specific indication of pneumothorax, since comet-tail artifacts are not always seen even during a normal examination. The examination is then repeated with the transducer oriented for sagittal or longitudinal views.

Accuracy. Several studies have documented the sensitivity and specificity of ultrasound for the detection of pneumothorax.[42] Recently, Dulchavsky and colleagues from Detroit Receiving Hospital showed that ultrasound can be successfully used by surgeons to detect a pneumothorax in injured patients.[43] Of the 382 patients (362 trauma, 18 spontaneous) evaluated with ultrasound, 39 had pneumothoraces, and ultrasound successfully detected 37 of them, yielding a 95% sensitivity. Not unexpected, pneumothoraces in two patients could not be detected because of the presence of subcutaneous emphysema because air reflects the sound wave and does not allow for through transmission. The authors recommended that when a portable chest radiograph cannot be readily obtained, the use of this bedside ultrasound examination for the identification of a pneumothorax can expedite the patient's management.

Sternal Fracture in Trauma Resuscitation

Fractures of the sternum are visualized on a lateral radiographic view of the chest, but this film may be difficult to obtain in a multisystem-injured patient. For this reason, an ultrasound examination of the sternum can rapidly detect a fracture while the patient is still in the supine position and therefore avoid the need to obtain a radiograph.

Technique. The ultrasound examination of the sternum is performed using a 5.0- or 7.5-MHz linear array transducer that is oriented for sagittal or longitudinal views. Ultrasound transmission gel is applied over the sternal area while the patient is in the supine position. Beginning at the suprasternal notch, the transducer is slowly advanced caudad to interrogate the bone for a fracture, and then the examination is repeated with the transducer oriented for transverse views. The examination of the intact sternum is shown in Figure 11-13. The sternal fracture is identified on the ultrasound examination as a disruption of the cortical reflex (Fig. 11-14).

Use of Ultrasound in the Intensive Care Unit

The surgeon's use of ultrasound is particularly applicable to the evaluation of critically ill patients for the following reasons: (1) many patients have a depressed mental status, making it difficult to elicit pertinent signs of infection; (2) physical examination is hampered by tubes, drains, and monitoring devices; (3) the clinical picture often changes, necessitating frequent reassessments; (4) transportation to other areas of the hospital is not without inherent risks; and (5) these patients frequently develop complications, which if diagnosed and treated early, may lessen their morbidity and length of stay in the ICU.[36]

Both diagnostic and therapeutic ultrasound examinations can be performed by the surgeon while on rounds in the ICU. These focused examinations should be done with a specific purpose and as an extension of the physical examination, not its replacement.[3]

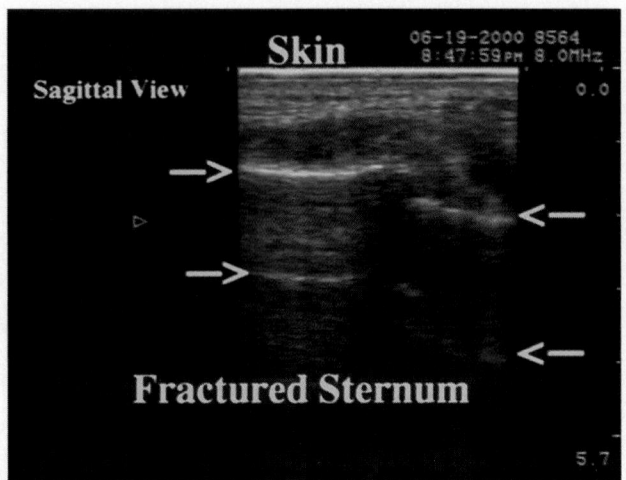

FIGURE 11-14. Sagittal view of fractured sternum. Note disrupted anterior and posterior cortex (arrows).

Several retrospective studies have documented the usefulness of portable ultrasound examinations performed in diverse groups of critically ill patients, most recently by Braxton and coworkers.[44] Surgeons most often use bedside ultrasound examination for the evaluation of patients in the ICU to detect pleural effusions, intra-abdominal and soft tissue fluid collections, hemoperitoneum, and femoral vein thrombosis and as a guide for the cannulation of central veins in patients with difficult access.

Advantages of interventional ultrasound as used by the surgeon in the ICU include the following: (1) visualization in real-time imaging to allow direct placement of a catheter and confirmation of complete drainage of a fluid collection; (2) performance at the patient's bedside so to avoid transport; and (3) safe, minimally invasive, and repeatable, if necessary. Contraindications to the performance of an ultrasound-guided interventional procedure include the lack of a safe pathway, presence of coagulopathy, and an uncooperative patient. The reader is referred to the Selected References section at the end of the chapter for techniques of interventional ultrasound.[45]

EDUCATION OF SURGEONS IN ULTRASOUND

Although many approaches have been shown to be effective in teaching these focused ultrasound examinations, surgeons should have a solid understanding of the physics principles of ultrasound imaging as an integral part of that education process. Furthermore, these principles should be emphasized each time the examinations are taught.

The first educational model for how surgeons can learn ultrasound was published by Han and colleagues from Emory University.[46] Incoming interns took a pretest and then attended a lecture and videotape about the FAST examination. After completion of the ATLS laboratory session, three pigs had diagnostic peritoneal lavage catheters reinserted to infuse fluid and produce "positive" ultrasound examinations. Two pigs were "negatives"; however, all five pigs were draped similarly to disguise interventions. Interns were tested individually by surgeon sonographers to determine whether the ultrasound image was "positive" or "negative." The interns completed a post-test that showed a statistically significant improvement from the pretest ($P < 0.001$). The authors concluded that incoming interns could learn the essential ultrasound principles of the FAST and that swine are feasible models for learning it.

Other paradigms that have been used as educational models include cadavers whose peritoneal cavities were instilled with saline[47] and simulators that had data stored in 3-dimensional images.[48] In the latter study, Knudson and Sisley conducted a prospective cohort study involving residents from two university trauma centers. They compared the post-test results between residents trained on a real-time ultrasound simulator versus those trained in a traditional hands-on format. The main outcome measured was the residents' performance on a standardized post-test, which included interpretation of ultrasound cases recorded on videotape. They determined no significant difference between those residents trained on the simulator and those trained on models or patients. From their study, the authors concluded that the use of a simulator is a convenient and objective method of introducing ultrasound to surgery residents.

Another issue is that of the learning curve. One of the best studies to address the issue of the learning curve for the FAST was conducted by Shackford and colleagues[2] from the University of Vermont. In this study, the authors questioned the recommendations that various numbers of ultrasound examinations should be done under supervision before a surgeon is considered qualified to perform them. The authors calculated the primary and adjusted error rates and then determined the potential clinical utility of the FAST. They found that although the clinician's (nonradiologists) initial error rate was 17%, it fell to 5% after the clinicians performed 10 examinations. Additionally, in that study, the authors proposed the following recommendations for credentialing:

1. The process for credentialing of surgeons in the use of ultrasound should occur within the department of surgery either by surgeons or a committee composed of surgeons and nonsurgeons that reports to the chairperson of the department of surgery.
2. A formal course with 4 hours of didactic and 4 hours of hands-on training is adequate. The curriculum for the performance of ultrasound in trauma, recently developed by the American College of Surgeons, is strongly recommended.
3. Competency in the performance of the FAST examination should be determined based on error rate with respect to the prevalence of the target disease in the series.
4. "Control" or repeat scans should be allowed during the proctored experience.
5. After completion of proctoring, an ongoing monitoring process of error rates and causes of indeterminate

studies using the department of surgery's quality improvement program is essential.[2]

SUMMARY

As the role of the general surgeon continues to evolve, the surgeon's use of ultrasound will surely influence practice patterns. With the use of real-time imaging, the surgeon receives "instantaneous" information to augment the physical examination, narrow the differential diagnosis, or initiate an intervention. This is of benefit in both elective, outpatient settings as well as acute inpatient settings. As surgeons become more facile with ultrasound, it is anticipated that other uses will develop to further enhance its value for the assessment of patients in various clinical settings.

Selected References

Dulchavsky SA, Schwarz KL, Kirkpatrick A, et al: Prospective evaluation of thoracic ultrasound in the detection of pneumothorax. J Trauma 50:201-205, 2001.

> This series establishes ultrasound's use beyond the FAST examination in trauma patients and serves as a springboard for the use of ultrasound in remote locations for the diagnosis of injuries outside the abdomen.

Han DC, Rozycki GS, Schmidt JA, et al: Ultrasound training during ATLS: An early start for surgical interns. J Trauma 41:208-213, 1996.

> One of the earlier descriptions of training surgical residents for the use of FAST examination, it establishes a steep learning curve even for trainees early in their career.

Hedrick WR, Hykes L, Starchman DE: Ultrasound Physics and Instrumentation. St. Louis, Mosby, 1995.

> This text is a comprehensive resource for readers interested in further information regarding the technical and theoretical background of ultrasonic principles.

Hildebrandt U, Feifel G: Preoperative staging of rectal cancer by intrarectal ultrasound. Dis Colon Rectum 28:42-46, 1985.

> This paper contains one of the earlier descriptions of ultrasound's use in staging rectal cancer, establishing endorectal ultrasound as a viable preoperative tool and paving the way for the use of ultrasound in both preoperative and intraoperative staging.

Rozycki GS, Ballard RB, Feliciano DV, et al: Surgeon-performed ultrasound for the assessment of truncal injuries: Lessons learned from 1,540 patients. Ann Surg 228:557-567, 1998.

> One of the largest series of FAST examinations published, this report highlights the technical aspects of FAST performance as well as its potential shortcomings.

Staren ED, Skjoldbye B: General interventional ultrasound. *In* Staren ED (ed): Ultrasound for the Surgeon. Philadelphia, Lippincott-Raven, 1997.

> A general reference for readers interested in learning more about techniques of interventional ultrasound applicable to the intensive care unit.

References

1. Rozycki GS, Feliciano DV, Ochsner MG, et al: The role of ultrasound in patients with possible penetrating cardiac wounds: A prospective multicenter study. J Trauma 46:543-552, 1999.
2. Shackford SR, Rogers FB, Osler TM, et al: Focused abdominal sonogram for trauma: The learning curve of nonradiologist clinicians in detecting hemoperitoneum. J Trauma 46:553-564, 1999.
3. Rozycki GS, Pennington SD, Feliciano DV: Surgeon-performed ultrasound in the critical care setting: Its use as an extension of the physical examination to detect pleural effusion. J Trauma 50:636-642, 2001.
4. Dolich M, McKenney MG, Varela J, et al: 2,576 ultrasounds for blunt abdominal trauma. J Trauma 50:108-112, 2001.
5. Dubinsky T, Horii S, Odwin CS: Ultrasonic physics and instrumentation. *In* Odwin CS, Dubinsky T, Fleischer AC (eds): Appleton & Lange's Review for the Ultrasonography Examination. Norwalk, CT, Appleton & Lange, 1993, p 8.
6. Hedrick WR, Hykes L, Starchman DE: Ultrasound Physics and Instrumentation. St. Louis, Mosby, 1995, p 55.
7. Sanders RC, Miner NS: Introduction. *In* Sanders RC (ed): Clinical Sonography: A Practical Guide. Boston, Little, Brown, 1991, p 10.
8. Kremkau F: Doppler ultrasound: Principles and instruments. *In* Ultrasound: Principles, Instrumentation, and Exercises. Philadelphia, WB Saunders, 1995, p 123.
9. Miller RS, Adelman RW, Espinosa MH: The early detection of non-palpable breast carcinoma with needle localization: Experience with 500 patients in a community hospital. Am Surg 58:193-198, 1992.
10. Schlecht L, Hadijuana J, Hosten N, et al: Ultrasonography of the female breast: Comparison of 7.5 MHz versus 13 MHz. Aktuelle Radiol 6:69-73, 1996.
11. Chang R, Kuo W, Chen D, et al: Computer-aided diagnosis for surgical office–based breast ultrasound. Arch Surg 135:696-699, 2000.
12. Saarela AO, Kiviniemi HO, Rissanen TJ, et al: Nonpalpable breast lesions: Pathologic correlation of ultrasonographically guided fine-needle aspiration biopsy. J Ultrasound Med 15:549-553, 1996.
13. Rizzatto G: Towards a more sophisticated use of breast ultrasound. Eur Radiol 11:2423-2435, 2001.
14. Gufler H, Buitrago-Tellez C, Madjar H, et al: Ultrasound demonstration of mammographically detected microcalcifications. Acta Radiol 41:217-221, 2000.
15. Vilmann P, Jacobsen GK, Henriksen FW, et al: Endoscopic ultrasonography with guided fine-needle aspiration biopsy in pancreatic disease. Gastrointest Endosc 38:172-173, 1992.
16. Chen C, Yang C, Yeh Y: Preoperative staging of gastric cancer by endoscopic ultrasound: The prognostic usefulness of ascites detected by endoscopic ultrasound. J Clin Gastroenterol 35:321-327, 2002.
17. Fu K, Eloubeidi M, Jhala N, et al: Diagnosis of gastrointestinal stromal tumor by endoscopic ultrasound guided fine-needle aspiration biopsy—a potential pitfall. Ann Diagn Pathol 6:294-301, 2002.
18. Hernandez L, Mishra G, Forsmarck C, et al: Role of endoscopic ultrasound (EUS) and EUS-guided fine-needle aspiration in the diagnosis and treatment of cystic lesions of the pancreas. Pancreas 25:222-228, 2002.
19. Kusunoki M, Yanagi H, Gondoh N, et al: Use of transrectal ultrasonography to select type of surgery for villous tumors in the lower two thirds of the rectum. Arch Surg 131:714-717, 1996.

20. Saclarides TJ: Endorectal ultrasonography for malignant disease. *In* Staren ED, Arregui ME (eds): Ultrasound for the Surgeon. Philadelphia, Lippincott-Raven, 1997, p 75.

21. Hildebrandt U, Feifel G: Preoperative staging of rectal cancer by intrarectal ultrasound. Dis Colon Rectum 28:42-46, 1985.

22. Herzog U, von Flue M, Tondelli P, et al: How accurate is endorectal ultrasound in the preoperative staging of rectal cancer? Dis Colon Rectum 36:127-134, 1993.

23. Hulsmans F, Tio TL, Fockens P, et al: Assessment of tumor infiltration depth in rectal cancer with transrectal sonography: Caution is necessary. Radiology 190:715-720, 1994.

24. Steele S, Martin M, Platt RJ: Flexible endorectal ultrasound for predicting pathologic stage of rectal cancers. Am J Surg 184:126-130, 2002.

25. Deen KI, Kumar D, Williams JG: Anal sphincter defects: Correlation between endoanal ultrasound and surgery. Ann Surg 218:201-205, 1993.

26. Falk PM, Blatchford GJ, Cali RL: Transanal ultrasound and manometry in the evaluation of fecal incontinence. Dis Colon Rectum 37:468-472, 1994.

27. Cook TA, Galland RB: A prospective study to define the optimum rescreening interval for small abdominal aneurysm. Cardiovasc Surg 4:441-444, 1996.

28. Bastounis E, Georgopoulos S, Maltezos C, et al: The validity of current vascular imaging methods in the evaluation of aortic anastomotic aneurysms developing after abdominal aortic aneurysm repair. Ann Vasc Surg 10:537-545, 1996.

29. Knudson MM, Collins JA, Goodman SB, et al: Thromboembolism following multiple trauma. J Trauma 32:2-11, 1992.

30. Barteau JA, Castro D, Arregui ME, et al: A comparison of intraoperative ultrasound versus cholangiography in the evaluation of the common bile duct during laparoscopic cholecystectomy. Surg Endosc 9:490-496, 1995.

31. Ravikumar TS, Kane R, Cady B: Hepatic cryosurgery with intraoperative ultrasound monitoring for metastatic colon carcinoma. Arch Surg 122:403-409, 1987.

32. Rafaelsen SR, Kronborg O, Larsen C, et al: Intraoperative ultrasonography in detection of hepatic metastases from colorectal cancer. Dis Colon Rectum 38:355-360, 1995.

33. Machi J, Sigel B: Operative ultrasonography in general surgery. Am J Surg 172:15-20, 1996.

34. American College of Surgeons Committee on Trauma: Advanced Trauma Life Support Course for Physicians. Chicago, American College of Surgeons, 1997.

35. Rozycki GS, Ochsner MG, Feliciano DV, et al: Early detection of hemoperitoneum by ultrasound examination of the right upper quadrant: A multicenter study. J Trauma 45:878-880, 1998.

36. Rozycki GS, Ballard RB, Feliciano DV, et al: Surgeon-performed ultrasound for the assessment of truncal injuries: Lessons learned from 1,540 patients. Ann Surg 228:557-567, 1998.

37. Mutabagani K, Coley B, Zumberge N, et al: Preliminary experience with focused abdominal sonography for trauma (FAST) in children: Is it useful? J Pediatr Surg 4:48-54, 1999.

38. Chiu WC, Cushing BM, Rodriguez A, et al: Abdominal injuries without hemoperitoneum: A potential limitation of focused abdominal sonography for trauma (FAST). J Trauma 42:617-625, 1997.

39. Huang M, Liu M, Wu J, et al: Ultrasonography for the evaluation of hemoperitoneum during resuscitation: A simple scoring system. J Trauma 36:173-177, 1994.

40. McKenney KL, McKenney MG, Cohn SM, et al: Hemoperitoneum score helps determine the need for therapeutic laparotomy. J Trauma 50:650-656, 2001.

41. Sisley AC, Rozycki GS, Ballard RB, et al: Rapid detection of traumatic effusion using surgeon-performed ultrasound. J Trauma 44:291-297, 1998.

42. Wernecke K, Galanski M, Peters P, et al: Pneumothorax: Evaluation by ultrasound—preliminary results. J Thorac Imaging 2:76-78, 2000.

43. Dulchavsky SA, Schwarz KL, Kirkpatrick A, et al: Prospective evaluation of thoracic ultrasound in the detection of pneumothorax. J Trauma 50:201-205, 2001.

44. Braxton CC, Reilly PM, Schwab CW: The traveling intensive care unit patient: Road trips. Surg Clin North Am 80:949-956, 2000.

45. Staren ED, Skjoldbye B: General interventional ultrasound. *In* Staren ED (ed): Ultrasound for the Surgeon. Philadelphia, Lippincott-Raven, 1997, pp 137-160.

46. Han DC, Rozycki GS, Schmidt JA, et al: Ultrasound training during ATLS: An early start for surgical interns. J Trauma 41:208-213, 1996.

47. Frezza EE, Solis RL, Silich RJ, et al: Competency-based instruction to improve the surgical resident technique and accuracy of the trauma ultrasound. Am Surg 65:884-888, 1999.

48. Knudson MM, Sisley AC: Training residents using simulation technology: Experience with ultrasound for trauma. J Trauma 48:659-665, 2000.

CHAPTER 12

SURGICAL INFECTIONS AND CHOICE OF ANTIBIOTICS

Daniel A. Anaya, M.D., and E. Patchen Dellinger, M.D.

Surgical Site Infections	**Pathogens in Surgical Infections**
Specific Surgical Infections	**Antimicrobials**

During the second half of the 19th century many operations were developed after anesthesia was introduced by Morton in 1846, but advances were few for many years because of the high rate of infection and the high mortality rate that followed infections. By the beginning of the 20th century, following the work of Ignaz Philipp Semmelweis and later on with the introduction of antisepsis into the practice of medicine by Joseph Lister, reduced infection rates and mortality in surgical patients were seen. The work of Holmes, Pasteur, and Kocher in infectious diseases as well as the operating room (OR) environment and discipline established by Halsted continued to prove the "aseptic and antiseptic" theory to be the first effective measure in preventing infections in surgical patients.

These initial principles helped to change surgical therapy from a dreaded event, with infection and death commonplace, to one that alleviates suffering and prolongs life with predictable success when carefully performed. With the introduction of antibiotic therapy in the middle of the 20th century a new adjunctive method to treat and prevent surgical infections was discovered, and hope for final elimination of infections was fostered. However, not only have postoperative wound and hospital-acquired infections continued, but widespread antibiotic therapy has often made prevention and control of surgical infections more difficult. The present generation of surgeons has seen increasing numbers of serious infections related to a complex combination of factors, including the performance of more complicated and longer operations; an increase in the number of geriatric patients with accompanying chronic or debilitating diseases; many new surgical procedures with implants of foreign materials; a rapidly expanding number of organ transplants requiring the use of immunosuppressive agents; and increased use of diagnostic and treatment modalities that cause greater bacterial exposures or the suppression of normal host resistance.

The modern surgeon cannot escape the responsibility of dealing with infections and in dealing with them, of having the knowledge for the appropriate use of aseptic and antiseptic technique, proper use of prophylactic and therapeutic antibiotics, and adequate monitoring and support with novel surgical and pharmacologic as well as nonpharmacologic aids. Basic understanding of how the body defends itself against infection is essential to a rational application of surgical and other therapeutic principles to the control of infection.

SURGICAL SITE INFECTIONS

Surgical site infections (SSIs) are those that present in any location along the surgical tract after a surgical procedure. In 1992 the Surgical Wound Infection Task Force published a new set of definitions for wound infections that included changing the term to *SSI*. Unlike surgical wound infections, SSIs involve postoperative infections presenting at any level (incisional or deep) of a specific procedure. SSIs are divided into incisional superficial (skin, subcutaneous tissue), incisional deep (fascial plane and muscles), and organ/space related (anatomic location of the procedure itself). Examples of organ/space SSIs would include intra-abdominal abscesses, empyema, or mediastinitis.[1]

SSI is the most common nosocomial infection in our population, reaching 38% of all infections in surgical patients. By definition it can present anytime from 0 to 30 days after the operation or up to 1 year after a procedure that has involved the implantation of a foreign material (such as mesh, vascular graft, or prosthetic joint). Incisional infections are the most common accounting for 60% to 80% of all SSIs and have a better prognosis than organ/space-related SSIs, the latter accounting for 93% of SSI-related mortalities.[1-3]

The microbiology of SSI is related to the bacterial flora present in the exposed anatomic area of a particular procedure and has been relatively fixed during the last 30 years as shown by the National Nosocomial Infection Surveillance System (NNIS) established by the Centers for Disease Control and Prevention (CDC). This study has shown that *Staphylococcus aureus* remains the most common pathogen of SSI followed by *Staphylococcus coagulase negative*, *Enterococcus,* and *Escherichia coli.* However for clean-contaminated and contaminated procedures, *E. coli* and other Enterobacteriaceae are the most common cause of SSI. Also in recent years some emerging organisms have become more common. Vancomycin-resistant enterococcus (VRE) and gram-negative bacilli with unusual patterns of resistance have been isolated more frequently. Of particular interest is the growing frequency of *Candida* spp as cause for SSI and surgical infections in general.[2]

Understanding the microbiology of SSI is important to guide initial empiric therapy of infections in a specific patient, as well as for identification of outbreaks and for strategies in the management of prophylactic antibiotics as discussed later in this chapter.

Causes and Risk Factors

Three areas have been identified as risk factors for SSI: bacterial factors, local wound factors, and patient factors (Table 12-1). The interaction between these three is what determines the risk of SSI as a complication in surgery. Most of these factors have been shown to be associated with SSI; however it has been difficult to show an independent association between each one of these and the presence of SSI.

Bacterial factors include virulence and bacterial load in the surgical site. The development of infection is affected by the toxins produced by the microorganism and the microorganism's ability to resist phagocytes and intracellular destruction. Several bacterial species have surface components that contribute to their pathogenicity by inhibiting phagocytosis (e.g., the capsules of *Klebsiella* and *Streptococcus pneumoniae,* slime of *Staphylococcus coagulase negative*). Gram-negative bacteria have surface components (endotoxin or lipopolysaccharide) that are toxic, and others, such as certain strains of clostridia and streptococci, produce powerful exotoxins. These exotoxins permit streptococci and clostridia to establish invasive infection after smaller inocula than other pathogens and to evolve much more rapidly. Thus, although most wound infections do not become evident clinically for 5 days or longer after the operation, infections due to streptococci or clostridia may become severe within 24 hours. Studies of traumatic wounds in healthy subjects have shown that bacterial contamination with more than 10^5 organisms frequently causes infection, whereas contamination with less than 10^5 organisms usually does not. The normal defense mechanisms therefore are of great importance in preventing infection at its inception, but wound infection is inevitable if the bacterial inoculum is sufficiently large. This observation led, in the 1990s, to the wound classification system in which wounds are classified and presumed to have different number and type of bacteria according to the anatomic areas entered and to the aseptic and antiseptic techniques used (Table 12-2). Length of preoperative stay, remote site infection at the time of operation, and duration of the procedure have also been associated with an increased SSI rate.[4] Preoperative shaving has been shown to increase SSI after clean procedures. This practice increases the infection rate about 100% compared with removing the hair by clippers at the time of the procedure or not removing it at all, probably secondary to bacterial growth in microscopic cuts. Therefore, the patient should not be shaved before an operation. Extensive removal of hair is not needed, and any that is done should be performed by electric clippers with disposable heads at the

TABLE 12-1.   Risk Factors for Surgical Site Infection (SSI) According to the Three Main Determinants of SSI

Microorganism	Local Wound	Patient
Remote site infection	Surgical technique:	Age
Long-term care facility	Hematoma/seroma	Immunosuppression
Duration of the procedure	Necrosis	Steroids
Wound class	Sutures	Malignancy
Intensive care unit patient	Drains	Obesity
Prior antibiotic therapy	Foreign bodies	Diabetes
Preoperative shaving		Malnutrition
Bacterial number, virulence, and antimicrobial resistance		Multiple comorbidities
		Transfusions
		Cigarette smoking
		Oxygen
		Temperature
		Glucose control

TABLE 12-2. Surgical Wound Classification According to Contamination

Wound Class	Definition
Clean	Uninfected operative wound in which no inflammation is encountered and the respiratory, alimentary, genital, or infected urinary tract are not entered. Wounds are primarily closed and, if necessary, drained with closed drainage. Surgical wounds following blunt trauma should be included in this category if they meet the criteria.
Clean-contaminated	Operative wound in which the respiratory, alimentary, genital or urinary tracts are entered under controlled conditions and without unusual contamination.
Contaminated	Open, fresh, accidental wounds. In addition, operations with major breaks in sterile technique or gross spillage from the gastrointestinal tract, and incisions in which acute, nonpurulent inflammation is encountered are included in this category.
Dirty	Old traumatic wounds with retained devitalized tissue and those that involve existing clinical infection or perforated viscera. This definition suggests that the organisms causing postoperative infection were present in the operative field before the operation.

time of the procedure and in a manner that does not traumatize the skin.[5]

Local wound factors are related to the fact that surgeons break basic barrier defense mechanisms such as skin and gastrointestinal mucosa while performing a procedure. In doing so there are specific factors associated with an increased rate of infection. Good surgical technique is the best way to avoid SSI while managing tissues (local wound) in the most appropriate manner and using sutures, drains, and foreign bodies only with adequate indications.

Patient-related factors include age, immunosuppression, steroids, malignancy, obesity, perioperative transfusions, cigarette smoking, diabetes, other preexisting illness and malnutrition, among others. It is hard to perform a study in which independent association with SSI can be proven while controlling for all other factors; however, patient-related factors seem to play an important role in SSI, and preventive measures are starting to focus on manipulating these, as discussed later in this section. Recent data suggest that maintaining normothermia and delivering an inspired fraction of oxygen (FiO_2) of 80% or more in the OR and postanesthesia care unit will reduce the rate of SSI by improving oxygen tension and white blood cell function in the surgical incision. Also, data suggest that control of glucose levels in the perioperative period and up to 48 hours later in both diabetic and nondiabetic patients can reduce the rates of SSI.[6-9]

SSI Risk Scores

SSI risk has traditionally been correlated to wound class. The accepted range of infection rate has been clean, 1% to 5%; clean-contaminated, 3% to 11%; contaminated, 10% to 17%; and dirty, higher than 27%. Wound class as discussed earlier is a significant risk factor for SSI; however, it assesses only the bacterial factors related to wound infection, and it is an imprecise method of including different types of procedures and different kinds of patients into one same category.

More recently the NNIS score, published by Culver and associates in 1991,[2] includes additional factors that have

TABLE 12-3. NNIS Score and Risk for Surgical Site Infection (SSI)

Risk Factors	Number of Positive Risk Factors	Risk of SSI (%)
Procedure time > 75th percentile	0	1.5
Contaminated or dirty wound	1	2.9
ASA III, IV, V	2	6.8
	3	13.0

SSI, surgical site infection; NNIS, National Nosocomial Infection Surveillance System; ASA, American Society of Anesthesiologists score.

TABLE 12-4. Comparison of NNIS Score and Wound Classification for Predicting Risk of SSI

Wound Class	NNIS Risk Score				
	0	1	2	3	All
Clean	1.0	2.3	5.4	—	5.4
Clean-contaminated	2.1	4.0	9.5	—	4.5
Contaminated	—	3.4	6.8	13.2	6.4
Dirty	—	3.1	8.1	12.8	7.1
All	1.5	2.9	6.8	13.0	—

SSI, surgical site infection; NNIS, National Nosocomial Infection Surveillance System.
Adapted from Dellinger EP, Ehrenkranz NJ: Surgical infections. *In* Bennett JV, Brachman PS (eds): Hospital Infections, 4th ed. Philadelphia, Lippincott-Raven, 1998.

an independent relation with SSI (Table 12-3). The NNIS score includes the wound class, the American Society of Anesthesiologists score, and the duration of the procedure measured by the duration of the operation compared with national averages for the same operation. This differentiates risk of SSI more accurately than the prior wound classification system used alone (Table 12-4).[2, 10]

Prevention

Understanding risk factors and preventive measures should promote better control with lower infection rates. Three primary measures have proven to have a significant impact on SSI. First, the aseptic and antiseptic technique introduced by Lister reduced SSI markedly. The second is the proper use of prophylactic antibiotics, and the third, the implementation of surveillance programs.[11-14]

Microorganisms are part of the human body microenvironment, and they will always be present. Even clean wounds have small numbers of bacteria present at the end of the operation. Most early prevention measures implemented were focused on controlling the bacterial factors for wound infections. In recent years research has focused on manipulating host (patient) factors to assist the body in dealing with fixed bacterial factors (assuming all preventive measures have been applied appropriately). The future in the control of infection will focus on patient factors and the body's ability to counteract the obligatory presence of microorganisms.

Preventive measures can be also classified according to the three determinants of wound infection and to the timing at which they are implemented (preoperatively, intraoperatively, postoperatively) (Table 12-5).

Microorganism Related

Microorganisms causing SSI can be either exogenous or endogenous. Exogenous microorganisms come from the operating team or from the environment around the surgical site (such as OR, equipment, air, and water). Endogenous microorganisms come either from the bacteria present in the patient at the surgical site or from bacteria present at a different location (e.g., remote site infection, nasal colonization). Two primary measures exist to control the bacterial load in the surgical site: aseptic and antiseptic methods and antimicrobial prophylaxis.[14]

Aseptic and Antiseptic Methods

Specific environmental and architectural characteristics of the OR help reduce the bacterial load in the OR itself, although it has not been proven to decrease the incidence of SSI except in refined clean procedures such as joint replacement. Basic principles include size of the OR, air management (filtered, flow, positive pressure toward the outside, and air cycles/hour), equipment handling (disinfection and cleansing), and traffic rules. All OR personnel should wear clean scrubs, caps, and masks, and traffic in and out of the OR should be minimized. Exogenous sources of bacteria causing SSI are rare when standard measures are followed and is only important in cases of outbreaks, such as those that follow failure of sterilization procedures or are traced to OR personnel who shed bacteria. Specific air-filtering mechanisms and other high-technology measures for environmental control in the OR play a significant role in wound infection control only in clean cases in which prostheses are implanted. However, a minimum of basic traffic, environment, and OR behavior rules should be followed by staff in the surgical pool as part of a discipline that keeps the team aware of potential causes of infections in surgical patients.

Surgical site preparation, however, is an important measure in preventing SSI. Preoperative showers the night before surgery with chlorhexidine have not proven to affect SSI, although they reduce the bacterial colony count in skin areas. The CDC recommends its use, and it is reasonable to use particularly in patients that have been in the hospital for a few days and in those in whom a SSI will

---

TABLE 12-5. Preventive Measures for Surgical Site Infection (SSI)

| Timing of Action | Determinant in Which Preventive Measure Acts | | |
	Microorganism	Local	Patient
Preoperative	Shorten preoperative stay Antiseptic shower preoperative Appropriate preoperative hair removal Avoid or treat remote site infections Antimicrobial prophylaxis	Appropriate preoperative hair removal	Optimize nutrition Preoperative warming Tight glucose control (insulin drip) Stop smoking

Intraoperative	Asepsis and antisepsis
	Avoid spill in gastrointestinal cases
		Surgical technique:
		  Hematoma/seroma
		  Good perfusion
		  Complete débridement
		  Dead spaces
		  Monofilament sutures
		  Justified drain use (closed)
		  Limit use of sutures/foreign bodies
		  Delayed primary closure when indicated
			Supplemental oxygen
			Intraoperative warming
			Adequate fluid resuscitation
			Tight glucose control (insulin drip)

Postoperative	Protect incision for 48-72 hr Remove drains ASAP Avoid postoperative bacteremia	Postoperative dressing for 48-72 hr	Early enteral nutrition Supplemental oxygen Tight glucose control (insulin drip) Surveillance programs

carry significant morbidity (cardiac, vascular, and prostheses procedures). Skin preparation of the surgical site should be done using a germicidal antiseptic such as tincture of iodine, povidone-iodine, or chlorhexidine. An alternate preparation is the use of antimicrobial incise drapes applied to the entire operative area. Traditionally the surgical team has scrubbed their hands and forearms for at least 5 minutes the first time in the day and for 3 minutes every consecutive time. Popular antiseptics used are povidone-iodine and chlorhexidine. Recent data have shown that the use of alcoholic hand-rub solutions are as effective while being faster and kinder to the skin of the surgical team. The use of sterile drapes and gowns is a way of maintaining every surface in contact with the surgical site as sterile as possible.

As many as 90% of an operative team puncture their gloves during a prolonged operation. The risk increases with time as does the risk for contamination of the surgical site if the glove is not changed at the moment of puncture. The use of double-gloving is becoming a popular practice that avoids contamination of the wound as well as exposure to blood by the surgical team. Double-gloving is recommended for all surgical procedures.[15] Instruments that will be in contact with the surgical site should be sterilized in a standard fashion and protocols for flash-sterilization and/or emergent sterilization must be well established to ensure the sterility of instruments and implants.

Antimicrobial Prophylaxis

Systemic antimicrobial prophylaxis is a potentially powerful preventive measure for SSI that is frequently delivered in an ineffective manner due more to the lack of a reliable process in the hospital and OR than to lack of understanding. Experience has shown that the effectiveness of antibiotic prophylaxis depends on an organized system to ensure its delivery in an effective manner. If a system is not in place, the results are haphazard failures. Recent national surveys have documented suboptimal prophylactic antibiotic use in 40% to 50% of operative procedures. It is clear that the administration of therapeutic doses of antimicrobial agents can prevent infection in wounds contaminated by bacteria sensitive to the agents. The decision to use prophylactic antibiotic therapy, however, must be based on balancing possible benefit against possible adverse effects. Indiscriminate use of antibiotics should be discouraged because it may lead to emergence of antibiotic-resistant strains of organisms or serious hypersensitivity reactions. In particular, prolonged use of *prophylactic* antibiotics may also mask the signs of established infections, making diagnosis more difficult, and causes an increase in the number of resistant pathogens recovered from surgical patients.[16]

Prophylactic systemic antibiotics are not indicated for patients undergoing low-risk, straightforward, clean surgical operations in which no obvious bacterial contamination or insertion of a foreign body has occurred. When the incidence of wound infections is less than 1% and the consequences of SSI are not severe, the potential for reducing this low infection rate does not justify the expense and side effects of antibiotic administration. Prophylactic antibiotic therapy is no substitute for careful surgical technique using established surgical principles, and its indiscriminate or general use is not in the best interest of the patient. Antibiotic agents can be used effectively only as adjuncts to adequate surgery.

In several clinical situations the administration of prophylactic systemic antibiotic therapy is usually beneficial. These situations almost always involve a brief period of contamination by organisms that can be predicted with reasonable accuracy. As examples, prophylactic systemic antibiotics reduce infection with clinical benefit in the following circumstances:

1. High-risk gastroduodenal procedures—these include operations for gastric cancer, ulcer, obstruction, or bleeding; those operations when gastric acid production has been suppressed effectively; and gastric operations for morbid obesity
2. High-risk biliary procedures—these include operations in patients older than 60 years of age; those for acute inflammation, common duct stones, or jaundice; and those with prior biliary tract operations or endoscopic biliary manipulation
3. Resection and anastomosis of the colon or small intestine (see later)
4. Cardiac procedures through a median sternotomy
5. Vascular surgery of the lower extremities or abdominal aorta
6. Amputation of an extremity with impaired blood supply, particularly in the presence of a current or recent ischemic ulcer
7. Vaginal or abdominal hysterectomy
8. Primary cesarean section
9. Operations entering the oral-pharyngeal cavity
10. Craniotomy
11. Implantation of any permanent prosthetic material
12. Any wound with known gross bacterial contamination
13. Accidental wounds with heavy contamination and tissue damage. In such instances, the antibiotic should be given intravenously as soon as possible after injury. The two best-studied situations are penetrating abdominal injuries and open fractures.
14. Injuries prone to clostridial infection because of extensive devitalization of muscle, heavy contamination, and/or impairment of blood supply
15. Presence of preexisting valvular heart damage, to prevent the development of bacterial endocarditis

Whether or not prophylactic antibiotics should be given for "clean" operations not involving the implantation of prosthetic materials has been controversial. A well-designed trial demonstrated reduction in infection risk when patients undergoing breast procedures or groin hernia repairs received prophylactic antibiotics compared to placebo.[17] However, these procedures are not universally considered valid indications for prophylaxis. Some have proposed that such clean operations with one or more NNIS risk points should be considered for prophylactic antibiotic administration.[18]

The administration of oral nonabsorbable antibiotics to suppress both aerobic and anaerobic intestinal bacteria before scheduled operations on the colon has also been successful in controlled trials. Neomycin plus erythromycin given only on the day before surgery, 19, 18, and 9 hours before the scheduled start of the procedure, is the most well-established combination at present. Neomycin and metronidazole is also an effective combination. Thorough mechanical cleansing of the intestinal tract is an important component of the oral regimen.[19] Several reports demonstrate a reduced infection rate with the combination of oral nonabsorbable and intravenous antibiotics, and this is the most common practice among colorectal surgeons in the United States.

Prophylactic antibiotic therapy is clearly more effective when begun preoperatively and continued through the intraoperative period, with the aim of achieving therapeutic blood levels throughout the operative period. This produces therapeutic levels of the antibiotic agents at the operative site in any seromas and hematomas that may develop. Antibiotics started as late as 1 to 2 hours after bacterial contamination are markedly less effective, and it is completely without value to start prophylactic antibiotics after the wound is closed. Failure of prophylactic antibiotic agents occurs in part through a neglect of the importance of the timing and dosage of these agents, which are critical determinants.

For most patients with elective surgery, the first dose of prophylactic antibiotics should be given intravenously at the time anesthesia is induced. It is unnecessary and may be detrimental to start them more than 1 hour preoperatively, and it is unnecessary to give them after the patient leaves the OR. A single dose, depending on the drug used and length of operation, is often sufficient. For operations that are prolonged, the prophylactic agent chosen should be given in repeated doses at intervals of one to two half-lives for the drug being used. It is never indicated to give prophylactic antibiotic coverage for more than 12 hours for a planned operation. There is no evidence to support the practice of continuing prophylactic antibiotics until central lines, drains, and/or chest tubes are removed. There is evidence that this practice increases the recovery of resistant bacteria.

Many patients fail to receive needed prophylactic antibiotics because the system for their administration is complex at the time of multiple events just before a major operation. This problem has been made worse by the trend of admitting patients directly to the OR for planned operations, which intensifies the pressures to accomplish a large number of procedures during a short interval before the operation. The possibility that prophylactic antibiotics will be unintentionally omitted can be minimized by establishing a system with a checklist. One member of the operative team (usually the preoperative nurse or a member of the anesthesia team) should be responsible for initialing a portion of the operative record that states either that the patient received indicated prophylactic antibiotics or that the surgeon has determined that antibiotics are not indicated for the procedure.

Many antibiotics effectively reduce the rate of postoperative SSIs when used appropriately for indicated procedures. No antibiotic has been reliably superior to another when each possessed a similar and appropriate antibacterial spectrum. The most important determinant is whether the planned procedure is expected to enter parts of the body known to harbor obligate colonic anaerobic bacteria (*Bacteroides* species). If anaerobic flora are anticipated, such as during operations on the colon or distal ileum or during appendectomy, then an agent effective against *Bacteroides* species, such as cefotetan, must be used. Cefoxitin is an alternative with a dramatically shorter half-life. If anaerobic flora are not expected, cefazolin is the prophylactic drug of choice.

For patients who are allergic to cephalosporins, clindamycin, or in settings where methicillin-resistant *S. aureus* (MRSA) is common, vancomycin can be used. The prophylactic use of vancomycin should be minimized as much as possible to reduce environmental pressures favoring the emergence of VREs and staphylococci. If an intestinal procedure is planned in such an allergic patient, a regimen with activity against gram-negative rods and activity against anaerobes, such as an aminoglycoside combined with clindamycin or metronidazole, or aztreonam combined with clindamycin, must be used.

The use of topical antibiotics often effectively diminishes the incidence of infection in contaminated wounds. However, the combination of topical agents and parenteral agents is not more effective than either one alone, and topical agents alone are inferior to parenteral agents in complex gastric procedures. As a general rule, topical agents do not cause any harm if one adheres to the following rules: (1) do not use any agent in wounds or in the abdomen that would not be suitable for parenteral administration; and (2) do not use more of the agent than would be acceptable for parenteral administration. In considering the amount used, any drug being given parenterally must be added to the amount being placed in the wound. Topical agents used for burn wounds (discussed elsewhere) may be used in large open wounds in selected patients.

Prophylactic antibiotic therapy is generally ineffective in clinical situations in which continuing contamination is likely to occur. Examples are as follows: (1) in patients with tracheostomies or tracheal intubation to prevent pulmonary infections; (2) in patients with indwelling urinary catheters; (3) in patients with indwelling central venous lines; (4) in patients with wound or chest drains; and (5) in most open wounds, including burn wounds.

Local Wound Related

Most of the preventive measures related to the local wound are determined by the good judgment and surgical technique of the surgeon. Intraoperative measures include appropriate handling of tissues and assurance of satisfactory final vascular supply but with adequate control of bleeding to prevent hematomas/seromas. Complete débridement of necrotic tissues and removal of unnecessary foreign bodies as well as avoiding the placement of foreign bodies in clean-contaminated, contaminated, or dirty cases is recommended. Monofilament sutures have proven in experimental studies to have a lower rate of SSI. Sutures are foreign bodies that should be used only when required. Suture closure of dead space has not been shown to prevent SSI. Large potential dead spaces can be treated with the use of closed-suction systems for short periods, since these provide a route for bacteria to reach the wounds and cause SSI. Open drainage systems (e.g., Penrose) increase rather than decrease infections in surgical wounds and should be avoided unless used to drain wounds that are already infected.

In heavily contaminated wounds or in wounds in which all the foreign bodies or devitalized tissues cannot be satisfactorily removed, delayed primary closure minimizes the development of serious infection in most instances. With this technique, the subcutaneous tissues and skin are left open and dressed loosely with gauze after fascial closure. The number of phagocytic cells at the wound edges progressively increases to reach a peak about 5 days after the injury. Capillary budding is intense at this time, and closure can usually be accomplished successfully even with heavy bacterial contamination because phagocytic cells can be delivered to the site in large numbers. Experiments have shown that the number of organisms required to initiate an infection in a surgical incision progressively increases as the interval of healing increases, up to the 5th postoperative day.

Finally, adequate dressing of the closed wound isolates it from the outside environment. Providing an appropriate dressing for 48 to 72 hours can decrease wound contamination. However, dressings after this period increase the subsequent bacterial count by altering the microenvironment underneath in the healing wound.

Patient Related

Host resistance is abnormal in a variety of systemic conditions and diseases, including leukemia, diabetes mellitus, uremia, prematurity, burn or traumatic injury, advanced malignancy, old age, obesity, malnutrition, and several diseases of inherited immunodeficiency. With surgical patients who have these or similar problems, extra precautions should be taken to prevent the development of wound infections, including correction or control of the underlying defect whenever possible.

Malnutrition and low albumin levels are associated with an increased rate of SSI. Optimizing nutritional status prior to surgery and early in the postoperative periods with specific immunonutrition (arginine, nucleotides, omega-3 fatty acids) formulas may decrease SSI in upper gastrointestinal tract cancer patients. Recent studies have also demonstrated that maintaining a higher partial pressure of oxygen by delivering higher FiO_2 with adequate fluid resuscitation is associated with decreased rate of SSI. The presumed mechanism is through more available oxygen for white blood cells to kill bacteria present in the wound at the time of the operation. Preoperative warming was also shown in two recent prospective, randomized, controlled trials to reduce SSI rates. Other studies have shown that increasing temperature results in increased perfusion and increased oxygen delivery to the incision. Finally, in critically ill patients, aggressive perioperative insulin therapy with the use of insulin drips to maintain glucose levels between 80 and 110 mg/dL was associated with decreased mortality in this set of patients. Other studies of cardiac and gastrointestinal surgery patients have demonstrated an increased rate of SSI when perioperative blood glucose levels exceeded 200 mg/dL whether the patients were diabetic or not.[6-9]

Although SSIs are still the most common nosocomial infection in surgical patients, knowledge regarding risk factors as well as methods for prevention are rapidly growing. Present and future investigations are focusing on the patient's ability to overcome the presence of microorganisms and avoid infection. It is the modern surgeon's responsibility to be up to date with this information and to implement all known and proven measures that reduce the presence of this complication. Wound infection surveillance systems have proven to be an important measure in controlling SSI rates, and perhaps this is achieved by permanent and continuous awareness from surgeons and surgical teams of the risk and the measures that can be used to avoid this common complication.[12] Surveillance of SSI should include a determination for each SSI of whether or not all accepted preventive measures were provided for that patient and procedure. If they were not, the SSI can be classified as "potentially preventable." If all appropriate preventive measures were provided, then the SSI is "apparently unpreventable." The goal of surgical practice and surveillance should be to have no potentially preventable SSI. As our knowledge regarding SSI prevention increases, the definition of potentially preventable can expand.

SPECIFIC SURGICAL INFECTIONS

Surgical infections are those that present as a result of a surgical procedure or those that require surgical intervention as part of their treatment. They are characterized by a breech of mechanical/anatomic defense mechanisms (barriers) and are associated with increased morbidity, significant mortality, and increased cost of care.[20]

Some generalizations can be made concerning typical differences between surgical and medical infections. In common community-acquired medical infections, such as primary pneumonia, general host defenses are usually intact. Some exceptions to intact host defenses occur in patients undergoing systemic treatment for malignancy or for transplant rejection and patients with human immunodeficiency virus (HIV) infection. Most surgical infections, in contrast, are the result of damaged host defenses, especially injury to the epithelial barrier that normally protects the sterile internal environment from endogenous and exogenous bacteria. Immunologic defects may be acquired, through either trauma (accidental or surgical) or tumor. Nonmechanical host defense defects are global, caused by nutritional deficiency and/or the systemic effects of trauma.

The pathogens found in medical infections are usually single and aerobic. They either derive from exogenous sources or are present only in a minority of asymptomatic normal hosts. Typically, they possess virulence properties, allowing them to invade and infect despite an intact epithelial barrier. Examples include β-hemolytic streptococci, *S. pneumoniae, Shigella, Salmonella,* and *Vibrio cholerae.* The pathogens causing surgical infections, in contrast, are frequently mixed, involving aerobes and anaerobes, and usually originate from the patient's own endogenous flora. These pathogens are opportunistic, often depending on an acquired epithelial defect to cause infection.

The primary principle when treating surgical infections is *source control*. This refers to drainage of the infection and/or correction of the predisposing cause. Typical types of source control include draining an abscess, resecting or débriding dead tissue, diverting bowel, relieving obstruction, closing a perforation, and so forth. Antibiotic treatment of a surgical infection without this mechanical solution will not resolve the infection. The most important aspect of the initial approach to a surgical infection is the recognition that operative intervention is required. Antibiotic treatment and systemic support are only adjunctive therapies that will help the patient overcome the infectious insult once the appropriate source control has been achieved.

Soft Tissue Infections

The distinction between surgical and medical infections in superficial tissues depends on the recognition of dead tissue in surgical infections. The most obvious example of a surgical infection is a subcutaneous abscess, an infectious process characterized by a necrotic center without a blood supply and composed of debris from local tissues, dead and dying white blood cells, components of blood and plasma, and bacteria. This semiliquid central portion (pus) is surrounded by a vascularized zone of inflammatory tissue. An abscess will not resolve unless the pus is drained and evacuated. It is recognized clinically as a localized swelling with signs of inflammation and tenderness. An abscess must be distinguished from cellulitis, which is a soft tissue infection with intact blood supply and viable tissue, marked by an acute inflammatory response with small vessel engorgement and stasis, endothelial leakage with interstitial edema, and polymorphonuclear leukocyte infiltration. Cellulitis resolves with appropriate antibiotic therapy alone if treatment is initiated before tissue death occurs.

An abscess may be mistaken for cellulitis when the central necrotic portion is located deep beneath overlying tissue layers and it cannot be readily detected by physical examination. It may also be disguised in anatomic locations where fibrous septa join skin and fascia, dividing subcutaneous tissue into compartments that limit the local expression of fluctuance while leading to high pressures that cause ischemia and promote early tissue death. Examples of such infections include perirectal abscesses, breast abscesses, carbuncles on the posterior neck and upper back, and infections in the distal phalanx of the finger (felon).

Knowledge of the local anatomy and pathophysiology of these special abscesses helps provide optimal treat-

ment. A perirectal abscess is often associated with a fistula communicating with the anus at a crypt. A fistula should be sought and, if found, unroofed at the time a perirectal abscess is drained. If a fistula is not found acutely, the surgeon should be alert for its occurrence in the postoperative period. A breast abscess is preferably drained by a circumferential incision in natural skin lines. A felon should be drained through a lateral incision to avoid a painful scar on the pressure-bearing distal pulp. At the time of incision and drainage for a felon, all fibrous septa in the infected pulp must be broken to resolve the infection.

Superficial abscesses on the trunk and head and neck are most commonly caused by *S. aureus,* often combined with streptococci. Abscesses in the axillae often have a prominent gram-negative component. Abscesses below the waist, especially on the perineum, are frequently found to harbor a mixed aerobic and anaerobic gram-negative flora.

Traumatic wounds when closed and infected become a surgical complication that needs to be opened, drained, and treated with antibiotics when associated with cellulitis or systemic compromise. Wounds older than 6 hours, those with significant contamination (dirty, including human and animal bites), with presence of necrotic and/or ischemic tissue, puncture wounds, those classified as stab wounds or gunshot wounds, and those caused by a significant crush mechanism or avulsion should not be closed. These wounds as well as those deeper than 1 cm and those caused by burns or frostbite mechanism should receive tetanus prophylaxis if the most recent tetanus booster was 5 or more years earlier. The use of antibiotics for simple extremity lacerations has not been proven to reduce the risk of infection after closure.

Necrotizing Soft Tissue Infections

Necrotizing soft tissue infections, both clostridial and nonclostridial, are less common than subcutaneous abscesses and cellulitis but much more serious conditions whose severity initially may be unrecognized. These infections are marked by the absence of clear local boundaries or palpable limits. This lack of clear boundaries accounts both for the severity of the infection and for the frequent delay in recognizing its surgical nature. Anatomically, these infections are marked by a layer of necrotic tissue, which is not walled off by a surrounding inflammatory reaction and thus does not present a clear boundary. In addition, the overlying skin has a relatively normal appearance in the early stages of infection, and the visible degree of involvement is substantially less than that of the underlying tissues. A clostridial infection typically involves underlying muscle and is termed *clostridial myonecrosis* or *gas gangrene.* Most nonclostridial and some clostridial necrotizing infections spread in the subcutaneous fascia, between the skin and the deep muscular fascia. These infections have been described under a variety of labels but are most commonly called *necrotizing fasciitis* (Table 12-6). Gas in a soft tissue infection has traditionally been recognized as a grave finding. It is important to under-

TABLE 12-6. Comparison of Clostridial and Nonclostridial Infections

Variable	Clostridial Myonecrosis	Nonclostridial Necrotizing Infections
Erythema	Usually absent	Present, often mild
Swelling/edema	Mild to moderate	Moderate to severe
Exudate	Thin	"Dishwater" to purulent
White blood cells	Usually absent	Present
Bacteria	GPR ± others	Mixed ± GPR
		May be GPC alone
Advanced signs	Hypesthesia	Hypesthesia
	Bronze discoloration	Ecchymoses
	Hemorrhagic bullae	Bullae
	Dermal gangrene	Dermal gangrene
	Crepitus	± Crepitus
Deep involvement	Muscle > skin	Subcutaneous tissue ± fascia ± muscle (uncommon) > skin
Histology	Minimal inflammation	Acute inflammation
	Muscle necrosis	Microabscesses
		Viable muscle
Physiology	Rapid onset of tachycardia, hypotension, volume deficit ± intravascular hemolysis	Variable—minimal to tachycardia, hypotension, and volume deficit
Treatment		
General	Aggressive cardiopulmonary resuscitation	Aggressive cardiopulmonary resuscitation
Antibiotics	Penicillin G plus broad-spectrum. Clindamycin may be useful for inhibiting toxin production	Third-generation cephalosporin or ciprofloxacin plus antianaerobic agent. Clindamycin may be useful for inhibiting toxin production
Hyperbaric O$_2$	If it does not delay other treatment	No
Surgery	Aggressive removal of infected tissue; amputation of extremity often required	Débridement and exposure; not much removal required; usually no amputation
Antitoxin	No	No

GPR, gram-positive rods; GPC, gram-positive cocci.
Adapted from Dellinger EP: Crepitus and gangrene. *In* Platt R, Kass EH (eds): Current Therapy in Infectious Diseases—3. Hamilton, Ontario, BC Decker, 1990.

stand that most soft tissue infections with gas are not "gas gangrene." Most bacteria, especially facultative gram-negative rods such as *E. coli,* make insoluble gases whenever they are forced to use anaerobic metabolism. Thus the presence of gas in a soft tissue infection implies anaerobic metabolism. Since human tissue cannot survive in an anaerobic environment, gas associated with infection implies dead tissue and therefore a surgical infection. The majority of gas-producing infections do not involve *Clostridium* species but are instead necrotizing infections involving other bacterial pathogens.

Rapid progression of a soft tissue infection, a marked hemodynamic response to infection, or the failure to respond to conventional nonoperative therapy may be the earliest signs of a necrotizing soft tissue infection. An apparent cellulitis with ecchymoses, bullae, any dermal gangrene, extensive edema, or crepitus suggests an underlying necrotizing infection and mandates operative exploration to confirm the diagnosis and definitively treat the infection. The critical step in diagnosis is to recognize the nonlocalized, necrotizing nature of the infection and the need for operative treatment. This is more important than applying a specific diagnostic label to the process. Operative treatment requires excision of involved tissues for clostridial myonecrosis. On an extremity this may mean amputation. Nonclostridial infections can often be managed by wide incision and débridement and do not

usually require amputation. In either case, all areas of necrotic tissue must be unroofed and débrided, which often produces large disfiguring wounds.

The most common organisms associated with clostridial infections are *Clostridium perfringens, Clostridium novyi,* and *Clostridium septicum.* Other bacteria are commonly found in association with the clostridial organisms. The only bacterium commonly reported as the sole cause of nonclostridial necrotizing soft tissue infections is β-hemolytic *S. pyogenes.* This is the most common pathogen recovered when no prior injury or operation is the cause of the infection. Postoperative and postinjury cases of necrotizing soft tissue infection are most often caused by mixed bacterial species, including aerobic and anaerobic pathogens, both gram positive and gram negative, a similar spectrum to that seen in intra-abdominal infections.

The treatment of necrotizing soft tissue infection should always include débridement, and additional support is given with broad-spectrum antibiotics and monitoring and systemic support. Antibiotic choices should include agents with broad activity against facultative gram-negative rods, gram-positive cocci, and anaerobes. More narrow antibiotic regimens can be given once a definitive culture with specific sensitivity results is available. Appropriate single agents include imipenem/cilastatin, meropenem, ertapenem, and piperacillin/tazobactam.

TABLE 12-7. Antibiotics with Predominantly Aerobic or Anaerobic Broad-Spectrum Activity

Aerobic Coverage	Anaerobic Coverage
Gentamicin	Clindamycin
Tobramycin	Metronidazole*
Amikacin	Chloramphenicol
Netilmicin	
Cefotaxime	
Ceftizoxime	
Ceftriaxone	
Ceftazidime	
Cefepime	
Aztreonam*	
Ciprofloxacin	
Ofloxacin	
Levofloxacin	

*Do not use aztreonam alone with metronidazole.

Combination regimens should include an aerobic and anaerobic agent as demonstrated in Table 12-7.

Intra-abdominal and Retroperitoneal Infections

Most serious intra-abdominal infections require surgical intervention for resolution. In this context, surgical intervention includes percutaneous drainage of intra-abdominal abscesses. The specific exceptions to the requirement for surgical intervention include pyelonephritis, salpingitis, amebic liver abscess, enteritis (e.g., *Shigella, Yersinia*), spontaneous bacterial peritonitis, some cases of diverticulitis, and some cases of cholangitis. However, all of these *exceptions* can be diagnosed presumptively with a rapid initial evaluation. If the diagnosis of one of these exceptions cannot be made, a patient with fever and abdominal pain should not be given antibiotics without a plan leading to operation or other drainage procedure. The administration of antibiotics in this setting before diagnosis may obscure subsequent findings and delay diagnosis and will certainly delay definitive operative management. If the patient is too sick to go without antibiotic therapy, he or she is also too sick to avoid operative intervention and definitive diagnosis and treatment.

Despite modern antibiotics and intensive care, mortality from serious intra-abdominal or retroperitoneal infection remains high (5% to 50%) and morbidity is substantial. The systemic response to intra-abdominal or retroperitoneal infection is accompanied by fluid shifts similar to those seen in patients with major burns. Fever, tachycardia, and hypotension are common, and a severe hypermetabolic, catabolic response is universal. If a corrective operation and effective antibiotics are not employed promptly, the sequence of events termed *multiple-organ dysfunction syndrome* may ensue and cause the death of the patient even after the primary focus of infection has been controlled. Regardless of the initial antibiotic choice and operative procedure, there is a significant chance that a change in antibiotics may be required and that a re-operation may be necessary. The physician caring for a patient with intra-abdominal infection must be alert to these possibilities and diligent in following and re-examining the patient and examining the antimicrobial susceptibilities of the recovered pathogens, so this decision can be made at the earliest possible time.

Outcome is improved by early diagnosis and treatment. The risk of death and of complications increases with increased age, preexisting serious underlying diseases, and malnutrition. The risk of death or failure to control the abdominal source of infection is also related to the normal homeostatic balance of the patient at the time of diagnosis and initiation of definitive therapy. This balance can be measured by scales designed to quantitate the number of physical findings and laboratory tests that are abnormal. One of the most widely used scales is the Acute Physiology and Chronic Health Evaluation (called *APACHE*) scoring system. The higher the score, the more abnormal tests and findings are present, and the greater the risk of death.[21]

When a patient is diagnosed with intra-abdominal infection, initial treatment consists of cardiorespiratory support, antibiotic therapy, and operative intervention. In most cases, the responsible bacteria are not known for at least 24 hours, and sensitivity information is not available for 48 to 72 hours after cultures are obtained during the operative procedure. Because most intra-abdominal infections yield three to five different aerobic and anaerobic pathogens, specific, targeted antibiotic therapy is not possible at first and the initial choice must be empiric, designed to cover a range of possible organisms. In recent years, numerous new antibiotics have widened the available choices. For infections acquired in the community with a small likelihood of resistant gram-negative rods and for a patient not severely ill, empiric therapy can be initiated with cefoxitin, cefotetan, ticarcillin/clavulanate, ertapenem, or ampicillin/sulbactam. For the more severely ill, or a patient who has been in the hospital or has recently been treated with antibiotics, a more comprehensive antimicrobial spectrum is needed. Imipenem, meropenem, piperacillin/tazobactam or a combination chosen from Table 12-7 is useful, taking one antibiotic from the aerobic column and one from the anaerobic column (see later for discussion of specific antibiotics).[22, 23]

Operative Intervention

The goal of operative intervention in patients with intra-abdominal infection is to correct the underlying anatomic problem that either caused the infection or perpetuates it. The cause of peritonitis must be corrected. Foreign material in the peritoneal cavity that inhibits white blood cell function and promotes bacterial growth (feces, food, bile, mucin, blood) must be removed. Large deposits of fibrin that entrap bacteria, allowing bacterial growth and preventing phagocytosis, should be removed.[24,25]

An intra-abdominal or retroperitoneal abscess requires drainage. Computed tomographic scans provide precise localization of intra-abdominal abscesses, permitting selected abscesses to be drained percutaneously under radiologic or ultrasound guidance. If the abscess is single and has a straight path to the abdominal wall that does not transgress bowel, it can be drained percutaneously. This is accomplished by needle puncture with aspiration of a small sample of pus to confirm the location and diagnosis. Subsequently, a guide wire is passed through the needle, which is then removed. The guide wire allows dilation of the tract, followed by placement of a drainage catheter. The progress of abscess closure can be followed by plain radiographs after instillation of contrast materials. If percutaneous drainage is not successful, an open operation may be required.[26]

If a patient has multiple abscesses or abscesses combined with underlying disease that requires operative correction, or if a safe percutaneous route to the abscess is not present, then open, operative drainage may be required. A single abscess in the subphrenic or subhepatic position may be drained by an extraperitoneal subcostal or posterior 12th-rib approach, which provides open drainage without exposing the entire peritoneal cavity to the abscess contents. Likewise, most retroperitoneal abscesses should be drained from a retroperitoneal approach. However, most pancreatic abscesses, which in reality more often consist of diffusely infected, necrotic, peripancreatic retroperitoneal tissue, require transabdominal operation and débridement. Recent reports demonstrate that some cases of necrotizing pancreatitis can be débrided and drained using minimally invasive techniques aided by laparoscopy. A pelvic abscess may be amenable to transrectal or transvaginal drainage.

Prosthesis Device-Related Infections

As the ability to replace parts of the body has increased, so has the potential for infectious complications associated with these replacement parts. Some of the most significant complications associated with vascular grafts, cardiac valves, pacemakers, and artificial joints are caused by infections at the site of implantation. The presence of the foreign material (the prosthetic device) impairs local host defenses, especially polymorphonuclear leukocyte function, and allows for certain bacteria with specific virulence factors (*Staphylococcus epidermidis*—slime) to stick to foreign surfaces colonizing and causing infections. Accordingly, most such infections resist treatment short of removing the offending device. Morbidity and mortality associated with infection is high. Some success can be obtained by intensive antibiotic therapy, removal of the infected device under antibiotic cover, and replacement with a new uninfected device followed by prolonged antibiotic treatment. This approach is warranted when the device is life sustaining, as in the case of a cardiac valve, or prevents severe disability, as in the case of a prosthetic joint.

Nonsurgical Infections in Surgical Patients

Postoperative patients are at increased risk for a variety of nonsurgical postoperative nosocomial infections. The most common of these is urinary tract infection (UTI). Any patient who has had an indwelling urinary catheter is at increased risk for a UTI. Despite the benign course of most UTIs, the occurrence of one in a surgical patient is associated with a threefold increase in death occurring during hospitalization. The best prevention is to use urinary catheters sparingly and for specific indications and short durations and to employ strict closed-drainage techniques for those that are used.

Lower respiratory tract infections are the third most common cause of nosocomial infection in surgical patients (after SSIs and UTIs) and are the leading cause of death due to nosocomial infection. Diagnosis is usually relatively straightforward in a patient who is breathing spontaneously. However, a patient who is intubated and being ventilated because of adult respiratory distress syndrome presents an extremely difficult diagnostic problem. Patients with this syndrome commonly have abnormal chest radiographic findings, abnormal blood gas values, and elevated temperatures and white blood cell counts even in the absence of infection. Both false-positive and false-negative diagnosis of pneumonia is common. New chest radiographic infiltrates with signs of infection constitute a good indication for bronchoalveolar lavage, a method being used to diagnose and identify bacteria causing ventilator-associated pneumonia, which has proven to minimize the indiscriminate use of antibiotics and possesses a higher specificity than previous methods.

As part of the work-up for fever in a surgical patient, central lines used for monitoring or treatment should always be considered. Catheter-related sepsis is diagnosed when an organism is isolated from blood cultures and from a segment of the catheter in question, without any other source of septicemia and with clinical findings consistent with sepsis. Infection of the catheter site is defined as presence of erythema, warmth, tenderness, and/or pus at the site of the catheter insertion. Both require removal of the catheter, and if a new central line is needed, a new puncture is warranted. Further treatment usually depends on the organism isolated. Placement of lines should be done following standard aseptic and antiseptic technique including wide drapes and full gown and glove for the inserting physician. Still the best way to minimize these infections is to avoid placement of unnecessary lines and to remove them once the indication is not present anymore. Routine change of central lines has not proven to reduce infection rates.

Other causes of nosocomial infections that can present in surgical patients include sinusitis and meningitis. These do not present as frequently but should always be considered, particularly in high-risk patients.

Postoperative Fever

Approximately 2% of all primary laparotomies are followed by an unscheduled operation for intra-abdominal infection, and roughly 50% of all serious intra-abdominal infections are postoperative. Wound infections are more common but less serious. Postoperative fever occurs frequently and may be a source of concern to physician and patient. Fever is associated with infection, and the empiric prescription of antibiotics is a common response to fever. However, most febrile postoperative patients are not infected, and indeed a significant proportion of infected patients may not be febrile, depending on the definition of *fever*. Because fever is common in the absence of infection, it is important to consider causes of postoperative fever other than infection and to make a presumptive diagnosis before instituting antibiotic treatment.[27]

The most common nonsurgical causes of postoperative infection and fever—UTI, respiratory tract infection, and intravenous catheter-associated infection—all are readily diagnosed. The other important causes of postoperative infection and fever—wound infection and intra-abdominal infection—require operative treatment and are not properly managed with antibiotics in the absence of operative treatment. The most sensitive test for detecting these infections and determining their location continues to be history taking and physical examination conducted by a conscientious physician. The physician with the most detailed understanding of the relevant history in a postoperative patient is the operating surgeon. Supportive laboratory and radiographic evaluation, including white blood cell count, blood cultures, and computed tomography, can supplement the physical examination. Fever in the first 3 days after operation most likely has a noninfectious cause. However, when the fever starts or continues 5 or more days postoperatively, the incidence of wound infections exceeds the incidence of undiagnosed fevers. Neither the prolongation of perioperative prophylactic antibiotics nor the initiation of empiric therapeutic antibiotics is indicated without a presumptive clinical diagnosis and a plan for operative intervention when needed.

Only two important infectious causes of fever are likely in the first 36 hours after a laparotomy. Both can be diagnosed readily if they are suspected and appropriate examinations are made. The first is an injury to bowel with intraperitoneal leak. This is characterized by marked hemodynamic changes—first tachycardia and then hypotension and a falling urine output. Fluid requirements are large, and physical examination reveals diffuse abdominal tenderness. The other early cause of fever and infection is an invasive soft tissue infection, beginning in the wound, caused either by β-hemolytic streptococci or by clostridial species (most commonly *C. perfringens)*. This event is diagnosed by inspection of the wound and Gram stain of wound fluid, which shows either gram-positive cocci or gram-positive rods. White blood cells are often present with streptococcal infections but are usually absent in cases of clostridial infection. A rare cause of infection in the first 48 hours after operation is wound toxic shock syndrome. This occurs when certain toxin-producing *S. aureus* species grow in a wound. Less than 1% of all toxic shock cases reported to the CDC were from wounds, and half of these presented within 48 hours of operation. Presenting symptoms include fever, diarrhea, vomiting, erythroderma, and hypotension. Desquamation follows later. Physical findings of wound infection were often unimpressive or absent. Wound drainage and antibiotics are recommended, but the best treatment is not known. Administration of clindamycin may be helpful for its inhibition of exotoxin production.

PATHOGENS IN SURGICAL INFECTIONS

This discussion of pathogens commonly responsible for surgical infections is not intended to be a complete review. Rather, it focuses on some broad distinctions and classifications that help organize the vast body of data concerning the usual bacterial flora of different surgical infections and the antibiotic susceptibility patterns of these pathogens. Bacteria important in surgical infections are broadly divided into aerobic and facultative bacteria in one group and anaerobic bacteria in the other; into gram-positive and gram-negative bacteria; and into bacilli (rods) and cocci.

Most infections presenting in surgical patients are caused by endogenous bacteria. Specific bacteria are found in specific parts of the body, and the exposed anatomic areas during a surgical procedure are usually the source of microorganisms that cause infection. It is helpful to know the normal microbial flora of the body, since this helps direct prophylactic antibiotics, start intelligent empiric therapy, and suspect the origin of an unknown source of infection in patients with positive blood cultures.

It is also helpful to be familiar with the different classifications of bacteria (Figs. 12-1 and 12-2) since it can take up to 72 hours for a final culture to give the result as a specific bacteria; however, Gram stain and biochemical tests can help in providing earlier guidance regarding which group of bacteria may be responsible for an infection.

Gram-Positive Cocci

Gram-positive cocci of importance to surgeons include staphylococci and streptococci. Staphylococci are divided into coagulase-positive and coagulase-negative strains. Coagulase-positive staphylococci are *S. aureus* and are the most common pathogen associated with infections in wounds and incisions not subject to endogenous contamination. Coagulase-positive staphylococci should be assumed resistant to penicillin and require treatment by a penicillinase-resistant antibiotic. Extensive use of penicillinase-resistant β-lactam antibiotics in the past has encouraged the emergence of MRSA. These organisms do not seem to have intrinsic pathogenicity greater than that of other staphylococci, but they are more difficult to treat because of antibiotic resistance. The prevalence of MRSA varies considerably by geographic region but has been increasing during the past 2 decades. MRSA initially was seen primarily in hospitalized patients but is now seen in an increasing number of community-acquired infections. The incidence of MRSA recovery is increased in patients coming from long-term care facilities, previously hospitalized or treated with antibiotics, and those with diabetes or on dialysis. These organisms are especially common in cases of endocarditis associated with intravenous drug use. MRSA must be treated with vancomycin, quinupristin/dalfopristin, or linezolid. Recent years have seen the introduction of *S. aureus* strains with decreased susceptibility to vancomycin, and, more recently, of *S. aureus* strains with high-level resistance to vancomycin. If the history of other pathogens and antimicrobial agents repeats itself, the number of such strains will increase in the future.

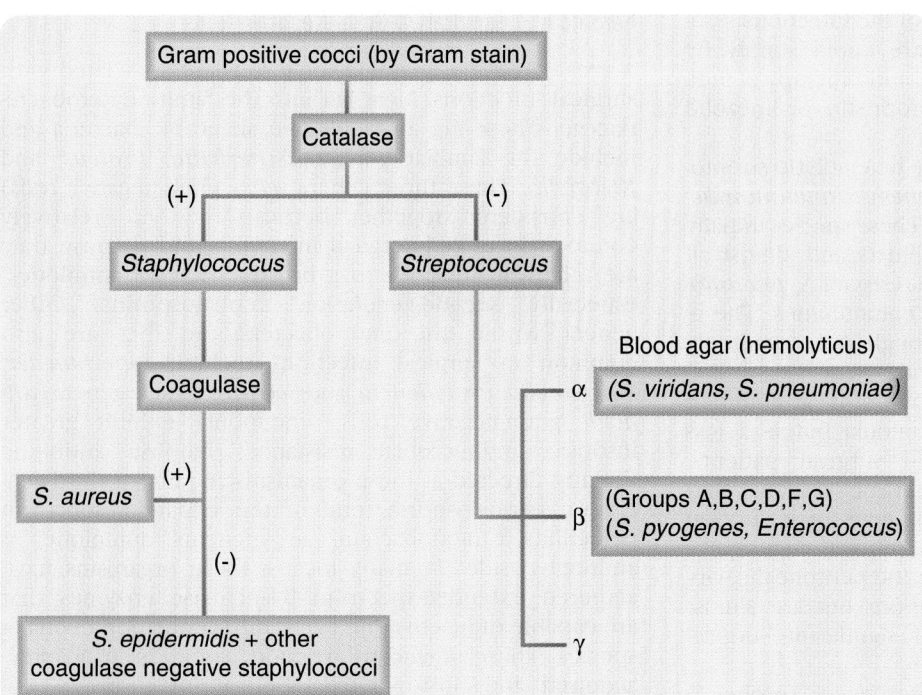

FIGURE 12-1. Biochemical tests used to identify specific pathogens within gram-positive cocci (GPC).

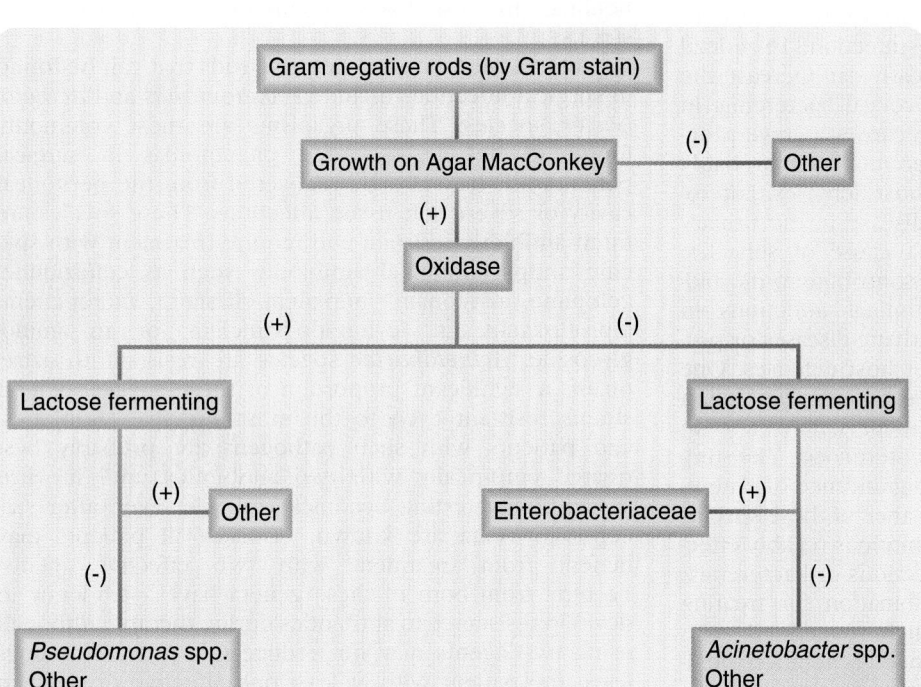

FIGURE 12-2. Biochemical tests used to identify specific pathogens within gram-negative rods (GNR).

For many years, coagulase-negative staphylococci were considered contaminants and skin flora incapable of causing serious disease. However, in the correct clinical setting, coagulase-negative staphylococci can cause serious disease. This is most common in patients who have been compromised by trauma, extensive surgery, or metabolic disease and who have invasive vascular devices in place. Coagulase-negative staphylococci are the most common organisms recovered in nosocomial bacteremia and are frequently associated with clinically significant infections of intravascular devices. Coagulase-negative staphylococci are also found in endocarditis, prosthetic joint infections, vascular graft infections, and postsurgical mediastinitis. Most coagulase-negative staphylococci are methicillin resistant. Although most of the infections associated with intravascular devices are cured simply by removing the device, if empiric antibiotic therapy is indicated, vancomycin, quinupristin/dalfopristin, or linezolid should be chosen.

The streptococcal species include β-hemolytic streptococci (especially group A or *S. pyogenes*), *S. pneumoniae*, and other α-hemolytic streptococci. These species initially were uniformly sensitive to penicillin G and almost all other β-lactam antibiotics. Penicillin-resistant *S. pneumoniae* are now found in most urban communities. The β-hemolytic streptococci alone, although not commonly recovered from soft tissue wounds, can cause life-threatening infections. *S. pneumoniae* is a common cause of community-acquired pneumonia but is a less common pathogen in hospitalized surgical patients. The other α-hemolytic streptococci or viridans streptococci rarely are significant pathogens in a surgical setting. They are commonly found on mucous membranes and skin and may be recovered from the peritoneal cavity after upper gastrointestinal perforations but are almost never found as the sole cause of significant surgical infections.

The precise significance of enterococci (group D streptococci) in surgical infections is controversial. Enterococci are commonly recovered as part of a mixed flora in intra-abdominal infections. It is rare to recover enterococci alone from a surgical infection. In animal models of infection, enterococci clearly can increase the virulence of other bacteria. Enterococcal bacteremia in association with a surgical infection carries a grave prognosis. The occurrence of the bacteremia itself probably signals a profound compromise of host defenses. Enterococci clearly do cause significant disease in the urinary tract and the biliary tract or as a cause of subacute bacterial endocarditis and probably contribute to morbidity and mortality from intra-abdominal infections in high-risk patients with serious underlying diseases or protracted illnesses with impairment of host defenses. One recent report of patients with intra-abdominal infection found a significantly higher treatment failure rate in patients who had initial isolation of enterococci. The stimulus for discussing the pathogenic significance of enterococci derives from the relative resistance of these species to antibiotic therapy. No single antibiotic is reliably effective for eradicating deep-seated infections or bacteremia. The most effective antibiotic combination for treating enterococcal infections is gentamicin combined with either ampicillin (or another advanced-generation penicillin) or vancomycin. However, enterococci resistant to all known antibiotics including gentamicin and vancomycin (VRE) have been isolated in increasing numbers in most major medical centers in the United States. The isolation of VRE is especially common and carries a grave prognosis in liver transplant patients. Between 1989 and 1993 the incidence of VRE reported to the CDC increased 26-fold, while the incidence in intensive care units (ICUs) increased 34-fold. The incidence of VRE infections and colonization in hospitalized patients is increased following therapy with third-generation cephalosporins and vancomycin.

Aerobic and Facultative Gram-Negative Rods

A great variety of gram-negative rods are associated with surgical infections. Most fall into the family Enterobacteriaceae. These are all facultative anaerobic bacteria and include the familiar genera *Escherichia, Proteus,* and *Klebsiella.* These three genera (*easy* gram-negative rods) are considered together because they are relatively common in mixed surgical infections and because they are relatively sensitive to a broad variety of antibiotics, especially second-generation cephalosporins. Other genera within the Enterobacteriaceae that are also common in surgical infections include *Enterobacter, Morganella, Providencia,* and *Serratia.* These genera (*difficult* gram-negative rods) commonly exhibit greater intrinsic antimicrobial resistance. Empiric antibiotic therapy directed at these organisms requires a third-generation cephalosporin, one of the expanded-spectrum penicillins, a monobactam, carbapenems, quinolone, or aminoglycoside. In many locales these organisms have acquired extended-spectrum β-lactamase enzymes that are capable of inactivating even third-generation cephalosporins. These organisms are more common in hospital-acquired and postoperative surgical infections. Gram-negative rods recovered from infections originating in the community, such as uncomplicated appendicitis or diverticulitis, are less likely to involve antibiotic-resistant strains.

Obligate aerobic gram-negative rods that can be found in surgical infections include *Pseudomonas* and *Acinetobacter* species. These organisms are most commonly found in hospital-associated pneumonias in surgical patients but may also be recovered from the peritoneal cavity or severe soft tissue infections. These species are often antibiotic resistant and require treatment with specific antipseudomonal antibiotics such as ceftazidime, cefepime, aztreonam, imipenem/cilastatin, meropenem, ciprofloxacin, an acylureido-penicillin, or an aminoglycoside. *Acinetobacter* species are resistant to aztreonam. A significant proportion of these species exhibit strains resistant even to the most effective antibiotics, and patients with such pathogens are probably best treated empirically with two antibiotics until in vitro susceptibility testing becomes available. Even after susceptibility data are known, critically ill patients may benefit from treatment with two effective agents. Bacteria from both of these genera have a tendency to develop resistance to antibiotics during therapy. Although using two agents may not reduce this process, it does leave the patient with at least one effective drug when it occurs. *Stenotrophomonas maltophilia* (previously *Pseudomonas* or *Xanthomonas maltophilia*) is uniformly resistant to imipenem and meropenem and is most commonly encountered as an emerging organism when one of these carbapenems is used for empiric treatment of a serious infection.

Anaerobes

Anaerobic bacteria are the most numerous inhabitants of the normal gastrointestinal tract, including the mouth.

The most common anaerobic isolate from surgical infections is *Bacteroides fragilis*. *B. fragilis* and *Bacteroides thetaiotaomicron* are two common anaerobic species with significant resistance to many β-lactam antibiotics. The most effective antibiotics against these species are metronidazole, clindamycin, chloramphenicol, imipenem, meropenem, and ertapenem and the combinations of a penicillin and a β-lactamase inhibitor (ticarcillin/clavulanate, ampicillin/sulbactam, and piperacillin/tazobactam). Other anaerobic species commonly recovered from surgical infections but with less significant bacterial resistance patterns include *Bacteroides melaninogenicus* and most of the anaerobic cocci.

The other important genus of anaerobic bacteria found in surgical infections is *Clostridium,* previously mentioned in the discussion of necrotizing soft tissue infections. Although they can survive for variable periods while exposed to oxygen, they require an anaerobic environment for growth and invasion and for elaboration of the toxins that account for their dramatic virulence in soft tissue infections. The *Clostridium* species are all gram-positive, spore-forming rods. However, when present in human infections, they do not form spores, so Gram-stained material from a soft tissue infection shows gram-positive rods without spores. *Clostridium difficile* belongs to this family, and *Clostridium tetani* is responsible for tetanus. The prevention of tetanus is accomplished solely through active and passive immunization, not through antibiotic administration.

Anaerobic bacteria have a special importance in relation to surgical infections. These strains grow only in settings with a low oxidation-reduction potential, which is incompatible with the survival of mammalian tissue. Thus, the recovery of anaerobes from a soft tissue infection or even from the blood implies their growth and multiplication in a focus of dead tissue. The predominant source of anaerobic bacteria is the gastrointestinal tract; thus, an anaerobic infection implies a defect in the anatomic integrity of the gastrointestinal tract. Both of these conditions (dead tissue and a defect in the gastrointestinal tract) require surgical correction, so most anaerobic infections (other than lung abscess) require surgical intervention. Certainly an anaerobic bacteremia should always prompt a search for an abscess or for an enteric lesion that requires surgical intervention.

Fungi

Fungi are infrequently the primary pathogens in deep-seated surgical infections. *Candida* infections, however, have become a relatively frequent pathogen in surgical infection over the last years. The NNIS data show that it is now the fourth cause of bacteremia in hospitalized patients in the United States and other studies show that it can be present as the source of intra-abdominal infection in 8% of the cases.

Pathogens from the *Candida* genus may be seen frequently as an opportunistic invader in patients with serious surgical infections who have received broad-spectrum antibiotic treatment suppressing normal endogenous flora. These infections are best avoided through judicious use of systemic broad-spectrum antibiotics and through prophylaxis with oral nystatin or ketoconazole when broad-spectrum antibacterial therapy is required. *Candida* species recovered from open wounds usually represent contamination, not true invasion. Recovery of *Candida* species from peptic ulcer perforations also does not usually require treatment. However, recovery of *Candida* from an established intra-abdominal abscess or from urine and sputum in an otherwise compromised patient may warrant therapy. Intra-abdominal *Candida* infections are more common in association with infections after severe pancreatitis.

Therapy of *Candida* infections in patients with multiple sites colonized or patients with well-drained abscesses formerly required the use of amphotericin at 3 to 5 mg/kg total dose over a 10- to 14-day period with all the intrinsic complications derived from the use of this nephrotoxic antimicotic. Fluconazole and the newly developed triazole voriconazole have allowed for a better control of *Candida* infections with more liberal indications for treatment and with less side effects or complications. Fluconazole is usually an adequate treatment for *C. albicans.* However, *Candida krusei, Candida glabrata,* and occasionally *Candida lusitaniae,* which are becoming more frequent in surgical infections, are species resistant to fluconazole, in which case the use of voriconazole or amphotericin is indicated.

Virus

Viruses do not cause any infections that require operation for resolution and thus are not discussed in any detail here. As a result of immune suppression to prevent rejection, transplant patients are at significant risk of viral infection, especially with cytomegalovirus. The viral infections of most relevance to routine surgical patients are the blood-borne viruses that may be transmitted through blood transfusion: the hepatitis B virus (HBV), the hepatitis C virus (HCV), and HIV. Transmission of HBV and HIV by transfusion is unusual because of the use of accurate tests for screening infected units of blood. Previously, HCV was one of the most common viruses transmitted by transfusion in the medical setting, but a new serologic test for HCV has greatly reduced that risk. Cytomegalovirus is also commonly transmitted by transfusions. However, other, currently unknown blood-borne viruses are likely to be described in the future. Therefore, it is good medical practice to limit blood transfusion to circumstances clearly requiring it.

ANTIMICROBIALS

This discussion of antibiotics is not intended to be exhaustive. Rather, it focuses on the antibiotics that are most commonly indicated in the treatment of patients with surgical infections. Table 12-8 lists these antibiotics with their relative half-lives, mechanism of action, important toxicities, and general antibacterial spectra. Several handy references are updated yearly and provide more detailed

TABLE 12-8.   Antibiotics Commonly Used in Surgical Infections

Drug Class and Name	Mechanism of Action	Comment	Half-Life	Toxicity	Antibacterial Spectrum
Penicillins					
Penicillin G	β-lactam mechanism: inhibits bacterial cell wall by binding to penicillin-binding proteins (PBP). It inhibits the final transpeptidation step of peptidoglycan synthesis in bacterial cell wall	Prototype; hydrolyzed by all β-lactamases	Short	Low, but rarely allergic reaction may be life-threatening	Streptococcal species except enterococcus and penicillin-resistant *Pneumococcus*; *Neisseria* spp, except lactamase-producing gonococci
Antistaphylococcal					
Methicillin	β-lactam mechanism; also penicillinase resistant and acid stable	First antistaphylococcal drug	Short	Interstitial nephritis	Staphylococcal species (methicillin sensitive) and streptococcal species except enterococcus. Narrow spectrum; usually used for staphylococcal infections only
Oxacillin			Short	Interstitial nephritis	
Nafcillin			Short	Interstitial nephritis	
"Easy" gram-negative					
Ampicillin	β-lactam mechanism	Hydrolyzed by all β-lactamases	Short	Diarrhea and rashes	Streptococcal species, including many enterococci, *Neisseria* species (non-lactamase producing), *Hemophilus influenzae* (non-lactamase producing), some *Escherichia coli* and *Proteus mirabilis*
Amoxicillin			Medium		
Expanded spectrum					
Carbenicillin	β-lactam mechanism	Hydrolyzed by all β-lactamases	Short	High sodium load; inhibition of platelet aggregation	Greatly expanded gram-negative spectrum while still active against streptococcal species including *Enterococcus*. Moderate antianaerobe activity. May not be reliable as sole agent for established gram-negative rod infections
Ticarcillin	β-lactam mechanism	Same	Short		Same, but less activity against *Enterococcus*
Very advanced spectrum					
Mezlocillin	β-lactam mechanism	Hydrolyzed by all β-lactamases	Short	Low	Same as expanded-spectrum penicillins with more activity against *Pseudomonas*, *Acinetobacter*, and *Serratia* species
Piperacillin		Same	Short	Low	
β-Lactamase Inhibitor Combination	β-lactam mechanism, plus			Low; same as constituent β-lactam	
Clavulanic acid plus	Clavulanic acid mechanism: β-lactamase inhibitor which increases the antibacterial activity of β-lactam antibiotics				
Ticarcillin			Short		Same as ticarcillin or amoxicillin plus *Staphylococcus* (methicillin sensitive), lactamase-positive *H. influenzae* and some lactamase-producing gram-negative rods, and anaerobes
Amoxicillin		Oral only	Medium		

TABLE 12-8.   Antibiotics Commonly Used in Surgical Infections—Cont'd

Drug Class and Name	Mechanism of Action	Comment	Half-Life	Toxicity	Antibacterial Spectrum
Sulbactam plus	β-lactam mechanism, plus	IV only	Short		
Ampicillin	Sulbactam mechanism: forms enzyme-sulbactam complex that inhibits β-lactamases				Similar to cefoxitin with activity against *Enterococcus*
Tazobactam plus	β-lactam mechanism, plus		Short		
Piperacillin	Tazobactam mechanism: Inhibits β-lactamases. More potent than sulbactam or clavulanic acid				Similar to piperacillin plus *Staphylococcus* (methicillin sensitive), some lactamase-producing gram-negative rods, and anaerobes
Cephalosporins					
"First" generation	β-lactam mechanism				Streptococcal species except *Enterococcus*, staphylococcal species (methicillin sensitive), and "easy" gram-negative rods
Short half-life					
Cephalothin		Prototype of class	Short	Low	
Cephapirin			Short	Low	
Longer half-life					
Cefazolin			Medium	Low	
"Second" generation	β-lactam mechanism				Same as first-generation cephalosporins with expanded gram-negative activity not including *Pseudomonas*, *Acinetobacter*, or *Serratia*
Poor anaerobic activity					
Shorter half-life					
Cefamandole			Short	Low	
Cefuroxime			Medium	Low	
Longer half-life					
Ceforanide		Reduced antistaphylococcal activity	Long		
Cefonicid		Reduced antistaphylococcal activity	Long		
Good anaerobic activity					Same as above, plus many anaerobes
Short half-life					
Cefoxitin			Short	Low	
Longer half-life					
Cefmetazole			Medium	Low	
Cefotetan			Long	Prolonged prothrombin times	
"Third" generation Poor *Pseudomonas* activity	β-lactam mechanism				Very active against most gram-negative rods except *Pseudomonas*, *Acinetobacter*, and *Serratia*. Poor against anaerobes. Less activity against streptococcal and staphylococcal species than first- and second-generation cephalosporins. Same as above plus activity against many *Pseudomonas*, *Acinetobacter*, and *Serratia* species
			Short	Low	
Short half-life			Medium	Low	
Cefotaxime					
Ceftizoxime					
Long half-life					
Ceftriaxone			Long	Low	

Continued

TABLE 12-8.   Antibiotics Commonly Used in Surgical Infections—Cont'd

Drug Class and Name	Mechanism of Action	Comment	Half-Life	Toxicity	Antibacterial Spectrum
Good *Pseudomonas* activity					Same as above with increased activity against gram-positive cocci
Cefoperazone			Medium	Low	
Ceftazidime			Medium	Low	
Cefepime			Medium	Low	
Monobactams					
Aztreonam	β-lactam mechanism: Preference to PBP 3 of gram-negative bacteria; very stable against β-lactamases	Safe for most patients with penicillin allergy	Short	Low	Good activity against most gram-negatives, including *Pseudomonas* and *Serratia*. Inactive against gram-positive cocci, anaerobes, and most *Acinetobacter* strains
Carbapenems	β-lactam mechanism, plus				
Imipenem/cilastatin	Cilastatin mechanism: inactivates dehydropeptidases, which normally would break the β-lactam ring of imipenem in the proximal tubule	Provided combined with cilastatin to prevent renal breakdown and renal toxicity	Short	Low; seizures in certain high-risk patients	Extremely broad gram-positive and gram-negative aerobic and anaerobic. Modest activity against *Enterococcus*. Inactive against *Stenotrophomonas* (formerly *Xanthomonas*) *maltophilia*
Meropenem		Provided alone without cilastatin	Short	Reduced potential for seizures	Same activity as imipenem
Ertapenem		Provided alone without cilastatin	Long	Low	Better activity against Enterobacteriaceae, less activity against gram-positive cocci, *Pseudomonas, Acinetobacter,* and anaerobes
Quinolones					
Poor anaerobic activity	Inhibit bacterial enzyme DNA-gyrase, thus inhibiting DNA replication				
Norfloxacin		Oral only; urine levels only	Long	Low; interaction leads to accumulation of theophylline	Very broad gram-negative activity; gram-positive and very broad gram-negative activity, including *Pseudomonas, Acinetobacter,* and *Serratia;* poor activity against anaerobes
Ciprofloxacin		Oral and intravenous (applies to all below)	Long		See above
Ofloxacin		Racemic mixture of levofloxacin (active) and dextrofloxacin (inactive)	Long		See above
Levofloxacin			Long		See above
Better anaerobic activity					
Gatifloxacin			Very long		As above plus better gram-positive, gram-negative and anaerobe coverage
Moxifloxacin			Very long		Broad-spectrum against gram positive, gram negative and anaerobes

TABLE 12-8.   Antibiotics Commonly Used in Surgical Infections—Cont'd

Drug Class and Name	Mechanism of Action	Comment	Half-Life	Toxicity	Antibacterial Spectrum
Aminoglycosides	Bind to a specific protein in the 30S subunit of bacterial ribosome, leading to faulty alignment or recognition by RNA during initiation of microbial peptide chain formation	All have low ratio* of therapeutic/toxic levels; all are frequently underdosed; all exhibit significant postantibiotic effect	Medium	Nephrotoxicity and 8th nerve toxicity, both auditory and vestibular	Extremely broad coverage of gram-negative rods. Poor activity against streptococci. Some synergism with penicillin or vancomycin against enterococci. No activity against anaerobes
Gentamicin		See above	Medium	See above	Most active against enterococci and *Serratia* spp
Tobramycin		See above	Medium	Statistically but questionably clinically significant decrease in nephrotoxicity	More active against *Pseudomonas* spp
Amikacin		See above	Medium	See above (aminoglycosides)	Active against a significant number of gentamicin- and tobramycin-resistant organisms
Netilmycin		See above	Medium	See above (aminoglycosides)	See above (aminoglycosides)
Other Antianaerobes					
Chloramphenicol	Inhibits bacterial protein synthesis by reversibly attaching to the 50S subunit of the 70S bacterial ribosome	Oral or IV	Long†	Dose-dependent, reversible bone marrow suppression; rare (1/25,000-40,000) irreversible bone marrow aplasia	Many gram-positive and easy gram-negative rods. *H. influenzae*, most anaerobes
Clindamycin	Inhibits bacterial protein synthesis by attaching to the 50S subunit of the bacterial ribosome	Oral or IV	Long†		Streptococcal species except enterococci, staphylococci, most anaerobes. Inactive against gram-negative rods
Metronidazole	Not fully elucidated; seems to produce cytotoxic effects on anaerobes by a reduction reaction (nitro group of metronidazole)	Oral or IV	Very long†	Disulfiram-type (Antabuse) reaction; peripheral neuropathy with prolonged use	Very active against most anaerobes. Inactive against facultative and aerobic bacteria. Active against protozoa (amoebae and *Giardia*)
Glycopeptides Vancomycin	Inhibits cell wall synthesis by binding to carboxyl subunits on peptide subunits containing free D-alanyl-D-alanine (different site to β-lactams, no cross resistance), plus may affect permeability of membrane, plus may inhibit RNA synthesis	Only IV, no oral absorption	Very long	Hypertension and histamine release phenomena (Redman syndrome) during infusion. Nephrotoxicity and ototoxicity	Streptococcal species, including many enterococci, staphylococci (including methicillin-resistant strains), *Clostridium* species. No activity against gram-negative rods
Streptogramins Quinupristin/dalfopristin	It binds to different sites on the 50S subunit of bacterial ribosomes; a 5-10-fold decrease in the dissociation constant of quinupristin is seen in the presence of dalfopristin	Significant postantibiotic effect*	Medium	Reversible transaminase elevations; must be given through central line	Most gram-positive pathogens, including vancomycin-resistant *E. faecium*, methicillin-resistant *S. aureus* and *S. epidermidis*, and penicillin-resistant *S. pneumoniae* but *not* *E. faecalis*

Continued

TABLE 12-8. Antibiotics Commonly Used in Surgical Infections—Cont'd

Drug Class and Name	Mechanism of Action	Comment	Half-Life	Toxicity	Antibacterial Spectrum
Macrolides					
Erythromycin	It attaches to the 50S subunit of the bacterial ribosome and may interfere with translocation reactions of the peptide chains.	Oral or IV	Medium	Cholestasis with estolate (IV) form	Most gram-positive *Neisseria, Campylobacter, Mycoplasma, Chlamydia, Rickettsia, Legionella*
Tetracyclines	Inhibit protein synthesis by attaching to 30S subunit of bacterial ribosome				
Tetracycline		Oral or IV	Long	Stain teeth of children	Many gram-positive, easy gram-negative rods, some anaerobes, *Rickettsia, Chlamydia, Mycoplasma*
Doxycycline		Oral or IV	Very long	Same	
Antifungal					
Triazoles					
Fluconazole	Inhibition of cytochrome p-450–dependent ergo-sterol synthesis	Oral or IV	Very long	Elevation of liver function tests	Most fungi except *Candida krusei, C. glabrata*
Voriconazole			Long	Visual disturbances, fever	Most fungi
Amphotericin B	Binds to sterols of cell wall and interferes with permeability	IV	Very long	Nephrotoxicity, fevers and chills	Most fungi
Caspofungin	Inhibits β-glucan synthase, disrupts the integrity of the cell wall and causes cell lysis	IV	Very long	Fever; infusion-related complications	Most fungi

Drugs have been grouped into those with short, medium, long, and very long half-lives. Short half-life drugs usually have a half-life of ≤1 hour and are commonly administered every 3-6 hours depending on the severity of the infection and the sensitivity of the pathogen. Medium half-life drugs usually have half-lives of 1-2 hours and are administered every 6-12 hours, most commonly every 8 hours. Long half-life drugs have half-lives >2 hours and are usually administered every 12-24 hours. Very long half-life drugs usually have half-lives >6-8 hours and can safely be administered every 24 hours in most cases. Amphotericin with a half-life of approximately 24 hours can be administered every other day.

*Postantibiotic effect is the effect of certain antibiotics that results in inhibition of bacterial growth for several hours *after* the antibiotic levels have fallen below the minimal inhibitory concentration.

†Chloramphenicol, clindamycin, and metronidazole all have half-lives >2 hours but traditionally have been administered at 6- to 8-hour intervals due to historical factors rather than pharmacokinetics.

IV, intravenous.

information regarding all commercially available antibiotics, including doses and dose ranges, pharmacokinetic data, sensitivity patterns, incompatibilities, and excretion data.

General Principles

Whichever antibiotics are employed, the goal of therapy is to achieve levels of antibiotic at the site of infection that exceed the minimum inhibitory concentration for the pathogens present. For mild infections, including most that can be handled on an outpatient basis, this may be achievable with oral antibiotics when appropriate choices are available. For severe surgical infections, however, the systemic response to infection may make gastrointestinal absorption of antibiotics unpredictable and thus antibiotic levels unreliable. In addition, for intra-abdominal infections, gastrointestinal function is often directly impaired. For this reason, most initial antibiotic therapy for surgical infections is begun intravenously.

Each patient with a serious infection should be evaluated daily or more frequently to assess response to treatment. If obvious improvement is not seen within 2 to 3 days, one often hears the question, "Which antibiotic should we add [switch] to?" That question is appropriate, however, only after the following question has been addressed: Why is the patient failing to improve? Likely answers include the following:

1. The initial operative procedure was not adequate.
2. The initial procedure was adequate but a complication has occurred.
3. A superinfection has developed at a new site.

4. The drug choice is correct, but not enough is being given.
5. Another or a different drug is needed.

The choice of antibiotics is not the most common cause for failure unless the original choice was clearly inappropriate, such as failing to provide coverage for anaerobes in an intra-abdominal infection.

As the patient improves, one must decide when to stop antibiotic therapy. For most surgical infections there is not a specific duration of antibiotics known to be ideal. Antibiotics generally support local host defenses until the local responses are sufficient to limit further infection. When an abscess is drained, the antibiotics prevent invasive bacterial infection in the fresh tissue planes opened in the course of drainage. After 3 to 5 days, the local responses of new capillary formation and inflammatory infiltrate provide a competent local defense. For deep-seated or poorly localized infections, longer treatment may be needed. A reliable guideline is to continue antibiotics until the patient has shown an obvious clinical improvement based on clinical examination and has had a normal temperature for 48 hours or more. Signs of improvement include improved mental status, return of bowel function, resolution of tachycardia, and spontaneous diuresis. A shorter course of antibiotics may be sufficient, but data supporting a specific duration are not available.

The recent availability of potent systemic antibiotics that can be given orally has led to some studies demonstrating that patients with intra-abdominal and other serious infections can be treated initially with parenteral antibiotics and then switched to oral antibiotics to complete their antibiotic course. This has the potential to reduce overall costs of antibiotic treatment, but it also has the risk to increase unnecessarily the duration of antibiotic treatment. Some physicians have succumbed to the temptation to send home patients with antibiotics by mouth because it is easy when previously the same patient would have been sent home without any antibiotics at all. This temptation should be resisted.

The white blood cell count may not have returned to normal when antibiotics are stopped. If the white blood cell count is normal, the likelihood of further infectious problems is small. If the white blood cell count is elevated, further infections may be detected but in most cases they will not be prevented by continuing antibiotics. Rather, a new infection requires drainage or different antibiotics for a new, resistant pathogen in a different location. In this case, the best approach is to stop the existing drugs and observe the patient closely for subsequent developments.

When choosing an antibiotic for empiric treatment, the following guidelines should be followed:

1. Coverage of the presumed microorganisms involved should be ensured. This usually means starting broad-spectrum antibiotics that can then be tailored and narrowed to the specific microorganism isolated. Anaerobic spectrum antibiotics should be avoided when possible since this group of bacteria plays an important role in maintaining the gastrointestinal tract microenvironment.

2. The antibiotic chosen should be able to reach the site of the infection. Specifically for UTI and for cholangitis, antibiotics with high renal and biliary concentrations, respectively, should be chosen. Skin, lungs, and central nervous system tissue concentration should also be considered for infections at these sites.

3. Toxicity should be considered, particularly in critically ill patients in which bioavailability and therapeutic and toxic level range are harder to predict. Once an antimicrobial with significant toxic side effects is started, blood levels and organ function should be closely monitored.

4. Whenever an infection that will need antibiotics is identified, these should be dosed aggressively. The volume of redistribution of these patients is unpredictable since they usually have aggressive fluid replacements as part of their support or resuscitation.

5. Whenever an antibiotic regimen is started, set a time limit for the period for which the antibiotic will be given.

Superinfection

A superinfection is a new infection that develops during antibiotic treatment for the original infection. Whenever antibiotics are used, they exert a selective pressure on the endogenous flora of the patient and on exogenous bacteria that colonize sites at risk. Bacteria that remain are resistant to the antibiotics being used and become the pathogens in superinfection. Respiratory tract infections are common superinfections that occur during the treatment of intra-abdominal infection. The greater the severity of the abdominal infection and the greater the risk of poor outcome, the greater the risk of pneumonia as well.

Careful surveillance of hospitalized patients reveals superinfections in 2% to 10% of antibiotic-treated patients, depending on the underlying risk factors. The best preventive action is to limit the dose and duration of antibiotic treatment to what is obviously required and to be alert to the possibility of superinfections. The use of increasingly powerful and broad-spectrum antibiotics during the past 2 decades has also led to an increasing incidence of fungal superinfections.

Antibiotic-associated colitis is another significant superinfection that can occur in hospitalized patients with mild to serious illness. This entity is caused by the enteric pathogen *C. difficile* and has been reported after treatment with every antibiotic except vancomycin. *C. difficile* colitis can vary from a mild, self-limited disease to a rapidly progressive septic process culminating in death. The most important step in treating this disease is to suspect it. Diagnosis is best accomplished by detecting *C. difficile* toxin in the stool. In severe cases, endoscopy, revealing the typical mucosal changes with inflammation, ulceration, and plaque formation can make a more rapid diagnosis of the severe form of the disease, pseudomembranous colitis. Treatment is supportive with fluid and electrolytes, withdrawal of the offending antibiotic if possible, and oral metronidazole to treat the superinfection. Vancomycin should be reserved for metronidazole failures. In rare instances when an overwhelming colitis does not respond to medical management, emergency colectomy may be required.

Antibiotic Resistance

Antibiotic resistance is an escalating problem presenting particularly in patients in ICUs. Its implications include increased length of stay, increased costs of care, and, more importantly, an increased morbidity and mortality derived from infections treated unsuccessfully.

Resistance has been broadly divided into two forms: (1) intrinsic resistance, in which a specific species is inherently resistant to a specific antibiotic (e.g., gram-negative bacteria to vancomycin) and (2) acquired resistance, in which a change of the genetic composition of the bacteria occurs. This acquired resistance can be the result of intrinsic changes within the native genetic material of the pathogen or can be transferred from another species.

The molecular mechanisms by which bacteria acquire resistance to antibiotics can be broadly classified into the following four categories[28]:

1. Decreased intracellular concentration of antibiotic, either by decreased influx or increased efflux— Most antibiotics are susceptible to this mechanism (*Pseudomonas*/Enterobacteriaceae to β-lactams).
2. Neutralization by inactivating enzymes—This is the most common mechanism of antibiotic resistance and affects all β-lactam antibiotics (e.g., β-lactamases from gram-positive and gram-negative bacteria).
3. Alteration of the target at which the antibiotic will act—It affects all antibiotics and is the main resistance mechanism for some specific bacteria (*Pneumococcus* to penicillin or MSRA to all β-lactam antibiotics).
4. Complete elimination of the target at which the antibiotic will act—Some specific bacteria develop the ability to create new metabolic pathways and completely eliminate a specific target (e.g., VRE).

Antibiotic resistance is usually achieved by the combination of these different mechanisms. However, the presence of one of them may confer resistance to one or more different groups of antibiotics.

The bacterial genome is divided into chromosomal DNA, which gives specific characteristics and metabolic pathways to the bacteria, and smaller, circular, and independent DNA elements (plasmids) that encode information for supplemental bacterial activities such as virulence factors and resistance mechanisms. Most resistance mechanisms are plasmid mediated, although they can interchange with chromosomal information (with the aid of transposons [mobile DNA elements]), conferring more fixed mechanisms that will be transmitted vertically. However, plasmids can also be transmitted horizontally through conjugation, transduction, and transformation processes in which different bacteria are exposed to a specific plasmid.

Risk factors for antibiotic resistance in a specific patient include use of antibiotics, prolonged hospital stays, use of broad-spectrum antibiotics, use of invasive devices (e.g.,

endotracheal tubes, central lines, Foley catheters) and the presence of outbreaks that may reflect ineffective infection control policies. The population at highest risk are ICU patients in which the potential absence of effective antibiotic treatments correlates with higher mortality rates.

Prevention strategies have been studied, and although it is difficult to establish a clear relation between their practice and decreased resistance, they should be part of a discipline that not only reduces the incidence of antibiotic resistance but also follows a logical practice for infection control and use of antibiotics. Some of these strategies include guidelines for use of antibiotics (hospital formulary restriction, use of narrow-spectrum antibiotics, antibiotic cycling, use of new antibiotics), assessment of infection risk and quantitative cultures, infectious disease specialists, and area-specific use of antibiotics (e.g., outpatients vs. nosocomial, hospital to hospital difference). Nonantibiotic strategies include prevention of nosocomial infections (general and specific measures) and prevention of hospital transmission (hand washing, contact precautions). The battle against antibiotic resistance is definitely multidisciplinary and involves the development of new antibiotics as well as strategies in the everyday care of patients from all the health care personnel.[28,29]

Specific Antimicrobials

Penicillins

The penicillins are broadly divided into those that are stable against staphylococcal penicillinase and all others. The antistaphylococcal penicillins are active against methicillin-susceptible staphylococcal species but have reduced activity against streptococcal species and essentially no activity against gram-negative rods or anaerobic bacteria. All the remaining penicillins are readily hydrolyzed by staphylococcal penicillinase and are therefore unreliable for treating staphylococcal infections. They all have excellent activity against other gram-positive cocci except for enterococci, which are variably resistant. The major difference among these penicillins is in their spectrum of aerobic and facultative gram-negative rod activity. The more advanced acylureido-penicillins are highly active against this group, including the *difficult* gram-negative rods.

Recently, various penicillins have been combined with one of the β-lactamase inhibitors, clavulanic acid, sulbactam, or tazobactam. These combinations provide antibiotic compounds that retain their broad gram-negative activity while also acting against methicillin-sensitive staphylococci and anaerobes, facultative species, and aerobic bacteria that are resistant to the penicillins by virtue of β-lactamase production. The β-lactamases produced by some *E. coli*, and by *Pseudomonas*, *Enterobacter*, *Citrobacter*, and *Serratia* species, however, are not susceptible to these inhibitors, so these organisms are not susceptible to antibiotic combinations that rely on β-lactamase inhibition unless they are susceptible to the antibiotic alone.

Cephalosporins

The cephalosporin class is the largest and most frequently used group of antibiotics. It is commonly divided into three *generations,* but there are also important differences between members within each generation. The first-generation cephalosporins have excellent activity against methicillin-susceptible staphylococci and all streptococcal species but not against enterococci. No cephalosporin in any generation has reliable activity against enterococci, and indeed many cephalosporins seem to encourage enterococcal overgrowth. The first-generation cephalosporins also have modest activity against the *easy* Enterobacteriaceae, such as *E. coli, Proteus mirabilis,* and many *Klebsiella* species. The only important difference between members of the first generation is in half-life. Cefazolin, with its longer half-life, can be given every 8 hours rather than every 4 to 6 hours and maintains more reliable serum and tissue levels when used for prophylaxis than do the other members of this class.

The second-generation cephalosporins have expanded gram-negative activity when compared with the first generation but still lack activity against many gram-negative rods. They can be used when susceptibility patterns are known or when community-acquired infections with a low probability of antibiotic-resistant bacteria are being treated. This class of antibiotics is not reliable for empiric treatment of hospital-acquired gram-negative rod infections. The most important distinction within the second generation is between those antibiotics with good activity against anaerobes (cefoxitin and cefotetan) and those without important anaerobic activity (cefamandole, ceforanide, and cefonicid). Within each of these groups are antibiotics with relatively short half-lives (cefamandole and cefoxitin) and with relatively long half-lives (cefotetan, ceforanide, and cefonicid).

The third-generation cephalosporins have greatly expanded activity against gram-negative rods, including many resistant strains, and rival the aminoglycosides in their coverage while having a much more favorable safety profile. In exchange for this gram-negative coverage, most members of this group have significantly less activity against staphylococci and streptococcal species than first- and second-generation cephalosporins. Anaerobic coverage is, generally, rather poor as well. The important distinction in the third-generation cephalosporins is between those with significant activity against *Pseudomonas* species (cefoperazone, ceftazidime, and cefepime) and those without (cefotaxime, ceftizoxime, and ceftriaxone). The use of third-generation cephalosporins has been associated with an increased incidence of VRE in critically ill patients. Their use against specific gram-negative rods has also been shown to promote the release of endotoxin and increase the concentration of tumor necrosis factor, which is related with a "septic response" after the antibiotic has been given. These are disadvantages that are becoming more important and that could potentially be avoided with the use of different kinds of antibiotics that have a similar or even broader spectrum and is something worth considering once an antibiotic is going to be chosen.

Monobactams

Aztreonam is the only currently available member of the class of monobactams. It has gram-negative coverage, including many *Pseudomonas* species, similar to the aminoglycosides, and like the aminoglycosides lacks significant activity against gram-positive cocci and anaerobes. It also lacks activity against most *Acinetobacter* species. It has the safety profile of other β-lactam antibiotics but does not cross-react in patients who are allergic to penicillins or cephalosporins.

Carbapenems

Imipenem and meropenem are the first representatives of the class of carbapenems. They have a very broad spectrum of antibacterial activity with excellent activity against all gram-positive cocci except for MRSA and only modest activity against enterococci. They are quite active against all anaerobic bacteria, with broad activity against gram-negative rods, including most *Pseudomonas* species, but are inactive against *Pseudomonas cepacia* and *S. maltophilia,* and strains of indole-positive *Proteus* are often resistant. As with all other antibiotics, *Pseudomonas* species have an unfortunate propensity to develop resistance during treatment. Imipenem is provided only in combination with the enzyme inhibitor cilastatin, which prevents its hydrolysis in the kidneys and resultant nephrotoxicity. Meropenem is given without a renal enzyme inhibitor. More recently ertapenem, a newer carbapenem, has become available. It differs from its predecessors in that it only has to be given once a day since it has a longer half-life. It does not require cilastatin since it is resistant to hydrolysis in the kidneys, and its spectrum seems to be better against most enterobacteria but less active than imipenem against some gram-positive cocci and *Pseudomonas* and *Acinetobacter* species.

Quinolones

In recent years a large number of new fluoroquinolone antibiotics have been developed, with six currently available. The currently available members of this class are norfloxacin, which has useful levels only in the urine, and ciprofloxacin, ofloxacin, levofloxacin, gatifloxacin and moxifloxacin, which are effective against sensitive pathogens throughout the body. As a class, the fluoroquinolones are marked by extremely broad activity against gram-negative rods, including many *Pseudomonas* species. Most also have relatively broad activity against gram-positive cocci, including some MRSAs, although there is insufficient clinical information to recommend their routine use against MSRA. Activity against anaerobes is poor for all fluoroquinolones except moxifloxacin, which has good activity in this area, as well as against gram-positive cocci (better than other quinolones), although its spectrum against some Enterobacteriaceae and *Pseudomonas* species may be reduced compared to ciprofloxacin. The fluoroquinolones other than norfloxacin are distinguished by excellent tissue penetration and comparable serum and tissue levels with either intravenous or oral administration. Heavy use of quinolones has led to increasing levels of quinolone-resistant pathogens.

Aminoglycosides

For many years the aminoglycoside class of antibiotics was the only reliable class of drugs for the empiric treatment of serious gram-negative infections. The availability of third-generation cephalosporins, advanced-generation penicillins, monobactams, carbapenems, and now fluoroquinolones has greatly reduced the instances when aminoglycosides must be used. As a class, aminoglycosides have very broad activity against aerobic and facultative gram-negative rods. They have relatively indifferent activity against gram-positive cocci but are an important component of synergistic therapy against enterococci when combined with a penicillin or vancomycin. Aminoglycosides have no activity against anaerobes or against facultative bacteria in an anaerobic environment.

Clinically, aminoglycosides are difficult to use because the ratio of therapeutic levels to toxic levels is low, approximately 2:3. The primary toxicities are nephrotoxicity and 8th cranial nerve damage, both auditory and vestibular. Aminoglycosides distribute in interstitial fluid, a body compartment that varies significantly with disease and is greatly enlarged in patients with life-threatening infections. Therefore, aminoglycoside doses and intervals of administration need to be tailored to the individual patient, and the results must be confirmed by determination of serum levels. No nomogram or dosing scheme has been sufficiently reliable to recommend without this testing. In routine clinical practice it has been far more common to find inadequate levels of aminoglycosides than toxic levels. Because of these difficulties, many clinicians now reserve aminoglycosides for specific therapy for known resistant organisms or as part of a synergistic combination to treat serious enterococcal infections or certain gram-negative rod infections. More recent data suggest that once-daily administration of aminoglycosides is as effective as the more traditional twice- or three-times-per-day administration and is less toxic.

Antianaerobes

The antibiotics with important antianaerobic activity are not logically grouped except by this characteristic. The oldest effective antianaerobic drug is chloramphenicol. It is still highly active against most anaerobic pathogens by in vitro testing but is uncommonly used because of its potential for bone marrow toxicity. Clindamycin possesses activity against most anaerobic bacteria as well as most gram-positive bacteria. Its complete lack of activity against gram-negative aerobic and facultative rods means that it must be used in combination with another antibiotic to cover the pathogens that commonly accompany anaerobes in clinical infections. Its spectrum against *Bacteroides* species is not as good as metronidazole. In animal models clindamycin improves the outcome of infections caused by toxin-producing clostridia, streptococci, or staphylococci, presumably by inhibiting the production and release of exotoxins.

Metronidazole currently possesses the most complete activity against all anaerobic pathogens. However, it has no activity against any aerobic or facultative pathogens, either gram negative or gram positive, so it must always be combined with another antibiotic for complete coverage. Because it has no activity against the gram-positive cocci, as clindamycin does, its combination with aztreonam in the treatment of mixed aerobic and anaerobic infections leaves this potentially important group of pathogens uncovered. For this reason, metronidazole is theoretically better combined with a third-generation cephalosporin or a fluoroquinolone. Metronidazole is active against *C. difficile*. Other antibiotics with important antianaerobic activity, including cefoxitin, cefotetan, the penicillin–β-lactamase inhibitor combinations, the carbapenems, and moxifloxacin, are discussed elsewhere.

Macrolides

Erythromycin is a macrolide antibiotic with only modest antianaerobic activity in the concentrations that can be achieved systemically. It has found widespread use, however, as an oral agent (erythromycin base) used in combination with an aminoglycoside to reduce numbers of bacteria in the lumen of the bowel before operations on the colon. In the concentrations achieved within the lumen of the colon, it markedly suppresses anaerobic growth. Erythromycin is also active against many gram-positive cocci and *Neisseria* species. For this reason it is sometimes used as an alternate agent for patients allergic to penicillins. In addition, it has significant activity against mycoplasmas, *Chlamydia*, *Legionella* species, and *Rickettsia*. It is also an effective antibiotic against *Campylobacter jejuni*. Clarithromycin and azithromycin are two more recent macrolides with expanded antimicrobial spectra that are available only in oral formulations.

Tetracyclines

Tetracyclines previously were an important class of antibiotics with significant antianaerobic activity. In addition to activity against anaerobes, tetracyclines possess modest activity against easy gram-negative rods and many gram-positive cocci. Currently other agents are preferable as first and second choices for most surgical infections.

Glycopeptides

Vancomycin is the only glycopeptide antibiotic available in the United States, whereas teicoplanin is also available in Europe. It is active against essentially all gram-positive cocci, especially the MRSA, for which it is one of only three reliable antibiotics. It also has moderate activity against enterococci. Vancomycin is active against most *Clostridium* species, especially *C. difficile*, the primary pathogen responsible for antibiotic-associated diarrhea. However, it should not be used as a first-line agent against *C. difficile* diarrhea, owing to the risk that this will increase the incidence of vancomycin-resistant enterococci. Several new glycopeptide antibiotics are in development, and some of these may be effective against vancomycin-resistant enterococci and staphylococci.

Streptogramins

The first water-soluble streptogramin antibiotic is actually a combination, quinupristin/dalfopristin. It is active against nearly all gram-positive pathogens, including vancomycin-resistant *Enterococcus faecium* (but not *Enterococcus faecalis*), multidrug-resistant *S. aureus*, and penicillin-resistant *S. pneumoniae*.

Oxazolidinones

The first representative of the class, oxazolidinone, is linezolid. This drug is also active against nearly all gram-positive bacteria, including VRE and vancomycin-intermediate *S. aureus*. Linezolid is also quite active against many anaerobic bacterial species. It is available in both parenteral and oral forms.

Antifungals

Triazoles are a type of antifungal that acts on cell wall function through inhibition of the cytochrome P-450–dependent ergosterol synthesis. Fluconazole is the triazole most commonly used in surgical patients. It has a good spectrum against *Cryptococcus* and most *Candida* species, although *C. krusei* and other subtypes have been reported as resistant to this drug. Its use in surgical patients includes treatment of systemic *Candida* infection as well as prophylaxis in high-risk patients. Voriconazole is a newly developed triazole with a broader spectrum than fluconazole. It has excellent activity against all *Candida* species, including *C. krusei, C. glabrata, C. tropicalis,* and *C. parapsilosis,* which often have significant resistance against fluconazole. This new antifungal has enabled appropriate treatment of some lethal fungal infections without the toxicity of amphotericin B. It also has very good activity against *Aspergillus* infections. Both of these triazoles are available in oral and parenteral preparations.

Amphotericin B is a polyene antifungal with broad activity but significant toxicity. It acts by binding to the sterols of the cell wall and interfering with membrane permeability. It has been used traditionally for the treatment of lethal infections only (given its toxicity), usually secondary to *Candida, Aspergillus,* and *Histoplasma*.

Caspofungin is an echinocandin derivative, systemic antifungal agent. It acts by inhibiting β-glucan synthase and thus disrupting the integrity of the cell wall causing cell lysis. It is indicated in the treatment of refractory systemic fungal infections caused by *Aspergillus* and *Candida*.

Selected References

Fry DE (ed): Surgical Infections. Boston, Little, Brown, 1995.

This is a complete textbook devoted to surgical infections—their prevention, diagnosis, and treatment. It is comprehensive, well written, and an invaluable resource for more detailed information regarding surgical infections.

Gilbert DN, Moellering RC, Sande MA: The Sanford Guide to Antimicrobial Therapy. Hyde Park, VT, Antimicrobial Therapy, 2003.

This handy guide to indications and doses of all available antimicrobial agents is updated every year. It comes in pocket-sized text or can be downloaded to personal digital assistants. It tends to be more up to date on doses and new indications than a regular textbook.

Gorbach SL, Bartlett JG, Blacklow NR, et al (eds): Infectious Diseases. Philadelphia, WB Saunders, 1998.

This is a comprehensive textbook of infectious diseases with specific chapters devoted to surgical site infections and to the evaluation of postoperative fever. It also has more extensive information regarding specific pathogens and specific antimicrobial drugs.

Wilmore DE, Cheung LY, Harken AH, et al (eds): American College of Surgeons Surgery. New York, WebMD Corporation, 2002.

This is a comprehensive, on-line, frequently updated surgical textbook emphasizing the perioperative care of the surgical patient. It has an entire section with multiple chapters devoted to all aspects of surgical infection.

References

1. Horan TC, Gaynes RP, Martone WJ, et al: CDC definitions of nosocomial surgical site infections, 1992: A modification of CDC definitions of surgical wound infections. Infect Control Hosp Epidemiol 13:606-608, 1992.
2. Culver DH, Horan TC, Gaynes RP, et al: Surgical wound infection rates by wound class, operative procedure, and patient risk index: National Nosocomial Infections Surveillance System. Am J Med 91:152S-157S, 1991.
3. Cruse PJE, Foord R: The epidemiology of wound infection: A 10-year prospective study of 62,939 wounds. Surg Clin North Am 60:27-40, 1980.
4. Haley RW, Culver DH, Morgan WM, et al: Identifying patients at high risk of surgical wound infection: A simple multivariate index of patient susceptibility and wound contamination. Am J Epidemiol 121:206-215, 1985.
5. Alexander JW, Fischer JE, Boyajian M, et al: The influence of hair-removal methods on wound infections. Arch Surg 118:347-352, 1983.
6. Melling AC, Ali B, Scott EM, et al: Effects of preoperative warming on the incidence of wound infection after clean surgery: A randomised controlled trial. Lancet 358:876-880, 2001.
7. Kurz A, Sessler DI, Lenhardt R: Perioperative normothermia to reduce the incidence of surgical-wound infection and shorten hospitalization: Study of Wound Infection and Temperature Group. N Engl J Med 334:1209-1215, 1996.
8. Greif R, Akca O, Horn EP, et al: Supplemental perioperative oxygen to reduce the incidence of surgical-wound infection. Outcomes Research Group. N Engl J Med 342:161-167, 2000.
9. van den Berghe G, Wouters P, Weekers F, et al: Intensive insulin therapy in the critically ill patients. N Engl J Med 345:1359-1367, 2001.
10. Emori TG, Culver DH, Horan TC, et al: National nosocomial infections surveillance system (NNIS): Description of surveillance methods. Am J Infect Control 19:19-35, 1991.

11. Haley RW, Culver DH, White JW, et al: The efficacy of infection surveillance and control programs in preventing nosocomial infections in U.S. hospitals. Am J Epidemiol 121:182-205, 1985.

12. Olson M, O'Connor M, Schwartz ML: Surgical wound infections: A 5-year prospective study of 20,193 wounds at the Minneapolis VA Medical Center. Ann Surg 199:253-259, 1984.

13. SHEA, APIC, CDC, SIS: Consensus paper on the surveillance of surgical wound infections. Infect Control Hosp Epidemiol 13:599-605, 1992.

14. Mangram AJ, Horan TC, Pearson ML, et al: Guideline for prevention of surgical site infection, 1999. Centers for Disease Control and Prevention (CDC) Hospital Infection Control Practices Advisory Committee. Am J Infect Control 27:97-132; quiz 133-134; discussion 196, 1999.

15. Quebbeman EJ, Telford GL, Wadsworth K, et al: Double-gloving: Protecting surgeons from blood contamination in the operating room. Arch Surg 127:213-216; discussion 216-217, 1992.

16. Dellinger EP, Gross PA, Barrett TL, et al: Quality standard for antimicrobial prophylaxis in surgical procedures. Infectious Diseases Society of America. Clin Infect Dis 18:422-427, 1994.

17. Platt R, Zaleznik DF, Hopkins CC, et al: Perioperative antibiotic prophylaxis for herniorrhaphy and breast surgery. N Engl J Med 322:153-160, 1990.

18. Page CP, Bohnen JM, Fletcher JR, et al: Antimicrobial prophylaxis for surgical wounds: Guidelines for clinical care. Arch Surg 128:79-88, 1993.

19. Clarke JS, Condon RE, Bartlett JG, et al: Preoperative oral antibiotics reduce septic complications of colon operations: Results of prospective, randomized, double-blind clinical study. Ann Surg 186:251-259, 1977.

20. Dellinger EP, Ehrenkranz NJ: Surgical infections. *In* Bennett JV, Brachman PS (eds): Hospital Infections, 4th ed. Philadelphia, Lippincott-Raven, 1998, pp 571-585.

21. Christou NV, Barie PS, Dellinger EP, et al: Surgical Infection Society Intra-abdominal Infection Study: Prospective evaluation of management techniques and outcome. Arch Surg 128:193-198; discussion 198-199, 1993.

22. Mazuski JE: The Surgical Infection Society guidelines on antimicrobial therapy for intra-abdominal infections: Evidence for the recommendations. Surg Infect (Larchmt) 3:175-233, 2002.

23. Mazuski JE, Sawyer RG, Nathens AB, et al: The Surgical Infection Society guidelines on antimicrobial therapy for intra-abdominal infections: An executive summary. Surg Infect (Larchmt) 3:161-173, 2002.

24. Koperna T, Schulz F: Relaparotomy in peritonitis: Prognosis and treatment of patients with persisting intra-abdominal infection. World J Surg 24:32-37, 2000.

25. Seiler CA, Brugger L, Forssmann U, et al: Conservative surgical treatment of diffuse peritonitis. Surgery 127:178-184, 2000.

26. Levison MA: Percutaneous versus open operative drainage of intra-abdominal abscesses. Infect Dis Clin North Am 6:525-544, 1992.

27. Dellinger EP: Approach to the patient with postoperative fever. *In* Gorbach S, Bartlett J, Blacklow N (eds): Infectious Diseases in Medicine and Surgery. Philadelphia, WB Saunders, 1998, pp 903-909.

28. Kaye KS, Fraimow HS, Abrutyn E: Pathogens resistant to antimicrobial agents: Epidemiology, molecular mechanisms, and clinical management. Infect Dis Clin North Am 14:293-319, 2000.

29. Kollef MH, Fraser VJ: Antibiotic resistance in the intensive care unit. Ann Intern Med 134:298-314, 2001.

SURGICAL PROBLEMS IN THE IMMUNOSUPPRESSED PATIENT

Donald E. Fry, M.D.

Clinical Immunosuppression	Acquired Immunosuppression
Primary Immunosuppression	

The scope of surgical care over recent decades has continued to expand. A multitude of different diseases is managed surgically, but the expanded scope of care has also encompassed an ever larger population of patients with underlying biologic conditions that render the host response inadequate. The immunosuppressed patient from numerous different causations may present with special surgical problems. Immunosuppression may be the result of specific treatments to avoid rejection of transplanted organs. Corticosteroid treatment with the specific goals of managing a patient's inflammatory condition (e.g., rheumatoid arthritis, inflammatory bowel disease) may have adverse systemic anti-inflammatory consequences that lead to delayed or obscure presentations of many surgical disease processes. Acquired immunocompromise may attend burns, trauma, protein-calorie malnutrition, and critical illness itself, which leads to a number of clinical complications following operation. The clinical reality of the new millennium in surgery is that an older, more complex patient population with fundamental compromise of host responsiveness will constitute a larger percentage of the overall patients seen and procedures that will be performed.

CLINICAL IMMUNOSUPPRESSION

The complex processes involved in host responsiveness and the human immune response are beyond the scope of this presentation and are covered elsewhere (see Chapter 24). A simplified view of the host response consists of the nonspecific and primitive inflammatory response, which has a "first responder" role for injury and potential infection, and is then followed by the process of specific immunity. Inflammation has an initial vasoactive phase, which is characterized by vasodilation, changes in vascular permeability, and edema. A second phagocytic phase of inflammation results in infiltration of the contaminated or injured area with neutrophils and monocytes. Neutrophils function to eradicate foreign proteins and microbes, whereas monocytes/macrophages orchestrate the intensity of the inflammatory response and initiate the process of specific immunity. Antigen processing and presentation by the monocyte begin specific immunity leading to differentiation of lymphocyte populations by both humeral and cell-mediated pathways.

The vast number of processes in the nonspecific and specific pathways of host defense can be studied by an array of intricate and sophisticated biologic methods. Specific rates of neutrophil chemotaxis, efficiency of antigen processing by monocytes, and lymphoproliferative responses can be defined in considerable analytical detail. Where specific therapy is available to combat specific defects in host responsiveness, then detailed definition of specific abnormalities would be a sound approach for the proven or suspected immunosuppressed patient. In reality, immunosuppression or compromise is suspected by any of a number of surrogate markers, and the surgeon proceeds with clinical management armed with the knowledge that specific patients pose special problems in diagnosis and management.

Surrogate markers of host and immune responsiveness may be as simple as measurement of the white blood cell (WBC) count, although this determination is quite insensitive and nonspecific. Profound leukopenia (WBC count <1000 cells/mm^3) would certainly have a high association with host compromise. Absolute lymphocyte counts are perhaps a more specific measure of immune compromise.[1] Delayed-type hypersensitivity skin test responses have certainly been used as a global marker of immune suppression but have limited clinical utility[2] and are infrequently done outside of a research setting. Albumin, prealbumin, and other short half-life serum proteins are indicators of nutritional insufficiency and as such are markers of host responsiveness.[3] These parameters are most commonly used as indications of the effectiveness of nutritional support (see Chapter 6) but are also considered barometers of current immunoresponsiveness.

Problems of immunosuppression may be assumed to exist by elements of the patient's history. Current or chronic steroid therapy or an immunosuppressive regimen that is taken by a patient to avoid organ rejection is certainly strong evidence for the clinician to presume that immune compromise exists. Human immunodeficiency virus (HIV) infection should be documented.

Finally, the identification of specific pathogens may be strong evidence that host responsiveness is impaired. Bacterial infections with organisms that have low virulence profiles, such as *Enterococcus* species and *Staphylococcus epidermidis*, are clinical evidence that efficient host defenses are not operational. Acute fungal infections with *Candida* species are not seen in a normal host. Atypical mycobacterial infections mean abnormalities in cellular immunity. Cytomegalovirus (CMV) infection, *Pneumocystis* infection, *Mucor* infection, and many other unusual infections mean that the host is compromised and that the clinician must be sensitive to the alterations in clinical presentation and recognition that will occur with other clinical problems in these patients.

In most situations, the state of "immunosuppression" and "immunocompromise" in the surgical patient is not objectively determined but are intuitive determinations. Understanding that immunosuppression is present arms the clinician with the special expectations that common diseases will present in uncommon ways and that uncommon illnesses will present more commonly.

PRIMARY IMMUNOSUPPRESSION

Primary immunosuppression refers to those groups of clinical conditions where the patient has a genetically predetermined abnormality in host responsiveness. There are large arrays of primary immunosuppressive illnesses that are seen very uncommonly. A detailed and more complex organization of the primary immunodeficiency states is presented elsewhere,[4] but it is important to have a brief familiarity with the scope of these illnesses (Table 13-1).

Defects of the primary inflammatory response result in a host that is extraordinarily susceptible to common bacterial infections. Complement deficiency states of any of a number of specific complement proteins means that chemotactic and opsonic functions of the complement cascade are deficient.[5] An allied series of deficiency syndromes to complement deficiency states are losses of regulatory proteins that coordinate and control complement function. These would include losses of C1 inhibitor or C3 inactivator functions.[6]

Specific neutrophil defects are well recognized. Alterations of chemotaxis and neutrophil motility are rarely recognized and are generally diagnosed in patients with increased rates of cutaneous infection following seemingly trivial injury. Impaired mechanisms of intracellular killing activity are best exemplified in the occasional patient seen with chronic granulomatosis disease,[7]

TABLE 13-1. General Categories of Primary Immunodeficiency States*

Host Defense Component	Specific Defect
PRIMARY INFLAMMATION	
Coagulation abnormalities	Congenital decrease in factor XII
Platelets	Congenital amegakaryocytic thrombocytopenia
Complement proteins	Specific protein component deficiencies
Contact activating system (bradykinin production)	Kininogen deficiency state
PHAGOCYTIC PHASE OF INFLAMMATION	
Neutrophils	Defective chemotaxis, mobility, microbicidal activity
Monocytes	Impaired mobility, generalized dysfunction
T-CELL DEFECTS	
Severe combined deficiency states	Reduced T cells and reduced antibody production
Thymoma/hypoplasia of thymus	T-cell deficiency state
B-CELL DEFECTS	
Congenital agammaglobulinemia	Reduction in all immunoglobulin classes
Specific subclass deficiencies	Selective deficiency of IgG, IgA, or IgM

*These abnormalities affect the initiator events of inflammation, inflammatory cell function, and specific T-cell/B-cell functions.

myeloperoxidase deficiency,[8] or Chédiak-Higashi syndrome.[9] All abnormalities of human inflammation are clearly recognized by increased rates of infection with common bacterial species (e.g., *Staphylococcus aureus*).

Abnormalities of cellular immunity are identified with increased rates of infection with uncommon pathogens but are also associated with increased rates of specific malignancies. Many of these T-cell abnormalities are associated with thymic abnormalities of hypoplasia of the thymus or with thymoma.[10] Dysfunction or absent T cells are the basis for the diagnosis. Chronic mucocutaneous candidiasis is a syndrome with sustained and recurrent infections with candidiasis species,[11] whereas the Wiskott-Aldrich syndrome patients have nearly a uniform development of malignancies by 30 years of age.[12]

Altered humoral immunity syndrome results from impaired maturation of B cells caused by specific deficiency states in the production of one or more immunoglobulins.[13] These patients have chronic and recurrent pulmonary infections; lymphomas and gastrointestinal malignancies are seen with increased frequency in this group of patients.

ACQUIRED IMMUNOSUPPRESSION

As noted in the prior discussion, a small number of patients are affected with primary immunosuppressive states. Most problems of immunosuppression are consequences of acquired illnesses that have compromised host defenses as a result.

Human Immunodeficiency Virus Infection

Infections with HIV leading to acquired immune deficiency syndrome (AIDS) have been the focus of considerable academic attention during the past 20 years. This infection is an indolent process that potentially requires a full decade, even in the untreated patient, from the time of acute infection before immunosuppression becomes clinically significant.[14] Surgical problems in the HIV patient include abnormal presentation of common illnesses but also include unique problems that are consequences of the acquired immunosuppression.

Pathogenesis

HIV is a blood-borne infection that is transmitted to the susceptible host after percutaneous or a mucus membrane exposure to infected blood or body fluids.[15] The virus attaches to specific receptors on the host CD4 lymphocytes. The virus is internalized with release of the viral RNA. The unique enzyme, reverse transcriptase, of the virus then results in the synthesis of complementary copies of DNA to the RNA template of the virus (cDNA). This cDNA then migrates into the nucleus of the infected cell, is incorporated into the chromosomal configuration of the host cell, and then initiates the synthesis of new viral particles. The viral burden within the infected cell reaches a critical level with lysis of the infected cell and release of viral particles to infect other cells. The result of this process over time is the systematic depletion of CD4 depressor cells with dominance of the CD8 cells and subsequent immunosuppression of the host.

The natural history of HIV infection passes through four phases. First there is the acute viral infection, which includes fever, malaise, pharyngitis, and other symptoms that would be nonspecific features of many viral infections.[16] Second, there is a sustained period of asymptomatic disease. It is during this asymptomatic disease period that active viral replication is occurring in a slow but progressive fashion, which slowly progresses to a state with significant reduction in CD4 cell counts.[17] This indolent second phase is highly variable in different patients and for many patients evolves over a decade or longer. A third phase, which was formerly referred to as AIDS-related complex, represents the first evidence of symptomatic AIDS. The patients present with evidence of regional adenopathy. During this early symptomatic period, the viral load in the patient is increasing and the CD4 count is progressively declining. Clinical AIDS is considered to exist when the patient has an indicator condition (Box 13-1) or has a CD4 count lower than 200.[18] The indicator conditions may present as problems requiring surgical care, or conventional illnesses may present with

---

Box 13-1. Clinical Conditions that Fulfill the Revised Case Definition of Clinical AIDS Diagnosis[18]

Any one of the following combined with a positive HIV serology:

- Candidiasis of the upper aerodigestive tract (e.g., esophagitis, lungs)
- Invasive cervical cancer
- Extrapulmonary coccidioidomycosis
- Extrapulmonary cryptococcosis
- Cryptosporidiosis
- Extralymphatic cytomegalovirus infection (e.g., non-lymph nodes, non-spleen or liver)
- Herpes simplex pneumonia or esophagitis
- Extrapulmonary histoplasmosis
- HIV-associated wasting or dementia
- Isosporiasis infection
- Kaposi's sarcoma
- Primary central nervous system lymphoma
- Any non-Hodgkin's or B-cell, or undifferentiated type of lymphoma
- Disseminated tuberculosis or atypical *Mycobacterium* infection
- Nocardiosis
- *Pneumocystis carinii* infection
- Progressive multifocal leukoencephalopathy
- *Salmonella* septicemia
- Extraintestinal *Strongyloides* infection
- Toxoplasmosis

an obscure presentation because of the patient's immuno-suppressed state, or conventional illnesses may be mistaken for nonsurgical illnesses associated with the primary HIV infection.

Acute Abdomen

The AIDS patient has an increased frequency of the clinical acute abdominal pain syndrome than does the age-matched non-AIDS population. AIDS patients undergo abdominal exploration for a host of different reasons. It is likely that AIDS patients actually have an increased rate of emergency abdominal procedures because they have the anticipated rates of operation for commonly seen indications (e.g., appendicitis) but have indications in addition to those that are specific for this disease. An increased probability of abdominal operation but also increased nonsurgical causes for abdominal pain means that a discriminating evaluation of these patients is always necessary.

Acute appendicitis in the AIDS patient occurs due to the conventional occlusion of the appendiceal orifice by a fecalith[19] but also due to occlusion of the orifice by Kaposi's sarcoma lesions[20] and acute CMV infections.[21] Accumulated appendicitis cases in aged patients indicate that 30% are caused by complications of AIDS-related conditions. Clinical presentation for the AIDS patient with appendicitis is with characteristic right lower pain but is commonly associated with normal WBC counts in most patients. Most have fever, but fever and nonspecific abdominal pain alone are common findings among AIDS patients without surgical illness. Although there is no clear definition in the published literature, there appears to be an increased rate of perforation, gangrenous appendicitis, and initial appendiceal abscess among AIDS patients. Delay in patient presentation because of frequent abdominal pain and fever, and delay by the physician because of the numerous nonsurgical causes of abdominal pain, may account for this apparent observation.

Perforation of the gastrointestinal tract not related to appendicitis is certainly increased in the AIDS patient. The mean age of the clinical onset of AIDS is in the late 30s. Other than appendicitis, this age group infrequently has a perforated viscus. AIDS patients have perforation of the gastroduodenum, small bowel, and colon due to CMV infection in particular.[22] The terminal ilium and colon are most common sites for CMV perforations. The diagnosis of CMV perforations is confirmed by identification of the intranuclear inclusion bodies on biopsy specimens from sites of perforation. Appropriate surgical management of the site of perforation requires suture plication of gastroduodenal perforations, resection and anastomosis of small bowel perforations, and colostomy for colonic perforations. Acute antiviral chemotherapy is initiated. CMV perforation is an indicator of advanced HIV disease and carries a grave prognosis owing to death from peritonitis or other AIDS-related complications.

Kaposi's sarcoma,[23] gastrointestinal lymphoma,[24] and severe ileocolitis from *Mycobacterium avium intracellulare*[25] are additional causes of AIDS-related perforations of the gastrointestinal tract. Biopsies of the site of perforation at operation are necessary to establish causation. Man-

agement of the perforated site is the same as for any other perforation due to infectious causes.

Gastrointestinal obstruction is seen secondary to AIDS-related disease.[26,27] Causes include gastric outlet obstruction secondary to lymphoma, small bowel obstruction due to mycobacterial disease, intussusception secondary to Kaposi's sarcoma, and an Ogilvie-like syndrome progressing to toxic megacolon due to CMV infection. The diagnosis of the AIDS-related events needs to be differentiated for more conventional causes of obstruction. In the usual age group for AIDS patients, particularly when prior abdominal operation and the risk of adhesions are not present, most intestinal obstruction events are AIDS related.

Gastrointestinal bleeding is similarly seen by the same array of disease processes that are responsible for perforation and obstruction. When bleeding arises from the gastroduodenum or colon, endoscopy procedures will assist diagnosis. Operation is required only when medical measures to control hemorrhage have failed.

Hepatobiliary Disease

Hepatobiliary disease is common in the HIV-infected patient. Chronic hepatitis B and C infections share common routes of transmission with HIV disease. Persistent elevation of hepatic enzymes from chronic hepatitis is common with cirrhosis as a frequent result. Once clinical AIDS has evolved, infection of the liver parenchyma from *Candida albicans* and *M. avium intracellulare* result in small hepatic abscesses, which may require liver biopsy for diagnosis. Although infections with *Entamoeba histolytica* among the male homosexual population with AIDS are common, amebic abscess is much less common.

A particularly interesting but infrequent infectious problem is AIDS-associated cholangiopathy.[28] This appears to be the consequence of infection of the actual bile ducts themselves with opportunistic pathogens including *Cryptosporidium* species, CMV, and *Microsporidia*. Inflammatory changes secondary to invasion of the ducts result in a sclerosis-like picture. The patients have new-onset right upper quadrant pain, fever, alkaline phosphatase elevations, but rarely jaundice, at the time of initial presentation. Jaundice becomes more of a feature of the disease as the process advances over time. Diagnosis is suggested by ultrasound demonstration of thickened ducts. Endoscopic retrograde cholangiopancreatography is used to culture the bile or obtain biopsies of the bile ducts. Specific antimicrobial chemotherapy is used for treatment. Surgical care for these patients is limited. An occasional patient may develop acute cholecystitis secondary to cystic duct occlusion. Radionuclide scans are used for diagnosis, and cholecystectomy may be necessary in the patient with acute cholecystitis.

Splenomegaly

Splenomegaly is a common finding among AIDS patients but may be the result of multiple causes.[29] Patients may have portal hypertension from severe liver disease or portal fibrosis. Parenchymal infection of the spleen may be secondary to CMV, *Microbacterium*, *Pneumocystis carinii*, and other pathogens. Splenic enlargement may be secondary to lymphoma or Kaposi's sarcoma. The patients commonly have left upper quadrant pain and the spleen is palpable and quite tender on physical examination. Splenectomy may infrequently be necessary secondary to spontaneous rupture or to rupture from incidental trauma.

Vascular Disease

Vascular infections are reported among AIDS patients. Some infected pseudoaneurysms are seen among the intravenous drug abuse population with common bacteria (e.g., *S. aureus*).[30] These infections among the AIDS population are difficult to eradicate. Perhaps more interesting and somewhat unique to the AIDS patient is *Salmonella* arteritis.[31] AIDS patients have a high incidence of *Salmonella* infection. Apparently *Salmonella* has a particular affinity for atherosclerotic plaque. Adherence of the microbe to an atheroma of the distal aorta or iliac arteries can result in invasive infection, pseudoaneurysm formation, and potential rupture. Surgical management prior to rupture is desired. Reconstruction of these patients following resection proceeds along guidelines for management of any mycotic aneurysm infection.

Neoplasms

B-cell lymphoma occurs commonly among AIDS patients.[32] These malignancies are commonly undifferentiated and aggressive. Operative intervention for the lymphoma patient is for the purpose of diagnosis of the disease (e.g., needle biopsy). More commonly surgical intervention is for the management of complications secondary to bleeding, obstruction, or perforation of the gastrointestinal tract. Primary management of the lymphoma disease is medical.

Kaposi's sarcoma is a neoplasm of the skin that was uncommon until the AIDS epidemic. Kaposi's sarcoma is the result of the patient having chronic infection with human herpesvirus-8,[33] but clinical disease occurs only when the patient's clinical immunosuppression reaches an advanced stage. Kaposi's sarcoma in the AIDS patients occurs at numerous different sites, including skin, gastrointestinal tract, lung, liver, and even the heart.[34] Surgical involvement is primarily for diagnosis and the management of complications, particularly in the gastrointestinal tract. As noted earlier, perforation, bleeding, and small bowel intussusception are noted gastrointestinal complications from Kaposi's sarcoma. Radiation and chemotherapy are the primary treatment modalities for this neoplasm.

Anorectal Disease

The immunosuppressed AIDS patient is at increased risk for human papillomavirus infection. Large condylomata acuminata are the result.[35] Very large condylomata commonly need to be surgically reduced to be followed by local topical therapy. Squamous cell carcinoma of the anus occurs with increased frequency presumably due to the role of papillomavirus in causing this disease.[36]

Occupational Risk of Infection

A major surgical concern about the HIV-infected patient was the potential of infection being occupationally acquired during the course of providing surgical care for these patients. Surgical exposure to patient blood during the performance of operative procedures has been well documented. With the knowledge that HIV is a blood-borne pathogen and that other blood-borne pathogens (e.g., hepatitis B) have been documented to be transmitted in the operating room, many surgeons have been concerned about this risk.

At this time it can be said that the risk of occupational transmission of HIV disease is low, but it is not zero. As of the last available Centers for Disease Control and Prevention report, 57 documented cases of occupational transmission of HIV have occurred and 138 cases of probable transmission among health care workers have been identified. No documented cases have been seen in surgeons (Table 13-2).[37] Most occupational infections have come from major percutaneous injuries from hollow needles. Solid-needle injuries have not been documented to occur in the United States. Current rates of transmission from hollow needles are about 0.2% to 0.3%. Surgeons should feel comfortable in providing care for HIV-infected patients but should use appropriate and standardized safeguards to prevent blood exposure in the care of all patients.

Transplant Patient

One of the remarkable accomplishments of medicine and surgery over the last 50 years has been the success of organ transplantation. Kidney, liver, heart, and lung transplantation are commonly performed in many areas of the United States. The success of transplantation has been the direct result of vastly improved tissue typing to optimize donor/recipient compatibility, better organ preservation techniques, better surgical techniques for the placement of the donor organs, and progressive improvement of immunosuppressive strategies for the prevention of graft rejection.

The number of immunosuppressive agents has steadily increased during the last 30 years of transplantation science. Corticosteroids, azathioprine, cyclosporine, tacrolimus, antithymocyte globulin, and monoclonal T-cell antibody (OKT3) all are in clinical use today. Many other agents are currently in development. The focus of transplantation research in immunosuppression is to design that strategy that will protect the transplanted graft from rejection but will not have pan-suppressive events that yield increased infectious complications or long-term neoplastic consequences. Until the ideal immunosuppressive strategy is developed or until specific immunotolerance becomes a reality, the surgeon must be prepared to manage the infectious and neoplastic sequelae of transplant immunosuppression.

TABLE 13-2. Current Documented and Possible HIV Infections Acquired by Health Care Workers Through Occupational Activity

Occupation	No. of Documented Cases	No. of Possible Cases
Nurses	24	35
Clinical lab technicians	16	17
Health aide/attendants	1	15
Emergency medical technicians	0	12
Housekeeping/maintenance personnel	2	13
Nonsurgical physicians	6	12
Surgical physicians	0	6
Others	8	28
Total	57	138

From Centers for Disease Control and Prevention: *www.cdc.gov/ncidod/hip/BLOOD/hivpersonnel.htm.*

Infection in Transplant Patients

Transplant patients are at risk to develop all of the infections that might be identified in any patient but are also at risk to an array of infections from minimally virulent potential pathogens that ordinarily would not be identified in patients with normal host and immune capacity. The spectrum of infection includes the surgical site immediately following the procedure, hospital-based nosocomial infection during the postoperative period or during rehospitalization because of complications, and community-acquired infections.

Infection at the surgical site occurs for the same reasons that infections occur in nontransplantation surgery. Excessive contamination from either exogenous microbes (e.g., *S. aureus*) or from endogenous colonists (e.g., *Escherichia coli*) will be responsible for surgical wound infections. The duration of liver transplantation procedures and the high-risk median sternotomy wound for heart transplants carry increased probabilities of wound infection. The presence of hematoma, necrotic tissue (i.e., excessive use of the electrocautery), and foreign bodies (e.g., suture material, bone wax) all contribute to wound infection morbidity. Deep-seated abscess and empyema are commonly secondary to technical complications of the procedure itself (e.g., leaking anastomoses). The effects of immunosuppression are minimal for the surgical site infection since it will have just been initiated immediately prior to, during, or immediately following the procedure. However, the consequences of the patient's fundamental chronic illness will have led to malnutrition, hypoalbuminemia, and other systemic variables that will increase infection rates.

The prevention, diagnosis, and treatment of surgical site infections are the same as would be employed for similar infections in nontransplant patients. Sound infection control practices in the operating room during the procedure, appropriate utilization of perioperative systemic antibiotics, hemostasis at the surgical site, and other routine preventive strategies are important. The diagnosis of wound infection follows clinical recognition with the understanding that several days into the postoperative period, the patient will have effects from immunosuppression and clinical evidence of inflammation within the wound may be obscured. Abdominal abscess and empyema are suspected in all patients with systemic evidence of postoperative infection and are confirmed with computed tomographic scans. The treatment of wound infection is drainage and débridement, whereas deep-seated infections within the visceral cavities require control of the technical source of infection in addition to drainage of the septic focus.

Postoperative infections following the initial transplant event most commonly is due to conventional nosocomial infections. Bacterial nosocomial pneumonia, urinary tract infection, and intravascular device infections are seen with equal or greater frequency compared to other surgical intensive care patients. Of these postoperative infections, pneumonia is the greatest risk since immunosuppression increases the host's vulnerability and preexistent antibiotic therapy will have dramatically changed the host's colonization with resistant microbes. Airborne resistant gram-negative bacteria are most common and can be seen particularly when the patient has had a complicated and/or protracted course in the intensive care unit. Prevention, diagnosis, and treatment of these bacterial nosocomial infections follow the same pattern in other patients, although physical findings commonly are more subtle as the effects of systemic immunosuppression begin to influence the host's responsiveness.

Beginning at approximately 1 month following transplantation and usually after discharge from the hospital, the community-acquired infection with unusual pathogens begins to be a problem as the accumulative effects of immunosuppression accrue. Infection may either be new pathogens from environmental exposure or may be activation of quiescent, but preexistent infection. Infection with the herpes group of viruses assumes considerable significance, of which CMV infection is most important. CMV infection results in direct consequences to the host of pneumonia, gastrointestinal ulceration, and with chronic infection leading to chorioretinitis.[38-40] CMV infection exacerbates host immunosuppression, leading to an array of other secondary opportunistic infections (e.g., *P. carinii*). Some evidence indicates that CMV infection also may aggravate graft rejection and can be of significance in immunosuppression-associated neoplasms.

CMV infection may occur by several mechanisms in the transplant patient. First, infection may have been present already. More than 50% of the population are estimated to have latent CMV infection.[41] For the transplant patient, it becomes active disease with immunosuppression. Second, the patient may become acutely infected with CMV from the donor organ or from transfusion therapy associated with the transplant procedure. Community-acquired infection from intimate contacts after transplant is also a risk for initial CMV infection. Third, superinfection with a second strain of the virus appears to also be possible with apparent synergy and more severe consequences to the host.[42]

Prevention of clinical CMV infection in the transplant patient is attempted by several methods. Screening blood products for anti-CMV antibody is considered to have some value.[43] Screening donor organs seems intellectually sound but is impractical with restricted donor availability. The use of CMV hyperimmune globulin is commonly employed and appears to have greatest benefit in kidney transplant recipients.[44] Both acyclovir and ganciclovir are used for prophylaxis within the initial 4 to 6 months following transplantation. Ganciclovir is used intravenously for the initial 2 weeks followed by high-dose acyclovir thereafter.[45]

Clinical infection is associated with fever, malaise, and myalgia. Other findings include tachypnea, cough, symmetrical infiltration on chest roentgenogram, evidence of a hepatitis syndrome, leukopenia, and atypical lymphocytes. Diagnosis is confirmed by virologic methods to identify viral antigens or DNA. Therapy for established infection is ganciclovir 5 mg/kg twice per day.[46]

Epstein-Barr (EB) virus infection begins in the oropharynx epithelial cells and subsequently infects B cells in transit through this area of infection.[47] The dissemination of infected B cells and the attendant cytotoxic T-cell response initiates the symptomatology of acute mononucleosis. Acute EB virus infection may be totally latent, relatively mild, or a florid mononucleosis syndrome before it then lapses into a chronic latent state.

For the transplant patient with immunosuppression, the latent infection is reactivated, although acute interval infection from intimate contacts or even from transfusion can occur. CMV infection is thought to activate EB virus infection.[48] A protein product of EB virus infection has chemical homology with interleukin (IL)-10 and may further immunocompromise the host.[49]

Reactivated EB virus infection may give either a mononucleosis or a hepatitis syndrome. More important, sustained EB virus infection may lead to post-transplant lymphoproliferative disease.[50] Fever, mononucleosis syndrome, lymphadenopathy, gastrointestinal symptoms, hepatosplenomegaly, and even central nervous system symptoms (e.g., seizures) are signs of the clinical presentation. Tissue biopsies may range from reactive hyperplasia at one site to B-cell lymphoma or immunoblastic sarcoma at another.

Prevention of EB virus activation remains undefined, but hope exists that chemoprophylaxis as is used for CMV will be effective for EB virus infection. Decrease in immunosuppression, antilymphoma chemotherapy, and surgery and/or radiation therapy to control local disease is the treatment for transplantation-associated lymphoproliferative neoplasms.

Other viral infections are seen in the immunosuppressed transplant patient, although they occur less frequently or are less of a threat to the patient. These infections are summarized in Box 13-2.

In addition to the large number of viral pathogens, other opportunistic infections from unusual bacteria, fungi, and even protozoans can occur. The list of these possible pathogens is extensive and must be kept in mind when evaluating the transplant patient with evidence of infection. They are summarized in Box 13-2.

Neoplasia in Transplant Patients

Sustained immunosuppression in the transplant patient is associated with increased rates of malignancies, although the types of malignancies differ among the patient groups receiving each type of transplant. An obvious explanation for the increased incidence is the impaired immunosurveillance that normally controls malignant transformation. However, viral infection such as CMV, EB virus, her-

---

Box 13-2. Unusual Viral, Bacterial, Fungal, and Protozoan Infections Encountered in Immunosuppressed Transplant Patients

Viral Infections

Herpes simplex virus-1 and -2
Human herpesvirus-6
Varicella-zoster
Hepatitis B and C
Human immunodeficiency virus
Papovavirus
Respiratory syncytial virus

Unusual Other Pathogens

Listeria monocytogenes
Salmonella sp.
Mycobacterium tuberculosis
Mycobacterium avium intracellulare
Cryptococcus neoformans
Coccidioides immitis
Nocardia asteroides
Candida albicans (also non-*albicans* sp.)
Aspergillus fumigatus
Histoplasma capsulatum
Pneumocystis carinii

pesvirus, and human papillomavirus results in increased malignancies in these patients. Some immunosuppressive agents may potentiate the effects of other carcinogens or may be carcinogens themselves (e.g., azathioprine, cyclosporine).

General strategies have been advocated to reduce the overall rates of malignancies among these patients. Avoidance of sun exposure should reduce skin cancer rates. Safe-sex practices reduce infections of the transplant patient with herpesvirus or papillomavirus infection, which is associated with cervical cancer. Patients with frequent immunosuppression rescue events to salvage organs threatened by rejection appear to be at increased risk and should have frequent physical examinations to identify early signs of malignant changes.

Specific cancers are seen more commonly in the transplant patient. Skin cancers are most common in the kidney transplant patient, whereas lymphomas are the most common among liver transplant patients. Other cancers with increased frequencies in transplant patients include Kaposi's sarcoma, lip cancer, carcinoma of the kidney, vulvar and perineal cancers, and hepatobiliary cancers.[51]

The treatment of transplantation-associated neoplasms is the same for cancer management under similar circumstances for nontransplant, non-immunosuppressed patients. A complex judgment is necessary for many of these patients as to whether immunosuppressive therapy should be changed, reduced, or even stopped in the interest of better management of the malignancy. The potential negative consequences of reducing or halting immunosuppression to the patient's transplant graft are obvious.

Malnutrition

Malnutrition becomes an associated condition for a large number of surgical illnesses, which compounds efforts to provide appropriate patient management. Malnutrition is an issue in patients with cancer, intestinal fistula, chronic pancreatitis and other malabsorption states, sustained catabolic illnesses, and yet many others. Malnutrition in the surgical patient may have many facets in that the patient may be deficient in total calorie intake, the patient may have primarily a protein intake deficiency, or deficiencies in vitamins and other nutrients may be the important issue. Patients may present for care in a malnourished state, or they may develop malnutrition as a consequence of disease (e.g., sepsis) or treatment (e.g., radiation and chemotherapy).

Virtually all components of the inflammatory and immune response are affected by malnutrition. Initiation of inflammation is impaired because of reductions in complement proteins.[52] Vitamin K deficiency states combined with inadequate protein intake impair synthesis of the proteins of the coagulation cascade, which functions as a major initiator of inflammation.[53] Neutrophil function, cell-mediated immunity, and humoral immunity are adversely affected by malnutrition.[54]

However, the most thoroughly studied immune function in the surgical patient is the delayed-type hypersensitivity (DTH) skin test reaction.[2] Numerous studies have demonstrated nonresponsiveness of DTH skin test to a battery of antigens in the malnourished patient. Decreased DTH seems greatest in malnourished children. Patients with depressed DTH skin test responsiveness have been shown to have both an increased rate and severity of infections after major operations.

The diagnosis of malnutrition can be difficult to establish. Few patients present as thin and emaciated, although the diagnosis of malnutrition is not difficult in patients with advanced cancer or those with severe malabsorption problems. Various anthropometric studies are used but lack consistency of application. Measurement of absolute lymphocyte counts, serum albumin or prealbumin, serum retinol proteins, and creatinine-height indices give potentially objective measures of malnutrition. However, these measures are affected by acute changes secondary to the patient's illness (e.g., acute peritonitis) and may not be completely accurate reflections of the patient's nutritional state. In general, patients with clinical weight loss or those with acute catabolic illnesses (e.g., trauma, sepsis) are presumptively considered to be either malnourished or in a state of rapidly diminishing nutritional reserve and must be considered for nutritional support.

Enormous strides have been made in the route and composition of nutritional support strategies to manage or prevent malnutrition in the clinical management of patients. Central venous feeding allowed the delivery of adequate protein and glucose calories to meet apparent needs, and they even ushered into clinical practice in the 1970s an era of "hyperalimentation" where patients were given protein and total caloric support in excess of need to achieve anabolic effects. The subsequent introduction of lipid preparations allowed fat calories to be added to the nonprotein support regimen. However, complications with parenteral support were significant, lipid calories proved to be potentially immunosuppressive, and overfeeding was harmful to the patient. A rejuvenation of interest in enteral feeding occurred in the 1980s, and nutritional support via nasojejunal, small-caliber feeding tubes or surgically placed jejunostomy tubes was demonstrated to be superior to parenteral feeding. Enteral feeding likely has provided better nutritional delivery to the enterocyte/colonocyte of the gut and caloric access through the physiologic portal route, and the sheer mechanics of the feeding process avoided overfeeding lest diarrhea became a complication. Many of the complications associated with parenteral feeding were avoided. Prospective, randomized clinical trials showed that patients experienced fewer nosocomial infectious complications when compared to parenteral feeding.[55,56]

Most recently, immunonutritional support has emerged as a promising new direction.[57] This strategy has taken conventional enteral feeding formulations and added arginine, nucleic acids, and omega-3 fatty acid. The addition of these nutrients experimentally was shown to enhance T-cell responsiveness. Several prospective, randomized trials have now been completed in cancer patients, trauma patients, and other critically ill surgical patients and have demonstrated lower nosocomial infection rates when compared to conventional enteral feeding formulations.

However, mortality rates have not been improved. Although improved patient outcome has yet to be fully proven with this newer strategy (i.e., improved survival), the direction of nutritional support in the immunocompromised surgical patient is moving away from quantitative considerations about the amount of delivered protein and calories and is moving toward better refinements in the composition of feeding.

Burn and Trauma Injury

Immunosuppression is an obligatory response of the host to thermal burns and to virtually any form of mechanical trauma.[58] Surgical intervention with the effects of general anesthesia constitutes a controlled injury but nevertheless is a traumatic event where the greater the magnitude of the invasiveness results in measurably greater immunosuppressive consequences. The suppressiveness of the traumatic event is measurable within hours of the event and is clearly not simply a malnutrition-associated complication that occurs after critical illness has been sustained over a period of several catabolic postinjury days without feeding.

The immunosuppression of burn and trauma is comprehensive across all measurable aspects of immune function. Reduced complement protein concentrations, reduced neutrophil chemotaxis/phagocytosis/intracellular killing, reduced B-cell function, and decreased cell-mediated immunity all have been demonstrated in a consistent fashion in the trauma patient. The loss of major histocompatibility class II expression on monocytes has been demonstrated as yet another acquired deficiency from trauma that appears to correlate with infectious morbidity and patient outcome.

A vast array of released humoral substances is being proposed as responsible agents for this immunosuppression.[59] Prostaglandins E and F and thromboxane B_2 from monocytes have been implicated. Soluble products released by suppressor T cells have been reported. Anti-inflammatory cytokines (e.g., IL-4, IL-10, and IL-13) are being recognized as antagonists to the human pro-inflammatory cytokines and have further added to the evolving concept that an exaggerated counter-inflammatory response following injury may suppress host responsiveness. Considerable clinical evidence indicates that the immunosuppression of trauma and burn injury increases the rates of infection but also increases the morbid consequences of infection. The nadir of immunosuppression occurs at 1 to 2 days after injury and lasts for 7 or more days in the absence of intercurrent events (e.g., shock, sepsis, severe catabolism) that add an additional immunosuppressive insult to the patient.

Considerable interest is presently being focused on the use of exogenous agents to reverse or attenuate the immunosuppression of acute traumatic injury. Interferon-γ has been shown to increased major histocompatibility expression on monocytes and has been studied in injured patients with encouraging but not statistically significant results.[60] Glucan[61] and granulocyte-monocyte colony-stimulating factor[62] are yet additionally proposed treatments to enhance immune function following injury.

Shock

Shock as a clinical event has been proposed to have immunosuppressive consequences.[63] Measurement of the same immunosuppressive parameters recognized in the trauma patient have similarly shown comprehensive effects across all measured facets of host responsiveness in experimental laboratories. Reduced complement protein concentrations, depressed neutrophil function studies, and altered B- and T-cell functions are consistently identified. Most observations about shock have been experimental and not human studies. Clinical shock is virtually impossible to study separate from trauma, major operations, and general anesthesia, all of which have immunosuppressive effects and are invariably present in the hypotensive patient. Experimental shock is associated with increased frequency and severity of infections.[64] Since experimental measures of immunosuppression in the shocked animal follow so closely with those seen in burn and trauma studies, it is assumed that common humoral mediators are operative.

Transfusion

Blood transfusion has been recognized for many decades as having immunosuppressive effects. Multiple units of transfusion with homologous blood was shown to improve the survival of transplanted kidney grafts and was used as a strategy for enhancement of graft survival.[65] However, a series of reports in the early 1980s demonstrated that blood transfusion was a negative independent variable in the outcomes of cancer patients receiving surgical management of their primary disease.[66] This negative effect on cancer survival appeared to be specific for different cancers and to even have different effects on the same cancer cell type, depending on the stage of the disease. Reported negative effects of transfusion included both a reduced disease-free interval following presumably curative procedures and reductions in patient survival. Whether cancer survival is truly affected has been disputed in other studies, and the effects of transfusion on cancer survival remain unsettled.

These observations in cancer patients led to similar investigations in patients receiving blood transfusions in other settings. Blood transfusion was identified as an independent variable for infection morbidity in patients with penetrating abdominal trauma.[67] Increased infection rates were independent of the coexistence of shock and were independent of the magnitude of injury (i.e., Injury Severity Score).

The exact mechanism of immunosuppression from transfusion remains unknown. Immunosuppression can be demonstrated to occur in experimental animals receiving compatible transfusion from genetically different animals.[68] Suppression has been theorized to occur from the release of prostaglandin E derivatives or from other suppressor cell products that are released in response to the transfusion. Mixed lymphocyte reaction studies have demonstrated immunosuppression with sera from transfused patients that was not present with sera from nontransfused patients.[69]

It is apparent that laboratory immunosuppression from transfusion is present, but its clinical consequences remain unclear. From this perspective, infections are probably increased with transfusion, but the consequences in cancer management require further definition. Given the specter of blood-borne pathogens in donated blood, immunosuppression is yet another reason to limit the use of transfusion when clinically practical.

Diabetes

The global consequences of diabetes to the patient are well recognized. Numerous clinical studies have noted increased rates of infection that occur in diabetic patients. Poor perfusion of tissues due to both macrovascular and microvascular disease, increased tissue fat in type II diabetic patients, and the consequences of hyperglycemia alone on the viability of the pathogen may enhance rates of infection.

Although increased rates and severity of infection in diabetic patients are generally accepted, specific immunosuppression as a cause for increased infectious morbidity remains unproved. Neutrophil chemotaxis and phagocytosis in diabetic patients have been demonstrated, but only when blood glucose is poorly controlled.[70] Correction of blood glucose to normal limits appears to reverse these defects of neutrophil function. Reduced CD4 cell counts have also been reported in diabetic patients, but as is the case with neutrophil function, this abnormality was not seen when normal glucose control was present.[71] Thus, it would appear that better blood sugar control will likely reduce rates of infection in diabetic patients. Because infection, when established, destabilizes blood sugar control in the diabetic patient, immunosuppressive effects from hyperglycemia may assume clinical significance.

Aging

Infections are more common and have greater consequences to the elderly patient. Rates of cancer at virtually all anatomic sites increase with aging of the host. These observations certainly suggest that immunosurveillance for the presence of neoplastic transformation may be defective and that responsiveness to bacterial challenge may be compromised with the aging process.

Several immune changes with aging have been reported that may address increased infection rates[72]:

- Reduced T-cell stimulation with low concentrations of mitogen
- Reduced IgG antibody response to vaccination
- Reduced DTH response to multiple skin test antigens
- Increased sensitivity of the host to prostaglandin E with aging

The aging process produces a number of changes that may increase infection rates but are independent of specific immunity. Reduced pulmonary compliance and reduced tidal volumes of ventilation increase pneumonia rates. Fragile skin may increase the local consequences of trauma and increase infection rates. Reduced cardiac output may affect infection and healing rates after major operation. Impaired thermal control and poor nutritional habits are significant problems that mediate immunosuppression but are not issues of aging per se. Separation of aging-specific from nonspecific elements of host defenses in the elderly patient is not easily done, but clearly the elderly have a number of factors that increase the risk of infection.

Postsplenectomy

Prior to the 1980s, a traditional strategy for the management of splenic injury was to perform splenectomy. However, evidence began to accumulate that patients, particularly in the pediatric and adolescent age groups, developed overwhelming postsplenectomy sepsis. This septic event was not common in the postsplenectomy trauma patient (<1%) but was somewhat higher in splenectomy for medical indications and occurred in older patients after medical splenectomy. This infection was associated with a fulminant course that resulted in death rates of 70% or higher. For surgeons, it resulted in the adoption of splenic salvage except for severe injuries in most patients. It also leads to considerable investigation into the specific immune mechanisms that increased the vulnerability of specific patients to postsplenectomy sepsis.

Splenectomy results in several specific immune consequences.[73] The removal of foreign proteins and particles from the circulation by the spleen does not require opsonization of the particle or the microbe. For the liver to replace this reticuloendothelial function of the spleen following splenectomy, the particle or microbe must be opsonized. In the absence of specific antibody for a specific microbe to serve as an opsonin, hepatic clearance of that microbe is defective. The encapsulated bacteria of *Streptococcus pneumoniae, Neisseria meningitidis,* and *Haemophilus influenzae* must be opsonized with specific antibody for hepatic clearance. These pathogens emerged as the significant bacterial pathogens of postsplenectomy sepsis. In addition, the spleen is important in acute antibody production. Splenectomized patients have decreased IgM antibodies.

Although greater attempts to salvage the spleen are part of current surgical practice, splenectomy is still required in specific circumstances. Specific immunization has been effective in reducing rates of postsplenectomy sepsis. Patients requiring splenectomy for trauma should receive the pneumococcal, meningococcal, and *H. influenzae* vaccine. The trauma patients usually show excellent antibody responses to vaccination, which is not true for patients with splenectomy for medical indications. This latter group of patients needs to be appropriately informed about the risks, signs, and symptoms of postsplenectomy sepsis.

Surgical Site Infection

Infection at the surgical site occurs as the biologic summation of the influences of the inoculum of contaminants, the virulence of the contaminants, adjuvant factors (e.g., hematoma, foreign bodies), and the integrity of the host. Assessments of host integrity and the opportunity to manipulate acquired deficiencies of host responsiveness have been elusive. Recent evidence indicates that specific aspects of host responsiveness can be manipulated in the care of the surgical patient and can reduce surgical site infections.

The surgical wound has been viewed as being a hypoxemic local environment. Experimental evidence has supported the use of supplemental systemic oxygenation as a means to combat this local reduction in oxygen tension.[74] Better oxygen delivery to the wound during the time of the operation and during the immediate postoperative period would enhance the production of reactive oxygen intermediates by the phagocytic cell.

A prospective, randomized trial in elective colon surgery has demonstrated a significant reduction in surgical site infection rates.[75] Patients received a fraction of inspired oxygen (FiO_2) of 0.3 versus 0.8 with all other clinical variables controlled. Since increased oxygen delivery required enhanced delivery by the plasma, patients received vigorous crystalloid volume support. Enhanced oxygen delivery was during the operation and for 2 hours into the postoperative period. The control infection rate of 11% in patients receiving the FiO_2 of 0.3 was significantly reduced to 5% ($P < 0.05$) in the 0.8 group.

Temperature control of the patient has been a source of concern for trauma surgeons because of coagulopathic complications. Intraoperative temperature control has similarly been used with increased frequency to reduce surgical blood loss. Reduction in the core body temperature of the host during operations may have an acquired immunosuppressive effect on the host.

Patients undergoing elective colon surgery were randomized to have their core body temperatures maintained above 36.5°C versus patients who were permitted to have the core body temperature decline to levels of 34.5°C during the operation.[76] All other clinical variables were similar between the two groups. Patients allowed to have their core temperatures drift to the lower level had a surgical site infection rate of 19%. Those who had the core temperature maintained higher than 36.5°C had an infection rate of 6% ($P < 0.01$). The efficiency of host responsiveness appears to be influenced by core body temperature.

The diabetic patient has been appreciated as having increased rates of surgical site infection, although efforts as noted earlier to identify specific defects of host responsiveness have not been successful. Furnary and associates[77] have studied large numbers of diabetic patients undergoing open heart surgery. They have put forth the hypothesis that better intraoperative and postoperative control of glucose would reduce sternal wound infection rates. In studies that have occurred over a decade, nearly 2500 diabetic patients have been studied. Maintenance of blood sugar concentrations below 200 mg/dL has reduced sternal wound infection rates to 0.8%, which is similar to the rate identified in nondiabetic patients. Diabetic patients without insulin infusion and rigorous glucose control had a sternal wound infection rate of 2%.

Thus, these studies of surgical site infection have demonstrated that supplemental oxygenation, temperature control, and glucose control can enhance host responsiveness. This raises the question of whether similar control of these variables in the surgical patient could actually affect nosocomial infection rates. The studies of van den Berghe and colleagues[78] would clearly indicate that glucose control has benefits for nondiabetic patients as well. Manipulation of other clinical variables in the surgical patient during the time of the operation may well present an opportunity to augment host responsiveness and reduce overall infectious complications.

References

1. Lewis RT, Klein H: Risk factors and postoperative sepsis: Significance of preoperative lymphocytopenia. J Surg Res 26:365-371, 1975.
2. Christou NV, Meakins JL, Gordon J, et al: The delayed hypersensitivity response and host resistance in surgical patients: 20 years later. Ann Surg 222:534-546, 1995.
3. Spiekerman AM: Proteins used in nutritional assessment. Clin Lab Med 13:353-369, 1993.
4. Scientific Group on Immunodeficiency: Primary immunodeficiency disease. Immunodefic Rev 1:173, 1989.
5. Whaley K, Schwaeble W: Complement and complement deficiencies. Semin Liv Dis 17:297-310, 1997.
6. Cicardi M, Bergamaschini L, Cugno M, et al: Pathogenetic and clinical aspects of C1 inhibitor deficiency. Immunobiology 199:366-376, 1998.
7. Ross D: The genetic basis of chronic granulomatous disease. Immunol Rev 138:121-157, 1994.
8. Lanza F: Clinical manifestations of myeloperoxidase deficiency. J Mol Med 76:676-681, 1998.
9. Milech HL, Nauseef WM: Primary inherited defects in neutrophil function: Etiology and treatment. Semin Hematol 34:279-290, 1997.
10. Morgenthaler TI, Brown LR, Colby TV, et al: Thymoma. Mayo Clin Proc 68:1110-1123, 1993.
11. Kirkpatrick CH: Chronic mucocutaneous candidiasis. J Am Acad Dermatol 31:S14-S17, 1994.
12. Ochs HD: The Wiskott-Aldrich syndrome. Semin Hematol 35:332-345, 1998.
13. Satterthwaite AB, Witte ON: Lessons from human genetic variants in the study of B-cell differentiation. Curr Opin Immunol 8:454-458, 1996.
14. Pantaleo G, Graziosi C, Fauci A: The immunopathogenesis of human immunodeficiency virus infection. N Engl J Med 328:327-335, 1993.
15. Curran JW, Morgan JW, Hardy AM: Epidemiology of HIV infection and AIDS in the United States. Science 239:610-616, 1988.
16. Tindall B, Barker S, Donovan B, et al: Characterization of the acute clinical illness associated with human immunodeficiency virus infection. Arch Intern Med 148:945, 1988.
17. Stein DS, Korvick JA, Vermund SH: CD4+ lymphocyte cell enumeration for prediction of clinical course of human immunodeficiency virus disease: A review. J Infect Dis 165:352-363, 1992.
18. Centers for Disease Control: 1993 Revised classification system for HIV infection and expanded surveillance case definition for AIDS among adolescents and adults. MMWR CDC Surveill Summ 41:1-19, 1992.

19. Whitney TM, Macho JR, Russell TR, et al: Appendicitis in acquired immunodeficiency syndrome. Am J Surg 164:467-471, 1992.
20. Ravalli S, Vincent RA, Beaton H: Primary Kaposi's sarcoma of the gastrointestinal tract presenting as acute appendicitis. Am J Gastroenterol 85:772-773, 1990.
21. Valerdiz-Casasola S, Pardo-Mindan FJ: Cytomegalovirus appendicitis in a patient with acquired immunodeficiency syndrome. Gastroenterology 101:247-249, 1991.
22. Kram HB, Shoemaker WC: Intestinal perforation due to cytomegalovirus infection in patients with AIDS. Dis Colon Rect 33:1037-1040, 1990.
23. Yoshida EM, Chan NH, Chan-yan C, Baird RM: Perforation of the jejunum secondary to AIDS-related gastrointestinal Kaposi's sarcoma. Can J Gastroenterol 11:38-40, 1997.
24. Heise W, Arasteh K, Mostertz P, et al: Malignant gastrointestinal lymphoma in patients with AIDS. Digestion 58:218-224, 1997.
25. Domingo P, Rio J, Lopez-Contreras J, et al: Appendicitis due to *Mycobacterium avium* complex in a patient with AIDS. Arch Intern Med 156:11-14, 1996.
26. Wilson SE, Robinson G, Williams RA: AIDS indications for abdominal surgery, pathology, and outcome. Ann Surg 210:428-433, 1989.
27. Deziel DJ, Hyser MJ, Doolas A, et al: Major abdominal operations in AIDS. Am Surg 56:445-450, 1990.
28. Benhamou Y, Caumes E, Gerosa Y, et al: AIDS-related cholangiopathy: Critical analysis of a prospective series of 26 patients. Dig Dis Sci 38:1113-1118, 1993.
29. Mathew A, Raviglione MC, Niranjan U, et al: Splenectomy in patients with AIDS. Am J Hematol 32:184-189, 1989.
30. Welch GH, Reid DB, Pollack JG: Infected false aneurysms in the groin of intravenous drug abusers. Br J Surg 77:330-333, 1990.
31. Dupont JR, Bonavita JA, DiGiovanni RJ, et al: Acquired immunodeficiency syndrome and mycotic abdominal aortic aneurysms. J Vasc Surg 10:254-257, 1989.
32. Herndier BG, Kaplan LD, McGrath MS: Pathogenesis of AIDS lymphomas. AIDS 8:1025-1049, 1994.
33. Fry DE: Herpesviruses: Emerging nosocomial pathogens? Surg Infect 2:121-130, 2001.
34. Krown SE: Acquired immunodeficiency syndrome–associated Kaposi's sarcoma: Biology and management. Med Clin North Am 81:471-494, 1997.
35. Quinn TC: Clinical approach to intestinal infection in homosexual men. Med Clin North Am 70:611-634, 1986.
36. Chadha M, Rosenblatt EA, Malamud S, et al: Squamous cell carcinoma of the anus in HIV-positive patients. Dis Colon Rect 37:861-865, 1994.
37. Centers for Disease Control and Prevention: Documented and possible occupationally acquired AIDS/HIV infection, by occupation. HIV/AIDS Surveill Rep 11:26, 1999.
38. Rubin RH: Infectious disease complications of renal transplantation. Kidney Int 44:221-236, 1993.
39. Vachon GC, Brown BS, Kim C, Chessin LN: CMV gastric ulcers as the presenting manifestation of AIDS. Am J Gastroenterol 90:319-321, 1995.
40. Skiest DJ: Cytomegalovirus retinitis in the era of highly active antiretroviral therapy. Am J Med Sci 317:318-335, 1999.
41. Smith MA, Brennessel DJ: Cytomegalovirus. Infect Dis Clin North Am 8:427-438, 1994.
42. Grundy JE, Lui SF, Super M, et al: Symptomatic cytomegalovirus infection in seropositive patients: Reinfection with donor virus rather than reactivation of recipient virus. Lancet 2:132-135, 1988.
43. Sayers MH, Anderson KC, Goodnough LT, et al: Reducing the risk for transfusion-transmitted cytomegalovirus infection. Ann Intern Med 116:55-62, 1992.
44. Rubin RH, Tolkoff-Rubin NE: Antimicrobial strategies in the care of organ transplant recipients. Antimicrob Agents Chemother 37:619-624, 1993.
45. Martin M, Manez R, Linden P, et al: A prospective randomized trial comparing sequential ganciclovir–high-dose acyclovir to high-dose acyclovir for prevention of cytomegalovirus disease in adult liver transplant recipients. Transplantation 58:779-785, 1994.
46. Dunn DL, Mayoral JL, Gillingham KJ, et al: Treatment of invasive cytomegalovirus disease in solid-organ transplant patients with ganciclovir. Transplantation 51:98-106, 1991.
47. Straus SE, Cohen JI, Tosato G, et al: Epstein-Barr virus infection: Biology, pathogenesis, and management. Ann Intern Med 118:45-58, 1993.
48. Aalto SM, Linnavuori K, Peltola H, et al: Immunoreactivity of Epstein-Barr virus due to cytomegalovirus primary infection. J Med Virol 56:186-191, 1998.
49. Vieira P, DeWaal-Malefyt R, Dang MN, et al: Isolation and expression of human cytokine inhibiting factor cDNA clones: Homology to Epstein-Barr open reading frame BCRF-1. Proc Natl Acad Sci U S A 88:1172-1176, 1991.
50. Preiskaitis JK, Diaz-Mitoma F, Mirzayans F, et al: Quantitative oropharyngeal Epstein-Barr virus shedding in renal and cardiac transplant recipients: Relationship to immunosuppressive therapy, serologic responses, and the risk of post-transplant lymphoproliferative disease. J Infect Dis 166:986-994, 1992.
51. Penn I: Malignancy. Surg Clin North Am 74:1247-1257, 1994.
52. Sakamoto M, Fujisawa Y, Nishioka K: Physiologic role of the complement system in host defense, disease, and malnutrition. Nutrition 14:391-398, 1998.
53. Hassanein EA, Tankovsky I: Disturbances of coagulation mechanism in protein-calorie malnutrition. Trop Geograph Med 25:158-162, 1973.
54. Santos JI: Nutrition, infection, and immunocompetence. Infect Clin North Am 8:243-267, 1994.
55. Moore FA, Moore EE, Jones TN, et al: TEN versus TPN following major abdominal trauma—reduced septic morbidity. J Trauma 29:916-923, 1989.
56. Kudsk KA, Croce MA, Fabian TC, et al: Enteral versus parenteral feeding: Effects on septic morbidity following blunt and penetrating abdominal trauma. Ann Surg 215:503-513, 1992.
57. Heys SD, Walker LG, Smith I, Eremin O: Enteral nutritional supplementation with key nutrients in patients with critical illness and cancer: A meta-analysis of randomized controlled clinical trials. Ann Surg 229:467-477, 1999.
58. Howard RJ: Effect of burn injury, mechanical trauma, and operation on immune defenses. Surg Clin North Am 59:199-211, 1979.
59. Faist E, Schinkel C, Zimmer S: Update on the mechanisms of immune suppression of injury and immune modulation. World J Surg 20:454-459, 1996.
60. Polk HC Jr, Cheadle WG, Livingston DH, et al: A randomized prospective clinical trial to determine the efficacy of interferon-gamma in severely injured patients. Am J Surg 163:191-196, 1992.
61. Babineau TJ, Hackford A, Kenlar A, et al: A phase II multicenter, double-blind, randomized, placebo-controlled study of three dosages of an immunomodulator (PGG-glucan) in high-risk surgical patients. Arch Surg 129:1204-1210, 1994.
62. Stern AC, Jones TC: Role of human recombinant GM-CSF in the prevention and treatment of leukopenia with special ref-

erence to infectious disease. Diag Microbiol Infect Dis 13:391-396, 1990.

63. Fry DE, Pearlstein L, Fulton RL, Polk HC Jr: Multiple-system organ failure: The role of uncontrolled infection. Arch Surg 115:136-140, 1980.

64. Esrig BC, Frazee L, Stephonson SF, et al: The predisposition to infection following hemorrhagic shock. Surg Gynecol Obstet 144:915-917, 1977.

65. Ramsey G, Sherman LA: Transfusion therapy in solid organ transplantation. Hematol Oncol Clin North Am 8:1117-1129, 1994.

66. Bordin JO, Blajchman MA: Immunosuppressive effects of allogeneic blood transfusion: Implications for the patient with a malignancy. Hematol Oncol Clin North Am 9:205-218, 1995.

67. Nichols R, Smith JW, Klein DB, et al: Risk of infection after penetrating abdominal trauma. N Engl J Med 311:1065, 1984.

68. Waymack JP, Yurt RW: The effect of blood transfusion on immune function: V. The effect on the inflammatory response to bacterial infection. J Surg Res 48:147-153, 1990.

69. Abraham E, Chang YH: Cellular and humoral bases of hemorrhage-induced depression of lymphocyte function. Crit Care Med 14:81, 1986.

70. Moutschen MP, Scheen AJ, Lefebvre PF: Impaired immune responses in diabetes mellitus—analysis of the factors involved: Relevance to the increased susceptibility of diabetic patients to specific infections. Diabetes Metab 18:187, 1992.

71. Rodier M, Andary M, Richard JL,et al: Peripheral blood T-cell subsets studies by monoclonal antibodies in type 1 (insulin-dependent) diabetes: Effect of blood glucose control. Diabetologia 27:136-138, 1984.

72. Charpentier B, Fournier C, Fries D, et al: Immunological studies in human aging: I. In vitro functions of T cells and polymorphs. J Clin Lab Immunol 5:87-93, 1981.

73. Lynch AM, Kapila R: Overwhelming postsplenectomy infection. Infect Dis Clin North Am 10:693-707, 1996.

74. Knighton DR, Halliday B, Hunt TK: Oxygen as an antibiotic: A comparison of the effects of inspired oxygen concentration and antibiotic administration on in vivo bacterial clearance. Arch Surg 121:191-195, 1986.

75. Greif R, Akca O, Horn EP, et al: Supplemental perioperative oxygen to reduce the incidence of surgical wound infection. N Engl J Med 342:161-167, 2000.

76. Kurz A, Sessler DI, Lenhardt R: Perioperative normothermia to reduce the incidence of surgical wound infection and shorten hospitalization. N Engl J Med 334:1209-1215, 1996.

77. Furnary AP, Zerr KJ, Grunkemeier GL, Starr A: Continuous intravenous insulin infusion reduces the incidence of deep sternal wound infection in diabetic patients after cardiac surgical procedures. Ann Thorac Surg 67:352-360, 1999.

78. van den Berghe G, Wouters P, Weekers F, et al: Intensive insulin therapy in the surgical intensive care unit. N Engl J Med 345:1359-1367, 2001.

CHAPTER 14

SURGICAL COMPLICATIONS

Merril T. Dayton, M.D.

Wound Complications	**Gastrointestinal Complications**
Complications of Thermoregulation	**Hepatobiliary Complications**
Respiratory Complications	**Neurologic Complications**
Cardiac Complications	**Ear, Nose, and Throat Complications**
Renal and Urinary Tract Complications	**Special Considerations**
Metabolic Complications	

Postoperative surgical complications represent one of the most frustrating and difficult occurrences experienced by surgeons who do a significant volume of surgery. Regardless of how technically gifted, bright, and capable a surgeon is, surgical complications are a virtually guaranteed aspect of life. The cost of surgical complications in the United States today runs into millions of dollars and is associated with lost work productivity, disruption of normal family life, and unanticipated stress to employers and society in general. Frequently, the functional results of the operation are compromised by complications; in some cases, the patient never recovers to the preoperative level of function. The most significant and difficult part of complications is the suffering borne by the patient who enters the hospital anticipating an uneventful operation but is left suffering and compromised by the complication.

Complications can occur for a variety of reasons. A surgeon can perform a technically perfect operation in a patient who is severely compromised by the disease process and still have a complication. Similarly, a surgeon who is sloppy, is careless, or hurries through an operation can make technical errors that account for the operative complications. Finally, the patient can be doing well nutritionally, have an operation performed meticulously, and yet suffer a complication because of the nature of the disease. The possibility of postoperative complications is a part of every surgeon's thought processes—something with which all surgeons will be required to deal.

Surgeons can do much to avoid complications by the careful preoperative screening process. When the surgeon sees the potential surgical candidate the first time, a host of questions come to mind, such as the nutritional status of the patient and questions about the health of the heart and lungs. The surgeon will make a decision regarding performing the correct operation for the appropriate disease. Similarly, the timing of the operation is often an important issue. Some operations can be performed in a purely elective fashion, whereas others have some urgency about an expeditious surgical solution. Occasionally, the surgeon will demand that the patient lose weight before the operation so that the likelihood of a successful outcome is improved. Occasionally, the wise surgeon will request preoperative consultation from a cardiologist or pulmonary specialist to make certain that the patient will be able to tolerate the stresses of a particular procedure.

Once the operation has begun, the surgeon can do much to influence the postoperative outcome. Surgeons learn to handle tissues gently, to dissect meticulously, and honor tissue planes. Performing the technical portions of the operation carefully will lessen the possibility of a significant complication. At all costs, surgeons must avoid the temptation to rush, cut corners, or accept marginal technical results. Similarly, the judicious use of antibiotics and other preoperative medications can influence the outcome. For the seriously ill patient, adequate resuscitation may be necessary to optimize the patient before giving a general anesthetic.

Once the operation is completed, compulsive postoperative surveillance is mandatory. Thorough and careful rounding on patients on a regular basis postoperatively gives the operating surgeon an opportunity to be vigilant and seek postoperative complications in an early stage when they can be most successfully addressed. During this process, the surgeon will carefully check all wounds, evaluate intake and output, check temperature profiles, ascertain what activity levels have been, evaluate nutritional status, and check pain levels. Over years of experience, the clinician can begin to assess the aforementioned parameters and detect deviations from the normal postoperative course. Expeditious response to a complication makes the difference between a brief, inconvenient complication and a devastating, disabling complication. In summary, the wise surgeon will deal with complications quickly, thoroughly, and appropriately.

WOUND COMPLICATIONS

Seroma

Etiology

One of the most benign but bothersome complications after an operative procedure is the development of a seroma. A seroma is the collection of liquefied fat, serum, and lymphatic fluid under the incision. The fluid is usually clear, yellow, and somewhat viscous. It is found in the subcutaneous layer just below the dermis. Seromas are particularly likely to occur when large skin flaps are developed in the course of the operation, as is often seen with mastectomy, axillary dissection, groin dissection, and large ventral hernias. The etiology of seromas is uncertain but may relate to liquefaction of fat in the subcutaneous layer as well as lymphatic drainage.

Presentation and Management

Seromas usually present as localized and well-circumscribed swelling, pressure discomfort, and occasional drainage of clear liquid from the immature wound. Seromas that develop in abdominal incisions and extremity incisions can usually be evacuated and packed with saline-moistened gauze to allow healing by secondary intention. However, seromas that develop under breast flaps or axillary or groin dissections often are much more difficult to manage. Placement of suction drains in wounds with skin flaps is indicated. Their premature removal often results in large seromas, which require repeated aspirations under sterile conditions followed by placement of a pressure dressing. On occasion, in spite of repeated aspirations, the seroma persists or becomes secondarily infected; in those cases the wound must be opened. Those that become secondarily infected have to be opened and packed to heal by secondary intention. It should be noted that seromas do not usually have the associated erythema and exquisite tenderness that a localized wound infection has.

Hematoma

Etiology

A hematoma is an abnormal collection of blood, usually in the subcutaneous layer of a recent incision. Hematomas are more worrisome than seromas because of the potential for secondary infection. Bleeding in the involved layer after the skin is closed causes a hematoma. The reason for the poor hemostasis may be manyfold. Inadequate hemostasis at the time of wound closure can account for a hematoma. Similarly, rough handling of the tissues during the closure can predispose to wound hematomas. Finally, a coagulopathy can lead to postoperative hematomas in the patient who has exhausted clotting factors during a large abdominal or thoracic procedure, has been taking aspirin or nonsteroidal anti-inflammatory agents, or who has been on warfarin (Coumadin) or heparin. A host of other disease processes can contribute to coagulopathy, including myeloproliferative disorders, liver disease, clotting factor deficiencies, and platelet disorders. Hematomas may cause significant pain to the patient as well as a poor cosmetic result and can even become secondarily infected. A wound hematoma often presents as physical findings of purplish/blue discoloration of the overlying skin, localized wound swelling, drainage of dark red fluid out of the fresh wound, and occasional pressure pain and discomfort. Hematomas can range from a small, localized collection in the abdominal incision to huge collections of blood and thrombus in the obese patient. Occasionally, in patients who have had a neck dissection, a hematoma can develop postoperatively that is life threatening owing to compression of the soft tissues surrounding the airway. Immediate and emergent evacuation of the hematoma may be a lifesaving maneuver. Large hematomas may collect in the retroperitoneal tissues, causing paralytic ileus, anemia, and ongoing bleeding due to consumption of clotting factors. Management of hematomas depends on the size and age of the wound. Those hematomas detected soon after surgery should be evacuated under sterile conditions and the wound packed with saline-moistened gauze. Hematomas developing under skin flaps usually have to be evacuated in the operating room. A small hematoma that occurs 2 weeks after an operation will often resorb with conservative management only and may not require an operation. Most retroperitoneal hematomas should be managed by expectant waiting after correction of all clotting factors.

Prevention

The most important principle in prevention of hematoma is careful hemostasis of the subcutaneous layer during closure. Whereas hematomas may occur in any tissue space in the body, they are most frequently encountered in the subcutaneous layer in a fresh incision. Prevention of the hematoma can also be facilitated by correcting all clotting abnormalities before surgery and discontinuing medications that can prolong bleeding times (e.g., warfarin and nonsteroidal anti-inflammatory agents). Wounds that require large skin flaps and have large potential spaces should be drained with closed suction drainage systems until output is nonbloody and scant.

Wound Dehiscence

Etiology

Wound dehiscence is among the most dreaded complications faced by surgeons. The term *dehiscence* has its greatest clinical significance in patients with a full-thickness abdominal incision. By definition, dehiscence is the separation of fascial layers early in the postoperative course, an event that usually leads to emergency action. Dehiscence is of greatest concern because of the possibility of evisceration, which is protrusion of the small intestines through the fascial layers and out onto the abdominal skin surface. Dehiscence that occurs soon after operation will usually require a return trip to the operating room. However, a small partial dehiscence 10 days after operation can often be watched and the wound packed without danger of evisceration. The etiology of dehiscence is often related to technical errors in placing sutures too close to the edge, too far apart, or under too much tension. A multitude of other factors may contribute to increased intra-abdominal pressure and poor healing, thus leading to dehiscence of the fascial closure (Box 14-1).[1] Wound dehiscence occurs in approximately 2% of patients who undergo an abdominal operation. Local wound complications such as hematoma and infection can also predispose to localized dehiscence. In fact, a deep wound infection is one of the most common causes of a localized wound separation. In healthy patients, there appears to be no difference in the wound dehiscence rates between those closed using a continuous technique versus an interrupted technique. However, one has to be concerned about a continuous closure in high-risk patients because suture breakage in one place in a continuous closure weakens the entire closure and, in high-risk patients, an interrupted closure may occasionally be a wise choice.

Presentation and Management

Wound dehiscence usually presents as a sudden, dramatic drainage of relatively large volumes of a clear, salmon-colored fluid. Most often, the dehiscence is a partial dehiscence that can be detected by opening the skin staples and probing the wound with a sterile, cotton-tipped applicator. If probing with the applicator reveals a large segment of the wound that is open all the way to the omentum and intestines, plans to take the patient back to the operating room immediately should be made. Evisceration is a surgical emergency and, if encountered, the eviscerated intestines should be covered with a sterile,

saline-moistened towel and preparations made to return to the operating room emergently.

Management of the dehisced wound once in the operating room is a function of the condition of the fascia. Where technical mistakes were made and the fascia is strong and intact, the fascia can merely be closed with caution and expected to do very well. However, if the fascia is infected or is weak or in poor condition, occasionally some of it must be débrided and retention sutures may be required. The surgeon should look for any evidence of anastomotic leak or intra-abdominal infection that may have predisposed to the dehiscence. Management of that infection is of critical importance before attempting to close. If significant amounts of fascia need to be débrided because of infection or poor tissue integrity, it is poor judgment to attempt to close the fascia under significant tension. Such an approach will universally lead to repeated dehiscence and necessitate another trip to the operating room. If the fascial layers cannot be closed without tension, an absorbable mesh may be placed in the wound and sewn to both fascial layers to bridge the gap until the underlying cause of the patient's dehiscence resolves.[2] This uniformly results in the development of a hernia, but the surgeon may always return at another date to put in a permanent mesh with skin coverage. Occasionally, if the dehiscence is small and fairly far postoperatively, the wound can be managed by conservative treatment including débridement of the wound, saline-moistened gauze packing of the wound, and keeping an abdominal binder on the patient. Certainly, a permanent mesh, such as Marlex, should not be placed in the field under conditions where there has been significant contamination.

Prevention

Preventing wound dehiscence is largely a function of careful attention to technical detail during the fascial closure. The technical details of fascial closure include such things as proper spacing of the suture, adequate depth of bite of the fascia, relaxation of the patient during fascial closure, and closing the fascial layer only when there is not excessive tension on the closure. For very high-risk patients, an interrupted figure-eight closure is often the wisest choice. While retention sutures were used extensively in the past, their use is less common today, with many surgeons opting to use an absorbable mesh or an interrupted closure. Reduction of massively distended bowel by milking air and fluid back up into the stomach also may facilitate a tension-free closure. This is particularly relevant in patients with bowel obstruction and ileus. While the manipulation takes some time and is tedious, it often results in a tension-free closure.

Wound Infection

Etiology

Wound infections continue to be a significant problem for surgeons in the modern era. Despite significant improve-

---

Box 14-1. Factors Associated With Wound Dehiscence

Technical error (fascial closure)
Intra-abdominal infection
Malnutrition
Advanced age
Chronic corticosteroid use
Wound complications (hematoma, infection, tension)
Underlying disease (diabetes, renal failure, cancer, immune deficiency, chemotherapy, irradiation)
Increased intra-abdominal pressure (ascites, distended bowel, coughing, straining, vomiting)

ments in antibiotics, improved anesthesia, superior instruments, earlier diagnosis of surgical problems, and improved techniques for postoperative vigilance, wound infections continue to occur. While some may view the problem as a merely cosmetic one, that view represents a very shallow understanding of this problem, which causes significant morbidity and expense, substantial patient suffering, and even occasional mortality. It has been estimated that a postoperative wound infection costs about $2000 per patient; and with an overall wound infection rate in healthy, nonobese patients of 2.5%, this translates into a significant cost of $320,000 per year in the United States to treat infected open abdominal surgical incisions. Currently, in the United States, wound infections account for almost 40% of hospital-acquired infections among surgical patients.

The surgical wound encompasses that area of the body both internally and externally that involves the entire operative site. Wounds are thus categorized into three general categories: (1) superficial, which includes skin and subcutaneous tissue, (2) deep, which includes fascia and muscle, and (3) organ space, which includes the internal organs of the body if the operation includes that area. Wound infections, which are also referred to as surgical site infections (SSIs) by the Centers for Disease Control and Prevention, have very specific criteria for diagnosis of both superficial and deep surgical site infections (Box 14-2). Wound infections obviously occur because of bacterial contamination of the surgical site. Bacterial contamination can occur in a variety of ways. One of the most common sources of bacterial contamination is transecting or entering the lumen of a hollow viscus in the abdominal cavity. A second source of bacteria is the skin flora present in all patients. Third, a break in the surgical technique may allow exogenous contamination from the operating surgeon, the equipment, or the surrounding environment.

A host of factors may contribute to the development of postoperative wound infection. In general, these risk factors may be divided into factors associated with the patient and factors associated with the operation. An example of some of the risk factors associated with the operation include a large spill of enteric contents at the time of surgery, failure to prepare the skin preoperatively, and tears in the surgeon's glove. Other operation risk factors are listed in Table 14-1. Similarly, the patient may have a number of risk factors that contribute to the increased operative risk.

The pathogens associated with a postoperative wound infection reflect the area that provided the inoculum for the infection to develop. *Staphylococcus aureus* and coagulase-negative *Staphylococcus* remain the most common bacteria colonized from wounds (Table 14-2).[3] However, where high volumes of gastrointestinal operations are done, the predominant bacteria species will include *Enterobacter* species and *Escherichia coli*. In most studies, group D *Enterococcus* continues to be a common pathogen isolated from postoperative wound infections.

Surgical wounds are classified according to the relative risk of postoperative wound infection occurring. The four

---

Box 14-2. CDC Criteria for Defining a Surgical Site Infection (SSI)

Superficial Incisional

- Infection less than 30 days after operation
- Involves skin and subcutaneous tissue only *plus* one of the following:
  - Purulent drainage
  - Diagnosis of superficial SSI by surgeon
  - Symptoms of erythema, pain, local edema

Deep Incisional

- Less than 30 days after operation with no implant and soft tissue involvement
- Infection less than 1 year after operation with implant and infection involves deep soft tissues (fascia and muscle) *plus* one of the following:
  - Purulent drainage from the deep space but no extension into organ space
  - Abscess is found in the deep space on direct or radiologic examination or on reoperation
  - Diagnosis of a deep space SSI by surgeon
  - Symptoms of fever, pain, and tenderness lead to dehiscence of wound or opening by a surgeon

Organ Space

- Infection less than 30 days after surgery with no implant
- Infection less than 1 year after surgery with implant and infection; involves any part of the operation opened or manipulated *plus* one of the following:
  - Purulent drainage from a drain placed into the organ space
  - Cultured organisms from material aspirated from the organ space
  - Abscess found on direct or radiologic examination or during reoperation
  - Diagnosis of organ space infection by a surgeon

Modified from Mangram AJ, Horan TC, Pearson ML, et al: Guidelines for prevention of surgical site infection. Infect Control Host Epidemiol 20:252, 1999.

---

categories are (1) clean, (2) clean contamined, (3) contaminated, and (4) dirty (Table 14-3).

Presentation and Management

Postoperative wound infections present as erythema, tenderness, edema, and occasionally drainage. The wound is often soft or fluctuant at the site of the infection, which is a departure from the firmness of the healing ridge present elsewhere in the wound. Wound infections most commonly occur 5 to 6 days postoperatively but may present sooner or later than that; the patient may have a leukocytosis and a low-grade fever. According to the Joint Commission on Accreditation of Healthcare Organizations (JCAHO), a surgical wound is considered infected if (1) there is drainage of grossly purulent material from the wound, (2) the wound spontaneously opens and drains purulent fluid, (3) the wound drains fluid that is culture positive or Gram stain positive for bacteria, and (4) the surgeon notes erythema or drainage and opens the wound after deeming it to be infected. A number of studies have indicated that 80% to 90% of all postoperative infections occur within 30 days after the operative procedure. With the increased utilization of outpatient surgery and decreased length of stay in hospitals, 30% to 40% of all wound infections have been shown to occur after hospital discharge. Nevertheless, while less than 10% of surgical patients are hospitalized for 6 days or less, 70% of post-discharge infections occur in that group. Management of a postoperative wound infection depends on the depth of the infection.[4] For a superficial wound infection that involves the subcutaneous tissue and skin, staples are removed over the area of the infection and a cotton-tipped applicator may be easily passed into the wound with

efflux of purulent material and pus. The wound should be gently explored and loculations broken up. After exploration, one should irrigate with normal saline solution in a syringe. Débridement of any nonviable tissue is also an important element of wound management after an infection. At this point, probing the wound with a cotton-tipped applicator will determine whether the fascia or muscle tissues are involved. In an abdominal incision, if the fascia is intact, there are no further concerns about this wound. However, if the fascia has separated and the

TABLE 14-1. Risk Factors for Postoperative Wound Infection

Patient	Operation
Advanced age	Inadequate preoperative preparation
Malnutrition	Duration of operation (long)
Diabetes	No prophylactic antibiotics when indicated
Morbid obesity	Contamination of instruments
Immunosuppression	Break in aseptic technique
Coexisting remote infection	Foreign body in wound
Colonization with bacteria	Ischemic or devitalized tissue
Prior radiation therapy	Amount of intraoperative contamination (spillage)
Smoking	

TABLE 14-2. Pathogens Isolated from Postoperative Surgical Site Infections at a University Hospital

Pathogen	% of Isolates
Staphylococcus (coagulase negative)	25.6
Enterococcus (group D)	11.5
Staphylococcus aureus	8.7
Candida albicans	6.5
Escherichia coli	6.3
Pseudomonas aeruginosa	6.0
Corynebacterium	4.0
Candida (non-*albicans*)	3.4
Alpha-hemolytic *Streptococcus*	3.0
Klebsiella pneumoniae	2.8
Vancomycin-resistant *Enterococcus*	2.4
Enterobacter cloacae	2.2
Citrobacter species	2.0

From Weiss CA, Statz CL, Dahms RA, et al: Six years of surgical wound surveillance at a tertiary care center. Arch Surg 134:1041, 1999.

TABLE 14-3. Classification of Surgical Wounds

Category	Criteria	Infection Rate
Clean	No hollow viscus entered Primary wound closure No inflammation No breaks in septic technique Elective procedure	1%-3%
Clean contaminated	Hollow viscus entered but controlled No inflammation Primary wound closure Minor break in aseptic technique Mechanical drain used Bowel preparation preop	5%-8%
Contaminated	Uncontrolled spillage from viscus Inflammation apparent Open, traumatic wound Major break in aseptic technique	20%-25%
Dirty	Untreated, uncontrolled spillage from viscus Pus in operative wound Open suppurative wound Severe inflammation	30%-40%

pus appears to be coming from deep to the fascia, there is obvious concern about an intra-abdominal wound that may require either computed tomographic (CT)-guided drainage or possible reoperation.

Careful evaluation of a wound infection that involves the fascia and muscle layer would include evaluating for the possibility of a fasciitis, which is associated with a grayish dishwater-colored fluid as well as frank necrosis of the fascial layer. If this process seems to be extensive, the wound needs to be opened and aggressively débrided. The presence of gram-positive rods suggests the presence of *Clostridia perfringens,* which constitutes an urgent or emergent surgical problem. The presence of crepitus in any surgical wound is a surgical emergency and signifies an aggressive clostridiomyonecrosis. Rapid and expeditious surgical débridement is indicated in this setting. After the wound has been adequately cleaned, the wound should be packed to its base with saline-moistened gauze to allow healing of the wound from the base anteriorly to prevent premature skin closure. If there is widespread cellulitis, additional intravenous antibiotics should be considered. A culture of the abscess should be sent in most cases, although that is controversial. If the wound appears to be a small superficial infection, culture may not be necessary. However, if fascial dehiscence and a more complex infection is present, a culture should be sent. Premature closure of the skin should rarely be considered in a wound infection, because it virtually always results in recurrent infection in the deeper spaces. Most postoperative infections should be treated using healing by secondary intention (allowing the wound to heal from the base anteriorly with epithelialization being the final event). In some cases when there is a question about the amount of contamination, a delayed primary closure may be considered. In this setting, close observation of the wound for 5 days may be followed by closure of the skin if the wound looks clean and the patient is otherwise doing well.

Prevention

The operating surgeon plays a major role in reducing or minimizing the presence of postoperative wound infections.[5] Patients who are heavy smokers should be encouraged to stop smoking around the time of the operation. Obese patients should be encouraged to lose weight if the procedure is elective and there is time to allow significant weight loss. There is good evidence that tight control of glucose levels, especially in diabetics, will lower the risk of wound infections. Similarly, patients who are on high doses of corticosteroids will have lower infection rates if weaned off of corticosteroids or are, at least, on a lower dose. The night before surgery, patients should be encouraged to take a shower or bath in which an antibiotic soap is used. Similarly, for patients who are undergoing intra-abdominal surgery, a bowel preparation should be strongly considered. Particularly in surgery of the colon and small bowel, preoperative bowel preparation lowers the patient's infection risk from that of a contaminated case (25%) to a clean-contaminated case (5%). A number of strategies for bowel preparation are available,

but among the most common is use of a large volume of nonabsorbable oral fluid (lavage). Similarly, placing the patient on clear liquids associated with magnesium-based cathartics for 2 days before surgery seems to work quite effectively. In addition to the cleansing of the bowel, oral antibiotics, including nonabsorbable neomycin and erythromycin, are used to lower the bacteria count. At the time of the operation, the surgeon should make certain that the patient undergoes a thorough skin preparation with appropriate antiseptic solutions such as iodine-based solutions and is draped in a very thorough and careful fashion. During every step of the operation, the surgeon can make certain that there is careful handling of the tissues. Meticulous hemostasis and débridement of devitalized tissue will be helpful. Similarly, compulsive control of all intraluminal contents is imperative. Ensuring that the operated organs have adequate blood supply for healing also seems to be an important element of preventing wound infections. Eliminating a foreign body from the wound is another factor that the surgeon can control. There is strong clinical evidence that keeping the patient euthermic during the operation plays a major role in avoiding postoperative infections. The surgeon also must be careful to ascertain that there are no breaks in sterile techniques, such as holes in the glove or use of instruments that have been contaminated. Similarly, care should be demonstrated to avoid environmental contamination, such as debris falling from an overhead light or extensive exposure to the contaminated organ. When purulent drainage is found, thorough drainage of the wound with voluminous warm saline irrigation seems to be an important element in preventing postoperative wound infections. Similarly, the surgeon's judgment at the end of the case with regard to closing skin or packing the wound plays a major role in lowering infection rates.

The role of antibiotic prophylaxis has been thoroughly studied in the general area of wound infections. Clearly, for dirty or contaminated wounds, the use of antibiotics is not prophylactic but, rather, therapeutic and any use of antibiotics in that setting would involve not only preoperative administration but also a full therapeutic course of the indicated antibiotics. The greatest controversy occurs in the area of clean surgery. Most surgeons do not believe that preoperative antibiotics are indicated for clean operations. However, there are some recent data that indicate a small but significant benefit may be achieved through prophylactic administration of a first-generation cephalosporin for certain types of clean surgery (e.g., mastectomy and herniorrhaphy). This remains controversial, and most surgeons at the present time do not give preoperative prophylactic antibiotics. However, there is convincing evidence that for clean-contaminated procedures, the administration of preoperative antibiotics is indicated. The appropriate preoperative antibiotic is a function of the most likely inoculum based on the area being operated on. For example, for patients who may have placement of a prosthesis in a clean wound, preoperative antibiotics would include something to protect against *Staphylococcus aureus* and *Streptococcus* species. A first-generation cephalosporin, such as cefazolin, would be appropriate in this setting. For patients undergoing upper gastrointestinal tract surgery, complex biliary tract operations, or elective colonic resections, administration of a second-generation cephalosporin such as cefoxitin or a penicillin derivative with a β-lactamase inhibitor would be suitable. Surgeons would give a preoperative dose, appropriate intraoperative doses approximately 4 hours apart, and two postoperative doses appropriately spaced. There is convincing evidence that the timing of the prophylactic antibiotic administration is critical. To be most effective, the prophylactic antibiotic agent should be administered intravenously before the incision is made so that the tissue levels are present at the time the wound is created and exposed to the bacterial contamination. A good time to administer the preoperative dose is when the patient arrives in the operating room. Most often, a period of anesthesia induction, prepping, and draping takes place that is adequate to allow tissue levels to build up to therapeutic levels before the incision is made. Of equal importance is making certain that the prophylactic antibiotic is not administered for extended periods postoperatively. To do so in the prophylactic setting is to invite the development of drug-resistant organisms as well as serious complications such as pseudomembranous colitis.

The use of drains remains somewhat controversial in preventing postoperative wound infections. In general, there is virtually no indication for drains in this setting. There is some evidence that in small wounds (e.g., appendectomy wounds with gangrenous appendicitis) a small rubber vessel loop placed in the wound of the thin patient may allow any drainage of contaminated fluid for the first few days while host defenses minimize the risk of infection. Similarly, some surgeons have placed closed suction drains in very deep, large wounds to prevent the accumulation of contaminated fluid. This seems to be particularly germane where large skin flaps are present.

Chronic Wounds

Etiology

Chronic wounds are wounds that by definition have not healed completely within 30 to 90 days of the operative procedure. A host of causes may be found for these large granulating wounds with shaggy granulation tissue. They are commonly found in patients on high doses of corticosteroids, cancer patients who are immune suppressed, patients who are undergoing chemotherapy, patients who have had radiation therapy, malnourished patients, morbidly obese patients with huge wounds, or patients in whom wound dehiscence occurred and there is a large granulating base. Nonhealing perineal wounds can occur in patients who have had previous irradiation, Crohn's disease, AIDS, or cancer.

Presentation and Management

Patients with large chronic wounds require a great deal of patience and willingness to work with them. Sometimes the wound is simply so large due to an abdominal dehiscence or massive wound infection that epithelization is difficult. In these patients, a fenestrated skin graft will often accelerate epithelization and help the wound to heal. Patients who have slow healing of a granulating wound otherwise will notice that the granulation tissue is often exuberant and has a purple color rather than a beefy red color. Often there is substantial exudation from chronic wounds of this nature that appears to impair their healing. Meticulous wound care in the way of frequent dressing changes or the use of a wound suction system may accelerate healing of these chronic wounds. Recent development of a negative pressure wound treatment device has shown promise in the treatment of these difficult, chronic wounds.[6] If the granulation is exuberant, occasionally débridement of the wound is helpful and provides a well-vascularized base from which healthy granulation can occur. Similarly, if there is underlying infection responsible for the nonhealing wound, surgical management of that infection is appropriate. Occasional rotation of a full-thickness skin flap over a chronic, nonhealing wound is indicated. This is particularly applicable in the perineum and pelvis, where wounds may be extremely hard to heal. Quantitative wound cultures may be helpful in identifying organisms that are not responding to current antibiotic use. Reducing corticosteroid doses and improving nutritional status may also help in wound healing. There is some evidence that epidermal growth factor preparations may help heal some types of chronic wounds.

Prevention

Preventing large chronic wounds is often difficult but, in situations where one can, avoiding an operation in a radiated field, encouraging an obese patient to lose weight before surgery or to improve nutritional status before surgery, and having the patient cease smoking may all contribute to preventing a chronic wound infection.

COMPLICATIONS OF THERMAL REGULATION

Hypothermia

Etiology

Optimal function of physiologic systems in the body occurs within a narrow range of body temperatures. A drop in body temperature of 2°C or an increase of 3°C signifies a health emergency that is life threatening requires immediate intervention. Hypothermia can result from a number of mechanisms preoperatively, intraoperatively, or postoperatively. A trauma patient involved with injuries in a cold environment can suffer significant hypothermia[7]; similarly, paralysis leads to hypothermia because of a loss of the shiver mechanism. Rapid resuscitation with cool intravenous fluids leads to hypothermia, and, intraoperatively, the patient who has a large, exposed area from the operation can have significant evaporative cooling. Rapid transfusions intraoperatively can lead to hypothermia as well as irrigation of intracavitary areas with cold saline and a prolonged operation with low ambient room temperature. Postoperatively, the patient can have problems with hypothermia secondary to cool ambient room temperatures, rapid administration of intravenous fluids or blood, and failure to keep the patient covered when he or she is only partially responsive.

The body's response to hypothermia includes a decrease in cardiac output, reduction in heart rate, and, at lower temperatures, cardiac arrhythmias. At temperatures below 35°C, coagulation is significantly affected as well as platelet function.[8] For this reason, bleeding becomes a more serious problem in the hypothermic patient. Patients in shock or with severe illnesses often have associated vasoconstriction, which results in poor perfusion of peripheral organs and tissues. The administration of anesthetics eliminates the shiver response and can also result in significant heat loss intraoperatively. Studies demonstrate that over 80% of elective operative procedures are associated with a drop in body temperature, and 50% of trauma patients are hypothermic on arrival in the operating suite.

Presentation and Management

Meticulous temperature monitoring is an important part of every operation. Most commonly, the monitoring is done with an esophageal thermometer, but a rectal thermometer and oral thermometer may be used as well. In severe cases the patient can have significant cardiac slowing and may be comatose with low blood pressure, bradycardia, and a very low respiratory rate.

Other complications include the previously mentioned cardiac alterations, a relative diuresis, compromised hepatic function, and some neurologic manifestations. Similarly, the patient's ability to manage acid-based abnormalities as well as his or her capacity to fight infection is compromised by hypothermia. There is significant literature suggesting that careful control of body temperatures intraoperatively significantly lowers infection rates postoperatively.

Whether emergency surgery for trauma or elective procedures are planned, a surgeon must be aware of the importance of maintaining euthermia from the very onset of management. A wide variety of modalities are available to assist in maintaining the euthermic patient during surgery or improving the hypothermic patient who arrives in the operating suite. If the patient does not require immediate operative intervention but is profoundly hypothermic, attention should be first directed to warming the patient before an operation. Modalities include (1) immediate placement of warm blankets as well as currently available forced air warming devices, (2) infusion of blood and intravenous fluids through a warming device, (3) heating and humidifying inhalation gases, (4) peritoneal lavage with warmed fluids, (5) rewarming infusion devices using an arteriovenous system,[9] and (6) in rare cases, cardiopulmonary bypass. Special attention should be paid to cardiac monitoring during the rewarming process, because cardiac irritability may be a significant problem. Similarly, acid-base disturbances should be corrected aggressively while the patient is being rewarmed. For elective operations, ambient room temperature should be increased while the patient is being anesthetized and during skin prepping, because significant evaporative cooling can take place. After the patient is draped, the room temperature can be lowered to a more comfortable setting. Similarly, warming devices should be placed on the patient, such as forced air warming devices. There is some evidence that significant amounts of heat loss occur through the head of the patient, so simply covering the patient's head during surgery may prevent significant heat loss.

Prevention

The simplest and easiest way to deal with problems of hypothermia is to prevent them from occurring in the first place. This requires an anxious and ready awareness of the problem and prevention in all elective operations and rapid correction in emergency cases as well as trauma cases.

Malignant Hyperthermia

Etiology and Presentation

Malignant hyperthermia is a rare autosomal dominant–inherited disorder of skeletal muscle. The condition is characterized by a hypermetabolic state triggered by exposure to certain inhalation agents or succinylcholine. The incidence is increased when succinylcholine is used but, in general, is thought to be in the range of 1 per 50,000 cases. The majority of cases occur in children and young adults. The condition is created when uncontrolled amounts of intracellular calcium accumulate in skeletal muscle. The anesthetic agents associated with this reaction include older anesthetics such as halothane and enflurane but also isoflurane, desflurane, and sevoflurane. The incidence may even be increased when the aforementioned agents are associated with the use of succinylcholine. The disorder may present within 30 minutes after administration of the anesthetic agents, and the clinical presentation is variable both in onset and severity. The most severe cases are associated with high fever, tachycardia, muscular rigidity, and cyanosis. However, it may occur at any time during anesthesia or as late as 24 hours postoperatively. The test for diagnosing malignant hyperthermia is the halothane-caffeine contracture test. This requires a muscle biopsy with exposure to halothane and caffeine, which cause significant muscle contraction. Similarly, patients with malignant hyperthermia may have extremely high levels of creatinine kinase, with peak levels occurring from 12 to 18 hours after the hyperthermia begins. Patients with malignant hyperthermia may also have a significant metabolic acidosis as well as hyperkalemia and hypercalcemia.

Treatment

Most cases of malignant hyperthermia will be diagnosed by the anesthesiologist while monitoring during the pro-

Box 14-3. Management of Malignant Hyperthermia

Stop inhalation agent.
Cancel or conclude surgery.
Administer dantrolene, 2.5 mg/kg (may repeat).
Start 100% oxygen.
Cool body with hypothermia blanket, cold intravenous solution, cool lavage of body cavity.
Correct metabolic acidosis with 2 mEq/kg bicarbonate.
Monitor with arterial line and central venous pressure line.
Monitor electrocardiogram and urinary output.
Reverse hyperkalemia with $CaCl_2$ (10 mg/kg) and insulin (0.2 unit/kg in 50% glucose solution).

From Landsman IS, Cook DR: Pediatric Anesthesia. *In* O'Neill JA, Rowe MI, Grosfeld JL, et al (eds): Pediatric Surgery, 5th ed. St. Louis, Mosby, 1998, pp 197-228.

TABLE 14-4.   Causes of Postoperative Fever

Infectious	Noninfectious
Abscess	Acute hepatic necrosis
Acalculous cholecystitis	Adrenal insufficiency
Bacteremia	Allergic reaction
Pseudomembranous colitis	Atelectasis
Device-related infections	Dehydration
Empyema	Drug reaction
Endocarditis	Head injury
Fungal sepsis	Hepatoma
Hepatitis	Hypothyroidism
Decubitus ulcers	Solid organ hematoma
Meningitis	Lymphoma
Soft tissue infection	Myocardial infarction
Osteomyelitis	Pancreatitis
Sinusitis	Pheochromocytoma
Parotitis	Pulmonary embolus
Perineal infections	Retroperitoneal hematoma
Peritonitis	Subarachnoid hemorrhage
Pharyngitis	Systemic inflammatory response syndrome
Pneumonia	Thrombophlebitis
Retained foreign body	Transfusion reaction
Tracheobronchitis	Withdrawal syndromes
Urinary tract infection	
Wound infection	

cedure. The anesthesiologist should immediately discontinue the use of the inhalation agent and administer dantrolene, 2.5 mg/kg, to treat this life-threatening condition. Correction of any electrolyte disturbances should be done as soon as possible. The patient should be hyperventilated with oxygen and the cardiac function monitored carefully. Sometimes this may involve discontinuing or ending an operation prematurely, but this should be done because of the life-threatening nature of this problem (Box 14-3). A cooling blanket should be used to lower the patient's core body temperature.

Postoperative Fever

Etiology

One of the most concerning clinical findings in a patient postoperatively is the development of a persistent fever. A host of infectious and noninfectious agents may cause a postoperative fever, and although most of them do not represent serious threats to the patient, those that do must be sought out and managed. Temperature modulation is managed by the anterior hypothalamus, which reacts to a variety of systemic stimuli. A slight postoperative fever is so common that in most patients it is not considered a serious threat and usually dissipates quickly. However, the patient who has a high, sustained fever with large fluctuations is a concern to all clinicians. Table 14-4 lists a number of the causes of clinical diseases that can result in a fever.

Presentation and Management

Postoperative fevers are less concerning for the first 48 to 72 hours postoperatively. During this interval, most fevers are believed to be caused by atelectasis, which can be managed by having the patient cough and breathe deeply, both of which open up the alveoli. Occasionally, clostridial or streptococcal wound infections can manifest as a fever within the first 72 hours, but this is extremely uncommon. Temperatures that are elevated 5 to 8 days postoperatively are a concern and are usually associated with something that needs to be evaluated or treated by the surgical team. Evaluation of the patient 5 to 8 days postoperatively usually involves studying the five "Ws" associated with postoperative fever. They include wind (lungs), wound, water (urinary tract), waste (lower gastrointestinal tract), and wonder drug. A chest radiograph to evaluate the lungs for evidence of pneumonia as well as urinalysis to look for urinary tract infection is a good place to start. Careful evaluation of the patient to look for evidence of wound infection or phlebitis is important. Similarly, deep vein thrombosis can be associated with fever as well as pulmonary embolus. A number of medications can be associated with fevers, and the patient's drug use should be reviewed. Similarly, if the patient has diarrhea and fever, clostridial infection associated with pseudomembranous colitis should be considered. Patients who continue to have a fever and slow clinical progress may require CT of the abdomen to look for occult, intra-abdominal infection accounting for the fever. Management of postoperative fevers is dictated by the results of the careful work-up. Although temperature elevation of 2°C to 3°C is not immediately life threatening, the persistence of the temperature elevation associated with slow clinical progress and general malaise of the patient usually signifies a significant problem that should stimulate an aggressive work-up.[10] More controversial is management of the elevated temperature itself. Although the temperature may not be life threatening, the patient is usually uncomfortable, and attempts to bring the temperature down using antipyretics are recommended by most surgeons.

Respiratory Complications

General Considerations

A host of factors contribute to the abnormal pulmonary physiology present after an operative procedure. First, a loss of functional residual capacity is present in virtually all patients. This loss may be due to a host of problems, including abdominal distention, a painful upper abdominal incision, obesity, a strong smoking history with associated chronic obstructive pulmonary disease, prolonged supine positioning, and fluid overload leading to pulmonary edema.

Virtually all patients who undergo an abdominal incision or a thoracic incision have a significant alteration of their breathing pattern. Vital capacity may be reduced up to 50% of normal for the first 2 days after surgery for reasons that are not completely clear. Use of narcotics substantially inhibits the respiratory drive, and anesthetics may take some time to wear off. The majority of patients who have respiratory problems postoperatively have mild to moderate problems that can be managed with aggressive pulmonary toilet. However, a portion of patients develop a severe postoperative respiratory failure, which may lead to intubation and ultimately be life threatening.

Two types of respiratory failure are commonly described. Type I, or hypoxic, failure results from abnormal gas exchange at the alveolar level.[11-13] This type is characterized by a low PaO_2 with normal $PaCO_2$. This type of hypoxemia is associated with ventilation-perfusion mismatching and shunting. Clinical conditions associated with type I include pulmonary edema and sepsis. Type II respiratory failure is associated with hypercapnia and is characterized by a low PaO_2 and a high $PaCO_2$. These patients are unable to adequately eliminate CO_2. This condition is often associated with excessive narcotic use, increased CO_2 production, altered respiratory dynamics, and adult respiratory distress syndrome (ARDS). The overall incidence of pulmonary complications exceeds 25% of surgical patients. Twenty-five percent of all postoperative deaths are due to pulmonary complications, and pulmonary complications are associated with a fourth of the other lethal complications. Thus, it is of critical importance that the surgeon anticipates and prevents serious respiratory complications from occurring.

One of the most important elements of this prophylaxis is careful preoperative screening of patients. The majority of patients have no pulmonary history and need no formal preoperative evaluation. However, a patient with a history of heavy smoking, a patient on home oxygen, a patient who is unable to walk one flight of stairs without severe respiratory compromise, a patient with a prior history of major lung resection, and an elderly patient who is malnourished all should be carefully screened with pulmonary function tests. Similarly, patients who are on chronic bronchodilator therapy for asthma or other pulmonary conditions should be carefully assessed as well. Although there is some controversy about the value of perioperative assessment, most careful clinicians will study a high-risk pulmonary patient before making an operative decision. The assessment may start with posteroanterior and lateral chest radiographs to evaluate the appearance of the lungs. It serves as a baseline if the patient should have problems postoperatively. Similarly, a patient with polycythemia or chronic respiratory acidosis warrants careful assessment. A room arterial blood gas analysis should be obtained on high-risk patients. Any patient with a PaO_2 less than 60 mm Hg is at increased risk. If the $PaCO_2$ is greater than 45 to 50 mm Hg, perioperative morbidity might be anticipated. Spirometry is a simple test that high-risk patients should have before surgery. Probably the most important parameter in spirometry is the forced expiratory volume in 1 second (FEV_1). Studies demonstrate that any patient who has an FEV_1 greater than 2 L will probably not have serious pulmonary problems. Conversely, patients with an FEV_1 less than 50% of the predicted value will likely have exertional dyspnea. If bronchodilator therapy demonstrates an improvement in breathing patterns by 15% or more, bronchodilatation should be considered. Consultation with the patient should include a discussion about cessation of cigarette smoking 48 hours before the operative procedure as well as a careful discussion about the importance of pulmonary toilet after the operative procedure.

Atelectasis and Pneumonia

The most common postoperative respiratory complication is atelectasis.[14] As a result of the anesthetic, an abdominal incision, and postoperative narcotics, the alveoli in the periphery collapse and a pulmonary shunt may occur. If appropriate attention is not directed to aggressive pulmonary toilet with the presenting symptoms, the alveoli remain collapsed and a build-up of secretion occurs that becomes secondarily infected with bacteria. The risk appears to be particularly high in patients who are heavy smokers, are obese, and have copious pulmonary secretions. Careful postoperative surveillance will detect the early signs and symptoms of atelectasis, and the prudent surgeon will immediately instigate aggressive pulmonary toilet to obviate the development of a frank pneumonia. While pneumonia acquired on the hospital ward accounts only for 5% of all patients, particularly in elderly patients, the process may rapidly progress to frank respiratory failure requiring intubation.

Presentation and Management

The most common cause of a postoperative fever in the first 48 hours after the procedure is atelectasis. The patients present with a low-grade fever, malaise, and diminished breath sounds in the lower lung fields. Very often the patient is uncomfortable from the fever but has no other overt pulmonary symptoms. Atelectasis is so common postoperatively that a formal work-up is usually not required. With the use of incentive spirometry, deep breathing, and coughing, the majority of cases of atelectasis will resolve without any difficulty. However, if aggressive toilet is not instituted or the patient refuses to participate, frank development of pneumonia is likely. The patient with pneumonia will have a high fever, occasionally mental confusion, and the production of a thick secretion with coughing, leukocytosis, and a chest radiograph that reveals infiltrates. If the patient is not expeditiously diagnosed and treated, this condition may rapidly progress to respiratory failure and require intubation. Simultaneous with initiation of aggressive pulmonary toilet, induced sputum for culture and sensitivity should be sent immediately to the laboratory. While awaiting the results of such a culture, broad-spectrum intravenous antibiotics should be instituted. Once the organisms are cultured from the sputum, a specific antibiotic should be used as indicated.

Prevention

Prevention of atelectasis and pneumonia is associated with pain control, which allows the patient to take deep breaths and cough. A patient-controlled analgesia device seems to be associated with better pulmonary toilet, as does the use of an epidural infusion catheter, particularly for patients with epigastric incisions. Respiratory care, otherwise, begins preoperatively. The patient should be instructed in use of the incentive spirometer and be held accountable by nurses and physicians during rounds. Encouraging the patient to breathe deeply and cough is the single most valuable management approach in resolving atelectasis and pneumonia. Encouraging the patient to cough while applying counter-pressure with a pillow on the abdominal incision site is most helpful. Rarely, other modalities such as intermittent positive-pressure breathing and chest physiotherapy may be required.

Aspiration Pneumonitis

Etiology

A host of iatrogenic maneuvers place the patient at increased risk for aspiration pneumonitis in a hospital setting. Very often the patient presents to the hospital with an acute clinical problem with a full stomach. During anesthesia induction, patients are sedated and lose control of the ability to clear the airway. The aforementioned setting is probably the most common cause of aspiration in a hospital setting. However, there are other scenarios in which aspiration is likely. They include the patient with a nasogastric tube, the patient with a recent stroke or debility making it difficult to swallow and clear the airway, the patient who is on extremely high doses of narcotics, and the patient who becomes obtunded during a deterioration of the medical condition. The pathophysiology of aspiration pneumonitis is associated with pulmonary intake of gastric contents at a low pH associated with particulate matter. The lower the pH, the greater the injury to the bronchiolar mucosa. The physiologic response to the injury is sloughing of the epithelium, influx of fluid, atelectasis and, on occasion, even hemorrhage. The patient will have a dramatic inflammatory response to the injury and usually develop a severe pulmonary infection, which is refractory to management because of the combination of infection occurring in an injured field. Aspiration pneumonitis often progresses very rapidly and may require intubation soon after the injury occurs.

Presentation and Management

The patient with aspiration often has associated vomiting at the time the aspiration occurs. This may occur during induction for anesthesia, on the ward with a nasogastric tube, or with the obtunded patient whose condition is deteriorating. Initially, the patient may have associated wheezes and labored respiration. However, it often rapidly progresses to frank respiratory failure associated with low oxygen saturation and a low PO_2. Patients who sustain this injury need to be immediately placed on oxygen and have a chest radiograph to confirm the clinical suspicions. A diffuse interstitial pattern is usually seen bilaterally that is often described as bilateral, fluffy infiltrates.

Close surveillance of the patient immediately after aspiration is absolutely essential. If the patient is maintaining oxygen saturation with a face mask and is not requiring excessively high work of breathing, intubation may not be required. However, if the patient's oxygenation deteriorates, the work of breathing increases as manifested by an increased respiratory rate; or if the patient is obtunded, prompt intubation should be accomplished. After intubation, aggressive suctioning of the bronchopulmonary tree will usually confirm the diagnosis. Although the use of antibiotics is controversial in aspiration pneumonitis, most clinicians would probably start the patient on broad-spectrum antibiotic therapy.

Prevention

Identification of the high-risk patient for aspiration pneumonitis is important. When one considers that anesthesia increases the risk of aspiration pneumonitis, strategies including adequate preoperative fasting, the use of H_2 blockers preoperatively, the use of pressure on the trachea during intubation, and even awake intubation may be warranted in high-risk patients. Similarly, in the postoperative period, identification of the elderly or overly sedated patient or the patient whose condition is deteriorating mandates maneuvers to protect the patient's airway. Postoperatively, it is important to avoid the overuse of narcotics, encourage the patient to ambulate, and cautiously feed a patient who is obtunded, elderly, or debilitated.

Pulmonary Edema, Acute Lung Injury, and Adult Respiratory Distress Syndrome

Etiology

A wide variety of injuries to the lungs and/or cardiovascular system may result in acute respiratory failure.[15] Three of the most common manifestations of such injury are pulmonary edema, acute lung injury (ALI), and ARDS. The clinician's ability to recognize and distinguish between these conditions is of critical importance because clinical management of these three entities varies significantly.

Pulmonary edema is a condition associated with accumulation of fluid in the alveoli. As a result of the fluid in the lumen of the alveoli, oxygenation cannot take place and hypoxemia occurs. As a consequence, the patient must increase the work of breathing, including an increased respiratory rate and exaggerated use of the muscles of breathing (Box 14-4). Pulmonary edema is usually due to increased vascular hydrostatic pressure associated with congestive heart failure and acute myocardial infarction. It is also commonly associated with fluid overload due to overly aggressive resuscitation.

A recent consensus conference identified ALI and ARDS as two separate grades of respiratory failure secondary to injury. In contrast to pulmonary edema, which is associated with increased wedge and right-sided heart pressures, ALI and ARDS are associated with hypo-oxygenation due to a pathophysiologic inflammatory response that leads to the accumulation of fluid in the alveoli as well as thickening in the space between the capillaries and the alveoli.[16] ALI is associated with a PaO_2/FIO_2 ratio of less than 300, bilateral infiltrates on chest radiography, and a wedge pressure of less than 18 mm Hg. It tends to be shorter in duration and not as severe. On the other hand, ARDS is associated with a PaO_2/FIO_2 ratio of less than 200 and also has bilateral infiltrates and a wedge pressure of less than 18 mm Hg.

Presentation and Management

Patients with pulmonary edema often have a corresponding cardiac history and/or a recent history of massive fluid administration. In the presence of the frankly abnormal chest radiograph, invasive monitoring in the form of a Swan-Ganz catheter to detect pulmonary capillary wedge pressure is indicated. The patient with an elevated wedge pressure should be managed with the administration of fluid restriction and aggressive diuresis. Administration of oxygen via face mask in mild cases, and intubation in more severe cases, is also clinically indicated. In most cases with diuresis and fluid restriction, pulmonary edema resolves quickly.

The patients presenting with ALI and ARDS usually have tachypnea, dyspnea, and increased work of breathing, as manifested by exaggerated use of the muscles of

---

> ### Box 14-4. Conditions Leading to Pulmonary Edema, Acute Lung Injury, and ARDS
>
> **Increased Hydrostatic Pressure**
>
> Acute left ventricular failure
> Chronic congestive heart failure
> Volume overload
> Thoracic lymphatic insufficiency
> Obstruction of left ventricular outflow tract
>
> **Altered Permeability State**
>
> Acute radiation pneumonitis
> Aspiration of gastric contents
> Drug overdose
> Near-drowning
> Pancreatitis
> Pneumonia
> Pulmonary embolus
> Shock states
> Systemic inflammatory response syndrome and multiple organ failure
> Sepsis
> Transfusion
> Trauma and burns
>
> **Mixed or Incompletely Understood Pathogenesis**
>
> Hanging injuries
> High-altitude pulmonary edema
> Narcotic overdose
> Neurogenic pulmonary edema
> Postextubation obstructive pulmonary edema
> Re-expansion pulmonary edema
> Tocolytic therapy
> Uremia

---

breathing. Cyanosis is associated with advanced hypoxia and is an emergency. Auscultation of the lung fields reveals very poor breath sounds associated with crackles and, occasionally, with rales. An arterial blood gas analysis will reveal the presence of a low PaO_2 and a high $PaCO_2$. Administration of oxygen alone usually does not produce an improvement in the hypoxia. In the presence of the clinical observation of impending respiratory failure, including tachypnea, dyspnea, and air hunger, management of ALI and ARDS should be initiated by immediate intubation associated with careful administration of fluids and invasive monitoring with a Swan-Ganz catheter to assess wedge pressures and right-sided heart pressures. The strategy should be one of maintaining the patient on the ventilator with assisted breathing while healing of the injured lung takes place. The patient with severe ALI or ARDS should be initially placed on an FIO_2 of 100% and then weaned to 60% as healing takes place. Positive end-expiratory pressure (PEEP) is a valuable addition to ventilator management of patients with this injury. Similarly, the tidal volume should be 6 to 8 mL/kg with peak pressures kept at 35 cm H_2O. Tidal volume should be set at 10 to 12 mL/kg of body weight and the respiratory rate chosen to produce a $PaCO_2$ near 40 mm Hg. Similarly, the inspiratory to expiratory ratio should be set at 1:2. Most patients will require heavy sedation and pharmacologic paralysis during the early phases of their recuperation.

Careful monitoring of oxygenation, respiratory rate with intermittent mandatory ventilation, and general alertness will suggest when the patient is ready to be extubated. Criteria for extubation are listed in Table 14-5.

Pulmonary Embolism

Etiology

Pulmonary embolus is a serious postoperative complication that represents a source of preventable morbidity and mortality in the United States. Approximately 500,000 cases of pulmonary embolus occur each year, 100,000 of which are fatal. Any operative procedure increases the risk of postoperative venous thromboembolic disease and pulmonary embolus by causing a perturbation of the homeostatic coagulation system with intimal injury, stasis of blood flow, and a hypercoagulable state. Risk factors for the development of pulmonary embolus are listed in Box 14-5.[17]

The iliofemoral venous system represents the site from which most clinically significant pulmonary emboli arise.

TABLE 14-5.	Criteria for Weaning from the Ventilator
Parameter	**Weaning Criteria**
Respiratory rate	<25 breaths/min
PaO_2	>70 mm Hg (FiO_2 < 40%)
$PaCO_2$	<45 mm Hg
Minute ventilation	8-9 L/min
Tidal volume	5-6 mL/kg
Negative inspiratory force	–25 cm H_2O

Box 14-5. Risk Factors for Pulmonary Embolus

Prior pulmonary embolus
Lengthy operative procedures
Oral contraceptives
Traumatic injuries
Malignancy
Immobilization
Paralysis
Inflammatory bowel disease
Chronic heart disease
Coagulation abnormalities
Obesity
Age
Inherited coagulation abnormalities

The clinical severity of the pulmonary embolus is a function of the clot size that separates from the peripheral venous system and travels to the pulmonary vasculature. Much rarer causes of pulmonary embolus include fat embolus associated with fractures of long bones and air embolism, often associated with operative procedures and central lines.

Presentation and Management

Patients who develop a clinically significant pulmonary embolus will most commonly have dyspnea, pleuritic chest pain, apprehension, and a cough. Massive pulmonary embolus may be associated with syncope and hemoptysis but is much less common. The most common physical signs are tachypnea and tachycardia. About one third of patients with pulmonary embolus will also demonstrate lower extremity findings consistent with deep vein thrombosis. In general, however, the signs and symptoms associated with pulmonary embolus are nonspecific and may suggest a host of clinical problems, including myocardial infarction, pneumothorax, pneumonia, and atelectasis.

When a patient presents with chest pain and shortness of breath on the wards, an immediate battery of nonspecific tests should be obtained, including room air arterial blood gas analysis, electrocardiography, and chest radiography. These tests will rule out other causes for the patient's symptoms. Any patient who has a room air arterial blood gas with a PaO_2 of less than 70 mm Hg should be considered a candidate for pulmonary embolus. ECG changes associated with pulmonary embolus are nondiagnostic and include T-wave inversions and nonspecific ST segment changes. With more severe pulmonary embolus, the ECG may be associated with an S1 Q3 T3 pattern, right bundle branch block, or right-axis deviation. Chest radiographic findings tend to be nonspecific but, occasionally, a pleural-based, wedge-shaped defect can been seen. Occasionally, with very large emboli obstructing the main pulmonary artery, there may be an abrupt cutoff of the pulmonary vascular markings on the affected side (Westermark's sign).

In any patient in whom the diagnosis of pulmonary embolus is seriously considered, an immediate course of treatment and work-up should be begun. The patient should be immediately placed on high-flow oxygen by face mask and, in more severe pulmonary embolus, may even require intubation. Additionally, the patient should be hydrated and sent for immediate diagnostic work-up. Pulmonary angiography for years has been considered the gold standard for making a diagnosis of pulmonary embolus. However, it is an invasive procedure with associated morbidity. For this reason, the ventilation-perfusion scan was developed. The ventilation portion of the scan was performed with the patient inhaling xenon, while the perfusion was performed after intravenous injections of technetium-labeled albumin. The scans were read as "high," "intermediate," or "low" probability. Patients with a high probability of pulmonary embolus required immediate medical management with anticoagulants. However, those with a low probability reading often required a pulmonary angiogram. The development of CT angiography represents a major step forward in diagnosis of pulmonary embolus in a noninvasive fashion and is a very promising new diagnostic modality.[18] This technique is rapid, has very low morbidity, and has 86% sensitivity and 92% specificity. Although it is not as accurate in identifying subsegmental pulmonary emboli, it is rapidly becoming the diagnostic modality of choice for larger pulmonary emboli. It will probably render the ventilation perfusion scan obsolete.

Patients who have a diagnosis of pulmonary embolus should be immediately anticoagulated with 10,000 units of heparin followed by approximately 1000 units per hour thereafter.[19] The partial thromboplastin time must be carefully monitored during the intravenous administration of heparin. In addition to administration of the heparin, patients should be observed in a surgical intensive care unit with high oxygen flow available as well as close monitoring. Patients should also be kept at bed rest for a few days after the pulmonary embolus. The patient should be kept on therapeutic doses of constant intravenous heparin until the clinician is able to institute warfarin therapy, which can be done as soon as the patient is stabilized and started on oral intake. The patient will require anticoagulation therapy for 6 months after development of a pulmonary embolus.

Rarely, a patient develops a massive pulmonary embolus characterized by shock, severe hypoxia, and, on occasion, cyanosis. Immediate treatment of these patients includes intravenous fluids, inotropic agents, and maintenance of a favorable cardiac rhythm. After the diagnosis is made, thrombolytic therapy should be considered in cases in which there has not been recent intracranial pathology or a major abdominal procedure within 10 days. Agents such as streptokinase, urokinase, and tissue plasminogen activator may be considered. On occasion, a decision must be made whether to administer thrombolytic therapy in the presence of a major operation, accepting the likelihood of bleeding to save the patient's life. Even more rarely, pulmonary embolectomy may be considered in a desperate attempt to save the patient's life.

For those patients who are placed on anticoagulation therapy and suffer a major hemorrhage, placement of a vena cava filter should be considered to prevent further pulmonary emboli.

Prevention

The best way to manage patients with potential for pulmonary embolus is to prevent them from occurring.[20,21] A host of agents have been demonstrated to be effective in inhibiting pulmonary embolus. They include elastic compression stockings, sequential pneumatic compression devices, low-molecular-weight heparin, and platelet inhibitors. Particularly, high-risk patients, including those with prior history of deep vein thrombosis and/or pulmonary embolus, should undergo compulsive prophylaxis both before and in the operation. This may include the use of low-molecular-weight heparin preoperatively, sequential pressure devices during the operation, and early institution of low-molecular-weight heparin after the operation. Although there is some risk of bleeding with the use of low-molecular-weight heparin in high-risk patients, the risk is justified. Any patient considered at moderate risk for pulmonary embolus after surgery should undergo the routine use of sequential pressure devices and early ambulation.

CARDIAC COMPLICATIONS

Postoperative Hypertension

Etiology

Hypertension is a serious problem that can cause devastating complications in the preoperative, intraoperative, and postoperative periods. If not adequately controlled, difficulties with perioperative hypertension can exacerbate an incipient aortic aneurysm rupture, result in cerebrovascular accidents, cause arrhythmias, lead to myocardial ischemia or infarction, cause bleeding into the operative wound, and even result in renal failure. It has been estimated that 25% of patients with a prior history of hypertension will develop postoperative hypertension in the postanesthesia periods. Preoperatively most hypertension is essential hypertension; much less common are cases associated with renovascular causes, and even rarer is preoperative hypertension due to vasoactive tumors. Intraoperatively, hypertension may be caused by pharmacologic agents. Postoperatively, a host of causes for hypertension include inadequately managed pain, fluid overload, and failure to administer hypertensive medications taken previously. The observant surgeon will consider hypertension in preoperative screening of patients, recognizing that failure to detect significant problems with hypertension can lead to needless hypertension-related complications.

Presentation and Management

Most cases of perioperative hypertension are detected during the routine preoperative work-up. Immediate attention to hypertension with pharmacologic agents or medications when pain is contributing to the hypertension is extremely important. Similarly, the development of new-onset postoperative hypertension is an urgent medical matter because of the concerns of stroke and bleeding from the operative wound. This appears to be particularly the case in a carotid endarterectomy, aortic aneurysm surgery, and many head and neck procedures. By definition, any patient who has a diastolic blood pressure greater than 110 mm Hg should be assessed and consideration given to medical management of the hypertension. Certainly, diastolic blood pressure levels at that magnitude should be managed and controlled preoperatively if elective surgery is contemplated. A large variety of pharmacologic agents are available for the management of preoperative and postoperative hypertension. Ideal agents would include those that have a rapid onset of action, short half-life, and few autonomic side effects. Medications most commonly used in this setting include β blockers and α₂ agonists. A number of prospective studies have demonstrated reduced perioperative myocardial complications with β blockade. Ideally, preoperative β blockade is optimal, but even intraoperative β blocker use seems to be effective. There is some evidence that α₂ agonists (clonidine) can reduce perioperative heart complications in some patients. There is also evidence that calcium-channel blockers, angiotensin-converting enzyme (ACE) inhibitors, and intravenous vasodilators such as nitroglycerin and nitroprusside might be protective. The latter two should be reserved for the severe, intractable hypertensive who has not responded to other medications.

Prevention

Tight control of the hypertensive patient who requires emergency surgery is usually not possible. More frequently, the medications administered during induction and utilized during the procedure will assist in bringing the blood pressure down. The anesthesiologist plays a major role in making certain that the intraoperative course is minimally labile and blood pressures stay at acceptable levels. However, patients undergoing elective surgery should have fairly rigorous control of their blood pressure before undergoing the operative procedure. Current recommendations include taking antihypertensive medications on the day of surgery with a sip of water. Intraoperatively, the anesthesiologist should carefully monitor blood pressure and make certain that it stays within acceptable limits. In the postoperative period, the patient should continue to receive antihypertensive medications as well as a pulse of analgesia administration and sedation as required to control his or her blood pressure. In most cases, within 24 to 48 hours postoperative hypertension becomes less labile and more predictable. The patient should continue to take antihypertensive medications during this period.

Perioperative Ischemia and Infarction

Etiology

Approximately 30% of all patients taken to the operating room have some degree of coronary artery disease. Although management of nonoperative myocardial infarctions has improved, the mortality of a perioperative myocardial infarction remains approximately 30%. Perioperative myocardial complications result in at least 10% of all perioperative deaths. There have been recent advances in improving the outcome of patients at risk for coronary artery disease via improved preoperative assessment and postoperative management and monitoring.[22] In the 1970s, the risk of a recurrent myocardial infarction within 3 months of a myocardial infarction was reported to be 30% and, if a patient had surgery between 3 to 6 months of infarction, reinfarction was 15%. If the patient was 6 months out from the operation, his or her rein-farction rate was only 5%. However, more recently, because of improvements in monitoring techniques, anesthesia, and more sophisticated intensive care unit monitoring, individuals undergoing an operation within 3 months of an infarction have an 8% to 15% reinfarction rate and those between 3 and 6 months only a 3.5% reinfarction rate. The general mortality rate for myocardial infarction in patients without a surgical procedure is 12%.

Presentation and Management

The classic presentation of acute myocardial infarction is chest pain often radiating into the jaw and left arm region.[23] However, in surgical patients, the presentation may be more subtle. Whereas left precardial pain is often seen in perioperative myocardial infarction, patients may present with shortness of breath, increased heart rate, hypotension, or respiratory failure. Certainly, shortness of breath and chest pain remain two postoperative symptoms that should always be carefully evaluated and never written off as postoperative discomfort.

Evaluation of the patient suspected of having an intraoperative or postoperative myocardial infarction include immediate ECG assessment as well as serum troponin levels. The majority of episodes of postoperative myocardial ischemia are silent with no clinical signs or symptoms. If the level of cardiac function is a concern, echocardiography may be considered. Similarly, in the clinical scenario in which more extensive cardiac assessment is indicated and the need for cardiac revascularization must be assessed, nuclear imaging studies and angiography should be considered.

Medical management of the infarction once ischemia has been documented includes immediate administration of high flow oxygen, transfer to the intensive care unit, and the early involvement of a cardiologist. Immediate administration of β blockers and aspirin should be instituted as well as systemic heparinization. In most cases thrombolytic therapy is contraindicated in the postoperative period and could be used only in the situation in which minor surgery was done. Judicious use of diuretic agents and antiarrhythmic agents should be considered.[24] There is some recent evidence that emergency stricture dilatation and coronary artery stenting may be more effective than thrombolytic therapy. Constant ECG is required so that the development of any potentially lethal arrhythmia can immediately be treated. Similarly, close assessment to detect early congestive heart failure should be considered.

Angiography should be strongly considered if the patient has ongoing myocardial ischemia that does not respond to pharmacologic therapy. Clearly, the goal of management of myocardial ischemia is to preserve the maximal amount of myocardial muscle possible as well as improving coronary blood flow and decreasing myocardial work.

Prevention

Preventing the complications of coronary ischemia is a function of prospectively identifying the patient at risk for a perioperative cardiac complication. A comprehensive history will identify the patient with a previous history of coronary artery disease, including recent myocardial infarction, presence of valvular heart disease, congestive heart failure, or arrhythmias. Unstable chest pain, especially crescendo angina, warrants a careful evaluation and probable postponing of an elective operation. The cardiac risk index system (CRIS) is a commonly utilized and accepted system of assessing preoperatively the relative risk of a patient undergoing noncardiac surgery (Table 14-6).[25-27]

The detection of a history of significant coronary artery disease or of ongoing symptoms from coronary artery disease mandates a preoperative cardiac work-up with either thallium scanning or angiography, with probable canceling of the elective operative procedure. Similarly, the patient who is found to have congestive heart failure on physical examination or history should have the problem treated before considering an elective operative procedure. An algorithm for perioperative cardiovascular evaluation has been proposed by Eagle and colleagues (Fig. 14-1). Patients identified as having high risk for myocardial events in the perioperative period should be managed with β blockers, careful monitoring intraoperatively, and continued pharmacologic management postoperatively, including the administration of adequate pain medication and even probable monitoring on a telemetry unit.

Cardiogenic Shock

Etiology

Cardiogenic shock is one of the most serious sequelae of an acute myocardial infarction. Presumably, 50% or more of the left ventricular muscle mass is irreversibly damaged, leading to substantial reduction in cardiac output and resulting hypoperfusion.[28] Other possible causes of cardiogenic shock include ruptured papillary muscle, ruptured ventricular wall, aortic valvular insufficiency, mitral regurgitation, or ventricular septal defect. However, the latter groups are seen less frequently. Cardiogenic shock is a highly lethal condition, which results in death to 75% of patients unless immediate management is instituted. Other serious sequelae from acute myocardial infarction include congestive heart failure, arrhythmias, and thromboembolic complications.

Presentation and Management

Observant physicians will watch a patient with an acute myocardial infarction closely for evidence of the aforementioned complications. Cardiogenic shock patients usually develop rapidly over a short period of time and present with hypotension and respiratory failure. Aggressive management is required to save the life of a patient with this devastating condition. The immediate institution

TABLE 14-6. Cardiac Risk Index System (CRIS)

Factors	Points
History	
Age > 70	5
Myocardial infarction <6 months ago	10
Aortic stenosis	3
Physical Examination	
S$_3$ gallop, jugular venous distention, congestive heart failure	11
Bedridden	3
Laboratory Findings	
Po$_2$ < 60 mm Hg	3
Pco$_2$ > 50 mm Hg	3
Potassium < 3 mEq/dL	3
Blood urea nitrogen > 50 mg/dL	3
Creatinine > 3 mg/dL	3
Operation	
Emergency	4
Intrathoracic	3
Intra-abdominal	3
Aortic	3

Incidence of Major Complications (%)					
	Baseline	I (0-5 pts)	II (6-12 pts)	III (13-25 pts)	IV (>26 pts)
Minor surgery	1	0.3	1	3	19
Major noncardiac surgery, age >40	4	1	4	12	48
Aortic surgery, age > 40 with other characteristics	10	3	10	30	75

Adapted from Goldman L: Cardiac risks and complications of non-cardiac surgery. Ann Intern Med 98:504,1983.

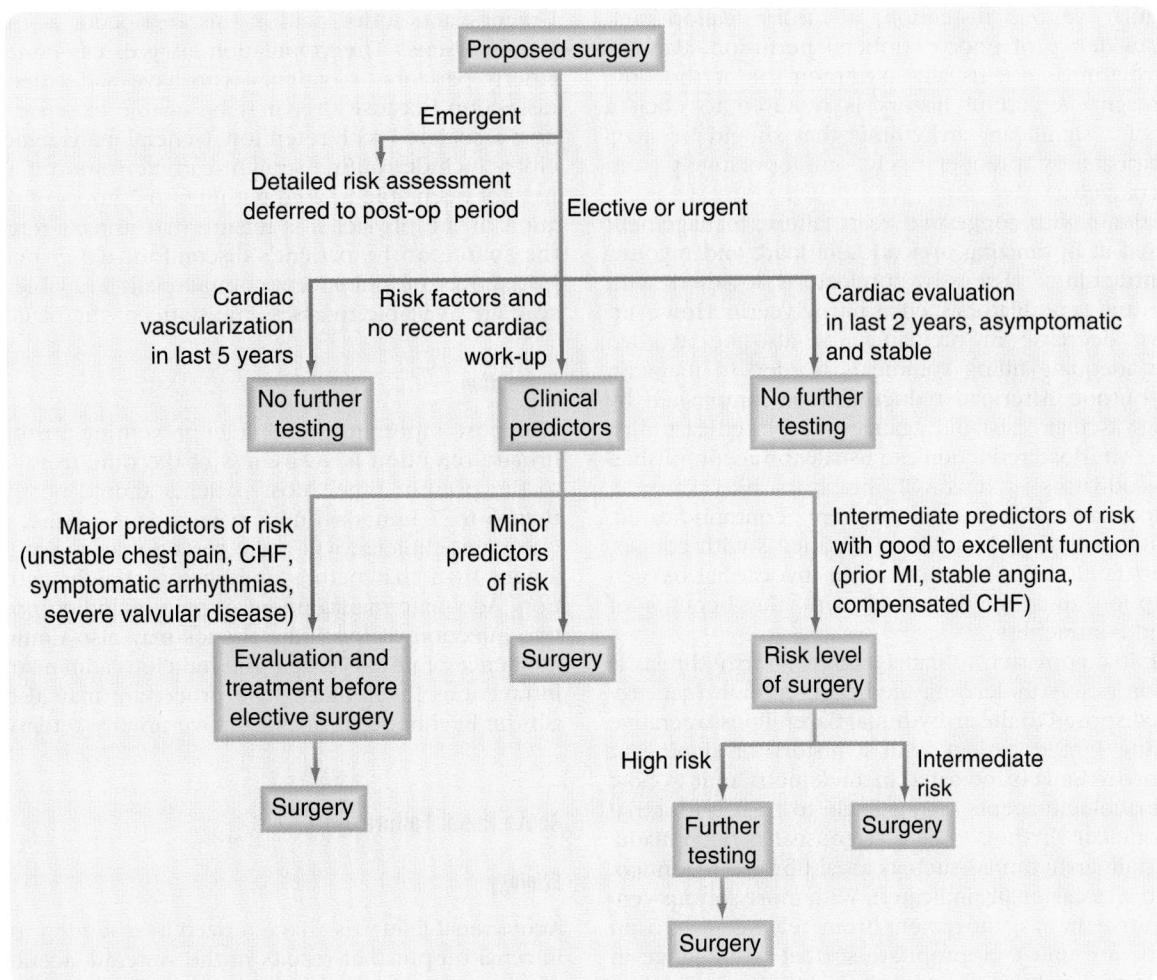

FIGURE 14-1. Algorithm for perioperative cardiovascular evaluations of noncardiac surgery. Patients with major predictors of risk and patients with intermediate predictors of risk and a planned high-risk procedure should undergo additional testing and resultant indicated treatment before elective surgery. MI, myocardial infarction; CHF, congestive heart failure. (Modified from Eagle KA, Brundage BH, Chaitman BR, et al: Guidelines for perioperative cardiovascular evaluation for noncardiac surgery. Report of the American College of Cardiology/American Heart Association Task Force on Practice Guidelines. J Am Coll Cardiol 27:910-945, 1996.)

of mechanical ventilation with high FIO$_2$, as well as monitoring with a Swan-Ganz catheter, is important. For patients who do not respond to pharmacologic and conservative management, intra-aortic balloon pumps and ventricular-assist devices may be lifesaving. For patients who have adequate myocardial reserves, a coronary artery bypass may occasionally be indicated.

Arrhythmias and Congestive Heart Failure

Etiology

Coronary artery disease is the most common cause of arrhythmias and congestive heart failure. It is estimated that 500,000 new cases of congestive heart failure develop each year, with a 2-year mortality of almost 50%. The standard definition of a cardiac arrhythmia is 30 seconds of abnormal cardiac activity, with intraoperative occurrence being 60% to 80%. However, the clinically significant inci-

dence of arrhythmias is probably significantly less than that. Arrhythmias can occur due to electrolyte abnormalities, medications, stress, endocrine abnormalities, and underlying cardiac disease.

Presentation and Management

Poorly controlled congestive heart failure represents one of the most serious cardiac risk factors for a preoperative patient. However, patients with well-managed congestive heart failure generally do well during an operation. Patients with congestive heart failure may present in a variety of ways. The well-managed congestive heart failure patient may have virtually no symptoms as long as he or she takes the prescribed medications. On the other hand, poorly controlled congestive heart failure is a serious clinical scenario, especially when combined with the need for surgery. Patients with uncontrolled congestive heart failure present with shortness of breath, edema, wheezing, jugular venous distention, a cardiac gallop, and general evidence of poor peripheral perfusion. Patients with arrhythmias are usually asymptomatic at the time they present. A careful history is required to elicit a history of a significant arrhythmia that should be managed expectantly preoperatively, intraoperatively, and postoperatively.

In patients with congestive heart failure, management is directed at optimizing preload, afterload, and myocardial contractility.[29] Excessive preload is lowered with diuretics and venodilators such as nitroglycerin. However, excessive decrease in preload must also be avoided because adequate filling volume is needed to maintain cardiac output. Afterload reduction is accomplished by lowering vascular resistance against which the heart must contract. Afterload reduction can usually be accomplished using vasodilators such as ACE inhibitors, nitroprusside, or hydralazine. Vasoconstrictors are contraindicated. Inotropic agents may be utilized in patients with congestive heart failure, but the increase in myocardial oxygen consumption must be balanced with the benefits of increased contractility.

The initial approach to management of arrhythmias is correction of any underlying medical condition that may have predisposed to the arrhythmia. Careful postoperative monitoring of the patient with a history of significant cardiac arrhythmia is indicated in a telemetry unit. A host of pharmacologic agents are available to treat both atrial and ventricular rhythms once a diagnosis has been made. With certain arrhythmias such as atrial fibrillation, anticoagulation is occasionally indicated. With more serious ventricular arrhythmias, movement from telemetry into an intensive care unit is appropriate so that any change in the status of the rhythm can be dealt with immediately.

RENAL AND URINARY TRACT COMPLICATIONS

Urinary Retention

Etiology

Inability to evacuate a urine-filled bladder is referred to as urinary retention. Urinary retention is a common postoperative complication seen in particularly high incidence in patients with perianal operations and hernia repairs. Urinary retention may also occur after operations for low rectal cancer when an injury to the nervous system affects bladder function. Most commonly, however, the complication is a reversible abnormality resulting from discoordination of the trigone and detrusor muscles as a result of increased pain and postoperative discomfort. Urinary retention is also occasionally seen after spinal or epidermal procedures and may occur after overly vigorous intravenous administration of fluid. Rarely, a urethral stricture may also be the cause of urinary retention.

Presentation and Management

Patients with postoperative urinary retention will complain of a dull, constant discomfort in the hypogastrium.

Urgency and actual pain in this area occur as the retention worsens. The population of greatest concern are elderly patients or patients who have had a deep rectal dissection because they may be unable to sense the fullness associated with retention. General management principles include routine straight catheterization if a patient has not been able to void within 6 to 7 hours of the operation. If the physician is unsure that urinary retention is the source of the patient's discomfort, either percussing just above the pubis or a commercially available bladder scan are available to assess the status of the bladder.

Prevention

The most important principle in preventing postoperative urinary retention is awareness of the time from last void to the present time. Most patients should not go more than 6 to 7 hours without passing some urine, and the observant clinician will make certain that no patient goes longer than that before undergoing straight catheterization. Adequate management of pain including postoperative injection of local anesthetics may also diminish the incidence of urinary retention. Judicious administration of intravenous fluids during the procedure may also diminish the likelihood of postoperative urinary retention.

Acute Renal Failure

Etiology

Acute renal failure is characterized by a sudden reduction in renal output that results in the systemic accumulation of nitrogenous wastes. Two types of renal failure have been identified: oliguric and nonoliguric.[30] Oliguric renal failure refers to urine in which volumes of less than 480 mL are seen in a day. Nonoliguric renal failure involves outputs exceeding 2 L/day and is associated with large amounts of isosthenuric urine that clears no toxins from the bloodstream. Most commonly, renal failure is divided into three general categories: prerenal, renal, or postrenal (Table 14-7).[31] Prerenal acute renal failure is usually caused by impaired renal perfusion. This may be due to severe hypovolemia, hemorrhage, dehydration, cardiac malfunction, and insufficient fluid administration during operative procedures and extensive third-space fluid losses during a large dissection. Renal vascular stenosis and thrombosis can also be causes although are much less common. Prerenal failure is often referred to as prerenal azotemia because of the build-up of nitrogenous wastes.

Renal failure usually involves actual injury to the nephrons, glomeruli, or tubules of the kidney. Common causes of renal failure include severe, prolonged prerenal azotemia including prolonged hypotension, toxins including radiographic contrast, medications[32] including aminoglycosides and amphotericin, and myoglobin injuries. Renal failure is frequently the most serious type of failure because, on occasion, it may be irreversible. Postrenal causes of acute renal failure involve obstruction of either the urinary excretory pathway or an injury to the bladder. Examples include ligation of the ureter intraoperatively,

TABLE 14-7. Causes of Postoperative Acute Renal Failure

Prerenal	Renal	Postrenal
Hemorrhage	Toxins (contrast, sepsis)	Ureter ligation
Hypovolemia	Drugs (aminoglycoside, amphotericin)	Bladder dysfunction
Cardiac failure	Pigment nephropathy (myoglobin, hemoglobin)	Urethral obstruction
Dehydration		

damage or injury to the urethra, and obstruction of the urethra due to thrombus or mucus.

Acute renal failure (ARF) is of particular relevance to surgeons because of the common association of ARF with complicated operative procedures. Approximately 10% of patients who undergo operations will have associated ARF during the perioperative course. Some operations appear to be particularly predisposed to associated ARF, including major vascular procedures (ruptured aneurysm, aortobifemoral bypass), renal transplants, cardiopulmonary bypass procedures, major abdominal cases associated with septic shock, and major urologic operations. Similarly, ARF may occur in cases in which there is major blood loss, with transfusion reactions, in serious diabetics undergoing operations, in life-threatening trauma, with major burn injuries, and in multiple organ system failure.

Special mention should be made of the risks of ARF in patients who receive contrast agents during the course of diagnostic work-ups. Particularly, diabetic patients with vascular disease are at risk for major renal injury when contrast agents are administered. If the patient is hypovolemic and already has some renal dysfunction, use of contrast dyes virtually guarantees some degree of renal injury. On occasion, the injury is severe and irreversible.

Blunt trauma with associated crush injuries places the surgery patient at risk because of high serum levels of hematin and myoglobin, both of which are nephrotoxic when found in high levels in the renal tubules. When visualizing "brown" urine, the clinician should rapidly hydrate the patient to induce a diuresis and alkalinize the urine to prevent myoglobin precipitation.

Another special category involves patients with preexisting renal dysfunction. Patients with elevated creatinine levels should be carefully managed in the perioperative period because any perturbation can result in the loss of the remaining renal function and resultant acute tubular necrosis. Judicious hydration, avoidance of nephrotoxic antibiotics, and use of contrast agents only if absolutely indicated can preserve the remaining renal function.

A final special category that can lead to ARF if not quickly diagnosed and treated is the abdominal compartment syndrome. Growing awareness of this problem has led surgeons to intervene surgically, often resulting in dramatic improvement in renal function and preservation of the filtering capacity of the kidneys. This syndrome is due to massive edema of intra-abdominal organs causing intra-abdominal hypertension (>25 cm H_2O as measured through the Foley catheter).[33] This causes decreased renal perfusion and significantly reduces venous and urinary outflow via prerenal and postrenal mechanisms. If this is not quickly diagnosed and treated, irreversible acute tubular necrosis can result. Treatment includes laparotomy with fascial closure using absorbable mesh, thus relieving intra-abdominal pressure.

Presentation and Management

Patients who had normal renal function preoperatively and have virtually no urine postoperatively almost always have postrenal dysfunction. Common causes include a kinked or occluded Foley catheter, and irrigation of the Foley catheter should be the first maneuver. If that is normal, one should suspect ligation of the ureter, often related to complex pelvic cases. If CT reveals hydronephrosis, immediate surgical treatment is indicated. Postrenal causes of ARF are the most dramatic, are the most straightforward to diagnose, and result in significant immediate improvement with treatment.

Distinguishing between prerenal and renal azotemia may be more complicated. Both are heralded by postoperative oliguria (<15 to 20 mL of urine/hr) with associated increases in blood urea nitrogen (BUN) and creatinine. A careful history and preoperative laboratory studies may reveal preexisting renal dysfunction. Patients with large fluid losses from the gastrointestinal tract (e.g., diarrhea, vomiting, fistula, high ileostomy output) often have associated profound dehydration. In such cases, the rise in BUN is usually greater than the rise in creatinine and the ratio of BUN:creatinine is greater than 20. In other patients, examination of the patient may reveal distended neck veins, rales in the lungs, and a cardiac gallop—all signs that a failing heart may be underperfusing the kidneys as the cause of the oliguria.

A few simple laboratory studies may help distinguish between prerenal and renal azotemia. In prerenal causes, the concentrating ability of the nephrons is normal, resulting in a normal urine osmolality and fractional excretion of sodium (>500 mOsm and an FE_{na}< 1, respectively). Conversely, with acute tubular necrosis, the concentrating ability of the kidney is lost and the patient produces urine with a concentration equal to serum and high urine sodium levels (>350 mOsm and >40 mg/L, respectively). See Table 14-8 for a comparison of laboratory tests in prerenal, renal, and postrenal azotemia. The best laboratory test for discriminating prerenal from renal azotemia is probably fractional excretion of sodium (FE_{na}). In prerenal patients, the FE_{na} is 1% or less whereas in renal azotemia patients, it often exceeds 3%.

TABLE 14-8. Diagnostic Evaluation of Acute Renal Failure

Parameter	Prerenal	Renal	Postrenal
Urine osmolality	>500 mOs/L	= Plasma	Variable
Urinary sodium	<20 mOs/L	>50 mOs/L	>50 mOs/L
Fractional excretion of sodium	<1%	>3%	Variable
Urine/plasma creatinine	>40	<20	<20
Urine/plasma urea	>8	<3	Variable
Urine osmolality/plasma osmolality	<1.5	>1.5	Variable

Management of acute renal failure obviously begins with making the correct diagnosis of the cause of the oliguria or anuria. As previously mentioned, postrenal problems are usually managed by clearing the Foley catheter or, in rare cases, reoperating to remove ureter or urethral obstructions. If prerenal azotemia is diagnosed, one has to ascertain whether the hypoperfusion of the kidney is due to hypovolemic or cardiac failure. Distinguishing the two is critical because giving congestive heart failure patients more fluid exacerbates an already failing system. Similarly, giving diuretics to a hypovolemia patient can worsen the renal failure.

If the prerenal patient has no history of cardiac disease, administration of isosmotic fluid (normal saline or lactated Ringer's solutions or blood in patients who have hemorrhaged) is indicated. The intravenous fluid can be given rapidly (1 L/20 to 30 min) in young patients with healthy hearts and a Foley catheter in place to measure hourly urine output and should be administered until the patient is producing a minimum of 30 to 40 mL urine/hr. If fluid administration does not result in improvement of the oliguria, placement of a central venous pressure or Swan-Ganz catheter is indicated to measure left- or right-sided heart filling pressures. In the presence of congestive heart failure, diuretics, fluid restriction, and appropriate cardiac medications are indicated.

If renal azotemia is diagnosed, the treatment must be supportive, with management of fluid and electrolyte imbalances, careful monitoring of fluid administration, avoidance of nephrotoxic agents, provision of adequate nutrition, and adjustment of the doses of renally excreted medications until the recovery of renal function. Most urgent in management of ARF is treating hyperkalemia and fluid overload. When one begins to see hyperkalemia-associated cardiac irritability (prolonged PR interval or peaked T waves), urgent treatment is indicated. Administration of a 10% calcium gluconate solution over 15 minutes as well as simultaneous intravenous administration of glucose and insulin (30 units regular insulin in 1 L of 10% dextrose) will rapidly lower serum potassium levels. Similarly, administration of an ion exchange resin (Kayexalate) in enema form will help lower potassium levels. Careful monitoring of intravenous fluids with emphasis on fluid restriction and occasional use of

Box 14-6. Indications for Hemodialysis

Serum potassium >5.5 mEq/L
Blood urea nitrogen >80 to 90 mg/dL
Persistent acidosis
Acute fluid overload
Uremic symptoms
Removal of toxins

catheters to measure right- and left-sided heart filling pressures is indicated.

When supportive measures fail, consideration must be given to hemodialysis. Indications for hemodialysis are listed in Box 14-6.[34] Although some hemodynamic instability may occur during dialysis, it is usually transient and may be treated with fluids. Dialysis may be continued on an intermittent basis until renal function has returned, which occurs in the vast majority of cases.

Prevention

The astute clinician can do much to prevent ARF in surgical patients. Close attention in the preoperative period will reveal the patient with elevated serum creatinine and preexisting renal dysfunction. Adequate hydration during bowel preparations, avoidance of nephrotoxins, hydration before the use of radiocontrast agents, and close postoperative fluid monitoring are essential.

Monitoring postoperative renal function closely in all surgery patients is a sound clinical practice. Early intervention in urinary retention, postrenal obstruction, and abdominal compartment syndrome can obviate the development of renal injury. Fluid administration must be particularly judicious in patients with a history of congestive heart failure.

If ARF due to acute tubular necrosis progresses despite careful supportive measures, aggressive management including dialysis may be required to prevent the complications of renal failure, including bleeding, infection, malnutrition, encephalopathy, and impaired healing.

TABLE 14-9. Relative Corticosteroid Potency Compared with Hydrocortisone

	Glucocorticoid Activity	Mineralocorticoid Activity
Short Acting		
Hydrocortisone	1	1
Cortisone	0.8	0.8
Intermediate Acting		
Prednisone	4	0.25
Prednisolone	4	0.25
Methylprednisolone	5	Trace
Triamcinolone	5	Trace
Long Acting		
Dexamethasone	20	Trace

Modified from Druck P, Andersen DK: Diabetes mellitus and other endocrine problems. *In* Stillman RM (ed): Surgery: Diagnosis and Therapy. New York, Lange, 1989, p 205.

Box 14-7. Diagnosis of Adrenal Insufficiency With Rapid ACTH Stimulation

Steps

1. Determine baseline serum cortisol.
2. Give 0.25 mg cosyntropin intravenously.
3. Administer glucocorticoid immediately.
4. Measure serum cortisol levels 30 minutes after cosyntropin is given

Results

1. Normal level is greater than 7 g/dL increase in cortisol after 30 minutes or absolute level greater than 18 g/dL.
2. Neither time of day nor glucocorticoid administration interfere with the cortisol assay.

METABOLIC COMPLICATIONS

Adrenal Insufficiency

Etiology

Adrenal insufficiency is an uncommon but potentially lethal condition associated with failure of the adrenal glands to produce adequate glucocorticoids. Primary adrenal insufficiency is due to autoimmune adrenal atrophy (Addison's disease), but the other uncommon causes of adrenal insufficiency include infectious diseases (e.g., tuberculosis), adrenal hemorrhage, metastases, and bilateral surgical resection. Secondary adrenal insufficiency may be caused by inadequate secretion of adrenocorticotropic hormone (ACTH) owing to disease of the pituitary or hypothalamus. However, by far the most common cause of adrenal insufficiency is administration of pharmacologic doses of glucocorticoids, which suppresses ACTH secretion and thus suppresses the adrenal glands. Abrupt cessation of pharmacologic doses of chronic glucocorticoid administration results in adrenal insufficiency, which is often very symptomatic and occasionally lethal. All patients on chronic glucocorticoids need to be thoroughly instructed in the dangers of an abrupt termination of their glucocorticoid medication (Table 14-9). These patients include those with rheumatoid arthritis or inflammatory bowel disease and transplant and autoimmune disease patients. A baseline cortisol level of less than 15 µg/dL is considered diagnostic, but the rapid administration of ACTH to determine adrenal responsiveness is the diagnostic procedure of choice (Box 14-7).

Prevention

Patients present with sudden cardiovascular collapse, including hypotension, fever, mental confusion, and abdominal pain. Laboratory work-up reveals hyponatremia, hyperkalemia, hypoglycemia, and azotemia. An ECG will occasionally reveal low voltage and peaked T waves. Patients at risk include the elderly who are critically ill,[35] patients on prior high doses of corticosteroids, patients who undergo adrenal resection, and patients with large retroperitoneal bleed. Prevention and avoidance of this problem are most desirable and result from a thorough preoperative history, adequate perioperative corticosteroid administration, and a high index of suspicion in elderly, high-risk patients. Treatment involves immediate, rapid administration of hydrocortisone or methylprednisolone with appropriate monitoring until clinical improvement is seen.

Hyperthyroidism

Etiology

Hyperthyroidism is caused by excess amounts of thyroid hormone in the systemic circulation. It is caused by Graves' disease, thyroid adenoma, toxic multinodular goiter, and self-administration of excessive amounts of thyroid hormone. The most serious manifestation of hyperthyroidism is thyroid storm, which is a medical emergency and is associated with mortality rates of 20%.

Symptoms associated with the hyperthyroidism include cardiac (tachycardia, atrial fibrillation, dyspnea, congestive heart failure, gastrointestinal (diarrhea, nausea, vomiting), nervous (anxiety, delirium, restlessness, and irritability), eye (exophthalmos), musculoskeletal (weakness), and cutaneous (warm, moist skin with heat intolerance) manifestations.

Diagnostic work-up includes thyroid function tests, thyroid scan using iodine-123 (^{123}I), and occasionally ultrasound. Thyroid-stimulating hormone (TSH) is the most accurate test for diagnosis of hyperthyroidism, with significant suppression noted in hyperthyroid states. In most cases, the three commonly used thyroid function tests are elevated, including free T_4, total T_4, and total T_3. Thyroid scan is useful in helping diagnose thyroid disease in patients with abnormal thyroid function (Graves' disease, adenoma, multinodular goiter). Patients with Graves' disease have increased uptake of ^{123}I in a diffuse pattern without evidence of nodules. Toxic multinodular patients have a scan that reveals several nodules with varying degrees of uptake. Toxic adenoma is seen as a single "hot spot" on the thyroid scan. Management of hyperthyroidism includes both medical and surgical options.[36] The initial treatment involves trying to establish a euthyroid state using one of the two medications, propylthiouracil (PTU) or methimazole. Caution must be exercised in using PTU because rash, fever, polyarteritis, agranulocytosis, and aplastic anemia can result. After medical treatment, most patients become euthyroid within 4 to 6 weeks. Use of a β blocker such as propranolol can help treat cardiac manifestations.

For Graves' disease, definitive therapy is accomplished with either radioactive iodine (RAI) or surgery. RAI has obvious advantages in elderly high-risk patients but should be avoided in children, pregnant women, and patients with large toxic adenomas. By using doses of ^{123}I in the range of 10 mCi and subsequent thyroxine, thyrotoxicosis can be successfully managed in 85% to 90% of patients. Surgery usually includes one of two operations, either total thyroidectomy or a lobectomy on one side with subtotal on the other side. Total thyroidectomy has a lower recurrence rate than subtotal thyroidectomy (4% to 15%) but does require lifelong thyroxine replacement postoperatively. For toxic adenoma, excision of the lesion is indicated whereas total thyroidectomy is indicated in toxic multinodular goiter. In both cases (and Graves' disease), the patient should be made euthyroid using medications and iodide preoperatively.

Although now an uncommon entity, thyroid storm still occurs, and rapid, expeditious management is critical. Medical treatment includes placement of an intravenous line with hydration and immediate cardiac monitoring. β-Adrenergic blockade is central to the management strategy, along with Lugol iodine solution and PTU administration. Recognition of the thyroid storm preoperatively is essential, because the mortality rates of those with thyroid storm who undergo surgery are very high.

Hypothyroidism

Etiology

Hypothyroidism is characterized by low systemic levels of thyroid hormone and is associated with cold intolerance, constipation, brittle hair, dry skin, sluggishness, weight gain, and fatigue. In its most severe form, it may manifest as myxedema coma with an associated mortality of 40% to 50%. The hypothyroidism may be primary (surgical removal, ablation, disease), secondary (hypopituitarism), or tertiary (hypothalamic disease) and must be distinguished as treatment varies. In patients with primary hypothyroidism, serum total T_4, free T_4, and free T_3 levels are low whereas TSH is elevated. In secondary disease, TSH, free T_4 index, and free T_3 are low. Distinguishing the two is important because adrenal insufficiency is present in secondary disease and administration of thyroxine

should be accompanied by cortisol or the disease could be exacerbated.

Severe postoperative hypothermia, hypotension, hypoventilation, psychosis, and obtundation may signal clinically significant hypothyroidism. Immediate treatment with thyroid hormone is indicated concomitant with intravenous administration of hydrocortisone to avoid an addisonian crisis. The dose is usually 200 to 300 μg daily until oral intake is possible. Prevention of postoperative hypothyroidism is the ideal with recognition of clinical symptoms and treatment until euthyroid before operating.

Syndrome of Inappropriate Antidiuretic Hormone Secretion (SIADH)

Etiology

SIADH occurs when ADH continues to be secreted by the pituitary despite sustained hyponatremia. Regulation of sodium occurs through ADH secretion in response to increasing sodium levels and results in increased water resorption in the kidneys. The diagnosis should be considered in any patient who remains hyponatremic despite all attempts to correct the imbalance. Disorders and conditions that predispose to this relatively rare condition include trauma, stroke, ADH-producing tumors, drugs (ACE inhibitors, dopamine, nonsteroidal anti-inflammatory medications), and pulmonary conditions.

Clinical characteristics of SIADH include anorexia, nausea, vomiting, obtundation, and lethargy. With more rapid onset, seizures, coma, and death can result. The clinical expression of the syndrome is caused by hyponatremia and is a function of the degree of hyponatremia as well as the rapidity of its onset.

Management of SIADH includes treatment of the underlying disease process eventually. However, immediate treatment includes fluid restriction (mild disease) and intravenous administration of normal saline (moderate). Correction should occur at a rate of 0.5 mmol/L/hr until the serum sodium concentration is 125 mg/dL or higher. Diuretics such as furosemide occasionally help to correct the imbalance. In some cases, intravenous administration of 3% saline solution may be required (severe) but correction must be done in a constant, sustained fashion because overly rapid correction can result in seizure activity.

GASTROINTESTINAL COMPLICATIONS

Ileus and Obstruction

Etiology

Ileus is a general term used to describe intestine that ceases contracting for a brief period of time. Most patients develop a transient ileus after a major abdominal operation. Within 3 to 5 days, however, the patient begins passing flatus, signaling the resolution of the temporary ileus. Although extensive operative manipulation, major small bowel injury, heavy narcotic use, intra-abdominal infection, and pancreatitis can prolong the ileus, most uncomplicated operative cases should resolve within 5 to 7 days. Those who do not resolve their ileus in that time period are believed to have either a prolonged ileus or a mechanical small bowel obstruction (SBO). Distinguishing between these two entities is imperative because their treatment is completely different.

Presentation and Management

Patients with postoperative ileus or SBO either do not pass flatus and bowel movements immediately postoperatively or they begin having bowel activity within the normal time frame but then have cessation of function. They develop abdominal distention, nausea, vomiting, obstipation, and varying amounts of abdominal pain depending on the cause.

Patients with postoperative ileus can be very difficult to distinguish from patients with postoperative SBO. Clinically, ileus patients have a distended abdomen with diffuse discomfort but no sharp colicky pain. They often have a quiet abdomen with few bowel sounds detected on auscultation with a stethoscope. Abdominal radiographs reveal diffusely dilated bowel throughout the intestinal tract with air in the colon and rectum. Air-fluid levels may be present and the amount of dilated bowel varies greatly. Common causes of prolonged postoperative ileus are listed in Box 14-8. A standard battery of laboratory tests to ascertain the possible cause of the ileus includes a complete blood cell count with differential, determinations of amylase, lipase, and electrolytes, including magnesium and calcium, and urinalysis. Treatment of any of the causes listed in the table usually results in resolution of the ileus with continuation of bowel function. In most cases, postoperative ileus is treated by resolving the abnormality and expectantly waiting for resolution, with surgery usually not being required.

On the other hand, mechanical SBO may result in operative therapy and an observant, experienced surgeon is necessary to ascertain when surgery may be required. Postoperative SBO occurs in 1% to 3% of all abdominal operations. Among all patients who develop SBO (preoperatively and postoperatively), the cause is most commonly adhesions (70%), malignancy (10%), and hernias (5% to 10%). In postoperative patients, however, the vast majority are due to adhesions, often resulting from operations in the lower abdomen and pelvis. These patients present with abdominal distention, nausea, vomiting, and obstipation and often (but not always) have intermittent, colicky pain. Patients with high intestinal obstruction vomit early in the course and usually have only mild distention. Distal obstructions are characterized by vomiting later in the course and much more abdominal distention.

The most important task for the involved surgeon is to decide which SBO requires operative management[37] and which can be observed and managed expectantly. The simplest category, from a decision standpoint, is patients who present to the emergency department with a massively distended abdomen, significant pain, and a 12- to 24-hour history of obstipation. Almost without exception, those patients need to be prepared to go to the operating room urgently. At the other extreme is the postoperative patient who is passing some flatus and liquid, has a mildly distended abdomen, but vomits whenever oral intake is attempted. These patients can be observed for a longer period of time with the likelihood that the SBO will resolve spontaneously. The group in between the two aforementioned extremes are the most difficult to deal with clinically. Generally, patients with partial SBO that fails to resolve after 3 to 5 days, those associated with increasing pain, and those associated with tachycardia should be taken to the operating room.

The diagnostic evaluation of SBO virtually always begins with a flat plate and upright abdominal radiograph. Patients with SBO have air-fluid levels, distended small bowel, and a cutoff resulting in no colonic or rectal air. Auscultation of the abdomen may reveal high-pitched, tinkling sounds in early obstruction but may reveal a quiet abdomen in more protracted disease. If sequential abdominal radiographs (every 12 to 24 hours) reveal no improvement, further diagnostic work-up is indicated with either enteroclysis or CT with contrast medium enhancement. Although enteroclysis was the test of choice for many years because of the detailed "map" it gave regarding the anatomy of the obstruction, recent studies have revealed that CT of the abdomen is highly accurate in diagnosing SBO.[38,39] CT is capable of revealing dilated bowel, decompressed bowel, and a cutoff at the obstruction site.

Management of all patients with SBO includes aggressive intravenous hydration to reverse the hypovolemia secondary to nausea, vomiting, and fluid sequestration into the bowel. Electrolyte imbalances, most commonly hypokalemic and hypochloremic metabolic alkalosis, should be corrected. The patient should be given nothing by mouth and a nasogastric tube placed to decompress the distended stomach and protect against aspiration. If surgery is anticipated, preoperative antibiotics are indicated. Operative therapy consists of laparotomy, decompression of the bowel, lysis of the offending adhesions, and closure.

Prevention

A concerted effort should be made during any abdominal operation to minimize the serosal injury to small bowel and other peritoneal surfaces—the recognized source of

---

Box 14-8. Causes of Intestinal Paralytic Ileus

Pancreatitis
Intra-abdominal infection
Electrolyte abnormality
Medications (narcotics, psychotropics)
Operative bowel manipulation
Retroperitoneal hemorrhage
Pneumonia
Inflamed viscera
Abdominal trauma

adhesion formation. During the operation, the surgeon should handle the tissues gently and limit peritoneal dissection to only that which is essential. Bowel should not be desiccated by prolonged exposure to air without protection. Laparotomy pads should be moistened before prolonged contact with bowel, and instrument injury to bowel should be avoided.

Because the scope and magnitude of serious problems related to adhesions are so large, recent attempts have been made to develop anti-adhesion barriers that can be placed in the abdomen after surgery. A number of agents are now approved by the U.S. Food and Drug Administration as anti-adhesion barriers, including an oxidized, cellulose product and a product that is a combination of sodium hyaluronate and carboxymethyl cellulose. Prospective, randomized studies have demonstrated that these agents effectively inhibit adhesions wherever they are placed.[40] However, to be completely effective in preventing adhesive bowel obstruction, they would need to be placed everywhere in the peritoneal cavity that injury occurred—a situation not clinically possible because of the physical characteristics of the agents. No prospective studies have demonstrated a decrease in SBO in patients receiving the agents, although a study is being done to evaluate this.

Abdominal Compartment Syndrome

Etiology

Abdominal compartment syndrome occurs in patients who have sustained massive abdominal trauma, had an operation for massive intra-abdominal infection, or undergone a complicated, prolonged abdominal operation. Because of significant bowel edema, fascial closure is extremely difficult and results in high intra-abdominal pressures exceeding 25 cm H_2O. The elevated intra-abdominal pressure causes pulmonary compromise owing to pressure on both diaphragms and severely compromises venous return from the kidneys as well as renal arterial perfusion.[41] The syndrome may be seen in up to 5% of surgical patients in intensive care units.

Presentation and Management

The syndrome is characterized by a distended, tense abdomen, hypoxia, inability to adequately ventilate, elevated peak airway pressures, and profound oliguria. If untreated, patients go on to develop renal failure, respiratory failure, acidosis, compromise of cardiac output, and eventual shock. The diagnosis is made by obtaining intra-abdominal pressure readings through the Foley catheter.[42] Ordinarily, intra-abdominal pressures are near or at 0 cm H_2O. With elevations to 15 cm H_2O pressure, the patient will become oliguric and experience respiratory compromise. At pressures of 25 cm H_2O or higher, the patient becomes anuric and begins the cycle of exacerbation of pulmonary failure, cardiac decompensation, and death. Abdominal compartment syndrome is a surgical emergency, and the patient should be taken immediately to the operating room and have the fascial closure opened and

subsequent fascial closure done using an absorbable mesh. As the edema resolves, the patient can be taken back to the operating room in 5 to 7 days for permanent fascial closure.

Prevention

Most cases of abdominal compartment syndrome cannot be prevented because they often develop in a setting of critically ill patients who undergo emergency operations. However, early diagnosis in the postoperative period by the discerning surgeon can be a lifesaving decision. Because most cases develop in the first 24 hours after operation, a high index of suspicion will result in a low threshold for performing the very simple measurement of intra-abdominal pressure via a Foley catheter. When an intravesical pressure exceeds 25 cm H_2O and is associated with renal and pulmonary compromise, emergency surgery must be performed to save the patient's life.

Postoperative Gastrointestinal Bleeding

Etiology

Postoperative gastrointestinal bleeding represents one of the most worrisome complications encountered by general surgeons. Possible sources in the stomach include peptic ulcer disease, stress erosion, Mallory-Weiss tear, and gastric varices. In the small intestine, arteriovenous malformations or bleeding from an anastomosis have to be considered. In the large intestine, anastomotic hemorrhage, diverticulosis, arteriovenous malformation, or varices should be considered.

Etiology

In considering the source of the hemorrhage, a prior history is important in assessing the patient.[43] A patient with a prior history of peptic ulcer disease and previous upper gastrointestinal bleeding leads one to consider a duodenal ulcer. Similarly, the patient who has been severely injured in trauma, major abdominal surgery, central nervous system injury, sepsis, or myocardial infarction may have associated stress erosions. An antecedent history of violent emesis should lead to consideration of Mallory-Weiss tear, and a patient with portal hypertension and prior problems with variceal bleeding should make one think about that as a possible source of the bleeding. Anastomotic bleeding is unpredictable and very uncommon but always must be considered. In the large intestine, bleeding that occurs postoperatively is usually bright red and an anastomotic hemorrhage has to be considered. In a patient with a prior history of diverticulosis, a diverticular hemorrhage must be considered as well as an arteriovenous malformation.

In general, bright red blood is considered to come from a colonic or distal small bowel source. Melanotic stools suggest a gastric cause of the bleeding. However, rapid bleeding at any site may result in bright red blood.

Presentation and Management

Postoperative bleeding can present as slow oozing or rapid hemorrhage that can lead to hypotension. Patients who appear to have lost a unit of blood, have associated tachycardia or hypotension, or have a significant drop in hematocrit should immediately be transferred to the intensive care unit for assessment. Resuscitation begins before any consideration of the diagnosis. Large-bore intravenous lines are placed, the patient is resuscitated with iso-osmotic crystalloids, and specimens should be immediately sent to assess hematocrit, platelet count, prothrombin time, and partial thromboplastin time. A nasogastric tube can be quickly placed into the stomach and placed on suction to determine if the bleeding is gastric in origin. A negative aspiration virtually rules out a gastric or upper duodenal source of the bleeding. Serial hematocrits are critical for assessing the patients with ongoing bleeding. If the bleeding is a slow, continuous ooze, transfusion does not usually need to be considered until the patient is in the low 20s. Obviously a more rapid bleed with tachycardia and hypotension should be associated with almost immediate transfusion. A critically ill patient due to the conditions mentioned previously should have been previously placed on H_2 blockers to keep the pH of gastric contents above 4. This will prevent activation of pepsinogen to pepsin, a condition associated with stress erosions.[44] Other possible strategies include the use of antacids and sucralfate.[45] In refractory conditions, proton pump inhibitors may be considered. Those patients with a prolonged prothrombin/partial thromboplastin time or low platelet count should immediately be corrected to normal to see if conservative management will stop the bleeding. If bleeding persists in spite of these conservative techniques, upper gastrointestinal endoscopy should immediately be considered to look for a possible Mallory-Weiss tear, stress erosions, varices. In the presence of ongoing bleeding, local therapy through the endoscope has been successful in a moderately large number of patients. This includes such techniques as epinephrine injection around bleeding ulcers and erosions, heater probe cautery of bleeding lesions, banding of varices, as well as injection of sclerosants. Risk factors for stress erosions are listed in Box 14-9. For the patient who appears to have lower gastrointestinal bleeding, emergency colonoscopy may be considered, although it is often dif-ficult to clear the colon enough to see adequately. Occasionally, a bowel preparation with lavage solutions may provide brief visualization to detect the bleeding lesion. If bleeding continues in the presence of a normal upper gastrointestinal endoscopy and colonoscopy, anastomotic bleeding should be considered. Rarely, the patient will require reoperation to resect the anastomosis and reconnect the bowel. Surgery for stress erosions in the stomach occurs very uncommonly and generally requires a generous gastrotomy to evacuate blood clot with cauterization of ulcers. A total gastrectomy should almost never be required.

Prevention

Of the lesions mentioned previously, stress ulceration appears to be of the greatest clinical significance. Maintaining the gastric pH above 4 with the medications mentioned earlier seems to protect the patient against stress erosions. This problem, which was common 25 years ago, is much less common today, and in 75% to 80% of patients the bleeding spontaneously resolves. Nevertheless, constant attention to maintaining a high pH in a critically ill patient in the intensive care unit is an important part of prophylaxis postoperatively. The administration of antacids has been shown to be equally effective to H_2 blockers in the prevention of bleeding from stress ulcerations. However, this requires a good deal more care by the intensive care unit nurses and has been less commonly practiced in recent years. Similarly, sucralfate, which is a topical mucosal protectant, has been administered in refractory bleeding and found to be successful in a high percentage of patients. It appears to work by binding to the ulcer site and stimulating bicarbonate and mucus production, which seem to be protective.

Stomal Complications

Etiology

One of the most frustrating and difficult complications occurring in patients who undergo gastrointestinal operations are stomal complications. These can range from a bothersome problem with fit of the stomal appliance to major skin erosion and bleeding around a stoma to a large fistula. A wide variety of complications occur, including prolapse of the stoma due to inadequate length obtained during the surgery, prolapse, stomal necrosis, stenosis of the stoma, peristomal hernia formation, rotation of the stoma in a crease, and high stoma output. Similarly, bleeding from a stoma, problems with bringing a massively dilated segment of bowel through the abdominal wall, and obstruction of the stoma outlet due to edema can occur.

It is important to realize that careful, thoughtful stoma placement and taking the required amount of time to get enough length to bring the stoma through the abdominal wall will prevent the majority of complications. The stoma should be below the anterior superior iliac crest, which is the usually the belt line, and should be brought through the rectus abdominal muscle. Large scars and indentations

---

Box 14-9. Risk Factors for the Development of Stress Erosions

Multiple trauma
Head trauma
Major burns
Clotting abnormalities
Severe sepsis
Systemic inflammatory response syndrome (SIRS)
Cardiac bypass
Intracranial operations

in the abdominal wall should be avoided so that fit of the stoma plate is not compromised. A common temptation at the end of a long operation is to mobilize an inadequate length of the stoma. This will virtually always result in one of two complications: stoma retraction or stenosis at the skin level. Similarly, overly aggressive mobilization can result in necrosis of the stoma. Stomal complications are most common in the first couple of weeks after surgery, but complications may occur 5 or 10 years later, including peristomal hernias, fistulas from Crohn's disease, prolapse, or stricture. Overall, approximately 20% of patients will require reoperation related to the stoma at some time.

Patients who have poor selection of the stoma site such as the stoma located next to a crease or a fold will have difficulty with fit of the appliance, resulting in excoriation of the skin around the stoma. In most patients, an enterostomal therapist will use a variety of skin protectants, paste, and additional layers of stoma adhesive to build up the area around the fold. Occasionally, the problem can be so severe that a patient will have to be admitted to the hospital and placed on total parenteral nutrition (TPN) while the skin around the stoma heals enough to allow subsequent placement of an appliance. Similarly, a patient who has massive stomal output should be particularly watched to make certain that the skin around the stoma is not excoriated.

Stoma prolapse is frightening to the patient but uncommonly becomes incarcerated or a surgical problem. Prolapse occurs most commonly after massively dilated bowel is brought through the abdominal wall in an emergency procedure; it also occurs commonly after a transverse colostomy. In most cases, the prolapse can be observed until time for the reversal of the colostomy. In patients who have the stoma as a permanent structure, resection of the redundant bowel can be accomplished with a layer of stitches attaching the two ends of the bowel together.

Frequently, in the immediate postoperative course, patients will have a mildly cyanotic stoma. If adequate time to get length on the bowel being brought through the abdominal wall was taken, a cyanotic stoma will usually become better perfused as the postoperative edema resolves. The most severe form of this problem is frank stomal ischemia in which the mucosa turns a grayish-white color and begins to slough. Use of a small penlight to look down into the stoma will indicate whether the mucosa is necrotic just at the skin level or if it extends down into the abdominal wall. If the ischemia and necrosis extend down into the abdominal wall, reoperation is usually necessary. On the other hand, if ischemia extends to the skin level, the patient can usually be observed. A high incidence of stricture occurs when this conservative management is used. In most cases, a pulsating artery within 3 cm of the end of the bowel will be compatible with survival of the stoma. In permanent stomas placed in a poor location and in large peristomal hernias with obstruction or cosmetic problems, reoperation will be likely. For the poorly placed stoma, takedown of the stoma with movement to the other side of the abdomen will be successful in most cases. Peristomal hernias occur commonly and are seen most frequently in obese patients, patients who have poor healing, and patients who receive a stoma under emergency conditions. Approximately 15% of patients will develop a peristomal hernia, which can develop within months of the operation but may develop 10 years later. Management of a peristomal hernia depends on the amount of herniation and the clinical course of the patient. If the peristomal hernia is small and the patient is asymptomatic, it may merely be observed. However, if the peristomal hernia causes partial obstruction, incarceration, or severe pain, repair of the hernia should be considered. Similarly, a peristomal hernia that becomes very large and cosmetically bothersome should be repaired. Options in the repair of a peristomal hernia include local repair, use of a prosthesis, and movement of the stoma to another location in the abdomen. The first choice of repair options is relocation of the stoma to a place on the opposite of the abdomen. One should make the opening of the abdominal wall only large enough to accommodate the bowel, carefully suture closed the gap between fascia and bowel, and move the stoma as far away from the abdominal incision as possible without going lateral to the rectus abdominis. In a very high-risk patient, local repair of the fascia with interrupted suture can be attempted, but it is associated with a high recurrence rate. Another option is use of Marlex mesh or a similar prosthesis to bridge the defect. However, prosthesis repairs are much less predictable and can be associated with erosion, bleeding, and high recurrence. Unfortunately, patients who have a first peristomal hernia develop are much more likely to develop a second hernia. Similarly, recurrence of a peristomal hernia is associated with a surprisingly high rate of recurrence on further repairs.

Pseudomembranous Colitis

Etiology

Use of antibiotics in the preoperative or postoperative period can lead to pseudomembranous colitis in up to 1% of inpatients. The etiology appears to be related to alteration of the intestinal flora by the antibiotic, resulting in emergence of *Clostridium difficile*. Because of the superinfection by *C. difficile*, and secretion of an exotoxin, the patient develops a profound inflammatory reaction in the mucosa of the colon.[46] The inflammatory reaction is characterized by the development of the pseudomembrane, which is a whitish membrane consisting of fibrin, white blood cells, necrotic mucosal cells, and mucus. Most frequently, the distal colon is involved, but involvement of the entire colon in serious cases can occur. Studies have demonstrated that virtually all antibiotics have the potential of causing pseudomembranous colitis, although broad-spectrum antibiotics are more commonly associated with this condition. Similarly, there is usually a close temporal relationship with the development of this condition and cessation of antibiotic use, but it may occur even as late as 6 weeks after the use of the antibiotics.

Presentation and Management

The clinician should be suspicious of pseudomembranous colitis in the postoperative patient when an individual continues to have copious diarrhea, cramping, and dehydration. The persistent nature of the diarrhea should alert the clinician that a deviation in the normal postoperative course has occurred. In more advanced cases, the patient may develop severe abdominal pain and a paralytic ileus. In the presence of leukocytosis and fever, the patient may, in rare cases, need to undergo an operation. In most cases, however, the diagnosis is made in a fairly early stage in the disease. The diagnosis is made when a stool sample is sent for detection of the exotoxin. In the presence of the toxin, the diagnosis is virtually assured and treatment should be initiated immediately.

Two antibiotics have commonly been used for the treatment of pseudomembranous colitis: vancomycin and metronidazole. For many years, oral vancomycin was considered the antibiotic of choice. Because vancomycin reaches the colon in high concentrations, it has been an effective agent for the treatment of these organisms. However, with the emergence of vancomycin-resistant *C. difficile*, metronidazole has become the agent of choice. In both cases, oral administration is always preferable to intravenous administration. Therapy should be continued for 2 weeks and, in some cases, may be required for 3 to 4 weeks if resistant strains are present. In patients with paralytic ileus who are unable to tolerate oral intake, intravenous metronidazole can be given; however, it may be less successful than when given via the oral route. In rare cases, if the disease progresses in spite of antibiotic use the patient may become dehydrated and febrile and may develop shock. If this is associated with an exquisitely tender abdomen, emergency colectomy is indicated and is associated with a mortality of 20% to 30%. Nevertheless, judicious clinical management leading to an operation can be lifesaving for severe, refractory pseudomembranous colitis.

Anastomotic Leak

Etiology

Leak of an anastomosis between two hollow organs is one of the most serious complications a surgeon will ever encounter. Extravasation of bacteria-laden fluids leads to local abscess, fistula formation, breakdown of the anastomosis, wound dehiscence, sepsis, and even death. Therefore, performing an intra-abdominal anastomosis must be done with optimization of the patient preoperatively, ascertaining that his or her nutritional status is normal if possible. The large and small bowel should be preoperatively prepared by using cathartic and oral antibiotics. Drainage of abscess or decompressing distended bowel also is helpful when possible. Careful, meticulous mobilization of the organ to undergo surgery is of critical importance, with caution demonstrated to preserve blood supply and minimize manipulative trauma to the organ being treated. Meticulous, careful placement of suture or staple lines under adequate visualization is imperative. An anastomotic leak usually suggests that there has been a technical misadventure that can be prevented by the following: (1) the organ to be treated must have an adequate blood supply up to the edge of the anastomosis so that adequate healing can occur; (2) the two attached organs must have a tension-free anastomosis, which means taking the time to mobilize so that they lie next to each other; (3) the technical placement of each suture or staple must be correct with very little variance; (4) matching of the lumina of the two organs to be connected must be accommodated by a variety of techniques; (5) the surgeon must handle tissue gently so that there is no crushing or injury to the tissue to be attached; and (6) optimal visualization is critical and may require additional work and mobilization.

Certain anastomoses are particularly difficult from a technical standpoint and, thus, more prone to anastomotic leak. A pancreaticojejunostomy after a Whipple procedure has a leak rate of 15% to 20%. Because the lumen of small bowel is manipulated to accommodate the pancreas size, less than perfect anastomoses may be created. Similarly, because the esophagus has no serosa, esophagoenterostomies are of much higher risk and must be done with particular care. Finally, anastomosis of the colon to a very low rectal stump is difficult and associated with a fairly high leak rate. Most colorectal surgeons recommend a temporary diverting ileostomy in the scenario just mentioned.

Presentation and Management

Patients presenting with anastomotic leak usually develop fever, abdominal pain, malaise, and general failure to thrive. Often, a paralytic ileus develops and the patient refuses to eat or vomits when attempting to eat. Occasionally, the anastomotic leak will present as fullness in the area of leak; similarly, wound dehiscence, development of a fistula, or extensive erythema raises the question of anastomotic leak. In the presence of any of the aforementioned findings, immediate CT is indicated to assess the patient for the possibility of an anastomotic leak. The diagnosis of an anastomotic leak must be considered in the presence of large fluid collections, air-fluid levels in an abscess cavity, a large amount of fluid in the peritoneal cavity, or a large amount of free air in the peritoneal cavity. In circumstances in which the anastomotic leak is small and a controlled fistula forms, conservative management may be utilized until the leak heals. If the patient is not septic but has development of a controlled fistula, the patient should be immediately placed on gut rest with TPN and antibiotics. Similarly, a bile duct leak or a pancreaticojejunostomy leak, if adequately drained and a controlled fistula forms, may respond to conservative management. However, if drains were not placed and the infection is uncontrolled, reoperation is indicated. If the anastomotic leak occurs at a colon anastomosis, a colostomy should be brought up and a mucous fistula left behind. In many cases of small intestinal anastomotic leak, the leaking section can be resected and an immediate primary anastomosis done if the process is localized and there is minimal edema. The patient who has a bile duct leak will require drainage of the infection and placement of a drain next to the leak or, in the case of a large leak, may require bile duct reconstruction. A pancreaticojejunostomy leak, if small, can probably be drained and a drain placed next to the leak. However, for an anastomosis that has virtually fallen apart, the patient will probably require completion pancreatectomy. Whatever the source of the anastomotic leak, immediate judicious management is required to prevent the cycle of sepsis, septic shock, and death.

Fistulas

Etiology

Management of gastrointestinal fistulas is a complex and challenging clinical scenario that many surgeons are likely to deal with. Most fistulas occur after an abdominal procedure and are frequently associated with sepsis, malnutrition, immune suppression, or a technical mistake. A fistula represents an abnormal communication between one hollow epithelialized organ and another epithelialized surface. Abnormal connections can occur between two hollow organs, a hollow organ and the skin, and a hollow organ and the bladder; the genital tract even can be involved. Postoperative fistula is a serious problem that carries a mortality of 15% to 20% if not aggressively managed. The overwhelming majority of fistulas occur after an abdominal operation involving either an anastomosis under difficult circumstances, a technical mistake, or inadvertent enterotomy during a lysis of adhesions. Crohn's disease also represents a common cause of fistula. Technical factors such as gentle handling of tissue, avoiding tension of an anastomosis, ensuring adequate blood supply, good visualization of the anastomosis, and proper bowel preparation can help avoid the development of a fistula.

Presentation and Management

A small bowel or colonic fistula to the skin usually presents as initial erythema, abscess, and the subsequent efflux of gastrointestinal contents. It is often associated with excoriation of the skin surrounding the fistula as well as pain and fever. Similarly, a fistula from bowel to bladder is associated with fecaluria and pneumaturia. If the fistula is a controlled fistula and is not leaking into the peritoneal cavity, the patient may have a low-grade fever but will usually not be overtly septic. A fistula associated with significant sepsis may require urgent surgical intervention. However, in most cases the fistula will not need to be dealt with on an urgent basis, but clinical management of the fistula requires aggressive treatment. Diagnostic modalities used in patients with intestinal fistulas include CT, which is used for establishment of underlying abscesses, cancer, or other abnormality. Although the CT will usually not reveal the exact fistula, it is helpful to understand the surrounding disease process. A simple diagnostic maneuver is placement of a catheter into the fistula with placement of contrast material to identify the exact site of the fistula. Similarly, an enteroclysis procedure may demonstrate the anatomy of the fistula.

Initial treatment of enterocutaneous fistulas includes fluid resuscitation in the presence of high output, institution of antibiotics to treat any underlying infection, and protection of the skin. Skin protection can usually be accomplished by the placement of stoma adhesive on the skin surrounding the fistula with a suction catheter to suction the contents if the output is high. Occasionally, a stoma bag can be placed on the stoma adhesive surrounding the wound. Early involvement of enterostomal therapists is important in protecting the skin and assisting with limiting the effect of the contents on the surrounding skin or wound. The patient should be placed NPO and immediate nutritional supplementation with TPN should be started in virtually all patients with an enterocutaneous fistula. If the patient is seen to have a low output fistula (less than 200 mL/24 hr), use of enteral feedings may be considered. If the feedings do not substantially increase output from the fistula, nutrition may be accomplished without TPN. However, if there is any question, TPN is the preferred route so that wound healing may be accelerated without additional pressure of high output. In patients with extremely high outputs exceeding 1 to 2 L/day, careful management of electrolytes is imperative. Replacement of enteric fluid with lactated Ringer's solution is a simple approach to dealing with the problem. Use of H_2 blockers and octreotide may decrease the volume of flow through the fistula and accelerate healing. In general, fistulas with an output less than 200 mL/day will heal with conservative management. However, those fistulas that are high in the gastrointestinal tract and have an output over 500 mL/day are less likely to heal with conservative management.

Pancreatic fistulas represent a special problem usually occurring after trauma to the pancreas or after an operative procedure associated with a bowel anastomosis. If a drain is left at the time of surgery, the output in the drain will increase over time and become a clear, watery material. Diagnosis of a fistula is confirmed by amylase measurement of the fluid, which is usually in the tens of thousands. The same strategy is utilized for treatment of pancreatic fistulas. Specifically, stopping oral intake, placing the patient on TPN, and administering subcutaneous octreotide is indicated initially. If the fistula is a low-volume fistula (75 mL/day or less), oral intake may often be instituted as long as the output does not increase significantly. The drain should be left in place until the output is down to 10 to 12 mL/day, at which time it may be removed. With conservative management, approximately 60% of pancreatic fistulas will close spontaneously.

Intestinal fistulas that fail to close are usually associated with an underlying risk factor that includes the presence of a foreign body, radiation injury to the fistula site, an abscess or infection of the fistula site, epithelialization of the fistula tract, a surrounding neoplasm,[47] and obstruction of the bowel distal to the fistula. If these underlying conditions are not surgically treated, the fistula may persist indefinitely. When a fistula from a bowel anastomosis or inadvertent enterotomy site is present, resuscitation, TPN, and skin management should continue for a couple of weeks. Reoperating on a patient with a controlled fistula early on is fraught with danger because of poor tissue planes, bleeding, and risk of creating additional injury to the bowel. In most circumstances, a fistula that fails to close should not undergo operative therapy for 4 to 6 weeks after the fistula has formed. Operating at that time will result in a safer, less bloody operation. Surgical treatment of a fistula that has failed to close involves entering the abdomen through any virgin area possible so that the planes can be identified and dissected. The process involves circular excision of the fistula site and mobilization of the intestine until it is freed from the fistula site. Resection of the bowel containing the fistula will be required, and a primary anastomosis can be done in most cases. Placing omentum between the anastomosis and fascial closure is a prudent thing to do to prevent refistulization. The fistula should never be closed locally because the incidence of suture line failure is virtually 100%.

Pancreatic fistulas that fail to close after conservative management represent a particularly difficult operative challenge. If the patient continues to have high output from the fistula site 2 to 3 months after the operation, reoperation may be required to take a Roux-en-Y limb up to the site of the fistula and suture it to the dense tissue surrounding the fistula site. If done carefully, this operation has a high likelihood of success.

HEPATOBILIARY COMPLICATIONS

Bile Duct Injuries

Etiology

The advent of laparoscopic cholecystectomy has resulted in a significant increase in the number of bile duct injuries treated.[48] The incidence of bile duct injuries after laparoscopic cholecystectomy at one time approached four times the incidence of open cholecystectomy. This was particularly true in the 5 years after the general acceptance of laparoscopic cholecystectomy and has decreased in frequency in the intervening years.[49] Nevertheless, the incidence of significant bile duct injury is approximately 0.5% today. Bile leaks due to other causes may occur including bile leak from a cystic duct whose clip comes off, but 25% of bile duct leaks are due to a major bile duct injury.

Presentation and Management

Patients with a bile duct injury present with right upper quadrant pain, fever, and malaise and occasionally have associated jaundice. Late presentation of a bile duct injury may simply be the presence of jaundice without associated fever, leukocytosis, and sepsis. Patients presenting with this constellation of symptoms should immediately undergo CT of the abdomen. In the presence of a large fluid collection in the right upper quadrant, a bile duct injury and leak is virtually ensured. Management of the problem begins with immediate percutaneous drainage of the bile collection with the drain left in place. Patients should then proceed to endoscopic retrograde cholangiopancreatography where the study will indicate the size of the leak, the location of the leak, and whether an obstructive component is present. In a patient with a small leak and an open common bile duct, placement of a stent past the area of injury will often result in dramatic decrease in the drainage of bile from the injury. In a cystic duct leak or a small injury, stenting and drainage may be adequate therapy. However, where there is a major obstruction of the bile duct or large injury, stenting is only supplementary to surgical therapy. After adequate resuscitation, placement on antibiotics, and adequate drainage, the patient should be watched for a few days to make certain he or she is not septic at the time of the operation. If there is evidence of adequate control of the leak, the surgeon may wait up to 5 to 7 days for inflammation in the area to subside before undertaking operative repair. The operation is approached through a generous upper abdominal incision, and meticulous and careful dissection is required in this area, because there is usually loss of common bile duct substance. After identifying the source of the bile extravasation, dissection in that area associated with débridement of nonviable common bile duct material is prudent. After ascertaining that there is tissue with good integrity, a Roux-en-Y limb can be brought up to do a hand-sewn anastomosis to the common bile duct. Multiple drains should be left around the site of the repair. Occasionally, the repair will require an attachment to two or three different lumina.

Prevention

The surgeon should approach each operation on the biliary tree with caution and respect because of the frequent anomalies and anatomic variations. The anatomic variability associated with severe inflammation should create a low threshold for doing an open cholecystectomy and converting from the laparoscopic approach. Liberal use of cholangiography may be helpful in defining anatomy. Some authors have advocated the use of intraoperative ultrasound to help establish the relationship between the common duct, cystic duct, and gallbladder.

NEUROLOGIC COMPLICATIONS

Delirium, Dementia, and Psychosis

Etiology

Management of cognitive disorders in postoperative patients is a frustrating and challenging clinical scenario. A planned operation with loss of the patient's routine schedule, stresses of the disease process, fear of the operation, loss of personal control, placement in an unfamiliar environment, the addition of mind-altering pain medications, and pain all can lead to dramatic alterations in behavior in postoperative patients. These problems can present as changes in memory, affect, and ability to reason. Patients who have particularly high risk for behavioral disorders in the postoperative period include the elderly, patients with a prior history of substance abuse, patients with a prior history of psychiatric disorders, and children. Patients in these high-risk categories should be carefully followed with attempts made to minimize interruptions in their normal schedule. The changes, which may be affective or cognitive, can result in disorientation, inappropriate response, depression, agitation, and catatonia. Clinical changes of that nature usually indicate delirium, dementia, or psychosis (Box 14-10).

The most immediately threatening disorder encountered by physicians is delirium tremens associated with acute alcohol withdrawal. Because of the serious underlying nutritional and medical deficiencies, these patients have a moderately high mortality that approaches 20% in some series. Other causes of delirium and psychosis include medications, sepsis, intracranial tumors, metabolic derangements, trauma, and toxins.

Presentation and Management

Patients may present on a spectrum from mild confusion and memory loss to full-blown delirium with confusion, irrational behavior, disorientation, and frank hallucinations. Patients may become noncommunicative, emotionally flat, and unresponsive and may withdraw from any emotional exchange. Particularly in older people, these symptoms may become cyclically worse at night with dramatic improvements during the day.

Patients who present with a sudden change in behavior should be immediately evaluated for the cause of the problem. A careful look at the recent medication history will assess whether the patient is on mind-altering medications. Clinical examinations should reveal whether there is evidence of sepsis or a recent neurologic event with localizing findings. Laboratory tests to look for evidence of metabolic, electrolyte, and nutritional abnormalities should be sent. A thorough, neurologic examination looking for evidence of ataxia, paresis, or paralysis is of critical importance. Part of the drug history evaluation should assess whether withdrawal from a certain medication may have caused the problems.

Patients who have an abrupt change in their behavior patterns should be considered for CT or magnetic resonance imaging (MRI) after the physical examination is done and the history is taken. Occasionally, a spinal tap may be indicated to make certain no central nervous system infection is the cause of the problem.

The patient should be assessed to ascertain whether they might be a physical threat to themselves or others. On occasion, physical restraints may be required until the patient can be quieted. Speaking to the patient in a reassuring and calm fashion will often do much to help him or her. Making certain that the patient sleeps well and is oriented on a regular basis with regard to time and place is also important. Family and staff members may be able to help the patient a great deal during periods of confusion. If sepsis is the cause of delirium, immediate administration of antibiotics and treatment of the source of infection should result in rapid improvement in the patient's function.

Medical management of the patient with delirium or psychosis involves administration of appropriate sedatives, treatment of underlying disorders, and careful observation.[50] On occasion, one-to-one nursing will be required. Patients with delirium tremens may have tachycardia, fever, diaphoresis, and cardiac arrhythmias. Initial restraints may be required while administering sedatives intravenously until the patient is quieted. This may be required for 24 to 48 hours until the patient's behavior improves somewhat. Similarly, thiamine and niacin should be administered intravenously as well as other vitamins.

Prevention

Awareness of the high-risk patient for postoperative delirium is the single most important principle in prevention. Minimizing the dose and use of medications that cause interruption in mental function should be considered.

Seizure Disorders

Etiology

Seizures are caused by paroxysmal electrical discharges from the cerebral cortex. They are associated with convulsions, rhythmic myoclonic activity, loss of consciousness, and a change in mental status. Seizures may be primary or secondary depending on the etiology. Primary causes of seizures include intracranial tumors, hemorrhages, trauma, or idiopathic seizure activity. Secondary causes of seizure include metabolic derangements, sepsis, systemic disease processes, and pharmacologic agents. Seizure activity is often associated with fecal and urinary incontinence, lack of neurologic responsiveness, and post-

---

Box 14-10. Causes of Acute Delirium

Drug intoxication (alcohol, antihistamines, sedatives)
Drug withdrawal (alcohol, narcotics, anxiolytics)
Acute cerebral disorders (edema, transient ischemic attack, stroke, neoplasm)
Metabolic disturbances (electrolyte imbalance, hypoglycemia)
Hemodynamic disturbances (hypovolemia, myocardial infarction, congestive heart failure)
Infections (septicemia, urinary tract infection, pneumonia)
Respiratory disorders (respiratory failure, pulmonary embolism)
Trauma (head injury, burns)

From Monks R: Cognitive and sensory deficits. *In* Wilmore DW, Brennan MF, et al (eds): Case of the Surgical Patient, vol 2. New York, Scientific American, 1991.

event amnesia. Patients at particularly high risk for postoperative seizure include those with a prior history of epilepsy as well as patients acutely withdrawing from alcohol or medications, and other pharmacologic agents including antidepressants, hypoglycemic agents, and lidocaine.

Presentation and Management

On recognizing evidence of seizure activity, the patient should be carefully restrained so as not to sustain injury during the course of the seizure. The patient should be placed on a bed or gurney with observation during the course of the seizure. Administration of intravenous benzodiazepines is the standard for immediate care of the patient undergoing seizure activity. Benzodiazepines stop the seizure activity acutely but are not used for long-term convulsion suppression. Phenytoin (Dilantin) is the most commonly used anticonvulsant for a new presentation of generalized or focal seizures. It may be administered intravenously during acute convulsion or orally for maintenance. Phenytoin does have some side effects, including a problem with development of rash, and may affect liver function. Occasionally, phenobarbital may be used but, because of sedation, is not an agent of choice. The two most commonly used agents for maintenance after seizure or for someone with status epilepticus are carbamazepine (Tegretol) and valproic acid. Neither of these agents can be given intravenously and, thus, can be used for maintenance but not for acute treatment. Gabapentin can be used when the patient's condition is refractory to other agents. After the seizure has been managed a diagnostic work-up for its cause should be initiated. This would include a detailed history and physical examination as well as a history of prior medication and drug use. An assessment of the white blood cell count to rule out occult infection as well as electrolyte and metabolic assessment is indicated. CT or MRI should be ordered in a patient with new onset of seizure activity, because tumors will often be the cause. Similarly, an electroencephalogram should be obtained at some point to look for abnormal waveform activity.

Stroke and Transient Ischemic Attacks

Etiology

Postoperative stroke is one of the most devastating complications witnessed by surgeons. In the truly irreversible injury, the impact on the patient's overall health is immeasurable and his or her ability to function and to enjoy a good quality of life is severely compromised. Fortunately, a high percentage of neurologic events are either transient (occurring for seconds to minutes) or reversible (occurring for minutes to hours). The most common causes of stroke include advanced atherosclerotic disease of the internal carotid artery, atrial fibrillation, a ventricular septal defect, acute hepatic failure, or excessive anticoagulation. Similarly, transient neurologic events can be caused by trauma, tumor, cerebral edema, and hematoma. In most cases of adult stroke, the cause is cardiovascular.

Presentation and Management

Patients with stroke or transient ischemic attack present with focal alteration in motor function, which is unilateral, alteration in mental status, aphasia, and occasionally unresponsiveness. In all cases, the neurologic changes represent a dramatic departure from normal patient function. On recognizing the clinical signs and symptoms of a stroke, the patient should have an intravenous line placed. Management beyond that point rests on distinguishing between hemorrhagic and nonhemorrhagic (usually embolic from the internal carotid or heart) strokes. Hemorrhagic strokes are commonly associated with poorly controlled hypertension or anticoagulation and can be accurately diagnosed with CT or MRI. Management includes pharmacologic reduction of blood pressure, mannitol given intravenously to reduce cerebral swelling, and administration of dexamethasone. Occasionally, an unsuspected cerebral aneurysm rupture or subarachnoid hemorrhage is detected and immediate surgical intervention can result in preservation of brain function.

If the lesion is nonhemorrhagic, the management principles are similar to those with hemorrhagic stroke but, in addition, anticoagulation is instituted. Treatment of any underlying cardiac arrhythmia is imperative to prevent recurrent embolization. There are encouraging recent preliminary studies that suggest that tissue plasminogen activator may be effective in restoring cerebral blood flow if given intravenously within 2 hours of the stroke.

EAR, NOSE, AND THROAT COMPLICATIONS

Epistaxis

Etiology

Epistaxis may be associated with primary disease conditions such as leukemia, hemophilia, excessive anticoagulation, and hypertension. The most frequent postoperative cause of epistaxis is injury during placement of a nasogastric tube, endotracheal tube, or temperature probe. Epistaxis is divided into two general categories: anterior and posterior. Anterior trauma is often associated with the manipulations just mentioned and results in a contusion or laceration to the nasal septum or turbinates. Firm pressure applied between the thumb and index finger to the nasal ala and held for 3 to 5 minutes is generally successful in stopping most cases of epistaxis. Occasionally, packing with strip gauze for 10 to 15 minutes will aid in a particularly refractory case. If the bleeding fails to stop, packing for an extended period of time with petroleum-covered strip gauze may be required. Removal of the packing in 1 to 3 days is usually associated with successful treatment of refractory epistaxis along with treatment of the underlying condition or reversal of anticoagulation.

A more serious scenario is posterior nasal septal bleeding that, on occasion, can even be life threatening. If all attempts to stop anterior nasal septal bleeding are unsuccessful, one may infer the probability of a posterior nasal hemorrhage, which may necessitate placement of a posterior pack of strip gauze covered in petrolatum ointment. For particularly refractory cases, a Foley catheter with a 30-mL balloon can be passed through the nasal passages and, after the pack is placed, pressure can be applied to the pack by pulling on the Foley catheter. This type of epistaxis may require concomitant anterior nasal packing to be successful. The packs on a difficult hemorrhage like this may need to be left in place for 2 to 3 days. For epistaxis that defies all attempts at conservative management, ligation of the sphenopalatine artery or the anterior ethmoidal artery may be required.

Acute Hearing Loss

Etiology

Abrupt loss of hearing in the postoperative period is an uncommon event. An immediate physical examination should be done to ascertain the degree of hearing loss. Unilateral hearing loss is usually associated with obstruction or edema associated with a nasogastric or feeding tube. Bilateral hearing loss is more often neural in nature and is usually associated with pharmacologic agents such as aminoglycosides and diuretics. Examination with an otoscope will often reveal the presence of cerumen impaction or edema due to a middle ear infection. If the otologic examination is completely normal, one should suspect neural injury related to the just-mentioned agents. Those agents should be discontinued immediately and hearing monitored over the ensuing 2 to 3 days to see if recovery occurs. For cerumen impactions, use of a delicate speculum is indicated under direct vision. If the hearing loss is associated with edema related to a nasogastric tube, merely removing the nasogastric tube will result in resolution of the edema.

Sinusitis

Etiology

Patients with sinusitis usually present with malaise, a dull aching pain in the maxillary or frontal sinus area, and often a low-grade fever. Because of edema associated with nasogastric tube use, sinusitis is often exacerbated or delayed in healing. Sinusitis in the acute postoperative patient is often missed because of the frequent use of analgesics and antipyretics as well as the presence of the nasogastric tube itself, which is uncomfortable. However, an unexplained fever in a patient with a nasogastric tube postoperatively should suggest the possibility of sinusitis.[51] As usual, an index of suspicion is required before one considers sinusitis in the differential diagnosis of a low-grade fever. CT of the head will demonstrate sinusitis, which may be treated with broad-spectrum antibiotics. Treatment is usually accelerated with removal of the nasogastric tube and decongestants. In rare cases, severe intractable sinusitis may require a drainage procedure using an operative technique.

Parotitis

Etiology

Parotitis most commonly occurs in an elderly man with poor oral hygiene and poor oral intake with associated decrease in saliva production. The pathophysiology involves obstruction of the salivary ducts or an infection in a diabetic or immune-compromised patient. The patient is noted to have significant edema and focal tenderness surrounding the parotid gland, which eventually progresses to involve edema of the floor of the mouth. If left undiagnosed and untreated, the parotitis can cause life-threatening sepsis. In the worst-case scenario, the infection can dissect into the mediastinum and cause stridor from partial airway obstruction. Patients who have advanced parotitis will have dysphagia and some respiratory occlusion. If the diagnosis of parotitis is entertained, the patient should be placed on intravenous, high-dose, broad-spectrum antibiotics with good coverage of *Staphylococcus* (the most common agent cultivated from this disease). In the presence of a fluctuant area, incision and drainage is indicated with care demonstrated to avoid the facial nerve. On rare occasions, advanced disease may even require an emergency tracheostomy. Most patients with parotitis will have the condition arise 4 to 12 days after the initial operation. Because of the rapid progression of this disease, one must be aware of the diagnosis and, when present, institute immediate therapy, including emergency surgery on occasion for patients with an obvious fluctuant area.

SPECIAL CONSIDERATIONS

Complications at the Extremes of Age

It is of critical importance that the surgeon understands the varying ability with which old people and very young people respond to postoperative complications. Although infants that are otherwise healthy can tolerate complications and seem to heal well, in the presence of impairments or congenital abnormalities there may be delay in healing and alteration in the presentation of the disease. The elderly vary in a number of ways with regard to their response to complications. The elderly patient frequently will mount very little white blood cell increase with serious infections. They often have less intra-abdominal pain and peritoneal tenderness with serious infections, they often present much later in the course of the disease because of lack of body awareness, and they frequently have comorbid factors that increase their risk for the operation and response to any postoperative complication. Because of those factors, one should be particularly careful in the preoperative period, screening the patients for comorbid diseases and getting a careful history from the patient regarding cardiac, pulmonary, and renal problems. In the presence of significant underlying disease, management of that disease process should be undertaken before proceeding with elective surgery. If the surgery is emergent or urgent surgery, maximizing the patient's medical condition before doing the operation is always indicated.

One must be aware that young children and elderly patients process medications in a different fashion than mature adults and, because of a lower lean body mass, may have an exaggerated response to any medications given. It is also important to understand that the young patient and elderly patient may require additional time and attention to explain the nature of the medical care they will be receiving and what the possible outcomes are. Sympathy, kindness, and patience are of critical importance in dealing with this patient population because of the special needs elucidated earlier. A few additional minutes spent in the preoperative period addressing these issues will result in a smoother postoperative course with a lower likelihood of serious postoperative complications.

Ethical Concerns

A patient interacts with the surgeon at a time of great concern. He or she may be preoccupied with the outcome of the procedure and may even have questions about quality of life after the operation. Because the medical issues are often very complicated and not easy to explain, some surgeons may be tempted to gloss over discussion with the patient. However, the preoperative period is an important time in not only developing a relationship with the patient but also for sitting down and talking with him or her in great depth regarding the operation, the potential risks, complications, alternatives, and possible benefits. During these discussions, it is of critical importance that the surgeon allows the patient time to ask questions, to explore fears, and to explain the likely outcome with possible minor and major complications. It may also be an important time to explain to the patient what the standard of care is and what the patient may expect from the operation. A frank explanation about possible complications and their management is also appropriate. Too often, the patients fear the surgeon to the point that they do not feel comfortable enough to ask the important questions that they may have. A calm, approachable, friendly demeanor on the part of the surgeon will do much to assuage those fears.

Operations that may result in distasteful complications or irreversible alterations in lifestyle should be explained in great detail. Glossing over any postoperative outcome that has such a significant impact on the patient invites concern, anger, and belligerence on the unsuspecting patient. Additional time should be taken to explain to the patient who will receive an abdominoperineal resection what a colostomy is and what the individual's lifestyle will be with it. The patient to receive a low anterior resection needs to understand there is a significant risk of loss of sexual function. A patient with an esophagogastrectomy will certainly have an alteration in eating lifestyle as will a patient with a bariatric procedure. The surgeon who takes great pains to explain in detail the expected outcome of the operation before the procedure will have many fewer calls postoperatively and a much more understanding patient in the long run. Similarly, respect and a nonjudgmental attitude toward patients who may have customs and mores that are different from the surgeon's and the local society are important.

Should complications occur postoperatively, or should the surgeon make an egregious error, the best way to deal with the patient is to be completely honest, frank, and open with regard to any questions that are asked. Most patients will respond with a fair amount of respect and sympathy to the surgeon who is openly honest and expresses frustration and sadness over the complication. The surgeon should deal with the complication or problem in an efficient, expeditious fashion and make certain the patient is restored to as normal a status as possible.

Occasionally, patients who have a bad outcome from an operation performed by another surgeon will request feedback from you as a consultant regarding whether a medical mistake was made in their management. This is a difficult ethical dilemma for the consulting surgeon because there are so many aspects of the patient's management to which the consultant will not have full understanding and access. In a situation in which the complication is a recognized risk of the operation with a surgeon who has a demonstrated track record as a competent, careful surgeon, the consultant can do much to allay a litigious attitude by recognizing the complication as such. However, on occasion, a clinical scenario will be presented that is so obviously a departure from the standard of care, the consultant is wise to communicate openly and frankly with the patient regarding the breaches of care that may have occurred. In general, it is unwise to denigrate another surgeon unless there is a clear-cut and obvious violation of medical standards.

In summary, ethics and ethical choices are a part of the practice of every busy surgeon's life. A practice of complete candor and honesty with the patient, genuine concern, open lines of communication involving the patient in decisions regarding his or her care, informed consent, and confidentiality regarding the patient's care will always place the surgeon in a positive position. The surgeon should strive to uphold the highest standards of care primarily because the patient benefits from such a posture and the surgeon is conducting his or her professional life the way a physician and healer should.

Public and Regulatory Concerns

A recent flurry of articles has been published regarding complication rates associated with complex operative procedures. Most of the papers demonstrate that centers where high volumes of complicated procedures are done have a lower morbidity and mortality rate. Industry and insurance payers have recognized these data and are beginning to become involved in a major way in deciding where they will send patients for care, particularly if there is a complicated medical problem. Increasingly, hospitals and medical institutions are beginning to compare surgeons with regards to morbidity, mortality, and functional outcome. It is likely that in the near future, only those physicians who have low morbidity and mortality rates will be permitted to do more complex operations. Additionally, with the formation of the National Physicians Data Bank, surgical complications play a major role in identifying surgeons who fall well below the standard of care with regard to surgical outcome. Those who consistently fall below that norm may even be denied operating room privileges in the future.

With the widespread use of the Internet, patients in the future will be able to evaluate a prospective surgeon even before the operation is scheduled to ascertain where the individual surgeon lies compared with a national norm. Those who fall below that norm will certainly be less busy than those who excel. For that reason and, more importantly, the care of the patient, surgeons will need to be even more meticulous and careful and strive to minimize error of any kind in the management of surgical patients. Whereas reporting of surgical complications and errors had been primarily a local event for the past 50 years, in the future, national data may be available on every surgeon.

Selected References

ACCP Consensus Committee on Pulmonary Embolism, American College of Chest Physicians: Opinions regarding the diagnosis and management of venous thromboembolic disease. Chest 113:499-504, 1998.

This paper is the result of a consensus conference held by the ACCP regarding pulmonary embolus. The paper discusses the appropriate way to manage pulmonary embolus and the current recommendations regarding diagnosis and prevention.

Alonso DR, Scheidt S, Post M, et al: Pathophysiology of cardiogenic shock: Quantification of myocardial necrosis, clinical, pathologic and electrocardiographic correlations. Circulation 48:588-596, 1973.

This classic paper describes in detail the management of cardiogenic shock after major myocardial infarction. It is a comprehensive and in-depth study of the clinical presentation, diagnostic approach, and natural history of the disease.

Barquist E, Kirton O: Adrenal insufficiency in the surgical intensive care unit patient. J Trauma 42:27-31, 1997.

This is a fairly recent paper that describes in detail the clinical presentation and management of an often unrecognized problem in intensive care unit patients—adrenal insufficiency.

Becker JM, Dayton MT, Fazio VW, et al: Prevention of postoperative abdominal adhesions by a sodium hyaluronate-based bioresorbable membrane: A prospective, randomized, double-blind multicenter study. J Am Coll Surg 183:297-306, 1996.

This is the first published report in the literature in prospective randomized fashion of an anti-adhesion membrane that does prevent postoperative abdominal adhesions. This study demonstrates that the membrane is effective in preventing adhesions, but it does not extend to show a decrease in clinical small bowel obstruction.

Bartlett JG, Chang TW, Gurwith M, et al: Antibiotic-associated pseudomembranous colitis due to toxin-producing clostridia. N Engl J Med 298:531-534, 1978.

This is an important paper that describes pseudomembranous colitis and the causal organism as well as clinical management. It is an important paper because it underscores the dangers of inappropriate antibiotic use.

Bizer LS, Liebling RW, Delany HM, et al: Small bowel obstruction: The role of nonoperative treatment in simple intestinal obstruction and predictive criteria for strangulation obstruction. Surgery 89:407-413, 1981.

This older paper is a good paper to use in management of the full spectrum of small bowel obstruction. It covers not only indications for operative therapy but also when nonoperative treatment is indicated.

Cohn JN: The management of chronic heart failure. N Engl J Med 335:490-498, 1996.

This is a fairly recent, comprehensive review of the management of both uncomplicated and complicated chronic heart failure.

Connors AFJ, Speroff T, Dawson NV, et al: The effectiveness of right heart catheterization in the initial care of critically ill patients. SUPPORT Investigators. JAMA 276:889-897, 1996.

There is controversy regarding the actual value of right-sided heart catheterization in management of critically ill patients. This study objectively assesses the contribution right-sided heart catheterization makes.

Cook DJ, Fuller HD, Guyatt GH, et al: Risk factors for gastrointestinal bleeding in critically ill patients. Canadian Critical Care Trials Group. N Engl J Med 330:377-381, 1994.

This review article looks at risk factors for patients in the intensive care unit, particularly addressing stress erosions and gastrointestinal bleeding in that high-risk population.

Eagle KA, Brundage BH, Chaitman BR, et al: Guidelines for perioperative cardiovascular evaluation for noncardiac surgery. Report of the American College of Cardiology/American Heart Association Task Force on Practice Guidelines (Committee on Perioperative Cardiovascular Evaluation for Noncardiac Surgery). J Am Coll Cardiol 27:910-948, 1996.

This is an important report from the American College of Cardiology that carefully outlines management of patients with cardiac risk factors who will undergo a noncardiac operation. There is a valuable algorithm in the paper that helps the surgeon understand the management of any patient with chest pain, angina, or other risk factors.

Frager DH, Baer JW, Rothpearl A, et al: Distinction between postoperative ileus and mechanical small-bowel obstruction: Value of CT compared with clinical and other radiographic findings. AJR Am J Roentgenol 164:891-894, 1995.

Recent studies suggest that CT has become an important modality in diagnosing small bowel obstruction. This paper describes ways to distinguish postoperative ileus from mechanical small bowel obstruction. Some believe that CT is now more valuable than enteroclysis in making this diagnosis.

Frager D, Medwid SW, Baer JW, et al: CT of small-bowel obstruction: Value in establishing the diagnosis and determining the degree and cause. AJR Am J Roentgenol 162:37-41, 1994.

> This is another paper that documents the value of CT in small bowel obstruction.

Goldman L: Cardiac risks and complications of noncardiac surgery. Ann Intern Med 98:504-513, 1983.

> This is the classic paper describing the relative cardiac risks for noncardiac surgery. It clearly documents that recent myocardial infarction and current congestive heart failure are the two highest cardiac risk factors before surgery. This is an invaluable paper for every surgeon's library.

Mangram AJ, Horan TC, Pearson ML, et al: Guideline for prevention of surgical site infection, 1999. Hospital Infection Control Practices Advisory Committee. Infect Control Hosp Epidemiol 20:250-278, 1999.

> This fairly comprehensive review article delineates guidelines for wound infections postoperatively. It thoroughly treats the topic of preoperative antibiotics and current recommendations regarding their use in various operations.

Stewart L, Way LW: Bile duct injuries during laparoscopic cholecystectomy. Factors that influence the results of treatment. Arch Surg 130:1123-1129, 1995.

> This is an important paper because it describes a classification system for patients who undergo bile duct injury during laparoscopic cholecystectomy. Because injuries at each of the different levels are managed slightly differently, this paper codifies them and makes suggestions regarding surgical management of each individual type.

References

1. Riou JP, Cohen JR, Johnson H Jr: Factors influencing wound dehiscence. Am J Surg 163:324-330, 1992.
2. Dayton MT, Buchele BA, Shirazi SS, et al: Use of an absorbable mesh to repair contaminated abdominal-wall defects. Arch Surg 121:954-960, 1986.
3. Mangram AJ, Horan TC, Pearson ML, et al: Guideline for prevention of surgical site infection, 1999. Hospital Infection Control Practices Advisory Committee. Infect Control Hosp Epidemiol 20:250-278, 1999.
4. Christou NV, Nohr CW, Meakins JL: Assessing operative site infection in surgical patients. Arch Surg 122:165-169, 1987.
5. Hunt TK, Hopf HW: Wound healing and wound infection: What surgeons and anesthesiologists can do. Surg Clin North Am 77:587-606, 1997.
6. Banwell PE: Topical negative pressure therapy in wound care. J Wound Care 8:79-84, 1999.
7. Gentilello LM, Jurkovich GJ, Stark MS, et al: Is hypothermia in the victim of major trauma protective or harmful? A randomized, prospective study. Ann Surg 226:439-449, 1997.
8. Rohrer MJ, Natale AM: Effect of hypothermia on the coagulation cascade. Crit Care Med 20:1402-1405, 1992.
9. Gentilello LM, Cobean RA, Offner PJ, et al: Continuous arteriovenous rewarming: Rapid reversal of hypothermia in critically ill patients. J Trauma 32:316-327, 1992.
10. O'Grady NP, Barie PS, Bartlett J, et al: Practice parameters for evaluating new fever in critically ill adult patients. Task Force of the American College of Critical Care Medicine of the Society of Critical Care Medicine in collaboration with the Infectious Disease Society of America. Crit Care Med 26:392-408, 1998.
11. Demling RH: Adult respiratory distress syndrome: Current concepts. New Horiz 1:388-401, 1993.
12. Kollef MH, Schuster DP: The acute respiratory distress syndrome. N Engl J Med 332:27-37, 1995.
13. Luce JM: Acute lung injury and the acute respiratory distress syndrome. Crit Care Med 26:369-376, 1998.
14. Strandberg A, Tokics L, Brismar B, et al: Atelectasis during anaesthesia and in the postoperative period. Acta Anaesthesiol Scand 30:154-158, 1986.
15. Moore FA, Haenel JB, Moore EE: Postoperative respiratory failure. In Cameron JL (ed): Current Surgical Therapy, 5th ed. St. Louis, Mosby, 1995, pp 968-972.
16. Dellinger RP: Clinical trials in adult respiratory distress syndrome. New Horiz 1:584-592, 1993.
17. Geerts WH, Code KI, Jay RM, et al: A prospective study of venous thromboembolism after major trauma. N Engl J Med 331:1601-1606, 1994.
18. Ferretti GR, Bosson JL, Buffaz PD, et al: Acute pulmonary embolism: Role of helical CT in 164 patients with intermediate probability at ventilation-perfusion scintigraphy and normal results at duplex US of the legs. Radiology 205:453-458, 1997.
19. ACCP Consensus Committee on Pulmonary Embolism. American College of Chest Physicians: Opinions regarding the diagnosis and management of venous thromboembolic disease. Chest 113:499-504, 1998.
20. Clagett GP, Anderson FA Jr, Geerts W, et al: Prevention of venous thromboembolism. Chest 114:531S-560S, 1998.
21. Goldhaber SZ, Morpurgo M: Diagnosis, treatment, and prevention of pulmonary embolism. Report of the WHO/International Society and Federation of Cardiology Task Force. JAMA 268:1727-1733, 1992.
22. Mangano DT, Hollenberg M, Fegert G, et al: Perioperative myocardial ischemia in patients undergoing noncardiac surgery: I. Incidence and severity during the 4 day perioperative period. The Study of Perioperative Ischemia (SPI) Research Group. J Am Coll Cardiol 17:843-850, 1991.
23. Fuster V, Badimon L, Badimon JJ, et al: The pathogenesis of coronary artery disease and the acute coronary syndromes (2). N Engl J Med 326:310-318, 1992.
24. Teo KK, Yusuf S, Furberg CD: Effects of prophylactic antiarrhythmic drug therapy in acute myocardial infarction: An overview of results from randomized controlled trials. JAMA 270:1589-1595, 1993.
25. Eagle KA, Brundage BH, Chaitman BR, et al: Guidelines for perioperative cardiovascular evaluation for noncardiac surgery. Report of the American College of Cardiology/American Heart Association Task Force on Practice Guidelines (Committee on Perioperative Cardiovascular Evaluation for Noncardiac Surgery). J Am Coll Cardiol 27:910-948, 1996.
26. Goldman L: Cardiac risks and complications of noncardiac surgery. Ann Intern Med 98:504-513, 1983.
27. Goldman L: Cardiac risk for vascular surgery. J Am Coll Cardiol 27:799-802, 1996.
28. Alonso DR, Scheidt S, Post M, et al: Pathophysiology of cardiogenic shock. Quantification of myocardial necrosis, clinical, pathologic and electrocardiographic correlations. Circulation 48:588-596, 1973.
29. Cohn JN: The management of chronic heart failure. N Engl J Med 335:490-498, 1996.
30. Anderson RJ, Schrier RW: Clinical spectrum of oliguric and non-oliguric acute renal failure. In Brenner BM, Stein JH (eds): Acute Renal Failure. New York, Churchill Livingstone, 1980.

31. Gamelli RL: Acute renal failure. *In* Cameron JL (ed): Current Surgical Therapy, 5th ed. St. Louis, Mosby, 1995, pp 972-975.

32. Thadhani R, Pascual M, Bonventre JV: Acute renal failure. N Engl J Med 334:1448-1460, 1996.

33. Ivatury RR, Diebel L, Porter JM, et al: Intra-abdominal hypertension and the abdominal compartment syndrome. Surg Clin North Am 77:783-800, 1997.

34. Pastan S, Bailey J: Dialysis therapy. N Engl J Med 338:1428-1437, 1998.

35. Barquist E, Kirton O: Adrenal insufficiency in the surgical intensive care unit patient. J Trauma 42:27-31, 1997.

36. Battathiry MM, Clark OH: Endocrinopathies in the critically ill patient. *In* Barie PS, Shires GD (eds): Surgical Intensive Care. Boston, Little, Brown, 1993, pp 861-892.

37. Bizer LS, Liebling RW, Delany HM, et al: Small bowel obstruction: The role of nonoperative treatment in simple intestinal obstruction and predictive criteria for strangulation obstruction. Surgery 89:407-413, 1981.

38. Frager D, Medwid SW, Baer JW, et al: CT of small-bowel obstruction: Value in establishing the diagnosis and determining the degree and cause. AJR Am J Roentgenol 162:37-41, 1994.

39. Frager DH, Baer JW, Rothpearl A, et al: Distinction between postoperative ileus and mechanical small-bowel obstruction: Value of CT compared with clinical and other radiographic findings. AJR Am J Roentgenol 164:891-894, 1995.

40. Becker JM, Dayton MT, Fazio VW, et al: Prevention of postoperative abdominal adhesions by a sodium hyaluronate-based bioresorbable membrane: A prospective, randomized, double-blind multicenter study. J Am Coll Surg 183:297-306, 1996.

41. Meldrum DR, Moore FA, Moore EE, et al: Prospective characterization and selective management of the abdominal compartment syndrome. Am J Surg 174:667-673, 1997.

42. Saggi BH, Sugerman HJ, Ivatury RR, et al: Abdominal compartment syndrome. J Trauma 45:597-609, 1998.

43. Cook DJ, Fuller HD, Guyatt GH, et al: Risk factors for gastrointestinal bleeding in critically ill patients. Canadian Critical Care Trials Group. N Engl J Med 330:377-381, 1994.

44. Cook DJ, Reeve BK, Guyatt GH, et al: Stress ulcer prophylaxis in critically ill patients: Resolving discordant meta-analyses. JAMA 275:308-314, 1996.

45. Cook D, Guyatt G, Marshall J, et al: A comparison of sucralfate and ranitidine for the prevention of upper gastrointestinal bleeding in patients requiring mechanical ventilation. Canadian Critical Care Trials Group. N Engl J Med 338:791-797, 1998.

46. Bartlett JG, Chang TW, Gurwith M, et al: Antibiotic-associated pseudomembranous colitis due to toxin-producing clostridia. N Engl J Med 298:531-534, 1978.

47. Chamberlain RS, Kaufman HL, Danforth DN: Enterocutaneous fistula in cancer patients: Etiology, management, outcome, and impact on further treatment. Am Surg 64:1204-1211, 1998.

48. Bonatsos G, Leandros E, Dourakis N, et al: Laparoscopic cholecystectomy: Intraoperative findings and postoperative complications. Surg Endosc 9:889-893, 1995.

49. Stewart L, Way LW: Bile duct injuries during laparoscopic cholecystectomy: Factors that influence the results of treatment. Arch Surg 130:1123-1129, 1995.

50. Weigelt JA: Fever, hypothermia, and delirium. *In* Levine BA, Copeland EM, et al (eds): Current Practice of Surgery. New York, Churchill Livingstone, 1993, pp 1-8.

51. Talmor M, Li P, Barie PS: Acute paranasal sinusitis in critically ill patients: Guidelines for prevention, diagnosis, and treatment. Clin Infect Dis 25:1441-1446, 1997.

CHAPTER 15

SURGERY IN THE ELDERLY

Ronnie A. Rosenthal, M.D.   and   Michael E. Zenilman, M.D.

Aging and Surgery	**Preoperative Assessment**
Physiologic Decline	**Specific Considerations**
Comorbid Disease	**Ethical Issues**

The population of the United States has increased significantly over the past generation, mostly as a result of decreases in mortality from medical and public health interventions. These interventions, many depicted in Figure 15-1,[1] impacted positively on the average *life expectancy* of humans, defined as the years of life remaining for a stated age. Whereas it is controversial whether they affected the overall human *life span,* defined as the maximum survival potential of our particular species, the interventions have allowed us to closely approach this value.

The portion of the population older than age 65 years is expected to grow from the present 12.7% to approximately 20% by the year 2030. The most rapidly growing segment of this older population is persons older than age 85. Their number is expected to increase sixfold, reaching nearly 20 million by 2050.[2] Social Security, Medicare, and Medicaid benefits to the elderly currently consume one third of U.S. spending and have the potential to consume the entire federal budget by 2012. Therefore, the simple increase in number of older persons is going to stress the health care industry. This will occur even though the actual cost for care of older persons is relatively low when compared with younger counterparts.[3]

As the number of older patients increases, it becomes increasingly important for every surgeon to have a clear understanding of the factors that influence the life expectancy of his or her older patients. This is essential when weighting the risks of operation against the benefits of survival time and quality of life. Life expectancy at various ages is shown in Figure 15-2A.[4] Although life expectancy is usually described in terms of a mean or median, the curve demonstrates that a significant fraction of even the oldest patients can be expected to survive many years. For example, 10% of those age 90 years can be expected to survive until age 99 years. When comorbid

disease is present, life expectancy decreases. The influence of congestive heart failure and dementia, two common comorbid conditions in older persons, on the years of life remaining for persons age 75 years is shown in Figure 15-2B. When making decisions about surgical treatment in older patients, it is important to consider the actual life expectancy of the individual patient based on his or her overall health. Patients with serious comorbidity may not live long enough to gain the benefit from surgery so the risk of surgery becomes an even greater concern.

AGING AND SURGERY

As the number of persons reaching old age continues to grow, there will be a concomitant need to provide surgical care to an increasing number of elderly patients. Over the past 2 decades alone, the percentage of operations in which the patient is older than age 65 increased from 19% of all operations to 37% (Fig. 15-3A).[5] When obstetric procedures are excluded, this portion rises to 43%. In 2000, the rate of surgery for persons older than age 65 was over two and a half times the rate for persons age 45 to 64 years (see Fig. 15-3B). Discharge data from short-stay hospitals in 2000 show that 36% of cholecystectomies, 52% of hernia repairs, 55% of coronary artery bypass grafts, and 57% of bowel resections were performed on patients older than age 65. It is now estimated that at least 50% of patients in most general surgical practices are older than age 65.

This increase in the percentage of operations in which the patient is older than age 65 is not entirely due to the increase in the number of older patients. It is also a reflection of a greater willingness to offer surgical treatment to the elderly. Over the past several decades, advances in surgical and anesthetic techniques have allowed us to

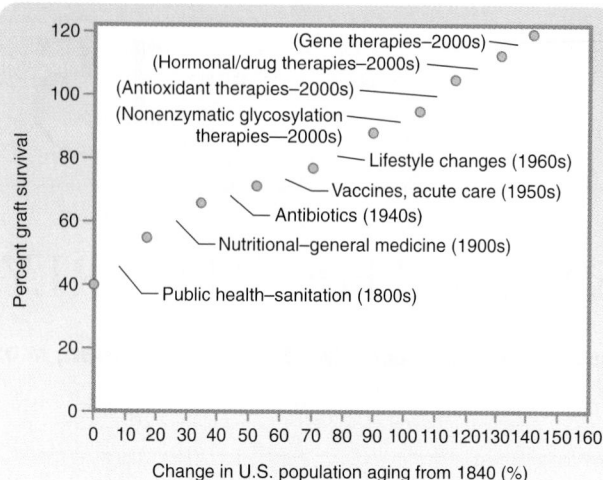

FIGURE 15-1. The changes in the life expectancy at birth for males and females in the United States plotted as a percent change from 1840. Factors thought to be responsible for the actual changes are shown below the line, whereas speculative factors associated with projected changes are shown above the line. The authors warn that "Projections in life expectancy are linear extrapolations and represent potential increases based on untested interventions." (From Baker GT III, Martin GR: Molecular and biological factors in aging: The origins, causes, and prevention of senescence. *In* Cassel CK, et al [eds]: Geriatric Medicine, 3rd ed. New York, Springer, 1997.)

operate with much greater control and safety. Operative mortality in older patients has declined sharply. As a result, the "risk" of surgery has become somewhat less of a concern than the need to provide maximal disease management.

The pattern of surgical management of malignant disease in the elderly is an example of the changing views on surgery in this age group. Data from the National Cancer Institute's Surveillance, Epidemiology and End Results (SEER) Program indicates a decrease in the gap between the percent of younger and older patients treated surgically for certain cancers.[6] The likelihood of receiving surgery for cancers of the breast, ovary, uterus, colon, and rectum has increased more rapidly among patients older than age 75 than in those younger than 55. For cancers that require extensive surgery and for those in which survival is poor even with surgery, there has been less of a change, even for early-stage disease. Figure 15-4 demonstrates that for early-stage colon and rectal cancer in which the chance of surgical cure is high, the percent of older patients receiving surgical treatment has approached that of younger patients. For gastric and pancreatic cancer, operative percentages still decline sharply with age. At present it is still unclear whether this is the result of appropriate decision making based on the overall health of the patient and patient treatment preference or whether this is a reflection of vestigial prejudice and age bias.

It is also important to remember that the pattern of symptoms and the natural history of the surgical disease in older patients may not be identical to that seen in their younger counterparts. The absence of "typical" signs and symptoms often leads to errors in diagnosis and delays in treatment. As a result, it is not unusual for an acute complication to be the first indication of disease. This is unfortunate because emergency operative mortality is 3 to 10 times higher than in comparable elective cases.

There is no doubt that increasing age appears to have a negative effect on the outcome of surgery. However, most studies indicate that chronologic age alone has little effect on outcome. It is rather the age-related decline in physiologic reserves and increase in comorbidity that is responsible for this observation.

PHYSIOLOGIC DECLINE

With aging there is a decline in physiologic function in all organ systems, although the magnitude of this decline is variable among organs and among individuals. In the resting state, this decline usually has minimal functional consequence, although physiologic reserves may be utilized just to maintain homeostasis. However, when physiologic reserves are required to meet the additional challenges of surgery or acute illness, overall performance may deteriorate. This progressive age-related decline in organ system homeostatic reserves, known as "homeostenosis," was first described by the physiologist Walter Cannon in the 1940s. Figure 15-5 is a graph of the present concepts of homeostenosis.[7] With increased age there is an increased utilization of physiologic reserves just to maintain normal homeostasis. Therefore, when these reserves are stressed there are fewer available to meet the challenge, and overall function may be pushed over the "precipice" of organ failure or death.

Over the past several decades, an enormous amount of research has been conducted to define the specific changes in organ function that are directly attributable to aging. This is an inherently difficult task because aging is also accompanied by an increased vulnerability to disease. It is often difficult to determine whether an observed decline in function is secondary to aging, per se, or to disease associated with aging. The overall effect, however, is still the same: a much small margin for error in the care of the older patient. Understanding the changes in organ function can help minimize these errors.

Cardiovascular

Morphologic changes are found in the myocardium, conducting pathways, valves and vasculature of the heart, and great vessels with increasing age. The number of myocytes declines as the collagen and elastin content increases, resulting in fibrotic areas throughout the myocardium and an overall decline in ventricular compliance. Nearly 90% of the autonomic tissue in the sinus node is replaced by fat and connective tissue, and fibrosis interferes with conduction in the intranodal tracts and bundle of His. These changes contribute to the high incidence of sick sinus syndrome, atrial arrhythmias, and bundle branch blocks. Sclerosis and calcification of the aortic valve is common but usually of no functional significance.

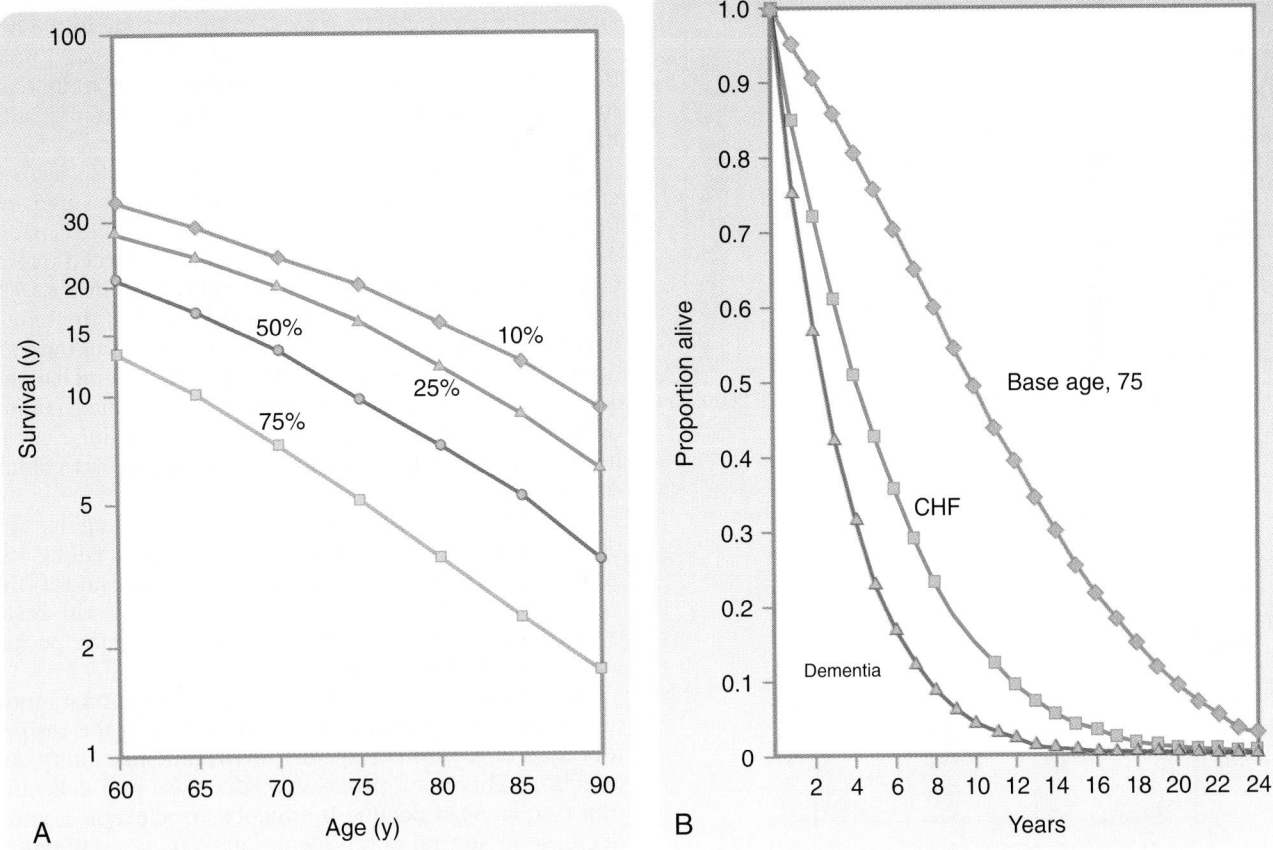

FIGURE 15-2. **A,** Percentiles for life expectancy at various ages. **B,** Survival at age 75 years base *(black diamonds)* and with congestive heart failure (CHF) *(black squares)* or dementia *(open triangles)*. Median survival is 10, 4, and 2.5 years, respectively. (From Robinson B, Beghe C: Cancer screening in the older patient. Clin Geriatr Med 13:97-118, 1997.)

Progressive dilation of all four valvular annuli is probably responsible for the multivalvular regurgitation demonstrated in healthy older persons. Finally, there is a progressive increase in rigidity and decrease in distensibility of both the coronary arteries and the great vessels. Changes in the peripheral vasculature contribute to increased systolic blood pressure, increased resistance to ventricular emptying, and compensatory loss of myocytes with ventricular hypertrophy.

The direct functional implications of these changes are difficult to accurately assess because age-related changes in body composition, metabolic rate, general state of fitness, and underlying disease all influence cardiac performance. It is now generally accepted that systolic function is well preserved with increasing age. Cardiac output and ejection fraction are maintained in spite of the increase in afterload imposed by the stiffening of the outflow tract.[8] The mechanism by which cardiac output is maintained during exercise, however, is somewhat different. In younger persons, output is maintained by increasing heart rate in response to β-adrenergic stimulation. With aging there is a relative "hyposympathetic state" in which the heart becomes less responsive to catecholamines, possible secondary to declining receptor function. The aging heart, therefore, maintains cardiac output not by increasing rate but by increasing ventricular filling (preload). Because of the dependence on preload, even minor hypovolemia can result in significant compromise in cardiac function.

Diastolic function, however, which depends on relaxation rather than contraction, is affected by aging. Diastolic dysfunction is responsible for up to 50% of the cases of heart failure in patients older than age 80 years.[9] Myocardial relaxation is more energy dependent and therefore requires more oxygen than does contraction. With aging there is a progressive decrease in the partial pressure of oxygen. As a result, even mild hypoxemia can result in prolonged relaxation, higher diastolic pressures, and pulmonary congestion. Because early diastolic filling is impaired, maintenance of preload becomes even more reliant on the atrial kick. Loss of the atrial contribution to preload can result in further impairment of cardiac function.

It is also important to remember that the manifestation of cardiac diseases in the elderly may be nonspecific and atypical. While chest pain is still the most common symptom of myocardial infarction, as many as 40% of older patients will present in a nonclassic manner with symptoms such as shortness of breath, syncope, acute confusion, or stroke.

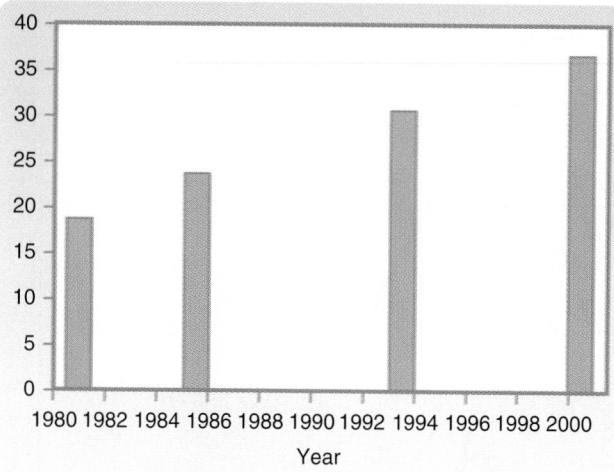

A

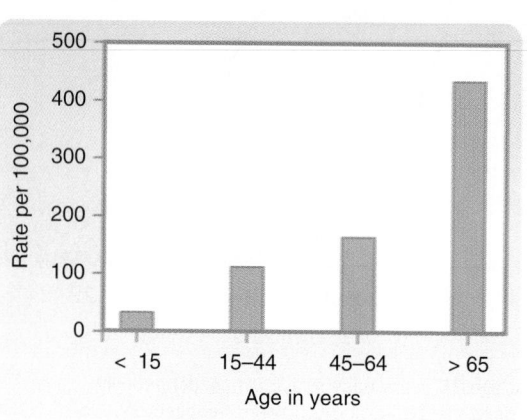

B

FIGURE 15-3. **A,** Increase in the percent of operations in which the patient is over age 65. In 1980, 19% of operations in nonfederally funded hospitals were performed on patients older than age 65. This percentage has increased to 37% by 2000. When obstetrical procedures are excluded, this percentage rises to 43%. **B,** Rate of operations per 100,000 persons, by age in year 2000. (Data from CDC Advance Data No. 329, June 19, 2002.)

The P_{CO_2} does not change, in spite of an increase in dead space. This may be due, in part, to the decline in the production of CO_2 that accompanies the falling basal metabolic rates. Air trapping is also responsible for an increase in the residual volume, or the volume remaining after maximal expiration.

The loss of support of the small airways also leads to collapse during forced expiration, which limits dynamic lung volumes and flow rates. Forced vital capacity decreases by 14 to 30 mL/yr and 1-second forced expiratory volume decreases by 23 to 32 mL/yr (in males.) The overall effect of loss of elastic inward recoil of the lung is balanced somewhat by the decline in chest wall outward force. Total lung capacity, therefore, remains unchanged, and there is only a mild increase in resting lung volume or functional residual capacity. Because total lung capacity remains unchanged, the increase in respiratory volume results in a decrease in vital capacity.

The control of ventilation is also affected by aging. Ventilatory responses to hypoxia and hypercapnia fall by 50% and 40%, respectively. The exact mechanism of this decline has not been well defined but may be the result of declining chemoreceptor function either at the peripheral or central nervous system level.[10]

In addition to these intrinsic changes, pulmonary function is affected by alterations in the ability of the respiratory system to protect against environmental injury and infection. There is a progressive decrease in T-cell function (see later), a decline in mucociliary clearance, and a decrease in several components of swallowing function. The loss of cough reflex secondary to neurologic disorders, combined with swallowing dysfunction may predispose to aspiration.[11] The increased frequency and severity of pneumonia in older persons has been attributed to these factors and to an increased incidence of oropharyngeal colonization with gram-negative organisms. This colonization correlates closely with comorbidity and with the ability of older patients to perform activities of daily living. This fact lends support to the idea that functional capacity is a crucial factor in assessing the risk of pneumonia in older patients (see later).

Respiratory

With aging there is a decline in respiratory function that is attributable to changes in both the chest wall and the lung. Chest wall compliance decreases secondary to changes in structure caused by kyphosis and exaggerated by vertebral collapse. Calcification of the costal cartilage and contractures of the intercostal muscles results in a decline in rib mobility. Maximum inspiratory and expiratory force decreases by as much as 50%, secondary to progressive decrease in the strength of the respiratory muscles.

In the lung, there is a loss of elasticity, which leads to increased alveolar compliance with collapse of the small airways and subsequent uneven alveolar ventilation with air trapping. Uneven alveolar ventilation leads to ventilation-perfusion mismatches, which, in turn, cause a decline in arterial oxygen tension of 0.3 or 0.4 mm Hg per year.

Renal

Between the ages of 25 and 85 there is a progressive decrease in the renal cortex in which approximately 40% of the nephrons become sclerotic. The remaining functional units hypertrophy in a compensatory manner. Sclerosis of the glomeruli is accompanied by atrophy of the afferent and efferent arterioles and by a decrease in renal tubular cell number. Renal blood flow also falls by approximately 50%.

Functionally, there is a decline in glomerular filtration rate of approximately 45% by age 80 years. This decrease is reflected in a decline in creatinine clearance of 0.75 mL/min/yr in healthy older men. The serum creatinine value, however, remains unchanged because there is a concomitant decrease in lean body mass and, thus, a decrease in creatinine production. Estimates of creatinine clearance in the healthy aged can be made from the serum

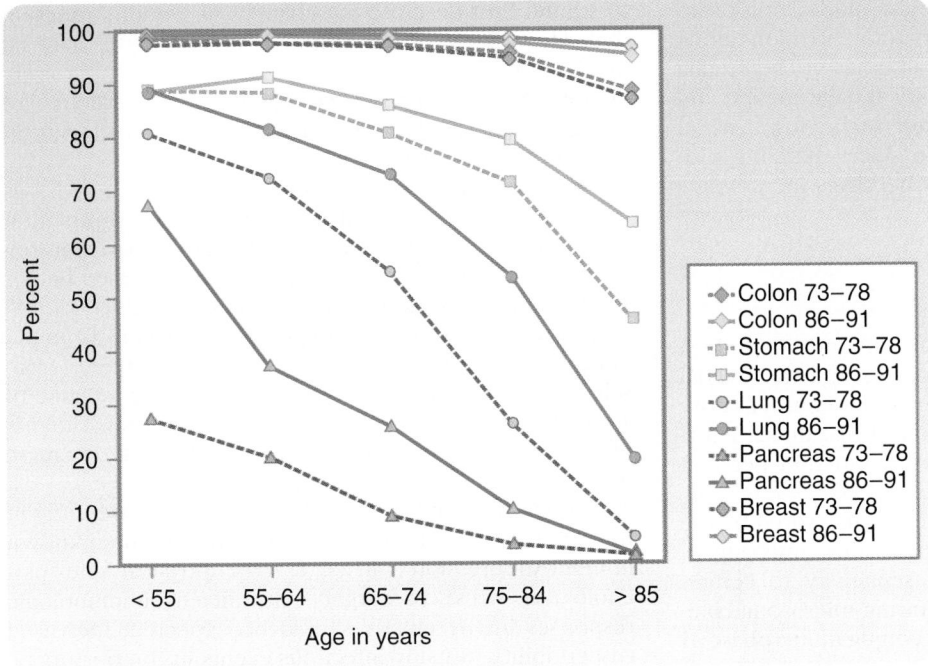

FIGURE 15-4. Temporal variation in the percent of patients treated surgically for local stage cancer, as a function of age. *Dashed lines* represent the earlier time period (1973-1978); *solid lines* represent the later time period (1986-1991). For operations in which surgical risk is high or postoperative survival overall is low, the gap between younger and older patients has not narrowed significantly over time. (From Farrow DC, Hunt WC, Samet JM: Temporal and regional variability in the surgical treatment of cancer among older people. J Am Geriatr Soc 44:559-564, 1996.)

Legend:
- Colon 73–78
- Colon 86–91
- Stomach 73–78
- Stomach 86–91
- Lung 73–78
- Lung 86–91
- Pancreas 73–78
- Pancreas 86–91
- Breast 73–78
- Breast 86–91

X-axis: Age in years — < 55, 55–64, 65–74, 75–84, > 85
Y-axis: Percent

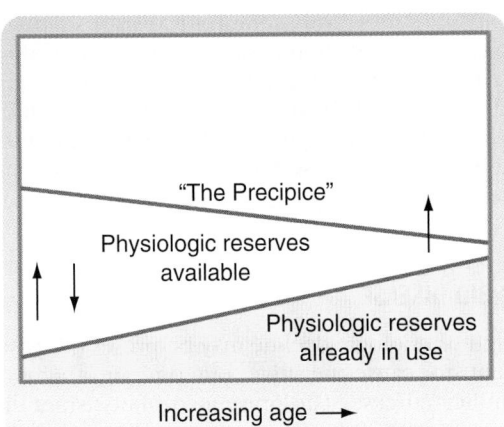

FIGURE 15-5. Graphic representation of "homeostenosis." With increasing age, physiologic reserves are increasingly utilized to maintain homeostasis. *Vertical arrows* represent challenges such as surgical stress or acute illness. Because reserves are already utilized, there are fewer available to meet these challenges. As a result, the "precipice" is crossed by a stress that would be easily tolerated in younger age. This "precipice" may be any relevant clinical marker such as organ dysfunction or failure or death. (From Taffett GE: Physiology of aging. *In* Cassel CK, Leipzig RM, Cohen HJ, et al [eds]: Geriatric Medicine: An Evidence-Based Approach, 4th ed. New York, Springer, 2003.)

Labels within figure: "The Precipice"; Physiologic reserves available; Physiologic reserves already in use; Increasing age →

creatinine by using the formula derived by Cockcroft and Gault.[12]

$$(140 - \text{age in years}) \times (\text{weight in kg}) \div [72 \times (\text{serum creatinine in mg/dL})]$$

Caution must be exercised when applying this formula to critically ill patients or those on medications that directly affect renal function.

Renal tubular function also declines with advancing age. The ability to conserve sodium and excrete hydrogen ion falls, resulting in a diminished capacity to regulate fluid and acid-base balance. Dehydration becomes a particular problem because losses of sodium and water from nonrenal causes are not compensated for by the usual mechanisms of increased renal sodium retention, increased urinary concentration, and increased thirst. The inability to retain sodium is believed to be due to a decline in the activity of the renin-angiotensin system. The increasing inability to concentrate the urine is related to a decline in end organ responsiveness to antidiuretic hormone. The marked decline in the subjective feeling of thirst is also well documented but not well understood. Alterations of osmoreceptor function in the hypothalamus may be responsible for the failure to recognize thirst in spite of significant elevations in serum osmolality.[13]

Alterations in renal function also have important implications for the type and dosage of drugs used in older patients. Although drugs are handled by the kidney in several different ways, most changes in renal drug processing parallel the decline in glomerular filtration rate. Therefore, creatinine clearance can be used to determine the appropriate clearance of most agents processed by the kidney.

The lower urinary tract also changes with increasing age. In the bladder, increased collagen content leads to limited distensibility and impaired emptying. Overactivity of the detrusor secondary to neurologic disorders or idiopathic causes has also been identified. In women, decreased circulating levels of estrogen and decreased tissue responsiveness to this hormone cause changes in the urethral sphincter that predispose to urinary incontinence. In males, prostatic hypertrophy impairs bladder emptying. Together, these factors lead to urinary incontinence in 10% to 15% of elderly persons living in the community and 50% of those in nursing homes.

There is also an increased prevalence of asymptomatic bacteriuria with age, which varies from 10% to 50%

depending on gender, level of activity, underlying disorders, and place of residence. Urinary tract infections alone are responsible for 30% to 50% of all cases of bacteremia in older patients. Alterations in the local environment and declining host defenses are thought to be responsible. Because of the lack of symptoms in elderly patients with bacteriuria, preoperative urinalysis becomes increasingly important.

Hepatobiliary

Morphologic changes in the liver with age include a decrease in the number of hepatocytes and the overall weight and size. There is, however, a compensatory increase in cell size and proliferation of bile ducts. Functionally, hepatic blood flow falls by 0.3% to 1.5% per year to 40% to 45% of earlier values after age 65.[14]

The synthetic capacity of the liver, as measured by the standard test of liver function, remains unchanged. However, the metabolism of and sensitivity to certain kinds of drugs is altered. Drugs requiring microsomal oxidation (phase I reactions) before conjugation (phase II reactions) may be metabolized more slowly, whereas those requiring only conjugation may be cleared at a normal rate. Drugs that act directly on hepatocytes, such as warfarin (Coumadin), may produce the desired therapeutic effects at lower doses in the elderly owing to an increased sensitivity of the cells to these agents.

The most significant correlate of altered hepatobiliary function in the aged is the increased incidence of gallstones and gallstone-related complications. Gallstone prevalence rises steadily with age, although there is variability in the absolute percentages depending on the population. Stones have been demonstrated in as many as 80% of nursing home residents older than age 90 years. Biliary tract disease is the single most common indication for abdominal surgery in the elderly population (see later).

Immune Function

Immune competence, like other physiologic parameters, declines with advancing age. This immunosenescence is characterized by an increased susceptibility to infections, an increase in autoantibodies and monoclonal immunoglobulins, and an increase in tumorigenesis. Also, like other physiologic systems, this decline may not be apparent in the nonchallenged state. For example, there is no decline in neutrophil count with age, but the ability of the bone marrow to increase neutrophil production in response to infection may be impaired.[15] Elderly patients with major infections frequently have normal white blood cell counts, but the differential count will show a profound shift to the left, with a large proportion of immature forms.

With aging, there is an involution of the thymus gland and a decline in the production of thymic polypeptide factors such as thymosin a-1. This and other thymic hormones control the differentiation and proliferation of thymocytes into mature T lymphocytes. The resulting alterations in T-cell populations, products, and response to stimuli best describe the changes in immune function that accompany aging. Although other factors may be involved, the decline in T-cell responsiveness to a variety of antigens is demonstrated by the high incidence of anergy to delayed hypersensitivity skin tests seen in persons older than age 60.

Some B-cell defects have been identified, although it is thought that the functional deficits in antibody production are related to altered T-cell regulation rather than to intrinsic B-cell changes.[16] In vitro, there is an increased helper T-cell activity for nonspecific antibody production and there is a decreased ability of suppressor T cells from old mice to recognize and suppress specific antigens from self. This is reflected in an increase in the prevalence of autoantibodies to more than 10% by age 80 years. The mix of immunoglobulins also changes: IgM levels decrease while IgG and IgA increase slightly.

The clinical implications of these changes are difficult to determine. When superimposed on the known immunosuppression caused by the physical and psychological stress of surgery, insufficient immunologic responses in the elderly should be expected. Increased susceptibility to many infectious agents in the postoperative period, however, is more likely a result of a combination of stress and comorbid disease rather than physiologic decline. Immunosenescence alone does not appear to be responsible for the observation that older patients are more likely to contract an infectious illness and less able to eradicate it quickly. The decline in physiologic reserve of other organ systems combined with comorbid illnesses, however, may impair and prolong recovery.

COMORBID DISEASE

Although physiologic decline may be present, it is seldom sufficient to cause negative outcome in the elective, uncomplicated case. The presence of coexisting disease, however, strongly influences outcome in any setting. With age, there is a clear rise in diseases of organ systems other than that for which the older patient seeks surgical care. In patients with colon cancer, for example, Yancik and coworkers documented a clear rise in concomitant conditions such that by age 75 patients had a mean of five disorders in addition to the primary malignancy.[17]

There are numerous studies that document the impact of comorbidity on outcome. In one such study, there were few adverse events in all age groups without additional illness. However, adverse events increased consistently with increasing comorbidity. This effect was most pronounced at both extremes of life (Fig. 15-6).[18] In another study of 21,000 cholecystectomies in the prelaparoscopic era, there was a fourfold rise in mortality from 1.5% in patients with no concomitant diseases to 6.1% in patients with more than three additional conditions.[19]

Like the surgical disease itself, the manifestations of comorbid illnesses in the elderly frequently are less "typical" than in younger patients. In the Framingham heart study, for example, over 40% of the myocardial infarctions in patients age 75 to 84 were unrecognized or silent compared with less than 20% in patients between

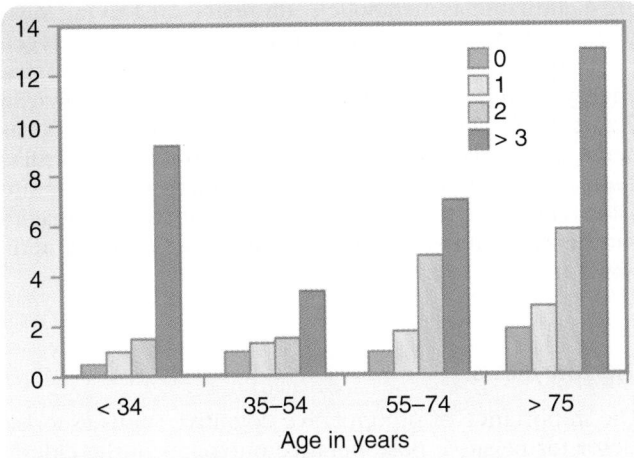

FIGURE 15-6. Rate of perioperative events associated with age and the number of comorbid conditions 0, 1, 2, or more than 3. (From Tiret L, et al: Complications associated with anaesthesia—a prospective survey in France. Can Anaesth Soc J 33:336-344, 1986.)

Box 15-1. Simple Preoperative Assessment Tools

Function

ASA classification
Activities of daily living (ADLs)
Exercise capacity in metabolic equivalents (METs)

Cognition

Three-item recall
Folstein Mini Mental Status exam if three-item recall is positive

Nutrition

Risk factor assessment
Subjective global assessment
Mini-nutritional assessment
Serum albumin

---

the ages of 45 and 54.[20] In another study of hospitalized patients older than age 70, 72% of moderate to severe cognitive disorders and 46% of moderate to severe nutritional deficits identified on formal admission assessment were unrecognized by the primary caregiver in the community. The search for comorbidity must therefore be thorough.

PREOPERATIVE ASSESSMENT

The goal of the preoperative assessment of the elderly patient is to define the extent of decline and identify the coexisting diseases or comorbidities. Extensive testing for disease in every organ system is not cost effective, practical, or necessary for most patients. A thorough history and physical examination will provide information to direct further work-up if necessary. It is important, however, to adjust the history and physical examination to carefully look for the risk factors and signs and symptoms of the more common comorbid conditions. The addition of simple tools for assessment of functional, cognitive, and nutritional status will significantly enhance the understanding of the individual patient's true operative risk (see later and Box 15-1). When initial evaluation identifies disease or risk factors for disease, further work-up may be indicated.

Of all comorbid conditions, cardiovascular disease is the most prevalent, and cardiovascular events are a leading cause of severe perioperative complications and death. For this reason the main thrust of preoperative evaluation, in general, has focused on identifying those patients at risk for cardiac complications. The American College of Cardiology (ACC) and the American Heart Association (AHA) Task Force on Practice Guidelines has published an in-depth set of guidelines for preoperative cardiac evaluation.[21] These guidelines provide a stepwise Bayesian strategy for determining which patients will need further testing to clarify risk or further treatment to minimize risk. Stratification is based on factors related to the patient and the type of surgery. For elderly patients

with known cardiac disease, a rigorous work-up may be necessary. A recent study cautions against using only an abnormal electrocardiogram (ECG) as a indication for extensive work-up, because ECG abnormalities are common in older patients but do not correlate with postoperative complications.[22] For most patients, an assessment of exercise tolerance and functional capacity is an accurate method for predicting the adequacy of cardiac and pulmonary reserves (see later).

Although the main focus of preoperative evaluation has been cardiac status, in older patients pulmonary complications are at least as common as cardiac complications, if not more so. Risk factors for pulmonary complications are not nearly as well studied as for cardiac complications, although many of the same issues apply to both. Poor exercise capacity and poor general health predict pulmonary as well as cardiac complications.[23] Preexisting pulmonary disease, smoking, obesity, and type of incision have also been implicated.[24] In the elderly, subtle cognitive, nutritional, and swallowing abnormalities are also common and are associated with aspiration, pneumonia, and other negative outcomes.

Functional Status

Assessment of functional status, by a variety of methods, is an extremely reliable means for predicting postoperative outcome. For decades, the American Society of Anesthesiologist (ASA) Physical Status Classification has been used successfully to stratify operative risk. This simple classification ranks patients according to the functional limitations imposed by coexisting disease. When curves for mortality versus ASA class are examined with regard to age, there is little difference between younger and older patients. This indicates that mortality is a function of coexisting disease rather than chronologic age. ASA classification has been shown to accurately predict postoperative mortality even in patients older than age 80. In a large, multicenter Department of Veterans Affairs study (The National Surgical Quality Improvement Program-NSQIP), surgical patients were assessed prospectively for operative risk and risk-adjusted models were then created to allow comparison of the quality of surgical care among different institutions.[25] Of the 68 variables studied, ASA functional classification was the most predictive factor of postoperative morbidity and the second most predictive factor for mortality.

Other standard measures of functional capacity, such as the ability to perform the activities of daily living (ADLs) (e.g., feeding, continence, transferring, toileting, dressing, and bathing), have also been correlated with postoperative mortality and morbidity. Inactivity has been associated with a higher incidence of all major surgical complications. Postoperative mortality for severely limited patients has been reported as nearly 10 times higher than for active patients. Preoperative functional deficits also contribute to postoperative immobility, with associated complications such as atelectasis and pneumonia, venous stasis and pulmonary embolism, and multisystem deconditioning. Deconditioning is an important clinical entity, which leads to further functional decline despite improvement in the acute illness.

Of all the methods of assessing overall functional capacity, exercise tolerance is the most sensitive predictor of postoperative cardiac and pulmonary complications in the elderly. In a frequently quoted study comparing exercise tolerance, and a variety of other assessment techniques, Gerson and colleagues demonstrated that the inability to raise the heart rate to 99 beats/min while doing 2 minutes of supine bicycle exercise was the most sensitive predictor of postoperative cardiac and pulmonary complications and death.[23]

Formal exercise testing, however, is not necessary in every elderly patient. The metabolic requirements for many routine activities have already been determined and are quantitated as metabolic equivalents (MET). One MET, defined as 3.5 mL/kg/min, represents the basal oxygen consumption of a 70-kg, 40-year-old man at rest. Estimated energy requirements for various activities are shown in Figure 15-7.[21] The inability to function above 4 METs has been associated with increased perioperative cardiac events and long-term risk. If appropriate questions are asked about the level of activity, then functional capacity can be accurately determined without the need for additional testing.

Cognitive Status

The importance of preoperative cognitive status as a risk factor for negative postoperative outcomes in the elderly patient is not well appreciated. Cognitive assessment is rarely a part of the preoperative history and physical examination, and there are no widely accepted guidelines for this evaluation in surgical patients. Postoperative delirium, defined as an acute confusional state, however, is associated with a significant increase in mortality, major morbidity, length of stay, and discharge to long-term care or rehabilitation facilities (Table 15-1).[26] In addition, recent studies on the long-term effects of surgery on cognition show that deficits can persist for as long as 3 months after operation.[27] The incidence of postoperative delirium in older patients varies with the type of procedure, reaching 20% to 25% for peripheral vascular cases and certain orthopedic procedures. Rates as high as 60% have been reported in operations for hip fracture.

Delirium must be distinguished from dementia, the more chronic type of baseline cognitive impairment. Preoperative dementia is a major risk factor for delirium in the postoperative period. There are several methods for evaluating baseline cognitive function in the elderly. Among them, the Folstein Mini Mental Status Evaluation

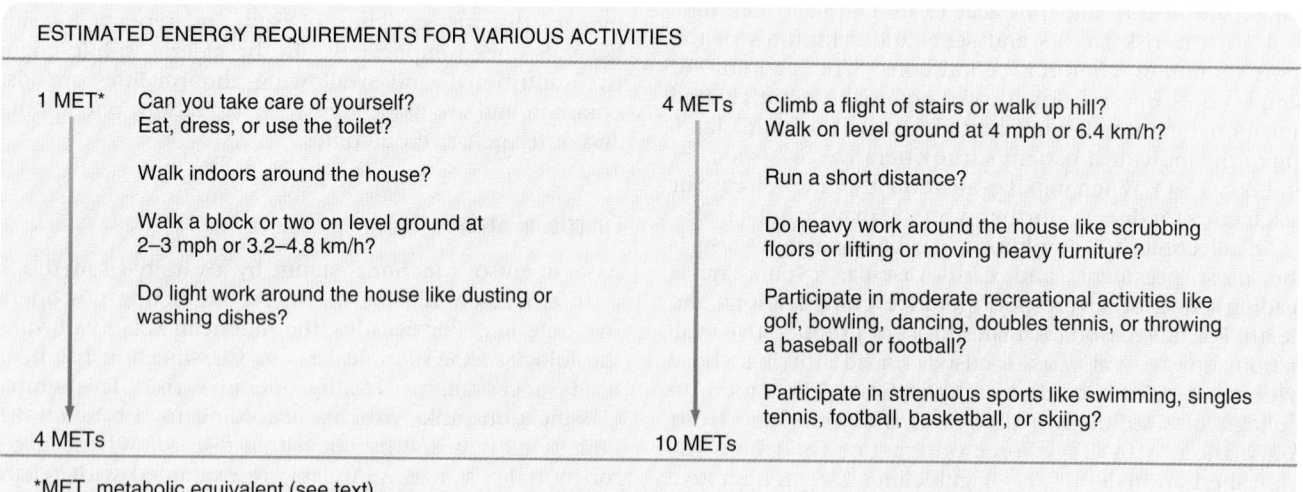

ESTIMATED ENERGY REQUIREMENTS FOR VARIOUS ACTIVITIES

1 MET*	Can you take care of yourself? Eat, dress, or use the toilet?	4 METs	Climb a flight of stairs or walk up hill? Walk on level ground at 4 mph or 6.4 km/h?
	Walk indoors around the house?		Run a short distance?
	Walk a block or two on level ground at 2–3 mph or 3.2–4.8 km/h?		Do heavy work around the house like scrubbing floors or lifting or moving heavy furniture?
	Do light work around the house like dusting or washing dishes?		Participate in moderate recreational activities like golf, bowling, dancing, doubles tennis, or throwing a baseball or football?
			Participate in strenuous sports like swimming, singles tennis, football, basketball, or skiing?
4 METs		10 METs	

*MET, metabolic equivalent (see text).

FIGURE 15-7. Estimated energy requirements for various activities. With increasing activity the number of metabolic equivalents (METs) increases. The inability to function above 4 METs has been associated with increased perioperative cardiac events and long-term risk. (From Eagle KA, et al: ACC/AHA Task Force Report: Guidelines for perioperative cardiovascular evaluation for noncardiac surgery. Circulation 93:1278, 1996.)

TABLE 15-1. Surgical Outcomes in Older Patients With and Without Delirium

Outcome	Delirium (n = 117)	No Delirium (n = 1224)	P
Major complication*	18 (15%)	28 (2%)	<.001
Death	5 (4%)	3 (0.2%)	<.001
Length of stay	15 ± 20	7 ± 5	<.001
Discharge to long-term care or rehabilitation	43 (36%)	136 (11%)	<.001

*Cardiac arrest, ventricular tachycardia or fibrillation, myocardial infarction, pulmonary edema, respiratory failure requiring intubation, renal failure requiring dialysis or stroke.
From Marcantonio ER, et al: A clinical prediction rule for delirium after elective noncardiac surgery. JAMA 271:134, 1994.

ETIOLOGY OF DELIRIUM

D ementia
E lectrolytes
L ungs, liver, heart, kidney, brain
I nfection
R x
I njury, pain, stress
U nfamiliar environment
M etabolic

FIGURE 15-8. Etiology of delirium. The etiology of delirium is multifactorial. It is not uncommon for several factors to exist simultaneously, increasing risk in the individual patient. (From Inouye SK: Delirium in hospitalized elderly patients: Recognition, evaluation and management. Conn Med 57:309-12, 1993.)

(MMSE) has become widely accepted for its ease of administration and reliability.[28] This instrument gives a total of 30 points to four areas: orientation, registration, attention/calculation, and language. A score below 24 is an indication of cognitive impairment. A formal MMSE may be too time consuming to administer in a busy surgical clinic setting, but simple clinical strategies for assessing mental status may be sufficient. The ability to remember and recall three objects after a short delay is the most sensitive of these strategies.

The etiology of delirium in hospitalized patients is multifactorial (Fig. 15-8).[29] Postoperative delirium may be the manifestation of unrecognized preexisting disease or the result of intraoperative or postoperative events. Over the past few years several studies have attempted to identify risk factors for delirium in hospitalized elderly surgical and medical patients. Among the factors associated with delirium, age, preoperative cognitive impairment, poor functional status, alcohol consumption, and polypharmacy are among the most frequently cited. A variety of medications including certain antibiotics, analgesics, antihypertensives, β blockers, and tranquilizers have also been shown to precipitate delirium.

Intraoperative and postoperative factors have also been studied. No association has been found with the route of anesthesia (epidural vs. general) or the occurrence of intraoperative hemodynamic complications. However, intraoperative blood loss, the need for blood transfusion, and postoperative hematocrit less than 30% are associated with a significant increased risk of postoperative delirium.[30] Alterations in the wake-sleep cycle after surgery has also been associated with delirium. In nonsurgical hospitalized elderly patients, independent precipitating factors for delirium include malnutrition, the use of physical restraints, the use of bladder catheters, the need for more than three medications, and any iatrogenic event during hospitalization.

It is most important to recognize that mental status changes in the elderly surgical patient are often the earliest signs of postoperative complication. Therefore, tests for cognitive impairment are essential components of the routine postoperative evaluation. If an adequate preoperative mental status examination has been conducted, postoperative assessment should require only brief observations of behavior and comparison to baseline.

Nutritional Status

The impact of poor nutrition as a risk factor for pneumonia, poor wound healing, and other postoperative complications has long been appreciated. A variety of psychosocial issues and comorbid conditions common to the elderly place this population at high risk for nutritional deficits. Malnutrition is estimated to occur in 0% to 15% of community-dwelling elderly persons, 35% to 65% of older patients in acute care hospitals, and 25% to 60% of institutionalized elderly. Factors that lead to the inadequate intake and utilization of nutrients in this population include the ability to get food (e.g., financial constraints, availability of food, limited mobility), the desire to eat food (e.g., living situation, mental status, chronic illness), the ability to eat and absorb food (e.g., poor dentition, chronic gastrointestinal disorders such as gastroesophageal reflux disease or diarrhea), and medications that interfere with appetite or nutrient metabolism (Box 15-2).[31]

The measurement of nutritional status in the elderly, however, is difficult. Standard anthropomorphic measures do not take into account the change in body composition and structure that accompanies aging. Immune measures of nutrition are influenced by age-related changes in the immune system in general. Furthermore, criteria for the

Box 15-2. Historical Findings Associated with an Increased Risk of Nutritional Deficiency

Recent weight loss
Restricted dietary intake (limited variety)
  Limited variety, food avoidances
Psychosocial situation
  Depression, cognitive impairment, isolation, economic difficulties
Problems with eating, chewing, swallowing
Previous surgery
Increased losses due to gastrointestinal disorders such as malabsorption and diarrhea
Systemic disease interfering with appetite or eating (chronic lung, liver, heart and renal disease, abdominal angina, cancer)
Excessive alcohol use
Medications that interfere with appetite and/or nutrient metabolism

From Rosenberg IH: Nutrition and aging. *In* Hazzard WR, Bierman EL, Blass JP, et al (eds): Principles of Geriatric Medicine and Gerontology, 3rd ed. New York, McGraw-Hill, 1994.

interpretation of biochemical markers in this age group have not been well established.

Complicated markers of malnutrition exist but are not necessary in the routine surgical setting. Subjective assessment by history and physical examination, in which risk factors and physical evidence of malnutrition are assessed, has been shown to be as effective as objective measures of nutritional status.[32] The Subjective Global Assessment (SGA) is a relatively simple, reproducible tool for assessing nutritional status from the history and physical examination. SGA ratings are most strongly influenced by loss of subcutaneous tissue, muscle wasting, and weight loss. The Mini Nutritional Assessment (MNA), which measures 18 factors, including body mass index, weight history, cognition, mobility, dietary history, and self assessment, among others, is also a reliable method for assessing nutritional status. Nutritional status, as determined by both the SGA and the MNA, has been shown to predict mortality in hospitalized geriatric medical patients.[33]

Serum albumin has been implicated as a strong predictor of outcome. Evidence demonstrates that low serum levels of albumin in elderly patients correlate with increased length of stay, increased rates of readmission, unfavorable disposition, and increased all-cause mortality. In surgical patients, low albumin has also been shown to correlate with postoperative morbidity and mortality. In the VA NSQIP study mentioned earlier,[25] low serum albumin was the most important predictive factor for mortality. This suggests that low serum albumin is an important marker of outcome, regardless of whether it is directly related to poor nutritional status or to unidentified complex chronic illness. In a study of patients undergoing elective gastrointestinal surgery both SGA and serum albumin were predictive of postoperative nutrition-related complications.[34]

SPECIFIC CONSIDERATIONS

Endocrine Surgery

Breast

In Western countries, the incidence of breast cancer increases with age. Forty-eight percent of new cases appear in patients older than the age of 65. The SEER database noted an incidence of 60 cases per 100,000 population for patients younger than the age of 65, of 322 cases per 100,000 population for patients older than the age of 65, and of 375 cases per 100,000 population for persons older than the age of 85.[35] The biologic behavior of breast cancer in older women may be less aggressive; a larger portion of tumors have estrogen receptors and other favorable tumor markers.[36] There is some controversy regarding the presentation and survival of breast cancer in elderly patients. Whereas some believe that elderly persons present at a later stage, others have shown that early breast cancer is equally common in all age groups. Some of these differences may be the result of inadequate staging; fewer older patients have axillary dissection, whereas more are reported as "stage undetermined." Similarly, some have shown that elderly patients with breast cancer seem to have poorer survival than younger patients whereas others studies have failed to show a statistical relationship between age and mortality from breast cancer. In studies in which all-cause mortality is considered, these differences are likely attributable to increased comorbidity in older patients. Approximately 30% of deaths in breast cancer patients older than age 85 are directly related to breast cancer, whereas nearly three fourths of deaths are cancer related in patients aged 50 to 54 years. What is not disputed, however, is the fact that elderly patients have been routinely excluded from most of the large clinical trials in the past. Therefore, accurate data on staging, treatment, and outcomes are still lacking.[36]

Elderly women are frequently not treated according to the protocols used for younger women. Up to 60% of elderly patients undergoing lumpectomy fail to follow through with radiation. However, even in elderly patients, radiation therapy after lumpectomy has been shown to reduce local failure rates at 5 years from 28% to 8%.[37] In addition, multiple studies have documented that performing lumpectomy in patients older than the age of 75 and not following with radiation therapy results in local recurrence rates ranging from 25% to 38% at 40 to 50 months.[38] Most of these local recurrences happen within 6 years of lumpectomy, well within the median life expectancy of women aged 80 years. Logistical reasons and patient preferences are often stated as reasons why radiation therapy is not pursued. Radiation therapy is well tolerated by older women and until data indicate which older patients can forego this treatment, recommendations for treatment should be much the same as they are for younger women.

In the past, axillary dissection was necessary for accurate staging before chemotherapy. Now, however, there is an increasing trend to treat both node-positive and node-negative women. For most patients older than the age of 70, tamoxifen is now frequently given regardless of node or receptor status and node dissection.[38] Local control of the axilla in these patients can be achieved by including the area in the port of radiation. Local control of clinically palpable nodes can be performed in a similar way. Nodal status in the axilla, however, is still an important prognostic indicator. In the past, nodal status was determined by axillary dissection, which carried a risk of lymphedema, pain, and shoulder immobility. These complications were particularly limiting in older patients with preexisting musculoskeletal problems. The introduction of sentinel node biopsy, which allows nodal sampling without axillary dissection, may offer older women the opportunity to have this prognostic information without additional risks.

Treatment of breast cancer in the frail elderly should be very different than in the healthy elderly. These patients typically present with clinically palpable lesions. Comorbid illness usually precludes operative intervention, and simple local control of the disease should be the goal of therapy. Tissue diagnosis can be made easily by bedside fine-needle aspiration or Tru-Cut needle biopsy, and treatment can then be individualized. Tamoxifen therapy alone can be used for these frail patients. Response rates range from 10% to 50%, and failure rates range between 23% and 58%.[38]

Thyroid

The incidence of thyroid nodules increases throughout life, whether detected by physical examination, ultrasound, or autopsy. The incidence of nodules in autopsy series is 50%. Most thyroid nodules are single when detected and are four times more common in women. Thyroid nodules change slowly over the short term. Prospective studies have shown, however, that up to one fourth of colloid nodules can shrink over 2 to 3 years and may disappear. Up to 35% of the glands removed at autopsy harbor small cancers, and these are typically of the papillary variety.

After exposure to ionizing radiation, the incidence of new nodules increases at 2% per year, reaching a peak incidence at 15 to 25 years. The highest risk is in patients younger than the age of 20, not the elderly. Because radiation treatment of benign diseases such as tonsillitis, hemangiomas, thymic enlargement, and lymphadenopathy has not been practiced for many years, the majority of patients presenting with this history are now in the elderly cohort. The effect of radiation-induced thyroid disease from atomic bombs or accidental discharges from nuclear power plants is being examined. Early data suggest a similar pattern.[39]

Sporadic papillary thyroid cancer has almost a bell-shaped distribution of age at presentation, with a decreasing trend in patients older than 60. Age is a negative prognostic factor for survival and other variables. Patients older than the age of 60 years have increased risk of local recurrence, and patients younger than 20 and older than 60 have a higher risk than others for developing distant metastasis.

Similar results have been noted for follicular cancer. Increasing patient age correlates with increased risk of death by 2.2 times per 20 years. Others have documented that age greater than 40 to 50 years as well as size greater than 2.5 cm are poor prognostic indicators.

Therefore, chronologic age alone appears to be a true independent predictor of survival from well-differentiated thyroid cancer.[40] The AMES classification (age, distant metastases, extent, and size) proposed by Cady[41] shows that age older than 41 years in men and 51 years in women is a poor prognostic indicator. This classification has been used to determine the extent of resection for patients undergoing surgery.

Parathyroid

Most cases of primary hyperparathyroidism in the elderly are the sporadic type. Today, diagnosis is usually made by increased serum calcium level and elevated parathyroid hormone level. It is believed that up to 1.5% to 3% of hospitalized geriatric persons may have this disease.

The incidence of asymptomatic hyperparathyroidism has increased, although the frequency of the overt complications has decreased. A careful history, however, will frequently reveal the presence of less obvious psychological and emotional symptoms. Presenting complaints are typically mild—lethargy (62%), neurologic complaint (44%), constipation (42%)—whereas overt symptoms such as peptic ulcer disease and renal lithiasis were less frequent. Other subtle symptoms of hyperparathyroidism in older persons include memory loss, personality changes, inability to concentrate, exercise fatigue, and back pain. All of these symptoms can disappear after surgical extirpation of an adenoma. Only 8% of patients are "truly asymptomatic."[42]

Primary hyperparathyroidism in postmenopausal women can also present as significant orthopedic disease. Up to 5% of patients can present with back pain and even vertebral fractures that are indistinguishable from those of senile or postmenopausal osteoporosis.

In response to the controversy regarding treatment of asymptomatic hyperparathyroidism, the National Institutes of Health consensus conference in 1990 offered parameters for care.[43] Participants agreed that truly asymptomatic patients with serum calcium levels that are only mildly elevated, no previous history of life-threatening hypercalcemia, and normal renal, bone, and mental status can be safely observed without surgery. Patients with decreased creatinine clearance of 30% over age-matched controls, 24-hour urinary calcium excretion of more than 400 mg, and decreased bone mass more than 2 standard deviations from age- and race-matched controls should be offered surgical treatment. Further indications for surgery include primary hyperparathyroidism in patients younger than age 50 and hyperparathyroidism in patients for whom close follow-up would be difficult or for whom significant concomitant illness complicates management.

Minimally invasive parathyroid surgery has gained acceptance with the adoption of sestamibi-directed surgery, intraoperative parathyroid hormone assay, and videoscopic surgery, but results are mixed regarding recurrence rates.[44]

Gastrointestinal

Esophagus

The esophagus undergoes characteristic changes with aging. There is a progressive decrease in amplitude of the primary peristaltic waves after deglutition, with octogenarians exhibiting only 50% the amplitude of younger controls, and nonagenarians, 20%. Although the lower esophageal sphincter resting pressure is normal and relaxes appropriately after deglutition, the sphincter fails to rapidly contract back to baseline, resulting in prolonged decreased tone. There is also an increased incidence of sliding hiatal hernia with aging, likely caused by laxity at the gastroesophageal junction. These conditions, in addition to delayed gastric emptying in elderly patients, predispose to gastroesophageal reflux disease.

Dysmotility of the cricopharyngeus (upper esophageal sphincter) with increasing age can result in Zenker's diverticulum (see Chapter 39). Failure of the cricopharyngeus to relax results in a herniation of mucosa above it and below the thyropharyngeus. Cricopharyngeal myotomy to relieve the underlying motor dysfunction is the treatment of choice. For large pouches, many surgeons combine myotomy with stapled resection of the diverticulum. Endoscopic approaches have also been used with excellent results.[45]

Resection for esophageal cancer is a complicated issue, owing to its low cure rate and high operative morbidity and mortality. In general, patients are at risk for pulmonary, cardiac, nutritional, and anastomotic complications, which are amplified in elderly patients. Most studies show no difference in morbidity related to age, although some have shown increased complication and death rates.[46] Overall 5-year survival rates for curative resection are 14% to 25%, similar to those observed in younger patients.

Stomach

A progressive cephalad migration of the antral-fundic junction occurs with age. Studies have shown that between 25% and 80% of elderly persons have fasting achlorhydria. This is due to progressive loss of parietal cells and decreased antral and serum concentrations of gastrin. Achlorhydria results in derangements in folate, iron, and vitamin B_{12} absorption.

The incidence of peptic ulcer disease increases with age. Up to 80% of peptic ulcer–related deaths occur in patients older than the age of 65. Other factors that increase the risk of peptic ulcer disease in the elderly population are use of nonsteroidal anti-inflammatory agents (NSAIDs) and infection with *Helicobacter pylori*. NSAIDs are well-established inducers of peptic ulcer disease, the mechanism being inhibition of formation of prostaglandins, essential components of the gastric mucosal barrier. NSAID use has increased markedly over the past few years, especially in the elderly population. Use of NSAIDs increases the risk of developing complicated peptic ulcer disease in the elderly, when compared with younger patients. Actual NSAID use is also a useful prognostic indicator: the mortality rate from peptic ulcer disease in elderly patients who take NSAIDs is twice that of those who do not. Similarly, 80% of all ulcer-related deaths were in patients taking NSAIDs. Despite this finding, NSAIDs are frequently prescribed to older patients, even those with previous gastrointestinal problems.

H. pylori infections are believed to occur at a rate of 1% per year, yielding a substantial percentage of the elderly population harboring infections. Some have postulated that a cohort of patients who were infected during childhood earlier in this century is now aged and developing complications of the infection. *H. pylori* screening and treatment has increased significantly in recent years, while counseling about the risks of NSAID therapy has not. Yet in one study, treatment for *H. pylori* did not reduce the risk of rehospitalization or death within 1 year of initial hospitalization whereas counseling about NSAIDs did both.[47]

Elderly patients typically present for surgical correction of peptic ulcer disease in a delayed fashion and with more advanced disease. This translates to statistically significant increases in operative mortality for elderly patients undergoing surgery for complicated peptic ulcer disease. Age alone has not been shown to be an independent predictor of surgical risk. Using multivariate analysis Boey and coworkers[48] identified three risk factors for operative mortality in perforated ulcer. They were the presence of concomitant disease, preoperative shock, and more than 48 hours of perforation. Age, amount of peritoneal soilage, and length of history of ulcer disease were not significant risks. When zero risk factors were present, the mortality was 0%. Mortality was 10%, 46%, and 100% with 1, 2, or 3 risk factors, respectively.

In a similar study of patients with bleeding duodenal ulcer by the same authors,[49] multivariate logistic regression analysis revealed that age played only a minor role in determining outcome. The presence of concomitant medical illness, a greater than 5-unit hemorrhage, and, to a lesser degree, ulcer size negatively affected outcome. If all three risk factors were present, the mortality rate was 47%; if none was present, the rate was 0.1%.

Gastric cancer is also a disease of aging. The peak incidence occurs at 60 to 70 years of age. Risks include diet (pickled vegetables, salted fish, nitrates, and nitrites), occupation (metal, asbestos, and rubber workers), and geography (Asia vs. Western Hemisphere). Chronic atrophic gastritis, previous gastric surgery, and chronic *H. pylori* infection, more frequently found in older patients, are associated with increased risk of gastric cancer. Chronic atrophic gastritis and *H. pylori* infection are also risk factors for gastric lymphoma and its precursor, mucosal-associated lymphoid tissue. These patients typically present in the sixth decade of life.

The presentation of gastric cancer is changing in older persons, leading toward the need for more aggressive surgery. Elderly patients present with a predominance of intestinal type tumors rather than the more aggressive diffuse type. There is also a progression of the location of the tumor to more proximal areas of the stomach. As a result, total gastrectomy for cure in this population is now required in 13% to 34% of cases. No difference in resectability or the rate of positive lymph nodes found at surgery (60% to 70%) has been noted between young and older patients.

Liver

Tumors of the liver are 20 times more likely to arise from metastatic disease than from primary cancers. Metastatic tumors from gastrointestinal tract primary tumors are the most common type referred for resection. Patients with colon cancer have a 35% risk of developing liver recurrence, and only 10% to 20% of those identified have resectable disease. Patients who undergo liver resection have upward of 30% 5-year survival versus 0% if surgery is not done.

In 1995, Karl and colleagues showed that persons older than the age of 70 can undergo liver resection with a morbidity of 31% and mortality of 0%.[50] A reduction in mortality for patients older than 65 has occurred over the past 20 years, and today the rates in young and older patients are comparable. This is now accepted to the level that recent reports indicate that simultaneous resection of colorectal malignancy and liver metastases is safe.[51]

In addition to surgical resection, treatment of hepatic cancer includes radiologic embolization, cryotherapy, and radiofrequency ablation therapy, which can be performed operatively or transcutaneously.

Biliary Tract Disease

Biliary tract disease is the single most common cause of acute abdominal complaints and accounts for approximately one third of all abdominal operations in the elderly. In nearly all populations, the prevalence of gallstones increases with increasing age, although the magnitude of this increase varies with the population. By age 65, 90% of female Pima Indians have gallstones, compared with 23% of female civil servants in Rome, Italy. In the United States about 75% of gallstones are composed primarily of cholesterol, although with increasing age there is an increased incidence of pigment-containing stones as well. There is also an increased incidence of common duct stones with advancing age. Choledocholithiasis is found at the time of cholecystectomy in as many as 30% of patients in the seventh decade of life and up to 50% of those in the eighth decade.

The increased development of gallstones in the elderly is thought to result from both changes in the composition of bile and from impaired biliary motility. Alterations in the composition of bile with advancing age include an increase in the activity of HMG-CoA (the rate-limiting enzyme in the synthesis of cholesterol) and a decrease in the activity of 7α-hydroxylase (the rate-limiting enzyme in the synthesis of bile salts from cholesterol).[52] This results in supersaturation of the bile with cholesterol and a decrease in the primary bile salt pool. The ratio of secondary to primary bile salts also increases. It is postulated that these secondary bile salts promote cholesterol gallstone formation by enhancing cholesterol synthesis, increasing protein content of the bile, decreasing nucleation time, and increasing the production of specific phospholipids that are thought to affect the production of mucin. It has also been suggested that the increase in secondary bile salts in the aged may promote a recycling of bilirubin, which in turn leads to the unconjugated bilirubin supersaturation necessary for pigment stone formation.

Alterations in gallbladder motility and bile duct motility are thought to be central to the development of cholesterol stones and brown pigment stones, respectively. The role of motility in black pigment stone formation, however, is less clear. Biliary motility is a complex interaction of hormonal and neural factors; however, the major stimulus of gallbladder emptying is cholecystokinin (CCK). The sensitivity of the gallbladder wall to CCK has been shown to decrease with increasing age in animal models. Exogenous administration of CCK to animals fed a lithogenic diet inhibits the age-dependent development of cholesterol gallstones.[53] In humans, gallbladder sensitivity to CCK is also decreased. However, there is a compensatory increase in the production of CCK in response to a stimuli that results in normal gallbladder contraction. The significance of this observation with regard to gallstone formation, however, is undetermined.

Regardless of the pathogenesis, gallstones are associated with complications in 40% to 60% of older patients requiring treatment of the disease, compared with less than 20% of younger patients. In the study by Escarce and associates,[19] nearly two thirds of the over 21,000 open cholecystectomies in elderly patients were performed under urgent or emergent conditions. The increased rate of complicated disease seen in this age group may be directly attributable to the increased severity of the disease and/or to increased prevalence of comorbid illnesses. It is more likely, however, due to a combination of factors, including delays in diagnosis and treatment caused by the frequent absence of typical biliary tract symptoms. Biliary colic, or episodic right upper quadrant pain radiating to the back, precedes the development of a complication only half as often in older than younger patients. Even in the presence of acute cholecystitis, one fourth of older patients may have no abdominal tenderness, one third no elevation in temperature or white blood cell count, and as many as one half no peritoneal signs in the right upper quadrant.[54] Unfortunately, mortality in the emergent setting is at least three times the elective mortality. Until predictors of impending complications other than symptoms are identified, improving the outcome of biliary tract disease in the elderly will be difficult. Increased awareness of the atypical presentation of gallstone-related illness in this age group is essential.

The presence of common bile duct (CBD) stones increases the likelihood of postoperative complications and death. In the prelaparoscopic era, bile duct stones were addressed at the time of cholecystectomy. Although open CBD exploration was extremely successful at clearing the bile duct of stones, it was associated with a significant increase in operative mortality and morbidity over simple cholecystectomy alone. Most clinicians now agree that if CBD stones are suspected, either from a dilated duct on ultrasound or abnormal liver or pancreatic chemistries, a preoperative attempt at sphincterotomy and extraction via endoscopic retrograde cholangiopancreatography should be made. Successful duct clearance by this approach is reported in over 90% on cases. Some caution should be exercised when recommending endoscopic sphincterotomy in elderly patients. The frequent presence of periampullary duodenal diverticula and multiple CBD stones in this age group makes cannulation and clearance of the duct more difficult. Postprocedure mortality, morbidity, and cholangitis rates are higher as well.

The management of the gallbladder after successful endoscopic treatment of CBD stones in patients without acute gallbladder disease is controversial. Several studies indicate that 9% to 21% of patients managed by endoscopic sphincterotomy alone will go on to develop a complication related to the gallbladder. Unfortunately, because the patients managed in this fashion are frequently the oldest and most frail, the mortality for acute cholecystitis in this setting is as high as 25%.

Special consideration must be given to the treatment of gallstones found at the time of laparotomy for an unrelated condition. The addition of cholecystectomy to the primary procedure usually adds little increased morbidity or mortality. Although some controversy still exists, many surgeons would proceed with incidental cholecystectomy if the patient were stable, exposure were appropriate, and the cholecystectomy added little additional operative time. In the past, stronger arguments for incidental cholecystectomy were based on concerns that the symptoms of acute postoperative cholecystitis might be unrecognized in the setting of a recent laparotomy incision. With better postoperative monitoring, more accurate imaging techniques, and percutaneous methods for decompressing the gallbladder should postoperative cholecystitis occur, these concerns have diminished.

Small Bowel Obstruction

Small bowel obstruction (SBO) is, by far, the most common and surgically relevant disorder of small intestinal function encountered in the aged. Although the exact incidence of small bowel obstruction in the elderly is difficult to ascertain, lysis of adhesion is the third most common gastrointestinal procedure after cholecystectomy and partial excision of the large bowel. Fifty percent of the deaths associated with SBO occur in patients older than age 70.

SBO can result from lesions or objects extrinsic to the bowel wall, intrinsic to the bowel wall, or within the bowel lumen (obturation). The vast majority of SBOs are caused by lesions extrinsic to the bowel wall, many of which increase with increasing age. In spite of frequent need for emergency operation in older patients with SBO, there are little recent data regarding etiology, treatment, or outcome of this disorder in this age group. Studies from more than 25 years ago show that just over half of the SBOs in older patients were caused by incarcerated abdominal wall hernias, with postoperative adhesions accounting for another 40%. More recent data indicate that adhesions are now responsible for over 50% of SBOs, hernias for 15% to 20% of cases, and neoplasms for another 15% to 20%. It has also been noted that the age of the patients with incarcerated hernias is slightly, although not significantly, older than patients with adhesive obstruction. In addition, certain kinds of hernias, such as those that occur through the obturator foramen, are found almost exclusively in the elderly and are particularly difficult to diagnose.

Luminal obstruction from other than deliberately swallowed foreign bodies, while uncommon, occurs most often in the elderly. Phytobezoars, or large concretions of poorly digested fruit and vegetable matter, form with increased frequency in the stomach of elderly patients with poor dentition, decreased gastric acid, and impaired gastric motility. In the stomach these masses can become enormous without any symptoms. However, when a portion breaks free and migrates into the small bowel, obstruction ensues. Obturation of the small bowel lumen by an aberrantly located gallstone, incorrectly termed *gallstone ileus,* is another uncommon cause of obstruction seen primarily in the elderly. Although it only accounts for 1% to 3% of all SBOs, it has been implicated in as many as 25% of obstructions in patients older than age 65 with no hernia or history of prior surgery.

The pathophysiology, diagnosis, and treatment of SBO have been discussed elsewhere in the text. It is important to note, however, that the three important management issues—distinguishing functional (ileus) from mechanical obstruction, distinguishing simple from strangulated obstruction, and determining the optimal timing of operation for partial obstruction—are even further exaggerated in elderly patients.[55]

Many of the factors associated with ileus (systemic infections, intra-abdominal infections, metabolic abnormalities and medications) are more common in older persons. The relevance of these factors to the finding of abdominal distention is not always appreciated. Signs and symptoms of underlying infections such as pneumonia, urinary tract infection, or appendicitis may be subtle. Bowel distention may be erroneously considered the primary problem rather than a secondary event. Vomiting from a variety of nonobstructive causes can rapidly lead to dehydration and subsequent electrolyte abnormalities in the elderly. The constellation of vomiting and bowel distention can easily be mistaken for obstruction. Finally, the elderly are more likely to be on multiple medications that may impair normal bowel motility.

The accurate distinction between strangulated and simple mechanical small bowel obstruction is difficult to make in all age groups but even more so in the elderly. Clinical findings of fever, tachycardia, elevated white blood cell count, and focal tenderness are notoriously misleading, particularly in the elderly in whom the risk of strangulation is the highest. In only 50% of patients of all ages with strangulation is the white blood cell count elevated. Unfortunately, because no laboratory tests are available that consistently differentiate strangulated from simple obstruction, the correct diagnosis is made in as few as 25% of cases preoperatively. Resection for strangulation is required in as many as 50% of older patients with adhesive SBO, compared with only 8% overall.

In patients suspected of having a partial adhesive SBO, nonoperative management with nasogastric decompression and intravenous hydration is standard. From two thirds to over three fourths of partial adhesive SBOs will resolve with conservative therapy, usually within 24 to 72 hours. Although some authors report that delays longer than 48 hours are associated with increased complications,[56] others disagree.[57]

In the elderly, several additional considerations are important. Although the natural reflex is to avoid unnecessary operations in sick older patients, prolonged conservative management can present new problems. Prolonged bed rest is associated with an increased incidence of venous stasis, pulmonary complications, and deconditioning. Prolonged nasogastric intubation is associated with an increased incidence of aspiration and pneumonia. Even a short period of nutritional deprivation may present a significant risk to the elderly patient with a baseline nutritional deficit. These factors together may result in a poor outcome should surgery become necessary after a prolonged attempt to avoid it.

In a review of patients treated for SBO, recurrence occurred in 34% at 4 years and 42% at 10 years.[58] Those who were operated on initially had a recurrence rate of 29% compared with 53% for those treated nonoperatively. In the operated group, the majority of the recurrences occurred in patients with malignant rather than adhesive obstruction.

For elderly patients with prior abdominal operations for malignant disease, the decision about when to operate is even more difficult. Metastatic obstruction presents several technical and ethical problems. Obstructing lesions are frequently found at multiple points in the bowel, and resection may not be possible. Bypass of long partially obstructed segments may be technically feasible but can leave the patient with a functionally short gut. Thirty-day operative mortality rates for this form of obstruction in elderly patients exceed 35%, and the majority of all patients die within 6 months. This discouraging outcome has led some to advocate prolonged periods of nonoperative decompression. Unfortunately, this approach produces only a transient relief of obstructive symptoms. Furthermore, a prior history of malignancy is not an absolute indication that the obstruction is due to metastatic disease. In 10% to 38% of patients with suspected malignant obstruction, a benign cause is found at the time of operation.

At first glance, the laparoscopic approach to diagnosis and treatment of SBO in the elderly has considerable appeal. Early intervention with minimal surgical stress would seem ideal. Although the numbers of patients treated was small, early studies show success in approximately three fourths of cases. However, laparoscopy in this setting can be technically challenging and not without complications. In one study by experienced laparoscopic surgeons, 80% of SBOs were approached laparoscopically and slightly over one half of those were successfully treated. However, the rate of unplanned reoperation was 14% in the laparoscopic group compared with 5% in the open group.[59] It is unclear at present whether the benefit of laparoscopy is offset by the risks of additional operative complications or the potential need for more than one procedure.

Colorectal

Appendicitis

Although appendicitis typically occurs in the second and third decades of life, 5% to 10% of cases present in old age. Appendicitis in the elderly has increased in recent decades while the incidence in younger patients is declining. Inflammation of the appendix now accounts for 2.5% to 5% of acute abdominal disease in patients older than age 60 to 70. The overall mortality from appendicitis is only 0.8%, but the vast majority of deaths occur in the very young and the very old. In patients younger than 65 the mortality rate is less than 0.5%, whereas for those older than 65 the overall mortality rate is nearly 5%.

The classic presentation of appendicitis—periumbilical pain that localizes over a period of several hours to the right lower quadrant—is present only half as often in older patients as in younger patients. Instead, abdominal pain tends to be vague and diffuse. In one study, only 55% of patients older than age 80 had right lower quadrant pain and 18% had no abdominal pain at all. In addition, because vague abdominal pain is a common complaint in older persons, its significance is frequently overlooked.

Other signs of acute appendicitis are also unreliable in the elderly. White blood cells counts are less than $10,000/mm^3$ in 20% to 50% of older patients with simple appendicitis. Similarly, temperature is less than 37.6°C in as many as half the cases. Nausea, vomiting, and anorexia are also found less frequently in older patients.[60]

The indolent nature of the initial symptoms of appendicitis in the elderly usually leads to delays of 48 to 72 hours before medical attention is sought. These delays are compounded by a delay in diagnosis once the patient reaches the hospital. In only 30% to 70% of cases is the correct diagnosis made on admission. Delays to operation of greater than 24 hours are three times as likely to occur in older than in younger patients.[60]

Perforated appendicitis is far more common in the elderly. Rates of perforation increase directly with age; by age 70 years, 70% to 90% of patients will present with perforation.[61] Although changes in the structure and blood supply of the appendix have been implicated in the high incidence of perforation, data supporting this contention are few. The theory that appendicitis progresses more rapidly in this age group is also unsubstantiated. The long duration of symptoms, errors in diagnosis, and long delays until operation are most likely responsible. Mortality rates for perforated appendicitis also increase with age from 0% in patients younger than age 50 to 11% for those age 50 to 70 and to 32% for those older than age 70.[61]

If there is a suspicion of perforation and periappendiceal abscess, CT should be obtained before operation.

Percutaneous drainage and intravenous antibiotics are often preferable to exploration in the presence of a large abscess. In younger patients, this approach is followed by interval appendectomy approximately 6 weeks after the abscess has resolved. In the elderly, recurrent appendicitis after resolution of the abscess is uncommon and interval appendectomy is, therefore, not necessary in all cases. However, the possibility of perforated cancer in this age group does mandate a thorough evaluation of the colon when the acute process is controlled.

Carcinoma of the Colon and Rectum

Colorectal cancer is the second leading cause of cancer mortality in the United States. The overall incidence of colon cancer is 17 cases per 100,000 population, but this incidence rises sharply after age 50. For persons age 40 to 44 the annual incidence of colon cancer is 6.2 and 8 cases per 100,000 men and women, respectively. For those older than 85 years, the annual incidence of colon cancer is 239 and 209, respectively, and the annual incidence of rectal cancer is 142 and 126, respectively. Carcinoma of the colon and rectum accounts for two thirds of all gastrointestinal malignancies in patients older than age 70.

With increasing age there is a progressive increase in percent of right-sided colon cancer, which is offset by a decrease in the percent of rectal cancers (Fig. 15-9).[62] There is some regional disagreement about the influence of age on stage of disease at diagnosis. A large prospective Israeli study found no significant difference in stage in patients older than or younger than age 70,[63] whereas data from the Trafford database in the United Kingdom showed patients older than age 75 were twice as likely to present

with advanced disease compared with those younger than age 65.[64] A report by the Commission on Cancer of the American College of Surgeons, using data from the U.S. National Cancer Data Base, shows a trend for earlier-stage colon cancer in patients older than age 80.[65]

The presenting signs and symptoms of colorectal cancer do not vary substantially with age, although some report more local symptoms in younger patients and more anorexia in older patients with rectal cancer. The response to these signs and symptoms, however, may be different. Right-sided lesions tend to cause microcytic anemia from occult bleeding, which may present as lassitude, weakness, syncope, or a fall. Left-sided neoplasms tend to present as changes in bowel habits or stool caliber. Because fatigue, falls, constipation, and bowel dysfunction are accepted as a common sequela of aging, these symptoms are frequently ignored by both the patient and the physician. The diagnosis, therefore, is often not made until a complication occurs.

The increased incidence of complications at presentation in the elderly leads to an increased need for emergent surgical treatment; over 50% of operations for colorectal cancer in patients older than age 70 are performed on an urgent/emergent basis compared with only one third in patients of all ages. Operative mortality for colorectal cancer is determined by the same two factors that influence operative mortality in the elderly in general: the presence of coexisting disease and the need for emergency surgery. In patients with little or no comorbidity, operative mortality is similar regardless of age. When surgery is performed as an emergency, mortality increases threefold to fourfold over elective mortality for similar procedures. Even in patients older than age 80 years elective operative

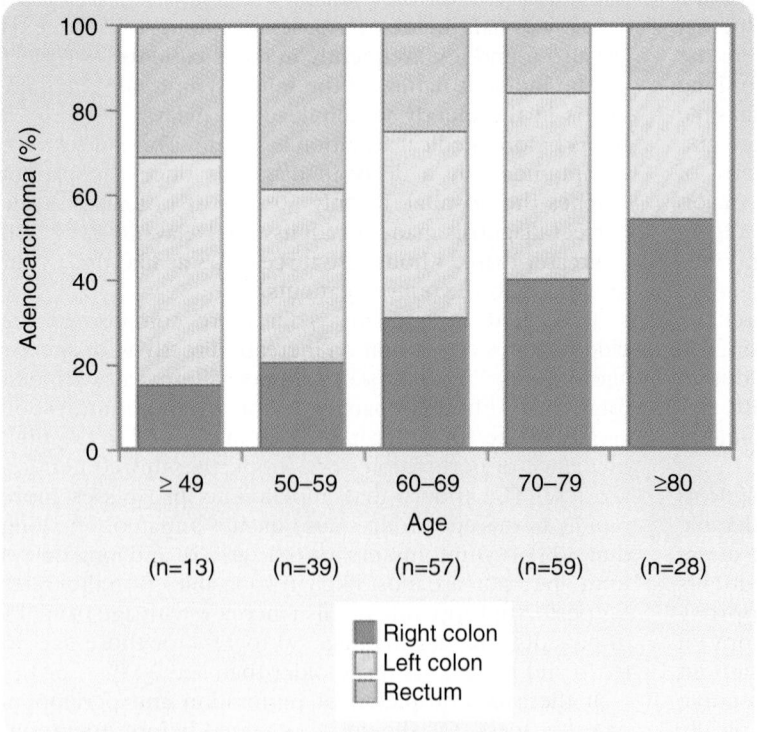

FIGURE 15-9. Location of colorectal carcinoma with increasing age. With age there is a progressive increase in right-sided colon cancer and decrease in rectal cancer. (From Okamoto M, et al: Relationship between age and site of colorectal cancer based on colonoscopy findings. Gastrointest Endosc 55, 2002.)

mortality rates are only approximately 2%. Length of hospital stay and hospital costs, however, are increased with advanced age and emergency setting. In addition, survivors of elective operations are twice as likely to return to independent living as are those surviving emergency surgery.

The long-term outcome of surgery for colorectal cancer in the elderly is good. Three- and five-year cancer-specific survival rates do not appear to be influenced by increasing age even in patients older than age 80. In a multivariate analysis of age, stage, tumor location, and type of operation, only stage and emergency operation negatively influenced survival.[63]

Screening for colorectal cancer in the elderly is essential. Several organizations including the American Cancer Society, the American College of Gastroenterology, the U.S. Preventive Services Taskforce, the Agency for Healthcare Policy and Research, and the American Society for Gastrointestinal Endoscopy, have made recommendations for screening.[66] For average-risk patients, screening should begin at age 50. Recommendations in general include annual fecal occult blood testing and flexible sigmoidoscopy every 5 years (with full colonoscopy for positive occult blood or adenomatous polyps on flexible sigmoidoscopy) or colonoscopy every 10 years. With increasing age the incidence of right-sided colon cancer increases. Over half of patients with right-sided cancers have no lesions within reach of the flexible sigmoidoscope. Therefore, colonoscopy may be a more effective screening tool in older patients. The interval of screening in the elderly should depend on the life expectancy of the individual and the length of time for which the screening tool is expected to be effective.

In general, surgical resection is the treatment of choice for resectable colorectal cancer regardless of age. For tumors of the abdominal colon, only prohibitive anesthetic risk secondary to severe comorbidity should influence this choice. There has been some concern, however, about the ability of elderly patients to tolerate resectional procedures for low rectal cancers. This includes abdominoperineal resection, low anterior resection, and sphincter-saving coloanal anastomosis. Over the past 15 years, resection and coloanal anastomosis with J pouch for low rectal tumors has been more widely accepted. While technically more demanding than the traditional abdominoperineal resection, coloanal anastomosis provides a sphincter-saving alternative that is well tolerated by the elderly, both in terms of operative mortality and postoperative complications.[67] Both are equally effective for cure provided there is at least a 2-cm distal resection margin. While abdominoperineal resection obligates patients to a permanent colostomy, coloanal reconstruction can achieve continence in nearly 80% of elderly individuals. Assessment of anal function is extremely important in patient selection for low rectal anastomosis. Fecal incontinence may be far worse for quality of life than a well-controlled end-sigmoid colostomy.

For the frail elderly or high-risk patient, lesser procedures including transanal excision and fulguration can provide local control of the tumor without disrupting continence. Transanal excision may also be curative in selected patients with small well-differentiated T1 or T2 lesions, although local recurrence rates are higher than with resection procedures. Local control of rectal tumors with chemoradiation is also possible to control pain and bleeding in poor-risk patients with metastatic disease and short life expectancy.

Adjuvant therapy is recommended for all patients at risk for recurrence after resection for colorectal carcinoma. Because elderly patients are often excluded from clinical trials, the efficacy and toxicity of various regimens in this age group are not well established. Less formal analyses do indicate that radiation therapy for pelvic malignancy including rectal cancer is well tolerated regardless of age. It is clear, however, that adjuvant therapy is not utilized as frequently in older patients with colon or rectal cancer as it is in younger patients with the same-stage disease (Fig. 15-10).[68] Whether this is secondary to a formal assessment of the risk of adjuvant therapy in the individual, ignorance of the utility of adjuvant therapy in older patients, or patient preference is not well defined.

Hernia

The estimated incidence of abdominal wall hernia in persons older than the age of 65 is 13 per 1000, with a fourfold to eightfold increase in incidence in men. Fifty percent of all hernias are indirect inguinal, 20% are direct inguinal, 10% are ventral, 6% are femoral, 3% are umbilical, and 1% are esophageal hiatal. Whereas 85% of all groin hernias occur in males, 84% of femoral hernias occur in females. The elderly are also at risk for the more occult types of hernias that do not become apparent until a complication has occurred. Typically, paraesophageal hernias may reach enormous size without symptoms and are only discovered when gastric volvulus or strangulation occurs. Similarly, herniation through the obturator canal is rarely diagnosed until SBO occurs (Fig. 15-11).[69]

Repair of groin hernia can be performed as an outpatient procedure using either epidural anesthesia or local anesthesia with intravenous sedation. Mortality rates are very low even in patients with concomitant medical disease, with many reports showing rates of 0%. Newer techniques in surgical repair include open tension-free repair, preperitoneal approach, and laparoscopic repair. In each, dissection is minimized, as is the incision, and operative time is shortened. These procedures are well tolerated as outpatient procedures even in the frail elderly, and recurrence rates are very low.[70]

Morbidity and mortality rates for emergency hernia repair are over 50% and 8% to 14%, respectively. This is largely because of the high incidence of bowel incarceration at presentation. Intestinal resection is required in up to 30% of cases. The markedly better outcome for elective repair should dictate evaluation for surgery in all newly diagnosed hernias.

Vascular Surgery

The most frequent vascular diseases seen in elderly patients are abdominal aortic aneurysms, carotid artery

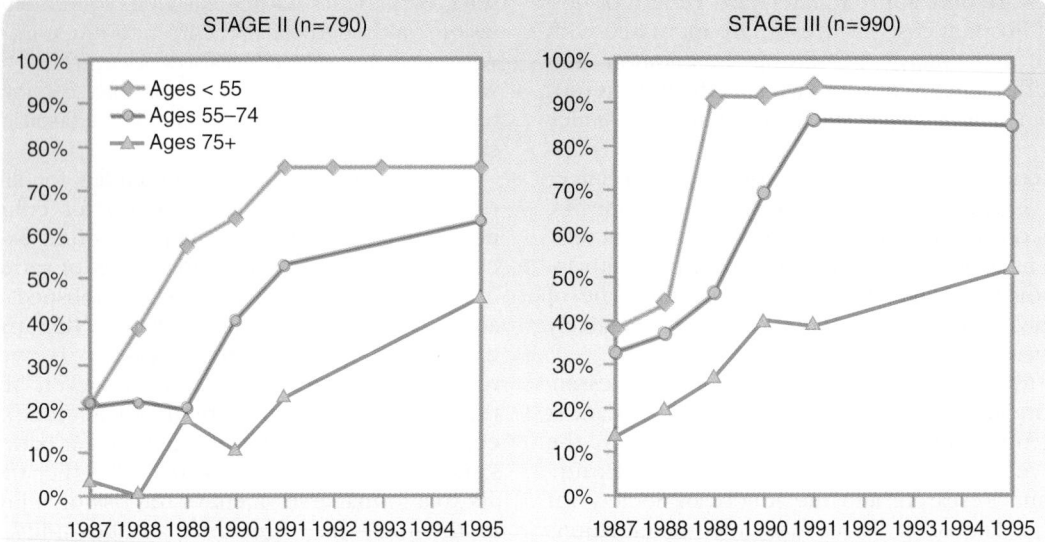

FIGURE 15-10.   Utilization of adjuvant therapy for rectal cancer by stage, age group, and year. **Left,** Stage II disease. **Right,** Stage III disease. (From Potosky AL, et al: Age, sex and racial differences in the use of standard adjuvant therapy for colorectal cancer. J Clin Oncol 20:1192-1202, 2002.)

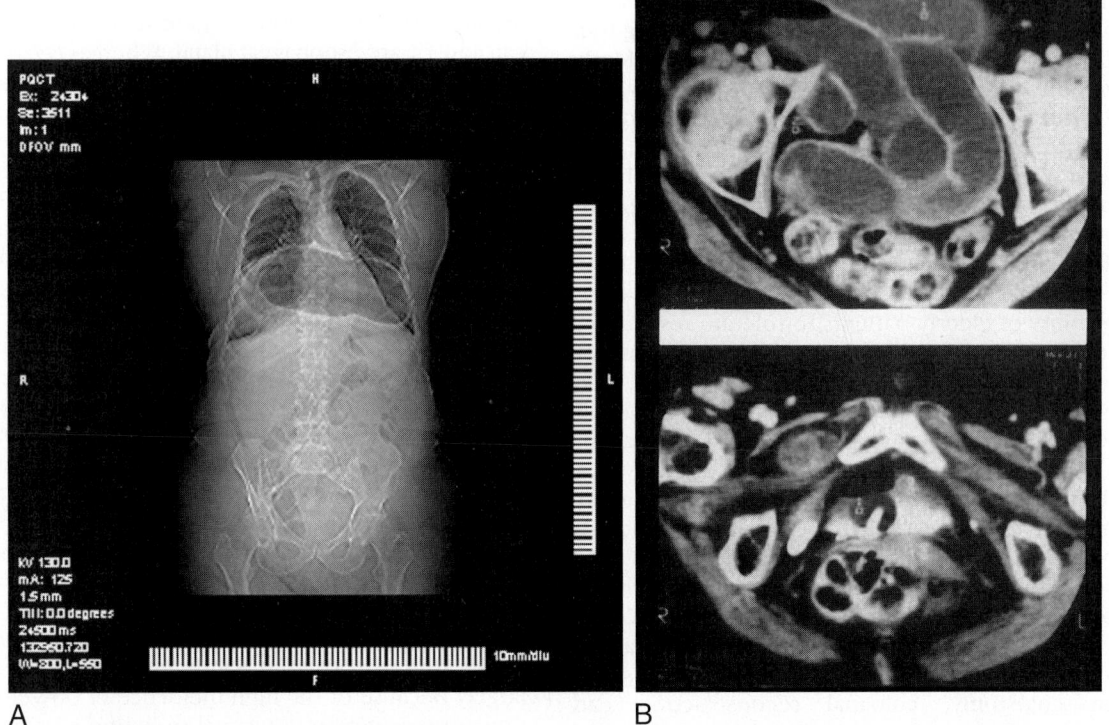

FIGURE 15-11.   **A,** CT scout film showing gigantic paraesophageal hernia with entire stomach rotated in the chest. **B,** CT of the pelvis showing small bowel obstruction *(top)* with loop of bowel through the obturator canal on the patient's right *(arrow, bottom).* (From Emory RE, Laporta AJ: Obturator hernia. Surg Rounds16:43, 1993.)

disease, and peripheral arterial occlusive disease. Under elective conditions and in patients with well-managed concomitant disease, vascular surgery is safe and effective.

In patients age 65 years and older, the mortality from elective aneurysm repair is less than 5% despite the high incidence of comorbidity in this age group.[71] Emergency repair for rupture carries an operative mortality rate of over 50% and an extremely high morbidity rate in those that do survive. Although elective surgery has been shown to be safe, older patients are still being treated conservatively. A study from 25 years ago showed that only 49% of internists and family practitioners would refer a patient with an aneurysm to surgery, and only one half of those would do so for an aneurysm smaller than 8 cm.[72] It is unclear whether that attitude has changed, although there have been many reports in the past 25 years suggesting aneurysm repair is safe, specifically in octogenarians. It is likely that the increased availability of minimally invasive techniques such as aortic endograft placement will encourage more referrals for early aneurysm repair.[73]

The perception of excess risk in the elderly patient by medical professionals is also present in cases of carotid artery disease. As many as 28% of internists do not refer an octogenarian for operation, despite the fact that multiple studies have shown that endarterectomy is safe, has minimal mortality, and can prevent strokes. In patients age 65 to 80 years, the stroke rate from surgery is 2.8% and the mortality rate is 2.4%. Survival after endarterectomy in octogenarians is similar to that in the general population of 80-year-olds. Similarly, the incidence of neurologic symptoms after endarterectomy is lower than in the unoperated patient (13% vs. 33%), and the incidence of late stroke is much lower as well (2% vs. 17%). Proper indications in the octogenarian include high-grade carotid lesions and hemispheric symptoms and well-controlled concomitant disease.[74] Recent application of endovascular stenting to the carotid artery may provide a less invasive method for treating carotid artery disease. At present, this procedure is only indicated for high-risk patients or complex technical situations. There is no evidence to suggest stenting should replace open surgery in the routine setting. In fact, octogenarians have been shown to experience a higher rate of stroke with carotid stenting compared with standard carotid endarterectomy.[75]

Peripheral vascular surgery for limb salvage is indicated for ischemic rest pain, nonhealing ulcers, or frank gangrene. This, too, can be safely done in the elderly patient. In patients older than 80 years, the mortality rate of surgery is 4.6% and limb salvage rates over 3 to 5 years are 50% to 87%.[74] Quality of life and preservation and/or restoration of functional independence are the most important considerations in older patients.

Cardiothoracic Surgery

Coronary Artery Bypass Grafting (CABG)

The number of coronary artery bypasses performed on patients older than age 65 years rose from 2.6 operations per 1000 population in 1980 to 13.0 operations per 1000

population in 1993. Over the past decade, with the increasing use of coronary artery stents, the rate for persons older than age 65 has fallen to 8.9 per 1000 population, whereas the rate for males older than age 75 in 2001 was 11.4 per 1000. Patients who are now referred for bypass usually have more complex disease or have failed alternative procedures. Over 55% of CABGs are now performed on patients older than age 65 years. As the mortality and morbidity of cardiac surgical procedures has decreased, there has been a growing willingness to offer surgical therapy to older patients with reconstructable coronary artery disease. The literature in the late 1980s and early 1990s described series of patients older than age 70. Now there are numerous reports of CABG in octogenarians. Unfortunately, elderly patients referred for cardiac surgery have a higher incidence of advanced disease (triple-vessel disease, left main or main equivalent disease, and poor left ventricular function), have more symptomatic disease (90% of octogenarians are preoperatively classified as NYHA functional class III or IV), and require emergent or urgent procedures more often.[76]

Several preoperative risk factors for mortality after coronary bypass surgery have been identified.[77] These include emergency procedure, severe left ventricular dysfunction, mitral insufficiency requiring combined procedure, NYHA functional class IV, elevated preoperative creatinine level, chronic pulmonary disease, anemia (hematocrit < 34%), and prior vascular surgery. Further risk factors for morbidity include obesity (weight > 65 kg), diabetes mellitus, aortic stenosis, and cerebrovascular disease. These risk factors have been assigned scores from 1 to 6 depending on the strength of the association. Emergency surgery receives a point score of 6, whereas age 65 to 74 receives a score of 1 and age greater than 75 a score of 2. When considered alone, the contribution of age to increased mortality is small and not sufficient to warrant withholding surgical therapy.[78]

Even in patients older than age 80 years, coronary artery bypass surgery is associated with an acceptable overall mortality of 7% to 12%, with mortality from elective procedures under 3%. Early elective operation is clearly preferable to emergency surgery, which is associated with a 2 to 10 times higher mortality. Unfortunately, because of a reluctance to offer elective operations to the very old, some series report as many as 40% of elderly patients require urgent or emergent operations.

Morbidity after coronary surgery in the elderly is quite high in many series. Pulmonary failure requiring prolonged intubation, neurologic events including cerebrovascular accident, delirium and other cognitive disorders, and sternal wound infections increase with age and are associated with postoperative mortality. Other complications including reoperation for bleeding, need for pacemaker insertion, perioperative myocardial infarction, and other wound infections occur with equal frequency in both age groups.

The effectiveness of coronary artery bypass surgery versus medical management in octogenarians has been assessed in terms of cost per quality of life year survival.[79] The cost per quality of life year saved was only $10,424, which was less than the cost for many common procedures such as screening mammography. The survival in the surgery group was 80% and 69% at 3 and 4 years, respectively, whereas in the medical group, comparable survival was 64% and 32%. Using the validated health status assessment tool, the EurQol Questionnaire, the authors assessed the quality of life in five domains: pain, activity, mobility, self care, and depression/anxiety. In all areas, quality of life was better in the surgically treated than in the medically treated groups. Quality of life in the group of 80-year-old patients who selected CABG was found to be equal to that of an average 55-year old in the general population.

Valve Replacement

Calcific aortic stenosis is a disease of the elderly. Over the past several years there have been more than 20 published series concerning valve replacement in older people. The growing willingness to offer aortic valve replacement to older patients comes, in part, from a better understanding of the natural history of aortic valvular disease. Once symptoms such as angina or syncope develop, average life expectancy is only 3 to 4 years. Once congestive heart failure occurs, death can be expected in 1.5 to 2 years and over 80% of patients with any of these symptoms will be dead in 4 years. Average life expectancy for a healthy 70-year-old is approximately 13 years; and for an 80-year-old, approximately 8 years. Clearly if aortic valve replacement could be accomplished with acceptable operative mortality, the benefit would justify the procedure. Since 1975, much data have accumulated that support the safety and efficacy of aortic valve replacement in the elderly. Operative mortality is 3% to 10% (mean 7.7%) and long-term survival is 75% to 80%. While the mortality in older patients in several series is slightly higher than the mortality in younger patients, most differences were not statistically significant. In addition, the vast majority of elderly patients receiving new aortic valves have great improvement in the quality of life. As many as 90% of elderly patients who were classified as NYHA functional class III or IV preoperatively and survive are reclassified postoperatively as class I or II.

Mitral valve disease in the elderly has been less well investigated, partly because it is less common but also because the natural history is less well defined and the outcome of surgical therapy is not as good as that of aortic valve disease. In one study, operative mortality after mitral valve replacement was 20.4%, compared with 5.3% for aortic valve replacement.[80] Left ventricular reserve is often compromised in the elderly with mitral insufficiency because of the frequently associated ischemic disease. Low cardiac output is a particular problem after mitral valve replacement. Frequently, both aortic and mitral valve replacement is accompanied by additional procedures. There is some debate about whether valve replacement plus CABG or multiple valve replacements in the very elderly are too "risky" to justify the combined procedures. Many believe that with appropriate patient selection even multiple procedures can be performed with relative safety, but the number of patients meeting selection criteria is small.

The choice of valve material is also an important consideration in older patients. Mechanical valves are extremely durable but require lifelong anticoagulation. In patients older than age 75, the mortality from long-term anticoagulation alone is nearly 10% per year. Bioprosthetic valves do not require anticoagulation but are somewhat less durable.

Trauma

The aging process puts older persons at increased risk for trauma. Central nervous system changes increase the risk for accident. Cerebral atrophy and decreased viscoelastic properties within the cranial vault make the brain more susceptible to blunt injury. Increased bone fragility results in increased tendency to fracture.

Trauma is currently the fifth leading cause of death in the elderly. Persons older than 65 years account for 4.4% to 29% of trauma cases and for 30% to almost 40% of trauma deaths, with more recent rates being highest.[81] Motor vehicle accidents are the most common form of fatal injury in patients younger than the age of 80, and after the age of 80 falls take the lead. Interestingly, the incidence of deaths from injuries sustained in motor vehicle accident is equal for the elderly person as passenger or as pedestrian.

Significant injury can result from even simple falls from a level surface on the ground. The incidence of fracture or serious injury from such a fall is as high as 40% in the older person. After a person sustains an injury in a fall there is significant morbidity. Of those hospitalized after a fall, up to 43% end up being discharged from the hospital to a nursing facility and only 50% are alive 1 year later.

Blunt head trauma in the elderly person carries a particularly frightening mortality. A recent study of blunt head trauma demonstrated that mortality for persons older than the age of 60 presenting with a Glasgow Coma Scale score of 5 was 79%, compared with 36% for similarly matched patients aged 20 to 40 years. Multivariate analysis showed that the elderly patient had 126 times the risk of mortality when compared with similar injuries in younger persons.[82] Mortality rates are as high as 57% to 100% for elderly patients presenting with Glasgow Coma Scale scores of 8 or less. Importantly, only 2% of the elderly patients had a "favorable" recovery, compared with 38% of the younger patients. Older patients take much longer to recover from head trauma than younger ones and require more intensive rehabilitation.

Injury from burns comprises 8% of elderly trauma. The elderly are at particular risk for burns due to impaired vision, decreased reaction time, depressed alertness, and decreased sensation of pain. In 81% of elderly burn victims, injuries occurred as a result of their own action and resulted in scalding, cooking accidents with flame, and electrical burns. While survival from burns is directly related to total body surface area affected, this is more pronounced in the elderly. In general, burns over 40% of total body surface area in older persons have very poor prognosis. Reasons for the increased mortality are concomitant medical disease, burn wound sepsis, and multisystem failure. For survivors of serious burns aged 59 or greater, fewer than half are discharged to independent living, one third to assisted living homes, and one fifth to nursing facilities.

Transplant

In 1946, the first successful renal transplant was performed. Early results with cadaveric renal transplant in patients older than age 45 were poor. The introduction of cyclosporine in the 1980s led to a dramatic improvement, particularly in high-risk patients. As experience at transplant centers has grown, the number of elderly patients who could potentially benefit from transplantation has also increased. With end-stage renal disease, for example, the percent of the dialysis population older than age 60 has increased from 39% in 1981 to 51% in 1990 and was projected to rise to 60% by last year. Correspondingly, the percent of patients on kidney transplant waiting lists has increased from 23.5% from age 50 to 64 and from 2.9% when older than 65 in 1988 to 38.3% when older than age 50 in 1995.[83] On the liver and lung transplant lists, the absolute number of older patients has increased 20 and 40 times, respectively, over the same time period.

The increase in the number of elderly patients needing and presenting for transplantation has translated into an increase in the portion of the transplant population older than age 65. In the United States, the percent of kidney transplant patients older than age 65 increased from 2.8% in 1988 to just under 6% in 1995. In Spain, the percent has increased from 8% in 1984 to 34.7% in 1995. At the University of California at San Francisco, 10.6% of kidney transplants and 11.6% of liver transplants performed over the past 5 and 8 years, respectively, were for patients older than age 60.[83]

The results of transplant in the elderly in terms of survival and quality of life justify the extension of the age limit for this procedure. In a Canadian study of patients with end-stage renal disease older than age 60, well controlled for comorbidity, calculated 5-year survival was 81% for those receiving transplants compared with 51% for those maintained on dialysis.[84] Others report that results of the SF36 Health Survey in transplant patients older than age 60 are similar to the national norms in most areas. These results are limited, however, because the time after transplant was not standardized in this analysis.

Although some centers report lower overall survival for older versus younger renal transplant patients, many report no significant differences with age.[83] Graft survival is also not significantly different. In fact, because patient death with a functioning graft is counted as graft loss and more older patients die with functioning grafts, some centers report even better graft survival in the elderly when death is excluded in the census.

As the number of elderly transplant patients has increased, one important factor has emerged. The rate of both acute and chronic rejection is clearly lower in older patients. This has been attributed to the overall decline in immunocompetence with age. However, this decline also renders the elderly patient more susceptible to infection and malignancy. The high incidence of lymphoproliferative disorders in older transplant patients in general and the high rate of recurrent hepatitis C in older liver transplant patients in particular may be the result of excessive immunosuppression in this already compromised population. Decreasing immunosuppression in older patients may, in fact, improve both long- and short-term survival.

ETHICAL ISSUES

Do Not Resuscitate Orders

As the technical ability to maintain life by artificial means has become increasingly evident, the issues of "do not resuscitate" (DNR) orders and withdrawing or withholding medical treatment have gained prominence. Whereas these issues have been addressed by the medical community fairly extensively, only recently have physicians discussed these issues in the surgical sense, specifically the incidence and practice of withdrawal of life support in critically ill intensive care patients, the concept of futility of care, and the issue of DNR orders for patients undergoing operative procedures.

Up to 90% of patients entering the hospital, even those with poor prognoses, have not had meaningful discussions with their physicians about life-sustaining treatments.[85] Although 80% to 90% of patients who die in tertiary care centers eventually do have DNR orders written, the orders are usually only written within days of the patient's death. This strongly suggests that writing DNR orders is still considered tantamount to delivering a patient's last rites. Adequate communication by the physician with the patient and family still needs work.

The Patient Self-Determination Act requires that hospitals and other health care facilities inform patients of their rights to appoint a proxy (or surrogate) decision maker to act on their wishes regarding life-sustaining care should they become incompetent. This usually results in advance directives and living wills, documents that appoint such a surrogate and define the patients' wishes. Unfortunately, only 3% to 15% of the population employs such documents. Interventions by nurse clinicians to enhance communication has been shown to increase the utilization of advance directives to 77%.[85] Unfortunately, even when employed, advance directives do not work: they are sometimes left behind when patients are transferred from nursing homes to the hospital or simply ignored or overridden by the patient's family. This has led to controversy whether any real benefit comes from the use of advance directives or health care proxies.

Medical Futility

The American Medical Association report[86] from its Council on Ethical and Judicial Affairs regarding decisions near the end of life states that there is "no ethical distinction between withdrawing and withholding life-sustaining treatment." For patients in whom medical care is believed futile, studies have shown that withholding care does not even decrease health care expenditures significantly. Aggressive interventions in these patients, however, usually prevent death but do not prolong life and have adverse effects on patients, physicians, and family members.

The problem really is in predicting futility of medical care. Prognostic indicators are being developed. A study of comatose patients has shown that if on the third day of coma there is no motor response to pain, a lack of verbal response, a serum creatinine value greater than 1.5 mg/dL, and age older than 70, mortality was 100% at 2 months. If three of the four factors were present, mortality was 95%.[87]

Prognostic indicators for survival are also available for critically ill patients who are not comatose, based on the Acute Physiology and Chronic Health Evaluation (APACHE) III scoring system. This system uses physiologic parameters, comorbid conditions, and age to predict outcome. Importantly, age alone accounts for only 3% of total explanatory power, whereas acute physiologic parameters account for 86%.[88] This is the extreme example of concomitant medical disease and emergency situations being more important than chronologic age.

Statistical analysis has shown that objective estimates for survival based on APACHE III scores correlate better with actual survival than estimates by experienced clinicians. For example, one study showed that when clinicians gave subjective probability of survival of 25.5% for a group of 850 critically ill patients, the APACHE III predicted 19.7% mortality and the actual mortality was 20.7%. Similarly, whereas only 62% of 45 patients died in a group that clinicians predicted to have a 90% death rate, 100% of 16 patients died in a group in which APACHE III predicted a 90% mortality rate.[88] Such objective probability estimates obviously should not dictate care, because both a patient's family and the physician may differ in personal religious beliefs and values, but it can help in physician counseling of a patient's family regarding prognosis.

Interacting With the Elderly Patient

Communication by the physician with the elderly patient should be approached in a much different way than with the younger one. In a session focusing on surgery in the elderly patient at the 1995 Clinical Congress of the American College of Surgeons, Eiseman outlined a number of unique facts about the elderly patient.[89] First, he noted that most elderly patients have some degree of hearing loss, so important conversations should occur in a quiet room, with the surgeon speaking in a strong voice, describing the plan slowly and deliberately. A family member should attend, to help clarify issues and communicate with other family members. If one is not available, it is important that one be contacted by telephone.

Second, even though elderly patients are often frightened by their illness, they usually do not like being told what to do. "Elderly patients do not like to be hurried." Third, elderly patients realize that they are old and therefore probably have a different outlook of their disease and

---

Box 15-3. Goals of Medical and Surgical Care for the Elderly Patient

1. Maximize or maintain potential life span.
2. Maintain dignity of life; maximize self-esteem.
3. Maximize independent function; minimize dependence.
4. Relieve suffering, giving particular attention to pain.
5. Although cure might not be possible, palliation and comfort are equally important.

Adapted from Zerilman ME: Surgery in the elderly. Curr Probl Surg 35:101-179, 1998.

---

longevity than we might think. We should in no way assume that the older patient equates life with happiness and therefore must realize that they may be completely uninterested in a long-term survival concept such as 5-year survival rates (Box 15-3). Elderly patients may be simply interested in shorter-term goals, such as getting home to their families.

Finally, elderly patients tolerate major surgery differently than younger ones. Even vigorous persons should be warned preoperatively that easy fatigability is expected after surgery, and it may last for weeks after discharge.

Similarly, Morgenstern outlined a "set of rules" regarding communication with the elderly patient.[90] The doctor should speak to the patient while sitting down on a chair (not the bed) close to the patient, in an unhurried manner, to put the frightened patient at ease. Direct eye contact with the patient, not the chart, and words of encouragement help. Finally, when leaving the patient, the physician should offer his or her hand, because even the act of touching alone is therapeutic.

References

1. Baker GT III, Martin GR: Molecular and biological factors in aging: The origins, causes, and prevention of senescence. *In* Cassel CK, et al (eds): Geriatric Medicine, 3rd ed. New York, Springer, 1997.
2. U.S. Census Bureau: Projections of the total resident population by 5-year age groups and sex with special age categories: Middle series 2025 to 2045, 2050 to 2070. Population Projections Program, U.S. Census Bureau, 2000.
3. Rowe JW: Health care myths at the end of life. Bull Am Coll Surg 81:11-18, 1996.
4. Robinson B, Beghe C: Cancer screening in the older patient. Clin Geriatr Med 13:97-118, 1997.
5. Centers for Disease Control and Prevention: Advance Data No. 329, June 19, 2002.
6. Farrow DC, Hunt WC, Samet JM: Temporal and regional variability in the surgical treatment of cancer among older people. J Am Geriatr Soc 44:559-564, 1996.
7. Taffett GE: Physiology of aging. *In* Cassel CK, Leipzig RM, Cohen HJ, et al (eds): Geriatric Medicine: An Evidence-Based Approach, 4th ed. New York, Springer, 2003.
8. Lewis JF, Maron BJ: Cardiovascular consequences of the aging process. *In* Lowenthal DT (ed): Geriatric Cardiology. Vol. 22 of Cardiovascular Clinics. Philadelphia, FA Davis, 1992.

9. Tresch DD, McGough MF: Heart failure with normal systolic function: A common disorder in older people. J Am Geriatr Soc 43:1035, 1995.

10. Campbell EJ: Physiologic changes in respiratory function. *In* Rosenthal RA, Zenilman ME, Katlic MR (eds): Principles and Practice of Geriatric Surgery. New York, Springer, 2000.

11. Marik PE: Aspiration pneumonitis and aspiration pneumonia. N Engl J Med 344:665-671, 2001.

12. Cockroft DW, Gault MH: Prediction of creatinine clearance from serum creatinine. Nephron 16:31, 1976.

13. Ryan JJ, Zawada ET Jr: Renal function and fluid and electrolyte balance. *In* Rosenthal RA, Zenilman ME, Katlic MR (eds): Principles and Practice of Geriatric Surgery. New York, Springer, 2000.

14. Mason DL, Brunicardi FC: Hepatobiliary and pancreatic function. *In* Rosenthal RA, Zenilman ME, Katlic MR (eds): Principles and Practice of Geriatric Surgery. New York, Springer-Verlag, 2000.

15. Currie MS: Immunosenescence. Compr Ther 18:26, 1992.

16. Burns EA, Goodwin JS: The effects of aging on immune function. *In* Rosenthal RA, Zenilman ME, Katlic MR (eds): Principles and Practice of Geriatric Surgery. New York, Springer, 2000.

17. Yancik R, et al: Comorbidity and age as predictors of risk for early mortality of male and female colon carcinoma patients: A population-based study. Cancer. 82:2123-2134, 1998.

18. Tiret L, et al: Complications associated with anaesthesia—a prospective survey in France. Can Anaesth Soc J 33:336-344, 1986.

19. Escarce JJ, et al: Outcomes of open cholecystectomy in the elderly: A longitudinal analysis of 21,000 cases in the prelaparoscopic era. Surgery 117:156, 1995.

20. Kannel WB, Dannenberg AV, Abbott RD: Unrecognized myocardial infarction and hypertension: Framingham Study. Am Heart J 109:581, 1985.

21. Eagle KA, et al: ACC/AHA Task Force Report: Guidelines for perioperative cardiovascular evaluation for noncardiac surgery. Circulation 93:1278, 1996.

22. Liu LL, Dzankic S, Lueng JM: Preoperative electrocardiogram abnormalities do not predict postoperative cardiac complications in geriatric surgical patients. J Am Geriatr Soc 50:1186-1191, 2002.

23. Gerson MC, et al: Prediction of cardiac and pulmonary complications related to elective abdominal and noncardiac thoracic surgery in geriatric patients. Am J Med 88:101-107, 1990.

24. Smetana GW: Current concepts: Preoperative pulmonary evaluation. N Engl J Med 340:937-944, 1999.

25. Khuri SF, et al: Risk adjustment of the postoperative mortality rate for the comparative assessment of quality of surgical care: Results of the National Veterans Affairs Surgical Risk Study. J Am Coll Surg 185:315-327, 1997.

26. Marcantonio ER, et al: A clinical prediction rule for delirium after elective noncardiac surgery. JAMA 271:134, 1994.

27. Moller JT, et al: Long-term postoperative cognitive dysfunction in the elderly: ISPOCD1 study. Lancet 351:857, 1998.

28. Folstein MF, Folstein SE, McHugh PR: The mini-mental state examination: A practical method for grading the cognitive state of patients for the clinician. J Psychiatr Res 12:189, 1975.

29. Inouye SK: Delirium in hospitalized elderly patients: Recognition, evaluation and management. Conn Med 57:309-212, 1993.

30. Marcantonio ER, Goldman L, Orav JE, et al: The association of intraoperative factors with the development of postoperative delirium. Am J Med 105:380, 1998.

31. Rosenberg IH: Nutrition and Aging. *In* Hazzard WR, Bierman EL, Blass JP, et al (eds): Principles of Geriatric Medicine and Gerontology, 3rd ed. New York, McGraw-Hill, 1994.

32. Souba WW: Nutritional Support. N Engl J Med 336:41, 1997.

33. Persson MD, et al: Nutritional status using mini nutritional assessment and subjective global assessment predict mortality in geriatric patients. J Am Geriatr Soc 50:1996-2002, 2002.

34. Detsky AS, et al: Predicting nutrition-associated complications for patients undergoing gastrointestinal surgery. JPEN J Parenter Enter Nutr 11:440-46, 1987.

35. Yancik R, Ries LG, Yates JW: Breast cancer in aging women: A population-based study of contrasts in stage, surgery, and survival. Cancer 63:976-81, 1989.

36. Wyld L, Reed MWR: The need for targeted research into breast cancer in the elderly. Br J Surg 90:388-399, 2003.

37. Fisher B, Bauer M, Margolese R, et al: Five-year results of a randomized clinical trial comparing total mastectomy and segmental mastectomy with or without radiation in the treatment of breast cancer. N Engl J Med 312:665-673, 1985.

38. Hansen N, Morrow M: Breast cancer in elderly women. *In* Rosenthal RA, Zenilman ME, Katlic MR (eds): Principles and Practice of Geriatric Surgery. New York, Springer-Verlag, 2000.

39. Nagataki S, Shibata S, Inoue S, et al: Thyroid diseases among atomic bomb survivors in Nagasaki. JAMA 272:364-370, 1994.

40. Shoup M, Stojadinovic A, Nissan A, et al: Prognostic indicators of outcomes in patients with distant metastases from differentiated thyroid carcinoma. J Am Coll Surg 197:191-197, 2003.

41. Sanders LE, Cady B: Differentiated thyroid cancer: Reexamination of risk groups and outcome of treatment. Arch Surg 133:419-425, 1998.

42. Chigot JP, Menegaux F, Achrafi H: Should primary hyperparathyroidism be treated surgically in elderly patients older than 75 years? Surgery 117:397-401, 1995.

43. Consensus Development Conference Panel: Diagnosis and management of asymptomatic primary hyperparathyroidism: Consensus development conference statement. Ann Intern Med 114:593-597, 1991.

44. Prager G, Czerny C, Ofluoglu S, et al: Impact of localization studies on feasibility of minimally invasive parathyroidectomy in an endemic goiter region. J Am Coll Surg 196:541-548, 2003.

45. Peracchia A, Bonavina L, Narne S, et al: Minimally invasive surgery for Zenker's diverticulum: Analysis of results in 95 consecutive patients. Arch Surg 133:695-700, 1998.

46. Gillison EW, Powell J, McConkey CC, Spychal RT: Surgical workload and outcome after resection for carcinoma of the oesophagus and cardia. Br J Surg 89:344-348, 2002.

47. Brock J, Sauaia A, Ahnen D, et al: Process of care and outcomes for elderly patients hospitalized with peptic ulcer disease. JAMA 286:1985-1993, 2001.

48. Boey J, et al: Risk stratification in perforated duodenal ulcers: A prospective validation of predictive factors. Ann Surg 205:22-26, 1987.

49. Branicki FJ, et al: Bleeding duodenal ulcer: A prospective evaluation of risk factors for rebleeding and death. Ann Surg 211:411-418, 1990.

50. Karl RC, Smith SK, Fabri PJ: Validity of major cancer operations in elderly patients. Ann Surg Oncol 2:107, 1995.

51. Martin R, Paty P, Fong Y, et al: Simultaneous liver and colorectal resections are safe for synchronous colorectal liver metastasis. J Am Coll Surg 197:233-241; discussion 241-242, 2003.

52. Bowen JC, et al: Gallstone disease: Pathophysiology, epidemiology, natural history, and treatment options. Med Clin North Am 76:1143, 1992.

53. Poston GJ, et al: Effect of age and sensitivity to cholecystokinin on gallstone formation in the guinea pig. Gastroenterology 98:993, 1990.

54. Morrow DJ, Thompson J, Wislon SE: Acute cholecystitis in the elderly: A surgical emergency. Arch Surg 113:1149, 1978.

55. Eagon JC: Small bowel obstruction in the elderly. *In* Rosenthal RA, Zenilman ME, Katlic MR (eds): Principles and Practice of Geriatric Surgery. New York, Springer, 2000.

56. Sosa J, Gardner B: Management of patients diagnosed as acute intestinal obstruction secondary to adhesions. Am Surg 59:125-128, 1993.

57. Cox MR, Gunn IF, Eastman MC, et al: The safety and duration of non-operative treatment for adhesive small bowel obstruction. Aust N Z J Surg 63:367-371, 1993.

58. Landercasper J, et al: Long-term outcome after hospitalization for small-bowel obstruction. Arch Surg 128:765-770: discussion 770-771, 1993.

59. Bailey IS, et al: Laparoscopic management of acute small bowel obstruction. Br J Surg 85:84-87, 1998.

60. Horattas MC, Guyton DP, Wu D: A reappraisal of appendicitis in the elderly. Am J Surg 160:291-293, 1990.

61. Franz MG, Norman J, Fabri PJ: Increased morbidity of appendicitis with advanced age. Am Surg 61:40-44, 1995.

62. Okamoto M, Shiratori Y, Yamaji Y, et al: Relationship between age and site of colorectal cancer based on colonoscopy findings. Gastrointest Endosc 55:548-551, 2002.

63. Avital S, et al: Survival of colorectal carcinoma in the elderly: A prospective study of colorectal carcinoma and a five-year follow-up. Dis Colon Rectum 40:523-529, 1997.

64. Kingston RD, et al: The outcome of surgery for colorectal cancer in the elderly: A 12-year review for the Trafford database. Eur J Surg Oncol 21:514-516, 1995.

65. Jessup JM, et al: National Cancer Data Base: A report on colon cancer. Cancer 78:918-926, 1996.

66. Peterson KA, DiSario GM: Secondary prevention: Screening and surveillance of persons at average and high risk for colorectal cancer. Hematol Oncol Clin North Am 16:841-856, 2002.

67. Leo E, et al: Total rectal resection and colo-anal anastomosis for low rectal tumours: Comparative results in a group of young and old patients. Eur J Cancer 30A:1092-1095, 1994.

68. Potosky AL, et al: Age, sex and racial differences in the use of standard adjuvant therapy for colorectal cancer. J Clin Oncol 20:1192-1202, 2002.

69. Emory RE, Laporta AJ: Obturator hernia. Surg Rounds 16:43, 1993.

70. Read RC: Recent advances in the repair of groin herniation. Curr Probl Surg 40:13-79, 2003.

71. Nehler MR, Taylor LM, Moneta GL, Proter JM: Indications for operation for infrarenal abdominal aortic aneurysms: Current guidelines. Semin Vasc Surg 8:108-114, 1995.

72. Petracek MR, Lawson JD, Rhea WG Jr: Resection of abdominal aortic aneurysms in the over-80 group. South Med J 73:579, 1980.

73. Ouriel K: Endovascular repair of abdominal aortic aneurysms: The Cleveland Clinic experience with five different devices. Semin Vasc Surg 16:88-94, 2003.

74. Perler BA: Vascular disease in the elderly patient. Surg Clin North Am 74:199-216, 1994.

75. Rockman CB, Jacobowitz GR, Adelman MA, et al: The benefits of carotid endarterectomy in the octogenarian: A challenge to the results of carotid angioplasty and stenting. Ann Vasc Surg 17:9-14, 2003.

76. Comacho MT, Plestis KA, Gold JP: Cardiac surgery in the elderly. *In* Rosenthal RA, Zenilman ME, Katlic MR (eds): Principles and Practice of Geriatric Surgery. New York, Springer, 2000.

77. Williams DB, et al: Determinants of operative mortality in octogenarians undergoing coronary bypass. Ann Thorac Surg 60:1038-1043, 1995.

78. Katz NM, Chase GA: Risks of cardiac operations for elderly patients: Reduction of the age factor. Ann Thorac Surg 63:1309-1314, 1997.

79. Sollano JA, Rose EA, et al: Cost-effectiveness of coronary artery bypass surgery in octogenarians. Ann Surg 228:297-306, 1998.

80. Davis EA, et al: Valvular disease in the elderly: Influence on surgical results. Ann Thorac Surg 55:333-338, 1993.

81. Antora TA, Trooskin SZ, Kaplan LJ: Care of the injured elderly. *In* Rosenthal RA, Zenilman ME, Katlic MR (eds): Principles and Practice of Geriatric Surgery. New York, Springer, 2000.

82. Pennings JL, Bachulis BL, Simons CT, Slazinski T: Survival after severe brain injury in the aged. Arch Surg 128:787-794, 1993.

83. Feng S, Tomlanovich SL, Fraser K, et al: Transplantation in elderly patients. *In* Rosenthal RA, Zenilman ME, Katlic MR (eds): Principles and Practice of Geriatric Surgery. New York, Springer, 2000.

84. Schaubel D, et al: Survival experience among elderly end-stage renal disease patients: A controlled comparison of transplant and dialysis. Transplantation 60:1389-1394, 1995.

85. Rowe JW: Health care myths at the end of life. Bull Am Coll Surg 81:11-18, 1996.

86. Council Report: Decisions near the end of life. JAMA 267:2229-2233, 1992.

87. Knaus WE, Harrel FE, Lynn J, et al: The SUPPORT prognostic model: Objective estimates of survival for seriously ill hospitalized adults. Ann Intern Med 122:191-203, 1995.

88. Knaus WA, Wagner DP, Lynn J: Short term mortality predictions for critically ill hospitalized adults: Science and ethics. Science 254:389-394, 1991.

89. Eiseman B: Surgical decision making and elderly patients. Bull Am Coll Surg 81:8-11, 1996.

90. Morgenstern L: The art of sitting. West J Med 161:93, 1994.

MORBID OBESITY

Bruce David Schirmer, M.D.

The surgical treatment of morbid obesity is known as bariatric surgery. It has its origin in the 1950s, when malabsorptive operations were first performed for severe hyperlipidemia syndromes. Subsequently, jejunoileal bypass to produce weight loss began to be performed sporadically during the 1960s, then more frequently in the 1970s. This produced unacceptable metabolic complications. Bariatric surgeons developed myriad operations, few of which proved effective in the long term for providing safe and durable weight loss.

This process has clearly pointed out two very unique aspects of the field of bariatric surgery. The first is that this is surgery that involves the alteration of metabolic processes, not just simply weight loss. The effects of any bariatric operation on metabolic processes need to be fully understood before the operation's effectiveness and safety can be determined. The second is that long-term follow-up is required to adequately assess the merits of an operation. Durability of weight loss is as important, ultimately, as the amount of weight loss achieved. Similarly, some consequences of an operation may only be fully appreciated after a long period of follow-up.

We now understand that morbid obesity is a disease affecting over 20 million Americans in 2004. Bariatric surgical operations are in more demand by patients than any other operation and have experienced the most rapid growth rate both of procedures performed and surgeons performing them than any area of general surgery over the past 3 years.

OBESITY: THE MAGNITUDE OF THE PROBLEM

Morbid obesity is defined as being either 100 pounds above ideal body weight, twice ideal body weight, or having a body mass index (BMI, measured as weight in kilograms divided by height in meters squared) of $40 \, kg/m^2$. The latter definition is more accepted internationally and has essentially replaced the former ones for all practical and scientific purposes. The National Institutes of Health (NIH) Consensus Conference,[1] in 1991, suggested that the term *severe obesity* is more appropriate to defining people of such size. This term shall be used interchangeably with *morbid obesity* in the remainder of this chapter.

It is estimated that between 3% and 5% of the adult population of the United States is morbidly obese, or clinically severely obese,[2] the highest percentage of population of any country. Patients undergoing bariatric surgery in the United States have average BMIs that are significantly higher than those reported in Europe. Australia, however, is not far behind, according to Australian bariatric surgeons. Even Europe, where severely obese individuals are not common among crowds, is now experiencing an overall enlargement of the population. Studies of adolescent obesity have estimated the incidence of obesity (being 40% above ideal body weight) as being in the 35% range for adolescents in the United States but over 20% in most European countries. The problem is also growing at an alarmingly rapid rate in the United States. In 1985, when statistics of national obesity were first measured by the Centers for Disease Control (CDC) according to individual states, many states had no available such data. Of the roughly half that did, more than half of those reported an incidence of people with BMI over 30 kg/m² of under 10%. By 1990, when most states' data were known, the incidence of BMI greater than 30 kg/m² of over 10% rose to 60% of states. By 1995, half the states had a BMI greater than 30 kg/m² incidence of over 15%. By 2000, 21 states reported that incidence had risen to over 20%, with all but one of the remaining states having an incidence over 15%.[3] This alarming rate of increasing obesity outstrips any theory that the disease has a solely genetic component to it.

Obesity is estimated to cause 280,000 deaths annually in the United States.[4] The total number of deaths annually from both breast and colon cancer is only about 90,000 per year. After tobacco use, obesity is the second leading cause of preventable death in the United States and is second to smoking on the list of preventable factors responsible for increased health care costs.

In 1995, it was estimated the cost of obesity for direct costs alone (not contributing to other costs) to the health care budget was $70 billion, or roughly 3% of the budget.[2] These costs have increased since then. There is speculation that within the next decade obesity may overtake tobacco as the leading cause of preventable medical expense in the United States.

PATHOPHYSIOLOGY AND ASSOCIATED MEDICAL PROBLEMS

The pathophysiology of severe obesity is poorly understood. Debate is ongoing as to the relative genetic versus environmental components of the disease. There is a clear familial predisposition; it is rare for a single family member to have severe obesity. The rapid increase in obesity from 1980 to 2003 emphasizes the considerable environmental component that contributes to the problem as well.

Although there is no definitive answer as to the pathophysiology of severe obesity, several observations from caring for such individuals are worthy of mention. It is clear that the severely obese individual has, in general, persistent hunger that is not satiated by amounts of food that satisfy the nonobese. This lack of satiety or maintenance of satiety may be the single most important factor in the process. The capacity to eat large amounts is greatly increased in the morbidly obese. Others eat or "nibble" for prolonged periods of the day, usually later in the day, to increase caloric intake, greatly in excess of metabolic needs.

Basic scientific understanding of the roles played by hormones, peptides, or other factors on satiety is incomplete. Cholecystokinin (CCK) and ghrelin, produced largely in the proximal stomach by food, are involved in satiety. Increased levels of ghrelin seem to produce increased food intake. Individuals who are on low-calorie diets develop increased levels of ghrelin. Patients with gastric inflow restricted but allowing food to pass through the stomach have normal to elevated ghrelin levels postoperatively. In contrast, patients undergoing gastric bypass have suppressed postoperative levels of ghrelin.[5] The role of ghrelin in the lack of hunger after gastric bypass or recovery of appetite is not clear.

Morbid obesity is a metabolic disease associated with numerous medical problems. Some are virtually unknown in the absence of obesity. Box 16-1 lists the most common problems. These must be carefully considered when one is contemplating offering a patient weight reduction surgery. The most frequent problem is the combination of arthritis and/or degenerative joint disease, present in at least 50% of patients seeking surgery for severe obesity. The incidence of sleep apnea is high. Asthma is present in over 25%, hypertension in over 30%, diabetes in over 20%, and gastroesophageal reflux in 20% to 30% of patients. The incidence of these conditions increases with the duration of severe obesity and age. Individuals beyond the age of 50 often have several associated conditions.

The "metabolic syndrome" includes type II diabetes mellitus, impaired glucose tolerance, dyslipidemia, and hypertension. Patients with this constellation of problems are generally obese, with central body obesity being the primary body feature. The syndrome is thought to result in impaired hepatic uptake of insulin, systemic hyperinsulinemia, and subsequent tissue resistance to insulin.

Not listed in Box 16-1 are the associated societal discriminatory problems that severely obese individuals face. Public facilities in terms of seating, doorways, and restroom facilities often make access to events held in such settings unavailable to the severely obese person. Travel on public transportation is sometimes difficult if not impossible. Employment discrimination clearly exists for these individuals. Finally, the combination of low self-esteem, the frequent history of sexual or physical abuse, and these social difficulties combine to create a very high incidence of depression in the severely obese patient population.

MEDICAL VERSUS SURGICAL THERAPY

Medical therapy for severe obesity has limited short-term success and almost nonexistent long-term success. Once a person is severely obese, the likelihood they will lose enough weight by dietary means alone and remain at a BMI below 35 is estimated as 3% or less. The NIH Consensus Conference recognized that, for this patient population, medical therapy has been uniformly unsuccessful in treating the problem.[1]

Despite this limited success, it is generally agreed that the severely obese patient should be given the chance to comply with a medically supervised diet program to see if any success can be achieved. Insurance funding for surgery has traditionally been linked to such an attempt, or, for some insurance companies, a well-documented history of several such attempts.

Very low calorie diets fall into two categories: those that restrict primarily fat intake and those that restrict primarily carbohydrate intake. The latter produce slightly more short-term weight loss than the former but no difference in long-term results.[6] Both diets produce weight

Box 16-1 Medical conditions associated with severe obesity

Cardiovascular

Hypertension
Sudden cardiac death
Cardiomyopathy
Venous stasis disease
Deep venous thrombosis
Pulmonary hypertension
Right-sided heart failure

Pulmonary

Obstructive sleep apnea
Hypoventilation syndrome of obesity
Asthma

Metabolic

Type II diabetes
Hyperlipidemia
Hypercholesterolemia
Nonalcoholic steatotic hepatitis

Gastrointestinal

Gastroesophageal reflux disease
Cholelithiasis

Musculoskeletal

Degenerative joint disease
Lumbar disc disease
Osteoarthritis
Ventral hernias

Genitourinary

Stress urinary incontinence
End-stage renal disease (secondary to diabetes and hypertension)

Gynecologic

Menstrual irregularities

Skin/Integumentary System

Fungal infections
Boils, abscesses

Oncologic

Cancers of the uterus, breast, colon, kidney, prostate

Neurologic/Psychiatric

Pseudotumor cerebri
Depression
Low self-esteem
Stroke

Social/Societal

History of physical abuse
History of sexual abuse

loss that is insufficient to affect any major change in health status.

Pharmacologic therapy in 2003 focused on two medications. Sibutramine blocks presynaptic receptor uptake of both norepinephrine and serotonin, potentiating their anorexic effect in the central nervous system. Orlistat inhibits pancreatic lipase and thereby reduces absorption of up to 30% of ingested dietary fat. A maximum weight loss of up to 10% of body weight has been noted in unselected individuals using either or both drugs; weight is regained within 12 to 18 months.[7] For the severely obese individual, neither drug has proven effective therapy alone. Their efficacy after weight reduction surgery is unknown.

In summary, nonsurgical weight loss programs have limited success for severely obese patients. However, owing to the potential for success, albeit low, they should be recommended for all patients before consideration for bariatric surgery. Unwillingness to follow such a course is unusual, for most patients who seek bariatric surgery have a history of trying many diet plans. Such lack of willingness may be a harbinger of poor postoperative compliance.

PREOPERATIVE EVALUATION AND SELECTION

Eligibility

The preoperative selection of patients for weight reduction surgery should be strictly based on currently accepted NIH guidelines.[1] Patients must have a BMI greater than 40kg/m^2 without associated comorbid medical conditions or a BMI greater than 35kg/m^2 with an associated comorbid medical problem. They must have also failed dietary therapy. Beyond this, the NIH guidelines are not specific. However, it has been our experience that several practical criteria must also be used as guidelines for indications for surgery. These include psychiatric stability, motivated attitude, and ability to comprehend the nature of the operation and its resultant changes in eating behavior and lifestyle. The criteria used for our institution for eligibility for bariatric surgery are given in Box 16-2. Inability to fulfill these criteria is a contraindication to bariatric surgery.

One criterion not listed in Box 16-2 that is, unfortunately, often a significant issue for the severely obese patient is that of insurance coverage for the operation. The cost of the hospitalization alone for bariatric surgery can easily approach $20,000, especially if any complications arise. This figure makes the cost prohibitive for most individuals without insurance coverage. The criteria of individual insurance companies are as varied as the number of companies in existence.

Medical contraindications are not clear. All patients with comorbidity conditions are at greater risk. The surgeon must ensure that these are well understood by all patients before bariatric surgery, especially those at high risk. Several family members should be included in these discussions. There are certain individuals who have

---

Box 16-2   Indications for bariatric surgery

Patients should meet the following criteria for consideration for bariatric surgery:

- BMI > 40 kg/m² or BMI > 35 kg/m² with associated medical comorbidity worsened by obesity
- Failed dietary therapy
- Psychiatrically stable
- Knowledgeable about operation and its sequelae
- Motivated
- Medical problems do not preclude likely survival from surgery

---

end-stage organ function of heart, lungs, or both. These patients are unlikely to gain the benefit of longevity and improved health.

Patients who cannot walk have greater risk than those who can ambulate, even for short distances. Whereas nonambulatory status is not an absolute contraindication for surgery, it does place the patient at increased risk for deep venous thrombosis, pulmonary failure, and sacral decubitus ulcers, among other problems.

Patients who weigh more than 600 pounds have even more complications. Many options for testing, such as computed tomographic (CT) scanners, are exceeded by this weight limit. At this weight operating room tables, moving and lift equipment and teams, blood pressure cuffs, sequential compression device boots, and any sort of invasive bedside procedures such as central venous catheters become extraordinarily difficult or problematic. It has been my practice to strongly encourage patients weighing over 600 pounds to lose weight down to that level by nonoperative means, even if that means enforced hospitalization.

The Prader-Willi syndrome is an absolute contraindication. No surgical therapy affects the constant need to eat.

Age is a controversial contraindication to bariatric surgery. For adolescents, most pediatric/bariatric surgeons recommend that the operation be performed after the major growth spurt (mid to late teens) and thus allowing for increased maturity on the part of the patient. Simple restrictive operations are thought to be most appropriate for patients in this age group. In the United States, one such procedure, the laparoscopic adjustable gastric banding procedure (LAP-BAND), has been approved by the Food and Drug Administration only for patients age 18 or over. Increasing experience will be required to determine which operation is most effective in adolescents.

While my colleagues and I in our practice have generally set the age of 60 as a rough cut-off for performing gastric bypass, patients between the ages of 60 and 65 have been individually evaluated. These evaluations focus on the patient's relative physiologic age and potential for longevity rather than on chronologic age. Duration and degree of obesity are the most important factors in evaluating the older patient. In general, the longer and more severe the degree of obesity, the more comorbid medical problems exist and the lower the potential for such individuals to benefit.

Preoperative Evaluation

Preoperative assessment of the bariatric surgical patient involves two distinct areas. One is the specific preoperative assessment of candidacy for bariatric surgery and assessment of comorbid conditions. The second is the general assessment and preoperative preparation as for any major abdominal surgery. This second area will not be extensively reviewed in this chapter and is discussed in depth in Chapter 10 of this textbook.

General Bariatric Preoperative Evaluation and Preparation

A team approach is required for optimal care of the morbidly obese patient. Box 16-3 lists the key personnel for the bariatric multidisciplinary team. Current guidelines of the Society of American Gastrointestinal Endoscopic Surgeons (SAGES)[8] and the American Society for Bariatric Surgery (ASBS)[9] reinforce the need for the multidisciplinary team approach.

Box 16-4 summarizes the steps and tests routinely performed for the preoperative evaluation of bariatric patients in the author's clinic. After the complete history and physical examination at the initial assessment, the patient is referred for other evaluations as required. Then final testing before surgery is performed. In this group of tests is included arterial blood gas analysis and upper endoscopy for those patients in whom it is indicated and ultrasound of the gallbladder.

Proper preoperative patient education is essential, and attendance at educational sessions is mandatory. Family members are encouraged to attend. After preoperative testing is completed, a final counseling session with the surgeon and an education session with the nurse educator are held.

Patients undergoing laparoscopic bariatric surgery have a 2-day mechanical bowel prep. This decompresses the

---

Box 16-3   The bariatric multidiscipline team

Surgeon
Assisting surgeon
Nutritionist
Anesthesiologist
Operating room nurse
Operating room scrub tech/nurse
Nurse care coordinator/educator
Secretary/administrator
Psychiatrist/psychologist
Primary care physician
Medical specialists for cardiac, pulmonary, gastrointestinal, endocrine, musculoskeletal, and neurologic conditions as indicated

Box 16-4 Preoperative Evaluation

Prior to Clinic Visit

- Documented medically supervised diet
- Counseling and referral from primary care physician
- Reading comprehensive written brochure regarding operative procedures, expected results, potential complications

Initial Clinic Visit

- Group presentation on information in booklet
- Group presentation on preoperative and postoperative nutritional issues by nutritionist
- Individual assessment by surgeon's team
- Individual counseling session with surgeon
- Individual counseling session with nutritionist
- Screening blood tests

Subsequent Events/Evaluations

- Full psychological assessment and evaluation as indicated
- Medical specialist evaluations as indicated
- Insurance approval for coverage of procedure
- Screening flexible upper endoscopy as indicated
- Screening ultrasound of gallbladder (if present)
- Arterial blood gas analysis

Second Clinic Visit

- Counseling session with surgeon (including choosing date for surgery)
- Education session with nurse educator
- Preoperative evaluation by anesthesiology
- Final paperwork by preadmissions center

---

bowel, making it safer for intraoperative handling by laparoscopic instruments. They are encouraged to drink liberally to avoid dehydration the day before surgery.

A first-generation cephalosporin, in a dose appropriate for weight, is given preoperatively, and antibiotics are continued for only 24 hours. Three major measures are used for prophylaxis against deep venous thrombosis (DVT) and pulmonary embolism: ambulation within 4 to 6 hours of surgery, sequential compression device stockings or shoe sleeves, and low-molecular-weight heparin subcutaneously on call to the operating room and then twice daily until discharge. High-risk patients (e.g., with history of DVT, venous stasis ulcers, known or highly suspected pulmonary hypertension, hypoventilation syndrome of obesity, or requiring reoperation during the initial hospitalization) are given subcutaneous injections of heparin at home for a full 2-week course. Data support the use of preoperative antibiotics, but there are no data that establish the optimal regimen for DVT prophylaxis. Despite aggressive prophylactic programs, pulmonary embolism remains the most common cause of death after bariatric surgery.

Evaluation of Specific Comorbidities

Cardiovascular evaluation of the bariatric patient must include a history of recent chest pain and functional assessment of activity with relation to cardiac function. Patients with a history of recent chest pain or change in exercise tolerance should have a formal cardiology assessment, including stress testing as indicated. I almost never resort to invasive central monitoring with a Swan-Ganz catheter; central venous and pulmonary hypertension are the norm and should not be interpreted as volume overload. The use of transesophageal echocardiography intraoperatively is occasionally helpful for patients with cardiomyopathy.

Pulmonary assessment includes a search of obstructive sleep apnea. The incidence of sleep apnea has been reported in 42% to 48% in morbidly obese men and 8% to 38% in severely obese women.[10] A history of falling asleep driving or while at work, or a history of feeling tired after a night's sleep, coupled with a history of snoring or even witnessed apnea, are all strongly suggestive of the condition. Patients with suggestive histories of clinically significant sleep apnea should undergo preoperative sleep study testing. If found to have the condition, the use of a continuous positive airway pressure (CPAP) or a bilevel positive airway pressure (BiPAP) apparatus while sleeping postoperatively can eliminate the otherwise stressful periods of hypoxia that would otherwise result in these patients. Although tolerated under normal circumstances, these hypoxic episodes in the immediate postoperative period are more dangerous, because other factors affecting hemodynamic stability are at work.

Reactive asthma is another common problem of the severely obese and one that is underrecognized. It requires less preoperative preparation in terms of testing than sleep apnea and is less dangerous. However, it is still often limiting in terms of patients' tolerance of activity and must be adequately addressed with inhalers as needed.

Hypoventilation syndrome of obesity (pickwickian syndrome) is a diagnosis that is often suspected by the patient's clinical appearance. The condition is usually limited to the superobese patient population with a BMI over 60 kg/m². Individuals with this diagnosis have plethoric faces, may appear clinically cyanotic, and clearly exhibit difficulty with normal respiratory efforts at baseline or mild exertion. The arterial blood gas analysis reveals $PaCO_2$ higher than PaO_2 and elevated hematocrit. Pulmonary artery pressures are greatly elevated. These patients have an extremely high cardiopulmonary morbidity and mortality and are among the few subsets of patients who, in my practice, require planned intensive care admission postoperatively. Prolonged ventilator support is often required and management of intravascular volume is based on the patient's baseline status. The incidence of postoperative respiratory failure, pneumonia, pulmonary embolism, and cardiac failure is high in this patient group.

Whereas most patients with hypoventilation syndrome of obesity are clinically obvious, those with less obviously compromised pulmonary status often are only detected by preoperative baseline arterial blood gases.

Because there is a considerable incidence of hypertension or diabetes in those patients with concomitant renal disease, the serum creatinine value is an excellent preoperative screening test for baseline renal function.

Musculoskeletal conditions, especially arthritis and degenerative joint disease, are the most common group of comorbidities found in the severely obese patient. Over half the patients have some form of these conditions, often to an advanced degree. Limited ambulation, joint replacement, severe back pain, and other sequelae are not uncommon. Before surgery, it is important for patients to understand that structural damage done cannot be reversed by weight loss. Fortunately, significant weight loss often alleviates or even reverses the chronic pain or disability from such conditions.

Metabolic problems are common in severely obese patients, particularly hyperlipidemia, hypercholesterolemia, and type II diabetes mellitus. All are easily screened for by simple blood tests. Twenty percent of severely obese patients undergoing bariatric surgery have clinically significant type II diabetes. Diabetes must be controlled.

Skin must be examined for fungal infection and venous stasis changes. Sugerman and colleagues[11] report that venous stasis disease is associated with a greatly increased incidence of postoperative DVT.

Umbilical or ventral hernias may be present. Preparations as to how to best deal with large hernias must be decided preoperatively; the approach and incision may be affected by their presence.

Cholelithiasis is the most prevalent of the several gastrointestinal conditions and must be sought before bariatric surgery. Gallstone formation occurs during time periods of rapid weight loss. Shiffman and colleagues[12] have shown the incidence of gallstone or sludge formation after gastric bypass is approximately 30%. If gallstones are present, most surgeons agree that simultaneous cholecystectomy should be performed at the time of bariatric surgery. For patients undergoing malabsorptive operations, gallstone formation is so frequent that prophylactic cholecystectomy is a standard part of those procedures. However, for patients undergoing restrictive operations, a screening ultrasound is recommended. This is particularly true of patients undergoing Roux-en-Y gastric bypass (RYGB), because endoscopic retrograde cholangiopancreatography (ERCP) is not possible. We have had no significant morbidity from adding cholecystectomy in over 500 RYGB cases; cholecystectomy adds 30 minutes of additional operating time.[13] Ursodeoxycholic acid, 300 mg twice daily for 6 months postoperatively, reduces the incidence of gallstone formation to 3% in patients who follow this treatment plan.[14] Our current recommendations for patients undergoing laparoscopic bariatric surgery are for simultaneous cholecystectomy if gallstones are present and ursodiol therapy for 6 months after surgery if the gallbladder is normal.

Gastroesophageal reflux disease (GERD) is common in severely obese patients due to the increased abdominal pressure and its shortened lower esophageal sphincter. Preoperative upper endoscopy is indicated for all patients who have GERD to detect Barrett's esophagus and to evaluate the lower stomach and duodenum in patients undergoing RYGB.[15]

The patient with nonalcoholic steatotic hepatitis (NASH) presents a potential problem. Ultrasound screening to determine the size of the left lobe of the liver is done because the enlarged liver may interfere with access or visualization of the stomach at operation. Size of the left lobe of the liver often determines the ability to complete an operation laparoscopically. Patients with known enlarged fatty livers may benefit from caloric restriction, especially carbohydrate restriction, for a period of several weeks preoperatively. Bariatric surgery is beneficial for NASH; weight loss improves the prognosis. NASH is not a contraindication for bariatric surgery if there is no cirrhosis and portal hypertension or hepatocellular decompensation. Liver biopsy should be performed at the time of bariatric surgery for any patient whose liver appears abnormal.

SPECIAL EQUIPMENT

Clinic

The clinic for evaluating bariatric patients must be constructed with the needs of the patient in mind. The waiting area must contain comfortable benches with backs, not standard size chairs. Doorways must be extra wide to accommodate wheelchairs. This is true for bathrooms as well, which must be equipped with toilets on the floor, not mounted on the wall. A scale that can weigh up to 1000 pounds is necessary. Large-sized gowns, wide examining tables stable enough for large patients, and wide blood pressure cuffs are needed. A large room with appropriate seating is needed for the patient group education session.

Operating Room

The operating room should contain a hydraulically operated operating room table that can accommodate up to 800 pounds. Side attachments to widen the table as needed are required. Foam cushioning, extra large SCD stockings, wide and secure padded straps for the abdomen and legs, and a footboard for the operating room table are all essential to safely secure the patient for placement in steep reverse Trendelenburg position during surgery.

Video telescopic equipment used for any laparoscopic abdominal procedure is necessary. Two monitors, one near each shoulder, are essential. I have found that two insufflators are helpful to maintain pneumoperitoneum.

The choice of laparoscopic instruments is based on surgeon preference. I have found a 45-degree telescope, extra long staplers, atraumatic graspers, and other instruments to be most useful. Extra-long trocars may be needed. The ultrasonic scalpel is most helpful in the gastric dissection, particularly along the lesser curvature of the stomach. I use the standard disposable drape used for cardiac surgical cases, which has side pockets for placement of instruments.

A fixed retractor device secured to the operating room table for clamping and holding the liver retractor is also essential. The left lobe of the liver must be retracted safely and atraumatically. This can pose one of the most difficult technical challenges for patients with a large thick liver. A variety of retractors all may achieve this purpose. Sometimes, two retractors may be necessary for the large liver.

OPERATIVE PROCEDURES

Bariatric operations are performed using either an open or laparoscopic approach. However, the clear trend for the future is to have most procedures done laparoscopically. Data already appear to confirm the advantages of the laparoscopic approach.[16-19]

Bariatric operations produce weight loss due to two factors. One is restriction of oral intake. The other is malabsorption of ingested food. There are operations that employ only one mechanism for weight loss, and there are others that combine the two. Box 16-5 lists the major procedures to be described.

Vertical Banded Gastroplasty

This procedure is mentioned for historic purposes only. It has now largely been abandoned in favor of other operations, owing to the poor long-term weight loss,[20] high rate of late stenosis of the gastric outlet,[21] and tendency of patients to adopt a high-calorie liquid diet, leading to regain of weight.[22]

Adjustable Gastric Banding

The adjustable gastric banding (AGB) procedure may be performed with any one of three types of adjustable bands. The only band approved for use by the FDA in the United States is the LAP-BAND (INAMED Health, Santa Barbara, CA). The Swedish Adjustable Gastric Band (Obtech Medical, Baar, Switzerland), the MIDBAND (Medical Innovation Development, Villeurbanne, France), and the Heliogast Band (Helioscopie, Vienne, France) are other banding systems used in Europe and elsewhere, with the Swedish band having a multiyear track record,

whereas the others are relatively new to the bariatric field. Worldwide experience is largest with the LAP-BAND. The techniques of placement of the bands are similar; only the locking mechanisms, band shape and configuration, and adjustment schedules vary somewhat for the different types of bands. They all work on the principle of restriction of oral intake by limiting the volume of the proximal stomach. The advantage over the traditional vertical banded gastroplasty is the adjustability.

Trocar placement for the AGB is shown in Figure 16-1. The surgeon stands to the patient's right, the assistant is to the patient's left, and the camera operator is adjacent to the surgeon. Most surgeons place the patient in the supine position, but some prefer to have the patient's legs spread, allowing the surgeon to stand between the legs. This is the so-called French position, described by Dubois[23] after the location of the surgeon in performing laparoscopic cholecystectomy. The trocars in Figure 16-1 are designed for the surgeon to be on the patient's right side.

The technique for AGB placement is described in detail by Fielding and Allen,[24] modified from the original laparoscopic approach of Belachew and coworkers,[25] who in turn used the technique as originally described using an open approach by Kuzmak.[26] The operation begins after pneumoperitoneum is obtained and trocars are placed. The left lobe of the liver is retracted. The peritoneum at the angle of His is divided, creating an opening in the peritoneum between the angle of His and the top of the spleen (Fig. 16-2A). The telescope is placed through the left upper quadrant port for this part of the operation, to maximally view the angle of His area.

The pars flaccida technique has become the approach of choice for placing the adjustable band. Placement of the band using this approach is preferred to the original description of placing the posterior aspect of the band into the free space of the lesser sac, high up on the posterior surface of the stomach.[27] Posterior placement of the band was associated with a high incidence of band slippage (13% in Zimmerman's series of 1090 patients[27]), which has decreased since adoption of the pars flaccida approach. The pars flaccida approach begins with dividing the gastrohepatic ligament in its thin area just over the caudate lobe of the liver. The anterior branch of the vagus is spared, and any aberrant left hepatic artery is preserved. The base of the right crus of the diaphragm is identified. Care must be taken that the crus is clearly identified, as occasionally the vena cava can lie close to the caudate lobe. There is almost always a fat pad lying directly on the base of the right crus. Division of the plane between the fat pad and the crus, on the medial side of the base of the crus, initiates the correct plane for band placement. The surgeon gently follows the surface of the right crus posterior and inferior to the esophagus, aiming for the angle of His (see Fig. 16-2B). A gentle spreading and pushing technique is used to create an avascular tunnel along this plane. Special tunneling devices designed for this part function well, but some surgeons use a grasping instrument. The distance of this tunnel is usually 3 to 4 cm. Once the tip of the tunneling instrument is seen near the top of the spleen, it is gently pushed through any

---

> **Box 16-5 Bariatric operations: mechanism of action**
>
> **Restrictive**
> Vertical banded gastroplasty (VBG) (historic purposes only)
> Adjustable gastric banding (AGB)
>
> **Largely Restrictive/Mildly Malabsorptive**
> Roux-en-Y gastric bypass (RYGB)
>
> **Largely Malabsorptive/Mildly Restrictive**
> Biliopancreatic diversion (BPD)
> Duodenal switch (DS)

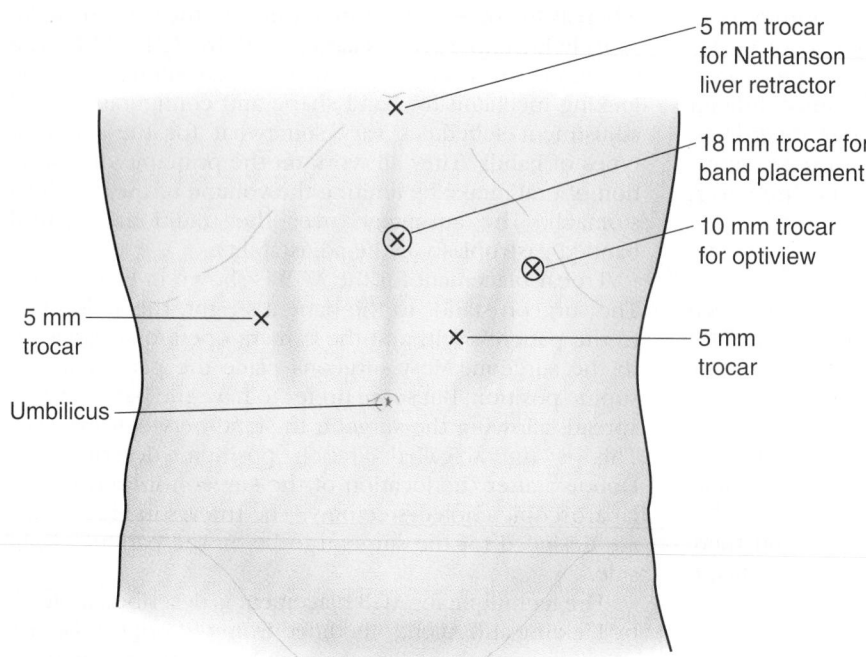

5 mm trocar
for Nathanson
liver retractor

18 mm trocar for
band placement

10 mm trocar
for optiview

5 mm
trocar

Umbilicus

5 mm
trocar

FIGURE 16-1.   Trocar location for adjustable gastric banding.

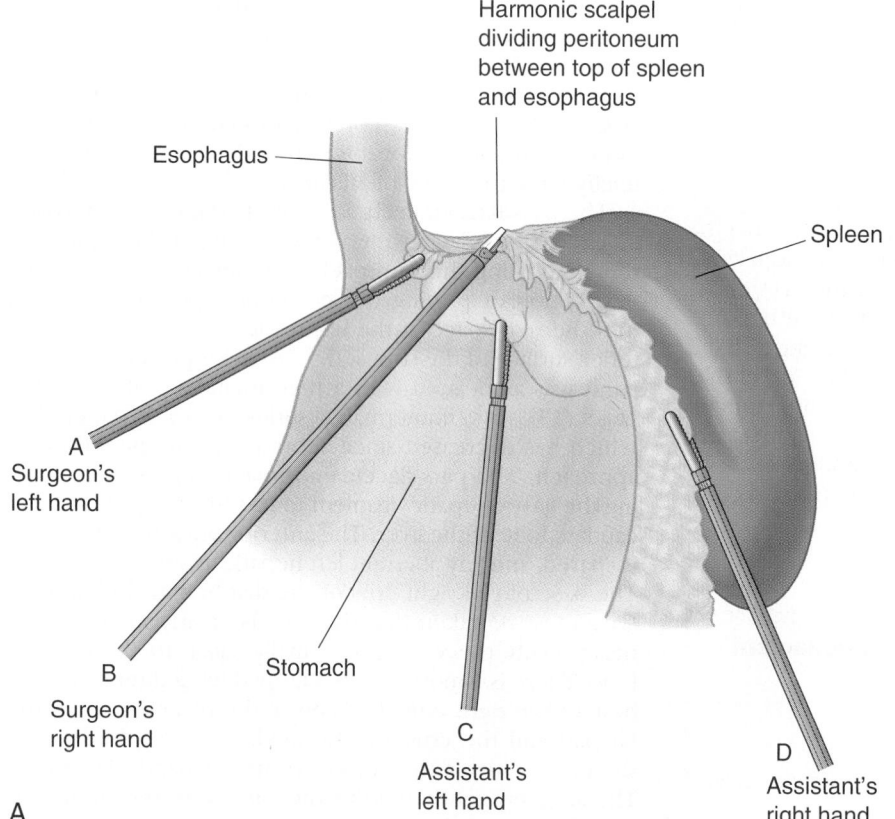

Harmonic scalpel
dividing peritoneum
between top of spleen
and esophagus

Esophagus

Spleen

A
Surgeon's
left hand

B
Surgeon's
right hand

Stomach

C
Assistant's
left hand

D
Assistant's
right hand

A

FIGURE 16-2.   **A,** Dividing the peritoneum at the angle of His.

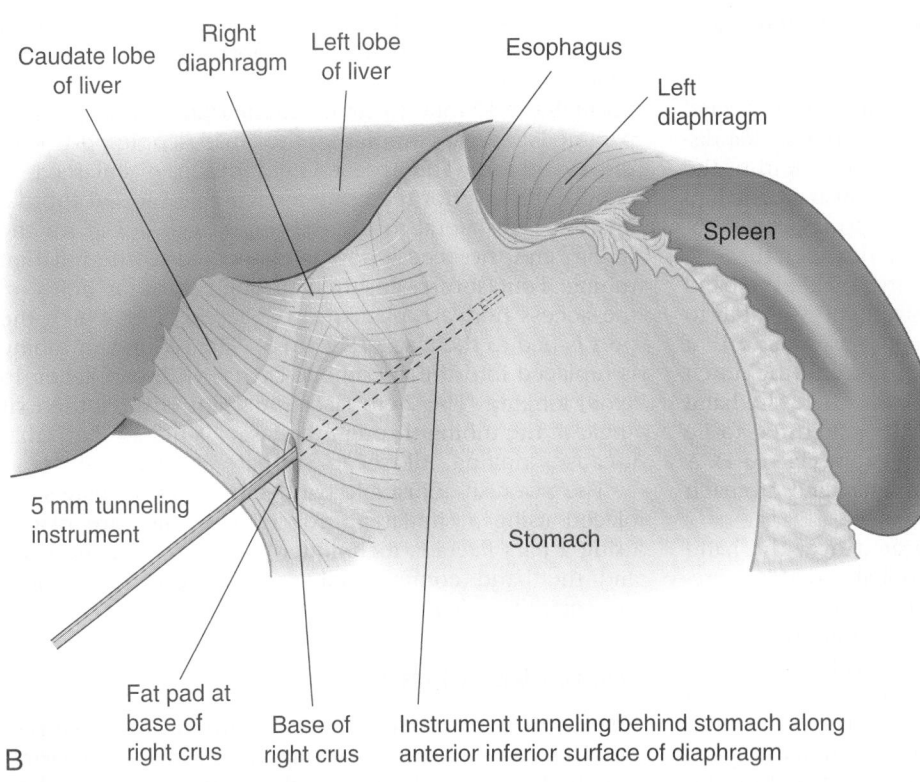

Caudate lobe of liver

Right diaphragm

Left lobe of liver

Esophagus

Left diaphragm

Spleen

Stomach

5 mm tunneling instrument

Fat pad at base of right crus

Base of right crus

Instrument tunneling behind stomach along anterior inferior surface of diaphragm

B

FIGURE 16-2—Cont'd **B,** Pars flaccida technique, dividing the fat pad at the base of the right crus. **C,** Tunnel posterior to stomach completed.

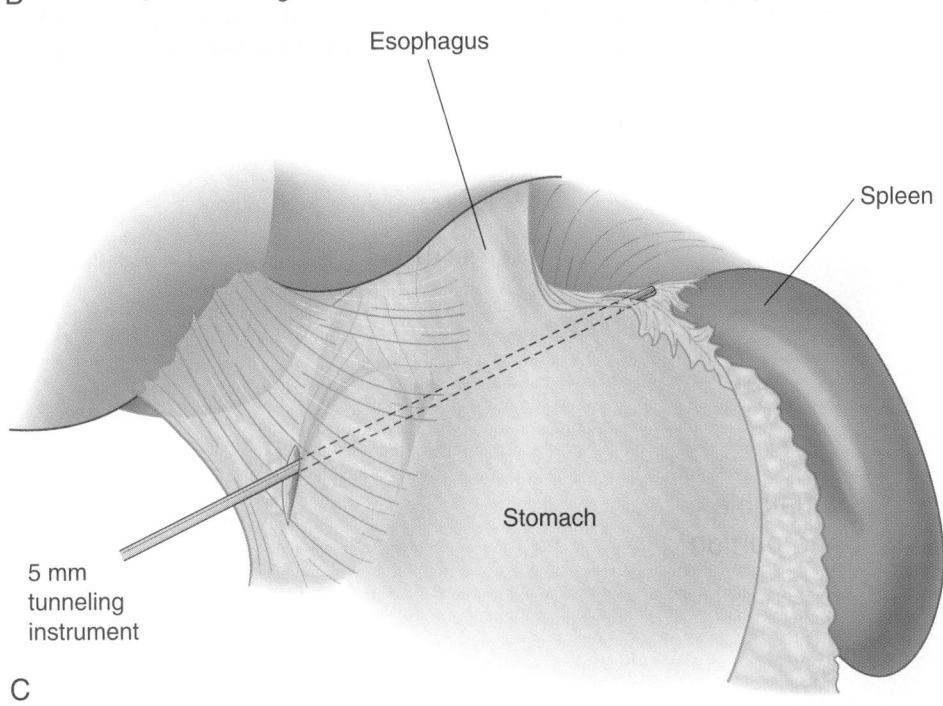

Esophagus

Spleen

Stomach

5 mm tunneling instrument

C

remaining peritoneal layers, completing the tunnel (see Fig. 16-2C).

The adjustable band has already been placed into the peritoneal cavity through the large 15-mm trocar located in the right upper quadrant, before the pars flaccida dissection. The band is not inflated. The narrow end of the band itself is grasped by the tunneling instrument and pulled through the tunnel, from greater to lesser side of the stomach (Fig. 16-3). That end is then threaded through the locking mechanism of the band, after which the band is locked. There is a specialized instrument available to lock the band, which some surgeons use instead of graspers. This instrument has a hook to fit into the notch of the band, facilitating locking the band. Once the band has been locked into place, the buckle is adjusted to lie on the lesser curvature side of the stomach (Fig. 16-4). A 5-mm grasper inserted between the band and stomach ensures the band is not too tight.

The anterior gastric wall is imbricated over the band with four interrupted sutures using nonabsorbable material (Fig. 16-5). There should be just enough stomach above the level of the band for incorporating that tissue into the suture. Suturing is performed with the camera in the umbilical or left upper quadrant port. Suturing is carried as far posterolateral as possible; this has been the most frequent area of fundus herniation through the band. The band ideally is thus secured about 1 cm below the gastroesophageal junction using this technique.

The final steps of the operation involve placement of the adjustable subcutaneous port used to inflate the band. The Silastic tubing leading from the band is pulled through the 15-mm trocar site in the right upper quadrant paramedian area, completing the laparoscopic portion of the operation. The trocar site incision is enlarged to expose the anterior rectus fascia, which is incised approximately 2 cm lateral to the existing fascial defect for the trocar, and the access port is connected to the inflation tubing. Four sutures inserted through the four holes on the access port are placed in the fascia after which the port is tied to the fascia (Fig. 16-6). The redundant tubing is replaced into the abdominal cavity, with care taken to avoid kinking. The 2-cm fascial incision ensures the exit angle of the tubing through the fascia is not so sharp that it causes kinking. All trocars sites are closed.

The Swedish adjustable band and the other bands are placed using a similar approach. They also are placed using a pars flaccida technique. The locking of the band and the band configurations are the only differences between these bands.

Roux-en-Y Gastric Bypass

The gastric bypass first described by Ito[28] in 1969 incorporated a loop of jejunum anastomosed to a proximal gastric pouch. This proved unacceptable, owing to bile reflux. Griffen and colleagues,[29] among others, popularized the

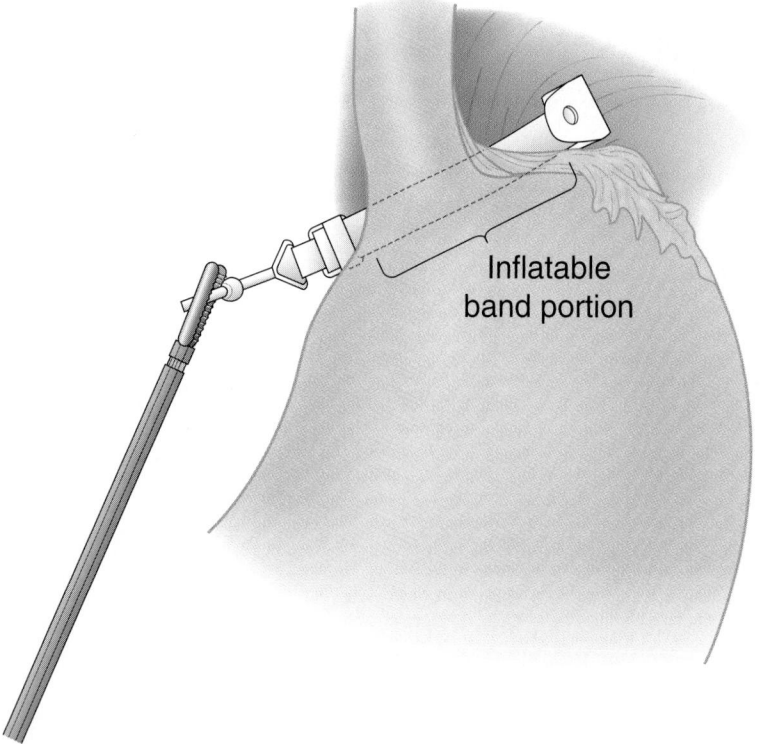

FIGURE 16-3. Pulling lap band through the tunnel.

Inflatable band portion

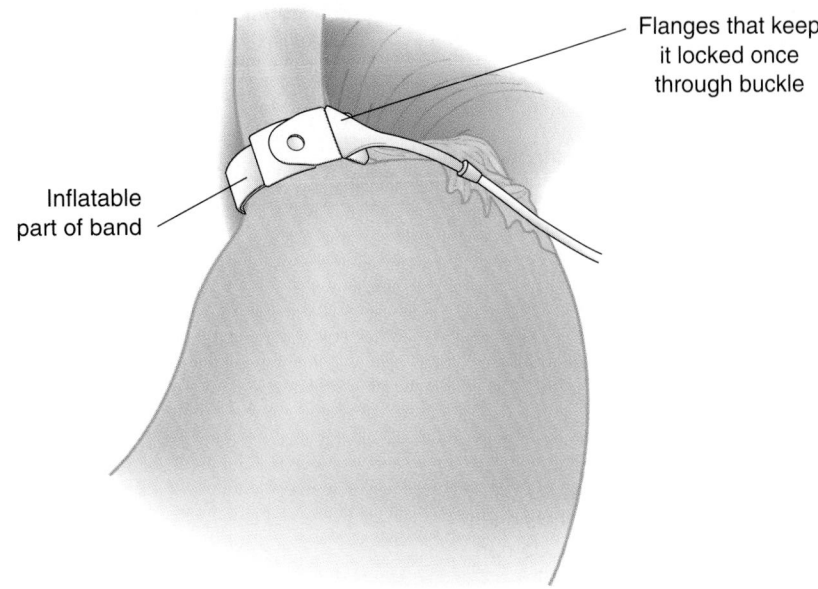

Flanges that keep
it locked once
through buckle

Inflatable
part of band

FIGURE 16-4.   Locking the band.

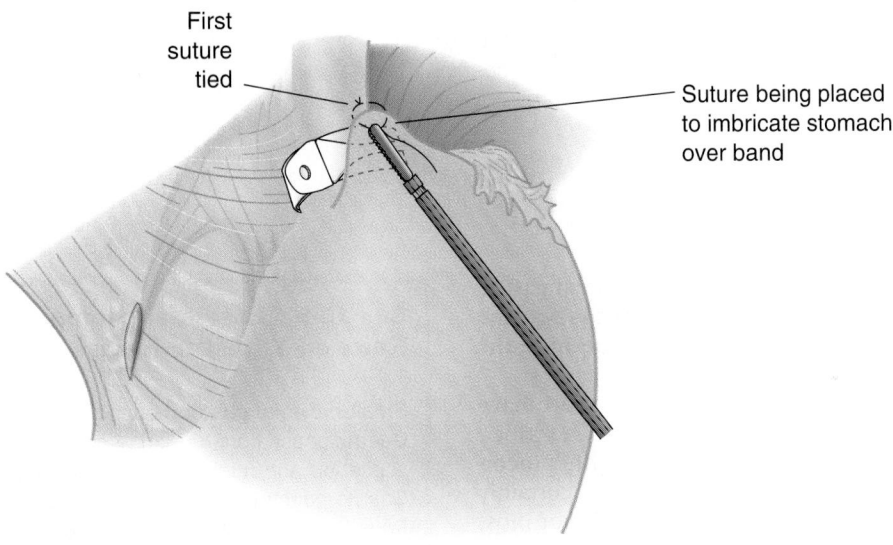

First
suture
tied

Suture being placed
to imbricate stomach
over band

FIGURE 16-5.   Imbricating the anterior stomach over the band.

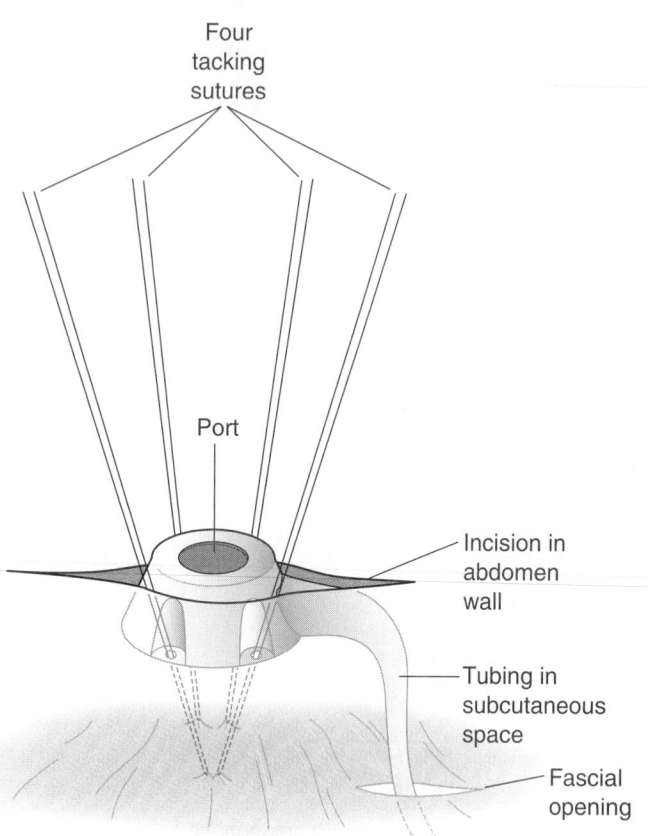

Four
tacking
sutures

Port

Incision in
abdomen
wall

Tubing in
subcutaneous
space

Fascial
opening

FIGURE 16-6.   Passing the inflation tubing through the abdominal wall adequately far from the port site to prevent acute kinking of the tubing.

use of the Roux limb as drainage for the proximal gastric pouch. The Roux-en-Y gastric bypass (RYGB) has become the most commonly performed bariatric operation in the United States.

Adjustments and modifications of the procedure have been made based on experience and results. Described here is the technique used at my institution, which incorporates many of those modifications. There are certainly many variations on this technique, and many if not most of these will give excellent results.[30-33] However, there seem to be certain essential principles of the operation. These are listed in Box 16-6.

The laparoscopic approach to RYGB begins with creation of a pneumoperitoneum. My colleagues and I have found the use of the left subcostal region, near the midclavicular line, to be an ideal place for retraction of the fascia with a tracheostomy hook and use of a Veress needle to create the pneumoperitoneum. The first trocar is placed there; a 45-degree telescope performs peritoneoscopy. Subsequent trocars are placed under laparoscopic vision to achieve the configuration shown in Figure 16-7. Any intra-abdominal adhesions preventing mobilization of the omentum or visualization of the upper abdominal organs must be divided as the trocars are being placed.

Once the omentum is mobilized, the ligament of Treitz is identified. A location approximately 40 cm distal to the ligament is chosen for division of the jejunum. This area

---

Box 16-6   Essential components of the Roux-en-Y gastric bypass

Small proximal gastric pouch
Gastric pouch constructed of cardia of stomach to prevent dilation and minimize acid production
Gastric pouch divided from distal stomach
Roux limb at least 75 cm in length
Enteroenterostomy constructed to avoid stenosis or obstruction
Closure of all potential spaces for internal hernias

---

of jejunum is more mobile than the more proximal jejunum. The bowel is divided with the stapler, using a vascular load. The mesentery is then further divided with staples or the harmonic scalpel. If the stapler is used, the presence of pulses to the bowel on each side of the stapler jaws is confirmed before firing (Fig. 16-8). Otherwise, ischemia to one of the bowel segments may result. The proximal end of the Roux limb is now marked by suturing a small (1/4 inch) Penrose drain to it.

The length of Roux limb is now measured. This length is arbitrary but influenced in my practice by patient weight. Patients with a BMI in the 40s will be well served

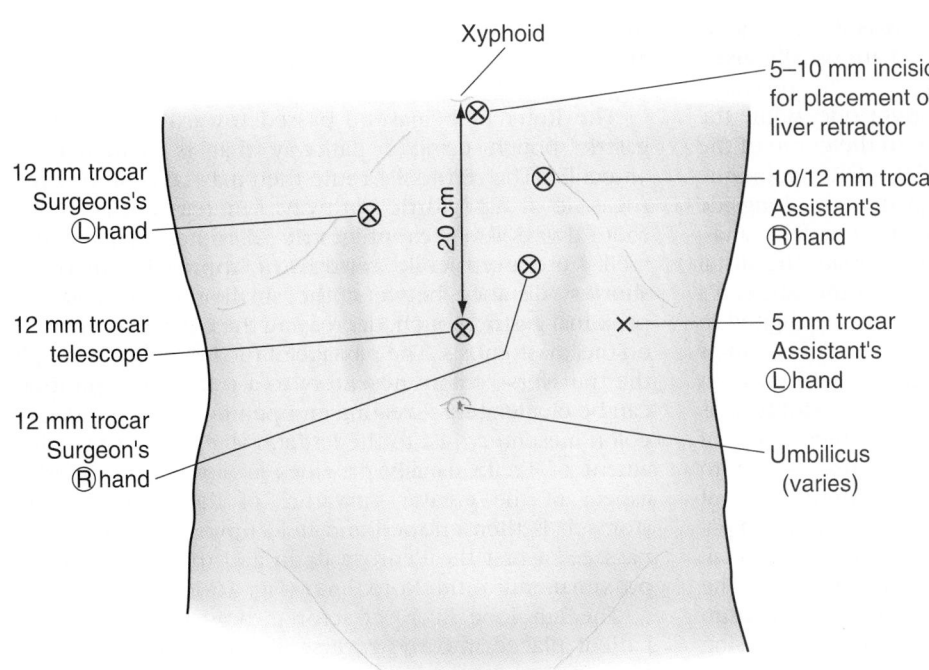

FIGURE 16-7. Trocar configuration for laparoscopic Roux-en-Y gastric bypass.

Xyphoid

5–10 mm incision for placement of liver retractor

12 mm trocar Surgeons's Ⓛ hand

10/12 mm trocar Assistant's Ⓡ hand

20 cm

12 mm trocar telescope

5 mm trocar Assistant's Ⓛ hand

12 mm trocar Surgeon's Ⓡ hand

Umbilicus (varies)

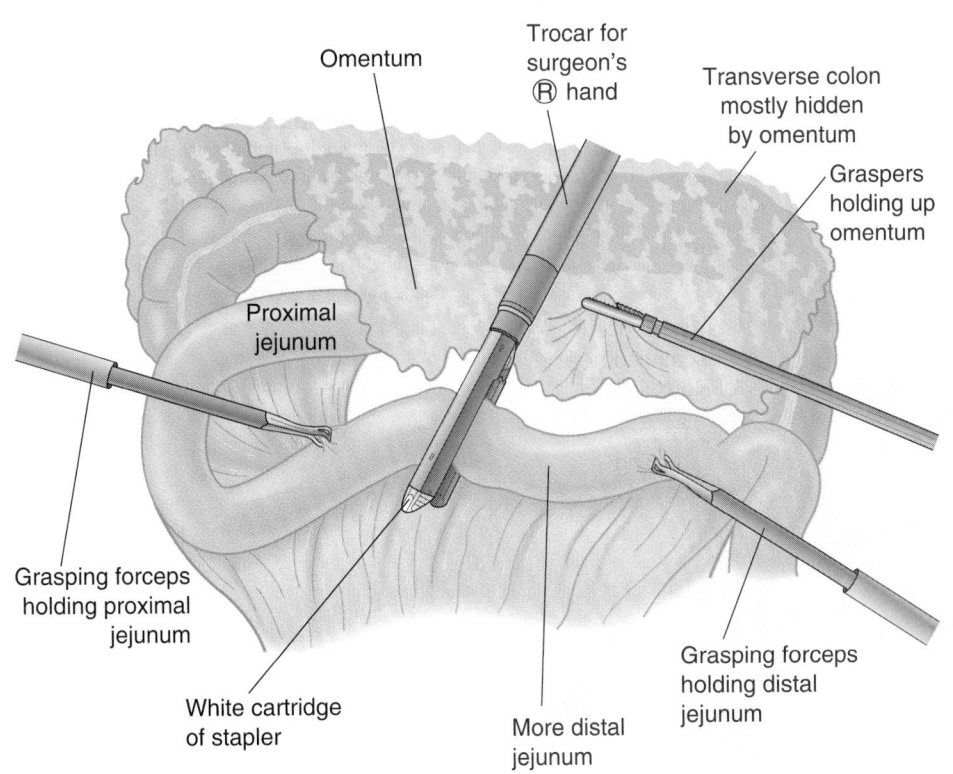

FIGURE 16-8. Placing stapler to divide jejunum to create Roux limb.

Omentum

Trocar for surgeon's Ⓡ hand

Transverse colon mostly hidden by omentum

Graspers holding up omentum

Proximal jejunum

Grasping forceps holding proximal jejunum

White cartridge of stapler

More distal jejunum

Grasping forceps holding distal jejunum

with a Roux limb of 80 to 120 cm, whereas those patients with a BMI significantly in excess of 50 are usually given a Roux limb of approximately 150 cm.[34] The proximal jejunum is left to lay to the patient's right side, while the Roux limb is lifted cephalad, coiling it in the curve of the transverse colon mesentery (Fig. 16-9). This technique allows the proximal jejunum to align directly alongside the designated point on the Roux limb for the distal anastomosis. The vascular stapler is used to create the distal anastomosis. The stapler is placed through the surgeon's left hand port, as the bowel segments are easily aligned to facilitate placement of the stapler into enterotomies created in each segment of bowel at the desired location of the anastomosis (Fig. 16-10). Once the anastomosis is created, the stapler defect is closed by a single layer of suture. I have found that stapling will predispose to obstruction or stenosis. Suturing from the inferior edge of the stapler defect to the superior edge facilitates exposure. The mesenteric defect between the loops of small bowel is now closed with running permanent suture. The defect is easily exposed by retracting the omentum toward the patient's right upper quadrant, exposing the base of the mesentery, and retracting the distal end of the proximal jejunum toward the patient's left side, putting tension on and displaying the mesentery. Its lower edge, stapled previously from the mesenteric division, is sutured to the mesentery directly beneath it, with the suture line being carried up to and includ-ing the bowel, aligning the bowel just distal to the anastomosis to prevent kinking of the distal limb (Fig. 16-11).[35]

The Roux limb may be passed toward the proximal gastric pouch using a pathway that is retrocolic or antecolic. The retrocolic route then may take either a retrogastric or antegastric pathway, whereas the antecolic route always also goes antegastric. All routes seem to work well. I use a retrocolic, retrogastric approach; this is the shortest distance between the small intestine and the proximal gastric pouch, decreasing the chance for tension on the anastomosis. The passage of the Roux limb through the transverse colon mesentery to a retrogastric position can be challenging. Creating an opening in the transverse colon mesentery just to the left and slightly above the ligament of Treitz usually provides a view of the inferior aspect of the greater curvature of the stomach. The stomach is then grasped and held upward, allowing the passage of first the Penrose drain and then the attached proximal end of the Roux limb (Fig. 16-12).

The left lobe liver retractor is now placed and the patient placed into the reverse Trendelenburg position. Exposure of the angle of His allows division of the peritoneum between the top of the spleen and the gastroesophageal junction using the ultrasonic scalpel. The lesser sac is entered through the gastrohepatic ligament, 2 cm below the gastroesophageal junction, and dissection is carried out with the ultrasonic scalpel. The blue load of

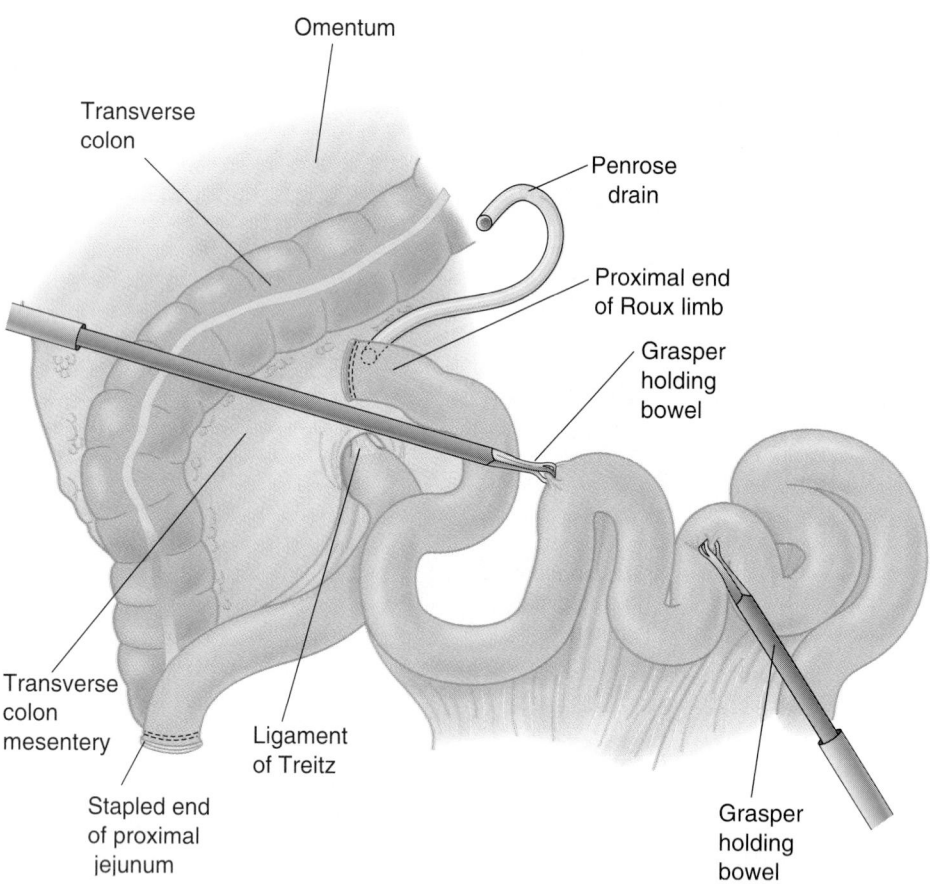

FIGURE 16-9. Measuring and laying out jejunum to set up distal anastomosis for length of Roux-en-Y gastric bypass.

Omentum

Transverse colon

Penrose drain

Proximal end of Roux limb

Grasper holding bowel

Transverse colon mesentery

Ligament of Treitz

Stapled end of proximal jejunum

Grasper holding bowel

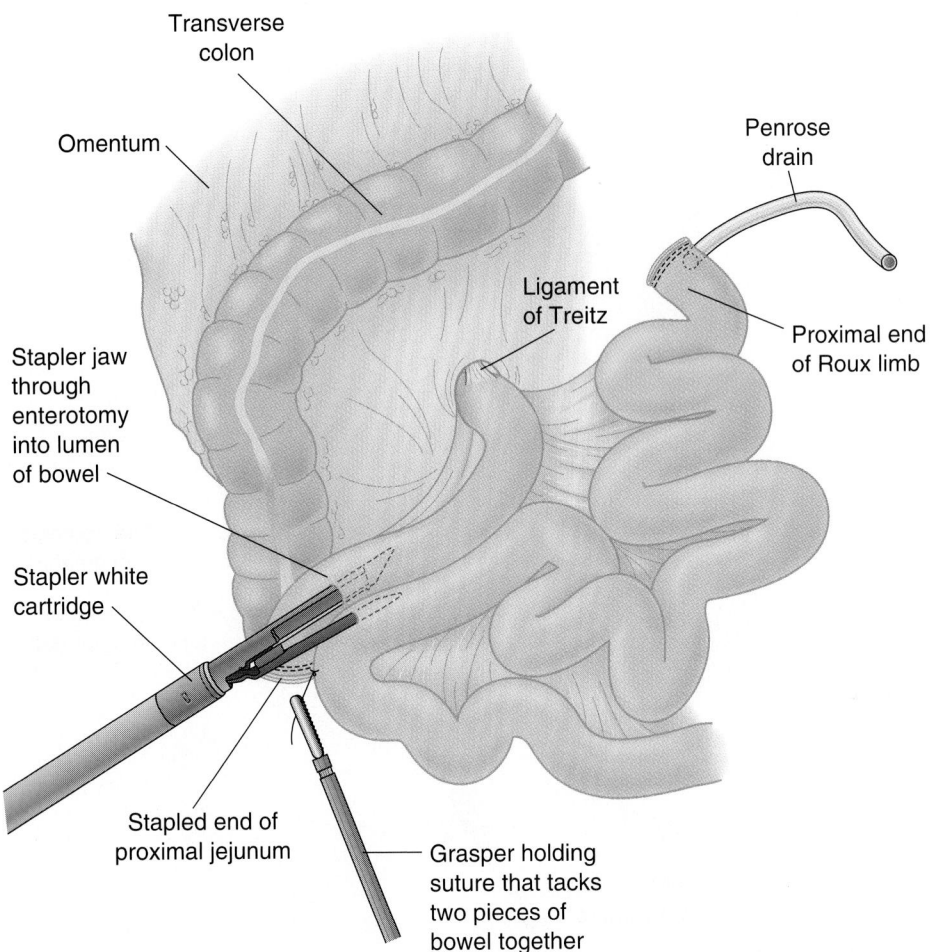

FIGURE 16-10.   Placing stapler to create enteroenterostomy.

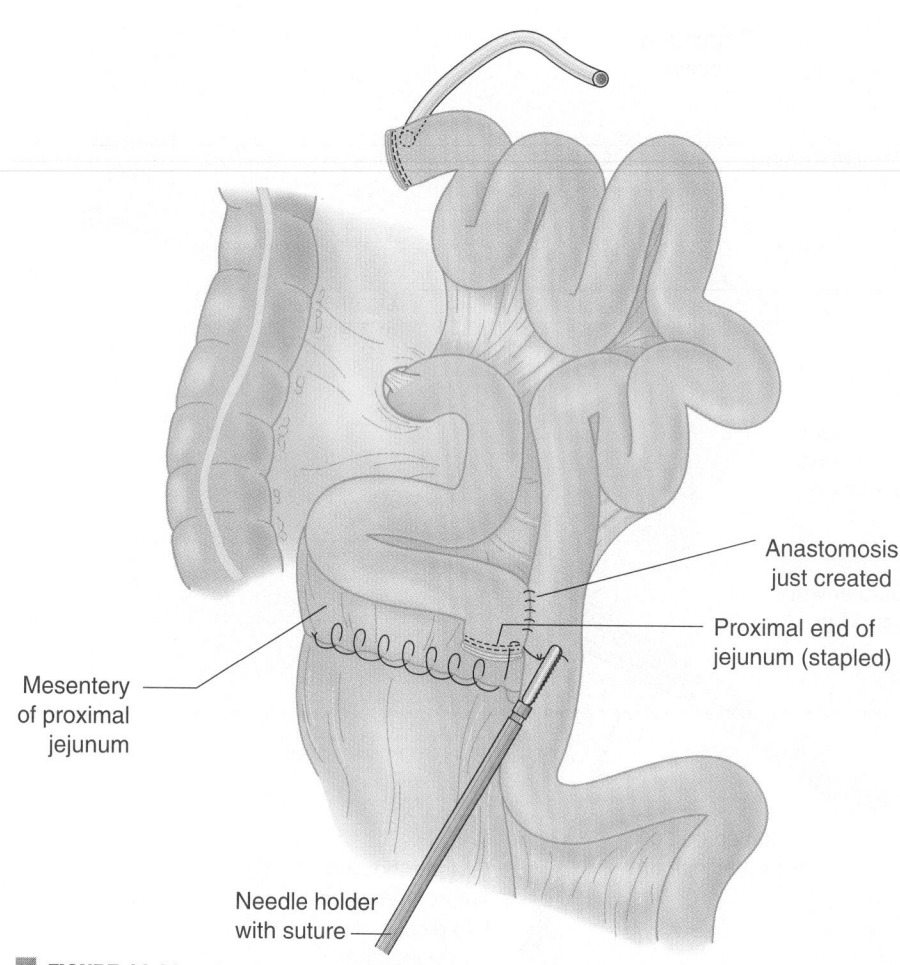

Anastomosis
just created

Proximal end of
jejunum (stapled)

Mesentery
of proximal
jejunum

Needle holder
with suture

FIGURE 16-11. Sewing mesenteric defect and placing anti-obstruction stitch.

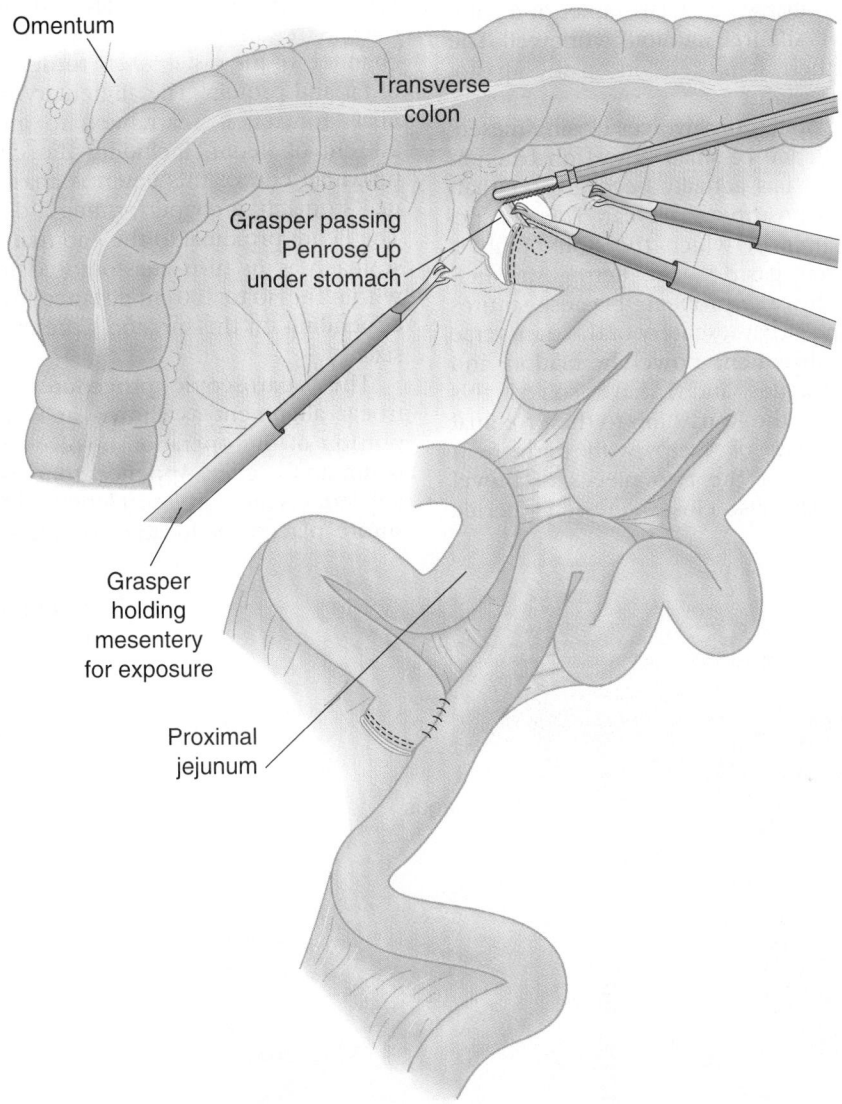

Omentum

Transverse
colon

Grasper passing
Penrose up
under stomach

Grasper
holding
mesentery
for exposure

Proximal
jejunum

FIGURE 16-12.   Passing the Roux limb into a retrocolic and retrogastric position.

the linear stapler is now fired multiple times to create a proximal gastric pouch of 10 to 15 mL, based on the upper lesser curvature of the stomach (Fig. 16-13). The final firing of the stapler is done using the divided area of peritoneum at the angle of His to facilitate stapler passage. Once the gastric pouch is created, the drain is used to help pass the Roux limb into a position adjacent to the proximal gastric pouch. The blue load of the linear stapler is then used to create the proximal anastomosis (Fig. 16-14). The stapler defect is closed, and methylene blue dye is used to check for leaks. Alternatively, the gastrojejunostomy may be performed using a circular stapler or a hand sutured technique.[30-33, 36] All three methods work well. The surgeon must ensure there is no tension on the anastomosis and that it is watertight.

The final step of the operation involves closing mesenteric defects. The incidence of small bowel obstruction after laparoscopic RYGB has actually been greater than open RYGB for the first postoperative year. This is especially true for procedures in which the Roux limb is passed in a retrocolic, retrogastric plane. Retrogastric herniation of the Roux limb was a problem, because sutures often pulled through the fatty mesentery of the transverse colon, allowing the subsequent bowel herniation and obstruction.[37] My colleagues and I have solved this problem through suturing the Roux limb to the proximal jejunum near the ligament of Treitz with permanent sutures to fix a segment of the two pieces of bowel together[38] (Fig. 16-15). This also closes Petersen's hernia defect.

Biliopancreatic Diversion

Biliopancreatic diversion (BPD) was first described and popularized by Scopinaro and colleagues.[39] The operation, like most bariatric operations that had been done using an open approach, is now done using a laparoscopic approach.[40] The BPD is based on largely malabsorption to produce weight loss but does have a mild restrictive component.

The anatomic configuration of the BPD is shown in Figure 16-16. The operation serves to promote malabsorption, particularly of fat and protein. The intestinal tract is reconstructed to allow only a short "common channel" of the distal 50-cm terminal ileum for absorption of fat and protein. The alimentary tract beyond the proximal stomach is rearranged to include only the distal 200 cm of ileum, including the common channel. The proximal end of this ileum is anastomosed to the proximal stomach, after performing a distal hemigastrectomy. The ileum proximal to the end that is anastomosed to the stomach is in turn anastomosed to the terminal ileum within the 50 to 100 cm distance from the ileocecal valve, depending on the surgeon's preference and the patient's size.

The laparoscopic procedure is performed using a trocar alignment as shown in Figure 16-17. The initial portion of the operation involves exposing the terminal ileum and cecum. Appendectomy is optional. The terminal ileum is measured to a length of 50 cm, with a marking suture placed for location of anastomosis. After placing

FIGURE 16-13. Firing the stapler to create the proximal gastric pouch.

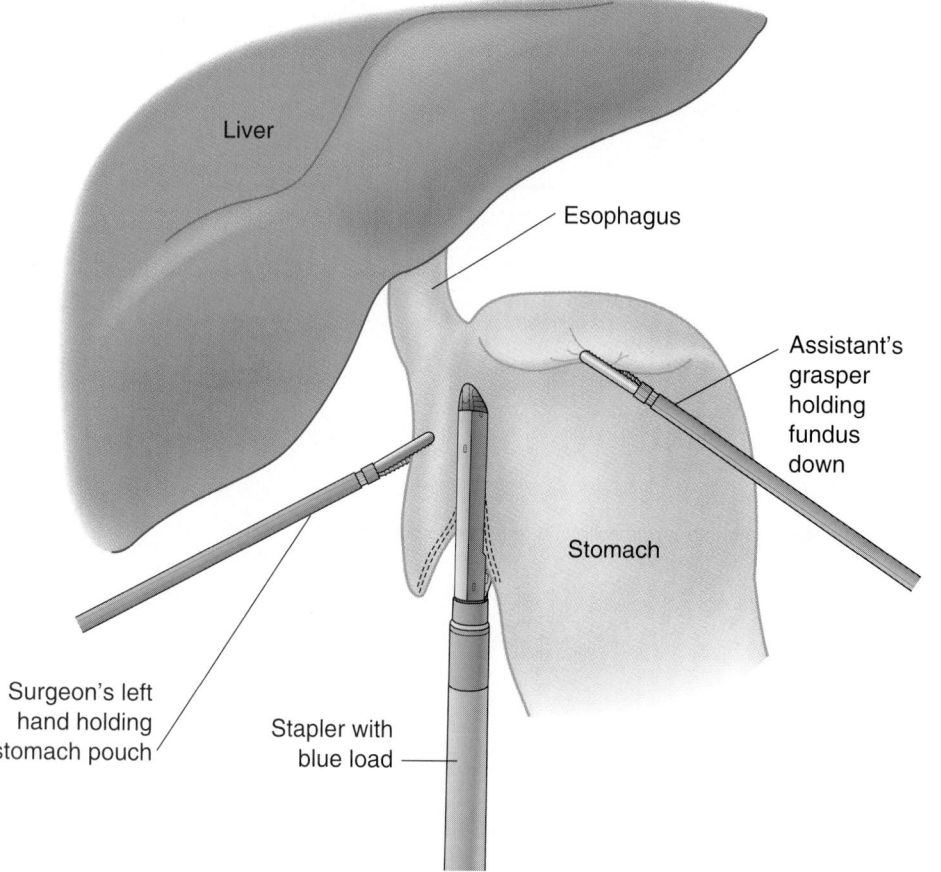

Liver

Esophagus

Assistant's grasper holding fundus down

Stomach

Surgeon's left hand holding stomach pouch

Stapler with blue load

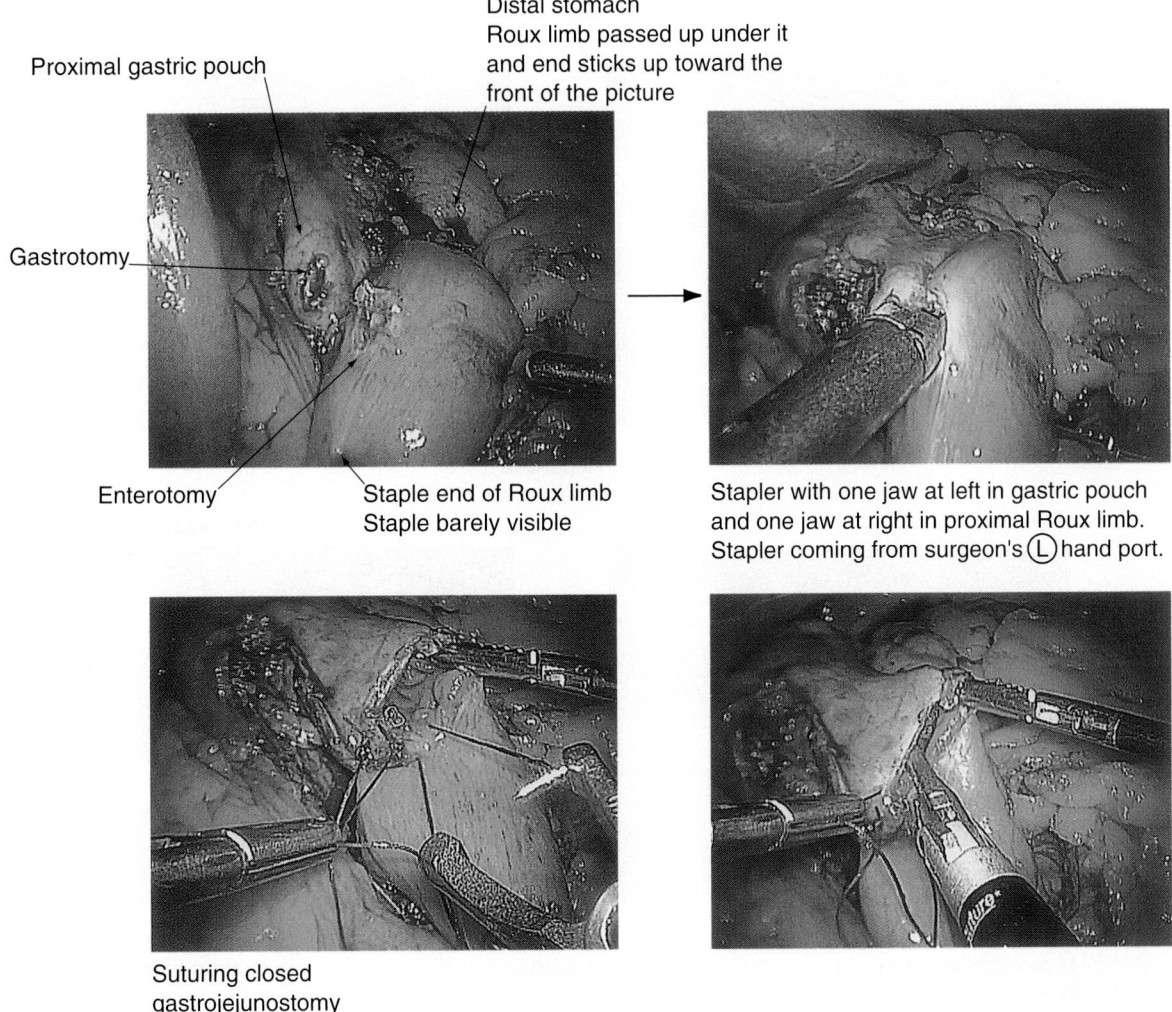

Proximal gastric pouch

Distal stomach
Roux limb passed up under it
and end sticks up toward the
front of the picture

Gastrotomy

Enterotomy

Staple end of Roux limb
Staple barely visible

Stapler with one jaw at left in gastric pouch
and one jaw at right in proximal Roux limb.
Stapler coming from surgeon's Ⓛ hand port.

Suturing closed
gastrojejunostomy
Stapler defect

FIGURE 16-14. Creating the proximal anastomosis.

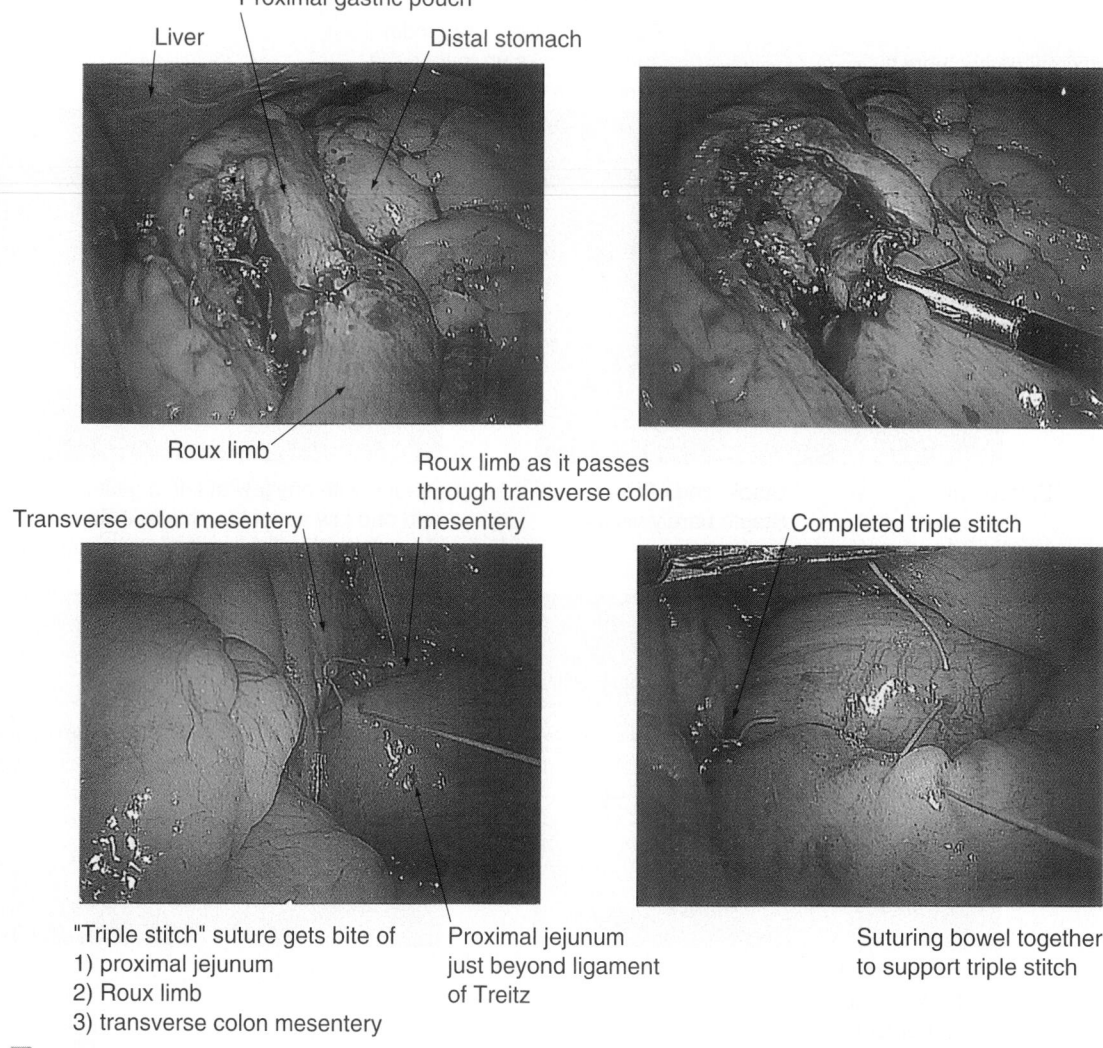

Liver

Proximal gastric pouch

Distal stomach

Roux limb

Transverse colon mesentery

Roux limb as it passes
through transverse colon
mesentery

Completed triple stitch

"Triple stitch" suture gets bite of
1) proximal jejunum
2) Roux limb
3) transverse colon mesentery

Proximal jejunum
just beyond ligament
of Treitz

Suturing bowel together
to support triple stitch

FIGURE 16-15.   Placing the "triple stitch" to close mesenteric defects.

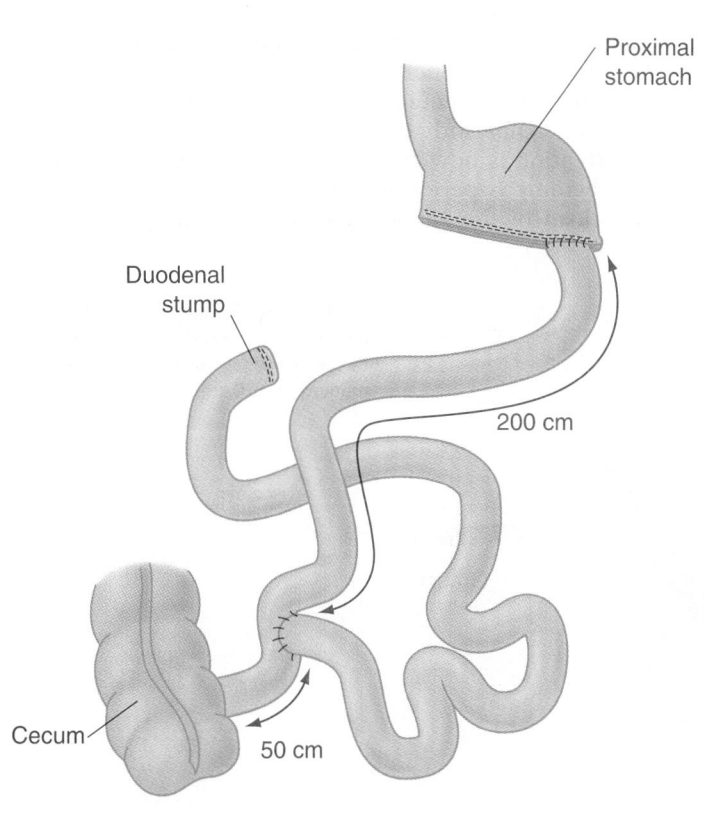

Proximal
stomach

FIGURE 16-16. Anatomic configuration of the biliopancreatic diversion.

Duodenal
stump

200 cm

Cecum

50 cm

Alimentary channel = 250 (± 50) cm
Common channel = 50 cm

Biliopancreatic diversion (BPD)

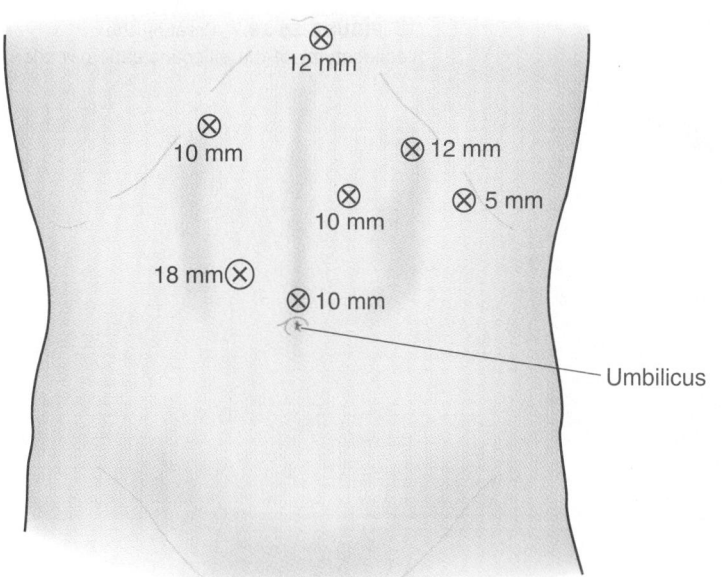

FIGURE 16-17. Location of trocars for performing laparoscopic biliopancreatic diversion.

12 mm

10 mm

12 mm

10 mm

5 mm

18 mm

10 mm

Umbilicus

the marking suture, a total length of 200 cm of ileum is measured and at this point the ileum is divided with the vascular staple load (Fig. 16-18). The proximal end of the bowel is then anastomosed to the terminal ileum at the site of the marking suture. This is done with a standard linear stapling technique, closing the stapler and mesenteric defects with sutures (Fig. 16-19). The alimen-

tary tract limb can be lengthened beyond 200 cm in total length if there is concern the patient may not eat a protein-rich diet. A maximum length of 300 cm has been used without significantly compromising weight loss.[41]

Attention is now turned toward the stomach. A distal gastrectomy is performed with serial applications of the blue load of the stapler (Fig. 16-20). The duodenum is

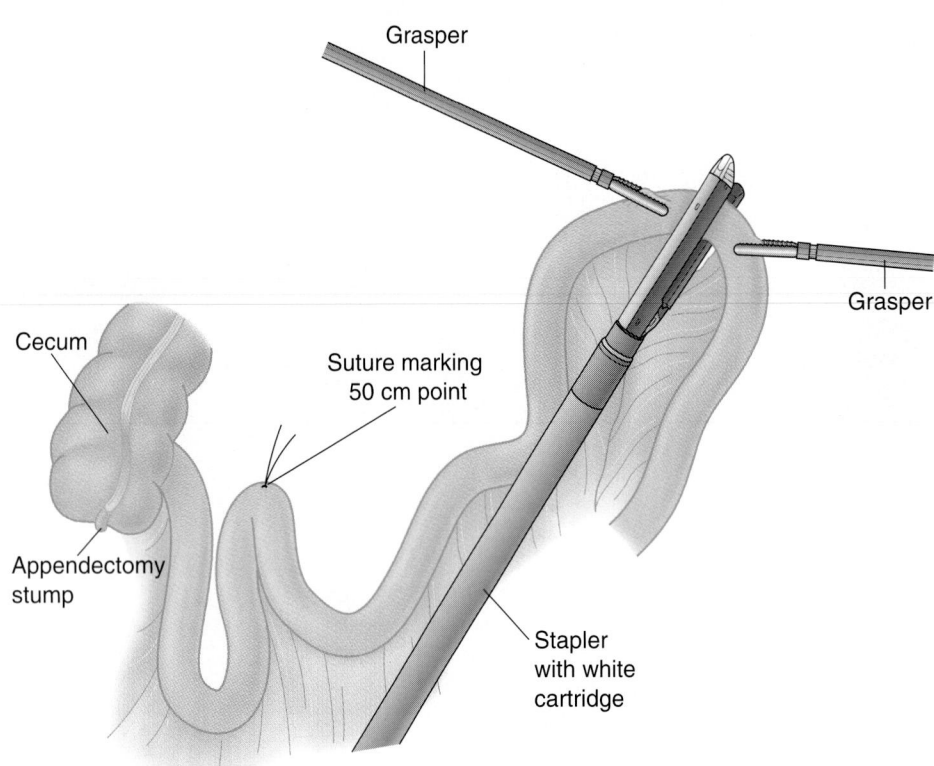

FIGURE 16-18. Dividing the ileum at the 200-cm location proximal to the ileocecal valve, having already marked the 50-cm location.

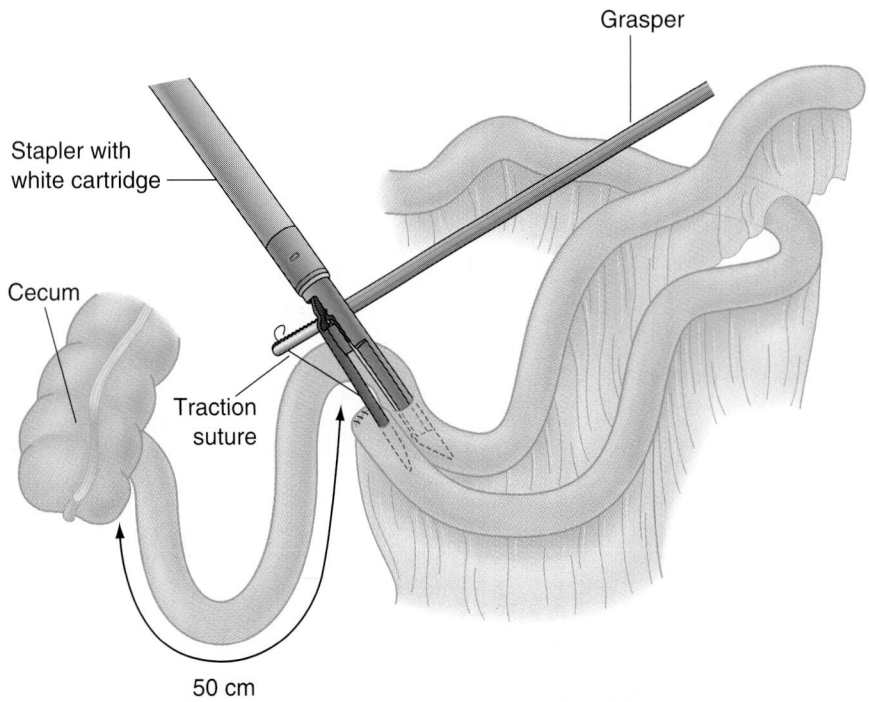

FIGURE 16-19. Creating the ileoileostomy of the biliopancreatic diversion.

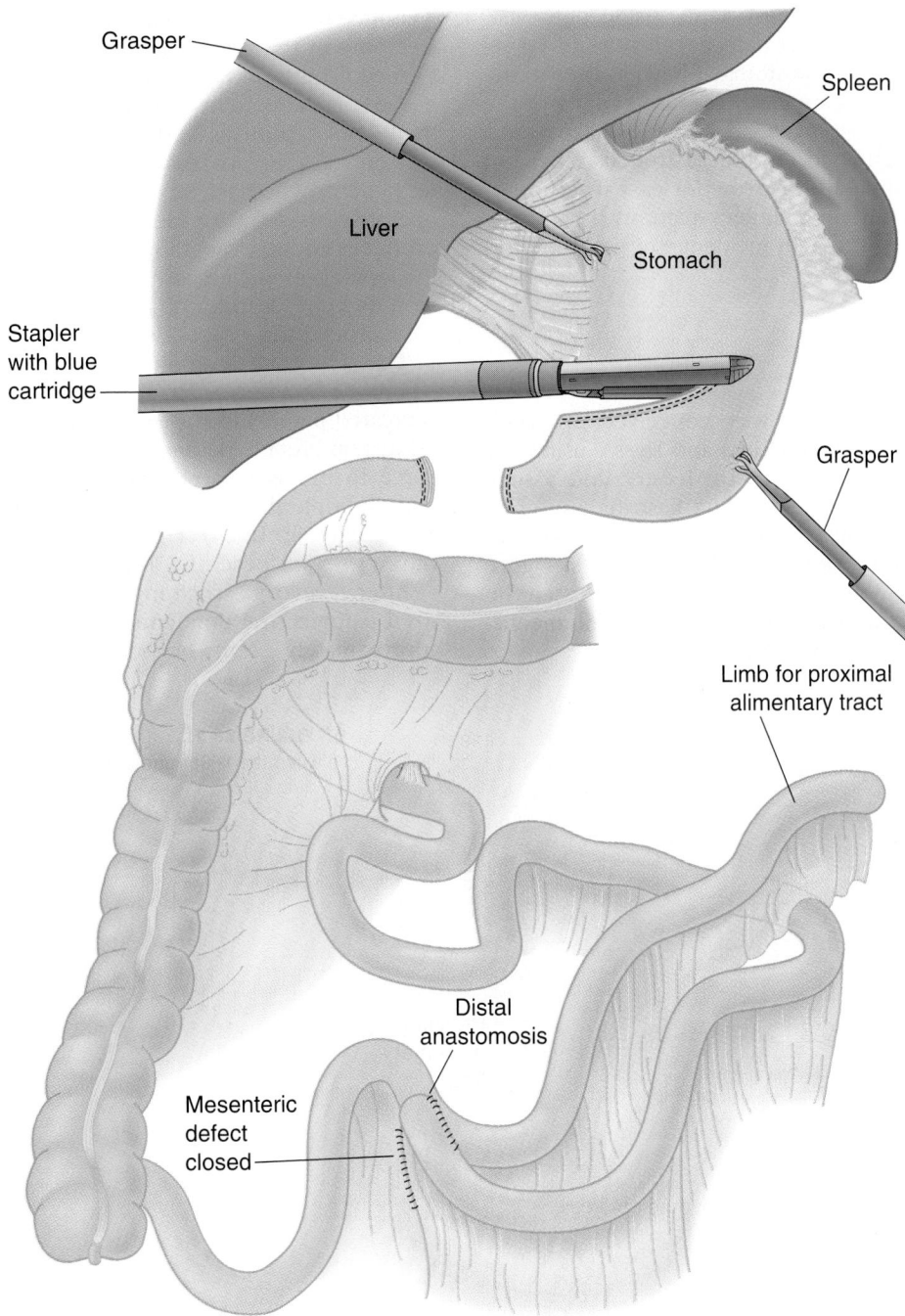

FIGURE 16-20. Performing the distal gastrectomy.

stapled and divided distal to the pylorus. Gastric volume may be tailored to the patient's degree of obesity, with larger volumes of 250 mL being created for patients with a BMI less than 50 kg/m^2 and smaller size pouches to a lower limit of 150 cm for patients with a BMI greater than 50 kg/m^2. The proximal end of the 200-cm length of terminal ileum is anastomosed to the posterior surface of the proximal stomach with the linear stapler using a blue cartridge (Fig. 16-21). The stapler defect is closed and bowel secured to the surface of the stomach beyond the anastomosis with an anchoring suture to prevent kinking of the bowel at the gastroileostomy. Some surgeons have used a circular stapling technique for the gastroileostomy, but the ileal lumen is often a bit narrow for easy insertion of the circular stapler device. A cholecystectomy is routinely performed, owing to the high incidence of gallstone formation after this operation.

Duodenal Switch

The duodenal switch (DS) was conceived by both Marceau and colleagues[42] and Hess and Hess[43] using the concept originally proposed by DeMeester and associates[44] for the treatment of bile reflux gastritis and combining it with the BPD concept of Scopinaro and coworkers. The configuration of a DS is shown in Figure 16-22. This modification was developed to help lessen the high incidence of marginal ulcers after BPD. The mechanism of weight loss is similar to that of a BPD.

Trocar locations for performing the operation laparoscopically are shown in Figure 16-17, as described by Ren and associates.[45] An appendectomy is followed by measurement of the terminal ileum. In the DS, however, the common channel is 100 cm and the entire alimentary tract is 250 cm. The major difference between the DS and the BPD, however, is the gastrectomy and the proximal anatomy. Instead of a distal hemigastrectomy, a sleeve gastrectomy of the greater curvature of the stomach is performed. This is done as the initial part of the operation, because if the patient exhibits any intraoperative instability the operation can be discontinued after the sleeve gastrectomy alone. A two-stage DS has been used by Gagner for patients who have an extremely high BMI and are high operative risks.[46] The sleeve gastrectomy alone usually produces enough weight loss to make the second stage of the operation technically easier. This approach lowers mortality rate despite the patient's undergoing two operative procedures.

The sleeve gastrectomy is performed using a stapling technique that begins at the mid antrum, and a staple line is created parallel to the lesser curvature of the stomach, using a 60 French Maloney dilator placed along the lesser curve to prevent narrowing. The staple line is created with multiple firings of the stapler until the angle of His is reached (Fig. 16-23). The goal is to produce a lesser curvature gastric sleeve of 150 to 200 mL in volume.

After sleeve gastrectomy, or preceding it in smaller sized patients, the duodenum is divided with the stapler approximately 2 cm beyond the pylorus. The distal

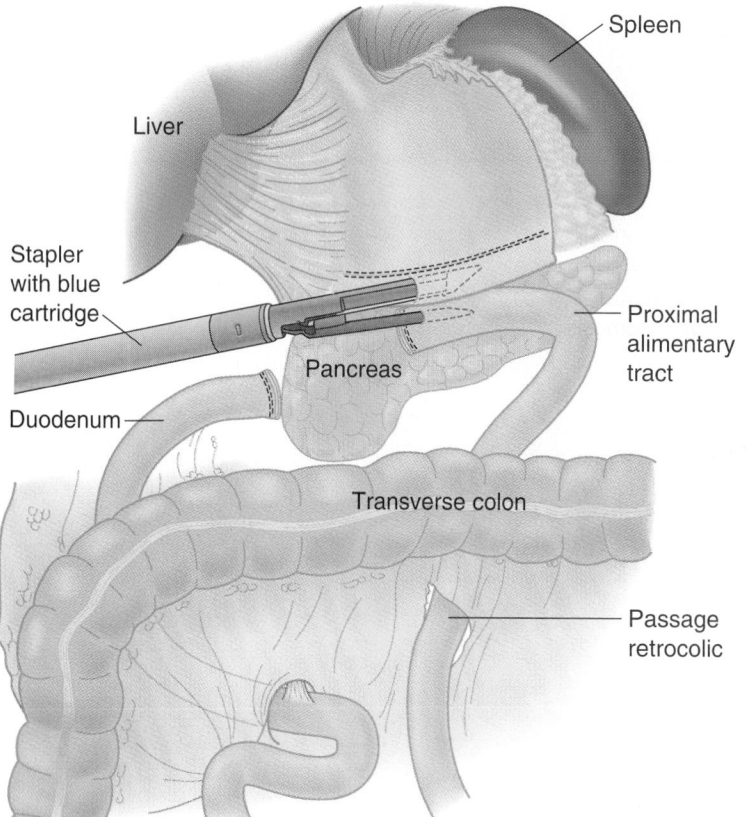

Liver

Spleen

Stapler with blue cartridge

Pancreas

Proximal alimentary tract

Duodenum

Transverse colon

Passage retrocolic

FIGURE 16-21. Creation of the gastrojejunostomy between the ileum and proximal stomach.

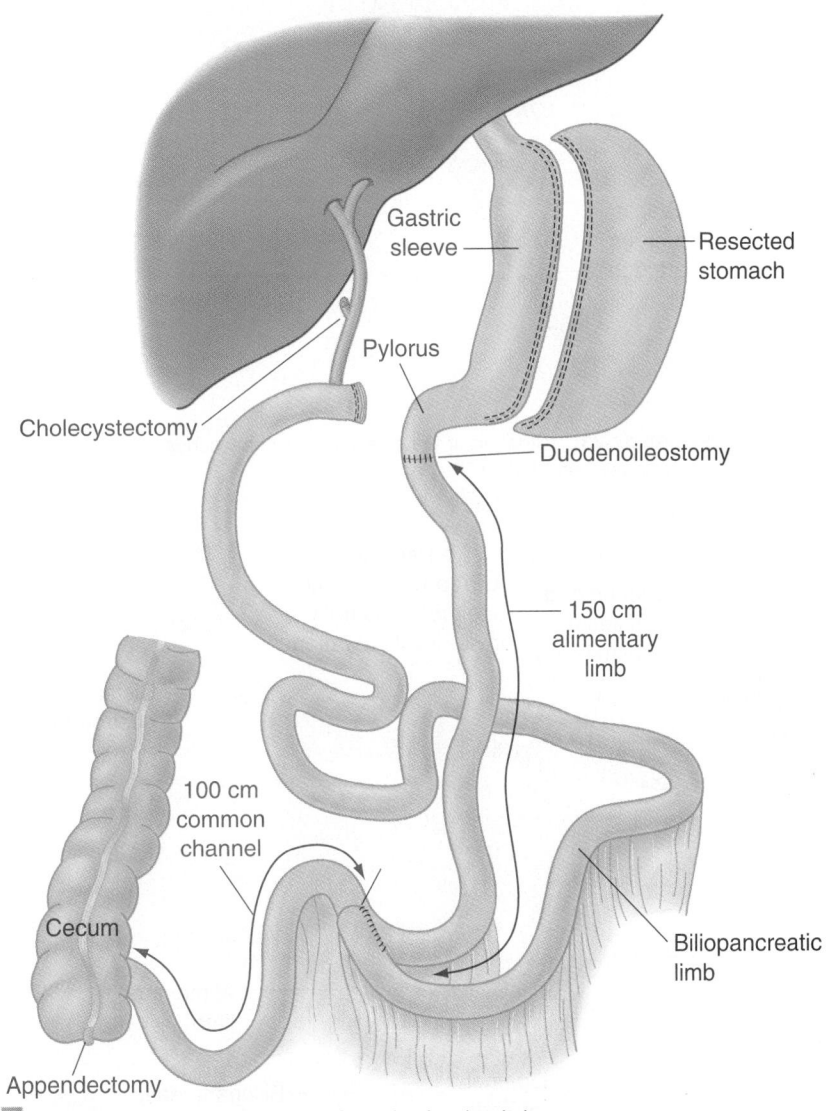

Gastric sleeve

Resected stomach

Pylorus

Cholecystectomy

Duodenoileostomy

150 cm alimentary limb

100 cm common channel

Cecum

Biliopancreatic limb

Appendectomy

FIGURE 16-22. Configuration of the duodenal switch.

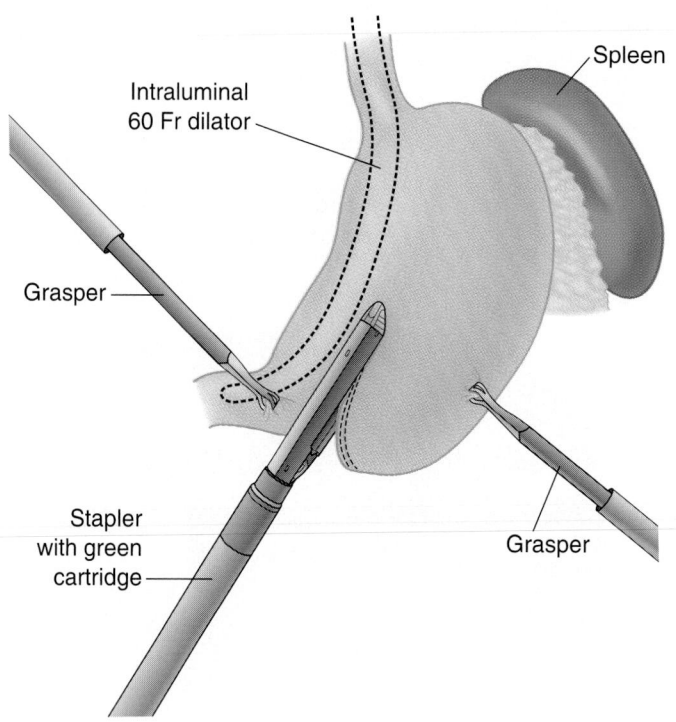

FIGURE 16-23. Creation of the sleeve gastrectomy during laparoscopic duodenal switch.

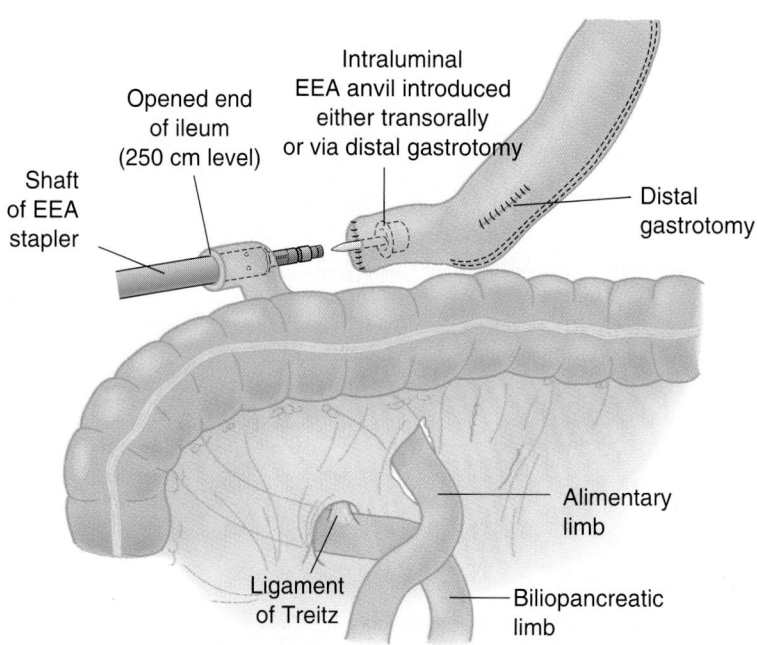

FIGURE 16-24. Creation of the duodenoenterostomy.

connections are performed as in BPD. The distal anastomosis is created at the 100-cm point proximal to the ileocecal valve. The proximal anastomosis is created between the proximal end of the 250-cm of terminal ileum and the first portion of the duodenum. The duodenoileostomy is an antecolic end-to-side duodenoenterostomy. This anastomosis is the most tenuous of the operation and is performed with a circular stapler, owing to the nature of the relatively narrow first portion of duodenum (Fig. 16-24).

The anvil is inserted through the duodenal stump staple line using a gastrotomy and direct insertion with suture guidance, or through an oral approach using a nasogastric tube, similar to the technique used for RYGB.[30] Cholecystectomy is a routine part of the DS operation, although Ren and associates[45] only performed cholecystectomy when gallstones were present.

A relative indication for selecting either a BPD (or possibly a DS) operation for patients includes those patients who are morbidly obese and who have undergone a previous fundoplication for the treatment of GERD. Such patients, because of the potential heavy scarring present in the gastroesophageal junction area, are more amenable to a BPD or DS, which can be performed with little (BPD) or less (DS) disturbance of the proximal gastric area than can either a banding type procedure or a gastric bypass.

POSTOPERATIVE CARE AND FOLLOW-UP

Excellent surgical outcomes require the appropriate selection of patients, thorough preoperative preparation, technically well-performed operations, and attentive postoperative care. The bariatric patient requires particularly attentive and special postoperative care in several areas above and beyond that of the average surgical patient. There are unique manifestations of intra-abdominal problems in severely obese patients.

Meticulous attention must be given to the vital signs, which are often the key to signaling problems. The most dreaded complication after bariatric surgery is a gastrointestinal tract leak. Tachycardia, at times accompanied by tachypnea or agitation, is often the only manifestation of this severe intra-abdominal problem. The severely obese patient may not develop a fever or signs of peritonitis, as would the patient with normal body habitus.

Appropriate fluid resuscitation is essential. A 200-kg patient who undergoes an open gastric bypass can easily require 6 to 10 L of fluid to achieve replacement of maintenance, third space, and operative fluid or blood losses. Our postoperative protocol calls for 400 mL/hr of balanced salt solution (usually lactated Ringer's) with boluses as needed for low urine output. A Foley catheter is used for the first 24 hours. Patients undergoing laparoscopic surgery usually have much less third space and operative blood loss than patients undergoing open surgery, shortening the period of high fluid resuscitation. Some patients who have been on diuretics for many years will not have adequate urine output without diuretic use, but the surgeon must ensure that the patient is adequately volume resuscitated before giving diuretics. Higher than expected fluid requirements, oliguria, and tachycardia are a constellation of postoperative findings suggesting intra-abdominal problems.

Adequate pain control is essential. Narcotic requirements are decreased with a laparoscopic approach. A patient-controlled analgesia pump is appropriate and helpful. The value of an epidural catheter for pain relief is controversial. It has been my experience that such catheters in the severely obese population are often difficult to place and easy to dislodge.

DVT prophylaxis is important. Pulmonary embolism is the leading cause of death after bariatric surgery. There are no data that substantiate one regimen of prophylaxis over another. I employ a combination of early ambulation (the same day as surgery, usually within 4 to 6 hours), use of SCDs, and subcutaneous low-molecular-weight heparin (Enoxaparin).

My standard practice procedure is to obtain a radiographic study of the gastrointestinal tract on the first postoperative day (although there are no data for randomized, prospective trials to evaluate this). It is valuable to document pouch size and to identify the patient with partial obstruction of the distal anastomosis, usually owing to edema but on occasion to technical reasons. The latter requires early reoperation.

Discharge, regardless of bariatric operation, occurs when the patient is mobile, is tolerating an oral liquid diet, has adequate pain control with oral analgesics, and has no signs of problems (e.g., fever or wound cellulitis). The timing of discharge, once these criteria are met, is often influenced by cultural issues or patient expectation. Thus the duration of hospitalization is not always an accurate one in reflecting optimal outcomes when comparing published studies in the literature.

Although the schedule of postoperative visits varies, all patients must undergo long-term follow-up. This guarantees the surgeon obtains feedback as to patient results and helps ensure that the patient avoids any preventable long-term metabolic or other procedure-related complications. The potential for such metabolic complications is inherently present for all the malabsorptive procedures. The restrictive procedures have minimal health risks from metabolic complications but have their own set of potential problems, such as band slippage or erosion for patients undergoing AGB.

A typical regimen for following the patient having AGB would be to have the first visit within the first month postoperatively, to evaluate oral intake, food tolerance, and wound healing, and to determine if appropriate restriction has resulted from placement of the noninflated band. Subsequent visits, usually scheduled monthly to bimonthly in the beginning then less frequently, involve counseling with a nutritionist and assessment of weight loss and determination for the need for band adjustment. A goal of 1 to 2 kg/wk of weight loss is adjusted for initial body weight. Less weight loss is an indication for instillation of additional saline into the band system via the port. This should initially be done under fluoroscopic control until the surgeon has sufficient experience and confidence to perform such adjustments in the office or clinic without fluoroscopic guidance. Blood tests are done periodically throughout the patient's follow-up based on metabolic indications, the patient's underlying medical illnesses, and other indications for them.

After RYGB, a typical postoperative checkup regimen would include a visit within the first 2 to 3 weeks postoperatively to assess wound healing, advance from a liquid to solid food diet, and check overall recovery. Subsequent visits are scheduled at 6 weeks, 3 months, 6 months, and 1 year after surgery, then annually. Visits during the first year monitor weight loss; those after the first year check maintenance of weight loss. Blood sampling for potential anemias or other metabolic changes to existing medical conditions is indicated. The risk of iron or vitamin B_{12} deficiency exists for life, necessitating annual blood checks.

Patients undergoing malabsorptive operations must understand the necessity of strict compliance with a strict follow-up plan. The BPD or DS patient should be seen within the first 2 weeks to be certain diarrhea is not too prolific and dehydration has not resulted. The patient should be taught the signs of dehydration and the plans for its treatment. Replacement of fat-soluble vitamins is mandatory, and patient compliance must be documented. Initial visits after the first month should be monthly for the first several months, until the risk of dehydration, poor protein intake, and significant metabolic consequences of rapid weight loss have lessened. The potential for protein-calorie malnutrition exists after these procedures and will manifest itself usually during this time. Thereafter, as weight loss slows, periodic visits separated by 3-month intervals are indicated for the first year, then semiannually thereafter. Weight loss will taper after the first 12 to 18 months. Lifelong follow-up to assess fat-soluble vitamin deficiencies as well as protein levels, liver function tests, and metabolic stability is indicated after BPD or DS.

Most bariatric practices employ patient support groups as a component of the postoperative support system. These groups are variously organized and managed but usually consist of patients having had weight reduction surgery or contemplating it who meet to discuss personal experiences with respect to their surgery, recovery from it, and the experience of losing weight and maintenance of lost weight. Although no data exist as to their medical benefit, those groups that are vigorous and successful seem to provide an excellent forum for patients to exchange information as well as provide psychological and emotional support and encouragement to patients both before and after surgery.

RESULTS

The operations discussed are effective for weight reduction and reversal of associated comorbidities of severe obesity. There is no consensus on the definition of success for any of these operations in terms of percentage of weight loss or extent of reversal of comorbidities. There are no scales for rating relative importance of outcomes including mortality, complications, reoperations, overall weight loss, and relief of medical comorbidities. However, increased mortality and serious complications as well as a

high reoperative rate would quickly lead to the abandonment of any operation. There are no data to show significantly improved disease-free or overall survival.

Results of operations can only be determined after adequate long-term follow-up and with adequate numbers of operations performed by a variety of surgeons. The applicability of some operations may vary based on patient factors, such as size or previous abdominal surgery.

Adjustable Gastric Banding

Patients undergoing AGB experience an operation that may last as little as 1 hour in experienced hands. Discharge from the hospital after an overnight stay is the norm, with a few reports of same-day discharge but more frequent reports of longer discharge based on cultural norms and acceptance. Table 16-1 gives the results of laparoscopic AGB in several large reported series in the literature with long-term follow-up.[47-52]

The band is initially placed without adding any saline to distend it. Additions of 1.0 to 1.5 mL of saline are added to produce a desired weight loss of 1 to 2 kg/wk. Excess weight loss may lead to actual removal of a small amount of saline, whereas inadequate weight loss is an indication for the addition of more saline to the system, increasing the restriction of the band. The incidence of metabolic problems is low after AGB because there is no disruption of the normal gastrointestinal tract. One potential problem is esophageal dilatation from chronic obstruction from band slippage.

Weight loss after AGB may average as high as 50% to 60% of excess weight loss after follow-up of 3 years or longer.[47-52] The pattern of weight loss is such that weight loss continues after the first year, up to a maximal amount usually by the third year (see Table 16-1). Series with 5-year follow-up confirm the weight loss may even improve slightly further after 3 years. The decrease in BMI in series with over 5-year follow-up[50-52] shows a decrease from baseline BMI average of 42 to 46 kg/m^2 to a BMI of 30 to 36 kg/m^2 at 5 years. The percentage of patients lost to

TABLE 16-1.   Results of Laparoscopic Adjustable Gastric Banding Procedures

	Study				
	O'Brien et al.[48]	Belachew et al.[50]	Dargent[49]	Vertruyen[51]	Favretti et al.[52]
No. Patients	709	763	500	543	830
Age	41	36	39.4	41	37.9
Body Mass Index	45	42	43	44	46.4
Operating Room Time (min)	56	65		60	
Conversion (%)	1.0	1.3	1.9	1.2	2.7
Length of Stay (days)			4.2		
Follow-up (yr)	0.25-6	1-3	1.75	3	7
% Excess Weight Loss/yr	54/5	50-60/5	65/2	53/5	
Body Mass Index/yr		<30/5		31.2/5	36/5

All numbers except number of patients represent percentages.

follow-up in some of these series has been remarkably low (under 2%).[47]

The success of AGB in treating existing medical comobidities for severely obese patients has been equally good.[53] The LAP-BAND has been shown to resolve type II diabetes in two thirds of cases. Improved blood glucose control resulted for all patients. Hypertension was resolved in 55% of one cohort of patients after this procedure. Patients also experienced a decrease in fasting triglyceride levels and elevation of high-density lipoprotein levels. Obstructive sleep apnea was reduced from an incidence of 33% preoperatively to 2% postoperatively.[54] Asthma symptom scores fell from 44.5 before operation to 14.3 at 1 year, with all patients showing improvement.[48] Gastroesophageal reflux was resolved or improved in 90% of patients with this problem in the Australian experience[48] and in all 12 patients in another report by Angrisani and colleagues.[55]

Quality of life testing measures parameters that include physical, mental, and psychological well-being of patients. There are several standard surveys that have been developed to calculate quality of life. A group of 459 patients undergoing a LAP-BAND procedure had scores at 1 year after surgery that were in the normal values for the community for the Medical Outcomes Trust Short Form-36 (SF-36) test.[53] Resolution of depression, as measured by the Beck Depression Inventory, has also been shown to result from weight loss after performance of an AGB procedure.[53]

Roux-en-Y Gastric Bypass

The RYGB has an established track record, longer than any other operation. Its performance has been modified over the years, and results presented reflect data from series in both the era of its performance as an open (Table 16-2)[15,34,56-60] and a laparoscopic procedure (Table 16-3).

With the use of a laparoscopic approach, the RYGB can be performed in 2 to 3 hours by an experienced team, with lower times after more extensive experience. The operative times for laparoscopic RYGB have decreased with increasing experience and improved laparoscopic instrumentation. They compare favorably to the times for open RYGB.[16]

Duration of hospitalization has decreased for all patients undergoing RYGB. Patients undergoing laparoscopic RYGB are usually hospitalized about 3 days. Since the advent of laparoscopic RYGB, in my own practice those few patients who undergo open RYGB or who require conversion to open RYGB are discharged within 1 day of the patients undergoing laparoscopic RYGB. This is likely due to protocols in place to encourage early ambulation and oral intake after RYGB that did not exist before the era of laparoscopic RYGB. However, some centers using traditional open surgery have reported routine discharge at 2 to 3 days postoperatively after open RYGB.

Excess weight loss from long-term follow-up studies shows that open RYGB provides a weight loss of over 65% at 1 year in many studies[15,16,34,56,57,59] Long-term follow-up

TABLE 16-2. Results of Open Roux-en-Y Gastric Bypass

	Study						
	Pories et al.[56]	Fobi et al.[15]	Capella and Capella[57]	Sugerman et al.[60]	MacLean et al.[58]	Hall et al.[59]	Brolin et al.[34]
No. Patients	1160	500	560	1025	243	99	90
Age				39	34		
Body Mass Index	50	46	50	51	49		62
% Ideal Body Weight						198	
Operating Room Time (min)						120	
Length of Stay (days)	5-6	4				8	
Follow-up (yr)	4	2	5	10-12	5.5	3	3.6
% Excess Weight Loss	49	80	77	52		67% lost >50%	64
Change in Body Mass Index				50 to 36	44 to 29		
Resolution/Improvement							
Diabetes Mellitus Type II				83			
Hypertension				69			
Gastroesophageal Reflux Disease				92			
Osteoarthritis				18			

All numbers except number of patients represent percentages.

TABLE 16-3. Results of Laparoscopic Roux-en-Y Gastric Bypass

	Study							
	Schauer et al.[61]	Wittgrove and Clark[18]	DeMaria et al.[69]	Higa et al.[37]	Nguyen et al.[16]	Westling and Gustavsson[68]	Papasavas et al.[70]	Schauer et al.[17]
No. Patients	191	500	281	1040	79	30	116	275
Age	40		41.6			36		42
Body Mass Index	50.4	40-45	48.1	47.8	47.6	42	49.3	48.3
Operating Room Time (min)			162		225	245	236	260
Conversion	1.6		2.8	3	0	23	6.9	1.1
Length of Stay (days)	3.3	2.5	4.0	1.9	3	4	3	2.6
Follow-up (yr)	4	5	1.0	1.9	1	1	1.5	2.5
% Excess Weight Loss	60	80	70	68	68	81	77	77
Resolution/Improvement								
Diabetes Mellitus Type II	83/17	98/2	93				50/	82/18
Hypertension	36/53	92/0	52				36/	70/18
Obstructive Sleep Apnea	33/47	98/0					100/	74/19
Cholesterol	37/41						62.5/	63/33
Gastroesophageal Reflux Disease		98/0	95				52/	72/24
Osteoarthritis			76				45.5	74/19

All numbers except number of patients represent percentages.

studies show that there is a tendency for patients to regain some weight after the first year. Pories and colleagues[56] have the longest reported follow-up, with a high percentage of patients being followed, and show that excess weight loss was 58% at 5 years and 49% at 14 years. Capella and Capella[57] reported a series of 560 patients followed for 5 years with an excess weight loss of 62%. MacLean and associates[58] reported a decrease in BMI from 44 to 29 kg/m^2 in 243 patients followed for an average of 5.5 years. Table 16-2 summarizes the weight loss achieved in large published series of open RYGB.

Resolution of comorbidities after open RYGB has been generally excellent. Pories and colleagues[56] reported an 85% incidence of resolution of type II diabetes after RYGB. Sugerman and associates[60] found a similar effect: 83% of patients resolved their diabetes after RYGB. Schauer and associates[61] showed glycosylated hemoglobin levels returned to normal in 83% of their patients, and reduction in the use of insulin was seen in 79% of patients. Patients with diabetes for more than 5 years, more severe forms of diabetes, or postoperative less weight loss were all factors that contributed to lack of resolution of the problem. All series demonstrate that resolution of diabetes begins after only modest weight loss and must be related to enteric factors regulating glucose metabolism rather than sheer weight loss alone, because a similar amount of weight loss after low calorie diets produces no such high incidence of resolution of diabetes. MacDonald and coworkers[62] showed that RYGB also reduces the subsequent progression of diabetes and the mortality associated with it. In comparing a group of morbidly obese patients who had

RYGB versus a group who did not, mean follow-up of 9 and 6 years showed a mortality rate of 9% in the surgically treated group versus 28% in the control group.

Hypertension was resolved in 69% of patients undergoing RYGB by Sugerman and associates[60] and resolved in 54% and improved in 15% of patients treated by Carson and coworkers.[63] Resolution of sleep apnea occurred in 67% of patients and resolution of obesity hypoventilation syndrome symptoms occurred in 76% of patients undergoing RYGB by Sugerman and associates.[64]

Hyperlipidemia syndromes improve. Brolin and coworkers[65] reported that 35% of patients had preoperatively elevated cholesterol or triglyceride levels and that RYGB resulted in a mean decrease of over 15% in cholesterol and over 50% in triglycerides, changes that remained stable for 5 years even if patients regained 15% of the 55% excess weight lost after 2 years. Jones[66] showed 24% of patients with preoperatively abnormal cholesterol levels decreased their cholesterol levels by an average of 24% and their triglyceride levels by an average of 40% 1 year after RYGB.

Sugerman and associates have demonstrated the excellent efficacy of RYGB in resolving the symptoms of pseudotumor cerebri as well as curing the difficult problem of venous stasis ulcers.[11]

Immediate resolution of symptoms of patients with GERD occurs in over 90% of cases. The extremely small gastric pouch has a limited reservoir for holding gastric juice, and the cardia is a low acid-producing area of the stomach.

Laparoscopic RYGB will likely produce results similar to open RYGB. However, just as there have been variable ways of performing a "typical" open RYGB, there are a similarly diverse number of minor variations on the laparoscopic version of the operation. The exact degree to which these modifications will affect outcomes is unknown. What can be stated is that there are no high-quality data with long-term follow-up after laparoscopic RYGB to confirm or refute this position.[67]

There is one prospective randomized study comparing open versus laparoscopic RYGB.[16] In that study, patients were followed for 1 year, at which time weight loss for both approaches was comparable (68% excess weight loss for laparoscopic RYGB vs. 62% excess weight loss for open RYGB). In another prospective randomized study, in which the authors had variable experiences in the two procedures, the weight loss was slightly higher with the laparoscopic approach.[68] Because many large case series of laparoscopic RYGB have reported excess weight loss in the 65% to 81% range (see Table 16-3)[16,18,37,61,68-70] (these short-term data mimic those reported for open RYGB), it is likely that the long-term weight loss produced by laparoscopic RYGB will be comparable to that of open RYGB.

One large comparison study of laparoscopic RYGB versus laparoscopic AGB showed that the laparoscopic RYGB achieved greater weight loss at all times during the comparison until 18 months postoperatively. At 12 months the laparoscopic RYGB patients had lost 67% of their excess weight versus 33% for AGB. However, the AGB series was older, and the long-term follow-up of the AGB group showed excess weight loss at 4 years of 58%.[71]

Resolution of comorbidities is less well documented than weight loss in all series of RYGB, whether laparoscopic or open (see Table 16-3).[17,18,61,69,70]

Recovery after RYGB does seem to be improved after a laparoscopic approach, as has been proven true for several other abdominal operations and strongly suggested for others. This is largely related to the decrease in postoperative pain experienced by patients after laparoscopic RYGB versus open RYGB.[72] Nguyen and colleagues[16] reported a shorter length of hospitalization and more rapid return to activities of daily living with laparoscopic RYGB. These factors, more so than other potentially more important long-term medical factors, currently make the initiation of any further prospective randomized trials of open versus laparoscopic RYGB almost impossible. Patient acceptance of such a trial is becoming increasingly difficult. Although the early (3 month postoperatively) improvement in quality of life reported by Nguyen and colleagues[16] after laparoscopic RYGB was greater than with open RYGB, the data were comparable for the two groups at 6 months after surgery, suggesting the major recovery benefit for a laparoscopic approach is limited to the first 3 months postoperatively.

One advantage of the laparoscopic approach for RYGB is a decrease in wound complications and incisional hernia seen after RYGB. My colleagues and I reported wound and hernia complications after our first 83 laparoscopic RYGB procedures compared with the previous 583 open RYGB operations and found a significant decrease in the complication rate from 32% to 7%.[73] We had no incisional hernia in over 400 patients who have undergone laparoscopic RYGB.

Biliopancreatic Diversion

Scopinaro and associates[41] reported weight loss after BPD of up to 78% at 12 years of follow-up. In an earlier report of over 2000 patients undergoing BPD, this group reported a mortality rate of 0.8% and a protein malnutrition rate of 12%.[74] The latter was higher in patients whose diets were traditionally higher in carbohydrates and in patients with smaller gastric volumes. A total of 4% of patients required reversal of the BPD or elongation of the common channel to reverse protein malnutrition.

Patients who undergo malabsorptive procedures such as BPD typically experience the highest weight loss of any of the standard bariatric procedures. This is particularly true of patients with higher BMI. In Scopinaro and associates' series there was no difference in the percentage of excess weight lost in patients with a BMI over $50 \, kg/m^2$ versus those with a BMI under $50 \, kg/m^2$. With AGB or RYGB, the effectiveness of weight loss tends to lessen slightly in patients who have a very high BMI, making BPD or DS a consideration for this patient population.

After BPD, patients typically have between two and four bowel movements per day. Excessive flatulence and foul-smelling stools are the rule. Relatively selective malabsorption of starch and fat provide the major mechanism of weight loss, but the partial gastric resection does contribute a restrictive component to the operation. In most patients, a "postcibal" syndrome is present immediately after surgery and resolves during the first year. It causes early satiety, often associated with vomiting and epigastric pain. According to Scopinaro, these symptoms are not true dumping, because the vasomotor response of dumping is absent.[41] The postcibal syndrome is instead attributed to rapid distention of the ileum and its resultant feedback on oral intake. The postcibal syndrome is said to be less problematic after the DS than the BPD, but data to confirm this are lacking. The postcibal syndrome seems to resolve by 1 year after surgery, and Scopinaro and associates report that patients undergoing BPD eat more at 1 year after surgery than preoperatively but the malabsorptive component of the operation prevents weight gain. They propose that the BPD causes an augmented bowel size and functional activity stimulus, which requires significant energy expenditure to achieve. This energy expenditure is theoretically offset by the loss of adipose and other soft tissue.[41]

The malabsorptive component of BPD causes selective malabsorption of fats and starches. Most patients can absorb adequate protein; however, protein malnutrition may occur, and patients must achieve adequate protein intake to prevent this; surgeons caring for these patients must be alert to measure protein levels to confirm adequate absorption. When protein malnutrition does occur, the common channel may need to be lengthened with reoperation. Patients must also be aware that their ability to absorb simple sugars, alcohol, and short-chain triglycerides is good and that overindulgence of sweets, milk products, soft drinks, alcohol, and fruit may produce excess weight gain.

The BPD has also been highly effective in treating comorbidities, including hypertension, diabetes, lipid disorders, and obstructive sleep apnea. Lipid disorders and type II diabetes are almost uniformly resolved after BPD in several reported series. Table 16-4 summarizes the results of patients treated with both BPD as well as DS procedures.[41-43,75]

Major considerations for achieving excellent results for patients offered a BPD include the ability to reliably follow those patients, as well as confirm they are being compliant with the recommendations to take appropriate vitamin supplements. These include multivitamins, as well as at least 2 g of oral calcium per day. Supplemental fat-soluble vitamins, including D, K and A, are indicated monthly as well.

Protein-calorie malnutrition is, however, the worst complication inherent in performance of either of the malabsorptive operations. Scopinaro and associates identified two subtypes of patients who developed "protein-energy malnutrition" (PEM). In the marasmic form, patients develop energy and nitrogen deficits but have hypoinsulinemia and development of lipolysis and proteolysis of skeletal muscle, which supplies needed amino acids for preservation of visceral muscle. In the hypoalbuminemic form of PEM, a lack of nitrogen is associated with normal energy supply, resulting in hyperinsulinemia. This leads to decreased visceral production of protein, with subsequent hypoalbuminemia and anemia and immune suppression. The marasmic form of PEM is much more desirable and not very unhealthy for patients in the immediate postoperative period undergoing rapid weight loss. Patients who eat a protein-rich diet after BPD will fall into the marasmic group, whereas those who concentrate on a carbohydrate-rich diet are at risk for developing the hypoalbuminemic form of PEM.

Oral intake after BPD can, if insufficient, result in a high incidence of PEM. Scopinaro's series contained a group of patients in whom they created a smaller volume stomach (150 mL), which resulted in a higher excess weight loss (near 90%) but a 30% incidence of PEM. Similarly, those few patients who developed a severe "postcibal syndrome" and had inadequate food intake were at high risk for developing PEM.[41]

The absorption of protein after either BPD or DS is dependent not just on the length of the common channel of intestine but more importantly on the total length of the alimentary tract limb, according to the results of Scopinaro and associates. Since 1992, this group has adjusted the length of the alimentary tract to be 200 cm for their patients from northern Italy, where protein-rich diets are the norm, while increasing the length of the common channel to 300 cm for patients from southern Italy, where carbohydrate-rich diets are standard. This resulted in a decrease in the incidence of early sporadic PEM and recurrent PEM in the southern Italian group from 17.5% and 6.5% to 2.4% and 2.4%, respectively.[41]

Careful monitoring of patient intake, compliance with appropriate vitamin supplementation, and a high degree of suspicion for potential protein-calorie malnutrition are all appropriate in following patients after BPD.

Duodenal Switch

Hess and Hess[43] reported a series of 440 patients undergoing DS who achieved a mean excess weight loss at 8 years of 70%. This was true if patients had a BMI either greater or less than 50 kg/m².

TABLE 16-4   Results of Malabsorptive Operations (Biliopancreatic Diversion and Duodenal Switch)

	Study			
	Scopinaro et al.[41]	Hess and Hess[43]	Anthone et al.[75]	Marceau et al.[42]
No. Patients	1356	440	701	259 (BPD)/465 (DS)
Age	37	40	42.3	37/37
Body Mass Index	47	50	52.3	46/47
Operating Room Time (min)		158-199		
Length of Stay (days)				
Follow-up (yr)	12	9	5	8.3/4.1
% Excess Weight Loss	78	80	66	61/73
No. Bowel Movements/day	2-4		2.8	3.7/3.0
Resolution/Improvement				
Diabetes Mellitus Type II	100	100		96
Hypertension	87			58
Cholesterol	100			

All numbers except number of patients represent percentages.

Marceau and colleagues[42] compared a group of patients undergoing BPD with a group subsequently operated on by them using DS. The excess weight loss after the BPD group, followed for 8.3 years, was 61%. The DS group, followed for only an average of 4.1 years, had achieved an excess weight loss averaging 73%. The DS patients also had less stool frequency than the BPD patients (the common channel being 100 cm vs. 50 cm for the BPD group). DS patients also had improved food variety tolerance, less vomiting, and improved appetite compared with BPD.

Anthone and colleagues[75] reported achieving an excess weight loss of 66% at 5 or more years after operation. The entire series reported was 701 patients, with average BMI of over 52 kg/m^2, and 50 of those patients were followed for over 5 years. Weight loss at 1 year for 333 patients was 69% of excess weight. Patients restricted oral intake after this operation: it was 50% (1 year post operation) and 65% (5 years post operation) of their preoperative intake. They averaged fewer than three bowel movements per day. At 3 years after operation, 98.3% of 58 patients had a normal albumin level, 51.7% had a normal hemoglobin level, and 70.7% had a normal serum calcium value.

The reported experience with laparoscopic DS has been limited. Ren and coworkers[45] reported results in 40 laparoscopic DS procedures. The patients in this series were larger than most selected series, averaging a BMI of 60 kg/m^2. Only one patient required conversion to open surgery, the median operating room time was only 210 minutes, and median length of hospitalization was 4 days. Median excess weight loss at 9 months after surgery was 58% of excess weight. There was a 2.5% mortality (one patient) and a complication rate of 15%.

Due to a high incidence of morbidity and mortality (23% and 6.5%) for patients with a BMI greater than 60 kg/m^2 undergoing laparoscopic DS, Gagner developed the two-stage DS, with the sleeve gastrectomy alone performed as the first stage to decrease morbidity in this superobese patient population. He reported a group of 18 patients done within 1 year, with a mean interval time between operations of 196 days and a mean decrease in BMI from 65 to 51 kg/m^2 between stages. Mean excess weight loss for the group at 6 months was 71% with no mortality and two complications (5.6%).[46]

COMPLICATIONS

The various procedures have complications that can occur with any intra-abdominal operation, such as pulmonary embolism. However, each operation has unique complications, as well as differing incidences of some of the shared common complications seen after any abdominal operation.

Adjustable Gastric Banding

Mortality for the AGB has been significantly lower than that for RYGB or either of the malabsorptive operations. O'Brien and Dixon report the mortality for 5827 patients undergoing AGB to be 0.05%.[47] Complications for the procedure are described in this section and summarized for some of the larger series in the literature in Table 16-5.[47,49-51,76]

Two large series of AGB procedures, those of the Australian Safety and Efficacy Register of New Interventional Procedures—Surgical[47] and the Italian Collaborative Study Group,[77] both report an overall complication rate of AGB of 11.3% and a LAP-BAND related complication rate of 11.3%, respectively. For the Australian experience, the rate of perioperative complications for laparoscopic AGB was 1.5%. The rate of band slippage or prolapse was 13.9%, of erosion was 3%, and of port access problems was 5.4%.

A common complication that plagued the AGB in the mid to late 1990s was the high incidence of band slippage. This was reported as 13% in one large series,[25] a figure that was comparable to other reports for patients done using

| | **Study** | | | | |
TABLE 16-5 Complications After Laparoscopic Adjustable Gastric Banding	O'Brien[47]	Belachew[50]	Dargent[49]	Vertruyen[51]	Weiner[76]
No. Patients	1120	763	500	543	184
Mortality	0	0	0	0	0
Postoperative complications	1.5	12.3	2.2	1.5	9
Slippage	13.9	8.0	5.0	4.6	2.2
Erosion	3	0.9	0.6		1.1
Port Complications	5.4	2.5	1.0	2.9	3.2
Reoperation Rate	25.3	10.5	6.6	4.2	6.4
Gastric Perforation	0	0.5	0.8	0	0
Pulmonary Embolism	0	0	0	0	0
Wound Infection	0.9	0.1	1.0		2.2

All numbers except number of patients represent percentages.

the initial perigastric band placement. Before the pars flaccida technique, the band was placed around the proximal stomach with the posterior portion of the band free within the lesser sac. This allowed much more movement of the stomach, and despite the anterior imbricating sutures, the fundus of the stomach herniated up through the band in a significant percentage of cases. This "slippage" usually manifested itself as the patient suddenly developing food intolerance, or occasionally gastroesophageal reflux. The latter symptom is also indicative of any form of obstruction at the site of the band. Slippage is by far the most common cause of obstruction, but on occasion erosion and fibrosis can also cause similar symptoms. The patient who presents with obstructive symptoms or food intolerance should undergo a plain radiograph of the abdomen. In its appropriate position, the band is oriented in a diagonal direction, along the 1 to 7 or 2 to 8 o'clock axis of a clock, in the epigastric region. When a plain film shows the band in a horizontal or 10 to 4 o'clock position, this is diagnostic for slippage and alteration in band position. Slippage or any other obstructive process at the band site will result in functional stenosis of the gastrointestinal tract at the proximal stomach. As a result, esophageal dilation can result if this situation is not fixed. Reversal of the obstruction will cure esophageal dilation. Reoperation is the appropriate treatment for band slippage.

Erosion of the band into the lumen of the stomach is a far less frequent complication but requires reoperation. The incidence of erosion may increase with the passage of time. At this time, however, the incidence remains below 1% for many large series, and up to 3% as noted above in the Australian collected experience.[47] Erosion may present as abdominal pain or as a port access site infection. In cases in which the band does erode into the stomach, it is presumed the band is either too tight or the stomach was imbricated too close to the buckle of the band, which will cause erosion with the passage of time. Surprisingly, this complication is rarely life threatening, and there are many reports in the literature describing removal of the eroded band, repair of the stomach, and replacement of a new band or even the same band at the same operative setting.

Port access site problems are the most numerous of the complications that occur after AGB. These also require reoperative therapy in most cases, but often the procedure can be done under local anesthesia and does not involve the peritoneal cavity. Leakage of the access tubing is a common problem, occurring in up to 11% of cases in the Italian experience, and less in most other series. Also, kinking of the tubing as it passes through the fascia is another relatively common reason for port access difficulties. Port site infection is the least common port access problem (under 1%) but should be evaluated with upper endoscopy to be certain that band erosion has not occurred.

Roux-en-Y Gastric Bypass

Mortality rates after RYGB have generally been in the 0.3% to 1.0% range for large reported series. Large reported series of laparoscopic RYGB have generally been reporting mortality rates of up to 1%.

Causes of mortality have varied but include pulmonary embolism, anastomotic leak, cardiac events, intra-abdominal abscess, and multiorgan failure. Mortality rates are obviously influenced heavily by patient selection. Livingston and associates[78] showed that the incidence of complications was not different for patients older than age 50 undergoing RYGB, but these patients were much more likely to have a fatal outcome. Male gender is also associated with an increased risk of morbidity and mortality in many published series where this has been analyzed.[78,79]

Overall complication rates from RYGB vary greatly, depending on the reporting. Liu and coworkers[79] reviewed the incidence of complications after RYGB in California, during which time the incidence of serious complications went from 15.1% to 7.6%. The authors identified male gender, presence of comorbidity, and low hospital volume of the procedure as independent predictors of complications. Overall complication rates in the authors' series of open RYGB approached 40%. This included a 15% to 24% incidence of incisional hernias, depending on the time of the series analysis, and a wound seroma/hematoma rate approaching 8%. The wound infection rate, of all severity, was in the 7% range. As noted earlier, the use of a laparoscopic approach has greatly lessened the incisional hernia rate and wound complication rate in my experience. DeMaria and associates[69] reported a similarly low incidence of wound infections (1.5%, all associated with open surgery for reoperation for complications) and incisional hernias (5 of 281 patients, with three of those involving open reoperations as well). Tables 16-6 and 16-7 summarize data regarding the complications of various published series in the literature for open[15,56-58,60,78] and laparoscopic[17,18,33,69,70,80,81] RYGB, respectively.

Pulmonary embolism is the most feared complication after any form of bariatric surgery, and its incidence in large reported series of RYGB approaches and sometimes exceeds 1%. The same is likely to be true for laparoscopic series, although the reported incidences thus far have been under 1%.

Postoperative atelectasis is relatively common after open RYGB but less frequently seen after laparoscopic RYGB. The incidence of pneumonia after either approach is in the 1% to 3% range. Major cardiovascular complications have less than a 1% incidence in most series of either approach.

Whereas nausea and vomiting are not unusual in isolated circumstances after RYGB, especially in relation to a patient's adaptation to food restriction, if persistent they can present the obvious problem of dehydration. This must be aggressively treated in the postoperative period or when associated with a viral or other gastrointestinal illness that is compounding the problem and further limiting oral intake. Intravenous fluids are indicated when in doubt. This is true for all bariatric operations, not just RYGB.

One specific problem that may arise with persistent vomiting after *any* of the bariatric operations and that is *imperative* for the surgeon to remember and treat is the

TABLE 16-6   Complications After Open Roux-en Y Gastric Bypass

	Study					
	Livingston et al.[78]	Fobi et al.[15]	MacLean et al.[58]	Pories et al.[56]	Sugerman et al.[60]	Capella and Capella[57]
No. Patients	1067	705	274	608	1025	652
Mortality	1.3	0.4	0.36		0.9	
Gastrointestinal Hemorrhage	0.66					
Leak	1.4	1.3			3	
Pulmonary Embolism	0.84	0.57	0.36		1.2	
Small Bowel Obstruction	0.94	4.0	2.2		4	
Stenosis	0.1	0.57			15	
Wound Infection					14	
Incisional Hernia		4.5	14.6			
Splenectomy		0.43				

All numbers except number of patients represent percentages.

TABLE 16-7   Complications After Laparoscopic Roux-en-Y Gastric Bypass

	Study						
	Schauer et al.[17]	Higa et al.[33]	Wittgrove and Clark[18]	DeMaria et al.[69]	Papasavas et al.[70]	Gould et al.[80]	Oliak et al.[81]
No. Patients	275	1500	500	281	116	223	300
Mortality	0.36	0.2	0	0	0.86	0	1.0
Gastrointestinal Hemorrhage	1.1	1.1			1.7		
Leak	4.4	0.9	2.2	5.1	2.6	1.8	1.3
Pulmonary Embolism	0.73	0.2		1.1	0.86		0.67
Small Bowel Obstruction	1.1	3.5	0.6	3.3	1.03	1.8	1.67
Stenosis	4.7	4.9	1.6	6.6	3.4	5.4	2.0
Wound Infection	8.7	0.13	5.6	1.1		7.6	6.67
Incisional Hernia	0.73	0.27	0	1.8		0.9	
Marginal Ulcer				5.1			
Splenectomy	0	0	0	0	0	0	0
Pneumonia	0.36	0.07					0.3

All numbers except number of patients represent percentages.

problem of Wernicke's encephalopathy from prolonged vomiting. This neurologic deficit is preventable with appropriate administration of parenteral thiamine (vitamin B_1) when the patient presents with persistent and severe vomiting. If the neurologic symptoms become significant, they may often not be fully reversed despite thiamine therapy.

Because depression is so frequent in the patient population undergoing bariatric surgery, severe postoperative depression may develop after any of the bariatric operations as well. When it does, the patient may totally stop eating, producing what at first seems like wonderful weight loss but soon, when gone beyond its desired endpoint, becomes a loss of critical visceral and musculoskeletal protein mass that can be life threatening. This is usually recognized by the family or friends and is a complaint worthy of the surgeon's attention.

Complications specific to the RYGB include anastomotic leaks from the proximal or distal anastomosis. Leaks from the gastrojejunostomy are more common and are generally the cause of a significant percentage of the life-threatening complications and deaths in any large series of patients. Data suggest a surgeon's experience will influence leak rate, especially early in the laparoscopic experience with RYGB.[82] Most large series of open RYGB procedures reported a leak rate of 1% to 2%, whereas some laparoscopic surgeons early in their experience were observing a leak rate approaching 5%.[69] Fortunately, this appears to be a not obligatory and transient phenomenon of learning for some surgeons; most large series of laparoscopic RYGB now report anastomotic leak rates of 1% to 2%. The fact that an anastomotic leak may present with nothing except isolated tachycardia as the only clinical symptom has made this postoperative complication one of the most feared ones among bariatric surgeons.

Another specific life-threatening complication that may result after RYGB is that of bowel obstruction. Patients who have had RYGB and present with a clinical or radiographic picture of small bowel obstruction need reoperation. The potential for internal hernias after this operation makes strangulation obstruction a frequent type of bowel obstruction. Patients who present with bowel obstruction and not ileus in the immediate postoperative period (I obtain CT with contrast or upper gastrointestinal series to confirm or rule out) *must* be promptly operated on. Retrograde distention of the biliopancreatic limb and distal stomach can result in rupture of the distal gastric staple line with subsequent peritonitis.

Stenosis of the gastrojejunostomy may occur after RYGB and has been reported in 2% to 14% in various series. The higher incidence seems associated with circular stapler versus sutured type anastomoses. Postoperative anastomotic stenosis usually presents at 4 to 6 weeks postoperatively as progressive intolerance to solids then liquids in a setting where these were previously tolerated. The problem is quite successfully treated with endoscopic or fluoroscopic balloon dilation. Unless marginal ulcer is associated with the stenosis, the problem does not require reoperation.[21,83]

Marginal ulcer occurs in 2% to 10% of RYGB. The incidence can be decreased by preoperative treatment of patients with *Helicobacter pylori* colonization of the stomach.[21] Patients with marginal ulcer typically present with continuous boring epigastric pain. The treatment is medical therapy, with proton pump inhibitors. Medical treatment resolves all marginal ulcers unless the ulcer has fistulized to the lower stomach, creating a source of ongoing acid to exacerbate the ulcer.

Short-term metabolic complications after RYGB can include dehydration. Another problem, both short- and long-term, may be severe dumping. This should be initially addressed by diet modification to avoid sweets and highly concentrated foods, as well as separating eating and drinking. Should the dumping be uncontrollable with these measures, subcutaneous octreotide is usually highly successful in reversing the symptoms of severe postoperative dumping. The medication may need to be administered for several months, but then usually patients may be tapered off it over a several-month interval.

Long-term metabolic complications of RYGB are limited to iron and vitamin B$_{12}$ deficiencies. The incidence of iron insufficiency varies among reported series. Iron is preferentially absorbed in the duodenum and proximal jejunum. Hence, RYGB bypasses the area of maximal iron absorption in the gut. Iron deficiency, based on serum values, is between 15% and 40%, whereas actual iron-deficiency anemia occurs in as many as 20% of patients after RYGB. This problem is easily treated in most cases with oral iron supplements. The gluconate form of iron is best absorbed in a nonacid environment. Brolin and colleagues[84] showed that daily multivitamin supplements are not sufficient to protect menstruating women from developing iron deficiency and anemia after RYGB. They showed that prophylactic oral iron supplements can prevent iron deficiency but not necessarily anemia in this patient population.[85] Prophylactic iron supplementation should be prescribed for premenstrual women.

The incidence of vitamin B$_{12}$ deficiency after RYGB is reported as being 15% to 20%, although it rarely causes anemia. Peripheral neural complications from low vitamin B$_{12}$ after RYGB are virtually unknown. Vitamin B$_{12}$ deficiency is due to inefficient absorption because of delayed mixing with intrinsic factor. The oral supplementation of vitamin B$_{12}$ usually suffices to treat deficits in vitamin B$_{12}$ levels. Other routes of vitamin B$_{12}$ administration include a sublingual medication, nasal spray, and parenteral injections. If injections are chosen, they are given at monthly or longer intervals.

Laparoscopic RYGB has had similar overall complications to open RYGB in many areas but has differed significantly in some. The major differences have been in the lower incidence of wound and hernia complications and splenectomy reported after laparoscopic RYGB versus open RYGB. On the other hand, the incidence of bowel obstruction, especially early bowel obstruction, appears higher in patients undergoing laparoscopic RYGB. Podnos and coworkers[86] found an increase in early and late bowel obstruction, stomal stenosis, and gastrointestinal tract hemorrhage after laparoscopic RYGB versus the incidence of those problems seen with open RYGB. On the other hand, they found the incidence of associated splenectomy, wound infection, incisional hernia, and mortality was lower with laparoscopic RYGB versus open RYGB. Laparoscopic RYGB appears to have similar metabolic postoperative complication rates of iron and vitamin B$_{12}$ deficiencies to open RYGB, but few data on the subject are available.

Biliopancreatic Diversion

Mortality rates after BPD have been reported as being 0.66% in the large series of Scopinaro and associates.[74] Surgical complications occur in 1.2% to 2.8% of patients, a remarkably low incidence relative to other experiences in the literature of open surgery to treat the morbidly obese.

The most significant and specific complication seen after BPD is protein malnutrition in 11.9% of patients.[74] The treatment is hospitalization with 2 to 3 weeks of parenteral nutrition. This particular problem usually manifests itself within the first few months after surgery, but it can occur sporadically, although less frequently, after operation. Scopinaro's group reported that 4% of the patients in their series eventually required reoperation to either reverse the BPD completely or to lengthen the common channel.

While the complication of protein malnutrition and poor intake is theoretically most likely to occur soon after BPD, the fact that Scopinaro and associates reported three late deaths from protein malnutrition and one case of Wernicke's encephalopathy suggests that these patients may always be at risk for these problems. They also revealed that there were three deaths from alcoholic cirrhosis and three cases of death from obstruction of the biliopancreatic limb, with all patients suffering from a lack of diagnosis of their problems by being seen by other physicians.

Other complications that are unique to BPD include those associated with excess amounts of diarrhea. Perianal irritation and hemorrhoids may occur. Dehydration may be a problem, particularly in the early days after operation.

Marginal ulcers are a distinct problem of BPD and occurred in 12.5% of the initial patient group treated by Scopinaro and associates but, with anastomotic technique revisions and use of H_2 blockers, was reduced to 3.2% by the end of their reported series, with the overall incidence being 5.6%.[41] Most marginal ulcers appeared within 1 year of surgery, and 75% were successfully treated with

medical therapy. There was a reported 20% incidence of stenosis with healing, requiring subsequent endoscopic dilatation or surgical revision.

Malabsorption of fat-soluble vitamins is one of the major problems associated with BPD. This may result in low levels of vitamins D and A. Scopinaro and associates reported all patients required calcium intake of 2 g/day to avoid bone resorption, along with weekly vitamin D supplementation. The incidence of bone resorption was otherwise very high, and the incidence of bone pain due to such problems was believed to be in the 6% range for patients after BPD.[41]

Perhaps it is the overall difficulty of the operation, as well as the potential dangers of the operation, that has left the BPD as the least popular operation performed in the United States. Even the DS modification does not represent more than 15% of bariatric operations.

Duodenal Switch

Mortality and complications after DS are similar to those seen after BPD but have a few distinct differences (Table 16-8). Anthone and colleagues[75] reported a 1.4% mortality for 701 patients, with pulmonary embolus being the

TABLE 16-8 Complications After Malabsorptive Operations (Biliopancreatic Diversion and Duodenal Switch)

	Study			
	Scopinaro et al.[41]	Hess and Hess[43]	Anthone et al.[75]	Marceau et al.[42]
No. Patients	1356	440	863	259 (BPD)/465 (DS)
Mortality	0.7	0.5	1.4	1.6/1.9
Revision		3.9	5.7	10.2/0.6
Gastrointestinal Hemorrhage		0.5	2/863	
Leak	2/1356	3.75	4/863	1.2/4.1
Pulmonary Embolism	9/1356	0.7	4/863	3.6*/1.7*
Gastric Ileus				9.1/6.2
Small Bowel Obstruction		1.8	1/863	
Stenosis		0.75		
Wound Infection				0.8/1.0
Splenectomy		24.5	3/863	
Pneumonia		0.5	1/863	With pulmonary embolism
Iron-Deficiency Anemia	40	9	48	9/6
Low Iron	>40			20/9
Low Vitamin B12			0	3/3
Low Calcium			29	16/8
High Parathyroid Hormone				30/17
Low Vitamin A				12/5

* Includes all pulmonary complications.
All numbers except number of patients represent percentages.

leading cause of death. Revisional surgery to increase the length of the common channel was performed in 5.7% of patients; in 4.8% it was for protein-calorie malnutrition. Major perioperative complications including gastrointestinal leaks, bleeding, gluteal rhabdomyolysis, bowel obstruction, and wound dehiscence represented a 2.9% complication rate. Half the patients at 3-year follow-up were anemic, and 30% were hypocalcemic.

Marceau and coworkers,[42] comparing both the DS and BPD approaches in their experience, reported that half the DS patients who initially had the operation performed by stapling and not dividing the duodenum required reoperation, owing to recanalization of the duodenum. The authors also reported that of all gallbladders left in situ during their early experience with either operation, 50% later required removal. Operative mortality for DS was 1.9%, and the operative complication rate was 16.3%. The most common complication was gastric retention postoperatively (6.2%). While the leak rate is not specifically given, the incidence of anastomotic fistula was 1.7% and that of intra-abdominal abscess was 2.4%, which together probably account for the total incidence of leaks. Pancreatitis occurred after 1.7% of DS operations. The revision rate was given as 0.1% annually for the first 6 years, and the rehospitalization rate for malabsorption or diarrhea was 0.93% annually during that time. The percentage of patients averaging over three bowel movements per day was 7%; 34% believed the unpleasant odor of stools and flatus was a problem. Abdominal bloating was experienced in one third of patients more than once weekly. Bone pain was reported in 29% of patients. Metabolic complications and side effects included iron deficiency in 9%, low ferritin level in 25%, low calcium concentration in 8%, and low levels of vitamin A in 5%. Elevated parathyroid hormone levels were present in 17%.

Ren and associates[87] showed that the levels of vitamins D and A 2 years after BPD were significantly depressed, with vitamin D deficiency being 36%, vitamin A deficiency 55%, elevated alkaline phosphatase level at 48%, and all patients having essential fatty acid deficiency. Lack of clinical correlation with these levels suggests that the problem may be more prevalent than originally reported or suspected based on past series.

REOPERATIVE SURGERY

A controversial topic is the appropriateness of performing repeat bariatric operations for failed previous ones. There are no specific rules to govern the appropriateness of repeat bariatric surgery. The absolute definition of a failed operation is unclear, but most surgeons would accept return to the criteria listed in Box 16-2 as appropriate for consideration for reoperation. If a patient has undergone an operation that has proven by mass experience to be ineffective, repeat operation for failure of that procedure is appropriate. Complications of procedures such as stenosis causing gastric outlet obstruction after vertical banded gastroplasty or metabolic complications after jejunoileal bypass are obvious indications for revisional surgery. One mistake frequently made by the nonbariatric surgeon in correcting a complication of a bariatric operation is to simply perform a procedure that corrects the complication but does not provide for continued weight restriction. In these circumstances, a typical long-term course is for the patient to slowly regain weight to their initial degree of obesity before the initial bariatric procedure and then seek further surgical assistance.

In assessing the patient for the appropriateness of reoperative surgery, the surgeon must determine whether the original bariatric operation is intact and anatomically still appropriate for maintaining weight loss. If not, consideration for reoperation is appropriate. However, a patient who has failed an anatomically intact and well-constructed bariatric operation is, in my opinion, at high risk to fail a second or revisional bariatric operation. Although little has been reported, there are no reports contradicting this logic. It is known that the incidence of infection, organ ischemia, anastomotic leakage, blood transfusion, and other severe intra-abdominal complications is increased in revisional surgery. Armed with this knowledge, the bariatric surgeon should be appropriately judicious and conservative in recommending reoperative bariatric surgery to patients, reserving such procedures for patients who have clear anatomic and not behavioral failure of a previous bariatric operation.

All bariatric operations have some incidence of failure. A figure of approximately 10% is often used in discussions regarding the "failure rate" of various well-established operations considered effective, including all of those described in this chapter. The definition of "failure" is varied and may include inadequate weight loss, inadequate resolution of medical comorbidities, development of side effects negatively influencing lifestyle and satisfaction, development of complications requiring medical or surgical intervention, or complications requiring alteration or reversal of the operation.

The jejunoileal bypass, a relic of history, still exists in a small number of patients, who appropriately may seek to have it reversed for dangers of complications. Any reversal should include a replacement weight reduction operation. Other operations that have failed the test of time include simple gastric partitioning or nonadjustable banding type operations, the most popular by far of which has been the vertical banded gastroplasty. The vertical banded gastroplasty was not discussed extensively in this chapter, despite its having been the most popular weight reduction operation in the 1980s both in the United States and worldwide. This is because its incidence of performance is sharply on the decline, with long-term follow-up data suggesting it is a poor long-term operation for the reasons discussed earlier in this chapter. However, many patients with previously performed vertical banded gastroplasties are now experiencing weight regain and requesting reoperative surgery. There is fairly extensive evidence that conversion of a vertical banded gastroplasty can be successfully performed, with a RYGB usually the operation preferred to replace it. Sugerman and associates[88] performed conversion of 53 vertical banded gastroplastic procedures with complications to RYGB, achieving 67% excess weight loss. The complication rate was approximately 50% for the series, including 20 marginal ulcers. Jones[89] reported only a 13% complication rate for a series of 141 patients undergoing reoperative surgery to convert from failed bariatric procedures to RYGB. However, high complications, such as the incidence of 33.8% early and 21.8% late complications reported by Cariani and colleagues[90] for reoperative performance of both vertical banded gastroplasty and RYGB in 47 patients are probably more the norm for reoperative surgery.

Use of the AGB as a revision procedure has been successful in several centers. O'Brien and coworkers[91] described using AGB via an open approach to revise failed gastroplasty and other procedures for 50 patients. The 3-year weight loss was 47% of excess weight, with increased early (17% vs. 1.1%) and decreased late (2% vs. 18%) complications as compared with placement of AGB as an initial procedure. Kyzer and colleagues[92] had a similar experience with placing AGB in 37 patients who had failed gastroplasty or RYGB, achieving good weight loss with low intraoperative and only five late reoperative complications.

Failed RYGB has been treated by adding a malabsorptive component to the original procedure by both Fobi and coworkers[93] and by Sugerman and associates.[94] Fobi's group performed a distal RYGB, reconnecting the efferent end of the RYGB halfway down the alimentary bowel length, decreasing the alimentary tract in half. The 65 patients experienced decrease in BMI from 42 to 35 kg/m^2, but at the cost of a 23% incidence of protein malnutrition. Sugerman and associates reported worse results. In their first 5 patients converted to distal RYGB a 50-cm common channel was created, resulting in protein-calorie malnutrition in all and eventual death in 2 from hepatic failure. In 22 patients given a 150-cm common channel as part of distal RYGB, 3 developed malnutrition requiring bowel lengthening.

Conversion of 27 patients with failed open or laparoscopic gastroplasty, AGB, or RYGB was all successfully done laparoscopically to RYGB by Gagner and colleagues.[95] A decrease in BMI from 43 to 36 kg/m^2 was achieved, and the complication rate was 22%. Other sporadic reports of small case series in the literature suggest that even reoperations can, under appropriate circumstances, be performed laparoscopically to give relatively good results, although not with as low a complication rate as initial surgery.

The use of a laparoscopic BPD to treat patients with failed weight loss after laparoscopic AGB was reported by Fielding and associates.[96] A laparoscopic (38) or open (20) BPD or a laparoscopic DS (21) was performed on the 5.4% of patients in their AGB series who had their bands removed for various reasons. A 40% excess weight loss at 2 years was achieved. No mortality was noted, and a 6.3% serious complication rate was observed.

Thus, the use of a variety of strategies and approaches has been reported for the patient who is an appropriate candidate for reoperative bariatric surgery. These experiences serve to emphasize that the weight loss achieved is not as large and that the complication rate is higher than that of initial bariatric procedures. The danger of combining too significant a malabsorptive procedure with an existing restrictive one, and the potential for protein-calorie malnutrition, must be appreciated as well.

THE BARIATRIC REVOLUTION

Bariatric surgery is literally in the midst of a revolution. Figure 16-25 shows the numbers of RYGB procedures performed in the United States based on data from the CDC.[97]

There are several reasons for this rapid "revolution." The primary ones are listed in Box 16-7. The most important one, which temporally corresponds with the rapid rise in patient demand for bariatric surgery, is the use of a laparoscopic approach for operations. While a laparoscopic approach was more commonplace in Europe and Australia in the mid 1990s with the advent of the popularity of the laparoscopic AGB in those continents, the use of laparoscopic approach for RYGB in the United States really only began in 1999. Before that, only a very few medical centers were offering that approach. The laparoscopic AGB was not performed in the United States until 2001, and insurance companies continue to limit patient access to this procedure by illogical denial of coverage. Patient perception and referring physician perception of any operation using a laparoscopic approach are that the procedure is less invasive and inherently less dangerous. While those perceptions are inaccurate, they nevertheless exist and contribute to the marked increase in demand and referrals for many operations once a laparoscopic approach is adopted. This was true for cholecystectomy in 1990 and antireflux surgery in the mid 1990s and is now true for bariatric surgery.

Mass media and the rapid dissemination of information is also a major factor in the bariatric revolution. Patients may now access many sites on the Internet where infor-

---

Box 16-7 Reasons for the bariatric revolution
■ The introduction of laparoscopy as a viable approach for procedures
■ The use of mass media to convey information to the public
■ The use of the Internet by patients to communicate about bariatric surgery
■ Evolution of advanced laparoscopy as a desirable focus for general surgical specialization
■ Patient demand fueled by the first three entries in this list

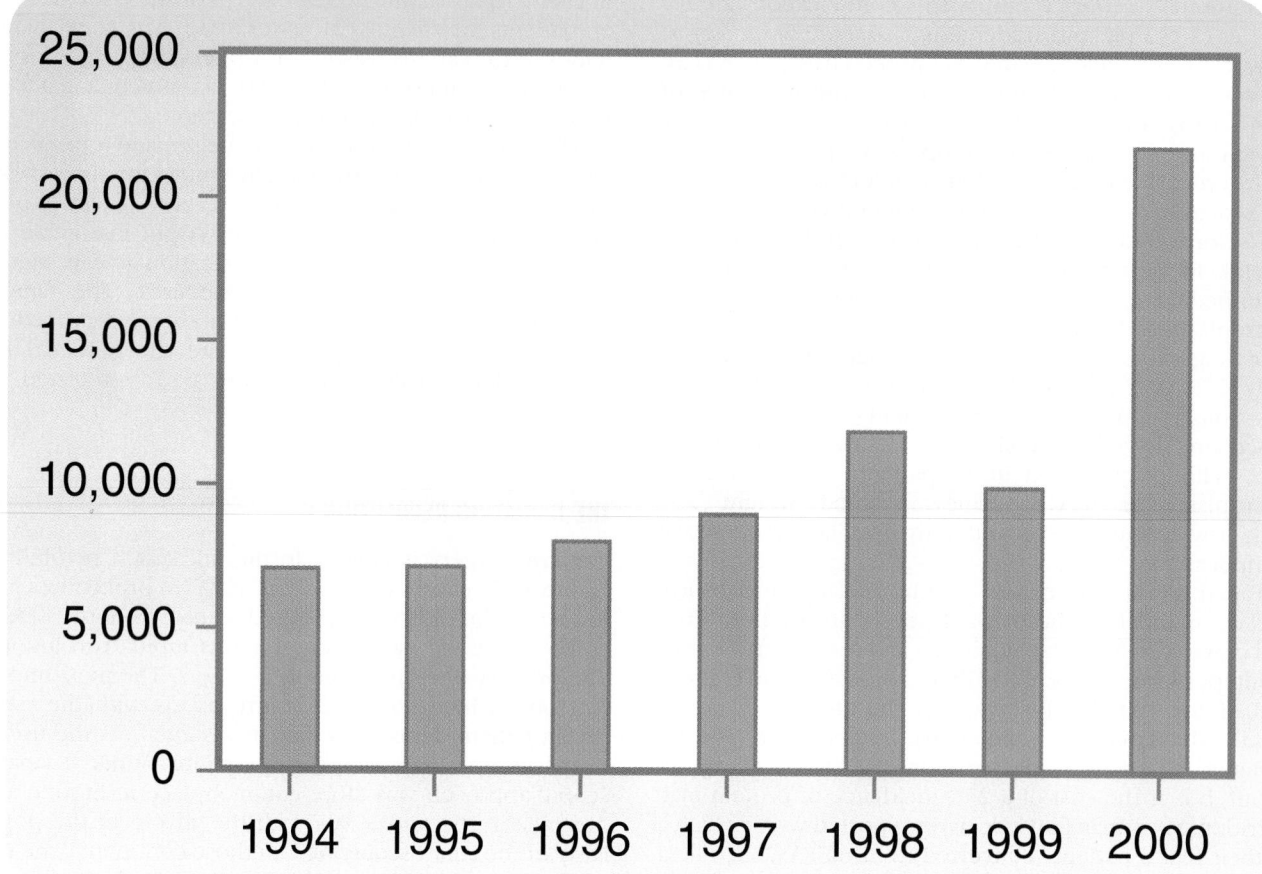

FIGURE 16-25. Number of laparoscopic Roux-en-Y gastric bypasses performed in the United States since 1995.

mation about bariatric surgery is available. Television stations show videos of actual operations. Internet "chat groups" between former and prospective patients on the topic of bariatric surgery are common, and many patients participate in these both before and after surgery. Media and television personalities have had bariatric surgery, with superb results that they have been quite willing to share with the public. The combination of all these factors has led to a patient population that is more informed and more aware of the potential of such surgery as a treatment of their morbid obesity. Demand for bariatric surgery has consequently escalated dramatically in the past 5 years.

Finally, the surgical community itself has adjusted its perception of bariatric surgery. It is now a desirable area of specialization for graduating residents, who enjoy the technical challenge of advanced laparoscopic surgery combined with the rewards of performing a life-altering and usually highly successful operation for their patients. It has been the young laparoscopic surgeons that have generated much of the change in perception of bariatric surgery among the surgical community.

CONCLUSION

The surgical treatment of morbid obesity is no longer considered out of the mainstream of general surgery and is now a component of most surgical resident's training programs. It represents the current fastest growing area of general surgery. Patient demand for the procedure has vastly increased, and currently surgeons are only operating annually on 1% of the eligible patients who would benefit from bariatric surgery. This chapter has discussed all aspects of the performance of bariatric surgery in current surgical practice, including the most commonly performed procedures at this time. The disease process of morbid obesity is unfortunately both poorly understood and rapidly increasing. Although operation will likely not represent the ultimate treatment for the disease, it currently remains the only effective treatment of morbid obesity. The incorporation of a laparoscopic approach to previously existing operations has not only offered the potential for improved patient outcomes but generated increased patient interest in choosing surgical therapy.

References

1. Gastrointestinal surgery for severe obesity: National Institutes of Health Consensus Development Conference Statement. Am J Clin Nutr 55(Suppl 2):S615-S619, 1992.

2. Mokhad AH, Serdula MK, Diketz WH, et al: The spread of the obesity epidemic in the United States 1991-1998. JAMA 282:1519-1522, 1999.

3. Mokdad AH, Bowman BA, Ford ES, et al: The continuing epidemics of obesity and diabetes in the United States. JAMA 286:1195-1200, 2002.

4. Allison DB, Fontaine KR, Manson JE, et al: Annual deaths attributable to obesity in the United States. JAMA 282:1530-1538, 1999.

5. Cummings DE, Weigle DS, Frayo RS, et al: Plasma ghrelin levels after diet-induced weight loss or gastric bypass surgery. N Engl J Med 346:1623-1629, 2002.

6. Samaha FF, Iqbal N, Seshadri P, et al: A low-carbohydrate as compared with a low-fat diet in severe obesity. N Engl J Med 348:2074-2081, 2003.

7. Weigle DS: Pharmacological therapy of obesity: Past, present, and future. J Clin Endocrinol Metab 88:2462-2469, 2003.

8. Society of American Gastrointestinal Endoscopic Surgeons: Guidelines for the clinical application of laparoscopic bariatric surgery. Surg Endosc 17:2037-2040, 2003.

9. American Society of Bariatric Surgeons: ASBS guidelines for granting privileges in bariatric surgery. Obes Surg 13:238-239, 2003.

10. Kyzer S, Charuzi I: Obstructive sleep apnea in the obese. World J Surg 22:998-1001, 1998.

11. Sugerman HJ, Sugerman EL, Wolfe L, et al: Risks and benefits of gastric bypass in morbidly obese patients with severe venous stasis disease. Ann Surg 234:41-46, 2001.

12. Shiffman ML, Sugerman HJ, Kellum JM, et al: Gallstone formation after rapid weight loss: A prospective study in patients undergoing gastric bypass surgery for treatment of morbid obesity. Am J Gastroenterol 86:1000-1005, 1991.

13. Ben-Meir A, Miller A, Holbrook C, Schirmer B: Feasibility of cholecystectomy at time of Roux-en-Y gastric bypass. Surg Endosc 16:S240, 2002.

14. Sugerman HJ, Brolin RE, Fobi MAL, et al: Prophylactic ursodeoxycholic acid prevents gallstone formation following gastric bypass induced rapid weight loss: A multicenter, placebo controlled, randomized, double-blinded, prospective trial. Am J Surg 169:91-97, 1995.

15. Fobi MAL, Lee H, Holness R, Cabinda D: Gastric bypass operation for obesity. World J Surg 22:925-935, 1998.

16. Nguyen NT, Goldman C, Rosenquist CJ, et al: Laparoscopic versus open gastric bypass: A randomized study of outcomes, quality of life, and costs. Ann Surg 234:279-291, 2001.

17. Schauer PR, Ikramuddin S, Gourash W, et al: Outcomes after laparoscopic Roux-en-Y gastric bypass for morbid obesity. Ann Surg 232:515-529, 2000.

18. Wittgrove AC, Clark GW: Laparoscopic gastric bypass, Roux en-Y—500 patients: Techniques and results, with 3-60 month follow-up. Obes Surg 10:233-239, 2000.

19. Higa KD, Boone KB, Ho T, Davies OG: Laparoscopic Roux-en-Y gastric bypass for morbid obesity: Technique and preliminary results of our first 400 patients. Arch Surg 135:1029-1034, 2000.

20. Balsinger BM, Poggio JL, Mai J, et al: Ten and more years after vertical banded gastroplasty as primary operation for morbid obesity. J Gastrointest Surg 4:598-605, 2000.

21. Flexible endoscopy in the management of patients undergoing Roux-en-Y gastric bypass. Obes Surg 12:634-638, 2002.

22. Brolin RE, Robertson LB, Kenler HA, et al: Weight loss and dietary intake after vertical banded gastroplasty and Roux-en-Y gastric bypass. Ann Surg 220:782-790, 1994.

23. Dubois F, Icard P, Berthelot G, Levard H: Coelioscopic cholecystectomy: Preliminary report of 36 cases. Ann Surg 211:60-62, 1990.

24. Fielding GA, Allen JW: A step-by-step guide to placement of the LAP-BAND adjustable gastric banding system. Am J Surg 184:26S-30S, 2002.

25. Belachew M, Legrand MJ, Defechereux TH, et al: Laparoscopic adjustable silicone gastric banding in the treatment of morbid obesity: A preliminary report. Surg Endosc 8:1354-1356, 1994.

26. Kuzmak LI: A review of seven years experience with silicone gastric banding. Obes Surg 1:403-408, 1991.

27. Belachew M, Zimmerman J-M: Evolution of a paradigm for laparoscopic adjustable banding. Am J Surg 184:21S-25S, 2002.

28. Mason EE, Ito C: Gastric bypass in obesity. Surg Clin North Am 47:345-351, 1969.

29. Griffen WO, Young VL, Stevenson CC: A prospective comparison of gastric and jejunoileal bypass procedures for morbid obesity. Ann Surg 2:500-509, 1977.

30. Wittgrove AC, Clark WG, Tremblay LJ: Laparoscopic gastric bypass, Roux en-Y: Preliminary report of five cases. Obes Surg 4:353-357, 1994.

31. De la Torre RA, Scott JS: Laparoscopic Roux-en-Y gastric bypass: A totally intra-abdominal approach—technique and preliminary report. Obes Surg 9:492-498, 1999.

32. Schauer P, Ikramuddin S, Hamad G, Gourash W: The learning curve for laparoscopic Roux-en-Y gastric bypass is 100 cases. Surg Endosc 17:212-215, 2003.

33. Higa KD, Ho T, Boone KB: Laparoscopic Roux-en-Y gastric bypass: Technique and 3-year follow-up. J Laparoendosc Adv Surg Tech 11:377-382, 2001.

34. Brolin RE, Kenler HA, Gorman JH, Cody RP: Long-limb gastric bypass in the superobese: A prospective randomized study. Ann Surg 215:387-395, 1992.

35. Brolin RE: The antiobstruction stitch in stapled Roux-en-Y enteroenterostomy. Am J Surg 169:355-357, 1995.

36. Gonzalez R, Lin E, Venkatesh KR, et al: Gastrojejunostomy during laparoscopic gastric bypass: Analysis of 3 techniques. Arch Surg 138:181-184, 2003.

37. Higa KD, Boone KB, Ho T: Complications of the laparoscopic Roux-en-Y gastric bypass: 1,040 patients: What have we learned? Obes Surg 10:509-513, 2000.

38. Scott JR, Miller A, Miller M, et al: Retrocolic herniation following laparoscopic Roux-en-Y gastric bypass: Potential prevention? Obes Surg 13:230, 2003.

39. Scopinaro N, Gianetta E, Civalleri D, et al: Two years of clinical experience with biliopancreatic bypass for obesity. Am J Clin Nutr 33:506-514, 1980.

40. Scopinaro N, Marinari GM, Camerini G: Laparoscopic standard biliopancreatic diversion: Technique and preliminary results. Obes Surg 12:362-365, 2002.

41. Scopinaro N, Adami GF, Marinari GM, et al: Biliopancreatic diversion. World J Surg 22:936-946, 1998.

42. Marceau P, Hould FS, Simard S, et al: Biliopancreatic diversion with duodenal switch. World J Surg 22:947-954, 1998.

43. Hess DS, Hess DW: Biliopancreatic diversion with a duodenal switch. Obes Surg 8:267-282, 1998.

44. DeMeester TR, Fuchs KH, Ball CS, et al: Experimental and clinical results with proximal end-to-end duodenojejunostomy for pathological duodenogastric reflux. Ann Surg 206:414-424, 1987.

45. Ren CJ, Patterson E, Gagner M: Early results of laparoscopic

biliopancreatic diversion with duodenal switch: A case series of 40 consecutive patients. Obes Surg 10:514-523, 2000.

46. Gagner M: Laparoscopic malabsorptive procedures. Presented at SAGES Scientific Session, Los Angeles, March 2003.

47. O'Brien PE, Dixon JB: Weight loss and early and late complications—the international experience. Am J Surg 184:42S-45S, 2002.

48. O'Brien PE, Dixon JB, Brown W, et al: The laparoscopic adjustable gastric band (Lap-Band): A prospective study of medium-term effects on weight, health, and quality of life. Obes Surg 652-660, 2002.

49. Dargent J: Laparoscopic adjustable gastric banding: Lessons from the first 500 patients in a single institution. Obes Surg 9:446-452, 1999.

50. Belachew M, Belva PH, Desaive C: Long-term results of laparoscopic adjustable gastric banding for the treatment of morbid obesity. Obes Surg 12:564-568, 2002.

51. Vertruyen M: Experience with LAP-BAND system up to 7 years. Obes Surg 12:569-572, 2002.

52. Favretti F, Cadiere GB, Segato G, et al: Laparoscopic banding: Selection and technique in 830 patients. Obes Surg 12:385-390, 2002.

53. Dixon JB, O'Brien PE: Changes in comorbidities and improvements in quality of life after LAP-BAND placement. Am J Surg 184:51S-54S, 2002.

54. Dixon JB, Schachter LM, O'Brien PE: Sleep disturbance and obesity. Arch Intern Med 161:102-106, 2001.

55. Angrisani L, Iovino P, Lorenzo M, et al: Treatment of morbid obesity and gastroesophageal reflux with hiatal hernia by Lap-Band. Obes Surg 9:396-398, 1999.

56. Pories WJ, Swanson MS, MacDonald KG, et al: Who would have thought it? An operation proves to be the most effective therapy for adult-onset diabetes mellitus. Ann Surg 222:339-350, 1995.

57. Capella JF, Capella RF: The weight reduction operation of choice: Vertical banded gastroplasty or gastric bypass? Am J Surg 171:74-79, 1996.

58. MacLean LD, Rhode BM, Nohr CW: Late outcome of isolated gastric bypass. Ann Surg 231:524-528, 2000.

59. Hall JC, Watts JM, O'Brien PE, et al: Gastric surgery for morbid obesity. The Adelaide study. Ann Surg 211:419-427, 1990.

60. Sugerman HJ, Wolfe LG, Sica DA, Clore JN: Diabetes and hypertension in severe obesity and effects of gastric bypass-induced weight loss. Ann Surg 237:751-758, 2003.

61. Schauer PR, Burguera B, Ikramuddin S, et al: Effect of Roux-en Y gastric bypass on type 2 diabetes mellitus. Ann Surg 238:467-484, 2003.

62. MacDonald KG Jr, Long SD, Swanson MS, et al: The gastric bypass operation reduces the progression and mortality of non-insulin-dependent diabetes mellitus. J Gastrointest Surg 1:213-220, 1997.

63. Carson JL, Ruddy ME, Duff AE, et al: The effect of gastric bypass surgery on hypertension in morbidly obese patients. Arch Intern Med 154:193-200, 1994.

64. Sugerman HJ, Fairman RP, Sood RK, et al: Long-term effects of gastric surgery for treating respiratory insufficiency of obesity. Am J Clin Nutr 55:597S-601S, 1992.

65. Brolin RE, Bradley LJ, Wilson AC, Cody RP: Lipid risk profile and weight stability after gastric restrictive operations for morbid obesity. J Gastrointest Surg 4:464-469, 2000.

66. Jones KB Jr: The effect of gastric bypass on cholesterol, HDL, and the risk of coronary heart disease. Obes Surg 2:83-85, 1992.

67. Schneider BE, Villegas L, Blackburn G, et al: Laparoscopic gastric bypass surgery: Outcomes. J Laparoend Adv Surg Tech 13:247-256, 2003.

68. Westling A, Gustavsson S: Laparoscopic versus open Roux-en-Y gastric bypass: A prospective, randomized trial. Obes Surg 11:284-292, 2001.

69. DeMaria EJ, Sugerman HJ, Kellum JM, et al: Results of 281 consecutive total laparoscopic Roux-en-Y gastric bypass to treat morbid obesity. Ann Surg 235:640-647, 2002.

70. Papasavas PK, Hayetian FD, Caushaj PF, et al: Outcome analysis of laparoscopic Roux-en-Y gastric bypass for morbid obesity: The first 116 cases. Surg Endosc 16:1653-1657, 2002.

71. Biertho L, Steffen R, Ricklin T, et al: Laparoscopic gastric bypass versus laparoscopic adjustable gastric banding: A comparative study of 1,200 cases. J Am Coll Surg 197:536-547, 2003.

72. Nguyen NT, Lee ST, Goldman C, et al: Comparison of pulmonary function and postoperative pain after laparoscopic versus open gastric bypass: A randomized trial. J Am Coll Surg 192:469-476, 2001.

73. Ben Meir A, Miller A, Schirmer B: Decreased incisional complications after laparoscopic versus open gastric bypass. Presented at annual meeting of Society for Surgery of the Alimentary Tract, San Francisco, May 2002.

74. Scopinaro N, Gianetta E, Adami GF, et al: Biliopancreatic diversion for obesity at eighteen years. Surgery 119:261-268, 1996.

75. Anthone GJ, Lord RVN, DeMeester TR, Crookes PF: The duodenal switch operation for the treatment of morbid obesity. Ann Surg 238:618-628, 2003.

76. Weiner R, Wagner D, Bockhorn H: Laparoscopic gastric banding for morbid obesity. J Laparoendosc Adv Surg Tech 9:23-30, 1999.

77. Angrisani L, Alkilani M, Basso N, et al: Laparoscopic Italian experience with the LAP-BAND. Obes Surg 11:307-310, 2001.

78. Livingston EH, Huerta S, Arthur D, et al: Male gender is a predictor of morbidity and age a predictor of mortality for patients undergoing gastric bypass surgery. Ann Surg 236:576-582, 2002.

79. Liu J, Zingmond D, Etzioni DA, et al: Characterizing the performance and outcomes of obesity surgery in California. Am Surg 69:823-828, 2003.

80. Gould JC, Bradley NJ, Ellison C, et al: Evolution of minimally invasive bariatric surgery. Surgery 132:565-572, 2002.

81. Oliak D, Ballantyne GH, Weber P, et al: Laparoscopic Roux-en-Y gastric bypass: Defining the learning curve. Surg Endosc 17:405-408, 2003.

82. Nguyen NT, Rivers R, Wolfe B: Factors associated with operative outcomes in laparoscopic gastric bypass. J Am Coll Surg 197:548-557, 2003.

83. Vance PL, de Lange EE, Shaffer HA Jr, Schirmer B: Gastric outlet obstruction following surgery for morbid obesity: Effect of fluoroscopically guided balloon dilation. Radiology 222:70-72, 2002.

84. Brolin RE, Gorman RC, Milgrim LM, Kenler HA: Multivitamin prophylaxis in prevention of post-gastric bypass vitamin and mineral deficiencies. Int J Obes 15:661-668, 1991.

85. Brolin RE, Gorman JH, Gorman RC, et al: Prophylactic iron supplementation after Roux-en-Y gastric bypass: A prospective, double-blind randomized study. Arch Surg 133:740-744, 1998.

86. Podnos YD, Jiminez JC, Wilson SE, et al: Complications after laparoscopic gastric bypass: A review of 3464 cases. Arch Surg 138:957-961, 2003.

87. Ren CJ, Siegel N, Williams T, et al: Fat-soluble nutrient deficiency after malabsorptive operations for morbid obesity. Presentation at annual meeting of the Society for Surgery of the Alimentary Tract, Orlando, May 2003.

88. Sugerman HJ, Kellum JM, DeMaria EJ, et al: Conversion of failed or complicated vertical banded gastroplasty to gastric bypass in morbid obesity. Am J Surg 171:263-269, 1996.

89. Jones KB Jr: Revisional bariatric surgery—safe and effective. Obes Surg 11:183-189, 2001.

90. Cariani S, Nottola D, Grani S, et al: Complications after gastroplasty and gastric bypass as a primary operation and as a reoperation. Obes Surg 11:487-490, 2001.

91. O'Brien P, Brown W, Dixon J: Revisional surgery for morbid obesity—conversion to the Lap-Band system. Obes Surg 10:557-563, 2000.

92. Kyzer S, Raziel A, Landau O, et al: Use of adjustable silicone gastric banding for revision of failed gastric bariatric operations. Obes Surg 11:66-69, 2001.

93. Fobi MAL, Lee H, Igew D Jr, et al: Revision of failed gastric bypass to distal Roux-en-Y gastric bypass: A review of 65 cases. Obes Surg 11:190-195, 2001.

94. Sugerman HJ, Kellum JM, DeMaria EJ: Conversion of proximal to distal gastric bypass for failed gastric bypass for super-obesity. J Gastrointest Surg 1:517-525, 1997.

95. Gagner M, Gentileschi P, deCsepel J, et al: Laparoscopic reoperative bariatric surgery: Experience from 27 consecutive patients. Obes Surg 12:254-260, 2002.

96. Fielding GA: Laparoscopic biliopancreatic diversion with or without duodenal switch as revision for failed lapband. Surg Endosc 17:S187, 2003.

97. Centers for Disease Control, National Hospital Discharge Summary Survey, 2001.

CHAPTER 17

ANESTHESIOLOGY PRINCIPLES, PAIN MANAGEMENT, AND CONSCIOUS SEDATION

Edward Sherwood, M.D., Ph.D., Courtney G. Williams, M.D. and Donald S. Prough, M.D.

The relatively brief history of anesthesiology began only a little more than 150 years ago with the administration of the first ether anesthetic. Throughout much of the subsequent history, the risk of anesthesia-related mortality and morbidity has been unacceptably high as a consequence of primitive equipment, complication-prone drugs, and lack of adequate monitors. However, during the past four decades, rapid technologic and pharmacologic progress has resulted in the ability to provide anesthesia safely for complex surgical procedures, even in patients with severe underlying diseases. The importance of continuously improving the safety of the practice of anesthesiology is evident in the practice guidelines developed by the American Society of Anesthesiologists (ASA). These guidelines are available at the ASA web site: *www.ASA.org*.

The most notable advances in anesthesia equipment have been anesthetic machines that reduce the possibility of providing hypoxic gas mixtures, vaporizers that provide more accurate doses of potent inhalational agents, and intraoperative anesthesia ventilators that provide more precise physiologic support. Pharmacologic advances have generally consisted of shorter-acting drugs with fewer important side effects. However, the greatest advances have been in monitoring devices. With currently

available monitoring devices, 40-year-old anesthesia machines and drugs could be used safely to provide anesthesia for many current procedures. Monitoring devices of particular value include in-circuit FIO_2 analyzers, capnometers, pulse oximeters, and agent-specific analyzers. Although these monitors do not guarantee a successful outcome, they markedly increase that probability. In this chapter the stage is set for discussing anesthetic management by first reviewing the unique aspects of the anesthetic environment: the drugs, equipment, and monitors that are the basis for safe practice. Subsequent sections address preanesthetic assessment and preparation for anesthesia, selection of anesthetic techniques and drugs, typical scenarios of regional and general anesthetic management, airway management, intraoperative fluid and blood management, postanesthetic care, and management of acute postoperative pain.

PHARMACOLOGIC PRINCIPLES

The initial practice of anesthesiology used single drugs such as ether or chloroform to abolish consciousness, prevent movement during surgery, ensure amnesia, and provide analgesia. In contrast, current anesthesia practice combines multiple agents, often including regional techniques, to achieve specific endpoints. Although inhalational agents remain the core of modern anesthetic combinations, most anesthesiologists initiate anesthesia with intravenous induction agents and then maintain anesthesia with inhalational agents supplemented by intravenous opioids and muscle relaxants. Benzodiazepines are often added to induce anxiolysis and amnesia. The choice of preoperative medications varies greatly among anesthesiologists, although benzodiazepines and antacids, including H_2 antagonists or proton pump inhibitors, are frequently chosen.

Inhalational Agents

The original inhalational anesthetics—ether, nitrous oxide, and chloroform—had important limitations. Ether was characterized by notoriously slow inductions and equally delayed emergence but could produce unconsciousness, amnesia, analgesia, and lack of movement without the addition of other agents. In contrast, both induction and emergence were rapid with nitrous oxide, but the agent lacked sufficient potency to be used alone. Nitrous oxide is still used in combination with other agents. Chloroform was associated with hepatic toxicity and occasionally fatal cardiac arrhythmias. Subsequent development has emphasized inhalational agents that facilitate rapid induction and emergence and that are nontoxic. These include halothane, isoflurane, enflurane, sevoflurane, and desflurane. The important aspects of each drug can be summarized in terms of key clinical attributes (Table 17-1). Two of the most important characteristics of inhalational anesthetics are the blood/gas (B/G) solubility coefficient and the minimal alveolar concentration (MAC). The B/G solubility coefficient is a measure of the uptake of an agent by blood. In general, less soluble agents (lower B/G solubility coefficients), such as nitrous oxide and desflurane, are associated with more rapid induction and emergence. The MAC is the concentration of agent required to prevent movement in response to a skin incision in 50% of patients. (A higher MAC represents a less potent agent.)

Nitrous Oxide

Although nitrous oxide provides only partial anesthesia at atmospheric pressure its MAC is 104% of inspired gas at sea level. Because nitrous oxide minimally influences respiration and hemodynamics, it often is combined with one of the potent volatile agents to permit a lower dose of the second agent, thus limiting side effects, reducing cost, and facilitating rapid induction and emergence. The most important clinical problem with nitrous oxide is that it is 30 times more soluble than nitrogen and diffuses into closed gas spaces faster than nitrogen diffuses out. Because nitrous oxide increases the volume or pressure of these spaces, it is contraindicated in the presence of closed gas spaces such as pneumothorax, small bowel obstruction, or middle ear surgery and in retinal surgery in which an intraocular gas bubble is created. Because nitrous oxide gradually accumulates in the pneumoperitoneum, some clinicians prefer to avoid its use during laparoscopic procedures. However, periodic venting can prevent buildup,[1] and some investigators have suggested that nitrous oxide might be preferable to CO_2 as the insufflated gas.[1]

Halothane

Introduced in the mid 1950s, halothane provided more rapid induction and emergence than ether. The drug has a pleasant odor that facilitates mask induction and has a variety of useful clinical characteristics (see Table 17-1). Halothane's MAC is 0.74 vol% in adults. Because the vapor pressure of halothane is 240 mm Hg (30% of atmospheric pressure), halothane can be administered at concentrations greatly exceeding MAC (a technique called overpressure) at the beginning of anesthesia to more quickly increase alveolar and blood concentration. A potent bronchodilator, halothane was previously the inhalational

TABLE 17-1.   Important Characteristics of Inhalational Agents

Anesthetic	Potency	Speed of Induction and Emergence	Suitability for Inhalational Induction	Sensitization to Catecholamines	% Metabolized
Nitrous oxide	Weak	Fast	Insufficient alone	None	Minimal
Diethyl ether	Potent	Very slow	Suitable	None	10
Halothane	Potent	Medium	Suitable	High	20+
Enflurane	Potent	Medium	Not suitable	Medium	<10
Isoflurane	Potent	Medium	Not suitable	Minimal	<2
Sevoflurane	Potent	Rapid	Suitable	Minimal	<5
Desflurane	Potent	Rapid	Not suitable	Minimal	0.02

agent of choice in patients at risk for bronchospasm, although other agents have subsequently been shown to provide equivalent bronchodilation.

Halothane has numerous shortcomings that have contributed to its almost complete replacement by newer agents. First, the drug is a powerful cardiac depressant that could potentially be beneficial in patients with ischemic heart disease but can precipitate acute decompensation in patients with severe left ventricular dysfunction (Table 17-2). Second, halothane sensitizes the myocardium to catecholamines, which is a particular problem in surgical procedures in which epinephrine is added to local anesthetic that is infiltrated into the surgical site. Third, halothane is associated with a rare form of fulminant hepatitis that presents as postoperative fever and jaundice and is microscopically indistinguishable from viral hepatitis. The incidence, about 1/35,000, is thought to be due to metabolites of halothane.

In contrast to chloroform, halothane is not a direct hepatotoxin. However, in adults, the incidence of hepatitis is increased sevenfold if halothane is repeated within 3 months. Therefore, halothane is best avoided in adults who have received the agent within the preceding year. Because halothane hepatitis has not been reported in children younger than 8 years of age, halothane can be used repeatedly in children. For medicolegal reasons, prudence also suggests that halothane should be avoided in cases in which there is a potential for postoperative liver problems (e.g., trauma, history of viral hepatitis, or liver surgery) or if the patient has taken enzyme-inducing drugs such as phenobarbital and isoniazid. Although the majority of halothane is eliminated through the lungs, as are other inhalational anesthetics, approximately 20% is metabolized, primarily to nontoxic compounds. Like all other potent inhalational agents, halothane occasionally triggers malignant hyperthermia.[2]

Enflurane

Introduced in the 1970s as an alternative to halothane, enflurane failed to achieve wide popularity. Although enflurane is less soluble than halothane and produces less cardiac sensitization to catecholamines, the drug is metabolized to fluoride (F^-) and, after prolonged administration, especially in obese patients, is associated with mild renal dysfunction. In addition, enflurane is relatively contraindicated in patients with seizure disorders because it induces epileptiform electroencephalographic (EEG) changes that are most pronounced at high inspired concentrations and with hypocapnia.

Isoflurane

Approved by the Food and Drug Administration in 1979, isoflurane rapidly replaced halothane as the most commonly used potent inhalational agent. Despite the recent release of sevoflurane and desflurane, isoflurane remains popular, at least in part because the cost of the now-generic compound is well below that of the newer agents. Isoflurane has several advantages over halothane, including less reduction of cardiac output, less sensitization to the arrhythmogenic effects of catecholamines, and minimal metabolism. However, isoflurane-induced tachycardia, a variable response, can increase myocardial oxygen consumption. Careful observation of the heart rate is necessary when it is used in patients with coronary artery disease (CAD). In concentrations of 1.0 MAC or less, isoflurane causes little increase in cerebral blood flow and intracranial pressure (ICP) and depresses cerebral metabolic activity more than halothane or enflurane. The pungent odor virtually precludes use for inhalational induction.

TABLE 17-2. Cardiopulmonary Effects of Inhalational Anesthetics

Inhalational Agent	Blood Pressure	Heart Rate	Cardiac Output	Sensitization to Catecholamines	Ventilatory Depression	Bronchodilation
Nitrous oxide	Little effect	Little effect	Little effect	No	Minimal	No
Halothane	Marked dose-dependent decrease	Moderate decrease	Marked dose-dependent decrease	Marked	Moderate dose-dependent	Moderate
Enflurane	Marked dose-dependent decrease	Moderate decrease	Moderate dose-dependent decrease	Moderate	Marked dose-dependent	Minimal
Isoflurane	Moderate dose-dependent decrease	Variable increase	Minimal decrease	Minimal	Marked dose-dependent	Moderate
Sevoflurane	Moderate dose-dependent decrease	Little effect	Moderate dose-dependent decrease	Minimal	Moderate dose-dependent	Moderate
Desflurane	Minimal decrease	Variable; marked increase with rapid increase in concentration	Minimal decrease	Minimal	Marked dose-dependent	Moderate

Sevoflurane

Sevoflurane's relatively low solubility facilitates rapid induction and emergence. Sevoflurane is associated with faster emergence than isoflurane, especially in longer cases, although slightly faster emergence does not result in earlier discharge after outpatient surgery. Sevoflurane is associated with low incidences of postoperative somnolence and nausea in the postanesthesia care unit (PACU) and in the first 24 hours after discharge than isoflurane. Unlike isoflurane, sevoflurane is pleasant to inhale, making it suitable for inhalational induction in children. However, the clinical differences between halothane and sevoflurane are subtle. In premedicated pediatric patients undergoing bilateral myringotomy and tube placement and randomized to receive sevoflurane or halothane, anesthesiologists correctly identified the agent (to which they were blinded) in only 56.6% of cases.[3]

Sevoflurane is clinically suitable for outpatient surgery, mask induction of patients with potentially difficult airways, and maintenance of patients with bronchospastic disease. When sevoflurane, halothane, and isoflurane were compared with thiopental/nitrous oxide anesthesia, all three of the potent agents decreased respiratory resistance in endotracheally intubated nonasthmatics; sevoflurane reduced airway resistance more than halothane or isoflurane.[4] Another advantage of sevoflurane is that the cardiovascular side effects are minimal.

However, considerable metabolic transformation takes place, resulting in increases in serum F^- and, in the presence of soda lime or Baralyme, production of "compound A," a metabolite that is toxic in experimental animals. Although nephrotoxicity secondary to the obsolete anesthetic methoxyflurane has clearly been linked to F^-, comparable plasma concentrations of F^- are not achieved with sevoflurane. β-Lyase, the enzyme responsible for formation of compound A,[5] has 8 to 30 times greater activity in rat kidneys than in human kidney tissue.[6] In humans, the toxicity of compound A appears to be theoretical and not clinically important.

Desflurane

Desflurane is rapidly taken up and eliminated. After anesthesia lasting more than 3 hours, desflurane was associated with more rapid recovery than isoflurane.[7] The most volatile of the potent inhalational agents, desflurane must be administered through electrically heated vaporizers that release pure desflurane vapor, which then mix with carrier gas to produce specific inspired concentrations. However, its pungent odor precludes inhalational induction. Generally benign hemodynamically, desflurane is associated with tachycardia and hypertension if the concentration is too rapidly increased.[8]

When exposed to dry CO_2 absorbent, desflurane, isoflurane, and enflurane are partially converted to carbon monoxide. Desflurane, enflurane, and isoflurane produce more carbon monoxide than halothane or sevoflurane. Carbon monoxide production is greater in dry CO_2 absorbent, in Baralyme in comparison to soda lime, at higher temperatures, and at higher anesthetic concentra-

tions.[9] Because continued gas flow in an unused machine will desiccate CO_2 absorbent, turning off gas flow in anesthesia machines after the last case of the day can reduce carbon monoxide production.

Intravenous Agents

Since the introduction of thiopental, intravenous agents have become an indispensable component of modern anesthetic practice. However, they are used without inhalational agents in only a minority of anesthetics. After intravenous agents are used only for induction of anesthesia, potent opioids are often used as part of a multidrug combination to produce anesthesia. Propofol, a newer intravenous anesthetic, has been combined with potent opioids for total intravenous anesthesia.

Induction Agents

Most adult patients and many older children prefer intravenous induction to inhalational induction. Intravenous inductions are rapid, pleasant, and safe for the vast majority of patients, although there are situations in which intravenous induction introduces hazards. The five intravenous agents most commonly used in the United States for induction of anesthesia are sodium thiopental, ketamine, propofol, etomidate, and midazolam.

Induction with thiopental, the oldest intravenous induction agent, is rapid and pleasant. Although the drug is remarkably well tolerated by a wide variety of patients, several clinical situations necessitate caution (Table 17-3). In hypovolemic patients and in those with congestive heart failure, thiopental-induced vasodilation and cardiac depression can lead to severe hypotension unless doses are markedly reduced. In such patients, etomidate or ketamine are alternative agents. Although thiopental does not directly precipitate bronchospasm, patients with reactive airway disease may develop bronchospasm in response to the intense airway stimulation produced by endotracheal intubation. Endotracheal intubation, but not laryngeal mask airway (LMA) insertion, is associated with reversible bronchoconstriction after induction with a combination of fentanyl, thiopental, and succinylcholine.[10] Consequently, propofol or ketamine are often chosen as alternatives for induction in patients with reactive airway disease.

In usual doses used for induction of anesthesia, thiopental is associated with rapid emergence because of redistribution of the agent from the brain to peripheral tissues, particularly fat. In higher doses, circulating blood levels increase and the action of thiopental must be terminated by hepatic metabolism, which eliminates only about 10% per hour.

Ketamine, which produces a dissociative state of anesthesia, is the only intravenous induction agent that increases blood pressure and heart rate and decreases bronchomotor tone. Usually associated with increased sympathetic tone, ketamine causes direct cardiac depression that may become evident if given to patients with high preanesthetic sympathetic tone, as in patients with

TABLE 17-3. Clinical Characteristics of Intravenous Induction Agents

IV Induction Agent	Dose (mg/kg)	Comments	Side Effects	Situations Requiring Caution	Relative Indications
Thiopental	2-5	Inexpensive; slow emergence after high doses	Hypotension	Hypovolemia; compromised cardiac function	Suitable for induction in many patients
Ketamine	1-2	Psychotropic side effects controllable with benzodiazepines; good bronchodilator; potent analgesic in subinduction doses	Hypertension, tachycardia	Coronary disease; severe hypovolemia	Rapid sequence induction of asthmatics, patients in shock (reduced doses)
Propofol	1-2	Burns on injection; good bronchodilator; associated with low incidence of postoperative nausea and vomiting	Hypotension	Coronary artery disease; hypovolemia	Induction of outpatients; induction of asthmatics
Etomidate	0.1-0.3	Cardiovascularly stable; burns on injection; spontaneous movement during induction	Adrenal suppression (with continuous infusion)	Hypovolemia	Induction of patients with cardiac contractile dysfunction; induction of patients in shock (reduced doses)
Midazolam	0.15-0.3	Relatively stable hemodynamics; potent amnesia	Synergistic ventilatory depression with opioids	Hypovolemia	Induction of patients with cardiac contractile dysfunction (usually in combination with opioids)

hemorrhagic shock. In markedly reduced doses (15% to 20% of the usual induction dose), ketamine is an appropriate choice for intravenous induction of severely hypovolemic patients in whom it causes the least fall in blood pressure of any of the induction agents. Ketamine is an appropriate agent for intravenous induction of asthmatic patients because it reduces the increase in bronchomotor tone associated with endotracheal intubation. Among the intravenous induction agents, ketamine also causes the least amount of ventilatory depression and loss of airway reflexes. However, owing to the induction by ketamine of copious oropharyngeal secretions a drying agent such as glycopyrrolate is usually administered with ketamine.

Ketamine can be used as the sole anesthetic for brief, superficial procedures because it produces profound amnesia and somatic analgesia. It is less useful, however, for abdominal cases or delicate surgery because it produces no muscular relaxation, does not control visceral pain, and may not completely control patient movement. The potent pain-relieving effects of ketamine have been exploited for preemptive analgesia. In patients in whom ketamine was infused continuously before incision and continued through wound closure, in contrast to patients to whom ketamine was administered only after wound closure, postoperative morphine consumption was significantly lower on postoperative days 1 and 2.[11]

In patients with CAD, ketamine usually is avoided because tachycardia and increased blood pressure may cause myocardial ischemia. In patients with increased ICP (e.g., after traumatic brain injury) ketamine may further increase ICP because it is the only intravenous agent that increases cerebral blood flow. Another clinically important side effect of ketamine is emergence delirium and bad dreams. In adults and older children, supplemental benzodiazepines or volatile agents are necessary to prevent emergence delirium.

Propofol, popular as an induction agent for ambulatory surgery, is a short-acting induction agent that is associated with smooth, nausea-free emergence. Small doses also are useful for short-term sedation during brief procedures such as performance of retrobulbar or peribulbar eye blocks. The primary limitations of propofol are pain on injection and blood pressure reduction. The latter precludes use in patients who may be hypovolemic and prompts caution in patients, such as those with severe CAD, who may tolerate hypotension poorly.

Propofol also produces excellent bronchodilation. In asthmatic patients, 0% (95% confidence interval 0%, 9%) of those who received propofol wheezed at 2 or 5 minutes after intubation versus 45% (23%, 67%) of those who received a thiobarbiturate and 26% (8%, 44%) of those who received an oxybarbiturate.[12] In nonasthmatic patients, three fourths of whom smoked, airway resistance was less after induction with propofol, 2.5 mg/kg, than after induction with thiopental, 5 mg/kg, or etomidate, 0.4 mg/kg.[13] Brown and colleagues[14] demonstrated that the bronchodilatory effects of propofol and ketamine are mediated through neural mechanisms, such as block of vagally mediated and cholinergically mediated bronchoconstriction.

Etomidate is an imidazole compound that produces minimal hemodynamic changes. Because it preserves blood pressure in most patients, etomidate is often chosen as an alternative for induction of patients with cardiovascular disease. Major drawbacks include burning pain on injection, abnormal muscular movements (myoclonus), and adrenal suppression when given as a prolonged infusion for sedation of critically ill patients.

Midazolam is sometimes used for induction because it usually causes minimal cardiovascular side effects and has a much shorter duration of action than diazepam. The onset of action is acceptably rapid and, even in smaller doses, induces profound amnesia for painful or anxiety-producing events. Midazolam is often selected for induction of patients for cardiovascular surgery. Because midazolam combines powerful anxiolytic and amnesic effects, smaller doses also are commonly used to premedicate anxious patients and as a component of a multidrug anesthetic.

Opioids

Opioids are used in the majority of patients undergoing general anesthesia and are given systemically to many patients receiving regional or local anesthesia. As a component of a multifaceted anesthetic, opioids produce profound analgesia and minimal cardiac depression. Their disadvantages include ventilatory depression and inconsistent hypnosis and amnesia that usually must be provided by other agents.

Several reasons explain the universal popularity of opioids in anesthetic management. First, they reduce the MAC of potent inhalational agents. For instance, fentanyl (3 ng/mL plasma concentration) decreased the MAC of sevoflurane by 59% and reduced MAC_{awake} (the alveolar concentration at which an emerging patient responds to commands) by 24%.[15] Second, opioids blunt the hypertensive and tachycardic response to endotracheal intubation and incision. Third, they provide analgesia that extends through the early postemergence interval and facilitates a smoother awakening from anesthesia. Fourth, in doses 10 to 20 times the analgesic dose, opioids act as complete anesthetics in a high proportion of patients, providing not only analgesia but also hypnosis and amnesia. This characteristic has prompted their use in cardiac surgery patients, sometimes as sole anesthetic agents and more often as a major component of the anesthetic. Finally, they are now often added to local anesthetic solutions in epidural and intrathecal blocks to improve the quality of analgesia.

Morphine, hydromorphone, and meperidine are inexpensive, intermediate-acting agents that are less commonly used for maintenance of anesthesia than for postoperative analgesia. Fentanyl, a synthetic opioid that is 100 to 150 times more potent than morphine, remains popular because of its proven record and because it is inexpensive. Newer synthetic, short-acting opioids, including sufentanil and alfentanil, are also quickly metabolized and excreted but are more expensive. Remifentanil, an opioid metabolized by serum esterases, is particularly short acting but is the most expensive narcotic in clinical use.

Neuromuscular Blockers

Fifty years ago, anesthesia typically was conducted using single potent inhalational agents that produced all of the components of general anesthesia, including whatever degree of muscle relaxation was necessary for the conduct of surgery. Among the drawbacks of this approach was the fact that the depth of anesthesia necessary to produce profound muscle relaxation was much deeper than that necessary to provide hypnosis and amnesia. The addition of muscle relaxants afforded the opportunity to deliver only enough of the inhalational and intravenous agents to achieve hypnosis, amnesia, and analgesia, while still providing satisfactory operating conditions.

The two categories of neuromuscular blockers in clinical use are depolarizing (noncompetitive) agents and nondepolarizing (competitive) agents. The depolarizing agents exert agonistic effects at the cholinergic receptors of the neuromuscular junction, initially causing contractions evident as fasciculations, followed by an interval of profound relaxation. The nondepolarizing neuromuscular blockers compete for receptor sites with acetylcholine, with the magnitude of block dependent on the availability of acetylcholine and the affinity of the agent for the receptor.

Succinylcholine, the only depolarizing agent still in use, remains popular for endotracheal intubation because of its rapid onset and its short duration of action. However, it is associated with serious hazards, including hyperkalemia and malignant hyperthermia, in a small proportion of patients. The drug can be administered in a relatively high dose for intubation because it is rapidly metabolized by plasma pseudocholinesterase except in a small fraction of patients with atypical or absent pseudocholinesterase. Because the duration of action is only 5 minutes, a patient who cannot be successfully intubated can be ventilated by mask for a short time until spontaneous respiration resumes. However, a patient who cannot be ventilated by mask will not resume spontaneous breathing before the onset of life-threatening hypoxemia.[16]

The side effects of succinylcholine include bradycardia, especially in children, and severe, life-threatening hyperkalemia in patients with burns, paraplegia, quadriplegia, and massive trauma. Succinylcholine, when combined with a volatile agent, is also implicated in triggering malignant hyperthermia in susceptible individuals. Therefore, it is best avoided in patients with a family history of malignant hyperthermia or those at risk for malignant hyperthermia, including patients with muscular dystrophy. Some anesthesiologists avoid succinylcholine in children because masseter spasm is a common occurrence that may presage malignant hyperthermia but usually is a benign occurrence. Because succinylcholine is a depolarizing agent that causes visible muscle fasciculations, it has been implicated in causing postoperative muscle pain that can be reduced by pretreatment with a small, "precurarizing" dose of a nondepolarizing agent. Because of the multiple sporadic problems associated with the use of succinylcholine, some anesthesiologists now reserve its use for only those situations in which an airway must be rapidly secured (i.e., a rapid sequence induction). In other situations, nondepolarizing agents, chosen largely on the basis of mode of excretion and duration of action are preferable. For instance, *cis*-atracurium is largely metabolized in the serum by Hoffman degradation and is suitable for patients with reduced renal function, in whom pancuronium and vecuronium would be unsuitable because they are partially eliminated by the kidneys.

Nondepolarizing relaxants are used when succinylcholine is contraindicated, as an alternative to succinylcholine for patients in whom easy endotracheal intubation is anticipated, and when intraoperative relaxation is required to facilitate surgical exposure. The older, longer-acting drugs *d*-tubocurarine, pancuronium, and metocurine are sometimes used for longer operations, whereas *cis*-atracurium, vecuronium, mivacurium, and rocuronium are used for shorter cases. The costs of muscle relaxants vary widely. Pancuronium is inexpensive but difficult to use in cases lasting less than 90 minutes. *cis*-Atracurium, vecuronium, mivacurium, and rocuronium are more expensive. Knowledge of the side effects of individual agents (often related to vagolysis or histamine release) and routes of metabolism plays a major role in the selection of specific agents for individual cases. Doses required to provide satisfactory operating conditions are summarized in Table 17-4.

Dosing of nondepolarizing agents requires knowledge of several important characteristics. First, the use of neuromuscular blockers prevents movement in response to noxious stimuli. Therefore, chemical paralysis can mask the signs of inadequate anesthesia (or sedation or analgesia in postoperative patients). Medicolegal claims of intraoperative awareness during general anesthesia were more than twice as frequent in patients receiving intraoperative muscle relaxants.[17] Second, higher doses are required to provide satisfactory conditions for intubation than for surgical relaxation. Therefore, if a nondepolarizer is used only after intubation, smaller doses are required. Third, other anesthetic drugs potentiate the actions of nondepolarizing agents. Succinylcholine used for intubation decreases subsequent requirements for nondepolarizers. Potent inhalational agents dose-dependently potentiate the effects of competitive neuromuscular blockers.[18] The newer inhalational agent desflurane potentiates the effects of vecuronium approximately 20% more than isoflurane.[19] Fourth, individual responses to muscle relaxants vary widely, with patients demonstrating both markedly increased and markedly decreased neuromuscular block in comparison to expected levels.

Fifth, and most importantly, subtle blockade can be difficult to detect and can be associated with postoperative problems. The importance of subtle residual paralysis has been quantified using the train-of-four (TOF) fade ratio, a semiquantitative monitoring technique used to assess the adequacy of neuromuscular blockade and the adequacy of pharmacologic reversal. At the conclusion of anesthesia, a TOF ratio of more than 0.70 has been considered adequate return of neuromuscular function. This ratio means that the fourth of four muscle twitches in response to supramaximal stimuli delivered at 0.5-second intervals to the ulnar nerve is at least 70% of the magnitude of the first twitch. A recent report characterized the symptoms of volunteers receiving graded doses of muscle relaxants in comparison to TOF ratios.[20] A sustained 5-second head-lift (a commonly used clinical index of adequate reversal) was achieved if the TOF ratio averaged more than 0.60. At TOF ratios less than 0.70, all subjects maintained patent airways and oxygen saturation greater than 96%. However, at TOF ratios less than 0.90, subjects had diplopia and had difficulty tracking objects in all directions. The ability to strongly oppose the incisors did not return until the TOF was more than 0.90. The authors concluded that satisfactory return of neuromuscular function requires return of the TOF to more than 0.90 and ideally to 1.0.[20] In patients who received the intermediate-acting neuromuscular blockers atracurium, vecuronium, or rocuronium only for endotracheal intubation, the TOF was lower than 0.9 in 37% of patients 2 hours after receiving the muscle relaxant.[21]

The use of neuromuscular blocking agents in general, and nondepolarizing agents in particular, necessitates a strategy to ensure adequate muscular function at the conclusion of anesthesia. Many of the complications associated with neuromuscular blockers relate to inadequate reversal at the conclusion of cases or inadequate assessment of reversal.

At the conclusion of anesthesia, nondepolarizing relaxants usually are pharmacologically reversed using an anticholinesterase (neostigmine or edrophonium), accompanied by atropine or glycopyrrolate to counteract the muscarinic effects of the anticholinesterase. However, recovery depends both on the intensity of neuromuscular blockade at the time that reversal is attempted and the effects of the reversal agent. At the end of anesthesia, profound neuromuscular block may preclude reliable antagonism by an anticholinesterase within 5 to 10 minutes.[22]

TABLE 17-4. Dose-Response Relationships of Nondepolarizing Neuromuscular Blocking Drugs in Humans

	ED_{50} (mg/kg)	ED_{95} (mg/kg)
d-Tubocurarine	0.23 (0.16-0.26)	0.48 (0.34-0.56)
Pancuronium	0.036 (0.022-0.042)	0.067 (0.059-0.080)
Vecuronium	0.027 (0.015-0.031)	0.043 (0.037-0.059)
Atracurium	0.12 (0.08-0.15)	0.21 (0.13-0.28)
Mivacurium	0.039 (0.027-0.052)	0.067 (0.045-0.081)
Rocuronium	0.147 (0.069-0.220)	0.305 (0.257-0.521)

ED_{50}, dose effective for surgical relaxation in 50% of patients; ED_{95}, dose effective for surgical relaxation in 95% of patients; means (95% confidence limits). Somewhat larger doses are required to facilitate endotracheal intubation. Modified from Savarese JJ, Caldwell JE, Lien CA, Miller RD: Pharmacology of muscle relaxants and their antagonists. *In* Miller RD, Cucchiara RF, Miller RG Jr, et al (eds): Anesthesia, 5th ed. Philadelphia, Churchill Livingstone, 2000, pp 412-490.

With the longer-acting muscle relaxants, residual blockade potentially can complicate postoperative recovery. In a clinical trial of reversal of muscle relaxation, 691 patients undergoing abdominal, gynecologic, or orthopedic surgery under general anesthesia were randomized to receive pancuronium, vecuronium, or atracurium. After reversal with neostigmine, a higher proportion (26%) of patients who had received pancuronium had residual neuromuscular blockade (TOF < 0.70) than did patients who had received vecuronium or atracurium (5.3% combined).[23] Patients who received pancuronium and had a TOF less than 0.70 had a higher incidence of atelectasis or pneumonia on postoperative chest radiography (16.9% of 59 patients in that category). There was no association between postoperative pulmonary complications and residual blockade with the other two muscle relaxants.

One key factor determining recovery from neuromuscular blockade is the ability to metabolize and excrete the drugs. In patients with renal disease, the half-lives of *d*-tubocurarine, rocuronium, vecuronium, and pancuronium are prolonged. In such patients, alternative drugs include atracurium or *cis*-atracurium, which are metabolized by Hoffman degradation and thus do not have prolonged half-lives in patients with renal dysfunction.

ANESTHESIA EQUIPMENT

Anesthesia equipment has undergone rapid development over the past few decades. Delivery systems for inhaled anesthetic agents have become more complex but also have become more difficult to misuse. Despite many years of improving design, hazards of gas delivery systems must still be considered.[24] Adverse anesthetic outcomes were associated with gas delivery equipment in 72 of 3791 claims in the ASA closed claims database. Misuse of equipment occurred in 75% of incidents, and 78% could have been detected with monitoring using pulse oximetry, capnography, or both devices.[25]

Major items of anesthesia equipment include the anesthesia machine, anesthesia vaporizers, monitoring devices (discussed in a later section), the anesthetic circuit, the anesthesia ventilator, the anesthetic gas scavenging system, and various smaller pieces of equipment generally related to vascular access and airway management.

The essential elements of an anesthesia machine are gas sources (oxygen, nitrous oxide, and air), flowmeters, and a flow proportioning device. In recent years, microprocessor controls have replaced some of the older mechanical components. The gas sources can be small, attached tanks that are pin-indexed to prevent accidental connection of incorrect tanks or can be wall outlets that provide gas from large remote tanks. The flowmeters allow independent adjustment of individual gases but are designed to minimize the chance of delivering a hypoxic gas mixture by both "fail-safe" valves that require pressurization of the oxygen line before nitrous oxide can be delivered and by flow-proportioning devices that automatically reduce the flow of nitrous oxide if the flow of oxygen is reduced below a safe concentration.

Most anesthetic vaporizers are agent-specific, temperature-compensated devices that divert a proportion of fresh gas through a system that saturates the diverted gas with anesthetic vapor before it rejoins the remainder of the gas flow. Desflurane, however, has a vapor pressure that is close to atmospheric pressure at room temperature. Therefore, the desflurane vaporizer heats a small quantity of liquid desflurane to generate a specific volume of vapor that then is added to the fresh gas flow.

The most commonly used anesthetic circuit is a circle system with one-way valves that direct inspired and expired gas flow. The typical circuit includes a CO_2 absorber containing either soda lime (sodium hydroxide, calcium hydroxide, and potassium hydroxide) or Baralyme (a combination of barium hydroxide and calcium hydroxide). As CO_2 flows through the absorber, insoluble carbonates are formed until the absorbent is exhausted. Gas flow is adjusted to provide sufficient oxygen for metabolism and to provide sufficient anesthetic vapor while limiting the expense of anesthetic that is lost through the gas scavenging system. In addition to adult and pediatric circle systems, there are a variety of systems that do not include a CO_2 absorber and that depend on the total volume of fresh gas flow to eliminate exhaled CO_2.

Most anesthesia machines have a built-in mechanical ventilator. Generally, these are volume-controlled, gas-driven ventilators that are capable of ventilating most anesthetized patients and can provide a limited amount of positive end-expiratory pressure. However, they have a limited range of features and are not suitable for ventilating the occasional patient with severe respiratory failure.

Gas scavenging systems are attached to the exhaust valve of anesthetic circuits to permit elimination of anesthetic gases and vapors that otherwise would contaminate the operating room environment. Although the health risks of operating room contamination are poorly quantified, the general consensus is that exhausting gases into the operating room risks potential harm to personnel and their offspring. The gas is exhausted into the air outside the hospital or ambulatory surgery center where the dilution with ambient air is so great that no health risks are considered to be present.

Although not yet a routine component of anesthesia equipment, the development of computerized anesthesia information systems promises to improve the accuracy of anesthesia records. Some systems integrate data from the anesthesia machine as well as monitoring devices to provide an on-line record of intraoperative events. In addition, automated record keeping can include information regarding the types and doses of agents used. One promised benefit of automated record keeping that has not yet been realized is time saving. Based on videotaping of anesthesiologists with and without an automated system, record keeping still occupies 10% to 15% of an anesthesiologist's time.[26] However, automated systems offer promise in improved detection of intraoperative events that have implications for quality and in improved cost containment. Electronic scanning of computerized anesthesia records markedly increased detection of intraoperative incidents, in comparison to voluntary reporting.[27]

PATIENT MONITORING DURING AND AFTER ANESTHESIA

Effective monitoring is a critical aspect of anesthesia care. The essential components of monitoring include observation and vigilance, instrumentation, data analysis, and institution of corrective measures, if indicated. The goal of patient monitoring is to provide optimal anesthetic management and to detect abnormalities early in their course so that corrective measures can be instituted before serious or irreversible injury occurs. Although it is difficult to directly relate improved patient outcomes with specific monitors, the reduction in anesthesia-related morbidity and mortality has paralleled the institution of current monitoring practices.

The indications as well as risks and benefits associated with the use of noninvasive and invasive electronic monitors must be assessed (Table 17-5). These decisions should be guided by the patient's medical condition, the type of surgery, and the potential complications associated with invasive monitoring. However, the proliferation of electronic monitoring devices does not circumvent the need for clinical skills such as observation, inspection, auscultation, and palpation. The ASA has established standards for basic anesthetic monitoring that are designed to integrate clinical skills and electronic monitoring with the goal of enhancing patient safety.[28]

Standard I asserts that a qualified anesthesia care provider must be continuously present in the operating

TABLE 17-5. Routine and Specialized Electronic Monitors Used in Anesthetic Practice and Their Indications

Type of Monitor	Indications
Routine Monitors	
Pulse oximetry	Measure blood oxygen saturation Heart rate
Automated blood pressure cuff	Blood pressure
Electrocardiography	Heart rhythm Heart rate Monitor of myocardial ischemia
Capnography	Adequacy of ventilation Intratracheal placement of endotracheal tube
Oxygen analyzer	Monitoring of delivered oxygen concentration
Ventilator pressure monitor	Ventilator disconnection during general anesthesia Monitoring of airway pressures
Thermometry	Temperature monitoring
Specialized Monitors	
Foley catheter	Monitoring of urine output Gross indicator of intravascular volume status and renal perfusion
Arterial catheter	Continuous measurement of arterial blood pressure Sampling of arterial blood
Central venous catheter	Continuous measurement of central venous pressure Delivery of centrally acting drugs Rapid administration of fluids and blood
Pulmonary artery catheter	Measurement of pulmonary artery pressures Measurement of left ventricular pressures Measurement of cardiac output Measurement of mixed venous oxygenation
Precordial Doppler	Detection of air embolism
Transesophageal echocardiography	Evaluation of myocardial performance Assessment of heart valve function Assessment of intravascular volume Detection of air embolism
Esophageal Doppler	Assessment of descending aortic blood flow Assessment of cardiac preload
Transpulmonary indicator dilution	Measurement of cardiac output Measurement of preload
Esophageal and precordial stethoscope	Auscultation of breathing and heart sounds

room during the administration of anesthesia. The practitioner must continuously monitor the status of the patient and alter anesthesia care based on the patient's response to the dynamic changes associated with anesthesia and surgery. Standard II, which mandates continuous assessment of ventilation, oxygenation, circulation, and temperature, specifically requires:

1. The use of an oxygen analyzer with a low concentration alarm during general anesthesia.
2. Quantitative assessment of blood oxygenation such as by pulse oximetry.
3. Continuous assurance of adequacy of ventilation by clinical evaluation. Quantitative monitoring of CO_2 content in expired gas is recommended.
4. Clinical assessment and the presence of CO_2 in expired gases to ensure correct tube placement after endotracheal intubation. Continuous use of a device capable of detecting disconnection of breathing system components is required during mechanical ventilation. This device must give an audible signal when its alarm threshold is exceeded.
5. Continuous electrocardiographic (ECG) monitoring during anesthesia and blood pressure and heart rate evaluation at least every 5 minutes. In patients undergoing general anesthesia, circulatory function must be continuously monitored by assessing the adequacy of peripheral circulation using electronic means, palpation, or auscultation.
6. Ready availability of means of temperature evaluation in the operating room that should be utilized during periods of intended or expected changes in body temperature.

Blood Pressure Monitoring

Blood pressure monitoring is required during all anesthetic procedures. Available techniques for noninvasive blood pressure monitoring include palpation, Doppler analysis, auscultation, plethysmography, and arterial tonometry. Most modern operating rooms are equipped with automated oscillometric blood pressure analyzers. Automated blood pressure devices sense changes in oscillation amplitude as the blood pressure cuff is deflated and calculate systolic, mean, and diastolic blood pressures using an algorithm. The accuracy of any noninvasive blood pressure measurement depends on an appropriate width of the blood pressure cuff, which should be 20% to 50% greater than the diameter of the extremity. A cuff that is too narrow will overestimate systolic blood pressure, and one that is too wide will underestimate systolic blood pressure. Blood pressure cuffs should only be cycled as frequently as necessary. Excessive inflation can result in nerve palsies, extremity edema, and extravasation of intravenous fluids. Application of blood pressure cuffs to extremities with vascular or neurologic abnormalities should be avoided.

Indications for invasive blood pressure monitoring include intraoperative use of deliberate hypotension, continuous blood pressure assessment in patients with significant end-organ damage or undergoing high risk surgical procedures, anticipation of wide perioperative blood pressure swings, need for multiple blood gas analyses, and inadequacy of noninvasive blood pressure measurements, such as in morbidly obese patients. Several sites for arterial cannulation are available, each with inherent advantages and potential for complications. The radial artery is most commonly cannulated because of its superficial location, relative ease of cannulation, and, in most patients, adequate collateral flow from the ulnar artery. Other potential sites for percutaneous arterial cannulation include the femoral, brachial, axillary, ulnar, dorsalis pedis, and posterior tibial arteries. Possible complications of intra-arterial monitoring include hematoma, neurologic injury, arterial embolization, limb ischemia, infection, and inadvertent intra-arterial injection of drugs. Intra-arterial catheters should not be placed in extremities with potential vascular insufficiency. However, with proper patient selection, the complication rate associated with intra-arterial cannulation is low and benefits can be important.

Central Venous Monitoring

Central venous cannulation is indicated for monitoring of central venous pressure, chronic intravenous therapy such as hyperalimentation, administration of centrally acting drugs, rapid administration of fluids, insertion of transvenous electrodes, treatment of intraoperative air embolism, and obtaining venous access in patients with difficult peripheral venous access. The internal jugular and subclavian veins are most commonly cannulated, although central access can also be obtained via the external jugular, femoral, and antecubital veins. Central venous pressure monitoring is used as one criterion for assessing fluid management in patients with unclear volume status. Potential complications include hematoma, neurologic injury, pneumothorax, hemothorax, inadvertent arterial cannulation, arrhythmias, cardiac rupture, and thrombosis.

Pulmonary Arterial Catheters

The use of pulmonary arterial catheters (PACs) has generated controversy regarding their safety and effectiveness. The PAC can provide important information regarding volume status, cardiac output, mixed venous oxygenation, pulmonary artery pressures, and left ventricular end-diastolic pressure. The key to utilizing PACs is a detailed knowledge of cardiovascular pathophysiology and understanding of the physiologic implications of generated data. However, many physicians do not have a sufficient understanding of the use and interpretation of PAC data. Of 535 critical care physicians in 86 intensive care units (ICUs) in Europe, only 50% correctly identified the pulmonary arterial occlusion pressure from a clear chart recording.[29] Nevertheless, experience suggests that in well-trained hands, data from PACs can guide the management of many life-threatening conditions, including congestive heart failure, heart valve dysfunction, adult respiratory distress syndrome, and complex fluid management problems such as sepsis, acute renal failure, and shock.[30] However, these benefits are not without risk. Many of the complications associated with PAC placement are secondary to obtaining central venous access. Additional complications include complete heart block, right bundle branch block, pulmonary arterial rupture, pulmonary infarction, cardiac valve injury, and line sepsis.

Transpulmonary Indicator Dilution

Used more commonly in Europe than in the United States, transpulmonary indication dilution (TID) requires the placement of a central venous catheter housing a thermistor that senses injectate temperature and an arterial catheter (usually in the femoral artery) containing a thermistor that senses changes in blood temperature. Cardiac output is determined by thermodilution as it is with PACs. However, because TID measures blood temperature distal to the aortic valve, this technique also estimates specific blood volumes such as intrathoracic blood volume and global end-diastolic cardiac blood volume. Cardiac output measurements made by TID correlated well with those made using PAC.[31] Intrathoracic blood volume measurements may more accurately indicate preload than central venous pressure or pulmonary arterial occlusion pressure. Potential complications are those associated with central venous and femoral arterial cannulation.

Transesophageal Echocardiography

Transesophageal echocardiography (TEE), although expensive and not readily available in all medical centers, is increasingly used as a valuable monitor of intraoperative circulation, particularly during cardiac surgery and in high-risk patients undergoing high-risk procedures. TEE can provide sensitive and accurate information regarding intravascular volume, myocardial function, myocardial ischemia, and valvular integrity. Complications mainly center on esophageal injury associated with probe placement.

Esophageal Doppler

Esophageal Doppler can provide useful information regarding circulation by providing continuous measurement of descending aortic blood flow and, by calculation of systolic time intervals, cardiac preload. Esophageal Doppler probes, approximately the diameter of nasogastric tubes, are easily placed in patients who are free of esophageal pathology. A study by Gan and colleagues[32] demonstrated that esophageal Doppler provided an effective means of directing perioperative fluid management during major surgery.

Electrocardiography

ECG monitoring is a standard of care during administration of anesthesia. Information regarding dysrhythmias and cardiac ischemia can be readily obtained from ECG data. Analysis of ECG tracings is the cornerstone of cardiopulmonary resuscitation protocols.

Ventilation Monitoring

Sedation and opioid administration and the induction of general or regional anesthesia can depress or abolish spontaneous ventilation, necessitating intraoperative ventilatory support. Several means are available to assess the adequacy of ventilation. Among these are physical assessment of chest expansion, auscultation of breath sounds, and evaluation for evidence of upper airway obstruction and stridor. Precordial and esophageal stethoscopes provide continuous input regarding air movement and development of wheezing. During mechanical ventilation, monitors of airway pressure and minute ventilation alert the anesthesiologist to conditions such as disconnection of the ventilatory circuit, dislodgement of the endotracheal tube, obstruction of the gas delivery system, and changes in airway resistance and/or compliance that can impair ventilation.

The advent of end-tidal carbon dioxide ($ETCO_2$) monitoring has greatly enhanced the monitoring of ventilation and the detection of esophageal intubation. In normal individuals, the difference between $ETCO_2$ and $PaCO_2$ is 2 to 5 mm Hg. The gradient between end-tidal and arterial CO_2 reflects dead space ventilation, which is increased in cases of decreased pulmonary blood flow such as pulmonary air embolism or thromboembolism and decreased cardiac output. Therefore, $ETCO_2$ monitoring can also provide important information regarding systemic perfusion.

Oxygenation Monitoring

Monitoring of FIO_2 and hemoglobin oxygen saturation are standards of care during all general anesthetics. Modern anesthesia machines are equipped with oxygen analyzers that detect the delivered oxygen concentration (FIO_2). This monitor, in combination with fail-safe devices, low oxygen delivery alarms, and oxygen ratio monitors greatly decreases the chance of delivering a hypoxic gas mixture during anesthesia.

Pulse oximetry is required during the use of all anesthetics. Oximetry is dependent on the observation that oxygenated and reduced hemoglobin differ in their absorbance of red and infrared light (Beer-Lambert law). To assess arterial oxygen saturation by pulse oximetry (SpO_2), readings are taken during arterial systole. Factors that can alter the accuracy of pulse oximeters include low oxygen saturations, peripheral vasoconstriction, excessive ambient light, malposition of the probe, and methemoglobinemia, carboxyhemoglobinemia, and certain injected dyes. Methemoglobin causes overestimation of SaO_2 at low saturations. Carboxyhemoglobin is interpreted as oxyhemoglobin. Methylene blue and indocyanine green artifactually lower pulse oximetry readings of oxygen saturation. Indigo carmine has a lesser effect. Motion artifact resulting in false alarms can be troubling but can be reduced by more recent technology.

When the accuracy of the pulse oximeter is suspect or when a more precise measurement of oxygen content is needed, pulse oximetry can be supplemented with blood gas analysis of PaO_2. In addition to oxygen saturation, pulse oximeters also provide information regarding tissue perfusion (pulse amplitude) and heart rate.

Temperature Monitoring

Temperature should be monitored in all patients undergoing general anesthesia. The site of measurement depends on the surgical procedure and the physical characteristics of the patient. Esophageal temperature is most commonly measured during general anesthesia. Other sites of temperature monitoring include rectal, cutaneous, tympanic membrane, bladder, nasopharynx, and, in patients with PACs, the pulmonary artery. Because of the potential morbidity associated with hypothermia and hyperthermia, it is important to monitor body temperature and to institute measures to maintain temperature as close to normal as possible.

Neuromuscular Blockade Monitoring

Because of the variability in sensitivity to neuromuscular blockers among patients, it is essential to monitor neuromuscular function in patients receiving intermediate- and long-acting muscle relaxants. The most common sites of monitoring are at the ulnar or orbicularis oculi muscles. The basis of neuromuscular monitoring is the assessment of muscle activity after proximal nerve stimulation (Box 17-1). This evaluation gives an indication of acetylcholine receptor blockade at the neuromuscular junction. The degree of neuromuscular blockade is indicated by decreased evoked response to twitch stimulation.

Central Nervous System Monitoring

Awareness during anesthesia is an uncommon but disturbing complication. Many years of experience with intraoperative EEG signal processing has resulted in the development of the bispectral array (BIS), which is believed to monitor awareness during anesthesia.[33] The monitor is essentially a modified EEG that assesses brain wave activity and reports numbers from 0 to 100 that correlate with level of awareness. A value of 100 represents complete awareness, and 0 indicates complete suppression of brain wave activity. Early data suggest that BIS is an accurate indicator of depth of anesthesia. Monitoring the depth of anesthesia may improve time to awakening and discharge in the outpatient setting.

PREOPERATIVE EVALUATION

The American Association of Anesthesiologists has developed basic standards for preanesthetic care that require that an anesthesiologist evaluate the medical status of the patient, derive a plan for anesthetic care, and discuss the plan with the patient.[34] The Joint Commission for the

---

Box 17-1. Techniques for Assessing Neuromuscular Blockade

Train-of-four: 4 successive 200 msec stimuli over 2 seconds
  Twitch height progressively fades with increasing blockade
  Loss of fourth twitch indicates 75% receptor blockade
  Loss of third twitch indicates 80% blockade
  Loss of second twitch indicates 90% blockade
  Loss of first twitch indicates 100% blockade
  Clinical relaxation requires 75% to 95% blockade
  Presence of four twitches without fade suggests adequate reversal of neuromuscular blockade

Double burst stimulation: 2 successive sets of 50-Hz bursts (3 stimuli/burst) separated by 750 msec (appears as 2 twitches)
  Easier to detect fade visually with this technique than train-of-four
  Loss of second twitch indicates 80% receptor blockade
  Presence of 2 twitches without fade suggests adequate reversal of neuromuscular blockade

Tetany: Sustained 50 or 100 Hz burst
  Duration of sustained contraction fades with increasing blockade
  Sustained contraction for 5 seconds suggests adequate reversal of neuromuscular blockade

---

Accreditation of Healthcare Organizations requires that all patients receiving anesthesia undergo a preanesthetic evaluation. Because a decreasing percentage of patients are admitted to the hospital on the day before surgery, preoperative testing clinics have been developed to facilitate preoperative evaluation. Optimally, preoperative clinics should be efficient, predictable, and thorough.

The anesthesia evaluation serves multiple purposes. First, the patient has the opportunity to meet an anesthesiologist and discuss the expected impact of anesthesia, including the patient's fears and concerns regarding anesthesia and postoperative pain management. The expected perioperative events should be discussed as well as the potential risks of anesthesia. This discussion should be guided by the patient's desire for information regarding the risks and benefits of anesthesia. A perioperative care plan should be developed, guided by patient choices.

Second, the preanesthetic interview should focus on the type of surgery, the underlying conditions necessitating surgery, the history of prior anesthetics, and the presence of coexisting diseases. The preoperative interview allows evaluation of preoperative medical status to determine whether additional medical evaluation or treatment is required before surgery. This process requires a focused history, physical examination, and laboratory evaluation. Current medications must be reviewed to anticipate potential drug interactions and manage medical problems during the perioperative period.

A well-focused history will allow the practitioner to perform targeted physical and laboratory examinations. Overall, the patient's age, gender, and the type of surgery should dictate the need for preoperative testing. Laboratory tests performed within 1 year of surgery probably do not need to be repeated unless a significant change in the patient's medical status has occurred. Healthy patients undergoing elective procedures may not need any preoperative laboratory testing (Table 17-6).

In the current climate of cost containment, preoperative testing must be minimized but effective. Therefore, a skilled preoperative evaluation minimizes unproductive testing yet uncovers and effectively evaluates conditions that have a high probability of resulting in perioperative morbidity or mortality. Fischer[35] has reported that development of an anesthesia preoperative evaluation clinic in a teaching hospital reduced day-of-surgery cancellations and produced a potential savings on preoperative testing of $1 million.

The investigation of conditions that are associated with increased perioperative morbidity is important for reducing the risks associated with anesthesia and surgery. Coexisting conditions that must be carefully evaluated include intravascular volume status, airway abnormalities, cardiovascular disease, pulmonary disease, neurologic disease, renal and hepatic disease, and disorders of nutrition, endocrinology, and metabolism. The performance of preoperative pregnancy testing is controversial. The rationale for performing preoperative pregnancy testing is the potential for spontaneous abortion and birth anomalies associated with surgery and anesthesia. There is no clear evidence to demonstrate an association of anesthetic drugs with the development of fetal anomalies in humans, but animal studies have shown that some anesthetics, such as nitrous oxide, may cause developmental abnormalities. A clear sexual history and documentation of last menstrual cycle should be obtained in women of childbearing age. In ambiguous situations, a preoperative pregnancy test is indicated.

Assessment of Intravascular Volume

Clinical signs that suggest hypovolemia include oliguria, supine hypotension, and a positive tilt test. Oliguria implies hypovolemia, although hypovolemic patients may be nonoliguric and normovolemic patients may be oliguric because of renal failure or stress-induced endocrine responses. Supine hypotension implies a blood volume deficit exceeding 30%. The tilt test adds little to preoperative assessment because of the large number of false positives, especially in elderly patients, and the large number of false negatives, especially in robust young patients. Laboratory evidence that suggests hypovolemia or extracellular volume depletion includes azotemia, low urinary sodium, metabolic alkalosis, and metabolic acidosis. Although hypovolemia does not generate metabolic alkalosis, extracellular volume depletion is a potent stimulus for the maintenance of metabolic alkalosis. Severe hypovolemia may result in systemic hypoperfusion and lactic acidosis. Hematocrit is unchanged by acute hemorrhage until fluid shifts from the interstitial to the intravascular space or until fluids are administered.

TABLE 17-6. Preoperative Testing Recommendations for Asymptomatic Patients Undergoing Elective Surgery

| Age (yr) | General Anesthesia | | MAC or Regional Technique (Men and Women) | Local (Men and Women) |
	Men	Women		
<40	None	Hb or Hct Pregnancy test?	None	None
40-50	ECG	Hb or Hct Pregnancy test?	None	None
50-64	Hb or Hct ECG	Hb or Hct ECG Pregnancy test?	Hb or Hct*	None
65-74	Hb or Hct ECG Creatinine/BUN	Hb or Hct ECG Creatinine/BUN	Hb or Hct* ECG	Hb or Hct*
>74	Hb or Hct ECG Creatinine/BUN Glucose Chest radiograph?	Hb or Hct ECG Creatinine/BUN Glucose Chest radiograph?	Hb or Hct* ECG Creatinine/BUN Glucose	Hb or Hct* ECG Creatinine/BUN

Hb, hemoglobin; Hct, hematocrit; ECG, electrocardiogram; BUN, blood urea nitrogen.
*Within 6 months.
Modified from Roizen M, Cohn S: Preoperative evaluation for elective surgery: What laboratory tests are needed? *In* Stoelting R, et al (eds): Advances in Anesthesia. Chicago, Mosby–Year Book, 1993, vol 10, pp 25-43.

Airway Examination

Airway abnormalities usually are asymptomatic and may not influence a patient's health status until they require expeditious establishment of an airway. Assessing the airway is a crucial step in developing an anesthetic plan. Even if regional anesthesia is planned, general anesthesia could be necessary. The goal of the airway examination is to identify characteristics that could hinder assisted mask ventilation or tracheal intubation. A history of diseases or conditions that are associated with airway closure or difficult laryngoscopy will alert the practitioner to potential airway difficulties. Review of prior anesthetic records can provide invaluable information regarding previous airway management. The airway examination should be completed by systematic inspection of the mouth opening, thyromental distance, neck mobility, and the size of the tongue in relation to the oral cavity (Box 17-2). The patient should be observed in both frontal and profile views. Many airway abnormalities, such as a receding mandible, will not be evident from a frontal view. The size of the tongue in relation to the oral cavity can be graded using the Mallampati classification (Fig. 17-1). The examination is performed with the patient sitting with the head in a neutral position, mouth opened as wide as possible and the tongue protruded maximally. The observer views the oral and pharyngeal structures that are evident. In general, a patient in which the uvula, tonsillar pillars, and soft palate are visible (class I), will be easy to mask ventilate and intubate. Patients with a class IV airway, only hard palate visible, have a higher likelihood of being difficult to mask ventilate and intubate. Of course the Mallampati classification is only one component of the airway examination and should be used in conjunction with other aspects of airway examination and the patient's history to provide a complete airway assessment.

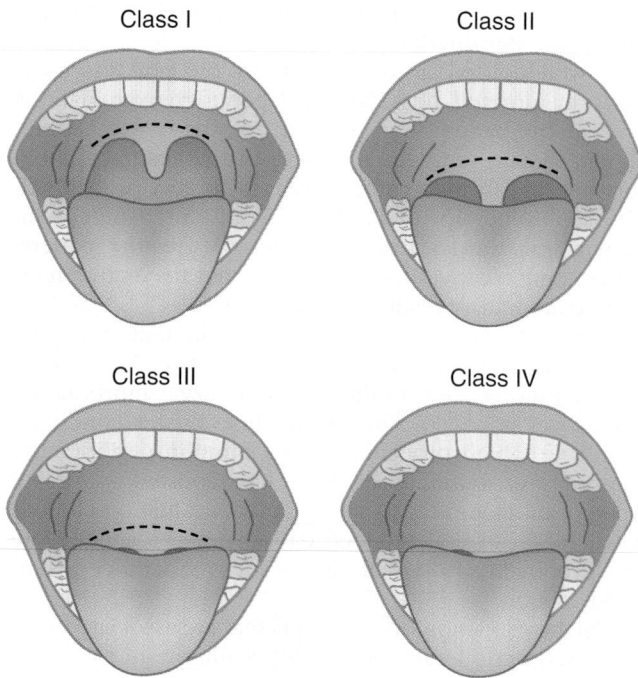

FIGURE 17-1. The Mallampati classification relates tongue size to pharyngeal size. This test is performed with the patient in the sitting position, the head held in a neutral position, the mouth wide open, and the tongue protruding to the maximum. The subsequent classification is assigned based on the pharyngeal structures that are visible. Class I = visualization of the soft palate, fauces, uvula, and anterior and posterior pillars. Class II = visualization of the soft palate, fauces, and uvula. Class III = visualization of the soft palate and the base of the uvula. Class IV = soft palate is not visible at all. From Mallampati SR, Gatt SP, Gugino LD, et al: A clinical sign to predict difficult tracheal intubation: A prospective study. Can Anaesth Soc J 32:429-434, 1985.

Cardiovascular Disease

The risks of perioperative myocardial ischemia and infarction and the risk of cardiac death have been major questions for several decades as progressively more complex surgery has been offered to patients with increasingly severe systemic disease. The apparent incidence of perioperative myocardial ischemia depends on the perspective of the study (prospective or retrospective), the sensitivity of the markers used, and the type of surgical procedure. Major predictors of postoperative myocardial ischemia include (1) ECG evidence of left ventricular hypertrophy; (2) history of hypertension; (3) diabetes mellitus; (4) definite CAD; and (5) use of digoxin. Chronic renal failure has also been shown to be associated with the development of perioperative myocardial ischemia.

The preanesthetic evaluation should identify potentially serious cardiovascular disorders, including CAD, congestive heart failure, and arrhythmias. The American College of Cardiology (ACC) and American Heart Association (AHA) have published guidelines for the evaluation and treatment of CAD in noncardiac surgical patients.[36] These guidelines focus on the patient's history of CAD, exercise tolerance, and the type of surgery (Fig. 17-2). Patients with known CAD are at increased risk for peri-

---

Box 17-2. Important Factors in Performing an Airway Examination

Patient history

Prior anesthetic history
Medical history (e.g., history of oropharyngeal mass, pharyngeal disease)
Review of chart to assess prior airway management in previous anesthetics

Physical examination

Mouth opening (should be 6-8 cm [3-4 fingerbreadths])
Cervical spine mobility
Mallampati classification
Thyromental distance (should be 6-8 cm [3-4 fingerbreadths])
Frontal and profile view
Assessment for disease-associated airway abnormalities

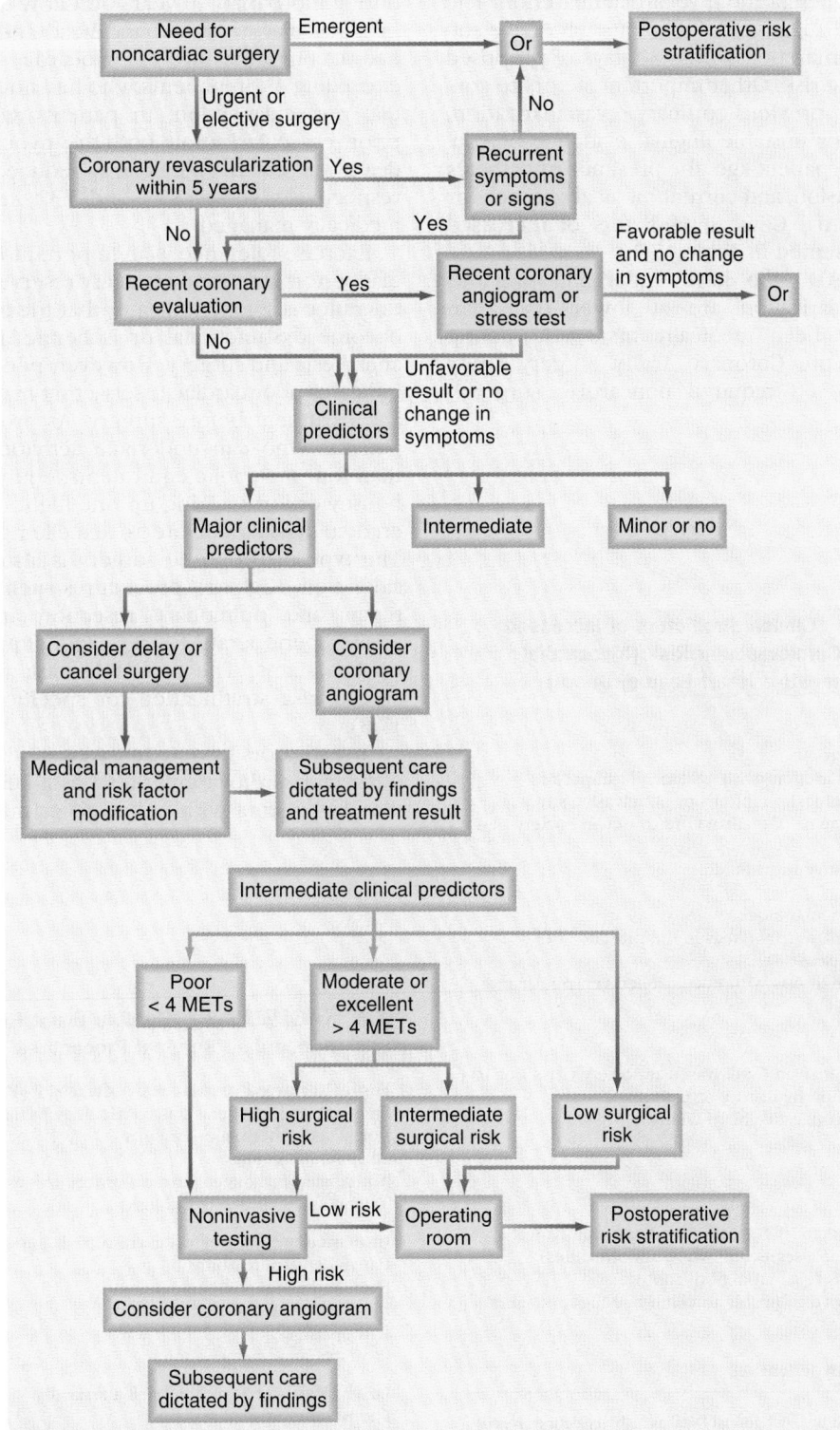

FIGURE 17-2. Algorithm for preoperative evaluation of patients with cardiac disease undergoing noncardiac surgery. From Eagle K, Brundage B, Chaitman B, et al: Guidelines for perioperative cardiovascular evaluation for noncardiac surgery: A report of the American College of Cardiology/American Heart Association Task Force on practice guidelines. Circulation 93:1278-1317, 1996. Copyright 1996, American Heart Association.

operative cardiac ischemia and myocardial infarction. The ACC/AHA task force suggests that patients who have suffered a myocardial infarction within 30 days of proposed surgery are at highest risk. Other important factors to consider are a history of previous coronary revascularization, presence of stable or unstable angina, evidence of congestive heart failure, patient age, the presence of diabetes mellitus or hypertension, and current medical regimen for the treatment of CAD. Clinical predictors of increased cardiac risk are presented in Table 17-7.

Patients with CAD who have undergone previous myocardial revascularization are at lower risk than patients who have been medically managed. Among 24,959 patients in the Coronary Artery Surgery Study (CASS) database, 3,368 required noncardiac surgery[37]

during more than 10 years of follow-up. Of these, abdominal, vascular, thoracic, and head and neck surgery each had a combined rate of myocardial infarction or death exceeding 4% in patients who had not undergone myocardial revascularization; in patients who had undergone prior revascularization, both the myocardial infarction and death rates were significantly reduced to 0.8% and 1.7%, respectively, versus 2.7% and 3.3% in patients who were medically managed.

Exercise tolerance is an important indicator of myocardial performance and coronary reserve. Excellent exercise tolerance is a good indicator that the myocardium will not become dysfunctional or ischemic during the stress of anesthesia and surgery. However, poor exercise tolerance indicates poor cardiac reserve that may require evaluation and treatment before surgery. As proposed by the AHA, patients who can undertake activities requiring greater than four metabolic equivalents, equivalent to doing light housework or walking up one flight of stairs, are considered to have moderate to excellent exercise tolerance. The type of proposed surgery is also an important consideration. High-risk procedures such as aortic aneurysm repair and pulmonary resection are associated with greater perioperative stress and require optimization of cardiac status. The ACC/AHA task force has proposed cardiac risk stratification for specific procedures (Table 17-8).

Investigators have extensively studied the implications of certain cardiovascular tests as a guide to perioperative risk. In patients with either no or mild angina, proceed-

TABLE 17-7.   Clinical Predictors of Increased Perioperative Cardiovascular Risk (Myocardial Infarction, Congestive Heart Failure, Death)

Major

Unstable coronary syndrome
   Recent myocardial infarction* with evidence of important
     ischemic risk by clinical symptoms or noninvasive study
   Unstable or severe† angina (Canadian Cardiovascular Society Class
     III or IV)‡
Decompensated congestive heart failure
Significant arrhythmias
   High-grade atrioventricular block
   Symptomatic ventricular arrhythmias in the presence of
     underlying heart disease
   Supraventricular arrhythmias with uncontrolled ventricular rate
Severe valvular disease

Intermediate

Mild angina pectoris (Canadian Cardiovascular Society Class I or II)
Prior myocardial infarction by history or pathologic waves
Compensated or prior congestive heart failure
Diabetes mellitus

Minor

Advanced age
Abnormal electrocardiogram (left ventricular hypertrophy, left
   bundle branch block, ST segment/T wave abnormalities)
Rhythm other than sinus (e.g., atrial fibrillation)
Low functional capacity (e.g., unable to climb one flight of stairs
   with a bag of groceries)
History of stroke
Uncontrolled systemic hypertension

*The American College of Cardiology National Database Library defines *recent myocardial infarction* as greater than 7 days but less than or equal to 1 month (30 month).
†May include "stable" angina in patients who are unusually sedentary.
‡Canadian Cardiovascular Society classification from Campeau L: Grading of angina pectoris. Circulation 54:522-523, 1976. Copyright 1976, American Heart Association.
From Eagle K, Brundage B, Chaitman B, et al: Guidelines for perioperative cardiovascular evaluation for noncardiac surgery: A report of the American College of Cardiology/American Heart Association Task Force on practice guidelines. Circulation 93:1278-1317, 1996. Copyright 1996, American Heart Association.

TABLE 17-8.   Cardiac Event Risk Stratification for Noncardiac Surgical Procedures

High (Reported cardiac risk often > 5%)*
Emergent major operations, particularly in the elderly
Aortic and other major vascular
Peripheral vascular
Anticipated prolonged surgical procedures associated with large
   fluid shifts and/or blood loss

Intermediate (Reported cardiac risk generally < 5%)*
Carotid endarterectomy
Head and neck
Intraperitoneal and intrathoracic
Orthopedic
Prostate

Low† (Reported cardiac risk generally < 1%)*
Endoscopic procedures
Superficial procedures
Cataract
Breast

*Combined incidence of cardiac death and nonfatal myocardial infarction.
†Further preoperative cardiac testing is not generally required.
From Eagle K, Brundage B, Chaitman B, et al: Guidelines for perioperative cardiovascular evaluation for noncardiac surgery: A report of the American College of Cardiology/American Heart Association Task Force on practice guidelines. Circulation 93:1278-1317, 1996. Copyright 1996, American Heart Association.

ing directly to vascular surgery without cardiac testing led to lower morbidity and cost unless patients had an estimated mortality from vascular surgery that was substantially higher than average. Of 302 patients scheduled for major vascular surgery who received clinical risk assessment and dobutamine-atropine stress echocardiography, 100 were considered low risk by clinical criteria and further testing was considered redundant.[5] Dobutamine-atropine stress echocardiography was positive in 72 patients, including all 27 patients who had a perioperative cardiac event (cardiac death, nonfatal myocardial infarction, unstable angina pectoris). Dobutamine-atropine stress echocardiography had a positive predictive value of 38% and a negative predictive value of 100%. Combining the heart rate at which ischemia occurred with stress echocardiography established a high-risk group with a low ischemic threshold and an intermediate-risk group with a high ischemic threshold. All 5 patients with fatal outcomes and 8 of 12 with nonfatal myocardial infarctions were in the group with low ischemic thresholds. The predictive values of ambulatory electrocardiography and dipyridamole thallium scanning were compared in 109 patients undergoing noncardiac surgery.[38] Ten patients died or suffered myocardial infarction or symptomatic ischemia. The positive predictive values for ambulatory electrocardiography and dipyridamole thallium scanning were 25% and 18%, respectively. A strongly positive thallium test had a somewhat greater likelihood ratio (3.5) for in-hospital events and was associated with significantly worse long-term cardiac survival, whereas positive ambulatory electrocardiography was not.

Another important preoperative question in patients at high risk for perioperative myocardial ischemia or myocardial infarction is whether to provide prophylactic drug treatment to decrease the risk of cardiac complications. Mangano and colleagues[39] first reported that perioperative β blockade decreased long-term mortality in patients with or at risk for CAD undergoing high-risk noncardiac surgery. Subsequent investigations have addressed both the efficacy of perioperative β blockers and of other agents that might decrease the likelihood of perioperative ischemia.

Wallace and associates[40] randomized 200 patients with, or at risk for, CAD to receive atenolol/placebo and showed that atenolol was associated with a reduction in the incidence of myocardial ischemia in the first 2 postoperative days from 34/101 to 17/99 and in the first 7 postoperative days from 39/101 to 24/99. Patients with perioperative myocardial ischemia were more likely to die within the next 2 years. Palda and coworkers,[41] in a systematic review of studies of preoperative assessment and management of perioperative risk from CAD, noted that β blockers were indicated in high-risk patients and that cancellation of such patients was occasionally necessary but that the role of catheterization and myocardial revascularization was unclear. Intermediate-risk patients undergoing vascular surgery are better stratified using pharmacologic stress testing or echocardiography, but such tests have not been shown to have a role in nonvascular surgery.

Hypertension is a common disorder that can be associated with end-organ damage, relative hypovolemia, and, if inadequately treated, intraoperative blood pressure lability. In hypertensive patients, assessment of cardiovascular, neurologic, and renal function quantify the extent of end-organ impairment. The preoperative antihypertensive regimen and compliance with that regimen should also be reviewed. In general, antihypertensive medications should be continued throughout the perioperative period.

Endocarditis Prophylaxis

Some patients with congenital or valvular heart disease are at increased risk of developing bacterial endocarditis.[42] The guidelines for endocarditis prophylaxis have changed several times during the past 15 years. The prophylaxis guidelines provided here are the most current recommendations of the American Heart Association. Dental procedures and surgery of the respiratory, gastrointestinal, and genitourinary tracts cause significant release of organisms into the circulation that have a high affinity for causing bacterial endocarditis (Box 17-3). Therefore, patients with high to moderate risk of developing endocarditis should receive antibiotics for prophylaxis during these procedures (Box 17-4).

Pulmonary Disease

Surgical patients often present with obstructive or restrictive pulmonary disease. The history should focus on functional status, exercise tolerance, severity of disease, and current medications. Recent worsening of symptoms should be closely evaluated. A thorough chest physical examination must be performed. Findings on history and physical examination, as well as an understanding of the planned surgical procedure, suggest appropriate preoperative testing, which may include chest radiography, arterial blood gas analysis, and pulmonary function testing. The goal of the preoperative evaluation is to detect and treat reversible pulmonary pathology, optimize medical management, and allow planning for postoperative ventilatory support, if indicated.

The perioperative risk associated with preexisting pulmonary disease has been extensively studied. Smetana,[43] reviewing the topic of preoperative pulmonary evaluation, noted that the topic is complicated by inconsistent definitions of pulmonary complications (Table 17-9). He identified patient-related risk factors, factors related to surgical site, and other factors related to surgery, such as the duration of surgery, choice of general anesthesia, and intraoperative use of pancuronium.

In a cohort of patients diagnosed as having asthma and subsequently requiring surgery at the Mayo Clinic (general or regional anesthesia), perioperative bronchospasm was documented in 1.7% (confidence interval, 0.9% to 3%).[44] All episodes were treated successfully and there were no episodes of pneumothorax, pneumonia, or death. The risk was greatest in patients who were older, had recently used antiasthmatic medications, had recent asthma

Box 17-3. Guidelines for Endocarditis Prophylaxis

Patients at risk for developing bacterial endocarditis

High risk

Prosthetic cardiac valves, including bioprosthetic and homograft valves

Previous bacterial endocarditis

Complex congenital heart disease (e.g., single ventricle states, transposition of the great arteries, tetralogy of Fallot)

Surgically constructed systemic pulmonary shunts or conduits

Moderate risk

Most other congenital cardiac malformations (other than above)

Acquired valvular dysfunction (e.g., rheumatic heart disease)

Hypertrophic cardiomyopathy

Mitral valve prolapse with valvular regurgitation and/or thickened leaflets

Procedures for which endocarditis prophylaxis is recommended

Dental

Dental extractions

Periodontal procedures including surgery, scaling and root planing, probing, and recall maintenance

Endodontic (root canal) instrumentation or surgery only beyond the apex

Subgingival placement of antibiotic fibers or strips

Initial placement of orthodontic bands but not brackets

Intraligamentary local anesthetic injections

Prophylactic cleaning of teeth or implants where bleeding is anticipated

Respiratory tract

Tonsillectomy and adenoidectomy

Surgical procedures that involve respiratory mucosa

Bronchoscopy with a rigid bronchoscope

Gastrointestinal tract

Sclerotherapy for esophageal varices

Esophageal stricture dilation

Endoscopic retrograde cholangiopancreatography

Biliary tract surgery

Surgical operations that involve intestinal mucosa

Genitourinary tract

Prostatic surgery

Cystoscopy

Urethral dilation

Box 17-4. Recommended Antibiotic Regimens for Endocarditis Prophylaxis

I. Standard general prophylaxis for patients at risk:
   Amoxicillin—Adults, 2 g (children, 50 mg/kg) given orally 1 hour before procedure

II. Unable to take oral medications:
   Ampicillin—Adults, 2 g (children, 50 mg/kg) given IM or IV 30 minutes before procedure

III. Amoxicillin/Ampicillin/Penicillin allergic patients:
   Clindamycin—Adults, 600 mg (children, 20 mg/kg) given orally 1 hour before procedure

   or

   Cephalexin or cefadroxil—Adults, 2 g (children, 50 mg/kg) orally 1 hour before procedure

   or

   Azithromycin or clarithromycin—Adults, 500 mg (children, 15 mg/kg) given orally 1 hour before procedure

IV. Amoxicillin/Ampicillin/Penicillin allergic patients that cannot take oral medications:
   Clindamycin—600 mg (children, 20 mg/kg) 30 minutes before procedure

   or

   Cefazolin—Adults, 1 g (children, 25 mg/kg) 30 minutes before procedure

   Cephalosporins should not be given to patients with immediate-type hypersensitivity to penicillins. A follow-up dose is no longer recommended.

TABLE 17-9. Patient-Related Risk Factors Associated with Postoperative Pulmonary Complications

Potential Risk Factor	Type of Surgery	Relative Risk Associated with Factor
Smoking	Coronary bypass	3.4
	Abdominal	1.4-4.3
ASA class > II	Unselected surgery	1.7
	Thoracic or abdominal	1.5-3.2
Age > 70 yr	Unselected surgery	1.9-2.4
	Thoracic or abdominal	0.9-1.9
Obesity	Unselected surgery	1.3
	Thoracic or abdominal	0.8-1.7
COPD	Unselected surgery	2.7-3.6
	Thoracic or abdominal	4.7

ASA, American Society of Anesthesiologists; COPD, chronic obstructive pulmonary disease.

Modified from Smetana GW: Preoperative pulmonary evaluation. N Engl J Med 340:937-944, 1999.

symptoms, and had recently required physician attention for bronchospasm or required hospitalization.[44]

Pulmonary function testing remains controversial, in part, because of changing expectations regarding the ability of patients with chronic pulmonary disease to tolerate extensive surgery. Pulmonary function testing has variable predictive value, cannot define a threshold above which the risk of surgery is prohibitive,[45] and identifies no group at high risk but without clinical evidence of pulmonary disease. Arterial blood gases also do not identify a group for whom the risk of surgery is prohibitive. Spirometry may be helpful in a patient who has unexplained cough, dyspnea, or exercise intolerance or if there is a question regarding optimal improvement of airflow obstruction. Warner and associates[46] compared 135 patients who had undergone spirometry, were undergoing abdominal surgery, and met objective criteria for obstructive pulmonary disease (mean $FEV_{1.0}$ 0.9 $\pm$ 0.2 L) with 135 patients matched for gender, surgical site, smoking history, and age. Although there was a significantly greater incidence of bronchospasm, the incidence of prolonged endotracheal intubation, prolonged intensive care unit admission, or readmission was no different.

Neurologic Disease

The neurologic assessment begins with a thorough history and neurologic examination. Careful documentation is required, particularly in patients with neurologic impairment or patients who will be undergoing regional anesthetic procedures that could be associated with postoperative neurologic injury. Identification of seizure disorders and upper motor neuron lesions has important anesthetic implications. A thorough history of the duration, type, and medical management of seizure disorders is important in developing a plan to prevent perioperative seizures. In some cases, consultation with the patient's neurologist is indicated. Many neuromuscular diseases markedly alter the response to both depolarizing and nondepolarizing muscle relaxants and can predispose patients to severe acute hyperkalemia after succinylcholine administration. Therefore, documentation of the type, duration, and severity of neuromuscular disease is imperative.

Renal and Hepatic Disease

Renal and hepatic dysfunction alters the metabolism and disposition of many anesthetic agents as well as impairing many systemic functions. Patients with acute renal or hepatic insufficiency should not undergo elective surgery until these conditions can be adequately stabilized. Chronic renal insufficiency (CRI) provides many perioperative management challenges, including acid-base abnormalities, electrolyte disturbances, and coagulation disorders. A thorough history must include the etiology of CRI and the presence of systemic complications related to CRI and other systemic diseases. Current daily urinary output, type and frequency of dialysis, and dialysis-related complications must also be evaluated. The physical examination should focus on identifying systemic complications of CRI, including evidence of altered volume status, coagulopathy, anemia, pericardial effusion, and encephalopathy. The laboratory evaluation should include evaluation of anemia, electrolyte abnormalities, coagulopathy, and cardiovascular disease. Dialysis should be performed 18 to 24 hours before surgery to avoid fluid and electrolyte shifts that occur immediately after dialysis.

The patient with chronic liver disease poses many perioperative challenges. The presence of liver disease alters anesthetic drug metabolism, and hypoalbuminemia increases the free fraction of many drugs, thus making these patients sensitive to both the acute and long-term effects of many anesthetics. The perioperative risks of anesthesia and surgery are dependent on the severity of hepatic dysfunction. The preoperative evaluation should focus on hepatic synthetic and metabolic function, the presence of coagulopathy, encephalopathy, and ascites as well as the nutritional status of the patient.

Nutrition, Endocrinology, and Metabolism

Nutritional status plays an important role in perioperative stress responses and wound healing. Like chronic liver disease, malnutrition can impair anesthetic drug metabolism and increase free drug levels by causing hypoalbuminemia. Therefore, every effort should be made to optimize nutritional status in surgical patients.

Diabetes mellitus warrants discussion because of its high prevalence and potential for comorbidity. Preanesthetic evaluation should focus on the duration and type of diabetes as well as the current medical regimen. Review of end-organ function with emphasis on autonomic dysfunction, cardiovascular disease, renal insufficiency, retinopathy, and neurologic complications is mandatory. Patients with diabetes are considered to have delayed gastric emptying and to be at risk for gastroesophageal reflux.

Perioperative plasma glucose levels should be well controlled yet hypoglycemia must be prevented. The appropriate control of perioperative blood sugar in diabetics is difficult to define. Over the long term, there is compelling evidence of a correlation between hyperglycemia and long-term diabetic complications. It is much less clear that blood sugar must be tightly controlled during the acute stress of surgery. However, there is a strong correlation between mortality and tight control of glucose in critically ill patients, including surgical patients.[47]

In diabetic patients undergoing surgery, several principles of management are generally accepted. First, substitute shorter-acting for longer-acting insulin. Second, provide a reduced dose of insulin on the morning of surgery. Third, once a diabetic who is receiving nothing by mouth is given insulin, provide glucose in intravenous fluids. Fourth, in type 2 diabetic patients, long-acting sulfonylurea drugs such as chlorpropamide should be stopped and shorter-acting agents should be substituted. Fifth, metformin should always be stopped because of the slight risk of perioperative drug-induced lactic acidosis. Perioperative insulin requirements vary based on body weight, liver disease, corticosteroid therapy, infection, and the use of cardiopulmonary bypass.

Patients who have received systemic glucocorticoids during the year before surgery may not be able to respond adequately to surgical stress. Because of the remote risk of adrenal insufficiency during anesthesia, patients who receive chronic glucocorticoids generally receive perioperative corticosteroid coverage. Recommendations regarding identification of patients at risk and appropriate dosing are based on anecdote. Newer recommendations are based on the preoperative dosage of glucocorticoid, the duration of therapy, and the type of surgery. For minor surgical stress, Salem and associates[48] recommend the equivalent of 25 mg of hydrocortisone on the operative day; for moderate surgical stress, 50 to 75 mg equivalent for 1 to 2 days; and for major surgical stress, 100 to 150 mg/day for 2 to 3 days.

Fasting Before Surgery

The pulmonary aspiration of gastric contents during anesthesia is an uncommon, but serious, complication. To prevent aspiration, *nil per os* (NPO) guidelines have been developed for patients scheduled for anesthesia and surgery. Traditionally, orders for "NPO after midnight" forbade any intake of liquids and solids. However, applying the same guidelines for clear liquids (gastric emptying time: 1 to 2 hours) and solids (gastric emptying time: 6 hours) has been questioned. The ASA adopted guidelines in 1998 that recommended a minimal fasting period of 2 hours after ingestion of clear liquids and 6 hours for solids and nonclear liquids such as milk or orange juice. Clear liquids are defined as liquids that you can see through and do not contain solids or particulates. The routine use of gastrointestinal stimulants, gastric acid secretion blockers, antacids, and antiemetics is not recommended. However, many patients have medical conditions that cause decreased gastric emptying. In these patients, the use of agents to improve gastric emptying and neutralize gastric acid may be warranted. In addition, precautions should be instituted to decrease the risk of aspiration during anesthesia for patients undergoing emergency procedures.

The reported incidence of aspiration during anesthesia in various studies has varied from 1.4 per 10,000 to 11 per 10,000 anesthetic procedures. A higher incidence has been noted during emergency surgery and in patients with underlying disease processes that cause decreased gastric emptying. Interestingly, some reports suggest that aspiration is at least as common during emergence from anesthesia as during the induction phase. Of patients who have suspected aspiration, fewer than half exhibit evidence of pulmonary injury. In one study, approximately one third of patients with suspected aspiration during anesthesia required postoperative intubation and ventilation. Most of these patients were extubated within 6 hours of surgery. About 10% of patients required intubation and ventilation for 24 hours or greater. Approximately half of the patients requiring ventilation for greater than 24 hours

after aspiration of gastric contents died of pulmonary complications.

Assessment of Physical Status

The ASA has developed a graded, descriptive scale as a means of categorizing preoperative comorbidity.[49] Classification is independent of operative procedure and serves as standardized method of communicating patient physical status among anesthesiologists and other health care providers. Patients are categorized as follows:

ASA I—No organic, physiologic, biochemical or psychiatric disturbance.

ASA II—A patient with mild systemic disease that results in no functional limitation. Examples: well-controlled hypertension, uncomplicated diabetes mellitus.

ASA III—A patient with severe systemic disease that results in functional impairment. Examples: diabetes mellitus with vascular complications, prior myocardial infarction, uncontrolled hypertension.

ASA IV—A patient with severe systemic disease that is a constant threat to life. Examples: congestive heart failure, unstable angina pectoris.

ASA V—A moribund patient who is not expected to survive with or without the operation. Examples: ruptured aortic aneurysm, intracranial hemorrhage with elevated intracranial pressure.

ASA VI—A declared brain dead patient whose organs are being harvested for transplantation.

E—Emergency operation is required. Example: *ASA IE* = otherwise healthy patient for emergency appendectomy.

SELECTION OF ANESTHETIC TECHNIQUES AND DRUGS

The selection of anesthetic techniques and drugs begins with the preoperative anesthetic evaluation. Recognition of important preexisting conditions and chronic medication use may suggest that certain approaches are preferable. Then, the requirements of the surgical procedure and surgeon are considered. What is the operative site? How will the patient be positioned? What is the expected duration of surgery? Is the patient expected to return home after an ambulatory procedure or is hospital admission anticipated? Finally, in this era of cost constraints, are the costs of newer drugs justified by likely clinical benefit? Evidence of the increasing safety of anesthesia is the fact that multiple options often can be used safely and effectively for the same procedure and the same patient.

After completing the preanesthetic evaluation, the anesthesiologist discusses various options regarding anesthetic care with the patient. Together, sometimes with input from the patient's surgeon, the anesthesiologist and the patient choose an anesthetic technique. Continued progress in the pharmacology of anesthetic drugs, improvements in the accuracy and applicability of monitoring devices, and parallel improvements in the management of chronic disease processes have resulted in the ability to extensively customize the anesthetic management of individual patients.

Risk of Anesthesia

Patients often desire information regarding the risk of death or major complications associated with anesthesia. However, because perioperative death and major complications have become so uncommon, the risk of anesthesia is difficult to quantify. The risk of cardiac arrest attributable to anesthesia appears to be less than 1 in 10,000 cases.[50,51] Schwilk and colleagues[52] prospectively studied preoperative risk factors as predictors of perioperative adverse events in 26,907 patients undergoing noncardiac surgery. Fourteen variables proved to be independent risk factors, including gender, age, ASA status, general condition, nutritional state, coronary disease, airway and lung pathology, Mallampati classification, fluid and electrolyte balance, metabolic state, grade of urgency, operative site, duration of operation, and anesthetic technique (regional lower risk than general). Using a point system, patients could be reliably separated into low- and high-risk groups.

Because so many surgical procedures now are performed without admission to the hospital, the risk associated with ambulatory anesthesia is particularly important. To assess this risk, 38,598 patients who had undergone 45,090 consecutive ambulatory surgical procedures were contacted within 72 hours and 30 days of surgery (99.94% and 95.9% of patients). No patient died of a medical complication within 1 week of surgery.[53] The total death rate was 1:11,273 (four deaths), and the total complication rate was 1:1,366.

Selection of Specific Technique (Box 17-5)

The first step in selecting a specific anesthetic technique for an individual patient is to consider if the procedure can appropriately be performed using monitored anesthesia care, regional anesthesia (including regional upper and lower extremity blocks, subarachnoid blocks, and epidural anesthesia), or general anesthesia. Monitored anesthesia care supplements local anesthesia performed by surgeons. Anesthesiologists usually participate because an individual patient or procedure requires higher doses of potent sedatives or opioids or because an acutely or chronically ill patient requires close monitoring and hemodynamic or respiratory support. Regional anesthesia (discussed in detail in a later section) is useful for operations on the upper and lower extremities, pelvis, and lower abdomen. Certain other procedures, such as carotid endarterectomy and "awake" craniotomy, can also be successfully performed under regional or field block. Patients receiving regional anesthesia usually can remain awake and, if needed, can receive intravenous sedation or analgesics. Although regional anesthesia avoids general anesthesia, and intuitively appears safer, hazards specific to regional anesthesia must be considered. These include, among others, postdural puncture headache, local anesthetic toxicity, and peripheral nerve injury. In addition, an

---

Box 17-5. Selection of Specific Techniques

Factors in selection

Skills of anesthesiologist
Requirements of surgery
Preferences of patient
Preferences of surgeon

Specific types of techniques
Monitored anesthesia care (MAC)

Individual patient or procedure requires more than moderate sedation. Severely ill patient requires close monitoring or hemodynamic or respiratory support

Regional anesthesia

Procedures in appropriate sites, e.g., extremities, lower abdomen (may be combined with general anesthesia in other sites)

General anesthesia

Most upper abdominal and thoracic procedures

---

inadequate regional anesthetic may require rapid transition to heavy sedation or general anesthesia.

General anesthesia is a reversible state of unconsciousness. Although the mechanism of general anesthetics remains speculative and controversial, the four components of general anesthesia (amnesia, analgesia, inhibition of noxious reflexes, and skeletal muscle relaxation) are usually achieved in modern anesthesia by a combination of intravenous anesthetics and analgesics, inhalational anesthetics, and often muscle relaxants. Because the drugs that produce these components cause both desirable and undesirable physiologic changes, the pharmacologic effects of the agents must be matched to the pathophysiology of the patient's medical problems. The major adverse changes associated with anesthetic drugs are respiratory depression, cardiovascular depression, and loss of airway maintenance and protection. Important complications of general anesthesia include hypoxemia (with possible central nervous system damage), hypotension, cardiac arrest, and aspiration of acidic gastric contents (which can lead to severe pulmonary damage). Dental damage is more frequent but not life threatening.

Regardless of the suitability of a specific technique for a specific surgical procedure, other factors, including the patient's preferences, must be considered. For instance, regional anesthesia might not be chosen if a patient were extremely anxious or could not communicate effectively because of a language barrier. Monitored anesthesia care might be inappropriate if a patient were unlikely to lie quietly during delicate or prolonged surgery. Any procedure planned under regional anesthesia or monitored anesthesia care can require conversion to general anesthesia if the original choice proves unsatisfactory.

GENERAL ANESTHESIA STRATEGIES

Key Considerations

If general anesthesia is chosen, the anesthesiologist must address several questions. First, does the patient's condition or the scheduled surgery suggest additional monitoring techniques beyond the monitors that are used in every patient? Second, does the patient have any conditions that contraindicate specific drugs? For example, does the patient have recently acquired paraplegia or quadriplegia that would contraindicate succinylcholine? Third, is endotracheal intubation necessary for this procedure? Fourth, if endotracheal intubation is required or desirable, are there any anticipated difficulties with oral translaryngeal intubation? Fifth, are neuromuscular blockers required for adequate exposure during surgery? Sixth, are there specific surgical requirements that mandate use of or avoidance of specific interventions? For instance, if a surgical procedure will include intraoperative nerve stimulation, neuromuscular blockers would interfere with assessment. If intraoperative somatosensory evoked potentials are to be used, as in certain spine procedures, an anesthetic regimen must be chosen that does not confound that monitoring modality. Seventh, are substantial blood loss or large fluid shifts anticipated?

Steps in a "Typical" General Anesthetic Procedure

Immediate Preoperative Preparation

Having resolved the answers to those questions, management of the typical general anesthetic procedure begins with arrival of the patient in the holding area before surgery. After ascertaining the identity of the patient, confirming that informed consent has been obtained, checking any pending diagnostic tests, and noting any acute changes in health status, an intravenous catheter is started in adult patients. Usually intravenous catheterization is deferred in small children undergoing elective surgery until after inhalational induction; older children may prefer intravenous cannulation to placement of a face mask for inhalational induction.

Intravenous premedication is then an option for apprehensive patients who have not received oral premedication. Although premedication practices are highly variable, many clinicians give intravenous medications before moving patients from the holding area into the operating room, especially if patients are undergoing procedures associated with considerable anxiety. Premedication with midazolam or diazepam reduced preprocedure anxiety before needle-guided breast biopsy, reduced discomfort during the procedure, and improved anxiety scores in the PACU without prolonging discharge times.[54]

In the operating room, a cooperative patient is asked to breathe oxygen from a face mask during application of monitoring devices, including a chest stethoscope, noninvasive blood pressure, ECG, and pulse oximetry. Capnography is initiated after the airway has been secured, and temperature monitoring may or may not be initiated before induction, depending on the type of temperature monitor to be used. Invasive monitors such as arterial or pulmonary arterial catheters may be placed before or after induction, depending on the specific situation. When the monitors have been applied and the surgeon is available, induction of anesthesia can begin.

Induction of Anesthesia

Induction of general anesthesia, like taking off in an airplane, is an especially critical interval. Complications of anesthesia are most likely during induction and emergence. During this brief interval, a patient rapidly loses consciousness, ceases to maintain a natural airway, abruptly reduces or ceases spontaneous ventilation, and receives drugs that depress the myocardium and change vascular tone. The specific sequence of interventions during induction varies depending on the patient and the type of surgery to be performed.

Awake Intubation

In a small fraction of patients, the risk of inducing anesthesia without first securing the airway may indicate an awake intubation. Depending on an individual patient's status, an awake intubation may be supplemented with sedatives and opioids and with topical or local anesthesia. Indications for awake intubation include inadequate mouth opening, facial trauma, known or suspected cervical spine injury, chronic cervical spine disease, and lesions in the upper airway. Awake intubation can be accomplished by the "blind" nasal route, by fiberoptic bronchoscopy, or by direct visualization. In the blind nasal approach, the endotracheal tube is inserted through the nose and guided into the trachea by listening to the patient's breath sounds as they are transmitted through the tube. An awake fiberoptic intubation is performed by passing an endotracheal tube through the nose or mouth into the pharynx and then passing a bronchoscope through the tube, visualizing the larynx and the trachea, and threading the tube over the bronchoscope. Regardless of the route chosen for awake intubation, induction drugs are given once the airway is secured.

Intravenous Induction

Intravenous induction is used commonly in elective adult cases. The patient is first preoxygenated with 100% oxygen to provide the patient with a reservoir of oxygen (equivalent to functional residual capacity) should mask ventilation or intubation be difficult. At the discretion of the anesthesiologist, opioids or benzodiazepines may be given immediately before induction. A rapidly acting, intravenous induction agent is then administered. Commonly used induction agents, in sufficient doses, quickly render patients unconscious and apneic. The anesthesiologist then determines whether the patient can be manually ventilated using an anesthesia face mask and the reservoir bag on the breathing circuit. If mask ventilation is satisfactory, the patient is given a neuromuscular blocker, such as succinylcholine or a nondepolarizing agent. After the patient is adequately relaxed, endotracheal intubation is performed. After endotracheal intubation, the position of the tube in the trachea is confirmed by auscultation and by capnographic evidence of exhaled CO_2. Endotracheal intubation maintains airway patency and limits the possibility of gastric aspiration.

There are two primary drawbacks associated with intravenous induction. The first is that spontaneous ventilation is abolished without certainty that manual ventilation can be accomplished. The second is that endotracheal intubation is performed while the patient is lightly anesthetized, thereby potentially precipitating hypertension, tachycardia, or bronchospasm. Adjuvant agents (e.g., lidocaine and opioids) may be used to blunt reflex responses to intubation. Preoperative airway evaluation reduces the possibility that a patient will be abruptly rendered "unable to ventilate, unable to intubate." (Management of the expected or unexpected difficult airway is discussed in greater detail later in the text.)

Rapid-Sequence Induction

Rapid-sequence induction is indicated for patients who are at high risk for acid aspiration. This includes obese patients, obstetric patients, patients with symptomatic gastroesophageal reflux, those who have recently eaten, and those with bowel obstruction. Patients for emergency surgery usually are considered to have "full stomachs" because of uncertainty regarding recent food ingestion and because pain or injury delay gastric emptying. The concept of rapid sequence induction is to progress rapidly from the awake state to the anesthetized, endotracheally intubated state. This is done by first preoxygenating the patient, then giving thiopental (or another intravenous induction agent), immediately followed by succinylcholine, waiting approximately 1 minute, and intubating the trachea without first ensuring that manual ventilation can be accomplished. From the time of injection of the induction drugs until confirmation that the endotracheal tube is properly positioned in the trachea, an assistant applies firm pressure on the cricoid cartilage (Sellick's maneuver) to prevent passive regurgitation from the stomach to the pharynx. The risk of rapid sequence induction is that the anesthesiologist gives a paralyzing dose of succinylcholine without proving that mask ventilation is possible. If intubation cannot be performed successfully, and if mask ventilation proves unsatisfactory, hypoxia and its accompaniments, including arrhythmias and cardiac arrest, may occur.

Inhalational Induction

Inhalational induction was the only option for inducing general anesthesia before the introduction of thiopental. In the early days of ether and chloroform anesthesia, induction consisted of having the patient inhale anesthetic through a face mask while the anesthesiologist gradually assumed maintenance of the airway. Inhalational induction with ether was often turbulent and hazardous because patients progressed slowly from an awake state (anesthetic stage 1) to a surgical level of anesthesia (stage

3). Patients would spend several minutes in stage 2 (the "excitement stage") and often become agitated and combative and require physical restraint. During this hazardous interval, patients were at risk for laryngospasm, vomiting, and aspiration. Although modern inhalational agents induce anesthesia more rapidly and safely, inhalational induction continues to be used in children, in adult patients at severe risk of bronchospasm, and in some patients in whom the airway may be difficult to secure. Children rapidly progress through stage 2, and postinduction intravenous catheterization avoids the trauma of insertion in awake, struggling children.

Combined Intravenous and Inhalational Induction

Features of intravenous and inhalational induction are often combined to gain the advantage of smooth, rapid hypnosis but still permit establishment of a deep level of inhalational anesthesia before airway instrumentation. With a combined technique, after preoxygenation, an intravenous induction agent is given to rapidly render the patient unconscious. A potent inhalational agent, often combined with nitrous oxide, is then administered by face mask to deepen the anesthetic. Maintenance of the airway by face mask, a skill that requires practice, is more difficult to master than intubation.

There are several techniques that can be used to manage the upper airway obstruction that typically develops as patients lose consciousness. The chin can be tilted, extending the neck, the mandible can be displaced anteriorly, and an oral or nasal airway can be inserted. If the procedure is brief and there are no contraindications, the case can be conducted using a face mask. More commonly, after demonstrating that the patient can be ventilated by mask, a short-acting muscle relaxant (succinylcholine) is given to facilitate intubation. An endotracheal tube is then placed in the trachea to help ensure a patent airway and prevent aspiration. An alternative, in cases that do not require endotracheal intubation, is the use of an LMA, which maintains airway patency and permits gentle ventilatory assistance but does not protect against aspiration of gastric contents. With a modest amount of experience, the LMA can be placed in proper position in most patients.[55] In patients undergoing carotid endarterectomy, use of an LMA rather than endotracheal intubation was associated with fewer hypertensive and tachycardic episodes and a lower incidence of required drug treatment for such episodes.[56]

Maintenance of Anesthesia

After inducing the patient and securing the airway, the maintenance phase of anesthesia begins, during which the patient is positioned, the surgical incision site is scrubbed with antiseptic soap and surrounded with sterile towels and drapes, and the surgery is performed. During this interval, the level of stimulation changes from minimal during cleansing of the incision site to intense during incision and retraction. Maintenance of anesthesia is usually accomplished with a titratable combination of intravenous opioids and hypnotics, nitrous oxide, and volatile anesthetic agents. If no potent inhalational agents are used, the technique becomes more dependent on opioids and amnesia from sedative-hypnotics such as midazolam and is often termed a *nitrous-narcotic* technique. Some anesthesiologists prefer to use total intravenous anesthesia, in which a short-acting hypnotic such as propofol is continuously infused in combination with a short-acting opioid. Changes in blood pressure and heart rate are most commonly used as indirect evidence of provision of adequate anesthesia. Muscle relaxants may be used to facilitate surgical exposure. The challenge during the maintenance phase is to ensure that the patient has no pain and no recall. The use of some agents (e.g., ketamine) during anesthesia may reduce subsequent postoperative requirements for analgesic drugs.

Titration of agents using indirect autonomic signs of anesthetic depth is usually satisfactory but can result in either inadequate anesthesia or in administration of more agent than is necessary, thus prolonging emergence and delaying tracheal extubation. Early evidence suggests that use of the BIS monitor might permit use of lower inspired concentrations of inhalational agent with little risk of inadequate anesthesia.[57] During anesthesia, monitoring of neuromuscular blockade permits adequate dosage of muscle relaxants to provide surgical relaxation while retaining the ability to reverse paralysis at the end of the case.

Emergence from Anesthesia

As surgery concludes, the patient must emerge from anesthesia. The process of emergence and extubation usually consists of timing the withdrawal of potent inhalational agents and nitrous oxide (if it is being used) or cessation of continuous infusion of intravenous agents. Reversal of neuromuscular blockade returns the ability to spontaneously ventilate and protect the airway. Emergence requires knowledge and experience with the pharmacokinetic and pharmacodynamic principles that underlie the elimination of inhalational and intravenous agents and that govern the reversal of neuromuscular blockade. The time required for emergence is a function of the solubility of a potent inhalational agent in blood and tissues and of the duration of anesthesia.[58] Reversal of neuromuscular blockade with anticholinesterases is dependent both on the characteristics of the relaxant and on the depth of blockade before giving the reversal agent (Fig. 17-3).[59]

Extubation usually occurs when the patient follows commands and demonstrates sufficient strength to spontaneously breathe and protect the airway. Alternatively, in a patient who is not at risk for aspiration, the endotracheal tube can be removed while the patient is still deeply anesthetized after which emergence occurs with a natural airway. Deep extubation is most commonly used in patients who are at risk for bronchospasm with stimulation of the trachea during emergence from anesthesia.

After extubation, monitors are removed and the patient is moved to a stretcher for transport to the PACU. Because of the risk of hypoxemia occurring during transport, oxygen will often be given or pulse oximetry will continue. If a patient received invasive monitors as part of

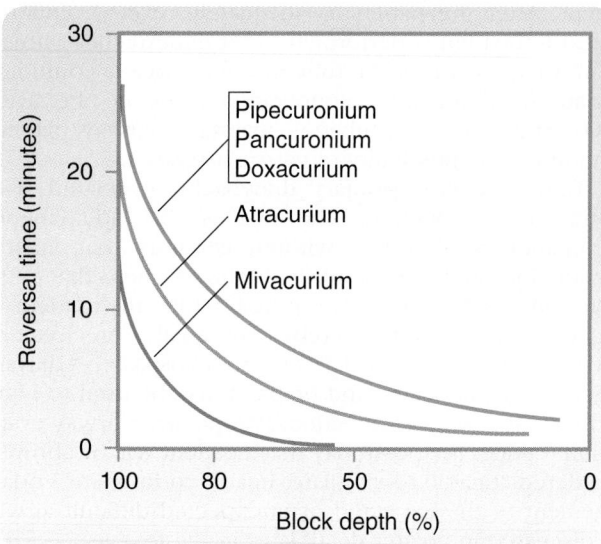

FIGURE 17-3. Comparative mean speed of antagonism by neostigmine of neuromuscular blockade induced by long-acting agents (doxacurium, pancuronium, pipecuronium), intermediate-acting drugs (atracurium and others), and the short-acting agent mivacurium. Antagonism is more rapid as processes of clearance increase. From Savarese JJ, Caldwell JE, Lien CA, Miller RD: Pharmacology of muscle relaxants and their antagonists. *In* Miller RD, Cucchiara RF, Miller RG Jr, et al (eds): Anesthesia, 5th ed. Philadelphia, Livingstone, 2000, pp 412-490.

perioperative management, the monitoring often will be continued en route to the PACU or ICU.

COMMON INTRAOPERATIVE PROBLEMS

Several of the most important problems, usually identified quickly from intraoperative monitoring devices, that arise after induction of anesthesia include inability to secure the airway (see extended discussion later), hypotension, hypoxemia, increased peak inspiratory pressure, and increased body temperature. Hypotension, which is operationally defined during anesthesia as a decrease in systolic or mean arterial pressure by more than 25%, occurs commonly and usually is easily treated. Especially during the interval between endotracheal intubation and surgical incision the lack of intense sensory stimulation may result in hypotension even in lightly anesthetized patients. In this situation, temporization with fluid boluses or short-acting pressors is appropriate, pending the beginning of surgical stimulation. Of course, hypotension arising during anesthesia may also indicate more serious complications, including myocardial ischemia, hypovolemia, and tension pneumothorax. Treatment of intraoperative hypotension should be accompanied by evaluation of these possible causes.

Hypoxemia severe enough to merit treatment occurs much less commonly. The differential diagnosis of intraoperative hypoxemia includes right mainstem intubation, pneumothorax, bronchospasm, and aspiration of gastric contents. Treatment should be directed at the primary pathologic process, if any is identified. Very rarely, an intraoperative chest radiograph is useful in diagnosing potential causes of hypoxemia that do not quickly respond to empirical therapy.

Myocardial ischemia is a particular risk in patients with known CAD or who have major risk factors for CAD. Most myocardial ischemia can be diagnosed from leads V_5 or II. Management of myocardial ischemia depends on the precipitating cause. Tachycardia can be managed with β blockers (esmolol is particularly useful because of its rapid onset of action and short half-life). Myocardial ischemia due to hypotension is usually managed by increasing blood pressure, often with an α agonist to avoid increases in myocardial consumption associated with increased heart rate or myocardial contractility.

Increased peak inspiratory pressure identified on the airway pressure monitoring gauge may have multiple causes, including bronchospasm, pneumothorax, and acute processes, such as aspiration pneumonia, that decrease pulmonary compliance. Auscultation of the lungs and occasionally a chest radiograph will guide therapy.

Increased body temperature may be due to release of cytokines from an area of infection as it is surgically drained or to overzealous attempts to prevent hypothermia, or it may be due to malignant hyperthermia. Confirmatory evidence of malignant hyperthermia includes increased CO_2 production (evidenced by increasing end-tidal CO_2 and by metabolic acidosis, either of which could also be the presenting sign, with fever being delayed). Muscle is variably noted. If malignant hyperthermia is strongly suspected, treatment should follow a specific protocol, the most important parts of which are to discontinue the triggering agent (usually an inhalational anesthetic), replace the existing anesthesia machine with a machine free of inhalational anesthetic, and begin intravenous administration of dantrolene. Patients who appear to have developed malignant hyperthermia should be observed in the hospital for at least 24 hours and should be instructed to wear medical-alert bracelets.

AIRWAY MANAGEMENT

Airway management is perhaps the most critical skill in anesthesia. As discussed earlier in this chapter, the preoperative evaluation focuses on recognition of patients who may be difficult to intubate. Facility with various techniques for establishment of a patent airway constitutes the central group of skills that are taught to anesthesia residents. Fortunately, the incidence of difficult intubations is low. Of all general anesthetic procedures, difficult direct laryngoscopy occurs in 1.5% to 8.5% and failed intubation occurs in 0.13% to 0.3%.

The LMA, the Combitube, the lighted stylet, and the Bullard laryngoscope are recent developments that make intubation possible in many patients who have failed intubation using a conventional laryngoscope. The fiberoptic bronchoscope is an additional tool for the management of the difficult airway.

Because of the importance of a prompt, effective response to difficult intubation, the ASA has developed guidelines for managing difficult airways (Fig. 17-4). A key factor is the initial airway examination and the recognition of patients with potentially difficult airways. If the practitioner suspects that mask ventilation and tracheal intubation will be difficult, it is recommended that spontaneous ventilation be preserved. Approaches to these patients include awake intubation or the use of anesthetic techniques that preserve spontaneous ventilation. In some cases, establishment of a surgical airway in the awake patient under local anesthesia may be indicated. However, some patients present with an unrecognized difficult airway after anesthesia and muscle relaxation have been induced. This is an emergency situation that must be rectified quickly to avoid hypoxemia, brain injury, or death. A variety of airway adjuncts are available to preserve ventilation and facilitate tracheal intubation. Of course, the practitioner should always call for assistance in these situations to optimize patient care and consider reestablishment of spontaneous ventilation.

INTRAOPERATIVE FLUID AND BLOOD MANAGEMENT

Perioperative fluid administration consists of both maintenance and replacement fluids.[60] Maintenance fluids in healthy, 70-kg adults consist of 2500 mL/day of water containing a sodium (Na^+) concentration of 30 mEq/L and a potassium (K^+) concentration of 15 to 20 mEq/L. Intraoperatively, fluids containing sodium-free water (i.e., $Na^+ < 130$ mEq/L) are rarely used in adults, because of the necessity for replacing isotonic losses and the risk of postoperative hyponatremia. Surgical patients require replacement of plasma volume and extracellular volume losses secondary to wound or burn edema, ascites, and gastrointestinal secretions. Wound and burn edema and ascitic fluid are protein rich and contain electrolytes in concentrations similar to plasma. Although gastrointestinal secretions vary greatly in composition, the composition of replacement fluid need not be closely matched if extracellular volume is adequate and renal and cardiovascular functions are normal.

Owing to the hyperglycemic response associated with surgical stress, glucose is usually not required intraoperatively. Iatrogenic hyperglycemia can limit the effectiveness of fluid resuscitation by inducing an osmotic diuresis and worsen outcome in both ischemic and traumatic brain injury in humans.

Replacement of intraoperative fluid losses must compensate for the acute reduction of functional extracellular volume that accompanies trauma, hemorrhage, and tissue manipulation. For example, otherwise healthy subjects who received no intraoperative sodium while undergoing gastric or gallbladder surgery demonstrated a decline in extracellular volume of nearly 2 L and a 13% decline in glomerular filtration rate.[61] Patients studied during the first 10 days after resuscitation from massive trauma demonstrated a 55% increase in interstitial fluid volume.[62] To replace the fluid losses accompanying various operations, the simplest formula provides, in addition to replacement

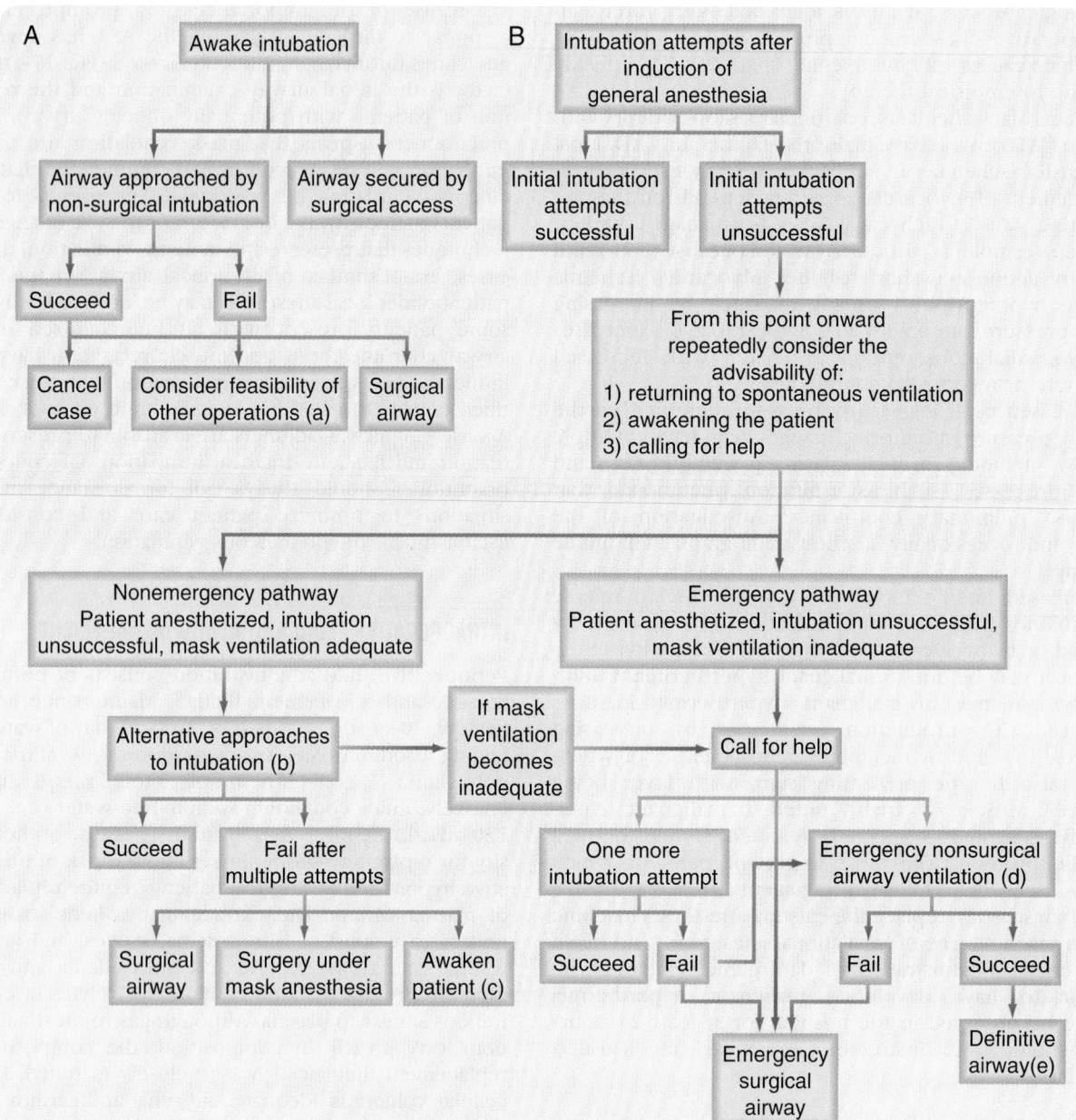

FIGURE 17-4. **A** and **B,** The ASA difficult airway algorithm. The likelihood and clinical impact of basic management problems such as difficult intubation, difficult mask ventilation, and difficulty with patient cooperation or consent should be assessed in all patients in which airway management is contemplated. The clinician should consider the relative merits and feasibility of basic management choices, including the use of awake intubation techniques, preservation of spontaneous ventilation, and the use of surgical approaches to establish a secure airway. Primary and alternative strategies should be established. (a) Other options include, but are not limited to, surgery under mask anesthesia, surgery under local infiltration or nerve block and intubation attempts after induction of general anesthesia. (b) Alternative approaches include use of different laryngoscope blades, awake intubation, blind oral or nasal intubation, fiberoptic intubation, use of intubating stylet or tube changer, light wand, retrograde intubation, and surgical airway access. (c) See awake intubation. (d) Options for emergency nonsurgical airway include transtracheal jet ventilation, laryngeal mask airway, and Combitube. From American Society of Anesthesiologists: Practice guidelines for management of the difficult airway: A report by the American Society of Anesthesiologists task force on management of the difficult airway. Anesthesiology 78:597-602, 1993.

of estimated blood loss, 4 mL/kg/hr for procedures involving minimal trauma, 6 mL/kg/hr for those involving moderate trauma, and 8 mL/kg/hr for those involving extreme trauma. An important implication of perioperative interstitial fluid expansion is the subsequent mobilization and return of accumulated fluid to the extracellular volume and the plasma volume. In most patients, mobilization occurs on approximately the third postoperative day. If the cardiovascular system and kidneys cannot effectively transport and excrete mobilized fluid, hypervolemia and pulmonary edema may occur.

Although fluid shifts associated with ambulatory surgery should be much less than in major surgical procedures in inpatients, fluid management appears to contribute to the overall quality of the perioperative experience. Of 200 ASA I to III patients undergoing ambulatory surgery, symptoms of thirst, drowsiness, and dizziness were significantly less frequent in patients randomized to receive 20 mL/kg rather than 2.0 mL/kg of balanced salt solution over 30 minutes before anesthesia.[63] Nausea on the first postoperative day was also decreased.

Monitoring of Intravascular Volume

For most surgical patients, conventional clinical assessment of the adequacy of intravascular volume is appropriate. For high-risk patients, goal-directed hemodynamic management may be superior.

Monitoring the adequacy of intraoperative fluid resuscitation integrates multiple clinical variables, including heart rate, blood pressure, urinary output, and arterial pH. During profound hypovolemia, indirect measurements of blood pressure may significantly underestimate true blood pressure. In patients undergoing extensive procedures, direct arterial pressure measurements may reflect increased systolic blood pressure variation accompanying positive-pressure ventilation in the presence of hypovolemia.[64-67] Urinary output usually declines precipitously during moderate to severe hypovolemia. Therefore, in the absence of glycosuria or diuretic administration, a urinary output of 0.5 to 1.0 mL/kg/hr during anesthesia suggests adequate renal perfusion. Arterial pH may decrease only when tissue hypoperfusion becomes severe. An important diagnostic point is differentiation of lactic acidosis secondary to hypoperfusion from hyperchloremic acidosis associated with infusion of 0.9% saline. Lactic acidosis is associated with a high anion gap and requires treatment, usually by improving perfusion. Hyperchloremic metabolic acidosis after administration of large volumes of 0.9% saline perioperatively or in critically ill hospitalized patients is not associated with an increased anion gap[68]; therefore, no specific treatment is required.

Visual estimation, the simplest technique for quantifying intraoperative blood loss, assesses the amount of blood absorbed by gauze squares and laparotomy pads and adds an estimate of blood accumulation on the floor and surgical drapes and in suction containers. Both surgeons and anesthesiologists tend to underestimate losses.

No currently available intraoperative monitor is sufficiently sensitive or specific to detect hypoperfusion in all patients. Cardiac output can be normal despite severely reduced regional blood flow. Mixed venous hemoglobin desaturation, a specific indicator of poor systemic perfusion, reflects average perfusion in multiple organs and cannot supplant regional monitors such as urinary output. Moreover, unrecognized, subclinical tissue hypoperfusion may progress to acute renal failure, hepatic failure, and sepsis.

One key variable that is assumed to reflect tissue perfusion and has been associated with increased survival in surgical patients is oxygen delivery greater than or equal to 600 mL/m^2/min (equivalent to a cardiac index of 3.0 L/m^2/min, a hemoglobin concentration of 14 g/dL, and 98% oxyhemoglobin saturation). At present, available data are consistent with several inferences. First, there is no apparent benefit for patients other than surgical patients.[69] Second, the benefit for surgical patients is variable, with the greatest improvement in outcome associated with the use of goal-oriented resuscitation in patients with a high predicted mortality.[70] Third, using a less aggressive goal for resuscitation is associated with a reduction in the total volume of fluid required but no difference in the hemodynamic values attained by trauma patients.[71]

Intraoperative Blood Administration

Because of widespread concern about the risks of allogeneic blood transfusion and because the majority of blood transfusions are administered intraoperatively, anesthesiologists have come under increasing pressure to decrease their use of homologous blood. Important developments related to intraoperative blood transfusion include impressive progress in limiting the infectious risks of blood transfusion, reducing the incidence of transfusion reactions, acceptance of lower hematocrits as "transfusion triggers," quantification of the costs and benefits of preoperative autologous blood donation, physiologic characterization of the risks and benefits of acute normovolemic hemodilution, improvement of the techniques of perioperative red cell salvage, declining interest in deliberate hypotension, and introduction of increasingly effective pharmacologic adjuvants to reduce bleeding in certain surgical patients.

Infectious Risks of Blood Transfusion

Sufficient progress has been made in reducing the risk of human immunodeficiency virus (HIV) infection, hepatitis B, and hepatitis C that the very low rates of infection can no longer be measured and rather must be modeled mathematically (Fig. 17-5).[72] In 1984, 714 cases of transfusion-associated HIV infection were reported to the Centers for Disease Control and Prevention; after institution of enhanced screening procedures and implementation, in March 1985, of HIV antibody testing, only 5 cases were reported.[72] Screening for hepatitis B surface antigen has been available since 1975; therefore, today it accounts for a small fraction of transfusion-related hepatitis. Non-A, non-B hepatitis was the most common form of post-transfusion hepatitis before the cumulative effects of four

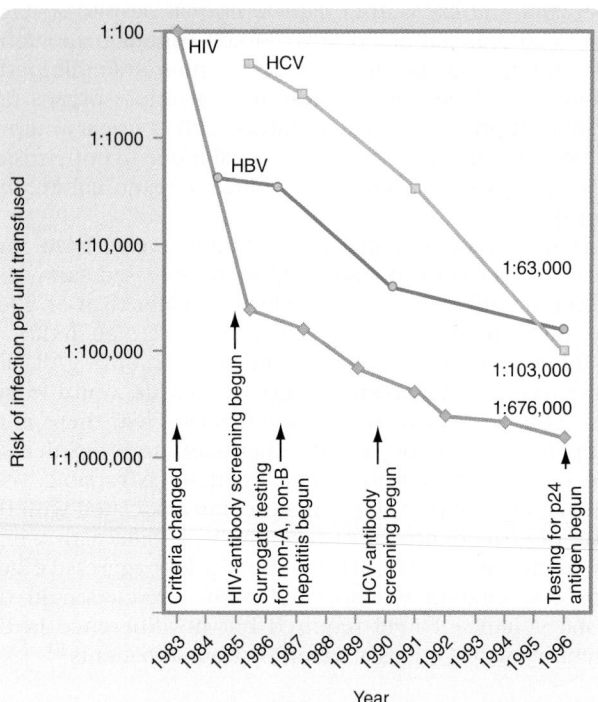

FIGURE 17-5. Risks of transfusion-related transmission of human immunodeficiency virus (HIV) in the United States. Each unit represents exposure to one donor. The risk of each of these infections has declined dramatically since 1983, the year the criteria for donor screening were changed; at that time the prevalence of HIV infection among donors was approximately 1%. Further declines have resulted from the implementation of testing of donor blood for antibodies to HIV beginning in 1985; surrogate testing for non-A, non-B hepatitis beginning in 1986-1987; testing for antibodies to HCV beginning in 1990; and testing for HIV p24 antigen beginning in late 1995. (Adapted from Buchon JP, Birkmeyer JD, Busch MP: Safety of the blood supply in the United States: Opportunities and controversies. Ann Intern Med 127:904-909, 1999.)

interventions: efforts to reduce potential HIV-positive donors, testing for alanine aminotransferase, testing for hepatitis B core antigen, and, finally, implementation of a test for hepatitis C antibody.[72]

"Transfusion Triggers"

Perhaps the most striking consequence of concerns about the risks of transfused blood is the growing consensus that the perioperative "transfusion trigger" should be at a lower hematocrit than the traditional 10 g/dL. In 1988, a National Institutes of Health Consensus Conference stated that "otherwise healthy patients with hemoglobin levels of [10 g/dL] or greater rarely require perioperative transfusion, whereas those with acute anemia with resulting hemoglobin values of less than [7 g/dL] frequently will require red blood cell transfusions."[73] In 1996 the Task Force on Blood Component Therapy of the ASA[74] concluded, based on available evidence, that transfusion should not be based on a single hemoglobin "trigger" but rather should be based on an individual patient's risk of

developing inadequate tissue oxygenation. The ASA Task Force further concluded that transfusion was rarely needed if hemoglobin exceeded 10 g/dL and was almost always needed if hemoglobin was less than 6 g/dL.[74] An important aspect of the gradual acceptance of lower transfusion triggers is that a reduction of hematocrit is associated with a reduction of viscosity; this helps to maintain systemic oxygen delivery by facilitating higher cardiac output. The other important acute compensation for anemia is increased oxygen extraction.

Acute normovolemic anemia (hemoglobin of 6.0 g/dL or less) is well tolerated in healthy young volunteers and is not associated with excess mortality at hemoglobin levels exceeding 8.0 g/dL in elderly patients undergoing repair of hip fractures; at hemoglobin levels of 7.0 to 9.0 g/dL it perhaps even improves outcome in critically ill patients. Of 11 healthy patients aged 35 to 69 years and in 21 volunteers aged 19 to 33 years in whom acute, severe, normovolemic anemia (5.0 ± 0.1 g/dL) was induced, oxygen transport was maintained at 79% of the prehemodilution baseline by a compensatory increase in cardiac index and no patient developed evidence of inadequate systemic oxygenation.[75] Of 8,787 consecutive patients, 57% of whom exceeded age 80, who had undergone emergent repair of hip fractures, there was no correlation between hemoglobin levels greater than 8.0 g/dL and mortality.[76] In critically ill patients, 30-day mortality was not statistically different between the two groups, one randomized to a restrictive transfusion strategy in which red cells were transfused to maintain a hemoglobin concentration between 7.0 and 9.0 g/dL and one randomized to a liberal strategy that maintained a hemoglobin concentration between 10.0 and 12.0 g/dL.[77] Of the patients in the restrictive strategy group, 33% received no red cells after randomization while no patient in the liberal strategy group avoided transfusion of red cells.

However, known cardiovascular disease may necessitate a higher transfusion trigger. Nelson and colleagues[78] reported a small case-controlled study of 27 patients with ischemic heart disease who underwent lower extremity vascular surgery. In patients with hematocrits of less than 28%, 10 developed myocardial ischemia and 6 died or had important morbidity; in contrast, in the 14 patients in whom hematocrit exceeded 28%, only 2 developed myocardial ischemia and none died or had severe morbidity. Nevertheless, in the retrospective series of patients undergoing repair of fractured hips[76] and the critically ill patients randomized to maintenance at lower hemoglobin levels,[77] there was no apparent influence of acute anemia on outcome in the fraction with cardiovascular disease.

Strategies to Reduce Blood Transfusion

A variety of strategies have been proposed to limit the use of allogenic red cell transfusion. These include preoperative autologous blood donation, acute normovolemic hemodilution, perioperative red cell salvage, deliberate hypotension, and administration of pharmacologic adjuvants. Although preoperative autologous blood donation effectively decreases or eliminates the need for homologous blood during and after surgery,[79] it is somewhat expensive, significantly lowers preoperative hematocrit, and results in more liberal transfusion practices.[80]

Acute intraoperative hemodilution is less expensive and administratively far simpler than preoperative donation. In addition, blood harvested intraoperatively provides active platelets, has minimal opportunity for bacterial contamination and overgrowth, because the units never leave the operating room, and is less prone to clerical errors such as administration to an incorrectly identified patient. Finally, the patient, or the surgical team, requires no additional time because the procedure is carried out during anesthesia.[81] However, Bryson and colleagues,[82] in a meta-analysis of 24 trials of acute normovolemic hemodilution, found no overall effect in trials that used a rigorous transfusion protocol. In other words, much of the benefit of acute normovolemic hemodilution can be achieved simply by using a lower hematocrit level as a transfusion trigger.

In surgical procedures associated with massive blood loss, red cell salvage is relatively simple and safe but cost-effectiveness is an issue. Unless more than 2 units of blood are recovered, red cell salvage is unlikely to be cost-effective or to reduce the number of homologous units transfused. However, intraoperative red cell salvage may be of value in surgical procedures involving rapid blood loss because it provides inexpensive blood that is immediately available.[81]

In general, the popularity of deliberate hypotension has waned as other techniques for transfusion avoidance have evolved. In cardiac surgery, pharmacologic agents used to limit blood loss include aprotinin, ε-aminocaproic acid, tranexamic acid, and desmopressin. In controlled studies, each has reduced the perioperative volume of transfused red cells. However, issues of cost-effectiveness have limited widespread use.

REGIONAL ANESTHESIA

Regional anesthesia is an attractive anesthetic option for many types of operative procedures and can provide excellent postoperative pain management in selected patients. However, like any anesthetic technique, the risks and benefits of regional anesthesia must be assessed for each individual. Several regional techniques are in common use, including spinal, epidural, and peripheral nerve blocks. Each technique has specific benefits and risks, which depend in part on the choice of local anesthetic drugs.

Local Anesthetic Drugs

Local anesthetics have played a critical part in intraoperative anesthesia almost since they were first described. The two classes of local anesthetic drugs in common use are the aminoesters and the aminoamides (often described as esters and amides). The mechanism of action of local anesthetics is dose-dependent blockade of sodium currents in nerve fibers. Local anesthetic drugs differ in terms of physicochemical characteristics. Of these, the most important are the pK_a, protein binding, and the degree of hydrophobicity.[83] The pK_a refers to the pH at which half of the drug exists in the basic unchanged form and half exists in the cationic form. In general, agents with a lower pK_a have an onset that is faster than agents with a higher pK_a, although some agents, such as chloroprocaine, can be given at much higher concentrations, thereby offsetting the effects of a high pK_a. Because all commonly used local anesthetics have relatively high pK_as, they are largely ineffective in acidotic (inflamed) environments, in which local anesthetics exist primarily in the ionized form that does not penetrate nerves. In general, greater hydrophobicity is associated with greater potency and increased protein binding correlates with a longer duration of action. The speed of onset, duration of action, and typical doses of agents commonly used for regional anesthesia or local anesthesia are summarized in Table 17-10.

In using local anesthetics clinically, the priority is to prevent local anesthetic toxicity. When used for regional anesthesia, the toxicity of local anesthetics is dependent on the site of injection and the speed of absorption. Inadvertent intravascular injection of local anesthetics will produce toxicity with much smaller doses. The main symptoms of local anesthetic toxicity involve the central nervous system and cardiovascular system (Fig. 17-6). The earliest signs of an overdose or inadvertent intravascular

---

TABLE 17-10.   Important Characteristics of Local Anesthetics for Major Nerve Blocks

Local Anesthetic	Aminoamide or Aminoester	Speed of Onset (min)	Duration of Action (min)	Maximal Dose* (Axillary Block; mg)
Lidocaine	Aminoamide	10-20	60-180	5 mg/kg
Mepivacaine	Aminoamide	10-20	60-180	5 mg/kg
Bupivacaine	Aminoamide	15-30	180-360	3 mg/kg
Chloroprocaine	Aminoester	10-20	30-50	(not usually used)

*Maximal dose without epinephrine; doses of lidocaine and mepivacaine can be increased to 7-8 mg/kg if epinephrine is added. Lower doses may be toxic if infiltrated subcutaneously, as in intercostal nerve blocks; larger doses of lidocaine and mepivacaine may be tolerated if given by epidural injection.

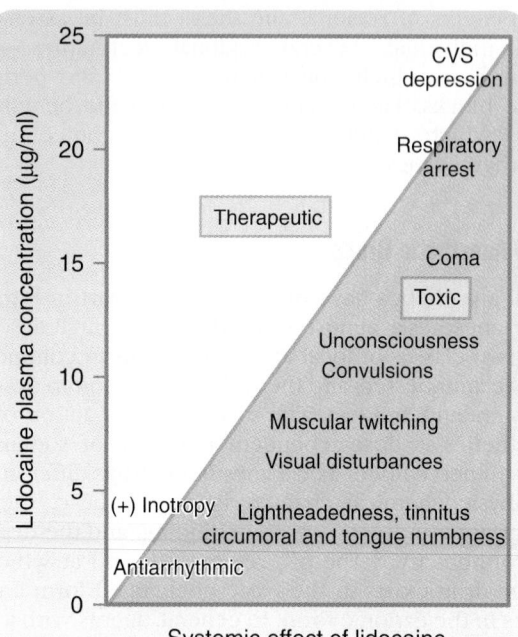

FIGURE 17-6.   Relationship between plasma concentration of lidocaine and various signs and symptoms of toxicity. CVS, cardiovascular system. From Berde CB, Strichartz GR: Local anesthetics. *In* Miller RD (ed): Anesthesia, 5th ed. Philadelphia, Churchill Livingstone, 2000, pp 491-522.

injection are numbness or tingling of the tongue or lips, a metallic taste, light-headedness, tinnitus, or visual disturbances. The signs of toxicity can progress to slurred speech, disorientation, and seizures. With higher doses of local anesthetics, cardiovascular collapse will ensue.

The best defenses against local anesthetic toxicity are aspiration to detect unplanned vascular entry before injecting large doses of local anesthetics and knowledge of the maximal safe dose of the drug being injected. Adding epinephrine, which slows absorption, also decreases the likelihood of a toxic response secondary to rapid absorption. The primary treatments of local anesthetic toxicity are oxygen and airway support. If a seizure does not terminate spontaneously, a benzodiazepine (e.g., midazolam) or thiopental should be given. Cardiovascular support may be needed.

Cardiovascular toxicity from bupivacaine may be particularly difficult to treat. One approach intended to reduce the cardiovascular toxicity of bupivacaine (a racemic mixture of the *levo*- and *dextro*-isomers) has been to produce a solution consisting only of the *levo*-isomer. In healthy male volunteers, a slow intravenous infusion of levobupivacaine reduced mean stroke index, acceleration index, and ejection fraction less than racemic bupivacaine.[84] Ropivacaine, a newer potent amide local anesthetic, was compared with bupivacaine and lidocaine in volunteers receiving a slow intravenous infusion until central nervous system symptoms first occurred. Echocardiography and ECG monitoring were used to quantify systolic, diastolic, and electrophysiologic effects. Bupivacaine increased QRS width during sinus rhythm compared with the other two treatments and reduced both systolic and diastolic function, whereas ropivacaine only reduced systolic function.[85]

An area of intense research interest has been the use of α_2-adrenergic agents to potentiate or substitute for local anesthetics. Production of regional anesthesia was first produced with cocaine (also a local anesthetic) for subarachnoid block in the late 1800s, although the specific receptors involved were not established until much later.[86] The α_2-adrenergic drug clonidine was first used epidurally in 1984 after extensive characterization in animals. Despite side effects, such as hypotension, bradycardia, and sedation, experience in thousands of patients demonstrates considerable safety when used alone or with local anesthetics or opioids for epidural anesthesia and analgesia, subarachnoid block, or peripheral nerve block. In general, clonidine prolongs or intensifies the effects of local anesthetics or opioids and produces pain relief when used alone.[86]

Spinal Anesthesia

Spinal anesthesia or subarachnoid block has many applications for urologic, lower abdominal, perineal, and lower extremity surgery. Spinal anesthesia is induced by injection of local anesthetic with or without opiates into the subarachnoid space. A well-performed subarachnoid block provides excellent sensory and motor blockade below the level of the block. The block generally has a relatively rapid and predictable onset. Several factors determine the level, speed of onset, and duration of spinal blocks.

1. Local anesthetic agent: Local anesthetics have varying potencies, durations of action, and speeds of onset after subarachnoid administration. Typical doses and durations of action are shown in Table 17-11. These properties are determined by the lipid solubility, protein binding, and pK_a of each agent.
2. Volume and dose of local anesthetic: Increasing the dose will generally increase the extent of cephalad spread and duration of subarachnoid block. Eighteen volunteers received one of three doses (4, 8, or 12 mg) of bupivacaine and one of three doses of ropivacaine for subarachnoid analgesia. Ropivacaine is half as potent and in equipotent doses has a similar profile with a higher incidence of side effects (such as a 28% incidence of pain on injection).[87] Rapidly injecting local anesthetic solutions leads to turbulent flow and unpredictable spread.
3. Patient position and local anesthetic baricity: Local anesthetic solutions can be prepared as hypobaric, isobaric, and hyperbaric solutions. Cerebrospinal fluid has a low specific gravity (i.e., only slightly greater than water). Local anesthetic solutions prepared in water have a slightly lower specific gravity than cerebrospinal fluid and will ascend within it. Plain local anesthetic solutions are isobaric, and local anesthetics mixed in 5% dextrose are hyperbaric, relative to cerebrospinal fluid. The baricity of the local anesthetic solution and

TABLE 17-11. Local Anesthetics Used for Subarachnoid Block

Drug	Usual Concentration (%)	Usual Volume (mL)	Total Dose (mg)	Baricity	Glucose Concentration (%)	Usual Duration (min)
Lidocaine	1.5, 5.0	1–2	30–100	Hyperbaric	7.5	30-60
Tetracaine	0.25–1.0	1–4	5–20	Hyperbaric	5.0	75-200
	0.25	2–6	5–20	Hypobaric	0	75-200
	1.0	1–2	5–20	Isobaric	0	75-200
Bupivacaine	0.5	3–4	15–20	Isobaric	0	75-200
	0.75	2–3	15–22.5	Hyperbaric	8.25	75-200

From Berde CB, Strichartz GR: Local anesthetics. *In* Miller RD (ed): Anesthesia, 5th ed. Philadelphia, Churchill Livingstone, 2000, pp 491-522.

the position of the patient at the time of injection and until the local anesthetic firmly binds to nervous tissue will determine the level of block. For example, administration of hyperbaric bupivacaine at the low lumbar level to a patient in the sitting position will result in an intense lumbosacral block. The longer the patient remains in the sitting position, the less the cephalad spread of the block.

4. Vasoconstrictors: The addition of epinephrine, particularly to short-acting local anesthetics, will increase the duration of action.
5. Addition of opioids: Addition of small doses of fentanyl (e.g., 20 µg) or morphine (e.g., 0.25 mg) will prolong the duration of analgesia and increase the duration of analgesia and tolerance for tourniquet pain.
6. Anatomic and physiologic factors: A higher than expected level of spinal anesthesia can result from anatomic factors, such as obesity, pregnancy, increased intra-abdominal pressure, prior spine surgery, and abnormal spinal curvature, that decrease the relative volume of the subarachnoid space. Elderly patients tend to be more sensitive to intrathecally injected local anesthetics.

Spinal anesthesia provides the advantage of avoiding manipulation of the airway and the potential complications of tracheal intubation, as well as the potential side effects of general anesthetics such as nausea, vomiting, and prolonged emergence or drowsiness. Spinal anesthesia also provides advantages for several types of surgery, including endoscopic urologic procedures, particularly transurethral resection of the prostate, in which an awake patient provides a valuable monitor for assessment of hyponatremia or bladder perforation. Less confusion and postoperative delirium have been reported in elderly patients after repair of hip fractures under spinal anesthesia. Intrathecal opiate administration can provide high-quality postoperative analgesia for patients undergoing abdominal, lower extremity, urologic, and gynecologic procedures.

In most cases, spinal anesthesia is administered as a single bolus injection. Therefore, the block is of limited

duration and is not suitable for prolonged procedures. The practice of continuous spinal anesthesia using small-bore catheters has been largely abandoned because of neurologic complications associated with local anesthetic toxicity. However, continuous spinal anesthesia with relatively large-bore epidural catheters can provide the advantages of incremental titration and the ability to administer additional doses in selected elderly patients. Unfortunately, this technique has a high likelihood of inducing a postdural puncture headache in young patients.

Complications of subarachnoid block include hypotension (sometimes refractory), bradycardia, postdural puncture headache, transient radicular neuropathy, backache, urinary retention, infection, epidural hematoma, and excessive cephalad spread resulting in cardiorespiratory compromise. Frank neurologic injury, although recently described with continuous techniques using small-bore catheters, is quite rare. Hypotension, occurring as a consequence of sympathectomy, usually responds readily to fluids and small doses of pressor, such as ephedrine. The efficacy of fluid preloading in providing prophylaxis against hypotension is controversial.

Postdural puncture headache occurs after a small proportion of subarachnoid blocks. Factors that increase the incidence include female gender, younger age, and larger needles. Epidural analgesia would appear to avoid the complication, but, if the dura is inadvertently punctured, leaves a much larger dural rent. Compared with epidural anesthesia, spinal anesthesia has a quicker onset, is more predictably satisfactory for surgery, and is less frequently associated with backache. Transient radicular neuropathy, a painful but usually self-limiting condition, recently became evident in association with an increase in enthusiasm for the use of lidocaine for subarachnoid block.

When cardiac arrest results from excessive cephalad spread of subarachnoid block or protracted hypotension, cardiopulmonary resuscitation is notoriously difficult. Patients who suffer cardiac arrest during subarachnoid block have poor survival, possibly because the profound sympathectomy causes difficulty in generating adequate coronary perfusion pressure. Relatively large doses of epinephrine may be necessary to achieve adequate perfusion pressure during cardiopulmonary resuscitation after spinal anesthesia. Absolute contraindications to spinal anesthesia include sepsis, bacteremia, infection at the site of injection, severe hypovolemia, coagulopathy, therapeutic anticoagulation, increased intracranial pressure, and patient refusal.

Epidural Anesthesia

Epidural block, another form of neuraxial regional block, has application in a wide variety of abdominal, thoracic, and lower extremity procedures. Induction of epidural anesthesia or analgesia results from injection of local anesthetics with or without opiates into the lumbar or thoracic epidural space. Generally, a catheter is inserted after the epidural space has been located with a needle. The presence of the catheter provides several advantages. First, local anesthetic can be added in a controlled fashion so that the time to block onset can be well controlled. Second, the catheter can be "redosed" repeatedly so that anesthesia can be provided for the duration of lengthy procedures. Third, local anesthetics or opiates can be administered for several days to provide postoperative analgesia.

Epidural anesthesia has specific advantages for thoracic surgery, peripheral vascular surgery, and gastrointestinal surgery. Epidural anesthesia also has been shown to decrease blood loss and deep venous thrombosis during total joint arthroplasty. Postoperative epidural analgesia for thoracic surgery provides superior pain control, less sedation, and better pulmonary function compared with parenteral opiates.

Christopherson and coworkers[88] randomized 100 patients undergoing major elective vascular reconstruction to receive either epidural anesthesia followed by postoperative epidural analgesia or general anesthesia followed by patient-controlled analgesia. Epidural anesthesia was associated with a lower rate of reoperation for vascular insufficiency (2 vs. 11 in the general anesthesia group). Other morbidity and mortality rates were similar. However, the choice of anesthesia does not apparently influence overall morbidity in patients undergoing peripheral vascular surgery.

The use of low concentrations of local anesthetics in conjunction with epidural opiates has been associated with earlier ambulation and less postoperative ileus after abdominal surgery. Thoracic epidural anesthesia, but not lumbar epidural anesthesia, appears to be associated with more rapid recovery of gastrointestinal function after major abdominal surgery.[89] However, because intraoperative intravenous lidocaine also resulted in more rapid return of bowel function (flatus and bowel movement), circulating systemic lidocaine may account for at least some of the effects of epidural anesthesia on postoperative bowel function. A continuing controversy relates to whether epidural or subarachnoid analgesia reduces subsequent analgesic requirements after the block has resolved ("preemptive analgesia").

The complications and contraindications for epidural anesthesia are similar to those for spinal anesthesia.

However, a special cautionary note is indicated regarding epidural anesthesia and anticoagulation. Because of the risk of spinal hematoma, the placement and removal of epidural catheters in patients receiving oral or parenteral anticoagulation should be performed in conjunction with an anesthesiologist. The recent advent of low-molecular-weight heparin (LMWH) for prophylaxis of deep venous thrombosis has resulted in an increase in the incidence of epidural hematomas associated with the removal or placement of epidural catheters. Although LMWH is effective as prophylaxis against venous thromboembolism, spinal hematomas have occurred in association with perioperative use of LMWH in patients given neuraxial anesthesia.[90] The timing of catheter placement and removal in the setting of LMWH use is critical to avoiding this rare but catastrophic complication. A high index of suspicion of epidural hematoma must be maintained in patients undergoing neuraxial block who have received or who will receive LMWH. All persons involved in the care of patients receiving continuous epidural analgesia should be aware of the signs of epidural hematoma, including back pain, lower extremity sensory and motor dysfunction, and bladder and bowel abnormalities. To reduce the risk, needle placement should not occur less than 10 to 12 hours after the last dose and subsequent dosing should be delayed at least 2 hours. Epidural catheters should be withdrawn at least 10 to 12 hours after the last dose of LMWH.

A final rare complication, epidural abscess, should be considered in patients who develop back pain after epidural injection; MRI is an effective diagnostic tool in such patients.

Peripheral Nerve Blocks

Blockade of the brachial plexus, lumbar plexus, and specific peripheral nerves is an effective means of providing surgical anesthesia and postoperative analgesia for many surgical procedures involving the upper and lower extremities. Typical doses of local anesthetics for a variety of regional nerve blocks are shown in Table 17-11.[83] The advantage of peripheral nerve blocks is the reduced physiologic stress compared to spinal or epidural anesthesia, the avoidance of airway manipulation and the potential complications associated with endotracheal intubation, and the avoidance of potential side effects associated with general anesthesia. However, successful nerve block anesthesia requires a cooperative patient, an anesthesiologist skilled in peripheral nerve blocks, and a surgeon who is accustomed to operating on awake patients. The success of nerve blocks depends on the type of block, the type of surgery, and the expertise of the block practitioner. All patients undergoing peripheral nerve block should receive full preoperative evaluation, with the assumption that general anesthesia could be utilized if the block is inadequate.

Improvements in nerve block equipment and methodology as well as the availability of a wide range of local anesthetics have greatly improved the effectiveness and safety of peripheral nerve blocks. In addition to providing surgical anesthesia, peripheral nerve blocks and the placement of indwelling catheters for prolonged nerve block provide excellent analgesia for many types of upper extremity surgery and after extremity injury. An additional application of indwelling catheters is the enhancement of blood flow after reattachment of amputated limbs and in patients with peripheral vascular disease. Each specific block has specific associated risks and benefits. However, general complications of peripheral nerve blocks include local anesthetic toxicity, neurologic injury, inadvertent neuraxial block, and intravascular injection of local anesthetics.

CONSCIOUS SEDATION

When anesthesiologists participate in sedation of patients undergoing surgical procedures, the procedure is termed *monitored anesthesia care.* Monitored anesthesia care encompasses a wide range of depths of sedation, ranging from minimal sedation to brief intervals of complete unconsciousness (for instance, during placement of a retrobulbar block by an ophthalmologist). When non-anesthesia personnel administer sedation for surgical procedures, the process is generally termed *conscious sedation,* although the term *moderate sedation* is preferable. Moderate sedation implies that the patient can respond purposefully to verbal or tactile stimulation, has a patent airway requiring no intervention, has adequate spontaneous ventilation, and has maintained cardiovascular function. There is a narrow margin between minimal sedation, which may be inadequate for surgery to continue, and deep sedation, which may result in airway compromise and cardiovascular and ventilatory depression. Because of the risks associated with moderate sedation, the Joint Commission on Healthcare Organizations requires that patients be managed using similar precautions to what they would receive if sedation were managed by an anesthesiologist. Important factors include the necessity for a preprocedure evaluation, continuous presence of a trained monitoring assistant who has no other responsibilities throughout the procedure, immediate availability of airway and resuscitation equipment, monitoring after the procedure until the effects of sedation have resolved, and specific written postoperative instructions. Physicians who perform procedures on patients under conscious sedation should be granted privileges based on training and experience in the appropriate resuscitative procedures.

Drugs used for moderate sedation usually consist of opioids such as fentanyl or morphine, often combined with an anxiolytic such as midazolam. Titration of these agents requires careful assessment of a patient's level of pain or anxiety and the requirements for the surgical procedure. In general, intravenous induction agents such as propofol introduce an added element of risk and increase the need for caution, because of the ease with which administration of additional agent may result in progression to deep sedation or even general anesthesia. Most hospitals now have specific policies and procedures governing moderate sedation. Those who use moderate sedation outside hospitals (e.g., in office-based surgical practices) should practice the same precautions as are practiced in the hospital environment.

POSTANESTHESIA CARE

The PACU is the area designated for the care of patients recovering from the immediate physiologic and pharmacologic consequences associated with anesthesia and surgery. The PACU should be located in close proximity to the operating rooms. Monitors for the assessment of ventilation, oxygenation, and circulation should be available for all recovering patients. The extent of monitoring will depend on the condition of the patient. The ASA has established standards of postanesthesia care, which mandate that:

1. All patients undergoing general, regional, or monitored anesthesia care will receive appropriate postanesthesia care as dictated by the responsible anesthesiologist.
2. An anesthesia provider who is aware of the patient's condition will accompany all patients to the PACU.
3. Upon arrival in the PACU, the patient's condition will be reassessed and reported to the care provider assuming responsibility for care.
4. The patient's condition will be evaluated continually in the PACU.
5. A physician is responsible for the discharge of the patient from the PACU.

Recovery from anesthesia is usually uneventful and routine. Most patients stay in the PACU for 30 to 60 minutes until they are fully reactive and can move to a second-stage recovery area (for ambulatory patients who are returning home that day) or to a bed on a surgical floor. However, several criteria should be met before the patient can be safely discharged from the PACU. All patients must be awake and oriented with stable vital signs. Patients must be breathing without difficulty and able to protect their airways and be oxygenating appropriately. Pain, shivering, nausea, and vomiting must be adequately controlled. Patients receiving regional anesthesia must be observed for resolution of the block. There should be no evidence of surgical complications such as postoperative bleeding.

Several types of anesthesia-related complications are commonly encountered in the PACU and must be promptly recognized and treated to prevent serious injury.

Postoperative Agitation and Delirium

Pain and anxiety are often manifested as postoperative agitation. However, agitation may also signal serious physiologic disturbances such as hypoxemia, hypercarbia, acidosis, hypotension, hypoglycemia, surgical complications, and adverse drug reactions. Serious underlying conditions must be excluded as the cause of agitation before empirically treating patients with pain medications, sedatives, or physical restraints.

Respiratory Complications

Respiratory problems are the most frequently occurring major complications in the PACU. Airway obstruction is most commonly due to obstruction of the oropharynx by the tongue or oropharyngeal soft tissues caused by the residual effects of general anesthetics, pain medications, or muscle relaxants. Other causes of airway obstruction include laryngospasm, blood, vomitus or debris in the airway, glottic edema, vocal cord paralysis, and external compression of the airway by a hematoma, dressing, or cervical collar. Oxygen must be administered to a patient with airway obstruction as measures are taken to relieve the obstruction. The characteristic physical signs of airway obstruction are sonorous respiratory sounds and paradoxical chest movement.

Many obstructions can be relieved by applying a head-tilt and jaw-thrust maneuver with or without placement of an oral or nasopharyngeal airway. Suctioning the airway may also be beneficial, and the patient should be examined for evidence of external airway compression. In cases of laryngospasm, continuous positive airway pressure (CPAP) should be applied, followed by administration of 10 to 20 mg of succinylcholine if CPAP is ineffective. Patients may require mask ventilation and endotracheal intubation if laryngospasm does not resolve promptly. In children, glottic edema or postextubation croup can result in airway obstruction. Mild cases are treated with humidified oxygen. Refractory obstruction may require the administration of systemic corticosteroids and racemic epinephrine by nebulization. Reintubation may also be required.

Hypoxemia is a surprisingly common problem. In one study, the incidence of mild hypoxemia (SpO_2 86% to 90%) and severe hypoxemia ($SpO_2 \leq 85\%$) was 7% and 0.7%, respectively, in the PACU for patients undergoing superficial elective plastic surgery, 38% and 3%, respectively, for patients undergoing upper abdominal surgery, and 52% and 20%, respectively, for patients undergoing thoracoabdominal surgery.[91] Hypoxemia can result from hypoventilation, ventilation-perfusion mismatching, or right to left intrapulmonary shunting. Reluctance to inspire deeply after abdominal or thoracic surgery may also result in hypoxemia. Clinically, hypoxemia must be suspected as an underlying problem in patients exhibiting restlessness, tachycardia, or cardiac irritability. Bradycardia, hypotension, and cardiac arrest are late signs. Hypoxemia in the PACU may be secondary to atelectasis, which may respond to incentive spirometry or vigorous encouragement to inspire deeply and cough. Treatment of hypoxemia requires administration of oxygen, assurance of adequate ventilation, and treatment of underlying causes.

Hypoventilation (synonymous with hypercarbia) can result from airway obstruction, central respiratory depression caused by the residual effects of anesthetic agents, hypothermia, or central nervous system injury, or restriction of ventilation caused by muscle relaxants, abdominal distention, and electrolyte abnormalities. Signs can include prolonged somnolence, slow (or rapid) respiratory rate, airway obstruction, shallow breathing, tachycardia, and arrhythmias. Severe hypoventilation can result in hypoxemia, although augmented inspired oxygen will limit the severity of hypoventilation-induced hypoxemia. Treatment is aimed at identification and treatment of the underlying problem. In all cases, ventilation must be supported until corrective measures are instituted. Obtundation, circulatory depression, and severe respiratory acidosis are indications for endotracheal intubation and ventilatory support.

Postoperative Nausea and Vomiting

Perhaps one of the most annoying problems for both patients and personnel in the PACU is postoperative nausea and vomiting. Agents used to prevent or treat postoperative nausea and vomiting include propofol for induction of anesthesia; droperidol, an inexpensive agent that is often effective in subsedative doses; ondansetron (and related drugs), which are expensive agents that are marginally more effective; and metoclopramide, which increases gastric motility. No technique has yet proven to be both uniformly therapeutic and cost effective. One important complication related to intravenous co-administration of ondansetron and metoclopramide has been the production of bradyarrhythmias, including a slow junctional escape rhythm and ventricular bigeminy.

The approach to the prophylaxis and treatment of postoperative nausea and vomiting should be guided by an understanding of the mechanisms causing nausea and vomiting. Areas in the brain stem such as the chemoreceptor trigger zone that control nausea and vomiting reflexes contain receptors for dopamine, acetylcholine, histamine, and serotonin. Binding of all of these receptors may precipitate nausea and/or vomiting. Effective pharmacologic approaches to the treatment of postoperative nausea and vomiting include the use of anticholinergics, serotonin receptor antagonists, antidopaminergics, and antihistamines (Table 17-12). The use of any particular agent should be based on efficacy, potential side effects, and cost.

Hypothermia

Hypothermia has been extensively studied as a perioperative complication. The most important issues related to perioperative hypothermia include the risk of increased oxygen consumption postoperatively and the possibility that hypothermia could increase the rate of surgical infections. Increased oxygen consumption could be a particular problem in patients with CAD in whom shivering could trigger myocardial ischemia. However, the risk of mild hypothermia has not been well defined in otherwise healthy patients.

Circulatory Complications

Hypotension in the PACU is most commonly due to hypovolemia, left ventricular dysfunction, or arrhythmias. Other causes include anaphylaxis, transfusion reactions,

TABLE 17-12. Commonly Used Antiemetic Agents

Drug Class	Drug Name	Common Side Effects
Dopamine receptor antagonists (DA-2)		
Phenothiazines	Fluphenazine	Sedation
	Chlorpromazine	Dissociation
	Prochlorperazine	Extrapyramidal effects
Butyrophenones	Droperidol	
	Haloperidol	
Substituted benzamide	Metoclopramide	
Antihistamines (H1)	Diphenhydramine	Sedation
	Promethazine	Dry mouth
Anticholinergics	Scopolamine	Sedation
	Atropine	Dry mouth
		Tachycardia
Serotonin receptor antagonists	Ondansetron	Headache
	Dolasetron	
Corticosteroids	Dexamethasone	Glucose intolerance
	Methylprednisolone	Altered wound healing
	Hydrocortisone	Immunosuppression
		Renal effects

cardiac tamponade, pulmonary emboli, adverse drug reactions, adrenal insufficiency, and hypoxemia. Treatment involves support of the circulation with fluids, inotropic agents, Trendelenburg position, and oxygen until the underlying cause is diagnosed and treated.

Hypertension is a common finding in the PACU. Common causes include pain, anxiety, and inadequately managed essential hypertension. Hypoxemia and hypercarbia should always be ruled out. Other less common causes include hypoglycemia, drug reactions, diseases such as hyperthyroidism, pheochromocytoma, or malignant hyperthermia, and bladder distention. The fundamental goal in control of postoperative hypertension is to identify and correct the underlying cause.

ACUTE PAIN MANAGEMENT

Pain, one of the most common symptoms experienced by surgical patients, has historically been poorly evaluated and frequently undertreated. Recently, there have been important changes in medical care with respect to pain management, including increased emphasis on pain management in medical school curricula, development of institutional protocols and procedures for pain management, development of the subspecialty of pain medicine, creation of organizations focused on pain, and increased interest on the part of governmental and third-party payers.[92-95] These changes will continue into the future, and medical personnel must continue to increase their knowledge of pain control and their commitment to provide optimal analgesia as a key component of patient care. A recent survey demonstrates that continued improvement is necessary to further reduce the high incidence of moderate to severe acute postoperative pain.[96]

Acute pain occurs frequently in the setting of surgery and trauma. The pain experience may be part of the symptom-complex that prompts the patient to seek medical care, or it may result from tissue injury sustained from surgery or trauma. The term *acute* refers to pain that is expected to be of relatively short duration and that should resolve with tissue healing or withdrawal of the noxious stimulus. Acute pain usually resolves within minutes, hours, or days. *Chronic* pain, which can persist for years, is defined as pain that persists for at least 1 month beyond the usual course of an acute disease or beyond a reasonable time in which an injury would be expected to heal. The acute stress response associated with acute pain serves a useful function, although undertreatment may result in harmful pathophysiologic changes. Chronic pain serves no useful function and is now recognized not only as a part of certain disease processes such as cancer but often as a disease itself.

Mechanisms of Acute Pain

Pain is defined by The International Association for the Study of Pain (IASP) as "an unpleasant sensory and emotional experience associated with actual or potential tissue damage or described in terms of such damage." This definition emphasizes not only the sensory experience but also the affective component of pain. The tissue injury that leads to the complaint of pain results in a process called nociception, which has four steps: transduction, transmission, modulation, and perception (Fig. 17-7). With transduction, the noxious stimulus is converted into an electrical signal at free nerve endings, which are also known as nociceptors. Nociceptors are widely distributed throughout the body in both somatic and visceral tissues.

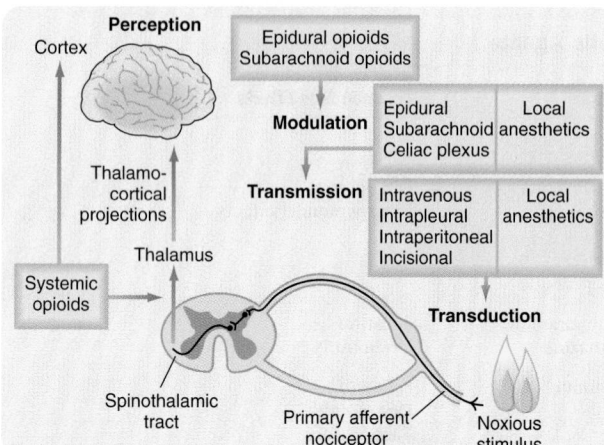

FIGURE 17-7. Schematic diagram outlines the nociceptive pathway for transmission of painful stimuli. Interventions that prevent nociceptive transmission are shown at the points in the pathway that are thought to be their sites of action. From Ferrante FM, VadeBoncouer TR: Postoperative Pain Management. New York, Churchill Livingstone, 1993.

With transmission, the electrical signal is sent in nerve pathways toward the central nervous system. Nerve pathways include primary sensory afferents (primarily $A\delta$ and C fibers) that project to the spinal cord, ascending pathways from the spinal cord to the brain stem and thalamus (including the spinothalamic tract), and thalamocortical pathways. Modulation, the process that either enhances or suppresses the pain signal, occurs primarily in the dorsal horn of the spinal cord, in particular the substantia gelatinosa. Perception, the final step in the nociceptive process, occurs when the pain signal reaches the cerebral cortex. The first three steps in nociception are important for the sensory and discriminative aspects of pain. The fourth step, perception, is integral to the subjective and emotional experience.

Methods of Analgesia

Multiple agents, routes of administration, and modalities are available for effective management of acute pain. Analgesic agents include opioids, nonsteroidal anti-inflammatory drugs, acetaminophen, and local anesthetics. Less traditional agents that may be used more frequently in the future include clonidine, dexmedetomidine, and dextromethorphan. Routes of administration include the oral, parenteral, epidural, and intrathecal routes. The oral route is the preferred route for analgesic delivery. Patients experiencing mild to moderate acute pain and who can receive agents orally can obtain effective analgesia. Parenteral administration is preferred for patients experiencing moderate to severe pain, patients who require rapid control of pain, and patients who cannot receive agents through the gastrointestinal tract. The intravenous route is preferred over intramuscular and subcutaneous injections when the parenteral route is indicated. Intramuscular injections are painful, result in erratic absorption, and lead to variable blood levels of the administered agent.

Opioids

Opioids are potent analgesic agents that are effective but frequently underused. By binding to opioid receptors in the central nervous system, and likely also in peripheral tissues, opioids modulate the nociceptive process. The best characterized opioid receptors are $\mu1$, $\mu2$, δ, κ, ε, and σ receptors. The $\mu1$ receptors are involved in supraspinal analgesia. The δ and κ receptors are involved in spinal analgesia. Opioids can be provided using multiple routes of administration, including oral, parenteral, neuraxial, rectal, and transdermal.

Opioids have varying degrees of potency. Strong opioids are ideal for moderate to severe pain and for pain that is constant in frequency. Weak opioid agents are suitable for mild to moderate pain that is intermittent in frequency. Morphine, the prototype strong opioid, can be delivered using a variety of routes and techniques. Other strong opioids include hydromorphone, fentanyl, and meperidine. Morphine is metabolized to morphine-3-glucoronide and morphine-6-glucoronide, which can accumulate in patients who have renal impairment. For moderate to severe pain in patients with renal dysfunction, fentanyl and hydromorphone are more suitable agents. Historically, meperidine has frequently been the preferred strong opioid; however, this practice has declined because meperidine is metabolized to normeperidine, a unique toxic metabolite that can accumulate and cause seizures. Particularly vulnerable patients include the elderly, patients who are dehydrated, and patients with renal impairment. Fentanyl is available in a transdermal preparation, but this route is not recommended for acute pain management.

Weak opioid agents, such as hydrocodone and codeine, are commonly combined with aspirin or acetaminophen. Tramadol is an analgesic that is a nonopioid but has some opioid-like effects. It is a centrally acting agent that is administered orally and can be used for mild to moderate pain. Common opioid-related side effects include nausea, pruritus, sedation, mental clouding, decreased gastric motility, urinary retention, and respiratory depression. Appropriate agent selection, monitoring, and treatment can prevent or ameliorate these side effects.

One major barrier to the effective use of opioid agents by patients, physicians, and other health care providers is the fear of addiction, which can be manifested as underdosing, use of excessively wide dosing intervals, use of weak opioids for moderate to severe pain, and underreporting of pain. In the setting of acute perioperative pain, use of opioids has not been shown to be a risk factor for the development of an addiction disorder. Key terms to understand include tolerance, addiction (psychological dependence), and physical dependence. Tolerance occurs when a previously effective opioid dose fails to provide adequate analgesia. Tolerance is a normal physiologic effect and should not be confused with addiction. Tolerance develops not only to the analgesic effect of opioids but also to opioid-related side effects. Duration of opioid exposure also plays a role in the development of tolerance. In tolerant patients, an increased dose is required to achieve effective analgesia. Addiction or psychological dependence is a compulsive disorder manifested by pre-occupation with obtaining and use of a substance, continued use despite harm, decreased quality of life, and denial. Psychological dependence should not be confused with physical dependence, which is a normal physiologic process. Physical dependence is manifested by the occurrence of a withdrawal syndrome when a drug is stopped suddenly or when an antagonist is given. The duration of opioid treatment is a factor in the development of physical dependence. The short-term use of opioids in the perioperative period should rarely result in physical dependence. Slow tapering of opioids usually prevents withdrawal symptoms.

Nonsteroidal Anti-inflammatory Agents

Nonsteroidal anti-inflammatory drugs (NSAIDs) are an important component of perioperative analgesia that, when used as a part of the analgesic regimen, reduce pain and can decrease opioid consumption. Their mechanism of action is through the inhibition of cyclooxygenase enzyme activity, resulting in a decreased production of prostaglandins. Prostaglandins are potent mediators of pain that act directly at nociceptors and also increase nociceptor sensitivity. Inhibition of prostaglandin production results in analgesia but can also lead to side effects such as gastric ulceration, bleeding, and renal injury. These side effects have limited the use of NSAIDs in the perioperative period. Contrary to previous evidence that NSAIDs act mainly in peripheral tissues, there is now evidence that NSAIDs also work in the central nervous system.

There is a wide range of compounds in this analgesic class with differing chemical structures. Most of these agents are for oral administration, which limits their use perioperatively. Ketorolac is available for parenteral administration and has been shown to be effective for analgesia and safe with appropriate patient selection. Ketorolac should be avoided in patients with a history of gastropathy, platelet dysfunction, or thrombocytopenia, in those with a history of allergy to the agent, and in patients with renal impairment or hypovolemia. It should be used with caution for elderly patients. A loading dose of 30 mg IV, followed by 15 mg IV every 6 hours for a short course, can provide effective analgesia for mild to moderate pain or can be a useful adjunct for moderate to severe pain when combined with opioids or other analgesic techniques.

The most recent advance in this analgesic category involves the introduction of agents that are selective in their inhibition of the subtypes of the cyclooxygenase enzyme. There are at least two subtypes of this enzyme: COX-1 (constitutive) and COX-2 (inducible). Traditional NSAIDs are nonselective inhibitors of COX. The newer agents (celecoxib, rofecoxib, valdecoxib) are selective COX-2 inhibitors. COX-2 inhibitors appear to offer similar analgesia with a somewhat reduced risk of causing gastrointestinal bleeding, bleeding diathesis, and renal compromise.[97] They have mostly been studied and used clinically in the management of arthritis-related pain but are becoming more frequently used in the perioperative period. Currently available COX-2 inhibitors are for oral administration. Parecoxib is being studied for parenteral use. There are indications that COX-2 inhibitors have a lower incidence of gastropathy. They are increasingly being used in the perioperative period and may have preemptive analgesic effects.[98] In patients undergoing total knee replacement, oral administration of rofecoxib from 24 hours before surgery through the fifth postoperative day increased knee flexion and decreased both pain and postoperative opioid consumption.[99] Concerns about the use of these selective NSAIDs include the risk for cardiovascular events and their effects on bone healing.

Local Anesthetics for Management of Acute Pain

Local anesthetics work by blocking conduction in nerve fibers, the second step in the process of nociception. These agents are used to provide regional anesthesia for surgery, but their effects last into the perioperative period and contribute to preemptive analgesia. Local anesthetics used in doses lower than that required for anesthesia can also provide analgesia by a variety of application techniques. These include local infiltration, topical application, epidural infusion, and peripheral nerve infusion. Local infiltration of local anesthetic before surgical incision may reduce sensitization of nociceptors resulting in reduced conduction of pain signals to the central nervous system. This may manifest as decreased postoperative pain and analgesic requirements.[100] Local infiltration on wound closure may also be helpful. Topical application of local anesthetic is obtained using agents such as EMLA cream, which contains prilocaine and lidocaine. This agent can be used for superficial procedures and can be placed before surgical incision. The placement of peripheral nerve catheters for local anesthetic infusion is becoming a frequently used technique for postoperative pain management. The development of disposable and light infusion pumps is leading to the increasing use of peripheral nerve infusion in the ambulatory setting.

Combination Analgesic Therapy

By combining agents from different analgesic classes, synergy may be obtained, resulting in potentiation of effect, reduced dosage of each individual agent, and fewer, less severe side effects from each agent. Common combinations include opioids and NSAIDS in an analgesic regimen or epidural administration of a local anesthetic with an opioid. The choice of agent and technique will depend on factors such as the patient's medical history, the patient's preference, the extent of surgery and expected degree of postoperative pain, the experience of the staff providing care for the patient, and the postoperative setting in which the patient will recover.

The concept of preemptive analgesia continues to be actively explored and used in the perioperative period.[101-104] Using a variety of agents and techniques, the goal is to influence the analgesic process before the initiation of the noxious stimulus (e.g., surgical incision). This minimizes the sensitization of the nervous system and moderates the process of nociception described previously. Effective preemptive analgesia results in decreased postoperative pain, decreased postoperative analgesic requirement, decreased side effects from analgesics, increased compliance with postoperative rehabilitation, and decreased incidence of chronic postsurgical pain syndromes.

Neuraxial Analgesia

Neuraxial routes of administration include the epidural and intrathecal (subarachnoid) routes. These modes of administration require consultation from acute pain specialists, usually anesthesiologists who receive specialized training in the use of the neuraxial route for the administration of anesthesia and analgesia. Neuraxial agents are delivered by a single injection into the epidural or subarachnoid space, by intermittent injections through an indwelling epidural catheter, by continuous infusion through an indwelling epidural catheter, or by patient-controlled epidural analgesia through an indwelling catheter. Indwelling subarachnoid catheters are rarely used for acute pain. An important consideration in selecting patients for neuraxial analgesia is the presence of abnormal coagulation, including concurrent use of antiplatelet and anticoagulant agents. This is important to minimize the risk of intraspinal bleeding and spinal hematoma formation, which can lead to severe neurologic injury. The neuraxial route requires education of the medical and nursing staff and the use of protocols and guidelines. In general, patients can be managed on surgical floors using these analgesic techniques. However, monitoring procedures should be in place to minimize the development of side effects and to enhance patient safety.

Agents such as opioids and local anesthetics are given via the neuraxial route to achieve analgesia. Other agents that have been used neuraxially include clonidine, neostigmine, and acetaminophen. Opioids, when delivered by the neuraxial route, provide analgesia by their action at opioid receptors located in the dorsal horn of the spinal cord. An important determinant of opioid action when delivered using the neuraxial route is the drug's degree of lipid solubility. Morphine is hydrophilic, which accounts for its slow onset of analgesia, long duration of action, its ability to provide analgesia over a wide dermatomal distribution, and the risk for late respiratory depression associated with the use of neuraxial morphine. Fentanyl is lipophilic, which accounts for its fast onset and short duration of action, its ability to provide segmental analgesia, and its limited risk of late respiratory depression. A hydrophilic opioid such as morphine, when delivered into the epidural or subarachnoid space, remains in the cerebrospinal fluid for a longer period of time than a lipophilic opioid. The drug can travel rostrally to the brain, influencing the respiratory centers hours after initial delivery.

Local anesthetics, when used for neuraxial analgesia, provide analgesia by blocking nerve conduction. To achieve neuraxial analgesia, local anesthetics are delivered in smaller doses and weaker concentrations than that which is required to achieve surgical anesthesia. This resulting sensory blockade is sufficient to provide analgesia but not sufficiently profound to interfere with motor function and to mask complications. Analgesic concentrations of local anesthetics also cause less impairment of sympathetic tone. Bupivacaine, the most common local anesthetic used for epidural analgesia, affects sensory fibers more than motor fibers (differential blockade) and has a lower incidence of tachyphylaxis (tolerance to local anesthetic action). Neuraxial analgesia for acute pain commonly combines opioids and local anesthetics. Each agent has a different mechanism of action; combining these agents produces synergistic analgesia, resulting in reduced doses of each agent and a decreased incidence and severity of side effects. A recent meta-analysis of the efficacy of postoperative epidural analgesia concluded that epidural analgesia, regardless of agent, location of catheter placement, and type of pain assessment, provided superior analgesia in comparison to parenteral opioids.[105]

Intravenous Patient-Controlled Analgesia

An increasingly popular and effective modality using the parenteral route of administration is intravenous patient-controlled analgesia (IV PCA). This modality minimizes the steps involved in the delivery of analgesia and increases patient autonomy and control. Opioids are the agent of choice for IV PCA. In comparing IV PCA to conventional, intermittent, nurse-administered opioid delivery, patients receive prompt analgesia, receive smaller doses of opioids at more frequent intervals, can maintain blood concentration of drug in the analgesic range, and have a lower incidence of drug-related side effects. Candidates for IV PCA are patients who can understand the basic steps involved in drug delivery, who are willing to assume control of their analgesia, and who are physically capable of activating the device. These include children as young as 4 years of age and most adults, including geriatric patients.

The preferred agents for IV PCA are opioids, with morphine sulfate most commonly chosen. Other opioids commonly used for IV PCA include hydromorphone, fentanyl, and meperidine. Methadone IV PCA has been described. Physicians' orders for IV PCA should specify the drug, drug concentration, loading dose, bolus dose, continuous infusion rate (basal rate), lockout interval, and dose limits. These parameters are chosen based on the patient's age, medical status, and level of pain. The routine use of a continuous basal infusion rate with IV PCA remains controversial. With a continuous infusion, drug is delivered to the patient regardless of demand, thus resulting in the potential for a higher incidence of drug-related side effects, including respiratory depression. It is safest to restrict the use of basal infusions to patients in special categories, including patients with severe pain due to extensive surgery or trauma and patients who are tolerant due to chronic opioid use.

The use of structured protocols and guidelines are encouraged for facilities using IV PCA. The medical and nursing staff should receive training in the care of patients using this modality. There is an increased risk of complications if staff are not trained to understand the concept of IV PCA; to perform appropriate patient selection, education, and assessment; to use appropriate drug and dose selection; and to establish appropriate monitoring requirements and protocols for management of side effects.

Selection of Methods of Postoperative Analgesia

The choice of postoperative pain management strategies is a function of patient factors, surgeons' preferences, anesthesiologists' skills, and availability of resources for postoperative care and monitoring. There is little evidence that the choice of postoperative analgesic regimen alters outcome other than variables related to patient satisfaction with analgesic management. Patient factors related to choice of postoperative analgesic strategies include tolerance for discomfort and willingness to cooperate with such postoperative maneuvers as deep breathing and coughing. In general, ambulatory surgical patients receive less intensive analgesic therapy than inpatients. Institutional factors of great importance include the number of qualified nursing personnel on wards in which patients recover and the ability to provide adequate monitoring, especially for patients who receive epidural infusions of local anesthetics and opioids.

Chronic Pain

In a subset of patients, pain persists after the expected healing time despite the lack of sufficient pathology to account for pain. Chronic pain persisting for 3 to 6 months is considered evidence of a chronic pain syndrome. Such patients with persistent pain frequently use words such as burning, shooting, and shocklike to describe their pain, which is usually associated with a neuropathic pain syndrome. Neuropathic pain syndromes occur when there has been injury to the nervous system (central, peripheral, or both). Central sensitization is believed to underlie the development of neuropathic pain. Examples include patients with persistent pain after head and neck surgery, thoracotomy, mastectomy, hernia repair, and amputation. Certain factors that may increase the risk for chronic pain include infection at the surgical site, intraoperative trauma to nerves, diabetes mellitus, and nerve entrapment by cancer. There is some evidence that preemptive analgesia may help to minimize the occurrence of these syndromes.

Because chronic pain syndromes can be difficult to diagnose in the early postoperative period it is important for physicians to perform appropriate pain assessment during postoperative follow-up. For instance, patients after amputation might consider it strange to continue to feel sensation and pain in the locations of amputated limbs and might be reluctant to volunteer information that they believe could suggest psychological instability. In such circumstances, appropriate questioning may elicit the complaint, resulting in patient reassurance and appropriate treatment. Referral to a pain medicine consultant is appropriate when the diagnosis of a chronic postoperative pain syndrome is made. Treatment modalities include the use of adjuvant medications such as antidepressants and anticonvulsants, nerve blocks, physical therapy, and psychological techniques.

Specific Types of Acute Pain Patients

Patients with a History of Chronic Pain

Patients who have a history of chronic pain may experience acute pain as a result of surgery or trauma differently from patients who have no history of chronic pain. Their experience of pain is affected by their experience with chronic pain. Some of these patients may be receiving chronic opioid therapy as a part of their chronic pain management. It is likely that these patients will manifest tolerance to opioid therapy and a decreased pain threshold. This may result in the patient reporting higher levels of pain and the physician increasing the opioid requirements. Appropriate analgesia can be achieved by obtaining a pain history preoperatively, choosing anesthetic and surgical techniques to minimize tissue trauma and the response to trauma, and appropriate planning for postoperative analgesia.

Patients with a History of Substance Abuse

Patients with a history of substance abuse are frequently undertreated for acute pain complaints. The stigma associated with drug abuse, misunderstanding on the part of health care providers, and inappropriate pain behaviors contribute to undertreatment in this patient population. Effective analgesia can be obtained with strict guidelines, patient education, and appropriate use of consultants and modalities such as regional analgesia.

Pediatric Patients

Pediatric patients experience similar severity of acute postoperative and post-traumatic pain compared with adults. A major historical myth that has been refuted is the belief that neonates, infants, and children do not perceive pain as adults do. Effective analgesia for the pediatric patient experiencing acute pain can be achieved with pain assessment tools that are tailored for this population and the use of modalities and agents similar to those used for adults. Dosage selection in the pediatric patient must be guided by calculations based on patient weight. With neonates, nurse-controlled analgesia is standard. Older children can effectively use patient-controlled analgesia. Regional anesthesia is increasingly used for pediatric surgery, with the benefits of analgesia extending into the postoperative period and reduced opioid requirements. Epidural analgesia, usually via a caudally placed catheter or a single injection into the caudal canal, can provide effective analgesia. Placement of a peripheral catheter for infusion of local anesthetics can also be used. Topical anesthesia with local anesthetics such as the application of EMLA (Eutectic Mixture of Local Anesthetics) cream can also minimize pain from intravenous catheter placement and superficial procedures.

Elderly Patients

As the proportion of the elderly in the general population increases, an increasing percentage of patients presenting for surgery or presenting for treatment after trauma will be geriatric. These patients will require pain assessment and evaluation tailored to their mental status and cognitive abilities. The modalities and agents used to manage acute pain in this population must take into consideration underlying disease states and decreased organ function.

CONCLUSION

Modern anesthesia is safe and effective for the vast majority of patients, in large part because of important advances in anesthesia equipment, monitors, and drugs. With a wide variety of choices of specific techniques, an anesthetic regimen and a postoperative pain regimen can be selected for each patient based on the requirements of the surgical procedure, the patient's preferences, and the experience and expertise of the anesthesiologist.

Selected References

Apfelbaum JL, Chen C, Mehta SS, et al: Postoperative pain experience: Results from a national survey suggest postoperative pain continues to be undermanaged. Anesth Analg 97:534-540, 2003.

> A survey of 250 adult patients who had undergone surgery found that 86% had moderate, severe, or extreme pain before or after hospital discharge.

Benumof JL, Dagg R, Benumof R: Critical hemoglobin desaturation will occur before return to an unparalyzed state following 1 mg/kg intravenous succinylcholine. Anesthesiology 87:979-982, 1997.

> Using a combination of pharmacologic and physiologic information from the literature, the authors provide a detailed discussion of factors that influence the rate at which clinically important hypoxemia occurs in relation to the expected duration of succinylcholine. This contributes an important counter to the common misconception that succinylcholine will be metabolized before hypoxemia-induced harm occurs.

Brown RH, Wagner EM: Mechanisms of bronchoprotection by anesthetic induction agents: Propofol versus ketamine. Anesthesiology 90:822-828, 1999.

> The choice of induction agents in patients with bronchospastic disease remains controversial because of the potentially lethal consequences of severe intraoperative bronchospasm. In this study in sheep, both propofol and ketamine, two preferred agents in patients at risk for bronchospasm, appear to act through neurally mediated mechanism and not through direct bronchodilation.

Debaene B, Plaud B, Dilly MP, et al: Residual paralysis in the PACU after a single intubating dose of nondepolarizing muscle relaxant with an intermediate duration of action. Anesthesiology 98:1042-1048, 2003.

> In a study of 526 patients who received a single dose of vecuronium, rocuronium, or atracurium to facilitate tracheal intubation, received no more relaxant thereafter and did not undergo reversal of neuromuscular blockade, residual paralysis was present in 45% overall and 37% after 2 hours. The authors emphasize the importance of quantitative measurement of neuromuscular transmission.

Eagle KA, Berger PB, Calkins H, et al: ACC/AHA guideline update for perioperative cardiovascular evaluation for noncardiac surgery—executive summary. A report of the American College of Cardiology/American Heart Association Task Force on Practice Guidelines (Committee to Update the 1996 Guidelines on Perioperative Cardiovascular Evaluation for Noncardiac Surgery). Circulation 105:1257-1267, 2002.

> In this extensive review, a joint task force of the American College of Cardiology and the American Heart Association report guidelines for evaluation of patients scheduled for surgery. They thoroughly examine the importance of history, physical findings, and available tests and the influence of various types of surgery. This is a valuable update of a consensus approach to this difficult topic.

Goodnough LT, Brecher ME, Kanter MH, et al: Transfusion medicine: I. Blood transfusion. II. Blood conservation. N Engl J Med 340:438-447, 525-533, 1999.

> In this two-part review, the authors provide an overview of the current risk associated with transfusion, the indications for transfusion, and strategies for avoiding perioperative transfusion.

Hébert PC, Wells G, Blajchman MA, et al: A multicenter, randomized, controlled clinical trial of transfusion requirements in critical care. N Engl J Med 340:409-417, 1999.

> In this randomized controlled trial, 838 critically ill patients were maintained either at a target range of hemoglobin concentration of 7 to 9 g/dL or 10 to 12 g/dL. The mortality was significantly lower (22.2% vs. 28.1%) in the group in which transfusions were restricted.

Mangano DT, Layug EL, Wallace A, et al: Effect of atenolol on mortality and cardiovascular morbidity after noncardiac surgery. N Engl J Med 335:1713-1720, 1996.

> This landmark study randomized 200 patients with coronary artery disease or who were at risk for coronary artery disease to receive placebo or atenolol intravenously preoperatively and postoperatively and orally for the remainder of hospitalization. Atenolol increased survival over the first 2 years of the study, an effect that was particularly evident in the first 6 months (0% vs. 8% in the first 6 months after hospital discharge).

Reuben SS, Bhopatkar S, Maciolek H, et al: The preemptive analgesic effect of rofecoxib after ambulatory arthroscopic knee surgery. Anesth Analg 94:55-59, 2002.

> Sixty patients undergoing arthroscopic meniscectomy were randomized to receive intra-articular bupivacaine 0.25% before and after surgery and IV sedation using midazolam and propofol plus either 50 mg of rofecoxib 1 hour before surgery (preincisional group); rofecoxib, 50 mg after completion of surgery (postincisional group), or placebo. Analgesic duration, defined as the time from completion of surgery until first opioid use, was significantly longer in those patients receiving preincisional (803 ± 536 min) versus postincisional (461 ± 344 min) rofecoxib or placebo (318 ± 108 min). The preincisional group also received less postoperative opioid analgesia. This report strongly suggests the efficacy of preemptive analgesia with nonsteroidal analgesics.

Sprung J, Warner ME, Contreras MG, et al: Predictors of survival following cardiac arrest in patients undergoing noncardiac surgery—a study of 518,294 patients at a tertiary referral center. Anesthesiology 99:259-269, 2003.

> Cardiac arrest occurred in 223 of 518,294 patients (4.3 per 10,000) undergoing noncardiac surgery between January 1, 1990, and December 31, 2000. Frequency of arrest for patients receiving general anesthesia decreased over time (7.8 per 10,000 during 1990-1992; 3.2 per 10,000 during 1998-2000). Immediate survival after arrest was 46.6%, and hospital survival was 34.5%. Twenty-four patients (0.5 per 10,000) had cardiac arrest related primarily to anesthesia.

References

1. Diemunsch PA, Van Dorsselaer T, Torp KD, et al: Calibrated pneumoperitoneal venting to prevent N_2O accumulation in the CO_2 pneumoperitoneum during laparoscopy with inhaled anesthesia: An experimental study in pigs. Anesth Analg 94:1014-1018, 2002.

2. Rosenbaum HK, Miller JD: Malignant hyperthermia and myotonic disorders. Anesthesiol Clin North Am 20:623-664, 2002.

3. Bacher A, Burton AW, Uchida T, et al: Sevoflurane of halothane anesthesia: Can we tell the difference? Anesth Analg 85:1203-1206, 1997.

4. Rooke GA, Choi JH, Bishop MJ: The effect of isoflurane, halothane, sevoflurane, and thiopental/nitrous oxide on respiratory system resistance after tracheal intubation. Anesthesiology 86:1294-1299, 1997.

5. Spracklin DK, Kharash ED: Evidence for metabolism of fluoromethyl 2,2-difluoro-1-(trifluoromethly)vinyl ether (compound A), a sevoflurane degradation product, by cysteine conjugate β-lyase. Chem Res Toxicol 9:696-702, 1996.

6. Iyer RA, Anders MW: Cysteine conjugate β-lyase–dependent biotransformation of the cysteine S-conjugates of the sevoflurane degradation product compound A in human, nonhuman primate, and rat kidney cytosol and mitochondria. Anesthesiology 85:1454-1461, 1996.

7. Beaussier M, Deriaz H, Abdelahim Z, et al: Comparative effects of desflurane and isoflurane on recovery after long lasting anaesthesia. Can J Anaesth 45:429-434, 1998.

8. Muzi M, Lopatka CW, Ebert TJ: Desflurane-mediated neurocirculatory activation in humans. Anesthesiology 84:1035-1042, 1996.

9. Fang ZX, Eger EIII, Laster MJ, et al: Carbon monoxide production from degradation of desflurane, enflurane, isoflurane, halothane, and sevoflurane by soda lime and baralyme. Anesth Analg 80:1187-1193, 1995.

10. Kim ES, Bishop MJ: Endotracheal intubation, but not laryngeal mask airway insertion, produces reversible bronchoconstriction. Anesthesiology 90:391-394, 1999.

11. Fu ES, Miguel R, Scharf JE: Preemptive ketamine decreases postoperative narcotic requirements in patients undergoing abdominal surgery. Anesth Analg 84:1086-1090, 1997.

12. Boldt J, Mueller M, Menges T, et al: Influence of different volume therapy regimens on regulators of the circulation in the critically ill. Br J Anaesth 77:480-487, 1996.

13. Eames WO, Rooke GA, Sai-Chuen R, et al: Comparison of the effects of etomidate, propofol, and thiopental on respiratory resistance after tracheal intubation. Anesthesiology 84:1307-1311, 1996.

14. Brown RH, Wagner EM: Mechanisms of bronchoprotection by anesthetic induction agents. Propofol versus ketamine. Anesthesiology 90:822-828, 1999.

15. Katoh T, Ikeda K: The effects of fentanyl on sevoflurane requirement for loss of consciousness and skin incision. Anesthesiology 88:18-24, 1998.

16. Benumof JL, Dagg R, Benumof R: Critical hemoglobin desaturation will occur before return to an unparalyzed state following 1 mg/kg intravenous succinylcholine. Anesthesiology 87:979-982, 1997.

17. Domino KB, Posner KL, Caplan RA, et al: Awareness during anesthesia: A closed claims analysis. Anesthesiology 90:1053-1061, 1999.

18. Miller RD, Way WL, Dolan WM, et al: The dependence of pancuronium- and d-tubocurarine–induced neuromuscular blockades on alveolar concentrations of halothane and forane. Anesthesiology 37:573-581, 1972.

19. Wright PMC, Hart P, Lau M, et al: The magnitude and time course of vecuronium potentiation by desflurane versus isoflurane. Anesthesiology 82:404-411, 1995.

20. Kopman AF, Yee PS, Neuman GG: Relationship of the train-of-four fade ratio to clinical signs and symptoms of residual paralysis in awake volunteers. Anesthesiology 86:765-771, 1997.

21. Debaene B, Plaud B, Dilly MP, et al: Residual paralysis in the PACU after a single intubating dose of nondepolarizing muscle relaxant with an intermediate duration of action. Anesthesiology 98:1042-1048, 2003.

22. Beemer GH, Bjorksten AR, Dawson PJ, et al: Determinants of the reversal time of competitive neuromuscular block by anticholinesterases. Br J Anaesth 66:469-475, 1991.

23. Berg H, Viby-Mogensen J, Roed J, et al: Residual neuromuscular block is a risk factor for postoperative pulmonary complications. Acta Anaesthesiol Scand 41:1095-1103, 1997.

24. Andrews JJ: Inhaled anesthetic delivery systems. In Miller RD, Cucchiara RF, Miller ED Jr, et al (eds): Anesthesia. Philadelphia, Churchill Livingstone, 2000, pp 174-206.

25. Caplan RA, Vistica MF, Posner KL, et al: Adverse anesthetic outcomes arising from gas delivery equipment. Anesthesiology 87:741-748, 1997.

26. Allard J, Dzwonczyk R, Yablok D, et al: Effect of automatic record keeping on vigilance and record keeping time. Br J Anaesth 74:619-626, 1995.

27. Sanborn KV, Castro J, Kuroda M, et al: Detection of intraoperative incidents by electronic scanning of computerized anesthesia records. Anesthesiology 85:977-987, 1996.

28. Standards for basic anesthetic monitoring. ASA Standards, Guidelines and Statements webpage. American Society of Anesthesiologists (Approved by House of Delegates on October 8, 1988 and last amended October 28, 2000). Accessed January 29, 2004.

29. Gnaegi A, Feihl F, Perret C: Intensive care physicians' insufficient knowledge of right-heart catheterization at the bedside: Time to act? Crit Care Med 25:213-220, 1997.

30. Pizov R, Brown RH, Weiss YS, et al: Wheezing during induction of general anesthesia in patients with and without asthma: A randomized, blinded trial. Anesthesiology 82:1111-1116, 1995.

31. Sakka SG, Reinhart K, Wegscheider K, et al: Comparison of cardiac output and circulatory blood volumes by transpulmonary thermo-dye dilution and transcutaneous indocyanine green measurement in critically ill patients. Chest 121:559-565, 2002.

32. Gan TJ, Soppitt A, Maroof M, et al: Goal-directed intraoperative fluid administration reduces length of hospital stay after major surgery. Anesthesiology 97:820-826, 2002.

33. O'Connor MF, Daves SM, Tung A, et al: BIS monitoring to prevent awareness during general anesthesia. Anesthesiology 94:520-522, 2001.

34. Basic standards of pre-anesthesia care: Standards, Guidelines, and Statements web page. American Society of Anesthesiologists (Approved by House of Delegates on October 14, 1987, and affirmed on October 18, 1998). Accessed January 29, 2004.

35. Fischer SP: Development and effectiveness of an anesthesia preoperative evaluation clinic in a teaching hospital. Anesthesiology 85:196-206, 1996.

36. Eagle KA, Berger PB, Calkins H, et al: ACC/AHA guideline update for perioperative cardiovascular evaluation for noncardiac surgery—executive summary—a report of the American College of Cardiology/American Heart Association Task Force on Practice Guidelines (Committee to Update the 1996 Guidelines on Perioperative Cardiovascular Evaluation for Noncardiac Surgery). Circulation 105:1257-1267, 2002.

37. Eagle KA, Rihal CS, Mickel MC, et al: Cardiac risk of noncardiac surgery: Influence of coronary disease and type of surgery in 3368 operations. Circulation 96:1882-1887, 1997.

38. Fleisher LA, Rosenbaum SH, Nelson AH, et al: Preoperative dipyridamole thallium imaging and ambulatory electrocardiographic monitoring as a predictor of perioperative cardiac events and long-term outcome. Anesthesiology 83:906-917, 1995.

39. Mangano DT, Layug EL, Wallace A, et al: Effect of atenolol on mortality and cardiovascular morbidity after noncardiac surgery. N Engl J Med 335:1713-1720, 1996.

40. Wallace A, Layug B, Tateo I, et al: Prophylactic atenolol reduces postoperative myocardial ischemia. Anesthesiology 88:7-17, 1998.

41. Palda VA, Detsky AS: Perioperative assessment and management of risk from coronary artery disease. Ann Intern Med 127:313-328, 1997.

42. Seto TB, Kwiat D, Taira DA, et al: Physicians' recommendations to patients for use of antibiotic prophylaxis to prevent endocarditis. JAMA 284:68-71, 2000.

43. Smetana GW: Preoperative pulmonary evaluation. N Engl J Med 340:937-944, 1999.

44. Warner DO, Warner MA, Barnes RD, et al: Perioperative respiratory complications in patients with asthma. Anesthesiology 85:460-467, 1996.

45. Wong D, Weber EC, Schell MJ, et al: Factors associated with postoperative pulmonary complications in patients with severe chronic obstructive pulmonary disease. Anesth Analg 80:276-284, 1995.

46. Warner DO, Warner MA, Offord KP, et al: Airway obstruction and perioperative complications in smokers undergoing abdominal surgery. Anesthesiology 90:372-379, 1999.

47. Van Den BG, Wouters P, Weekers F, et al: Intensive insulin therapy in the critically ill patients. N Engl J Med 345:1359-1367, 2001.

48. Salem M, Tainsh RE, Jr., Bromberg J, et al: Perioperative glucocorticoid coverage. Ann Surg 219:416-425, 1994.

49. American Society of Anesthesiologists: New classification of physical status. Anesthesiology 24:111, 1963.

50. Newland MC, Ellis SJ, Lydiatt CA, et al: Anesthetic-related cardiac arrest and its mortality: A report covering 72,959 anesthetics over 10 years from a US teaching hospital. Anesthesiology 97:108-115, 2002.

51. Sprung J, Warner ME, Contreras MG, et al: Predictors of survival following cardiac arrest in patients undergoing noncardiac surgery—a study of 518,294 patients at a tertiary referral center. Anesthesiology 99:259-269, 2003.

52. Schwilk B, Muche R, Treiber H, et al: A cross-validated multifactorial index of perioperative risks in adults undergoing anaesthesia for non-cardiac surgery. J Clin Monit Comput 14:283-94, 1998.

53. Warner MA, Shields SE, Chute CG: Major morbidity and mortality within 1 month of ambulatory surgery and anesthesia. JAMA 270:1437-1441, 1993.

54. van Vlymen JM, Sá Rêgo MM, White PF: Benzodiazepine premedication. Anesthesiology 90:740-747, 1999.

55. Benumof JL: Laryngeal mask airway and the ASA difficult airway algorithm. Anesthesiology 84:686-699, 1996.

56. Marietta DR, Lunn JK, Ruby EI, et al: Cardiovascular stability during carotid endarterectomy: Endotracheal intubation *versus* laryngeal mask airway. J Clin Anesth 10:54-57, 1998.

57. Song D, Joshi GP, White PF: Titration of volatile anesthetics using bispectral index facilitates recovery after ambulatory anesthesia. Anesthesiology 87:842-848, 1997.

58. Eger E III: Uptake and distribution. *In* Miller RD, Cucchiara RF, Miller ED Jr, et al (eds): Anesthesia. Philadelphia, Churchill Livingstone, 2000, pp 74-95.

59. Savarese JJ, Caldwell JE, Lien CA, et al: Pharmacology of muscle relaxants and their antagonists. *In* Miller RD, Cucchiara RF, Miller RG Jr, et al (eds): Anesthesia. Philadelphia, Churchill Livingstone, 2000, pp 412-490.

60. Prough DS, Mathru M: Acid-base, fluids, and electrolytes. *In* Barash P, Cullen B, Stoelting R (eds): Clinical Anesthesia. Philadelphia, Lippincott Williams & Wilkins, 2000.

61. Roberts JP, Roberts JD Jr, Skinner C, et al: Extracellular fluid deficit following operation and its correction with Ringer's lactate: A reassessment. Ann Surg 202:1-8, 1985.

62. Böck JC, Barker BC, Clinton AG, et al: Post-traumatic changes in, and effect of colloid osmotic pressure on, the distribution of body water. Ann Surg 210:395-405, 1989.

63. Yogendran S, Asokumar B, Cheng DCH, et al: A prospective randomized double-blinded study on the effect of intravenous fluid therapy on adverse outcomes on outpatient surgery. Anesth Analg 80:682-686, 1995.

64. Perel A: Assessing fluid responsiveness by the systolic pressure variation in mechanically ventilated patients. Anesthesiology 89:1309-1310, 1998.

65. Stoneham MD: Less is more...using systolic pressure variation to assess hypovolaemia. Br J Anaesth 83:550-551, 1999.

66. Tavernier B, Makhotine O, Lebuffe G, et al: Systolic pressure variation as a guide to fluid therapy in patients with sepsis-induced hypotension. Anesthesiology 89:1313-1321, 1998.

67. Rooke GA, Schwid HA, Shapira Y: The effect of graded hemorrhage and intravascular volume replacement on systolic pressure variation in humans during mechanical and spontaneous ventilation. Anesth Analg 80:925-932, 1995.

68. Scheingraber S, Rehm M, Sehmisch C, et al: Rapid saline infusion produces hyperchloremic acidosis in patients undergoing gynecologic surgery. Anesthesiology 90:1265-1270, 1999.

69. Heyland DK, Cook DJ, King D, et al: Maximizing oxygen delivery in critically ill patients: A methodologic appraisal of the evidence. Crit Care Med 24:517-524, 1996.

70. Kern JW, Shoemaker WC: Meta-analysis of hemodynamic optimization in high-risk patients. Crit Care Med 30:1686-1692, 2002.

71. Bolsin SNC: Detection of neurological damage during cardiopulmonary bypass. Anaesthesia 41:61-66, 1986.

72. Goodnough LT, Brecher ME, Kanter MH, et al: Transfusion medicine: I. Blood transfusion. N Engl J Med 340:438-447, 1999.

73. Consensus Conference. Perioperative red blood cell transfusion. JAMA 260:2700-2703, 1988.

74. Practice guidelines for blood component therapy: A report by the American Society of Anesthesiologists Task Force on

Blood Component Therapy. Anesthesiology 84:732-747, 1996.

75. Weiskopf RB, Viele MK, Feiner J, et al: Human cardiovascular and metabolic response to acute, severe isovolemic anemia. JAMA 279:217-221, 1998.

76. Carson JL, Duff A, Berlin JA, et al: Perioperative blood transfusion and postoperative mortality. JAMA 279:199-205, 1998.

77. Hébert PC, Wells G, Blajchman MA, et al: A multicenter, randomized, controlled clinical trial of transfusion requirements in critical care. N Engl J Med 340:409-417, 1999.

78. Nelson AH, Fleisher LA, Rosenbaum SH: Relationship between postoperative anemia and cardiac morbidity in high-risk vascular patients in the intensive care unit. Crit Care Med 21:860-866, 1993.

79. Toy PT, Strauss RG, Stehling LC, et al: Predeposited autologous blood for elective surgery: A national multicenter study. N Engl J Med 316:517-520, 1987.

80. Kanter MH, van Maanen D, Anders KH, et al: Preoperative autologous blood donations before elective hysterectomy. JAMA 276:798-801, 1996.

81. Goodnough LT, Brecher ME, Kanter MH, et al: Transfusion medicine: II. Blood conservation. N Engl J Med 340:525-533, 1999.

82. Bryson GL, Laupacis A, Wells GA: Does acute normovolemic hemodilution reduce perioperative allogeneic transfusion? A meta-analysis. Anesth Analg 86:9-15, 1998.

83. Berde CB, Strichartz GR: Local anesthetics. In Miller RD (ed): Anesthesia. Philadelphia, Churchill Livingstone, 2000, pp 491-522.

84. Bardsley H, Gristwood R, Baker H, et al: A comparison of the cardiovascular effects of levobupivacaine and rac-bupivacaine following intravenous administration to healthy volunteers. Br J Clin Pharmacol 46:245-249, 1998.

85. Knudsen K, Beckman Suurkula M, Blomberg S, et al: Central nervous and cardiovascular effects of i.v. infusions of ropivacaine, bupivacaine and placebo in volunteers. Br J Anaesth 78:507-514, 1997.

86. Eisenach JC, de Kock M, Klimscha W: α_2-Adrenergic agonists for regional anesthesia: A clinical review of clonidine (1984-1995). Anesthesiology 85:655-674, 1996.

87. McDonald SB, Liu SS, Kopacz DJ, et al: Hyperbaric spinal ropivacaine. Anesthesiology 90:971-977, 1999.

88. Christopherson R, Beattie C, Frank SM, et al: Perioperative morbidity in patients randomized to epidural or general anesthesia for lower extremity vascular surgery. Anesthesiology 79:422-434, 1993.

89. Steinbrook RA: Epidural anesthesia and gastrointestinal motility. Anesth Analg 86:837-844, 1998.

90. Horlocker TT, Heit JA: Low molecular weight heparin: Biochemistry, pharmacology, perioperative prophylaxis regimens, and guidelines for regional anesthetic management. Anesth Analg 85:874-885, 1997.

91. Xue FS, Li BW, Zhang GS, et al: The influence of surgical sites on early postoperative hypoxemia in adults undergoing elective surgery. Anesth Analg 88:213-219, 1999.

92. American Pain Society: Quality assurance standards for relief of acute and cancer pain. In Bond MR, Charlton JE, Woolf CJ (eds): Proceedings of the VIth World Congress on Pain. Amsterdam, Elsevier, 1991, pp 185-189.

93. US Department of Health and Human Services: Acute Pain Management: Operative or Medical Procedures and Trauma, publication No. 92-0032. Rockville, MD, AHCPR, 1992.

94. ASA Task Force on Pain Management: Practice guidelines for acute pain management in the perioperative setting: A report by the American Society of Anesthesiologists Task Force on Pain Management, Acute Pain Section. Anesthesiology 82:1071-1081, 1995.

95. Quality improvement guidelines for the treatment of acute pain and cancer pain. American Pain Society Quality of Care Committee. JAMA 274:1874-1880, 1995.

96. Apfelbaum JL, Chen C, Mehta SS, et al: Postoperative pain experience: Results from a national survey suggest postoperative pain continues to be undermanaged. Anesth Analg 97:534-540, 2003.

97. Gilron I, Milne B, Hong M: Cyclooxygenase-2 inhibitors in postoperative pain management: Current evidence and future directions. Anesthesiology 99:1198-1208, 2003.

98. Reuben SS, Bhopatkar S, Maciolek H, et al: The preemptive analgesic effect of rofecoxib after ambulatory arthroscopic knee surgery. Anesth Analg 94:55-59, 2002.

99. Buvanendran A, Kroin JS, Tuman KJ, et al: Effects of perioperative administration of a selective cyclooxygenase 2 inhibitor on pain management and recovery of function after knee replacement: A randomized controlled trial. JAMA 290:2411-2418, 2003.

100. Hannibal K, Galatius H, Hansen A, et al: Preoperative wound infiltration with bupivacaine reduces early and late opioid requirement after hysterectomy. Anesth Analg 83:376-381, 1996.

101. Tverskoy M, Cozacov C, Ayache M, et al: Postoperative pain after inguinal herniorrhaphy with different types of anesthesia. Anesth Analg 70:29-35, 1990.

102. Woolf CJ, Chong MS: Preemptive analgesia—treating postoperative pain by preventing the establishment of central sensitization. Anesth Analg 77:362-379, 1993.

103. Kissin I: Preemptive analgesia. Anesthesiology 93:1138-1143, 2000.

104. Kehlet H: Controlling acute pain: Role of preemptive analgesia, peripheral treatment, balanced analgesia, and effects on outcome. In Max M (ed): Pain 1999: An Updated Review. Seattle, IASP Press, 1999, pp 459-462.

105. Block BM, Liu SS, Rowlingson AJ, et al: Efficacy of postoperative epidural analgesia: A meta-analysis. JAMA 290:2455-2463, 2003.

CHAPTER 18

MINIMALLY INVASIVE SURGERY

CRAIG CHANG, M.D.   and   ROBERT V. REGE, M.D.

Laparoscopic Surgery **Video-Assisted Thoracoscopic Surgery**	**Conclusion**

When you do the common things in life in an uncommon way, you will command the attention of the world.

George Washington Carver (1864–1943)

LAPAROSCOPIC SURGERY

Indications

Laparoscopic surgery was first performed early in the 20th century when surgeons adapted cystoscopes to examine the peritoneal cavity. At first, this technique was limited to diagnosis of intraperitoneal tuberculosis and disseminated cancer. Later, modification of equipment allowed simple biopsy of suspicious lesions and eventually accomplishment of simple operations such as tubal ligation and appendectomy. However, the extent of operation was limited by the need for the surgeon to view the abdomen through an eyepiece and to hold the laparoscope with one hand. The view for assistants was nonexistent or limited by a teaching attachment, precluding active participation in the operation. Complex procedures were not even considered to be possible.

The marriage of the laparoscope with a video camera in the mid 1980s expanded the potential of laparoscopy by freeing both of the surgeon's hands to manipulate instruments. Assistants could simultaneously view the procedure and actively participate by helping the surgeon perform the operation. In 1985, the first cholecystectomy was performed in France. Patients had less pain and recovered more quickly, and cholecystectomy was transformed from an inpatient procedure requiring 5 to 7 days of hospitalization to an outpatient or short-stay procedure. This procedure rapidly became the method of choice for removal of the gallbladder worldwide.

These results led surgeons to devise methods for performance of more complex intra-abdominal and thoracic procedures. The process was fueled by industry, which saw great business potential in minimally invasive surgery. "Advanced" laparoscopic surgery and its counterpart in the chest, video-assisted thoracoscopic surgery (VATS), were born. Over the past decade, equipment, instrumentation, and surgical skills have markedly improved and surgeons are now capable of using these techniques to safely perform a multitude of procedures. Patients realize the benefits of minimally invasive approaches for many operations, and many more patients now actively seek operative treatment for several diseases that they would not have previously considered (gastroesophageal reflux and obesity). This chapter reviews the current state of laparoscopic and VATS and briefly describes techniques currently available to accomplish sophisticated surgical procedures in the abdominal and thoracic cavities.

Physiology

Although laparoscopy causes fewer untoward effects than open surgery, physiologic functions are altered during performance of any surgical procedure. Insufflation of gas into the peritoneum, preperitoneal space, or retroperitoneal space increases intra-abdominal pressure, impairing ventilation, decreasing venous return, depressing circulation, reducing renal perfusion, and increasing intracranial pressure (ICP). The process is analogous to, although less marked than, abdominal compartment syndrome. The type of gas used for insufflation is important. Most surgeons use CO_2, but CO_2 is poorly tolerated by patients with impaired pulmonary function. Alternately, helium, air, nitrous oxide, and abdominal wall lifting (with no gas

445

TABLE 18-1. Physiologic Effects of Pneumoperitoneum and Potential Clinical Outcomes

Organ System	Physiologic Effects	Potential Outcomes
Pulmonary	↑ peak airway pressures ↓ pulmonary compliance and vital capacity Superior displacement of the diaphragm ↑ end-tidal CO_2	Barotrauma/pneumothorax ↑ P_{CO_2} and/or ↓ P_{O_2} ↑ P_{CO_2} and/or ↓ P_{O_2} Acidosis
Circulatory	Direct effects—increased CVP, CWP, SVR, MAP Indirect effects of CO_2—arteriolar dilation and myocardial depression Indirect effects on the sympathetic system, renin-angiotensin system, and vasopressin	↑ cardiac work; effects on cardiac output dependent on volume status ↓ blood pressure ↑ blood pressure and cardiac output ↓ urine output
Renal	↓ renal blood flow	↓ urine output
Coagulation	Lower extremity venous stasis	DVT and PE
Immunity and inflammation	Preserved systemic immunity Impaired local immunity	Greater resistance to infection and tumor seeding ↓ resistance to infection or tumor seeding
Central nervous system	↑ ICP	↓ central perfusion pressure
Intestinal	Attenuated sympathetic response	Less ileus

CVP, central venous pressure; CWP, capillary wedge pressure; SVR, systemic vascular resistance; MAP, mean arterial pressure; DVT, deep venous pressure; PE, pulmonary embolus; ICP, intracranial pressure.

insufflation) have been used but have not clearly demonstrated significant advantages. Obesity magnifies the effects of pneumoperitoneum and complicates patient positioning. The patient's size and weight place stress on pressure points, increase the difficulty of securing the patient to the table, and increase intra-abdominal pressure.

Patient positioning is also important, especially its effects on the circulatory system. Adequate visualization of pelvic and lower abdominal structures requires steep Trendelenburg, whereas those in the upper abdomen require modified lithotomy (or split-leg) position and reverse Trendelenburg. Other procedures such as splenectomy, adrenalectomy, renal surgery, and thoracic operations require lateral decubitus positions. All of these positions place particular stress on pressure points, necessitating careful padding. The patient must also be reliably secured to the operating table to avoid shifting if the table is repositioned during surgery. Excessive localized pressure and shifting of the center of gravity increase the risk for development of pressure sores and nerve compression syndromes postoperatively.

Although intraoperative management of patients undergoing laparoscopy can be challenging, benefits are derived postoperatively. Decreased pain, an attenuated stress response, and earlier return to ambulation after laparoscopic procedures decrease postoperative complications and lead to a quicker return to full activity. The efficacy of a minimally invasive procedure, compared to its open counterpart, therefore depends on its relative effects during and after the procedure. A detailed description of specific perioperative effects of laparoscopy on pulmonary, cardiac, immune function, and other organ systems follows.

Pulmonary Effects

Peritoneal insufflation causes an increase in intra-abdominal volume and pressure, both of which impede diaphragmatic excursion (Table 18-1). Peak airway pressures rise, whereas pulmonary compliance and vital capacity fall in proportion to intra-abdominal pressure, but patient positioning does not significantly alter the effects of insufflation on pulmonary function.[1] Upward displacement of the diaphragm compresses basilar lung segments, decreasing functional residual capacity and increasing alveolar dead space. The resultant effects on the ventilation-perfusion equation are complex. Volatile anesthetics and positive-pressure ventilation alone result in shunting and alveolar collapse. Initially, establishment of pneumoperitoneum may improve pulmonary shunting by increasing airway pressure (intrinsic positive end-expiratory pressure), partially compensating for mechanical compression of alveoli and anesthetic effects. Although early improvement of oxygenation may be realized, the beneficial effect of pneumoperitoneum is short-lived and shunting actually increases after about 30 minutes.[2]

Absorption from the peritoneum increases delivery of CO_2 to the lung as much as 50% during CO_2 pneumoperitoneum. If CO_2 exchange across the alveoli is impaired, serum CO_2 (P_{CO_2}) levels may rise and overload the serum bicarbonate buffering system, since CO_2 is readily converted to carbonic acid ($CO_2 + H_2O \leftrightarrow H_2CO_3 \leftrightarrow H^+ + HCO_3^-$). Acid-base balance disturbances may ensue. Patients at risk for acidosis include those with high metabolic and cellular respiratory rates (i.e., septic patients), impaired regional blood flow, a large ventilatory "dead space" (i.e., patients with chronic obstructive pulmonary disease), or poor cardiac output. Close monitoring of end-tidal CO_2 and arterial blood gases is essential for at-risk patients during laparoscopy. Since elevated P_{CO_2} levels continue for approximately 30 minutes after release of the pneumoperitoneum, monitoring must extend into the postoperative period. Some patients may require assisted ventilation postoperatively. In contrast, helium pneumoperitoneum does not increase ventilatory requirements, but like CO_2, it alters airway pressure, increases the alveolar-arterial gradient for oxygen, and is less soluble in water, increasing the risk of gas embolism.

Pneumoperitoneum also induces locoregional acidosis, in the absence of systemic acidosis, by impairing micro-circulation and decreasing organ blood flow. Increased intra-abdominal pressure decreases blood flow to the stomach, jejunum, colon, and liver. The amount of depression is proportional to the duration of the procedure.[3] The most significant drop in pH occurs in the abdominal cavity. Intra-abdominal pH rises with helium insufflation, but there is no change with air pneumoperitoneum—the significance of these differences is not known.[4] Impaired microcirculation and local acidosis are more likely due to changes in cardiac output and local effects of increased intra-abdominal pressure. Nonetheless, the resultant decrease in organ blood flow superimposed on preexisting intestinal vascular disease might explain reported cases of fatal intestinal ischemia after laparoscopic cholecystectomy.

On the other hand, laparoscopic surgery results in less pain, and subsequently less pulmonary embarrassment, postoperatively compared to the corresponding open procedure. For example, pulmonary function tests including forced vital capacity, forced expiratory volume in 1 second, midexpiratory phase of forced expiratory flow, and peak expiratory flow rates show smaller decrements postoperatively in patients undergoing laparoscopic cholecystectomy compared with those undergoing open cholecystectomy. More important, these benefits translate into a lower incidence of atelectasis and improved oxygenation.

Circulatory Effects

The cardiovascular effects of laparoscopy are well tolerated by healthy individuals but pose a threat to patients with comorbid conditions that impair compensatory mechanisms. Fortunately, careful monitoring, optimization of patient fluid balance, and prompt correction of problems allow most patients to undergo laparoscopic surgery safely. However, an open operation may be safer in patients with severely impaired cardiac function or sepsis.

Analogous to pulmonary effects, the consequences of laparoscopy on the cardiovascular system are due to increased intra-abdominal pressure, but patient positioning has a more striking effect. Pneumoperitoneum increases central venous pressure, capillary wedge pressure (preload), mean arterial pressure, and systemic vascular resistance (afterload). These changes have a dual effect: increased preload tends to augment cardiac output, whereas increased afterload decreases it and increases

cardiac work. Transesophageal echocardiography demonstrates a 45% increase in the two-dimensional area of the ventricles (a surrogate for end-diastolic volume) in healthy women after induction of 10 mm CO_2 pneumoperitoneum, but the cross-sectional area of the common iliac veins decreases, suggesting decreased flow of blood returning from the lower extremities. There appears to be shifting of blood toward the thorax as a result of the pneumoperitoneum.[5] Although arterial pressure and venous resistance increase proportionally with intraperitoneal pressure, the ultimate effects on cardiac output are highly dependent on patient volume status. For example, an increase in intraperitoneal pressure to 40 mm Hg results in a 53% decrease in cardiac output in hypovolemic, a 17% decrease in normovolemic, and a 50% increase in hypervolemic animals. It is speculated that high intraperitoneal pressure compresses the inferior vena cava and markedly impedes venous return, when low right heart filling pressures are present. The effect is diminished with normovolemia, and reversed by hypervolemia, which allows intraperitoneal pressure to augment venous return by compressing the splanchnic and venous systems.[6] The net result of the cardiovascular changes on cardiac output therefore depends on the patient's volume status, autonomic response, and cardiac reserve (Fig. 18-1).

The physiologic changes associated with patient positioning and repositioning are equally important. Trendelenburg position increases intrathoracic pressure, central venous pressure, capillary wedge pressure, and mean arterial pressure, increasing cardiac work. Reverse-Trendelenburg position leads to reductions in cardiac output by decreasing preload and may cause hypotension. Hypercarbia, due to CO_2 absorption, causes arteriolar dilation and myocardial depression, which tend to lower blood pressure. These effects are counteracted by an autonomic

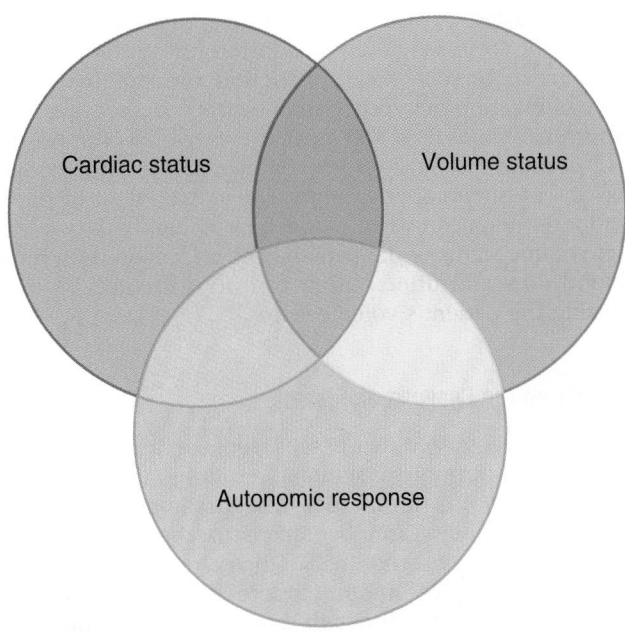

FIGURE 18-1. Factors influencing tolerance of laparoscopic surgery.

response, mostly due to the sympathetic nervous system, that elevates heart rate, systolic blood pressure, central venous pressure, left ventricular stroke volume, and cardiac output.[7] The roles of serum catecholamines, the renin-angiotensin system, and vasopressin are less clear. Increased serum catecholamine levels during the pneumoperitoneum may not be detected; possibly, there is selective vascular activation without catecholamines. Vasopressin may be responsible for the reduced diuresis and blood pressure elevations during long laparoscopic operations but plays little role under usual circumstances. The renin-angiotensin system may play a minor role in the elevation of blood pressure if the pneumoperitoneum is maintained for long periods.

Patients with cardiac disease tolerate the effects of laparoscopy poorly. Only 15 mm Hg of intra-abdominal pressure causes elevated mean arterial pressure, increased systemic vascular resistance, and significant reductions in cardiac output in patients with preexisting heart disease. The reduction in cardiac output, associated with elevated central venous pressure, increased pulmonary artery pressure, and decreased systemic venous O_2, suggests cardiac decompensation. Although transient, this decompensation in cardiac function does not return to normal immediately after deflation of the abdomen. Patients with cardiac disease are therefore at increased risk for complications such as myocardial infarction during and after laparoscopic surgery.

Renal Effects

Randomized studies demonstrate that urine output is lower with a pneumoperitoneum versus either open techniques or gasless laparoscopy and that intraoperative oliguria is common during long laparoscopic operations. This finding is usually ascribed to increased intra-abdominal pressure leading to reduced renal blood flow. In addition to decreasing cardiac output, pneumoperitoneum activates the renin-angiotensin-aldosterone system, which may promote renal vasoconstriction via angiotensin II.[8] The interaction between systemic effects decreasing total and renal blood flow and local effects such as renovascular constriction is complex but similar to the cardiac effects of pneumoperitoneum. The actual effect of pneumoperitoneum on renal blood flow is highly dependent on volume status of the patient. The effects on both renal blood flow and urine output can be overcome by optimizing the patient's volume status.

Effects on the Coagulation System

It is well recognized that tissue trauma activates the coagulation and fibrinolytic systems, resulting in an increased risk for venous thromboses and pulmonary embolus. Hypercoagulability can be linked to three physiologic abnormalities: (1) endothelial injury, (2) stasis, or (3) increased viscosity and/or abnormalities of circulating blood components. Although tissue trauma is thought to be less with minimally invasive procedures, increasing intra-abdominal pressure with pneumoperitoneum and

patient positioning, especially reverse Trendelenburg position, decreases femoral venous flow. These changes suggest that increased intra-abdominal pressure contributes to lower extremity venous stasis and increases the risk for thromboses. However, current studies do not document significant differences in the incidence of venous thrombosis between laparoscopic versus open operations. This may be because the deleterious effects of pneumoperitoneum may be offset by earlier return to full activity. The effects of laparoscopy on coagulation factors have been studied in obese patients undergoing gastric bypass, a group at particular risk for deep venous thrombosis and pulmonary embolus.[9] D-dimer levels increase significantly more after open as compared to laparoscopic gastric bypass. Antithrombin III and protein C levels decrease in both groups, although the decreases are less after laparoscopic gastric bypass. These findings suggest less activation of the coagulation system with laparoscopic patients. Although the risk appears less, patients may still develop venous thrombosis and pulmonary embolus. Therefore, deep venous thrombosis prophylaxis is indicated during laparoscopic procedures (Table 18-2).

Immune Function and Inflammatory Response

The systemic and local immune responses to surgery that afford resistance to infection and metastatic spread of tumors are mediated by a variety of cellular components (neutrophils, natural killer [NK] cells, lymphocytes, plasma cells, and macrophages), humoral factors (antibodies, complement, and cortisol), and acute-phase reactants (C-reactive protein [CRP], cytokines). In general, surgical procedures are immunosuppressive, but compared to open surgery, laparoscopy appears to be less so.

Delayed-type hypersensitivity (DTH) reactions are representative of overall immune function. Experimental evidence shows that open surgery results in significantly more immunosuppression, as assessed by DTH reaction, than laparoscopic techniques. The response after minilaparotomy is not significantly different from laparoscopy, suggesting that the degree of immunosuppression is related to the length of the abdominal incision and the amount of abdominal wall trauma.[10] More recently, changes in leukocyte subpopulations have been examined after surgical stress. Stress increases the number of granulocytes in the peripheral blood and decreases the number of lymphocytes. Specifically, NK cells and CD4+ cells are reduced after surgery, which may have important implications in the treatment of malignant disease since NK cellular immunity is important for resistance to tumor spread. Reductions tend to be less severe after laparoscopic procedures (Fig. 18-2).[11] Although there is some conflict between studies, other measures of systemic immune function generally demonstrate less immune depression with laparoscopy. These changes are summarized in Table 18-3.

Local intraperitoneal immunity also depends on mechanical clearance of bacteria, cellular immunity due to NK cells,

TABLE 18-2. Recommendations for Prevention of Venous Thromboembolism in Patients Undergoing General Surgical Procedures

Risk Category	Recommended Operative Treatment	Recommended Postoperative Treatment
Low risk (age < 40 yr, minor operations, no clinical risk factors*)	No specific prophylaxis	Early ambulation
Moderate risk (age > 40 yr, major operation, but no clinical risk factors)	IPC + ES *or* ES + LDUH (given 2 hr before and q 12 hr after operation)	IPC + ES *or* ES + LDUH
High risk (age > 40 yr, major operation, with 1 clinical risk factor)	LDUH (given q 8 hr) + IPC *or* LMWH + IPC	LDUH (given q 8 hr) + IPC *or* LMWH + IPC
Very high risk (age > 40 yr, major surgery, with multiple clinical risk factors)	LDUH, LMWH, or dextran + IPC (LDUH or LMWH started preoperatively; dextran and IPC given intraoperatively)	LDUH (given q 8 hr) + IPC *or* LMWH + IPC *or* warfarin (INR, 2.0–3.0)

Includes prolonged immobility; paralysis; prior venous thromboembolism; cancer; obesity; varicose veins; congestive heart failure; myocardial infarction; stroke; fractures of the pelvis, hip, or leg; congenital and acquired hypercoagulable states.
IPC, intermittent pneumatic compression; ES, elastic stockings; LDUH, low-dose unfractionated heparin; LMWH, low-molecular-weight heparin.
From Clagett GP, Anderson FA, Heit J, et al: Prevention of venous thromboembolism. Chest 108:312S-331S, 1995.

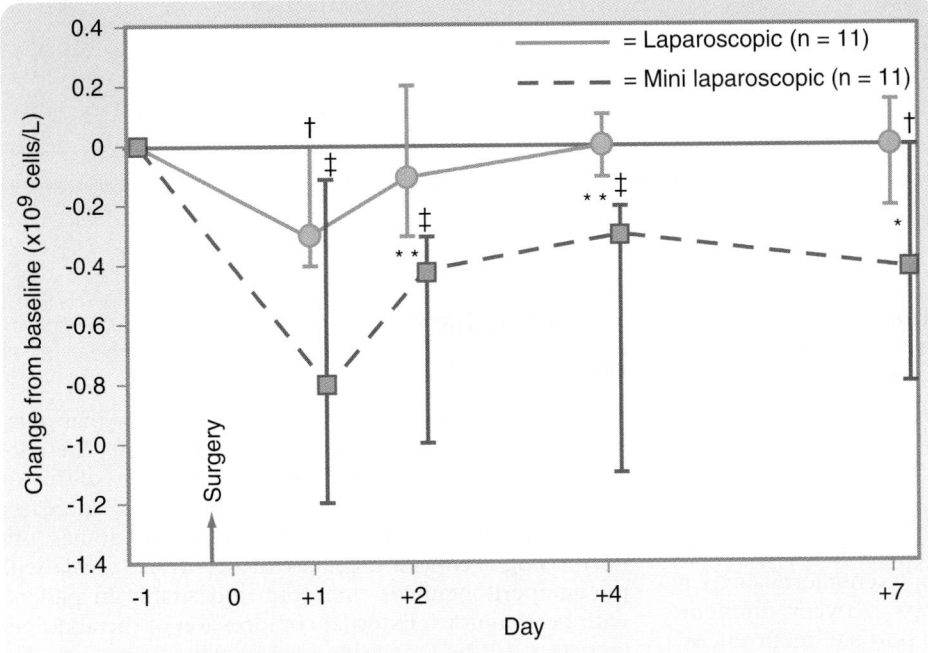

FIGURE 18-2. Variations in the lymphocyte count of patients undergoing elective laparoscopic *(horizontal bar)* or minilaparotomy *(quintuple dash)* cholecystectomy. Statistical analysis: †, $P < 0.05$, ‡, $P < 0.01$ (Wilcoxon matched-pairs test); *, $P < 0.05$, **, $P < 0.01$ (Mann-Whitney U test). (From Walker CB, Bruce DM, Heys SD: Minimal modulation of lymphocyte and natural killer cell subsets following minimal access surgery. Am J Surg 177:50, 1999.)

polymorphonuclear neutrophils and macrophages, and a specific immune system mediated by T- and B-cell lymphocytes. Peritoneal macrophages play a primary role in this inflammatory response. The scavenging action of macrophages is mediated in part by the production of inflammatory cytokines such as tumor necrosis factor-alpha (TNF-α). High CO_2 results in less interleukin-1 and TNF-α production by peritoneal macrophages challenged with lipopolysaccharide, and less peritoneal macrophage TNF-α production in a tumor model.[12] Helium pneumoperitoneum and gasless laparoscopy groups did not exhibit these changes. Likewise, mice inoculated intraperitoneally with a sublethal dose of *Listeria monocytogenes* (cleared by cell-mediated immunity) clear bacteria faster if insufflated with helium compared to CO_2.[13]

CRP is the most extensively studied marker of the inflammatory response following trauma and surgery. CRP levels rise 4 to 12 hours after operation, peak at 24 to 72 hours, and remain elevated for about 2 weeks. After laparoscopic procedures including cholecystectomy, inguinal hernia repair, colectomy, and gastric bypass, postoperative CRP levels are significantly lower than after open surgery but are not significantly different from those undergoing minilaparotomy, supporting the hypothesis that abdominal wall trauma influences immunologic function. There is insufficient data examining the physiologic

TABLE 18-3. Effect of Surgery on Components of Systemic Immune Response

Marker of Systemic Immune Response	Changes Following Open Surgery	Changes Following Laparoscopy
CRP	↑↑↑	↑
IL-1	↑↑	↑
IL-6	↑↑↑	↑
IL-8	↑↑	↑
IL-10	Data unclear	Data unclear
TNF	Data unclear	Data unclear
Fibrinogen, transferrin	Data unclear	Data unclear
Elastase	↑	↑ (returns to preop. levels early)
Albumin	Data unclear	Data unclear
PMN number	↑↑	↑
PMN function	↓↓	↓
Delayed hypersensitivity	↓↓↓	↓
T_H1, T_H2	↓↓	↓
$CD4^+/CD8^+$	↓↓	↓
Monocyte HLA-DR expression	↓↓↓	↓
Monocyte-mediated cytotoxicity	↓↓	↓
Kupffer cell activity	Data unclear	Data unclear
NK cell number and function	↓	↓

CRP, C-reactive protein; HLA, human leucocyte antigen; IL, interleukin; PMN, polymorphonuclear neutrophil; NK, natural killer; T_H, T-helper cell; TNF, tumor necrosis factor.
From Gupta A, Watson DI: Effect of laparoscopy on immune function. Br J Surg 88:1301, 2001.

changes of small-instrument laparoscopy ("minilaparoscopy") compared to laparoscopy with standard instrumentation. It is also not clear whether changes in these parameters translate into significant clinical benefits for patients or whether they are simply markers of what is already known—patients recover more quickly after laparoscopic surgery.

Intraperitoneal immunity and local factors play vital roles in cancer recurrence. Initial reports of increased trocar site tumor recurrences prompted numerous experiments examining the relationships between immune response, pneumoperitoneum, and port site recurrences. Currently, there is an abundance of conflicting information, but most investigators agree that tumor implantation is more likely after CO_2 pneumoperitoneum and increases with higher pneumoperitoneum pressures and more extensive tumor manipulation. A variety of experiments have shown reduced port site recurrences with instillation of cytotoxic agents (methotrexate, 5-fluorouracil, and heparin), helium pneumoperitoneum, and greater experience. Indeed, several authors cite surgeon experience as the key factor in recurrence rates. Despite the risk of tumor implantation with laparoscopy, recent large series now show that port site recurrence rates approximate wound recurrence rates from open surgery (Table 18-4).

Miscellaneous Effects

Intracranial Pressure

Several clinical and experimental studies show that pneumoperitoneum is associated with elevated ICP. The etiology is likely twofold—the vasoactive properties of CO_2 on the cerebral circulation and transmission of increased central venous pressure to ICP. Carbon dioxide has long been recognized as a mediator of ICP. Hypercarbia with pneumoperitoneum is therefore undesirable in patients with head injuries. External compression of the abdomen increases ICP by increasing central venous pressure. The effect of pneumoperitoneum on ICP is likely the same. Trendelenburg position is associated with elevations of ICP, whereas reverse Trendelenburg is not associated with lowered ICP in laparoscopic operations.

Intestinal Function

Multiple randomized studies demonstrate that bowel function returns quicker after laparoscopic procedures. However, little is known about the etiology of this finding. It is suspected that reduced surgical trauma in laparoscopy results in less sympathetic activity. The sympathetic nervous system inhibits motility through a spinal reflex.

TABLE 18-4. Colon Cancer Recurrences: Laparoscopy Versus Open

Authors	Year	No. of Patients	No. of Port Site Metastases	Percentage of Port Site Metastases
Guillou et al	1993	59	1	1.7
Franklin et al	1996	191	0	0
Gellman et al	1996	58	1	1.7
Kwok et al	1996	83	1	1.2
Vukasin et al	1996	451	5	1.1
Fleshman et al	1996	372	4	1.1
Lacy et al	1997	106	0	0
Fielding et al	1997	149	2	1.3
Larach et al	1997	108	0	0
Croce et al	1997	134	1	0.9
Khalili et al	1998	80	0	0
Bouvet et al	1998	91	0	0
Kawamura et al	1999	67 (gasless)	0	0
Leung et al	1999	217	1	0.65
Poulin et al	1999	172	0	0
Schiedeck et al	2000	399	1	0.25
Total		**1737**	**17**	**1**

From Zmora O, Gervaz P, Wexner SD: Trocar site recurrence in laparoscopic surgery for colorectal cancer. Surg Endosc 15:790, 2001.

Experimental studies show that this reflex is lessened after epidural local anesthetics (but not opioid anesthetics) and sympathectomy. Nitric oxide, vasoactive intestinal peptide, and substance P are inhibitory neurotransmitters in the intrinsic gut nervous system. Elevations of these substances may be attenuated in laparoscopy.

Technical Considerations

Laparoscopic operations are technically demanding procedures necessitating specific surgical skills, sophisticated state-of-the-art equipment, and well-trained, coordinated operative teams. A poorly designed operating room, incorrect patient positioning, poor-quality images of the operative field, malfunctioning equipment, or inexperienced members of the operative team can make the difference between a safe, efficient operation and a long, difficult procedure that puts the patient at risk for complications. Certainly, the length of the procedure and, therefore, the cost of laparoscopic surgery are highly dependent on these factors.

Laparoscopic surgery is most efficiently performed in rooms specifically designed for such surgery, so-called endosuites. At a minimum, endosuites include ceiling-mounted, mobile booms holding monitors and laparoscopic equipment. These booms can be moved into several configurations to accommodate the various positions and operating room layouts necessary to perform a multitude of laparoscopic (and other minimally invasive) procedures and to provide an unobstructed, comfortable view of monitors by the entire operative team. Equipment is always connected and ready for use and can be repositioned during cases quickly if needed. When not in use, the booms holding the monitors and equipment are moved out of the path of operating room traffic, maximizing usable space and decreasing the risk of damage to the equipment. Recently, more sophisticated laparoscopic suites have incorporated state-of-the-art electronics such as high-definition monitors, flat-screen technology, digital rather than analog cameras, image-capture devices, heated gas insufflators, and voice-activated and touch-screen remote control of all equipment from the operative field, enhancing picture quality and efficient task performance.

The specific equipment required for advanced laparoscopic surgery varies from surgeon to surgeon, but some general principles hold. Laparoscopic instrument trays should be designed to allow versatility by providing several types of graspers to handle and retract different tissues, dissectors with and without angled tips, scissors, needle holders for suturing, knot pushers, electrocautery hooks, and instrument handles with and without locking devices. Most instruments should be compatible with electrocautery and adequately insulated to ensure that coagulation occurs only at the active tip. Instrument designs with interchangeable handles and "semidisposable" tips allow greater versatility in a single tray.

Controversy exists concerning the prudence and cost of reusable, limited-use, and disposable instruments, and the role of each may vary by institution. At a minimum, disposable instruments may be an excellent option as back-up instruments for reusable trays or to fill a gap in instrumentation for rarely performed procedures. Bariatric procedures may require longer instruments and scopes. Laparoscopes should be available with several viewing angles, ranging from 0 to 45 degrees, and extra-long scopes are also sometimes required for surgery in larger patients.

Special devices that enhance the surgeon's ability to perform complex laparoscopic operations include linear and end-to-end staplers, bipolar scissors, ultrasonically activated scissors, laparoscopic clipping devices in several sizes, laparoscopic ultrasound probes, an argon coagulator with laparoscopic tips, and, if tumor ablation is to be done, laparoscopic radiofrequency ablation probes. Staplers that can be reloaded with cartridges and refired several times are essential when complex operations requiring several anastomoses are performed. Likewise, clipping devices that deliver several clips are helpful and avoid loss of exposure of key structures while clips are reloaded.

Positioning of the patient and layout of the room are crucial for exposure of the operative field, comfort of the operative team, and safety of the patient. Repositioning of the patient during the operation is essential at times. Patients should be placed on an operating room table with automated controls. Tables with higher weight limits are needed for obese patients. All pressure points should be well padded, and the patient must be secured to the table to avoid shifting during repositioning. As discussed previously, patient position influences cardiopulmonary function. Surgeons and anesthesiologists must work closely together to ensure that the patient is optimally positioned without compromising cardiopulmonary stability. Many problems can be avoided simply by attention to the patient's volume status. Specific comments about positioning are made elsewhere in this chapter.

Although surgeons who initially developed laparoscopic surgery had little formal training in laparoscopic techniques, it is now clear that the skills and knowledge required for safe, efficient, and efficacious performance of advanced laparoscopy are quite different from those required for open surgery. If trainees have not acquired basic laparoscopic skills, training in the operating room is expensive and may lead to increased numbers of complications. Therefore, basic laparoscopic skills training is essential to decrease learning curves and operative times. Skills training taught outside the operating room improves operative task performance.[14] At the authors' institution, skills training is an essential part of the curriculum for all residents. Currently, laparoscopic trainers, inanimate models, and first-generation virtual-reality trainers are used. There is still a need for realistic simulators that teach actual operations. Such devices are currently under development. Laparoscopic fellowships are also available for individuals who wish to concentrate their practice in advanced procedures.

Laparoscopy During Pregnancy

Surgery during pregnancy carries an increased risk of fetal loss. Therefore, surgery is generally limited to urgent situations such as appendicitis, acute cholecystitis, or adnexal torsion. Each of these disorders can be treated laparoscopically, but like open surgery, laparoscopic surgery presents a risk to the fetus. With laparoscopy, the surgeon must be aware of the general risks imposed by anesthesia, operative manipulation, and the physiologic effects of pneumoperitoneum and patient positioning. Altered anatomy within the peritoneal cavity also affects placement of trocars and manipulation of instruments. The operation should be performed in such a way to minimize the effects of pneumoperitoneum on the uterus and fetus.

The gravid uterus may encroach on the usual sites where trocars are placed and intra-abdominal organs such as the appendix may be displaced. An open approach is recommended for placement of the first trocar and establishment of pneumoperitoneum, because of the risk of injury to the gravid uterus by misplacement of a Veress needle. Intra-abdominal pressure should be maintained at the lowest possible limit to preserve uterine blood flow and prevent maternal and fetal acidosis, a risk factor for fetal loss. Careful monitoring of end-tidal CO_2 must also be performed. With increasing gestational size, compression of the inferior vena cava may impede venous return and predispose to thromboembolic complications. Intraoperative positioning may further aggravate this situation. Therefore, a left lateral decubitus position is recommended to alleviate venous obstruction. Finally, intraoperative fetal monitoring is recommended so that if fetal distress develops, the pneumoperitoneum pressures can be decreased or the patient can be hyperventilated in an attempt to correct the problem. There is general agreement that surgery should be performed in the second trimester, when possible, because the risks of spontaneous abortion and preterm labor are lower.

Complications

Laparoscopic and open operations share many of the same complications and problems associated with pneumoperitoneum already discussed in the physiology section, and they are not discussed here. On the other hand, the mode of abdominal access, the presence of pneumoperitoneum, and the method of specimen removal lead to specific complications of laparoscopy not often encountered in open operations (Box 18-1).

The most serious complication of abdominal access is injury to a major vascular structure. Although the reported incidence ranges from only 0.02% to 0.3%, the mortality of 15% from the injury is quite significant.[15] The injury most commonly occurs from placement of a Veress needle or primary trocar that punctures or lacerates the aorta, common iliac artery, or inferior vena cava. Although usually due to "blind" placement of the device, major vascular injury has been reported with the open approach. Injury is more common in thin patients where the distance between vascular structures and the abdominal wall

Box 18-1. General Complications of Laparoscopy

Injury to adjacent organs
  Bleeding from solid organs (liver and spleen)
  Vascular injuries
  Puncture/perforation/cauterization of the bowel
  Transection/perforation of bile ducts
  Perforation of the bladder
  Puncture/perforation of the uterus
Complications of abdominal access
  Port site hernia
  Wound infection
  Also see Injury to adjacent organs
Complications of specimen removal
  Port site recurrence of cancer
  Splenosis
  Endometriosis
Complications of the pneumoperitoneum
  Pneumothorax
  Pneumomediastinum
  Gas embolus
  Subcutaneous emphysema

Box 18-2. Factors Responsible for Large-Vessel Injury During Laparoscopic Access

Inexperienced or unskilled surgeon
Failure to sharpen the trocar
Failure to place the patient in Trendelenburg position
Failure to elevate or stabilize the abdominal wall
Perpendicular insertion of the needle or trocar
Lateral deviation of the needle or trocar
Inadequate pneumoperitoneum
Forceful thrust
Failure to note anatomic landmarks
Inadequate incision size

From Philips PA, Amaral JF: Abdominal access complications in laparoscopic surgery. J Am Coll Surg 192:526, 2001.

is as little as 2 cm. The right common iliac artery lies directly below the umbilicus and is the most commonly injured vessel. Other contributing factors are listed in Box 18-2. Injuries are recognized by free blood in the peritoneal cavity, retroperitoneal hematoma, or otherwise unexplained hypotension.

Bowel injury is the second most common cause of death from laparoscopic surgery. About one third of these injuries occur during abdominal access by mechanisms similar to those described earlier for vascular injuries. However, injury to the bowel during open access is also common, especially in patients with previous surgery and adhesions. Bowel can also be injured as instruments are placed into or removed from the abdomen through any port site, during dissection of structures in the operative field, and by electrocautery burns. Cautery burns can be quite vexing since they may not present immediately. Symptoms may not appear until several days later, once full-thickness necrosis of the bowel wall occurs. The small bowel is the most commonly injured segment, but injuries may occur in the stomach, duodenum, colon, and rectum. If recognized at the time of surgery and repaired, morbidity is low. However, many injuries are not recognized until the patient presents with peritonitis.

The reported incidence of bowel injury during abdominal access ranges from 0.04% to 0.3%, but the true incidence may be higher secondary to under-reporting.[15] Although injuries are typically reported with the Veress approach, randomized, controlled trials are insufficiently powered to reach clear conclusions about major injuries. When minor injuries are included, the open approach may be faster and safer (Table 18-5). Access injuries can largely be prevented with careful technique. With the Veress needle, the surgeon should hold the grasping edges of the device. Placing one's hand over the external end causes the sharp portion of the needle to be continually engaged. Countertraction on the skin brings the abdominal wall away from the bowel and retroperitoneum and avoids "overshooting" with the needle. When the Veress is placed at the umbilicus, the needle should be angled toward the pelvis to avoid the retroperitoneal vessels. With the Hassan approach, the surgeon divides the fascia and bluntly enters the peritoneum with a finger or blunt instrument. Care must be taken when the fascia is divided, because the bowel may be adhesed to the abdominal wall. Injuries are prevented by opening the fascia under direct vision and digitally entering the peritoneum. Optical-viewing trocars, dilatable ports, and trocar shields are used by most surgeons with good results, but a clear advantage is not demonstrated in the literature.

Potential complications of specimen removal are infection, recurrence (port site and regional intra-abdominal recurrence), splenosis, and endometriosis. The pathophysiology is similar in all during the dissection or specimen extraction; viable bacteria or cells are released within the abdomen or at the port site. Bacteria may then result in intra-abdominal abscesses or wound infections. Splenic, endometrial, and neoplastic cells may take residence, forming a discrete mass. When splenosis occurs after splenectomy for idiopathic thrombocytopenic purpura (ITP), the platelet count may not rise or it may fall after a period of weeks. Port site recurrences have been described for essentially all intra-abdominal malignancies. Implantation of cells can be avoided by placing the specimen into a specially designed sac, or "endobag," before removal.

The most serious complication of the pneumoperitoneum is gas embolism. Although clinically rare, when it occurs, it may be fatal. In a meta-analysis of nearly 500,000 closed-entry laparoscopic procedures, the incidence of significant CO_2 embolism was 0.0014%.[16] The mortality is approximately 30%. In 60% of cases, it results from direct entry of gas into the arterial or venous systems during the establishment of the pneumoperitoneum. In the remainder, it occurs during the course of the operation. Experimental models show that laparoscopic liver resection is

TABLE 18-5.   Randomized Clinical Trials of Veress Needle and Open Approaches for Laparoscopic Access

Reference (Year)	No. of Patients	Procedure	Access Time (min)	Complications	Results
Gullà et al (2000)	262	Diagnostic and operative laparoscopy	Not mentioned	Needle: 11/101 Open: 0/161	Open technique is safer
Saunders et al (1998)	176	Diagnostic laparoscopy in abdominal trauma	Needle: 2.7 Open: 7.3	Needle: 0/98 Open: 0/78	Veress technique is faster
Cogliandolo et al (1998)	150	Laparoscopic cholecystectomy	Needle: 4.5 Open: 3.2	Needle: 5/75 Open: 5/75	Open technique is faster
Peitgen et al (1997)	50	Diagnostic and operative laparoscopy	Needle: 3.8 Open: 1.8	Needle: 0/25 Open: 0/25	Open technique is faster
Byron et al (1993)	252	Diagnostic and operative laparoscopy	Needle: 5.9 Open: 2.2	Needle: 19/141 Open: 4/111	Open technique is safer and faster
Nezhat et al (1991)	200	Diagnostic and operative laparoscopy	Not mentioned	Needle: 22/100 Open: 3/100	Open technique has fewer complications
Borgatta et al (1990)	212	Laparoscopic tubal sterilization	Needle: 9.6 Open: 7.5	Needle: 7/110 Open: 4/102	Open technique is safer and faster

From The European Association for Endoscopic Surgery clinical practice guideline on the pneumoperitoneum for laparoscopic surgery. Surg Endosc 16:1127, 2002.

prone to gas embolism. Clinically, gas embolus presents as bradycardia, hypotension, arrhythmia, or a "mill wheel" heart murmur, during or shortly after insufflation. Transesophageal echocardiography definitively establishes the diagnosis. Treatment includes immediate desufflation of the abdomen and placing the patient in the head-down, left lateral decubitus position.

Pneumothorax and pneumomediastinum may occur when gas passes through the diaphragm or with iatrogenic diaphragmatic injury during upper abdominal surgery. It is recognized by the surgeon who notes bulging of the diaphragm into the abdominal cavity or by the anesthesiologist who has difficulty ventilating the patient. Most often, it is of little consequence since patients are on positive-pressure ventilation. Large pneumothoraces resolve spontaneously and quickly because of the diffusible nature of CO_2. If due to diaphragmatic hernia, the defect can usually be closed using laparoscopic suturing techniques. The pneumothorax requires no treatment or can be aspirated using a red rubber tube placed transabdominally through the defect, which is removed as the last stitch is tied. If tension pneumothorax occurs during any laparoscopic procedure, the abdomen and pneumothorax must be decompressed and the procedure should be converted to an open approach. Using the lowest insufflation pressure that allows adequate working space minimizes both pneumothorax and pneumomediastinum. In general, pressure greater than 15 mm Hg should be avoided.

Specific Procedures

Diagnostic Laparoscopy

Despite sophisticated methodology to image abdominal contents, establishment of a diagnosis prior to surgery remains difficult for several conditions. Unnecessary laparotomy is painful, increases hospital stay, increases hospital costs, and is associated with a morbidity of 5% to 22%.[17] Diagnostic laparoscopy effectively establishes a diagnosis, can be therapeutic, and causes less morbidity than laparotomy. Laparoscopy diagnoses 81% to 96% of patient problems accurately. Most important, the information obtained changes the planned operation to a more limited approach in at least two thirds of cases. However, laparoscopy does not visualize retroperitoneal structures well and may miss subtle findings within the peritoneal cavity. A negative laparotomy is preferable to missing a serious abdominal process and should be performed if laparoscopy does not visualize all potential causes of the patient's symptoms.

Gynecologic surgeons have long used diagnostic laparoscopy to determine the causes of pelvic/abdominal pain. Adnexal torsion, ovarian cysts, pelvic inflammatory disease, ectopic pregnancy and gastrointestinal diseases such as appendicitis and diverticulitis present with similar symptom complexes. These diseases continue to be diagnostic dilemmas despite increasingly sophisticated imaging modalities. Diagnostic laparoscopy remains a useful tool in women with lower abdominal pain but is now more likely to be used by general abdominal surgeons also. Complications of ovarian cysts, tubo-ovarian abscess, ruptured ectopic pregnancy in hemodynamically stable patients, and appendicitis all can be managed effectively and efficiently with the laparoscope. Diagnostic laparoscopy is also useful for accurate staging of malignant intra-abdominal tumors to ensure optimal treatment of the patient and to avoid unnecessary exploration to exclude unresectable disease.

The use of diagnostic laparoscopy in trauma patients is increasing but is restricted to hemodynamically stable patients. In a study of 28 patients with blunt abdominal trauma, diagnostic laparoscopy performed prior to planned surgical exploration was accurate in 100% of cases and reduced the incidence of nontherapeutic laparotomy by 60%.[18] Laparoscopy is ideally suited to evaluation and repair of diaphragmatic and isolated visceral injuries.

It reduces negative laparotomy rates, morbidity, length of hospital stay, and costs when employed in evaluation of stable penetrating abdominal trauma. The greatest gains are derived in patients with isolated abdominal stab wounds, especially if ultrasound or local exploration indicates that the posterior fascia of the abdomen is violated. Smaller advantages are seen with gunshot wounds to the abdomen. In the past, the primary role of diagnostic laparoscopy was to determine the presence or absence of peritoneal violation. Today, many surgeons use laparoscopy to thoroughly evaluate the entire abdominal cavity for injury and, in select cases, repair injuries without laparotomy.

Biliary Disease

Laparoscopic cholecystectomy, and its rapid acceptance by surgeons and patients alike, radically altered abdominal surgery. Although biliary tract diseases and their treatment are discussed fully elsewhere, several aspects of laparoscopic biliary operations are appropriately discussed here. Despite general acceptance of laparoscopic techniques, several controversies remain.

Although laparoscopic cholecystectomy is the procedure of choice today, the rate of common bile duct injury is higher than with open operation. A learning curve for laparoscopic cholecystectomy, with high rates of bile duct injury, reflected inexperience with the procedure. Several studies now show that the risk of bile duct injury by experienced laparoscopic surgeons is much lower than initially reported and approaches rates for open operation. Guidelines to minimize bile duct injury during laparoscopic cholecystectomy are now well defined and listed in Box 18-3.

Studies also demonstrate that laparoscopic cholecystectomy is appropriate for most patients with acute, including gangrenous, cholecystitis. The surgeon must have a low threshold for conversion to open operation if anatomy is unclear or the operation does not progress. Conversion rates vary from about 7% to 30% for emergent operation and largely depend on the duration of symptoms experienced by the patient. Elderly patients, male patients, and patients with symptoms for longer than 72 hours, a history of cardiac disease, white blood cell counts greater than 16,000, or gangrenous cholecystitis are at the highest risk for conversion.[19]

Although it is generally agreed that liberal use of cholangiography is helpful when anatomy is unclear, routine cholangiography during laparoscopic cholecystectomy continues to be debated. Critics site the low yield for common duct stones and ductal injuries and the expense of routine cholangiography. Advocates claim that routine cholangiography adds no more than 10 minutes to the operation, reduces the risk and severity of bile duct injury, and reveals ductal stones in up to 17% of cases. Recent meta-analysis suggests that routine intraoperative cholangiography lowers the incidence of duct injury by approximately 50%. Ludwig and associates[20] demonstrated an overall incidence of common bile duct injury in 0.36% of patients but only 0.21% incidence with routine intraoperative cholangiography versus 0.43% without it.

Box 18-3. Guidelines for Prevention of Bile Duct Injuries During Laparoscopic Cholecystectomy

Recognize "at-risk" situations
  Severe cholecystitis
  Fibrotic, shrunken gallbladder
  Aberrant anatomy
    Absent or short cystic duct
    Cystic duct arising from the right hepatic duct
    Aberrant or accessory right hepatic duct
    Aberrant right hepatic artery
Retract gallbladder fundus superiorly and infundibulum to the right and inferior to open triangle of Calot
  Dissect lateral to medial
  Meticulously dissect the cystic duct and artery close to the gallbladder
  Make judicious use of cautery
  Do not clip, divide, or cauterize structures unless clearly identified
Perform intraoperative cholangiography if anatomy in doubt
  Cholangiography must visualize the entire intrahepatic and extrahepatic to ensure that the catheter is in the cystic duct
  Visualize both right and left hepatic ducts
  Reposition patient and repeat cholangiogram if poor filling
Convert to open if
  Operation is not progressing
  Anatomy in doubt
  Cholangiogram does not clearly define anatomy

More important, the injury was diagnosed at the time of cholecystectomy in 87% undergoing operative cholangiography but only in 45% without it. Some surgeons suggest that the cost of routine intraoperative cholangiography is less than the cost of treating additional common bile duct injuries. Surgeons agree that fluorocholangiography facilitates the procedure and is useful if ductal exploration is needed (see later). Alternately, some surgeons advocate routine use of laparoscopic ultrasound. The advantages of laparoscopic ultrasound include a lack of adverse effects, lower costs, less time to perform compared with cholangiography, and the possibility of unlimited repetition. It is, however, operator dependent. In one prospective study comparing laparoscopic ultrasound and intraoperative cholangiography, sensitivities were 83.3% and 100%, and specificities were 100% and 98.9%, respectively, with an overall accuracy of 99.2% and 98.9%.[21]

During the era of open cholecystectomy, treatment of common bile duct stones was straightforward. Surgeons were adept at open common bile duct exploration and readily performed it in conjunction with cholecystectomy. However, surgeons now are generally less experienced in performing laparoscopic duct explorations and are reticent to convert laparoscopic to open procedures to treat common duct stones. During the last decade, most bile duct stones have been treated using endoscopic retrograde cholangiography (ERCP) and endoscopic extraction. Paradigms for treatment of common bile duct calculi therefore shifted from operative to endoscopic management.

Preoperative ERCP is commonly performed for transient episodes of pancreatitis or jaundice, persistently elevated liver function tests, or a dilated bile duct. However, it identifies pathology in 20% or less of patients with such presentations. The cost of two procedures, ERCP followed by laparoscopic cholecystectomy, has recently been questioned. Cholangiography, followed by laparoscopic transcystic duct exploration or laparoscopic exploration via a choledochotomy when stones are identified, is reliable in clearing the common duct of stones, has low complication rates, is cost effective, and is rapidly gaining acceptance as surgeons become facile with the technique. In a randomized, prospective study comparing two-stage treatment of ductal calculi versus single-staged laparoscopic treatment, stone clearance (84% and 83%) and morbidity were equal between groups. Although there was a trend toward more conversions in the single-stage group, patients had a significantly shorter hospital stay.[22] When clinical, laboratory, and radiographic signs of persistent cholestasis or pancreatitis are present, the incidence of ductal stones is much higher (50% to 80%) and preoperative ERCP may be more cost effective. Postoperative ERCP is reserved for patients in whom common duct exploration is not possible or was unsuccessful.

Laparoscopic Common Bile Duct Exploration

Laparoscopic common bile duct exploration is an advanced endoscopic procedure requiring coordination of several instruments. Multivariate analysis shows that experience of the individual surgeon is the only significant factor predicting successful outcome.[23] Exploration may be performed via a transcystic approach or choledochotomy, but most surgeons use the transcystic approach because it is simpler. Generally, the transcystic approach allows visualization only of the distal bile duct and cannot be used for intrahepatic stones.

Transcystic duct exploration is best accomplished with a large cystic duct (>4 mm), but smaller ducts can be dilated to accommodate instruments. Cholangiography is performed first to identify and determine the number of stones. In some cases, simple flushing of the duct with 50 to 200 mL of saline after administration of 1 to 2 mg of glucagon intravenously to relax the sphincter of Oddi will suffice in pushing small stones into the duodenum. Clearance of all stones is verified by repeat cholangiography.

If flushing is unsuccessful, instruments are passed through the opening created in the cystic duct for the cholangiocatheter, which must be enlarged. In some cases, a longitudinal cut may be made on the cystic duct to enlarge the opening into the common bile duct. Care is taken to place the port for the choledochoscope laterally so that the instruments enter the common bile duct via a relatively straight course. If the cystic duct is less than 2.5 mm, it will not allow insertion of instruments or withdrawal of stones. Enlargement of the cystic duct may be performed by successive dilation with mechanical over-the-wire dilators under fluoroscopic control or by use of a pneumatic (balloon) dilator that exerts a radial force, thereby enlarging the cystic duct. Once access to the common bile duct is obtained, stones are removed using a spiral stone basket under fluoroscopic or choledochoscopic control.[24]

Transcystic choledochoscopy is generally chosen because of its ability to directly visualize stones. The choledochoscope is introduced through a port and is guided into the cystic duct with a combination of the scope controls, rotational movements, and internal manipulation with atraumatic forceps. Prepackaged kits containing a soft sheath through which the choledochoscope is inserted, a soft-tipped guide wire, a stone-extraction basket, and coaxial or balloon dilators for enlarging the cystic duct simplify preparation for the operating room team. Once stones are visualized, the scope may be used to push the stone into the duodenum, but more commonly, a wire basket is inserted through the working channel to capture stones. The choledochoscope and wire basket are then removed from the cystic duct as a unit and the stone is deposited on the omentum for later retrieval. Impacted stones or stones too large for extraction through the cystic duct may be fractured with electrohydraulic or laser lithotripsy, and pieces extracted.[24] At the end of the procedure, the gallbladder is then removed and the cystic duct stump is controlled with clips or sutures.

Choledochotomy is used for large stones when the bile duct is dilated. It is more difficult than transcystic duct exploration because it requires significant expertise at laparoscopic suturing. About 1 to 2 cm of the anterior distal bile duct above the duodenum is cleared of tissue. A 1-cm choledochotomy is then made either longitudinally or transversely across the duct. Extraction of stones is then similar to the transcystic duct approach, although the choledochotomy allows insertion of larger instruments, removal of large stones, and exploration of the proximal biliary tree. Choledochotomy is not prudent with a small common bile duct (<6 mm) because subsequent healing and fibrosis may cause stricture. The choledochotomy may be closed primarily without drainage using 4-0 or 5-0 absorbable sutures or be decompressed by inserting an internal (antegrade) stent, T tube, or transcystic duct drainage catheter. Recently, primary duct closure without T-tube placement has gained popularity. Some surgeons place a drainage catheter in proximity to the choledochotomy. Again, cholecystectomy is performed at the end of the procedure if the gallbladder is still present.

Gastroesophageal Reflux Disease

Successful surgical treatment of gastroesophageal reflux disease (GERD), using either open or laparoscopic approaches, requires reduction of sliding or paraesophageal hernias to bring the distal esophagus below the diaphragm, closure of the diaphragmatic crura, and some form of a fundoplication to form a high-pressure zone ("valve") at the esophagogastric junction. The fundoplication may either be partial (Belsey, Toupet, and Dor procedures) or complete (Nissen procedure). The goal is to eliminate reflux of gastric contents into the esophagus while allowing normal swallowing to occur. In patients with well-established stricture or those who have had previous surgery, the esophagus may be "shortened" and cannot be brought back into the abdomen without tension. A lengthening procedure involving creation of a medial-based gastric tube (Collis gastroplasty) may be required. Although complex procedures such as this are usually performed by open surgical techniques, techniques have been developed to perform them both thorascopically and laparoscopically.

Before 1990, all antireflux operations were performed using open surgical techniques. Surgeons argued the benefits and risks of thoracic and abdominal approaches versus medical treatment, and patients were reticent to undergo operative therapy even when medical treatment was less than optimal. Today, more than 90% of antireflux operations are performed laparoscopically, and surgical treatment competes effectively with medical therapies for patients. Laparoscopic antireflux operations result in less postoperative pain, shorter hospital stays, and quicker recovery to full activity when compared to open approaches. Several trials show comparable relief of symptoms by laparoscopic and open antireflux surgery. Although data are still evolving, laparoscopic operations afford equivalent durability when compared to open surgery. Laparoscopic surgery is now the preferred option for young, low-risk patients requiring multiple or high-dose medications. It also improves asthma associated with free reflux in children and adults. Laparoscopy improves acceptance of reflux surgery, in lieu of chronic medical treatment, and is responsible for the exponential growth in the surgical treatment of GERD that has occurred during the past decade.

The benefits of laparoscopic approaches have now almost completely obviated the need for thoracic and open abdominal surgery. Open surgery is reserved for rare patients needing complex reoperative procedures, those with dense upper abdominal adhesions, or for complications during laparoscopic surgery requiring conversion to an open operation. Controversy still exists as to which operation yields the best results with the fewest complications (Nissen, Nissen-Rosetti, Toupet, or Dor). However, the most common operation performed is a Nissen fundoplication. Currently, a short 2- to 3-cm, loosely constructed fundoplication is preferred since it is as effective as longer, "tighter" variants but is associated with fewer complications.

The most common and significant complications are analogous to those encountered with open operations, including dysphagia, fundoplication slippage, and "gas-bloat" syndrome. A fundoplication that is too tight may result in the inability to belch or vomit, and gas-bloat syndrome or may be manifest as dysphagia. Dysphagia is typically associated with inadequate esophageal peristalsis or obstruction by a poorly constructed or slipped plication. If preoperative distal esophageal peristaltic amplitudes are 30 mm Hg or greater, and the fundoplication is in proper position, dysphagia is uncommon. On the other hand, peristaltic pressures below 30 mm Hg have a higher incidence of dysphagia. Many surgeons prefer a partial fundoplication (Toupet or Dor operation) under these circumstances. Although partial fundoplications theoretically afford less control of reflux symptoms and may be less durable than a Nissen, excellent results are reported with these operations.[25]

Complications are minimized after laparoscopic reflux surgery if several key technical elements are included in each operation. A "shoeshine" maneuver ensures that there is sufficient laxity of the plication and that the esophagus is invaginated into the stomach rather than the stomach being twisted around the esophagus. A Babcock clamp grasps the posterior wall of the stomach through the posterior esophageal window. A second clamp is used to grasp the anterior stomach and the wrap is placed into its final position. If the stomach moves freely around the esophagus when gentle traction is applied alternately to each Babcock, the fundoplication will be properly constructed and will not be too tight. When properly performed, the short gastric vessels (greater curve of the stomach) will remain in their natural position. Although not mandatory, use of a 54- to 58-French bougie assists with calibration of the hiatal closure and construction of a nonobstructive wrap. Some surgeons construct the wrap with the bougie in the esophagus; others use it after the wrap is complete to calibrate the hiatus, but some experienced surgeons report excellent results and reduced operative times by not using a bougie. The latter surgeons also suggest iatrogenic esophageal injuries are less common if a bougie is not used.

Fundoplication slippage results in recurrent reflux and/or dysphagia. The most common type of slippage is migration of the stomach into the chest, but the plication can also slip downward, entrapping a portion of the proximal stomach. The latter disorder causes early satiety, dysphagia, and heartburn because acid from the partially obstructed pouch refluxes through the hypotonic lower esophageal sphincter (LES). Dehiscence of the plication may also occur with return of the patient's reflux symptoms. Construction of the fundoplication without tension, mobilization of the distal esophagus to place more than 6 cm of esophagus intra-abdominally, ensuring that the entire hiatal hernia sac is divided, meticulous repair of the hiatal defect, division of the short gastric vessels, and incorporation of the esophageal muscular layer with the gastric sutures minimize slippage and dehiscence. The need for division of short gastric vessels remains controversial. Prospective studies show satisfactory control of reflux and shorter operative times when the short gastric vessels are not divided. Others believe that dysphagia and dehiscence are higher if the short gastric vessels are not divided. It is the authors' preference to divide three to five short gastric vessels to mobilize the fundus and ensure a tension-free fundoplication. Mesh hiatoplasty has been suggested as another method to prevent wrap migration, although there have been reports of dysphagia due to the presence of mesh and an inflammatory reaction around the esophagus.

Recently, the U.S. Food and Drug Administration approved two endoscopic procedures—the Stretta

System* and the Bard Interventional Endoscopic Suturing System†—for treatment of GERD. The Stretta System delivers radiofrequency energy to the gastroesophageal junction. Treatment with this device causes histopathologic muscular wall thickening, a modest increase in LES pressure at 6 months after the procedure, and a 25% to 44% decrease in transient lower esophageal relaxation.[26] Transoral endoscopic suture plication is performed using the Bard device. An overtube is placed transorally using an endoscope and the system is advanced through the tube. A fold of the gastric wall is suctioned into the sewing capsule and a suture is placed by the system. The device is removed and a half-hitch is created extracorporeally. A knot-pusher is used to secure the plication. A total of five half-hitches are recommended. The plications are configured linearly or circumferentially at the gastroesophageal junction to create a valvelike effect. Direct comparisons of these procedures with laparoscopic antireflux surgery have not yet been performed.

Achalasia

Achalasia is an esophageal disorder characterized by loss of ganglion cells in the submyenteric plexus of the esophagus. This results in loss of peristalsis in the esophageal body and impaired relaxation of the LES. The patient experiences dysphagia and inability to take adequate nutrition. Since esophageal peristalsis cannot be improved, treatment of the disorder focuses on decreasing LES pressure, allowing food to pass into the stomach more easily.

Three effective treatments are available for achalasia. Injection of botulinum toxin (Botox) into the distal esophageal muscle decreases LES pressure approximately 30% and provides clinical relief in about a third of patients. However, the response is short-lived (several months to a year), and repeat treatments are less successful. Most physicians now reserve botulinum treatments for patients who are poor surgical risks. Forceful pneumatic dilation with a specially designed balloon disrupts the lower esophageal muscle and improves swallowing in about 80% of patients. Repeat dilations may be required and increase the rate of success. Success rates also increase as the size of the balloon used increases from 30 to 40 mm, but so does the incidence of esophageal perforation. Surgical disruption of the lower esophageal muscle, or myotomy, is also effective but previously required an open surgical procedure through the chest or abdomen. Currently, minimally invasive approaches using VATS or a laparoscopic approach are available. Most surgeons find the laparoscopic approach to be less difficult compared to VATS. Laparoscopic myotomy is associated with shorter operative times, shorter hospital stays, and decreased time to full recovery.[27] The laparoscopic approach also yielded the best response rates when data in the literature were analyzed by meta-analysis.[28]

Retrospective studies suggest that surgical failures are often secondary to inadequate myotomy or, alternately, to

progression of disease. Success clearly requires decompression of the entire high-pressure zone in the distal esophagus, but care must be taken to ensure that the myotomy is not too long, increasing gastroesophageal reflux. In general, the myotomy is extended onto the cardia of the stomach 1 to 2 cm and is at least 4 to 6 cm long. Some surgeons circumferentially mobilize the esophagus to allow longer proximal myotomy and a posterior fundoplication. Others divide the muscular layer only up to the level of the crura and do fully mobilize the esophagus. Sharp and colleagues[27] suggest that performance of the myotomy without full mobilization of the esophagus preserves the angle of His and eliminates the need for concomitant reflux procedures. Most surgeons use intraoperative endoscopy to gauge the length of the myotomy and to test the integrity of the esophageal mucosa at the conclusion of the procedure. The endoscope light is used to transilluminate the esophagus, exposing bands of intact muscle that must be divided. The lumen of the esophagus is easily dilated with insufflated air when the myotomy is complete. Air insufflation may reveal small perforations, allowing them to be repaired before the operation is completed. Some surgeons also report that intraoperative manometry is useful in ensuring complete myotomy.

Myotomy effectively alleviates symptoms in 90% of patients, but 10% to 15% of patients develop significant reflux. Debate continues concerning the importance of fundoplication in addition to the myotomy. Some surgeons routinely perform fundoplication with myotomy. Others do a fundoplication only if an intraoperative perforation is identified to reinforce the repair. Certain surgeons advocate use of a full wrap (Nissen), but others worry about dysphagia in a patient with no esophageal peristalsis. The advantages of the anterior Dor fundoplication are that it is relatively easy to perform and it buttresses the myotomy. A Toupet fundoplication can also be sutured to the edges of the myotomy to keep it open and prevent contracture of the myotomy.

Laparoscopic approaches are also used for patients who perforate during balloon dilation. Results are best if the perforation is recognized promptly and addressed quickly. The principles are the same as with open surgery: the perforation is meticulously closed with fine suture, a myotomy is performed on the esophagus opposite to the side of perforation, and the perforation is reinforced with a partial or complete wrap. Closure of the perforation with suture and performance of fundoplication to buttress the repair is also the method of choice for perforations identified during myotomy.

Appendicitis

There have been more than 1100 articles on laparoscopic appendectomy published worldwide since Semm performed the first laparoscopic appendectomy in Germany in 1981. Several meta-analyses comparing laparoscopic and open appendectomy demonstrate fewer wound infections, less pain, and earlier return to normal activities, with an average increase in operative time of 16 minutes. Rates of intra-abdominal abscess and length of hospital stay appears similar, although patients are

*Curon Medical, Sunnyvale, CA.
†Bard Interventional Products, Billerica, MA.

discharged earlier today with both procedures than in the past.

Generally, the operation is performed using three ports placed radially about the right lower quadrant. A common mistake is placing a right-sided trocar too close to the appendix, thus preventing full utilization of the port. Most surgeons mobilize the appendix, elevate it anteriorly, and then transect the mesoappendix with one or two firings of a vascular endoscopic stapler. The base of the appendix is clearly identified and subsequently transected with a bowel endoscopic stapler. The mesoappendix may also be divided using clips and cautery, and the appendiceal stump controlled with an endoloop. The latter technique takes longer but is more economical. Irrigation of the right lower quadrant is required if an abscess is present. However, irrigation of the entire abdomen has shown no benefit in the absence of diffuse contamination.

Colorectal Procedures

For benign colonic pathology, there is general agreement that a laparoscopic approach confers a benefit to patients, but it may take longer and cost more. Laparoscopic treatment of prolapse of the rectum, colon resection for benign polyps or for recurrent diverticulitis, and ileoanal pouch with anal anastomosis for ulcerative colitis are now routinely performed in select patients. Initial enthusiasm for laparoscopic treatment of colon carcinoma decreased after early reports that lymph node dissection was not complete and port site recurrences were common (as high as 21%).

Recently, there has been a resurgence of interest in laparoscopic colorectal cancer surgery. Data now demonstrate no difference between laparoscopic and open operation when performed by experienced surgeons. In fact, one study suggests that local recurrence is lower after laparoscopic colectomy.[29] Randomized, prospective studies by Milsom[30] and Stage[31] and their coworkers show that laparoscopic patients have less pain, earlier return of bowel function, earlier discharge from the hospital, and no increase in the rate of wound or port site recurrences, although follow-up was short. Multiple prospective, non-randomized, and retrospective studies support these conclusions. There are now several large prospective, randomized studies underway, which should clarify the roles of laparoscopic and open colectomy for cancer. Preliminary results suggest that the laparoscopic operation is similar to open surgery and results in comparable disease-free survival.[32,33]

There is an increasing body of literature supporting laparoscopic abdominoperineal resection. These reports suggest that laparoscopic abdominoperineal resection results in shorter hospital stays, less postoperative analgesia, and less blood loss, but the operation takes significantly longer to perform. Studies also suggest that the local and distant recurrence rates and survival are no different. Fleshman and associates[34] suggest that although overall morbidity is lower in the laparoscopic group, the rate of perineal infection is significantly higher. Other studies report equivalent morbidity and mortality. Randomized, prospective studies are currently lacking.

Bariatric Surgery

Obesity is a major health problem in the United States. An estimated $140 billion is spent each year on the treatment of obesity-related medical problems, and medical approaches to obesity have not been successful. Several operations, including Roux-en-Y gastric bypass and biliopancreatic diversion with or without duodenal switch, are successful for long-term treatment of weight-related comorbidities in select patients. In the past, all operations required long laparotomy incisions with attendant wound infection rates of approximately 10% and hernia rates ranging between 20% and 30%. Today, many of these operations may be performed laparoscopically. Randomized, prospective studies demonstrate that laparoscopic gastric bypass results in less blood loss, less pain, shorter hospital stays, faster convalescence, and lower rates of incisional hernia than open surgery. This operation is, however, technically demanding and has a significant learning curve. With experience, complications and operative times approach those for open surgery.

Laparoscopic gastric bypass is usually performed using five or six upper abdominal ports and stapling devices for all anastomoses, although some surgeons report excellent results with hand-sewn techniques. A 15- to 20-mL gastric pouch based on the lesser curve is created by inserting the anvil of a 21-mm EEA stapler into the stomach via separate gastrotomy. Linear staplers are then used to transect the stomach around the anvil. A 75-cm Roux limb (150 cm in the superobese) is constructed by dividing the bowel below the ligament of Treitz. It is placed in a retrocolic, antegastric position and intestinal continuity is re-established by creating a stapled side-to-side jejunojejunostomy. The proximal end of the Roux limb is anastomosed to the pouch with an EEA stapler brought through a 12-mm port site on the patient's left side. The EEA device is placed into the proximal end of the Roux limb and the side of the jejunum is anastomosed to the gastric pouch by engaging the anvil. The open end of the Roux limb is stapled closed and all mesenteric defects are carefully closed.

Laparoscopic biliopancreatic diversion is a malabsorptive procedure in which a 65% distal gastrectomy is performed. The gastric remnant is anastomosed to a 250-cm alimentary limb. The biliopancreatic limb is in turn anastomosed to this alimentary limb 50 cm proximal to the ileocecal valve, creating a 50-cm common channel (Fig. 18-3). Laparoscopic duodenal switch is a modification of biliopancreatic diversion (Fig. 18-4). In duodenal switch, a sleeve gastrectomy is performed instead of a distal gastrectomy and the duodenum is transected distal to the pylorus with a linear stapler. A 250-cm alimentary limb is anastomosed to the proximal duodenal stump with a circular 21-mm stapler or by hand-sewing. The proximal bowel is sewn to the alimentary limb proximal to the ileocecal valve creating a 75- to 100-cm common channel. Both techniques can be accomplished laparoscopically using six ports in the upper abdomen. Linear endoscopic staplers are used to fashion the anastomoses and to perform the distal gastrectomy. Long-term follow-up and randomized comparison to the open techniques are lacking.

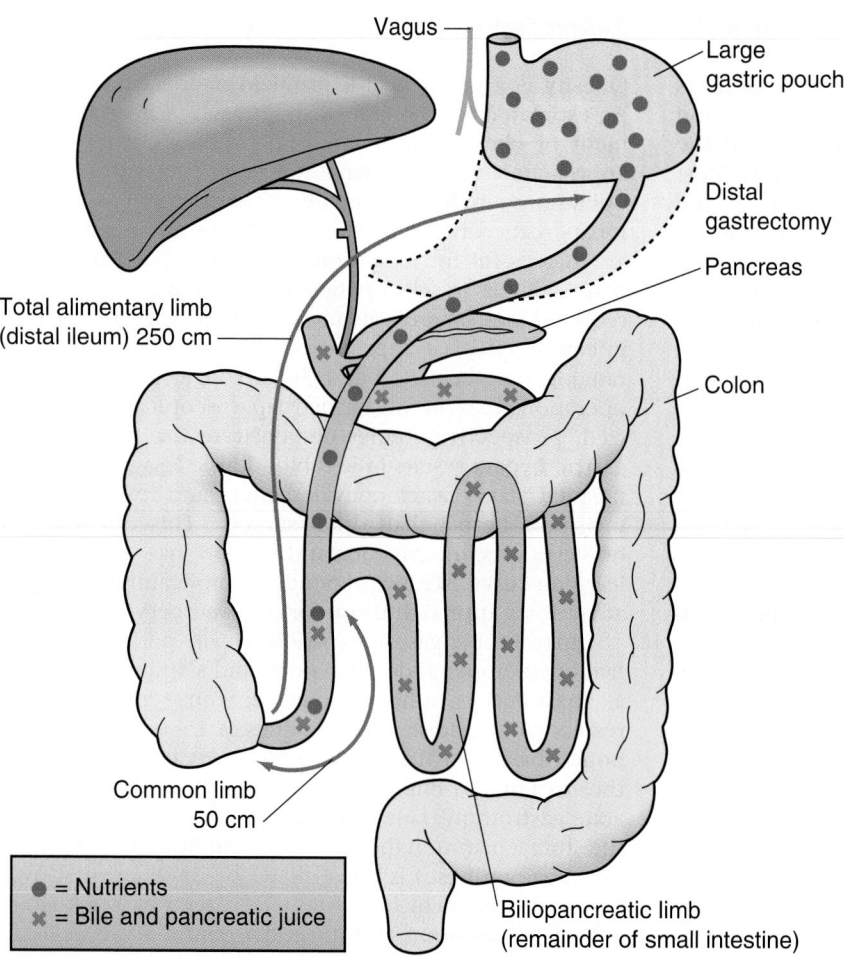

Vagus

Large gastric pouch

Distal gastrectomy

Pancreas

Colon

Total alimentary limb (distal ileum) 250 cm

Common limb 50 cm

● = Nutrients
✖ = Bile and pancreatic juice

Biliopancreatic limb (remainder of small intestine)

FIGURE 18-3. Configuration of the biliopancreatic diversion. (From Marceau P, Hould FS, Lebel S, et al: Malabsorptive obesity surgery. Surg Clin North Am 81:1113-1127, 2001.)

Recently, the adjustable gastric band (Lap-Band and the Swedish Adjustable Gastric Band) has gained favor because of its simplicity. The band is a soft, circular, inflatable device placed around the upper part of the stomach to restrict oral intake (Fig. 18-5). It is connected to an implanted port placed on the abdominal fascia that can be serially inflated or deflated to adjust oral intake. Although overall weight loss is not as great as in gastric bypass, the adjustable band avoids the risks of multiple anastomoses. Complications include infection necessitating band removal, erosion into the stomach, and slippage. Typically, these complications can be managed laparoscopically.

Laparoscopic Splenectomy

Splenectomy is an effective treatment for ITP, autoimmune hemolytic anemia, hereditary spherocytosis, Felty's syndrome, splenomegaly, and splenic cysts, and it is useful in staging of select patients with Hodgkin's and non-Hodgkin's lymphoma. Laparoscopic splenectomy may also be advantageous in select patients with splenic tumors, both primary and metastatic. Several retrospective and non-randomized, prospective studies show that there is less pain and blood loss, quicker return of bowel function, and shorter hospital stay, but a longer operative time with laparoscopic splenectomy performed for nontraumatic splenic diseases. With experience, operative times approach those for open operation. In general, laparoscopic splenectomy is as effective as open operation in treating hematologic disorders, and there has been no difference in the detection of accessory spleens.[35] On the other hand, controversy still exists concerning the benefits and potential for untoward outcomes if laparoscopic splenectomy is used to treat hypersplenism, malignant lesions, splenic artery aneurysms, and traumatic injuries of the spleen. The latter disorders are thus considered relative contraindications to the procedure, although they may be applicable for select patients by experienced surgeons.

The operation is most commonly performed in the lateral ("hanging spleen") position, but may be performed in modified lithotomy position. As with open operation, it is important to examine the abdomen for accessory spleens that are located, in descending order of frequency, in the splenic hilum and vascular pedicle, gastrocolic ligament, pancreatic tail, greater omentum, greater curve of the stomach, splenocolic ligament, small and large bowel mesentery, left broad ligament in women, and left spermatic cord in men. There is evidence that missed accessory spleens can be removed with a second laparoscopic operation. In one series, three patients were laparoscopically re-explored after performing tagged red blood cell scintigraphy for localization. All reoperations successfully removed the accessory spleen and induced a second remission of ITP.[36]

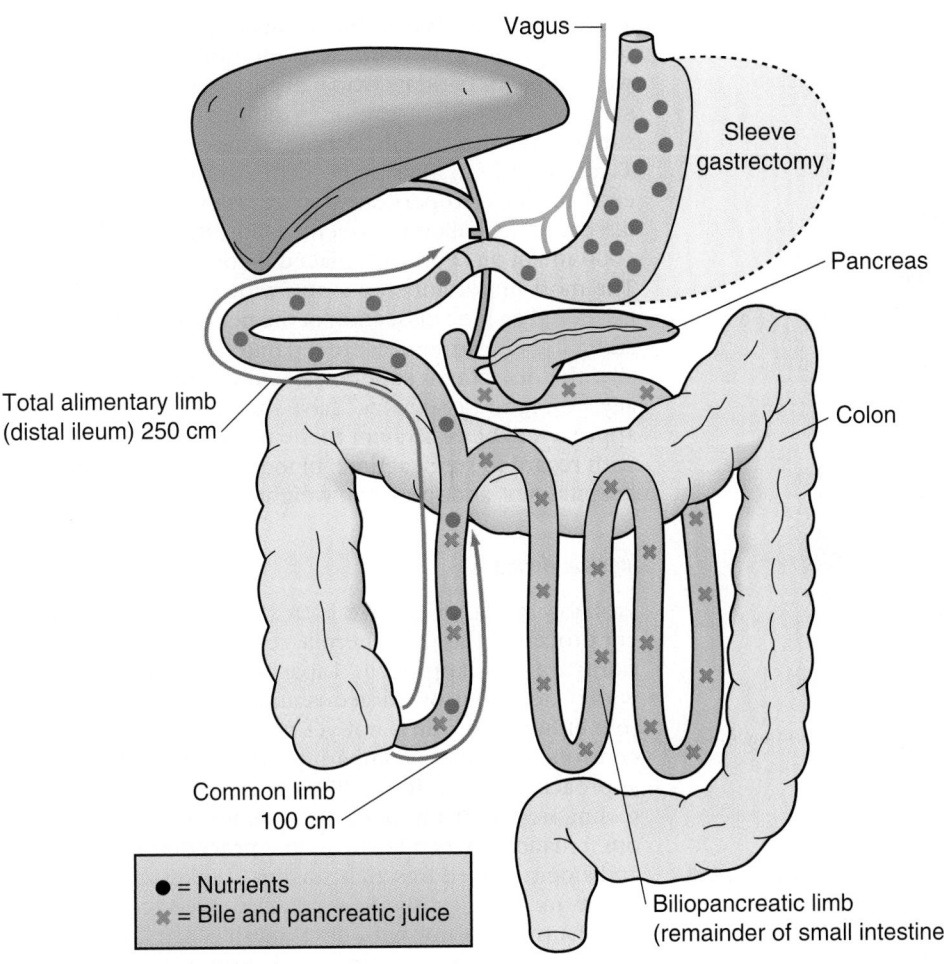

Vagus

Sleeve gastrectomy

Pancreas

Colon

Total alimentary limb (distal ileum) 250 cm

Common limb 100 cm

● = Nutrients
✖ = Bile and pancreatic juice

Biliopancreatic limb (remainder of small intestine)

FIGURE 18-4. Configuration of the duodenal switch. (From Marceau P, Hould FS, Lebel S, et al: Malabsorptive obesity surgery. Surg Clin North Am 81:1113-1127, 2001.)

After inspection, the dissection proceeds in five stages: (1) division of the short gastric vessels with ultrasonic shears, (2) division of the splenocolic ligament, (3) ligation of the inferior polar vessels, (4) transection of the hilum usually with staples, and (5) division of the phrenic attachments. Two common variations of the hilar vasculature are common. In the distributed pattern, multiple branches arise from the main vascular trunks 2 to 3 cm from the hilum. In the magistral pattern, the vascular pedicle formed by the artery and vein enters the hilum as a compact bundle and is transected en bloc with a single application of the linear stapler. In either case, it is important to dissect and visualize the tail of the pancreas to avoid injury when the hilum is transected.

Complications of laparoscopic splenectomy include bleeding, left pneumothorax, pleural effusion, pneumonia, splenosis, subphrenic abscess, pancreatic injury, and urinary retention. It is also postulated that the positions required for laparoscopic splenectomy promote venous stasis and deep venous thrombosis, but there are no data to support this.

Adrenalectomy

During the last decade, the development of laparoscopy has markedly improved outcomes for patients undergoing adrenalectomy. In the past, open transabdominal, flank, and posterior approaches used for adrenalectomy were associated with significant postoperative pain and necessitated prolonged periods of convalescence. Laparoscopic adrenalectomy, on the other hand, is associated with earlier resumption of enteral feedings, shorter hospital stay, lower infection rates, and faster return to normal activity, although it may take longer to perform. Laparoscopic adrenalectomy is particularly well suited for the resection of nonmalignant adrenal lesions such as aldosteronomas, pheochromocytomas, Cushing's disease with adrenal hyperplasia, nonfunctional adenoma, and rare entities such as cyst or myelolipoma.

Lesion size appears to be important for two reasons: (1) technical difficulty and (2) the increased risk of malignancy in larger lesions. Patients with adrenocortical carcinoma are currently not considered candidates for the minimally invasive approach because of the risk of tumor seeding and local recurrence. In addition, laparoscopy is not advisable for tumors larger than 6 cm because of technical difficulties associated with excision of these tumors, though this approach is not universally accepted. A few reports of laparoscopic excision of solitary, small, contained adrenal metastases are available. Some surgeons believe that an adequate operation can be performed for cancer when lesions are less than 6 cm.

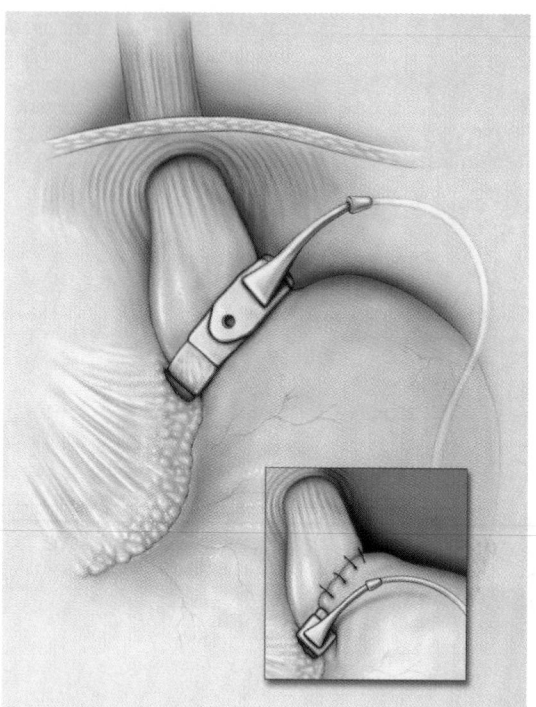

FIGURE 18-5. Proper position of the Lap-Band. (Courtesy of Inamed Health, Inc, Santa Barbara, CA, 2002.)

Currently, there are three laparoscopic transperitoneal and two retroperitoneal approaches to the adrenal gland. The most commonly used transperitoneal technique is the lateral approach. The patient is placed in a 45- to 90-degree flank position with the side to be resected facing upward. A camera port is placed either in the midline at or above the umbilicus, and two or three ports are placed along the ipsilateral costal margin. On the left, the lateral attachments of the colon and spleen are divided. The spleen, tail of the pancreas, splenic flexure, and descending colon are then mobilized and allowed to fall toward the midline. The adrenal gland is visualized over the medial upper kidney and the adrenal vein is found as it exits obliquely from the inferomedial aspect of the gland draining into the renal vein. On the right, some mobilization of the hepatic flexure is required but, more important, the right triangular ligament of the liver is divided and the liver retracted to expose the vena cava and the area of entry of the right adrenal vein. The right adrenal vein is found as it exits horizontally from the superomedial aspect of the gland draining into the inferior vena cava. Some surgeons mobilize the gland first and isolate the right vein as the final part of the procedure. In either case, lateral retraction on the gland must be performed with caution because the right vein is short and fragile. The vein is then controlled using clips or vascular stapling devices. On both sides, dissection can be performed on the anterior, posterior, and inferolateral aspects with ultrasonic shears, or with electrocautery because these areas are relatively avascular.

The other two transperitoneal approaches—the anterior and the supragastric—are used less commonly. They appear to yield comparable results to the lateral approach but take longer to perform. Retroperitoneal approaches are well suited for patients who had previous upper abdominal surgery. The patient can be positioned either laterally or supine, but the lateral position is more commonly used. Typically, a 2-cm incision is created at the level of the iliac crest and the retroperitoneal space is developed with finger dissection. A balloon dissector is inserted and filled with 1000 mL of air. Ports are placed below the costal margin. The most important step is the wide opening of Gerota's fascia and en bloc dissection of the perinephric fat with the adrenal gland. Structures are separated from the psoas laterally, the diaphragm superiorly, and the peritoneum medially.[37] Sung and associates[38] have shown the retroperitoneal approach to be equivalent to the transperitoneal approach with regard to surgical time, blood loss, pain management, hospital stay, and specimen weight.

Inguinal Hernia

Probably no other disease is treated with as many different procedures as groin hernia, reflecting the lack of superiority of any approach. Laparoscopic hernia repair is widely accepted by surgeons and patients, but its exact role in hernia repair is not yet fully defined. Randomized, controlled studies comparing open and laparoscopic approaches suffer from difficulties in standardizing the techniques used for both approaches. Comparisons are often made between laparoscopic procedures using mesh and open procedures that do not. Laparoscopic repairs result in significantly fewer recurrences compared to open suture but not with open mesh repairs. Recurrence and complication rates vary widely leading to variable conclusions. Meta-analysis does not improve comparisons because study flaws cannot be mathematically eliminated. Comparisons of open and laparoscopic mesh repairs indicate that laparoscopic repairs take longer to perform and cost more but result in fewer infections and allow patients to return to work slightly earlier (small but significant decreases). With increasing experience, operative times decrease to less than 1 hour. Although overall complication rates do not differ, major complications such as injury to adjacent organs, including bowel perforation, may be more common. Laparoscopic hernia repair appears to afford more benefit for patients undergoing bilateral simultaneous repair or repair of recurrent inguinal hernia.

Currently, there are two common laparoscopic approaches: the transabdominal preperitoneal (TAPP) or totally extraperitoneal (TEP). Both require working knowledge of pelvic vascular and nerve anatomy viewed from the posterior approach (Fig. 18-6). In the TAPP approach, the peritoneal cavity is insufflated with CO_2 and a camera port and two working ports are placed into the peritoneal cavity. Important structures and the hernia defect are identified. Peritoneum superior to the hernia is incised, and superior and inferior peritoneal flaps are created by blunt dissection. The hernia sac is separated from cord structures, avoiding trauma to the spermatic cord and genital branches of the genitofemoral nerve. The field of dissection should allow a 10×15 cm piece of mesh to lie flatly over the entire myopectineal orifice of Fruchaud (Fig. 18-7). Although the

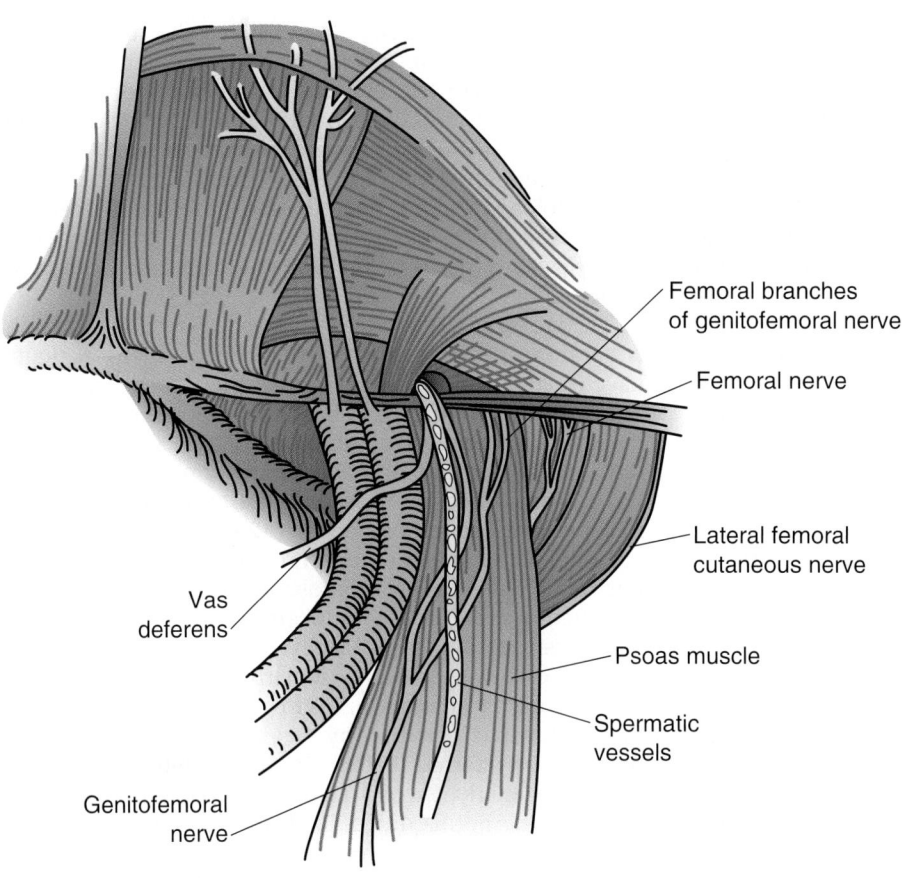

FIGURE 18-6. Locations of nerves at risk for entrapment with mesh fixation. (From Lucas SW, Arregui ME: Minimally invasive surgery for inguinal hernia. World J Surg 23:351, 1999.)

Femoral branches of genitofemoral nerve

Femoral nerve

Lateral femoral cutaneous nerve

Psoas muscle

Spermatic vessels

Vas deferens

Genitofemoral nerve

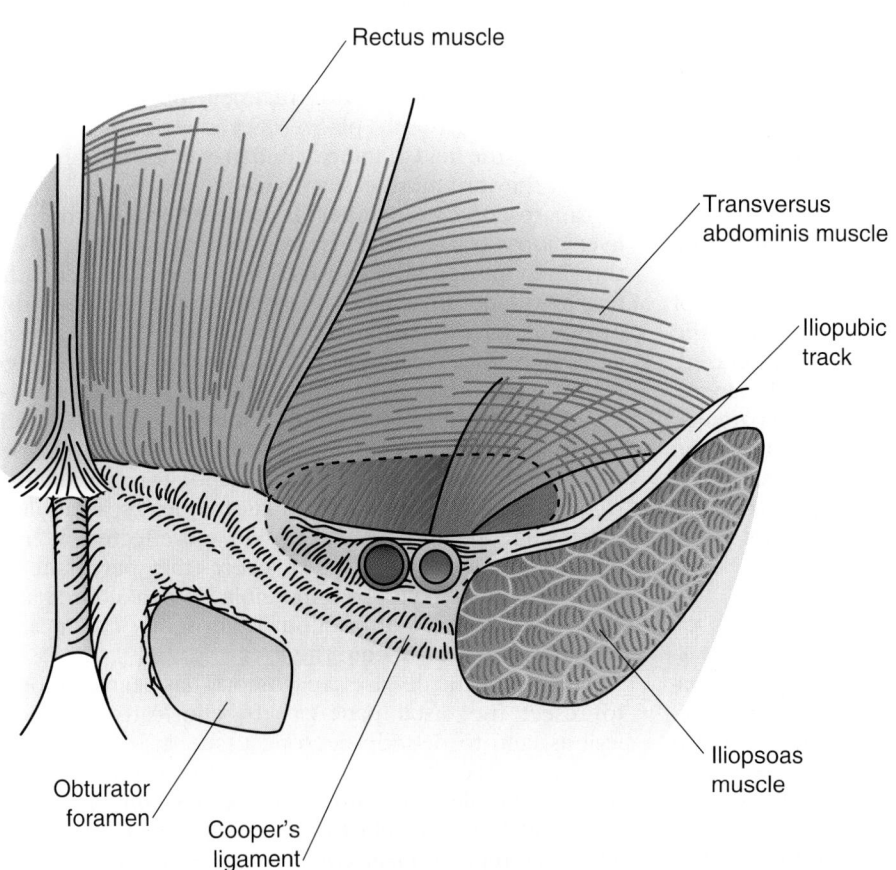

FIGURE 18-7. Myopectineal orifice of Fruchaud. (From Lucas SW, Arregui ME: Minimally invasive surgery for inguinal hernia. World J Surg 23:351, 1999.)

Rectus muscle

Transversus abdominis muscle

Iliopubic track

Obturator foramen

Cooper's ligament

Iliopsoas muscle

mesh is usually held in place using a few staples or tacks, randomized studies show no difference in hernia recurrence if staples are not used.

In the TEP repair, an incision is made just below the umbilicus. The anterior rectus fascia is incised just lateral to the midline and rectus muscle fibers are split to visualize the posterior fascia. Dissection is then begun inferiorly along the fascia, and the preperitoneal space is entered at the semilunar line. The preperitoneal space is then bluntly developed with laparoscopic instruments or a balloon dissector. Typically, a dissector is passed inferiorly to the mid pubis and insufflated to enlarge the preperitoneal space. Hernia repair then proceeds as in the TAPP. The preperitoneal space does not expand properly during TEP when the patient has had lower abdominal surgery, particularly prostatectomy. Complications such as bladder injury are also more common. TAPP or open repair may be preferable in this situation or with incarcerated hernias because the bowel can be reduced and inspected for viability.

Incisional Hernia

Direct suture repair of incisional hernias results in high recurrence rates (30% to 49%), but repairs using prosthetic materials (Mersilene, Prolene, and expanded polytetrafluoroethylene) decrease recurrence rates to 0% to 10%. Successful laparoscopic incisional hernia therefore requires placement of a prosthetic material, which should overlap the edges of the fascial defect by at least 3 cm. The introduction of composite ("double-sided") mesh, which is coated/covered by polytetrafluoroethylene on one side allowing ingrowth of abdominal wall tissues into the mesh but minimal adhesions to bowel, has facilitated this procedure. Nonabsorbable sutures are placed at the corners of the prosthesis and approximately every 5 cm around the perimeter. The mesh is inserted into the peritoneal cavity with suture tails attached, and suture tails are retrieved through small (3-mm) abdominal wounds using a suture closure device. The passer is reinserted via the same incision at a different angle and the opposing suture tail is brought through the fascia 1 cm away. The tails are tied and tacks are placed 1 cm apart along the edge of the mesh to eliminate space between the mesh and the abdominal wall. To date, there is only one randomized, prospective study comparing open mesh with laparoscopic incisional hernia repair. In this study of 60 patients, two developed recurrences in the open group and none were noted in the laparoscopic group.[39] Several small retrospective studies suggest that laparoscopic incisional hernia repair results in similar recurrence rates with fewer complications and shorter hospital stays.

Miscellaneous Procedures

Many general surgical, urologic, and gynecologic operations, in addition to those specifically outlined previously, are now performed laparoscopically. Often the exact role for and the patients who clearly benefit from these laparoscopic approaches have not been fully defined. For example, experienced transplant teams perform laparoscopic donor nephrectomy each day across the country.

This approach decreases donor pain, shortens time to full recovery, and improves cosmesis. Patients are more willing to donate kidneys, expanding the kidney donor pool. However, concerns about warm ischemic time and the duration of the operation tempered the initial enthusiasm, although significant differences in graft function and histology have not been demonstrated. Modifications of the procedures, such as hand-assisted laparoscopy, may allow faster retrieval of the donor kidney and decreased ischemic time.

The laparoscopic treatment of small bowel obstruction is another area of controversy. Although many patients have isolated bands responsible for their obstruction, it is not possible to distinguish them preoperatively from patients with extensive adhesions. Patients who are the best candidates for primary laparoscopic treatment of bowel obstruction are those with a history of only one or two previous operations, early (<24 hours) obstruction, and minimal to moderate distention of the bowel.[40] Bowel obstruction after recent laparoscopic surgery, early bowel obstruction associated with incarcerated inguinal hernias, and obstruction after localized operations such as appendectomy may be particularly good candidates for laparoscopic exploration. With incarcerated hernias, transabdominal laparoscopy (vs. the preperitoneal approach) is preferred to free the incarcerated bowel and assess its viability. Careful manipulation of inflamed friable bowel in the hernia defect, and use of atraumatic instruments, is essential to prevent iatrogenic perforations. Trocars should be placed by open technique and an initial assessment should be made with the laparoscope. If adhesions are dense or bowel is of questionable viability, the operation should be converted to an open procedure. Rotating the table so that the area of obstruction is at the highest point facilitates the treatment of bowel obstruction. Gravity naturally places distended loops of bowel away from the field of interest and may elongate adhesions so that they are more easily divided.

Laparoscopic liver surgery is in evolution. Laparoscopic liver biopsy is a straightforward tool that has lowered the threshold for operative biopsy. Multiple reports detail the feasibility and advantages of laparoscopic hepatectomy, but none have been randomized studies. There is some agreement that laparoscopic hepatectomy is best suited for patients with small, peripheral liver lesions that can be managed by wedge resection or by removal of the left lateral lobe. Proponents suggest that laparoscopy causes significantly less morbidity and that long-term prognosis is unchanged. Laparoscopic radiofrequency ablation is increasingly being used. It is a safe and effective alternative for hepatic neoplasms where the percutaneous approach is difficult or impossible. When coordinated with intraoperative ultrasound, laparoscopy can localize virtually all lesions within the liver.

For pancreatic disease, laparoscopy has been employed to resect the distal pancreas, to enucleate superficial lesions, and to débride necrotic tissue. It has also been used in pancreatitis to create a cystogastrostomy. Laparoscopic Whipple procedures have been accomplished but have not shown benefit to the patient. These are largely anecdotal reports; clear conclusions cannot be drawn.

VIDEO-ASSISTED THORACOSCOPIC SURGERY

Indications

Thoracoscopic surgery, also known as *VATS*, requires equipment and techniques similar to, and has undergone parallel advances with, laparoscopy. Today, approximately 20% of general thoracic procedures are performed videoscopically. The benefits of VATS include less postoperative pain, less pulmonary trauma, shorter hospitalizations, and improved patient satisfaction. As with laparoscopy, surgeon skills and application of VATS vary widely. The greatest controversy surrounds the suitability of VATS for definitive resection of pulmonary malignant lesions.

VATS is widely accepted as a diagnostic procedure. Half of all operative biopsies are currently obtained with VATS. VATS is especially useful for definitive diagnosis of indeterminate pulmonary nodules and for undiagnosed effusions. It is increasingly used to stage cancer and to evaluate mediastinal masses and adenopathy. This technique provides a broad view of the entire thoracic cavity and mediastinum when the patient is well positioned; the inferior pulmonary ligament is divided, and single lung ventilation is used (Box 18-4). Its unmatched ability to visualize and biopsy every lymph node station in the ipsilateral thorax, including those unapproachable by mediastinoscopy, makes it particularly useful for assessment of tumor resectability and, in cases of suspected lymphoma, large pieces of tissue are obtainable to make a definitive diagnosis. VATS allows direct assessment of mediastinal invasion, inspection for pleural implants, and sampling of small effusions for malignant cells. Wedge and anatomic pulmonary resections, evacuation of the pleural space, and pleurodesis (for malignant effusion and pneumothorax) are commonly performed, and resection of mediastinal cysts and tumors can be accomplished with VATS.

Physiology

The working space for VATS is established by collapse of the ipsilateral lung using a double-lumen endotracheal tube and one-lung ventilation. Alternately, the hemithorax can be insufflated with CO_2 in conjunction with two-lung anesthesia, but the self-supporting ribcage and partial collapse of the lung limit the operative field. This technique is rarely used. Physiologic changes during VATS largely result from one-lung ventilation and patient positioning.

One-lung ventilation decreases the surface area available for gas exchange and results in loss of normal pulmonary autoregulation in which hypoxic pulmonary vasoconstriction results in redistribution of blood flow to better-ventilated segments improving arterial oxygenation. These compensatory mechanisms are obliterated when 70% of the lung is atelectatic and are further suppressed by volatile anesthetics.[41] VATS may thus cause a significant decrease in the PaO_2. Partial ventilation of the operative lung and administration of intrapulmonary nitrous oxide or almitrine, a peripheral chemoreceptor agonist, may maintain this reflex, but this remains inves-

---

> **Box 18-4. Potential Indications of Video-Assisted Thoracoscopic Surgery**
>
> **Diagnostic**
> Indeterminate pleural effusion (benign vs. malignant)
> Tissue diagnosis
>   Pleural-based masses (metastatic adenocarcinoma vs. mesothelioma)
>   Diffuse interstitial lung disease
>   Indeterminate peripheral pulmonary nodule
>   Mediastinal lymph node biopsy
>   Mediastinal mass biopsy
>
> **Therapeutic**
> Pleuropulmonary
>   Pleural effusion/empyema
>   Pleurodesis (thermal/mechanical/chemical/talc)
>   Bullous disease ablation/resection
>   Wedge resection for early-stage lung cancer in selected high-risk patients
>   Anatomic resection for lung cancer
> Esophageal
>   Resection of leiomyomata
>   Resection of enteric cysts
>   Esophagomyotomy
>   Antireflux surgery for intractable gastroesophageal reflux disease
>   Video-assisted esophagectomy
> Mediastinal
>   Thymectomy for myasthenia gravis
>   Thymectomy for stage I thymoma
>   Resection of benign mediastinal tumors (teratoma)
>   Resection of posterior mediastinal (neurogenic) masses
>   Excision of bronchogenic, enteric, or pericardial cysts
>   Drainage of pericardial effusion
>   Pericardiectomy
>
> **Miscellaneous**
>   Dorsal sympathectomy or splanchnicectomy
>   Drainage of paravertebral abscess
>   Orthopedic discectomy
>   Internal mammary artery harvest for coronary artery bypass grafting

From Lin JC, Landreneau RJ: Instruments and techniques of video-assisted thoracic surgery. *In* Shields TW, LoCicero J, Ponn RB (eds): General Thoracic Surgery. Philadelphia, Lippincott Williams & Wilkins, 2000, p 440.

---

tigational. Single-lung ventilation also increases pulmonary vascular resistance and right heart work.

Lateral decubitus positioning minimizes the effects of one-lung ventilation. There is an obligatory right-to-left transpulmonary shunt through the nonventilated lung. The lateral decubitus position causes a gravity-induced decrease in blood flow through this lung, improving the ventilation-perfusion relationship. Ultimately, the tolerance of one-lung anesthesia is dependent on preparation of the patient for surgery, the patient's pulmonary reserve, and comorbidities.

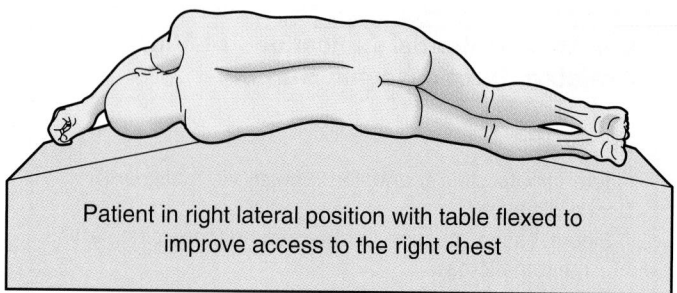

FIGURE 18-8. Patient position for right-sided thoracoscopy. (From Shah A, Davis R, Harpole D: Thorascopic lung volume reduction surgery. *In* Pappas T, Cheken E, Eubanks W [eds]: Atlas of Laparoscopic Surgery. Philadelphia, Current Medicine, 1999.)

> **Box 18-5. Complications of Video-Assisted Thoracoscopic Surgery**
>
> Air leak with persistent/recurrent pneumothorax
> Atelectasis
> Pneumonia
> Barotrauma
> Re-expansion pulmonary edema
> Dissemination of malignant disease
> Infection
>   Pulmonary abscess
>   Empyema
>   Wound infection
> Hemorrhage
> Myocardial infarct
> Arrhythmias
> Hypotension/hypertension
> Intercostal neuritis

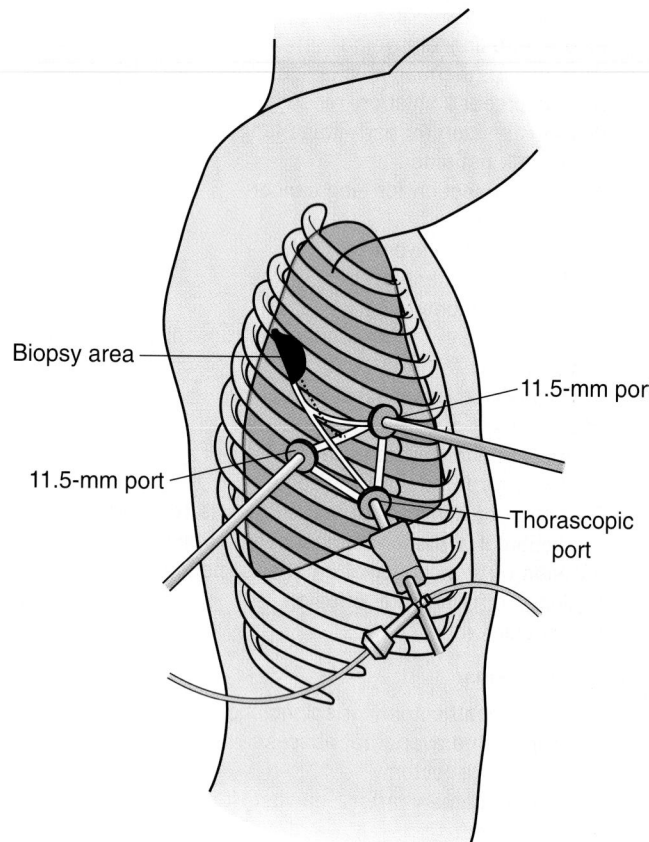

FIGURE 18-9. Port placement for right-sided thoracoscopy. (From Shah A, Davis R, Harpole D: Thorascopic lung volume reduction surgery. *In* Pappas T, Cheken E, Eubanks W [eds]: Atlas of Laparoscopic Surgery. Philadelphia, Current Medicine, 1999.)

Technical Considerations

The outcome of VATS is highly dependent on anesthetic technique and positioning of the patient. It is crucial that the anesthesia and surgical team be well acquainted with double-lumen endotracheal intubation, bronchial blockers, and bronchoscopy to support single-lung ventilation. Typically, double-lumen endotracheal intubation is accomplished with the patient in the supine position. The patient is then turned to the lateral decubitus position. Careful padding of pressure points is essential to avoid

peripheral nerve injuries. The table is flexed to maximize the size of the intercostal spaces on the operative side (Fig. 18-8) and the patient is secured to the table to allow for position changes. A beanbag works well. The patient is then prepped and draped to allow for a prompt thoracotomy if necessary.

As with laparoscopic procedures, port position significantly affects the ease of procedure performance. Ports are placed a sufficient distance from the lesion to optimize working space. Port triangulation allows instruments to converge on the operative field (Fig. 18-9). The incision for the primary viewing port is placed directly over the chosen intercostal space and a finger is inserted into the pleural space to assess for adhesions. Tunneling is discouraged because this limits movement of instruments and excessive torquing of instruments may result in intercostal neuritis. Other ports are placed under thoracoscopic vision after assessing the position of the lesion. All ports are placed immediately superior to the ribs to avoid injury to the neurovascular bundles.

Perhaps the most challenging element of VATS is accurate location of parenchymal lesions, especially those deep within the lung. An appreciation of the three-dimensional anatomy and correlation with plain films and computed tomographic (CT) scans is essential. Complete collapse of the operative lung is mandatory for locating deep lesions. Subtle puckering on the pleural surface of the lung may help locate the lesion. In many cases, direct digital palpation is still possible. The surgeon's finger is inserted through the port site and the area in question is brought to it. The lesion may also be detected by sweeping a blunt instrument over the surface of the lung to detect irregularities in texture. Alternately, wire-guided needle localization, subpleural dye injection, and intraoperative ultrasound have been used as adjuncts. Experience decreases the need for these adjuncts. Subpleural lesions greater than 1 cm often appear as discolored areas or as a faint bulge on the visceral pleura and are easier to detect. Once the lesion, lobe, or entire lung is resected, it is brought out through the largest port. Larger specimens should be placed within a specimen bag to avoid fracture or tumor spillage. Alternately, a limited thoracotomy is performed to remove a large specimen. A chest tube is placed through one port site and the other incisions are closed with absorbable sutures. Often, the chest tube can be removed in the postanesthesia care unit after ensuring adequate lung expansion by chest radiograph and absence of an air leak.

Complications

Several large series of VATS report perioperative morbidity ranging from 2% to 10% and mortality less than 2%, results comparable to or less than historical open controls. Complications are similar to those encountered during thoracotomy. The most common problems are atelectasis, prolonged air leak, hemorrhage, and infection (Box 18-5). Persistent atelectasis may lead to hypoxia and pneumonia. Patients require aggressive pulmonary toilet (ambulation, bronchodilators, and coughing) to hasten its resolution. Air leaks lasting longer than 7 days occur in 2% to 6% of cases and are a common reason for reoperation, often requiring a formal thoracotomy. Infections and hemorrhage each comprise 1% to 2% of the early complications and may also be a reason for further intervention.

Complications specific to thoracoscopy include trocar injuries, intercostal neuritis, and port site recurrence of malignancy. Nearly every organ in the hemithorax can be injured with blind trocar placement. Placing the first port under direct vision, and others under thoracoscopic guidance, best prevents trocar injuries. Port site recurrence has been reported in several series of VATS procedures and tends to be more common when specimens are not placed within a protective bag prior to removal from the chest. They are more common with mesothelioma, metastatic sarcoma, melanoma, or malignant effusion.

Specific Procedures

Pulmonary Resection/Cancer

Indeterminate pulmonary nodules are one of the most common problems facing the thoracic surgeon. Overall, 60% to 70% of nodules identified by chest radiography are benign. When lesions are greater than 3 cm and noncalcified, the risk of malignancy is greater than 90%. However, most lesions are smaller and less clear-cut. Diagnostic procedures such as bronchoscopy, sputum cytology, and fine-needle aspiration together establish a definitive diagnosis in 10% to 20% of these latter lesions, and false-negative results occur in up to 25% with malignant lesions. Resection of parenchymal lesions is definitive but until recently required thoracotomy. VATS is a less invasive, less morbid method of resection, especially when the lesion is superficial and at the lung margin. Approximately one half of VATS procedures are pulmonary resections for diagnosis. Thoracoscopic wedge resection may not be possible or prudent if there is dense pleural symphysis, inability to tolerate one-lung ventila-

tion, lesion size is greater than 3 cm, or if there is known cancer. A patient requiring anticoagulation is also a relative contraindication to the procedure.

Techniques for wedge biopsy are straightforward. The lesion is localized on preoperative plain films and/or CT scan, and ports are strategically placed to allow triangulation of instruments. The lesion is identified and resection performed by successive applications of an endoscopic stapler around the lesion. Specimens should be placed within a bag prior to extraction to prevent tumor seeding in the event that the lesion is malignant. For patients with T1 tumors and/or limited lung function (forced expiratory volume in 1 second [FEV_1] < 40%), wedge resection may provide the best option, although some reports indicate that tumor recurrence is three times more likely following wedge resection or segmentectomy when compared to lobar resection. If, at the time of VATS wedge resection, the lesion is found to be malignant, ipsilateral lymph node sampling should be performed to rule out stage III disease. A decision must then be made about the performance of lobectomy or pneumonectomy and whether definitive resection should be done by minimally invasive or open techniques.

Anatomic resections are performed less commonly because of concern about adequate tumor margins with minimally invasive approaches and chest wall (port site) recurrence. However, disease-free survival appears to be equivalent in nonrandomized studies. Randomized, prospective studies are lacking, and controversy remains concerning the role of VATS for definitive tumor resection. It is generally agreed that bulky mediastinal lymphadenopathy, endobronchial extension, chest wall or mediastinal invasion, and use of neoadjuvant therapy are either relative or absolute contraindications to minimally invasive surgery.[42] Pneumonectomy is rarely performed using VATS because most tumors needing a pneumonectomy are either T3 or large hilar tumors.

Biopsy may be required in up to one third of patients with diffuse interstitial disease of the lung to establish a diagnosis. In the past, bronchoscopy and transbronchial and transthoracic needle biopsies were used to avoid the morbidity associated with open lung biopsy. However, the diagnostic yield is less than 60%. VATS has a diagnostic accuracy (≥94%), operating time comparable to open biopsy, but less morbidity. If both lungs are affected equally, the right chest presents more free edges for biopsy, whereas the left lung tends to collapse more completely during one-lung ventilation.

Lung Volume Reduction

Emphysema, a chronic obstructive pulmonary disease (COPD), results in loss of alveolar and capillary surface area, elastic recoil of the lung, air trapping, and hyperexpansion of the lungs. Clinically, this is manifest by a prolonged expiratory phase (decreased FEV_1), poor exercise tolerance, and oxygen dependence in those with severe changes. Radiographically, lungs are hyperinflated and the hemidiaphragms are flattened. On CT, blebs of various sizes are usually seen in the upper lobes but may be distributed throughout the lung. Compression of normal parenchyma by blebs results in further impairment of gas exchange. Medical management, including pulmonary rehabilitation, reduces oxygen requirements during exercise but does not improve pulmonary function.

On the other hand, excision of large blebs (lung reduction surgery) reduces compression and may improve function by restoring elastic recoil and expanding functioning lung. Ideal candidates for lung reduction surgery have a localized pattern of parenchymal destruction with hypoperfusion in the diseased segments by pulmonary perfusion scanning. Lung volume reduction surgery offers a 60% chance of oxygen independence, 85% chance of steroid independence, and 60% to 70% improvement in pulmonary function in the 20% to 30% severe COPD patients who meet criteria, especially with upper lung bullae.[43]

Lung volume reduction surgery was initially performed through a median sternotomy but now is effectively performed with VATS. Unlike sternotomy, VATS provides access to inferior lobes and posterior aspect of the lungs. Decubitus position is preferred, especially for patients with adhesions or who require bilateral lower lobe resection (α_1-antitrypsin deficiency). Lung volume reduction by VATS can also be performed with the patient in supine position to shorten the time by allowing bilateral operation with a single skin preparation. This approach works well for uncomplicated resections of upper lobe emphysema, but it has the same disadvantages as median sternotomy. There are limited data directly comparing lung volume reduction by thoracotomy and VATS. One study of 42 patients showed that lung volume reduction by VATS takes longer to perform but resulted in fewer days on the ventilator, in the intensive care unit, and with an air leak. Patients also experienced shorter hospital stays and lower hospital costs.[44]

The area of diseased lung is localized preoperatively and ports are placed accordingly. Successive applications of an endoscopic stapler are used to remove the diseased, unperfused portions of lung. Typically, about 50% of each upper lobe is removed, but more extensive resections may be required for lower lobe emphysema or when the there are extensive areas without perfusion. Prolonged air leaks occur in 35% to 50% of patients. A randomized, prospective trial showed that buttressing of staple/suture lines with bovine pericardium reduced the duration of chest tube drainage by 2.5 days and hospitalization by 2.8 days. The savings in hospital days was offset by the increased cost of the operation.[45] Placing chest tubes to water seal without suction immediately may decrease this complication.

Pneumothorax

More than 20,000 nontraumatic pneumothoraces occur every year in the United States. Primary and secondary pneumothoraces differ in the presence or absence of underlying pulmonary disease, most often COPD. Although there is significant variability in the timing of operative intervention, most authors agree that VATS is the preferred approach for dealing with persistent air leaks (>4 days), recurrent pneumothorax, and selected patients whose activities put them at high risk if the pneumothorax recurred (scuba divers and aviators). Often the responsible bleb or diseased lung is at the apex. Stapled bullectomy yields a 95% to 100% success rate compared to 78% to 91% success with chemical pleurodesis alone.[46] Parietal pleurectomy or talc poudrage can be added to reduce recurrence.

Pleural Effusion

Pleural effusion is one of the most common indications for VATS. Thoracentesis and closed pleural biopsy do not yield an etiology in as many as 20% of patients. VATS is diagnostic in 95% of these cases, including distinguishing between poorly differentiated adenocarcinoma and mesothelioma in patients with malignant effusions. During the procedure, a generous pleural biopsy is obtained and specific pleural lesions are biopsied. Consideration should be given to mechanical or chemical pleurodesis to deal with the effusion. VATS, in this setting, is performed with low morbidity and essentially no mortality.

Thoracoscopy is also indicated for selected cases of empyema and hemothorax. In acute empyema, VATS allows evacuation and lavage of the pleural space, thus removing the fibrin that prevents lung re-expansion. In complex empyema, VATS disrupts loculations between the lung and chest wall and removes fibrinopurulent debris. However, the success rate for VATS decreases from near 100% to 50% when empyema reaches the fibrotic stage. Similarly, VATS is used in clotted hemothoraces that have failed tube thoracostomy. Localization of the bleeding source and removal of blood clots prevent trapped lung and fibrothorax.

Mediastinal Disease

VATS allows the surgeon to widely inspect the entire mediastinum and hemithorax and to obtain generous biopsies. This improves diagnostic accuracy and staging of mediastinal masses by detecting tumor invasion or metastatic spread not apparent on preoperative imaging. It is also useful for restaging of medically treated lesions. For well-encapsulated benign tumors, VATS allows definitive resection. Excision of neurogenic tumors, mediastinal cysts, and teratomas has been described. VATS can be used for pericardial effusive disease as well. Effusions can be approached from either side and pericardial resection is more extensive compared to the subxiphoid technique.

Total thymectomy for myasthenia gravis is highly effective compared to medical treatment alone. However, the success of the operation is dependent on complete removal of the gland. Total thymectomy can be achieved with VATS, but the choice between a right, left, or bilateral approach is still debated, and thoracoscopic excision of thymoma remains controversial. If the lesion is small (<3 cm), it can be removed thoracoscopically en bloc with all the adjacent thymic tissue. Invasiveness represents an absolute contraindication to VATS resection.[47]

Sympathectomy/Splanchnicectomy

Thoracic sympathectomy is indicated for patients with palmar and axillary hyperhidrosis, selected patients with reflex sympathetic dystrophy, and those with vasculopathies such as Raynaud's or Buerger's disease. Portions of the sympathetic chain are excised or ablated. For palmar hyperhidrosis, only the T2 segment needs to be excised, but if axillary hyperhidrosis is present, the level of ablation needs to be extended to the T4 level. Success rates for the treatment of hyperhidrosis range from 85% to 95%, although compensatory truncal hyperhidrosis may occur in 20% to 50% of patients and is difficult to treat. Other complications including Horner's syndrome and rhinitis from injury to the stellate ganglion and T1, respectively, pneumothorax, and hemothorax occur in less than 5% of patients.

Thoracic splanchnicectomy is an attractive alternative to abdominal sympathectomy for patients with intractable visceral pain arising in the upper abdomen. Abdominal sympathectomy generally requires a celiotomy, whereas thoracic splanchnicectomy is readily performed via VATS. The greater splanchnic nerve arises from T5 to T10 and the lesser splanchnic nerve from T10 to T11. These nerves are ablated or excised between these levels. Unilateral treatment is successful in approximately half of patients.[48]

CONCLUSION

With each year that passes, the limitations of laparoscopy have decreased. Ten years ago, few would have believed that complex laparoscopic operations such as adrenalectomy, colectomy, and gastric bypass would be commonplace. However, advances in optics and instrumentation have opened new horizons. Yet, it is the ingenuity and vision of surgeon scientists that are ultimately responsible for progress within the field.

Selected References

Low DE: The short esophagus: Recognition and management. J Gastrointest Surg 5:458-461, 2001.

This paper discusses the predictors and clinical management of short esophagus in the context of reflux surgery.

Lucas SW, Arregui ME: Minimally invasive surgery for inguinal hernia. World J Surg 23:350-355, 1999.

The authors review the common techniques of laparoscopic inguinal hernia repair, the internal anatomy, and their experience.

Odeberg-Wernerman S: Laparoscopic surgery: Effects on circulatory and respiratory physiology—an overview. Eur J Surg Suppl 585:4-11, 2000.

This review focuses on the cardiopulmonary effects of laparoscopy. The author highlights changes with patient positioning and physiologic compromise.

Park A, Marcaccio M, Sternbach M, et al: Laparoscopic versus open splenectomy. Arch Surg 13:1263-1269, 1999.

This study compares laparoscopic splenectomy to historical open controls. It provides a good review of the techniques, complications, and costs.

Stocchi L, Nelson H: Wound recurrences following laparoscopic-assisted colectomy for cancer. Arch Surg 135:948-958, 2000.

The authors provide a comprehensive review of the world literature on wound recurrences after laparoscopic colorectal cancer surgery. Pathogenesis, experimental studies, and prevention are discussed.

Yim APC: VATS major pulmonary resection revisited: Controversies, techniques, and results. Ann Thorac Surg 74:615-623, 2002.

This paper provides a detailed review of the items listed in the title. It also discusses instrumentation and reviews the largest series of VATS lobectomy.

References

1. Rauh R, Hemmerling TM, Rist M, et al: Influence of pneumoperitoneum and patient positioning on respiratory system compliance. J Clin Anesth 13:361-365, 2001.
2. Andersson L, Lagerstrand L, Thorne A, et al: Effect of CO_2 pneumoperitoneum on ventilation-perfusion relationships during laparoscopic cholecystectomy. Acta Anaesthesiol Scand 46:552-560, 2002.
3. Schilling MK, Redaelli CR, Krahenbuhl L, et al: Splanchnic microcirculatory changes during CO_2 laparoscopy. J Am Coll Surg 184:378-382, 1997.
4. Kuntz C, Wunsch A, Bodeker C, et al: Effect of pressure and gas type on intra-abdominal, subcutaneous, and blood pH in laparoscopy. Surg Endosc 14:367-371, 2000.
5. Rist M, Hemmerling TM, Rauh R, et al: Influence of pneumoperitoneum and patient positioning on preload and splanchnic blood volume in laparoscopic surgery of the lower abdomen. J Clin Anesth 13:244-249, 2001.
6. Kashtan J, Green JF, Parsons EQ, et al: Hemodynamic effects of increased abdominal pressure. J Surg Res 30:249-255, 1981.
7. Aneman A, Svensson M, Stenqvist O, et al: Intestinal perfusion during pneumoperitoneum with carbon dioxide, nitrogen, and nitric oxide during laparoscopic surgery. Eur J Surg 166:70-76, 2000.
8. Nguyen NT, Perez RV, Fleming N, et al: Effect of prolonged pneumoperitoneum on intraoperative urine output during laparoscopic gastric bypass. J Am Coll Surg 195:476-483, 2002.
9. Nguyen NT, Owings JT, Gosselin R, et al: Systemic coagulation and fibrinolysis after laparoscopic and open gastric bypass. Arch Surg 136:909-916, 2001.
10. Allendorf JD, Bessler M, Whelan RL, et al: Postoperative immune function varies inversely with the degree of surgical trauma in a murine model. Surg Endosc 11:427-430, 1997.
11. Walker CB, Bruce DM, Heys SD: Minimal modulation of lymphocyte and natural killer cell subsets following minimal access surgery. Am J Surg 177:48-54, 1999.
12. Neuhaus SJ, Watson DI, Ellis T, et al: Influence of gases on intraperitoneal immunity during laparoscopy in tumor-bearing rats. World J Surg 24:1227-1231, 2000.
13. Checkan EG, Nataraj C, Clary EM, et al: Intraperitoneal immunity and pneumoperitoneum. Surg Endosc 13:1135-1138, 1999.
14. Scott DJ, Bergen PC, Rege RV, et al: Laparoscopic training on bench models: Better and more cost effective than operating room experience? J Am Coll Surg 191:272-283, 2000.
15. Philips PA, Amaral JF: Abdominal access complications in laparoscopic surgery. J Am Coll Surg 19:525-536, 2001.

16. Bonjer HJ, Hazebroek EJ, Kazamier G, et al: Open versus closed establishment of pneumoperitoneum in laparoscopic surgery. Br J Surg 84:599-602, 1997.

17. Memon MA, Fitzgibbons RJ: The role of minimal access surgery in the acute abdomen. Surg Clin North Am 77:1333-1353, 1997.

18. Taner AS, Topgul K, Kucukel F, et al: Diagnostic laparoscopy decreases the rate of unnecessary laparotomies and reduces hospital costs in trauma patients. J Laparoendosc Adv Surg Tech A 11:207-211, 2001.

19. Merriam LT, Kanaan SA, Dawes LG, et al: Gangrenous cholecystitis: Analysis of risk factors and experience with laparoscopic cholecystectomy. Surgery 126:680-686, 1999.

20. Ludwig K, Bernhardt J, Steffen H, et al: Contribution of intraoperative cholangiography to incidence and outcome of common bile duct injuries during laparoscopic cholecystectomy. Surg Endosc 16:1098-1104, 2002.

21. Birth M, Ehlers KU, Delinikolas K, et al: Prospective randomized comparison of laparoscopic ultrasonography using a flexible-tip ultrasound probe and intraoperative dynamic cholangiography during laparoscopic cholecystectomy. Surg Endosc 12:30-36, 1998.

22. Chang L, Lo S, Stabile BE, et al: Preoperative versus postoperative endoscopic retrograde cholangiopancreatography in mild to moderate gallstone pancreatitis: A prospective randomized trial. Ann Surg 231:82-87, 2000.

23. Catheline J, Rizk N, Champault G: A comparison of laparoscopic ultrasound versus cholangiography in the evaluation of the biliary tree during laparoscopic cholecystectomy. Eur J Ultrasound 10:1-9, 1999.

24. Petelin JB: Laparoscopic common bile duct exploration: Transcystic duct approach. *In* SAGES Manual: Fundamentals of Laparoscopy and GI Endoscopy. New York, Springer-Verlag, 1999, pp 167-177.

25. Hagedorn C, Lönroth H, Rydberg L, et al: Long-term efficacy of total (Nissen-Rossetti) and posterior partial (Toupet) fundoplication: Results of a randomized clinical trial. J Gastrointest Surg 6:540-545, 2002.

26. Tam WCE, Schoeman MN, Zhang Q, et al: Delivery of radiofrequency energy (RFe) to the lower esophageal sphincter (LES) and gastric cardia inhibits transient LES relaxations and gastroesophageal reflux in patients with reflux disease. Gastroenterology 120:16, 2001.

27. Sharp KW, Khaitan L, Scholz S, et al: One hundred consecutive minimally invasive Heller myotomies: Lessons learned. Ann Surg 235:631-639, 2002.

28. Spiess AE, Kahrilas PJ: Treating achalasia: From whalebone to laparoscope. JAMA 280:638-642, 1998.

29. Lezoche E, Feliciotti F, Paganini AM, et al: Laparoscopic colonic resections versus open surgery: A prospective non-randomized study on 310 unselected cases. Hepatogastroenterology 47:697-708, 2000.

30. Milsom JW, Bohm B, Hammerhofer KA, et al: A prospective, randomized trial comparing laparoscopic versus conventional techniques in colorectal cancer surgery: A preliminary report. J Am Coll Surg 187:46-55, 1998.

31. Stage JG, Schulze S, Moller P, et al: Prospective randomized study of laparoscopic versus open colonic resection for adenocarcinoma. Br J Surg 84:391-396, 1997.

32. Nelson H: Laparoscopic colectomy for colon cancer: A trial update. Swiss Surg 7:248-251, 2001.

33. Hazebroek EJ, The Color Study Group: COLOR: A randomized clinical trial comparing laparoscopic and open resection for colon cancer. Surg Endosc 16:949-953, 2002.

34. Fleshman JW, Wexner SD, Anvari M, et al: Laparoscopic versus open abdominoperineal resection for cancer. Dis Colon Rect 42:930-939, 1999.

35. Cogliandolo A, Berland-Dai B, Pidoto PP, et al: Results of laparoscopic and open splenectomy for nontraumatic diseases. Surg Laparosc Endosc Percutan Tech 11:256-261, 2001.

36. Morris KT, Hovarth KD, Jobe BA, et al: Laparoscopic management of accessory spleens in immune thrombocytopenic purpura. Surg Endosc 13:520-522, 1999.

37. Suzuki K, Kageyama S, Hirano Y, et al: Comparison of three surgical approaches to laparoscopic adrenalectomy: A nonrandomized, background matched analysis. J Urol 166:437-443, 2001.

38. Sung GT, Gill IS, Hobart MG: Laparoscopic adrenalectomy: Prospective, randomized comparison of transperitoneal versus retroperitoneal approaches (abstract). J Urol 161S:21, 1999.

39. Carbajo MA, Martin del Olmo JC, Blanco JI, et al: Laparoscopic treatment versus open surgery in the solution of major incisional and abdominal wall hernias with mesh. Surg Endosc 13:250-252, 1999.

40. Levard H, Boudet MJ, Msika S, et al: Laparoscopic treatment of acute small bowel obstruction: A multicenter retrospective study. Aust N Z J Surg 71:641-646, 2001.

41. Fredman B: Physiologic changes during thoracoscopy. Anesthesiol Clin North Am 19:141-152, 2001.

42. McKenna RJ: The current status of video-assisted thoracic surgery lobectomy. Chest Surg Clin North Am 8:775-785, 1998.

43. McKenna RJ, Gelb A, Brenner M: Lung volume reduction surgery for chronic obstructive pulmonary disease: Where do we stand? World J Surg 25:231-237, 2001.

44. Ko CY, Waters PF: Lung volume reduction surgery: A cost and outcomes comparison of sternotomy versus thoracoscopy. Am Surg 64:1010-1013, 1998.

45. Hazelrigg SR, Naunheim K: Effect of bovine pericardial strips on air leak after stapled pulmonary resection. Ann Thorac Surg 63:1573, 1997.

46. Baumann MH, Strange C: Treatment of spontaneous pneumothorax: A more aggressive approach? Chest 112:789-804, 1997.

47. Roviaro GC, Varoli F, Vergani C, et al: State of the art in thoracoscopic surgery: A personal experience of 2000 video-thoracoscopic procedures and an overview of the literature. Surg Endosc 16:881-892, 2002.

48. Yim APC, Lee TW, Izzat MB, et al: Place of video-thoracoscopy in thoracic surgical practice. World J Surg 25:157-161, 2001.

CHAPTER 19

EMERGING TECHNOLOGY IN SURGERY: INFORMATICS, ELECTRONICS, ROBOTICS

Guillermo Gomez, M.D.

Minimally Invasive Surgery and Robotics
The Concept and Functions of Surgical Robots

Classification of Surgical Robots

Informatics, electronics, and robotics are intermingled fields that constantly change the way we experience our lives and practice medicine. For instance, we order and receive our journals through Internet connections, we enter orders on computerized sheets, we go on rounds with the pharmacopeia in a pocket PC, we obtain scrubs from a dispensing robot, our patients are imaged by robotic computed tomography (CT) and magnetic resonance imaging (MRI) scanners, and we read clinical results on high-resolution, interactive video displays (just to mention some examples of our reliance on technology). From the user's point of view, it is not practical to discuss these fields separately. Despite many decades of technologic developments, the performance of surgical operations (the cutting and suturing of the artisan) remained unchanged. The advent of minimally invasive surgery (MIS), however, brought about a major deviation from traditional surgery.[1,2] The traditional premise that large surgical problems require large incisions for adequate treatment is no longer sustainable. MIS is here to stay and will continue to embody a growing portion of surgery. At the forefront of MIS is robotics.[3,4] Robotic surgery is aimed at improving surgical outcomes through increased precision in a setting of minimal invasiveness. In addition, robotics is creating fertile ground for the gestation of telementoring and telepresence in the surgery of the 21st century.[3,4] The focus in this chapter is on concepts and technologic developments that have reached clinical applications. The description of different robotic systems provides insight for the understanding of surgical robotics and its applications.

MINIMALLY INVASIVE SURGERY AND ROBOTICS

The principle *first do not harm* is central to the practice of medicine. In surgery, however, wounding is an inseparable component of the operation itself. Indeed, in many instances the trauma inflicted by the surgical access alone is greater or adds significantly more injury than the tissue damage caused by the dissection of the organ to be operated on. Significant pain and morbidity derive at large from the surgical access (e.g., laparotomy, thoracotomy) alone. The development of MIS (or minimal access surgery), therefore, has been a logical and ethically justified process. Advantages of MIS were clearly demonstrated by pioneer surgeons such as Kurt Semm, who performed the first laparoscopic appendectomy in a human in 1980, and Eric Mühe, who performed the first laparoscopic cholecystectomy in a human in 1985.[5] Technologic and dogmatic limitations of that time, however, placed constraints on the progress of MIS. In 1985, a major technologic leap took place with the invention of the solid-state, charged couple device (CCD), which allowed for the manufacturing of the miniature video camera. Digital video transformed the operating room, allowing the entire team to observe simultaneously, in the same direction, a magnified surgical field. In 1987, laparoscopic cholecystectomy was reintroduced by Philippe Mouret and other pioneers[5] but in a new environment—the digital era; from there on, the so-called laparoscopic revolution took place around the world. In a relatively short period of time, several operations were adapted to MIS technique (e.g., appendectomy, antireflux procedures, hernia repairs, adrenalectomy, splenectomy).[1,2] In many aspects these MIS operations yielded better outcomes when compared with their open counterparts: less pain, decreased blood loss, less wound complications, shorter hospital stay, faster recovery, and better cosmetics. In general, a better quality of life was obtained without compromising the primary outcome of the surgical procedure. In addition, reduced surgical stress, less impairment of physiologic functions, and improved immune responses with MIS expanded the indications for MIS to include the elderly and the high-risk patient.[6] Not unexpectedly, the educated public has become a major advocate of MIS. However, other more complex operations have not found an easy transition to MIS (e.g., colectomy, pancreatectomy, coronary bypass). In part, the problem has been due to the technical limitations inherent to the videoscopic platforms. In brief, videoscopic surgery is hindered by (1) replacement of the normal open three-dimensional (3-D) sight by a two-dimensional (2-D) vision of the field displayed on a monitor, (2) unstable video camera positioning, (3) inferior operative ergonomics compared with open surgery, and (4) loss of the normal degrees of freedom for manipulation of surgical instruments.[4,6,7] Robotic technology has been envisioned as the way to overcome physical obstacles of MIS and improve on the surgeon's natural limitations.[6,7] In relation to these advances, the research on surgical robots was begun before the advent of videoscopic MIS.[8]

THE CONCEPT AND FUNCTIONS OF SURGICAL ROBOTS

The term *robot* is derived from the Czechoslovakian word *robata*, which is translated as "forced labor" or "worker."[4] The term *surgical robot* is refuted by some because a robot is generally considered a machine that is programed to perform tasks autonomously. The terms *computer-enhanced* and *computer-assisted* have been coined in reference to surgical systems that operate without autonomy. However, the idea of having a humanoid machine (as seen in books and movies of science fiction) replacing the surgeon is not the intent of a surgical robot. For instance, surgical robots are not capable of clinical judgment. Robots do not have the compassion to establish a humane patient-physician relationship or the requirement to earn continuous medical education credits. A surgical robot has been defined as a powered, computer-controlled device that can be programed to aid in the positioning and manipulation of surgical instruments.[8] The central requirement for a surgical system to be classified as a robot is to be self-powered.[9] In a broad sense, surgical robots represent sophisticated powered instruments that enable the surgeon to carry out more complex tasks.

Common tasks given to industrial robots include the execution of repetitive, tiresome, or hazardous motions and the handling of specialized tools with high precision. Similar applications have been given to surgical robots, but the development of these robots has been more complex owing to constraints imposed by human safety and functionality (e.g., sterilization, interference with medical equipment, restricted room space). Examples of surgical tasks assigned to robotic systems include percutaneous biopsy of solid organs (e.g., brain, prostate, kidney), high-precision drilling or cutting (e.g., bone), automated resection of solid organs (e.g., prostate), image processing (e.g., magnification) and reproduction of 3-D vision, microsurgery (e.g., motion scaling), suturing in MIS, endoscope holding, and operation under biohazardous conditions (e.g., radiosurgery, brachytherapy).[9] Furthermore, surgical robots are becoming integral components of a more comprehensive network of clinical information.[10,11] Integrated robotic systems will be capable of assisting in the preoperative, intraoperative, and postoperative management of the surgical patient. A surgical robot linked to another robotic system such as a CT or MRI scanner can have access to imaging studies to be imported into the operative theater. Robots have the potential to assist not only with the preoperative planning but also with the rehearsal of individualized operations.[10,11] In fact, current robots such as Robodoc (see later) function by using the actual patient's anatomy obtained by preoperative imaging examinations.

Surgical training has changed little in more than a century despite several lapses of technologic progress. Surgical training remains lengthy because there are a "minimal" number of cases to complete to achieve competency. Surgical experience continues to be, to a significant extent, the product of a trial-error exercise in patients. The learning curves are said to be steep, and there is an "inherent" rate of morbidity and mortality for each operation. Most residency programs do not offer training in cutting-edge MIS. The relative magnitude of these problems should not be seen as "acceptable" for an indeterminate amount of time. Robotic technologies offer feasible solutions for updating our methods of surgical training and improve the outcomes in patient care. New technologic disciplines such as virtual reality have emerged and approach a practical realm thanks to a rapid growth in computational power and software capabilities. Similar to the aerospace industry (e.g., aircraft simulators), purpose-designed robots in surgical simulation may become invaluable tools for surgical training and licensing procedures.[11-13]

Progress in telecommunications has brought telemedicine into fruition. Telementoring, a class of telemedicine, has been carried out successfully in surgery using standard means of transmission and over various distances. Short-distance telementoring (e.g., between adjacent operating theaters) has been accomplished by the link of video monitors with fixed coaxial cables.[13] Short-distance telementoring has been shown to be a feasible and safe method for the supervision and assessment of competency of trainees during laparoscopic cholecystectomy.[14] Long-distance telementoring (e.g., over thousands of miles apart) has been accomplished successfully using standard telephone, cellular, and satellite systems. For example, laparoscopic inguinal hernia repairs were performed aboard the aircraft carrier USS *Abraham Lincoln* under telementoring from land-based laparoscopic surgeons[15] and laparoscopic cholecystectomy was performed in Ecuador under expert telementoring from New Haven,

Connecticut.[16] A more active system of surgical telementoring has been attained by linking a robot to a telecommunication system. Using custom software and fast data transfer (ISDN lines), a telementor had control over a robotic arm, video cameras, electrosurgical generator, and a drawing pen/pad assembly that were used by a mentored surgeon operating several thousand miles away.[17] Using this setup, advanced laparoscopic operations (e.g., varicocelectomy, nephrectomy, and adrenalectomy) were telementored from Baltimore, Maryland, to Bangkok (Thailand), Innsbruck (Austria), Rome (Italy), and Singapore.[17] Telementoring represents a feasible method of conveying proctorship and expert consultation in MIS.

Telepresence surgery has traversed the portal of the MIS suite in the 21st century. In telepresence surgery, the surgeon does not operate in direct contact with, but rather at a distance from, the patient (see Fig. 19-1). The distance can be a few meters or thousands of kilometers away. The surgeon is immersed in a virtual representation of the surgical field by observing a video display mounted in an ergonomic console. In return, the surgeon telecasts his manual commands to the robotic instruments, which are positioned over the surgical field at the patient's side.[18] The robots used for telepresence surgery are called telerobots. Jacques Marescaux and coworkers have provided an elegant demonstration of telepresence surgery.[19] They successfully performed a transatlantic telerobotic cholecystectomy in July 2001. In that operation, the operating surgeon was in New York City and the patient was in Strasbourg, France (appropriately supervised by assistant surgeons). The surgeon-side and the patient-side components of the telerobot were connected by a high-speed terrestrial optic fiber (asynchronous transfer mode [ATM] technology); the mean total delay time of the circuit was 155 ms. Remote telepresence surgery is not intended to interfere with the art of the patient-physician relationship or with local and international regulations for medical practice. Telepresence surgery, however, stands as a viable channel to outreach underserved areas in need of surgical expertise.[18] Today, telepresence surgery is readily conducted within the same operative theater (i.e., single operative room). On a daily basis, telerobots can be used to overcome shortcomings of traditional MIS. Telerobots enable the surgeon to (1) take personal control of the optical system (e.g., camera positioning, zooming, and magnification); (2) operate with 3-D vision; (3) increase precision (e.g., dumping of tremor and scaling of motion; and (4) improve dexterity (e.g., increased degrees of freedom).[9] The term *degrees of freedom* refers to the maximum possible motions at a joint. Furthermore, telerobots may be used to maximize the surgeon's safety when operating in hazardous environments (infectious, radioactive).[4,9]

CLASSIFICATION OF SURGICAL ROBOTS

Passive Robots

In passive robots, the energy to propel the system is provided by the surgeon; in turn, the system provides information about the tracking and relative position of the device with regard to the target.[8,9] Passive robots function to hold a fixture at a desired location through which the surgeon introduces an instrument into an area of difficult access. The first passive robot appeared in 1985; it was a modified industrial robot, "Puma 560" (Unimation Limited), and was used to guide drills and needles for intracranial biopsies. Another early surgical robot was a modified "Scara" robot (IBM) and was used to cut bone in the proximal femur for total hip replacement; this robot found veterinarian applications only.

In the beginning of laparoscopy, existing passive retractors were adapted to assist with the holding of the camera and other laparoscopic instruments. These devices, however, are considered prerobotic devices.[20] In general, these prerobots attach to the side rail of the table and have joints and links to be deployed in the most unobtrusive manner; positioning, locking, and release functions are facilitated by mechanical, electromagnetic, or pneumatic brakes controlled by hand or foot pedals. Examples of prerobots include the Omni-Lapo Tract (Omnitract), the Iron Intern (Automated Medical Products), the Surgassistant (Solos Endoscopy), the Trocar Sleeve Stabilizer (Richard Wolfe), the Bookwalter retraction systems (Codman), the Robotrac system (Aesculap), the First Assistant (Leonard Medical Inc.), and the Endex laparoscopic holder (Andronic Medical Ltd.). Prerobots are useful because they can be used as adjuncts to current robotic devices.

Semi-Active and Synergistic Robots

Semi-active robots are devices that combine the capability of some autonomous function with other actions carried out by the surgeon.

One example is LARS (Laparoscopic Assistant Robotic System, Johns Hopkins University and IBM).[9,21] LARS is a robotic arm that has four degrees of freedom for positioning of video camera or retracting instruments and is fitted with sensors that monitor forces and torque. The arm is driven by the operator, but should the forces exceed the programmed safety thresholds (e.g., tissue resistance), the robot halts the motion until the operator corrects the position. The arm is mounted in a cart that is rolled to the side of the operating table. LARS has been used in experimental surgery only.

Synergistic robots are devices simultaneously powered by both the robot's engine and the surgeon. This hybrid platform establishes a partnership between the skills and experience of the surgeon and the geometric accuracy of a tireless machine. ACROBOT (Active Constraint Robot, Imperial College, London, UK) is an example of a synergistic robot.[22] ACROBOT was designed to cut bone with maximum precision and safety in preparation for knee replacement. After the knee is immobilized and the robot is registered to the target, the area of resection is calculated and transferred to ACROBOT. Then, the surgeon manually drives a motorized cutter, thus having complete force feedback of the procedure but restricted to move within a preprogramed spatial framework. Another example of synergistic robot is the Steady Hand robot

(Johns Hopkins).[23] The Steady Hand robot is a device under development with the purpose of enhancing the ability of the human hand to perform micromanipulations.

Active Robots

Active surgical robots are powered devices that can function with significant independence from the surgeon. These robots carry the greatest safety concerns and have been developed for specific purposes.

Camera Holder Robots

Often, in traditional laparoscopy, the camera person is a less acquainted member in the team who stands in an uncomfortable position. The result is an unstable, improperly centered, and rotated picture that misses important anatomic details and causes motion sickness (among other things). If the surgeon has to take over the camera, he loses one of his hands needed for two-handed maneuvers. Therefore, robots for camera holding were the first active robots to be developed for commercial use. Furthermore, these robots have fewer safety concerns since the telescope is not a cutting tool and they can also be operated in a passive mode. AESOP (Automated Endoscopic System for Optimal Positioning, Computer Motion, Inc.)[24] and EndoAssist (Armstrong Healthcare, Ltd.)[25] are the better-known robotic camera holder systems around the world. They have successfully replaced the camera assistant and have allowed for the performance of solo surgery.

AESOP was the first laparoscopic robot to gain approval by the U.S. Food and Drug Administration. This system is composed of a control computer, a power system, and an articulated, electromechanical arm for holding and maneuvering the telescope.[24] The arm attaches to the operating table, and its action can be controlled via foot pedals, hand controls, or a voice activation/recognition system. The voice activation platform has been the preferred technique.[26] The arm provides 7 degrees of freedom and centers at the point where the telescope enters the patient (e.g., abdominal or chest cavity). AESOP has been used extensively to assist in urologic (e.g., nephrectomy, prostatectomy), gynecologic (e.g., hysterectomy), gastrointestinal (e.g., cholecystectomy, colectomy, Nissen fundoplication), and thoracic (e.g., internal mammary artery) videoscopic operations. Several authors have reported that the use of AESOP significantly reduces smudging, fogging, need for cleaning, and inadvertent movements of the telescope.[27-29] The use of a robot camera holder has not increased but sometimes has reduced the operative time.[27]

EndoAssist is another robot for camera holding that differs from AESOP in the commanding mechanism. EndoAssist is a head-mounted navigation system that allows the laparoscopic camera to follow the surgeon's head movements by tracking a headband sensor.[30] The robot is in active mode only when a foot switch is pressed by the surgeon. In active mode, any glance of the operator in one direction on the video monitor causes the camera to pan in the same direction (left/right, up/down, zoom in/out).

Orthopedic Robots

One of the first active robots was designed for orthopedic surgery. Orthopedic operations are especially suited for automated tasks because the target site can be effectively stabilized. Among the goals for using robots in orthopedic surgery include decreased frequency of iatrogenic fractures, more precise bone drilling, better alignment of fragments and prostheses, improved contact areas, better bone ingrowth, and, hopefully, improved long-term performance.

Robodoc (Integrated Surgical Systems) has been developed for primary total hip replacement, revision hip replacement, and total knee replacement.[31,32] Manual bone milling produces a rough and uneven cavity for cementless implantation of prosthesis. An average contact area created by manual drilling is about 23%. In contrast, the contact area achieved with Robodoc is 98% (or better). Robodoc is a computer-controlled mechanical arm capable of 5 degrees of freedom and force sensing in all axes. The tip of the arm holds a rotary bone cutter. Robodoc functions in coordination with a preoperative planning station, Orthodoc (Integrated Surgical Systems).[31-33] Orthodoc is a computer workstation that converts actual CT images of the patient to create a 3-D reconstruction of the joint to be replaced. Using computer modeling, the surgeon can choose the prosthesis (from a software library) with the best fit and can simulate the joint replacement (virtual surgery). At the time of the operation, the patient is clamped to a rigid framework and the joint is exposed by conventional means. Robodoc is then moved next to the patient and is "registered" (using preoperative imaging and fiducial markers) to the intraoperative location of the target. The robot then cuts and shapes the bone for a precise fit of the prosthesis following a decided preoperative plan. The procedure is constantly monitored for the sequence of motions, applied force, and any misdisplacement of the bone. The robot stops immediately if there is any deviation to the preoperative plan.

There are other computer-assisted robotic systems under development for different orthopedic applications that integrate image reconstruction and guidance; some examples include CASPAR,[34] CRIGOS,[35] and Loughborough manipulator.[36]

Neurosurgery Robots

The rigid structure of the skull and the delicateness of access to specific regions in the cranial cavity stimulated the use of robots in neurosurgery since the early 1980s. Initially, passive robots were employed as stereotactic frames only. Today, powered, computer-assisted, image-guided devices have been developed to assist with active, frameless neuronavigation.

Minerva is a powered neurosurgery robot that functions under the guidance of a dedicated CT imaging system.[37] Specifically designed instruments loaded onto a rotary carrousel can carry out the entire operation without assistance from the surgeon.[37] Minerva was developed at the University of Lausanne and has not been commercialized.

NeuroMate (Integrated Surgical Systems) is a computer-assisted, image-guided device for stereotactic procedures in neurosurgery.[38,39] It consists of a mechanical arm, an image-planning computer station, and a head stabilizer. Preoperatively, CT, MRI, or other images are correlated to the individual characteristics of the patient. With the use of a system of spatial coordinates, the robot is registered to the patient at the time of the operation. During the operation, the robot moves and positions the instruments as programmed preoperatively. The surgeon can manually drive instruments to preselected areas of the central nervous system using the fixture provided by the robot (semantically, because the surgeon takes active part in portions of the operation, NeuroMate also classifies as a semi-active robot).

PathFinder (Armstrong-Healthcare, Ltd.) is a powered, image-guided robot for accurate positioning of stereotactic instruments.[40] PathFinder consists of a planning workstation and a gyratory mechanical arm mounted on a wheeled trolley. The workstation accepts standard output formats from CT and MRI scanners and enables the surgeon to view and mark images to plan the path to a designated target within the brain; the preoperative planning also includes a demarcation of "no-go" zones for safety purposes. To allow for registration, preoperative images have to be acquired with titanium fiducial markers placed on the surface of the head. The robotic arm has 6 degrees of freedom and a camera. PathFinder uses the preoperative images and the camera picture for registration and intraoperative navigation. The algorithm also calculates the error of fit, and the surgeon can instruct for a re-registration, if necessary. Other safety built-in features in PathFinder include an interlock mechanism (to prevent motion of the robot when an instrument is active) and contact sensors (to stop motion in case of collision). The robot moves and positions the arm and the effector using its own power according to the preoperative plan. Then, the surgeon can proceed in a semiactive mode by inserting an instrument manually or he or she can mount motorized drivers to let the robot complete the procedure autonomously. The maximum error between the specified position and the obtained position of a tool is 1 mm.

CyberKnife (Accuray) is an advanced system for stereotactic radiosurgery.[41,42] It is composed of a computer-controlled robotic arm, a compact 6-MV linear accelerator, and an image guidance system. The linear accelerator is mounted on the robot arm, and the arm has 6 degrees of freedom. The maneuverability of the system enables for nonisocentric delivery of radiotherapy, thus limiting radiation of normal tissue. The imaging system (built into the treatment room) uses the body's skeletal structure and small implanted fiducial markers as a reference frame, thus avoiding the pinning of external rigid stereotactic frames. The image guidance system utilizes preoperative CT or MR scans, along with intraoperative radiographs and video cameras, to register the target and monitor any movements of the patient; any displacement of the target is compensated by repositioning of the robot arm. CyberKnife can be used for any other parts of the body.[9,42]

Urology Robots

The prostate and the kidney are relatively fixed solid organs amenable for minimally invasive access.

The prostate is readily accessible through the urethra. Transurethral resection of the prostate (TURP) is accomplished by passing a diathermy cutter under endoscopic guidance (resectoscope). TURP is a repetitive, manual "debulking" procedure. Preventable complications from TURP include incontinence, damage to sphincter muscles and nerves, bleeding from the capsule, and rectal injury. Therefore, TURP is a good candidate procedure for automation in order to improve precision.

Probot (Mechatronics in Medicine, Imperial College)[43,44] is a powered, image-guided, computer-controlled robot for TURP. It moves in four axes to carry out TURP within the constraints of the prostate's size exclusively. The surgeon docks Probot to the patient and measures the length of the prostate under direct endoscopic visual cues. The prostate is then imaged using transurethral, thin-cut ultrasound scanning. In a computer station, specific software uses the ultrasound images to create a 3-D reconstruction of the prostate and the surgeon can specify the cavity to be cut. Probot carries out TURP by cutting tissue cones in a sequence of concentric rings, starting at the bladder neck and moving toward the verumontanum. The operation is completely performed by Probot under the supervision of the surgeon. The surgeon follows the progression of the procedure at the workstation and can adjust the cutting parameters or can stop the robot at any time. If there is a system failure, the surgeon can complete the operation. Further refinements may render Probot an invaluable tool for training in TURP.

Percutaneous access of the kidney is a common procedure. The RCM robot (Remote Center of Motion, Brady Urological Institute, Johns Hopkins University)[45,46] was developed for radiologic percutaneous access for MIS interventions and delivery of therapy. Initially developed for percutaneous access of the kidney (PAKY), the device also has been referred to as the PAKY-RCM robot. The RCM robot is a three-module system consisting of the RCM unit, the PAKY unit, and a passive mechanical arm. The mechanical arm mounts on the operating table, confers 7 degrees of freedom for positioning, and accommodates both the RCM and the PAKY units. The RCM unit has 2 degrees of freedom for motorized rotation in two planes (x and y directions) around the RCM point. The PAKY unit is a motorized needle driver that holds and inserts the trocar needle. PAKY is radiolucent, thus making it compatible with radiographic imaging. The low and flexible profile of the robot makes it compatible with CT scanners and C-arms in operating rooms. The RCM and PAKY units are activated in sequence. The RCM unit is used first to align the needle under radiologic guidance. After alignment is complete, the RCM unit is deactivated and the PAKY unit is activated to insert the needle. The RCM robot is able to insert a needle to a precise depth with minimal deflection and in shorter time than the traditional manual procedure. Therefore, the radiation exposure of the patient and surgical team is reduced. The RCM robot can be used in manual or automatic mode.

Master-Slave Robots

Master-slave robots are powered, computer-controlled devices that do not perform autonomous tasks but are completely governed by the surgeon, thus the term *master-slave* system where the surgeon is the "master" and the robot is the "slave." The master surgeon is seated at a control console, and the slave robotic arm is located at the surgical field over the patient (Fig. 19-1). They are also called *telemanipulators,* implying that the master and the slave are separated from each other by a distance but communicate through data cables. At the console, the surgeon observes the surgical field on a video display and actuates his or her hands not on traditional surgical instruments but on mechanical transducers (masters or joysticks) (Fig. 19-2). The surgeon's motions are telecasted from the console to the robotic arms, which, in turn, manipulate instruments (needle drivers, forceps, scissors) and the telescope (Fig. 19-3). The surgeon's console also holds commands for special functions (e.g., focusing, motion scaling) and accessory equipment (e.g., electrosurgical and ultrasonic units). The separation between master and slave components may vary, from a few meters (e.g., inside the same operating room) to several kilometers apart (e.g., transatlantic operation).[19] These systems provide unique advantages for MIS when compared with conventional laparoscopic or thoracoscopic surgery: (1) the surgeon holds control of a stable camera-telescope platform, eliminating the dependence from a camera assistant; (2) the surgical field is presented to the surgeon in a 3-D display; (3) the robotic instruments have articulations

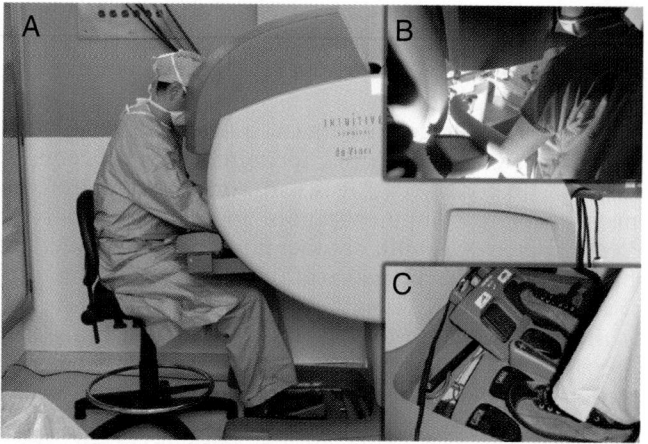

FIGURE 19-2. Surgical console of a master-slave robot (da Vinci system). **A,** The surgeon sits at the console in an ergonomic position and observes the surgical field in a 3-D video display; his eyes and hands are aligned with the field. **B,** The surgeon actuates his hands on mechanic transducers or "masters"; the surgeon's motions are telecasted to the robotic arms, which, in turn, manipulate the instruments and the telescope. **C,** Foot pedals function in concert to transfer the action of the "masters" to take control of the instruments or the telescope, to realign the masters, or to activate energy sources.

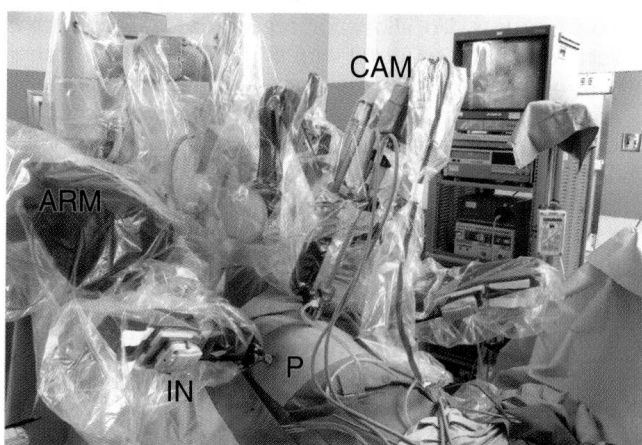

FIGURE 19-3. Arms of a master-slave robot (da Vinci system). The robotic arms covered with sterile drapes are positioned over the patient (P). The arms are connected to laparoscopic cannulas; the center arm holds the telescope and camera (Cam), and the lateral arms (Arm) hold exchangeable instruments (In).

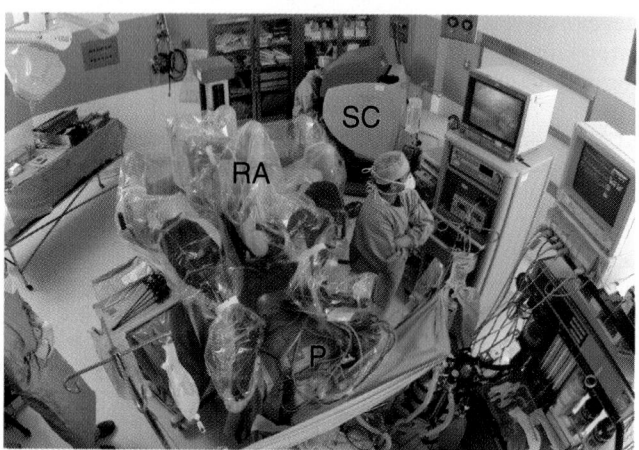

FIGURE 19-1. Telepresence surgery at the University of Texas Medical Branch. The surgeon operates at a distance from the patient, seated at the surgeon's console (SC). The robotic arms (RA) are positioned and docked to the patient (P). The assistants stand at the patient's side, sterile and ready to perform the changes of instruments.

near the tip that increase the degrees of freedom to function more like a human hand; (4) the computer eliminates hand tremor and the scale of motion is programmable; and (5) the console provides a more ergonomic operating position for the surgeon. All together, these computer-enhanced functions add precision and dexterity to the MIS surgeon, particularly when performing microsurgical procedures.[47] Master-slave robots of today, however, have significant limitations: (1) the major drawback is the lack of tactile feedback and, therefore, the force applied in tissue dissection and suturing must rely on visual cues exclusively; (2) there is a scant number of instruments available; and (3) the hardware is extremely bulky, heavy, and clutters the operating room easily.[47] Special technical features of current systems are presented below.

The da Vinci robotic surgical system (Intuitive Surgical)[48] gives a "true" 3-D view of the surgical field by using a dual-lens, three-chip digital camera system. The dual-lens system is bundled into one large telescope. Each camera transmits to separate CRT screens located inside the console, and each screen projects separately to an individual eye (i.e., binocular system). A synchronizer keeps both cameras in phase. At the surgeon's console, the binocular viewer is anatomically aligned with the position of the masters (i.e., the hands). Such an arrangement creates the feeling of being immersed into the surgical field, much like in open surgery. Both the instruments and the telescope are driven via the masters, switching control from one to the other with the press of a clutch. The robotic arms of the da Vinci system are floor mounted and, therefore, the patient cannot be moved after the robotic arms become attached to the cannulas. Any repositioning of the patient requires undocking of the system. Initially developed for cardiovascular surgery, both thoracic and abdominal operations have been performed using the da Vinci system.

The Zeus robotic surgical system (Computer Motion)[49] produces 3-D views of the field by merging right and left video frames (from right and left cameras) over a single video monitor fitted with an active matrix and polarizing filters. The broadcast alternates between right and left frames that synchronize with clockwise or counterclockwise polarization filters, respectively. The surgeon wears glasses fitted with different polarizing filters, a clockwise filter for the right eye, and a counterclockwise filter for the left eye. This causes the right eye to see right video frames only and the left eye to see left video frames only. The telescope is driven by a voice-activation system. The robotic arms are mounted on the operating table and, therefore, it is possible to change the patient's position without undocking the robot. Thoracic and abdominal operations have been performed with Zeus.

The ARTEMIS (Advanced Robotics and Telemanipulator System for Minimally Invasive Surgery, Karlsruhe Research Center) consists of two master-slave units for manipulation of surgical instruments and a guiding system for a 3-D endoscope. ARTEMIS is still a project under development for both abdominal as well as thoracic MIS.[50,51]

Robotic Abdominal Surgery

The technical pitfalls of laparoscopic surgery have been discussed before; robotic technology promises to solve these hindrances. In fact, the increased dexterity and fidelity conferred by master-slave telemanipulators is giving them increased acceptance for abdominal MIS. The first telerobotic operation was a cholecystectomy performed with an early version of the da Vinci system in 1997. Since then, both the da Vinci and Zeus systems have been successfully utilized for a broad spectrum of interventions in general surgery, gynecology, and urology.

Telerobotic operations described in general surgery include cholecystectomy,[52-54] antireflux procedures,[54-57] Heller's cardiomyotomy,[57-59] distal pancreatectomy,[57] gastrojejunostomy,[59] esophagectomy,[57,59] gastric bypass,[59] gastric banding,[60] pyloroplasty,[58] colectomy,[61] adrenalectomy,[59] and splenectomy.[57,62] Pediatric operations include Thal fundoplication, Nissen fundoplication, cholecystectomy, and salpingo-oophorectomy.[63] Telerobotic operations in gynecology include hysterectomy[64] and tubal reanastomosis.[65,66] Telerobotic urologic procedures include nephrectomy,[59,67] radical prostatectomy,[68-70] and pelvic lymph node dissection.[71]

Robotic Cardiothoracic Surgery

Despite well established benchmarks of safety and technical outcomes of current open chest surgery, there is still significant morbidity from median sternotomy used for access (e.g., thoracic cage deformation and fractures, pain, prolonged rehabilitation time, large amount of blood loss, ventilatory problems, sternitis, mediastinitis) and from the cardiopulmonary bypass (CPB) needed to obtain a stable and dry operative field (e.g., hemolysis, complement activation, immunosuppression, and impairments of visual, memory, and intellectual functions, among others). Therefore, MIS techniques have been actively pursued in cardiovascular surgery to improve on both the access and the dependence of CPB.[72-74]

A major obstacle to minimize the size of access in cardiothoracic surgery is the inherent rigidity of the chest wall and mediastinum. Mediastinal structures cannot be displaced to be exposed or exteriorized through a small thoracotomy. Working through small thoracic incisions greatly limits exposure and technical dexterity. Digital technology, however, has facilitated substantial progress in cardiothoracic MIS (CT-MIS). A high-resolution videoscope introduced into the chest can reach targets and replace or even improve the classic open exposures. For instance, the 10× to 20× optic magnification capability of the digital video-camera is more powerful than the typical 2.5× to 3× magnification provided by conventional surgical glasses. Furthermore, 3-D video displays have been refined to eliminate the lack of depth perception given by the conventional 2-D videoscopic systems. In addition, when the videoscope is mounted on a robotic arm, the control of the visual field is at the personal command of the surgeon via voice- or hand-mediated mechanisms. Finally, robotic-articulated instruments (e.g., da Vinci and Zeus systems) have been developed that permit working at a distance with the natural 7 degrees of freedom of the human hand; indeed, scaling of motion and filtering of tremor can augment hand dexterity. Current digital technology has made totally endoscopic and closed-chest cardiothoracic operations a reality. Loulmet and coworkers,[75] from Paris, France, and Mohr and coworkers,[76] from Leipzig, Germany, have reported the first human cases of robot-assisted CT-MIS since 1998; the procedures include repair of atrial septal defect, repair or replacement of mitral valve, and coronary artery bypass.

Carpentier and Loulmet have proposed a classification of increasing complexity for the development and implementation of CT-MIS. In level I CT-MIS or the direct-vision/mini-incision approach, the procedure is performed under direct vision through small incisions by conventional means. A number of mini access approaches have been developed and described under different acronyms, such as LAST (Limited Anterior Small Thoracotomy) and MIDCAB (Minimally Invasive Direct Coronary Artery Bypass); these techniques, however, suffer from the limited access itself and have obvious restricted applications.[72,77] In level II CT-MIS or the video-assisted/micro-incision approach, a videoscope is passed through the incision to function as a secondary visual aid for portions of the operation; an intracardiac minicamera has been used to add lighting and a magnified view of anatomic details. Accessory operative ports can be added to pass surgical instruments. This type of videoscopic assistance has been used successfully for mitral valve surgery and harvesting the internal mammary artery. In level III CT-MIS or the video-directed/port-incision approach, most of the operation is conducted videoscopically and instruments are passed through operative ports. A helmet-mounted 3-D videoscopic system (Vista Medical Technologies, Becton, MA) driven by an assistant or docked to an AESOP mechanical arm has been used successfully to improve visualization and dexterity.[77] This video-directed/port-incision technique has been used in mitral valve surgery with outcomes that challenge the conventional open approach but achieve faster recovery times and significant cost savings.[78] The level IV, or video-directed/robot-assisted, approach represents the current cutting edge of CT-MIS; at this level of technologic sophistication and skill, complex procedures are performed through port incisions only using 3-D video displays and robotic-articulated microinstruments (e.g., DeBakey forceps, Potts scissors, microclips). A sternotomy or limited thoracotomy has been included in preliminary trials for safety purposes. Surgical robots have been used for heart valve surgery, dissection of the internal mammary artery, anastomosis of coronary bypass grafting, and correction of atrial septal defect; both the da Vinci and Zeus systems have been employed in various phases of development of these procedures.[78,79] In fact, robotic telemanipulators were initially targeted for CT-MIS. At the cutting edge of CT-MIS is the totally endoscopic coronary artery bypass or TECAB, where both conduit preparation (e.g., for dissection of the internal mammary artery) and anastomosis for a single- or two-vessel disease are completed through a three-port operation.[80]

Important to mention here are the alternatives to conventional CPB that have been developed to permit closed-chest CT surgery. The Port-Access (Heartport, Redwood City, CA) is a device for femoro-femoral CPB and endovascular balloon clamping of the aorta. The Heartport system allows for antegrade as well as retrograde perfusion for systemic and coronary circulation. The proper positioning of the Heartport is guided by contrast fluoroscopy or by transesophageal echocardiography. The Heartport technology has proved an invaluable adjunct to accomplish videoscopic valve surgery as well as coronary bypass.[78,79] Another more striking alternative is the off-pump or beating-heart technique; at this moment, however, this technique has been applicable to coronary bypass only. For this purpose, a myocardial stabilizer (e.g., Genzyme, Intuitive Surgical) is deployed over the target coronary artery to be anastomosed. Kappert and coworkers from Dresden, Germany, have already achieved off-pump TECAB with bilateral harvest of the internal mammary artery for single-and double-vessel coronary disease.[80]

In summary, robotic technology has the great promise to expand the spectrum of MIS—not only on the technical aspects of surgery but also in areas such as training and telesurgery. Furthermore, surgery will merge with diagnostic imaging whereby image-guided procedures will be performed after preoperative planning and rehearsal has been completed using the actual patient's anatomic data. To this point, however, all the studies have documented and proved the feasibility and safety of these emerging technologies as employed under ideal conditions. Although early results are encouraging, the cost-effectiveness of them has not been established, and they do not represent the standard of care. One major hurdle to overcome in cost analysis is the high cost of the technology itself. Another major technical problem pending solution is providing the surgeon with some sort of tactile feedback information. Expansion of the instrument armamentarium for the different specialties is also needed. The rapidly growing computational power and dedicated instrument design are expected to address unresolved technical pitfalls. Finally, future controlled trials with outcome and cost analysis will help determine the place of surgical robots in MIS. However, it is said that one picture may be worth a thousand words. Today, performing just one operation at the console of a surgical robot may be all that is needed to recognize that MIS with 3-D vision and 7 degrees of freedom is better surgery.

Selected References

Ballantyne GH: The pitfalls of laparoscopic surgery: Challenges for robotics and telerobotic surgery. Surg Laparosc Endosc Percutan Tech 12:1-5, 2002.

> **A concise presentation of the triumph and pitfalls of laparoscopic surgery; how robotic technology offers solutions for the advancement of MIS.**

Chitwood WR Jr: Endoscopic robotic coronary surgery: Is this reality or fantasy? J Thorac Cardiovasc Surg 118:1-3, 1999.

> **Objective review of the use of current robotic systems (da Vinci and Zeus) in coronary bypass surgery.**

Davies B: A review of robotics in surgery. Proc Inst Mech Eng [H] 214:129-140, 2000.

> **A comprehensive introduction to the world of surgical robots, their history, and classification.**

Kappert U, Cichon R, Schneider J, et al: Robotic coronary artery surgery—the evolution of a new minimally invasive approach in coronary artery surgery. Thorac Cardiovasc Surg 48:193-197, 2000.

> **Remarkable pioneering work towards totally endoscopic, robotic and off-pump coronary bypass surgery.**

Marescaux J, Leroy J, Gagner M, et al: Transatlantic robot-assisted telesurgery. Nature 413:379-380, 2001.

A landmark publication that illustrates the introduction of modern digital technology into the art and science of surgery.

Périssat J, Collet D, Monguillon N: Advances in laparoscopic surgery. Digestion 59:606-618, 1998.

Comprehensive and authoritative review of the origins of MIS and its projections for the modern practice of surgery.

Reynolds W Jr: The first laparoscopic cholecystectomy. JSLS 5:89-94, 2001.

The real story of the operation that revolutionized the practice of surgery; a tribute to our pioneers.

Vanermen H, Wellens F, De Geest R, et al: Video-assisted Port-Access mitral valve surgery: From debut to routine surgery. Will Trocar-Port-Access cardiac surgery ultimately lead to robotic cardiac surgery? Semin Thorac Cardiovasc Surg 11:223-234, 1999.

Comprehensive review and analysis of the progress in minimally invasive mitral valve surgery including the techniques for minimizing the access and the alternatives for cardiopulmonary bypass.

References

1. Périssat J, Collet D, Monguillon N: Advances in laparoscopic surgery. Digestion 59:606-618, 1998.
2. Himal HS: Minimally invasive (laparoscopic) surgery. Surg Endosc 16:1647-1652, 2002.
3. Fitzgibbons R Jr: 1999 SLS presidential address. JSLS 4:1-4, 2000.
4. Kavic MS: Robotics, technology, and the future of surgery. JSLS 4:277-279, 2000.
5. Reynolds W Jr: The first laparoscopic cholecystectomy. JSLS 5:89-94, 2001.
6. Fuchs KH: Minimally invasive surgery. Endoscopy 34:154-159, 2002.
7. Ballantyne GH: The pitfalls of laparoscopic surgery: Challenges for robotics and telerobotic surgery. Surg Laparosc Endosc Percutan Tech 12:1-5, 2002.
8. Davies B: A review of robotics in surgery. Proc Inst Mech Eng [H] 214:129-140, 2000.
9. Stoianovici D: Robotic surgery. World J Urol 18:289-295, 2000.
10. Mack MJ: Minimally invasive and robotic surgery. JAMA 285:568-572, 2001.
11. Satava RM: Emerging technologies for surgery in the 21st century. Arch Surg 134:1197-1202, 1999.
12. Satava RM: Virtual reality, telesurgery, and the new world order of medicine. J Image Guid Surg 1:12-16, 1995.
13. Kaufmann C, Rhee P, Burris D: Telepresence surgery system enhances medical student surgery training. Stud Health Technol Inform 62:174-178, 1999.
14. Byrne JP, Mughal MM: Telementoring as an adjunct to training and competence-based assessment in laparoscopic cholecystectomy. Surg Endosc 14:1159-1161, 2000.
15. Cubano M, Poulose BK, Talamini MA, et al: Long distance telementoring: A novel tool for laparoscopy aboard the USS Abraham Lincoln. Surg Endosc 13:673-678, 1999.
16. Rosser JC Jr, Bell RL, Harnett B, et al: Use of mobile low-bandwith telemedical techniques for extreme telemedicine applications. J Am Coll Surg 189:397-404, 1999.
17. Lee BR, Moore R: International telementoring: A feasible method of instruction. World J Urol 18:296-298, 2000.
18. Bowersox JC: Telepresence surgery. Br J Surg 83:433-434, 1996.
19. Marescaux J, Leroy J, Gagner M, et al: Transatlantic robot-assisted telesurgery. Nature 413:379-380, 2001.
20. Moran ME: Stationary and automated laparoscopically assisted technologies. J Laparoendosc Surg 3:221-227, 1993.
21. Poulose BK, Kutka MF, Mendoza-Sagaon M, et al: Human vs robotic organ retraction during laparoscopic Nissen fundoplication. Surg Endosc 13:461-465, 1999.
22. Davies BL, Harris SJ, Lin WJ, et al: Active compliance in robotic surgery—the use of force control as a dynamic constraint. Proc Inst Mech Eng [H] 211:285-292, 1997.
23. Taylor R, Jensen P, Whitcomb L, et al: A steady-hand robotic system for microsurgical augmentation. Int J Robotics Res 18:1201-1210, 1999.
24. Sackier JM, Wang Y: Robotically assisted laparoscopic surgery: From concept to development. Surg Endosc 8:63-66, 1994.
25. Yavuz Y, Ystgaard B, Skogvoll E, et al: A comparative experimental study evaluating the performance of surgical robots AESOP and EndoAssist. Surg Laparosc Endosc Percutan Tech 10:163-167, 2000.
26. Allaf ME, Jackman SV, Schulam PG, et al: Laparoscopic visual field: Voice vs foot pedal interfaces for control of the AESOP robot. Surg Endosc 12:1415-1418, 1998.
27. Mettler L, Ibrahim M, Jonat W: One year of experience working with the aid of a robotic assistant (the voice-controlled optic holder AESOP) in gynaecological endoscopic surgery. Hum Reprod 13:2748-2750, 1998.
28. Omote K, Feussner H, Ungeheuer A, et al: Self-guided robotic camera control for laparoscopic surgery compared with human camera control. Am J Surg 177:321-324, 1999.
29. Merola S, Weber P, Wasielewski A, et al: Comparison of laparoscopic colectomy with and without the aid of a robotic camera holder. Surg Laparosc Endosc Percutan Tech 12:46-51, 2002.
30. EndoAssist. Armstrong Healthcare. Accessed March 3, 2003, from *http://www.armstrong-healthcare.com/endoassist.html.*
31. Paul HA, Bargar WL, Mittlestadt B, et al: Development of a surgical robot for cementless total hip arthroplasty. Clin Orthop 57-66, 1992.
32. Robodoc. Integrated Surgical Systems. Accessed February 27, 2003, from *http://robodoc.com/eng/robodoc.html.*
33. Orthodoc. Integrated Surgical Systems. Accessed February 27, 2003, from *http://www.robodoc.com/eng/orthodoc.html.*
34. Siebert W, Mai S, Kober R, et al: Technique and first clinical results of robot-assisted total knee replacement. Knee 9:173-180, 2002.
35. Brandt G, Zimolong A, Carrat L, et al: CRIGOS: A compact robot for image-guided orthopedic surgery. IEEE Trans Inf Technol Biomed 3:252-260, 1999.
36. Bouazza-Marouf K, Browbank I, Hewit JR: Robotic-assisted internal fixation of femoral fractures. Proc Inst Mech Eng [H] 209:51-58, 1995.
37. Glauser D, Fankhauser H, Epitaux M, et al: Neurosurgical robot Minerva: First results and current developments. J Image Guid Surg 1:266-272, 1995.
38. Li QH, Zamorano L, Pandya A, et al: The application accuracy of the NeuroMate robot—a quantitative comparison with frameless and frame-based surgical localization systems. Comput Aided Surg 7:90-98, 2002.
39. NeuroMate. Integrated Surgical Systems. Retrieved February 27, 2003, from *http://robodoc.com/eng/neuromate.html.*

40. Finlay PA, Morgan P: PathFinder image guided robot for neurosurgery. Armstrong Healthcare. Accessed February 27, 2003, from *http://www.armstrong-healthcare.com/pathfinder.html.*

41. Adler JR Jr, Chang SD, Murphy MJ, et al: The Cyberknife: A frameless robotic system for radiosurgery. Stereotact Funct Neurosurg 69:124-128, 1997.

42. CyberKnife. Accuray. Accessed February 28, 2003, from *http://www.accuray.com/cyberknife.html.*

43. The Probot. Mechatronics in Medicine—Imperial College. Accessed March 1, 2003, from *http://www.me.ic.ac.uk/case/mim/projects/probot/index.html.*

44. Arambula Cosio F, Davies BL: Automated prostate recognition: A key process for clinically effective robotic prostatectomy. Med Biol Eng Comput 37:236-243, 1999.

45. The RCM Robot. URobotics Brady Urological Insititue, Johns Hopkins Medical Institutions. Accessed March 1, 2003, from *http://urology.jhu.edu/urobotics/projects/rcm/.*

46. Stoianovici D, Whitcomb LL, Anderson JH, et al: A modular surgical robotic system for image guided percutaneous procedures. *In* Lecture Notes in Computer Science. New York, Springer, 1998, pp 404-410.

47. Hashizume M, Konishi K, Tsutsumi N, et al: A new era of robotic surgery assisted by a computer-enhanced surgical system. Surgery 131:S330-333, 2002.

48. da Vinci Surgical Systems. Intuitive Surgical. Accessed March 1, 2003, from *http://www.intuitivesurgical.com/products/da_vinci.html.*

49. Zeus Robotic Surgical System. Computer Motion Inc. Accessed March 1, 2003, from *http://www.computermotion.com/zeus.html.*

50. Schurr MO, Buess G, Neisius B, et al: Robotics and telemanipulation technologies for endoscopic surgery: A review of the ARTEMIS project. Advanced Robotic Telemanipulator for Minimally Invasive Surgery. Surg Endosc 14:375-381, 2000.

51. Rininsland H: ARTEMIS: A telemanipulator for cardiac surgery. Eur J Cardiothorac Surg 16(Suppl 2):S106-111, 1999.

52. Marescaux J, Smith MK, Folscher D, et al: Telerobotic laparoscopic cholecystectomy: Initial clinical experience with 25 patients. Ann Surg 234:1-7, 2001.

53. Ruurda JP, Broeders IA, Simmermacher RP, et al: Feasibility of robot-assisted laparoscopic surgery: An evaluation of 35 robot-assisted laparoscopic cholecystectomies. Surg Laparosc Endosc Percutan Tech 12:41-45, 2002.

54. Chitwood WR Jr, Nifong LW, Chapman WH, et al: Robotic surgical training in an academic institution. Ann Surg 234:475-484; discussion 484-476, 2001.

55. Cadiere GB, Himpens J, Vertruyen M, et al: Evaluation of telesurgical (robotic) NISSEN fundoplication. Surg Endosc 15:918-923, 2001.

56. Gould JC, Melvin WS: Computer-assisted robotic antireflux surgery. Surg Laparosc Endosc Percutan Tech 12:26-29, 2002.

57. Melvin WS, Needleman BJ, Krause KR, et al: Computer-enhanced robotic telesurgery: Initial experience in foregut surgery. Surg Endosc 16:1790-1792, 2002.

58. Shah J, Rockall T, Darzi A: Robot-assisted laparoscopic Heller's cardiomyotomy. Surg Laparosc Endosc Percutan Tech 12:30-32, 2002.

59. Horgan S, Vanuno D: Robots in laparoscopic surgery. J Laparoendosc Adv Surg Tech A 11:415-419, 2001.

60. Cadiere GB, Himpens J, Vertruyen M, et al: The world's first obesity surgery performed by a surgeon at a distance. Obes Surg 9:206-209, 1999.

61. Weber PA, Merola S, Wasielewski A, et al: Telerobotic-assisted laparoscopic right and sigmoid colectomies for benign disease. Dis Colon Rectum 45:1689-1694; discussion 1695-1686, 2002.

62. Chapman WH III, Albrecht RJ, Kim VB, et al: Computer-assisted laparoscopic splenectomy with the da Vinci surgical robot. J Laparoendosc Adv Surg Tech A 12:155-159, 2002.

63. Gutt CN, Markus B, Kim ZG, et al: Early experiences of robotic surgery in children. Surg Endosc 16:1083-1086, 2002.

64. Diaz-Arrastia C, Jurnalov C, Gomez G, et al: Laparoscopic hysterectomy using a computer-enhanced surgical robot. Surg Endosc 16:1271-1273, 2002.

65. Falcone T, Goldberg JM, Margossian H, et al: Robotic-assisted laparoscopic microsurgical tubal anastomosis: A human pilot study. Fertil Steril 73:1040-1042, 2000.

66. Degueldre M, Vandromme J, Huong PT, et al: Robotically assisted laparoscopic microsurgical tubal reanastomosis: A feasibility study. Fertil Steril 74:1020-1023, 2000.

67. Guillonneau B, Jayet C, Tewari A, et al: Robot assisted laparoscopic nephrectomy. J Urol 166:200-201, 2001.

68. Abbou CC, Hoznek A, Salomon L, et al: Laparoscopic radical prostatectomy with a remote controlled robot. J Urol 165:1964-1966, 2001.

69. Guillonneau B, Vallancien G: Laparoscopic radical prostatectomy: The Montsouris experience. J Urol 163:418-422, 2000.

70. Rassweiler J, Frede T, Seemann O, et al: Telesurgical laparoscopic radical prostatectomy. Initial experience. Eur Urol 40:75-83, 2001.

71. Guillonneau B, Cappele O, Martinez JB, et al: Robotic assisted, laparoscopic pelvic lymph node dissection in humans. J Urol 165:1078-1081, 2001.

72. Goldstein DJ, Oz MC: Current status and future directions of minimally invasive cardiac surgery. Curr Opin Cardiol 14:419-425, 1999.

73. Chitwood WR Jr: Endoscopic robotic coronary surgery: Is this reality or fantasy? J Thorac Cardiovasc Surg 118:1-3, 1999.

74. Vanermen H, Wellens F, De Geest R, et al: Video-assisted Port-Access mitral valve surgery: From debut to routine surgery. Will Trocar-Port-Access cardiac surgery ultimately lead to robotic cardiac surgery? Semin Thorac Cardiovasc Surg 11:223-234, 1999.

75. Loulmet D, Carpentier A, d'Attellis N, et al: Endoscopic coronary artery bypass grafting with the aid of robotic assisted instruments. J Thorac Cardiovasc Surg 118:4-10, 1999.

76. Mohr FW, Falk V, Diegeler A, et al: Computer-enhanced coronary artery bypass surgery. J Thorac Cardiovasc Surg 117:1212-1214, 1999.

77. Reichenspurner H, Boehm D, Reichart B: Minimally invasive mitral valve surgery using three-dimensional video and robotic assistance. Semin Thorac Cardiovasc Surg 11:235-243, 1999.

78. Chitwood WR Jr: Video-assisted and robotic mitral valve surgery: Toward an endoscopic surgery. Semin Thorac Cardiovasc Surg 11:194-205, 1999.

79. Damiano RJ Jr, Reichenspurner H, Ducko CT: Robotically assisted endoscopic coronary artery bypass grafting: Current state of the art. Adv Card Surg 12:37-57, 2000.

80. Kappert U, Cichon R, Schneider J, et al: Robotic coronary artery surgery—the evolution of a new minimally invasive approach in coronary artery surgery. Thorac Cardiovasc Surg 48:193-197, 2000.

III

TRAUMA AND CRITICAL CARE

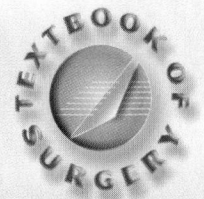

CHAPTER 20

MANAGEMENT OF ACUTE TRAUMA

David B. Hoyt, M.D., Raul Coimbra, M.D., Ph.D., and Bruce Potenza, M.D.

The Surgeon's Role in a Trauma System	**Management of Specific Injuries**
Initial Management	

Trauma is a major worldwide public health problem. It is one of the leading causes of death and disability in both industrialized and developing countries. Globally, injury is the seventh leading cause of death, resulting in 5.8 million deaths in 2000. In the United States, trauma is the leading cause of death in children and adults up to age 44 years and kills more Americans age 1 to 34 than all diseases combined. Fatalities from injury only represent a small fraction of the scope of injury. During 2000, there were 147,000 injury fatalities in the United States. Another 2.5 million patients were hospitalized for their injuries, whereas 40.4 million were treated at local emergency departments and released. An estimated 89.9 million patients were treated by primary care physicians or "self doctored" at home. The total cost of injury in the United States is estimated to be about $200 billion per year, and these costs only continue to rise.

Mortality after Traumatic Injury

Trauma deaths occur at traditionally recognized time points after injury (Fig. 20-1). Approximately one half of trauma deaths occur within seconds or minutes after injury and are caused by injury to the aorta, heart, brain stem, or spinal cord or by acute respiratory distress. Very few of these patients can be saved by trauma systems, and these deaths must be addressed by improved injury prevention and control strategies.[1]

The second mortality peak occurs within hours of injury and accounts for approximately 30% of deaths. Half of these are caused by hemorrhage, and the other half are caused by central nervous system injury. Most of these deaths can be averted by treatment during the "golden hour." Trauma systems with acute patient care have the greatest impact on this group of injured patients. Recent analysis of trauma system efficacy suggests at least a 10% reduction in preventable death. Mortality reduction through a statewide trauma system has been demon-

strated, yet despite this only approximately 50% of the United States is served by trauma systems.[2-4]

The third peak in mortality represents deaths that occur 24 hours after injury and include late mortality due to infection and multiple organ failure. Traditionally, this peak has included 10% to 20% of trauma-related deaths.[1] More recently, analyses suggest that this incidence is closer to 10%. Death due to pulmonary embolus has emerged as an important late cause of death as well.[1]

Further improvements in mortality reduction will require a different strategy for each peak. Early deaths will be reduced by injury prevention and control programs, active legislation, and behavior modification. Regional planning and trauma system development will impact the second mortality peak most effectively. Late deaths will be impacted only as we better understand the pathophysiology of multiple organ failure and delayed treatment of secondary brain injury.

Development of Trauma Care

Modern trauma care has evolved from the close association of surgery and casualty management in times of war. Many important concepts, including prehospital transport, volume resuscitation, wound management, enteric injury management, and critical care, have been advanced based on observations during military conflict. These management principles have been refined in the civilian sector and have led to advances such as the primary repair of colonic injuries rather than colostomy and early revascularization of ischemic limbs rather than amputation.[5]

Major progress in the development of trauma systems has occurred in civilian practice owing to the efforts of federal agencies, professional organizations, and individual institutions that have led to the development of regional trauma centers. Advancements in acute care, critical care, and rehabilitation have been realized because of these specialized centers.

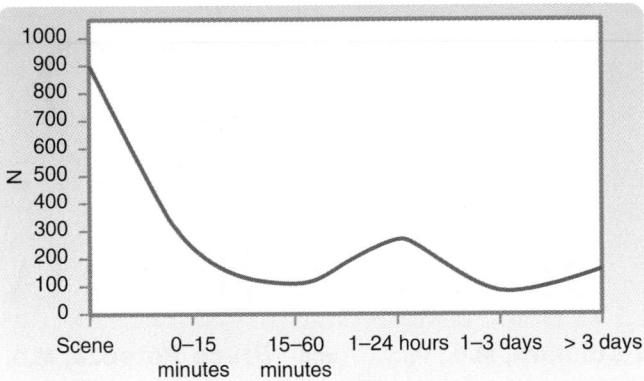

FIGURE 20-1. Trimodal distribution of death. The time to mortality for a population of trauma patients admitted to a single trauma center from a unified geographic area over a 10-year period is shown. All deaths at the scene and hospital deaths are included. (From Committee on Trauma: Resources for Optimal Care of the Injured Patient: 1999. Chicago, American College of Surgeons, 1999.)

The American College of Surgeons, with the establishment of the Committee on the Treatment of Fractures, recognized the importance of injury more than 80 years ago. Formal recognition of multidisciplinary trauma and the establishment of the American College of Surgeons Committee on Trauma have occurred only during the past 50 years. The first organized trauma unit opened in 1961 at the University of Maryland. It was not until 1966 that the National Academy of Sciences and the National Research Council published, "Accidental Death and Disability: The Direct Disease of Modern Society."[6] This landmark paper documented how little progress in applying what was known had been made in injury control. In 1985, the National Research Council again analyzed the status of trauma care in the United States in the report, "Injury in America: A Continuing Health Problem." Injury was once again identified as "the principal health problem in America," highlighted by the fact that over 2.5 million Americans had died of injuries since the 1966 report. Most recently, the Institute of Medicine again documented the importance of injury in the report, "Reducing the Burden of Injury: Advancing Prevention and Treatment." Each of these reports over the past 35 years emphasized the same essential elements to effectively reduce and treat injury. Despite these clear mandates, and although much progress has been made, we still have much to accomplish.

These analyses have acknowledged the need for a coordinated national approach to trauma care. Regional trauma centers integrated with public education, injury prevention, prehospital care, quality assurance, and rehabilitation form the basis of a trauma system's approach to trauma care.

Historically, trauma centers were inner city county hospitals that had de facto trauma center status. In the 1970s an evolution in the initial development of trauma systems began. The elements necessary to establish a trauma system have been defined. These include four primary patient needs: (1) access to care, (2) prehospital care, (3) hospital care, and (4) rehabilitation. Additional issues that require both social and political solutions to supplement the medical efforts include prevention, disaster medical planning, patient education, research, and rational financial planning. Through recent reappropriation of federal legislation and the Health Resources and Services Administration (HRSA) technical assistance program, an organized process for trauma system planning has occurred. The Trauma Office of the HRSA now works to complete trauma system development throughout the United States. The American College of Surgeons has also developed a trauma system consultation process based on a multidisciplinary collaboration. The trauma systems consultation document defines the elements of a trauma system, including administrative, operational, and clinical components.

Access and Emergency Medical Services Response

The vital components of prehospital care include committed medical control, established lines of communication, tested triage criteria, effective transportation, and a cadre of prehospital providers well trained in specific field intervention. Hospitals were first developed by the Romans for care of the military legions, however, prehospital care or field care of the injured victim can be traced back to the *Edwin Smith Surgical Papyrus* (3000-1600 BC), in which procedures for treatment of injuries are specifically described.

Most of the history of medicine pertains to field care of the injured patient, consisting primarily of first aid. Modern emergency medical services (EMS) training, perhaps, can be traced to 1962 when the Chicago Committee on Trauma and the Chicago Fire Department collaborated to develop a prehospital trauma school. In 1966, the National Highway Safety Act authorized the U.S. Department of Transportation to fund ambulance services, communications systems, and training programs to address the needs of the trauma victim before reaching the hospital. In 1969, the U.S. Department of Transportation published the first manual for emergency medical technician—ambulance (EMT-A) training based on the Chicago Trauma School program. Subsequent programs were developed in collaboration with the American Academy of Orthopedics for the training of paramedics (EMT-P).

An integral component of the EMS system is active physician involvement in establishing, directing, and monitoring emergency medical care. The 1973 Emergency Medical Services Systems Act (EMSS) authorized federal funding for EMS that regionalized prehospital emergency care through a series of interrelated components and identified physician involvement as an essential element. Since this time, state and community governments have assumed responsibility for EMS development and its medical control. There still remains wide regional variability in policies, procedures, and authority of medical control of EMS. The basic premise of medical control is physician-directed assurance of quality emergency care. In caring for the trauma patient, surgeons must be involved along with emergency physicians to ensure quality trauma care, based on knowledge and active participation. The NHSTA's EMS "Agenda for the Future" attempts to further define and set standards for each aspect of medical control.

After the events of September 11, 2001, the need for an organized approach to mass casualty events has increased. This commitment to readiness will increase the focus to complete the process of EMS and trauma system implementation.

Triage

The term *triage,* derived from the French word "to sort," in its military application involves prioritizing victims into categories based on severity of injury, likelihood of survival, and urgency of care. The goal of civilian prehospital triage is to identify high-risk injured patients who would benefit from the resources available in a trauma center. This is debated to be between 5% and 10% of all injured patients. As such, a second goal of triage is to limit the excessive transport of non–severely injured patients so as not to overwhelm the trauma center.

The ideal tool to accomplish these two divergent tasks does not exist. Assessment must be made quickly, often under difficult conditions with limited resources, and current schemes are of limited accuracy. Although it is easy to identify patients with severe injuries based on abnormal physiology, a more difficult problem is the identification of high-risk patients whose initial physiologic status is normal. Perhaps the most useful currently available system is that advocated by the Committee on Trauma of the American College of Surgeons, which assesses four components simultaneously: physiologic response, injury anatomy, injury biomechanics, and comorbid factors (Fig. 20-2).

The goal of a trauma system is to prevent unnecessary death, and, thus, a certain degree of over-triage is acceptable, and even desirable. Under-triage, however, is always to be avoided because the benefits of trauma center care are withheld from a patient who is so misclassified. Many studies have tried to determine and adjust the optimal ratio of under-triage and over-triage. Conventional wisdom suggests that a 50% over-triage rate may be required to minimize under-triage. Although this seems high, the additional number of patients going to trauma centers

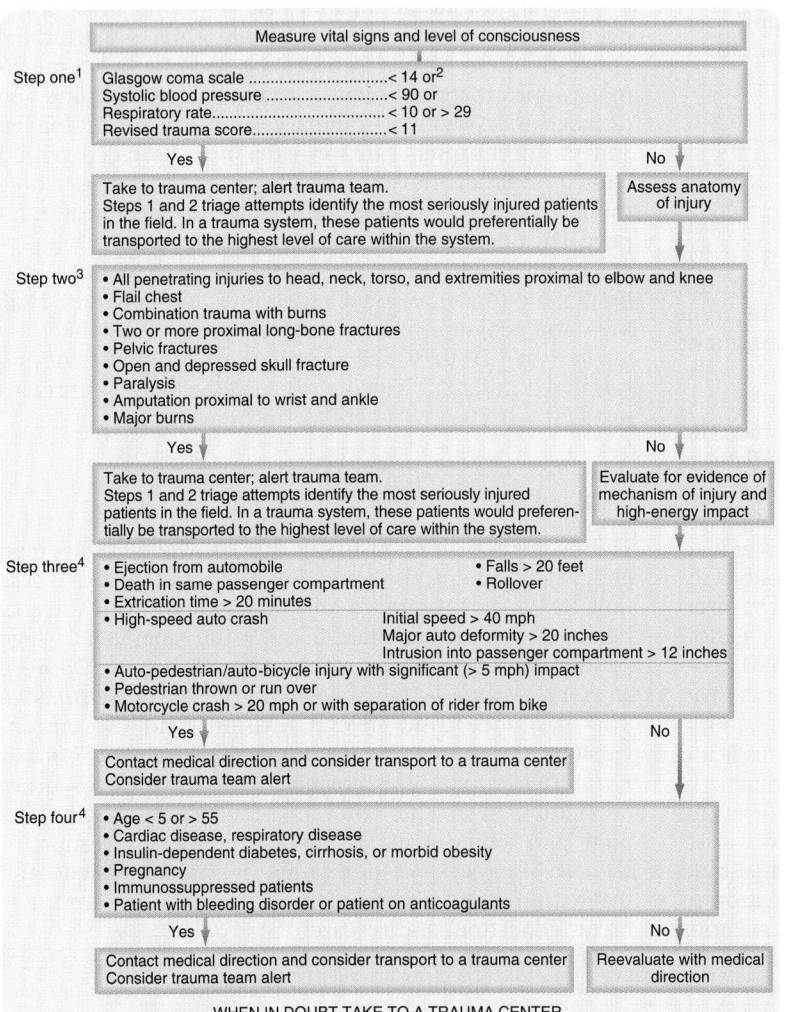

FIGURE 20-2. American College of Surgeons field triage algorithm.

represents only about 5% of all paramedic transports when analyzed over a large geographic area. The accepted norm for under-triage is less than 3%.

Triage can take on differing forms as the situation demands. As medical care resources become limited, alternative triage schemes may be employed so the greatest number of patients may be treated. These may be seen in situations of multiple or mass casualties. In these cases the "most good is applied to the greatest number of patients." This is different than our present triage scheme in which the most seriously injured patient receives the majority of the medical care while the less seriously injured patients wait for care.

The military uses a triage scheme in which patients are classified for transport as immediate, delayed, or expectant.

The method of triage widely used by municipalities is the START triage scheme, which stands for *simple triage and rapid treatment*. This is accomplished by color "tagging of patients." The color red is first priority and signifies a "critical" patient, yellow (urgent) is a second priority, green (minor) is a third priority patient, whereas black represents expectant or dead patients. The initial triage assessment components include the ability of the patient to ambulate, respiratory function, systemic perfusion, and level of consciousness. Patients are classified into the transport categories based on these assessments.

Prehospital Care

The principles of prehospital care of the trauma victim are (1) securing the area, (2) determining the need for emergency treatment, (3) initiating treatment according to protocols for medical direction, (4) communicating with medical control, and (5) rapid transfer of the patient to a trauma center. The treatment at the scene varies according to the severity of injury, local medical practice, and training experience of prehospital providers. The complexity of prehospital care that is appropriate is debated but is generally agreed to be different from that of the medical arrest victim. The goal in prehospital care of the trauma patient is to deliver the trauma patient to the hospital for definitive care as rapidly as possible. In this context, the role of advanced life support (ALS) interventions is debated. The efficacy of immediate evacuation (scoop and run) versus scene resuscitation (stay and play) has been argued repeatedly over the past 20 years. The use of prehospital airway control with endotracheal intubation continues to be debated. Several studies indicate endotracheal intubation, and excessive ventilation may increase mortality.[7] Nonetheless, adequate control of the airway, when indicated, to include suctioning, jaw thrust, oral pharyngeal airway, and bag mask ventilation should be applied as needed to ensure adequate oxygenation to the injured patients. The need for prehospital intravenous fluid administration has been challenged recently and the use of MAST garments has been largely abandoned.[8,9] New strategies to provide fluid resuscitation including hyperosmolar solutions, modified crystalloids, and hemo-globin solutions will require study before being put into practice.

Transportation

Rapid transportation of patients to a trauma center probably originated with Napoleon's chief surgeon, Dominic Jean Larrey. He developed horse-drawn carts, or "flying ambulances," to transport the wounded to medical care behind the battle lines. By World War I, horse-drawn ambulances had been replaced by motorized vehicles, although the first use of motorized ambulances was during the 1906 San Francisco earthquake. The helicopter was introduced during the Korean Conflict, and this was expanded during the Vietnam War. Civilian aeromedical transport has been possible via military helicopters since 1970 due to the Military Assistance to Safety and Traffic Program. The first hospital-based aeromedical transport program in the United States was established in Denver in 1972 and has led to the rapid development of helicopter access to virtually every region in the United States.

The best method for transportation depends on the patient's condition, distance to the regional trauma center, accessibility of the scene, and weather conditions. In general, ground ambulances serve the majority of the needs in the urban setting, although at times with traffic congestion and natural barriers the use of a helicopter is more appropriate. In rural or remote areas, the time and distance to a regional trauma center may be prolonged and the prehospital care provider may be faced with a choice of either transporting the patient to a closer non-trauma hospital or calling for a remote aeromedical transport. The development of transportation guidelines is part of a regionalized trauma care system. Such guidelines must be flexible to the regional variabilities in personnel, facilities, and geography. In general, if transport distances are greater than 20 to 30 miles, or if 15 to 20 minutes of prehospital time can be saved, the use of the helicopter seems justified.

Hospital Care

Trauma center care consists of care provided in the emergency department, the operating room, the intensive care unit (ICU), and the ward and may extend even to rehabilitation in some hospitals. In 1979, the American College of Surgeons Committee on Trauma published the *Optimal Hospital Resources for the Care of the Seriously Injured*. This has undergone several revisions and the current version, *Resources for Optimal Care of the Injured Patient: 1999* stratifies hospitals into levels of resources depending on specific criteria. These include specific hospital and equipment resources, personnel resources, volume of experience in treating the trauma patient, and the requirements for programs such as quality improvement, education, and research.

The general approach to the multiply injured victim is addressed through a trauma team that determines the specific needs of nursing, other paramedical support staff, consulting physicians, and intensive care programs. The

American College of Surgeons' document has been adopted by many state legislatures either directly or in some derived form and truly forms the basis of current trauma center care in the United States. A verification review program of the American College of Surgeons utilizes this document as a basis for individual trauma center assessment and verification. Use of this document and the external review process ensures that the trauma patient, who usually is delivered by local prehospital protocol, will have the demands for diagnostic services, operating rooms, laboratory services, critical care beds, and professional services met at that hospital. There is little question that the standardization of these resources has led to major improvements in the care of injured patients.

The importance of predesignated "trauma team" members with assigned duties cannot be overemphasized. Equally important is the team leader who accepts the responsibility of leadership and is responsible for making overall assessment and management decisions. This "team approach" enables the resuscitative process to be continually coordinated and ensures that no details are neglected or overlooked, so that the resuscitation is timely and focused. The overall coordinated team approach to the critically ill trauma patient is one of the most significant and compelling examples of excellence in modern health care. The effects of a trauma care program on a hospital are far reaching, and the decision to commit to becoming a trauma center is one of the most challenging and satisfying decisions a hospital will ever make.

Rehabilitation

Rehabilitation, the long-term component of trauma care, is as important as prehospital and hospital care, although it is traditionally undeveloped. Too often rehabilitation is ignored in regional plans, despite the fact that it ultimately plays an integral role in returning the patient to productive life. For each trauma-related death, two or three patients experience associated permanent or partial disability, accounting for 350,000 patients annually. The long-term functional recovery of patients after injury is poorly understood. Recent data suggest that post-traumatic depression is a significant problem even for moderately injured patients.

Many patients have difficulty returning to their preinjury activities. Those who return to work after a serious injury may function at a lower level than before. Quality of life evaluations are lower in this group of patients.[10]

A challenge to those practicing trauma care is that despite the development of sophisticated prehospital and hospital care systems, too many patients obtain post-traumatic rehabilitation in inadequate facilities. One exception is the excellent spinal cord rehabilitation centers that have been developed. The rehabilitation of spinal cord injuries can significantly reduce the number of patients requiring institutionalization and decrease associated costs. This example should serve as a model for incorporating regionalized rehabilitation into global trauma center care.

Disaster Management

As the world population increases, people are crowding into areas that are prone to natural disasters. The risk of a disaster increases as villages develop on the hillside of volcanoes and cities flourish in hurricane- and earthquake-prone areas. Cities have many industrial sites that have the potential for a catastrophic event. The threat of terrorism is now ever present.

While natural disasters tend to occur infrequently, the loss of life and property tend to be high. The World Health Organization defines a disaster as "a sudden ecological phenomenon of sufficient magnitude to require external assistance." In more common terms a disaster may be any event that overwhelms a local or regional EMS system. Patients may present as multiple or mass casualties.

Multiple casualties involve a number of injured patients who may require triage and medical attention. The local and regional EMS and hospitals should have the capacity to receive and treat all of the patients. With minor modifications, patient flow and medical care is preserved. A mass casualty situation is one in which the local EMS and hospital system is overwhelmed and triage and transportation of the injured is modified so that the "most good can be provided to the greatest number" of injured patients. In this scenario, the most seriously injured patients may not receive medical care because they will consume too many medical resources. This is in contradistinction to the usual method of treating the most seriously injured patients first while the less seriously injured wait for their care.

With the events of the World Trade Center attacks and the ensuing threat of ongoing terrorism, disaster management has become critical to minimize the loss of life and property. The threat of chemical, biologic, or nuclear attack mandates a multifaceted approach to recognition, care, and management of victims of a terrorist attack.[11] The medical response to a disaster involves a mix of personnel not typically associated with the management of trauma. These personnel include fire, police, public works, and safety and governmental officials as well as public health officers. All must be coordinated into a functioning entity ready to adapt to the situation at hand. An organizational schema designed to assimilate these differing groups is the incident command structure. This was originally utilized by the forest service to fight large multijurisdictional fires and has evolved into a command structure that has been adapted by most municipalities in the United States.

The incident command structure has five main organizational groups. They include the command staff, operations, planning, logistics, and finance. The command staff is headed by the incident commander, who is in charge of the entire disaster scene. Participating agencies include public safety, public information, and emergency medical services. The operations staff controls fire fighting, trauma triage, transportation, and the on-scene EMS. The planning section includes situational and resource management, damage assessment, and demobilization. The logistics section coordinates the movement of goods and personnel in and out of the disaster site. The finance section tracks costs of the disaster and ensures the allocation of funds to keep the disaster scene operational. Each of these five arms of the incident command structure function to ensure vital resources are brought to bear on the most pressing problems at the disaster site.

Numerous agencies at the city, state, and federal level must coordinate their efforts to meet a disaster situation. This requires predetermined arrangements between the agencies for the command and control of the disaster scene. Regional assessment of manpower and equipment must be undertaken. Practice scenarios must be rehearsed and fine tuned so that the various units may function together. This requires an intense effort because communications equipment may be dissimilar between agencies. As seen in the World Trade Center attack, typical ground and radio communications were overwhelmed and there were periods when vital information could not be relayed to the field personnel. Disaster management requires planning, organization, equipment, and personnel that are continually training for a "high impact, yet low probability event."

Research and Education

Future direction in trauma care and injury research is dependent on regional trauma centers because these facilities are the most likely places to make potential care improvements and to identify the need for development and improvement. The responsibility for maintaining a research and education agenda goes along with the opportunity to see the most significantly injured patients who are concentrated in higher-level trauma centers. The National Center for the Prevention and Control of Injury is the lead division within the Centers for Disease Control and Prevention (CDC) that spearheads injury research. It is a good resource for injury data at the federal, state, and regional level. Research grants are funded through this agency covering many injury-related areas, including data collection, acute and rehabilitative care, as well as injury prevention and control. It has created regional injury prevention centers that work on specific areas in research of injury prevention and control and acts as a clearinghouse for regional data. Projects include the biomechanics of fractures and injury, injury scoring systems, prevention of intentional injury and interpersonal violence, as well as outcomes for traumatic brain injury. Extensive injury data may be obtained from the CDC. In addition to CDC, acute care, research has been funded by the National Institutes of Health. Recent efforts by several agencies, including the National Institute of General Medical Sciences, National Health, Lung, & Blood Institute, National Institute of Neurological Disorders and Stroke, and Agency for Healthcare Research and Quality, have increased both basic and clinical opportunities for funding projects that support research in all aspects of acute care, including resuscitation, sepsis, and multiple organ failure.

Prevention and Injury Control

Because 50% of trauma deaths occur within seconds or minutes of injury, with little chance of organized trauma system care reducing this mortality, programs in prevention and injury control must be a priority. The term *accident prevention* is no longer used because it leads one to conclude that injuries are a result of events that we cannot control or modify. This is not true, because most injuries are preventable or the results of the injury are modifiable. The field of injury prevention focuses on the reduction of events that may result in injury. Injury control is an area concerned with the modification of the event so as to minimize traumatic injury.

There are four main tenets of injury prevention and control. They include education, engineering, enactment, and enforcement. The target population must be educated to the problem of a specific type of injury and how to prevent it from occurring. Engineering improvements help to reduce the likelihood of an injury as well as the severity of injury. For example, better street lighting may reduce motor vehicle crashes or pedestrians struck by a motor vehicle. Padded dashes and front and side air bags have lessened the potential for injury during a motor vehicle crash. Enactment of laws to improve the safety of products aids in injury prevention. In-home smoke detectors and flame-retardant children's wear are examples of legislated prevention initiatives. Enforcement of existing safety standards and laws is central to injury prevention and control. For example, at least half of motor vehicle–related deaths in the United States involve intoxicated drivers, and as many as 80% of intentional penetrating trauma deaths occur in intoxicated individuals. The relationship of handgun availability and homicide rates is well established and should be addressed by legislation. The mandatory use of seatbelts has resulted in a significant reduction in fatalities from motor vehicle collisions.

To alert researchers to the factors contributing to injury incidence and severity and the timing involved in those factors, Haddon devised a matrix of broad categories of factors and phases of injury (Table 20-1). The Haddon matrix analyzes each injury by phase and factors and uses this methodology to identify potential opportunities for intervention.

Concurrent with the broadening of the scope of injury control is a shift from active to passive approaches to prevention. Active strategies are those requiring active, continued cooperation on the part of the individual, whereas, in contrast, passive strategies are effective without requiring special response from an individual. Passive approaches, or a combination of passive and active approaches, on the whole have proved to be much more successful in reducing the toll from injuries than has sole reliance on active strategies. Whereas motor vehicle occupant injuries can be prevented by the use of seatbelts or airbags, the latter is a much more effective option, particularly for teenagers or intoxicated drivers, because it works automatically and does not require action by the individual. Similarly, tap water scalds to young children can be prevented by constant and close parental supervision for the first 5 years of life or, alternatively, by water heater temperature regulation lower than 125° F preset in the water heater at the factory.

Legislation can be successful in injury control. Motorcycle and bicycle helmet laws have been successful in

TABLE 20-1. Haddon Matrix

Phases	Factors			
	Host	Agent	Physical Environment	Sociocultural Environment
Pre-event	Alcohol treatment programs	Antilock brakes	Safer roads	55 mph speed limit
Event	Seat belt use	Airbags	Guard rails	Automatic call systems
Post-event	General physical condition	Explosion-resistant gas tanks	Distance to trauma center	Trauma systems

A matrix made by arraying the factors and phases of an injury allows for the analysis of potential interventions.

increasing helmet use. Increasingly, states have adopted mandatory child seat restraint legislation and mandatory seatbelt use for drivers and other passengers. It is estimated that these laws have resulted in a 9% to 12% reduction in occupant fatalities. Recent studies have shown that postinjury intervention is effective in reducing alcohol consumption and recurrent injury over time.

THE SURGEON'S ROLE IN A TRAUMA SYSTEM

The key individual in the development of a system of trauma care is the general surgeon. The general surgeon is the best suited and most widely trained person capable of participating in and supervising all aspects of trauma care. The surgeon should be involved in the development of trauma systems, the local needs assessment, prehospital management protocols, and evaluation of prehospital services. During the resuscitation the surgeon should maintain involvement in the initial management of injured patients and the application of advanced trauma life support protocols while working together with emergency physicians and other members of the trauma team in resuscitation areas. It is essential for the surgeon to maintain active involvement in the initial resuscitation and to prioritize and orchestrate the sequence of evaluation and management of complex injuries. Because the greatest source of preventable death and morbidity occurs during the initial phase of care related to rapid operative intervention, the essential role of the surgeon is obvious. Equally important, postinjury critical care, including ventilatory management, hemodynamic support, management of organ failure, and nutrition are within the armamentarium of the general surgeon and further defines this surgeon's essential involvement.[12]

INITIAL MANAGEMENT

The initial management of the severely injured patient requires the surgeon to make rapid choices between various diagnostic and therapeutic interventions. In patients with a single severe injury there is a single set of priorities. In sharp contrast, a patient with critical injuries to several different organ systems often presents conflicting priorities in management. The thoughtful and accurate ordering of diagnostic and therapeutic interventions is critical to provide the optimal outcome and is perhaps the most important task of the trauma surgeon.[13]

Priorities in Initial Management

It is essential to begin with the assumption that the physiologic state of the patient is likely to deteriorate, perhaps abruptly, and that there is more than one serious injury present. It is also essential to realize that the most obvious or most dramatic injury may not be the most critical one. The trauma surgeon must adopt a very focused approach in which problems are addressed in strict order of their threat to life and function. Even a small delay for the treatment of a more minor injury cannot be tolerated. Within this focused approach, the surgeon must be constantly reassessing the situation as new data are obtained and be able to instantly change the focus and the order of priorities as new injuries or new findings are brought to light. The necessity to balance various conflicting priorities and accurately direct the initial diagnosis and treatment requires an approach to the patient as a whole, not as isolated organ systems. The overall management of the patient is best directed by one person who has the experience and authority to make difficult immediate decisions under stressful circumstances.

The correct prioritization of diagnostic and therapeutic interventions requires an assessment of the criticality of the intervention, the time frame in which action must be taken, and the cost of delay imposed on other injured systems. In general, establishing a patent airway with adequate oxygenation and ventilation are the primary concerns during resuscitation. Next the physiologic stabilization of the patient and control of significant hemorrhage must be addressed. Under these circumstances, optimal resuscitation of the patient is the best resuscitation for any specific organ system. Once immediately life-threatening problems have been controlled, management of possible brain injury is the next priority. Patients with a high likelihood of intracranial mass lesion requiring surgical intervention should undergo computed tomography (CT) of the head as soon as practicable. This group would include patients with Glasgow Coma Scale (GCS) score less than 8, especially in the presence of lateralizing signs. After management of brain injury has been undertaken, injuries causing less immediate threat to life and function should be addressed. Damage-control laparotomy for control of visceral injury, angiography for control of pelvic bleeding or to assess potential aortic injury, revascularization of an ischemic extremity, or management of a contaminated open fracture are examples of this type of problem. Treatment of injuries that present no immediate threat to life or function should be deferred until all other more critical issues have been resolved. This group of injuries is often orthopedic and includes closed-extremity fractures, spine fractures without neurologic compromise, facial fractures, and most soft tissue injuries.

Initial Evaluation of the Trauma Patient

The initial evaluation of the trauma patient consists of a rapid primary survey, aimed at identifying and treating immediately life-threatening problems. The primary survey should be completed in no more than 5 to 10 minutes. After all critical issues in the primary survey have been addressed, a full head-to-toe secondary survey is undertaken, with the goal of carefully examining the entire patient and identifying all injuries. The primary survey is conducted according to the mnemonic ABCDE: Airway, Breathing, Circulation, Disability, Exposure.

Airway

The crucial first step in managing an injured patient is securing an adequate airway. The mechanical removal of debris and the chin lift or jaw thrust maneuver, both of which pull the tongue and oral musculature forward from the pharynx, are often useful in clearing the airway of less severely injured patients. However, if there is any question about the adequacy of the airway, if there is evidence of severe head injury, or if the patient is in profound shock, more definitive airway control is necessary and appropriate. In the majority of patients this is accomplished by endotracheal intubation. Endotracheal intubation must be done rapidly, under the assumption of cervical spine instability, and in a fashion that does not induce increased intracranial pressure (ICP) in patients with head injury. This is best accomplished through a technique borrowed from surgical anesthesia known as rapid-sequence induction. In rapid-sequence induction, the patient is given a fast-acting anesthetic agent followed by a neuromuscular blocking agent. This combination of deep sedation and muscular relaxation allows careful intubation without cervical hyperextension and with minimal physiologic impact. The technique can be used with a number of different pharmacologic agents, depending on the knowledge and preferences of the individual practitioner. It is incumbent on the individual responsible for the procedure to be fully aware of the dosage, risks, and indications associated with the agents chosen. Excessive ventilation must be avoided after intubation, particularly in the hypovolemic patient, because it will increase mean intrathoracic pressures and compromise cardiac filling.

Although nasotracheal intubation has been widely suggested as a central modality, if not the primary modality, for emergency airway control in the past, we believe that nasotracheal intubation now should be used only rarely in the initial management of the injured patient. Nasotracheal intubation has a number of drawbacks, and the goal of safe endotracheal intubation with cervical spine precautions can be better accomplished using orotracheal

intubation after rapid-sequence induction. Our approach to airway control is outlined in Figure 20-3.

In a few patients, endotracheal intubation is either impractical or impossible and a surgical airway is required. Indications for a surgical airway include massive maxillofacial trauma, anatomic distortion due to neck injury, and inability to visualize the vocal cords because of the presence of blood, secretions, or airway edema. Cricothyroidotomy is the preferred emergency procedure in the majority of circumstances. Actual tracheotomy may be indicated in select patients, such as those with laryngeal injuries. Either surgical procedure may be preceded by needle cricothyroidotomy with jet insufflation to improve oxygenation and allow the surgical procedure to be performed in a more orderly fashion. Emergency airway procedures are one of the few immediately lifesaving

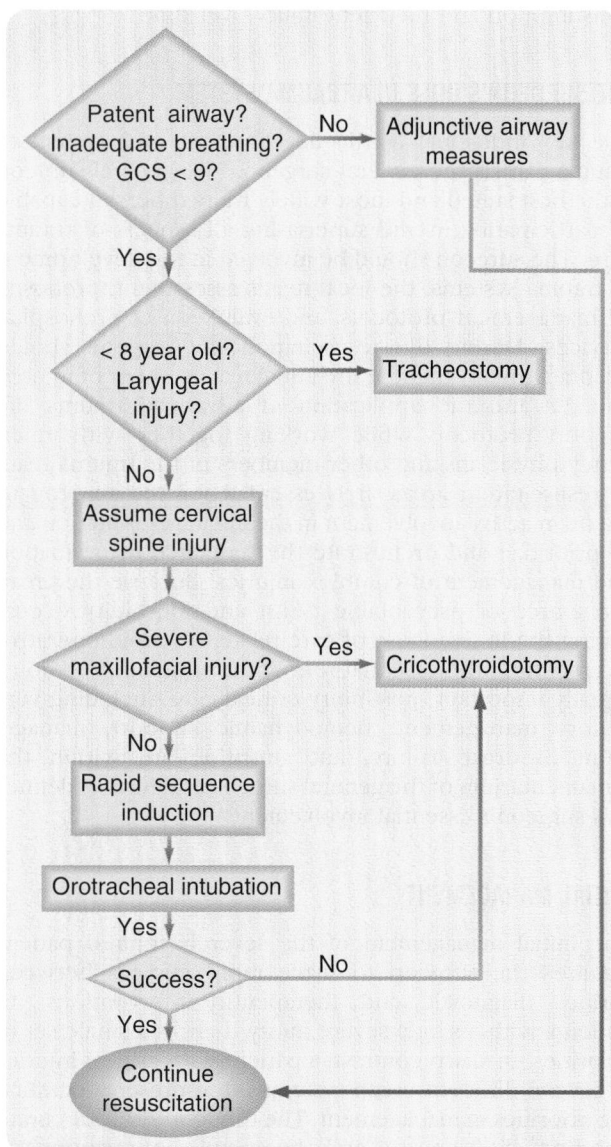

FIGURE 20-3.   Approach to airway management in the trauma patient.

interventions that a surgeon is likely to be called on to perform. By their nature, such procedures are always done under suboptimal conditions and under high stress. It is important for the trauma surgeon to have fully planned the approach to secure a surgical airway before being called on to actually perform the procedure.

Breathing

After a secure airway has been established, the nature and adequacy of tidal ventilation is assessed. Inspection, palpation, and auscultation of the chest will demonstrate the presence of normal, symmetrical ventilatory effort and adequate bilateral tidal exchange. A supine anteroposterior chest radiograph is the primary diagnostic adjunct, demonstrating chest wall, pulmonary parenchymal, and pleural abnormalities. If there is decreased respiratory drive or severe chest wall injury, assisted ventilation is usually necessary. In addition to these mechanical factors, pulmonary parenchymal injury may lead to poor gas exchange and inadequate oxygenation, which necessitates mechanical ventilation. In either circumstance, the decision to provide assisted ventilation should be made early, as soon as it appears likely that the patient will not be able to sustain adequate oxygenation and ventilation, rather than at the point of overt ventilatory failure. Serial measurement of arterial blood gases should be used to monitor patients who are at risk and to assist in appropriate adjustment of the ventilator. It is especially important to prevent episodes of hypoxemia and hypoventilation in patients with associated head injury. There is also a body of evidence that suggests that hyperventilation may be detrimental to cerebral perfusion, accentuating the need for accuracy in ventilator management and vigilance in monitoring pH and $PaCO_2$.

Circulation

Once the airway is secured, and adequate breathing has been established, the focus shifts to the circulatory system. The primary goal is the identification and control of the hemorrhage. External hemorrhage is controlled by direct pressure on the wound, while the possibility of hemorrhage into the chest, abdomen, or pelvis is rapidly assessed. In patients with known pelvic fracture, a pneumatic antishock garment may be applied or circumferential compression can be accomplished with a bed sheet wrapped around the pelvis. While steps are being taken to control hemorrhage, at least two large-bore intravenous lines should be placed to allow fluid resuscitation. These lines are usually placed percutaneously in the vessels of the arm. If peripheral upper extremity access is inadequate, alternative routes include the placement of a large-bore venous line in the femoral vein at the groin or cutdown on the greater saphenous vein at the ankle. The subclavian vein is a poor site for emergency access in the hypovolemic patient and should be used only when other sites are not available. In small children, intraosseous infusion is the preferred alternative route if peripheral access cannot be established. Fluid resuscitation begins with a 1000-mL bolus of lactated Ringer's solution for an adult or 20 mL/kg for a child. Response to therapy is monitored by clinical indicators, including blood pressure, skin perfusion, urinary output, and mental status. If there is no response or only transient response to the initial bolus, a second bolus should be given. If ongoing resuscitation is required after two boluses, it is likely that transfusion will be required, and blood should be administered early. The primary goal is the control of hemorrhage, and fluid resuscitation is of value only if active measures to control hemorrhage are in progress.

The clinician must be vigilant for possible causes of hypotension that require immediate intervention during the primary survey, such as pericardial tamponade or tension pneumothorax. If the pattern of injury and clinical presentation raise suspicion of such injuries, immediate steps must be taken, often before the chest radiograph is available. For example, if a patient presents with profound hemodynamic instability and there is a high suspicion of tension pneumothorax, a needle catheter decompression of the affected hemithorax should be performed immediately, without radiologic confirmation. Needle catheter decompression can be done with relative impunity, even bilaterally, in patients who are intubated and on positive-pressure ventilation. Much greater care must be taken in patients who are breathing spontaneously, because the process of needle catheter decompression can induce pneumothorax and worsen ventilatory dysfunction, especially if done on both sides of the chest.

Disability

The next step is a rapid examination to determine the presence and severity of neurologic injury. Level of consciousness measured by the Glasgow Coma Scale (GCS) score (Table 20-2), pupillary response, and movement of extremities are evaluated and recorded. The assessment of

TABLE 20-2. The Glasgow Coma Scale

Eye Opening	
No response	1
To painful stimulus	2
To verbal stimulus	3
Spontaneous	4
Best Verbal Response	
No response	1
Incomprehensible sounds	2
Inappropriate words	3
Disoriented, inappropriate content	4
Oriented and appropriate	5
Best Motor Response	
No response	1
Abnormal extension (decerebrate posturing)	2
Abnormal flexion (decorticate posturing)	3
Withdrawal	4
Purposeful movement	5
Obeys commands	6
Total	3-15

neurologic function can be complicated by endotracheal intubation and administration of neuromuscular blocking agents. Pupillary response still can be assessed in the paralyzed patient, but the GCS measured under these circumstances is of no value. Intubation interferes with the assessment of the verbal component of the GCS, and there is no standard method for interpretation. If the GCS is used in intubated and paralyzed patients, notation should be made about the circumstances of the assessment to signify that the score may be inaccurate.

Exposure

The final step in the primary survey is to completely undress the patient and do a rapid head-to-toe examination to identify any injuries to the back, perineum, or other areas that are not easily seen in the supine, clothed position. Evidence of blunt trauma, fracture, and unexpected penetrating injuries is likely to be discovered.

After completion of the primary survey and after all immediately life-threatening injuries have been addressed, a complete physical examination is performed. This secondary survey is often done in a head-to-toe manner and includes ordering and collecting data from appropriate laboratory and radiologic tests. This time period also allows for the placement of additional lines, catheters (e.g., nasogastric tube or Foley), and monitoring devices. Data accumulated then can be used to reset priorities and plan definitive management of all injuries.

A number of minor injuries may not become apparent until the patient has been under medical care for 12 to 24 hours. By this time, competing pain from other major injuries has often subsided, and the patient has had an opportunity to take inventory of all bodily complaints. It is very important for the physician to return and perform a tertiary survey, which is another complete head-to-toe physical examination aimed at identifying injuries that may have escaped notice in the first several hours.

MANAGEMENT OF SPECIFIC INJURIES

Head Injury

Brain injury, either alone or in combination with other injuries, is the major determinant of survival and functional outcome in most cases of blunt trauma. Traumatic brain injury (TBI) affects 1.5 million patients a year in the United States. Approximately 50,000 patients will die of TBI, whereas another 80,000 to 90,000 will have long-term neurologic impairment.[14] TBI is the leading cause of death in trauma patients and is responsible for over 50% of all traumatic deaths.[1] Falls and motor vehicle crashes account for 80% of TBI.

It is critical to optimize the early care of the patient with head injury. The overall trauma to the brain is believed to consist of a primary injury and subsequent secondary injuries. The primary injury is the anatomic and physiologic disruption that occurs as a direct result of the external trauma. Secondary injury consists of extension of the primary injury that may result from local swelling, increased intracranial pressure, hypoperfusion, hypoxemia, or other factors. The type and severity of primary injury can be affected only through measures aimed at injury prevention and through the increased use of safety equipment. The acute care of the patient with head injury is focused on the prompt recognition and treatment of TBI and the prevention of secondary injury.

Resuscitative Priorities

Secondary TBI is primarily due to cerebral ischemia. Hypotension and hypoxemia have proven to be the most significant factors leading to a poor neurologic outcome or death. Hypotension appears to be more deleterious than hypoxemia and in one study resulted in a twofold increase in the mortality from closed-head injuries. A goal of a systolic blood pressure of 90 mm Hg or greater is of prime importance.[15] Adequate oxygenation and ventilation are essential to the management of these patients. A PaO_2 of greater than 60 mm Hg and the prevention of an elevated $PaCO_2$ also are essential to management. An elevated $PaCO_2$ may lead to cerebral vasodilation and an increased cerebral blood volume. In patients with an elevated ICP, this small increase in blood volume may result in a sharp increase in the ICP (Monro-Kellie doctrine). Both the initial treatment and later definitive care are primarily intended to prevent these secondary injuries.

The approach to initial resuscitation is the same in all trauma patients, because optimal resuscitation of the patient constitutes the best initial resuscitation for the brain. In patients with severe brain injury the airway should be secured immediately, taking care to remember that spinal cord injury is present in as many as 10% of patients with head injuries. Definitive control of the airway is increasingly controversial in the prehospital phase of care. Because the brain is extremely susceptible to lowered perfusion states after injury, it is essential that adequate cardiac output, arterial pressure, blood volume, and oxygenation be maintained. Resuscitation fluids should be administered and blood loss corrected to maintain adequate perfusion while avoiding volume overload.

The nature of definitive care depends on the presence of surgically correctable lesions (e.g., epidural, subdural, or intraparenchymal hematoma). Patients with these lesions may require prompt operative evacuation, often as the top management priority. Knowledge of the anatomic location of the lesion is necessary to optimize surgical therapy. Patients with diffuse injury do not benefit from surgical intervention, and precise anatomic information is not required for optimal management. Therefore, the urgency for early CT of the head is a function of the likelihood of a surgically correctable lesion. Patients with a GCS score of 8 or less and patients with lateralizing neurologic findings are at particularly high risk and should undergo head CT as soon as they are hemodynamically stable.

Assessment of Injury Severity

The severity of brain injury can be rapidly estimated by determining the level of consciousness and presence or absence of lateralizing signs of central nervous system dysfunction, including pupillary changes and motor findings.

Level of consciousness is most commonly assessed by the GCS score. Although this system was initially developed for the evaluation of chronic coma, it has been almost universally applied to patients with acute brain injury. The GCS score is based on an evaluation of eye opening, best motor response, and verbal response (see Table 20-2). The GCS score is determined by summation of the best response in each category (motor, verbal, and eye movement) and ranges from 3 to 15. Head injury is often classified as severe, moderate, or mild based on the GCS score, as illustrated in Table 20-3. The level of GCS score is an indicator of overall prognosis and also is predictive of the likelihood of neurosurgical intervention. In a study done at an urban level I trauma center, patients with a GCS score less than 8 had a 19% rate of craniotomy, those with a GCS score between 8 and 13 had a 9% rate, and those with a GCS score more than 13 required craniotomy in only 3% of cases.

The GCS score is useful because it is simple and objective and can be repeated serially. A decrease of even 1 or 2 points in the GCS score is indicative of a significant change in neurologic status and demands prompt reevaluation and treatment. The GCS score should be assessed in the field or by the first responders and then reassessed frequently during resuscitation and treatment. Endotracheal intubation complicates assessment of the verbal score. Some assign a verbal score of 1 and apply the modifier "T," as in GSC-10T, under these circumstances. Further, assignment of a value of 1 to the verbal component is not an accurate reflection of underlying function. Such usage is not standardized and therefore of limited value. It is often possible, and generally more useful, to make an estimate of what the patient's verbal ability would be if the endotracheal tube were not in place. Neuromuscular blockade precludes assessment of the GCS. Some advocate the use of the modifier "P," as in GCS-3P, but it is more accurate to state that the GCS could not be evaluated, because the numeric score of 3 is not reflective of underlying function. In either circumstance, the key is to document the conditions and assumptions under which the assessment was made.

The GCS is heavily weighted toward higher cognitive function, and the presence of acute drug or alcohol intoxication can greatly lower scores in the eye opening and verbal categories, even in the absence of brain injury. Changes in the motor component of the GCS are most predictive of serious anatomic injury to the brain and correlate most strongly with outcome. It is impossible to have a GCS score in the severe head injury range (GCS < 8) without changes in the motor component.

Signs of central nervous system dysfunction that are unilateral or asymmetrical, so-called lateralizing signs, are highly suggestive of focal intracranial lesions that may require surgical intervention. Pupillary function is assessed by the size, equality, and response to bright light. Regardless of whether there has been ocular injury, any pupillary asymmetry greater than 1 mm must be attributed to intracranial injury unless proved otherwise. Often, the largest pupil is on the side of the mass lesion, but this information is inadequate for accurate surgical planning. CT of the head should be done as rapidly as possible to ensure accurate localization of the lesion. Lateralized extremity weakness is detected by testing motor power in patients able to cooperate or by observing symmetry of movement in response to painful stimulus. In patients with a markedly decreased level of consciousness, lateralized weakness can be quite difficult to appreciate and small differences in response to stimuli may be important. Lateralizing signs of either type, motor or pupillary, are relatively uncommon, but when seen they must lead to a very high priority for CT of the head and subsequent neurosurgical evaluation, even in patients with other severe injuries.

Definitive Management Strategy

The key to therapy for patients with severe head injury is the maintenance of existing cerebral function and the prevention of further secondary injury. Evidence-based guidelines for the management of severe head injury were published in 1995 and revised in 2000.[16] Institutions that adhere to these guidelines and are aggressive in their management principles may have better outcomes than those institutions with a more empirical approach. Multiply-injured patients with both TBI and extracranial trauma have been considered to be at increased risk for secondary brain insults. Recently, there are institutions reporting similar outcomes in both groups of patients. Close neurologic monitoring guiding goal-directed therapy of ICP and cerebral perfusion pressure and delayed operative management of extracranial lesions are cornerstones of this management strategy.[17]

In an effort to standardize institutional approaches to the management of severe TBI, clinical pathways and guidelines have been developed. A decrease in ICU ventilator days, length of hospital stay, patient morbidity, and overall cost expenditures has been demonstrated.

Patients with focal intracranial pathology that is causing significant mass effect require urgent surgical evacuation of the mass lesion. The outcome in these patients is improved by rapid decompression; therefore, time is of the essence. Craniotomy takes precedence over, or must be done simultaneously with, any other necessary interventions. In general, any epidural or subdural hematoma that is causing significant mass effect, especially in a patient with poor mental status, should be evacuated. The threshold for surgical evacuation of intraparenchymal contusions causing mass effect is somewhat more controversial, but large lesions or smaller frontal, temporal contusions that are likely to increase in size should be approached

TABLE 20-3.	Classification of Head Injury Severity
Classification	**Range of Glasgow Coma Scale Score**
Mild	GCS ≥ 13
Moderate	GCS 9 to 12
Severe	GCS ≤ 8

aggressively. Failure of nonoperative management from CNS trauma is more common in frontal and temporal contusions and occipital hemorrhages. Serial neurologic assessment in the ICU with liberal use of head CT is mandatory for nonoperative management of these lesions.[14]

The management of diffuse axonal injury and the postoperative management of patients undergoing surgical decompression involves measures aimed at maintaining cerebral perfusion and at maintaining overall homeostasis. ICP monitoring is widely used in patients with severe injury, as are other invasive means of monitoring, including arterial catheters and pulmonary artery catheters.

Therapy is directed at two major goals. First is general supportive care of the patient, maintenance of pulmonary and cardiovascular function to provide adequate oxygen delivery, treatment of infection, and early use of enteral nutrition. Second is to optimize cerebral perfusion, which is primarily achieved through control of ICP. Therapeutic interventions are added sequentially to provide an adequate degree of ICP control. Simple measures such as adequate sedation and pain control, neuromuscular paralysis, and the elevation of the head of the bed by 30 degrees are utilized. In general, strenuous efforts are made to keep ICP below 20 cm H_2O. If a ventriculostomy is in place, drainage of cerebrospinal fluid is the first and most direct route. Under current guidelines, only modest degrees of hyperventilation are used, with $PaCO_2$ in the range of 30 to 35 mm Hg. There is a lack of data showing efficacy of hypocapnia, and recent concerns have arisen about hypocapnia resulting in decreased cerebral perfusion. The next step is the use of mannitol to induce an osmotic diuresis. In a patient who is intravascularly resuscitated, mannitol is given as needed, or on a scheduled basis, as long as the serum osmolality remains below 305 to 315 mOsm/L. The potential deleterious effects of hyperosmolality above this level generally are believed to outweigh the therapeutic benefits. In circumstances in which large amounts of mannitol are given, it is important to provide free water replacement, both to prevent hypovolemia and to control hypernatremia. High urine output caused by mannitol administration can complicate management and creates a situation in which the diagnosis of diabetes insipidus is raised. In patients with severe anatomic injuries believed to be at high risk for diabetes insipidus, early pharmacologic therapy is warranted, whereas in other cases careful fluid management will usually suffice.

Patients who do not respond to this increasing gradation of therapy are candidates for barbiturate use. The use of barbiturates in patients with severe head injury and uncontrollable ICP is supported strongly by some but is not of benefit to the majority of patients. It is a reasonable strategy in selected patients who are unresponsive to conventional therapy. Potential complications include myocardial depression and severe pneumonia.

Vertebrae and Spinal Cord

There are approximately 11,000 new cases of spinal cord injury diagnosed each year. The permanent nature of some of these injuries has resulted in 200,000 patients living with spinal cord disability in the United States. A study published in 1990 reported that approximately 6% of hospitalizations for injury result from vertebral injuries, whereas only 1% are the result of spinal cord injury. Despite this low incidence, spinal cord injuries are often devastating in both socioeconomic and psychological impact. Patients with high spinal cord injuries require intensive initial hospital care, long-term rehabilitation, and life-long care. The prognosis for patients with incomplete neurologic injury can be fairly good, and many patients will regain significant function with appropriate rehabilitation. In addition, great progress has been made in the field of rehabilitation for patients with spinal cord injury, allowing them to optimize functional recovery even after the cord injury has become stable. Because a patient's ultimate level of function is highly dependent on the degree and level of spinal cord injury, it is absolutely essential that early care be focused on identification of the patient with a potentially unstable vertebral injury, prevention of any progression of neurologic injury, and optimization of chances for neurologic recovery.

Resuscitative Priorities

High cervical spinal injuries can result in acute ventilatory decompensation due to loss of phrenic nerve function (roots C3-C5) and intercostal muscle function (primarily thoracic roots). As always, the patency of the airway must be ensured and the adequacy of ventilation assessed. Patients with injuries above C3 are often completely apneic, necessitating early intubation in the field as a lifesaving measure. Patients with injuries between C3 and C5 may initially have good ventilatory function, but this is likely to deteriorate because of the patient's fatigue and difficulty in clearing secretions. An aggressive approach to early endotracheal intubation is warranted, especially if the patient has other injuries.

High spinal cord injuries also can result in systemic hypotension owing to loss of sympathetic tone. The patient will usually have hypotension and relative bradycardia and will have evidence of good peripheral perfusion on physical examination. The term *neurogenic shock* is used, but it is somewhat of a misnomer, because the patients are typically hyperdynamic, with high cardiac output due to a loss of sympathetic vascular tone. After hemorrhagic causes of hypotension have been ruled out, the hypotension associated with high spinal injury can be treated by administration of an α agonist such as phenylephrine.

The essential priority in initial care of patients with potential spinal cord injury is to maintain strict immobilization of the entire spine. This immobilization is most often initiated in the field. As soon as practical, and often before extrication is complete, the neck is immobilized in a cervical collar and the patient is secured to a full-length backboard. The head is maintained in neutral position in the midline. Before transportation, the patient's body is securely strapped at all major joints, the head is taped to the board, and sandbags may be applied alongside the head. On arrival in the emergency department, the pro-

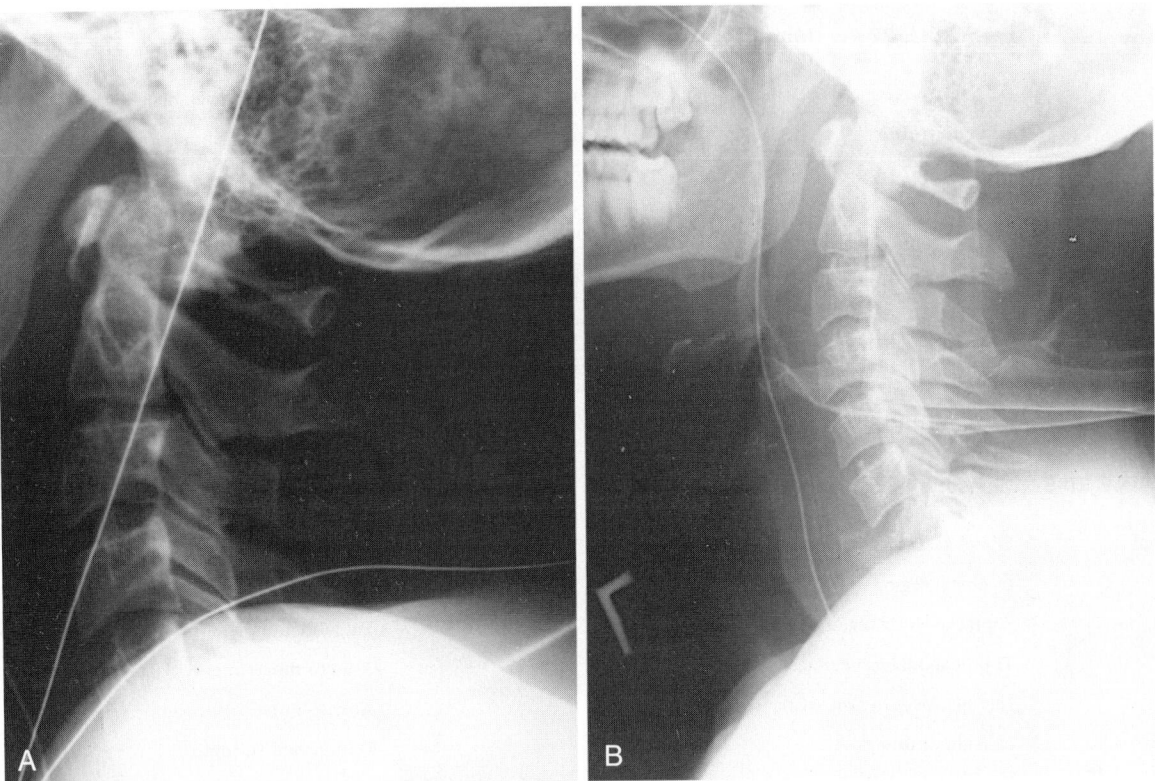

FIGURE 20-4. The importance of completely visualizing all seven cervical vertebrae in a cross-table lateral cervical spine radiograph is illustrated in these two photoradiographs. **A,** An inadequate cross-table lateral cervical spine radiograph (C7 not visualized). **B,** The repeat lateral film demonstrates a burst fracture of C7.

tective cocoon must be partially removed to allow assessment of the patient, but it is critical that the immobilization of the spine be maintained until an unstable injury has been ruled out both by radiologic and clinical examination. In the cervical spine, it is essential for the radiographs to include all seven cervical vertebrae, down to and including the articulation between C7 and T1. The lower portion of the cervical spine is often difficult to visualize well on lateral views, especially in large patients. If the region of C7 to T1 is not visualized, there is potential for dramatic missed injury (Fig. 20-4). Under these circumstances, or in situations in which the findings on plain films are equivocal, CT is a useful adjunct. Likewise, if a cervical fracture is identified on any cervical spine radiograph, further evaluation of the neck should be accomplished with CT. Subtle movement of the cervical spine has been demonstrated while obtaining further films, including the lateral swimmer's view. There is a small group of patients who will have spinal cord injury without radiographic abnormality. Originally described in pediatric patients, it is now seen more frequently in adult patients. The use of magnetic resonance imaging (MRI) in these patients will reveal the cause of injury in many patients.

Vertebral fractures and vertebral instability can be easily missed if vigilance is not maintained. This is especially true in patients with altered level of consciousness due to head injury or intoxication or in patients with multiple injuries and competing pain. Spinal immobilization must be maintained until a careful follow-up clinical exam-

ination can be done and all areas of pain or tenderness have been fully evaluated to rule out occult fracture or ligamentous injury. In patients who cannot cooperate with a clinical examination, it may be necessary to maintain spinal immobilization for a considerable period of time. Clearance of a cervical spine injury in the obtunded patient is problematic. There are many algorithms that address this issue and include complete cervical CT, MRI, and dynamic flexion and extension films in an otherwise radiographically normal appearing spine.

Assessment of Injury Severity

Injury to the spinal cord may occur with direct compression from a bony fragment, subluxation of a vertebra onto the cord, distraction, disc protrusion, cord contusion, hematoma, or ischemia. Whenever possible, injury assessment begins with determination of the history, including mechanism of injury and any weakness, loss of sensation, and tingling or other neurologic symptoms noted in the field. A careful physical examination of the spine is done, including palpation of the entire dorsal spine looking for areas of tenderness, deformity, or swelling. All patients at risk for spinal injury should undergo a thorough neurologic examination, assessing both motor and sensory function for all major nerve roots. Table 20-4 illustrates the basic physical examination steps for motor evaluation, and Table 20-5 illustrates the steps for sensory evaluation. Motor strength is measured on a scale of 0 to 5, as

TABLE 20-4.   Motor Function of Spinal Roots

	Nerve Root	Muscle	Motor Examination
Upper Extremity	C5	Deltoid	Shoulder abduction
	C6	Biceps	Elbow flexion
	C7	Triceps	Elbow extension
	C8	Flexor carpi ulnaris	Wrist flexion
	T1	Lumbricales	Finger abduction
Lower Extremity	L2	Iliopsoas	Hip flexion
	L3	Quadriceps	Knee extension
	L4	Tibialis anterior	Ankle dorsiflexion
	L5-S1	Extensor hallucis longus	Great toe extension
	S1	Gastrocnemius	Ankle plantarflexion

TABLE 20-5.   Sensory Assessment of Spinal Roots

Nerve Root	Site of Assessment
C2	Occipital region
C3	Supraclavicular region, near head of clavicle
C4	Top of shoulder, near acromion
C5	Lateral aspect of arm, just above elbow
C6	Dorsum of thumb
C7	Dorsum of middle finger
C8	Dorsum of little finger
T1	Medial arm, just above elbow
T2	Axilla
T4	Thorax at level of nipples
T10	Abdomen at level of umbilicus
L1	Region of femoral pulse
L2	Medial thigh, mid femur
L3	Medial aspect of knee
L4	Medial leg, above medial malleolus
L5	Dorsum of great toe
S1	Lateral aspect of heel
S2	Popliteal fossa
S3	Medial gluteal region
S4-S5	Perianal region

TABLE 20-6.   Assessment of Motor Strength

Score	Functional Ability
0	No contraction of muscle
1	Palpable muscle contraction, no limb movement
2	Able to move in gravity-neutral plane
3	Able to move against gravity
4	Diminished strength
5	Normal strength

outlined in Table 20-6. Sensation is generally assessed with a combination of pinprick and light touch. In patients with neurologic deficits, the presence of low spinal cord reflexes is also assessed. This examination includes testing for anal sphincter tone, anal wink, and bulbocavernosus reflex. The motor and sensory findings should be fully documented in the medical record, including the time of the assessment, because changes compared with this baseline examination are of critical importance in determining the course of therapy.

The sensory and motor deficits that occur in spinal cord injury often fit into recognizable patterns. Most commonly, patients with severe trauma to the cord will have a complete loss of both motor and sensory function below the level of injury. The motor deficits are the most critical to the patient's long term functional outcome. In correlating the physical examination finding with injuries identified on the radiographs of the spine, it is important to remember that vertebral body level and the spinal cord level may not correlate exactly. They are fairly close in the cervical spine, but in the thoracic and lumbar spine the nerve roots descend within the spinal canal, exiting through foramina that are more caudad. These nerve roots are fairly mobile and much less susceptible to injury. Thus, a fracture at the level of the L1 vertebral body will affect motor function in the cord at the L3 or L4 level, and fractures below L4 will not involve the spinal cord at all.

If the injury appears to be complete, the presence of spinal cord reflexes, especially the sacral reflexes, yields important prognostic information. After acute spinal cord injury, a transient phenomenon known as "spinal shock" is seen, in which all cord function is absent below the level of injury. The affected muscle groups are flaccid and areflexic. As time progresses, the spinal reflex arcs return, and the muscle groups become hyperreflexic owing to loss of inhibition. Therefore, lack of reflexes, particularly sacral reflexes such as the bulbocavernosus, indicates the presence of spinal shock and leaves hope that the actual degree of anatomic injury may be less than initially perceived. Once spinal reflexes have returned, the examination is more likely to represent the true extent of cord damage.

As a general rule, complete cord lesions are fixed and permanent, with little hope for major recovery of distal function. Restoration of the spinal canal anatomy and decompression of the spinal cord do not improve neurologic outcome because the lesion in the spinal cord is fixed. These are devastating injuries, especially in the high cervical spine. A change of a single motor level in the cervical spine has an enormous impact on functional outcome, and so every effort must be made to ensure that the level of injury does not ascend as the result of therapeutic intervention. In the thoracic and lumbar spine the precise level is of less importance, because ventilatory function and upper extremity function are unaffected.

The second pattern of spinal cord injury is the incomplete injury. Under these circumstances, the patient will exhibit some sensory and motor function below the level of injury. Incomplete injuries have a much better prognosis for recovery of function, and most will improve with time. In addition, under certain circumstances, restoration of the anatomy of the spinal canal and decompression of the spinal cord may lead to improved outcome. Therefore, in a patient with an incomplete injury it is essential that careful sequential neurologic examinations be done to determine if the deficit is worsening, stable, or improving. Patients with a condition that is stable or improving are monitored closely, whereas patients with a condition that is deteriorating are candidates for emergency surgical intervention.

Incomplete cord injuries most often present a mixed picture of sensory and motor findings. In the minority of cases, the findings represent well-defined clinical syndromes that are related to the type of injury. Most common is the central cord syndrome. A patient with central cord syndrome will present with motor weakness and sensory loss primarily involving the distal muscles of the upper extremity. The proximal muscles of the upper extremity and the full function of the lower extremities are preserved. Often, there is no radiologically identifiable fracture of the spinal column. Central cord syndrome is thought to be an ischemic lesion, in which hyperflexion or hyperextension of the neck leads to interference with blood flow in the spinal arteries. This leads to hypoperfusion of the cord and loss of function in a watershed distribution, most affecting the tissue in the central portion of the cord. These anatomic data provide the rationale for the clinical presentation. The neurologic elements controlling the distal portion of the upper extremity are in the most central portions of the cord and are most affected, whereas the structures controlling the lower extremity are more lateral and nearly always preserved. The function of the proximal upper extremity is variable. Central cord syndromes can be functionally quite significant because the muscles most affected are the small muscles of the hand and the distal arm. Usually, the neurologic changes are transient and will improve with time, but there still may be a degree of permanent impairment.

A second clinical syndrome is the Brown-Séquard syndrome, which is anatomically interesting but uncommon in clinical practice. This syndrome results from partial transection of the cord and yields a split motor and sensory deficit. Motor function is lost on the ipsilateral side, and sensory loss is on the contralateral side. This is caused by an anatomic difference in the level of midline crossing between motor and sensory neural tracts. Motor tracts cross over at the level of the brain stem, whereas sensory tracts cross near the level of the spinal root.

The assessment of the severity of injury to the spinal column itself is independent of the nature and type of spinal cord injury. The primary question that must be answered is one of stability. Initial evaluation should be based on at least three views of the cervical spine (lateral, anteroposterior, and odontoid) and two views (lateral and anteroposterior) of the thoracolumbar spine. In alert patients with normal plain radiographs but persistent symptoms, flexion-extension views, especially in the cervical spine, can be obtained to look for ligamentous instability.

The spinal column is generally conceptualized as having three "columns:" the anterior spinal ligament and anterior walls of the vertebral bodies, the posterior spinal ligament and posterior walls of the vertebral bodies, and the posterior elements of the vertebral column. Injuries involving only one column are believed to be stable, and those involving two or three columns are unstable. Many spine fractures are difficult to visualize with standard radiographs. CT of the spine, and more recently MRI, provide much better detail of bony and ligamentous structures, respectively. These more detailed studies should be used whenever there is a suspicion of injury on plain radiographs. Careful examination of the plain radiographs, augmented by CT or MRI of the spine, provides the data, but the final assessment of stability is based on the judgment of the physician.

Definitive Care

There is little that can be done to repair the anatomic injury done to the spinal cord, and acute therapy for spinal cord injury is targeted at preservation of remaining function. General support of the patient's cardiovascular function is important to optimize spinal cord perfusion and prevent ischemic secondary injury. Some advocate the use of inotropic support or vasoactive infusions to maintain spinal cord perfusion pressure in a manner analogous to that used in brain injury, although data for the efficacy of this approach are lacking. The use of high doses of corticosteroids for the first 24 hours after spinal cord injury has become nearly universal in the United States as a result of a placebo-controlled clinical trial published in 1990. This trial showed a statistically significant improvement in function for the corticosteroid group, although the practical significance of the improvement is open to debate. To be efficacious, the corticosteroid therapy must be initiated within a few hours of injury and consists of a bolus of 30 mg/kg of methylprednisolone infused over 1 hour, followed by an infusion of 5.4 mg/kg/hr for the next 23 hours. If the injury has occurred for greater than 3 hours but less than 8 hours, corticosteroids should be continued for a total of 48 hours.[18]

Although the study only addressed patients with documented neurologic deficits, the use of corticosteroids is often generalized to all patients with known or suspected spinal cord injury. The rate of complications is low and, hence, this aggressive approach can be justified, but the likelihood of a clinically significant functional improvement is also low.

Surgical therapy for lesions of the spinal cord is limited to the restoration of spinal canal anatomy, removal of foreign bodies, and removal of any bone, disc, or hematoma that may be compressing the cord. Therefore, decompressive surgery is unlikely to be of benefit in complete lesions and is rarely done. In patients with incomplete injury, the decision to operate requires mature judgment. In general, if the examination shows the patient's condition is stable or improving, urgent surgical decompression is unlikely to improve the situation and it is usually delayed until all acute physiologic problems have been fully stabilized. The patient with an incomplete examination whose condition is deteriorating may benefit from acute decompression to prevent further loss of cord function. There is interesting work being done on the rapid decompression (<24 hr) of patients with cervical cord injury. Emergent MRI is obtained, and if there is evidence of cord compression, decompression and stabilization is undertaken. There have been documented improvements in the preoperative and postoperative examination of patients who present with complete motor tetraplegia and improve to independent ambulation. Further study is needed in this area because the older literature suggests that early operative intervention does not improve the outcome compared with delayed fixation.

The need for surgical intervention for the injury to the spinal column itself is dictated by the degree of deformity and the perceived stability of the injury. Displaced fractures of the cervical spine are usually treated with careful application of traction, using a halo brace or Gardner-Wells tongs. Weight is gradually added to the traction apparatus until the spine is realigned. The rule of thumb is that a weight of about 5 pounds per cervical level will be required for reduction. The neurologic examination must be followed very closely as weight is added to the traction. Serial radiographs are used to determine when adequate reduction has been obtained. The inability to obtain adequate reduction is usually an indication for surgical intervention.

Those injuries believed to be relatively stable, or with instability in only one column, can be managed with immobilization only. For significant fractures, this involves the use of a halo brace in the cervical spine and an orthosis, usually a molded jacket, in the thoracic and lumbar spine. Unstable injuries usually require surgical stabilization. Stabilization can be achieved by placement of hardware posteriorly, by use of hardware and bone grafting anteriorly, or in some cases, using both techniques simultaneously. The anterior approach allows better access to the vertebral body and better decompression of the spinal canal. Three-column injuries generally will require both anterior and posterior stabilization.

The benefits of early spinal stabilization in patients with complete injury are primarily related to the prevention of complications of long-term immobilization. Data show fewer complications in patients whose spinal injuries are fixed early, although there are no compelling survival differences. Therefore, spinal column injuries should be fixed as early as practical, once the patient is physiologically stable and no longer at risk to suffer deterioration of neurologic function, either from exacerbation of brain injury or as a result of manipulation of the spinal cord.

Neck Injuries

The neck contains multiple vital structures with little anatomic protection from overlying bone, muscle, and soft tissue. Most severe neck injuries are the result of penetrating wounds and may present an immediate threat to life due to airway compromise or hemorrhage. Neck injuries can also result from blunt trauma, and the diagnosis is often more difficult owing to the more subtle presentation of blunt injuries. Because of the high likelihood of injury to the airway or major blood vessels, accurate and aggressive initial evaluation and treatment is required to optimize outcome.

In evaluating penetrating injuries of the neck, it is important to consider location in both an anteroposterior direction as well as a craniocaudad direction. On an anatomic basis, the neck is divided into anterior and posterior triangles (Fig. 20-5). The major vascular and aerodigestive structures in the neck are located in the anterior triangle, and all are deep to the platysma. Therefore, the platysma and the sternocleidomastoid muscle are useful anatomic boundaries. Injuries that do not penetrate the platysma can be considered superficial, and no further investigation is needed. Wounds that penetrate the platysma must be further evaluated. Injuries that are anterior to the sternocleidomastoid present a high likelihood of significant injury, whereas those that track posterior to the sternocleidomastoid are unlikely to involve major vascular or aerodigestive injury.

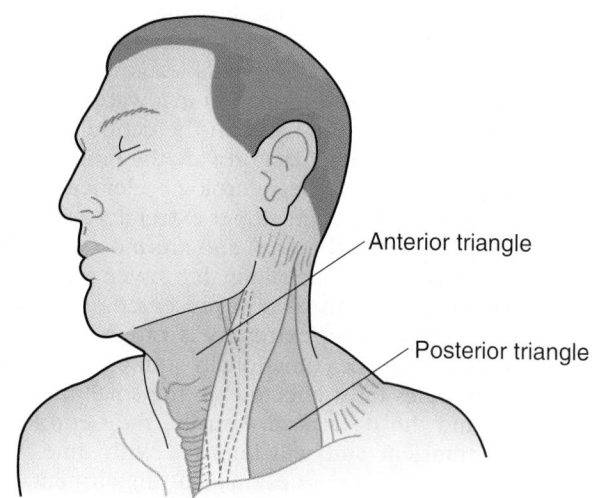

FIGURE 20-5. The anterior and posterior anatomic triangles of the neck are defined by the sternocleidomastoid muscle. The major vascular and aerodigestive structures in the neck are contained in the anterior triangle. Wounds involving only the posterior triangle have a low probability of injury requiring urgent surgical intervention.

Anterior triangle

Posterior triangle

In analyzing wounds based on craniocaudad location, the neck is commonly divided into three horizontal zones (Fig. 20-6). Zone I is the thoracic inlet, extending roughly from the sternal notch to the cricoid cartilage. Injuries in this zone carry the highest mortality, owing to the presence of the great vessels and the difficulty of surgical approach. Zone II is the midportion of the neck, extending from the cricoid cartilage to the angle of the mandible. Injuries in this zone are usually clinically apparent, and vascular control is relatively straightforward. Zone III extends from the angle of the mandible to the base of the skull. Exposure in this zone, particularly of the distal carotid artery, can be quite difficult to manage.

Resuscitative Priorities

Significant injuries to the neck often present with immediate threat to life from airway compromise. Airway obstruction can be caused by direct injury to the larynx or trachea, expanding hematoma within the neck, or bleeding into the airway. Patients may present initially with a patent airway that becomes compromised a short time later. It is essential to obtain early definitive control of the airway as the top priority in all patients with major neck injuries. Progressive bleeding or neck swelling may produce a circumstance in which orotracheal intubation is no longer possible. What might have been a routine intubation in the first 15 minutes of the resuscitation may become a difficult emergency surgical airway procedure. If the airway is not in jeopardy, intubation may be deferred, but this course should be chosen only if the perceived likelihood of significant injury is very low.

Neck injuries also present the threat of hemorrhage from the carotid artery, jugular vein, and great vessels. After the airway has been controlled, the potential for major vascular injury must be assessed. Injuries in zone II are usually clinically apparent, with significant hematoma or frank external hemorrhage. These injuries are approached by immediate surgical exploration, using direct pressure to maintain hemostasis until vascular control can be obtained. Based on the potential for great vessel injury, and the difficulties in vascular exposure in both zone I and zone III, angiography is mandatory before surgical exploration in all but the most unstable patients. If no vascular injury is found, angiography may preclude the need for surgical exploration.

The potential for blunt injury to the larynx, trachea, or carotid arteries must be kept in mind in any patient with evidence of a blunt impact to the neck. Such injuries are often subtle in presentation, and work-up must be based on appropriate clinical suspicion based on mechanism of injury.

Assessment of Injury Severity

Patients with overt clinical signs of vascular or aerodigestive tract injury require surgical exploration of the neck. Such clinical signs include significant external hemorrhage, large or expanding hematoma, air movement through the wound with breathing, crepitance in the neck, voice changes, dysphagia, and odynophagia (Box 20-1). Preoperative work-up in this subset of patients is minimal. Those patients with penetrating injuries in zone II are generally taken directly to surgery, whereas patients with injuries in zone I and zone III should undergo preoperative angiography, if possible. Work-up of the aerodigestive tract is undertaken at the time of surgical exploration. Those neck injuries not requiring operative exploration may need to have the aerodigestive track worked up with bronchoscopy, upper endoscopy, or esophagography to exclude injury.

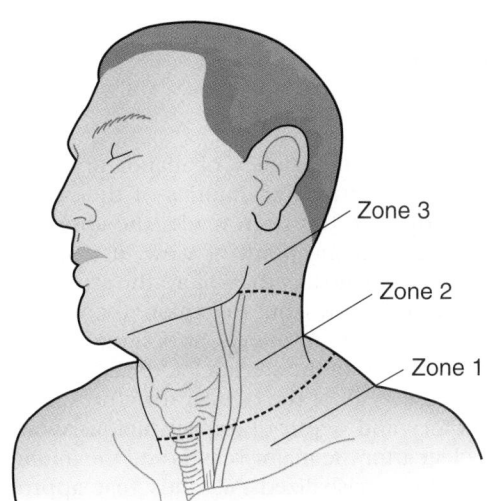

FIGURE 20-6. The zones of the neck. The border between zone I and zone II is at the level of the cricoid cartilage. The border between zone II and zone III is at the angle of the mandible. These zones are primarily useful in management of injuries in the anterior triangles of the neck.

Zone 3
Zone 2
Zone 1

Box 20-1 Clinical Indications for Neck Exploration

Vascular

Expanding hematoma
External hemorrhage
Diminished carotid pulse

Airway

Stridor
Hoarseness
Dysphonia/voice change
Hemoptysis
Subcutaneous air

Digestive Tract

Dysphagia/odynophagia
Subcutaneous air
Blood in oropharynx

Neurologic

Lateralized neurologic deficit consistent with injury
Altered state of consciousness not due to head injury

Significant controversy exists regarding the optimal approach to patients with injuries that penetrate the platysma but who exhibit no suspicious clinical findings.[19] One school of thought favors mandatory surgical exploration for all penetrating injuries, citing a low rate of complications and the potentially devastating effect of delay in diagnosis of aerodigestive tract injuries. The second school of thought favors selective exploration based either on the results of extensive evaluation including angiography, esophagoscopy, and esophagography or on progression of clinical symptoms. Proponents of this course of action cite the high rate of negative exploration in asymptomatic patients and the low incidence of devastating complications of delay. Current data show similar outcome for both approaches and do not favor one approach over the other. There are centers that advocate thin-sliced CT of the neck with intravenously administered contrast medium to determine the track of a penetrating object, such as a knife or bullet. Knowledge of the track of penetration permits a determination of anatomic structures at risk for injury. The presence of contrast medium extravasation, nonvisualization of vascular structures, or free air in the tissue planes suggests injury.[20] Proponents cite that this method is no better than serial physical examination for injuries occurring in zone II.[21] We favor an aggressive approach to neck exploration, especially in patients with zone II injuries. Patients with zone I and zone III injuries, and patients believed to be at very low risk of injury, undergo further clinical evaluation and are observed if studies are negative.

The nonsurgical evaluation of potential vascular injury is relatively straightforward. In penetrating injuries, and blunt injuries with clinical evidence of carotid injury, full four-vessel evaluation of the neck must be done and the arch and great vessels included in the wound trajectory considered suspicious. Careful biplanar films are mandatory, because the signs of vascular injury can be quite subtle. In asymptomatic patients with blunt injuries, duplex ultrasound is used as a screening examination before angiography. Duplex ultrasound has been evaluated for use in penetrating trauma but is not in widespread application.

Nonsurgical evaluation of the aerodigestive tract must include the pharynx, larynx, trachea, and esophagus. In penetrating injuries, this is accomplished by a combination of direct laryngoscopy, bronchoscopy, and esophagoscopy. Early endotracheal intubation may complicate the evaluation of the larynx and proximal trachea. There has been some controversy regarding the use of rigid versus flexible esophagoscopy, but the utility of either approach appears to be operator dependent. Clinical data support the efficacy of both modalities. Contrast esophagography is a complementary examination, and its use probably improves diagnostic accuracy over esophagoscopy alone.

Blunt injury to the neck often involves the larynx, and these injuries are difficult to assess by direct laryngoscopy. Furthermore, the examination itself has the risk of worsening the injury. Therefore, CT of the neck is commonly used to assess the larynx in blunt injury (Fig. 20-7). Blunt injury to the esophagus is exceedingly uncommon, and

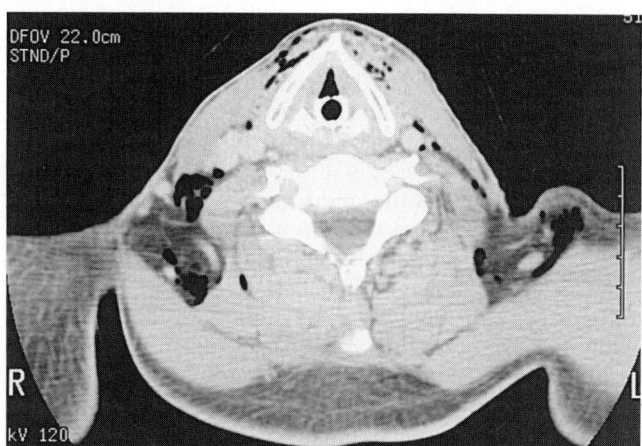

FIGURE 20-7. CT of the neck after blunt trauma shows fracture of the thyroid cartilage, with significant airway swelling and air in the soft tissues surrounding the larynx.

clinical observation is probably sufficient in asymptomatic patients with no clinical signs of esophageal injury. Patients with symptoms referable to the aerodigestive tract must be aggressively evaluated. Blunt vascular injuries to the carotid or vertebral arteries are more difficult to diagnose. These lesions may be asymptomatic on presentation. These injuries tend to be arterial dissections, flaps, or thrombosis rather than frank bleeding. A suspicion of injury based on mechanism or the association of adjacent injuries may be the only clue to an occult vascular injury. Diagnosis by angiography, MRI angiography, or duplex color flow Doppler imaging may be used to evaluate these potential lesions.[22]

Patients with evidence of either significant vascular injury or injury to the aerodigestive tract will likely require surgical repair. Patients with no clinical findings, and negative evaluation of both vascular and aerodigestive systems, can be safely observed.

Definitive Therapy

Technique of Neck Exploration

Whether one adopts a policy of mandatory or selective exploration for penetrating injuries of the neck, once a decision to operate has been made, the approach is the same. From a strategic point of view, it is important to remember that the goal is to explore the structures of the neck to identify injuries, not to explore the wound per se. In the case of unilateral injury, an oblique incision along the anterior border of the sternocleidomastoid muscle will provide access to all of the critical structures in the neck. The trajectory and depth of any suspicious wounds will become clear after the major vessels and the midline structures have been visualized. Wounds that approach the carotid sheath or the midline must be followed to the end of the wound tract to rule out injury. Those that do not approach the carotid sheath or the midline do not need to be fully explored. If bilateral exploration is necessary, a modified collar-type incision, carried up along the sternocleidomastoid muscle on both sides, will allow complete bilateral exposure.

Intraoperative endoscopy is a very useful adjunct in cases in which there is a high suspicion of aerodigestive injury but no injury is immediately identified during surgical exploration. The ability to simultaneously observe the esophagus or trachea from both inside and outside allows the surgeon to most reliably identify an injury or exclude the possibility of injury.

Vascular Injuries

Vascular injuries are common in penetrating wounds of the neck, occurring in approximately 20% of cases. Blunt injuries to the carotid are relatively uncommon, accounting for only about 3% of all carotid injuries and comprising a small percentage of all patients with blunt neck injuries. The general approach to major vascular injuries in the neck is the same as that for vascular injuries elsewhere in the body.[23] In brief, hemostasis should be maintained by direct pressure or digital occlusion until proximal and distal control of the vessel can be obtained. If possible, proximal and distal control should be obtained before a large contained hematoma is entered. Arterial injuries should be débrided and repaired primarily, if possible. In most circumstances, primary repair will not be practical owing to loss of length, and a short interposition graft should be used. Choice of graft material should be based primarily on size match. Although there is a small theoretical preference for autologous vein, it is often difficult to find an appropriate match for the common carotid or proximal internal carotid. In practice, a correctly sized synthetic graft, usually of polytetrafluoroethylene, will be commonly used. Major injuries of the external carotid can be safely treated with ligation. Ligation of the common or internal carotid carries much more functional significance and should be done only for uncontrollable hemorrhage or if repair is technically impossible. The advisability of revascularization after a period of ischemia has been debated, but the concerns appear to be primarily theoretical. Existing clinical data show improved outcome with repair in all subsets of patients except those with frank coma, in whom both repair and ligation groups do poorly. Extracranial-intracranial bypass has been suggested in patients requiring ligation of the common or internal carotid artery, but experience is limited. Major venous injuries should be repaired primarily when practical and ligated under other circumstances. There is probably no role for interposition grafting to repair a unilateral internal jugular injury.

Airway Injuries

Penetrating injuries to the airway are either clinically overt, with bubbling and air movement through the wound, or they are found at the time of neck exploration done for other indications. In blunt laryngotracheal injuries, the diagnosis is generally established through a combination of neck CT, direct laryngoscopy, and bronchoscopy. Almost all tracheal lacerations and disruptions should be repaired. The need for operative intervention in laryngeal trauma is determined by the degree of anatomic derangement and the mucosal integrity in the larynx.

In general, tracheal injuries should be débrided and closed primarily. Simple lacerations of the trachea often can be repaired by direct suture. The use of nonabsorbable suture is often suggested, but absorbable suture can be used in this setting as well. If there is significant tissue loss, the trachea usually can be mobilized sufficiently to allow for the loss of about two tracheal rings without undue difficulty. Loss of a larger portion of trachea may necessitate tracheostomy or complex reconstructive procedures. Injuries of the larynx are treated with closure of mucosal lacerations and reduction of cartilaginous fractures. The structure of the larynx is important to glottic function, and careful anatomic reconstruction if possible, is critical. Injuries involving the larynx can be difficult to treat, and there is significant controversy regarding the timing of repair, operative technique, and the use of adjuncts such as stents or systemic corticosteroids.

Pharynx and Esophagus

Injuries of the esophagus present a difficult problem. If early diagnosis is made, primary surgical repair is usually possible. If the diagnosis is delayed for more than 12 hours, primary repair may be impractical, leaving diversion and drainage as the only alternative. The major morbidity and mortality associated with esophageal injuries is the result of delays in diagnosis. This underscores the necessity to aggressively exclude esophageal injury during initial evaluation of the patient with neck injury. Any positive findings mandate operative exploration.

The basic approach to injuries of the esophagus is to achieve primary repair of the majority of injuries. The esophagus must be sufficiently mobilized to allow full evaluation of the wound and careful débridement of devitalized tissue. The injury should be repaired primarily if possible, either by the one-layer or two-layer technique. If there is sufficient tissue loss to preclude primary repair, a cervical esophagostomy should be done as a temporizing measure, with plans for complex reconstruction of the esophagus after the initial trauma has resolved. A drain should be left in place after all esophageal repairs. Leakage from the repair is not an uncommon complication. If the fistula is well controlled, the clinical course is generally benign, whereas uncontrolled leakage into the neck can lead to devastating infection. In cases operated on after the first 12 hours, there is established infection and inflammation. Under these circumstances primary repair is usually impossible. Wide drainage is established, and flow of oropharyngeal secretions is diverted through a cervical esophagostomy. This course of action commits the patient to a complex reconstructive procedure after the initial trauma has resolved.

Injuries of the pharynx above the level of the constrictor muscles do not seem to be as critical as injuries of the esophagus. Pharyngeal injuries are treated with débridement and primary closure whenever practical. However, much of the pharynx, especially the posterior aspect, cannot be approached through the neck without great difficulty. In these areas, the mucosal lacerations can be closed from within the pharynx and the cervical area drained. The patient is generally kept NPO for 5 to 7 days. The majority of such wounds will heal without difficulty, and those that develop a fistula will generally heal if drainage is adequate. Isolated small pharyngeal lacerations do not mandate neck exploration if other cervical injuries have been ruled out.

Nerve Injury

There are many important nerves that run through the neck and are at risk, both from the primary injury and from operative attempts to repair the primary injury. It is important to document a full neurologic examination before operative intervention, including cranial nerve function, vocal cord function, and peripheral nerve function, whenever possible. In the routine course of neck exploration, it is critical to avoid injury to the main trunk of the vagus in the carotid sheath and to the recurrent laryngeal nerves that run in the tracheoesophageal groove. In addition, the marginal mandibular nerve is at risk in exploration of the upper aspect of the neck, under the angle of the mandible. Obvious primary injuries to major nerves should be noted. In the majority of trauma cases, primary repair of such injuries is impractical. In selected cases with clean transection of the nerve and no significant associated injuries, there may be a role for primary repair of the injured nerve.

Maxillofacial Injuries

Maxillofacial injuries are quite common and can have significant functional and cosmetic impact. Most maxillofacial injuries do not present with initial threat to life, and definitive evaluation and care are often deferred in patients with multiple injuries. Nevertheless, it is important to carefully evaluate and appropriately treat maxillofacial injuries in a timely fashion to optimize functional outcome and provide the best cosmetic result.

Resuscitative Priorities

Severe maxillofacial injuries have the potential to lead to airway obstruction, either as a direct result of anatomic derangement or secondarily due to the presence of blood and debris in the upper airway. These factors can make orotracheal intubation difficult or impossible, and the presence of significant midface injuries is an absolute contraindication to nasotracheal intubation. Immediate consideration must be given to the need for surgical airway in the course of initial resuscitation. If the patient has a patent airway, but is at risk, it is reasonable to consider an attempt at orotracheal intubation, but any significant difficulty in visualizing the cords, either due to anatomy or airway debris, should lead to immediate placement of a surgical airway.

Once the airway has been secured, the patient should be assessed for the presence of brisk ongoing bleeding from the oropharynx. Facial fractures can lead to significant hemorrhage from maxillary and palatine arteries,

which are branches of the external carotid artery. Basilar skull fracture can lead to injury to the internal carotid artery as well. Initial control should be obtained by anterior and posterior nasal packing as well as direct packing of the oropharynx. Careful packing will temporarily control maxillofacial bleeding in almost all cases. Direct surgical approach is difficult, leaving the options of angiography and selective embolization or ligation of the external carotid. In most circumstances, angiography and embolization will be the most efficacious.

All other injuries in the maxillofacial region, though potentially of great functional significance, do not present a threat to life. Major maxillofacial injuries often have a very dramatic appearance and can easily divert the attention of the resuscitation team. The physician must be careful to maintain the correct focus in the overall care of the patient and not be distracted by obvious injuries in the maxillofacial region until all potentially life-threatening problems in other body areas have been fully evaluated.

Evaluation of Injury Severity

During the primary survey, evaluation of the maxillofacial region is limited to evaluation and control of the airway and control of significant ongoing bleeding. All other diagnostic measures are of secondary importance and should not be undertaken until the patient is fully stabilized.

Physical examination of the face should include a careful evaluation of all lacerations, noting depth and proximity to functionally important structures such as the main parotid duct or the lacrimal apparatus. The bony structure of the face should be palpated, feeling for obvious deformity or bony stepoffs. In a cooperative patient, a careful neurologic examination, including function of all cranial nerves and facial motor nerves, should be conducted. The eyes should be carefully examined, assessing visual acuity as well as evidence of injury to the globe itself. Signs suggestive of globe injury include hyphema, scleral lacerations, and deformity of the globe. Extraocular movement is carefully assessed as well. The stability of the bite and presence of malocclusion are also of importance.

The diagnosis of facial fractures is now largely done through the use of computed tomography (CT). CT of the face is far more accurate than plain radiographs in determining the presence and significance of fractures of the facial bones (Fig. 20-8). Obvious fractures can be seen on the lower cuts of the CT performed for the evaluation of head trauma, and important suggestive findings, such as opacification of the maxillary or ethmoidal sinuses, also can be seen. To fully evaluate the bony structure of the face, CT is performed in a coronal plane, using 1-mm cuts. This requires that the patient be able to flex and extend the cervical spine and also requires a relatively long scanning time. Neither condition is often met in the early care of patients with significant associated injuries, and full delineation of maxillofacial fracture often must be deferred.

Fractures of the maxilla are classified as according to a system proposed by Le Fort in 1901. There are three types, Le Fort I, II, or III (Fig. 20-9), determined by the type and location of fractures. In a Le Fort I fracture (also

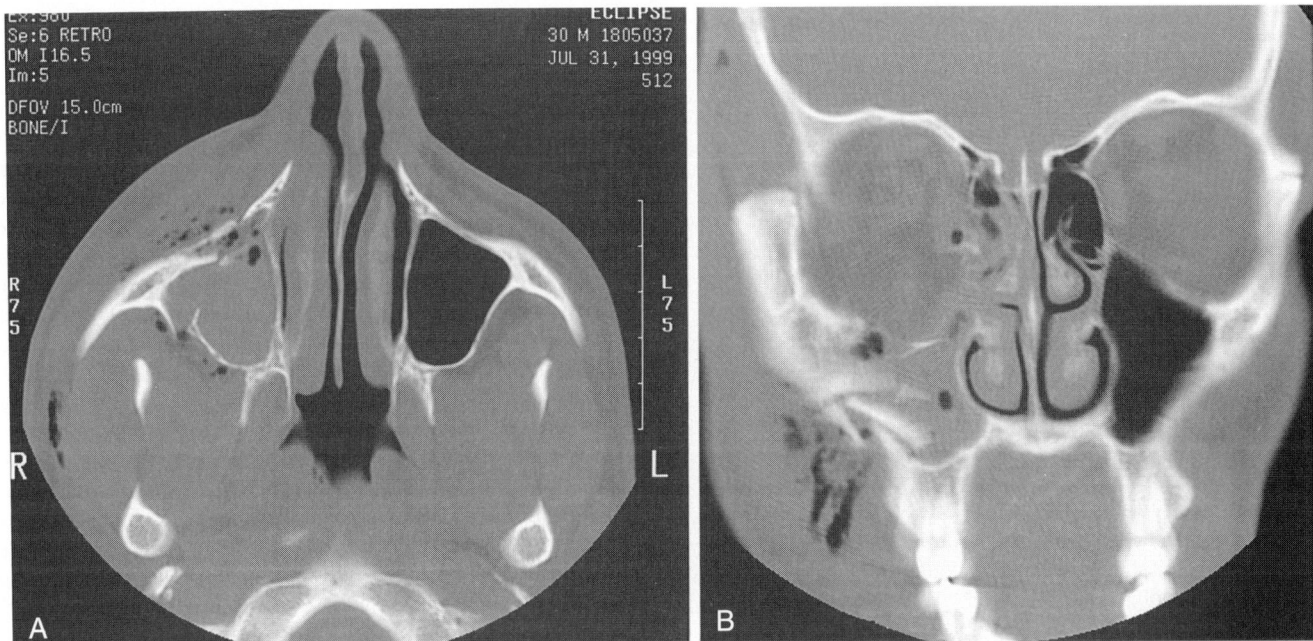

FIGURE 20-8. Use of CT for diagnosis of facial fractures. Axial views (**A**) and coronal views (**B**) demonstrate complex fractures involving the right maxilla as well as lateral, inferior, and medial walls of the right orbit. Note opacification of the maxillary and ethmoidal sinuses.

known as Guérin's fracture, or dentoalveolar dysjunction), the fracture lines are transverse through the pyriform aperture above the alveolar ridge and run posteriorly to the pterygoid region. The dental alveolar supporting bone and palate of the maxilla are involved as a single detached block. In Le Fort II fractures, the superior fracture lines are transverse through the nasal bones or through the articulation of the maxillary and nasal bones with the frontal bones. The fracture line extends laterally from that superior point into the medial orbital wall, travels through the lacrimal and ethmoid bones, and exits the orbital floor

anteriorly at the medial to middle portions of the infraorbital rim. Occasionally, the right and left maxilla are completely separated at the midline of the hard palate, with each unit containing maxillary and palatal bones. This fracture line, or palatal split, may splay the maxillary alveolar ridge laterally and outside the occlusal arch of the mandible. The Le Fort III fracture is the highest level of midface injury. The central third of the face is literally displaced from its attachments to the cranial base. The transverse superior fracture line is similar to that of the Le Fort II fracture, but at the medial orbital wall it extends pos-

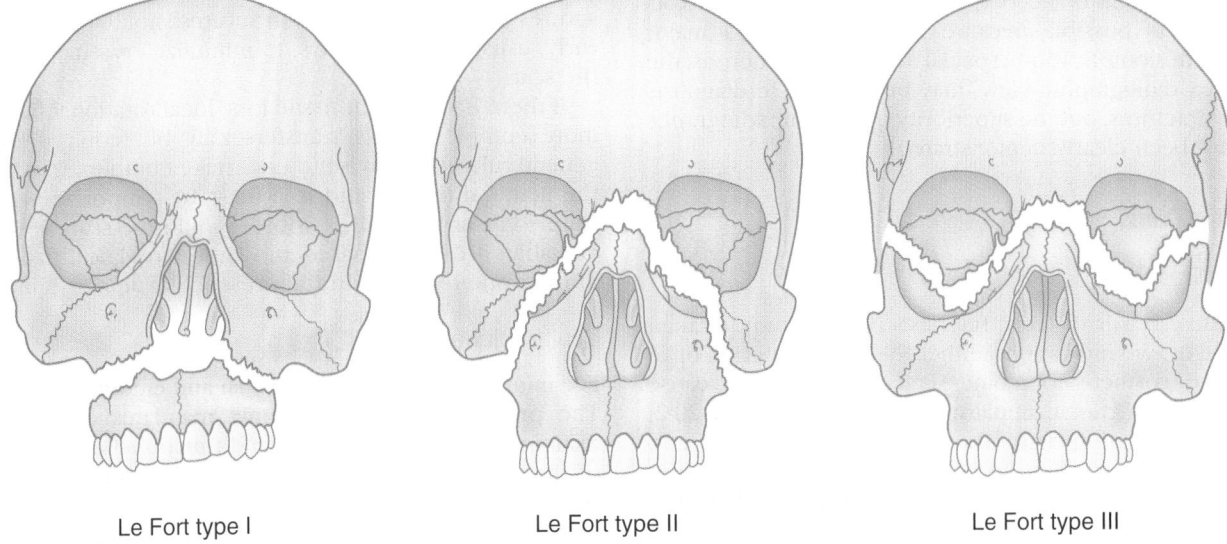

Le Fort type I   Le Fort type II   Le Fort type III

FIGURE 20-9. Le Fort I, II, and III fracture lines as seen in frontal view.

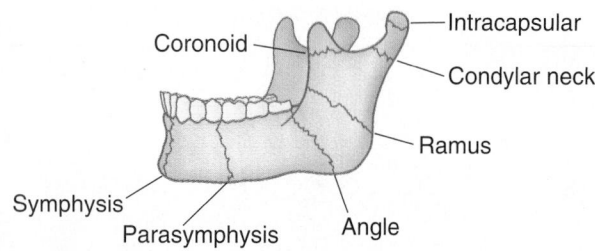

FIGURE 20-10. Anatomy of the mandible and common lines of fracture.

Box 20-2 Facial Fractures of Functional Significance

Fracture Type	Functional Impairment
Blowout fracture of muscles inferior orbital floor	Entrapment of extra-ocular muscles
Maxilla, alveolar ridge	Malocclusion
Mandible	Malocclusion
Depressed zygomatic arch fracture	Entrapment of temporalis muscle

---

teriorly or laterally, rather than anteriorly, and continues across the orbital floor to the inferior orbital fissure. From that point, the lines run through the lateral orbital wall and rim to the pterygoid fossa, zygomatic arch, and pterygoid process. An important component is a fracture line through the septum and the perpendicular plate of the ethmoid. This fracture may extend into the cribriform plate of the anterior cranial fossa and produce cerebrospinal fluid rhinorrhea.

Fractures of the mandible are also classified by anatomic location (Fig. 20-10). The need for surgical intervention and its nature are determined by the type and location of the fracture, so complete radiographic evaluation is important. Reduction and fixation of mandibular fractures should be accomplished as precisely and expeditiously as possible because malocclusion is a major long-term complication. Special techniques, such as the Panorex radiographic view, may be valuable in diagnosis of jaw fractures, but the superiority over plain radiographs has not been clearly demonstrated.

Definitive Care

Facial Fractures

Operative repair of facial fractures is usually undertaken for one of two indications, either to restore function or to improve cosmetic outcome. Fractures that can cause significant functional impairment are listed in Box 20-2. The determination that a fracture must be fixed for cosmetic reasons is often an aesthetic one and sometimes cannot be made until significant facial swelling has decreased. Because there are no compelling physiologic indications, many of these operations will be undertaken late in the course, after acute injury and swelling have decreased.

Facial fractures are stabilized internally, using fine screws and plates. Bone graft may be required if there is bone loss or a high degree of comminution. External fixators are occasionally used for fractures of the mandible. In some circumstances, intermaxillary fixation alone provides sufficient stabilization of fracture fragments, without the need for formal internal fixation. Fractures in the upper portion of the face, involving the frontal and upper ethmoidal sinuses, may extend into the cranium and involve the dura. Under these circumstances, operative repair should be done in conjunction with neurosurgical intervention.

Optimal timing of operation is controversial. Some advocate early fixation, citing minimal edema formation, shorter hospital stay, and decreased patient discomfort. Others opt to provide operative fixation later in the hospital course, after facial edema has resolved and full diagnostic evaluation has been completed. In patients with severe associated injuries, the low priority of facial reconstruction often mandates a delayed approach.

Facial Lacerations

Facial lacerations are quite common and must be treated carefully because of their cosmetic significance and because of the danger to underlying structures. All lacerations should be carefully evaluated before closure. It is important to determine if deeper structures are at risk and to identify any such injuries before closure of the laceration. Examples would include involvement of the facial nerve or parotid duct with injuries in the preauricular and cheek region, involvement of the nasolacrimal system in the medial orbit, through-and-through lacerations of the cheek and lip, or injuries involving the tarsal plate in the eyelid.

In general, facial lacerations should be carefully cleaned and gently débrided of obviously devitalized tissue. In most circumstances, primary closure is done, using deep stitches as required and using fine, carefully placed sutures in the skin. These skin sutures should be removed early, usually within 3 days, to minimize crosshatching of the scar.

If there is significant tissue loss, local rotational flaps or more complex tissue transfers may be required. As a general rule, it is unwise to undertake complex repairs in the acute situation, and it is best to temporize with a simple closure if at all possible. Should the scar be unacceptable, it can be revised at a later date. Local flaps are more prone to failure in the presence of acute trauma.

Ocular Injuries

Eye injuries have a high functional and emotional impact. The presence of ocular trauma mandates a thorough examination of the structural and functional components of the eye. Patients with maxillofacial trauma may have significant periorbital soft tissue edema. Although difficult to perform, the initial ophthalmologic examination may be the only examination obtained until the edema resolves. Removal of contact lenses and debris and examination of the anterior structures of the eye may reveal proptosis, hyphema, corneal abrasions, or lacerations. The globe may be lacerated or ruptured. Compression of the optic nerve due to bone fragments, retinal detachment, vitreous hemorrhage, and acute traumatic glaucoma should be identified and treated. A functional eye examination includes visual acuity testing, pupillary response, and assessment of extraocular eye movements.

Severe blunt trauma may result in an orbital hematoma, proptosis, and an elevation of the intraocular pressure. Penetrating eye injuries are more serious as the injury extends more posteriorly. Simple lacerations to the cornea, lens, or anterior chamber may be repaired using microsurgical techniques. Rupture of the globe requires débridement and suture repair. Early in the examination it is imperative to identify conditions that may lead to blindness if untreated. Traumatic glaucoma, central retinal occlusion, and optic nerve compression are examples of this. In the worst case, traumatic blindness may result from a serious eye injury. Traumatic optic neuropathy may be detected by the presence of an afferent papillary defect. High doses of corticosteroids are recommended in these patients. Those patients with optic nerve compression may benefit from high doses of corticosteroids or bony decompression depending on the location of the orbital fracture fragments. Patients presenting with complete blindness without a correctable etiology are typically followed for a number of days before the decision to enucleate the eye is made. A rare, but devastating complication of unilateral traumatic blindness is sympathetic ophthalmia. This is a bilateral inflammatory condition initiated by the injured eye. It may progress and damage the contralateral eye and result in blindness. Enucleation of an injured blind eye is usually performed within 2 weeks to avoid this problem.

Repair of the periorbital structures such as the eyelid, lacrimal duct, and canaliculus should be meticulous to preserve functional integrity. A lateral canthotomy may be indicated in those patients with acute posterior orbital hematoma resulting in elevated intraocular pressures. Inferior orbital wall fractures should raise the possibility of entrapment of the inferior oblique and rectus muscles. A slightly retracted and downward gaze of the involved globe is typical of this injury. Early recognition of serious ocular trauma followed by ophthalmologic consultation is essential for the preservation of function and vision.

Thoracic Trauma

Thoracic injuries account for 20% to 25% of all trauma-related deaths, and complications of chest trauma contribute to another 25% of all deaths. Considering immediate deaths after motor vehicles accidents, the most frequent injuries leading to a fatal outcome include blunt cardiac injuries with chamber disruption and injuries to the thoracic aorta. Early deaths (within the golden hour) are caused by airway obstruction, major respiratory problems (e.g., tension pneumothorax), massive hemothorax, and cardiac tamponade. These clinical situations are easily managed if recognized promptly. Chest wall trauma is the most frequent injury after blunt thoracic trauma. The majority of thoracic injuries are managed with simple procedures such as clinical observation, thoracentesis, respiratory support, and adequate analgesia. The remaining 15% to 20% of patients sustaining chest trauma will require a thoracotomy for definitive repair of major intrathoracic injuries.

Pathophysiology

The pathophysiology of chest trauma includes three factors: hypoxia, hypercarbia, and acidosis. Hypoxia can be caused by airway obstruction, changes in intrathoracic pressure, ventilation-perfusion mismatches, and hypovolemia. Hypercarbia is caused by inadequate ventilation, either due to the presence of a collapsed lung, associated head injuries with altered mental status, or exogenous intoxication (drugs and alcohol). Acidosis is caused mainly by hypoperfusion due to blood loss.

Initial Evaluation

The initial evaluation of a patient sustaining chest trauma follows the same principles and guidelines outlined under advanced trauma life support. The first priority is the maintenance of a patent airway. This may be obtained by simply repositioning the head, anteriorizing the mandible (chin lift and jaw thrust), or removing foreign bodies from the oropharynx. Some patients with more severe injuries or with severe head injuries will require tracheal intubation either by a nasal or oral route or by means of a surgical airway. The physical examination of the chest is extremely important in identifying life-threatening situations that will require immediate attention. These include tension pneumothorax, massive hemothorax, open pneumothorax, flail chest, and cardiac tamponade.

The chest radiograph is of the utmost importance in thoracic trauma; however, the just-mentioned life-threatening injuries preclude the necessity of a chest radiograph for diagnosis and should be identified clinically. The chest radiograph is useful to identify pneumothorax, hemothorax, rib fractures, widened mediastinum, pneumomediastinum, and clavicular and scapular fractures. Other diagnostic modalities include ultrasound, chest CT, esophagography, esophagoscopy, bronchoscopy, and angiography.

The use of ultrasound in the evaluation of chest trauma has been less frequent than for abdominal trauma. However, recent reports have shown that the pleural spaces can be evaluated by ultrasound to diagnose or exclude hemothorax and pneumothorax. Two ultrasonographic signs have been used to rule out pneumothorax. One is the lung sliding sign, which is a to-and-fro movement of the hyperechoic line between the chest wall and aerated lung with respiration. The other is the "comet-tail artifacts," which are ray-like hyperechoic reverberation artifacts that arise from the visceral pleural line and spread to the edge of the screen, indicating the absence of a pneumothorax.[24]

With the development of the helical scanners, CT has been used more liberally in the evaluation of chest trauma and some authors have recommended its routine use despite the results of plain chest films.

The routine use of CT in the evaluation of blunt chest injury was recently evaluated in 93 patients. In 25 patients the chest radiograph was normal and chest CT identified multiple injuries in 13 (52%), including two aortic lacerations, three pleural effusions, and one pericardial effusion. The routine use of helical CT in patients with high-risk deceleration injuries in the chest has also been proposed. The accuracy of CT is higher when compared with plain chest radiographs. However, CT may diagnose minor injuries unappreciated by plain films but without clinical significance. Further prospective studies are necessary to decide whether routine CT is cost effective after blunt chest trauma.

Tube Thoracostomy

Tube thoracostomy is the most common procedure performed in the management of thoracic trauma. In fact, 85% of the patients sustaining chest injuries will require only clinical observation or tube thoracostomy. A large-bore (36 to 40 French) chest tube should be used in adolescents and adult patients. The proper site of insertion is in the fifth or sixth intercostal space in the midaxillary line. The index finger should be inserted into the pleural space before tube placement to ensure that the pleural cavity has been entered and is free of adhesions and that intra-abdominal organs have not herniated through the diaphragm. The tube should be advanced posteriorly and superiorly in the pleural cavity. After insertion, the tube should be secured in the skin of the chest wall and connected to a collection system under suction. A chest radiograph is usually obtained after chest tube insertion to confirm adequate placement and positioning. General criteria for chest tube removal include absence of air leak and less than 100 mL of fluid drainage over a 24-hour period.

Thoracotomy

An emergent thoracotomy is indicated after chest trauma in the following situations: (1) cardiac arrest (resuscitative thoracotomy), (2) massive hemothorax (greater than 1500 mL of blood through the chest tube acutely or greater than 200 to 300 mL/hr after initial drainage), (3) penetrating injuries of the anterior chest with cardiac tamponade, (4) large open wounds of the thoracic cage, (5) major thoracic vascular injuries in the presence of hemodynamic instability, (6) major tracheobronchial injuries, and (7) evidence of esophageal perforation.

Nonemergent indications for thoracotomy include (1) empyema not resolved with tube thoracostomy, (2) clotted hemothorax, (3) lung abscess, (4) thoracic duct injuries, (5) tracheoesophageal fistulas, and (6) chronic sequelae of vascular injuries (pseudoaneurysms and arteriovenous fistulas).

Specific Injuries

Rib Fractures

Rib fractures are the most common injuries after blunt chest injuries. Ribs 4 through 10 are usually fractured. One or two rib fractures without pleural or lung involvement are usually treated on an outpatient basis. However, in the elderly, owing to decreased bone density, reduced chest wall compliance, and increased incidence of underlying parenchymal disease, rib fractures may lead to decreased ability to cough, reduced vital capacity, and infectious complications. Pain on inspiration is usually the primary clinical manifestation after rib fractures. Other clinical signs associated with rib fractures include tenderness to palpation and crepitus. Rib fractures are confirmed with a chest radiograph (Fig. 20-11).

Poor pain control significantly contributes to complications such as atelectasis and pneumonia. Pain control is attempted initially with oral or intravenous analgesics. Intercostal nerve blocks with bupivacaine are effective for pain control; however, it is not feasible for multiple fractures and it requires frequent injections. Epidural analgesia is adequate for patients with multiple or bilateral fractures and provides adequate pain control and appropriate pulmonary toilette, decreasing the number of complications.

Multiple rib fractures are the hallmark of a severe trauma due to high-energy transfer. Patients with multiple rib fractures should have intrathoracic and abdominal injuries investigated. In fact, fractures of the lower ribs (9 through 12) are associated with an increased incidence of hepatic and splenic injuries, and fractures of the upper ribs (1 through 3), clavicle, or scapula are associated with major vascular injury.

Flail Chest

By definition, a flail chest occurs in the presence of two or more fractures in three or more consecutive ribs,

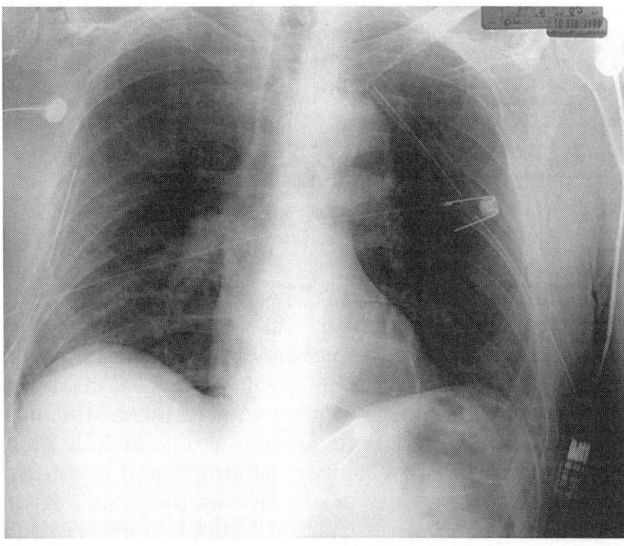

FIGURE 20-11. Chest radiograph shows multiple rib fractures.

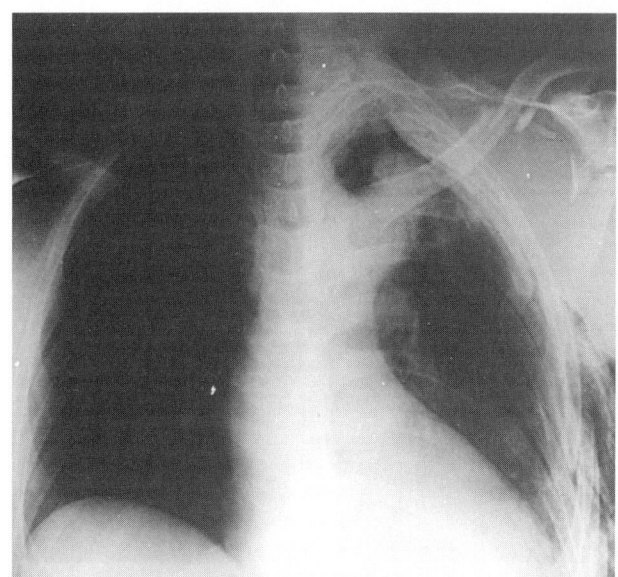

FIGURE 20-12. Chest radiograph shows a flail chest.

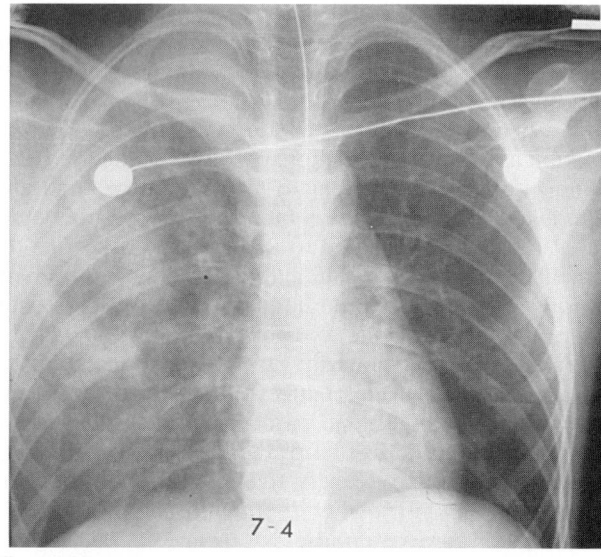

FIGURE 20-13. Chest radiograph shows a pulmonary contusion.

causing instability of the chest wall; however, it can also occur after costochondral separation (Fig. 20-12). It is characterized by paradoxical motion of the chest wall (inward with inspiration and outward with expiration). Fractures can be located in the anterior, lateral, or posterior chest wall. Flail chest occurs in 10% to 15% of patients sustaining major chest trauma, and the chance of having an intrathoracic injury in this situation increases several-fold. Closed-head injury is the most frequently associated extrathoracic injury, contributing to higher morbidity and mortality rates. Isolated flail chest carries a low mortality rate in younger patients.

The paradoxical motion increases the work of breathing, and the most important consequence of flail chest is respiratory failure. Until recently, it was believed that ineffective air movement between both lungs caused by the paradoxical motion of the chest wall was the main cause of respiratory distress. It is now understood that underlying pulmonary contusion and pain during inspiration are the most important components in the pathophysiology of respiratory failure (Fig. 20-13). Sequential measurements of forced vital capacity, tidal volume, and inspiratory force are useful to predict which patients will require ventilatory support. The pathophysiologic effects may be present immediately or may progress over several hours and present as late respiratory decompensation.

Care should be taken not to fluid overload these patients because it may further impair respiratory function. Patients without evidence of respiratory distress can be managed only with analgesia. Pain control can be provided by intercostal nerve block or more adequately by epidural anesthesia.

If respiratory distress develops, endotracheal intubation and mechanical ventilation with peak-end expiratory pressure (PEEP) are usually indicated, provided pain control is adequate. Open reduction and internal fixation of sternal or rib fractures is rarely needed.

Sternal Fractures

Although rare, sternal fractures may occur after motor vehicle accidents. The presence of a fractured sternum implies a significant trauma to the anterior chest wall with high-energy transfer. Signs and symptoms include chest pain, particularly over the sternum, and crepitus. A hematoma over the sternum may be seen eventually (caused by the steering wheel) or across the chest (seat belt sign). A lateral radiograph should be obtained in these circumstances and usually confirms the diagnosis. Sternal fractures also constitute a marker for serious associated injuries, including myocardial contusion, myocardial rupture, esophageal perforation, airway injury, and thoracic aortic rupture.

Treatment is usually conservative, although patients with significant chest wall instability may require open reduction and internal fixation.

Pulmonary Contusion

Pulmonary contusion occurs more frequently after blunt chest trauma; however, penetrating injuries may also cause significant lung parenchymal contusions. This has been defined as a pathologic state in which hemorrhage and edema of the lung parenchyma occur without parenchymal disruption. Mortality rates vary according to age, associated injuries, and chronic underlying lung disease. Pathophysiology involves decreased lung compliance and the development of ventilation-perfusion mismatch, leading to hypoxemia and increased work of breathing.

Respiratory failure occurs more often in patients with large contusions, in the elderly, and in those with underlying chronic lung disease, aggravated by inadequate pain control. Diagnosis is confirmed by low PaO_2 and by a chest radiograph demonstrating a well-defined infiltrate underlying the contused area on the chest wall. It is important to realize, however, that radiologic findings may not be present on admission and may develop 24 to 48 hours after the initial injury. Pulmonary contusion may be confused with the adult respiratory distress syndrome or may even be associated with it.

Management is directed toward maintaining good oxygenation and adequate pulmonary toilette. Judicious crystalloid infusion is important to avoid fluid overload and pulmonary edema; however, intravascular volume depletion also should be avoided to decrease the risk of global ischemia and multiple organ failure. Patients with persistent low PaO_2 levels who do not respond to supplemental oxygen, pulmonary toilette, and pain control should be intubated and mechanically ventilated. Correction of acute anemia and coagulopathy, by means of transfusing packed red blood cells and blood products, is important to minimize blood loss and increase oxygen-carrying capacity and oxygen delivery to the tissues. No benefits have been demonstrated with the use of prophylactic antibiotics or corticosteroids.

Pneumonia is the most frequent complication, particularly in the elderly, aggravating chronic lung diseases, increasing ventilator days, and significantly contributing to mortality.

Pneumothorax

A pneumothorax occurs when air from an injured lung or airway is trapped within the pleural cavity, increasing the normal negative intrapleural pressure. It may be caused by penetrating or blunt mechanisms. After blunt trauma, pneumothorax is caused by rib fractures penetrating the lung parenchyma or by lung injuries without chest wall involvement. Deceleration injuries and sudden increases in intrathoracic pressure also may cause pneumothorax.

Clinical findings suggestive of a pneumothorax include decreased breath sounds, hyperresonance to percussion, and decreased expansion of the affected lung during inspiration. Pneumothoraces are classified according to the volume of lung loss or collapse identified on chest radiography or by respiratory and systemic signs. In a small pneumothorax, the volume loss is one third of the normal lung volume. In a large pneumothorax, the lung is completely collapsed but there is no mediastinal shift or associated hypotension. A tension pneumothorax is characterized by complete lung collapse, tracheal deviation, mediastinal shift leading to decreased venous return to the heart, hypotension, and respiratory distress. It usually occurs in patients with parenchymal lung injury under positive-pressure ventilation (Fig. 20-14). Clinical signs and symptoms include dyspnea, tachypnea, hypotension, diaphoresis, and distended neck veins. It is diagnosed clinically, constituting a life-threatening emergency. Chest radiographs are not necessary to confirm the diagnosis, and delays to definitive treatment significantly increase the risk of circulatory collapse and cardiorespiratory arrest. Treatment includes chest decompression initially with a large-bore needle inserted in the second intercostal space on the midclavicular line and subsequent tube thoracostomy. Re-expansion of the lung and reapproximation of the pleural surfaces usually seal the lung defect. All patients with a pneumothorax, regardless of its size,

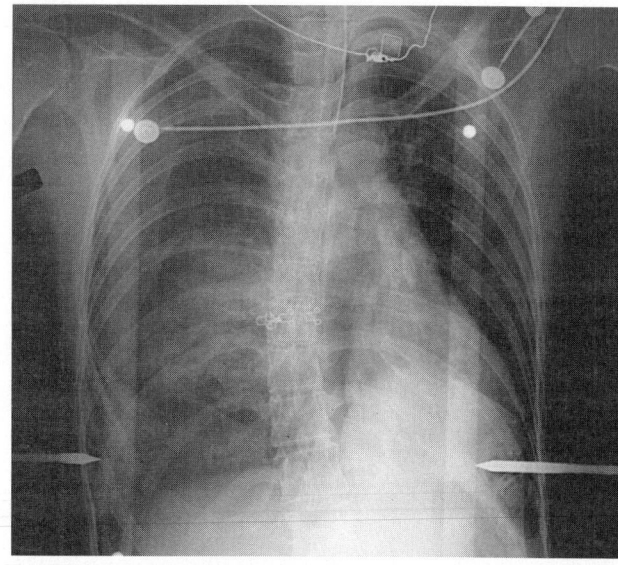

FIGURE 20-14. Chest radiograph shows a right pneumothorax.

who will undergo positive-pressure ventilation should have a chest tube placed before the start of mechanical ventilation.

Open Pneumothorax

Open pneumothorax, also known as sucking chest wound, occurs when there is a significant defect in the chest wall (e.g., large-caliber gunshot wounds, traumatic thoracotomy) large enough to exceed the laryngeal cross-sectional area, allowing the air to enter from the exterior into the pleural cavity and leading to lung collapse due to a rapid equilibration between the intrathoracic (pleural) pressure and the atmospheric pressure. The increased intrathoracic pressure also causes mediastinal shift and decreased venous return. Signs and symptoms include hypoxia, hypercarbia, hypotension, and respiratory and circulatory failure.

Management includes applying an occlusive dressing and placement of a chest tube before closure of the chest wall defect to avoid the development of a tension pneumothorax.

Hemothorax

Blood may accumulate in the pleural cavity after blunt or penetrating injuries. Depending on the nature of the injury, bleeding may vary from minor to massive. Symptoms depend on the amount of blood accumulated in the pleural space. On physical examination, breath sounds may be decreased on the side of the injury. A chest radiograph obtained in the supine position may reveal accumulations of blood greater than 200 mL; however, a supine film may demonstrate a diffuse haziness or none at all. The pleural space can accumulate up to 3 L of blood. Massive hemothorax is usually the result of major pulmonary vascular injury or major arterial wounds, whereas minor lung injuries cause a small hemothorax (Fig. 20-15).

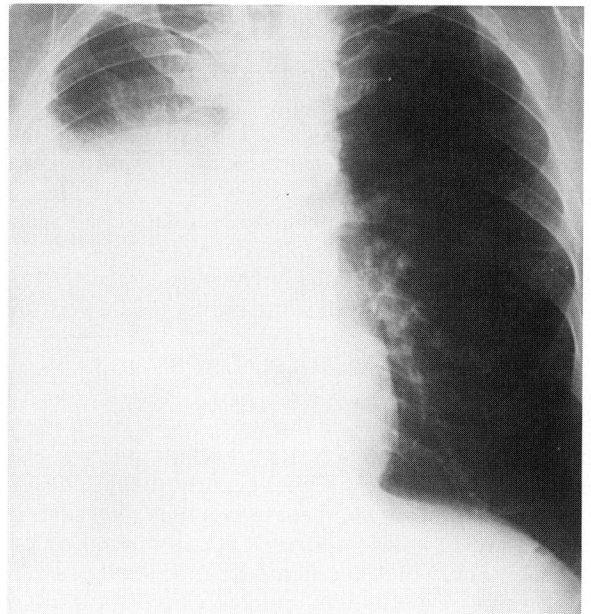

FIGURE 20-15.   Chest radiograph shows a right hemothorax.

Hemothoraces are initially treated by chest tube placement (36 French), and in approximately 85% of the cases, the bleeding will stop as the lung is re-expanded owing to the low pressure in the systemic circulation. A small number of cases will have continued bleeding and will require a thoracotomy. These are usually injuries in systemic arteries (intercostal arteries or internal mammary artery) or veins or major pulmonary vessels or are cardiac in origin, and autotransfusion should be considered in these circumstances.

As previously described, indications for emergent thoracotomy are initial chest tube output of 1500 mL of blood or persistent drainage of 200 to 300 mL/hr.

Pulmonary Parenchyma Injury

Simple lacerations of the lung are common after penetrating injuries and rare after blunt trauma. Patients usually present with variable degrees of pneumothorax and hemothorax. Management usually includes chest tube placement to drain blood collection in the pleural space and re-expand the lung.

Occasionally, some patients will develop major and persistent air leaks. This situation is sometimes identified immediately after chest tube placement but may be more evident when mechanical ventilation with positive pressure is started. Massive air leaks should raise suspicion for major tracheal bronchial injuries.

Although less than 10% of patients with severe chest injuries will require thoracotomy and some degree of pulmonary resection, recent studies have reported better results with lung-sparing techniques (nonanatomic resections and tractotomy) than with formal lobectomy or pneumonectomy.[25,26]

Massive hemorrhage from extensive lung injuries can be treated by oversewing or stapling the wound or, more rarely, by performing wedging or lobar resections.[27]

Gunshot wounds causing through-and-through injuries to the lung can be managed by opening up the missile trajectory (tractotomy), communicating with both entrance and exit wounds to obtain hemostasis. Wedge resections of peripheral injuries to the lung parenchyma that is actively bleeding can be accomplished by using staples. Complications associated with large injuries in the lung parenchyma, as well as after tractotomy include increased bleeding and air embolism, which may be controlled by stapling the lung parenchyma. Air embolism can be minimized by decreasing the peak inspiratory pressure and cross clamping the pulmonary hilum.

Tracheobronchial Injuries

Tracheobronchial injuries are uncommon. Most patients with these injuries die at the scene or during transport because of poor ventilation and severe associated injuries. Blunt injuries occur after direct compression of the airway with a closed glottis or after decelerating injuries causing partial or complete avulsion of the right mainstem bronchus from the carina or tracheal lacerations. Penetrating wounds may cause tracheobronchial injuries at any level.

Patients may present with pneumothorax, massive air leak, subcutaneous emphysema, hemoptysis, pneumomediastinum, and respiratory distress. Bronchoscopy is always required if one of these signs is present and should be performed, ideally, before intubation. Minor injuries of the upper airway after blunt trauma should be treated by placing the endotracheal tube beyond the injury. If this is not possible, a tracheostomy should be performed.

More extensive wounds, greater than one third of the circumference of the airway, are primarily repaired after the contralateral bronchus has been selectively intubated.

Small injuries usually heal spontaneously; however, late complications such as stricture formation at the injury site, recurrent pulmonary infection, and atelectasis may occur.

Blunt Cardiac Injuries

Significant trauma to the anterior chest wall may cause injury to the heart. Blunt cardiac injury encompasses a wide spectrum of injuries from contusion of the cardiac wall to cardiac chamber or valvular rupture. Most patients sustaining rupture of cardiac chambers do not reach the hospital alive; however, it should be suspected in patients sustaining severe chest trauma who develop pericardial tamponade. The right ventricle is most frequently involved, owing to its proximity to the sternum.

Myocardial contusion may occur in less severe chest trauma. Its definition, diagnosis, clinical significance, and management are still subject to debate. It has been estimated that 15% to 20% of patients sustaining severe chest trauma have some degree of cardiac involvement. Small myocardial contusions may produce wall motion abnormalities and lead to the development of arrhythmias. There are no classic findings suggestive of myocardial contusion, and there is no consensus in terms of diagnostic criteria. Increased central venous pressure in the absence of obvious cause may indicate right ventricular dysfunction secondary to cardiac contusion, provided the appropriate mechanism has occurred. The electrocardiogram (ECG) is the first diagnostic test. Patients are usually monitored for a period varying from 8 to 24 hours. If the initial ECG is normal, no further work-up is usually necessary. The most frequent arrhythmias are ST segment and T wave changes and sinus tachycardia. Right bundle branch block is common. Supraventricular and ventricular arrhythmias should be treated accordingly in an ICU setting. Measurements of the MB band of creatine kinase (CK), expressed as a percentage of the total CK, has been used as a diagnostic tool. The specificity of this test is low, because other muscle injuries can falsely elevate the MF band. A two-dimensional echocardiogram may demonstrate a wall motion abnormality, but its clinical significance without hemodynamic instability or arrhythmias is unknown. Radionuclide scans may be more specific than the just-described methods, but these are impractical in clinical use.

Recently, the combination of electrocardiography and serum troponin I (TnI) levels was evaluated as predictors of blunt cardiac injury in 333 consecutive patients sustaining blunt chest trauma. Significant blunt cardiac injury as defined by the presence of cardiogenic shock, arrhythmias requiring treatment, or post-traumatic structural deficits was diagnosed in 44 patients. Of 80 patients with an abnormal ECG and TnI, 27 developed significant blunt cardiac injury. Of patients with an abnormal ECG, only 22% developed significant blunt cardiac injury. The same occurred in 7% of those with altered TnI. If the admission ECG or TnI was abnormal, 43 of 44 patients developed significant blunt cardiac injury. The only patient with significant blunt cardiac injury and normal ECG and TnI on admission had an abnormal test 8 hours after admission. The combination of ECG and TnI at admission and 8 hours after injury rules out the diagnosis of significant blunt cardiac injury. Patients with normal tests at both times can be safely discharged from the hospital.[28]

Recently, the short-term and long-term prognosis of blunt myocardial injury was investigated prospectively in 118 patients sustaining blunt chest trauma. Fourteen patients met the diagnostic criteria of blunt cardiac injury, and none developed acute cardiac complications. Long-term follow-up (12 months) by exercise testing revealed no ECG abnormalities or exercise limitations.

Penetrating Cardiac Injuries

Penetrating cardiac injuries are still a great challenge for trauma surgeons. Adequate prehospital care, rapid transportation, aggressive resuscitation, immediate diagnosis, and prompt treatment are of fundamental importance and constitute the basis for improvements in survival rates in the past decade. All patients with penetrating injuries within an area determined by the midclavicular line bilaterally, a line at the level of the clavicles superiorly, and a line at the level of the costal margins inferiorly potentially have a cardiac injury until proven otherwise.

Hemodynamically unstable patients should be taken to the operating room for an emergent thoracotomy. Stable patients should have a chest radiograph to identify other injuries and to determine the trajectory of the missile in the case of gunshot wounds. Diagnosis usually is made by echocardiography, identifying abnormal amounts of pericardial fluid, or more accurately by performing a subxiphoid pericardial window. If the result is positive, a median sternotomy is performed for definitive cardiac repair.

Sequelae or complications after cardiac repair include valvular insufficiency or septal defects. Repair of these acquired lesions may involve valve replacement or repair or patch closure of septal lesions and should be performed at a later time.

Mortality rates vary from 8.5% to 81.3%. Approximately 80% of all patients sustaining a penetrating injury to the heart die at the scene or during transportation. Of the remaining 20% who reach the hospital with any sign of life, mortality is still very high. Recently, many series have reported a significant decrease in mortality rates after penetrating cardiac injuries. Survival is determined by many factors, among which the hemodynamic status on admission, prompt resuscitation, and aggressive application of emergency department thoracotomy for patients in extremis have gained special emphasis.

Lack of standardization regarding terminology and injury classification has lead to discrepancies in the results reported in the literature.[29] An index for the quantification of anatomic severity in penetrating cardiac injuries associated with a physiologic index has been proposed.

Mortality is directly related to the mechanism of injury. Victims of gunshot wounds have more severe physiologic impairment than those with stab wounds. Gunshot wounds cause larger defects in the myocardium, through-and-through wounds, and a larger number of injuries in other vital organs leading to hemorrhage and exsanguination. Stab wounds are more likely to produce small injuries that seal off during systole, leading to cardiac tamponade.

The presence of shock or hemodynamic instability has been cited as an important determinant of mortality. The characterization of the physiologic status on admission using a score such as the RTS seems to be more appropriate.[29] The survival rate is greater than 70% if vital signs are present on admission.

Pericardial tamponade must be suspected in all patients sustaining penetrating injuries to the anterior chest. Classic signs of pericardial tamponade include muffled heart tones, distended neck veins, and hypotension, also known as Beck's triad. All these signs are present in 30% to 40% of patients with a cardiac injury. Neck vein distention reflects increases in central venous pressure and is the most useful clinical sign; however, hypotensive patients with associated injuries may not have neck vein distention because of excessive blood loss. Volume resuscitation transiently improves cardiac output by increasing venous return; however, treatment consists of evacuating small amounts of blood (pericardiocentesis), followed by immediate repair of the underlying injury. It is generally agreed, at least, that tamponade is more frequent in stab wounds. It seems reasonable to assume that tamponade leads to "temporary" hemodynamic compensation, playing a role in survival.

Diaphragmatic Injuries

Diaphragmatic injuries are often caused by penetrating injuries. Patients sustaining penetrating injuries below the nipples and above the costal margins should be investigated to rule out diaphragmatic injury. The work-up includes peritoneal lavage in those with stab wounds to the epigastrium, thoracoscopy in patients with hemothorax or pneumothorax, or laparoscopy in those with a normal chest radiograph and an external wound in the thoracoabdominal transition. Chest and abdominal radiographs should be obtained in hemodynamically stable patients sustaining a gunshot wound in an attempt to determine the trajectory of the missile. If the bullet is in the abdomen, the patient will undergo an exploratory laparotomy and the diagnosis of a diaphragmatic injury will be done intraoperatively.

After blunt trauma, injury to the diaphragm involves both sides equally, as reported in autopsy and CT studies, although in clinical practice left-sided injuries are more frequent. The diagnosis is suspected when respiratory distress develops after a severe blow to the abdomen without apparent chest injury or when an upright chest radiograph demonstrates visceral herniation. In fact, herniation of intra-abdominal contents may not occur immediately or may not be evident on initial chest radiography, delaying the diagnosis. Herniation occurs due to the pressure differential between the thoracic and abdominal cavity (Fig. 20-16).

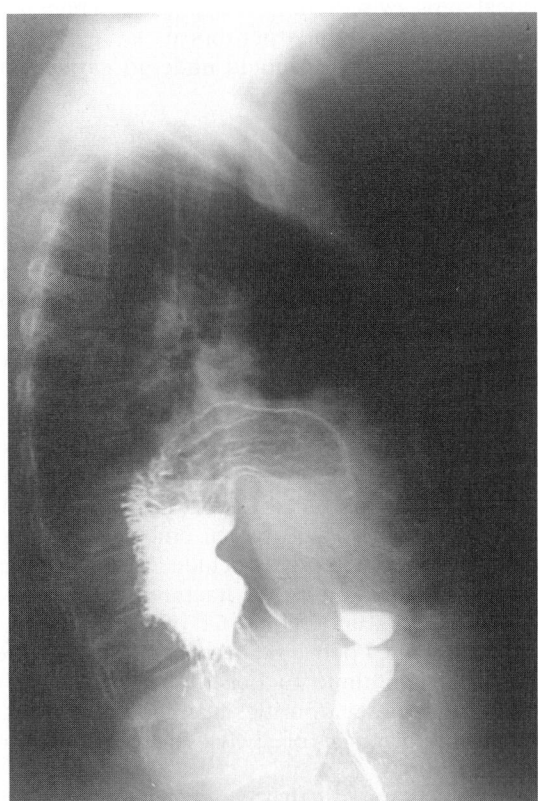

FIGURE 20-16. Lateral chest radiograph shows a herniation of the stomach into the left pleural cavity.

At the time of surgical exploration the entire diaphragm should be inspected. Diaphragmatic injuries are repaired with interrupted horizontal sutures. Larger defects may eventually require use of a prosthetic material.

Acute diaphragmatic rupture is usually repaired through a midline abdominal incision owing to the increased incidence of associated intra-abdominal injuries. Chronic defects discovered months or years after the initial injury can be treated through a transthoracic, an abdominal, or a combined approach.

Esophageal Injuries

Most esophageal injuries are secondary to penetrating trauma and may occur at any level. The esophagus is well protected in the posterior mediastinum and injuries after blunt trauma are rare. Sudden increases in intraesophageal pressure due to a direct blow to the epigastrium may cause rupture of the distal esophagus. Associated injuries are the rule. Esophageal injury after blunt trauma should be considered in patients with a pleural effusion without rib fractures, pain out of proportion to the clinical findings, subcutaneous emphysema or pneumomediastinum without an obvious source, and gastric contents in the chest tube. All mediastinal traversing gunshot wounds or stab wounds near the posterior midline should be evaluated for possible esophageal injury.

The diagnosis is confirmed with esophagography and esophagoscopy. These tests have a reported sensitivity varying from 50% to 90%.[30]

Delay in diagnosis of traumatic esophageal injuries is accompanied by high morbidity and mortality rates. A recent multicenter study was carried out to define the period of time after which delays in management of penetrating esophageal injuries increased morbidity and mortality. Patients were divided into two groups: those operated on immediately after arrival to the trauma center and those who underwent preoperative work-up. The average length of time to the operating room was 1 hour and 13 hours, respectively. The overall incidence of complications, as well as the incidence of esophageal-related complications, was significantly higher in the preoperative work-up group. The optimal time interval between admission and operative intervention in these patients remains to be defined; however, rapid assessment and early operative intervention are accompanied by decreased complications.

Treatment consists of early débridement, primary repair, and drainage if identified within 24 hours after injury. Injuries diagnosed after 24 hours with mediastinal contamination are treated by cervical esophagostomy and distal feeding access. Esophageal resection is rarely needed but may be indicated in esophageal necrosis or severe mediastinitis.

Transmediastinal Gunshot Wounds

Transmediastinal gunshot wounds constitute a significant challenge for trauma surgeons. Hemodynamically unstable patients are treated with exploratory thoracotomy, and the diagnosis of specific injuries will be made during the operation. Hemodynamically stable patients can be evaluated by multiple diagnostic modalities, and significant controversy remains regarding the best methods and the most appropriate sequence of tests used.

Traditionally, evaluation often includes angiography, esophagoscopy, esophagography, bronchoscopy, cardiac two-dimensional echocardiography, and pericardial window. More recently, contrast medium–enhanced CT has been used as a screening modality to determine the trajectory of the projectile, to identify specific injuries, and to determine the need of further evaluation by other diagnostic modalities.[31]

Abdominal Trauma

The abdomen is frequently injured after both blunt and penetrating trauma. Approximately 25% of all trauma victims will require an abdominal exploration. The clinical evaluation of the abdomen by means of physical examination is inadequate to identify intra-abdominal injuries. This is due to the high number of patients with altered mental status secondary to head trauma, alcohol, or drugs and because of the inaccessibility of the pelvic, upper abdominal, and retroperitoneal organs to palpation. For these reasons, several diagnostic modalities evolved during the past three decades, including diagnostic peritoneal lavage, ultrasound, CT, and laparoscopy, all of them with advantages, disadvantages, and limitations.

Mechanism of Injury

Blunt trauma secondary to motor vehicle accidents, motorcycle accidents, falls, assaults, and pedestrians struck remain the most frequent mechanisms of abdominal injury. Penetrating abdominal wounds are usually caused by either gunshot or stab wounds and by a significantly smaller number of shotgun wounds.

Based on the high frequency of intra-abdominal organ injury after gunshot wounds, mandatory abdominal exploration, with rare exceptions, remains the standard form of management. Stab wounds to the abdomen, however, carry a significantly lower risk of intra-abdominal organ injury when compared with gunshot wounds, and recently several studies have favored a more selective approach, as opposed to mandatory exploratory laparotomy.

In children, besides the previously mentioned mechanisms of injury, child abuse and trauma secondary to recreational activities, such as bicycling, swimming, and roller skating, should also be considered.

Diagnosis

The history of the traumatic event is particularly important in determining the likelihood of an intra-abdominal organ injury. All possible information should be obtained from the prehospital personnel, including mechanism of injury, height of a fall, damage to the interior and exterior of a vehicle in a motor vehicle accident, other deaths at the accident scene, ejection, vital signs, mental status, presence of external bleeding, type of weapon, and so on.

On arrival to the hospital, history and physical examination are usually accurate in determining intra-abdominal injury in the awake and responsive patient, although the limitations of the physical examination are significant. Many patients with moderate intra-abdominal bleeding will present in a compensated hemodynamic condition and will not have peritoneal signs. Furthermore, retroperitoneal and pelvic injuries cannot be ruled out based only on physical findings. We consider that an objective abdominal evaluation is necessary and should be obtained by utilizing any of the available diagnostic modalities in addition to the physical examination. The test of choice will depend on the hemodynamic stability of the patient and the severity of associated injuries.

Hemodynamically stable patients sustaining blunt trauma are adequately evaluated by an abdominal ultrasound study or CT, unless other severe injuries take priority and the patient needs to go to the operating room before the objective abdominal evaluation. In such instances, a diagnostic peritoneal lavage is usually performed in the operating room to rule out intra-abdominal injury requiring an immediate surgical exploration.

Blunt trauma patients with hemodynamic instability should be evaluated by ultrasound in the resuscitation room, if available, or by peritoneal lavage to rule out intra-abdominal injuries as the source of blood loss and hypotension.

Patients with isolated penetrating abdominal trauma who are admitted hypotensive, in shock, or with peritoneal signs should go to the operating room despite the mechanism of injury. Stab wound victims without peritoneal signs, evisceration, or hypotension benefit from wound exploration and peritoneal lavage. Gunshot wound victims generally should undergo exploration of the wound.

Plain Radiographs

The chest radiograph is a useful test to reveal pneumoperitoneum, abdominal contents in the chest (ruptured hemidiaphragm), or lower rib fractures. Fractures increase the probability of splenic and hepatic injuries.

An intravenous pyelography and a retrograde cystogram are useful tests in the evaluation of a trauma patient with hematuria.

With the current frequent use of CT to objectively evaluate the abdomen after blunt trauma in stable patients, the use of routine anteroposterior pelvic radiographs, as recommended by the advanced trauma life support course, has been questioned. One recent study examining the utility of pelvic radiography concluded that it has limited sensitivity for detecting pelvic fractures compared with CT. Stable patients undergoing CT of the abdomen and pelvis do not need a pelvic radiograph. Unstable patients, however, may continue to benefit from a pelvic radiograph because other priorities may take place that will require prompt diagnosis of a pelvic fracture in the trauma resuscitation room.

Other studies suggest that clinical factors could accurately identify patients at high risk for pelvic fractures, making routine films unnecessary.[32]

Diagnostic Peritoneal Lavage

Diagnostic peritoneal lavage is a rapid and accurate test used to identify intra-abdominal injuries after blunt trauma in the hypotensive or unresponsive patient without obvious indication for abdominal exploration. Standard criteria for a positive peritoneal lavage include aspiration of at least 10 mL of gross blood, a bloody lavage effluent, a red blood cell count greater than $100,000/mm^3$, a white blood cell count greater than $500/mm^3$, an amylase value greater than 175 IU/dL, or the detection of bile, bacteria, or food fibers. The indications and contraindications for peritoneal lavage are listed in Box 20-3. This test is highly sensitive to the presence of intraperitoneal blood; however, specificity is low and because a positive test prompts surgical exploration, a significant number of explorations will be nontherapeutic.

Significant injuries also may be missed by diagnostic peritoneal lavage. Diaphragmatic tears, retroperitoneal hematomas, and renal, pancreatic, duodenal, minor intestinal, and extraperitoneal bladder injuries are frequently underdiagnosed by peritoneal lavage alone. Complications are infrequent and are mostly related to iatrogenic injuries caused during insertion of the catheter into the abdominal cavity. A semi-open or open technique should be the preferred method to avoid or reduce the incidence of such complications.

Diagnostic peritoneal lavage results can be misleading in the presence of a pelvic fracture. False-positive results are expected owing to bleeding from the retroperitoneum into the peritoneal cavity.

Anterior abdominal and flank wounds can be accurately evaluated by peritoneal lavage. False-positive results are frequent after peritoneal lavage owing to bleeding of the abdominal wall, thus increasing the number of negative explorations. Another potential disadvantage of peritoneal lavage is the low accuracy in the diagnosis of hollow viscus injuries. Debate still exists regarding the most appropriate positive criteria to determine the threshold for surgical exploration after a stab wound to the abdomen. If a red blood cell count of $1000/mm^3$ is considered, the number of negative explorations may be above 20%. If a count of $100,000/mm^3$ is considered, the missed injury rate will approach 5%. There is no consensus on this matter, although most trauma centers use a low threshold (cell count between 1000 and $5000/mm^3$) for exploration.

Diagnosis of abdominal penetration in anterior abdominal stab wounds has been evaluated by diagnostic peritoneal lavage in an attempt to determine who should potentially be discharged from the emergency department. Hemodynamically stable patients with normal physical examination were entered in the study and evaluated with closed peritoneal lavage. If the red blood cell count in the lavage fluid was greater than $1000/mm^3$, patients were admitted for observation. Hemodynamically stable patients with evisceration but without abdominal tenderness had the viscera reduced to the peritoneal cavity in the emergency department and they were admitted for observation. In 44 patients the red cell count was less than $1000/mm^3$, 34 were discharged home; and none required laparotomy or developed complications. Thirty-eight patients were observed because of a red blood cell count greater than $1000/mm^3$. Eight developed peritoneal signs and underwent exploratory laparotomy, which was positive in five. The authors concluded that patients sustaining stab wounds can be safely discharged home if the red blood cell count is less than $1000/mm^3$, provided that they are hemodynamically stable and have no clear indication, based on physical examination, for operative intervention. This approach needs further validation.

Ultrasound

Ultrasound has been used more frequently in recent years in the United States for evaluation of the patient with blunt abdominal trauma. The objective of ultrasound evaluation is to search for free intraperitoneal fluid. It can be done expeditiously, and it is as accurate as diagnostic peritoneal lavage to detect hemoperitoneum. It can also evaluate the liver and the spleen once free fluid is identified, however, that is not its main purpose. Portable machines can be used in the resuscitation area or in the emergency department in the hemodynamically unstable patient without delaying the resuscitation. Another advantage of ultrasound over peritoneal lavage is its noninvasiveness. No further work-up is necessary after a negative ultrasound in a stable patient. CT of the abdomen usually follows a positive ultrasound in a stable patient. The advantages and disadvantages of abdominal ultrasound are listed in Box 20-4. The sensitivity ranges from 85% to 99%, and the specificity from 97% to 100%.[33]

The use of ultrasound for the evaluation of penetrating abdominal trauma has been reported only in limited, small series. Recently, a prospective study was carried out to evaluate the usefulness of ultrasound as a screening test in penetrating trauma to the same extent it is used in blunt trauma. The study included stab as well as gunshot wounds. The overall sensitivity of ultrasound was 46% and the specificity was 94%. This study shows that ultrasound in penetrating trauma is not as reliable as it is in blunt trauma. If ultrasound is positive, the patient should be operated on. If it is negative, further studies should be performed.

Box 20-3 Indications and Contraindications for Diagnostic Peritoneal Lavage

Indications

Equivocal pulmonary embolism
Unexplained shock or hypotension
Altered sensorium (e.g., closed-head injury, drugs)
General anesthesia for extra-abdominal procedures
Cord injury

Contraindications

Clear indication for exploratory laparotomy
Relative:
  Previous exploratory laparotomy
  Pregnancy
  Obesity

Box 20-4 Advantages and Disadvantages of Ultrasound

Advantages

Noninvasive
Does not require radiation
Useful in the resuscitation room or emergency department
Can be repeated
Used during initial evaluation
Low cost

Disadvantages

Examiner dependent
Obesity
Gas interposition
Lower sensitivity for free fluid <500 mL
False-negatives: retroperitoneal and hollow viscus injuries

Box 20-6 Advantages and Disadvantages of Abdominal Computed Tomography

Advantages

Adequate assessment of the retroperitoneum
Nonoperative management of solid organ injuries
Assessment of renal perfusion
Noninvasive
High specificity

Disadvantages

Specialized personnel
Hardware
Duration: helical vs. conventional
Hollow viscus injuries
Cost

Box 20-5 Indications and Contraindications for Abdominal Computed Tomography

Indications

Blunt trauma
Hemodynamic stability
Normal or unreliable physical examination
Mechanism: duodenal and pancreatic trauma

Contraindications

Clear indication for exploratory laparotomy
Hemodynamic instability
Agitation
Allergy to contrast media

Abdominal CT

CT is the most frequently used method to evaluate the stable patient with blunt abdominal trauma. The retroperitoneum is best evaluated by CT. The indications and contraindications of abdominal CT are listed in Box 20-5. The drawback of CT is that the patient needs to be transported to the radiology department, and it is expensive compared with other tests. CT also evaluates solid organ injury, and in the stable patient with a positive ultrasound it is indicated to grade organ injury and to evaluate contrast medium extravasation. If contrast medium extravasation is seen, even in minor hepatic or splenic injuries, an exploratory laparotomy or, more recently, angiography and embolization are indicated. Another indication for CT is in the evaluation of patients with solid organ injuries initially treated nonoperatively who present with a falling hematocrit. The most important disadvantage of CT is its inability to reliably diagnose hollow viscus injury (Box 20-6). Usually, the presence of free abdominal fluid on CT without solid organ injury should raise the suspicion of mesenteric, intestinal, or

bladder injury, and an exploratory laparotomy is often warranted.

One of the most intriguing problems regarding the objective evaluation of blunt abdominal trauma by CT is what to do when free fluid without signs of solid organ or mesenteric injury is found. Coupled with the relatively poor sensitivity of CT to diagnose hollow viscus injury, it creates a dilemma for most trauma surgeons. The options are either to surgically explore all patients and accept a significant rate of nontherapeutic laparotomies or to observe and "act" when peritoneal signs develop, keeping in mind that a delay in diagnosis of bowel injury may be catastrophic. A recent survey of trauma surgeons who were asked what would be the appropriate management of patients in this circumstance showed a variety of responses: 42% would do peritoneal lavage, 28% would observe the patient, 16% would surgically explore, and 12% would repeat an abdominal CT. The accuracy of CT ranges from 92% to 98% with low false-positive and false-negative rates.

Although the use of abdominal CT in the evaluation of penetrating abdominal trauma has been limited owing to low sensitivity in diagnosing bowel and diaphragmatic injury, newer technology (spiral CT) has been evaluated in this circumstance and thus has led to considering nonoperative management in selected cases.[34] Nonoperative management of stab wounds to the anterior abdomen has been emphasized because of the high morbidity rate after nontherapeutic laparotomies.

In one study, triple-contrast helical CT was evaluated as a diagnostic tool after penetrating injuries to the torso. The authors concluded that CT accurately predicted the necessity of laparotomy in 95% of the patients.

Other Diagnostic Modalities

Despite the initial enthusiasm, the use of diagnostic laparoscopy in the patient with blunt trauma is very limited. It is an invasive and expensive method and does not seem to be superior to other methods used for decision making. Missed small bowel, splenic, and retroperitoneal injuries have been reported. It seems that laparoscopy is the best method to evaluate diaphragmatic injuries after thoracoabdominal penetrating injuries.

A study analyzing laparoscopy as a diagnostic modality in patients sustaining penetrating abdominal trauma revealed a progressive reduction in the incidence of negative laparotomies. These findings are in accordance with previous observations showing that laparoscopy has a place in the diagnosis of peritoneal penetration after stab wounds to the anterior abdominal wall. It is particularly useful in thoracoabdominal stab wounds for detecting occult diaphragmatic wounds in the hemodynamically stable patient.

Angiography is used to evaluate renal artery thrombosis and to manage pelvic hemorrhage in patients with pelvic fractures and bleeding from minor hepatic and splenic injuries.

Gastric Injuries

Gastric injuries often result from penetrating trauma. Less than 1% of such wounds are due to blunt trauma secondary to motor vehicle accidents, falls, cardiopulmonary resuscitation, or interpersonal violence.[35]

The stomach is partially protected by the rib cage, making blunt injuries rare occurrences and relatively difficult to diagnose. Causes of blunt gastric rupture include vigorous ventilation with an endotracheal tube placed inadvertently in the esophagus, crushing against the spine, cardiopulmonary resuscitation, the Heimlich maneuver, and other causes leading to sudden increase in intraluminal pressure.

Blunt gastric trauma includes a wide range of injuries, from mucosal lacerations to full-thickness disruption and gastric necrosis due to avulsion of vascular pedicles. Other intra-abdominal and extra-abdominal injuries are frequently present. Diagnostic peritoneal lavage or CT of the abdomen may confirm the diagnosis; however, in most instances the diagnosis will be made during surgical exploration.

Any penetrating abdominal injury, particularly in the upper abdomen, should be suspected of causing injury to the stomach. During initial evaluation a nasogastric tube should be inserted; and if the aspirate is positive for blood, an injury to the stomach should be suspected. The intraoperative evaluation includes good visualization of the esophagogastric junction, examination of the anterior gastric wall, opening of the gastrocolic ligament, and complete visualization of the posterior gastric wall. Minor injuries may not be identified and require distention of the organ with saline or methylene blue to evaluate for leaking.

Most penetrating wounds are treated by means of débridement of the wound edges and primary closure in layers. Injuries with major tissue loss may be best treated by gastric resection. Postoperative complications include bleeding, usually from the submucosal vessels, intra-abdominal abscesses, and, more rarely, gastric fistula.

Due to its proximity with the diaphragm, the stomach is frequently injured after thoracoabdominal wounds. Depending on the severity of contamination due to spillage of gastric contents, empyema is another frequent complication.[35]

The role of the extravasation of gastric contents in the genesis of postoperative complications is closely related to the dynamics of the gastric flora. Usually many microorganisms originating from the nasopharynx and oropharynx reach the stomach through the saliva and nasal mucus. Changes in gastric pH are frequent after eating, drinking, and saliva ingestion, which act in an attempt to neutralize gastric acidity. When gastric pH is below 4, gastric juice has bactericidal properties that act to inhibit bacterial enzymatic activity. In this situation, microorganisms such as *Streptococcus salivarium, Streptococcus viridans, Lactobacillus, Bacteroides, Veillonella, Micrococcus, Staphylococcus,* and *Neisseria* are found in very low concentrations, usually below 1000/mL. Inversely, when the gastric pH is neutralized, bactericidal properties of the gastric juice are extremely suppressed, which leads to prompt bacterial growth. Concentrations can reach as high as 10^6/mL and remain there for approximately 1 hour before returning to normal levels. If the neutralization occurs for prolonged periods of time, bacteria from the lower digestive tract such as *Bacteroides fragilis, Escherichia coli, Streptococcus faecalis,* and enterobacterias can be found inside the stomach. This fact is especially important in trauma patients who frequently have great amounts of food and liquid inside the stomach.

Morbidity and mortality rates after penetrating abdominal injuries associated with gastric wounds have been reported close to 27% and 14%, respectively, in most cases due to the associated injuries, although the risk of morbidity from gastric injury itself is close to 6%.[35]

Injuries to the Duodenum

The majority of duodenum injuries are caused by penetrating trauma; however, blunt injuries, although infrequent, are difficult to diagnose because patients may present with subtle findings on admission. The incidence of duodenal injuries varies from 3% to 5%. Most of duodenal injuries are accompanied by other intra-abdominal injuries. This occurs owing to its close anatomic relationship with other solid organs and major vessels.

A motor vehicle accident causing a steering wheel blow to the epigastrium is the most common mechanism of blunt duodenal injuries. Other mechanisms, such as assault and falls, also cause duodenal injuries. A closed loop compression of an air-filled loop after a direct blow can account for duodenum rupture.

The retroperitoneal location of the duodenum (second and third portions) exerts a protective effect against injuries but also prevents an early diagnosis. Isolated injury to the duodenum is rare and usually does not cause significant clinical signs of peritonitis or hemodynamic instability. A thorough search based on mechanism of injury is necessary to prevent delays in diagnosis. Failure to recognize this injury is associated with the development of intra-abdominal abscesses, sepsis, and high mortality rates.

Hyperamylasemia occurs in about 50% of patients with blunt injury to the duodenum, and although it is not

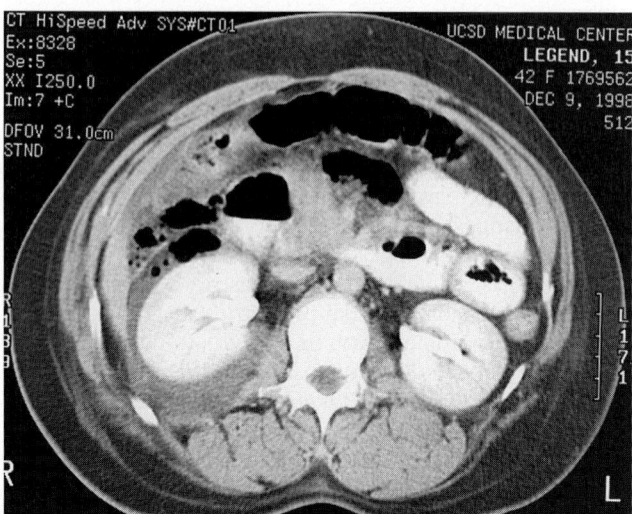

FIGURE 20-17. CT shows blunt duodenal injury with retroperitoneal air.

TABLE 20-7.   Duodenum Injury Scale

Grade*	Type of Injury	Description of Injury
I	Hematoma	Involving single portion of duodenum
	Laceration	Partial thickness, no perforation
II	Hematoma	Involving more than one portion
	Laceration	Disruption <50% of circumference
III	Laceration	Disruption 50%-75% of circumference of D2
		Disruption 50%-100% of circumference of D1, D3, D4
IV	Laceration	Disruption >75% of circumference of D2 involving ampulla or distal common bile duct
V	Laceration	Massive disruption of duodenopancreatic complex
	Vascular	Devascularization of duodenum

*Advance one grade for multiple injuries up to grade III. D1, first position of duodenum; D2, second portion of duodenum; D3, third portion of duodenum; D4, fourth portion of duodenum.
From Moore EE, Cogbill TH, Malangoni MA, et al: Organ injury scaling: II. Pancreas, duodenum, small bowel, colon, and rectum. J Trauma 30:1427-1429, 1990, with permission.

diagnostic of an injury, its presence should raise suspicion and further diagnostic studies should be obtained.

Plain films of the abdomen may suggest duodenal injury showing mild scoliosis, obliteration of the right psoas shadow, absence of air in the duodenal bulb, or air in the retroperitoneum outlining the kidney. Definitive diagnosis requires a Gastrografin upper gastrointestinal series or CT of the abdomen with oral and intravenous contrast medium in the hemodynamically stable patient (Fig. 20-17). Extravasation of contrast material is an absolute indication for laparotomy. The radiographic finding of a duodenal hematoma (coil spring or stacked coin sign) is not an indication for surgical exploration. If this causes obstruction that fails to resolve, then operative management is indicated. If CT findings are equivocal, an upper gastrointestinal series with diluted barium is the test of choice.

The utility of duodenography in the diagnosis of blunt duodenal injury was recently evaluated and compared with abdominal CT. Duodenography in patients with CT findings suggestive of blunt duodenal trauma was found to be of minimal utility. The most important sign of duodenal perforation was retroperitoneal extraluminal air seen on CT.

Diagnostic peritoneal lavage is unreliable in detecting retroperitoneal injuries, and a negative test does not rule out duodenal injury. The test is useful in the hemodynamically unstable patient with blunt duodenal rupture; and because of the high number of associated injuries, a positive test will prompt surgical exploration and the duodenal injury will be found during the laparotomy. In penetrating abdominal wounds the diagnosis of duodenal injury offers no difficulty and will be made during surgical exploration.

Intraoperative evaluation of the duodenum requires an adequate mobilization of the duodenum by means of a Kocher maneuver. The hepatic flexure of the colon is also mobilized to provide adequate exposure of the anterior wall of the second portion, and examination of the third

and fourth portions of the duodenum should also be done. The presence of retroperitoneal hematomas around the duodenum should raise the suspicion of an associated pancreatic injury.

The appropriate repair of duodenal injuries depends on injury severity (Table 20-7) and elapsed time from injury to treatment. Eighty to 85% of duodenal wounds can be primarily repaired. The remaining 15% to 20% are severe injuries that require more complex procedures.

For most of minor injuries (grade I to II) diagnosed within 6 hours of injury, a simple primary repair is suitable. After 6 hours, the risk of leak increases and any form of duodenal decompression (e.g., transpyloric nasogastric tube, tube jejunostomy, or tube duodenostomy) is advisable.

Grade III injuries involving major disruption of the duodenal circumference are best treated by primary repair, pyloric exclusion, and drainage or, alternatively, by a roux-en-Y duodenojejunostomy.

Grade IV injuries (involving the ampulla or distal common bile duct) are difficult to repair. In this situation, primary repair of the duodenum, repair of the common bile duct, and placement of a tracheostomy tube with a long transpapillary limb or a choledochoenteric anastomosis may be attempted when possible. If repair of the common bile duct is impossible to be performed, ligation and a second intervention for a biliary enterostomy can be done. Pancreaticoduodenectomy, although rarely needed, is reserved for grade V injuries, including massive disruption of the duodenum and pancreatic head or for massive devascularization of the duodenum.

Duodenal hematomas are expected to resolve between 10 to 15 days, and management consists of nasogastric suction until peristalsis resumes and after slow introduction of solid food. Exploration is indicated in the event of persistent duodenal obstruction.

The incidence of complications after duodenal injuries is high, ranging from 30% to more than 100%.[36] The most significant complication after duodenal injury is the development of a duodenal fistula, which occurs in 5% to 15% of patients. Duodenal fistulas are generally managed nonoperatively with nasogastric suction, intravenous nutritional support, and aggressive stoma care. Usually, closure will occur within 6 to 8 weeks. Abscess formation occurs in 10% to 20% of the patients and may or may not be associated with a duodenal fistula. Abscesses are initially managed by percutaneous drainage. Surgical drainage is indicated when multiple abscesses are present or when located between small bowel loops.

Pancreatic Injuries

Pancreatic injury is rare, accounting for 10% to 12% of all abdominal injuries. The great majority of such injuries are caused by penetrating mechanisms and are often associated with significant injuries involving other intra-abdominal organs. Blunt trauma to the abdomen caused by direct blow or seatbelt injury may compress the pancreas over the vertebral column and cause pancreatic disruption. Major abdominal vascular injuries are present in more than 75% of cases of penetrating pancreatic trauma, and injuries to the solid organs and hollow viscus are common after blunt trauma.

Mortality rates range from 10% to 25%, mostly due to associated intra-abdominal injuries. Approximately 50% of the overall mortality after a pancreatic injury is caused by associated major abdominal vascular injuries. Sepsis and multiple organ failure account for most of the late deaths. Pancreatic-related mortality ranges from 2% to 5% in large urban trauma series.

Diagnosis of a pancreatic injury is made by having a high index of suspicion based on history, mechanism of injury, and associated clinical findings. However, owing to its retroperitoneal location, the pancreas is a well-protected organ, and signs and symptoms may appear late, thus delaying diagnosis. Increased levels of serum and urinary amylase after blunt injury are not diagnostic, but a persistent elevation suggests pancreatic injury. Contrast duodenography may reveal widening of the C-loop. Diagnostic peritoneal lavage is not sensitive enough for the diagnosis of retroperitoneal injuries, but this test may be positive owing to the high frequency of associated injuries, prompting an abdominal exploration. Abdominal CT is of potential value but its role is still unclear. The diagnosis of a pancreatic injury with the use of newer-generation CT scanners has improved significantly; however, some injuries may be identified only during follow-up scans obtained for changes in the clinical status (Fig. 20-18).

Isolated pancreatic injuries are rare. Diagnosis is difficult to make, and patients may complain of vague abdominal pain radiating to the back several hours after the incident. Frequently, patients develop mild abdominal tenderness and some will eventually develop peritoneal signs. A delay in diagnosis correlates with increased incidence of severe complications.

Patients are generally operated on because of intraperitoneal blood loss or peritonitis, and the diagnosis of a pan-

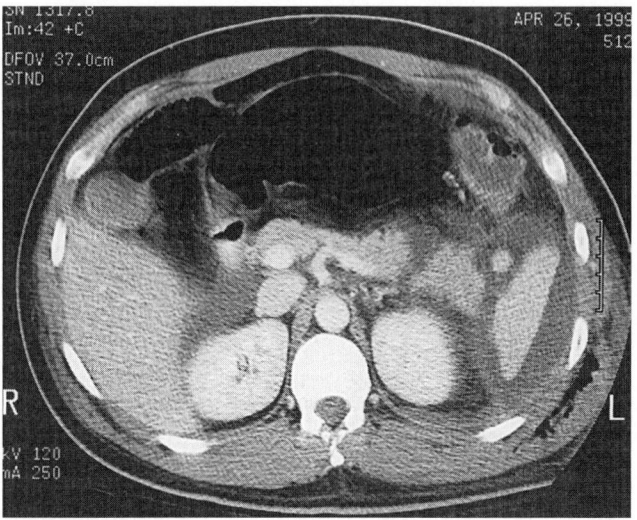

FIGURE 20-18. CT shows a pancreatic transection.

creatic injury is usually an incidental finding. However, patients with questionable CT findings, persistent abdominal pain, or elevated serum amylase levels may benefit from repeat CT. At laparotomy, a careful examination of the pancreas should be carried out. All retroperitoneal hematomas surrounding the pancreas should be explored.

The presence of a pancreatic duct injury appears to be a key factor in postoperative morbidity.[37] There is still controversy regarding the best method to evaluate the main pancreatic duct during laparotomy. Several authors are in favor of aggressively pursuing the identification of ductal injury by obtaining an intraoperative pancreatography. Others favor a more conservative approach and base their management on location and on surgical identification of ductal injuries. In fact, a more conservative approach in the diagnosis and management of pancreatic injuries has been advocated recently.

Pancreatic injuries are divided into proximal or distal according to the location on the right or left of the superior mesenteric vessels. The classification of pancreatic injuries according to injury severity is described in Table 20-8.

In the recent past, most distal pancreatic injuries with suspected ductal injuries were treated by distal resection with or without splenectomy. More recently, it has been shown that the form of treatment (i.e., drainage or resection) does not influence the incidence of a pancreatic fistula in patients with indeterminate ductal status during laparotomy. There is no question that if a distal ductal injury is identified during the operation, distal resection is the treatment of choice, although the associated morbidity with this procedure is not dismal.

If there is any evidence that the pancreas has been contused, independent of the location, it should be drained. Complete transections of the midportion of the pancreas theoretically can be treated with pancreaticojejunostomy, but there are no prospective data to support this approach when compared with distal pancreatectomy.

Penetrating wounds to the right of the superior mesenteric vein should be treated with débridement and direct

TABLE 20-8.   Pancreas Injury Scale

Grade*	Type of Injury	Description of Injury
I	Hematoma	Minor contusion without duct injury
	Laceration	Superficial laceration without duct injury
II	Hematoma	Major contusion without duct injury or tissue loss
	Laceration	Major laceration without duct injury or tissue loss
III	Laceration	Distal transaction or parenchymal injury with duct injury
IV	Laceration	Proximal transaction or parenchymal injury involving ampulla†
V	Laceration	Massive disruption of pancreatic head

*Advance one grade for multiple injuries up to grade III. II631.51, 863.91—head; 863.99, 862.92—body; 863.83, 863.93—tail.
†Proximal pancreas is to the patient's right of the superior mesenteric vein.
From Moore EE, Cogbill TH, Malangoni MA, et al: Organ injury scaling: II. Pancreas, duodenum, small bowel, colon, and rectum. J Trauma 30:1427-1429, 1990, with permission.

suture ligation of areas of bleeding. Extensive injuries to the pancreatic head or to the right of the superior mesenteric vessels are usually associated with a probability of temporary pancreatic fistula greater than 40%. In these circumstances, drainage seems to be the best treatment option, particularly when compared with a proximal pancreatectomy or to a Whipple procedure, which is reserved for severe combined pancreaticoduodenal injuries. Severe trauma to the duodenum and head of the pancreas may be treated with débridement of the pancreas, closure of the duodenal wound, and pyloric exclusion. Wide drainage is also mandatory in this situation.

The most frequent complications after pancreatic trauma are pancreatic fistula and peripancreatic abscess. These complications occur in 35% to 40% of the patients sustaining pancreatic injuries. Pancreatic fistulas, if well drained, in the majority of the patients will close spontaneously. Somatostatin has been used to expedite healing of pancreatic fistulas, but the results are controversial. Peripancreatic abscesses are treated with surgical débridement and drainage. The incidence of pancreatitis after a pancreatic injury is 8% to 18%. Pancreatic pseudocysts are infrequent.

Small Intestine Injuries

The small bowel is the most frequently injured organ after penetrating injuries. After blunt trauma, the incidence of small bowel injuries ranges from 5% to 20% of the patients who require surgical exploration. The postulated mechanisms involved in blunt intestinal injuries include (1) crushing injury of the bowel between the vertebral bodies and the blunt object, such as a steering wheel or handlebars; (2) deceleration shearing of the small bowel at fixed points such as the ligament of Treitz, the ileocecal valve, and around the mesenteric artery; and (3) closed loop rupture caused by sudden increase in intra-abdominal pressure.

The presence of a seatbelt sign should raise the suspicion for enteric and mesenteric injuries. The majority of patients with blunt intestinal trauma will present with signs of peritoneal irritation; however, small lacerations may present with mild abdominal pain without peritoneal signs. If peritoneal signs or hemodynamic instability are present, the patient should be taken to the operating room for surgical exploration, and the diagnosis of intestinal rupture will be intraoperative. Hollow viscus injuries are often characterized by delay in diagnosis after blunt abdominal trauma. Delays in diagnosis and management of blunt hollow viscus injuries are associated with increased morbidity and mortality, as shown by recent studies.

Several tests may help in the diagnosis of blunt intestinal trauma in patients without a clear indication for surgical exploration. Plain films of the abdomen may reveal free air; however, this is an uncommon finding. Diagnostic peritoneal lavage is not a reliable test to identify small bowel injuries, particularly small injuries with a minimum leak. CT with intravenous and oral contrast medium enhancement also carries a significant false-negative rate, and suggestive findings include free fluid in the abdomen without solid organ injury, free air, and thickening of the small bowel wall or mesentery.

Before the advent of CT as the primary tool for the evaluation of blunt abdominal trauma, peritoneal lavage was the gold standard and the diagnosis of hollow viscus injury was usually made in the operating room during an exploratory laparotomy. For this reason, delay in diagnosis of hollow viscus injury was uncommon. With the more frequent use of CT and the development of nonoperative management protocols for solid organ injuries, the diagnosis of hollow viscus injury may be effected. False-negative rates of up to 15% have been reported with the use of CT to diagnose hollow viscus injury. A recent multi-institutional study analyzing a large number of patients revealed that current diagnostic modalities lack sensitivity in the diagnosis of hollow viscus injury and 13% of patients with perforated small bowel have a normal CT. A negative abdominal CT is inadequate to safely rule out perforated small bowel injury.[38]

Occasionally, a large tear in the mesentery occurs without bowel involvement. In these instances bowel necrosis and subsequent perforation occurs hours or even days after the initial injury and the patients may present with frank peritoneal signs, acidosis, and sepsis.

At laparotomy, a careful examination of the entire small bowel should be performed. Bleeding should be initially controlled and clamps or sutures should be applied to prevent further leakage of intestinal contents into the peritoneal cavity. Penetrating injuries caused by firearms should be débrided, and usually small tears are closed primarily. If two adjacent holes are found, they can be connected across the bridge of normal bowel and closed transversally to avoid narrowing of the intestinal lumen. Extensive lacerations, devascularized segments, or multiple lacerations in a short segment of bowel are better treated by resection and reanastomosis. All mesenteric hematomas should be explored, because these can hide small bowel injuries.

During the initial postoperative period, patients are usually maintained with a nasogastric tube for decompression until peristalsis resumes and feeding is started. Postoperative complications include intra-abdominal abscess and sepsis, anastomotic leakage, wound infection, enteric fistula, and intestinal obstruction. Enteric leakage caused by suture breakdown is rare and manifests as fever, leukocytosis, leak through the surgical wounds, or peritonitis.

Intra-abdominal abscesses are suspected in the presence of fever, tachycardia, and abdominal pain and confirmed by ultrasound or CT. The development of postoperative abscesses depends on the amount of contamination or spillage and the location of the injury. Proximal injuries carry a lower risk for subsequent infection due to a decreased number of enteric bacteria present in the lumen of the jejunum as compared with the distal ileum. Intra-abdominal abscesses may be secondary to gross contamination, repair breakdown, or missed injuries. Drainage, either surgical or percutaneous, is the treatment of choice after identification of the abscess by CT. Prompt re-exploration is indicated if percutaneous drainage fails to resolve infection or if abscesses are located between loops of small bowel.

Fistulas may be treated operatively or nonoperatively. Re-exploration is indicated in the presence of sepsis, peritonitis, distal obstruction, and inadequate drainage around the area of the fistula or if nonoperative treatment fails to control fistula output and persistent fluid and electrolyte imbalances occur. Proximal small bowel fistulas require total parenteral hyperalimentation as opposed to distal ones, which can be treated by oral nutrition.

Short bowel syndrome is a devastating complication after extensive resection of the small bowel. It is characterized by persistent diarrhea, loss of protein and fat in the stool, and weight loss. Ileal resections are less well tolerated than jejunal resections because the ileum is the site for absorption of bile salts and vitamin B_{12} and has a greater adaptive capacity. The presence of the ileal cecal valve is also of paramount importance because it slows the intestinal transit time, providing a prolonged exposure of the nutrients to the intestinal mucosa. Treatment of short bowel syndrome includes adequate fluid intake, parenteral hyperalimentation, vitamin B_{12} replacement, cholestyramine to reduce diarrhea, H_2 blockers to reduce gastric secretion, and oral narcotics to reduce intestinal motility. Isosmotic oral elemental diets are used after the acute phase when wound healing has occurred. Surgical procedures to slow intestinal transit time have been used, but their effectiveness remains unknown. Small bowel transplantation is a promising alternative for the treatment of this complication.

Injuries to the Colon

Colon injuries are usually the result of penetrating trauma. The colon is the second most frequently injured organ after gunshot wounds and the third after stab wounds to the abdomen. Colon injuries after blunt trauma are relatively infrequent (only 5% of all colonic injuries).

Recent studies have shown that morbidity rates after colonic injuries vary from 20% to 35% and mortality rates range from 3% to 15%. The incidence of infectious complications after a colonic injury is related to inadequate treatment or delay in diagnosis, and several reports have confirmed that repair of a colonic injury within 2 hours dramatically reduces the incidence of infectious complications.

Physical examination is particularly useful to establish that a laparotomy is necessary after a stab wound to the abdomen if peritoneal signs are present; however, a negative physical examination does not rule out the presence of a colonic injury, particularly in patients with stab wounds to the back and flanks. An objective evaluation of the abdomen is warranted after stab wounds and may include a diagnostic peritoneal lavage or a triple-contrast (oral, intravenous, and rectal) CT. Gunshot wounds to the abdomen usually indicate the necessity of a laparotomy, and with few exceptions, no further work-up is necessary and the colonic injury will be diagnosed during the abdominal exploration.

Laboratory studies usually are not helpful, and plain abdominal films may, eventually, show a pneumoperitoneum. The rectal examination may show the presence of blood, which is strong evidence of colon or rectal injury. Patients undergoing abdominal exploration should receive preoperative antibiotics, and this measure is an important adjunct to decrease infectious complications.

The operative management of colonic injury is still controversial. During World War I, primary repair of colonic injuries was the treatment of choice; however, mortality rates reached 60%. During World War II, surgeons concerned about the high rates of postoperative infection considered diversion of fecal contents by means of a colostomy and delayed colostomy closure to be safer than primary repair. In fact, the mortality rates reported during World War II for colonic injuries were approximately 35%. These results influenced the way colonic injuries were treated until recent years. Recently, this concept has been challenged because colonic injuries in civilian practice are caused by low-velocity missiles and stab wounds, mechanisms different than those present in the military practice. This led to a resurgence of primary repair as an adequate alternative to colostomy for the treatment of most (but not all) colonic injuries.

Primary repair can be selected when known associated complicating factors have been excluded. General criteria for primary repair include early diagnosis (within 4 to 6 hours), absence of prolonged shock or hypotension, absence of gross contamination of the peritoneal cavity, absence of associated colonic vascular injury, less than 6 units of blood transfusion, and no requirement for the use of mesh to permanently close the abdominal wall. Increased complication rates after primary repair include prolonged hypotension, massive intraperitoneal hemorrhage, more than two associated organs injured, significant fecal spillage, or delayed diagnosis. Most patients with low risk penetrating colonic injuries can be treated with primary closure or resection and primary anastomosis after these guidelines. High-risk colon injuries or those associated with severe injuries will benefit from resection and colostomy. The exteriorization of the colonic repair has been done infrequently, owing to extremely high rates of failure, repair breakdown, and infectious complications. Some surgeons will have different approaches to treat injuries on the right side as compared with the left side of the colon; however, no prospective randomized data are available to compare primary repair performed on right-sided colonic injuries with end-colostomy for left-sided injuries.

The comparison of results between primary repair versus colostomy for colonic injuries should include complications that occur during or after colostomy takedown. Some studies analyzing complications and deaths after colostomy takedown have reported an overall incidence of 10% to 50% of complications.

Penetrating colon injuries requiring resection (colostomy vs. primary anastomosis) were recently evaluated in a prospective multicenter study. The type of colon management was not found by multivariate analysis to be a risk factor for abdominal complications. The authors concluded that, once resection is necessary, the surgical method of colon management does not affect the incidence of abdominal complications irrespective of the associated risk factors and that primary anastomosis should be considered in all patients.[5]

The type of anastomosis used in the colon (hand sewn vs. stapled) has been also a subject of controversy. A multicenter prospective study comparing the staples with hand-sewn anastomosis after penetrating colon trauma concluded that the method of colonic anastomosis does not affect the incidence of abdominal complications.

In summary, stab and low velocity wounds to the colon with minimal contamination and hemodynamic stability can be managed by primary repair.

Postoperative complications include abscess formation, anastomotic leak, peristomal hernia, and the morbidity and mortality associated with colostomy closure.

Rectum

Rectal injuries are uncommon. Most of the rectal injuries result from gunshot wounds; however, other causes, such as foreign body, impalement, pelvic fractures, and iatrogenic (after proctosigmoidoscopy) should be considered. Transpelvic gunshot wounds as well as any penetrating injury to the lower abdomen and buttocks should raise suspicion for a rectal injury even if the physical examination is unremarkable. Rectal injuries can be intraperitoneal or extraperitoneal. The rectal examination may reveal blood, or an injury may be palpable. The work-up of rectal injuries includes anoscopy and rigid proctosigmoidoscopy.

Primary closure of extraperitoneal rectal injuries, particularly those located in the inferior third of the rectum, should be attempted, although this is not always possible. A diverting colostomy, washout of the distal rectal stump, and wide presacral drainage are mandatory. Rectal stump irrigation in this setting decreases the incidence of pelvic abscess, rectal fistulas, and sepsis. Intraperitoneal rectal injuries are usually managed by primary closure and by a diverting colostomy. A primary abdominal perineal resection is indicated in extensive rectal injuries.

Complications after rectal injuries include sepsis, pelvic abscesses, urinary or rectal fistulas, rectal incontinence and stricture, loss of sexual function, and urinary incontinence.

Liver Injuries

Because of its size and location in the abdominal cavity, the liver is frequently injured in both blunt and penetrating trauma. Despite progress in the management of trauma patients in the past two decades, mortality after hepatic trauma has remained stable.[39] Spontaneous hemostasis is observed in more than 50% of small hepatic lacerations at the time of laparotomy. In fact, most liver injuries will require only documentation and no drainage. Although most liver injuries can be properly managed with simple procedures, control of profuse bleeding from deep hepatic lacerations remains a formidable challenge for trauma surgeons. Overall mortality rate ranges from 8% to 10%, and overall morbidity rate varies from 18% to 30%, depending on the number of associated injuries and the severity of injury. The classification of liver injuries is shown in Table 20-9. In less severe hepatic injuries (grades

TABLE 20-9.   Liver Injury Scale (1994 Revision)

Grade*	Type of Injury	Description of Injury
I	Hematoma Laceration	Subcapsular, <10% surface area Capsular tear, <1-cm parenchymal depth
II	Hematoma Laceration	Subcapsular, 10%-50% surface area: intraparenchymal <10 cm in diameter Capsular tear, 1-3-cm parenchymal depth <10 cm in length
III	Hematoma Laceration	Subcapsular, >50% surface area of ruptured subcapsular or parenchymal hematoma, intraparenchymal hematoma >10 cm or expanding 3-cm parenchymal depth
IV	Laceration	Parenchymal disruption involving 25%-75% hepatic lobe or 1-3 Couinaud segments
V	Laceration Vascular	Parenchymal disruption involving >75% of hepatic lobe or >3 Couinaud segments within a single lobe Juxtahepatic venous injuries (i.e., retrohepatic vena cava/central major hepatic veins)
VI	Vascular	Hepatic avulsion

*Advance one grade for multiple injuries up to grade III.
From Moore EE, Cogbill TH, Jurkovich GJ, et al: Organ injury scaling: Spleen and liver (1994 revision). J Trauma 38:323-324, 1995, with permission

1 to 3), mortality is related to associated injuries, which are more frequently seen after blunt trauma, although in high-grade liver injuries mortality is related to the injury itself, regardless of the mechanism. The mortality rate of isolated liver trauma is 3%, increasing to 24% in the presence of three associated injuries.

Some small non-deep bleeding lacerations are easily controlled with simple suture or with the use of hemostatic agents. More severe liver injuries will require more complex procedures, including deep mattress sutures, packing, débridement, resection, mesh hepatorrhaphy, and so on. The resurgence of packing and the emergence of damage control, as an alternative for the treatment of severe hepatic injuries in patients in shock, metabolic derangement, and coagulopathy, have been incorporated in the armamentarium of trauma surgeons in recent years. A 34% survival rate was reported when packing was used as an adjunct to other measures to control bleeding.

A patient with a history of shock at the scene after blunt trauma should be suspected of having a major liver injury. Hemodynamically unstable patients, those with altered mental status, or those that will undergo general anesthesia for extra-abdominal procedures should be evaluated with diagnostic peritoneal lavage. However, stable patients without peritoneal signs are better evaluated by CT due to the possibility of nonoperative treatment and injury severity grading.

Injuries vary from capsular tears and nonbleeding lacerations to large fractures and lobar destruction with extensive parenchymal disruption and hepatic artery and venous injuries. The type of injury dictates surgical management. The principles of surgical management of liver injury are the same, regardless of the severity of injury. They involve control of bleeding, removal of devitalized tissue, and establishment of adequate drainage.

Simple lacerations, which are not bleeding at the time of surgery, do not require drainage unless they are deep into the parenchyma with the possibility of postoperative biliary fistula. Subcapsular hematomas can be simply observed or surgically evacuated if there is no associated parenchymal injury. Lacerations that continue to bleed despite attempts at local control will require a more extensive approach, usually opening the liver wound and directly approaching the bleeding vessels, a procedure known as tractotomy. Bleeding vessels and biliary radicals should be individually ligated. In the event that bleeding continues despite directly ligating small vessels, a vascular clamp or vessel loops can be placed around the porta hepatis (Pringle maneuver) (Fig. 20-19). If bleeding stops after clamping the portal triad, it can be assumed to be from the portal veins or hepatic artery branches. If the bleeding continues despite clamping the portal triad, an injury of the hepatic veins or the retrohepatic vena cava is suspected. The portal triad also can be intermittently clamped to allow visualization during placement of sutures as parenchymal vessels are ligated. If a Pringle maneuver is applied, caution regarding the duration of inflow occlusion is necessary. Hypothermic patients do not tolerate liver ischemia for prolonged periods of time and significant damage to the liver parenchyma due to ischemia may occur. The exact length of warm ischemia

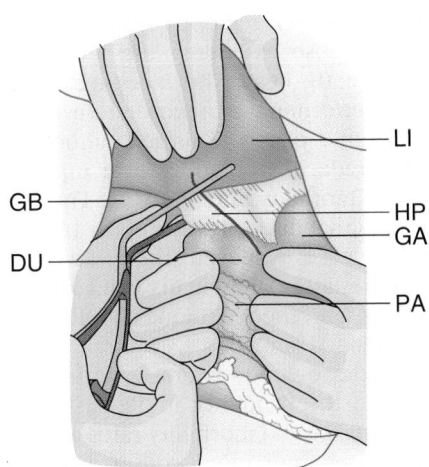

FIGURE 20-19. Diagram shows the Pringle maneuver. DU, duodenum; GA, gastric antrum; GB, gallbladder; HP, hepatic pedicle; LI, liver; PA, pancreas. (From Aun F, Birolini D: Critical maneuvers in trauma surgery. In Editora Pedagogica e Universitaria (E. P. U.) LTDA. New York, Springer-Verlag, 1982.)

time tolerated by the human liver is not known; however, some authors have reported inflow occlusion for up to 1 hour with the use of adjuvant corticosteroid therapy without major consequences.

Packing the liver wound is used when the just-described techniques fail in controlling hemorrhage. The results of temporary packing must be analyzed in the light of its relation to timing. Perihepatic packing was once condemned because of the high incidence of intra-abdominal abscesses. Recently, temporary packing has been used particularly in patients with hypothermia, coagulopathy, and severe acidosis with severe injuries in other intra-abdominal organs.

Usually, these patients are taken to the ICU for rewarming and resuscitation. Re-exploration for packing removal is performed within 48 to 72 hours after the initial operation. After hemostasis is achieved and the packs are removed, copious irrigation of the abdominal cavity is performed and closed-suction drains are placed. The incidence of intra-abdominal abscess in survivors of liver packing is generally less than 15%.

One recent study compiled several clinical series addressing the use of packing. Hepatic packing was used in 230 patients; mortality ranged from 10% to 58%, averaging 34%. Packing does not seem to be as effective for bleeding from the hepatic veins, retrohepatic vena cava, or arterial bleeding as compared with parenchymal injuries not involving major vessels. Arteriography is a useful adjunct to locate the arterial bleeding, and embolization may be of benefit before re-exploration for packing removal.

Despite the use of any method to obtain hemostasis, all necrotic tissue should be débrided before closure. If bleeding in the raw surface of the liver after resectional débridement is not significant, an omentum flap can be used to cover or fill the defect in the liver parenchyma.

Deep liver lacerations should not be simply closed, because of the risk of abscess formation and hemobilia. As an alternative approach for deep liver lacerations, some investigators propose extending the liver laceration to expose and directly ligate the bleeding vessel. This is achieved by performing a finger fracture hepatotomy along nonanatomic planes. This technique was used in patients with grade III to grade V liver injuries with the remarkably low mortality rate of 10.7%. The advantage of this technique is that direct ligation of the bleeding vessels and biliary radicals is achieved; the disadvantage is that the defect in the liver parenchyma is usually bigger than the initial injury, and the technique should be performed only by experienced surgeons.

Formal hepatic resection is unusual after liver injuries and has been mostly abandoned in the past decade owing to the high mortality and morbidity rates after this procedure and because other more conservative approaches have proven to be as effective to control hemorrhage with significantly lower complication rate and mortality.

In a 5-year multi-institutional review of 1335 liver injuries, resectional débridement was performed in 36 patients (2.6%), hepatotomy and vessel ligation in 50 patients (3.7%), and segmentectomy in 18 patients (1.3%). Formal hepatic lobectomy was performed in only 12 patients (0.9%).

Another technique described recently encompasses the use of an absorbable mesh, individually wrapping each lobe of the liver and attaching the mesh to the falciform ligament. This technique is useful in multiple superficial lacerations of the liver with active bleeding; however, it is not effective when major vascular injuries are present. The reported mortality rate in hepatic trauma patients managed by mesh wrapping is 25% to 37.5%.

Major hepatic injuries including retrohepatic and juxtahepatic venous injuries are discussed in the section on major abdominal vascular injuries.

Ligation of the hepatic artery is also an alternative for continued bleeding; however, with the use of modern cautery (electric or argon beam coagulators), topical hemostatic agents, and fibrin glue, this is seldom required. It should be reserved for the occasional stab wound or the gunshot wound involving one lobe where exposure of the wound will require extensive incision of the liver. The proper hepatic artery must never be ligated. Injudicious hepatic artery ligation may result in liver infarction, particularly if associated with portal vein injury.[40] Packing the liver is a reasonable alternative to hepatic artery ligation.

Nonoperative Treatment

Blunt hepatic injuries in hemodynamic stable patients without other indications for exploration are best served by a conservative, nonoperative approach. These stable patients without peritoneal signs are better evaluated by ultrasound, and, if abnormalities are found, a CT scan with contrast medium enhancement should be obtained (Fig. 20-20). In the absence of contrast agent extravasation during the arterial phase of the CT, most injuries can be potentially treated nonoperatively. The classic criteria for nonoperative treatment of liver injuries include hemodynamic stability, normal mental status, absence of a clear indication for laparotomy such as peritoneal signs, low-

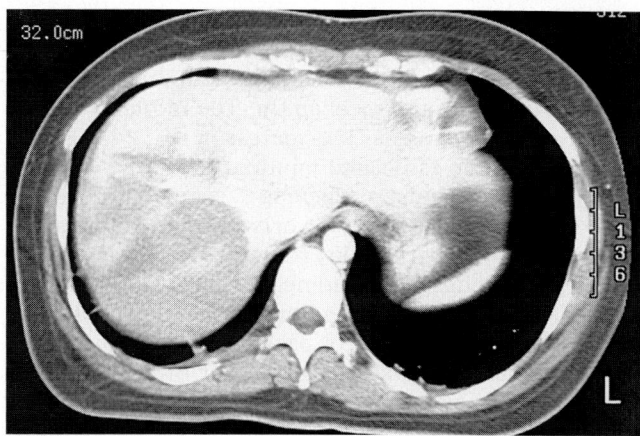

FIGURE 20-20.   CT shows a grade IV liver laceration.

grade liver injuries (grade 1 to 3), and transfusion requirements of less than 2 units of blood. Recently, these criteria have been challenged and a more broad indication for nonoperative management has been used. It has been demonstrated that most of these patients are followed by serial hematocrit and vital signs rather than by serial abdominal examinations. For this reason an intact mental status is not mandatory for nonoperative management. Furthermore, most patients will undergo a repeat CT if the hematocrit drops to evaluate and quantify the hemoperitoneum. The overall reported success of nonoperative management of blunt hepatic injuries is greater than 90% in most series. Breaking it down by injury grade, the success rate of nonoperative treatment for injuries grade 1 to 3 approaches 95%, whereas for injuries grade 4 and 5, the success rate decreases to 75% to 80%. With the use of angiography and superselective embolization in patients with persistent bleeding, the success rate may, in fact, be higher.

Angiographic embolization has been added to the protocol of nonoperative management of liver injuries in some institutions in an attempt to decrease the necessity of blood transfusions and the number of operations.[41,42]

Patients are admitted to the ICU unit for monitoring of vital signs and serial hematocrit. Usually, after 48 hours, patients are transferred to an intermediate-care unit where they are started on an oral diet but remaining on bed rest until post-injury day 5. A repeat CT before discharge does not seem to be necessary. Normal physical activity resumes in 3 months post-injury.

Porta Hepatis

A recent multicenter retrospective study including data from eight trauma centers reported an incidence of portal triad injuries of only 0.07%.[40] Penetrating trauma is the most frequent mechanism associated with porta hepatis injuries, although 30% of the porta hepatis injuries in the just-mentioned study followed blunt trauma. Isolated injuries to the porta hepatis are uncommon. Because of the proximity of other organs, porta hepatis injuries are usually associated with hepatic, duodenal, gastric, colonic, and other major vascular injuries. The overall mortality rate is 50%, increasing to 80% in patients with associated injuries.

Management is difficult because of life-threatening hemorrhage and associated organ injury. If the patient survives the operation, complications such as biliary fistula, portal vein thrombosis, and hepatic ischemia may contribute to morbidity. The management of portal vein and hepatic artery injuries is discussed later in the chapter in the section on major abdominal vascular injuries.

The management of common bile duct injury is challenging. Primary repair and placement of a tracheostomy tube should be attempted in partial or minor injuries involving less than 50% of the duct's circumference. Major injuries or complete transections of the common bile duct are best managed by means of a choledochoenteric anastomosis. This procedure significantly reduces the incidence of late postoperative complications, in particular, the development of strictures.

A closed-suction drain always should be placed in the vicinity of the repair to allow adequate drainage of an eventual biliary fistula. Missed extrahepatic bile duct injuries occurred in nine patients in a recent multicenter review, with a 75% complication rate in those who survived.[40]

Gallbladder injury is also an uncommon injury after both blunt and penetrating trauma. Cholecystectomy is the procedure of choice.

Postoperative Complications

Significant complications after liver injury include pulmonary complications, postoperative bleeding, coagulopathy, biliary fistulas, hemobilia, and subdiaphragmatic and intraparenchymal abscess formation.

Postoperative bleeding occurs in less than 10% of patients sustaining liver injuries. It may occur due to inappropriate hemostasis, postoperative coagulopathy, or both. Considering the patient is not hypothermic, coagulopathic or acidotic, re-exploration should be undertaken. Bleeding vessels should be directly visualized and ligated, even if a more extensive disruption of the hepatic parenchyma is necessary for adequate exposure. If diffuse oozing is found, packing and a planned re-exploration are performed.

Intra-abdominal abscesses have accounted for late deaths after hepatic trauma. A 7.2% incidence of perihepatic abscesses was reported in a prospective analysis of 482 injuries. We found that 27% of the deaths were due to the presence of intra-abdominal abscesses. The population at increased risk included patients in prolonged shock, extensive parenchymal disruption, associated hollow viscus injuries, hepatic ischemia due to ligation of major vessels, and those who underwent open drainage. Several studies have criticized the use of drains after liver injury because of the risks of intraperitoneal infection.[39] It seems that grade 1 and 2 injuries do not require drain placement. However, in severe injuries, drainage, although controversial, is frequently used.[39]

The presence of nonviable hepatic tissue is also an important cause of postoperative abscess formation and points to the fact that adequate débridement of all devitalized tissue is an important step before closing the abdomen. CT is the method of choice to diagnose intra-abdominal abscesses. Percutaneous drainage is the treatment of choice for nonloculated abscesses. However, patients with peritoneal signs, persistence of fever despite percutaneous drainage, or multiple abscesses should be surgically re-explored through the same incision used for the initial operation.

The incidence of biliary fistulas after hepatic trauma varies from 7% to 10%.[39] In a recent multicenter review of hepatic injuries, an 8% incidence of biliary fistula was noted in 210 patients with grade 3, 4, and 5 hepatic injuries. The group at risk includes patients with severe hepatic injuries (grade 3 and higher) and those requiring hepatic resection or extensive débridement. Usually, biliary fistulas close spontaneously after a period of 2 to 4 weeks of closed drainage.

Hemobilia is a rare complication, usually after blunt intrahepatic hematomas are formed, which presents as bleeding into the bile ducts and subsequently into the small bowel. Patients usually complain of jaundice, right upper quadrant pain, malaise, and melena. Hemobilia can be diagnosed by upper gastrointestinal endoscopy and treated with angiographic embolization. Surgery is rarely required.

Splenic Injuries

The spleen is the intra-abdominal organ most frequently injured in blunt trauma. Suspicion of a splenic injury should be raised in any patient with blunt abdominal trauma. History of a blow, fall, or sports injury to the left chest, flank, or left upper abdomen is usually associated with splenic injury. The diagnosis is confirmed by abdominal CT in the hemodynamically stable patient or during exploratory laparotomy in the unstable patient with a positive diagnostic peritoneal lavage.

For several decades splenectomy was considered the only acceptable surgical option for splenic injuries. With the significant experience in nonoperative management of splenic injuries in the pediatric population, and with the recognition of the overwhelming postsplenectomy syndrome as a serious postoperative threat, other options have emerged in the past decades. Initially, splenic repair and, more recently, nonoperative management in the adult population have been considered adequate options in selected patients. The pediatric surgeons initiated this more conservative approach and their experience was later applied to the adult trauma population.

The spleen is responsible for the production of immunoglobulins and the cellular immune response. Phagocytosis and clearance of blood-borne particles and the antigen-antibody response are impaired in asplenic patients. After splenectomy, the immune response to bacterial capsular type II polysaccharide antigens, which are the antigenic component of the capsule of the encapsulated bacteria (*Streptococcus pneumoniae, Haemophilus influenzae,* and *Neisseria meningitidis*), is decreased. These immunologic alterations, although transient, determine an indefinite risk of increased susceptibility to sepsis.

In 1952, a postsplenectomy syndrome of severe, some-times fatal meningitis and sepsis in four of five children splenectomized before the age of 6 months for congenital hemolytic anemia was reported. The term *overwhelming postsplenectomy infection* was introduced in 1969.

The true incidence of overwhelming postsplenectomy sepsis is not well defined, although a commonly used estimation of its incidence is 0.6% in children and 0.3% in adults, which may be a low estimate. The courses of 688 patients (388 children, 300 adults) who underwent splenectomy for injury to the spleen were reviewed. Among these were 10 patients with sepsis (incidence of 1.45%), 4 of whom died, resulting in a mortality rate of 0.58%. When combined with four deaths from sepsis after splenectomy for trauma in another series of 342 children, the incidence rate of mortality from sepsis is 0.78%, for a total of 78 times the expected rate in the general population. The risk of postsplenectomy septicemia, pneumonia, and meningitis was estimated to be 8.3% in trauma patients, or 166 times the 0.05% rate expected in the general population. The longest follow-up of splenectomy patients is of 740 World War II veterans who underwent splenectomy between 1939 and 1945. Six patients in this group (0.8%) died of pneumonia, whereas none of the 740 matched control patients died.

This syndrome is unlike fulminating bacteremias and septicemias in patients with normal splenic function. The overwhelming postsplenectomy infection syndrome is distinct from the septicemia in patients with normal immune function and is characterized by a sudden onset of symptoms and a rapid and fulminating course that often lasts only 12 to 18 hours. Patients usually complain of fever, nausea, vomiting, headache, and altered mental status. It is mainly caused by pneumococcus, but other species such as *Escherichia coli, H. influenzae, Meningococcus, Staphylococcus,* and *Streptococcus* may also be found in decreasing frequency. The disease is complicated by shock, electrolyte imbalance, hypoglycemia, and disseminated intravascular coagulation. The overall mortality rate is as high as 50% to 80%. Because of the severity of the disease process and the high mortality rates, the universal use of polyvalent pneumococcal vaccine (Pneumovax 23, Merck; Pnu-Immune, Lederle) and close follow-up after trauma splenectomy is routine. Patients should receive the vaccine before discharge. The effectiveness of the vaccine in splenectomized patients is unclear. The use of prophylactic antibiotics in asplenic patients is also controversial; however, minor infections in this group should be treated with antibiotics.

Management

Hemodynamic stable patients now undergo ultrasound examination. If ultrasound is positive for free fluid and the patient remains stable, an abdominal CT is obtained to identify the source of bleeding, evaluate for contrast agent extravasation and other intra-abdominal injuries that would require an operation, and grade the severity of the splenic injury (Fig. 20-21). The finding of contrast agent extravasation or "contrast blush" observed during the

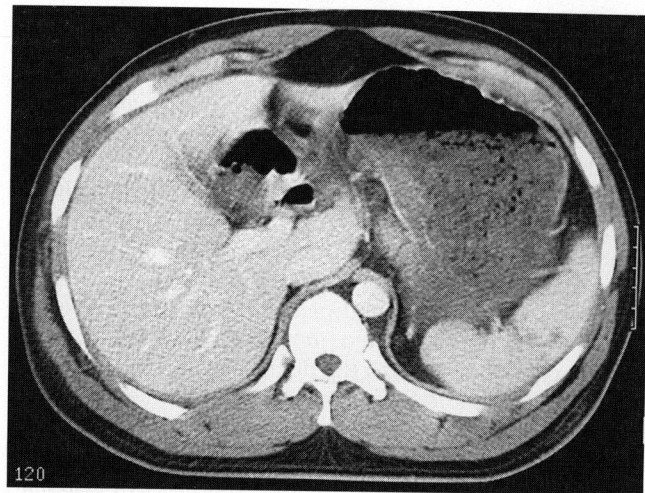

FIGURE 20-21. CT shows a splenic laceration.

arterial phase of the intravenous contrast agent abdominal CT is indicative of persistent bleeding. Some authors would argue that when present in the spleen, contrast blush should prompt operative intervention, whereas others argue that there is an opportunity for angiographic embolization and continuation of nonoperative management provided that the patient remains hemodynamically stable. In a recent study, the authors found contrast blush in 11% of patients with splenic injuries. No correlation between contrast blush and operative intervention was found. The authors concluded that the presence of contrast blush is not an absolute indication for an operative or angiographic intervention.[43]

Some institutions advocate for more routine use of angiography, but overall splenic salvage rates are similar to institutions following more selective use of angiography. Prospective studies should clarify this issue in the future.[44]

More than 70% of all stable patients are being treated by means of a nonoperative approach.[45] The classic criteria for nonoperative treatment include hemodynamic stability, negative abdominal examination, absence of contrast extravasation on CT, absence of other clear indications for exploratory laparotomy or associated injuries requiring a surgical intervention, absence of associated health conditions that carry an increased risk of bleeding (coagulopathy, hepatic failure, use of anticoagulants, specific coagulation factor deficiency), and grade 1 to 3 injuries.

Recent series have also indicated that nonoperative management should be done in patients older than age 55 years, with a large hemoperitoneum, and with injuries grades 4 and 5, which in the past have been relative contraindications.[46,47]

It has been shown that inclusion of high-risk patients increases the nonoperative management rate without changing the failure rate significantly. Age older than 55 years and grades 4 and 5 splenic injuries are predictors but do not constitute contraindications for nonoperative management of splenic injuries.[48]

Patients are usually admitted to the ICU and kept on bed rest with a nasogastric tube in place. Serial abdomi-

TABLE 20-10. Spleen Injury Scale (1994 Revision)

Grade*	Type of Injury	Description of Injury
I	Hematoma	Subcapsular, <10% surface area
	Laceration	Capsular tear, <1-cm parenchymal depth
II	Hematoma	Subcapsular, 10%-50% surface area: intraparenchymal, <5 cm in diameter
	Laceration	Capsular tear, 1- to 3-cm parenchymal depth that does not involve a trabecular vessel
III	Hematoma	Subcapsular, >50% surface area or expanding; ruptured subcapsular or parenchymal hematoma; intraparenchymal hematoma >5 cm or expanding
	Laceration	>3-cm parenchymal depth or involving trabecular vessels
IV	Laceration	Laceration involving segmental or hilar vessels producing major devascularization (>25% of spleen)
V	Laceration	Completely shattered spleen
	Vascular	Hilar vascular injury that devascularizes spleen

*Advance one grade for multiple injuries up to grade III.

From Moore EE, Cogbill TH, Jurkovich GJ, et al: Organ injury scaling: Spleen and liver (1994 revision). J Trauma 38:323-324, 1995, with permission.

nal examinations and hematocrit are obtained during the initial 48 to 72 hours. The necessity of blood transfusion is recorded. At 48 to 72 hours, stable patients are transferred to an intermediate care unit, start walking and eating, and are followed clinically. A repeat CT is obtained in cases of falling hematocrit, hypotension, or persistent ileus. If contrast agent extravasation is observed or a pseudoaneurysm is found, a selected group of patients benefit from angiography and selective embolization.

A repeat CT before discharge does not seem to be necessary. Patients are instructed to avoid intense physical activity and contact sports for 3 months. The success rate of nonoperative treatment is greater than 90%.[45] Several reports have reported that nonoperative treatment of splenic injuries is safe and effective.[45]

The surgical treatment of a splenic injury will vary depending on its severity (Table 20-10), the presence of shock, and associated injuries.

The spectrum of injury may vary from a simple laceration or contusion without capsular disruption to total fragmentation of the spleen. During laparotomy, the spleen is evaluated for active bleeding. If active hemorrhage is present, the surgeon must decide to perform either a total splenectomy or a splenic salvage procedure. Careful adequate mobilization of the spleen is essential to prevent further injury. Ongoing bleeding can be controlled from the spleen during mobilization by digital compression. Capsular tears of the spleen can be controlled by compression only or by using topical hemostatic agents. Deeper lacerations can be controlled with horizontal mattress absorbable sutures. Major lacerations involving less than 50% of the splenic parenchyma and not extending into the hilum can be treated with segmental or partial splenic resection. This is indicated only if the patient is stable, and in the absence of other major injuries. More extensive injuries involving the hilum or the central portion of the spleen may be managed by splenectomy; however, alternative procedures have been described. The technique of implanting thin splenic fragments in an omental pouch (autotransplantation) remains experimental and controversial but may provide significant long-term

splenic function. The use of a Dexon or Vicryl mesh wrapping the spleen or the utilization of the argon beam coagulator and fibrin glue have been described in selected patients. The success rate of splenic salvage procedures varies from 40% to 60%. This increases to 90% if nonoperative treatment is included.

Complications

Inadequate hemostasis, massive transfusion, or coagulation may cause bleeding after splenectomy or splenic salvage procedures. Other complications include transient thrombocytosis, pancreatitis, and intra-abdominal abscess.

Urinary Tract Injuries

Injuries to the genitourinary tract are often clinically unsuspected and frequently overlooked. Gross hematuria is the most frequent sign associated with urinary tract injuries. An understanding of the mechanism of injury and the forces involved is essential to identify urologic trauma and avoid missed injuries. In blunt trauma, fractures of the lower ribs or spinous processes fractures, crush abdominal or pelvic injuries, direct blows to the back and flanks, or decelerating injuries, such as in falls or motor vehicle accidents, have been associated with urologic injuries. Upper urologic tract injuries frequently present as gross or microscopic hematuria. Lower urinary tract injuries usually present as blood in the urethral meatus, a floating or displaced prostate on rectal examination, bladder distention, inability to void, and large perineal hematomas or other perineal injuries.

Penetrating injuries to the back or the flank have the potential to cause significant renal injury without obvious clinical manifestations.

The work-up of patients with suspected urinary tract injuries will depend on the hemodynamic status. Patients sustaining penetrating abdominal injuries requiring immediate exploratory laparotomy may undergo a one-shot intravenous pyelogram. Victims of blunt trauma with blood at the urethral meatus should undergo a urethro-

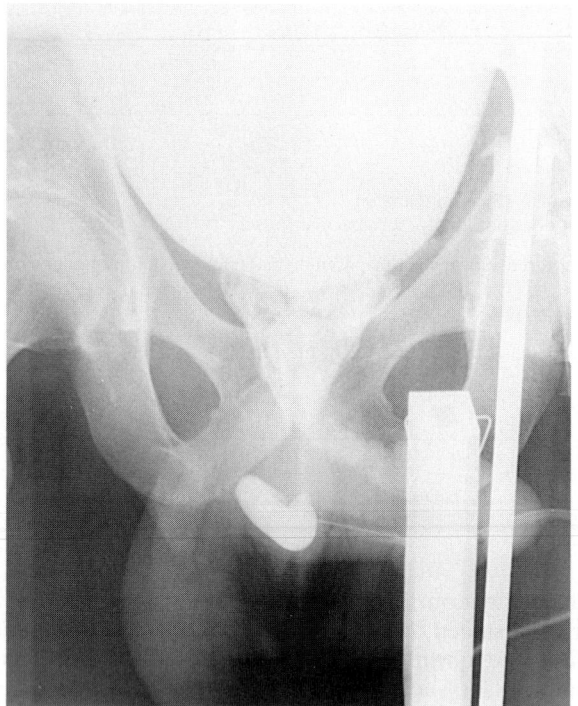

FIGURE 20-22. Urethrogram shows a complete urethral injury.

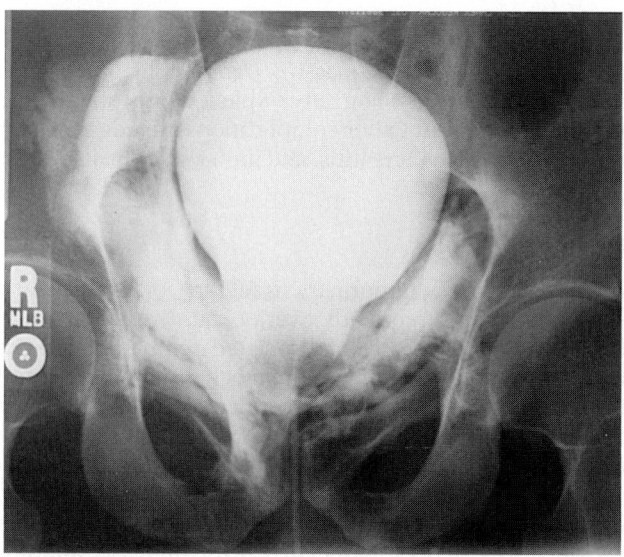

FIGURE 20-23. Cystogram shows a bladder injury.

cystogram to rule out the presence of a urethral injury before bladder catheterization (Fig. 20-22). Once urethral injury has been ruled out, a cystogram is performed by injecting 250 to 300 mL of contrast medium through the Foley catheter to maximally distend the bladder. Films should be obtained after full distention and after emptying the bladder. This post-void film is important to identify posterior extravasation of contrast agent that is not seen in anteroposterior films obtained when the bladder is maximally distended (Fig. 20-23). Patients with pelvic fractures involving the anterior arch are particularly prone to have an associated bladder injury.

CT is as effective as intravenous pyelography to evaluate the urinary tract; however, its major advantage over pyelography is its ability to evaluate potential intra-abdominal injuries and the retroperitoneum. It is also useful to stage renal injuries and to evaluate renal perfusion and function. Absence of kidney perfusion is an indication for renal artery angiography.

Specific Injuries

Renal Injuries. The kidney is the most commonly injured part of the urinary tract. Penetrating wounds causing small parenchymal injuries are generally treated with débridement, primary repair, and drainage. More extensive wounds may require a partial or total nephrectomy. An important technical aspect to keep in mind is that in major perinephric hematomas, proximal control of the renal pedicle before opening Gerota's fascia is advisable. Injuries involving the hilum are seldom repaired primarily, and in most circumstances a total nephrectomy is necessary. More than 80% of patients sustaining penetrating renal injuries have other intra-abdominal injuries.

Blunt renal injuries are generally divided into minor and major injuries (Fig. 20-24). Minor injuries comprise approximately 85% of cases. A classification system for renal injuries proposed by the American Association for the Surgery of Trauma was recently validated. It found that the severity of organ injury correlates with the need for operative intervention.[49]

Renal contusions encompass the vast majority of minor renal trauma and can almost invariably be treated nonoperatively. Major renal trauma includes deep cortical medullary lacerations with extravasation, large perinephric hematomas, and vascular injuries of the renal pedicle. These injuries should be explored because of the high incidence of complications, such as bleeding, abscess formation, hypertension, and so on. At laparotomy, the major problem is the decision to explore a perinephric hematoma.

It is our opinion that all perinephric hematomas caused by penetrating mechanisms, not previously evaluated by intravenous pyelography, should be explored. If a preoperative intravenous pyelogram shows renal pedicle injury, extensive parenchymal laceration, or urinary extravasation, surgical exploration remains the best option.

Ureteral Injuries. Injury to the ureter is uncommon and occurs mostly after penetrating trauma. The presence of hematuria in ureteral injury is the exception rather than the rule. Ureteral injury is suspected preoperatively by the location of the entrance site of penetrating injuries, or in the case of blunt injury by the presence of concomitant intra-abdominal or other genitourinary tract injuries. Nondiagnosed ureteral injuries may lead to complications such as fistulas, urinomas, and abscess formation. In the majority of cases, intravenous pyelography will confirm the diagnosis. In 15% to 20% of ureteral injuries a retrograde ureterography will be required to confirm the diagnosis. In hemodynamically unstable patients the diagnosis of ureteral injury may be made at the time of laparotomy by intravenously injecting 5 mL of methylene blue or indigo carmine dye. Extravasation of the blue-stained urine

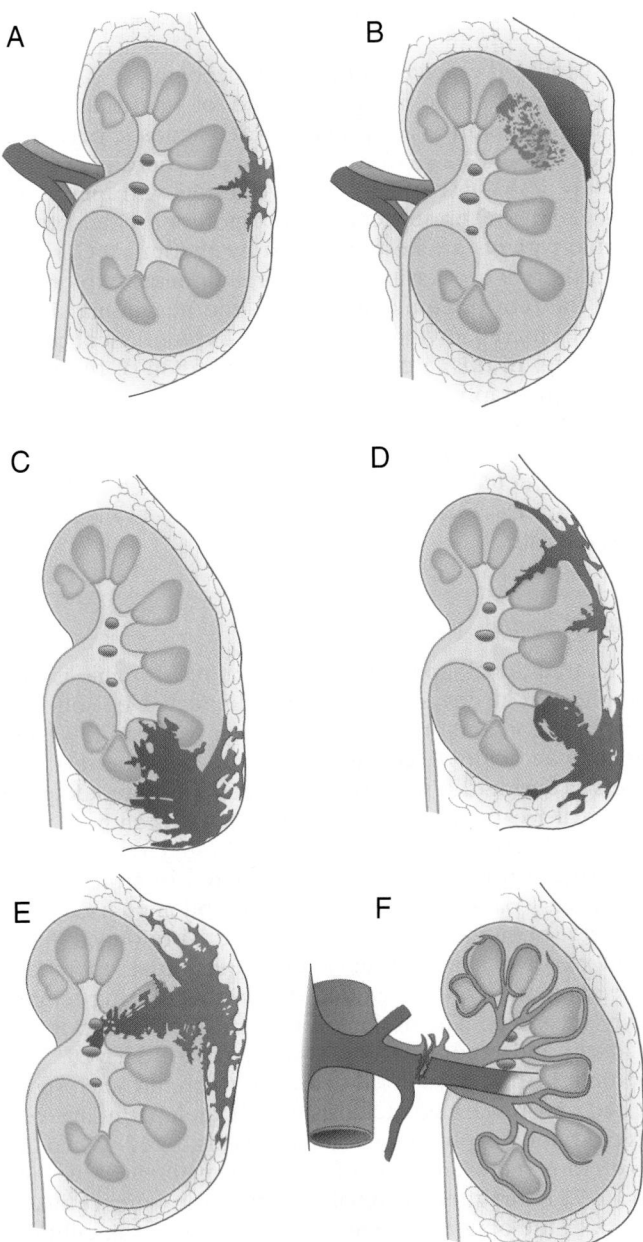

FIGURE 20-24. Different types of renal injuries. **A,** Small renal laceration with contained subcapsular hematoma. **B,** Minor subcapsular and parenchymal hematoma. **C,** Parenchymal laceration extending through the renal cortex without involvement of the collecting system. **D,** Multiple parenchymal lacerations; the inferior one extends through the cortex and collecting system, **E,** Parenchymal laceration extending through the cortex, medulla, and collecting system, with major subcapsular hematoma and urine extravasation. **F,** Injury to the renal vessels at the hilum. (From Peterson NE: Genitourinary trauma. *In* Feliciano DV, Moore EE, Mattox KL [eds]: Trauma, 3rd ed. Norwalk, CT, Appleton & Lange, 1996, p 667, with permission of the McGraw-Hill Companies.)

confirms the presence of a ureteral injury. The principles of ureteral repair are adequate débridement, tension-free repair, spatulated anastomosis, watertight closure, ureteral stenting, and drainage. Surgical options include ureteroureterostomy for injuries located in the upper and middle thirds of the ureter. The use of a double-J stent is indicated because it seems to decrease the incidence of postoperative fistulas. More distal injuries may require ureteral reimplantation in the bladder. A percutaneous nephrostomy is indicated to divert urinary flow in cases when primary repair is not feasible, either due to the overall clinical condition of the patient or when there is loss of a long segment of the ureter. Other options in the presence of extensive ureteral injuries include a transureteroureterostomy or kidney autotransplantation into the iliac fossa.

Bladder Injuries. The majority of bladder injuries occur as a result of blunt trauma, and the association of bladder rupture and pelvic fractures is extremely frequent. In fact, approximately 70% of patients with bladder rupture have associated pelvic fractures. Hematuria is the most frequent sign and in the presence of a pelvic fracture should increase the suspicion for bladder injury. Bladder rupture may be extraperitoneal or intraperitoneal. Extraperitoneal ruptures usually result from perforations by adjacent bony fragments. Intraperitoneal rupture of the bladder results from injuries located in the dome, which occur when a full bladder sustains a direct blow. Diagnosis is made by cystography. As stated previously, a post-void film is necessary to identify lateral or posterior injuries.

Intraperitoneal injuries are primarily repaired via a transabdominal approach, including a three-layer closure. A suprapubic cystostomy may be necessary in large wounds.

The management of extraperitoneal rupture of the bladder is primarily nonoperative by leaving the Foley catheter in place for 10 to 14 days, provided that the patient has no intra-abdominal injuries requiring surgical exploration. Patients with severe pelvic fractures and massive retroperitoneal bleeding are always initially managed nonoperatively. Once the retroperitoneal bleeding is controlled and the patient's condition is stable, a delayed repair of the extraperitoneal rupture can be performed, if necessary. Complications of bladder rupture include hemorrhage, urinoma, abscess formation, and sepsis.

Injuries to the Urethra. Disruption of the urethra is a rare injury in women. It is found mostly in men, frequently following either pelvic fractures or straddle injuries. Posterior urethral injuries are present in approximately 10% of pelvic fractures. Anterior urethral injuries are generally associated with straddle injuries and are often isolated lesions. Urethral injuries are suspected on the basis of mechanism of injury, associated pelvic fracture, perineal hematoma or perineal injury, blood at the urethral meatus, and displacement of the prostate gland. A retrograde urethrogram is essential for diagnosis. Currently, patients sustaining urethral injuries should be managed initially by bladder decompression via a suprapubic cystostomy and delayed urethroplasty.

Complications of urethral injuries include stricture, incontinence, and impotence, with disruptions of the urethra.

Pelvic Fractures. Pelvic fractures are the prototype of a severe trauma and account for less than 5% of all fractures after trauma. The most frequent mechanisms that cause pelvic fractures are motor vehicle accidents, motorcycle accidents, falls, and pedestrians struck. Unstable pelvic fractures are accompanied, most of the time, by major retroperitoneal hemorrhage. The incidence of associated injuries is high, particularly intra-abdominal, thoracic, and head injuries.

Mortality rates vary depending on the amount of bleeding and number of associated injuries. The mortality rate directly attributed to pelvic fracture is less than 15% in most series.

Pain is frequently present in the awake and alert patient. Urethral injury in males is also frequent and may manifest as urethral bleeding or inability to void with a distended bladder. A careful examination of the perineum is imperative, because mortality of open pelvic fractures is severalfold higher than that of closed fractures. A rectal examination should be carefully performed to identify rectal bleeding, to evaluate the position of the prostate gland, and to assess mucosal lacerations. If the prostate is misplaced or urethral bleeding is present, a retrograde urethrogram is mandatory before placement of a Foley catheter.

An anteroposterior film of the pelvis usually shows the fracture and asymmetry of the pelvis, if present. The radiographic evaluation in these circumstances should be complemented by inlet and outlet views of the pelvis. CT of the pelvis provides information on displacement of the sacroiliac joint, acetabular fractures, and sacral fractures; however, it should not be obtained in the hemodynamically unstable patient.

Pelvic fractures can be classified according to the resultant vector force (anteroposterior compression, lateral compression, and vertical shear), anatomy of the fracture lines, and pelvic stability.

The problem trauma surgeons face with pelvic fracture is related to retroperitoneal bleeding. Hemorrhage can be arterial, venous, or osseous in origin.

Fractures involving the posterior ring are generally believed to have more associated injuries and complications, require more resuscitation fluid, and have a higher mortality rate than do pure anterior fractures. Unstable pelvic fractures are usually associated with increased blood loss.

The objectives of the initial management of pelvic fractures are directed to control hemorrhage. This can be accomplished in unstable fractures, and particularly in those known as the open book type, with external fixation in the acute setting. Posterior fractures with involvement of the sacroiliac joint are frequently associated with arterial bleeding, which can be controlled with embolization of the bleeding vessel (usually branches of the internal iliac artery). Indications for angiography are recurrent hypotension after initial resuscitation attributed to the pelvic fracture or if the transfusion requirements exceed 4 to 6 units within the first 2 hours after injury. Blood infusion should be started early during resuscitation in the hemodynamically unstable patient. As a temporizing measure, the abdominal component of the MAST suit can be inflated during transport or in the resuscitation room to stabilize the pelvis and control bleeding.

Because of the high incidence of associated intra-abdominal injuries, a supraumbilical diagnostic peritoneal lavage should be performed; however, there is approximately a 35% rate of false-positive results with peritoneal lavage in the presence of a retroperitoneal hematoma. Stable patients are best evaluated by abdominal CT.

If there is a clear indication for abdominal exploration and the retroperitoneum is intact, the hematoma should not be entered, owing to an increased risk of uncontrolled bleeding. In this circumstance, stabilization of the pelvis and angiographic embolization should be performed. If the retroperitoneum is ruptured and active bleeding is found during an exploratory laparotomy, packing the pelvis and temporarily closing the abdomen, followed by external fixation and angiographic evaluation is appropriate.

Damage Control

The traditional approach to abdominal trauma is not applicable in devastating injuries. Repeated episodes of hypotension and organ hypoperfusion will lead to severe metabolic acidosis, coagulopathy, and hypothermia that persist during the postoperative period despite adequate surgical treatment of multiple injuries. Recently, a new approach has been proposed in these circumstances. Damage control includes an abbreviated laparotomy and temporary packing and closure of the abdomen used as an effort to blunt the physiologic response to prolonged shock and massive hemorrhage. During the initial operation, bleeding and contamination are controlled using temporary measures. The abdomen is packed and temporarily closed, and reconstruction and repair are delayed. The patient is then transferred to an ICU to be further resuscitated and rewarmed; acidosis and coagulopathy are corrected, and full physiologic support is instituted. When the patient is stable and organ function is maintained, usually 48 to 72 hours after the initial operation, the patient is taken back to the operating room for packing removal, débridement of nonviable tissue, and definitive repair.[50]

Abdominal Compartment Syndrome

Abdominal compartment syndrome occurs predominantly in patients presenting in profound shock who require large amounts of resuscitation fluids and blood and in patients with major visceral or vascular abdominal injuries.

This syndrome is characterized by a sudden increase in intra-abdominal pressure, increased peak inspiratory pressure, decreased urinary output, hypoxia, hypercarbia, and hypotension due to decreased venous return to the heart. Diagnosis is confirmed by measuring bladder pressure that ultimately represents the intra-abdominal pressure. Treatment includes a rapid decompression of the elevated intra-abdominal pressure by opening the abdominal wound and performing a temporary closure of the abdominal wall with mesh or with a plastic bag (Bogota's Bag). The

Box 20-7 Physiologic Consequences of Increased Intra-abdominal Pressure

Decreased

Cardiac output
Central venous return
Visceral blood flow
Renal blood flow
Glomerular filtration

Increased

Cardiac rate
Pulmonary capillary wedge pressure
Peak inspiratory pressure
Central venous pressure
Intrapleural pressure
Systemic vascular resistance

physiologic consequences of persistent elevated intra-abdominal pressure are listed in Box 20-7.

Selected References

Acosta JA, Yang JC, Winchell RJ, et al: Lethal injuries and time to death in a level I trauma center. J Am Coll Surg 186:528, 1998.

> This paper describes a 10-year experience of death after injury and delineates the time to death in a level I trauma center. It serves as a good reference for assessing outcome of injured patients and helps define the priorities for ongoing research in hemorrhage control, resuscitation, and management of head injury and multiple organ failure.

Bonnie RJ, Fulco CE, Liverman CT (eds) and the Committee on Injury Prevention and Control, Division of Health Promotion and Disease Prevention, Institute of Medicine: Reducing the Burden of Injury: Advancing Prevention and Treatment. Washington, DC, National Academic Press, 1999.

> This monograph is the most recent evaluation of current problems with regard to development of trauma systems and the challenges for acute care. The study was commissioned by the Institute of Medicine and represents the most current synthesis of what is known and what is left to be done in trauma care in the United States.

The Brain Trauma Foundation, The American Association of Neurological Surgeons, The Joint Section on Neurotrauma and Critical Care: Guidelines for the management of severe head injury. J Neurotrauma 17:471-91, 2000.

> This article represents the recommendations of the Brain Trauma Foundation based on its evidence-based assessment and development of guidelines for the management of head injury. This is the second revision of this important work and represents the most complete example to date of the use of evidence-based medicine in trauma. It has changed the way in which most people approach head injury, and there is some evidence to suggest that following these guidelines improves overall outcome.

Committee on Trauma: Resources for Optimal Care of the Injured Patient: 1999. Chicago, American College of Surgeons, 1999.

> This monograph defines the resources for the optimal care of the injured patient. It is rewritten every 4 to 5 years and has evolved as the standard for trauma care in the United States and for much of the world. The members of the Committee on Trauma are national authorities on trauma care. The current version is the basis for assessing trauma centers and verifying them against these standards.

Ivatury RR, Cayton CG: Textbook of Penetrating Trauma. Philadelphia, Lea & Febiger, 1996.

> This is the first book devoted exclusively to the management of penetrating trauma. The authors are leading authorities throughout the country, and the text covers all aspects of trauma care for penetrating injuries.

MacKenzie EJ, Hoyt DB, Sacra JC, et al: National inventory of hospital trauma centers. JAMA 289:1515-1522, 2003.

> This article describes a national inventory of trauma centers and reflects the current status of trauma center distribution and readiness. It describes how far we have come since the last time of this assessment (in the early 1990s) and how far we have to go. This is particularly important given the fact that a trauma system is the basis for an organized response to disasters.

Mattox KL, Feliciano DV, Moore EE: Trauma, 4th ed. New York, McGraw-Hill, 1999.

> This text is written by authors who truly represent the leaders in trauma care. The material presented is comprehensive and covers the history of trauma centers to the critical care of trauma patients. This is the standard textbook in trauma care.

Mullins RJ (ed): The Skamania conference. J Trauma 47(3):S2, 1999.

> This conference at Skamania evaluated the overall status of trauma system development and developed a consensus regarding the efficacy of trauma systems on reducing mortality. The entire reference is up to date and discusses essentially every issue. It has been effectively used to help encourage development of trauma systems nationwide.

References

1. Acosta JA, Yang JC, Winchell RJ, et al: Lethal injuries and time to death in a level I trauma center. J Am Coll Surg 186:528-533, 1998.
2. Simons R, Kasic S, Kirkpatrick A, et al: Relative importance of designation and accreditation of trauma centers during evolution of a regional trauma system. J Trauma 52:827-834, 2002.
3. Nathens AB, Jurkovich GJ, Maier RV, et al: Relationship between trauma center volume and outcomes. JAMA 285:1164-1171, 2001.
4. MacKenzie EJ, Hoyt DB, Sacra JC, et al: National inventory of hospital trauma centers. JAMA 289:1515-1522, 2003.
5. Demetriades D, Murray JA, Chan L, et al: Penetrating colon injuries requiring resection: Diversion or primary anastomosis? An AAST prospective multicenter study. J Trauma 50:765-775, 2001.

6. Accidental Death and Disability: The Neglected Disease of Modern Society. Washington, DC, National Academy of Sciences, National Research Council, 1966.

7. Bochicchio GV, Ilahi O, Joshi M, et al: Endotracheal intubation in the field does not improve outcome in trauma patients who present without an acutely lethal traumatic brain injury. J Trauma 54:307-311, 2003.

8. Mattox KL, Brundage SI, Hirshbert A: Initial resuscitation. New Horizons 7:4, 1999.

9. Bickell WH, Wall MJ Jr, Pepe PE, et al: Immediate versus delayed fluid resuscitation for hypotensive patients with penetrating torso injuries. N Engl J Med 331:1105-1109, 1994.

10. Holbrook TL, Anderson JP, Sieber WJ, et al: Outcome after major trauma: 12-month and 18-month follow-up results from the Trauma Recovery Project. J Trauma 46:765-773, 1999.

11. Macintyre AG, Christopher GW, Eitzen E Jr, et al: Weapons of mass destruction events with contaminated casualties: Effective planning for health care facilities. JAMA 283:242-249, 2000.

12. Hoyt DB, Moore EE, Shackford SR, et al: Trauma surgeon's leadership role in the development of trauma systems [editorial]. J Trauma 46:1142, 1999.

13. Shackford SR, Mackersie RC, Hoyt DB, et al: Impact of a trauma system on outcome of severely injured patients. Arch Surg 122:523-527, 1987.

14. Patel NY, Hoyt DB, Nakaji P, et al: Traumatic brain injury: Patterns of failure of nonoperative management. J Trauma 48:367-375, 2000.

15. Lee LA, Sharar SR, Lam AM: Perioperative head injury management in the multiply injured trauma patient. Int Anesthesiol Clin 40:31-52, 2002.

16. The Brain Trauma Foundation, The American Association of Neurological Surgeons, The Joint Section on Neurotrauma and Critical Care: Resuscitation of blood pressure and oxygenation. J Neurotrauma 17:471-478, 2000.

17. Sarrafzadeh AS, Peltonen EE, Kaisers U, et al: Secondary insults in severe head injury—do multiply injured patients do worse? Crit Care Med 29:1116-1123, 2001.

18. Bracken MB, Shepard MJ, Holford TR, et al: Administration of methylprednisolone for 24 or 48 hours or tirilazad mesylate for 48 hours in the treatment of acute spinal cord injury: Results of the Third National Acute Spinal Cord Injury Randomized Controlled Trial. National Acute Spinal Cord Injury Study. JAMA 277:1597-1604, 1997.

19. Asensio JA, Valenziano CP, Falcone RE, et al: Management of penetrating neck injuries: The controversy surrounding zone II injuries. Surg Clin North Am 71:267-296, 1991.

20. Mazolewski PJ, Curry JD, Browder T, et al: Computed tomographic scan can be used for surgical decision making in zone II penetrating neck injuries. J Trauma 51:315-319, 2001.

21. Gonzalez RP, Falimirski M, Holevar MR, et al: Penetrating zone II neck injury: Does dynamic computed tomographic scan contribute to the diagnostic sensitivity of physical examination for surgically significant injury? A prospective blinded study. J Trauma 54:61-65, 2003.

22. McKevitt EC, Kirkpatrick AW, Vertesi L, et al: Blunt vascular neck injuries: Diagnosis and outcomes of extracranial vessel injury. J Trauma 53:472-476, 2002.

23. Hoyt DB, Coimbra R, Potenza BM, et al: Anatomic exposures for vascular injuries. Surg Clin North Am 81:1299-1330, xii, 2001.

24. Sisley AC, Rozycki GS, Ballard RB, et al: Rapid detection of traumatic effusion using surgeon-performed ultrasonography. J Trauma 44:291-297, 1998.

25. Cothren C, Moore EE, Biffl WL, et al: Lung-sparing techniques are associated with improved outcome compared with anatomic resection for severe lung injuries. J Trauma 53:483-487, 2002.

26. Karmy-Jones R, Jurkovich GJ, Shatz DV, et al: Management of traumatic lung injury: A Western Trauma Association Multicenter review. J Trauma 51:1049-1053, 2001.

27. Wall MJ Jr, Hirshberg A, Mattox KL: Pulmonary tractotomy with selective vascular ligation for penetrating injuries to the lung. Am J Surg 168:665-669, 1994.

28. Velmahos GC, Karaiskakis M, Salim A, et al: Normal electrocardiography and serum troponin I levels preclude the presence of clinically significant blunt cardiac injury. J Trauma 54:45-51, 2003.

29. Coimbra R, Pinto MC, Razuk A, et al: Penetrating cardiac wounds: Predictive value of trauma indices and the necessity of terminology standardization. Am Surg 61:448-452, 1995.

30. Weigelt JA, Thal ER, Snyder WH III, et al: Diagnosis of penetrating cervical esophageal injuries. Am J Surg 154:619-622, 1987.

31. Stassen NA, Lukan JK, Spain DA, et al: Reevaluation of diagnostic procedures for transmediastinal gunshot wounds. J Trauma 53:635-638, 2002.

32. Duane TM, Tan BB, Golay D, et al: Blunt trauma and the role of routine pelvic radiographs: A prospective analysis. J Trauma 53:463-468, 2002.

33. Healey MA, Simons RK, Winchell RJ, et al: A prospective evaluation of abdominal ultrasound in blunt trauma: Is it useful? J Trauma 40:875-885, 1996.

34. Demetriades D, Velmahos G, Cornwell E III, et al: Selective nonoperative management of gunshot wounds of the anterior abdomen. Arch Surg 132:178-183, 1997.

35. Coimbra R, Pinto MC, Aguiar JR, et al: Factors related to the occurrence of postoperative complications following penetrating gastric injuries. Injury 26:463-466, 1995.

36. Ivatury RR, Nallathambi M, Gaudino J, et al: Penetrating duodenal injuries: Analysis of 100 consecutive cases. Ann Surg 202:153-158, 1985.

37. Jurkovich GJ, Carrico CJ: Pancreatic trauma. Surg Clin North Am 70:575-593, 1990.

38. Fakhry SM, Watts DD, Luchette FA: Current diagnostic approaches lack sensitivity in the diagnosis of perforated blunt small bowel injury: Analysis from 275,557 trauma admissions from the EAST multi-institutional HVI trial. J Trauma 54:295-306, 2003.

39. Cogbill TH, Moore EE, Jurkovich GJ, et al: Severe hepatic trauma: A multi-center experience with 1,335 liver injuries. J Trauma 28:1433-1438, 1988.

40. Jurkovich GJ, Hoyt DB, Moore FA, et al: Portal triad injuries. J Trauma 39:426-434, 1995.

41. David Richardson J, Franklin GA, Lukan JK, et al: Evolution in the management of hepatic trauma: A 25-year perspective. Ann Surg 232:324-330, 2000.

42. Hagiwara A, Murata A, Matsuda T, et al: The efficacy and limitations of transarterial embolization for severe hepatic injury. J Trauma 52:1091-1096, 2002.

43. Omert LA, Salyer D, Dunham CM, et al: Implications of the "contrast blush" finding on computed tomographic scan of the spleen in trauma. J Trauma 51:272-278, 2001.

44. Haan J, Scott J, Boyd-Kranis RL, et al: Admission angiography for blunt splenic injury: Advantages and pitfalls. J Trauma 51:1161-1165, 2001.

45. Pachter HL, Guth AA, Hofstetter SR, et al: Changing patterns in the management of splenic trauma: The impact of nonoperative management. Ann Surg 227:708-719, 1998.

46. Myers JG, Dent DL, Stewart RM, et al: Blunt splenic injuries: Dedicated trauma surgeons can achieve a high rate of non-operative success in patients of all ages. J Trauma 48:801-806, 2000.

47. Cocanour CS, Moore FA, Ware DN, et al: Age should not be a consideration for nonoperative management of blunt splenic injury. J Trauma 48:606-612, 2000.

48. Harbrecht BG, Peitzman AB, Rivera L, et al: Contribution of age and gender to outcome of blunt splenic injury in adults: Multicenter study of the Eastern Association for the Surgery of Trauma. J Trauma 51:887-895, 2001.

49. Santucci RA, McAninch JW, Safir M, et al: Validation of the American Association for the Surgery of Trauma organ injury severity scale for the kidney. J Trauma 50:195-200, 2001.

50. Rotondo MF, Schwab CW, McGonigal MD, et al: "Damage control": An approach for improved survival in exsanguinating penetrating abdominal injury. J Trauma 35:375-383, 1993.

CHAPTER 21

EMERGENT CARE OF MUSCULOSKELETAL INJURIES

Bruce D. Browner, M.D., Frank G. Alberta, M.D.,
Patricia C. Furey, M.D., Douglas Goumas, M.D., and Vikas Varma, M.D.

Epidemiology of Orthopedic Injuries	Orthopedic Emergencies
Terminology	Common Long Bone Fracture
Fixation Principles	Complications
Patient Evaluation	Postoperative Mobilization
Initial Management	Summary

EPIDEMIOLOGY OF ORTHOPEDIC INJURIES

Accidents are a prominent cause of death and disability throughout the world today. They account for more deaths in people in their first 5 decades of life than any other cause. They are the fifth leading cause of death in all age groups in the United States today. Commonly, the multiply injured patient will have musculoskeletal injuries owing to the significant amounts of energy absorbed in accidents. Because of the high energy involved, fractures and soft tissue injuries are common. Of the more than 174,000 patient records in the Major Trauma Outcomes Study, 48.6% had one or more musculoskeletal injuries between 1982 and 1990.[1] Disability and its ensuing costs following accidents are staggering. Hundreds of billions of dollars per year are lost when medical expenses, productivity losses, and property damage are tabulated.

At the national and global levels, significant strides have been made to provide for safer transportation and better, more efficient emergency medical care. Seatbelt and helmet laws, enforcement of drunk driving laws, mandates for improved safety features in automobiles, rapid deployment of emergency medical teams, and the establishment of trauma centers have decreased the number of accident scene fatalities. Victims are now more likely to survive accidents that might have been fatal in the recent past. As more accident victims survive their major life-threatening injuries, caregivers will be challenged with caring for more complex fractures and soft tissue wounds. These realities demand that trauma teams be aware of the frequency and the consequences of musculoskeletal injuries in every patient. An appreciation for the unique features of skeletally injured patients who may also have severe head, thoracic, or intra-abdominal injuries is essential. This mandates a cohesive, integrated approach to the diagnosis and treatment of musculoskeletal injuries in the multiply injured patient.

TERMINOLOGY

Communication among collaborating specialists is integral to optimal patient care. Trauma and emergency department findings need to be represented accurately to consulting specialists. This is particularly challenging when describing the variety of anatomic locations and multiple fracture patterns encountered in orthopedic injuries. Although many injuries are identified by eponyms among orthopedists, the most practical and universally understood characterizations of injuries are those that adhere to basic anatomic and mechanical principles.

Fracture Types

A *fracture* is a disruption of the normal architecture of bone. In pediatric injuries, this can include an injury to, or through, the cartilaginous growth plate that may not be evident radiographically. *Acute* fractures have sharp, well-defined edges to the fragments. *Chronic* fractures have a rounded and sclerotic appearance after resorption of bone has occurred at the fracture ends. This distinction can usually be made on clinical examination. Incomplete disruptions of bone are termed *greenstick fractures* in children or *infractions* in adults. Chronic, repetitive trauma can also cause microscopic disruptions when bone is stressed beyond its failure point. These injuries are termed *stress fractures* and are considered overuse injuries.

When a bone fails through an area weakened by pre-existing disease, it is termed a *pathologic fracture*. Causes may include weakness from primary bone tumors, metastatic lesions, infection, metabolic disease, and injuries at old fracture sites. Although not commonly referred to in this way, fractures in osteoporotic bone are technically considered to be pathologic. The term *insufficiency fracture* is most frequently used to describe these injuries. In distinction to acute fractures in healthy bone, these normally occur after much lower energy injuries. Hip fractures, compression fractures of the vertebral bodies, and distal radius fractures in the elderly are common examples.

A fracture is considered *open* when an overlying wound produces communication between the fracture site and the outside environment. These can range from an inside-to-outside poke hole in the skin to severe crushing injuries. High-energy fracture patterns indicate that the soft tissues, as well as the bones, have absorbed large forces. Although the skin laceration is the most obvious component, the energy of the fracture, the degree of contamination, and the soft tissue injury all must be taken into account when grading the severity of the injury. Contamination of bone can lead to the development of osteomyelitis and all of its catastrophic consequences, necessitating emergent treatment.

An *intra-articular* fracture extends into a joint. When there is significant cartilage damage, late degenerative changes are likely. These injuries normally occur from a compressive, or axial, load across the joint. Displaced intra-articular fractures require urgent, anatomic reduction and rigid fixation to avoid post-traumatic arthritis.

Long bone fractures are characterized by anatomic location. The *epiphysis* includes the area between the growth plate (physis) or physeal scar and the articular surface. The *metaphysis* is located between the epiphysis and the shaft and includes the growth plate. The bone in this area is softer and more vascular owing to its cancellous nature. The *diaphysis* encompasses the shaft of the bone between the proximal and the distal metaphyses. Fractures can be described based on location within these three sections or based on location with the bone being divided into thirds (proximal, middle, and distal). Distally, the humerus and femur flare to form their articular surfaces. These flares are termed the *epicondyles*. Fractures

in these areas are referred to as *supracondylar*. The articular surfaces are known as *condyles*. Condylar fractures are intra-articular and may extend proximally. These are important distinctions because these injuries present difficult treatment challenges.

A fracture may also be described by the pattern of cortical disruption. The orientation of the primary fracture line may be transverse, oblique, or spiral. *Transverse* and *oblique fractures* occur when a bending moment is applied. *Spiral fractures* generally result from a rotational force about the long axis of the bone. *Comminution* is the presence of multiple fragments involved in a fracture and usually connotes a higher energy injury or weakened bone in an elderly patient. A *butterfly fragment* is an area of comminution in one of the simple fracture patterns previously described (Fig. 21-1*D*).

Displacement, if present, is described from a combination of principles. These deformities may occur in any plane. When viewed on plain radiographs, all injuries will be resolved into pure coronal or sagittal displacement. However, it is important to realize that the true displacement usually occurs in a plane that is somewhere in between. *Translation* is the relationship of the proximal fracture fragment to the distal one. It is described in terms of percent overlap. A fracture 100% translation in any plane is said to be totally displaced. *Angulation* is simply the angle created by the displaced fracture fragments. It is described by the direction of the apex that the fracture fragments form (e.g., 20-degree apex lateral). The final component is *rotation*. To truly describe rotation, a full-length film of the limb segment involved including the joints above and below must be examined. A fracture may appear nondisplaced on one radiographic view yet be significantly displaced on another.

Once a fracture has been identified, it must be described in a consistent, systematic manner. All descriptions begin with whether or not the fracture is open and its grade. A closed fracture is assumed if no indication is given otherwise. The presence of an intra-articular fracture is communicated next. The side of the body and the injured bone are stated next. A description of the pattern followed by its location in the bone is then indicated. Finally, the displacement as described previously is related. Adherence to this scheme will allow for uniform understanding of the fracture.

Other Injuries

Ligamentous injuries are commonly encountered in all areas of orthopedics. When a ligament is damaged but is still in continuity, it is termed a *sprain*. Sprains can range in severity from minimal injuries to moderate instability about a joint. Grade I ligamentous injuries result from stretching of a ligament or ligament complex. They normally do not result in instability. A simple ankle sprain is the typical example of this type of injury. Partial ruptures of ligaments can result in minor instability and are considered grade II injuries. Complete ruptures, or grade III injuries, lead to significant instability at the associated joint. Avulsion fractures at the insertion of ligamentous

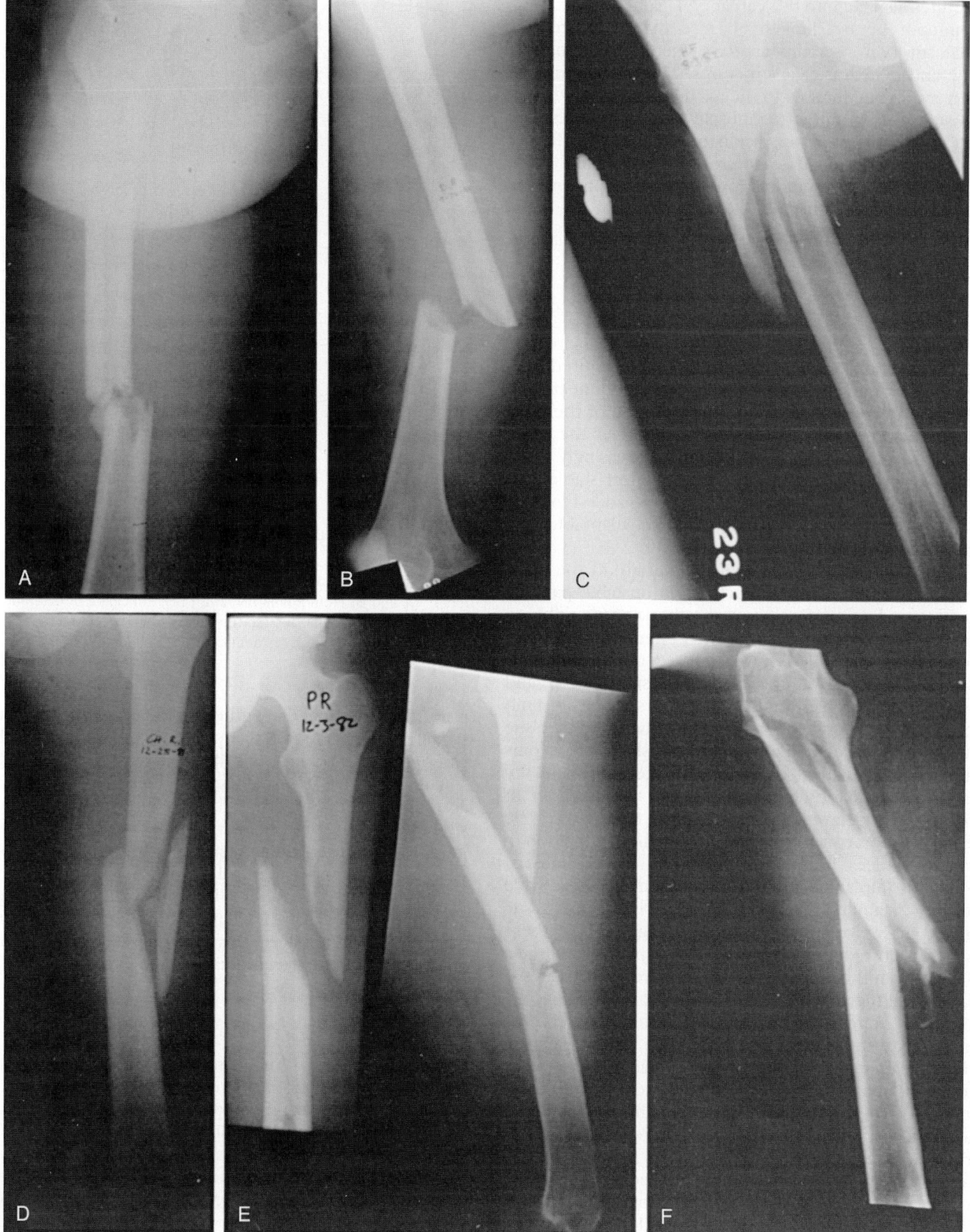

FIGURE 21-1.   Descriptive terms used to characterize femoral shaft fractures. **A,** Transverse mid-shaft fracture. **B,** Short oblique fracture. **C,** Long oblique fracture. **D,** Butterfly (or wedge) fragment in a mid-shaft femur fracture. **E,** Segmental fracture. **F,** Comminuted fracture. (**A** to **F,** From Wolinsky PR, Johnson KD: Femoral shaft fractures. *In* Browner BD, Jupiter TB, Levine AM, Trafton PG [eds]: Skeletal Trauma, 2nd ed. Philadelphia, WB Saunders, 1998.)

structures also fall into this category. Ligamentous injuries should not be overlooked because they can produce significant joint instability and endanger surrounding soft tissue and neurovascular structures. This is most critical when evaluating injuries to the axial skeleton.

A *strain* is an injury to a muscle or tendon. These are most commonly of an overuse nature. Further loading of the already weakened structure can compound these injuries. Rest, ice, compression, and elevation are the mainstays of treatment.

FIXATION PRINCIPLES

External Fixation

External fixation provides stabilization of an injured limb segment through the use of pins or wires connected to rods via clamps or rings. With the exception of the pins, the entire construct is external to the body, as the name implies. Recent designs have become increasingly more complex, yet they are easier to apply and more stable than ever before. The addition of modularity has added to their prospective uses and has led to more adaptable and adjustable constructs.

The primary uses of external fixation are in the treatment of open fractures, of fractures in unstable patients who cannot tolerate significant anesthesia times or blood loss, of complex fractures in which open reduction and internal fixation (ORIF) is not warranted, of fractures with associated vascular injuries requiring stabilization and urgent vascular repair, and of those in specialized limb reconstruction surgery. In fractures with soft tissue injuries, the placement of percutaneously inserted pins that minimize further soft tissue damage and avoid the area of contamination helps to decrease the incidence of infection and delayed unions. External fixators may be used as temporary stabilization or for definitive fixation in certain instances. In complex fractures around joints, fixation with implanted plates or screws may not provide adequate stability. Sometimes, overlying soft tissue damage makes operative exposure dangerous. In these instances, an external fixator with the pins placed at a distance from the fracture—and the injured soft tissues—can provide the stability necessary for healing.

External frames are constructed from three components: pins, connectors, and rods (Fig. 21-2). Pins are either threaded or smooth and vary in size. They serve to connect the bone to the rest of the device. Pin placement is chosen to best stabilize the fracture while not compromising the viability of the fragments. Pins are never placed through compromised or infected skin. A variety of different clamps serve as connectors and secure pins to the rods that form the external frames. Most are universal joints that allow multiple degrees of freedom. Connecting clamps have advanced to the point that they now snap into place onto the pins and the rods. They may be combined with rings or hinged rods and allow for almost limitless permutations of frame constructs. Stabilizing rods are nearly universally radiolucent to allow radiographic examination after application. Threaded rods, bone trans-

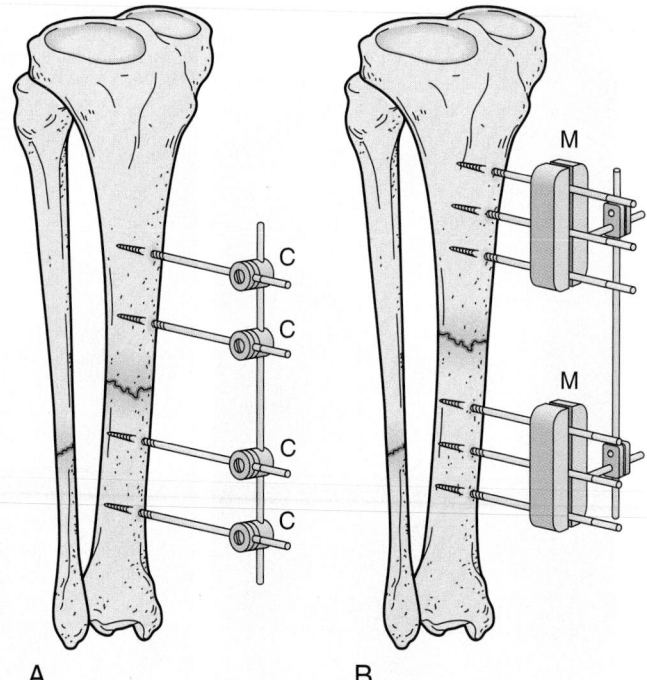

FIGURE 21-2. Frame types. **A,** Simple frame clamps (C) connect a single pin individually to the rod(s). **B,** Modular frame clamps (M) connect clusters of two or three pins to the connecting rod(s). (**A** and **B,** From Pollak AN, Ziran BH: Principles of external fixation. *In* Browner BD, Jupiter TB, Levine AM, Trafton PG [eds]: Skeletal Trauma, 3rd ed. Philadelphia, WB Saunders, 2003.)

port rails, motorized lengthening devices, and dynamic struts represent a small sample of the types of rods that can be used to achieve specific results.

Once applied, external fixators require persistent care and monitoring. Pin care is begun immediately and consists of cleansing with either normal saline or half-strength peroxide solution. Drainage must be addressed with local care, antibiotics, pin removal and replacement, or a combination of these modalities. Pins are checked after 1 to 2 weeks to ensure that they have not loosened. Depending on the fracture pattern, the fixator construct, and the goals of treatment, weight-bearing status is adjusted.

Internal Fixation

ORIF implies that an incision is made at or near the site of injury with reduction of the fracture under direct vision (open reduction) and rigid stabilization with plates, screws, wires, or combinations thereof (internal fixation). ORIF is frequently used to treat periarticular fractures and fractures of the axial skeleton. This technique allows for anatomic reduction and the creation of highly stable constructs. Multiple types of implants can be used to achieve these results.

Pins and Screws

Pins and screws are the simplest implants. They can be placed in a variety of areas and are often placed percutaneously. Kirschner wires may be temporary and are often used in the stabilization of small fragments. They can also be used to provisionally hold a reduction while more stable fixation is applied. Screws can be used for interfragmentary compression when placed with a lag technique (Fig. 21-3). This technique uses a gliding hole in the one fragment that allows the screw to pull the opposite fragment toward the near fragment, achieving compression.

Tension Bands

When the forces applied across a fracture site tend to displace it in tension, the tension band technique can be applied. This technique uses a variety of implants to convert tension forces on one side of a fracture into a compressive force across the entire contact area (Fig. 21-4). Typically, wires or cables are used to create tension bands. However, nonabsorbable suture and plates can also be used. Tension bands are most frequently used in fractures of the olecranon, patella, and greater trochanter.

Plates

Plates are used frequently in the internal fixation of fractures. They allow for the distribution of forces evenly across their length and can serve a variety of biomechanical functions.

A *neutralization plate* is used to protect another form of fixation from excessive forces. Often used in combination with lag screws, these plates add torsional and bending stability. Addition of a neutralization plate allows earlier mobilization than what would have been possible with less stable fixation.

Buttress plates are used to counteract forces that occur through a fracture site with axial loading. Longitudinal and oblique fractures near joints tend to displace along the line of the fracture when subjected to axial loads. Plates placed in a longitudinal fashion can form an axilla with the intact cortex that prevents this axial displacement. There are plates specifically designed for buttressing; however, any plate can be applied in a buttress mode.

Compression plating is used to increase the stability of fixation when the two major fracture fragments can be brought into contact. This technique allows for the direct compression of the fracture ends. Specific compression plates have oval screw holes that allow for the eccentric placement of screws. When applied in this fashion, the plate (and the bone fragment fixed to it) can be translated as the screw tightens down against the plate. Compression through a plate can also be achieved by overbending or with the use of a tensioning device.

Highly comminuted or segmental fractures may not allow for the anatomic reduction and direct fixation of all the fragments. In these situations, a *bridge plate* can be used to rigidly stabilize a long bone. The proximal and distal intact fragments are rigidly fixed to each other through the plate while the fracture site is bypassed. This concept has been popularized lately because it allows for minimal dissection at the fracture site that will decrease the devitalization of the fragments.

Special plates have been designed for specific fracture patterns and anatomic locations. Blade plates, dynamic condylar screws, and pelvic reconstruction plates are examples of these specialized plates.

Intramedullary Nails

In contrast to wires, plates, and screws, intramedullary (IM) nails are placed in the medullary canal of long bones. They are used to splint or bridge a fracture while still controlling axial, bending, and rotational forces. IM nailing also permits the fixation of a fracture through an incision distant from the fracture site. This technique has been described as *closed nailing* because the fracture site is not opened. Nails are made of a variety of materials and can be fluted, smooth, solid, or cannulated (Fig. 21-5). When transverse screws are placed through the proximal and distal ends of the nail, it is considered to be locked. Locked nails better control rotation and maintain bone length in the presence of comminution or bone loss. The locking holes in nails may be round or oval. Using a nail with an oval hole or leaving the nail unlocked at one end allows the bone fragment to slide axially along the nail, producing compression at the fracture site. Nails locked in this fashion are said to be *dynamically locked*. When screws are inserted through round holes in both ends of the nail, they are considered to be *statically locked* (Fig. 21-6).

IM nails can be inserted either from proximal to distal or vice versa, and are termed *antegrade* and *retrograde,* respectively. Nails may be inserted with or without canal preparation by reaming. *Reaming* involves passing a large drill down the medullary canal with the intent of removing the cancellous bone and effectively widening the canal. This allows for the insertion of a larger diameter nail that will substantially increase the strength and stiffness of the nail. Reaming leads to increased pressure in the medullary canal, increased temperatures in the cortical bone, and embolization of marrow contents into the vascular system. This embolization is not well tolerated in patients with severe derangement of pulmonary function or hemodynamic instability. However, reaming causes morcellization of cancellous and cortical bone in the canal, which is subsequently deposited at the fracture site and provides exceptional autogenous bone graft.

Unreamed nails are inserted without reaming of the canal. Destruction of the cortical blood supply from the medullary system is largely avoided when no reaming is performed. In fractures in which there is a large degree of soft tissue loss or periosteal stripping, an unreamed nail is typically used.

PATIENT EVALUATION

History

Obtaining a detailed history of the skeletally injured patient is essential to facilitate accurate diagnosis and treatment. This becomes challenging in the trauma setting with multiply injured and elderly patients. However, it is

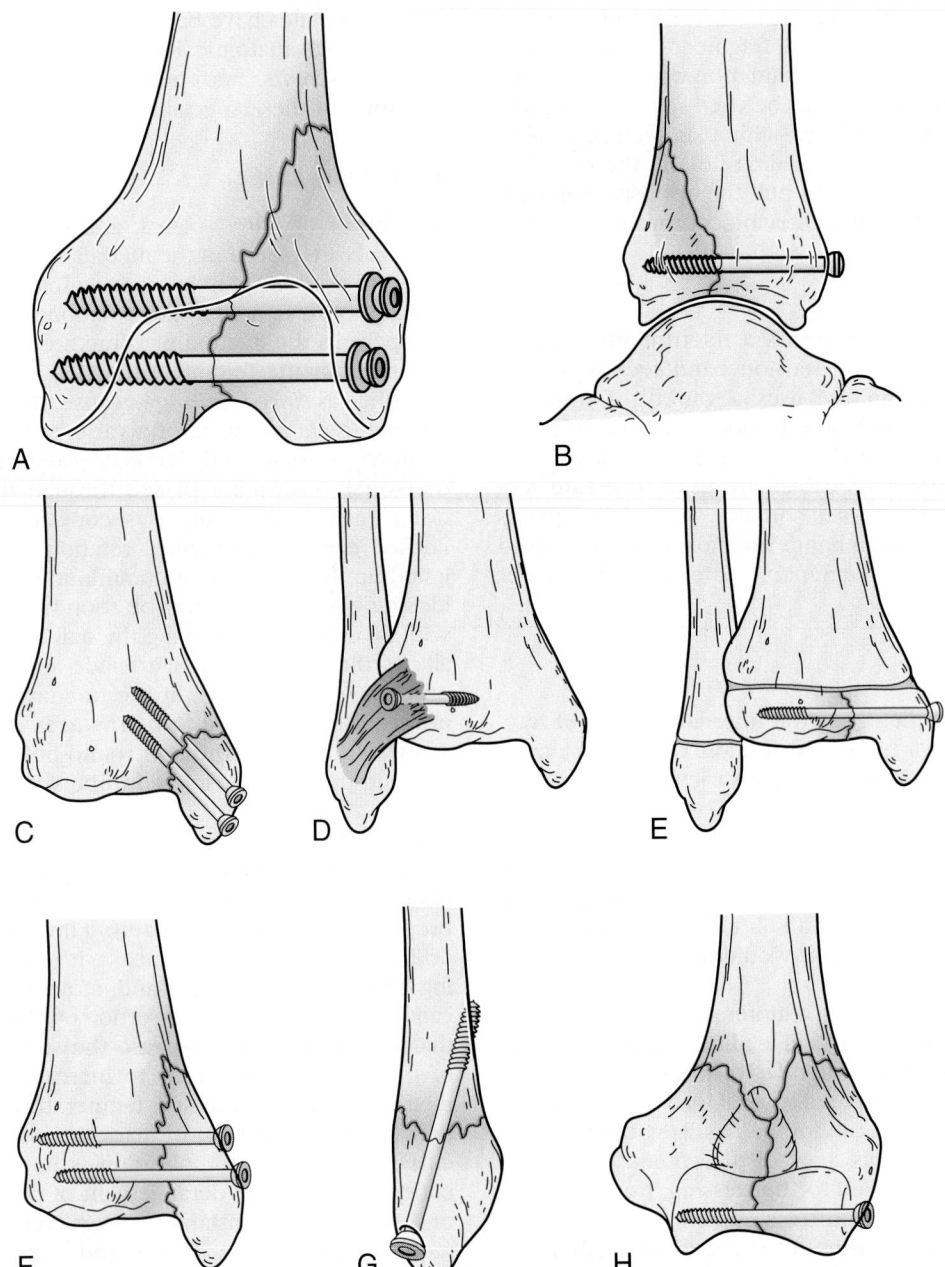

FIGURE 21-3. Typical indications for cancellous lag screws. **A,** Two 6.5-mm cancellous screws with a 32-mm thread, used with washers to fix a lateral femoral condyle fracture. **B,** A 4.0-mm cancellous screw inserted from front to back to fix the posterior lip fragment of the distal tibia. **C,** Two 4.0-mm cancellous screws used to fix a medial malleolus fracture. **D,** A 4.0-mm cancellous screw used to fix a fragment from the anterior aspect of the distal tibia carrying the syndesmotic ligament. **E,** A 4.0-mm cancellous screw used to fix an epiphyseal fracture of the distal tibia. **F,** Two 4.0-mm cancellous screws used to fix an oblique fracture of the medial malleolus. **G,** A malleolar screw inserted obliquely to fix a short, oblique fracture of the distal fibula. This direction of insertion allows cortical purchase with an increased compression force. **H,** A 4.0-mm cancellous screw used to fix the vertical component of a supracondylar Y fracture of the distal humerus. (**A** to **H,** From Mazzocca AD, Caputo AE, Browner BD, et al: Principles of internal fixation. *In* Browner BD, Jupiter TB, Levine AM, Trafton PG [eds]: Skeletal Trauma, 3rd ed. Philadelphia, WB Saunders, 2003.)

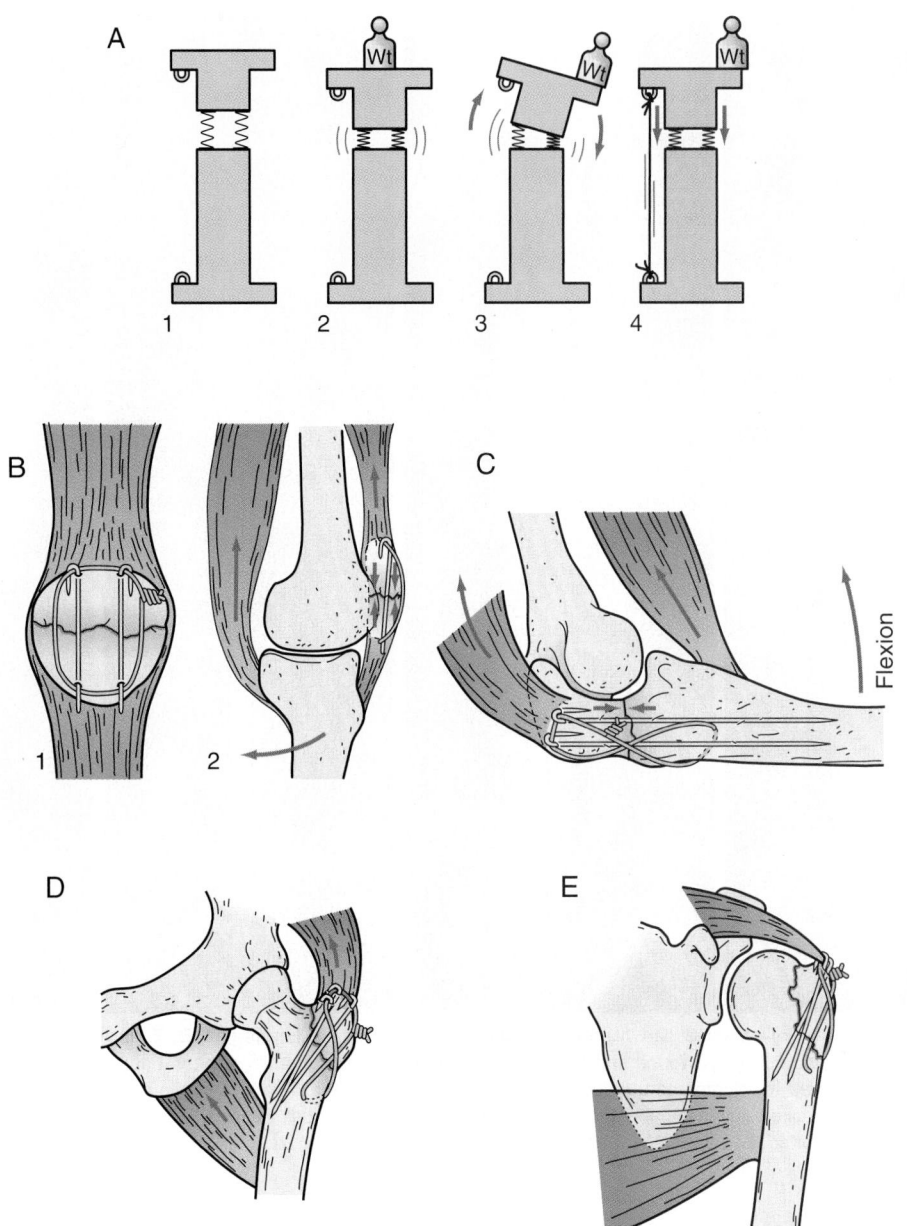

FIGURE 21-4.   Tension band principles. **A,** (1) An interrupted I-beam connected by two springs. (2) The I-beam is loaded with a weight (Wt) placed over the central axis of the beam; there is uniform compression of both springs at the interruption. (3) When the I-beam is loaded eccentrically by placing the weight at a distance from the central axis of the beam, the spring on the same side compresses, whereas the spring on the opposite side is placed in tension and stretches. (4) If a tension band is applied prior to the eccentric loading, it resists the tension that would otherwise stretch the opposite spring and thus causes uniform compression of both springs. **B,** The tension band principle applied to fixation of a transverse patellar fracture. (1) The anteroposterior view shows placement of the parallel Kirschner wires and anterior tension band. (2) The lateral view demonstrates antagonistic pull of the hamstrings and quadriceps, causing a bending moment of the patella over the femoral trochlea. An anterior tension band transforms this eccentric loading into compression at the fracture site. **C,** The tension band principle applied to fixation of a fracture of the ulna. The antagonistic pull of the triceps and brachialis causes a bending moment of the ulna over the humeral trochlea. The dorsal tension band transforms this eccentric load into compression at the fracture site. **D,** The tension band principle applied to fixation of a fracture of the greater trochanter. With the hip as a fulcrum, the antagonistic pull of the adductors and abductors causes a bending moment in the femur. The lateral tension band transforms this eccentric load into compression at the greater trochanteric fracture site. **E,** The tension band principle applied to fixation of a fracture of the greater tuberosity of the humerus. Using the glenoid as a fulcrum, the antagonistic pull of the pectoralis major and supraspinatus causes a bending moment of the humerus. The lateral tension band transforms this eccentric load into compression at the greater tuberosity fracture site. (**A** to **E,** From Mazzocca AD, Caputo AE, Browner BD, et al: Principles of internal fixation. *In* Browner BD, Jupiter TB, Levine AM, Trafton PG [eds]: Skeletal Trauma, 3rd ed. Philadelphia, WB Saunders, 2003.)

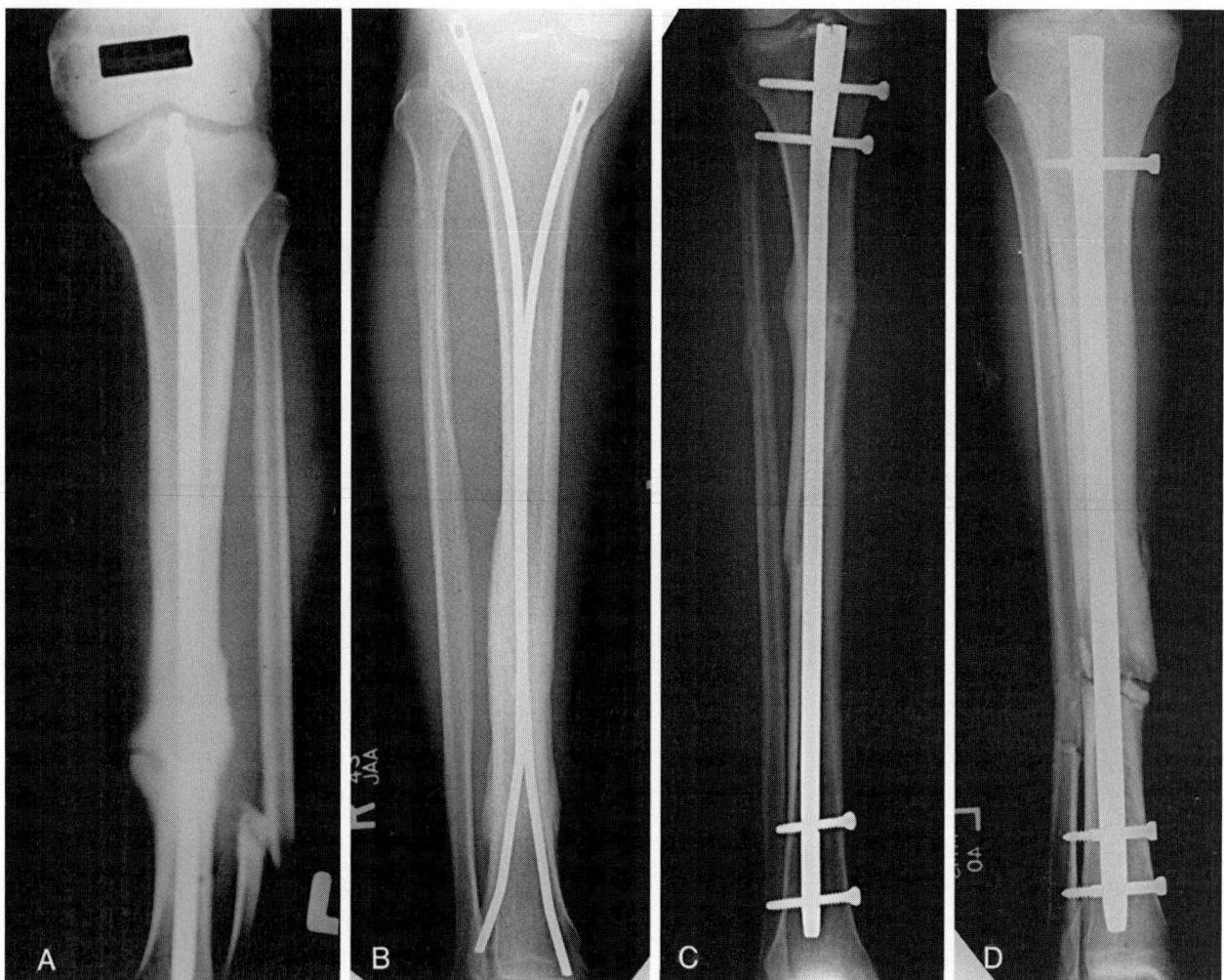

FIGURE 21-5.   Examples of intramedullary fixation for tibial shaft fractures. **A,** Lottes nail. **B,** Ender nails in a patient with a major-severity, open, comminuted injury. Wound and fracture healed benignly. The prominent lateral nail was associated with some knee pain until it was removed. **C,** Nonreamed, static, locked intramedullary nail in a patient with a healing, comminuted, major-severity injury. **D,** Reamed, locked nail in a patient with a closed, major-severity injury. (**A** to **D,** From Trafton PF: Tibial shaft fractures. *In* Browner BD, Jupiter TB, Levine AM, Trafton PG [eds]: Skeletal Trauma, 2nd ed. Philadelphia, WB Saunders, 1998.)

important to gather as much information as possible regarding the mechanism of injury. Descriptions from the accident or injury scene can be most helpful because common patterns of injury follow from specific mechanisms (Table 21-1).

A general history including demographic information, past medical history, past surgical history, and social history should be obtained. Allergies, current medications, and time since last oral intake are useful in guiding treatment. In addition, it is important to obtain information about the position of the limb before and after the injury. Ambulatory status before the injury helps determine realistic goals for functional recovery. Any transient neurologic symptoms, such as loss of consciousness, numbness, paresthesias, and spasm, must be documented. Loss of bowel or bladder control in patients with back or neck pain must also be noted. The elapsed time since injury becomes critical information in the patient with a vascular injury, an open wound, or a dislocation.

Trauma Room Evaluation

Examination of the multiply injured patient must follow Advanced Trauma Life Support protocols in a systematic fashion and must be accompanied by treatment. The first 5 minutes of trauma resuscitation secures an airway, establishes ventilation, and maintains circulatory support. Hemodynamically unstable patients are assumed to be in hemorrhagic shock until proved otherwise. A search for occult hemorrhage is undertaken and may include the pleural cavities, abdomen, retroperitoneum, or pelvis. Diagnostic peritoneal lavage or serial transabdominal ultrasound examinations are performed in unstable patients with suspected intra-abdominal injuries. A plain chest radiograph quickly reveals hemothorax. Chest tubes are placed, if necessary. The width of the mediastinum is noted, and arteriography is undertaken after life-threatening hemorrhage is controlled. Pelvic instability, and the need for rapid external pelvic fixation, is addressed. The

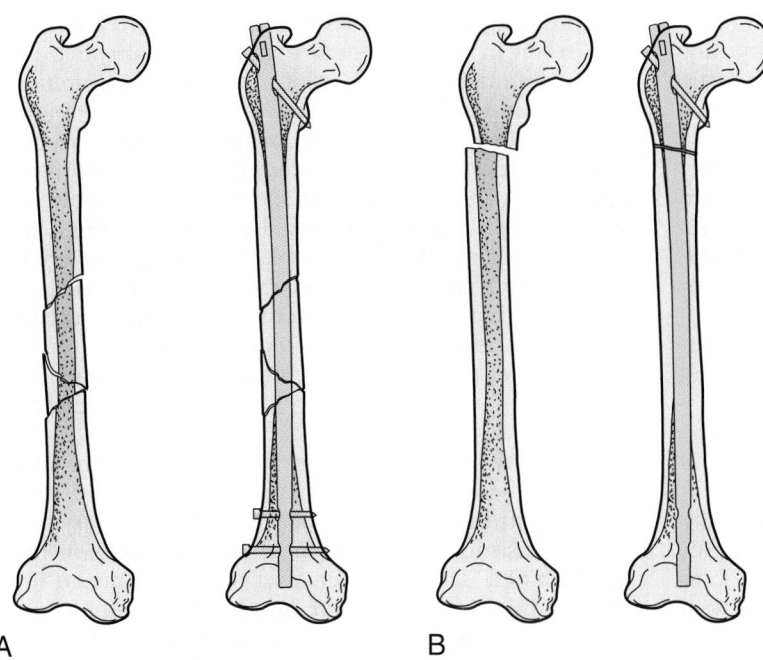

A   B

FIGURE 21-6. **A,** *Static* locked intramedullary nail fixed to *both* the proximal and the distal fragments. **B,** *Dynamic* locked intramedullary nail fixed to *either* the proximal (as shown) or the distal fragment, but not to both. (**A** and **B,** From Wolinsky PR, Johnson KD: Femoral shaft fractures. *In* Browner BD, Jupiter TB, Levine AM, Trafton PG [eds]: Skeletal Trauma, 2nd ed. Philadelphia, WB Saunders, 1998.)

patient's neurologic status is noted on admission, and the Glasgow Coma Scale is calculated. Patients with suspected head injury should be evaluated as soon as possible by computed tomography (CT). Peripheral vascular injuries and musculoskeletal injuries are next in priority, followed by maxillofacial injuries. All open fractures should be treated within the first 8 hours.[2] Early trauma room management includes antibiotics, tetanus prophylaxis, splinting, and wound coverage. *Sterile dressings* placed at the scene or in the trauma room should be left in place until the patient reaches the operating room. This practice has led to decreased infection rates when compared with routinely redressing wounds in the trauma area.[3] Urgent stabilization of fractures, vascular repair, débridement, and fasciotomy in severely injured extremities has reduced the incidence of adult respiratory distress syndrome (ARDS) and multisystem organ failure.[2,4] In less severe injuries, once the patient is stabilized, wound closure, complex joint reconstruction, and repair of maxillofacial injuries can be completed.

Severe pelvic fractures are addressed in the primary survey owing to the possibility of exsanguination. Cervical spine injuries, with associated neurologic compromise, also deserve immediate attention. These exceptions aside, the examination and management of the extremities are deferred to the secondary survey after the airway has been controlled and hemodynamic stability is obtained. In the team approach, these examinations and treatments are happening simultaneously. Throughout the resuscitation phase and the remainder of the hospital course, re-examination will ensure that no injuries go unrecognized (tertiary survey).

Evidence of pelvic fractures is assessed early in the resuscitative effort. Massive flank or buttock contusions and swelling are indicative of significant bleeding. The Morel-Lavale lesion is an ecchymotic lesion over the greater trochanter that represents a subcutaneous degloving injury. This lesion is frequently associated with acetabular fractures. Blood at the urethral meatus, signifying injury to the genitourinary tract, may be a sign of underlying pelvic fracture. Palpation of the symphysis as well as the sacroiliac joints can help determine the presence of gapping. Gentle rocking and lateral compression through the anterior iliac crests can provide helpful clues to the stability of the pelvic ring. Any opening or looseness signifies instability and may represent a source of hemorrhage. Rectal and vaginal examinations are performed,

TABLE 21-1. **Common Patterns and Their Associated Injuries**

Injury Pattern/Mechanism	Associated Injuries
Fall from height	Calcaneus fracture Tibial plateau fracture Fractures around the hip (proximal femur, acetabulum) Vertebral burst fracture
Ejection from vehicle	Closed head injury Spine fractures
"T-bone" motor vehicle accident	Lateral compression–type pelvic fracture Closed-head injury Thoracic injury
Head-on motor vehicle accident	Abdominal visceral injury "Open-book" pelvic fracture Retroperitoneal bleeding
Posterior knee dislocation	Popliteal artery injury
Supracondylar humerus fracture	Brachial artery injury Nerve injury (median or radial)
Anterior shoulder dislocation	Axillary nerve injury
Posterior hip dislocation	Sciatic (peroneal division) nerve injury

noting any bleeding, lacerations, bony fragments, hematomas, or masses. Wounds and palpable bony fragments on either of these examinations are diagnostic of an open pelvic fracture, which carries with it a poor prognosis.

At all times, the trauma team must take steps to protect the patient from self-inflicted or iatrogenic spinal cord injury. This includes observing full spine precautions until it is confirmed that the patient's vertebral column is intact, either by physical examination and clinical suspicion, or by radiologic confirmation when warranted.

The cervical spine is stabilized by fitting the patient with a hard cervical collar, and the thoracic, lumbar, and sacral spine are protected by maintaining the patient in the flat supine position at all times. If the patient is to be moved, strict log-roll technique is employed. At times a patient may have to be physically restrained to prevent potential self-inflicted injury by head or lower extremity movements that may impart rotational, translational, or bending moments on the vertebral column. Special care must be taken in combative patients or in patients with altered mental status who may have lost the ability to protect themselves from further injury.

The presence of deformity, edema, or ecchymosis is noted by the examiner. Tenderness elicited on palpation of the spine is noted for the level at which the patient complains of pain and any associated findings at that level. A distinction should be made as to whether the pain is midline or paraspinal. In patients with known neurologic deficit or back or neck pain, perianal sensation and rectal sphincter tone must be evaluated. Deep tendon reflexes and pathologic reflexes, such as the bulbocavernosus and Babinski, should be tested. The presence of sacral sparing (intact perianal sensation, rectal tone, or great toe flexion) represents at least partial continuity of the white matter long tracts. In one large series,[5] sacral sparing was predictive of the completeness of injury in 97% of patients with spinal cord injury. Radiographs of the thoracolumbar spine are indicated when the patient reports pain; when there are ecchymoses, abrasions, or step-off; or when ejection from a vehicle or a fall from a significant height has occurred. In *all* trauma patients anteroposterior, lateral, and odontoid radiographs of the cervical spine must be obtained. Radiographs are not considered adequate unless the entire cervical spine can be visualized from the superior tip of the dens distally to the superior endplate of the first thoracic vertebra.

Cervical spine injuries can occur by several mechanisms and can be divided into three main categories. The first involves direct trauma to the neck itself. The second method is by motion of the head relative to the axial skeleton. This can occur either by direct trauma to the head, or by continued movement of the head relative to the fixed body, as often occurs in blunt trauma, such as motor vehicle collisions where the body is restrained. In attempting to tether the head against motion, the cervical spine endures a large bending or twisting moment, resulting in flexion-extension injuries or rotational injuries, respectively.

A third mechanism of cervical spine injury involves a direct axial load imparted on the cranium causing axial compression forces across the cervical vertebrae. This may result in a *burst fracture* and potential spinal cord injury, although this pattern of injury is more commonly seen in the lumbar spine. Burst fractures, by definition, involve injury to the middle column of the vertebrae. These fractures are to be differentiated from *compression fractures*, which involve the anterior column only, and are rarely associated with spinal cord injury. Burst fractures are commonly found in falls from height where the feet transmit an axial load to the upper axial skeleton, resulting in a common pattern of calcaneal fractures and lumbar burst fractures. Depending on the fracture pattern, treatment of spine injuries may range from observation, to bracing, surgical fixation, or external halo fixation.

Extremity examination in isolated injuries or the multitrauma patient follows a simple, systematic, and reproducible pattern. Even if an isolated extremity injury is the primary reason for evaluation, the entire skeleton must be examined. The examiner must not be distracted from the task by obvious or severe injuries. Deformity, edema, ecchymosis, crepitus, tenderness, and pain with motion are the cardinal signs of acute fracture. Each limb segment should be examined for lacerations and the previously described signs of trauma. All joints should be put through a passive range of motion at minimum. Active range of motion should be tested whenever possible. Joint effusions are evidence of intra-articular pathology (e.g., ligament or cartilage damage or intra-articular fracture). The joints should then be manually stressed to assess integrity of ligamentous structures. A neurovascular examination is performed and documented. Pulses are recorded and compared with the opposite, uninvolved extremity when possible. Doppler signals are obtained when palpable pulses are not present or are weak. Motor function and sensation must be documented for the extremity dermatomes as well as the trunk in the patient with thoracic spine pain. To avoid the complications of a missed compartment syndrome, palpation of the involved compartments should be performed. Any firm or tense compartments are checked for increased pressure if time and the patient's condition allow. Fasciotomies are performed urgently if pressures are elevated. Gross alignment and interim immobilization of long bone fractures are achieved before the transportation of the patient from the trauma room. This will facilitate transfer, decrease pain, decrease soft tissue trauma and hemorrhage, reduce the chance of turning a closed fracture into an open one, improve the quality of radiographic studies, and prevent potential neurovascular injury. Traction splints or skeletal traction is applied when indicated.

Diagnostic Imaging

Radiographic examination should be used to supplement and enhance the information gathered during the primary survey, history, and physical examination. In the multiply injured patient, Advanced Trauma Life Support protocol calls for a lateral cervical spine film and anteroposterior views of the pelvis and chest. The secondary survey then dictates which extremity radiographs are necessary. When filming long bone injuries, it is important to verify the integrity of the adjacent limb segments. Therefore, the joints above and below the level of injury are always included in the films. They should be filmed separately if the cassette is not large enough to accommodate the entire view. Similarly, when pathology is suspected in a joint, the long bones above and below should be imaged as well. This practice helps identify commonly associated injuries to the adjacent limb segments that might otherwise be missed.

Since bone is a three-dimensional object, a single two-dimensional radiograph cannot describe a fracture. To understand the position and direction of the fracture fragments, orthogonal views (true anteroposterior and lateral films of the bone taken at 90 degrees to one another) must be obtained. All extremities with deformity should be rotated to the anatomic position prior to taking radiographs. This leads to decreased confusion when describing the fracture.

The goal of radiographic assessment of intra-articular fractures is the quantitation of articular incongruity. Orthogonal views of the joint and adjacent long bones are obtained. Radiographs made parallel to the articular surface best display any step-off that may be present. In complex intra-articular fractures, a CT scan is usually necessary to fully understand the position and displacement of all articular fragments. CT scans provide fine detail, help locate small fragments in the joint, and can further describe the extension of intra-articular fracture lines. These should not be used in lieu of acceptable plain radiographs, however. Plain radiographs are better suited to accurately describe overall fracture characteristics and limb alignment.

Additional imaging is undertaken in specific circumstances only after acceptable plain radiographs have been thoroughly reviewed. Stress radiographs are made when ligamentous or growth plate injuries are suspected after clinical examination but are not evident on plain films. Gapping of the joint or physis while stressing the structure in question is diagnostic (Fig. 21-7). Cervical spine ligamentous injuries are often diagnosed this way, using *active* flexion-extension radiographs. *Passive* flexion-extension should not be attempted. Oblique views are sometimes necessary to evaluate more complex structures such as the shoulder, proximal tibia, and acetabulum. True anteroposterior and lateral views of the shoulder must be taken in relation to the scapula owing to the orientation of the joint. The most useful lateral view is an axillary film. The tube is angled cephalad with the plate on the superior aspect of the shoulder and the arm in abduction and external rotation. This view is often difficult to obtain owing to pain or instability at the proximal end of the humerus. Judet views or 45-degree oblique views of the pelvis are used to evaluate the acetabuli. Owing to the spatial orientation of the acetabulum, these represent orthogonal views when the x-ray tube is canted toward or away from the affected side. Similarly, inlet and outlet views of the pelvis allow for closer examination of the sacroiliac joints and the sacrum itself. The inlet view is taken with the beam angled 30 degrees caudad, making

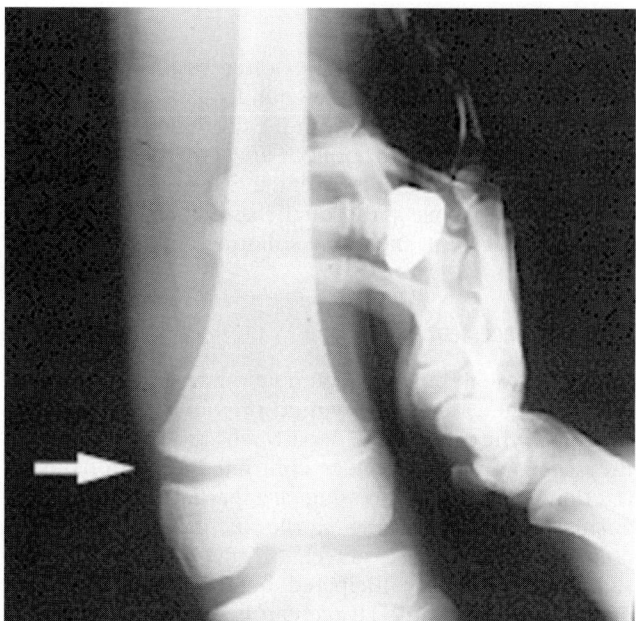

FIGURE 21-7. Stress radiograph of a physeal injury of the distal femur. An anteroposterior radiograph with valgus stress applied reveals unstable physeal disruption.

the beam perpendicular to the pelvic brim. The sacral ala and displacement of the sacroiliac joints in the anteroposterior plane are easily seen. The outlet view is a 45-degree oblique view with the tube angled cephalad. The sacrum is pictured en face, and the foramina are easily evaluated.

Magnetic resonance imaging (MRI) has become a particularly useful imaging modality. It is used to evaluate soft tissue, acute fractures, stress fractures, spinal cord injuries, and intra-articular pathology. Its role in the trauma setting has expanded as well, and it is particularly useful in the setting of spinal cord injury. More frequently, MRI is used in the outpatient setting to evaluate soft tissue injuries and pathologic lesions. MRI is now commonly used in the diagnosis of acute fracture when plain films are negative. In elderly patients with osteopenic femoral neck fractures, bone scans, although accurate, are unreliable within 48 hours after injury. MRI has been shown to be at least as accurate as bone scans in the diagnosis of acute fracture. Additionally, the sensitivity and specificity of MRI were the same within 24 hours of admission when compared with its use later.[6] Earlier diagnosis can potentially lead to shorter hospital stays and therefore more than offset the additional cost of the MRI.

Arteriography is another important modality used in the evaluation of extremity and pelvic injuries. It is indicated any time signs of distal ischemia are noted in an extremity. Knee dislocations are a common cause of arterial injury secondary to the proximity of the popliteal vessels. Prompt reduction of these injuries is mandatory followed by reevaluation of the vascular status. In cases in which pulses return after reduction, arteriography is still indicated owing to the probability of intimal damage to the artery and late thrombosis.

INITIAL MANAGEMENT

Care of musculoskeletal injuries often begins in the field. The extent of fracture and wound management differs with the level of training and experience of the first responders (lay people, police) and emergency medical personnel. Therefore, it is essential that the initial treating physician performs a thorough assessment and begins initial management, including splinting and wound care.

Wound Management

After a thorough physical examination, treatment is immediately begun. All sterile wound dressings placed in the field or in the emergency department are left intact until they can be removed under controlled conditions. Nontraction splints and dressing are partially removed by a single examiner using sterile technique. Superficial contamination by dirt, gravel, or grass is removed. If a significant delay is anticipated before formal operative débridement, pulsatile lavage can be used in the trauma room. Sterile saline solution or povidone-iodine–soaked dressings are then applied. Careless wound management in the emergency department has been shown to increase the ultimate infection rate by 300% to 400%.[7] Tetanus prophylaxis and broad-spectrum intravenous antibiotics are administered. Immobilization is then undertaken in the same manner as for a closed injury. External bleeding in the extremities is controlled with direct manual pressure.

Following wound care in the initial period, subsequent early débridement and reassessment of wounds with *frequent dressing changes* can prevent secondary infection and subsequent bacterial translocation. Avoidance of protein malnutrition, in addition, can protect against gut translocation and systemic infection. Earlier range of motion and muscle strengthening can result in decrease in length of hospitalization, rehabilitative time, and long-term disability.[8,9]

Reduction and Immobilization

All displaced fractures and dislocations are gently reduced to regain gross limb alignment. If the patient's condition allows, formal reductions are performed and the extremities are splinted to hold their position. Difficulty of reduction increases, as does edema and muscle spasm. Therefore, reduction should be attempted as soon as possible and with the patient as relaxed as possible. This often requires the use of narcotic analgesics and sedatives. This becomes particularly important with dislocations. Muscle spasm obstructs atraumatic reduction of these injuries. If after adequate sedation and relaxation, a joint is still dislocated, general anesthesia may become necessary.

Reduction maneuvers follow the same principles for all fracture and dislocation types. First, inline traction is applied to the limb. If the soft tissue envelope surrounding the fracture fragments is intact, this may be all that is required to obtain satisfactory alignment. The deformity is then recreated and exaggerated to unhook the fragment ends. Finally, the mechanism of injury is reversed and the fracture immobilized. Neurovascular status is again checked after any reduction maneuver or splint application. Once satisfactory reduction or alignment is achieved, it must be maintained by immobilization through casting, splinting, or continuous traction. The joints above and below the fracture must be included to provide the greatest control against displacement. Postreduction radiographs are required to confirm alignment and rotation.

Nondisplaced fractures are treated in the same manner as displaced ones, except that no reduction is necessary. It is still important to obtain adequate radiographs and to fully evaluate the injured limb. The same principles of immobilization apply. Most nondisplaced fractures do not require surgical treatment. Splints are placed initially and then changed to circumferential casts after swelling is allowed to subside.

Ligamentous injuries require similar immobilization. The joint is fully evaluated as described previously, and a thorough neurovascular examination is performed on the limb. Frequently, pain, effusions, or hemarthroses occur and represent intra-articular pathology. The limb is then immobilized and re-evaluated after the acute pain and swelling decrease.

The rationale of immobilization is threefold. First, splinting, particularly with traction or compression devices, reduces bleeding. Second, additional soft tissue injury may be averted. The chance of converting a closed to an open fracture is reduced. Third, immobilization of the fracture leads to reduced pain. This facilitates patient transportation and radiographic evaluation.[10] All fractures and dislocations should be splinted or immobilized in the emergency department. Most frequently, splints are fashioned from padded plaster or fiberglass. Splints can be secured with bias-cut stockinette, Ace wraps, and gauze bandage provided they are wrapped in a nonconstrictive fashion. The role of circumferential casting in the acute setting is questionable. Because swelling of the injured extremity increases for 48 to 72 hours, a circular cast would be too constrictive and can lead to pressure necrosis or compartment syndrome. In cases in which the cast will be the definitive treatment, a circumferential cast is applied and then split longitudinally to allow for swelling. The padding is not split, however. This maintains reduction more effectively than an open splint.

Traction

Traction is used to immobilize fractures or dislocations displaced by muscle forces that cannot be adequately controlled with simple splints. The most common indications are vertical shear injuries of the pelvis, hip dislocations, acetabular fractures, and fractures of the upper two thirds of the femur. Traction may be applied through the skin or skeletally through a pin inserted distal to the injury site. Traction of greater than 8 pounds through the skin for any extended period causes skin damage. Skin traction is prac-

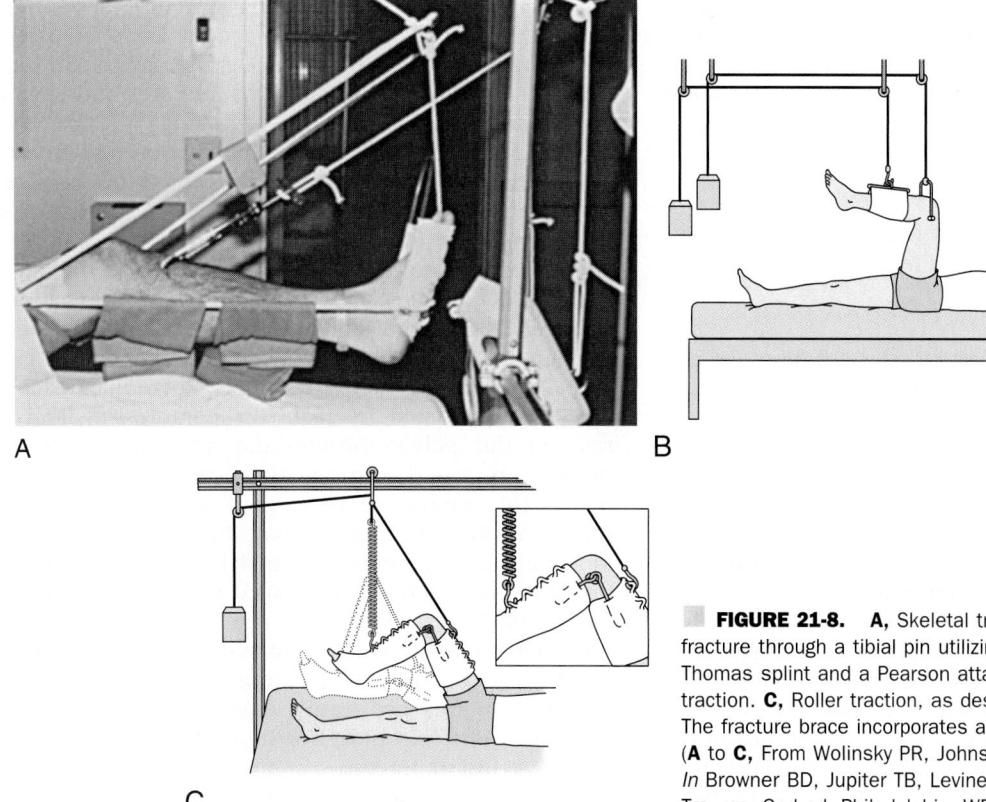

A

B

C

FIGURE 21-8. **A,** Skeletal traction applied to a femoral shaft fracture through a tibial pin utilizing balanced suspension with a Thomas splint and a Pearson attachment. **B,** 90-90 skeletal traction. **C,** Roller traction, as described by Neufeld and Mooney. The fracture brace incorporates a traction pin in the tibial tubercle. (**A** to **C,** From Wolinsky PR, Johnson KD: Femoral shaft fractures. *In* Browner BD, Jupiter TB, Levine AM, Trafton PG [eds]: Skeletal Trauma, 2nd ed. Philadelphia, WB Saunders, 1998.)

tical only for geriatric hip fractures and pediatric injuries requiring limited distraction force. The Hare temporary traction splint, which applies a distraction force through an ankle stirrup, can provide effective immobilization for femoral shaft fractures. It can be applied in the field and helps facilitate transport and mobilization.

Skeletal traction may be maintained for longer periods and with greater weight than skin traction (Fig. 21-8). Neurovascular structures must be avoided during placement of pins. Once pins are placed, the skin should be checked for tension and relieved with incisions if necessary. The wounds are then dressed with povidone-iodine–soaked sponges. Pin tract infection is a common complication and can lead to osteomyelitis in the worst cases. Pin care is begun every nursing shift and includes cleaning of the pin sites with 0.5% hydrogen peroxide and sterile dressings.

Prioritization of Surgical Care

After the secondary survey is completed and necessary diagnostic studies are obtained, the multiple trauma patient is moved to the operating room. Operative decisions are made on a continuous basis as the patient's condition evolves. The trauma surgeon is the coordinator of care and prioritizes all surgical procedures after consulting with the anesthesiologist, neurosurgeon, and orthopedic surgeon. Critical procedures are carried out first, and each additional step is reviewed as the patient's status changes. Intra-abdominal, thoracic, retroperitoneal, and intracranial hemorrhage are immediate surgical priorities. These include acute visceral hemorrhage, aortic or caval injuries, injuries to the heart or pulmonary vessels, intracranial mass lesions, depressed skull fractures, and pelvic fractures with associated instability. In addition to hemorrhage, immediate surgery is also indicated for the prevention of the pulmonary failure septic state; the prevention of local and systemic infections from open, devitalized wounds; and limb salvage. Stabilization of severe open and femoral shaft fractures may be performed simultaneously or after hemodynamic stabilization of the surgical patient. Limb-threatening vascular injuries are managed emergently because warm ischemia time is limited to 6 hours for optimal limb salvage. Decisions regarding limb viability, compartment syndrome, and the need for amputation of the mangled extremity are made in the same setting. Consideration must also be given to emergency capsulotomy and ORIF of femoral head fractures as well as reduction of posterior hip dislocations to prevent avascular necrosis. Definitive care of complex upper extremity fractures or intra-articular fractures is undertaken if the patient's condition permits. Spine, acetabular, and upper extremity injuries are next addressed. Operative repair of maxillofacial injuries may usually be delayed several days, depending on the status of the patient.

ORTHOPEDIC EMERGENCIES

Pelvic Ring Disruptions

Pelvic ring disruptions are a major cause of mortality and morbidity in multiply injured patients. Whereas fatalities result from uncontrolled retroperitoneal hemorrhage and other associated injuries, disabilities such as low back pain, leg-length discrepancies, dyspareunia, difficulties with childbearing, and impotence are caused by the anatomic disruption of the pelvic ring. Pelvic fractures can be particularly lethal when they occur in combination with significant injuries to other major organ systems.[11] Because of the high force necessary to disrupt the pelvic ring in young patients, it is not surprising that up to 80% of these patients have additional musculoskeletal injuries. Mortality rates in the patient with high-energy pelvic ring injuries are approximately 15% to 25%. These deaths are generally a result of the injuries commonly associated with this injury pattern. Mortality increases nearly 13 times when the patient presents with hypotension. When combined with either a head or an abdominal injury that requires surgical intervention, the mortality increases to 50%. When both procedures are necessary, mortality increases to 90%.

Classification

Orthopedic surgeons and traumatologists broadly classify pelvic ring disruptions into two major groups: stable and unstable. A *stable* pelvis is defined as one that can withstand normal physiologic forces without displacing. This stability depends on the integrity of bony and ligamentous structures (Fig. 21-9). *Instability* is generally divided into rotational and vertical components (Fig. 21-10). These displacements can be appreciated on the initial anteroposterior screening radiograph. Stable injuries include nondisplaced fractures of the pelvic ring and anterior displacements of less than 2.5 cm. Rotational instability is characterized by widening of the symphysis pubis or displacement of pubic rami fractures of greater than 2.5 cm. Superior translation of a hemipelvis through fractures of the sacrum or ilium and disruption of the sacroiliac joint by more than 1 cm constitute vertical instability. Serial sectioning studies reveal that division of the symphyseal ligaments alone leads to diastasis of 2.5 cm or less, maintaining stability.[12] Further sectioning of the anterior sacroiliac ligaments and sacrospinous and sacrotuberous ligaments (pelvic floor) permits rotational instability. Vertical instability results only after the posterior sacroiliac ligaments are also sectioned. Displaced fractures (superior and inferior pubic rami fractures, sacral or iliac wing fracture) can also result in similar instability patterns.

Because the pelvis is a true ring structure, a significant anterior displacement must be accompanied by a corresponding posterior disruption. Disruptions in the pelvic ring are usually a combination of fractures and ligamentous injuries.

Early recognition of unstable pelvic ring disruptions is essential because they are more likely to be associated with fatal hemorrhage. Likewise, these injuries require stabilization to restore the pelvic ring anatomy and decrease late disability. Determination of the stability of the injured hemipelvis must be established through a combination of physical examination and review of the anteroposterior radiograph. An anterior defect can sometimes be detected by palpation at the symphysis pubis. Rotational instability can be appreciated by manually compressing and distracting the pelvis through the anterior iliac spines. Because repeated manipulation can cause iatrogenic injury, this should be performed a limited number of times. Vertical instability may be appreciated when movement of the hemipelvis is detected as manual compression and traction are applied through an extended, uninjured lower extremity. The screening anteroposterior radiograph is then examined. In 90% of cases, this is sufficient to assess stability and guide initial treatment. Anterior injuries are easily identified on this projection. Most unstable posterior injuries can also be appreciated. Avulsion fractures at the L5 transverse process and the ischial spines indicate ligamentous disruption and are usually identifiable. Large posterior gapping or displacement of the hemipelvis superiorly by more than 1 cm indicates complete posterior disruption and instability.[12]

Detailed classification systems have been developed based on the direction of force, stability of the pelvis, location of fracture, or whether it is an open or closed injury. The Comprehensive Pelvic Disruption classification of the Arbeitsgemeinschaft fur Osteosynthesefragen (AO) combines the mechanism of injury with the degree of pelvic instability. Type A injuries preserve the integrity of the posterior ligamentous and bony structures. These injuries maintain a stable pelvic ring and usually require no further treatment unless neurologic injury is associated with a sacral fracture. Type B injuries represent incomplete disruption of the posterior pelvis. These injuries result in rotational instability of the pelvis. A varying degree of sacroiliac joint or sacral disruption is characteristic. These injuries occur with both anterior and lateral compression mechanisms. In type C pelvic injuries, the hemipelvis is vertically, rotationally, and posteriorly unstable.

Lateral compression as well as vertical shear-type fractures are associated with intra-abdominal and head injuries. The most common cause of death in a lateral compression injury to the pelvis is associated closed head trauma.[3] The anteroposterior compression-type injuries have the greatest risk for retroperitoneal hemorrhage. Intrapelvic visceral injuries are also more common in the anteroposterior patterns. Mortality in anteroposterior compression-type injuries relates to a combination of retroperitoneal bleeding and visceral injuries.[3]

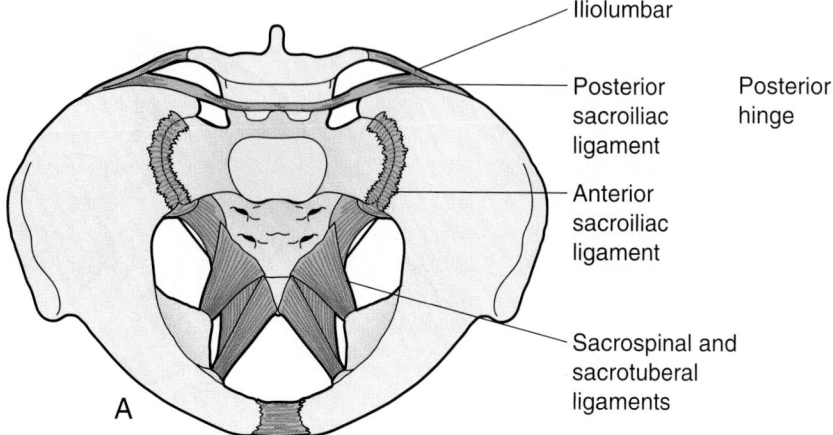

Iliolumbar

Posterior sacroiliac ligament

Posterior hinge

Anterior sacroiliac ligament

Sacrospinal and sacrotuberal ligaments

A

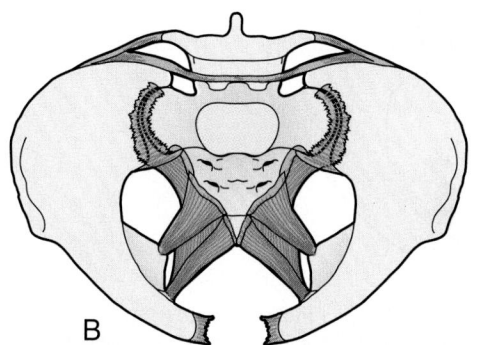

B

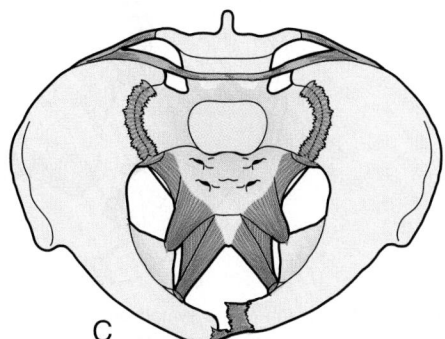

C

FIGURE 21-9. Pelvic stability. **A,** The intact ligamentous bony structures of the pelvis maintain its integrity with regard to stability. The posterior hinge, consisting of the posterior sacroiliac ligaments and the iliolumbar ligaments, is imperative to maintain vertical stability. The sacrospinous prevents rotation, and the sacrotuberous prevents vertical migration. As long as these, the anterior sacroiliac, and the symphysis are intact, the pelvis will remain stable. If, however, the anterior symphysis is separated or the sacrum is crushed posteriorly, as seen in **B** and **C,** the posterior hinge remains intact and the pelvis is usually stable vertically. The sacrospinous ligaments are intact, and rotatory abnormalities are thus prevented. (**A** to **C,** From Kellam JF, Mayo K: Pelvic ring disruptions. *In* Browner BD, Jupiter TB, Levine AM, Trafton PG [eds]: Skeletal Trauma, 3rd ed. Philadelphia, WB Saunders, 2003.)

Hemorrhage in Pelvic Fracture

The usual cause of hemorrhage in pelvic fractures is from the posterior pelvic venous plexus and bleeding cancellous bone surfaces. Rarely, in less than 10% of cases, it may be caused by bleeding from a named artery (Fig. 21-11).[13-15] Bleeding from a larger artery is even less frequent. Two large series[16] demonstrated rates of bleeding from femoral or iliac vessels in 1% and 0% of patients. In light of these studies, initial treatment should focus on the control of venous bleeding. Reduction and stabilization of the displaced pelvic ring help achieve this. Reduction leads to a decrease in pelvic volume and tamponade of the bleeding vessels through compression of the viscera and pelvic hematoma. Stabilization maintains the reduction and avoids movement of the hemipelvis, reducing pain and limiting the disruption of organizing clots. Since reduction and stabilization alone usually control venous bleeding, patients who do not respond to these maneuvers are more likely to have arterial bleeding.

Stabilization

Reduction and stabilization of the pelvis can be achieved by a variety of mechanical means (Fig. 21-12). When field personnel detect unstable pelvic ring disruptions on physical examination, they can begin treatment by binding the pelvis with a rolled sheet or applying pneumatic antishock garments (PASGs). Like the air splints applied to the extremities, the garment functions by compressing the pelvis. If applied in the field, PASGs should not be deflated until the patient is actively being resuscitated in the trauma room. The PASG has as its advantages ease of use, application in the field, and reusability. However, it blocks access to the patient and restricts excursion of the diaphragm, and there have been reports of gluteal and thigh compartment syndromes developing after its extended use in hypotensive patients.

The standard method for controlling pelvic hemorrhage has been the application of an anterior external fixation frame. Proper application of an anterior pelvic

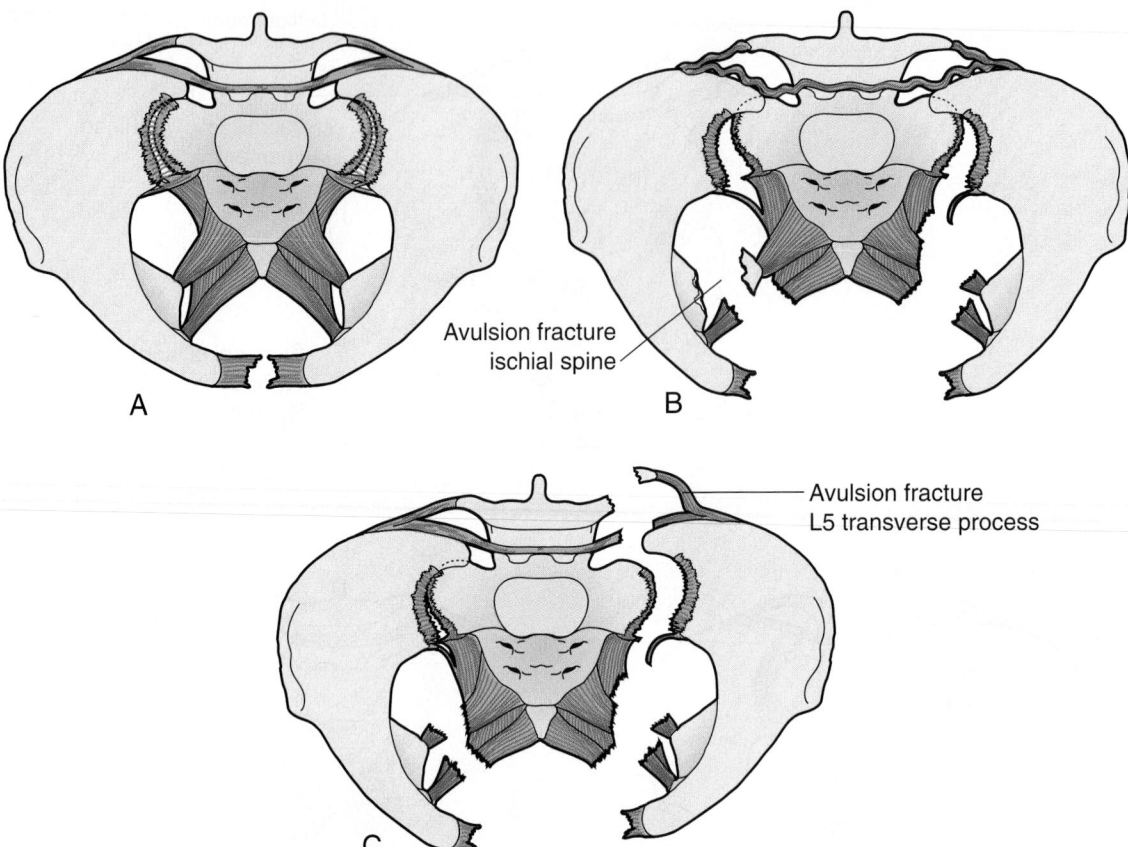

Avulsion fracture
ischial spine

Avulsion fracture
L5 transverse process

FIGURE 21-10.   **A,** Division of the symphysis pubis will allow the pelvis to open to approximately 2.5 cm with no damage to any posterior ligamentous structures. **B,** Division of the anterior sacroiliac and sacrospinous ligaments, either by direct division of their fibers (*right*) or by avulsion of the tip of the ischial spine (*left*), allows the pelvis to rotate externally until the posterior superior iliac spines abut the sacrum. Note, however, that the posterior ligamentous structures (e.g., the posterior sacroiliac and iliolumbar ligaments) remain intact. Therefore, no displacement in the vertical plane is possible. **C,** Division of the posterior tension band ligaments, that is, the posterior sacroiliac, as well as the iliolumbar, depicted here on the left side, plus an avulsion of the transverse process of L5 causes complete instability of the hemipelvis. Note that posterior displacement is now possible. (**A** to **C,** From Kellam JF, Mayo K: Pelvic ring disruptions. *In* Browner BD, Jupiter TB, Levine AM, Trafton PG [eds]: Skeletal Trauma, 3rd ed. Philadelphia, WB Saunders, 2003.)

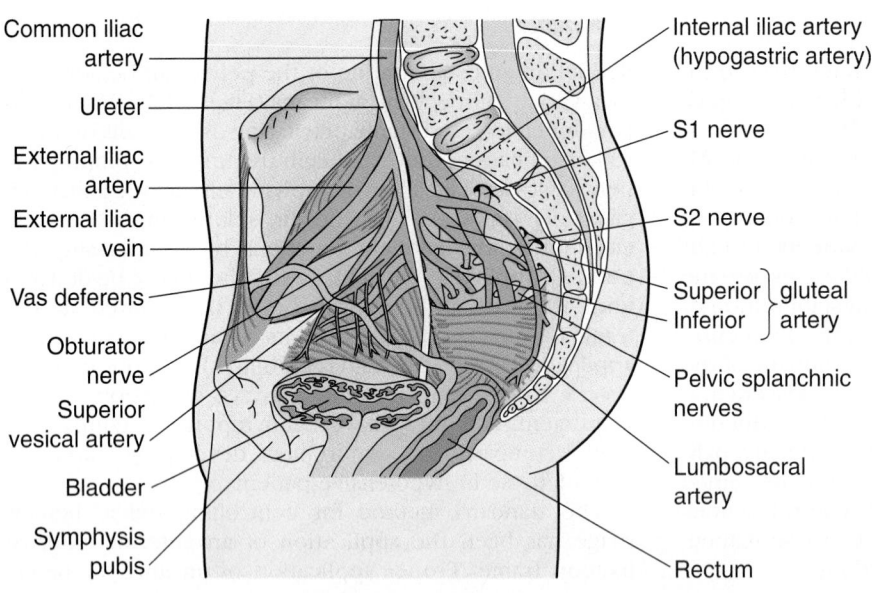

Common iliac
artery

Ureter

External iliac
artery

External iliac
vein

Vas deferens

Obturator
nerve

Superior
vesical artery

Bladder

Symphysis
pubis

Internal iliac artery
(hypogastric artery)

S1 nerve

S2 nerve

Superior } gluteal
Inferior } artery

Pelvic splanchnic
nerves

Lumbosacral
artery

Rectum

FIGURE 21-11.   Internal aspect of the pelvis shows the great vessels in the lumbosacral plexus as well as the pelvic floor and the pelvic contents, bladder, and rectum. (From Kellam JF, Mayo K. Pelvic ring disruptions. *In* Browner BD, Jupiter TB, Levine AM, Trafton PG [eds]: Skeletal Trauma, 3rd ed. Philadelphia, WB Saunders, 2003.)

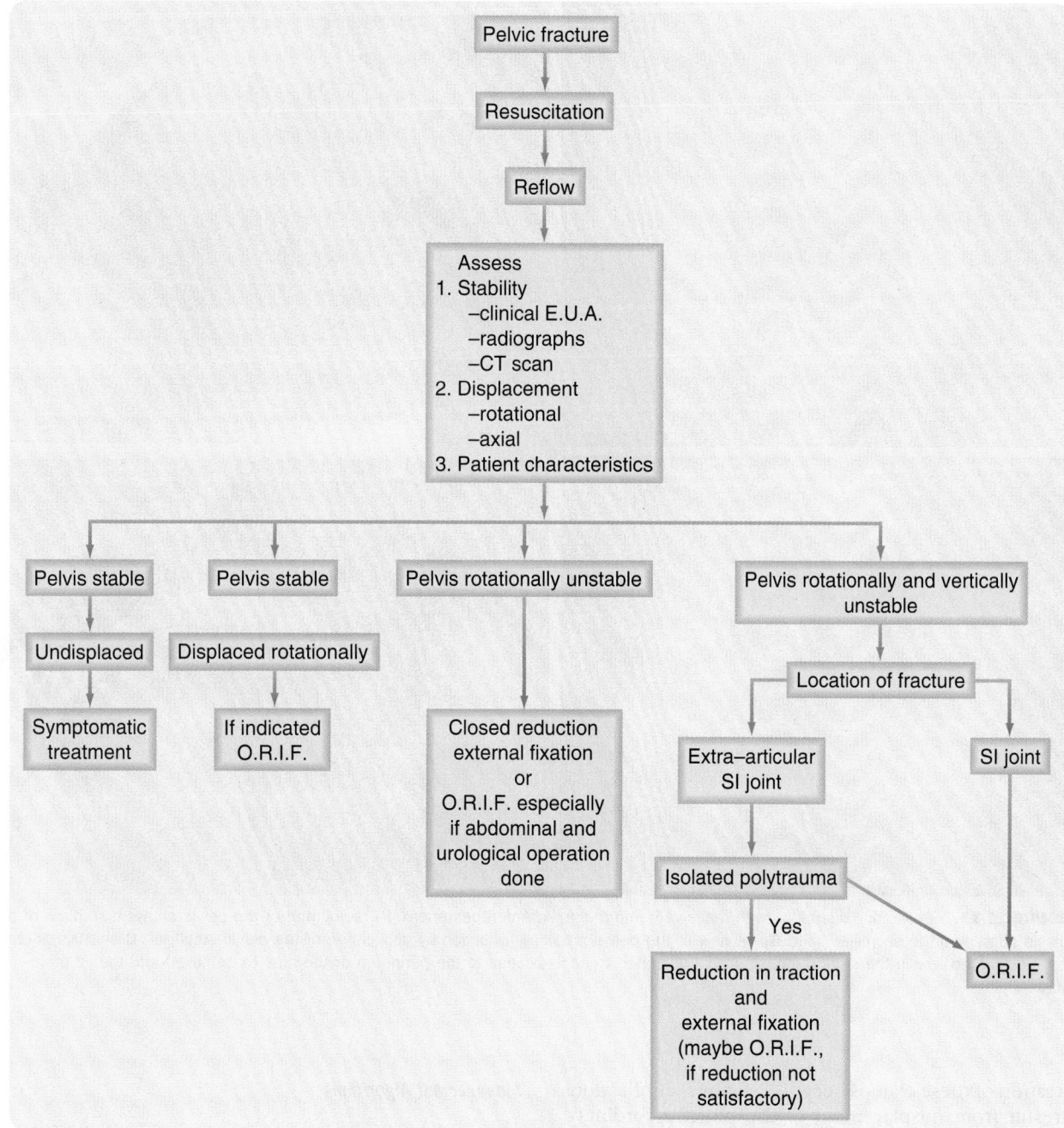

FIGURE 21-12. Algorithm of pelvic fracture management. CT, computed tomography; E.U.A., examination under anesthesia; O.R.I.F., open reduction and internal fixation; SI, sacroiliac. (From Kellam JF, Mayo K: Pelvic ring disruptions. *In* Browner BD, Jupiter TB, Levine AM, Trafton PG [eds]: Skeletal Trauma, 3rd ed. Philadelphia, WB Saunders, 2003.)

external fixator should provide stability to the pelvis and hematoma, while allowing access to the abdomen for surgical procedures. Multiple studies have shown that outcomes can improve with their routine use.[14,15,17] Although this device can be applied in the emergency department, it is frequently deferred until the patient is brought to the operating suite. In these circumstances, the pelvis can remain displaced for many hours with venous bleeding continuing uncontrolled. If an external fixator cannot be applied expeditiously, another method of provisional stabilization must be employed. Recently, devices called

pelvic C-clamps have been developed that can be rapidly applied to reduce and provisionally stabilize the pelvis in the emergency department. The design allows for compression of the pelvis through percutaneously inserted pins applied to the outer surface of the ilium. They provide adequate stabilization and easy access to the abdomen or extremities without removal of the device (Fig. 21-13). The C-clamps can remain in place throughout the resuscitation phase and then be replaced by definitive stabilization methods when the patient is able to undergo these procedures. Care must be taken in the

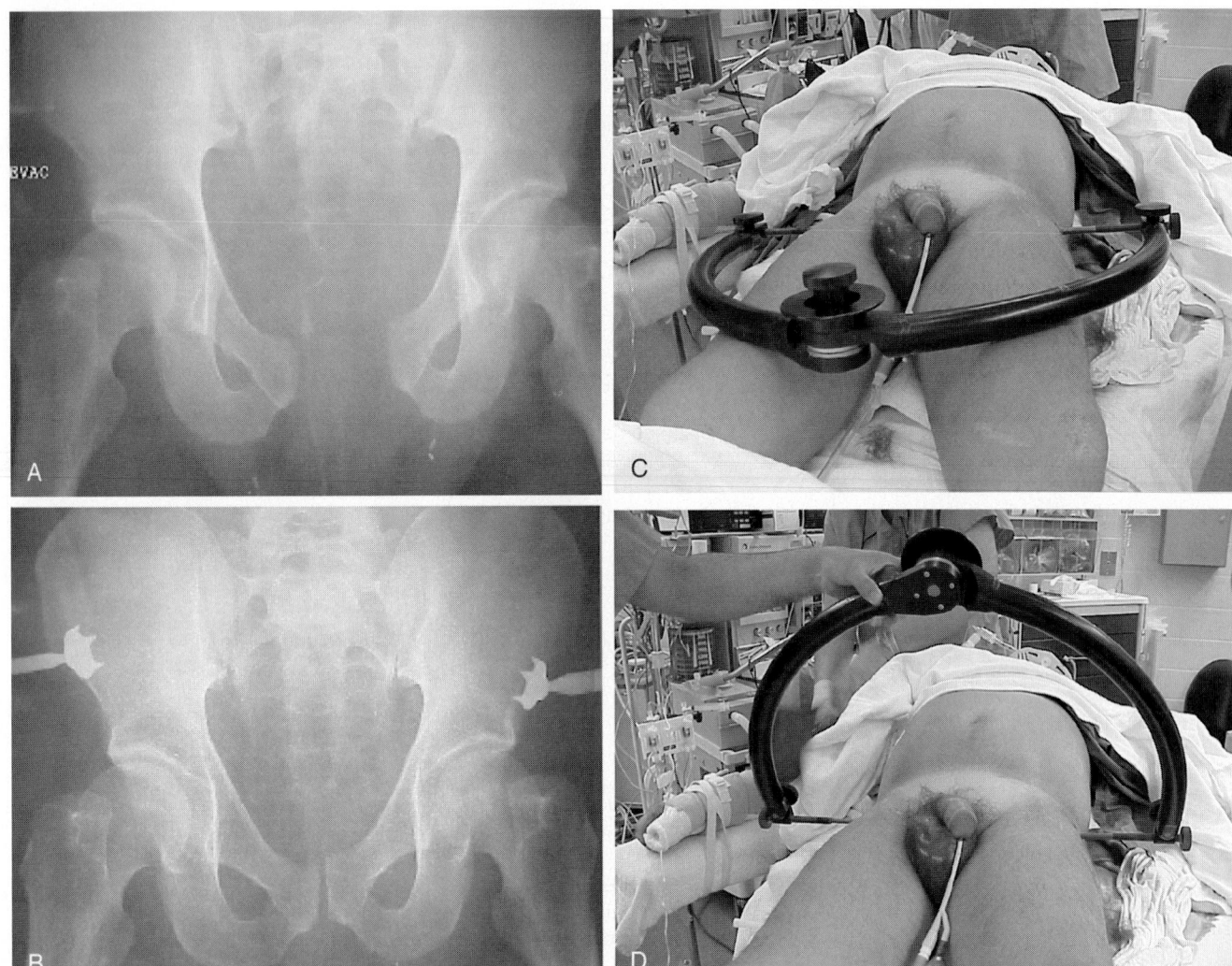

FIGURE 21-13.   Pelvic ring disruption with massive hemorrhage. **A,** Anteroposterior (AP) radiograph of the pelvis shows disruption of the symphysis pubis and the sacroiliac joint. **B,** AP view of the pelvis following reduction by application of the pelvic stabilizer. **C** and **D,** Patient with the pelvic stabilizer in the standard position and elevated to allow access to the perineum or the hips to be flexed into the lithotomy position.

application of these clamps because serious complications can result from misplacement of the pins. Accordingly, these devices are utilized only in rotationally and vertically unstable pelvic ring disruptions and not in stable injury patterns.

The role of angiography in the diagnosis and management of pelvic hemorrhage is controversial. Large series have demonstrated the incidence of arterial hemorrhage amenable to embolization to be approximately 10%.[13,14] Furthermore, it is even less common for the bleeding to be the result of an injury to a large or named artery. In these cases, arteriography with embolization can be lifesaving. However, catheterization and embolization of vessels in the pelvis are technically difficult and time consuming. The use of these techniques should be reserved for those cases when all other methods of control of hemorrhage have been exhausted.[13]

Management Algorithms

Algorithms for management of the hypotensive patient with a pelvic fracture all should begin with a search for the cause of the shock (Fig. 21-14). All possible causes of bleeding are explored. Auscultation of the chest and review of the chest radiograph determine the presence of hemothorax and the need for thoracostomy. Once the hemothorax is either ruled out as a cause of shock or is controlled by chest tubes, a diagnostic peritoneal lavage or ultrasound of the abdomen is performed. Examination of the pelvis is performed as described previously. Any wounds are noted around the pelvis and in the perineum. Bleeding from the rectum, vagina, or urethral meatus is noted. Digital vaginal and rectal examinations are performed, feeling for tears and fracture fragments.

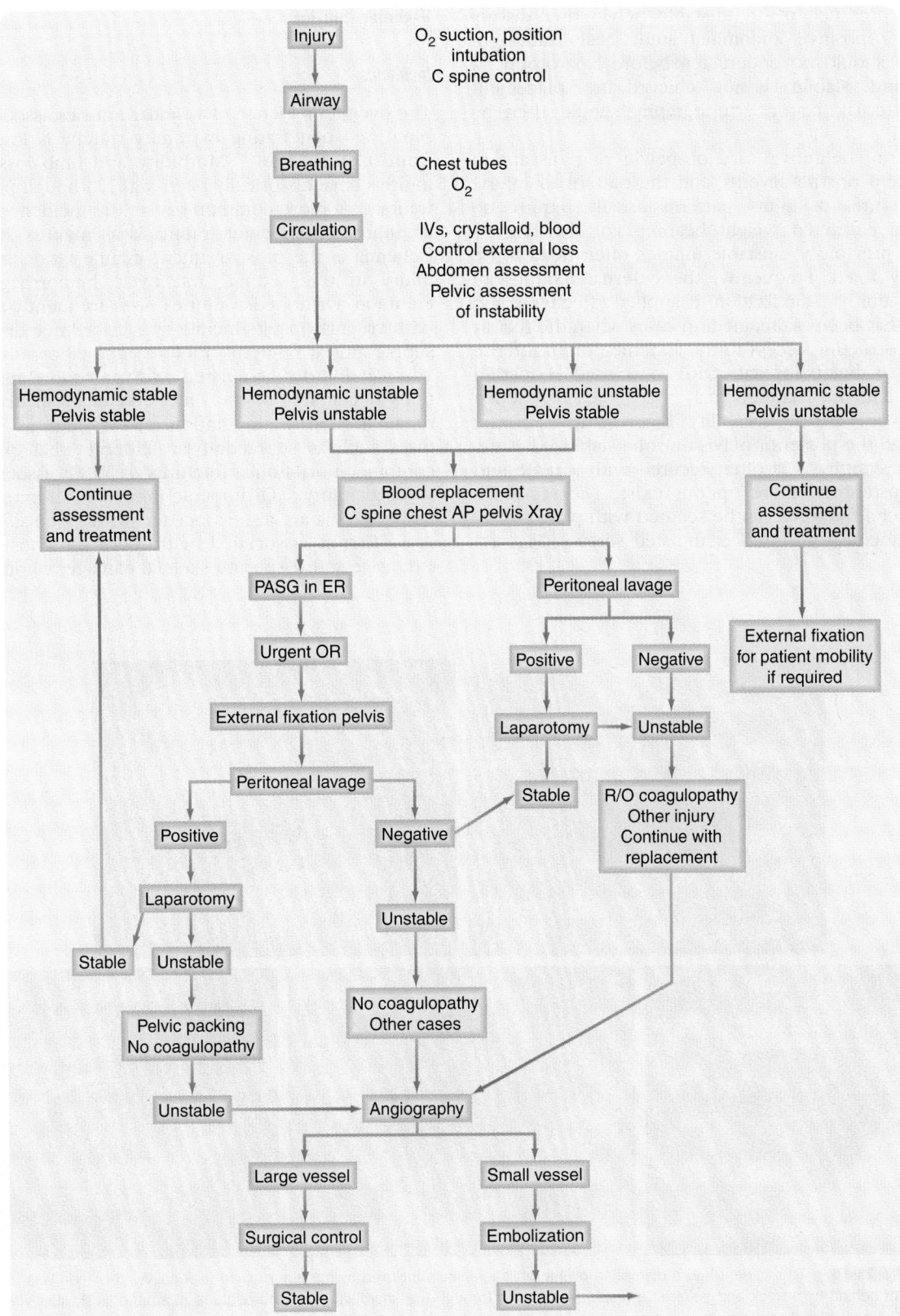

FIGURE 21-14. Algorithm for resuscitation after pelvic disruption. C spine, cervical spine; ER, emergency room, Fx, fracture; IVs, intravenous lines; OR, operating room; PASG, pneumatic antishock garment; RPH, retroperitoneal hematoma; R/O, rule out. (From Kellam JF, Mayo K.: Pelvic ring disruptions. *In* Browner BD, Jupiter TB, Levine AM, Trafton PG [eds]: Skeletal Trauma, 3rd ed. Philadelphia, WB Saunders, 2003.)

In the presence of an unstable pelvic ring disruption and a positive abdominal study, stabilization of the pelvis should be undertaken before laparotomy. If hemodynamic stability is not achieved after placement of the external fixator, arteriography should then be performed.

Long-term, definitive care of pelvic ring disruption is dependent on the severity and the pattern of injury. Stable fractures or injury patterns usually require no more than restricted weight bearing. For the reasons described previously, unstable injuries often need to be definitively fixed. Frequently, the external fixator can provide definitive stabilization, if applied effectively and reduction has been maintained. In cases when the fixator may be obstructing access to the abdomen or an interim C-clamp has been applied, ORIF or closed reduction and percutaneous fixation may be indicated. When rotational or vertical instability is present, both the anterior and the posterior pelvis must be stabilized. Anteriorly, the symphysis is often secured with a plate and screws. Posteriorly, more options exist. The sacroiliac joint or sacral fractures can be secured with plates, bars, or percutaneously inserted cannulated screws (Fig. 21-15).

Vascular Injuries

Incidence

The overall incidence of vascular injuries associated with blunt and penetrating extremity trauma is low, ranging from 0.2% to 1.5%.[18] Morbidity and limb loss in these injuries have historically been high. Although penetrating trauma is a more common cause, the incidence of vascular injuries from blunt trauma is as high as 20%. Distal ischemia is the most frequent manifestation of vascular injury in this setting, and overt hemorrhage is less common. Orthopedic injuries most frequently associated with vascular insults include posterior knee dislocations, supracondylar humerus fractures, and elbow dislocations. Vascular injuries associated with posterior knee dislocations occur 40% of the time, and delay in diagnosis or repair has led to amputation rates as high as 85%. Fractures such as supracondylar femoral, tibial plateau, or combined tibial-fibular fractures are rarely associated with vascular injury.[18] Orthopedic injuries with extensive soft tissue trauma are also associated with vascular abnormalities. Factors associated with poor prognosis include extensive soft tissue and skeletal damage, warm ischemic

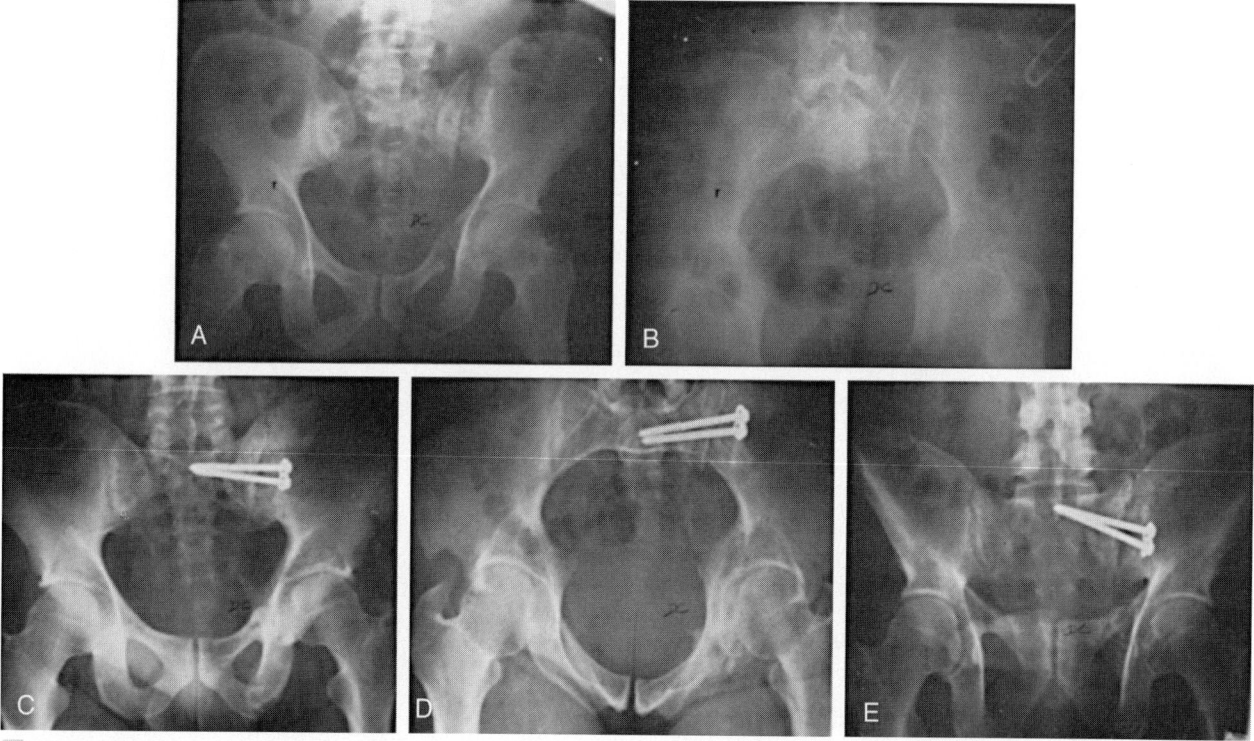

FIGURE 21-15.   This patient had a disruption of his left sacroiliac joint fixed by posterior screw fixation. **A,** This man was struck from behind by a truck and suffered a displaced fracture through the sacroiliac joint and pubic rami anteriorly. **B,** Inlet view confirms the posterior displacement at the sacroiliac joint on the left side. **C,** Anteroposterior view demonstrates posterior screw fixation of the pelvis. Note how the screws have been placed across and into the body of the sacrum. This is necessary for sacral fractures, but it also gains good purchase in sacroiliac joint dislocations. The screws are above the first sacral foramen sitting in the ala. **D,** Good screw placement is noted on the inlet view, showing that the reduction has been obtained and adequate fixation has occurred with the screws in the ala and body of the sacrum. **E,** Outlet view again confirms proper positions of the screws. (**A** to **E,** From Kellam JF, Mayo K: Pelvic ring disruptions. *In* Browner BD, Jupiter TB, Levine AM, Trafton PG [eds]: Skeletal Trauma, 3rd ed. Philadelphia, WB Saunders, 2003.)

time greater than 6 hours, mangled extremity severity score (MESS) greater than 7, and tibial nerve injury.[19]

Although upper extremity injuries account for approximately 30% of all peripheral vascular injuries, lower extremity vascular trauma carries a poorer prognosis and is potentially more serious. The popliteal region, in particular, is prone to ischemia for several reasons. Although there is abundant collateral circulation around the knee, these vessels are fragile and can easily be damaged from direct soft tissue trauma or adjacent swelling. The popliteal artery begins at the adductor hiatus, and its movement is restricted at this location. The soleus muscles also restrict movement of the popliteal artery, making it prone to injury with knee dislocation (Fig. 21-16). In the setting of popliteal artery thrombosis, lack of high-flow collaterals may lead to end-vessel in situ thrombosis secondary to low flow. Patency of these vessels is critical in limb salvage. Injuries to the common femoral or superficial femoral artery rarely result in amputation because of the presence of collateral circulation and the profunda femoris artery. This vessel is rarely injured; however, when it is injured, it is usually clinically silent and the diagnosis is made angiographically.

Management

Optimal results in combined vascular and orthopedic injuries depend on a high index of suspicion and expeditious intervention (Fig. 21-17). A thorough vascular examination is performed in the trauma room, and all upper and lower extremity pulses are evaluated. Color, temperature, and the presence of pain or paresis are noted. The systolic pressure in the arm as well as at the ankle is recorded, and the ankle/brachial index is calculated by dividing the ankle pressure by the brachial pressure. In the absence of chronic peripheral vascular disease, the index should normally be greater than 0.95. Usually ankle/brachial indices and pulses are bilaterally symmetrical. Audible bruits over blood vessels at affected areas may signify arterial injury or traumatic fistula. Abnormal swelling may indicate injury or rupture of a deep vessel. Any pulse deficit warrants formal arteriography. Prolonged or severe ischemia mandates immediate operative exploration. An ankle/brachial index less than 0.95 also warrants arteriography. Intraoperative arteriography may be useful in planning vascular reconstruction if overt injury is present but there is no sign of critical ischemia. Direct arterial exploration of suspected injuries is warranted in open fractures.

The staging of skeletal stabilization and vascular repair should be individualized. Generally, vascular reconstruction precedes fracture fixation. Disruption of the vascular repair after orthopedic fixation is rare, provided the repair is performed with limb length restored. The ipsilateral and contralateral limbs are prepared widely to allow access to distal vessels, fasciotomy, and contralateral saphenous vein harvest. Fasciotomy is employed before vascular repair if compartment syndrome is suspected. In knee dislocations, it is advisable to release the compartments of the lower leg owing to the chance of reperfusion injury and the development of compartment syndrome. Proximal and distal control are obtained before exploration of the hematoma. The artery and vein are carefully inspected, and an assessment of the injury is made.

The use of indwelling intraoperative shunts is appropriate in selected unstable skeletal lesions.[20] Standard carotid endarterectomy shunts are often used in this setting. Proximal and distal thrombectomy are performed before shunt

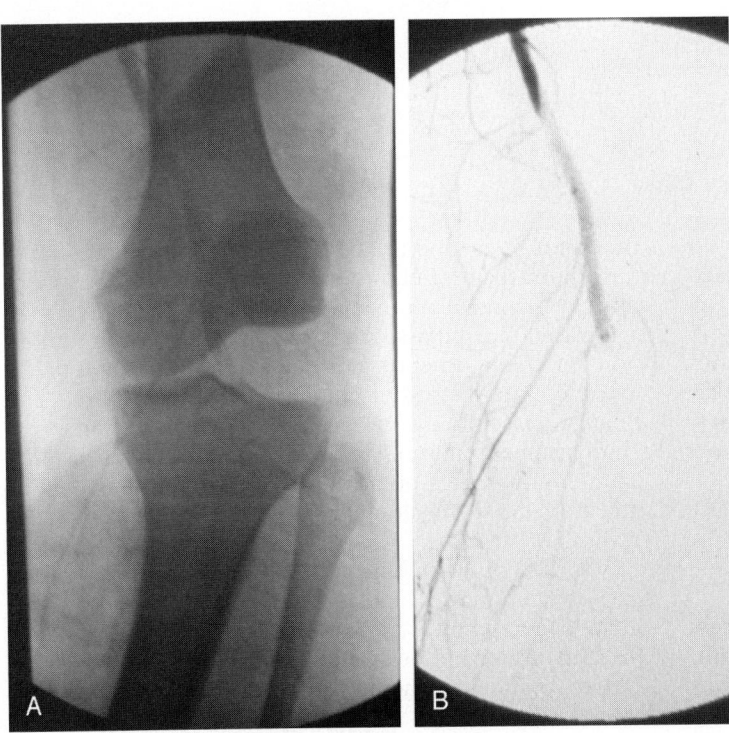

FIGURE 21-16. Angiogram of the lower extremity after posterior knee dislocation. **A,** The fluoroscopic image shows significant displacement after a posterior knee dislocation. **B,** Disruption of popliteal blood flow at the level of the dislocation is clearly appreciated on the angiogram.

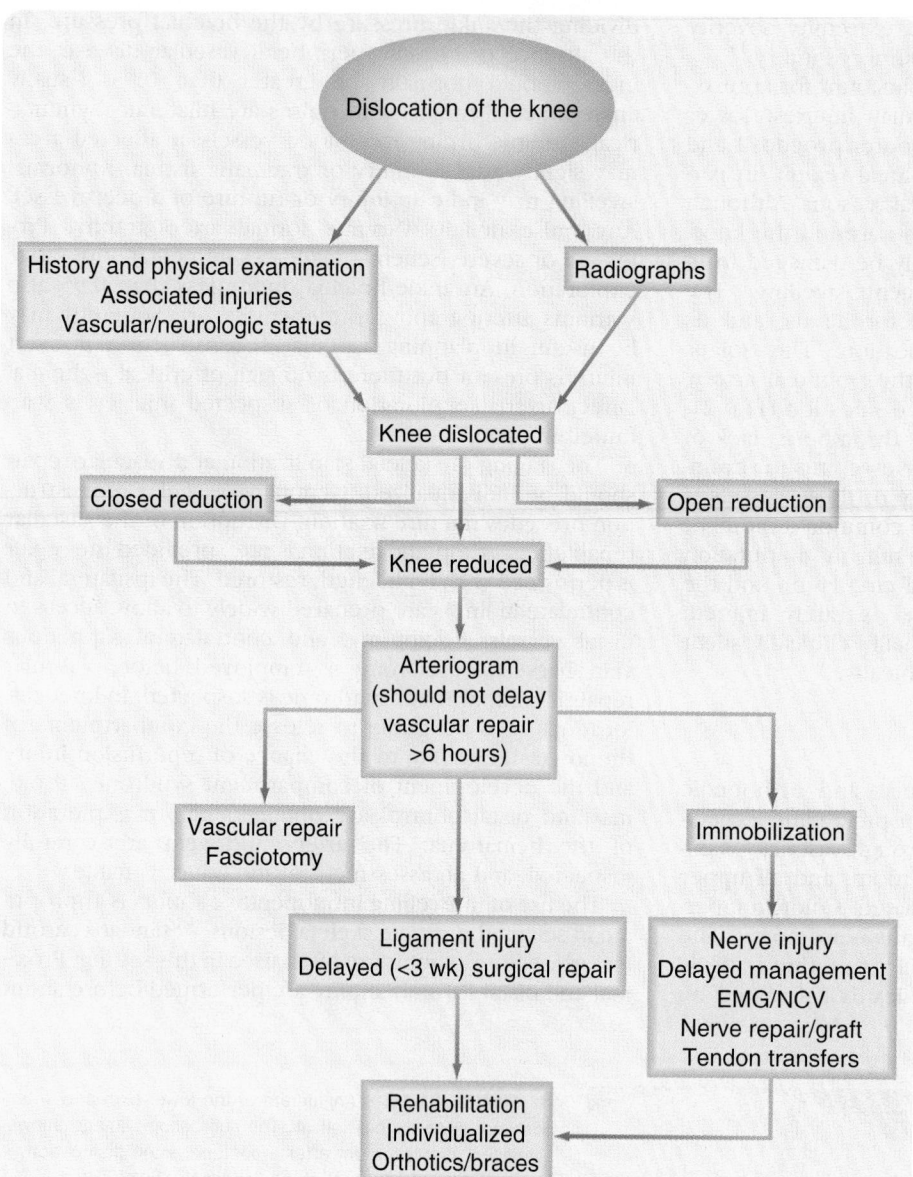

FIGURE 21-17.   Treatment algorithm for dislocation of the knee. EMG/NCV, electromyography nerve conduction velocity. (From Siliski JM: Dislocations and soft tissue injuries of the knee. *In* Browner BD, Jupiter TB, Levine AM, Trafton PG [eds]: Skeletal Trauma, 3rd ed. Philadelphia, WB Saunders, 2003.)

placement or repair. Often, arterial resection is necessary to obtain acceptable margins, and saphenous vein graft is used if primary repair without tension is not possible. Completion arteriogram is performed routinely because limb salvage depends on arterial patency. All major vein injuries are repaired to increase the patency rate of the arterial repair and prevent the sequelae of chronic venous insufficiency. Completion arteriography should be routinely performed to assess the adequacy of repair.

Acute Compartment Syndrome

Early recognition and treatment of compartment syndrome is critical in the trauma patient to avoid death, early amputation, and limb dysfunction. Volkmann was the first to describe the results of postischemic contracture more than a century ago. He attributed permanent muscle contracture to trauma, swelling, and tight bandaging. Seddon and associates reviewed the late complications of compartment syndrome of the upper and lower extremities and stressed the importance of early recognition and fasciotomy.[20a,20b] Failure to diagnose and treat compartment syndrome in the trauma patient has resulted in numerous cases of preventable morbidity, as well as litigation, often resulting in settlements in favor of the plaintiff.[21]

Various compartment syndromes have been described in both the upper and the lower extremities. These include compartment syndromes of the shoulder, arm, forearm, hand, buttocks, thigh, lower leg, and foot. The causes of compartment syndrome are numerous and include, but are not limited to, open and closed fractures, arterial injury, gunshot wounds, snake bites, extravasation at venous and arterial access sites, limb compression, burns, constrictive dressings, and tight casts. The rapid diagnosis and management of compartment syndrome is paramount to achieving a successful clinical outcome. This section addresses the pathogenesis, diagnosis, and management of acute compartment syndrome, specifically of the forearm and lower leg.

Pathogenesis

Compartment syndrome occurs secondary to increased pressure in the enclosed osseofascial space. The most common cause of compartment syndrome in the orthopedic patient is muscle edema, resulting from direct trauma to the extremity or from reperfusion after vascular injury. This edema causes an increase in compartment pressure, which prevents venous outflow from the affected extremity, causing backflow congestion and furthering the cycle of increasing pressure and muscle ischemia. In the case of the orthopedic trauma patient with a long bone fracture, the situation is exacerbated by fracture bleeding, which produces a space-occupying hematoma. On reduction of the fracture, compartment pressures increase secondary to a decrease in the volume of the osseofascial space. External compressive casts or bandages further reduce the ability of the compartment to expand.

Controversy exists regarding the level of compartment pressure that requires surgical intervention. Whitesides and Heckman[22] recommend a fasciotomy in any patient in whom the intracompartmental pressure approaches 20 mm Hg below the diastolic pressure in the presence of a worsening general condition, documented rising tissue pressure, significant tissue injury, or history of 6 hours of total ischemic time of an extremity. Mubarak and coworkers determined that absolute tissue pressure of 30 mm Hg is the critical cut-off at which fasciotomy should be performed.[22a] They conclude that because normal capillary pressure is 30 mm Hg, any pressure higher will result in tissue necrosis. Finally, Matsen and associates state that the critical compartment pressure requiring fasciotomy is 45 mm Hg.[22b] They note that as compartment pressure develops, capillary pressure must increase as the venous pressure rises within the compartment. As a result of this, they believe that normal baseline capillary pressure is irrelevant in the case of determining compartment syndrome.

Although there is controversy regarding when a fasciotomy should be performed, there is little debate regarding the effect prolonged ischemic time has on skeletal muscle and nerve tissue. Investigators have established that peripheral nerve and muscle can survive for as long as 4 hours under ischemic conditions without irreversible damage. However, total ischemic time for longer than 8 hours resulted in irreversible nerve and muscle injury. Ischemic time of 6 hours resulted in a variable return to function in both muscle and nerve tissue.[22]

Diagnosis

The diagnosis of acute compartment syndrome requires a high degree of clinical suspicion, a full understanding of the mechanism of injury, and careful serial physical examinations (Fig. 21-18). Tscherne and Gotzen[7] stated that the more severe the initial soft tissue injury, the greater the probability that soft tissue complications, including compartment syndrome, will develop. The diagnosis of compartment syndrome relies on an understanding of the patient at risk, subjective complaints, and an appreciation of early and late physical and clinical findings.

The presence of distal pulses and the absence of pallor cannot exclude the diagnosis of compartment syndrome because tissue perfusion in a compartment is dependent on both arterial and capillary perfusion gradients. Paralysis and paresthesias are unreliable because studies have shown that peripheral nerves can conduct impulses after 1 hour or more of total ischemic time. Ischemia of muscles, however, causes pain. Patients are typically said to have "pain out of proportion to that expected for the injury." Unusual requests for frequent narcotic analgesics are another indication of ischemic pain. Passive stretching of the ischemic muscle of the compartment in question causes exquisite pain and is the most sensitive clinical finding in developing compartment syndrome. Clinical palpation of the compartment in question and comparing with the contralateral limb is also useful in the determination of compartment syndrome. Any evidence of increased tension or fullness of the compartment should raise suspicion of an impending compartment syndrome.

Although pain out of proportion to the injury sustained is a cardinal clinical finding of an impending compartment syndrome, it must be emphasized that, over time, this pain will diminish as further ischemia occurs. In addition, in a patient heavily medicated with narcotics, this "window" to make a clinical diagnosis may be obscured. Therefore, if there is any clinical suspicion of an impending compartment syndrome, narcotic administration should be closely monitored.

Systemic hypotension, vascular injury, external limb compression, coagulopathy, and deep venous thrombosis predispose trauma patients to the development of compartment syndrome. In an uncooperative, intoxicated, intubated, or neurologically impaired patient, the diagnosis of compartment syndrome may depend more on the measurement of compartment pressures.

Tissue Pressure Measurements

Four methods have been described to measure compartment pressures. These include the wick catheter, the slit catheter, Whitesides' infusion technique,[22] and the Stic (Stryker) catheter (Fig. 21-19). Although the first three techniques are still utilized, the most common method of measurement utilizes the Stryker Stic device. This hand-held electronic device is easily calibrated and used. Pressures are obtained by inserting the needle into each compartment. It is generally used to make meas-

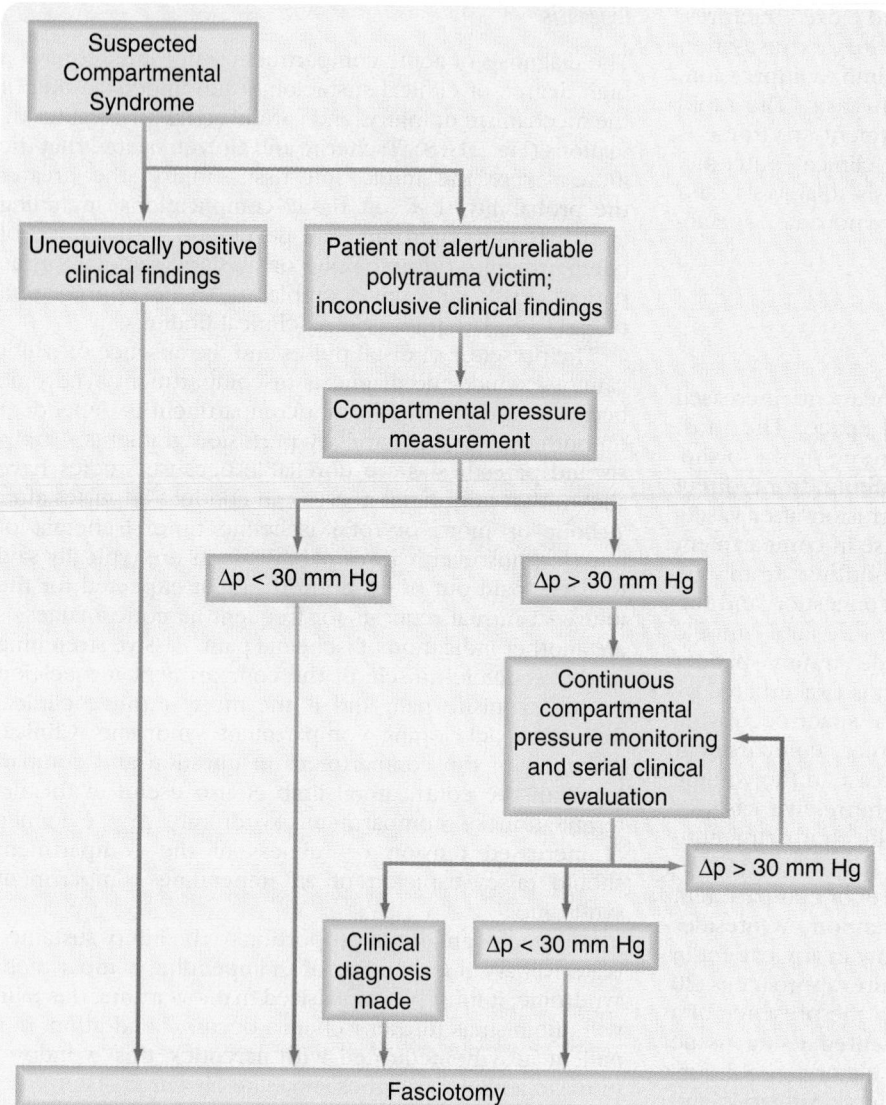

FIGURE 21-18.   Algorithm for the management of a patient with suspected compartment syndrome. (From Amendola A, Twaddle BC: Compartment syndromes. *In* Browner BD, Jupiter TB, Levine AM, Trafton PG [eds]: Skeletal Trauma, 3rd ed. Philadelphia, WB Saunders, 2003.)

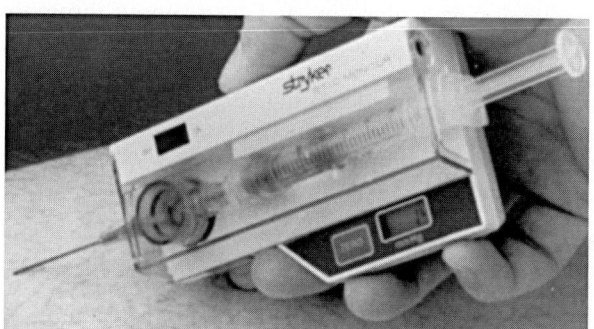

FIGURE 21-19.   The Stic catheter. (Courtesy of Stryker Mississauga, Ontario, Canada.)

urements at one point in time and is not an indwelling device.

Heckman and colleagues,[23] in a prospective study of tibia fractures, reviewed the correlation between the site at which the Stic device is introduced into the compartment and the proximity of the fracture site. They reported that the highest compartment pressures were usually at the level of the fracture or within 5 cm of it. Tissue pressure decreased at an increasing distance proximal and distal to the fracture site. It is important to take this into consideration when using the Stryker Stic device to measure compartment pressures in the presence of a long bone fracture.

Surgical Treatment

The two-incision approach to fasciotomy (Fig. 21-20) of the lower leg is a reliable and straightforward procedure, given that the anatomy is well understood (Table 21-2). It

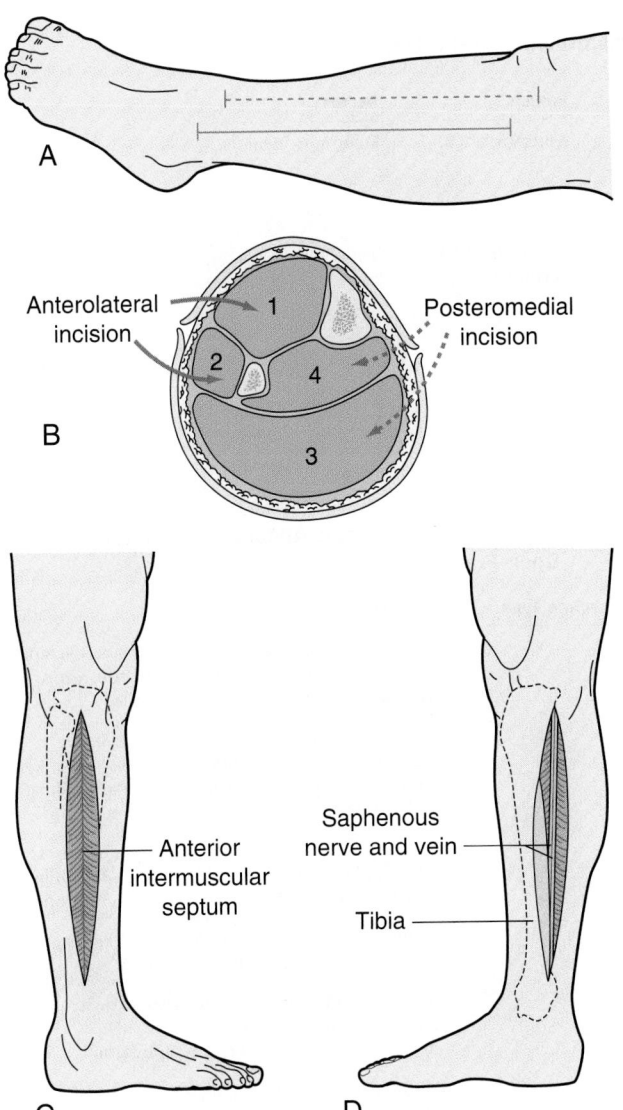

FIGURE 21-20. **A,** The double-incision technique for performing fasciotomies of all four compartments of the lower extremity. **B,** Cross section of the lower extremity shows a position of anterolateral and posteromedial incisions that allows access to the anterior and lateral compartments (1 and 2) and the superficial and deep posterior compartments (3 and 4). **C,** A vertical anterior incision is centered midway between the tibia and the fibula. The anterior intermuscular septum is identified, and two fasciotomy incisions are made: one anterior and one posterior to the septum. **D,** A vertical posteromedial incision is centered 2 cm to the rear of the tibia. Care is taken to avoid injury to the saphenous vein and nerve. (**A** to **D,** Modified from AAOS Instructional Course Lectures, Vol. 32. St. Louis, CV Mosby, 1983, pp 519-520.)

involves an anterolateral incision over the anterior and lateral compartments and a medial incision just posterior to the medial aspect of the tibia. Generous skin incisions are important to protect the underlying nerve and prevent compartment syndrome from skin. The anterolateral incision is centered halfway between the fibular shaft and the tibia. Once the fascia is identified, a small transverse incision is made to identify the anterior and lateral compartments. This is also important to help protect the

superficial peroneal nerve because it runs in this location from the lateral compartment. It is important to release the entire compartment at its most distal and proximal aspects while maintaining preservation of the superficial peroneal nerve. The posteromedial incision is used to decompress the deep and superficial posterior compartments. The incision is made approximately 2 cm posterior to the posterior aspect of the tibial shaft. Care must be taken in preserving the saphenous vein and nerve that can usually be retracted anteriorly. Once the fascia is identified, a transverse incision is made to delineate the superficial and deep compartments. The superficial posterior compartment is released first, both proximally and distally to behind the medial malleolus. In a similar fashion, the deep posterior compartment is released both proximally and distally. To completely decompress the deep compartment, the soleus muscle must be taken down off the medial side of the tibia.

Skin closure of the fasciotomy is best accomplished utilizing vessel loops laced through staples along the skin edges. These can be tightened daily at the bedside as the soft tissue swelling diminishes. Often, this eliminates the need for skin grafting and enables secondary wound closure.

Open Fractures

Open fractures are surgical emergencies. The long-term complications are limb threatening, and in cases of systemic sepsis, are life threatening. The difficult treatment challenges of open fractures have been recognized for centuries. Amputation had been the mainstay of treatment until the mid 1800s when antiseptic technique came into use. Antisepsis, combined with débridement of all contaminated and devitalized tissue, provided the first reduction in mortality. Contemporaneous advances in antibiotic prophylaxis, aggressive débridement and open wound management, rotational muscle flaps, free tissue transfer, and bone grafting techniques provided a dramatic enhancement in our capability to treat severe open fractures that resulted from motor vehicle accidents and gunshot wounds.

Classification

A fracture is considered open when the fracture site communicates with the environment. Whereas the laceration or skin avulsion is the most obvious component, the entire zone of injury must be fully appreciated at the time of surgical exploration to adequately assign a severity grade (Fig. 21-21). Gustilo and Andersen and coworkers[24] described the most commonly cited classification of fractures with soft tissue injury (Table 21-3). They divided fractures into three types and subdivided the type III lesions into three subgroups based on length of skin opening, degree of comminution, soft tissue injury, and contamination. The classification scheme represents a continuum. Sharp divisions between groups are difficult, particularly among the intermediate types; thus, interobserver variation occurs. Soft tissue destruction in closed injury can be worse than in comparable open injuries.

TABLE 21-2.   Contents of Fascial Compartments in the Leg

Compartment	Muscles	Vessels	Nerves
Anterior	Tibialis anterior Extensor hallucis longus Extensor digitorum communis	Anterior tibial	Deep peroneal
Deep posterior	Tibialis posterior Flexor hallucis longus Flexor digitorum longus	Posterior tibial Peroneal	Tibial
Superficial posterior	Gastrocnemius Soleus Plantaris		
Lateral	Peroneals		Superficial peroneal

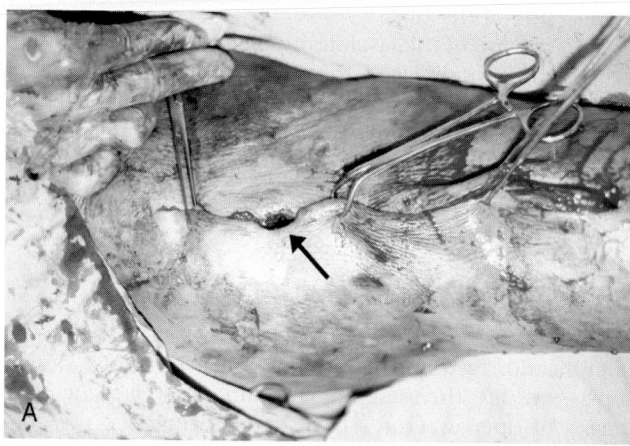

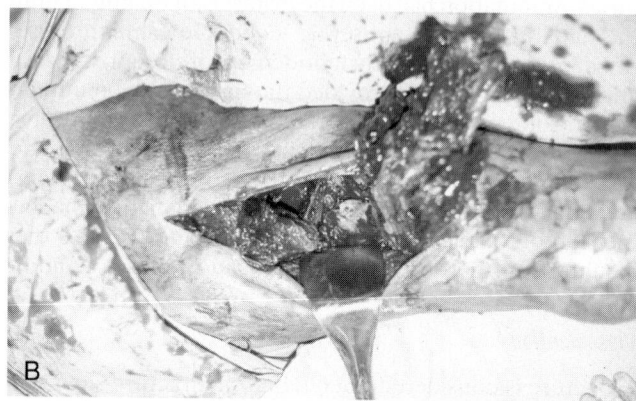

FIGURE 21-21. Débridement of open wound. **A,** The small original skin wound *(arrow)* is shown in the center of a surgical incision. **B,** The full extent of underlying soft tissue damage cannot be appreciated until after exploration.

Tscherne and associates[7] classified closed fractures (Table 21-4), creating a spectrum similar to that recognized in open fractures. Although this system has not been critically validated with outcome measures, it provides a baseline to gauge the significance of the soft tissue damage in injuries in which it may not be apparent. When these tissues become necrotic, or if a surgical approach is carried out through them, infection rates could potentially increase.

TABLE 21-3.   Gustilo-Andersen Classification of Open Fractures

Fracture Type	Description
I	Skin opening of ≤1 cm, clean; most likely inside-to-outside lesion; minimal muscle contusion; simple transverse or oblique fracture
II	Laceration >1 cm with extensive soft tissue damage, flaps, or avulsion; minimal-to-moderate crushing; simple transverse or short oblique fracture with minimal comminution
III	Extensive soft tissue damage, including muscle, skin, and neurovascular structures; often high-velocity injury with severe crushing component
IIIA	Extensive laceration, adequate bone coverage; segmental fracture, gunshot injuries
IIIB	Extensive soft tissue damage with periosteal stripping and bone exposure; usually associated with massive contamination
IIIC	Vascular injury requiring repair

From Gustilo R, Mendoza R, Williams DN: Problems in the management of type III (severe) open fractures. J Trauma 24:742-746, 1984.

The Gustilo-Andersen classification provides useful information regarding the prognosis and treatment of the injured extremity. Infection rates tend to increase from type I fractures through type III. Seven percent of type I fractures, 11% of type II, 18% of type IIA, and 56% of type IIIB/C became infected in one series. Wound cultures taken in the emergency department are positive in 60% to 70% of open fractures,[25] with most growing saprophytic organisms.[7] More useful cultures can be obtained after formal irrigation and débridement of the wounds. Forty-three percent of these cultures taken from types I, II, and IIIA fractures grew *Staphylococcus aureus*, whereas another 14% grew facultative or aerobic gram-negative rods. In types IIIB and C lesions, *S. aureus* was recovered only 7% of the time, whereas gram-negative rods accounted for 67% of the recovered organisms. Regardless of type, antimicrobials and tetanus prophylaxis are administered in the trauma room for any open fracture. In types I and II open fractures and in closed fractures with soft

TABLE 21-4. Tscherne Classification of Fractures with Soft Tissue Injuries

Fracture Type	Description
0	Minimal soft tissue damage; indirect violence; simple fracture patterns; *example:* torsion fracture of the tibia in skiers
I	Superficial abrasion or contusion caused by pressure from within; mild to moderately severe fracture configuration; *example:* pronation fracture-dislocation of the ankle joint with soft tissue lesion over the medial malleolus
II	Deep, contaminated abrasion associated with localized skin or muscle contusion; impending compartment syndrome; severe fracture configuration; *example:* segmental "bumper" fracture of the tibia
III	Extensive skin contusion or crush; underlying muscle damage may be severe; subcutaneous avulsion; decompensated compartment syndrome; associated major vascular injury; severe or comminuted fracture configuration

From Tscherne H, Oestern H: Die klassifizierung des weichteilschadens bei offenen und geschlossenen frakturen. Unfallheikunde 85:111-115, 1982.

tissue injuries, a first-generation cephalosporin is preferred. In type III fractures, an aminoglycoside is added. For any fracture with suspected soil contamination, high-dose penicillin is added to the regimen to cover *Clostridium* species. Duration of treatment remains controversial.

Management

Early irrigation and débridement are the mainstays of treatment. Once the patient is in the operating room, dressings can be removed with all loose debris. Débridement is the meticulous removal and resection of all foreign and nonviable material from a wound. The goal is reduction of the bacterial count by leaving only clearly viable tissue behind. The wound is aggressively explored because the zone of injury is always larger than initially apparent. Areas in which the extent of injury is commonly misjudged include the thigh and the posterior leg secondary to thick muscle bulk. Fascial compartments are not completely decompressed by open fractures. Therefore, fasciotomies are liberally performed during débridement. Irrigation with saline solution in copious amounts is then performed. Repeat débridement is performed 48 to 72 hours later, as tissue may demarcate and necrose. Surgical incisions used to enlarge the wound for exploration are closed. The original wound created by the injury is usually left open. Saline solution–soaked dressings are applied and changed at least daily. In contrast to temporary dressings applied for transport from the emergency department, definitive wound management dressings should not be soaked in povidone-iodine because this causes tissue destruction.

Planning for wound coverage is begun at the initial débridement. Early plastic surgery consultation may be helpful and will play a key role in determining the timing and method of soft tissue reconstruction. If skin grafting or muscle flap coverage is necessary, it should be performed within the first week before secondary colonization and wound fibrosis develop.[26] Desire to avoid nosocomial infections has encouraged a trend toward immediate coverage of open fracture wounds.

Limb Salvage Versus Primary Amputation

The choice between primary amputation and limb salvage in the severely injured extremity is difficult. Successful salvage depends on multiple factors including vascular status, extent of soft tissue injury, degree of comminution and bone loss, and neurologic function. In addition to these local factors, the outcome is dependent on systemic and psychological elements. Patients with poor nutrition, multisystem injuries, psychoses, and those not able to cooperate with a lengthy reconstructive process may not be candidates for limb salvage. Several scoring systems have been developed to help objectively assess the need for primary amputation. These systems were developed in a retrospective manner, with most limited to injuries involving the lower leg. Severely injured upper extremities have a far greater impact on the overall functioning status of the patient. Likewise, the indications for upper extremity amputation are significantly more limited.

Lange and colleagues described indications for primary below-knee amputation in 1985. Absolute indications were defined as anatomically complete disruption of the tibial nerve in an adult and warm ischemia time longer than 6 hours in a crush injury. The relative indications are serious associated polytrauma, severe ipsilateral foot trauma, and anticipated protracted course to obtain soft tissue coverage and bony reconstruction. The authors suggested that if either of the absolute indications or two of the three relative indications were met, amputation was indicated. Although no further studies have been performed to validate this scheme, these guidelines have been widely adopted and are used as the standard of care.

The MESS, the most widely validated classification system, emerged from the retrospective review of 25 charts of patients with severe open fractures of the lower extremity (Table 21-5).[27] Investigators found that limb salvage was related to vascular status, patient age, duration of ischemia, and absorbed energy. A score of 7 or higher consistently predicted the need for amputation, whereas all limbs with initial scores of 6 or less remained viable in the long term. This system was also validated prospectively.[19] Further studies have nearly uniformly supported the specificity of the MESS in evaluating the severely injured lower leg.

Salvage has routinely been accepted as preservation of a viable extremity, with no concern given to the functional status of the limb. Few studies have compared the functional outcome of below-knee amputation with salvaged limbs. Those that have, showed that patients with below-knee amputations returned to function and work more rapidly and had high levels of satisfaction. In contrast, limb salvage requires significantly more operative procedures and disability time. Although some patients in

TABLE 21-5. Mangled Extremity Severity Score

Component	Points
SKELETAL AND SOFT TISSUE INJURY	
Low energy (stab, simple fracture, "civilian" gunshot wound)	1
Medium energy (open or multiplex fractures, dislocation)	2
High energy (close-range shotgun or "military" gunshot wound; crush injury)	3
Very high energy (same as above plus gross contamination, soft tissue avulsion)	4
LIMB ISCHEMIA (DOUBLED WHEN >6 hr)	
Pulse reduced or absent but perfusion normal	1
Pulseless; paresthesias, diminished capillary refill	2
Cool, paralyzed, insensate, numb	3
SHOCK	
Systolic blood pressure always >90 mm Hg	0
Hypotensive transiently	1
Persistent hypotension	2
AGE (yr)	
<30	0
30–50	1
>50	2

From Johansen K, Daines M, Howey T, et al: Objective criteria accurately predict amputation following lower extremity trauma. J Trauma 30:568-573, 1990.

this group were more dysfunctional than amputees, others were extremely satisfied and highly functional.

When presented with a severely mangled extremity, it is important to document all pertinent local and systemic factors accurately. A MESS should be calculated for each patient and used as a guideline to supplement the clinical findings. Whenever possible, pictures should be taken and added to the permanent medical record. Primary amputation should be performed when injuries include complete tibial or sciatic nerve injury in an adult or unreconstructible bone or arterial injury. When the indications are not absolute, it is essential that several surgeons—who must each document their opinion in the medical record—independently evaluate the patient.

Treatment

Skeletal stabilization has been shown to be crucial to soft tissue healing. When compared with cast and splints, internal or external fixation permits greater access for wound care and is more effective in controlling pain during mobilization. At the cellular level, the inflammatory response is shortened and the spread of bacteria is diminished. The decision to employ one mode of fixation versus another is dependent on fracture pattern, degree of contamination, and surgeon preference.

The most widely accepted method of fixation has been external fixation. Advances in design have made these devices lighter, yet more stable, and easier to apply. External fixation minimizes additional dissection and avoids insertion of large metallic implants by utilizing percutaneously inserted pins that are interconnected by external stabilizing devices. They are easily removed, replaced,

and adjusted and can be combined with other means of fixation.

External fixators are not without their problems. Pin tract osteomyelitis has become rare with changes in design and technique of pin insertion. However, superficial infection with drainage occurs in approximately 30% of all patients. Owing to their size and location, further débridement and coverage can be cumbersome. In the tibia, for instance, pin insertion through the subcutaneous anteromedial border reduces pin tract infection but often results in obstructed access for plastic and reconstructive surgery. In other cases, more extensive fracture patterns may require more complex frame constructs that further limit access. Although effective for providing skeletal stabilization during soft tissue reconstruction, external fixation is not ideal for achieving fracture union. Additional surgery, including bone grafting or conversion to internal fixation, is often necessary.

For these reasons, IM nailing appears to be an attractive option. Definitive fracture care usually can be accomplished in a single operation. There are no bulky external frames to work around, and mobilization and daily care are facilitated. However, several early series[28] reported an unacceptably high incidence of infection when reamed IM nailing was employed in type III open tibia fractures. For this reason, external fixation remained the standard of care for these serious fractures throughout the 1980s. Originally, this was believed to be due to destruction of cortical blood flow by reaming. Animal studies showed a 70% reduction compared with only a 30% decrease when a nail is placed without reaming.[29] Although the injury itself caused periosteal stripping and significant soft tissue loss, the loss of the medullary blood supply further weakened the bone's healing potential and resistance to infection.

When unreamed, small diameter nails were employed in open fracture care, deep infection and nonunion rates were found to be the same as with external fixation. Studies have shown that with aggressive irrigation and débridement, closed unreamed nailing can be carried out immediately in even severe, type III open tibia fractures.[4,30,31]

Although the benefits of unreamed nailing have been documented, problems with their application have led to a significant reoperation rate for removal of screws, fibular osteotomies, exchange with larger diameter reamed nails, or bone grafting. Use of small-diameter rods and cross-locking screws has led to some implant failure, particularly with premature weight bearing. Intraoperative malalignment and subsequent malunion of proximal fractures has been a continuing problem. Despite these issues, unreamed locked IM nailing has supplanted external fixation for most open tibia fractures.[4]

Another approach to the treatment of open tibia fractures has been the initial use of external fixation followed by reamed IM nailing or plating. Many investigators have reported a high incidence of infection when reamed IM nailing was attempted after a substantial period of external fixation. Osteomyelitis after IM nailing was associated with long periods of external fixation and history of pin tract infection. If this technique is to be employed, the

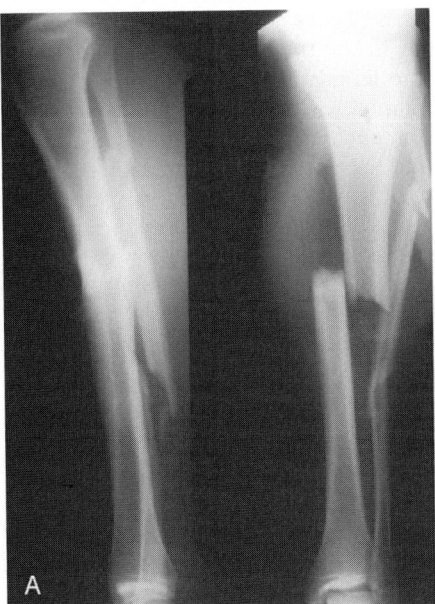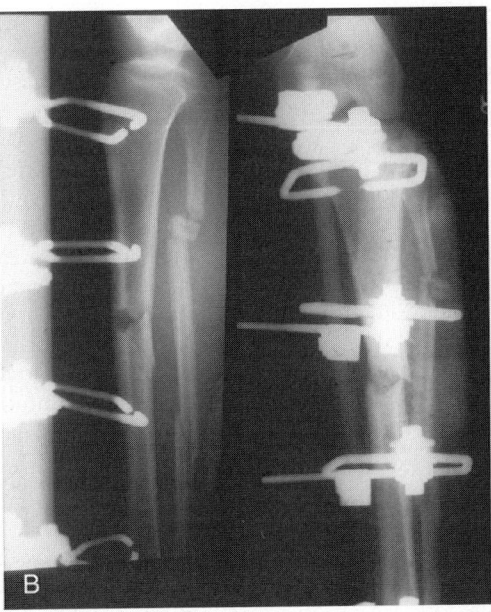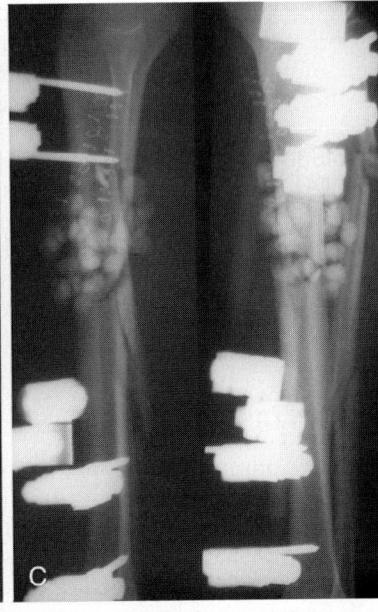

FIGURE 21-22. Management of open tibia/fibula fracture with external fixators. **A,** Anteroposterior (AP) and lateral views of tibia/fibula fracture. **B,** Interim stabilization is achieved with a pinless external fixator. Note that the pins do not traverse the medullary canal. **C,** Conversion to a definitive external fixator (owing to severe open wound and significant bone loss precluding intramedullary nailing) and insertion of antibiotic-impregnated beads after débridement of necrotic bone.

external fixator should be left on no longer than 2 weeks.[32]

To avoid these problems, the pinless external fixator was developed. This device allows the tibial fragments to be fixed with a series of C-clamps that grasp the outer cortex without penetrating the medullary canal (Fig. 21-22). This reduces the IM contamination and provides another route for safe conversion to reamed IM nails.[33] Because the pins do not penetrate the canal, the device may even be left in place to help maintain alignment and stability during the subsequent IM nailing. However, early investigations have shown problems with soft tissue necrosis from the current clamp design that may be eliminated by subsequent design improvements.

Despite the discussions regarding skeletal fixation, the hallmarks of successful treatment of open femur fractures are still antibiotic prophylaxis, irrigation, débridement, compartment decompression, stabilization, and early wound coverage. Although external fixation is a safe and useful tool, its use in types I, II, and IIIA open fractures of the tibia has been replaced by unreamed IM nailing. Although evidence suggests that this is a safe practice in type IIIB fractures,[30] some are reluctant to adopt it. Until further evidence is available, some form of external fixation should be applied initially and then converted to a reamed, locked nail within 2 weeks in these difficult fractures. Coverage for all wounds is accomplished within 1 week, whenever possible. Using these guidelines, the amputation rate has fallen dramatically.

Dislocations

Dislocations of major joints (e.g., shoulder, elbow, hip, knee, ankle) are considered orthopedic emergencies.

Prolonged dislocation can lead to the development of cartilage cell death, posttraumatic arthritis, neurovascular injury, ankylosis, and avascular necrosis. These injuries, which are more likely to occur in young, active patients, can have devastating consequences.

Most dislocations have characteristic physical findings. After a dislocation, muscles around the joint typically become spasmotic, limiting range of motion. This often causes the limb to assume a distinctive position. In posterior hip dislocations, the thigh is held flexed and internally rotated. The affected limb is often shortened and cannot be passively extended. An anterior shoulder dislocation causes an externally rotated and adducted arm position. Elbow and knee dislocations (most commonly posterior) result in an extremity locked in extension. As with all extremity injuries, a meticulous neurovascular examination must be performed and documented before and after manipulation.

Dislocations of the hip require special discussion because of the extreme consequences of failing to recognize and address them in a timely fashion. Sciatic nerve injury, cartilage cell death, and avascular necrosis can result from delay in treatment of these injuries. Of these, avascular necrosis is the most devastating owing to its propensity to cause collapse of the femoral head and subsequent development of degenerative joint disease. This problem can lead to total hip replacement or hip fusion at a young age. After these procedures, multiple major reconstructive operations are common during the patient's lifetime.

Avascular necrosis usually develops in a time-dependent fashion. In the dislocated position, tension on the capsular blood vessels restricts blood flow to the femoral head. If the hip remains dislocated for 24 hours, avascular necrosis will ensue in 100% of cases. Although irreversible damage to the blood supply may occur at the time of injury, reduction by 6 hours is generally accepted as the window to reduce the incidence of ischemic changes.

Reduction of dislocations often requires intravenous sedation to reduce the muscle spasm at the joint. If a joint cannot be reduced by closed methods with adequate sedation, general anesthesia is required. Attempts are made to reduce the joint with closed techniques in the operating room with staff available for open reduction procedures if this fails.

COMMON LONG BONE FRACTURES

With all injuries it is important to identify not only the presence of a fracture but also the energy involved in causing it. The fracture pattern offers clues to the mechanism of injury: a low-energy twisting injury typically yields a simple spiral fracture; and a direct impact typically causes a bending moment yielding a transverse fracture, whereas the most severe fractures (resulting from crush injuries) will often have complex segmental, or highly comminuted patterns. Ultimately, fracture patterns help identify mechanisms of injury, which further help assess the amount of kinetic energy ($0.5 \, mv^2$) that is absorbed by the fractured and surrounding soft tissues. Often it is the injury to surrounding skin, muscle, microvasculature and macrovasculature, and periosteum that collectively determine the ability of the bone to heal successfully and rapidly.

Femur Fractures

Epidemiology and Significance

Femoral shaft fractures deserve special attention. Femur fractures occur at a rate of 1 per 10,000 people per year. A closed femoral shaft fracture is considered a "major" injury when calculating the Injury Severity Score (ISS). Therefore, another major injury in any other organ system qualifies the patient as multiply injured. Except for the rare pathologic or insufficiency fracture in the elderly, these fractures are always the result of a high-energy injury, and in the trauma setting are predictive of small bowel injury. Often, these injuries lead to significant bleeding. Because of the geometry of the thigh, several units of blood can be hidden in the tissues with little external evidence of bleeding. Transfusion with packed red blood cells is frequently necessary, with 40% of patients needing 2.5 units or more.

Initial Management

All femur fractures must be immobilized before the patient is transported from the trauma setting. Leaving a displaced fracture unsplinted leads to increased edema and bleeding and risks further damage to the surrounding soft tissues and neurovascular structures. Continued motion at the fracture site also leads to increased fat

embolization and contributes to the development of ARDS. Traction is key in the treatment of these fractures. Traction increases the length of the thigh compartment, and, therefore, its diameter is decreased. The soft tissues are then under tension and can impart a tamponade effect to the bleeding fracture site. Immobilization can be achieved in a variety of ways. If the patient is in extremis, a posterior splint alone will suffice until formal traction or immobilization can be achieved. If time allows, a traction pin can be placed through the proximal tibia to provide the necessary traction and allow access to the distal femur. A Hare traction splint, either with skin traction through the ankle or attached to a skeletal traction pin, is quite effective at immobilizing a femur fracture (Fig. 21-23).

Definitive Stabilization

Definitive stabilization of femur fractures within the first 24 hours is essential in the polytrauma victim.[8] Some studies have shown deleterious effects when fracture fixation is delayed only 2 to 4 days.[34,35] Immediate fixation leads to earlier mobilization, prevention of deep venous thrombosis and decubitus ulcers, easier nursing care, and decreased need for analgesia. Furthermore, the magnitude of fat embolus is also decreased.[8] Taken together, these factors can significantly improve pulmonary status and decrease the incidence of ARDS. This benefit is magnified as the ISS increases. In patients with severe trauma (ISS > 40), delayed fixation of femoral shaft fractures leads to a fivefold increase in the incidence of ARDS. In addition, immediate stabilization of femoral fractures significantly decreases the cost of the hospital stay.[8]

These studies have proved definitively that early, immediate stabilization of femoral fractures is essential in the multiply injured patient. Contraindications to immediate stabilization include hypothermia, coagulopathy, excessive intracranial pressure, and high pulmonary shunting. The findings in the femoral fracture studies have been broadened to support immediate fixation of all long bone fractures, but definitive studies have not yet been performed. In isolated long bone fractures, the need for immediate fixation is not evident. However, if the institution is capable of performing the stabilization within 24 hours, there is no reason to delay. Early fixation shortens hospital stays and decreases overall costs and patient morbidity.

The method of fixation of femoral shaft fractures has become fairly standardized. The treatment of choice for closed fractures and types I through IIIA open fractures is closed, locked IM nailing. In contrast to open reduction methods, this practice reduces bleeding and soft tissue disruption at the fracture site. These minimally invasive techniques reduce perioperative stress and decrease the incidence of infection and nonunion. Types IIIB and IIIC open femoral shaft fractures are usually managed with immediate external fixation.

Tibial Shaft Fractures

Tibial shaft fractures are among the most common injuries in the trauma setting. They are the most common dia-

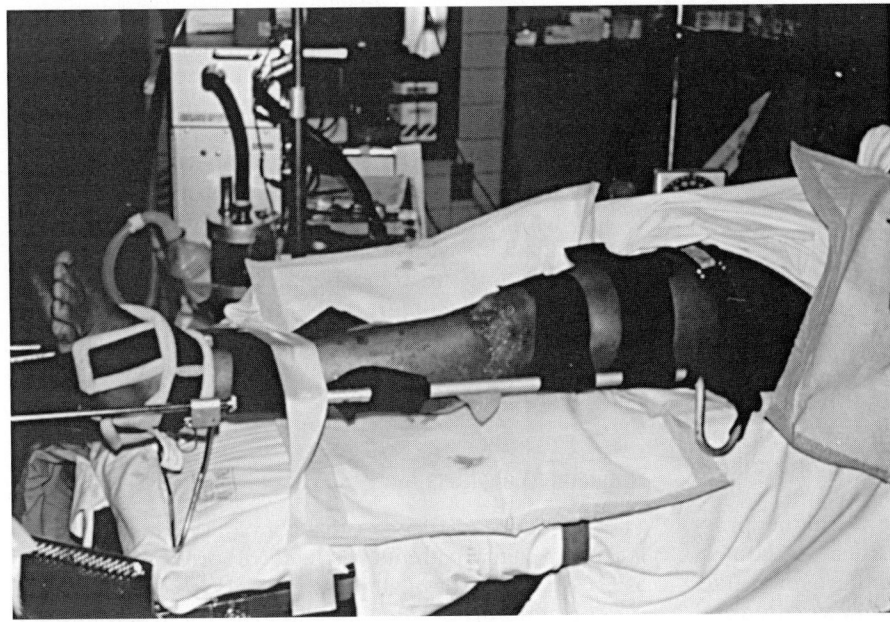

FIGURE 21-23. Patient in the emergency department with a Hare temporary traction splint in place to stabilize a femoral shaft fracture and aid in transport. (From Wolinsky PR, Johnson KD: Femoral shaft fractures. *In* Browner BD, Jupiter TB, Levine AM, Trafton PG [eds]: Skeletal Trauma, 2nd ed. Philadelphia, WB Saunders, 1998.)

physeal long bone fractures. The worst of such fractures are typically sustained by pedestrians struck by motor vehicles, and by motorcyclists. Their successful treatment is fraught with difficulties owing to the varying anatomical demands and fixation limitations as one moves from proximal to distal.

Blood Supply

Tibia shaft fractures tend to be slow healing, in part, due to the tenuous blood supply. Diaphyseal blood supply is via a single nutrient artery that branches off of the posterior tibial artery and enters the medullary canal, coursing proximally and distally to anastomose with metaphyseal endosteal vessels. There is also some contribution from penetrating periosteal arteries that supply the outer one third of the cortex. However, a diaphyseal fracture can easily compromise nutrient arterial blood supply, and concomitant soft tissue stripping may leave an entire segment of tibia devascularized. This predisposes tibia shaft fractures to impaired healing, and in open fractures, to osteomyelitis.

Associated Soft Tissue Injuries

Aside from injuries to the overlying skin and muscle, tibia shaft fractures often have other associated soft tissue injuries. Ligamentous injuries causing knee instability and future morbidity or disability are not uncommon and are often identified later.

Neurovascular injury must always be suspected and a careful examination must always be performed. Both dorsalis pedis and posterior tibial arterial pulses are palpated and capillary refill is assessed. If injury is suspected, a Doppler probe can be used to further assess arterial blood flow. When used with a blood pressure cuff proximally,

arterial pressures can be measured and compared to brachial artery pressure. This test is a sensitive and specific indicator of significant arterial injury. An ankle/brachial index less than 0.9 indicates a high probability of vessel injury.

Neurologic examination includes all four major nerves that travel distally in the leg. Deep peroneal nerve can be assessed by testing first dorsal web space sensation and foot and toe dorsiflexion. Superficial peroneal nerve function can be assessed by testing sensation along the dorsum of the foot as well as foot eversion. Tibial nerve function can be assessed by testing sensation along the sole of the foot as well as foot and toe plantar flexion. The sural nerve is a pure sensory nerve and its function can be assessed by testing sensation to the lateral heel.

Management and Treatment

Management and treatment of tibia shaft fractures has evolved over the years. Closed, minor-severity fractures can be treated well with cast immobilization and functional bracing. However, almost all moderate and severe fractures benefit from surgical stabilization. Reamed IM nailing is the technique of choice when possible. Previously it was thought that open fractures were a contraindication to IM stabilization. However, studies have indicated that nonreamed IM nailing is successful in open fractures, as well. There is still debate regarding the use of reamed IM nailing in these circumstances. External fixation remains an option for treatment of tibia shaft fractures, although it is usually reserved for temporary stabilization or for treatment of open fractures. Plate fixation has fallen out of favor due to the high risk of wound healing complications with the surgical incision passing through the zone of acutely injured soft tissues. However, it remains a valuable treatment option for diaphyseal fractures that extend proximally or distally into the meta-physics and would be less amenable to IM stabilization. Newer percutaneous plating techniques have further allowed plate fixation to remain a viable option for tibia shaft fractures due to the surgical insertion site being distanced from the region of injury.

Humeral Shaft Fractures

Humeral shaft fractures consist of 3% of all fractures. Many of these can be treated nonoperatively owing to the internal splinting effects of intramuscular septa. In addition, the mobility of the shoulder and elbow joints allows for acceptance of 15 degrees of malrotation, 20 degrees of flexion-extension deformity, 30 degrees of varus-valgus deformity, and 3 cm of shortening without compromising function or appearance.

Transverse diaphyseal fractures pose a unique problem in that they are significantly harder to control than spiral oblique fractures. With distal-third spiral fractures, radial nerve function must be carefully assessed and documented owing to the high incidence of associated radial nerve injury (Holstein-Lewis fracture) as a result of the intimate anatomic relationship of the radial nerve with the humerus shaft as it courses distally in the spiral groove. In the trauma setting, right-sided humerus shaft fractures are significantly predictive of concomitant liver injury.

Treatment

Various nonoperative options exist for treating these humeral shaft fractures: hanging arm cast, coaptation splint, Velpeau dressing, sling, and swathe. Typically, a coaptation splint is placed in the acute setting, and subsequently replaced by a functional fracture brace after the initial painful fracture period has passed (3 to 7 days). Patients are then allowed free elbow flexion-extension and arm abduction to 60 degrees. Motion is encouraged to stimulate fracture healing because it is the hydraulic compression created by muscle contraction that helps achieve fracture union.

In certain circumstances operative intervention is indicated: failed closed reduction, intra-articular fractures, concomitant neurologic or vascular injury, ipsilateral forearm or elbow fractures ("floating elbow"), segmental fractures, open fractures, and polytrauma patients. Operative options include IM nailing, plate and screw fixation, and external fixation.

COMPLICATIONS

Missed Injuries

Missed musculoskeletal injuries account for a large proportion of delays in diagnosis made within the first few days of care of the critically injured patient.[36] Clinical reassessment of trauma patients within 24 hours has reduced the incidence of missed injuries by nearly 40%.

Patients should be reexamined as they regain consciousness and resume activity. Repeated assessment should be routinely performed in all patients, including unstable and neurologically impaired patients. This tertiary trauma survey includes a comprehensive complete re-examination and, in addition, a re-evaluation of all laboratory results and radiographs within 24 hours of admission. Specific injury patterns should be reviewed closely, including those in patients with multiple injuries and severe injuries. External soft tissue trauma may be indicative of more severe underlying injury. Missed cervical spine trauma occurs in 5% of all spine injuries and can potentially lead to paralysis and death.[9] Formal radiology rounds can lead to greater recognition of occult injuries.[36,37]

Drug and Alcohol Use

The incidence of drug and alcohol use among musculoskeletal injury patients has been reported to be as high as 50%. Nearly 25% of all these patients tested positive for two or more drugs. Alcohol and drug use result in more severe orthopedic injuries and in an increased frequency of injuries requiring longer hospitalizations. Associated complications include those from cocaine use, such as fever, hypertension, acute myocardial ischemia, arrhythmias, and stroke. Cocaine can also facilitate cardiac arrhythmias when combined with halothane, nitrous oxide, and ketamine. Furthermore, the use of alcohol or drugs can adversely affect the administration of premedicating drugs. Proper monitoring and preparation should accompany the administration of any intravenous premedicating drug. Prophylaxis for delirium tremens in postoperative patients should be performed when indicated. Inpatient detoxification consultation should be obtained before patient discharge.

Thromboembolic Complications

Multiply injured patients have an increased incidence of thromboembolic complications, including deep venous thrombosis and pulmonary embolism, when compared with patients with isolated injuries.[8] The incidence of pulmonary embolism in major trauma patients ranges from 2% to 22% and is the third leading cause of death among these patients (Fig. 21-24).[38] Multiply injured patients represent a high-risk group for venous thromboembolism, along with patients undergoing elective neurosurgical, orthopedic, cancer, and spinal cord surgery. In particular, long bone fractures, pelvic fractures, advanced age, spinal cord injuries, and surgical procedures are associated with an increased risk of deep venous thrombosis in trauma patients.[6] The use of indwelling venous catheters also leads to an increase in thromboembolic complications. There have been few randomized trials evaluating deep venous thrombosis prophylaxis in multiple trauma patients, and therefore, no specific recommendations have evolved. The most common forms of pharmacologic prophylaxis include adjusted-dose unfractionated heparin, low-molecular-weight heparin, warfarin, and aspirin. In addition, hirudin, a selective thrombin inhibitor, has been

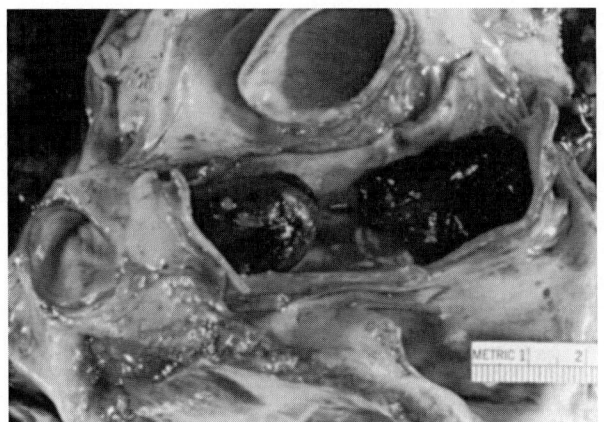

FIGURE 21-24.   A large embolus in the pulmonary artery, which was the cause of death. (Courtesy of James E. Parker, MD, University of Louisville, Louisville, KY.)

used in elective hip surgery prophylaxis. Other forms of prophylaxis include mechanical devices, such as foot pumps, sequential calf compression pumps, and barrier devices, such as vena cava filters.

It is generally agreed that in the high-risk trauma patient, prophylaxis is critical in preventing thromboembolic complications. Two controversial issues in the prevention of venous thromboembolism in the trauma patient are currently being debated. The first is the role of venous surveillance. Several authors[39,40] recommend routine duplex surveillance and formal institutional protocols to detect thromboembolic events, arguing that the incidence of proximal deep venous thrombosis is higher than formerly suspected. The second issue is that of appropriate prophylaxis. No single form of anticoagulation has proved maximally efficacious in minimizing the incidence of deep venous thrombosis in trauma patients. Adjusted-dose heparin and low-molecular-weight heparin are currently the most common forms of prophylaxis. In a randomized study comparing low-dose unfractionated heparin with low-molecular-weight heparin, Geerts and coworkers[41] documented an overall 44% incidence of deep venous thrombosis in trauma patients receiving low-dose unfractionated heparin versus 31% in those receiving enoxaparin. There was a slight increase in major bleeding in the enoxaparin group; however, none of the patients' hemoglobin dropped by more than 2 g/dL. Further research in this area is needed to determine appropriate prophylaxis for trauma patients with orthopedic injuries.

Frequently, there are multiple contraindications to using anticoagulation therapy in the multiply injured trauma patient, and mechanical compression devices are an alternative form of prophylaxis. Patients with significant head injury, coagulopathic patients, or those at risk for ongoing bleeding may not be appropriate candidates for anticoagulation. Intermittent pneumatic compression devices deliver sequential rhythmic compression to the calf and thigh and can help in reducing rates of deep venous thrombosis in trauma patients. Unfortunately, one third of patients with orthopedic injuries are not candidates for intermittent pneumatic compression because of long bone fractures or open wounds. In this setting, foot compression devices are a reasonable alternative to calf compression.[42]

Vena cava filters offer pulmonary embolism prophylaxis in high-risk patients who have failed anticoagulation, who are not appropriate candidates for anticoagulation, or who are at very high risk secondary to the severity of injury. These devices are not routinely placed because of potential morbidity including migration of the filter, bleeding during or after placement, or filter thrombosis. Selected patients who may benefit from prophylactic filter placement include those with severe spinal cord injuries with neurologic deficit, multiple long bone fractures, or long bone fractures associated with pelvic fractures or those with severe head injury who cannot be anticoagulated.

Pulmonary Failure: Fat Emboli Syndrome and Adult Respiratory Distress Syndrome

Fat emboli syndrome (FES) is a condition characterized by respiratory distress, altered mental status, and skin petechiae. First described as a syndrome in 1873, it occurs in multiply injured patients, especially those with orthopedic injuries. Clinical signs are evident hours to days after trauma involving multiple long bone fractures or isolated femoral, tibial, and pelvic fractures. Although fat globule embolization may occur in nearly 100% of traumatized patients, the incidence of FES ranges from 1% to 17% in traumatized individuals.[43] In patients with isolated long bone fractures, the incidence is between 2% and 5%. In the multiply injured patient with long bone fractures or pelvic fractures, the incidence is as high as 15%. Marrow fat from the fracture site after musculoskeletal trauma can enter into the pulmonary vasculature. This causes activation of the coagulation cascade and platelet dysfunction with the subsequent release of vasoactive substances.[44] The histopathologic diagnosis of FES is difficult. The presence of lipid within alveolar macrophages obtained by bronchoalveolar lavage may help in the early diagnosis of FES.[45] Morbidity from FES may be anywhere between 0 and 20%.[43] In an autopsy study of more than 5000 deaths, FES was causative in 16% of injury-related deaths. FES may represent a clinical entity related to or a subset of ARDS. ARDS is a pulmonary failure state defined as a Pao_2/Fio_2 less than 200 for greater than 5 consecutive days or bilateral diffuse infiltrates on chest radiograph in the absence of congestive heart failure.[46] FES may be causative in the development of ARDS. This is important because the timing of surgical care has been correlated with outcome. Early fixation has resulted in a reduction of FES and ARDS in several studies.[47,48] Johnson and associates[49] reported a 17% incidence of ARDS with early fracture stabilization compared with 75% with delayed fixation. Both clinical and experimental studies suggest that the method of fracture fixation plays a minor role in the development of pulmonary complications.[50] The early ventilatory dependency, which occurs immediately after severe trauma, is secondary to the effects of any thoracic trauma or fluid resuscitation that may accompany such cases. ARDS occurs several days after the primary insult and can be lessened with early fixation, débridement of necrotic soft tissue and hematoma, and maintenance of the upright position.

POSTOPERATIVE MOBILIZATION

The benefits of early fixation and mobilization of multiply injured patients have already been discussed. The distinction between mobilization and weight bearing should be made clear, however. *Mobilization* is the transfer of the patient from the supine position, either under her or his own power or with the help of nurses and therapists. This includes turning every shift by the nurses, sitting up in bed, or transferring the patient to a chair. All patients whose general condition allows should be mobilized by the second postoperative day. Mobilization helps prevent the development of pulmonary and septic complications.

Weight bearing, in contrast, is the transmission of load by an injured extremity. For a patient to be allowed to bear weight on an injured extremity, the following three conditions must be met.

1. There must be bone-to-bone contact at the fracture site. This is appreciated either intraoperatively or on the postreduction radiographs after closed treatment. Without contact of the fracture ends, the fixation devices will be subjected to all the stresses applied to the extremity. This will frequently result in failure of the fixation.
2. Stable fixation of the fracture must be achieved. By definition, stable fixation is not disrupted when subjected to normal physiologic loads. Stable fixation is dependent on multiple factors. Fixation may be less than ideal in patients with osteopenic bone or severely comminuted fractures. When excessive loads are anticipated, such as with heavy or obese patients, typical fixation may not be adequate.
3. The patient must be able to comply with the weight-bearing status. Often, the reliability of the patient is a significant consideration in the determination of weight-bearing status. Social, psychological, or emotional circumstances can affect a patient's ability to comply with weight-bearing restrictions.

Unless all of these criteria are met, the fixation will need to be protected with restricted weight-bearing status. *Touch-down weight bearing* allows for the weight of the leg to be applied with the foot flat on the floor. Touch-down status is often allowed in patients with injuries around the hip. Touch-down weight bearing allows for extension of the hip and knee and dorsiflexion at the ankle. This natural position relaxes the hip musculature and minimizes the joint forces. Crutch walking with the foot off the floor (non-weight bearing) leads to a significant increase in the forces across the hip joint, greater than in the touch-down weight-bearing state. *Toe-touch weight bearing*, a term often used synonymously with touch-down weight bearing, is an unfortunate use of terminology. Most patients attempt to walk while touching only the toe of the injured extremity to the ground. In this position, the hip and knee are flexed and the ankle is held in equinus. When this status is maintained for any significant amount of time, contractures at the hip, knee, and ankle are common.

Partial weight bearing is defined in terms of the percentage of body weight on an injured extremity. It is gradually increased as a fracture gains stability through healing. Using a scale, the patient can learn what different amounts of body weight feel like. When a fracture and patient are stable enough to withstand normal loads, *weight bearing as tolerated* is instituted. It is believed that reliable patients limit their own weight bearing based on their pain.

Even when weight bearing is not allowed, mobilization of affected and adjacent joints is typically performed within a few days. After surgical treatment, joints are typically immobilized briefly and then allowed either passive or active range of motion in bed if weight bearing is not prudent. Early joint mobilization decreases the likelihood of fibrosis and, therefore, increases early mobility. Furthermore, joint motion is necessary for good health of articular cartilage. Cartilage is nourished from synovial fluid most efficiently when the joint is moving. Early joint mobilization has become a basic tenet of orthopedic care and has led to decreased stiffness and improved cartilage health.

SUMMARY

In all trauma settings, the preservation of life takes precedent over the preservation of limb. Injuries of the extremities and axial skeleton may be life threatening in rare circumstances. However, once the patient is stabilized through the critical period, these injuries are a major cause of post-traumatic morbidity that manifests itself in health care costs, lost work days, physical disability, emotional distress, and diminished quality of life. Accordingly, it is essential that a detailed and complete extremity and axial musculoskeletal survey is performed on every patient, that injuries are identified early, and that the consulting orthopedic surgical team is notified of the specifics of these injuries in a timely fashion. This allows them the opportunity to make the necessary arrangements to address the specific injury. Moreover, the patient should not be transported from the trauma room, unless for life-saving interventions, until the orthopedic team has evaluated and stabilized the involved extremity so as to protect against further injury and morbidity.

Selected References

Bone LB, Johnson KD, Weigelt J, et al: Early versus delayed stabilization of femoral shaft fractures: A prospective randomized study. J Bone Joint Surg Am 71-A:336-340, 1989.

This classic article has shaped the treatment of the multiply injured patient. It was the first to clearly define the benefits of early stabilization of femoral shaft fractures prospectively.

Browner, BD, Jupiter JB, Levine AM, Trafton PG (eds): Skeletal Trauma: Fractures, Dislocations, Ligamentous Injuries, 3rd ed. Philadelphia, WB Saunders, 2003.

This is one of the premiere, comprehensive texts covering traumatic musculoskeletal injuries. This two-volume set is now in its third edition with the most recent update in 2003. It is clearly written and visually appealing. The chapter authors comprise the elite orthopedic trauma surgeons in the world. It is an excellent reference for any surgical resident dealing with the multiply injured patient.

Gustilo R, Anderson J: Prevention of infection in the treatment of 1025 open fractures of long bones: Retrospective and prospective analyses. J Bone Joint Surg Am 58-A:453-458, 1976.

This classic article in 1976 defined the classification and proposed management guidelines in patients with open fractures. It includes greater than 300 cases reviewed retrospectively and another 600 prospective cases where the new classification was applied.

Tile M (ed): Fractures of the Pelvis and Acetabulum, 2nd ed. Baltimore, Williams & Wilkins, 1988.

This text covers pelvic and acetabular trauma in depth. This book is written for the orthopedic trauma surgeon but includes a clear description of the mechanisms of injuries and the classification of pelvic ring injuries.

Tscherne H, Gotzen L: Fractures with Soft Tissue Injuries. Berlin, Springer-Verlag, 1984.

This fracture textbook is comprehensive in its coverage of open and closed fractures with soft tissue injuries. It covers all classifications, immediate management, fracture care, and wound care of these injuries. It employs the team approach to dealing with these complicated injuries.

References

1. Copes W: Musculoskeletal injuries in the major trauma outcome study. Personal Communication, Trianalytics, Inc, Baltimore, 1999.
2. Committee on Trauma: ATLS Instruction Manual. Chicago, American College of Surgeons, Committee on Trauma, 1993.
3. Burgess A, Eastridge BJ, Young JW, et al: Pelvic ring disruption: Effective classification system and treatment protocols. J Trauma 30:848-856, 1990.
4. Court-Brown C, Keating J, McQueen MM: Infection after intramedullary nailing of the tibia: Incidence and protocol for management. J Bone Joint Surg Br 74-B:770-774, 1992.
5. Waters RL, Adkins RH, Yakura JS: Definition of complete spinal cord injury. Paraplegia 29:573-581, 1991.
6. Geerts W, Code K, Jay RM, et al: A prospective study of venous thromboembolism after major trauma. N Engl J Med 331:1601-1606, 1994.
7. Tscherne H, Gotzen L: Fractures with Soft Tissue Injuries. Berlin, Springer-Verlag, 1984.
8. Bone L, Johnson KD, Weigelt J, et al: Early versus delayed stabilization of femoral shaft fractures: A prospective randomized study. J Bone Joint Surg Am 71-A:336-340, 1989.
9. Latenser B, Gentilello L, Tarver AA, et al: Improved outcome with early fixation of skeletally unstable pelvic fractures. J Trauma 31:28-31, 1991.
10. Harkess J, Ramsey W, et al: Principles of fractures and dislocations. In Rockwood C, Green D, Bucholz R, Heckman J (eds): Rockwood and Green's Fractures in Adults, 4th ed. Philadelphia, Lippincott-Raven, 1996.
11. Ochsner MG Jr, Hoffman AP, DiPasquale D, et al: Associated aortic rupture–pelvic fracture: An alert for orthopaedic and general surgeon. J Trauma 33:429-434, 1992.
12. Tile M: Pelvic ring fractures: Should they be fixed? J Bone Joint Surg Br 70-B:1-12, 1988.
13. Ben-Menachem Y: Exploratory angiography and transcatheter embolization for control of arterial hemorrhage in patients with pelvic ring disruption. Tech Orthop 9:271-274, 1995.
14. Buckle R, Browner B, et al: Emergency reduction for pelvic ring disruptions and control of associated hemorrhage using the Pelvic Stabilizer. Tech Orthop 9:258-266, 1995.
15. Ganz R, Krushell M, Jakob RP, et al: The antishock pelvic clamp. Clin Orthop 267:71-78, 1991.
16. Klein S, Saroyan M, Baumgartner F, et al: Management strategy of vascular injuries associated with pelvic fractures. J Cardiovasc Surg 33:349-357, 1992.
17. Riemer BL, Butterfield SL, Diamond DL, et al: Acute mortality associated with injuries to the pelvic ring: The role of early patient mobilization and external fixation. J Trauma 35:671-677, 1993.
18. Breest T, Moody M: Frequency of vascular injury with blunt trauma–induced extremity injury. Am J Surg 160:226-228, 1990.
19. Helfet D, Howey T, Sanders R, et al: Limb salvage versus amputation: Preliminary results of the MESS. Clin Orthop 256:80-86, 1990.
20. Nichols J, Svoboda J, Parks SN, et al: Use of temporary intraluminal shunts in selected peripheral arterial injuries. J Trauma 26:1094-1096, 1996.
20a. Seddon H: Volkmann's contracture treatment of excision of the infarct. J Bone Joint Surg Br 38-B: 152-174, 1956.
20b. Seddon H: Volkmann's ischemia of the lower limb. J Bone Joint Surg Br 48-B:627-636, 1966.
21. Orthopaedic Trauma Association: Economic costs of missed compartment syndrome. Eighth Annual Orthopaedic Trauma Association Meeting, Minneapolis, MN, Nov. 6-10, 1992.
22. Whitesides T, Heckman M: Acute compartment syndrome: Update on diagnosis and treatment. J Am Acad Orthop Surg 4:209-218, 1996.
22a. Mubarak S, Hargens A (eds): Compartment Syndromes and Volkmann's Contracture. Philadelphia, WB Saunders, 1981.
22b. Matsen FA III, Winquist R, Krugmire RB Jr: Diagnosis and management of compartment syndromes. J Bone Joint Surg Am 62-A:286-291, 1980.
23. Heckman MM, Whitesides TE Jr, Grewe SR, et al: Compartment pressure in association with closed tibial fractures: The relationship between tissue pressure, compartment, and distance from the site of fracture. J Bone Joint Surg Am 76-A:1285-1292, 1994.
24. Gustilo R, Anderson J: Prevention of infection in the treatment of 1025 open fractures of long bones: Retrospective and prospective analyses. J Bone Joint Surg Am 58-A:453-458, 1976.
25. Patzakis M: Management of open fractures. Instr Course Lect 31:62-64, 1982.
26. Patzakis M, Wilkins J, Moore TM, et al: Considerations in reducing the infection rate of open tibia fractures. Clin Orthop 178:36-41, 1983.
27. Johansen K, Daines M, Howey T, et al: Objective criteria accurately predict amputation following lower extremity trauma. J Trauma 30:568-573, 1990.
28. Jenny J, Jenny G, Kempf I: Infection after reamed intramedullary nailing of lower limb fractures: A review

of 1464 cases over 15 years. Acta Orthop Scand 65:94-96, 1994.

29. Schemitsch E, Kowalski MJ, Swiontkowski MF, et al: Cortical bone blood flow in reamed and unreamed locked intramedullary nailing: A fractured tibia model in sheep. J Orthop Trauma 8:373-382, 1994.

30. Tornetta P III, Bergman M, Watnik N, et al: Treatment of type IIIB open tibial fractures: A prospective randomized comparison of external fixation and non-reamed locked nailing. J Bone Joint Surg Br 76-B:13-19, 1994.

31. Tu Y, Lin C, Su JI, et al: Unreamed interlocking nail versus external fixator for open type III tibia fractures. J Trauma 39:361-367, 1995.

32. Blachut P, Meek R, O'Brien PJ: External fixation and delayed intramedullary nailing of open fractures of the tibial shaft: A sequential protocol. J Bone Joint Surg Am 72-A:729-735, 1990.

33. Schutz M, Sudkamp N, Frigg R, et al: Pinless external fixator: Indications and preliminary result in tibial shaft fractures. Clin Orthop 347:35-42, 1998.

34. Fakhry S, Rutledge R, Dahners LE, et al: Incidence, management, and outcome of femoral shaft fracture: Statewide population-based analysis of 2805 adult patients in a rural state. J Trauma 37:255-260, 1994.

35. Reynolds M: Is the timing of fracture fixation important for the patient with multiple trauma? Ann Surg 222:470-481, 1995.

36. Janjua K, Sugrue M, Deane SA: Prospective evaluation of early missed injuries and the role of tertiary survey. J Trauma 44:1000-1007, 1998.

37. Rizoli SB, Boulanger BR, McClellan BA, Sharkey PW: Injuries missed during initial assessment of blunt trauma. Accid Anal Prev 26:681-686, 1994.

38. O'Malley K, Ross S: Pulmonary embolism in major trauma patients. J Trauma 30:748-750, 1990.

39. Montgomery K, Geerts W, Potter HG, et al: Practical management of venous thromboembolism following pelvic fractures. Orthop Clin North Am 28:397-404, 1997.

40. Velmahos G, Nigro J, Tatevossian R, et al: Inability of an aggressive policy of thromboprophylaxis to prevent deep venous thrombosis (DVT) in critically injured patients: Are current methods of DVT prophylaxis insufficient? J Am Coll Surg 187:529-533, 1998.

41. Geerts W, Jay R, Code KI, et al: A comparison of low-dose heparin with low-dose unfractionated heparin as prophylaxis against venous thromboembolism after major trauma. N Engl J Med 335:701-707, 1996.

42. Spain D, Bergamini T, Hoffmann JF, et al: Comparison of sequential compression devices and foot pumps for prophylaxis of deep venous thrombosis in high risk trauma patients. Am Surg 64:522-525, 1998.

43. Ganong RB: Fat emboli syndrome in isolated fractures of the tibia and femur. Clin Orthop 291:208-214, 1993.

44. Turen C, Dube M, LeCroy MC, et al: Approach to the polytraumatized patient with musculoskeletal injuries. J Am Acad Orthop Surg 7:154-165, 1999.

45. Benzer A, Offner D, Totsch M, et al: Early diagnosis of fat embolism syndrome by automated image analysis of alveolar macrophages. J Clin Monit 10:213-215, 1994.

46. Bernard G, Artigas A, Brigham KL, et al: The American-European Consensus Conference on ARDS: Definitions, mechanisms, relevant outcomes, and clinical trial coordination. Am J Resp Crit Care Med 149:818-824, 1994.

47. Pape H, Aufmkolk M, Paffrath T, et al: Primary intramedullary femur fixation in multiple trauma patients with associated lung contusion: A cause of posttraumatic ARDS? J Trauma 34:540-548, 1993.

48. Seibel R, LaDuca J, Hassett JM, et al: Blunt multiple trauma (ISS 36), femur traction, and the pulmonary-failure septic state. Ann Surg 202:283-295, 1985.

49. Johnson K, Cadambi A, Seibert GB, et al: Incidence of adult respiratory distress syndrome in patients with multiple musculoskeletal injuries: Effect of early operative stabilization of fractures. J Trauma 25:375-384, 1985.

50. Richards R: Fat embolism syndrome. Can J Surg 40:334-339, 1997.

CHAPTER 22

BURNS

Steven E. Wolf, M.D. and **David N. Herndon, M.D.**

General Considerations	Minimizing Complications
Burn Units	Nutrition
Pathophysiology of Burns	Outcomes
Initial Treatment of Burns	Electrical Burns
Inhalation Injury	Chemical Burns
Wound Care	Summary

GENERAL CONSIDERATIONS

More than 1.2 million people are burned in the United States every year; most cases are minor and treated in the outpatient setting. However, approximately 50,000 burns per year in the United States are moderate to severe and require hospitalization for appropriate treatment. Of these cases, more than 3900 people die of complications related to burns *(www.cdc.gov/ncicp/wisqars)*.[1] The societal significance of severe burns is supported by the finding that only motor vehicle collisions cause more trauma-related deaths. Burn deaths generally occur in a bimodal distribution, either immediately after the injury or weeks later as a result of multiorgan failure, a pattern similar to all trauma-related deaths. Two thirds of all burns occur at home and commonly involve young adult men, children younger than 15 years of age, and the elderly.[2] Seventy-five percent of all burn-related deaths occur in house fires. Young adults are frequently burned with flammable liquids, whereas toddlers are often scalded by hot liquids. A significant percentage of burns in children are due to child abuse. Other risk factors include low socioeconomic class and unsafe environments.[3] These generalizations emphasize that most of these injuries are preventable and therefore amenable to prevention strategies.

Morbidity and mortality rates associated with burns are decreasing. Recent reports reveal a 50% decline in burn-related deaths and hospital admissions in the United States over 20 years.[1] This rate of decline was similar in sample statistics for all burns above a reportable level of severity.[4] The declines were likely the result of prevention efforts resulting in decreased number of patients with potentially fatal burns, as well as improved clinical management of persons sustaining severe burns.

Prevention strategies have decreased the number and severity of injuries. Successful approaches included legislation mandating nonflammable children's sleepwear, changes in the National Electrical Code decreasing oral commissure burns, elevation of hot water heaters from the ground, and increased smoke alarm use.[5,6] In addition, mortality rate has improved for patients sustaining severe injuries. In 1949, Bull and Fisher from the Birmingham Burns Centre in the United Kingdom[7] first reported a 50% mortality rate for children 14 years old and younger with burns of 49% of the total body surface area (TBSA); 50% mortality was reached for those 15 to 44 years old with burns of 46% TBSA, those aged 45 to 64 years with burns of 27% TBSA, and those 65 years and older with burns of 10% TBSA. These dismal statistics have improved,[8] with the latest studies reporting a 50% mortality rate for 98% TBSA burns in children 14 years old and younger, and 75% TBSA burns in other young age groups.[9] Therefore, a healthy young patient with almost any size burn might be expected to live using modern treatment techniques. Advances in treatment are based on improved understanding of resuscitation, enhanced wound coverage, better support of the hypermetabolic response to injury, more appropriate infection control, and improved treatment of inhalation injuries. Further improvements can be made in these areas, and investigators are active in all these fields to discover means to further improve survival and outcomes.

BURN UNITS

Improvements in burn care originated in specialized units specifically dedicated to the care of burned patients. These units consist of experienced personnel with resources to maximize outcome from these devastating injuries (Box 22-1). Because of these specialized resources, burned patients are best treated in such places. Patients with the following criteria should be referred to a designated burn center[10]:

1. Partial thickness burns greater than 10% TBSA
2. Burns involving the face, hands, feet, genitalia, perineum, or major joints
3. Any full-thickness burn
4. Electrical burns, including lightning injury
5. Chemical burns
6. Inhalation injury
7. Burns in patients with preexisting medical disorders that could complicate management, prolong recovery, or affect outcome
8. Any patient with burns and concomitant trauma (such as fractures) in which the burn injury poses the greater immediate risk of morbidity and mortality. In such cases, if the trauma poses the greater immediate risk, the patient may be initially stabilized in a trauma center before being transferred to a burn unit. Physician judgment is necessary in such situations and should be in concert with the regional medical control plan and triage protocols.
9. Burned children in hospitals without qualified personnel or equipment to care for children
10. Burns in patients who will require special social, emotional, or long-term rehabilitative intervention.

PATHOPHYSIOLOGY OF BURNS

Local Changes

Burn causes coagulative necrosis of the epidermis and underlying tissues, with the depth depending on the temperature to which the skin is exposed and the duration of exposure. The specific heat of the causative agent also affects the depth. For example, the specific heat of fat is higher than that of water; thus, a grease burn is deeper than a scald burn from water with the same temperature and duration of exposure.

Burns are classified into five different causal categories and depths of injury (Box 22-2). The causes include injury from flame, hot liquids (scald), contact with hot or cold objects, chemical exposure, and conduction of electricity. The first three induce cellular damage primarily by the transfer of energy, inducing coagulative necrosis. Chemicals and electricity cause direct injury to cellular membranes in addition to the transfer of heat.

The skin provides a robust barrier to transfer of energy to deeper tissues; therefore, much of the injury is confined to this layer. However, after the inciting focus is removed, the response of local tissues can lead to injury in the deeper layers. The area of cutaneous injury has been divided into three zones: zone of coagulation, zone of stasis, and zone of hyperemia (Fig. 22-1). The necrotic area of burn where cells have been disrupted is termed the *zone of coagulation*. This tissue is irreversibly damaged at the time of injury. The area immediately surrounding the necrotic zone has a moderate degree of insult with decreased tissue perfusion. This is termed the *zone of stasis* and, depending on the wound environment, can either survive or go on to coagulative necrosis. The zone of stasis is associated with vascular damage and vessel leakage.[11] Thromboxane A_2, a potent vasoconstrictor, is present in high concentrations in burn wounds, and local application of inhibitors improves blood flow and decreases the zone of stasis. Antioxidants, bradykinin antagonists, and subatmospheric wound pressures also improve blood flow and affect the depth of injury.[12-14] Local endothelial interactions with neutrophils mediate some of the local inflammatory responses associated with the zone of stasis. Blocking leukocyte adherence with

---

Box 22-1. Burn Unit Organization and Personnel

Experienced burn surgeons (burn unit director and qualified surgeons)
Dedicated nursing personnel
Physical and occupational therapists
Social workers
Dietitians
Pharmacists
Respiratory therapists
Psychiatrists and clinical psychologists
Prosthetists

Box 22-2. Burn Classifications

Causes

Flame—damage from superheated, oxidized air
Scald—damage from contact with hot liquids
Contact—damage from contact with hot or cold solid materials
Chemicals—contact with noxious chemicals
Electricity—conduction of electrical current through tissues

Depths

First degree—injury localized to the epidermis
Superficial second degree—injury to the epidermis and superficial dermis
Deep second degree—injury through the epidermis and deep into the dermis
Third degree—full-thickness injury through the epidermis and dermis into the subcutaneous fat
Fourth degree—injury through the skin and subcutaneous fat into underlying muscle or bone

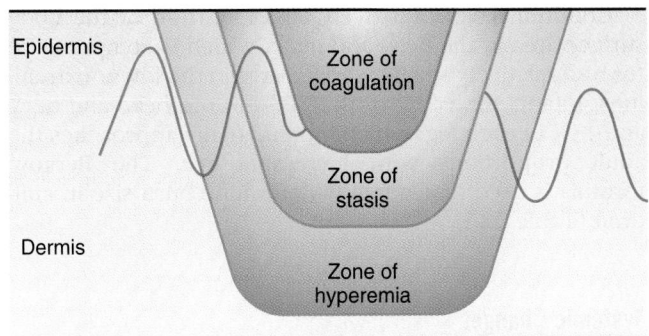

FIGURE 22-1.   Zones of injury after burn. The zone of coagulation is the portion irreversibly injured. The zones of stasis and hyperemia are defined in response to the injury.

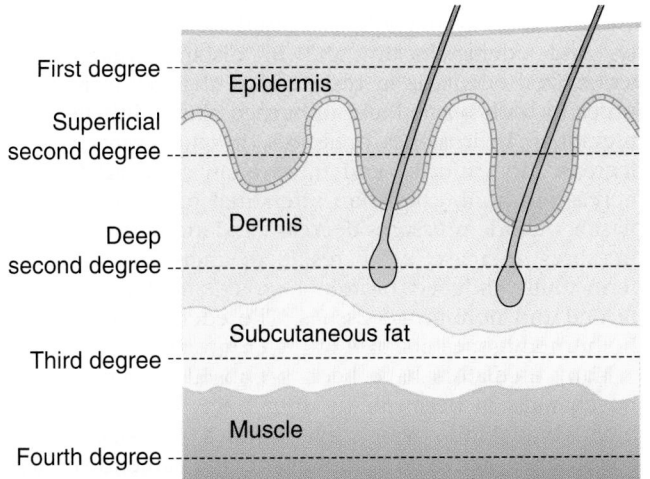

FIGURE 22-2.   Depths of burn. First-degree burns are confined to the epidermis. Second-degree burns are into the dermis (dermal burns). Third-degree burns are "full thickness" through the epidermis and dermis. Fourth-degree burns involve injury to underlying tissue structures such as muscle, tendons, and bone.

anti-CD18 or anti-intercellular adhesion molecules monoclonal antibodies improves tissue perfusion and tissue survival in animal models, indicating that treatment directed at the control of inflammation immediately after injury may spare the zone of stasis.[15] The last area is termed the *zone of hyperemia,* which is characterized by vasodilation from inflammation surrounding the burn wound. This region contains the clearly viable tissue from which the healing process begins and is generally not at risk for further necrosis.

Burn Depth

The depth of burn varies depending on the degree of tissue damage. Burn depth is classified into degree of injury in the epidermis, dermis, subcutaneous fat, and underlying structures (Fig. 22-2). First-degree burns are, by definition, injuries confined to the epidermis. These burns are painful, erythematous, and blanch to the touch with an intact epidermal barrier. Examples include sunburn or a minor scald from a kitchen accident. These

burns do not result in scarring, and treatment is aimed at comfort with the use of topical soothing salves with or without aloe and oral nonsteroidal anti-inflammatory agents.

Second-degree burns are divided into two types: superficial and deep. All second-degree burns have some degree of dermal damage, and the division is based on the depth of injury into this structure. Superficial dermal burns are erythematous, painful, blanch to touch, and often blister. Examples include scald injuries from overheated bathtub water and flash flame burns from open carburetors. These wounds spontaneously re-epithelialize from retained epidermal structures in the rete ridges, hair follicles, and sweat glands in 7 to 14 days. After healing, these burns may have some slight skin discoloration over the long term. Deep dermal burns into the reticular dermis appear more pale and mottled, do not blanch to touch, but remain painful to pinprick. These burns heal in 14 to 35 days by re-epithelialization from hair follicles and sweat gland keratinocytes, often with severe scarring as a result of the loss of dermis.

Third-degree burns are full thickness through the epidermis and dermis and are characterized by a hard, leathery eschar that is painless and black, white, or cherry red. No epidermal or dermal appendages remain; thus, these wounds must heal by re-epithelialization from the wound edges. Deep dermal and full-thickness burns require excision with skin grafting from the patient to heal the wounds in a timely fashion.

Fourth-degree burns involve other organs beneath the skin, such as muscle, bone, and brain.

Currently, burn depth is most accurately assessed by judgment of experienced practitioners. Accurate depth determination is critical because wounds that will heal with local treatment are treated differently than those requiring operative intervention. Examination of the entire wound by the physicians ultimately responsible for their management then is the gold standard used to guide further treatment decisions. New technologies, such as the multisensor heatable laser Doppler flowmeter, hold promise for quantitatively determining burn depth. Several recent reports claim superiority of this method over clinical judgment in the determination of wounds requiring skin grafting for timely healing (Fig. 22-3), which may lead to a change in the standard of care in the near future.[16-18]

Burn Size

Determination of burn size estimates the extent of injury. Burn size is generally assessed by the "rule of nines" (Fig. 22-4). In adults, each upper extremity and the head and neck are 9% of the TBSA, the lower extremities and the anterior and posterior trunk are 18% each, and the perineum and genitalia are assumed to be 1% of the TBSA. Another method of estimating smaller burns is to equate the area of the open hand (including the palm and the extended fingers) of the patient to be approximately 1% TBSA and then to transpose that measurement visually onto the wound for a determination of its size. This method is helpful when evaluating splash burns and other burns of mixed distribution.

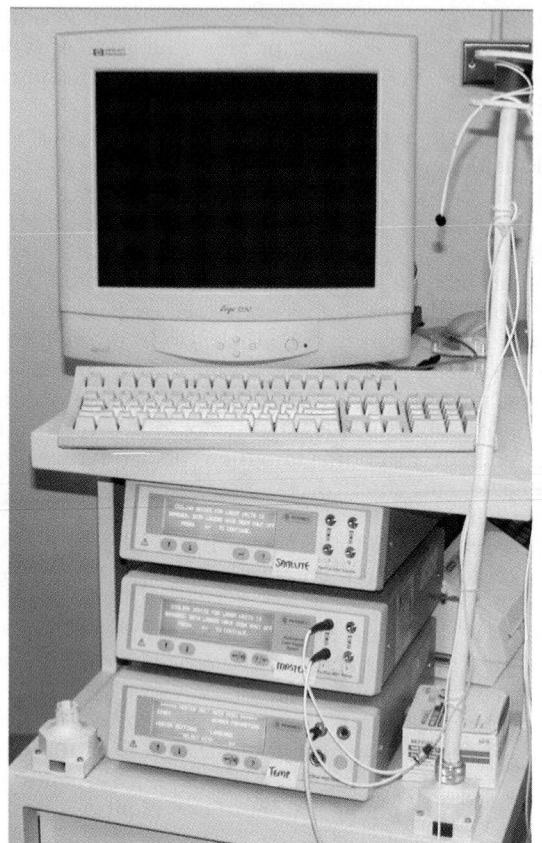

FIGURE 22-3. Laser Doppler flowmeter. The sensor is placed on the skin in question, which returns a value of perfusion units. A value of 0 is obviously necrotic, whereas values about 80 indicate viable skin that will heal.

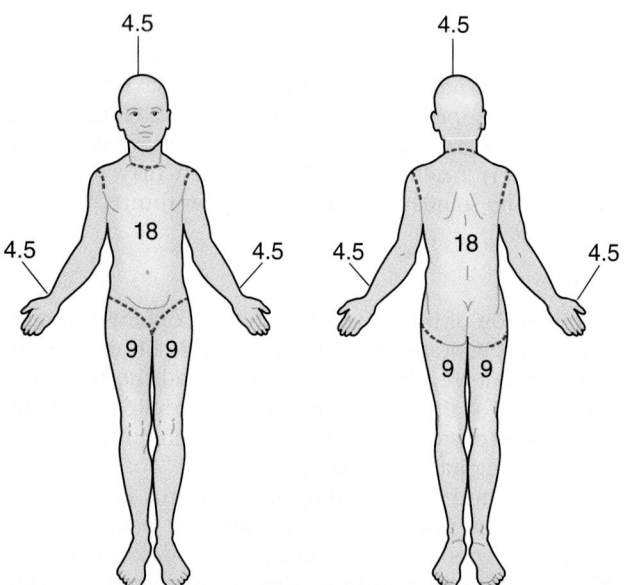

FIGURE 22-4. Body surface area diagram. This figure depicts the relative percentage of the total body surface area of defined anatomic areas.

Children have a relatively larger portion of the body surface area in the head and neck, which is compensated for by a relatively smaller surface area in the lower extremities. Infants have 21% of the TBSA in the head and neck and 13% in each leg, which incrementally approaches the adult proportions with increasing age. The Berkow formula is used to accurately determine burn size in children (Table 22-1).

Systemic Changes

Inflammation and Edema

Significant burns are associated with massive release of inflammatory mediators, both in the wound and in other tissues (Fig. 22-5). These mediators produce vasoconstriction and vasodilation, increased capillary permeability, and edema locally and in distant organs. The generalized edema is in response to changes in Starling forces in both burned and unburned skin.[19] Initially, the interstitial hydrostatic pressures in the burned skin decrease dramatically, and there is an associated slight increase in nonburned skin interstitial pressures. As the plasma oncotic pressures decrease and interstitial oncotic pressures increase as a result of increased capillary permeability-induced protein loss, edema forms in the burned and nonburned tissues. The edema is greater in the burned tissues because of lower interstitial pressures.

Many mediators have been proposed to account for the changes in permeability after burn, including histamine, bradykinin, vasoactive amines, prostaglandins, leukotrienes, activated complement, and catecholamines, among others. Mast cells in the burned skin release histamine in large quantities immediately after injury, which elicits a characteristic response in venules by increasing intercellular junction space formation. The use of antihistamines in the treatment of burn edema, however, has had limited success. In addition, aggregated platelets release serotonin to play a major role in edema formation. This agent acts directly to increase pulmonary vascular resistance, and it indirectly aggravates the vasoconstrictive effects of various vasoactive amines. Serotonin blockade improves cardiac index, decreases pulmonary artery pressure, and decreases oxygen consumption after burn.[20] When the antiserotonin methysergide was given to animals after scald injury, wound edema formation decreased as a result of local effects.[21] In addition, decreases in resuscitation fluid requirements are seen with high-dose vitamin C therapy immediately after burn, presumably because of its anti-inflammatory effects.[22]

Another mediator likely to play a role in changes in permeability and fluid shifts is thromboxane A_2. Thromboxane increases dramatically in the plasma and wounds of burned patients. This potent vasoconstrictor leads to vasoconstriction and platelet aggregation in the wound, contributing to expansion of the zone of stasis. It also caused prominent mesenteric vasoconstriction and decreased gut blood flow in animal models that compromised gut mucosal integrity and decreased gut immune function.[23]

TABLE 22-1. Berkow Diagram to Estimate Burn Size (%) Based on Area of Burn in an Isolated Body Part*

Body Part	0–1 yr	1–4 yr	5–9 yr	10–14 yr	15–18 yr	Adult
Head	19	17	13	11	9	7
Neck	2	2	2	2	2	2
Anterior trunk	13	13	13	13	13	13
Posterior trunk	13	13	13	13	13	13
Right buttock	2.5	2.5	2.5	2.5	2.5	2.5
Left buttock	2.5	2.5	2.5	2.5	2.5	2.5
Genitalia	1	1	1	1	1	1
Right upper arm	4	4	4	4	4	4
Left upper arm	4	4	4	4	4	4
Right lower arm	3	3	3	3	3	3
Left lower arm	3	3	3	3	3	3
Right hand	2.5	2.5	2.5	2.5	2.5	2.5
Left hand	2.5	2.5	2.5	2.5	2.5	2.5
Right thigh	5.5	6.5	8	8.5	9	9.5
Left thigh	5.5	6.5	8	8.5	9	9.5
Right leg	5	5	5.5	6	6.5	7
Left leg	5	5	5.5	6	6.5	7
Right foot	3.5	3.5	3.5	3.5	3.5	3.5
Left foot	3.5	3.5	3.5	3.5	3.5	3.5

*Estimates are made and recorded, then summed to gain an accurate estimate of the body surface area burned.

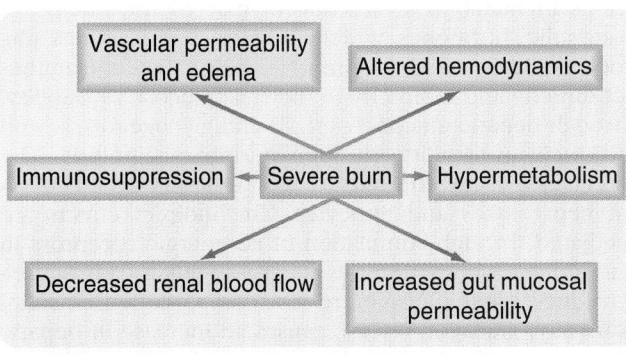

FIGURE 22-5. Systemic effects of severe burn.

Microvascular changes induce cardiopulmonary alterations characterized by loss of plasma volume, increased peripheral vascular resistance, and subsequent decreased cardiac output immediately after injury.[24] Cardiac output remains depressed from decreased blood volume and increased blood viscosity, as well as decreased cardiac contractility. Ventricular dysfunction in this period is attributed to a circulating myocardial depressant factor present in lymphatic fluid, although the specific factor has never been isolated.[25] Cardiac output is almost completely restored with resuscitation.[26]

Effects on the Renal System

Diminished blood volume and cardiac output result in decreased renal blood flow and glomerular filtration rate. Other stress-induced hormones and mediators such as angiotensin, aldosterone, and vasopressin further reduce renal blood flow immediately after the injury. These effects result in oliguria, which, if left untreated will cause acute tubular necrosis and renal failure. Before 1984, acute renal failure in burn injuries was almost always fatal; after 1984, however, newer techniques in dialysis became widely used to support the kidneys during recovery.[27] The latest reports indicate an 88% mortality rate for severely burned adults and a 56% mortality rate for severely burned children in whom renal failure develops in the postburn period.[28,29] Early resuscitation decreases renal failure and improves the associated mortality rate.[9]

Effects on the Gastrointestinal System

The gastrointestinal response to burn is highlighted by mucosal atrophy, changes in digestive absorption, and increased intestinal permeability.[30] Atrophy of the small bowel mucosa occurs within 12 hours of injury in proportion to the burn size and is related to increased epithelial cell death by apoptosis.[31] The cytoskeleton of the mucosal brush border undergoes atrophic changes associated with vesiculation of microvilli and disruption of the terminal web actin filaments. These findings were most pronounced 18 hours after injury, which suggests that changes in the cytoskeleton, such as those associated with cell death by apoptosis, are processes involved in the changed gut mucosa.[32] Burn also causes reduced uptake of glucose and amino acids, decreased absorption of fatty acids, and reduction in brush border lipase activity.[33] These changes peak in the first several hours after burn and return to normal at 48 to 72 hours after injury, a timing that parallels mucosal atrophy.

Intestinal permeability to macromolecules, which are normally repelled by an intact mucosal barrier, increases after burn.[34] Intestinal permeability to polyethylene glycol 3350, lactulose, and mannitol increases after injury, correlating to the extent of the burn.[35] Gut permeability increases even further when burn wounds become infected. A study using fluorescent dextrans showed that larger molecules appeared to cross the mucosa between the cells, whereas the smaller molecules traversed the mucosa through the epithelial cells, presumably by pinocytosis and vesiculation.[36] Mucosal permeability also paralleled increases in gut epithelial apoptosis.

Changes in gut blood flow are related to changes in permeability. Intestinal blood flow was shown to decrease in animals, a change that was associated with increased gut permeability at 5 hours after burn.[37] This effect was abolished at 24 hours. Systolic hypotension has been shown to occur in the hours immediately after burn in animals with a 40% TBSA full-thickness injury. These animals showed an inverse correlation between blood flow and permeability to intact *Candida*.[38]

Effects on the Immune System

Burns cause a global depression in immune function, which is shown by prolonged allograft skin survival on burn wounds. Burned patients are then at great risk for a number of infectious complications, including bacterial wound infection, pneumonia, and fungal and viral infections. These susceptibilities and conditions are based on depressed cellular function in all parts of the immune system, including activation and activity of neutrophils, macrophages, T lymphocytes, and B lymphocytes. With burns of more than 20% TBSA, impairment of these immune functions is proportional to burn size.

Macrophage production after burn is diminished, which is related to the spontaneous elaboration of negative regulators of myeloid growth. This effect is enhanced by the presence of endotoxin and can be partially reversed with granulocyte colony-stimulating factor (G-CSF) treatment or inhibition of prostaglandin E_2.[39] Investigators have shown that G-CSF levels actually increase after severe burn. However, bone marrow G-CSF receptor expression is decreased, which may in part account for the immunodeficiency seen in burns.[40] Total neutrophil counts are initially increased after burn, a phenomenon that is related to a decrease in cell death by apoptosis.[41] However, neutrophils that are present are dysfunctional in terms of diapedesis, chemotaxis, and phagocytosis. These effects are explained, in part, by a deficiency in CD11b/CD18

expression after inflammatory stimuli, decreased respiratory burst activity associated with a deficiency in p47-phox activity, and impaired actin mechanics related to neutrophil motile responses.[42,43] After 48 to 72 hours, neutrophil counts decrease somewhat like macrophages with similar causes.[40]

T-helper cell function is depressed after a severe burn that is associated with polarization from the interleukin-2 and interferon-γ cytokine-based T-helper 1 (T_H1) response toward the T_H2 response.[44] The T_H2 response is characterized by the production of interleukin-4 and interleukin-10. The T_H1 response is important in cell-mediated immune defense, whereas the T_H2 response is important in antibody responses to infection. As this polarization increases, so does the mortality rate.[45] Administration of interleukin-10 antibodies and growth hormone has partially reversed this response and improved mortality rate after burn in animals.[46,47] Burn also impairs cytotoxic T-lymphocyte activity as a function of burn size, thus increasing the risk of infection, particularly from fungi and viruses. Early burn wound excision improves cytotoxic T-cell activity.[48]

Hypermetabolism

After severe burn and resuscitation, *hypermetabolism* develops, which is characterized by tachycardia, increased cardiac output, elevated energy expenditure, increased oxygen consumption, proteolysis and lipolysis, and severe nitrogen losses. Even though this response is seen in all major injuries, it is present in its most dramatic form in severe burn, in which it may be sustained for months, leading to weight loss and decreased strength (particularly when strength is needed to recover from the complications associated with the injury). These alterations in metabolism are due in part to the release of "catabolic" hormones, which include catecholamines, glucocorticoids, and glucagons (Fig. 22-6). Catecholamines act directly and indirectly to increase glucose availability, through hepatic gluconeogenesis and glycogenolysis, and fatty acid availability, through peripheral lipolysis. The direct effects are through α- and β-adrenergic receptors on hepatocytes and lipocytes. The indirect effects are mediated through stimulation of adrenergic receptors in endocrine tissue within the pancreas, which causes a relative increase in glucagon release compared with insulin. Normally, glucagon release causes an increase in hepatic glucose production and peripheral lipolysis, whereas insulin has the opposite effects on decreasing hepatic glucose production and peripheral lipolysis. Catecholamine stimulation of β-adrenergic receptors within the pancreas increases the release of both glucagon and insulin, but concurrent stimulation of α-receptors has a greater inhibitory effect on insulin than on glucagon, resulting in a greater net release of glucagon compared with insulin. The effects of catecholamine-stimulated glucagon release then outweigh the effects of insulin on glucose and fatty acid production and release. Glucocorticoid hormones, released by way of the hypothalamic-pituitary-adrenal axis, are mediated through neural stimulation. Cortisol has similar actions on energy substrates, and it induces insulin resistance, which is additive

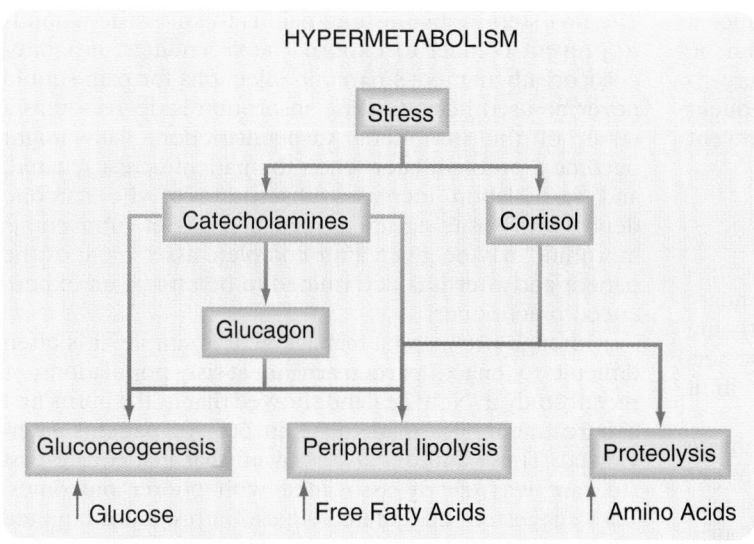

HYPERMETABOLISM

FIGURE 22-6. Results of hypermetabolism. A stress such as severe burn induces the release of inflammatory hormones, resulting in gluconeogenesis, lipolysis, and proteolysis.

to the hyperglycemia because of the release of liver glucose. Catecholamines, when combined with glucagon and cortisol, augment glucose release, which, initially, could be beneficial because glucose is the principal fuel of inflammatory cells as well as neural tissue.

Substrate supply for hepatic gluconeogenesis is produced through proteolysis and to some extent by peripheral lipolysis. Structural and constitutive proteins, degraded to amino acids, enter into (1) the tricarboxylic acid cycle for energy production, (2) the liver to be used as substrate for gluconeogenesis, or (3) the synthesis of acute-phase proteins. Most available body protein for this process is located in the musculature, thus depleting the muscle of its basic building blocks. Lactate and alanine are important intermediates that are released in proportion to the extent of injury. Glutamine is also released in massive quantities and can deplete muscle tissue stores to 50% of normal concentrations. After conversion to pyruvate or oxaloacetate, these amino acids form glucose with a net loss of adenosine triphosphate. Eighteen of the 20 amino acids are glucogenic and can be used for glucose synthesis. The increased acute-phase protein synthesis in the liver includes compounds such as C-reactive protein, fibrinogen, α_2-macroglobulin, and some complement factors.

Peripheral lipolysis, mediated through the catabolic hormones, is another principal component of the metabolic response to severe burn. Elevation of catecholamines, glucagon, and cortisol levels stimulates the same or similar intracellular hormone-sensitive lipases in the adipocyte to release free fatty acids. These are circulated to the liver where they are oxidized for energy, re-esterified to triglyceride, and deposited in the liver or further packaged for transport to other tissues by way of very low-density lipoproteins. Glycerol from fat breakdown enters the gluconeogenic pathway at the glyceraldehyde 3-phosphate level after phosphorylation. In injured patients, the rates of lipolysis are dramatic, and the processing of lipid by the liver can be compromised from the increasing amounts of circulating fat. Fatty liver development in this situation is thought to be secondary to the overload of normal processing enzymes or perhaps to a

downregulation of fatty acid handling mechanisms as a result of hormonal or cytokine manipulation associated with the injury.[49]

The classic description of the ebb and flow phases of response to illness and trauma deserve mention. The ebb phase is characterized by low metabolic rate, hypothermia, and low cardiac output. This is often temporally related to the onset of disease or time of injury. After resuscitation, this state gives way to the flow phase, which is characterized by high cardiac output and oxygen consumption, increased heat production, hyperglycemia, and an elevated metabolic rate. Moore has expanded these definitions to the *catabolic* and *anabolic* portions of the flow phase of recovery.[50] Duration of the catabolic flow phase is also dependent on the type of injury and the efficacy of therapeutic interventions. The frequency and severity of complications also have a bearing on the length of time of this phase of recovery, which in critically ill patients can last for weeks. The anabolic flow phase is characterized by a slow reaccumulation of protein and fat. This phase continues for months after injury.

INITIAL TREATMENT OF BURNS

Prehospital

Before undergoing any specific treatment, burned patients must be removed from the source of injury and the burning process stopped. Inhalation injury should always be suspected and 100% oxygen should be given by facemask. While removing the patient from the source of injury, care must be taken so that the rescuer does not become another victim. All caregivers should be aware that they might be injured by contact with the patient or the patient's clothing. Universal precautions including wearing gloves, gowns, mask, and protective eyewear should be used whenever there is likely contact with blood or body fluids. Burning clothing should be extinguished and removed as soon as possible to prevent further injury. All rings, watches, jewelry, and belts should be removed because they retain heat and can produce a tourniquet-like effect. Room temperature water can be poured on the wound within 15 minutes of injury to decrease the depth of the wound, but any subsequent measures to cool the wound should be avoided to prevent hypothermia during resuscitation.

Initial Assessment

As with any trauma patient, the initial assessment of a burned patient is divided into a primary and secondary survey. In the primary survey, immediate life-threatening conditions are quickly identified and treated. In the secondary survey, a more thorough head-to-toe evaluation of the patient is undertaken.

Exposure to heated gases and smoke results in damage to the upper respiratory tract. Direct injury to the upper airway results in edema, which, in combination with generalized whole-body edema associated with severe burn, may obstruct the airway. Airway injury must be suspected with facial burns, singed nasal hairs, carbonaceous sputum, and tachypnea. Upper airway obstruction may develop rapidly, and respiratory status must be continually monitored to assess the need for airway control and ventilatory support. Progressive hoarseness is a sign of impending airway obstruction, and endotracheal intubation should be instituted early before edema distorts the upper airway anatomy. This is especially important in patients with massive burns, who may appear to breathe without problems early in the resuscitation period until several liters of volume are given to maintain homeostasis, resulting in significant airway edema.

The chest should be exposed to assess breathing; airway patency alone does not ensure adequate ventilation. Chest expansion and equal breath sounds with CO_2 return from the endotracheal tube ensure adequate air exchange.

Blood pressure may be difficult to obtain in burned patients with edematous or charred extremities. Pulse rate can be used as an indirect measure of circulation; however, most burned patients remain tachycardic even with adequate resuscitation. For the primary survey of burned patients, the presence of pulses or Doppler signals in the distal extremities may be adequate to determine adequate circulation of blood until better monitors, such as arterial pressure measurements and urine output, can be established.

In those patients who have been in an explosion or deceleration accident, a possibility exists for spinal cord injury. Appropriate cervical spine stabilization must be accomplished by whatever means necessary, including using cervical collars to keep the head immobilized until the condition can be evaluated.

Wound Care

Prehospital care of the burn wound is basic and simple because it requires only protection from the environment with application of a clean dry dressing or sheet to cover the involved part. Damp dressings should not be used. The patient should be wrapped in a blanket to minimize heat loss and for temperature control during transport.

The first step in diminishing pain is to cover the wounds to prevent contact to exposed nerve endings. Intramuscular or subcutaneous narcotic injections for pain should never be used because drug absorption is decreased as a result of the peripheral vasoconstriction. This might become a problem later when the patient is resuscitated, and vasodilation increases absorption of the narcotic depot with resulting apnea. Small doses of intravenous morphine may be given after complete assessment of the patient and after it is determined to be safe by an experienced practitioner.

Although prehospital management is simple, it is often difficult to enact, particularly in at-risk populations. A recent study in New Zealand showed that initial burns first aid treatment was inadequate in 60% of patients interviewed. These authors also showed that inadequate first aid care was clearly associated with poorer outcomes. They suggested that defined education programs targeted on at-risk populations might improve these outcomes.[51]

Transport

Rapid, uncontrolled transport of the burn victim is not a priority, except when other life-threatening conditions coexist. In most incidents involving major burns, ground transportation of victims to the receiving hospital is appropriate. Helicopter transport is of greatest use when the distance between the accident and the hospital is 30 to 150 miles. For distances of more than 150 miles, transport by fixed-wing aircraft is most appropriate. Whatever the mode of transport, it should be of appropriate size and have emergency equipment available, with trained personnel on board, such as nurses, physicians, paramedics, or respiratory therapists who are familiar with multiply injured trauma patients.

Resuscitation

Adequate resuscitation of the burned patient depends on the establishment and maintenance of reliable intravenous access. Increased times to beginning resuscitation of burned patients result in poorer outcomes, and delays should be minimized. Venous access is best attained through short peripheral catheters in unburned skin; however, veins in burned skin can be used and are preferable to no intravenous access. Superficial veins are often thrombosed in full-thickness injuries and, therefore, are not suitable for cannulation. Saphenous vein cutdowns are useful in cases of difficult access and are used in preference to central vein cannulation because of lower complication rates. In children younger than 6 years of age, experienced practitioners can use intramedullary access in the proximal tibia until intravenous access is accomplished. Lactated Ringer's solution without dextrose is the fluid of choice except in children younger than 2 years, who should receive 5% dextrose Ringer's lactate. The initial rate can be rapidly estimated by multiplying the TBSA burned by the patient's weight in kilograms and then dividing by 8. Thus the rate of infusion for an 80-kg man with a 40% TBSA burn would be

$$80 \text{ kg} \times 40\% \text{ TBSA}/8 = 400 \text{ mL/hour}$$

This rate should be continued until a formal calculation of resuscitation needs is performed.

Many formulas have been devised to determine the proper amount of fluid to give a burned patient, all originating from experimental studies on the pathophysiology of burn shock. Baxter[52] and others established the basis for modern fluid resuscitation protocols. They showed that edema fluid in burn wounds is isotonic and contains the same amount of protein as plasma and that the greatest loss of fluid is into the interstitium. They used various volumes of intravascular fluid to determine the optimal amount in terms of cardiac output and extracellular volume in a canine burn model, and this was applied to the clinical realm in the Parkland formula. Plasma volume changes were not related to the type of resuscitation fluid in the first 24 hours, but thereafter colloid solutions could increase plasma volume by the amount infused. From these findings, they concluded that colloid solutions should not be used in the first 24 hours until capillary permeability returned closer to normal. Others have argued that normal capillary permeability is restored somewhat earlier after burn (6 to 8 hours), and therefore colloids could be used earlier.[53]

Concurrently, Pruitt and associates[24] showed the hemodynamic effects of fluid resuscitation in burns, which culminated in the Brooke formula. They found that fluid resuscitation caused an obligatory 20% decrease in both extracellular fluid and plasma volume that concluded after 24 hours. In the second 24 hours, plasma volume returned to normal with the administration of colloid. Cardiac output was low in the first day despite resuscitation, but it subsequently increased to supernormal levels as the flow phase of hypermetabolism was established. Since these studies, it has been found that much of the fluid needs are due to "leaky" capillaries that permit passage of large molecules into the interstitial space to increase extravascular colloid osmotic pressure. Intravascular volume follows the gradient to tissues, both into the burn wound and the nonburned tissues. Approximately 50% of fluid resuscitation needs are sequestered in nonburned tissues in 50% TBSA burns.[54]

Hypertonic saline solutions have theoretical advantages in burn resuscitation. These solutions decrease net fluid intake, decrease edema, and increase lymph flow, probably by the transfer of volume from the intracellular space to the interstitium. When using these solutions, hyperna-

tremia must be avoided, and it is recommended that serum sodium concentrations should not exceed 160 mEq/dL. However, it must be noted that for patients with more than 20% TBSA burns who were randomized to either hypertonic saline or lactated Ringer's solution, resuscitation did not have significant differences in volume requirements or changes in percentage of weight gain.[55] Other investigators found an increase in renal failure with hypertonic solutions that has tempered further efforts in this area of investigation.[56] Some burn units successfully use a modified hypertonic solution of 1 ampule of sodium bicarbonate (50 mEq) in 1 L of lactated Ringer's solution. Further research should be done to determine the optimal formula to reduce edema formation and to maintain adequate cellular function.

Most burn units use something akin to either the Parkland or Brooke formula, which calls for administering varying amounts of crystalloid and colloid for the first 24 hours (Table 22-2). The fluids are generally changed in the second 24 hours with an increase in colloid use. These are guidelines to direct resuscitation of the amount of fluid necessary to maintain adequate perfusion. In fact, recent studies have shown that the Parkland formula often underestimates the volume of crystalloid received in the first 24 hours after severe burn,[57] indicating that monitoring of the resuscitation is crucial to insure acceptable outcome. This is easily monitored in burned patients with normal renal function by following the volume of urine output, which should be at 0.5 mL/hour in adults and 1.0 mL/kg per hour in children. Changes in intravenous fluid infusion rates should be made on an hourly basis determined by the response of the patient to the particular fluid volume administered.

For burned children, formulas are commonly used that are modified to account for changes in surface area-to-mass ratios. These changes are necessary because a child with a comparable burn to that of an adult requires more resuscitation fluid per kilogram. The Galveston formula uses 5000 mL/TBSA burned (in m^2) + 1500 mL/m^2 total for maintenance in the first 24 hours. This formula accounts for both maintenance needs and the increased fluid requirements of a child with a burn. All of the formulas listed in Table 22-2 calculate the amount of volume given in the first 24 hours, one half of which is given in the first 8 hours.

Recently, the use of albumin during intravenous resuscitation has come under criticism. The Cochrane group showed in a meta-analysis of 31 trials that the risk of death

TABLE 22-2. Resuscitation Formulas

Formula	Crystalloid Volume	Colloid Volume	Free Water
Parkland	4 mL/kg per % TBSA burn	None	None
Brooke	1.5 mL/kg per % TBSA burn	0.5 mL/kg per % TBSA burn	2.0 L
Galveston (pediatric)	5000 mL/m^2 burned + 1500 mL/m^2 total	None	None

These are used as guidelines for the initial fluid management after burn. The response to fluid resuscitation should be continuously monitored, and adjustments in the rate of fluid administration should be made accordingly.
TBSA, total body surface area.

was higher in burned patients receiving albumin compared to those receiving crystalloid, with a relative risk of death at 2.40 (95% confidence interval, 1.11 to 5.19).[58] Another meta-analysis of all critically ill patients refuted this finding, showing no differences in relative risk between albumin-treated and crystalloid-treated groups.[59] In fact, as quality of the trials improved, the relative risks were reduced. Additional recent evidence suggests that albumin supplementation even after resuscitation does not affect the distribution of fluid among the intracellular/extracellular compartments.[60] What we can conclude from these trials and meta-analyses is that albumin used during resuscitation is at best equal to crystalloid and at worst detrimental to the outcome of burned patients. For these reasons, we cannot recommend the use of albumin during resuscitation.

To combat any regurgitation with an intestinal ileus, a nasogastric tube should be inserted in all patients with major burns to decompress the stomach. This is especially important for all patients being transported in aircraft at high altitudes. Additionally, all patients should be restricted from taking anything by mouth until the transfer has been completed. Decompression of the stomach is usually necessary because the apprehensive patient will swallow considerable amounts of air and distend the stomach.

Recommendations for tetanus prophylaxis are based on the condition of the wound and the patient's immunization history. All patients with burns of greater than 10% TBSA should receive 0.5 mL of tetanus toxoid. If prior immunization is absent or unclear, or the last booster dose was more than 10 years ago, 250 units of tetanus immunoglobulin is also given.

Escharotomies

When deep second- and third-degree burn wounds encompass the circumference of an extremity, peripheral circulation to the limb can be compromised. Development of generalized edema beneath a nonyielding eschar impedes venous outflow and eventually affects arterial inflow to the distal beds. This can be recognized by numbness and tingling in the limb and increased pain in the digits. Arterial flow can be assessed by determination of Doppler signals in the digital arteries and the palmar and plantar arches in affected extremities. Capillary refill can also be assessed. Extremities at risk are identified either on clinical examination or on measurement of tissue pressures greater than 40 mm Hg. These extremities require escharotomies, which are releases of the burn eschar performed at the bedside by incising the lateral and medial aspects of the extremity with a scalpel or electrocautery unit. The entire constricting eschar must be incised longitudinally to completely relieve the impediment to blood flow. The incisions are carried down onto the thenar and hypothenar eminences and along the dorsolateral sides of the digits to completely open the hand, if it is involved (Fig. 22-7). If it is clear that the wound will require excision and grafting because of its depth, escharotomies are safest to restore perfusion to the underlying nonburned tissues until formal excision. If vascular compromise has

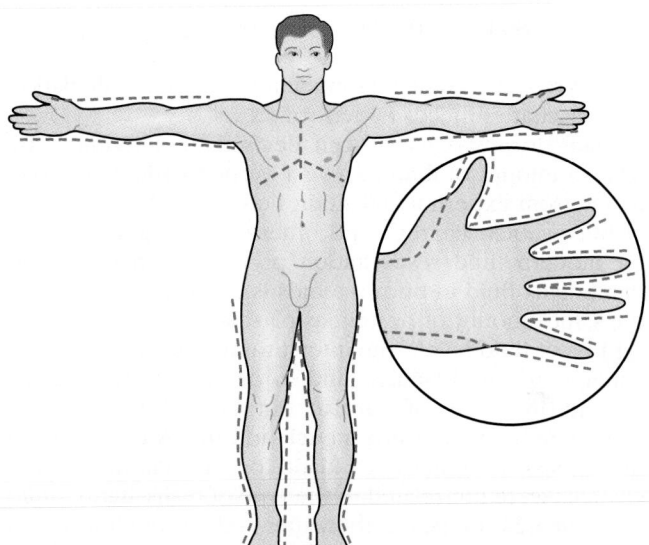

FIGURE 22-7.   Recommended escharotomies. In limbs requiring escharotomies, the incisions are made on the medial and lateral sides of the extremity through the eschar. In the case of the hand, incisions are made on the medial and lateral digits and on the dorsum of the hand.

been prolonged, reperfusion after an escharotomy may cause reactive hyperemia and further edema formation in the muscle, making continued surveillance of the distal extremities necessary. Increased muscle compartment pressures may necessitate fasciotomies. The most common complications associated with these procedures are blood loss and the release of anaerobic metabolites, causing transient hypotension. If distal perfusion does not improve with these measures, central hypotension from hypovolemia should be suspected and treated.

A constricting truncal eschar can cause a similar phenomenon, except the effect is to decrease ventilation by limiting chest excursion. Any decrease in ventilation of a burned patient should produce inspection of the chest with appropriate escharotomies to relieve the constriction and allow adequate tidal volumes. This need becomes evident in a patient on a volume-control ventilator whose peak airway pressures increase.

INHALATION INJURY

One major factor contributing to death in burn injury patients is the presence of inhalation injury. Smoke damage adds another inflammatory focus to the burn and impedes normal gas exchange vital for critically injured patients. Inhalation injury increases the amount of time spent on mechanical ventilation, which is a predictor of mortality.[9] Early diagnosis and prevention of complications are necessary to decrease morbidity and mortality rates related to this condition.

With inhalation injury, damage is caused primarily by inhaled toxins. Heat is dispersed in the upper airways, whereas the cooled particles of smoke and toxins are carried distally into the bronchi. Thus, the injury to the airways is principally chemical in nature. Direct thermal damage to the lung is seldom seen because of dispersal of

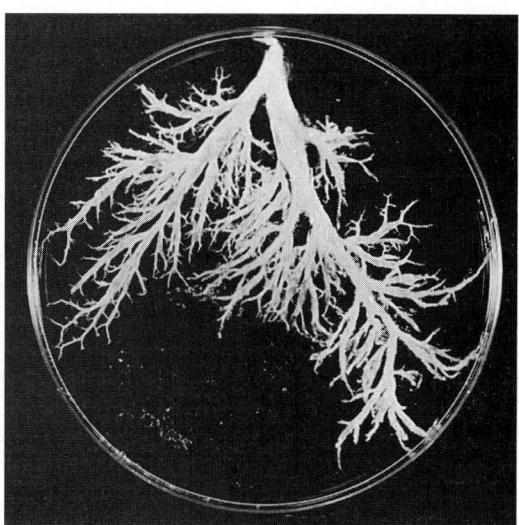

FIGURE 22-8. Bronchial cast found at autopsy from a patient with inhalation injury.

the heat in the pharynx. The exception is high-pressure steam inhalation, which has 4000 times the heat-carrying capacity of dry air.

The response to smoke inhalation is an immediate dramatic increase in blood flow in the bronchial arteries to the bronchi with edema formation and increases in lung lymph flow. The lung lymph in this situation is similar to serum, indicating that permeability at the capillary level is markedly increased. The edema that results is associated with an increase in lung neutrophils, and it is postulated that these cells may be the primary mediators of pulmonary damage with this injury. Neutrophils release proteases and oxygen free radicals that can produce conjugated dienes by lipid peroxidation. High concentrations are present in the lung lymph and pulmonary tissues after inhalation injury, suggesting the increased concentration of neutrophils is active in producing cytotoxic materials. When neutrophils are depleted before injury by nitrogen mustard, increases in lung lymph flow and conjugated diene levels are markedly reduced.[61]

Another hallmark of inhalation injury is separation of the ciliated epithelial cells from the basement membrane followed by exudate formation within the airways. The exudate consists of proteins found in the lung lymph and eventually it coalesces to form fibrin casts (Fig. 22-8). Clinically, these fibrin casts can be difficult to clear with standard airway suction techniques, requiring bronchoscopic removal. These casts also add barotrauma to localized areas of lung by forming a "ball-valve." During inspiration, the airway diameter increases, and air flows past the cast into the distal airways. During expiration, the airway diameter decreases, and the cast effectively occludes the airway, preventing the inhaled air from escaping. Increasing volume leads to localized increases in pressure that are associated with numerous complications, including pneumothorax and decreased lung compliance.

Smoke inhalation injury is often seen with a clinical history of closed space smoke exposure, hoarseness, wheezing, and carbonaceous sputum. It may also be associated with facial burns and singed nasal hairs. Each of

these findings has poor sensitivity and specificity; therefore, the definitive diagnosis must be established by the use of bronchoscopy or less commonly by [133]xenon ventilation scanning. Bronchoscopy can reveal early inflammatory changes such as erythema, ulceration, and prominent vasculature in addition to infraglottic soot. The findings of airway erythema and ulceration alone are also nonspecific, and these findings must be placed with the entire clinical presentation to verify significant inhalation injury. Ventilation scanning with [133]xenon reveals areas of the lung retaining isotope 90 seconds after intravenous injection, indicating segmental airway obstruction resulting from inhalation injury. Many of these patients require mechanical ventilation to maintain gas exchange, and repeated bronchoscopy may reveal continued ulceration of the airways with granulation tissue formation, exudate formation, inspissation of secretions, and focal edema. Eventually, the airway heals by replacement of the sloughed cuboidal ciliated epithelium with squamous cells and scar.

The clinical course of patients with inhalation injury is divided into three stages. The first is acute pulmonary insufficiency. Patients with severe lung injuries may begin to show signs of pulmonary failure from the time of injury with asphyxia, carbon monoxide poisoning, bronchospasm, and upper airway obstruction. Clinical signs of parenchymal damage with hypoxia are not common during this phase. The second stage occurs from 72 to 96 hours after injury and is associated with hypoxia and development of diffuse lobar infiltrates. This condition is similar clinically to the adult respiratory distress syndrome (ARDS) that occurs in nonburned injured and critically ill patients. In the third stage, clinical bronchopneumonia dominates. These infections generally occur 3 to 10 days after inhalation injury and are associated with the expectoration of large mucous casts formed in the tracheobronchial tree. The differentiation of pneumonia from tracheobronchitis is difficult at this stage, and bronchoscopy with lavage may be of assistance. Early pneumonias are usually caused by penicillin-resistant *Staphylococcus* species, whereas after 5 to 7 days, the changing flora of the burn wound is reflected in the appearance in the lung of gram-negative species, especially *Pseudomonas*. Ball-valve effects and ventilator-associated barotrauma are also hallmarks of this period.

Management of inhalation injury is directed at maintaining open airways and maximizing gas exchange while the lung heals. A coughing patient with a patent airway can clear secretions effectively, and efforts should be made to manage patients without mechanical ventilation if possible. If respiratory failure is imminent, intubation should be instituted, with frequent chest physiotherapy and suctioning performed to maintain pulmonary toilet (Table 22-3). Frequent bronchoscopy may be needed to clear inspissated secretions. Mechanical ventilation should be used to provide gas exchange with as little barotrauma as possible. "Permissive hypercapnia" and the current ARDS Network ventilation protocols can be used with lower ventilatory rates and volumes to maintain the arterial pH greater than 7.25, thus minimizing positive airway pressures delivered by the ventilator.[62] Arterial oxygen

TABLE 22-3.   Clinical Indications for Intubation

Criteria	Value
PaO_2 (mm Hg)	<60
$PaCO_2$ (mm Hg)	>50 (acutely)
PaO_2/FiO_2 ratio	<200
Respiratory/ventilatory failure	Impending
Upper airway edema	Severe

TABLE 22-4.   Inhalation Treatments for Smoke Inhalation Injury

Treatment	Time/Dosage
Bronchodilators (Albuterol)	q 2 hr
Nebulized heparin	5000 to 10,000 units with 3 mL normal saline q 4 hr
Nebulized acetylcysteine	20%, 3 mL q 4 hr
Hypertonic saline	Induce effective coughing
Racemic epinephrine	Reduce mucosal edema

tensions of greater than 60 (or an oxygen saturation of 92%) are also tolerated to minimize oxygen toxicity to the lungs. When the clinical condition improves to the point that the patient can be weaned from ventilatory support, oxygen concentration, positive end-expiratory pressure, and ventilator volumes and rate should be decreased in a graduated manner until the patient can be extubated. This may take several weeks.

Inhalation treatments have been effective in improving the clearance of tracheobronchial secretions and decreasing bronchospasm (Table 22-4). Intravenous heparin has been shown to reduce tracheobronchial cast formation, minute ventilation, and peak inspiratory pressures after smoke inhalation.[63] When heparin was administered directly to the lungs in a nebulized form, it had similar effects on casts without causing systemic coagulopathy. When N-acetylcysteine treatments are added to nebulized heparin in burned children with inhalation injury, reintubation rates and mortality rates are decreased.[64] In addition to the measures already discussed, adequate humidification and treatment of bronchospasm with β-agonists are indicated. Steroids have not been shown to be of benefit in inhalation injury and should not be given unless the patient is steroid dependent before injury or if the patient has bronchospasm resistant to standard therapy.

In addition to conventional ventilator methods, novel ventilator therapies have been devised to minimize barotrauma, including high-frequency percussive ventilation. This method combines standard tidal volumes and respirations (ventilator rates 6 to 20/minute) with smaller high-frequency respirations (200 to 500/minute) and permits adequate ventilation and oxygenation in patients who failed conventional ventilation. One reason for the greater utility of this method is that it recruits alveoli at lower airway pressures.[65] This ventilator method may also have a percussive effect that loosens inspissated secretions and improves pulmonary toilet. Prospective, randomized trials comparing this method to conventional therapies are underway, the first of which has shown improved oxygenation in the first 3 days after inhalation injury. Liquid ventilation using perfluorocarbons and use of inhaled nitric oxide as a selective pulmonary vasodilator are also being studied as adjuncts to current methods. Recent animal studies with perfluorocarbons, however, have had disappointing results, leading to decreased enthusiasm for this treatment.[66]

Several clinical studies have shown that pulmonary edema is not prevented by fluid restriction. Indeed, fluid resuscitation appropriate for the patient's other needs results in a decrease in lung water, has no adverse effect on pulmonary histology, and improves survival rate. Although overhydration could increase pulmonary edema, inadequate hydration increases the severity of pulmonary injury by sequestration of polymorphonuclear cells, leading to increased risk of death. In both animal and clinical studies, resuscitation was adequate if normal cardiac index or urine output was maintained.

Prophylactic antibiotics for inhalation injury are not indicated but are clearly needed for documented lung infections. Empirical choices for treatment of pneumonia before culture results are returned should include coverage of methicillin-resistant *Staphylococcus aureus* and gram-negative organisms (especially *Pseudomonas*). Systemic antibiotic regimens are based on serially monitored sputum cultures, bronchial washings, or transtracheal aspirates.

As patients recover from lung injury, they should be extubated as soon as possible. Patients are able to clear their own airways through coughing more effectively than suction through an endotracheal tube; therefore, those patients without the need for ventilatory support should be extubated. This is preferably done as soon as upper airway edema has resolved (injury days 1 to 2) in those who were intubated to control the airway or for burn excision. It is our experience that patients who are extubated with the same degree of inhalation injury do better than those who are intubated. Standard extubation criteria can be used, although many patients who do not meet these criteria may also do well without mechanical ventilation. If the airway is easily accessible, a trial of extubation might be of benefit in patients with borderline weaning parameters.

WOUND CARE

After the airway is assessed and resuscitation is underway, attention must be turned to the burn wound. Treatment depends on the characteristics and size of the wound. All treatments are aimed at rapid and painless healing. Current therapy directed specifically toward burn wounds can be divided into three stages: assessment, management, and rehabilitation. Once the extent and depth of the wounds have been assessed and the wounds have been thoroughly cleaned and débrided, the management phase begins. Each wound should be dressed with an appropriate covering that serves several functions. First, it should protect the damaged epithelium, minimize bacterial and fungal colonization, and provide splinting action to maintain the desired position of function. Second, the dressing should be occlusive to reduce evaporative heat loss and minimize cold stress. Third, the dressing should provide comfort over the painful wound.

The choice of dressing is based on the characteristics of the treated wound (Table 22-5). First-degree wounds are minor with minimal loss of barrier function. These wounds require no dressing and are treated with topical salves to decrease pain and keep the skin moist. Systemic nonsteroidal anti-inflammatory agents given by mouth assist in pain control. Second-degree wounds can be treated with daily dressing changes with topical antibiotics, cotton gauze, and elastic wraps. Alternatively, the wounds can be treated with a temporary biological or synthetic covering to close the wound. Deep second-degree and third-degree wounds require excision and grafting for sizable burns, and the choice of initial dressing should be aimed at holding bacterial proliferation in check and providing occlusion until the operation is performed.

Antimicrobials

The timely and effective use of antimicrobials have revolutionized burn care by decreasing invasive wound infections. The untreated burn wound rapidly becomes colonized with bacteria and fungi because of the loss of normal skin barrier mechanisms. As the organisms proliferate to high wound counts ($>10^5$ organisms per gram of tissue), they may penetrate into viable tissue. Organisms then invade blood vessels, causing a systemic infection that often leads to the death of the patient. This scenario has become uncommon in most burn units because of the effective use of antibiotics and wound care techniques. The antimicrobials that are used can be divided into those given topically and those given systemically.

Available topical antibiotics can be divided into two classes: salves and soaks. Salves are generally applied directly to the wound with cotton dressings placed over them, and soaks are generally poured into cotton dressings on the wound. Each of these classes of antimicrobials has advantages and disadvantages. Salves may be applied once or twice a day but may lose their effectiveness between dressing changes. Frequent dressing changes can result in shearing with loss of grafts or underlying healing cells. Soaks remain effective because antibiotic solution

TABLE 22-5. Burn Wound Dressing Descriptions

Burn Wound Dressings	Advantages and Disadvantages
ANTIMICROBIAL SALVES	
Silver sulfadiazine (Silvadene)	Broad-spectrum antimicrobial; painless and easy to use; does not penetrate eschar; may leave black tattoos from silver ion; mild inhibition of epithelialization
Mafenide acetate (Sulfamylon)	Broad-spectrum antimicrobial; penetrates eschar; may cause pain in sensate skin; wide application may cause metabolic acidosis; mild inhibition of epithelialization
Bacitracin	Ease of application; painless; antimicrobial spectrum not as wide as the above agents
Neomycin	Ease of application; painless; antimicrobial spectrum not as wide
Polymyxin B	Ease of application; painless; antimicrobial spectrum not as wide
Nystatin (Mycostatin)	Effective in inhibiting most fungal growth; cannot be used in combination with mafenide acetate
Mupirocin (Bactroban)	More effective staphylococcal coverage; does not inhibit epithelialization; expensive
ANTIMICROBIAL SOAKS	
0.5% Silver nitrate	Effective against all microorganisms; stains contacted areas; leaches sodium from wounds; may cause methemoglobinemia
5% Mafenide acetate	Wide antibacterial coverage; no fungal coverage; painful on application to sensate wound; wide application associated with metabolic acidosis
0.025% Sodium hypochlorite (Dakin's solution)	Effective against almost all microbes, particularly gram-positive organisms; mildly inhibits epithelialization
0.25% Acetic acid	Effective against most organisms, particularly gram negative; mildly inhibits epithelialization
SYNTHETIC COVERINGS	
OpSite	Provides a moisture barrier; inexpensive; decreased wound pain; use complicated by accumulation of transudate and exudate requiring removal; no antimicrobial properties
Biobrane	Provides a wound barrier; associated with decreased pain; use complicated by accumulation of exudate risking invasive wound infection; no antimicrobial properties
Transcyte	Provides a wound barrier; decreased pain; accelerated wound healing; use complicated by accumulation of exudate; no antimicrobial properties
Integra	Provides complete wound closure and leaves a dermal equivalent; sporadic take rates; no antimicrobial properties
BIOLOGICAL COVERINGS	
Xenograft (pig skin)	Completely closes the wound; provides some immunologic benefits; must be removed or allowed to slough
Allograft (homograft, cadaver skin)	Provides all the normal functions of skin; can leave a dermal equivalent; epithelium must be removed or allowed to slough

can be added without removing the dressing; however, the underlying skin can become macerated.

Topical antibiotic salves include 11% mafenide acetate (Sulfamyalon), 1% silver sulfadiazine (Silvadene), polymyxin B, neomycin, bacitracin, mupirocin, and the antifungal agent nystatin. No single agent is completely effective, and each has advantages and disadvantages. Silver sulfadiazine is the most commonly used. It has a broad spectrum of activity because its silver and sulfa moieties cover gram-positive, most gram-negative, and some fungal forms. Some *Pseudomonas* species possess plasmid-mediated resistance. Silver sulfadiazine is relatively painless on application, has a high patient acceptance, and is easy to use. Occasionally, patients complain of a burning sensation after it is applied, and, in a few patients, a transient leukopenia develops 3 to 5 days following its continued use. This leukopenia is generally harmless and resolves with or without treatment cessation.

Mafenide acetate is another topical agent with a broad spectrum of activity owing to its sulfa moiety. It is particularly useful against resistant *Pseudomonas* and *Enterococcus* species. It also can penetrate eschar, which silver sulfadiazine cannot. Disadvantages include painful application on skin, such as in second-degree wounds. It also can cause an allergic skin rash, and it has carbonic anhydrase inhibitory characteristics that can result in a metabolic acidosis when applied over large surfaces. For these reasons, mafenide sulfate is typically reserved for small full-thickness injuries.

Petroleum-based antimicrobial ointments with polymyxin B, neomycin, and bacitracin are clear on application, painless, and allow for easy wound observation. These agents are commonly used for treatment of facial burns, graft sites, healing donor sites, and small partial-thickness burns. Mupirocin is a relatively new petroleum-based ointment that has improved activity against gram-positive bacteria, particularly methicillin-resistant *S. aureus* and selected gram-negative bacteria. Nystatin either in a salve or powder form can be applied to wounds to control fungal growth. Nystatin-containing ointments can be combined with other topical agents to decrease colonization of both bacteria and fungus. The exception is the combination of nystatin and mafenide acetate; each inactivates the other.

Available agents for application as a soak include 0.5% silver nitrate solution, 0.025% sodium hypochlorite (Dakin's), 0.25% acetic acid, and mafenide acetate as a 5% solution. Silver nitrate has the advantage of being painless on application and having complete antimicrobial effectiveness. The disadvantages include its staining of surfaces to a dull gray or black when the solution dries. This can become problematic in deciphering wound depth during burn excisions and in keeping the patient and his or her surroundings clean of the black staining. The solution is hypotonic as well, and continuous use can cause electrolyte leaching, with rare methemoglobinemia as another complication. A new commercial dressing containing biologically potent silver ions (Acticoat) that are activated in the presence of moisture is available. This dressing holds the promise to retain the effectiveness of silver nitrate without the problems of silver nitrate soaks.

Dakin's solution (0.25% sodium hypochlorite) has effectiveness against most microbes; however, it also has cytotoxic effects on the healing cells of patients' wounds. Low concentrations of sodium hypochlorite (0.025%) have less cytotoxic effects while maintaining most of the antimicrobial effects. Hypochlorite ion is inactivated by contact with protein, so the solution must be continually changed. The same is true for acetic acid solutions, which may be more effective against *Pseudomonas*. Mafenide acetate soaks have the same characteristics of the mafenide acetate salve, except in liquid form.

The use of perioperative systemic antimicrobials also has a role in decreasing burn wound sepsis until the burn wound is closed. Common organisms that must be considered when choosing a perioperative regimen include *S. aureus* and *Pseudomonas* species, which are prevalent in burn wounds.

Synthetic and Biological Dressings

Synthetic and biological dressings are an alternative to antimicrobial dressings. These types of dressings provide stable coverage without painful dressing changes, provide a barrier to evaporative losses, and decrease pain in the wounds. They do not inhibit epithelialization, which is a feature of most topical antimicrobials. These coverings include allograft (cadaver skin), xenograft (pig skin), Transcyte, Biobrane, and Integra. These should generally be applied within 72 hours of the injury, before high bacterial colonization of the wound occurs. Most often, synthetic and biological dressings are used to cover second-degree wounds while the underlying epithelium heals or it is used to cover full-thickness wounds for which autograft is not yet available. Each type of dressing has its advantages and disadvantages.

Biobrane consists of collagen-coated silicone manufactured into a sheet (Fig. 22-9). This is placed on the wound and becomes adherent in 24 to 48 hours with dried wound transudate. This sheet then provides a barrier to moisture loss, and it provides a relatively painless wound bed that does not require dressing changes.[67] When the epithelium is complete under the Biobrane sheet, it is easily peeled off the wound. Caution must be exercised when using this product to ensure that copious exudate does not form under the Biobrane, which provides an optimum environment for bacterial proliferation and eventual invasive wound infection. Biobrane has no antimicrobial activities. Biobrane then should be used primarily in superficial second-degree burns and split-thickness skin graft donor sites.

Transcyte is a product that is similar to Biobrane with the addition of growth factors from lysed fibroblasts grown in culture that has been shown to decrease hospital stay and the incidence of autografting.[68] This product has the theoretical advantages of Biobrane with the additional advantage of stimulated wound healing. The applications are the same for Transcyte and Biobrane, with the

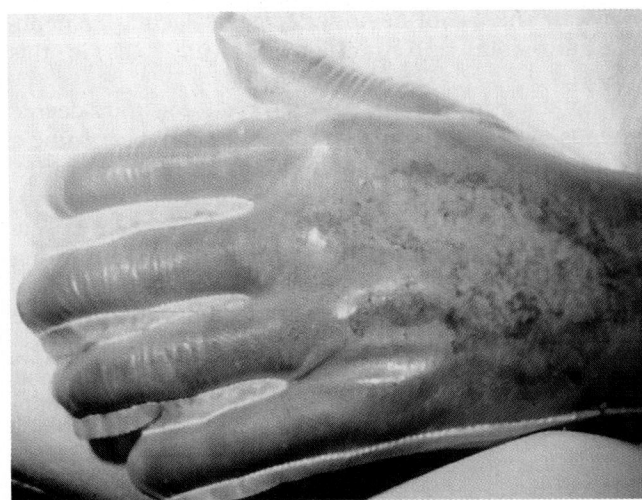

FIGURE 22-9. Biobrane in the form of a glove. This artificial dressing has elastic properties, forming a seal with the wound. Once wound exudate has dried to form a barrier, epithelialization takes place under the dressing in partial-thickness wounds in 1 to 2 weeks.

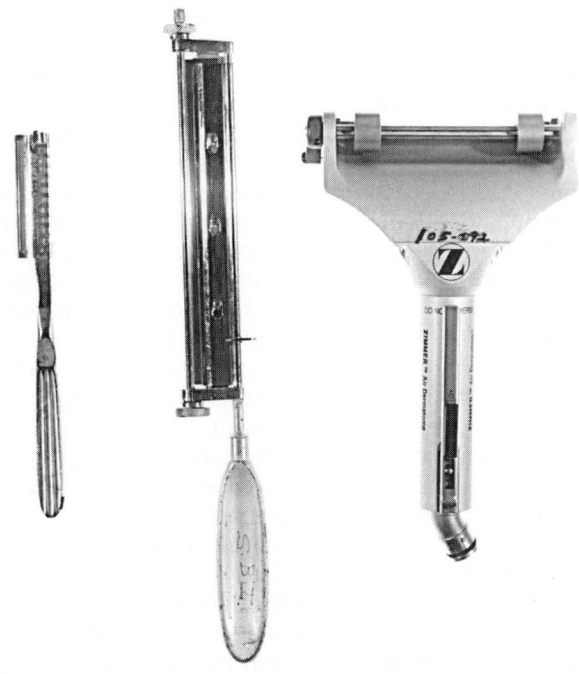

FIGURE 22-10. Instruments for tangential excision of burn wounds. Each of these may be used to excise the burn wound in layers until viable tissue is reached. Powered dermatomes such as the Zimmer instrument shown here (right) require either nitrogen or electricity. The others (Watson blade, which is the larger blade, and Weck blade) are hand instruments.

additional use of Transcyte in deeper second-degree wounds that will heal with stimulation.

Integra is a product that combines a collagen matrix (dermal substitute) with a silicone sheet outside layer (epidermal substitute). The collagen matrix engrafts into the wound, and after 2 weeks the silicone layer is removed and replaced with available autograft. The advantages of this product are that it can be used in full-thickness burns to close the wound. It also provides a dermal equivalent that has the theoretical advantage of inhibiting future scarring of the burn wound. The disadvantages are similar to those of all synthetic products, in that it has no antimicrobial properties and, thus, its use can be complicated by invasive wound infections. Additionally, it takes two operations for wound coverage because the silicone layer simulating the epidermis must be replaced 2 to 3 weeks after application with autograft. Recent reports on the use of Integra purport acceptable take rates and infection rates.[69] One of the potential advantages of this product is the limitation of scarring because of the presence of the dermal substitute; however, this has not been borne out in the initial reports.[70,71] Further studies with larger numbers of patients are required to test whether decreased scarring is an additional benefit with the use of this product.

Biological dressings include xenografts from swine and allografts from cadaver donors. These human skin equivalents are applied to the wounds in the manner of skin grafts, where they engraft and perform the immunologic and barrier functions of normal skin. Thus, these biological dressings are the optimal wound coverage in the absence of normal skin. Eventually, these biological dressings will be rejected by usual immune mechanisms, causing the grafts to slough. They can then be replaced, or the open wound can be covered with autograft skin from the patient. Generally, severely burned patients are immunosuppressed, and biological dressings that have adhered will not reject for several weeks. Biological dressings can be used to cover any wound as a temporary dressing. They are particularly well suited to massive partial-thickness injuries (>50% TBSA) to close the wound and allow for healing to take place underneath the dressing. Disadvantages include the possible transmission of viral diseases with allograft and the possibility that a residual mesh pattern will be left from engrafted cadaver dermis if meshed allograft is used.

Excision and Grafting

Deep second- and third-degree burns do not heal in a timely fashion without autografting. In fact, the practice of leaving these dead tissues only serves as a nidus for inflammation and infection that could lead to the patient's death. Early excision and grafting of these wounds is currently done by most burn surgeons since reports have shown benefit over serial débridement in terms of survival, blood loss, incidence of sepsis, and length of hospitalization.[72,73] The technique of early excision and grafting has made conservative treatment of full-thickness wounds a practice to be used only in the elderly and in the infrequent cases in which anesthesia and surgery are contraindicated. Attempts are made to excise tangentially to optimize cosmetic outcome. A number of instruments are commonly used to perform these excisions (Fig. 22-10). Rarely, excision to the level of fascia is necessary to remove all nonviable tissue, or it may become necessary at subsequent operations for infectious complications. These excisions can be performed with tourniquet control or with application of topical epinephrine and thrombin to minimize blood loss.

After a burn wound has been excised, the wound must be covered. This covering is ideally the patient's own skin. Wounds covering 20% to 30% TBSA can usually be closed at one operation with autograft split-thickness skin taken from the patient's available donor sites. In these operations, the skin grafts are not meshed, or they are meshed with a narrow ratio (≤2:1), to maximize cosmetic outcome. In major burns, autograft skin may be limited to the extent that the wound cannot be completely closed. The availability of cadaver allograft skin has changed the course of modern burn treatment for these massive wounds. A typical method of treatment is to use widely expanded autografts (≥4:1) covered with cadaver allograft to completely close the wounds for which autograft is available. The 4:1 skin heals underneath the cadaver skin in approximately 21 days, and the cadaver skin falls off (Fig. 22-11). The portions of the wound that cannot be covered with even widely meshed autograft are covered with allograft skin in preparation for autografting when donor sites are healed. Ideally, areas with less cosmetic importance are covered with the widely meshed skin to close most of the wound before using nonmeshed grafts at later operations for the cosmetically important areas, such as the hands and face.

Most surgeons excise the burn wound in the first week, sometimes in serial operations by removing 20% of the burn wound per operation on subsequent days. Others remove the whole of the burn wound in one operative procedure; however, this can be limited by the development of hypothermia or continuing massive blood loss. It is our practice to perform the excision immediately after stabilization of the patient after burn injury, because blood loss diminishes if the operation can be done the first day after injury. This may be due to the relative predominance of vasoconstrictive substances such as thromboxane and catecholamines and the natural edema planes that develop immediately after the injury. When the wound becomes hyperemic after 2 days, blood loss can be a considerable

problem. The use of hemostatic agents such as epinephrine, thrombin, and tourniquets greatly aids in this approach.

Early excision should be reserved for third-degree wounds. A deep second-degree burn can appear to be a third-degree wound at 24 to 48 hours after injury, particularly if it has been treated with topical antimicrobials, which combine with wound fluid to form a dense pseudoeschar. A randomized, prospective study comparing early excision versus conservative therapy with late grafting of deep second-degree wounds showed that those excised early had more wound excised, more blood loss, and more time in the operating room. No difference in hospital length of stay or infection rate was seen.[74] Long-term scarring and functional outcome, however, have not been examined in detail.

Occasionally, split-thickness skin grafts do not adhere. Loss of skin grafts is due to one or more of the following reasons: fluid collection under the graft, shearing forces that disrupt the adhered graft, presence of infection causing graft lysis, or an inadequate excision of the wound bed with remaining necrotic tissue. Meticulous hemostasis, appropriate meshing of grafts, or "rolling" of sheet grafts or bolsters over appropriate areas minimizes fluid collections. Shearing is decreased by immobilization of the grafted area. Infection is controlled by the appropriate use of perioperative antibiotics and covering the grafts with topical antimicrobials at the time of surgery. Inadequately excised wound beds are diminished by careful excision to viable tissue by experienced surgeons. Punctate bleeding or color of the dermis or fat in areas excised under tourniquet denotes the proper level of excision. Tissues that retain a red color after excision typically do not take grafts.

One alternative to split-thickness autografts typically used for skin grafting is cultured keratinocytes from the patient's own skin. Keratinocytes can be cultured in sheets from full-thickness skin biopsies, which are used as autografts. This technology has been used to greatly expand the capacity of a donor site, such that most of the body can be covered with grafts from a single small, full-thickness biopsy sample. Cultured epithelial autografts are of use in truly massive burns (>80% TBSA) because of their limited donor sites. The disadvantages of cultured epithelial autografts are the length of time required to grow the autografts (2 to 3 weeks), a 50% to 75% take rate of the grafts after initial application, the low resistance to mechanical trauma over the long term, and a proposed increase in scarring potential associated with the lack of dermis. These grafts are also quite expensive to produce. When a group of patients with greater than 80% TBSA burns receiving cultured epithelial autografts were compared with a group receiving conventional treatment, the acute hospitalization length of stay and the number of subsequent reconstructive operations was lower in the conventional group.[75] These results demonstrate that more research and experience are needed to further optimize this technique. Technologies like cultured epithelial autografts hold the promise to radically limit donor sites, and it may be the optimal closure in combination with a dermal equivalent in the future.

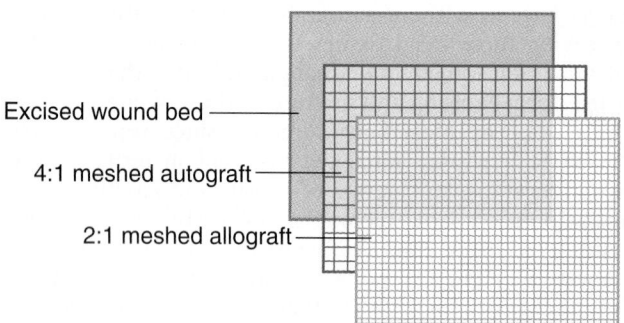

Excised wound bed

4:1 meshed autograft

2:1 meshed allograft

FIGURE 22-11. Diagram of skin closure using widely meshed autografts. The widely meshed autograft is placed on a freshly excised viable wound bed. The remaining open wound between the interstices of the autograft is closed with an overlying layer of allograft, which can also be meshed to allow transudate, exudate, and hematoma to escape.

The use of anabolic agents to accelerate wound healing has been investigated. The most effective agent to date has been systemic administration of recombinant human growth hormone.[76] The use of growth hormone has stimulated donor sites to heal faster, allowing more frequent donor site harvest and thus less time between operations. Growth hormone decreased donor site healing time by an average of 2 days with therapy that was associated with a reduction in length of hospital stay from 0.8 days per percent TBSA burn to 0.54 days per percent TBSA burn. This improved healing time was associated with a cost saving of 23% for a typical 80% TBSA burn, including the cost of the growth hormone. This effect is thought to be due to stimulation of insulin-like growth factor-1 release as well as upregulation of insulin-like growth factor-1 receptors in the wound.[77] It has recently been shown that insulin in pharmacologic doses may have similar effects on wound healing. Insulin given at 30 μU/kg/min for 7 days decreased donor site healing time from 6.5 plus or minus 0.9 days to 4.7 plus or minus 2.3 days.[78] In this study, the caloric intake necessary to maintain euglycemia during the insulin infusion was double that of the placebo time period. The effects of insulin on wound healing also seem to be potentiated with additional amino acids.[79] Studies are underway using much lower doses to determine whether a significant effect is still present at doses that would be clinically safer to use.

In all burned patients, every effort should be made to maximize the long-term appearance of the wound, because almost all patients will survive to bear the scars of their injury. Burn wound scarring causes both functional and cosmetic deficits associated with wound contracture. Experience has shown that full-thickness skin grafts that include the entire dermal and epidermal layer provide the best outcomes in wound coverage, with diminished contracture and superior skin appearance compared with split-thickness skin grafts. Split-thickness and full-thickness grafts both have a complete epidermal layer; therefore, the superior function and appearance of full-thickness grafts must lie in the uninterrupted complete dermal layer. Thickness of split thickness skin grafts should also be addressed because it is thought by extension that thicker skin grafts carrying more dermis will diminish the amount of contracture and scarring. A recent study comparing standard thickness grafts (0.015 inches) to thick grafts (0.025 inches) applied to full-thickness hand wounds revealed no differences in range of motion, appearance, or patient satisfaction.[80] Therefore, it is reasonable to conclude that standard-thickness skin grafts are appropriate for acute coverage of burn wounds. The challenge to burn surgeons in terms of minimizing scarring, then, is to provide complete dermis during wound coverage.

Full-thickness skin grafts to supply the dermal layer are not plentiful and cannot be used more than once. The use of tissue expanders to increase available full-thickness donor skin is conceivable, but impractical, for most injuries. For these reasons, these grafts are not commonly used in burn wound coverage. Engrafted cadaver dermis that has the epidermis removed by dermabrasion 1 to 2 weeks after placing it on the wound has been used with some success to provide the dermal layer. Presumably, the sparse cellular component of the dermis is removed by immunologic processes, leaving the dermal matrix in place as scaffolding for the ingrowth of normal dermal cells. A commercially available product of decellularized preserved cadaver dermis (AlloDerm) has also been used to provide a dermal equivalent in wound coverage. As discussed earlier, the product Integra also has a dermal equivalent component to form a neodermis. All these have the potential to minimize scarring contractures and to maximize the cosmetic appearance of burn scars. The long-term results with the use of these techniques are not yet known.

Recently, the use of vacuum-assisted closure of wounds has been reported. These vacuum-assisted devices have been used successfully for closure of complicated decubitus ulcers, among other uses, and have now been tried in burn wounds to secure skin grafts and improve take rates.[81] Those treated with vacuum-assisted devices compared to standard bolster securement of skin grafts had significantly improved rates of reoperation for failed skin grafts without differences in complications.

MINIMIZING COMPLICATIONS

Early, aggressive resuscitation regimens have improved survival rates dramatically. With the advent of vigorous fluid resuscitation, irreversible burn shock has been replaced by sepsis and subsequent multiorgan failure as the leading cause of death associated with burns. In our pediatric burn population with burns more than 80% TBSA, sepsis defined by bacteremia developed in 17.5% of the children.[9] The mortality rate in the whole group was 33%; most of these deaths were attributable to multiorgan failure. Some of the patients who died were bacteremic and "septic," but most were not. These findings highlight the observation that development of multiorgan failure is often associated with infectious sepsis, but infection is by no means required to develop multiorgan failure. What is required is an inflammatory focus, which in severe burns is the massive skin injury that requires inflammation to heal. It has been postulated that the progression to multiorgan failure exists in a continuum with the systemic inflammatory response syndrome.[82] Nearly all burned patients meet the criteria for systemic inflammatory response syndrome as defined by the consensus conference of the American College of Chest Physicians and the Society of Critical Care Medicine.[83] It is therefore not surprising that multiorgan failure is common in burned patients.

Etiology and Pathophysiology

The progression from the systemic inflammatory response syndrome to multiorgan failure is not well explained, although some of the responsible mechanisms are recognized. Most of these are found in patients with inflammation from infectious sources. In the burned patient, these infectious sources most likely emanate from invasive wound infection or from lung infections (pneumonia). As organisms proliferate out of control, endotoxins are liberated from gram-negative bacterial walls, and exotoxins from gram-positive and gram-negative bacteria are released. Their release causes the initiation of a cascade of inflammatory mediators that can result, if unchecked, in organ damage and progression toward organ failure. Occasionally, failure of the gut barrier with penetration of organisms into the systemic circulation may incite a similar reaction. However, this phenomenon has only been demonstrated in animal models, and it remains to be seen whether this is a cause of human disease.[34]

Inflammation from the presence of necrotic tissue and open wounds can incite a similar inflammatory mediator response to that seen with endotoxin. The mechanism by which this occurs, however, is not well understood. Regardless, it is known that a cascade of systemic events is set in motion either by invasive organisms or from open wounds that initiates the systemic inflammatory syndrome, which may progress to multiorgan failure. Evidence from animal studies and clinical trials suggests that these events converge to a common pathway, which results in activation of several cascade systems. Those circulating mediators can, if secreted in excessive amounts, damage organs distal from their site of origin. Among these mediators are endotoxin, the arachidonic acid metabolites, cytokines, neutrophils and their adherence molecules, nitric oxide, complement components, and oxygen free radicals.

Prevention

Because different cascade systems are involved in the pathogenesis of burn-induced multiorgan failure, it is so far impossible to pinpoint a single mediator that initiates the event. Thus, because the mechanisms of progression are not well known, prevention is currently the best solution. The current recommendations are to prevent the development of organ dysfunction and to provide optimal support to avoid conditions that promote the onset.

The great reduction of mortality rate from large burns was seen with early excision and an aggressive surgical approach to deep wounds. Early removal of devitalized tissue prevents wound infections and decreases inflammation associated with the wound. In addition, it eliminates small, colonized foci, which are a frequent source of transient bacteremia. Those transient bacteremias during surgical manipulations may prime immune cells to react in an exaggerated fashion to subsequent insults, leading to whole body inflammation and remote organ damage. We recommend complete early excision of clearly full-thickness wounds within 48 hours of the injury.

Oxidative damage from reperfusion after low-flow states makes early, aggressive fluid resuscitation imperative. This is particularly important during the initial phases of treatment and operative excision with its attendant blood losses. Furthermore, the volume of fluid may not be as important as the timeliness with which it is given. In the study of children with more than 80% TBSA burns, it was found that one of the most important contributors to survival was the time required to start intravenous resuscitation, regardless of the initial volume given.

Topical and systemic antimicrobial therapy have significantly diminished the incidence of invasive burn wound sepsis. Perioperative antibiotics clearly benefit patients with injuries greater than 30% TBSA burns. Vigilant and scheduled replacement of intravascular devices minimizes the incidence of catheter-related sepsis. We recommend changes of indwelling catheters every 3 days. The first can be done over a wire using sterile Seldinger technique, but the second change requires a new site. This protocol should be kept as long as intravenous access is required. Where possible, peripheral veins should be used for cannulation, even through burned tissue. The saphenous vein, however, should be avoided because of the high risk of thrombophlebitis.

Pneumonia, which contributes significantly to death in burned patients, should be vigilantly anticipated and aggressively treated. Every attempt should be made to wean patients as early as possible from the ventilator to reduce the risk of ventilator-associated nosocomial pneumonia. Furthermore, early ambulation is an effective means of preventing respiratory complications. With sufficient analgesics, even patients on continuous ventilatory support can be out of bed and in a chair.

The most common sources of sepsis are the wounds and/or the tracheobronchial trees; efforts to identify causative agents should be concentrated there. Another potential source, however, is the gastrointestinal tract, which is a natural reservoir for bacteria. Starvation and hypovolemia shunt blood from the splanchnic bed and promote mucosal atrophy and failure of the gut barrier. Early enteral feeding reduces septic morbidity and prevents failure of the gut barrier. At our institution, patients are fed immediately through a nasogastric tube. Early enteral feedings are tolerated in burned patients, preserve the mucosal integrity, and may reduce the magnitude of the hypermetabolic response to injury. Support of the gut goes along with carefully monitored hemodynamics.

Organ Failure

Even with the best efforts at prevention, the presence of the systemic inflammatory syndrome that is ubiquitous in burned patients may progress to organ failure. It was recently found that approximately 28% of patients with greater than 20% TBSA burns will develop severe multiorgan dysfunction, of which 14% will also develop severe sepsis and septic shock.[84] The general development begins either in the renal or pulmonary systems and can progress through the liver, gut, hematologic system, and central nervous system. The development of multiorgan failure does not predict mortality, however, and efforts to support the organs until they heal is justified.

Renal Failure

With the advent of early aggressive resuscitation, the incidence of renal failure coincident with the initial phases of recovery has diminished significantly in severely burned patients. However, a second period of risk for the development of renal failure 2 to 14 days after resuscitation is still present.[29] Renal failure is hallmarked by decreasing urine output; fluid overload; electrolyte abnormalities, including metabolic acidosis and hyperkalemia; the development of azotemia; and increased serum creatinine level. Treatment is aimed at averting complications associated with these conditions.

Urine output of more than 1 mL/kg is an adequate measure of renal perfusion in the absence of underlying renal disease. Decreasing the volume of fluid being given can alleviate volume overload in burned patients. These patients have increased insensible losses from the wounds, which can be roughly calculated at 1500 mL/m^2 TBSA + 3750 mL/m^2 TBSA burned. Further losses are accrued on airbeds (1 L/day in an adult). Decreasing the infused volume of intravenous fluids and enteral feedings to less than the expected insensate losses alleviates fluid overload problems. Electrolyte abnormalities can be minimized by decreasing potassium administration in the enteral feedings and giving oral bicarbonate solutions such as Bicitra. Almost invariably, severely burned patients require exogenous potassium because of the heightened aldosterone response that results in potassium wasting; therefore, hyperkalemia is rare even with some renal insufficiency.

If the problems listed earlier overwhelm the conservative measures, some form of dialysis may be necessary. The indications for dialysis are volume overload or electrolyte abnormalities not amenable to other treatments. Peritoneal dialysis is effective in burned patients to remove volume and correct electrolyte abnormalities. Occasionally, hemodialysis is required. Continuous venovenous hemodialysis is often indicated in these patients because of the fluid shifts that occur.[27] All hemodialysis techniques should be done in conjunction with experienced nephrologists who are well versed in the techniques.

After beginning dialysis, renal function may return, especially in patients who maintain some urine output. Therefore, patients requiring such treatment may not require lifelong dialysis. It is a clinical observation that whatever urine output was present will decrease once dialysis is begun, but it may return in several days to weeks once the acute process of closing the burn wound nears completion.

Pulmonary Failure

Many burned patients require mechanical ventilation to protect the airway in the initial phases of their injury. We recommend that these patients be extubated as soon as possible after the risk is diminished. A trial of extubation is often warranted in the first few days after injury, and reintubation in this setting is not a failure. To perform this technique safely, however, requires the involvement of experts in obtaining an airway. The goal is extubation as soon as possible to allow the patients to clear their own airways, because they can perform their own pulmonary toilet better than through an endotracheal tube or tracheostomy. The first sign of impending pulmonary failure

is a decline in oxygenation. This is best followed up with continuous oximetry, and a decrease in saturation to less than 92% is indicative of failure. Increasing concentrations of inspired oxygen are necessary, and when ventilation begins to fail, denoted by increasing respiratory rate and hypercarbia, intubation is needed.

Some have stated that early tracheostomy (within the first week) might be indicated in those with significant burn who are likely to require long-term ventilation. In one study, it was found in severely burned children who underwent early tracheostomy that the peak inspiratory pressures were lower after tracheostomy with higher ventilatory volumes and pulmonary compliance, and higher PaO$_2$/FiO$_2$ ratios.[85] No instances of tracheostomy site infections or tracheal stenoses were identified in the 28 patients studied. Another randomized study comparing those severely burned patients who underwent early tracheostomy with those who did not found similar improvements in oxygenation; however, no significant differences could be found in outcome measures such as ventilator days, length of stay, incidence of pneumonia, or survival. In fact, 26% of those not undergoing tracheostomy were successfully extubated within 2 weeks of admission, implying that they would not have required tracheostomy at all.[86] It seems that although tracheostomy may be required in some severely burned patients on ventilatory support, the advantages of early tracheostomy do not outweigh the disadvantages. Further data from other centers may change this conclusion in the future.

Hepatic Failure

The development of hepatic failure in burned patients is a challenging problem without many solutions. The liver synthesizes circulating proteins, detoxifies the plasma, produces bile, and provides immunologic support. When the liver begins to fail, protein concentrations of the coagulation cascade decrease to critical levels and the patient becomes coagulopathic. Toxins are not cleared from the bloodstream, and concentrations of bilirubin increase. Complete hepatic failure is not compatible with life, but a gradation of liver failure with some decline of the function is common. Efforts to prevent hepatic failure are the only effective methods of treatment.

With the development of coagulopathies, treatment should be directed at replacement of factors II, VII, IX, and X until the liver recovers. Albumin replacement may also be required. Attention to obstructive causes of hyperbilirubinemia, such as acalculous cholecystitis, should be considered as well. Initial treatment of this condition should be gallbladder drainage, which can be done percutaneously.

Hematologic Failure

Burned patients may become coagulopathic through two mechanisms: (1) depletion and impaired synthesis of coagulation factors or (2) thrombocytopenia. Factors associated with factor depletion are through disseminated intravascular coagulation associated with sepsis. This process is also common with coincident head injury. With breakdown of the blood-brain barrier, brain lipids are exposed to the plasma, which activates the coagulation cascade. Varying penetrance of this problem results in differing degrees of coagulopathy. Treatment of disseminated intravascular coagulation should include infusion of fresh frozen plasma and cryoprecipitate to maintain plasma levels of coagulation factors. For disseminated intravascular coagulation induced by brain injury, following the concentration of fibrinogen and repleting levels with cryoprecipitate are the most specific indicators. Impaired synthesis of factors from liver failure is treated as alluded to earlier.

Thrombocytopenia is common in severe burns from depletion during burn wound excision. Platelet counts lower than 50,000 are common and do not require treatment. Only when the bleeding is diffuse and is noted from the intravenous sites should consideration for exogenous platelets be given.

Paradoxically, it was found that severely burned patients are also at risk for thrombotic and embolic complications likely related to immobilization. It was found that complications of deep venous thrombosis were associated with increasing age, weight, and TBSA burned.[87] These data intimate that deep venous thrombosis prophylaxis would be prudent for adult patients in the absence of bleeding complications.

Central Nervous System Failure

Obtundation is one of the hallmarks of sepsis, and in burns this is not excepted. The new onset of mental status changes not attributed to sedative medications in a severely burned patient should incite a search for a septic source. Treatment is supportive.

NUTRITION

The response to injury known as *hypermetabolism* occurs dramatically after severe burn. Increases in oxygen consumption, metabolic rate, urinary nitrogen excretion, lipolysis, and weight loss are directly proportional to the size of the burn. This response can be as high as 200% of the normal metabolic rate and returns to normal only with the complete closure of the wound. Because the metabolic rate is so high, energy requirements are immense. These requirements are met by mobilization of carbohydrate, fat, and protein stores. Because the demands are prolonged, these energy stores are quickly depleted,

leading to loss of active muscle tissue and malnutrition. This malnutrition is associated with functional impairment of many organs, delayed and abnormal wound healing, decreased immunocompetence, and altered cellular membrane active transport functions. Malnutrition in burns can be subverted to some extent by delivery of adequate exogenous nutritional support. The goals of nutrition support are to maintain and improve organ function and prevent protein-calorie malnutrition.

Several formulas are used to calculate caloric requirements in burned patients. One formula multiplies the basal energy expenditure determined by the Harris-Benedict formula by 2 in burns 40% TBSA, assuming a 100% increase in total energy expenditure. When total energy expenditure was measured by the doubly labeled water method, actual expenditures were found to be 1.33 times the predicted basal energy expenditure for pediatric patients with burns greater than 40% TBSA.[88] To meet the minimal needs of all the patients in this study, 1.55 times the predicted basal energy expenditure would be required; however, giving caloric loads in excess of this probably leads to fat accumulation without affecting lean mass accretion. This correlated to 1.4 times the measured resting energy expenditure by indirect calorimetry. These studies indicate that the calculation of 2 times the predicted basal energy expenditure might be too high.

Other commonly used calculations include the Curreri formula, which calls for 25 kcal/kg/day plus 40 kcal per percent TBSA burned per day. This formula provides for maintenance needs plus the additional caloric needs related to the burn wounds.[89] This formula was devised as a regression from nitrogen balance data in severely burned adults. In children, formulas based on body surface area are more appropriate because of the greater body surface area per kilogram of weight. We recommend the formulas depending on the child's age shown in Table 22-6. These formulas were determined to maintain body weight in severely burned children.[90] The formulas change with age based on the body surface area alterations that occur with growth.

The composition of the nutritional supplement is also important. The optimal dietary composition contains 1 to 2 g/kg/day of protein, which provides a calorie-to-nitrogen ratio at around 100:1 with the earlier suggested caloric intakes. This amount of protein provides for the synthetic needs of the patient, thus sparing to some extent the proteolysis occurring in the active muscle tissue. Nonprotein calories can be given either as carbohydrate or as fat. Carbohydrates have the advantage of stimulating

TABLE 22-6. Formulas to Predict Caloric Needs in Severely Burned Children

Age Group	Maintenance Needs	Burn Wound Needs
Infants (0–12 mo)	2100 kcal/% TBSA burned/24 hr	1000 kcal/% TBSA burned/24 hr
Children (1–12 yr)	1800 kcal/% TBSA burned/24 hr	1300 kcal/% TBSA burned/24 hr
Adolescents (12–18 yr)	1500 kcal/% TBSA burned/24 hr	1500 kcal/% TBSA burned/24 hr

TBSA, total body surface area.

endogenous insulin production, which may have the beneficial effects on muscle and burn wounds as an anabolic hormone. In addition, it was recently shown that almost all of the fat transported in very low-density lipoprotein after severe burn is derived from peripheral lipolysis and not from de novo synthesis of fatty acids in the liver from dietary carbohydrates.[91] Additional fat to deliver noncarbohydrate calories then has little support.

The diet may be delivered in two forms: either enterally through enteric tubes or parenterally through intravenous catheters. Parenteral nutrition may be given in isotonic solutions through peripheral catheters or with hypertonic solutions in central catheters. In general, the caloric demands of burned patients prohibit the use of peripheral parenteral nutrition. Total parenteral nutrition delivered centrally in burned patients has been associated with increased complications and mortality rate compared with enteral feedings.[92] Total parenteral nutrition is reserved only for those patients who cannot tolerate enteral feedings. Enteral feeding has been associated with some complications, however, which can be disastrous. These include mechanical complications, enteral feeding intolerance, and diarrhea.

Recently, interest in nutritional adjunctive treatment with anabolic agents has received attention as a means to decrease lean mass losses after severe injury. Agents used include growth hormone,[93] insulin-like growth factor,[94] insulin,[95] oxandrolone,[96] testosterone,[97] and propranolol.[98] Each of these agents has different actions to stimulate protein synthesis through an increase in protein synthetic efficiency. Put simply, the free amino acids available in the cytoplasm from stimulated protein breakdown with severe injury or illness are preferentially shunted toward protein synthesis rather than export out of the cell (Fig. 22-12). Some of these agents such as insulin and oxandrolone have shown efficacy not only in improving protein kinetics but also in improving lean mass after severe burn. Further research will reveal whether these biochemical and physiologic measures translate to improved function.

OUTCOMES

Many of the treatments for burn are directed at improving functional psychologic and work outcomes, which are only now being systematically studied. Authors are now

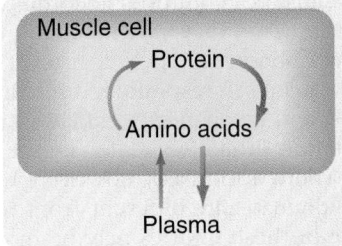

FIGURE 22-12. Amino acids from stimulated protein breakdown in the neurocele cell are routed out of the cell to provide substrate for recovery. Anabolic agents attenuate this by directing these amino acids back into protein synthesis.

reporting new methods to evaluate outcomes through Burn Specific Health Scales[99] and measures of adjustment. Authors found that severely burned adult patients adjust relatively well, although some develop clinically significant psychological disturbances such as somatization and phobic anxiety. Children with severe burns were found to have similar somatization problems as well as sleep disturbances, but in general were well adjusted.[100,101] Time off work in adult patients was found to be associated with increasing percent TBSA burned, psychiatric history, and extremity burns with considerable job disruption.[102] These data intimate that major burns can lead to significant disturbances in psychiatric health and outcomes, but in general, these can be overcome.

ELECTRICAL BURNS

Initial Treatment

Three percent to 5% of all admitted burned patients are injured from electrical contact. Electrical injury is unlike other burn injuries in that the visible areas of tissue necrosis represent only a small portion of the destroyed tissue. Electrical current enters a part of the body, such as the fingers or hand, and proceeds through tissues with the lowest resistance to current, generally the nerves, blood vessels, and muscles. The skin has a relatively high resistance to electrical current and is therefore mostly spared. The current then leaves the body at a "grounded" area, typically the foot. Heat generated by the transfer of electrical current and passage of the current itself then injures the tissues. During this exchange, the muscle is the major tissue through which the current flows, and thus it sustains the most damage. Most muscle is in close proximity to bones. Blood vessels transmitting much of the electricity initially remain patent, but they may proceed to progressive thrombosis as the cells either die or repair themselves, thus resulting in further tissue loss from ischemia.

Injuries are divided into high- and low-voltage injuries. Low-voltage injury is similar to thermal burns without transmission to the deeper tissues; zones of injury from the surface extend into the tissue. Most household currents (110 to 220 V) produce this type of injury, which causes only local damage. The worst of these injuries are those involving the edge of the mouth (oral commissure) sustained when children gnaw on household electrical cords.

The syndrome of high-voltage injury consists of varying degrees of cutaneous burn at the entry and exit sites, combined with hidden destruction of deep tissue. Often, these patients also have cutaneous burns associated with ignition of clothing from the discharge of electrical current. Initial evaluation consists of cardiopulmonary resuscitation if ventricular fibrillation is induced. Thereafter, if the initial electrocardiogram findings are abnormal or there is a history of cardiac arrest associated with the injury, continued cardiac monitoring is necessary along with pharmacologic treatment for any dysrhythmias. The most serious derangements occur in the first 24 hours after injury. If patients with electrical injuries have no cardiac dysrhythmias on initial electrocardiogram or recent history of cardiac arrest, no further monitoring is necessary.

Patients with electrical injuries are at risk for other injuries, such as being thrown from the electrical jolt or falling from heights after disengaging from the electrical current. In addition, the violent tetanic muscular contractions that result from alternating current sources may cause a variety of fractures and dislocations. These patients should be assessed as any other patient with blunt traumatic injuries.

The key to managing patients with an electrical injury lies in the treatment of the wound. The most significant injury is within the deep tissue, and subsequent edema formation can cause vascular compromise to any area distal to the injury. Assessment should include circulation to distal vascular beds, because immediate escharotomy and fasciotomy may be required. If the muscle compartment is extensively injured and necrotic, such that the prospects for eventual function are dismal, early amputation may be necessary. We advocate early exploration of affected muscle beds and débridement of devitalized tissues, with attention given to the deeper periosteous planes, because this is the area with the most muscle tissue. Fasciotomies should be complete and may require nerve decompressions, such as carpal tunnel and Guyon canal releases. Tissue that has questionable viability should be left in place, with planned re-exploration in 48 hours. Many such re-explorations may be required until the wound is completely débrided. Electrical damage to vessels may be delayed, and the extent of necrosis may extend after the initial débridements. After the devitalized tissues are removed, closure of the wound becomes paramount. Although skin grafts suffice as closure for most wounds, flaps may offer a better alternative, particularly with exposed bones and tendons. Even exposed and superficially infected bones and tendons can be salvaged with coverage by vascularized tissue. Early involvement by reconstructive surgeons versed in the various methods of wound closure is optimal.

Muscle damage results in release of hemochromogens (myoglobin), which are filtered in the glomeruli and may result in obstructive nephropathy. Therefore, vigorous hydration and infusion of intravenous sodium bicarbonate (5% continuous infusion) and mannitol (25 g every 6 hours for adults) are indicated to solubilize the hemochromogens and maintain urine output if significant amounts are found in the serum. These patients also require additional intravenous volumes over predicted amounts based on the wound area because most of the wound is deep and cannot be assessed by standard physical examination. In this situation, urine output should be maintained at 2 mL/kg/hr.

Delayed Effects

Neurologic deficits may occur. Serial neurologic evaluations should be performed as part of routine examination to detect any early or late neuropathology. Central nervous system effects such as cortical encephalopathy, hemiplegia, aphasia, and brain stem dysfunction injury have been reported up to 9 months after injury; others report delayed peripheral nerve lesions characterized by demyelination with vacuolization and reactive gliosis. Another devastating long-term effect is the development of cataracts, which can be delayed for several years. These complications may occur in up to 30% of patients with significant high-voltage injury, and patients should be made aware of their possibility even with the best treatment.

CHEMICAL BURNS

Most chemical burns are accidental from mishandling of household cleaners, although some of the most dramatic presentations involve industrial exposures. Thermal burns are, in general, short-term exposures to heat, but chemical injuries may be of longer duration, even for hours in the absence of appropriate treatment. The degree of tissue damage as well as the level of toxicity is determined by the chemical nature of the agent, concentration of the agent, and the duration of skin contact. Chemicals cause their injury by protein destruction, with denaturation, oxidation, formation of protein esters, or desiccation of the tissue. In the United States, the composition of most household and industrial chemicals can be obtained from the Poison Control Center in the area, which can give suggestions for treatment.

Speed is essential in the management of chemical burns. For all chemicals, lavage with copious quantities of clean water should be done immediately after removing all clothing. Dry powders should be brushed from the affected areas before irrigation. Early irrigation dilutes the chemical, which is already in contact with the skin, and timeliness increases effectiveness. Several liters of irrigant may be required. For example, 10 mL of 98% sulfuric acid dissolved in 12 L of water decreases the pH to 5.0, a range that can still cause injury. If the chemical composition is known (acid or base), monitoring of the spent lavage solution pH gives a good indication of lavage effectiveness and completion. A good rule of thumb is to lavage with 15 to 20 L of tap water or more for significant chemical injuries. The lavage site should be kept drained to remove the earlier, more concentrated effluent. Care should be taken to drain away from uninjured areas to avoid further exposure.

All patients must be monitored according to the severity of their injuries. They may have metabolic disturbances, usually from pH abnormalities, because of exposure to strong acids or caustics. If respiratory difficulty is apparent, oxygen therapy and mechanical ventilation must be instituted. Resuscitation should be guided by the body surface area involved (burn formulas); however, the total fluid needs may be dramatically different from the calculated volumes. Some of these injuries may be more superficial than they appear, particularly in the case of acids, and therefore require less resuscitation volume. Injuries from bases, however, may penetrate beyond that which is apparent on examination and therefore require more volume. For this reason, patients with chemical injuries should be observed closely for signs of adequate perfusion, such as urine output. All patients with significant chemical injuries should be monitored with indwelling bladder catheters to accurately measure outputs.

Operative débridement, if indicated, should take place as soon as a patient is stable and resuscitated (Fig. 22-13). Following adequate lavage and débridement, burn wounds are covered with antimicrobial agents or skin substitutes. Once the wounds have stabilized with the indicated treatment, they are taken care of as with any loss of soft tissue. Skin grafting or flap coverage is performed as needed.

Alkali

Alkalis, such as lime, potassium hydroxide, bleach, and sodium hydroxide, are among the most common agents involved in chemical injury. Accidental injury frequently occurs in infants and toddlers exploring cleaning cabinets. There are three factors involved in the mechanism of alkali burns: (1) saponification of fat causes the loss of insulation of heat formed in the chemical reaction with tissue; (2) massive extraction of water from cells causes damage because of the hygroscopic nature of alkali; and (3) alkalis dissolve and unite with the proteins of the tissues to form alkaline proteinates, which are soluble and contain hydroxide ions. These ions induce further chemical reactions, penetrating deeper into the tissue.[103] Treatment involves immediate removal of the causative agent with lavage of large volumes of fluid, usually water. Attempts to neutralize alkali agents with weak acids are not recommended, because the heat released by neutralization reactions induces further injury. Particularly strong bases should be treated with lavage and consideration for the addition of wound débridement in the operating room. Tangential removal of affected areas is performed until the tissues removed are at a normal pH.

Cement (calcium oxide) burns are alkali in nature, occur commonly, and are usually work-related injuries. The critical substance responsible for the skin damage is the hydroxyl ion. Often, the agent has been in contact with the skin for prolonged periods, such as underneath the boots of a cement worker who seeks treatment hours after the exposure, or after the cement penetrates clothing and, when combined with perspiration, induces an exothermic reaction. Treatment consists of removing all clothing and irrigating the affected area with water and soap until all the cement is removed and the effluent has a pH of less than 8. Injuries tend to be deep because of exposure times, and surgical excision and grafting of the resultant eschar may be required.

Acids

Acid injuries are treated initially like any other chemical injury, with removal of all chemicals by disrobing the affected area and copious irrigation. Acids induce protein breakdown by hydrolysis, which results in a hard eschar that does not penetrate as deeply as the alkalis. These agents also induce thermal injury by heat generation with contact of the skin, further causing soft tissue damage. Some acids have added effects, which are discussed here.

Formic acid injuries are relatively rare, usually involving an organic acid used for industrial descaling and as a hay preservative. Electrolyte abnormalities are of great concern for patients who have sustained extensive formic acid injuries, with metabolic acidosis, renal failure, intravascular hemolysis, and pulmonary complications (acute respiratory distress syndrome) being common. Acidemia detected by a metabolic acidosis on arterial blood gas analysis should be corrected with intravenous sodium bicarbonate. Hemodialysis may be required when extensive absorption of formic acid has occurred. Mannitol diuresis is required if severe hemolysis occurs

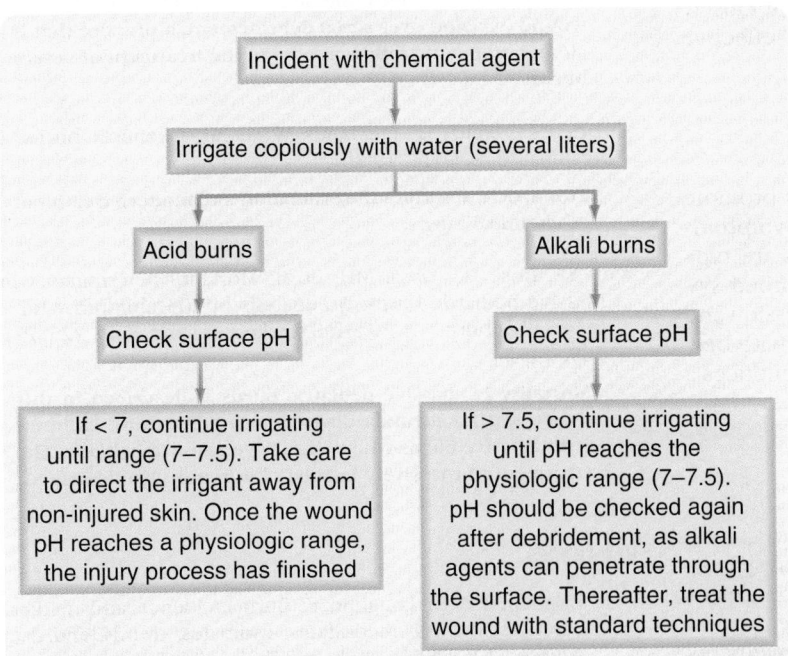

FIGURE 22-13. Treatment of acid and alkali burns.

after deep injury. A formic acid wound typically has a greenish appearance and is deeper than what it initially appears to be; it is best treated by surgical excision.

Hydrofluoric acid is a toxic substance used widely in both industrial and domestic settings and is the strongest inorganic acid known. Management of these burns differs from other acid burns in general. Hydrofluoric acid produces dehydration and corrosion of tissue with free hydrogen ions. In addition, the fluoride ion complexes with bivalent cations such as calcium and magnesium to form insoluble salts. Systemic absorption of the fluoride ion then can induce intravascular calcium chelation and hypocalcemia, which causes life-threatening arrhythmias. Beyond initial copious irrigation with clean water, the burned area should be treated immediately with copious 2.5% calcium gluconate gel. These wounds in general are extremely painful because of the calcium chelation and associated potassium release. This finding can be used to determine the effectiveness of treatment. The gel should be changed at 15-minute intervals until the pain subsides, an indication of removal of the active fluoride ion. If pain relief is incomplete after several applications or if symptoms recur, intradermal injections of 10% calcium gluconate (0.5 mL/cm^2 affected), intra-arterial calcium gluconate into the affected extremity, or both may be required to alleviate symptoms. If the burn is not treated in such a fashion, decalcification of the bone underlying the injury and extension of the soft tissue injury may occur.

All patients with hydrofluoric acid burns should be admitted for cardiac monitoring, with particular attention paid to prolongation of the QT interval. A total of 20 mL of 10% calcium gluconate solution should be added to the first liter of resuscitation fluid, and serum electrolytes must be closely monitored. Any electrocardiographic changes require a rapid response by the treatment team with intravenous calcium chloride to maintain heart function. Several grams of calcium may be required in the end until the chemical response has run its course. Serum magnesium and potassium also should be closely monitored and replaced. Speed is the key to effective treatment.

Hydrocarbons

The organic solvent properties of hydrocarbons promote cell membrane dissolution and skin necrosis. Symptoms include erythema and blistering, and the burns are typically superficial and heal spontaneously. If absorbed systemically, toxicity can produce respiratory depression and eventual hepatic injury thought to be associated with benzenes. Ignition of the hydrocarbons on the skin induces a deep full-thickness injury.

SUMMARY

The treatment of burns is complex. Minor injuries can be treated in the community by knowledgeable physicians. Moderate and severe injuries, however, require treatment in dedicated facilities with resources to maximize the outcomes from these often devastating events. Improvements in care of patients have markedly improved such that most patients even with massive injuries survive. Challenges for the future will be in the areas of scar modulation and acceleration of the healing time to result in functional and visually appealing outcomes in a prompt fashion.

Selected References

Baxter CR: Fluid volume and electrolyte changes in the early post-burn period. Clin Plast Surg 1:693-703, 1974.

> **This is the classic article describing the development and use of the Parkland formula for resuscitation of burned patients.**

Bull JP, Fisher AJ: A study in mortality in a burn unit: Standards for the evaluation for alternative methods of treatment. Ann Surg 130:160-173, 1949.

> **Bull and Fisher first described the incidence of burn mortality in this classic article. Mortality has significantly improved since these statistics.**

Cioffi WG, DeMeules JE, Gamelli RL: The effects of burn injury and fluid resuscitation on cardiac function in vitro. J Trauma 26:638-645, 1986.

> **This paper describes the effect of severe burn on cardiac dynamics and explains the effects we see on hemodynamics early in resuscitation.**

Curreri PW: Nutritional support of burn patients. World J Surg 2:215-222, 1978.

> **This was the seminal manuscript describing the Curreri formula, which is still used in many burn units for the prescription of nutritional needs after severe burn.**

Herndon DN, Parks DH: Comparison of serial débridement and autografting and early massive excision with cadaver skin overlay in the treatment of large burns in children. J Trauma 26:149-152, 1986.

> **This paper describes the use and superiority of early wound excision over serial débridement, a practice that is almost uniformly followed now in the treatment of severe burns.**

Mozingo D, Smith A, McManus W, et al: Chemical burns. J Trauma 28:642-647, 1988.

> **This article describes the evaluation and modern treatment of chemical burns.**

Wolf SE, Rose JK, Desai MH, et al: Mortality determinants in massive pediatric burns: An analysis of 103 children with ≥ 80% TBSA burns (≥ 70% full-thickness). Ann Surg 225:554-569, 1997.

> **Mortality in massive pediatric burns is described in this paper, with a formula devised to predict those children with massive burns who will survive and who will die. The treatment of massively burned children is also described.**

References

1. Brigham PA, McLoughlin E: Burn incidence and medical care use in the United States: Estimates, trends, and data sources. J Burn Care Rehabil 17:95-107, 1996.

2. Barillo DJ, Goode R: Fire fatality study: Demographics of fire victims. Burns 22:85-88, 1996.

3. Kemp A, Sibert J: Childhood accidents: Epidemiology, trends, and prevention. J Accid Emerg Med 14:316-320, 1997.

4. McGwin G Jr, Cross JM, Ford JW, et al: Long-term trends in mortality according to age among adult burn patients. J Burn Care Rehabil 24:21-25, 2003.

5. Cusick JM, Grant EJ, Kucan JO: Children's sleepwear: Relaxation of the Consumer Product Safety Commission's flammability standards. J Burn Care Rehabil 18:469-476, 1997.

6. Mallonee S, Istre GR, Rosenberg M, et al: Surveillance and prevention of residential-fire injuries. N Engl J Med 335:27-31, 1996.

7. Bull JP, Fisher AJ: A study in mortality in a burn unit: Standards for the evaluation for alternative methods of treatment. Ann Surg 130:160-173, 1949.

8. Rashid A, Khanna A, Gowar JP, et al: Revised estimates of mortality from burns in the last 20 years at the Birmingham Burns Centre. Burns 27:723-730, 2001.

9. Wolf SE, Rose JK, Desai MH, et al: Mortality determinants in massive pediatric burns: An analysis of 103 children with ≥80% TBSA burns (≥70% full-thickness). Ann Surg 225:554-569, 1997.

10. Committee on Trauma, American College of Surgeons: Resources for Optimal Care of the Injured Patient. Chicago, American College of Surgeons, 1999.

11. Vo LT, Papworth GD, Delaney PM, et al: A study of vascular response to thermal injury on hairless mice by fibre optic confocal imaging, laser Doppler flowmetry, and conventional histology. Burns 24:319-324, 1998.

12. Demling RH, LaLonde C: Early postburn lipid peroxidation: Effect of ibuprofen and allopurinol. Surgery 107:85-93, 1990.

13. Morykwas MJ, David LR, Schneider AM, et al: Use of subatmospheric pressure to prevent progression of partial-thickness burns in a swine model. J Burn Care Rehabil 20:15-21, 1999.

14. Nwariaku FE, Sikes PJ, Lightfoot E, et al: Effect of a bradykinin antagonist on the local inflammatory response following thermal injury. Burns 22:324-327, 1996.

15. Chappell VL, LaGrone L, Mileski WJ: Inhibition of leukocyte-mediated tissue destruction by synthetic fibronectin peptide (Trp-9-Tyr). J Burn Care Rehabil 20:505-510, 1999.

16. Atiles L, Mileski W, Spann K, et al: Early assessment of pediatric burn wounds by laser Doppler flowmetry. J Burn Care Rehabil 16:596-601, 1995.

17. Holland AJ, Martin HC, Cass DT: Laser Doppler imaging prediction of burn wound outcome in children. Burns 28:11-17, 2002.

18. Kloppenberg FW, Beerthuizen GI, ten Duis HJ: Perfusion of burn wounds assessed by laser Doppler imaging is related to burn depth and healing time. Burns 27:359-363, 2001.

19. Kinsky MP, Guha SC, Button BM, et al: The role of interstitial Starling forces in the pathogenesis of burn edema. J Burn Care Rehabil 19:1-9, 1998.

20. Holliman CJ, Meuleman TR, Larsen KR, et al: The effect of ketanserin, a specific serotonin antagonist, on burn shock hemodynamic parameters in a porcine burn model. J Trauma 23:867-871, 1983.

21. Ferrara JJ, Westervelt CL, Kukuy EL, et al: Burn edema reduction by methysergide is not due to control of regional vasodilation. J Surg Res 61:11-16, 1996.

22. Matsuda T, Tanaka H, Reyes HM, et al: Antioxidant therapy using high-dose vitamin C: Reduction of postburn resuscitation fluid volume requirements. World J Surg 19:287-291, 1995.

23. Ramzy PI, Wolf SE, Irtun O, et al: Gut epithelial apoptosis after severe burn: Effects of gut hypoperfusion. J Am Coll Surg 190:281-287, 2000.

24. Pruitt BA Jr, Mason AD Jr, Moncrief JA: Hemodynamic changes in the early postburn patient: The influence of fluid administration and of a vasodilator (hydralazine). J Trauma 11:36-46, 1971.

25. Ferrara JJ, Franklin EW, Kukuy EL, et al: Lymph isolated from a regional scald injury produces a negative inotropic effect in dogs. J Burn Care Rehabil 19:296-304, 1998.

26. Cioffi WG, DeMeules JE, Gamelli RL: The effects of burn injury and fluid resuscitation on cardiac function in vitro. J Trauma 26:638-642, 1986.

27. Leblanc M, Thibeault Y, Querin S: Continuous haemofiltration and haemodiafiltration for acute renal failure in severely burned patients. Burns 23:160-165, 1997.

28. Chrysopoulo MT, Jeschke MG, Dziewulski P, et al: Acute renal dysfunction in severely burned adults. J Trauma 46:141-144, 1999.

29. Jeschke MG, Barrow RE, Wolf SE, et al: Mortality in burned children with acute renal failure. Arch Surg 133:752-756, 1998.

30. LeVoyer T, Cioffi WG Jr, Pratt L, et al: Alterations in intestinal permeability after thermal injury. Arch Surg 127:26-30, 1992.

31. Wolf SE, Ikeda H, Matin S, et al: Cutaneous burn increases apoptosis in the gut epithelium of mice. J Am Coll Surg 188:10-16, 1999.

32. Ezzell RM, Carter EA, Yarmush ML, et al: Thermal injury–induced changes in the rat intestine brush border cytoskeleton. Surgery 114:591-597, 1993.

33. Carter EA, Udall JN, Kirkham SE, et al: Thermal injury and gastrointestinal function: I. Small intestinal nutrient absorption and DNA synthesis. J Burn Care Rehabil 7:469-474, 1986.

34. Deitch EA, Rutan R, Waymack JP: Trauma, shock, and gut translocation. New Horiz 4:289-299, 1996.

35. Deitch EA: Intestinal permeability is increased in burn patients shortly after injury. Surgery 107:411-416, 1990.

36. Berthiaume F, Ezzell RM, Toner M, et al: Transport of fluorescent dextrans across the rat ileum after cutaneous thermal injury. Crit Care Med 22:455-464, 1994.

37. Horton JW: Bacterial translocation after burn injury: The contribution of ischemia and permeability changes. Shock 1:286-290, 1994.

38. Gianotti L, Alexander JW, Fukushima R, et al: Translocation of *Candida albicans* is related to the blood flow of individual intestinal villi. Circ Shock 40:250-257, 1993.

39. Gamelli RL, He LK, Liu H, et al: Burn wound infection–induced myeloid suppression: The role of prostaglandin E_2, elevated adenylate cyclase, and cyclic adenosine monophosphate. J Trauma 44:469-474, 1998.

40. Shoup M, Weisenberger JM, Wang JL, et al: Mechanisms of neutropenia involving myeloid maturation arrest in burn sepsis. Ann Surg 228:112-122, 1998.

41. Chitnis D, Dickerson C, Munster AM, et al: Inhibition of apoptosis in polymorphonuclear neutrophils from burn patients. J Leukoc Biol 59:835-839, 1996.

42. Rosenthal J, Thurman GW, Cusack N, et al: Neutrophils from patients after burn injury express a deficiency of the oxidase components p47-phox and p67-phox. Blood 88:4321-4329, 1996.

43. Vindenes HA, Bjerknes R: Impaired actin polymerization and depolymerization in neutrophils from patients with thermal injury. Burns 23:131-136, 1997.

44. Hunt JP, Hunter CT, Brownstein MR, et al: The effector component of the cytotoxic T-lymphocyte response has a biphasic pattern after burn injury. J Surg Res 80:243-251, 1998.

45. Zedler S, Bone RC, Baue AE, et al: T-cell reactivity and its predictive role in immunosuppression after burns. Crit Care Med 27:66-72, 1999.

46. Kelly JL, Lyons A, Soberg CC, et al: Anti-interleukin-10 antibody restores burn-induced defects in T-cell function. Surgery 122:146-152, 1997.

47. Takagi K, Suzuki F, Barrow RE, et al: Recombinant human growth hormone modulates T_H1 and T_H2 cytokine response in burned mice. Ann Surg 228:106-111, 1998.

48. Hultman CS, Yamamoto H, deSerres S, et al: Early but not late burn wound excision partially restores viral-specific T-lymphocyte cytotoxicity. J Trauma 43:441-447, 1997.

49. Martini WZ, Irtun O, Chinkes DL, et al: Alteration of hepatic fatty acid metabolism after burn injury in pigs. JPEN J Parenter Enteral Nutr 25:310-316, 2001.

50. Moore FD: Bodily changes during surgical convalescence. Ann Surg 137:289-295, 1953.

51. Skinner A, Peat B: Burns treatment for children and adults: A study of initial burns first aid and hospital care. N Z Med J 115:U199, 2002.

52. Baxter CR: Fluid volume and electrolyte changes of the early postburn period. Clin Plast Surg 1:693-703, 1974.

53. Carvajal HF, Parks DH: Optimal composition of burn resuscitation fluids. Crit Care Med 16:695-700, 1988.

54. Demling RH, Mazess RB, Witt RM, et al: The study of burn wound edema using dichromatic absorptiometry. J Trauma 18:124-128, 1978.

55. Gunn ML, Hansbrough JF, Davis JW, et al: Prospective, randomized trial of hypertonic sodium lactate versus lactated Ringer's solution for burn shock resuscitation. J Trauma 29:1261-1267, 1989.

56. Huang PP, Stucky FS, Dimick AR, et al: Hypertonic sodium resuscitation is associated with renal failure and death. Ann Surg 221:543-557, 1995.

57. Cartotto RC, Innes M, Musgrave MA, et al: How well does the Parkland formula estimate actual fluid resuscitation volumes? J Burn Care Rehabil 23:258-265, 2002.

58. Alderson P, Bunn F, Lefebvre C, et al: Human albumin solution for resuscitation and volume expansion in critically ill patients. Cochrane Database Syst Rev CD001208, 2002.

59. Wilkes MM, Navickis RJ: Patient survival after human albumin administration: A meta-analysis of randomized, controlled trials. Ann Intern Med 135:149-164, 2001.

60. Zdolsek HJ, Lisander B, Jones AW, et al: Albumin supplementation during the first week after a burn does not mobilise tissue oedema in humans. Intensive Care Med 27:844-852, 2001.

61. Basadre JO, Sugi K, Traber DL, et al: The effect of leukocyte depletion on smoke inhalation injury in sheep. Surgery 104:208-215, 1988.

62. Ventilation with lower tidal volumes as compared with traditional tidal volumes for acute lung injury and the acute respiratory distress syndrome. The Acute Respiratory Distress Syndrome Network. N Engl J Med 342:1301-1308, 2000.

63. Cox CS Jr, Zwischenberger JB, Traber DL, et al: Heparin improves oxygenation and minimizes barotrauma after severe smoke inhalation in an ovine model. Surg Gynecol Obstet 176:339-349, 1993.

64. Desai MH, Mlcak R, Richardson J, et al: Reduction in mortality in pediatric patients with inhalation injury with aerosolized heparin/N-acetylcysteine [correction of acetylcystine] therapy. J Burn Care Rehabil 19:210-212, 1998.

65. Cioffi WG, Graves TA, McManus WF, et al: High-frequency percussive ventilation in patients with inhalation injury. J Trauma 29:350-354, 1989.

66. Harrington DT, Jordan BS, Dubick MA, et al: Delayed partial liquid ventilation shows no efficacy in the treatment of smoke inhalation injury in swine. J Appl Physiol 90:2351-2360, 2001.

67. Lal S, Barrow RE, Wolf SE, et al: Biobrane improves wound healing in burned children without increased risk of infection. Shock 14:314-319, 2000.

68. Lukish JR, Eichelberger MR, Newman KD, et al: The use of a bioactive skin substitute decreases length of stay for pediatric burn patients. J Pediatr Surg 36:1118-1121, 2001.

69. Heimbach DM, Warden GD, Luterman A, et al: Multicenter postapproval clinical trial of Integra® dermal regeneration template for burn treatment. J Burn Care Rehabil 24:42-48, 2003.

70. Dantzer E, Braye FM: Reconstructive surgery using an artificial dermis (Integra): Results with 39 grafts. Br J Plast Surg 54:659-664, 2001.

71. van Zuijlen PP, Vloemans JF, van Trier AJ, et al: Dermal substitution in acute burns and reconstructive surgery: A subjective and objective long-term follow-up. Plast Reconstr Surg 108:1938-1946, 2001.

72. Herndon DN, Parks DH: Comparison of serial débridement and autografting and early massive excision with cadaver skin overlay in the treatment of large burns in children. J Trauma 26:149-152, 1986.

73. Xiao-Wu W, Herndon DN, Spies M, et al: Effects of delayed wound excision and grafting in severely burned children. Arch Surg 137:1049-1054, 2002.

74. Desai MH, Rutan RL, Herndon DN: Conservative treatment of scald burns is superior to early excision. J Burn Care Rehabil 12:482-484, 1991.

75. Barret JP, Wolf SE, Desai MH, et al: Cost-efficacy of cultured epidermal autografts in massive pediatric burns. Ann Surg 231:869-876, 2000.

76. Herndon DN, Barrow RE, Kunkel KR, et al: Effects of recombinant human growth hormone on donor-site healing in severely burned children. Ann Surg 212:424-431, 1990.

77. Herndon DN, Hawkins HK, Nguyen TT, et al: Characterization of growth hormone–enhanced donor site healing in patients with large cutaneous burns. Ann Surg 221:649-659, 1995.

78. Pierre EJ, Barrow RE, Hawkins HK, et al: Effects of insulin on wound healing. J Trauma 44:342-345, 1998.

79. Zhang XJ, Chinkes DL, Irtun O, et al: Anabolic action of insulin on skin wound protein is augmented by exogenous amino acids. Am J Physiol Endocrinol Metab 282:E1308-E1315, 2002.

80. Mann R, Gibran NS, Engrav LH, et al: Prospective trial of thick versus standard split-thickness skin grafts in burns of the hand. J Burn Care Rehabil 22:390-392, 2001.

81. Scherer LA, Shiver S, Chang M, et al: The vacuum-assisted closure device: A method of securing skin grafts and improving graft survival. Arch Surg 137:930-934, 2002.

82. Bone RC, Grodzin CJ, Balk RA: Sepsis: A new hypothesis for pathogenesis of the disease process. Chest 112:235-243, 1997.

83. Muckart DJ, Bhagwanjee S: American College of Chest Physicians/Society of Critical Care Medicine Consensus Conference definitions of the systemic inflammatory response syndrome and allied disorders in relation to critically injured patients. Crit Care Med 25:1789-1795, 1997.

84. Cumming J, Purdue GF, Hunt JL, et al: Objective estimates of the incidence and consequences of multiple organ dys-

function and sepsis after burn trauma. J Trauma 50:510-515, 2001.

85. Palmieri TL, Jackson W, Greenhalgh DG: Benefits of early tracheostomy in severely burned children. Crit Care Med 30:922-924, 2002.

86. Saffle JR, Morris SE, Edelman L: Early tracheostomy does not improve outcome in burn patients. J Burn Care Rehabil 23:431-438, 2002.

87. Harrington DT, Mozingo DW, Cancio L, et al: Thermally injured patients are at significant risk for thromboembolic complications. J Trauma 50:495-499, 2001.

88. Goran MI, Peters EJ, Herndon DN, et al: Total energy expenditure in burned children using the doubly labeled water technique. Am J Physiol 259:E576-E585, 1990.

89. Curreri PW: Nutritional support of burn patients. World J Surg 2:215-222, 1978.

90. Hildreth MA, Herndon DN, Desai MH, et al: Current treatment reduces calories required to maintain weight in pediatric patients with burns. J Burn Care Rehabil 11:405-409, 1990.

91. Aarsland A, Chinkes D, Wolfe RR, et al: Beta-blockade lowers peripheral lipolysis in burn patients receiving growth hormone: Rate of hepatic very low-density lipoprotein triglyceride secretion remains unchanged. Ann Surg 223:777-789, 1996.

92. Herndon DN, Barrow RE, Stein M, et al: Increased mortality with intravenous supplemental feeding in severely burned patients. J Burn Care Rehabil 10:309-313, 1989.

93. Hart DW, Wolf SE, Chinkes DL, et al: Beta-blockade and growth hormone after burn. Ann Surg 236:450-457, 2002.

94. Debroy MA, Wolf SE, Zhang XJ, et al: Anabolic effects of insulin-like growth factor in combination with insulin-like growth factor binding protein-3 in severely burned adults. J Trauma 47:904-911, 1999.

95. Thomas SJ, Morimoto K, Herndon DN, et al: The effect of prolonged euglycemic hyperinsulinemia on lean body mass after severe burn. Surgery 132:341-347, 2002.

96. Hart DW, Wolf SE, Ramzy PI, et al: Anabolic effects of oxandrolone after severe burn. Ann Surg 233:556-564, 2001.

97. Ferrando AA, Sheffield-Moore M, Wolf SE, et al: Testosterone administration in severe burns ameliorates muscle catabolism. Crit Care Med 29:1936-1942, 2001.

98. Herndon DN, Hart DW, Wolf SE, et al: Reversal of catabolism by beta-blockade after severe burns. N Engl J Med 345:1223-1229, 2001.

99. Kildal M, Andersson G, Fugl-Meyer AR, et al: Development of a brief version of the Burn Specific Health Scale (BSHS-B). J Trauma 51:740-746, 2001.

100. Blakeney P, Meyer W III, Robert R, et al: Long-term psychosocial adaptation of children who survive burns involving 80% or greater total body surface area. J Trauma 44:625-634, 1998.

101. Meyer WJ III, Robert R, Murphy L, et al: Evaluating the psychosocial adjustment of 2- and 3-year-old pediatric burn survivors. J Burn Care Rehabil 21:178-184, 2000.

102. Brych SB, Engrav LH, Rivara FP, et al: Time off work and return to work rates after burns: Systematic review of the literature and a large two-center series. J Burn Care Rehabil 22:401-405, 2001.

103. Mozingo DW, Smith AA, McManus WF, et al: Chemical burns. J Trauma 28:642-647, 1988.

CHAPTER 23

BITES AND STINGS

Robert L. Norris, M.D., Paul S. Auerbach, M.D., M.S. and Elaine E. Nelson, M.D.

Snakebites	Arthropod Bites and Stings
Mammalian Bites	Marine Bites and Stings

SNAKEBITES

Epidemiology

An estimated 50,000 to 100,000 individuals die each year worldwide from venomous snakebites. Those at greatest risk include agricultural workers and hunters living in tropical countries.[1] In the United States, approximately 8000 bites by venomous snakes occur,[2] with approximately six deaths each year.[3] Venomous species indigenous to the United States can be found in all states except Alaska, Maine, and Hawaii. The typical victim is a young male, often intoxicated, bitten on an extremity. Lower extremity bites tend to result from stepping near a snake, whereas purposeful handling of a snake is more likely to produce a bite to the upper extremity. Snakes are poikilothermic, which accounts for the higher incidence of bites during warmer months.[2]

Species

In the United States, bites by snakes of the subfamily Crotalinae (pit vipers), which include the rattlesnakes (Fig. 23-1), copperheads, and cottonmouths, account for 99% of medically significant bites. Only 1% of bites are attributable to the other family of venomous snakes in the United States, the Elapidae (coral snakes).[4]

Several characteristics distinguish pit vipers from nonvenomous snakes. Pit vipers tend to have relatively triangular heads; elliptical pupils; heat-sensing facial pits; large, retractable anterior fangs; and a single row of subcaudal scales. Nonvenomous snakes often have more rounded heads, circular pupils, no fangs, and a double row of subcaudal scales (Fig. 23-2). Coral snakes possess a red, black, and yellow–banded pattern. In the United States, the alignment of red bands next to yellow reliably differentiates coral snakes from nonvenomous mimics. There are three species of coral snakes in the United States—the eastern and Texas coral snakes (*Micrurus fulvius fulvius* and *Micrurus fulvius tenere,* respectively) and the Arizona coral snake (*Micruroides euryxanthus*).

Toxicology

Snake venoms are complex, possessing many peptides and enzymes. Peptides can damage vascular endothelium, increasing permeability and leading to edema and hypovolemic shock. Enzymes include proteases and L-amino acid oxidase, which cause tissue necrosis; hyaluronidase, which facilitates the spread of venom through tissues; and phospholipase A_2, which damages erythrocytes and muscle cells. Other enzymes include endonucleases, alkaline phosphatase, acid phosphatase, and cholinesterase.[4,5] Besides causing local injury, these components also have deleterious effects on the cardiovascular, pulmonary, renal, and neurologic systems.[6] Other components of the venom profoundly affect coagulation, fibrinolysis, platelet function, and vascular integrity, sometimes producing hemorrhagic or thrombotic sequelae.[7]

Clinical Manifestations

Local

Approximately 20% of bites by pit vipers lack any venom injection ("dry bites").[8] The only findings in such cases include puncture wounds or lacerations and minimal pain. Actual venom poisoning produces burning pain within

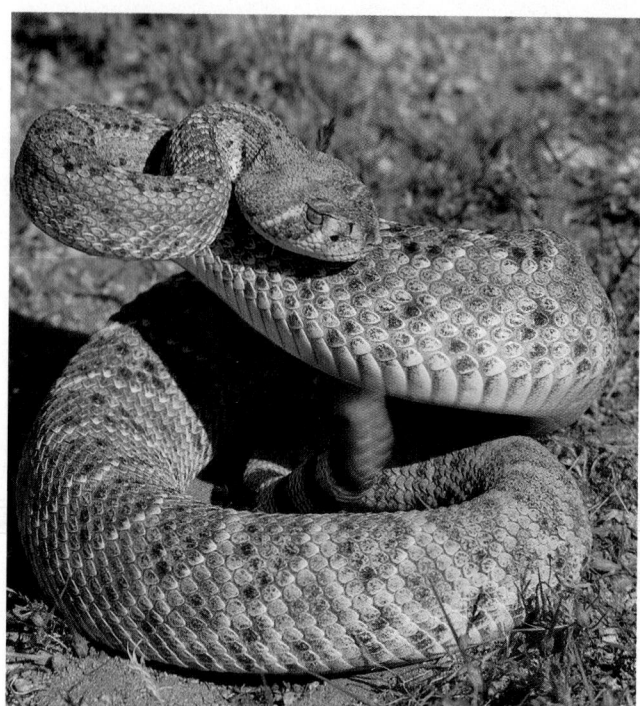

FIGURE 23-1. A typical North American pit viper—the western diamondback rattlesnake, *Crotalus atrox.* (Courtesy of Michael Cardwell.)

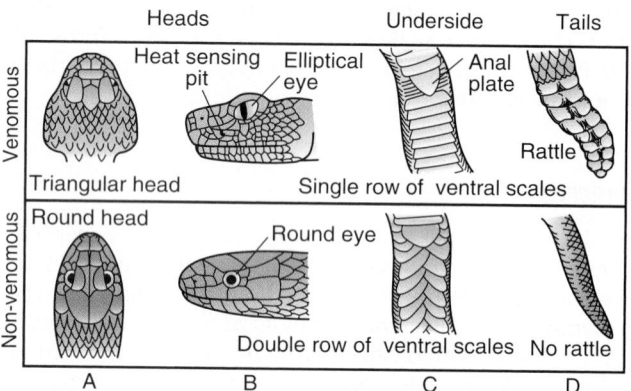

FIGURE 23-2. Comparison of pit vipers and nonvenomous snakes. Rattle in *D (top panel)* applies to rattlesnakes only. (**A** to **D**, From Sullivan JB, Wingert WA, Norris RL: North American venomous reptile bites. *In* Auerbach PS [ed]: Wilderness Medicine: Management of Wilderness and Environmental Emergencies, 3rd ed. St. Louis, Mosby–Year Book, 1995, p 684.)

minutes, followed by edema and erythema. Swelling progresses over the next few hours, and ecchymoses and hemorrhagic bullae may appear (Fig. 23-3). Involvement of the lymphatic system is common, causing lymphangitis and lymphadenopathy.[4,6] With delayed or inadequate treatment, severe tissue necrosis can occur.

Systemic

Patients may complain of weakness, nausea, vomiting, perioral paresthesias, metallic taste, and muscle twitch-

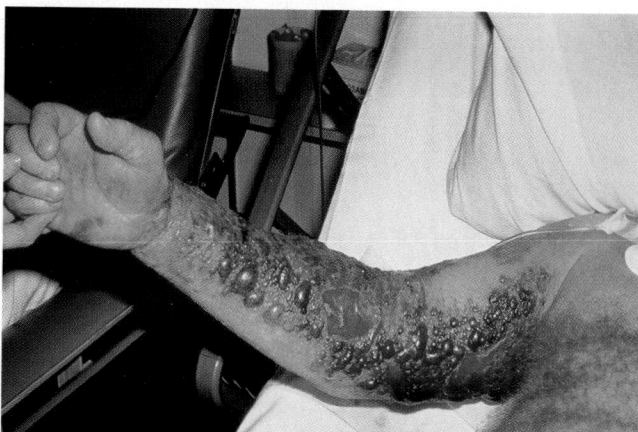

FIGURE 23-3. A case of severe venom poisoning by a western diamondback rattlesnake (*Crotalus atrox*) at four days following the bite. Note the soft tissue swelling, and hemorrhagic and serum-filled vesicles. (Courtesy of David Hardy, MD.)

ing.[6,9] Diffuse capillary leakage leads to pulmonary edema, hypotension, and eventually shock. In victims of severe bites, a consumptive coagulopathy can develop within an hour.[7] Such patients can spontaneously bleed from almost any anatomic site, though clinically significant bleeding is uncommon, even in the face of significantly abnormal coagulation tests. Acute renal failure resulting from direct nephrotoxins, circulatory collapse, myoglobinuria, and consumptive coagulopathy are possible. Laboratory abnormalities may include hypofibrinogenemia, thrombocytopenia, prolonged prothrombin and partial thromboplastin times; increased fibrin split products; elevated creatinine and creatine phosphokinase; proteinuria; hematuria; and anemia or hemoconcentration.[7,9]

Unlike pit viper venoms, which tend to affect multiple-organ systems, coral snake venom is primarily neurotoxic. Local injury is generally minimal or absent. Systemic signs of coral snake bites, including cranial nerve dysfunction and loss of deep tendon reflexes, may progress to respiratory depression and paralysis over several hours.[4] Differences in therapy make it important to distinguish between coral snake and pit viper bites.

Management

Field Treatment

The patient should be removed from the vicinity of the snake and placed at rest. The wound should be cleansed and immobilized at approximately heart level if possible. Cryotherapy, incision and suction, tourniquets, and electric shock therapy are harmful and must be avoided. Although syringe-type suction devices have been recommended for field management of snakebites in the past, there are no data available to suggest any beneficial effect, and some preliminary research suggests that they could, in fact, be harmful.[10] Most pit viper bites in the United States pose more of a threat to local tissues than to the life of the victim, and the use of any method to limit venom to the bite site may be ill advised. The use of a lymphoveno-occlusive constriction band should be considered following a pit viper bite only if the victim has been bitten by a large, dangerous snake, is more than 1 hour from medical care, and with the realization that local tissue effects could be worsened by these measures. The Australian pressure-immobilization technique in which the entire bitten extremity is snugly wrapped with a bandage, beginning at the bite site, and splinted has been demonstrated in small studies to significantly limit systemic spread of various snake venoms.[3] This technique is the field treatment of choice for a non-necrotizing bite such as a coral snake but again could make the local necrosis worse following a pit viper bite. Field measures must not delay transport to the nearest hospital appropriately equipped to handle a venomous snakebite.

Hospital Management

Any snake brought in with the patient for identification should be handled cautiously. Even dead snakes and severed heads can still have a bite reflex for up to an hour.

A rapid, detailed history of the incident, type of snake, field management, and previous antivenom exposure is important. Physical assessment should emphasize vital signs, cardiopulmonary status, neurologic examination, and wound appearance and size. The bitten extremity should be marked in two or three locations so that circumferences can be measured every 15 minutes to judge progression of local findings. Such measurements should continue until swelling has clearly stabilized.

Necessary laboratory analyses include a complete blood count, coagulation studies (prothrombin time, partial thromboplastin time, fibrin degradation products, fibrinogen level), electrolytes, blood urea nitrogen, creatinine, creatine phosphokinase, and urinalysis. No laboratory studies are necessary for a coral snake bite. A chest radiograph and electrocardiogram should be obtained in older patients and in any patient with severe poisoning.

If the patient is completely asymptomatic 6 hours after a pit viper bite or 24 hours after a coral snake bite, and all laboratory results are normal, it is unlikely that venom poisoning occurred, and discharge is acceptable. All envenomed patients are best observed for at least 24 hours in the hospital.

Antivenom Therapy

Deciding when to administer antivenom to a victim of venomous snakebite requires significant clinical judgment. The treating physician must quickly weigh the potential benefits of giving a heterologous antiserum to the victim in an effort to halt progression of venom poisoning against the risks inherent in administration of such a product—anaphylaxis, anaphylactoid reaction, or serum sickness. Furthermore, as snake venom poisoning is a dynamic process, the decision for or against antivenom must be re-evaluated as the syndrome declares its severity over time. Currently, antivenom should be administered to any patient with evidence of venom poisoning and clear progression in severity after arrival at the hospital, or without delay in any patient with clearly serious poisoning (i.e., severe swelling, hypotension, respiratory distress).

In the United States, there are currently two pit viper antivenoms commercially available. Antivenin (Crotalidae) Polyvalent (ACP) (Wyeth-Ayerst Laboratories, Philadelphia, PA) has been available for more than 40 years, but its future production is in doubt. Until existing supplies are exhausted, it can be administered as per the package insert. In 2000, the U.S. Food and Drug Administration (FDA) approved a second pit viper antivenom for use in this country, CroFab (Protherics, Inc., London). This product, produced in sheep and purified using Fab technology, appears to be more effective and safer to use than ACP (see later).[11-13] It also has the advantage of not requiring any skin testing or pretreatment of the victim with antihistamines before administration.

CroFab is given intravenously as four to six vials in 250 mL of diluent over approximately an hour. If, after the initial dose, there is progression of venom poisoning severity over the next hour, the loading dose should be repeated. This sequence should be repeated as needed until the victim has stabilized. Following stabilization, to prevent recurrence of venom effects, repeat dosing of CroFab should occur at a dose of two vials intravenously every 6 hours for three additional doses.[13] The same dosing regimen is used for children, and pregnancy is not a contraindication to antivenom therapy.

A separate antivenom, North American Coral Snake Antivenin, also produced by Wyeth-Ayerst, is available for eastern and Texas coral snake bites. Administration is similar to that for ACP except that therapy should be initiated in all cases in which a positively identified coral snake bite has occurred—even in the absence of local or systemic symptoms—because these may be delayed many hours in onset. Once established, venom poisoning can be hard to reverse, even with the use of antivenom. There is no antivenom produced to treat Arizona coral snake bites, but there have been no reported fatalities following bites by this small animal. The future availability of coral snake antivenom in the United States is in doubt because it appears that Wyeth-Ayerst may cease its production.

Any currently available snakebite antivenom carries some risk of acute allergic reaction (either anaphylactic or anaphylactoid) and delayed serum sickness. Epinephrine should always be immediately available when such products are being administered, and patients should be warned of the symptoms of serum sickness prior to discharge from the hospital. Serum sickness is generally easily treated with steroids and antihistamines.

Poison control centers and zoos can provide important information regarding management of the occasional exotic snakebite that occurs in the United States to a zookeeper or private hobbyist. The University of Arizona Poison and Drug Information Center (telephone, 520-626-6016) is a useful source of information for physicians needing help in managing venomous snakebite.

Wound Care/Blood Products

The bite site should be cleansed thoroughly and the extremity splinted and elevated. Good conservative wound care is indicated, with surgical débridement of clearly necrotic tissue performed as necessary after any coagulopathy has resolved. Tetanus toxoid and tetanus immune globulin should be administered as appropriate. Antibiotics should be reserved for the rare wound that develops secondary infection.[14,15]

Blood products are needed only in the rare setting of clinically significant bleeding that is not reversed with antivenom. Patients with serious bleeding (e.g., gastrointestinal bleeding, intracranial bleeding, hemoptysis) may need packed red cells, platelets, or fresh frozen plasma, depending on the scenario and the results of serial complete blood counts and coagulation studies. Antivenom must be started before these second-line agents are infused, however.[16] Patients who developed a coagulopathy while in the hospital following a pit viper bite should be warned that coagulation abnormalities can recur for up to 2 weeks following the bite, even after antivenom therapy.[17] They should be warned to look for signs of bleeding and to avoid any elective surgery during this period.

Fasciotomy

Most snakebites result in subcutaneous deposition of venom. Venom that is deposited by larger snakes into muscle compartments, however, can result in an increase in intracompartmental pressures. Clinically differentiating a true compartment syndrome from the typical swollen, painful extremity seen in subcutaneous poisoning is difficult and may require the measurement of compartmental pressures. Fasciotomies should be considered only if pressures are documented to exceed 30 to 40 mm Hg despite antivenom treatment and elevation (Fig. 23-4). In a hemo-

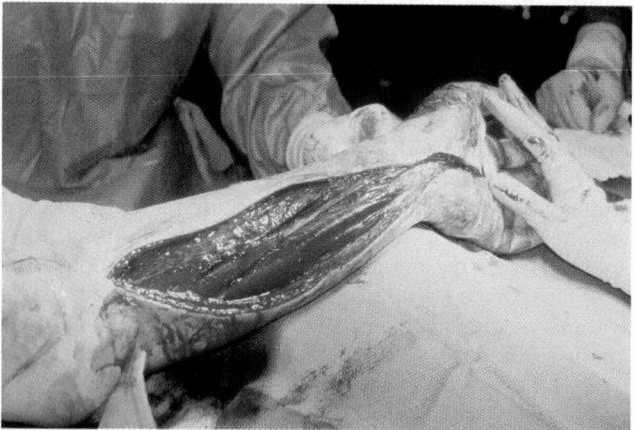

FIGURE 23-4. Fasciotomy of the forearm compartments in a victim of severe rattlesnake bite to the hand. The intracompartmental pressures were documented to be exceedingly elevated in this patient despite limb elevation and large doses of antivenom. (Courtesy of Robert Norris, MD.)

dynamically stable patient, a trial of intravenous mannitol in addition to antivenom and elevation may obviate the need for surgery if intracompartmental pressures can be reduced within approximately 1 hour. In areas too small to measure pressures (e.g., the digits), increased pressure may be suspected when pricking the skin of the affected digit yields dark venous blood flow.[18] There is no role for routine or prophylactic fasciotomy in venomous snakebite.[19]

MAMMALIAN BITES

Epidemiology

The actual incidence of mammalian bite injuries is unknown because most patients with minor wounds never seek medical care. Although death from animal bites is uncommon in the United States, thousands of people are killed around the world each year, primarily by large animals such as lions and tigers. Dogs are responsible for 80% to 90% of animal bites in the United States, followed by cats and humans.[20] An estimated 4 million dog bites occur annually, accounting for 1% of emergency department visits.[20,21] Animal bites occur most frequently to the extremities in adults and to the head, face, and neck in children.[21] More than 60% of the reported cases of bites occur in children, especially boys 5 to 9 years of age.[21]

Treatment

Evaluation

Humans attacked by animals are at risk for blunt and penetrating trauma. Animals produce blunt injuries by striking with their head or extremities, biting with powerful jaws, and crushing with their body weight. Teeth and claws can puncture body cavities, including the cranium, and amputate extremities. Patients with serious injuries should be managed as major trauma victims, with special attention being given to wound management. Useful laboratory tests include a hematocrit when blood loss is of concern and cultures when an infection is present. Radiographs should be obtained to diagnose potential fractures, joint penetration, severe infections, and presence of foreign bodies, such as teeth. The patient's tetanus status should be updated as necessary.

Wound Care

Local wound management prevents infection and maximizes functional and aesthetic outcomes. Early wound cleansing is the most important therapy for preventing infection and contracting rabies. Intact skin surrounding dirty wounds can be scrubbed with a sponge and 1% povidone-iodine solution. Contamination of the wound with skin flora should be minimized. Copious irrigation of the wound with normal saline or tap water using a 19-gauge needle and syringe significantly decreases the likelihood of infection.[20] Alternatively, a 1% povidone-iodine solution can be used, as long as the wound is irrigated afterward with normal saline or water. Scrubbing the wound surface itself can increase tissue damage and infection and should be avoided. Wounds that are dirty or contain devitalized tissue should be cleansed lightly with gauze or a porous sponge and débrided.[20]

Options for wound repair include primary, delayed primary, and secondary closure. The anatomic location of the bite, the source of the bite, and the type of injury determine the appropriate method. Contrary to past beliefs, primary closure of selected bites produces the best outcome for patients without increasing the risk of infection.[20,22] This is especially true for head and neck wounds, for which aesthetic results are more important and infection rates are low.[23] Severe human bites and avulsion injuries of the face that require flaps have been successfully repaired with primary closure; however, this technique remains controversial.[23] Healing by secondary intention generally produces unacceptable scars in cosmetic areas.

Bites involving the hands or feet have a much greater chance of becoming infected and should be left open initially.[20] The primary goal in repairing bite wounds to the hand is to maximize functional outcome. Approximately one third of dog bites to the hand become infected, even with adequate therapy.[24] Healing by secondary intention is recommended for most hand lacerations.[20] After a thorough exploration, irrigation, and débridement, the hand should be immobilized, wrapped in a bulky dressing, and elevated.

A common human bite wound associated with a high morbidity rate is the clenched fist injury. Regardless of the history obtained, injuries over the dorsum of the metacarpophalangeal joints should be treated as clenched fist injuries resulting from striking another person's mouth. The extensor tendon retracts when the hand is opened, so evaluation needs to be done with the hand in both the open and the clenched positions. Minor injuries should be irrigated, débrided, and left open. Potentially deeper injuries and infected bites that are seen after 24 hours require exploration and débridement in the operating room and administration of intravenous antibiotics.[25]

The method of repair used for bite wounds to other body parts depends on the risk factors associated with the particular injury (Box 23-1). Delayed primary repair or healing by secondary intention should be considered for high-risk bites, whereas early primary closure can be performed safely in low-risk bites.[20] Primary closure can be used for low-risk wounds to the arms and legs presenting within 6 to 12 hours and for the face presenting in 12 to 24 hours or possibly days.[20] Puncture wounds have an increased incidence of infection and should not be sutured. Deep irrigation of small puncture wounds and wide excision have not proved to be beneficial. Larger puncture wounds can benefit from irrigation and débridement, however.[20,24] Sterile, dry dressings should be placed over all wounds. Wounds should be re-evaluated in 2 days if considered low risk or in 1 day if considered high risk or infected.

Box 23-1. Animal Bite Risk Factors for Infection

High Risk

Location
   Hand, wrist, or foot
   Scalp or face in infants (high risk of cranial perforation; skull radiograph mandatory)
   Over a major joint (possible perforation)
   Through-and-through bite of cheek
Type of wound
   Puncture (difficult to irrigate)
   Tissue crushing that cannot be débrided
   Carnivore bite over vital structure (artery, nerve, joint)
Patient
   Older than 50 years
   Asplenic
   Chronic alcoholic
   Altered immune status
   Diabetic
   Peripheral vascular insufficiency
   Chronic corticosteroid therapy
   Prosthetic or diseased heart valve or joint
Species
   Domestic cat
   Large cat (deep punctures)
   Human (hand bites)
   Primates
   Pigs

Low Risk

Location
   Face, scalp, ears, or mouth
Type of wound
   Large, clean lacerations that can be thoroughly irrigated
Species
   Rodents

Adapted from Keogh S, Callaham ML: Bites and injuries inflicted by domestic animals. In Auerbach PS (ed): Wilderness Medicine: Management of Wilderness and Environmental Emergencies, 4th ed. St. Louis, Mosby, 2001, pp 961-978.

Microbiology

Given the large variety and concentration of bacteria in mouths, it is not surprising that wound infection is the main complication of bites, occurring in 3% to 18% of dog bites and in approximately 50% of cat bites.[26] Infections are usually polymicrobial, with both aerobic and anaerobic bacteria (Box 23-2). *Staphylococcus* and *Streptococcus* species and anaerobes are present in most infections. *Pasteurella multocida* is the primary microorganism responsible for infections in cat bites (including large, wild cats) and is isolated in 25% of infected dog bites.[27] *Eikenella corrodens* has been isolated from human bites.[20,25] Many microorganisms that are present locally can progress to

Box 23-2. Common Bacteria Found in Animals' Mouths

Actinobacillus species
Peptococcus species
Propionibacterium species
Bacteroides species
Micrococcus species
Leptotrichia bacillus
Staphylococcus aureus
Streptococcus species
Bacillus species
Corynebacterium species
Eubacterium species
Pasteurella aerogenes
Pseudomonas species
Eikenella corrodens
Neisseria species
Clostridium perfringens
Brucella canis
Haemophilus haemolyticus

Fusobacterium species
Peptostreptococcus species
Veillonella parvula
Escherichia coli
Moraxella species
Staphylococcus epidermidis
Acinetobacter species
Enterobacter species
Serratia marcescens
Proteus mirabilis
Aeromonas hydrophila
Pasteurella dagmatis, canis
Pasteurella multocida
Haemophilus aphrophilus
Klebsiella species
Capnocytophaga canimorsus
Bordetella species

Data from: Dire DJ: Emergency management of dog and cat bite wounds. Emerg Med Clin North Am 10:719-736, 1992; and Keogh S, Callaham ML: Bites and injuries inflicted by domestic animals. In Auerbach PS (ed): Wilderness Medicine: Management of Wilderness and Environmental Emergencies, 4th ed. St. Louis: Mosby, 2001, pp 961-978.

TABLE 23-1. Atypical Organisms Associated With Bite Wounds and Unusual Sources

Source	Pathogen*
Alligator	Aeromonas hydrophila
Bear	Similar to dogs
Cat	Afpia felis (cat scratch disease) Rochalimaea (bacillary angiomatosis) Cowpox
Cat family (wild)	Pasteurella species
Coyote	Francisella tularensis
Human	Syphilis Tuberculosis Herpes Hepatitis B and C Human immunodeficiency virus (?)
Lion	Pasteurella species
Livestock	Brucella (brucellosis) Pasteurella species
Opossum	Pasteurella species
Platypus	Venomous spurs
Primate	Eikenella corrodens
Rabbit	Francisella tularensis
Rodent	Streptobacillus moniliformis, Spirillum minus (rat bite fever)
Short-tailed shrew	Venomous bites
Squirrel	Francisella tularensis

*In addition to organisms listed in Box 23-2 and excluding rabies.

systemic disease such as rabies, cat scratch, cowpox, tularemia, leptospirosis, brucellosis and human immunodeficiency virus (HIV)-1.[20] Although HIV-1 transmission from human bites is rare, several case reports suggest that this occurs.[28] Seroconversion is possible when a person with an open wound either from a bite or preexisting injury is exposed to saliva containing HIV-1–positive blood.[28] In this scenario, baseline HIV testing should be obtained and prophylactic treatment with anti-HIV-1 viral agents should be considered. Atypical pathogens and organisms from unusual sources of bites are listed in Table 23-1.

Antibiotics

Prophylactic antibiotics are recommended for patients with high-risk bites.[20,24] Initial antibiotic choice and route should be based on the type of animal and the severity and location of the bite. Cat bites often cause puncture wounds that require antibiotics. Patients with low-risk dog bites do not benefit from prophylactic antibiotics unless the hand or foot is involved. Initial antibiotic selection should cover Staphylococcus and Streptococcus species and anaerobes for all bites, in addition to Pasteurella species for dog and cat bites and E. corrodens for human bites. Amoxicillin-clavulanate is an acceptable first-line antibiotic for most bites. Alternatives include second-generation cephalosporins, such as cefoxitin, or a combination of penicillin and a first-generation cephalosporin. Penicillin-allergic nonpregnant woman can receive clindamycin and ciprofloxacin together.[20,27] Infections developing within 8 hours of the bite are usually caused by Pasteurella species. Patients seen 24 hours after a bite without signs of infection usually do not need prophylactic antibiotics. Antibiotics should be administered early and, in serious bites, parenterally. Routine cultures of uninfected wounds have not proved useful and should be reserved for infected wounds that fail antibiotic therapy.[20,24]

Rabies

Worldwide, approximately 30,000 people die of rabies annually, with dog bites or scratches being the major source.[29] Immunization of pets against rabies has decreased the number of cases to approximately one to three a year in the United States, where skunks, raccoons, and bats are the most common sources.[30] Rabies virus from bats accounts for greater than 80% of the rabies cases reported in this country during the last 20 years, with a majority of the patients unaware of contact with a bat.[30]

Rabies is caused by a rhabdovirus found in the saliva of animals and is transmitted through bites or scratches. Patients with rabies develop acute encephalitis and almost invariably die. The disease usually begins with a prodromal phase of nonspecific complaints and paresthesias, itching, or burning at the bite site. Local symptoms may spread to involve the entire bitten extremity.[29] The disease then progresses into an acute neurologic phase. This phase usually takes one of two forms: The more common encephalitic, or furious, form is typified by fever and hyperactivity that can be stimulated by internal or external stimuli such as thirst, fear, light, or noise. This is followed by fluctuating levels of consciousness, aerophobia or hydrophobia, inspiratory spasm, and abnormalities of the autonomic nervous system. The paralytic form of rabies manifests with fever, progressive weakness, loss of deep tendon reflexes, and urinary incontinence. Both forms progress to paralysis, coma, circulatory collapse, and death.[29]

Adequate wound care and postexposure prophylaxis can prevent the development of rabies. Wounds should be washed with soap and water and irrigated with a viricidal agent such as povidone-iodine solution. If suspicion is high for a rabid bite, consider leaving the wound open. The decision to administer rabies prophylaxis following an animal bite or scratch depends on the offending species and the nature of the event. Guidelines for administering rabies prophylaxis can be obtained from local public health agencies or from a recent publication by the Advisory Committee on Immunization Practices.[31] A recent study indicates that rabies prophylaxis is not being administered according to guidelines resulting in either costly overtreatment or potentially life-threatening undertreatment.[30] Unprovoked attacks are more likely to occur by rabid animals. All wild carnivores should be considered rabid, but birds and reptiles do not contract rabies. In cases of bites by domestic animals, rodents, or lagomorphs, the local health department should be consulted before beginning rabies prophylaxis.[31] A bite from a healthy-appearing domestic animal does not require prophylaxis if the animal can be observed for 10 days.[31]

Rabies prophylaxis consists of both passive and active immunization. Passive immunization consists of administering 20 IU per kg of rabies immunoglobulin (Ig). As much of the dose as possible should be infiltrated into and around the wounds.[31] The rest can be given intramuscularly at an anatomic site remote from the site of vaccine administration. Active immunization consists of administering 1 mL of human diploid cell vaccine, purified chick embryo cell vaccine, or rabies vaccine absorbed intramuscularly into the deltoid in adults and into the anterolateral thigh in children on days 0, 3, 7, 14, and 28. Patients with pre-exposure immunization do not need passive immunization and need active immunization only on days 0 and 3.[31]

ARTHROPOD BITES AND STINGS

Black Widow Spiders

Widow spiders (genus *Latrodectus)* are found throughout the world. At least one of five species inhabits all areas of the United States except Alaska.[32] The best-known widow spider is the black widow (*Latrodectus mactans*). The female has a leg span of 1 to 4 cm and a shiny black body with a distinctive red ventral marking (often hourglass shaped) (Fig. 23-5). Variations in color occur among other species, with some appearing brown or red and some without the ventral marking. The nonaggressive, female widow spider bites in defense. Males are too small to bite through human skin.

Toxicology

The black widow spider produces a neurotoxic venom with minimal local effects. The venom acts at the presynaptic terminal, enhancing neurotransmitter release. Excess acetylcholine at the neuromuscular junction causes muscle spasms, and release of norepinephrine and epinephrine produces adrenergic stimulation.[33]

Clinical Manifestations

Although it is not uncommon for the bite to go unnoticed, initially the site may be painful and slightly red with two small puncture wounds.[32,34] The patient may, however, have only systemic complaints, making the diagnosis challenging. Neuromuscular symptoms may occur as early as 30 minutes after the bite and include severe pain and spasms of large muscle groups. Abdominal cramps and rigidity could mimic a surgical abdomen, but rebound is absent. Dyspnea can result from chest wall tightness. Autonomic stimulation produces hypertension, diaphoresis, and tachycardia. Other symptoms include muscle twitching, nausea and vomiting, headache, paresthesias,

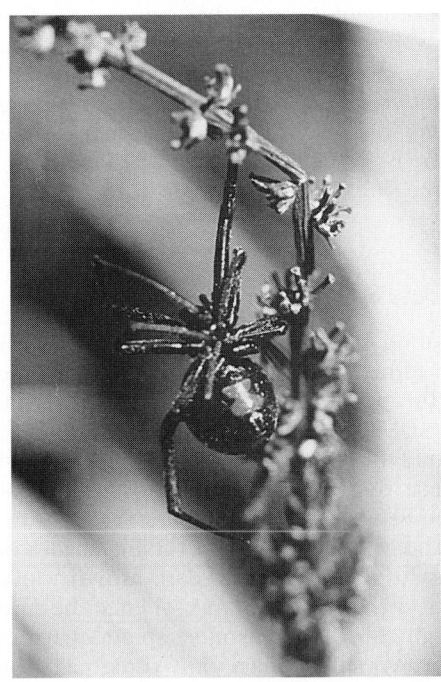

FIGURE 23-5. Female black widow spider (*Latrodectus mactans*) with the characteristic hourglass marking. (Courtesy of Paul Auerbach, MD.)

fatigue, and salivation.[32,34] Symptoms typically peak at several hours and resolve in 1 to 2 days. Mild pain and nonspecific symptoms, primarily neurologic, can persist for several weeks. Death is an unusual result of widow spider bites.

Treatment

Mild bites are managed with local wound care—cleansing, applying ice, and administering tetanus prophylaxis as needed. The possibility of delayed, severe symptoms makes an observation period of several hours prudent. The optimal therapy for severe envenomation is controversial. Intravenous calcium gluconate, previously recommended as a first-line drug to relieve muscle spasms following widow spider bite, has no significant efficacy.[32,34] Narcotics and benzodiazepines are more effective agents to relieve muscular pain.

In the United States, antivenom derived from horse serum is available (Black Widow Spider Antivenin, Merck & Co., Inc., West Point, PA). Because it can cause anaphylaxis and serum sickness, however, it should be reserved for serious cases. Antivenom is currently recommended for pregnant women, children younger than 16 years, individuals older than 60 years, and patients with severe poisoning manifesting uncontrolled hypertension or respiratory distress.[32] Skin testing (outlined in the package insert) may predict individuals who are allergic to antivenom. Patients to receive antivenom may be pretreated with antihistamines to reduce the likelihood or severity of a systemic reaction to the serum. The initial recommended dose is one vial intravenously or intramuscularly, repeated as necessary (although it is exceedingly rare for more than two vials to be required). Studies have demonstrated that antivenom can decrease a patient's hospital stay, with discharge occurring as early as several hours following administration.[34] A high-quality antivenom is also available in Australia for *Latrodectus* bites. It appears that any widow spider antivenom is effective regardless of which species inflicted the bite.[35]

Brown Recluse Spiders

Envenomation by the brown spiders of the genus *Loxosceles* is termed *necrotic arachnidism* or *loxoscelism.* These arthropods primarily inhabit North and South America, Africa, and Europe. Several species of *Loxosceles* are found throughout the United States, with the greatest concentration in the Midwest. Most significant bites in the United States are by *Loxosceles reclusa*—the brown recluse. The brown spiders are varying shades of brownish gray, with a characteristic dark brown, violin-shaped marking over the cephalothorax—hence the name *violin spider* (Fig. 23-6). Whereas most spiders have four pairs of eyes, brown spiders have only three pairs. Both male and female specimens can bite and may do so when threatened.

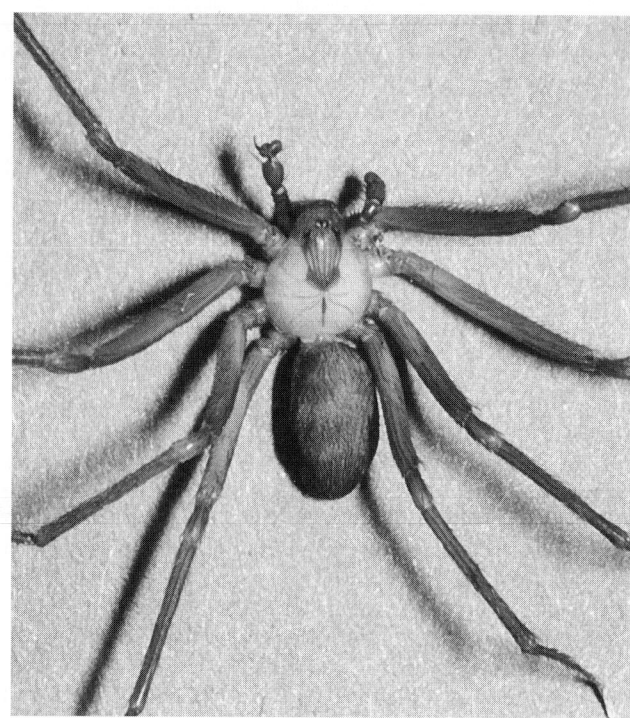

FIGURE 23-6. Brown recluse spider (*Loxosceles reclusa*) with a violin-shaped marking on the cephalothorax. (Courtesy of Sherman Minton, MD, Indiana University.)

Toxicology

Although several enzymes have been isolated from the venom, sphingomyelinase D is the major deleterious factor, causing both dermonecrosis and hemolysis.[32,36] It is a phospholipase that interacts with cell membranes of erythrocytes, platelets, and endothelial cells and causes hemolysis, coagulation, and platelet aggregation. Host responses have some significance in determining the severity of venom poisoning because functioning polymorphonuclear leukocytes and complement are necessary for the venom to have maximal effect.[36,37]

Clinical Manifestations

Local findings at the bite site range from mild irritation to severe necrosis with ulceration.[38] The patient is often completely unaware of the bite or may have felt a slight stinging. It is unusual for the victim to actually see or capture the spider. Within several hours in some patients, local tissue ischemia develops with resulting pain, itching, swelling, and erythema. A blister may form at the site. In more severe bites, the central area turns purple as a result of microvascular thrombosis. Peripheral vasoconstriction can also create a pale border surrounding the central region of necrosis. Over the next several days, the widening necrotic area develops an eschar. The eschar separates, leaving an ulcer that usually heals over many weeks to months, but occasionally requires skin grafting.[32,39] Necrosis is most severe in fatty areas such as the abdomen and thigh.[33,39]

Systemic features can include headache, nausea and vomiting, fever, malaise, arthralgias, and maculopapular rash.[32] Additional findings may include thrombocytopenia, disseminated intravascular coagulation, hemolytic anemia, coma, and, possibly, death. Renal failure can result from intravascular hemolysis.[36,39]

In patients with lesions consistent with brown spider bites, a search for evidence of systemic involvement (viscerocutaneous or systemic loxoscelism) should be initiated, particularly if the victim has any systemic complaints. Appropriate laboratory tests include a complete blood count (with platelet count) and a bedside urine test for blood. If any of these are abnormal, electrolytes, liver function studies, and coagulation studies are in order, but there are no truly diagnostic studies available. Systemic loxoscelism is more common in children and can occur with minimal local findings.[32]

Treatment

Recommended management remains controversial. The bite site should be splinted, elevated, and treated with cold compresses. Cold therapy inhibits venom activity and reduces inflammation and necrosis. Heat application, on the other hand, enhances tissue damage and ulcer development.[32,33] Although controversial, a lipophilic, prophylactic antibiotic can be administered,[33] and tetanus status should be updated. Brown spider bites in which necrosis does not develop within 72 hours usually heal well and require no additional therapy. There is no commercial antivenom available in the United States.

Some research suggests that more severe lesions may benefit from dapsone administration if given within the first few days after the bite, even though the drug is not approved for this indication.[40] Dapsone may reduce local inflammation and necrosis by inhibiting neutrophil function. The suggested adult dose is 100 mg/day. Dapsone can cause methemoglobinemia and is contraindicated in patients with glucose-6-phosphate dehydrogenase deficiency. Thus, a level of this enzyme should be checked as therapy begins and dapsone discontinued if found to be deficient.

Early surgical intervention, other than simple, conservative débridement of obviously necrotic tissue should be avoided. It is difficult or impossible to predict with any certainty the extent of eventual necrosis, and early surgery is apt to be overaggressive and needlessly disfiguring.[32] Pyoderma gangrenosum, presenting as nonhealing ulcers and failure of skin grafts, occurs more often in patients undergoing early excision and débridement, possibly as a result of the rapid spread of venom.[36] After 1 to 2 weeks, when eschar margins are defined, débridement can be performed as necessary. In severe cases, wide excision and split-thickness skin grafting are necessary while dapsone therapy is continued.[33]

Steroid administration, by any route, has never been shown to be beneficial in limiting dermonecrosis. A short course (few days) of oral steroids can help stabilize red blood cell membranes and reduce hemolysis in the setting of viscerocutaneous loxoscelism.

Patients with rapidly expanding, necrotic lesions or a clinical picture suggesting systemic loxoscelism should be admitted for close observation and management. Patients with less serious lesions can be followed up on an outpatient basis with frequent wound checks. Visits during the first 72 hours should include a reassessment for any evidence of systemic involvement.

Scorpions

Significant scorpion envenomations occur worldwide by species belonging to the family Buthidae. In this group, the bark scorpion *(Centruroides exilicauda)* is the only potentially dangerous species in the United States. It is found throughout Arizona and, occasionally, in immediately contiguous areas of surrounding states. It is a yellow to brown crablike arthropod, up to 5 cm in length. Approximately 7000 scorpion stings are reported yearly in the United States, with one third of these occurring in Arizona. Scorpions tend to be nocturnal and sting when threatened.

Clinical Manifestations

Most scorpion stings in the United States result in short-lived, searing pain and mild, local irritation with slight swelling. The bark scorpion, whose sting can, in rare cases, be lethal, produces a neurotoxin that prevents sodium channel closure. When stung, a patient typically experiences local paresthesias and burning pain. Systemic manifestations may include cranial nerve and neuromuscular hyperactivity and respiratory distress.[41,42] Signs of adrenergic stimulation, accompanied by nausea and vomiting, may also develop. Young children are at greatest risk of severe stings from the bark scorpion.

Treatment

All patients should receive tetanus prophylaxis if indicated, cold compress application to the sting site, and analgesics for pain. Victims of bark scorpion sting with signs of systemic envenomation require supportive care, with close monitoring of cardiovascular and respiratory status in an intensive care setting. Although an antivenom for this arthropod has been available in the past, production has currently ceased. The product was goat derived (with resultant risks of allergic sequelae), lacked FDA approval, and was available for use only within Arizona. Its use was highly controversial. There is an antivenom produced for related scorpions in Mexico that could eventually find application in the United States.

Ticks

Several potentially serious diseases occur from tick bites. Timely and adequate removal of the tick is important.

Common tick removal remedies, such as application of gasoline, methylated spirits, and fingernail polish, are ineffective. Proper removal involves grasping the tick by the body as close to the skin surface as possible with an instrument and applying gradual, gentle axial traction, without twisting. Commercial tick removal devices are superior to standard tweezers for this purpose.[43] Crushing the tick should be avoided because this may squeeze potentially infectious secretions into the wound. After extraction, the wound should be cleansed with alcohol or povidone-iodine. If the tick was embedded for less than 24 hours, the risk of infection transmission is very low. Tetanus immunization should be current. Occasionally, a granulomatous lesion requiring steroid injection or surgical excision may develop at the tick bite site a few weeks after the incident.[44] Patients in whom a local rash or systemic symptoms develop within 4 weeks of exposure to tick-infested areas (even in the absence of a known bite) should be evaluated for infectious complications such as Lyme disease (LD),[43] the most common vector-borne disease in the United States.

LD is caused by the spirochete *Borrelia burgdorferi* and may present at any of three stages—early localized (stage 1), early disseminated (stage 2), or late/persistent (stage 3). Stage 1 findings of limited infection include a skin rash in at least 80% of patients that develops after an incubation period of approximately 3 to 30 days[45,46] The rash, termed *erythema migrans* (EM), is typically a round or oval erythematous lesion that begins at the bite site and expands at a relatively rapid rate (up to 1 cm each day) to a median size of 15 cm in diameter.[47] As the rash expands, there may be evidence of central clearing, and less commonly, a central vesicle or necrotic eschar.[47] The rash may be accompanied by fatigue, myalgias, headache, fever, nausea, vomiting, regional lymphadenopathy, sore throat, photophobia, anorexia, and arthralgias.[45,46] Without treatment, the rash fades in approximately 4 weeks.[45] If untreated, the infection may disseminate, and between 30 and 120 days, the victim may develop multiple EM lesions (generally smaller than the primary lesion) and neurologic, cardiac, or joint abnormalities.[45] Neuroborreliosis occurs in approximately 15% of untreated patients and presents with central or peripheral findings such as lymphocytic meningitis, subtle encephalitis, cranial neuritis (especially facial nerve palsy which may be unilateral or bilateral), cerebellar ataxia, and motor neuropathies.[48] Cardiac findings occur in approximately 5% of untreated patients and usually presents with atrioventricular nodal block or myocarditis.[46] Oligoarticular arthritis is a common presentation of early, disseminated LD and occurs in approximately 60% of untreated victims.[46] There is a particular propensity for larger joints such as the knee, which becomes recurrently and intermittently swollen and painful.[46] Findings of early disseminated LD eventually disappear with or without treatment.[46] Over time, as much as a year following the initial tick bite, LD can progress to its chronic form manifested by chronic arthritis, chronic synovitis, neurocognitive disorders, and/or chronic fatigue.[45]

Diagnosis of LD is largely based on the presence of a classic EM rash in a patient with a history of possible tick exposure in an endemic area or the presence of one or more findings of disseminated infection (nervous system, cardiovascular system, and/or joint involvement) and positive serology on acute and convalescent plasma samples (enzyme-linked immunosorbent assay and Western blot testing for IgM and IgG antibodies to *B. burgdorferi*). If the patient has been ill for longer than a month, an isolated positive IgM antibody level is likely a false positive, and a positive IgG level is required for diagnosis.

First-line treatment of early or disseminated LD, in the absence of neurologic involvement, is oral doxycycline for 14 to 21 days. The second-line agent for use in children 8 years of age or younger and pregnant women is amoxicillin. An equally effective third choice is cefuroxime axetil. Each of these oral agents provides a cure in better than 90% of patients.[46] If the patient has any evidence of neuroborreliosis, treatment should be with daily intravenous ceftriaxone for 14 to 28 days.[46] Likewise patients with cardiac manifestations should be treated via the intravenous route for at least part of their course and should receive cardiac monitoring if atrioventricular nodal block is significant (i.e., PR interval > 0.3 sec).[46] Oral antibiotics for 30 to 60 days or intravenous therapy for 30 days are usually effective for Lyme arthritis, though approximately 10% of patients will have persistent joint complaints following treatment.[46,47] Persistent arthritis in these nonresponders after antibiotic therapy is thought to be autoimmune mediated because the spirochete has been eradicated.[46] Treatment of persistent arthritis following antibiotics should consist of anti-inflammatory agents or arthroscopic synovectomy.[46]

Decisions to prophylactically treat a victim of tick bite to prevent LD are controversial. Some authors condemn such an approach given the low (approximately 1.4%) risk of transmission following a tick bite, even in an endemic area.[47] Research has shown, however, that a single dose of doxycycline, 200 mg orally, given within 72 hours of a tick bite can further reduce the already low risk of disease transmission.[46] A vaccine is available for use in patients at significant risk for LD—adults living or traveling regularly to endemic regions.[46] Even if immunized, however, people entering a tick habitat should use appropriate preventive measures such as insect repellents and frequent body checks for ticks since the vaccine is only approximately 76% effective, and it does not protect against other tick-borne diseases.[47]

Hymenoptera

Most arthropod envenomations occur by species belonging to the order Hymenoptera, which includes bees, wasps, yellow jackets, hornets, and stinging ants. The winged Hymenoptera are located throughout the United States, whereas the so-called fire ants are currently limited to the southeastern and southwestern regions. The Africanized honeybee, which characteristically attacks in massive numbers, has recently migrated into the southern United States.

Envenomation

Hymenoptera sting humans defensively, especially if their nests are disturbed. The stingers of most Hymenoptera are attached to venom sacs located on the abdomen and can be used repeatedly. Some bees, however, have barb-shaped stingers, preventing detachment from the victim and rendering them capable of only a single sting. Hymenoptera venom contains vasoactive compounds such as histamine and serotonin, which are responsible for the local reaction and pain. They also contain peptides, such as melitin, and enzymes (primarily phospholipases and hyaluronidases), which are highly allergenic and elicit an IgE-mediated response in some victims.[49] Fire ant venom consists primarily of nonallergenic alkaloids that release histamine and cause mild, local necrosis. Allergenic proteins constitute only 0.1% of fire ant venom.

Clinical Reactions

A Hymenoptera sting in a nonallergic individual produces immediate pain followed by a wheal-and-flare reaction. Fire ants characteristically produce multiple pustules from repetitive stings at the same site. Multiple Hymenoptera stings can produce a toxic reaction characterized by vomiting, diarrhea, generalized edema, cardiovascular collapse, and hemolysis, which can be difficult to distinguish from an acute, anaphylactic reaction.[50]

Large, exaggerated, local reactions develop in approximately 17% of envenomed subjects.[49] These reactions present as erythematous, edematous, painful, and pruritic areas larger than 10 cm in diameter and may last 2 to 5 days. The precise pathophysiology of such reactions remains unclear, although they may be, in part, IgE mediated.[51] Patients in whom large local reactions develop are at risk for similar episodes with future stings, but they do not appear to be at increased risk of systemic allergic reactions.[49]

Bee sting anaphylaxis develops in 0.3% to 3% of the general population and causes approximately 40 reported deaths annually in the United States.[49,50] Fatalities occur most often in adults, usually within 1 hour of the sting. Symptoms usually occur within minutes, ranging from mild urticaria and angioedema to respiratory arrest secondary to airway edema and cardiovascular collapse. A positive IgE-mediated skin test to Hymenoptera extract helps predict an allergic sting reaction.

Unusual reactions to Hymenoptera stings include late-onset allergic reactions (>5 hours after the sting), serum sickness, renal disease, neurologic disorders such as Guillain-Barré syndrome, and vasculitis.[52] The etiology of these reactions is thought to be immune mediated.

Treatment

Local therapy has traditionally been to remove any retained stinger by gentle scraping, avoiding compression of the venom sac. Current information, however, suggests that the most important factor is to get the stinger out as quickly as possible by whatever means necessary to reduce the total amount of venom that is injected.[53] The sting site should be cleansed and locally cooled. Topical or injected lidocaine can help decrease pain from the sting. Antihistamines administered orally or topically can decrease pruritus. Blisters and pustules (typically sterile) from fire ant stings should be left intact.

Treatment of an exaggerated, local envenomation includes the aforementioned therapy in addition to elevation of the extremity and analgesics. A 5-day course of oral prednisone (1 mg/kg/day) is also recommended.[49] Isolated local reactions (typical or exaggerated) do not require epinephrine or referral for immunotherapy.

Mild anaphylaxis can be treated with 0.3 to 0.5 mL of 1:1000 subcutaneous or intramuscular epinephrine (0.01 mL/kg in children, up to 0.5 mL) and an oral or parenteral antihistamine. More severe cases should also be treated with steroids and may require oxygen, endotracheal intubation, intravenous epinephrine infusion, bronchodilators, intravenous fluids, or vasopressors. These patients should be observed for approximately 24 hours in a monitored environment for any recurrence of severe symptoms.

Venom immunotherapy effectively prevents recurrent anaphylaxis from subsequent stings in certain patients with positive skin tests.[50] All persons with previous severe, systemic, allergic reactions to Hymenoptera stings or in whom serum sickness develops should be referred for possible immunotherapy. Referral is also recommended for adults with purely systemic, dermal reactions, such as diffuse hives. Children with systemic skin manifestations alone appear to be at relatively low risk for more serious anaphylaxis on subsequent stings and do not need referral.[50] Patients with a history of anaphylaxis resulting from Hymenoptera stings should carry injectable epinephrine with them at all times; they should also wear an identification medallion identifying their medical condition.

MARINE BITES AND STINGS

Four fifths of all living creatures reside underwater.[54] Hazardous marine animals are encountered by humans primarily in temperate or tropical seas. Increased exposure to marine life through recreation, research, and industry leads to frequent encounters with aquatic organisms. Injuries generally occur through bites, stings, or punctures, and infrequently from electrical shock from creatures such as the torpedo ray.

Initial Assessment

Injuries from marine organisms can range from mild local skin reactions to systemic collapse from major trauma or severe envenomation.[55] Several aspects unique to marine trauma make the treatment of these patients challenging. Immersion in cold water predisposes patients to hypothermia and near drowning. Rapid ascent after an encounter with a marine organism can cause air embolism or decompression illness in a scuba diver. Anaphylactic reaction to venom further complicates an envenomation. Late complications include unique infections caused by a wide variety of aquatic microorganisms.

Microbiology

Most marine isolates are gram-negative rods.[54] *Vibrio* species are of primary concern, particularly in the immunocompromised host. In fresh water, *Aeromonas* species can be particularly aggressive pathogens. *Staphylococcus* and *Streptococcus* species are also frequently cultured from infections. The laboratory should be notified that cultures are sent from aquatic-acquired infections to alert them of the need for appropriate culture media and conditions.

GENERAL MANAGEMENT

Initial management is focused on airway, breathing, and circulation. Anticipate anaphylaxis and treat the victim accordingly. Patients with extensive blunt and penetrating injuries should be managed as major trauma victims. Patients who have been envenomed should receive specific intervention directed against a toxin (discussed separately, according to marine creature) in addition to general supportive care. Antivenom can be administered if available. Antitetanus immunization should be updated following a bite, cut, or sting. Radiographs should be obtained to locate foreign bodies and fractures. Magnetic resonance imaging is more useful than ultrasound to identify small spine fragments.

Selection of antibiotics is tailored to marine bacteriology. Third-generation cephalosporins provide adequate coverage for the gram-positive and gram-negative microorganisms found in ocean water, including *Vibrio* species.[54] Ciprofloxacin, cefoperazone, gentamicin, and trimethoprim-sulfamethoxazole are acceptable antibiotics. Outpatient regimens include ciprofloxacin, trimethoprim-sulfamethoxazole, or doxycycline.[54] Patients with large abrasions, lacerations, puncture wounds, or hand injuries, as well as immunocompromised patients, should receive prophylactic antibiotics. Infected wounds should be cultured. If a wound, commonly on the hand after a minor scrape or puncture, appearance is erysipeloid in nature, infection by *Erysipelothrix rhusiopathiae* should be suspected. A suitable initial antibiotic based on the presumptive diagnosis would be penicillin, cephalexin, or ciprofloxacin.

Wound Care

Meticulous wound care is necessary to prevent infection and to optimize aesthetic and functional outcome.[56] Wounds should be irrigated with normal saline. Débridement of devitalized tissue can decrease infection and promote healing. Large wounds should be explored in the operating room. The decision to close a wound primarily must balance the cosmetic result against the risk of infection. Wounds should be loosely closed and drainage

allowed. Primary closure should be avoided in distal extremity wounds, punctures, and crush injuries.

Antivenom

Antivenom is available for several envenomations, including those from the box jellyfish, sea snake, and stonefish.[57] Patients demonstrating severe reactions to these envenomations benefit from antivenom. Skin testing to determine which patients would benefit from pretreatment with diphenhydramine or epinephrine can be performed before antivenom is administered but is not an absolute predictor for severe reactions. Ovine-derived antivenom to treat severe *Chironex fleckeri* (box jellyfish) envenomation has been administered intramuscularly by field rescuers at least 60 to 70 times without report of a serious adverse reaction. Serum sickness is a complication of antivenom therapy and can be treated with corticosteroids. Regional poison control centers or major marine aquariums can sometimes assist in locating antivenoms.

Injuries From Nonvenomous Aquatic Animals

Sharks

Approximately 50 to 100 shark attacks are reported annually. However, these attacks cause fewer than 10 deaths each year.[56,58] The tiger, great white, gray reef, and bull sharks are responsible for most attacks.[56] Most incidents occur at the surface of shallow water within 100 feet of shore.[58] Sharks locate prey by detecting motion, electrical fields, and sounds, and by sensing body fluids through smell and taste. Most sharks bite the victim one time and then leave.[56,58] Most injuries occur to the lower extremities.

Powerful jaws and sharp teeth produce crushing, tearing injuries. Hypovolemic shock and near drowning are lifethreatening consequences of an attack.[56] Other complications include soft tissue and neurovascular damage, fractures, and infection.[58] Massive blood transfusion may predispose the patient to disseminated intravascular coagulation. Most wounds require exploration and repair in the operating room (see the section on wound care). Occasionally, "bumping" by sharks can produce abrasions, which should be treated as second-degree burns.[54]

Moray Eels

Morays are savage bottom dwellers, residing in holes or crevices. Eels bite defensively, producing multiple small puncture wounds and rare gaping lacerations. The hand is most frequently bitten. Occasionally, the eel remains attached to the victim, requiring decapitation of the animal for release. Puncture wounds and bites to the hand from all animals, including eels, are at high risk for infection and should not be closed primarily if the capability exists for delayed primary closure.[54]

Alligators and Crocodiles

Crocodiles can attain a length of more than 20 feet and travel at speeds of 20 miles per hour in water and on land. Like sharks, alligators and crocodiles attack primarily in shallow water. These animals can produce severe injuries by grasping victims with their powerful jaws and dragging them underwater. Injuries from alligator and crocodile attacks should be treated like shark bites.

Miscellaneous

Other nonvenomous animals capable of attacking include the barracuda, giant grouper, sea lion, and needlefish. Except for the needlefish, which spears a human victim with its elongated snout, these animals bite. Barracuda are attracted to shiny objects and have bitten dangling legs adorned with reflective jewelry.

Envenomation by Invertebrates

Coelenterates

The phylum Coelenterata consists of hydrozoans, which include fire coral, hydroids, and Portuguese man-of-wars; scyphozoans, which include jellyfish and sea nettles; and anthozoans, which include sea anemones. Coelenterates carry stinging cells called nematocytes, which in turn carry the nematocysts.[59]

Mild envenomations, typically inflicted by fire coral, hydroids, and anemones, produce skin irritation.[57] The victim notices immediate stinging followed by pruritus, paresthesias, and throbbing pain with proximal radiation. Edema and erythema develop in the involved area, followed by blisters and petechiae. This can progress to local infection and ulceration.

Severe envenomations are caused by anemones, sea nettles, and jellyfish.[57] Patients have systemic symptoms in addition to the local manifestations. An anaphylactic reaction to the venom may contribute to the pathophysiology of envenomation. Fever, nausea, vomiting, and malaise can develop. Any organ system can be involved, and death is attributed to hypotension and cardiorespiratory arrest. One of the most venomous sea creatures, found primarily off the coast of northern Australia, is the box jellyfish, *C. fleckeri*. In the United States, *Physalia physalis*, *Chiropsalmus quadrigatus*, and *Cyanea capillata* are substantial stingers.

Therapy consists of detoxification of nematocysts and systemic support. The wound should be rinsed in seawater and gently dried.[57] Fresh water and vigorous rubbing can cause nematocysts to discharge. Dilute (5%) acetic acid (vinegar) can inactivate the toxin and should be applied for 30 minutes or until the pain is relieved.[57] This is critical with the box jellyfish. For a sting from this creature, Australian authorities also recommend the pressure-immobilization technique (see earlier section on snakebites). This is achieved by wrapping the envenomed limb with an elastic or cloth wrap to compress and occlude the superficial veins and lymphatics; the arterial circulation should be maintained. The limb is then splinted (immobilized). This maneuver is maintained until the victim can be brought to a setting where antivenom and advanced life support are available.

To decontaminate other jellyfish stings, isopropyl alcohol should be used only if vinegar is ineffective. Baking soda may be more effective than acetic acid for inactivating the toxin of U.S. eastern coastal Chesapeake Bay sea nettles.[57] Do not apply baking soda after vinegar without a brisk saline or water rinse in between the two substances to avoid an exothermic reaction. Powdered or solubilized papain (meat tenderizer) may be more effective than other remedies for seabather's eruption (often misnomered "sea lice"), caused by thimble jellyfishes or larval forms of certain sea anemones.

After the skin surface has been treated, remaining nematocysts must be removed. One method is to apply shaving cream or a flour paste and shave the area with a razor. The affected area should again be irrigated, dressed, and elevated. Medical care providers should wear gloves for self-protection. Cryotherapy, local anesthetics, antihistamines, and steroids can relieve pain after the toxin is inactivated. Prophylactic antibiotics are usually unnecessary. The ocean bather should be advised to apply Safe Sea jellyfish safe sun block (Nidaria Technology Ltd., Jordan Valley, Israel) as a preventive measure prior to entering the water.

Sponges

Two syndromes occur after contact with sponges[57]: The first is an allergic plantlike contact dermatitis characterized by itching and burning within hours of contact. This can progress to soft tissue edema, vesicle development, and joint swelling. Large areas of involvement can cause systemic toxicity with fever, nausea, and muscle cramps. The second syndrome is an irritant dermatitis after penetration of the skin with small spicules. Sponge diver's disease is actually caused by anemones that colonize the sponges rather than by the sponges themselves.

Treatment consists of washing the affected area and drying gently. Dilute (5%) acetic acid (vinegar) should be applied for 30 minutes three times daily.[57] Remaining spicules can be removed with adhesive tape. A steroid cream can be applied to the skin after decontamination. Occasionally, a systemic glucocorticoid and an antihistamine are required.

Echinodermata

Starfish, sea urchins, and sea cucumbers are members of the phylum Echinodermata. Starfish and sea cucumbers produce venoms that can cause contact dermatitis.[59] Sea cucumbers occasionally feed on coelenterates and secrete nematocysts; therefore, local therapy for coelenterates should also be considered. Sea urchins are covered with venomous spines capable of producing local and systemic reactions similar to those from coelenterates.[59] First aid consists of soaking the wound in hot, but tolerable, water.

Residual spines can be located with soft tissue radiographs or magnetic resonance imaging. Purple skin discoloration at the site of entrance wounds may be indicative of dye leached from the surface of an extracted urchin spine. This temporary tattoo disappears in 48 hours, which generally signifies the absence of a retained foreign body. A spine should be removed only if it is easily accessible or if it is closely aligned to a joint or critical neurovascular structure. Reactive fusiform digit swelling attributed to a spine near a metacarpal bone or flexor tendon sheath may be alleviated by a high-dose glucocorticoid administered in an oral 14-day taper.

Mollusks

Octopuses and cone snails are the primary envenoming species in the phylum Mollusca. Most harmful cone snails are found in Indo-Pacific waters. Envenomation occurs from a detachable tooth injected into the victim.[57,59] Blue-ringed octopuses can bite and inject tetrodotoxin, a paralytic agent. Both species can produce local symptoms such as burning and paresthesias. Systemic manifestations are primarily neurologic. Management of the bite site is controversial. Options include pressure and immobilization to contain the venom. Treatment of systemic complications is supportive.

Envenomation by Vertebrates

Stingrays

Rays are bottom dwellers ranging from a few inches to 12 feet long (tip to tail). Venom is stored in whiplike appendages. Stingrays react defensively by thrusting spines into a victim, producing puncture wounds and lacerations. The most common site of injury is the lower leg and top of the foot. Local damage can be severe, with occasional penetration of body cavities.[60] This is worsened by vasoconstrictive properties of the venom, producing cyanotic-appearing wounds. The venom is often myonecrotic. Systemic complaints include weakness, nausea, diarrhea, headache, and muscle cramps. The venom can cause vasoconstriction, cardiac dysrhythmias, respiratory arrest, and seizures.[61]

The wound should be irrigated and then soaked in non-scalding hot water (up to 45°C) for an hour.[61,62] Débridement, exploration, and removal of spines should occur during or after hot water soaking. Immersion cryotherapy is detrimental. The wound should not be closed primarily. Lacerations should heal by secondary intention or be repaired by delayed closure. The wound should be dressed and elevated. Pain should be relieved locally or systemically. Radiographic studies should be obtained to locate remaining spines. Acute infection with aggressive pathogens should be anticipated.[57] In the event of a non-healing, draining wound, suspect foreign body retention.

Miscellaneous

Other spined fish that can produce injuries similar to those of stingrays include lionfish, scorpionfish, stonefish, catfish, and weeverfish. Each can produce envenomation, puncture wounds, and lacerations, with spines transmitting venom. Clinical manifestations and therapy are similar to those pertaining to stingrays. In the case of the lionfish, vesiculations are sometimes noted. An equine-derived antivenom exists for administration in the event of a significant stonefish envenomation.

Sea Snakes

Sea snakes of the family Hydrophiidae appear similar to land snakes. They inhabit the Pacific and Indian Oceans. Venom produces neurologic signs and symptoms, with possible death from paralysis and respiratory arrest. Local manifestations can be minimal or absent. Therapy is similar to that for coral snake (Elapidae) bites. The pressure-immobilization technique is recommended in the field. Antivenom should be administered if any signs of envenomation develop.[61,62] The initial dose is 1 ampule, repeated as needed.

Selected References

Auerbach PS (ed): Wilderness Medicine: Management of Wilderness and Environmental Emergencies, 4th ed. St. Louis, Mosby–Year Book, 2001.

> This textbook is an in-depth review of wilderness medicine. Bites and stings by many organisms are discussed in detail by experts from each field. Many recent, pertinent studies are reviewed.

Dire DJ: Emergency management of dog and cat bite wounds. Emerg Med Clin North Am 10:719, 1992.

> This is a comprehensive and practical review of dog and cat bites. The author discusses the epidemiology, bacteriology, and management of these injuries. A section on rabies is included.

Gold BS, Dart RC, Barish RA: Bites of venomous snakes. N Engl J Med 347:347-356, 2002.

> This article is a concise, practical review of snake venom poisoning in the United States. Proper use of the new North American antivenom is well summarized.

Reisman RE: Insect stings. N Engl J Med 331:523-527, 1994.

> The reactions to Hymenoptera stings are well organized in this practical monograph. The natural history of stinging insect allergy is reviewed. Therapeutic considerations are discussed.

Steere AC: Medical progress: Lyme disease. N Engl J Med 345:115-125, 2001.

> This manuscript is a thorough review of the current understanding of Lyme borreliosis and clearly outlines diagnosis and treatment.

Williamson JA, Fenner PJ, Burnett JW (eds): Venomous and Poisonous Marine Animals. Sydney, Australia, University of New South Wales Press, 1996.

> This book is a superb reference with a complete discussion of all common and uncommon toxic marine animals.

Wilson DC, King LE: Spiders and spider bites. Dermatol Clin North Am 8:277, 1990.

> **This is a thorough review of spider bites. Various aspects of managing spider bites are presented, including areas of controversy.**

References

1. Warrell DA, Fenner PJ: Venomous bites and stings. Br Med Bull 49:423-439, 1993.
2. Parrish HM: Incidence of treated snakebites in the United States. Public Health Rep 81:269-276, 1966.
3. Norris RL, Bush SP: North American venomous reptile bites. *In* Auerbach PS (ed): Wilderness Medicine: Management of Wilderness and Environmental Emergencies, 4th ed. St. Louis, Mosby–Year Book, 2001, pp 896-926.
4. Gold BS, Wingert WA: Snake venom poisoning in the United States: A review of therapeutic practice. South Med J 87:579-589, 1994.
5. Ownby CL: Pathology of rattlesnake envenomation. *In* Tu AT (ed): Rattlesnake Venoms. New York, Marcel Dekker, 1982, pp 164-169.
6. Russell FE: Snake Venom Poisoning. New York, Scholium International, 1983.
7. Hutton RA, Warrell DA: Action of snake venom components on the haemostatic system. Blood Rev 7:176-189, 1993.
8. Russell FE, Carlson RW, Wainschel J, et al: Snake venom poisoning in the United States: Experiences with 550 cases. JAMA 233:341-344, 1975.
9. Wingert WA, Chan L: Rattlesnake bites in southern California and rationale for recommended treatment. West J Med 148:37-44, 1988.
10. Bush SP, Hegewald KG, Green SM, et al: Effects of a negative pressure venom extraction device (Extractor) on local tissue injury after artificial rattlesnake envenomation in a porcine model. Wilderness Environ Med 11:180-188, 2000.
11. Consroe P, Egen NB, Russell FE, et al: Comparison of a new ovine antigen binding fragment (Fab) antivenin for United States Crotalidae with the commercial antivenin for protection against venom-induced lethality in mice. Am J Trop Med Hyg 53:507-510, 1995.
12. Dart RC, Seifert SA, Carroll L, et al: Affinity-purified, mixed monospecific crotalid antivenom ovine Fab for the treatment of crotalid venom poisoning. Ann Emerg Med 30:33-39, 1997.
13. Gold BS, Dart RC, Barish RA: Bites of venomous snakes. N Engl J Med 347:347-356, 2002.
14. Clark RF, Selden BS, Furbee B: The incidence of wound infection following crotalid envenomation. J Emerg Med 11:583-586, 1993.
15. Kerrigan KR, Mertz BL, Nelson SJ, et al: Antibiotic prophylaxis for pit viper envenomation: prospective, controlled trial. World J Surg 21:369-373, 1997.
16. Burgess JL, Dart RC: Snake venom coagulopathy: Use and abuse of blood products in the treatment of pit viper envenomation. Ann Emerg Med 20:795-801, 1991.
17. Bogdan GM, Dart RC, Falbo SC, et al: Recurrent coagulopathy after antivenom treatment of crotalid snakebite. South Med J 93:562-566, 2000.
18. Vigasio A, Battiston B, De Filippo G, et al: Compartmental syndrome due to viper bite. Arch Orthop Trauma Surg 110:175-177, 1991.
19. Garfin SR, Castilonia RR, Mubarak SJ, et al: Role of surgical decompression in treatment of rattlesnake bites. Surg Forum 30:502-504, 1979.
20. Keogh S, Callaham ML: Bites and injuries inflicted by domestic animals. *In* Auerbach PS (ed): Wilderness Medicine: Management of Wilderness and Environmental Emergencies, 4th ed. St. Louis, Mosby–Year Book, 2001, pp 961-978.
21. Overall KL, Love M: Dog bites to humans—demography, epidemiology, injury, and risk. J Am Vet Med Assoc 218:1923-1934, 2001.
22. Chen E, Hornig S, Shepherd SM, et al: Primary closure of mammalian bites. Acad Emerg Med 7:157-161, 2000.
23. Kountakis SE, Chamblee SA, Maillard AA, et al: Animal bites to the head and neck. Ear Nose Throat J 77:216-220, 1998.
24. Callaham M: Prophylactic antibiotics in common dog bite wounds: A controlled study. Ann Emerg Med 9:410-414, 1980.
25. Perron AD, Miller MD, Brady WJ: Orthopedic pitfalls in the ED: Fight bite. Am J Emerg Med 20:114-117, 2002.
26. Talan DA, Citron DM, Abrahamian FM, et al: Bacteriologic analysis of infected dog and cat bites. Emergency Medicine Animal Bite Infection Study Group. N Engl J Med 340:85-92, 1999.
27. Garcia VF: Animal bites and *Pasturella* infections. Pediatr Rev 18:127-130, 1997.
28. Vidmar L, Poljak M, Tomazic J, et al: Transmission of HIV-1 by human bite. Lancet 347:1762, 1996.
29. Hemachudha T, Phuapradit P: Rabies. Curr Opin Neurol 10:260-267, 1997.
30. Moran GJ, Talan DA, Mower W, et al: Appropriateness of rabies postexposure prophylaxis treatment for animal exposures. Emergency ID Net Study Group. JAMA 284:1001-1007, 2000.
31. Human rabies prevention—United States, 1999. Recommendations of the Advisory Committee on Immunization Practices (ACIP). MMWR Recomm Rep 48:1-21, 1999.
32. Boyer LV, McNally JT, Binford GJ: Spider bites. *In* Auerbach PS (ed): Wilderness Medicine: Management of Wilderness and Environmental Emergencies, 4th ed. St. Louis, Mosby–Year Book, 2001, pp 807-838.
33. Wilson DC, King LE Jr: Spiders and spider bites. Dermatol Clin North Am 8:277-286, 1990.
34. Clark RF, Wethern-Kestner S, Vance MV, et al: Clinical presentation and treatment of black widow spider envenomation: A review of 163 cases. Ann Emerg Med 21:782-787, 1992.
35. Wong RC, Hughes SE, Voorhees JJ: Spider bites. Arch Dermatol 123:98-104, 1987.
36. Futrell JM: Loxoscelism. Am J Med Sci 304:261-267, 1992.
37. Smith CW, Micks DW: The role of polymorphonuclear leukocytes in the lesion caused by the venom of the brown spider, *Loxosceles reclusa*. Lab Invest 22:90-93, 1970.
38. Sams HH, Dunnick CA, Smith ML, et al: Necrotic arachnidism. J Am Acad Dermatol 44:561-573; quiz 573-576, 2001.
39. Ingber A, Trattner A, Cleper R, et al: Morbidity of brown recluse spider bites: Clinical picture, treatment, and prognosis. Acta Derm Venereol 71:337-340, 1991.
40. King LE Jr, Rees RS: Dapsone treatment of a brown recluse bite. JAMA 250:648, 1983.
41. Connor DA, Seldon BS: Scorpion envenomations. *In* Auerbach PS (ed): Wilderness Medicine: Management of Wilderness and Environmental Emergencies, 3rd ed. St. Louis, Mosby–Year Book, 1995, pp 831-842.
42. Gateau T, Bloom M, Clark R: Response to specific *Centruroides sculpturatus* antivenom in 151 cases of scorpion stings. J Toxicol Clin Toxicol 32:165-171, 1994.
43. Stewart RL, Burgdorfer W, Needham GR: Evaluation of three commercial tick removal tools. Wilderness Environ Med 9:137-142, 1998.

44. Metry DW, Hebert AA: Insect and arachnid stings, bites, infestations, and repellents. Pediatr Annu 29:39-48, 2000.

45. Montiel NJ, Baumgarten JM, Sinha AA: Lyme disease: II. Clinical features and treatment. Cutis 69:443-448, 2002.

46. Steere AC: Lyme disease. N Engl J Med 345:115-125, 2001.

47. Shapiro ED, Gerber MA: Lyme disease. Clin Infect Dis 31:533-542, 2000.

48. Steere AC: A 58-year-old man with a diagnosis of chronic Lyme disease. JAMA 288:1002-1010, 2002.

49. Wright DN, Lockey RF: Local reactions to stinging insects (Hymenoptera). Allergy Proc 11:23-28, 1990.

50. Reisman RE: Stinging insect allergy. Med Clin North Am 76:883-894, 1992.

51. Reisman RE: Insect stings. N Engl J Med 331:523-527, 1994.

52. Reisman RE: Unusual reactions to insect venoms. Allergy Proc 12:395-399, 1991.

53. Visscher PK, Vetter RS, Camazine S: Removing bee stings. Lancet 348:301-302, 1996.

54. Auerbach PS, Halstead BW: Injuries from nonvenomous aquatic animals. *In* Auerbach PS (ed): Wilderness Medicine: Management of Wilderness and Environmental Emergencies, 4th ed. St. Louis, Mosby–Year Book, 2001, pp 1418-1449.

55. Williamson JA, Fenner PJ, Burnett JW (eds): Venomous and Poisonous Marine Animals. Sydney, University of New South Wales Press, 1996.

56. Howard RJ, Burgess GH: Surgical hazards posed by marine and freshwater animals in Florida. Am J Surg 166:563-567, 1993.

57. Barber GR, Swygert JS: Necrotizing fasciitis due to *Photobacterium damsela* in a man lashed by a stingray. N Engl J Med 342:824, 2000.

58. Guidera KJ, Ogden JA, Highhouse K, et al: Shark attack: A case study of the injury and treatment. J Orthop Trauma 5:204-208, 1991.

59. McGoldrick J, Marx JA: Marine envenomations: II. Invertebrates. J Emerg Med 10:71-77, 1992.

60. Cooper MNK: Stone fish and stingrays—some notes on the injuries that they cause to man. J R Army Med Corps 137:136-140, 1991.

61. McGoldrick J, Marx JA: Marine envenomations: I. Vertebrates. J Emerg Med 9:497-502, 1991.

62. Auerbach PS: Envenomation by aquatic vertebrates. *In* Auerbach PS (ed): Wilderness Medicine: Management of Wilderness and Environmental Emergencies, 4th ed. St. Louis, Mosby–Year Book, 2001, pp 1488-1505.

CHAPTER 24

SURGICAL CRITICAL CARE

Walter L. Biffl, M.D.,   **Tomomi Oka**, M.D.
and   **William G. Cioffi**, M.D.

Central Nervous System
Cardiovascular System
Respiratory System
Gastrointestinal System
Acute Renal Failure

Hepatic Dysfunction
Endocrine System
Hematologic System
Sepsis and Multiple Organ Failure

The definitive management of illness is the essence of surgical practice. In the vast majority of cases, patients are returned to their usual health status after surgery. However, there is a subset of patients whose insult is so catastrophic, or whose baseline health status so marginal, that the acute illness, trauma, or elective surgical procedure results in critical illness. Although critical care is increasingly being delivered by nonsurgeon critical care specialists ("intensivists") in closed intensive care units (ICUs), it is important that surgeons have an understanding of critical care concepts. The purpose of this chapter is to provide an overview of critical care issues that pertain to surgical patients and outline a practical approach to them.

CENTRAL NERVOUS SYSTEM

Neurologic Dysfunction

There are many potential causes of altered consciousness in the ICU, including drugs and toxins, metabolic disorders, sepsis, meningitis/encephalitis, subarachnoid hemorrhage, head trauma, seizure, stroke, intracranial hypertension, and intracranial mass lesion. "ICU psychosis" should be considered strictly a diagnosis of exclusion. The term *altered mental status* is nonspecific; more descriptive definitions were offered by Plum and Posner[1] more than 20 years ago and still apply today. *Confusion* refers to bewilderment, with difficulty following commands, disturbed memory, and drowsiness or night-time

agitation. *Delirium* is "a floridly abnormal mental state characterized by disorientation, fear, irritability, misperception of sensory stimuli, and, often, visual hallucinations." *Obtundation* is defined as mental blunting associated with slowed psychological responses to stimulation. *Stupor* is described as "a condition of deep sleep or behaviorally similar unresponsiveness in which the patient can be aroused only by vigorous and repeated stimuli." *Coma* is "a state of unarousable psychologic unresponsiveness in which the subject lies with eyes closed and shows no psychologically understandable response to external stimuli or inner need." A *vegetative state* is a state of wakefulness but with apparent total lack of cognitive function. *Death* in the presence of cardiopulmonary function ("brain death") refers to the absence of function of the brain, including brainstem reflexes. There are specific criteria for the diagnosis of death: absence of cerebral function and of pupillary light reflex, corneal reflex, vestibulo-ocular reflex, and oropharyngeal reflex and apnea in the presence of "adequate stimulation" ($Paco_2 > 60$ mm Hg for 30 seconds). Generally, two clinical examinations must be documented, separated by a defined time interval (e.g., 6 hours) and confirmed by two physicians. It is important that there be a reason sufficient to cause death and no complicating conditions (e.g., sedative or anesthetic agents, hypothermia, hypoglycemia or hyperglycemia, or hypernatremia). If such complicating conditions preclude the completion of a clinical examination with apnea test, additional tests are required. Electroencephalography, radioisotope "brain scanning," and transcranial Doppler ultrasonography may provide supportive evidence, but the diagnostic gold standard for death is cerebral arteriography with documentation of absent flow.

When there is an alteration in a patient's neurologic status, assessment should be thorough yet rapid, with initial management and corrective measures instituted concurrently to minimize irreversible central nervous system (CNS) damage. The patient's level of consciousness may be described as alert, responsive to verbal stimuli, responsive to painful stimuli, or unresponsive. Acute loss of consciousness (seconds to minutes) is consistent with a cerebrovascular accident or head trauma. A subacute course (many minutes to hours) may suggest intoxication, infection, or a metabolic disturbance, whereas a more prolonged course may suggest a CNS tumor. The pupillary examination is informative. Damage to the midbrain affects the reticular activating system (and thus consciousness) as well as pupil reactivity; on the other hand, metabolic disease may produce coma but usually leaves the light reflex intact. Small reactive pupils are the hallmark of drug (particularly opioid) intoxication and metabolic disease. Large unreactive pupils may be associated with anticholinergic or glutethimide administration as well as anoxia. A unilateral fixed dilated pupil suggests third nerve dysfunction or uncal herniation. In the absence of purposeful eye movements, spontaneous roving eye movements imply intact cortical control of the brain stem. If no spontaneous eye movement is found, the cervical ocular reflex ("doll's eyes" maneuver) should be tested after excluding a cervical cord or spine lesion. The reflex is tested by rapidly turning the head from midline to one side. Contralateral conjugate eye movement, keeping the eyes seemingly fixed on a point in space, suggests an intact brain stem. The head should be turned in the opposite direction to check for symmetry. Failure of the reflex in either direction implies brain stem dysfunction. If this maneuver cannot be done, the vestibulo-ocular reflex may be assessed ("cold caloric" testing). This is done by elevating the head to 30 degrees and rapidly instilling 50 mL of ice water into the external auditory canal. This results in reflex slow eye movement toward the stimulus. In an intact brain the frontal eye fields attempt to override this stimulus, producing rapid saccades away from the stimulus (nystagmus). On the other hand, if there is cortical damage the eyes will maintain a fixed deviation. A fixed deviation implies a hemispheric lesion on the side toward which the eyes deviate. Assessment of motor function helps to identify the location and severity of deficits. Asymmetry of motor function suggests a focal cerebral lesion contralateral to the deficit. Decorticate (flexion of arms and extension of legs) and decerebrate (extension of both arms and legs) posturing are poor prognostic signs.

Laboratory studies will help to identify metabolic derangements, infection, or hypothyroidism. A urine toxicology screen should be routine, because drug intoxication is one of the most common causes of coma of unknown etiology. Arterial blood gas (ABG) analysis should be performed to look for hypoxia, hypercarbia, or acidosis. Computed tomography (CT) is indicated in any patient with coma or focal neurologic findings and many patients with depressed level of consciousness. A lumbar puncture should be performed on any patient for whom the cause of coma is still unknown, as well as in patients in whom meningitis, encephalitis, or occult subarachnoid hemorrhage is suspected.

Initial management begins with assurance of a patent *A*irway and adequate *B*reathing and *C*irculation (the "ABCs"). Comatose patients are intubated for airway protection. Before intubation the stability of the cervical spine must be ensured, and if there is a possibility of increased intracranial pressure (ICP), 100 mg of lidocaine or 300 mg of thiopental should be administered. Hypotension should be corrected with fluids and/or vasopressors. A dose of 50 mL of 50% dextrose should be given immediately to any patient with coma of unknown etiology. This will produce no detrimental effect on any causes of coma except Wernicke's encephalopathy (see later) and may correct the underlying problem. Even in the case of hyperglycemia producing coma, a marginal increase in the glucose concentration will not adversely affect the patient. In alcoholic patients or others with poor general nutrition, thiamine (1 mg/kg) should be administered before glucose. This may avoid acute Wernicke's encephalopathy (confusion, ataxia, ophthalmoplegia) with necrosis of midline gray matter. Narcotic overdose is a common cause of coma; shallow respirations, small reactive pupils, and hypotension are often seen. Naloxone (0.4 to 2 mg) should be given to patients with coma of unknown etiology. Flumazenil (0.2 mg) should be administered for suspected benzodiazepine intoxication, and activated charcoal (25 to 50 mg) given for ingestion of other drugs and toxins. Empirical antibiotic therapy is warranted if bacterial meningitis is suspected.

If increased ICP is suspected, treatment should be initiated immediately. The head of the bed should be elevated to 30 to 45 degrees and the patient should be hyperventilated to a target $PaCO_2$ of 35 to 40 mm Hg. Mannitol (0.5 to 1 g/kg) should be administered and may be repeated every 4 to 6 hours as long as the serum sodium level and osmolarity remain less than 155 and 320 mmol/L, respectively. Other factors involved in managing ICP include adequate sedation, suppression of fever, and seizure prophylaxis. If the patient has refractory intracranial hypertension, second-tier therapies should be employed that include ventriculostomy drainage, neuromuscular blockade, barbiturate coma, vasopressors to increase cerebral perfusion pressure, and, possibly, decompressive craniectomy.

Seizure activity is often the first sign of a CNS complication. Because most seizures terminate rapidly, the most important intervention is protecting the patient from harm. The etiology should be sought and treated. CT or magnetic resonance imaging (MRI) is usually indicated for new seizures, and an electroencephalogram should be obtained to exclude status epilepticus in patients who have persistent or recurrent seizures or who do not awaken after seizure activity. Patients with status epilepticus generally respond to lorazepam (0.1 mg/kg) within 5 minutes. If they do not, phenytoin (1 g) should be administered, followed by high-dose benzodiazepines, high-dose barbiturates, or propofol. The major systemic complications of seizures are rhabdomyolysis and hyperthermia and cerebral edema.

Analgesia, Sedation, and Neuromuscular Blockade

Pain and anxiety are common among ICU patients. Pain may be related to the underlying disease state, trauma, or invasive procedures; however, nursing interventions, monitoring and therapeutic devices, and immobility exacerbate discomfort. Unrelieved pain can provoke a sympathetic stress response as well as contribute to agitation. Consequently, a universal goal for critical care practitioners is providing an optimal level of comfort and safety for patients.

Pain Assessment and Management

Perception of pain is influenced by prior experiences, expectations, and the cognitive capacity of the patient. The patient and family should be advised of the potential for pain and strategies to communicate pain. Patient self-reporting is the "gold standard" for the assessment of pain and the adequacy of analgesia. Pain assessment tools such as the visual analogue scale or numeric rating scale (NRS) are most useful. The NRS may be preferable because it is applicable to many age groups and does not require verbal responses. In noncommunicative patients, assessment of behavioral (movements, facial expressions, posturing) and physiologic (heart rate, blood pressure, respiratory rate) indicators is necessary.

Nonpharmacologic interventions (e.g., a comfortable environment with attention to positioning and arrangement of tubing and drains) should be employed initially, but analgesics are often required. Opioids are the mainstay of pain management in the ICU. Desired properties of an opiate include rapid onset of action, ease of titration, lack of accumulation of parent drug or active metabolites, and low cost. The most commonly prescribed opioids are fentanyl, morphine, and hydromorphone. Fentanyl has a rapid onset of action and short half-life and generates no active metabolites. It is ideal for use in hemodynamically unstable patients or in combination with benzodiazepines for short procedures. Continuous infusion may result in prolonged effect owing to accumulation in lipid stores, and high dosing has been linked to muscle rigidity syndromes. Morphine has a slower onset of action and longer half-life. It may not be suitable for hemodynamically unstable patients because associated histamine release may lead to vasodilatation and hypotension. An active metabolite can accumulate in renal insufficiency. Morphine can also cause spasm of the sphincter of Oddi, which may discourage its use in patients with biliary disease. Hydromorphone has a half-life similar to morphine but generates no active metabolites and no histamine release. All opioid analgesics are associated with varying degrees of respiratory depression, hypotension, and ileus.

Preventing pain is more effective than treating established pain; thus, continuous or scheduled intermittent dosing is preferable to "p.r.n." administration. To avoid variable absorption, analgesics should be given intravenously to critically ill patients. A patient-controlled analgesia device can decrease opioid consumption, sedation, and other adverse effects while providing good pain control. Alternatives to opioids include acetaminophen and nonsteroidal anti-inflammatory agents (NSAIDs). Ketorolac is the only available intravenous NSAID. It is an effective analgesic agent used alone or in combination with an opioid. It is primarily eliminated by renal excretion, so it is relatively contraindicated in patients with renal insufficiency. Prolonged (>5 days) use has been associated with bleeding complications.

Many benefits of epidural anesthesia have been reported, including better suppression of surgical stress, more stable hemodynamics, better peripheral circulation, and reduced blood loss. A prospective, randomized study of 1021 abdominal surgery patients demonstrated that epidural opioid analgesia provides better postoperative pain relief compared with parenteral opioids.[2] Furthermore, in patients undergoing abdominal aortic operations, overall morbidity and mortality were improved and intubation time and ICU length of stay were shorter.

Sedation

Inability to communicate, constant noise and light, frequent sleep interruptions, and lack of mobility contribute to increased anxiety among ICU patients. This is exacerbated by mechanical ventilation. Sedation may be necessary to alleviate anxiety and provide comfort, as well as to prevent accidental removal of lines, catheters, and other crucial devices. A predetermined sedation goal should be established, and the level of sedation should be documented objectively based on a sedation scale such as the Ramsay sedation scale or Riker sedation/agitation scale (Table 24-1). The ideal level of sedation depends on the clinical situation; generally, a patient who is calm, is easily arousable, and follows commands is appropriately sedated. Benzodiazepines have both sedative and hypnotic effects, and some possess anterograde amnestic effects. They may also moderate the pain response when used in combination with opioids. Diazepam, lorazepam, and midazolam are the most frequently used agents in the ICU. Diazepam has a short onset of action and short half-life, but its long-acting metabolite may accumulate after repetitive dosing. Lorazepam has a slow onset and intermediate half-life, making it most useful for medium- to long-term sedation. Lorazepam can accumulate in elderly patients with hepatic and renal dysfunction, resulting in prolonged sedation. Midazolam is a rapid-onset, short-acting drug with amnestic properties, and thus is the agent of choice for acutely agitated patients. Prolonged sedation with midazolam results in accumulation of the agent and less reliable arousal. Propofol is a general anesthetic agent with significant sedative and hypnotic properties but no analgesic effect. Propofol has rapid onset and ultra-short duration of action. Its phospholipid vehicle can cause hypertriglyceridemia as well as pain on injection. Propofol is most often used for sedation of neurosurgical patients, because it allows rapid awakening for neurologic assessments and may decrease cerebral metabolism and reduce ICP. The main disadvantages of prolonged use are high cost and dose-related hypotension. Figure 24-1 is an algorithm for the provision of analgesia and sedation in the ICU.[3]

TABLE 24-1.   Sedation/Agitation Scales

Scale	Score	Description	Definition / Examples
Riker Sedation-Agitation Scale	7	Dangerous agitation	Pulls at endotracheal tube, climbs out of bed, thrashes, strikes at staff
	6	Very agitated	Bites at endotracheal tube, requires restraints, does not respond to verbal calming
	5	Agitated	Attempts to sit up, responds to verbal calming
	4	Calm and cooperative	Calm, awakens easily, follows commands
	3	Sedated	Awakens to gentle shaking or verbal stimuli but drifts off; follows simple commands
	2	Very sedated	Arouses to physical stimuli, does not follow commands
	1	Unarousable	Minimal or no response to noxious stimuli
Ramsay Scale	1	Awake	Anxious, agitated/restless
	2		Cooperative, oriented, tranquil
	3		Responds to commands only
	4	Asleep	Brisk response to light glabellar tap or loud auditory stimulus
	5		Sluggish response to light glabellar tap or loud auditory stimulus
	6		No response to light glabellar tap or loud auditory stimulus

Adapted from Jacobi J, Fraser GL, Coursin DB, et al: Clinical practice guidelines for the sustained use of sedatives and analgesics in the critically ill adult. Crit Care Med 30:119-141, 2002.

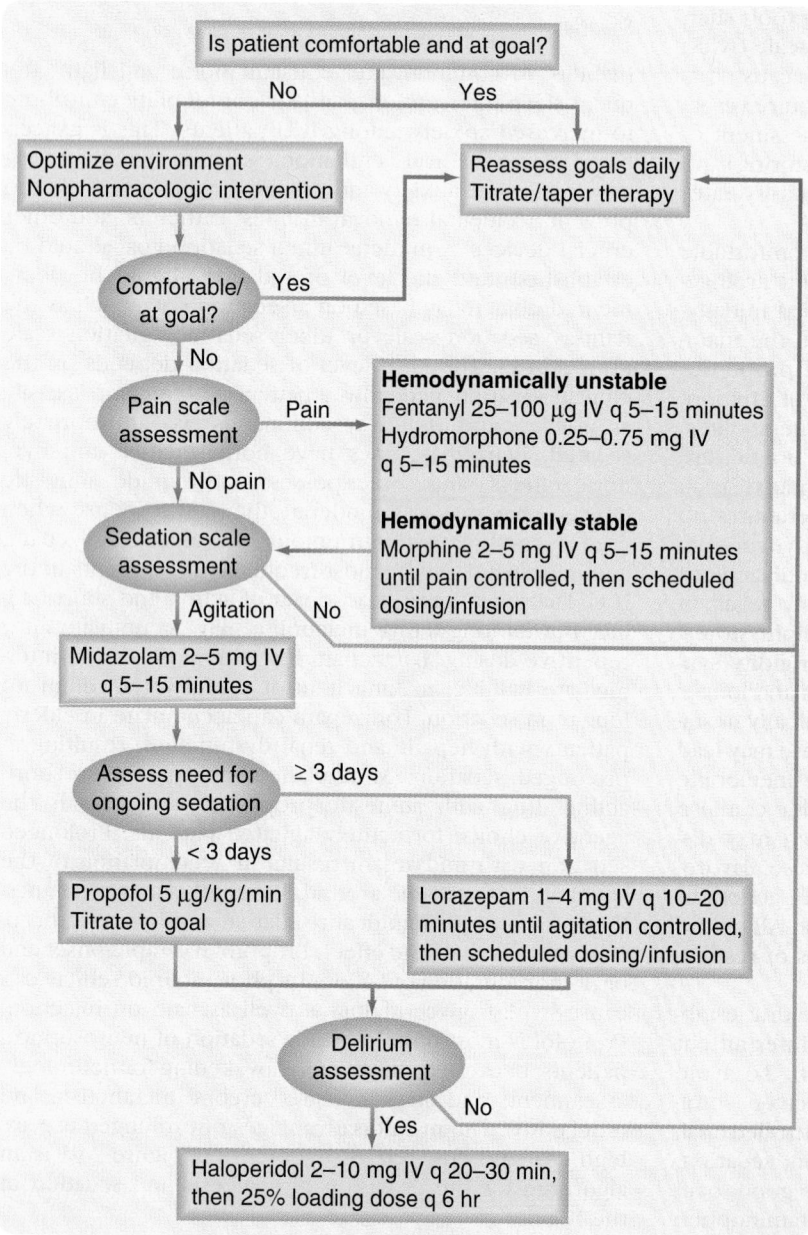

FIGURE 24-1. Algorithm for analgesia and sedation in the ICU. (Adapted from Jacobi J, Fraser GL, Coursin DB, et al: Clinical practice guidelines for the sustained use of sedatives and analgesics in the critically ill adult. Crit Care Med 30:119-141, 2002.)

Neuromuscular Blockade

Muscle relaxation may be warranted to minimize O_2 consumption (VO_2) or facilitate patient-ventilator synchrony, particularly when employing nonconventional modes of ventilation or positioning. There are two major categories of neuromuscular blockers. Depolarizing neuromuscular blockers mimic acetylcholine, binding the acetylcholine receptors and causing depolarization (clinically seen as muscle fasciculations). Succinylcholine is the only depolarizing neuromuscular blocker available for use and is characterized by a rapid onset and short half-life; it is most useful for short invasive procedures. Succinylcholine is degraded by plasma pseudocholinesterase, and in patients with this enzyme deficiency the drug can have a prolonged effect. The nondepolarizing neuromuscular blockers bind acetylcholine receptors but do not activate them. The aminosteroidal neuromuscular blocker compounds include rocuronium, vecuronium, and pancuronium. Rocuronium has a rapid onset and intermediate duration of action, making it useful for short procedures as well as prolonged relaxation. Vecuronium is an intermediate-acting agent, achieving neuromuscular blockade within 1 to 2 minutes and lasting about 30 minutes, but it can also be infused continuously. Patients with renal or hepatic dysfunction may have prolonged effect, because vecuronium is cleared by both the kidneys and liver. Pancuronium is long acting (up to 90 minutes). It is relatively contraindicated in patients with coronary artery disease because it is associated with a vagolytic effect and frequent tachycardia. Similar to vecuronium, pancuronium is eliminated through both the kidneys and liver. The benzylisoquinolonium neuromuscular blocker compounds include atracurium, cisatracurium, tubocurarine, and mivacurium. Of these, atracurium and cisatracurium are the two agents most commonly used in the ICU. Both are metabolized by plasma ester hydrolysis and Hofmann elimination and thus are useful in patients with hepatic and renal dysfunction. Atracurium is intermediate acting with minimal cardiovascular effects, but a metabolite may precipitate seizure activity at high doses. Cisatracurium is an isomer of atracurium, with less tendency to produce histamine release. An algorithm for the provision of neuromuscular blockers in the ICU is outlined in Figure 24-2.[4]

Monitoring of neuromuscular blockade is accomplished by train-of-four testing, with one to two twitches considered the optimal depth. In paralyzed patients, assessment of adequate analgesia and sedation is extremely difficult, and patients must be presumptively medicated. Prolonged recovery from paralysis is associated with the corticosteroidal neuromuscular blockers, and critical-illness myopathy syndromes have been reported in patients receiving neuromuscular blockers and corticosteroids. While not seemingly related to specific neuromuscular blocking agents, prolonged exposure to neuromuscular blockers appears to be the key risk factor. Consequently, patients should have daily medication withdrawal to reassess the need for neuromuscular blockers and allow some muscle activity.[4]

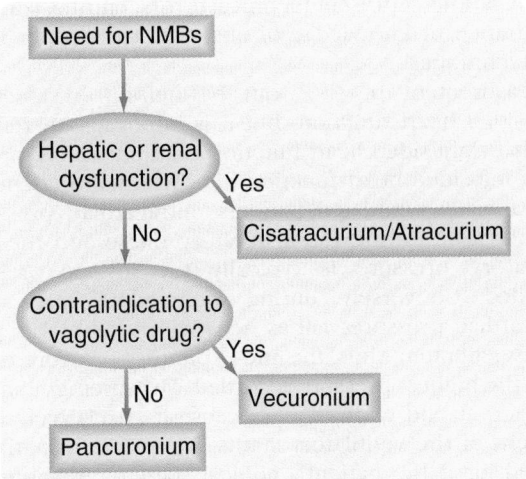

FIGURE 24-2. Algorithm for neuromuscular blockade (NMB) in the ICU. (Adapted from Murray MJ, Cowen J, DeBlock H, et al: Clinical practice guidelines for sustained neuromuscular blockade in the adult critically ill patient. Crit Care Med 30:142-156, 2002.)

CARDIOVASCULAR SYSTEM

Hemodynamic Monitoring

Arterial Catheters

Systemic arterial catheter placement is indicated if vasoactive or cardiotonic drugs are being administered or for frequent or continuous monitoring of systemic arterial pressure or ABGs. The primary complications associated with arterial catheter use include line infection and arterial thrombosis. The infection risk associated with an arterial catheter is much lower than that of a central venous catheter, but arterial catheters must still be placed under sterile conditions. Thrombosis with distal ischemia can be minimized by placing catheters in arteries with good collateral circulation. Thus, the radial or dorsalis pedis arteries are preferred to the brachial or femoral arteries. An Allen test should be performed before placement of a radial artery catheter to document adequate collateral flow from the ulnar artery. Stiffness and resistance of a catheter and measuring system, catheter whip, and the distance from the heart all contribute to variance between the actual and measured systolic (SBP) and diastolic (DBP) blood pressures. Thus, the mean arterial pressure (MAP) is the most accurate measurement obtained:

$$MAP = DBP + \{1/3\}(SBP - DBP).$$

Central Venous Catheters

Central venous catheter placement may be indicated for long-term venous access, to provide parenteral nutrition or chemotherapeutic agents, or to measure central venous pressure (CVP). The most common complications associated with central venous catheter insertion include dysrhythmias; pneumothorax (up to 5% to 10% after subclavian vein placement); arterial puncture with resultant intimal flap, pseudoaneurysm formation, or hemorrhage; and air or catheter embolism. These complications represent technical errors, emphasizing the importance of knowledge of anatomy and proper insertion techniques.

Measurement of CVP can be helpful in assessing right-sided heart function, but it is important to remember that right-sided heart function is an unreliable predictor of left-sided heart function in critically ill patients. In mechanically ventilated patients, intracardiac pressures are increased during the inspiratory phase and the end-expiratory pressure is typically the lowest pressure recorded. Conversely, during spontaneous respiration, intracardiac pressures fall as negative intrathoracic pressure is generated; thus, the end-expiratory pressure is typically the highest pressure recorded. Measurement should be made at end expiration, because it is relatively independent of the ventilatory status. If more information is desired, or if the patient's clinical status or response to therapy seems incongruous, a pulmonary arterial catheter may be useful.

Pulmonary Arterial Catheters

Pulmonary artery catheters allow the measurement of CVP, pulmonary arterial pressure (PAP), pulmonary arterial wedge pressure (PAWP), cardiac output (CO), and mixed venous blood gases. Insertion of a pulmonary artery catheter is warranted in any patient with severe cardiopulmonary derangement. It provides information about volume status as well as cardiac performance and helps to determine the need for volume, inotropic support, and vasoactive drugs. Complications associated with pulmonary artery catheter placement include those associated with central venous catheter placement, plus intracardiac knotting of the catheter, valvular damage, and chamber rupture. Pulmonary artery rupture has been reported owing to prolonged positioning or balloon inflation in the distal pulmonary vasculature. Prophylactic lidocaine may help prevent dysrhythmias in patients with irritable myocardium. Floating a pulmonary artery catheter in a patient with left heart block can be particularly hazardous, because the catheter may interfere with conduction in the right side of the heart, resulting in complete heart block. A pacemaker should be immediately available.

Placement of a pulmonary artery catheter relies on the correct interpretation of pressure tracings from the distal catheter transducer. The catheter should be inserted between 15 and 20 cm and the balloon inflated. Passage into the right ventricle is usually obvious because it is accompanied by wide excursions in the pressure tracing. As the catheter is continuously advanced, exit into the pulmonary artery is heralded by much higher diastolic pressures, with gradually decreasing pressure waves during diastole. A dampened waveform usually signals the "wedge" position. This occurs at 45 to 50 cm in the average-sized adult. The catheter should be inched back to achieve a minimal distance required for a proper position. A chest radiograph should confirm position of the catheter in the pulmonary arterial trunk.

Cardiovascular Dysfunction

Shock

Shock is defined as perfusion that is inadequate to meet metabolic needs. Management of the patient in shock is focused on (1) identifying the presence of shock; (2) searching for and treating immediately life-threatening conditions; and (3) treating shock based on the underlying pathophysiology (see Chapter 5). Shock commonly presents as hypotension, but it is important to recognize that it can exist in the face of normal blood pressure. Other signs of shock may include tachycardia, bradycardia, tachypnea, mental status changes, cutaneous hypoperfusion (cool skin, sluggish capillary refill), oliguria, myocardial ischemia, hypoxemia, and metabolic acidosis. Once shock is identified, the first step is to identify and correct immediately life-threatening abnormalities. These might include loss of airway or inadequate ventilation, compression of the heart or great vessels, dysrhythmias, hemorrhage, or anaphylaxis. A rapid assessment of the ABCs can help direct life-saving interventions such as endotracheal intubation/mechanical ventilation, tube thoracostomy, pericardiocentesis, transfusion, fluid resuscitation, or administration of antidysrhythmic or vasoactive medications.

After addressing immediate threats to life, one must identify and treat the underlying cause of shock. Shock may be classified into five categories: hypovolemic, cardiac compressive, neurogenic, septic, and cardiogenic. Hypovolemic shock may be due to third-spacing of fluid, gastrointestinal or insensible losses, or hemorrhage. A crystalloid bolus (20 mL/kg) should be administered immediately and repeated if necessary. Glucose-containing fluids should be avoided, because they may provoke an osmotic diuresis. If hemorrhage is suspected and the hemodynamic response to crystalloid is not satisfactory, blood transfusion should be initiated without delay and a search for the source of hemorrhage aggressively undertaken. The rapidity of resuscitation is predicated on the patient's condition: restoration of normal blood pressure, heart rate, skin color, mentation, and urine output signify a reversal of hypoperfusion. The need for continued resuscitation may be estimated by additional measurements (see "Endpoints of Resuscitation," later). In the setting of hemorrhagic shock, it is prudent to restore hemoglobin to near-normal levels.

Cardiac/great vessel compressive shock may be due to tension pneumothorax or massive hemothorax, which can impede venous return by shifting the mediastinum, or pericardial tamponade, which prohibits cardiac diastolic filling. Tube thoracostomy relieves mediastinal shift associated with tension pneumothorax or hemothorax, and it may provide definitive management of the problem. Pericardial tamponade may be due to blood, transudative fluid, or air in the pericardium. A hemodynamically unstable patient should undergo immediate decompression, either via thoracotomy or pericardiocentesis. Pericardiocentesis may be performed under ultrasound guidance, and a catheter can be left in with a stopcock to allow intermittent drainage while transporting the patient for definitive management (thoracotomy or pericardial window). The appearance of hemodynamic "stability" must be interpreted with caution, however, because ongoing subendocardial ischemia may compromise long-term recovery from the insult. Thus, the confirmation of pericardial tamponade calls for action (fluid resuscitation and plans for decompression) without undue delay. Neurogenic shock is typically seen in the setting of a spinal cord injury resulting in loss of vasomotor tone. The treatment is fluid administration, with vasopressors as needed. Septic shock represents cardiovascular collapse associated with an infectious process; management involves treating the underlying infectious process ("source control") and administering appropriate antibiotics (see "Sepsis," later). Cardiogenic shock refers to pump failure. Inflammatory and cardiogenic shock often require specific support of the circulation.

Support of the Circulation

To reverse shock, one must ensure adequate perfusion of tissues. The factors that determine perfusion are the O_2 content of the blood (CaO_2), the pumping function of the heart, and the tone of the vasculature. The O_2 delivery (DO_2) is the product of CaO_2 (mL O_2/dL blood) and the CO (L/min). The DO_2 is usually indexed to body surface area, so the cardiac index (CI) is used in the calculation and the result is reported in milliliters of O_2/min/m^2:

$$DO_2 = CaO_2 \times CI \times 10$$

The CaO_2 consists of that which is carried by hemoglobin (Hb) and that which is dissolved:

$$CaO_2 = [Hb \times SaO_2 \times 1.39] + [0.003 \times PaO_2]$$

where Hb is the concentration in g/dL, SaO_2 is the arterial O_2 saturation (%), and PaO_2 is the partial pressure of O_2 (mm Hg) in arterial blood. Usually, the fraction of O_2 that is dissolved in blood is inconsequential; an exceptional circumstance is a patient with a critically low hemoglobin value (e.g., a Jehovah's witness who has bled). To optimize DO_2 to tissues, one should try to maximize the SaO_2 and provide a normal concentration of hemoglobin. The usual guidelines for transfusion (see later) do not apply to the patient in shock. Once the CaO_2 is maximized, CO must be addressed. The CO is equal to stroke volume times heart rate and is influenced by cardiac rhythm and contractility, as well as vascular tone. The approach to augmenting CO begins with ensuring a perfusing heart rate and rhythm and good contractility of the heart.

Dysrhythmias

Dysrhythmias are common in the ICU, and correct interpretation of the rhythm is the key to proper treatment. In a patient with cardiopulmonary arrest, first diagnose the rhythm with quick-look paddles and treat according to the guidelines in Box 24-1.[5] Symptomatic bradycardia (heart rate < 60 beats/min) should be treated with atropine (0.5 to 1 mg) or cardiac pacing. Dopamine or epinephrine may be required. Unstable patients with tachycardia (heart rate > 100 beats/min) should undergo cardioversion (100-200-

Box 24-1. Guidelines for Management of Cardiopulmonary Arrest

Ventricular Fibrillation/Pulseless Ventricular Tachycardia

Defibrillation 360 J × 3; initiate CPR
Epinephrine, 1 mg every 3 to 5 minutes, *or* vasopressin, 40 IU single dose
Defibrillation: 360 J
Consider amiodarone, lidocaine, magnesium sulfate, procainamide.

Asystole

Verify by rotating leads.
Transcutaneous pacemaker
Epinephrine, 1 mg every 3 to 5 minutes
Atropine, 1 mg every 3 to 5 minutes, to total 0.04 mg/kg

Pulseless Electrical Activity

Diagnose and treat underlying cause.
Epinephrine, 1 mg every 3 to 5 minutes
Atropine, 1 mg every 3 to 5 minutes, to total 0.04 mg/kg
Consider calcium chloride and sodium bicarbonate.
Consider pacing and thoracotomy/cardiac massage.

From International guidelines 2000 conference on cardiopulmonary resuscitation and emergency cardiovascular care. Circulation 102(Suppl I): I136-I165, 2000. Copyright 2000, the American Heart Association.

300-360 J). When stable, a 12-lead ECG and rhythm strip should be obtained. If the QRS complex is wide, cardiovert and give amiodarone or procainamide. If the QRS is narrow, attempt to establish a specific diagnosis by employing vagal maneuvers or adenosine (6 mg, repeated once). For junctional tachycardia, amiodarone is favored; it may be used in patients with normal ejection fraction. For ectopic or multifocal atrial tachycardia, amiodarone or diltiazem is recommended if the ejection fraction is less then 40%; otherwise, calcium-channel blockers or β blockers may be tried first. Paroxysmal supraventricular tachycardia may be treated with calcium-channel blockers, β blockers, or digoxin, but in the setting of an ejection fraction less than 40%, digoxin or amiodarone is preferred first.[5]

The most common sustained dysrhythmia is atrial fibrillation (A-Fib), with a prevalence of 5% in people older than age 65 years. Numerous stresses in the perioperative period may trigger new-onset A-Fib or loss of rate control in the patient with chronic A-Fib. Cardioversion should be performed for hemodynamic instability. Otherwise, rate control and rhythm conversion are attempted while the underlying cause (e.g., myocardial ischemia, fluid overload, electrolyte imbalances, hypoxemia, acidosis, pulmonary embolism) is identified and treated. Intravenous calcium-channel blockers or β blockers are usually effective in rapid conversion; digoxin takes several hours for maximal effect. If the rhythm has been present for less than 48 hours, conversion to normal sinus rhythm should be attempted with cardioversion; alternatively, amiodarone may be used. If A-Fib has been present for more than 48 hours or an unknown duration, cardioversion is contraindicated unless the patient is anticoagulated.[5]

Pump Dysfunction

In patients with inflammatory or cardiogenic shock, cardiac pump function may be disturbed owing to circulating myocardial depressants or ischemia. The clinical manifestations of the failing heart may include pulmonary edema (left-sided heart failure), peripheral edema, distended neck veins (right-sided heart failure), or both. Once CaO_2 has been maximized and a perfusing rhythm has been ensured, the next step is to optimize CO. The principal determinants of CO are preload, afterload, and contractility. At a minimum, CVP monitoring should be instituted. If CVP and MAP are both low, volume replacement is warranted. If CVP is high and MAP is low, however, a pulmonary artery catheter should be inserted for monitoring of PAWP and CI. If PAWP and CI are both high, the patient may have been over, resuscitated; fluids should be slowed and diuretic therapy considered. Low PAWP and high CI may be associated with inflammatory shock, anaphylaxis, and hepatic or autonomic dysfunction, and fluid resuscitation is warranted. If the PAWP and CI are both low, administer fluid boluses of crystalloid to increase PAWP by 3 to 5 mm Hg and re-measure the CI; if it improves, repeat this therapy until the patient's condition stabilizes. If PAWP is high and CI is low, then either an inotropic agent or an afterload-reducing agent may be warranted. If the patient is normotensive, then an afterload reducer may be helpful. Sodium nitroprusside and nitroglycerin are most frequently employed, but angiotensin-converting enzyme inhibitors (ACE-I) or ganglionic blocking agents (e.g., trimethaphan) may be considered. Nitroprusside (0.5 µg/kg/min) is desirable because of its rapid onset and reversibility and rare tolerance or tachyphylaxis. A byproduct is cyanide, which is converted to thiocyanate and excreted by the kidneys.

Cyanide toxicity may be heralded by increasing mixed venous oxygen saturation (S{vbar}O₂), and is treated by administering 3% sodium nitrite (10 mL) followed by methylene blue (1 mg/kg). Thiocyanate levels greater than 10 mg/dL may necessitate hemodialysis. Nitroglycerin (0.25 to 0.5 µg/kg/min) is a good choice in patients with elevated preload as well as afterload and especially in those with pulmonary edema.

Hypotensive patients may require medication to augment cardiac contractility, increase systemic arterial vasoconstriction, or both. There are several agents that may be used, each having a unique profile of activity on adrenergic receptors (Table 24-2). The α_1 receptors have a primary effect on systemic arterial vasoconstriction and lesser effects on systemic veins and pulmonary arteries. The β_1 receptors act primarily on the heart, increasing heart rate, contractility, and atrioventricular conduction. The β_2 receptors increase heart rate and contractility but are also vasodilatory to the systemic and pulmonary vasculature. Dopaminergic receptors modulate arterial vasodilatation; the D_2 subtype decreases heart rate.

Three of the most commonly used medications for hypotensive patients are epinephrine, norepinephrine, and dopamine. Epinephrine is a potent α- and β-adrenergic agonist and thus increases myocardial contractility as well as vasoconstriction. It increases myocardial Vo_2 and is arrhythmogenic, so its usefulness in the ICU is limited to patients with profound hypotension. Norepinephrine's primary value is to increase MAP; it has deleterious effects on CO, so its use is limited to patients with elevated CO (e.g., patients in inflammatory shock). Dopamine is most useful when an increase in MAP is needed to better perfuse the brain, heart, or kidneys. Low doses (3 to 5 µg/kg/min) may improve renal and mesenteric perfusion. Up to 8 µg/kg/min, its effect is primarily inotropic, but at higher doses peripheral vasoconstriction and increased myocardial work predominate.

In patients who have an adequate MAP but who need help with myocardial contractility, inotropic drugs are

TABLE 24-2. Effects of Selected Vasoactive Agents

Drug	Dosage (µg/kg/min)	Receptor Activity			Hemodynamic Response			
		α	β1	β2	HR	MAP	CO	SVR
Dopamine	3-5	(−)	++	(−)	↑	↑	↑	→
	5-20	++	++	(−)	↑↑	↑↑	↑	↑↑
Dobutamine	2-20	(−)	++	+	↑↑	↑	↑	↓
Norepinephrine	1-20 µg/min	++	+	(−)	↑	↑↑	↑	↑↑
Phenylephrine	10-100 µg/min	++	(−)	(−)	→	↑↑	↓	↑↑
Epinephrine	0.005-0.02	(−)	++	++	↑↑	↑	↑	↓
	0.01-0.1	++	++	+	↑↑	↑↑	↑	↑↑
Isoproterenol	0.03-0.15	(−)	++	+	↑↑	→	↑	↓
Amrinone	5-10				→	→	↑↑	↓
Milrinone	0.3-1.5				→	→	↑↑	↓

HR, heart rate; MAP, mean arterial blood pressure; CO, cardiac output; SVR, systemic vascular resistance.

useful. For the most part, these drugs have vasodilatory effects, so it is important to ensure adequate preload before infusion. Dobutamine (5 to 15 µg/kg/min) can be very effective and is less arrhythmogenic than dopamine. Isoproterenol is a powerful β-adrenergic agonist. It is a potent inotrope with vasodilatory properties, but its usefulness is outweighed by its arrhythmogenicity. The phosphodiesterase inhibitors amrinone and milrinone are believed to act by inhibiting the breakdown of cyclic adenosine monophosphate. They increase the CI and reduce preload and afterload without significant dysrhythmias. Amrinone may cause profound vasodilation, and long-term administration is associated with thrombocytopenia and gastrointestinal side effects. Milrinone is a more potent inotrope with fewer side effects.

Resuscitation

Fluids

Fluid resuscitation is a key maneuver to institute as soon as shock is recognized. Crystalloid is administered to expand the intravascular volume, acknowledging that only about one third of the fluid will remain in the intravascular space. Although it may be tempting to administer colloid solutions, they should not be used in the acute phase of shock resuscitation. Cellular dysfunction may result in loss of capillary integrity and extravasation of water as well as colloid, resulting in widespread tissue edema. Prospective randomized clinical trials (PRCTs) have demonstrated that survival is no better—and possibly worse—when albumin is given instead of crystalloid.[6,7] In the case of hemorrhagic shock, the usual "transfusion triggers" do not apply, and hemoglobin should be restored to near-normal levels.

Endpoints of Resuscitation

While resuscitation may normalize many clinical signs (e.g., heart rate, blood pressure, respiratory rate, skin color, mentation, urine output), it does not ensure that the O_2 debt has been repaid. For that reason, there should be an objective measure of the success of resuscitation in meeting tissue metabolic needs.[8] In the early 1990s, Bishop and colleagues[9] identified values for CI (4.5 L/min/m^2), DO_2 (600 mL O_2/min/m^2), and VO_2 (170 mL O_2/min/m^2) above which survival could be predicted in critically ill patients. Subsequent PRCTs testing these resuscitation goals offered mixed results. Recently, Kern and Shoemaker[10] reviewed published data and concluded that if hemodynamic optimization is applied to subgroups with an expected mortality of 20% or greater, prior to the development of organ failure, and the goal of increased DO_2 is achieved, then survival will be improved. While it is difficult to argue that early aggressive resuscitation benefits critically ill patients, it must be recognized that not all patients respond in the same way. For example, Moore and colleagues[11] reported that 38% of severely injured patients were unable to attain a VO_2 of 150 mL O_2/min/m^2, despite supranormal DO_2. This group, appearing to have

defective aerobic metabolism, had a higher incidence of multiple organ failure (MOF). Thus, routine resuscitation to "supranormal" targets may be unnecessary in some patients (whose shock is readily reversed) and fruitless in others (who cannot respond).

Alternative parameters that may serve as resuscitation endpoints include S{vbar}O_2, end-tidal carbon dioxide (ETCO_2), gastric intramucosal pH (pHi), base deficit, and arterial lactate. The S{vbar}O_2 is an indicator of O_2 extraction and is used to calculate VO_2. Continuous monitoring of S{vbar}O_2 can provide an early warning of complications (e.g., hemorrhage or myocardial ischemia), but intermittent measurements are not as reliable. Furthermore, a low value is helpful, but a normal or high S{vbar}O_2 may be misleading. For example, in severe sepsis or preterminal shock there can be significant shunting with little O_2 being delivered to tissue beds. The ETCO_2 reflects alveolar CO_2. Decreased CI or increased pulmonary dead space may decrease ETCO_2 and increase the arterial-ETCO_2 difference; this has been associated with death.[12] The mesenteric circulation is the first to be compromised in shock and the last to be restored. Gastric tonometry measures the pHi in the stomach, which reflects mesenteric ischemia. A pHi greater than 7.3 has compared favorably with supranormal DO_2 and VO_2 (600 and 150 mL/min/m^2, respectively) as an endpoint.[13] The major drawbacks to the widespread use of gastric tonometry are technologic limitations, cost, and convenience. A number of investigators have measured transcutaneous O_2 and CO_2 levels, as well as skeletal muscle oxyhemoglobin. Early results were encouraging, but these techniques have not gained broad acceptance. Arterial lactate and base deficit are measures of global tissue perfusion. Elevated levels of either are predictive of adverse outcomes; moreover, the time to normalization strongly correlates with mortality and morbidity.[14,15] In addition to their prognostic significance, these parameters allow the degree of physiologic derangement to be quantified, and they serve as targets for ongoing resuscitation.

With few exceptions, every prospective, goal-directed clinical trial that has shown a survival advantage has espoused the principles of the "supranormal DO_2" strategy—volume loading with or without transfusion and inotropic support as needed to meet a predetermined goal. The optimal algorithm for fluids and inotropes has not been determined; however, it is clear that a defined endpoint is important. Rather than selecting a goal that simply confirms the act of resuscitation, it is best to choose an endpoint that confirms a response to resuscitation.

Perioperative Cardiac Support

Cardiac Risk Assessment

Cardiovascular complications are frequent after noncardiac surgery. In 1996 it was estimated that, annually, 50,000 patients will have a perioperative myocardial infarction and another 1 million patients will have a cardiac complication.[16] These figures stand to increase as

TABLE 24-3.   Risk Factors for Perioperative Cardiac Complications in Patients Undergoing Noncardiac Surgery

Risk Factor	Odds Ratio
Diabetes mellitus	3.0 (1.3-7.1)
Renal insufficiency	3.0 (1.4-6.8)
High-risk surgery	2.8 (1.6-4.9)
Ischemic heart disease	2.4 (1.3-4.2)
Congestive heart failure	1.9 (1.1-3.5)
Poor functional status	1.8 (0.9-3.5)

Adapted from Fleisher LA, Eagle KA: Lowering cardiac risk in noncardiac surgery. N Engl J Med 345:1677-1682, 2001.

our population ages, calling for increased vigilance in assessing and minimizing cardiac risk. In an acute surgical emergency, the preoperative risk assessment is limited to vital signs, volume status, and an ECG. There is no opportunity for further risk assessment or risk reduction. In less urgent circumstances, evaluation proceeds based on the presence of risk factors (Table 24-3). If the patient has no risk factors, no further testing or treatment is necessary. One or two risk factors do not by themselves warrant additional testing, but in the presence of a history consistent with coronary artery disease, noninvasive testing is prudent. Three or more risk factors mandate noninvasive testing.[16] The optimal noninvasive test is debated.[17] Exercise ECG is generally advocated as the first test. However, it is not suitable for patients who have uninterpretable ECGs or who are unable to exercise. In those cases, an imaging test is necessary. Imaging is also preferable in patients with poor myocardial function or previous revascularization, to assess regional myocardial viability. The choice of imaging—radionuclide perfusion imaging versus echocardiography—depends primarily on local expertise. An abnormal noninvasive test mandates cardiac catheterization with coronary arteriography. Three-vessel or left main coronary artery disease may be an indication for coronary artery bypass surgery; one- or two-vessel disease may be treated by coronary angioplasty. Revascularization should be limited to those patients with a clear need, independent of the need for noncardiac surgery.

Patients who will not be referred for revascularization but who harbor cardiac risk factors should receive medical therapy aimed at minimizing perioperative risk. Randomized clinical trials have not proven a benefit to perioperative monitoring with a pulmonary artery catheter. β Blockers should be administered to all patients at risk for cardiac events who are scheduled to undergo surgery.[16] If possible, therapy should be instituted in advance, with shorter-acting agents such as metoprolol and by targeting a resting heart rate less than 60 beats/min.

Heart Failure

Heart failure may be encountered in the perioperative period, manifest by tachycardia, low CO, and pulmonary (if left-sided failure) or peripheral (if right-sided failure) edema. The most common cause of heart failure in the surgical ICU is myocardial ischemia, but it may represent decompensation of chronic heart failure. Thus, history and physical examination should be supplemented with ECG and possibly a cardiac enzyme panel. Chest radiographs may be helpful to identify pulmonary pathology. Invasive monitoring with a PAC allows determination of right- and left-sided filling pressures, CI, and afterload. It may help distinguish cardiogenic from noncardiogenic pulmonary edema but not systolic from diastolic dysfunction. Echocardiography may be a more useful tool in patients with acute heart failure, providing information on chamber size, ventricular function, valvular function, and indirect measurements of pressure, as well as extracardiac problems such as pericardial effusion. Diuretics and vasodilators are the mainstays of treatment of heart failure. Diuretics improve pulmonary congestion and reduce ventricular end-diastolic volume, improving myocardial VO_2. Loop diuretics are the class of choice in the acute setting, owing to reliable efficacy, short onset, and potency. Vasodilators including ACE-I, hydralazine, and nitrates are also used. The ACE-I prevent the formation of angiotensin II, a potent vasoconstrictor and stimulus for aldosterone secretion. In addition to decreasing afterload, they augment stroke volume and thus are generally preferred, particularly in patients with a depressed (<40%) left ventricular ejection fraction. They provide symptomatic improvement as well as a long-term survival advantage.[18] Hydralazine and nitroglycerin are second-line agents for patients who cannot tolerate ACE-I therapy. The cardiac glycoside digoxin has a limited role in the treatment of acute heart failure. In patients with diastolic failure, inotropes may exacerbate failure, and treatment with a negative inotrope may be needed. β Blockers help attenuate the sympathetic overactivity associated with heart failure and decrease myocardial VO_2. Mechanical support including an intra-aortic balloon pump or left ventricular assist device may be required in patients in post-bypass cardiogenic shock or as a bridge to transplant.

RESPIRATORY SYSTEM

Respiratory Failure

Respiratory failure is relatively common in surgical ICUs for a variety of reasons. Preexisting cardiopulmonary or neuromuscular disease may compromise respiratory mechanics, gas exchange, or ventilatory drive. A number of factors also affect postsurgical or critically ill patients: respiratory mechanics may be compromised by the acute disease process, the surgical intervention, or pain; gas exchange may be adversely affected by fluid shifts, lung injury, or systemic inflammation with resultant acute lung injury; and ventilatory drive or airway protection may be depressed from analgesics or sedatives. To minimize morbidity and mortality associated with respiratory failure, it is critically important to recognize it, ascertain the cause, and treat it.

Symptoms and signs of acute respiratory failure include dyspnea, anxiety, altered mental status, cyanosis, the use of accessory muscles of respiration, stridor, tachypnea, tachycardia, and hypoxia. The initial evaluation includes a rapid assessment to ensure airway patency and air movement. Vital signs, including pulse oximetry, should be obtained and supplemental O_2 should be provided immediately, as causes of failure are sought. A chest radiograph and ABG analysis are mandatory; other studies such as ECG, bronchoscopy, ventilation-perfusion ($\dot{V}/\dot{Q}$) scanning, and CT should be considered. There are several options for delivery of supplemental O_2: nasal cannula, face tent, face mask, noninvasive positive-pressure systems, and endotracheal intubation with mechanical ventilation. The choice is dictated by the patient's condition and ventilatory needs. Indications for intubation and mechanical ventilation include "SOAP": excessive *Secre*tions requiring pulmonary toilet; impaired *Oxygenation* requiring positive-pressure ventilation; *Airway* obstruction or inability to protect the airway; compromised *Pulmonary* function (i.e., inability to generate adequate respiratory effort or to meet minute ventilatory needs).

The amount of O_2 that must be supplied is the lowest amount that provides adequate CaO_2 in the blood. As discussed earlier, this is directly related to the hemoglobin concentration and SaO_2. Therefore, as in the setting of shock, consideration should be given to restoring near-normal hemoglobin levels in patients with acute respiratory failure. Pulse oximetry and ABG analysis will yield information on PaO_2 and SaO_2. Although related, PaO_2 and SaO_2 have a complex relationship, as indicated by the hemoglobin-O_2 dissociation curve (Fig. 24-3). At low levels of O_2 tension (point A to point B), increases in PaO_2 translate into only small increases in the percentage of O_2 bound to hemoglobin. During mid-range O_2 tension (point B to point C), however, the relationship of PaO_2 to O_2-hemoglobin binding is nearly linear, with significant increases in SaO_2 resulting from increases in PaO_2. The curve plateaus at higher O_2 tension (point C to point D), such that continued increases in PaO_2 result in very little increase in SaO_2. The goal in acute respiratory failure is to achieve a PaO_2 that lies on the upper plateau of the curve.

Hypoxemia is affected by inspired O_2, ventilation, and $\dot{V}/\dot{Q}$ matching. $\dot{V}/\dot{Q}$ matching is the balance between ventilation and perfusion at the alveolar level. It is a continuum, ranging from complete shunt (perfused but nonventilated space) to dead space (ventilated but nonperfused space). Alveolar collapse (e.g., atelectasis, alveolar flooding with fluid and/or proteinaceous debris) results in a shunt. Blood that perfuses such an alveolus returns to the left atrium with low CaO_2—essentially the same as that of mixed venous blood. Dead space ventilation occurs in the conducting airways, where perfusion is limited and essentially no gas exchange occurs. Ultimately, PaO_2 represents the sum total of gas exchange (Fig. 24-4). Defects can be quantified as the alveolar-arterial O_2 gradient ($AaDO_2$):

$$AaDO_2 = PAO_2 - PaO_2$$

where $PAO_2 = [FiO_2 \times (PATM - PH_2O)] - PaCO_2$

PATM is the atmospheric pressure (760 mm Hg at sea level; 627 mm Hg at 5280 feet); PH_2O is the vapor pressure of water (47 mm Hg); and $PaCO_2$ is the alveolar pressure of CO_2, which can be calculated from $PaCO_2$ divided by the respiratory quotient (normally 0.8). Thus, as an example, for a person breathing room air at sea level and having $PaCO_2 = 40$ mm Hg:

$$PAO_2 = [0.21 \times (760 - 47)] - (40/0.8) =$$
$$(0.21 \times 713) - 50 = 150 - 50 = 100 \text{ mm Hg}$$

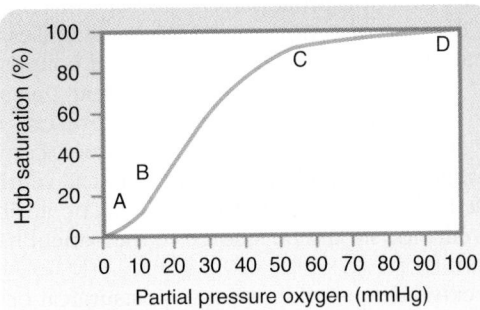

FIGURE 24-3. Oxygen and hemoglobin (Hgb) dissociation curve. A sigmoid-shaped curve shows maximal oxygen loading in the lung and unloading of O_2 in the periphery occurring over a very narrow range of PaO_2.

FIGURE 24-4. A model of the two-alveolus theory of lung function. In the presence of alveolar collapse or alveolar flooding (hatched area), nonoxygenated venous blood on the right is allowed to shunt pass the alveolus with no oxygen transfer, yielding a PaO_2 of 40 mm Hg and oxygen content of 15 mL%. Despite a normal alveolus on the left and normal oxygen content after passing by the alveolus (O_2 content 22 mL%), the mixing of right and left gives the systemic blood a PO_2 of 60 mm Hg and a low oxygen content of 18.5 mL%. (From Hall JB, Wood LD: Acute hypoxemic respiratory failure. *In* Hall JB, Schmidt GA, Wood LDH [eds]: Principles of Critical Care. New York, McGraw-Hill, 1992, with permission of the McGraw-Hill Companies.)

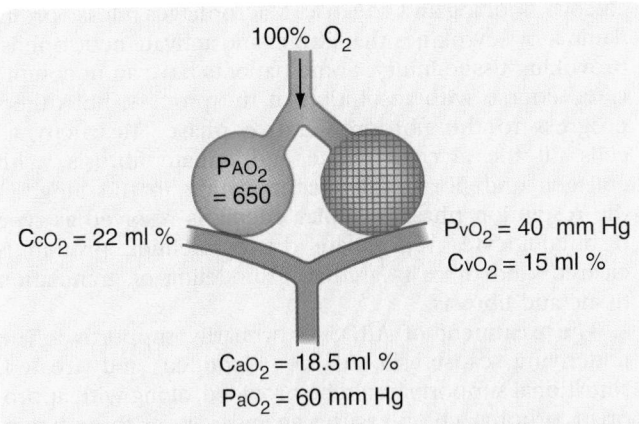

At 5280 feet, $PaO_2 = 72$ mm Hg, and at sea level breathing 100% O_2, $PaO_2 = 663$ mm Hg. Subtracting the PaO_2 from PAO_2 quantifies the $AaDO_2$. In healthy individuals, ventilation and perfusion are well matched and the $AaDO_2$ is low (10 to 25 mm Hg), reflecting only dead space ventilation in the conducting airways and shunting of small amounts of blood via bronchial vessels and thebesian veins. An elevated $AaDO_2$ suggests impaired gas exchange. Nonpulmonary causes of right-to-left shunting include atrial septal defect, pulmonary arteriovenous malformations, severe sepsis, and cirrhosis. There are numerous pulmonary causes of pulmonary dysfunction. These include aspiration, atelectasis, pneumonia, pulmonary contusion, pulmonary embolism, pulmonary edema, and acute lung injury/acute respiratory distress syndrome (ARDS).

Up to 50% of patients who have an aspiration event develop pneumonia, with a subsequent mortality as high as 50%. Aspiration may occur from impairment in laryngeal competence and glottic closure or from gastric reflux due to ileus or gastric outlet obstruction. The initial manifestations of aspiration are caused by mechanical effects of airway obstruction. Obtunded patients will not typically cough to expel the aspirate, and the effects may be more severe. Soon after, the chemical injury becomes evident, with bronchoconstriction and fluid sequestration in the alveoli. An inflammatory response follows, with release of leukocyte- and platelet-derived inflammatory mediators and leak of protein-rich fluid into the alveoli. Pulmonary function progressively worsens through these phases. Because of compromised airway defenses, bacterial pneumonia is a risk during the clinical course. Treatment of aspiration is to mechanically clear the airways of debris, decompress the stomach to prevent further events, and provide supportive respiratory care (e.g., bronchodilators, bronchoscopy, mechanical ventilation) as needed. There is no role for prophylactic antibiotics, but surveillance should be tailored to the patient's overall condition.

Atelectasis is most often seen in postsurgical or immobilized patients. As alveoli collapse, there is increased shunting with resultant hypoxemia. Additional findings are related to the degree of atelectasis and include diminished breath sounds and reduced lung volume, elevated hemidiaphragm, or consolidation on chest radiography. Associated fever usually abates with re-inflation, but the collapsed alveoli are prone to bacterial colonization with the development of pneumonia. Treatment is aimed at re-expansion of collapsed alveoli. Maintenance of airway patency and pulmonary toilet are of primary importance. Pain management is pivotal to balance splinting with sedation and hypoventilation. Pneumonia is common in the ICU, particularly among ventilated patients and those with direct lung injury. The clinical presentation involves fever, leukocytosis, hypoxia, a distinct radiographic infiltrate, and purulent sputum with bacterial colonization. Respiratory support, pulmonary toilet, and antibiotics are the fundamentals of treatment. It is discussed further in Chapter 12. Pulmonary contusion is usually associated with chest wall injury, and so pulmonary dysfunction stems from disruption in respiratory mechanics, hypoventilation secondary to pain, and disruption of lung tissue with alveolar hemorrhage and fluid sequestration. The initial presentation varies widely, and the condition typically worsens during the ensuing 24 to 48 hours with evolution of the inflammatory response and fluid shifts from resuscitation. Management is supportive, with respiratory support and pulmonary toilet as needed. This is discussed further in Chapter 20. A pulmonary embolism is a potentially catastrophic event, initially manifested by hypoxemia. It is discussed in detail later in the section on the hematologic system. Clinical signs of pulmonary edema include dyspnea, tachypnea, hypoxemia, and bilateral rhonchi/rales. Patients may have signs of hypervolemia or congestive heart failure such as distended neck veins or peripheral edema. Radiographic findings include redistribution of blood flow ("cephalization"), perivascular cuffing, enlarged cardiac silhouette, and pleural effusions. The underlying cause may be either fluid overload or left-sided heart failure. Young, healthy patients may be managed by fluid restriction and/or diuresis. In patients with cardiopulmonary or renal dysfunction, invasive hemodynamic monitoring may be warranted to clarify the diagnosis. Hypoxemia and hypercapnia are treated supportively, and inotropic support is provided as needed. A diuretic should be administered, and nitroprusside or nitroglycerin infused to promote afterload reduction.

Acute Lung Injury/Acute Respiratory Distress Syndrome

Acute lung injury and ARDS are clinical syndromes of pulmonary dysfunction that may result from any number of infectious, inflammatory, or tissue injury or cellular shock conditions. Criteria for the diagnosis of ARDS include acute onset, bilateral pulmonary infiltrates on chest radiography, the absence of cardiogenic pulmonary edema (i.e., PAWP < 18 mm Hg), and hypoxemia ($PaO_2:FIO_2 <$ 200). On the same continuum, acute lung injury is a milder form, with $PaO_2:FIO_2 = 201 - 300$.[19] The mortality of ARDS approaches 40% to 50%, with most deaths attributed to MOF. The pathogenesis of ARDS involves three stages. The first stage, coinciding with the acute onset of respiratory failure, is known as the exudative phase. Disruption of the alveolar epithelium results in the influx of protein-rich edema fluid and a leukocytic infiltrate. Destruction of type II pneumocytes disrupts normal alveolar fluid transport and surfactant production, leading to alveolar flooding and collapse. Macrophages release proinflammatory cytokines that attract and activate neutrophils, provoking tissue injury. Some patients have an uncomplicated course with resolution of the process, but others progress to the fibroproliferative phase. Mesenchymal cells fill the alveolar space and initiate fibrosis, with collagen and fibronectin accumulating in the lung. In the resolution phase, alveolar edema is resolved as type II pneumocytes repopulate the epithelium; protein is cleared; and there is gradual remodeling of granulation tissue and fibrosis.

The treatment of ARDS is primarily supportive. The underlying cause should be identified and treated. Nutritional support should be provided, along with appropriate prophylactic measures against venous thromboembolism and stress gastritis. Adequate oxygenation and ventilation must be provided; this generally requires intubation and mechanical ventilation. A number of novel adjunctive therapies have been studied in ARDS.

Preliminary clinical studies suggest that fluid management aimed at lowering filling pressures may decrease pulmonary edema; whether this improves outcome remains to be seen. Surfactant-replacement therapy has been successful in neonates but not yet proven beneficial in adults with ARDS. Despite encouraging results in observational studies, nitric oxide has not proven beneficial in PRCTs; the same goes for other vasodilators. Corticosteroids were never found to be beneficial when administered early in ARDS. However, as the pathophysiology became better understood, the therapy was applied to the fibroproliferative phase. Encouraging results were reported in observational studies[20] as well as in a small PRCT.[21] Corticosteroids warrant consideration as salvage therapy for severe ARDS that is not resolving but must be used with caution because they predispose patients to the risk of infection.

The optimal ventilatory strategy for ARDS patients remains elusive. A number of methods have been employed, including extracorporeal membrane oxygenation (ECMO); extracorporeal carbon dioxide removal; high-frequency jet ventilation; high-frequency oscillatory ventilation; liquid ventilation; permissive hypercapnia; and inverse-ratio ventilation. None of these has been associated with a mortality reduction. Prone positioning has been proposed as a means to improve oxygenation by increasing end-expiratory lung volume, improving $\dot{V}/\dot{Q}$ matching, and changing chest wall mechanics. In a multicenter PRCT, prone positioning improved oxygenation but not survival.[22] Although this intervention may be useful in treating severe hypoxemia for short periods, care must be exercised to minimize complications such as pressure ulceration, accidental extubation, and loss of vascular catheters and feeding/drainage tubes. Low tidal volume (VT) ventilation has been the focus of a number of PRCTs. The National Institutes of Health ARDS Network study group performed a multicenter PRCT in which patients were randomized to a VT of 12 mL/kg vs 6 mL/kg, with plateau pressures maintained at less than 50 versus less than 30 cm H_2O, respectively. After enrolling 861 patients, the trial was stopped because in-hospital mortality was reduced from 40% to 31% in the low VT group.[23] The results of this study were discrepant from earlier, smaller trials. Whether the benefit was attributable solely to lower VT is unclear; nevertheless, this approach has gained widespread support.

Positive end-expiratory pressure (PEEP) can improve oxygenation by recruiting collapsed alveoli and reducing functional residual capacity. "Conventional" ventilation generally calls for the minimal PEEP necessary to provide acceptable oxygenation. However, in the setting of ARDS, there may be benefit to increasing PEEP to improve oxygenation as well as to protect the lung by preventing repetitive recruitment/de-recruitment of alveoli, reducing cyclic reopening and stretch during mechanical breaths. The optimal level of PEEP may be determined by incrementally increasing PEEP to maximize the PaO_2:FIO_2 ratio;

however, some argue that this ignores lung mechanics. A lung pressure-volume curve may be generated for a given patient, and the lower inflection point (P_{FLEX})—the point at which the slope increases in steepness, representing a pressure at which the majority of alveolar units are open—identified. Alternatively, the PEEP may be titrated to maximal compliance, which may be easier to measure at the bedside.[24] A "lung-protective" strategy employed in a PRCT included a VT less than 6 mL/kg, PEEP above P_{FLEX}, driving pressures less than 20 cm H_2O above the PEEP level, pressure-limited ventilation, and permissive hypercapnia. Compared with conventional ventilation, there was improved 28-day survival, less barotrauma, and a higher rate of weaning from mechanical ventilation.[25] This trial was small and had a higher than expected mortality in the conventional ventilation group, but it has stimulated further study into the use of higher PEEP levels.

Ventilatory Support

Noninvasive Ventilatory Support

Many patients require more support than a passive O_2 delivery device. There are several noninvasive interventions that can support oxygenation and ventilation and possibly obviate the need for endotracheal intubation and mechanical ventilation. Intermittent positive-pressure breathing (IPPB) aids in clearance of secretions but is labor intensive and, because it is not continuously applied, does not permanently recruit air spaces. Continuous positive airway pressure (CPAP) applied by a tight-fitting mask can maintain and restore functional residual capacity and, therefore, provides a temporary salutary effect on oxygenation as the underlying cause of hypoxia is treated. This intervention has no effect on ventilation and requires a nasogastric tube due to associated aerophagia. Bilevel positive airway pressure (BiPAP) also employs a tight-fitting mask, but it requires a ventilator to deliver a high airway pressure during spontaneous patient-initiated breaths and a lower baseline pressure during exhalation (like PEEP). It may provide enough assistance to prevent fatigue and stave off endotracheal intubation. Like CPAP, BiPAP should be considered a short-term therapy that allows for the identification and treatment of the underlying derangement. Continued close monitoring is necessary for patients on CPAP and BiPAP because their condition may deteriorate precipitously.

Mechanical Ventilation

As outlined earlier, there are four primary indications for endotracheal intubation and mechanical ventilation: excessive *Secretions*, impaired *Oxygenation*, *Airway* obstruction or inability to protect the airway, and compromised *Pulmonary* function. Once mechanical ventilation is instituted, the ventilator must be programmed to meet the patient's needs. The first variable to set is the trigger, that is, the variable that will initiate inspiration. The trigger may be a time interval or a threshold rate of air flow. The second variable to set is an inspiratory limit, which may be a volume, a pressure, or a maximum air flow rate. The third variable to set is the cycle, which may be a volume, pressure, or time. Based on these variables, the ventilator will deliver one of three types of breaths: mandatory, assisted, or spontaneous. A mandatory breath is triggered, limited, and cycled by the machine. An assisted breath is triggered by the patient but is limited and cycled by the ventilator. A spontaneous breath is triggered, limited, and cycled by the patient.

Volume-Cycled Ventilation

This type of ventilation delivers a preset V_T with each breath. Advantages include delivery of a reliable minute volume and ease of use. The major disadvantage is potential for high airway pressures and resulting lung injury. The different modes of volume-cycled ventilation include controlled mandatory ventilation (CMV), assist control ventilation (ACV), and intermittent mandatory ventilation (IMV). With CMV, the patient receives a set number of fixed-volume breaths but is unable to increase minute ventilation by triggering additional breaths. CMV is used only in the operating room under general anesthesia. ACV differs from CMV in that the patient is able to trigger additional breaths. Every triggered breath will be a full machine-cycled breath. ACV is used when full ventilatory support is required but is not suitable for the agitated patient who is tachypneic because it may lead to severe respiratory alkalosis. IMV allows spontaneous breathing. It delivers intermittent fixed-volume breaths and allows the patient to breathe spontaneously between mechanical breaths. Synchronized IMV (SIMV) allows the mechanical breaths to be triggered by the patient's own respiratory effort and avoids stacking of breaths. Varying degrees of pressure support may be added to the spontaneous breaths to assist the patient. SIMV is a useful mode of ventilation when attempting to wean or when there is patient-ventilator asynchrony.

Pressure-Cycled Ventilation

Pressure-controlled ventilation (PCV) is designed to protect the lung from alveolar overdistention and epithelial injury. A set pressure is applied to the ventilatory circuit during each breath, allowing the lungs to expand. The major advantages are lower mean and peak airway pressures and an exponential decelerating flow pattern that tends to be more comfortable for the patient. The major disadvantage is fluctuating minute ventilation in the face of changing lung compliance. Pressure-cycled breaths can be delivered in an analogous fashion to volume-cycled breaths, in either an AC or SIMV mode. Pressure-support ventilation (PSV) is a spontaneous ventilatory mode. A negative inspiratory force created by the patient will trigger the ventilator to apply a certain pressure to the ventilator circuit. PSV is the most comfortable mode of ventilation because the patient is able to control all elements of inspiration and expiration. PSV is rapidly becoming the mode of choice for weaning patients off of mechanical ventilation. The major disadvantage of PSV is that minute ventilation cannot be ensured and hypoven-

tilation and apnea can occur. Thus, patients must have an intact respiratory drive.

The Difficult-to-Ventilate Patient

Patients with severe lung disease can be a challenge to oxygenate and ventilate. On volume-cycled ventilator modes, airway pressures may climb; on pressure-cycled modes, the delivered V_T may decrease. The goals include maintaining airway pressures less than 35 to 40 cm H_2O and SaO_2 more than 90%. Definitive recommendations for optimal ventilator strategies are not available, but there are a number of maneuvers that may be attempted. Prone positioning can improve oxygenation as discussed earlier, but it can be associated with loss of tubes and lines, as well as sequelae of positioning and cutaneous pressure. Inhaled nitric oxide can also improve oxygenation transiently but is expensive and not readily available. Permissive hypercapnia attempts to minimize barotrauma and volutrauma to the lung. Hypercapnia and respiratory acidosis are usually tolerated, but tracheal gas insufflation may be employed to attenuate them. It involves the positioning of a small-caliber catheter just above the carina, with 2 to 10 L/min of 100% O_2 delivered to "wash out" the anatomic dead space. Inverse ratio ventilation involves lengthening inspiratory time to more than 50% of the respiratory cycle. This increases mean airway pressure and recruits air spaces by auto-PEEP in a manner similar to applied PEEP. Inverse ratio ventilation should be used with caution in patients with known severe chronic obstructive pulmonary disease and asthma, given their propensity for air trapping. Pharmacologic paralysis relaxes the chest wall musculature and allows for synchronization of ventilator and patient while decreasing VO_2 and CO_2 production. High-frequency ventilation typically delivers a V_T of 1 to 3 mL/kg at rates of 100 to 3000 cycles/min and allows adjustment of mean airway pressures to maintain oxygenation. Extracorporeal membrane oxygenation or CO_2 removal may offer enough lung protection to salvage critically ill patients, but expertise and availability are variable. Partial liquid ventilation, in which the lung is filled with perfluorocarbon and then subjected to standard mechanical ventilation, may be efficacious in preserving lung histology, lung compliance, and systemic oxygenation. Anecdotal success has been reported for each of these innovations, but it is unlikely that any one of them will be a panacea for the treatment of severe respiratory failure. Appropriate treatment of these patients will require an arsenal of several of these techniques.

Weaning from Mechanical Ventilation

Patients who are intubated for pulmonary failure usually require a period of weaning, to regain strength and to prove their ability to support themselves. To consider liberating a patient from the ventilator, it is important to first ensure that the underlying problem leading to intubation has been rectified and the patient is hemodynamically stable. Then, one may make the same "SOAP" assessment as in determining the need for intubation: (1) Are the Secretions too much for the patient to handle? (2) Is the patient *Oxygenating* adequately (i.e., PaO_2:FIO_2 >150; requiring FIO_2 < 0.40 to 0.50 and PEEP < 5 to 8 cm H_2O)? (3) Can the patient protect his or her *Airway*? (4) Is *Pulmonary* function adequate? Ideally, the patient may be assessed while breathing spontaneously. A number of parameters may be obtained to assess pulmonary function. Negative inspiratory force (>−20 to −30 cm H_2O), minute ventilation (<10 to 15 L/min), V_T (>5 mL/kg), and respiratory rate (<30/min) are all useful indicators. Perhaps the most reliable single test is the f/V_T ratio, or the "Rapid Shallow Breathing Index."[26] A value more than 105 predicts failure of extubation with a 95% likelihood, whereas a value less than 80 predicts success in 95%. There are four primary methods of weaning. Multiple daily tracheostomy-piece trials may be performed, with extubation once the patient tolerates several hours. This is labor intensive. A single daily tracheostomy-piece trial may be performed, with extubation if it is successful; if not, the patient is rested for 24 hours. IMV and PSV weaning are popular, without a proven advantage of one over the other. It is clear that trials of spontaneous breathing shorten weaning time. Thus, the preferred strategy may be to assess parameters daily and perform a single tracheostomy-piece trial for at least 30 minutes.

GASTROINTESTINAL SYSTEM

Stress Gastritis

Stress-related mucosal lesions are the result of gastric acid acting on compromised (i.e., poorly perfused and/or immunologically incompetent) gastric mucosa. These lesions have been reported to develop in 25% to 100% of ICU patients within 24 to 48 hours of admission, with clinically significant bleeding in 5% to 10% of patients. Based on these data, routine stress ulcer prophylaxis is provided in most ICUs. However, it is probably not necessary in every ICU patient. The evolution of care in ICUs has provided earlier and better resuscitation and nutritional support, resulting in improved mucosal perfusion and preserved integrity. Risk factors for stress gastritis include mechanical ventilation longer than 48 hours, coagulopathy, significant burns, and head injury. Patients with risk factors should receive prophylaxis until they are taking an enteral diet at more than 50% of caloric intake goals. Prophylactic agents include antacids, sucralfate, histamine-2 (H_2) receptor antagonists, and proton pump inhibitors. Antacids have not been proven effective in ICU patients at risk and should not be considered first-line agents. Sucralfate is a sucrose-based polymer that is activated in an acidic environment. It binds to exposed gastric mucosa and ulcer craters, forming a protective barrier, and stimulates local prostaglandin synthesis. It is given as an elixir by mouth or via nasogastric tube (1 g every 6 hours). Early trials suggested a lower risk of nosocomial pneumonia compared with H_2 receptor antagonists, owing to the preservation of an acidic gastric environment and less bacterial proliferation. The major disadvantage of sucralfate is its interference with absorption of other medications, such as antibiotics, warfarin, and phenytoin. The H_2 receptor antagonists have potent acid-reducing properties. Concerns regarding H_2 receptor antagonists include the development of tachyphylaxis and increased gastric bacterial colonization, leading to development of pneumonia. A large, multicenter PRCT comparing the use of sucralfate to ranitidine in ICU patients with risk factors determined that H_2 receptor antagonists were superior to sucralfate in preventing clinically important bleeding. The rate of ventilator-associated pneumonia was similar between the groups.[27] With the recent development of intravenous proton pump inhibitors, further trials may demonstrate the superiority of these agents compared with H_2 receptor antagonists. In the meantime, choice of an agent is dependent on institutional preference.

Abdominal Compartment Syndrome

The abdomen is a closed space, bound by the relatively nonexpansile fascia of the abdominal musculature, and hence is susceptible to a compartment syndrome analogous to that seen in the lower extremities. The abdominal compartment syndrome (ACS) is fundamentally defined as an increased intra-abdominal pressure (IAP) that is associated with adverse physiologic consequences.[28] The ACS has most commonly been described in patients with massive abdominal or pelvic hemorrhage, often following damage control laparotomy, but it may be encountered in numerous scenarios. Circumferential burn eschar, reduction of a large ventral hernia, or military anti-shock trousers may significantly increase IAP. Bowel distention due to obstruction or ileus or pneumoperitoneum may lead to the ACS. Pancreatitis or surgical dissection may result in profound retroperitoneal edema. Edema of the bowel may result from prolonged evisceration during surgery, which elongates and narrows mesenteric veins and lymphatics; it may also be related to ischemia/reperfusion of the bowel aggravated by resuscitation with large volumes of crystalloid solutions. "Secondary" ACS refers to ACS in the absence of abdominal or pelvic pathology and is entirely due to edema and ascites after shock and aggressive resuscitation.[29] In this setting—particularly in nontrauma patients—it may represent a state of irreversible shock, with loss of capillary integrity.

The organ systems that appear most affected are the cardiovascular, pulmonary, and renal systems. Cardiovascular effects of increased IAP include decreased CI owing to diminished venous return; therefore, adequate volume resuscitation is a key feature of management of ACS. A markedly increased systemic vascular resistance has also been recognized. Increased IAP pushes up on the diaphragm, decreasing pulmonary compliance and creating high airway pressures. Resultant hypoventilation leads to hypoxia and hypercarbia. Renal dysfunction (oliguria, anuria) due to ACS appears to be caused by direct parenchymal compression and shunting of renal plasma flow. Visceral blood flow is similarly affected, leading to intestinal necrosis, hepatic dysfunction, and gut anastomotic breakdown. Intracranial hypertension is also observed owing to decreased venous outflow. Decompression of the abdominal cavity can immediately reverse these changes. However, if untreated, ACS leads to lethal organ failure, with collective mortality rates exceeding 50%.[28]

The recognition of ACS is not difficult once the diagnosis is considered. Those at highest risk include severely injured patients who require abdominal packing for abbreviated/staged laparotomy and particularly those with a coagulopathy, such as core hypothermia and cirrhosis. It may be prudent to screen patients at high risk for developing ACS; this should include patients acutely resuscitated from shock, particularly if requiring vasopressors and receiving more than 6 L of crystalloid or 6 units of packed red blood cells over a 6-hour period.[29] The findings of a tensely distended abdomen, progressive oliguria in spite of adequate CO, or hypoxia with increasing airway pressures are sufficient to justify abdominal decompression. However, physical findings alone may be inaccurate in the critically ill patient, and for less obvious scenarios bladder pressure can be measured to ascertain the degree of IAP elevation and correlate with physiologic parameters. Bladder pressure has become accepted as the objective standard for measuring IAP. The level of IAP at which ACS occurs is patient specific. The diagnosis (and treatment) is therefore based on the patient's physiologic responses to increased IAP. Nevertheless, rough correlations can be made between the level of IAP elevation and the need for decompression (Table 24-4). Although significant alterations in physiology can be demonstrated with IAP between 10 and 15 mm Hg (grade I), it is doubtful that abdominal decompression is warranted at this level. With IAP between 15 and 25 mm Hg (grade II), the need for treatment should be based on the patient's clinical condition. In the absence of oliguria, hypoxia, or significantly elevated airway pressures, abdominal decompression is difficult to justify. However, this group requires close monitoring. Most patients with IAP between 25 and 35 mm Hg (grade III) ultimately require decompression, although signs and symptoms of ACS may develop insidiously. All patients with IAP greater than 35 mm Hg (grade IV) require immediate decompression; this group of patients may deteriorate to cardiac arrest at any time. Percutaneous drainage of ascitic fluid may be an effective temporizing maneuver, but operation is usually required. At the time of decompression, an abdominal closure that can compensate for additional intra-abdominal volume is indicated. Of the various meshes and plastic or rubber sheets that are available, the most cost effective

is a sterilized, opened 3-L genitourinary irrigation bag known to many as the "Bogota bag." Every reasonable effort should be made to achieve a definitive abdominal closure within 3 or 4 days. If this is not accomplished, the lateral tractive forces of the broad, flat muscles of the abdominal wall preclude a primary closure in most instances. This condition relegates the patient to split-thickness skin grafts or mesh closure that risks intestinal fistulas. Vacuum-assisted wound closure may facilitate early definitive abdominal closure.[30]

Nutritional Support

The neuroendocrine response to critical illness includes the release of stress hormones (epinephrine, glucagon, and cortisol) and inflammatory mediators that culminate in a hypercatabolic state (see Chapter 7). Endogenous substrates are mobilized, depleting glucose and fat stores and "auto-cannibalizing" lean muscle mass. Visceral protein is subsequently eroded, resulting in organ system and immune dysfunction. Because we are still unable to modulate the systemic inflammatory response (see Chapter 4), the preferred therapeutic strategy is to administer exogenous substrate in the form of nutritional therapy. Nutritional support should be considered if (1) the patient has been without nutrition for 5 to 7 days; (2) the duration of illness is expected to exceed 10 days; or (3) the patient is malnourished. Malnutrition may be assessed by recent weight loss (15% body weight). Serum protein levels may be measured, but they may be affected by severe illness. Once the decision is made to provide support, the next step is to determine the nutritional needs of the patient. A practical rule of thumb is based on weight. For normal weight patients, 30 kcal/kg/day should be adequate; 35 kcal/kg/day may be targeted for underweight patients and 25 kcal/kg/day advised for overweight patients. A more precise number for the basal energy expenditure (BEE, kcal/day) may be estimated by the Harris-Benedict equations:

$$BEE = 66 + (13.7 \times weight) + (5 \times height) - (6.8 \times age) \text{ (males)}$$

$$BEE = 665 + (9.6 \times weight) + (1.8 \times height) - (4.7 \times age) \text{ (females)}$$

where weight is measured in kilograms, height in centimeters, and age in years. The BEE estimate is then multiplied by a "stress factor" ranging from 1.25 to 1.75, depending on the severity of illness. In stable mechanically ventilated patients in whom overfeeding or underfeeding would be particularly detrimental, whose energy expenditure is significantly altered from expected values, or who are not responding as expected to calculated regimens, indirect calorimetry can be used to calculate measured energy expenditure (MEE):

$$MEE = [(3.9 \times Vo_2) + 1.1 + Vco_2] \times 1.44 - (2.8 \times UUN)$$

where Vo_2 and CO_2 production (Vco_2) reflect a 30-minute period. The preferred ratio of nonprotein calories:nitrogen varies with stress level. In minimally stressed patients, 200 to 300:1 is appropriate, but it should be decreased to 150:1 in moderately stressed and to 100:1 or less in

TABLE 24-4.   Grading System for the Abdominal Compartment Syndrome

Grade	Intra-abdominal Pressure (mm Hg)	Treatment
I	10-14	Normovolemic resuscitation
II	15-24	Hypervolemic resuscitation
III	25-35	Decompression
IV	>35	Emergent re-exploration

severely stressed patients. Protein should be restricted in patients with hepatic or renal failure. Another way to determine protein needs is weight and stress based: 1.5 for mild, 2.0 for moderate, and 2.5 g protein/kg for severe stress. Alternatively, measurement of urine urea nitrogen (UUN) can help determine protein needs. As stress-related catabolism increases, nitrogen excretion (and UUN) increases. The UUN represents 90% of excreted nitrogen. Protein losses (g/day) may be calculated based on 24-hour UUN:

$$\text{Protein loss} = [\text{UUN} + (4 \text{ g insensible} + \text{nonurea nitrogen loss})]$$

The goal of nutritional support is to provide positive nitrogen balance of 3 to 5 g/day, so additional protein must be added beyond the calculated requirements. To calculate the protein requirements, multiply nitrogen requirements by 6.25.

The optimal route for delivery of nutritional support is debated. Enteral feeding preserves gut mucosal integrity and barrier function, IgA production, and normal flora. These mechanisms may explain reduced septic complications and improved survival in patients with severe injuries, acute pancreatitis, inflammatory bowel disease, and after liver transplantation. Furthermore, the safety and feasibility of early postoperative enteral feeding have been proven. On the other hand, there are some conflicting data, and clear superiority over parenteral nutrition has not been demonstrated. Parenteral delivery of nutrition can ensure adequate provision of nutrients and should be employed when enteral feeding is not tolerated or in the presence of short gut or high output/proximal gastrointestinal fistulas. In critically ill patients, postpyloric feeding is believed to be safer than gastric feeding in terms of aspiration risk. While several trials have suggested that gastric feeding with promotility agents is equally safe, these studies have been underpowered to reflect the occasional catastrophic event.

"Immune-enhancing" diets provide specific nutrients (glutamine, arginine, nucleotides, and ω-3 fatty acids) that exert favorable immunomodulatory effects. Glutamine is an oxidative fuel for enterocytes and other rapidly replicating cells. Arginine promotes normal T-cell distribution and function and aids in wound healing. Nucleotides enhance the replication of rapidly dividing cells as well as immune responsiveness. The ω-3 fatty acids compete with ω-6 fatty acids (specifically, arachidonic acid) in cyclooxygenase metabolism, resulting in production of prostaglandins of the three series and leukotrienes of the five series. These are less inflammatory and immunosuppressive eicosanoids compared with the two-series prostaglandins and four-series leukotrienes produced by arachidonic acid. Although several clinical trials have suggested significant benefits with these diets, the literature is mixed.[31]

ACUTE RENAL FAILURE

Acute renal failure (ARF) is a deadly problem, with mortality rates exceeding 50%. It is typically heralded by oliguria (<0.5 mL/kg/hr or <400 mL/24 hr) or rising serum creatinine concentration, which should prompt a search for its cause (prerenal, renal parenchymal, or postrenal). The first step is physical examination to look for signs of hypovolemia, heart failure, shock, renovascular obstruction, ACS, or urinary tract obstruction. The most common problem in surgical ICU patients is hypovolemia. A Foley catheter should be inserted to exclude outlet obstruction and follow the urine output closely, and a fluid bolus (approximately 500 mL, or 10% of the circulating blood volume) should be administered. An exception is the patient in whom heart failure is suspected; in that case, early measurement of CVP or PAWP may be prudent to help direct therapy. If the patient does not respond to fluid administration, a more extensive evaluation must be undertaken. Invasive hemodynamic monitoring may be warranted to measure filling pressures and assess cardiac function. A spot urine sodium (U_{Na}) level may be helpful in distinguishing prerenal from renal parenchymal causes of ARF: a U_{Na} less than 20 mEq/L is consistent with a prerenal cause and one of more than 40 mEq/L is consistent with a renal parenchymal cause. By measuring both sodium and creatinine in the urine as well as plasma, the fractional excretion of sodium (FE_{Na}) as a percentage may be calculated:

$$FE_{Na} = [(U_{Na} \times P_{Cr})/(P_{Na} \times U_{Cr})] \times 100$$

An FE_{Na} less than 1% indicates a prerenal etiology of ARF, whereas FE_{Na} greater than 3% suggests a renal parenchymal or postrenal problem. The patient's medication list should be reviewed for nephrotoxic agents. Identification of postrenal pathology may be made by renal ultrasonography. Urinalysis can also provide clues to the underlying etiology. A high urine specific gravity and low pH are consistent with prerenal ARF. Tubular casts are indicative of renal parenchymal dysfunction; hemoglobinuria is consistent with a transfusion reaction, vasculitis, or rhabdomyolysis; myoglobinuria is suggestive of rhabdomyolysis; and eosinophilia is associated with interstitial nephritis. These laboratory investigations are less helpful in the elderly, those with chronic renal dysfunction, or patients who have received diuretics or osmotic agents in the previous 24 hours.

The management of prerenal causes is to augment renal perfusion. Volume loading ensures adequate preload, and inotropic support is provided as needed. Renal vasoconstriction may be an unwanted side effect of inotropic agents. Low doses (0.3 to 3 μg/kg/min) of dopamine can selectively dilate the renal vasculature and stimulate diuresis. However, this agent should be used with caution because it may be dysrhythmogenic and has not been proven to affect the incidence or ultimate outcome of ARF.[32] Nephrotoxic drugs, including contrast agents, should be avoided, and all renal-excreted drugs should be dose adjusted. The creatinine clearance (C_{Cr}; mL/min) can be used for medication dose adjustment:

$$C_{Cr} = (U_{Cr} \times V)/P_{Cr}$$

where U_{Cr} is urine creatinine concentration (mg/dL), V is urine volume (mL/min), and P_{Cr} is plasma creatinine concentration (mg/dL). A 24-hour collection is most accurate, but a 4-hour sample may be used. An immediate calculation may be made by the following equation:

$$C_{Cr} = [(140 - age) \times weight]/(P_{Cr} \times 72)$$

where weight is measured in kilograms. In females, the value is multiplied by 0.85. Normal C_{Cr} is 95 mL/min in females and 120 mL/min in men. Clearance of circulating myoglobin or hemoglobin may be achieved by forcing diuresis (>100 mL/hr) with crystalloids. Obstructing lesions should be treated. Comorbid conditions need to be addressed and nutritional support provided. Although the conversion of oliguric to nonoliguric ARF may facilitate volume management, there is insufficient evidence that it improves outcomes.[33] In fact, a recent cohort study suggested an increased risk of nonrecovery of renal function and mortality associated with diuretic use.[34]

Renal replacement therapy (RRT) may be indicated for symptomatic fluid overload, severe electrolyte or acid-base disorders, sepsis, or uremic complications such as encephalopathy or pericarditis. There are several options for RRT. Intermittent techniques include peritoneal dialysis and hemodialysis. Peritoneal dialysis is appropriate in chronic renal failure patients who do not have peritonitis or recent abdominal surgery. Hemodialysis provides efficient removal of fluid, solutes, and filtrate but may be associated with hemodynamic instability and is relatively resource intensive. One report claimed that daily hemodialysis offers a survival advantage, but this needs to be confirmed by further studies.[35] Continuous RRT techniques offer the advantage of improved hemodynamic stability and relatively less resource utilization, but they require some anticoagulation and have not been proven superior to hemodialysis in improving outcomes. Continuous hemofiltration may be used to remove fluid and solutes only, in patients who only suffer from fluid overload. Continuous venovenohemodialysis (CVVHD) is the most commonly used method in the ICU. It employs a double-lumen central venous catheter and pumps blood through a filter against the flow of dialysate before returning it to the patient. Continuous arteriovenous hemodiafiltration (CAVHD) is essentially the same, except that a large-bore arterial cannula is required.

Given the significant morbidity and mortality associated with ARF, prevention is an ideal strategy. This involves careful attention to fluid balance and perfusion, proper dosing of medications, and avoidance of nephrotoxic drugs. Radiographic contrast material causes 10% to 15% of hospital-acquired ARF. Hydration and use of nonionic contrast agents may help reduce this occurrence. Additional adjuncts include *N*-acetylcysteine and possibly the dopaminergic agonist fenoldopam.

HEPATIC DYSFUNCTION

Liver disease is often suspected on the basis of a history of alcohol or intravenous drug abuse, blood transfusions, sexual promiscuity, or the presence of tattoos. Physical signs associated with liver disease include jaundice, ascites, muscle wasting, malnutrition, encephalopathy, gynecomastia, testicular atrophy, bitemporal muscle wasting, vascular spiders, palmar erythema, and caput medusae. Laboratory findings consistent with liver dysfunction include elevated liver function tests, prolonged prothrombin time, and hypoalbuminemia.

Critically ill patients may develop secondary liver failure, manifested by cholestatic jaundice, impaired synthetic activity, and altered mental status. Treatment is aimed at the underlying condition; failure to correct the underlying problem often results in MOF and death. Primary liver failure may represent an exacerbation of chronic liver disease or an acute problem caused by viral illness, drugs, or other toxins. In cases of acute liver failure, both the etiology and the extrahepatic complications (e.g., fluid, electrolyte, and coagulation abnormalities; renal, pulmonary, and immune dysfunction) are generally treated medically. Cerebral edema is present in 80% of patients dying of fulminant hepatic failure, so aggressive management, including early ICP monitoring, is critical. Orthotopic liver transplantation may prove lifesaving but must be considered before irreversible brain damage or organ failure develops.

Patients with an exacerbation of chronic liver disease usually present with a complication that must be treated. Variceal hemorrhage is the most dramatic presentation; its management is addressed in Chapter 44. Patients with ascites and acute physiologic decompensation should undergo diagnostic paracentesis to exclude bacterial peritonitis and possibly large volume paracentesis to alleviate symptoms. A white blood cell count greater than 500/mm³ suggests bacterial peritonitis. Spontaneous bacterial peritonitis occurs in over 20% of cirrhotic patients with ascites. It is typically monomicrobial and can be treated by antibiotics (third-generation cephalosporin or fluoroquinolone) alone, although it is associated with 50% 1-year mortality. Polymicrobial peritonitis is indicative of intra-abdominal abscess or perforated viscus. Medical management of ascites includes sodium restriction (1 to 2 g/day), water restriction in patients with hyponatremia, and diuresis. Spironolactone is preferred because it inhibits sodium reabsorption, but furosemide may be required as well. Large-volume paracentesis is generally well tolerated, but albumin replacement (7 to 9 g/L) may decrease renal insufficiency and encephalopathy. Management of hepatic encephalopathy begins with reversal of precipitating factors, such as removal of drugs with CNS effects, treating infections, and correcting fluid/electrolyte abnormalities. Ammonia formation and elimination are addressed by administering lactulose and neomycin. Branched-chain amino acid–enriched nutritional formulas have been promoted to decrease encephalopathy.

The hepatorenal syndrome is a functional renal problem that probably results from a combination of systemic vasodilation, relative hypovolemia, and increased activity of the renin-angiotensin-aldosterone system. It is characterized by azotemia, oliguria, low urinary sodium (<10 mEq/L), and high urinary osmolality. Prognosis is poor, but recent trials suggest some improvement in outcomes with systemic vasoconstriction using terlipressin or ornipressin.[36] Nutritional support should limit protein to 1 to 1.2 g/kg/day and provide 25 to 35 kcal/kg/day, with 30% to 40% of nonprotein calories in the form of fat. Coagulopathy is addressed by administration of clotting factors and platelets.

ENDOCRINE SYSTEM

Adrenal Insufficiency

The hypothalamic-pituitary-adrenal axis is stimulated by stress, resulting in proportional increases in corticotropin-releasing hormone (CRH), adrenocorticotropic hormone (ACTH), and cortisol. An impairment in this stress response may result in adrenal insufficiency, with potentially catastrophic consequences. Patients with potential adrenal insufficiency may be identified based on a history of chronic or recent corticosteroid administration or clinical findings consistent with hypercortisolism/Cushing's syndrome (hypertension, diabetes, truncal obesity, hirsutism, buffalo hump) or primary adrenal insufficiency/Addison's disease (thin, hyperpigmented, constitutional complaints). In this setting, corticosteroids should be administered based on the anticipated degree of stress. For minor surgical procedures, a patient should receive 25 mg of hydrocortisone equivalent daily (Table 24-5) and for moderate stress, 50 to 75 mg/day. In the ICU, it is safe to assume higher stress and so the targeted dose should be 100 to 150 mg daily.[37]

It may be difficult to recognize adrenal insufficiency in the ICU. An acute adrenal crisis may present as unexplained hypotension, fever, abdominal pain, or weakness. If adrenal crisis is suspected, administer hydrocortisone, 200 mg, along with glucose and saline while awaiting confirmatory laboratory values (hyponatremia, hyperkalemia, hypoglycemia, azotemia, cortisol less than 20 μg/dL). If adrenal insufficiency is present, hydrocortisone should be continued at 100 mg every 8 hours for 2 days, and then the dosage should be tapered. If there is a concern about adrenal insufficiency, the serum cortisol level should be measured. This may be a random level, because there is loss of diurnal variation of cortisol secretion in critical illness. A level greater than 34 μg/dL suggests normal adrenal function, and no further testing is required. On the other hand, less than 15 μg/dL is consistent with hypoadrenalism and corticosteroids should be administered (hydrocortisone, 50 mg every 6 hours). For cortisol levels between 15 and 34 μg/dL, a cosyntropin stimulation test should be performed. Cosyntropin, 250 μg, is administered, with plasma cortisol measured at 0, 30, and 60 minutes. An increase less than 9 μg/dL is consistent with hypoadrenalism and should prompt corticosteroid therapy.[38]

Glucose Disorders

Diabetic ketoacidosis (DKA) is typically seen in patients with type I diabetes mellitus (DM), owing to noncompliance with insulin therapy or an illness or injury. Patients may present with symptoms such as nausea, abdominal pain, excessive thirst, or fatigue. They may be hemodynamically unstable, with altered level of consciousness, including coma. A classic finding is Kussmaul breathing (rapid, deep respirations) and an acetone breath odor. Laboratory findings include hyperglycemia (400 to 800 mg/dL), a high anion gap metabolic acidosis, and the presence of serum and urine ketones. Hyperkalemia is common despite total body potassium deficit. Mortality from DKA can approach 10% to 15%, so aggressive treatment is critical. Normal saline is infused to replace intravascular volume, along with regular insulin (0.1 to 0.2 U/kg bolus followed by 0.1 U/kg/hr). Glucose should be monitored frequently, and once it is below 250 mg/dL the intravenous fluid should be changed to 5% dextrose in hypotonic saline. The insulin infusion should be titrated but continued until ketoacidosis abates. Hypokalemia and hypophosphatemia commonly develop during therapy and should be corrected.

Hyperosmolar nonketotic dehydration syndrome (HONK) is more common in patients who have sufficient insulin to prevent ketoacidosis but not hyperglycemia. Its precipitating factors and clinical presentation are similar to those of DKA, but mental status changes are more common and more severe. The hyperglycemia of HONK is more extreme, generally exceeding 800 mg/dL, and ketoacidosis is absent. Dehydration often results in hypernatremia, but the sodium level can be misleading because of osmotic fluid shifts due to hyperglycemia. The free water deficit may be calculated based on the corrected serum sodium level (add 1.6 mmol/L for every 100 mg/dL elevation in glucose):

TABLE 24-5. Relative Potency of Corticosteroid Preparations

Drug	Equivalent Dose (mg)	Glucocorticoid Potency*	Mineralocorticoid Potency*	Half-Life (hr)
Cortisone	25	0.8	0.8	8-12
Hydrocortisone	20	1	1	8-12
Prednisone	5	4	0.8	12-36
Prednisolone	5	4	0.8	12-36
Methylprednisolone	4	5	0	12-36
Triamcinolone	4	5	0	12-36
Betamethasone	0.80	25	0	36-54
Dexamethasone	0.67	30	0	36-54

*Relative to hydrocortisone.

Free water deficit = 0.6 × weight [1 − (140/serum Na)]

where weight is in kilograms and free water deficit is in liters. Treatment of HONK is similar to that of DKA except that fluid resuscitation is necessarily more aggressive.

Hyperglycemia (defined as blood glucose level greater than 200 mg/dL) in the absence of a diagnosis of diabetes mellitus is quite common in critically ill patients. The phenomenon of stress-related hyperglycemia appears to be related to insulin resistance resulting from the release of counter-regulatory hormones (e.g., glucagon, epinephrine, norepinephrine, glucocorticoids, growth hormone) and cytokines (e.g., tumor necrosis factor, interleukins-1 and -6). It is typically seen shortly after admission to an ICU and resolves as the catabolic illness subsides. However, ongoing metabolic dysregulation and protracted hyperglycemia may persist in some patients, particularly those with untreated infection or ongoing injury. The consequences of protracted hyperglycemia include increased postoperative infectious complications[39] and worse outcomes following myocardial infarction, stroke, and head injury.[40] Increasing attention has been directed toward insulin as a therapeutic drug in critical illness. It has potent anabolic as well as immunomodulatory effects that may favorably impact the course of critical illness. A large prospective, randomized clinical trial in a surgical ICU demonstrated improved survival associated with intensive insulin therapy (i.e., maintenance of glucose between 80 and 110 mg/dL, compared with 180 to 200 mg/dL).[41] It is unknown whether the benefit was attributable to lower glucose levels or to relative hyperinsulinemia; further studies are anticipated in this area.

HEMATOLOGIC SYSTEM

Venous Thromboembolism

Deep Venous Thrombosis

Virchow's triad of stasis, endothelial injury, and hypercoagulability is common among ICU patients; indeed, deep venous thrombosis (DVT) occurs in 30% of them.[42] Consequently, every institution should have a formal prevention strategy for venous thromboembolism (VTE). High risk factors that justify prophylaxis include major general surgery (thoracic or abdominal operations under general anesthesia lasting more than 30 minutes); neurosurgical procedures; coronary artery bypass surgery; surgery for gynecologic malignancies; major urologic surgery; multiple trauma; hip fracture; spinal cord injury; surgery or chemotherapy for malignancy; congestive heart failure; and respiratory failure. There are additional risk factors that are not sufficient to justify prophylaxis but that may, in combination, warrant or alter prophylaxis: prior VTE; age older than 40; obesity; prolonged immobility; hormone replacement therapy; antiphospholipid antibody syndrome; and hereditary risk factors. Because ICU patients typically have at least one risk factor and often more, prophylaxis should be considered routine. Patients who are at risk for bleeding should have intermittent pneumatic compression devices applied. If there is no contraindication, low-molecular-weight heparin (LMWH), low-dose unfractionated heparin (LDUH), adjusted-dose heparin, or oral anticoagulants should be administered.[42] Fondaparinux sodium, a synthetic pentasaccharide that inhibits activated factor X, appears promising in major orthopedic surgery.[43] The use of prophylactic inferior vena caval filters is controversial and should be limited to high-risk patients who have contraindications to anticoagulation or to those with recurrent pulmonary embolisms.

The clinical signs and symptoms (leg pain, swelling, rubor, fever) of DVT are unreliable in the ICU. Venography is considered the gold standard for diagnosis, but it is invasive and requires a contrast load. Imaging with CT or MRI is expensive and requires moving the patient. On the other hand, duplex ultrasonography is noninvasive, is portable, and has sensitivity and specificity of more than 95%, making it an excellent screening tool. Recent literature has supported use of the D-dimer assay, pointing to its high negative predictive value. An evidence-based literature review concluded that D-dimer is insufficient to exclude DVT in patients who have moderate to high clinical probability based on pretest assessment.[44] On the other hand, the combination of a normal D-dimer concentration and a low pretest probability is safe to rule out DVT.

Treatment of DVT generally begins with heparin. Because of its more consistent and predictable response, once-daily dosing without the need for monitoring, and equivalent efficacy with fewer bleeding complications, LMWH is preferred over LDUH. In addition, it allows the option of long-term treatment, obviating the need for warfarin. Treatment is generally recommended for 6 months, although this is debated.[45] Thrombolytic therapy should be considered for limb-threatening thrombosis of the iliofemoral system, but otherwise it offers little additional benefit to offset its bleeding risk.[44] Upper extremity DVT should be treated as aggressively as lower extremity DVT, because the rate of pulmonary embolism exceeds 10%.

Pulmonary Embolism

Pulmonary embolism is common and probably underdiagnosed. Its clinical manifestations are nonspecific, and it is likely that the majority of episodes are clinically insignificant. The most common signs of pulmonary embolism are tachypnea, hypoxemia, and tachyarrhythmias; hypotension is associated with moderate-sized pulmonary embolism. If pulmonary embolism is suspected clinically, heparin may be administered empirically while a diagnosis is pursued. Lytic therapy should be considered for moderate to severe cases. If pulmonary embolism is deemed clinically unlikely, diagnostic testing is performed. If the clinical suspicion is very low, a noninvasive study such as D-dimer assay or duplex ultrasonography may be used. However, if the pulmonary embolism was moderate to severe, a more definitive test is needed. Pulmonary angiography is considered the gold standard, but it requires mobilizing the interventional radiology team.

Ventilation-perfusion scanning, the former first-line test, is only valuable if it is either negative or of high probability. CT pulmonary angiography is reportedly accurate, in addition to demonstrating additional/alternative pathology. Catastrophic pulmonary embolism may cause sudden death. Immediate cardiopulmonary resuscitation is required, with large doses of heparin or thrombolytics. Trendelenburg's procedure is an option but is rarely indicated and more rarely successful.

Heparin-Induced Thrombocytopenia

Up to 15% of patients who receive heparin experience acute thrombocytopenia, which spontaneously reverses and has no clinical sequelae. It is caused by transient sequestration of platelets and is termed HIT I. Heparin-associated antiplatelet antibodies (HAAb) develop in 2% to 4% of patients and lead to platelet activation and aggregation. Thrombocytopenia (HIT II) occurs an average of 8 days after the beginning of heparin administration (5 days if a patient was previously sensitized). Because HIT cannot be predicted, patients receiving heparin should be monitored with serial platelet counts. The diagnosis should be suspected if a patient develops resistance to anticoagulation, thromboembolic events, a fall in the platelet count greater than 30%, or a platelet count less than 100,000/mm^3. If HIT is suspected, heparin should be stopped and the patient tested for HAAb. If there are no antibodies, heparin can be resumed. If the patient has HAAb, options for anticoagulation include nonreactive heparins and heparinoids (LMWH formulations have 25% to 35% cross-reactivity), direct thrombin inhibitors (lepirudin, argatroban), defibrinogenating agents (ancrod), and platelet function inhibitors (glycoprotein IIb/IIIa inhibitors). The direct thrombin inhibitors should be considered the preferred agents. The HAAb typically disappear in a few weeks to months, but patients should be retested for antibodies before subsequent heparin administration.[46]

Blood Transfusions

Anemia is very common in critically ill patients; among its many causes are blood loss (including phlebotomy) and decreased erythropoietin production. A multicenter observational study reported that 29% of patients admitted to ICUs had hemoglobin levels less than 10 g/dL and 37% were transfused during their stay.[47] In clinical trials looking at restrictive transfusion strategies, hemoglobin consistently drifts down to 8.5 g/dL.[48,49] Moderate anemia (hemoglobin, 7 to 10 g/dL) is well tolerated in healthy individuals, but ICU patients with excessive metabolic demands may not tolerate the associated decrease in Do_2. On the other hand, blood is altered during storage, such that transfusion may incite electrolyte and acid-base disturbances, coagulopathy, and dysfunctional Do_2. And although the current blood supply is safer than ever, there are still potential risks associated with transfusion. These include transmission of viral infections to both the patient and health care provider, incompatibility resulting in hemolytic reactions, and anaphylactic and febrile reactions.[50] Moreover, transfusions have significant immunomodulatory properties: they can improve the survival of transplanted kidneys but are also associated with recurrence of cancers and increased rates of postoperative infections. In addition, blood transfusion has been identified as a robust independent predictor of postinjury MOF.[51] Recognition of these effects has led clinicians to scrutinize the "transfusion trigger" in ICUs.

A multicenter, prospective randomized clinical trial examined the effects of a restrictive transfusion strategy—transfusing for hemoglobin less than 7 g/dL and maintaining hemoglobin at 7 to 9 g/dL—compared with a liberal strategy (maintaining hemoglobin at 10 to 12 g/dL).[48] The in-hospital mortality was lower among the restrictive-strategy group. In this same group, 30-day mortality was lower among the subsets who were less acutely ill (APACHE scores < 20) and younger (<55 years old) but not those with clinically significant cardiac disease. Based on the current literature, a rational set of transfusion guidelines may be constructed. These are listed in Box 24-2 along with transfusion guidelines for other blood products.

Recognizing the detrimental effects of low Do_2, transfusion alternatives are actively being investigated. In the setting of elective surgery, practicable alternatives include

---

Box 24-2. Transfusion Guidelines

Packed Red Blood Cells

Hemoglobin <7 g/dL
Acute blood volume loss >15%
Greater than 20% drop in blood pressure, or blood pressure <100 mm Hg due to blood loss
Hemoglobin <10 g/dL accompanied by symptoms (chest pain, dyspnea, fatigability, lightheadedness, orthostatic hypotension) or in the presence of significant cardiac disease
Hemoglobin <11 g/dL for patients at risk for multiple organ failure

Fresh Frozen Plasma

Prothrombin time > 17 sec
Partial thromboplastin time > 50 sec
Clotting factor deficiency (<25% normal value)
Massive transfusion (1 unit/5 units red blood cells), or if clinically bleeding
Severe traumatic brain injury

Platelets

Platelet count <10,000/μL
Platelet count <10,000 to 20,000/μL with bleeding
Platelet count <50,000/μL acutely after severe trauma
Bleeding time >15 min

Cryoprecipitate

Fibrinogen <100 mg/dL
Hemophilia A, von Willebrand's disease
Severe traumatic brain injury

preoperative autologous blood donation, normovolemic hemodilution, and induced hypotension to reduce blood loss. These are not feasible in the ICU, however. Auto-transfusion involves the recovery and re-administration of shed blood from body cavities, wounds, and drains. The blood is collected in a reservoir containing an anticoagulant and reinfused after washing and/or filtering. There is virtually no risk of transmission of infectious disease, and transfusion reactions are essentially eliminated. On the other hand, shed blood recovered from body cavities is defibrinated and essentially depleted of clotting factors, and thus a dilutional coagulopathy results after major auto-transfusion. In addition, because the blood has been partially clotted with subsequent lysis, transfusion of the serum containing the products of fibrinolysis can activate the patient's coagulation system and result in disseminated intravascular coagulation. In addition, there is a risk of contamination of the shed blood. Inability to predict who will benefit from it limits its cost effectiveness.

The anemia of critical illness is associated with a blunted increase in circulating erythropoietin concentrations in response to physiologic stimuli. A multicenter PRCT found that weekly administration of 40,000 units of recombinant human erythropoietin increases hemoglobin and decreases transfusions.[49] It is unclear whether this expensive therapy improves clinical outcomes.

Blood Substitutes

Blood products require typing and crossmatching and have a limited shelf life; economics and logistics preclude the immediate availability of stored blood in all health care facilities. A worldwide chronic shortage of blood products is not likely to correct itself. Consequently, Hb substitutes are a focus of ongoing investigation. The ideal blood substitute should provide physiologic O_2-carrying capacity and volume expansion without adverse effects or risks (Box 24-3). Over the past 20 years, two fundamental formulations of blood substitutes have been developed and tested clinically: perfluorocarbon (PFC) emulsions and hemoglobin (Hb) solutions. The PFCs have a solubility for O_2 that is 10 to 20 times that of blood but have no special affinity for O_2, and thus their efficacy relies on maintaining a high PaO_2. To date, they have not been found to offer benefit to injured patients compared with crystalloid solutions. In addition, they have been associated with unacceptable toxicities and a new generation is being developed.

Box 24-3. The Ideal Blood Substitute

- Physiologic loading and unloading of O_2
- Volume expansion capability
- Immediate availability
- Universal compatibility
- No adverse physiologic effects
- Freedom from disease transmission
- Long-term storage capability

The hemoglobin tetramer is the "active ingredient" of the red blood cell; it is quite durable and can function independently to transport O_2 outside its cell membrane. Unfortunately, unmodified tetrameric hemoglobin has proven to be unsafe clinically as it dissociates into heterodimers and extravasates, scavenging nitric oxide and attenuating physiologic vasodilatation. Unmodified tetrameric hemoglobin is further compromised, owing to a low P_{50} and relatively high osmotic activity. Modification of hemoglobin, therefore, has at least four major objectives: (1) to minimize toxicity; (2) to prolong intravascular retention; (3) to decrease O_2 affinity; and (4) to reduce colloid osmotic pressure. There are at least four hemoglobin-based red blood cell substitutes that have been investigated in clinical trials. The primary differences in the hemoglobin solutions lie in the source and the technical aspects of polymerization. Diaspirin cross-linked hemoglobin (HemAssist, Baxter Healthcare, Round Lake, IL), derived from outdated human blood, has been one of the most widely studied solutions. Unfortunately, clinical experience has been disappointing. A multicenter randomized trial in patients with hemorrhagic shock found that mortality was higher in the HemAssist group (46%) compared with a saline resuscitation comparison group (17%).[52] The cause of the excessive death rate is not known. The solution, a known pressor, could have accelerated hemorrhage or scavenged nitric oxide, decreasing cellular perfusion. Another product derived from human blood is an O-raffinose polymerized hemoglobin (HemoLink, Hemosol, Inc., Etobicoke, Ontario, Canada). A phase II clinical trial concluded that it may be effective in reducing transfusions in patients undergoing coronary artery bypass grafting; however, this trial confirmed phase I findings of a pressor effect.[53] A glutaraldehyde-polymerized bovine hemoglobin product (Hemopure or HBOC-201, Biopure Corporation, Cambridge, MA) has a reduced O_2 affinity that promotes O_2 unloading in the tissues. In clinical trials, it has been able to reduce the need for transfusions, but at the cost of increased systemic vascular resistance and methemoglobinemia.[54] A human hemoglobin-based glutaraldehyde-polymerized pyridoxylated stroma-free hemoglobin (Poly SFH-P) solution (PolyHeme, Northfield Laboratories, Chicago, IL) has a near-normal P_{50}, and essentially all unreacted tetramer is removed in a purification process. Clinical trials have demonstrated the safety and physiologic function of PolyHeme, as well as the ability to avoid transfusions of allogeneic blood.[55,56] Unlike the other solutions, there is no evidence that PolyHeme increases systemic or pulmonary vascular resistance.[57] Moreover, the transfusion-related hyperinflammatory response is attenuated with PolyHeme.[58]

SEPSIS AND MULTIPLE ORGAN FAILURE

Sepsis

The MOF syndrome was first described in the 1970s, and early reports linked it directly to sepsis. In the mid-to-late 1980s, however, it was becoming increasingly recognized that the systemic manifestation of gram-negative sepsis could result from noninfectious stimuli. To clarify terminology in this area, the American College of Chest Physicians and the Society of Critical Care Medicine published a consensus description and definition of the systemic inflammatory response syndrome (SIRS) (Box 24-4).[59] These definitions are important in determining which patients might be candidates for new adjunctive therapies.

An epidemiologic study based on hospital discharge databases from seven states (25% of the United States population) in 1995 determined that severe sepsis affects 751,000 patients annually (2.3 per 100 hospital discharges) with a 29% mortality.[60] Based on anticipated population growth and the incidence of sepsis in older patients, it was estimated that the incidence of severe sepsis will increase 1.5% per year. Not every infection causes sepsis. The occurrence of sepsis depends on bacterial virulence factors (e.g., adherence properties, resistance to phagocytosis or antibiotics, endotoxin from gram-negative bacteria, exotoxin from gram-positive bacteria) and host factors (immune status and immune response, epithelial barrier function, gender, genetic factors).

The fundamental strategy in managing septic patients involves resuscitation and treatment of the underlying infection. The two major components are the provision of appropriate antibiotics (see Chapter 12) and source control of the septic focus. Appropriate empirical monotherapy for severe sepsis includes a carbapenem or a third- or fourth-generation cephalosporin. Glycopeptides might be appropriate monotherapy if there is high suspicion of methicillin-resistant *Staphylococcus aureus* or catheter-related sepsis. Source control refers to drainage of abscesses, débridement of devitalized tissue and removal of infected foreign bodies, and definitive

management of the source (e.g., appendectomy, colectomy for diverticular abscess). Resuscitation of patients should follow the principles outlined earlier. The benefits of early goal-directed therapy—targeting CVP, 8 to 12 mm Hg; MAP, 65 to 90 mm Hg; and central venous SO_2 greater than 70%—have been demonstrated.[61] In-hospital mortality was reduced in all patients, as well as the subgroups with severe sepsis and septic shock.

Septic shock is an abnormal vasodilatory distribution of CO in which CO may be normal or increased. Septic shock is often hyporesponsive to catecholamines and may be related to vasopressin deficiency. Thus, there may be a role for vasopressin administration in patients with septic shock. Indeed, an early clinical trial found that in 14 of 16 patients who had catecholamine-refractory septic shock had an immediate and sustained increase in the mean arterial pressure associated with vasopressin infusion.[62]

Increasing recognition of adrenal insufficiency in critically ill patients has prompted a resurgence in interest in corticosteroids as an adjunct in severe sepsis. Two separate meta-analyses in 1995 concluded that there was no survival benefit to the use of corticosteroids. However, more recently, a number of clinical trials have focused on patients with severe sepsis and found that corticosteroids reverse shock, reduce vasopressor days and organ dysfunction scores, and may improve survival. Patients with documented adrenal insufficiency stand to benefit the most. A recent multicenter PRCT demonstrated that patients with septic shock who have adrenal insufficiency have significant reductions in 28-day ICU mortality and hospital mortality if they receive a course of corticosteroids.[63]

There are a number of adjunctive therapies that have shown promise in preclinical studies or small clinical trials, but large multicenter PRCTs have not demonstrated survival benefits.[64,65] These include ibuprofen, prostaglandin E_1, pentoxifylline, *N*-acetylcysteine, selenium, antithrombin-3, intravenous immunoglobulins, hemofiltration, recombinant tissue factor pathway inhibitor, p55 TNF receptor fusion protein, and antibodies to TNF-α and endotoxin.

One of the only compounds that has been shown to improve survival in patients with severe sepsis is recombinant human activated protein C (APC). APC is an endogenous protein that promotes fibrinolysis and inhibits thrombosis and inflammation and is an important modulator of the coagulation and inflammation associated with severe sepsis. In a multicenter PRCT of 1690 randomized severe sepsis patients, APC reduced mortality from 31% to 25%.[66] The only significant adverse effect was an increase in bleeding complications in the APC group (3.5% vs 2.0%, $P = .06$).

Multiple Organ Failure

MOF has been called a "syndrome of surgical progress," because its emergence was the result of advances in treating circulatory shock, renal failure, and pulmonary insufficiency. The description of MOF as a distinct entity dates back to the 1970s, when a number of groups described

---

Box 24-4. Systemic Inflammatory Response Syndrome and Sepsis: Definitions

Systemic Inflammatory Response Syndrome (SIRS)

Two or more of the following:
  Temperature > 38°C or <36°C
  Heart rate > 90 beats/min
  Respiratory rate >20 or $Paco_2$ <32 mm Hg
  White blood cell count >12,000 or <4000/mm³

Sepsis

SIRS + documented infection

Severe Sepsis

Sepsis + organ dysfunction or hypoperfusion (lactic acidosis, oliguria, or altered mental status)

Septic Shock

Sepsis + organ dysfunction + hypotension (systolic blood pressure < 90 mm Hg or > 90 mm Hg with vasopressors)

THE "TWO EVENT" MODEL OF MOF

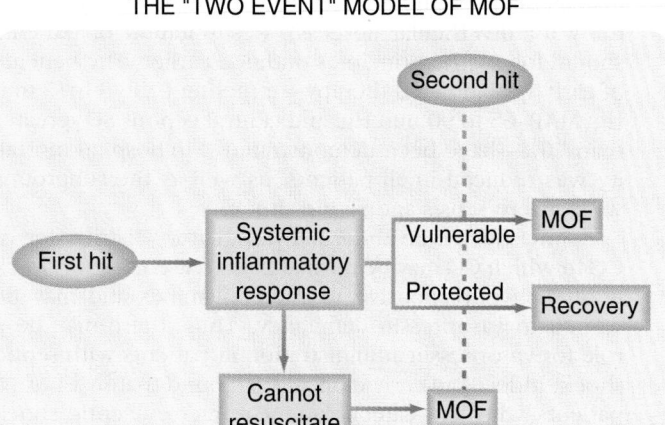

FIGURE 24-5. The "two-event" model of multiple organ failure (MOF). An initial insult results in systemic hyperinflammation. If either the insult or the inflammatory response is exaggerated or perpetuated, patients may develop overt MOF. More commonly, the host endures multiple sequential insults. A second insult during a vulnerable period amplifies the systemic inflammatory response to produce MOF.

DYSFUNCTIONAL INFLAMMATORY/IMMUNE RESPONSE

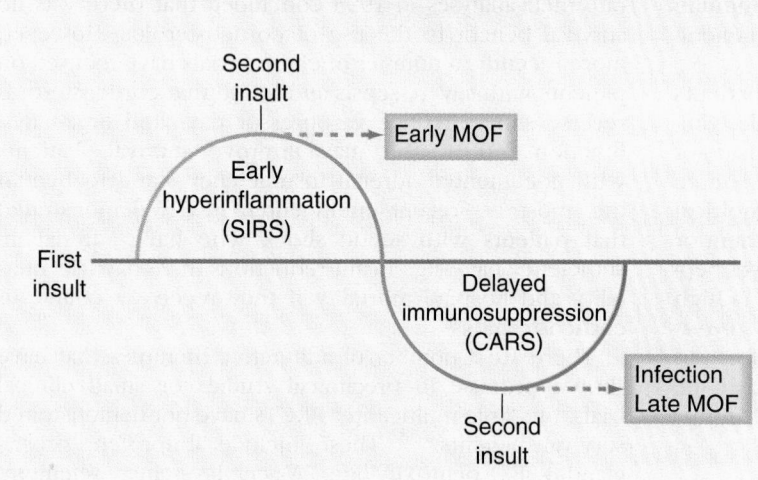

FIGURE 24-6. A dysfunctional inflammatory/immune response leads to multiple organ failure (MOF). The amplitude of the early systemic inflammatory response syndrome (SIRS) is related to the initial insult. A compensatory anti-inflammatory response (CARS) may result in delayed immunosuppression. Sequential insults superimposed on either the hyperinflammatory state or the immunosuppressed state may result in MOF.

the progressive failure of organ systems with a sequential pattern.[67,68] Mortality associated with MOF ranges from 40% to 100% and is related directly to the number and duration of organ failures. Unfortunately, neither the incidence nor the mortality of the syndrome has improved significantly in recent years, and MOF remains the leading cause of delayed mortality in the ICU.[69]

Early reports of MOF implicated infection as the primary etiologic factor,[70] but subsequent studies emphasized that overt clinical infections were not a requisite to MOF. The current thought is that MOF represents the culmination of a generalized and excessive neuroendocrine, immune, and inflammatory response. The cascade may be precipitated by a wide variety of insults, broadly classified as tissue injury, cellular shock, inflammation, and infection. Based on a large body of clinical as well as basic science research, it appears that multiple insults are likely responsible for MOF. In the "two-event" model of MOF (Fig. 24-5), the host sustains sequential insults in such a manner that the subsequent systemic inflammatory response exceeds the typical response elicited by either insult alone. The initial insult primes the inflammatory

response, and patients enter a state of systemic hyperinflammation (i.e., SIRS). If the insult or the inflammatory response is exaggerated or perpetuated, patients enter a state of malignant systemic hyperinflammation (severe SIRS) that can evolve into overt MOF, independent of other factors. The more common scenario involves multiple sequential insults. A second insult during a vulnerable period amplifies SIRS to produce MOF. The progression appears to be dependent on the type of insult, with a bimodal pattern to the development of MOF. Early MOF (occurring within 72 hours of the initial insult) seems to be precipitated by cellular shock. In contrast, late MOF (typically 6 to 8 days post event) is typically related to an infection.[69] While the initial insult determines the patient's susceptibility, there is little direct evidence that any one insult is more likely than another to lead to MOF. It seems that the pivotal risk factor is a dysfunctional inflammatory/immune response (Fig. 24-6). The amplitude of the early systemic inflammatory response is related to the initial insult. Negative feedback mechanisms downregulate this response in an attempt to limit potentially autodestructive inflammation; this compensatory anti-inflammatory response may result in delayed immuno-suppression and thus susceptibility to infection. In this paradigm, a second hit during either early hyperinflammation or delayed immunosuppression will have the same net effect: deterioration into MOF.

Given the disappointing results of "antimediators," alternative approaches to MOF prevention must focus on attenuating the hyperinflammation associated with the first hit and avoiding second hits. Aggressive resuscitation to endpoints such as lactate and base deficit minimizes the cellular injury resulting from shock. The choice of resuscitation fluids may impact the inflammatory response. Hypertonic saline (HTS) appears to have favorable immunomodulatory properties and is worthy of further study as a resuscitation fluid. Given its immunomodulatory effects, transfusion of stored blood may serve as a second hit. While we await the development of an ideal blood substitute, there may be ways in which stored blood can be processed that will minimize its effects.[71] The optimal timing for fracture fixation has yet to be determined; it may be possible to measure markers of systemic hyperinflammation and distinguish "vulnerable" from "protected" periods. Early nutritional support may enhance the immune system and minimize the delayed immunosuppressive effects of the compensatory anti-inflammatory response.

Selected References

Fleisher LA, Eagle KA: Lowering cardiac risk in noncardiac surgery. N Engl J Med 345:1677-1682, 2001.

An up-to-date review of cardiac risk factors and risk reduction strategies for the surgical patient.

International guidelines 2000 conference on cardiopulmonary resuscitation and emergency cardiovascular care. Circulation 102 (Suppl I):I136-I165, 2000.

The latest algorithms for management of cardiopulmonary arrest and dysrhythmias are presented in detail, along with narrative and references. The remainder of the supplement addresses related topics.

Jacobi J, Fraser GL, Coursin DB, et al: Clinical practice guidelines for the sustained use of sedatives and analgesics in the critically ill adult. Crit Care Med 30:119-141, 2002.

An up-to-date evidence-based review and guidelines for sedation and analgesia in the ICU.

Singri N, Ahya SN, Levin ML: Acute renal failure. JAMA 289:747-751, 2003.

A concise yet thorough review of the management of acute renal failure.

Tobin MJ: Advances in mechanical ventilation. N Engl J Med 344:1986-1996, 2001.

A review of ventilator management and weaning strategies.

References

1. Plum F, Posner J: The Diagnosis of Stupor and Coma. Philadelphia, FA Davis, 1980.
2. Park WY, Thompson JS, Lee KK, et al: Effect of epidural anesthesia and analgesia on perioperative outcome: A randomized, controlled Veteran Affairs cooperative study. Ann Surg 234:560-571, 2001.
3. Jacobi J, Fraser GL, Coursin DB, et al: Clinical practice guidelines for the sustained use of sedatives and analgesics in the critically ill adult. Crit Care Med 30:119-141, 2002.
4. Murray MJ, Cowen J, DeBlock H, et al: Clinical practice guidelines for sustained neuromuscular blockade in the adult critically ill patient. Crit Care Med 30:142-156, 2002.
5. International guidelines 2000 conference on cardiopulmonary resuscitation and emergency cardiovascular care. Circulation 102 (Suppl I):I136-I165, 2000.
6. Wilkes MM, Navickis RJ: Patient survival after human albumin administration: A meta-analysis of randomized, controlled trials. Ann Intern Med 135:149-164, 2001.
7. Bunn F, Alderson P, Hawkins V: Colloid solutions for fluid resuscitation. Cochrane Database Syst Rev 2003.
8. Elliot DC: An evaluation of the endpoints of resuscitation. J Am Coll Surg 187:536-547, 1998.
9. Bishop MH, Shoemaker WC, Appel PL, et al: Relationship between supranormal circulatory values, time delays, and outcomes in severely traumatized patients. Crit Care Med 21:56-63, 1993.
10. Kern JW, Shoemaker WC: Meta-analysis of hemodynamic optimization in high-risk patients. Crit Care Med 30:1686-1692, 2002.
11. Moore FA, Haenel JB, Moore EE, et al: Incommensurate oxygen consumption in response to maximal oxygen availability predicts postinjury multiple organ failure. J Trauma 33:58-66, 1992.
12. Tyburski JG, Collinge JD, Wilson RF, et al: End-tidal CO_2-derived values during emergency trauma surgery correlated with outcome: A prospective study. J Trauma 53:738-743, 2002.
13. Ivatury RR, Simon RJ, Islam S, et al: A prospective randomized study of endpoints of resuscitation after major trauma: Global oxygen transport indices versus organ specific gastric mucosal pH. J Am Coll Surg 183:145-154, 1996.
14. Sauaia A, Moore FA, Moore EE, et al: Early predictors of postinjury multiple organ failure. Arch Surg 129:39-45, 1994.
15. Davis JW, Kaups KL, Parks SN: Base deficit is superior to pH in evaluating clearance of acidosis after traumatic shock. J Trauma 44:114-118, 1998.
16. Fleisher LA, Eagle KA: Lowering cardiac risk in noncardiac surgery. N Engl J Med 345:1677-1682, 2001.
17. Lee TH, Boucher CA: Noninvasive tests in patients with stable coronary artery disease. N Engl J Med 344:1840-1845, 2001.
18. Smith WHT, Ball SG: ACE inhibitors in heart failure: An update. Basic Res Cardiol 95(Suppl 1):I8-I14, 2000.
19. Ware LB, Matthay MA: The acute respiratory distress syndrome. N Engl J Med 342:1334-1349, 2000.
20. Biffl WL, Moore FA, Moore EE, et al: Are corticosteroids salvage therapy for refractory acute respiratory distress syndrome? Am J Surg 170:591-596, 1995.
21. Meduri GU, Headley AS, Golden E, et al: Effect of prolonged methylprednisolone therapy in unresolving acute respiratory distress syndrome: A randomized controlled trial. JAMA 280:159-165, 1998.
22. Gattinoni L, Tognoni G, Pesenti A, et al: Effect of prone positioning on the survival of patients with acute respiratory failure. N Engl J Med 345:568-573, 2001.
23. ARDS Network: Ventilation with lower tidal volumes as compared with traditional tidal volumes for acute lung

injury and the acute respiratory distress syndrome. N Engl J Med 342:1301-1308, 2000.

24. Ward NS, Lin DY, Nelson DL, et al: Successful determination of lower inflection point and maximal compliance in a population of patients with acute respiratory distress syndrome. Crit Care Med 30:963-968, 2002.

25. Amato MBP, Barbas CSV, Medeiros DM, et al: Effect of a protective-ventilation strategy on mortality in the acute respiratory distress syndrome. N Engl J Med 338:347-354, 1998.

26. Tobin MJ: Advances in mechanical ventilation. N Engl J Med 344:1986-1996, 2001.

27. Cook D, Guyatt G, Marshall J, et al: A comparison of sucralfate and ranitidine for the prevention of upper gastrointestinal bleeding in patients requiring mechanical ventilation. N Engl J Med 338:791-797, 1998.

28. Burch JM, Moore EE, Moore FA, et al: The abdominal compartment syndrome. Surg Clin North Am 76:833-842, 1996.

29. Biffl WL, Moore EE, Burch JM, et al: Secondary abdominal compartment syndrome is a highly lethal event. Am J Surg 182:645-648, 2001.

30. Garner GB, Ware DN, Cocanour CS, et al: Vacuum-assisted wound closure provides early fascial reapproximation in trauma patients with open abdomen. Am J Surg 182:630-638, 2001.

31. Biffl W, Moore E, Haenel J: Nutrition support of the trauma patient. Nutrition 18:960-965, 2002.

32. Kellum JA, Decker JM: Use of dopamine in acute renal failure: A meta-analysis. Crit Care Med 29:1526-1531, 2001.

33. Singri N, Ahya SN, Levin ML: Acute renal failure. JAMA 289:747-751, 2003.

34. Mehta RL, Pascual MT, Soroko S, et al: Diuretics, mortality, and nonrecovery of renal function in acute renal failure. JAMA 288:2547-2553, 2002.

35. Schiffl H, Lang SM, Fischer R: Daily hemodialysis and the outcome of acute renal failure. N Engl J Med 346:305-310, 2002.

36. Solanki P, Chawla A, Garg R, et al: Beneficial effects of terlipressin in hepatorenal syndrome: A prospective, randomized placebo-controlled clinical trial. J Gastroenterol Hepatol 18:152-156, 2003.

37. Salem M, Tainsh RE, Bromberg J, et al: Perioperative glucocorticoid coverage: A reassessment 42 years after emergence of a problem. Ann Surg 219:416-425, 1994.

38. Cooper MS, Stewart PM: Corticosteroid insufficiency in acutely ill patients. N Engl J Med 348:727-734, 2003.

39. Golden SH, Perat-Vigilance C, Kao WH, et al: Perioperative glycemic control and the risk of infectious complications in a cohort of adults with diabetes. Diabetes Care 22:1408-1414, 1999.

40. Walia S, Sutcliffe AJ: The relationship between blood glucose, mean arterial pressure and outcome after severe head injury: An observational study. Injury 33:339-344, 2002.

41. van den Berghe V, Wouthers P, Weekers F, et al: Intensive insulin therapy in critically ill patients. N Engl J Med 345:1359-1367, 2001.

42. Geerts WH, Heit JA, Clagett GP, et al: Prevention of venous thromboembolism. Chest 119:132S-175S, 2001.

43. Turpie AGG, Bauer KA, Eriksson BI, et al: Fondaparinux vs enoxaparin for the prevention of venous thromboembolism in major orthopedic surgery. Arch Intern Med 162:1833-1840, 2002.

44. American College of Emergency Physicians: Clinical policy: Critical issues in the evaluation and management of adult patients presenting with suspected lower-extremity deep venous thrombosis. Ann Emerg Med 42:124-135, 2003.

45. Tovey C, Wyatt S: Diagnosis, investigation, and management of deep vein thrombosis. BMJ 326:1180-1184, 2003.

46. Warkentin TE, Kelton JG: Temporal aspects of heparin-induced thrombocytopenia. N Engl J Med 344:1286-1292, 2001.

47. Vincent JL, Baron JF, Reinhart K, et al: Anemia and blood transfusion in critically ill patients. JAMA 288:1499-1507, 2002.

48. Hebert PC, Wells G, Blajchmann MA, et al: A multicenter, randomized, controlled clinical trial of transfusion requirements in critical care. N Engl J Med 340:409-418, 1999.

49. Corwin HL, Gettinger A, Peral RG, et al: Efficacy of recombinant human erythropoietin in critically ill patients: A randomized controlled trial. JAMA 288:2827-2835, 2002.

50. Goodnough L, Brecher M, Kanter M, et al: Transfusion medicine. First of two parts. Blood transfusion. N Engl J Med 340:438-447, 1999.

51. Moore FA, Moore EE, Sauaia A: Blood transfusion: An independent risk factor for postinjury multiple organ failure. Arch Surg 132:620-625, 1997.

52. Sloan EP, Koenigsberg M, Gens D, et al: Diaspirin cross-linked hemoglobin (DCLHb) in the treatment of severe traumatic hemorrhagic shock. JAMA 282:1857-1864, 1999.

53. Hill SE, Gottschalk LI, Grichnik K: Safety and preliminary efficacy of hemoglobin raffimer for patients undergoing coronary artery bypass surgery. J Cardiothorac Vasc Anesth 16:695-702, 2002.

54. Sprung J, Kindscher JD, Wahr JA, et al: The use of bovine hemoglobin glutamer-250 (Hemopure) in surgical patients: Result of a multicenter, randomized, single-blinded trial. Anesth Analg 94:799-808, 2002.

55. Gould SA, Moore EE, Hoyt DB, et al: The first randomized trial of human polymerized hemoglobin as a blood substitute in acute trauma emergent surgery. J Am Coll Surg 187:113-122, 1998.

56. Gould SA, Moore EE, Hoyt DB, et al: The life-sustaining capacity of human polymerized hemoglobin when red cells might be unavailable. J Am Coll Surg 195:445-455, 2002.

57. Johnson JL, Moore EE, Offner PJ, et al: Resuscitation of the injured patient with polymerized stroma-free hemoglobin does not produce systemic or pulmonary hypertension. Am J Surg 176:612-617, 1998.

58. Johnson JL, Moore EE, Offner PJ, et al: Resuscitation with a blood substitute abrogates pathologic postinjury neutrophil cytoxic function. J Trauma 50:449-456, 2001.

59. American College of Chest Physicians/Society of Critical Care Medicine Consensus Conference: Definitions for sepsis and organ failure and guidelines for the use of innovative therapies in sepsis. Crit Care Med 20:864-874, 1992.

60. Angus DC, Linde-Zwirble WT, Lidicker J, et al: Epidemiology of severe sepsis in the United States: Analysis of incidence, outcome, and associated costs of care. Crit Care Med 29:1303-1310, 2001.

61. Rivers E, Nguyen B, Havstad S, et al: Early goal-directed therapy in the treatment of severe sepsis and septic shock. N Engl J Med 345:1368-1377, 2001.

62. Tsuneyoshi I, Yamada H, Kakihana Y, et al: Hemodynamic and metabolic effects of low-dose vasopressin infusions in vasodilatory septic shock. Crit Care Med 29:487-493, 2001.

63. Annane D, Sebille V, Charpentier C, et al: Effect of treatment with low doses of hydrocortisone and fludrocortisone on mortality in patients with septic shock. JAMA 288:862-871, 2002.

64. Arndt P, Abraham E: Immunological therapy of sepsis: Experimental therapies. Intensive Care Med 27:S104-S115, 2001.

65. Carlet J: Immunological therapy in sepsis: Currently available. Intensive Care Med 27:S93-S103, 2001.
66. Bernard GR, Vincent JL, Laterre PF, et al: Efficacy and safety of recombinant human activated protein C for severe sepsis. N Engl J Med 344:699-709, 2001.
67. Baue A: Multiple, progressive, or sequential systems failure: A syndrome of the 1970s. Arch Surg 110:779-781, 1975.
68. Eiseman B, Beart R, Norton L: Multiple organ failure. Surg Gynecol Obstet 144:323-326, 1977.
69. Sauaia A, Moore FA, Moore EE, et al: Epidemiology of trauma deaths: A reassessment. J Trauma 38:185-193, 1995.
70. Fry DE, Pearlstein L, Fulton RL, et al: Multiple system organ failure: The role of uncontrolled infection. Arch Surg 115:136-140, 1980.
71. Biffl WL, Moore EE, Offner PJ, et al: Plasma from aged stored red blood cells delays neutrophil apoptosis and primes for cytotoxicity: Abrogation by post-storage washing but not prestorage leukodepletion. J Trauma 50:426-432, 2001.

CHAPTER 25

THE SURGEON'S ROLE IN UNCONVENTIONAL CIVILIAN DISASTERS

David B. Hoyt, M.D., **Donald E. Fry**, M.D., and **Jay Doucet**, M.D.

Disasters, especially terrorist attacks, have the potential to produce mass casualties and destroy infrastructure needed to sustain the health care system. Surgeons have traditionally played a leadership role in mass casualty incidents. In North America, the emergency medical system (EMS) and the trauma system represent the resources most ready to respond rapidly to the injured patient. It is a natural extension that the trauma system will form the backbone of the medical response to terrorism, and in some U.S. states this has already become part of the system's mandate.

Terrorist attacks differ from most natural disasters in the capacity to rapidly produce very large numbers of dead and injured. Table 25-1 illustrates how the attacks of September 11, 2001, in a few hours produced more fatalities for a single day than had been seen in a century of U.S. disasters.[1] Historically, terrorist attacks usually involve conventional weapons such as high explosive bombs detonated in public places. Such attacks produce significant numbers of dead and injured and are termed *mass trauma events* by the Centers for Disease Control

and Prevention (CDC). The situation is complicated by the potential for terrorist attacks using weapons of mass destruction (WMD), which include chemical, biological, or radiological weapons producing large numbers of dead and injured persons. The sarin nerve agent attack on the Tokyo subway in 1995 used 1-L intravenous fluid bags of relatively impure nerve agent placed on the seats on five different subway cars that were then punctured with an umbrella tip.[2-5] Despite the crude dispersal system, the attack resulted in 5,510 casualties, including 12 dead and 160 casualties among responding police, fire, and medical personnel. Such incidents overwhelm local medical systems and can place providers at risk. A plan to cope with large numbers of patients must be already in place to limit preventable deaths and morbidity.

The evolution of political events in recent years has brought attention to terrorist acts that have targeted civilian populations. While these events have generally employed conventional explosive devices, there is considerable concern that WMD originally designed for military applications would be accessed by private groups of

TABLE 25-1. U.S. Disasters With Deaths in 1 Day Exceeding 1000

April 27, 1865. Steamship *Sultana* explosion on the Mississippi River near Memphis, Tennessee	1547
October 8, 1871. Forest Fire, Peshtigo, Wisconsin	1182
May 31, 1889. Flood, Johnstown, Pennsylvania	2200
August 27, 1900. Hurricane, Galveston, Texas	5000
June 15, 1904. Fire on Steamship *General Slocum* on the East River, New York	1021
September 13, 1928. Hurricane, Lake Okeechobee, Florida	2000
December 7, 1941. Attack on Pearl Harbor, Hawaii	2338
September 11, 2001. Terrorist hijackings in New York City, Washington, DC, and Pennsylvania	3021

From Auf der Heide E: Principles of hospital disaster planning. *In* Hogan DE, Burstein JL (eds): Disaster Medicine. Philadelphia, Lippincott Williams & Wilkins, 2002, pp 57-89.

individuals and that civilians would be targeted. The 1995 incident involving sarin gas in the Japanese subway system is an example that provides substance to this concern.[6]

During the 20th century, the military of many countries developed different arrays of WMD. Chemical weapons were developed and deployed in World War I. Nuclear weapons were used with mass casualties in World War II. Following World War II, many governments, including the United States, launched extensive programs to develop biological weapons. Although a Biological Weapons Convention was signed in 1972 by most countries to discontinue these programs and to forbid stockpiling such weapons, considerable concern remains to this day that biological agents have fallen into the hands of rogue political groups. The threat of all of these various WMD is not so much that governments will use them but rather that nongovernmental groups will.

Surgeons must be informed and have reasonable knowledge about the various agents of mass destruction. Community-based disaster plans will likely use the preexistent format of the trauma disaster planning scheme and state trauma networks for managing casualties from these unconventional events. It is likely that physical injuries to large numbers of victims will be associated with biological or chemical agents and will certainly be present with even a small nuclear detonation. Surgeons will be part of managing the patients because of physical injury and for critical care management. Finally, risks will exist for health care providers from these unconventional casualties. The best protection against occupationally associated exposure to radiation, biological, or chemical injury during the care of these patients will be having knowledge about the agents involved and the real or perceived risks that they pose. Surgeons should also be knowledgeable about the various disaster planning structures that exist at local, regional, and federal levels to optimize the available resources to assist them in the care of casualties from one of these events. Preparedness is essential. It is not a matter

of "if" one of these events will occur but "when" will it happen.

DIFFERENCES IN THE EMS AND TRAUMA SYSTEM RESPONSE TO WEAPONS OF MASS DESTRUCTION

The EMS and the trauma system are designed to be a combined, organized response to injury.[7,8] As such, it has many of the elements needed for a disaster response. These include identification of injury, transport of the injured, communications, designation of receiving facilities or hospitals, and delivery of appropriate, timely medical care at the point of injury and at receiving hospitals. These systems can cope with incidents involving multiple casualties using just the local resources within the hospital. Such events are multiple casualty incidents and not mass casualty events. A disaster producing a mass casualty event overwhelms local medical resources.

The response required for a disaster due to WMD may be proportionally different but, in principle, is still an organized response to injury. Differences would include the magnitude and types of injury, the numbers of injured, and the risk to providers of exposure and personal injury. Chemical and biological disasters may not be covered by planning of trauma systems in a local community, and a disaster response will differ from a traditional response of a trauma system and EMS in several ways. It is imperative that surgeons and their communities understand these differences and become educated and participate in disaster planning and training.

DISASTER RESPONSE PLANNING

Poorly prepared institutions and communities have difficult questions to answer after disaster strikes. Joint Committee on Accreditation of Healthcare Organization standards require hospitals to have a disaster plan and prepare for patients contaminated by hazardous materials.[9] To avoid the "paper plan syndrome" the plan must be read, revised, and exercised regularly.[1] Box 25-1 refers

---

Box 25-1. Problems with Disaster Plans

- Not based on valid assumptions of what happens in disasters
- Planned in isolation, not taking an interorganizational perspective
- Not accompanied by resources necessary to carry out the plan, including time, money, space, personnel, and supplies
- Not accompanied by an effective training plan to ensure end-users understand plan
- End-users do not participate in planning and lose the chance to become familiar with and enable the plan.

From Auf der Heide E: Disaster Response: Principles of Preparation and Coordination. St Louis, Mosby, 1989.

to some of the problems related to disaster planning. Surgeons need to participate in planning and training for disasters. Meeting the players in other departments and in the prehospital system will smooth operations when disasters strike. Within their own hospitals, surgeons should participate in planning to define and develop the internal response capabilities of their hospital for WMD injury. Surgeons should consider joint hospital representation to community disaster planning committees. Study of past incidents allows future potential problems to be identified and addressed in planning (Box 25-2).

PREDICTING CASUALTY LOAD AND SEVERITY

Casualties tend to arrive quickly at the nearest hospital after a mass trauma event. Typically, half of the casualties a hospital can expect will arrive within 1 hour of the arrival of the first casualty.[10-12] Meanwhile, hospitals outside the affected area will receive few casualties, if any. Casualties arriving first often are ambulatory and less severely injured than casualties who are triaged through the EMS system arriving later.

Bombings of public places produce a typical distribution of casualties in which one third of casualties are critically injured and are killed outright, die of injuries, or require admission to hospital or emergency surgery.[11] Two thirds of casualties are noncritical and are treated and released from the emergency department. Ninety-two percent of admitted victims from bombings will require surgery.

PREDICTING HOSPITAL CAPACITY

The number of available trauma bays and operating rooms is a major factor in determining a hospital's capacity to care for critically injured casualties.[13-15] If the number of predicted or actual critical casualties exceeds the number of operating rooms that are available, consider diverting further critical casualties to other hospitals. Noncritical casualties typically take 3 to 6 hours to discharge from the emergency department. A significant bottleneck in evaluating these patients is obtaining radiographs and computed tomographic scans. On average, each casualty will require about 10 minutes of x-ray machine time. Therefore, one determinant of the hourly capacity to care for noncritical casualties is the number of x-ray machines with technicians multiplied by six. A guide to planning disaster response is available from the U.S. Department of Health and Human Services (DHHS) at the CDC's bioterrorism website at www.bt.cdc.gov.[16]

INITIAL RESPONSE TO TERRORIST ATTACK: METROPOLITAN MEDICAL RESPONSE SYSTEM

The Federal Response Plan (FRP) describes the mechanism by which the federal government will respond to provide defense and mobilize resources during national security emergencies and major domestic emergencies.[17,18] Under the FRP annex Emergency Services Func-

---

Box 25-2. Historical Problems in Disaster Response[a,b]

- Communications systems (including radios and cell phones) are impaired, overwhelmed, or incompatible.[c]
- Widespread panic is uncommon.[a]
- The surviving hospital closest to the event receives the most patients.[d]
- Information is scarce and often unreliable.[e,f]
- Less severely injured often arrive first.[d,e]
- Most patients will not require sophisticated medical treatment.[g]
- Overtriage impairs ability to care for the most critically injured and increases mortality.[h,i]
- Need to manage many non-trauma casualties and need for access to routine care and prescription medications are not anticipated.[j]
- Hospital staff will assemble in emergency receiving area or at the disaster scene unless directed to muster elsewhere.[k]
- Volunteers may be numerous or overwhelming; emergency credentialing becomes an issue.[j,l]
- Hospital security may need help from police in maintaining perimeter.[j]
- Requests for information from public and media may overwhelm hospital resources.[a]
- Hospitals must be responsible for decontamination of casualties without immediate fire department assistance.

[a]Auf der Heide E: Disaster Response: Principles of Preparation and Coordination. St Louis, Mosby, 1989.
[b]Roccaforte JD, Cushman JG: Disaster preparation and management for the intensive care unit. Curr Opin Crit Care 8:607-615, 2002.
[c]Chaloner E, Ryan J: Weapons and the law. Lancet 353:2078, 1999.
[d]Ryan J, Gavalas M: What goes wrong at a disaster or major incident? Hosp Med 59:944-946, 1998.
[e]Quarentelli EL: Delivery of Emergency Medical Care in Disasters: Assumptions and Realities. New York, Irvington, 1983.
[f]Nakajima T, Ohta S, Morita H, et al: Epidemiological study of sarin poisoning in Matsumoto City, Japan. J Epidemiol 8:33-41, 1998.
[g]Cushman JG, Pachter HL, Beaton HL: Two New York City Hospitals' surgical response to the September 11, 2001, terrorist attack in New York City. J Trauma 54:147-154, 2003.
[h]Frykberg ER, Tepas JJ III. Terrorist bombings: Lessons learned from Belfast to Beirut. Ann Surg 208:569-576, 1988.
[i]Holcomb JB, Helling TS, Hirshberg A: Military, civilian, and rural application of the damage control philosophy. Mil Med 166:490-493, 2001.
[k]Roccaforte JD: The World Trade Center Attack: Observations from New York's Bellevue Hospital. Crit Care 5:307-309, 2001.
[l]Rozovsky F: Emergency credentialing helps disaster response. Hosp Peer Rev 27:63-64, 2002.

tion 8—Health and Medical Services, the DHHS is designated as the lead agency responsible for providing assistance for public health and medical care needs.

Within the DHHS, the Office of Emergency Preparedness has contracted with the 72 most heavily populated U.S. cities to develop the Metropolitan Medical Response System (MMRS) initiative. The traditional field response by EMS is with an emergency medical technician provider. MMRS is fundamentally integrated with the traditional local EMS system and provides an enhanced local health and medical response to victims in the first 90 minutes after a terrorist incident or other disaster. MMRS allows a metropolitan area to manage the event until state or federal response resources are mobilized. MMRS provides a team capable of initial response to terrorist attack or other disaster, including emergency medical services, decontamination of victims, mental health services, plans for the disposition of nonsurvivors, and activation of plans for the forward movement of patients to regional hospitals via the National Disaster Medical System (NDMS).

NATIONAL DISASTER MEDICAL SYSTEM

The NDMS provides federal level resources to any incident that exceeds the capability of any local, state, or federal health care system, with a planned capacity of up to 100,000 victims. NDMS is the responsibility of the Departments of Homeland Security (DHS), Defense (DOD), Veterans Affairs, and Health and Human Services (DHHS), with the DHS as the lead agency. NDMS may be activated by presidential decree or by DHS or the DOD.[19] States may activate components of NDMS under emergency conditions to augment local resources.

NDMS has three primary functions:

- Medical response: NDMS responds to the disaster with disaster medical response teams (DMAT) of physicians, nurses, technicians and ancillary personnel, specialty DMATs, disaster mortuary operational response teams (DMORTs), management support teams (MSTs), and medical supplies and equipment.
- Patient evacuation: Arrangements are coordinated for patients who need to be evacuated to other locations in the United States.
- Hospitalization: NDMS has designated a network of hospitals in major urban centers that have agreed to accept evacuated patients in a national emergency.

DMATS are composed of volunteer civilian personnel who become temporary federal employees when deployed. This avoids issues such as torts, license jurisdiction, and workers' compensation. In large-scale disasters, teams typically come from a distant city or town and not from the area involved in the incident. DMATs arrive within 8 to 16 hours of activation. Team composition varies with need from 20 to 200 people but is typically about 35 people. Teams are airlifted by the DOD, and each team is expected to be self sufficient for 72 hours after arrival at the site. Specialty DMATs may have expertise in specific areas such as chemical or biological weapons decontamination, pediatrics, burns, or international disas-

ters. These teams may work at the scene or supplement or replace existing medical facilities (Fig. 25-1).[20]

Another component of the NDMS is the Strategic National Stockpile (SNS) (formerly the National Pharmaceutical Stockpile) composed of critical drugs, chemical weapon antidotes, antibiotics, vaccines, and medical supplies.[21] The SNS is transported to the incident by DOD airlift. During the September 11, 2001, attack, 50 tons of SNS supplies were transported to New York City within 7 hours for trauma or WMD victims. State governments hold exercises to demonstrate their ability to receive and distribute vaccines and supplies from the SNS.

TRIAGE—START SYSTEM

Triage, from the French "sorting," can be characterized as doing the greatest good for the greatest number. Triage is a continual process and starts with the first responder.

A widely accepted field triage system used in prior U.S. disasters is the Simple Triage & Rapid Treatment (START) system consisting of evaluating four physiologic variables (Fig. 25-2).[22] All casualties are sorted into 1—immediate (red), 2—delayed (yellow), 3—minor (green), or 0—dead (black) groups. Each is tagged with the appropriate field tag at the scene. Identification information, vital signs, medications administered, and decontamination status can also be recorded on the tag. The patient is re-triaged at each level of care, including hospital entrance, emergency department, and preop area because the patient's condition may change. Surgeons re-triage their patients before sending them for imaging or surgery.

INCIDENT COMMAND

In 1970 an immense series of wildfires in Southern California occurred in multiple jurisdictions and burned 1000 square miles and 772 buildings with 16 deaths.[1] Difficulties responding in an organized fashion with over 100 government agencies led the U.S. Congress to fund analysis and documentation of the problem. The result is the Incident Command System (ICS). ICS provides an organizational framework of a common, modular design that allows for unified command and control of a fire emergency. Over 6000 emergency services agencies and hospitals have adopted ICS without modification of the basic concepts because it provides a common structure for management of any disaster.

Structure and Function of Incident Command

The incident command center structure is composed of seven key groups. If the disaster is small in scope, then a single person may fill all seven areas. As the disaster increases in scope, more personnel are required to fulfill these functions and more typical command organization structures are utilized. First and foremost, the incident commander is responsible for the entire rescue and recovery operation. Under the direction of the incident commander are seven group chiefs: operations, logistics,

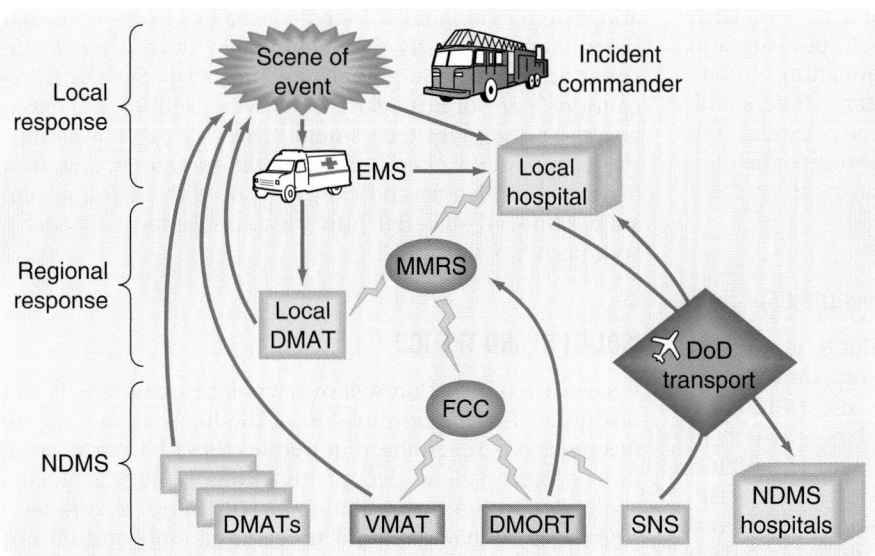

FIGURE 25-1. The National Disaster Medical System (NDMS) and Metropolitan Medical Response System (MMRS) make teams available capable of initial response to a terrorist attack or other disasters that work at the scene or supplement or replace existing medical facilities when the capability of any local, state, or federal health care system is exceeded, providing an enhanced local health care and medical response to victims.

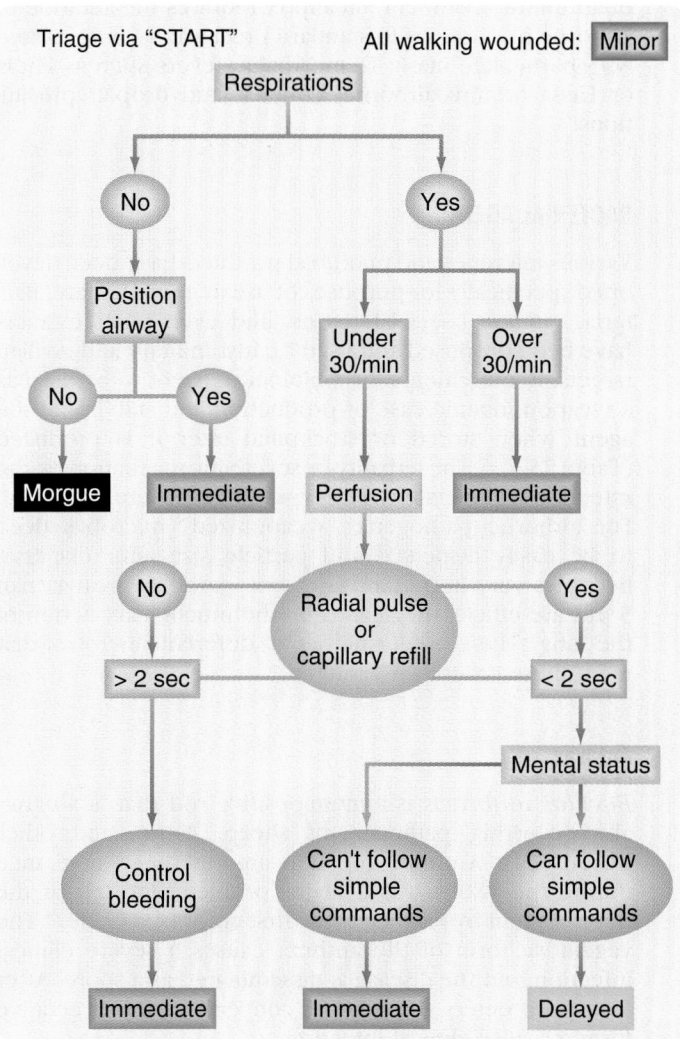

FIGURE 25-2. Simple Triage & Rapid Treatment (START) system, a widely accepted field triage system used in previous U.S. disasters. (From Super G, Groth S, Hook R: START: A Triage Training Module. Newport Beach, CA, Hoag Memorial Hospital Presbyterian, 1994, with permission.)

planning, finance, safety, information, and liaison. Each of these chiefs has a well-defined area of authority and responsibility. Continuous on-scene information is communicated through the command center. Understanding these differences and accepting the ICS model will prevent confusion and give a much clearer role to the individual trauma surgeon or individual hospital or field provider.[23]

Hospital Emergency Incident Command System (HEICS)

The hospital version of ICS, known as HEICS, was developed in 1991 in hospitals in Orange County, California.[24] The majority of California hospitals now use HEICS and this free-of-charge system is being adopted more widely in the United States and Canada as well as overseas. HEICS follows the ICS model in that it employs a logical management structure, defined responsibilities, prioritized checklists, clear reporting channels, and a common nomenclature to help unify the hospital with other emergency responders. As a disaster evolves, surgeons will need an organized management structure to allow care for increasing numbers of injured patients to be sustained. Adoption of HEICS into the hospital disaster plan will provide an ICS-based response that reduces the amount of chaos by improving communication within the facility and with outside agencies.

ROLE OF THE SURGEON AT THE SCENE

Although surgeons may be experienced in medical team leadership and concepts such as triage, most have little preparation or training for the prehospital environment. Surgeons are more effectively employed away from the incident site at a facility where patients are sorted to a level where surgical intervention is required. An exception may be in rare structural collapse incidents that require a field amputation to extricate a victim.

HOSPITAL RESPONSE

Hospitals need to reassess their disaster plans to include response to WMD. Before 2001, a survey of all U.S. level I trauma centers found only 3% adequately prepared to handle hazardous material–contaminated casualties.[25] Hospitals must now develop this capability to avoid contamination of hospital staff.[26,27] Decontamination support from the fire department may not be available immediately to the hospital during a disaster, and the hospital should have its own hazardous material system composed of a team in personal protective equipment with decontamination gear.[28] Also required are mechanisms for locking down the hospital, maintaining security around the parameter, and maintaining "shelter-in-place."[29,30]

THE OPERATING ROOM

Removing contaminated clothing and decontamination with water is sufficient for most WMD exposures. Operating room personnel who treat casualties from WMD that have been previously decontaminated do not need personal protective equipment beyond usual "Standard Precautions" of surgical garb of gloves, tight-fitting mask, gown, and goggles/face shield. The risk of "off-gassing" from embedded chemical agent on foreign bodies in a living patient is low and can be dealt with by immersing such removed material into bleach solution (3% to 6% sodium hypochlorite).[31,32]

ISOLATION AND THE ICU

Excess use of isolation will overwhelm isolation beds and resources. Early determination of the likely agents simplifies decisions regarding required levels of barrier precautions. After patient decontamination, biological agents such as anthrax, botulinum toxin, and *Francisella tularensis* require standard precautions only and do not require the patient to undergo isolation (Table 25-2). Plague requires the addition of droplet precautions to standard precautions with the use of masks until 72 hours of antibiotic treatment. Smallpox requires the addition of airborne precautions to standard precautions, with a fitted N95 particulate mask. Hemorrhagic fevers such as Ebola or Lassa require airborne, contact, and droplet precautions.

BACTERIAL AGENTS

Various microbes and microbial products have been developed specifically for purposes of use in germ warfare. Bacteria, viruses, bacterial toxins, and even plant extracts have been proposed and used against military and civilian targets. Requirements for a biological agent to be used as a weapon include ease of production and stability of the agent when stored or stockpiled after it is produced (Table 25-3).[33] The lethality or severe incapacitation by the infection will dictate which types of agents are produced. For airborne pathogens, "weaponized" microbes need to be easily dispersed and particle size after dispersal becomes very important. Airborne particles greater than 5 μm are efficiently cleared by the mucociliary action of the lung. There are a number of different microbes that meet these criteria.

Anthrax

Bacillus anthracis is a gram-positive rod that is a naturally occurring pathogen of sheep, cattle, and other quadrupeds. Anthrax infection among sheep in France during the 1800s was a major problem and led to the development by Pasteur of the first anthrax vaccine.[34] The vegetative form of the anthrax causes a severe clinical infection, but the disease is disseminated as a spore. After the spore enters the host, it converts to the vegetative form to cause clinical infection.

Infection with anthrax can occur via three different routes.[35] Cutaneous anthrax, or woolsorter's disease, occurs when open wounds or abrasions become inocu-

TABLE 25-2.   Infection Control Measures Required For Bioterrorism Agents

Bioagent	Type of Isolation Required	Patient Placement	Provider Measures
Anthrax Botulism Tularemia	Standard precautions	Private room only if noncompliant in maintaining appropriate hygiene or environmental control	Hand washing, gloving; if sprays of body fluids possible, then masks, goggles. or face shield.
Infectious diarrheas (e.g., cholera)	Contact precautions	Private room or with a patient(s) who has active infection with the same microorganism but with no other infection (cohorting).	Gown and gloves. Goggles or face shield per standard precautions.
Plague	Droplet precautions	Private room or with a patient(s) who has active infection with the same microorganism but with no other infection (cohorting).	Wear a surgical mask when working within 3 ft of the patient. When patient contact is likely, use contact precautions: gown and gloves.
Smallpox Tuberculosis	Airborne precautions	Private room that has negative air pressure and 6 to 12 air changes per hour, and high-efficiency filtration of room air before discharge to other areas in the hospital.	Standard precautions plus N95 respirator. When patient contact is likely, use contact precautions: gown and gloves. Use goggles or face shield per standard precautions.
Hemorrhagic fevers (e.g., Ebola, Lassa, Marburg)	Airborne, contact, and droplet precautions	Private room that has negative air pressure and 6 to 12 air changes per hour, and high-efficiency filtration of room air before discharge to other areas in the hospital.	Standard precautions and wear N95 respirator, gown, gloves, and goggles. Treat all body fluid-stained material as infective.

From Centers for Disease Control and Prevention. Department of Health and Human Services. CDC Public Health Emergency Preparedness & Response Site. Available from www.bt.cdc.gov. Accessed 6-29-2003.

lated with anthrax spores. This is the most common naturally occurring form of anthrax infection in humans. A papule forms at the site, followed by the coal-black necrotic lesion that is characteristic of the cutaneous infection. Proliferating microorganisms invade the lymphatics locally, but the disease is rarely systemic and it is rarely (<1%) fatal given appropriate recognition and treatment. Cutaneous anthrax is not an objective of terrorists, but identification of cutaneous anthrax infections would be a clinical indicator for concern about the presence of anthrax in a given community.

Oropharyngeal/gastrointestinal anthrax occurs from ingestion of the spore from uncooked or poorly cooked meat products. The patient with oropharyngeal disease will have intraoral ulcerations, cervical adenopathy, and dysphagia. A patient with gastrointestinal anthrax will have abdominal pain, nausea, vomiting, and fever, features that rapidly proceed to systemic toxemia. Mortality rates may exceed 50% with this form of anthrax infection because diagnosis is not easily made. In fatal cases, only postmortem blood cultures and pathologic findings at autopsy would confirm anthrax infection. Identification of a case of gastrointestinal anthrax should similarly raise concerns about the source of the pathogen.

Inhalational anthrax has been the proposed use for the spores as a biological weapon.[35,36] It requires inhalation of as few as 2500 spores to cause the infection. Inhaled anthrax does not cause pneumonia. Rather, the inhaled spores are ingested by the pulmonary macrophages and are transported to the regional lymph nodes. The spore transforms to the vegetative state within the lymph nodes, resulting in toxin production and access of the proliferating pathogen to the systemic circulation. The period of incubation from inhalation to clinical disease is 1 to 6 days. The disease is fulminant with a picture of rapidly developing systemic sepsis without a readily apparent source. The subsequent pulmonary failure that develops is the result of the septic process and not pulmonary infection.

The diagnosis of inhalational anthrax is very difficult because the fulminant septic course is without disease-specific signs or symptoms. Most literature on the diagnosis emphasizes having a high index of suspicion that

TABLE 25-3. Desired Characteristics of Biological Weapons

Characteristic	Comment
Ease of production	Generally favors bacterial pathogens over viral agents.
Incapacitation/lethality	Incapacitation of large numbers of casualties saturates the health care system.
Particle size	Adherence of bacterial cells together make for too large a particle; anthrax spores are about 1 μm in diameter.
Ease of dissemination	Dry powders or aerosols are speculated as the most efficient means.
Stability after production	Both anthrax spores and smallpox virus meet these criteria.
Communicability	Plague bacillus and smallpox result in human-to-human transmission after primary dissemination.
Delay in symptoms	Delay before clinical disease means a greater dissemination of the microbe and greater numbers of exposed individuals.

anthrax is a disease of concern. Recent cases of any form of anthrax infection should heighten awareness. The septic process in these patients is fulminant in nature. The chest radiograph will provide evidence of a widened mediastinum because of hemorrhagic mediastinitis. A bloody pleural effusion may be seen. Blood cultures are positive but are usually reported too late to be of any value in patient management. In experimental models of primate inhalational anthrax, Gram stains of the blood itself may demonstrate microorganisms. The bacteremia is seen within 48 to 72 hours of clinical symptoms. Index cases of anthrax infection may not be identified until postmortem examination.

The treatment of inhalational anthrax infection is the usual supportive care of the septic patient and specific antibiotic therapy. The antibiotic treatment of anthrax is based on in vitro and experimental studies because no clinical trials of human infection are available. Only 18 cases were reported from 1900 to 1978,[37] and none were reported since 1978 until the cases of October 2001 involving dissemination of the spores via the U.S. mail system. Both penicillin and doxycycline are approved for the management of this infection. Ciprofloxacin appears effective in animal models, and its favorable oral pharmacology has made it a choice for early presumptive therapy or for postexposure prophylaxis. Penicillin and doxycycline are also recommended for postexposure prophylaxis.

A vaccine for anthrax is available.[38] It is an antigen from attenuated cultures of *B. anthracis.* Successful vaccination requires six doses to be administered subcutaneously over an 18-month period. Annual booster doses are rec-

ommended to maintain protection. It remains unclear whether the vaccination would be effective against a large inoculum of inhaled spores, given the fulminant nature of these infections.

Standard infection control practices are satisfactory for handling patients who are infected with anthrax. Infected patients are not infectious to others. Health care workers could contract the infection from injured casualties presenting to the hospital with unknown spore contamination and without prehospital decontamination. Health care workers and surgeons are not at risk from the actively infected patient. Standard disinfection of instruments and equipment with chlorine-based solutions is appropriate because of known sporicidal activity. Standard steam sterilization for surgical instruments is sufficient.

Plague

Yersinia pestis is the plague bacillus. It is a gram-negative bacterium that is responsible for several of the most deadly pandemics in recorded history. It is a naturally occurring infection of rodents. Fleas become the vector that transmits the disease from rats to humans. A few naturally occurring plague infections are seen annually in the United States.[39]

Infection with *Yersinia pestis* can occur in three separate scenarios.[40] Bubonic plague occurs with cutaneous inoculation, usually on an extremity. With dissemination of the bacteria into a civilian population, bubonic plague might occur by inoculation through nonintact skin. The pathogen proliferates locally at the site of introduction and then passes via the lymphatics to the regional lymph nodes where the organism is phagocytosed but not killed. The inflammatory response within the regional lymph node results in swelling and the characteristic "buboes" of this infection. Necrosis, and even suppuration with drainage, may occur though the skin over the swollen lymph glands. The plague bacillus may gain systemic access from the inflamed lymph nodes. Bubonic plague infection is associated with a 50% mortality rate in the absence of treatment.

Primary septicemic plague occurs when the site of cutaneous infection actually bypasses the regional lymph nodes and gains systemic access directly. These fulminant infections are associated with disseminated intravascular coagulation and purpuric skin lesions. Small vessel necrosis is associated with the ischemic digits that are seen. Both bubonic plague and primary septicemic plague are associated in a minority of cases with secondary pneumonic infection, in which the pulmonary infection arises from the bacteremic state. Primary septicemic plague is nearly 100% fatal.

Primary pneumonic plague was less common than bubonic infection during the pandemics of years ago but could be seen whenever circumstances might result in aerosolization of the plague bacillus. Patients with secondary pulmonary infection could disseminate the organism with coughing, and airborne transmission would occur from one human to another. It is the airborne pulmonary form of the disease that poses the greatest threat for a civilian biological attack. Inhalation of the pathogen would result in symptoms 1 to 6 days later. Patients would develop acute respiratory symptoms not unlike a myriad of other pulmonary infections. A pneumonia develops with systemic dissemination of the microbe from the lung tissue. Invasion of the pathogen into the regional lymph nodes of the lung also occurs.

The diagnosis of pulmonary plague is very difficult because of the nonspecific nature of the symptoms. Fever, chills, hemoptysis, and a systemically toxic condition characterize the clinical presentation. Chest radiographs demonstrate acute bronchopneumonia. The patients develop a rapidly evolving picture of pulmonary failure and hypoxemia. Circulatory collapse with a disseminated intravascular coagulopathy is the terminal event. Laboratory findings are characteristic of patients with severe bacterial sepsis. The organism is readily cultured from blood, sputum, or aspirates from the enlarged lymph nodes. Like other potential pathogens from a biological attack, recognition of index cases from cultures or from postmortem identification requires distribution of the information to increase the index of suspicion for additional cases to occur.

The Food and Drug Administration–approved treatment for infection secondary to *Y. pestis* has been streptomycin.[41] This antibiotic is not likely to be available in most hospitals in the United States. Gentamicin is recommended as the alternative treatment. There are both experimental and a small amount of clinical data to support gentamicin treatment. The plague bacillus is actually sensitive in vitro to many different antibiotics, including tetracycline, doxycycline, fluoroquinolones, and sulfonamides. Some resistance to the nonaminoglycoside antibiotic choices has been seen and still makes gentamicin the agent of choice. The alternative choices become desirable to use in a mass casualty situation because supplies of gentamicin would likely be short. If postexposure prophylaxis were deemed necessary, those antibiotic choices that are effective oral agents (e.g., fluoroquinolones) would be good choices for large-scale administration.

A vaccine for *Y. pestis* has been used in the past but currently is not available.[42] The vaccine was made from formalin-killed virulent strains of bacteria. It was believed to prevent or blunt bubonic infection, but it was not effective in the prevention of pulmonic infection.

Tularemia

The bacterial pathogen of tularemia is *Francisella tularensis*. It is a gram-negative intracellular pathogen. Like the plague bacillus, this bacterium is a pathogen of rodents that is transmitted to humans by insect vectors. Naturally occurring tularemic infections are seen in humans and are thought to most commonly occur among hunters handling carcasses of infected dead animals. *F. tularensis* has been the focus of potential germ warfare applications because a very low number of inhaled bacteria are necessary to cause infection. Engineered plasmids that will promote resistance to many different antibiotics have been used to enhance the virulence of wild strains of this species to make it a more formidable weapon.[43]

There are four different types of clinical infection with this microbe.[44] Ulceroglandular tularemia occurs at the local site of an insect bite. It may also infect the host by contamination of an open wound or nonintact skin. Incubation time from inoculation until clinical infection is 3 to 6 days. Local necrosis commonly occurs at the site of inoculation, and the regional lymph nodes become involved in a pattern similar to bubonic plague. The lymph node groups may ulcerate, suppurate, and/or drain. The infection can become systemic from the regional node groups. Mortality rates from this form or tularemia are about 5%.

Oropharyngeal tularemia comes from the ingestion of contaminated water or food. The pharyngitis may have an array of pathologic findings, including erythema and exudative pharyngitis and, in some cases, frank ulceration. Lymphadenopathy may or may not occur. Tularemic pneumonia may accompany the pharyngitis, presumably owing to aspiration of aerosol from the infected upper aerodigestive tract.

Gastrointestinal tularemia is uncommon. The acidity of the stomach may reduce the viable inoculum that is delivered to the intestines after ingestion of the organism. Diarrhea and crampy abdominal pain are common presenting symptoms.

Pulmonary tularemia is the greatest concern for a biological attack. Very few organisms need be inhaled to result in clinical infection.[45] The microbe causes a pleuropneumonitis 3 to 5 days after inhalation. The natural history of pulmonary tularemia is quite variable and may be dependent on the inoculum of contamination. The clinical picture is one of severe pneumonia and is not easily differentiated from any of a number of gram-negative pneumonias. Pulmonary tularemia, like the other agents of biological warfare, is so uncommon as a naturally occurring infection that any identified case should generate an increased index of suspicion for the infection in other patients. Mortality rates from pulmonary tularemia are about 35%.

The diagnosis is a difficult one. Gram-negative bacteria will be seen on Gram stain. Hilar adenopathy is seen on the chest radiograph. Cultures of the sputum establish the diagnosis, but special media containing cysteine or other sulfhydryl compounds are necessary to enhance rates of recovery. Serologic methods are also available through reference laboratories but are seldom useful for the timely diagnosis necessary to effect treatment.

The drug of choice for the treatment of tularemia is streptomycin, but in all likelihood other aminoglycosides will be used (e.g., gentamicin). Chloramphenicol and tetracycline have also been used.[46] Because a patient with tularemia can pursue a chronic and protracted course with weight loss, malaise, and so on, antibiotic therapy should be given and continued even if the patient appears to be improving from the acute infection. Oral tetracycline is recommended for postexposure prophylaxis. No vaccine is under evaluation.

Transmission of infection from human to human is thought to be very low. Standard infection control practices are believed to be sufficient. No isolation of patients with acute infection is necessary. Standard sterilization and disinfection of equipment, instruments, and devices is sufficient.

Brucellosis

Brucellosis is caused by an aerobic coccobacillus that is gram negative. Infection in humans is caused by *Brucella melitensis, B. suis, B. abortus,* and *B. canis.* Infection with *Brucella* species may occur from direct skin contact with the organism, from ingestion, or by inhalation.[47] Cutaneous infection is quite rare. The pathogenesis of gastrointestinal and inhalation brucellosis is similar. Small inocula (<100 organisms) are required to cause clinical infection. The organism is ingested by the macrophage cell and transported to the regional lymph nodes. The microbe proliferates intracellularly and destroys the macrophage. They may then replicate extracellularly. Whereas airborne *Brucella* species would be the most likely route in a biological attack, the infection is a systemic illness rather than a pneumonia. Invasive infection results in dissemination of the organism with metastatic foci developing at remote sites. The sites of infection remote from the gastrointestinal or pulmonary portal of entry include abscess of the liver and spleen, arthritis and osteomyelitis, meningitis and encephalitis, orchitis, pyelonephritis, and even endocarditis. The disease usually has an onset 2 to 4 weeks after transmission, but the delay in clinical infection may be as long as 2 months. The disease has about a 5% mortality rate, but its value in terrorism is the chronic incapacitation that affects the host. Symptoms may last for 6 months or more without treatment. High relapse rates are noted if there has been an insufficient length of therapy.

The diagnosis of brucellosis is difficult because of the lack of specific findings that are characteristic of the disease. Leukocyte counts are generally normal. The diagnosis is suggested when patients present with a generally debilitating illness with local infections at remote sites. Blood and bone marrow cultures, especially the latter, are most useful.[48] Joint aspirates[49] and solid organ abscess[50] collections will allow recovery of the organism. Cultures are slow to yield the organism and may need to be kept for 60 days. Because of the problems with culturing the organism, serologic tests to detect antibody are of greatest value in making the diagnosis.

The recommended treatment for brucellosis is combination therapy with doxycycline and rifampin.[51] Streptomycin with tetracycline has formerly been used with success. Many still think that the addition of an aminoglycoside to the treatment regimen is important. Duration of antibiotic therapy should be for 6 weeks. Specific types of infection (e.g., endocarditis or osteomyelitis) may require a much longer course of therapy. Recommendations on postexposure antibiotic use are not currently available. No vaccine is available.

Standard precautions are believed to be adequate for infected patients. Person-to-person transmission has been reported, but the risk of such an event is very low given the small numbers of pathogens that are found in the lung in the patient with brucellosis. Standard practices of environmental decontamination of equipment with hypochlorite solution are adequate.

Other Bacteria

Other bacteria that have been proposed as potential agents of a biological attack are summarized in Table 25-4. A guiding feature for surgeons and other health care personnel is to constantly be sensitive to the occurrence of unusual pathogens emerging in a given area or location. These clusters of unusual infections deserve an epidemiologic evaluation to assess whether deliberate infections are being transmitted.

VIRUSES

Viruses have been sources of concern as potential biological weapons. Viruses are more difficult to generate in large quantities, and storage of viruses is more problem-

---

TABLE 25-4. Other Agents That Have Been Proposed for Acts of Bioterrorism

Disease	Organism	Route of Transmission	Treatment
Cholera	*Vibrio cholerae*	Oral	Rehydration; doxycycline; quinolones
Salmonellosis	*Salmonella typhi*	Oral	Quinolones
Glanders	*Burkholderia mallei*	Airborne	Quinolones, doxycycline, rifampin
Q fever	*Coxiella burnetii*	Airborne	Quinolones
Shigella dysentery	*Shigella dysenteriae*	Oral	Quinolones
Cryptosporidiosis	*Cryptosporidium parvum*	Oral	No effective chemotherapy

atic than that of bacteria. Nevertheless, specific viruses continue to be sources of concern and fear as agents to be used in unconventional civilian disasters.

Smallpox

Of all of the potential biological weapons, none has generated more debate than smallpox. Variola is the virus of smallpox. Following the intensive efforts of the World Health Organization to eradicate smallpox,[52] there has not been a case of smallpox infection identified in the world since 1977. Vaccination against smallpox has ceased for about the past 20 years. It is currently thought that only the CDC, in Atlanta, and the Institute for Viral Preparation, in Moscow, have cultures of smallpox at this time. However, concern exists that the security of these remaining cultures may have been breeched or that viral cultures of smallpox may have existed other than those just cited.[43]

Smallpox creates grave concern as a biological weapon for several reasons. The population of the world is unvaccinated or received vaccination against the virus more than 20 years ago. The natural transmission of the virus is as an airborne pathogen, so that aerosolization would efficiently infect many individuals. Furthermore, the virus is quite stable for a period of time in aerosol form. Of greatest significance is that infected smallpox patients are highly infectious to others, thus making a large outbreak in a densely populated urban area an infection control nightmare.[53]

Smallpox infection begins with inhalation of a small inoculum of the virus.[54] The virus adheres to the oropharyngeal and respiratory epithelium and migrates to the regional lymph nodes. On the third or fourth day after inoculation, the patient has an asymptomatic viremia that results in dissemination of the virus throughout the reticuloendothelial system. On approximately the eighth day after inoculation the patient has clinical symptoms of fever and toxicity that herald the second viremia. Systemic viral symptoms increase, with even abdominal pain and delirium being present. From day 12 to 14, a maculopapular rash begins that forms vesicles and then pustules. The rash finally evolves to the crusted, umbilicated rash of smallpox. Mortality rates from smallpox infection are 30%, with those of the hemorrhagic and malignant forms of the disease being higher.

The diagnosis is made by the recognition of the characteristic rash of smallpox, which could potentially be confused with that of chickenpox. The rash of chickenpox is usually dense and appears on the trunk, whereas that of smallpox is most dense on the face and extremities. The virus itself can be identified on electron microscopy of scrapings from the lesions, whereas scrapings will show Guarnieri bodies under light microscopy when appropriately stained. The virus can be cultured.

There is no established antiviral therapy for smallpox infection, although some are being investigated (e.g., cidofovir).[55] Acutely infected individuals require supportive care as the only meaningful treatment. Vaccinia immune globulin is thought to be of value in the first week after exposure. Vaccination is also recommended within the first postexposure week.

The infection control management of patients with smallpox is a very difficult problem. Because smallpox patients are infectious until the scabs from the rash separate, inpatient transmission to other patients and to hospital personnel is a major risk. Personnel will need to be vaccinated. Patients will need to be in negative-pressure rooms. Full barrier protection with gloves/gowns/masks will need to be employed. Laundry and waste must be incinerated when discarded. Large outbreaks will saturate hospital and personnel capacity to care for the patient load. Community disaster plans need to consider designated temporary facilities that can be activated for care of patients in the event of this or other large infectious attacks.

The concern about the return of smallpox infection as a biological weapon against civilian populations has stimulated interest in the renewal of public vaccination. The vaccination process is with the vaccinia virus, which has similar antigenic properties to variola. Vaccination is achieved by giving the naive host an infection with the vaccinia virus. While this vaccination process is safe for the vast majority of the population, it is not without risk. In Table 25-5, the rates of major complications with smallpox vaccination are summarized.[56] A resumption of large-scale public vaccination will have significant numbers of individuals sustain major neurologic injury and even death.

The Advisory Committee on Immunization Practice (ACIP) has made the following recommendations to the CDC with respect to smallpox vaccination.[57]

- Vaccination of the general population is not recommended because of risk-benefit concerns.
- Vaccination is recommended for smallpox response teams that are designated to investigate cases of smallpox. Each state should have one team.
- Vaccination is recommended for selected personnel in designated referral centers that will care for smallpox patients.

The initial adoption of these recommendations for selected vaccination of health care personnel has had a lukewarm reception. Deaths associated with the vaccine have already been reported. Given that it has been over

TABLE 25-5. Complication Rates from Vaccination for Smallpox per Million Patients for All Age Groups from a 10-State Survey In 1968

Complication	Primary Vaccination	Secondary Vaccination
Generalized vaccinia	241.5	9.0
Progressive vaccinia	1.5	3.0
Postvaccinal encephalitis	12.3	2.0
Eczema vaccinatum	38.5	3.0

From Lane JM, Ruben FL, Neff JM, Miller JD: Complications of smallpox vaccination, 1968: Results of ten statewide surveys. J Infect Dis 122:303-309, 1970.

25 years since the last case of smallpox has been identified anywhere in the world, and given that deaths and major neurologic incapacitation will surely happen with the vaccination process, it would seem appropriate to await further evidence that smallpox infection will re-emerge.

Other Viruses

Many other viruses have been the subjects of interest as potential biological weapons. Particular interest has focused on the hemorrhagic fever viruses.[58] These viruses are summarized in Table 25-6.

TOXINS

Biological toxins have also been hypothesized as potential agents for biological attacks on civilian populations. Bacterial and plant toxins have been the principal ones to be sources of concern at present.

Botulinum Toxin

Botulinum toxin refers to the accumulated seven different neurotoxins that are specifically produced by *Clostridium botulinum*. Botulinum toxin is actually used at the present time for medical indications, but it was also used by the Japanese against the Chinese as a weapon in World War II.[59]

Botulinum toxin prevents the release of acetylcholine from the presynaptic nerve terminal at the neuromuscular junction. The result is paralysis. Clinical infection with *C. botulinum* in wounds or within the gastrointestinal tract can make "botulism" a naturally occurring event.

Ingestion of food stuffs contaminated with the toxin can produce illness without live bacterial infection. The greatest concern for botulinum toxin is for it to be inhaled as a finely dispersed powder. The toxin has incredible toxicity in small quantities. The lung becomes an efficient absorptive surface to result in systemic paralysis very quickly.[60]

The diagnosis of botulism is a clinical one. The patients have progressive clinical paralysis that is not associated with fever. Botulism has clinical characteristics that are similar to Guillain-Barré syndrome or myasthenia gravis. In an acute setting that appeared to be an unconventional civilian attack, botulism and nerve agent poisoning would have some common features. The features of botulism are diplopia, ptosis, dilated pupils, dysphagia, and dysarthria. Nerve agent poisoning would be associated with miosis and copious pulmonary secretions. The mouse bioassay study has been the diagnostic study for botulinum poisoning but has limited availability to establish the diagnosis. Serum, stool, and gastric aspirate specimens are saved for reference laboratory determination of the presence of the toxin.

The initial management of the patient with botulism is to use the antitoxin.[61] This preparation is an equine antitoxin. It will only influence potential effects from botulinum toxin that has not been absorbed systemically. Thus, it will have benefit in neutralizing that toxin that may have been orally ingested but not yet absorbed from the intestinal tract. It likely will have limited or no value for toxin that has been inhaled. Because the antitoxin is from horses, skin testing should be performed before administration to avoid anaphylaxis. Because the illness is due to toxin and not bacterial infection, antibiotics have no role other than to manage nosocomial infections that will attend the care of these patients. Aminoglycosides in

TABLE 25-6. Viruses of Viral Hemorrhagic Fever*

Disease	Genus	Natural Locale
Viral Equine Encephalitis		
Eastern equine encephalitis	Alphavirus	North/South America
Western equine encephalitis	Alphavirus	North America
Venezuelan equine encephalitis	Alphavirus	Northern South America
Viral Hemorrhagic Fever		
Argentine hemorrhagic fever	Arenavirus	South America
Bolivian hemorrhagic fever	Arenavirus	South America
Brazilian hemorrhagic fever	Arenavirus	South America
Crimean-Congo hemorrhagic fever	Nairovirus	Africa, Asia, Europe
Dengue fever	Flavivirus	Africa, Americas, Asia
Ebola/Marburg hemorrhagic fever	Filovirus	Africa
Hantavirus infection	Hantavirus	Asia, Europe, Southwest United States
Kyasanur forest disease	Flavivirus	Africa, South America
Lassa fever	Arenavirus	Africa
Omsk hemorrhagic fever	Flavivirus	Eastern Europe
Rift Valley fever	Phlebovirus	Africa
Venezuelan hemorrhagic fever	Arenavirus	South America
Yellow fever	Flavivirus	Africa, South America

*All of these viruses are of potential concern as biological weapons.

particular need to be avoided, because they will potentially exacerbate the neuromuscular blockade.

A botulinum toxoid is under investigational use.[62] It is a pentavalent toxoid. It would likely have application for military use or for individuals at occupational risk of botulinum toxin exposure.

No isolation of patients is required. The toxin is not active on intact skin, and secondary exposures from affected patients are not an issue. Standard precautions and disinfection of equipment in the health environment are recommended.

Ricin

Ricin is a complex toxin that is extracted from the castor bean. The process for extraction is relatively simple, and large quantities of the toxin can be produced and stored, which makes this a source of concern for use as an agent for a biotoxin attack. It was actually evaluated by the United States and the United Kingdom jointly for use in bombs in World War II but was never deployed. On a weight basis it does not have near the toxicity of botulinum toxin. Ricin has highly variable toxicity for different animal species.

The ricin protein has an A-chain and a B-chain.[63] The B-chain when administered systemically binds to the cell membrane and results in endocytosis of the toxin. The toxin is released within the cytoplasm. The A-chain then binds to a specific ribosome in the cytoplasm and inhibits protein synthesis. It appears to affect most cell populations. Its greatest effects are in the tissues at the portal of entry into the body.

Oral ingestion is less toxic than other routes.[64] Evidence from castor bean ingestion indicates that patients have rapid onset of nausea, vomiting, abdominal pain, and diarrhea. Gastrointestinal bleeding, fever, hypotension, and death over a 72-hour period happen in severe cases. A 6% mortality has been reported in castor bean ingestion. Autopsies showed extensive necrosis of the gastrointestinal mucosa.

Parenteral injection was employed in a political assassination in London in 1978.[65] There was marked tissue necrosis at the site of injection. Gastrointestinal bleeding, hepatic necrosis, nephritis, and systemic reticuloendothelial changes are noted.

Inhalation has been studied in animals only. It is associated with a severe fibrinopurulent pneumonia. Extensive tissue necrosis and inflammatory changes are noted. Purulent lymphadenitis was seen in mediastinal nodes. Causes of death due to ricin appear to be pulmonary damage and failure after inhalation, with activation of the systemic inflammatory response and the septic syndrome.

Inhalation would appear to be the most likely scenario for a terrorist incident. An acute pulmonary insult would suggest the diagnosis among the numerous other inhaled agents that would cause an acute pulmonary crisis. Ricin can be identified from a nasal swab specimen within 24 hours of the episode. Ricin identified from blood would be unlikely because of its mechanism of action. Antibodies could be identified in survivors at 2 weeks.

Therapy would be supportive care for the patient with a severe pulmonary insult. Intubation and ventilator support would be required. A large number of agents are being investigated as treatments for ricin. None has been tested clinically. Ricin remains at this point as an agent of concern but one with which there has been minimal clinical experience to assist in making a diagnosis or providing specific treatment.

Other Toxins

The potential toxins that could be derived from bacterial cultures or other plants are numerous. Staphylococcal enterotoxin B and the vast array of potential mycotoxins are examples. The presentation of patients with toxic conditions without explanation should create an index of suspicion about malicious use of toxins. Whereas culturing patients with clinical syndromes that resemble infection is a standard, the presentation of patients with an unexplained toxic condition should stimulate the observant physician to obtain nasal swabs, blood samples, and other body fluids for subsequent analysis. The large number of toxins that could potentially be used will commonly not benefit the specific patient who is being evaluated, but subsequent evaluation of the specimens may allow identification of the agent in question.

CHEMICAL AGENTS

Chemical agents have been used in World War I and other military conflicts. Chemicals are generally more easily produced and stored than are biological agents. Most are dispersed as gases or vapors and have posed problems of delivery because of environmental conditions at the time they are used. Chemical agents dispersed into public meeting rooms and arenas have the potential to make them very dangerous for use in unconventional civilian attacks.

Cyanide

Cyanide is an ubiquitous substance that occurs by natural processes. It is found in bitter almonds, peach stones, cherry leaves, and sorghum. Cyanide was used as a military weapon by the French during World War I. It was used to exterminate millions during the Holocaust, it has been used for capital punishment executions, it was used to contaminate acetaminophen products, and it has been used as an agent in mass religious suicides.

Cyanide may be present as a sodium or potassium salt, but military applications have focused on the volatile liquids of hydrogen cyanide or cyanogen chloride. Ingestion of a cyanide salt results in rapid death when a large enough dose is absorbed. Inhalation of the gas has rapid onset of symptoms. Conjunctival and skin surfaces can absorb fatal doses of cyanide solutions.

The cyanide ion binds to the iron of cytochrome oxidase within the mitochondria of the cell.[66] This results in complete inhibition of electron transport and adenosine triphosphate synthesis. Oxygen is available as the electron acceptor of oxidative phosphorylation, but cyanide inhibits the process.

Onset of symptoms from acute cyanide exposure are rapid.[67] An odor of bitter almonds at the scene may be reported by individuals experiencing minor exposures. Acute symptoms of cyanide poisoning include weakness, fatigue, anxiety, dyspnea, nausea and vomiting, headache, and confusion. Large exposures are associated with rapid onset of convulsions, coma, and death. Cyanosis is not present, because the patient has adequate hemoglobin saturation.

A chemical attack on a civilian population could occur with the use of this agent by several means. Contamination of food, water, or medicines is a possibility, although the almond odor would be a clue that contamination had occurred. Release of the volatile liquid or vapor into a room or confined space would be another method. Sources of undelivered cyanide were actually found in the Tokyo subway system subsequent to the sarin gas attack of 1995. Deaths under such circumstances would be rapid for many victims, and the opportunity to treat and reverse the chemical poisoning would be quite brief.

Treatment of acute cyanide poisoning requires immediate administration of an antidote; these are numerous and have different modes of action:

- Methemoglobin-forming drugs[68]: Amyl nitrite and sodium nitrite are antidotes that work by generating methemoglobin, which has a higher affinity for cyanide ion than does cytochrome oxidase. Because the binding of cyanide to cytochrome oxidase is reversible, the elimination of free cyanide in plasma results in dissociation of the bound cyanide and a resumption of oxidative phosphorylation. Nitrites are also vasodilators, which some authors believe adds to therapeutic effect, but overexuberant administration can lead to hypotension. Methemoglobin should not exceed 40% of total hemoglobin, because higher levels will interfere with oxygenation and delivery.
- Sulfur donors[68]: Sodium thiosulfate is usually given with a methemoglobin-forming agent. Thiosulfate com-

pounds bind the cyanide into a stable compound that attenuates the action of the cyanide but then facilitates clearance of the cyanide via urinary excretion.

- Cobalt salts[69]: The cobalt salt of ethylenediaminetetraacetic acid binds the cyanide ion and is clinically used for cyanide poisoning in Europe. Toxicity of this treatment has resulted in it not being used in the United States.
- Hydroxocobalamin (vitamin B_{12a})[70]: This compound directly binds cyanide ion. It has been used with sodium thiosulfate, but this has been limited because of hypersensitivity reactions, tachyphylaxis, and its considerable cost.

The recommended treatment of cyanide poisoning at the present time is the combination of sodium nitrite (10 mL of solution of 30 mg/mL) and sodium thiosulfate (50 mL of 250 mg/mL solution, or 12.5 g). The patients also require the usual elements of vigorous supportive care. Monitoring oxygenation and cardiac output during and after antidote therapy are important. Hemodynamic management may include blood pressure support and management of arrhythmias. These patients will have significant lactic acidosis, which may require management, although monitoring lactate concentrations also becomes an important part of monitoring the effectiveness of anti-cyanide antidotes.[71]

Nerve Agents

The nerve agents are a group of organophosphate compounds.[72] These agents include sarin, tabun, soman, and VX. The agents are liquids at room temperature. The nerve agents were produced but not used for military applications in World War II. Sarin has been used in terrorist incidents in Japan. The proposed dispersal of the agent as a weapon has been as a vapor to be inhaled by the victims. Because the methods used to disperse nerve gases and cyanide are similar, the physiologic effects of these two agents are compared in Table 25-7.

TABLE 25-7. Comparison of Physiologic Effects of Cyanide and Nerve Agents by Organ System

Organ System	Cyanide	Nerve Agents
Skin	Sweating, flushing	Sweating
Muscle	Weakness	Fasciculations, twitching
Eye	Mydriasis, irritation	Miosis
Nose	Irritation of mucous membranes	Profuse rhinorrhea
Mouth	Irritation of mucous membranes	Salivation
Pulmonary	Acute hyperventilation	Bronchoconstriction, wheezing, rhonchi, increased secretions
Cardiovascular	Tachycardia	Increased blood pressure, variable rate changes
Gastrointestinal	Nausea and vomiting	Nausea, vomiting, cramping, diarrhea
Central nervous system	Headache, agitation, unconsciousness	Seizures, loss of consciousness

These agents are potent and irreversible inhibitors of acetylcholinesterase.[73] Acetylcholine is the neurotransmitter for the cholinergic nervous system. Presynaptic nerve impulses arrive at the synapse and stimulate the release of presynthesized acetylcholine, which depolarizes the postsynaptic target. The enzyme acetylcholinesterase hydrolyzes the acetylcholine transmitter. Thus, each presynaptic impulse is associated with a discrete postsynaptic effect. Blockade of the cholinesterase enzyme results in accumulation of the acetylcholine and continuous postsynaptic stimulation, which results in a cholinergic crisis.

The effects on human physiology after inhalation of nerve agents are extensive.[74] Profound sweating, rhinorrhea, and excessive salivation begin quickly. Severe miosis and eye pain are experienced. The patient experiences copious secretions, wheezing, rhonchi, dyspnea, and cough. Nausea, vomiting, and cramping abdominal pain followed by diarrhea are the results of increased smooth muscle constriction in the gut. Weakness, flaccid muscles, and fasciculations are seen. Pulse changes are variable, but blood pressure commonly rises. Severe exposures result in loss of consciousness and seizures, followed by respiratory arrest and death. Dermal contact can produce many of these same effects, depending on the magnitude of the exposure. Large dermal exposures can be as lethal as inhaled vapor, although there may be as long as a 30-minute delay before physiologic changes occur.

The treatment of the individual exposed to nerve agents begins by removing them from the exposure, quick decontamination of the skin if there is dermal exposure (not necessary for vapor exposure), and adherence to fundamental principles of airway, breathing, and immediate cardiovascular support while the individual is being transported.

The antidotal treatment of nerve agent exposure is atropine and pralidoxime chloride.[75] Atropine blocks the effects of the acetylcholine by competitive inhibition for the postsynaptic receptor sites but does not affect the amount of acetylcholine that is present. The amount of atropine that is given depends on the severity of the exposure event. Because no clinician will have any direct experience in treating one of these exposure cases, making the determination of the severity of the insult is a problem. Convulsing or unconscious patients are obvious examples of this severity. In awake casualties, atropine should be given in 2-mg doses every 10 to 15 minutes until hypersecretion and shortness of breath resolve. Up to 15 mg of atropine may need to be given to unconscious patients. The goal of atropine therapy is reversal of life-threatening symptoms but not the reversal of all symptoms (e.g., miosis). A comfortably breathing and conscious exposure victim with stable vital signs does not need additional atropine at that moment.

Oximes are compounds that will break the organophosphate-to-acetylcholinesterase bond and regenerate active enzyme activity. Unfortunately, "aging" of the organophosphate-to-acetylcholinesterase bond influences the effectiveness of oxime therapy. The aging process is also different for each of the different nerve agents. Early

administration of the oxime compound is obviously important. Furthermore, the oximes tend to reverse nicotinic effects (e.g., muscle fasciculations) rather than muscarinic effects (e.g., hypersalivation). Atropine has principally muscarinic effects. The selective effects of each treatment likely reflect activity of nerve agents that are not yet understood.

Pralidoxime chloride is the oxime of choice by the U.S. military. The dosage should be 15 to 25 mg/kg. Ideally, the dose should be given intravenously, but in military or in a recognized unconventional civilian attack it may be given intramuscularly in the field. When given intravenously, it should be administered over 20 to 30 minutes. It is considered important to give pralidoxime and atropine at the same time.

Supportive care will need to be given consistent with the patient's level of exposure. Ventilation management and management of transient arrhythmias are necessary in severe cases. Control of seizures has been successfully managed with diazepam in organophosphate insecticide poisonings.[76]

Lung Toxicants

Phosgene gas is the prototype agent in this category.[77] This small molecule of carbonic dichloride has been used as a military chemical agent by the Germans in World War I, by the Japanese against the Chinese in World War II, and by Iran against Iraq in the 1980s. It is a colorless gas that is heavier than air. It has the odor of newly mown hay to the discriminating observer.

Phosgene gas as a chemical agent for human injury is delivered for inhalation. Skin or eye exposure to dense vapor can cause local irritation. The mechanism of injury of phosgene is local toxicity and inflammatory injury. It wounds and kills people by injury to the respiratory epithelium and lung tissue.[78] Severe, noncardiogenic pulmonary edema and suffocation are the result.

Symptoms from inhaled phosgene may occur within 30 minutes but can be delayed.[79] Symptoms begin with chest pain, dyspnea, bronchospasm, and then hypoxemia as the pulmonary edema syndrome evolves. Hemoptysis is seen in severe cases. Pulmonary hypertension and death follow. Even if patients have had exposure but do not seem affected, they should be monitored in a hospital setting because the onset of dyspnea and pulmonary edema is reported to not start for 48 hours after exposure.

Initial management of the suspected phosgene casualty is to remove the person from the contaminated environment. The gas layers across the floor of a building or confined space, so casualties and rescue personnel need to evacuate the area. Clothing should be removed and the skin should be cleansed with tepid water as soon as possible to avoid continued skin injury or secondary risk to emergency personnel. There is some evidence that would support the use of ibuprofen after exposure.[80]

The treatment of phosgene poisoning is supportive care until the injured lung recovers.[81] Ventilation management to maintain oxygenation and appropriate cardiovascular support are clearly necessary. Ventilation support can be protracted, and a small number of patients may even require tracheostomy. Nosocomial pneumonia is a major risk for the prolonged ventilator patient. There is no antidote for phosgene poisoning.

The major dilemma from large phosgene gas attack within a large auditorium or public place would be the potential number of acute casualties. The presentation of hundreds of lung injuries that required ventilator management would eclipse the critical care capacity of all but a few communities. Triage of injuries would be a difficult and painful proposition.

Vesicants

The vesicants are a group of military chemicals that were designed to injure and incapacitate the enemy rather than to kill them. Inflicting large numbers of nonlethal but serious injuries on a civilian population would have serious psychosocial as well as health management problems.

The most recognized vesicant is sulfur mustard.[82] It was used in World War I and again by Iraq in the war with Iran in the 1980s. Nitrogen mustard proved to not be as good as sulfur mustard for military purposes. Death rates from sulfur mustard used as a military weapon have been about 5%.

Sulfur mustard is a liquid at room temperature. It has been delivered as a vapor in military use but may condense under cooler environmental conditions. Its mechanism of action remains unclear.[83] It is topically toxic to the tissues that it contacts. The principal organs injured from sulfur mustard are the skin, eyes, and lung. Systemic absorption of significant amounts of mustard through the skin and lung may cause gastrointestinal, hematopoietic, and central nervous system injury.

Injury after mustard exposure is evident within 1 to 2 hours. Severe exposures are associated with partial thickness blistering of large surface areas of the skin. Eye injuries include a conjunctival inflammation, severe pain, swelling, and possible permanent corneal damage. Inhalation has a mild lung toxicant effect that is associated with cough and dyspnea. Severe cases may have pulmonary edema.

Management of the casualties is largely supportive. The severity of injury can be reduced by rapid decontamination within minutes of the injury. Any delay means that fixation of the chemical to the tissues has already occurred and that significant absorption may well have occurred. Extensive soft tissue wounds are handled in the same fashion as burn injuries. Severe eye injuries require local analgesics, topical mydriatic therapy, and antibiotic eye drops.[84] Pulmonary management may include supplemental oxygen, bronchodilation, and chest physiotherapy. Severe injuries of the lung may require ventilator support. Nosocomial pneumonia is a risk for these severe injuries because of the lung injury and because of immunosuppression that attends significant systemic absorption of the mustard.

Lewisite is an arsenical vesicant that is mentioned only for completeness.[85] It has never been actually used as a chemical weapon. It is toxic like mustard when employed as a vapor. It has skin, eye, and lung actions very similar to mustard. Management of lewisite exposure is the same as would be employed with mustard injuries. Lewisite does not have the systemic immunosuppression of mustard.

RADIATION TERRORISM

The use of radioactive contamination or even a nuclear detonation as an unconventional civilian act of terrorism looms as a perceived threat.[86,87] Radioactivity is feared by the population in general, and it is not well understood by most practicing physicians. Dissemination of radioactivity could occur by several different means, each of which would have a different risk to the exposed population.

First, radioactive particles, liquids, or gases could be released at a public place or gathering. The contamination of the physical grounds at a meeting place, a public source of drinking water, or airborne dissemination by a spray or via an aircraft would deliver small amounts of radioactivity. Physical harm from acute radiation exposure would not occur because of the limited dose that could be delivered by such means, but the psychosocial impact would be considerable.

Second, radioactive materials could be loaded into a conventional explosion—the so-called "dirty bomb." Conventional explosions used to target nuclear power plants or nuclear waste facilities would be a similar strategy. The effects of the radioactivity within the conventional explosion would be to exposed casualties, to exposed rescue personnel, and to people where radioactivity would be carried to sites distant from the primary explosion. The actual delivered dose of radioactivity is small, but the psychosocial consequences would be great.

The third scenario would be a detonation of a nuclear device. A 1-kiloton (1000 kg of TNT in explosive impact) device is thought to be a possibility for production by a terrorist group. That compares to 15 to 20 kilotons as the force of the bombs used in Japan in World War II. A nuclear detonation would be associated with massive physical injuries, significant numbers of irradiated casualties, and downwind fallout of radioactive contamination.

Basics of Radioactivity

Each atom of the periodic table theoretically has an equal number of electrons, protons, and neutrons.[88] Isotopes exist in nature in which variations may occur in the number of neutrons and thus isotopes may be stable or unstable. Unstable isotopes undergo decay and emit radiation. The emitted radioactivity is electromagnetic (e.g., x-rays, gamma rays) or particulate (e.g., alpha, beta, or neutron) or combinations for each different type of unstable isotope.

As emitted radioactivity proceeds along a pathway, there is energy transfer into the medium (e.g., air, liquid, tissue) until there is complete dissipation of the energy. Energy transfer when the radiation proceeds through tissue results in ionization or the production of free radicals from oxygen or water in the cell. Free radicals mediate immediate- and long-term injury to the cell.

The measured units of radiation are gray units (Gy), formerly know as rads (1 Gy = 100 rads). Cellular injury is likely to occur as a function of the amount of radiation dose, the degree of active replication of the cells (e.g., bone marrow vs. muscle), the oxygen content of the tissue (e.g., brain vs. adipose tissue), and the water content (e.g., liver vs. bone). The risks of ionization will depend on the type of radiation, because particulate types will more likely have energy transfer in tissue than will electromagnetic types. The time interval of delivery of the dose is also important.

Radiation Injury

Acute radiation exposure will give a variable pattern of illness depending on the exposure dose.[89] The rapidity and severity of symptoms will directly relate to the dose of exposure. Acute exposures of less than 1 Gy will usually have minimal or no symptoms and complete recovery is expected. Exposures greater than 1 Gy would ordinarily only be expected with an actual nuclear detonation as opposed to mechanical dissemination of radioactivity or radiation contaminants that are included with conventional explosives.

Long-term effects of radiation exposure are generally identified as oncogenic effects that may occur after a lengthy latent period of many years. Leukemia appears 7 to 10 years later and solid tumors 20 to 30 years later. From the exposures of the Japanese populations of World War II, a 50% increase in leukemia rates has been observed with a 10% increase in solid tumors.

Medical Management of Irradiated Patients

In the "dirty bomb" scenario, management is relatively simple. Surface decontamination is achieved by removal of clothing, surface rinsing of the skin, and washing the hair. Physical injuries are then managed by conventional methods. Radiation exposure to the patient and the health care team is not considered to be significant.

With a nuclear detonation, patient management requires effective triage of those with significant exposure into groups of those with and those without physical injuries from the kinetic force of the explosion.[90,91] A 1-kiloton device would have an LD_{50} radius of about 300 m from the effects of the blast. Debris, glass, and fires will create large numbers of physical injuries even outside of this radius. Thermal energy will likely have an LD_{50} radius of 600 m. The acute radiation exposure plus fallout exposure will likely create a 5.5-km radius for a 4-Gy dose. Obviously, wind conditions will affect that distribution. Thus, a 10-km radius from a 1-kiloton detonation will have significant casualties with physical injury and severe radiation exposure close to the center of the event and large numbers of irradiated but not physically injured patients in the outer perimeter. In-the-field triage may be necessary to determine which patients should be transported to the health care facilities, which should go to designated decontaminated facilities, and which have injuries that are beyond recovery and receive only symptomatic care. Field decontamination is desirable but may not be practical. Decontamination will likely be necessary at the receiving acute care facility.

After decontamination, physical injuries are treated according to standard guidelines. Advanced trauma life support guidelines are used and care is completed following primary and secondary surveys. With effective decontamination, the patients should not pose a risk to health care personnel. *Irradiated patients who have been decontaminated are not radioactive.*

In following injured and noninjured patients for acute radiation injury, the initial 48 hours of observation are important. Signs and symptoms of nausea, vomiting, diarrhea, and fever are predictive of the magnitude of exposure using the data of Table 25-8. Neutrophil, lymphocyte, and platelet counts are followed. Patients are treated in a supportive fashion for all symptoms that develop. There is no antidote to ameliorate or diminish the effects of acute radiation exposure.

Internal contamination from inhaled or ingested contamination is a significant concern with a nuclear detonation. Major fission products would include radioactive isotopes such as ^{131}I, ^{137}Cs, and ^{90}Sr. Early administration (within 48 hours of exposure) of potassium iodide may reduce long-term risks of thyroid cancer. Ferric hexacyanoferrate (Prussian blue) adsorbs cesium and may enhance elimination. Aluminum phosphate decreases strontium absorption from the gastrointestinal tract.

Acute immunosuppression can be anticipated among all patients with exposures in excess of 1 Gy. Infection control practices are important. Preventive antibiotics should only be used consistent with accepted principles of trauma care. The febrile response of acute radiation exposure should not be used as justification for empirical antibiotic use. The use of granulocyte-colony-stimulating factor, granulocyte-macrophage colony-stimulating factor, and selective gut decontamination has been proposed as possible therapies for these patients but no data are available to support their use.

CONCLUSION

Surgeons can ensure a successful response to terrorist attack by taking a proactive role in the planning, training, and management of terrorist incidents involving mass trauma and WMD (Box 25-3).

TABLE 25-8.   Clinical Manifestations After Different Doses of Radiation Exposure

Organ System	Amount of Radiation Dose				
	1-2 Gy	2-4 Gy	4-6 Gy	6-8 Gy	>8 Gy
Temperature control Frequency	Normal	Febrile (1-3 hr) 50-80%	Febrile (1-2 hr) 80-100%	High fever 100%	High fever 100%
Skin Timing	None	Hair loss ≥15 days	Hair loss 11-21 days	Complete hair loss ≤ 11-15 days	Complete hair loss <10 days
Vomiting Incidence	At 2 hr <50%	1-2 hr 70-90%	<1 hr 100%	<30 min 100%	<10 min 100%
Diarrhea Timing	None	None	Mild 3-8 hr	Severe 1-3 hr	Severe <1 hr
Headache Timing	Slight	Mild	Moderate 4-24 hr	Severe 3-4 hr	Severe 1-2 hr
Mental status	Normal	Normal	Normal	Altered	Unconscious
Granulocytes (3-6 days) (10^9 cells/L)	>2.0	1.5-2.0	1.0-1.5	≤0.5	≤0.1
Lymphocytes (3-6 days) (10^9 cells/L)	0.8-1.5	0.5-0.8	0.3-0.5	0.1-0.3	<0.1
Platelets (3-6 days) (10^9 cells/L) Incidence	60-100 10-25%	30-60 25-40%	25-35 40-80%	15-25 60-80%	<20 80-100%
Mortality rates Timing	0	<50% 6-8 wk	20-70% 4-8 wk	50-100% 1-2 wk	100% 1-2 wk

Adapted from Guskova AK: Radiation sickness classification. *In* Gusev IA, Guskova AK, Mettler FA (eds): Medical Management of Radiation Accidents. Boca Raton, FL, CRC Press, 2001, pp 23-31.

Box 25-3.   Things Surgeons Can Do to Enhance Their Response to Terrorist Attack

■ Participate in the development of your MMRS

Understand the model of incident command that exists within your community so that in the event of a disaster you will know your role and participate accordingly. Determine if your hospital uses an ICS-based disaster plan. Appropriate people to contact can be identified by linking to your state or local EMS agency at the National Association of Emergency Medical Directors at www.nasemsd.org

■ Participate in hospital WMD planning

Within each hospital, surgeons should participate to define and develop the internal response capabilities of their hospital for injury from biological and chemical agents using the DHHS OEP guide at www.bt.cdc.gov or www.ahapolicyforum.org

■ Learn WMD effects and treatment

Individual surgeons need to expand their own knowledge of biological and chemical agents by learning: (1) agents that are most likely to be used, (2) appropriate initial injury control and risk reduction and barrier precaution procedures, (3) presenting signs and symptoms and the natural history of exposure, and (4) definitive treatment. A primary resource for didactic information is at the CDC web site at www.bt.cdc.gov

■ Surgeons' role in education on WMD—local

The surgeon should participate in the education of colleagues, hospital staff, and administration. Surgeons should partner with local public health officials to educate the public regarding the thoroughness of the local disaster response, the need for specific prevention measures, and the comprehensiveness of our national systems for disaster response and management.

■ Surgeons' role in response to WMD—national

Beyond participating in the local hospital and community plan, surgeons should ask how they might participate at the national or international level in either a homeland disaster or war. They may participate in the NDMS by joining a local DMAT team. Further information is provided at www.ndms.dhhs.gov

From Committee on Trauma, American College of Surgeons: Disasters from Biological and Chemical Terrorism—What Should the Individual Surgeon Do?: A Report from the Committee on Trauma. Available at http://www.facs.org/civiliandisasters/trauma.html. Accessed 6-28-2003.

Selected References

Auf der Heide E: Disaster Response: Principles of Preparation and Coordination. St Louis, Mosby, 1989. Available online at http://216.202.128.19/dr/flash.htm.

This reference is a classic description of principles of disaster response, and an accompanying website makes for easy access.

California Department of Health Services: California Hospital Bioterrorism Response Planning Guide. Sacramento, 2001. Available online at http://www.dhs.cahwnet.gov.

The California Hospital Bioterrorism Response Planning Guide describes the incident command system. It was originated by the U.S. Force Service, and it is a standard reference for describing the components and responsibilities of an incident command structure.

Darling RG, Mothershead JL, Waeckerle JF, Eitzen EE (eds): Bioterrorism. Emerg Med Clin North Am 20(2):1-535, 2002.

This is a very nice review article of the aspects of bioterrorism that has been written since the events of September 11, 2001 and is up to date.

Hogan DE, Burstein JL (eds): Disaster Medicine. Philadelphia, Lippincott Williams & Wilkins, 2002.

This reference was recently published as a definitive textbook and is widely referenced with essentially all chapters up to date and with relevant content.

Sidell FR, Takafuji ET, Franz DR (eds): Textbook of Military Medicine: Medical Aspects of Chemical and Biological Warfare. Washington, DC, Office of The Surgeon General, at TMM Publications Borden Institute, 1997.

This is a comprehensive text published by the military covering all aspects of chemical and biological warfare as a classic reference for referral with regard to any topic in this area.

References

1. Auf der Heide E: Disaster Response: Principles of Preparation and Coordination. St. Louis, Mosby, 1989.
2. Okumura T, Suzuki K, Fukuda A, et al.: The Tokyo subway sarin attack: Disaster management: III. National and international responses. Acad Emerg Med 5:625-628, 1998.
3. Okumura T, Suzuki K, Fukuda A, et al: The Tokyo subway sarin attack: Disaster management: II. Hospital response. Acad Emerg Med 5:618-624, 1998.
4. Okumura T, Suzuki K, Fukuda A, et al: The Tokyo subway sarin attack: Disaster management: I. Community emergency response. Acad Emerg Med 5:613-617, 1998.
5. Okumura T, Takasu N, Ishimatsu S, et al: Report on 640 victims of the Tokyo subway sarin attack. Ann Emerg Med 28:129-135, 1996.
6. Nozaki H, Aikawa N, Shinozawa Y, et al: Sarin poisoning in Tokyo subway. Lancet 345:980-981, 1995.
7. Bazzoli GJ, MacKenzie EJ: Trauma centers in the United States: Identification and examination of key characteristics. J Trauma 38:103-110, 1995.
8. MacKenzie EJ, Hoyt DB, Sacra JC, et al: National inventory of hospital trauma centers. JAMA 289:1515-1522, 2003.
9. Joint Commission on Accreditation of Healthcare Organizations: Emergency Management Standard. Oak Brook Terrace, IL, Joint Commission on Accreditation of Healthcare Organizations, 2001.
10. Quarentelli EL: Delivery of Emergency Medical Care in Disasters: Assumptions and Realities. New York, Irvington, 1983.
11. Auf der Heide E: Disaster planning: II. Disaster problems, issues, and challenges identified in the research literature. Emerg Med Clin North Am 14:453-480, 1996.
12. Feliciano DV, Anderson GV Jr, Rozycki GS, et al: Management of casualties from the bombing at the centennial Olympics. Am J Surg 176:538-543, 1998.
13. Hirshberg A, Holcomb JB, Mattox KL: Hospital trauma care in multiple-casualty incidents: A critical view. Ann Emerg Med 37:647-652, 2001.
14. Hirshberg A, Stein M, Walden R: Surgical resource utilization in urban terrorist bombing: A computer simulation. J Trauma 47:545-550, 1999.
15. Levi L, Bregman D, Geva H, et al: Does number of beds reflect the surgical capability of hospitals in wartime and disaster? The use of a simulation technique at a national level. Prehospital Disaster Med 12:300-304, 1997.
16. Centers for Disease Control, Department of Health and Human Services, CDC Public Health Emergency Preparedness & Response Site. Accessed June 29, 2003 from www.bt.cdc.gov.
17. National Security Decision Directive 47. Emergency Mobilization Preparedness. 7-22-1983; Bill/Resolution.
18. Federal Emergency Response Plan, Federal Response Plan. 9230.1-PL ed, Washington, DC, 1999.
19. Public Health Service Act. 42 USC 243 (c)(2); 42 USC 319. 2003; Statute. 1985.
20. Department of Health and Human Services, Office of Emergency Preparedness: Team Handbook. Rockville, MD, U.S. Public Health Service, 2001.
21. Havlak R, Gorman SE, Adams SA: Challenges associated with creating a pharmaceutical stockpile to respond to a terrorist event. Clin Microbiol Infect 8:529-533, 2002.
22. Super G, Groth S, Hook R: START: A Triage Training Module. Newport Beach, CA, Hoag Memorial Hospital Presbyterian, 1994.
23. Schultz CH, Mothershead JL, Field M: Bioterrorism preparedness: I. The emergency department and hospital. Emerg Med Clin North Am 20:437-455, 2002.
24. California Emergency Medical Services Authority, Hospital Emergency Incident Command System III Project, 2003.
25. Ghilarducci DP, Pirrallo RG, Hegmann KT: Hazardous materials readiness of United States level 1 trauma centers. J Occup Environ Med 42:683-692, 2000.
26. Horton DK, Berkowitz Z, Kaye WE: Secondary contamination of ED personnel from hazardous materials events, 1995-2001. Am J Emerg Med 21:199-204, 2003.
27. Nozaki H, Hori S, Shinozawa Y, et al: Secondary exposure of medical staff to sarin vapor in the emergency room. Intensive Care Med 21:1032-1035, 1995.
28. American College of Emergency Physicians, Department of Health and Human Services, et al: Developing Objectives, Content, and Competencies for the Training of Emergency Medical Technicians, Emergency Physicians, and Emergency Nurses to Care for Casualties Resulting from Nuclear, Biological, or Chemical (NBC) Incidents. Dallas, TX, American College of Emergency Physicians, April 23, 2001.
29. NATO Civil Defense Committee. NATO Handbook on Standards and Rules for the Protection of the Civil Population Against Chemical Toxic Agents, 2nd rev ed. Report No. AC/23-D/680. 1983.
30. Sorensen JH, Vogt BM: Will Duct Tape and Plastic Really Work? Issues Related to Expedient Shelter-In-Place. Oak

Ridge, TN, The Oak Ridge National Laboratory, August 1, 2001.

31. Hurst CG: Decontamination. *In* Sidell FR, Takafuji ET, Franz DR (eds): Textbook of Military Medicine: Medical Aspects of Chemical and Biological Warfare, Washington, DC, Office of the Surgeon General at TMM Publications Borden Institute, 1997, pp 351-359.

32. Cooper GJ, Ryan JM, Galbraith KA: The surgical management in war of penetrating wounds contaminated with chemical warfare agents. J R Army Med Corps 140:113-118, 1994.

33. Medical Management of Biological Casualties, 3rd ed. Fort Detrick, Frederick, MD, U.S. Army Medical Research Institute of Infectious Diseases, 1998.

34. Fry DE: In vino veritas. Surg Infect (Larchmt) 2:185-191, 2001.

35. Inglesby TV, Henderson DA, Bartlett JG, et al: Anthrax as a biological weapon: Medical and public health management. Working Group on Civilian Biodefense. JAMA 281:1735-1745, 1999.

36. Friedlander A: Anthrax. *In* Zajtchuk R, Bellamy RF (eds): Textbook of Military Medicine: Medical Aspects of Chemical and Biological Warfare. Washington, DC, Office of the Surgeon General, U.S. Department of the Army, 1997, pp 467-478.

37. Brachman PS: Inhalation anthrax. Ann NY Acad Sci 353:83-93, 1980.

38. Stepanov AV, Marinin LI, Pomerantsev AP, et al: Development of novel vaccines against anthrax in man. J Biotechnol 44:155-160, 1996.

39. Centers for Disease and Prevention: Human plague—United States 1993-1994. MMWR Morbid Mortal Wkly Rep 43:242-246, 1994.

40. McGovern TW, Friedlander A: Plague. *In* Zajtchuk R, Bellamy RF (eds): Textbook of Military Medicine: Medical Aspects of Chemical and Biological Warfare. Washington, DC, Office of the Surgeon General, U.S. Department of the Army, 1997, pp 479-502.

41. Inglesby TV, Dennis DT, Henderson DA, et al: Plague as a biological weapon: Medical and public health management. Working Group on Civilian Biodefense. JAMA 283:2281-2290, 2000.

42. Centers for Disease Control and Prevention: Prevention of plague: Recommendations of the Advisory Committee on Immunization Practice (ACIP). MMWR Morbid Mortal Wkly Rep 45:1-15, 1996.

43. Albibek K, Handelman S: Biohazard. New York, Random House, 1999.

44. Evans ME, Friedlander AM: Tularemia. *In* Zajtchuk R, Bellamy RF (eds): Textbook of Military Medicine: Medical Aspects of Chemical and Biological Warfare. Washington, DC, Office of the Surgeon General, U.S. Department of the Army, 1997, pp 503-512.

45. Saslaw S, Eigelsbach HT, Prior JA, et al: Tularemia vaccine study: II. Respiratory challenge. Arch Intern Med 107:134-146, 1961.

46. Dennis DT, Inglesby TV, Henderson DA, et al: Tularemia as a biological weapon: Medical and public health management. JAMA 285:2763-2773, 2001.

47. Hoover DL, Friedlander AM: Brucellosis. *In* Zajtchuk R, Bellamy RF (eds): Textbook of Military Medicine: Medical Aspects of Chemical and Biological Warfare. Washington, DC, Office of the Surgeon General, U.S. Department of the Army, 1997, pp 513-521.

48. Gotuzzo E, Carrillo C, Guerra J, et al: An evaluation of diagnostic methods for brucellosis—the value of bone marrow culture. J Infect Dis 153:122-125, 1986.

49. Mousa AR, Muhtaseb SA, Almudallal DS, et al: Osteoarticular complications of brucellosis: A study of 169 cases. Rev Infect Dis 9:531-543, 1987.

50. Ibrahim AI, Awad R, Shetty SD, et al: Genito-urinary complications of brucellosis. Br J Urol 61:294-298, 1988.

51. Hall WH: Modern chemotherapy for brucellosis in humans. Rev Infect Dis 12:1060-1099, 1990.

52. World Health Organization: The Global Eradication of Smallpox: Final Report of the Global Commission for the Certification of Smallpox Eradication. Geneva, Switzerland, World Health Organization, 1980.

53. Wehrle PF, Posch J, Richter KH, et al: An airborne outbreak of smallpox in a German hospital and its significance with respect to other recent outbreaks in Europe. Bull World Health Organ 43:669-679, 1970.

54. Henderson DA, Inglesby TV, Bartlett JG, et al: Smallpox as a biological weapon: Medical and public health management. Working Group on Civilian Biodefense. JAMA 281:2127-2137, 1999.

55. Bradbury J: Orally available cidofovir derivative active against smallpox. Lancet 359:1041, 2002.

56. Lane JM, Ruben FL, Neff JM, et al: Complications of smallpox vaccination, 1968: Results of ten statewide surveys. J Infect Dis 122:303-309, 1970.

57. Advisory Committee on Immunization Practices: Draft Supplemental Recommendation of the ACIP-Use of Smallpox (Vaccinia) Vaccine. Submitted to CDC and DHHS for approval, June 2002.

58. Borio L, Inglesby T, Peters CJ, et al: Hemorrhagic fever viruses as biological weapons: Medical and public health management. JAMA 287:2391-2405, 2002.

59. Middlebrook JL, Franz DR: Botulinum toxins. *In* Zajtchuk R, Bellamy RF (eds): Medical Aspects of Chemical and Biological Warfare. Washington, DC, U.S. Department of the Army, 1997, pp 643-654.

60. Arnon SS, Schechter R, Inglesby TV, et al: Botulinum toxin as a biological weapon: Medical and public health management. JAMA 285:1059-1070, 2001.

61. Robinson RF, Nahata MC: Management of botulism. Ann Pharmacother 37:127-131, 2003.

62. Siegel LS: Human immune response to botulinum pentavalent (ABCDE) toxoid determined by a neutralization test and by an enzyme-linked immunosorbent assay. J Clin Microbiol 26:2351-2356, 1988.

63. Lord JM, Roberts LM, Robertus JD: Ricin: Structure, mode of action, and some current applications. FASEB J 8:201-208, 1994.

64. Rauber A, Heard J: Castor bean toxicity re-examined: A new perspective. Vet Hum Toxicol 27:498-502, 1985.

65. Crompton R, Gall D: Georgi Markov—death in a pellet. Med Leg J 48:51-62, 1980.

66. Baskin SI, Brewer TG: Cyanide poisoning. *In* Zajtchuk R, Bellamy RF (eds): Textbook of Military Medicine: Medical Aspects of Chemical and Biological Warfare. Washington, DC, Office of the Surgeon General, U.S. Department of the Army, 1997, pp 271-286.

67. Hall AH, Rumack BH: Clinical toxicology of cyanide. Ann Emerg Med 15:1067-1074, 1986.

68. Chen KK, Rose CL: Nitrite and thiosulfate therapy in cyanide poisoning. JAMA 149:113-119, 1952.

69. Evans CL: Cobalt compounds as antidotes for hydrocyanic acid. Br J Pharmacol 23:455-475, 1964.

70. Sauer SW, Keim ME: Hydroxocobalamin: Improved public health readiness for cyanide disasters. Ann Emerg Med 37:635-641, 2001.

71. Baud FJ, Borron SW, Megarbane B, et al: Value of lactic aci-

dosis in the assessment of the severity of acute cyanide poisoning. Crit Care Med 30:2044-2050, 2002.

72. Sidell FR: Nerve agents. *In* Zajtchuk R, Bellamy RF (eds): Textbook of Military Medicine: Medical Aspects of Chemical and Biological Warfare. Washington, DC, Office of the Surgeon General, U.S. Department of the Army, 1997, pp 129-179.

73. Volans AP: Sarin: Guidelines on the management of victims of a nerve gas attack. J Accid Emerg Med 13:202-206, 1996.

74. Lee EC: Clinical manifestations of sarin nerve gas exposure. JAMA 290:659-662, 2003.

75. Yokoyama K, Yamada A, Mimura N: Clinical profiles of patients with sarin poisoning after the Tokyo subway attack. Am J Med 100:586, 1996.

76. Holstege CP, Kirk M, Sidell FR: Chemical warfare: Nerve agent poisoning. Crit Care Clin 13:923-942, 1997.

77. Borak J, Diller WF: Phosgene exposure: Mechanisms of injury and treatment strategies. J Occup Environ Med 43:110-119, 2001.

78. Diller WF: Pathogenesis of phosgene poisoning. Toxicol Ind Health 1:7-15, 1985.

79. Evison D, Hinsley D, Rice P: Chemical weapons. BMJ 324:332-335, 2002.

80. Sciuto AM, Stotts RR, Hurt HH: Efficacy of ibuprofen and pentoxifylline in the treatment of phosgene-induced acute lung injury. J Appl Toxicol 16:381-384, 1996.

81. Diller WF, Zante R: A literature review: Therapy for phosgene poisoning. Toxicol Ind Health 1:117-128, 1985.

82. Sidell FR, Urbanetti JS, Smith WJ, et al: Vesicants. *In* Zajtchuk R, Bellamy RF (eds): Textbook of Military Medicine: Medical Aspects of Chemical and Biological Warfare. Washington, DC, Office of the Surgeon General, U.S. Department of the Army, 1997.

83. Karnofsky DA, Graef I, Smith HW: Studies on the mechanism of action of the nitrogen and sulfur mustards in vivo. Am J Pathol 24:275-291, 1948.

84. Safarinejad MR, Moosavi SA, Montazeri B: Ocular injuries caused by mustard gas: Diagnosis, treatment, and medical defense. Mil Med 166:67-70, 2001.

85. Goldman M, Dacre JC: Lewisite: Its chemistry, toxicology, and biological effects. Rev Environ Contam Toxicol 110:75-115, 1989.

86. Mettler FA Jr, Voelz GL: Major radiation exposure—what to expect and how to respond. N Engl J Med 346:1554-1561, 2002.

87. Leikin JB, McFee RB, Walter FG, et al: A primer for nuclear terrorism. Dis Mon 49:485-516, 2003.

88. Mettler FA Jr, Kelsey CA: Fundamentals of radiation accidents. *In* Gusev IA, Guskova AK, Mettler FA (eds): Medical Management of Radiation Accidents. Boca Raton, FL, CRC Press, 2001, pp 1-13.

89. Guskova AK: Radiation sickness classification. *In* Gusev IA, Guskova AK, Mettler FA (eds): Medical Management of Radiation Accidents. Boca Raton, FL, CRC Press, 2001, pp 23-31.

90. Glasstone S, Dolan PJ: The Effects of Nuclear Weapons, 3rd ed. Washington, DC, U.S. Department of Defense and U.S. Department of Energy, 1977.

91. Jacocks J: Medical Management of Radiation Casualties: Handbook. Bethesda, MD, Armed Forces Radiobiology Research Institute, 2003.

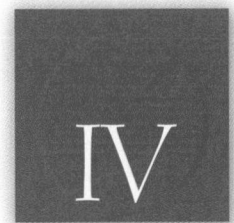

TRANSPLANTATION AND IMMUNOLOGY

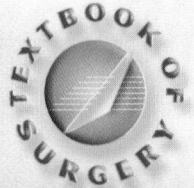

CHAPTER 26

Transplantation Immunology and Immunosuppression

Darla K. Granger, M.D.,   Michele A. Domenick, M.D.,

and   Suzanne T. Ildstad, M.D.

Conceptual Approaches to Immunosuppressive Therapy	Clinical Immunosuppression
The Cells Involved in Alloreactivity	Xenotransplantation
Cell-to-Cell Interactions	Tolerance
Major Histocompatibility Locus: Transplantation Antigens	New Areas of Transplantation
	Conclusion

Transplantation of solid organs has become the treatment of choice for end-stage renal, hepatic, cardiac, and pulmonary disease. The field has progressed rapidly in the past 5 decades, primarily because of the development of safer and more effective immunosuppressive agents. After Carrel described a reliable technique for vascular anastomoses in the early 1900s, the technical problems confronting surgeons seeking to replace diseased kidneys or other solid organs were largely resolved. However, the crucial advance that made clinical organ transplantation feasible between unrelated individuals was the development of immunosuppressive drugs to prevent or control rejection. The combination of azathioprine with corticosteroids, introduced in 1962, was the first effective clinical immunosuppressive regimen. It is still used in many patients today. The introduction of cyclosporine in 1978, a specific and nonmyelotoxic immunosuppressant, changed heart and liver transplantation from research to service procedures and dramatically increased the success rates of renal transplantation. Continued improvements in the control of rejection at both the cellular and molecular levels have been possible, owing to increased understanding of the complexity of the immune system and of the events that constitute the rejection process. Because outcomes may vary with the type of graft and the patient's clinical history, the choice of immunosuppression depends on a complete understanding of the interrelationship between host and graft. In the past decade a diverse armamentarium of immunosuppressive

agents targeting various aspects of the immune system has emerged.

CONCEPTUAL APPROACHES TO IMMUNOSUPPRESSIVE THERAPY

Lymphocytes have an essential, central role in the immune response and mediate its specificity.[1] The rejection reaction begins when T lymphocytes recognize foreign histocompatibility antigens on cells of the transplanted tissue.[2] The foreign antigen is thought to be presented directly to host lymphocytes by antigen-presenting cells (APCs), most notably dendritic cells and macrophages, which phagocytose and then display the processed antigenic epitope on their surface. Whatever the APC, the ability to differentiate *self* from *nonself* resides with the lymphocytes.[1] Early in the development of the body's immune system, groups or clones of lymphocytes are formed that have discrete target specificity. A lymphocyte, therefore, can recognize only one or a few closely related antigens. The range of possible antigen configurations is matched by a panoply of lymphocyte clones arrayed against them. Immune specificity is acquired during early development, and it is postulated that fully competent clones of small resting lymphocytes await immunologic stimulation by foreign tissue antigens (Fig. 26-1). Among the vast variety of antigens that can be recognized are the foreign anti-

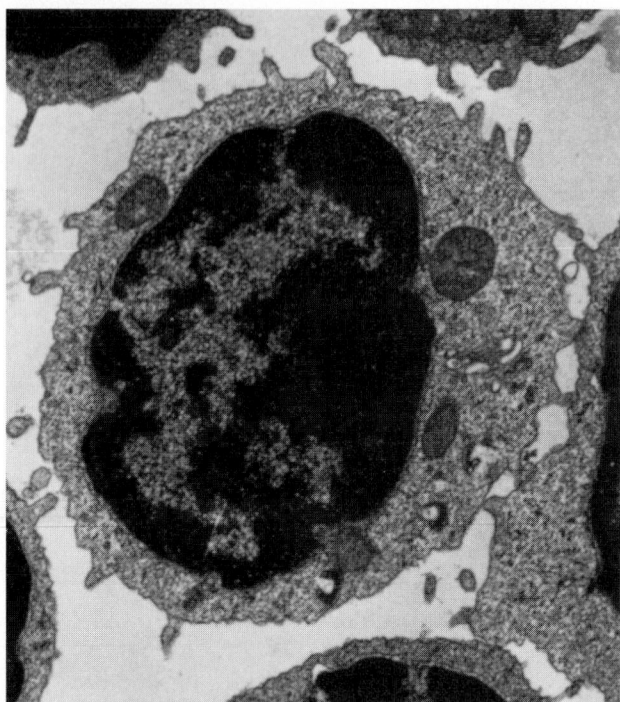

FIGURE 26-1. The morphology of this small lymphocyte is typical of mammalian peripheral small lymphocytes from the blood, thoracic duct, lymph nodes, or spleen. The dense, inactive nucleus occupies much of the intracellular occasional mitochondria. The small lymphocytes are resting cells, awaiting immunologic stimulation that transforms them into large active cells. If resting lymphocytes do not encounter antigen, they probably die within a few days or weeks (×12,000).

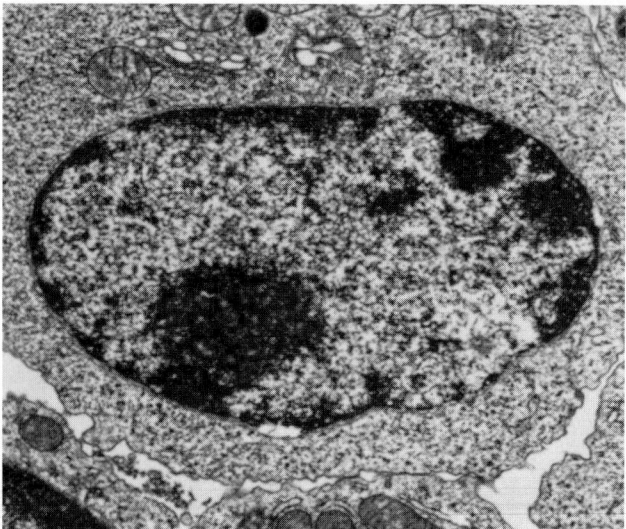

FIGURE 26-2. The transformed lymphocyte, 24 hours after stimulation, is a much larger, more active cell. The open nucleus is the site of increased RNA synthesis, and the enlarged cytoplasm contains abundant polysomes and mitochondria. Many subcellular changes take place in the conversion from resting to active lymphocytes. These biosynthetic events are vulnerable to the antimetabolites used to prevent allograft rejection. In addition, these cells begin to synthesize DNA at this time, increasing their susceptibility to antimetabolites, alkylating agents, and radiation (×12,000).

gens, which are governed by the major histocompatibility complex (MHC).[3]

Stimulation of a resting lymphocyte by the antigen for which it is specific causes it to transform into a large active cell that secretes chemical communicators called *cytokines.* These are soluble proteins or glycoproteins (Table 26-1) that are effective across short distances and that, in turn, amplify the response and activate other cells.[4] Before the antigen is disposed of, however, myriad cellular and subcellular events ensue. Interference with this complex series of events at one or more stages offers many opportunities for therapeutic intervention to suppress the rejection response.[5] For the transplant patient, the encounter of the APC and the T lymphocyte is generally considered to be the first point of possible immunosuppressive attack.

Once the lymphocyte has responded to foreign antigen and become activated (Fig. 26-2), immunosuppressive therapy is less effective. Many cells and molecules are involved. Specific effectors, such as preformed antibodies and activated killer (cytotoxic) lymphocytes as well as nonspecific agents such as platelets, neutrophils, complement, and coagulation factors, are difficult to suppress. The suppression of only one or two effectors is ineffective.[6]

In the early days of organ transplantation, the major problem was suppression of allograft rejection. Even

though this can be achieved, its consequences and potential dangers are apparent. Immunosuppressive agents that are in widespread use today act largely in a broad, *nonspecific manner* to suppress the entire immune response. As a result, there is increased risk of opportunistic infections and malignancy. Effective general immunosuppression can cripple the host response to infections or suppress other proliferating cells (e.g., bone marrow and intestinal mucosal cells). Infections with agents such as cytomegalovirus (CMV) and *Pneumocystis carinii,* which are not life threatening to normal individuals, frequently become lethal to the transplant recipient.

At present, clinical immunosuppression relies on three general approaches. The first is to simply deplete circulating lymphocytes by destroying them. The second is to use an inhibitor of lymphocyte activation (cyclosporine or tacrolimus) to interrupt the early events of antigen-induced T-lymphocyte activation and cytokine production crucial for the subsequent cascade of immunologic events leading to graft rejection. The third is to use various metabolic inhibitors (e.g., azathioprine, mycophenolate mofetil) to interfere with lymphocyte proliferation essential to amplify the response. These agents are biochemically specific but do not distinguish between dividing lymphocytes and other proliferating cells.[7-9]

Future progress in immunosuppressive therapy concerns the successful implementation of an *antigen-specific approach* in which the goal is to induce long-lasting *donor-specific unresponsiveness* (immunologic tolerance) in the host while preserving general immunocompetence.[10] The full promise of transplantation will not be

TABLE 26-1. Summary of Cytokines and Their Associated Functions*

Cytokine		Cell Source	Functions
Interleukin-1	IL-1	Mononuclear phagocytes; T and B cells; NK cells; fibroblasts; neutrophils; smooth muscle cells	Proliferation of T and B cells; fever, inflammation; endothelial cell activation; increases liver protein synthesis. Binds to CD121
Interleukin-2	IL-2	Activated T cells	T-cell growth factor, cytotoxic T-cell generation; B-cell proliferation/differentiation; growth/activation of NK cells. Binds to CD122
Interleukin-4	IL-4	CD4$^+$ T cells; mast cells	B-cell activation/differentiation; T and mast cells growth factor. Binds to CDw124
Interleukin-5	IL-5	T cells	Eosinophil proliferation/activation. Binds to CD125
Interleukin-6	IL-6	Mononuclear phagocytes; T cells; endothelial cells	B-cell proliferation/differentiation; T-cell activation; increases liver acute phase reactants; fever, inflammation. Binds to CD126
Interleukin-7	IL-7	Bone marrow, thymic stromal cells, and spleen cells	Stimulates growth of progenitor B and T cells and mature T cells
Interleukin-8	IL-8	Lymphocytes, monocytes, and multiple other cell types	Stimulates granulocyte activity, chemotactic activity; potent angiogenic factor
Interleukin-9	IL-9	Activated T$_H$2 lymphocytes	Enhances proliferation of T cells, mast cell lines, erythroid precursors, and megakaryoblastic cell lines
Interleukin-10	IL-10	Mononuclear phagocytes; T cells	B-cell activation/differentiation; inhibition; mononuclear phagocyte
Interleukin-11	IL-11	Fibroblasts, bone marrow stromal cell lines	Stimulates growth of hematopoietic multipotential and committed megakaryocytic and macrophage progenitors; stimulates growth of plasmacytomas; inhibits adipogenesis
Interleukin-12	IL-12	Mononuclear phagocytes; dendritic cells	INF-γ synthesis; T-cell cytolytic function; CD4$^+$ T-cell differentiation
Interleukin-13	IL-13	Activated T cells	Inhibits cytokine and nitric oxide production by activated macrophages; induces B-cell proliferation; stimulates IgE and IgG isotype switching
Interleukin-14	IL-14	T cells and some B cell tumors	Enhances proliferation of activated B cells; inhibits immunoglobulin synthesis
Interleukin-15	IL-15	Mononuclear phagocytes; others	NK-cell and T-cell proliferation
Interferon gamma	IFN-γ	NK and T cells	Increased expression of class I and class II MHC; activates macrophages and endothelial cells; augments NK-cell activity; antiviral. Binds to CDw119
Interferon alfa and beta	IFN-α, -β	Mononuclear phagocyte-α; fibroblast-β	Mononuclear phagocyte increases class I MHC expression; antiviral; NK-cell activation. Binds to CD118
Tumor necrosis factor-alpha and beta	TNF-α, -β	NK and T cells; mononuclear phagocytes	B-cell growth/differentiation; enhances T-cell function; macrophage activator; neutrophil activator. Binds to CD120
Transforming growth factor-beta	TGF-β	T cells; mononuclear phagocytes	T-cell inhibition
Lymphotoxin		T cell	Neutrophil activator; endothelial activation

*Cytokines are secreted polypeptides that mediate *autocrine* (act on self) and *paracrine* (nearby) cellular communication but do not bind antigen. They include those compounds previously termed *interleukins* and *lymphokines*.
MHC, major histocompatibility complex; NK, natural killer.
Adapted from Abbas AK, Lichtman AH, Pober JS: Cellular and Molecular Immunology, 4th ed. Philadelphia, WB Saunders, 2000.

fulfilled until graft rejection can be specifically and safely prevented while the integrity of the immune system as a whole is maintained. Such tolerance of the recipient to allografted organs without the requirement for nonspecific immunosuppression is the ultimate goal in clinical transplantation.[10] Approaches to achieve this state are discussed later. Finally, because the number of individuals who can benefit from a transplant far exceed the number of donors available, xenotransplantation is considered by some to hold promise for the future.

TABLE 26-2. Summary of Cell Surface CD Markers

Marker	Main Cellular Expression	Function
T-CELL ASSOCIATED		
CD3	T cells, thymocytes	Cell surface expression and signal transduction with TCR; ε is required for both expression and signal transduction
CD4	Class II restricted T cells, thymocyte subsets, monocytes, and macrophages	Adhesion molecule, binds to class II MHC; signal transduction; thymocyte development; primary receptor for HIV retroviruses
CD5	T cells, B-cell subset	Ligand for CD72
CD8	Class I restricted T cells, thymocyte subsets	Adhesion molecule, binds to class I MHC; signal transduction, thymocyte development
CD28	T cells (most CD4$^+$, some CD8$^+$)	T-cell receptor for co-stimulatory molecules CD80 (B7-1) and CD86 (B7-2)
CD152	Activated T lymphocytes	Inhibitory signaling in T cells, binds CD80 (B7-1) and CD86 (B7-2) on antigen-presenting cells
CD154	Activated CD4$^+$ T cells	Activates B cells, macrophages, and endothelial cells; ligand for CD40
B-CELL ASSOCIATED		
CD10	Immature and some mature B cells, granulocytes	Cell surface metallopeptidase
CD19	Most B cells	B-cell activation, forms co-receptor with CD21 and CD81 to synergize with signals from B-cell antigen receptor complexes
CD20	Most or all B cells	? B cell activation or regulation, calcium ion channel
CD21	Mature B cells, follicular dendritic cells	B-cell activation; receptor for C3d, forms a co-receptor with CD19 and CD81 to deliver activated signals in B cells; EBV receptor
CD40	B cells, macrophages, dendritic cells, endothelial cells, epithelial cells	Role in B-cell activation by T-cell contact; receptor for CD154 (CD40 ligand); macrophage, dendritic cell, and endothelial cell activation
CD80 (B7-1)	Dendritic cells, activated B cells, macrophages	Co-stimulator for T-cell activation; ligand for CD28 and CD152 (CTLA-4)
CD86 (B7-2)	B cells, monocytes	Co-stimulator for T-cell activation; ligand for CD28 and CD152 (CTLA-4)
MYELOID-CELL ASSOCIATED		
CD11a	Leukocytes	Adhesion, binds to CD54 (ICAM-1), CD102 (ICAM-2), CD50 (ICAM-3)
CD11b	Granulocytes, monocytes, NK cells	Adhesion; phagocytosis of iC3b-coated particles
CD11c	Granulocytes, monocytes, NK cells, dendritic cells	Similar to CD11b; major CD11, CD18 integrin on macrophages and dendritic cells
NK-CELL ASSOCIATED		
CD16a	Macrophages, NK cells	Low-affinity Fc receptor; activation of NK cells, ADCC
CD16b	Neutrophils	Immune complex–mediated neutrophil activation
CD57	NK cells, subset of T cells	? Adhesion
PLATELET ASSOCIATED		
CD31	Platelets, monocytes, granulocytes, B cells, endothelial cells, T cells	Adhesion molecule in leukocyte diapedesis
CD41	Platelets, megakaryocytes	Platelet aggregation and activation; binds to fibrinogen
MISCELLANEOUS		
CD25	Activated T cells and B cells	Complexes with IL-2R, high-affinity IL-2 receptor
CD34	Precursors of hematopoietic cells	Ligand for L-selectin; cell-to-cell adhesion
CD55	Broad	Regulation of complement activation; binds C3b, C4b
CD58	Broad	Adhesion; ligand for CD2
CD59	Broad	Inhibits formation of complement MAC
CDw70	Activated T and B cells, macrophages	Binds CD27, co-stimulatory signals
CD95	Multiple cell types	Binds Fas ligand, mediates activation-induced cell death
CD102 (ICAM-2)	Endothelial cells, monocytes, other leukocytes	Ligand for CD11a; CD18 (LFA-1), cell-cell adhesion
CD105	Endothelial cells, activated macrophages	Binds TGF-β, modulates cell response to TGF-β

ADCC, antibody-dependent cellular cytotoxicity; EBV, Epstein-Barr virus; INF, interferon; ICAM, intracellular adhesion molecule; IL, interleukin; LFA, leukocyte function-associated; MAC, membrane attack complex; MHC, major histocompatibility complex; NK, natural killer; TCR, T-cell receptor.
Adapted from Abbas AK, Lichtman AH, Pober JS: Cellular and Molecular Immunology, 4th ed. Philadelphia, WB Saunders, 2000.

THE CELLS INVOLVED IN ALLOREACTIVITY

The key components of the immune system—T cells, B cells, and APCs—are produced by the hematopoietic stem cell. The development of the lymphoid system begins with pluripotential stem cells in the liver and bone marrow of the fetus. As the fetus matures, the bone marrow becomes the primary site for lymphopoiesis. The pre–T cells migrate to the thymus, which becomes the primary lymphoid organ wherein CD3$^+$ T lymphocytes mature and become "educated" to self. The mature T cells are then released to populate the peripheral lymphoid tissues, including lymph nodes, spleen, and gut. It is in the thymus that T cells acquire their cell surface antigen–specific receptors (T-cell receptors [TCRs]) (Table 26-2), which, in turn, confer specificity to the immune system and immune responses.[1] Another lymphocyte subpopulation produced by the hematopoietic stem cell is the B cell. B cells derive their name from the primary lymphoid organ that produces B cells in birds, the bursa of Fabricius. In the human and other mammals, the bone marrow is the primary site of B-cell development.[11]

The T cells, B cells, and APCs have unique roles in orchestrating the immune response. It is a very tightly controlled network, with most communication mediated by cytokines. B cells have the unique capacity to synthesize antibody. A behavioral difference between B and T cells reflects their functional abilities. B cells are specialized to respond to whole antigen and synthesize and secrete antibody that can interact with antigen at distant sites. The T cells that are responsible for cell-mediated immunity are of necessity more peripatetic and must migrate to the periphery to neutralize or eliminate foreign antigens. From the peripheral blood, T cells enter the lymph nodes or spleen through highly specialized regions in the postcapillary venules. After exiting the lymphoid tissue through the efferent lymph, they percolate through the thoracic duct and return to the blood to begin recirculation in quest of antigen. When an organ is transplanted, responsive clones of T cells are activated in the organ itself. In addition, donor dendritic cells leave the graft, home to host lymph nodes, and stimulate both host T cells and B cells therein. Activated T cells leave the lymph nodes and can augment the cellular response in the graft. B cells send out antibody molecules that bind to antigens in the graft within a few days, mediating destructive reactions.[1]

Considerable progress has been made in dissecting the mechanisms of T-cell maturation in the thymus. Precursor T cells migrate to the thymus where they undergo maturational changes. All T cells express on their surface an antigen-specific TCR, which is the site for antigen binding. The majority of T cells are $\alpha\beta$-TCR$^+$. A smaller subpopulation, which primarily resides in the gut, is $\gamma\delta$-TCR$^+$. There are also transmembrane proteins (CD3) with the TCR. Collectively, these complexes compose the TCR complex and provide the signaling molecules needed to respond to foreign antigens.

The thymic stromal cells produce two types of molecules that are important for T-cell maturation. The first type is thymic hormones (e.g., thymopoietin and thymosin) and the cytokine interleukin-7 (IL-7), which regulate the functional differentiation of the peripheral T-cell system. The second type is MHC molecules that are important for selection of the T-cell repertoire. Fundamental properties of a mature T-cell repertoire include (1) restriction to self-MHC and (2) tolerance to self-antigens.[1]

The development of self-tolerance occurs through both central and peripheral mechanisms. Each of these mechanisms is vital for the discrimination of self/nonself. Central tolerance is achieved through clonal deletion occurring in the thymus.[6] The acquisition of the TCR complex takes place through a series of genetically programmed maturational steps. Pre–T cells, not expressing CD4 or CD8 molecules, enter the thymus and proliferate to an intermediate stage of development where they become double positive (CD4$^+$ and CD8$^+$) cells. These cells are educated by self-MHC class I or class II (present on host stromal cells). T cells expressing TCR molecules that interact at an intermediate affinity with self-MHC survive whereas those with too low or too high affinities for MHC do not. This phenomenon is termed *positive selection*. Cells that do not bind to class I or class II undergo programmed cell death or death by neglect. After positive selection occurs, the developing T cells are exposed to self-antigens. If they react too strongly to self-antigen MHC complexes, they are deleted from the immune repertoire, a phenomenon termed *negative selection* (Fig. 26-3).[6]

Programmed Cell Death

Not all progeny of stimulated T cells proliferate but instead die by a process called *apoptosis.* Apoptosis is a form of regulated cell death. In apoptosis, the nucleus of the cell condenses and becomes fragmented, the plasma membrane becomes vesiculated, and the dead cell is rapidly phagocytosed. There is subsequently no release of the cellular contents, and an inflammatory response does not occur. This programmed cell death is an important homeostatic mechanism that limits the lymphoid pool, allowing it to remain relatively constant throughout a lifetime.

Activation-induced cell death (AICD) is an apoptotic pathway that is important in the maintenance of self-tolerance in the periphery. The hallmark of this system is Fas(CD95)/FasL(CD95 ligand) interactions. The physiologic importance of this system is to prevent uncontrolled T-cell activation and resulting autoimmune disease. The importance of Fas/FasL to peripheral tolerance was first discovered in two mouse strains: *lpr* and *gld.* The *lpr* mutation occurs in the gene that encodes Fas and results in a lack of Fas expression. The *gld* mutation results in a defective FasL protein that lacks the ability to bind to the Fas receptor. Either of these mutations results in severe, accelerated autoimmune diseases.[12]

Fas is a surface receptor expressed on activated T cells. The expression of FasL occurs in response to increased levels of IL-2 secreted by activated T cells. This expression of Fas and FasL leads to cell death through apoptosis.[12] The Fas/FasL system is believed to be one mechanism to control immune responses from being too robust. Binding of FasL to Fas results in the activation of intracellular cysteine proteases, which ultimately results in the fragmentation of nucleoproteins and apoptotic cell death. CD4$^+$ T cells appear to be more sensitive to the Fas/FasL interaction than CD8$^+$ T cells. Not all apoptosis is the direct result of activation; some forms occur when activated cells are exposed to an environment without needed growth factors or cytokines necessary for T-cell function; this is termed *growth factor withdrawal.*[1]

CELL-TO-CELL INTERACTIONS

Once confronted with an antigen, the response of the lymphocytes is complex. Multiple cell-to-cell interactions are required to produce the immune response. T cells, B cells,

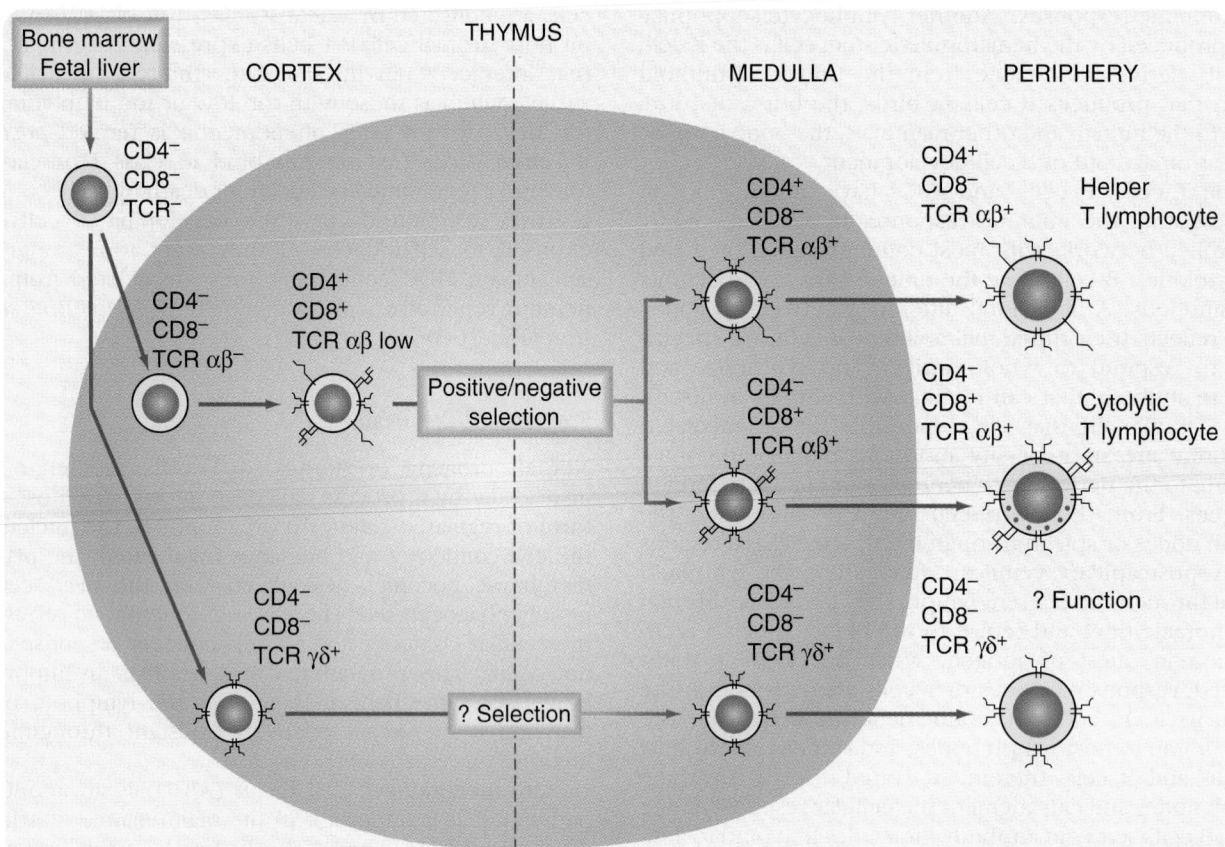

FIGURE 26-3. Lineage relationships of maturing T cells. γδ-T-cell receptor (TCR) and αβ-TCR–expressing cells are separate lineages that develop from a common precursor. In the αβ lineage, the majority of thymocytes express both CD4 and CD8. TCR expression commences in this double-positive stage, beginning with low numbers of receptors on each cell and increasing as maturation proceeds. Single-positive (i.e., CD4 or CD8 αβ-TCR–expressing mature cells) are selected from this population. Some αβ cells express CD4 or CD8. (From Abbas AK, Lichtman AH, Pober JS: T cell maturation in the thymus. *In* Cellular and Molecular Immunology, 3rd ed. Philadelphia, WB Saunders, 1997.)

APCs, and cytokines all play a role. Critical to this response are the professional APCs—dendritic cells and macrophages—that bind antigen and present it to T and B cells. Protein antigens need to be digested by phagocytic cells before the antigenic information can be presented to the lymphocyte for self and nonself recognition by MHC. In addition, activated macrophages produce and secrete IL-1, a cytokine that further amplifies the response and stimulates T- and B-cell activation.[1] For a productive immune response to be generated, the TCR complex must bind to the MHC on the APC, be stabilized by costimulatory molecules, and cause intracellular signaling, resulting in activation of the lymphocyte and production of cytokines.

T-Lymphocyte Activation

T-cell activation is an elegant series of events that are still in the process of full delineation (Fig. 26-4). Antigen recognition by T cells is the initiating stimulus for their activation, proliferation, cytokine production, and performance of regulatory or cytolytic effector functions. The TCR is composed of membrane proteins expressed only on T lymphocytes. The TCR does not recognize soluble antigens; rather, it must recognize antigen in the context of peptide (6-13 amino acids in length)/MHC complexes on the surface of APCs. Associated with the TCR is the CD3 molecule. Together they constitute the *TCR complex.*[1]

Most TCRs are heterodimers, consisting of two transmembrane polypeptide chains designated α and β, which are bonded covalently. All TCRs have a variable region that confers antigen specificity. The αβ-TCR is noncovalently associated with CD3. This highly conserved complex of proteins is responsible for providing the signaling components to the antigen-binding TCR heterodimer, which binds the antigen. Binding of a foreign antigen results in the conformational change in the complex. The associated CD3 molecules transduce the intracellular signals after antigen binding occurs. The development of monoclonal antibodies directed against CD3, such as OKT3, which interfere with T-cell function by altering or inhibiting the intracellular signaling, have played a significant clinical role in organ transplantation.[1,13]

Both MHC molecules and αβ-TCR are expressed on resting T cells; however, the IL-2 receptor (IL-2R) is expressed at only very low levels. When T-cell activation

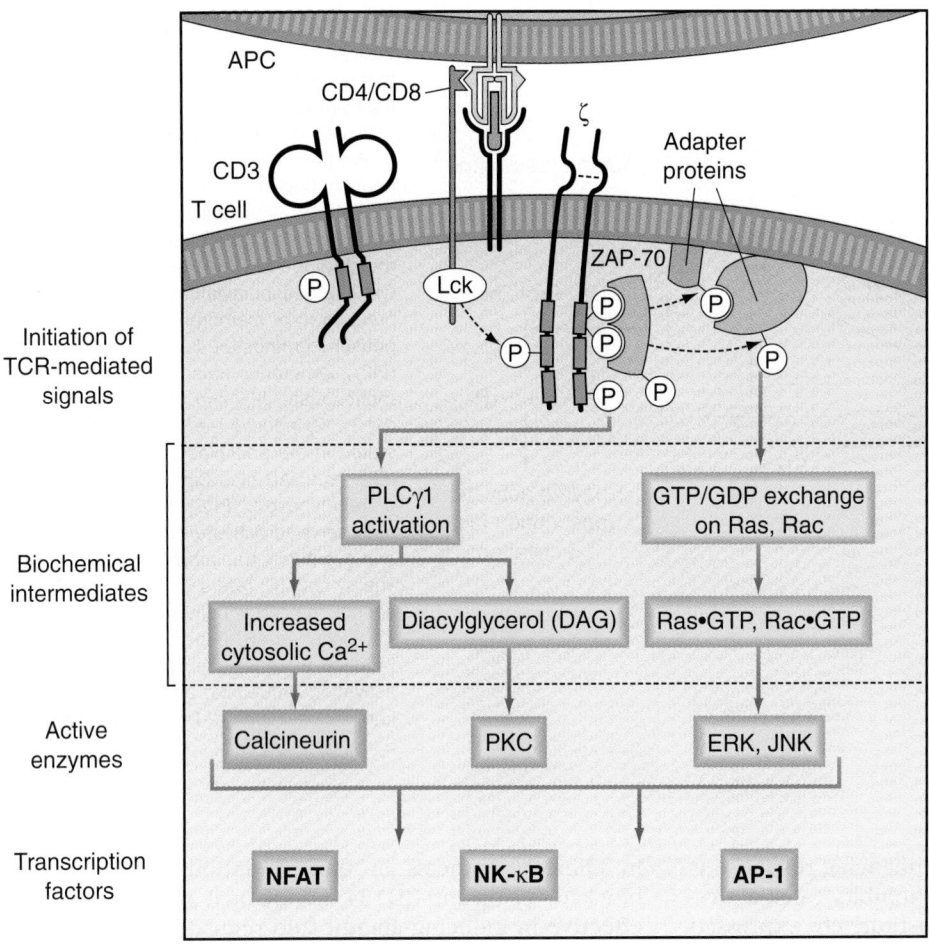

FIGURE 26-4. Overview of intracellular signaling events during T-cell activation. Immediately after the T-cell receptor (TCR) binds antigen on an antigen-presenting cell (APC), several protein tyrosine kinases are activated, and these enzymes phosphorylate substrates, which leads to activation of guanosine triphosphate (GTP)–binding proteins such as Ras and activation of enzymes that break down membrane phospholipids. (From Abbas AK, Lichtman AH, Pober JS: Intracellular signaling events during T cell activation. *In* Cellular and Molecular Immunology, 4th ed. Philadelphia, WB Saunders, 2000.)

occurs, there is a decrease in the number of TCRs expressed on the T cell, accompanied by an increase in IL-2R expression. Activated T cells produce and secrete IL-2, exerting an autocrine and paracrine response. Only those T cells that have been activated by their specific antigen and express the high-affinity IL-2R can respond to IL-2. After IL-2R bind IL-2, T-cell proliferation begins. After the antigenic stimulus is removed, the number of surface IL-2R starts to decrease, and the TCR complex is re-expressed on the cell surface. This inverse relationship between the TCR and IL-2R suggests a negative feedback mechanism. This is an elegant system, which is reactive only in the presence of an antigen and ceases to function as the antigen is removed.

Molecular signaling via the TCR/CD3 complex and its relationship with IL-2 production and IL-2R expression have been characterized. Antigen binding initiates the activation of two signal-transduction pathways through a conformational change in the TCR complex. The beta chain of the complex is phosphorylated by means of a CD4- or CD8-associated tyrosine-kinase–dependent pathway. The activated TCR complex is coupled via a G-binding protein to phospholipase C. The activation of phospholipase C results in the hydrolysis of phosphatidylinositol 4,5 biphosphate (PIP_2) to produce diacylglycerol (DAG) and inositol 1,4,5-triphosphate (IP_3). These are the second messengers that are responsible for the mobilization of intracellular and extracellular Ca^{2+} that activate protein kinase C. The result of these changes is the transcription of early-activation genes (*NFAT* and c-*fos*) and the production of messenger RNA (mRNA) for IL-2 and its receptor (Fig. 26-5).[1]

Co-stimulatory Pathways

Two signals are required for T-cell activation: an antigen-specific signal and a co-stimulatory signal. The TCR/CD3 interaction (signal 1) required for cell activation has been well defined. The co-stimulatory pathways present on APC surface molecules provide the second signal for T-cell activation (signal 2). If these co-stimulatory pathways are interrupted or blocked, such as with monoclonal antibodies directed at the receptors, the result of signal 1 alone is clonal anergy. In the presence of TCR/CD3 complex providing the primary signal, without the secondary signal, the T cell is rendered anergic or functionally inactive. Co-stimulatory molecules on the T-cell surface specifically interact with molecules on the APC surface. The most well characterized co-stimulatory important pathway involves the T-cell surface molecule CD28. This molecule binds to both CD80 (B7-1) and CD86 (B7-2) found on APCs (dendritic cells, monocytes, B cells), and signaling through CD28 enhances the T-cell response

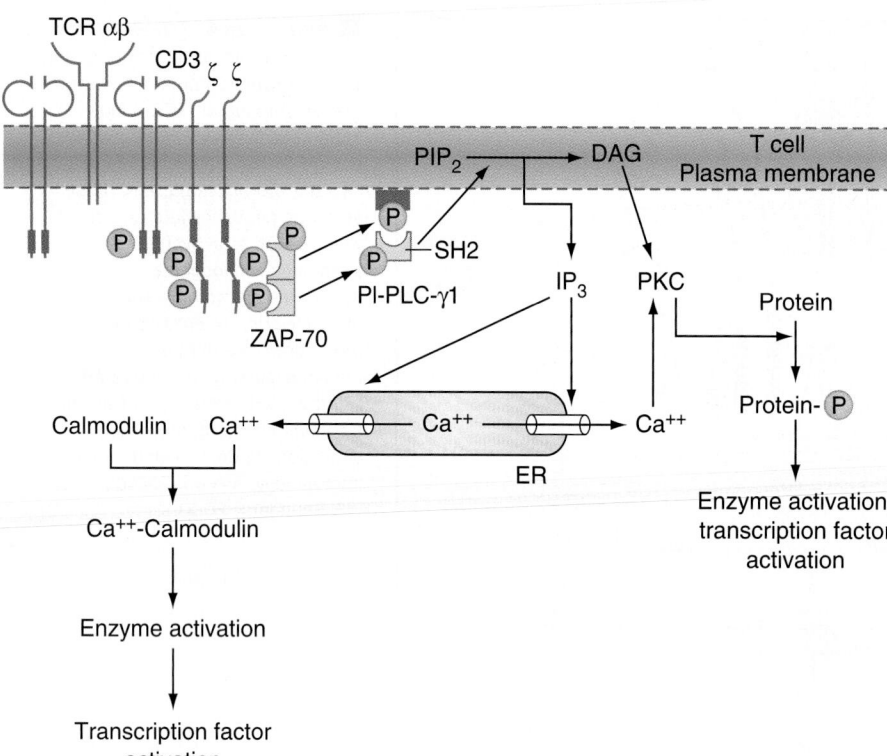

FIGURE 26-5. T-cell signaling through membrane inositol lipid metabolism. T-cell receptor (TCR)–associated protein tyrosine kinases activated by antigen presentation lead to the phosphorylation of phosphatidylinositol phospholipase C-γ1 (PI-PLC-γ1) as well as docking sites for PI-PLC-γ1 on the plasma membrane. PI-PLC-γ1, activated tyrosine phosphorylation, catalyzes the breakdown of membrane phosphatidylinositol 4, 5-bisphosphate (PIP$_2$), generating inositol 1,4,5-triphosphate (IP$_3$) and diacylglycerol (DAG). IP$_3$ induces the release of Ca^{2+} stored in the endoplasmic reticulum (ER), and DAG plus Ca^{2+} activate protein kinase C (PKC). Ca^{2+} and PKC both serve to activate other enzymes and eventually transcription factors. The symbol (P) refers to phosphorylated tyrosine. (From Abbas AK, Lichtman AH, Pober JS: T lymphocyte antigen recognition and activation. *In* Cellular and Molecular Immunology, 3rd ed. Philadelphia, WB Saunders, 1997.)

to antigens (Fig. 26-6). To balance enhancing response is another T-cell surface molecule that inhibits T-cell activation, CD152 (CTLA-4). CD28 is constitutively expressed on all CD4$^+$ T cells and on about 50% of CD8$^+$ T cells. CD28 is upregulated after the T cell receives signal 1. In contrast, CD152 is not expressed on any resting T cells but is induced after T-cell activation, reaching highest concentrations 48 hours after stimulation. The postulated mechanism for this inhibitory function is through abrogation of the tyrosine kinase activity required for TCR signaling.[1,14]

The exact mechanism by which CD28 promotes T-cell activation has not been fully defined. Proposed mechanisms include CD28-mediated expression of T-cell IL-2. This expression is enhanced at the level of mRNA production, resulting in increased production. Another mechanism involving CD28 is the protection of T cells from programmed cell death, or apoptosis. CD28 is associated with an increased expression of Bcl-x$_L$, a survival protein. The expression of this gene results in the resistance to T-cell death by apoptosis.[1]

Closely related to this CD28/CD152/CD80/CD86 pathway is the CD40/CD154 (also known as CD40 ligand) pathway. CD40 is a surface molecule constitutively expressed on B cells. After antigen recognition by the B cells, there is upregulation of CD80 (B7-1) and CD86 (B7-2), which interacts with the T-cell CD28, causing an increased expression of CD154 by the activated T cell, which binds to CD40 receptor on the B cells. This interaction of CD40/CD154 provides the stimulus for B cells to continue activation and proliferation.[15] Manipulation of both of these important pathways is under investigation

in clinical protocols in transplantation. Co-stimulatory blockade using anti-CD154 monoclonal antibodies is very effective in inducing anergic and regulatory T cells. This further emphasizes the importance of the CD40/CD154 pathway in providing co-stimulation and upregulates the effects of CD28/B7 pathway.

T-Cell Effector Functions

In addition to acquiring the TCR complex during thymic maturation, T cells also acquire differentiation receptors called *cluster of differentiation (CD) antigens.* CD4 and CD8 are the best-known CD markers. Other frequently occurring CD markers can be found in Table 26-2. The subpopulations of T cells have several different functional activities. T cells bearing the CD8$^+$ molecule interact with MHC class I/peptide complexes and can directly lyse a foreign or tumor cell on activation. These activated CD8$^+$ T cells are the cytotoxic T lymphocytes (CTLs). In contrast, CD4$^+$ T cells recognize antigen in the context of MHC class II molecules. CD4$^+$ T cells become T helper (T$_H$) cells after activation and primarily function through the secretion of distinct cytokines to induce either a cell-mediated response (T$_H$1) or a humoral response (T$_H$2).[1]

Even the recognition of foreign cells is a complex process. The initial responding and proliferating cells do not destroy foreign grafts; rather, they activate another group of T cells (cytotoxic), which in turn damage the graft. The first group of T cells are CD4$^+$ T$_H$ cells. T$_H$-cell proliferation is an important step in the amplification of the immune response, and these actively dividing cells are particularly vulnerable

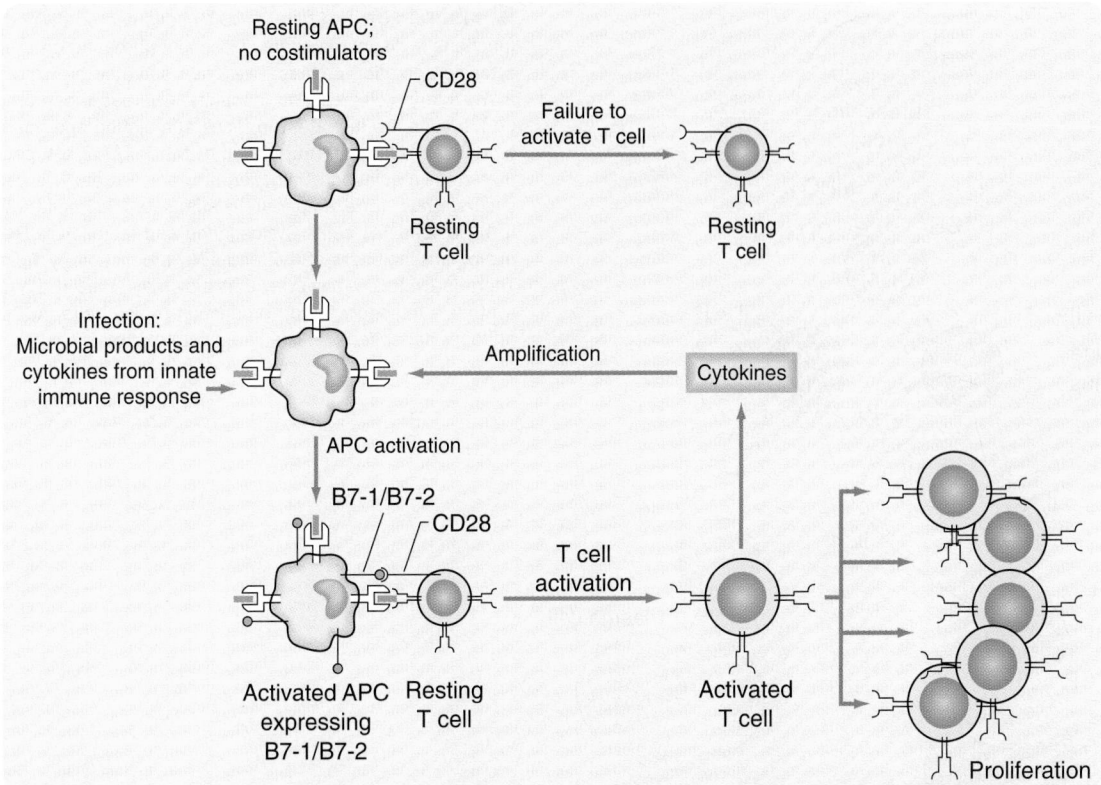

FIGURE 26-6. Co-stimulators on antigen-presenting cells (APCs) are required for effective T-cell activation. Resting macrophage APCs do not express co-stimulatory molecules such as B7-1 (CD80) or B7-2 (CD86), and they fail to activate T cells during antigen presentation. In the setting of an infection, microbial products such as endotoxin or cytokines elaborated by innate immune responses can upregulate B7-1 (CD80) and B7-2 (CD86) expression on the macrophage. Antigen presentation by the activated macrophage will then lead to T-cell activation characterized by cytokine production and proliferation. Cytokines secreted by the activated T cell, such as interferon-γ, can induce co-stimulator expression on other macrophages, enabling them to serve as effective APCs and thereby amplifying the immune response. (From Abbas AK, Lichtman AH, Pober JS: T lymphocyte antigen recognition and activation. *In* Cellular and Molecular Immunology, 3rd ed. Philadelphia, WB Saunders, 1997.)

to antimetabolites. The activities of the $CD4^+$ T_H cells are thus one of the major targets of clinical immunosuppression using drugs or monoclonal antibodies.[5]

T_H cells have a central role in response to alloantigen. Once antigen has been processed and presented in the context of cell surface MHC class II molecules on an APC, the T_H cell proliferates. The two distinct T_H populations have been characterized (T_H1 and T_H2 subsets) based on their pattern of cytokine synthesis (Fig. 26-7).[16] In T_H1 responses, the main cytokines are IL-2 and interferon-gamma (IFN-γ). IL-2 is produced by activated T cells and is a potent T-cell growth factor. IL-2 enhances B-cell and natural killer (NK)-cell differentiation. IFN-γ activates macrophages and is involved in B-cell isotype switching. These responses are important for cell-mediated immunity. T_H1 response is balanced by the T_H2 response. The T_H2 response results in the production of IL-4, IL-5, and IL-10. IL-4 is the T_H2-polarizing cytokine and is required for the production of immunoglobulin E. In addition, IL-4 is an essential growth factor for T cells, and it stimulates the expression of MHC class II and adhesion molecules. An important feature of these $CD4^+$ T_H cells is the ability of one subset to regulate the activities of the other. Thus,

IFN-γ directly inhibits the proliferation of T_H2 cells, whereas IL-10 (and IL-4) inhibits cytokine production by T_H1 cells. This cross-regulation occurs at the level of the effector cells triggered by these subsets. Thus, IFN-γ inhibits IL-4–induced B-cell activation, whereas IL-4 suppresses IL-2–induced T- and B-cell proliferation. The current theory postulates that differentiation of naive $CD4^+$ T cells, down either pathway, is directly related to the neighboring cells and the cytokines that these neighboring cells produce.[16]

Regulatory T cells (T_{reg}) have received a great deal of recent attention and may hold significant promise for strategies to achieve antigen-specific tolerance in the clinic. T_{reg} are defined by their function: to suppress alloreactivity in vitro (a state reversed by exogenous IL-2) and downregulate the proliferation of other T-cell populations via IL-10.[17] Initially, they are cell (antigen) contact dependent but on maturation become contact independent to amplify the response. The most important subset of T_{reg} is $CD4^+/CD25^+$.[18] In animal models T_{reg} have been shown to play a role in the maintenance of tolerance and prevention of graft-versus-host disease (GVHD) after marrow transplantation.[19,20]

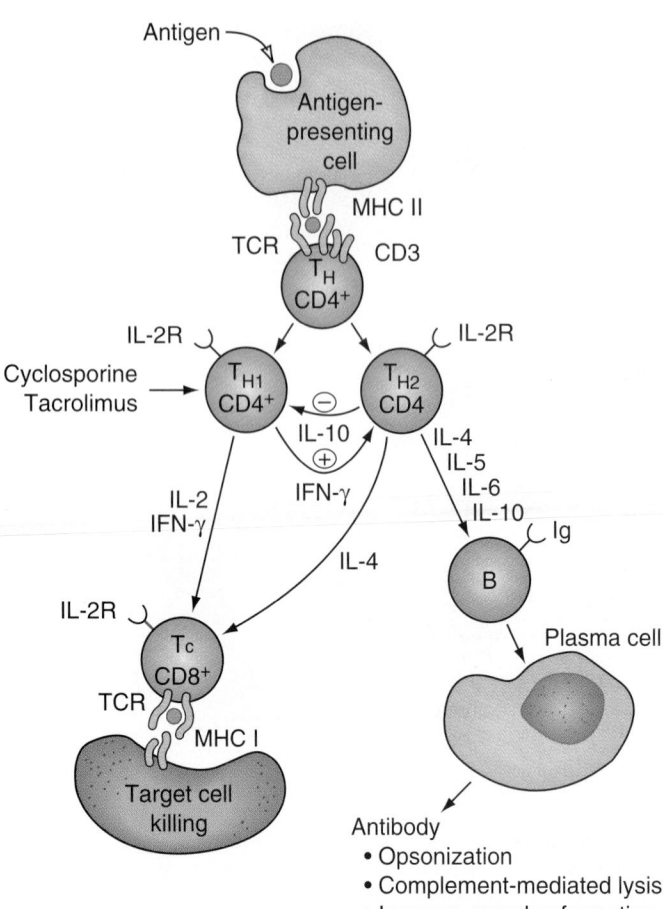

FIGURE 26-7.   T-helper (CD4⁺) cells can be divided into functionally distinct subsets (T$_H$1 and T$_H$2) based on their cytokine secretion profiles. Cytokines secreted by T$_H$1 cells play a key role in cell-mediated immunity, whereas those produced by T$_H$2 cells are important in B-cell stimulation and antibody production. An important feature of the T$_H$1/T$_H$2 cell paradigm is that cross-regulation of function between T$_H$1 and T$_H$2 cells occurs. Thus, for example, IFN-γ stimulates T$_H$2 cells whereas IL-10 inhibits T$_H$1 cells. Cyclosporine and tacrolimus (FK-506) are potent inhibitors of IL-2 and IFN-γ production by T$_H$1 cells. There is evidence, however, that they may spare IL-10 (cytokine synthesis inhibitory factor) production by T$_H$2 cells. ADCC, antibody-dependent cell-mediated cytotoxicity.

B Lymphocytes

Similar to all other cells in the immune system, B cells are derived from the pluripotent bone marrow stem cell. IL-7, produced by bone marrow stromal cells, is a growth factor for pre–B cells, whereas IL-4, IL-5, and IL-6 are cytokines that stimulate the maturation and proliferation of mature primed B cells.[1] B cells are responsible for the humoral or antibody-mediated immune response against foreign antigen. B cells express immunoglobulin antibody on their cell surface. These membrane-bound immunoglobulins are the B-cell antigen receptors and allow for specific antigen recognition. Only one antigen-specific antibody is produced from each mature B cell. Each antibody is composed of two heavy chains and two light chains. Both heavy and light chains have a constant region (Fc), as well as a variable, antigen-binding region. The antibody-binding site is composed of both the heavy- and light-chain–variable regions.[11] There are two antigen-binding sites per antibody molecule.

In the human there are nine different immunoglobulin subclasses: IgM, IgD, IgG₁, IgG₂, IgG₃, IgG₄, IgA₁, IgA₂, and IgE. Resting naive B cells express IgD and IgM on their cell surface. On antigen stimulation and T-cell cytokine, B cells undergo isotype switching. Distinct immune effector functions are assigned to each isotype. IgM and IgG anti-bodies provide a pivotal role in the endogenous or intravascular immune response. The first isotype produced in response to a foreign antigen is IgM, which is very efficient at binding complement to facilitate phagocytosis or cell lyses. B cells undergo isotype switching with the maturation of the immune response against a specific antigen. This results in a decrease in IgM titers with a concomitant rise in IgG titers (Fig. 26-8).[1,11] A primed B cell may undergo further mutations within the variable regions that lead to increased affinity of antibody; this is termed *somatic hypermutation.*

Monocytes

Mononuclear phagocytes, which also have an integral role in the immune response, are derived from bone marrow. This cell type initially emerges as a monocyte while in peripheral blood. On settling in tissues, the mononuclear phagocytes are called *macrophages* or *histocytes.* The main function of monocytes and macrophages is phagocytosis. After phagocytosis, they process antigen, present the antigen to lymphocytes, and produce various cytokines (see Table 26-2) that regulate the immune response.[21]

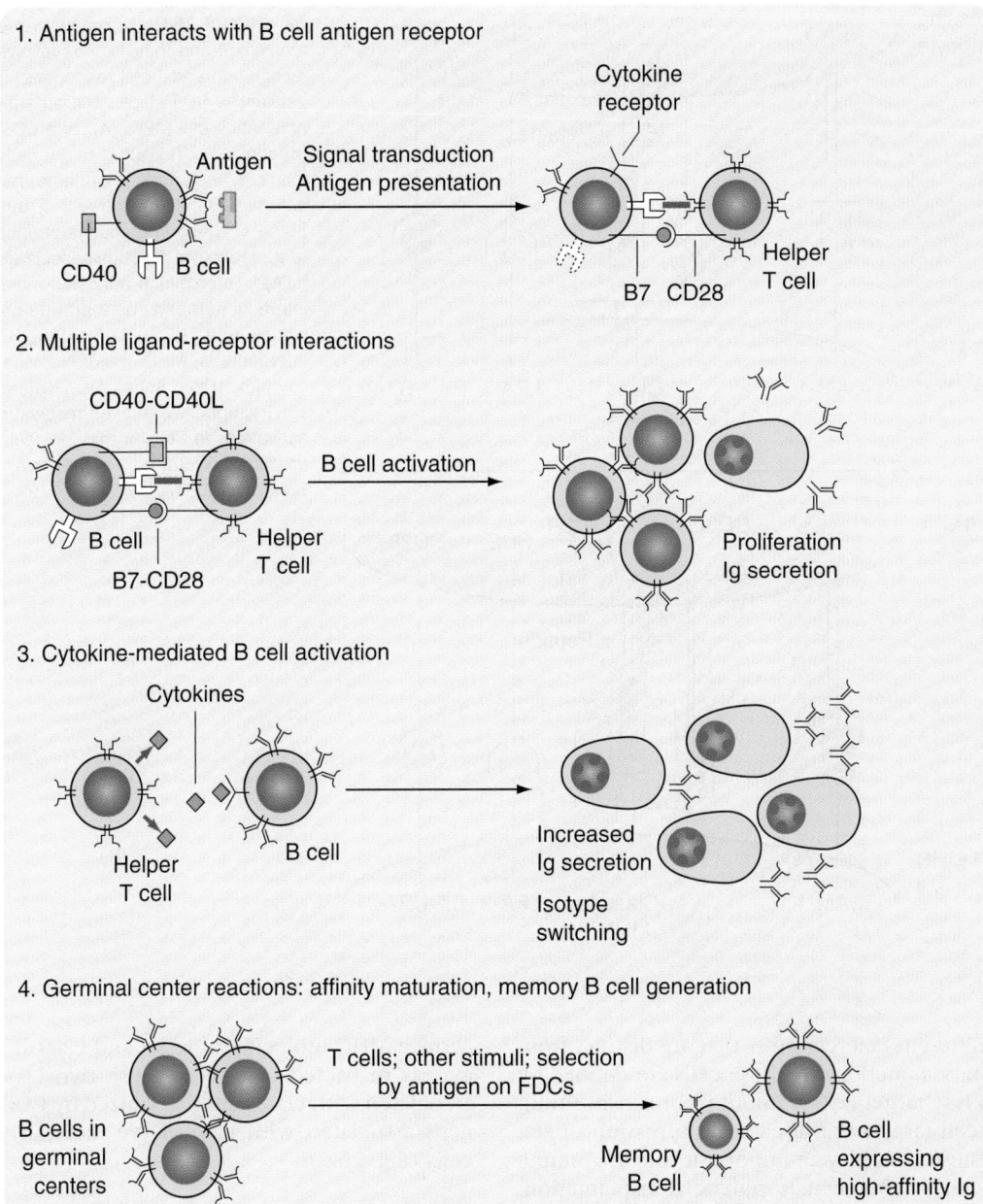

1. Antigen interacts with B cell antigen receptor

Cytokine receptor

Antigen   Signal transduction
Antigen presentation

CD40   B cell

B7 CD28   Helper T cell

2. Multiple ligand-receptor interactions

CD40-CD40L

B cell   Helper T cell

B7-CD28

B cell activation

Proliferation
Ig secretion

3. Cytokine-mediated B cell activation

Cytokines

Helper T cell   B cell

Increased Ig secretion

Isotype switching

4. Germinal center reactions: affinity maturation, memory B cell generation

B cells in germinal centers

T cells; other stimuli; selection by antigen on FDCs

Memory B cell

B cell expressing high-affinity Ig

FIGURE 26-8. Phases of helper T-cell–dependent antibody responses. Ig, immunoglobulin; FDCs, follicular dendritic cells. (From Abbas AK, Lichtman AH, Pober JS: T lymphocyte antigen recognition and activation. *In* Cellular and Molecular Immunology, 3rd ed. Philadelphia, WB Saunders, 1997.)

Dendritic Cells

The most potent APCs are CD11c+ bone marrow–derived dendritic cells, which are distributed ubiquitously throughout the lymphoid and nonlymphoid tissues of the body. Immature dendritic cells are located along the gut mucosa and other sites of antigen entry. Antigen presentation by immature dendritic cells leads to TCR signaling without co-stimulation and induces T-cell anergy. On contact with antigen, dendritic cells are activated to mature, increasing expression of both MHC and co-stimulatory molecules. As dendritic cells mature, they migrate to peripheral lymphoid tissue, where they can activate T cells. Dendritic cells provide signals that initiate clonal expansion of T cells as well as provide signals to promote naive T cells to either T_H1 or T_H2 response.[22] Two lineages of dendritic cells have been described, the myeloid and lymphoid. It is speculated that myeloid dendritic cells (DC1) are more immunogenic whereas lymphoid dendritic cells (DC2) are more tolerogenic. Recent data in animals suggest that DC2, under specific conditions, can be potently tolerogenic in vivo and may therefore present the future for cell-based therapies.

Natural Killer Cells

Natural killer cells are bone marrow–derived cells capable of killing specific tumor cells and virally infected cells. NK

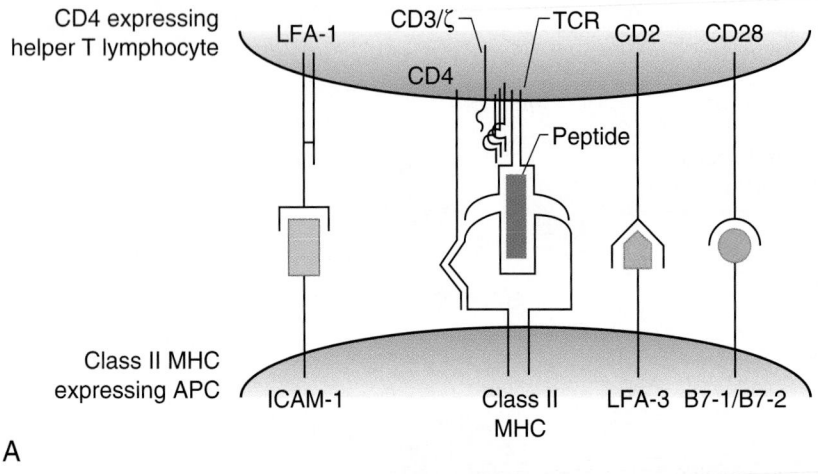

CD4 expressing
helper T lymphocyte

LFA-1   CD3/ζ   TCR   CD2   CD28
           CD4
                          Peptide

Class II MHC
expressing APC   ICAM-1   Class II   LFA-3   B7-1/B7-2
                                   MHC

A

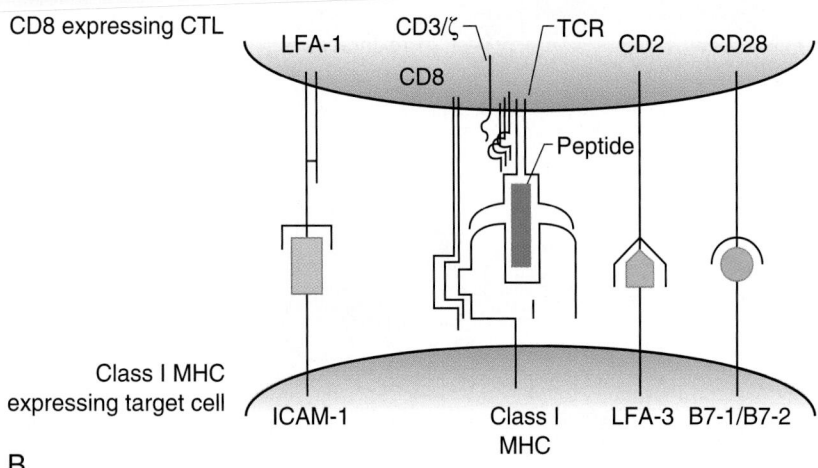

CD8 expressing CTL

LFA-1   CD3/ζ   TCR   CD2   CD28
           CD8
                          Peptide

Class I MHC
expressing target cell   ICAM-1   Class I   LFA-3   B7-1/B7-2
                                           MHC

B

FIGURE 26-9. T-lymphocyte surface molecules and their ligands involved in antigen recognition and T-cell responses. Interactions between a CD4+ T cell and an antigen-presenting cell (APC) (**A**), or a CD8+ cytolytic T lymphocyte (CTL) and a target cell (**B**), involve multiple T-cell surface proteins that recognize different ligands on the APC or target cell. Some of these interactions promote adhesion (e.g., leukocyte function-associated antigen [LFA]-1–intercellular adhesion molecule [ICAM]-1 interactions), and some provide co-stimulatory signals (e.g., CD28-B7-1[CD80]/B7-2[CD86] interactions). MHC, major histocompatibility complex. (From Abbas AK, Lichtman AH, Pober JS: T lymphocyte antigen recognition and activation. *In* Cellular and Molecular Immunology, 3rd ed. Philadelphia, WB Saunders, 1997.)

cells express different cell receptors that are distinct from the TCR complex. Functionally, these cells are defined by their ability to lyse target cells without prior sensitization. NK cells lyse cell targets that lock the expression of self MHC class I. These cells play an important role in immune defenses, especially after hematopoietic transplantation. They also contribute to the defenses against virus-infected cells, graft rejection, and neoplasia, and they participate in the regulation of hematopoiesis through cytokine production and cell-to-cell interaction. NK cells also mediate rejection in xenotransplantation.[23]

MAJOR HISTOCOMPATIBILITY LOCUS: TRANSPLANTATION ANTIGENS

The MHC is a region of highly conserved polymorphic genes. The products of these genes are expressed on the cell surface of a wide array of cell types. MHC genes play a pivotal role in immune response. MHC is so important because antigen-specific T lymphocytes do not recognize antigens in the free form or in soluble form but only as small peptides, products of protein digestion, that are bound to MHC molecules. There are two types of cell

surface MHC molecules: class I and class II. Any lymphocyte is restricted to one of these two classes. Antigens associated with class I are recognized by CD8+ T cells; antigens associated with class II are recognized by CD4+ T cells (Fig. 26-9).[1]

Human Histocompatibility Complex

The strongest antigens present in transplantation are the MHC molecules and the peptides they hold. The MHC in humans is located on chromosome 6. The gene products of the MHC molecules in humans are called human leukocyte antigens (HLA). Class I molecules important to transplantation in humans are expressions of HLA-A, HLA-B, and HLA-C genes. HLA-E, HLA-F, and HLA-G are more conserved but may later demonstrate importance in transplantation. The class II molecules are expressions of HLA-DR, HLA-DQ, HLA-DP, and HLA-DM genes.[1] There are class III molecules, but they are not cell surface proteins involved in antigen recognition. Instead, class III molecules contain mainly soluble mediators of immune function and include tumor necrosis factor (TNF)-α and -β, complement components, heat shock protein, and nuclear transcription factor β.

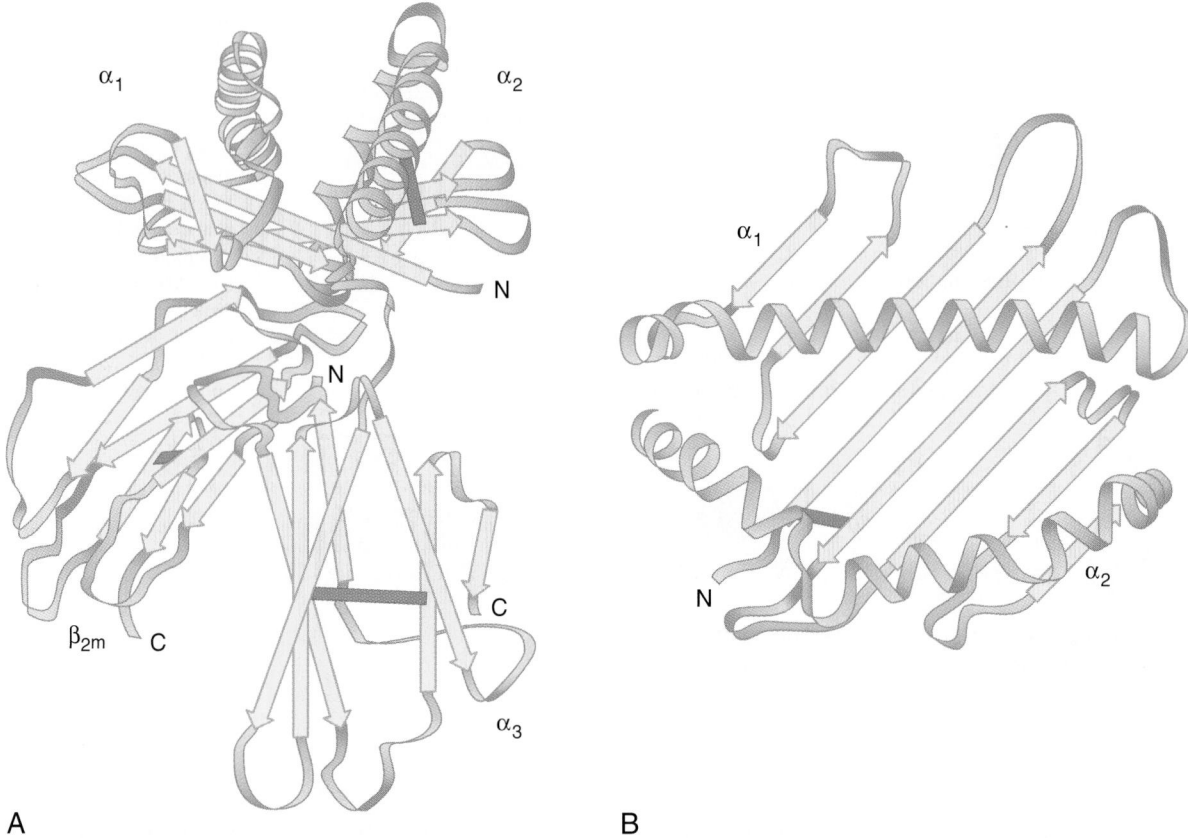

■ **FIGURE 26-10.** Polypeptide folding pattern of a human class I major histocompatibility complex molecule. A side view (**A**) and a top view (**B**) reveal the peptide-binding cleft. The *yellow arrows* represent polypeptide folded as β-pleated sheet, the *green coils* represent polypeptide folded as a-helix, and the *bars* represent disulfide bonds. N and C refer to the amino and carboxyl termini of the polypeptide chains, respectively. (**A** and **B,** Adapted with permission from Bjorkman PJ, Saper MA, Samraoul B, et al: Structure of the human class I histocompatibility antigen HLA-A2. Nature 329:506-512, 1987. Copyright 1987, Macmillan Magazines Ltd.)

Class I and class II molecules were previously considered antigens. They are, however, vital to T-cell and B-cell interactions. HLA class I molecules are present on all nucleated cells. In contrast, class II molecules are found almost exclusively on cells associated with the immune system (macrophages, dendritic cells, B cells, and activated T cells). Resting T cells do not express class II molecules. Both class I and II MHC molecules are similar in their structures. The structures have been elucidated using x-ray crystallography. This important advance added much to the understanding of antigen recognition (Fig. 26-10). MHC molecules are composed of four domains: a peptide-binding domain, immunoglobulin-like domain, transmembrane domain, and cytoplasmic domain. The immunoglobulin-like domain has limited polymorphism and contains the interaction region for CD8/class I and CD4/class II molecules. There is considerable homology between class I and class II molecules, suggesting a common evolutionary origin.[1]

Class I MHC

Class I molecules in humans are expressions of HLA-A, HLA-B, and HLA-C genes, which are recognized by cyto-

toxic CD8+ T cells. The class I molecules are composed of a 44-kD transmembrane glycoprotein in a noncovalent complex with a nonpolymorphic 12-kD polypeptide called β2-microglobulin. The peptide-binding region of class I, composed of the first and second domains of a protein, forms a binding cleft. The α3 immunoglobulin-like domain, which is the domain closest to the membrane and interacts with CD8, demonstrates limited polymorphism and contains conserved interactions limited to CD8+ T cells. The expression of class I molecules occurs on nearly all cells of the adult; however, this expression can be increased by cytokines. This is important as an amplification mechanism. Interferons (INF-α, INF-β, INF-γ) induce an increase in the expression of class I molecules by increasing levels of gene transcription.[1] Interestingly, the areas specific for antigen binding are not conserved, whereas the non–antigen-binding regions are conserved.

Class II MHC

The class II molecules are expressions of HLA-DR, HLA-DQ, HLA-DP, and HLA-DM genes. The class II molecules contain two MHC-encoded polymorphic chains, one

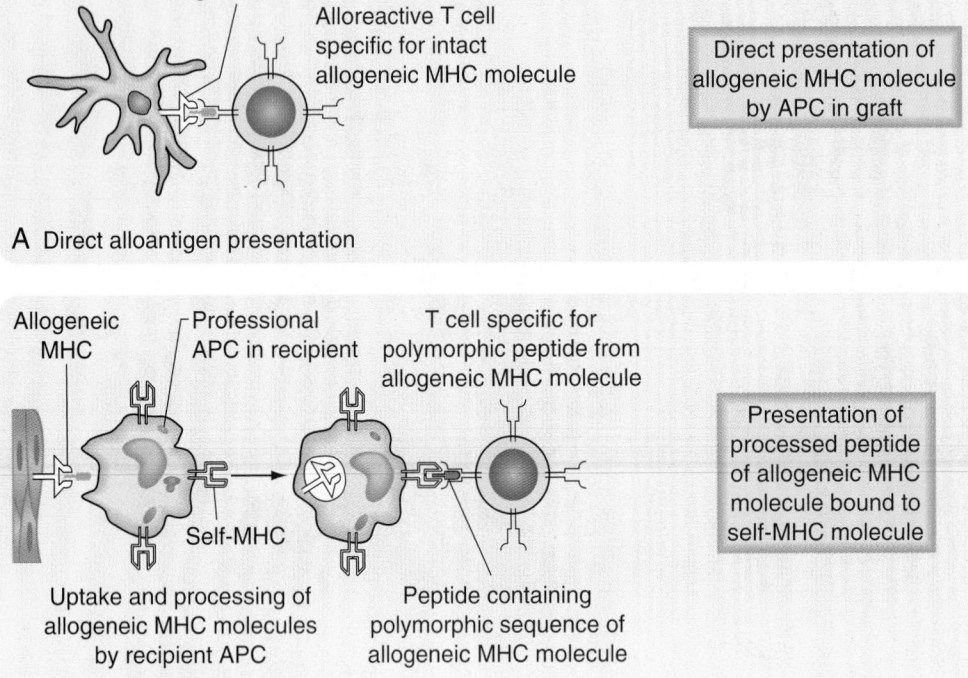

A Direct alloantigen presentation

B Indirect alloantigen presentation

FIGURE 26-11. *Direct recognition* occurs when alloantigen is presented by donor antigen-presenting cells (APCs). *Indirect recognition* occurs when alloantigen is processed by recipient APCs. MHC, major histocompatibility complex. (Adapted from Abbas AK, Lichtman AH, Pober JS: Direct and indirect alloantigen presentation. *In* Cellular and Molecular Immunology, 4th ed. Philadelphia, WB Saunders, 2000.)

approximately 32 kD and the other approximately 30 kD. The peptide-binding region is composed of the α1 and β1 domains. The immunoglobulin-like domain is composed of the α2 and β2 segments. Similar to the class I immunoglobulin-like domain, there is limited polymorphism, and interactions are limited to CD4+ T cells. The class II molecules are constitutively expressed on professional APCs, including dendritic cells, B lymphocytes, and macrophages.[1,3] Expression can be induced on endothelial cells with cytokine stimulation and on other cells in certain disease states such as bile duct epithelium in primary sclerosing cholangitis and beta islet cells in diabetes.

Expression of MHC Molecules

The presence of MHC molecules is essential for recognizing interactions between cells. This presence of MHC molecules is the primary determinant of whether T lymphocytes can interact with foreign antigens. For the most part, class I molecules contain peptides that originate inside the cell whereas class II molecules hold peptides that were outside the cell, have been internalized, and were degraded in lysozymes. Importantly in the regulation of cytotoxic effector cell function, neither class I nor class II molecules can be expressed on the cell surface without a bound peptide. Therefore, the peptide-binding groove is always occupied with either self or foreign peptides. The class I and class II genes can generally be expressed in one of several states in a particular cell. First, the genes can be constitutively expressed and further upregulation can occur with the presence of cytokines. Second, the genes cannot be expressed but rather are induced by

cytokines. Third, the genes are not expressed and not inducible. These states are of tremendous importance in clinical transplantation and in determining the antigenicity of the transplanted allograft. The expression of MHC molecules is important in T-cell–mediated rejection, owing to the recognition of nonself.

Antigen Presentation: Direct Versus Indirect Recognition

In conventional antigen recognition, the foreign antigen is ingested by the host APC, digested into small peptides, and presented to T cells that recognize the antigen as well as class I or class II of the APC. This is termed *indirect antigen presentation* or the *indirect pathway*. In addition, when a solid organ is transplanted, the professional (dendritic cells, macrophages) and nonprofessional (activated vascular endothelial cells) APCs of the donor can present themselves. This is termed *direct recognition* (Fig. 26-11). In a solid organ transplant, both pathways play an important role. Recent studies in knock-out mice show that tolerance induction through mechanisms of co-stimulatory blockade may be selective for the indirect pathway, since elimination of the direct antigen presentation alone does not induce tolerance when combined with co-stimulatory blockade. Tolerance is relatively easily achieved by blockade of the CD28/B7 or CD154/CD40 co-stimulatory pathways in mice.[24]

HLA Typing: Prevention and Rejection

Organ transplantation in a recipient with a fully functional immune system may result in rejection. To minimize rejection, approaches that make the graft less antigenic to the host can be applied. The major strategy to achieve this is through minimizing alloantigen differences between donor and host. ABO compatibility is determined to avoid hyperacute rejection. Another determining factor is HLA typing or *tissue typing*. Potential donors and recipients are HLA-typed for HLA-A, HLA-B, and HLA-DR molecules. On close examination of graft survival, HLA matching is the best means of prolonging allograft survival. The larger the number of HLA-A, HLA-B, and HLA-DR alleles that are matched between both donor and recipient, the better the survival rate, particularly in the first year after transplantation. Current immunosuppressive regimens negate much of the impact of matching, however. Humans have two different HLA-A, HLA-B, and HLA-DR alleles (one from each parent, six alleles in total). Large, single-center trials have shown significant survival benefits for only six of six antigen matches. Matching remains controversial in the transplant community. It may be that historically imprecise tissue typing led to the contradictory results of some studies.

Historically, serologic testing that used the microcytotoxicity technique was used for both crossmatching and antibody testing. A gradual transition to molecular typing has occurred because of its greater accuracy. Poor HLA class II resolution, limitations in cell viability, and broad cross reactivity for different cross-reactive antigens limit the utility of serologic testing, especially for bone marrow transplantation. The serologic method uses an antigen-specific serum that binds to the cells expressing that particular antigen. The functional method measures the reactivity of the lymphocytes of a potential recipient to a donor. When antigens are recognized as foreign, lymphocyte proliferation results.[1]

Molecular techniques for performing HLA typing that use polymerase chain reaction (PCR) have been developed. PCR permits a more complete typing of class II loci (HLA-DR, HLA-DQ, and HLA-DP subsets) as well as precise typing of HLA-A and HLA-B. This DNA typing has become the predominant method because it better defines the crucial sequence of amino acids around the peptide-binding groove. Studies have been conducted that compare HLA-DR typing using traditional serologic methods and PCR methods. Serologic typing will likely be abandoned over time.

In clinical transplantation, crossmatching is performed using microcytotoxicity or flow cytometric techniques. Crossmatching differs from tissue typing. Crossmatching uses the serum from the recipient and is tested for preformed antibodies against donor cells to exclude the possibility of hyperacute rejection. Despite excellent histocompatibility matching, hyperacute rejection can still occur if preformed antibodies are present.[1] Preservation time is more severely limited in heart, lung, and liver transplantation; therefore, in those organs, crossmatching is performed before organ recovery only for recipients with known antibody titers.

Rejection

Graft rejection requires the participation of various combinations of immunologically specific and nonspecific cells. Three types of graft rejection occur (Fig. 26-12). *Hyperacute rejection* occurs within minutes to days after transplantation and is mediated primarily by preformed antibody. This type of rejection is prevented by screening the recipient for preformed antibodies, not by classic anti-rejection pharmaceuticals. *Acute rejection* is mediated primarily by T lymphocytes and first occurs between 1 and 3 weeks after solid organ transplantation without immunosuppression. Acute rejection episodes are most common in the first 3 to 6 months after transplantation but can occur at any time. Acute rejection can quickly destroy a graft if left untreated. The new immunosuppressive agents have made acute rejection increasingly less common. *Chronic rejection* occurs over months to years and is the most common cause of graft loss after 1 year. From an immunologic standpoint, chronic rejection is mediated by both T- and B-cell responses.[1,25]

Hyperacute rejection is mediated by preformed antibodies that bind to endothelium and subsequently activate complement. This rejection is characterized by a rapid thrombotic occlusion of the vasculature of the transplanted allograft. The thrombotic response occurs within minutes to hours after host blood vessels are anastomosed to donor vessels. Hyperacute rejection is mediated predominantly by IgG antibodies directed toward foreign protein molecules, such as MHC molecules. These IgG antibodies are the result of prior exposure to alloantigens from blood transfusions, pregnancy, or previous transplantation.[25]

There are two forms of acute rejection: acute vascular rejection and acute cellular rejection. *Acute vascular rejection* is the more severe form, with greater potential for long-term complications for the graft. In the setting of acute vascular rejection, the response is mediated by IgG molecules that develop in response to the graft against the endothelial antigens and involves the activation of complement. T cells contribute to the acute vascular rejection episode by responding to the foreign antigen. This response leads to direct lysis of the endothelial cells or the production of cytokines that further recruit and activate inflammatory cells. The end result is endothelial necrosis. This process occurs within the first week of allograft transplantation in the absence of immunosuppression.[25]

In the setting of *acute cellular rejection* there is necrosis of parenchymal cells caused by the infiltration of T cells and macrophages. The exact mechanism that underlies this process has not been fully delineated. An effector mechanism in the macrophage-mediated lysis is similar to a delayed-type hypersensitivity response. The T-cell effector mechanism is mediated by a CTL-mediated lysis. Much of the evidence emerging has implicated the alloreactive CD8+ CTL. The CD8+ CTL recognizes and lyses foreign cells. To support this mechanism, the cellular infiltrate present in acute rejection is enriched for CD8+ CTL.[1]

The mechanism for chronic rejection is less clearly defined and is an area of intense study. Chronic rejection appears as fibrosis and scarring in all organs currently transplanted, although the specific histopathologic lesions vary with the organ. It presents as accelerated atherosclerosis in heart recipients, as bronchiolitis obliterans in lung recipients, as "vanishing bile duct syndrome" in liver

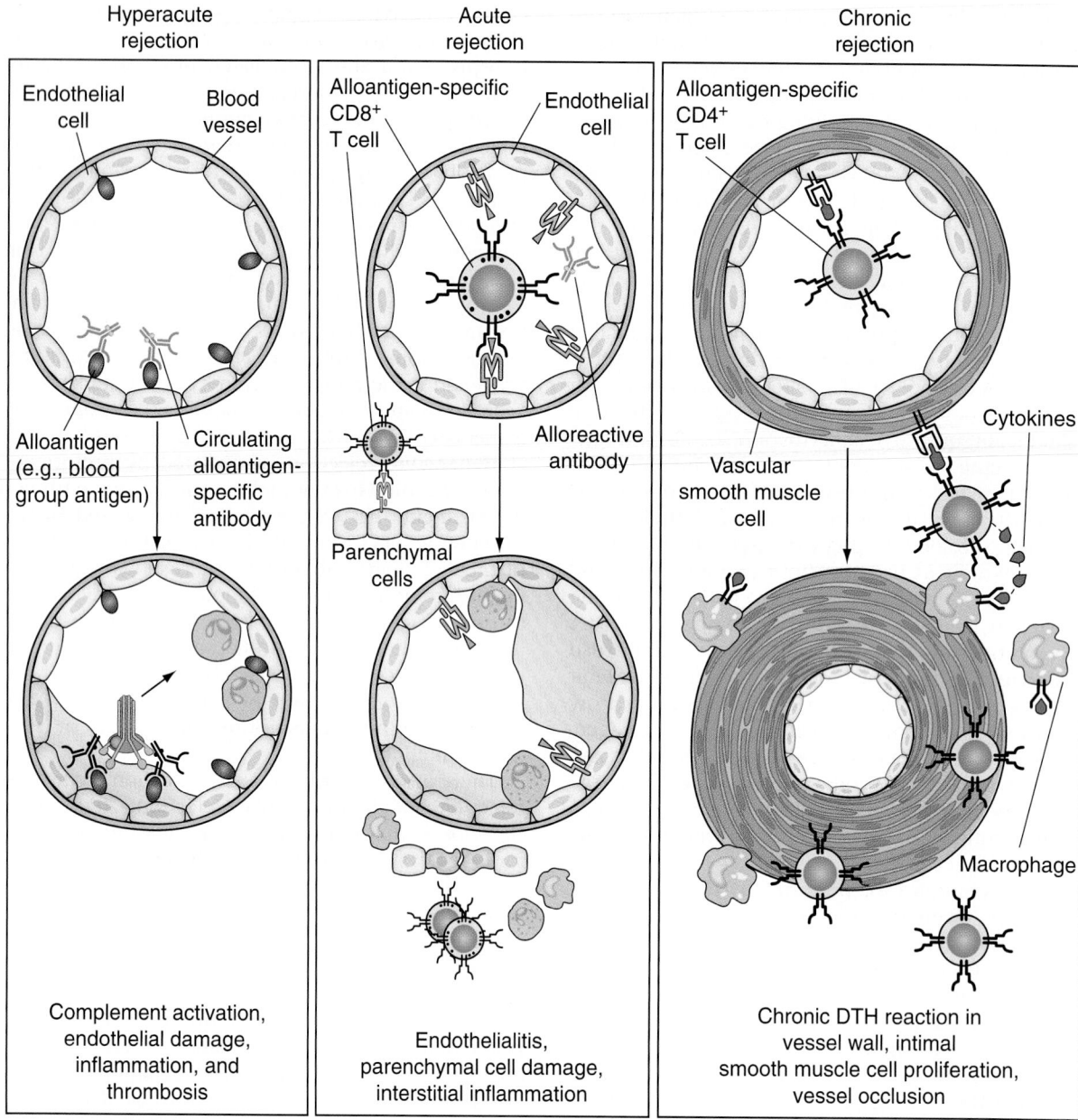

FIGURE 26-12. *Hyperacute rejection* results when preformed antibodies bind to vascular endothelium and activate complement. In *acute rejection,* CD8⁺ T cells attack alloantigens in parenchyma and vessels. *Chronic rejection* has a multifactorial etiology but leads to smooth muscle proliferation and fibrosis. (Adapted from Abbas AK, Lichtman AH, Pober JS: Immune mechanisms of graft rejection. *In* Cellular and Molecular Immunology, 4th ed. Philadelphia, WB Saunders, 2000.)

recipients, and as fibrosis and glomerulopathy in kidney recipients. It is unlikely that chronic rejection is strictly an immunologic phenomenon: ischemia and inflammation, among other processes, also play a role. Risk factors for development of the lesions of chronic rejection include (1) previous acute rejection episodes, with increased severity and increased number of episodes further increasing risk of chronic rejection; (2) inadequate immunosuppression, including patient noncompliance; (3) initial delayed graft function; (4) donor issues such as age and hypertension; (5) organ recovery–related issues including preservation and reperfusion injury; and (6)

recipient diabetes, hypertension, or post-transplant infections. In essence, almost any injury to the organ in the donor or post transplant can contribute to the development of chronic rejection.[26] Therefore, given the multifactorial basis of chronic rejection, the transplant is not completely protected with currently available immunosuppression. Episodes of acute rejection are a very significant risk factor, however, for the subsequent development of chronic rejection.[26] To the extent immunosuppressive agents prevent acute rejection episodes, the drugs do clearly decrease chronic rejection. New immunosuppressive drugs are evaluated not only by their ability to prevent acute rejection episodes and their safety profiles but also by their ability to prevent chronic rejection and improve the recipient's quality of life. Improved side-effect profiles may improve recipient compliance with immunosuppressive regimens.

The preceding, abbreviated description of the development of allograft immunity discloses many processes that may potentially be manipulated to suppress the immune response: (1) destroying the immunocompetent cells that would otherwise react to donor antigen *before* transplantation; (2) minimizing histoincompatibility or altering the antigen to make it unrecognizable or even toxic to the reactive lymphocyte clones; (3) interfering with antigen processing and presentation by the recipient cells; (4) inhibiting antigen recognition by lymphocytes; (5) inhibiting production or release by macrophages or lymphocytes of the signal substances or cytokines involved in differentiating lymphocytes into cytotoxic or antibody-synthesizing cells; (6) suppressing clonal expansion of lymphocytes; (7) activating sufficient numbers of suppressor lymphocytes; (8) interfering with the binding of immunoglobulins to graft target antigens; (9) preventing tissue damage by the nonspecific cells and molecules that are activated by sensitized cells or antigen-antibody complexes; and (10) inducing donor-specific transplantation tolerance.[10] Potential sites for regulation are discussed in detail below.

CLINICAL IMMUNOSUPPRESSION

Immunosuppressive agents are, for the most part, essential to graft survival. It is rare for a transplant recipient to become drug free, even over a prolonged period of time. Shortly after cardiac transplantation, recipients must orchestrate taking approximately 60 pills per day. Over time, fewer numbers of medications are required, but the medication regimen still takes its toll. The relatively nonspecific mechanism of action with the currently available immunosuppressive agents is associated with increased rate of infections (particularly viral infections) and malignancy. In addition, the individual agents themselves have specific toxicities. The overall risks of immunosuppression, the individual agents used in modern-day immunosuppression, and possible immunosuppressive drug regimens are each discussed separately. As the effector mechanisms responsible for graft rejection have been increasingly well defined, strategies to develop immunosuppressive agents with increasingly specific actions have emerged. Although tolerance remains the unattained goal of research in transplantation, significant improvements in immunosuppressive medication regimens have occurred in the past few years as newer agents and newer protocols have been developed.

Overall Risks of Immunosuppression

Risks of Infection

Prevention of rejection in any recipient is possible, but prevention itself is achieved at a high cost in terms of increased risk of infections and malignancies due to increased immunosuppression. Immunosuppressive drugs do not specifically block alloreactivity, and a certain degree of increased susceptibility to opportunistic infection plagues all transplant recipients (Fig. 26-13). This increased risk is caused not only by environmental pathogens but also by reactivation of previously controlled internal pathogens. An important example of the latter is CMV infection. CMV infection can result in pneumonia, hepatitis, pancreatitis, and gastrointestinal side effects, among others, in the transplant recipient (Fig. 26-14). CMV has been implicated in the lesions of heart transplant recipients with chronic rejection. Risk of reactivation is highest 6 to 12 weeks after transplantation and again after periods of increased immunosuppression for rejection episodes.[27]

Prevention of CMV reactivation is one of the areas in which prophylaxis is used to prevent post-transplant infections. Transplant programs use various prophylactic regimens, depending on the specific organs transplanted. Many regimens include pneumococcal vaccine, hepatitis B vaccine, trimethoprim-sulfamethoxazole for *Pneumocystis* pneumonia and urinary tract infections (pentamidine nebulizers may be substituted in the sulfa-allergic patient), acyclovir, ganciclovir, or valganciclovir for CMV, and clotrimazole troche or nystatin for oral and esophageal fungal infections. Hyper-CMV immunoglobulins are also used to prevent Epstein-Barr virus (EBV)–derived lymphomas in some high-risk populations. Although outcomes have definitely improved, infections remain a major problem in transplantation despite prophylaxis.[27]

Increased attention has focused on the potential role of BK virus in the development of renal allograft dysfunction. Studies previously have reported the role of the virus in ureteral stenosis. BK virus–associated nephropathy is diagnosed by viral inclusion bodies on biopsy, along with urine and plasma PCR testing. Sixty to 80 percent of the adult population may be seropositive for the BK virus, so determining the true role of the virus as a pathogen may be difficult. The nephropathy has reportedly improved with decreases in immunosuppression. Studies also recount success in eradicating the virus with low doses of cidofovir.[28]

Risks of Malignancy

Malignancy is also a complication of chronic immunosuppressive therapy. Penn,[29] in reporting results from his transplant tumor registry over 30 years, found no increase in lung, breast, prostate, colon, or uterine cancer in transplant recipients. Most post-transplant malignancies are easily treatable in situ carcinomas of the cervix or low-grade skin tumors. Virus-mediated tumors occur in greater frequency in transplant recipients, similar to those found in patients with AIDS. Human papillomavirus is associated with cancers of the cervix, hepatitis B and C with hepatomas, and human herpesvirus 8 with Kaposi's sarcoma. Lymphomas, particularly those associated with EBV, have an increased incidence in immunosuppressed transplant patients. Recipients treated repeatedly for

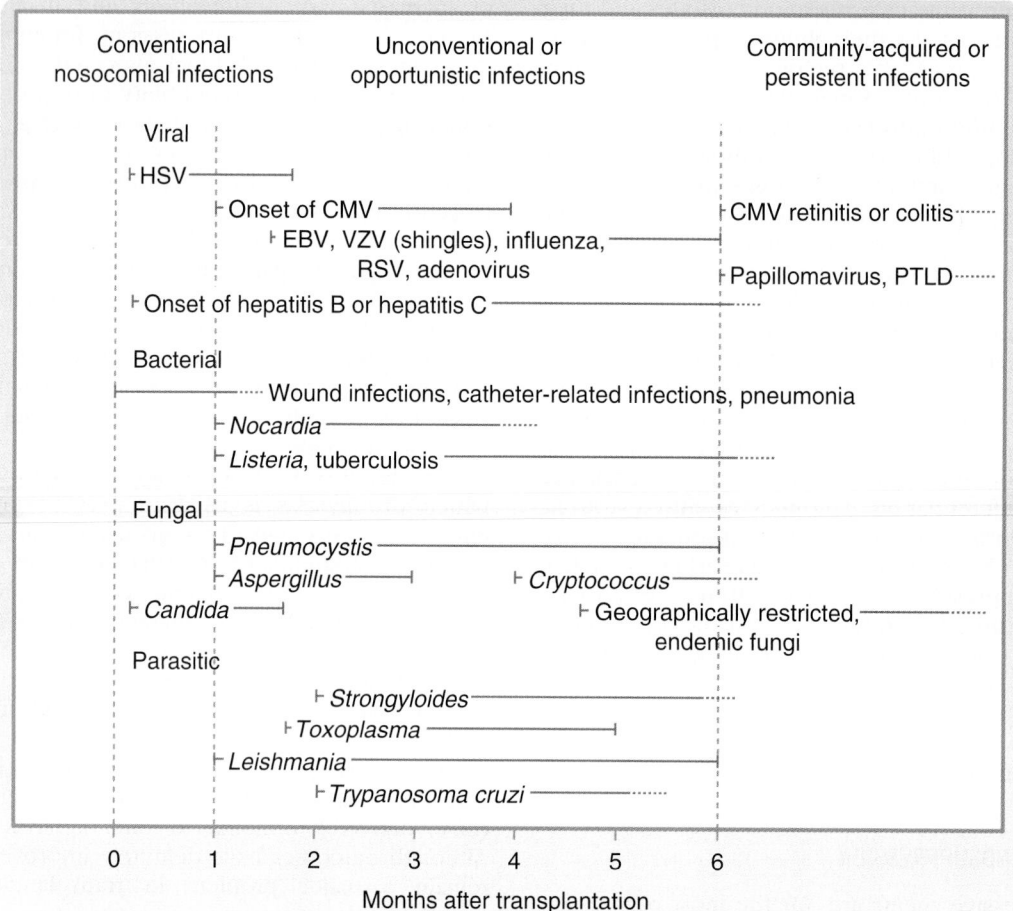

FIGURE 26-13. Usual sequence of infections after organ transplantation. Exceptions suggest the presence of unusual epidemiologic exposure or excessive immunosuppression. CMV, cytomegalovirus; EBV, Epstein-Barr virus; HSV, herpes simplex virus; PTLD, post-transplantation lymphoproliferative disease; RSV, respiratory syncytial virus; VZV, varicella-zoster virus. *Zero* indicates the time of transplantation; *solid lines* indicate the most common period for the onset of infection; *dotted lines* and *arrows* indicate periods of continued risk at reduced levels. (Reprinted from Rubin RH, Wolfson JS, Cosimi AB, Tolkoff-Rubin NE: Infection in the renal transplant patient. Am J Med 70:405-411, 1981. Copyright 1981, with permission from Excerpta Medica, Inc.)

acute rejection are at increased risk, as are young recipients of liver and small-bowel transplants. The EBV-associated lymphomas are often referred to as post-transplant lymphoproliferative disorders (PTLD) to better distinguish the differences in etiology and treatment from lymphomas in non-immunocompromised populations. PTLD varies from asymptomatic to life threatening, and treatment varies from no treatment, to reduction or withdrawal of immunosuppression in non-lifesaving transplants, to treatment with antiviral agents, to traditional chemotherapy.[29] Rituximab, an anti-CD20 monoclonal antibody that results in depletion of B cells, has been successfully used in the treatment of EBV-PTLD in solid organ transplant recipients.[30] Hyper-CMV immunoglobulin has also been used as prophylaxis in high-risk recipient groups.

Risks of Cardiovascular Disease

Cardiovascular disease remains a significant cause of morbidity and mortality in transplant recipients. After the first year, the most common causes of death in transplant recipients are (1) allograft loss from chronic rejection and (2) death of the patient with a functioning graft, secondary to cardiovascular death, disease, or infection. Atherosclerotic disease in heart transplant recipients is multifactorial. It can be related to chronic rejection, CMV infection, or classic hyperlipidemia. Pancreas allograft recipients suffer from the increased cardiovascular risk factors associated with diabetes, and renal allograft recipients are at increased risk for cardiovascular events as a result of underlying diseases, including diabetes or hypertension with concomitant left ventricular hypertrophy. These pre-transplant risk factors are amplified by post-transplant immunosuppression. Cyclosporine and corticosteroids, in particular, are associated with increased coronary artery disease. Adequate pre-transplant assessment of coronary artery disease, including liberal use of coronary angiography, helps identify those patients at risk. Post-transplant manipulation of immunosuppression in high-risk recipients should be undertaken. For instance,

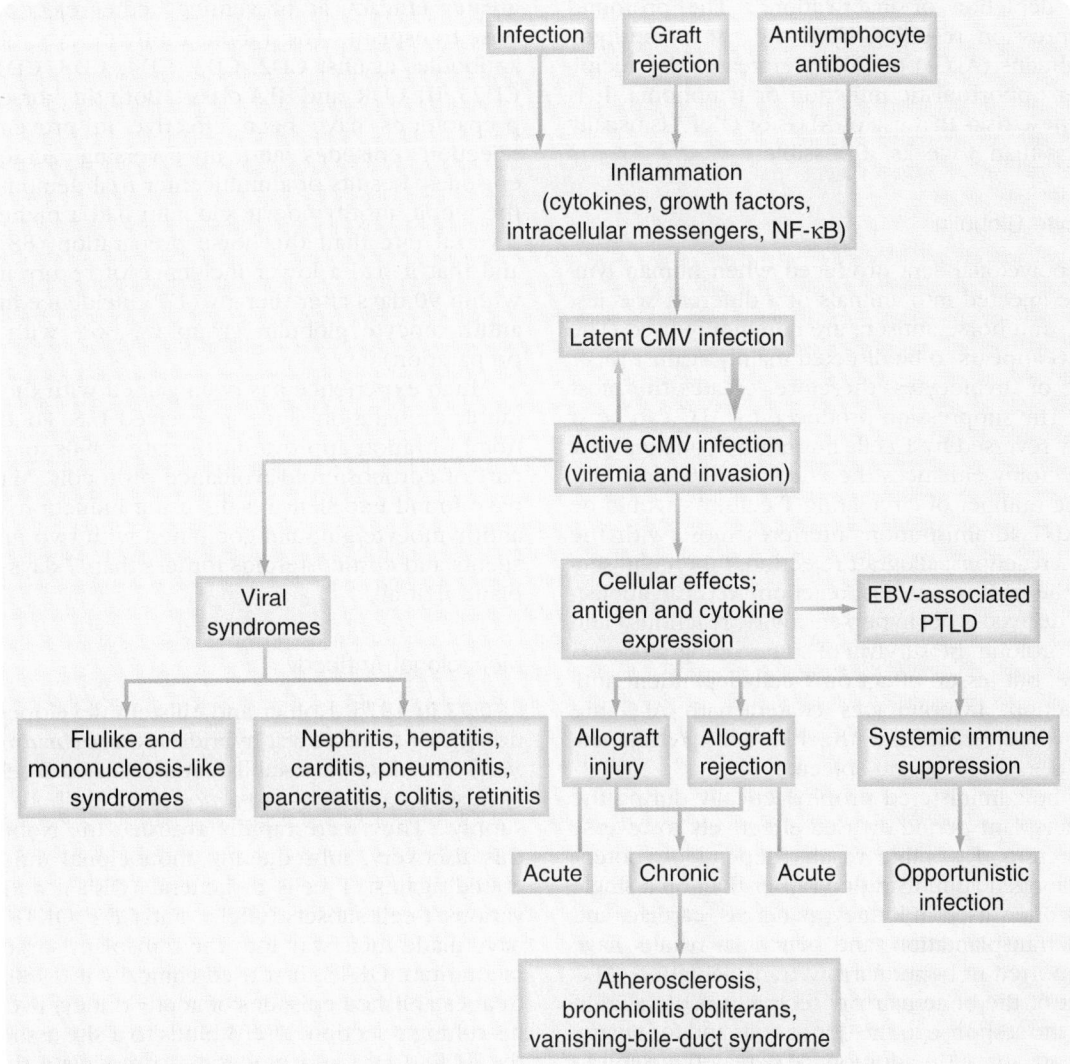

FIGURE 26-14. Role of cytomegalovirus (CMV) infection in transplant recipients. Mediators of systemic inflammation link the activation of CMV infection to allograft injury and rejection, to infection with opportunistic pathogens, and to the development of cancer in organ-transplant recipients. EBV, Epstein-Barr virus; PTLD, post-transplant lymphoproliferative disease. (From Fishman JA, Rubin RH: Infection in organ transplant recipients. N Engl J Med 338:1741-1751, 1998. Copyright © 1998 Massachusetts Medical Society. All rights reserved.)

switching from cyclosporine to tacrolimus should be considered, as well as avoiding or withdrawing corticosteroids in selected patients. HMG-CoA reductase inhibitors may lower lipid levels in transplant recipients, in addition to protecting the graft. Exercise and smoking cessation should also be emphasized.[31,32]

Induction Agents

Immunosuppressive drugs are divided naturally into two groups: those agents used for *induction therapy* immediately after transplant (often used also for treatment of rejection) and those drugs used for *maintenance therapy*. In contrast to the past decade, the first group includes primarily various antibody preparations.

There are currently five commercially available agents used primarily for induction. These include two poly-

clonal antilymphocyte agents, two monoclonal antibodies against the IL-2 receptor, and a monoclonal antibody against CD3 cells. Three other agents are also being tested experimentally in the perioperative period: an anti-CD20 monoclonal antibody, an anti-CD52 monoclonal antibody, and intravenous immunoglobulin (IVIG). These types are each discussed.

Lymphocyte Depletion Measures

Many clinically important immunosuppressive agents are effective because they deplete the host of lymphocytes. As the mechanism of action of these agents becomes better understood, a more sophisticated classification system may evolve; but, for the present, antilymphocyte globulin therapy, irradiation, and traditional monoclonal antibody therapy appear to act by relatively nonselective lymphocyte depletion or inactivation.[10] The profound immunosuppression resulting from the use of antilymphocyte globulins (ALGs) or OKT3 increases the recipient's risk for opportunistic infection or lymphoma. It is because of these risks that use of ALGs or OKT3 is usually limited to less than 3 weeks, if possible.

Antilymphocyte Globulin

ALGs are a polyclonal sera produced when human lymphocytes are injected into animals of a different species. Rabbit, goat, and horse antisera are commonly used. The action of ALG appears to be directed mainly against the T cell; the use of thymocytes, therefore, creates the most potent sera. The suppression produced by ALG can be at least partially reversed by T cells but not by bone marrow cells. Thymectomy enhances the effect of ALG, and ALG decreases the number of circulating T cells. As would be expected, ALG administration interferes most with the cell-mediated reactions: allograft rejection, tuberculin sensitivity, and the graft-versus-host reaction. ALG can abolish preexisting delayed-type hypersensitivity reactions, and larger doses prolong the survival of some xenografts. ALG has a definite, but lesser, effect on T-cell–dependent antibody production. Lymphocytes coated with ALG are either lysed or cleared from the blood by reticuloendothelial cells in the liver and spleen.

ALG may be administered prophylactically during the early post-transplant period or used effectively to reverse ongoing rejection. Favorable results depend on potent ALG and prolonged administration rather than on a single dose. ALG is often used in kidney, pancreas, cardiac, and small bowel transplantation, and beneficial results have also been reported in bone marrow transplantation. ALG pretreatment of the bone marrow recipient is of value in suppressing the response to the donor cells and for enlarging the marrow space. In addition, ALG may be useful in preventing the graft-versus-host reactions that arise in these patients.

The toxicity of any heterologous serum prepared against human tissue depends on two factors: (1) its cross-reactivity with other tissue antigens and (2) the ability of the patient to make antibodies against the foreign protein. Anemia and thrombocytopenia can occur and are presumably caused by a reaction between the ALG and host erythrocytes and platelets. Although prior absorption with human platelets and red cell stroma reduces its severity, some cross-reactivity with these cells persists in all ALG preparations.

Allergic reactions to the antiserum itself are the most common clinical problems associated with the use of ALG. Urticaria, anaphylactoid reactions, and serum sickness, including joint pain, fever, and malaise, all follow development of immunity to the heterologous globulin. These reactions are reduced, however, in the presence of the other immunosuppressive drugs used in transplantation.

Currently, there are two commercially available antithymocyte globulins. The first is a horse antithymocyte globulin, and the second is a rabbit antithymocyte globulin, which is much more commonly used. Clinical trials have demonstrated that the rabbit antithymocyte globulin has greater efficacy at preventing acute rejection episodes post transplant. The rabbit antithymocyte globulin has antibodies against CD2, CD3, CD4, CD8, CD11a, CD18, CD25, HLA-DR, and HLA class I. Both the horse and rabbit preparations have been effective in preventing acute rejection episodes and in reversing acute rejection episodes. Results of a multicenter trial demonstrated that the rabbit antithymocyte globulin had a higher rejection reversal rate than the horse preparation (88% vs. 76%) and that it had a lower incidence of recurrent rejection within 90 days after therapy (17% incidence in the rabbit antithymocyte globulin group vs. 36% with the horse preparation).[33]

Much experience has been gained with the use of the rabbit preparation since it received U.S. Food and Drug Administration approval in the late 1990s, particularly as part of corticosteroid-avoidance protocols. Many centers have found excellent results using induction with rabbit antithymocyte globulin combined with two maintenance agents and corticosteroids for less than 7 days after transplant, if at all.

Monoclonal Antibody

OKT3 In 1975, Kohler and Milstein developed the technology for somatic cell hybridization (*hybridoma formation*), which could establish immortalized B-cell lines that each secrete a single, or *monoclonal*, antibody in limitless supply.[1] They were rapidly awarded the Nobel Prize for this discovery. Subsequently, monoclonal antibodies generated against T cells in general (OKT3, anti-CD3) and various T-cell subsets (OKT4, anti-CD4; OKT8, anti-CD8) have made their way into the transplant surgeon's armamentarium. OKT3, first used clinically in 1980, is used to treat established episodes of acute kidney, liver, heart, or heart-lung rejection. OKT3 binds to a site associated with the TCR (CD3) and functions to modulate the receptor and inactivate T-cell function.[13,34]

By engaging the TCR complex, OKT3 blocks not only the function of naive T cells but also the function of established cytotoxic T cells, thereby blocking cell-mediated cytotoxicity. OKT3 blocks the T-cell effector functions involved in allograft rejection. After intravenous administration, OKT3 binds to T cells. As a result, the TCR complex is internalized and no longer expressed on the cell surface. These key T cells are then removed by the reticuloendothelial cells that reside in liver and spleen. Circulating T cells decrease abruptly (30 to 60 min) after the first OKT3 injection. Once OKT3 is stopped, CD3+ cells rapidly return to their normal levels, probably owing to re-expression of the TCR complex on the cell surface.[34]

The major limitation to use of OKT3 is that it is immunogenic and can elicit immune reactions.[13] After prolonged use, OKT3 becomes less effective, owing to the production of human anti-mouse antibodies that bind to the circulating OKT3. An acute cytokine release syndrome can also be seen, usually with the first or second dose of the drug. Concomitant administration of corticosteroids or indomethacin can ameliorate this problem. Because of these problems the use of rabbit antithymocyte globulin has essentially replaced the use of OKT3 at many centers.

Interleukin-2 Receptor Inhibitors The IL-2R is a complex of several transmembrane polypeptide chains. Three IL-2R binding chains, alpha (CD25, 55 kD), beta (75 kD), and gamma (64 kD) have been characterized. Noncovalent association of these chains forms the high-affinity binding site for IL-2. The alpha chain (IL-2Ra) is present only on activated T cells and a subset of activated B cells and APCs. Thus, anti-CD25 monoclonal antibody treatment targets the minor population of cells enriched for antigen-activated T cells. Two agents became available in 1998 that share as their mechanism of action binding of the alpha chain of the IL-2R. These monoclonal antibodies, basiliximab and daclizumab, are thought to decrease rejection by binding to IL-2R without activating it, leaving the cell with no free receptors for IL-2 to bind. The two agents differ in that daclizumab is a humanized anti-CD25 monoclonal antibody, whereas basiliximab is a chimeric anti-CD25 monoclonal antibody. The immunogenicity of these molecules, as measured by in vivo circulating half-life and by the appearance of antibodies against the agents, is significantly reduced when compared with strictly murine anti-CD25 monoclonal antibodies. Early studies demonstrated a decrease in acute rejection episodes without a concomitant increase in infections or malignancy. Both of these agents are well tolerated and can be administered through a peripheral intravenous line. Neither agent results in the type of cytokine-release syndrome occasionally found with OKT3 administration, nor the serum sickness seen with ALGs.[35,36] Neither agent, however, provides adequate immunosuppression on its own to prevent rejection, because T-cell proliferation can occur through IL-2 $\beta\gamma$ receptors or by other pathways. Therefore, both agents must be used in conjunction with other immunosuppressive drugs.

Anti-CD20 Monoclonal Antibody (Rituximab) Rituximab, as mentioned earlier, has been used as an anti-PTLD agent owing to its depleting effect on B cells. CD20 is a surface molecule expressed on B cells. The antibody has also been used in some centers to decrease antibody production in recipients with high panel reactive antibody (PRA) or as part of positive crossmatch protocols. Additionally, rituximab has been used to treat humoral rejection in cardiac recipients.[37]

Anti-CD52 Monoclonal Antibody (Alemtuzumab or Campath 1H) Early results are available now in the use of alemtuzumab as a depleting induction agent in renal transplantation. Alemtuzumab is a humanized monoclonal antibody against CD52, which is expressed on B cells, T cells, monocytes, and macrophages. Administration of the agent results in a dramatic, prolonged depletion of lymphocytes lasting 2 to 6 months. Alemtuzumab has been used in the treatment of lymphoid malignancies, rheumatoid arthritis, and multiple sclerosis. Used with low-dose cyclosporine or sirolimus monotherapy, alemtuzumab has prevented rejection in renal allograft recipients. It has also been used to treat lung transplant rejection and as an induction agent in small bowel transplantation. Long-term results are not yet known, but the benefits of this type of protocol are exciting in terms of potential decrease in immunosuppressive risks and cost.[38,39]

Intravenous Immunoglobulin

IVIG is made from the pooled plasma of thousands of screened donors and should contain all the antibodies found normally in humans. IVIG works through many mechanisms to modulate the immune system, including neutralization of circulating autoantibodies by anti-idiotypes and selective downregulation of antibody production. The preparation can also regulate production of T-cell cytokines, inhibit lymphocyte proliferation, and regulate apoptosis.

IVIG has been used primarily in positive crossmatch and ABO-incompatible protocols, often in combination with plasmapheresis. Additionally, IVIG has successfully treated humoral rejection in all types of organ transplants, including some rejection episodes resistant to corticosteroids and antithymocyte globulin.[40,41]

Maintenance Agents

A general rule in the management of immunosuppression is that the greatest amount of drug is required early after transplantation. Usually, agents can be slowly tapered in dosages after the graft has been in place for a period of time. However, it is highly unusual for a transplant recipient to become drug free even after a prolonged time interval. The mainstay of human organ transplantation is daily immunosuppression with oral pharmaceuticals. Prednisone and azathioprine have been used for many years. In those early years of transplantation, though, severe complications with corticosteroid therapy were common when the high doses were used. Currently, many agents are available, all with different side-effect profiles. Multidrug therapy using immunosuppressive agents with a nonoverlapping mechanism of action is used in most organ recipients to decrease the side effects associated with any individual drug in doses large enough to adequately prevent rejection (Box 26-1).

Box 26-1. Maintenance Agents

Adrenal Corticosteroid

Prednisone

Antiproliferative Agents

Azathioprine
Mycophenolate mofetil
Leflunomide

T-Cell–Directed Immunosuppressants

Calcineurin inhibitors: cyclosporine, tacrolimus
Cell cycle arrest: sirolimus

Lymphocyte Sequestration

FTY720

Adrenal Corticosteroids

Adrenal corticosteroids are the immunosuppressive agents most commonly used in clinical practice.[42] Glucocorticoids have many diverse anti-inflammatory actions, which make them potent immunosuppressants. A major effect of corticosteroids appears to be the inhibition of cytokine gene transcription in, and cytokine secretion (IL-1, IL-6, TNF) by, macrophages. Corticosteroids also suppress the production and the effect of T-cell cytokines, which amplify the responses of lymphocytes and macrophages. Thus, IL-2 production and binding of IL-2 to its receptor is inhibited by glucocorticoids. Moreover, the ability of macrophages to respond to lymphocyte-derived signals such as migration inhibition factor and macrophage activation factor is blocked by corticosteroids. This may underlie the marked inhibition of delayed-type hypersensitivity reactions observed with use of these agents. An additional effect is the suppression of prostaglandin synthesis. Corticosteroids have little net effect on antibody production.

Some of the molecular mechanisms by which glucocorticoids exert their effect have been elucidated. Much activity is initiated at the subcellular level by means of hormone receptors. Unlike polypeptide mediators with receptors on the cell surface, corticosteroids move freely through the cell membrane to bind receptors in the cytoplasm, producing a steroid-receptor complex. This complex then moves into the nucleus, where it attaches to the DNA. There it acts on gene promoters to either depress or activate part of the genome and cause transcription of specific mRNA. Thus, some protein synthesis is downregulated and other proteins are synthesized. These changes are the presumed effectors of glucocorticoid action.

Specific intracytoplasmic receptors for glucocorticoids have been identified in normal human lymphocytes, monocytes, neutrophils, and eosinophils. In addition, varying degrees of receptor density have been demonstrated in different lymphoid cell subpopulations. Presumably, the sensitivity of a particular subpopulation of lymphocytes relates to the relative density of the intracytoplasmic receptors for the corticosteroids. These messengers can inhibit DNA, RNA, and protein synthesis. Glucose and amino acid transport can also be affected.

The effectiveness of cortisone in suppressing allograft rejection was first recognized in the 1950s by its ability to prolong skin graft survival in rabbits. In organ allografts, corticosteroids are not effective by themselves, but they are valuable in combination with other agents. Corticosteroids, in high doses, are especially effective at interrupting ongoing rejection reactions in clinical practice, but prolonged use leads to unacceptable side effects, such as hypertension, weight gain, peptic ulcers and gastrointestinal bleeding, euphoric personality changes, cataract formation, hyperglycemia that could progress to steroid diabetes, pancreatitis, muscle wasting, and osteoporosis with avascular necrosis of the femoral head and other bones. Susceptibility to pyogenic and opportunistic infections is a direct result of the suppression of phagocytic microbial killing by macrophages and neutrophils.

Cushingoid features are the external signs of these dangerous processes. Clinical transplantation will be improved tremendously when more specific means of immunosuppression are developed and current corticosteroid dosages are reduced substantially or eliminated. These significant side effects have led many centers to develop steroid-avoidance protocols. Earlier attempts at steroid withdrawal have resulted in unacceptably high rejection rates. Current protocols, many using rabbit antithymocyte globulin for induction and less than 7 days of steroids, have had much better results. A possible explanation for the success of steroid avoidance over steroid withdrawal may be the prevention of upregulation of steroid receptors in the avoidance protocols; this is just conjecture at this point.[31]

Antiproliferative Agents

Antiproliferative agents inhibit the full expression of the immune response by preventing the differentiation and division of the immunocompetent lymphocytes after their encounter with antigen.[8] They either structurally resemble essential metabolites or combine with certain cellular components, such as DNA, and thereby interfere with molecular function.

The antimetabolites, the former group, either inhibit enzymes that regulate a particular metabolic pathway or are incorporated during synthesis to produce *faulty* molecules. They include purine, pyrimidine, and folic acid analogues that are most effective against proliferating and differentiating cells. These drugs are given at the time of transplantation when the immunocompetent cells are first stimulated, and for the life of the graft, to inhibit the continuing response of the immune system.

Azathioprine

Until the mid 1990s, the purine analogue azathioprine was the most widely used immunosuppressive drug in clinical organ transplantation. In fact, Hitchings and Elion were awarded the Nobel Prize for a simple modification that made the drug safe for use in transplantation. Azathioprine is 6-mercaptopurine (6-MP) plus a side chain to protect the labile sulfhydryl group. In the liver, the side chain is split off to form the active compound 6-MP. The mechanism of action of these two compounds is similar, although azathioprine appears to have the advantage of slightly lower toxicity.[8]

Full metabolic activity occurs in the cell with the addition of ribose-S6-phosphate from phosphoribosyl pyrophosphate to form 6-MP ribonucleotide. The structural resemblance of this molecule to inosine monophosphate is obvious, and 6-MP ribonucleotide inhibits the enzymes that begin to convert inosine nucleotide to adenosine and guanosine monophosphate. In addition, the presence of 6-MP ribonucleotides slows the entire purine biosynthetic pathway by fraudulent feedback inhibition of an early step. The steric similarity to either adenosine or guanine nucleotides is not sufficient to allow significant incorporation into DNA or RNA and synthesis of faulty molecules. The result of inhibiting these several enzymes, however, is to block the synthesis of cellular DNA, RNA, certain cofactors, and other active nucleotides.

The biologic activity of azathioprine and 6-MP is greatest when nucleic acid synthesis is most required.[8] These agents thus strongly inhibit the development of both humoral and cellular immunity by interfering with the differentiation and proliferation of the responding lymphocytes. When the expansion of fully immunocompetent cells is complete, nucleic acid synthesis is less important, and the drug is less effective. An additional benefit of azathioprine is that it can also reduce neutrophil production and macrophage activation effects that suppress the nonspecific inflammatory components of the immune reaction.

The toxicity of azathioprine derives from the same antimetabolite action.[8] The primary effect is bone marrow suppression, leading to leukopenia. Liver toxicity may also occur, possibly because of the high rate of RNA synthesis by hepatocytes. Because hepatic dysfunction does not appear to be dose related, the mechanism is unclear.

Mycophenolate Mofetil

Mycophenolate mofetil (MMF) is another immunosuppressant that functions by the inhibition of purine metabolism. MMF inhibits inosine monophosphate dehydrogenate and serves to block the proliferation of lymphocytes late in the cell cycle. MMF has almost completely replaced azathioprine as part of traditional triple-therapy immunosuppression. The U.S. Renal Transplant Mycophenolate Mofetil Study demonstrated that in primary cadaver renal transplant recipients randomized either to azathioprine, MMF 2 g/day, or MMF 3 g/day, the incidence of rejection decreased from 38% in the first group to 19.8% in the 2-g/day group and to 17.5% in the 3-g/day group. The 3-g/day group, however, had significant gastrointestinal side effects. Most recipients currently receive 2 g/day. The major clinical side effects of this medication are leukopenia and gastrointestinal upset, particularly diarrhea.[7]

Leflunomide

Approved for use in the United States in the treatment of rheumatoid arthritis, leflunomide has been used experimentally and clinically in solid organ transplantation. The drug reversibly blocks dihydroorotate dehydrogenase, an enzyme necessary for de novo pyrimidine synthesis in lymphocytes. Experimentally, the drug demonstrates synergy with calcineurin inhibitors and inhibits herpesvirus (including ganciclovir-resistant CMV). Major toxicities appear to vary by organ transplant type. Liver transplant recipients have had significant increases in transaminases; renal transplant recipients have suffered gastrointestinal upset and anemia. Because of sizable variations patient-to-patient in rates of metabolism, drug levels need to be monitored. Not enough experience with leflunomide has been gained to determine whether successes reported experimentally in preventing chronic rejection will translate into the clinical arena.[9]

T-Cell–Directed Immunosuppressants

Cyclosporine

Borel's discovery in 1972 of the immunosuppressive properties of cyclosporine, a fungal metabolite extracted from *Tolypocladium inflatum* Gams, contributed enormously to the rapid and successful growth of the field of clinical organ transplantation, especially of livers and hearts.[43] It represented a completely new class of clinically important immunosuppressive agents. Many of its selective, suppressive effects on T cells appear to be related to its selective inhibition of TCR-mediated activation events (Fig. 26-15). It inhibits cytokine production by T_H cells in vitro and impairs the development of mature $CD4^+$ and $CD8^+$ T cells in the thymus. Cyclosporine is a cyclic peptide (11 amino acids, molecular weight: 1202 daltons).

Cyclosporine was discovered to be immunosuppressive by its ability to suppress antibody production in mice. Other in vivo properties include inhibition of antibody plaque-forming cell production, GVHD, skin graft rejection, delayed solid organ allograft rejection, and delayed-type hypersensitivity reactions. Absence of myelosuppression was a major advance over other immunosuppressive agents and indicated that the mechanism of action was relatively specific for lymphocytes.[8,43] Other inflammatory cells are much less sensitive to its inhibitory effects. Clinically, prophylactic administration of cyclosporine suppresses allograft rejection and GVHD.

Analyses of the effect of cyclosporine on T lymphocytes have shown (1) inhibition of both IL-2–producing T lymphocytes and cytotoxic T lymphocytes; (2) inhibition of IL-2 gene expression by activated T lymphocytes; (3) no inhibition of activated T lymphocytes in response to exogenous IL-2; (4) inhibition of resting T-lymphocyte activation in response to alloantigen and exogenous lymphokine; (5) inhibition of IL-1 production; and (6) inhibition of mitogen (concanavalin A) activation of IL-2–producing T lymphocytes. These T-cell responses involve both $CD4^+$ (T_H) and/or $CD8^+$ (T-cytotoxic/suppressor) cells, and the inhibition appears to occur at the level of activation, and perhaps even maturation, of the resting cell. In mice, maturation of T cells that occurs in the thymus is significantly suppressed by cyclosporine, thus enriching a population of immature and less responsive T cells.

Cyclosporine induces potent immunosuppression without myelosuppression. The addition of corticosteroids to cyclosporine permitted a lowering of the cyclosporine dosage and decreased nephrotoxicity (the principal clinical side effect of the drug). The introduction of cyclosporine into widespread clinical use in 1983 led to a substantial improvement in the outcome of cadaveric renal transplantation and permitted the widespread practice of heart and liver grafting.

Cyclosporine is metabolized in the liver by cytochrome p450 enzymes. Medications that increase or decrease cytochrome p450 function can dramatically increase or decrease cyclosporine or tacrolimus levels. The narrow therapeutic windows of these immunosuppressants require care in prescribing practices. Antibiotics, seizure

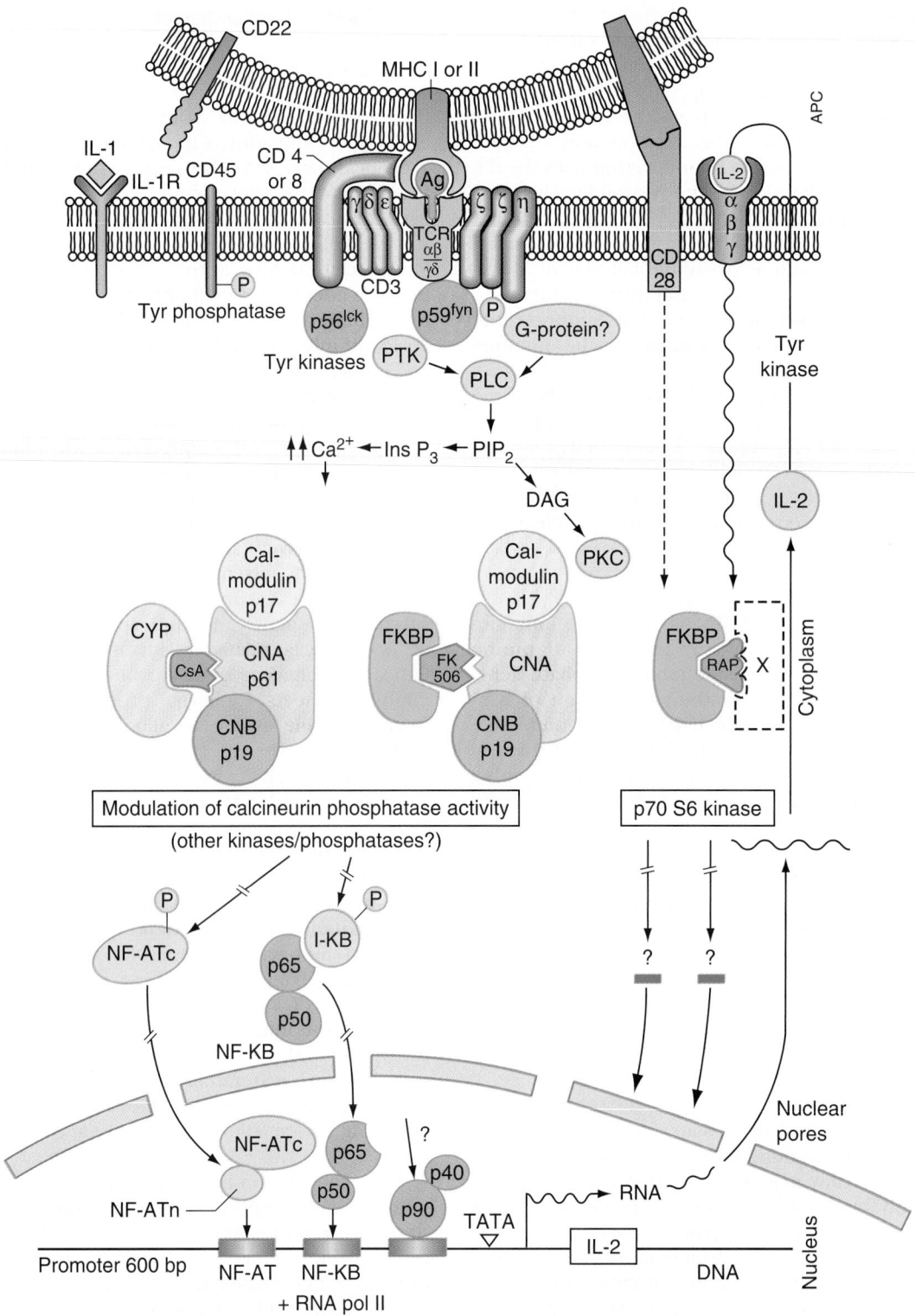

FIGURE 26-15. Signal transduction in activated T cells and the sites (center of figure) at which cyclosporine (CsA), tacrolimus (FK-506), and sirolimus (rapamycin [RAP]) are believed to act. CsA or FK-506 bound to their respective immunophilins (cyclophilin [CYP]) or FKBP form pentameric complexes with calmodulin and calcineurin A (CAN) and B. Inhibition of the phosphatase activity of calcineurin is believed to inhibit translocation to the nucleus of the cytoplasmic component of the nuclear factor of activated T cells (NF-ATc) that is required for activation of the interleukin-2 (IL-2) gene. RAP, which also binds to FKBP, inhibits phosphorylation and activation of a 70-kD, ribosomal S6-protein kinase (p70S6), which normally occurs within minutes of cell activation by cytokine receptors. RAP also targets other kinases (not shown) that are essential for cell cycle progression. X refers to target of rapamycin. (From Schreier M, Quesniaux VFJ, Baumann G, et al: Molecular basis of immunosuppression. Transplant Sci 3:185, 1993.)

medications, and some calcium-channel blockers are major culprits, but interactions should be verified before prescribing any new medication to a transplant recipient.

The potential adverse effects of cyclosporine include nephrotoxicity, hypertension, hyperkalemia, hirsutism, gingival hyperplasia, tremor and other neurotoxicities, diabetogenicity, and hepatotoxicity. As with other immunosuppressive agents, cyclosporine therapy increases the risk of infection and malignancy; but by reducing corticosteroid requirements, an overall general decrease in infection rates is seen compared with historical immunotherapy.

Tacrolimus

Tacrolimus (formerly known as FK-506) is a potent immunosuppressive agent isolated in 1984 in Japan from the soil fungus *Streptomyces tsukubaensis*. It is a macrocyclic lactone with a molecular weight of 822 daltons. Although structurally distinct from cyclosporine, it exhibits a very similar molecular action. Both drugs are regarded as *pro-drugs*. Their antilymphocytic effects result from the formation of active complexes between the drug and its respective intracellular binding protein or *immunophilin* (cyclophilin or FK-506 binding protein [FKBP]) (see Fig. 26-15).[44] The drug-immunophilin complex blocks the phosphatase activity of calcineurin that is important in regulation of IL-2 gene transcription.[45] The activity of tacrolimus in vitro, however, is approximately 100 times greater than that of cyclosporine. Like cyclosporine, tacrolimus functions to inhibit (1) IL-2 gene expression and IL-2 production; (2) mixed lymphocyte culture cellular proliferation, which is mediated by T_H cells; (3) the generation of cytotoxic T cells; and (4) the appearance of IL-2R on human lymphocytes. In vivo, tacrolimus prolongs the survival of MHC-disparate skin, as well as cardiac, renal, hepatic, and small bowel allografts. Tacrolimus has been approved for the treatment of liver allograft rejection. It also has efficacy in rescue therapy for recurrent acute allograft rejection in renal allograft recipients. The side effects of cyclosporine and tacrolimus are similar, but tacrolimus does not cause hirsutism or gum hypertrophy. It does, however, cause alopecia and has an increased incidence of post-transplant diabetes when compared with cyclosporine, particularly at higher doses. Drug levels must be monitored.

Sirolimus

Similar to tacrolimus, the immunosuppressant sirolimus (also known as rapamycin) is a macrolide antibiotic. It is a close structural analogue of tacrolimus and binds to the same cytoplasmic receptor (FKBP). Unlike tacrolimus or cyclosporine, however, sirolimus does not block T-cell cytokine gene expression but instead inhibits the transduction of signals from the IL-2R to the nucleus.[3,44] Binding of sirolimus to FKBP inhibits p70S6 protein kinase activity, which is essential for ribosomal phosphorylation and cell cycle progression (see Fig. 26-15). Sirolimus potently inhibits allograft rejection. Two additional, important properties of this drug are that it acts synergis-

tically with cyclosporine and that it prevents rejection in rat transplant models.[45] Sirolimus has been combined with cyclosporine, tacrolimus, or mycophenolate mofetil in attempts to decrease or avoid calcineurin inhibitors with their associated nephrotoxicity. Clinical trials are ongoing to assess its impact on chronic rejection in human renal allograft recipients. Sirolimus is also being used as a coating in cardiac stents to prevent restenosis. Clinical trials have demonstrated that sirolimus is not significantly nephrotoxic; however, it has been demonstrated to increase triglycerides and decrease platelets and hemoglobin in some recipients. Increased incidence of lymphoceles and delays in wound healing have also been reported with the use of sirolimus.[46]

Lymphocyte Sequestration

FTY720

FTY720 uniquely works by sequestering lymphocytes in peripheral nodes and Peyer's patches, preventing them from migrating to the graft. FTY720 administration results in a decreased lymphocyte count, which reverses when the drug is discontinued. Bradycardia, associated with the first or second dose, has been the major side effect. Activation of sphingosine-1-phosphate receptors on atrial myocytes, with which FTY720 shares structural homology, is likely the cause of the bradycardia. Clinical trials are ongoing. FTY720 is being used in combination with cyclosporine and other agents.[47]

Local Immunosuppression

One approach toward reducing the drug-specific and general adverse consequences of systemic immunosuppression is the use of local drug administration systems to establish more selective presence of immunosuppressive agents in the transplanted organ. Experimental drug-targeting approaches include intra-arterial drug infusion, implantable infusion pumps, controlled-release matrices, drug-impregnated polymer rods, liposomes, topical application (skin or cornea), and aerosol inhalation (lung). Details on this topic are reviewed elsewhere.[48] Currently, this approach is only used in composite tissue allotransplant recipients in whom topical immunosuppression is added to systemic immunosuppression to boost levels to the skin.[49]

Positive Crossmatch Protocols

Previous transfusion, pregnancy, or transplant can prevent successful transplantation in sensitized individuals. Left ventricular assist devices also can result in high panel reactive antibody titers in potential heart recipients. These preformed antibodies can result in hyperacute rejection of transplanted organs. In the case of sensitized potential kidney recipients, such people may languish on the lists for years while waiting for their "perfect match."

New protocols have been developed utilizing various combinations of plasmapheresis, intravenous immunoglobulin administration, splenectomy, and anti-CD20 monoclonal antibodies, combined with conventional immunosuppression to allow for successful transplantation in these otherwise "untransplantable" individuals. These protocols have been successful, particularly for recipients with living donors, allowing for pretreatment before a scheduled transplant. Antibody levels can be measured and transplants undertaken when antibody levels decrease appropriately. A few potential recipients will not decrease their antibody levels, however, and will remain "untransplantable."[40,50]

Possible Immunosuppressive Regimens

In the past, immunosuppression has been of a "one-size-fits-all" mentality. Most allograft recipients received an induction agent of either ALG or OKT3, followed by cyclosporine, azathioprine, and prednisone as maintenance therapy. The new agents now available have allowed for many more options and finally for some tailoring of immunosuppression to the recipient's situation. Although tolerance, or a drug-free state, remains the long-term goal in transplantation, the addition of new agents to the pharmacologic armamentarium has reduced the incidence of acute allograft rejection while decreasing the side effects for individual recipients. Decreasing side effects increases the likelihood that a recipient will actually continue the immunosuppressive medications. Noncompliance with medications remains a significant issue in long-term graft survival. A young woman with severe hirsutism may think twice about continuing her cyclosporine therapy; switching her to tacrolimus may be a more appropriate option. A recipient with inadequate financial resources may be more appropriately continued on prednisone and azathioprine than being switched to the more costly MMF. We are beginning to reach an era in transplantation in which we can "custom fit" immunosuppression to the recipient based on donor and recipient factors, as well as the organ transplanted. A greater emphasis is also being placed on withdrawal of corticosteroids in all organs.[31] From experimental "tolerizing" protocols using alemtuzumab or rabbit antithymocyte globulin followed by low-dose monotherapies with tacrolimus, cyclosporine, or sirolimus, to more traditional triple-therapy regimens with or without induction agents, to corticosteroid avoidance, no "standard" protocols exist today.

Treatment of Acute Rejection

Although there is great debate about the most appropriate agents and duration of therapy in the treatment of acute rejection, there is little debate over the importance of a prompt and accurate diagnosis, which usually requires biopsy. Most often, therapy is tailored to the degree of rejection. Mild rejections are usually treated with high-dose methylprednisolone with or without a subsequent oral prednisone taper. Mild liver allograft rejection is often treated with increased tacrolimus doses. Moderate to severe rejection is treated with either rabbit antithymocyte globulin or the monoclonal antibody OKT3; failing that, alemtuzumab, rituximab, and intra-

venous immunoglobulin have all been used with some success.[13,33,37,39,41] CMV prophylaxis with ganciclovir or valganciclovir is usually administered concurrently with therapy for acute rejection. Repeated treatments for acute rejection increase the risk both of infection and malignant complications, particularly post-transplant lymphoproliferative disease.

Antirejection therapy is achieved at a high cost to the recipient, both financially and physically. Complete treatment of rejection is critically important, however, because inadequately treated acute rejection is a leading cause of chronic rejection and subsequent graft loss.[26] Chronic rejection remains the primary cause of late graft loss. Even with perfect patient compliance, there is a fixed rate of graft loss for all transplanted organs. For example, whereas some graft loss is due to technical problems or patient death, at 5 years only 67% of transplanted hearts, 61% of transplanted cadaver kidneys, and 64% of transplanted livers function (OPTN/SRTR data). It has become clear that the immunosuppressive agents that are so effective at controlling acute rejection are not as effective at controlling chronic rejection.

XENOTRANSPLANTATION

There is a critical shortage of organs available for transplantation. Over 80,000 potential recipients are currently listed and awaiting organ transplantation. Many more patients could benefit from transplantation but, given the current shortage of organs, are not even considered for transplantation. Since 1990, over 20% of listed potential heart recipients have died while awaiting a heart transplant. Many experts in the field have concluded that the supply of human donors will never meet the demand. Currently, about 6,000 cadaver donors are recovered each year (UNOS data). This number has increased somewhat over the years as older donors have been included, but organ donation in the United States has reached a plateau. This shortage forces continued interest in xenotransplantation, which remains hotly debated. A possibility for expansion of the donor pool includes the use of nonhuman sources as donors. However, the mechanisms of xenoreactivity differ from alloreactivity, and the resulting rejection is vigorous. The principal barrier to the widespread use of xenotransplantation is the presence of natural antibodies. Similar to ABO blood groupings, natural IgM antibodies develop against nonself carbohydrate moieties. These naturally occurring antibodies are reduced in number as the species are more closely related, such as with humans and chimpanzees. These naturally occurring antibodies mediate the hyperacute rejection typically found with transplantation across species. The majority of the naturally occurring antibodies are against a carbohydrate moiety α-galactose.[10,51] The preferred xenogeneic species for human clinical transplantation is the pig, because of size and availability. The pig also has the potential for less transmission of zoonoses than a primate species, but porcine endogenous retroviruses have been discovered in human cells used to reconstitute SCID mice after transplantation with pig tissue.[52]

Xenogeneic hyperacute rejection has many similar features to the allogeneic hyperacute rejection seen immediately post transplant with ABO incompatibility. This reaction is dependent on complement with the generation of procoagulants and platelet aggregating substances. Unlike with allogeneic organ transplantation, in xenotransplantation the ability to limit or control the complement cascade is lost. In humans, a decay factor (CD55) is present that limits the complement-induced injury. In the pig cells, CD55 is not expressed. Strategies are emerging in which soluble factors such as human CD55 and complement receptors are administered that will limit the extent of the hyperacute rejection.[53] Transgenic pigs that express human CD55 have been developed. Additionally, pigs have been cloned that do not produce the galactosyl transferase enzyme.[51]

On inhibition of the soluble agents to eliminate the complement-mediated hyperacute rejection, the next problem is with delayed xenograft rejection. Research models that inhibit the complement system have made delayed xenograft rejection available for study. This form of rejection involves both NK cells and macrophages as mediators of the inflammatory process. NK-cell activities are initiated, and owing to the lack self-MHC molecules that normally provide the inhibitory signals for NK cells, the NK function remains unopposed. These activated NK cells secrete cytokines such as TNF and INF-γ that both recruit and activate macrophages.[1,10,23]

TOLERANCE

Historical Background

The cherished goal of the transplant scientist and clinician is to induce donor-specific tolerance and eliminate the need for exogenous immunosuppressants. Although tolerance has been achieved in numerous species, including humans, the widespread clinical application is incumbent on improving the safety and reducing the risk of such an approach. Nevertheless, there are rare instances of the establishment of drug-free unresponsiveness to organ allografts in humans who have discontinued immunosuppressive therapy for various reasons. Moreover, some humans have been rendered drug free for acceptance of kidney allografts after a bone marrow transplant from the same donor for leukemia.[54,55] Contemporary developments in our understanding of cellular and molecular immunology and of the basis of experimental tolerance induction hold promise for the development of clinically effective approaches. Authentic transplantation tolerance is antigen specific. It is induced as the result of prior exposure to antigen and does not depend on the continuous administration of exogenous antigen-nonspecific immunosuppressive agents.

In 1953, in a seminal study, Billingham and colleagues[56] were among the first to demonstrate actively acquired donor-specific tolerance. They performed historic experiments in which they exchanged reciprocal skin grafts between Freemartin cattle twins. Freemartin cattle are genetically different cattle twins that share a common placenta. Billingham and colleagues predicted that the cattle would reject those grafts because they were genetically different. However, the grafts were accepted. This result was explained by Owen's observation that the Freemartin cattle strain shared a common placenta; they are actually red blood cell chimeras.[57] With this observation, the researchers returned to the laboratory to demonstrate that when they transplanted bone marrow–derived cells from a donor into a fetal mouse they could actively transfer acquired tolerance to the recipient. If a skin graft from the same bone marrow donor was transplanted, the graft was permanently accepted. The tolerance was donor specific, because when a third-party skin graft was transplanted the graft was rejected.[56] An important lesson learned from this experiment was that the acquired tolerance was due to the immunologic incompetence of the graft recipient and not to any alteration in the grafted tissue itself. Similar mixed chimerism and tolerance was established in adult mice with the addition of conditioning.[58]

Mechanisms

Reliable, nontoxic methods of inducing transplantation tolerance are needed to overcome the problems of chronic organ graft rejection and immunosuppression-related toxicity. Potential approaches for the induction of tolerance in *adults* include (1) cell depletion protocols using total body irradiation or total lymphoid irradiation or depleting monoclonal antibodies; (2) reconstitution protocols using allogeneic bone marrow; (3) a combination of (1) and (2); (4) cell surface molecule–targeted therapy (e.g., use of anti-CD4 or anti-intercellular adhesion molecule monoclonal antibodies); (5) immunosuppressive drugs (e.g., cyclosporine, sirolimus); (6) donor-specific blood transfusion combined with drug or monoclonal antibody therapy; and (7) manipulation of specific cell populations.

The principal hypotheses proposed for the cellular basis of transplantation tolerance are *clonal deletion* (cell death for donor-reactive T cells) and *clonal anergy* (functional inactivation without cell death). Clonal deletion of antigen-reactive lymphocytes occurs either in the thymus or peripherally. Clonal anergy of lymphocytes is caused by the delivery of the antigenic signal alone without co-stimulatory signals or suppressor mechanisms. Suppressor mechanisms involve anti-idiotypic regulatory cells directed against the TCR idiotype of the responsive T lymphocytes, veto cells, or suppressor cytokines, such as tumor growth factor-beta (TGF-β). It has yet to be definitely established whether clonal deletion and clonal anergy are stages along a continuum in the T-cell interactions or whether these are two independent pathways produced by exposure to different toleragens under different conditions. An individual's immune system may develop unresponsiveness to a particular antigen, despite the presence of normally responsive lymphocytes. The normally responsive cells may be inhibited by other mechanisms, such as suppressor cells. Thus, any combination of deletion or inactivation of T cells and B cells could result in the failure of the immune system to respond to an antigen.

Monoclonal Antibodies

One of the major goals in therapeutic immunosuppression has been to achieve a long-term benefit from a short-term therapy. A variety of monoclonal antibodies to cell surface molecules, in particular anti-CD4, used alone or in combination with other immunosuppressive modalities such as cyclosporine or total lymphoid irradiation, induce tolerance in rodents.[5,59] Development of CD4 monoclonal antibodies that can induce immunologic tolerance without depleting CD4+ T cells has reawakened interest in the use of nondepleting monoclonal antibodies for reprogramming the immune system in autoimmunity and in transplantation. The mechanisms that are involved in tolerance induction and its maintenance are under debate. In a number of allogeneic transplant models (heart, skin, bone marrow), anti-CD4 (+CD8) antibodies block the rejection process by selectively promoting the development of CD4+/CD25+ regulatory T cells. As a result "infectious tolerance" occurs via these potent regulatory cells. This promotion of CD4+ provides a link between suppression and tolerance. In these models T cells that have never been exposed to CD4 antibodies become tolerant to grafted antigens when exposed to antigen in the microenvironment of regulatory T cells.[5] In addition to anti-CD4 monoclonal antibodies, antibodies targeting adhesion molecules, other molecules on T cells, or other molecules on APCs have emerged as important approaches to promoting tolerance induction. Monoclonal antibody therapy has been used in attempts at tolerance induction in primates using combinations of anti-CD154, anti-CD80, and anti-CD86 monoclonal antibodies.[60]

Donor Bone Marrow

Donor bone marrow has been shown to have a strong regulatory effect. The induction of unresponsiveness, with a combination of antilymphocyte serum and donor bone marrow, has been achieved in mice, dogs, and monkeys. It is thought that, under these circumstances, a naturally occurring regulatory cell (veto or suppressor cell) induces tolerance within the bone marrow inoculum. The development of these cells may be facilitated by appropriate growth factors, such as granulocyte-macrophage colony-stimulating factor and IL-3. In a limited human study conducted by Barber and colleagues,[10] transfusion of donor-specific bone marrow was performed a week after a course of ALG in cadaveric renal allograft recipients. These patients received conventional immunosuppressive drugs—cyclosporine, prednisone, and azathioprine—and most subjects were also administered cyclophosphamide at the time of marrow cell infusion. Even though the number of rejection episodes and renal function were not affected, graft survival at 1 year was improved significantly.

Ciancio and colleagues have demonstrated a significant decrease in the incidence of chronic rejection in human cadaveric renal recipients receiving donor bone marrow at the time of renal transplant. Acute rejection episodes were similar in the group receiving bone marrow infusion when compared with controls. In 6 years of follow-up, only 2 of 63 recipients receiving bone marrow developed biopsy-proven chronic rejection compared with 41 of 219 control recipients. Immunosuppressive drug therapy was identical in both groups. A similar study in living donor recipients did not demonstrate the same differences.[61,62]

Starzl and colleagues[63] have reported long-lasting donor-cell chimerism in conventionally immunosuppressed human organ allograft recipients. Augmentation of this *natural chimerism* by infusion of donor bone marrow at the time of organ transplantation is being performed in patients who do not receive any form of cytoreductive therapy. The procedure has been shown to be safe and effective in augmenting chimerism, but the chimerism is not yet accompanied by donor-specific tolerance.[61,62]

Suppressor Cells and Tolerance Induction

Suppressor cells have been implicated in a number of experimental models of tolerance induction.[2,64] Thus, the existence of suppressor T cells generated in the presence of cyclosporine can be demonstrated by the adoptive transfer of tolerance from cyclosporine-treated allograft recipients. It has not been possible, however, to show that cyclosporine can induce authentic tolerance in human organ transplantation. In experimental animals, donor-specific blood transfusion before transplantation induces antigen-specific unresponsiveness associated with dysregulation of IL-2 production and the generation of suppressor cells. Donor-specific blood transfusion with cyclosporine has been shown clinically to reduce sensitization and improve renal allograft outcome.

Hematopoietic Stem Cell Chimerism and Tolerance

The most robust form of donor-specific tolerance is that associated with hematopoietic stem cell chimerism. As previously mentioned, the first association between chimerism and tolerance was observed in the 1940s when Dr. Owen reported that Freemartin cattle were red blood cell chimeras.[57] The common placenta that they shared allowed exchange with hematopoietic stem cells. Although genetically disparate, these cattle accepted skin grafts from the other twin. Billingham and colleagues[56] demonstrated that this active transfer of tolerance to donor antigens was due to bone marrow hematopoietic stem cells from the donor. Subsequently, chimerism has been demonstrated to be associated with tolerance in mice, rats, pigs, nonhuman primates, and humans. Until recently, the risk of conventional bone marrow transplantation was too great to tolerate in clinical attempts to induce tolerance. However, a number of advances have made the clinical application of hematopoietic stem cell chimerism to induce tolerance a clinical reality. Reconstitution of mice with mixtures of T-cell–depleted syngeneic and allogeneic bone marrow (pioneered by Ildstad and

Sachs) produces mixed hematopoietic bone marrow chimerism and donor-specific tolerance to skin grafts. Most importantly, 1% donor chimerism is sufficient to provide robust deletional tolerance, opening the door to nonmyeloablative partial conditioning strategies to establish mixed chimerism. These nonmyeloablative approaches, using anti–T-cell monoclonal antibodies, cyclophosphamide, ALG, and tacrolimus, in addition to sublethal total body irradiation plus donor bone marrow, have been shown to induce tolerance in mice. Recent improvements in bone marrow processing and graft engineering to decrease the toxicity associated with GVHD may increase interest in this approach.

Mixed lymphopoietic chimerism has induced tolerance in humans treated by nonmyeloablative bone marrow transplantation for myeloma who also received a renal allograft. Both were free of myeloma and of rejection after receiving a nonmyeloablative conditioning regimen of cyclophosphamide, horse antithymocyte globulin, thymic irradiation with donor bone marrow infusion, kidney transplantation, and a 12-day course of cyclosporine. Chimerism was maintained for approximately 100 days before it became undetectable. Lack of durability of chimerism did not impact on the result; both recipients remain free of rejection without immunosuppressive drugs.[65]

Manipulation of Dendritic Cells

In addition to traditional concepts regarding the role of the thymus in negative and positive selection in the development of tolerance, recent work has focused on other cell populations and mechanisms of tolerance induction. There is mounting evidence that other nonparenchymal cells may play a role in the development of donor-specific tolerance. In a recent review, Coates and coworkers emphasized the potential role of passenger dendritic cells as mediators of allorecognition and as a potential target to induce donor-specific tolerance.[66] Dendritic cells are an excellent population to use for cell-based antirejection therapy in transplantation because they specifically target the T-cell–rich regions of draining lymph nodes. Immature dendritic cells can be driven to produce immunoregulatory properties by presentation of donor antigen in the absence of a second signal, inducing anergy in donor-specific recipient T cells.[66]

Additionally, another new and potentially important immune modulating strategy is the alternation of the antidonor response from a T_H1 to a T_H2 response. The vast majority of aggressive rejection immune responses are associated with a T_H1 phenotype, whereas animals with demonstrated allograft acceptance generally have T cells with a predominant T_H2 phenotype. It is thought that dendritic cells may promote this immune deviation from a T_H1 rejection profile by selective activation of the T_H2 cells. In the clinic, mobilization of hematopoietic stem cells with granulocyte colony-stimulating factor also mobilizes higher concentrations of precursor tolerogenic (plasmacytoid) dendritic cells. Studies to analyze the effect of these populations on tolerance induction in the clinic are in progress.[66]

NEW AREAS OF TRANSPLANTATION

Composite Tissue Allotransplantation

Composite tissue transplantation could benefit millions worldwide with lost limbs and extensive tissue defects. Since the first hand transplant was performed in Lyon, France, in September 1998, much excitement has been generated in the area of composite tissue allotransplantation. Within 4 years, 12 recipients received single hand transplants and 4 recipients received double hand transplants. All have had good functional recovery; the first recipient, however, required amputation after he elected to stop immunosuppression. The longest surviving hand recipient received his transplant in Louisville, Kentucky, in January 1999. His current abilities include tying his shoes, dialing his cell phone, turning doorknobs, throwing a ball, and sensitivity to hot and cold.[49]

Hand transplantation combines two well-established procedures: hand reimplantation and immunosuppressive therapy (Figs. 26-16 and 26-17). These transplant recipients have been maintained on standard immunosuppressive regimens of tacrolimus, mycophenolate mofetil, and prednisone. Tacrolimus speeds nerve regeneration in animal models, which also seems to be the case in the hand transplant recipients in whom nerve regeneration has proceeded more rapidly than would be expected from replant experience.[49] Despite the transplantation of vascularized bone marrow with the hand transplant, no evidence of donor chimerism or GVHD has been observed in the recipients.[67]

The success with hand transplantation has spurred research into other composite tissue allografts. Larynx transplantation successfully restored the voice of a 40-year-old man 20 years after a laryngeal crush injury.[68] If success is seen with tolerance protocols, further use of composite tissue allotransplants in areas of reconstructive surgery can be expected.

Islet Cell Transplantation

Nowhere in the field of transplantation are the advances in immunosuppression clearer than in the area of islet cell transplantation. Attempts at islet transplantation uniformly failed until the development of the so-called Edmonton protocol. A group in Edmonton, Alberta, reported their success in rendering recipients insulin free by using an immunosuppressive protocol of daclizumab, low-dose tacrolimus, and sirolimus. Corticosteroids and high doses of tacrolimus were avoided because both are known to be toxic to islets.[69]

Initially, islets from between two to four pancreata were needed to achieve insulin independence in these recipients. Subsequent progress in islet isolation technique at the University of Minnesota and other centers has achieved insulin independence using a single pancreas. Approximately 9,000 islet equivalents per kilogram of recipient body weight have been necessary to attain insulin independence.[69] The success with the Edmonton

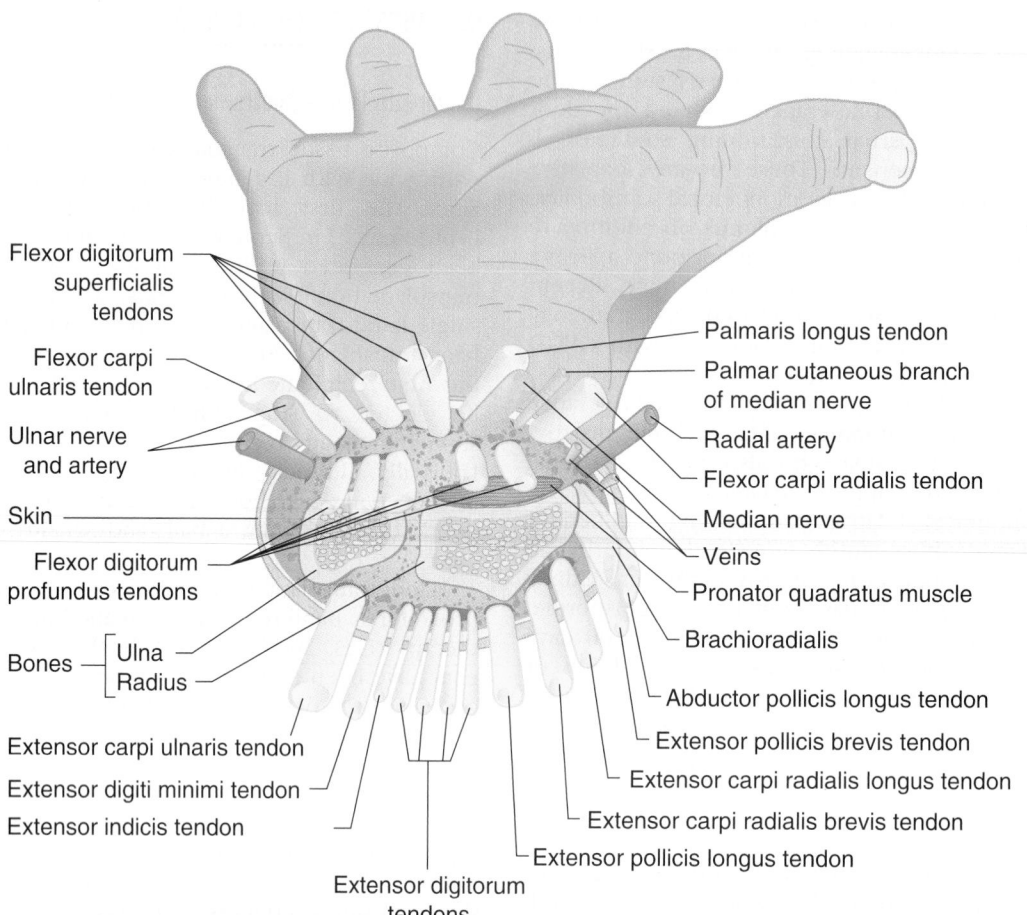

Flexor digitorum superficialis tendons

Flexor carpi ulnaris tendon

Ulnar nerve and artery

Skin

Flexor digitorum profundus tendons

Bones
- Ulna
- Radius

Extensor carpi ulnaris tendon

Extensor digiti minimi tendon

Extensor indicis tendon

Extensor digitorum tendons

Palmaris longus tendon

Palmar cutaneous branch of median nerve

Radial artery

Flexor carpi radialis tendon

Median nerve

Veins

Pronator quadratus muscle

Brachioradialis

Abductor pollicis longus tendon

Extensor pollicis brevis tendon

Extensor carpi radialis longus tendon

Extensor carpi radialis brevis tendon

Extensor pollicis longus tendon

FIGURE 26-16. Schematic of hand transplant. (Copyright 1998, Elaine Bammerlin.)

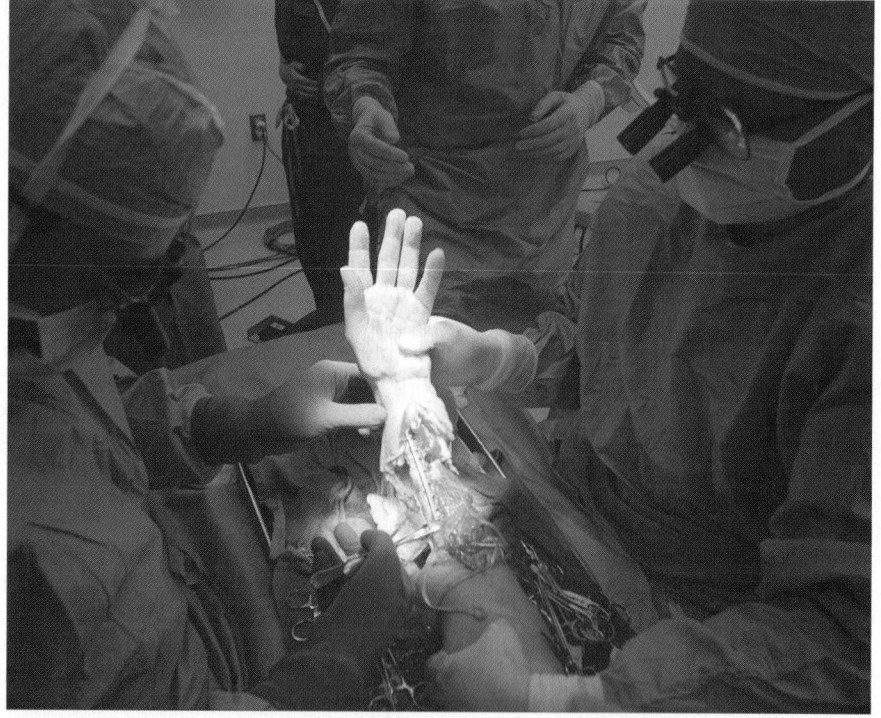

FIGURE 26-17. Dr. Warren Breidenbach and colleagues begin to attach the hand transplant. (Photograph courtesy of Patrick Pfister, Jewish Hospital, Louisville, KY.)

protocol has focused interest in corticosteroid avoidance regimens in other organ transplants.[31]

Tissue Engineering

The loss or failure of an organ or tissue is devastating. Current treatment methods include transplantation of organs, surgical reconstruction, use of mechanical devices, or supplementation of metabolic products. However, the ultimate goal of transplantation should reside in the ability to restore living cells to maintain or even enhance existing tissue function. This is emerging through the process of tissue engineering. Initial discoveries in engineered tissues were made in the mid-1980s with skin-based products. By developing replacement tissues that remain intact with bioactive properties after implantation, retaining physiologic functions as well as structure to the tissue or organ damaged by disease or trauma, tissue engineering could provide an alternative to transplantation and other forms of reconstruction. Skin replacement products are the most advanced, with several tissue-engineered wound care materials currently on the market worldwide. The potential impact of this field is endless, offering unique solutions to the medical field for tissue and organ replacement. Tissue engineering may eventually be applied to the regeneration of diverse tissues such as the liver, small intestine, cardiovascular structures, nerve, and cartilage. Work on bioartificial liver devices has been under way for several years.

The sources of cells required for tissue engineering are summarized by three categories: autologous cells (from the patient), allogeneic cells (from a donor, but not immunologically identical), and xenogeneic cells (donor from a different species). Each category may be further delineated in terms of stem cells (adult or embryonic) or "differentiated" cells obtained from tissue, where the cell population obtained from tissue dissociation comprises a mixture of cells at different maturation stages and includes rare stem and progenitor cells. Recent discoveries have indicated that stem cells of one type can *transdifferentiate* to repair damaged tissue of another type (i.e., hematopoietic stem cells home to infarcted myocardium and repair the tissue). Tissue engineering will remain an area of intense research. Advances in the areas of growth factors, stromal matrices, gene encapsulation, and gene delivery will all play a role.

CONCLUSION

Progress continues in the areas of immunosuppressive therapy, xenotransplantation, transplant tolerance induction, tissue engineering, and our overall understanding of the immune system. Much remains to be learned, however, before patients with end-organ failure can live free of the risks and expenses now associated with solid organ transplantation. Still, it is an exciting time to be involved in transplantation: the "Holy Grail" of transplantation,[70] namely, transplantation tolerance, does appear much closer.

ACKNOWLEDGMENT

The authors wish to acknowledge the technical assistance of Carolyn DeLautre in preparation of the manuscript.

Selected References

Abbas AK, Lichtman AH, Pober JS: Cellular and Molecular Immunology, 4th ed. Philadelphia, WB Saunders, 2000.

This is a concise, well-illustrated textbook of immunology.

Auchincloss H Jr: In search of the elusive Holy Grail: The mechanism and prospects for achieving clinical transplantation tolerance. Am J Transplant 1:6, 2001.

Auchincloss succeeds in simplifying a rather complex topic in this minireview.

Coates PTH, Calvin BL, Hackstein H, Thomas AW: Manipulation of dendritic cells as an approach to improved outcomes in transplantation. Exp Rev Mol Med, 2002. http://www-ermm.cbcu.cam.ac.uk/02004283h.htm.

Online review discusses the impact of dendritic cells on transplantation. It includes a helpful list of other online resources.

Dorling A: Clinical xenotransplantation: Pigs might fly? Am J Transplant 2:695, 2002.

This review delineates the current barriers to xenotransplantation.

Foster CE, Philosophe B, Schweitzer EJ, et al: A decade of experience with renal transplantation in African Americans. Ann Surg 236:794, 2002.

The group from the University of Maryland touches upon the many issues facing clinical transplantation today, including donor shortages, viral infections, long waiting times, and immunosuppression, as well as advances over 10 years.

References

1. Abbas AK, Lichtman AH, Pober JS: Cellular and Molecular Immunology, 4th ed. Philadelphia, WB Saunders, 2000.
2. Sayegh MH, Watschinger B, Carpenter CB: Mechanisms of T cell recognition of alloantigen: The role of peptides. Transplantation 57:1295, 1994.
3. Thomson AW, Catto GRD (eds): Major and minor histocompatibility antigens. *In* Immunology of Renal Transplantation. Boston, Little, Brown, 1993.
4. Arai K, Tsuruta L, Watanabe S, et al: Cytokine signal networks and a new era in biomedical research. Mol Cells 7:1, 1997.
5. Waldmann H, Cobbold S: How do monoclonal antibodies induce tolerance? A role for infectious tolerance? Annu Rev Immunol 16:619, 1998.
6. Kappler JW, Roehm N, Marrack P: T cell tolerance by clonal elimination in the thymus. Cell 49:273, 1987.
7. Sollinger HW: Mycophenolate mofetil for the prevention of acute rejection in primary cadaveric renal allograft recipients. U.S. Renal Transplant Mycophenolate Mofetil Study Group. Transplantation 60:225, 1995.
8. Gruber SA, Chan GLC, Canafax DM, et al: Immunosuppression in renal transplantation: I. Cyclosporine and azathioprine. Clin Transplant 5:65, 1991.

9. Williams JW, Mital D, Chong A, et al: Experiences with leflunomide in solid organ transplantation. Transplantation 73:358, 2002.

10. Brouha PC, Ildstad ST: Mixed allogeneic chimerism. Past, present, and prospects for the future. Transplantation 72:S36, 2001.

11. Burrows PD, Cooper MD: B cell development and differentiation. Curr Opin Immunol 9:239, 1997.

12. Nagata S, Suda T: Fas and Fas ligand: *lpr* and *gld* mutations. Immunol Today 16:39, 1995.

13. de Mattos AM, Norman DJ: OKT3 for treatment of rejection in renal transplantation. Transplantation 7:374, 1993.

14. Guinan EC, Gribben JG, Boussiotis VA, et al: Pivotal role of the B7:CD28 pathway in transplantation tolerance and tumor immunity. Blood 84:3261, 1994.

15. Greenfield EA, Nguyen KA, Kuchroo VK: CD28/B7 costimulation: A review. Crit Rev Immunol 18:389, 1998.

16. Romagnani S: The T_H1/T_H2 paradigm. Immunol Today 18:263, 1997.

17. Drobyski W, Ash R, Casper JT, et al: Effect of T-cell depletion as graft-versus-host-disease prophylaxis on engraftment, relapse, and disease-free survival in unrelated marrow transplantation for chronic myelogenous leukemia. Blood 83:1980, 1994.

18. Ildstad ST, Vecchini F, Johnson PC, et al: Mixed allogeneic chimeras (A+B→A): Evidence for syngeneic and allogeneic donor stem cell co-engraftment and stable multilineage chimerism. Transplant Sci 3:123, 1993.

19. Akashi K, Kondo M, Freeden-Jeffry U, et al: Bcl-2 rescues T lymphopoiesis in interleukin-7 receptor-deficient mice. Cell 89:1033, 1997.

20. Thomas ED: Frontiers in bone marrow transplantation. Blood Cells 17:259, 1991.

21. van Furth R: Human monocytes and cytokines. Res Immunol 149:719, 1998.

22. Rissoan MC, Soumelis V, Kadowaki N, et al: Reciprocal control of T helper cell and dendritic cell differentiation. Science 283:1183, 1999.

23. Manilay JO, Sykes M: Natural killer cells and their role in graft rejection. Curr Opin Immunol 10:532, 1998.

24. Rulifson IC, Szot GL, Palmer E, et al: Inability to induce tolerance through direct antigen presentation. Am J Transplant 2:510, 2002.

25. Orosz CG, VanBuskirk AM: Immune mechanisms of acute rejection. Transplant Proc 30:859, 1998.

26. Halloran PF, Melk A, Barth C: Rethinking chronic allograft nephropathy: The concept of accelerated senescence. J Am Soc Nephrol 10:167, 1999.

27. Fishman JA, Rubin RH: Infection in organ-transplant recipients. N Engl J Med 338:1741, 1998.

28. Vats A, Shapiro R, Singh RP, et al: Quantitative viral load monitoring and cidofovir therapy for the management of BK virus-associated nephropathy in children and adults. Transplantation 75:105, 2003.

29. Penn I: Post-transplant malignancies. Transplant Proc 31:1260, 1999.

30. Verschuuren EA, Stevens SJ, van Imhoff GW, et al: Treatment of post-transplant lymphoproliferative disease with rituximab: The remission, the relapse, and the complication. Transplantation 73:100, 2002.

31. Matas AJ, Ramcharan T, Paraskevas S, et al: Rapid discontinuation of steroids in living donor kidney transplantation: A pilot study. Am J Transplant 1:278, 2001.

32. Sells RA: Cardiovascular complications following renal transplantation. Transplant Review 11:111, 1997.

33. Gaber AO, First MR, Tesi RJ, et al: Results of the double-blind, randomized, multicenter, phase III clinical trial of Thymoglobulin versus Atgam in the treatment of acute graft rejection episodes after renal transplantation. Transplantation 66:29, 1998.

34. Goldstein G: Overview of the development of Orthoclone OKT3: Monoclonal antibody for therapeutic use in transplantation. Transplant Proc 19:1, 1987.

35. Kahan BD, Rajagopalan PR, Hall M: Reduction of the occurrence of acute cellular rejection among renal allograft recipients treated with basiliximab, a chimeric anti-interleukin-2-receptor monoclonal antibody. United States Simulect Renal Study Group. Transplantation 67:276, 1999.

36. Vincenti F, Kirkman R, Light S, et al: Interleukin-2-receptor blockade with daclizumab to prevent acute rejection in renal transplantation. Daclizumab Triple Therapy Study Group [comment]. N Engl J Med 338:161, 1998.

37. Aranda JM Jr, Scornik JC, Normann SJ, et al: Anti-CD20 monoclonal antibody (rituximab) therapy for acute cardiac humoral rejection: A case report. Transplantation 73:907, 2002.

38. Calne R, Moffatt SD, Friend PJ, et al: Campath IH allows low-dose cyclosporine monotherapy in 31 cadaveric renal allograft recipients. Transplantation 68:1613, 1999.

39. Reams BD, Davis RD, Curl J, et al: Treatment of refractory acute rejection in a lung transplant recipient with campath 1H. Transplantation 74:903, 2002.

40. Glotz D, Antoine C, Julia P, et al: Desensitization and subsequent kidney transplantation of patients using intravenous immunoglobulins (IVIg). Am J Transplant 2:758, 2002.

41. Luke PP, Scantlebury VP, Jordan ML, et al: Reversal of steroid- and anti-lymphocyte antibody-resistant rejection using intravenous immunoglobulin (IVIG) in renal transplant recipients. Transplantation 72:419, 2001.

42. Gruber SA, Chan GLC, Canafax DM, et al: Immunosuppression in renal transplantation: II. Corticosteroids, antilymphocyte globulin, and OKT3. Clin Transplant 5:219, 1991.

43. Kahan BD: Cyclosporine. N Engl J Med 321:1725, 1989.

44. Sigal NH, Dumont FJ: Cyclosporin A, FK-506, and rapamycin: Pharmacologic probes of lymphocyte signal transduction. Annu Rev Immunol 10:519, 1992.

45. Kahan BD, Koch SM: Current immunosuppressant regimens: Considerations for critical care. Curr Opin Crit Care 7:242, 2001.

46. Langer RM, Kahan BD: Incidence, therapy, and consequences of lymphocele after sirolimus-cyclosporine-prednisone immunosuppression in renal transplant recipients. Transplantation 74:804, 2002.

47. Vincenti F: What's in the pipeline? New immunosuppressive drugs in transplantation. Am J Transplant 2:898, 2002.

48. Gruber SA: The case for local immunosuppression. Transplantation 54:1, 1992.

49. Jones JW, Gruber SA, Barker JH, et al: Successful hand transplantation: One-year follow-up. N Engl J Med 343:468, 2000.

50. Gloor JM, Moore SB, Pineda AA, et al: Living donor kidney transplantation in positive crossmatch patients [abstract]. Am J Transplant 2, 2002.

51. Dorling A: Clinical xenotransplantation: Pigs might fly? Am J Transplant 2:695, 2002.

52. van der Laan LJ, Lockey C, Griffeth BC, et al: Infection by porcine endogenous retrovirus after islet xenotransplantation in SCID mice. Nature 407:90, 2000.

53. Auchincloss H Jr, Sachs DH: Xenogeneic transplantation. Annu Rev Immunol 16:433, 1998.

54. Spitzer TR, Delmonico F, Tolkoff-Rubin N, et al: Combined histocompatibility leukocyte antigen-matched donor bone marrow and renal transplantation for multiple myeloma with end stage renal disease: The induction of allograft tol-

erance through mixed lymphohematopoietic chimerism. Transplantation 68:480, 1999.

55. Sayegh MH, Fine NA, Smith JL, et al: Immunologic tolerance to renal allografts after bone marrow transplants from the same donors. Ann Intern Med 114:954, 1991.

56. Billingham RE, Brent L, Medawar PB: Actively acquired tolerance to foreign cells. Nature 172:603, 1953.

57. Owen RD: Immunogenetic consequences of vascular anastomoses between bovine twins. Science 102:400, 1945.

58. Ildstad ST, Sachs DH: Reconstitution with syngeneic plus allogeneic or xenogeneic bone marrow leads to specific acceptance of allografts or xenografts. Nature 307:168, 1984.

59. Strober S, Dhillon M, Schubert M, et al: Acquired immune tolerance to cadaveric renal allografts: A study of three patients treated with total lymphoid irradiation. N Engl J Med 321:28, 1989.

60. Montgomery SP, Xu H, Tadaki DK, et al: Combination induction therapy with monoclonal antibodies specific for CD80, CD86, and CD154 in nonhuman primate renal transplantation. Transplantation 74:1365, 2002.

61. Ciancio G, Burke GW, Garcia-Morales R, et al: Effect of living-related donor bone marrow infusion on chimerism and in vitro immunoregulatory activity in kidney transplant recipients. Transplantation 74:488, 2002.

62. Ciancio G, Miller J, Garcia-Morales RO, et al: Six-year clinical effect of donor bone marrow infusions in renal transplant patients. Transplantation 71:827, 2001.

63. Starzl TE, Demetris AJ, Murase N, et al: Cell migration, chimerism and graft acceptance. Lancet 339:1579, 1992.

64. Bloom BR, Salgame P, Diamond B: Revisiting and revising suppressor T cells. Immunol Today 13:131, 1992.

65. Buhler LH, Spitzer TR, Sykes M, et al: Induction of kidney allograft tolerance after transient lymphohematopoietic chimerism in patients with multiple myeloma and end-stage renal disease. Transplantation 74:1405, 2002.

66. Coates PT, Thomson AW: Dendritic cells, tolerance induction and transplant outcome. Am J Transplant 2:299, 2002.

67. Granger DK, Breidenbach WC, Pidwell DJ, et al: Lack of donor hyporesponsiveness and donor chimerism after clinical transplantation of the hand. Transplantation 74:1624, 2002.

68. Nelson M, Fritz M, Lorenz R, et al: Update on laryngeal transplantation. Graft 5:437, 2002.

69. Ryan EA, Lakey JR, Paty BW, et al: Successful islet transplantation: Continued insulin reserve provides long-term glycemic control. Diabetes 51:2148, 2002.

70. Auchincloss H Jr: In search of the elusive Holy Grail: The mechanism and prospects for achieving clinical transplantation tolerance. Am J Transplant 1:6, 2001.

CHAPTER 27

TRANSPLANTATION OF ABDOMINAL ORGANS

James F. Markmann, M.D., PH.D., Kenneth L. Brayman, M.D., PH.D., Ali Naji, M.D., PH.D., Kim M. Olthoff, M.D., Abraham Shaked, M.D., PH.D., and Clyde F. Barker, M.D.

Renal Transplantation	**Transplantation of Isolated Pancreatic Islets**
Liver Transplantation	**Intestinal Transplantation**
Pancreatic Transplantation	**Socioeconomic and Ethical Considerations**

The earliest attempts at organ transplantation in humans were made during the first decade of the 20th century.[1] Since animal donors were used for these grafts, they functioned either briefly or not at all. However, the therapeutic promise of allografts became apparent from animal experiments also performed during the same decade by Alexis Carrel, who successfully transplanted kidneys and other organs into animals, utilizing this model to develop the technique of modern blood vessel surgery. This brilliant work resulted in a Nobel Prize in 1912 but was so far ahead of its time that it was not followed by further clinical trials for another 40 years. Not until the early 1950s did Medawar's detailed description of rejection, and his discovery with Billingham and Brent that it could be prevented in mice by tolerance, stimulate surgeons to resume attempts at human renal transplantation.[2] Medawar's work was rewarded with a Nobel Prize in 1960. Some of the clinical trials that followed it were technically successful, but because immunosuppressive drugs were yet to be discovered the transplanted kidney allografts were all destroyed by rejection. However, transplants from identical twins begun in 1954 by Murray in Boston were successful. In the late 1950s, rejection was first circumvented in several patients by Murray, in Boston, and Hamburger, in Paris, by the use of whole-body irradiation. Murray was later (1990) awarded the Nobel Prize for his role in these pioneering studies. When immunosuppressive drugs became available in the early 1960s, prolonged allograft survival became more common, although not yet consistent. Progress in histocompatibility typing, immunosuppressive therapy, organ preservation, and the accumulation of clinical experience gradually resulted in improved results of transplantation, which now frequently allows successful replacement not only of failing kidneys but of the other vital organs as well.

This chapter describes transplantation of abdominal organs (kidney, liver, pancreas, small bowel). Because the kidney was the first organ to be transplanted extensively, experience acquired in renal transplantation programs has been the basis of much of the current management of other organ transplants as well. Therefore, renal transplantation is considered first; contained in this section are discussions of several topics, which are also relevant to all other organ transplants: histocompatibility, immunosuppression, management of cadaveric donors, and the possibilities of xenotransplantation.

RENAL TRANSPLANTATION

Indications

The three diseases most commonly leading to renal failure and treated by kidney transplantation are insulin-dependent diabetes mellitus, glomerulonephritis, and hypertensive nephrosclerosis, accounting for about 60% of the total.[3] Other important causes include polycystic kidney disease, Alport's disease, immunoglobulin (Ig) A nephropathy, systemic lupus erythematosus, nephrosclerosis, interstitial nephritis, pyelonephritis, and obstructive uropathy. In African Americans, hypertensive nephrosclerosis is the most common of all causes of renal failure.

The best recipients are young individuals whose renal failure is not due to a systemic disease that will damage the transplanted kidney or cause death from extrarenal causes. With the increasing appreciation that the results of transplantation are superior to those of chronic dialysis, the indications for transplantation have been broadened. The presence of infection or malignancy that cannot be eradicated remains an absolute contraindication to transplantation because immunosuppression encourages both microbial and tumor growth. Although history of a successfully treated cancer is not a contraindication to transplantation, it is a general rule to wait at least 2 years before transplantation is justified. Even then recurrent cancer may still occur, possibly encouraged by immunosuppression. In fact, 13% of recurrent cancers take place in recipients who were tumor free for over 5 years before their transplants. Predicted noncompliance is another contraindication because careful adherence to immunosuppression is necessary. Advanced age and severe cardiovascular disease, such as unreconstructable coronary artery or aortoiliac disease, are also deterrents. However, even in such patients, the long-term cumulative risks of dialysis are at least as great as those of transplantation. Therefore, because of improvements in perioperative care and immunosuppression, many patients who would previously have been denied transplantation are now considered acceptable. For example, diabetics, once considered poor candidates, clearly do better with transplantation than with dialysis. In fact, both graft and patient survival for 1 to 2 years are reported to be as good in diabetics as in other patients, whereas on chronic dialysis less than 20% of diabetics survive 5 years.[3] Even patients with diseases in which the transplanted kidney may eventually be damaged by recurrent disease (e.g., lupus erythematosus, cystinosis, amyloidosis, diabetes, and some forms of glomerulonephritis) are often better palliated by transplantation than by dialysis. Indeed, the current results of transplantation mandate serious consideration of this therapy in virtually any patient with terminal renal disease. Not only is the quality of life far better with transplantation than with dialysis, but because the mortality of patients in the first year after transplantation is now less than 5%, survival is also superior. Unfortunately, however, the insufficient availability of donors keeps many appropriate transplant candidates on chronic dialysis. In fact, the number of patients awaiting transplantation is increasing more rapidly than the number of transplants done per year.[3]

Recipient Evaluation and Preparation

The evaluation of all transplant candidates, in addition to a standard medical work-up, should include cytomegalovirus (CMV) antibody titer; creatinine clearance; serology for syphilis, human immunodeficiency virus (HIV), and hepatitis B (HBV) and C (HCV) viruses; evaluation of parathyroid status; coagulation profile; Papanicolaou smear; ABO and histocompatibility typing; urologic evaluation (including a voiding cystourethrogram in selected patients to assess outlet obstruction and reflux);

gastrointestinal evaluation (as warranted by history of ulcer, diverticulitis, or other symptoms); and psychiatric evaluation.

The proper timing of transplantation is a delicate decision because the progression of renal dysfunction is variable and premature imposition of the risks of transplantation is not justified. However, dialysis or transplantation should not be withheld until advanced uremic symptoms, such as pericarditis, cardiac failure, severe anemia, osteodystrophy, and neuropathy, ensue because these complications may become irreversible. Even when a donor is readily available, pretransplant dialysis is often necessary, at least briefly, to optimize the patient's general condition (nutrition, electrolyte balance, and coagulation status). Careful attention must be given to eradication of all infections, including those of the urinary tract, lungs, teeth, and skin (especially at the site of the planned incision). Because cardiovascular complications are as common as infection as a cause of posttransplantation mortality, the patient's cardiovascular status should be carefully evaluated and optimized. In older patients and diabetics, this might require stress testing, cardiac catheterization, or even pretransplant coronary artery bypass.

Histocompatibility Typing and Crossmatching

Although opinions vary regarding the significance of histocompatibility testing for selection of unrelated donors, its importance is unquestionable for selection of the optimal donor within a family. Regardless of the donor source, compatibility for ABO blood groups and a negative leukocyte crossmatch are mandatory.

ABO BLOOD GROUPS

Because the major blood group antigens are not expressed by human leukocytes, it was initially assumed that they might be unimportant in transplant rejection. However, experimental and clinical evidence soon indicated that ABO antigens function as important histocompatibility antigens.[4] In animals, prior exposure to erythrocytes from incompatible donors provoked accelerated rejection of skin grafts from donors of the same blood group. In the early days of renal transplantation, it was noted that ABO incompatibility often led to acute or hyperacute rejection, a finding that resulted in adherence to the rule of blood group compatibility. Because of the donor organ shortage and reports of some success with ABO-incompatible liver and heart allografts, attempts have been made at breaching the ABO barrier for kidney allografts. Successful transplantation is quite possible in blood group O or B recipients of kidneys from A2 donors (who have a lower number of A antigenic determinants on their cells than A1 donors).[5] Successful ABO-incompatible transplants have also been reported in recipients whose ABO isoagglutinins have been removed by plasmapheresis or immunoadsorption. Because isoagglutinins eventually reappear and the long-term outcome of these transplants is likely to be inferior, most centers do not employ this strategy. However, it is an intriguing approach, especially for allowing utilization of ABO-incompatible family donors. One report of 67 ABO-incompatible kidney donor transplants indicates that 75% of such grafts can survive after 6 years.[6]

LYMPHOCYTOTOXIC CROSSMATCHING

Sensitization to human leukocyte antigen (HLA), as indicated by the presence of lymphocytotoxic antibodies in the recipient's serum, may occur as a result of pregnancy, blood transfusions, or prior transplantation. Presence of donor-reactive antibodies, detected by incubation of recipient serum with donor cells in the presence of complement (a positive "crossmatch"), is a contraindication to renal transplantation because of its strong association with hyperacute renal allograft rejection. Serum from patients awaiting cadaveric renal transplantation is periodically screened against a panel of randomly selected HLA-typed lymphocyte donors. Nonreactivity of the patient's serum to the panel cells indicates a high likelihood of obtaining a crossmatch-compatible donor, whereas uniform reactivity of the patient's serum with panel cells greatly reduces this probability. The number of highly sensitized patients on most transplant waiting lists is increasing as less-sensitized patients receive transplants while sensitized individuals remain on the list and those with failed renal allografts (frequently sensitized) are returned to the list.

Successful transplantation can often be achieved despite positivity of certain types of crossmatch, a finding that allows transplantation of some apparently sensitized patients. For example, lymphocytotoxic autoantibodies do not cause rejection. In some patients, the titers of bona fide lymphocytotoxic antibodies decline or disappear with time. In the past, it was a common practice to store serum from the period of peak sensitization for later use in crossmatching, and if it was found positive, transplantation was denied, even if current serum was negative. Several reports now indicate that a positive crossmatch using peak serum may be disregarded with only a minimal risk of hyperacute rejection, provided that the current serum is negative. The conditions that allow transplantation in a patient with a "historical" positive but current negative crossmatch are not clearly defined. Most centers require a certain interval (1 to 12 months) between the last positive serum and transplantation. There is controversy whether the most sensitive crossmatching methods such as antiglobulin and flow cytometry techniques should be used because they may exclude donors that might have been used successfully. In addition, the clinical relevance of positive crossmatches to B lymphocytes (especially if performed in the cold) and those caused only by IgM antibodies is questionable. Attempts have also been made to define the role of antibodies against minor (non-HLA) specificities. For example, there is evidence that antibodies reactive to determinants on vascular endothelial cells can damage renal allografts.

To allow transplantation of sensitized patients, several methods have been tried to remove cytotoxic antibody (including thoracic duct drainage, total lymphoid irradiation, and plasmapheresis). Recently, several groups have explored the ability of intravenous immunoglobulin (IVIG) to inhibit anti-HLA antibodies by an anti-idiotypic mechanism. They have shown in a limited number of patients that IVIG can reduce the levels of antibody in highly sensitized transplant candidates, thus increasing the likelihood of finding a crossmatch-negative donor and allowing successful transplantation.[7] Because none of these maneuvers has yet gained wide acceptance, the increasingly large sensitized patient pool remains a formidable problem.

Attempts to Induce Specific Unresponsiveness

Blood Transfusions

In the first two decades of renal transplantation, transfusions were avoided whenever possible to minimize the formation of lymphocytotoxic antibodies, which might exclude patients from transplantation or damage the allograft. However, in 1973, Opelz and colleagues[8] made the surprising observation in a multi-institutional survey that renal allograft survival was actually 10% to 15% better in transfused than in nontransfused recipients. This resulted in a worldwide policy of deliberate pretransplant blood transfusions, which was subsequently credited with a substantial improvement in the outcome of renal transplants that occurred over the next decade.

Reasons for this beneficial "transfusion effect" were unclear. Some thought that transfusions simply prevented "high-responder" patients from being transplanted by sensitizing them so that they were crossmatch positive to most available donors, causing more kidneys to go instead to "low-responder" patients, who remained crossmatch negative despite transfusions and were likely to have a successful transplant, but for reasons unrelated to the transfusions. Another possible explanation was that transfusions had a true immunosuppressive effect, mediated through induction of suppressor T lymphocytes or enhancing alloantibodies.

With the improvement in graft survival that occurred when the new immunosuppressive agent cyclosporine became available in 1984, the need for blood transfusions was questioned. For a few years, there was disagreement as to whether cyclosporine-treated patients still benefited from transfusions, but within the ensuing 5 to 6 years it became apparent that whatever the mechanism of the transfusion effect, it was no longer discernible because of the improved outcome in all patients.[9] Because of this finding and the risks of transmitting infection (HIV and hepatitis) or of sensitizing patients to prospective donors, pretransplant transfusions have largely been abandoned at most centers.

Bone Marrow Conditioning

Although pretransplant blood transfusions are now rarely practiced, there has been an interest in conditioning recipients with bone marrow from the organ donor. Although this procedure might act by the same (unexplained) mechanism as blood transfusions, an additional intriguing rationale is the self-replicating ability of bone marrow and the resultant potential for persistent microchimerism. For many years, animal experiments have shown that administration of donor bone marrow is an especially effective method of conditioning transplant recipients. Bone marrow was found by Billingham, Brent, and Medawar in the 1950s to be an ideal inoculum for induction of acquired donor-specific immunologic tolerance.[2] Monaco[10] later found that donor bone marrow promotes skin allograft survival in adult rodents if combined with a brief course of antilymphocyte serum. In 1987, Barber and colleagues initiated a randomized study in which cryopreserved donor bone marrow was administered 10 to 14 days after kidney transplantation to recipients who were treated with antilymphocyte serum (ALS) and other standard immunosuppressive agents. Because the incidence of acute rejection was decreased, the early results were intriguing. However, improvement in long-term patient and graft survival was not impressive and, disappointingly, chronic rejection was not prevented.[11]

Other investigators continue to study the administration of donor bone marrow as a possible method of inducing "tolerance" to human recipients of renal and pancreas transplants.[12] Although they have reported that the incidence of rejection episodes is less and that there is greater likelihood that the patient can successfully be weaned from corticosteroid therapy, the long-term graft survival was not different than that of non–bone marrow–treated recipients. Microchimerism for donor cells can often be found in successful bone marrow–treated recipients (and also in tissues of non–bone marrow–treated recipients), but it remains controversial whether this is an epiphenomenon or the cause or effect of successful organ transplantation.

Pretransplant Operations

Any necessary urinary tract reconstructions must be carried out before transplantation (e.g., lysis of posterior urethral valves, transurethral resection for obstructing prostatic hypertrophy). The patient's own bladder should be utilized for ureteroneocystostomy, even if this necessitates bladder reconstruction or augmentation of a small bladder by ileocecocystoplasty. Careful intermittent catheterization of a neurogenic bladder three or four times daily after transplantation is preferable to the use of an intestinal conduit. In the absence of an alternative strategy, ileal conduits should be constructed at least 6 weeks before the transplant operation to avoid risk of infection.

Bilateral nephrectomy of recipients was once routine, the rationale being that even if current urine was sterile, pyelonephritic kidneys would remain a dangerous focus of infection and that glomerulonephritic kidneys, if retained, would be a stimulus for autoimmune destruction of the allograft. Because evidence to support these hypotheses was never forthcoming, bilateral nephrectomy is now performed only for special indications, such as recalcitrant urinary tract infections (especially in the presence of stones, reflux, or obstruction), uncontrollable hypertension, massive proteinuria, bilateral renal tumors, or large polycystic kidneys, especially if they are bleeding or infected.

Splenectomy was at one time widely practiced on an empirical basis for its nonspecific immunosuppressive effect. A large randomized study eventually indicated that the procedure modestly improved early, but not late, graft survival.[13]

Selection and Management of Living Donors

For the prospective recipient, there are major advantages to obtaining a living donor that obviates the discomfort, expense, and risks of prolonged dialysis while waiting for a cadaver kidney. Post-transplant morbidity is also minimized by decreasing the chances of acute tubular necrosis (ATN). Since the advent of cyclosporine therapy, short-term results of cadaveric transplantation now approach those with living related donors. Nevertheless, because of better histocompatibility, long-term results of related donor transplantation remain superior to those of cadaveric grafts.[3] Thus, most authorities believe the use of living donors is still justified, and in the United States, they account for about 35% of kidney transplants.

Histocompatibility Considerations in Living Donor Selection

The HLA antigens are gene products of alleles at a number of closely linked loci on the short arm of chromosome 6 in humans. At least six HLAs (A, B, C, DQ, DP, DR) have been defined, and the existence of several others has been deduced from family studies and immunochemical findings. The extreme polymorphism of the HLA system, which is the basis of infinite genetic variability of the human species, plays a pivotal role in regulation of the immune response. The gene products of the HLA-A, -B, and -C loci are referred to as class I major histocompatibility complex (MHC) antigens, and the products of the D region are class II MHC antigens. Class I MHC antigens are expressed on all nucleated cells and can be readily detected serologically using lymphocytotoxicity assays. Class II MHC antigens are important in antigen presentation and are expressed on B lymphocytes, dendritic cells, endothelium, and activated T cells.

HLA antigens are inherited as codominant alleles, and because of the relatively low recombinant frequency, the HLA genes are usually inherited en bloc from each parent. In immediate families, inheritance of the HLA, which is of overriding importance in transplant outcome, can be determined serologically and falls into four different combinations of haplotypes. Any two siblings have a 25% chance of being HLA identical, that is, of having inherited the same chromosome 6 (haplotype) from each parent, a 50% chance of sharing one haplotype, and a 25% chance of sharing neither haplotype. Parent-to-child donation always involves a one-haplotype identity.

The importance of matching HLA antigens in the selection of living related donors for renal transplantation is well established. Excellent graft survival (>95%) can be expected when a related donor and a recipient are HLA identical. There is a progressively lower graft survival associated with one or zero haplotype matches, although even totally mismatched related living donor grafts have a significantly better outcome than cadaveric grafts.[3]

Risks to the Living Donor

Despite the major advantages of related donors, their use is justified only if the risks to the donor are minimal. Nevertheless, it is important to frankly present these risks to the donor. In addition to discomfort and morbidity associated with any operation, there is an operative mortality of about 0.05%. Concern for even a small mortality rate has led to a traditional policy of accepting as donors only individuals between 18 and 55 years of age and in virtually perfect health. Because donor age limits are now being extended at most centers, it is important to exercise even greater care to avoid unacceptable risks.

Obviously, the donor must have two normal kidneys, as confirmed by standard renal function tests, intravenous pyelography, and imaging of the renal arteries. Magnetic resonance angiography is now substituted for contrast arteriography at many centers. This minimizes the risk of the procedure to the donor, although it has the disadvantage that small accessory renal arteries may not be visualized by this technique. Despite the knowledge that unilateral nephrectomy is followed by compensatory hypertrophy of the remaining kidney, near-normal renal function, and normal life expectancy, concern has been expressed regarding the long-term status of living donors. This concern is based on the finding that ablation of renal tissue in an experimental rat model leads to hyperfiltration by the remaining kidney tissue and eventual functional deterioration owing to sclerosis. Ten years after nephrectomy, some human donors have also been noted to exhibit proteinuria and hypertension, and a small number have exhibited renal failure, although in the largest single-center study with more than 20 years' follow up this number did not differ from the control population.[14]

The identification of a donor from a family group is preferably based on histocompatibility factors, although selection of a less well-matched donor by a well-informed family must be respected. It is important that potential candidates be protected from pressure to donate against their will, especially if they are minors. However, most family members willingly donate, and the psychological benefits of doing so are often profound.

Living Unrelated Donors

Until recently, unrelated volunteers were excluded from donation because the results were assumed not sufficiently advantageous compared with those of cadaver grafts to warrant the risk. However, the improvement in unrelated kidney allograft survival with cyclosporine and the shortage of cadaver donors provoked re-examination of this issue. Whereas the use of paid donors is unlawful, genetically unrelated but emotionally related donors (especially spouses) are now considered acceptable by most centers and, by 2002, accounted for about 25% of living donor transplants (Fig. 27-1).[3] Surprisingly, these transplants have graft survival as good at 5 and 10 years as living related transplants, except for those from HLA-identical sibling donors, and were significantly better than the survival of cadaveric transplants.

Techniques of Living Donor Nephrectomy

The left kidney is chosen if possible because its longer renal vein facilitates the recipient operation. However, if the arteriogram shows multiple renal arteries on one side, the kidney with a single artery is usually selected to facilitate the anastomosis. A flank incision is used. After incising the Gerota fascia, the greater curvature of the kidney and upper pole are mobilized, and the hilar structures are exposed. On the left side, the adrenal and gonadal veins are ligated so that the full length of the renal vein can be utilized. Traction on the renal artery should be avoided because it causes spasm and decreased kidney perfusion, possibly compromising early function. The ureter should be mobilized along with its blood supply and a generous amount of periureteric tissue. It is divided close to the

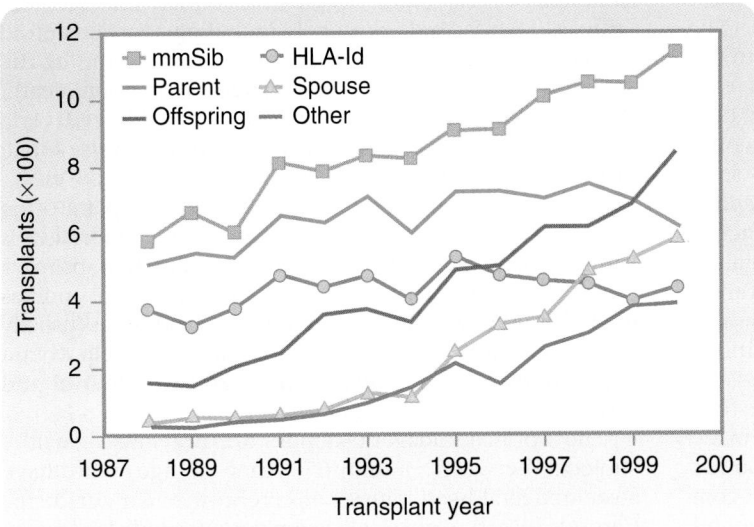

FIGURE 27-1. The shortage of cadaveric donors and the recognition that renal transplants from unrelated donors fare as well as those from genetic relatives (except HLA identical siblings) have encouraged the use of genetically unrelated but emotionally related donors, which now account for 25% of living donor kidneys.

bladder after ligating the distal end. If the donor is well hydrated, urine should be seen issuing from the proximal end of the divided ureter. Mannitol and furosemide are useful in promoting a diuresis. At this stage, attention is given to coordinating with the recipient operation (which is performed simultaneously by a separate team). When the recipient iliac vessels have been prepared, the donor renal artery and vein are clamped and divided in that order. Blood is flushed from the kidney via the artery with 4°C heparinized preservative solution, and the kidney is immersed in a basin of cold solution to protect it during the brief interval before transplantation. The donor blood vessels are oversewn, and the incision is closed without drainage. The traditional open surgical procedure for procuring kidneys from living donors has documented efficacy and safety. In addition, graft survival in the recipient is superior to that with cadaveric donors. Despite these advantages, live kidney donation accounts for only about 30% of U.S. renal transplants each year. One reason for this is the reluctance of some potential donors to submit to the expected discomfort and inconvenience of the procedure, which may result in a significant hospital stay and a lengthy recovery period before return to work or resumption of normal physical activity. In addition, although fatality from the open procedure is unusual (approximately 1 in 10,000), it is not without morbidity such as wound complications (10%) and chronic pain syndromes.

Laparoscopic Nephrectomy

In an effort to make the procedure more acceptable to prospective donors by reducing morbidity, minimally invasive kidney recovery is now commonly practiced at many centers.[15] The laparoscopic approach was first employed in 1995 by Ratner and associates.[16] The largest single-center experience with the technique has been accrued at the University of Maryland, where the results of more than 300 laparoscopic nephrectomies indicate that in experienced hands, the procedure is safe and effective at yielding high-quality organs.[17] Donors undergoing the laparoscopic operation had a shorter hospital stay (2.2 vs. 4.5 days), a decrease in parenteral narcotic usage postoperatively, and earlier return to work (15.9 vs. 51.5 days). Serious operative morbidity was comparable to that of open nephrectomy. There was an increase in early ureteral complications, but this had no impact on long-term results. Graft function after laparoscopic versus open nephrectomy was also examined in detail. Whereas some early (day 7 to 30) graft dysfunction was evident in kidneys removed laparoscopically, the long-term function of these grafts was equal or superior to those obtained by the conventional approach.[18] More recent advances utilizing a "hand-assist" laparoscopic approach may further improve on these results and provide an additional margin of safety for the procedure.[19]

Despite these encouraging results, several questions remain about the laparoscopic technique. First, an inadequate number of cases have been performed and too few centers have applied the technique for conclusive comparisons of open and laparoscopic procedures. Second,

the laparoscopic removal of right-sided kidneys is problematic and is infrequently employed. The shorter and thinner-walled right renal vein complicates the procedure, especially because the stapling devices used to transect vessels shorten them by 1 to 1.5 cm. These impediments to right nephrectomy could lead to a decision to utilize the left kidney, which for other reasons, such as multiple renal arteries, might be suboptimal. However, the increasing employment of the laparoscopic approach appears justified and many are convinced that it has increased the number of living donors. Although the rate of serious complications is not statistically different than that from open donor nephrectomy, the two deaths reported in a U.S. survey of living donors between January 1, 1999, and July 1, 2000, both occurred in the 5186 laparoscopic donors while no death occurred in the 5660 open donors.

Selection and Management of Cadaveric Donors

In the absence of a family donor, cadaveric renal transplantation is a satisfactory alternative. In most countries, acceptance of the concept of brain death allows removal of viable organs from heart-beating donors. The donor shortage is perhaps the most important impediment to transplantation. Although in the United States the Uniform Anatomical Gift Act has been adopted in all 50 states, few cadaver kidneys are actually removed on the basis of donor cards alone without permission of the next of kin. Only about half of U.S. citizens currently consent to donation of organs from deceased relatives, and organs are in fact recovered from fewer than half of potentially acceptable donors. In the United States, it has been estimated that only about 20,000 brain-dead patients per year are acceptable donors. However, only approximately 9000 cadaveric kidney transplants are performed annually, a number that has changed little over the past decade. Even a modest increase was primarily the result of utilizing suboptimal or "marginal" donors, raising the concern that outcomes may be compromised by donor senescence, inadequate renal mass, or increased sensitivity of poor-quality kidneys to damage from drug toxicity, ischemia, or rejection. Aggressive donor management with a standarized protocol including corticosteroid therapy may have the potential to reverse some of the pathophysiologic changes associated with brain death, thus increasing somewhat the pool of suitable cadaveric donors.[20] Nevertheless, waiting lists continue to rise for all organs out of proportion to cadaveric organs recovered,[3] and the waiting time for a cadaveric renal transplant often exceeds 5 years (Fig. 27-2). The donor shortage is similarly severe in Europe. It is important that primary physicians, neurosurgeons, and intensive care nurses identify potential donors. Procurement personnel (usually part of a regional team) are then available to help obtain permission from the family and coordinate removal and distribution of viable organs.

The optimal cadaveric donors are previously healthy subjects between 3 and 65 years of age who have sustained fatal head injuries or cerebrovascular accidents. Careful history, physical examination, and laboratory

MANAGING THE WAITING LISTS

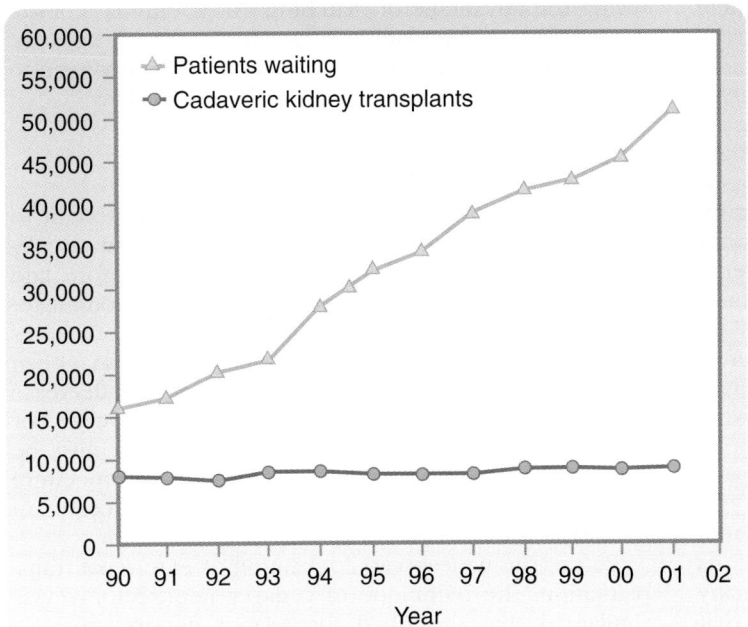

FIGURE 27-2. The supply of cadaveric organs has not increased substantially while waiting lists for transplants continue to grow. Illustrated here are the waiting list and the number of cadaveric and related donor kidneys transplanted.

surveys should be carried out to uncover factors that are contraindications to organ donation, such as the presence of generalized infections (including occult ones, such as human immunodeficiency virus, hepatitis B virus, and hepatitis C virus) or high risk of these (such as the use of intravenous drugs), malignancy other than nonmetastasizing brain tumors, and known renal disease, hypertension, or advanced arteriosclerosis. Donors older than 65 years of age may also sometimes be suitable, but the likelihood of vascular disease makes them less attractive. The use of bilateral adult renal transplants has been proposed as a means to salvage kidneys from older cadaver donors with suboptimal nephron mass that would otherwise be discarded.[21] The use of kidneys from infants is also possible, but technical aspects are exacting, and both kidneys may need to be implanted into a single recipient, a procedure that is associated with an increased incidence of technical complications.

The use of cadaver donors raises the ethical and legal problems of defining brain death. Consideration of transplantation should never be allowed to influence the treatment of patients who have any chance to survive or the definition or declaration of death, which must always be the responsibility of the patient's primary physician or of a neurologic consultant, with the full understanding and permission of the family. To avoid any conflict of interest, the transplant team must never be involved with care of the donor or with decisions regarding prognosis or therapy. Commonly accepted criteria for brain death include two in-hospital examinations at least 12 hours apart by a neurologist or neurosurgeon documenting loss of function of the entire brain. Loss of cerebral function is documented by lack of response to painful stimuli or movement except for spinal reflexes. The loss of brain stem function is documented by fixed pupils, absence of

corneal, oculovestibular, and oculocephalic reflexes, loss of gag reflex, and absence of movement or spontaneous respiration off the respirator for 3 minutes, a test that is done only after other criteria indicate no brain function. The declaration of brain death may be accelerated by 6 hours if a confirmatory test is performed such as a flat electroencephalogram. Strict adherence to these criteria is not always possible. For example, electroencephalographic confirmation is not required to declare brain death in the presence of angiographic evidence for complete lack of blood flow to the brain, which may occur with severe brain swelling. The use of brain scans to document lack of blood flow is also an acceptable criterion for brain death, which may facilitate this decision.[22] The diagnosis of brain death should not be made in the presence of severe hypothermia, marked hypovolemia, or toxic levels of depressant drugs such as barbiturates because these factors can produce an isoelectric electroencephalogram, a pattern that is reversible.

Donor Pretreatment

An interesting procedure that has been recommended, but never widely adopted, is donor pretreatment with immunosuppressive drugs, a strategy that could be employed only for cadaver donors. The rationale is that interstitial cells of hematopoietic origin normally present in the transplant organ ("passenger" cells) contribute importantly to graft immunogenicity and that their removal is beneficial. Conflicting results with pretreatment of donors with such agents as methylprednisolone, cyclophosphamide, or cyclosporine emphasize that circulating passenger cells are not the only source of transplantation antigens within kidney allografts. Interstitial dendritic cells and vascular endothelial cells, which cannot be removed, are probably also important in antigen presentation. It is conceivable that more complete eradication of passenger cells by vigorous prolonged treatment of donors or treatment of the ex vivo kidney might be more beneficial. However, current attention is focused on the possibly more likely benefits of employing an exactly opposite strategy, that is, augmenting passenger cell transfer. This is based on the recent observation by Starzl and Zinkernagel that in many successful organ transplant recipients of many years' standing, persistent donor lymphoid cells (especially dendritic cells) can be identified in various organs of the recipient (skin, thymus, brain).[23,24] It remains to be seen whether these cells are the cause of successful organ transplantation or merely accompany it. Several trials are under way to condition transplant recipients with donor bone marrow.

HLA Considerations in Cadaver Donor Selection

Although the benefit of matching for HLA-A and -B antigens in selection of family donors is well established, its value for cadaveric grafts remains controversial. For many years, reports from European centers have indicated that matching has a beneficial effect.[25] Not only was there a significant difference between grafts fully matched and totally mismatched for HLA-A and -B, but graded improvements in outcome could be related to the extent of the match. The value of HLA-A and -B typing has been confirmed by some reports from North America but not by others. The benefit of matching is more apparent in long-term rather than short-term results.[3] Several possible explanations have been put forth for differences in American and European results, such as the greater genetic heterogeneity of the U.S. population and the uniformity of tissue typing, which in Europe is performed in only the select and highly experienced laboratories of Eurotransplant. Both in Europe and in the United States, class II (HLA-DR) matching appears to be of greater benefit than class I matching.[26] However, some, especially in the United States, believe the improved survival of kidney allografts in patients treated with cyclosporine and newer agents, such as tacrolimus and mycophenolate mofetil (MMF), largely overrides the effect of HLA matching. It appears that the DR matching is still important in selecting donors for patients who have rejected previous transplants.

Even in the United States, the benefits of six antigen-matched (or zero antigen-mismatched) kidney transplants are now uncontested, causing UNOS to mandate their sharing on a national basis.[27] Whether lesser degrees of matching are important is controversial (especially since the introduction of cyclosporine and other potent new immunosuppressive agents) and is the central issue of an ongoing debate whether to change UNOS's point system for cadaveric kidney allocation, which currently emphasizes HLA matching. Two analyses on the outcomes of over 30,000 renal transplants led to opposite conclusions. Takemoto and coworkers[28] noted that HLA matching and transplant success were correlated, whereas Held and colleagues,[29] who stratified other risk factors, found little benefit and argued that the ischemic damage inherent in transportation necessary for national sharing would outweigh the advantage of matching. An additional consideration in sharing nationally is the potential negative impact on a second kidney that will subsequently need to be shipped to "pay back" the first shipped kidney.[30]

Operative Technique for Cadaveric Donors

After declaration of brain death, the donor is brought to the operating room and optimal respiration and circulation are maintained during the procedure. Before and during the operation, it is often necessary to administer large volumes of intravenous fluids because of diabetes insipidus or to restore blood volume that may have been depleted during the premortem attempts to decrease brain swelling and achieve neurologic recovery. For non–heart-beating donors, the recovery team must be poised in the operating room ready to start the procedure as soon as death is pronounced on the basis of cessation of cardiac function.

Before the widespread application of extrarenal transplantation, the technique of cadaver nephrectomy was similar to that described for related donors. Because multiorgan recovery has now become almost routine, the following technique of in situ perfusion and en bloc dissection has evolved as the standard (Fig. 27-3). The peritoneal cavity is entered through a midline incision, usually extended to the suprasternal notch to facilitate heart, lung, and liver donation. After exploration for unsuspected neoplasia or infection, the small bowel is retracted and the posterior peritoneum is incised in the midline up through the ligament of Treitz to expose the aorta and inferior vena cava. The peritoneal reflection around the cecum is incised and continued cephalad, allowing visualization of the retroperitoneum. By retraction of the duodenum and pancreas superiorly, the proximal aorta and vena cava are exposed. After dissection of the vascular structures of the extrarenal organs to be concomitantly recovered (liver, pancreas, heart, lung), the aorta and vena cava are divided just above their bifurcations after proximal insertion of large-bore cannulas for retrograde in situ perfusion. Anticoagulation is achieved by intravenous heparin, and the aorta is clamped proximally (at the aortic arch for cardiac recovery, above the celiac axis for liver and pancreas, and just above the renal arteries if only the kidneys are to be removed), and infusion of cold (4°C) preservation solution via the aortic cannula is initiated along with simultaneous decompression via the caval cannula. The kidneys, which rapidly become pale and cold, are then mobilized while avoiding damage to the hilar structures or ureters. The divided distal aorta and vena cava are mobilized cephalad by securing the lumbar vessels between clips, and the aorta is divided above the renal arteries. The entire bloc of kidneys, ureters, aorta, and vena cava are transferred to a basin of cold solution where careful dissection of the renal vessels is performed. The kidneys are then separated by division of the vena cava and aorta and packaged for cold storage to allow time for recipient selection, tissue typing, and transportation. Additional "bench surgery" for accurate dissection of the renal vessels and ureter is usually

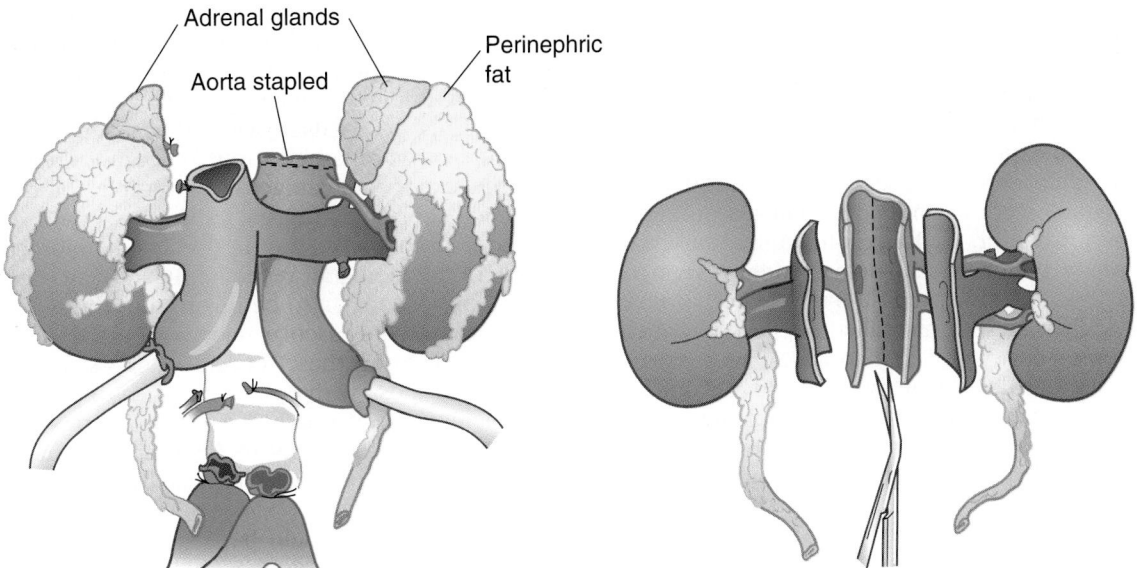

Adrenal glands

Aorta stapled

Perinephric
fat

■ FIGURE 27-3.   Dissection for cadaver kidney donation. Cannulas are placed in the aorta and vena cava for hypothermic perfusion to protect the kidneys during the terminal phases of the operation and for short-term storage. Segments of the aorta and vena cava are left intact when the kidneys are separated. The use of a Carrel patch of aorta is especially helpful when there are multiple renal arteries.

carried out later under continued hypothermic conditions just before transplantation.

Preservation of Cadaveric Kidneys

Two methods of kidney preservation (simple cooling and continuous pulsatile perfusion) have been widely utilized. Both allow sufficient time for transportation of kidneys to distant transplant centers. Simple cooling is achieved by flushing the allograft with a cold iso-osmolar or hyperosmolar buffered solution followed by storage at 4° to 10°C. Additives to the solutions include various ratios of K^+, Na^+, Cl^-, citrate, PO_4^-, SO_4^-, glucose, sucrose, mannitol, bicarbonate, and magnesium. These solutions are used for short-term (<48 hours) preservation. Although some disagreement exists, it is generally held that if longer preservation of organs is necessary (48 to 72 hours), it would require the use of a pulsatile perfusion apparatus, which circulates through the kidney either cryoprecipitated homologous plasma or a preservation solution.

In the late 1970s, there was a trend away from machine pulsatile preservation (which previously was used by about two thirds of centers) toward simple cooling, which is now employed at almost all centers. Responsible for the change were the greater costs and inconvenience of machine perfusion, including the need for a trained attendant during transportation to distant centers. In addition, it was shown that for short preservation times (<24 hours), pulsatile perfusion probably had little advantage. In 1987, Belzer and Southard introduced a solution (University of Wisconsin [UW] solution) containing several new components (lactobionate, raffinose, hydroxyethyl starch) that substantially extended the period of storage possible for liver and pancreas to 24 hours. Although the

solution is in wide usage by others for simple cold storage of kidneys, it has also been used by Belzer and Southard with excellent results as a perfusate for machine preservation. Because, even with improved preservation solutions, simple cooling has a finite time limit, it seems likely that major progress in preservation can come only from advances in perfusion techniques. Several groups that resisted the trend toward simple cooling and that continue to use machine perfusion have reported an extremely low incidence of ATN. The additive adverse effects of ischemia, nephrotoxic immunosuppressive drugs, and the use of older and suboptimal donors has induced some centers to resume pulsatile preservation. In fact, from 1996 to 2000 this method was utilized for 12% of kidneys transplanted in the United States.[2] These kidneys had a significantly lower rate of delayed graft function than those preserved by cold storage, but so far no graft survival advantage is apparent.

Xenogeneic (Interspecies) Grafts

The growing shortage of human organs for transplantation has rejuvenated interest in using donors of alien species. Although the success of cross-species organ grafts could revolutionize the field of transplant surgery, uncertainty exists as to when this will be feasible.[31] The xenograft barrier consists of several components: humoral, cellular, and physiologic. In the first two components, experimental advances were considerable during the 1990s. Most striking was the prevention of humorally based hyperacute rejection of organ from distantly related donor species by genetic engineering of donors.[32] Progress has also been made in defining and overcoming the cellular aspects of xenorejection. In fact, no specific evidence exists that in the absence of humoral response, the cellular response to xenografts would be substantially more formidable than to allografts or any less susceptible to conventional immunosuppression.

Despite these experimental advances, experience with clinical xenografts is less encouraging. About 40 whole-organ xenografts were performed in humans during the 20th century. However, the longest functional survival (9 months) was a chimpanzee-to-human kidney xenograft performed by Reemtsma in 1964.[33] Other primate-to-human kidney transplants failed earlier in patients immunosuppressed with azathioprine and cortico-steroids.[31] Careful studies done by Starzl and coworkers in 1992[34] in which baboon livers were transplanted to two human patients were quite informative. These xenografts were transplanted with the optimal immunologic advantages of the day: (1) a concordant donor species, (2) the known relative resistance of the liver to antibody-mediated damage, and (3) potent immunosuppression. Despite the well-conceived nature of this trial, graft and patient survival were short lived (25 days and 70 days, respectively). Moreover, the development of graft dysfunction in the absence of significant histologic evidence of rejection raises concerns that some as-yet-undefined physiologic incompatibility existed between graft and recipient.

Considering that the outcomes that could now be obtained with clinical xenografts might well be comparable with those of allografts of the 1950s and 1960s and that recent progress in experimental xenobiology has been considerable, one might predict that eventual clinical success is likely. In fact, limited success might be within reach now if primate donors could be used. However, the shortage of these animals in most parts of the world, the difficulty of breeding them in captivity, and the ethical question of their use are major deterrents. Another important cautionary note deserves mention: the possible dangers of zoonoses.[35] The consequences of transferring microorganisms from other species into immunosuppressed humans via organ xenografts is unknown. However, it seems likely that the origin of the HIV epidemic in humans was a transfer of a virus originating in nonhuman primates.

In view of the problems noted, further attempts at clinical xenotransplantation with primate donors seems unlikely. However, progress in controlling hyperacute rejection in nonhuman primates of organs transplanted from more distantly related species (i.e., pigs) suggests that these discordant donors could be used successfully. Specific carbohydrate epitopes have been defined that serve as the dominant targets of the natural antibody response in the primate antiporcine response. Progress has been made in preventing preformed and induced antibody-mediated graft damage with immunosuppressive regimens that blunt the induced response and with the novel strategy of inducing transgene-encoded regulators of complement activation to avoid the attack of natural antibodies.[36] The survival for several months in nonhuman primates of heart and kidney xenograft from pigs (genetically engineered to express human proteins on endothelial cells) is quite encouraging because preformed

antibody and complement activation otherwise destroys xenografts from normal pigs in 60 to 90 minutes.[32] Possibly even more promising is another genetic engineering approach. In pigs, both alleles of the gene responsible for synthesizing α1,3-galactosyltransferase epitopes on the cell surface were knocked out.[37] Because these epitopes are the major xenoantigens responsible for hyperacute rejection in pig-to-human transplants, their complete removal from pig organs is predicted to preclude this phase of the xenograft response. In addition, because the same epitopes may also be involved in the next formidable barrier (acute vascular rejection), the results of xenotransplants from these porcine donors could be far superior to those with donors modified to express human complement regulators. The value of this potentially important work remains to be tested by transplanting nonhuman primates with organs from these modified porcine donors.

Porcine donors would have several important advantages over primate donors, including greater supply and less ethical concern. However, the possibility of zoonoses has been raised, particularly with regard to the porcine endogenous retrovirus, which is present in all pigs and which has been shown to infect human cells in vitro.[38] However, it is reassuring that in a survey of 160 patients treated with living porcine tissue (skin, cells, heart valves), there has been no evidence of virus transmission.[39]

The Recipient Operation

General anesthesia is usually employed, although spinal anesthesia is also satisfactory. Good relaxation is important during the vascular and ureteral anastomosis, but excessive use of muscle relaxants (especially succinyl-choline) must be avoided because low cholinesterase levels in dialysis patients may otherwise lead to prolonged apnea. The muscle relaxant atracurium can be used safely because this agent has a short half-life and its degradation is independent of renal and hepatic metabolism.

The iliac vessels are exposed retroperitoneally through an oblique incision just above the inguinal ligament (Fig. 27-4). The dissection is slightly easier on the right, but a more important consideration in selecting the appropriate side is avoiding sites of previous transplants, other operations (e.g., appendectomy, herniorrhaphy, or bladder or ureteral operations), or peritoneal dialysis catheters. Lymphatics that must be divided to expose the iliac vessels are ligated to prevent prolonged lymph drainage or lymphocele formation. Exposure of the bladder is facilitated by dividing the inferior epigastric vessels and, in females, the round ligament. Division of the spermatic cord should be avoided because this may cause epididymitis, testicular ischemia, and atrophy.

Historically, vascular anastomoses were performed between the end of the donor renal artery and the proximal end of the recipient's divided internal iliac artery and between the end of the donor renal vein and the side of the external iliac vein. More commonly, an end-to-side anastomosis of renal artery to external iliac artery is now used, especially if there is significant atheromatous disease

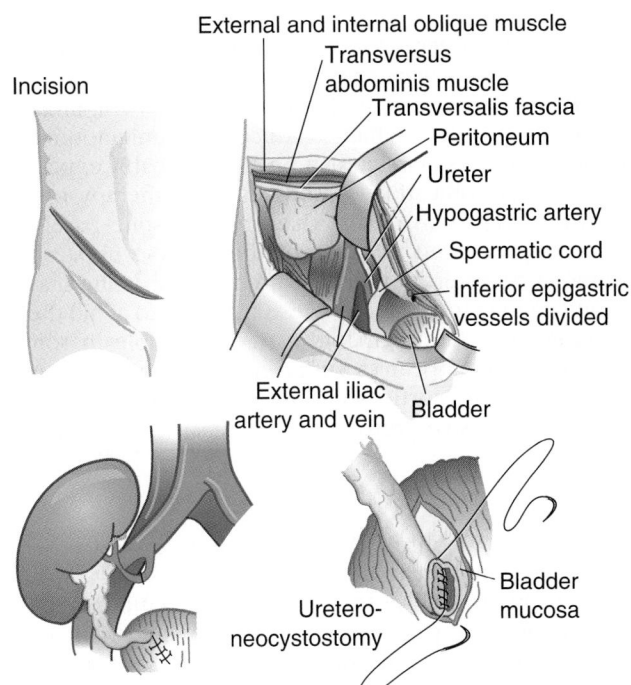

Incision

External and internal oblique muscle
Transversus abdominis muscle
Transversalis fascia
Peritoneum
Ureter
Hypogastric artery
Spermatic cord
Inferior epigastric vessels divided

External iliac artery and vein

Bladder

Uretero-neocystostomy

Bladder mucosa

FIGURE 27-4. The recipient operation is done through a retroperitoneal incision using the iliac vessels to revascularize the kidney and a ureteroneocystostomy to establish urinary continuity.

in the internal iliac artery, as there often is in older or diabetic recipients, or if the contralateral internal iliac artery has been ligated during a previous transplant operation. Most transplant surgeons routinely favor the end-to-side procedure because exposure of the external iliac artery requires less dissection and because stenosis at the anastomosis may be less likely, especially if a Carrel patch of donor aorta is used (as is usually the case for cadaveric but not living donors).

If there are multiple donor renal arteries that are not on an aortic cuff, we favor anastomosis of the end of the smaller renal arteries to the side of the largest renal artery. These anastomoses can be performed deliberately under magnification while the ex vivo kidney is protected by immersion in a basin of cold saline solution. Revascularization in the recipient can then be accomplished rapidly by a single anastomosis. The sacrifice of even small accessory donor renal arteries should be avoided because occlusion of these end arteries will cause renal infarcts. Preservation of accessory arteries to the lower portion of the kidney is especially important because they may constitute the blood supply of a segment of collecting system or ureter and their ligation may lead to necrosis and urinary fistula. In 470 living related donors studied at the University of Pennsylvania, multiple renal arteries were found to be present in one kidney in 30% and bilaterally in 9%.[40] In 42 patients in whom the type of ex vivo anastomosis described previously was performed for multiple arteries, only one kidney was lost, owing to a technical complication, and the 1-year survival of 76% was no

different from that of single-artery kidneys in the precyclosporine period. Venous collateral circulation is almost always adequate, so that in instances of multiple renal veins (which are even more common than multiple arteries), only one large vein need be saved for anastomosis. If a large adult kidney is to be transplanted into a small child, a transperitoneal approach is used to provide adequate room for the kidney, which is revascularized via the aorta and vena cava.

Urinary tract continuity is usually established by ureteroneocystostomy. The ureter should pass beneath the spermatic cord to avoid obstruction. Ureteropyelostomy (anastomosis of the recipient's ureter to the pelvis of the donor kidney) is an alternative procedure, which should be used in instances of donor ureteral devascularization or injury. A few surgeons prefer this procedure to ureteroneocystostomy, but it is associated with a higher incidence of urinary fistula.

Meticulous technique and hemostasis are particularly important because of the coagulopathy and susceptibility to infection of uremic immunosuppressed patients. We prefer to close the wound without drains, but if hemostasis is suboptimal, closed suction catheters may be used.

Post-transplant Management

If the transplanted kidney has not suffered ischemic damage, a brisk diuresis is likely to begin within minutes of revascularization. Responsible for the diuresis (which may reach 1000 mL/hr) are (1) osmotic factors secondary to uremia or high glucose concentrations in intravenous fluids, (2) total body fluid and electrolyte overload secondary to chronic uremia, and (3) mild proximal tubular damage resulting from allograft ischemia. Early in the postoperative period, mild diuresis is reassuring and should be encouraged by replacement of urine volumes and, if necessary, by diuretics. Initial under-replacement of fluid may lead to oliguria or impaired transplant function interfering with diagnosis of vascular occlusion, urinary obstruction, or early rejection. Severe dehydration can be the outcome of inadequate replacement of losses during a massive diuresis, especially in children. During the first few days, there may also be a need for colloid or blood replacement because of losses into the wound.

Serious problems may also result from over-replacement of volume, especially if the transplant is not producing urine. Hyperkalemia is particularly dangerous in this setting and may necessitate administration of an ion exchange resin (sodium polystyrene sulfonate [Kayexalate], 25 to 50 g orally or by enema). In more emergent circumstances, administration of intravenous glucose and insulin or prompt dialysis may be necessary to control hyperkalemia. Suggested replacement fluids include 0.45% saline solution, with or without isotonic glucose, and sodium bicarbonate (30 mEq/L) and potassium (10 to 15 mEq/L), depending on the status of the serum electrolytes and blood glucose. If diuresis continues, fluid replacement should lag behind the urine output, allowing gradual return to normal urine volumes over the next 12 to 24 hours.

Because of the retroperitoneal approach, the transplant operation is relatively nondisruptive to intestinal function, and medications and fluids can usually be given by mouth within 12 to 24 hours. Ambulation on the first postoperative day is beneficial. The Foley catheter can be removed within the first few days. Hypertension, which is common, should be managed conventionally with drugs such as hydralazine, β blockers, calcium channel blockers, or angiotensin-converting enzyme inhibitors. Antacids are given to prevent ulcers, and nystatin (Mycostatin) is used for prophylaxis against candidal infections. Perioperative antibiotics (which should be given for no more than 48 hours) decrease the incidence of wound infection. Trimethoprim and sulfamethoxazole are used routinely by most centers for prophylaxis against urinary tract infections and *Pneumocystis carinii*. If rejection and other postoperative complications do not occur, the subsequent care is relatively simple because the restoration of renal function is associated with a rapid return to normal health in patients previously suffering from single-organ system failure.

Immunosuppression

Thus far, the success of solid organ transplantation has been dependent on lifelong administration of nonspecific pharmacologic immunosuppressants. Since the early 1980s, advances in understanding mechanisms of T-cell activation have facilitated the development of more powerful and somewhat more selective immunosuppressive drugs that target the distinctive cell surface molecules of T cells, which initiate rejection.

Azathioprine

Prevention of rejection of human renal allograft rejection was first attempted by whole-body irradiation in the 1950s. Although one irradiated patient retained his allograft for 25 years without ever receiving immunosuppressive drugs, 11 others died of infections owing to the profound immunodepression caused by this treatment.[1] In 1959, Schwartz and Dameshek discovered that the antimetabolite 6-mercaptopurine inhibited humoral immunity in rabbits. Shortly thereafter, Calne and associates and Zukowski and colleagues found that the drug could prevent kidney allograft rejection in dogs.[2] This drug and its derivative azathioprine had more predictable, reversible, and safer action than radiation and were soon used with considerable success in human renal allograft recipients. In 1988, the Nobel Prize was awarded to Gertrude Elion and George Hitchings for the development of these drugs.

Adrenal Corticosteroids

The previously known immunosuppressive effects of adrenal corticosteroids, although not sufficient in themselves to prevent rejection, were noted in the early 1960s to be synergistic with those of azathioprine. The combination of azathioprine and corticosteroids then became standard therapy for the next two decades. The complex impact of corticosteroids on the immune system involves blockade of postreceptor events occurring after engagement of the T-cell receptor with antigen and the inhibition of certain cytokine gene activation such as interleukin (IL)-1 and IL-6. Corticosteroids also possess potent anti-inflammatory properties, which reduce the migration of monocytes to sites of inflammation. This probably explains why brief intensification of corticosteroid therapy often aborts the "rejection crises" that ensue despite baseline immunosuppression. Because of the adverse impact of chronic corticosteroid therapy, attempts are being made at many centers to withdraw these agents or to avoid their use altogether. Although this may be possible in some patients, others appear to suffer either acute or chronic refection when corticosteroids are withdrawn from immunosuppressive protocols.[41]

Antilymphocytic Antibodies

In the 1960s, Woodruff, Medawar, Monaco, and others studied antilymphocyte serum (ALS), which in animals proved to be a more potent and more specific immunosuppressant than azathioprine. ALS contained xenoantibody raised by immunization of heterologous animals (e.g., rabbits, horses) with lymphoid cells of the prospective allograft recipient species. In rodents, small doses of ALS strikingly reduced the number of circulating lymphocytes and often prevented rejection of allografts. Although ALS also proved to be a potent immunosuppressant in humans, several problems limited its usefulness. Even the purified globulin fraction (antilymphocyte globulin [ALG]) of the foreign serum sometimes provoked allergic reactions. The therapeutic window of ALG was quite small, and large doses or prolonged therapy often led to leukopenia, thrombocytopenia, and serious infections, especially of viral origin (e.g., herpesvirus, cytomegalovirus, varicella-zoster). In addition, patients formed antibodies to the heterologous protein, diminishing the feasibility of prolonged or repeated courses. Thus, ALS or antilymphocyte globulin (ALG) could be given only for a limited time, at marginal doses, and only as an adjunct to "conventional" immunosuppressive agents. ALS was also found to be very effective in reversing rejection crises, even those resistant to high-dose corticosteroid therapy, and this has become a common indication.[42] Thymoglobulin (a rabbit antihuman thymocytoglobulin [Sangstat]), available in Europe since 1985, has also been effective in preventing or reversing acute rejection and has become the most commonly used polyclonal agent.[43]

The effectiveness of ALS was the basis for the introduction by Cosimi and coworkers[44] of monoclonal mouse antihuman anti–T-cell antibodies. Monoclonal anti–T-cell antibodies induce rapid depletion of T lymphocytes from peripheral blood while having little detrimental effect on other populations, such as red blood cells, platelets, or granulocytes, all of which are affected by cross-reacting antibodies present in the polyclonal ALG preparations. Because of lower cost and greater availability, specificity, and standardization of the preparation, monoclonal antibodies such as OKT3 have largely replaced ALS and ALG in many centers. The structure recognized by OKT3, the CD3 antigen, is linked to the T-cell antigen receptor, which is critical for the activation of human T cells. In vivo depletion of T cells after exposure to OKT3 is believed to be mediated by mechanisms such as complement-mediated lympholysis or opsonization of cells. In the presence of bound OKT3, the CD3 T-cell receptor complex is internalized by the cell, further rendering the T-cell population inactive. Multi-institutional, randomized prospective trials revealed the efficacy of OKT3 in reversal of acute rejection in 94% of cadaveric renal allograft rejections, a figure significantly better than that obtained with corticosteroid treatment.[45]

Side effects associated with OKT3 therapy (particularly the initial doses) include fever, shaking chills, headache, nausea, vomiting, diarrhea, wheezing, and pulmonary edema. These phenomena are probably due to release of cytokines, especially tumor necrosis factor, and have been termed the *cytokine release syndrome*. Fortunately, such side effects can often be ameliorated by pretreatment with methylprednisolone, acetaminophen, and antihistamines or, more recently, antibodies against tumor necrosis factor or its receptor. As with polyclonal ALG, the use of monoclonal antibody OKT3 may induce rapid sensitization to mouse antibody, which results in the neutralization of OKT3 and reappearance in the peripheral blood of CD3[+] cells. Concomitant administration of azathioprine and corticosteroids may delay the production of anti-OKT3 antibody and prolong its immunosuppressive effect. Beyond return of graft function, in vivo efficacy of OKT3 may be monitored by sequential analyses of the CD3[+] T-cell populations in the peripheral blood and the circulating level of OKT3 and by measurement of human antibodies to the murine immunoglobulin.

Other monoclonal antibodies that have been developed for the prevention or treatment of rejection are under clinical investigation. These include mouse antihuman monoclonal antibodies directed against various T-cell surface markers, including the IL-2 receptor, adhesion molecules (e.g., anti-intercellular adhesion molecule [ICAM]-1), and CD52.[46] Also promising is the development of monoclonal antibodies in which the entire protein backbone structure of the antibody molecule is replaced with corresponding human sequences, except for the idiotypic specific region. Such engineered molecules, termed *humanized* antibodies, appear to retain their in vivo efficacy for T-cell depletion but may have limited side effects (diminished cytokine release syndrome) and prolonged effectiveness because their elimination through the development of human antimurine immunity is less.

Cyclosporine

The introduction of cyclosporine in the early 1980s revolutionized transplantation by facilitating successful extrarenal transplants and improving cadaveric kidney graft survival. Cyclosporine is a fungal derivative that appears to block T-lymphocyte production of the lymphokine IL-2 through inhibition of the production of its messenger RNA. Like azathioprine, cyclosporine is most useful for prophylaxis rather than reversal of rejection. Calne, using it for single-drug immunosuppression in 1979, found it to be potent but also quite toxic at higher doses and its administration to be associated with infections, tumors, and renal failure. By reducing the dose of cyclosporine and combining it with small doses of prednisone, Starzl subsequently reported spectacular improvement in the outcome of liver and kidney allografts. Similarly improved results were confirmed by multicenter randomized studies in Europe and Canada. After its release for general use in 1983, cyclosporine was adopted by virtually all centers.

Cyclosporine has the major advantage over azathioprine of lacking bone marrow toxicity but the disadvantage of nephrotoxicity, which is its major side effect. Nephrotoxicity may be manifest as a delay in function of a newly transplanted kidney or impairment of function of a well-established renal allograft. Although therapeutic drug monitoring and maintenance of blood levels in the therapeutic range are helpful, these do not eliminate the possibility of nephrotoxicity, which may occur even at "subtherapeutic" levels or after prolonged, stable dosage.[47] Elevated blood levels of the agent and toxicity may appear, especially during concurrent use of certain drugs (such as erythromycin, cimetidine, diltiazem, and ketoconazole) that increase bioavailability through inhibition of hepatic metabolism. Conversely, decreased blood levels may result from patient noncompliance or interactions with drugs such as phenobarbital, phenytoin, and trimethoprim-sulfamethoxazole, which activate the hepatic P-450 cytochrome system and increase conversion of the parent compound to immunologically less active metabolites. In addition to nephrotoxicity, other side effects attributable to cyclosporine include hypertension, hepatotoxicity, seizures, tremor, hypertrichosis, nausea, vomiting, and diarrhea. Delayed renal allograft function from ischemic damage of cadaveric kidneys may be accentuated by nephrotoxic drugs. Therefore, many centers avoid the use of cyclosporine until delayed function has resolved. A prophylactic course of polyclonal or monoclonal anti–T-cell antibodies is advocated by some, along with corticosteroids to delay rejection until graft function allows institution of cyclosporine therapy. Even without initial ischemic renal damage, patients on cyclosporine tend to have persistently higher serum creatinine levels than azathioprine-treated patients and histologic changes of interstitial fibrosis in the kidney over the long term. Because of uncertainty regarding the risk of permanent renal damage from long-term cyclosporine therapy, most centers use lower doses of cyclosporine in combination with prednisone and azathioprine or MMF. The risks of chronic renal damage appear to be outweighed by the substantial advantages of cyclosporine, including the possibility that in selected cyclosporine-treated patients, corticosteroid therapy could eventually be minimized or completely withdrawn. Doses are determined by trough levels in whole blood, which are maintained at 100 to 200 µg/L (as determined by high-performance liquid chromatography). Absorption and bioavailability of cyclosporine were found to be quite variable after oral administration, complicating regulation of blood levels. A microemulsion formulation of cyclosporine (Neoral) allows faster and more consistent absorption and facilitates management.[48]

Patient survival has also been improved by the introduction of cyclosporine, probably because of a decrease in incidence and severity of infections. Many believe that histocompatibility matching is less important than in the precyclosporine era. Disappointingly, the impact of cyclosporine on long-term results has not been nearly as favorable as its influence on early outcome. Both U.S. and European multicenter reports indicate a continuing attrition in late graft survival from chronic rejection, which unfortunately is not avoided by cyclosporine. Despite these shortcomings of cyclosporine, the introduction of the agent represented a major advance.

Tacrolimus (FK-506)

Tacrolimus has properties similar but perhaps superior to those of cyclosporine. The antilymphocytic effect of tacrolimus results from the formation of active complexes between the drug and the respective intracellular binding protein or immunophilin. The FK-506 immunophilin complex inhibits the phosphatase activity of calcineurin, which is important in the regeneration of IL-1 gene transcription. Tacrolimus was first described by Kino and colleagues in 1987 and introduced clinically in the United States at the University of Pittsburgh in 1989. It is about 100 times more potent as an anti–T-cell agent than is cyclosporine (on a per-milligram basis). Initially, tacrolimus was used to "rescue" liver transplants observed to be failing on cyclosporine-based immunosuppression. Subsequent trials have assessed the efficacy of tacrolimus as primary immunosuppression. Prospective randomized trials in the United States and Europe initially showed that patient and graft survival were comparable with tacrolimus and cyclosporine but that the incidence of rejection, both acute and corticosteroid-refractory, was significantly lower with tacrolimus.[49] A subsequent randomized study in the United States comparing the efficacy and safety of tacrolimus with cyclosporine immunosuppression in patients receiving cadaveric kidney transplants revealed 1-year graft survival rates of 91.2% for tacrolimus and 87.9% for cyclosporine. Acute rejection episodes were significantly reduced for tacrolimus patients, as was the requirement for antilymphocyte therapy for rejection. Tremor and paresthesias were more frequent in patients on tacrolimus, and the incidence of post-transplant diabetes was 19.9% for tacrolimus versus 4% for cyclosporine. Several studies have addressed the use of tacrolimus induction and rescue therapy after kidney or kidney-pancreas transplantation.[50] These observations have encouraged the adoption of tacrolimus-based primary immunosuppressive regimens for kidney-pancreas transplant recipients.[51] The adverse effects of tacrolimus are similar to those of cyclosporine: nephrotoxicity, neurologic problems (tremor, headache), and diabetes.

Mycophenolate Mofetil

Mycophenolate mofetil (MMF), the morpholino-ethyl ester of mycophenolic acid (MPA), which in vivo is hydrolyzed to free MPA (the active immunosuppressive moiety), is a potent and specific inhibitor of de novo purine synthesis. MPA blocks the proliferation of both T and B lymphocytes because these cells lack a significant purine biosynthetic salvage pathway activity.[52] The use of MMF in combination with cyclosporine dramatically reduced both the incidence and the severity of acute rejection.[53] Subsequent trials combining MMF with cyclosporine indicated that the risk of biopsy-proven acute rejection declined to less than 20% and the frequency of resistant rejection was markedly decreased.[3] As a result, MMF has virtually replaced azathioprine at many transplant centers. The trials indicated a slight increase in the risk of viral infection in MMF-treated patients, although this can usually be controlled by prophylactic drugs. Unfortunately, MMF has not altered the rate of chronic graft rejection, despite the lower incidence of acute rejection episodes after use of this combination. Its most common side effects involve the gastrointestinal tract. MMF has also been extremely effective in pancreas transplantation. In a single-center study, simultaneous pancreas and kidney transplant (SPK) recipients demonstrated a markedly improved survival of allografts, with 2-year renal and pancreas graft survival rates increasing from 86% to 95% and 83% to 95%, respectively, with the use of MMF rather than azathioprine.

Sirolimus (Rapamycin)

Sirolimus, which is structurally similar to tacrolimus, was discovered in a search for novel antifungal agents. It is a macrocyclic triantibiotic produced by *Streptomyces hygroscopicus,* an *Actinomyces* that was isolated from a soil sample collected from Rapa Nui (Easter Island). Although sirolimus also binds to FKBP25, its effect is distinct from the calcineurin-based activity of tacrolimus or cyclosporine. Sirolimus and cyclosporine were found to be strikingly synergistic in experimental animal studies of heart and kidney transplantation.[54] Phase II studies in human kidney transplantation show that the incidence of acute rejection may be reduced to approximately 10% by using both drugs.[55] Phase III studies are now under way to determine the risks and benefits of this combination. Sirolimus is not nephrotoxic but may cause thrombocytopenia and hypercholesterolemia. It also appears to be associated with delayed wound healing.

Other Immunosuppressive Agents

Development of new, less toxic immunosuppressive therapies is very important. A new class of biological agents that target co-stimulatory molecules necessary for T-cell activation holds great promise for this purpose. Unlike conventional agents such as tacrolimus and cyclosporine that inhibit T-cell activation by blocking the effects of T-cell receptor triggering by antigen (termed *signal I*), these agents target the interaction of T cell CD28 with antigen-presenting cell (APC) B7 molecules, or T cell CD154 with APC CD40 *(signal II).* The theoretical attractiveness of this approach is based on considerable experimental research indicating that T cells receiving signal I in the absence of signal II are rendered anergic. This may allow for the design of immunosuppressive protocols with a greater probability of inducing a state of tolerance to the graft. In large animal studies, Kirk and coworkers[56] reported long-term survival of kidney allografts utilizing simultaneous blockade of CD154 and B7. In subsequent work, even monotherapy with anti-CD154 alone administered for a 5-month course resulted in prolonged function of all grafts without graft loss owing to rejection. Interesting in these studies was the finding that combination therapy with conventional agents and anti-CD154 produced inferior results to monotherapy with anti-CD154, perhaps indicating that conventional therapy inhibits anergy induced by co-stimulatory blockade.

Rejection

Considerable effort has been made to correlate allograft morphology with the clinical course of rejection. However, histologic study of a kidney biopsy can never provide more than a narrowly focused "snapshot" of the target of a complex systemic process that is in continuous evolution while also being modified by immunosuppression. Rejection is conveniently categorized as hyperacute, acute, or chronic, but there are overlapping features and transitions among these categories. The introduction of newer potent immunosuppressive agents has also changed the classic histologic changes of rejection. The outcome of an interventional conference in Banff was the proposal of new criteria for the semiquantitative analysis of rejection and the development of standardized nomenclature.[57]

Hyperacute Rejection

In the 1960s, several instances were noted in which transplanted kidneys that initially seemed viable were rejected within minutes of revascularization, as evidenced by bluish discoloration of the kidney, deterioration of perfusion, and cessation of function. Histologically, extensive intravascular deposits of fibrin and platelets and intraglomerular accumulation of polymorphonuclear leukocytes, fibrin, platelets, and red blood cells along with accumulation of leukocytes in the peritubular and glomerular capillaries were seen.[58] This process proved refractory to immunosuppressive or anticoagulant therapy and inevitably led to rapid destruction of the kidney. It soon became evident that the occurrence of hyperacute rejection was usually correlated with the presence of preformed circulating antibodies against donor antigens and that these could be identified by a pretransplant crossmatch. The classic form of hyperacute rejection has become rare because transplants are no longer performed when the crossmatch is positive.

Acute Cellular Rejection

Acute cellular rejection most commonly becomes evident during the early days or weeks after transplantation, although it may occasionally occur months or years later. The diagnosis of acute rejection is based on a constellation of findings that include clinical signs and symptoms, laboratory assays of blood and urine, radioisotope studies, and allograft biopsies.[59] Classic signs and symptoms are malaise, fever, oliguria, hypertension, and tenderness from swelling of the allograft. However, most of these symptoms are rarely seen in patients receiving newer immunosuppressive agents, such as cyclosporine and tacrolimus. Under the influence of these agents, rejection takes on a more subtle clinical picture in which fever and allograft swelling are absent and impaired renal function may be the only signal. Under these circumstances, we usually obtain a radioisotope renal perfusion scan, a test that cannot provide specific evidence of rejection, but that helps to exclude several other conditions that can cause impaired renal function, such as vascular occlusion, ureteric obstruction, or urinary fistula.

Because the diagnosis of rejection on clinical grounds alone may be difficult, a biopsy is often performed when rejection is suspected. This procedure may be performed transcutaneously with little risk. Early microscopic signs of acute rejection include the adherence of lymphocytes to the endothelium of peritubular capillaries and venules, which then progresses to disruption of these vessels, tubular necrosis, and interstitial infiltrates. Cellular infiltration, which is the hallmark of rejection, is composed at first of small lymphocytes and later consists of a variety of cells such as large lymphocytes and macrophages. As rejection proceeds toward irreversibility, there is greater involvement of the vascular elements of the graft. Swelling of the intima and focal fibrinoid necrosis of the media take place, followed by endothelial cell proliferation and obliteration of the lumina of small arteries by fibrin, platelets, and lymphoid cells.

In the Banff schema, glomerular, interstitial, tubular, and vascular lesions are graded 0 to 3+, depending on whether they are absent (0), mild (1), moderate (2), or severe (3).[57] Total reliance cannot be placed on a biopsy as the "gold standard" for diagnosing acute rejection. Not only are biopsies subject to sampling error, but lymphocytic infiltration in itself cannot be taken as conclusive evidence of rejection because, for obscure reasons, even perfectly functioning renal allografts may exhibit some degree of mononuclear infiltration.

Distinguishing impairment of renal function owing to rejection from nephrotoxicity induced by cyclosporine or tacrolimus is a challenging problem. In cyclosporine nephrotoxic states, variable degrees of lymphocytic infiltration in the interstitium of the kidney have been observed. Careful attention to trends and fluctuations of cyclosporine blood levels may aid in decision making. Cyclosporine nephrotoxicity characteristically causes smaller increments in serum creatinine than rejection does, and these are usually reversible within a few days after dose reduction. Arteriolar hyalinosis is another factor considered in the Banff criteria because this is thought to be a feature of cyclosporine toxicity.

A particularly challenging clinical problem is the diagnosis of rejection in the setting of ATN. Under this circumstance, a biopsy may be the only aid to diagnosis. Unfortunately, however, even a skilled pathologist cannot always distinguish the histologic picture of rejection from that of ATN (or cyclosporine toxicity). Therefore, enthusiasm for repeated biopsies varies, some transplant surgeons being content in most instances to rely on their clinical judgment. At times, empirical antirejection therapy is employed as a diagnostic test for suspected rejection. In the presence of acute rejection (and the absence of ATN), this usually promptly lowers the creatinine value.

When the diagnosis of acute rejection is made, prompt institution of antirejection therapy (corticosteroids, anti–T cell antibodies) is necessary to prevent permanent damage to the allograft. This treatment is usually capable of reversing the process, although it may recur. Intravenous high-dose corticosteroids (0.5 to 1.0 g methylprednisolone) are used as first-line therapy for rejection at most centers. We find that about 65% of acute rejections will respond to three to five doses. Corticosteroid-resistant rejection may respond to anti–T-cell antibodies in an additional 30% of cases. Rejection refractory to both corticosteroid and antilymphocyte antibody therapy may still respond to treatment with newer agents such as tacrolimus or MMF.

It is important that antirejection therapy not be employed needlessly or for a prolonged period, because this is the cause of most morbidity and mortality. During the 1970s (before the introduction of cyclosporine), a progressive improvement in patient survival took place in most centers. This was probably the result of the realization that overly intense immunosuppression and repeated courses of antirejection therapy were unwise and dangerous and that better long-term results could be accomplished by more conservative therapy. Many groups adopted the policy of refusing to aggressively treat more than two episodes of acute rejection. Experience taught the important lesson that eventual loss of some grafts could not be avoided. Early recognition and acceptance of this eventuality, transplant nephrectomy, reinstitution of dialysis, and the chance of a later successful transplant were obviously preferable to pushing heavy immunosuppression to the point of serious infection and death.

Chronic Rejection

The border between acute and chronic rejection is not always sharply defined, but the typical course of chronic rejection is gradual, progressive loss of renal function. It may begin after years of stable function but is more often seen in patients who have had multiple early and incompletely reversible episodes of acute rejection. Humoral injury (thought to be a more important factor in this condition than in acute cellular rejection) is manifested histologically by intimal fibroproliferative arterial lesions that probably stem from repetitive cycles of immune injury to the endothelium with focal thrombosis and incorporation of thrombus into the arterial wall. Also seen in chronic rejection are glomerular changes. Histologically, increased mesangial matrix and mesangial proliferation are seen. The glomerular basement membrane is thickened, and focal deposition of IgM, IgG, and complement may be identified along capillary walls and within the mesangium. Clinically, these are manifested by proteinuria, microscopic hematuria, and slowly deteriorating function. As with acute rejection, a semiquantitative analysis of assessing renal progress for chronic rejection has been proposed under the Banff schema.[57]

In the presence of these morphologic vascular and glomerular changes, antirejection therapy is ineffective. Employment of high-dose corticosteroid or ALS or OKT3 therapy in hopes of reversing the process should not be risked because this will be of no benefit and may lead to opportunistic infection or other serious sequelae. An abrupt cessation of immunosuppression is also unwarranted early in the course of chronic rejection because its progression may be slow and significant periods of useful, although diminishing, transplant function may be possible. However, immunosuppression should generally be reduced as renal failure progresses because the additive immunodepressive effects of uremia and immunosuppressive drugs are particularly dangerous.

It is important to remember that acute cellular rejection is also occasionally encountered after years of stable transplant function, sometimes as the result of discontinuation of immunosuppression by the careless or noncompliant patient. This must be distinguished from chronic rejection if possible, although a timely diagnosis of late acute rejection is usually fortuitous because symptoms are uncommon. A prompt biopsy is warranted in cases of unexpected or precipitous deterioration in stable function because late cellular rejection (unlike chronic rejection) can often be reversed if treated before severe damage occurs.

Recurrent Disease in Transplanted Kidneys

Because transplantation does not modify the underlying etiology of the renal disease, it is not surprising that the transplanted kidney is sometimes regarded by the host as an appropriate new target for destruction by the original disease process, especially in autoimmune or metabolic diseases.

Glomerulonephritis

In identical twin donor transplants performed in the 1950s, Murray recognized recurrent glomerulonephritic damage, which sometimes became apparent within only a few months.[60] Late follow-up of 30 twin grafts indicated that 8 had failed from recurrent glomerulonephritis, making a strong case for the use of mild immunosuppression even in recipients of twin grafts.[61] Fortunately, recurrent disease is less common in allografts, but in this setting it is more difficult to diagnose because its clinical manifestations and even histologic changes may be confused with those of chronic rejection. A recent report from Australia indicates that recurrent glomerulonephritis may be a more important cause of allograft loss than previously recognized.[62] All 1505 renal transplants performed in that country between 1988 and 1997 were analyzed. Graft loss from biopsy-proven recurrent glomerulonephritis occurred in 52 patients (8.4%). It was more common than acute rejection and in fact was the third most common cause of allograft loss after chronic rejection and death with a functioning transplant. Independent risk factors included peak levels of panel reactive antibodies and the type of glomerulonephritis, especially mesangiocapillary type I, focal segmental membranous nephropathy, IgA nephropathy, and immune crescentic glomerulonephritis. Recurrent disease is most likely in patients whose original disease process has run a rapid course. It appears to be most likely in twins and next most likely in recipients of closely matched related donor allografts. However, the other advantages of related living donors seem to override the risks of recurrent glomerulonephritis and their graft survival remained superior to that of mismatched cadaveric grafts in a large U.S. study of transplants in patients with glomerulonephritis. The graft loss from recurrent glomerulonephritis appears to be quite low (2% to 4%), at least for the first several years, and in an Australian series even at 10 years it was no higher than in patients who had other causes of renal failure. Thus, the risk of recurrent glomerulonephritis should not be considered a contraindication to transplantation, although its very long-term impact is not fully known.

Collagen Diseases

Collagen diseases such as lupus erythematosus are possible but unlikely causes of recurrent damage and are often well palliated by transplantation.

Metabolic Diseases

Cystinosis causes intracellular deposition of cysteine crystals in various organs, usually leading to end-stage renal disease by age 10 years. Although recurrent renal disposition may occur after transplantation, its effects appear to be mild.

Oxalosis is likely to reappear and destroy transplanted kidneys very rapidly (although these changes may be delayed by prolonged pretransplant dialysis and post-transplant diuresis). However, hepatic transplantation, which will reverse the metabolic defect, and concomitant renal transplantation are the ideal treatments, especially in patients with renal and other systemic oxalate damage.[63]

Diabetes, when it causes end-stage nephropathy, has become one of the most common indications for renal transplantation. Diabetic nephropathy is thought to be caused by protracted abnormal glucose homeostasis that, of course, is not corrected by successful renal transplantation. Thus, in diabetic patients, it is not surprising that Kimmelstiel-Wilson lesions may be found on biopsies of the transplanted kidney within 2 years. However, because 10 to 20 years are probably required for these changes to cause functional deterioration, the threat of recurrence is certainly not a contraindication to renal transplantation, which gives diabetics a better chance of survival than chronic dialysis. Successful pancreatic transplantation, if performed concomitantly with renal transplantation, may prevent the early morphologic changes of diabetes in the transplanted kidney.[64]

Complications of Renal Transplantation

Technical Complications

Complications occurring in the first few hours or days after transplantation are commonly related to technical problems in establishing vascular and urinary continuity or to damage that occurs during donor nephrectomy or preservation. Because rejection may also be an early event, its differentiation from various other causes of poor function may be difficult.

VASCULAR COMPLICATIONS

Arterial obstruction, although less common than ATN or urinary tract complications as a cause of early postoperative oliguria or anuria, should be considered promptly if an established diuresis suddenly ceases. A diseased hypogastric artery is likely to thrombose and should never be used to vascularize the transplant. Instead, the usually more normal common or external iliac artery that is also accessible with less dissection should be utilized. Partial occlusion of the transplant vessels may be caused by kinking from unfortunate positioning of the kidney. Although radioisotopic scanning and arteriography will confirm suspected vascular occlusion, immediate reoperation without delay for diagnostic studies is usually the only chance for salvaging such a graft because only a few minutes of total ischemia can be tolerated before damage becomes irreversible.

Occlusion of the transplant renal vein, although rare, can result from technical anastomotic errors or from kinking or compression. Iliofemoral thrombosis occasionally follows renal transplantation, presumably because of clamping of the vein or compression by the transplant. The thrombus rarely extends into the renal vein, and standard anticoagulant treatment is generally effective. In a few cases, therapy with urokinase has been successfully employed to lyse clots occluding the renal vein. If pulmonary embolus occurs despite adequate anticoagulation, caval interruption should be performed by standard techniques such as a Greenfield filter and rarely compromises transplant function.

HEMORRHAGE

Imperfect operative hemostasis in the setting of uremic coagulopathy or anticoagulation during hemodialysis is the usual cause of early postoperative bleeding. Fracture and frank rupture of the transplanted kidney are unusual causes of bleeding, but these may occur from rapid swelling of the transplant during acute rejection. Rupture is more common in kidneys from infant or child donors, in which the small organ is sometimes unable to tolerate adult levels of blood pressure and flow.

Bleeding from the arterial suture line, except in the early hours postoperatively, should bring to mind the strong possibility of infection. Resuturing of an infected suture line is futile because recurrent disruption is virtually ensured. The kidney should be removed and the hypogastric artery securely ligated. If the anastomosis is in the common or external iliac artery, the problem is more serious. Even removal of the kidney necessitates a suture line to close the iliac arteriotomy. This then becomes a potential site of arterial disruption. Ligation of the iliac artery and extra-anatomic bypass (femorofemoral or axillofemoral) may be necessary.

HYPERTENSION AND RENAL TRANSPLANT ARTERY STENOSIS

More than half of renal transplant recipients are hypertensive. Impaired allograft function and administration of cyclosporine and corticosteroids are the major causes. In about 10%, the native kidneys may be the source, and alleviation can be accomplished by nephrectomy. A source of hypertension, which is important to diagnose, is renal transplant artery stenosis (RTAS). This condition may be confused with rejection because both may result in hypertension and diminished renal function. Although RTAS is a relatively unusual cause of decreased renal function, which is more commonly the result of rejection or cyclosporine toxicity, a high index of suspicion should be maintained because it is correctable. The usual time of presenting symptoms is between 3 months and 2 years after transplant (peak, 6 months). The true incidence of RTAS is not known, but in patients suspected on clinical grounds of having renal artery stenosis, confirmation of the diagnosis by biplanar arteriography occurs in 4% to 12%. However, when 100 consecutive transplant patients were subjected to routine postoperative arteriography by Lacombe,[65] a surprising prevalence of stenosis was found (23%).

The etiology of RTAS is frequently technical: improper anastomosis, injury of the intima of the renal artery during washout, or perfusion or kinking at the anastomotic site from redundancy or twisting of the arteries. Arteriosclerotic lesions of the donor or recipient vessels may be a contributing factor, especially in recent years as the donor shortage has mandated the use of older donors. An immunologic pathogenesis also seems likely because intimal proliferation and subintimal fibrotic changes seen in RTAS are similar to small vessel changes caused by rejection. About 70% of the lesions are at the anastomotic site, but 20% are beyond the anastomosis in the transplant renal artery proper. Thus, even the use of a Carrel patch does not preclude this complication. Fortunately, not all instances of RTAS are clinically relevant. Because the incidence of at least mild hypertension is as high as 50% in transplant patients, RTAS is by no means always its cause. Thus, its correction cannot always be expected to be followed by normotension.

We presently advocate percutaneous transluminal angioplasty in most instances of RTAS. Of 547 consecutive renal allograft recipients, 39 suspected of RTAS because of refractory hypertension had the diagnosis confirmed by arteriography and underwent balloon dilatation.[66] Seventy-six percent of percutaneous transluminal angioplasties were successful, whereas only one graft was lost as a result. Three patients initially treated successfully developed recurrent stenosis, which was corrected operatively by patch angioplasty. Although some authors favor operation over percutaneous transluminal angioplasty,[67] the surgical treatment is difficult and not always successful. The long-term results of percutaneous transluminal angioplasty and surgery are probably roughly comparable, but because of simplicity and patient acceptability, most surgeons advocate percutaneous transluminal angioplasty as the initial approach, with surgery reserved for persistent or recurrent stenosis. If surgery is necessary, preserved cadaveric iliac artery may be useful in the repair.[68]

Urinary Tract Complications

The most common cause of sudden cessation of urinary output in the immediate postoperative period is the presence of a blood clot in the bladder or urethral catheter, which can be relieved by irrigation. Other more serious causes of urinary obstruction are unusual and should be investigated simultaneously with consideration of vascular occlusion, ATN, or rejection. A ureteroneocystostomy may become occluded by a hematoma at the site of the submucosal tunnel in the bladder or by a technically unsatisfactory anastomosis. An adynamic ureter or edema at the orifice in the bladder can also cause temporary partial obstruction.

Devascularization of the ureter during donor nephrectomy is a more serious problem that may lead to ureteral necrosis and fistula within the first few days or weeks. Mild ureteral ischemia is the probable cause of an occasional late distal ureteral stenosis, which may lead to partial or total occlusion. Fluid obtained from wound drains or needle aspiration can be identified as urine by its urea content, which is severalfold higher than that of serum or lymph. Ultrasound studies (for fluid collections), radioactive scans, and cystograms (which via reflux may visualize the ureter) are other helpful studies. However, ureterography is usually necessary to define the status of the ureter and is best accomplished by percutaneous fine-needle puncture of the kidney and antegrade catheterization of the pelvis and ureter. Treatment must be individualized and may consist either of reconstruction of the ureteroneocystostomy (if it is not ischemic) or of ureteropyelostomy using the patient's own ureter.

Acute Tubular Necrosis

Ischemia occasionally precipitates ATN in a related donor transplant, but in cadaver transplants the incidence is much higher. Even in transplants from "heart-beating cadavers," some degree of ATN occurs in 5% to 30%. Therefore, in the absence of vascular or ureteral problems, initially nonfunctional cadaver kidneys may be assumed to suffer from ATN, especially if technetium and iodohippurate scans demonstrate good blood flow and poor tubular function. At times, however, a kidney has adequate urine output briefly and then lapses into ATN. Estimating the true output of the transplanted kidney may be difficult if the patient's own kidneys are producing substantial amounts of urine.

Oliguria in the early transplant period should be treated with aliquots of fluid and colloid to exclude hypovolemia, while care is taken not to fluid-overload the patient. Mannitol, 12.5 to 25 g, and furosemide, 100 to 200 mg, intravenously in divided doses may be used to increase the output but are unlikely to alter the course of true ATN. The impact of ATN is definitely an adverse one. Delayed graft function reduces the 5-year graft survival by 10%.[3] Some kidneys that never produce urine (termed *primary nonfunction*) are no doubt lost because potentially reversible damage from ATN is compounded by undiagnosed rejection before function returns, with the result that antirejection therapy is delayed until immunologic damage progresses to an irreversible stage. In an attempt to avoid this sequence, many authors employ ALG or monoclonal anti-T-cell antibodies prophylactically in all instances of ATN. Because there is no specific treatment for ATN, the return of function (usually within 1 to 4 weeks) must be patiently awaited while adequate but safe immunosuppression and good general condition are maintained, if necessary, by dialysis. If there is reasonable clinical confidence in the diagnosis of ATN, it is best to minimize the use of invasive studies such as cystoscopy, arteriography, or biopsy, none of which will provide positive evidence of ATN. Serial renal scans to identify decreases in blood flow may be helpful in making the difficult diagnosis of rejection during ATN, but biopsy is often necessary for confirmation. Even in the absence of rejection, management of immunosuppression is difficult during ATN. The nephrotoxic potential of cyclosporine is particularly disturbing when renal function cannot be assessed. Blood levels of this agent should be carefully monitored during ATN. Many centers avoid cyclosporine entirely during ATN because of the additive damage of ischemia and cyclosporine toxicity.

LYMPHOCELES

Extensive mobilization of the iliac vessels during the transplant operation or failure to ligate lymphatics crossing them may predispose to lymphoceles, which have a variable reported incidence (0.6% to 18%). Possible manifestations that can occur weeks or months postoperatively are swelling of the wound; edema of the scrotum, labia, and lower extremity; and urinary obstruction from pressure on the collecting system or ureter. Ultrasound to identify a fluid-filled mass is the most useful diagnostic study. Aspiration of the cyst will be of only temporary benefit because lymph rapidly reaccumulates. External drainage should be avoided because this will place the kidney and vascular suture line at risk from infection. The treatment of choice is fenestration of the cyst into the peritoneal cavity. This can often be accomplished by laparoscopic technique. We have also successfully employed a nonoperative treatment of percutaneous drainage followed by repeated instillation of tetracycline or povidone-iodine to sclerose and obliterate the cyst.

Nontechnical Complications

INFECTIONS

Factors predisposing to infection of transplant recipients include a major surgical operation involving the urinary tract, infection carried over from the donor, and indwelling catheters in the bladder, bloodstream, and peritoneal cavity. Because of these and the immunodepression associated with uremia and antirejection therapy, 30% to 60% of patients suffer some type of infection during the first transplant year; and in half of the deaths that occur during the first year, infection is an important contributing feature. More cautious use of immunosuppression in the 1980s and the introduction of cyclosporine have reduced the magnitude of this problem, but infection remains the most common and most lethal complication of renal transplantation.

Bacterial Infections. During the first month after transplantation, conventional bacterial infections are the most common, and the urinary tract, respiratory system, and wound are the most prevalent sites. These infections usually respond to prompt vigorous conventional antibiotic therapy. Acute bacterial infections may have a clinical presentation that can be confused with rejection: fever, malaise, swelling, and tenderness of the wound, or even rising creatinine level in the case of a urinary tract infection. It is especially important to exclude the possibility of infection before instituting antirejection therapy because, during infection, immunosuppression should be decreased rather than intensified, even though this action may lead to acute rejection. The incidence of wound infections (reported to be anywhere from 1% to 10%) can probably be reduced by preoperative or intraoperative prophylaxis with a cephalosporin, which should not be continued for more than 24 to 48 hours. Even more important, however, is meticulous surgical technique to avoid hematomas, urinary fistulas, and lymphoceles. Transplant recipients are subject to the usual respiratory infections that occur in normal or hospitalized individuals, and acute bacterial pneumonitis is a potentially lethal infection in these patients. Urinary tract infections, which are the most common bacterial infections in transplant recipients, can be decreased by 50% by using trimethoprim-sulfamethoxazole for the first 6 months after transplantation. This is also helpful in decreasing the incidence of *P. carinii.*

Opportunistic Infections. The period between 30 and 180 days after transplantation, usually the time of most intense immunosuppression, is the most common time for infection with opportunistic organisms, which in normal individuals rarely cause significant illness. In recent years, it has become evident that viral infections are even more important than bacterial ones in this regard, in terms of prevalence, diagnostic and therapeutic difficulty, and immunologic and neoplastic ramifications. This epidemiologic change is probably due to cyclosporine therapy, which allows lower doses of azathioprine and corticosteroids and has decreased the incidence of bacterial infections. At the same time, the use of antibodies against T lymphocytes, which cause seriously impaired antiviral defenses, has increased.

Cytomegalovirus (CMV). CMV, a member of the herpesvirus family, is the most important viral pathogen. This ubiquitous agent infects most normal people at some point in their lives.[69] Although in healthy individuals CMV infections are either clinically silent or mild, the presence of the latent virus and seropositivity persists for life. After renal transplantation, previously seropositive patients usually excrete CMV and exhibit elevations of antibody titer, on the basis of either reactivation of latent virus during immunosuppression or transmission of virus latent in the donor tissues. Under these circumstances, symptomatic illness sometimes occurs (20%) and is usually mild, supporting the hypothesis that previous exposure and immunity to the virus confer protection.[70] However, seronegative recipients who receive a kidney from a seropositive donor are subject to a three times greater incidence of symptomatic illness, and of affected patients 25% have severe disease. CMV "disease" (as distinguished from asymptomatic seroconversion) varies in severity from mild fever and malaise to a debilitating syndrome marked by leukopenia, hepatitis, interstitial pneumonia, arthritis, central nervous system changes including coma, gastrointestinal ulceration and bleeding, renal insufficiency, bacterial or fungal infection, and even death.

Distinguishing CMV disease, which has its usual onset 4 to 6 weeks after transplant, from rejection can be especially difficult because the viral infection can cause renal insufficiency. Seroconversion may not occur for an additional 3 to 6 weeks, and viral cultures consume several weeks. A rapid diagnosis can be made by utilizing tests for antigenemia or polymerase chain reaction assays using blood samples or the demonstration of virus on biopsy of infected tissues. Possible causes of renal malfunction during CMV infections include direct damage from the virus ("glomerulopathy") and triggering of rejection.[69] This is a dilemma because delay in institution of antirejection therapy may lead to irreversible renal damage, but intensification of immunosuppression may lead to lethal superinfection. In cases of decreasing renal function, a decision for or against antirejection therapy must often be based on clinical grounds; however, biopsy should probably be done first if CMV is suspected because it may distinguish rejection from CMV.

Because CMV disease has an adverse impact on morbidity, mortality, and graft loss, it is important to find ways of avoiding it. One obvious partial solution would be to avoid transplantation of all kidneys from seropositive donors to seronegative recipients. Although this might substantially improve graft survival as well as avoid morbidity in seronegative recipients, it would have the disadvantage of greatly reducing the donor pool for seronegative recipients because most adult donors are CMV seropositive. Another possibility would be active immunization for CMV because the most severe disease occurs in seronegative recipients. A live attenuated CMV vaccine was developed that, although not totally preventing infection after transplantation, strikingly reduced the incidence of symptomatic and severe illness.[71] However, it is not available commercially. Passive immunization with immune globulin has also been used effectively by some centers.[72]

Fortunately, both the incidence and the severity of CMV disease appear to be diminished in cyclosporine- or tacrolimus-treated patients. There is impressive evidence that preemptive ganciclovir therapy decreases the incidence of CMV disease.[73] In established clinical CMV disease, intravenous ganciclovir is required for 2 to 4 weeks; viremia should be cleared before discontinuance of therapy.

Polyomavirus Nephropathy. Primary infections with the polyomavirus (type BK) are known to occur in up to 90% of the population, typically without specific signs or symptoms. This virus persists in the kidney where reactivation and shedding into the urine may be detected in 0.5% to 20% of healthy individuals depending on the sensitivity of the assay (polymerase chain reaction vs. detection of viral inclusion bearing "decoy cells" on urinary cytology). Before 1996, BK virus nephropathy was either unrecognized or virtually nonexistent in many transplant centers. Whether the increasing recognition of its prevalence since then is a function of new risk factors such as new immunosuppressive agents, emergence of more virulent viral gene types, or simply greater awareness is uncertain.[74] In any event, it now appears that up to 5% of renal allograft recipients can be affected. The diagnosis can be suspected on the basis of screening urinary cytology, but definitive diagnosis requires allograft biopsy to demonstrate nuclear inclusions in tubular epithelial cells and to rule out rejection or drug toxicity. Progression from an inflammatory stage to a fibrotic stage and finally to sclerosis and irreversible allograft failure has been observed in as many as 45% of affected cases. Current management is based on judicious decreases in immunosuppression to allow clearance of viral replication. In a few instances, the antiviral agent cidofovir has been used with success.

Other opportunistic infections such as aspergillosis, blastomycosis, nocardiosis, toxoplasmosis, and cryptococcosis are particularly likely to occur in transplant patients. The protozoan *P. carinii,* which has infected most individuals by age 10 years, is a pulmonary pathogen only in immunodepressed patients. It is the organism most commonly causing fatal pneumonia in this group. A prompt diagnosis by aggressive measures such as bronchoscopic alveolar lavage and brushing or percutaneous transbronchoscopic or open-lung biopsy is important in cases of *P. carinii* infection because effective treatment exists (trimethoprim and sulfamethoxazole). Prophylaxis with the same agents is warranted in the early postoperative period and also reduces the incidence of bacterial urinary tract infections. Mycobacterial infections are unusual, but their potential lethality mandates constant vigilance.

HYPERGLYCEMIA

For reasons not entirely clear, but generally attributed to intensive or persistent corticosteroid administration, previously normoglycemic patients may become diabetic in the post-transplant period. Uncontrolled hyperglycemia may cause "pseudorejection" on the basis of interference with the laboratory determination for creatinine and increased serum osmolality with resultant intracellular and extracellular dehydration and impaired renal function. In this condition, control of the blood glucose level promptly results in correction of the elevated creatinine value.

GASTROINTESTINAL COMPLICATIONS

Ulceration and perforation of the stomach, duodenum, and small and large intestine are relatively common after transplantation. The colon is especially vulnerable to perforation, and in immunosuppressed patients, abdominal pain or signs of peritoneal irritation merit very close attention if not immediate laparotomy.[75] Diverticulitis is the most common cause of perforation (36%) followed by ischemic colitis (24%). Pancreatitis is another recognized complication of both azathioprine and corticosteroid therapy in transplant patients, in which its course is frequently fulminating and fatal. Infectious gastrointestinal complications such as *Candida* stomatitis and esophagitis, pseudomembranous colitis, and CMV ulceration are also common. Symptoms and signs of these conditions may be masked by corticosteroid therapy.

HYPERPARATHYROIDISM

Secondary hyperparathyroidism from chronic renal failure usually subsides after a successful transplant. However, its persistence ("tertiary hyperparathyroidism") has been reported in 2.6% to 70% of patients, with the smaller number being closer to the true incidence. In cases in which significant hypercalcemia and elevated parathyroid hormone levels persist for more than 12 months after transplant despite normal renal function, we advocate total parathyroidectomy and autotransplantation of fragments from a portion of one gland into the muscle of the forearm, where they are easily accessible for further resection without neck exploration should hypertrophy persist and recurrent hypercalcemia ensue. The sequelae of hyperparathyroidism, such as renal calculi, bone pain, and muscle weakness, are usually benefited by this procedure. In some unfortunate patients, a devastating complication of persistent hyperparathyroidism has been seen in which diffuse cutaneous vascular calcification leads to extensive ulceration and gangrene.[76] Despite total parathyroidectomy, most such patients never heal their ischemic ulcers, which eventually lead to sepsis and death. Common to these patients is persistent post-transplant elevation of serum calcium and radiographic evidence on xerography of extensive small- and medium-vessel calcification. Fortunately, this complication is uncommon, but in the face of nonhealing ulceration that occurs in unusual areas such as the upper extremities, elevation of serum calcium level, and increased parathyroid hormone levels, this diagnosis should be entertained.

TUMORS

In the early days of transplantation, it was found that utilization of apparently uninvolved kidneys from donors with known cancer sometimes resulted in transmission of the malignancy. Since then, in occasional instances, tumors have inadvertently been transplanted from donors with unrecognized cancer. If this complication is recognized early, cessation of immunosuppression is sometimes followed by rejection not only of the transplanted kidney but also of the allogeneic tumor. However, once the transplanted tumor becomes well established, it may continue to flourish and cause death even in the absence of immunosuppression.

It has been known for many years that both naturally occurring and iatrogenic states of immunodeficiency are accompanied by an increased risk of neoplasia. For example, chronic dialysis patients have an increased risk of malignancy that causes death in 1% to 4%. One hypothesis invoked to explain the more striking prevalence of malignancies in immunosuppressed patients is a breakdown of normal immunologic surveillance mechanisms that allows persistence of mutant malignant cells that would be recognized and destroyed by an intact immune system. It is theorized that such "forbidden clones" are particularly likely to go unrecognized in the brain, an immunologically privileged site. Other etiologic possibilities for the increased neoplasia are chronic immunologic stimulation of the lymphoreticular system by the transplant, direct carcinogenic action of immunosuppressive drugs, and oncogenesis by the viral pathogens whose growth is encouraged by immunosuppression. The latter possibility is supported by the finding that tumors in which a viral pathogenesis seems likely (lymphoma, skin, lip, uterine cervix, and perineal cancers) are especially prevalent in transplant patients. Since 1968, Israel Penn's Cincinnati Transplant Tumor Registry has collected data from around the world on tumors in transplant patients.[77] This registry has received reports on 11,663 post-transplant malignancies, 8,868 of them in renal transplant patients. In renal transplant recipients, the reported incidence of 6% de novo malignant neoplasms represents a risk approximately 100 times greater than that in normal age-matched populations. The increased incidence of tumors appears to be related to the degree and duration of immunosuppression rather than to any particular agent. These tumors often occur in young patients, and their behavior is unusually aggressive. Cancers common in the general population (lung, breast, prostate, and colon) are not increased, but certain uncommon neoplasms are extremely prevalent (lymphomas, lip cancers, renal cancers, various other sarcomas, hepatobiliary carcinomas, Kaposi's sarcoma, and carcinomas of the vulva and perineum). Carcinomas of the uterine cervix are also very common, although most of these are in situ lesions. Most common of all are squamous cell carcinomas of skin and lip, which are especially prevalent in sunny areas such as Australia and New Zealand, where their incidence is increased 21-fold and patients who survive 15 years after transplantation have a striking 44% incidence of skin cancer. These cancers kill 5.1% of their victims.

Transplant recipients in all parts of the world have a disproportionately high incidence of lymphomas (350 times normal) that constitute 20% of all tumors in this population.[78] Of the 1953 post-transplant lymphomas and lymphoproliferations reported to the Cincinnati registry, well-defined entities such as Hodgkin's disease and plasmacytoma/myeloma were less common than in the general population, accounting for 2.8% and 3.9% of lymphomas, respectively, compared with 10% and 19% in nonimmunosuppressed populations. There has been considerable disagreement regarding the classification of the more usual lymphomatous lesions of transplant patients. As a result, the nonspecific term *post-transplant lymphoproliferative disease* (PTLD) is now widely used, covering a spectrum of lesions ranging from benign hyperplasia to frankly malignant lymphomas. According to the UNOS database of 205,114 recipients transplanted between 1988 and 1999, 2,365 (1.15%) developed PTLD.[79] The highest incidence was in intestinal transplants (6.0%). The hyperplasias include infectious mononucleosis and plasma cell hyperplasia, whereas the neoplasias include polymorphic PTLD, monomorphic PTLD, myeloma, plasmacytoma, and lymphomas with Hodgkin's disease–like features. Hyperplastic PTLDs are polyclonal in origin, whereas neoplastic PTLDs contain a monoclonal component that can be detected by sensitive assays. Of 765 PTLDs in the Penn registry that were studied immunologically, 85% were of B-cell origin, 15% were of T-cell origin, and rare cases were of null-cell origin or were combined B- and T-cell lymphomas. In patients with these tumors, extranodal involvement is unusually common (69%) and the transplanted kidney is often involved (23%). Twenty-two percent of these tumors are in the central nervous system, an unusual site for lymphomas.

De novo lymphomas may begin as lymphoproliferative lesions induced by viruses. Although other viruses may also be involved, growing evidence implicates infection with the Epstein-Barr virus as the most important factor in PTLD. Compelling evidence of this is the finding of Epstein-Barr virus incorporated into the genome of lymphoma cells. These patients often have a syndrome resembling mononucleosis with fever, pharyngitis, and diffuse lymphadenopathy. Indicating polyclonal B-cell proliferation rather than true malignancy is the finding in these early lesions of a diversity of cellular immunoglobulins.[80] During the stage of polyclonality, cessation of immunosuppression may allow regression of the lesions. The use of the antiviral agent acyclovir, which blocks Epstein-Barr virus-inhibited oropharyngeal shedding of the virus, has also been reported to contribute to remissions. Tumors that are initially polyclonal may eventually undergo a cytogenetic alteration, leading to malignant transformation and the monoclonality characteristic of true B-cell lymphomas. Monoclonal tumors do not regress after cessation of immunosuppression or acyclovir therapy. They are aggressive malignancies that can be treated only by surgery and irradiation, neither of which is very effective. The outcomes were studied in 1366 patients with PTLD reported to the Cincinnati registry. Of these, 224 patients had no treatment; the tumor was discovered at autopsy in 104 of them. No treatment data were available in 62 patients. Treatment was given to 1080 patients (79%), and, of these, 411 (38%) had complete remissions. In 69 of these recipients (17%), the only treatment was reduction or cessation of immunosuppressive therapy, and in 50 (12%) the only treatment was chemotherapy.

Results of Renal Transplantation

The outcome of each renal transplant depends on a number of complex and interrelated variables. The cumulative influence of these variables is analyzed annually by the UNOS Scientific Registry, which by federal law receives data on all transplants performed in the United States.[3] The most recent registry report details the outcome of the 53,055 primary transplants done from 1996 to 2000, including 19,692 living and 33,363 cadaveric transplants. The results in this era of the current immunosuppression were also compared with those of earlier eras and especially to the 84,982 transplants performed from 1988 to 1995.

Because rejection is the chief deterrent to success, it is not surprising that histocompatibility remains an influential factor. During the early days of transplantation, the success of HLA-identical sibling donor grafts was twice that of cadaveric transplants. Since then, the short-term results of cadaveric grafts have improved greatly and now, at least for a year, approach the success of HLA identical sibling grafts (89% vs. 96%) (Fig. 27-5). However, when long-term survival is examined, the importance of histocompatibility remains obvious. At 5 years, 90% of HLA-identical sibling grafts survive and at 10 years, 65%, but despite striking advances in immunosuppressive therapy, the survival of cadaveric grafts at 5 years is only 65% and

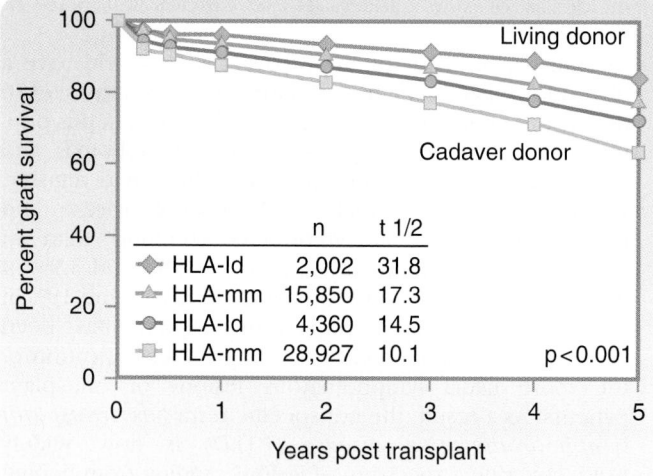

FIGURE 27-5. Although the short-term success of kidneys transplanted from cadaveric donors approaches that of related donors, the long-term survival increasingly favors related donor grafts. The half-life of HLA-identical living donor grafts is three times longer than that of HLA-mismatched cadaveric donor grafts.

at 10 years less than 40% unless they are matched for the recipient's HLA antigens, which improves their 5-year survival to about 73% (see Fig. 27-5).

Many other factors also influence the results of transplantation. Those compromising outcomes include unusually young or old recipients or donors (<5 or >50 years); interracial grafts; broadly sensitized recipients as identified by preformed antibodies against a panel of donor lymphocytes; previous failed transplants, especially if lost from early rejection; delayed transplant function, requiring dialysis; poor early function (serum creatinine > 3 at time of hospital discharge); and certain disease states (e.g., hypertensive nephrosclerosis, oxalosis). There is considerable evidence that donor brain death itself is accompanied by physiologic and immunologic changes that may cause or predispose to further renal damage. This may account in part for the fact that about one fourth of cadaveric grafts have delayed function.

Despite improvements in crossmatching and immunosuppression, sensitized recipients of first cadaveric kidneys had a 14% greater incidence of delayed graft function and an 8% lower graft survival at 5 years. Loss of a previous transplant was also a negative predictor. For recipients of cadaveric grafts, 5-year graft survivals were 66% for a primary graft but only 62% and 56% for second and third grafts, respectively.

Recipient race was another important factor in graft survival. Late graft loss was twice as frequent in blacks as in nonblack recipients whether the donor was living or cadaveric. Because of racially associated histocompatibility differences, blacks have also been at a disadvantage for allocation of cadaveric kidneys (the majority of which come from white donors) since the distribution algorithm has been heavily influenced by matching. To address this inequity, the UNOS Board of Directors recently voted to discontinue matching at the B locus as a consideration in allocation of cadaveric donor organs.

Factors associated with favorable outcome include relatively young donors (especially those 6 to 50 years old);

good histocompatibility (especially complete HLA identity); and living donors (even if not related to the recipient by blood) (Fig. 27-6). The addition of tacrolimus and MMF to the immunosuppressive armamentarium as well as availability of a variety of antilymphocytic antibodies utilized for induction therapy appears to have greatly diminished the incidence of early rejection crises and improved graft survival at least for the first few years. The impact of these agents on chronic rejection and very long-term graft survival is more difficult to assess.

Since about 1980, the 1-year survival of first cadaveric grafts has gradually improved from 50% to almost 89%. The 20% improvement, which occurred between 1973 and 1984, was attributed to the policy of deliberate pretransplant blood transfusions (a strategy that was abandoned with the availability of cyclosporine). The additional 19% improvement since then was due to the introduction of cyclosporine in 1983 and the subsequent introduction of tacrolimus, MMF, and newer antilymphocytic antibodies. Cumulative experience and improvements in the art and science of transplantation undoubtedly also played a role in these impressive and progressively better short-term results. The 1-year survival of patients who receive cadaveric grafts has improved even more dramatically than graft survival and now for 1 year closely approaches that seen for recipients of related donor grafts at greater than 90%. But at 10 years, it is only 63% versus 80% for recipients of living donor grafts.[3]

A disappointing aspect of the results of renal transplantation is evident from examining long-term cadaveric graft survival. Despite the dramatic short-term improvements in both patient and graft survival since about 1980, substantive attrition of cadaveric grafts continues after 1 year. Until 1988, this attrition remained almost constant at about 7% per year despite the introduction of cyclosporine. Since then, the half-life of cadaveric grafts has improved to 14.5 years if they were HLA-matched with the recipient but to only 10.2 years for other cadaveric grafts. Patients who received cadaveric grafts in 1967 had

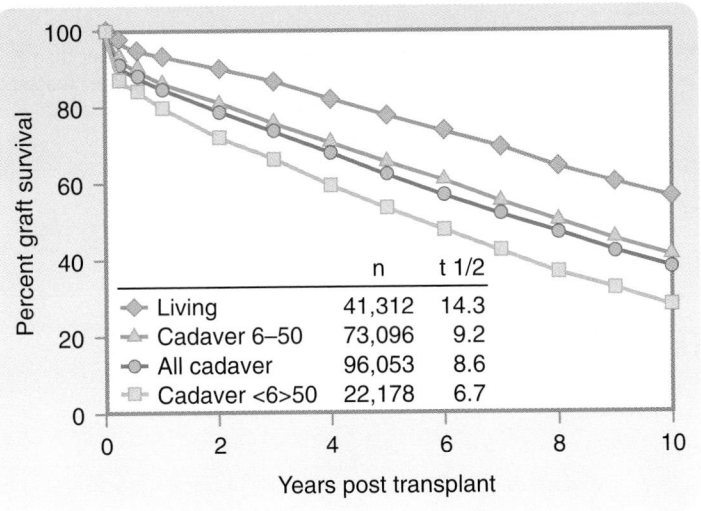

FIGURE 27-6. Renal transplants from living donors have the best survival, even if the donor is not genetically related to the recipient.

a 10-year graft survival of 23%, whereas those being performed today are still not expected to have a better than 40% 10-year graft survival, leaving considerable room for further improvement.[3] Continuing damage of grafts appears to be the result of chronic rejection, and in some patients recurrence of glomerulonephritis, entities for which we still lack effective therapy.

The excellent results of transplantation relative to dialysis and the donor shortage have resulted in a growing list of patients awaiting transplantation. By 2001 more than 50,000 candidates awaited cadaveric kidneys, in the United States whereas only about 9,000 renal transplants were done. For older patients, a 3- to 5-year waiting time represented a significant portion of their remaining life.

Impatience with long waiting times for cadaveric donor kidneys (during which many dialysis patients die) has led to a considerable increase in the use of living donors, which now exceed the number of cadaveric donors in the United States compared with less than 20% a decade ago. Unfortunately, donation of cadaveric kidneys has increased little, and most of this minimal increase has been from suboptimal donors; either younger than 5 or older than 50 years. The surprisingly good success of unrelated living donor transplants and the introduction of laparoscopic donor nephrectomy are responsible for much of this increase (Fig. 27-7). Overall results of transplantation have benefited from this shift to living donors because, at 10 years, there is an 18% better survival of living donor versus cadaveric grafts. For HLA-identical sibling donors, better than 90% 1-year graft survival has been reported since the mid 1970s and is now over 96%. The 1-year graft survival of parental or one-haplotype sibling transplants has also steadily improved since about 1980 from about 70% to the current 90% to 93%.[3]

Another impact of the donor shortage has had an adverse effect on overall results: the utilization of kidneys from suboptimal donors. The percentage of cadaveric kidneys from donors older than 50 years of age increased from 26% in 1988 to 46% in 2000. Unfortunately, age has a profound effect on 5-year graft survival, which was 72% for donors 6 to 18 years old but only 50% for donors older than 60 years (see Fig. 27-6). The use of kidneys from non–heart-beating donors might also have been expected to result in inferior outcomes, and indeed the incidence of delayed graft function was nearly double that of transplantation from heart-beating brain-dead donors (43% vs. 22%). Surprisingly, the 1- and 5-year survivals of 509 of these grafts transplanted between 1996 and 2000 were the same as for the heart-beating donors, perhaps because there donors were selected more carefully for other criteria, such as age.

LIVER TRANSPLANTATION

Indication for Liver Transplantation

Liver transplantation is the procedure of choice for a wide range of diseases that result in acute or chronic end-stage liver disease (ESLD), as well as for several diseases in which a major genetic error affects production of an essential liver protein.[81] It may also be considered as a treatment for a limited number of carefully selected patients who have nonresectable liver tumors that have not metastasized outside the liver.

Indications for liver transplantation in adults and children are summarized in Table 27-1. Despite the differences in the etiology of these diseases, their shared pathophysiology leads to a common set of symptoms and signs typical of end-stage liver failure.[82,83] The Child-Turcote-Pugh (CTP) score was established in an attempt to standardize the severity of chronic liver failure by using a reliable set of criteria that reflect the residual function of the liver (Table 27-2).[84] A combination of clinical

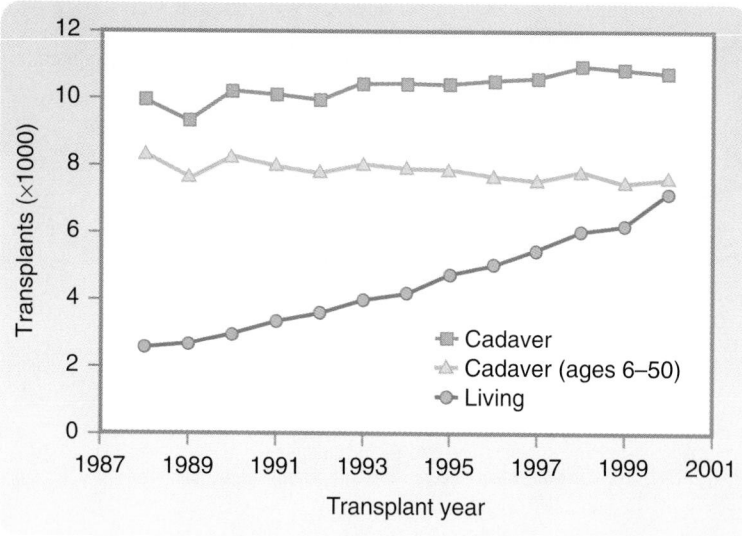

FIGURE 27-7.   Only a minor increase has occurred in the number of cadaveric donors over the past 15 years (and this only in suboptimal ages younger than 6 and older than 50 years). Living donors have increased on the basis of acceptance of genetically unrelated donors and the perceived lesser morbidity of laparoscopic donor operations.

TABLE 27-1. Indications for Liver Transplantation

Adults		Children	
Noncholestatic cirrhosis	65	Biliary atresia	58
Viral hepatitis B and C		Inborn errors of metabolism	11
Alcoholic*		Cholestatic	9
Cryptogenic		Primary sclerosing cholangitis	
Cholestatic	14	Alagille's syndrome	
Primary biliary cirrhosis		Autoimmune	4
Primary sclerosing cholangitis		Viral hepatitis	2
Autoimmune	5	Miscellaneous	16
Malignant neoplasm	2		
Miscellaneous	14		

*Most alcoholic patients are co-infected with the hepatitis C virus.

TABLE 27-2. Child-Turcote-Pugh Score of Severity of Liver Disease*

Points	1	2	3
Encephalopathy	None	1-2	3-4
Ascites	Absent	Slight	Moderate
Bilirubin (mg/dL)	<2	2-3	>3
For PBC/PSC	<4	4-10	>10
Albumin (g/dL)	>3.5	2.8-3.5	<2.8
PT (INR)	<1.7	1.7-2.3	>2.3

INR, International Normalized Ratio; PBC, primary biliary cirrhosis; PSC, primary sclerosing cholangitis; PT, prothrombin time.
*Patient can be placed on the transplant waiting list when the score is > 7. Higher status is assigned when the score is > 10 or when patients are developing severe life-threatening complications related to liver failure.

TABLE 27-3. Concordance with 3-Month Mortality: MELD and CTP

Score	Concordance	95% Confidence Interval
Model for End-Stage Liver Disease (MELD)	0.88	0.85, 0.90
Child-Turcote-Pugh (CTP)	0.79	0.75, 0.83

symptoms and laboratory data are used to provide insight into the severity of the disease and the residual function of the liver. In the absence of more reliable methods, the CTP scoring system was adopted as the standard method for the placement of patients suffering from ESLD on the transplant waiting list. Because categorization based on CPT was not a continuous scale, waiting time on the list was used to stratify patients within a CPT score group.

In 2002 the United Network for Organ Sharing put into place a new system for allocation that did not suffer from emphasis on waiting time and subjective clinical parameters (such as degree of ascites or encephalopathy) integral to the CPT base system. The overall goal of this major revision to liver allocation was to give priority to the sickest patients using a system based on objective variables. To accomplish this, a statistical model for end-stage liver disease (MELD) was employed for adult patients that had been shown to have a high predictive capacity in identifying those patients with ESLD at greatest risk of mortality within 3 months.[85] The MELD score was based on three laboratory values: total bilirubin, International Normalized Ratio, and creatinine value and demonstrated a better correlation with 3-month survival than the CPT score (Table 27-3). A similar approach was developed for pediatric patients, although the relevant variables suffer slightly (PELD score).[86]

This approach is not applied to urgent patients with fulminant liver failure (status 1 patients) but appears to work well for those with chronic liver disease. It is modified for certain conditions that express unique variables, such as small and potentially curable but nonresectable hepatocellular carcinomas and inborn errors of metabolism. The system is also adjusted to meet the special needs of children whose liver disease may be characterized by failure to thrive or recurrent cholangitis. It is recognized that no scoring system is perfect at identifying those at greatest risk; however, multiple laboratory tests such as serum levels of hyaluronate, amino-terminal propeptide collagen type III, indocyanine green clearance, or galactose elimination proved no better in quantitating hepatocyte function or in correlation with the progression of liver disease.[87,88]

Specific exclusion criteria for liver transplantation are not formally established, although it is generally agreed that the presence of active sepsis or the findings of extrahepatic malignancy should be considered absolute contraindications. Still controversial are conditions such as human immunodeficiency virus infection in the absence of the acquired immunodeficiency syndrome, large-size hepatocellular cancer (>6 cm), or cholangiocarcinoma. Several other entities such as portal vein thrombosis once considered contraindications for transplantation are no longer so categorized.

It is essential for the general surgeon to recognize the dynamics of chronic liver disease and to be able to assess the residual liver function in the presence of chronic liver disease. It is not uncommon for minor surgical procedures to exhaust the residual reserve and precipitate the development of acute on chronic failure. Management of these complications is extremely difficult. If liver transplantation must be performed during such circumstances it is associated with higher morbidity and mortality.

Diseases Treated by Liver Transplantation

The conditions that result in an end-stage acute or chronic liver failure are different in the pediatric and adult populations. Whereas the incidence of most liver diseases has remained relatively constant over recent times, the prevalence of liver failure from viral hepatitis is increasing, reflecting the increased rate of infection in the past two decades. It is expected that the relatively recent availability of the hepatitis B vaccine and the ability to detect the hepatitis C virus in donated blood will lower the rate of new infections and the number of individuals who subsequently develop chronic disease.

Hepatitis B

HBV belongs to a family of closely related DNA viruses called the hepadnaviruses. Chronic HBV infection afflicts 1.25 million people in the United States and is characterized serologically by the persistent presence of HBV DNA and usually HBV antigen in serum.[89] Treatment with recombinant interferon alfa-2b leads to remission in 40% of the patients.[90] Persistent infection is associated with the continuous host immune attack against HBV proteins expressed on the surface of the hepatocyte and results in the development of cirrhosis. HBV infection is also a risk factor for hepatocellular carcinoma, which arises almost exclusively in patients with cirrhosis.[91] As with other forms of liver cancer, tumors associated with hepatitis B result from chronic inflammation and repeated cellular regeneration, typically occurring only after 25 to 30 years of infection. Most patients with chronic hepatitis B undergoing liver transplantation will reinfect the hepatic graft, and some undergo rapidly progressive liver failure. Fortunately, prophylaxis consisting of high-titer hepatitis B immune globulin and/or lamivudine is highly effective in the control of viral replication and recurrent disease post transplant.[92]

Hepatitis C

The hepatitis C virus is an RNA virus of the flavivirus family that leads to chronic inflammation of the liver in about 85% of infected individuals. It is detected by the persistence of anti-HCV antibodies, serum viral proteins, and HCV RNA. Virtually all patients with chronic HCV infection develop histologic features of chronic hepatitis, and as many as 20% of patients develop cirrhosis within 10 to 20 years of HCV infection.[93] They develop the typical complications of chronic liver disease including portal hypertension, hepatocellular failure, and hepatic encephalopathy. Hepatocellular carcinoma may ensue in 1% to 4% per year of chronic active hepatitis C patients with established cirrhosis.[94] Serial liver biopsies every few years may be an important tool for following the course of chronic hepatitis C because they determine the degree of inflammation and the amount of fibrosis present.[95] For patients with advanced liver disease, liver transplantation is often the only therapeutic option. The initial results of transplantation are good, with patient and graft survivals of 85% and 90%, respectively, at 1 year. However, virtually all patients become reinfected with HCV after transplantation and about half of them develop histologic evidence of chronic hepatitis within a few months.[96] There is growing concern regarding the eventual recurrence of liver failure in these patients 5 to 10 years after transplantation, and recent evidence indicates that the long-term survival for patients transplanted for HCV may be significantly inferior in comparison to transplantation for other causes of liver disease.[97]

Alcoholic Liver Disease

Alcoholic liver injury results from toxic effects of ethanol to hepatocytes, the accumulation of fatty acids within the cells, and subsequent degeneration and necrosis.[98] The intensity of the inflammatory process is directly related to the amount of alcohol consumed and is associated with fibrosis and subsequent cirrhosis. The coexistence of hepatitis C infection accelerates liver injury in most cases.[99] Discontinuation of alcohol consumption may arrest hepatocyte destruction and allow regeneration and relatively compensated cirrhosis. Continued deterioration of liver function in the absence of alcohol and an appropriate CTP score is an indication for transplantation, just as in other liver diseases. Transplant candidates with alcoholic cirrhosis should undergo careful psychosocial evaluation in an attempt to document their sobriety for at least 6 months and the likelihood of post-transplant recidivism. Careful selection results in a low rate of recidivism in most centers. Outcomes of the transplant procedure are similar to those in other disease processes.

Primary Biliary Cirrhosis and Primary Sclerosing Cholangitis

Primary biliary cirrhosis (PBC) and primary sclerosing cholangitis (PSC) share many clinical, biochemical, and pathologic features.[100] Clinically, both give rise to characteristic symptoms and signs of chronic biliary tract disease (e.g., pruritus and jaundice). In both conditions, the most characteristic biochemical abnormality is an increased serum alkaline phosphatase level. Central to the pathologic changes in both PBC and PSC is damage to bile ducts; in the case of PBC, this involves mainly the smaller intrahepatic ducts, whereas in PSC it also affects large ducts outside the liver as well as the gallbladder and even pancreatic ducts. Unique to PSC is its association with inflammatory bowel disease, which occurs in 70% of the patients. There is an increased incidence of cholangiocarcinoma in PSC patients. Liver failure in both diseases is manifested by hyperbilirubinemia. Transplantation is highly successful in both groups leading to long-term survival of more than 90% and an insignificant incidence of recurrence.[101]

Hepatocellular Carcinoma

The rationale for liver transplantation in patients with nonresectable hepatocellular carcinoma is based on the logical potential of complete removal of disease that is confined to the liver. Unfortunately, it has become evident that in most cases the tumor recurs.[102] However, the procedure can provide significant benefit in a specific subpopulation of patients identified by the following characteristics: histologic grading of G1-2 and tumor size less than 5 cm, limited multifocally. The initial work-up in all transplant candidates must exclude extrahepatic metastases and macrovascular invasion of the liver on imaging. The results of transplantation for this selected group are variable but have been reported to have a disease-free survival of 60% to 85% at 3 years. It is yet to be determined whether the addition of adjuvant chemotherapy after transplantation could be an important factor in the control of recurrence.

Biliary Atresia

Extrahepatic biliary atresia is an obliterative cholangiopathy affecting all or part of the extrahepatic biliary tree.[103] The condition occurs in 1 of 10,000 neonates. The diagnosis is suggested in neonates who remain jaundiced for 6 weeks or more after birth and have pale stools and dark urine. By then, the liver is enlarged and firm or hard, a reflection of the presence of underlying portal fibrosis. The Kasai procedure (hepatic portoenterostomy with resection of the obliterated bile ducts and reestablishment of biliary drainage to the intestine) can increase survival rates at the early stage.[104] However, progressive intrahepatic bile duct destruction by chronic inflammation, fibrosis, and cirrhosis commonly occurs. Failure of the Kasai procedure is manifested by failure to thrive, recurrent cholangitis, and typical signs of ESLD. These are indications for transplantation.

Failure of Previous Liver Graft

An important and growing indication for transplantation is the failure of a previous graft. This occurs in the acute setting immediately post transplant arising from technical failures discussed later or chronically because of chimeric rejection or disease reoccurrence. Retransplantation can be particularly complex in the chronic setting owing to the usual factors associated with reoperative surgery. Overall, the results of retransplantation are inferior to those achieved with primary grafts and each subsequent transplant is associated with an additional decrement in survival.[105]

Patient Selection and Preoperative Consideration

Patients who experience progressive deterioration or acute decompensation of preexisting chronic liver disease, or previously normal patients who suddenly develop fulminant liver failure, are candidates for transplantation and should be promptly referred for evaluation to a transplant center. An extensive work-up is done to assess the degree of liver disease and the potential for recovery, as well as to determine the existence of other extrahepatic conditions that might compromise the outcome of a transplant. Comprehensive medical assessment is mandatory to establish the candidate's ability to withstand complex major surgery and to determine the potential for long-term survival. Only a few specific contradictions totally preclude transplantation in high-risk candidates (i.e., extrahepatic malignancy, irreversible brain damage, severe cardiopulmonary failure, or uncontrollable sepsis). In patients with liver failure, deterioration of the kidneys (hepatorenal) or the lungs (hepatopulmonary) are well-defined syndromes that may be reversible in the presence of a functioning liver and should not exclude candidates from liver transplantation. Irreversible kidney damage can be well managed by combined liver-kidney transplantation.

Assessment of Acute Liver Failure

The hallmarks of fulminant liver failure include the development of encephalopathy, coagulopathy, and hypoglycemia. Careful neurologic evaluation must determine the stage of hepatic coma. Progression from a state of confusion to one of unresponsiveness is associated with an increased likelihood that brain damage is irreversible. At this stage, assessment must include brain imaging with CT or MRI, and monitoring of intracranial pressure (ICP) should be considered. An attempt should be made to help promote cerebral perfusion (above 60 mm Hg) by reducing ICP and maintaining high mean arterial pressure. Irreversible injury is associated with persistent elevation of ICP, which leads to the development of severe brain edema and herniation. Other variables that define the extent of liver injury and predict chances of recovery relate to changes in prothrombin time, levels of factor V, phosphorus levels, and persistence of hypoglycemia. Coagulopathy may be resistant to correction but is best treated with transfusion of fresh frozen plasma. Plasmapheresis may be beneficial in small children in whom administration of large fluid volumes is problematic. Severe hypoglycemia is usually controlled by a dextrose infusion. Interestingly, changes in liver transaminases are not reliable indicators of the potential for recovery.

Superimposed acute liver failure in patients with chronic liver disease may have a clinical presentation similar to that of fulminant liver failure in previously normal patients. In most cases the precipitating factor is related to acute bleeding or infection. Management should be directed toward resuscitation and control of the bleeding or infection. Ideally, successful stabilization and clinical improvement should be followed by urgent transplantation. However, these candidates are at higher risk of morbidity and mortality, mostly owing to the development of bacterial and fungal infections. The surgeon must use clinical judgment to determine the presence of irreversible multiorgan system failure and avoid an unnecessary or futile transplant.

In the absence of a definitive therapy for most types of liver diseases, it must be expected that the natural course of decompensated liver disease will lead to worsening of the patient's general condition and development of life-threatening complications, including variceal bleeding, hepatic encephalopathy, spontaneous bacterial peritonitis, and hepatorenal syndrome. Unfortunately, there are few effective means to prevent such complications. Thus, patients who are judged to be at risk for decompensating should be given priority for urgent transplantation.

Donor Assessment

A major limitation to clinical transplantation is the availability of organ donors. Appropriate management of brain dead donors and the avoidance of potential injuries during the procurement procedure are essential to good function of the transplanted graft. It is important to establish aggressive donor management protocols to minimize the adverse physiological consequences of brain death. These protocols should include respiratory and hemodynamic support, adequate fluid resuscitation, and the initiation of hormone replacement. Brain death is associated with significant instability, and minute-to-minute management by experienced personnel in the intensive care unit (ICU) is necessary to ensure adequate perfusion of all organs. Simultaneously, the donor's liver function must be determined. A rapid screening and a serial follow-up of liver enzymes and synthetic functions are indicative of the degree of liver injury and predict the potential for recovery. Routine assessment for diseases, which might be transmitted by the liver graft, must include hepatitis screening as well as the history of use of toxic substances such as long-standing alcohol consumption.

The donor shortage has led to the more frequent use of livers that would have been discarded in the past. The terms *marginal donor* and *expanded criteria donor* have evolved as transplant programs have been forced to utilize suboptimal donors. These include older donors, hepatitis C and hepatitis B core Ab-positive donors, and livers with a moderate amount of steatosis. Although donor age has been shown to have an adverse impact on outcome, most programs now consider the use of donors up to 75 years of age. This approach has been necessary because of the desperate need for lifesaving organs and is supported by scientific evidence of a relatively slow aging process occurring within the liver parenchyma. It appears that grafts from donors with serologies positive for a pathogen present in the recipient (i.e., hepatitis B or C) can be utilized with results equal to those of transplantation with uninfected grafts as long as the liver does not have established severe hepatitis or fibrosis.[97] Severe steatosis in liver grafts is associated with a high degree of primary nonfunction, but acceptable results can be obtained if steatosis is mild to moderate (10% to 30%). Whenever a marginal graft is used, controllable variables, such as cold ischemic time, should be kept to a minimum.

Donor and recipient matching are based on ABO blood group compatibility and size. However, these barriers may be crossed when transplantation is urgent. Most surgeons try to match donor-recipient age for pediatric recipients, because variation may have an impact on long-term graft survival.[106]

Donor Operation

Liver procurement is almost always part of a multi-team approach aiming to maximize the number of transplantable organs that can be recovered from a single donor. A midline incision extending from the suprasternal notch to the symphysis pubis allows access to thoracic and abdominal organs. The round ligament is ligated and divided, the falciform ligament is incised, and the left lateral segment is freed from the diaphragm. Inspection of the gastrohepatic ligament will reveal a replaced left hepatic artery. Medial reflection of the right colon and small bowel allows the exposure of the infrahepatic vena cava and renal veins, control of the distal aorta, and identification of the inferior mesenteric vein. The attention is turned to the hepatoduodenal ligament, where a variable order of dissection is performed with the aim to identify one or more of the structures, including the common hepatic artery, common bile duct, and portal vein. Attention must be directed toward preservation of abnormal and/or accessory arteries to the liver. Technique varies between procurement surgeons, with some preferring to perform the majority of the dissection while the heart is still beating, whereas others first identify basic anatomy and then complete the dissection after cold perfusion. After all teams complete dissection of all organs, the donor is heparinized, followed by perfusion with cold preservation solution via cannulas inserted in the distal aorta and a branch of the portal vein and placement of topical ice. The liver is then removed with the entire length of the celiac artery and/or any other accessory or replaced arteries, a significant length of the portal vein, the common bile duct, and the entire retrohepatic vena cava (Fig. 27-8). Further preparation of the graft before transplantation is done on the bench while the liver is kept immersed in ice. This will usually include removal of the diaphragm and the excess tissue around the blood vessels and, if necessary, reconstruction of replaced hepatic arteries to one common trunk.

The tolerance of liver grafts to extended periods of cold ischemia is directly dependent on the composition of the preservation solution, donor age, the presence of steatosis, and hemodynamic stability before procurement. In theory, preservation in University of Wisconsin solution may extend cold ischemia time up to 24 hours before revascularization. However, most experienced surgeons prefer to minimize the length of cold ischemia to less than 10 hours.

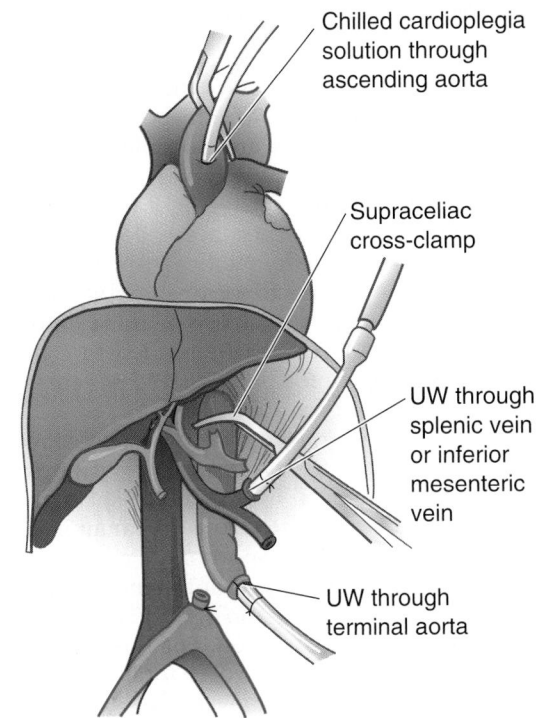

Chilled cardioplegia solution through ascending aorta

Supraceliac cross-clamp

UW through splenic vein or inferior mesenteric vein

UW through terminal aorta

FIGURE 27-8. The donor procedure. UW, University of Wisconsin solution.

Recipient Operation

The unpredictable nature of organ availability dictates that most liver transplants must be done without extensive preoperative preparation of the recipient. Most patients do not need complete bowel preparation, but they should receive preoperative prophylaxis with antibiotics to cover gram-positive and -negative bacteria. The administration of pretransplant immunosuppression is dictated by the specific immunosuppressive protocol being employed.

Anesthesia management in most cases should begin by preparation for continuous monitoring of arterial blood pressure, pulmonary artery pressure, and cardiac output. Large-bore intravenous cannulas and a rapid infuser may be inserted in anticipation of possible major blood loss. Correction of coagulopathy and replacement of blood loss should be initiated early in the operation before any possible extensive bleeding or the development of significant circulatory compromise.

Orthotopic liver transplantation is a three-step surgical procedure, each step of which presents different unique challenges for the surgeons and anesthesiologists.

Recipient Hepatectomy

The abdominal cavity is entered via a bilateral subcostal incision with a midline extension toward the xiphoid. The round ligament is clamped, divided, and ligated. Exploration of the abdominal cavity is performed, and ascites is removed. The falciform ligament is divided down to the suprahepatic vena cava. Placement of an appropriate mechanical retractor should allow adequate exposure of

the liver and its attachments. At this stage, the left lateral segment is separated from the diaphragm and the hepatogastric ligament is divided. The rest of the dissection is done on the hepatoduodenal ligament. The right and left branches of the hepatic artery are then ligated and divided at the hilum. Similarly, the common bile and cystic ducts are ligated and divided. At this stage, the portal vein is skeletonized. The rest of the dissection includes detachment of the liver from the retroperitoneum (bare area) and exposure of the infrahepatic and suprahepatic vena cava. At this stage, clamps are placed on the portal vein and suprahepatic vena cava and the liver is removed. To keep the blood loss to a minimum, the majority of the dissection is carried out using the electrocautery and hemostasis achieved with the use of the argon beam coagulator.

This standard technique is slightly modified in some centers, specifically with regard to the surgeon's preference for the use of venovenous bypass. The reduction of venous blood return from the portal system and the infrahepatic inferior vena cava may result in hemodynamic instability and portal venous congestion. This can be avoided by inflow cannulation of the portal and femoral/iliac veins (either by percutaneous or cut-down techniques) and outflow via a cannula in the internal jugular vein, allowing return of more than 2.5 L/min. Additional important advantages of this technique include control of body temperature with the use of a warming circuit and the potential for ultrafiltration using attached filters. Many surgeons do not advocate the routine use of the venovenous bypass, contending that most patients can tolerate clamping the portal vein and that the entire vena cava may be preserved without interrupting blood flow.

Anhepatic Phase

After hemostasis, the retroperitoneum may be reapproximated to cover the bare area. The suprahepatic vena caval cuff is prepared by opening the orifice of the right, middle, and left hepatic veins and oversewing of the phrenic branches. Transplantation is done by end-to-end anastomosis of the donor's to the recipient's suprahepatic vena cava, followed by similar end-to-end anastomosis of the infrahepatic vena cavae. Alternatively, an end-to-side anastomosis of the vena cavae may be utilized in a "piggyback" fashion in which the recipient's entire vena cava is left intact. The preservation solution is next flushed out with lactated Ringer's solution, the portal bypass cannula is removed, and portal vein anastomosis is carried out using a continuous suture, utilizing a "growth factor" to prevent stenosis at this anastomosis. The clamps are then released, and the liver is reperfused with portal blood. This part of the procedure is critical and is characterized by varying degrees of "reperfusion syndrome," which is manifested by hypotension, bradycardia, arrhythmias, and, rarely, cardiac arrest, owing to a sudden influx of cold, hyperkalemic, acidotic blood into the heart.

Arterial Revascularization and Biliary Reconstruction

After hemostasis reperfusion, the recipient hepatic artery is freed from surrounding tissue. The preferred method

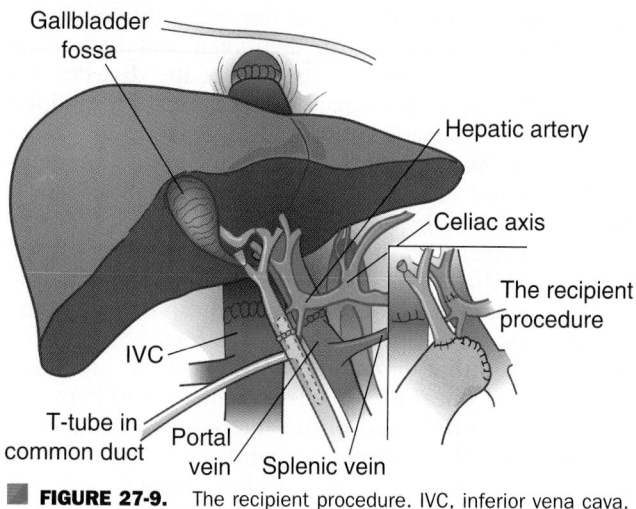

FIGURE 27-9.   The recipient procedure. IVC, inferior vena cava.

Segmental and Lobar Liver Transplantation

The necessity to maximize the number of liver grafts has led to several surgical innovations, including the transplantation of "split livers" from cadaveric and living donors.[107] These procedures are possible owing to the unique segmental anatomy of the liver and its regenerative capacity. For pediatric recipients, transplantation of left-lateral segments split from cadaveric donors or a living donor has become a standard practice. Especially for very young children for whom cadaveric grafts of the appropriate size are rare, the availability of these options in addition to whole cadaveric grafts has led to significant reduction in waiting time for pediatric patients and a reduction in waiting-list mortality.

Translating this experience to benefit adults awaiting transplantation required development of new approaches. The limitation of segmental liver graft transplantation for larger adult recipients is related to a minimum liver mass necessary for the adequate support of the recipient in the immediate post-transplant period. It is generally accepted that the graft to body weight ratio of more than 1% would allow adequate synthetic function. For this reason, right lobe grafts have recently been favored for live-donor transplantation to adults.[108] The removal of up to 60% of the donor's liver mass is naturally associated with greater potential for morbidity and mortality than with a left-lateral segmentectomy used for small children. This had led to cautious application of the procedure at experienced centers to target patients who are at risk of waiting-list mortality before a cadaveric donor liver becomes available. Frequent recipients in this group have been patients with hepatocellular carcinoma. Motivated by the ever-increasing number of patients waiting, the increase in living donor liver transplantation has been steady and over 400 such procedures were performed in 2001 (Fig. 27-10).

for reconstruction is an end-to-end anastomosis using an aortic Carrel patch of the donor celiac artery and a branch-patch of the recipient artery at the level of the gastro-duodenal bifurcation. This method allows for the creation of a relatively wide anastomosis and minimizes the potential for hepatic artery thrombosis. In most cases, biliary drainage can be achieved using a duct-to-duct anastomosis with or without placement of a T tube. Alternatively, pathology of the bile duct such as in the presence of PSC or biliary atresia requires biliary drainage via a choledo-chojejunostomy. The completion of this phase is demonstrated in Figure 27-9. After adequate hemostasis, three drains are placed around the liver and the abdominal cavity is closed.

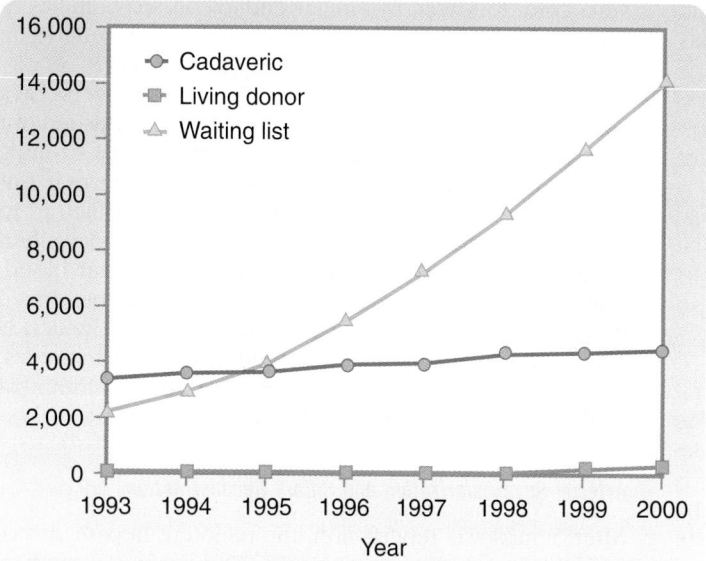

FIGURE 27-10.   The growth in living donor liver transplantation has been steady, and over 400 such procedures were performed in 2001.
(From University Renal Research and Education Association; United Network for Organ Sharing. 2002 Annual Report of the U.S. Organ Procurement and Transplantation Network and the Scientific Registry of Transplant Recipients: Transplant Data 1992-2001 [Internet]. Rockville, MD: Department of Health and Human Services, Health Resources and Services Administration, Office of Special Programs, Division of Transplantation; 2003 [modified 2003 Feb 18; cited YYYY MMM D]. Available from: *http://www.optn.org/data/annual Report.asp.*

Recent analysis of recipients of live-donor right lobe grafts documents that a massive amount of regeneration occurs in the first 1 to 2 weeks. Recipients of partial grafts have rapid proliferation of liver mass, with the majority reaching a calculated standard liver volume by 1 month. The donors, however, do not reach their complete starting volume, even by 1 year. This is contrary to what was believed and different from rodent models and remains to be studied in detail in the human setting. It also became apparent that graft size to recipient ratio was critical, in that grafts that were too small had decreased survival. These findings correlated with clinical experience in that small-for-size grafts regenerate to an appropriate size for the recipient; however, there was significant functional impairment of grafts that were less than 50% of expected weight, demonstrated by prolonged cholestasis and histologic changes consistent with ischemic injury. Liver grafts with a graft weight/standard liver volume of less than 40% have poor graft survival and prolonged hyperbilirubinemia.

Removal of a segment from a living donor, or the attempt to split a cadaveric liver for use in two recipients, is a complex procedure that requires precise knowledge of hepatic anatomy of the donor. In the case of the living donor, the surgeon's primary responsibility is to remove the donated segment without harming the donor. Similarly, splitting a cadaveric liver should be done without compromising either segment. Preoperative assessment of the live or cadaveric donor is similar to that previously described. In addition, it is helpful to use imaging studies in the living donor before surgery, aiming to determine the volume of the donated segment and its vascular supply.

The living donor operation is begun before the recipient hepatectomy and includes isolation of the individual branches of the hepatic artery, portal vein, and bile duct leading to the donated segment. The liver is separated from the vena cava that is left intact, and all small hepatic vein branches are ligated. Further preparation includes isolation of the main hepatic vein that provides the outflow tract. Completion of hepatic division is done via careful parenchymal dissection along the anatomic planes, using finger fracture technique, the harmonic scalpel, or the Cavitron ultrasonic aspirator (CUSA) (Fig. 27-11). It is important to preserve an intact blood flow to the segment until after transection of the hepatic parenchyma, when the vessels are clamped and transected and the segment is flushed with cold preservation solution. To minimize cold ischemia, the recipient operation is started once the donor anatomy is clearly identified to be favorable and the parenchyma is dissected. The diseased liver is then completely removed from the recipient when the donated segment is available for transplantation.

Transplantation of the donated lobe is performed by techniques similar to those developed for whole liver grafts, with a few modifications: The entire length of the recipient vena cava is preserved, and the lobe is transplanted in a "piggyback" fashion. The graft is placed in the usual anatomic position. This allows anastomoses of the portal vein and the hepatic artery without the need for interposition grafts. In most cases, bile duct reconstruction is done using hepaticojejunostomy.

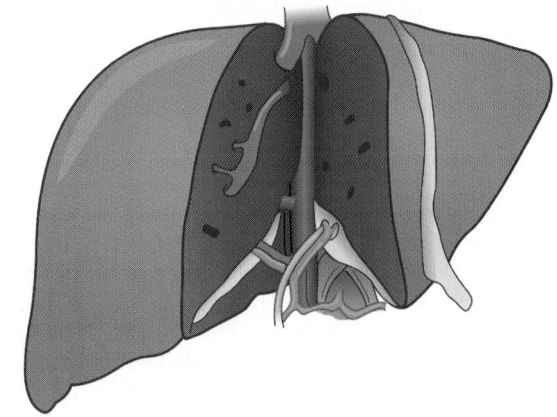

FIGURE 27-11. The living donor right lobe procedure.

Safety issues are of the highest priority for the living donor. Careful selection of the candidate, combined with fastidious surgical technique should minimize the potential complications. Early data regarding donor morbidity or mortality in the adult-to-adult cases suggest that the procedure can be performed with a high degree of safety. Despite this, donor mortality from the procedure has been reported. In addition, the recipient of these grafts may have an increased risk of postoperative complications such as bleeding or bile leak from the cut surface and potential short- and long-term problems with the biliary-enteric anastomosis. This reinforces the notion that living donor transplantation for adult recipients should be reserved for those who are unlikely to undergo transplant in time with conventional cadaveric transplantation.

Operative Complexities and Complications

Operative Bleeding

Excessive bleeding from portal hypertension may occur during hepatectomy and is likely to be accentuated by coagulopathy or adhesions from previous surgery. The removal of the cirrhotic organ, transplantation of a graft with normal function, and correction of coagulopathy by the appropriate use of platelets and fresh frozen plasma best control bleeding during hepatectomy and after reperfusion.

Thrombosis of the Portal Vein

The dissection may be more complex in the presence of a partially or totally thrombosed portal vein. In most cases, the thrombosed portion extends to the bifurcation of the splenic/superior mesenteric vein confluence, and the thrombus can be removed using endarterectomy techniques while preserving an intact main portal vein. Rarely, a vein graft may need to be placed to the superior mesenteric vein. Complete occlusion of the portal venous system is not an absolute contraindication for transplantation, because the infrahepatic vena cava can be split and anastomosed to the donor portal vein, providing adequate venous flow. At times, a large collateral vein, such as the coronary, may be used for inflow.

Hepatic Arterial Reconstruction

The surgeon is faced with arterial complexities more often than venous abnormalities. Intimal dissection or other pathology of the hepatic artery may necessitate the placement of an allogeneic vascular graft to the recipient's supraceliac or infrarenal aorta. The potential need for venous or arterial grafts for revascularization mandates that the procuring team always obtains adequate donor blood vessels for potential extension grafts. In addition, any unused blood vessel grafts must be kept refrigerated under sterile conditions for a few days after transplantation in case of emergent need for subsequent vascular reconstruction.

Post-transplant Management

Liver transplant recipients may require a short stay in the ICU after surgery. This period should be used to observe the recovery of the graft and ensure hemodynamic and respiratory stability as well as adequate kidney function. The principles of care are similar to those for other critically ill patients in the ICU setting but are rendered more complex by the necessity for immunosuppressive therapy. Common complications encountered in the early postoperative period are related to the initial graft function, technical misadventures, infections, and rejection. Treatment with anti-rejection drugs may be associated with the expression of several serious side effects such as metabolic encephalopathy, hypertension, and diabetes.

Common Complications

PRIMARY NONFUNCTION

The mechanisms of immediate graft failure after successful revascularization of the transplanted liver are not completely understood but may relate to donor variables, inadequate preservation, prolonged cold ischemia, or the humoral immune response. This problem is encountered in 2% to 5% of liver grafts. It is characterized by clinical and laboratory findings indicating poor synthetic function and severe hepatocytes injury. The recipient may present postoperatively with progressive hemodynamic instability, multiorgan system failure, and encephalopathy. Laboratory findings demonstrate worsening acidosis, coagulopathy, and extremely elevated liver enzymes (lactate dehydrogenase, aspartate aminotransferase, and alanine aminotransferase). The development of primary nonfunction is a surgical emergency and can be successfully treated by early retransplantation. The failure to find a suitable graft within 7 days is associated with high morbidity and mortality. Delayed nonfunction of the graft is characterized by failure of all liver functions, leading to persistent coagulopathy and progressive hyperbilirubinemia. Under these circumstances vital organs fail and/or

infection ensues, in most cases rapidly leading to death from bacterial or fungal sepsis.

INTRA-ABDOMINAL BLEEDING

The persistence of immediate post-transplant coagulopathy, fibrinolysis, and the presence of multiple vascular anastomoses places these patients at high risk for postoperative bleeding. However, coagulopathy spontaneously corrects itself in the presence of recovering liver graft function and with infusion of platelets. A persistent drop in hemoglobin and the need for transfusion of more than 6 units of packed red blood cells are usually indications for re-exploration and evacuation of the hematoma. In most cases, removal of the clot will be sufficient to arrest further fibrinolysis and will stop bleeding. Occasionally, it will be necessary to repair bleeding sites.

VASCULAR THROMBOSIS

Vascular complications after liver transplantation are more common in the pediatric population and are directly related to the small size of the vessels that are used for reconstruction. The most frequent complication is the occurrence of hepatic artery thrombosis. The pathology can present as rapid or indolent worsening of graft function or as necrosis of the bile duct and dehiscence of the biliary enteric anastomosis. Early recognition and successful thrombectomy may salvage the graft. However, deteriorating liver function and bile duct necrosis indicate the need for immediate retransplantation.

BILIARY LEAK

Reconstruction of the biliary system with either duct-to-duct anastomosis or choledochojejunostomy may be complicated with a bile leak, usually secondary to technical error or ischemia of the donor duct. Early leaks can be diagnosed by the appearance of bile in the drains and are confirmed by a T-tube cholangiogram or HIDA scan. Surgical exploration and revision of the anastomosis are mandatory and will solve the problem in most cases. Ischemic bile duct injury secondary to early hepatic artery thrombosis is an indication for retransplantation.

INFECTIONS

Infections remain the most significant complications in liver transplantation and are responsible for most of mortalities in the early postoperative period. There seems to be a direct correlation between the preoperative status of the recipient, the pattern of recovery after transplantation, and the incidence of bacterial and fungal infections. The probability for the development of such complications is the highest among patients who await a transplant in an ICU. These are chronically ill and malnourished patients who are unusually susceptible to resistant hospital flora before surgery and then are placed at further risk of infection by high-dose immunosuppression after the procedure. The development of organ system failure or graft malfunction further contributes to the morbid outcome. The spectrum of infection is evolving to more common occurrences of infections by resistant gram-positive bacteria (enterococci and staphylococci) rather than those caused by gram-negative bacteria. The deliberate use of broad-spectrum antibiotics in the immunosuppressed patient contributes in part to the development of systemic fungal infection (*Candida*, *Aspergillus*). It is wise to begin antibiotic therapy for common bacteria as soon as a patient's clinical status suggests the presence of infection. The treatment can then be modified when and if results of culture and sensitivity studies dictate a change.

Immunologic Aspects of Liver Transplantation

The relatively low immunogenicity of liver allografts and the unique ability of the liver to regenerate are probably the main reasons for the excellent long-term outcome. Good results are achieved when graft and recipient are ABO blood group compatible. Preoperative human leukocyte antigen (HLA) matching does not appear to be necessary. Most recipients are treated with combination therapy, which includes a calcineurin inhibitor (cyclosporine or tacrolimus), along with prednisone, with or without azathioprine or mycophenolate mofetil. The protocols are adjusted for a rapid taper of the corticosteroids within the first 3 to 6 months after surgery and significant reduction in the calcineurin inhibitor. Long-term maintenance of immunosuppression seems to be necessary in most recipients because complete cessation of immunosuppression carries significant risk for the development of acute and chronic rejection.

Acute Rejection

T-cell–mediated acute rejection is seen at a rate of 30% to 50% within the first 6 months after transplantation, most often within the first 10 days. Its clinical presentation is variable and may include the development of fever, abdominal pain, elevated liver enzymes, and bilirubin. Patients with a T tube may manifest a decrease in quantity and change in character of the bile. The diagnosis is confirmed by a liver biopsy that will demonstrate the presence of periportal lymphocytic infiltrate that extends into the liver parenchyma, as well as the invasion of inflammatory cells into the vascular endothelium. Most rejection episodes are responsive to the administration of high-dose corticosteroids. More potent monoclonal or polyclonal anti–T-cell antibodies are effective against corticosteroid-resistant rejection, leading to the reversal of the acute episode in more than 90% of the recipients. Rejection seems to be less responsive if an acute episode occurs long after transplant and/or in the case of chronic rejection.

Chronic Rejection

This type of rejection is seen months or years after transplantation. It is manifested by poor synthetic liver function and hyperbilirubinemia. It is usually characterized histologically by paucity of the bile ducts, thus often described as "vanishing bile duct syndrome." The etiology for this phenomenon is not well understood and may be related to a humoral reaction involving antibodies and fibrogenic cytokines. The treatment of chronic rejection is limited, and some of these patients may be considered as candidates for retransplantation.[109]

Recurrent Disease

Replacement of the liver may not permanently cure recipients of their original disease.[110] Recurrence of viral hepatitis is likely within a short time after transplantation in infected recipients. Control of active hepatitis B infection is possible in most patients using lamivudine, which inhibits the virus DNA polymerase, as well as hepatitis B immunoglobulin. In contrast, interferon alfa and/or ribavirin are less effective in hepatitis C infection. Reinfection of the liver graft may be mild and in many cases will not result in liver failure. Retransplantation for recurrent hepatitis B or C remains controversial. The obvious recurrence of viral hepatitis contrasts to reports describing the pattern of early pathologic findings seen in patients transplanted for PBC and PSC. The significance of these findings is not clear, because it rarely results in liver failure necessitating retransplantation.

Most liver transplant recipients who survive the immediate post-transplant period enjoy full functional recovery. However, restoration of a fully functional status depends on the patient's preoperative condition, an appropriate support system, and his or her attitude to rehabilitation.

Long-Term Results

UNOS registry data on nearly 30,000 liver transplants demonstrate impressive long-term survival. At 10 years, patient and graft survival for adults is 59% and 51%, respectively. The results in children are even better, with 78% of patients and 63% of grafts surviving at 10 years (Fig. 27-12).

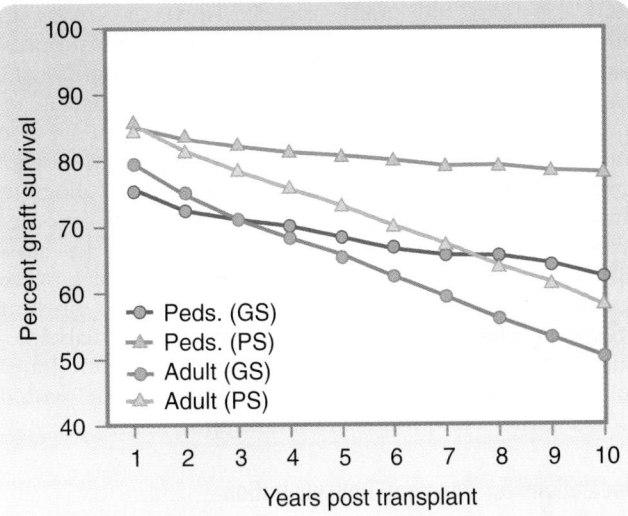

FIGURE 27-12. Survival curves: patient percentage survival (PS) and graft survival (GS) of primary liver transplants in over 4000 pediatric and 8000 adult patients.

Morbidity and mortality after orthotopic liver transplantation is directly correlated with the recipient preoperative status and the immediate function of the liver allograft. A higher mortality has been reported for recipients whose UNOS status was categorized as urgent and those who had multiorgan system failure (see Fig. 27-10).[111] Other variables associated with decreased survival include older age group, ventilator dependency, the need for dialysis, and retransplantation.[112,113] Controversy exists whether scarce livers should be utilized under these circumstances, because there would be greater chance of their long-term function in patients less seriously ill. However, the rationale for continuing to offer the procedure to these high-risk patients is based on their inability to survive if a transplant is not performed.

Overall, long-term survival after liver transplantation is excellent; however, recipients may suffer from significant side effects of the immunosuppressive drugs. Physical and psychosocial growth may be inhibited in the pediatric group.[114,115] In contrast, most adults will experience an average gain in weight of 15 to 20 lb. Recognized outcomes of corticosteroid and calcineurin inhibitors include osteoporosis, hypertension, hyperglycemia, and hyperlipidemia. Recipients have an increased incidence of malignancies, particularly in the form of post-transplant lymphoproliferative disease, an entity resembling lymphoma. This condition can often be resolved by reduction or complete withdrawal of corticosteroids and significant reduction in the cyclosporine or tacrolimus. However, attempts to stop all immunosuppression usually results in the development of acute and/or chronic rejection.

PANCREATIC TRANSPLANTATION

The purpose of pancreas transplantation is normalization of the diabetic recipient's blood glucose, thus preventing eventual microvascular complications, a goal unlikely to be possible with exogenous insulin therapy. The outcome of pancreas transplantation in the 1960s and 1970s was far inferior to that with other organs (frequent fatalities and less than 20% graft survival). However, owing to improvements in surgical technique and immunosuppression, the results of the procedure have progressively improved to the level of other transplants. The usual candidates for pancreas transplants are patients with diabetic nephropathy who are obligated to chronic immunosuppression to prevent rejection of a kidney allograft. Ironically, those diabetics who have no renal or other complications of their disease would be the ones most likely to benefit from the procedure because if it were carried out at that stage it would be likely to prevent microvascular complications. However, most diabetologists have been reluctant to recommend pancreatic transplantation in nonuremic diabetics because it would obligate them to chronic immunosuppression.

Indications for Pancreas Transplantation and Patient Selection

Because insulin is effective therapy for most diabetics (except for its failure to prevent eventual microvascular complications), pancreas transplantation is not considered a lifesaving procedure unless the patient is experiencing episodes of severe hypoglycemic unawareness. Thus, in considering pancreas transplantation, the requisite dangers of a major operation and lifelong immunosuppression must be balanced against the possible benefits. The evidence is now convincing that optimizing exogenous insulin therapy favorably influences microvascular complications.[116] That successful pancreas transplantation would also do so is based on softer evidence, although the assumption seems quite safe that the even better control of hyperglycemia associated with this method would provide optimal protection from complications. Microvascular sequelae, such as ocular, neurologic, and renal disabilities, will eventually occur in over 50% of diabetics on insulin therapy. Thus, the possibility of achieving glucose homeostasis by pancreas transplantation and avoiding microvascular complications is very attractive to patients, including many with advanced complications in whom objective analysis of the risks and benefits does not support its use. It is important for patients to understand that advanced complications (e.g., blindness, pregangrenous extremities, end-stage nephropathy) will not be reversed. Transplant surgeons are in the best position to understand the risks and benefits and, along with their diabetologist colleagues, should serve as the patients' advisors and advocates in considering transplantation. Because of the poor results of transplantation in the precyclosporine era, most clinicians then considered the risk unacceptable. Even now that success is more common, only a relatively small proportion of the world's many diabetics are appropriate candidates for pancreatic transplantation. In most centers, the procedure is usually employed only in patients who require immunosuppression for a kidney transplant necessitated by diabetic nephropathy.

Because of the prevalence in diabetics of microvascular disease, especially in the coronary arteries, evaluating the risks of major surgery is especially important. Indeed, one of the most common causes of pancreas transplant failure is death from myocardial infarction. Therefore, if substantial coronary artery disease is identified, it may need to be corrected before transplantation is undertaken.

Uremic type I diabetics who are candidates for cadaver donor kidney transplants are the most usual patients to be considered for pancreas transplantation, which is most often carried out simultaneously with the kidney transplant. Also appropriate for pancreas transplantation are diabetics who harbor a previously transplanted functioning kidney allograft because they are already committed to immunosuppression. In nonuremic diabetics who either do not need a kidney transplant or have not previously had one, the indications for pancreas transplantation are controversial. However, extremely labile diabetics who are at substantial risk from repeated episodes of dangerous hypoglycemia should be considered for transplantation even if they are not uremic.

In patients with seemingly early diabetic nephropathy, macroalbuminemia or microalbuminuria indicates that significant renal disease exists and that it will eventually progress to end stage, if they remain diabetic.[117] In these cases, it seems likely that progression of nephropathy could be halted, or at least slowed, by a successful pancreas transplant, although actual evidence for this is scarce because the procedure has been uncommon in this early stage.[118] Between 1988 and 2000, 10,562 pancreas transplants were performed: 83% of these were simultaneous pancreas-kidney transplants, 12% pancreas after kidney, and only 5% pancreas alone transplants. In other parts of the world, 93% of pancreas transplants were performed simultaneously with a kidney transplant.[119]

Donor Selection and Management

Selection of acceptable cadaveric donors of pancreas allografts is based on the standard criteria, avoiding donors who are aged, infected, hemodynamically unstable, or afflicted with malignancies. Hyperglycemia occurring after brain death is not necessarily a deterrent because this finding may be the result of an insulin-resistant state that often develops after head trauma. Serum amylase levels are not particularly helpful in evaluating prospective donors. Inspection of the pancreas by an experienced observer at the time of organ recovery is probably the best indicator of whether the pancreas is suitable for transplantation. The outcome of the transplant also appears to be strongly influenced by the care and expertise with which the donor operation is conducted.

The Donor Operation

Whenever possible, multiorgan en bloc excision is performed so that several transplantable organs can be obtained from the same donor. Through a midline abdominal incision (extending from the midline thoracic incision usually present for removal of the heart or lungs), the abdominal viscera are inspected. The blood supply to the liver is evaluated because anomalies in its arterial circulation sometimes prevent utilization of both the pancreas and the liver. If both organs cannot be safely used, priority must be granted to the liver because it is a lifesaving organ.

Once the decision is made that both pancreas and liver can be recovered, the gastrocolic ligament is divided, exposing the anterior surface of the pancreas. The transverse colon is mobilized, allowing the pancreas to be freed from the surrounding retroperitoneal tissues. The short gastric vessels are ligated and divided. The left gastric vessels are ligated and divided near the stomach, to preserve the blood supply to the liver via the celiac axis. After a povidone-iodine/amphotericin/antibiotic solution is instilled into the duodenal segment through a nasogastric tube, the duodenum is divided just distal to the pylorus.

Division of the lienophrenic ligament allows the mobilization of the pancreaticoduodenal allograft. The pancreas is freed from its posterior attachments to the left kidney and the left adrenal gland. The spleen is left in continuity with the pancreas to serve as a handle to minimize manipulation of the pancreas. The celiac axis, superior mesenteric, and splenic arteries are dissected from the surrounding lymphatic tissue and celiac ganglion. The infra-

hepatic inferior vena cava is exposed above the renal veins to facilitate dividing the inferior vena cava after the in situ irrigation of the donor organs with a cooled preservation solution. If both liver and pancreas are to be used, the gastroduodenal artery is ligated and divided. If only the pancreas is to be transplanted, this artery is left intact. The common bile duct is ligated and divided close to the pancreas. Through an opening in the gallbladder, the biliary ducts are irrigated with normal saline solution until clear of bile. A Kocher maneuver is performed to mobilize the head of the pancreas. The hepatic artery is freed from the surrounding lymphatics, and the proximal 1 to 2 cm of the splenic artery is dissected to complete exposure of the portal triad structures.

The donor is then systemically heparinized. The jejunum at the level of the ligament of Treitz is divided with a GIA stapler. The abdominal aorta is ligated at its bifurcation and cannulated for perfusion. The supraceliac aorta is then clamped and the portal vein divided about 1 cm cephalad to the superior margin of the pancreas. An in situ arterial flush with cooled UW solution at 4°C is begun, and the suprahepatic vena cava is divided. The liver can also be flushed through the open end of the portal vein (Fig. 27-13). Topical cooling of the liver and pancreas is also employed. If the liver and pancreas are procured en bloc, the portal vein is not divided in situ and the portal circulation can be flushed through the inferior mesenteric vein.

The pancreas and the liver can be separated in situ or ex vivo. If the liver is to be used, the celiac axis is usually left in continuity with the hepatic artery. The splenic artery is divided about 0.5 cm beyond its origin from the

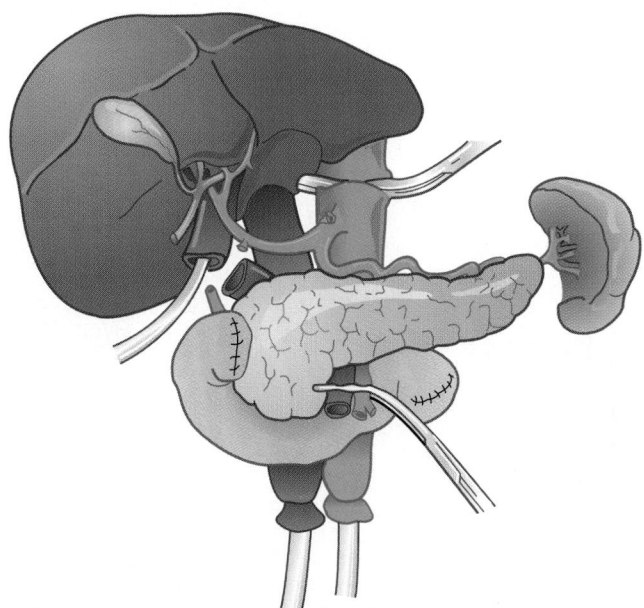

FIGURE 27-13. The pancreas and liver have been removed en bloc from a cadaveric donor. The portal vein, inferior vena cava, and aorta have been divided and cannulated for infusion of cold preservation solution.

celiac trunk. The mesentery of the small intestine, which courses through the parenchyma of the pancreas, is divided inferior to the pancreas either by individual ligature of the mesenteric vessels or en mass occlusion by a TA90 stapler. This completes the pancreas dissection. Long segments of the common, internal, and external iliac arteries and veins are also removed to use as vascular extension grafts if necessary.

Ex Vivo Preparation of the Donor Pancreas for Transplantation

The pancreaticoduodenal graft is submerged in a basin of cold UW solution for further preparation. The splenic hilar vessels are ligated and the spleen removed, avoiding injury to the tail of the pancreas. About 5 cm of duodenum beyond the ampulla of Vater should be retained with the graft. It is important to be sure that the proximal duodenum was divided distal to the pylorus and that no gastric mucosa is transplanted with the graft. If the mesenteric axis was divided with staples, the staple line is reinforced with a running suture. Commonly, an arterial extension Y graft is used to facilitate the transplant operation so that only one arterial anastomosis will be required in the recipient. The external iliac artery of the extension graft is anastomosed to the superior mesenteric artery of the pancreas graft, and the internal iliac artery of the extension graft is anastomosed to the stump of the splenic artery of the pancreas graft (Fig. 27-14). If there is sufficient length on both arteries, the splenic artery of the pancreas graft can be anastomosed end-to-side to the superior mesenteric artery. If the donor liver was not procured or if the liver team allowed the celiac axis to remain with

the pancreas graft, a patch of aorta, including the origins of the celiac axis and the superior mesenteric artery, is available for anastomosis directly to the recipient's vessels. An extension of the portal vein can be fashioned utilizing the external iliac vein of the donor, but this is rarely necessary and may be associated with increased risk of thrombosis of the portal vein.

The Recipient Operation

Although segmental grafts (consisting of only the pancreatic body and trail) were once common, the entire pancreas and its associated duodenal segment are now almost always transplanted (unless a living donor is used). Ligation or obliteration of the pancreatic duct was also once commonly practiced, but these techniques have also been abandoned. Instead, the pancreatic exocrine secretions are drained internally into either the small intestine or the bladder. Until recently, most centers employed only the bladder drainage technique, but since the late 1990s, enteric drainage has become the most common method in simultaneous kidney-pancreas grafts. The kidney and the pancreas grafts can both be placed within the peritoneal cavity through a midline incision. However, we have sometimes utilized two lateral incisions because they provide easier access to the iliac vessels and allow the kidney to be transplanted to its usual extraperitoneal location more easily. To avoid the consequences of fluid collection around the pancreas, the pancreas graft is placed intraperitoneally.

If a combined kidney-pancreas transplant is done, the pancreas is usually transplanted first to minimize ischemia time for the pancreas. However, if two teams are operating, the kidney can be transplanted while the pancreas is prepared for transplantation on a separate back table.

The external iliac arteries and veins are mobilized, preferably on the right side. The anatomic relationship of the vessels, as well as the presence of the colon, makes placement of a pancreas graft on the left more difficult, possibly resulting in a higher incidence of vascular thrombosis. Some surgeons advocate systemic heparinization, although others believe that this is not necessary in uremic recipients, whose clotting mechanisms are impaired. The arterial anastomosis is performed end to side to the external iliac artery, using either the aortic patch (containing the ostia of the celiac axis and superior mesenteric artery) or the common iliac artery portion of the Y-graft extension or the superior mesenteric if the splenic artery was anastomosed to it. The portal vein of the graft is anastomosed to the side of the external iliac vein of the recipient. A venous interposition graft is rarely needed and may increase the chance of thrombosis. The venous anastomosis is facilitated by complete mobilization of the common and external iliac veins with ligation of all venous branches; alternatively, the graft can be implanted to the aorta and vena cava and oriented with the head facing cephalad. The latter orientation may facilitate enteric drainage. Alternatively, portal venous drainage is accomplished by anastomosing the portal vein of the pancreas allograft to branches of the superior mesenteric vein.

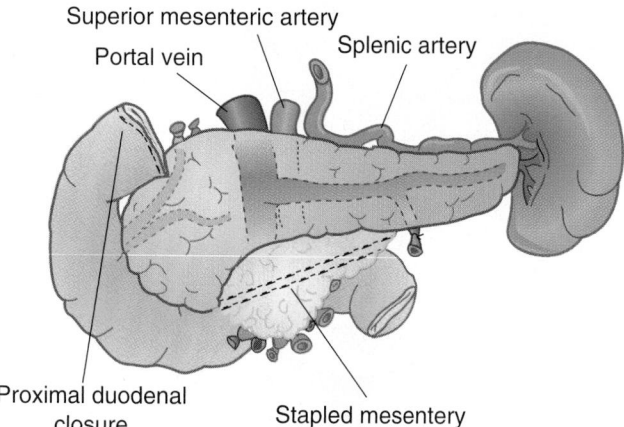

FIGURE 27-14. The pancreas has been separated from the liver and is ready for further ex vivo dissection on the back table while immersed in cold solution. The spleen will be removed and the distal duodenum shortened. The superior mesenteric and splenic arteries will be anastomosed to a Y-shaped extension graft of the donor's common, internal, and iliac arteries so that only a single arterial anastomosis will be needed in the recipient.

For bladder drainage of pancreaticoduodenal secretions, a horizontal cystotomy is made on the posterosuperior aspect of the bladder and a two-layer anastomosis is constructed between the bladder and the duodenum (Fig. 27-15A). Absorbable sutures are used for the inner layer to avoid leaving a nidus for stone formation. If enteric drainage is chosen, this can be performed as a simple side-to-side anastomosis of the donor duodenal segment to a convenient loop of small bowel or to a roux-en-Y loop (see Fig. 27-15B). Because the procedure involves opening the intestine, the wound is irrigated with antibacterial and antifungal agents. Drains are generally unnecessary. A Foley catheter is left in the bladder for 5 to 7 days.

An additional technical factor of possible importance is whether venous drainage should be systemic (via the iliac vein) or by the portal system. Portal venous drainage prevents the hyperinsulinemia resulting from systemic venous drainage but whether normal serum insulin and the somewhat more physiologic lipoprotein profile seen in patients with portal vein drained grafts have meaningful benefits is uncertain.[120] In view of the well-documented but subtle immunologic advantage of portal vein drainage of allografts in rodent models, it is intriguing that in a larger retrospective study at the University of Maryland portal vein–drained pancreas grafts had fewer acute rejection episodes and better survival than those systemically drained.[121] Interest in these findings resulted in 22% of all U.S. pancreas transplants between 1997 and 2000 being performed with portal drainage. However, the 1-year survival of these grafts was the same as for those with systemic venous drainage.

Biologic Factors Influencing the Outcome of Pancreas Transplantation

Histocompatibility Matching

That donor-recipient histocompatibility is advantageous for pancreas transplants has been shown by the somewhat superior outcome of the 142 living related donor pancreas transplants that had been reported as of October 2001 compared with cadaveric pancreas grafts. Despite this immunologic advantage of related donors, they have been used in only 0.8% of pancreas transplants because of the potential risks to the donor. These risks include not only morbidity of the operation itself but also the possibility of impairing the donor's glucose metabolism.[122] In addition, there is a theoretical concern that a pancreas transplanted from an HLA-matched related donor may be subject to increased susceptibility for the development of recurrent autoimmune diabetes in the graft, a risk analogous to that for development of recurrent autoimmune glomerulonephritis in kidney transplants from identical twin or HLA-identical sibling donors.

Most of the information regarding living donor transplants comes from the University of Minnesota, where 120 such transplants have been done, constituting 8.5% of that institution's pancreas transplants.[122] The graft survival of living donor transplants was 6% to 11% better at 1 year than that of cadaveric transplants done at the same institution.

For cadaveric transplants, the advantage of matching is subtle. Analysis of the results from 1997 to 2001 indicated no benefit of HLA matching for simultaneous pancreas kidney grafts, although with the pancreas after kidney and the pancreas alone transplants there was slightly better survival for HLA-A and HLA-B matching but surprisingly not for the HLA-DR matching.[119]

Immunosuppression

The immunosuppressive therapy used for pancreas transplant recipients is very similar to that employed for other solid organ transplants. Between 1983 and 1994, cyclosporine, in combination with azathioprine and prednisone, was employed in most centers. Between 1997 and 2000, 80% of recipients were treated with tacrolimus and MMF, instead of azathioprine and cyclosporine. More recently, sirolimus has been used in some patients. Most centers also continue to employ corticosteroids, although because of their known diabetogenic effect some groups

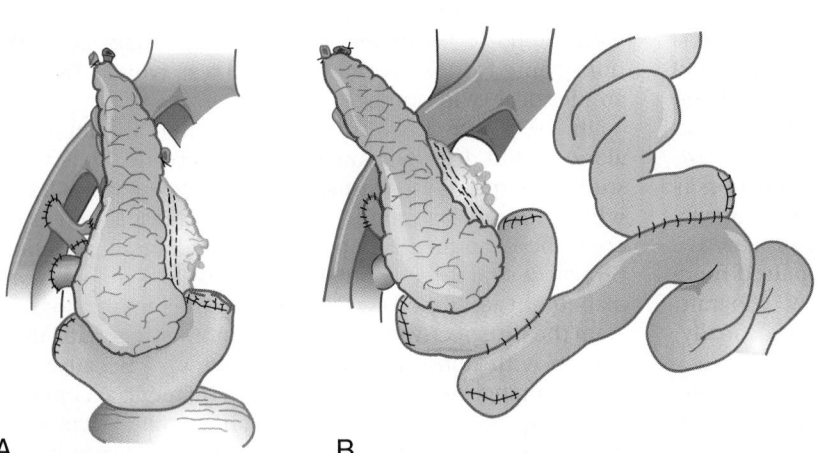

A   B

FIGURE 27-15. **A,** The extension Y graft has been anastomosed to the recipient's iliac artery and the portal vein of the graft to the iliac vein. The donor duodenum is anastomosed to the recipient's bladder to drain endocrine secretions of the graft. **B,** An alternative to bladder drainage of exocrine secretions is anastomosis of the donor duodenum to the recipient small bowel. Some surgeons prefer to make this anastomosis to a roux-en-Y loop, as shown here.

have tried to withdraw them. Anti–T-cell antibodies are also commonly used for induction immunosuppression because of the prevalence of early rejection and the difficulty of diagnosing it.

An interesting new immunosuppressive strategy being employed in pancreas transplantation at several centers is the administration of donor bone marrow cells. Stimulated by Starzl's emphasis on the role of microchimerism in the long-term success of some allografts, several groups inoculate donor bone marrow cells to recipients of pancreas transplants to augment the chimerism normally caused by migration of passenger leukocytes from the transplant. Although the Pittsburgh group did not find that bone marrow augmentation improved the 1-year graft survival they obtained without it (83%), they succeeded in maintaining graft survival after discontinuing corticosteroid therapy in two thirds of their bone marrow–treated patients, suggesting to them that a tolerant state may have been promoted by this treatment.[123]

Rejection

Prevalence and Severity

Whether human vascularized pancreas allografts are more or less vulnerable to rejection than vascularized allografts of other organs is a difficult question, especially because the pancreas is a composite organ with distinct exocrine and endocrine components, which may not be equally subject to rejection. Rejection of a kidney and pancreas transplanted simultaneously from the same donor is often manifested at the same time. However, either organ may undergo earlier or more severe rejection. In patients who receive pancreas and kidney transplants, rejection episodes tend to be more frequent than in those receiving only a kidney. Yet pancreatic graft loss from rejection is more frequent if the pancreas alone is transplanted than if both kidney and pancreas are transplanted.[119]

Diagnosis of Rejection

The early diagnosis of pancreatic allograft rejection is particularly important because physiologic evidence of islet damage (hyperglycemia) is a late indicator of rejection. Once islet damage is advanced, it is often difficult or impossible to reverse it by intensifying immunosuppression. The importance of identifying early rejection has led to exploration of a number of methods, such as imaging techniques and blood and urine tests. None of these has proved to be very reliable. Thus, in the effort to recognize early rejection, a combination of nonspecific indicators is utilized. These include increases in serum amylase, lipase, and anodal trypsinogen; decreases in urinary amylase (in the case of bladder-drained allografts); impaired function of a concomitantly transplanted kidney allograft; biopsy of the kidney or pancreas allograft; and, finally, hyperglycemia.

Particularly useful in patients receiving a simultaneous kidney-pancreas transplant is careful monitoring of kidney function. Because increased serum creatinine level is a sensitive indicator of kidney rejection, an increase in this value often takes place before manifestations of pancreas damage occur. Patients with pancreas-alone transplants lack the diagnostic advantage of monitoring function of a concomitant kidney transplant. In these patients, if bladder drainage of the pancreatic secretions was employed, decreased urinary amylase values are the best index of rejection. In patients with enteric drainage, and without a concomitant kidney transplant, the diagnosis of rejection must rely on serum amylase value, biopsy, and hyperglycemia (a late sign).

Histologic evidence of rejection is, of course, the most definitive indicator of rejection. Biopsy of the concomitantly transplanted kidney or the duodenum associated with the pancreas may be helpful, but most specific of all is a biopsy of the pancreatic allograft itself,[124] which can be obtained by ultrasound-guided transcutaneous or transcystoscopic techniques. If necessary, open biopsies can also be performed safely.

Treatment of Rejection Episodes

Although early initiation of antirejection therapy is more important in pancreas than in kidney transplantation, the treatment of rejection episodes is similar to that utilized for kidney allograft rejection, high-dose corticosteroids and anti–T-cell antibodies. Early rejection episodes can usually be reversed, but if extensive islet damage is allowed to occur there is much less chance of rescue than in the case of kidney or liver transplants. Because corticosteroids, cyclosporine, tacrolimus, and OKT3 all have a propensity for islet damage, increasing antirejection or heavy-maintenance immunosuppression should be avoided if possible. In this regard, Laftavi and coworkers found that utilization of biopsy in cases of questionable rejection avoided needless antirejection treatment in 44% of patients.[125]

Autoimmune Recurrence

In addition to rejection, an immunologic threat to pancreas transplants is the autoimmune response to islets, which was responsible for elimination of the native pancreatic beta cells. In the case of kidney transplants, an analogous vulnerability of transplanted kidneys was noted in the early 1960s when patients with glomerulonephritis were found to be subject to autoimmune damage of the transplanted kidney even if rejection was avoided by using an identical twin donor.

In 1979, we first examined whether autoimmunity alone would destroy transplanted pancreatic islets.[126] To study this question, we used an experimental model, in which the autoimmune response to transplanted islets could be examined independently of allograft rejection. BB rats (a strain that spontaneously develops autoimmune diabetes in adulthood) were rendered tolerant to allografts from the prospective normal islet donors by neonatal inoculation with donor strain bone marrow.[127] Because specific tolerance was confirmed by permanent acceptance of donor strain skin allografts, donor strain islets were exempt from rejection. Although in these tolerant recipients islet transplantation reversed diabetes, hyperglycemia recurred rapidly, indicating that transplanted islets are susceptible to destruction by autoimmunity.[128]

Several years after this demonstration that in animals recurrent autoimmunity could rapidly destroy transplanted islets in the absence of allogeneic rejection, it was found in humans that an analogous process could damage the islets of whole-organ pancreatic grafts transplanted from identical twin donors.[129] However, in these patients islet destruction occurred only after many weeks. This suggested that a vascularized pancreas graft might differ in its immunologic vulnerability from that of isolated islets, a question we also studied in immunologically tolerant BB rat recipients.[130] Whereas isolated islet grafts were routinely destroyed by autoimmunity within a few days, only a minority of whole-organ recipients became diabetic within 100 days, indicating that recurrent autoimmunity, although a substantial threat to isolated islet transplants, might be easy to overcome with immunosuppression in the case of vascularized pancreas.

A unique experience at the University of Minnesota with identical twin donor pancreas transplants provides definitive information on this issue.[129] Seven technically successful identical twin segmental pancreas transplants have been done there. The first three recipients were transplanted before the risks of recurrent disease were recognized. They received no immunosuppression. Biopsy-proven recurrent disease took place in 1 to 4 months. The fourth patient received only azathioprine and suffered recurrence at 5 years post transplant. The last three twins transplanted between 1987 and 1990 received induction and cyclosporine-based maintenance immunosuppression. Two remained normoglycemic for more than 10 years. One who received only low-dose immunosuppression experienced recurrence at 4 years and graft failure at 8 years. This experience confirms the autoimmune etiology of diabetes and indicates that low dose immunosuppression cannot prevent recurrence in twin transplants.

Recurrence of autoimmune diabetes with selective beta cell destruction has also been observed in pancreas transplants from living related HLA-identical donors.[131] Until recently, it was thought that it would be unlikely to occur in HLA-mismatched cadaveric transplants, either because the disease was major histocompatibility complex restricted or because the more intensive immunosuppression routinely utilized to prevent rejection of mismatched allografts would easily prevent autoimmune islet damage. Recently, however, in several recipients of cadaveric pancreas transplants, failures have been reported in which histologic evidence indicates that autoimmunity, rather than rejection, was the cause. The transplanted pancreas in these patients exhibited selective destruction of beta cells with preservation of alpha and delta cells, a pattern characteristic of patients with insulin-dependent diabetes.[132]

Complications of Pancreas Transplantation

Pancreas transplant patients are susceptible to the complications common to all immunosuppressed patients (e.g., infection, malignancy, corticosteroid-induced osteonecrosis). In addition, they are subject to several nonimmunologic complications specific to this type of transplant.

Vascular Thrombosis

The most common nonimmunologic cause of pancreas allograft failure is vascular thrombosis.[133] This complication is most frequent during the first 7 days. It almost always results in loss of the graft and is responsible for about 70% of technical failures. The reported incidence of this complication varies from 10% to 30%. Its etiology appears to be the relatively sluggish blood flow to the pancreas, estimated as only 1% of cardiac output, compared with the rapid blood flow through kidney, heart, or liver transplants. Risk factors were analyzed in a large experience (438 patients) at the University of Minnesota, where at various times most of the technical variations have been evaluated with regard to duct management, vascular reconstruction, and segmental versus whole-organ transplants.[134] Their overall thrombosis rate was 12% (5% arterial, 7% venous). There were no instances of obvious technical problems such as faulty vascular anastomoses. Thromboses did not appear to be caused by mechanical obstruction of the major vessels of the allograft but instead by abnormalities or changes in the microcirculation of the pancreas. Therefore, it is not surprising that strategies devised to increase blood flow in the major vessels (e.g., arteriovenous fistulas) have failed to decrease the incidence of thrombosis. Other findings of the Minnesota study were that the risk of thrombosis was highest in pancreas after kidney transplant patients (20%). Segmental grafts also had a propensity for thrombosis. Other risk factors identified were advanced donor age, cardiocerebral cause of donor death, prolonged preservation time (greater than 30 hours), the use of donor artery reconstructions other than Y-extension grafts, portal vein extension grafts, allograft pancreatitis, and transplantation of the pancreas graft to the left rather than the right iliac vessels. Although some centers advocate the use of anticoagulants, this remains of unproven benefit and, at least for the former, is associated with bleeding complications in the perioperative period.

Allograft Pancreatitis

Allograft pancreatitis in the early post-transplant period occurs in 10% to 20% of recipients. Predisposing factors are donor abnormalities (hemodynamic instability, vasopressor administration), procurement injury, perfusion injury (excessive pressure or volume), ischemic damage during preservation, and reperfusion injury. In severe pancreatitis, compromised pancreatic microcirculation causes necrosis and then arterial thrombosis. Mild edematous pancreatitis may be obvious at the time of allograft revascularization, but the diagnosis of significant pancreatitis and determination of its severity and progression are difficult. Serum amylase levels may not accurately reflect the degree of pancreatitis. Allograft pancreatitis may be difficult to differentiate from rejection or other complications such as extravasation of pancreatic juice, urine, or enteric contents. All of these can present as abdominal pain and tenderness, leukocytosis, hyperamylasemia, and computed tomographic abnormalities demonstrating graft edema. Unlike major leaks, however, graft pancreatitis should be treated nonsurgically, with Foley catheter drainage for bladder-drained grafts and, perhaps, with octreotide.

Fistula and Abscess

Extravasation of pancreatic juice from the pancreatic anastomosis is a more serious complication in enteric-drained than in bladder-drained allografts. During an era of more dangerous immunosuppression, this accounted for a substantial difference in survival from the two methods between 1987 and 1992 (for bladder-drained pancreas transplants, survival was 75% compared with only 54% for those enterically drained).[134] However, as immunosuppression and patient management have improved, this difference has become minimal and from 1997 to 2001 in enteric-drained grafts the 1-year survival was 82% versus 85% in bladder-drained grafts.[119] At least in the short term, bladder drainage may still be the safer procedure for several reasons. First, extravasation of succus entericus is much more serious than leakage of urine, not only because of microbial contamination but also because it activates pancreatic proenzymes. Second, minor leaks from bladder-drained pancreata can usually be controlled with Foley catheter drainage until they heal. However, there is unlikely to be an alternative to operative therapy for a leaking duodenoenterostomy. In addition, enteric leakage is often difficult to diagnose and differentiate from pancreatitis, whereas in bladder drainage the problem can usually be visualized on cystogram. In leaks occurring within the first month, leakage is usually from one of the anastomoses. Later leaks may also occur at suture lines, but perforated ulcers in the duodenal pouch are another source of leakage because of ischemia, rejection, or CMV infection.

Leakage in bladder-drained patients causes abdominal pain and tenderness, ileus, leukocytosis, elevated amylase and lipase levels, and computed tomographic abnormalities. A normal serum amylase value essentially rules out a leak in bladder-drained patients unless a Foley catheter is in place. In bladder-drained patients, leaks can often be treated successfully with Foley catheter decompression; if they are large or persistent, they may require enteric conversion, whereby the duodenal segment is anastomosed to an appropriate loop of small intestine or a roux-en-Y loop.

Urologic Complications

Urologic complications, such as urethritis, urethral disruption, hematuria, and recurrent urinary tract infections, are quite common in bladder-drained recipients. These problems, and bicarbonate losses, are the major disadvantages of this technique. Urethritis often resolves after a period of Foley catheter drainage, but, if not, enteric conversion is required to prevent scarring or disruption of the urethra. Hematuria may sometimes respond to simple bladder irrigation. If it persists, fulguration of the bleeding site may be effective; if not, enteric conversion is necessary.

Results of Pancreas Transplantation

Impact on Metabolic Defects of Diabetes

Successful pancreatic transplantation restores normo-glycemia and normal levels of hemoglobin A1c. The response to glucose challenge and to intravenous arginine and secretin is also normalized. The counter-regulation of glucose, which occurs in instances of insulin-induced hypoglycemia, is also improved by pancreatic transplantation.[135] Although recipients of successful pancreatic transplants may occasionally experience hypoglycemia, this is not nearly as severe or dangerous as it is in insulin-treated diabetics.

Successful recipients exhibit hyperinsulinemia owing to the systemic venous drainage of the allograft and insulin resistance caused by corticosteroid therapy. These abnormalities cause no symptoms. Their long-term significance is unknown, although hyperinsulinemia can elevate triglyceride levels, which could accelerate atherosclerosis. However, pancreas transplantation generally has a beneficial impact on the abnormal lipid profiles of diabetics. Although systemic venous drainage of the graft via the donor's iliac vein has been the standard method, several groups have evaluated the alternative of directing the venous effluent into the recipient's portal vein. Because this is the physiologic route there has been speculation that it would have a metabolic advantage. It does, in fact, prevent hyperinsulinemia. However, the procedure is more complex and there is little evidence that it has a meaningful advantage.

Graft Survival

After disappointing outcomes during the early years of pancreas transplantation, patient and graft survival rates for the procedure now approach those of other solid organ transplants.[51] From December 1966 to August 2002, more than 17,800 pancreas transplants were reported to the International Pancreas Transplant Registry.[119] For the more than 12,900 transplants in the United States, reporting was complete because since 1988 it has been mandatory for all centers in this country to submit regular reports on their activity and outcomes. In the most recent registry report of August 31, 2002, the 1997-2001 cases were analyzed.[119] Patient survival at 1 year was over 95%. For graft survival several important variables were studied, including recipient selection, donor factors, graft ischemia time, immunosuppressive regimen, recipient category (i.e., simultaneous pancreas and kidney [SPK] vs. pancreas after kidney [PAK] or pancreas alone [PTA]), and duct management.

Recipient Category

SPK recipients were the largest category, accounting for 83% of U.S. transplants (Fig. 27-16). For all U.S. SPK trans-

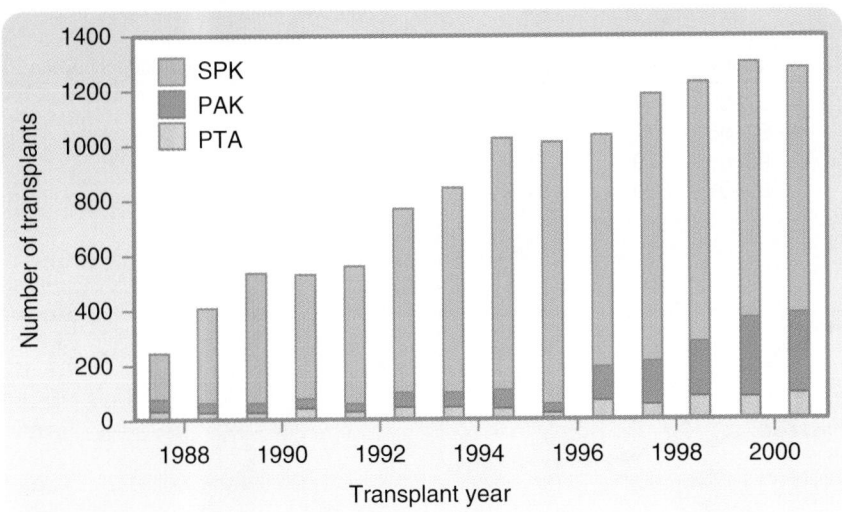

PANCREAS TRANSPLANT CATEGORIES
USA SPK, PAK AND PTA TRANSPLANTS

FIGURE 27-16.   Improvement in results of pancreas transplantation during the later part of the 1980s and in the 1990s led to increasing application of the procedure. Although simultaneous pancreas and kidney (SPK) transplants are still the most common, improved outcomes of pancreas-after-kidney (PAK) transplants have also encouraged an increase in this category. PTA, pancreas-alone transplants.

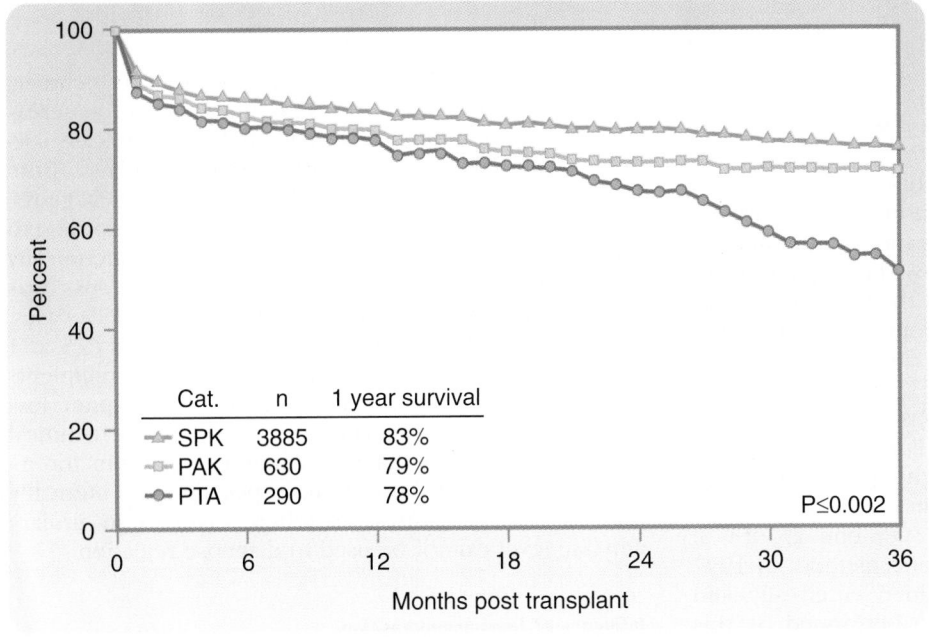

PANCREAS GRAFT FUNCTION
USA CAD PRIMARY PANCREAS TRANSPLANTS 1/1/1997–10/10/2001

Cat.	n	1 year survival
SPK	3885	83%
PAK	630	79%
PTA	290	78%

P≤0.002

FIGURE 27-17.   Graft survival continues to remain somewhat better for simultaneous pancreas and kidney (SPK) grafts than for pancreas-alone (PTA) transplants, probably because the diagnosis of rejection is facilitated by monitoring the function of the kidney transplant. PAK, pancreas-after-kidney transplants; Cad, cadaver.

plants performed between 1997 and 2001, 1-year patient and pancreas graft survival rates were 95% and 83%, respectively. Fortunately, kidney graft survival (92%) was not compromised by combining this procedure with a pancreas transplant. For PAK cases, 1-year patient and pancreas graft survival rates were 95% and 79%, respectively. For all PTA cases, 1-year patient and pancreas graft survival rates were 95% and 78%, respectively. Thus, although patient survival was essentially the same for the three groups, pancreas graft survival remained somewhat higher in SPK recipients than for PTA transplants (Fig. 27-17). That pancreas rejection can be diagnosed by monitoring kidney function in SPK recipients (when both

organs are from the same donor) is the likely explanation for the higher functional survival rates in this category. However, the difference was less than in earlier eras. In the 1994-1998 analysis, the PAK graft survival was 71% and the PTA survival was only 64%.

The improvement in results by era was particularly evident in the outcome of PAK transplants (Fig. 27-18). The factor that seemed most likely to be responsible for the improvement was the introduction of tacrolimus immunosuppression. That pancreas rejection can be diagnosed by monitoring kidney function in SPK recipients (when both organs are from the same donor) is the likely explanation for the higher functional survival rates in this category.

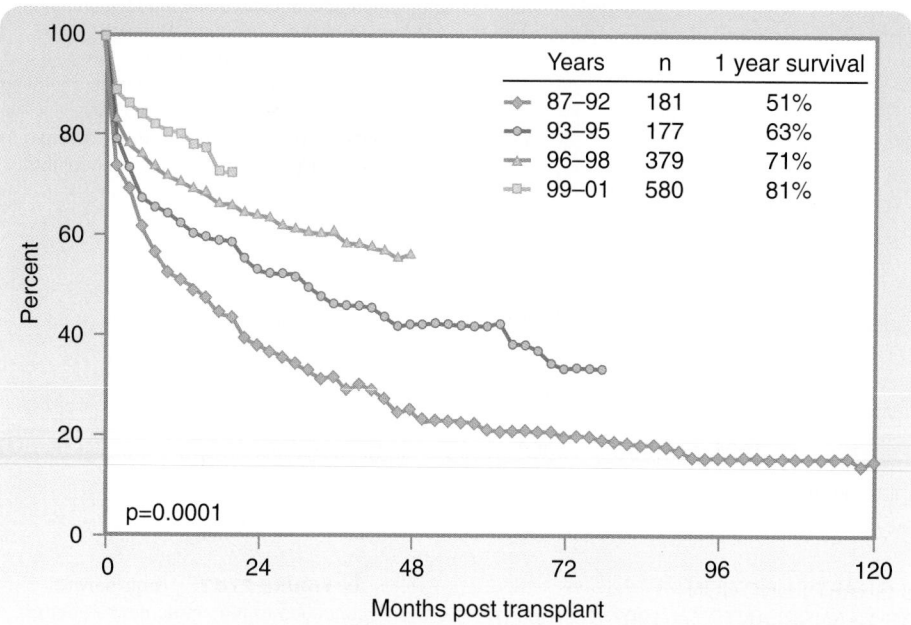

PAK GRAFT FUNCTION BY ERA
USA CAD PANCREAS TRANSPLANTS 10/1/1987–10/10/2001

Years	n	1 year survival
87–92	181	51%
93–95	177	63%
96–98	379	71%
99–01	580	81%

p=0.0001

FIGURE 27-18. Pancreas graft survival by era is probably due to improved immunosuppression. It is particularly evident in the pancreas-after-kidney (PAK) category. Cad, cadaver.

Impact of Duct Management Technique

In the United States, bladder drainage was until recently by far the most common technique for duct management because of its relative safety and because it facilitates early diagnosis of rejection by serial measurement of urinary amylase, which decreases if the graft suffers immunologic damage. From 1989 to 1996, over 90% of transplants were done by this method. Unfortunately, the bladder-drainage technique carries its own urologic and metabolic morbidities, including cystitis, urethritis, and chronic acidosis from bicarbonate loss. In fact, in 15% of bladder-drained transplants, these problems are serious enough to warrant enteric conversion within 3 years. Formerly the second most common duct management technique in the United States, the use of enteric drainage has now become the most common method. Whereas in 1988 only 2% of U.S. transplants were performed by enteric method, in 1997 48% of SPK transplants were drained enterically and between 1999 and 2001 71% were performed by this method.

Although in earlier years bladder-drainage grafts fared substantially better, from 1997 to 2001 the 1-year graft survival of SPK transplants was nearly the same for bladder drained (85%) versus enteric drained (82%) (Fig. 27-19). Complications remained somewhat more common in enteric-drained grafts (11% vs. 8%). In PAK transplants (in which the simultaneous kidney could not be used to monitor rejection), bladder-drained grafts continued to have a significantly better survival at 1 year (85%) than did enteric-drained grafts (74%). In this category, complications were twice as frequent in enteric-drained grafts (22% vs. 12%). For PTA transplants, pancreas graft survival rates were significantly higher at 1 year with bladder-drainage (81%) versus enteric-drainage grafts (74%).

Interestingly, when early graft losses due to technical problems were avoided, the subsequent loss of pancreas transplants was surprisingly small. In 2978 technically successful SPK cases, the pancreas graft failure rate from immunologic causes was only 2% at 1 year. In SPK grafts, the immunologic risk of failure did not differ according to duct management technique. However, for technically successful PAK cases, the immunologic graft loss was higher (5% at 1 year). For technically successful PTA cases, the risk for immunologic graft loss was highest (7% at 1 year). Transplantation of SPK grafts into uremic recipients may in part explain the lower immunologic graft loss in this category. Some failures categorized as technical (thrombosis) may actually be immunologic from thrombosis secondary to rejection, especially in enterically drained solitary transplants where changes in urinary amylase level cannot be used to diagnose rejection.

Influence of Immunosuppression

New immunosuppressive regimens, especially tacrolimus, appear to be responsible for the improvement noted in pancreas graft survival rates in the 1997-2001 era.

Impact of Pancreas Transplantation on the Microvascular Complications

Evaluating the impact of successful pancreas transplantation on the secondary complications of diabetes is difficult because randomized control studies are for the most part lacking. Defining appropriate control groups is also complicated because, in SPK recipients, uremia and diabetes are corrected at the same time. Some complications of diabetes such as neuropathy are likely to be improved

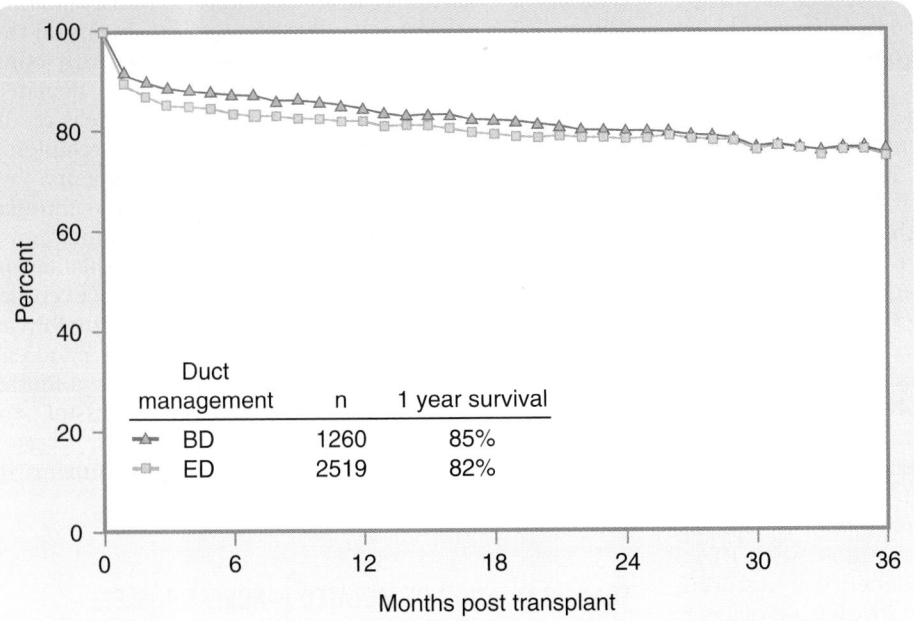

SPK GRAFT FUNCTION BY DUCT MANAGEMENT
USA CAD PRIMARY PANCREAS TRANSPLANTS 1/1/1997–10/10/2001

Duct management	n	1 year survival
BD	1260	85%
ED	2519	82%

FIGURE 27-19. The importance of duct management seen in earlier eras has disappeared. Enteric-drained (ED) transplants and bladder-drained (BD) transplants have virtually the same survival. SPK, simultaneous pancreas and kidney; Cad, cadaver.

by kidney transplantation alone. Thus, uremic diabetics who receive only a kidney transplant are a necessary control group for assessing the benefits of pancreas transplantation on microvascular complications.

NEUROPATHY

In nonuremic diabetic PTA recipients at the University of Minnesota Hospital, improvement in nerve conduction velocities was documented after 1 year.[136] Evoked muscle and nerve action potentials and amplitudes remained stable or improved in patients with long-standing pancreas grafts whereas amplitudes continued to decrease in diabetic recipients whose pancreas transplants failed early.[137] Thus, in the Minnesota patients, restoration of normoglycemia by successful pancreas transplantation appeared to halt the progression of diabetic neuropathy fairly promptly.[138] However, other investigators believe that improvement in neuropathy including autonomic neuropathies is delayed by as much as 2 years.[139,140]

RETINOPATHY

Several investigators have reported improvement in retinopathy in uremic diabetic patients after a successful pancreas transplant, but most of these studies have been poorly controlled. In nonuremic patients at the University of Minnesota Hospital, the retinas of successful pancreas recipients were compared over a 5-year period with those of patients with early graft failure.[141] In the first 3 posttransplant years, the probability of progression of retinopathy was the same (30%) in both groups. However, after 3 years, retinopathy appeared to stabilize in patients with successful pancreas transplants while it continued to worsen in those with failed grafts. After 5 years, 55% of patients with failed grafts had progressed to a more severe

state of retinopathy, whereas in successful recipients, similar progression in retinopathy had occurred in only 30%. In contrast to these patients with mild retinopathy, it seems unlikely that a pancreas transplant will benefit those with advanced retinal change.[142]

NEPHROPATHY

Microscopic lesions of diabetic nephropathy commonly appear within 1 to 2 years in kidneys from normal donors transplanted to diabetic patients who are treated only with insulin.[143,144] However, in recipients of successful SPK transplants in the Minnesota study, development of diabetic nephropathy in the transplanted kidney was generally prevented, presumably because the blood glucose level was normalized.[145] The ability of a pancreas transplant to prevent nephropathy was also suggested in serial biopsies by the Stockholm group.[146]

The Minnesota group has also contended that a PAK transplant may halt the progression of lesions that evolved in the renal graft before pancreas transplantation was done.[145] In patients whose kidneys were sampled an average of 8 years after transplantation, the mean glomerular mesangial volume was significantly less in those patients who had a successful pancreas transplant than in those who did not.

Whether restoration of normoglycemia with a pancreas transplant can influence the course of early lesions of diabetic nephropathy in the native kidneys of nonuremic, diabetic patients remains controversial. In a preliminary report from the University of Minnesota, native kidneys were sampled in seven nonuremic pancreas recipients who had early to moderately advanced diabetic nephropathy (albuminuria was present in all; mean creatinine clearance was 90 ± 20 mL/min) 2 years after a successful pancreas transplant. Mean glomerular mesangial volume was significantly reduced post transplant, compared with pretransplant biopsies. However, despite this histologic improvement the creatinine clearance had deteriorated in these pancreas transplant patients from 90 ± 15 mL/min to 60 ± 14 mL/min over the same 2-year period. The nephrotoxic effect of cyclosporine may explain this apparent paradox. The lesions of diabetic nephropathy in the patient's native kidneys were not ameliorated by pancreas transplantation, even after 5 years of normoglycemia.[118] However, neither of these studies proves that restoring normoglycemia after a pancreas transplant cannot prevent or retard progression of diabetic nephropathy.

Several other PTA recipients have been observed to progress to a uremic state in spite of a successful pancreas graft,[136,147] but in most nonuremic diabetic PTA recipients, serum creatinine and creatinine clearance values at 1 to 5 years post transplant did not deteriorate from those obtained 6 months post transplant. In summary, in all three categories of diabetic pancreas graft recipients (those with SPK, those with PAK, and those with PTA), there is encouraging histologic evidence that restoring euglycemia can prevent or halt progression of diabetic nephropathy. Whether this benefit is sufficient to offset the nephrotoxic effect of immunosuppressive agents such as cyclosporine or tacrolimus is a critical question.

Whereas these studies strongly suggest that pancreas transplantation may improve diabetic retinopathy, nephropathy, and neuropathy, no controlled or randomized studies have yet confirmed these. Whether transplantation can also prevent diabetic complications in otherwise unaffected patients, as tight insulin control has been shown to do, has not been investigated because pancreas transplantation, before the onset of any complications, is rarely performed. Therefore, the potential benefits of pancreas transplantation over other forms of intensive diabetic treatment cannot be fully assessed at this time, although it seems likely that the optimal control of blood glucose possible from a pancreas transplant would be the optimal prophylaxis for microvascular complications.

Conclusion

The results of pancreas transplantation have improved remarkably since the mid 1980s, and the likelihood of success now approaches that of other solid organ transplants.[136] Because pancreas transplants are not immediately lifesaving, except in patients with profound hyperglycemic unawareness, the serious side effects of lifelong immunosuppression must be weighed against the somewhat unpredictable sequelae of insulin-managed diabetes. Currently, transplantation is limited at most centers to diabetics who require a kidney transplant or have already had one. Prevention of microvascular complications of diabetes by pancreas transplantation seems likely but has not been proved by randomized studies. Advanced complications are much less likely to be stabilized or reversed.

Recent reports indicate that a successful kidney-pancreas transplant is associated with improved long-term patient survival relative to successful renal transplantation alone.[148-150] A 10-year follow-up of 13,467 diabetics on the UNOS waiting list indicated that despite more early complications and deaths in pancreas recipients the calculated life expectancy was 23.4 years for kidney-pancreas recipients versus 20.9 years for related kidney alone recipients and 12.6 years for cadaveric kidney alone recipients.

The morbidity and monetary expense of conventional insulin therapy, along with its complicating factors, must also be compared with those of successful transplantation and immunosuppression to determine the eventual place of pancreatic and islet transplantation. Possibly as important a consideration as the impact of a pancreas transplant on microvascular complications is its potential for improving quality of life. Recipients of successful pancreatic allografts usually report increased vitality, greater capability for self-care, and general improvement in quality of life.[151]

TRANSPLANTATION OF ISOLATED PANCREATIC ISLETS

The advantage of transplanting isolated pancreatic islets rather than the pancreas is the avoidance of the complex vascular reconstruction required with whole-pancreas transplantation and elimination of the unnecessary transplantation of the associated exocrine component of the gland. In the early 1970s, the initial descriptions of partial[152] and complete[153] reversal of experimental diabetes in animals by transplantation of isolated islets of Langerhans excited considerable interest because the risks of this procedure seemed minimal, whereas pancreatic transplants of that era were dangerous and rarely successful. It was also theorized that because some endocrine tissues were known to have minimal immunogenicity, islet allografts might succeed without immunosuppression. However, initial human islet transplants during the 1970s all failed, probably from technical difficulty in producing preparations with adequate islet yield or purity or because of immune destruction. Although considerable knowledge has been accumulated since then, both in the techniques of islet isolation and in preventing damage to the transplant by rejection or autoimmunity, much of the progress has been in experimental models. Until very recently, successful human islet transplantation has been exceedingly rare.

With the report in the year 2000 of 7 consecutive successful human islet transplants by an investigator in Edmonton, Alberta, a new era appears to have begun for this field. Within 3 years of this report almost 300 islet transplants have been performed worldwide. The results of these transplants are much better than before. One-year islet graft survival rates in many of the approximately 30 centers performing them are comparable to those of pancreas transplantation. If this persists, islet transplantation will gradually assume a greater role in treatment of patients' type I diabetes. Briefly summarized below are the history of islet transplantation, the barriers that remain, and the recent clinical results.

Lessons Learned from Experimental Islet Transplantation

Techniques of Islet Preparation

Separating the islets from the pancreas is begun by distending the pancreas by infusing a collagenase enzyme solution into the pancreatic duct. After mechanical disruption, islets are separated from acinar, ductal, lymph nodal, and vascular elements by handpicking under magnification or by density gradient centrifugation.[154] Although most non-islet tissue is thus eliminated, many islets are destroyed or discarded in the process.

Sites of Islet Transplantation

A potentially important advantage of a free graft, such as isolated islets graft, is the flexibility that exists in selecting a site for transplantation. Surprisingly, unlike the situation with other free grafts of endocrine tissue, only a few transplant sites will support engraftment and adequate function of transplanted islets. The peritoneal cavity is advantageous because remaining exocrine tissue that has not been separated from the islets can be tolerated there, but this transplant site is also relatively inefficient, requiring large numbers of islets for reversal of diabetes. For reasons not completely understood, the most easily accessible sites (subcutaneous or intramuscular) have not proved successful unless extremely large numbers of islets from multiple donors were transplanted. The spleen has been used successfully as a transplant site; however, the risk of splenic injury and bleeding is a deterrent. Thus, somewhat surprisingly, the liver via portal vein embolization has become the most commonly employed transplant site.[155] The liver's dual vascular supply allows embolized islets to completely occlude portal venules without infarcting the transplant site, which remains nourished by hepatic arterial blood (Fig. 27-20). The renal subcapsular space is another excellent islet transplant site in rodents, but it has rarely been used in humans.[156,157]

A number of immunologically privileged transplantation sites have been evaluated, including the anterior chamber of the eye, the brain, the pregnant uterus, the placenta, the testis, and the thymus. Several of these sites have been shown to provide at least partial sanctuary for allogeneic islets while allowing normal physiologic function.[158,159] However, the technical considerations and potential morbidity of engraftment into these sites discourage their clinical use.

In animal models, genetic alteration of islets to delete important alloantigens has allowed successful transplantation without immunosuppression.[160] Genetic modifications of islet allografts have also been attempted to create a protective environment that would be similar to a privileged site. An example of this strategy would be to induce the transplanted islets to produce immunosuppressive cytokines such as IL-10 and transforming growth factor. To test this method, Min transfected isolated murine islets with the genes encoding these factors. When the transfected islets were transplanted to allogeneic hosts, their survival was significantly prolonged.[161]

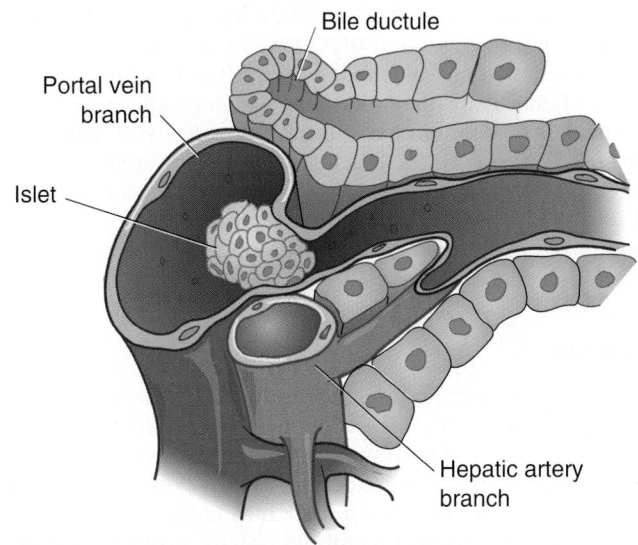

FIGURE 27-20. The liver's dual vascular supply allows transplantation of isolated pancreatic islets by embolization via the portal vein. The terminal portal venule can be occluded without infarcting the transplant site.

Islet Allograft Immunogenicity

Contrary to the early hope that islet tissue would be immunologically privileged like certain other endocrine tissues (e.g., parathyroid), the earliest reversal of experimental diabetes by islet transplantation indicated that unless the donor was genetically identical to the recipient, rejection was prompt.[162] Subsequent experiments indicated that rejection could be overcome by immunosuppression and also identified several other unusual strategies by which rejection can be avoided. For example, pretransplant storage of islets in tissue culture was found to reduce their immunogenicity, sometimes allowing successful transplantation without immunosuppression. This outcome was found to depend on depleting the islets of passenger leukocytes, especially class II major histocompatibility complex antigen-presenting cells (APCs) such as macrophages and dendritic cells.[163] Prolonged tissue culture of islets (1 to 2 weeks) allowed selective survival of the endocrine cells but not the antigen-presenting lymphoid cells.[164] Other methods that deplete or render nonfunctional APCs from islets include ultraviolet irradiation,[165] gamma irradiation,[166] and treatment with antibodies directed against APCs along with complement.[167-169] So far, these methods have been shown effective only in rodent models.

Immunosuppression

Conventional pharmacologic immunosuppressive agents, such as cyclosporine or tacrolimus, are relatively ineffective in prolonging islet allograft survival, requiring dangerously higher doses to prolong islet allograft survival beyond what is necessary for surgically vascularized solid organ allografts.[170] In addition, cyclosporine, tacrolimus, and corticosteroids have been found to have toxic effects on islets.[171] Antilymphocytic antibodies and specific anti–T-cell agents such as anti-CD4 have proved far more successful in preventing islet allograft rejection.

Co-stimulatory blockade (see Immunosuppression under Renal Transplantation) has also been applied to islet transplants with encouraging results. Kenyon and colleagues[172] reported the results of anti-CD154 treatment on the survival of isolated islet allografts in rhesus monkeys. Each of six monkeys treated with anti-CD154 antibody monotherapy demonstrated prolonged restoration of normoglycemia.

Tolerance

Classic immunologic tolerance induced by neonatal intravenous administration of allogeneic lymphoid cells from a prospective donor strain was shown many years ago to prevent skin allograft rejection.[2] Only donor lymphoid cells, but not other cell types such as kidney cells, which cannot migrate to host lymphoid organs, proved effective as tolerogens. Knowledge that the thymus serves as the primary site for self-tolerance initiation led Posselt and associates to investigate whether nonlymphoid donor cells such as islets might also possess tolerogenic properties if introduced directly into the thymus.[173] They injected allogeneic islets into the thymus of adult rats that were briefly immunosuppressed with a single dose of ALS to delete their mature T cells. Not only did these islets survive in the thymus, but they also allowed a second islet allograft from the same donor strain to be successfully transplanted under the kidney capsule 100 to 200 days later without any additional immunosuppression.[174] Attempts to induce tolerance by this method in larger animal models are not as encouraging.[175]

Autoimmune Recipients

Successful islet transplantation in human type I diabetics requires avoidance not only of rejection but also of damage by the autoimmune process, which causes failure of the native islets in this disease. Insight into this possible importance of autoimmune recurrence in transplant islet failure has been provided by studies in two rodent models of spontaneous autoimmune diabetes: the Bio-Breeding (BB) rat and the nonobese diabetic (NOD) mouse. These animals are similar to human type I diabetics in many ways, including abrupt disease onset in early adulthood and the presence of both cellular and humoral immune responses directed specifically against the beta cells of the islets. Without insulin therapy, ketoacidosis and death are inevitable. Thus, NOD mice and BB rats are suitable models for determining the vulnerability of transplanted islets in autoimmune recipients and possible methods for avoiding it. Studies in BB rats demonstrated that islets are more vulnerable to autoimmune recurrence after transplantation when they are isolated than they are if transplanted as part of a whole pancreas.[130]

Xenografts

Even if the technical and immunologic difficulties of islet transplantation were overcome, the donor shortage would leave millions of diabetics waiting for a transplant because of the donor shortage. An often discussed solution to a demand of this magnitude would be the use of xenogeneic tissues.

Porcine insulin is effective in the treatment of human diabetics, suggesting that the pig may be a promising source of islet tissue for xenotransplantation. Preformed antibodies are present in humans against porcine histocompatibility antigens, and these antibodies have been shown to bind islets and activate complement. However, unlike the situation for vascularized xenografts, there is apparently no hyperacute rejection of islets. Instead, the problems of cellular immunity seem to play a more prominent role in islet xenograft rejection.

Clinical Islet Transplantation

In theory, islet transplantation is the ideal treatment for patients with insulin-dependent diabetes because it has the potential to completely normalize blood glucose without the substantial risks associated with the operation of whole-pancreas transplantation. In rodent models, the technical and immunologic problems of islet transplantation have been overcome, routinely allowing consistent success. Recent improvement in the success of clinical islet transplantation suggests that islet transplantation could eventually replace both insulin therapy and whole-pancreas transplantation as the optimal treatment for type I diabetes.[176]

Isolation Methods

Digestion of the compact fibrous pancreas and isolation of viable islets is more difficult in humans than it is in rodents. In addition, hemodynamic instability and hyperglycemia of cadaveric human donors and prolonged pancreatic ischemia before initiation of the separation process have compromised efforts to obtain islet preparations of high quality. The fact that pancreata from the best donors are likely to be utilized for whole-organ grafts further reduces the likelihood of optimal islet recovery. Most centers now use an automated method of islet isolation described by Ricordi and coworkers.[177] The pancreas is digested enzymatically by collagenase in a chamber. During a period of agitation, islets and small fragments of the contaminating exocrine tissue fall through a screen and are collected, remaining in the bottom of the chamber. After the collagenase solution is washed from the islets, they are separated from acinar fragments and ductal elements by centrifugation through density gradients. Islets account for about 2% of the mass of an intact pancreas. Current islet separation methods are sometimes capable of yielding preparations composed of 90% pure islets, while at other times the same procedure may yield a preparation of less than 50% purity. The more manipulation carried out in an effort to reduce acinar tissue contamination, the more islets are lost. Even with the best techniques, many islets are lost or damaged. An important variable that contributes to inconsistency in the isolation process is the collagenase enzyme that is used to digest the pancreas. Recent refinement of the enzyme preparation has led to a marked improvement in isolation yield, purity, and number.

Another important technical achievement is islet preservation. Short-term preservation (days to several weeks) can be achieved by in vitro tissue culture. Islet culture has been shown to diminish the immunogenicity of islets in animal experiments, but this has not been evaluated in humans. Although even short-term culture (12 to 24 hours) also helps to decrease the acinar tissue contaminating islet preparations, this is at the expense of substantial loss of viable islets. Frozen islets can probably be stored permanently and, after thawing by appropriate techniques, appear to have virtually normal function. Cryopreservation allows islet preparations from multiple donors to be pooled, so that a sufficient number of islets for reversal of diabetes could be utilized for every transplant, obviating the possibility of performing a transplant with an inadequate number of islets from a single donor.[178]

Surgical Technique and Complications

In human transplants, the islets have usually been transplanted by embolization to the liver via the portal vein. Other transplant sites, proven effective in animals, such as the peritoneal cavity and the renal subcapsular space, have rarely been employed in humans.[179] Islets can be inoculated into the portal venous system by cannulating the umbilical vein via a minilaparotomy, or by transcutaneous, transhepatic cannulation of the portal vein itself. Islets are suspended in a heparinized solution for portal vein infusion. Portal venous pressure is monitored during islet infusion because the development of portal hypertension may be an indication of intravascular clotting. Although most patients tolerate the inoculation of intraportal islets, severe complications have been reported in a few, including portal vein thrombosis and disseminated intravascular coagulation.[180] These complications are probably related to rapid infusion of insufficiently pure islet preparations containing large amounts of enzymatically rich acinar tissue. With islet preparations of high purity, these sequelae have been rare. However, the procedure is not without other risks. Even in the recent experience, a mortality has been reported as a result of a hepatic arterial injury during transhepatic portal vein cannulation.

Metabolic Factors Influencing Success

During islet engraftment in the immediate post-transplant period, it is believed that maintenance of normal blood glucose levels is important to avoid islet damage. During the early post-transplant period, to avoid even brief episodes of hyperglycemia, patients are treated with continuous intravenous infusions of insulin. In most cases, after several days, this regimen is converted to subcutaneous insulin therapy, which may be maintained for several more weeks, even if the transplanted islets appear to be capable of maintaining normoglycemia. This intensive early insulin therapy is thought to be critical because islets traumatized by recent isolation may be particularly sensitive to increases in metabolic demand. Hyper-

glycemia might damage the beta cells by stimulating them to produce insulin until they became "exhausted." However, no randomized studies have been done to support this theory, and it should also be noted that successful islet engraftment in rodents does not require concomitant insulin therapy.

Islet Autotransplantation

Transplantation of pancreatic fragments to diabetics was attempted (unsuccessfully) as early as 1893. Modern human islet transplantation began in 1977 when Sutherland and colleagues at the University of Minnesota performed an intraportal autotransplant of islets in a patient who was undergoing a near-total pancreatectomy for the persistent pain of chronic pancreatitis.[181] This patient remained insulin independent for 6 years after the transplant, proving that transplanted islets could function in humans. Since then, more than 20 institutions have reported a combined series of 170 human islet autotransplants to the International Registry.[181] The largest experience is at the University of Minnesota, where between 1977 and 1995, 59 patients with chronic pancreatitis were subjected to total or near-total pancreatectomy for relief of pain. Islets, isolated from the excised organ, were transplanted into the pancreatectomized patient's liver via the portal vein to prevent the otherwise inevitable diabetes.[182] Because the exocrine pancreas in such patients is almost always atrophic, no purification of the digested pancreas is necessary. Because the islets were autologous, rejection was not a possibility; and because these patients were not type I diabetics, there was no concern over recurrent autoimmune damage. In these patients, the incidence of insulin independence after 2 years was 34%. Since they adopted the automated islet isolation method of Ricordi to increase their islet yield, the Minnesota group have increased their success to 55%. Furthermore, of those autograft recipients who received at least 300,000 islets, 74% were insulin independent after 2 years.[183]

Islet Allografts After Total Pancreatectomy for Patients With Malignant Disease

Prior to the Edmonton report in 2000,[176] the most consistent success with pancreatic islet allografts may have been in patients at the University of Pittsburgh who had their pancreas and liver removed as part of an upper abdominal exenteration for malignant disease.[184] Eleven such patients were treated with combined liver and islet allotransplantation. Six of them exhibited sustained insulin independence after the procedure. Although they all eventually died of recurrence of their malignancy, one remained insulin independent for 58 months and had normal insulin–C-peptide levels at 18, 30, and 57 months post transplantation and, at autopsy, had histologically normal intrahepatic islets. In these cases, the transplanted islets were from the same cadaveric donor as the liver (although several of them received islets from third-party donors in addition). The substantially better result of islet transplantation in these patients than other islet transplants of that era has two possible explanations that are not mutually exclusive: (1) The recipients were not type I diabetics and thus autoimmune damage of the transplanted islets was not a threat, and (2) successful liver allografts are known to have a protective influence that prevents rejection of allografts of other tissues transplanted from the same donor.[185]

Islet Allografts for Insulin-Dependent Diabetes

By far the largest number of candidates for allogeneic transplantation are type I diabetics. Ironically, it is in such patients that a successful outcome has until recently been so difficult to achieve. Between 1990 and 2000 over 300 type I diabetics were transplanted worldwide at 35 institutions, but insulin independence at 1 year was less than 10%.[183] During the 1990s, results improved somewhat, especially at the University of Giessen where 27 islet transplants were done between 1992 and 1996. These patients had a previous or concurrent kidney transplant except for five nonuremic type I diabetics, in whom the indication for islet transplantation was dangerous hypoglycemic unawareness. Three months after transplantation, 64% of the kidney- and islet-transplanted patients had discernible function of the transplanted islets. Later on, those patients who exhibited initial function had a significant reduction in their daily insulin requirement and maintained normal hemoglobin A1c levels. One patient eventually became insulin independent 400 days after transplantation and has remained so for over 2 years, whereas two others became insulin independent at 312 and 363 days post transplant, and both have remained so for more than 100 days. In the nonuremic recipients of islet transplants without kidney transplants, all five initially exhibited islet function. However, because chronic immunosuppression was considered an unacceptable risk in these patients who had no kidney allograft to be protected, the immunosuppression was eventually stopped in all. When immunosuppression was withdrawn, all five soon lost all evidence of islet function.[183,186]

Others also reported occasional success during this period,[178] including a series of a simultaneous islet-kidney transplants performed in Edmonton. In these patients, freshly isolated islets were added to cryopreserved islets from other donors to increase the total number of islets transplanted. One patient became insulin independent after 69 days and remained so for more than 2 years before eventual return of diabetes. A second patient was briefly insulin independent between 155 and 166 days post transplant and again between 837 and 990 days post transplant. Eventually, insulin dependence recurred in this patient, although for only 1 to 5 units daily.[1] Of note, both of the Edmonton patients had biopsy-proven evidence of chronic rejection of their renal allografts, which were from the same cadaveric donor as the non-cryopreserved transplanted islets. Although the mechanisms causing the eventual failure of initially successful islet allografts are unclear, chronic rejection and autoimmune islet damage seem the best possibilities.

A multivariate analysis of all islet transplants reported to the International Transplant Registry identified four characteristics that were associated with success (defined as achievement of insulin independence or at least some evidence of islet engraftment).[183] These were (1) preservation of the donor pancreas for less than 8 hours before islet isolation, (2) transplantation of at least 6000 islets per kilogram of body weight, (3) choice of the liver via the portal vein as the transplant site, and (4) the use of ALG or ATG for induction immunosuppression. In cases in which all four of these positive predictive parameters were present, 70% of patients had some evidence of transplant islet function, 83% had normal hemoglobin A1c levels, and 20% were insulin independent 1 year after transplantation.[183] Although this analysis is based on a small number of successful cases, it provided a framework for design of further trials of islet transplantation including the landmark 2000 report by the Edmonton workers.[176]

A problem in devising optimal immunosuppressive protocols for islet transplantation is the known diabetogenic nature of the commonly employed immunosuppressive drugs. Prednisone may cause insulin resistance and hyperglycemia, whereas both cyclosporine and tacrolimus suppress insulin secretion. The diabetogenic effect of these drugs may in part explain the requirement for a larger than anticipated number of islets needed for successful allografts and the longer than expected time to engraftment. That induction immunosuppression with anti–T-cell antibodies has a positive correlation with islet allograft success may be explained by the lack of islet toxicity of these agents. However, the use of OKT3 for induction therapy may cause islet cell damage from the cytokine release associated with this agent. Induction therapy with a new agent, antihuman thymocyte immunoglobulin, rabbit (Thymoglobulin), has been found to provide superior protection from rejection compared with ALG in renal allografts without the severe cytokine release syndrome common with OKT3. This agent may be ideal for use with isolated islet allografts.

In the setting of the usual failure of islet transplantation even in the 1990s, the report by the Edmonton group of seven consecutive successes gained much attention.[176] The approach employed by these investigators relied on several innovations. First, corticosteroids, the mainstay of traditional immunosuppression regimens, were completely avoided because of their known diabetogenic properties. Also novel was the immunosuppressive regimen selected that included induction therapy with anti–IL-2 receptor antibody and maintenance therapy with a combination of low-dose tacrolimus and sirolimus. Although the reasons for success still remain to be fully explained, it seems likely that this unique combination of agents is unusually effective against both the autoimmune and alloimmune threats to transplanted islets. Perhaps the most important factor in the success achieved by what is now routinely termed the *Edmonton protocol* is that multiple infusions of islets were administered. Whereas many prior investigators had achieved evidence of islet transplant function by detectable C-peptide levels following an infusion of islets from a single donor, unless their patients became insulin independent they usually considered the transplant a failure and discontinued immunosuppression. These earlier patients were not maintained on immunosuppression and regrafted with more islets. Shapiro and colleagues, on the other hand, maintained the immunosuppression and administered second and even third doses of islets from additional donors until insulin independence was achieved. As in the rodent experiments detailed earlier, the inefficiencies of the isolation process and engraftment in the recipient may make the islet yield obtained from a single donor insufficient to completely reverse hyperglycemia.

Based on the encouraging results in Edmonton, numerous centers in the United States and abroad have initiated islet transplant programs, usually copying the Edmonton approach to immunosuppressive protocol and retransplantation. Early results from several other centers are promising. In our own experience, each of nine consecutive patients completing the protocol have gained insulin independence. A result of improvements in isolation technique in four of these, success was achieved with single infusion, whereas in the others a repeat islet transplant was required.

Despite the encouraging nature of recent successes in the field, the frequent need for multiple infusions from multiple cadaveric donors poses practical problems. At present only about 5500 cadaveric donors are available each year in the United States, of which approximately 1500 pancreata are utilized for whole-organ transplantation. Even if the remainder were suitable for islet isolation, this would allow only 2000 diabetics to be successfully treated if two organs are needed for each recipient. Because there are nearly 1.5 million type I diabetics in the United States, other sources of transplantable beta cells would be necessary for transplantation to have its full impact in the treatment of type I diabetes.

Several possible alternative sources of beta cells have been suggested, including xenogeneic donors, genetically altered tissues, stem cells, and living donors. None of these sources is immediately at hand except living donors who volunteer to donate part of their pancreas. Living donors have been used successfully for segmental pancreatic grafts. That islets from two entire cadaveric pancreata are generally required for success using today's isolation techniques makes the utility of a half an organ doubtful unless the function and/or engraftment of the recovered islets could be markedly improved.

Autoimmune Damage of Islet Allografts

Recurrence of autoimmune disease, that is, the destruction of the transplanted islets by the original diabetogenic immune process, has been postulated as an important contributor to the poor results previously seen in type I diabetics. This hypothesis is based on extensive animal studies in the BB rat[127] and the NOD mouse[187] and a few humans who have received pancreas transplants from identical twin donors.[129] Definitive proof of recurrence of autoimmune disease has been difficult to find in humans because biopsies of islet grafts are not practical. The important success of islet allografts in patients who lost their pancreatic function not from autoimmune diabetes but from pancreatectomy during upper abdominal exenteration suggest that if autoimmune recurrence is not an

issue, islet allografts might be more successful.[184] The experience with whole-pancreas transplantation indicates that autoimmune damage of the allograft is usually controlled by intensive immunosuppression with conventional agents. However, pancreatic grafts from identical twin donors have failed from recurrence of autoimmunity even if immunosuppression was given.[129] In addition, recurrence of autoimmunity has been described in two recipients of whole-pancreas allografts from cadaveric donors.[132] In these patients, autoimmune recurrence was assigned as the cause of graft failure because histologic examination of the pancreatic grafts revealed clear patterns of selective beta cell destruction with sparing of alpha and delta cells of the islets.

Islet grafts are fully susceptible not only to T-lymphocyte–mediated rejection and to damage by the autoimmune process of diabetes but also to the phenomenon of primary nonfunction. The causes of this problem are obscure. Although inadequate numbers of transplanted islets and ischemic damage of islets before transplantation play a role in some cases, there may be other reasons. Islets are vulnerable not only to a variety of cytokines but also to inflammatory mediators and oxygen free radicals. Antibody- or macrophage-mediated islet damage could also recur before or during the engraftment phase.[188]

Fetal Islet Allografts and Xenografts

It is believed that over 5000 transplants of fetal islets have been performed, mostly in Russia and China. Apparently, most of these patients either received no immunosuppression or were treated with agents of unknown immunosuppressive activity (e.g., Chinese "traditional medicines").[189] Information of any sort is available on fewer than 200 of these procedures. Thus far, it is doubtful that insulin independence has been achieved in any of the recipients who were type I diabetics, although increases in C-peptide levels have been reported.[183]

Lafferty and associates performed 16 human fetal pancreas allografts in type I diabetic patients who were receiving simultaneous renal transplants.[190,191] They cultured fetal pancreatic fragments (1 mm^3) for 5 to 10 days before transplantation under the renal subcapsule of the kidney transplant. They obtained histologic evidence that the grafted fetal pancreas became revascularized within 14 days and by 3 months after implantation had differentiated into islets. Eight patients received tissue from a single fetal donor, and eight others received tissue from two to four donors. The latter group exhibited some reduction in their insulin requirements compared with a control group of diabetics who received a kidney transplant alone. One patient had a 65% reduction in insulin requirement, measurable serum C-peptide levels, and a normal hemoglobin A1c level 2 years after transplantation. Evidence of meaningful islet function was never evident sooner than 3 to 6 months after transplantation. Even if insulin independence could be achieved with fetal pancreas allografts, the political and ethical issues surrounding the use of human fetal tissues remain a substantial barrier to widespread use of this method.

The use of animal donors for fetal islet transplants might circumvent ethical issues, an interesting possibility that has been explored by Groth and coworkers.[192] They transplanted fetal porcine islets into 10 type I diabetic patients. In 8 patients with functional renal transplants, the grafts were placed in the liver, and 2 patients had the fetal islets placed in the renal subcapsular space of a concomitantly transplanted kidney. The presence of preformed antibodies to this discordant xenogeneic tissue, as well as strong cellular rejection, would be expected to cause rapid destruction of these transplants. Surprisingly, porcine C-peptide was detectable in the urine of 4 patients from 200 to 400 days after transplantation; however, no change was observed in the insulin requirement of these patients.

Postoperative Monitoring for Rejection

A management problem nearly unique to islet transplantation is lack of a reliable marker for early graft rejection. Hyperglycemia is likely to be a late indication of rejection that becomes apparent when the graft is not salvageable by anti-rejection therapy. More sensitive measures of insulin reserve, such as Sustacal stimulation tests or arginine-induced insulin-release assays, are cumbersome and not practical for serial monitoring of graft function.

Immune markers of graft dysfunction have been sought. Olack and colleagues[193] reported a rise in panel-reactive antibody in patients with islet graft dysfunction. Islet grafts in this series were from multiple donors, which may have been responsible for the marked increases in panel-reactive antibody that were observed. Elevations in islet autoantibodies have also been reported after transplant, and their presence before transplant may correlate with poorer graft survival.[194] Whether either alloreactive or autoreactive humoral responses have an important role in islet graft destruction is unknown but would not be surprising given the liver's potential for antibody-dependent cytotoxicity with its large population of resident phagocytes. However, it is unlikely that serologic markers are of promise for routine graft monitoring.

INTESTINAL TRANSPLANTATION

The introduction of intravenous hyperalimentation by Dudrick and associates[195] in 1968 allowed long-term survival of patients with complete intestinal failure who would previously have died rapidly. However, total parenteral nutrition (TPN) severely affects quality of life and may be associated with a number of highly morbid and sometimes fatal complications. In addition, it is estimated that the annual cost of total intravenous nutrition exceeds $200,000.[196]

An alternative to lifelong intravenous nutrition is restoration of enteral absorptive function by intestinal replacement. The earliest experimental transplants of the intestine performed by Lillehei in the 1960s indicated that success of intestinal grafts would be more difficult to achieve than that reported for other solid organ grafts.[197] In fact, it was not until the availability of cyclosporine that

even occasional success was achieved. However, since then the results have greatly improved. Three varieties of intestinal transplantation have been reported: (1) small bowel with or without a portion of the colon (SI), (2) combined liver-small bowel grafts (LI), and (3) multivisceral grafts in which up to five organs are transplanted simultaneously (MV). Nearly equal numbers of SI and LI grafts have been reported, whereas only a few MV grafts have been done (about 10% of the total). It is speculated that a concomitantly transplanted liver graft from the same donor would provide immunologic protection to the more immunogenic intestinal graft, as shown in some animal models.[198] Although the issue is far from resolved, recent clinical results indicate that in humans, this protective effect is minor. This and the fact that failure of a small bowel graft alone may be successfully treated by removal of the graft and reinstitution of TPN, whereas a failed liver graft is fatal without urgent liver retransplantation, cause most groups to perform combined transplants only if both organs are failing. Selection of an isolated small intestinal graft would allow the possibility of utilizing a living related donor, a procedure with considerable technical and immunologic advantages.[199]

The most frequent etiology of intestinal failure is the "short gut" syndrome, which follows extensive resection for intestinal ischemia or disease. At present, the most common indication for intestinal replacement is inability to sustain successful TPN owing to lack of intravenous access sites or because of severe complications from chronic TPN, such as liver failure. That successful intestinal transplantation allows resumption of normal oral intake would make intestinal transplantation the preferred method of therapy for intestinal failure, if the risks of this relatively new procedure can be further decreased.

The principal barrier to widespread application of intestinal replacement at present is the unusually vigorous rejection response elicited by intestinal grafts. Unlike other solid organ grafts such as kidney or liver, which may incite a rejection crisis in 10% to 40% of recipients, 90% to 100% of small bowel grafts undergo rejection crisis within the first 6 months.[194] The reasons for this difference are not entirely clear, but it is assumed that the large amount of gut-associated lymphoid tissue is responsible. Which of the transferred lymphoid cells may be most important in this regard or the antigenic characteristic of these cells has not been elucidated.

A uniquely dangerous consequence of intestinal transplantation rejection is the loss of the protective mucosal barrier of the gut, consequent bacterial translocation, and systemic sepsis in an immunocompromised host. Thus, it is not surprising that the most common cause of death after small bowel transplantation is sepsis and multiorgan failure. Early diagnosis of rejection is therefore crucial. Ironically, intestinal rejection is associated only with nonspecific clinical signs and symptoms, such as fever, anorexia, abdominal pain, and changes in the output and character of intestinal content (often observable as output from an ostium). Even endoscopic biopsies are not entirely reliable in diagnosing rejection because the histologic manifestations of rejection can be patchy, with some areas of the graft appearing entirely normal.

Because the intestine is the largest lymphoid organ in the human body, an intestinal graft can mount a formidable immune response against the graft-versus-host (GVH) disease. In the simplest manifestation of GVH disease, the immune cells and antibody produced by blood group-compatible but nonidentical grafts mediate a severe hemolytic reaction by targeting foreign blood group antigens on the host's red blood cells. A more severe form of GVH disease occurs when T cells of the graft respond to foreign histocompatibility antigens of diverse host tissues, leading to a spectrum of pathology, the most fulminant form including destruction of host hematopoiesis. Interestingly, despite the outcome predicted by animal experiments, GVH disease has not been a severe problem in most clinical cases.[200,201] Perhaps the potent immunosuppressive regimens administered to human patients are especially effective in preventing GVH disease. If so, development of tolerogenic protocols to obviate heavy immunosuppression would ironically be counterproductive for intestinal grafting because in experimental bowel transplant models induction of tolerance leads to dramatically more severe GVH disease.

Results

Data from the most recent International Intestinal Transplant Registry accumulated from 33 programs indicate that by February 1997 there were 273 transplants performed in 260 patients. Forty-one percent of grafts were isolated bowel, and 48% included a simultaneous liver graft.[201] Only 11% of grafts were multivisceral. For grafts transplanted since 1995, 1-year graft survival was nearly equivalent in all three groups (SI, 55%; LI, 63%; MV, 63%), as was patient survival. Better survival was observed in patients transplanted after 1991 and in those transplanted at centers with the greatest experience (>10 transplants). The importance of experience was emphasized by the superior results at the University of Pittsburgh.[202] This center has performed more than 165 intestinal transplants. It reported an actuarial patient survival rate of 75% at 1 year, 54% at 5 years, and 42% at 10 years. For the 93 patients transplanted since 1994, results were substantially improved. One-year survival was 78%, and 5-year survival was 63%. The improvement was attributed to several changes in the immunosuppressive regimen, including cyclophosphamide anti–IL-2 receptor antibody therapy, and, in some recent recipients, to administration of donor bone marrow cells to and/or pretransplant irradiation of the graft. If this early success is sustained and is attainable by other groups as well, transplantation would become the preferred therapy for patients with intestinal failure.[203]

SOCIOECONOMIC AND ETHICAL CONSIDERATIONS

Transplantation is an expensive treatment, although in many cases not as expensive as medical treatment of end-stage organ failure. For example, the median charge for renal transplantation is $38,487 in 1988 U.S. dollars, including hospital charges, professional fees, and charges for the acquisition of donor organs.[204] Second or subse-

quent kidney transplantations cost even more ($41,980). Although dialysis costs remain constant over the years, those for transplantation decrease to about $4,000 after the first year, which is about one third the cost of dialysis. Thus, after 3 years, patients with functioning grafts represent a net savings to the Medicare program, which funds the treatment of end-stage renal disease in most patients. In addition to its cost effectiveness and better survival, renal transplantation is superior to dialysis because it returns 75% of patients to work (compared with 25% to 60% of dialysis patients), with substantial consequent saving in expenses of dialysis and welfare payments, not to mention benefit to patients' families. During the 1990s, improved survival and other advantages of transplantation over dialysis have been widely recognized by the public and nephrologists, greatly increasing the demand for transplants. Only elderly or very poor risk patients are now treated preferentially by dialysis rather than transplantation. Despite this, because of the donor shortage, the number of patients awaiting a cadaveric kidney continues to increase (to nearly 40,000 by 1998), while the number of cadaveric renal transplants performed remains relatively constant at about 9000 per year. The total number of renal transplants has increased since the mid 1990s mainly on the basis of utilizing living unrelated donors and suboptimal cadaveric donors.[3]

With regard to intestinal transplantation versus chronic TPN, it appears there would also be a substantial cost advantage of successful transplantation.[196] Pancreas transplantation is more expensive than the annual cost of insulin therapy, but over several decades, it could be cost effective if it prevents blindness and renal failure. This is perhaps the rationale in the Health Care Financing Administration's recent decision for Medicare to provide coverage of pancreas transplants, which were previously considered by them to be experimental.

For other organs, costs of transplantation versus medical therapy are more difficult to analyze. Successful liver or heart transplantation may be more expensive than repeated prolonged hospitalizations for liver failure and bleeding esophageal varices or multiple bouts of heart failure. However, other transplant-associated costs, such as a long period of support with ventricular-support devices before heart transplant, would greatly increase the total expense. Failure of a vital organ and rapid death are no doubt less expensive than transplantation, but few patients would prefer this option, if a reasonable chance of survival is possible with transplantation.

Public interest in transplantation during the 1980s led to appointment of a national task force to address issues such as the donor shortage, establishment of standards, and provision of transplant services to all citizens. As a result, the National Organ Transplant Act was passed by Congress, which mandated a national Organ Procurement and Transplantation Network.[205] In 1986, a government contract to provide these services was awarded to UNOS, a private nonprofit organization that had been formed by representatives of the majority of transplant centers in anticipation of these governmental actions.

UNOS's board of directors includes representatives of 11 regions that have been established in the United States and is composed of transplant surgeons and physicians, nurses, representatives of voluntary health organizations, transplant recipient families, lawyers, ethicists, theologians, and health care financing representatives. UNOS has established criteria for accreditation of transplantation centers, histocompatibility laboratories, and local organ procurement organizations. All patients awaiting transplants must now be registered with UNOS. A central computer and a point system based on medical criteria determine the assignment of kidneys, which local organ procurement organizations distribute first locally, then regionally, and then nationally. Because hospitals performing transplantation must be members of UNOS to be eligible for Medicare funding, the organization has assumed a powerful role. Each center must now submit outcome data on every transplant performed, and these data are published regularly.

The severe donor shortage, which limits application of transplantation as a lifesaving treatment, causes an ethical dilemma. Criteria for distribution of cadaveric kidneys are the subject of continuing debate. By law, age, race, and socioeconomic status can play no role. Should scarce organs go to high-risk patients, for example, older, highly sensitized individuals whose need might be more pressing but who are unlikely to experience long-term benefit because of rejection or death? Or should younger, better-risk patients whose need is less acute be transplanted because they will have a more lasting benefit? An additional related issue is whether organ allocation should be based on national or regional listing of patients.

The sale of human organs has been condemned by the (International) Transplantation Society and is forbidden by law in most Western countries. It remains an issue because needy individuals in many parts of the world are sometimes willing to sell one of their kidneys for the high price it will bring. Of additional concern are reports of use of organs from executed criminals in China. These tarnish the image of transplantation.

The number of patients dying while awaiting an organ transplant grows every year. This increase in mortality is the result of an expanding number of candidates listed for organ transplants, coupled with a continuing shortage of donor organs. In the United States, obtaining organs from a cadaver donor relies on voluntary consent of a family to donate the organs of a deceased relative or, less commonly, the documented intent of the deceased. In the past 10 years the number of cadaveric organs recovered has increased by only 10%, clearly inadequate to meet the demand. The inadequacy of the current system is based on a decrease in the number of dying individuals suitable for organ donation and on the low rate of family consent for donation from suitable donors (40% to 60%).

A panel of ethicists, organ procurement organization executives, physicians, and surgeons was recently convened by the American Society of Transplant Surgeons to consider whether to recommend a pilot trial to provide a financial incentive for a family to consent to organ donation from a deceased relative. Currently, financial compensation for donation of organs is against the law in the United States. Another concern is that an offer of payment for donated organs might be offensive to some families and decrease their inclination to make an altruistic donation. The panel was unanimously opposed to the exchange of money for donor organs because it would violate the standard of altruism and commercialize the value of human life. However, a majority of the panel supported reimbursement for funeral expenses or a charitable contribution as an ethically permissible approach. The concept of a pilot project of this sort has been supported by the UNOS Board of Directors and the AMA, but this remains controversial, as shown by the opposition of others, including the American College of Surgeons.

The evolution of transplantation from an experimental curiosity to a highly successful therapy represents one of the remarkable achievements of 20th century medicine. Terminal diseases of the kidney, liver, and other organs were uniformly fatal until the 1960s but can now be treated with greater success than most cancers. Because many victims of these diseases are relatively young and productive, the achievement of a successful transplant is one of the most gratifying of all surgical therapies.

References

1. Moore FD: The Give and Take of Tissue Transplantation. New York, Simon & Schuster, 1972.
2. Billingham RE, Brent L, Medawar PB: Actively acquired tolerance of foreign cells. Nature 172:603, 1953.
3. Cecka JM: The UNOS Scientific Transplant Registry, 2001. In Cecka JM, Terasaki PI (eds): Clinical Transplants. Los Angeles, UCLA Tissue Typing Laboratory, 2001, pp 1-18.
4. Bannett A, Brynger H, McAlack RF, et al: Experiences with known ABO-mismatched renal transplants. In Bannett A, Brynger H, Samuellson B, et al (eds): ABO Incompatibility and Transplantation. New York, Grune & Stratton, 1987.
5. Monaco A: Review of transplantation. In Terasaki PI, Cecka JM (eds): Clinical Transplantation. Los Angeles, UCLA Tissue Typing Laboratory, 1998, pp 349-397.
6. Tanabe K, Takahashi K, Sonda K, et al: Long-term results of ABO-incompatible living kidney transplantation: A single-center experience. Transplantation 65:224-228, 1998.
7. Glotz D, Antoine C, Julia P, et al: Desensitization and subsequent kidney transplantation of patients using intravenous immunoglobulins (IVIg). Am J Transplant 2:758-760, 2002.
8. Opelz G, Sengar DP, Mickey MR, et al: Effect of blood transfusions on subsequent kidney transplants. Transplant Proc 5:253-259, 1973.
9. Amed Z, Terasaki PI: Effect of transfusions. In Terasaki PI, Cecka JM (eds): Clinical Transplants. Los Angeles: UCLA Tissue Typing Laboratory, 1991, pp 305-312.
10. Monaco AP: Antilymphocyte serum, donor bone marrow and tolerance to allografts: The journey is the reward. Transplant Proc 31:67-71, 1999.
11. Barber WH, Mankin JA, Laskow DA, et al: Long-term results of a controlled prospective study with transfusion of donor-specific bone marrow in 57 cadaveric renal allograft recipients. Transplantation 51:70-75, 1991.
12. Garcia-Morales R, Carreno M, Mathew J, et al: Continuing observations on the regulatory effects of donor-specific bone marrow cell infusions and chimerism in kidney transplant recipients. Transplantation 65:956-965, 1998.
13. Sutherland DE, Fryd DS, So SK, et al: Long-term effect of splenectomy versus no splenectomy in renal transplant

patients. Reanalysis of a randomized prospective study. Transplantation 38:619-624, 1984.

14. Ramcharan T, Matas AJ: Long-term (20-37 years) follow-up of living kidney donors. Am J Transplant 2:959-964, 2002.
15. Bartlett ST: Laparoscopic donor nephrectomy after seven years. Am J Transplant 2:896-897, 2002.
16. Ratner LE, Ciseck LJ, Moore RG, et al: Laparoscopic live donor nephrectomy. Transplantation 60:1047-1049, 1995.
17. Flowers JL, Jacobs S, Cho E, et al: Comparison of open and laparoscopic live donor nephrectomy. Ann Surg 226:483-490, 1997.
18. Philosophe B, Kuo PC, Schweitzer EJ, et al: Laparoscopic versus open donor nephrectomy: comparing ureteral complications in the recipients and improving the laparoscopic technique. Transplantation 68:497-502, 1999.
19. Velidedeoglu E, Williams N, Brayman KL, et al: Comparison of open, laparoscopic, and hand-assisted approaches to live-donor nephrectomy. Transplantation 74:169-172, 2002.
20. Rosendale JD, Chabalewski FL, McBride MA, et al: Increased transplanted organs from the use of a standardized donor management protocol. Am J Transplant 2:761-768, 2002.
21. Johnson LB, Kuo PC, Dafoe DC, et al: The use of bilateral adult renal allografts—a method to optimize function from donor kidneys with suboptimal nephron mass. Transplantation 61:1261-1263, 1996.
22. Jenkins DH, Reilly PM, Schwab CW: Improving the approach to organ donation: A review. World J Surg 23:644-649, 1999.
23. Starzl TE, Zinkernagel RM: Antigen localization and migration in immunity and tolerance. N Engl J Med 339:1905-1913, 1998.
24. Starzl TE, Zinkernagel RM: Transplantation tolerance from a historical perspective. Nat Rev Immunol 1:233-239, 2001.
25. Opelz G, Mytilineos J, Scherer S, et al: Survival of DNA HLA-DR typed and matched cadaver kidney transplants. The Collaborative Transplant Study. Lancet 338:461-463, 1991.
26. Taylor CJ, Welch KI, Grey CM, et al: Clinical and socioeconomic benefits of serological HLA-DR matching for renal transplantation over 3 eras of immunosuppression regimens at a single center. In Terasaki PI, Cecka JM (eds): Clinical Transplants. Los Angeles: UCLA Tissue Typing Laboratory, 1993, pp 233-241.
27. Takemoto S, Terasaki PI, Cecka JM, et al: Survival of nationally shared, HLA-matched kidney transplants from cadaveric donors. The UNOS Scientific Renal Transplant Registry. N Engl J Med 327:834-839, 1992.
28. Takemoto S, Terasaki PI, Gjertson DW, et al: Equitable allocation of HLA-compatible kidneys for local pools and minorities. N Engl J Med 331:760-764, 1994.
29. Held PJ, Kahan BD, Hunsicker LG, et al: The impact of HLA mismatches on the survival of first cadaveric kidney transplants. N Engl J Med 331:765-770, 1994.
30. Mange KC, Cherikh WS, Maghirang J, et al: A comparison of the survival of shipped and locally transplanted cadaveric renal allografts. N Engl J Med 345:1237-1242, 2001.
31. Markmann JF, Barker CF: Basic and clinical considerations in the use of xenografts. Curr Probl Surg 31:387-460, 1994.
32. Bhatti FN, Schmoeckel M, Zaidi A, et al: Three-month survival of HDAFF transgenic pig hearts transplanted into primates. Transplant Proc 31:958, 1999.
33. Reemtsma K: Heterotransplantation. In Rapaport FT, Dausset J (eds): Human Transplantation. New York, Grune & Stratton, 1968, pp 357-366.
34. Starzl TE, Valdivia LA, Murase N, et al: The biological basis of and strategies for clinical xenotransplantation. Immunol Rev 141:213-244, 1994.
35. Michaels MG, Simmons RL: Xenotransplant-associated zoonoses: Strategies for prevention. Transplantation 57:1-7, 1994.
36. Squinto SP: Genetically modified animal organs for human transplantation. World J Surg 21:939-942, 1997.
37. Phelps CJ, Koike C, Vaught TD, et al: Production of alpha 1,3-galactosyltransferase-deficient pigs. Science 299:411-414, 2003.
38. Specke V, Denner J: [Porcine endogenous retroviruses (PERVs) and xenotransplantation. A risk for the recipient and for society?]. Dtsch Med Wochenschr 128:1301-1306, 2003.
39. Paradis K, Langford G, Long Z, et al: Search for cross-species transmission of porcine endogenous retrovirus in patients treated with living pig tissue. The XEN 111 Study Group. Science 285:1236-1241, 1999.
40. Roza AM, Perloff LJ, Naji A, et al: Living-related donors with bilateral multiple renal arteries: A twenty-year experience. Transplantation 47:397-399, 1989.
41. Hricik DE: Steroid-free immunosuppression in kidney transplantation: An editorial review. Am J Transplant 2:19-24, 2002.
42. Hardy MA, Nowygrod R, Elberg A, et al: Use of ATG in treatment of steroid-resistant rejection. Transplantation 29:162-164, 1980.
43. Brennan DC, Flavin K, Lowell JA, et al: A randomized, double-blinded comparison of Thymoglobulin versus Atgam for induction immunosuppressive therapy in adult renal transplant recipients. Transplantation 67:1011-1018, 1999.
44. Cosimi AB, Colvin RB, Burton RC, et al: Use of monoclonal antibodies to T-cell subsets for immunologic monitoring and treatment in recipients of renal allografts. N Engl J Med 305:308-314, 1981.
45. A randomized clinical trial of OKT3 monoclonal antibody for acute rejection of cadaveric renal transplants. Ortho Multicenter Transplant Study Group. N Engl J Med 313:337-342, 1985.
46. Calne R, Moffatt SD, Friend PJ, et al: Prope tolerance with induction using Campath 1H and low-dose cyclosporin monotherapy in 31 cadaveric renal allograft recipients. Nippon Geka Gakkai Zasshi 101:301-306, 2000.
47. Shaw LM, Kaplan B, Kaufman D: Toxic effects of immunosuppressive drugs: Mechanisms and strategies for controlling them. Clin Chem 42:1316-1321, 1996.
48. Cole E, Keown P, Landsberg D, et al: Safety and tolerability of cyclosporine and cyclosporine microemulsion during 18 months of follow-up in stable renal transplant recipients: A report of the Canadian Neoral Renal Study Group. Transplantation 65:505-510, 1998.
49. Pirsch JD, Miller J, Deierhoi MH, et al: A comparison of tacrolimus (FK506) and cyclosporine for immunosuppression after cadaveric renal transplantation. FK506 Kidney Transplant Study Group. Transplantation 63:977-983, 1997.
50. Jordan ML, Shapiro R, Vivas CA, et al: FK506 "rescue" for resistant rejection of renal allografts under primary cyclosporine immunosuppression. Transplantation 57:860-865, 1994.
51. Sutherland DE: Pancreas and pancreas-kidney transplantation. Curr Opin Nephrol Hypertens 7:317-325, 1998.
52. Sollinger HW, Deierhoi MH, Belzer FO, et al: RS-61443—a phase I clinical trial and pilot rescue study. Transplantation 53:428-432, 1992.
53. Halloran P, Matthew T, Tomlanovich S, et al: Mycophenolate mofetil in renal allograft recipients: A pooled efficacy analysis of three randomized, double-blind, clinical studies

in prevention of rejection. The International Mycophenolate Mofetil Renal Transplant Study Group. Transplantation 63:39-47, 1997.

54. Stepkowski SM, Tian L, Napoli KL, et al: Synergistic mechanisms by which sirolimus and cyclosporin inhibit rat heart and kidney allograft rejection. Clin Exp Immunol 108:63-68, 1997.

55. Kahan BD: Concentration-controlled immunosuppressive regimens using cyclosporine with sirolimus or brequinar in human renal transplantation. Transplant Proc 27:33-36, 1995.

56. Kirk AD, Burkly LC, Batty DS, et al: Treatment with humanized monoclonal antibody against CD154 prevents acute renal allograft rejection in nonhuman primates. Nat Med 5:686-693, 1999.

57. Solez K, Axelsen RA, Benediktsson H, et al: International standardization of criteria for the histologic diagnosis of renal allograft rejection: The Banff working classification of kidney transplant pathology. Kidney Int 44:411-422, 1993.

58. Kissmeyer-Nielsen F, Olsen S, Petersen VP, et al: Hyperacute rejection of kidney allografts, associated with pre-existing humoral antibodies against donor cells. Lancet 2:662-665, 1966.

59. Fisher JS, Woodle ES, Thistlethwaite JR Jr: Kidney transplantation: Graft monitoring and immunosuppression. World J Surg 26:185-193, 2002.

60. Matthew TH: Recurrent disease after renal transplantation. Transplant Rev 5:31, 1991.

61. Tilney NL: Renal transplantation between identical twins: A review. World J Surg 10:381-388, 1986.

62. Briganti EM, Russ GR, McNeil JJ, et al: Risk of renal allograft loss from recurrent glomerulonephritis. N Engl J Med 347:103-109, 2002.

63. Watts RW, Calne RY, Rolles K, et al: Successful treatment of primary hyperoxaluria type I by combined hepatic and renal transplantation. Lancet 2:474-475, 1987.

64. Bilous RW, Mauer SM, Sutherland DE, et al: The effects of pancreas transplantation on the glomerular structure of renal allografts in patients with insulin-dependent diabetes. N Engl J Med 321:80-85, 1989.

65. Lacombe M: Arterial stenosis complicating renal allotransplantation in man: A study of 38 cases. Ann Surg 181:283-288, 1975.

66. Greenstein SM, Verstandig A, McLean GK, et al: Percutaneous transluminal angioplasty: The procedure of choice in the hypertensive renal allograft recipient with renal artery stenosis. Transplantation 43:29-32, 1987.

67. Roberts JP, Ascher NL, Fryd DS, et al: Transplant renal artery stenosis. Transplantation 48:580-583, 1989.

68. Shames BD, Odorico JS, D'Alessandro AM, et al: Surgical repair of transplant renal artery stenosis with preserved cadaveric iliac artery grafts. Ann Surg 237:116-122, 2003.

69. Sageda S, Nordal KP, Hartmann A, et al: The impact of cytomegalovirus infection and disease on rejection episodes in renal allograft recipients. Am J Transplant 2:850-856, 2002.

70. Fishman JA, Rubin RH: Infection in organ-transplant recipients. N Engl J Med 338:1741-1751, 1998.

71. Plotkin SA, Starr SE, Friedman HM, et al: Effect of Towne live virus vaccine on cytomegalovirus disease after renal transplant: A controlled trial. Ann Intern Med 114:525-531, 1991.

72. Snydman DR, Werner BG, Tilney NL, et al: Final analysis of primary cytomegalovirus disease prevention in renal transplant recipients with a cytomegalovirus-immune globulin: Comparison of the randomized and open-label trials. Transplant Proc 23:1357-1360, 1991.

73. Hibberd PL, Tolkoff-Rubin NE, Conti D, et al: Preemptive ganciclovir therapy to prevent cytomegalovirus disease in cytomegalovirus antibody-positive renal transplant recipients: A randomized controlled trial. Ann Intern Med 123:18-26, 1995.

74. Hirsch HH: Polyomavirus BK nephropathy: A (re-)emerging complication in renal transplantation. Am J Transplant 2:25-30, 2002.

75. Perloff LJ, Chon H, Petrella EJ, et al: Acute colitis in the renal allograft recipient. Ann Surg 183:77-83, 1976.

76. Perloff LJ, Spence RK, Grossman RA, et al: Lethal post-transplantation calcinosis. Transplantation 27:21-25, 1979.

77. Penn I: Some problems with posttransplant lymphoproliferative disease. Transplantation 69:705-706, 2000.

78. Penn I: Occurrence of cancers in immunosuppressed organ transplant recipients. In Terasaki PI, Cecka JM (eds): Clinical Transplants, Los Angeles: UCLA Tissue Typing Laboratory, 1998, pp 147-158.

79. Dharnidharka VR, Tejani AH, Ho PL, et al: Post-transplant lymphoproliferative disorder in the United States: Young Caucasian males are at highest risk. Am J Transplant 2:993-998, 2002.

80. Hanto DW, Gajl-Peczalska KJ, Frizzera G, et al: Epstein-Barr virus (EBV) induced polyclonal and monoclonal B-cell lymphoproliferative diseases occurring after renal transplantation: Clinical, pathologic, and virologic findings and implications for therapy. Ann Surg 198:356-369, 1983.

81. Rosen HR, Shackleton CR, Martin P: Indications for and timing of liver transplantation. Med Clin North Am 80:1069-1102, 1996.

82. Belle SH, Beringer KC, Detre KM: An update on liver transplantation in the United States: Recipient characteristics and outcome. Clin Transpl 19-33, 1995.

83. Cox KL, Berquist WE, Castillo RO: Paediatric liver transplantation: Indications, timing and medical complications. J Gastroenterol Hepatol 14 Suppl:S61-66, 1999.

84. Keeffe EB: Summary of guidelines on organ allocation and patient listing for liver transplantation. Liver Transpl Surg 4:S108-114, 1998.

85. Malinchoc M, Kamath PS, Gordon FD, et al: A model to predict poor survival in patients undergoing transjugular intrahepatic portosystemic shunts. Hepatology 31:864-871, 2000.

86. McDiarmid SV, Anand R, Lindblad AS: Development of a pediatric end-stage liver disease score to predict poor outcome in children awaiting liver transplantation. Transplantation 74:173-181, 2002.

87. Garello E, Battista S, Bar F, et al: Evaluation of hepatic function in liver cirrhosis: Clinical utility of galactose elimination capacity, hepatic clearance of D-sorbitol, and laboratory investigations. Dig Dis Sci 44:782-788, 1999.

88. Pimstone NR, Stadalnik RC, Vera DR, et al: Evaluation of hepatocellular function by way of receptor-mediated uptake of a technetium-99m–labeled asialoglycoprotein analog. Hepatology 20:917-923, 1994.

89. Lee WM: Hepatitis B virus infection. N Engl J Med 337:1733-1745, 1997.

90. Hoofnagle JH, Di Bisceglie AM: The treatment of chronic viral hepatitis. N Engl J Med 336:347-356, 1997.

91. Buendia MA: Hepatitis B viruses and cancerogenesis. Biomed Pharmacother 52:34-43, 1998.

92. Ben-Ari Z, Shmueli D, Mor E, et al: Beneficial effect of lamivudine in recurrent hepatitis B after liver transplantation. Transplantation 63:393-396, 1997.

93. Di Bisceglie AM: Hepatitis C. Lancet 351:351-355, 1998.

94. Di Bisceglie AM: Hepatitis C and hepatocellular carcinoma. Hepatology 26:34S-38S, 1997.

95. Guechot J, Poupon RE, Giral P, et al: Relationship between procollagen III aminoterminal propeptide and hyaluronan serum levels and histological fibrosis in primary biliary cirrhosis and chronic viral hepatitis C. J Hepatol 20:388-393, 1994.

96. Feray C, Gigou M, Samuel D, et al: The course of hepatitis C virus infection after liver transplantation. Hepatology 20:1137-1143, 1994.

97. Velidedeoglu E, Desai NM, Campos L, et al: The outcome of liver grafts procured from hepatitis C-positive donors. Transplantation 73:582-587, 2002.

98. Diehl AM: Alcoholic liver disease: Natural history. Liver Transpl Surg 3:206-211, 1997.

99. Yoshihara H, Noda K, Kamada T: Interrelationship between alcohol intake, hepatitis C, liver cirrhosis, and hepatocellular carcinoma. Recent Dev Alcohol 14:457-469, 1998.

100. Scheuer PJ: Ludwig Symposium on biliary disorders—part II: Pathologic features and evolution of primary biliary cirrhosis and primary sclerosing cholangitis. Mayo Clin Proc 73:179-183, 1998.

101. Wiesner RH: Liver transplantation for primary biliary cirrhosis and primary sclerosing cholangitis: Predicting outcomes with natural history models. Mayo Clin Proc 73:575-588, 1998.

102. Klintmalm GB: Liver transplantation for hepatocellular carcinoma: A registry report of the impact of tumor characteristics on outcome. Ann Surg 228:479-490, 1998.

103. Lefkowitch JH: Biliary atresia. Mayo Clin Proc 73:90-95, 1998.

104. Kasai M: Treatment of biliary atresia with special reference to hepatic porto-enterostomy and its modifications. Prog Pediatr Surg 6:5-52, 1974.

105. Markmann JF, Gornbein J, Markowitz JS, et al: A simple model to estimate survival after retransplantation of the liver. Transplantation 67:422-430, 1999.

106. McDiarmid SV, Davies DB, Edwards EB: Improved graft survival of pediatric liver recipients transplanted with pediatric-aged liver donors. Transplantation 70:1283-1291, 2000.

107. Busuttil RW, Goss JA: Split liver transplantation. Ann Surg 229:313-321, 1999.

108. Wachs ME, Bak TE, Karrer FM, et al: Adult living donor liver transplantation using a right hepatic lobe. Transplantation 66:1313-1316, 1998.

109. Markmann JF, Markowitz JS, Yersiz H, et al: Long-term survival after retransplantation of the liver. Ann Surg 226:408-420, 1997.

110. Davern TJ, Lake JR: Recurrent disease after liver transplantation. Semin Gastrointest Dis 9:86-109, 1998.

111. Eghtesad B, Bronsther O, Irish W, et al: Disease gravity and urgency of need as guidelines for liver allocation. Hepatology 20:56S-62S, 1994.

112. Markmann JF, Markmann JW, Markmann DA, et al: Preoperative factors associated with outcome and their impact on resource use in 1148 consecutive primary liver transplants. Transplantation 72:1113-1122, 2001.

113. Zetterman RK, Belle SH, Hoofnagle JH, et al: Age and liver transplantation: A report of the Liver Transplantation Database. Transplantation 66:500-506, 1998.

114. Kennard BD, Stewart SM, Phelan-McAuliffe D, et al: Academic outcome in long-term survivors of pediatric liver transplantation. J Dev Behav Pediatr 20:17-23, 1999.

115. Goss JA, Shackleton CR, McDiarmid SV, et al: Long-term results of pediatric liver transplantation: An analysis of 569 transplants. Ann Surg 228:411-420, 1998.

116. The effect of intensive treatment of diabetes on the development and progression of long-term complications in insulin-dependent diabetes mellitus. The Diabetes Control and Complications Trial Research Group. N Engl J Med 329:977-986, 1993.

117. Viberti GC, Hill RD, Jarrett RJ, et al: Microalbuminuria as a predictor of clinical nephropathy in insulin-dependent diabetes mellitus. Lancet 1:1430-1432, 1982.

118. Fioretto P, Steffes MW, Sutherland DE, et al: Reversal of lesions of diabetic nephropathy after pancreas transplantation. N Engl J Med 339:69-75, 1998.

119. Sutherland DE, Gruessner A, Bland B, et al: International Pancreas Transplant Registry (IPTR) Annual Report for 2001. News Letter IPTR 14:August 2002.

120. Reddy KS, Stratta RJ, Shokouh-Amiri MH, et al: Surgical complications after pancreas transplantation with portal-enteric drainage. J Am Coll Surg 189:305-313, 1999.

121. Philosophe B, Farney AC, Schweitzer EJ, et al: Superiority of portal venous drainage over systemic venous drainage in pancreas transplantation: A retrospective study. Ann Surg 234:689-696, 2001.

122. Gruessner RW, Sutherland DE: Living donor pancreas transplantation. Transplant Rev 16:108-119, 2002.

123. Corry RJ, Chakrabarti PK, Shapiro R, et al: Simultaneous administration of adjuvant donor bone marrow in pancreas transplant recipients. Ann Surg 230:372-381, 1999.

124. Benedetti E, Najarian JS, Gruessner AC, et al: Correlation between cystoscopic biopsy results and hypoamylasuria in bladder-drained pancreas transplants. Surgery 118:864-872, 1995.

125. Laftavi MR, Gruessner AC, Bland BJ, et al: Diagnosis of pancreas rejection: Cystoscopic transduodenal versus percutaneous computed tomography scan-guided biopsy. Transplantation 65:528-532, 1998.

126. Naji A, Silvers WK, Plotkin SA, et al: Successful islet transplantation in spontaneous diabetes. Surgery 86:218-226, 1979.

127. Naji A, Silvers WK, Bellgrau D, et al: Spontaneous diabetes in rats: Destruction of islets is prevented by immunological tolerance. Science 213:1390-1392, 1981.

128. Alinaji, Silvers WK, Bellgrau D, et al: Prevention of diabetes in rats by bone marrow transplantation. Ann Surg 194:328-338, 1981.

129. Sutherland DE, Sibley R, Xu XZ, et al: Twin-to-twin pancreas transplantation: Reversal and reenactment of the pathogenesis of type I diabetes. Trans Assoc Am Physicians 97:80-87, 1984.

130. Roza A, Markmann J, Brayman KL, et al: Isolated islet cells are more vulnerable to recurrent diabetes than vascularized pancreas grafts. Surg Forum 38:373-375, 1987.

131. Sutherland DE, Gruessner R, Dunn D, et al: Pancreas transplants from living-related donors. Transplant Proc 26:443-445, 1994.

132. Tyden G, Reinholt FP, Sundkvist G, et al: Recurrence of autoimmune diabetes mellitus in recipients of cadaveric pancreatic grafts. N Engl J Med 335:860-863, 1996.

133. Troppmann C, Gruessner AC, Benedetti E, et al: Vascular graft thrombosis after pancreatic transplantation: Univariate and multivariate operative and nonoperative risk factor analysis. J Am Coll Surg 182:285-316, 1996.

134. Sutherland DE, Gruessner RW, Gores PF, et al: Pancreas transplantation: An update. Diabetes Metab Rev 11:337-363, 1995.

135. Diem P, Redmon JB, Abid M, et al: Glucagon, catecholamine and pancreatic polypeptide secretion in type I diabetic recipients of pancreas allografts. J Clin Invest 86:2008-2013, 1990.

136. Sutherland DE: Effect of pancreas transplants on secondary complications of diabetes: Review of observations at a single institution. Transplant Proc 24:859-860, 1992.

137. Kennedy WR, Navarro X, Goetz FC, et al: Effects of pancreatic transplantation on diabetic neuropathy. N Engl J Med 322:1031-1037, 1990.

138. Gaber AO, Hathaway DK, Abell T, et al: Improved autonomic and gastric function in pancreas-kidney vs kidney-alone transplantation contributes to quality of life. Transplant Proc 26:515-516, 1994.

139. Hathaway D, Abell T, Cardoso S, et al: Improvement in autonomic function following pancreas-kidney versus kidney-alone transplantation. Transplant Proc 25:1306-1308, 1993.

140. Solders G, Tyden G, Tibell A, et al: Improvement in nerve conduction 8 years after combined pancreatic and renal transplantation. Transplant Proc 27:3091, 1995.

141. Ramsay RC, Goetz FC, Sutherland DE, et al: Progression of diabetic retinopathy after pancreas transplantation for insulin-dependent diabetes mellitus. N Engl J Med 318:208-214, 1988.

142. Wang Q, Klein R, Moss SE, et al: The influence of combined kidney-pancreas transplantation on the progression of diabetic retinopathy: A case series. Ophthalmology 101:1071-1076, 1994.

143. Mauer SM, Steffes MW, Connett J, et al: The development of lesions in the glomerular basement membrane and mesangium after transplantation of normal kidneys to diabetic patients. Diabetes 32:948-952, 1983.

144. Steffes MW, Barbosa J, Basgen JM, et al: Quantitative glomerular morphology of the normal human kidney. Lab Invest 49:82-86, 1983.

145. Bilous RW, Mauer SM, Sutherland DE, et al: Glomerular structure and function following successful pancreas transplantation for insulin-dependent diabetes mellitus. Diabetes 36:43A, 1987.

146. Bohman SO, Wilczek H, Tyden G, et al: Recurrent diabetic nephropathy in renal allografts placed in diabetic patients and protective effect of simultaneous pancreatic transplantation. Transplant Proc 19:2290-2293, 1987.

147. Morel P, Sutherland DE, Almond PS, et al: Assessment of renal function in type I diabetic patients after kidney, pancreas, or combined kidney-pancreas transplantation. Transplantation 51:1184-1189, 1991.

148. Ojo AO, Meier-Kriesche HU, Hanson JA, et al: The impact of simultaneous pancreas-kidney transplantation on long-term patient survival. Transplantation 71:82-90, 2001.

149. Smets YF, Westendorp RG, van der Pijl JW, et al: Effect of simultaneous pancreas-kidney transplantation on mortality of patients with type-1 diabetes mellitus and end-stage renal failure. Lancet 353:1915-1919, 1999.

150. Tyden G, Bolinder J, Solders G, et al: Improved survival in patients with insulin-dependent diabetes mellitus and end-stage diabetic nephropathy 10 years after combined pancreas and kidney transplantation. Transplantation 67:645-648, 1999.

151. Piehlmeier W, Bullinger M, Nusser J, et al: Quality of life in type 1 (insulin-dependent) diabetic patients prior to and after pancreas and kidney transplantation in relation to organ function. Diabetologia 34(Suppl 1):S150-157, 1991.

152. Ballinger WF, Lacy PE: Transplantation of intact pancreatic islets in rats. Surgery 72:175-186, 1972.

153. Reckard CR, Barker CF: Transplantation of isolated pancreatic islets across strong and weak histocompatibility barriers. Transplant Proc 5:761-763, 1973.

154. Lacy PE, Kostianovsky M: Method for the isolation of intact islets of Langerhans from the rat pancreas. Diabetes 16:35-39, 1967.

155. Kemp CB, Knight MJ, Scharp DW, et al: Effect of transplantation site on the results of pancreatic islet isografts in diabetic rats. Diabetologia 9:486-491, 1973.

156. Brown J, Clark WR, Molnar IG, et al: Fetal pancreas transplantation for reversal of streptozotocin-induced diabetes in rats. Diabetes 25:56-64, 1976.

157. Jindal RM, Sidner RA, McDaniel HB, et al: Intraportal vs kidney subcapsular site for human pancreatic islet transplantation. Transplant Proc 30:398-399, 1998.

158. Barker CF, Billingham RE: Immunologically privileged sites. Adv Immunol 25:1-54, 1977.

159. Levy MM, Ketchum RJ, Tomaszewski JE, et al: Intrathymic islet transplantation in the canine: I. Histological and functional evidence of autologous intrathymic islet engraftment and survival in pancreatectomized recipients. Transplantation 73:842-852, 2002.

160. Markmann JF, Bassiri H, Desai NM, et al: Indefinite survival of MHC class I–deficient murine pancreatic islet allografts. Transplantation 54:1085-1089, 1992.

161. Min JK: Adenoviral-mediated gene transfer of TGF-beta1 and vIL-10 promotes long-term survival of islet allografts. Surg Forum 46:438-440, 1995.

162. Reckard CR, Ziegler MM, Barker CF: Physiological and immunological consequences of transplanting isolated pancreatic islets. Surgery 74:91-99, 1973.

163. Lafferty KJ, Prowse SJ, Simeonovic CJ, et al: Immunobiology of tissue transplantation: A return to the passenger leukocyte concept. Annu Rev Immunol 1:143-173, 1983.

164. Bowen KM, Lafferty KJ: Reversal of diabetes by allogenic islet transplantation without immunosuppression. Aust J Exp Biol Med Sci 58:441-447, 1980.

165. Lau H, Reemtsma K, Hardy MA: Prolongation of rat islet allograft survival by direct ultraviolet irradiation of the graft. Science 223:607-609, 1984.

166. James RF, Lake SP, Chamberlain J, et al: Gamma irradiation of isolated rat islets pretransplantation produces indefinite allograft survival in cyclosporine-treated recipients. Transplantation 47:929-933, 1989.

167. Faustman D, Coe C: Prevention of xenograft rejection by masking donor HLA class I antigens. Science 252:1700-1702, 1991.

168. Faustman D, Coe C: Xenograft acceptance by masking donor antigens. Transplant Proc 24:2854-2855, 1992.

169. Faustman DL, Steinman RM, Gebel HM, et al: Prevention of rejection of murine islet allografts by pretreatment with anti-dendritic cell antibody. Proc Natl Acad Sci U S A 81:3864-3868, 1984.

170. Gray DW, Morris PJ: Cyclosporine and pancreas transplantation. World J Surg 8:230-235, 1984.

171. Ricordi C, Zeng YJ, Alejandro R, et al: In vivo effect of FK506 on human pancreatic islets. Transplantation 52:519-522, 1991.

172. Kenyon NS, Chatzipetrou M, Masetti M, et al: Long-term survival and function of intrahepatic islet allografts in rhesus monkeys treated with humanized anti-CD154. Proc Natl Acad Sci U S A 96:8132-8137, 1999.

173. Posselt AM, Barker CF, Tomaszewski JE, et al: Induction of donor-specific unresponsiveness by intrathymic islet transplantation. Science 249:1293-1295, 1990.

174. Naji A: Induction of tolerance by intrathymic inoculation of alloantigen. Curr Opin Immunol 8:704-709, 1996.

175. Une S, Kenmochi T, Miyamoto M, et al: Induction of donor-specific unresponsiveness in NIH minipigs following

intrathymic islet transplantation. Transplant Proc 27:142-144, 1995.

176. Shapiro AM, Lakey JR, Ryan EA, et al: Islet transplantation in seven patients with type 1 diabetes mellitus using a glucocorticoid-free immunosuppressive regimen. N Engl J Med 343:230-238, 2000.

177. Ricordi C, Lacy PE, Finke EH, et al: Automated method for isolation of human pancreatic islets. Diabetes 37:413-420, 1988.

178. Warnock GI, Tsapogas P, Ryan EA, et al: Natural history of insulin independence after transplantation of multidonor cryopreserved pancreatic islets in type 1 diabetic humans. Transplant Proc 27:3159-3160, 1995.

179. Hering BJ, Brendel MD, Schultz AO, et al: International islet transplant registry. (newsletter) 16:1-20, 1996.

180. Mehigan DG, Bell WR, Zuidema GD, et al: Disseminated intravascular coagulation and portal hypertension following pancreatic islet autotransplantation. Ann Surg 191:287-293, 1980.

181. Moudry-Munns KC, Gruessner A, Sutherland DE: International Pancreas Transplant Registry Report, 1993. J Transplant Coord 4:18, 1994.

182. Wahoff DC, Papalois BE, Najarian JS, et al: Autologous islet transplantation to prevent diabetes after pancreatic resection. Ann Surg 222:562-579, 1995.

183. Hering BJ, Ricordi C: Graft islet transplantation for patients with type I diabetes. Graft 2:12-27, 1999.

184. Rilo HL, Carroll PB, Tzakis A, et al: Insulin independence for 58 months following pancreatic islet cell transplantation in a patient undergoing upper abdominal exenteration. Transplant Proc 27:3164-3165, 1995.

185. Kamada N, Davies HS, Roser B: Reversal of transplantation immunity by liver grafting. Nature 292:840-842, 1981.

186. Bretzel RG, Hering BJ, Brandhorst D, et al: Islet transplantation in three different categories of type I diabetic patients: The Giessen experience. Exp Clin Endocrinol Diabetes 104:A16, 1996.

187. Mullen Y, Fujiya H, Motojima K, et al: Autoimmune destruction of syngeneic pancreatic cells in nonobese diabetic mice. Transplant Proc 28:831-833, 1986.

188. Kaufman DB, Platt JL, Rabe FL, et al: Differential roles of Mac-1+ cells, and CD4+ and CD8+ T lymphocytes in primary nonfunction and classic rejection of islet allografts. J Exp Med 172:291-302, 1990.

189. Satake M, Korsgren O, Ridderstad A, et al: Immunological characteristics of islet cell xenotransplantation in humans and rodents. Immunol Rev 141:191-211, 1994.

190. Lafferty KJ, Hao L, Babcock SK, et al: Is there a future for fetal pancreas transplantation? Transplant Proc 21:2611-2613, 1989.

191. Stegall MD, Lafferty KJ, Kam I, et al: Evidence of recurrent autoimmunity in human allogeneic islet transplantation. Transplantation 61:1272-1274, 1996.

192. Groth CG, Korsgren O, Tibell A, et al: Transplantation of porcine fetal pancreas to diabetic patients. Lancet 344:1402-1404, 1994.

193. Olack BJ, Swanson CJ, Flavin KS, et al: Sensitization to HLA antigens in islet recipients with failing transplants. Transplant Proc 29:2268-2269, 1997.

194. Jaeger C, Brendel MD, Hering BJ, et al: Progressive islet graft failure occurs significantly earlier in autoantibody-positive than in autoantibody-negative IDDM recipients of intrahepatic islet allografts. Diabetes 46:1907-1910, 1997.

195. Dudrick SJ, Wilmore DW, Vars HM, et al: Long-term total parenteral nutrition with growth, development, and positive nitrogen balance. Surgery 64:134-142, 1968.

196. Howard L, Heaphey L, Fleming CR, et al: Four years of North American registry home parenteral nutrition outcome data and their implications for patient management. JPEN J Parenter Enteral Nutr 15:384-393, 1991.

197. Khan FA, Tzakis AG: Intestinal and multivisceral transplantation. In Ginns LC, Cosimi AB, Morris PJ (eds): Transplantation. Malden, MA, Blackwell, 1999, pp 422-437.

198. Sun J, Sheil AG, Wang C, et al: Tolerance to rat liver allografts: IV. Acceptance depends on the quantity of donor tissue and on donor leukocytes. Transplantation 62:1725-1730, 1996.

199. Gruessner RW, Sharp HL: Living-related intestinal transplantation: First report of a standardized surgical technique. Transplantation 64:1605-1607, 1997.

200. Lee KK, Schraut WH: In vitro allograft irradiation prevents graft-versus-host disease in small-bowel transplantation. J Surg Res 38:364-372, 1985.

201. Kumar N, Grant D: Small bowel transplantation. Graft 2:149-153, 1999.

202. Abu-Elmagd K, Reyes J, Bond G, et al: Clinical intestinal transplantation: A decade of experience at a single center. Ann Surg 234:404-417, 2001.

203. Fishbein TM, Florman S, Gondolesi G, et al: Intestinal transplantation before and after the introduction of sirolimus. Transplantation 73:1538-1542, 2002.

204. Evans RW, Manninen DL, Dong FB, et al: Is retransplantation cost effective? Transplant Proc 25:1694-1696, 1993.

205. McDonald JC: The National Organ Procurement and Transplantation Network. JAMA 259:725-726, 1988.

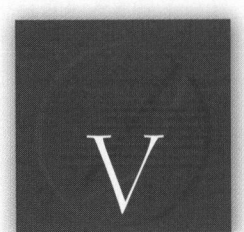
SURGICAL ONCOLOGY

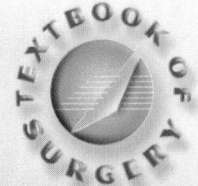

CHAPTER 28

TUMOR BIOLOGY AND TUMOR MARKERS

**Peter S. Goedegebuure, Ph.D.,   Udaya Liyanage, M.D.
and   Timothy J. Eberlein, M.D.**

TUMOR BIOLOGY	TUMOR MARKERS

TUMOR BIOLOGY

Tumors are characterized by an uncontrolled growth of transformed cells. Although tumors, also called *neoplasms,* do not arise spontaneously, once triggered, the proliferation of the tumor is independent of the presence of the stimulus. Tumors can be benign or malignant; the malignant ones are often referred to as *cancer* and can be further distinguished based on origin. All tumors can be either classified as hematopoietic or nonhematopoietic in origin. Within each category, tumors can be further divided into those of similar histologic origin, for example, tumors derived from the same organ, such as lung cancers and colon cancers, or tumors from the same cell type, such as epithelial cell–derived tumors.

The development of a tumor from a single transformed cell into metastatic tumor is categorized by stages and grades and involves three phases: initiation, promotion, and progression. The initiation phase is characterized by the series of genetic mutations that occur in sequence. For initiated cells to become tumor cells, exposure to promoting agents or conditions is required (promotion phase). The end of the promotion phase is characterized by the appearance of the first neoplastic cells. Before the appearance of neoplastic cells, the abnormal cells are called *preneoplastic* or *premalignant* cells. The progression phase is characterized by invasive growth of the transformed cells and progression of the tumorous lesion into a highly metastatic tumor that may ultimately kill the host.

A well-documented example of tumor development is presented in Table 28-1.[1,2] The transformation of melanocytes into malignant melanoma can be divided into five major histopathologically and clinically identifiable

steps (see Table 28-1). This chapter discusses the initiation and development of tumors as well as the expression of genotypic and phenotypic markers associated with these processes.

How Do Tumors Arise?

The formation, or genesis, of a tumor is a complex process primarily because tumors are not a single disease. The progression of a single transforming event in a cell toward the formation of a tumor requires multiple mutations that occur in sequence. The whole sequence occurs over a period that may exceed 20 years. Additionally, cancer is multifactorial: the cancer-inducing mutations may be induced by external factors (somatic mutations), such as exposure to physical or chemical carcinogens, or they may be germline mutations that are more likely to result in certain types of cancer.

Exposure to physical or chemical carcinogens is responsible for most cancers in industrialized countries and includes smoking, ingesting alcohol or particular foods, and exposure to sunlight and chemicals. Epidemiologic studies have shown strong correlations between several internal and external factors, although the exact sequence of events is still unknown. Smoking is associated with lung cancer, bladder cancer, and cancer of the mouth, pharynx, larynx, and esophagus. Immunosuppression is associated with lymphomas, and x-rays and gamma rays are associated with the development of leukemia. Chemical carcinogens include asbestos and polycyclic aromatic hydrocarbons, which increase the risk for lung cancer; benzene, which may induce leukemia; and aromatic amines, which may induce bladder cancer.

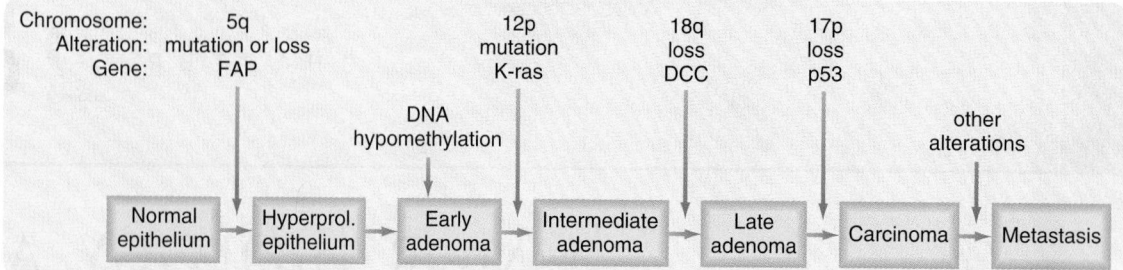

FIGURE 28-1. A genetic model for colorectal tumorigenesis. Tumorigenesis proceeds through a series of genetic alterations involving oncogenes (*ras*) and tumor suppressor genes (particularly those on chromosomes 5q, 12p, 17p, and 18q). The three stages of adenomas in general represent tumors of increasing size, dysplasia, and villous content. In patients with familial adenomatous polyposis (FAP), a mutation on chromosome 5q (*APC* gene) is inherited. This alteration may be responsible for the hypoproliferative epithelium present in these patients. Hypomethylation is present in very small adenomas in patients with or without polyposis, and this alteration may lead to aneuploidy, resulting in the loss of suppressor gene alleles. The *ras* gene mutation appears to occur in one cell of a preexisting small adenoma and, through clonal expansion, produces a larger and more dysplastic tumor. Allelic deletions of chromosome 17p and 18q usually occur at a later stage of tumorigenesis than do deletions of chromosome 5q or *ras* gene mutations. The order of these changes is not invariant, however, and accumulation of these changes, rather than their order with respect to one another, seems most important. Tumors continue to progress once carcinomas have formed, and the accumulated loss of suppressor genes on additional chromosomes correlates with the ability of the carcinomas to metastasize and cause death. (From Fearon ER: A genetic model for colorectal tumorigenesis. Cell 61:759, 1990.)

TABLE 28-1.	Stepwise Progression From Melanocyte to Metastatic Melanoma
Step*	**Characteristics**
1	Common melanocytic nevus
2	Dysplastic nevus
3	Radial growth phase of melanoma
4	Vertical growth phase of melanoma
5	Metastatic melanoma

*Common acquired and congenital nevi without cytologic atypia (step 1) may progress into dysplastic nevi with clear atypical histologic and cytologic features (step 2). Most of these lesions are stable, but a few may progress to a malignant melanoma that tends to grow outward along the radius of the plaque (step 3). Within the plaque, a nodule develops of fast-growing cells that expand in a vertical direction, invading the dermis and elevating the epidermis (step 4). Finally, the tumor metastasizes (step 5).

Adapted from Clark WH: A study of tumor progression: The precursor lesions of superficial spreading and nodular melanoma. Hum Pathol 15:1147, 1984; and Clark WH: The biologic forms of malignant melanoma. Hum Pathol 17:443, 1986.

An example of a germline mutation leading to (colon) carcinoma was proposed by Fearon and Vogelstein.[3] They postulated that the morphologic changes from normal mucosa to early, intermediate, and late adenoma and finally to colorectal carcinoma are associated with certain essential mutations that occur in sequence (Fig. 28-1). Patients with germline mutations in the tumor suppressor gene adenomatous polyposis coli (*APC* gene) are prone to develop familial adenomatous polyposis. Tumor suppressor genes can be regarded as negative regulators of growth-promoting signaling pathways. The *APC* gene product is involved in cellular adhesion and intercellular communication, and both functions are absent after gene mutations. Mutations in the *APC* gene can frequently be found in adenomas, including small adenomas, suggesting that they are an early event. The second important mutation may occur in the K-*ras* oncogene, a cell membrane–bound signal-transduction molecule. Oncogenes are positive regulators of growth-promoting signaling pathways. Mutations in K-*ras* resulting in continuous activation of *ras* occur in about half of colorectal cancers and adenomas larger than 1 cm but are found less frequently in small adenomas. Thus, K-*ras* mutations are early events but occur later than *APC* gene mutations. Late adenomas and colorectal cancer frequently show loss of the tumor suppressor gene *DCC* (deleted colon cancer). *DCC* deletion is, however, uncommon in early adenomas, placing this event after the K-*ras* mutations. The *DCC* gene product is a cell surface molecule involved in adhesion. Finally, deletion of the tumor suppressor gene *p53* is observed in 75% of colorectal cancers but is infrequently observed in adenomas and is therefore a late event in carcinogenesis. The mutations and deletions of the *APC*, K-*ras*, *DCC*, and *p53* genes are the most commonly detected genetic alterations in colon cancer.

In general, mutated genes in transformed cells include tumor suppressor genes and oncogenes. Both types of genes play an essential role in the regulation of cell cycle progression. Cell proliferation is a series of tightly controlled biochemical processes divided into an interphase and a mitotic (M) phase (Fig. 28-2). The interphase is further subdivided into two gap phases (G_1 and G_2), separated by a phase of DNA synthesis (S phase). Central to cell cycle progression are the cyclin-dependent kinases that bind to the cyclin proteins. These proteins are regulated by numerous other proteins including tumor suppressors and oncogenes that induce stimulatory or inhibitory signals. Both tumor suppressors and oncogenes can be part of the same signaling pathway, and some of these pathways are disrupted in virtually every tumor.[4]

Stimulation of Tumor Development

Even though tumors are characterized by unlimited growth, tumors are dependent on their environment for growth and development. The immediate tumor environment (the stroma) contains residing nonmalignant cells such as parenchymal cells, epithelial cells, fibroblasts, endothelial cells, and mast cells. In addition, most tumors are characterized by infiltrating immune cells such as lymphocytes, polymorphonuclear cells, and macrophages. Finally, basement membranes form the extracellular matrix (ECM) that forms a scaffold for proliferation of fibroblast and endothelial cells. The ECM consists of multiple different proteins and carbohydrates that together are responsible for the organization of cells into organs. ECM components, such as collagens, fibronectins, laminins, vitronectins, and proteoglycans, interact with cellular receptors, such as integrins and heparan sulfate proteoglycans. Each ECM molecule may bind to two or more receptors and may also bind other ECM molecules. The matrix molecule-receptor interaction leads to an "attachment" signal, which activates certain genes. It is believed that adhesion to ECM is required for cell growth and differentiation. The adhesion is cell-type specific. The specificity is mediated primarily through integrin receptor specificity. Integrins consist of an alpha subunit and a beta subunit, but a particular beta subunit can dimerize with several different alpha subunits. In addition, alternative splicing of the primary transcripts of several subunits has been described. Additional specificity is mediated through the cytoskeletal organization within the cell and through the array of genes being expressed in cells.

Together, tumor cells, ECM, stroma, and infiltrate produce factors (autocrine and paracrine factors) that, in cell-bound, matrix-bound, or soluble form, directly or indirectly influence tumor development. Proliferating tumors invade neighboring cell populations, thereby breaking down boundaries designed to keep normal tissue architecture. These boundaries consist of basement membranes, ECM communication with neighboring cells, and cell-cell communication preventing cells from inappropriately mixing. Tumor cells resistant to the regulatory signals can successfully expand into surrounding tissues. There is evidence that at the molecular level, signaling pathways regulating tumor cell motility are linked to pathways leading to proliferation and survival. For example, integrin-mediated signaling involved in disengagement from ECM (essential for motility) is associated with additional proinvasive signaling and proliferative and antiapoptotic signaling.

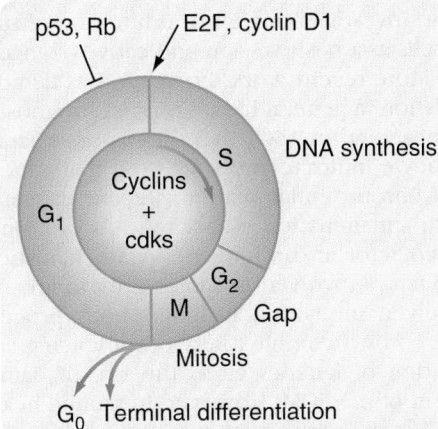

FIGURE 28-2. Schematic overview of the cell cycle. Cell division is governed by cyclin proteins and cyclin-dependent kinases (cdks). After mitosis, a cell can terminally differentiate, enter a quiescent state, or re-enter the cell cycle. A critical point in the cell-cycle control is the transition from G_1 to S. After passing this checkpoint, the cell is committed to division. Tumor suppressor genes such as the retinoblastoma (*Rb*) gene and *p53* block G_1 to S transition, whereas oncogenes such as *cyclin D1* and *E2F* promote transition.

Paracrine and Autocrine Growth Mechanisms

Autocrine factors secreted by tumor cells promote growth of tumor cells but may also stimulate neighboring cells. In addition, tumor cells secrete paracrine factors that act on host cells or ECMs. For example, transforming growth factor (TGF)-β may induce angiogenesis, production of ECM molecules, and production of other cytokines by fibroblasts and endothelial cells. Simplified, tumor growth is dependent on the response of tumor cells to paracrine and autocrine factors[5] (Fig. 28-3). These factors include

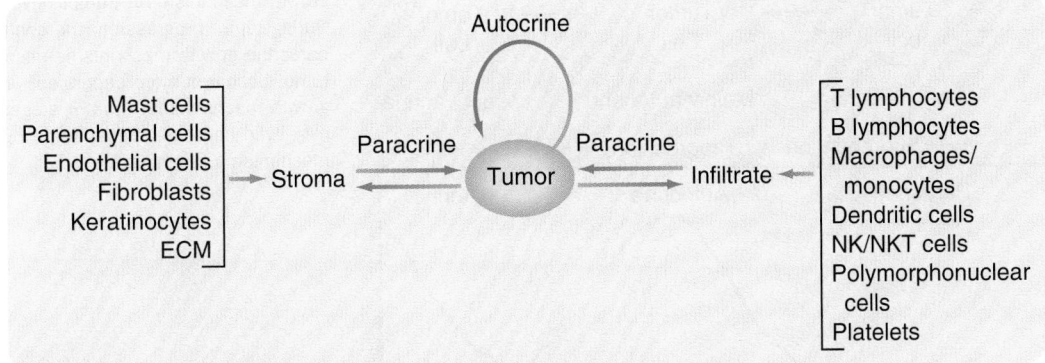

FIGURE 28-3. Paracrine and autocrine growth mechanisms. Both stromal cells and infiltrate secrete paracrine factors that affect tumor development. Additionally, tumor cells secrete autocrine as well as paracrine factors that, in turn, act on stromal cells and infiltrating cells. ECM, extracellular matrix; NK, natural killer.

angiogenesis factors secreted by tumor cells, growth factors, chemokines (polypeptide signaling molecules originally characterized by their ability to induce chemotaxis), cytokines, hormones, enzymes, cytolytic factors, and so forth, which may promote or reduce tumor growth (Table 28-2). Even though most paracrine factors promote tumor growth, growth inhibitors have also been found. TGF-β may inhibit tumor growth, as was found for kidney cells that secrete TGF-β$_1$, which inhibits formation of tumor metastases in the kidney. In melanoma, interleukin (IL)-6 produced by stromal cells (keratinocytes, endothelial cells, and fibroblasts), or infiltrate (monocytes and macrophages) may inhibit the growth of early lateral growth phase melanoma cells, but more progressed melanoma cells have lost responsiveness to IL-6.

During the evolution of a tumor, changes in growth and other properties occur. Paracrine growth mechanisms are dominant during tumor initiation and tumor promotion. Early stages of metastasis are characterized by a preferential outgrowth at restricted sites, suggesting that paracrine growth mechanisms are essential. However, autocrine growth mechanisms become more prominent in later stages. The observation that during tumor progression tumor cells tend to spread more randomly through the body suggests that autocrine growth mechanisms may be more dominant than paracrine growth mechanisms. Tumors become resistant to paracrine growth inhibitors and lose responsiveness to paracrine growth promoters. Progressing breast cancers, for example, lose hormone responsiveness. It is even possible for a tumor to grow completely autonomous (acrine state) and to be independent of growth factors and inhibitors (Fig. 28-4).

Role of Inflammation in Cancer

In the past, investigators viewed infiltration of tumors by immune cells as a positive sign, indicative of an antitumor response. More recent work, however, has demonstrated that infiltration in general has no proven prognostic value. Virchow observed in 1863 that tumors are characterized by a leukocyte infiltrate and suggested that cancers arise at sites of chronic inflammation. Recent data have confirmed that inflammation associated with chronic infections is a cofactor in carcinogenesis. Mechanistically, the cells and factors involved in tumor growth are similar to those involved in wound healing.[6] Both processes are characterized by a complex network involving activation and migration of leukocytes to the site of damage and involvement of the ECM. However, in wound healing proliferation of cells and inflammation subside when the tissue is successfully regenerated, but tumor cells maintain their proliferative capacity and as such are "wounds that do not heal."

The tumor infiltrate may include macrophages, dendritic cells, neutrophils, eosinophils, mast cells, and lymphocytes (see Table 28-2).[6] Macrophages generally

TABLE 28-2.   Cells and Soluble Factors Affecting Tumor Development*

Cells	Soluble Factors
STROMA	
Parenchymal cells	Growth factors, growth inhibitors,
Endothelial cells	nutritional factors, hormones,
Fibroblasts	degradative enzymes, cytokines,
Mast cells	angiogenesis factors
Extracellular matrix	
Keratinocytes	
INFILTRATE	
T lymphocytes	Cytokines, chemokines, cytolytic
B lymphocytes	factors, angiogenesis factors, growth
NK cells	(inhibitory) factors, degradative
NKT cells	enzymes, cytostatic factors,
Macrophages/monocytes	antibodies
Dendritic cells	
Polymorphonuclear cells	
Platelets	
TUMOR	Chemokines, cytokines, angiogenesis
	factors, degradative enzymes, growth
	(inhibitory) factors

*The list of cells and soluble factors is not meant to be complete but to illustrate the complexity of factors affecting tumor development.

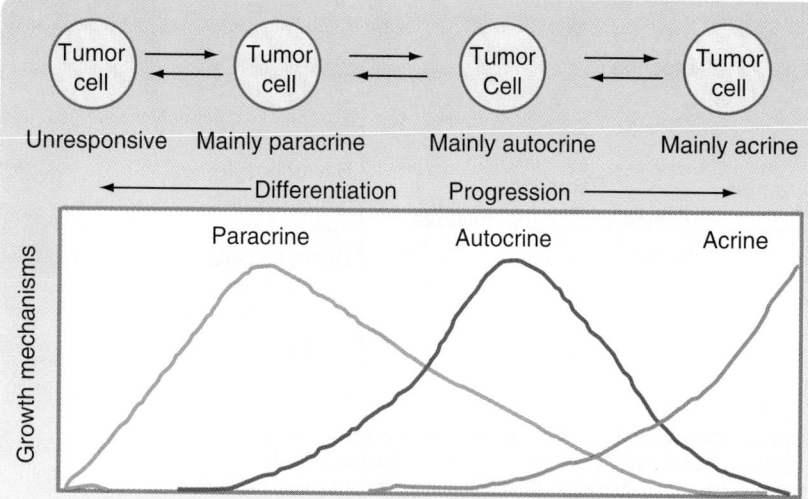

FIGURE 28-4.   Changes in contribution of growth mechanisms to tumor development. During tumor progression, the contribution of paracrine growth mechanisms decreases, and the tumor becomes more dependent on autocrine growth mechanisms. At later stages, the tumor may even become independent of growth mechanisms (acrine state).

comprise the majority of the leukocyte infiltrate, recruited by chemokines such as members of the macrophage inflammatory protein family secreted by tumor cells. The tumor-associated macrophages can produce proteolytic enzymes that degrade ECM, growth factors, and angiogenic factors such as vascular endothelial growth factor (VEGF) and prostaglandin E_2. Prostaglandin E_2 also stimulates tumor growth and blocks IL-12 production (IL-12 is an inducer of $CD4^+$ T helper 1 [T_H] cell differentiation, which supports a cellular immune response). Just as macrophages, dendritic cells are recruited to sites of inflammation such as tumors. Dendritic cells are essential for uptake and presentation of antigen, and stimulation of naive T lymphocytes. However, their ability to stimulate immune effector cells is often compromised in tumors and instead they may contribute to tumor development through stimulation of immune suppressor cells and suppressor cytokines.

Of the tumor-infiltrating lymphocytes (TILs), the vast majority are T lymphocytes expressing the antigen-specific T-cell receptor consisting of an alpha and beta chain. Tumor-derived T cells have received lots of attention because of their potential to recognize tumor antigen and destroy tumor cells ex vivo.[7] On the other hand, however, it has been demonstrated that signaling via the T-cell receptor is partially defective in freshly isolated tumor-derived T cells. It was also demonstrated in vitro that under starvation conditions TILs secrete basic fibroblast growth factor and heparin-binding epidermal growth factor (EGF), two factors that promote angiogenesis.[8]

Sustained production by tumor cells of certain cytokines, angiogenesis factors, and chemokines (e.g., IL-8, TGF-β, colony-stimulating factor [CSF], and macrophage chemotactic proteins) causes macrophages and other host cells to be continuously attracted and activated to further benefit growth and survival of tumor cells. The examples listed here and in Table 28-2 focus on only a few factors secreted by only a few cell types that have infiltrated tumors, to illustrate the complexity of the system.

Tumor Progression

The formation of tumor metastases is characterized by detachment of some tumor cells from the primary tumor and infiltration into the bloodstream or lymphatics (intravasation). The reciprocal process occurs at other locations in the body (extravasation). Both intravasation and extravasation are characterized by changes in ECMs and their interactions with tumor cells (reviewed in Reference 9). Like tumor promotion, tumor progression may also be dependent on infiltration. The difference between the growth of tumor at an earlier stage and that at later stages may be that at later stages, more tumor cells have acquired a stimulatory paracrine loop of growth factors as a result of the continuous transformations in tumor cells and the selection for survival. Overexpression of the EGF receptor in breast, lung, and bladder cancers and melanomas, for example, is often associated with poor survival and enhanced metastasis. Within the tumor, certain tumor cells may secrete chemokines that attract

inflammatory cells. These inflammatory cells may in turn secrete growth factors, promoting angiogenesis, or cytokines that directly promote tumor growth. As mentioned previously, at later stages of tumor development, tumor cells may start secreting these factors themselves.

Intravasation and Extravasation

In addition to adhesion to ECM, detachment from ECM is required for migration of cells. Detachment, like attachment, is an active process that requires signal transduction. Examples of ECM molecules that mediate detachment are hyaluran, which binds to hyaluran-binding cellular receptors such as CD44, and tenascin, which neutralizes adhesion to fibronectin; and certain proteoglycans. Tumor cells have acquired the ability to modify ECM-cell interactions to permit detachment from the primary tumor, intravasation into the circulation, attachment to endothelial cells throughout the body, and extravasation through the endothelial basement membrane. In addition to the attachment-mediating and detachment-mediating ECM molecules, tumor cells modulate ECM-bound proteases that regulate ECM turnover.

It is clear from the variety of processes that tumor progression may involve an increased expression of proteases, decreased expression of protease inhibitors, and enhanced expression of certain ECM-receptor interactions, whereas other matrix-receptor interactions are decreased. The latter may promote detachment of tumor cells. For example, in colorectal cancer, deficiencies in expression of collagen at the edges of the tumor may facilitate the invasiveness of this type of tumor. Expression of the protease tenascin is increased 10-fold in invasive breast carcinoma compared with normal breast tissue, and matrix metalloproteases are overexpressed in melanoma, invasive breast carcinoma, and invasive squamous cell carcinoma. In addition, aberrant expression of cellular receptors may contribute to extravasation and homing in tissues that highly express the ligand for the aberrant receptor. Because most receptors for ECM molecules are integrins, alterations in integrin expression are most frequent. Expression of $\alpha_4\beta_6$ integrin is reduced in breast carcinoma, whereas expression of $\alpha_4\beta_1$, which binds fibronectin, correlates with progression of melanoma. There is evidence that activation and overexpression of oncogenes, such as N-*myc*, results in downregulation of integrins such as $\alpha_2\beta_1$, which binds collagen and laminin, and $\alpha_3\beta_1$, which binds fibronectin in neuroblastomas. However, there is no clear pattern for the effects of alterations in ECM molecule and receptor expression. Nonetheless, all alterations eventually result in tumor progression. In this context, it is important to realize that most cancers are clonal in origin.

Both during tumor promotion and tumor progression, additional genetic mutations occur in tumor cells. These result in the formation of subpopulations of tumor cells that may or may not grow out, dependent on natural selection processes, and cause heterogeneity within a tumor. The clonal and genetic diversity of tumors permits adhesion and detachment from the same matrix. Some tumor cells within a primary tumor may have the correct genotype and phenotype to permit detachment from the surrounding tissue and intravasate blood vessels or lymphatic vessels. Likewise, extravasation may be mediated by a few tumor cells that express the required receptors for certain ECM molecules. In general, those mutations that confer escape from homeostatic control mechanisms in the host or that give the tumor cell a growth advantage over others are favorably selected. Thus, tumor clones that best complement the environment with expression of particular ECM receptors may thrive because this provides an advantage over other clones. The continuous evolution of a tumor has far-reaching consequences for antitumor therapies (discussed later).

Outgrowth at Preferred Sites

Invasion and metastatic spread of tumor cells do not appear to be random processes. Paget observed in 1889 that breast carcinoma often metastasized to the liver, lungs, bone, adrenals, or brain. He hypothesized that tumor cells (the "seed") would grow only in selective environments (the "soil"), where conditions supported tumor growth, hence the so-called seed-and-soil hypothesis. Since then, additional studies have confirmed this hypothesis. For example, malignant melanoma metastasizes to the brain, but ocular malignant melanoma frequently metastasizes to the liver. Prostate cancer metastasizes to the bone and colon carcinoma to the liver.

Molecular analysis has provided three major theories to explain preferential outgrowth of tumor cells. The first theory, the growth factor theory, proposes that tumor cells in the blood or lymphatics invade organs at pretty much the same frequency, but only those that find favorable growth factors multiply. Transferrins, for example, are iron-transferring ferroproteins required for cell growth that have additional mitogenic properties beyond their iron-transporting function. Increased concentrations of transferrin are found in lung, bone, and the brain and are associated with elevated levels of transferrin receptors on metastasizing tumor cells. The second theory, the adhesion theory, proposes that endothelial cells lining the blood vessels in certain organs express adhesion molecules that bind tumor cells and permit intravasation. The third theory is that chemokines secreted by the target organ can enter the circulation and selectively attract tumor cells that express receptors for the chemokines. Evidence for the importance of chemokines in tumor progression was recently obtained for breast cancer cells preferentially metastasizing in bone marrow, liver, lymph nodes, and lung. These organs were found to secrete CXCL12, which is the ligand for the chemokine receptor, CXCR4, enriched on breast cancer cells compared to normal breast epithelial cells. A similar phenomenon was observed for melanoma cells that were found to express elevated levels of the receptors CXCR4, CCR7, and CCR10 compared to normal melanocytes. Lymph nodes, lung, liver, bone marrow, and skin express the highest levels of the ligands for these receptors and are the preferred sites for metastatic spread of melanomas. Since chemokines are now known to affect angiogenesis and expression of cytokines, adhesion molecules, and proteases in addition to inducing migration, it appears that chemokines and their receptors play an essential role in the successful outgrowth of tumors at preferential sites.

Immune Surveillance

If tumors grow uncontrolled, what causes tumor cell death? In addition to physical constraints and lack of nutrients, the immune system is capable of eradication of tumor cells. In the early 1900s, it was proposed that the frequency of cancerous transformations would be very high if it were not for the defense system of the host. This concept was later substantiated in the 1950s and 1960s and the term *immunosurveillance* was introduced by Burnet in 1970.[10] Burnet hypothesized that the development of T-lymphocyte–mediated immunity during evolution was specific for elimination of transformed cells. He further proposed that there is a continuous surveillance of the body for transformed cells, hence the term *immunosurveillance*. During the subsequent years, experiments in immunosuppressed and immunodeficient mice demonstrated that T-cell–mediated immunity provides protection against virally induced tumors. However, no conclusive evidence was obtained for immune surveillance of cancer.

More recent discoveries have made it clear that the earlier studies were limited by incomplete knowledge of the models. When tested more accurately in more appropriate mouse models, evidence for immune surveillance of cancer was obtained: immunodeficient mice were significantly more susceptible to formation of chemically induced tumors and spontaneous tumors than immunocompetent mice.[11] This suggests that the unmanipulated immune system is capable of recognizing and eliminating primary tumors. Does immune surveillance of cancer exist in humans? Evaluation of long-term studies in transplant patients who were immunosuppressed and patients with immunodeficiencies showed an increased incidence of virally induced tumors such as non-Hodgkin's lymphoma, Kaposi's sarcoma, and carcinoma of the genitourinary and anogenital regions. However, they also showed a higher incidence of tumors with no apparent viral etiology such as malignant melanoma, lung cancer, pancreatic cancer, colon cancer, and kidney cancer. In addition, it was found that the presence of lymphocytes in such tumors is positively correlated to increased patient survival, especially in malignant melanoma. This finding should not be confused with the earlier mentioned correlation between inflammation and origin of cancer that applies mostly to tumors caused by chronic infections. The data from mouse and human studies combined suggest that immune surveillance of cancer does exist, mediated through immune cells and soluble factors. It also suggests that continuous pressure of the immune system in an immunocompetent host determines to a great degree if and how tumors evolve, a process called *immunoediting*.[12]

Immune Effector Cells

The immune system can be divided into two arms: natural or innate immunity and acquired or adaptive immunity.

TABLE 28-3. Immune Effector Cells

Effector Cell	Primary Effector Function
INNATE	
Macrophage/monocyte/ dendritic cell	Phagocytosis, processing and presentation of tumor antigens to T cells
NK cell	Direct tumor cell lysis, ADCC
Neutrophil	Direct tumor cell lysis, ADCC
NKT cell	Direct tumor cell lysis
ACQUIRED	
CD8 T lymphocyte	Direct tumor cell lysis
CD4 T lymphocyte	Regulate function of other immune cells, e.g., CD8 T cells (T_H1) and B cells (T_H2)
B lymphocyte	Secretion of tumor-specific antibodies

ADCC, antibody-dependent cell-mediated cytotoxicity.

The innate immune system often works "hand in hand" with the acquired immune system. Of the two arms of the immune system, acquired immunity (mediated through B and T lymphocytes) may be the most potent against tumors. A number of immune effector cells have the ability to eradicate tumor cells directly or indirectly (Table 28-3).

Innate Immune Cells

Innate immune cells, such as macrophages, dendritic cells, natural killer (NK) cells, NKT cells, and polymorphonuclear cells, characteristically do not need sensitization to respond to an immunogen. Macrophages and neutrophils are generally not cytotoxic to tumor cells unless activated by bacterial products. Activated macrophages and dendritic cells may exert direct antitumor activity through members of the tumor necrosis factor (TNF) family such as TNF, Fas ligand, and TNF-related apoptosis inducible ligand (TRAIL), or through oxyradicals such as nitric oxide. More important is perhaps the ability of macrophages and neutrophils to phagocytose and destroy antibody-coated tumor cells. In addition, macrophages and, more so, dendritic cells can process and present tumor antigens to T cells, thereby bridging innate and adaptive immunity. In this process, cytokines (primarily IL-12) and chemokines secreted by macrophages and dendritic cells are essential, too.

NK cells are a distinct population of lymphocytes that can efficiently lyse tumor cells. Inhibitory and stimulatory receptors regulate the activation of NK cells. Inhibitory receptors specifically bind certain major histocompatibility complex (MHC) class I molecules; downregulation or loss of expression of these MHC molecules removes the "brake" and makes tumor cells susceptible to NK-mediated lysis. Stimulatory receptors on NK cells recognize ligands encoded by genes that are selectively expressed or upregulated in tumor cells or virally infected cells. Some of these receptors such as NKG2D are also expressed in macrophages, and CD8 and γδ T cells (see "acquired immune cells"), and binding of a ligand induces secretion of interferon (IFN)-γ (NK cells) or TNF-α and nitric oxide (macrophages).

Finally, NKT cells resemble NK cells and T cells in phenotype and functional characteristics, hence their name. The population of NKT cells is heterogeneous and its exact function in vivo is unknown. NKT cells recognize antigen presented by MHC or MHC-like molecules through an antigen-specific T-cell receptor but at the same time express NK-cell receptors. Cross-linking of the T-cell receptor induces rapid secretion of large amounts of cytokines such as IL-4 and IFN-γ. Since IL-4 and IFN-γ generally induce opposing effects, controversy exists about the exact role of NKT cells in tumor surveillance.

Acquired Immunity

Acquired immunity is mediated by antigen-specific effector cells that recognize tumor antigens. Tumor-specific antigens have been discovered that are either unique or shared by other tumors and can be recognized by antibodies or T cells. The role of B cells and antibodies in antitumor responses is poorly understood. Antibodies specific for tumor antigens such as Her2/neu are often present in serum of patients but generally without correlation to clinical status. Possible mechanisms of tumor cell lysis through antibodies involve complex formation between antibody and tumor cells, followed by opsonization by macrophages (phagocytosis). The presence of complement may enhance this process. Alternatively, the Fc part of the antibody may be bound by Fc-receptor–positive immune cells, such as NK cells, macrophages, and neutrophils. This process is called *antibody-dependent cellular cytotoxicity*.

T cells, in contrast to antibodies, may directly lyse tumor cells. "Spontaneous" regression of solid tumors has sporadically been observed and may be mediated by tumor-specific T cells.[7,13] T-cell–mediated lysis is dependent on recognition of tumor antigens by the T-cell receptor on the T cell on which the lytic machinery of T cells is activated. The T-cell receptor is the antigen receptor expressed on every T cell. The T-cell receptor is encoded by genetically uniquely rearranged gene fragments, yielding a large repertoire of T-cell receptor molecules with a different antigen specificity.[14] The T-cell receptor molecule is designed to bind to molecules of the MHC. The

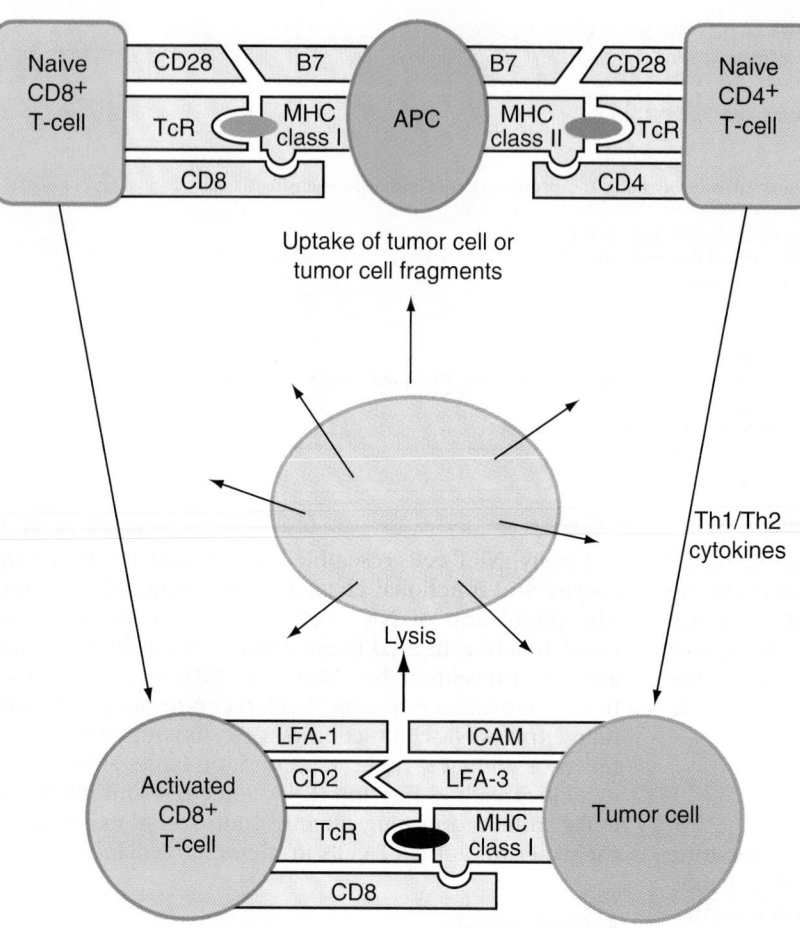

■ **FIGURE 28-5.** Schematic representation of the T-cell–mediated immune response to tumor cells. CD4+ T cells recognize tumor antigen presented by MHC class II molecules on antigen-presenting cells (APC). The activation of CD4+ T cells is dependent on costimulation through CD28. Activated CD4+ T cells secrete cytokines that regulate, among other things, activation of CD8+ T cells. Resting CD8+ T cells recognize MHC class I molecules on APC-presenting tumor antigen. When costimulated through CD28, CD8 T cells become activated and are capable of recognizing tumor cells. Lysed tumor cells are processed by antigen-presenting cell (APC).

T-cell receptor on CD8+ T cells binds to MHC class I molecules that are expressed on all nucleated cells, whereas the T-cell receptor on CD4+ T cells generally binds to MHC class II molecules, which are expressed predominantly on cells of the immune system (Fig. 28-5). The MHC molecules contain a groove in which protein fragments or peptides can be bound.[15] The peptides are derived from either endogenous (binding MHC class I) or exogenous proteins (binding primarily to MHC class II) after processing by proteolytic enzymes. After peptide binding, the MHC-peptide complex is transported to the cell surface for presentation to T cells. Because of the enormous diversity of different T-cell receptor molecules, it is predicted that for every possible MHC-antigen complex (including tumor antigens), one or more complementary T-cell receptor molecules exist.

T-cell activation is a two-signal process. In addition to the T-cell receptor binding to the MHC-peptide complex, a second or costimulatory signal is required (see Fig. 28-5). This signal is provided through interaction of certain ligands on the antigen-presenting cell and their receptors (costimulatory molecules) expressed on the T cell. A number of such interactions have been identified, including the T-cell molecules CD28 and CD11a/CD18 (leukocyte function–associated molecule-1 [LFA-1]), which bind to molecules of the CD80 (B7) family and CD54 (intercellular adhesion molecule-1 [ICAM-1]), respectively.[15]

Lack of costimulation induces unresponsiveness or even cell death. When properly activated, T cells undergo cell division (clonal expansion) and become functionally active. Expansion of T cells is also dependent on the availability of growth factors, such as IL-2. Most CD8+ T cells do not produce sufficient amounts of IL-2 to sustain proliferation and are dependent on CD4+ T cells for their IL-2, in particular the T_H1 subset of CD4+ T cells. Whereas CD8+ T cells recognize antigens presented by MHC class I molecules, CD4+ T cells are generally MHC class II restricted. Because most tumors of nonhematopoietic origin do not express MHC class II, CD4+ T cells are dependent on presentation of tumor antigen by professional antigen-presenting cells, such as dendritic cells and macrophages. B cells, on the other hand, are dependent on IL-4 that is produced by CD4+ T_H2 cells instead of T_H1 cells.

Escape From Immune Surveillance

With the availability of both innate and acquired immunity, one wonders why these systems have failed in cancer patients. Extensive research has demonstrated the existence of multiple escape mechanisms that permit tumor cells to escape from elimination by immune effector cells. Only those transformed cells that have a sufficiently dis-

TABLE 28-4. Tumor Escape Mechanisms	
Mechanism	**Characteristics**
TUMOR RELATED	
Tumor is not immunosensitive	No expression of tumor-specific antigens
	No or low expression of MHC molecules
	No antigen processing/presentation
	Resistance to immune cell-mediated killing
Tumor is not immunogenic	Lack of costimulatory molecules
	Secretion of immunosuppressive factors
	Shedding of tumor antigens
	Induction of T-cell tolerance
	Induction of T-cell apoptosis
HOST RELATED	Tumor grows too fast for the immune system
	Inherited or acquired immunodeficiency
	Treatment- or carcinogen-related immunosuppression
	Deficiency in antigen presentation by *APC*
	No access to tumor
	Expression of immunodominant antigens on parental tumor cells
	Age

tinct phenotype from normal cells are expected to induce an immune response. At the early stages of tumor development, the tumor cells may not (or may at insufficient levels) express tumor antigens that can be recognized by T cells and/or B cells, and at the same time escape from innate immune effector cells. After subsequent mutations, however, tumor cells may become more distinct from normal cells, but this may still not lead to eradication by immune effectors because of tumor-related issues, host-related issues, or both (summarized in Table 28-4).

Tumor-Related Immune Escape

The tumor cells may not, for example, be immunosensitive because they lack antigens that induce an immune response. With the exception of malignant melanoma, most tumors do not induce a strong T-cell response in vitro. Even though this could be related to many factors, circumstantial evidence suggests that lack of expression of dominant tumor antigens is an important factor. In addition, the expression of certain or all MHC alleles on the tumor cells may be lower or completely lacking, thereby escaping from MHC-restricted lysis by T cells. It is estimated that at least 40% of solid tumors show a loss of one or more MHC alleles. In a growing number of cases, loss of MHC expression has been positively correlated with tumor aggressiveness and metastatic potential.[16] Furthermore, the tumor cells may not be able to process or present tumor antigens, or antigens may be masked or modulated. The latter was shown in leukemia cells in which specific antibody binding led to modulation of the antigen from the cell surface. Finally, tumor cells may be resistant to tumoricidal activity by immune cells.

Different from immunosensitivity is immunogenicity. For example, tumor cells may express tumor antigens but still not induce an immune response because the tumor cells lack expression of costimulatory molecules. It has been shown that lack of expression of (CD54) ICAM-1 or (CD58) LFA-3 confers resistance to T-cell–mediated lysis.

Further, tumor cells may produce immunosuppressive factors such as TGF-β and IL-10 that directly or indirectly inhibit T-cell function. Additionally, tumor cells may secrete soluble factors that downregulate T-cell molecules involved in signal transduction, such as the zeta chain of the T-cell receptor/CD3 complex and the tyrosine phosphatases $p56^{lck}$ and $p59^{fyn}$. Signaling defects were first demonstrated in TILs isolated from renal cell carcinoma but were later demonstrated in many advanced cancers and even autoimmune diseases.[17] Soluble factors secreted by tumor cells may also redirect immune responses, activating immune cells that do not harm tumor cells. For example, secretion of IL-4 may shift the T_H1/T_H2 balance in favor of T_H2, whereas secretion of VEGF may block maturation and function of dendritic cells. Finally, the recently described regulatory CD4 T cells (T_{reg}) may be upregulated by factors and cells in the tumor environment. T_{reg} are a subset of CD4 T cells that inhibit autoreactive T cells and B cells to prevent autoimmune disease.[18] As antitumor effector cells are in some respects autoreactive since tumor antigens can be nonmutated self-antigens, T_{reg} inhibit antitumor effector cells. It was recently observed that the prevalence of T_{reg} in peripheral blood and the tumor environment of cancer patients was significantly increased compared to that in normal individuals.[19]

As another example of lack of immunogenicity, the antigen may be shed (e.g., carcinoma antigen [CA] 125 in ovarian cancer and carcinoembryonic antigen [CEA] in colon cancer), or it may induce T-cell tolerance. Tolerance induction may be related in some cases to the low avidity of the T cell–tumor cell interaction. Finally, the tumor cells may induce apoptosis in activated T cells. *Apoptosis*, or programmed cell death, is a special type of physiologic cell death and should not be mistaken with nonphysiologic accidental cell death or necrosis. In certain tumors, such as lung cancer, pancreatic cancer, melanoma, and others, tumor cells may express the apoptosis-inducing molecule, Fas ligand, on the cell surface that can bind to the Fas receptor (FasR) expressed on activated but not on resting T cells, and thereby induce apoptosis in T cells.[20]

Host-Related Immune Escape

Host-related factors that induce tumor escape include immunodeficiency (either inherited or acquired) that may increase the incidence of virally associated tumors; immunosuppression induced by radiation treatment, chemotherapeutic drugs, or chemical or physical carcinogens; tumor progression that may outpace tumor regression; deficient presentation of tumor antigens by antigen-presenting cells; lack of access of effector cells to the tumor (there is experimental evidence that the stroma can form a barrier); or expression of immunodominant antigens on parental tumor that prevents stimulation by other tumor antigens. The last mentioned is an intriguing phenomenon that was described in the 1980s but has so far not been explained. There appears to be a hierarchy in the immune response to various tumor antigens because the host fails to recognize all antigens simultaneously. The expression of an immunodominant antigen would prohibit the immune system from responding to antigen-negative tumor cells. A less clear failure of the host to mount an antitumor immune response is related to age. Over time, there may be a decrease in effectiveness of the immune response. The incidence of cancer may also rise over time, however, because certain carcinogens may have a long latency period or because exposure to certain carcinogens is accumulated over many years.

Antitumor Therapies

Therapies to treat cancer include conventional therapies such as surgery, chemotherapy, and radiation therapy, and a large variety of alternative treatments (Table 28-5) most of which are still experimental. Because surgery is extensively discussed in other chapters, it is not discussed further here. All therapies, apart from surgery, have in common that they directly or indirectly target the destruction of tumor cells. Mechanistically the various strategies differ widely. Some strategies attempt to interfere with intracellular signaling pathways to block cell division and/or induce apoptosis (e.g., chemotherapy and radiation), others target growth factors or cell surface receptors for growth factors, the tumor vasculature, or attempt to induce/enhance an antitumor immune response. Rather than discussing all possible therapies, we briefly discuss some of the main strategies in the following sections.

Chemotherapy

In chemotherapy, the goal is to kill rapidly dividing cells with drugs and leave other cells unharmed. Unfortunately, certain normal cells also divide rapidly; these cells include hair cells, bone marrow cells, and epithelial cells lining the digestive tract. Most anticancer drugs cause DNA damage or inhibit DNA replication and transcription (cytostatic drugs). In addition to the direct damage effects, however, certain genes may be triggered that are involved in apoptosis, leading to cell death.[21] Apoptosis plays a pivotal role in homeostasis of human cell proliferation. The general apoptosis signaling pathway involves the release of cytochrome c from mitochondria that activates various caspases (a family of at least 10 proteases) in sequence (Fig. 28-6). Activation of caspase cascades leads to DNA fragmentation and apoptosis. Induction of apoptosis by anticancer drugs is either death receptor dependent (extrinsic pathway) or independent (intrinsic pathway). The two best understood death receptor pathways include the Fas receptor and death receptor (DR)-5 that bind the extracellular Fas ligand and the TRAIL, respectively. Binding of the ligands triggers activation of caspase 8, which indirectly leads to release of cytochrome c from mitochondria and eventually apoptosis. Receptor-independent pathways involve translocation of proapoptotic molecules from the cytoplasm to the mitochondria, causing mitochondrial damage and release of cytochrome c. Cytochrome c is directly involved in the activation of

TABLE 28-5.	Antitumor Therapies
Treatments	**Characteristics**
CONVENTIONAL	
Surgery	Excision of malignancy
Chemotherapy	Drug-induced tumor cell lysis
Radiation	Radiation-induced tumor cell death
ALTERNATIVE	
Oncoviral	Tumor cell lysis through selectively replicating virus
Gene	Restore/add or inhibit expression of particular genes in tumor cells
Antiangiogenesis	Blockade of tumor vasculature
Immune	Tumor lysis through manipulation of the host's immune system
Stem cell	Graft-versus-malignancy response through stem cell transfer

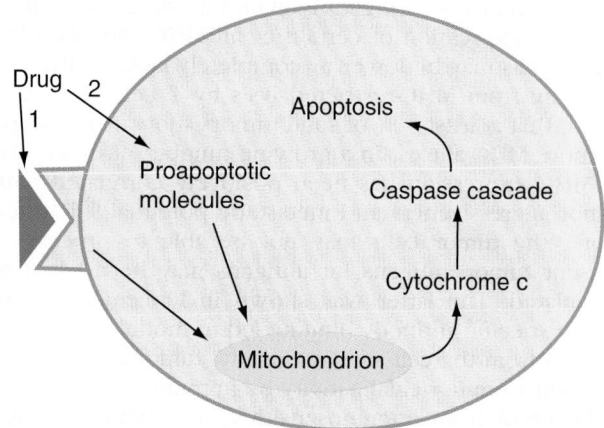

FIGURE 28-6. Apoptotic pathways. Chemotherapeutic drugs can induce apoptosis in tumor cells through a receptor-dependent (1) or receptor-independent (2) pathway. Both pathways induce release of cytochrome c from mitochondria, which triggers activation of various caspases in sequence, ultimately leading to apoptosis.

caspase 9, which activates caspase 3, which then leads to apoptosis.

Physiologic apoptosis appears to be regulated by multiple genes, but promotion of cell death by cytostatic drugs is usually regulated by a select number of genes. These genes include both tumor suppressor genes such as *p53* and oncogenes such as *myc, E2F, c-jun,* and *bcl-2* (B-cell leukemia/lymphoma gene-2).[22] The *p53* gene is rapidly upregulated after DNA damage and induces growth arrest by blocking cell cycle progression from G_1 to S phase to allow repair of the DNA. If the repair is unsuccessful (as may be the case after treatment with certain drugs), the cells undergo apoptosis.[4] However, the tumor suppressor gene, *p53*, is mutated in about 55% of tumor types, which may contribute to resistance to apoptosis-inducing drugs.[23]

Both *myc* and *c-jun* encode transcription factors that play a central role in regulating cell proliferation, differentiation, and apoptosis. The E2F gene family is a family of transcription factors that promote S-phase entry and thus with respect to cell growth appears to have the opposite function as *p53*. The role of transcription factors in apoptosis may differ depending on cell type and stimulus. In addition, more than 100 transcription factors have been identified and their biologic roles are not yet fully understood. Further enhancing the difficulty of understanding their role in apoptosis is the fact that several transcription factors activate downstream target genes, whereas others downregulate expression in response to DNA damage. The target genes play important roles in the overall outcome of the cell's fate.

The *bcl-2* gene is a member of a family of proteins that induce *(bax, bak, bcl-Xs)* or inhibit *(bcl-2, bcl-Xl, bag1)* apoptosis. High levels of *bcl-2* are found in tumor cells and may confer resistance to anticancer drugs. Initially, dysregulation of *bcl-2* was found in B-cell malignancies, but overexpression has also been noted in solid tumors, including prostate, lung, colon, and stomach cancers.

It has become apparent that cell-cycle progression is under tight genetic control. Growth factors or other stimuli activate oncogenes or inactivate tumor suppressor genes to allow progression through the cell cycle. Cells that receive conflicting, excessive, or unbalanced mitogenic signals undergo apoptosis. A similar deregulated cell cycle control and induction of apoptosis is observed after treatment with certain chemotherapeutic drugs.

Some anticancer drugs are effective as single agents (e.g., cisplatin for treatment of testicular cancer), but combination therapy with multiple drugs is common practice. The major advantage with combination chemotherapy is the increased chance to overcome drug resistance. Drug resistance may be inherent to the tumor cells or may arise after exposure to anticancer drugs. Certain types of cancers, such as pancreatic, renal, and non-small cell lung cancer, are known to be poor responders to chemotherapy. In contrast, cancers such as breast, ovarian, and small cell lung cancers and acute leukemias and lymphomas show a high initial response rate, but durable responses are rare because of the acquisition of drug-resistance mechanisms.

Cellular resistance mechanisms can be distinguished from extracellular mechanisms. Cellular mechanisms of drug resistance include decreased intracellular drug accumulation resulting from impaired transport through the membrane, or active efflux of drugs (multidrug resistance [MDR] phenotype) through the *MDR-1*[21] and multidrug resistance–associated protein (*MRP*) gene products or other drug transporters.[24] Alternatively, alterations may occur in intracellular drug metabolism, or the target of the drug may change, reducing the effectiveness of the drug. For example, drugs such as 5-fluorouracil and cyclophosphamide are dependent on conversion from an inactive to an active form by drug-activating enzymes. A common feature of drug-resistant cells is decreased activity or loss of drug-activating enzymes. Intracellular drugs can also be detoxified; for example, glutathione-S transferases are implicated in resistance to alkylators, and cytosolic retinoic acid–binding proteins may neutralize retinoic acid used for treatment of promyelocytic leukemia. A different mechanism is resistance resulting from changes in the target of the drug. Because of mutations in the target affecting the binding affinity of the drug, or overexpression of the drug target, enzymes involved in DNA synthesis or DNA multiplication are less sensitive to drugs. Other escape mechanisms include enhanced DNA repair capacity and disruption of the apoptotic pathway normally activated by drugs (e.g., overexpression of *bcl-2* or *MDM-2* [*p53* inhibitor] or mutation of either *p53* or the retinoblastoma gene).[23] Finally, insufficient penetration of the drug to and into the tumor may affect treatment outcome unfavorably.

Radiation Therapy

Radiation therapy is used alone or in conjunction with surgery, chemotherapy, or both. About half of cancer patients receive radiation therapy at some time during their treatment. Despite the successes in tumors such as seminomas, carcinomas of the skin, cervix, prostate, anus, and head and neck, it is not entirely clear why certain tumors are preferentially sensitive to radiation and why other tumors are resistant. Cell differentiation, proliferation, and maturation all are potentially affected by ionizing radiation. The effects of ionizing radiation are obvious at different levels of organization. At the cellular level, the most sensitive target for radiation is DNA, in which single-strand or double-strand breaks or cross-links are induced. Alternatively, sugars, nucleotides, or both are damaged. In addition to DNA damage, transcription of certain genes is induced. These genes can be distinguished into early-response genes, which mostly encode transcription factors, and late-response genes, which encode cytokines and growth factors. The physiologic significance of gene activation through radiation is not entirely clear yet.

Other than the nucleus, the cell membrane is radiosensitive, and damage involves lipid peroxidation by radiation-induced oxyradicals. Lipid peroxidation alters membrane fluidity and permeability and may affect ion fluxes and membrane-mediated transport processes. Ionizing radiation may also affect cell-cell interactions, which, for yet unknown reasons, occur more frequently in tumors than in normal tissues. To control radiation-induced damage, cells are equipped with DNA repair mechanisms and mechanisms to detoxify oxygen-containing radicals.

Radiation has recently been correlated with the induction of apoptosis (e.g., in thymocytes and the parotid gland, but also in tumors).[25] Recent work in the nematode *Caenorhabditis elegans,* however, suggests that the apoptotic pathway induced through radiation is different from that induced by physiologic triggers. Radiation may also induce delays in cell division through interference with the cell-cycle processes (see Fig 28-2). Most common is G_2-phase arrest, but G_1-phase arrest and S-phase delay have also been noted. Interference with the cell cycle is most likely related to the effect of radiation on tumor suppressor genes and oncogenes encoding cell-cycle regulatory proteins, such as *p53* and cdks.[25] For example, radiation induces the G_1 checkpoint through stabilization of the p53 protein and through induction of the cdk inhibitor p21. Chemotherapeutic drugs may increase the effectiveness of radiation.

More complicated is the evaluation of radiation damage in organs because of the presence of multiple cell types that may be differentially sensitive to radiation. The response of organs to radiation may in the early stages be characterized by a rapidly renewing stem cell population, early manifestation of damage, and complete healing; late stages are characterized by the lack of a separate stem cell population, late manifestation of damage, and irreversible damage. Intermediate stages are characterized by some early reactions and some late reactions. Tumors mostly resemble early-responding tissues, although the distorted physiology, vasculature, necrosis, and out-of-cycle cells make the situation more complex.

Alternative Treatments

The alternative treatment strategies can roughly be divided into five types ranging from entirely experimental such as oncoviral and genetic therapy to standard adjuvant therapy such as bone marrow or stem cell therapy (see Table 28-5). Oncoviral therapy involves injection of replicating virus into cancer patients. Replication of the virus is genetically engineered to be tumor selective, leading to destruction of tumor cells while sparing normal tissue. The most advanced in clinical testing is ONYX-015, an adenovirus that selectively replicates in cells deficient for the tumor suppressor gene *p53*.[26] In addition to selective targeting, the oncolytic virus may contain a therapeutic gene. Examples are the enzymes thymidine kinase and cytosine deaminase that convert the prodrugs ganciclovir and 5-fluorocytosine, respectively. Alternatively, oncolytic viruses encode immune-stimulatory genes such as cytokine genes. The use of therapeutic genes in oncolytic viruses combines oncoviral therapy and genetic therapy or immune therapy.

The transfer of copies of wild-type genes into tumor cells is referred to as *gene therapy* and aims to restore (e.g., tumor suppressor gene) or add (e.g., immune-stimulatory gene or chemoresistance gene) expression of genes. In contrast, the transfer of antisense oligonucleotides or small interfering RNA into tumor cells aims to inhibit expression of a particular gene such as that of an oncogene. Transfer of DNA or RNA into cells is a relatively simple procedure in vitro, and a variety of methods can be used with a high efficiency. Clinical application, however, requires the efficient transfer of potentially billions of tumor cells in a safe manner that is nondestructive to normal tissues. Thus, choice of vector (Table 28-6), transgene, and method of delivery all are crucial parameters. The use of viral vectors is common because of the ability of pathogenic viruses to transfer genes in an efficient way. Unlike in oncoviral therapy, the viral genes responsible for viral replication are removed, and the transgene is inserted.[27] Different applications may favor one vector over another.

Nonviral vectors are either cell based or non–cell based (see Table 28-6). Using cell lines, the genetic modification is relatively easy to perform in vitro, and successful modification can be monitored before the vector is used therapeutically. The non–cell-based nonviral vectors include liposomes and plasmid DNA. The artificial lipophilic vesicles fuse with the cell membrane, and the contents are released into the host cell. This application is often used to transfer antisense oligonucleotides. The other non–cell-based nonviral vector that is gaining interest is plasmid DNA, in particular for DNA vaccines. Direct injection of DNA into muscle cells, especially skeletal and cardiac muscle cells, has proved more effective than was predicted based on in vitro experiments. The immune response resulting from DNA vaccines appears to be mediated through dendritic cells that have taken up the DNA and express the transgene. Nonviral, non–cell-based vectors are sometimes preferred because of biosafety concerns: larger DNA sequences can be transferred and the vector has greater stability. In general, the problems with gene therapy are the poor targeting and the low efficiency of gene transfer in vivo.

Attempts to block the vasculature of tumors (anti-angiogenesis therapy) have shown encouraging results in mice but have thus far been less successful in cancer patients. The outgrowth of new blood vessels from pre-existing ones is essential for tumor growth and metastasis. Angiogenesis is mediated by both stimulatory (VEGF and basic fibroblast growth factor) and inhibitory factors (endostatin, angiostatin). Both naturally occurring angiogenesis inhibitors such as endostatin and angiostatin as well as synthetic agents or antibodies against angiogenesis factors are currently being tested in clinical trials.

The primary goal of immune therapy is to restore the imbalance between tumor growth and tumor destruction.

TABLE 28-6.	Vectors Used for Genetic Therapy
System	**Vector**
Viral	Retrovirus, adenovirus, adeno-associated virus, herpesvirus, pox virus
Nonviral	
Cell based	Tumor cells, fibroblasts, dendritic cells, T cells
Non-cell based	Liposomes, plasmid DNA

The secondary goal of immune therapy is to induce protective immunity.[7,28] Immune therapy is a relatively new treatment modality for cancer patients despite sporadic attempts made more than 100 years ago. Strategies may target innate as well as acquired immune components. Bacterial vaccines, such as bacille Calmette-Guérin (BCG) and *Corynebacterium parvum* stimulate innate immunity and are used as single agents (e.g., BCG is effective against residual bladder cancer) or in combination with specific stimulants. Likewise, cytokines, such as ILs, may boost innate immunity. Systemic administration of IL-2, for example, is used for the treatment of renal cell carcinoma and malignant melanoma. Durable cancer regressions have been induced by treatment with IL-2 alone. Systemic administration, however, usually requires a high dosage, which may explain the associated severe toxicity that sometimes occurs. Certain cytokines such as IFNs may also directly act on tumor cells and inhibit tumor growth.[11]

Strategies that target acquired immunity can be divided into active therapeutic immunization, passive therapy with antibodies, and adoptive transfer of immune effector cells (Table 28-7). Of these, most emphasis is placed on active therapeutic immunization.[29] The large variety of immunization approaches can roughly be grouped into three strategies. First, autologous or histologically matched allogeneic tumor cells genetically modified ex vivo to express a cytokine, a costimulatory molecule, or other immune-stimulatory molecule. Alternatively, autologous dendritic cells modified to express tumor antigen(s) are used. Tumor antigens can be introduced into dendritic cells through coculture or through transduction or transfection. Dendritic cells can also be fused with tumor cells in vitro. Finally, tumor antigen(s) in the form of DNA, peptide, or protein can directly be injected into patients with either an adjuvant or by using viral or nonviral vectors (see Table 28-6).

For hematopoietic tumors, immunization can be achieved with anti-idiotypic antibodies, which have the internal image of a tumor antigen. The B-cell receptor, just like the T-cell receptor, consists of a heavy chain and a light chain covalently linked through disulfide bonds. Both the heavy chain and the light chain are genetically encoded by a unique combination of DNA segments (variable, diverse [heavy chain only], and joining regions). The genetic rearrangement provides a unique antigen-binding site determined by the sets of variable domains. This creates unique regions or epitopes within the variable domains that are called *idiotopes*. The set of idiotopes expressed by a given immunoglobulin molecule is called an *idiotype*. Because of their uniqueness, antibodies can be generated against idiotypes; these are termed *anti-idiotype antibodies*. Thus, antibodies against tumor-specific antibodies can be used as immunogens to induce an antitumor immune response.

Passive antibody therapy focuses on molecules that are either uniquely expressed on tumor cells or overexpressed on tumor cells relative to normal cells. Examples include gangliosides and mucins. By using IgM antibody, complement-mediated cytotoxicity is induced, as well as inflammation and phagocytosis of tumor cells by the reticuloendothelial system. On the other hand, IgG antibodies may trigger antibody-mediated cytotoxicity. A variation of this theme is the use of bispecific antibodies. These antibodies are engineered to have specific binding sites for two different antigens. Consequently, bispecific antibodies can simultaneously bind to immune effector cells and tumor cells and thereby bridge effector cells and tumor cells. By cross-linking receptors such as CD3 or T-cell receptors, the effector mechanism of the immune cells is activated and the tumor cell is lysed. Antibody therapy may be successful against free tumor cells and micrometastases.

Although not strictly used to target acquired immunity, there are a number of antibody-based therapies worth mentioning. They involve the use of antibodies directed against growth factor receptors or angiogenesis factors expressed on tumor cells or in the tumor environment. It was recently reported at the 36th Annual Meeting of the American Society of Clinical Oncology that anti-VEGF antibody effectively blocked angiogenesis in metastatic colon cancer patients and significantly prolonged survival. Likewise, the IL-2 receptor on T-cell tumors is targeted by anti-IL-2 receptor antibodies. Recently, it was observed that certain antibodies may activate apoptosis in tumor cells through a yet undetermined mechanism, such as the anti-Her2/neu antibody for treatment of breast cancer. Finally, tumor-specific antibodies are used as vehicles for delivery of toxins or radionuclides to tumors.

Adoptive transfer of immune effector cells was made popular in the early 1980s.[28] Initially, a high concentration (1000 IU/mL) of IL-2 was used to generate lymphokine-

TABLE 28-7. Strategies of Immunotherapy	
Strategy	**Characteristics**
Active therapeutic immunization	Attempts to boost a host immune response through: 1. Gene-modified tumor cells 2. Dendritic cells expressing tumor antigen 3. Direct injection of tumor antigen Attempts to decrease tumorigenicity
Passive antibody therapy	Attempts to induce tumor cell cytolysis or cytostasis
Adoptive transfer of immune effector cells	Attempts to increase the number of specific antitumor effector cells in the host

activated killer (LAK) cells in vitro from peripheral blood mononuclear cells (PBMCs) obtained by leukapheresis. LAK cells and IL-2 were administered to patients. PBMCs were replaced by tumor-derived lymphocytes when it was found that these cells activated with IL-2 were more effective than IL-2–activated PBMCs in animal models. Both strategies, however, showed a fairly similar efficacy in patients with metastatic disease, primarily in patients with metastatic melanoma. Response rates, including complete and partial remissions, ranged from 25% to 35%.[30]

These studies illustrate some of the complexities related to immune therapy of cancer. For example, thus far, there are no good in vitro parameters that predict in vivo efficacy of the transferred cells. The number of adoptively transferred cells and the tumor load do not appear to correlate with clinical responses. Likewise, tumor-specific cytolytic activity or tumor-specific cytokine release in vitro does not guarantee a clinical response. The adoptively transferred T cells of clinical responders, however, usually do show a tumor-specific response in vitro. This points to the importance of inducing or selecting for tumor-specific effector cells and raises the question of which strategy should be used. Another question is which immune effector cells should be activated. Increased understanding of how NK and NKT cells recognize their target cells may change the focus from T cells to NK and NKT cells. Because loss of MHC expression is a common phenomenon in many solid tumors, NK cells could be an important component in immune therapy.

For many years, controversy has existed about how adoptively transferred T cells induce tumor eradication. The most common thought has been that the transferred tumor-specific T cells find their way back to the tumor and eradicate it. In a mouse sarcoma tumor model, however, evidence was obtained that suggests a different scenario.[31] A proportion of the adoptively transferred T cells indeed traffic back to the tumor, but they induce a successful *host* antitumor response. The induction is mediated through secretion of inflammatory cytokines, such as IFN-γ and granulocyte-macrophage CSF, that are secreted in response to reactivation of tumor-specific *donor* T cells by tumor cells.

Strategies aimed at promoting immune responses can potentially be combined with strategies aimed at blocking immune suppression. The documented benefit of cyclophosphamide to eliminate suppressor cells prior to therapy dates back many years, and cyclophosphamide is still presently used. Recently, $CD4^+CD25^+$ regulatory T cells (T_{reg}) were identified as suppressor cells of autoreactive CD4 and CD8 T cells, which includes tumor-reactive T cells.[18] T_{reg} can be depleted in the host through anti-CD25 antibody, and in animal tumor models this has led to significant tumor regression.

Finally, stem cell therapy is a standard treatment for hematologic malignancies. Prior to stem cell transfer, high doses of cytotoxic agents with or without total-body irradiation is used to eradicate malignant disease and reduce graft-versus-host disease in case of an allogeneic stem cell transfer. The goal is to induce a graft-versus-malignancy response mediated by donor T cells. This response is more pronounced after allogeneic stem cell transfer than autologous stem cell transfer and is likely mediated by donor CD4 and CD8 T cells that recognize tumor-specific proteins, overexpressed normal proteins in malignant cells, and minor histocompatibility antigens.

Conclusion

Even though scientists have learned a great deal about tumor biology since the early 1990s, a detailed understanding of how tumors arise, develop, and progress into highly metastatic tumors is still lacking. We are still at the stage at which finding the answer to one question raises several new questions. Nonetheless, our increased knowledge will most certainly lead to the design of better and more refined treatment modalities. Additionally, as more is learned about the biology of tumors, more tumor markers will become available that can be successfully applied to the diagnosis and treatment of cancer.

TUMOR MARKERS

What Is a Tumor Marker?

Tumor markers are molecules that can be detected in blood, body fluids, or tissue of a host with underlying cancer. It is not unusual for tumor cells to secrete or shed molecules or parts of a molecule. Occasionally, these molecules can be useful tumor markers, as evidenced by the monitoring of prostate-specific antigen (PSA) or prostate serum acid phosphatase (PSAP) levels in serum.[32] Elevated levels of PSA or PSAP are indicative of prostate cancer. PSA is a proteolytic enzyme that is secreted by the prostate into the glandular lumina, where it is contained and excreted with prostatic fluid. Cancer in the prostate can cause PSA to leak out of the gland into the blood. Note that other disease forms in the prostate, such as benign hyperplasia of the prostate and prostatitis, may also induce leakage of PSA. PSAP is another proteolytic enzyme that may leak into the blood, but it is associated with a more advanced disease stage. Likewise, elevated levels of CA 125 and mucin (MUC)-1 are associated with disease progression of ovarian and breast carcinoma, respectively.[33]

Classically, tumor markers are macromolecules such as proteins, carbohydrates, and DNA released by the tumor and detected in blood. For example, CEA is a modified protein secreted by multiple tumor types such as colorectal, pancreatic, breast, and lung cancers.[34] However, tumor markers may also be molecules released by the normal host tissue in response to the invasion of cancer. The first tumor marker described "acid phosphatase" was such a normal host enzyme secreted by bone in response to invading prostate carcinoma.

The ideal tumor marker should have several characteristics to be useful clinically. First, a simple test should detect a tumor marker long before the malignancy spreads widely. In many occasions, tumors are diagnosed by microscopic examination after obtaining a biopsy specimen of the tumor. However, by the time a tumor becomes clinically apparent enough to prompt a biopsy examination, the tumor has already spread widely. This can be avoided by using a tumor marker that can be detected long before a biopsy is possible, allowing the clinician to alter the natural history of the tumor in the host. Second, testing for a tumor marker should be sensitive; that is, the test for the tumor marker should be positive in all patients with a particular cancer (no false-negative results). Third, the test for the tumor marker should be specific, meaning that the test should be positive for the marker only when the patient has that particular cancer (no false-positive results). Fourth, the level of the tumor marker detected in the biologic sample should correlate with the size of the tumor. Fifth, the test for the tumor marker should be cheap enough to allow use of the marker in screening of large numbers of individuals.

The *sensitivity* of a tumor marker is determined by three interrelated factors: (1) the ability of the assay to reliably detect the tumor marker in a given biological sample; (2) the critical tumor mass that should be present before the marker can be detected; and (3) the percentage of tumors that expresses the particular tumor marker being tested. Development of highly sensitive immunoassays has decreased the threshold concentration of detection as well as the size of the tumor needed to achieve that concentration. However, discovering tumor markers that are uniformly expressed by all tumors with the same classification has been more of a problem.

The *specificity* of a tumor marker is also dependent on three factors: (1) the fidelity with which the assay detects only the tumor marker; (2) presence of other tumors that test positive for the same marker; and (3) other nonmalignant conditions in which the tumor marker is elevated.

The ideal tumor marker with all the desired characteristics has not been found yet. Despite advances in molecular biologic techniques and discovery of many new markers, all known tumor markers have characteristics that limit their clinical utility. Clinical applications of tumor markers in screening, diagnosis, prognosis, evaluation of success of therapy, and monitoring for recurrence are limited by problems in sensitivity and specificity. However, a marker that is not ideal for one application may be useful in another application. For example, a marker such as CEA may not be ideal for screening for colorectal cancer in large populations of people, but it may be useful in detecting recurrence in a patient who has undergone resection of the primary tumor. Examples of tumor markers with their clinical utility and potential limitations are listed in Table 28-8.

Molecular Basis of Tumor Markers

Tumor markers are a result of genetic alterations that occur in tumor cells that directly or indirectly affect the gene expression pattern of the tumor cells or the surrounding tissue. Molecular changes that occur in a cell that leads to the expression of a tumor marker can stem from incorporation of viral genes into the tumor cell, chromosomal translocations in the tumor cell, changes in the DNA methylation pattern, or any other genetic change such as point mutations and deletions.

Two categories of abnormalities can be distinguished based on their importance in oncogenesis: primary abnormalities that are essential at the tumor initiation stage, and secondary abnormalities that occur later and are thought to play a role during tumor progression. The primary abnormalities, such as the Philadelphia chromosome,[35] are specific for a particular tumor, whereas the secondary abnormalities are less specific. Primary abnormalities are mostly detected in leukemias, non-Hodgkin's lymphoma, and mesenchymal solid tumors and are of diagnostic value. In general, the genetic changes are reciprocal translocations leading to disruption of genes controlling growth, differentiation, and apoptosis. In epithelial solid tumors, the high incidence of chromosomal rearrangements with gross aneuploidy complicates karyotyping. In addition, these tumors are usually studied at later stages of development, at which time the tumor cells have undergone many additional genetic changes. Nonetheless, several primary abnormalities have been proposed in lung carcinoma, nonpapillary renal cell carcinoma, transitional cell carcinomas of the bladder, and adenocarcinoma of the prostate. Most chromosomal aberrations in these tumors involve deletions, unbalanced translocations, and loss of entire chromosomes. This may suggest that loss or inactivation of tumor suppressor genes plays an important role in these tumors.

Viral Genes

Tumors induced by viruses such as the Epstein-Barr virus (EBV) implicated in Burkitt's lymphoma, human papillomavirus (HPV) linked to cervical cancer, hepatitis B virus (HBV) associated with hepatocellular carcinoma, and human T-lymphotropic virus type 1 (HTLV-1) associated with T-cell leukemia may express viral gene products that are easily detectable because they are not expressed in normal cells. The viral DNA may be inserted into the host genome or exist in the cytoplasm, but in both cases, the cellular mechanisms of the host are manipulated to serve the virus. Papillomavirus DNA, for example, encodes genes of which the product inactivates the *p53* and the *Rb* genes. In addition, viral genes are transcribed that are involved in viral replication.

Chromosomal Translocations

Chromosomal translocations occur frequently and often nonrandomly. Because of the breakpoint and annealing at a different location, hybrid proteins may be expressed that could be used as markers.[36] Good examples of hybrid proteins with diagnostic value are the Philadelphia chromosome in chronic myeloid leukemia (CML) (90% of cases) and the EGF receptor in glioblastomas. The Philadelphia chromosome is a shortened version of chromosome 22 that resulted from the reciprocal translocation of part of chromosomes 9 and 22, resulting in a longer chromosome 9 and shorter chromosome 22.[35] The EGF receptor, which is expressed in about 40% of gliomas, has an internal deletion resulting in a characteristic fusion protein that con-

TABLE 28-8.   Tumor Markers in Clinical Application

Tumor Marker	Type of Molecule	Tumor Type	Type of Application	Nonmalignant Conditions with Elevated Levels
CEA	Glycoprotein	Stomach, liver, pancreas, breast, and colorectal cancer	Prognosis and monitoring therapeutic response	Hepatitis, cirrhosis, jaundice, COPD, inflammatory bowel disease, smoking
CA 19-9	Mucin-type glycoprotein	Pancreas cancer	Diagnosis, prognosis, and monitoring therapeutic response	Hepatitis, cirrhosis, sclerosing cholangitis, and extrahepatic biliary stasis
AFP	Oncofetal glycoprotein	Liver and testicular cancer	Diagnosis, prognosis, and monitoring therapeutic response	Hepatitis, cirrhosis, pregnancy, inflammatory bowel disease
PSA	Oncofetal glycoprotein	Prostate cancer	Screening, diagnosis, prognosis, and monitoring therapeutic response	BPH, prostatic massage or biopsy
β-HCG	Trophoblastic protein	Choriocarcinoma, hydatidiform mole, and invasive mole	Diagnosis, prognosis, and monitoring therapeutic response	Pregnancy
CA 125	Ovarian cell surface protein	Ovarian cancer	Prognosis and monitoring therapeutic response	Pregnancy, endometriosis, menstruation, jaundice, and pancreatitis
CA 15-3	Membranes of breast cancer cells	Breast cancer	Prognosis	Cirrhosis, hepatitis, and benign breast disease
Prostatic acid phosphatase	Prostate cellular protein	Prostate cancer	Prognosis and monitoring therapeutic response	BPH, dermatologic disorders
5-Hydroxyindoleacetic acid	Peptide metabolite of indoleacetic acid	Carcinoid	Diagnosis	—
Calcitonin	Hormone	Medullary thyroid cancer	Diagnosis, prognosis, and monitoring therapeutic response	—
Metanephrine	Catecholamine metabolite	Pheochromocytoma	Diagnosis, prognosis, and monitoring therapeutic response	—

CEA, carcinoembryonic antigen; CA, carcinoma antigen; AFP, α-fetoprotein; PSA, prostate-specific antigen; β-HCG, beta-human chorionic gonadotropin; COPD, chronic obstructive pulmonary disease; BPH, benign prostatic hypertrophy.

tains one or more new amino acids at the fusion point.[37] The fusion protein still has the ability to bind EGF and may in fact be more stable than the wild-type EGF receptor, resulting in overexpression. The overexpression may give glioma cells an advantage over normal cells when the amount of available EGF is limiting.

DNA Methylation

Altered DNA methylation patterns are also common in cancer cells and may be responsible for expression of some types of tumor antigens such as oncofetal antigens. Methylation of DNA at restricted cytosine phosphate guanine (CpG) sequences is a mechanism of regulating expression of certain genes. Genes that are expressed in fetal development are later silenced in adult life by methylating areas known as CpG islands near the promoter regions.[38] Methylation of CpG sequences in promoter regions blocks directly or indirectly the binding of transcription factors and thereby blocks transcription. When the distribution of methylation sites was evaluated in tumors, it was found that areas of hypomethylation exist as well as areas of hypermethylation. Hypomethylation may increase gene expression and may also decrease chromosome stability and lead to allelic loss. Hypermethylation, on the other hand, could suppress gene transcription.

With the isolation and characterization of oncogenes and tumor suppressor genes, another feature of DNA methylation became apparent. Point mutations in those genes are frequently associated with CpG sites. The methylation of cytosine is thought to increase the chance for a C-to-T or C-to-A transition by 12-fold to 30-fold. Thus, 5-methylcytosine is considered an endogenous mutagen that contributes to about 30% of all point mutations despite the fact that 5-methylcytosine constitutes only 1% of human DNA. For example, when all human tumors are considered together, one third of all inactivating point mutations in the tumor suppressor gene *p53* occur at methylation sites. Note that the point mutations related to methylation are not restricted to *p53* only but rather occur in many genes.

Point Mutations and Deletions

Gene mutations have been identified in various human cancers, and the list of mutated genes includes tumor suppressor genes (*BRCA-1*, *BRCA-2*, *APC*, *p53*, *nm23*), oncogenes (*ret*, β-catenin, *ras*, *bcl*), and genes involved in cell growth (*cdk4*).

Other genetic changes affect the transcription level of genes: transcription of previously silent genes may be induced; the transcription level may be enhanced over the normal level, leading to overexpression of the gene product; or transcription may be reduced or entirely blocked. Mutations occur at various locations in genes, but often "hot spots" are present. These hot spots are gene restricted and not specific for the type of tumor. Nonetheless, certain of these mutations have diagnostic value, such as mutated *ras*, *p53*, and others, because they confirm the malignant state of a cell.

Detection Methods of Tumor Markers

Immunologic Detection

Immunologic techniques have long been used to identify existing specific tumor markers and to discover new markers. The discovery of monoclonal antibodies and the generation of antibody-producing hybridomas[39] have greatly expanded the repertoire of clinicians and pathologists in the detection of malignant cells. More recently, the immunologic discoveries of tumor-specific T cells further expanded the available techniques to identify new tumor markers. Tumor-specific T cells are currently not used for detection purposes since the generation and maintenance is too labor intensive. However, the use of tumor-specific T cells, in particular cytotoxic T lymphocytes, in vitro has clearly helped to identify tumor antigens in a variety of tumors and has formed the rationale for immune-based therapies (see Tumor Biology section).

In general, monoclonal antibodies that bind specifically to epitopes on tumor markers are used for detection of tumor cells in biopsy specimens, blood cells, or other body fluids. The first and still most commonly used method for the initial diagnosis of cancer is through microscopic evaluation of tissue sections or cytologic preparations. Routinely, tissue is fixed in formalin to preserve morphologic structures and is embedded in paraffin or plastic. The fixation process, however, may negatively affect the three-dimensional structure of antigens recognized by antibodies. An alternative method involves the snap-freezing of tissue, which does not include a fixation step and does not denature antigens. The downside of this method, however, is that the morphology is poorly preserved. To use antibodies in paraffin sections, second-generation antibodies are developed that are selected to recognize antigens that are not destroyed by the fixation process.

Antibodies that recognize interesting epitopes in cryostat sections are used to identify the gene encoding the antigen. Subsequently, animals are immunized with the recombinant protein or protein fragments, and hybridomas are generated. The hybridomas are tested for secretion of antibodies that are reactive with the antigen of interest in paraffin sections. Second-generation antibodies have been made, for example, against the cell cycle–dependent nuclear proliferation marker, Ki67, expressed in many cancers.

Instead of immunohistology, flow cytometric analysis of antibody-stained cells is usually performed on hematopoietic tumors, mainly to facilitate classification. This method permits evaluation of the percentage of positive cells in a population of cells in suspension. In situ hybridization can be used to detect specific antigens in paraffin-embedded tissues. Specific oligonucleotide probes are incubated with the tissue slide to permit hybridization with the messenger RNA of the antigen of interest. The probe is labeled with a fluorescent or other dye to permit detection. Finally, enzyme-linked immunosorbent assays or radioimmunoassays are antibody-based detection methods to quantify the level of a particular marker in blood or other body fluids. Both procedures take less than a day and can detect quantities in the nanogram to picogram range (10^{-6} to 10^{-9} g). These types of assays are used for routine measurement of known markers, such as CA 15–3 in serum from breast cancer patients.

Cytogenetic Analysis

Another screening method used primarily to support the diagnosis of hematopoietic cancers is cytogenetic analysis. Chromosome aberrations can be the result of incorrect separation of chromosome pairs during mitosis (numerical chromosome change). One of the daughter cells may end up with an additional copy of the chromosome, whereas the other daughter cell is one copy short. Structural chromosome changes are initiated with DNA damage and incorrect DNA repair, leading to abnormal reconfiguration of broken chromosome ends. There is evidence that cancer-associated chromosomal aberrations are not random, although exact mechanisms are not fully understood. The first specific chromosome abnormality was observed in 1960 in patients with CML. The abnormality involves the earlier mentioned, unusually small chromosome 22.[35] Since the discovery was made in Philadelphia, the chromosome was named *Philadelphia chromosome*. It was subsequently found that chromosomal aberrations in hematopoietic cancers are restricted to a few chromosomes with an otherwise normal diploid karyotype.

Cytogenetics, especially in solid tumors, is used to identify possible locations of new tumor suppressor genes. By comparing numerous chromosomal aberrations in tumors of a particular histologic type, certain abnormalities may show up with an elevated frequency, which may indicate a common loss of a tumor suppressor gene. This mapping strategy has helped significantly in identification of the *BRCA-1* and *BRCA-2* genes in breast carcinoma.[40]

Genetic Analysis

In addition to immunologic techniques, molecular biologic techniques have been developed for detection of tumor markers. One such technique is based on gene analysis for detection of mutations in known molecules suspected of carrying a mutation. Generally, messenger RNA is isolated from the tumor cells and reverse transcribed into complementary DNA. The complementary DNA is incubated with an oligonucleotide specific for the tumor marker of interest, and the DNA is amplified by polymerase chain reaction (PCR), introduced in 1985.[41] Because of the specific primer, only the gene of interest is amplified by PCR. The PCR product is subsequently analyzed using a variety of techniques, such as analysis by gel electrophoresis, Southern blotting, and sequencing. Mutations in oncogenes (ras) and tumor suppressor genes (p53), are easily detected with these procedures. The PCR amplification method of genetic material can also be performed on formalin-fixed, paraffin-embedded tissues.

Clinical Applications of Tumor Markers

Diagnosis

Routinely, the first diagnosis of tumor is performed by the pathologist based on histologic and cellular characteristics (morphologic markers). Histopathologic classification is essential because not all tumors are equal, and they require differential treatment. In addition, within a particular histologic type, treatment strategies vary depending on the grade and stage of the tumor. Immunohistology using antibodies to detect specific markers is helpful for classification of the problem cases, such as apparently undifferentiated tumors. These tumors include large cell tumors, such as anaplastic carcinoma, and round cell tumors, such as Ewing's sarcoma.

Antibodies reactive to components of the intermediate-sized filaments can be helpful to classify tumors because their expression is tissue specific and is often preserved in malignancies. The intermediate-sized filaments are part of the intracellular matrix and comprise cytokeratins (carcinoma), vimentin (lymphoma, sarcoma, melanoma), desmin (myosarcoma), neurofilaments (neuroblastoma), and glial fibrillary acidic protein (astrocytoma). Within the more than 18 different keratins, cell-type–specific combinations occur, and antibodies against individual keratins may help in subclassification. Likewise, antibodies have been generated against a number of cell-lineage–associated markers, such as CD45 (common leukocyte antigen), PSA and PSAP (prostate epithelium), G250 (renal cell carcinoma), gp100 (melanoma), and polymorphic epithelial mucins (secretorial epithelia). Antibodies reactive with leukocyte-associated antigens are used for the subclassification of lymphomas and leukemias.

The list of clusters of differentiation, or CD, numbers contains more than 250 different antigens and keeps growing.[42] A similar, albeit much smaller, list of clusters has been prepared for differentiating antigens in lung cancer.

Prognosis

Prognosis is related to treatment. Morphologic criteria and the extent of metastatic disease are important prognostic parameters. Thus, factors that determine tumor growth, such as expression of particular growth factor receptors, the rate at which the tumor is growing, metastatic potential mediated through expression of certain receptors for ECM molecules, and sensitivity to therapy, all are important for prognosis. A marker indicative of tumor growth is the cell-cycle–dependent proliferation marker Ki-67. A high proportion of Ki-67–positive cells is inversely correlated with survival. Likewise, overexpression of Her2/neu and the EGF receptor on breast cancer cells and high levels of MUC-1 in the serum of breast cancer patients is associated with poor prognosis. A high expression of integrin molecules (involved in attachment to ECM molecules) is related to poor prognosis. Many factors are found to be involved in tumor development, and therefore many are related to prognosis.

Monitoring Efficacy of Therapy

Tumor markers such as CEA, PSA, and CA 125 are easily detectable in serum. Their expression levels in serum correlate with tumor volume, which means that levels that are significantly higher than average baseline levels indicate the presence of malignancy. By evaluating levels pretherapy and post-therapy, the clinician can monitor the efficacy of therapy and detect recurrences. For example, a patient with very high CEA level will experience a drastic decrease in that level immediately after the successful removal of his or her colon cancer. Thereafter, any significant increase in that level in the years after the operation may signify recurrent colon cancer or metachronous cancer, and the patient's physician can have a higher index of suspicion to prompt a cancer detection test such as colonoscopy early.

Guiding Choice of Therapy

Some tumor markers that can be easily evaluated through immunohistology may provide clinically important information, such as the evaluation of hormone receptor status in breast carcinoma. Estrogen receptor status has been for years the basis of selecting patients for potential therapy. Estrogen receptor–positive patients (especially postmenopausal patients) have been treated with tamoxifen. In contrast, estrogen receptor–negative patients (especially premenopausal patients) have been treated with chemotherapy. Although physicians rely on a number of markers, such as CEA, PSA, and α-fetoprotein (AFP), to treat patients, they do not necessarily select treatment on the basis of the level of expression.

Prevention of Cancer

Examples of markers that may help prevent tumor development are the genes with inheritable mutations such as BRCA-1, BRCA-2, ret (associated with multiple endocrine neoplasia),[43] and APC, or other genes that are commonly mutated in the initial stages of tumor development. Mutations in these genes are likely to cause cancer at some stage in life. Early screening for the known gene mutations (i.e., before the development of cancer) may permit corrective therapy, such as prophylactic surgery. Another such treatment may be gene therapy in which an intact copy of the mutated gene is transferred into cells with the defective gene.

Some Tumor Markers Most Frequently Used in Surgical Oncology

CEA is among frequently used markers in surgical oncology and is discussed here as a representative example (see also Table 28-8). CEA is an oncofetal protein with a molecular weight of 200,000 kD that is expressed in embryonic tissue. In adults, CEA is found in the mucous membranes of stomach, small intestine, and the biliary tree as a component of the glycocalix. Malignant epithelial type tumors such as colon cancer, lung cancer, and others may express higher levels of CEA on the cell surface and release CEA into blood. CEA in the normal cell is thought to function as a cell adhesion molecule. For cancer cells, CEA may offer a survival advantage by allowing adhesion into other cells and allowing metastasis. It may also offer some refuge from immune attack of the host due to the large glycosylated nature of the molecule creating a physical barrier between the immune effector cells and the cancer cell.

CEA is detected in serum by commercially available immunoassay kits that very specifically measure the level of CEA. However, the measured level can vary depending on the brand of kit used, although the measured level is reproducible within the brand and the laboratory. In general, normal individuals have less than 2.5 ng/mL. Benign conditions listed in Table 28-8 can raise this level to higher than 10 ng/mL. CEA is cleared from serum by hepatocytes and Kupffer cells. Any benign liver condition that affects hepatocellular function or causes cholestasis can decrease clearance of CEA, resulting in higher plasma levels.

Serum CEA level is not a useful test for screening for colorectal cancer for several reasons. In large studies, only about 40% patients with localized, potentially curable cancers had serum CEA levels higher than 5 ng/mL (sensitivity of 40%). This results in a large false-negative rate. If one uses the same 5-ng/mL level as cutoff for a normal CEA level, the test is 95% specific. However, due to the very low prevalence of colorectal cancer in large populations (1/1000), that 95% specificity still yields a large frequency of false-positive tests.

Although CEA is not useful in screening large populations, the level of CEA in colorectal cancer patients is of prognostic value. In general, the higher the preoperative CEA level, the poorer the rate of long-term survival. Patients with normal preoperative CEA levels have lower recurrence rate than patients with elevated CEA levels. If the CEA level does not decrease to normal levels after resection of the cancer, the risk of recurrence is higher.

Related to CEA are CA 125, CA 15-3, and CA 19-9, serum markers for detection of ovarian cancer, breast cancer, and pancreas cancer, respectively. All four molecules are high-molecular-weight molecules expressed on the respective tumors but not on normal tissues. Their expression levels correlate with tumor volume and as such they are useful indicators to monitor response to therapy and recurrence.

As mentioned earlier, estrogen and progesterone receptor status is routinely determined on breast biopsies to determine choice of treatment. Additionally, Her2/neu status is evaluated using specific antibodies. Patients with disseminated Her2/neu-positive tumors are potentially eligible for treatment with the anti-Her2/neu antibody, Herceptin.

PSA and AFP are the standard markers for detection of prostate cancer and hepatocellular carcinoma, respectively, and for monitoring the response to therapy.

Finally, neuron-specific enolase (NSE), CEA, and squamous cell carcinoma (SCC) antigen are commonly used markers for lung cancer. NSE detected in serum helps to support a diagnosis of small cell lung carcinoma and a postoperative decrease of serum level of NSE is the first sign of curative resection. SCC antibody measurement in serum of lung cancer patients is an aid to histologic analysis: Patients with an SCC antibody level higher than 2 µg/L have a 95% probability of having non–small cell lung cancer and 80% probability of having a squamous tumor.

In spite of the usefulness of many markers as outlined earlier, caution should be taken with the interpretation of the observed values. In addition to malignancy, several benign conditions may increase the value of serum markers. For example, many acute and chronic conditions of the biliary tract as well as cancers of the pancreas, colon, and stomach result in increased levels of CA 19-9. Likewise, the level of AFP is elevated in serum during pregnancy and cancers such as hepatocellular carcinoma and nonseminomatous testicular cancer. Nonmalignant conditions such as inflammatory bowel disease, hepatitis, and cirrhosis can also give rise to elevated AFP levels. Finally, benign conditions such as pregnancy, menstruation, endometriosis, pelvic inflammatory disease, hepatitis, cirrhosis, and renal failure may increase CA 125 levels.

Conclusion

Many tumor markers exist, and most are diagnostic markers. There is still a need for additional markers, however, especially those that indicate the presence of a tumor at very early stages. The completion of the sequencing of the human genome may increase the number and quality of available markers for all possible applications. The availability of markers for early diagnosis can be combined with more refined treatment modalities (e.g., gene therapy, vaccine therapy, and others) or with finding new indications for old treatments (e.g., prophylactic surgery).

Selected References

Burnet FM: The concept of immunological surveillance. Prog Exp Tumor Res 13:1, 1970.

> **An introduction to the concept of immunologic surveillance.**

Davis MM: T-cell antigen receptor genes and T-cell recognition. Nature 334:395, 1988.

A review on structural features and genetic organization of the T-cell receptor in the context of antigen recognition.

Fearon ER: A genetic model for colorectal tumorigenesis. Cell 61:759, 1990.

The first genetic model for tumorigenesis.

Kohler G: Continuous cultures of fused cells secreting antibody of predefined specificity. Nature 256:495, 1975.

An introduction to hybridoma technology.

Saiki RK: Enzymatic amplification of beta-globin genomic sequences and restriction site analysis for diagnosis of sickle cell anemia. Science 230:1350, 1985.

An introduction to polymerase chain reaction technology.

References

1. Clark WH Jr, Elder DE, Guerry DT, et al: A study of tumor progression: The precursor lesions of superficial spreading and nodular melanoma. Hum Pathol 15:1147-1165, 1984.
2. Clark WH Jr, Elder DE, Van Horn M: The biologic forms of malignant melanoma. Hum Pathol 17:443-450, 1986.
3. Fearon ER, Vogelstein B: A genetic model for colorectal tumorigenesis. Cell 61:759-767, 1990.
4. Munger K: Disruption of oncogene/tumor suppressor networks during human carcinogenesis. Cancer Invest 20:71-81, 2002.
5. Nicolson GL: Autocrine and paracrine growth mechanisms in cancer progression and metastasis. In Bertino JR (ed): Encyclopedia of Cancer, vol 1, 2nd ed. San Diego, Academic Press, 2002, pp 165-177.
6. Coussens LM, Werb Z: Inflammation and cancer. Nature 420:860-867, 2002.
7. Rosenberg SA: Progress in human tumour immunology and immunotherapy. Nature 411:380-384, 2001.
8. Peoples GE, Blotnick S, Takahashi K, et al: T lymphocytes that infiltrate tumors and atherosclerotic plaques produce heparin-binding epidermal growth factor–like growth factor and basic fibroblast growth factor: A potential pathologic role. Proc Natl Acad Sci U S A 92:6547-6551, 1995.
9. Culp LA: Extracellular matrix and matrix receptors: Alterations during tumor progression. In Bertino JR (ed): Encyclopedia of Cancer, vol 2, 2nd ed. San Diego, Academic Press, 2002, pp 215-233.
10. Burnet FM: The concept of immunological surveillance. Prog Exp Tumor Res 13:1-27, 1970.
11. Shankaran V, Ikeda H, Bruce AT, et al: IFN-gamma and lymphocytes prevent primary tumour development and shape tumour immunogenicity. Nature 410:1107-1111, 2001.
12. Dunn GP, Bruce AT, Ikeda H, et al: Cancer immunoediting: From immunosurveillance to tumor escape. Nat Immunol 3:991-998, 2002.
13. Rosenberg SA: A new era for cancer immunotherapy based on the genes that encode cancer antigens. Immunity 10:281-287, 1999.
14. Davis MM, Bjorkman PJ: T-cell antigen receptor genes and T-cell recognition. Nature 334:395-402, 1988.
15. van der Merwe PA, Davis SJ: Molecular interactions mediating T-cell antigen recognition. Annu Rev Immunol 21:659-684, 2003.
16. Garrido F, Ruiz-Cabello F, Cabrera T, et al: Implications for immunosurveillance of altered HLA class I phenotypes in human tumours. Immunol Today 18:89-95, 1997.
17. Finke J, Ferrone S, Frey A, et al: Where have all the T cells gone? Mechanisms of immune evasion by tumors. Immunol Today 20:158-160, 1999.
18. Shevach EM: Regulatory T cells in autoimmunity. Annu Rev Immunol 18:423-449, 2000.
19. Liyanage UK, Moore TT, Joo HG, et al: Prevalence of regulatory T cells is increased in peripheral blood and tumor microenvironment of patients with pancreas or breast adenocarcinoma. J Immunol 169:2756-2761, 2002.
20. O'Connell J, Bennett MW, O'Sullivan GC, et al: The Fas counterattack: Cancer as a site of immune privilege. Immunol Today 20:46-52, 1999.
21. Tsuruo T, Naito M, Tomida A, et al: Molecular targeting therapy of cancer: Drug resistance, apoptosis, and survival signal. Cancer Sci 94:15-21, 2003.
22. Brantley-Finley C, Lyle CS, Du L, et al: The JNK, ERK, and p53 pathways play distinct roles in apoptosis mediated by the antitumor agents vinblastine, doxorubicin, and etoposide. Biochem Pharmacol 66:459-469, 2003.
23. Brown JM, Wouters BG: Apoptosis, p53, and tumor cell sensitivity to anticancer agents. Cancer Res 59:1391-1399, 1999.
24. Persidis A: Cancer multidrug resistance. Nat Biotechnol 17:94-95, 1999.
25. Zhivotovsky B, Joseph B, Orrenius S: Tumor radiosensitivity and apoptosis. Exp Cell Res 248:10-17, 1999.
26. Biederer C, Ries S, Brandts CH, et al: Replication-selective viruses for cancer therapy. J Mol Med 80:163-175, 2002.
27. Wu N, Ataai MM: Production of viral vectors for gene therapy applications. Curr Opin Biotechnol 11:205-208, 2000.
28. Rosenberg SA: Adoptive immunotherapy for cancer. Sci Am 262:62-69, 1990.
29. Berinstein N: Overview of therapeutic vaccination approaches for cancer. Semin Oncol 30:1-8, 2003.
30. Goedegebuure PS, Douville LM, Li H, et al: Adoptive immunotherapy with tumor-infiltrating lymphocytes and interleukin-2 in patients with metastatic malignant melanoma and renal cell carcinoma: A pilot study. J Clin Oncol 13:1939-1949, 1995.
31. Nagoshi M, Goedegebuure PS, Burger UL, et al: Successful adoptive cellular immunotherapy is dependent on induction of a host immune response triggered by cytokine (IFN-gamma and granulocyte/macrophage colony-stimulating factor) producing donor tumor-infiltrating lymphocytes. J Immunol 160:334-344, 1998.
32. Sauvageot J, Epstein JI: Immunoreactivity for prostate-specific antigen and prostatic acid phosphatase in adenocarcinoma of the prostate: Relation to progression following radical prostatectomy. Prostate 34:29-33, 1998.
33. de Bruijn HWA, ten Hoor KA, Boonstra H, et al: Cancer-associated antigen CA 195 in patients with mucinous ovarian tumours: A comparative analysis with CEA, TATI, and CA 125 in serum specimens and cyst fluids. Tumour Biol 14:105-115, 1993.
34. Mitchell EP: Role of carcinoembryonic antigen in the management of advanced colorectal cancer. Semin Oncol 25:12-20, 1998.
35. Shtivelman E, Lifshitz B, Gale RP, et al: Fused transcript of abl and bcr genes in chronic myelogenous leukaemia. Nature 315:550-554, 1985.
36. Rabbitts TH: Chromosomal translocations in human cancer. Nature 372:143-149, 1994.

37. Humphrey PA, Gangarosa LM, Wong AJ, et al: Deletion-mutant epidermal growth factor receptor in human gliomas: Effects of type II mutation on receptor function. Biochem Biophys Res Commun 178:1413-1420, 1991.

38. Jones PA: The DNA methylation paradox. Trends Genet 15:34-37, 1999.

39. Kohler G, Milstein C: Continuous cultures of fused cells secreting antibody of predefined specificity. Nature 256:495-497, 1975.

40. Marx J: A second breast cancer susceptibility gene is found. Science 271:30-31, 1996.

41. Saiki RK, Scharf S, Faloona F, et al: Enzymatic amplification of beta-globin genomic sequences and restriction site analysis for diagnosis of sickle cell anemia. Science 230:1350-1354, 1985.

42. Zola H, Swart B, Boumsell L, et al: Human leucocyte differentiation Antigen nomenclature: Update on CD nomenclature. Report of IUIS/WHO Subcommittee. J Immunol Methods 275:1-8, 2003.

43. Ponder BA: The phenotypes associated with *ret* mutations in the multiple endocrine neoplasia type 2 syndrome. Cancer Res 59:1736s-1742s, 1999.

CHAPTER 29

MELANOMA AND CUTANEOUS MALIGNANCIES

Marshall M. Urist, M.D. and **Seng-jaw Soong, Ph.D.**

Melanoma	Cutaneous Malignancies: Nonmelanoma Skin Cancer

Skin cancers account for more than 40% of all malignancies in the United States, and the incidence continues to rise. This increase is attributed to environmental exposure, principally sunlight. The majority of skin cancers are basal cell carcinoma (BCC), squamous cell carcinoma (SCC), and melanoma, which account for more than 95% of the total. This chapter focuses on these three major types and briefly discusses the identification and management of less common cutaneous malignancies.

MELANOMA

Melanocytes are cells of neural crest origin that migrate during fetal development to multiple sites in the body, principally the skin. Positioned along the basement membrane at the dermoepidermal junction, these cells are exposed to carcinogenic stimuli that result in malignant transformation to become melanoma. This event is relatively rare compared to the transformation rate for the neighboring basal keratinocytes that become SCC and BCC. Melanoma accounts for only 4% to 5% of all skin cancers but causes the majority of deaths from skin malignancies. It is the eighth most common cancer in the United States, and the incidence is rising faster than any other type of cancer. It is estimated that there will be 54,200 new cases diagnosed and 7600 deaths from melanoma in 2003.[1] The lifetime probability of developing melanoma is 1 in 57 for males and 1 in 81 for females. In whites, the 5-year relative survival rate has risen from 80% for 1974-1976 to 89% for 1992-1998.[2] This impressive progress has resulted from increased public awareness and education programs.

Epidemiology and Etiology

The incidence and outcome of melanoma are related to multiple factors. Melanoma is principally a disease of whites, particularly those of Celtic ancestry. The disease occurs much less commonly in Asian and black populations. It is estimated that melanoma occurs 20 times more often in whites than in blacks. The reason for this difference is unknown. The disease occurs slightly more often in men than women, and the prognosis is slightly better for women when other prognostic factors are taken into account. The anatomic distribution of melanoma varies between the two genders. Melanomas arise more commonly on the lower extremity in women and more often on the trunk and head and neck in men. These differences in distribution are not accounted for by sun exposure alone. Melanoma can occur at any age from birth to advanced age. The median age of diagnosis is in the range of 45 to 55 years. Tumors rarely develop before the age of puberty; however, there is a significant incidence in the 3rd and 4th decades of life.

It is well established that exposure to sunlight increases the risk of developing melanoma in susceptible populations. This is specifically attributed to solar ultraviolet (UV) radiation.[3] UVA and UVB cause different patterns of effect in the skin; however, both are considered to be carcinogenic. UVB induces the effects of sunburn and increases melanin production and is the most carcinogenic part of the UV spectrum. UVA has a deeper level of penetration resulting in dermal connective tissue damage, loss of elasticity, and skin wrinkling. It is not clear whether it is the total amount of UV exposure or the pattern in which individuals receive UV irradiation that leads to development of melanoma. It is reported that people incurring severe burns in childhood appear to be at higher risk for development of melanoma years later. In contrast, those who receive exposure on a regular basis may not be at as high a risk. There is also a role for skin type since individuals who tan easily are not at as high a risk for the development of melanoma even with prolonged exposure. The highest risk population appears to be those individuals with a fair complexion who receive intermittent doses of radiation resulting in severe sunburns.

Additional factors that increase the risk for development of melanoma include dysplastic nevus (DN) syndrome, xeroderma pigmentosum, a history of non-melanoma skin cancer (NMSC), and a family history of melanoma.

The risk of melanoma increases with age; however, the role of aging is not clear. With increasing age there is more opportunity for the initiation of new tumors, either through exposure to carcinogens (UV irradiation) or through the decreasing ability of individual cells to repair DNA damage.[4]

Precursor Lesions and Risk Factors

Congenital nevi, DNs, Spitz nevi, and familial patterns all raise the risk of developing melanoma. Individuals with congenital nevi have an increased risk that is proportional to the size and number of nevi. Small congenital nevi represent a low risk and are therefore observed unless local changes appear. Giant congenital nevi are rare (1 in 20,000 newborns) and carry an increased risk for development of melanoma within the nevi (Fig. 29-1). This lifetime risk has been estimated to be in the range of 5% to 8%, which has led some authors to recommend complete excision if possible. At minimum, these patients should be examined regularly throughout life.

In general, a DN is a large (6- to 15-mm) pigmented flat skin lesion with indistinct margins and variable color. This simple definition belies the difficulty in making the diagnosis because precise criteria may vary both clinically and histologically. DNs may occur sporadically or in a familial pattern. Individuals with DNs and a family history of melanoma have an extremely high risk of developing melanoma. Patients with DN syndrome (B-K mole syndrome, familial atypical mole–malignant melanoma syndrome) have multiple nevi (>100) that present a great challenge to the patient and physician. There is a lack of consensus regarding the management of DNs since it may

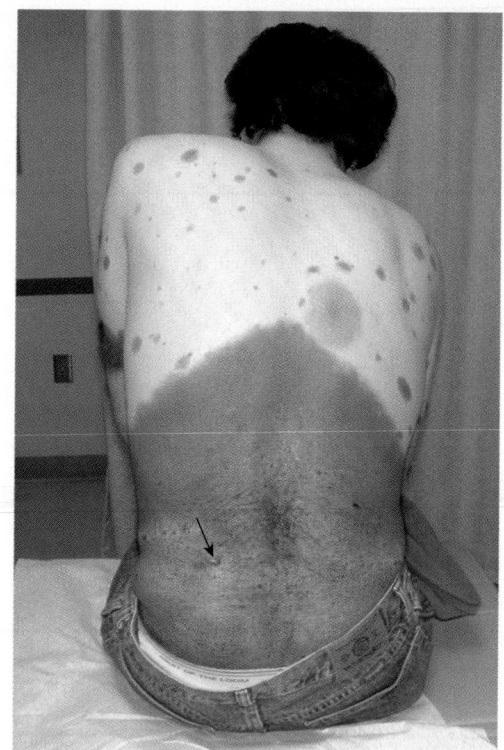

FIGURE 29-1. Giant congenital nevus of the trunk with a melanoma *(arrow)* arising on the lower back.

be difficult to follow changes in multiple nevi over time and most DNs will not become melanoma. Excision of all nevi might be reassuring for the patient and physician, but this still requires surveillance for the appearance of new lesions. In most instances, physician examinations are scheduled at 3- to 6-month intervals in addition to monthly patient self-examinations. When multiple nevi are present, reference photographs provide an excellent way to compare the appearance of nevi over time.[5]

Spitz nevi (juvenile melanoma, spindle cell melanoma, epithelioid cell melanoma) are rapidly growing, pink or brown, benign skin lesions arising most often in children and adolescents, although adult skin lesions may also have spitzoid features. They may be difficult to distinguish histologically from melanoma. Consultation with an experienced pathologist is often required to accurately diagnose these lesions. Complete local excision is the treatment of choice. In borderline cases, it may be necessary to excise the areas as a melanoma to ensure adequate treatment.[6] Sentinel lymph node (SLN) biopsy has been proposed as a mechanism to clarify the malignant potential in indeterminate cases.[7] If the diagnosis of *melanoma arising within a Spitz nevus* is made, the treatment should be based on the same criteria as other types of melanoma.

Familial Melanoma

Approximately 5% to 10% of melanoma patients have a family history of the disease. Compared to patients with sporadic melanoma, the age of onset is earlier, the incidence of DNs is higher, and multiple primary melanomas are more common. Chromosome mapping studies have shown evidence of linkage and heterogeneity to chromosomes 1p and 9p. Chromosome 1p contributes to both sporadic and familial melanoma, whereas 9p contributes more to sporadic melanoma alone. All reported kindreds are white.

Clinical Features

Cutaneous Melanoma

Melanoma commonly presents as a changing pigmented skin lesion. Patients typically describe a flat lesion that spreads over the surface of the skin and later becomes elevated. If the lesion is allowed to progress, itching, bleeding and ulceration will follow. In some instances, melanomas arise in preexisting nevi; however, the majority arise de novo. The most important aspect of the history is "change." Even experienced clinicians may not recognize a melanoma; therefore, physicians should have a low threshold for performing a diagnostic biopsy on any changing lesion. There are several other pigmented benign skin lesions that can mimic the appearance of melanoma: nevi (congenital and acquired), blue nevus, solar lentigo, keratosis, hemangioma, and pyogenic granuloma. The common features of melanoma are summarized in the mnemonic ABCDE: *A*symmetrical outline, changing irregular *B*orders, variation in *C*olor, *D*iameter greater than 6 mm, and *E*levation. In early melanoma, the changes may be limited to two or three features.

Not all melanomas are pigmented. These amelanotic lesions appear as raised papules that can be pink, red, purple, or of normal skin colors. Their atypical appearance frequently leads to a delay in diagnosis and therefore a poorer prognosis. Desmoplastic melanoma is a specific type of amelanotic melanoma that commonly arises on the face and can be associated with a lentigo maligna melanoma (LMM). Desmoplastic melanomas exhibit neurotropism, which is also a poor prognostic factor.[8]

In summary, any changing skin lesion should be carefully evaluated, and clinicians should have a low threshold to perform a diagnostic biopsy. This is especially true in individuals who have multiple pigmented lesions, a history of atypical or dysplastic lesions, or a family history of skin cancer.

Unknown Primary Melanoma

Melanoma may present as a nodal or distant metastasis as the first evidence of the disease. This occurs in less than 2% of all melanoma cases and less than 5% of all patients who present with metastatic melanoma.[9] Under these circumstances, the prognosis may be as good or better than if the primary were present. A thorough search for the primary lesion should include a histologic review of all previously removed skin lesions; questions regarding skin lesions that resolved without treatment; and inspection of areas that may have been missed in initial examination, including the scalp, external auditory canal, oral and nasal mucosa, nail beds, genitalia, anal canal, perianal skin, and the eye. In the case of a lymph node metastasis, a completion regional lymph node dissection is performed on the assumption that it is a regional node and therefore represents stage III, rather than stage IV, disease.[10] The patient should then be evaluated for adjuvant therapy, especially for participation in investigational protocols. For metastases at other sites see Surgical Considerations for Metastases, later in this chapter.

Noncutaneous Melanoma

In embryogenesis, melanocytes arise in the neural crest area and migrate to many sites other than the skin. Fewer than 10% of melanomas arise in these areas, which include the eye, mucosal surfaces, and unknown primary sites. A review from the National Cancer Database from 1985 to 1994 reports on a population of more than 80,000 melanomas: Whereas 91% were found in the skin, 5.2% occurred in the eye, 1.3% on mucosal surfaces, and 2.2% were considered of unknown primary origin.[9] Although melanoma has been reported to arise from many tissues and organs throughout the body, there is often the possibility that these are actually metastases from an unknown primary site on the skin. One exception may be in the esophagus, where melanocytic atypia and melanoma in situ have been shown to occur.

Ocular melanoma is the most common malignancy arising in the eye. Within the eye, melanocytes are found in the retina and uveal tract (iris, ciliary body, and choroids). The options for treatment are photocoagulation, partial resection, radiation, or enucleation. Although ocular and cutaneous melanomas have several common histologic features, their clinical course is quite different. Ocular melanoma rarely metastasizes to lymph nodes since the uveal tract has no lymphatic vessels. The most common site of distant metastases is the liver, and this may be the presenting site of disease for patients with retinal melanoma.

The most common sites of origin for melanomas arising on the mucous membranes are the head and neck (oral cavity, oropharynx, nasopharynx, and paranasal sinuses), anal canal, rectum, and the female genitalia. Compared to melanomas arising on the skin, mucosal melanomas are more advanced and have a uniformly poor prognosis. These tumors should be excised to negative margins. Extensive local resections do not affect survival, although locoregional control may be improved.[11] In general, lymph node dissections are not indicated unless patients have clinically evident lymphadenopathy. The one exception is for patients with vulvar melanomas—SLN biopsy is now being performed for this group of patients.[12] The overall prognosis for patients with mucosal melanomas is poor, with less than 10% of patients surviving 5 years.

Clinical Management

Choice of Biopsy

The clinical management of melanoma begins with an accurate diagnosis. The classic signs of melanoma include a skin lesion with changing characteristics such as irregular borders, varying degrees of pigmentation, an irregular surface, bleeding, itching, and ulceration. The decision to perform a biopsy is frequently based on clinical experience; however, even senior dermatologists and surgeons may underdiagnose melanoma. Concern on the part of either the physician or the patient is a valid indication for the biopsy. The specific method for the biopsy depends on the size of the lesion and anatomic location. Regardless of the method, biopsies should be full thickness into the subcutaneous tissues. For small lesions, an excisional biopsy is commonly performed that includes a narrow (1- to 2-mm) margin of surrounding skin. The biopsy area should not be enlarged to permit a better cosmetic appearance since this may lead to an unnecessary expansion of the final wide excision. Although shaved biopsies are commonly performed for benign-appearing lesions, this technique should not be used when melanoma is suspected. A shave biopsy may lead to a pathology report showing extension of the tumor to the deep margins of excision. Under these circumstances, the most important prognostic factor, tumor thickness, will not be accurate. This may lead to incorrect decisions regarding wide local excision (WLE), SLN biopsy, and adjuvant therapy. The clinical appearance of melanoma may be deceptively benign. This is why the use of cautery or cryoablation may lead to a delay in the diagnosis of melanoma. If a skin lesion appears at the site of a previously cauterized or frozen skin lesion, excisional biopsy and histopathologic analysis are mandatory.

The technique of a surgical biopsy is straightforward. The biopsy removes the full thickness of skin, taking a layer of the underlying fatty tissue and all the visible tumor. Care should be taken not to crush or otherwise traumatize the specimen since this may hinder the histologic interpretation. These biopsies are performed under local anesthesia in the office or outpatient setting. The wound is closed in one or two layers in an orientation that is consistent with a possible wider excision. There may be circumstances in which complete surgical excision is not appropriate. This may be because of a large primary lesion or proximity of the lesion to important structures such as the eye, nose, or ear. Under these circumstances, a punch biopsy or excision of a segment of the lesion is appropriate. Again, this should be a full-thickness biopsy and include a margin of adjacent normal skin if possible. When a biopsy of a large lesion is performed, at least one punch should be placed through the most elevated portion to accurately classify the thickness.

When performing a diagnostic biopsy, orientation of the biopsy closure may affect the options for closure of the WLE. For this reason, biopsy excisions on the extremities should be closed longitudinally to maximize the possibility for a primary wound closure and lower the use of skin grafts. Larger tissue defects may be closed with local rotational/advancement skin flaps or a skin graft.

Histologic Features of Cutaneous Melanoma

Histologically, melanoma is divided into four major types based on growth pattern and location. These forms are LMM, superficial spreading melanoma (SSM), acral lentiginous melanoma (ALM), and nodular melanoma (NM). Melanomas arise as proliferations of melanocytes in the basal layer of the skin. As they multiply, these cells expand radially in the epidermis and superficial dermal layer. With time, the growth begins in a vertical direction as the skin lesion may become palpable. NMs are an exception to this pattern wherein the vertical growth phase is present from an early point in tumor development. It is the vertical growth phase that more than any other histologic parameter of the primary tumor determines prognosis.

LMM (~10%) has distinctive clinical and histologic features. It occurs most commonly in older individuals with sun-damaged skin and presents as a flat, darkly pigmented lesion with irregular borders and a history of slow development. It is not uncommon to see LMMs that are several centimeters in diameter owing to the patient's inability to detect slow progress of the lesion. (Fig. 29-2). Overall, the prognosis of LMM is better than for the other histopathologic types; however, this is primarily related to the superficial nature of these lesions.

The most common histologic type is SSM (~70%). It is not necessarily associated with sun-exposed skin. As the name SSM suggests, these lesions initially appear as a flat, pigmented lesion growing in the radial pattern (Fig. 29-3). If left in place, the lesion begins to thicken as it develops a vertical growth phase.

ALM (~5%) is classified principally by its anatomic site of origin, although it does have a characteristic histologic appearance. These tumors are confined to the subungual

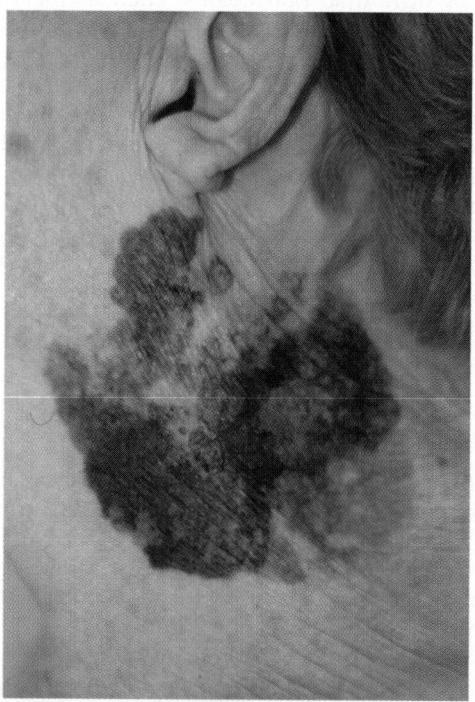

FIGURE 29-2. Lentigo maligna melanoma covering the left side of the neck. Despite a long history of growth, the tumor thickness remained less than 1 mm.

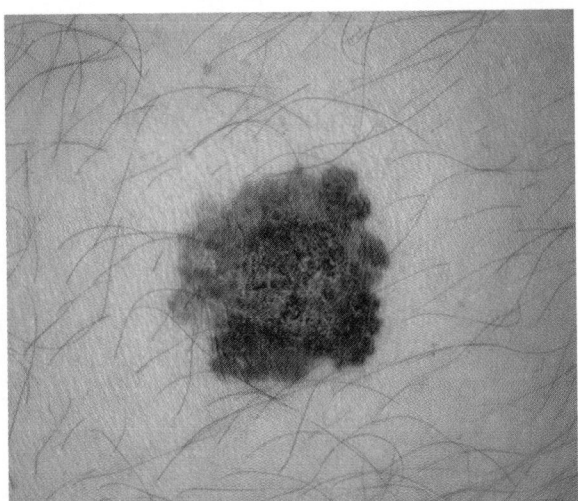

FIGURE 29-3. Superficial spreading melanoma. The 2-cm-diameter melanoma developed over a 2-year period.

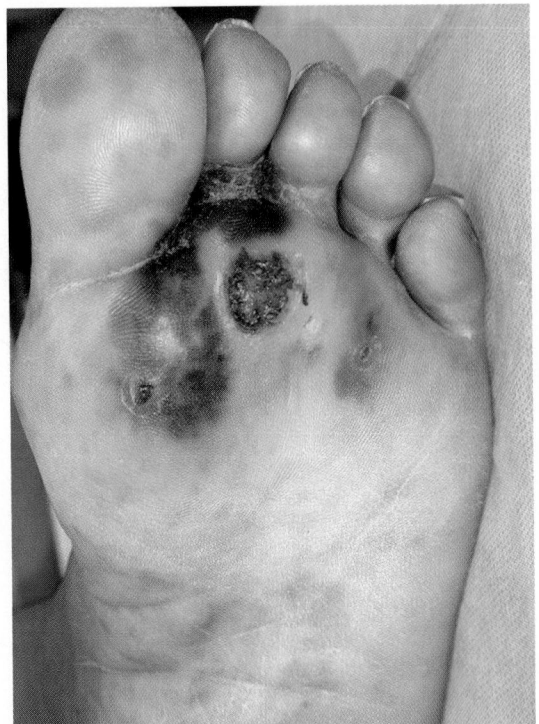

FIGURE 29-4. Acral lentiginous melanoma. The extensively pigmented areas on the sole were predominately melanoma in situ. The single invasive area was ulcerated.

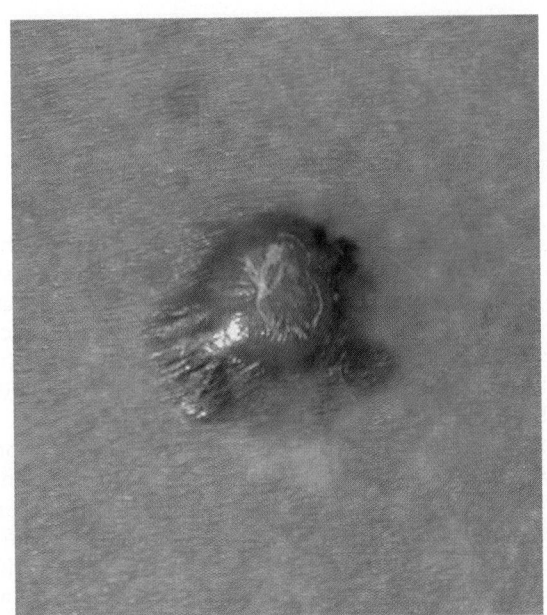

FIGURE 29-5. Nodular melanoma. This raised lesion had no radial growth phase.

areas and the glabrous skin of the palms and soles (Fig. 29-4). This is the most common histologic variant arising in blacks, and the diagnosis is often delayed because of the common appearance of irregular benign pigmentation on the surfaces. For this reason, the overall prognosis is poor. Melanomas arising in subungual areas also are frequently ignored because of their similar appearance to subungual hematomas secondary to trauma. The histologic appearance of ALMs is similar to melanomas arising on the mucous membranes.

NMs (~15%) develop a vertical growth pattern early in their history and may be devoid of junctional changes (Fig. 29-5). Melanomas in this group have the worst prognosis based on a higher average tumor thickness.

Historically, the classification of melanoma into various histologic types had a role in clinical management. With improved understanding of prognostic factors, management is based primarily on thickness and ulceration.

Prognostic Factors

Until the 1960s, invasive melanoma was considered to be a high-risk disease that required an extensive local excision for *all* tumors. In 1969, Clark and associates[13] described a classification of melanoma based on the extent of tumor invasion relative to the anatomic layers of the skin and showed that this level of invasion was related to survival (Fig. 29-6). Level 1 tumors are limited to the epidermis, are in situ, and theoretically have no risk of metastasis. Level 2 lesions extend into the papillary dermis and also have an excellent prognosis. Clark level 3 tumors fill the papillary dermis and are associated with a significant risk of tumor metastases. Extension into the reticular dermis defines a Clark 4 lesion and growth into the subcutaneous fat characterizes a Clark level 5, both of which signify a high mortality risk. In some cases, determining the Clark level was found to be difficult, and readings of the same slides could differ between pathologists

(especially in the level 3 to 4 range). In 1970, Breslow described a more straightforward system based on measuring the vertical thickness of the tumor in millimeters.[14] This was found to be accurately reproducible between pathologists, and there was an excellent correlation with

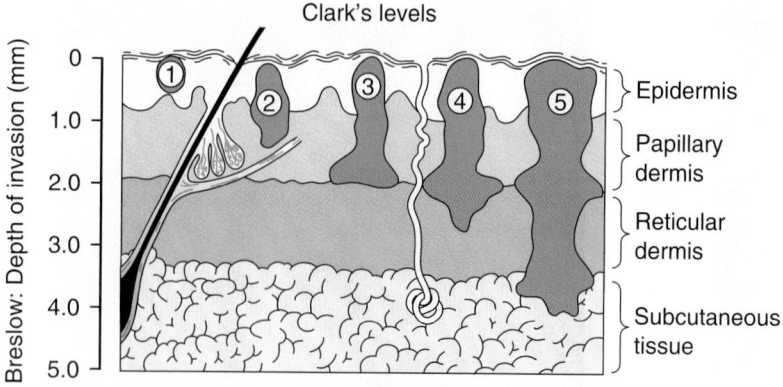

FIGURE 29-6. Schematic representation of Clark's levels of tumor penetration in relation to the normal layers of the skin.

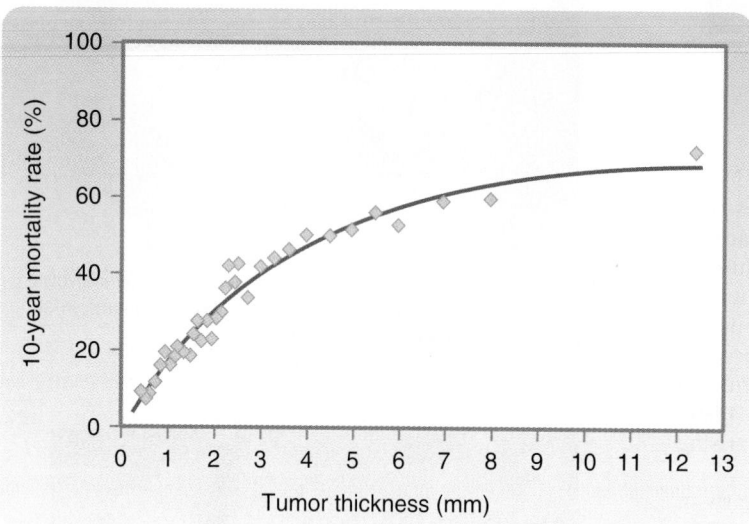

FIGURE 29-7. Observed (solid squares) and predicted (solid line) 10-year mortality rate for patients with clinically localized melanoma. This is based on a mathematical model derived from the American Joint Committee on Cancer melanoma database of 15,230 patients. (From Balch CM, Soong S-j, Gerschenwald JE, et al: Prognostic factors analysis of 17,600 melanoma patients: Validation of the American Joint Committee on Cancer melanoma staging system. J Clin Oncol 19:3622-3634, 2001.)

5-year survival. Prognosis worsens with increasing thickness as a continuous logarithmic function without stairstep areas or natural breakpoints (Fig. 29-7). The mortality rate begins to plateau at about 8 mm and never reaches 100%. Comparison of the two systems showed that the Clark level added little to the prognosis as determined by the Breslow thickness.

In melanoma, analysis of factors contributing to prognosis has led to a remarkably accurate prediction of outcome. Balch and collaborators from 13 institutions[15] collected a complete data set on 17,600 patients to form the American Joint Committee on Cancer (AJCC) Melanoma Database. In an analysis of 13,581 patients with localized melanoma, they defined the relative contribution of multiple known prognostic factors including age, gender, level, site, thickness, and ulceration. The findings of their multifactorial analysis are summarized in Table 29-1. As in all previous studies, tumor thickness was found to be the strongest predictor of outcome. Melanoma thickness is also associated with an increasing risk of local recurrence, regional metastases, distant metastases, and survival. The findings were the same at participating institutions in Australia, Europe, and North America.

Based on the findings just discussed, a complete pathologic report of a cutaneous melanoma should include the following: Breslow thickness, presence or absence of ulceration, Clark level, status of the surgical margins, histologic type, presence or absence of satellitosis, and presence or absence of regression. The report may also describe tumor-infiltrating lymphocytes, lymphovascular invasion, vertical growth phase, neurotropism, and mitotic rate.

Staging

Staging for melanoma uses the tumor-node-metastasis (TNM) system of classification as defined by the AJCC staging system for cutaneous melanoma (Box 29-1). The 6th edition (2002) of the *AJCC Cancer Staging Manual* contains important changes from the 1977 edition.[16] These changes are based on the in-depth prognostic factors analysis cited earlier.[15]

Changes in the 2002 AJCC staging system for cutaneous melanoma include the following:

TABLE 29-1.   Cox Regression Analysis for 13,581 Patients With Melanoma Without Evidence of Nodal or Distant Metastases

Variable	DF	Chi-Square Value	P	Risk Ratio	95% CL
Thickness	1	244.3	<0.00001	1.558	1.473–1.647
Ulceration	1	189.5	<0.00001	1.901	1.735–1.083
Age	1	45.6	<0.00001	1.101	1.071–1.132
Site	1	41.0	<0.00001	1.338	1.224–1.463
Level	1	32.7	<0.00001	1.214	1.136–1.297
Gender	1	15.1	0.001	0.836	0.764–0.915

DF, degrees of freedom; CL, confidence limits.
Revised from Balch CM, Soong S-j, Gerschenwald JE, et al: Prognostic factors analysis of 17,600 melanoma patients: Validation of the American Joint Committee on Cancer Melanoma Staging System. J Clin Oncol 19:3622-3634, 2001.

Box 29-1.   American Joint Committee on Cancer TNM Melanoma Classification—2002

Primary Tumor (T)

TX   Primary tumor cannot be assessed (e.g., shave biopsy or regressed melanoma)
T0   No evidence of primary tumor
Tis Melanoma in situ
T1   Melanoma ≤ 1.0 mm in thickness, with or without ulceration
T1a Melanoma ≤ 1.0 mm in thickness and level II or III, no ulceration
T1b Melanoma ≤ 1.0 mm in thickness and level IV or V or with ulceration
T2   Melanoma 1.01–2.0 mm in thickness, with or without ulceration
T2a Melanoma 1.01–2.0 mm in thickness, no ulceration
T2b Melanoma 1.01–2.0 mm in thickness, with ulceration
T3   Melanoma 2.01–4.0 mm in thickness, with or without ulceration
T3a Melanoma 2.01–4.0 mm in thickness, no ulceration
T3b Melanoma 2.01–4.0 mm in thickness, with ulceration
T4   Melanoma >4.0 mm in thickness, with or without ulceration
T4a Melanoma >4.0 mm in thickness, no ulceration
T4b Melanoma >4.0 mm in thickness, with ulceration

Regional Lymph Nodes (N)

NX   Regional lymph nodes cannot be assessed
N0   No regional lymph node metastasis
N1   Metastasis in one lymph node
N1a Clinically occult (microscopic) metastasis
N1b Clinically apparent (macroscopic) metastasis
N2   Metastasis in two or three regional nodes or intra-lymphatic regional metastasis without nodal metastases
N2a Clinically occult (microscopic) metastasis
N2b Clinically apparent (macroscopic) metastasis
N2c Satellite or in-transit metastasis *without* nodal metastasis
N3   Metastasis in four or more regional nodes, or matted metastatic nodes, or in-transit metastasis or satellites) with metastasis in regional node(s)

Distant Metastasis (M)

MX   Distant metastasis cannot be assessed
M0   No distant metastasis
M1   Distant metastasis
M1a Metastasis to skin, subcutaneous tissues, or distant lymph nodes
M1b Metastasis to lung
M1c Metastasis to all other visceral sites or distant metastasis at any site associated with an elevated serum lactic dehydrogenase

1. Clark's level of invasion is now used only for defining T1 melanomas.
2. The thickness categories are now simplified to change at 1.0, 2.0, and 4.0 mm.
3. Ulceration is included in all T stages and classified as (a) without ulceration and (b) with ulceration.
4. Satellite metastases are now included in the N category.
5. Thick melanomas larger than 4 mm are now staged as IIc.
6. The dimensions of lymph nodes are no longer included.
7. N stage is determined by number of positive lymph nodes.
8. N staging includes the size of metastases within the node to account for microscopic disease found at SLN biopsy.
9. Lung metastases are defined as a separate category of M1 disease because they are associated with a longer survival than other visceral metastases.
10. SLN biopsy results are included in the staging (Table 29-2).

As is true for other malignancies, the patient presenting with melanoma should undergo a systematic evaluation for metastatic disease. This begins with a history focused on constitutional, central nervous system, pulmonary, gastrointestinal, and soft tissue symptoms. A standard physical examination includes a detailed inspection and palpation of the skin and subcutaneous tissues to detect satellites, in-transit metastases, other primary tumors, and lymph node enlargement. When present, all symptoms and signs of metastasis require further radiologic evaluation. Clinical stages 0 and I patients do not require any further tests. Stages II and III patients may have a chest radiograph and serum lactate dehydrogenase level determined; however, these are rarely abnormal in the asymptomatic patient.

This 2002 version of the AJCC staging system provides excellent separation of prognostic groups by stage as is shown in Figure 29-8. The presence of ulceration indicates a significantly worse prognosis and can result in a change in stage (Table 29-3). The new system also provides useful substaging within the N categories based on the number of positive lymph nodes and the presence or absence of ulceration as is shown in Table 29-4.

Surgical Management of the Primary Lesion

The fundamental principle in the management of primary melanoma is to resect the tumor and minimize the risk of local recurrence. Historically, the resection of the primary site and surrounding skin was based on recommendations proffered by William Sampson Handley in 1907. From observations made on the autopsy of a single patient with locally advanced melanoma, he recommended WLE and regional lymph node dissection. This became the standard treatment except in anatomic locations where major adjacent structures (especially head and neck) were spared. With the insightful contributions of Wallace Clark[13] and Alexander Breslow[14] in the late 1960s, the natural history of melanoma became better understood. From many retrospective studies, it was clear that the risk of local recurrence and overall survival rates were related to tumor thickness. Four randomized studies were carried out to test whether narrow margins of excision could achieve the same results as wide margins. The current guidelines for WLE (Table 29-5) are based on these studies. The first trial, published in 1991, was the World Health Organization Melanoma Study[17] comparing WLE using a 1-cm margin versus a 3-cm margin in patients with primary tumors less than 2 mm in thickness.[18] This trial included 612 patients, and all local recurrences occurred in the group of patients undergoing a 1-cm radius of excision for tumors measuring 1.1 to 2 mm in thickness. The overall survival for all major groups and subgroups showed no differences. These findings confirm that melanomas measuring 1 mm or less in diameter can be resected with a 1-cm margin with a low subsequent risk for local recurrence. Melanomas between 1 and 2 mm in thickness have an equally low risk of local recurrence when a 2-cm margin is used. These margins may be lowered to 1 cm when this change facilitates primary closure of the wound. A narrower margin may result in a small increase in the number of patients who develop local recurrence but no difference in overall survival rates.

The Melanoma Intergroup Trial compared margins of 2 versus 4 cm for patients whose tumors measured 1 to 4 mm in thickness.[19] This prospective trial randomized 462 patients with melanomas of the trunk or proximal

TABLE 29-2. American Joint Committe on Cancer Melanoma Stage Classification

| Pathologic Stage | Grouping | | |
	Tumor	Node	Metastasis
0	Tis	N0	M0
IA	T1a	N0	M0
IB	T1b	N0	M0
	T2a	N0	M0
IIA	T2b	N0	M0
	T3a	N0	M0
IIB	T3b	N0	M0
	T4a	N0	M0
IIC	T4b	N0	M0
IIIA	T1-4a	N1a	M0
	T1-4a	N2a	M0
IIIB	T1-4b	N1a	M0
	T1-4b	N2a	M0
	T1-4a	N1b	M0
	T1-4a	N2b	M0
	T1-4a/b	N2c	M0
IIIC	T1-4b	N1b	M0
	T1-4b	N2b	M0
	Any T	N3	M0
IV	Any T	Any N	M1

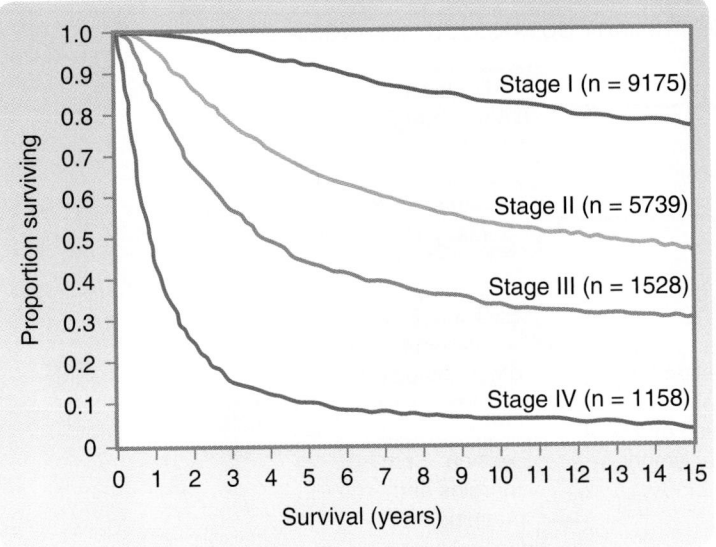

■ **FIGURE 29-8.** Fifteen-year survival curves for the melanoma staging system, comparing localized melanoma (stages I and II), regional metastases (stage III), and distant metastases (stage IV). The numbers in parentheses are the numbers of patients from the American Joint Committee on Cancer melanoma staging database used to calculate the survival rates. The differences between the curves are highly significant (*P* < 0.0001). (From Balch CM, Buzaid AC, Soong S-j, et al: Final version of the American Joint Committee on Cancer Staging System for cutaneous melanoma. J Clin Oncol 19:3635-3648, 2001.)

TABLE 29-3. Ten-Year Survival Rates for Stages I and II Melanomas

Stage	Tumor Ulceration	T-Stage	Approximate 10-Year Survival (%)
IA	No	T1a	90
IB	Yes	T1b	80
	No	T2a	80
IIA	Yes	T2b	65
	No	T3a	65
IIB	Yes	T3b	50
	No	T4a	55
IIC	Yes	T4b	35

TABLE 29-4. Five-Year Survival Rates for Stage III Melanoma Patients

Stage	Tumor Ulceration	N-Stage	Approximate 5-Year Survival (%)
IIIA	No	N1a	70
	No	N2a	60
IIIB	Yes	N1a	55
	Yes	N2a	50
	No	N1b	55
	No	N2b	45
IIIC	Yes	N1b	30
	Yes	N2b	25
	Yes or No	N3	30

TABLE 29-5. Recommended Margins for Surgical Resection of Primary Melanoma

Tumor Thickness (mm)	Margin Radius (cm)*
In situ	0.5
<1.0	1.0
1–2	2.0
>2.0	≥2.0

*Recommended margins may be adjusted to accommodate anatomic or cosmetic circumstances.

The Swedish Melanoma Trial[20] and the French Melanoma Trial[21] compared 2-cm versus 5-cm margins for tumors less than 2-mm thickness. Both trials show no significant differences in disease-free or overall survival between treatment groups. When melanomas are greater than 4 mm in thickness, recommendations for management are based on retrospective analyses in which there does not appear to be any advantage to extending the resection beyond 2 cm.[22]

The members of the Melanoma Committee of the National Comprehensive Cancer Network, a consortium of oncologists from National Cancer Institute–designated cancer centers, annually update their consensus-based guidelines for the treatment of cancer. The guidelines for the management of primary melanoma are summarized in Figure 29-9. (The complete guidelines algorithm is available on-line).

The operative procedure of WLE is often performed under local anesthesia using intravenous sedation if necessary. In most cases, the margin for a WLE is measured from the edges of the biopsy scar. This again emphasizes the importance of a minimal excision for the original biopsy to limit the size of the final resection. The incision is made through the skin and subcutaneous tissues to the level of the superficial fascia. The specimen is oriented for

extremities to receive either a 2- or 4-cm radius of excision. After a median follow-up of 10 years the incidence of local recurrence was the same for both groups (2.1% vs. 2.6%). The factor that most closely correlated with the appearance of a local recurrence was primary tumor ulceration. The conclusion from this trial was that all patients with tumors 1 to 4 mm in thickness should undergo WLE with a 2-cm margin.

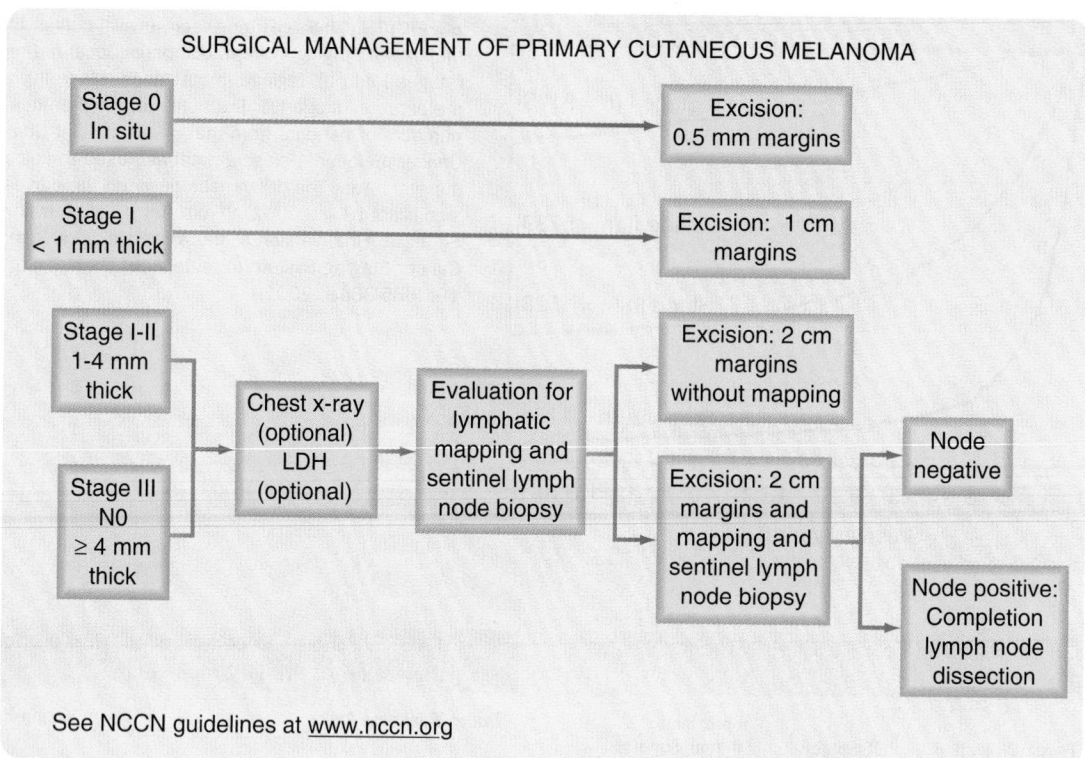

FIGURE 29-9. Management algorithm for primary cutaneous melanoma derived from the National Comprehensive Cancer Network guidelines (*www.nccn.org*). LDH, lactate dehydrogenase.

the pathologist and submitted for permanent section. In many cases, the resulting wound can be closed by elevation and advancement of skin edges or the use of local skin flaps. Skin grafts may be required on the hands, feet, and distal extremities. Tumors arising in proximity to structures such as the nose, eye, and ear may require a compromise of the conventional margins to avoid deformities or disabilities. Subungual melanomas are treated with amputation of the distal digit to provide 1 cm of margin from the tumor. For fingers, this commonly involves only the distal phalanx; ray amputations are unnecessary. In all cases, resection should reach histologically normal margins.

Most mucosal melanomas are locally extensive before becoming symptomatic. Oral cavity melanomas are an exception to this rule because they may be discovered during routine dental examinations. The diagnosis can be delayed in this area because of similarities to amalgam stains. Tumors should be resected with histologically clear margins; however, there is no evidence that WLE increases the chance for cure. Anorectal melanomas are excised to clear margins. For extensive tumors, abdominoperineal resection may be necessary. Abdominoperineal resection reduces the incidence of local and regional recurrence but does not result in an improvement in overall survival.

Radiation therapy has been recommended for patients with head and neck melanomas as well as mucosal melanomas in the pelvic region. Retrospective analyses suggest that this will reduce the incidence of local recurrence.[23]

Melanoma and Pregnancy

Early reports suggested an adverse relationship between pregnancy and outcome in patients with melanoma. This was reinforced by the finding of estrogen receptors in some melanoma tumors. More recent comprehensive analyses have not confirmed any differences in the course of the disease in gravid versus nongravid patients when all relevant prognostic factors are taken in account. Unfortunately, recommendations derived from these early reports included early termination of pregnancy when the diagnosis was made and delaying pregnancy for 2 years after treatment for melanoma. The data do support these recommendations. The decision regarding pregnancy is no different in melanoma than other malignancies. These decisions should be made between the patient and her physicians after an in-depth discussion of prognosis and options for treatment.

Management of Regional Lymph Nodes

After WLE of the primary tumor, the most common sites of first recurrence are regional (lymph nodes, in-transit metastases, and local recurrences). Nodal metastases generally appear in the basin(s) draining from the primary site. This is a predictable pattern for extremity melanomas; however, truncal and head and neck melanomas may drain to more than one site. The lines of drainage for truncal melanomas are divided by the midline and the line of Sappey that extends from the umbilicus across the iliac crest and around to the spine at the level of L2. The sequence of recurrence led surgeons to conclude that resection of nodal basins containing occult metastases could provide an increase in survival. This procedure, termed *elective lymph node dissection* (ELND), was commonly practiced but was often accompanied by significant morbidity including lymphedema, muscle weakness, and restricted range of motion. As prognostic factors became better understood, it was postulated that patients with thin tumors (<1-mm thickness) would have a low risk of metastases at any site and patients with thick tumors (>4-mm thickness) had a high risk of distant as well as regional metastases. In contrast, patients with intermediate-thickness melanoma (1 to 4 mm) would have an elevated risk of nodal metastases without a high risk of distant disease. The intermediate-thickness group formed the population of patients who would, in theory, benefit from ELND. Early retrospective analyses supported this hypothesis and provided the rationale for prospective, randomized trials comparing WLE alone versus WLE with ELND. Subsequent larger retrospective series reported no benefit.[24,25] Four phase III prospective, randomized trials have failed to provide convincing evidence to support ELND. Two early trials were criticized for being underpowered and uncontrolled for important prognostic factors. The Intergroup Melanoma Trial accessioned 740 patients with well-balanced treatment groups but did not show a survival benefit for the ELND population. In subgroup analysis, however, patients with tumors 1 to 2 mm in thickness were found to have a survival benefit.[26] The Intergroup investigators defend the criticism of subgroup analysis by reason of the detailed stratification used in their trial. A fourth trial, the World Health Organization Melanoma Programme Trial of melanomas arising on the trunk, randomized 240 patients with tumor greater than 1.5 mm in thickness to WLE or WLE plus ELND. The 5-year survival rates were 51.3% and 61.7% (*P* = 0.09), respectively.[17] In this trial, patients with occult nodal metastases did have a statistically significantly longer 5-year survival, suggesting that this may be true for SLN biopsy patients (see later).

The development of the SLN concept ended one debate over ELND, changed clinical management, and opened a new series of questions about the tumor biology of melanoma. In the mid-1970s, Dr. Donald Morton and colleagues described a radionuclide mapping technique to define the lymphatic drainage area from the primary site on the skin. This was designed to answer a perplexing problem for surgeons planning elective lymphadenectomy to resect occult metastases, that is, the at-risk lymph nodes. Primary sites, especially on the trunk and head and neck, could potentially drain to multiple lymphatic basins. This technique used technetium 99m–labeled colloid, injected intradermally at the primary site, to flow through lymphatic vessels and was taken up in regional nodes. This simple outpatient procedure identified the lymphatic basin(s) to be resected. More than 15 years later, Dr. Morton's group utilized blue dye injected intradermally at the primary site to show that the first blue node in the regional lymphatic basin(s) was the node that would contain a metastasis if any tumor were present. This node was termed the *SLN*. The theory was tested by performing the sentinel node biopsy in conjunction with a complete regional dissection.[27] Early reports showed several important findings, as follows:

1. Using a combination of isotope lymphatic mapping, an intraoperative hand-held gamma probe, and intraoperative blue dye, the SLN could be identified in more than 95% of cases.
2. There was great anatomic variation resulting in drainage to multiple or uncommon sites.[28-30]
3. A detailed pathologic analysis of the node using step sections enabled detection of micrometastases that could be missed by the standard techniques.[31]
4. In most cases a positive sentinel node was the only positive node.[32]
5. There were no prognostic factors that accurately identified a subpopulation of SLN-positive patients not requiring completion lymphadenectomy.[33,34]
6. When regional nodal metastases appear after a negative SLN biopsy, in the majority of cases micrometastases can be found in the original SLN by further histologic sectioning and examination.

Additional studies have confirmed that the hottest lymph node (most radioactive) is not always the positive sentinel node. For this reason it is recommended that all nodes with radioactive counts greater than 10% of the hottest node be resected for analysis.[35,36] The details of the SLN biopsy process requires close communication between all members of the team (radiologist, pathologist, and surgeon). The lymphoscintigram can be scheduled on the afternoon before or the day of the operative procedure. Multiple intradermal injections of Tc-99 sulfur colloid (total dose ~ 1 mCi) are made at the perimeter of the biopsy scar. All regional node–bearing areas are scanned under the gamma camera and the sites of uptake are labeled on the lymphoscintigram (and on the patient's skin if necessary) (Fig. 29-10). In the operating room, a hand-held gamma probe is used to precisely localize the most radioactive areas. Prior to the skin prep, isosulfan blue (lymphozurin) dye is injected intradermally at the biopsy margins. During the procedure, a 2- to 3-cm incision is made over the previously identified area and the dissection is performed by blunt dissection until a dye-colored lymphatic vessel is seen (Fig. 29-11). This vessel is traced down to the blue node that is removed. Using a combination of inspection and the gamma probe, the wound is examined for all blue and/or hot nodes. The wound is also palpated because nodes obliterated with tumor may not take up blue dye or radioisotope.

SLN biopsy has rapidly become the standard of care for patients with tumors greater than 1 mm in thickness to accurately stage the disease and provide guidance for treatment planning (see Fig. 29-9).[37] In a retrospective analysis, SLN biopsy appeared to provide a survival benefit compared to WLE alone.[38] The therapeutic benefit is now being evaluated in the Multicenter Selective Lymphadenectomy Trial (MSLT) in which patients with melanomas greater than 1 mm in thickness were randomized to undergo WLE alone or WLE plus SLN biopsy. Patients with positive lymph nodes then underwent completion lymph node dissection. Accessions to this trial

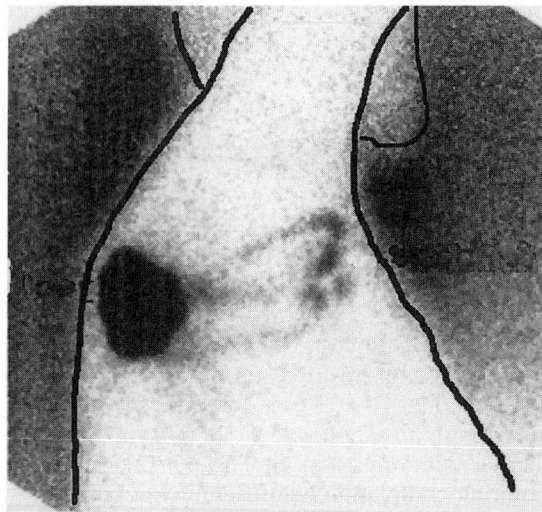

FIGURE 29-10.   Lymphoscintigram showing the lateral view of a patient with a primary melanoma of the back. Note the three parallel lymphatic vascular pathways leading to the axillary sentinel lymph nodes.

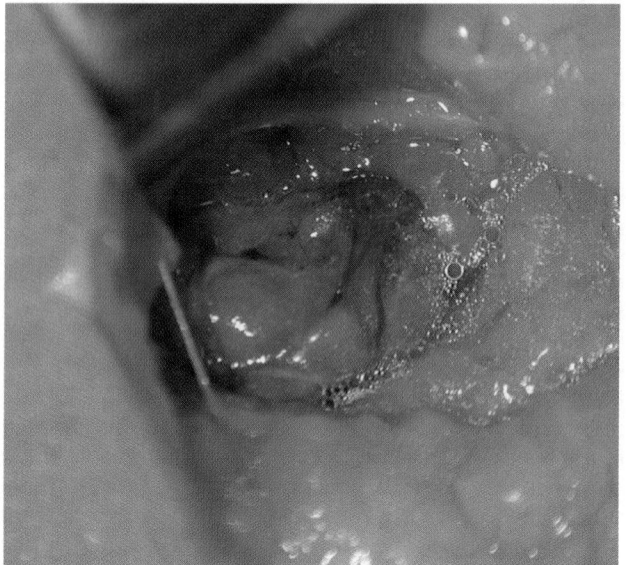

FIGURE 29-11.   Operative view of a sentinel lymph node stained with isosulfan blue dye. Note two parallel afferent vessels leading the sentinel node.

were closed at the end of March 2002 after 2001 patients were enrolled. The primary outcome is melanoma-related death with secondary outcomes being disease-free survival, and local, regional, and distant recurrence rates.

The trial was designed to answer three questions.

1. What is the false-negative rate for SLN biopsy?
2. Is there a survival benefit for patients with micrometastases diagnosed by SLN biopsy?
3. Is there a therapeutic benefit for all patients who undergo SLN biopsy compared to those who have WLE alone?

In so doing, it addresses one of the most fundamental questions in oncology: Is there a therapeutic benefit from the diagnosis and treatment of early lymphatic metastases? If a benefit is observed, it challenges the "modern" theory of Fisher and others who maintain that cancer is systemic from the onset of the metastatic process. If the early detection and resection of metastatic disease makes no difference in the long-term outcome, SLN biopsy will remain an important procedure for the purpose of establishing a prognosis and identifying patients who are candidates for subsequent systemic therapy. The MSLT investigators are planning a second trial to test the value of completion lymph node dissection in patients who are SLN positive.

A second large trial currently examining the value of SLN biopsy is the Sunbelt Melanoma Trial. In this ongoing study, all patients with melanoma greater than 1 mm in thickness undergo SLN biopsy. Patients whose SLN is positive for metastasis by hemotoxylin/eosin, immunohistochemistry (S-100 and HMB-45), or reverse transcriptase polymerase chain reaction (tyronaise, MAGE1, MART3, gp100) may participate in further randomization of surgery (completion lymph node dissection) and/or adjuvant interferon therapy. The role of interferon in stage III patients with melanoma remains controversial. The Sunbelt Melanoma Trial will determine if interferon has a beneficial role to play in the treatment of stage III patients with a minimal burden of metastatic disease.

Monitoring of Patients After Surgical Therapy

After the primary treatment of melanoma, the pattern of recurrences is predictable based on the same factors used to estimate survival (tumor thickness, ulceration, and lymph node status). The risk of the first metastasis being at a distant site increases with thick primary tumors and resected regional positive nodes. Follow-up examinations should focus on the detection of treatable metastases. The most common sites of initial recurrence are local and regional. Patients should be informed about the common symptoms and signs of recurrence so that they can report important changes arising between scheduled examinations. These include local swelling, itching, new lesions in and beneath the skin, enlargement of lymph nodes, central nervous system changes, and pulmonary and gastrointestinal symptoms.

The physical examination is the most important aspect of the return visit. A complete skin examination is performed with inspection and palpation of the primary site and skin surfaces leading to regional nodal basins. In-transit metastases may be palpable but not visible.

The follow-up examination schedule should reflect the risk of developing a recurrence. Initially patients are seen at 3- to 6-month intervals until they have reached the 3-year anniversary. By this time 75% of patients who would ever develop a metastasis would have had that event occur. Annual examinations are scheduled thereafter. Patients with early melanoma, stage IA, are followed without radiologic or laboratory studies. For asymptomatic patients, a chest radiograph and serum lactate dehydrogenase tests may be performed at 6- to 12-month intervals, although there is no evidence that the routine use of these follow-up tests results in a survival benefit. The routine use of screening computed tomographic (CT), magnetic resonance imaging, or positron emission tomographic (PET) scans has not been shown to be cost effective[39] and remains a subject of investigation.[40] In stage III patients, PET scan results change treatment decisions in up to 20% of cases. Scans and other tests may be required for patients participating in clinical protocols.

Surgical Considerations for Metastases

Approximately 80% of patients who develop melanoma are cured of their disease. Recurrent disease appears locally, regionally, or systemically or in a combination of these sites.

Regional Nodal Recurrence

Regional nodal metastases are the most common site of first recurrence in patients who undergo WLE alone. When patients develop palpable lymph nodes, the most rapid form of diagnosis is through the use of fine-needle aspiration (FNA) performed during the office visit. If positive, complete resection of the nodal basin will control regional disease in a large proportion of patients. If the FNA is negative or insufficient, an excisional biopsy should be performed to verify the diagnosis. If nodes are positive, unfortunately the long-term survival is low. Even with a single palpable nodal metastasis, the 5-year survival rate is 40% to 50% (see Table 29-4).

Prior to complete regional lymphadenectomy, a full metastatic work-up is performed. This includes CT scans of the head, chest, abdomen and pelvis, although these scans are normal in the majority of patients who are otherwise asymptomatic. The risk of further locoregional recurrence after complete lymph node basin dissection is increased in the presence of multiple positive nodes, especially those containing extracapsular extension. Postoperative irradiation of the involved areas has been advocated in some centers as a way to further reduce recurrences; however, this has not been tested in a prospective, randomized trial.

Local and Regional Recurrences

True local recurrence (N2c, stage III) is defined as tumor appearing in the skin or subcutaneous tissues within a 5-cm radius of the primary wide excision site (Fig 29-12). The factors that predict local recurrence are the same as those predicting overall survival. Local recurrence risk has been reported to be 0.2% for primary tumors less than 0.76 mm, 2% for those 0.76 to 1.49 mm, 6% for lesions 1.5 to 3.99 mm, and 13% for thick melanomas greater than 4 mm. Local recurrence is a poor prognostic sign: less than 20% of patients survive long term after local recurrence.

The treatment of local recurrence is surgical resection. This should be performed to reach histologically clear margins. WLE guidelines for primary tumors do not apply for local recurrences.

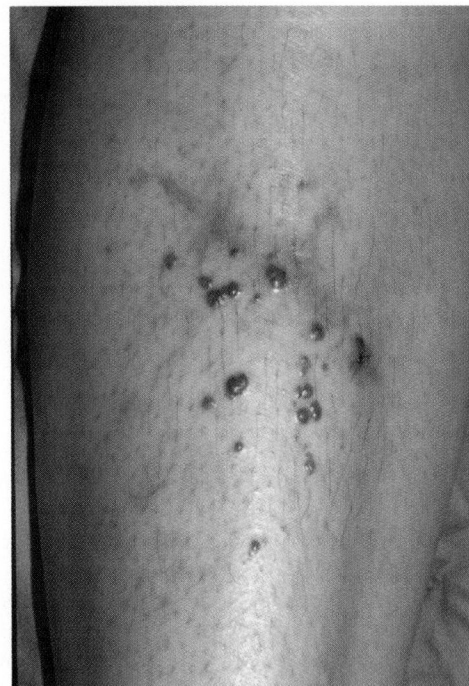

FIGURE 29-12. Multiple local recurrences growing around the scar on the leg of a patient who had undergone wide local excision 4 years earlier.

Amputation for extensive local regional recurrence is seldom indicated. These patients have a high risk of having other distant metastases and therefore long-term disease-free survival is not achieved by resection. Occasionally patients have indolent locoregional disease for which amputation is indicated only after other attempts at locoregional tumor control have been unsuccessful.

Patients with multiple recurrences on the limbs may be candidates for isolated hyperthermic limb perfusion (IHLP). This technique, introduced in the 1950s, uses cannulation of the principal extremity artery and vein, a tourniquet, and hyperthermic perfusion (~40°C) with L-phenylalanine mustard. Interleukin-2, tumor necrosis factor, and multiple other chemotherapeutic agents have also been utilized. Response rates exceed 80%, and complete responses are seen in 10% to 15% of patients. Unfortunately many of these complete responses are short-lived. Reperfusion of extremities can be performed for patients who have an excellent initial response.[41] Based on encouraging results using therapeutic IHLP, a randomized trial was designed to test the value of prophylactic perfusion in patients with high risk (>1.5-mm thickness) melanoma. More than 800 patients participated in this trial comparing WLE to WLE with IHLP. After more than 6 years' median follow-up, there was no improvement in overall survival, although the number of in-transit metastases were reduced from 6.6% to 3.3%.[42] Therefore, IHLP is recommended only for patients with established multiple in-transit metastases.

TABLE 29-6.   One-Year Survival Rates for Patients With Distant Metastases

Stage	Metastatic Site(s)	Approximate 1-Year Survival (%)
M1a	Skin, subcutaneous tissues, lymph nodes	60
M1b	Lung	55
M1c	Other visceral sites	40

Distant Metastases

The most common sites of initial distant metastases are in the brain, lung, and liver and less commonly in the skin, bone, and other gastrointestinal tract sites. The prognosis varies significantly with the site of first metastases (Table 29-6). In the majority of cases, metastases appear at multiple sites simultaneously. Under these circumstances, systemic therapy is indicated for palliation. Occasionally patients develop metastases that are apparently isolated to a single site. These patients should be evaluated for surgical resection because the long-term disease-free survival rate after metastasectomy is reported in the range of 10% to 20%.[43] Patients being considered for resection of visceral metastases should undergo complete staging, including CT and PET scans. In general, the prognosis for metastases to distant sites is related to the number of metastases and the disease-free interval between primary therapy and recurrent disease. Highly selected patients may undergo excision of multiple intra-abdominal metastases with a favorable outcome.[44]

For patients with isolated lung metastases, a period of observation (which may include chemotherapy or investigational protocols) has been recommended to determine if additional metastases are to appear in a short period (4 to 6 weeks). Pulmonary resection is then indicated for patients with no evidence of further recurrence. Melanoma is one of the most frequent tumors that metastasizes to the gastrointestinal tract. These metastases are commonly intramural lesions that may grow to form an intussusception leading to obstruction. Patients who undergo resection of visceral metastases from occult primary sites have been shown to have a better survival than when the primary site has been identified.[45]

Isolated metastases may appear in the adrenal glands, which, if stable, are also appropriately treated by resection. Symptomatic skeletal metastases can be effectively palliated with radiation. Metastases resulting in fractures of weight-bearing bones require internal fixation prior to radiation.

Melanoma patients also present with central nervous system metastases that are commonly multiple lesions at the time of diagnosis. At the time of autopsy, the majority of patients have central nervous system metastases. When single brain metastases cause symptoms, long-term favorable results have been obtained through surgical resection followed by radiation. The most successful form of radiation therapy is a stereotactic program (gamma knife).[46]

Systemic Treatment for Melanoma

Most of the increase in the incidence of melanoma comprises thin melanomas with an excellent prognosis. Unfortunately, the number of deaths from melanoma is also rising. Although melanoma has been reported to metastasize to almost any tissue site, the most common areas are lung, liver, bone, and brain. The most commonly used drug for systemic therapy is dacarbazine (DTIC) which has a response rate of 15% to 30%; however, complete responses are rare. A large number of clinical trials have investigated combinations of chemotherapy in an attempt to improve response rates and prolong survival. A doubling of the response rate has been observed with CVD (cisplatin, vinblastine, dacarbazine) combined with interferon-alfa or interleukin-2 or a combination of these two biologicals. Unfortunately, the increases in survival have been either nonsignificant or less than 6 months. A randomized trial comparing CVD to DTIC indicated a doubling of the response rate and no effect on overall survival. The combination of CVD + interferon + interleukin-2 (frequently called "biochemotherapy") has a response rate of 50% and a complete response rate of 15%; however, several trials of this combination have not resulted in a significant prolongation in survival.[47]

Stage IV patients are also candidates for investigational protocols using immunotherapy.[48,49] It is postulated that stage IV patients who can undergo resection of all detectable disease will be the group of patients who have the best chance of responding to immunotherapy.

Adjuvant Systemic Therapy

Adjuvant systemic therapy has proven to be a distinct advance in the treatment of common cancers such as those arising in the breast and colon. Clinical investigators have been attempting to identify an effective adjuvant therapy for melanoma for more than 40 years and yet there is no treatment regimen that has shown a conclusive benefit. In the mid-1990s the U.S. Food and Drug Administration approved interferon-alfa-2b for adjuvant therapy in treating patients with nodal metastases or thick melanomas in whom the expected survival rate is less than 50%. This approval was based on results from a single trial showing a significant increase in disease-free and overall survival. Subsequent randomized trials of interferon therapy have failed to confirm the initial observation. An updated analyses of randomized trials[50,51] in addition to a meta-analysis[52] do not show a consistent benefit for interferon adjuvant therapy. At the present time, stages IIc and III patients should be evaluated for and invited to participate in randomized clinical trials of adjuvant therapy, when available.

CUTANEOUS MALIGNANCIES: NONMELANOMA SKIN CANCER

SCC and BCC are the most common types of malignant neoplasms in the world. Just as in melanoma, the incidence of these cancers is rising each year. The current predictions are that one in five Americans will develop this disease during his or her lifetime. Fortunately mortality rates for NMSCs are falling, and this is attributed to early detection and effective treatment. Patients who develop any type of skin cancer should have long-term periodic surveillance. After the initial diagnosis of BCC or SCC, the risk of developing an additional skin cancer is estimated to be 35% in 3 years and 50% in 5 years. In addition, there is a risk of developing other common malignancies such as lung cancer.

Squamous Cell Carcinoma Epidemiology and Etiology

By some estimates more than 1 million people develop NMSC annually; however, accurate statistics are problematic for a disease that is often treated without a histologic diagnosis. Although BCC is the most common type of NMSC, SCC has a higher mortality rate. As is true with other types of skin cancer, the incidence of SCC is increasing. There is a disproportionate increasing risk for women compared to men.

The causes of SCC include the following: sunlight, susceptible phenotype, and compromise of immunity, in addition to environmental conditions and diseases. Sunlight is thought to be the major causative factor because most SCCs occur on the sun-exposed surfaces of the head and neck. In susceptible individuals (fair skin, blonde hair, blue eyes), increasing sun exposure carries a growing risk to develop SCC. Individuals with dark complexions have a lower risk even with prolonged sun exposure. Specifically, UVB is thought to be the form of UV radiation causing this disease. Most of the evidence for UV radiation comes from population-based studies in Australia where individuals of Celtic origin moved to a geographic area resulting in higher sun exposure. The pattern of skin cancer appearing in this population indicated that exposure to UV radiation earlier in life was a major risk factor since individuals who moved to Australia after adolescence had a lower incidence of skin cancer than those who moved in childhood. The risk of skin cancer increases with occupational or recreational sun exposure, advancing age, and proximity to the equator. The amount of sun exposure is also proportional to the incidence of precursor skin changes to a SCC, namely nevi, atrophy, and actinic keratosis.

It is postulated that UV radiation affects the skin in two ways that result in an increased incidence of SCC: There is a direct carcinogenic effect on frequently dividing keratinocytes in the basilar layer of the epidermis. Unrepaired mutations result in tumor promotion and growth. The second mechanism relates to the depression of the cutaneous immune surveillance response that in turn inhibits tumor rejection. The *P53* tumor suppressor gene is mutated in more than 90% of SCCs.[4]

Occupational and environmental exposure to arsenic, organic hydrocarbon, ionizing radiation, and cigarette smoke all have been associated with the increasing risk for SCCs. Genetic disorders including xeroderma pigmentosum and albinism are associated with increased risk of many types of skin cancer. Chronic conditions of the skin such as burn scars (Marjolin's ulcer), draining sinuses, infections, and ulcers can predate the development of SCCs. Previously healed wounds that break down or chronic wounds that will not heal should be biopsied for the presence of SCC.

Impaired immunity, especially cell-mediated immunity, is a well-established cause of SCCs of the skin. The largest population of chronically immunosuppressed patients are those undergoing organ transplantation (Fig. 29-13). Immunosuppressive drugs such as eosothyoprin, cyclosporine, and prednisone have been linked to a greater than 50% increase in the risk of SCC. Both the intensity of immunosuppression and the duration of therapy are associated with the risk of development of malignancies. After 10 years of immunosuppression, 10% of patients develop malignancies, and this increases to 40% risk after 20 years.[53] The conditions associated with acquired impaired cell-mediated immunity including lymphomas, leukemias, and autoimmune diseases all increase the risk of development of SCCs. Human papillomavirus, an infection associated with immunosuppression, is proposed as a causative factor of SCCs. Most SCCs begin with a proliferation of keratin cells in the basal layer of epidermis that appear as red or pink areas, clinically termed *actinic keratoses* (solar keratoses). Local symptoms may wax and wane over a period of many months. Lesions are scaling with an uneven surface and an erythematous base. Individual lesions are usually less than 1 cm in diameter and appear in chronically sun-damaged skin. The diagnosis is both clinical and histologic since actinic keratoses have many features in common with SCC in situ microscopically. The overall risk of malignant conversion to an invasive SCC is low and estimated to be in the range of 1 in 1000 per lesion per year.[54] When the reddened area begins to develop a plaque-like thickening, it is termed *Bowen's disease*, which appears histologically as SCC in situ and may vary from small lesions less than 1 cm to large areas of the anogluteal region.

Invasive SCCs are palpable scaling lesions that become ulcerated centrally and have elevated edges (Fig. 29-14).

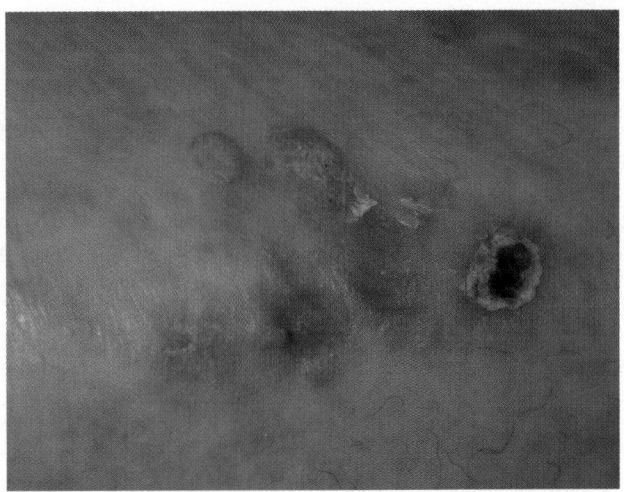

FIGURE 29-13. Squamous cell carcinoma appearing as areas of thickened, red, scaling skin.

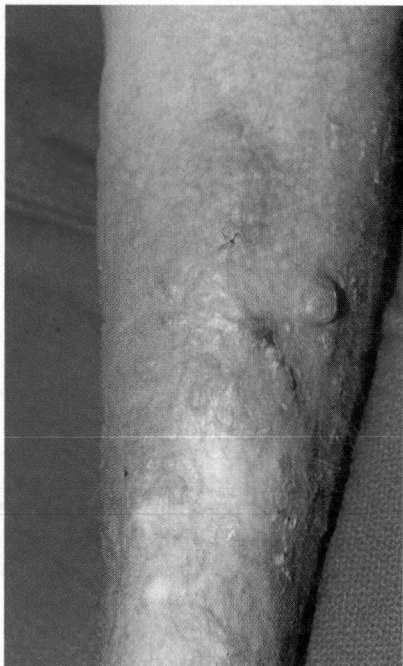

FIGURE 29-14.   Multiple squamous cell carcinomas on the upper extremity of a patient 11 years after kidney transplantation.

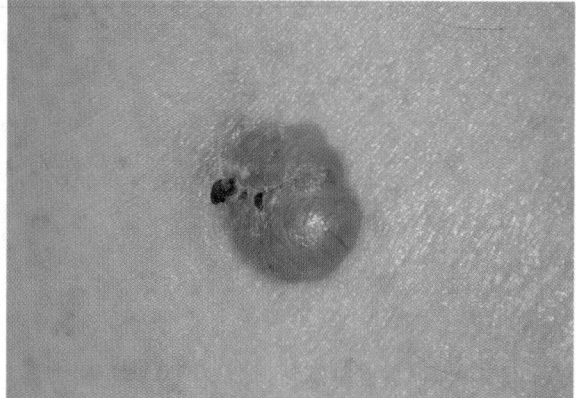

FIGURE 29-15.   Nodular basal cell carcinoma.

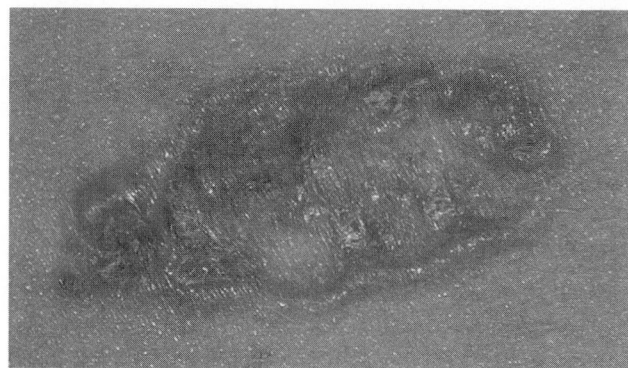

FIGURE 29-16.   Basal cell carcinoma simulating the appearance of psoriasis.

These may be confused with keratoacanthoma, a benign lesion that can also thicken and ulcerate. Biopsy may be required to differentiate between these two conditions.

Most SCCs can be treated locally with excellent results. (see treatment options). Recurrence is associated with tumor size, degree of differentiation, depth of invasion, perineural involvement, immune status of the patient, and anatomic site. Local recurrence is associated with increased risk for regional and distant metastases. The first site of metastases is usually in regional lymph nodes.

Basal Cell Carcinoma

In contrast to SCCs and actinic keratoses, there is no precursor skin lesion for BCCs. These lesions may have an appearance that varies from nodules in the skin to a large nonhealing sore with drainage and crusting. In comparison to SCCs, they have a slow growth rate, which can lead to a delay in diagnosis.

BCCs grow in distinct patterns described as nodular, pigmented, cystic, and superficial. The nodular growth pattern is characterized by a well-defined, elevated lesion with a waxy appearance (Fig. 29-15). As the lesion grows, it develops "pearly" opalescent nodules along the margins. A central depression with umbilication is a classic sign. Distinct blood vessels (telangiectasia) may be seen across the surface of the tumor mass. Although most BCCs are pink or skin colored, they may also have shades of brown or black pigmentation, thereby mimicking a benign mole or melanoma. Cystic BCCs are less common but have a distinctive appearance. Their surface is translucent and may appear blue or gray and be confused with a blue

nevus. Superficial BCCs (20%) are more macular than other growth patterns and may extend over the surface of the skin in a multicentric pattern (Fig. 29-16). The center can ulcerate and the margins become ill defined. These lesions may appear very similar to psoriasis, tenia, or eczema. They may also be multiple pink or red, small slightly elevated lesions that pepper the skin. This is a more aggressive growth pattern that is associated with extension well beyond visible changes in the skin surface and can penetrate deep into the underlying subdermis. The white scarring varieties of this growth pattern are termed *morpheaform*.

BCCs commonly infiltrate locally but rarely metastasize. Metastases are associated with advanced patient age and neglected large lesions. The primary site has often been resected on multiple occasions before metastases appear. The median survival time for patients with metastatic disease is less than 1 year.

Treatment Options for Squamous and Basal Cell Carcinoma

NMSC is staged by different criteria than melanoma. The T stage is determined by the largest diameter of the lesion

Box 29-2. American Joint Committee on Cancer System for Classification and Staging of Carcinomas of the Skin—2002

Primary Tumor (T)

TX	Primary tumor cannot be assessed
T0	No evidence of primary tumor
Tis	Carcinoma in situ
T1	Tumor ≤2 cm in greatest dimension
T2	Tumor >2 cm, but not >5 cm, in greatest dimension
T3	Tumor >5 cm in greatest dimension
T4	Tumor invades deep extradermal structures (i.e., cartilage, skeletal muscle, or bone)

Regional Lymph Nodes (N)

NX	Regional lymph nodes cannot be assessed
N0	No regional lymph node metastasis
N1	Regional lymph node metastasis

Distant Metastasis (M)

MX	Distant metastasis cannot be assessed
M0	No distant metastasis
M1	Distant metastasis

Stage Grouping

Stage 0	Tis	N0	M0
Stage I	T1	N0	M0
Stage II	T2	N0	M0
	T3	N0	M0
Stage III	T4	N0	M0
	Any T	N1	M0
Stage IV	Any T	Any N	M1

TABLE 29-7. Nonmelanoma Skin Cancer: Risk Factors for Local Recurrence Based on Characteristics of the Primary Tumor

Factor	Low Risk	High Risk
Location		
Trunk and extremities	<20 mm	≥20 mm
Forehead and neck	<10 mm	≥10 mm
Central face	<6 mm	≥6 mm
Borders	Well defined	Poorly defined
Incidence	Primary	Recurrent
Immunosuppression	Negative	Positive
Prior radiation therapy/ chronic inflammation	Negative	Positive
Rapid growth rate	Negative	Positive
Neurologic symptoms	Negative	Positive
Differentiation	Well	Moderate or poorly
Perineural/vascular invasion	Negative	Positive

Modified from National Comprehensive Cancer Network Practice Guidelines in Oncology. *www.nccn.org.*

on the skin surface and invasion of extradermal structures (Box 29-2).[16] The overall favorable prognosis and the fact that many patients develop multiple primary skin cancers make this staging system less useful in planning treatment compared to the melanoma staging system.

Actinic keratoses and the precursor lesions of SCC are most often treated with cryotherapy; however, alternate treatments include topical 5-fluorouracil, electrodesiccation and curettage, CO_2 laser, dermabrasion, and chemical peel. A tissue biopsy is indicated when the actinic keratosis is raised or recurrent after topical therapy.

Since multiple techniques are available, the strategy for surgical treatment of SCCs and BCCs begins with an assessment for high-risk factors (Table 29-7). Considerations include size, location, primary versus recurrent, histology, and individual patient factors. All appropriate options should be reviewed with the patient in addition to making a specific recommendation. Surgical resection techniques include a histopathologic analysis to define the margins of resection. In contrast, field therapies treat a generalized area but do not define the status of margins. These approaches include radiation therapy, cryosurgery, curettage, and electrodesiccation.

Standard surgical excision is the preferred treatment for the majority of SCCs and BCCs.[55] This procedure is usually performed under local anesthesia. The margin for resection is not as well defined as in the treatment of melanoma. A minimum acceptable margin is one that is found to be histologically free of carcinoma. This commonly involves a 3- to 4-mm area of normal-appearing skin. The risk of local recurrence is less when wider margins are obtained, especially in the presence of micronodular, infiltrative, and morpheaform histologic patterns. Using these methods, a local "cure" rate should be greater than 90%. An alternative surgical approach is the use of Mohs micrographic excision (MME) in which there is a high rate of local tumor control with the use of horizontal frozen sections. The high success rate of MME is attributed to examination of a greater proportion of the margin of excision in addition to mapping the precise location of any margins found to be positive. Excisions in positive areas continue until clear margins are obtained. MME is ideal under "high-risk" conditions and for anatomic areas where it is important to preserve as much tissue as possible such as around the eye, nose, mouth, and ear.[56]

Although field therapy techniques (cryotherapy, topical fluorouracil, electrodesiccation) do not histologically define the margins of treatment, they may still be effective in local tumor control. Cryotherapy is best suited for small superficial lesions and can be expected to have local control rates of greater than 90%. Treated areas may heal slowly by secondary intention and leave pale scars.

Radiation therapy is highly effective in the treatment of BCC and SCC, especially for preserving wide areas of skin in the head and neck region. Radiation is also useful in treating areas that are at high risk for recurrence after extensive surgical excision.

Uncommon Cutaneous Malignancies

Among the hundreds of specific types of skin conditions and tumors, there are four uncommon skin malignancies that are important for the general surgeon to understand and be prepared to manage.

Cutaneous angiosarcoma is a rare, aggressive soft tissue sarcoma derived from blood or lymphatic endothelium. It is most often seen on the face and scalp of older white men. Angiosarcoma has also been observed as a consequence of chronic lymphedema following axillary dissection for breast cancer (Stewart-Treves syndrome). Angiosarcoma may also arise in irradiated tissues after intervals of 10 to 20 years. The typical presentation is a flat, painless, often pruritic macule or plaque with a red, blue, or purple color that develops into a mass and ulcerates if left in place. Histologically they are high grade and often multifocal with skip areas of normal-appearing skin. Compared to other sarcomas, there is a high incidence of lymph node metastases (~15%). Treatment consists of resection with histologically negative margins and radiation therapy to the involved field. Lymph node dissection is indicated if adenopathy appears before distant metastases are identified. There is no consensus about the role of adjuvant chemotherapy. The 5-year survival rate is less than 40%.

Dermatofibrosarcoma protuberans is a low-grade sarcoma arising from dermal fibroblasts. The lesion appears as a smooth nodule in or immediately beneath the skin (trunk 40% and head/neck 40%) in mid-adult life. Due to their slow growth, lesions are commonly 1 to 2 cm at diagnosis. The external appearance belies the true character because tumor cells frequently invade the underlying soft tissues, leading to incomplete excision and local recurrence. Treatment consists of WLE with 3- to 4-cm margins. Specimen orientation and pathologic analysis of margins are required. Distant metastases are uncommon and are preceded by two or more local recurrences. Radiation therapy has been used effectively after resection of recurrences.

Extramammary Paget's disease (EMPD) is a rare form of adenocarcinoma arising from apocrine glands of the skin most commonly in the perianal area, vulva, and scrotum. The clinical appearance is that of an erythematous plaque but may also be white or depigmented with crusts and scaling. The size is variable from less than 1 cm to an entire area in the anogenital region. Since EMPD can share many clinical characteristics in common with eczema, bacterial and fungal infections, and nonspecific dermatitis, the diagnosis is often made by biopsy of lesions not responding to standard therapies. In the majority of cases EMPD is confined to the epidermis and is well controlled with excision. When invasion of the deeper structures appears, the disease becomes increasingly difficult to control and the mortality rate increases to about 50%. Since EMPD is also associated with an increased risk of simultaneous internal malignancies of the genitourinary and gastrointestinal tracts (~40%), a complete work-up should include a survey of these locations. The standard treatment is surgical resection extending to histologically clear margins. This may require multiple procedures because the histologic changes are best seen on permanent section. Patients require close clinical follow-up because local recurrences are common.[57] Radiation therapy has been reported to reduce local recurrences after excision.

Kaposi's sarcoma, a low-grade soft tissue malignancy, arises from lymphatic vascular endothelial cells in the skin. The incidence is rising because it is most often seen in patients with acquired immunodeficiency syndrome (AIDS) and other immunosuppressed states such as organ transplantation. In patients with human immunodeficiency virus, human herpesvirus-8 (HHV-8) has been identified as the causative agent. There is also a "classic" variant seen on the lower extremities of older men of Eastern European and Mediterranean descent. The clinical picture is variable, beginning as asymptomatic purple to brown bruises and progressing to spots, plaques, or nodules on both lower extremities. Local symptoms appear late as the tumors become advanced. In AIDS patients, skin changes respond best to aggressive antiretroviral therapy. Symptomatic skin lesions can be treated with radiation therapy, intralesional injection of chemotherapeutic agents, cryotherapy, or excision.

Merkel cell carcinoma, derived from neuroendocrine cells, is histologically indistinguishable from small cell carcinoma arising in the lung or any other site. The initial work-up should include a chest radiograph to rule out a pulmonary primary. From any site of origin, a small cell carcinoma is a highly malignant tumor with a propensity to spread locally and regionally to nodes and distant sites. In the skin it presents as a rapidly growing red-blue nodule most frequently in the head and neck area of elderly individuals. The diagnosis is confirmed on biopsy, and the primary treatment is WLE (2 to 3 cm) with histologically confirmed negative margins. SLN biopsy has been used successfully to identify patients with occult regional lymphatic metastases (10% to 30%); however, there is no evidence that patients benefit other than by improved regional tumor control. Involved-field radiation has been shown to reduce the local recurrence rate, and some reports have suggested a survival benefit; however, all studies are too small and uncontrolled to draw definitive conclusions.[58] Although metastases may be responsive to chemotherapy, there is little evidence to support adjuvant systemic therapy. Overall, the prognosis is poor, with variable mortality rates of 55% to 79%.[59]

There are many other forms of cutaneous malignancies and cutaneous conditions associated with malignancy. These are beyond the scope of this chapter; however, the important principles in the management of these entities, as follows, are the same as reviewed earlier:

1. Clinicians should have a low threshold for biopsy of new or changing skin lesions.
2. The diagnosis is made by biopsy and histologic analysis.
3. If appropriate, surgical excision should be performed with histologically defined negative margins.
4. Further treatment and follow-up schedules will be determined by the specific diagnosis.

Selected References

Allen PJ, Coit DG: The surgical management of metastatic melanoma. Ann Surg Oncol 9:762-770, 2002.

> In selected patients, surgical resection of distant melanoma metastases will result in long-term disease-free survival. This is a comprehensive review of indications and results.

Balch CM, Soong S-j, Gerschenwald JE et al: Prognostic factors analysis of 17,600 melanoma patients: Validation of the American Joint Committee on Cancer Melanoma Staging System. J Clin Oncol 19:3622-3634, 2001.

> This detailed analysis of a large melanoma database provides the basis for the new 2002 melanoma staging system.

Balch CM, Soong S-j, Smith T, et al: Long-term results of a prospective surgical trial comparing 2-cm versus 4-cm excision margins for 740 patients with 1–4-mm melanomas. Ann Surg Oncol 8:101-108, 2001.

> This paper summarizes the results of the first randomized trial, balanced for all important prognostic factors, to test the hypothesis that elective lymph node dissection has a therapeutic benefit. No advantage was found.

Chang AE, Karnell LH, Menck HR: The National Cancer Data Base report on cutaneous and noncutaneous melanoma: A summary of 84,836 cases from the past decade. Cancer 83:1664-1678, 1998.

> This patterns of care study from the National Cancer Data Base summarizes the results of the current practice patterns in the United States.

Feldman AL, Alexander HR, Bartlett DL, et al: Management of extremity recurrences after complete responses to isolated limb perfusion in patients with melanoma. Ann Surg Oncol 6:562-567, 1999.

> With standardization of techniques, isolated limb perfusion has become an effective tool in the management of metastatic melanoma in the small number of patients with disease limited to an extremity. This is an excellent summary with complete references.

Hersey P: Adjuvant therapy for high-risk primary and resected metastatic melanoma. Int Med J 33:33-43, 2003.

> This is a well-written summary of all interferon-alfa-2 trials and discussion of the controversy.

National Comprehensive Cancer Network (NCCN) Practice Guidelines in Oncology. *www.nccn.org.*

> The NCCN updates these on-line consensus-based guidelines annually or more often whenever major clinical information becomes available to change practice recommendations. Guidelines are described for all major types of malignancies. A CD-ROM can be ordered free of charge from NCCN.

Rosenberg SA: Progress in the development of immunotherapy for the treatment of patients with cancer. J Int Med 250:462-475, 2001.

> The Rosenberg laboratory is a major center for immunotherapy research for the treatment of melanoma.

Thompson, JF, Shaw HM: The prognosis of patients with thick primary melanomas: Is regional lymph node status relevant, and does removing positive regional nodes influence outcome [editorial]? Ann Surg Oncol 9:719-722, 2002.

> Drs. Thompson and Shaw from the Sydney Melanoma Unit present a well-balanced discussion about the role of lymphatic metastases in patients with a high risk of disease.

References

1. Jemal A, Murray T, Samuels A, et al: Cancer Statistics, 2003. CA Cancer J Clin 53:5-26, 2003.
2. Rigel DS, Carucci JA: Malignant melanoma: Prevention, early detection, and treatment in the 21st century. CA Cancer J Clin 50:215-236, 2000.
3. Gilchrest BA, Eller MS, Geller AC, et al: The pathogenesis of melanoma induced by ultraviolet radiation. N Engl J Med 340:1341-1347, 1999.
4. Brash DE, Ziegler A, Jonason AS, et al: Sunlight and sunburn in human skin cancer: p53, apoptosis, and tumor promotion. J Investig Dermatol Symp Proc 1:136-142, 1996.
5. Tucker MA, Fraser MC, Goldstein AM, et al: A natural history of melanomas and dysplastic nevi: An atlas of lesions in melanoma-prone families. Cancer 94:3192-3209, 2002.
6. Murphy ME, Boyer JD, Stashower ME, et al: The surgical management of Spitz nevi. Dermatol Surg 28:1065-1069, 2002.
7. Su LD, Fullen DR, Sondak VK, et al: Sentinel lymph node biopsy for patients with problematic spitzoid melanocytic lesions. Cancer 97:499-507, 2003.
8. Quinn MJ, Crotty KA, Thompson JF, et al: Desmoplastic and desmoplastic neurotropic melanoma: Experience with 280 patients. Cancer 83:1128-1135, 1998.
9. Chang AE, Karnell LH, Menck HR: The National Cancer Data Base report on cutaneous and noncutaneous melanoma: A summary of 84,836 cases from the past decade. Cancer 83:1664-1678, 1998.
10. Schlagenhauff B, Stroebel W, Ellwanger U, et al: Metastatic melanoma of unknown primary origin shows prognostic similarities to regional metastatic melanoma: Cancer 80:60-65, 1997.
11. Thibault C, Sagar P, Nivatvongs S, et al: Anorectal melanoma—an incurable disease? Dis Colon Rectum 40:661-668, 1997.
12. Abramova L, Parekh J, Irvin WP Jr, et al: Sentinel node biopsy in vulvar and vaginal melanoma: Presentation of six cases and a literature review. Ann Surg Oncol 9:840-846, 2002.
13. Clark WH Jr, From L, Bernadino EA, et al: The histogenesis and biologic behavior of primary human malignant melanomas of the skin. Cancer Res 29:705-727, 1969.
14. Breslow A: Thickness, cross-sectional areas and depth of invasion in the prognosis of cutaneous melanoma. Ann Surg 172:902-908, 1970.
15. Balch CM, Soong S-j, Gerschenwald JE, et al: Prognostic factors analysis of 17,600 melanoma patients: Validation of the American Joint Committee on Cancer melanoma staging system. J Clin Oncol 19:3622-3634, 2001.
16. Greene FL, Page DL, Fleming ID, et al (eds): AJCC Cancer Staging Manual, 6th ed. New York, Springer-Verlag, 2002.
17. Cascinelli N, Morabito A, Santinami M, et al: Immediate or delayed dissection of regional nodes in patients with melanoma of the trunk: A randomized trial. WHO Melanoma Programme. Lancet 351:793-796, 1998.
18. Veronesi U, Cascinelli N: Narrow excision (1-cm margin): A

safe procedure for thin cutaneous melanoma. Arch Surg 126:438-441, 1991.

19. Balch CM, Soong S-j, Smith T, et al: Long-term results of a prospective surgical trial comparing 2-cm versus 4-cm excision margins for 740 patients with 1–4-mm melanomas. Ann Surg Oncol 8:101-108, 2001.

20. Cohn-Cedermark G, Rutquist LE, Andersson R, et al: Long-term results of a randomized study by the Swedish Melanoma Study Group on 2-cm versus 5-cm resection margins for patients with cutaneous melanoma with tumor thickness 0.8–2.0 mm. Cancer 89:1495-1501, 2000.

21. Banzet P, Thomas A, Vuillermin E, et al: Wide versus narrow excision in thin (<2 mm) stage I primary cutaneous melanoma: Long-term results of a French multicentric prospective randomized trial of 319 patients [abstract]. Proc Am Assoc Clin Oncol 12:387, 1993.

22. Heaton KM, Sussman JJ, Gershenwald JE, et al: Surgical margins and prognostic factors in patients with thick (>4 mm) primary melanoma. Ann Surg Oncol 5:322-328, 1998.

23. Irvin WP Jr, Bliss SA, Rice LW, et al: Malignant melanoma of the vagina and locoregional control: Radical surgery revisited. Gynecol Oncol 71:476-480, 1998.

24. Slingluff CL Jr, Stidham KR, Ricci WM, et al: Surgical management of regional lymph nodes in patients with melanoma: Experience with 4682 patients. Ann Surg 219:120-130, 1994.

25. Coates AS, Ingvar CI, Peterson-Schaefer K, et al: Elective lymph node dissection in patients with primary melanoma of the trunk and limbs treated at the Sydney Melanoma Unit from 1960 to 1991. J Am Coll Surg 180:402-409, 1995.

26. Balch CM, Soong S-j, Ross MI, et al: Long-term results of a multi-institutional randomized trial comparing prognostic factors and surgical results for intermediate thickness melanomas (1.0–4.0 mm). Intergroup Melanoma Surgical Trial. Ann Surg Oncol 7:87-97, 2000.

27. Kelley MC, Ollila DW, Morton DL: Lymphatic mapping and sentinel lymphadenectomy for melanoma. Semin Surg Oncol 14:283-290, 1998.

28. Thompson JF, Uren RF, Shaw HM, et al: Location of sentinel lymph nodes in patients with cutaneous melanoma: New insights into lymphatic anatomy. J Am Coll Surg 189:195-206, 1999.

29. Schmalbach CE, Nussenbaum F, Rees RS, et al: Reliability of sentinel lymph node mapping with biopsy for head and neck cutaneous melanoma. Arch Otolaryngol Head Neck Surg 129:61-65, 2003.

30. Chao C, Wong SL, Edwards MJ, et al: Sentinel lymph node biopsy for head and neck melanomas. Ann Surg Oncol 10:21-26, 2003.

31. Clary BM, Brady MS, Lewis JJ, et al: Sentinel lymph node biopsy in the management of patients with primary cutaneous melanoma: Review of a large single-institutional experience with an emphasis on recurrence. Ann Surg 233:250-258, 2001.

32. Chao C, Wong SL, Ross MI, et al: Patterns of early recurrence after sentinel lymph node biopsy for melanoma. Am J Surg 184:520-524, 2002.

33. McMasters KM, Wong SL, Edwards MJ, et al: Frequency of non–sentinel lymph node metastasis in melanoma. Ann Surg Oncol 9:137-141, 2002.

34. Reeves ME, Delgado R, Busam KJ, et al: Prediction of non–sentinel lymph node status in melanoma. Ann Surg Oncol 10:27-31, 2003.

35. McMasters KM, Reintgen DS, Ross MI, et al: Sentinel lymph node biopsy for melanoma: How many radioactive nodes should be removed? Ann Surg Oncol 8:192-197, 2001.

36. McMasters KM, Reintgen DS, Ross MI, et al: Sentinel lymph node biopsy for melanoma: Controversy despite widespread agreement. J Clin Oncol 19:2851-2855, 2001.

37. Thompson JF, Shaw HM: The prognosis of patients with thick primary melanomas: Is regional lymph node status relevant, and does removing positive regional nodes influence outcome [editorial]? Ann Surg Oncol 9:719-722, 2002.

38. Dessureault S, Soong SJ, Ross MI, et al: Improved staging of node-negative patients with intermediate to thick melanomas (>1 mm) with the use of lymphatic mapping and sentinel lymph node biopsy. Ann Surg Oncol 8:766-770, 2001.

39. Swetter SM, Carroll LA, Johnson DL, et al: Positron emission tomography is superior to computed tomography for metastatic detection in melanoma patients. Ann Surg Oncol 9:646-653, 2002.

40. Prichard RS, Hill AD, Skehan SJ, et al: Positron emission tomography for staging and management of malignant melanoma. Br J Surg 89:389-396, 2002.

41. Feldman AL, Alexander HR, Bartlett DL, et al: Management of extremity recurrences after complete responses to isolated limb perfusion in patients with melanoma. Ann Surg Oncol 6:562-567, 1999.

42. Koops HS, Vaglini M, Suciu S, et al: Prophylactic isolated limb perfusion for localized, high-risk limb melanoma: Results of a multicenter randomized phase III trial, European Organization for Research and Treatment of Cancer Malignant Melanoma Cooperative Group Protocol-18832, the World Health Organization Melanoma Program Trial-15, and the North American Perfusion Group Southwest Oncology Group-8593. J Clin Oncol 16:2906-2912, 1998.

43. Allen PJ, Coit DG: The surgical management of metastatic melanoma. Ann Surg Oncol 9:762-770, 2002.

44. Wood TF, DiFronzo LA, Rose DM, et al: Does complete resection of melanoma metastatic to solid intra-abdominal organs improve survival? Ann Surg Oncol 8:658-662, 2001.

45. Vijuk G, Coates AS: Survival of patients with visceral metastatic melanoma from an occult primary lesion: A retrospective match cohort study. Ann Oncol 9:419-422, 1998.

46. Douglas JG, Margolin K: The treatment of brain metastases from malignant melanoma. Semin Oncol 29:518-524, 2002.

47. Eton O, Legha SS, Bedikian AY, et al: Sequential biochemotherapy versus chemotherapy for metastatic melanoma: results from a phase III randomized trial. J Clin Oncol 20:2045-2052, 2002.

48. Dudley ME, Wunderlich JR, Robbins PF, et al: Cancer regression and autoimmunity in patients after clonal repopulation with antitumor lymphocytes. Science 298:850-854, 2002.

49. Rosenberg SA: Progress in the development of immunotherapy for the treatment of patients with cancer. J Int Med 250:462-475, 2001.

50. Hersey P: Adjuvant therapy for high-risk primary and resected metastatic melanoma. Int Med J 33:33-43, 2003.

51. Lens MB, Dawes M: Interferon-alfa therapy for malignant melanoma: A systematic review of randomized controlled trials. J Clin Oncol 20:1818-1825, 2002.

52. Wheatley K, Hancock B, Fore M, et al: Interferon-α as adjuvant therapy for melanoma: A meta-analysis of the randomized trials. Proc Am Soc Clin Oncol 20:1394, 2001.

53. Jensen P, Hansen S, Moller B, Leivestad T, et al: Skin cancer in kidney and heart transplant recipients with different long-term immunosuppressive therapy regimens. J Am Acad Dermatol 40:177-186, 1999.

54. Fu W, Cockerell CJ: The actinic (solar) keratosis. Arch Dermatol 139:66-70, 2003.

55. National Comprehensive Cancer Network Practice Guidelines in Oncology. *www.nccn.org.*

56. Kuijpers DI, Thissen MR, Neumann MH: Basal cell carcinoma: Treatment options and prognosis, a scientific approach to a common malignancy. Am J Clin Dermatol 3:247-259, 2002.

57. Pierie JP, Choudry U, Muzikansky A, et al: Prognosis and management of extramammary Paget's disease and the association with secondary malignancies. J Am Coll Surg 196:45-50, 2003.

58. Medina-Franco H, Urist MM, Fiveash J, Heslin MJ, et al: Multimodality treatment of Merkel cell carcinoma: Case series and literature review of 1024 cases. Ann Surg Oncol 8:204-208, 2001.

59. Goessling W, McKee PH, Mayer RJ: Merkel cell carcinoma. J Clin Oncol 20:588-598, 2002.

CHAPTER 30

SOFT TISSUE SARCOMAS AND BONE TUMORS

SOFT TISSUE SARCOMAS

Samuel Singer, M.D.   and   Murray F. Brennan, M.D.

Predisposing Factors and Molecular Genetics	**Management**
Pathologic Evaluation	**Treatment of Recurrent Disease**
Clinical Evaluation and Diagnosis	**Prognostic Factors and Results**
Evaluation of Extent of Disease	**Long-Term Follow-Up**
Staging	**Summary**

Soft tissue sarcomas are rare and unusual neoplasms, accounting for about 1% of adult human cancers and 15% of pediatric malignancies. However, sarcomas continue to carry biologic and clinical interest and significance disproportionate to their clinical frequency because of the often clearly defined molecular genetic basis and the challenges they pose in diagnosis and management. Although these tumors may develop in any anatomic site, approximately 50% occur in the extremities, followed in order of frequency by the abdominal cavity/retroperitoneum, trunk/thoracic region, and head and neck.[1] This section focuses on the biology and management of soft tissue sarcomas among adults (>16 years old).

PREDISPOSING FACTORS AND MOLECULAR GENETICS

In most patients, no specific etiologic agent is found. Multiple predisposing factors have been identified (Box 30-1). Genetic syndromes such as neurofibromatosis, familial adenomatous polyposis, and the Li-Fraumeni syndrome have all been shown to be associated with the development of soft tissue sarcoma.[2-4] Ionizing radiation and lymphedema are well-established but uncommon antecedents to the development of soft tissue sarcoma.[5,6] The association with trauma is uncertain as a true causal factor. Chemical carcinogens have also been widely implicated, but the data to support their association are not well founded.[7-9]

Genetic alterations that play a role in the development of soft tissue sarcoma segregate into two major types. The first type consists of sarcomas with specific genetic alterations that include simple karyotypes, including fusion genes due to reciprocal translocations and specific point mutations such as *KIT* mutations in gastrointestinal stromal tumors and *APC*/β-catenin mutations in desmoid tumors. The second type consists of sarcomas with nonspecific genetic alterations and typically complex unbalanced karyotypes, representing numerous genetic losses and gains. A significant subset of soft tissue sarcoma, as well as most types of adipocytic tumors, are characterized by specific chromosomal aberrations, most commonly reciprocal translocations, which can be diagnostically[10-13] and occasionally prognostically useful (Table 30-1).[14,15] The fusion gene translocations include 11 different gene fusions involving the *EWS* gene or *EWS* family members *(TLS, TAF2N)* found in five different sarcomas and 10 other types of fusions in seven other sarcoma types.[16] If conventional cytogenetics is not available, molecular genetic techniques (e.g., reverse transcription polymerase chain reaction and fluorescence in situ hybridization) are very useful as diagnostic adjuncts. In addition, investigation of molecular changes of genes at the sites of chromosomal alterations has led to the identification of novel genes and the characterization of their mechanisms of deregulation. The tumor suppressor genes best studied in sarcomas are *p53* and *RB1*. Inactivation of both genes is involved in the tumorigenesis of several sarcomas.[12,17,18]

Box 30-1. Predisposing Factors for Sarcomas

Genetic Predisposition

Neurofibromatosis (von Recklinghausen's disease)
Li-Fraumeni syndrome
Retinoblastoma
Gardner's syndrome (familial adenomatous polyposis)

Radiation Exposure

Ortho- and megavoltage therapeutic radiation

Lymphedema

Postsurgical
Postirradiation
Parasitic infection (filariasis)

Trauma

Post parturition
Extremity

Chemical

2,3,7,8-Tetrachlorodibenzodioxin (TCDD)
Polyvinyl chloride
Hemachromatosis
Arsenic

The relevance of the *p53* gene to sarcoma tumorigenesis is underscored by the frequent occurrence of soft tissue sarcomas in the Li-Fraumeni syndrome; all families studied have *p53* germline mutations. The major mechanisms of *p53* pathway inactivation in sarcomas include *p53* point mutations, homozygous deletion of *CDKN2A*, which encodes both *p14ARF* and *p16,* and *MDM2* amplification. In sarcomas with specific reciprocal translocations, *p53* pathway alteration is a rare event, but when present it is a strong prognostic factor, associated with significantly decreased survival in synovial sarcoma,[19,20] myxoid liposarcoma,[21] and Ewing's sarcoma/peripheral neuroectodermal tumor (PNET).[22,23] Decreased survival in Ewing's sarcoma/ PNET was associated with deletion of *CDKN2A*, representing a type of *p53* pathway alteration through loss of the *CDKN2A* alternative product p14ARF.[24,25] In contrast, in sarcomas with nonspecific genetic alterations and complex karyotypes, *p53* pathway alteration is more common and has weaker prognostic value, often requiring large numbers of patients to achieve statistical significance, as demonstrated in several studies of mixed adult soft tissue sarcoma.[26,27] Its high prevalence in this class of sarcomas may account for its limited ability to define distinct clinical prognostic subsets in these tumors.

In addition to serving as very specific and powerful diagnostic markers, fusion genes resulting from translocations encode chimeric proteins that are important determinants of tumor biology, acting as abnormal transcription factors that alter the transcription of multiple

TABLE 30-1. Cytogenetic and Molecular Abnormalities in Sarcomas

Histologic Type	Cytogenetic Changes	Gene Rearrangement/Molecular Abnormality
Synovial sarcoma	t(X;18)(p11.2;q11.2)	*SYT-SSX1* fusion *SYT-SSX2* fusion
Myxoid/round cell liposarcoma	t(12;16)(q13;q11) t(12;22)(q13;q11-12)	*CHOP-TLS* fusion *CHOP-EWS* fusion
Ewing's sarcoma	t(11;22)(q24;q12) t(21;22)(q22;q12) t(7;22)(p22;q12) t(17;22)(q12;q12) t(2;22)(q33;q12)	*FLI1-EWS* fusion *ERG-EWS* fusion *ETV1-EWS* fusion *EIAF-EWS* fusion *FEV-EWS* fusion
Alveolar rhabdomyosarcoma	t(2;13)(q35;q14) t(1;13)(p36;q14)	*PAX3-FKHR* fusion *PAX7-FKHR* fusion
Extraskeletal myxoid chondrosarcoma	t(9;22)(q22;q12)	*TEC-EWS* fusion
Dermatofibrosarcoma protuberans	t(17;22)(q22;q13)	*PDGFB-COL1A1* fusion
Desmoplastic small round cell tumor	t(11;22)(p13;q12)	*WT1-EWS* fusion
Clear cell sarcoma	t(12;22)(q13;q12)	*ATF1-EWS* fusion
Infantile fibrosarcoma	t(12;15)(p13;q25)	*ETV6-NTRK3* fusion
Alveolar soft part sarcoma	17q25 rearrangement	Unknown
Atypical lipomatous tumor/well-differentiated liposarcoma	12q rings and giant markers	*HMGI-C, CDK4,* and *MDM2* amplification
Leiomyosarcoma	complex	*RB1* point mutations or deletions
Malignant fibrous histiocytoma	complex	*p53* point mutations or deletions
Malignant peripheral nerve sheath tumor	t(11;22) (q24;q11.2-12)	

downstream genes and pathways.[28] The structure of these chimeric proteins play a prominent role in the pathogenesis of sarcoma, as evidenced by the impact of relatively minor cytogenetic variability, as a result of variant molecular breakpoints, on tumor phenotype and clinical behavior.[15,29-31] A recent analysis of synovial sarcoma has clearly identified a characteristic *SYT-SSX* fusion gene resulting from the chromosomal translocation t(x;18)(p11;q11) detectable in almost all synovial sarcomas. Translocation fuses the *SYT* gene from chromosome 18 to either of two highly homologous genes at Xp11, SSX1, or SSX2. *SYT-SSX1* and *SYT-SSX2* are thought to function in aberrant transcriptional regulation. Recent analysis has suggested that these fusion products may influence outcome. It does appear that all biphasic synovial sarcomas have an *SYT-SSX1* fusion transcript, and tumors that were positive for *SYT-SSX2* were monophasic. Conversely, monophasic sarcomas may have either transcript.[14]

PATHOLOGIC EVALUATION

There are more than 50 histologic subtypes, many of which are associated with distinctive clinical, therapeutic, or prognostic features. Detailed descriptions of the histopathologic classification and guidelines for the histologic reporting of soft tissue sarcoma have been published elsewhere.[32] To summarize, the most commonly found are liposarcoma, malignant fibrous histiocytoma (MFH), and leiomyosarcoma (Fig. 30-1). Histopathology is anatomic site dependent: the common subtypes in the extremity are liposarcoma or MFH; in the retroperitoneal location liposarcoma and leiomyosarcoma are the most common histiotypes, whereas in the visceral location, gastrointestinal stromal tumors are found almost exclusively (Fig. 30-2). Age is also a factor in histopathology. In childhood, embryonal rhabdomyosarcoma is most common; synovial sarcoma is more likely to be seen in young adults (<35 years old); and there is an even distribution of liposarcoma and MFH as the predominant types in the older popula-

tion (Fig. 30-3). Sarcoma histiotype is generally an important determinant of prognosis and a predictor of distinctive patterns of behavior, because none of the existing grading systems is ideal and applicable to all tumor types. Biologic behavior is currently best predicted based on histologic type, histologic grade, tumor size, and depth. Although many published series have combined all the histologic types of sarcoma, the significance of such subtyping is exemplified by liposarcoma in which the five subsets (well differentiated, dedifferentiated, myxoid, round cell, and pleomorphic) have totally different biologies and patterns of behavior.[32] A further clear demonstration is the importance of myogenic differentiation in pleomorphic sarcomas, which is associated with a substantially increased risk of metastasis.[33] In a postoperative

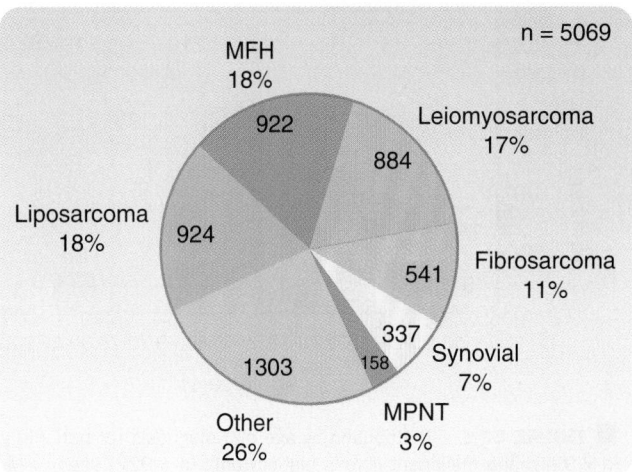

FIGURE 30-1.   Histopathologic subtype distribution of 5069 patients with soft tissue sarcoma treated at Memorial Sloan-Kettering Cancer Center from July 1, 1982, through June 30, 2002. These data include extremity, trunk, visceral, and retroperitoneal tumors. MFH, malignant fibrous histiocytoma; MPNT, malignant peripheral nerve tumor.

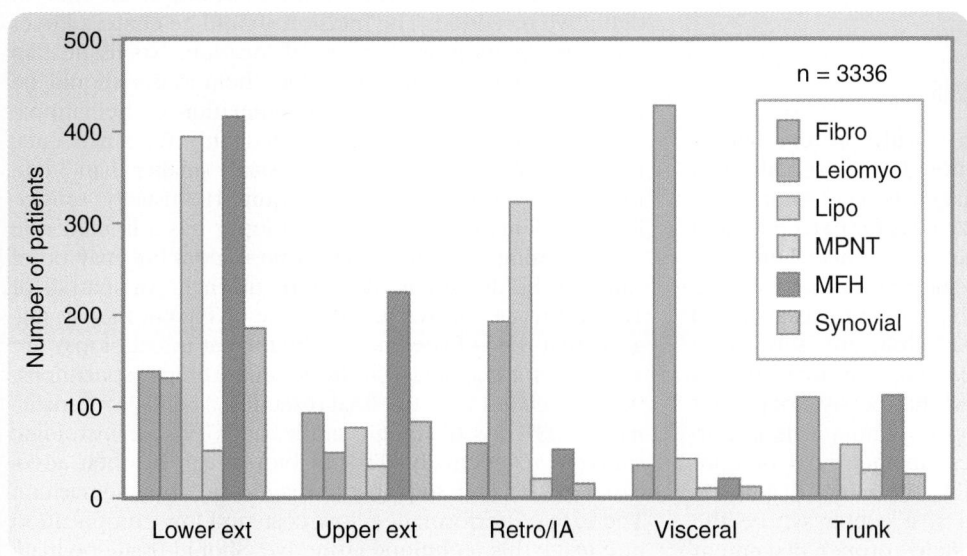

FIGURE 30-2.   Site-specific histopathologic subtype distribution of 3336 patients with soft tissue sarcoma treated at Memorial Sloan-Kettering Cancer Center from July 1, 1982, through June 30, 2002. MFH, malignant fibrous histiocytoma; MPNT, malignant peripheral nerve tumor.

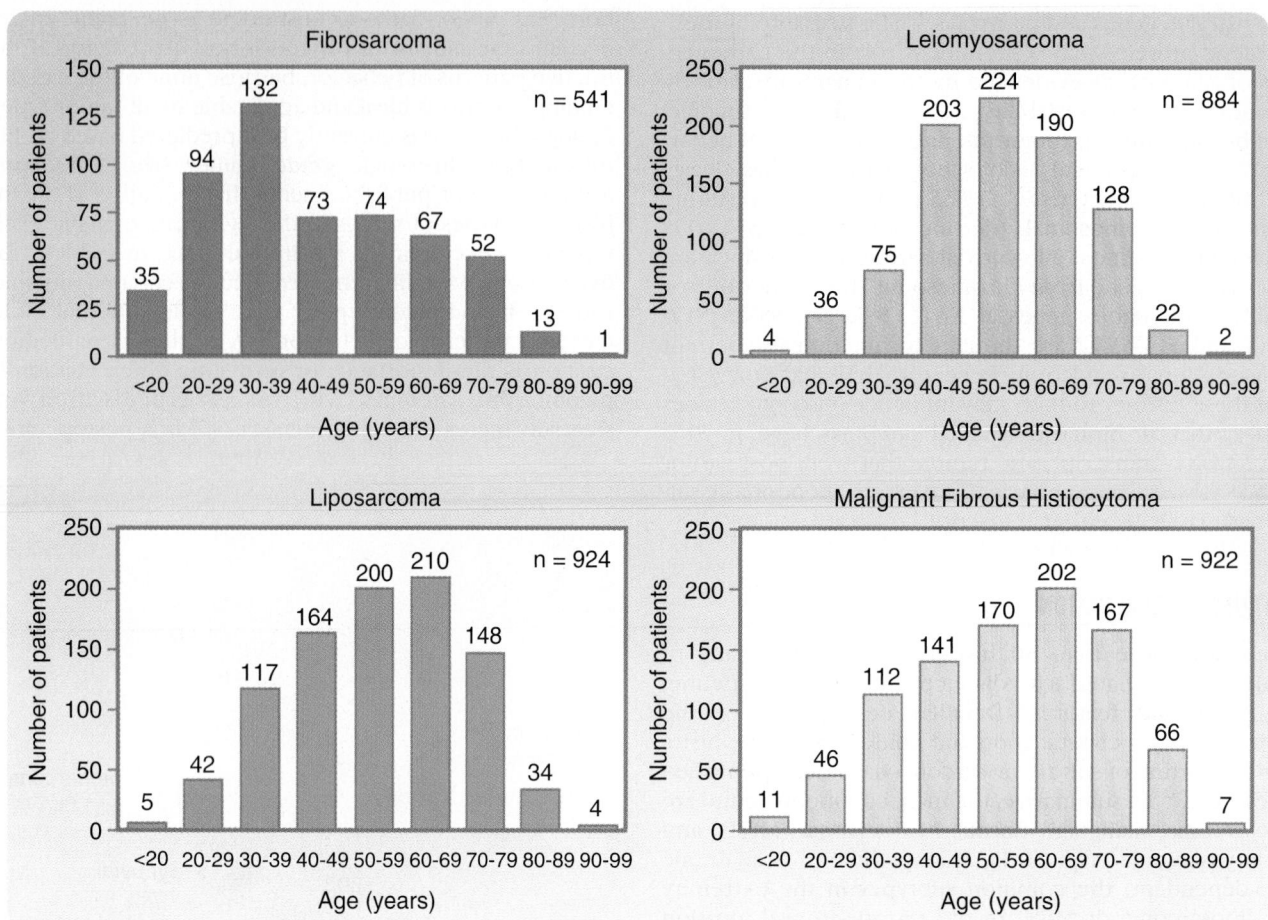

FIGURE 30-3.   Distribution by age and diagnosis for patients with fibrosarcoma (n = 541), leiomyosarcoma (n = 884), liposarcoma (n = 924), and malignant fibrous histiocytoma (n = 922) seen at Memorial Sloan-Kettering Cancer Center from July 1, 1982, through June 30, 2002.

nomogram based on a database of 2136 adult patients from MSKCC, histologic type was found to be one of the most important predictors of sarcoma-specific death, with malignant peripheral nerve sheath tumors having the highest risk of mortality.[34]

CLINICAL EVALUATION AND DIAGNOSIS

Patients with extremity sarcoma usually present with a painless mass, although pain is noted at presentation in up to 33% of patients. Delay in diagnosis is common, with the most common differential diagnosis for extremity and trunk lesions being a hematoma or a "pulled" muscle. Physical examination should include assessment of the size of the mass and its relationship to neurovascular and bony structures. Generally, in an adult, any soft tissue mass that is symptomatic or enlarging, any mass that is larger than 5 cm, or any new mass that persists beyond 4 weeks should be sampled.[35] Biopsy technique is important. For most soft tissue masses, an incisional or core biopsy is usually preferred. Ideally, the initial diagnostic procedure should be performed at a center where the patient will be treated. This facilitates proper placement

of the biopsy site (or incision) and also avoids the complications and diagnostic difficulties that can arise if such biopsy samples are handled infrequently. Limb masses are generally best sampled through a longitudinal incision so that the entire biopsy tract can be excised at the time of definitive resection. The incision should be centered over the mass in its most superficial location. No tissue flap should be raised, and meticulous hemostasis should be ensured to prevent cellular dissemination by hematoma. Excisional biopsy is recommended only for small cutaneous or subcutaneous tumors, usually smaller than 3 cm, in which a wide re-excision (if required) is usually straightforward. Fine-needle aspiration biopsy has a limited role in diagnosing extremity soft tissue tumors but may be of value in the documentation of recurrence. An analysis of 164 soft tissue masses for the value of Tru-cut biopsy suggests that 83% of specimens obtained at initial biopsy are adequate for diagnosis. Of the adequate biopsy specimens, 95% correlated with the final resection diagnosis for malignancy, 88% for histologic grade, and 75% for histologic subtype, respectively. Tru-cut biopsy can be then advocated as the first step in the diagnostic armamentarium. The ease of performance, low cost, and low complication rate make this technique attractive. Should tissue be inad-

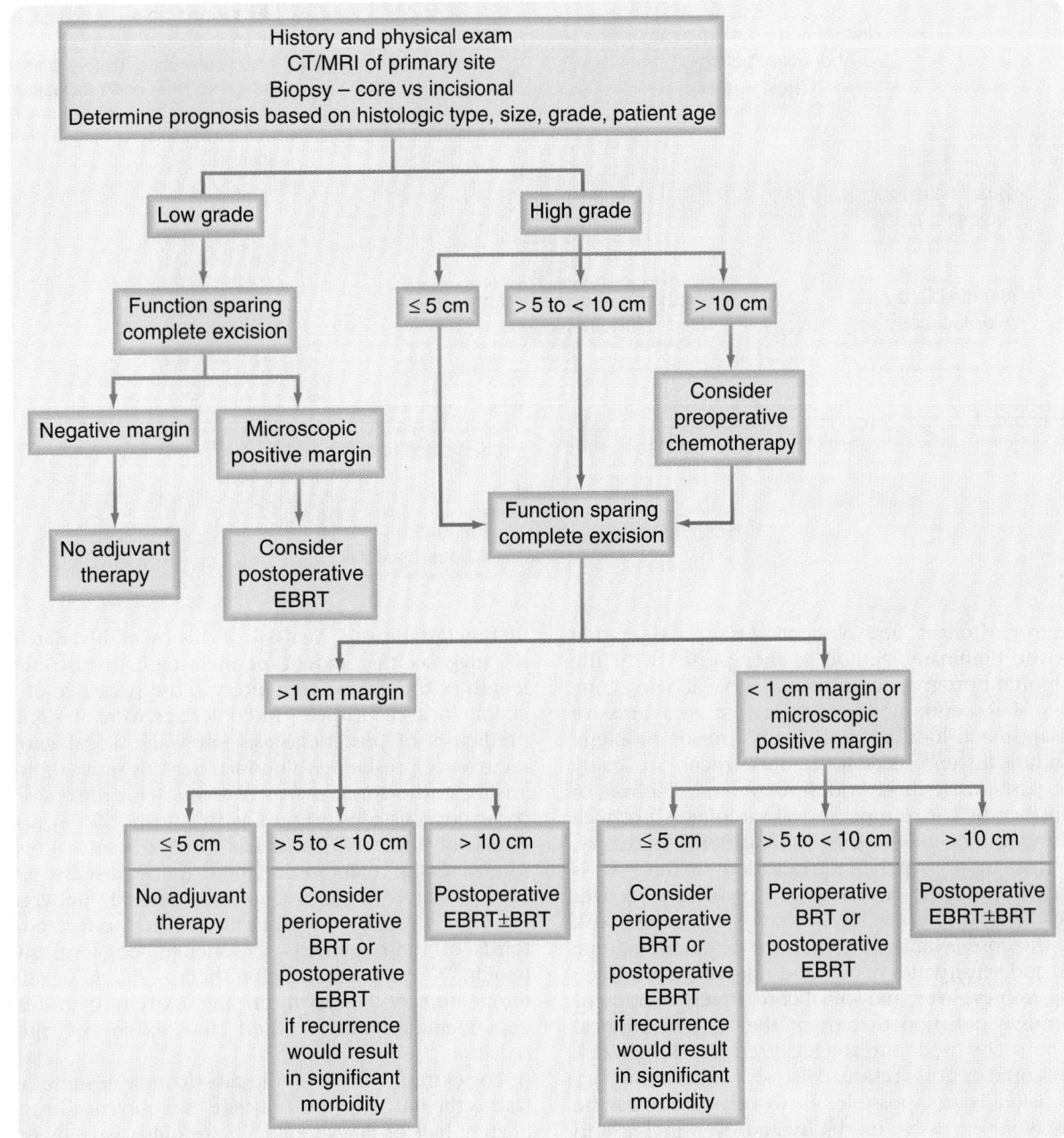

FIGURE 30-5. Algorithm for management of primary (with no metastases) extremity or trunk soft tissue sarcoma, using a biologic rationale (i.e., size and grade of tumor). CT, computed tomography; MRI, magnetic resonance imaging; EBRT, external beam radiation therapy; BRT, brachytherapy.

amputation, then adjuvant radiation therapy should be added to the surgical resection to reduce the probability of local failure.[51] However, irrespective of grade, we believe that postoperative irradiation is probably used more than is strictly necessary. In fact, several studies have shown that a significant subset of subcutaneous and intramuscular sarcomas can be treated by wide excision alone, with a local recurrence rate of 5% to 10%.[53,54]

The value of chemotherapy depends on the histologic type of sarcoma. Neoadjuvant chemotherapy is usually indicated for the treatment of Ewing's sarcoma (PNET) and rhabdomyosarcoma, because of the high risk of microscopic metastasis at diagnosis and high response rate seen

to such therapy.[55,56] The potential for cure is inversely proportional to the volume and spread of disease. For other histologic subtypes of sarcoma the role of chemotherapy remains controversial. Adjuvant chemotherapy has had no measurable impact on overall survival, with a small 10% to 15% improvement in disease-free survival.[57,58] Thus, adjuvant chemotherapy for soft tissue sarcoma should be regarded as investigational and is rarely indicated, except in a clinical trial. The preoperative use of neoadjuvant combination chemotherapy (usually with doxorubicin [Adriamycin] and ifosfamide) may be justified in carefully selected high-risk patients with large, high-grade tumors.

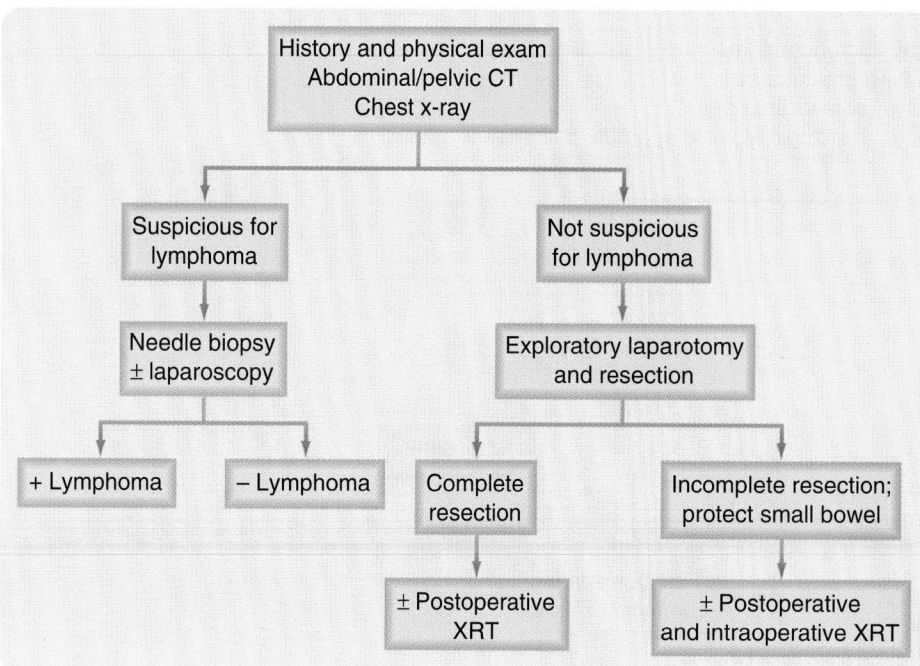

FIGURE 30-6. Algorithm for management of primary retroperitoneal or visceral soft tissue sarcoma. Fine-needle aspiration biopsy is not routinely used. CT, computed tomography; XRT, x-ray therapy.

In retroperitoneal and visceral lesions, operation remains the dominant method of therapy,[38,59] with the most important prognostic factors for survival being completeness of resection and grade. Despite an aggressive surgical approach local control is still a major problem, and multifocal, unresectable tumors recur in many patients, particularly those with liposarcoma. The role of radiation therapy for retroperitoneal sarcoma is not well defined and is in need of further investigation.[60] In theory, preoperative or postoperative irradiation to this site is desirable, but in reality it is often not possible to deliver full-dose radiation therapy (60 to 66 Gy) to areas at risk because the dose is limited by the large treatment volume required and sensitivities of adjacent normal tissues, such as bowel, kidney, liver, and spinal cord. Brachytherapy or intraoperative radiation therapy at the time of surgical resection may be used to treat a localized area at high risk of microscopic or gross residual disease when further surgical excision is not possible. However, care must be taken to avoid excessive morbidity and even increase in mortality that may result from aggressive brachytherapy, particularly when combined with external-beam radiation therapy.[61] Trials of preoperative radiation therapy with or without intraoperative irradiation are underway.

TREATMENT OF RECURRENT DISEASE

Despite optimum multimodality limb-sparing treatment for extremity soft tissue sarcoma, a significant number of patients continue to develop distant metastasis. In a recent analysis of 994 patients with primary extremity soft tissue sarcomas and a median follow-up of 33 months, distant metastasis developed in 230 patients (23%). Median survival after the development of metastasis was 11.6 months, and in 73% of these patients the lungs were the first metastatic site. Analysis of this by multivariate analysis suggests that extent of metastatic disease and the length of the disease-free interval, the presence of a preceding local recurrence, and older age were all significant predictors of post-metastasis survival.[62] Local extremity recurrence presents as a nodular mass or series of nodules arising in the surgical scar. Patients with retroperitoneal recurrence usually present with nonspecific symptoms, often only after the lesion has reached a substantial size. After work-up to determine the extent of disease, patients with isolated local recurrence should undergo re-resection. When re-resection can be performed, two thirds of these patients experience long-term survival benefit.[63,64] Adjuvant radiation therapy should be administered after re-operation on the extremity, if feasible, dependent on the method and extent of previous radiation.

For extremity lesions, the most common site of metastasis is the lung. It is the only site of recurrence in approximately half of all patients.[65] Extrapulmonary metastases are relatively uncommon and usually occur as a late manifestation of widely disseminated disease. Patients whose primary tumors are controlled or controllable, who have no extrathoracic disease, who are medically fit for thoracotomy, and in whom complete resection of all lung disease appears possible should undergo thoracotomy with the intent of resecting all disease.[62,65] Patients with unresectable pulmonary metastases or extrapulmonary metastatic sarcoma in more than a single site have a uniformly poor prognosis and are best treated with systemic chemotherapy. The role of chemotherapy in advanced sarcoma is controversial[66] and, at present, the treatment of metastatic sarcoma represents palliative, not curative, therapy. Current active drugs that have significant response rates include doxorubicin, ifosfamide, and dacarbazine (DTIC), but none has had a major impact on long-term survival.[67] The combination of mesna, ifosfamide, doxorubicin, and dacarbazine (MAID) has been shown to have a 47% response rate and a 10% complete response rate.[68] Randomized prospective clinical trials on combination chemotherapy regimens such as MAID and other ifosfamide-doxorubicin combinations with cytokine support have been shown to yield statistically improved rates of antitumor response.[67,69] However, these do not translate into improvements in survival and come at the cost of increased toxicity and a decrease in quality of life.

Given the limitations and toxicities associated with cytotoxic chemotherapy, emphasis has been to develop novel drugs against rational drug targets such as the *KIT* receptor tyrosine kinase, which is constitutively activated in most gastrointestinal stromal tumors (GISTs). GISTs are mesenchymal neoplasms showing differentiation toward the interstitial cells of Cajal and are typically characterized by the expression of the receptor tyrosine kinase *KIT* (CD117).[70] Recent studies have established that activating mutations of *KIT* are present in up to 92% of GISTs and likely play a key role in the development of these tumors.[71,72] Along with mitotic activity, histologic subtype, and size, the type and the location of *KIT* mutation are prognostic for survival in patients with GIST.[73] Imatinib is a competitive inhibitor of *BCR-ABL, KIT, PDGFR* tyrosine kinases.[74] In preclinical studies, imatinib was active against mutant isoforms of *KIT* commonly found in GIST.[75] A recently completed phase II trial has shown substantial response rates as well as clinical benefit of imatinib in patients with advanced and metastatic GIST,[76] a group typically highly resistant to convention doxorubicin/ifosfamide-based chemotherapy. A total of 147 patients were randomly assigned to receive 400 mg or 600 mg of imatinib daily. Overall, 79 patients (53.7%) had a partial response, 41 patients (27.9%) had stable disease, and, for technical reasons, response could

not be evaluated in 7 patients (4.8%). No patient had a complete response to the treatment. The median duration of response had not been reached after a median follow-up of 24 weeks after the onset of response. Early resistance to imatinib was noted in 20 patients (13.6%). Therapy was well tolerated, although mild-to-moderate edema, diarrhea, and fatigue were common. Gastrointestinal or intra-abdominal hemorrhage occurred in approximately 5% of patients. There were no significant differences in toxic effects or response between the two doses. Thus, inhibition of the *KIT* signal-transduction pathway is a promising treatment for gastrointestinal stromal tumors. Trials are presently underway to evaluate the efficacy of adjuvant imatinib therapy for patients with primary GIST larger than 2.5 cm.

PROGNOSTIC FACTORS AND RESULTS

A prospective collected series of over 1000 patients has characterized the risk factors for outcome in patients with extremity soft tissue sarcoma.[77] Overall 5-year survival for this cohort of patients was 76% with a median follow-up time of 4 years. Significant independent adverse prognostic factors are outlined in Table 30-4. The important prognostic factors for local recurrence were age greater than 50, recurrent disease at the time of presentation, microscopically positive surgical margins, and the histologic subtypes fibrosarcoma and malignant peripheral nerve tumor.

For distant recurrence, large tumor size, deep location, high histologic grade, recurrent disease at presentation, and leiomyosarcoma and nonliposarcoma histology were all independent adverse prognostic factors, as was depth. For disease-specific survival, large tumor size, high grade, deep location, recurrent disease at presentation, histologic subtypes leiomyosarcoma and malignant peripheral

TABLE 30-4. Multivariate Analysis of Prognostic Factors for Outcome, in 1041 Patients with Extremity Soft Tissue Sarcoma Managed at a Single Institution

	Local Recurrence	Distant Recurrence	Disease-Specific Survival
Age > 50	0.001		
Recurrent presentation	0.0001	0.015	0.003
Size > 10 cm		0.03	0.0001
Size > 5 cm		0.0001	
Deep location		0.0007	0.0002
Grade high		0.0001	0.0001
Histology: fibrosarcoma	0.006		
Not liposarcoma		0.003	
Leiomyosarcoma		0.024	0.012
Malignant peripheral nerve tumor	0.001		0.008
Margin positive	0.0001		0.011

Modified from Pisters P, Leung D, Woodruff J, et al: Analysis of prognostic factors in 1041 patients with localized soft tissue sarcomas of the extremity. J Clin Oncol 14:1679, 1996.

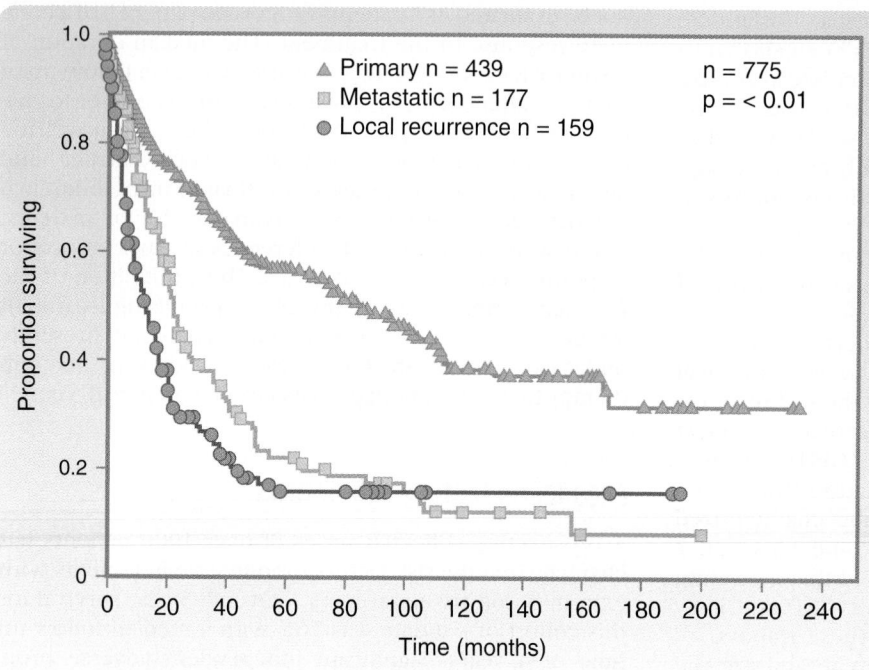

FIGURE 30-7. Disease-specific survival for patients with retroperitoneal/intra-abdominal soft tissue sarcoma grouped by presentation status. Of the 775 patients, 439 (56%) had primary disease, 159 (21%) had local recurrence, and 177 (23%) had metastasis. Median survival was 86 months for those with primary disease, 23 months for those with local recurrence, and 12 months for those with metastasis. Patients were seen at Memorial Sloan-Kettering Cancer Center from July 1, 1982, to June 30, 2002.

nerve tumor, and microscopically positive margins were all adverse prognostic factors. This emphasizes that there are numerous independent adverse prognostic factors for distant recurrence and disease-specific survival and that these are clearly different from those involved in local recurrence.

For retroperitoneal soft tissue sarcoma, an analysis of 500 patients with retroperitoneal soft tissue sarcoma treated and followed at a single institution has been reported.[38] Two hundred seventy-eight of these patients presented with a primary tumor, and 422, or 44%, presented with recurrent disease with a median follow-up of 28 months (1 to 172 months with 40-month follow-up for all survivors); this suggests a median survival of 72 months for patients with primary disease, 28 months for those with local recurrence and 10 months for those presenting with metastasis. Patients with locally recurrent tumors, unresectable disease, or incomplete resection and high-grade tumors all had a diminished survival time. Both for primary and locally recurrent tumors, the ability to completely resect the tumor was a predominant factor in outcome. After complete resection, the presence of a low-grade tumor was a favorable factor for outcome. Disease-specific survival is illustrated in Figure 30-7. It was of value to re-resect patients who experienced recurrence, the complete resectability rate falling with progressive recurrence with few tumors ever being able to be completely resected after a third or subsequent recurrence.

An analysis of 200 patients identified as having GISTs morphologically but not by expression of *KIT* by immunohistochemistry has suggested that complete surgical resection is the only factor that makes a significant outcome benefit for the patient.[44] Size but not microscopic margin appears to be a factor in predicting survival. A more recent analysis of 49 patients with GIST,[73] all confirmed by significant immunohistochemical expression of *KIT*, has demonstrated the prognostic importance of both mitotic activity and GIST mutation type in predicting sarcoma-specific survival in a group of patients with GISTs before the availability of imatinib therapy. In contradistinction to retroperitoneal sarcomas, recurrence occurs equally both locally (throughout peritoneal cavity) and systemically in the liver. Unfortunately, almost half of all patients will present with metastasis, usually to the liver. If complete surgical resection of gross disease in patients with a primary presentation can be achieved, then these patients will have a 5-year actuarial survival of 54%.

LONG-TERM FOLLOW-UP

It is essential to emphasize that long-term follow-up for all patients with soft tissue sarcoma is important. A recent analysis of long-term follow-up for patients followed more than 5 years showed that approximately 9% of patients who were disease free at the end of 5 years would go on to have further recurrence of the primary extremity sarcoma.[78]

SUMMARY

Soft tissue sarcomas are relatively rare, with an annual incidence of 6000 to 6500 in the United States. Primary therapy is predicated on surgical resection with an adequate margin of normal tissue. For high-risk patients, local control is improved with postoperative adjuvant irradiation. Local recurrence rates vary, depending on anatomic site. In extremity lesions, one third of patients develop locally recurrent disease, with a median disease-free interval of 18 months. Treatment results for localized extremity local recurrence may approach those for primary disease. Isolated pulmonary metastases may be resected with 20% to 30% 3-year survival rates after complete resection. In patients with retroperitoneal and visceral sarcoma, complete resection remains the dominant factor in outcome. As opposed to extremity sites, local recurrence in this site is a common cause of death. Patients with unresectable pulmonary metastases or extrapulmonary metastatic sarcoma have a uniformly poor prognosis and are best treated with systemic chemotherapy.

Selected References

Baldini EH, Goldberg J, Jenner C, et al: Long-term outcomes after function-sparing surgery without radiotherapy for soft tissue sarcoma of the extremities and trunk. J Clin Oncol 17:3252-3259, 1999.

> This study suggests that there may be a select subset of patients with soft tissue sarcoma in whom carefully performed function-sparing surgery may serve as definitive therapy and in whom adjuvant radiotherapy may not be necessary.

Brennan MF, Lewis JJ: Diagnosis and Management of Soft Tissue Sarcoma. London, Martin Dunitz, 2002.

Lewis JJ, Brennan MF: Soft tissue sarcomas. Curr Probl Surg 33:817-880, 1996.

Singer S, Demetri GD, Baldini EH, Fletcher CDM: Management of soft-tissue sarcomas: An overview and update. Lancet Oncol 1:75-85, 2000.

> These reviews summarize the subject in a single monograph/book.

Demetri GD, von Mehren M, Blanke CD, et al: Efficacy and safety of imatinib mesylate in advanced gastrointestinal stromal tumors. N Engl J Med 347:472-480, 2002.

Singer S, Rubin BP, Lux ML, et al: Prognostic value of KIT mutation type, mitotic activity, and histologic subtype in gastrointestinal stromal tumors. J Clin Oncol 20:3898-3905, 2002.

> These studies demonstrate the importance of KIT activation and mutations in GIST pathogenesis and rationale and application of KIT tyrosine kinase inhibitors for targeted therapy of GIST.

Ladanyi M, Bridge JA: Contribution of molecular genetic data to the classification of sarcomas. Hum Pathol 31:532-538, 2000.

> This thorough review details the significant progress made in recent years in characterizing chromosomal changes associated with soft tissue sarcomas. In addition, recent molecular analyses of several sarcoma-associated translocations and the identification of novel genes and mechanisms of dysregulation are discussed. The role of cytogenetics and molecular changes, in the context of diagnosis and future investigation, is discussed.

Lewis JJ, Leung D, Woodruff JM, Brennan MF: Retroperitoneal soft tissue sarcoma: Analysis of 500 patients treated and followed at a single institution. Ann Surg 228:355-365, 1998.

> This manuscript provides an extensive description of outcome for patients with retroperitoneal sarcoma.

Pisters P, Leung D, Woodruff J, et al: Analysis of prognostic factors in 1041 patients with localized soft tissue sarcomas of the extremity. J Clin Oncol 14:1679-1689, 1996.

> This manuscript provides data on prognostic factors for extremity soft tissue sarcoma, from a large single institution series.

Pisters PWT, Harrison LB, Leung DH, et al: Long-term results of a prospective randomized trial evaluating the role of adjuvant brachytherapy in soft tissue sarcoma. J Clin Oncol 14:859-868, 1996.

Yang JC, Chang AE, Baker AR, et al: Randomized prospective study of the benefit of adjuvant radiation therapy in the treatment of soft tissue sarcomas of the extremity. J Clin Oncol 16:197-203, 1998.

> These studies confirm the benefit of adjuvant radiation therapy in patients with completely resected localized extremity sarcoma.

References

1. Lewis JJ, Brennan MF: Soft tissue sarcomas. Curr Probl Surg 33:817, 1996.
2. Barken D, Wright E, Nguyen D: Gene for von Recklinghausen neurofibromatosis is in the pericentromeric region of chromosome 17. Science 236:1100, 1987.
3. Li FP, Fraumeni JF: Soft-tissue sarcomas, breast cancer, and other neoplasms: A familial syndrome? Ann Intern Med 71:747, 1969.
4. Sorensen SA, Mulvihill JJ, Nielsen A: Long-term follow-up of von Recklinghausen neurofibromatosis: Survival and malignant neoplasms. N Engl J Med 314:1010, 1986.
5. Brady MS, Gaynor JJ, Brennan MF: Radiation-associated sarcoma of bone and soft tissue. Arch Surg 127:1379, 1992.
6. Brennan MF, Lewis JJ: Diagnosis and Management of Soft Tissue Sarcoma. London, Martin Dunitz, 2002.
7. Bertazzi PA, Zocchetti C, Guercilena S, et al: Dioxin exposure and cancer risk: A 15-year mortality study after the "Seveso accident." Epidemiology 8:646, 1997.
8. Dich J, Zahm SH, Hanberg A, Adami HO: Pesticides and cancer. Cancer Causes Control 8:420, 1997.
9. Mundt KA, Dell LD, Austin RP, et al: Historical cohort study of 10,109 men in the North American vinyl chloride industry, 1942-72: Update of cancer mortality to 31 December 1995. Occup Environ Med 57:774, 2000.
10. Fletcher JA: Cytogenetics of soft tissue tumors. Cancer Treat Res 91:9, 1997.
11. Fletcher CD: Soft tissue tumours: The impact of cytogenetics and molecular genetics. Verh Dtsch Ges Pathol 81:318, 1997.
12. Sreekantaiah C, Ladanyi M, Rodriguez E, Chaganti RS: Chromosomal aberrations in soft tissue tumors: Relevance to diagnosis, classification, and molecular mechanisms. Am J Pathol 144:1121, 1994.
13. Meis-Kindblom JM, Sjogren H, Kindblom LG, et al: Cytogenetic and molecular genetic analyses of liposarcoma and its soft tissue simulators: Recognition of new variants and differential diagnosis. Virchows Arch 439:141, 2001.

14. Kawai A, Woodruff J, Healey JH, et al: *SYT-SSX* gene fusion as a determinant of morphology and prognosis in synovial sarcoma. N Engl J Med 338:153, 1998.

15. Ladanyi M, Antonescu CR, Leung DH, et al: Impact of SYT-SSX fusion type on the clinical behavior of synovial sarcoma: A multi-institutional retrospective study of 243 patients. Cancer Res 62:135, 2002.

16. Bennicelli JL, Barr FG: Chromosomal translocations and sarcomas. Curr Opin Oncol 14:412, 2002.

17. Cance WG, Brennan MF, Dudas ME, et al: Altered expression of the retinoblastoma gene product in human sarcomas. N Engl J Med 323:1457, 1990.

18. Dei Tos AP, Doglioni C, Piccinin S, et al: Molecular abnormalities of the p53 pathway in dedifferentiated liposarcoma. J Pathol 181:8, 1997.

19. Antonescu CR, Leung DH, Dudas M, et al: Alterations of cell cycle regulators in localized synovial sarcoma: A multifactorial study with prognostic implications. Am J Pathol 156:977, 2000.

20. Oda Y, Sakamoto A, Satio T, et al: Molecular abnormalities of p53, MDM2, and H-*ras* in synovial sarcoma. Mod Pathol 13:994, 2000.

21. Antonescu CR, Tschernyavsky SJ, Decuseara R, et al: Prognostic impact of P53 status, TLS-CHOP fusion transcript structure, and histological grade in myxoid liposarcoma: A molecular and clinicopathologic study of 82 cases. Clin Cancer Res 7:3977, 2001.

22. Abudu A, Mangham DC, Reynolds GM, et al: Overexpression of p53 protein in primary Ewing's sarcoma of bone: Relationship to tumour stage, response and prognosis. Br J Cancer 79:1185, 1999.

23. de Alava E, Antonescu CR, Panizo A, et al: Prognostic impact of P53 status in Ewing sarcoma. Cancer 89:783, 2000.

24. Wei G, Antonescu CR, de Alava E, et al: Prognostic impact of INK4A deletion in Ewing sarcoma. Cancer 89:793, 2000.

25. Lopez-Guerrero JA, Pellin A, Noguera R, et al: Molecular analysis of the 9p21 locus and p53 genes in Ewing family tumors. Lab Invest 81:803, 2001.

26. Drobnjak M, Latres E, Pollack D, et al: Prognostic implications of p53 nuclear overexpression and high proliferation index of Ki-67 in adult soft-tissue sarcomas. J Natl Cancer Inst 86:549, 1994.

27. Wurl P, Meye A, Lautenschlager C, et al: Clinical relevance of pRb and p53 co-overexpression in soft tissue sarcomas. Cancer Lett 139:159, 1999.

28. Ladanyi M, Bridge JA: Contribution of molecular genetic data to the classification of sarcomas. Hum Pathol 31:532, 2000.

29. Zoubek A, Dockhorn-Dworniczak B, Delattre O, et al: Does expression of different EWS chimeric transcripts define clinically distinct risk groups of Ewing tumor patients? J Clin Oncol 14:1245, 1996.

30. de Alava E, Kawai A, Healey JH, et al: EWS-FLI1 fusion transcript structure is an independent determinant of prognosis in Ewing's sarcoma. J Clin Oncol 16:1248, 1998.

31. Sorensen PH, Lynch JC, Qualman SJ, et al: *PAX3-FKHR* and *PAX7-FKHR* gene fusions are prognostic indicators in alveolar rhabdomyosarcoma: A report from the children's oncology group. J Clin Oncol 20:2672, 2002.

32. Fletcher CD, Unni KK, Mertens F: Pathology and genetics of tumors of soft tissue and bone. *In* Kleihues P, Sobin LH (eds): World Health Organization Classification of Tumors, vol 1. Lyon, IARC Press, 2002.

33. Brown FM, Fletcher CD: Problems in grading soft tissue sarcomas. Am J Clin Pathol 114(Suppl):S82, 2000.

34. Kattan MW, Leung DH, Brennan MF: Postoperative nomogram for 12-year sarcoma-specific death. J Clin Oncol 20:791, 2002.

35. Lewis J, Brennan MF: Soft tissue sarcomas. Curr Probl Surg 33:817, 1996.

36. Heslin MJ, Lewis JJ, Woodruff JM, Brennan MF: Core needle biopsy for diagnosis of extremity soft tissue sarcoma. Ann Surg Oncol 4:425, 1997.

37. Lewis JJ, Brennan MF: The management of retroperitoneal soft tissue sarcoma. Adv Surg 33:329, 1999.

38. Lewis JJ, Leung D, Woodruff JM, Brennan MF: Retroperitoneal soft-tissue sarcoma: Analysis of 500 patients treated and followed at a single institution. Ann Surg 228:355, 1998.

39. Varma DG: Optimal radiologic imaging of soft tissue sarcomas. Semin Surg Oncol 17:2, 1999.

40. Panicek DM, Go SD, Healey JH, et al: Soft-tissue sarcoma involving bone or neurovascular structures: MR imaging prognostic factors. Radiology 205:871, 1997.

41. Panicek DM, Gatsonis C, Rosenthal DI, et al: CT and MR imaging in the local staging of primary malignant musculoskeletal neoplasms: Report of the Radiology Diagnostic Oncology Group. Radiology 202:237, 1997.

42. Fong Y, Coit DG, Woodruff JM, Brennan MF: Lymph node metastasis from soft tissue sarcoma in adults: Analysis of data from a prospective database of 1772 sarcoma patients. Ann Surg 217:72, 1993.

43. Gadd MA, Casper ES, Woodruff JM, et al: Development and treatment of pulmonary metastases in adult patients with extremity soft tissue sarcoma. Ann Surg 218:705, 1993.

44. DeMatteo RP, Lewis JJ, Leung D, et al: Two hundred gastrointestinal stromal tumors: Recurrence patterns and prognostic factors for survival. Ann Surg 231:51, 2000.

45. Gaynor JJ, Tan CC, Casper ES, et al: Refinement of clinicopathologic staging for localized soft tissue sarcoma of the extremity: A study of 423 adults. J Clin Oncol 10:1317, 1992.

46. Fleming I, Cooper J, Henson D, et al (eds): AJCC Cancer Staging Manual, 5th ed. Philadelphia, Lippincott-Raven, 1997.

47. Brennan MF: Staging of soft tissue sarcomas. Ann Surg Oncol 6:8, 1999.

48. Greene F, Page D, Fleming I, Fritz A, et al (eds): AJCC Cancer Staging Manual, 6th ed. Heidelberg, Springer-Verlag, 2002.

49. Rosenberg SA, Tepper J, Glatstein E, et al: The treatment of soft-tissue sarcomas of the extremities: Prospective randomized evaluations of (1) limb-sparing surgery plus radiation therapy compared with amputation and (2) the role of adjuvant chemotherapy. Ann Surg 196:305, 1982.

50. Williard WC, Collin C, Casper ES, et al: The changing role of amputation for soft tissue sarcoma of the extremity in adults. Surg Gynecol Obstet 175:389, 1992.

51. Yang JC, Chang AE, Baker AR, et al: Randomized prospective study of the benefit of adjuvant radiation therapy in the treatment of soft tissue sarcomas of the extremity. J Clin Oncol 16:197, 1998.

52. Pisters PW, Harrison LB, Leung DH, et al: Long-term results of a prospective randomized trial of adjuvant brachytherapy in soft tissue sarcoma. J Clin Oncol 14:859, 1996.

53. Baldini EH, Goldberg J, Jenner C, et al: Long-term outcomes after function-sparing surgery without radiotherapy for soft tissue sarcoma of the extremities and trunk. J Clin Oncol 17:3252, 1999.

54. Alektiar KM, Leung D, Zelefsky MJ, Brennan MF: Adjuvant radiation for stage II-B soft tissue sarcoma of the extremity. J Clin Oncol 20:1643, 2002.

55. Baldini EH, Demetri GD, Fletcher CD, et al: Adults with Ewing's sarcoma/primitive neuroectodermal tumor: Adverse effect of older age and primary extraosseous disease on outcome. Ann Surg 230:79, 1999.

56. Esnaola NF, Rubin BP, Baldini EH, et al: Response to chemotherapy and predictors of survival in adult rhabdomyosarcoma. Ann Surg 234:215, 2001.

57. Bramwell V, Rouesse J, Steward W, et al: Adjuvant CYVADIC chemotherapy for adult soft tissue sarcoma—reduced local recurrence but no improvement in survival: A study of the European Organization for Research and Treatment of Cancer Soft Tissue and Bone Sarcoma Group. J Clin Oncol 12:1137, 1994.

58. Tierney JF, Stewart LA, Parmar MKB, et al: (Sarcoma Meta-analysis Collaboration): Adjuvant chemotherapy for localised resectable soft-tissue sarcoma of adults: Meta-analysis of individual data. Lancet 350:1647, 1997.

59. Singer S, Corson JM, Demetri GD, et al: Prognostic factors predictive of survival for truncal and retroperitoneal soft-tissue sarcoma. Ann Surg 221:185, 1995.

60. Brennan MF: Retroperitoneal sarcoma: Time for a national trial? Ann Surg Oncol 9:324, 2002.

61. Alektiar KM, Hu K, Anderson L, et al: High-dose-rate intraoperative radiation therapy (HDR-IORT) for retroperitoneal sarcomas. Int J Radiat Oncol Biol Phys 47:157, 2000.

62. Billingsley KG, Lewis JJ, Leung DH, et al: Multifactorial analysis of the survival of patients with distant metastasis arising from primary extremity sarcoma. Cancer 85:389, 1999.

63. Singer S, Antman K, Corson JM, Eberlein TJ: Long-term salvageability for patients with locally recurrent soft-tissue sarcomas. Arch Surg 127:548, 1992.

64. Brennan MF: The enigma of local recurrence. The Society of Surgical Oncology. Ann Surg Oncol 4:1, 1997.

65. Billingsley KG, Burt ME, Jara E, et al: Pulmonary metastases from soft tissue sarcoma: Analysis of patterns of diseases and post-metastasis survival. Ann Surg 229:602, 1999.

66. Benjamin RS, Rouesse J, Bourgeois H, van Hoesel QG: Should patients with advanced sarcomas be treated with chemotherapy? Eur J Cancer 34:958, 1998.

67. Antman K, Crowley J, Balcerzak S: An Intergroup phase III randomized study of doxorubicin and dacarbazine with or without ifosfamide and mesna in advanced soft tissue and bone sarcomas. J Clin Oncol 11:1276, 1993.

68. Elias A, Ryan L, Sulkes A: Response to mesna, doxorubicin, ifosfamide, and dacarbazine in 108 patients with metastatic or unresectable sarcoma and no prior chemotherapy. J Clin Oncol 7:1208, 1989.

69. Elias AD: High-dose therapy for adult soft tissue sarcoma: Dose response and survival. Semin Oncol 25:19, 1998.

70. Fletcher CD, Berman JJ, Corless C, et al: Diagnosis of gastrointestinal stromal tumors: A consensus approach. Hum Pathol 33:459, 2002.

71. Hirota S, Isozaki K, Moriyama Y, et al: Gain-of-function mutations of c-kit in human gastrointestinal stromal tumors. Science 279:577, 1998.

72. Rubin BP, Singer S, Tsao C, et al: KIT activation is a ubiquitous feature of gastrointestinal stromal tumors. Cancer Res 61:8118, 2001.

73. Singer S, Rubin BP, Lux ML, et al: Prognostic value of KIT mutation type, mitotic activity, and histologic subtype in gastrointestinal stromal tumors. J Clin Oncol 20:3898, 2002.

74. Druker BJ, Tamura S, Buchdunger E, et al: Effects of a selective inhibitor of the Abl tyrosine kinase on the growth of Bcr-Abl positive cells. Nat Med 2:561, 1996.

75. Tuveson DA, Willis NA, Jacks T, et al: STI571 inactivation of the gastrointestinal stromal tumor c-KIT oncoprotein: Biological and clinical implications. Oncogene 20:5054, 2001.

76. Demetri GD, von Mehren M, Blanke CD, et al: Efficacy and safety of imatinib mesylate in advanced gastrointestinal stromal tumors. N Engl J Med 347:472, 2002.

77. Pisters PW, Leung DH, Woodruff J, et al: Analysis of prognostic factors in 1,041 patients with localized soft tissue sarcomas of the extremities. J Clin Oncol 14:1679, 1996.

78. Lewis JJ, Leung D, Casper ES, et al: Multifactorial analysis of long-term follow-up (more than 5 years) of primary extremity sarcoma. Arch Surg 134:190, 1999.

BONE TUMORS

John H. Healey, M.D.

Primary Bone Tumors	Metastatic Bone Disease

PRIMARY BONE TUMORS

General Concepts

Bone tumors have a low incidence but a high significance. All surgeons should have a basic understanding of them to avoid errors and provide optimal care. In this chapter, the most common benign and malignant bone tumors are discussed; these tumors serve as paradigms for the management of other lesions in their category of bone tumors.

There is a wide spectrum of bone lesions for which benign and malignant tumors are in the differential diagnosis. Surgeons should seek appropriate radiologic and orthopedic help to diagnose and treat the lesions. The two basic questions to address are who needs a biopsy and who should perform the biopsy.

Who needs a biopsy? Any person with a lesion that cannot be diagnosed by clinical and radiographic means or whose lesion requires treatment is a biopsy candidate. A tissue diagnosis is needed when the history, examination, and imaging studies cannot be reconciled. Proper preliminary investigation includes plain radiographs and not just magnetic resonance imaging (MRI). These tests are complementary. Discriminating evaluation of the plain radiographs is still the most specific way to diagnose bone tumors. Get another opinion if doubt exists. Orthopedic, oncologic, and imaging expertise is available in most medical centers.

Generally, if the physician is not comfortable treating the possible tumors that could be diagnosed from a biopsy, it is better to refer the patient to a specialist. The treating surgeon should have the opportunity to biopsy and analyze the tumor. This principle is crucial to diagnose bone tumors accurately and avoid inopportune biopsies that could compromise or preclude definitive surgical treatment.[1] If there is inconsistency between the biopsy results and other clinical features, further analysis is needed. This may be another test, rebiopsy, or clinical follow-up.

Clinical Features

The medical history helps to exclude infection and congenital conditions. Focused examination may reveal the source of metastatic cancers. Rarely, the family history is diagnostic, as in multiple hereditary exostosis (osteochondromatosis).

Slow-growing benign tumors may not be painful, although they often are tender. Malignant and aggressive benign bone tumors usually hurt. They grow inside a rigid bony compartment, painfully increasing intraosseous pressure, or break out through the cortex and painfully stretch the periosteum. Exceptions include slowly growing tumors such as low-grade chondrosarcomas, which may be painless in one third of patients. Tumor pain may be worse at night. Mechanical pain, exacerbated by weight bearing, reflects structural insufficiency and may herald a fracture.

Coincidental findings are common. Thirty percent of patients report that they sustained trauma to the area, bringing a lesion to the patient's attention. A frequent source of confusion is periarticular or intra-articular pathology. Sources of referred pain must be considered and excluded. The physician must exhibit great restraint and avoid diagnosing the obvious comorbid condition and miss the offending primary lesion or tumor. If symptoms do not resolve in a predictable fashion, patients should have a radiographic (re)examination.

Physical examination findings such as a palpable mass, painful or restricted joint motion, tenderness, or an effusion are nonspecific. Vascular and neurologic findings are uncommon but may reflect compression or invasion of these structures. Lymph node involvement is rare, pointing toward a diagnosis of lymphoma, infectious, or metastatic disease. General examination of the chest, abdomen, and pelvis may reveal the site of a primary cancer in cases of metastatic disease.

Benign Tumors

Up to 43% of normal children have developmental or neoplastic bony defects during growth, the most common of which is a fibrous cortical defect.[2] This lesion usually is found incidentally and is asymptomatic. It is important to distinguish it from a true neoplasm that requires a biopsy.

The most common benign bone tumor (12% of all tumors and 50% of benign bone tumors) is the solitary osteochondroma (Fig. 30-8). Nearly one half of these develop about the knee. Symptomatic osteochondromas and those growing after skeletal maturity warrant excisional biopsy if the diagnosis is ensured. Incisional biopsy and staged resection are reserved for osteochondromas with a thick (e.g., 1.5 cm) cartilage cap on MRI. Such lesions could have converted to chondrosarcomas. Prophylactic excision of osteochondromas rarely is indicated, because the surgical risks exceed the risk of sarcomatous degeneration (estimated at 0.1%). One should not operate simply because a lesion is present.

Several of the less common tumors merit comment. Giant cell tumors are the most worrisome benign aggressive tumors (Fig. 30-9). They are lytic epiphyseal tumors that frequently (65%) occur in the distal femur or proximal tibia in young adults. Approximately 3% metastasize to lung despite their benign histologic appearance. Chondroblastomas have the same epiphyseal distribution but occur in skeletally immature patients and usually have a rim of reactive bone radiographically. The humeral head and tuberosities are frequent sites. One third of cases occur around the knee. Aneurysmal bone cysts are benign aggressive tumors that have a diaphyseal or metaphyseal distribution and may develop as secondary lesions on top of other benign or even malignant bone tumors. Treatment of these conditions is as described for giant cell tumor (see later).

There are several tumors that are treated differently. Unicameral bone cysts are common lytic lesions in the metaphysis that have a predilection for the proximal humerus and femur in children and often present as a

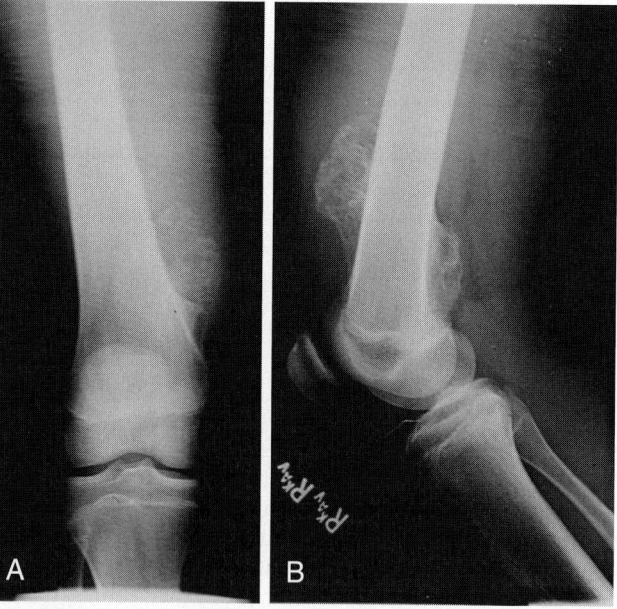

FIGURE 30-8. **A** and **B,** Benign osteochondroma. Note the continuity between the cortex of the shaft and that of the lesion. Similarly, the cancellous bone spaces are continuous.

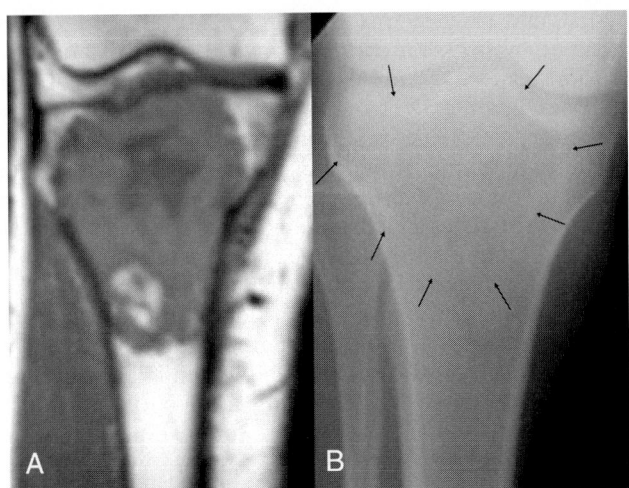

FIGURE 30-9. **A** and **B,** Giant cell tumor of bone. This is typically a lytic epiphyseal lesion in a young adult without surrounding bone reaction radiographically. MRI may show more extensive disease than is apparent on plain radiographs.

fracture. Repetitive injections of corticosteroid or bone marrow and demineralized bone matrix can cure these, with recurrence rates similar to after open curettage and grafting.[3] Osteoid osteomas are exquisitely painful lesions that provoke a large amount of reactive bone formation and are very responsive to aspirin or nonsteroidal anti-inflammatory drugs. Percutaneous radiofrequency ablation may obviate surgical excision for lesions that do not burn out during a 3- to 12-month medication trial.[4] Finally, enchondromas are benign cartilage deposits in long bones

that are rarely painful and do not require surgery. One to 10 percent can progress to chondrosarcoma, so they should be monitored.[5] When they are found by a bone scan during the work-up for possible metastases of a primary breast, prostate, or lung cancer, they may necessitate a biopsy to exclude a metastasis and allow treatment of the primary cancer to proceed.

Malignant Tumors

Sarcomas, metastatic carcinomas, and hematologic malignancies affect bone. Primary sarcomas of bone are rare. Only 2100 cases per year occur in the United States. The most common tumors are mentioned here.

Osteogenic sarcoma is the most common primary bone malignancy, occurring predominantly in teenagers and young adults. Approximately one half occur about the knee, usually in a metaphyseal site (Fig. 30-10). It provides the paradigm for treatment of spindle cell sarcomas. Chondrosarcomas, malignant fibrous histiocytomas, and fibrosarcomas are the other spindle cell mesenchymal tumors. Their incidence is approximately one half to two thirds that of osteogenic sarcomas, and they occur in an older population. Ewing's family tumors classically are diaphyseal tumors in youth, yet nearly 50% of them occur in nondiaphyseal locations, and about 20% may occur in young to middle-aged adults. Ewing's tumor is particularly common in the femur and pelvis and is the most common malignancy of the fibula. It serves as the prototype for treatment of round cell tumors.

Metastatic deposits in bone are much more common than primary sarcomas, especially in older individuals. Hematologic malignancies affect bone. Lymphoma may

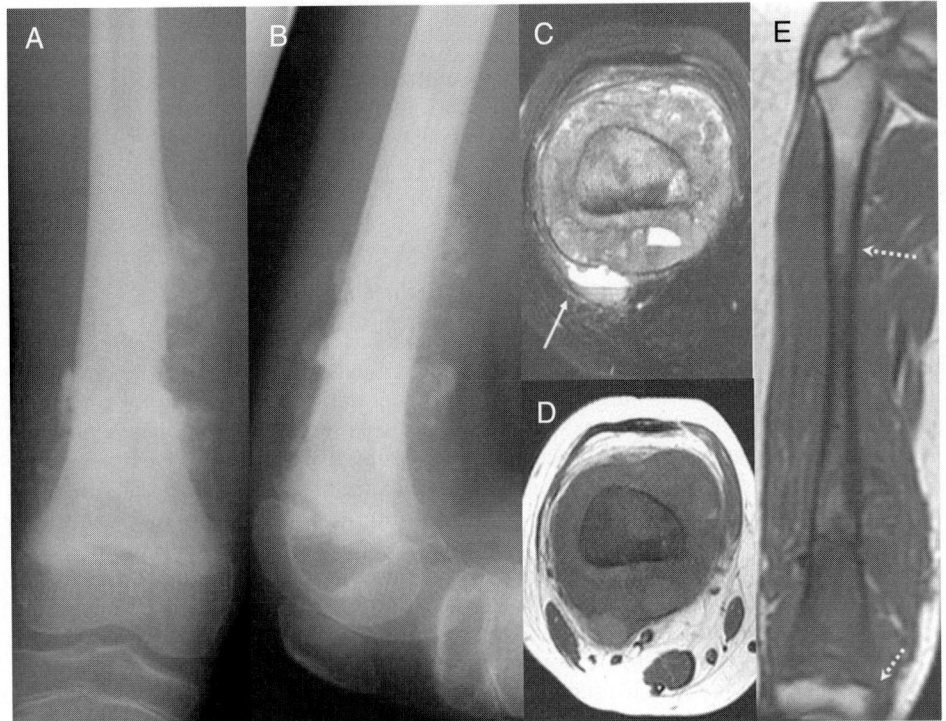

FIGURE 30-10. Osteogenic sarcoma. This is the most common primary bone sarcoma. It is typically a destructive bone formative lesion of the metaphyseal area of the distal femur or proximal tibia in an adolescent; however, it may occur in any bone at any age. **A,** Anteroposterior radiograph shows the extensive bone formation in the soft tissue and marrow space. **B,** Lateral radiograph. **C,** Axial gradient-echo MR image shows the huge soft tissue mass. The *arrow* shows the fluid-fluid levels typical of an aneurysmal bone cyst. **D,** Axial T1-weighted MR image shows the marrow margin present near the popliteal vessels. **E,** Coronal MR image shows the extent of the disease up into the proximal femur *(arrow)* and disease traversing the distal femoral growth plate *(arrow).*

develop as a primary bone tumor and seems to have a predilection for the femur in children or adults. If lymphoma is a possibility, then ample biopsy tissue should be taken so that studies such as cytogenetics and lymphoma markers can be performed. Multiple myeloma and metastatic lesions are the most common neoplasms in older adults. Breast, renal, and lung cancers are the usual culprits. The bone lesions should be sampled if they are the first site of presumed metastatic disease.

Diagnostic and Imaging Studies

Conventional biplane radiography is the most specific diagnostic test to determine if the tumor is benign or malignant. Benign lesions have sharp margins, narrow transition to the adjacent normal bone, and well-developed surrounding reactive bone. They may expand the bone cortex and rarely extend into the soft tissue. Malignant lesions lack sharp margins and are more permeative with a wide zone of transition, and their growth outstrips the bone's ability to wall off the lesion. Cortex is destroyed, and there is periosteal elevation and usually soft tissue extension. The matrix within the lesion can suggest a specific diagnosis, such as osteogenic sarcoma, which produces a white cloud of bony matrix, or chondrosarcoma, which has broken rings of calcified cartilage matrix.

Serum tests should be ordered selectively. Biochemical studies should be ordered when a metabolic disease or high-grade malignancy is suspected. The erythrocyte sedimentation rate (ESR) is elevated mildly in most malignant tumors and does not distinguish them from infections. Multiple myeloma causes significant elevations of the ESR and abnormal protein electrophoresis, as well as anemia, azotemia, and even hypercalcemia in widespread disease. The alkaline phosphatase level is elevated in 80% of osteogenic sarcomas and in most patients with Paget's disease of bone. Serum lactate dehydrogenase typically is elevated in round cell tumors such as Ewing's family tumors and lymphoma, with values correlating with tumor burden. Serum calcium and parathyroid hormone levels are elevated in brown tumors of hyperparathyroidism and may help differentiate them from giant cell tumor. Other tests are rarely helpful.

When a lesion displays benign and latent characteristics, no further imaging is warranted. When the diagnosis is unclear, or if a malignant lesion is suspected, advanced imaging should be done to aid the diagnosis and treatment. Systemic work-up (chest computed tomography [CT] for primary sarcomas and chest and abdominal CT for suspected bone metastases) should be done selectively. A whole-body technetium-99m pyrophosphate bone scan is essential to bone tumor staging and screening for multicentric disease or metastases. Occasionally, it will identify an easier lesion to biopsy.

Imaging of the lesion can be by MRI or CT. MRI provides valuable diagnostic information about both benign and malignant lesions yet remains imprecise. The technique excels at defining normal and pathologic anatomy. It is particularly accurate at detecting soft tissue, vascular,

neural, and marrow space involvement.[6] CT is the most effective in assessing cortical bone and endosteal cortical erosions caused by tumors such as low-grade chondrosarcomas. CT detects cortical breakthrough and is sensitive to identify soft tissue calcification (e.g., synovial sarcoma).

All bone tumors should be staged to define the extent and behavior of the lesion. Benign tumors are staged most easily by the Campanacci system, based solely on the radiograph.[7] Latent lesions (stage 1) are contained within bone and do not affect the surrounding cortex. Active lesions (stage 2) are also within bone but evoke cortical thinning, expansion, or thickening. Aggressive lesions (stage 3) breach the cortex and extend into the surrounding soft tissue. The technique chosen for tumor ablation is governed by the stage, symptoms, and potential for recurrence. Asymptomatic stage 1 lesions can be curetted and bone grafted; it may be appropriate merely to follow some regularly with examination and radiographs. Symptomatic lesions should be treated. Stage 2 lesions can be managed with similar intralesional therapy but have a higher recurrence rate; therefore, local adjuvants such as cement, phenol, or cryosurgery may be warranted to enhance local control. Stage 3 lesions usually should be excised, or, if intralesional therapy is chosen, a local adjuvant should be strongly considered.

Malignant bone tumor staging is standardized and prognostically accurate. Bone cancers are graded as either low grade (grade I) or high grade (grade II) based on histologic criteria and metastatic potential. The American Joint Committee on Cancer (AJCC) recently changed the subclassification of bone cancers. Substage A denotes that the tumor is less than 8 cm, whereas substage B signifies that the tumor is greater than 8 cm. Containment within the bone compartment remains an important prognostic factor and guides treatment decisions but is no longer part of the official staging system. Grade III identifies all metastatic tumors, whether high or low grade. Most malignant tumors are high grade and large grade IIB lesions that are also extracompartmental. The staging of Ewing's family tumor also includes bone marrow assessment. Refinements that take into account biologic measures of aggressiveness may be incorporated into future staging systems.

Staging and Biopsy Techniques

The most appropriate biopsy method is determined by practical considerations, such as the experience of the surgeon and pathologist and the availability of operating room space. Lesions that are virtually diagnostic radiographically can be sampled with a needle, whereas atypical radiographic presentations usually mandate an open biopsy (Box 30-2). Ample fresh tissue increasingly is needed for genetic testing of primary bone tumors; thus an open biopsy is required to obtain adequate tissue. This may be obviated in the future with advances in fluorescent in situ hybridization that will allow a genetic profile to be obtained from scant material. Biopsy and treatment are staged unless a definitive diagnosis can be obtained by frozen section analysis. Antibiotics should not be admin-

entire femur for a lesion of the distal femur or the entire quadriceps for a lesion in the distal vastus medialis.

Giant Cell Tumors

Benign Tumors

Treatment of giant cell tumor embodies the methods and common technical variations that are used for other benign tumors of similar virulence, such as aneurysmal bone cyst, chondroblastomas, and chondromyxoid fibroma. Most giant cell tumors occur in the epiphyseal distal femur or proximal tibia and often extend to the subchondral surface. Curettage and bone grafting has approximately a 50% recurrence rate. At the other extreme, wide excision cures most cases, but this treatment has more morbidity and reconstructive difficulty and does not eliminate the chance of developing a metastasis. Modern treatment addresses the tumor aggressiveness and has reduced the historically high recurrence rate to less than 10% by using intralesional treatment and adjuvants.[9] This approach is oncologically sound and preserves joint function. The method consists of the following steps: (1) fully exteriorize the tumor through a cortical bone window large enough to allow direct vision into all areas of the tumor; (2) curet the lesion aggressively; and (3) use a high-speed bur to eliminate tumor permeating cancellous bone and eradicate the subchondral tumor. Chemical and physical modalities extend the margin of tumor excision and improve tumor control. Acrylic cement is used most frequently. Cement polymerization is exothermic and thermally kills residual tumor cells, and the cement mechanically supports the defect. Despite expert technique, recurrence remains a problem. A study from the Massachusetts General Hospital reported recurrence in 7 of 25 tibial and 3 of 23 distal femoral giant cell tumors treated by these methods.[10] These disappointing results highlight the need for more aggressive treatment. Cryosurgery can dramatically extend the volume of bone sterilized and reduce the recurrence rate further. Prophylactic internal fixation prevents most fractures through the previously frozen bone. Malawer and colleagues reported a local recurrence rate of 2% for primary tumors and 8% for recurrent tumors treated with cryosurgery; the fracture rate was 6%.[9] Pathologic fracture or recurrence may disrupt the knee joint. Endoprosthetic knee replacement or allografts can salvage many such cases. Wide excision and replacement of a single condyle (or plateau) with an allograft is an excellent solution for large, eccentric tumors that destroy one tibial plateau or femoral condyle. This type of "hemi-joint" replacement replaces the articular cartilage, preserves joint alignment, stability, and structure and has a high success rate.

Malignant Tumors

Lesions that were once considered rapidly fatal now potentially are curable. Advances in sarcoma therapy have helped to establish and validate many of the concepts of modern surgical oncology, including principles of wide en bloc surgical excision, adjuvant multiagent

---

<table>
<tr><td>

Box 30-2.   Bone Biopsy Technique

Needle biopsy if radiograph is diagnostic
Open biopsy if radiograph is nondiagnostic
  No preoperative antibiotics
  Exsanguinate by gravity—not compression bandage ± tourniquet
  Small, extensile incision
  Radiographic localization if necessary
  Soft tissue biopsy if possible
  Round bone hole
  Frozen section for adequacy
  Fresh tissue for genetics studies
  Culture (fungus, tuberculosis, bacteriology)
  Absolute hemostasis
  Drain (if necessary) in line with definitive incision
  Protect weight bearing

</td></tr>
</table>

istered before the biopsy so that microorganisms may be recovered. A tourniquet is desirable to minimize bleeding, but avoid using a compression bandage to exsanguinate the limb because this can embolize tumor. Use gravity and patience instead.

The biopsy incision must be planned to be in continuity with the definitive resection incision. Generally, biopsy incisions should be extensile, avoid contaminating adjacent joints, and minimize unnecessary extracompartmental contamination. A frozen section analysis should confirm sufficiency of the biopsy. Meticulous hemostasis is very important to avoid local dissemination of tumor in hematoma. Absorbable gelatin sponge (Gelfoam) and thrombin or cementation of the cortical bone window prevents postoperative hemorrhage. If a drain is used, it should be placed in line with the incision, so that the tract of the drain can be excised easily in continuity with the biopsy incision. Fracture through the pathologic bone, which may preclude limb salvage, must be prevented. A typical biopsy weakens the bone 50%, so crutches are needed for at least 6 weeks to allow healing and prevent fracture.

Treatment of Primary Tumors

A four-part staging system specifies the nature of any tumor excision and defines the surgical margin.[8] An *intralesional margin* passes through the tumor; for example, curettage is an intralesional procedure suitable for benign lesions. A *marginal margin* courses through the layer of reactive, inflammatory tissue around a cancer. An *excisional biopsy* goes through the tumor pseudocapsule and almost always leaves microscopic disease behind. A *wide margin* removes the tumor and some surrounding normal tissue. Most limb-sparing en bloc excisions for sarcomas have a wide surgical margin. A *radical margin* removes the entire soft tissue and bone compartments that contain the tumor; examples are removing the

chemotherapy, and a multidisciplinary team approach to patient care.

Surgery remains the primary curative modality for sarcomas. Wide excision is appropriate for low-grade sarcoma. When an *effective* adjuvant is available, a wide local excision is appropriate for high-grade cancers; radical resection or amputation may not be necessary. The effectiveness of adjuvant therapy must be considered. If the cancer is not responding to chemotherapy, for example, then it is prudent to obtain a wider surgical resection margin. Sarcomas occur throughout the body. The anatomic and functional aspects of resection and reconstruction warrant specialized surgical care. These diseases should be treated in major centers, and outcome depends on the surgeon's experience. Because of the rarity of bone sarcomas, collaboration between large centers is necessary for advances to be made. Cases treated at nonparticipating centers off protocol compromise the ability to improve outcome for patients with these diseases.

Clinical Manifestations

The presenting symptoms of pain and swelling were described earlier. The patient's medical and family history occasionally provides valuable information such as conditions that may predispose the patient to a secondary sarcoma, such as prior radiation, Paget's disease, bone infarct, and fibrous dysplasia. Patients with hereditary retinoblastoma or Li-Fraumeni syndrome have a genetic predisposition to developing sarcomas (particularly osteogenic sarcoma) as a result of a germline mutation in the *RB* tumor suppressor gene or *TP53* gene, respectively. The pediatric patient with a sarcoma of bone is occasionally the index case for a family with Li-Fraumeni syndrome.

Imaging

Although the plain radiograph may seem unsophisticated, it remains the single most important radiographic test to diagnose bone sarcomas. The work-up of a sarcoma of bone also should include a plain chest radiograph and chest CT, because the lung is the most common site of metastasis. A technetium bone scan should be obtained to assess both the primary tumor and to screen for distant metastases. Other nuclear medicine scans, such as thallium scans (usually for osteogenic sarcoma) have some utility in monitoring the response to chemotherapy.[11] Proton emission tomography (PET) is being used for diagnosis, staging, and assessment of response to chemotherapy.[12] Although there is occasionally merit to using this test, it is not yet established for the routine use in bone tumor imaging.

Biopsy

Biopsy is mandatory before treating bone sarcoma and should follow the guidelines described earlier. Bone-forming lesions are especially difficult to sample percutaneously. The most dependable biopsies are open biopsies.

Surgical Management

It is vital to have a clear concept of whether the operation is performed for diagnostic, palliative, adjunctive, or curative intent. Both low- and high-grade cancers can be cured by local excision, and each requires at least a wide surgical resection margin to adequately ensure that all cancer was resected. Nevertheless, there is usually another opportunity to cure patients who sustain a recurrence of low-grade sarcoma, whereas most recurrences of high-grade sarcomas result in the death of the patient. Oncologic goals should take precedence over reconstructive goals, but they often are interrelated.

Limb-preserving surgery is currently appropriate for over 85% of patients with a sarcoma of the bone.[13] It is important to evaluate the relationship of the tumor with the vascular and neurologic structures to establish that limb-preserving surgery can be done. The primary indication for amputation is the inability to obtain an adequate margin of normal tissue around the tumor and still retain a useful limb. Conditions that commonly lead to amputation include widespread contamination of soft tissue by previous surgery, fracture, and infection. Another broad indication for amputation is the anticipated loss of vascular or nervous supply to the extremity that cannot be adequately restored. Finally the interrelationship between surgical margin and the effectiveness of adjuvant therapies must be taken into account.[14] If the chemotherapy is ineffective or compromised, then a wider surgical margin should be considered. An amputation is both an ablative and reconstructive procedure. Advances in prosthetics such as energy-conserving feet and ischial containment sockets have increased the potential function of amputees. Tellingly, young amputees are more likely to be able to participate in sports than sarcoma patients treated by endoprosthetic or allograft reconstructions of their limb. Disadvantages of amputations include (1) the psychological burden of losing a limb, (2) the considerable expense of maintaining and replacing prosthetic limbs, (3) the increased cardiac demand and oxygen consumption needed for lower extremity amputees to ambulate, and (4) phantom pain and sensations.

Limb-preserving surgery has become possible for many patients due to improved imaging, surgical technique, reconstructive materials, and adjuvant therapy. Reconstructions should address deficiencies of bone, joint, and soft tissue. Limb-sparing procedures usually require large bone grafts, endoprosthetic replacement, or a combination of biologic and artificial materials. There is no perfect reconstructive strategy, and there are advantages and disadvantages for each approach. Bone segmental replacements include autologous or allogeneic bone grafts. Single sides of joints can be replaced by osteoarticular allografts. When both sides of the joint are missing, an endoprosthesis, alloprosthetic composite, arthrodesis, or rotationplasty is needed. The majority of patients will enjoy long-term survival, and the long-term quality and durability of the limb reconstructions must be assessed critically.

Autogenous Grafts

Autogenous bone grafts are inexpensive, are biologically compatible, and avoid potential transmission of infectious diseases. They are used to replace short defects, to supplement allografts, and in specialized techniques such as free fibular transfer and bone transport (Ilizarov). Large bone grafts are used to provide structural support, and these usually are harvested from the fibula, iliac crest, and rib. The amount of bone available from these sites is limited. If the structural integrity of the diseased bone is preserved, it may be possible to remove the tumor, sterilize the bone, and reinsert it into the defect. This approach has been popular in many parts of the world where large bone banks do not exist and where endoprostheses are prohibitively expensive.

Vascularized autogenous grafts can be either local pedicular grafts or free grafts, the most versatile being the free fibular graft. Vascularized grafts have several theoretical advantages as the result of an intact blood supply. The limited experience with vascularized grafts after tumor excision shows that they have not yet fulfilled expectations. Complication rates are high: infection (16%), nonunion rate (6% to 19%), and fracture (8% to 43%).[15] The limb must be protected with a cast, brace, or external fixator until hypertrophy occurs, often 2 years or longer. Innovative approaches, such as combining vascularized fibular grafts with allografts, may expand indications for the procedure in the future. Bone transport uses an external fixation device and advances a cut bone segment across the defect at 1 mm daily, inducing new bone formation in its wake. Joint stiffness, pin-track infection, and nonunion are among the complications seen from this treatment.

Rotationplasty

The Van Nes rotationplasty typically is done for a distal femoral lesion in a child younger than 10 years old.[16,17] The procedure involves intercalary amputation of the knee and either distal femur or proximal tibia. The distal segment is rotated 180 degrees so that the foot faces backward and the tibia is secured to the proximal femur. This brings the ankle joint up to the level of the knee and allows it to bend in the direction of a normal knee. It effectively converts what would have been a high above-knee amputation into a below-knee amputation. Function is usually quite good, and most patients ambulate without crutches. The procedure allows for continued growth of the limb.

Endoprosthetic Replacement

Endoprostheses usually are employed in situations involving joint reconstruction where the primary advantage is immediate skeletal stability and restoration of function, an important consideration in patients who may not have very long to live. Prosthetic infection results in removal of the implant in 2% to 9% of cases and is highest for the proximal tibia, where the soft tissue coverage is poorest. Aggressive use of muscle flaps and free flaps has significantly reduced the rate of infections. Amputation may be needed to cure refractory infections or those for which treatment would delay resumption of postoperative chemotherapy or jeopardize the patient's life. Limb retention rates after initial limb preservation for sarcoma averages 90% at 10 years.[18] The major cause of late failure is aseptic loosening related to numerous factors.[19-22] The rate of loosening is highest for the proximal tibia, followed by the distal femur, proximal humerus, and finally proximal femur. Younger, more active patients have significantly higher failure rates than older, sedentary patients. The amount of bone resected also affects the rate of loosening. The use of less-constrained implants has improved longevity of implants. The newer, rotating hinge prostheses for knee replacement dissipate forces by allowing multiplanar motion.[23] The implants have long stems, secured to the host bone either by traditional cemented technique or with porous coated stems that rely on bone ingrowth for fixation. At this time it is not clear which method is better.

Extendible prostheses have been used primarily for tumors around the knee in adolescent children to maintain growth and prevent leg-length discrepancy.[24] The extendible portion of the device is weak in some designs and subject to fracture. The lengthening must be done in small, incremental steps to avoid nerve palsy and joint contracture, thereby necessitating multiple procedures. The rates of aseptic loosening and overall failure are higher than the corresponding rates for nonexpandable prostheses.[25]

Allografts

Bulk allografts of bone are versatile biologic implants that are available in all types and sizes. They can be ordered with soft tissue attachments to reattach ligaments, restore muscle function, and provide joint stability. Allograft tissue is dead, with the exception of limited preservation of articular cartilage. They can be used to replace a bone segment (intercalary) or one side of a joint (osteoarticular graft.) Allografts can transmit viruses, but processing seems to reduce this risk significantly. The biomechanical and biologic properties of allografts are affected by the method of processing. Freezing in liquid nitrogen reduces immunogenicity with little effect on mechanical strength. Freeze-drying dramatically reduces immunogenicity of the grafts and simplifies storage but results in a significant loss (10% to 61%) of bending and torsional strength.

The clinical results of allografts vary according to the situation in which they are employed. Replacement of a part of the diaphysis with an intercalary graft has the best outcome, and long-term graft survival is between 80% and 100%.[26,27] The worst results have occurred with allograft arthrodesis, and where only 40% of the grafts were retained at 10 years. Osteoarticular allografts have had intermediate results. These frozen allografts cryopreserve the chondrocytes with dimethyl sulfoxide or ethylene glycol. Although 40% to 70% of cells survive the experimental freeze-thawing process acutely, few survive long-term. Degenerative arthritis is inevitable over time. The major complications with allografts include fracture, 16% to 19%; nonunion, 17%; and infection, 13%. Because the graft is not vascularized, infections are difficult to eradicate and, in most instances, necessitate removal of the graft. The rate of infection is especially high for large pelvic allografts. To minimize the risk of infection, coverage of the graft with vital muscle and soft tissue is important. Impregnation of antibiotic bone cement into the medullary cavity may reduce the rate of infection while at the same time retarding bone resorption and preventing fractures.

Alloprosthetic Composite Reconstruction

Composite reconstructions use a combination of biologic and man-made materials. Most involve alloprostheses, which are a combination of allografts and endoprostheses (Fig. 30-11). This approach is advantageous because it provides tendinous and other soft tissue attachments to the endoprosthesis, as well as restoration of bone stock.[28] In the future, custom combinations of artificially engineered biological materials and implants will be used for limb reconstructions.

Adjuvant Therapies

Multiagent chemotherapy has been successful for primary sarcomas of bone and is now the standard treatment for

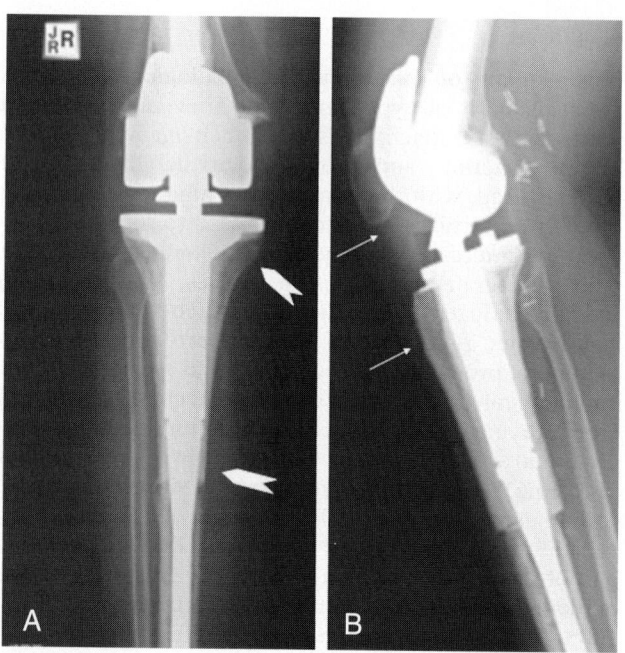

FIGURE 30-11.   Allograft-prosthetic composite reconstruction. This is an example of one of the many possible reconstructions. **A,** Anteroposterior radiograph shows the allograft *(arrows)* and the rotating hinge knee replacement. **B,** Lateral radiograph shows how the bone provides the patellar tendon attachment *(arrows).*

osteogenic sarcoma and Ewing's sarcoma, and possibly for malignant fibrous histiocytoma of bone. Unfortunately, chondrosarcoma does not respond to traditional agents. New cytotoxic or biologic agents are needed to treat these sarcomas. Most sarcomas, apart from Ewing's sarcoma, are resistant to radiation at tolerable doses.

Osteogenic Sarcoma

Osteogenic sarcoma is the most common primary bone sarcoma, with an incidence of 2 to 3 per million people per year, and 600 to 800 cases occur every year in the United States. The most commonly affected sites are the distal femur, proximal tibia, and proximal humerus. The peak incidence is in the adolescent years, with a second peak around the age of 60 years. Osteogenic sarcoma is composed of distinct disorders with different causes and outcomes. Primary, high-grade "conventional" osteogenic sarcoma is the most common. It is a highly malignant tumor, arising in the medullary canal and metastasizing in over 80% of cases treated by surgery alone. Secondary osteogenic sarcoma develops in Paget's disease, bone infarct, fibrous dysplasia, or previously radiated bone. Secondary osteogenic sarcoma is rare in young patients but accounts for over half of the cases in patients older than 60 years of age. Juxtacortical osteogenic sarcomas arise from the external surface of a bone, most commonly on the posterior aspect of the distal femur. The majority of tumors are low grade and have a favorable prognosis, but some are high grade, invade the medullary canal, and metastasize rapidly. They should be designated as high or low grade. Patients with low-grade osteogenic sarcomas of all varieties should not receive chemotherapy, whereas high-grade tumors warrant chemotherapy.

The genetic basis of osteogenic sarcoma is only partially understood.[29] Complex karyotypes are present in most tumors. Ring chromosomes have been noted in a substantial number of cases of juxtacortical osteogenic sarcoma. Every case seems to have an alteration of cell cycle regulation. Abnormalities of *TP53* or *RB* fail to be prognostic under these conditions. It has recently been established that a telomere maintenance mechanism is essential for the cancer to persist. Uniquely, a high percentage of osteogenic sarcoma cases have an alternative, nontelomerase mechanism to remain immortal.[30] Dominant oncogenes also may be involved, including *RAS, MET, FOS,* and *MYC.*[31] Recently, the *erb*-B oncogene (epidermal growth factor receptor) was found to be present in 42% of cases and may present a therapeutic opportunity to modulate tumor growth.

Diagnosis

The lesion usually arises in the metaphysis of a long bone and grows outward from the medullary canal. On plain radiographs, classic osteogenic sarcoma produces a characteristic osteoblastic lesion in about 60% of cases. Lytic osteogenic sarcomas are composed of predominantly fibrous or telangiectatic tissue. Typical malignant features include a permeative growth pattern, poorly defined borders, and erosion through the cortex. MRI is excellent for imaging lesions in the marrow, screening for skip lesions, and identifying intramedullary extension of juxtacortical tumors and penetration of the physeal cartilage. The essential histologic feature of osteogenic sarcoma is the production of osteoid by malignant, spindle-shaped cells.

Prognosis

Factors other than stage (discussed earlier) have possible prognostic importance [32]:

- Site: axial and pelvic tumors fare worse than appendicular tumors.
- Biochemistry: elevation of alkaline phosphatase above institutional normal and lactate dehydrogenase above institutional normal are independent predictors of an unfavorable outcome.
- Race: African Americans have a worse outcome.
- Secondary osteogenic sarcomas have a worse prognosis.
- Skip lesions, which may represent bone-to-bone metastases, are associated with a poor patient prognosis.
- Histologic necrosis: the extent of necrosis in the primary tumor reflects the response to chemotherapy and predicts long-term disease-free survival.

Treatment

For high-grade osteogenic sarcoma, surgical excision of the primary, and any metastatic tumor must be combined with adjuvant chemotherapy. An oncologically sound operation must be performed to prevent local recurrence. Data support the success of limb-preserving surgery. Overall survival matches that achieved after amputation, despite an increase in local recurrence rates. In North America, Rougraff and colleagues reported that the rate of local recurrence was 0% for hip disarticulation, 7.8% for transfemoral amputation, and 11% for limb-sparing surgery.[33] Internationally, the COSS group reported local recurrence in 2.2% of cases of amputation or rotationplasty, in contrast to 11.1% for limb-sparing procedures.[34] At the Rizzoli Institute, local recurrence was 0% for rotationplasty and radical amputation, 8% for wide amputation, and 10% for limb-sparing surgery.[35] Poor responders to chemotherapy who also had narrow surgical margins suffered local recurrence in 20% of cases. They showed the interrelationship between good surgery and successful chemotherapy and, more importantly, between inadequate surgery and ineffective chemotherapy. After local recurrence, the 5-year survival rate is only 10%. Taken together, these studies indicate that amputation is more likely to control local disease than limb-sparing surgery. Nevertheless, it is not established that amputation is any better at curing patients. Limb preservation is oncologically appropriate if coupled with effective adjuvant chemotherapy. Patients who present with metastatic disease have a poor prognosis, and only 30% survive for 5 years.[36] With aggressive treatment, including resection of pulmonary metastases and intensive chemotherapy, survival can be extended for most patients, and some patients can be cured. Complete resection of recurrences seems to be the most important factor for a successful outcome.

Adjuvant Therapy

Systemic adjuvant chemotherapy is required to eradicate metastatic deposits. Several randomized studies settled the issue definitively. High-dose methotrexate (HDMTX) has been used in most protocols for osteogenic sarcoma and continues to be a major component of current multiagent regimens. Several agents in addition to HDMTX subsequently were found to have efficacy, most notably doxorubicin and cisplatin. Multiagent chemotherapy is superior to single-agent adjuvant therapy. The T4, 5, 7, 10, and 12 protocols, used previously at Memorial Sloan-Kettering, resulted collectively in a 65% disease-free survival for 279 patients with stage II (nonmetastatic) disease, now after 13 years of follow-up.[37]

The search for more effective combinations of chemotherapy continues. Adding more drugs to current regimens will compromise the dose intensity of the active agents already being used. The Children's Oncology Group/Pediatric Oncology Group (CCG/POG) study investigated two agents: ifosfamide and muramyl tripeptide phosphoethanolamine (MTP-PE). The 2×2 factorial design allowed for complex interactions between the experimental agents, so no definitive conclusions can be drawn. However, the use of ifosfamide without MTP-PE had the worst outcome, so this approach should probably not be taken.

Chemotherapy for osteogenic sarcoma has included preoperative neoadjuvant chemotherapy. Benefits of preoperative chemotherapy include immediate treatment of micrometastatic disease, enhancement of the margin of resection, and provision of time for surgical planning; however, there has not been a clear survival benefit.[38] A major advantage of preoperative chemotherapy is the ability to assess the histologic response to chemotherapy in the surgical specimen. Patients with more than 90% tumor necrosis after chemotherapy have significantly higher disease-free survival. Response to preoperative chemotherapy is highly dependent on which agents are used and the length of neoadjuvant therapy. Conceptually, it is attractive to administer different agents postoperatively if a patient does not respond well to the initial drug selections. Unfortunately, tailoring of chemotherapy does not improve survival for patients that do not respond well to first-line therapy.[37] Nevertheless, even patients who fail to show a dramatic response to preoperative chemotherapy still have a survival advantage compared with not receiving chemotherapy. Thus, chemotherapy should not be abandoned if necrosis is less than 90%.

Understanding the mechanisms of drug resistance is of paramount importance. Finally, it is hoped that elucidation of the genetic mutations underlying osteogenic sarcoma ultimately will lead to gene-based therapy.

Ewing's Family Tumors

Ewing's tumor is a malignant tumor of small round cells that arises in bone. Cytogenetic and molecular studies show that Ewing's sarcoma is a member of a family of tumors that includes primitive neuroectodermal tumors, peripheral neuroepithelioma, Askin's tumor of the chest wall, and extraosseous Ewing's tumor. The cause is related to a reciprocal translocation t(,22)(q24,q12) in over 90% of cases, which results in a fusion of the *EWS* gene to the *FLI1* gene. In approximately 5% of cases there is a 21,22 translocation that fuses the *EWS* gene to the *ERG* gene, and in rare cases the *EWS* gene may be fused to other genes, such as the *E1A* gene and the *ETV1* gene. The chimeric proteins affect other genes that transform the cell.

Ewing's tumor is one half as common as osteogenic sarcoma in the United States. Among patients under 15 years old, Ewing's tumor is nearly as common as osteogenic sarcoma. The disease is distinctly uncommon in blacks and Asians. The pelvis and femur are favored locations, but any bone may be involved.

Clinical Manifestations

Most patients have pain and swelling at the affected site. Growth of the tumor is rapid, a substantial, firm mass is present, and some patients have constitutional symptoms. Pathologic fractures occasionally occur.

Diagnosis

Ewing's tumor has protean radiographic manifestations. Onionskin periosteal changes are characteristic but often lacking. Ewing's tumor usually produces an ill-defined, lytic defect that permeates up and down the medullary canal, giving the bone a moth-eaten appearance. A large, soft tissue mass usually is adjacent to the bone. It is important to note the lactate dehydrogenase level because it is correlated to the disease burden and has prognostic importance. Osteomyelitis, Langerhans cell granuloma, and lymphoma are in the differential diagnosis. The tumor is composed of sheets of small, round, blue cells with hyperchromatic nuclei, scant cytoplasm, and little extracellular matrix. The monoclonal antibodies HBA71 and O13 show strong membranous staining for Ewing's tumor in 91% of cases. However, the antibody is not 100% specific. Reverse transcriptase-polymerase chain reaction (RT-PCR) detects the chimeric pseudogenes.

Ewing's tumor can disseminate widely in the marrow so the bone marrow should be sampled during staging for Ewing's tumor. Lungs and other bones are the usual sites of metastases.

Treatment

Treatment consists of multiagent chemotherapy and definitive local therapy. The mainstays of chemotherapy are doxorubicin, cyclophosphamide, vincristine, and dactinomycin. Ifosfamide and etoposide also have been shown to be effective in phase II and preliminary phase III trials. There has been an effort to stratify patients into high-risk versus standard-risk categories based on tumor size, location, and metastases.[39-41]

Definitive local therapy of the primary tumor consists of surgery, radiation therapy, or a combination of both modalities. Approximately 50% of patients with Ewing's tumor in the United States undergo surgery. The response to chemotherapy also affects the likelihood of local recurrence. Patients who responded well to chemotherapy had significantly better local control than patients who respond poorly.[42] Patients who had an objective response to chemotherapy and small tumors (<8 cm) achieved 90% local control, despite being given only a low radiation dose (35 Gy). Patients with large tumors and an objective response to chemotherapy were given a high radiation dose (50 to 60 Gy) but only achieved 52% local control. Finally, patients who had no objective response to chemotherapy had only 17% local control, despite being given high-dose radiation (50 to 60 Gy). Sometimes after induction chemotherapy and the administration of radiation the lesion may regress and become resectable.

Surgery controls local disease better than radiation. Despite improvements in imaging and radiation technology, radiotherapy shows disappointing results. Bacci reported that local recurrence was only 5% after primary surgical treatment, with or without radiation, and 41% after radiation without surgery.[43] The CESS study reported only 77% local control at 5 years. Ozaki and associates reported 15% local recurrence with radiation therapy alone, compared with 4% local recurrence with surgery alone and 4% with surgery and radiation therapy.[44] Surgery is often a superior alternative to remove a focus of radioresistant and chemoresistant cells that resides within a large tumor and to avoid the risk of radiation sarcoma. The cumulative risk of secondary sarcoma increases with time and has been estimated to be 8.6% at 20 years, with a mean latency of 7.6 years.[45] Surgery should no longer be reserved for expendable bones, such as the ribs, clavicle, and fibula. With modern surgical techniques, all bones are potentially resectable and can be reconstructed.

The appropriate margin of resection is debated between (1) outside of the original tumor, (2) outside of the tumor after induction chemotherapy, or (3) outside of the tumor after induction chemotherapy and radiation. It is likely that no single therapeutic strategy will be ideal for all patients. The early and late morbidity of surgery varies with each tumor. Treatment efficacy and morbidity must be balanced when deciding how to manage the primary Ewing's tumor site.

METASTATIC BONE DISEASE

More than one third of the 965,000 new cancer patients annually in the United States will develop skeletal metastases. Bone metastases outnumber primary bone cancers 100 to 1. Bone disease and fractures cause most of the pain and disability endured by cancer victims. Patients deserve the highest quality diagnostic and therapeutic care to ameliorate symptoms and preserve their independence in the terminal phase of their illnesses. Metastatic bone cancer should be cared for in as knowledgeable and sensitive a fashion as primary sarcomas, even though most intervention is palliative. Patients have complex end-of-life issues to deal with, and the surgeon has an important role to play in the diagnosis and management of this most-feared sequela of cancer.

Treatment should be multidisciplinary and address the systemic disease as well as the local manifestations. Metabolic complications of hypercalcemia, bone pain, and fractures can be prevented or ameliorated with bisphosphonates, particularly in multiple myeloma, breast cancer, and other forms of lytic metastatic disease.

Fracture prevention is a major goal. Appropriate use of rest, crutches, and braces provides the protection necessary while medications and radiation control the disease. Radiation therapy is usually appropriate for patients with symptomatic metastatic bone lesions. Even the so-called radioresistant tumors respond in at least 30% of cases. Surgery benefits those who fail radiation and medical management and those who sustain fractures. Bones at risk for fracture should be identified and treated early for the best results.

Epidemiology

Every cancer can metastasize to bone, but breast, prostate, lung, and kidney cancer do so most frequently. Bone metastases can occur in any bone, but clinically significant metastases are most common in the femur, humerus, and spine. Certain bones are more likely to develop metastases from particular primary tumors, that is, scapula for kidney cancer and hand metastases from lung and stomach primary tumors. Metastatic deposits are found most often in the metaphyses of long bones; they usually are multiple. The so-called solitary metastasis is usually the first of many lesions to be identified. Thyroid cancer, renal cancer, and myeloma (plasmacytoma) are the most likely to present as isolated metastases. Even these favorable cases typically develop widespread disease, suggesting that there is unrecognized dissemination of cancer at the time the first bone metastasis is identified. Metastases to the cortex alone are unusual, most commonly occur in lung cancer patients, and rapidly cause fracture. Surgical treatment of pathologic fractures is needed for approximately 9% of patients with clinically identifiable metastatic bone disease. The proximal femur and humerus are the most frequent sites operated on.

Pathogenesis

Metastatic cancer cells localize in bone because of bone's unique microvasculature and microenvironment. Interactions between the tumor cell and the host bone are critical. Bone lacks lymphatic channels, and metastases are hematogenous in origin. A complex interconnecting valveless network of vertebral, epidural, and perivertebral veins, also known as Batson's plexus, influences the distribution of blood flow and metastases. Tumor cells extravasate easily from the marrow vasculature, and small implants develop. Local angiogenesis promotes implant growth. Anti-angiogenesis may block this critical stage. Bone turnover may release growth factors that promote tumor growth. Osteopontin and bone sialoprotein help to fix tumor cells within the matrix and recruit osteoclasts that release interleukin, tumor growth factor-β, and other proteins. Cytokine feedback between the cancer and stromal cells conspires to destroy local bone and stimulate growth of the tumor deposit. Bone lysis is mediated by osteoclasts.[46] Potentially, the eccrine and autocrine loops could be interrupted, preventing further tumor growth and bone destruction. Microarray techniques show promise in identifying a metastatic genetic profile of cells that spread to bone.[47]

General Considerations

Pain is the principal symptom of bone metastases. It is composed of a biologic and a mechanical aspect. Although sometimes difficult to distinguish clinically, both must be treated. The mechanical properties of bone correlate best with the plain radiograph. Radiographs should be obtained of every symptomatic area. Lytic metastases are seen with lung and renal cancer. Mixed lytic and blastic metastases occur most often in breast cancer. Breast lesions may vary throughout the skeleton and over the course of the disease. Osteoblastic metastases are less common and typically occur with prostate and breast cancer. Bone scans are the most efficient way to screen the entire skeleton for metastatic disease. Cancers that are progressing very rapidly and overwhelm the bone reparative response may not be identified by the bone scan. MRI may be helpful diagnostically in selected cases, especially in the spine and to distinguish pathologic fracture due to osteoporosis from that caused by tumor. There is no biochemical test that is specific for bony metastases. Breakdown of bone collagen can be evaluated by measuring pyridinium or pyridinoline crosslinks. Biopsy is needed to diagnose the first bone metastasis. Special histochemical stains are helpful to define the site of origin of the unknown primary metastasis. In addition to the specific markers typically used, such as prostate-specific antigen and thyroglobulin, rare markers can be crucial in guiding treatment. For example, lymphoma can masquerade as metastatic carcinoma and can be identified only by Ki-1 stains. Biopsy or tumor defects larger than $1/4$ inch create stress risers that decrease torsional strength by 50% to 70%. Defects larger than the diameter of the bone are termed *open segment defects* and may reduce strength by as much as 90%. The nature of a metastatic lesion affects the overall bone strength.

Treatment Goals

The goals of patient comfort and independence usually are met nonoperatively by radiation therapy and chemotherapy. Most patients without a fracture do not require surgery for the bone metastasis. Fractures are best treated by operative procedures to allow immediate weight bearing. If this cannot be achieved, then surgery should be avoided. Pathologic fractures through weight-bearing bones (e.g., femur) should be treated if the patient has more than 1 month to live and through non–weight-bearing bones if life expectancy is more than 3 months. Joint replacement and stabilization with polymethyl methacrylate (PMMA) is usually the most effective.

Imaging identifies areas of impending fracture that may require prophylactic surgery to fix the bone defect, prevent fracture, and maximize function. CT very effectively distinguishes between the *presence* of disease and *structurally significant* disease. Mirels and associates have proposed a graduated scoring system.[48] Four clinical and radiographic factors—anatomic site, pain pattern, radiographic nature, and lesion size—are each graded 0 to 3. The sum creates a composite score (0 to 12) that correlates with fracture risks (Table 30-5).

The rapid growth of metastatic cancers may overwhelm the healing response. Gainor and Buchert evaluated 129 long-bone fractures.[49] Healing occurred in 45 cases (36%). Among patients who lived 6 months or more, 50% of fractures healed. The best healing rates were in multiple myeloma (67%), kidney (44%), and breast cancer (37%). No patients with lung cancer healed their fractures. Chemotherapy effects in animal models are difficult to extrapolate to humans because of variation in dose intensity and treatment scheduling. Most studies suggest that healing is reduced 50% by common agents such as methotrexate or doxorubicin. Radiation suppresses osteoblast function and adversely affects fracture healing. Doses as low as 2000 cGy begin to interfere with normal fracture healing, and healing is very difficult to achieve after doses exceeding 5000 cGy.

Treatment: Surgery, Radiation, Systemic Therapy

Surgery

Metastatic deposits should be removed whenever possible in the course of fixing a pathologic fracture. This achieves an immediate partial response that could take weeks to achieve by other methods. Intralesional curettage is the typical method. Bleeding may be profuse but generally stops when the lesional tissue is removed back to normal bone so the tumor vessels can contract and stop bleeding. Preoperative angiography and tumor embolization greatly reduces blood flow and intraoperative hemorrhage. Adjuvants such as cryosurgery with liquid nitrogen can be helpful in treating metastatic disease. Cryosurgery extends the surgical margin and is indicated for tumors that are no longer responsive to other treatments. Radiation therapy is the principal surgical adjuvant. It should be delivered to the entire surgical field and extend the length of any internal fixation device. Surgery has an important role to play in the terminal care of cancer patients. Amputation continues to have a role in the management of metastatic cancer for (1) an unreconstructable extremity lesion, (2) treatment failures or complications such as a fungating infected lesion, and (3) intractable pain. Distal sites are most suitable for amputation to relieve symptoms and resume function. Occasionally, rhizotomy and cordotomy provide good pain relief of unilateral disease.

Stabilization of a fracture requires control of the proximal and distal fracture fragments. The considerations are different for epiphyseal, metaphyseal, diaphyseal, and apophyseal locations. The different regions are discussed in sequence. Epiphyseal fractures present the easiest problem. Fracture healing is not a consideration. Resection of the epiphyseal fractures is appropriate, and arthroplasty should be performed. Metaphyseal fractures have more complex geometry and require more complex surgical decision making. Defects on the tension side of the bone may be secured by plating techniques, particularly for pathologic fractures that have a decent chance to heal or those in very sick patients. Plating techniques are more prone to failure, however, than rodding methods. Eleven percent of plated pathologic fractures fail within 7 weeks, and a cumulative 40% failed after 5 years in a series of 167 fractures. Diaphyseal lesions are best treated by intramedullary fixation, combining an intramedullary rod

---

TABLE 30-5.   Scoring System to Predict Rate of Pathologic Fracture

Variable	Points		
	1	**2**	**3**
Site	Upper extremity	Lower extremity	Pertrochanteric
Pain	Mild	Moderate	Mechanical
Radiograph	Blastic	Mixed	Lytic
Size (% of shaft)	0-33	34-67	68-100

Score	Patients (n)	Fracture Rate (%)
0-6	11	0
7	19	5
8	12	33
9	7	57
10-12	18	100

with interlocking screws and cement. Intramedullary rods restore flexion and bending strength beautifully and torsional strength and stiffness poorly. Closed intramedullary rodding should be reserved for fractures that will heal when stabilized and supplemented by radiation or for patients with rapidly advancing preterminal disease in whom the proximal and distal fixation will outlast the patient's projected survival.

Radiation

Radiation effectively treats the pain of metastatic cancer affecting the bone. Radiation also arrests local tumor growth and permits functional improvement in most patients.[50] Seventy percent of patients have pain relief within 2 weeks, and 90% experience relief after 3 weeks. Fifty-five to 70 percent of patients who initially respond do not develop recurrent pain in the treatment field, according to the Radiation Therapy Oncology Group study.[51,52] There is no convincing evidence that different histologic cancers respond differently to radiation. Despite its efficacy, radiation should not be used indiscriminately because it can be expensive, does not address mechanical disease, and can have complications such as marrow fibrosis and neutropenia or thrombocytopenia that could preclude chemotherapy. Radiation is best thought of as an effective trump card to be played at an appropriate occasion in the course of the cancer patient's treatment for metastatic disease.

Systemic Therapy

Patients with widespread skeletal involvement require systemic therapy. Chemotherapy or endocrine therapy is the most appropriate. This is tailored to the nature of the metastasis. Monthly bisphosphonate treatment does not interfere with systemic chemotherapy and effectively prevents fractures, progression of existing bone lesions, and development of new symptomatic lesions; it is a well-established treatment of breast cancer and multiple myeloma. Although controversial, there is a rationale for extending the use of these drugs to patients with other lytic bone diseases. Despite enthusiasm for this approach among medical oncologists, there is sparse evidence that established lesions will heal during bisphosphonate therapy. It is preferable to treat most symptomatic lesions surgically, rather than have the patient endure a protracted course of bisphosphonates and crutches while waiting for undependable bone healing.[53]

Selected References

Clohisy DR, Ogilvie CM, Carpenter RJ, Ramnaraine ML: Localized, tumor-associated osteolysis involves the recruitment and activation of osteoclasts. J Orthop Res 14:2-6, 1996.

> This careful study conclusively shows that all tumor-related bone loss occurs via osteoclastic bone resorption. Treatment of bone loss, be it from metastatic disease or around prostheses, is geared to block the osteoclasts. Bisphosphonate therapy is based on these observations.

Malawer MM, Bickels J, Meller I, et al: Cryosurgery in the treatment of giant cell tumor: A long-term follow-up study. Clin Orthop 359:176-188, 1999.

> Local adjuvants are very helpful when intralesional therapy is chosen to reduce the amount of local resection required to control the bone tumor. This is particularly important when it means that a joint can be spared, thereby avoiding resection and reconstruction. Epiphyseal tumors such as giant cell tumor, some low-grade chondrosarcomas, and metastases are good candidates for cryosurgery treatment. This large study shows that stable internal fixation can reduce the rate of fracture complications.

Mankin HJ, Mankin CJ, Simon MA: The hazards of the biopsy, revisited. Members of the Musculoskeletal Tumor Society (see comments). J Bone Joint Surg Am 78:656-663, 1996.

> Inappropriate or careless biopsies complicate cancer care greatly. Biopsies performed in community centers had much higher complication rates than those performed in tumor centers. The conclusion is that bone biopsies should be done by a surgeon who will provide the definitive surgical treatment.

Mirels H: Metastatic disease in long bones: A proposed scoring system. Clin Orthop 249:256-265, 1989.

> Prediction of fracture is important to optimize the care of patients with metastatic bone disease. This popular system is simple, inexpensive, and reasonably accurate. It should be used by all oncologists and surgeons who deal with metastatic bone disease until a better system is devised.

Picci P, Sangiorgi L, Rougraff BT, et al: Relationship of chemotherapy-induced necrosis and surgical margins to local recurrence in osteosarcoma. J Clin Oncol 12:2699-2705, 1994.

> Effective chemotherapy and good surgery reduce the chance of local recurrence. This study documents the complex relationship between these variables. It is provocative in implying that cases that have a poor response to chemotherapy need more effective surgical treatment to avoid local recurrence.

Rougraff BT, Simon MA, Kneisl JS, et al: Limb salvage compared with amputation for osteosarcoma of the distal end of the femur: A long-term oncological, functional, and quality-of-life study. J Bone Joint Surg Am 76:649-656, 1994.

> This retrospective review is hailed as the evidence that limb preservation achieves equivalent results as amputation in the treatment of osteogenic sarcoma. Although it remains the best there is, the study is flawed by selection bias and low power, among other things.

Unwin PS, Walker PS: Extendible endoprostheses for the skeletally immature. Clin Orthop 322:179-193, 1996.

> Limb preservation in young children must take into consideration the anticipated growth of the extremities. Extendible implants have been a major advance that has allowed limb preservation to become a reality for children 6 to 10 years old. The implants suffer from high failure and revision rates, as documented in this, the largest, series.

References

1. Mankin HJ, Lange TA, Spanier SS: The hazards of biopsy in patients with malignant primary bone and soft-tissue tumors. J Bone Joint Surg Am 64A:1121-1127, 1982.
2. Caffey J: On fibrous defects in cortical walls of growing tubular bones. Adv Pediatr 7:13, 1955.
3. Wilkins RM: Unicameral bone cysts. J Am Acad Orthop Surg 8:217-224, 2000.
4. Rosenthal DI, Hornicek FJ, Wolfe MW, et al: Percutaneous radiofrequency coagulation of osteoid osteoma compared with operative treatment. J Bone Joint Surg Am 80A:815-821, 1998.
5. Marco RA, Gitelis S, Brebach GT, et al: Cartilage tumors: Evaluation and treatment. J Am Acad Orthop Surg 8:292-304, 2000.
6. Saifuddin A: The accuracy of imaging in the local staging of appendicular osteosarcoma. Skeletal Radiol 31:191-201, 2002.
7. Campanacci M, Capanna R, Picci P: Unicameral and aneurysmal bone cysts. Clin Orthop 25-36, 1986.
8. Enneking WF: A system of staging musculoskeletal neoplasms. Clin Orthop Rel Res 204:9-24, 1986.
9. Malawer MM, Bickels J, Meller I, et al: Cryosurgery in the treatment of giant cell tumor: A long-term follow-up study. Clin Orthop Rel Res 359:176-188, 1999.
10. O'Donnell RJ, Springfield DS, Motwani HK, et al: Recurrence of giant-cell tumors of the long bones after curettage and packing with cement. J Bone Joint Surg Am 76:1827-1833, 1994.
11. Murata H, Kusuzaki K, Takeshita H, et al: Assessment of chemosensitivity in patients with malignant bone and soft tissue tumors using thallium-201 scintigraphy and doxorubicin binding assay. Anticancer Res 20:3967-3970, 2000.
12. Franzius C, Bielack S, Flege S, et al: Prognostic significance of (18)F-FDG and (99m)Tc-methylene diphosphonate uptake in primary osteosarcoma. J Nucl Med 43:1012-1017, 2002.
13. Bacci G, Ferrari S, Lari S, et al: Osteosarcoma of the limb: Amputation or limb salvage in patients treated by neoadjuvant chemotherapy. J Bone Joint Surg Br 84:88-92, 2002.
14. Picci P, Sangiorgi L, Rougraff BT, et al: Relationship of chemotherapy-induced necrosis and surgical margins to local recurrence in osteosarcoma. J Clin Oncol 12:2699-2705, 1994.
15. Minami A, Kasashima T, Iwasaki N, et al: Vascularised fibular grafts: An experience of 102 patients. J Bone Joint Surg Br 82:1022-1025, 2000.
16. Gottsauner-Wolf F, Kotz R, Knahr K, et al: Rotationplasty for limb salvage in the treatment of malignant tumors at the knee: A follow-up study of seventy patients. J Bone Joint Surg Am 73:1365-1375, 1991.
17. Hillmann A, Hoffmann C, Gosheger G, et al: Malignant tumor of the distal part of the femur or the proximal part of the tibia: Endoprosthetic replacement or rotationplasty: Functional outcome and quality-of-life measurements. J Bone Joint Surg Am 81:462-468, 1999.
18. Horowitz SM, Glasser DB, Lane JM, et al: Prosthetic and extremity survivorship after limb salvage for sarcoma. How long do the reconstructions last? Clin Orthop, Aug (293):280-286, 1993.
19. Kawai A, Backus SI, Otis JC, et al: Interrelationships of clinical outcome, length of resection, and energy cost of walking after prosthetic knee replacement following resection of a malignant tumor of the distal aspect of the femur. J Bone Joint Surg Am 80:822-831, 1998.
20. Kawai A, Healey JH, Boland PJ, et al: A rotating-hinge knee replacement for malignant tumors of the femur and tibia. J Arthroplasty 14:187-196, 1999.
21. Mittermayer F, Krepler P, Dominkus M, et al: Long-term followup of uncemented tumor endoprostheses for the lower extremity. Clin Orthop 388:167-177, 2001.
22. Unwin PS, Cannon SR, Grimer RJ, et al: Aseptic loosening in cemented custom-made prosthetic replacements for bone tumours of the lower limb. J Bone Joint Surg Br 78:5-13, 1996.
23. Wunder JS, Leitch K, Griffin AM, et al: Comparison of two methods of reconstruction for primary malignant tumors at the knee: A sequential cohort study. J Surg Oncol 77:89-99, 2001.
24. Wilkins RM, Soubeiran A: The Phenix expandable prosthesis: Early American experience. Clin Orthop, Jan (382):51-58, 2001.
25. Unwin PS, Walker PS: Extendible endoprostheses for the skeletally immature. Clin Orthop, Jan (322):179-193, 1996.
26. Donati D, Di Liddo M, Zavatta M, et al: Massive bone allograft reconstruction in high-grade osteosarcoma. Clin Orthop, Aug (377):186-194, 2000.
27. Mankin HJ, Gebhardt MC, Jennings LC, et al: Long-term results of allograft replacement in the management of bone tumors. Clin Orthop, Mar (324):86-97, 1996.
28. Gitelis S, Piasecki P: Allograft prosthetic composite arthroplasty for osteosarcoma and other aggressive bone tumors. Clin Orthop Rel Res 270:197-201, 1991.
29. Gokgoz N, Wunder JS, Mousses S, et al: Comparison of p53 mutations in patients with localized osteosarcoma and metastatic osteosarcoma. Cancer 92:2181-2189, 2001.
30. Ulaner GA, Huang HY, Otero J, et al: Absence of a telomere maintenance mechanism as a favorable prognostic factor in patients with osteosarcoma. Cancer Res 63:1759-1763, 2003.
31. Sandberg AA, Bridge JA: Updates on the cytogenetics and molecular genetics of bone and soft tissue tumors: Osteosarcoma and related tumors. Cancer Genet Cytogenet 145: 1-30, 2003.
32. Bacci G, Ferrari S, Bertoni F, et al: Histologic response of high-grade nonmetastatic osteosarcoma of the extremity to chemotherapy. Clin Orthop, May (386):186-196, 2001.
33. Rougraff BT, Simon MA, Kneisl JS, et al: Limb salvage compared with amputation for osteosarcoma of the distal end of the femur: A long-term oncological, functional, and quality-of-life study. J Bone Joint Surg Am 76:649-656, 1994.
34. Fuchs N, Bielack SS, Epler D, et al: Long-term results of the co-operative German-Austrian-Swiss osteosarcoma study group's protocol COSS-86 of intensive multidrug chemotherapy and surgery for osteosarcoma of the limbs. Ann Oncol 9:893-899, 1998.
35. Picci P, Sangiorgi L, Bahamonde L, et al: Risk factors for local recurrences after limb-salvage surgery for high-grade osteosarcoma of the extremities. Ann Oncol 8:899-903, 1997.
36. Bielack SS, Kempf-Bielack B, Delling G, et al: Prognostic factors in high-grade osteosarcoma of the extremities or trunk: An analysis of 1,702 patients treated on neoadjuvant cooperative osteosarcoma study group protocols. J Clin Oncol 20:776-790, 2002.
37. Meyers PA, Gorlick R, Heller G, et al: Intensification of preoperative chemotherapy for osteogenic sarcoma: Results of the Memorial Sloan-Kettering (T12) protocol. J Clin Oncol 16:2452-2458, 1998.
38. Goorin AM, Schwartzentruber DJ, Devidas M, et al: Presurgical chemotherapy compared with immediate surgery and adjuvant chemotherapy for nonmetastatic osteosarcoma: Pediatric Oncology Group Study POG-8651. J Clin Oncol 21:1574-1580, 2003.
39. Bacci G, Mercuri M, Longhi A, et al: Neoadjuvant chemotherapy for Ewing's tumour of bone: Recent experi-

ence at the Rizzoli Orthopaedic Institute. Eur J Cancer 38:2243-2251, 2002.

40. Cotterill SJ, Ahrens S, Paulussen M, et al: Prognostic factors in Ewing's tumor of bone: Analysis of 975 patients from the European Intergroup Cooperative Ewing's Sarcoma Study Group. J Clin Oncol 18:3108-3114, 2000.

41. Paulussen M, Ahrens S, Dunst J, et al: Localized Ewing tumor of bone: Final results of the cooperative Ewing's Sarcoma Study CESS 86. J Clin Oncol 19:1818-1829, 2001.

42. Wunder JS, Paulian G, Huvos AG, et al: The histological response to chemotherapy as a predictor of the oncological outcome of operative treatment of Ewing sarcoma. J Bone Joint Surg Am 80:1020-1033, 1998.

43. Bacci G, Ferrari S, Longhi A, et al: Local and systemic control in Ewing's sarcoma of the femur treated with chemotherapy, and locally by radiotherapy and/or surgery. J Bone Joint Surg Br 85:107-114, 2003.

44. Ozaki T, Hillmann A, Hoffmann C, et al: Significance of surgical margin on the prognosis of patients with Ewing's sarcoma. A report from the Cooperative Ewing's Sarcoma Study. Cancer 78:892-900, 1996.

45. Kuttesch JF Jr, Wexler LH, Marcus RB, et al: Second malignancies after Ewing's sarcoma: radiation dose-dependency of secondary sarcomas. J Clin Oncol 14:2818-2825, 1996.

46. Clohisy DR, Ogilvie CM, Carpenter RJ, et al: Localized, tumor-associated osteolysis involves the recruitment and activation of osteoclasts. J Orthop Res 14:2-6, 1996.

47. Kang Y, Siegel PM, Shu W, et al: A multigenic program mediating breast cancer metastasis to bone. Cancer Cell 3:537-549, 2003.

48. Mirels H: Metastatic disease in long bones: A proposed scoring system for diagnosing impending pathologic fractures. Clin Orthop, Dec (249):256-264, 1989.

49. Gainor BJ, Buchert P: Fracture healing in metastatic bone disease. Clin Orthop 178:297-302, 1983.

50. Rose CM, Kagan AR: The final report of the Expert Panel for the Radiation Oncology Bone Metastasis Work Group of the American College of Radiology. Int J Radiat Oncol Biol Phys 40:1117-1124, 1998.

51. Blitzer PH: Reanalysis of the RTOG study of the palliation of symptomatic osseous metastasis. Cancer 55:1468-1472, 1985.

52. Ratanatharathorn V, Powers WE, Moss WT, et al: Bone metastasis: Review and critical analysis of random allocation trials of local field treatment. Int J Radiat Oncol Biol Phys 44:1-18, 1999.

53. Diel IJ, Mundy GR: Bisphosphonates in the adjuvant treatment of cancer: Experimental evidence and first clinical results. International Bone and Cancer Study Group (IBCG). Br J Cancer 82:1381-1386, 2000.

HEAD AND NECK

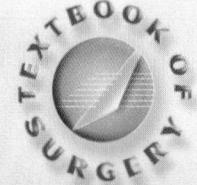

CHAPTER 31

HEAD AND NECK

Robert R. Lorenz, M.D., James L. Netterville, M.D., and Brian B. Burkey, M.D.

Normal Histology	Anatomic Sites
Epidemiology	Tracheotomy
Carcinogenesis	Vocal Cord Paralysis
Staging	Reconstruction
Clinical Overview	

NORMAL HISTOLOGY

The normal histology of the upper aerodigestive tract varies within each site.[1] A review of the thyroid and parathyroid glands is beyond the scope of this chapter. The nasal vestibule is considered a cutaneous structure and is lined by keratinizing squamous epithelium. The limen nasi or mucocutaneous junction is where the epithelium changes to a ciliated pseudostratified columnar (respiratory) epithelium to line the nasal cavities. The exception is the olfactory epithelium at the roof of the nasal cavity that is composed of bipolar, spindle-shaped olfactory neural cells with surrounding supporting cells. The paranasal sinuses are also lined by respiratory epithelium, but it tends to be thinner and less vascular than that of the nasal cavity. The nasopharynx lining varies from squamous epithelium to respiratory in an inconsistent manner. The adenoidal pad is composed of lymphoid tissue containing germinal centers without capsules or sinusoids. The oral cavity is lined by a nonkeratinized stratified squamous epithelium with minor salivary glands throughout the submucosa and within the muscular tissue of the tongue. Although the oropharynx is lined by squamous epithelium, Waldeyer's ring is formed by the lymphoid tissues of the palatine tonsils, adenoids, lingual tonsils, and the adjacent submucosal lymphatics. The tonsils contain germinal centers without capsules or sinusoids, but unlike the adenoids, the tonsils have crypts lined by stratified squamous epithelium.

The hypopharynx is lined by a nonkeratinizing, stratified squamous epithelium. Seromucous glands are found throughout the submucosa of the hypopharynx, in the lower two thirds of the epiglottis, and in the potential space between the true and false vocal folds known as the *ventricle*. A nonkeratinizing stratified squamous epithelium lines the epiglottis and true vocal fold. A pseudostratified, ciliated respiratory epithelium lines the false vocal fold, ventricle, and subglottis. Although the thyroid, cricoid, and arytenoid cartilages are composed of hyaline cartilage, the epiglottis, cuneiform, and corniculate cartilages are composed of elastic-type cartilage. The external ear is a cutaneous structure lined with keratinizing squamous epithelium and associated adnexal structures. The external third of the external auditory canal is unique in that it contains modified apocrine glands that produce cerumen. The middle ear is lined with respiratory epithelium.

Numerous noncancerous changes to the squamous epithelium can be seen in the upper aerodigestive tract. Leukoplakia, which describes any white mucosal lesion, and erythroplasia, describing any red mucosal lesion, are both clinical descriptions and should not be used as diagnostic terms (Fig. 31-1). Erythroplakia is more often indicative of an underlying malignant lesion. *Hyperplasia* refers to a thickening of the epithelium secondary to an increase in the total number of cells. *Parakeratosis* is an abnormal presence of nuclei in the keratin layers, whereas *dyskeratosis* refers to any abnormal keratinization of epithelial

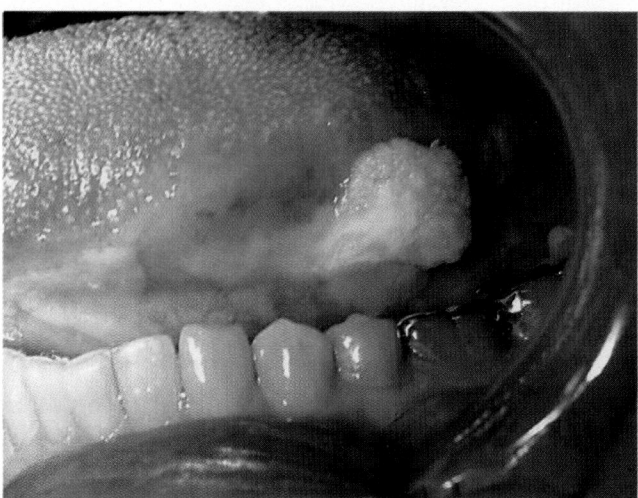

FIGURE 31-1. A leukoplakic lesion of the left mobile tongue. This lesion was determined to be hyperkeratosis on biopsy without invasive cancer.

whereas alcohol abuse carries an odds ratio of 2.11.[4] Combined abuse of alcohol and tobacco is not additive in terms of odds ratio but is multiplicative. Worldwide, incidence rates of cancer in the head and neck vary, usually in association with alcohol and tobacco use. The highest incidence rates among males exceeds 30/100,000 in areas of France, Hong Kong, India, Central and Eastern Europe, Spain, Italy, Brazil, and among U.S. blacks.[5] The highest female rates are greater than 10/100,000 and are found in India, where the chewing of betel quid and tobacco is common. Although aggregate rates are slowly declining in select areas such as India, Hong Kong, Brazil, and among U.S. whites, rates are increasing in most other regions of the world. In addition to alcohol and tobacco consumption as causative factors, other risk factors include human papillomavirus and Epstein-Barr virus infection, Plummer-Vinson syndrome, metabolic polymorphisms, malnutrition, and occupational exposure to mutagenic agents. According to the National Cancer Data Base, squamous cell carcinoma (HNSCC) is the most common head and neck malignant diagnosis (55.8%), followed by adenocarcinoma (19.4%) and lymphoma (15.1%).[6]

cells and is found in dysplastic lesions. *Koilocytosis* is a descriptive term for vacuolization of squamous cells and is suggestive of viral infection, especially human papillomavirus.

EPIDEMIOLOGY

The American Joint Committee on Cancer (AJCC) staging system divides the malignancy sites originating in the head and neck into six major groups: lip and oral cavity, pharynx, larynx, nasal cavity and paranasal sinuses, major salivary glands, and thyroid.[2] Of the sites arising from the aerodigestive tract, laryngeal cancer remains the most common cause of death (Table 31-1). Although there clearly remains a male predominance in aerodigestive tract malignancies, the ratio of male to female has been steadily decreasing owing to a direct association between tobacco as a causative agent and the increased incidence of female smokers. Tobacco abuse increases the odds ratio of developing laryngeal cancer by 15.1,

CARCINOGENESIS

Carcinogenesis is a multistep process consisting of a sequential accumulation of genetic alterations. These alterations, or mutations, are expressed phenotypically in the cancer cells as clonal outgrowth, increased proliferative capacity, immortality, cell motility, and invasion. Additionally, the tumor cells induce changes in the nontumor host cells to create paracrine growth feedback loops, inhibit host immunity, and cause neovascularization. Direct damage to DNA can be caused by either exogenous factors such as radiation, chemical carcinogens, oxidative stress, or viral insertions or by intrinsic factors such as spontaneous deletions, missense mutations, insertions, and chromosomal translocations. It is estimated that between 3 (early-onset nasal cancer) and 11 (laryngeal cancer) separate mutations are required to allow a head and neck tumor to develop.[7] Mutations then affect the two types of genes involved in carcinogenesis: protooncogenes and tumor suppressor genes.

Table 31-1. Head and Neck Cancer 2002 Statistics: Upper Aerodigestive Tract

Site	Estimated Incidence			Estimated Deaths		
	Both Sexes	Male	Female	Both Sexes	Male	Female
Tongue	7100	4700	2400	1700	1100	600
Mouth	9800	5200	4600	2000	1100	900
Pharynx	8600	6500	2100	2100	1500	600
Other oral cavity	3400	2500	900	1600	1200	400
Larynx	8900	6900	2000	3700	2900	800

From Jemal A, Thomas A, Murray T, et al: Cancer statistics, 2002. CA Cancer J Clin 52:23-47, 2002.

Protooncogenes normally encode for proteins involved in cell regulatory function, but when mutated, cause malignant characteristics such as increased proliferation, decreased apoptosis, and increased angiogenesis. The protooncogenes studied in association with HNSCC include cyclin D1 (PRAD1), VEGF, TGF-α, TGF-β, and EGF-R. Vascular endothelial cell growth factor (VEGF) is an endothelial cell mitogen and also promotes cell mobility and penetration of endothelium. In a study of 77 patients with either oral or oropharyngeal carcinoma, VEGF was found to be present in 41% of tumors, and its presence was the most significant predictor of poor patient prognosis.[8] The cyclin family of proteins is responsible for driving cellular proliferation. Cyclin D1 is encoded at the 11q13 chromosomal locus and is overexpressed in approximately 68% of tongue cancers. Although some studies are contradictory, increased expression of cyclin D1 has been shown to be an independent prognostic indicator of recurrence.[9] Epidermal growth factor receptor (EGF-R) overexpression or increased activation is ubiquitous in HNSCC and has also been shown to correlate with poor survival.

Tumor suppressor genes normally encode for proteins that inhibit tumor development. Typically, tumorigenesis is allowed only with the loss of both alleles, but p53 is the exception to this rule. As the most commonly altered tumor suppressor in human tumors, p53 is also the most studied tumor suppressor gene. Because mutated p53 is not degraded as rapidly as wild-type p53, overexpression is actually a signal that p53 has been altered and is nonfunctional. A steady increase in the number of p53 abnormalities occurs during the progression of HNSCC, with p53 being overexpressed in 19% of normal epithelia, 29% of hyperplastic lesions, 45% of dysplastic lesions, and 58% of invasive cancers.[10] p53 mutations also are correlated with tobacco and alcohol abuse. In analyses of different HNSCC tumors, 58% of tumors in patients who abused both alcohol and tobacco contained p53 mutations, as compared to 33% of lesions in patients who abused tobacco alone and 17% of cancers in patients who abused neither alcohol nor tobacco.[11] p53 has been shown to not only be inactivated by mutation and deletion but also by protein products of both Epstein-Barr virus associated with the majority of nasopharyngeal carcinomas and human papilloma virus associated with 50% of oropharyngeal squamous cell carcinomas. In addition to being inactivated by viral proteins, deletions, and mutations, p53 is also intimately connected with the tumor suppressor gene that is most frequently altered in HNSCC, the *p16-ARF* gene. The p16-ARF gene locus uniquely encodes two proteins translated in different reading frames, p16 and ARF. p16 is an inhibitor of cyclin-dependent kinase and therefore can be considered an activator of retinoblastoma with the biologic effect of stopping cellular proliferation. ARF, the other protein encoded by this gene locus, is an activator of p53 and can cause either cell cycle arrest or apoptosis. The p16-ARF gene locus is altered in more than 50% of head and neck squamous cell cancers, suggesting that inactivation of both retinoblastoma and p53 is important for formation of these tumors.

The ultimate clinical goal of deciphering the molecular abnormalities that result in head and neck cancer is to aid in the development of targeted molecular therapy. The recent success of imatinib mesylate (Gleevec), an inhibitor of the abl tyrosine kinase, in treatment of chronic myelogenous leukemia and gastrointestinal stromal tumors has advanced the cause of biologic therapy. The concept is that seemingly homogeneous head and neck cancers differ in their gene and protein expression profiles and therefore will differ in their response to biologic therapy. By identifying patterns of molecular abnormalities for a given tumor, specific therapy that will be most effective for a particular patient's tumor can be recommended. Biologic treatments may be solo therapy, but efficacy may be increased by combining novel biologicals with traditional surgery, radiation, or chemoradiation allowed by nonoverlapping toxicities.

Carcinogenesis in HNSCC also includes the development of second primary tumors, with patients having a 3% to 7% yearly incidence of secondary lesions in the upper aerodigestive tract, esophagus, or lung. A synchronous second primary lesion is defined as a tumor detected within 6 months of the index tumor. The occurrence of a second primary lesion more than 6 months after the initial lesion is referred to as *metachronous*. There is debate as to whether second lesions represent "reseeding" of the primary tumor or genetically separate lesions caused by the "field-cancerization" effect due to carcinogen exposure. When analyzing p53 mutations in patients with second primary tumors, up to 100% of p53 changes are different between the primary lesion and secondary cancer, strongly suggesting that these lesions arise as independent events.[12] Conversely, when analyzing synchronous oral carcinomas, both identical alterations (60%) and discordant alterations (40%) have been identified, suggesting that synchronous lesions can be of independent origin in some patients, but may be of clonal origin in others.[13] Fourteen percent of HNSCC patients will develop a second primary in the aerodigestive tract over the course of their lifetime, with more than half of these lesions occurring within the first 2 years of the index tumor. Owing to the incidence of either second lung primaries or metastatic lung lesions, both a posteroanterior and lateral chest radiograph are obtained at the time of diagnosis and annually for the patient's post-treatment cancer surveillance.

STAGING

The staging of head and neck cancer follows the TNM classification established by the AJCC.[2] The T classification refers to the extent of the primary tumor and is specific to each of the six sites of origin, with subclassifications within each site. The N classification refers to the pattern of lymphatic spread within the neck nodes and is the same for most head and neck sites (Table 31-2). Clinical staging of the neck is based primarily on palpation, although radiographic studies including computed tomography (CT) or magnetic resonance imaging (MRI) have been shown to be accurate in detecting positive nodes. If the CT criteria of nodes with central necrosis or size greater than 1.0 cm is used to determine positivity, only 7% of

Classification	Description
NX	Regional lymph nodes cannot be assessed
N0	No regional lymph node metastasis
N1	Metastasis in a single ipsilateral lymph node, ≤ 3 cm in greatest dimension
N2	Metastasis in a single ipsilateral lymph node, > 3 cm but not > 6 cm in greatest dimension; or in multiple ipsilateral lymph nodes, none > 6 cm in greatest dimension; or in bilateral or contralateral lymph nodes, none > 6 cm in greatest dimension
N2a	Metastasis in single ipsilateral lymph node > 3 cm but not > 6 cm in greatest dimension
N2b	Metastasis in multiple ipsilateral lymph nodes, none > 6 cm in greatest dimension
N2c	Metastasis in bilateral or contralateral lymph nodes, none > 6 cm in greatest dimension
N3	Metastasis in a lymph node > 6 cm in greatest dimension

From Greene FL, Page DL, Fleming ID, et al (eds): AJCC Cancer Staging Manual, 6th ed. New York, Springer-Verlag, 2002.

pathologically positive lymph nodes would be missed and these smaller nodes are most often in necks with more extensive disease.[13] Metastatic disease is reported simply as Mx (cannot be assessed), M0 (no distant metastases are present), or M1 (metastases present). The most common sites of distant spread are the lungs and bones, whereas hepatic and brain metastases occur less frequently. The risk of distant metastases is more dependent on the nodal staging than on the primary tumor size.

After complete resection of the primary and nodal disease, pathologic staging may be reported. This is designated by a preceding "p," as in pTNM. It must be remembered when measuring a pathologic mucosal specimen that the tumor size may decrease up to 30% after resection. Although clinical T staging is of primary concern, pathologic N staging allows detection of occult microscopic disease and is useful in determining prognosis. Site-specific staging systems are discussed according to primary site. The major change in the 2002 edition of the AJCC staging system for the HNSCC sites is the staging of T4 disease, which has been divided into T4a (resectable) and T4b (unresectable), leading to the division of stage IVA (advanced resectable), Stage IVB (advanced unresectable), and Stage IVC (advanced distant metastatic disease).

CLINICAL OVERVIEW

Evaluation

Proper treatment of HNSCC requires careful evaluation and accurate staging, both clinically and radiographically.

Patients with HNSCC are initially evaluated in a similar manner regardless of the site of tumor. Patient histories focus on symptomatology of the tumor, including duration of symptoms, detection of masses, location of pain, and the presence of referred pain. Special attention is paid to numbness, cranial nerve weakness, dysphagia, odynophagia, hoarseness, disarticulation, airway compromise, trismus, nasal obstruction, epistaxis, or hemoptysis. Alcohol and tobacco use histories are obtained. Office examination includes nasopharyngeal and laryngeal visualization, either with a mirror or fiberoptic endoscopy. The examiner should be especially vigilant for second primary tumors and not be preoccupied by the obvious primary lesion. CT and MRI scanning of the head and neck with contrast media may be obtained for tumor evaluation and occult lymphadenopathy detection. CT scanning is best at evaluating bony destruction, whereas MRI can determine soft tissue involvement and is excellent for evaluating the parotid and parapharyngeal space tumors. Chest radiography or chest CT scanning is obtained to rule out synchronous lung lesions. Serum tumor markers such as alkaline phosphatase and calcium may be obtained but are not standard.

Direct laryngoscopy and examination under anesthesia are commonly performed as part of the evaluation of HNSCC. These procedures allow the physician to evaluate tumors without patient discomfort and with muscle paralysis, as well as evaluate the oropharynx, hypopharynx, and larynx and obtain biopsies. Pathologic confirmation of cancer is mandatory prior to initiating treatment. Concurrent bronchoscopy and esophagoscopy have been historically recommended for detection of synchronous second primaries of the aerodigestive tract that occur in 4% to 8% of patients who have one head and neck malignancy. In the face of a normal chest radiograph or CT scan, bronchoscopy has a low yield for discovering bronchial tree second primaries. A barium esophagogram may substitute for esophagoscopy in patients at low risk to develop esophageal tumors.

Pet Scan

Fluorodeoxyglucose F18 is a glucose analogue that is preferentially absorbed by neoplastic cells and can be detected by positron emission tomography (PET) scanning. Recently, the role of PET scanning has been investigated in the initial evaluation of the HNSCC patient. PET scanning is more sensitive than CT in identifying the primary lesion but is not able to detect unknown primary tumors with more than 50% sensitivity (possibly because the unknown primary tumor may have spontaneously involuted).[14] PET evaluates neck metastases with equal sensitivity as CT but with fewer false-positive results. PET is able to detect a higher percentage of lung metastases than chest radiograph, bronchoscopy, or CT scan, but the specificity ranges from 50% to 80%, and how to treat a patient with a positive PET and an otherwise negative lung work-up is still in question.[15] Patients with tumors that demonstrate high uptake on PET imaging have a worse prognosis than patients with less avid tumors and

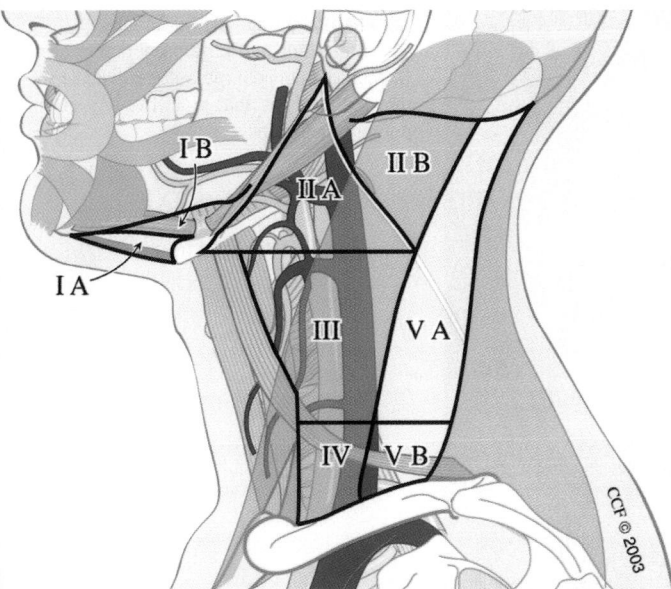

FIGURE 31-2. Diagram of the cervical lymph node levels I through V. Level II is divided into regions A and B by the spinal accessory nerve. (©Cleveland Clinic Foundation, 2003.)

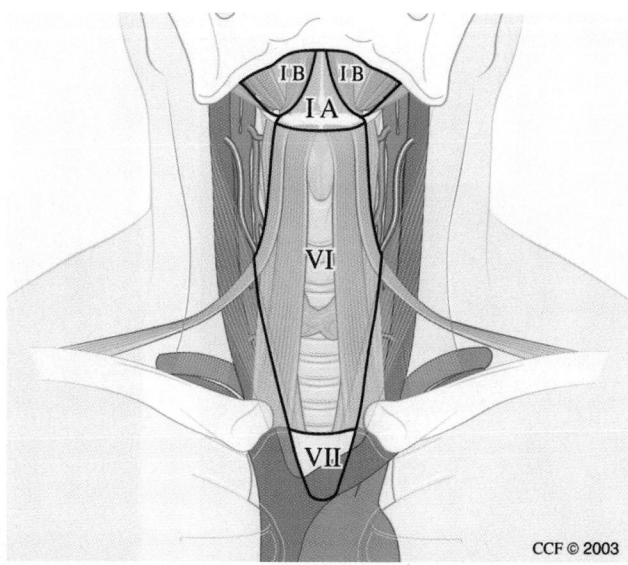

FIGURE 31-3. Diagram of the anterior lymph node levels: I, VI, and VII. Although large in area, the majority of level VI lymph nodes are confined to the paratracheal region. (©Cleveland Clinic Foundation, 2003.)

also have less response to radiation therapy. The exact role of PET scanning in the initial evaluation of HNSCC is still under investigation, and its routine use is not within the current standard of care.

Lymphatic Spread

The cervical lymphatic nodal basins contain between 50 to 70 lymph nodes per side and are divided into seven levels (Figs. 31-2 and 31-3). Level I is divided into IA bounded by the anterior belly of the digastric muscle, the hyoid bone, and the midline, whereas level IB is bounded by the anterior and posterior bellies of the digastric muscle and the inferior border of the mandible. Level IB contains the submandibular gland. Level II is bounded superiorly by the skull base, anteriorly by the stylohyoid muscle, inferiorly by a horizontal plane extending posterior from the hyoid bone, and posteriorly by the posterior edge of the sternocleidomastoid muscle. Level II is further divided into level IIA, which is anterior to the spinal accessory nerve and level IIB or the "submuscular triangle" which is posterior to the nerve. Level III begins at the inferior edge of level II and is bounded by the laryngeal strap muscles anteriorly, the posterior border of the sternocleidomastoid muscle posteriorly, and by a horizontal plane extending posteriorly from the inferior border of the cricoid cartilage. Level IV begins at the inferior border of level III and is bounded anteriorly by the strap muscles, posteriorly by the posterior edge of the sternocleidomastoid muscle, and inferiorly by the clavicle. Level V is posterior to the posterior edge of the sternocleidomastoid muscle, anterior to the trapezius muscle, superior to the clavicle, and inferior to the base of skull (Fig. 31-4). Level VI is bounded by the hyoid bone superiorly, the common

carotid arteries laterally, and the sternum inferiorly. Although level VI is large in area, the few lymph nodes it contains are mostly in the paratracheal regions near the thyroid gland. Level VII (superior mediastinum) lies between the common carotid arteries and is superior to the aortic arch and inferior to the upper border of the sternum.

Patterns of lymphatic drainage generally occur from superior to inferior and follow predictable patterns based on the primary site. Primary tumors from the lip and oral cavity generally metastasize to the nodes in levels I, II, and III, although skip metastases may occur to lower levels. The upper lip primarily metastasizes ipsilaterally, whereas the lower lip has both ipsilateral and contralateral drainage. Tumors in the oropharynx, hypopharynx, and larynx most commonly metastasize to levels II, III, and IV. Tumors of the nasopharynx spread to the retropharyngeal and parapharyngeal lymph nodes, as well as levels II through V. Other sites that metastasize to the retropharyngeal lymph nodes are the soft palate, posterior and lateral oropharynx, and hypopharynx. Tumors of the subglottis, thyroid, hypopharynx, and cervical esophagus spread to levels VI and VII. In addition to the lower lip, the supraglottis and soft palate have high incidences of bilateral metastases.

Therapeutic Options

The therapeutic options for patients diagnosed with HNSCC include surgery, radiation therapy, chemotherapy, and combination regimens. In general, early-stage disease (stage I or II) is treated by either surgery or radiation. Late-stage disease (stage III or IV) is best treated by a combination of either surgery and radiation, or chemotherapy

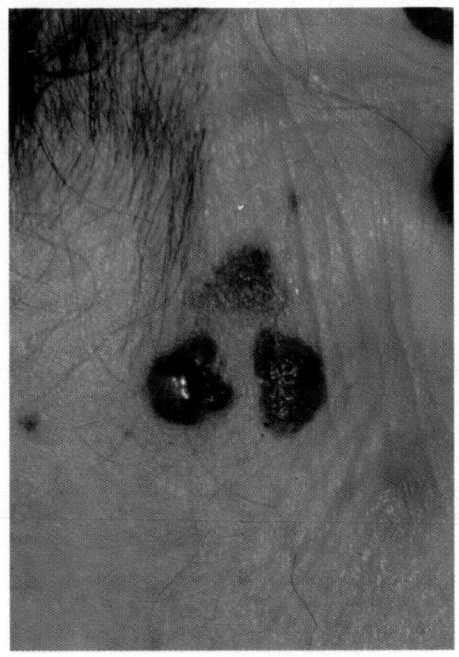

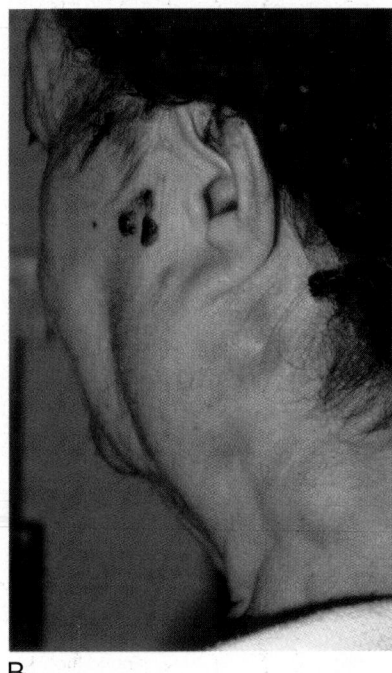

A   B

FIGURE 31-4.   **A,** Cutaneous melanoma arising in the preauricular area. **B,** Multiple cervical metastases visible in the nodal basins that drain the site of the primary malignancy.

and radiation, or all three modalities, depending on the site of the primary. Since surgery was the first therapeutic option available to physicians, it has the longest track-record of the three options and established the head and neck surgeon as the leader of the treatment team for HNSCC. Photon irradiation is superior to surgery in eradicating microscopic disease and is an excellent alternative to surgery for early lesions. Tonsil, tongue base, and nasopharyngeal primary tumors are especially responsive to photon irradiation. Neutron and proton irradiation are used much less often in the head and neck, although there are growing experiences with their role in salivary gland malignancies and skull base cancers, respectively. Electrons are not commonly used in the head and neck for noncutaneous tumors. With the advent of intensity-modulated radiation therapy, which is able to reduce photon dosage to surrounding normal tissues through computer three-dimensional planning, the dogma that patients may not receive greater than 7200 rads to tissue of the head and neck is being called into question. Hyperfractionation is the practice of administering radiation more than once per day and recent results of the European Organization for Research and Treatment of Cancer have determined that hyperfractionation in HNSCC sites produces greater locoregional control than conventional once-a-day regimens.[16] Radiation therapy is not as effective in treating large-volume, low-grade neoplasms, or tumors in close proximity to the mandible, due to the risk of osteoradionecrosis. The loss of salivary function with irradiation of the oral and oropharyngeal cavity can be quite disabling to patients, and its impact should not be minimized in the decision-making process.

The most heralded chemotherapy trial in HNSCC was the Veterans Affairs (VA) Larynx Trial, published in 1991.[17] Although chemotherapy alone has never been shown to be curative for HNSCC, its role as a "radiation sensitizer" was established in this study. Two thirds of the patients treated with both radiation and chemotherapy were able to keep their larynx, whereas survival was equal to patients treated with laryngectomy and radiation. Although "organ preservation" treatment with chemoradiation is currently being investigated in other head and neck subsites, its use (except in laryngeal cancer) outside of standardized protocols should be discouraged, given our current knowledge. Recurrences after radiation have been shown to be multifocal in the bed of the original tumor and the salvage surgeon should be familiar with the original tumor location and volumes. Chemotherapy is commonly used in the treatment of incurable HNSCC such as unresectable and metastatic disease and can have excellent symptom control in these patients.

The neck should be treated when there are clinically positive nodes or the risk of occult disease is greater than 20% based on the location and stage of the primary lesion. The decision to perform a neck dissection or radiate the neck is related to the treatment of the primary lesion. If the index tumor is being treated with radiation and the neck is N0 (no clinically detectable disease) or N1, the nodes are usually treated with irradiation. For surgically treated primary lesions, N0 or N1 neck disease may be treated surgically as well. Negative prognostic factors such as extracapsular spread of tumor, perineural invasion, vascular invasion, fixation to surrounding structures, and multiple positive nodes are indicators for postoperative adjuvant radiation. For N2 or N3 neck disease, a neck dissection with planned postoperative radiation therapy is performed. When chemoradiation therapy protocols are used in treating the primary lesion and there is a complete response in both the primary tumor and in an N2 or N3 neck, a planned neck dissection 8 weeks after chemoradiation will contain cancer in up to one third of specimens.[18] If the neck mass persists, the percentage of residual disease increases to two thirds. When patients present with advanced neck disease that involves the carotid artery or the deep neck musculature, radiation or chemoradiation is given preoperatively with the hope that the tumor reduces in size and becomes resectable. CT scans notoriously carry a high false-positive rate for determining carotid encasement. When carotid resection is necessary, the associated morbidity is high (17% major neurologic injury) with a 22% 2-year survival rate, and the decision to resect should be weighed carefully.[19]

The radical neck dissection (RND) was described by Crile in 1907 and was considered the gold standard for removal of nodal metastases. Through close reading of Crile's later surgical notes, it has been revealed that he had begun to modify his surgical technique to remove only selected regions of the neck dependent on the site of primary tumor. Today, this has become common surgical practice in HNSCC. All modifications of neck dissection are described in relation to the standard RND, which removes nodal levels I through V, the sternocleidomastoid muscle (SCM), the internal jugular vein (IJ), cranial nerve XI, the cervical plexus, and the submandibular gland. Preservation of the SCM, IJ, or cranial nerve XI in any combination is referred to as a *modified radical neck dissection* (MRND), and the structures preserved are specified for nomenclature. A modified neck dissection may also be referred to as a "Bocca" neck dissection after the surgeon who demonstrated that not only is the MRND equally as effective in controlling neck disease as a RND when structures are preserved that are not directly involved in tumor, but the functional outcomes of the patients after MRND are superior to RND.[20] Although resection of the SCM muscle or one IJ is relatively nonmorbid, loss of cranial nerve XI leaves a denervated trapezius muscle, which can cause a painful chronic "frozen" shoulder.

Either a RND or MRND can be performed for removal of detectable nodal disease. Preservation of any of levels I through V during a neck dissection is referred to as a *selective neck dissection* (SND) and is based on the knowledge of the patterns of spread to neck regions. A SND is performed on a clinically negative (N0) neck with preservation of nodal groups carrying less than a 20% chance of being involved with metastatic disease. Regional control has been shown to be as effective after SND as MRND in the patient with the clinically negative neck. Recent studies evaluating the treatment of the N0 neck have investigated the use of sentinel lymph node biopsy, which attempts to predict the disease status of the neck based on the first echelon of nodes that drain the tumor. Although sentinel lymph node biopsy has been used extensively with melanoma, its use in HNSCC has come about more gradually. Early results using isosulfan blue dye alone suggested that this technique could not consistently identify the sentinel node in HNSCC. More recent results using a gamma probe have been more encouraging, although there appears to be a learning curve in the ability to identify the node identified as the primary drainage pathway.[21]

ANATOMIC SITES

Lip

Anatomically, the lip is considered a subsite of the oral cavity. The lip begins at the junction of the vermilion border with the skin and is composed of the vermilion surface, which refers to the mucosa that contacts the opposing lip. It is divided into the upper lip, lower lip, and oral commissures. Most lip cancers occur on the lower lip (90% to 95%) and less often on the upper lip (2% to 7%) and commissures (1%). The most common group to develop lip cancer are white men 50 to 80 years of age. Sun exposure and pipe smoking are associated with lip cancer. Although squamous cell carcinoma is the most common lip cancer (90%), the most common cancer of the upper lip is basal cell carcinoma. Other lip cancers include variants of squamous cell carcinoma such as spindle cell and adenoid squamous carcinoma, as well as malignant melanoma and minor salivary gland cancers.

The most common clinical presentation of lip cancer is an ulcerative lesion on the vermilion or skin surface. Palpation is necessary to determine the submucosal extent of the lesion and possible fixation to underlying bone. Sensation of the chin should be tested to determine involvement of the mental nerve. Poor prognostic indicators include nerve involvement, fixation to the maxilla or mandible, cancer arising on the upper lip or commissure, positive nodal disease and age less than 40 years when diagnosed. The most commonly involved nodal basins are the submental and submandibular levels. Depth of tumor invasion of 5 mm has been shown to be a cutoff, above which the incidence of cervical nodal disease is significantly increased.[22]

Like the rest of the oral cavity, staging of lip cancer is based on size at presentation. Early-stage disease may be treated with surgery or radiation with equal success. Local surgery (wide local excision) with negative margin control of at least 3 mm is the preferred treatment, with a supraomohyoid neck dissection for tumors with clinically negative necks but deeper primary invasion or size greater than 3 cm. Neck dissection with postoperative radiation therapy for patients with clinically evident neck disease has an acceptable regional control rate of the neck of 91%.[23] The overall 5-year cure rate of 90% drops to 50% in the presence of neck metastases. Postoperative radiation is also indicated in advanced stage primary disease, tumors with perineural involvement, or "close" or positive margins at the time of resection.

The goals of lip reconstruction include re-creating oral competence, cosmesis, and maintenance of *dynamic* function while allowing adequate access for oral hygiene. Fortunately, the surgeon is able to remove up to one half of the lip and still close the defect primarily, particularly

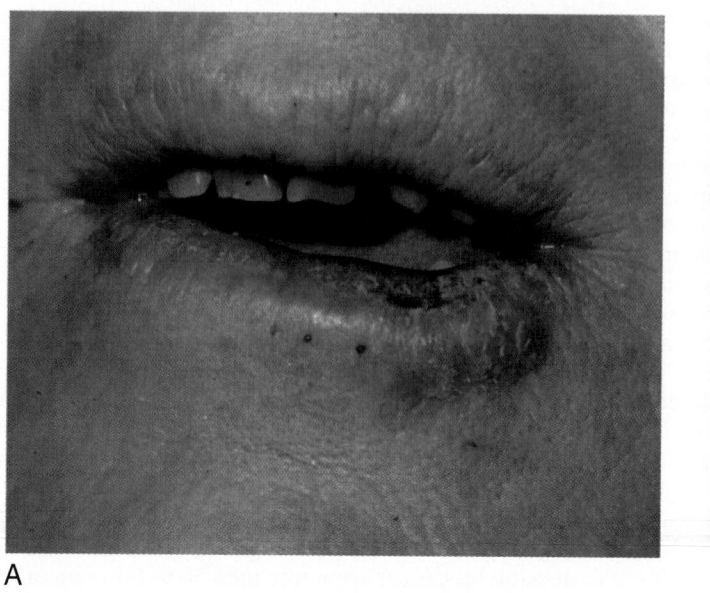

A

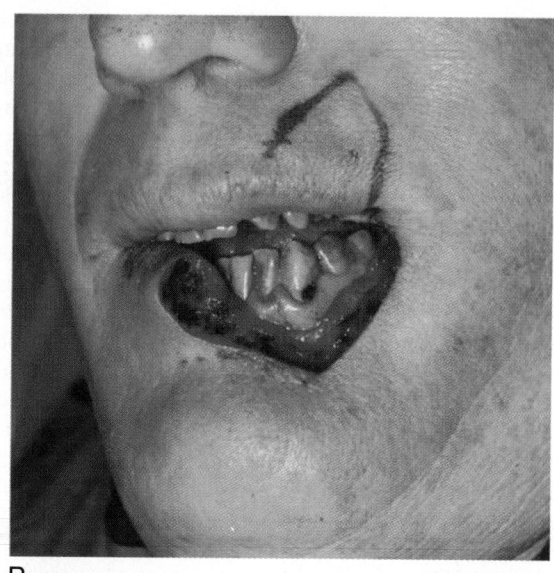

B

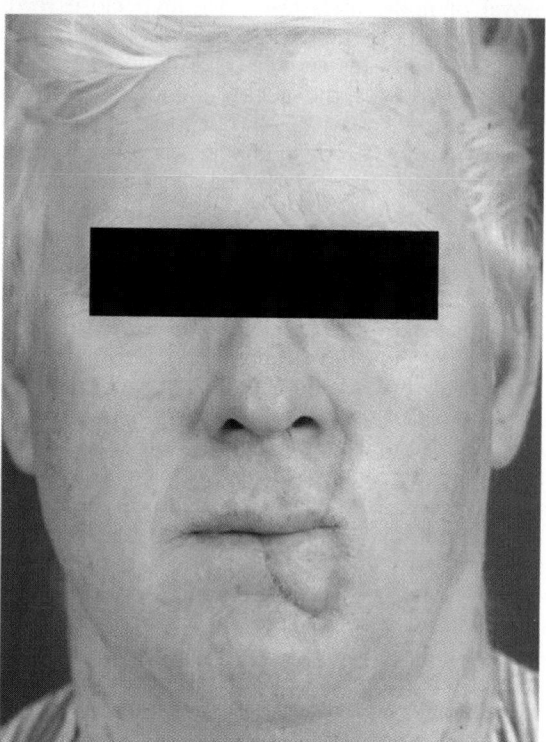

C

■ FIGURE 31-5. **A,** Squamous cell carcinoma involving the lower lip and encroaching on the oral commissure. **B,** Full-thickness excision and outlined Estlander flap for reconstruction based on the contralateral superior labial artery. **C,** Reconstructive result 3 months postoperatively.

in the lower lip, which contains more excess tissue than the upper lip. A lower lip wedge excision should not be carried below the mental crease unless the tumor dictates its excision. Care is taken for close approximation of the "white line" on either side of the defect at the vermilion border, because the eye is drawn to any mismatch that exists at this critical aesthetic location.

Defects between one half and two thirds of the lip require augmentation. The Estlander and Abbé flaps are lip-switch flaps based on the sublabial or superior labial artery. The Estlander is used when the defect involves the commissure, whereas the Abbé flap is used for more midline defects and requires a second-stage division of the pedicle (Fig. 31-5). The Karapandžić flap consists of circumoral incisions with circular rotation of the skin flaps while maintaining innervation of the orbicularis oris musculature. This one-stage procedure is used for defects involving more than two thirds of the lip. Microstomia is a potential complication from these types of flap reconstructions, and denture use may not be possible. For defects greater than two thirds, the Webster, Gilles, or Bernard types of repairs may also be used.

Oral Cavity

Since the oral cavity begins at the skin-vermilion junction, the lips are considered part of the oral cavity for staging purposes. The other subsites within the oral cavity include the buccal mucosa, the upper and lower alveolar ridges, the retromolar trigone, the floor of mouth, the hard palate, and the oral tongue. Staging of the oral cavity is based on size: 0 to 2 cm are T1; 2 to 4 cm are T2; 4 to 6 cm are T3; and T4 tumors are greater than 6 cm or invade adjacent structures including bone (cortical bone of mandible or maxilla, not superficial erosion or tooth sockets), deep tongue musculature, or facial skin. Squamous cell carcinoma accounts for 90% of the tumors located in these subsites, with a male predominance in the 5th and 6th decades of life. There is a close association with alcohol and tobacco abuse.[4]

Oral Tongue

The oral tongue begins at the junction between the tongue and the floor of mouth and extends posteriorly to the circumvallate papillae. Tumors present as exophytic, ulcerative, or submucosal masses that may be associated with tenderness or irritation with mastication. Benign tumors tend to be submucosal and include leiomyomas, neurofibromas, and granular cell tumors. Although granular cell tumors can arise in the larynx, they occur more frequently in the tongue and can be confused with SCC due to an overlying pseudoepitheliomatous hyperplasia. Complete excision is curative, but histologic borders are notorious for extending beyond gross disease and negative intraoperative margins are mandatory.

Squamous cell carcinoma is by far the most common type of malignancy, but leiomyosarcomas and rhabdomyosarcomas are also rarely encountered. Neurotropic malignancies may involve the lingual or hypoglossal nerves and tongue deviation or loss of sensation should be examined closely. Treatment of oral tongue cancers is primarily surgical, with wide local excision and negative margin control. The development of cervical metastases is related to the depth of invasion, perineural spread, advanced T stage, and tumor differentiation. Infiltration of more than 5 mm into the tongue musculature has been shown by several investigators to increase the incidence of occult cervical metastases.[24] Metastases from the anterior tongue most frequently spread to the submental and submandibular regions. Tumors more posteriorly often metastasize to levels II and III. Indications for postoperative radiation therapy include evidence of perineural or angiolymphatic spread, depth greater than 5 mm, or positive nodal disease.

Small tumors may be removed with wide local excision and primary closure or closure by secondary intention. Excision of larger tumors requires partial or hemiglossectomies. Extirpation may result in significant dysfunction in terms of disarticulation and dysphagia from inability to contact the palate, sense oral contents, or manipulate the tongue against the alveolus or lips. Reconstructive efforts should focus on maintaining tongue mobility without excess bulk. Split-thickness skin grafts, primary closure, or healing by secondary intention of larger tongue defects often results in tongue tethering. Thin, pliable, fasciocutaneous flaps (such as the radial forearm free flap) are the preferred reconstructive technique for such defects. A palatal augmentation prosthesis may assist in maintaining palatal contact, important in both speech and posterior propulsion of food boluses.

Floor of Mouth

The floor of mouth extends from the inner surface of the mandible medially to the ventral tongue and from the anterior-most frenulum posteriorly to the anterior tonsillar pillars. The mucosa of the floor of mouth contains the openings of the sublingual gland and submandibular gland (via Wharton's ducts). The muscular floor is composed of the genioglossus, mylohyoid, and hyoglossus muscles, with the lingual nerve located immediately submucosally.

Bimanual palpation can often determine fixation of floor of mouth tumors to the mandible. CT scanning demonstrates the depth of mandibular bony invasion and widening of cranial neural foramen, such as foramen ovale, suggests neurotropic intracranial spread in advanced tumors. Determining mandibular invasion is of utmost importance in preoperative planning (Fig. 31-6). Invasion into the tongue musculature necessitates partial glossectomy concurrently with removal of the floor of mouth lesion.

Treatment of floor of mouth lesions is primarily surgical with excision of involved tongue or mandible as necessary to obtain negative margins. Removal of bone with soft tissue in continuity is commonly referred to as a "commando" or composite resection. Involvement of the neck may occur either by direct tumor extension through the floor of mouth musculature or through lymphatic spread. The primary lesion and neck specimen should be taken in continuity such that accompanying lymphatic channels are resected. Adjuvant radiation therapy has similar

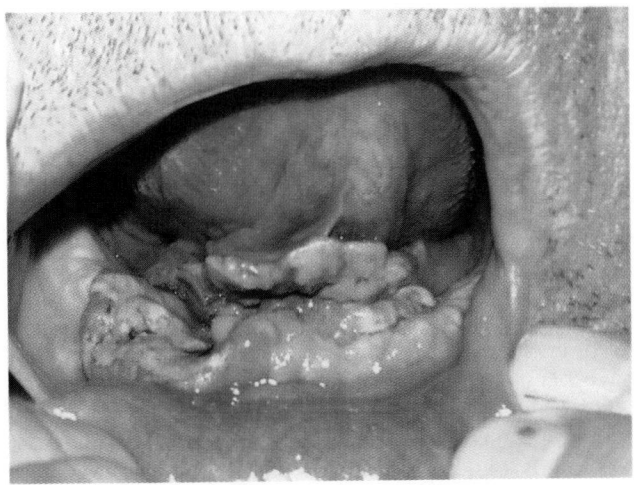

FIGURE 31-6. A 62-year-old man with squamous cell carcinoma of the anterior floor of mouth invading the mandible.

indications as in oral tongue cancers. The primary goal of reconstruction is the separation of the oral cavity from the neck by creating a "water-tight" oral closure. This prevents orocutaneous salivary fistula formation. Secondary goals are maintaining tongue mobility, creating a lingual-alveolar sulcus, and maintaining mandibular continuity. Local flaps for soft tissue reconstruction include the platysmal and submental myocutaneous pedicled flaps. Larger defects including mandibular resection require complex reconstruction most often performed with free flaps.

Alveolus

The alveolus and its accompanying gingiva constitute the dental surfaces of the maxilla and mandible, from the gingivobuccal sulcus laterally to the floor of mouth and hard palate medially. Posteriorly, the alveolus extends to the pterygopalatine arch and the ascending ramus of the mandible (also referred to as the *retromolar trigone*). Because of the tight attachment between the mucosa and underlying bone, treatment of alveolar SCC often involves treatment of the maxilla or mandible. Seventy percent of gingival carcinomas occur on the lower gum. The periosteum of the mandible is a strong tumor barrier, and tumors that abut the bone may often be resected along with the adjacent periosteum only. Tumors adherent to the periosteum should undergo excision with marginal mandibulectomy, which involves resection of the superior or inner cortical portions of the mandible, preserving a continuous rim. Even superficial tumors that invade the outermost mandible may be resected with a marginal mandibulectomy, although this is not oncologically sound if the tumor is a recurrence after radiation.[25] A segmental mandibulectomy entails excision of the full thickness of mandible, thus interrupting mandibular continuity, and is indicated when there is gross bone invasion by tumor. Primary radiation therapy for mandibular tumors is not a viable option for treatment due to the high likelihood of osteoradionecrosis and the poor response of involved bone to radiation therapy treatment.

Buccal Mucosa

The buccal mucosa extends from the inner surface of the opposing surfaces of the lips to the alveolar ridges and pterygomandibular raphe. Buccal cancer is an uncommon cancer, representing 5% of oral cavity carcinomas. Smoking, alcohol abuse, lichen planus, dental trauma, snuff dipping, and tobacco chewing are etiologic agents associated with buccal cancer. Approximately 65% of patients with buccal cancer present with extension beyond the cheek mucosa. Lymphatic drainage is to the submandibular lymph nodes; however, tumors of the posterior cheek may spread to level II initially. Stage I cancers have been historically treated with surgery and did not receive an elective neck dissection due to the low rate of occult metastases. More recent studies have suggested high rates of local recurrence for lesions treated with surgery alone, and adjuvant radiation has been suggested even for early-stage lesions.[26] Deep invasion may require

a through-and-through excision of cheek skin, necessitating both internal and external lining, usually by a fasciocutaneous free flap.

Palate

The hard palate is defined as the area medial to the maxillary alveolar ridges extending posterior to the edge of the palatine bone. Chronic inflammatory lesions such as viral lesions, zoster, and pemphigoid can mimic neoplasms and a biopsy is indicated for persistent lesions. Necrotizing sialometaplasia is a benign, self-limiting process of minor salivary glands that has a predilection for the palate and can clinically mimic a malignancy. The most common intraoral site for Kaposi's sarcoma is the palate in immunosuppressed patients. Torus palatini are benign exostosis of the midline hard palate that may require surgery if they interfere with denture wearing.

Minor salivary gland tumors, along with squamous cell carcinoma, make up the majority of hard palate tumors. Adenoid cystic carcinoma, mucoepidermoid carcinoma, adenocarcinoma, and polymorphous low-grade adenocarcinoma are common malignancies of salivary gland origin that tend to arise at the junction of the hard and soft palates. Malignancies of the hard palate are treated with local excision if early, but most commonly require resection of bone due to the close adherence of the mucosa to the palate. Inferior maxillectomies, subtotal maxillectomies, or total maxillectomies are indicated for progressively destructive tumors extending into the maxillary antrum. Adjuvant radiation therapy is given for advanced lesions. Reconstruction may be accomplished with soft tissue flap reconstruction for small defects, obturation with dental prosthesis for defects with some remaining hard palate, or bony free-tissue transfer for extensive palatal resections.

Oropharynx

The borders of the oropharynx include the circumvallate papillae anteriorly, the plane of the superior surface of the soft palate superiorly, the plane of the hyoid bone inferiorly, the pharyngeal constrictors laterally and posteriorly, and the medial aspect of the mandible laterally. The oropharynx includes the base of tongue, the inferior surface of the soft palate and uvula, the anterior and posterior tonsillar pillars, the glossotonsillar sulci, the pharyngeal tonsils, and the lateral and posterior pharyngeal walls. Similar to the oral cavity, T staging in the oropharynx is size dependent. T4 tumors may extend out of the oropharynx posteriorly into the parapharyngeal space, inferiorly to the larynx, or laterally to invade the mandible.

Ninety percent of tumors of the oropharynx are squamous cell carcinomas. Other tumors include lymphoma of the tonsils or tongue base or salivary gland neoplasms arising from minor salivary glands in the soft palate or tongue base. Presenting symptoms include sore throat, bleeding, dysphagia and odynophagia, referred otalgia, and voice changes, including a muffled quality or "hot potato" voice. Trismus suggests involvement of the pterygoid musculature. Imaging studies should focus on invasion through the pharyngeal constrictors, bony involvement of the pterygoid plates or mandible, invasion of the parapharyngeal space or carotid artery, involvement of the prevertebral fascia, and extension into the larynx. Lymph node metastases generally occur in the upper jugular chain (levels II to IV), although "skip" lesions to lower levels may occur and spread to level V and are more common with oropharyngeal tumors than with the oral cavity. Bilateral metastases are more common with tongue base and soft palate lesions, especially with midline lesions.

Treatment of oropharyngeal SCC has focused increasingly on "conservation therapy" with chemotherapy and radiation. Many tumors of the oropharynx are poorly differentiated and respond well to radiation. The use of chemotherapy as a radiation sensitizer has been demonstrated in numerous recent studies and the local control rate has achieved 90% even in stage IV disease, although overall survival has not improved over more traditional surgery and radiation therapy.[27] Surgery is necessary for primary disease that involves the mandible and resectable recurrent disease and has a role in very early, superficial tumors that do not justify a full course of radiation. Extensive surgery of the tongue base significantly alters a patient's ability to swallow. Reconstruction of the tongue with preservation of the larynx requires surgical techniques that maintain tongue mobility and suspend the larynx and neotongue to prevent aspiration.

Resection or contracture after radiation therapy of the soft palate may result in velopharyngeal insufficiency (VPI), which is manifested clinically as nasal regurgitation of liquids and solids and hypernasal speech. Augmentation of the soft palate may be performed surgically or with palatal obturation. Although a palatal obturator requires cleaning and is not permanent, patients are able to remove them during sleep. With surgical augmentation of the palate, the balance between reducing VPI and causing obstructive sleep apnea is difficult to achieve. For patients with tongue base resection, an inferiorly directed palatal obturator assists in achieving contact at the tongue base that is necessary for the projection of food posteriorly during the oral and pharyngeal phases of swallowing.

Hypopharynx

The hypopharynx is that portion of the pharynx that extends inferiorly from the horizontal plane of the top of the hyoid bone to a horizontal plane extending posteriorly from the inferior border of the cricoid cartilage. The hypopharynx includes both piriform sinuses, the lateral and posterior hypopharyngeal walls, and the postcricoid region. The postcricoid area extends inferiorly from the two arytenoid cartilages to the inferior border of the cricoid cartilage, thereby connecting the piriform sinuses and forming the anterior hypopharyngeal wall. The piriform sinuses are inverted, pyramid-shaped potential spaces medial to the thyroid lamina that begin at the pharyngoepiglottic folds and extend to the cervical esophagus at the inferior border of the cricoid cartilage.

Hypopharyngeal cancer is more common in men, age 55 to 70 years, with histories of alcohol abuse and smoking. The exception is in the postcricoid area, in which cancers are more common worldwide in women. This is directly related to Plummer-Vinson syndrome, a combination of dysphagia, hypopharyngeal and esophageal webs, weight loss, and iron deficiency anemia, usually in middle-aged women. Patients who fail to undergo treatment with dilation, iron replacement, and vitamin therapy may develop postcricoid carcinoma just proximal to the web.

Hypopharyngeal tumors present as a chronic sore throat, dysphagia, referred otalgia, and a foreign body sensation in the throat. A high index of suspicion should be maintained as similar symptoms may be seen with the more common gastroesophageal reflux disease. In advanced disease, patients may develop hoarseness from direct involvement of the arytenoid, the recurrent laryngeal nerve, or the paraglottic space. The rich lymphatics that drain the hypopharyngeal region contribute to the fact that 70% of patients with hypopharyngeal cancer present with palpable lymphadenopathy. Patients with hypopharyngeal cancer have the highest rate of metachronous malignancies and the highest rate of development of second HNSCC primaries of any of the head and neck sites. Staging for hypopharyngeal cancer is based on either the number of involved subsites or the size of the tumor.

Physical examination for hypopharyngeal lesions includes fiberoptic endoscopy. Having the patient blow against closed lips and pinching the nose closed will inflate the potential spaces of the piriforms and assist in tumor visualization. Palpation of the larynx may demonstrate loss of laryngeal crepitus. A fixed larynx suggests posterior extension into the prevertebral fascia and unresectability. Barium swallow may demonstrate mucosal abnormalities associated with an exophytic tumor and is useful in determining involvement of the cervical esophagus. It also assists in determining the presence and amount of aspiration present. CT scanning determines the presence of thyroid cartilage invasion, direct extension into the neck, and pathologic lymphadenopathy. Biopsy of the hypopharynx usually requires direct laryngoscopy under general anesthesia.

The most common area for lymphatic spread is the upper jugular nodes, even for inferior tumors. Other regions include the paratracheal and retropharyngeal nodes. The presence of contralateral cervical metastases or level V involvement is a grave prognostic indicator. Treatment of hypopharyngeal cancer yields poor results compared to other sites in the head and neck, presumably due to the late presentation of disease. For early lesions confined to the medial wall of the piriform or posterior pharyngeal wall, radiation or chemoradiation is effective as a primary treatment modality. Seldom is laryngeal-sparing partial pharyngectomy surgery possible. Small tumors of the medial piriform wall or pharyngoepiglottic fold may be amenable to conservation surgery but must not involve the piriform apex, and the patient must have mobile vocal cords and adequate pulmonary reserve.

The most common treatment of hypopharyngeal cancer is laryngopharyngectomy and bilateral neck dissections, including the paratracheal compartments, with adjuvant radiation therapy. Trials with neoadjuvant chemotherapy followed by concomitant chemotherapy and radiation therapy have shown promise in organ preservation in hypopharyngeal cancer.[28] The estimated 5-year laryngeal preservation rate is 35%, and induction chemotherapy appears to decrease the rate of death by distant metastases.

Following total laryngectomy and partial pharyngectomy, primary closure may be possible if at least 4 cm of viable pharyngeal mucosa remains. Primary closure utilizing less than 4 cm generally leads to stricture and inability to swallow effectively. Pedicled cutaneous flap such as a pectoralis myocutaneous flap can be used to augment any remaining mucosa in these cases. When a total laryngopharyngectomy with an esophagectomy has been performed, a gastric pull-up may be used for reconstruction. More recently, free flap reconstruction with enteric flaps or tubed cutaneous flaps, such as radial forearm or anterolateral thigh flaps, have been used to reconstruct the total pharyngectomy defect.

Larynx

The three-dimensional boundaries of the larynx are complex, and exacting definitions are necessary prior to understanding the pathologies affecting this organ system. The anterior border of the larynx is composed of the lingual surface of the epiglottis, the thyrohyoid membrane, the anterior commissure, and the anterior wall of the subglottis, which is composed of the thyroid cartilage, the cricothyroid membrane, and the anterior arch of the cricoid cartilage. The posterior and lateral limits of the larynx are composed of the arytenoids and interarytenoid region, the aryepiglottic folds, and the posterior wall of the subglottis that is composed of the mucosa covering the cricoid cartilage. The superior limits are composed of the tip and lateral borders of the epiglottis. The inferior limit is made up of the plane passing through the inferior edge of the cricoid cartilage.

For staging purposes, the larynx is divided into three regions: the supraglottis, the glottis, and the subglottis. The supraglottis is composed of the epiglottis, the laryngeal surfaces of the aryepiglottic folds, the arytenoids, and the false vocal folds. In addition to these supraglottic subsites, the epiglottis is divided into the suprahyoid and infrahyoid epiglottis for a total of five supraglottic subsites. The inferior limit of the supraglottis is a horizontal plane through the ventricles, which is the lateral recess between the true and false vocal folds. This plane is also the superior border of the glottis, which is composed of the superior and inferior surfaces of the true vocal folds and extends inferiorly from the true vocal folds 1cm in thickness. Also included in the glottis are the anterior and posterior commissures. The subglottis extends from the lower border of the glottis to the lower margin of the cricoid cartilage.

The innervation of the larynx includes the superior laryngeal nerve, which supplies the cricothyroid and inferior constrictor muscles and contains afferent sensory fibers from the mucosa of the false vocal folds and piriform sinuses. The recurrent laryngeal nerve supplies motor innervation to all the intrinsic muscles of the larynx as well as sensation to the mucosa of the true vocal folds, the subglottic region, and adjacent esophageal mucosa. The normal functions of the larynx are to provide airway patency, protect the tracheobronchial tree from aspiration, provide resistance for Valsalva and cough, and allow for phonation. Tumors that involve the larynx impair these functions to a variable degree, depending on location, size, and depth of invasion.

Glottic tumors often present early with hoarseness since the vibratory edge of the true vocal fold is normally responsible for the quality of voice and is sensitive to even small lesions. Signs of airway compromise occur later in disease progression when tumor bulk obstructs the glottic opening. Impaired movement of the vocal fold may cause hoarseness, aspiration, impaired cough, or obstructive symptoms. Impaired movement is caused by tumor bulk, direct invasion of the thyroarytenoid muscle, invasion of the cricoarytenoid joint, or invasion of the recurrent nerve. Hemoptysis occurs with hemorrhagic lesions.

In comparison to glottic tumors, supraglottic lesions are relatively indolent and present at a later stage of disease (Fig. 31-7). Patients often complain of sore throat or odynophagia. Referred otalgia is caused by Arnold's nerve, the vagal branch that supplies part of ear sensation. Bulky tumors of the epiglottis often present with a "hot potato" or muffled voice quality due to airway compromise. Dysphagia may cause weight loss and malnutrition. Subglottic tumors are rare and most often present with airway obstruction, vocal fold immobility, or pain.

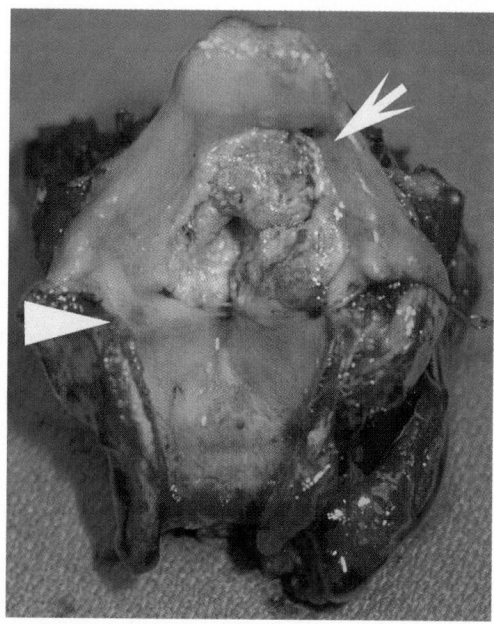

FIGURE 31-7. A pathologic specimen of supraglottic squamous cell carcinoma. The tumor's epicenter is in the region of the infrahyoid epiglottis and petiole *(arrow)* and is superior to the level of the true vocal folds *(arrowhead).*

The respiratory and squamous epithelium of the larynx are most often the etiology of laryngeal neoplasms, both benign and malignant. Laryngeal papillomatosis is a benign, exophytic growth of squamous epithelium with a tendency to recur despite surgical excision. It has a bimodal distribution, referred to as "juvenile" type and "adult" type. Granular cell tumors are also benign but may be confused with squamous cell carcinoma owing to a characteristic pseudoepitheliomatous hyperplasia that overlies this subepithelial lesion. Less frequent benign lesions include chondromas and rhabdomyomas. Non-neoplastic lesions of the larynx include vocal fold nodules and polyps, contact ulcers, subglottic stenosis, amyloidosis, and sarcoidosis. Finally, with exposure to carcinogens (tobacco), the epithelium of the larynx may undergo a series of precancerous changes clinically referred to as *leukoplakia* (any white lesion of the mucosa) or erythroplakia (a red lesion) composed of either hyperplasia, metaplasia, or variable degrees of dysplasia.

The most common malignant lesion of the larynx is squamous cell carcinoma, which is often classified into squamous cell carcinoma in situ, microinvasive SCC, or invasive SCC. Spindle cell carcinoma and basaloid squamous cell carcinoma are rare and represent more aggressive variants of squamous cell carcinoma. Verrucous carcinoma is a highly differentiated variant of squamous cell carcinoma that is locally destructive but does not metastasize and should respond to complete surgical excision. The nonepithelial components of the larynx may also undergo malignant transformation, leading to tumors of salivary origin such as adenocarcinoma, adenoid cystic carcinoma, and mucoepidermoid carcinoma. Other tumors include neuroendocrine carcinoma, adenosquamous carcinoma, chondrosarcoma, synovial sarcoma, and distant metastases from other organ systems.

The staging system for laryngeal cancers is based on subsite involvement and vocal fold mobility. Office examination includes flexible laryngoscopy to assess location and functional impairment. Stroboscopic laryngoscopy can detect subtle impairment of true fold mucosal waves that suggest significant tumor penetration. Direct laryngoscopy under anesthesia allows examination of all laryngeal subsites along with the ability to biopsy. Specific sites that are important to examine in supraglottic tumors include the ventricle, anterior commissure, the vallecula, the base of tongue, the piriform sinus, and the pre-epiglottic space. Key areas of glottic involvement include the false vocal fold, the ventricle, the anterior commissure, the arytenoids, the subglottis, and involvement of the posterior commissure or postcricoid mucosa. Under general anesthesia fixation of the vocal fold is differentiated from arytenoid fixation by palpation of the vocal process portion of the arytenoid.

CT scanning is routinely performed for laryngeal lesions and images the pre-epiglottic and paraglottic regions, the extent of cartilage involvement, as well as determines direct extension into the deep neck structures. For the natural barriers and pathways of direct tumor spread, the reader is referred to the landmark histopathologic work of Kirchner.[29] CT examination should be performed with contrast agents and thin (1.5-mm) cuts through the larynx. Lymph node metastases are identified on CT scanning as well. The lymphatic drainage of the larynx differs between the supraglottic and glottic regions. Supraglottic epidermoid cancers metastasize early, with up to 50% of lesions presenting with positive nodes.[30] Contralateral and bilateral nodal metastases are common with supraglottic lesions due to the embryologic development of the supraglottis as a midline structure. Lymphatic drainage exits along the course of the superior laryngeal neurovascular pedicle that pierces the thyrohyoid membrane to drain to the subdigastric and superior jugular groups of nodes (levels II and III). Lymphatic drainage of tumors in the glottic and subglottic areas exit via the cricothyroid ligament and drain to the prelaryngeal (delphian) node, the paratracheal nodes, and deep cervical nodes in the region of the inferior thyroid artery. Tumors confined to the glottis only rarely present with regional disease (4%), and positive nodes when present are most often ipsilateral.

Decision making in the treatment of laryngeal cancer is governed by tumor location and characteristics of tumor aggressiveness, as well as the patient's overall constitution and lifestyle. Poor prognostic factors include size, nodal metastasis, perineural invasion, and extracapsular spread. Low-grade epidermoid lesions of the larynx such as dysplasia and carcinoma in situ can be managed with local excision such as microscopic excision of the mucosa. Concurrent denuding of the mucosa of both vocal folds near the anterior commissure can lead to the formation of an anterior web that reduces voice quality and is a difficult complication to correct. Successful treatment of low-grade lesions includes close follow-up with repeat office or operative laryngoscopy as well as strict smoking cessation. For invasive disease, multiple treatment options are available, including both conservation surgery and aggressive surgery, radiation therapy, and chemoradiation therapy. In general, conservation of the larynx in early-stage disease is key, which can be accomplished with either laryngeal preservation surgery or with radiation. Later-stage disease that is still confined to the larynx is more commonly treated with chemoradiation therapy with total laryngectomy used for salvage.

Laryngeal preservation surgery includes endoscopic surgery with "cold steel," endoscopic laser resection, and open surgery with preservation of some portion of the larynx that maintains the ability to voice. Peretti and associates reported CO_2 laser excision in 140 patients with either carcinoma in situ (CIS) or T1 or T2 glottic lesions.[31] Local control at 5 years was achieved in 95% CIS, 87% T1, and 91% T2. Involvement of the anterior vocal fold, false vocal fold, and deep muscle invasion were associated with poor outcome. Transoral laser resection of supraglottic lesions has recently increased in frequency. Ambrosch and colleagues have demonstrated 100% 5-year control rates for T1 and 89% for T2 for supraglottic lesions with excellent functional outcomes including minimal aspiration and short recovery periods.[32]

Open conservation laryngeal surgery entails maintaining a conduit for airflow through the remnant of larynx allowing the ability to voice without aspiration. When deciding if a patient is a candidate for laryngeal preservation surgery, factors such as pulmonary function and cardiovascular status must be examined since these patients will often have to tolerate some amount of aspiration or airway compromise. Pulmonary function testing such as spirometry and arterial blood gases are obtained preoperatively. An excellent functional test is to have the patient climb two flights of stairs successively without becoming short of breath. The least invasive of the open procedures is the open cordectomy, which is indicated for small midfold lesions and has reported 100% and 97% 5-year control rates for T1 and T2 lesions, respectively.[33] Reconstruction is performed with a false vocal fold flap. For lesions involving the anterior commissure with less than 10 mm of inferior extension, an anterior frontal partial laryngectomy may be performed.

Conservation surgery options for more extensive tumors include vertical partial laryngectomy, supracricoid laryngectomy, and supraglottic laryngectomy. For T1 or T2 glottic lesions, a vertical partial laryngectomy with reconstruction with a false vocal cord pull-down or local muscle flap is indicated as long as the cartilage is not involved. For T3 lesions not involving the pre-epiglottic space or arytenoid cartilages, a supracricoid laryngectomy with cricohyoidopexy or cricohyoidoepiglottopexy is possible. Excellent disease control has been achieved with this technique largely due to the removal of the paraglottic space and the thyroid cartilage. Naudo and coworkers have shown that removal of feeding tubes and respiration without tracheotomy can be achieved in 98% of patients.[34] The standard supraglottic laryngectomy preserves both true vocal folds, both arytenoids, the tongue base, and the hyoid bone. Since there are numerous "extensions" of this operation that resect more than the standard structures, cure rates are difficult to compare, but in general T1 and T2 local control rates are range from 85% to 100%, with decreased control for higher-stage lesions.

If the decision is to undergo nonsurgical therapy, the patient must be able to complete the full course of radiation therapy that usually includes 5 to 7 weeks of continuous daily therapy visits. Previous irradiation is a contraindication to further radiation. Lastly, the patient must be able to follow-up reliably for years to come since recurrences may be indolent and difficult to detect. For neoadjuvant or concurrent chemotherapy, the patient must be of sufficient constitutional health to withstand the chemotherapeutic agents. For early laryngeal cancers (T1 or T2), irradiation provides excellent disease control with good to excellent post-therapy voice quality. For professional voice users with early lesions, radiation is most often the choice of therapy. The combination of chemotherapy and radiation for advanced stage disease (stages III and IV) was first brought into the mainstream with the VA larynx trial in 1991.[17] Induction chemotherapy followed by radiation therapy was found to have equal 2-year survival as total laryngectomy with postoperative radiation therapy while being able to preserve the larynges of 64% of patients. More recently, trials with concurrent chemotherapy and radiation have demonstrated even better local control of advanced laryngeal cancers.

For patients who present with disease extending outside the larynx or who fail conservative therapy (although some failures may still be amenable to conservation surgery), or are not otherwise candidates for organ-preserving strategies, total laryngectomy is still commonly performed. This involves a permanent tracheostoma and the loss of voice with permanent separation of the upper respiratory and digestive tracts. Patients may experience a period of depression or social withdrawal after becoming aphonic. Speech and swallowing rehabilitation has become an integral part of laryngeal cancer treatment and should begin preoperatively. Speech rehabilitation options include speech with an electrolarynx, esophageal speech, and tracheoesophageal puncture (TEP). The electrolarynx is considered the easiest of the three methods to use and comprises a vibratory sound wave generator that is usually placed either directly on the submandibular area or cheek. The patient "mouths" words to produce a monotone, electronic-sounding speech. Becoming understandable can take considerable time and patience. Esophageal speech is produced by the patient swallowing air into the esophagus and expulsing the air back through the pharynx, which vibrates as the air passes. The ability to master esophageal speech takes a motivated patient to be able to control the release of air through the upper esophageal sphincter and occurs in only 20% of laryngectomized patients. Lastly, the TEP is a surgically created conduit between the tracheal stoma and the pharynx made either at the time of laryngectomy or secondarily. This conduit is fitted with a one-way valve that allows passage of air posteriorly from trachea to pharynx but prevents food and liquid from entering anteriorly into the airway. By occluding the stomal opening with the thumb during exhalation, the patient can pass air into the pharynx that vibrates and allows remarkable clarity of speech. Patients who are good candidates for a TEP placement have an 80% success rate of achieving fluent speech.

Swallowing rehabilitation is a second role of the speech therapist in rehabilitating the laryngeal cancer patient, whether treated surgically or nonsurgically. Partial laryngectomy patients may have impaired pharyngeal movement and sensation, impaired vocal fold movement, decreased laryngeal elevation, and decreased subglottic pressure with poor cough, all contributing to possible aspiration. Specially designed swallowing maneuvers and training in regard to food consistencies are offered by the speech therapist to maintain oral diet, although some patients may require gastric feeding or conversion to total laryngectomy if aspiration persists. Even laryngectomized patients have difficulty relearning the act of swallowing. Radiation and chemotherapy, although "organ preserving," cause fibrosis, decreased sensation and movement, and decreased lubrication that negatively impact swallowing. Further, owing to the exposed circumferential ulcerated mucosa of the pharynx that occurs with chemoradiation, patients may develop pharyngeal stenosis during the recovery phase, necessitating dilation and even pharyngeal augmentation surgery with healthy, nonradiated tissue. Thus, the speech therapist and surgeon must work as a team to rehabilitate the larynx cancer patient.

Nasal Cavity and Paranasal Sinuses

The nasal cavity consists of the nares, vestibule, septum, lateral nasal wall, and roof. The paranasal sinuses include the frontal sinuses, maxillary sinuses, ethmoid sinuses, and the sphenoid sinus. The lateral nasal wall includes the highly vascular inferior, middle, superior, and occasionally supreme turbinates, as well as the osteomeatal complex and nasolacrimal duct and orifice. The frontal sinuses are two asymmetrical air cavities within the frontal bone that drain into the nasal cavity via the frontal recesses. The ethmoid sinuses are a complex bony labyrinth directly beneath the anterior cranial fossa. The lamina papyracea is the paper-thin lateral wall of the ethmoid sinus that constitutes the medial wall of the orbit. The anterior ethmoids drain into the middle meatus (inferior to the middle turbinate), whereas the posterior ethmoids drain via the sphenoethmoidal recess. The sphenoid sinus lies in the middle of the sphenoid bone and also drains via the sphenoethmoidal recess. The vital structures of the optic nerves, carotid arteries, and cavernous sinuses are contained within the lateral walls of the sphenoid sinus, whereas the sella turcica and optic chiasm lie superiorly within the roof. The maxillary sinuses drain into the middle meatus and are bound posteriorly by the pterygopalatine fossa and infratemporal fossa.

Tumors of the nasal cavity and paranasal sinuses tend to present at a late stage since their presenting symptoms are often attributed to more mundane etiologies. Symptoms include epistaxis, nasal congestion, headache, and facial pain. Orbital involvement produces proptosis, orbital pain, diplopia, epiphora, and even vision loss. Nerve involvement is heralded by numbness in the distribution of the infraorbital nerve. A variety of benign tumors occur in the nasal region. Sinonasal papilloma (or schniderian papilloma) is classified into three groups: (1) septal papilloma (50%) arise on the septum and are exophytic and are not associated with malignant degeneration; (2) inverted papilloma (47%) and (3) cylindrical cell papilloma (3%) arise on the lateral nasal wall or from the paranasal sinuses and are associated with malignant degeneration (10% to 15%), usually into squamous cell carcinoma. Previously thought to require radical extirpation, sinonasal papillomas require only local surgical excision with negative margins. Other benign nasal lesions include hemangioma, benign fibrous histiocytoma, fibromatosis, leiomyoma, ameloblastoma, myxoma, hemangiopericytoma (a benign, aggressive lesion with a tendency to metastasize), fibromyxoma, and fibro-osseous and osseous lesions such as fibrous dysplasia, ossifying fibroma, and osteoma. Intracranial tissues may extend into the nasal area and present as encephaloceles, meningoceles, and pituitary tumors. CT scans and MRI demonstrate the intracranial connection, and biopsy without prior imaging is unwarranted due to the risk of cerebrospinal fluid (CSF) leakage or uncontrollable bleeding from vascular tumors.

Malignancies of the sinonasal tract represent only 1% of all cancers or 3% of upper respiratory tract malignancies with a 2:1 male-to-female ratio. Since respiratory epithelium can differentiate into squamous or glandular histologies, squamous cell carcinoma and adenocarcinoma represent two of the most common sinonasal cancers.[35] Sinonasal carcinoma is related to exposure to nickel, Thorotrast, and softwood dust. Chronic exposure to hardwood dust or leatherworking has been associated with adenocarcinoma of the sinonasal tract. Other malignancies include olfactory neuroblastoma, malignant fibrous histiocytoma, midline malignant reticulosis (also known as lethal midline granuloma or polymorphic reticulosis), osteosarcoma, chondrosarcoma, mucosal melanoma, lymphoma, fibrosarcoma, leiomyosarcoma, angiosarcoma, teratocarcinoma, and metastases from other organ systems, especially renal cell carcinoma.

Staging of sinonasal tumors has been recently altered in the 2002 AJCC staging manual. The nasal cavity and ethmoid sinuses are now considered separate primary sites in addition to the maxillary sinus. The staging system is only for carcinomatous malignancies and does not include the frontal or sphenoid sinuses as separate sites due to the rarity of tumors arising in these sites. Staging is partly dependent on local spread of tumor. Ohngren's line extends from the medial canthus to the mandibular angle. Maxillary tumors superior to Ohngren's line have a poorer prognosis compared to those inferior to the line due to the proximity to the orbit and cranial cavity. Local spread of tumors may occur along nerves, vessels, or directly through bone. Advanced tumors of the maxillary sinuses commonly involve the pterygopalatine and infratemporal fossae. Widening of foramen rotundum (V2) or foramen ovale (V3) on imaging suggests neural spread with intracranial involvement (Fig. 31-8). Since olfactory neuroblastomas are thought to arise from the olfactory neuroepithelium, these tumors commonly involve the cribriform plate and spread intracranially toward the frontal lobes. Sphenoidal tumors may include extension to the cavernous sinuses, carotid arteries, optic nerves, or the ophthalmic or maxillary branches of the trigeminal nerves. Lymph node metastases are in general uncommon (15%), and elective neck dissection or radiation of a

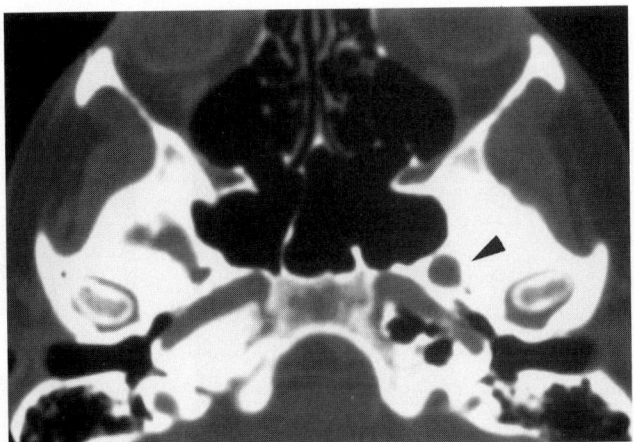

FIGURE 31-8. A 38-year-old woman with adenoid cystic carcinoma demonstrating perineural spread along V3 and widening of the foramen ovale on CT scan *(arrowhead)*.

clinically negative neck is most often unwarranted. Involved nodal groups include the retropharyngeal, parapharyngeal, submental, and upper jugulodigastric nodes.

The standard treatment for sinonasal malignancies is surgical resection, with postoperative radiation or chemoradiation for high-grade histologies or advanced local disease. Because these cancers can involve the dentition, orbits, or brain, treatment requires a multidisciplinary team including the head and neck surgeon, neurosurgeon, ophthalmologist, prosthodontist, oral surgeon, and reconstructive surgeon. After the preoperative work-up of imaging, endoscopy, and biopsy, a tumor map and operative plan are formulated. Vascular tumors are embolized by an interventional radiologist, preferably within 24 hours of surgery. Patients with tumors requiring skull base exploration may need a lumbar drain to decompress the dura from the cranium and reduce the risk of postoperative CSF leakage. Routine prophylactic use of tracheotomies for craniofacial surgery to reduce the risk of postoperative pneumocephalus is controversial.

Low-grade tumors limited to the lateral nasal wall, ethmoid sinuses, or septum are increasingly being removed with endoscopic techniques.[36] The lateral rhinotomy incision is the classic "open" approach for a medial maxillectomy that entails removal of the lateral nasal wall. If the tumor involves the inferior maxilla, an inferior maxillectomy including the hard palate and the medial, lateral, and posterior maxillary sinus walls is performed. For tumors more superior in the maxillary sinus, a total maxillectomy including the roof is performed. If the bone of the floor of the orbit is involved, removal with postoperative reconstruction is indicated. If orbital periosteum is involved with tumor, it may be resected with orbital preservation, although more extensive involvement of fat or muscle necessitates orbital exenteration (Fig. 31-9).[37]

If the anterior cranial floor is involved with tumor as it often is in olfactory neuroblastomas, a craniofacial resection is indicated. This combines a craniotomy approach with a transfacial approach. Surgical disruption of the cribriform region causes postoperative anosmia. Reconstruction of the anterior cranial fossa requires separation of the cranial vault from the nasal cavity with either a pericranial flap, temporoparietal fascial flap, fascia lata free graft, or when extensive resection has been performed, a microvascular free flap.[38] Unresectable lesions include those with brain involvement, carotid artery encasement, or bilateral optic nerve involvement.

Radiation therapy and chemotherapy for sinonasal malignancies are being used with increasingly frequency. Sinonasal undifferentiated carcinoma, rhabdomyosarcoma, and midline reticulocytosis are examples of aggressive cancers in which neoadjuvant chemotherapy and radiation play an integral role. Combining chemotherapy with radiation and surgery for treatment of advanced sinonasal squamous cell carcinoma has met with variable success.

Nasopharynx

The nasopharynx begins at the posterior nasal choana and ends at the horizontal plane between the posterior edge of the hard palate and the posterior pharyngeal wall. The nasopharynx includes the vault, the lateral walls that contain the eustachian tube orifices and the fossae of Rosenmüller, the roof made up of the sphenoid rostrum, and the posterior wall made up of the basiocciput or clivus. Both malignant and benign tumors of the nasopharynx are usually related to the normal histology that includes squamous and respiratory epithelium; the lymphoid tissues of the adenoids; and deeper tissues including fascia, cartilage, bone, and muscle. Benign tumors of the nasopharynx are rare and include fibromyxomatous polyps, papillomas, teratomas, and pedunculated fibromas. Angiofibroma is a benign tumor that affects young

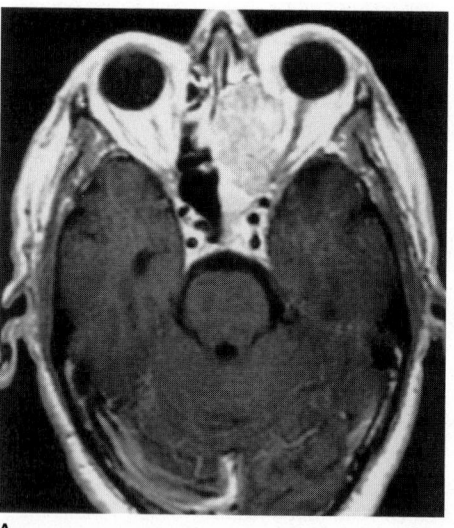

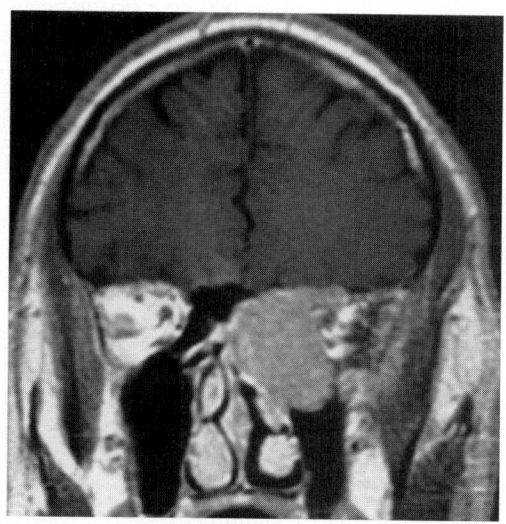

A

B

FIGURE 31-9. A, Axial MRI of a patient with adenosquamous carcinoma of the ethmoids involving the orbital fat, necessitating orbital exenteration. **B,** Coronal MRI of same patient demonstrating tumor extension to the floor of the anterior cranial fossa.

males and is the most common benign tumor of the nasopharynx. Rathke's pouch cysts arise high in the nasopharynx at the sphenovomer junction. The cyst arises from a remnant of ectoderm that normally invaginates to form the anterior pituitary and may become infected later in life. Thornwaldt's bursa is located more inferiorly and arises from a remnant of the caudal notochord that can contain a jelly-like material. It too may become infected in later life and marsupialization is most often all that is required to treat both it and Rathke's pouch cysts. Craniopharyngiomas, extracranial meningiomas, encephaloceles, hemangiomas, paragangliomas, chordomas (which can cause extensive destruction), and antral-choanal polyps can also be seen in the nasopharynx.

Clinical presentation of nasopharyngeal tumors include symptoms of nasal obstruction, serous otitis with effusion with associated conductive hearing loss, epistaxis, and nasal drainage. Symptoms such as cervical mass, headache, otalgia, trismus, and cranial nerve involvement suggest malignancy. Examination of the nasopharynx was historically performed with the mirror and has been greatly improved with the use of either rigid or flexible nasopharyngoscopes in the office. CT scanning is excellent for determining bony destruction and widening of foramina. MRI examines soft tissue involvement and intracranial extension, as well as nerve, cavernous sinus, and carotid involvement.

Angiofibromas are vascular lesions found exclusively in males, usually presenting during puberty, and are commonly referred to as *juvenile nasopharyngeal angiofibromas*. Although they are benign tumors, angiofibromas often erode bone and cause significant structural and functional dysfunction, as well as bleeding. CT findings of a nasopharyngeal mass, anterior bowing of the posterior wall of the antrum, erosion of the sphenoid bone, erosion of the hard palate, erosion of the medial wall of the maxillary sinus, and displacement of the nasal septum in an adolescent male are highly suggestive of angiofibromas (Fig. 31-10). Surgery after embolization represents the primary treatment modality, and understanding the location of origin is critical for complete tumor extirpation. Tumors originate at the posterolateral wall of the roof of the nasal cavity, at the sphenopalatine foramen. Whether performed endoscopically or via an "open" approach such as lateral rhinotomy or Caldwell-Luc, complete removal of all tumor and bone in the sphenopalatine region is crucial to decrease the possibility of recurrence. Radiation has been successfully used as treatment of these tumors but, given the young age of presentation and the lifelong risks associated with radiation exposure, is usually reserved for unresectable angiofibromas and recurrences.

Possible malignancies include nasopharyngeal carcinoma, low-grade nasopharyngeal papillary adenocarcinoma, lymphoma, rhabdomyosarcoma, malignant schwannoma, liposarcoma, and aggressive chordomas. The staging system of malignant tumors of the nasopharynx is for epithelial tumors only and is based on confinement to the nasopharynx or spread to surrounding structures. Although nasopharyngeal carcinoma accounts for only 0.25% of all cancers in North America, it accounts for approximately 18% of all malignancies in China. There

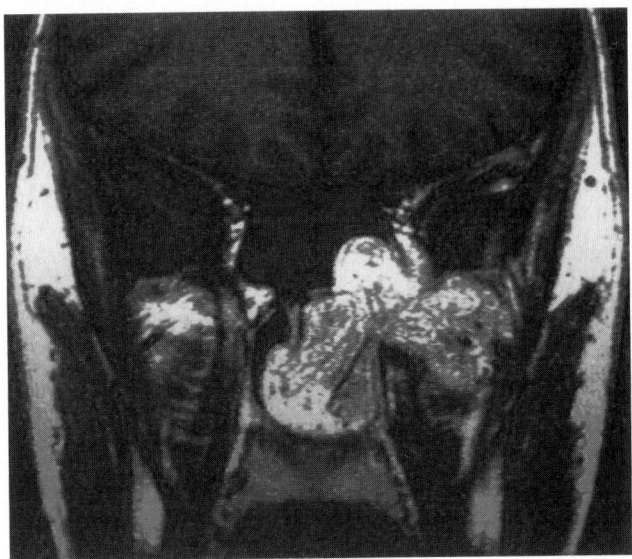

FIGURE 31-10. An MRI of a 16-year-old boy with a left-sided juvenile angiofibroma. The tumor arises in the pterygomaxillary region and has extended into the nasopharynx and infratemporal fossa.

is a strong correlation with Epstein-Barr virus that has been demonstrated in all histologic subtypes of nasopharyngeal carcinomas.[39] The World Health Organization has divided nasopharyngeal carcinomas into three histologic variants: keratinizing (25%), nonkeratinizing (15%), and undifferentiated (60%), although more recent classifications combine nonkeratinizing and undifferentiated tumors. The most common presenting symptom is neck node metastases, especially to the posterior cervical triangle, and low positive nodes predict poor outcomes. Treatment is based on radiation therapy both to the primary site and bilateral necks. With the addition of cisplatin and 5-fluorouracil, the rate of distant metastases decreases and both disease-free and overall survival increases.[40] Intracavitary radiation is used to provide a boost at the primary site for advanced tumors and is used in cases of re-irradiation. Surgery is reserved for persistent neck disease or in selected cases of local recurrences. It is unique that the risk of recurrence with nonkeratinizing and undifferentiated carcinoma appears to be chronic and does not level off at 5 years as it does with most other cancers. Rhabdomyosarcoma is the most common soft tissue sarcoma in the pediatric population and is the most common sarcoma occurring in the head and neck. Excluding the orbit, the most common site in the head and neck is the nasopharynx. Treatment is based on multimodality therapy of nonradical surgery and radiotherapy plus multiagent chemotherapy.

Although surgery of the nasopharynx is used primarily for benign pathologies, multiple approaches have been described, both endoscopic and open, to the surrounding skull base region. Little has been reported regarding the use of endoscopic removal of nasopharyngeal and medial skull base neoplasms.[36] Endoscopic techniques not only avoid facial incisions but allow shorter hospital stays. The most commonly described tumor removed via transnasal techniques is inverting papilloma excised in a piecemeal fashion. Success has also been reported with the endoscopic removal of mucoceles. Numerous open surgical approaches have been described to obtain access to the central skull base. For tumors of the nasopharynx, the transpalatal approach offers excellent visualization. The transfacial approach of lateral rhinotomy with unilateral or bilateral medial maxillectomies creates a facial incision but offers greater lateral exposure. The midfacial degloving procedure allows excellent exposure of bilateral maxillas, paranasal sinuses and the nasopharynx without facial incisions. The posterior wall of the maxillary sinus may be removed, allowing access to the pterygomaxillary fossa and deeper infratemporal fossa. For disease located more laterally, the approaches described by Fisch of transmastoid, transcochlear, and translabyrinthine are employed alone or in combination with more anterior approaches. More extensive approaches include the lateral facial split and mandibular swing, the fronto-orbital or fronto-orbital-zygomatic approach, the maxillary swing, and for disease of the high nasopharynx, the subfrontal approach affords excellent medial exposure (Fig. 31-11).

Ear and Temporal Bone

When referring to tumors of the "ear," the structures commonly involved include the external ear, the middle ear, and the inner ear. The external ear consists of the auricle or pinna and the external auditory canal to the tympanic membrane. The middle ear contains the tympanic cavity proper, the ossicles, the eustachian tube, the epitympanic recess, and the mastoid cavity. The borders of the middle ear include the tympanic membrane and squamous

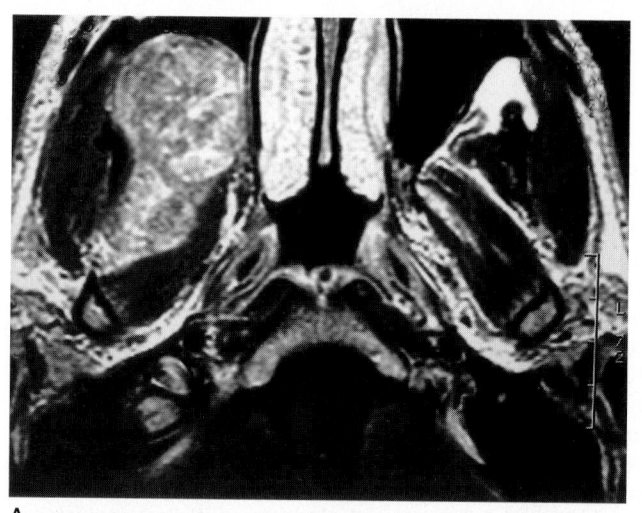

A

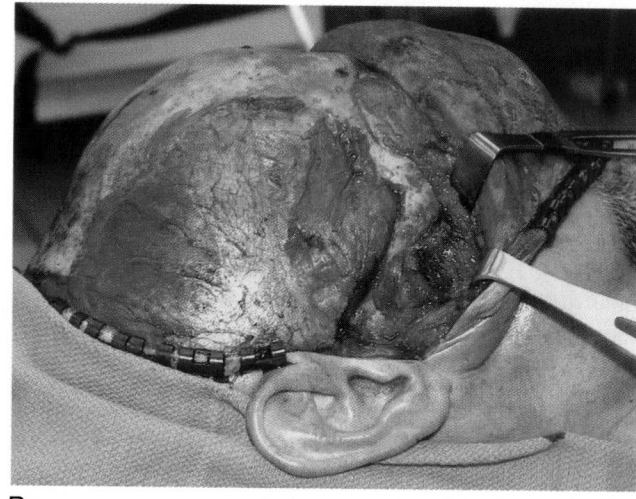

B

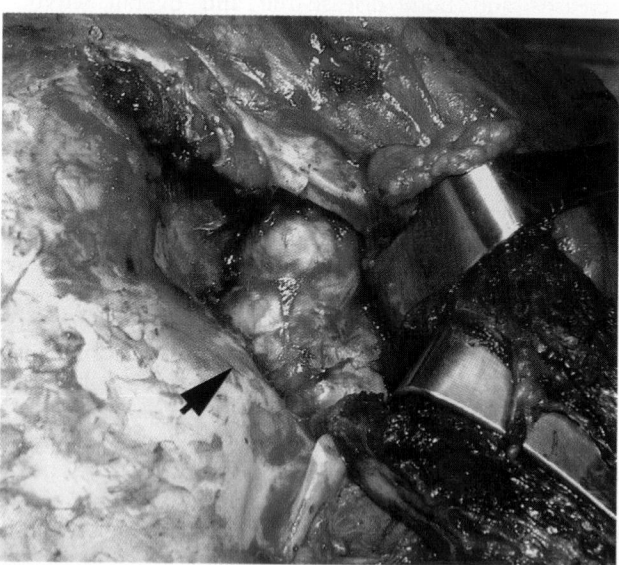

C

FIGURE 31-11. **A,** MRI of a 60-year-old man with a right-sided neuroma of V3 extending into the infratemporal fossa and parapharyngeal space. **B,** A bicoronal incision with a transzygomatic approach is used to approach the tumor (**C**), which is visualized after reflecting the temporalis muscle emanating from the foramen ovale region (*arrow*).

portion of the temporal bone laterally, the petrous temporal bone medially, the tegmen tympani or roof superiorly, the carotid canal anteriorly, the mastoid posteriorly, and floor of the tympanic bone inferiorly. The inner ear is contained within the petrous portion of the temporal bone and consists of the membranous and osseous labyrinth and the internal auditory canal.

Evaluation of ear and temporal bone neoplasms requires appropriate physical examination and audiologic and vestibular testing, as well as radiologic assessment. Findings of hearing loss, vertigo, eustachian tube dysfunction with serous otitis media, cranial nerve deficits, pulsatile tinnitus, drainage, and deep "boring" pain are often associated with tumors and must be thoroughly evaluated. CT scanning plays a crucial role in evaluating the temporal bone due to the complex anatomy contained within bony confines. MRI with gadolinium is complementary and is used to define soft tissue anatomy (Fig. 31-12).

Neoplasms of the pinna are most often related to sun exposure and are basal cell and squamous cell carcinomas. Keratoacanthoma is a benign tumor characterized by rapid growth and spontaneous involution that may be confused with a squamous cell carcinoma. In the external auditory canal, ceruminal gland adenocarcinomas, adenoid cystic carcinoma, and atypical fibroxanthomas may arise. Within the temporal bone, benign neoplasms include adenomas, paragangliomas (both at the tympanic membrane and the jugular bulb), acoustic neuroma, and meningioma. Squamous cell carcinoma is the most common cancer of the temporal bone, which also includes adenocarcinoma of either the middle ear or endolymphatic sac origin. In the pediatric population, soft tissue sarcomas such as rhabdomyosarcomas predominate. Metastases are an under-recognized cause of petrous bone tumors.

Malignancies of the pinna are treated similarly to skin cancers elsewhere on the face. Mohs microsurgery with frozen section control of margins minimizes the amount of normal tissue resected with the cutaneous malignancy. Involvement of underlying cartilage leads to more disseminated growth necessitating partial or total auriculectomy. If the extent of disease is great, a lateral temporal bone resection may be indicated with attempted preservation of the facial nerve and inner ear. When the facial nerve or parotid gland are involved, a lateral temporal bone resection with a parotidectomy is performed. Radiation therapy may be used uncommonly for primary treatment, or more commonly for adjuvant treatment in the case of perineural spread or poorly differentiated tumors.

The treatment of tumors involving the middle ear and bony canal is en bloc resection of those structures at risk for involvement. Rarely, when the tumor involves only the external canal without bony destruction, a sleeve resection of the canal can be performed. A lateral temporal bone resection removes the bony and cartilaginous canal, tympanic membrane, and ossicles. A subtotal temporal bone resection involves removal of the ear canal, middle ear, petrous bone, temporal mandibular joint, and facial nerve. Involvement of the petrous apex necessitates total temporal bone resection with removal of the carotid artery. Squamous cell carcinoma within the petrous apex is considered incurable, although adenoid cystic carcinoma and select low-grade sarcomas may be resected with a total temporal bone resection. The goals of reconstruction of temporal bone defects are protection from CSF leaks and coverage of vital structures and remaining bone to prepare for postoperative radiation therapy. Facial nerve rehabilitation is covered in salivary gland malignancies. Pedicled myocutaneous flaps, such as the lower

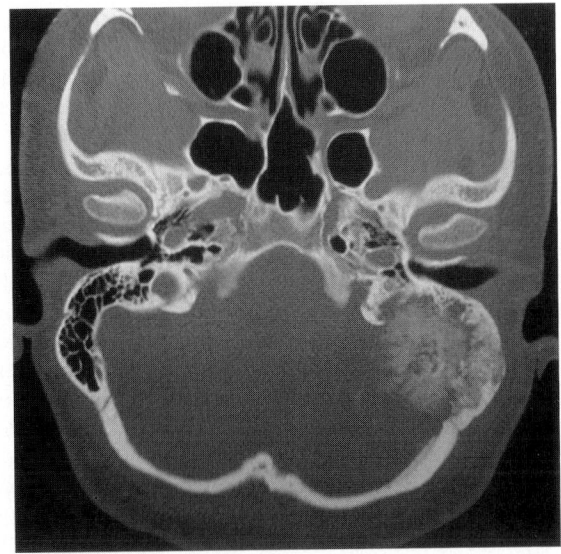

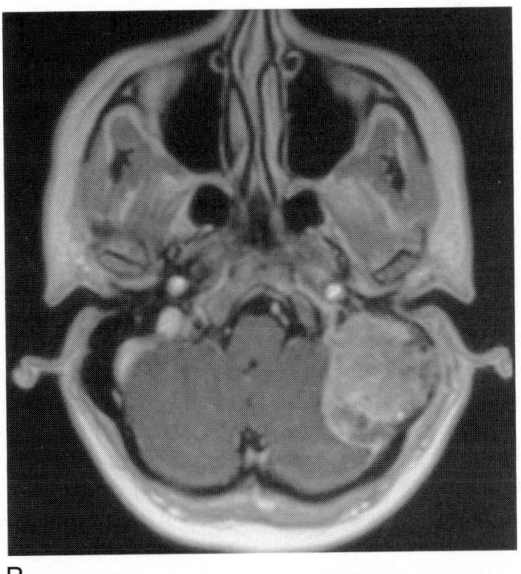

A   B

FIGURE 31-12. **A,** CT scan of a 19-year-old woman with osteosarcoma of the left temporal bone with bony destruction of the mastoid. **B,** MRI is useful in determining the extent of the tumor and the lack of brain invasion.

trapezius flap, have been used to accomplish these goals and provide bulk to restore some cosmesis to the area.[41] A prosthetic ear provides acceptable rehabilitation when total auriculectomy has been performed.

Salivary Gland Neoplasms

The major salivary glands include the parotid glands, the submandibular glands, and the sublingual glands. There are also approximately 750 minor salivary glands scattered throughout the submucosa of the oral cavity, oropharynx, hypopharynx, larynx, parapharyngeal space, and nasopharynx. Salivary gland neoplasms are rare, constituting 3% to 4% of head and neck neoplasms. The majority of neoplasms arise in the parotid gland (70%), whereas tumors of the submandibular gland (22%), and sublingual gland and minor salivary glands (8%), are less common. The ratio of malignant to benign tumors varies by site as well: parotid gland 80% benign, 20% malignant; submandibular gland and sublingual gland 50% benign, 50% malignant; minor salivary glands 25% benign, 75% malignant.

The parotid gland is the largest salivary gland and is divided into the superficial lobe and deep lobe by the facial nerve. On imaging, the lobes can be differentiated by the retromandibular vein that is commonly found at the division of the lobes. Deep lobe tumors lie within the parapharyngeal space. Stensen's duct is approximately 5 cm long and pierces the buccal fat pad to open in the oral cavity opposite the second maxillary molar. The submandibular glands are closely associated with the lingual nerve in the submandibular triangle and empty via Wharton's duct into the papilla just lateral to the frenulum. The sublingual gland lies on the inner table of the mandible and secretes via tiny openings (ducts of Rivinus) directly into the floor of mouth or via several ducts which unite to form the common sublingual duct (Bartholin), which then merges with Wharton's duct.

Numerous non-neoplastic diseases commonly affect the salivary glands. Sialadenitis is an acute, subacute, or chronic inflammation of a salivary gland. Acute sialadenitis commonly affects the parotid and submandibular glands and can be caused by bacterial (most frequently *Staphylococcus aureus*) or viral (mumps) infection. Chronic sialadenitis results from granulomatous inflammation of the glands commonly associated with sarcoidosis, actinomycosis, tuberculosis, or cat-scratch disease. Sialolithiasis is the accumulation of obstructive calcifications within the glandular ductal system, more common in the submandibular gland (90%) than the parotid (10%). When the calculi become obstructive, stasis of saliva may cause infection creating a painful, acutely swollen gland. Benign lymphoepithelial lesions of the salivary glands are non-neoplastic glandular enlargements associated with autoimmune diseases such as Sjögren's syndrome.

Salivary gland neoplasms most often present as slow-growing, well-circumscribed masses. Symptoms such as pain, rapid growth, nerve weakness, and paresthesias, and signs of cervical lymphadenopathy and fixation to skin or underlying muscles suggest malignancy. When the presenting symptom is complete unilateral facial paralysis, Bell's palsy may be misdiagnosed as the etiology and it is important to remember that all Bell's palsy patients will show some improvement in facial movement within 6 months of the onset of weakness. Trismus is associated with involvement of the pterygoid musculature by deep parotid lobe malignancies. Bimanual palpation of submandibular masses assists in determining fixation to surrounding structures. CT and MRI scans of salivary malignancies tend to show irregular tumor borders and obliteration of fat planes in the parapharyngeal space with deep parotid lobe cancers. The accuracy of fine-needle aspiration cytology of the salivary glands has been well established. Sensitivity, specificity, and accuracy of parotid gland aspirates in one series were 92%, 100%, and 98%, respectively.[42] Excision of the gland is used to confirm the final diagnosis.

Benign tumors of the salivary glands include pleomorphic adenomas, a variety of monomorphic adenomas (including Warthins's tumors, oncocytomas, basal cell adenomas, canalicular adenomas, and myoepitheliomas), a variety of ductal papillomas, and capillary hemangiomas. Pleomorphic adenomas account for 40% to 70% of all tumors of the salivary glands, most commonly occurring in the tail of the parotid. Like all benign parotid tumors, the treatment of choice is surgical excision with a margin of normal tissue (e.g., superficial parotidectomy). In the parotid gland, if this is possible without complete removal of the affected lobe, cosmetic postoperative appearance will be superior to patients in whom a complete lobe is removed. Shelling out of pleomorphic adenomas is to be avoided because it has been shown to correlate with increased rates of recurrence.[43] The facial nerve should not be sacrificed in removing a benign lesion (Fig. 31-13). Warthin's tumor, or papillary cystadenoma lymphomatosum, is the second most common benign parotid tumor and occurs most often in older, white men. Owing to the high mitochondrial content within oncocytes, the oncocyte-rich Warthin's tumor and oncocytomas will incorporate technetium Tc 99m and appear as "hot spots" on radionuclide scan. If fine-needle aspiration suggests a slow-growing Warthin's tumor with confirmatory technetium scanning in a patient with contraindications to surgery, the tumor may be closely followed, because this tumor has no malignant potential.

Malignant salivary tumors are staged according to size: T1 is less than 2 cm, T2 is 2 to 4 cm, T3 is greater than 4 cm or any tumor with macroscopic extraparenchymal extension, and T4 involves invasion of surrounding tissues. Malignant salivary tumors are listed in Table 31-3. Mucoepidermoid carcinoma is the most common malignant tumor of the parotid gland, and can be divided into low-grade and high-grade tumors. High-grade lesions have propensities for both regional and distant metastases and corresponding shorter survival rates than low-grade mucoepidermoid carcinomas. Adenoid cystic carcinoma constitutes 10% of all salivary neoplasms, with two thirds occurring in the minor salivary glands. The histologic types of adenoid cystic carcinoma are tubular, cribriform, and solid, listed from best prognosis to worst. An indolent growth pattern and a relentless propensity for perineural invasion characterize adenoid cystic carcinoma. Regional

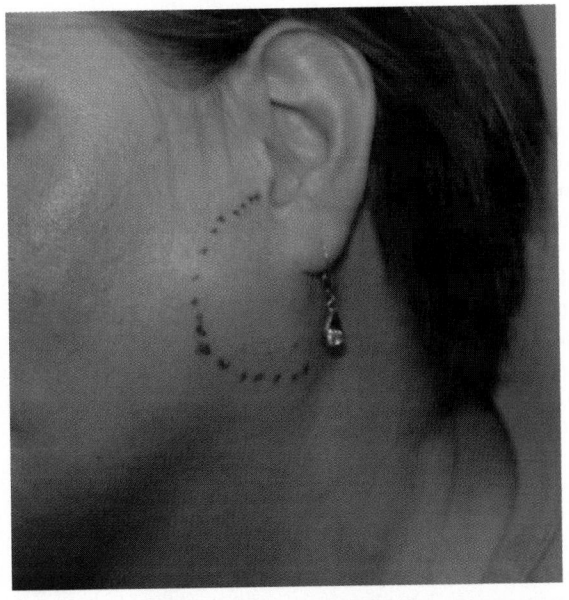

A

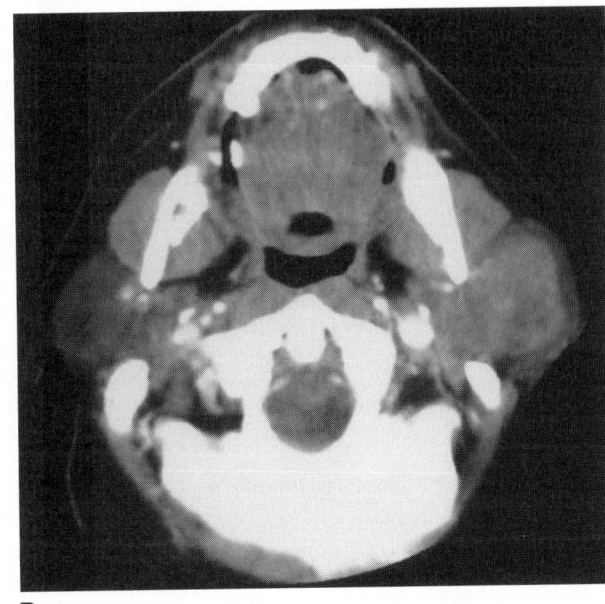

B

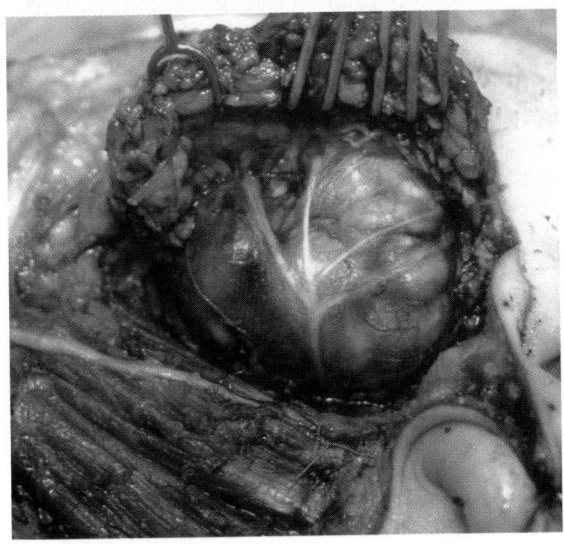

C

FIGURE 31-13. **A,** A 34-year-old woman with an asymptomatic left parotid mass. **B,** CT scan demonstrating a rim of normal parotid tissue superficial to a deeper, heterogeneous mass. **C,** The facial nerve stretched over the deep-lobe pleomorphic adenoma with preservation of the superficial lobe that was raised along with the skin flap for better postoperative cosmesis and prevention of postoperative Frey's syndrome or gustatory sweating.

lymphatic spread is uncommon, although distant metastases occur within the first 5 years after diagnosis and may remain asymptomatic for decades. Malignant mixed tumors include both cancers originating from pleomorphic adenomas, termed *carcinoma ex pleomorphic adenoma*, and de novo malignant mixed tumors. The risk of malignant transformation of benign pleomorphic adenomas is 1.5% within the first 5 years but increases to 9.5% once the benign tumor has been present for more than 15 years.[44] Most salivary gland lymphomas are of the non-Hodgkin's variety (85%). The risk of malignant lymphoma in patients with Sjögren's syndrome is 44-fold higher than the normal population. Metastatic tumors are most often from cutaneous carcinomas and melanomas from the scalp, temporal area, and the ear. Distant metastatic tumors are rare but may arise from the lung, kidneys, and breasts.

Treatment of salivary gland malignancies is en bloc surgical excision. Radiation therapy is administered postoperatively for high-grade malignancies demonstrating extraglandular disease, perineural invasion, direct invasion of surrounding tissues, or regional metastases. For tumors confined to the superficial lobe of the parotid gland, a lateral lobectomy with preservation of the facial nerve may be performed. Gross tumor should not be left in situ, but if the facial nerve is able to be preserved by "peeling" tumor off the nerve, the nerve should be preserved and radiation therapy given for microscopic residual disease. For cancers of the deep lobe, a total parotidectomy is performed. Elective neck dissections are performed for high-grade malignancies such as high-grade mucoepidermoid carcinoma. For gross facial nerve involvement, a temporal bone resection is performed and the nerve is sacrificed proximally to obtain a negative

TABLE 31-3. Tumors of the Major and Minor Salivary Glands

Benign	Malignant
Pleomorphic adenoma	Acinic cell carcinoma
Warthin's tumor	Mucoepidermoid carcinoma
Capillary hemangioma	Adenoid cystic carcinoma
Oncocytoma	Polymorphous low-grade adenocarcinoma
Basal cell adenoma	Epithelial-myoepithelial carcinoma
Canalicular adenoma	Basal cell adenocarcinoma
Myoepithelioma	Sebaceous carcinoma
Sialadenoma papilliferum	Papillary cystadenocarcinoma
Intraductal papilloma	Mucinous adenocarcinoma
Inverted ductal papilloma	Oncocytic carcinoma
	Salivary duct carcinoma
	Adenocarcinoma
	Myoepithelial carcinoma
	Malignant mixed tumor
	Squamous cell carcinoma
	Small cell carcinoma
	Lymphoma
	Metastatic carcinoma
	Carcinoma ex pleomorphic adenoma

margin. When the facial nerve is removed, rehabilitation with a simultaneous nerve graft may be performed with the hope of producing facial muscular tone. Although the primary goal of facial nerve rehabilitation is protection of the cornea from chronic exposure, other concerns include oral competency, nasal valve maintenance, and cosmesis. Upper lid gold weights, lateral tarsorrhaphies, static facial slings, dynamic muscular slings, and delayed reinnervation procedures are also used for facial rehabilitation. Submandibular gland and minor salivary gland malignancies are treated similarly to parotid gland cancers via en bloc resection. Submandibular gland malignancies are removed with level I contents and an accompanying modified radical neck dissection. Gross involvement of the hypoglossal or lingual nerves requires sacrifice and obtaining a negative margin by following the nerves toward the skull base. Adenoid cystic cancers are highly neurotropic and treatment comprises removal of gross tumor with radiation therapy for microscopic disease that is assumed to exist at the tumor periphery.

Neck and Unknown Primary

The work-up of a neck mass is different in children than it is in adults due to differing etiologies. Cervical masses are common in children and most often represent inflammatory processes or congenital abnormalities. Of pediatric neck masses that are persistent, 2% to 15% that are removed will be malignant. Pediatric evaluation requires thorough head and neck examination, including endoscopy of the nasopharynx and larynx. The most

common etiology of cervical adenopathy is viral upper respiratory tract infections. The associated lymphadenopathy generally subsides within 2 weeks, although mononucleosis lymphadenopathy may persist for 4 to 6 weeks. Location of the mass, as well as its character, most often lead to the diagnosis. Lymphadenopathy not due to viral infections may represent a less common infectious process. Bacterial cervical adenitis is most often caused by group A, β-hemolytic streptococcus or *S. aureus*. Scrofula is cervical adenitis due to tuberculosis and is relatively uncommon in industrialized countries, although atypical mycobacteria may also cause cervical adenitis. Cat-scratch disease should be suspected if there is a history of cat contact, and indirect fluorescence antibody testing for *Rochalimaea henselae* should be performed. Midline masses include thyroglossal duct cysts, enlarged lymph nodes, dermoid cysts, hemangiomas, or pyramidal lobes of thyroid. Nonlymphoid masses anterior to the sternocleidomastoid muscle are most commonly branchial cleft cysts. A soft, compressible mass of the posterior triangle may represent a lymphangioma (or cystic hygroma), which usually presents prior to the age of 2 years. Cervical teratomas are present at birth and may involve compression of the airway or esophagus. Malignancies most commonly encountered in pediatric neck masses include sarcomas, lymphomas, and metastatic thyroid carcinoma.

In the adult, neck masses more often represent malignancies than in children. *Persistent masses larger than 2 cm represent cancer in 80% of cases.* In addition to the head and neck examination, CT scanning assists in evaluating not only the masses but potential primary sites. Fine-needle aspiration (<22 gauge) is performed as one of the initial steps in the work-up of neck masses with an overall accuracy of 95% for benign neck masses and 87% for malignant masses.[45] As in children, the location of the masses bear on the likelihood of diagnosis: Midline masses may represent thyroglossal duct cysts, dermoid tumors, delphian nodes, thyroid masses, lipomas, or sebaceous cysts. Thyroglossal duct cysts represent the vestigial tract of descent that the thyroid followed from the foramen cecum to normal location below the cricoid. The cyst may become enlarged later in life concurrent with an upper respiratory tract infection. Surgical excision should include the central portion of the hyoid bone (Sistrunk procedure) or recurrence is more likely.

Persistent lateral neck masses in adults may represent enlarged benign or malignant lymph nodes, neuromas or neurofibromas, carotid body tumors, branchial cleft cysts, lipomas, sebaceous cysts, parathyroid cysts, or a primary soft tissue tumor. Enlarged lymph nodes may be secondary to infection of etiology similar to those in the pediatric population, as well as lymphoma, regional metastases from squamous cell carcinoma, melanomas, thyroid carcinomas or salivary gland tumors, or distant metastases. Most common, lymphadenopathy in an adult is indicative of metastatic HNSCC, with lymphoma less likely. Metastatic squamous cell carcinoma is most commonly from the nasopharynx, oropharynx, or hypopharynx and its presence is a negative prognostic indicator. In all cases of metastases to the neck, lymphadenectomy as treatment is valuable only in cases of squamous cell carcinoma, salivary gland tumors, melanoma, and thyroid carcinoma. Otherwise, removal of metastatic lymph nodes is indicated for diagnosis only and systemic treatment must be initiated. In cases of multiple lymph node enlargement, diagnoses of human immunodeficiency virus, toxoplasmosis, and fungal infection should be investigated.

Less frequently, benign neck masses do occur in adults. The branchial cleft apparatus that persists after birth may give rise to a number of neck masses. First, branchial cleft cysts present in the preauricular or submandibular areas and are intimately associated with the external auditory canal and parotid gland and may require dissection of the facial nerve during excision. Second and third branchial cleft cysts and tracts present anterior to the sternocleidomastoid muscle and often become symptomatic following upper respiratory tract infections. Although the second branchial cleft communicates with the ipsilateral tonsillar fossa, the third communicates with the piriform sinus. Removal of the cyst and tract necessitates dissection along the course of embryologic descent. Second branchial cleft tracts course between the internal and external carotid arteries. Third branchial cleft tracts course posterior to both branches of the carotid artery. Occasionally, a carcinoma may be found within the cyst. Debate continues as to whether the carcinoma represents a cystic metastasis from the tongue base or tonsil or whether cancer may occur de novo within a branchial cleft cyst.[46]

Carotid body tumors or chemodectomas are more properly referred to as *paragangliomas* and arise from the branchiomeric paraganglia at the carotid body. Tumors are usually benign, unifocal, and nonhereditary and present as a nonpainful mass at the carotid bifurcation and have a characteristic "lyre" sign on carotid arteriogram (Fig. 31-14). Due to their highly vascular nature, biopsy is contraindicated. Preoperative embolization is performed with tumors greater than 3 cm. The most common sequela from resection is cranial nerve injury, most commonly of the superior laryngeal nerve but also the vagal nerve or hypoglossal nerve with large tumors. Tumors larger than 5 cm are associated with a need for concurrent carotid artery replacement.[47] "First-bite syndrome" has been coined to describe the phenomenon of pain with the initiation of mastication thought due to removal of sympathetic nerves surrounding the carotid bifurcation and reinnervation of the parotid secretory glands by parasympathetic fibers. Excision of bilateral carotid body tumors may lead to baroreceptor failure with wide fluctuations in blood pressure.

Tumors of the parapharyngeal space are distinguished by their location: either prestyloid, usually of salivary gland origin, or poststyloid, usually vascular or neurogenic in origin. Presenting symptoms may be superior neck mass, a fullness to the parotid gland or tonsillar fossa, trismus, dysphagia, Horner's syndrome, or cranial nerve impairment. Tumors include paraganglioma, salivary

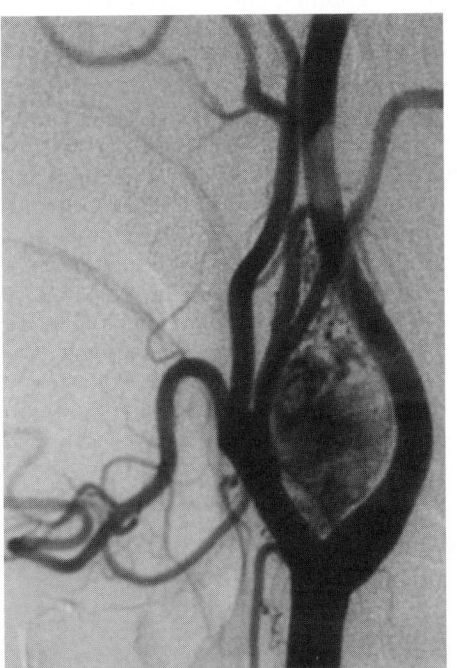
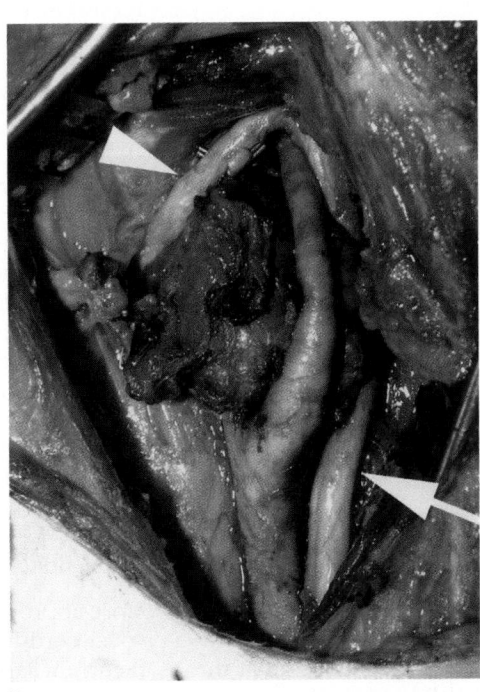
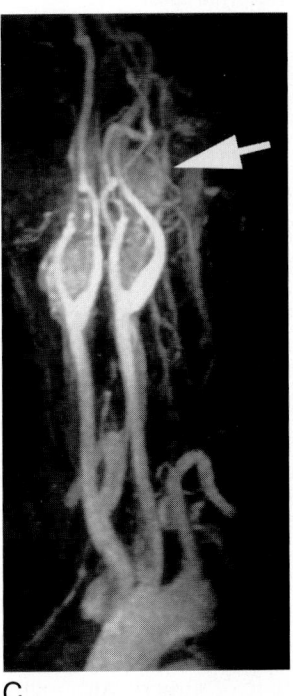

A   B   C

FIGURE 31-14. **A,** The characteristic "lyre" sign on arteriogram of a carotid body paraganglioma, splaying the internal and external carotid arteries. **B,** The tumor lies between the arteries, superficial to the vagus nerve *(arrow)* and deep to the hypoglossal nerve *(arrowhead).* **C,** Magnetic resonance angiography of a different patient demonstrating bilateral carotid body tumors, in addition to a separate, more superior left vagal paraganglioma *(arrow).*

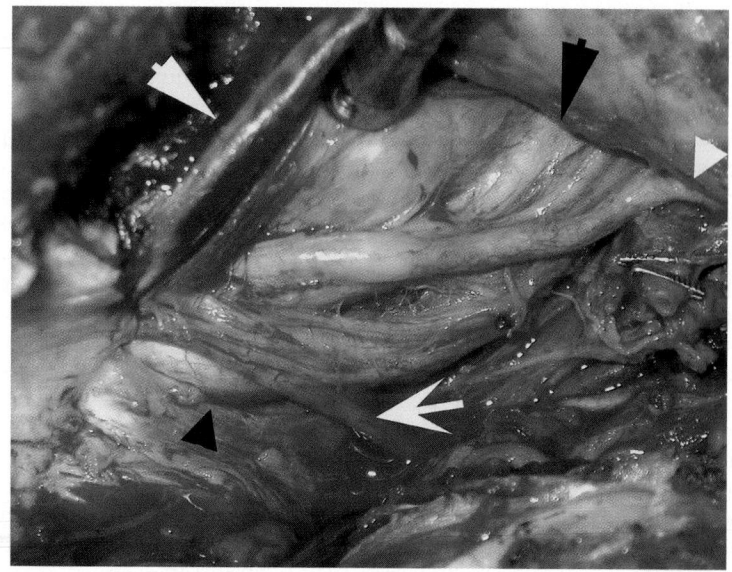

FIGURE 31-15. The left post-styloid space after removal of a parapharyngeal space tumor and a lateral temporal bone resection. The carotid is seen anteriorly *(black arrowhead)* where it enters the skull base, while the internal jugular vein *(large white arrowhead)* is retracted posteriorly. The vagus nerve *(large black arrowhead)* is intimately associated with the hypoglossal nerve *(small white arrowhead)* and separation of the two nerves at this level often leads to a vocal cord paralysis. The glossopharyngeal nerve is seen anteriorly *(large white arrow).*

gland neoplasms, schwannoma or neurilemoma, lipoma, sarcomas, or lymphadenopathy. Access to these tumors is most commonly performed transcervically, and care must be taken to preserve uninvolved structures such as the carotid artery and major cranial nerves (Fig. 31-15). Rarely is a mandibulotomy approach required.

TRACHEOTOMY

Tracheotomy is most commonly used today in patients requiring prolonged mechanical ventilation to reduce the risk of damage to the larynx, assist ventilation and pulmonary hygiene, and improve patient comfort and oral care. There is no hard rule as to how long a translaryngeal endotracheal tube can be left in place. Some laryngologists recommend conversion to tracheotomy after 3 days of intubation, although most use 2 to 3 weeks as a limit. Other common reasons for tracheotomy include chronic aspiration and acute airway obstruction secondary to facial or laryngeal trauma or oral or deep neck space infections or perioperatively during radical cancer ablation.

The term trache*otomy* implies formation of an opening that will close spontaneously once the tracheotomy tube is decannulated. This closure via secondary intention usually occurs over 5 to 7 days, and the healing process should not be hastened by suturing the overlying skin closed or an abscess may form in this highly contaminated wound. The term trache*ostomy* implies formation of a permanent opening that remains open after removal of the tube. The surgeon can form a tracheostomy by suturing an inferiorly based tracheal ring flap to the skin at the time of surgery. Although this flap allows for safer replacement of the tracheal tube should it become accidentally decannulated, once the mucocutaneous junction forms, a surgical procedure with rotational skin flaps is required to close the tracheostomy. A permanent tracheostomy

should be considered in cases of extended mechanical ventilation, chronic aspiration, obstructive sleep apnea, and uncorrectable upper airway obstruction.

Preoperative assessment should include a history of previous tracheotomy or neck surgery, laryngeal pathology, bleeding difficulties, or cervical spine injuries. Perioperative complications of tracheotomy include bleeding, aspiration, pneumothorax and pneumomediastinum, recurrent laryngeal nerve injury, and hypoxia. Long-term problems include formation of granulation tissue both at the skin and within the trachea, collapse of tracheal cartilage and airway obstruction, and tracheoinnominate artery and tracheoesophageal fistulas.

Although the traditional open tracheotomy technique is still primarily used and preferred, recently the percutaneous tracheotomy has gained in usage. There are reports of both increased and decreased complication rates with the percutaneous technique compared to the open technique.[48,49] Although one may suspect that the trauma from dilating the tracheal rings in the percutaneous technique may be associated with a substantial increase in long-term tracheal stenosis, this does not always seem to be the case, and percutaneous tracheotomies have become common in many intensive care units in patients with favorable anatomy and supportive clinical settings.

VOCAL CORD PARALYSIS

More appropriately termed *vocal cord immobility*, loss of vocal cord function remains a common occurrence. The recurrent laryngeal nerve supplies all laryngeal musculature except for the cricothyroid muscle, which is supplied by the superior laryngeal nerve. Paralysis of the laryngeal muscles may occur from a lesion in the central nervous system or, more commonly, with peripheral nerve involvement (90%). Once the vagal nerve exits the jugular foramen, the superior laryngeal nerve divides superiorly in the parapharyngeal space and passes deep to the carotid artery. On the left side, the recurrent laryngeal nerve separates from the vagal nerve in the thorax and passes around the aortic arch at the ductus arteriosus to travel superiorly in the tracheoesophageal groove to the cricothyroid joint. Likely due to the left recurrent nerve's longer course, left vocal cord paralysis is more common than right. The right recurrent nerve separates from the vagus to pass around the right subclavian artery and back to the larynx. A nonrecurrent recurrent laryngeal nerve is a rare finding (0.5% to 1.0%) on the right side, in which the nerve separates from the vagus prior to descending into the chest and passes directly to the larynx, and is associated with a retroesophageal right subclavian artery. Approaches to the cervical spine should generally be performed from the left to reduce traction injury to the recurrent nerve since right-sided approaches have been associated with a higher rate of laryngeal nerve injuries.[50]

Dysfunction of the superior laryngeal nerve most commonly occurs after thyroidectomy, where the nerve is in close proximity to the superior thyroid vascular pedicle, and may leave the patient with difficulty in achieving precision in pitch, noticeable most commonly in professional voice users. Injury to the recurrent laryngeal nerve results in vocal fold paresis or paralysis. Patients with unilateral vocal cord immobility may present with hoarseness, ineffective cough, dysphagia, aspiration, or airway compromise or may be completely asymptomatic based on their ability to compensate. Definitive diagnosis is made through laryngoscopy, and subtle weakness may require stroboscopic examination. Etiologies of paralysis include surgical trauma (most commonly thyroidectomy), malignancies of the thyroid, mediastinum, esophagus, or larynx, mediastinal compression, viral neuropathy, collagen vascular disease, sarcoidosis, and diabetic neuropathy, as well as a multitude of other reported causes. The etiology remains unknown in 20% of patients. Since re-creating volitional abduction and adduction of the vocal cord is not currently feasible, the goal of treatment entails creating sufficient medialization of the involved vocal cord to allow for efficient voicing and cough, as well as reduce hoarseness and aspiration. Medialization may be accomplished with intracordal injection with a variety of substances including fat, Gelfoam, and human cadaveric collagen preparations. Due to the risk of granuloma formation, Teflon injection is rarely used today. Medialization thyroplasty, with or without concurrent arytenoid adduction, consists of a surgically created window in the thyroid cartilage with the insertion of Silastic, hydroxyapatite, or Gore-Tex and has shown excellent results.[51] Laryngeal reinnervation via an ansa cervicalis–recurrent laryngeal nerve anastomosis provides medialization with tone to the paralyzed cord but takes several months to become effective. Bilateral vocal fold paralysis is an uncommon scenario, manifested by both vocal folds remaining near the midline position. Patients maintain a strong voice since the vocal folds continue to vibrate, but they may suffer from life-threatening airway obstruction and stridor and may require immediate reintubation or tracheotomy.

RECONSTRUCTION

Perhaps the area of head and neck surgery that has undergone the most advancement in the past 25 years is reconstruction, fueled largely by the advent of microvascular free flaps. Today, there is almost no defect which cannot be repaired, and this has afforded the ablative surgeon more leeway in obtaining tumor-free margins. The head and neck is unique in the intricacy of its form and function, and careful reconstruction is needed to return the patient back to his or her premorbid condition. Speech, swallowing, and cosmesis are most commonly focused on when considering rehabilitative goals. Swallowing may be impaired by resection of local tissues of the oral cavity, oropharynx, hypopharynx, larynx, and cervical esophagus. Loss of innervation, either sensory or motor, locally or at the skull base, can severely impair swallowing. Irradiation leads to fibrosis of local tissues as well as loss of saliva and taste and may cause stenosis years after treatment is finished. Rehabilitation of speech is covered in the larynx section. Due to the proximity and complexity of the airway and digestive tracts at the oral cavity, oropharynx, larynx, and hypopharynx, the ability to maintain the two functions is closely related. Often, aspiration occurs when the swallowing process is impeded. Although a tracheotomy tube helps protect the airway somewhat from aspiration and allows for increased pulmonary suctioning, it also tethers the larynx to the skin and often exacerbates dysphagia. Once dysfunction has occurred, the physician is hampered by trying to maintain the balance between airway, speech, and swallowing, and one function may have to be further impaired to improve another. In the severely dysfunctional upper airway, total sacrifice of one function may have to be accepted and a laryngectomy or permanent gastric tube may be required.

Cosmetic deformities are most obvious in the head and neck area. Functional deficits not only occur with speech and swallowing but also affect eyelid function, oral competence, and maintenance of a nasal and oral airway. General principles include reconstructing underlying bony framework, replacing skin with skin of matching quality, minimizing scar visibility and contracture, and reconstructing in zones of facial units. Skin should be matched by color, thickness, and hair-bearing units where possible. The aesthetic facial units include the forehead, eyes and periorbital area, midface, nose (which itself contains several subunits), and the lips and mentum. A spectrum of reconstructive options exists with healing by secondary intention and primary closure at one end, and extensive reconstruction such as microvascular free flaps at the other. Which option is selected depends on the location and severity of the defect, the overall health of the patient, the available donor sites for flaps, the status of the tissue adjacent to the defect (irradiated, infected, previously operated), and the functionality of the area to be reconstructed. Not only must the reconstructive surgeon choose which option is best for a given defect, but secondary and tertiary options should be planned, in case of flap failure or recurrent disease.

Healing by secondary intention is an excellent option in several clinical scenarios. Mucosal defects with an underlying layer of vascularized muscle or bone that will not contract to the point of impeding function may be left to close via secondary intention. Examples include tonsillectomy defects, tongue resections, and some laryngeal mucosal defects. Primary closure is likely to be the most commonly used option for cutaneous defect closure. Attempts should be made to keep incisions within the lines of relaxed skin tension. These lines are caused by muscular insertion into the skin and form when mimetic motion occurs. Incisions that parallel the lines of relaxed skin tension not only respect the aesthetic units of the face but also have the least amount of tension along them, which decreases scarring. A Z-plasty may be used to reorient an unfavorable line of closure into a relaxed skin tension line.

Skin grafts are most commonly used in the oral cavity, ear, or maxillectomy defects, as well as for coverage for donor sites like the radial forearm and fibular free flaps and the deltopectoral flap. Skin grafts are completely dependent for nutrition on the tissue over which they are placed and can heal well over muscle, perichondrium, and periosteum. They do not take well over bone or cartilage, nor on tissue which has been irradiated or infected or is hypovascular. Split-thickness skin grafts (STSGs) contain the epidermis and a portion of the dermis and are harvested with a dermatome at approximately 12 to 18/1000-inch thickness. Thinner grafts require less nutrients to remain viable but also will contract more when healing. Grafts may be meshed to allow greater surface coverage, but these are generally restricted to the scalp or over muscle owing to a less cosmetic result. A nonadherent antibiotic-impregnated bolster is commonly used to maintain stability between the STSG and the recipient bed for 5 days to allow for nutrient transmission and capillary ingrowth while healing. Harvest sites include the anterior and lateral thighs and buttocks.

Full-thickness skin grafts (FTSGs) are characterized by a better color match, texture, contour, and less contracture but decreased success rates compared to STSGs. Commonly used donor sites include the postauricular, the upper eyelid, and the supraclavicular fossa skin. Composite grafts are occasionally needed for cartilage and skin reconstruction of the nasal ala and may be harvested from the conchal bowl without significantly affecting the appearance of the pinna. Acellular cadaveric human dermis that has been prepared by removing immunogenic cells while leaving intact the collagen matrix has recently been growing in popularity as a skin graft substitute and avoids the need for a donor site.

Local skin flaps have excellent tissue match due to their proximity to the defect. Commonly used designs include the advancement, rotation, transposition, rhomboid, and bilobed flaps. Similar to primary closure, local flaps should be designed to be incorporated into the lines of relaxed skin tension. Although local flaps depend upon the subdermal plexus of capillaries, regional flaps have an axial blood supply. This latter vascular pedicle is necessary for flap viability because greater distances are spanned by the flap and is either contained within the subcutaneous fascia as in a fasciocutaneous flap, or within an underlying muscle as in a myocutaneous flap. The deltopectoral flap or "Bakamjian" flap was one of the early regional flaps and was used extensively in head and neck reconstruction. Based on the intercostal perforating branches from the internal mammary artery, the flap is based medially and designed over the upper pectoralis and deltoid regions. Due to the pliability of the transferred skin, it can be swung upward for skin defects or pharyngeal reconstruction. Perhaps the development with the most significant impact on head and neck reconstruction was the introduction of the pectoralis myocutaneous flap in 1978. Based on the pectoral branch of the thoracoacromial artery, the artery pierces the pectoralis muscle from the deep surface. A skin paddle designed over the muscle, or simply the muscle itself, may be transferred to reconstruct defects up to the nasopharynx. Historically, the pectoralis muscle is tunneled under the intervening skin to preserve the ipsilateral deltopectoral flap in case of the need for future coverage. Division of the pectoral nerve branches ensures atrophy of the muscle and reduces the bulge over the clavicle. In addition to the reconstruction of mucosal defects with the vascularized skin, coverage of an exposed carotid artery is an excellent usage of the myogenous flap. The trapezius muscle offers multiple soft tissue flaps that may be rotated into head and neck defects. The lower trapezius myocutaneous flap, based on the dorsal scapular artery, has already been referred to as an excellent choice for lateral temporal bone defects.[41] Finally, the submental and platysmal flaps are based on the facial artery and offer excellent local flap coverage for oral and oropharyngeal defects.

A "free flap" entails removal of composite tissue from a distant site along with its blood supply and reimplantation of the vasculature in the reconstructive field. Although the first successful human microvasculature transfer was a jejunal interposition flap in 1959, the modern era of microvasculature reconstruction did not arise until the 1970s with improvements in instrumentation and technique. Today's selection of donor sites allows the benefit of choosing between sites with large-caliber, long vascular pedicles that are anatomically consistent. In addition to favorable vascularity, optimal donor sites allow for a simultaneous two-team approach of ablation and harvesting, the possibility of a sensate flap, the composite transfer of bone stock capable of accepting osseointegrated implants, and/or the transfer of secretory mucosa. Patient selection for free flap reconstruction is of critical importance. Advanced age is not a contraindication to microvascular reconstruction, although previous recipient bed irradiation, contraction of tissues in cases of secondary reconstruction, or previous free flap failure should raise concern to the reconstructive surgeon. Complete loss of a free tissue transfer should occur in less than 5% of cases.

The radial forearm has emerged as the workhorse of soft tissue free flaps in head and neck reconstruction. A fasciocutaneous flap with sensate capabilities, the radial forearm flap is based on the radial artery and its venae comitantes and/or cephalic vein for drainage. Variations of the flap include harvest of partial radius bone or palmaris longus tendon for bony or suspensory reconstruction, respectively. The main advantage of the radial

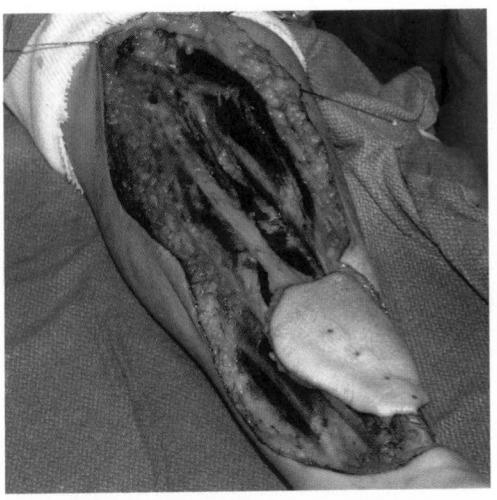

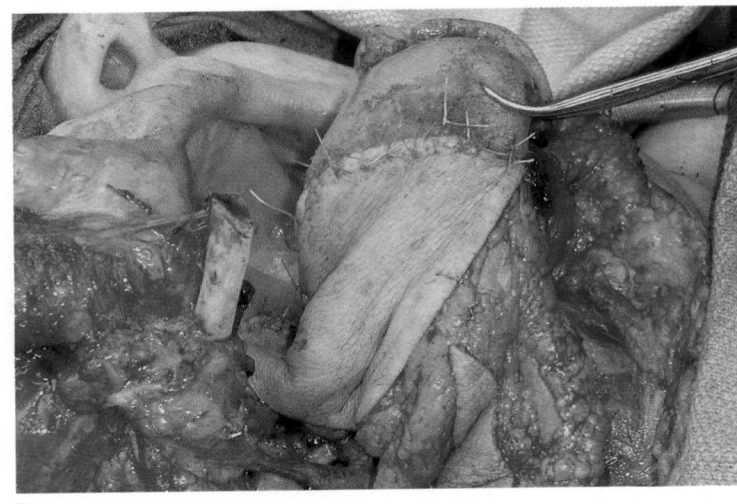

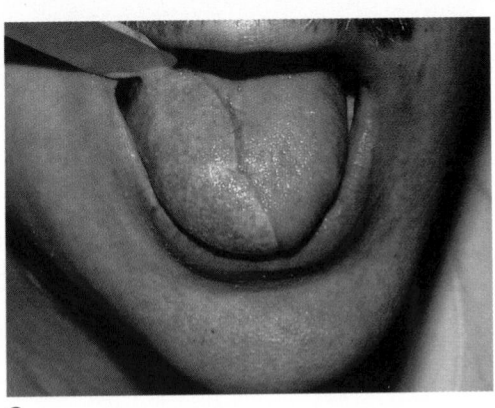

FIGURE 31-16. **A,** Harvest of a radial forearm fasciocutaneous free flap, based on the radial artery. **B,** A right hemiglossectomy for squamous cell carcinoma of the right, mobile tongue, reconstructed with a radial forearm flap. **C,** Postoperative result 1 year later demonstrating excellent contour and tongue mobility.

forearm flap is the thinness and pliability of the harvested skin that makes it ideal not only for external cutaneous defects but also reconstruction of the floor of mouth or tongue (Fig. 31-16), soft palate and oropharyngeal wall, and pharynx, as well as skull base reconstruction.[52] Although the donor site is more cosmetically obvious than other donor sites, long-term morbidity of the harvest is minimal. Other soft tissue flaps include the lateral arm flap, anterolateral thigh and lateral thigh flaps, latissimus dorsi flap, and rectus abdominis flap. The lateral arm flap is an excellent alternative to the radial forearm when the patient exhibits a dominant radial artery supply to the hand, which is a contraindication to the forearm site. The lateral arm flap is based upon the posterior branches of the radial collateral vessels. It offers slightly more bulk than the radial forearm flap, but is slightly compromised by vessels which are smaller in caliber. Experience with the thigh flaps has shown excellent results with tubed reconstruction of the pharynx. Both the latissimus dorsi and rectus abdominis flaps can be transferred as myogenous or myocutaneous flaps. Although skin match is not ideal, these flaps are best suited to large defects including skull base repair or maxillectomy defects with orbital exenteration (Fig. 31-17). Harvest of the rectus abdominis

may lead to the complication of postoperative hernia formation.

Enteric flaps include the gastro-omental flap and the jejunal flap. The disadvantages of these donor sites includes the need for a laparotomy, which may preclude a two-team approach. In addition, the allowed ischemia time is the shortest with the enteric flaps due to high tissue oxygen and nutrient demand. Unlike other donor sites, the pedicle of these flaps cannot be divided even years postoperatively since the flap tissues do not incorporate blood supply from the surrounding tissue bed. The main advantages of enteric flaps are their pliability and ability to continue secreting mucus. In the radiated patient who suffers from xerostomia, enteric reconstruction of recurrent oral or oropharyngeal tumors affords the opportunity to significantly improve quality of life. The omentum of the gastro-omental flap may be draped into the neck to provide contour and bulk to a neck that has been previously dissected.

The most commonly used osseous free flaps include the fibula, scapula, and iliac crest. The fibular free flap is based on the peroneal artery and vein, and the blood supply to the foot should be investigated prior to harvesting this flap.[53] Up to 25 cm of fibula may be harvested

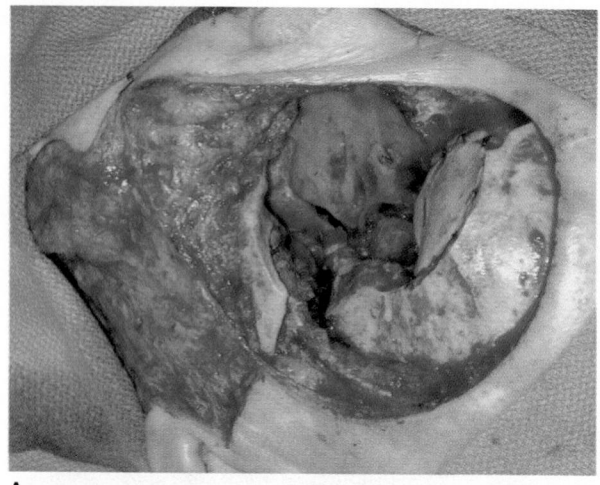

A

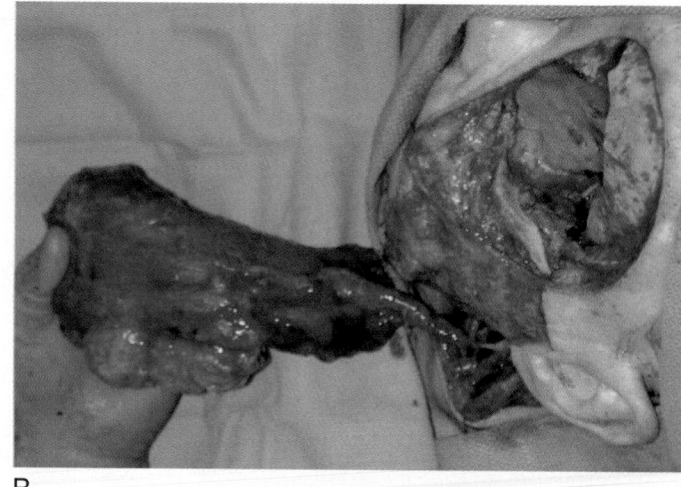

B

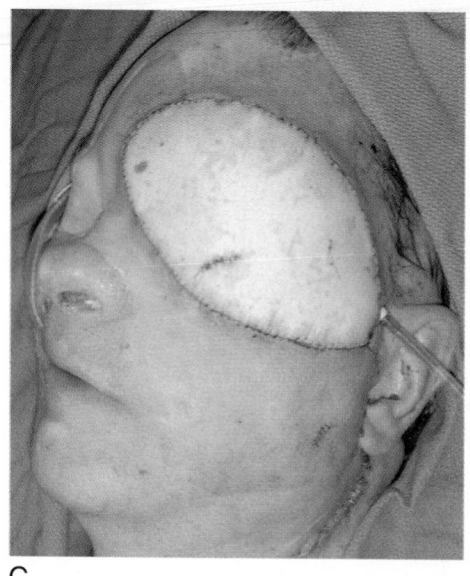

C

■ FIGURE 31-17.   A, Resection of recurrent skin squamous cell carcinoma, invading the left orbit, paranasal sinuses, and frontal lobe dura. **B,** A rectus abdominis myocutaneous free flap has been revascularized with microvascular techniques into the recipient vessels of the neck, with the flap inset into place (**C**) for cutaneous and skull base reconstruction.

for mandibular or maxillary reconstruction with an osseous or osteocutaneous harvest, with minimal donor site morbidity (Fig. 31-18). The bone stock of the fibula is sufficient to allow for osseointegrated implantation for dentition or prosthetic anchors. The iliac crest osteocutaneous free flap allows for even greater bone stock and is naturally shaped to approximate the mandibular angle. Like the rectus abdominis flap, the iliac crest is hampered by the potential for postoperative hernias and has a relatively short vascular pedicle. Although the scapular free flap has the least bone stock of the three osseous flaps, it offers the advantage of simultaneous muscular, cutaneous, and bony reconstruction based on separate pedicles that allow for tremendous versatility in flap orientation. The "mega-flap" includes the lateral border of the scapula based on the angular artery or periosteal branch of the circumflex scapular artery, the scapular or parascapular skin paddle based on the cutaneous branches of the circumflex scapular artery, and the latissimus dorsi and serratus anterior muscles supplied by the thoracodorsal artery. All arterial branches lead to the subscapular artery where it branches from the axillary artery and revascularization of all segments may be accomplished with a single arterial anastomosis.

Perhaps the ultimate in head and neck reconstruction lies in the possibility of replacing ablated tissue with identical cadaveric donor tissue. In 1998, the first successful human laryngeal transplantation was performed with microvascular reconstruction.[54] Not only was the larynx transplanted, but also the pharynx, thyroid, parathyroids, and trachea. While work continues in creating immunosuppressive regimens with minimal comorbidities, transplantation of nonvital organs is likely not to become commonplace until nontoxic immunosuppressive drugs and protection against fostering tumor recurrence have been developed.

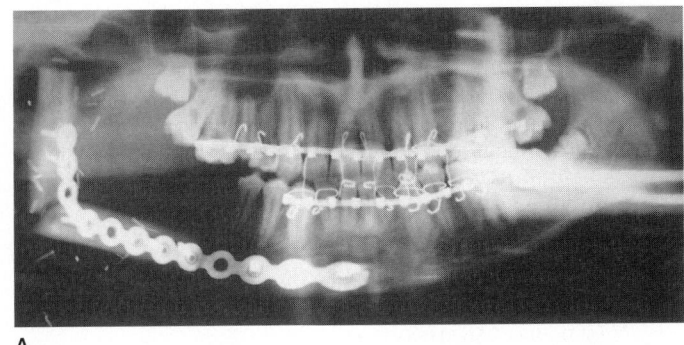

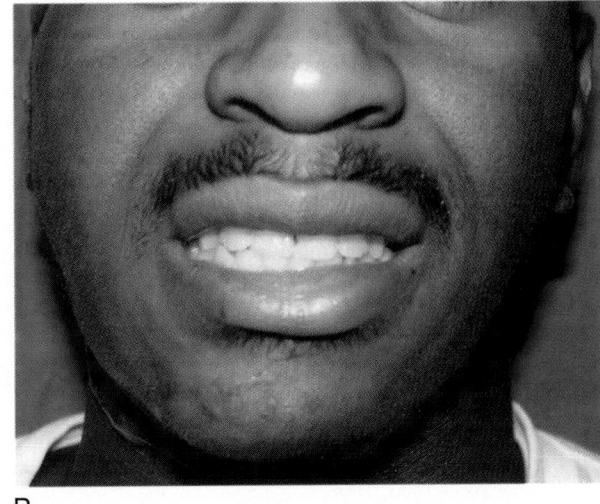

FIGURE 31-18.   A, The immediate postoperative radiograph of a 35-year-old man after resection of an osteosarcoma of the mandibular ramus and reconstruction with a fibular osseocutaneous free flap. **B,** Six months postoperatively, the patient's dental occlusion has been preserved along with excellent facial contour.

Selected References

Bocca E, Pignataro: A conservation technique in radical neck dissection. Ann Otol Rhinol Laryngol 76:975-987, 1967.

> A landmark paper demonstrating equal control of metastatic neck disease between the radical neck dissection and the modified radical neck dissection while avoiding the morbidity of the unnecessary removal of neck structures.

Kirchner JA: Vocal Fold Histopathology: A Symposium. San Diego, College-Hill Press, 1986.

> The culmination of a lifetime of study of the patterns of squamous cell carcinoma spread within the larynx, forming the histopathologic rationale for laryngeal preservation surgery.

Naudo P, Laccourreye O, Weinstein G, et al: Complications and functional outcome after supracricoid partial laryngectomy with cricohyoidoepiglottopexy. Otolaryngol Head Neck Surg 118:124-129, 1998.

> This paper describes the outstanding functional results of supracricoid laryngectomy in terms of speech and swallowing while obtaining excellent local control of disease.

Netterville JL, Koriwchak MJ, Winkle M, et al: Vocal fold paralysis following the anterior approach to the cervical spine. Ann Otol Rhinol Laryngol 105:85-91, 1996.

> A practice-changing paper reporting the higher incidence of vocal cord paralysis after right-sided cervical spine approaches and describing the anatomic rationale for approaching the C spine from the left side.

The Department of Veterans Affairs Laryngeal Cancer Study Group: Induction chemotherapy plus radiation compared with surgery plus radiation in patients with advanced laryngeal cancer. N Engl J Med 324:1685-1690, 1991.

> This multi-institutional, randomized trial demonstrated equal success between chemoradiation therapy and surgery with radiation for laryngeal carcinoma, while allowing patients who responded to the conservation treatment to keep their larynx.

References

1. Wenig BM: Atlas of Head and Neck Pathology. Philadelphia, WB Saunders, 1993.
2. Greene FL, Page DL, Fleming ID, et al (eds): AJCC Cancer Staging Manual, 6th ed. New York, Springer-Verlag, 2002.
3. Jemal A, Thomas A, Murray T, et al: Cancer statistics, 2002. CA Cancer J Clin 52:23-47, 2002.
4. Spitz MR: Epidemiology and risk factors for head and neck cancer. Semin Oncol 21:281-288, 1994.
5. Sankaranarayanan R, Masuyer E, Swaminathan R, et al: Head and neck cancer: A global perspective on epidemiology and prognosis. Anticancer Res 18:4779-4786, 1998.
6. Hoffman HT, Karnell LH, Funk GF, et al: The National Cancer Data Base report on cancer of the head and neck. Arch Otolaryngol Head Neck Surg 124:951-962, 1998.
7. Renan MJ: How many mutations are required for tumorigenesis? Implications from human cancer data. Mol Carcinog 7:139-146, 1993.
8. Smith BD, Smith GL, Carter D, et al: Prognostic significance of vascular endothelial growth factor protein levels in oral and oropharyngeal squamous cell carcinoma. J Clin Oncol 18:2046-2052, 2000.

9. Michalides R, van Veelen N, Hart A, et al: Overexpression of cyclin D1 correlated with recurrence in a group of forty-seven operable squamous cell carcinomas of the head and neck. Cancer Res 55:975-978, 1995.

10. Shin DM, Charuruks N, Lippman SM, et al: p53 protein accumulation and genomic instability in head and neck multistep tumorigenesis. Cancer Epidemiol Biomarkers Prev 10:603-609, 2001.

11. Brennan JA, Boyle JO, Koch WM, et al: Association between cigarette smoking and mutation of the *p53* gene in squamous cell carcinoma of the head and neck. N Engl J Med 332:712-717, 1995.

12. Chung KY, Mukhopadhyay T, Kim J, et al: Discordant *p53* gene mutations in primary head and neck cancers and corresponding second primary cancers of the upper aerodigestive tract. Cancer Res 53:1676-1683, 1993.

13. Scholes AGM, Woolgar JA, Boyle MA, et al: Synchronous oral carcinomas: Independent or common clonal origin? Cancer Res 58:2003-2006, 1998.

14. Hannah A, Scott AM, Tochon-Danguy H, et al: Evaluation of ^{18}F-fluorodeoxyglucose positron emission tomography and computed tomography with histopathologic correlation in the initial staging of head and neck cancer. Ann Surg 236:208-217, 2002.

15. Wax MK, Myers LL, Gabalski EC, et al: Positron emission tomography in the evaluation of synchronous lung lesions in patients with untreated head and neck cancer. Arch Otolaryngol Head Neck Surg 128:703-707, 2002.

16. Bourhis J, Wibault P, Lusinchi A, et al: Status of accelerated fractionation radiotherapy in head and neck squamous cell carcinomas. Curr Opin Oncol 9:262-266, 1997.

17. The Department of Veterans Affairs Laryngeal Cancer Study Group: Induction chemotherapy plus radiation compared with surgery plus radiation in patients with advanced laryngeal cancer. N Engl J Med 324:1685-1690, 1991.

18. Roy S, Tibesar RJ, Daly K, et al: Role of planned neck dissection for advanced metastatic disease in tongue base or tonsil squamous cell carcinoma treated with radiotherapy. Head Neck 24:474-481, 2002.

19. Snyderman CH, D'Amico F: Outcome of carotid artery resection for neoplastic disease: A meta-analysis. Am J Otolaryngol 13:373-380, 1992.

20. Bocca E, Pignataro O: A conservation technique in radical neck dissection. Ann Otol Rhinol Laryngol 76:975-987, 1967.

21. Ross GL, Shoaib T, Soutar DS, et al: The First International Conference on Sentinel Node Biopsy in Mucosal Head and Neck Cancer and adoption of a multicenter trial protocol. Ann Surg Oncol 9:406-410, 2002.

22. Onercl M, Yilmaz T, Gedikolu G: Tumor thickness as a predictor of cervical lymph node metastasis in squamous cell carcinoma of the lower lip. Otolaryngol Head Neck Surg 122:139-142, 2000.

23. Gooris PJ, Vermey A, de Visscher JG, et al: Supraomohyoid neck dissection in the management of cervical lymph node metastases of squamous cell carcinoma of the lower lip. Head Neck 24:678-683, 2002.

24. Fukano H, Matsuura H, Hasegawa Y, et al: Depth of invasion as a predictive factor for cervical lymph node metastasis in tongue carcinoma. Head Neck 19:205-210, 1997.

25. McGregor AD, MacDonald DG: Patterns of spread of squamous cell carcinoma to the ramus of the mandible. Head Neck 15:440-444, 1993.

26. Strome SE, To W, Strawderman M, et al: Squamous cell carcinoma of the buccal mucosa. Otolaryngol Head Neck Surg 120:375-379, 1999.

27. Adelstein DJ, Saxton JP, Lavertu P, et al: Maximizing local control and organ preservation in stage IV squamous cell head and neck cancer with hyperfractionated radiation and concurrent chemotherapy. J Clin Oncol 20:1405-1410, 2002.

28. Lefebvre JL, Chevalier D, Luboinski B, et al: Larynx preservation in piriform sinus cancer: Preliminary results of a European Organization for Research and Treatment of Cancer phase III trial. EORTC Head and Neck Cancer Cooperative Group. J Natl Cancer Inst 88:890-899, 1996.

29. Kirchner JA: Vocal Fold Histopathology: A Symposium. San Diego, College-Hill Press, 1986.

30. Zeitels SM, Vaughan CW, Domanowski GF: Endoscopic management of early supraglottic cancer. Ann Otol Rhinol Laryngol 99:951-956, 1990.

31. Peretti G, Nicolai P, Redaelli De Zinis L, et al: Endoscopic CO_2 laser excision for Tis, T1, and T2 glottic carcinomas: Cure rate and prognostic factors. Otolaryngol Head Neck Surg 123:124-131, 2000.

32. Ambrosch P, Kron M, Steiner W: Carbon dioxide laser microsurgery for early supraglottic carcinoma. Ann Otol Rhinol Laryngol 107:680-688, 1998.

33. Muscatello L, Laccourreye O, Biacabe B, et al: Laryngofissure and cordectomy for glottic carcinoma limited to the mid third of the mobile true vocal cord. Laryngoscope 107:1507-1510, 1997.

34. Naudo P, Laccourreye O, Weinstein G, et al: Complications and functional outcome after supracricoid partial laryngectomy with cricohyoidoepiglottopexy. Otolaryngol Head Neck Surg 118:124-129, 1998.

35. Myers LL, Nussenbaum B, Bradford CR, et al: Paranasal sinus malignancies: An 18-year single-institutional experience. Laryngoscope 112:1964-1969, 2002.

36. Roh HJ, Bolger W, Citardi MJ, et al: Endoscopic resection of sinonasal malignancies: A preliminary report. Am J Rhinol (in press).

37. Imola MJ, Schramm VL: Orbital preservation in surgical management of sinonasal malignancy. Laryngoscope 112:1357-1365, 2002.

38. Teknos TN, Smith JC, Day TA, et al: Microvascular free tissue transfer in reconstructing skull base defects: Lessons learned. Laryngoscope 112:1871-1876, 2002.

39. Vasef MA, Ferlito A, Weiss LM: Clinicopathological consultation: Nasopharyngeal carcinoma, with emphasis on its relationship to Epstein-Barr virus. Ann Otol Rhinol Laryngol 106:348-356, 1997.

40. Al-Sarraf M, LeBlanc M, Giri PB, et al: Chemoradiotherapy versus radiotherapy in patients with advanced nasopharyngeal cancer: Phase III randomized intergroup study 0099. J Clin Oncol 16:1310-1317, 1998.

41. Netterville JL, Wood DE: The lower trapezius flap: Vascular anatomy and surgical technique. Arch Otolaryngol Head Neck Surg 117:73-76, 1991.

42. Stewart CJ, MacKenzie K, McGarry GW, et al: Fine-needle aspiration cytology of salivary gland: A review of 341 cases. Diagn Cytopathol 22:139-146, 2000.

43. Witt RL: The significance of the margin in parotid surgery for pleomorphic adenoma. Laryngoscope 112:2141-2154, 2002.

44. Seifert G: Histopathology of malignant salivary gland tumours. Eur J Cancer B Oral Oncol 28B:49-52, 1992.

45. Amedee RG, Dhurandhar NR: Fine-needle aspiration biopsy. Laryngoscope 111:1551-1557, 2001.

46. Zimmermann CE, von Domarus H, Moubayed P: Carcinoma in situ in a lateral cervical cyst. Head Neck 24:965-969, 2002.

47. Netterville JL, Reilly KM, Robertson D, et al: Carotid body tumors: A review of 30 patients with 46 tumors. Laryngoscope 105:115-126, 1995.

48. van Heurn LW, Goei R, de Ploeg I, et al: Late complications of percutaneous dilatational tracheotomy. Chest 110:1572-1576, 1996.

49. Dulguerov P, Gysin C, Perneger TV, et al: Percutaneous or surgical tracheostomy: A meta-analysis. Crit Care Med 27:1617-1625, 1999.

50. Netterville JL, Koriwchak MJ, Winkle M, et al: Vocal fold paralysis following the anterior approach to the cervical spine. Ann Otol Rhinol Laryngol 105:85-91, 1996.

51. Netterville JL, Stone RE, Luken ES, et al: Silastic medialization and arytenoid adduction: The Vanderbilt experience—a review of 116 phonosurgical procedures. Ann Otol Rhinol Laryngol 102:413-424, 1993.

52. Burkey BB, Gerek M, Day T: Repair of the persistent cerebrospinal fluid leak with the radial forearm free fascial flap. Laryngoscope 109:1003-1006, 1999.

53. Lorenz RR, Esclamado R: Preoperative magnetic resonance angiography in fibular free flap reconstruction of head and neck defects. Head Neck 23:844-850, 2001.

54. Strome M, Stein J, Esclamado R, et al: Laryngeal transplantation and 40-month follow-up. N Engl J Med 344:1676-1679, 2001.

SECTION

VII

BREAST

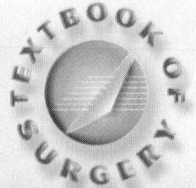

CHAPTER 32

DISEASES OF THE BREAST

J. Dirk Iglehart, M.D., and Carolyn M. Kaelin, M.D., M.P.H., F.A.C.S.

ANATOMY

Understanding the anatomy of the breast and its relation to underlying chest structures is important for the successful management of breast diseases. The mature breast lies cushioned in adipose tissue between the subcutaneous fat layer and the superficial pectoral fascia (Fig. 32-1). Between the breast and the pectoralis major muscle lies the retromammary space, a thin layer of loose areolar tissue that contains lymphatics and small vessels. During removal of the breast, the breast is separated from the pectoral muscle and includes the retromammary space and deep fascia over the muscle.

Located deep to the pectoralis major muscle, the pectoralis minor muscle is enclosed in the clavipectoral fascia, which envelops it and extends laterally to fuse with the axillary fascia. Dissection along the lateral border of the pectoralis minor muscle divides the axillary fascia and exposes the contents of the axilla. Within the loose areolar fat of the axilla are a variable number of lymph nodes grouped as shown in Figure 32-2. The number of lymph nodes found in the axilla depends on the extent of dissection and the diligence used to identify these nodes. An upper limit is established by the work of Durkin and Haagensen using ethanol clearing. These investigators found an average of 50 nodes in 100 specimens obtained in the course of a Halsted-type radical mastectomy. The current approach to less radical procedures has reduced the number of nodes retrieved.

To standardize the extent of axillary dissection, the axillary nodes are arbitrarily divided into three levels, as shown in Figure 32-3. Level I nodes are located in the external mammary, scapular, axillary vein, and central axillary groups, which lie lateral to the lateral border of the pectoralis minor muscle. Level II nodes are in the central axillary group located under the pectoralis minor muscle. Level III nodes include the subclavicular nodes medial to the pectoralis minor muscle and are difficult to visualize and remove unless the pectoralis minor muscle is sacrificed or divided. The apex of the axilla is defined by the costoclavicular ligament (Halsted's ligament), at which point the axillary vein passes into the thorax and becomes the subclavian vein. Lymph nodes in the space between the pectoralis major and minor muscles are known as the *interpectoral group*, or *Rotter nodes*, as described by Grossman and Rotter. Unless this group is specifically exposed, they are not encompassed in surgical procedures that preserve the pectoral muscles.

Lymphatic channels are abundant in the breast parenchyma and dermis. Specialized lymphatic channels collect under the nipple and areola, forming Sappey's plexus, named for the anatomist who described them in 1885. Lymph flows from the skin to the subareolar plexus and then into interlobular lymphatics of the breast parenchyma. Appreciation of lymphatic flow is important for performing successful sentinel node biopsy, described later. Seventy-five percent of lymphatic flow from the breast is into the axillary lymph nodes, and a minor amount goes through the pectoralis muscle and into more medial lymph node groups, shown in Figures 32-2 and 32-3. A major route of breast cancer metastasis is through lymphatic channels, and the anatomy of the lymphatic

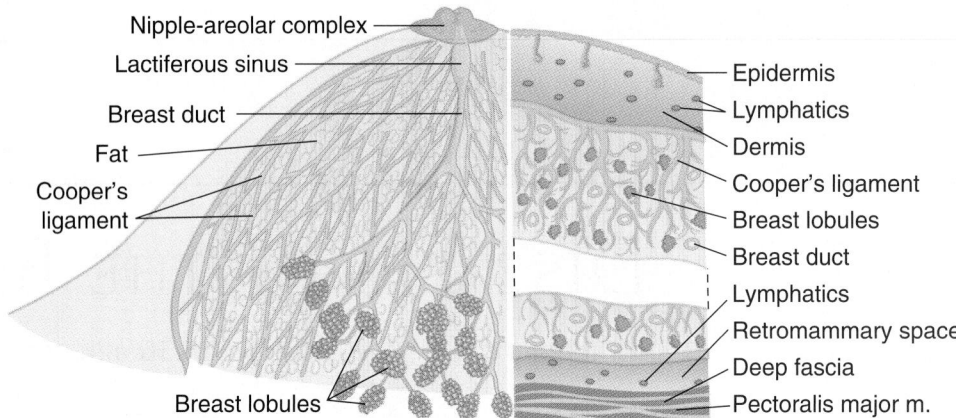

FIGURE 32-1. Cut-away diagram of the mature resting breast. The breast lies cushioned in fat between the overlying skin and the pectoralis major muscle. Both the skin and retromammary space under the breast are rich with lymphatic channels. Cooper's ligaments, the suspensory ligaments of the breast, fuse with the overlying superficial fascia just under the dermis, coalesce as the interlobular fascia in the breast parenchyma, and then join with the deep fascia of breast over the pectoralis muscle. The system of ducts in the breast is configured like an inverted tree, with the largest ducts just under the nipple and successively smaller ducts in the periphery. After several branching generations, small ducts at the periphery enter the breast lobule, which is the milk-forming glandular unit of the breast.

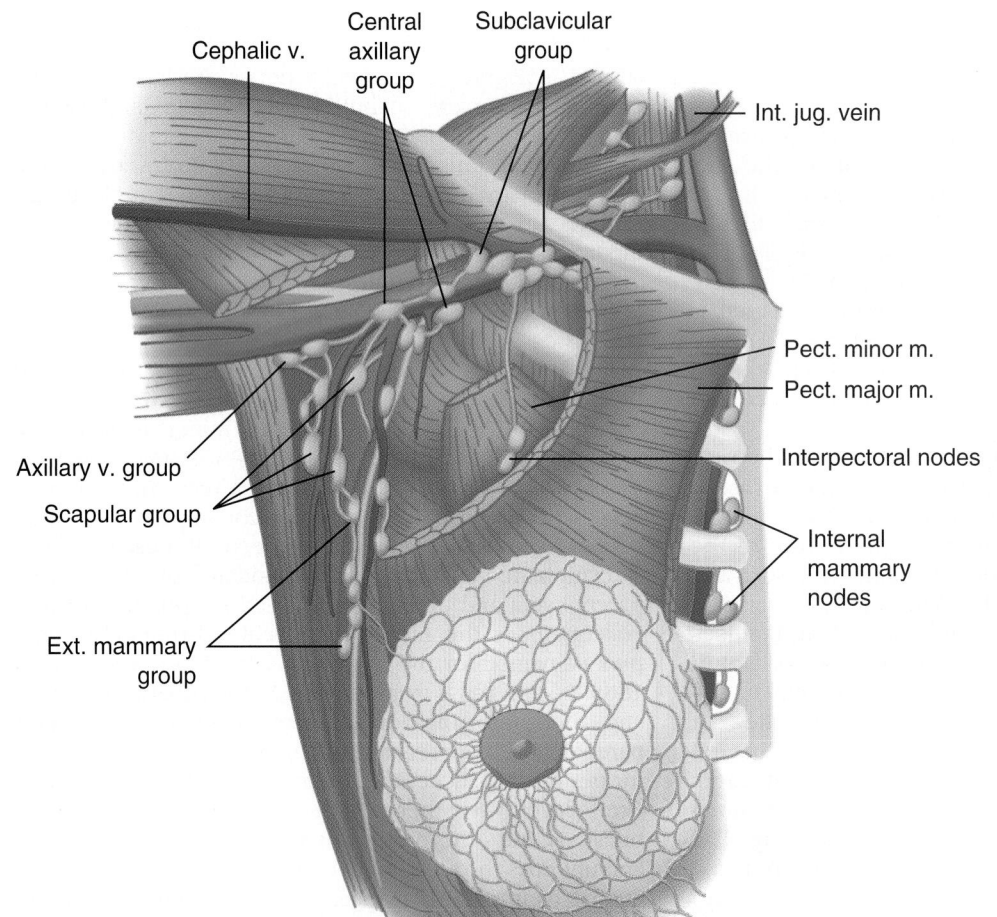

FIGURE 32-2. Contents of the axilla. In this diagram, there are five named and contiguous groupings of lymph nodes in the full axilla. A complete axillary dissection, as done with the historical radical mastectomy, removes all of these nodes. However, note that the subclavicular nodes in the axilla are continuous with the supraclavicular nodes in the neck and nodes between the pectoralis major and minor muscles, called the *interpectoral nodes* in this diagram, and also named *Rotter's lymph nodes*. The internal mammary nodes probably drain independently from the breast. The sentinel lymph node, located in modern sentinel biopsy, is functionally the first and lowest node in the axillary chain and anatomically usually found in the external mammary group. (From Donegan WL, Spratt JS: Cancer of the Breast, 3rd ed. Philadelphia, WB Saunders, 1988, p 19.)

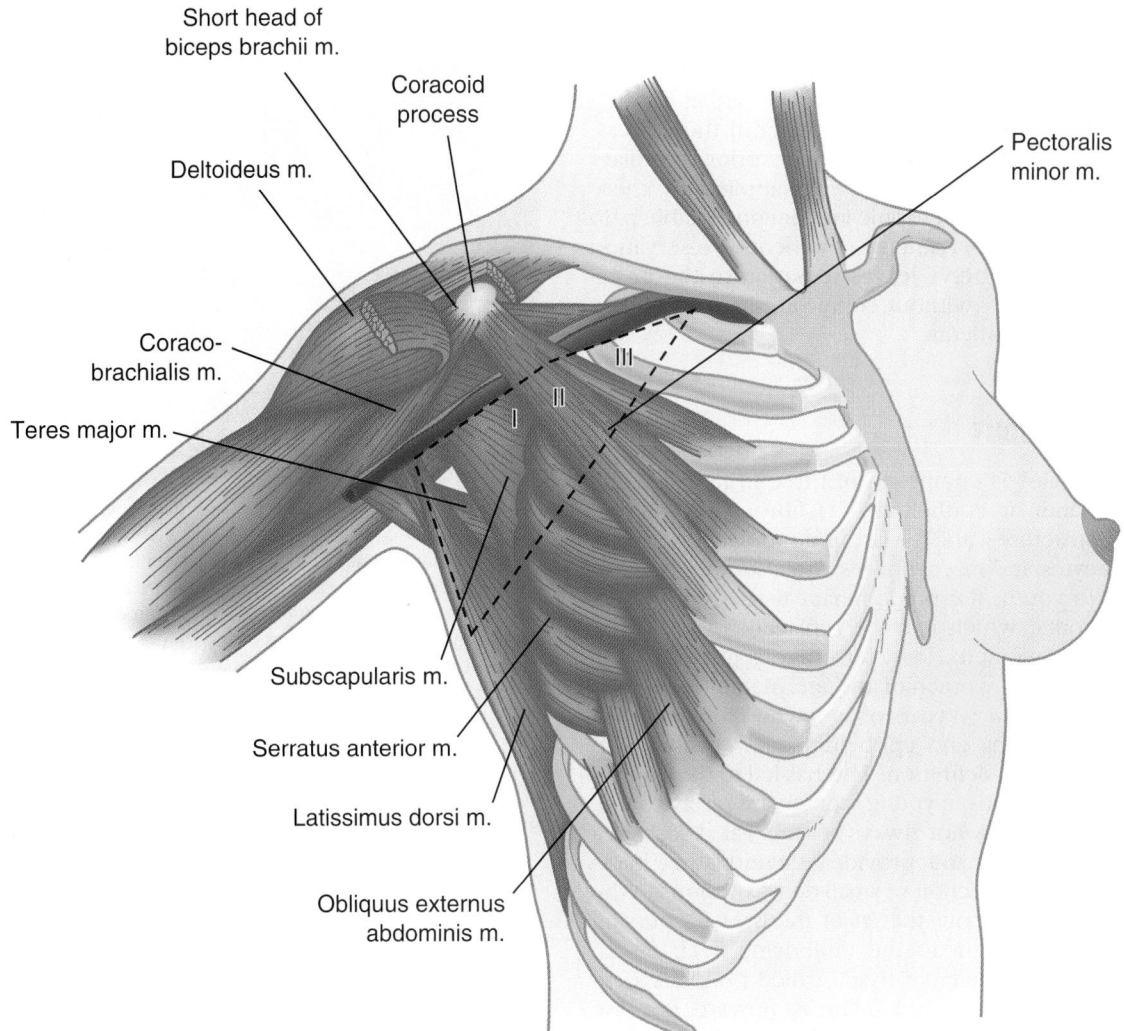

FIGURE 32-3.   Division of the axillary nodes into arbitrary levels. Current terminology defines the level I axillary lymph nodes as those nodes lying lateral to the lateral border of the pectoralis minor muscle (probably dividing the central axillary group, as shown in Fig. 32-2). The level II nodes are those under the pectoralis minor muscle, between its lateral and medial borders (probably the central axillary group). The level III nodes lie medial to the medial margin of the pectoralis minor muscle and are the subclavicular nodes shown in Figure 32-2. Not shown is the clavipectoral fascia, which invests the pectoralis minor muscle and covers the axillary nodes. Access to the axillary nodes requires penetration of this investing layer, usually evident during axillary surgery. (From Donegan WL, Spratt JS: Cancer of the Breast, 3rd ed. Philadelphia, WB Saunders, 1988, p 20.)

system determines the favored locations of regional cancer spread.

Knowledge of major nervous structures in the axilla is required to avoid their sacrifice during surgery. Coursing close to the chest wall on the medial side of the axilla is the long thoracic nerve, or the external respiratory nerve of Bell, which innervates the serratus anterior muscle. This muscle is important for fixating the scapula to the chest wall during adduction of the shoulder and extension of the arm, and its division may result in the winged scapula deformity. For this reason, the long thoracic nerve is preserved during standard axillary dissection. The second major nerve trunk encountered during axillary dissection is the thoracodorsal nerve to the latissimus dorsi muscle at the lateral border of the axilla. This nerve arises from the posterior cord of the brachial plexus and enters

the axillary space under the axillary vein, close to the entrance of the long thoracic nerve. It then crosses the axilla to the medial surface of the latissimus dorsi muscle. The thoracodorsal nerve is usually preserved during dissection of axillary nodes. Its sacrifice leads to loss of latissimus function and atrophy of the muscle.

A neurovascular bundle wrapping around the lateral border of the pectoralis minor muscle innervates the pectoralis major muscle. Although anatomists have called these nerves the *medial* pectoral nerves, many surgeons refer to them as the *lateral* pectoral nerves, reflecting their position during surgery. Exposure of the pectoral neurovascular bundle is a good landmark, indicating the position of the axillary vein just above and deep to (superior and posterior) the bundle. This neurovascular bundle should be preserved during standard axillary dissection.

The large sensory intercostal brachial or brachial cutaneous nerves span the axillary space and supply sensation to the undersurface of the upper arm and skin of the chest wall, along the posterior margin of the axilla. Cutting these nerves causes cutaneous anesthesia in these areas, which is helpful to emphasize to patients prior to axillary dissection. Denervation of the areas supplied by these sensory nerves can cause chronic and uncomfortable pain syndromes in a small percentage of patients. Preservation of the superior-most nerve leaves sensation to the posterior upper arm intact, without compromising the axillary dissection in most patients.

MICROSCOPIC ANATOMY

The mature breast is composed of three principal tissue types: (1) glandular epithelium, (2) fibrous stroma and supporting structures, and (3) fat. Infiltrating cells, including lymphocytes and macrophages, are also found within the breast. In youth, the predominant tissues are epithelium and stroma, which may be replaced by fat in the breasts of older women. However, there is great variability among individual women of any age. Mammography in women younger than 30 years of age, whose breast tissue is dense with stroma and epithelium, may produce an image without much definition. This has led to the impression that mammograms in young women are rarely useful, an impression that may not always be true. Fat absorbs relatively little radiation and provides a contrasting background that favors detection of small-density lesions in the older patient. Throughout the fat of the breast, coursing from the overlying skin to the underlying deep fascia, strands of dense connective tissue called *Cooper's ligaments* provide shape and hold the breast upward. Because they are anchored into the skin, tethering of these ligaments by a small scirrhous carcinoma commonly produces a dimple or subtle deformity on the otherwise smooth surface of the breast.

The glandular apparatus of the breast is composed of a branching system of ducts, roughly organized in a radial pattern, spreading outward and downward from the nipple-areolar complex (see Fig. 32-1). It is possible to cannulate individual ducts and visualize the lactiferous ducts with contrast agents. Figure 32-4 shows a ductogram, sometimes used to evaluate discharge from the nipple. This example is particularly useful in showing the arborizing tree of branching ducts, ending in terminal lobules. Also, the contrast dye opacifies only a single ductal system, showing the functional independence of each ductal tree. At the summit of the arborizing ductal system, the subareolar ducts widen to form the lactiferous sinuses, which then exit through 10 to 15 orifices on the nipple. These large ducts close to the nipple are lined with a low columnar or cuboidal epithelium that abruptly meets the squamous epithelium of the nipple surface, invading the duct for a short distance. This relationship is important for the discussion of Paget's disease of the nipple (see later).

At the opposite end of the ductal system and after progressive generations of branching, the ducts end blindly in clusters of spaces that are called *terminal ductules* or

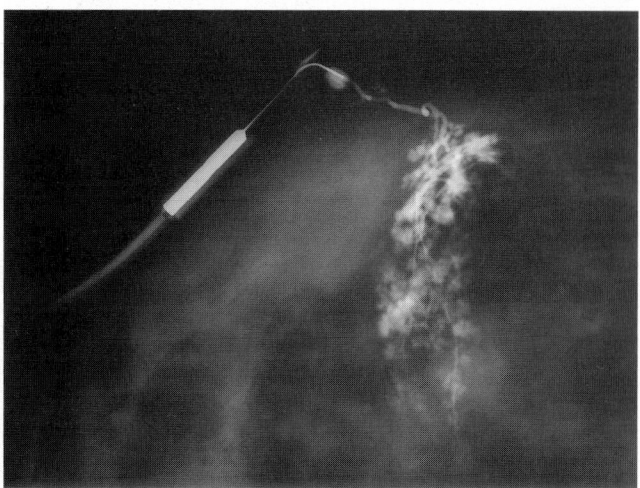

FIGURE 32-4. Contrast injection of a single ductal system (ductogram). Occasionally used to evaluate surgically significant nipple discharge, ductography is performed by cannulation of an individual duct orifice and injection of contrast material. This ductogram opacifies the entire ductal tree from the retroareolar duct to the lobules at the end of the tree. This picture also demonstrates the functional independence of each duct system; there is no cross-communication between independent systems.

acini (Fig. 32-5). These are the milk-forming glands of the lactating breast, and, together with their small efferent ducts or ductules, are known as the *lobular units* or *lobules*. As shown in Figure 32-5, the terminal ductules are invested in a specialized loose connective tissue that contains capillaries, lymphocytes, and other migratory mononuclear cells. This intralobular stroma is clearly distinguished from the denser and less cellular interlobular stroma and from the fat within the breast.

Under the luminal epithelium, the entire ductal system is surrounded by a specialized myoepithelial cell of ductal epithelial origin that has contractile properties and serves to propel secretion of milk toward the nipple. Outside the epithelial and myoepithelial layers, the ducts of the breast are surrounded by a continuous basement membrane containing laminin, type IV collagen, and proteoglycans. The basement membrane layer is extremely important in differentiating in situ from invasive breast cancer. Continuity of this layer around proliferations of ductal cells identifies ductal carcinoma in situ (DCIS), or noninvasive breast cancer (discussed later in the section on Pathology of Breast Cancer).

BREAST DEVELOPMENT AND PHYSIOLOGY

Development and Physiology[1-4]

Appreciation of the stages of breast development facilitates the understanding of many benign and malignant states that come to clinical attention. During adolescence, the breast is composed primarily of dense fibrous stroma and scattered ducts lined with epithelium. In the United States, puberty as measured by age of breast development

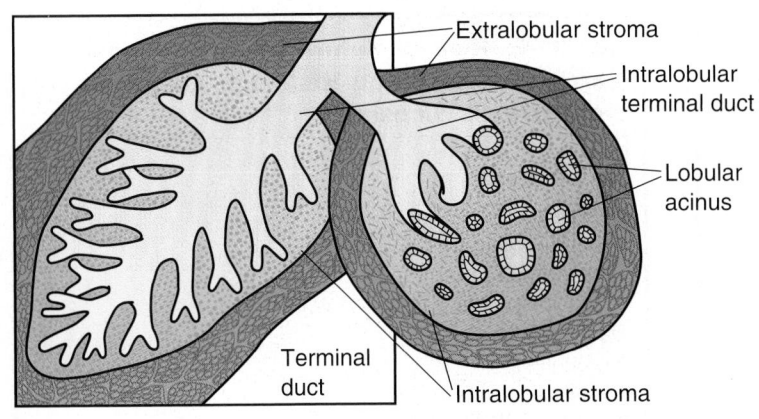

Extralobular stroma

Intralobular terminal duct

Lobular acinus

Terminal duct

Intralobular stroma

FIGURE 32-5. The mature resting lobular unit. At the distal end of the ductal system is the lobule. This structure is formed by multiple branching events at the end of terminal ducts, each ending in a blind sac or acini, and is invested with specialized stroma. The lobule is a three-dimensional structure, but seen in two-dimensions in a histologic thin section, shown in the lower right. The intralobular terminal ductule and the acini are invested in loose connective tissue containing a modest number of infiltrating lymphocytes and plasma cells. The lobule is distinct from the denser interlobular stroma, which contains larger breast ducts, blood vessels, and fat.

and onset of pubic hair begins between ages 9 and 12, and menarche begins about 12 to 13 years of age. These events are initiated by low-amplitude nocturnal pulses of gonadotropin, which raise serum estradiol concentrations. In the breast, this hormone-dependent maturation (*thelarche*) entails increased deposition of fat, formation of new ducts by branching and elongation, and the first appearance of lobular units. This process of growth entails cell division and is under the control of estrogen, progesterone, adrenal hormones, pituitary hormones, and trophic effects of insulin and thyroid hormone. There is evidence that local growth factor networks are also important, including epidermal growth factor, which can replace estrogen in breast development. The exact timing of these events and the coordinated development of both breast buds may vary from the average in individual patients. The term *prepubertal gynecomastia* refers to the symmetrical enlargement and projection of the breast bud in a young girl before the average age of 12 years, unaccompanied by the other changes of puberty. This process, which may be unilateral, should not be confused with neoplastic growth and should not be subjected to biopsy.

The postpubertal mature or *resting* breast contains fat, stroma, lactiferous ducts, and lobular units. During phases of the menstrual cycle or in response to exogenous hormones, the breast epithelium and lobular stroma undergo cyclic stimulation. It appears that the dominant process is hypertrophy and alteration of morphology rather than hyperplasia. In the late luteal (premenstrual) phase, there is an accumulation of fluid and intralobular edema. It is probable that this edema produces both pain and breast engorgement.

On physical examination, and even by mammography, this fluid accumulation leads to increased nodularity and may be mistaken for a dominant tumor. Ill-defined masses in premenopausal women are correctly observed through the course of one or two menstrual cycles. Finally, any alteration in the periodicity of the menstrual cycle, such as anovulatory cycles, can cause accentuation of engorgement, pain, and nodularity.

With pregnancy, there is diminution of the fibrous stroma to accommodate the hyperplasia of the lobular units. This formation of new acini or lobules is termed the *adenosis of pregnancy* and is influenced by high

circulating levels of estrogen and progesterone and by levels of prolactin that steadily increase during gestation. After birth, there is a sudden loss of the placental hormones. A continued high level of prolactin is the principal trigger for lactation. The actual expulsion of milk is under hormonal control and is caused by the contraction of the myoepithelial cells that surround breast ducts and terminal ductules. There is no evidence for innervation of the myoepithelial cells; their contraction appears to be in response to the pituitary-derived peptide oxytocin. Stimulation of the nipple appears to be the physiologic signal for both the continued pituitary secretion of prolactin and for the acute release of oxytocin. When breast-feeding ceases, there is a fall in prolactin and no stimulus for release of oxytocin. The breast then returns to a resting state and to the cyclic changes induced when menstruation begins again. During breast-feeding, there are frequently questions about which drugs are safe and do not harm the feeding infant. Drug safety during lactation is presented in Box 32-1.

With the approach of menopause, phases of the menstrual cycle may not be as symmetrical and regular. This irregularity can induce functional nodularity and breast pain in areas where there was none in earlier years. Menopause is defined by a cessation in menstrual flow for 1 year. In the United States, it usually occurs between ages 40 and 55, with a median age of 51 years. It may be accompanied by constitutional systems such as diaphoresis, vaginal dryness, urinary tract infections, and cognitive impairment (possibly secondary to interruption of sleep by hot flashes). For the breast, menopause results in involution and a general decrease in the epithelial elements of the resting breast. These changes include increased fat deposition, diminished connective tissue, and the disappearance of lobular units.

The persistence of lobules, hyperplasia of the ductal epithelium, and even cyst formation all can occur under the influence of exogenous ovarian hormones, usually in the form of postmenopausal hormone replacement therapy (HRT). Most commonly, hormones are given to relieve the symptoms of menopause or to prevent demineralization of bone, with potential additional benefits including a decreased risk of colon cancer and a lower risk of Alzheimer's disease. Risks of hormone replacement therapy include increased rates of breast cancer, heart

---

Box 32-1. Drug Safety During Breast-Feeding

Use with Concern or Caution

Antianxiety agents—diazepam, lorazepam
Antidepressants—amitriptyline, doxepin
Antipsychotics—chlorpromazine, haloperidol
Other—aspirin, clemastine, phenobarbital, primidone, sulfasalazine

Use Strongly Discouraged

Amphetamine, heroin, marijuana, nicotine, phencyclidine

Use with Temporary Interruption of Breast-feeding

Tocopharmaceuticals—copper 64 (50 hours), gallium 67 (2 weeks), indium 111 (20 hours), iodine 23 (36 hours), iodine 125 (12 days), iodine 131 (2–14 days), technetium 99m (15–36 hours)

Use Contraindicated

Bromocriptine, cocaine, cyclophosphamide, cyclosporine, doxorubicin, ergotamine, lithium, methotrexate, phencyclidine, phenindione

From Donegan WL, Spratt JS: Cancer of the Breast, 5th ed. Philadelphia, WB Saunders, 2002, p 47.

Box 32-2. Risk of Future Invasive Breast Carcinoma Based on Histologic Diagnosis from Breast Biopsies*

No Increase

Adenosis
Apocrine metaplasia
Cysts, small or large
Mild hyperplasia (>2 but <5 cells deep)
Duct ectasia
Fibroadenoma
Fibrosis
Mastitis, inflammatory
Periductal mastitis
Squamous metaplasia

Slightly Increased (relative risk, 1.5-2)

Moderate or florid hyperplasia, solid or papillary
Duct papilloma with fibrovascular core
Sclerosing adenosis, well-developed

Moderately Increased (relative risk, 4-5)

Atypical hyperplasia, ductal or lobular

*Compared with women with no breast biopsy.
From Donegan WL, Spratt JS: Cancer of the Breast, 5th ed. Philadelphia, WB Saunders, 2002, p 93.

---

attacks, pulmonary emboli, stroke, and gallbladder disease. The increased risk of breast cancer was observed after 5 years of combined estrogen and progesterone (Prempro) use and was not observed in women who had undergone hysterectomy and who were taking estrogen without progesterone replacement. Physicians should inquire about the menstrual history, establish the cessation of menses in postmenopausal women, and record the use of hormone replacement therapy. A history of hormone use is important to the radiologist looking at a mammogram and to the pathologist evaluating a breast biopsy.

Fibrocystic Changes[5]

Fibrocystic condition (FCC), previously referred to as *fibrocystic disease,* represents a spectrum of clinical, mammographic, and histologic findings and is present in one of its many forms in up to 90% of women. FCC appears to represent an exaggerated response of breast stroma and epithelium to a variety of circulating and locally produced hormones and growth factors and frequently presents with the constellation of breast pain, tenderness, and nodularity. Symptomatically, the condition presents as premenstrual cyclical mastalgia with pain and tenderness to touch. Patients with fibrocystic change have clinical breast examinations that range from mild, bilaterally symmetrical alterations in texture—most notable in the upper-outer quadrants where the majority of breast glandular tissue exists—to dense, firm breast tissue with palpable lumps, to the frequent appearance of gross cysts.

Mammographically, FCC is usually seen as bilaterally symmetrical diffuse or focal radiologically dense tissue. By ultrasound, cysts exist in up to one third of women 35 to 50 years of age, with most of these being nonpalpable. In women older than 60 years of age, cysts are uncommon (5%), with half occurring in women taking hormone replacement therapy.

Histologically, in addition to macrocysts and microcysts, identified solid elements include adenosis, sclerosis, apocrine metaplasia, stromal fibrosis, and epithelial metaplasia and hyperplasia. Depending on the presence of epithelial hyperplasia, FCC is observed as nonproliferative or proliferative without atypia. All these changes can occur alone or in combination and are seen in 90% of women at postmortem examination. Thus, to a variable degree, they comprise the normal female breast. However, the epithelial hyperplasia can be atypical (atypical ductal hyperplasia) and display some feature of more advanced in situ neoplasia. Box 32-2 summarizes the risk of developing a future breast cancer based on histologic findings from a benign breast biopsy as determined during a 1985 consensus meeting chaired by the College of American Pathologists and supported by the American Cancer Society. Based on data from 16,692 women from the Breast Cancer Detection Demonstration Project, Carter and associates quantified the relative risk (RR) of developing breast cancer as 1.5 for those whose breast biopsy demonstrated nonproliferative disease, 1.9 for those with proliferative disease without atypia, and as 3 for atypical hyperplasia. As described later, it is those women whose increased breast cancer risk is defined by atypical ductal or lobular hyperplasia who may consider tamoxifen for chemoprevention risk reduction.

Breast Pain[1,6]

Breast pain is common and a symptom that brings a woman to her physician. Usually it is of functional origin and uncommonly is it a symptom of breast cancer. Fortunately, most patients with pain do not have breast cancer. Conversely, Haagensen carefully recorded the symptoms of women presenting with breast carcinoma and found pain as an unprompted symptom in 5.4% of patients. For those women with breast pain and an associated palpable mass, the presence of the mass should be the focus of evaluation and treatment. For patients without a mass, the evaluation should be guided by whether the pain is cyclical or noncyclical.

Normal ovarian hormonal influences on breast glandular elements frequently produce *cyclical mastalgia*. Cyclic breast pain is dull, diffuse, and commonly bilaterally symmetrical in the upper outer quadrants. It is predominantly experienced in the luteal phase of the menstrual cycle and abates with menstruation. It is most common in women in their mid-30s. In addition, women commencing oral contraceptive use or hormone replacement therapy at menopause often experience mastalgia, with the pain usually subsiding within three cycles or months.

Noncyclical mastalgia is more likely to be the result of a nonbreast etiology or of a specific significant breast condition. A careful history and physical examination should eliminate musculoskeletal causes such as cervical radiculopathy, costochondritis, or intercostal muscle strain. Gastroesophageal reflux disorder, symptomatic gallstones, cardiovascular disease, and pulmonary pathology are fairly obvious after a brief patient interview. A breast cyst may cause focal pain and tenderness. Breast cellulitis (*mastitis*) causes breast pain with skin changes characteristic of a bacterial infection and may be associated with systemic symptoms of chills, fever, and malaise, particularly if an underlying abscess is present. If the presumed mastitis does not fully clear with a course of oral antibiotics, inflammatory breast cancer, where the dermal lymphatics are congested with tumor cells, should be considered, and the patient should be referred for surgical evaluation.

Although uncommon, breast pain may be the first symptom to suggest an underlying breast cancer. Women 30 years of age and older with cyclical or noncyclical mastalgia should undergo mammography. The exception to this rule is when the clinical breast examination reveals focal tenderness or a mass, and breast ultrasound detects a simple cyst. In this instance the work-up can be terminated with reassurance and without a mammogram. If the mammogram is abnormal or the ultrasound reveals a complex cyst or solid lesion, further evaluation of the mass should commence. For patients younger than 30 years of age with focal pain, ultrasound may be performed first, and, if negative, perhaps followed by a mammogram. For patients younger than 30 years of age without focal breast pain, the initial management should be symptomatic.

If the clinical breast examination and mammography are normal, 85% of women respond to reassurance that mastalgia is a common, benign condition. For the 15% of women who do not, wearing a supportive bra and taking ibuprofen 600 to 800 mg every 8 hours during symptomatic days may be adequate to relieve symptoms. There is little evidence that eliminating caffeine or taking vitamin E or B_6 supplements eases mastalgia.

Although painful cystic mastopathy is attributed to excessive intake of caffeine, nicotine, or commonly used antihistamines, careful investigation has cast doubt on these associations. Evening primrose oil results in symptomatic relief in 58% of patients with cyclical and 38% of patients with noncyclical mastalgia. Patients are treated with 1.5 g (three 500-mg capsules) twice daily for up to 1 year, but should respond within the first 4 months of therapy. Fifty percent of women relapse after cessation of therapy, but symptoms are usually more tolerable. More aggressive therapies include danazol, a synthetic androgen that decreases ovarian function (100 to 400 mg/day in two divided daily doses for 4 to 6 months). Bromocriptine, a long-acting dopaminergic drug that suppresses prolactin, is approved in Great Britain for the treatment of cyclical mastalgia (5 to 7.5 mg/day in 2.5 mg divided doses for 3 to 6 months). Tamoxifen 10 mg/day administered from day 15 to 25 of the menstrual cycle provided symptomatic relief in 75% of 297 patients in an Argentine trial. Breast specialists or reproductive endocrinologists should be involved in the decision to administer these latter therapies.

ABNORMAL DEVELOPMENT AND PHYSIOLOGY[3]

Absent or Accessory Breast Tissue

Absence of breast tissue (amastia) and absence of the nipple (athelia) are rare anomalies. Unilateral rudimentary breast development is much more common, as is adolescent hypertrophy of one breast with lesser development of the other. In contrast, accessory breast tissue (polymastia) and accessory nipples (supernumerary nipples) are both common. Supernumerary nipples are usually rudimentary and occur along the milk line from the axilla to the pubis in both males and females. They may be mistaken for a small mole. However, accessory nipples are removed only for cosmetic reasons. *True polythelia* refers to more than one nipple serving a single breast, which is rare.

Accessory breast tissue is commonly located above the breast in the axilla. Rudimentary nipple development may be present, and lactation is possible with more complete development. Accessory breast tissue, which may present as an enlarging mass in the axilla during pregnancy, is treated by surgical removal if it is large or cosmetically deforming, or it is removed to prevent enlargement during future pregnancy.

Gynecomastia

Hypertrophy of breast tissue in men is a common clinical entity for which there is frequently no identifiable cause.

Haagensen distinguishes *pubertal hypertrophy*, occurring in young boys between the ages of 13 and 17 years, from *senescent hypertrophy*, which occurs in men older than 50 years. The enlargement in teenage boys is common and is frequently bilateral, although it may be unilateral. Unless it is unilateral or painful, it may pass unnoticed and regresses with adulthood. Pubertal hypertrophy is generally treated by reassurance without operation. Surgical excision may be discussed if the enlargement fails to regress or is cosmetically unacceptable.

Hypertrophy in older men is also common and may regress spontaneously. It is frequently unilateral, although the contralateral breast may enlarge with time. The discoid mass is smooth, firm, and symmetrically distributed beneath the areola. It may be tender, and patients occasionally complain of breast discomfort. A number of commonly used medications, such as digoxin, thiazides, estrogens, phenothiazines, and theophylline, may exacerbate senescent gynecomastia. In addition, gynecomastia may be a systemic manifestation of hepatic cirrhosis, renal failure, and malnutrition. There should be little confusion with carcinoma occurring in the male breast. Carcinoma is usually not tender, it is asymmetrically located either beneath or beside the areola, and it may be fixed to the overlying dermis or to the deep fascia. As with pubertal hypertrophy, gynecomastia in older men is usually left untreated. A dominant mass suspected of carcinoma should be sampled or carefully observed.

Nipple Discharge

The appearance of a discharge from the nipple of a non-lactating woman is frequently frightening to the patient and misunderstood by the physician. Nipple discharge is common and is rarely associated with an underlying carcinoma. It is important to establish whether the discharge comes from one breast or from both breasts, whether it comes from multiple duct orifices or from just one, and whether the discharge is grossly bloody or contains blood. A milky discharge from both breasts is termed *galactorrhea*. In the absence of lactation or history of recent lactation, galactorrhea may be associated with increased production of prolactin. Radioimmunoassay for serum prolactin is diagnostic. However, true galactorrhea is rare and is diagnosed only when the discharge is milky (contains lactose, fat, and milk-specific proteins).

Unilateral, nonmilky discharge coming from one duct orifice is surgically significant and warrants special attention (Fig. 32-6). However, the underlying cause is rarely a breast malignancy. In one review of 270 subareolar biopsies for discharge coming from one identifiable duct and without an associated breast mass, carcinoma was found in only 16 patients (5.9%). In each of these cases, the fluid either was bloody or tested strongly positive for occult hemoglobin. In another series of 249 patients, including both multiple-duct and single-duct discharges, breast carcinoma was found in 10 (4%). In 8 of these patients, a mass lesion coexisted with the discharge. Nipple discharge that comes from a single duct and contains blood must be investigated further. However, in the absence of a palpable mass or a suspicious mammogram, this symptom is usually not associated with cancer.

The most common cause of spontaneous nipple discharge from a single duct is a solitary intraductal papilloma in one of the large subareolar ducts directly under the nipple. Fibrocystic change, or cystic mastopathy, typically produces multiple-duct discharge and is another commonly associated finding. Subareolar duct ectasia, producing inflammation and dilation of large collecting ducts under the nipple, is a common finding that usually produces multiple-duct discharge. In summary, nipple discharge that is bilateral and comes from multiple ducts is usually not a surgical problem. Bloody discharge from a single duct, depicted in Figure 32-6, does require surgical biopsy to establish a diagnosis. Intraductal papilloma is found in most of these cases. If an occult cancer is found, it is usually an intraductal carcinoma.

Galactocele

A galactocele is a milk-filled cyst that is round, well circumscribed, and easily movable within the breast. It usually occurs after the cessation of lactation or when feeding frequency has been curtailed significantly. Haagensen states that galactoceles may occur up to 6 to 10 months after breast-feeding has stopped. The pathogenesis of galactocele is not known, but it is thought that inspissated milk within ducts is responsible. The tumor is usually located in the central portion of the breast or under the nipple. Needle aspiration produces thick, creamy material that may be tinged dark-green or brown. Although it appears purulent, the fluid is sterile. Treatment is needle aspiration. Withdrawal of thick milky secretion confirms the diagnosis; operation is reserved for cysts that cannot be aspirated or that become infected.

DIAGNOSIS OF BREAST DISEASE

History

For patients with benign breast conditions, the history is an important part of the overall evaluation and frequently points to the underlying cause of a symptom or physical finding. For patients suspected of having cancer, the history aids in the approach to the patient, and the ultimate treatment if cancer is confirmed. A history may also uncover risk factors that help the clinician evaluate suspicious findings on physical examination or on mammogram. The examiner should determine the patient's age and obtain a reproductive history. The age of menarche, menstrual irregularities, and the age at menopause should be sought. Previous surgical procedures should be recorded, including previous breast biopsies and their pathologies and whether the ovaries were removed if a hysterectomy was performed. Because hysterectomy is a common procedure, accurate determination of menopause may be difficult. It is useful to inquire about menopausal symptoms in these patients. In younger

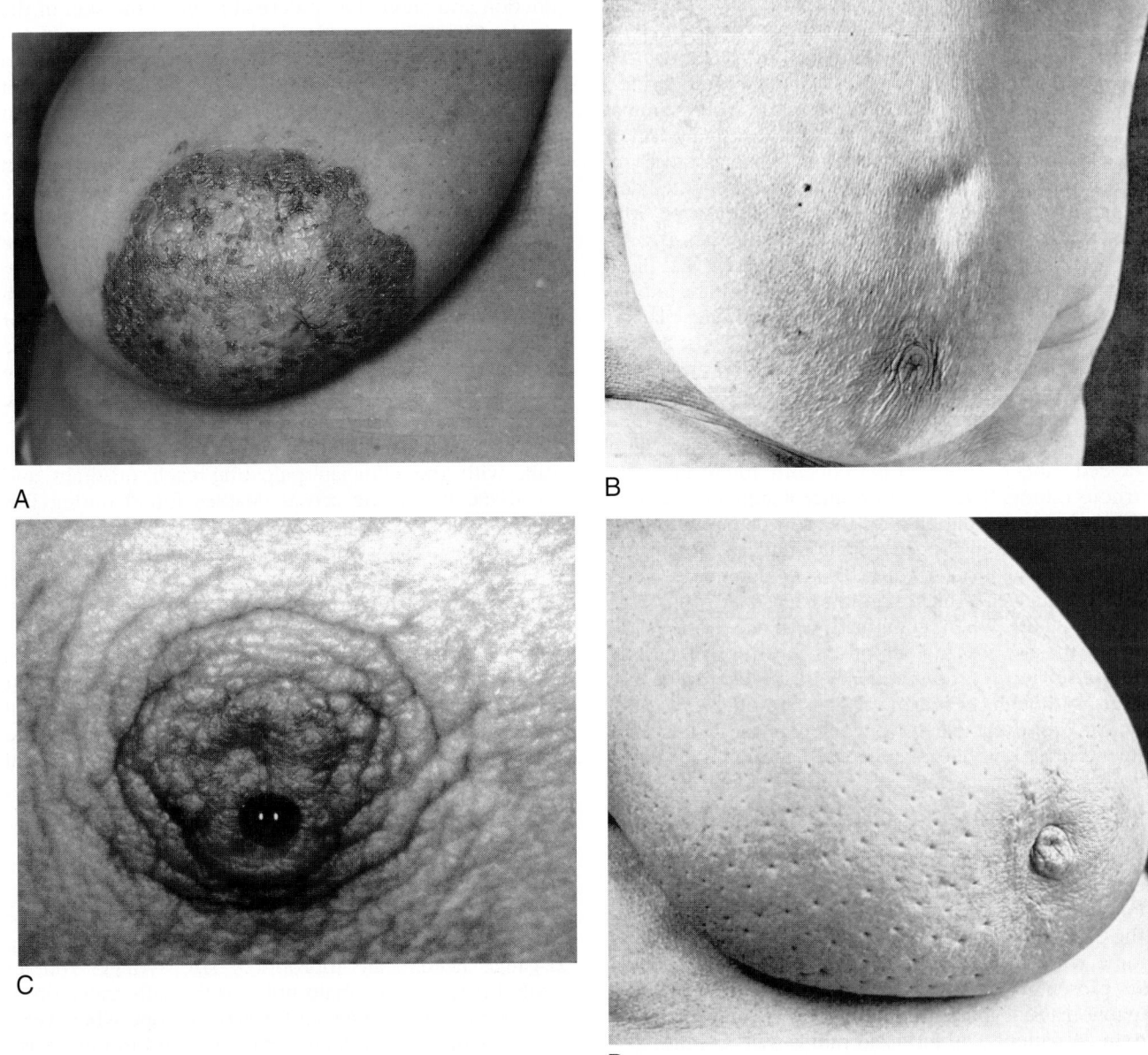

FIGURE 32-6. Common physical findings during breast examination. **A,** Paget's disease of the nipple. Malignant ductal cells invade the epidermis, without traversing the basement membrane of either the subareolar duct or the epidermis. The disease appears as a psoriatic rash that begins on the nipple and spreads off onto the areola and into the skin of the breast. **B,** Skin dimpling. Traction on Cooper's ligaments by a scirrhous tumor distorts the surface of the breast, producing the dimple best seen with angled indirect lighting during abduction of the arms upward. **C,** Nipple discharge. Discharge from multiple ducts or bilateral discharge is a common finding in healthy breasts. In this case, the discharge is from a single duct orifice and may signify underlying disease in the discharging duct. In this patient, a papilloma was the source of her symptoms. **D,** Peau d'orange (skin of the orange) or edema of the skin of the breast. This finding may be due to dependency of the breast, lymphatic blockage (from surgery or radiation), or mastitis. The most feared cause is inflammatory carcinoma, in which the malignant cells plug dermal lymphatics (the pathologic hallmark of the disease).

women, a recent history of pregnancy and lactation should be recorded. A drug history should pay attention to hormone replacement therapy or the use of hormones for contraception. As discussed later, the family history should be directed to cancer of the breast and ovaries in primary relatives (parents, siblings, and offspring).

In questioning the patient about the specific breast problem, it is worthwhile to inquire about breast pain, nipple discharge, and new masses in the breast. If a mass is present, it helps to know how it was found, how long it has been present, what has happened since its discovery, and if it changes with the menstrual cycle. If cancer is likely, inquiry about constitutional symptoms, bone pain, weight loss, respiratory changes, and similar clinical indications of metastatic disease may occasionally reveal unsuspected distant spread.

Physical Examination

Breast examination should be done with respect for privacy and patient comfort in a well-lighted room, preferably with an available indirect light source. The examination begins with the patient in the upright sitting position with careful visual inspection for obvious masses, asymmetries, and skin changes. The nipples are inspected and compared for the presence of retraction, nipple inversion, or excoriation of the superficial epidermis in Paget's disease (shown in Figure 32-6). The use of indirect lighting can unmask subtle dimpling of the skin or nipple caused by the scirrhous reaction of a carcinoma placing Cooper's ligaments under tension (see Fig. 32-6). Simple maneuvers such as stretching the arms high above the head, tensing the pectoralis muscles, or gently lifting the patient's breast may accentuate asymmetries and dimpling. It is a misconception to equate skin dimpling with advanced cancer. This sign is frequently found in small, scirrhous tumors that do not produce a large mass effect. If carefully sought, dimpling of the skin or nipple retraction is a sensitive and specific sign of underlying cancer.

Edema of the skin, frequently accompanied by erythema, produces a clinical sign known as *peau d'orange* (see Fig. 32-6). When combined with tenderness and warmth, these signs and symptoms are the hallmark of *inflammatory carcinoma* and may be mistaken for acute mastitis. Although these clinical signs are often dramatic, they can be overlooked in women with darker skin pigment in a room with inadequate lighting. The inflammatory changes and edema are caused by obstruction of dermal lymphatic channels with emboli of carcinoma cells. Occasionally, a bulky tumor may produce obstruction of large lymph channels that results in overlying skin edema. This is not, strictly speaking, an inflammatory carcinoma, in which the visible signs are out of proportion to the palpable mass. In 40 patients with inflammatory carcinoma who underwent treatment with Haagensen, all cases presented with erythema and edema of the skin; a palpable mass or localized induration was present in 19; and, in 21 patients, no localized tumor was present.

Involvement of the nipple and areola is a common histologic finding in breasts removed for carcinoma. Direct involvement may accompany tumors originating in breast tissue under the areola and may result in retraction of the usually protruding nipple. Flattening or actual inversion of the nipple can be caused by fibrosis in certain benign conditions, especially subareolar duct ectasia. In these cases, the finding is frequently bilateral and the history confirms that the condition has been present for many years. Unilateral retraction or retraction that develops over weeks or months is more suggestive of carcinoma. Centrally located tumors may directly invade and ulcerate the skin of the areola or nipple. Peripheral tumors may distort the normal symmetry of the nipples by traction on Cooper ligaments.

The second clinical feature of carcinoma that directly involves the nipple was described by Sir James Paget in 1874 and named *Paget's disease*. Histologically, this disease is produced by intraductal carcinoma occurring in the large sinuses just under the nipple (see Fig. 32-6). Carcinoma cells invade across the epidermoepithelial junction and enter the epidermal layer of the skin of the nipple. Clinically, this histologic variant produces a dermatitis that may appear eczematoid and moist or dry and psoriatic. It is usually confined to the nipple, although it can spread to the skin of the areola. Haagensen points out that benign skin conditions such as eczema frequently begin on the areola, whereas Paget's disease originates on the nipple and secondarily involves the areola.

Palpation follows visual inspection. While the patient is still in the sitting position, the examiner supports the patient's arm and palpates each axilla to detect the presence of enlarged axillary lymph nodes. The supraclavicular and infraclavicular spaces are similarly palpated for enlarged nodes. Palpation of the breast is always done with the patient lying supine on a solid examining surface with the arm stretched above the head. Palpation of the breast while the patient is sitting is insensitive and inaccurate. The breast should be compressed against the chest wall, with the clinician palpating each quadrant and the tissue under the areola. Masses found during this examination are characterized according to their size, shape, consistency, and location. Benign tumors, such as fibroadenomas and cysts, can be as firm as carcinoma; most commonly, these benign entities are usually distinct, well circumscribed, and movable. Carcinoma is typically firm but less circumscribed, and its movement produces a drag of adjacent tissue. Neither benign nor malignant tumors are usually tender; tenderness is rarely a helpful diagnostic sign. Generally, 75% of palpable masses are self-discovered by patients during casual or intentional self-examination.

Fine-Needle Aspiration

Fine-needle aspiration has become a routine part of the physical diagnosis of breast masses. It can be done with a 22-gauge needle, an appropriate size syringe, and an alcohol prep pad. Its main utility is the differentiation of solid from cystic masses, but it may be done whenever a new dominant, unexplained mass is found in the breast. This simple procedure is postponed only if mammography is necessary and there is worry that a small hematoma, resulting from needle puncture, might confuse the radiographic evaluation. Cyst fluid is usually turbid dark green or amber and can be discarded if the mass totally disappears and the fluid is not bloody. By using fine-needle aspiration in the routine examination of the breast, unnecessary open biopsy of cystic change is avoided. As a result of adding fine-needle aspiration to the routine examination of breast masses, a restating of criteria for open biopsy is helpful. Carcinoma will not be missed if a surgical biopsy is done when (1) needle aspiration produces no cyst fluid and a solid mass is diagnosed, (2) the cyst fluid produced is thick and blood tinged, and (3) fluid is produced but the mass fails to resolve completely. Other surgeons have added the frequent reappearance of the cyst in the same location and the rapid accumulation of fluid after initial aspiration (<2 weeks).

If the mass is solid and the clinical situation is consistent with carcinoma, a cytologic examination of the aspirated material is performed. The needle is repeatedly inserted into the mass while constant negative pressure is applied to the syringe. Suction is released and the needle is withdrawn. The scanty fluid and cellular material within the needle are either submitted in physiologically buffered saline (Normosol) or fixed immediately on slides in 95% ethyl alcohol. Most authors do not recommend definitive treatment based on a cytologic examination. In addition, the presence of carcinoma cells on fine-needle aspiration does not differentiate between in situ and invasive breast cancer. However, a positive result allows for informed discussions with the patient, definite plans for treatment, and appropriate consultations or second opinions.

BREAST IMAGING[7-9]

Breast radiographic imaging is used to detect small, non-palpable breast abnormalities, to evaluate clinical findings, and to guide diagnostic procedures. *Mammography* is the most sensitive and specific imaging test currently available, though 10% to 15% of clinically evident breast cancers have no mammographic correlate. *Digital mammography* is a technology that acquires digital images and stores them electronically. This allows users to manipulate images of the breast to enhance certain structures or densities while reducing the background of others. Film screen and digital mammography are equivalent in their ability to detect breast cancers. *Ultrasonography* is not used as a screening tool or in the evaluation of mammographic microcalcifications, but in a directed fashion to evaluate a breast mass and characterize it as cystic or solid. *Computed tomography* appears to be the best way to image internal mammary nodes and to evaluate the chest and axilla after mastectomy.

Magnetic resonance imaging (MRI) is the imaging method of choice to evaluate implant rupture. It may be used in efforts to identify the primary site of cancer in the breast of a woman who presents with malignant axillary adenopathy in the context of an unrevealing breast physical examination and mammogram (*occult breast cancer*). Particularly for an invasive lobular breast cancer diagnosed by core needle biopsy, where physician examination and mammography may underestimate the extent of disease, MRI may facilitate the decision as to whether the patient is an appropriate candidate for breast conservation. Its efficacy as a screening tool remains unproven, though studies in populations at increased risk for breast cancer appear promising. MRI sensitivity for invasive cancers approaches 100% but is only 60% at best for DCIS. Specificity remains low, with significant overlap in the appearance of benign and malignant lesions.

Screening Mammography[10]

The underlying principle of a screening strategy is the assumption that earlier detection reduces mortality and morbidity rates. *Screening mammography* is performed in efforts to detect breast cancer that is not clinically evident. It identifies women whose mammograms contain an abnormality and separates these women from those whose mammograms are clearly normal. In a National Health Interview Survey, the proportion of women 40 years of age and older reporting undergoing mammography over the previous 2 years increased from 29% in 1987 to 67% in 1998 to 76% in 2000. Modern film-screen mammography detects approximately eight breast cancers per 1000 women screened for the first time, the prevalent cases in the population. Subsequent screening detects about two or three new or incident cases per 1000 women screened.

Film-screen mammography uses compression of the breast between Plexiglas plates to lessen the thickness of the tissue through which the radiation must pass, to separate adjacent structures, and to improve resolution. Two views of each breast are obtained: the mediolateral oblique (MLO) and the craniocaudal (CC). The image, like standard radiographs, is viewed using transmitted light and is a negative image. Film-screen mammography delivers an average glandular dose of radiation that is less than 100 mrad (0.1 cGy or 0.1 rad). In comparison, the average dose to the center of the breast for patients undergoing barium swallow is more than 10-fold the dose of two-view mammography.

The prospective, randomized clinical trial is theoretically the most powerful method of demonstrating superiority of one diagnostic strategy over another. Randomized trials of screening with death as the principal end-point avoid lead time and length bias, the two most common biases of nonprospective trials. Eight prospectively randomized trials of screening mammography, which together randomized nearly 500,000 women, are summarized in Table 32-1. Seven of these trials included women in their 40s, and the eighth enrolled women beginning at age 50. No trial enrolled women after age 74. In each of these trials, approximately half of the women were invited to receive regular mammograms and the other half were assigned to usual care as recommended by their physicians. Some studies specified only one single mammographic view and others extended the screening interval to 2 years rather than annually. Table 32-1 shows the results of each trial depicted as the RR of mortality in the screened cohort compared with women randomized to receive usual care. An RR of 1.0 signifies no difference between the screened women and those receiving usual care, an RR greater than 1.0 signifies a survival advantage for women receiving usual care, and an RR less than 1.0 signifies improved survival for those randomized to compulsory screening.

In response to periodic controversies, the evolving results from the randomized trials with breast cancer mortality as the primary endpoint were reviewed, and the National Cancer Institute (NCI) issued a statement in 1994 that advised annual screening for women aged 50 and older. In 1997 and in 2002 the NCI added to this recommendation that women in their 40s should undergo screening every 1 to 2 years. The 2002 statement was in response to the controversy generated by the October 2001 *Lancet* article in which a meta-analysis was performed using two of the eight randomized clinical mammography screening trials, with the remaining six trials

TABLE 32-1. Prospective, Randomized Trials of Screening Mammography*

Study	Years Conducted	Age	Median Follow-up (yr)	Screening Interval (mo)	Mammograph Views (n)	RR for Death from Br Ca (95% CI)	Absolute Risk Reduction per 1000 Women	Women (n) Invited	Women (n) Control
Mammography Alone									
Stockholm	1981–1986	40–64	13.8	24–28	1	0.91 (0.65–1.27)	0.288	40,318	19,943
Gothenburg	1983–1988	39–59	12.8	18	1, 2	0.76 (0.56–1.04)	0.878	20,724	28,809
Malmo	1977–1990	45–70	17.1	18–24	1, 2	0.82 (0.67–1.00)	1.712	21,088	21,195
Swedish Two-County Trial†	1977–1989	40–74	17	24–33	1	0.68 (0.59–0.80)	1.809	77,080	55,985
Mammography plus CBE									
CNBSS-1‡	1980–1985	40–49	13	12	2	0.97 (0.74–1.27)	0.12	25,214	25,216
CNBSS-2‡	1980–1985	50–59	13	12	2	1.02 (0.78–1.33)	0.097	19,711	19,694
HIP§	1963–1966	40–64	16	12	2	0.79	1.438	30,239	30,256
Edinburgh	1978–1985	45-64	13	24	1, 2	0.79 (0.60–1.02)	1.020	28,628	26,015

*Results of eight randomized trials summarized in National Institutes of Health Consensus Development Panel: National Institutes of Health Consensus Development Conference Statement: Breast Cancer Screening for Women Ages 40-49, January 21-23, 1997. J Natl Cancer Inst Monogr 22:vii-xii, 1997, and updated in Humphrey LL, Helfand M, Chan BK, et al: Breast cancer screening: A summary of the evidence for the U.S. Preventive Services Task Force. Ann Intern Med 137:347, 2002.
†The Swedish Two-County Trial combines data from Ostergotland and Kopparberg.
‡Canadian National Breast Screening Study.
§Health Insurance Plan (HIP) of New York.
RR, relative risk; Br Ca, breast cancer; CI, confidence interval; CBE, clinical breast examination.

identified by the authors as too flawed to be included in the analysis. Olsen and Gotzsche concluded that screening mammography was not justified at any age. In March 2002, the U.S. Preventive Service Task Force reviewed the eight trials and considered only one seriously flawed. A meta-analysis using a Bayesian random effects model was used to evaluate the effectiveness of screening mammography after 14 years of observation. In the analysis of all age groups, screening mammography reduced the risk of breast cancer by 16% (RR, 0.84; confidence interval [CI], 0.77 to 0.91). Among women age 50 and older, this risk reduction was 15% (RR, 0.85; CI, 0.73 to 0.99) with the inclusion of the Canadian trial and 22% (RR, 0.78; CI, 0.67 to 0.96) with exclusion of this study. For women ages 40 to 49, screening mammography reduced the risk of breast cancer by 15% (RR, 0.85; CI, 0.73 to 0.99). Thus, the number of women needed to be screened to prevent one death from breast cancer after 14 years of observation would be 1224 women for all ages, 838 women for ages 50 and older, and 1792 for women ages 40 to 49. It has been suggested that women who participate in screening during their 40s are more likely to continue screening after age 50, when the magnitude of benefit may be higher. At present, screening mammography should be offered annually to women age 50 and older, and at least biennially in women age 40 to 49 with the screening interval made on an individual basis and considering the risk factors for breast cancer. Younger women with a significant family history, histologic risk factors, or a history of prior breast cancer should be offered annual screening.

Diagnostic Mammography[11,12]

Diagnostic mammography is performed when there is a breast abnormality on clinical examination or screening mammography. It includes magnifications and

TABLE 32-2. Breast Imaging Reporting and Data System (BI-RADS): Final Assessment Category

Category	Definition
0	Incomplete assessment; need additional imaging evaluation
1	Negative; routine mammogram in 1 year recommended
2	Benign finding; routine mammogram in 1 year recommended
3	Probably benign finding; short-term follow-up suggested
4	Suspicious abnormality; biopsy should be considered
5	Highly suggestive of malignancy; appropriate action should be taken

Adapted from Liberman L, Abramson AF, Squires FB, et al: The Breast Imaging Reporting and Data System: Positive predictive values of mammographic feature and final assessment categories. AJR Am J Radiol 171:35, 1998; and Liberman L, Menell JH: Breast imaging reporting and data systems (BI-RADS). Radiol Clin North Am 40:409, 2002.

compression imaging in addition to the MLO and CC views obtained with screening mammography, and is frequently supplemented by ultrasound. The mammographic features of malignancy can be broadly divided into density abnormalities (masses, architectural distortions, and asymmetries) and microcalcifications. Each mammogram is also assessed for the presence of abnormalities in the axillary nodes and for the presence of skin or nipple changes, such as thickening or retraction. The final interpretation is categorized according to the BI-RADS system (Breast Imaging Reporting and Data System) of the American College of Radiology, and reflects the likelihood of malignancy (Table 32-2 shows BI-RADS Categories and Table 32-3 illustrates the predictive power of BI-RADS classification). Selected pictures of mammographic

TABLE 32-3. Final Assessment Categories: Positive Predictive Value

Investigator	BI-RADS Category		
	3	**4**	**5**
	No. of Lesions Referred for Biopsy (%)		
Liberman	8/492 (2)	355/492 (72)	129/492 (26)
Orel	141/1312 (11)	936/1312 (71)	170/1312 (13)
Lacquement	322/688 (47)	234/688 (34)	106/688 (15)
	PPV (%)		
Liberman	0/8 (0)	120/355 (34)	105/129 (81)
Orel	3/141 (2)	279/936 (30)	165/170 (97)
Lacquement	9/322 (3)	54/234 (23)	97/106 (92)
Summary	12/471 (2.55)	453/1525 (29.7)	367/391 (93.9)

PPV, positive predictive value, which is equal to the number of cancers divided by total number of lesions that underwent biopsy in that category; Breast Imaging Reporting and Data Systems, BI-RADS.
Data from Liberman L, Menell JH: Breast Imaging Reporting and Data Systems (BI-RADS). Radiol Clin North Am 40:409, 2002; Liberman L, Abramson AF, Squires FB, et al: The Breast Imaging Reporting and Data System: Positive predictive values of mammographic feature and final assessment categories. AJR Am J Radiol 171:35, 1998; Orel SG, Kay N, Reynolds C, et al: BI-RADS categorization as a predictor of malignancy. Radiology 211:845, 1999; Lacquement MA, Mitchell D, Hollingsworth AB: Positive predictive value of the Breast Imaging Reporting and Data System. J Am Coll Surg 189:34, 1999.

abnormalities are displayed in Figure 32-7, illustrating common findings of malignancy.

Nonpalpable Mammographic Abnormalities

Mammographic abnormalities that cannot be detected by physical examination are classified in three broad categories: (1) lesions consisting of microcalcifications only, (2) density lesions (masses, architectural distortions, and asymmetries), and (3) those with both calcifications and density abnormalities (the first two findings are illustrated in Fig. 32-7). The incidence of malignancy after biopsy depends on the characteristics of the radiographic finding. Lesions with microcalcifications with an associated mass and linear branching calcifications carry the highest probability of being malignant. However, even well-defined, smooth densities can be malignant. Not every abnormality should undergo biopsy (BI-RADS 2 and 3), and recommendations should be made by surgeons in consultation with an experienced radiologist. For some patients not undergoing biopsy (BI-RADS 3), a mammogram repeated in a shorter interval (6 months) may be recommended to establish stability of the abnormality.

The two methods available to evaluate a nonpalpable mammographic abnormality include wire localization with surgical excisional biopsy and image-guided stereotactic or ultrasound-guided large-core needle biopsy (LCNB). Prior to either method of histologic diagnosis, mammographic magnification views should be performed to most accurately define the radiologic extent of the calcifications should these be present alone or in combination with a mammographic density.

Needle Localization Breast Biopsy

Until the early 1990s, the only method available to evaluate a nonpalpable mammographic abnormality involved an open surgical breast biopsy with preoperative image-guided wire localization. In addition to the permanent surgical scar on the breast skin, there is the possibility of a cosmetic contour change to the breast and the chance of not excising the site in question (2%). Typically, 75% of patients have a benign finding. Of the 25% (15% to 30%) diagnosed with a breast cancer, the majority require a second breast surgery to obtain negative surgical margins. For both calcifications and masses, a specimen radiograph is usually done to confirm the presence of the mammographic finding in the resected tissue.

Large-Core Needle Biopsy (LCNB)[8,13]

Since the early 1990s, LCNB increasingly is the diagnostic method of choice to histologically evaluate nonpalpable mammographic abnormalities. In experienced centers, it is considered the standard of care. LCNB can be performed using either mammographic (stereotactic) or ultrasound guidance. Mammographic calcifications are typically sampled using stereotactic capabilities. As with needle-directed surgical biopsy, imaging the cores removed by the procedure guarantees adequate sampling of calcifications. Mammographic densities can be sampled by ultrasound guidance when the density can also be visualized by ultrasound and by stereotactic guidance when the density is seen by mammography only.

Stereotactic LCNB involves the patient lying prone on the stereotactic core biopsy table with the breast in compression. After local anesthetic is injected, a 3-mm skin incision is made, and an 11-gauge core biopsy needle with vacuum assistance is inserted into the lesion to obtain the tissue sample. A robotic arm and biopsy gun is positioned by computed analysis of triangulated mammographic images. Firing the machine obtains a core biopsy through the abnormality.

In experienced centers, 65% of women who undergo the procedure are found to have a benign diagnosis and can resume annual mammographic screening. For instance, if the mammogram shows that the lesion is a smooth, round mass without distortion of the surrounding breast and the core shows a benign fibroadenoma, the patient can be reassured and returned to routine care. Twenty-five percent of patients are found to have a malignancy. The diagnosis of the malignancy by core biopsy affords the opportunity to proceed with one definitive surgery, with efforts toward breast preservation when appropriate and chosen by the patient. The remaining 10% of patients are found to have inconclusive histology, including (1) atypical cells on pathology (atypical ductal hyperplasia vs. DCIS); (2) biopsy results that are discordant from the mammography findings (e.g., mammographic appearance of a cancer with benign findings on core biopsy); (3) increased cellularity within a fibroadenoma (fibroadenoma vs. a phyllodes tumor); or (4) inadequate sampling of the site (calcifications do not appear on the core biopsy specimen images). In these cases where

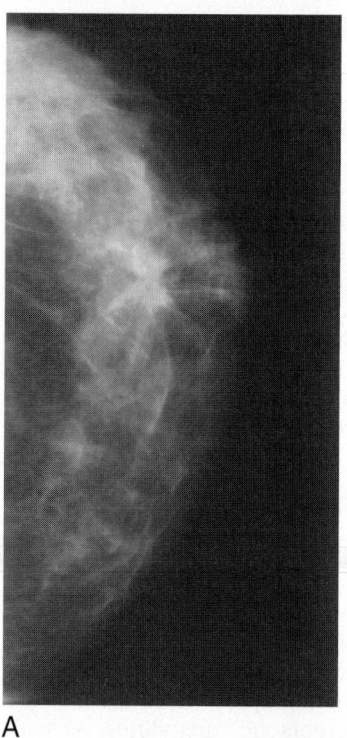

A

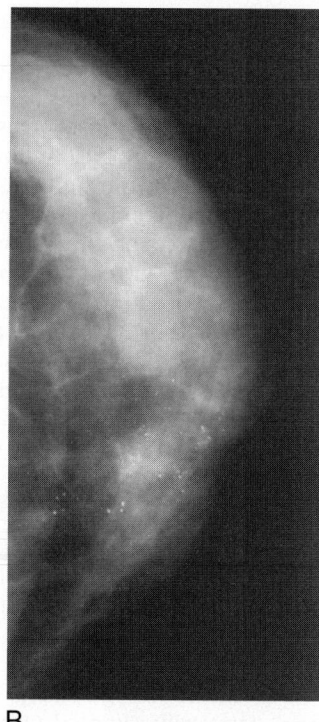

B

FIGURE 32-7.   Mammogram and ultrasound findings of breast disease. **A,** A stellate mass in the breast. The combination of a density with spiculated borders and distortion of surrounding breast architecture suggests a malignancy. **B,** Clustered microcalcifications. Fine, pleomorphic, and linear calcifications that cluster together suggest the diagnosis of ductal carcinoma in situ (DCIS). **C,** An ultrasound image of breast cancer. The mass is solid, containing internal echoes, and displaying an irregular border. Most malignant lesions are taller than they are wide. **D,** Ultrasound image of a simple cyst. By ultrasound, the cyst is round with smooth borders, there is a paucity of internal sound echoes, and there is increased through-transmission of sound with enhanced posterior echoes.

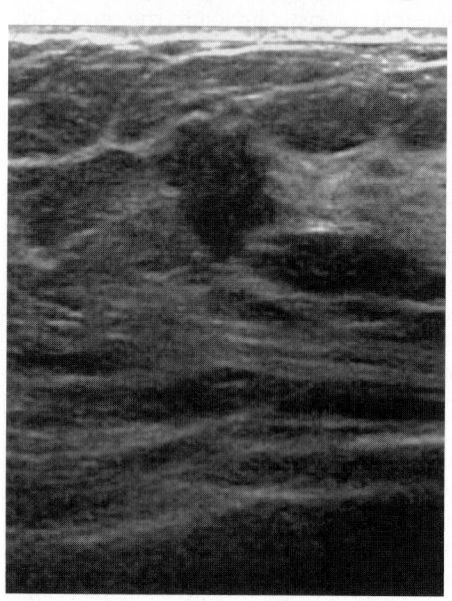

C

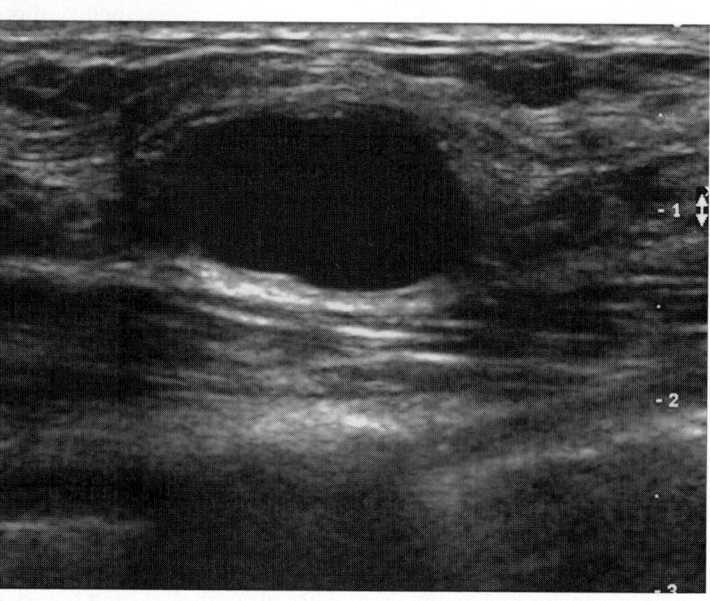

D

the core obtained does not contain cancer, and the histology does not entirely explain the mammographic finding, surgical biopsy is recommended. The false-negative rate of stereotactic biopsy should be extremely low if these guidelines are followed.

Atypia on Core Needle Biopsy

For patients with atypia on core needle biopsy, a wire localization and excisional biopsy are performed to clarify the histology. In the Brigham and Women's Hospital experience presented by Darling and associates, wire localization and excisional biopsy performed to evaluate atypical ductal hyperplasia found the site contained atypical hyperplasia and nothing more in 81% of patients, DCIS in 13%, or an invasive breast cancer in 6%. In the case of core biopsy demonstrating atypical *lobular* hyperplasia, at most an "upgrade" of this lesion would be to lobular carcinoma in situ (LCIS), and excisional biopsy is not mandated.

DCIS on Core Needle Biopsy

For patients with a core needle biopsy diagnosis of DCIS, 7% have had the lesion fully excised with the core needle.

At the time of surgical excision, an upgrade of the DCIS is seen in 12% of patients who had undergone core needle biopsy using an 11-gauge, vacuum-assisted needle device. As reported by Bonnett, the likelihood of an invasive breast cancer diagnosed at the time of surgical excision increases with the grade of DCIS seen in the core biopsy specimen: for low grades, 0 of 26 patients contained invasive cancer; for intermediate-grade DCIS, 2 of 31 (6%) contained invasive cancer; and for high grades, 10 of 36 (28%) were upstaged.

IDENTIFICATION AND MANAGEMENT OF THE HIGH RISK PATIENT[4,6,14-16]

Risk Factors for Breast Cancer

Identification of factors responsible for increasing the chance of developing breast cancer is important in daily clinical practice for clinicians who care for women. Risk factors used in clinical practice, the degree of risk conferred, and screening recommendations based on this risk are presented in Table 32-4.

Age

Age is probably the most important risk factor that clinicians use in everyday clinical practice. The age-adjusted incidence of breast cancer continues to increase with advancing age of the female population. Breast cancer is rare in persons younger than 20 years of age, and cases in women younger than 30 constitute less than 2% of the total cases. Thereafter, the incidence increases to 1 in 93 by age 40, 1 in 50 by age 50, 1 in 24 by age 60, 1 in 14 by age 70, and 1 in 10 by age 80. Alternatively stated, the annual frequency of breast cancer in the 8th decade of life is greater than 300 cases per 100,000. Gender is also an important risk factor. Males are at risk for breast cancer, although the incidence in males is less than 1% of the incidence in females, with 1300 cases anticipated in 2003. Lumps in the male breast are much more likely to be benign and the result of gynecomastia (discussed earlier) or other noncancerous tumors.

Histologic Risk Factors[17]

Histologic abnormalities diagnosed by breast biopsy comprise a category of breast cancer risk factors. A history of mammary cancer in one breast increases the likelihood of a second primary cancer in the contralateral breast. In many studies, the RR (ratio of observed cases over expected cases) ranges between 3 and 4. The magnitude of RRs depends on age at diagnosis of the first primary cancer. For patients younger than 45, risk for the cancer in the remaining breast is five or six times that of the general population. In older patients, this risk decreases to a twofold or less increased risk. In absolute terms, the actual risk varies between 1% per year in young patients to 0.2% in older patients.

LCIS is a relatively uncommon condition that is observed predominantly in younger, premenopausal women. It is typically an incidental finding at biopsy for another condition, and itself does not form a palpable mass or manifest as calcifications mammographically. Haagensen has collected the largest series of patients, all of whom were identified by review of biopsy material. In this review, LCIS was found in 3.6% of more than 5000 biopsies performed for benign disease. In his review of 297 patients with LCIS treated by biopsy and careful observation, Haagensen determined that the actuarial probability of developing carcinoma at the end of 35 years was 21.4%. Compared with the Connecticut Tumor Registry data, a risk ratio (observed-to-expected cases) of 7:1 was calculated. Significantly, 40% of the carcinomas that subsequently developed were purely in situ lesions, the invasive cancers that developed were predominantly ductal and not lobular in histology, and half of the carcinomas occurred in the contralateral breast. Thus LCIS is not a breast cancer but rather a histologic marker for increased breast cancer susceptibility, estimated at slightly less than 1% per year longitudinally. Management options are presented in Table 32-4.

Although no direct survey of surgical practice has been done, a conservative approach, rather than mastectomy, is more commonly practiced with LCIS patients. Certainly, a policy of close observation with or without tamoxifen chemoprevention is widely recognized as standard care. Patients must be informed that LCIS predisposes to subsequent carcinoma and that their risk is life-long and increases over passage of time. Because the risk of subsequent breast cancer is equal for both breasts, biopsy of the opposite breast adds little useful information. As described in the Chemoprevention section (later), a 5-year course of tamoxifen provides a 56% reduction in breast cancer risk. For those who elect surgery in preference to observation, bilateral total mastectomy remains the procedure of choice. Subcutaneous mastectomy, preserving the nipple-areolar complex, retains breast glandular cells in the nipple and behind the areola and is not an appropriate method of cancer prevention.

Fibrocystic changes are a spectrum of histologic changes that include nonproliferative and proliferative conditions. Nonproliferative changes include mild-to-moderate hyperplasia and do not appear to significantly increase a women's lifetime breast cancer risk. The excess risk of breast cancer concentrates in women whose specimens show proliferative changes. Dupont and Page have divided the proliferative lesions into those with atypical epithelial hyperplasia and those without atypia. The RR of cancer in women with *atypical ductal* or *lobular hyperplasia* was 4.4 times the risk of development of breast cancer in a control population of women. The coexistence of a positive family history with atypia on biopsy increased the risk to nearly nine times the general population. Thus, the annual risk of developing breast cancer for a woman with LCIS is slightly less than 1% per year, with atypical lobular hyperplasia 0.75% per year, and with atypical ductal hyperplasia 0.5% per year.

TABLE 32-4. The RMF Breast Care Management Algorithms: Risk Assessment and Potential Interventions

| Definitions of Risk | Screening Recommendations[1] | | Other Options |
	Clinical Breast Exam	Mammogram	
Usual • Two or more reproductive risk factors (see checklist) with no family history • Weak family history (i.e., two or fewer distant relatives with breast cancer, or 1st degree relative with postmenopausal breast cancer.)	Annual after age 20	Annual after age 40	
Moderate—Histology • Atypical ductal hyperplasia (ADH) • Atypical lobular hyperplasia (ALH) • Lobular carcinoma in situ (LCIS) • Previous history of ductal carcinoma in situ (DCIS) • Previous history of invasive breast cancer	At least once per year	Annual after diagnosis	
Moderate—Radiation[2] • Thoracic radiation before age 30	Annual after age 20	Annual after age 40 or 10 years after radiation	
Moderate—Strong family history • Any 1st or 2nd degree relative with breast cancer < age 50 • Two or more relatives with early onset breast cancer in the same lineage	At least once per year	Annual after 40 or 5–10 years earlier than youngest affected relative, but not before age 25.	
High—Features associated with 10% or greater prior probability of carrying a BRCA1/BRCA2 mutation • Personal history of breast cancer diagnosed ≤40 or ovarian cancer • Family history of breast cancer ≤40 in 1st degree relative • Family history of breast cancer ≤40 in paternal 2nd degree relative • Family history of breast cancer in two 1st degree relatives, at least one diagnosed ≤50	At least once per year	Annual after 40 or 5–10 years earlier than youngest affected relative, but not before age 25.	• Referral to high-risk counseling • Chemoprevention

Risk Factors Checklist

Aytpia or Cancer on Previous Biopsy

☐ Atypical ductal hyperplasia (ADH)
☐ Atypical lobular hyperplasia (ALH)
☐ Lobular carcinoma in situ (LCIS)
☐ Previous history ductal carcinoma in situ (DCIS)
☐ Previous history of invasive breast cancer

Thoracic Radiation Before Age 30[2]

☐ e.g., Hodgkin's
☐ Infant thymus radiation
☐ Frequent fluoroscopy for TB
☐ Multiple x-rays for scoliosis

Family History—Three Generations Maternal and Paternal

☐ Known or suspected gene mutation
☐ Early age onset <40
☐ Bilateral breast cancer
☐ Breast and/or ovarian cancer
☐ Male breast cancer
☐ Ethnicity[3], e.g., Jewish ancestry with family history
☐ Cluster of rare tumors in a biological family

Reproductive Risk Factors[4]

☐ >5 years of combined estrogen/ progesterone hormone replacement therapy
☐ Age at menarche <12
☐ Nulliparity
☐ Age at firstborn >30
☐ Age at menopause >55

- Prophylactic mastectomy and/or oophorectomy

- Family history of ovarian cancer and breast cancer in one 1st or 2nd degree relative or in close relatives in the same lineage
- One or more male relatives with breast cancer

- Known carrier of a *BRCA1* or *BRCA2* mutation or close relative with known mutation
  Note: Women of Ashkenazi Jewish ancestry may be included despite fewer affected relatives or later age onset

After age 25, at least once per year. Consider twice yearly

Annual after age 25 or individualized based on earliest stage onset in family. Preliminary data suggest that adding MRI to mammography in high risk patients may be helpful.
Note: More intensive screening for mutation carriers

Gail Model—the Gail model calculates actuarial estimates of future breast cancer risk based on race, age, reproductive risk factors, maternal family history, and previous biopsy status. The computerized version of the Gail model is available at: http://brca.nci.nih.gov/brc/. The Gail model score represents the cumulative risk of developing cancer over the next five years. For values >2, consider high-risk counseling. However, the Gail model may underestimate the risk for those with a strong family history of breast cancer.

Claus Model—the Claus model is an empiric risk model that predicts a woman's chance of developing breast cancer based on her family history. In these cases the Claus model may provide more useful information. This model considers the number for affected relatives in both the maternal and paternal lineages (up to two), their relationship to the patient (whether they are first or second degree relatives) and the age of onset of breast cancer in each relative. It does not factor in ethnic background, whether the cancer was bilateral, or a family history of ovarian cancer. All eight Claus model tables are available at: www.rmf.harvard.edu/rmlibrary/clinical-guidelines/breast-algo/bca/index.htm.

1 Based on the NCCN guidelines.

2 Risk from theraputic radiation is much greater than risk from diagnostic radiation.

3 The prevalence of *BRCA1* or *BRCA2* mutation is about 2% in the Ashkenazi Jewish population.

4 Reproductive risk factors alone are generally insufficient to put a patient in the "high risk" category.

Family History and Genetic Risk Factors[18]

Many studies have examined the relationship of family history and the risk of breast cancer. These studies can be summarized as follows: (1) there is a twofold to threefold excess risk of the disease in first-degree relatives (mothers, sisters, and daughters) of patients with breast cancer; (2) risk decreases quickly in women with distant relatives who are affected with breast cancer (cousins, aunts, grandmothers); and (3) the risk is much higher if affected first-degree relatives had premenopausal onset and bilateral breast cancers. In families with multiple affected members, particularly with bilateral and early-onset cancers, the absolute risk to first-degree relatives approaches 50%, consistent with an autosomal dominant mode of inheritance in these particular pedigrees. Because the disease is so common in North American and European populations, constellations of breast cancer in families are more often an expression of random occurrence than a genetic defect in these families.

Genetic factors are estimated to cause 5% to 10% of breast cancer cases. These factors may account for 25% of cases in women younger than 30 years of age. In 1988, a group led by Mary-Claire King provided evidence for transmission of a gene in high-risk families and by 1990 had identified a region on the long arm of chromosome 17 (17q21) that contained a susceptibility gene. The gene, BRCA1, was intensively sought by several international groups and finally discovered in the summer of 1994. It accounts for up to 40% of familial breast cancer syndromes. In addition to an increased breast cancer risk, those with this mutation are also at increased risk for ovarian cancer (15% to 45%), colon cancer, and for men, prostate cancer. Founder mutations include the 185delAG and 5382insC mutations found in 1.05% and 0.11% of the Ashkenazi Jewish population (Jews of Eastern European descent), and the C4446T mutation in French Canadian families. BRCA1 is a large gene, with 22 coding exons and more than 500 mutations, many unique and limited to a given family, which makes genetic testing a technically difficult procedure. BRCA1 is a tumor suppressor oncogene inherited in an autosomal dominant fashion. Germline mutation inactivates a single inherited allele of BRCA1 and precedes a somatic event, which occurs in breast epithelial cells, and eliminates the remaining BRCA1 allele. The gene product may provide negative regulation of cell growth or perhaps is involved in recognition and repair of genetic damage or spontaneous mutation.

At the same time BRCA1 was identified, a second susceptibility locus was mapped to chromosome 13. This gene, known as BRCA2, accounts for up to 30% of familial breast cancer and is associated with increased breast cancer risk in males. Women with a mutation in BRCA2 also have a 20% to 30% lifelong risk of ovarian cancer. Men have increased risks for prostate cancer, and men and women have increased risks for pancreatic and laryngeal cancers as well. Founder mutations of BRCA2 include the 617delT mutation present in 1.4% of the Ashkenazi population, the 8765delAG in the French Canadian population, and the 999del15 mutation in the Icelandic population. In Iceland, 7% of unselected female breast cancer patients and 0.6% of the general population carries the 999del15 mutation.

Deleterious mutations in BRCA1 or BRCA2 are rare in the general population. The frequency of mutations is about 1 in 1000 people in the American population. The penetrance of BRCA1 and BRCA2 refers to the chance that carriers of mutations in these genes will actually get breast cancer. The initial estimates of this chance were high, in the range of 80% to 90% based on the striking families used to link these genes to breast cancer. A more recent estimate, based on a larger population of gene carriers, is lower. In this study, the penetrance of BRCA1 and BRCA2 mutations was 56%, with a 95% confidence interval between 40% and 73%. It is reasonable to quote lifelong rates of breast cancer between 50% and 70% for carriers of BRCA1 or BRCA2 mutations.

The histopathology for BRCA1-associated cancers is unfavorable when compared with BRCA2 cancers and includes tumors that are high grade, hormone receptor negative, aneuploid, and have an increased S-phase fraction. BRCA2 tumors are most commonly hormone receptor positive. Overall mortality rates for the BRCA1 and BRCA2 groups are probably similar to those of sporadic breast cancers. Because the risk of breast cancer is high for carriers of a mutation, the question of increased screening versus chemoprevention, and these strategies versus prophylactic mastectomy is raised, and is discussed in detail in the subsequent sections.

Reproductive Risk Factors

Reproductive milestones that increase a woman's lifetime estrogen exposure are thought to increase her breast cancer risk and include menarche prior to age 12, first live childbirth after age 30, nulliparity, and menopause after age 55. There is a 10% reduced breast cancer risk for each 2-year delay in menarche. There is a doubling of risk with menopause after age 55. Those having a full-term first pregnancy prior to age 18 have half the risk of developing breast cancer than those whose first such pregnancy is after age 30. There is no known increase or decrease in breast cancer risk associated with induced abortion.

Exogenous Hormone Usage[4]

Women often ask whether the use of either oral contraceptives or postmenopausal hormone replacement therapy increases the chance of breast cancer. In the population-based case-control study by Marchbanks, for women ages 35 to 64 years of age, there was no increased risk of breast cancer seen in current (RR, 1; CI, 0.8 to 1.3) or past (RR, 0.9; CI, 0.8 to 1.0) users of oral contraceptives. With regard to the use of hormone replacement therapy, the prospective, randomized control trial from the Women's Health Initiative enrolled 16,608 healthy postmenopausal women ages 50 to 79. The study assessed the benefits and risks of hormone replacement therapy, low-fat diet, and calcium and vitamin D supplementation on rates of cancer, cardiovascular disease, and osteo-porosis-related fractures and reached its stopping rules at 5.2 years of follow-up. For 1000 healthy postmenopausal women taking Prempro for 10 years, when compared to those taking placebo, there were 8 more cases of breast cancer, 8 more strokes, 8 more pulmonary emboli, and 7 more events from coronary heart disease. In addition, there were 6 fewer cases of colon cancer and 5 fewer hip fractures. The study is still ongoing for women who previously underwent hysterectomy and randomized to estrogen alone versus placebo. Hormone replacement therapy in the form of estrogen and progesterone is currently recommended for less than 5 years in efforts to ameliorate menopausal symptoms.

Risk Assessment Tools—the Gail Model[19]

To assist medical counseling, a model for breast cancer risk has been developed from case-control data in the Breast Cancer Detection Demonstration Project (BCDDP) by Gail and coworkers. By examining many variables, these investigators were able to reject many factors that did not contribute to breast cancer risk. Factors that did contribute to risk in this model included age, race, age at menarche, age at first live birth, number of previous breast biopsies, atypia on biopsy, and the number of first-degree female relatives with breast cancer. Not included in the model are the age of diagnosis of female first-degree family members with breast cancer, history of breast cancer in the paternal lineage, and family history of ovarian cancer. Thus, for a woman from a family with a *BRCA1* or *BRCA2* mutation, the model may underestimate risk for a mutation carrier and overestimate risk in a noncarrier. The Gail model for breast cancer risk was used in the design of the Breast Cancer Prevention Trial, which randomly assigned women at high risk to receive tamoxifen or a placebo, and in the ongoing STAR trial, which is randomly assigning women at high risk to receive tamoxifen or raloxifene.

Management of the High-Risk Patient[20]

In practice, reproductive risk factors alone are insufficient to place a woman in the "high-risk" category for breast cancer. However, a strong family history suggestive of a genetic mutation or a previous breast biopsy demonstrating LCIS, atypical ductal hyperplasia, or atypical lobular hyperplasia can significantly raise a woman's breast cancer risk and prompt concern or treatment. For individuals at increased breast cancer risk, options include close surveillance with clinical breast examination, mammography, and possibly breast MRI; chemoprevention using tamoxifen; or bilateral prophylactic mastectomies.

Close Surveillance

Surveillance guidelines for individuals at high risk for breast cancer were established in 2002 by the National Comprehensive Cancer Network and the Cancer Genetics Studies Consortium. These guidelines are based primarily on expert opinion; the frequency of screening guidelines for high-risk individuals have not been well established by prospective, randomized trials. Recommendations for women in a breast-ovarian cancer syndrome family include monthly breast self-examination beginning at age 18, semiannual clinical breast examination beginning at age 25, and annual mammography beginning at age 25 or 10 years prior to the earliest age of onset of a family member. Several studies have demonstrated that within the context of similar screening guidelines, for women with known *BRCA1* or *BRCA2* mutations, half of breast cancers were diagnosed as interval cancers not detected during the course of routine screening. Coupled with evolving evidence of the superiority of screening MRI in the mutation carrier, this has prompted many groups to add annual screening MRI at a 6-month interval from screening mammography (although not yet of proven benefit). If not performed previously, genetic counseling should be offered to those with a strong family history or early-onset breast and ovarian cancer, including a discussion of genetic testing for *BRCA1* and *BRCA2* mutations.

Chemoprevention for Breast Cancer[16,21]

The only drug currently approved for reducing breast cancer risk is tamoxifen. Tamoxifen is an estrogen antagonist with proven benefit for the treatment of estrogen hormone receptor–positive breast cancer. Furthermore, tamoxifen reduces the incidence of second primary breast cancer in the contralateral breast of women who received the drug as adjuvant therapy for a first breast cancer. In the Early Breast Cancer Trialists' Collaborative Group (EBCTCG), adjuvant tamoxifen reduced the risk of a second breast cancer in the unaffected breast by 47%. Therefore, four prospective, randomized trials of preventive tamoxifen were initiated in healthy women, as summarized in Table 32-5.

The Italian Prevention Trial randomized 5408 women who had previously undergone hysterectomy to receive either tamoxifen or placebo and has not achieved adequate follow-up to establish a clear result. Participants were not required to be at increased risk for breast cancer and were allowed to take hormone replacement therapy. Because 26% of participants discontinued therapy, accrual was terminated earlier than planned. Within this construct, the trial has failed to show a protective effect of tamoxifen at a median follow-up of 46 months, except in a subgroup of women who used concurrent hormone replacement therapy while in the study.

The smallest trial is from the Royal Marsden Hospital in the United Kingdom; it randomized 2494 women with a family history of breast cancer to receive either tamoxifen or placebo. In this trial, 40% of women also received hormone replacement therapy. With a median follow-up of 120 months this European trial also failed to show a benefit from the use of tamoxifen in reducing the incidence of breast cancer. Women with LCIS or atypia on breast biopsy were excluded from this trial, the subgroup in whom tamoxifen risk reduction is shown to be most effective in the National Surgical Adjuvant Breast and Bowel Project (NSABP) P-1 trial, as described subsequently.

TABLE 32-5.   Randomized Trials of Breast Cancer Chemoprevention

Study	No. of Randomized Tam/Placebo (age range)	Accrual Years	Eligibility	% Postmenopausal	HRT Use	Median Follow-up (mo)	Summary Results*
NSABP P-1[1]	6576/6599 (>34)	1992–1997	High risk†	61	No	69	Positive
Italian National Trial[2]	1871/1966 (35–70)	1992–1997	Usual risk‡	Hysterectomy, 100; Oophorectomy, 74	Yes	94	Negative
Royal Marsden Trial[3]	1238/1233 (30–70)	1986–1996	Family history	34	Yes	120	Negative
IBIS[4]	3578/3566 (35–70)	1992–2001	High risk§	50	Yes	50	Positive

[1]Data from Fisher B, Constantino JP, Wichersham DL, et al: Tamoxifen for prevention of breast cancer: Report of the National Surgical Adjuvant Breast and Bowel Project P-1 study. J Natl Cancer Inst 90:1371, 1998.

[2]Data from Veronesi U, Masionneuve P, Costa A, et al: Prevention of breast cancer with tamoxifen: Preliminary findings from the Italian randomized trial among hysterectomised women. Lancet 352:93, 1998; and Veronesi U, Maisonneuve P, Sacchini V, et al: Tamoxifen for breast cancer among hysterectomised women. Lancet 359:1122, 2002.

[3]Data from Powels T, Eeles R, Ashley S, et al: Interim analysis of the incidence of breast cancer in the Royal Marsden Hospital tamoxifen randomized chemoprevention trial. Lancet 352:98, 1998.

[4]Data from IBIS Working Party and Principal Investigators: First results from the International Breast Cancer Intervention Study (IBIS-I): A randomized prevention trial. Lancet 360:817, 2002.

*Positive, tamoxifen superior to placebo; negative, tamoxifen equal to placebo.

†High risk based on Gail model of risk.

‡All women previously underwent hysterectomy and were recruited to participate.

§High risk based on family history, histology (lobular carcinoma in situ and atypia), and nulliparity.

Tam, tamoxifen; HRT, hormone replacement therapy.

Adapted from Powels TJ: Antioestrogenic prevention of breast cancer—the make or break point. Natl Rev Cancer 2:787, 2002.

The International Breast Intervention Trial (IBIS) enrolled 7140 women who had undergone hysterectomy and the majority of whom also had their ovaries removed. With a median follow-up of 50 months, there was a statistically significant breast cancer risk reduction of 33% for tamoxifen users, seen primarily in those women taking hormone replacement therapy. Given that breast cancer risk is reduced with oophorectomy and increased with prolonged use of hormone replacement therapy, it may be expected the benefits of tamoxifen in this population are less robust than in the NSABP P-1 trial.

The U.S. trial was performed by the NSABP and randomized 13,388 women age 35 to 59 with a diagnosis of LCIS or whose risk for breast cancer was moderately increased (RR of 1.66 over 5 years) or who were 60 or older. The risk estimates were based on the Gail model of risk, which includes age, reproductive factors, and the presence of atypical ductal hyperplasia on biopsy. In this study, tamoxifen reduced the risk of invasive breast cancer by 49% through 69 months of follow-up, with a risk reduction of 59% in the subgroup with LCIS and of 86% with atypical ductal or lobular hyperplasia. The reduction in risk was noted only for estrogen receptor–positive cancers. Tamoxifen treatment for 5 years was not devoid of complications. In the tamoxifen treatment arm, endometrial cancers resulting from the estrogen-like effects of the drug on the endometrium were increased by a factor of about 2.5. Pulmonary embolism (RR, 3), and deep venous thrombosis (RR, 1.7) were also more common. Data as to the efficacy of tamoxifen on breast cancer risk reduction in *BRCA1* and *BRCA2*

mutation carriers are currently too limited to quantify in this population.

Currently, the NSABP is conducting a randomized trial comparing tamoxifen to raloxifen, a selective estrogen receptor modulator (NSABP P-2, STAR trial). In a meta-analysis of more than 10,000 women who participated in placebo-controlled trials evaluating the efficacy of raloxifen with respect to osteoporosis, with an average of 3 years of follow-up, there is a 54% reduction in the incidence of breast cancer and no increase in uterine cancers.

Prophylactic Mastectomy[22]

To summarize the accumulating evidence, prophylactic mastectomy probably reduces the chance of breast cancer in high-risk women by 90%. However, women who are screened by mammograms annually have an overall 80% chance of surviving the occurrence of breast cancer. Coupled with penetrance figures in the range of 50% to 60% for mutation carriers, the chance of dying of breast cancer for carriers of *BRCA1* or *BRCA2* mutations is approximately 10%, without undergoing preventive mastectomy.

In a retrospective study by Hartman, 639 women with a family history of breast cancer underwent prophylactic mastectomy. Based on family pedigrees, the women were divided into high (*n* = 214) and moderate (*n* = 425) risk groups, with high-risk patients defined as those with a family history suggestive of an autosomal dominant predisposition to breast cancer. For women of moderate risk, the number of expected breast cancers was calculated using the Gail model. Based on this model, 37.4 breast cancers were expected to have developed and 4 cancers actually did, for an incidence risk reduction of 89%. For women in the high-risk cohort, the Gail model would underestimate the risk of developing breast cancer. Thus, the expected number of breast cancers was calculated using three different statistical models from a control study of the high-risk probands (sister). Three breast cancers developed after prophylactic mastectomy, for an incident risk reduction of at least 90%.

Two groups have reported prospective results in *BRCA1* and *BRCA2* mutation carriers followed after prophylactic mastectomy versus surveillance. Meijers-Heijboer reported that at 2.9 years of follow-up none of 76 mutation carriers who underwent preventive mastectomy had a breast cancer occurrence, whereas 8 of 63 women choosing surveillance did. Scheuer reported that at 24.2 months of follow-up, none of 29 women who underwent mastectomy had a breast cancer occurrence and 12 of 165 high-risk women not choosing preventive mastectomy did develop breast cancer. There is an underlying assumption that reduction in risk of breast cancer incidence will translate into survival benefits, though this is currently unproven.

BENIGN BREAST TUMORS AND RELATED DISEASES[3]

Breast Cysts

Cysts within the breast are fluid-filled, epithelium-lined cavities that may vary in size from microscopic to large, palpable masses containing as much as 20 to 30 mL of fluid. Cysts are generally discovered by physical examination and confirmed by ultrasound or needle aspiration. A palpable cyst develops in at least 1 of every 14 women, and 50% of cysts are multiple or recurrent. Cysts occur as solitary abnormalities, called *macrocysts* or *gross breast cysts*, or as part of a generalized process of microscopic cyst formation. This latter disease process is frequently bilateral and the cystic transformation can be extensive. The pathogenesis of cystic formation is not well understood; however, cysts appear to arise from destruction and dilation of lobules and terminal ductules. Microscopic studies have shown that fibrosis at or near the lobule, combined with continued secretion, results in the unfolding of the lobule and expansion of an epithelium-lined cavity containing fluid.

Cysts are influenced by ovarian hormones, a fact that explains their sudden appearance during the menstrual cycle, their rapid growth, and their spontaneous regression with completion of the menses. Most women with new cyst formation are first seen after the age of 35 and rarely before the age of 25 years. The incidence of cyst development steadily increases until the age of menopause and sharply declines after menopause; cysts are tumors of women in their late reproductive years. New cyst formation in older women commonly is explained by the use of exogenous hormone replacement.

When encountered during operation, cysts are frequently dark. These are often referred to as *blue dome cysts,* reflecting the dark cyst fluid contained within. Grossly, they are usually unilocular and lined by a smooth and glistening surface, although larger cystic structures may be trabeculated and multiloculated. Histologically, simple cysts are lined by a flattened epithelium. However, the epithelial layer may display apocrine metaplasia or may have papillary features. Intracystic carcinoma is exceedingly rare. Rosemond was able to report only three cancers in more than 3000 cyst aspirations (0.1%). Other investigators confirmed this exceedingly low incidence. Regarding the risk of cancer development for women with cystic disease, there are no convincing studies showing an increased risk of breast cancer, based solely on the presence of gross or microscopic cysts.

The management of palpable cysts is straight-forward; needle aspiration is both diagnostic and therapeutic. If the palpable abnormality totally disappears after aspiration, the cyst fluid can be discarded. There is little support for the *routine* submission of cyst fluid for cytology. Cyst fluid can be straw colored, opaque, dark-greenish, and even contain flecks of debris. The character of the cyst fluid is not an indication for sending the fluid for cytology. The only reliable indication for submitting fluid for cytology is the presence of a residual mass after aspiration of the fluid. If the cyst recurs multiple times (more than two times is a reasonable rule), cytology is justified. Finally, surgical removal of a cyst may be indicated if the cytology is suspicious or the cyst recurs multiple times.

Fibroadenoma and Related Tumors

Fibroadenoma (adenofibroma) is a benign tumor composed of stromal and epithelial elements. After carcinoma, fibroadenoma is the second most common solid tumor in the breast and is the most common tumor in women younger than age 30 years. In contrast to cysts, fibroadenomas appear in teenage girls and women during their early reproductive years; they are rarely seen as a new tumor in women after age 40 or 45. The benign nature of this lesion was recognized in 1840 by Cooper, who referred to the lesions as *chronic mammary tumors.* Clinically, they present as firm, solitary tumors that may increase in size over several months of observation. They may be lobulated but slip easily under the examining fingers. At operation, fibroadenomas appear to be well-encapsulated masses that may easily detach from the surrounding breast tissue. By history, fibroadenoma is favored over cyst in the adolescent or young adult; on examination, these tumors are distinguished from cysts by the needle aspiration that yields no fluid. Mammography is of little help in distinguishing between cysts and fibroadenomas; however, ultrasound usually clearly shows the cavity of a cyst. The gross appearance and histopathology are distinctive of fibroadenoma. Grossly, the tumor appears well encapsulated, with smooth borders that may be lobulated. Histologically, a variable proportion of epithelial and stromal proliferation is present, and the stroma may be quite cellular or replaced by acellular swirls of collagen. Although fibroadenomas are not considered to have a malignant potential, the epithelial elements appear to be at risk for neoplasia just as epithelium elsewhere in the breast. More than 100 invasive and noninvasive carcinomas have been reported in preexisting fibroadenomas since 1985. Most of these (50%) have been LCIS, 35% were infiltrating carcinomas, and 15% were intraductal carcinoma. Cancer in a newly discovered fibroadenoma is exceedingly rare. A modest risk of subsequent carcinoma in women who have previously undergone treatment for fibroadenoma has been reported, but the magnitude is about two times that in the general population. This is only slightly higher than the reported excess risk for all women who underwent previous breast biopsy.

The treatment of fibroadenoma follows that for any unexplained solid mass within the breast. Most patients in the United States undergo excisional biopsy to remove the tumor and establish the diagnosis. However, trends in treatment are changing. For the woman in her teens or 20s, with a typical fibroadenoma on physical examination, many surgeons counsel against surgery in favor of leaving this benign tumor undisturbed. An alternative approach, probably widely used, is to obtain a core needle biopsy. If the diagnosis is fibroadenoma, and the lesion is typical, it can be left in the breast. If excision is recommended, the approach to removal of a typical fibroadenoma in a young woman is different than the approach in older women with indeterminate masses. Cosmetic incisions around the areola with a modest amount of tunneling to remove the lesion is a commonly used technique and is proper for the treatment of fibroadenoma. Emphasis should be placed on removing a minimal amount of breast tissue adjacent to a typical fibroadenoma. Frozen section is rarely used or needed, and patients can be reassured based on the gross appearance, pending results of permanent sections.

Juvenile Fibroadenoma and Giant Fibroadenoma

Clinicians treating breast masses should be aware of the two terms juvenile fibroadenoma and giant fibroadenoma, which are sometimes confusing. *Giant fibroadenoma* is a descriptive term that applies to a fibroadenoma that attains an unusually large size, typically greater than 5 cm. Haagensen calls these lesions *massive adenofibromas in youth* to denote their common occurrence in adolescent women. *Juvenile fibroadenoma* refers to the occasional large fibroadenoma that occurs in adolescents and young adults and histologically is more cellular than the usual fibroadenoma. Both these lesions overlap, and both may display remarkably rapid growth within the breast. Although alarming to the patient and physician, prompt surgical removal is always curative. The differential diagnosis for a cellular juvenile fibroadenoma is benign phyllodes tumor, and the two may be difficult to distinguish. However, if the tumor has been completely removed, the diagnosis of benign cystosarcoma should reassure the surgeon and the patient that the risk of recurrence is low, particularly if the patient is an adolescent or young adult.

Malignant phyllodes is a distinctive and aggressive tumor that is discussed later.

Hamartoma and Adenoma

Although probably not of the same histogenesis as fibroadenoma, these tumors are benign proliferations of variable amounts of epithelium and stromal supporting tissue. The hamartoma is a discrete nodule that contains closely packed lobules and prominent, ectatic extralobular ducts. By physical examination, mammography, and gross inspection, the hamartoma is indistinguishable from fibroadenoma. The nodule is entirely benign, and removal is curative. The mammary adenoma or tubular adenoma has been a more elusive entity to define. Page and Anderson describe this tumor as a cellular neoplasm of ductules packed closely together forming a sheet of tiny glands without supporting stroma. During pregnancy and lactation, these tumors may increase in size, and histologic examination shows secretory differentiation. Malignancy is not a feature of tubular adenoma or lactating adenoma, but biopsy is required to establish the diagnosis.

Breast Abscess and Infections

Breast abscess commonly occurs in the subareolar breast tissue and may be recurrent and difficult to treat. Although the exact cause is not known, subareolar duct ectasia and obstruction of major ducts may lead to proliferation of bacteria and subsequent abscess. Further destruction of the normal ductal openings leads to fistula formation and chronic recurrent abscess. *Mammary duct ectasia*, first named by Haagensen, is an inflammatory condition that causes distortion and dilation of the lactiferous sinuses under the nipple. It is a common entity and is frequently responsible for nipple inversion in older women. In understanding subareolar abscess and probably mastitis in general, it is useful to remember that the nipple and areolar complex contain secretory ducts that are exposed to the environment. Chronic inflammation, duct dilation, and obstruction may combine at the nipple to produce circumstances that favor bacterial invasion.

The treatment of acute abscess of periareolar tissue should be conservative if possible. Antibiotics with broad-spectrum coverage should be used initially. More severe infections may require hospitalization and intravenous antibiotics. A small incision with drainage is preferred if the process cannot be controlled by antibiotics alone. Needle aspiration may be attempted, but the abscess cavity is usually multiloculated. Haagensen described excision of the involved ducts to prevent recurrence. However, recurrence is common and leads to chronic, recurring infection and fistula formation.

Mastitis describes a more generalized cellulitis of breast tissue that may involve a large area of the breast but may not form a true abscess. The etiology appears to be an ascending infection beginning in subareolar ducts and extending outward from the nipple. Occasionally, mastitis involves areas of cystic disease and may be sterile. Mastitis presents with erythema of the overlying skin, pain, and tenderness to palpation. There is induration of the skin and underlying breast parenchyma. Mastitis commonly complicates lactation, possibly as a result of bacteria ascending in ductal tree of the breast through the nipple. Local measures such as application of heat, ice packs, or use of a mechanical breast pump on the affected side all have been recommended. If conservative measures are not effective, administration of broad-spectrum antibiotics is usually indicated. In many situations, the differential diagnosis of acute mastitis includes inflammatory carcinoma. It is important to follow up patients with mastitis and confirm that there has been a complete resolution of symptoms and signs. The erythema produced by an inflammatory carcinoma does not resolve with conservative measures and generally worsens in a short period of follow-up.

Papilloma and Related Ductal Tumors

Solitary intraductal papillomas are true polyps of epithelium-lined breast ducts. Solitary papillomas are located under the areola in most cases but may present in peripheral ducts and can grow to a large size and present as a breast mass. When papillomas attain a large size, they may appear to arise within a cystic structure, probably representing a greatly expanded duct. In general, these lesions are less than 1 cm but can grow to as large as 4 or 5 cm.

Papillomas under the nipple and areolar complex often present with bloody nipple discharge. Less frequently, they are discovered as a palpable mass under the areola or as a density lesion on the mammogram. Treatment is total excision through a circumareolar incision. For peripheral papillomas, there is a differential diagnosis between a papilloma and invasive papillary carcinoma. Because these lesions can infarct, scar, and even develop squamous metaplasia, they can appear bizarre and disordered. Most pathologists urge evaluation on permanent sections for the majority of papillary lesions before more extensive surgery is undertaken.

It is important not to confuse the commonly used term *papillomatosis* with either solitary or multiple papillomas. Papillomatosis refers to epithelial hyperplasia that commonly occurs in younger women or is associated with fibrocystic change. This lesion is not composed of true papillomas. Hyperplastic epithelium in papillomatosis may fill individual ducts like a true polyp but has no stalk of fibrovascular tissue nor the frondlike growth. Solitary papillomas are entirely benign and do not predispose to development of cancer in the patients who have them. Page and Anderson state the degree of subsequent risk for breast cancer in patients with either papillomatosis or with true papillomas relates to the degree of atypical epithelial proliferation associated with them.

Sclerosing Lesions[23,24]

Sclerosing Adenosis

Adenosis refers to an increased number of small terminal ductules or acini. It is frequently associated with a proliferation of stromal tissue producing a histologic lesion, sclerosing adenosis, which can simulate carcinoma both grossly and histologically. There may be deposition of calcium, which can be seen on mammography in a pattern indistinguishable from microcalcifications in intraductal carcinoma. Sclerosing adenosis is the most common pathologic diagnosis in patients undergoing needle-directed biopsy of microcalcifications in many series. Sclerosing adenosis is frequently listed as one of the component lesions of fibrocystic disease; it is quite common and has no malignant potential.

Radial Scar

Radial scar belongs to a group of related abnormalities known as complex sclerosing lesions. They are important to the surgeon and pathologist because they can simulate carcinoma mammographically and on physical examination. These lesions contain microcysts, epithelial hyperplasia, adenosis, and a prominent display of central sclerosis. The gross abnormality is rarely more than 1 cm in diameter. The larger lesions form palpable tumors and appear as a spiculated mass with prominent architectural distortion on the mammogram. These tumors can even produce skin dimpling by traction on surrounding fibrous bands that become involved in the cicatrix. Biopsy is always recommended for tumors with these signs and symptoms. Although these lesions are benign, at least one recent study has uncovered a link between radial scars and the risk of eventual breast cancer. This study examined 1396 women in the Nurses' Health Study from Boston. The women with a history of radial scars had a risk of breast cancer almost twice the risk in women without radial scars, making this diagnosis a modest risk factor for breast cancer. Furthermore, the risk of radial scar was independent of atypical hyperplasia, adding risk both to women with atypical hyperplasia and to those without evidence of atypical histology.

Fat Necrosis

As with the other sclerosing abnormalities, fat necrosis can mimic cancer by producing a mass, a density lesion on mammography that can calcify, and surrounding distortion of the normal breast architecture. Fat necrosis may follow an episode of trauma to the breast but frequently there is no such history. Histologically, the lesion is composed of lipid-laden macrophages, scar tissue, and chronic inflammatory cells. This is not a lesion of epithelial tissue and has no malignant potential. It is usually sampled because of the signs it produces on examination or on mammogram.

PATHOLOGY OF BREAST CANCER (Box 32-3)[23,24]

Noninvasive Breast Cancer

Noninvasive neoplasms are broadly divided into two major types: LCIS and DCIS (or intraductal carcinoma). As noted in the introduction to breast pathology, histology

Box 32-3. Classification of Primary Breast Cancer

Noninvasive Epithelial Cancers

Lobular carcinoma in situ (LCIS)
Ductal carcinoma in situ (DCIS) or intraductal carcinoma
   Papillary, cribriform, solid, and comedo types

Invasive Epithelial Cancers (percentage of total)

Invasive lobular carcinoma (10–15)
Invasive ductal carcinoma
   Invasive ductal carcinoma, NOS (50–70)
   Tubular carcinoma (2–3)
   Mucinous or colloid carcinoma (2–3)
   Medullary carcinoma (5)
   Invasive cribriform (1–3)
   Invasive papillary (1–2)
   Adenoid cystic carcinoma (1)
   Metaplastic carcinoma (1)

Mixed Connective and Epithelial Tumors

Phyllodes tumors, benign and malignant
Carcinosarcoma
Angiosarcoma

NOS, nothing otherwise specified.

and nomenclature do not always accurately reflect biology. LCIS, once considered a malignant lesion, is now regarded more as a risk factor for development of breast cancer. LCIS is recognized by its conformity to the outline of the normal lobule, with expanded and filled acini (Fig. 32-8). DCIS is a more heterogeneous lesion morphologically, and pathologists recognize four broad categories: papillary, cribriform, solid, and comedo, the latter three types shown in Figure 32-8. DCIS is recognized as discrete spaces, surrounded by basement membrane, filled with malignant cells, and usually with a recognizable basally located cell layer made up of presumably normal myoepithelial cells. The four morphologies are prototypes of pure lesions, but in reality these appearances blend into one another. However, the papillary and cribriform DCIS probably transform to invasive cancer over a longer time frame and are of lower grade. Solid and comedo DCIS are generally higher-grade lesions and probably invade over a shortened natural history.

As the cells inside the ductal membrane grow, they have a tendency to undergo central necrosis, perhaps because the blood supply to these cells is located outside the basement membrane. The necrotic debris in the center of the duct undergoes coagulation and finally calcification, leading to the tiny, pleomorphic, and frequently linear forms seen on high-quality mammograms. In some patients, an entire ductal tree seems to be involved with the malignancy, and the mammogram shows typical calcifications from the nipple extending posteriorly into the interior of the breast (termed *segmental calcifications*). For reasons not understood, DCIS transforms into an invasive cancer, usually recapitulating the morphology of the cells inside the duct. In other words, low-grade cribriform DCIS tends to invade as a low-grade lesion retaining some cribriform features. There is not, as may be thought, a tendency for grade to advance with the invasion. Finally, DCIS frequently coexists with otherwise invasive cancers, and again the two phases of the malignancy are in step with each other morphologically.

Invasive Breast Cancers

Invasive cancers are recognized by their lack of overall architecture, by the infiltration of cells haphazardly into a variable amount of stroma, or by forming sheets of continuous and monotonous cells without respect for form and function of a glandular organ. Clinicians and pathologists broadly divide invasive breast cancers into *lobular* and *ductal* histology, which probably does not reflect histogenesis and only imperfectly predicts clinical behavior. However, invasive lobular cancer tends to permeate the breast in a single-file nature, which explains why it remains clinically occult, escaping detection on a mammogram or by physical exam until the total extent of the disease is large. Likewise, ductal cancers tend to grow as a more coherent mass, forming discrete abnormalities on mammograms and appearing sooner as a lump in the breast. The growth pattern of these lesions is shown in Figure 32-9; invasive ductal cancer in panel A and invasive lobular cancer in panel B.

Invasive ductal cancer, or infiltrating ductal carcinoma, is the most common presentation of breast cancer, accounting for 50% to 70% of invasive breast cancers. When this cancer does not take on special features, it is called *infiltrating ductal carcinoma, NOS* (which is an abbreviation for *nothing otherwise specified*). Invasive lobular carcinoma accounts for 10% to 15% of breast cancer, and mixed ductal and lobular cancers are increasingly recognized and described in pathology reports. When infiltrating ductal carcinomas take on differentiated features, they are named according to the features they display. If the infiltrating cells form small glands, lined by a single row of bland epithelium, they are called *infiltrating tubular carcinoma*, drawn in Figure 32-9. The infiltrating cells may secrete copious amounts of mucinous material and appear to float in this material. These lesions are called *mucinous* or *colloid tumors*. Both the tubular and mucinous tumors are low-grade (grade I) lesions and make up about 2% or 3%, each, of invasive ductal carcinomas. In contrast, bizarre invasive cells with high-grade nuclear features, many mitoses, and the lack of an in situ component characterize medullary cancer. The malignancy forms sheets of cells, in an almost syncytial fashion, and are surrounded by an infiltrate of small mononuclear lymphocytes. The borders of the tumor "push" into the surrounding breast rather than infiltrate or permeate the stroma. This tumor is drawn in Figure 32-9A, emphasizing the bizarre and pleomorphic nuclear features of the cells. In its pure form, it accounts for only

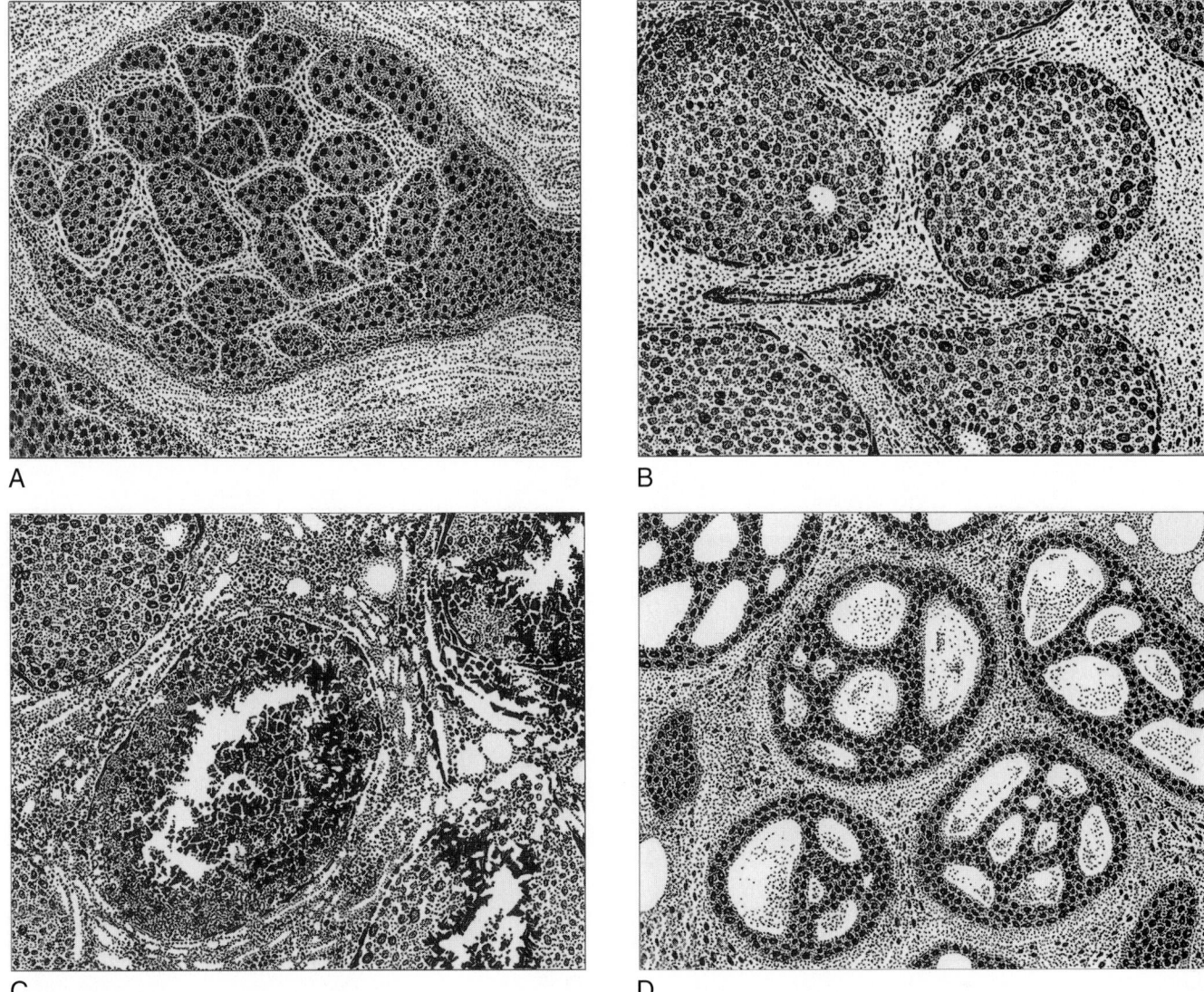

FIGURE 32-8. Noninvasive breast cancer. **A,** Lobular carcinoma in situ (LCIS). The neoplastic cells are small with compact, bland nuclei and distend the acini but preserve the cross-sectional architecture of the lobular unit. **B,** Ductal carcinoma in situ (DCIS), solid type. The cells are larger than in LCIS and fill ductal rather than lobular spaces. However, the cells are contained within the basement membrane of the duct and do not invade the breast stroma. **C,** DCIS, comedo type. In comedo DCIS, the malignant cells in the center undergo necrosis, coagulation, and calcification. **D,** DCIS, cribriform type. In this type, bridges of tumor cells span the ductal space leaving round, punched-out spaces.

about 5% of breast cancers; however, various pathologists describe a "medullary variant" that has some features of the pure form of the cancer.

It is commonly held that infiltrating ductal carcinoma, NOS is the most common form of breast cancer and carries the worst outcome (although modulated by modified Bloom-Richardson grade). Infiltrating lobular and pure medullary cancers carry an intermediate prognosis, whereas tubular and mucinous cancers are the least clinically aggressive cancers. However, these generalizations are useful only in context of tumor size, grade, and receptor status and are subject to many exceptions to these rules.

Other Tumors Primary to the Breast

Phyllodes Tumors

Tumors of mixed connective tissue and epithelium constitute an important group of unusual primary breast cancers. On one extreme, these tumors are exemplified by the benign fibroadenoma, characterized by a proliferation of connective tissue and a variable component of ductal elements, which may appear "compressed" by the swirls of fibroblastic growth. More perplexing are the intermediate neoplastic growths comprising phyllodes tumors, containing a biphasic proliferation of stroma and

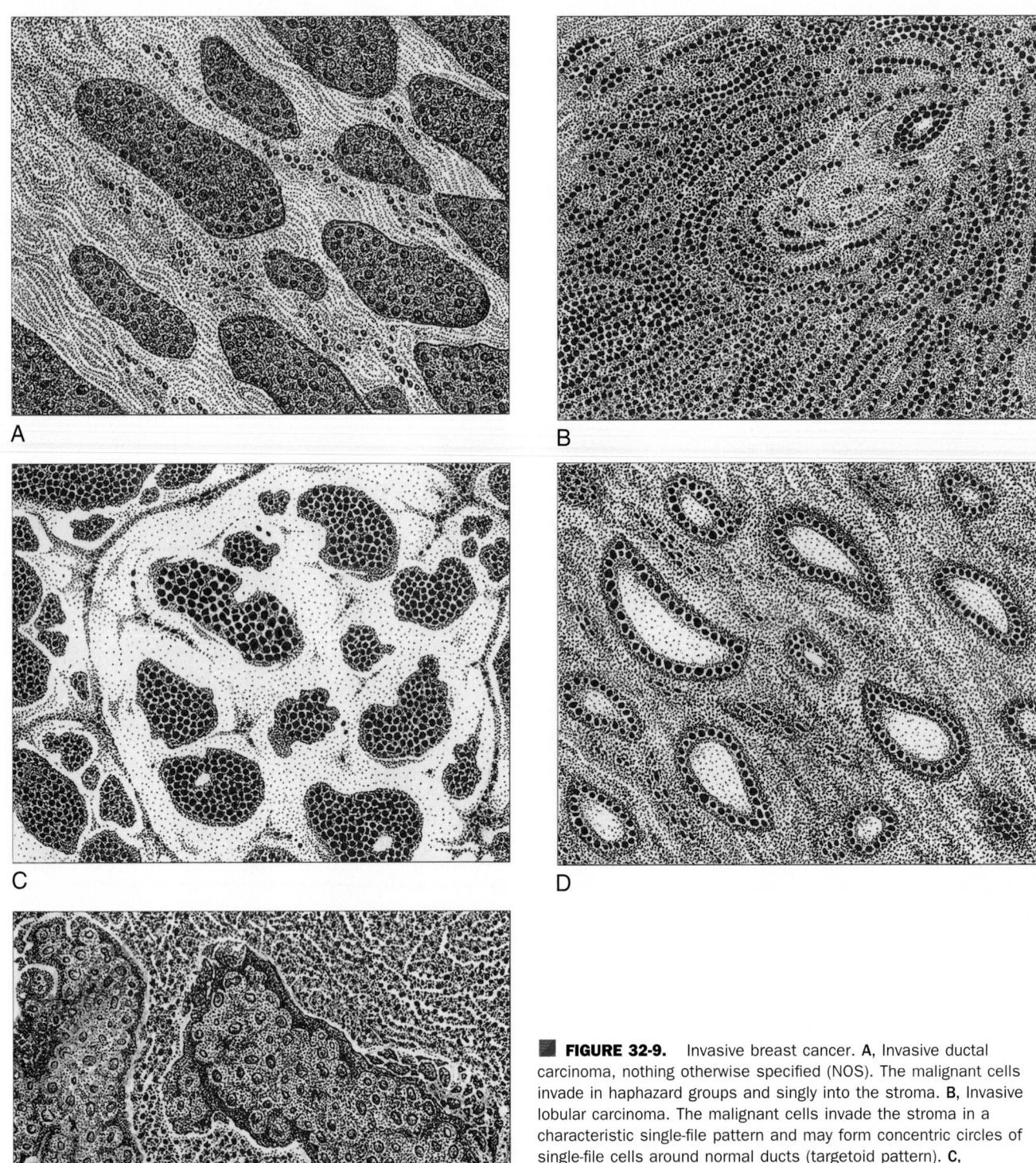

■ FIGURE 32-9.   Invasive breast cancer. **A,** Invasive ductal carcinoma, nothing otherwise specified (NOS). The malignant cells invade in haphazard groups and singly into the stroma. **B,** Invasive lobular carcinoma. The malignant cells invade the stroma in a characteristic single-file pattern and may form concentric circles of single-file cells around normal ducts (targetoid pattern). **C,** Mucinous or colloid carcinoma. The bland tumor cells float like islands in lakes of mucin. **D,** Invasive tubular carcinoma. The cancer invades as small tubules, lined by a single layer of well-differentiated cells. **E,** Medullary carcinoma. The tumor cells are large, very undifferentiated with pleomorphic nuclei. The distinctive features of this tumor are the infiltrate of lymphocytes and the syncytial-appearing sheets of tumor cells.

mammary epithelium. First called *cystosarcoma phyllodes*, the name has been changed to *phyllodes tumor* in recognition of its usual benign course. However, with increasing cellularity, an invasive margin, and truly sarcomatous appearance, these tumors may be classified as malignant phyllodes tumors. Benign phyllodes tumors are recognized as firm, lobulated masses between 2 and up to 40 cm in size, with an average size of about 5 cm (larger than average fibroadenomas). Histologically, these tumors resemble fibroadenomas, but the whorled stroma forms larger clefts lined by epithelium, and resembling clusters of leaflike structures. The stroma is more cellular than a fibroadenoma, but the fibroblastic cells are bland and mitoses are infrequent.

Local excision of a benign phyllodes tumor is curative, and clearly benign tumors are treated like a fibroadenoma. There is a group of intermediate tumors, so-called borderline phyllodes tumors, in which there is difficulty assigning a benign label. These tumors should be treated by excision with wide margins and patients placed under observation. Finally, at the other end of the spectrum are frankly malignant stromal sarcomas. Malignant phyllodes tumors are treated like sarcomas on the trunk or extremities. En bloc surgical excision of the entire affected part, in this case a total mastectomy, is advised. As with sarcomas in general, regional lymph node dissection is not required.

Angiosarcoma

This vascular tumor may occur de novo in the breast, but the clinically important presentation is in the dermis after breast radiation or in the lymphedematous upper extremity, historically following radical mastectomy. Angiosarcoma arising in the absence of previous radiation or surgery may form a mass within the parenchyma of the breast, in contrast to radiation-induced angiosarcoma, which arises in irradiated skin. Vascular proliferations in the skin are common following radiation to any part of the body, and the differential diagnosis is frequently between malignant angiosarcoma and atypical vascular proliferations in irradiated skin. Histologically, the tumor comprises an anastomosing tangle of blood vessels in the dermis and superficial subcutaneous fat. The atypical and crowded vessels invade through the dermis and into subcutaneous fat. These cancers are graded by the appearance and behavior of the endothelial cells, which comprise it. Pleomorphic nuclei, frequent mitoses and stacking up of the endothelial cells lining neoplastic vessels are features seen in higher grade lesions. Rarely seen in hemangiomas, necrosis is common in high-grade angiosarcomas. Clinically, radiation-induced angiosarcoma presents as a reddish-brown to purple, raised rash within the radiation portals and on the skin of the breast. As the disease progresses, or with high-grade sarcomas, tumors protruding from the surface of the skin may predominate. The treatment of angiosarcoma is described in the subsequent section of Modern Surgical Treatment for Breast Cancer.

STAGING BREAST CANCER[25]

The most widely used system for staging primary breast cancer has evolved from classifications proposed by the International Union Against Cancer (UICC) and the American Joint Committee on Cancer (AJCC). It is important to recognize that staging systems represent abbreviations to describe a heterogeneous disease and a clinical continuum from the earliest malignancy to fatal metastasis. In 2002, the AJCC issued its revised TNM classification system. This system is based on the description of the primary tumor (T), the status of regional lymph nodes (N), and the presence of distant metastases (M). The breast cancer staging system is complex, reflecting the introduction of sentinel node biopsy, the scrutiny of axillary nodes by immunohistochemistry and the polymerase chain reaction (PCR), and evolving views of internal mammary and supraclavicular node metastasis. Staging systems constantly change and reflect current trends in treatment, in changing outcomes after therapy, and new diagnostic technology. A four-part staging system should evolve toward an even distribution of likely outcomes (a survival rate of 100%, 75%, and so forth).

Because the 2002 system is complicated and may not apply to common practice in every hospital, readers should refer to the published staging tables, available in print and on the Internet (*www.cancerstaging.org*). Table 32-6 presents the TNM working guide, and stage groups are shown in Table 32-7. To use these guides, practitioners determine descriptors for the tumor (T), regional nodes (N), and the presence of metastatic disease (M). The current system attempts to incorporate the use of advanced technology, particularly in the evaluation of nodes removed by sentinel node biopsy. These newer techniques are not widely used nor approved and should be viewed as experimental. Immunohistochemistry uses antibodies against epithelial cell markers, such as keratins expressed in mammary gland cells, to find microscopic deposits of tumor cells in lymph nodes. PCR refers to the polymerase chain reaction, which amplifies extant RNA transcripts unique to epithelial cells, and is used to detect minute components of epithelial cells in nodes, which escape routine detection. The significance of these findings, for both immunohistochemistry and PCR, is not certain and these techniques should be used with caution. Furthermore, the use of sentinel node biopsy for evaluation of internal mammary nodes is not widely practiced and is uncertain. The current AJCC staging system recognizes the uncertainty of these new techniques. For instance, lymph nodes containing microscopic clusters of cells less than 0.2 mm (approximately 20 cells across) found by immunohistochemistry are still considered N0 lymph nodes. Until proven otherwise, practitioners are urged to rely on standard histologic evaluation of axillary lymph nodes and avoid sentinel biopsy of other regional nodes, unless the clinical situation dictates otherwise.

As an example of standard usage, consider a patient with a 2.2-cm invasive cancer in the breast and the presence of two positive lymph nodes after a standard level 1 or levels 1 and 2 lymph node dissection. Routine clinical

TABLE 32-6.   American Joint Committee on Cancer Staging System for Breast Cancer, 2002

(p)T (Primary Tumor)

Tis	Carcinoma in situ (lobular or ductal)
T1	Tumor ≤ 2 cm
T1a	Tumor ≥ 0.1 cm; ≤ 0.5 cm
T1b	Tumor >0.5 cm; ≤ 1 cm
T1c	Tumor >1 cm; ≤ 2 cm
T2	Tumor >2 cm; ≤ 5 cm
T3	Tumor >5 cm
T4	Tumor any size with extension to chest wall or skin
T4a	Tumor extending to chest wall (excluding pectoralis)
T4b	Tumor extending to skin with ulceration, edema, satellite nodules
T4c	Both T4a and T4b
T4d	Inflammatory carcinoma

(p)N (Nodes)

N0	No regional node involvement, no special studies
N0(i −)	No regional node involvement, negative IHC
N0(i +)	Negative node(s) histologically, positive IHC
N0(*mol* −)	Negative node(s) histologically, negative PCR
N0(*mol* +)	Negative node(s) histologically, positive PCR
N1	Metastasis to 1–3 axillary nodes *and/or* int. mammary positive by biopsy
N1(mic)	Micrometastasis (>0.2 mm, none >2.0 mm)
N1a	Metastasis to 1–3 axillary nodes
N1b	Metastasis in int. mammary by sentinel biopsy
N1c	Metastasis to 1–3 axillary nodes *and* int. mammary by biopsy
N2	Metastasis to 4–9 axillary nodes *or* int. mammary clinically positive, without axillary metastasis
N2a	Metastasis to 4–9 axillary nodes, at least 1 >2.0 mm
N2b	Int. mammary clinically apparent, negative axillary nodes
N3	Metastasis to ≥ 10 axillary nodes *or* combination of axillary and int. mammary metastasis
N3a	≥ 10 axillary nodes (>2.0 mm), or infraclavicular nodes
N3b	Positive int. mammary clinically with ≥ 1 axillary node *or* >3 positive axillary nodes with int. mammary positive by biopsy
N3c	Metastasis to ipsilateral supraclavicular nodes

M (Metastasis)

M0	No distant metastasis
M1	Distant metastasis

(p), pathologic staging of the tumor or axillary nodes; IHC, immunohistochemistry; PCR, polymerase chain reaction; int. mammary, internal mammary lymph nodes.

TABLE 32-7.   American Joint Committee on Cancer Stage Grouping

Stage	TNM
0	Tis, N0, M0
I	T1, N0, M0
IIA	T0, N1, M0
	T1, N1, M0
	T2, N0, M0
IIB	T2, N1, M0
	T3, N0, M0
IIIA	T0, N2, M0
	T1, N2, M0
	T2, N2, M0
	T3, N1, M0
	T3, N2, M0
IIIB	T4, N0, M0
	T4, N1, M0
	T4, N2, M0
IIIC	Any T, N3, M0
IV	Any T, any N, M1

studies rule out clinically apparent metastasis. In this case, the T score is T2, the N score is N1, and the M score is M0. Consultation of the Stage Grouping (see Table 32-7) places this hypothetical patient in the stage II category. If the staging system performs as desired, standard current treatment should yield a cure rate in the range of 50%. In fact, review of the results of clinical trials conducted in the last 25 years does yield an outcome measurement in this range (see later). It is important to recognize that this is an estimate and an average outcome; treatment responses vary, treatments for breast cancer are changing, and every patient, and her tumor, is individual.

In the modern era of adjuvant therapy, it is helpful to review the natural history of patients with operable cancer treated by surgery alone. A cooperative Natural History Database was established at the NCI in Milan, at the Royal Marsden Hospital, and at the M. D. Anderson Hospital, which included 1971 patients carefully staged and followed up for at least 10 years. These patients, with modern stage I or II breast cancer, underwent either radical or modified radical mastectomy before 1975, when adjuvant chemotherapy was first widely used. Figure 32-10 displays the overall survival results by Kaplan-Meier estimation and shows the effect of tumor size (T) and

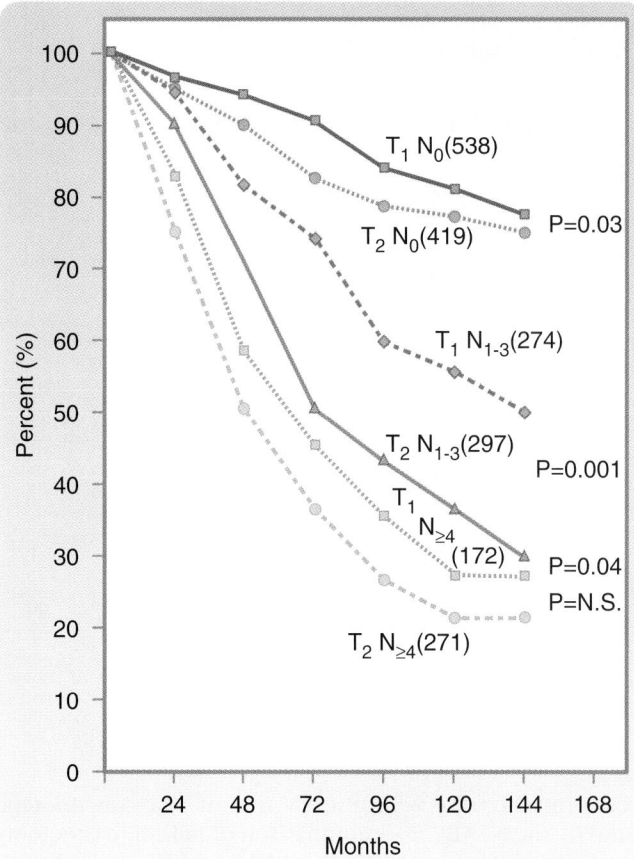

FIGURE 32-10. Survival by nodal status and by tumor size. These data are from a natural history database of 1971 patients treated at three large centers in the United States and Europe. None of these patients received postoperative systemic therapy (hormones or chemotherapy), and these results serve as a reference for comparison to modern trials, presented later in the chapter. (From Moon TE, et al: Development of a natural history data base of breast cancer studies. In Jones SE, Salmon SE (eds): Adjuvant Therapy of Cancer IV. Orlando, Grune & Stratton, 1984.)

nodal status (N). Metastasis to ipsilateral axillary nodes predicts outcome after surgical treatment more powerfully than tumor size. This relationship between nodal status and outcome is underscored by a survey of the management and survival of female breast cancer sponsored by the American College of Surgeons. Five-year end results of absolute survival and recurrence were tabulated in this survey, according to the number of pathologically positive axillary nodes, and revealed an almost linear decrement in survival rate with increasing nodal involvement (Table 32-8).

The survival of patients presenting with locally advanced or metastatic disease is heterogeneous. The median survival rate of patients with stage IV metastatic disease is 24 months or less from time of diagnosis but may vary considerably. Stage III disease is also heterogeneous and includes women with large tumors (>5 cm in size), inflammatory cancers (T4d), or fixed nodes (N2). Modern treatment for these cancers usually involves preoperative systemic chemotherapy, surgery, and postoperative radiation.

MODERN SURGICAL TREATMENT FOR BREAST CANCER

Brief Introduction to Breast Cancer[26]

Among women, the three most common cancers are those of the breast, the lung and bronchus, and the colon and rectum. In men, cancer of the prostate is the most common malignancy, with lung and colorectal cancers following. Cancers of the breast, lung, and colon and rectum account for 55% of the new cases of malignancy in women, and breast cancer alone is responsible for 32% of the cancer burden in women. In the United States, there were 211,300 new cases of breast cancer diagnosed in 2003. Because of the changing demographics in the United States (aging of the "baby boom" generation), combined with the increased incidence of breast cancer in older women, the prevalence of breast cancer will increase dramatically in the next decade. Surgical practitioners can expect to diagnose and treat larger numbers of women, and men, with this disease.

Cancer is the leading cause of death in women aged 40 to 79, in contrast to the burden of cardiovascular disease in men. Breast cancer alone is the most common cause of death in women aged 40 to 49, and the most common cause of cancer death in women for 4 decades, between age 20 and 59. In the year 2003, there were 39,800 deaths due to cancer of the breast in women. As a percentage of new cases, this is less than 20% of the new cases in the same year. Although this proportion is diluted by cases of noninvasive, in situ cancers, the mortality due to breast cancer has been decreasing in recent years, owing in part to early diagnosis and to improvements in treatment.

For early stages of breast cancer, surgical removal provides a reasonable chance for cure. Although the approach to operable breast cancer has changed dramatically over the past century, so, too, has the clinical presentation of breast tumors. In 1894, Halsted presented his first 50 patients treated by the "complete operation," which became the radical mastectomy. Over the next 75 years, radical mastectomy was used to treat virtually every breast malignancy operated on for cure in the United States. Examination of Halsted's first cases found at least two thirds with locally advanced disease and 60% with clinically evident axillary nodal metastases. By comparison, a 1980 survey by the American College of Surgeons found that 85% of patients presented with stage I or II disease. The frequency of cases with positive axillary lymph nodes was 40%, and by the 1970s the average tumor presenting for surgical treatment measured 2 cm. or less. In addition to these fundamental changes, realization that 90% of treatment failures will be systemic or visceral recurrences has led surgeons to explore alternatives to radical mastectomy.

Surgical Procedures, Past and Present[2,3]

In 1982, the American College of Surgeons investigated surgical practice in cases of operable breast cancer and compared results with practice in earlier years. A change in surgical practice occurred in the mid 1970s, with an

TABLE 32-8.   Five-Year End-Results (Absolute Survival, Cure, and Recurrence Rates) in 20,547 Patients With Breast Cancer According to Number of Pathologically Positive Axillary Nodes*

Positive Axillary Lymph Nodes (n)	Total Observed	Survival (%)	Cure (%)	Recurrence (%)
0	12,299	71.8	59.7	19.4
1	2,012	63.1	48.4	32.9
2	1,338	62.2	45.4	39.9
3	842	58.8	39.3	43.0
4	615	51.9	38.4	43.9
5	478	46.9	29.1	54.2
6–10	1,261	40.7	23.0	63.4
11-15	562	29.4	14.8	71.5
16-20	301	28.9	13.3	75.1
21+	225	22.2	9.8	82.2
All nodes or some nodes positive	614	40.4	26.9	58.6
Total, positive nodes	8,248	50.9	35.0	49.2

*Excluding cases with distant metastasis.
From Nemoto T, Vana J, Bedwani RN, et al: Management and survival of female breast cancer: Results of a national survey by the American College of Surgeons. Cancer 45:2917-2924, 1980.

abrupt shift from radical mastectomy to modified radical mastectomy. Procedures that preserved the breast, as described later, were performed in only 7.2% of cases in this survey. Current estimates of conservative breast procedures range between 40% and 60%, and this procedure continues to increase in popularity. The approach to the axillary nodes is also evolving. Many specialists are becoming more selective about the need for axillary dissection, and the use of sentinel node biopsy is replacing routine axillary dissection for women with clinically negative lymph nodes. The following paragraphs describe procedures in widespread use.

Radical Mastectomy

Radical mastectomy is a procedure that is rarely performed but remains the basis of several important clinical trials and registries of women treated by surgery only. In the radical mastectomy, the breast and underlying pectoralis muscles are sacrificed and regional lymph nodes along the axillary vein to the costoclavicular ligament (Halsted's ligament) are removed. This procedure may require a skin graft and uses incisions placed either vertically or obliquely. Prosthetic reconstruction is impossible unless muscle flaps are mobilized to cover the anterior chest defect.

Cure of breast cancer can be achieved by this procedure, as shown in Figure 32-10 from a natural history database of surgically treated patients. The personal series of Haagensen reports results from treatment of 1036 patients; 727 patients with clinically negative nodes (stage A, Columbia clinical staging) had a survival of 72.4% at 10 years. In contrast, only 42.3% of clinically node–positive patients (stage B) survived at 10 years. These figures were

confirmed by the NSABP early trial of adjuvant thiotepa and by the NSABP B0-4 comparison of radical mastectomy to total mastectomy with or without radiation (see later). In the trial of adjuvant chemotherapy, 76% of patients with histologically positive nodes suffered recurrence of breast cancer and one fourth of patients with negative nodes failed surgical treatment after 10 years of follow-up. In contrast, *local failure* rates are low, generally between 5% and 7%.

Modern Mastectomy

These procedures include total or simple mastectomy and the modified radical mastectomy. The boundaries of these two operations are depicted in Figure 32-11. *Mastectomy* refers to complete removal of the mammary gland, including the nipple and areola. An elliptical skin incision is used, as shown in Figure 32-11*A*. A variable amount of surrounding skin is sacrificed, depending on the location, size, and characteristics of the primary tumor. For highly selected patients with small tumors, some surgeons perform a "skin-sparing mastectomy," in which only the nipple-areolar complex is removed. Skin flaps are raised to separate the underlying gland from the overlying skin, as shown in Figure 32-11*B* and *C*. The gland is separated from the underlying pectoralis muscle in a plane just under the pectoral fascia and over the fibers of the muscle and swept off laterally. Division of the gland from the axillary contents, shown in Figure 32-11*B*, defines the extent of a simple mastectomy. Extension of the operation under the pectoralis major muscle and extending up to the axillary vein, removing the axillary lymph nodes, is called a *modified radical mastectomy*. This procedure is depicted in Figure 32-11*C*, showing further retraction of the pec-

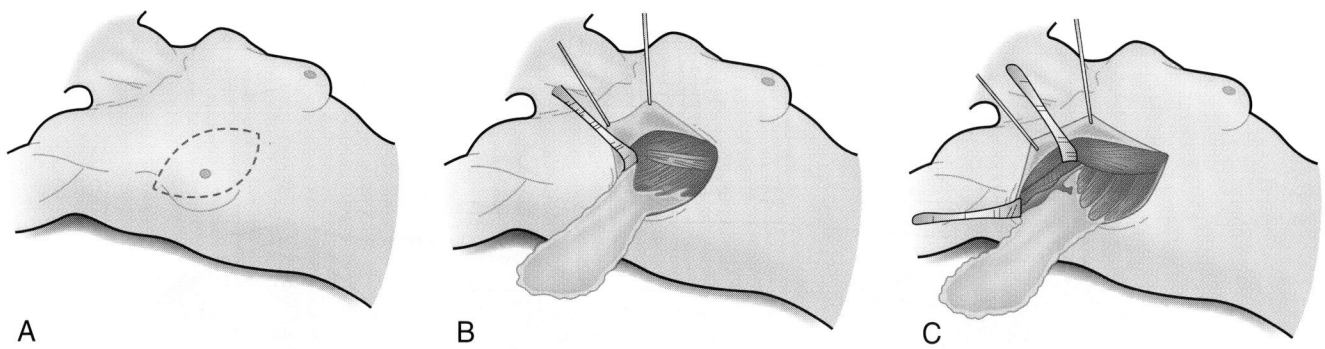

A   **B**   **C**

■ **FIGURE 32-11.** Total mastectomy with and without axillary dissection. **A,** Skin incisions are generally transverse and surround the central breast and nipple-areolar complex. **B,** Skin flaps are raised sharply, separating the gland from the overlying skin, and then the gland from the underlying muscle. Simple mastectomy divides the breast from the axillary contents and stops at the clavipectoral fascia. **C,** In the modified radical mastectomy, dissection continues into the axilla and generally extends up to the axillary vein, removing the level I or level I and II nodes. Division of a branch of the axillary vein is shown in this panel, separating the node-bearing axillary fat from the axillary vein at the superior aspect of the dissection.

toralis major muscle and exposure of the axillary vein. The level I nodes are those inferior to the axillary vein and lateral to the pectoralis minor muscle. With the pectoralis major and minor retracted medially, the level II nodes are exposed under the pectoralis minor. A modified radical mastectomy includes level I or levels I and II lymph nodes. Studies have shown that finding 10 lymph nodes in the axillary tissues (found and assessed by the pathologist), provides a suitable specimen to accurately stage the axillary nodes. The important distinction of the modern operation from the radical mastectomy is preservation of the pectoralis major muscle and, in general, a less extensive axillary procedure.

Two forms of the modified radical mastectomy are in use by surgeons: the Patey procedure and modifications described by Scanlon and the procedure described by Auchincloss. Patey, at the Middlesex Hospital in London, developed a procedure that preserves the pectoralis major muscle and sacrifices the underlying pectoralis minor muscle to remove levels I, II, and III lymph nodes in the axilla. A large number of Patey procedures performed by Handley, who wrote extensively about this procedure, were reviewed independently and reported by Donegan and associates. The survival of patients with negative axillary nodes was 82% at 10 years with a local recurrence rate of 5%. For patients with positive nodes, the survival was 48%, similar to results with radical mastectomy. Thus, preservation of the pectoralis major muscle did not produce inferior results. Scanlon modified the Patey procedure by dividing but not removing the pectoralis minor muscle, allowing removal of apical (level III) nodes and preservation of the lateral pectoral nerves to the major muscle.

The procedure described by Auchincloss differs from the Patey procedure by not removing or dividing the pectoralis minor muscle. This modification limits the complete removal of high axillary nodes but is justified by Auchincloss, who calculated that only 2% of patients benefit by removal of the highest-level nodes. It is probable that the Auchincloss mastectomy was the most popular procedure for breast cancer in the United States during the past decade.

Wide Local Excision and Primary Radiation Therapy

Excision of the primary tumor with preservation of the breast has been referred to by many names, including *partial mastectomy, segmentectomy,* or *lumpectomy.* *Wide local excision* seems to be the most descriptive term for the procedure, which removes the malignancy with a surrounding rim of grossly normal breast parenchyma. An even more aggressive local procedure designed to remove 1 to 2 cm of adjacent breast and overlying skin is called *quadrantectomy.* In modern practice, these more limited surgical procedures are applied as part of a multidisciplinary approach to breast cancer and nearly always includes postoperative radiation therapy, giving at least 4500 cGy to the whole breast and frequently including an additional boost of radiation to the excision site (the tumor bed). This procedure is depicted in Figure 32-12*A,* which shows the completed lumpectomy and the skin incision for the axillary component of the procedure.

Surgery to remove ipsilateral lymph nodes (axillary node dissection) continues to evolve in the United States. The purpose of removing nodes is twofold. First, removal of 10 or more nodes provides protection against future recurrence of cancer in those nodes (local control of breast cancer). Second, removal of 10 or more lymph nodes provides accurate information about the stage of the cancer, as described earlier, and about prognosis as documented in Table 32-8. Today, sentinel lymph node biopsy is used increasingly to provide staging information and guides the selective use of addition regional therapy. A positive sentinel node biopsy is an indication for either further node surgery or radiation (the use of sentinel node biopsy is described in detail later).

Axillary dissection is done through a separate incision in the majority of patients undergoing breast conservation. As shown in Figure 32-12*A,* the extent of the dissection is identical to the axillary component of the

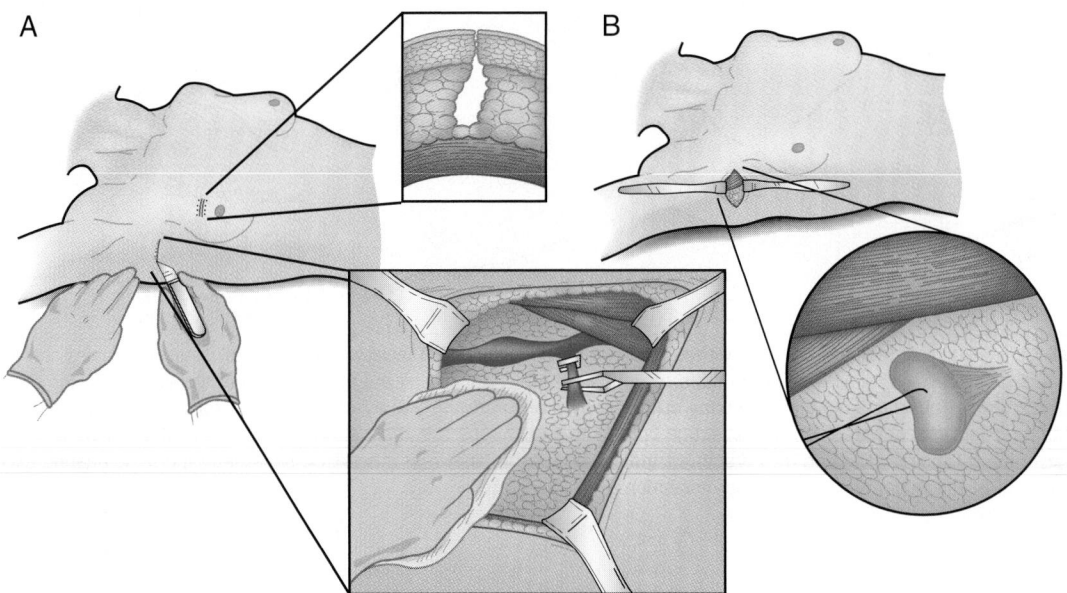

FIGURE 32-12. Breast-conserving surgery. **A,** Incisions to remove malignant tumors are placed directly over the tumor, without tunneling. A transverse incision in the low axilla is used for either the sentinel node biopsy or the axillary dissection. The axillary dissection is identical to the procedure in a modified radical mastectomy. The boundaries of the operation are the axillary vein superiorly, the latissimus dorsi muscle laterally, and the chest wall medially. The inferior dissection should enter the tail of Spence (the axillary tail) of the breast. The *inset* shows the excision cavity of the lumpectomy; no attempt is made to approximate the sides of the cavity, which fills with serous fluid and shrinks gradually. **B,** In the sentinel node biopsy, a similar transverse incision is made (it may be located by percutaneous mapping with the gamma probe if radiolabeled colloid is used) and extended through the clavipectoral fascia and the true axilla entered. The sentinel node is located by virtue of its staining with dye or radioactivity, or both, and dissected free as a single specimen.

modified radical mastectomy. Sentinel node biopsy (described later, and depicted in Fig. 32-12*B*) is replacing anatomic axillary node dissection. Therefore, *conservative breast surgery* or *breast preservation* usually refers to wide local excision of the primary tumor, whole breast radiation, and a separate axillary dissection and/or sentinel node biopsy.

Older Surgical Trials of Local Therapy for Operable Breast Cancer[27]

In 1971, the NSABP initiated a large prospective trial to examine different approaches to the local and regional control of breast cancer. NSABP B-04 used radical mastectomy as its control arm and randomized patients with and without clinically positive axillary lymph nodes to receive alternative approaches to regional lymph nodes. Patients with clinically negative nodes were randomized to one of three treatment regimens: *Arm 1*, Halsted's radical mastectomy (362 patients); *Arm 2*, total mastectomy (simple mastectomy) with radiation treatment of the ipsilateral nodes (352 patients); and *Arm 3*, total mastectomy alone with delayed axillary dissection if nodes became enlarged (365 patients). Clinically node-positive patients were randomly allocated to two randomized arms: *Arm 1*, radical mastectomy (292 patients) or *Arm*

2, total mastectomy with radiation of the enlarged nodes (294 patients). This study is widely cited for its contribution to understanding the significance of axillary and regional nodal metastases.

A final update of NSABP B-04 was published in 2002, with complete 25-year follow-up for the entire study. No significant differences in either overall survival or disease-free survival were noted for 1079 clinically node–negative patients treated by random allocation to radical mastectomy, total mastectomy plus nodal radiation, or total mastectomy and delayed axillary dissection. Likewise, for 586 clinically node–positive patients receiving either radical mastectomy or total mastectomy and nodal radiation, survival and recurrence statistics were identical (Fig. 32-13). The only differences were local and regional failures experienced by clinically node–negative patients. Patients receiving radical mastectomy or total mastectomy plus regional radiation had local failures of less than 10%, whereas about 15% of those treated by mastectomy experienced only local or regional recurrence as a first event. Several important conclusions have been reached as a result of this ground-breaking study:

1. Variations in local and regional treatments that involve total mastectomy do not alter the frequency or pattern of distant treatment failures. Although local treatment failures are influenced, overall survival is unaffected.

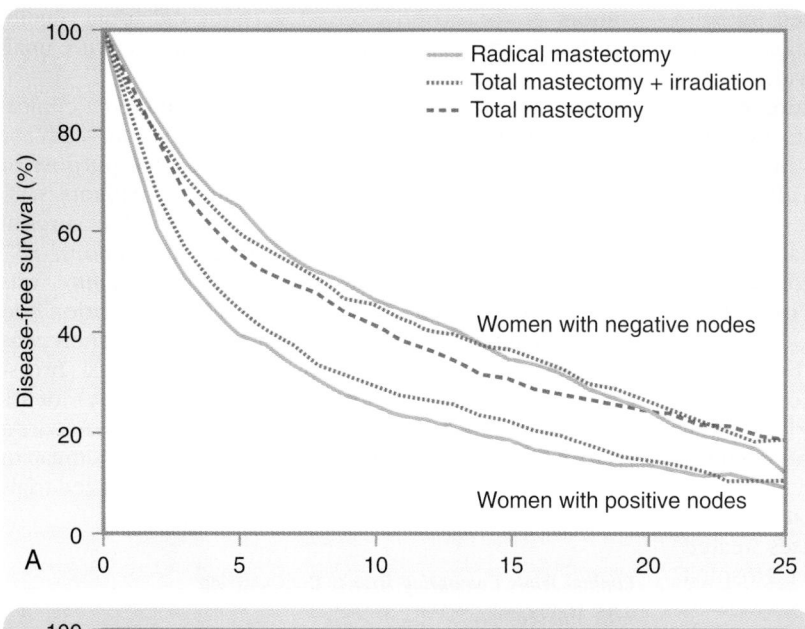

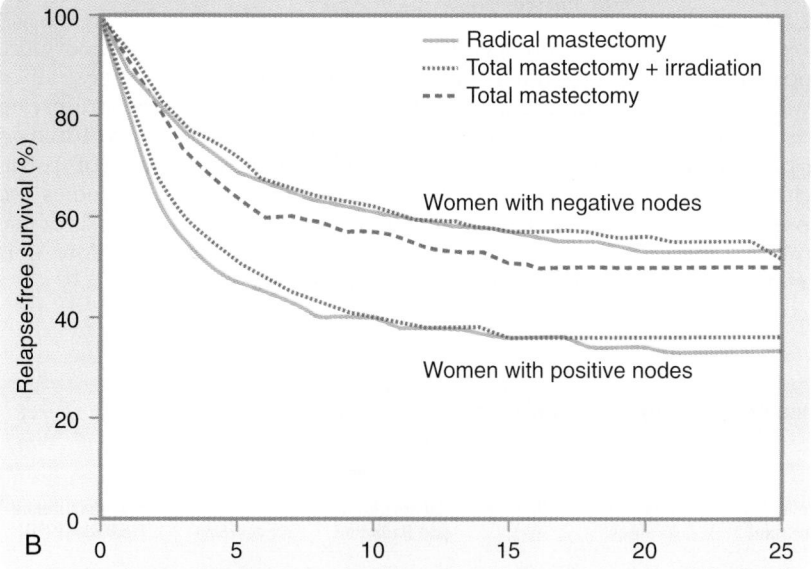

FIGURE 32-13. Disease-free survival (**A**) and relapse-free survival (**B**) at 25 years of continuous follow-up after surgery in NSABP B-04. There were no differences in the experience of three randomized groups of clinically node–negative patients and of two randomized groups of clinically node–positive patients. (**A** and **B**, From Fisher B, Jeong J-H, Anderson S, et al: Twenty-five-year follow-up of a randomized trial comparing radical mastectomy, total mastectomy, and total mastectomy followed by irradiation. N Engl J Med 347:567-575, 2002. Copyright 2002, Massachusetts Medical Society.)

2. The mode and time of treatment of axillary nodes do not alter disease-free survival or overall survival. Immediate removal, delayed removal, or radiation produced equivalent clinical results. However, removal and enumeration of positive lymph nodes provide the best indication of eventual relapse.

3. Results of breast cancer treatment trials can reliably be assessed at 5 years; however, 25% of distant recurrences occurred after 5 years, and 50% of contralateral breast cancers were detected during follow-up 5 years or longer from treatment of the incident breast cancer. After 10 years, there were few recurrences. Patients with positive nodes who were free of disease at 5 years had about the same probability of remaining disease-free as did the negative-node group.

4. The location of the primary tumor in the breast does not influence outcome. Furthermore, there was no justification for irradiation of internal mammary nodes solely based on the medial location of the breast cancer.

The Shift to Breast-Conserving Procedures[2,28]

The gradual shift away from radical surgery toward breast and soft tissues preservation was influenced by the results of several large trials of lesser surgical procedures. These influential studies are also valuable for the information they contain about the biology of breast cancer progression. The concept of breast-conserving treatment (BCT) refers to wide excision of the cancer, leaving the breast largely intact, with or without postsurgical radiation therapy and with or without surgery on axillary nodes (see Fig. 32-12).

Progress toward modern BCT began with individual surgeons and small, and sometimes bold, departures from contemporary norms. In 1928, Sir William Keynes at St. Bartholomew's Hospital in London reported leaving the tumor in situ, without surgery, and treating it with only radiation. Calle and colleagues at the Foundation Curie in France reported disease-free survival of 43% at 10 years for patients with tumors 3 cm or larger treated initially by radiation only. These results were confirmed in large series of patients from France; however, up to 55% of these patients required secondary surgery for persistent or recurrent disease. There seems to be little justification for leaving invasive cancer in the breast unless it technically cannot be removed (as with locally advanced or inflammatory cancers) or unless the patient has documented metastatic disease that is considered more immediately threatening. There are no clinical trials that omit surgical excision of early-stage breast cancers.

Noncontrolled series of patients treated by limited surgery with or without radiation followed. Cope, Crile, Adair, and others demonstrated the possibility that excision alone of certain breast cancers did result in long-term cures. Patients undergoing very limited surgery had local recurrence rates that generally exceeded 20% at intervals of 3 to 5 years. In a series of more than 800 cases treated without mastectomy at the Princess Margaret Hospital between 1958 and 1980, 177 were treated by excision without radiation. One hundred four tumors treated in this fashion were small T1 (<2 cm) lesions. Most patients receiving conservative treatment received postsurgical radiation to the breast, with or without radiation of regional nodal groups. At 5 years, there was an 8.7% relapse rate in the breast treated by excision plus radiation. Patients who underwent excision only, with no radiation, experienced an ipsilateral breast relapse rate of 24.9%. By 10 years, local failure had occurred in 13.3% and 28.3%, respectively, despite the preponderance of smaller tumors in the group excised without radiation. Significantly, distant relapse and overall survival rate were unaffected by the choice of local therapy.

The province of Ontario, Canada, conducted a clinical trial of lumpectomy and axillary dissection with or without postoperative radiation therapy. One purpose of this study was to identify a subgroup of patients who might be spared breast irradiation after complete surgical excision of the ipsilateral breast cancer. Among 837 patients randomized, the ipsilateral breast failure was 25.7% in the patients who did not receive radiation and was reduced to 5.5% in the irradiated patients. There was no subgroup of patients with sufficiently low-risk breast cancers (e.g., small tumors, low histologic grade) identified that could be spared radiation and still maintain a relapse rate of less than 5%. These results are similar in magnitude and direction to prospective, randomized trials of breast-conserving surgery and mastectomy.

Clinical Trials Comparing Breast Conservation with Mastectomy[29-31]

Seven prospective clinical trials have randomized more than 4500 patients to various surgical strategies, all of which include a mastectomy arm and a breast-preserving arm. Six trials using modern radiotherapy are listed in Table 32-9, including survival figures and rates of ipsilateral breast recurrences. Endpoints of these studies are local failure, distant failure, and survival. A synopsis of five trials with between 10 and 25 years of actual follow-up is included in the following sections.

TABLE 32-9. Prospective Trials Comparing Mastectomy with Lumpectomy Plus or Minus Radiation

Surgical Trial	No. of Patients (n)	Maximum Tumor Size (cm)	Systemic Therapy	Follow-up (yr)	Survival (%) Lumpectomy and Radiation	Mastectomy	Local Recurrence (radiation) (%)
NSABP B-06[1]	1851	4	Yes	20	47	46	14*
Milan Cancer Institute[2]	701	2	Yes	20	44	43	8.8*
Institute Gustave-Roussy[3]	179	2	No		73	65	13
National Cancer Institute, U.S.[4]	237	5	Yes	10	77	75	16
European Organization for Research and Treatment of Cancer (EORTC)[5]	868	5	Yes	10	65	66	17.6
Danish Breast Cancer Group[6]	905	None	Yes	6	79	82	3

[1]Data from Fisher B, Anderson S, Bryant J, et al: Twenty-year follow-up of a randomized trial comparing total mastectomy, lumpectomy, and lumpectomy plus irradiation for the treatment of invasive breast cancer. N Engl J Med 347:1233, 2002.
[2]Data from Veronesi U, Cascinelli N, Mariani L, et al: Twenty-year follow-up of a randomized study comparing breast-conserving surgery with radical mastectomy for early breast cancer. N Engl J Med 347:1227, 2002.
[3]Data from Arriagada R, Le M, Rochard F, et al: Conservative treatment versus mastectomy in early breast cancer: Patterns of failure with 15 years of follow-up data. J Clin Oncol 14:1558, 1996.
[4]Data from Jacobson J, Danforth D, Cowan K, et al: Ten-year results of a comparison of conservation with mastectomy in the treatment of stage I and II breast cancer. N Engl J Med 332:907, 1995.
[5]Data from van Dongen J, Voogd A, Fentiman I, et al: Long-term results of a randomized trial comparing breast-conserving therapy with mastectomy: European Organization for Research and Treatment of Cancer 10801 Trial. J Natl Cancer Inst 92:1143-1150, 2000.
[6]Data from Blichert-Toft M, Rose C, Andersen J, et al: Danish randomized trial comparing breast conservation therapy with mastectomy: Six years of life-table analysis. Danish Breast Cancer Cooperative Group. J Natl Cancer Inst Monogr 11:19, 1992.
*Includes only women whose excision margins were negative.

NSABP B-06 TRIAL OF MASTECTOMY, LUMPECTOMY, AND LUMPECTOMY WITH RADIATION

This trial began in 1976 and finished accrual in 1984. The trial included women with tumors up to 4 cm in diameter and that had clinically negative lymph nodes. A total of 1851 patients were randomized to receive a modified radical mastectomy, a lumpectomy alone, or a lumpectomy with postoperative radiation to the breast but without an extra boost to the lumpectomy site. All patients with histologically positive axillary nodes received chemotherapy with melphalan (an older alkylating agent) and fluorouracil. With 25 years of follow-up, final results were reported in 2002. Overall survival was the same in all three randomly assigned arms, with about 46% of women surviving at 25 years. Disease-free survival (survival without a recurrence of breast cancer) was also the same across the entire trial and about 35% for the three groups. These outcomes are depicted over 20 years of follow-up in Figure 32-14. As much a test of treatment strategies, the long-term results offer a modern look at overall and disease-specific outcome of stages I and II breast cancer. For pathologically node-negative women, death after recurrence of breast cancer occurred in 32% of women (with equal distribution among treatment selection). For pathologically node-positive women, death with breast cancer occurred in 54.2% of women. In both groups, breast cancer recurrence included women with new contralateral cancers.

The emphasis of NSABP B-06 was on the incidence of ipsilateral breast cancer recurrence in women treated by BCT, with or without breast radiation. At 20 years of follow-up, 14.3% of women treated with lumpectomy and radiation suffered a recurrence of cancer in the treated breast and 39.2% of women treated only with lumpectomy suffered a recurrence ($P = 0.001$ for the difference, shown in Fig. 32-15). For patients with positive nodes, the recurrence in the treated breast was 44.2% for lumpectomy only compared to 8.8% for women receiving postoperative radiation. For women receiving modern BCT with radiation, a useful number to remember is a recurrence rate of about 0.5% to 1% per year of follow-up, with a steady rate of events (recurrences and new cancers) over 20 years. For women treated by BCT, follow-up of the breast should be continued for an indefinite period; there is no point at which women with a conserved breast reach a baseline level of breast cancer risk.

MILAN CANCER INSTITUTE TRIAL OF BREAST-CONSERVING SURGERY

This trial in Italy was begun in 1973 and finished accrual in 1980. Twenty-five-year results were published in 2002. It is quite different from the NSABP trial in American women. The Italian trial employed more extensive surgery and advocated use of a quadrantectomy, which removes a large amount of breast tissue and overlying skin to achieve widely clear margins around the cancer. Furthermore, cancers in the Italian trial were smaller than in the American work; the Milan trial permitted only tumors up to 2 cm in size, and all patients with palpable lymph nodes in the ipsilateral axilla were excluded. Seven hundred one women were randomly divided to receive radical mastectomy (349) verses quadrantectomy plus postoperative

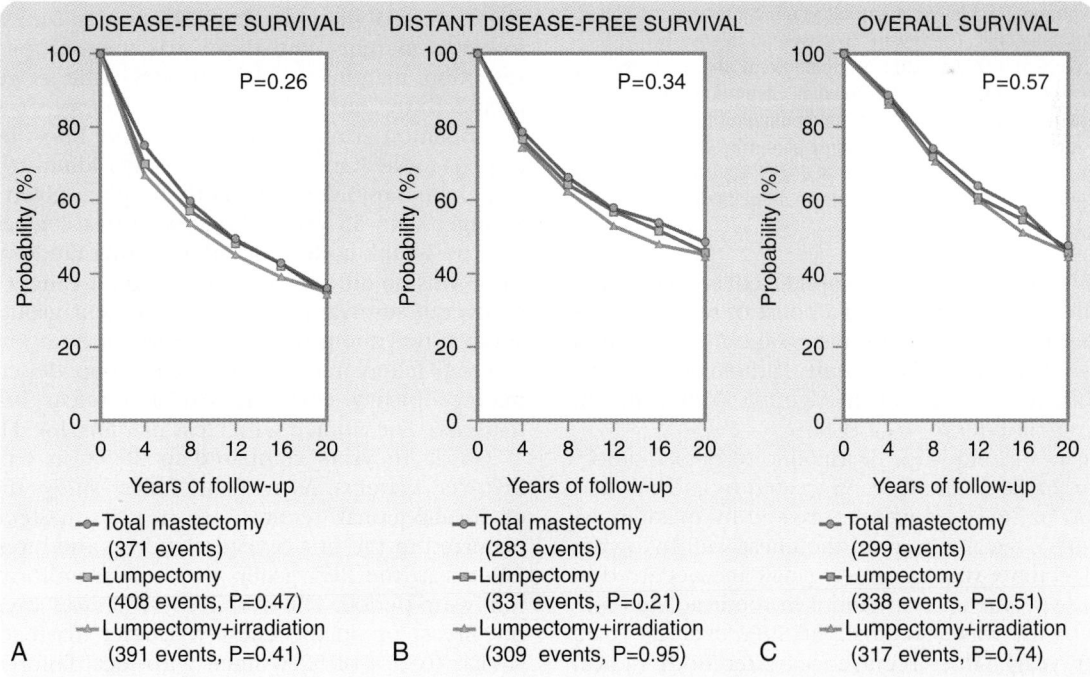

FIGURE 32-14. Disease-free survival (**A**), distant disease-free survival (**B**) and overall survival (**C**) after 20 years of follow-up in the NSABP Protocol B-06. There were no significant differences in the three randomized arms of this trial. (**A** to **C**, From Fisher B, Anderson S, Bryant J, et al: Twenty-year follow-up of a randomized trial comparing total mastectomy, lumpectomy, and lumpectomy plus irradiation for the treatment of invasive breast cancer. N Engl J Med 347:1237, 2002. Copyright 2002 Massachusetts Medical Society.)

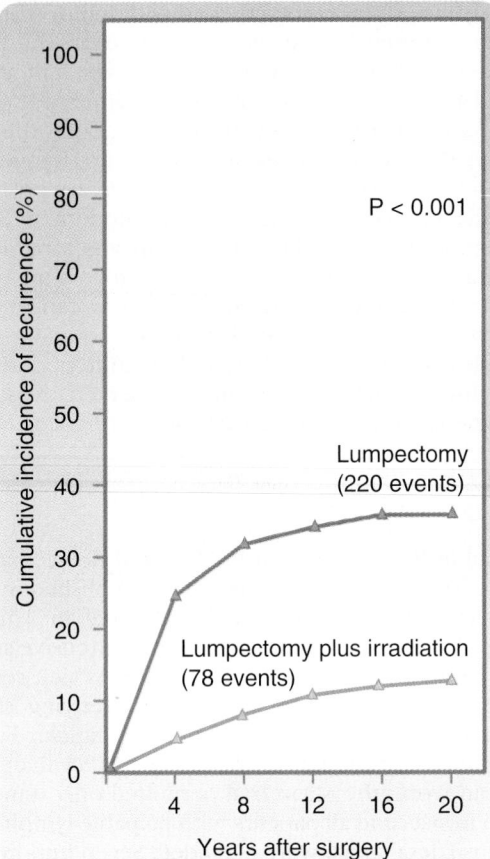

FIGURE 32-15. Cumulative incidence of a first recurrence of cancer in the treated, conserved breast during 20 years of follow-up in the NSABP Protocol B-06. The data presented here are for those patients achieving a pathologically tumor-free margin after lumpectomy. There were 570 women treated by lumpectomy alone and 567 treated by lumpectomy and ipsilateral breast radiation. (From Fisher B, Anderson S, Bryant J, et al: Twenty-year follow-up of a randomized trial comparing total mastectomy, lumpectomy, and lumpectomy plus irradiation for the treatment of invasive breast cancer. N Engl J Med 347:1233, 2002. Copyright 2002 Massachusetts Medical Society.)

radiation (352 received BCT). Complete axillary dissection was done in the BCT group, and a boost of radiation was given to the tumor bed, in contrast to the American trial that used whole breast radiation only. Pathologically node-positive patients received chemotherapy with cytoxan, methotrexate, and fluorouracil (CMF).

At 20 years of follow-up, deaths due to breast cancer occurred in 24.3% of the women treated by radical mastectomy and in 26.1% of women treated by quadrantectomy ($P = 0.8$). Local failure on the chest wall following radical mastectomy was extremely small and occurred in 2.3% of these women. Local failure in the irradiated and conserved breast was also small, at 8.8% over 20 years (<1/2% per year). Most recurrences after both radical mastectomy and BCT occurred in the first 5 years; thereafter, the event-rate in the conservatively treated group exceeded radical mastectomy. This implies the most aggressive cancers, persisting after both radical surgery and after radiation, became evident early on. Thereafter,

the majority of events were new breast cancers in the conserved breast. Contralateral breast cancer rates were identical at about 0.66% per year for all women, contradicting the hypothesis that radiation increases the incidence of contralateral cancers. Overall survival at 20 years was 41.2% in the group treated with radical mastectomy and 41.7% in the quadrantectomy group ($P = 1.0$).

The chest wall recurrence rate of 2.3% in the radical mastectomy group represents a lower target level of local failures in surgically treated women; modern rates of local failure in patients treated by modified radical mastectomy are in the range of 5%. However, at least some patients with local failure have aggressive cancers that resist all attempts at control, a local recurrence rate of 2.3% after mastectomy is probably a true biologic floor. The local failure in the conserved breast of women treated by quadrantectomy is highly dependent on age in the Italian series. Failure in women younger than 45 years of age was 1% per year, whereas for older women the failure in the breast was 0.5% per year.

EUROPEAN ORGANIZATION FOR RESEARCH AND TREATMENT OF CANCER TRIAL

This was another large trial and compared two modern treatments for breast cancer from 1980 until 1986. The trial compared modified radical mastectomy to a lumpectomy and post-operative breast radiation (BCT). Ten-year results from the European Organization for Research and Treatment of Cancer (EORTC) 10801 Trial were reported in 2001. The peculiar difference of this trial was the inclusion of women with large breast cancers (≤5 cm). In fact, 80% of women had tumors larger than 2.0 cm. Furthermore, the trial did not specify re-excision for even grossly involved margins, and there was microscopic tumor at resection margins in 217 of 448 patients receiving a lumpectomy and radiation. The majority of women in the radiation group did receive a large boost of radiation (25 Gy) to the lumpectomy site using iridium 192 implants (brachytherapy). CMF chemotherapy was given to women younger than 55 years of age with histologically proven positive lymph nodes. As with the other randomized trials, there was no difference in either breast cancer metastasis or overall survival in the two treatment groups. Overall survival was about 65% at 10 years for both groups.

Local failure rates in the BCT group depended on a microscopically complete excision (clear lumpectomy margins). For women with clear margins, local failure was 17.6% at 10 years compared to 26.5% in women with involved margins. As with the Italian study, the majority of local-regional recurrences in the mastectomy arm occurred in the first 5 years, whereas the rates of breast failures in the BCT group were more uniform over the follow-up period. The overall survival rates after failure in the breast or on the chest wall after mastectomy were similar (63.5% of 52 women with local failure after BCT died during follow-up, and 61% of 28 women with local-regional failure after mastectomy died). Because the EORTC trial involved centers across Europe and England, the effect of treatment variation could be examined. Local failure rates in both the conserved breast and on the chest wall after mastectomy varied widely, from 4.6% to 21.3% after mastectomy and from 10.5% to 36.0% in the conserved breast after BCT. This is a remarkable finding and emphasizes the importance of the initial evaluation and treatment of women with breast cancer. Undoubtedly, experience, technique, and clinical judgment are important components determining treatment outcomes.

INSTITUT GUSTAVE-ROUSSY TRIAL OF BREAST CONSERVATION VERSUS MASTECTOMY

This small study was begun in 1972 and entered patients with tumors less than 2.0 cm until closure in 1979. One hundred seventy-nine patients were randomly allocated to receive either modified radical mastectomy or a complete tumorectomy (lumpectomy) with a generous 2-cm margin of normal tissue around the cancer. In this study, women with pathologically positive lymph nodes in both groups were further randomized to receive nodal irradiation. Patterns of radiotherapy were similar, including an external-beam boost to the tumor bed in the tumorectomy group.

No differences were observed between the two surgical groups for risk of death, metastases, contralateral breast cancer, or local-regional recurrence at 15 years of follow-up time. Survival was about 75% for both groups of patients and was related to prognostic factors determined at the time of surgery. In fact, a prognostic score based on age, tumor size, tumor grade, and the number of involved lymph nodes was the most powerful determinant of overall survival, with an RR for dying of breast cancer of 4.5 for the worst prognostic group as compared to the best group. In contrast to other studies of nodal radiation, this addition to the initial treatment of women with node-positive disease did not result in improved survival or a lower rate of local recurrence.

NATIONAL CANCER INSTITUTE (USA) TRIAL OF BREAST CONSERVATION VERSUS MASTECTOMY

The NCI began a trial in 1979 to compare lumpectomy, axillary dissection, and postoperative radiation therapy to modified radical mastectomy. This was a small study; 237 patients with invasive breast cancer were enrolled into its two arms and included patients with T1 and T2 primary tumors (≤5 cm in size) and with clinically N0 or N1 axillary nodes. The NCI study had statistical power to detect a disease-free survival difference of 15% at 5 years. Results were published in 1995 after a median follow-up of 10 years. No differences were seen in overall survival rates at 10 years (75% for patients receiving lumpectomy and 77% for patients in the mastectomy arm). There were no differences in the 10-year disease-free survival rates (72% for breast conservation patients and 69% for patients randomized to receive mastectomy). The actuarial risk of in-breast relapse for the group undergoing lumpectomy and radiation therapy was 18% at 10 years of follow-up. As with other studies, the risk of relapse in the treated breast appears constant over time and was between 1% and 2% per year after treatment. The complication rate after breast radiation was low, but it was evaluated in the NCI trial. Common complications were rib fracture, chest wall and breast pain, and a higher incidence of seroma formation in the axillary wound or breast lumpectomy site.

SUMMARY AND SUGGESTED GUIDELINES

With the exception of the NCI in America and the EORTC in Europe, four of the six trials in Table 32-9 required negative margins for the lumpectomy specimen. Whole-breast radiation after surgical removal of the primary tumor delivered 45 to 50 Gy in all of these trials. With the exception of the NSABP, six of seven trials used a boost to the tumor location. All of the studies required axillary dissection, and adjuvant chemotherapy was prescribed for most node-positive patients. Follow-up times from 10 to 25 years have elapsed in all of these studies, allowing firm conclusions to be drawn. For patients treated in the last 25 years of the 20th century, 10-year survival for stage I breast cancer is 75% to 80%, and for stage II breast cancer overall survival is 50% to 60% and is not influenced by the choice of breast conservation in place of mastectomy. In the NSABP B-06 trial, lumpectomy alone, without postoperative radiation therapy, was the assigned treatment for 565 patients. After 25 years of actual follow-up, nearly 50% of patients treated in such a fashion suffered ipsilateral breast recurrence even though clear gross and histologic margins were required (although survival was not significantly compromised). The incidence of contralateral breast cancer is not increased in women assigned to receive radiation. In the NCI trial, complications of radiation were infrequent; trials with very long follow-up have not reported radiation complications. Depending on many factors, including tumor size, breast size, location, and preference, patients can safely be offered modified radical mastectomy (with immediate or delayed reconstruction) or wide excision to negative margins and postoperative radiation.

The following are guidelines for counseling patients about breast conservation: Patients can be told the following:

1. The appearance of cancer in the treated breast (recurrence plus new tumors) is steady over many years after treatment and in the range of 1% per year.
2. The cure rate from breast conservation is equal to mastectomy.
3. Complication rates from radiation are low (between 2% and 5%) and include spontaneous rib fracture, transient pericarditis for left-sided cancers, and some added distortion of the breast and tissues around the wide excision.

In our practice at the Brigham and Women's Hospital, the tumor is excised completely if possible, although we do not obtain frozen sections on the excision margins, nor do we use other experimental techniques to monitor margin status. Meticulous hemostasis is obtained in the tumor bed, and no attempt is made to approximate the lumpectomy defect. In the absence of a hematoma, the wound will temporarily fill with serous fluid and slowly contract over a period of several weeks. The specimen that is removed should be oriented and ink applied before it is bisected. If a histologically positive margin is found, reoperation to remove more tissue will frequently achieve a clear margin and allow conservation of the breast. A gross or histologically positive margin is the only unerring contraindication to recommending breast conservation. Extensive intraductal carcinoma may be associated with a higher recurrence rate but does not negate lumpectomy and radiation therapy as long as a negative margin can be obtained.

Postsurgical Radiation Therapy[32]

While the value of radiation therapy as part of breast conservation is not questioned, the addition of radiation after mastectomy is not widely recommended. Recent studies have caused reassessment of radiation therapy to the chest wall and lymph nodes following mastectomy. Two studies from the Danish Breast Cancer Cooperative Group (DBCCG) and one study from British Columbia were influential in altering the approach to women with positive axillary nodes or a high risk for recurrence after mastectomy. The Danish studies examined women with pathologic stage II or III breast cancer. Premenopausal women received adjuvant chemotherapy (DBCCG protocol 82b) and postmenopausal women received adjuvant tamoxifen (protocol 82c). Both age groups were randomized to receive systemic therapy alone or systemic therapy plus chest wall and regional node irradiation. The British Columbia study was confined to premenopausal women with lymph node–positive disease receiving chemotherapy, randomizing these women to receive chemotherapy alone or chemotherapy plus radiation to the chest wall and nodes. Table 32-10 summarizes the results of these three studies. There was both a significant decrease in the rate of local-regional recurrences but also an improvement in overall survival among women receiving the additional radiation in all three trials.

Although these three studies are flawed in ways peculiar to their design and execution, two recent meta-analyses have confirmed their findings. Chest wall and node irradiation after mastectomy reduces the odds of local or regional recurrence. In the analysis from the Early Breast Cancer Trialists (EBCT), this reduction was approximately two thirds and extended across most patients, stages, and radiation methods. Both meta-analyses showed improved breast cancer–specific mortality after radiation. However, in the EBCT analysis, the improved death rates from breast cancer were opposed by increased mortality from other causes, in particular vascular events. In the EBCT, the result of opposing radiation effects was to leave all-cause mortality unchanged by the addition of radiation to surgery. In the analysis from McMaster University there was a survival advantage to radiation after mastectomy, with an odds ratio (OR) of 0.83 (mortality in the radiation groups was 83% of mortality in the mastectomy-only groups).

Many centers now recommend chest wall and nodal irradiation after mastectomy for patients with multiple positive nodes (e.g., >3 nodes positive), for patients with extranodal extension of breast cancer, and for patients with large cancers or very aggressive histology (e.g., diffuse vascular invasion). For women undergoing BCT, postlumpectomy radiation can be extended to include the central axillary nodes (for women with positive sentinel nodes not undergoing axillary dissection) and full regional nodal irradiation for women with high-risk nodal metastases as noted earlier.

Sentinel Lymph Node Biopsy[33,34]

Morton first described the sentinel node in patients with melanoma, defined as the first node to receive lymphatic drainage from the site of the primary tumor. The concept has since been extended to breast cancer; the sentinel node is the first node in the ipsilateral axilla or internal mammary chain to drain the tumor in the breast. The sentinel node is located by injection of technetium-radiolabeled sulfur colloid, isosulfan blue dye, or both. If radiolabeled colloid is used, the node in the axilla is located using a handheld gamma detector. If only blue dye is used to identify the sentinel node, the node is located by meticulous dissection into the axillary space until either a blue-stained node or afferent lymphatic is located.

TABLE 32-10. Trials of Systemic Therapy with or without Radiation after Mastectomy

Radiation Trials	No. of Patients			Local Recurrence Rate (%)			Overall Survival (%)		
	Systemic + Radiation	Systemic Alone	TOTAL	Systemic + Radiation	Systemic Alone	P Value	Systemic + Radiation	Systemic Alone	P Value
DBCG 82b Trial (chemotherapy)[1]	852	856	1708	9	32	<0.001	54	45	<0.001
DBCG 82c Trial (tamoxifen)[2]	686	689	1375	8	35	<0.001	45	38	0.03
British Columbia Trial[3]	164	154	318	13	25	0.003*	64	54	0.003*

[1]Data from Overgaard M, Hansen Per S, Overgaard J, et al: Postoperative radiotherapy in high-risk premenopausal women with breast cancer who receive adjuvant chemotherapy. N Engl J Med 337:949, 1997.
[2]Data from Overgaard M, Jensen M-B, Overgaard J, et al: Postoperative radiotherapy high-risk postmenopausal breast cancer patients given adjuvant tamoxifen: Danish Breast Cancer Cooperative Group DBCG 82c randomized trial. Lancet 353:1641, 1999.
[3]Data from Ragaz J, Jackson S, Le N, et al: Adjuvant radiotherapy and chemotherapy in node-positive premenopausal women with breast cancer. N Engl J Med 337:956,1997.
*Aggregate P value for comparisons at various follow-up intervals; this is the 10-year result.

If the sentinel node is histologically negative, the patient is spared a complete axillary dissection.

This technique is contraindicated for patients with suspicious palpable axillary adenopathy, prior axillary surgery, locally advanced disease, and in the pregnant or lactating woman. There are insufficient data to advocate its use for patients with multicentric breast cancers or following neoadjuvant chemotherapy.

The application of sentinel node mapping to the breast cancer patient is an effort to minimize the complications and side effects that may occur with axillary dissection, including lymphedema, shoulder dysfunction, intercostobrachial nerve injury, injury to the long thoracic or thoracodorsal motor nerves and axillary vein thrombosis. The acceptance of sentinel node biopsy depends on the false-negative rate of the procedure, that is, the chance that positive nodes will be found in the axilla if the sentinel node is negative. A review of the published literature by Cox and colleagues found a worldwide false-negative rate of 3.1%. Investigators in experienced centers performing a large surgical volume have reported even lower rates of missed disease.

Nodal metastases have been termed *macrometastases* if the tumor deposit is larger than 0.2 cm and *micrometastases* if the deposit is 0.2 cm or smaller. This size cut-off was originally chosen because it can be measured on a glass slide with a ruler, it is about the width of a thinly sliced lymph node, and it is the width of tissue that easily fits into a histology cassette. The ability to identify a nodal metastatic deposit is directly proportional to the number of sections performed by the pathologist. Bisecting a node and examining a single slice will enable identification of metastases greater than 0.5 cm, but 14% to 40% of smaller macrometastases may be missed. If the node is sliced every 0.2 to 0.3 cm, and each slice is examined with one hematoxylin and eosin (H&E) stain, all macrometastases are detected, though micrometastases may be missed. This is the method currently recommended by the College of American Pathology. If three equally spaced levels of each slice are evaluated in addition to slicing the node every 0.2 cm, it is likely that 0.1-cm metastases will be found in routine practice. Table 32-11 summarizes the number of levels required per 0.2-cm lymph node slice to identify a metastasis of a given size.

TABLE 32-11. Finding a Metastasis Using Multiple Levels (0.2-cm slice)

Size of Metastasis Detected	No. of Levels Required
>0.2 cm (macro)	1
0.1 cm	3
0.05 cm	6
0.02 cm (~20 cells)	20
Single cell	500

Adapted from Dowlatshahi K, Fan M, Bloom KJ, et al: Occult metastases in the sentinel lymph nodes of patients with early-stage breast carcinoma: A preliminary study. Cancer 86:990, 1999.

In a compilation by the author of 14 peer-reviewed studies, in a cohort of 2046 patients with a positive sentinel node, 873 (43%) had at least one additional positive node (Table 32-12). In a 2001 report by Wong from the University of Louisville, of their 389 patients with a positive sentinel node, 92 (24%) had four or greater positive additional axillary nodes. When the sentinel node contains metastatic disease, the likelihood of additional nodes also containing metastatic disease is directly proportional to the size of the breast primary; the presence of lymphatic vascular invasion; the size of the lymph node metastasis; and, if the node metastasis is a micrometastasis (<2 mm), whether the micrometastasis was detected by H&E or by immunohistochemistry. In the presence of a positive sentinel node, current medical practice dictates additional treatment to the axilla. This is most commonly performed with a completion level I and II axillary dissection. In the context of clinical trials, it is being performed with axillary radiation, omitting the axillary dissection.

The presence of axillary micrometastatic disease is of growing importance in guiding therapy options. In a retrospective study, 373 node-negative patients treated at Memorial Sloan-Kettering Cancer Center between 1976 and 1978 and with a median follow-up of 17 years were identified. Additional evaluation of the lymph nodes was performed to identify those having a micrometastasis by H&E and immunohistochemistry. The breast cancer–specific death rates were reported as 20% for those who were node negative (N = 289), 37% for those who were node positive by immunohistochemistry (N = 28), and 50% for those who were node positive by H&E.

The integration of the sentinel node biopsy into surgical management is being addressed in ongoing prospective clinical trials by the American College of Surgeons (ACOSOG Z0010 and Z0011) and by the NSAPB (B-32).

Ductal Carcinoma In Situ or Intraductal Carcinoma[35,36]

Before modern mammography, DCIS represented less than 5% of newly diagnosed breast cancers. Patients with clinically evident DCIS presented with a palpable mass or asymmetrical thickening, nipple discharge, or Paget's disease of the nipple (as shown in Fig. 32-6). With the advent of screening mammography, between 1973 and 1992 there was a 587% increase in the incidence of DCIS, with most patients identified by a nonpalpable mammographic finding. In women undergoing annual mammography, DCIS represents 20% to 40% of newly diagnosed breast cancers and presents as clustered calcifications without an associated density in 75% of these patients, as calcifications coexisting with an associated density in 15%, and as density alone in 10%. The calcifications seen on a mammogram are deposited within the central necrotic debris in the involved duct. The calcifications tend to cluster closely together; are pleomorphic; and may be linear or branching, suggesting their ductal origin.

Treatment recommendations for patients with DCIS are based on consideration of several factors, including (1) the extent of disease within the breast, (2) the existence of

TABLE 32-12. Sentinel Node Biopsy Positive: Additional Affected Nodes

Study	Year	Site of Study	No. with Positive Sentinel Node	No. (%) with Positive Nonsentinel Node
Sachdev[1]	2002	Mt. Sinai	55	21 (38)
Weiser[2]	2001	Memorial	206	66 (32)
Abdessabum[3]	2001	Ohio State	100	40 (40)
Tafra[4]	2001	Annapolis	326	204 (63)
Wong[5]	2001	U. Louisville	389	144 (37)
Chua[6]	2001	Australia	51	24 (47)
Cox[7]	2000	Moffitt	315	125 (40)
Haigh[8]	2000	John Wayne	90	38 (42)
Hill[9]	1999	Memorial	114	45 (39)
Kollias[10]	1999	Australia	31	18 (58)
Reynolds[11]	1999	Mayo	60	28 (47)
Veronesi[12]	1999	Milan	168	95 (57)
Borgstein[13]	1998	Amsterdam	44	18 (41)
Krag[14]	1998	Multicenter	101	41 (41)
Total				873/2046 (43)

[1]Data from Sachdev U, Murphy K, Derzie A, et al: Predictors of nonsentinel lymph node metastasis in breast cancer patients. Am J Surg 183:213, 2002.

[2]Data from Weiser MR, Montgomery LL, Tan LK, et al: Lymphovascular invasion enhances the prediction of nonsentinel node metastases in breast cancer patients with positive sentinel nodes. Ann Surg Oncol 8:145, 2001.

[3]Data from Abdessalam SF, Zervos EE, Prasad M, et al: Predictors of positive axillary lymph nodes after sentinel lymph node biopsy in breast cancer. Am J Surg 182:316, 2001.

[4]Data from Tafra L, Lannin DR, Swanson MS, et al: Multicenter trial of sentinel node biopsy for breast cancer using both technetium sulfur colloid and isosulfan blue dye. Ann Surg 233:51, 2001.

[5]Data from Wong SL, Edwards MJ, Chao C, et al: Predicting the status of the nonsentinel axillary nodes. Arch Surg 136:563, 2001.

[6]Data from Chua B, Ung O, Taylor R, et al: Treatment implications of a positive sentinel lymph node biopsy for patients with early-stage breast carcinoma. Cancer 92:1769, 2001.

[7]Data from Cox CE, Bass SS, McCann CR, et al: Lymphatic mapping and sentinel lymph node biopsy in patients with breast cancer. Ann Rev Med 51:525, 2000.

[8]Data from Haigh PI, Hansen NM, Qi K, et al: Biopsy method and excision volume do not affect success rate of subsequent sentinel lymph node dissection in breast cancer. Ann Surg Oncol 7:21, 2000.

[9]Data from Hill AD, Tran KN, Akhurst T, et al: Lessons learned from 500 cases of lymphatic mapping for breast cancer. Ann Surg 229:528, 1999.

[10]Data from Kollias J, Gill PG, Chatterton BE, et al: Reliability of sentinel node status in predicting axillary lymph node involvement in breast cancer. Med J Aust 171:461, 1999.

[11]Data from Reynolds C, Mick R, Donohue JH, et al: Sentinel lymph node biopsy with metastasis: Can axillary dissections be avoided in some patients with breast cancer? J Clin Oncol 17:1720, 1999.

[12]Data from Veronesi U, Paganelli G, Viale G, et al: Sentinel lymph node biopsy and axillary dissection in breast cancer: Results in a large series. J Natl Cancer Inst 91:368, 1999.

[13]Data from Borgstein PJ, Pijpers R, Comans EF, et al: Sentinel lymph node biopsy in breast cancer: Guidelines and pitfalls of lymphoscintigraphy and gamma probe detection. J Am Coll Surg 186:275, 1998.

[14]Data from Krag D, Weaver D, Ashikaga T, et al: The sentinel node in breast cancer: A multicenter validation study. N Engl J Med 339:941, 1998.

multicentricity, (3) occult invasive cancer coexisting with the in situ lesion, and (4) the natural history after diagnosis by BCT. *Multifocal* refers to disease within the vicinity or same quadrant as the dominant lesion. *Multicentric* refers to disease in distant sites or quadrants within the same breast. Occult invasive cancer, or microinvasion, is defined in the AJCC classification (see earlier sections about staging and pathology) as invasive disease 1 mm or less in dimension (PTmic). When microinvasion exists, it is frequently present in several locations throughout the intraductal process.

Treatment options for DCIS include mastectomy, wide excision with radiation, and wide excision alone. With the choice of breast conservation, there is also the option of adjuvant tamoxifen. The breast cancer mortality rate following treatment by total mastectomy is 1% and represents the standard against which breast conservation techniques are compared (Table 32-13). Local recurrences

TABLE 32-13. Recurrence and Mortality Rates Following Mastectomy for Ductal Carcinoma in Situ

Study	Dates	No. of Patients	Follow-up (yr)	Percent Nonclinical	No. of Recurrences	No. Dead of Disease
Farrow[1]	1949–1967	181	5–20	0	6	4
Brown[2]	1952–1975	39	1–15	10	0	0
Carter[3]	1960–1975	28	1–14 (6.2)	—	1	1
Sunshine[4]	1960–1980	73	10-yr minimum	0	4	3
Von Rueden[5]	1960–1981	45	Not stated	8	1	0
Ashikari[6]	1965–1975	92	11-yr maximum	40	0	0
Schuh[7]	1965–1984	49	5.5 mean	33	1	1
Kinne[8]	1970–1976	101	11.5 median	58	1	1
Lagios[9]	1975–1980	42	Not stated	—	0	0
Fisher[10]	1976–1984	27	5	—	1	1
Arnesson[11]	1978–1984	28	6.4 median	100	0	0
Ward[12]	1979–1983	123	10	11	1	?
Silverstein[13]	1979–1990	98	4.9 median	62	1	0
Total		926			17 (2%)	11 (1%)

[1]Data from Farrow JH: Current concepts in the detection and treatment of the earliest of the early breast cancers. Cancer 25:468, 1970.

[2]Data from Brown PW, Silverman J, Owens E, et al: Intraductal "noninfiltrating" carcinoma of the breast. Arch Surg 111:1063, 1976.

[3]Data from Carter D, Smith RL: Carcinoma in situ of the breast. Cancer 40:1189, 1977.

[4]Data from Sunshine JA, Moseley MS, Fletcher WS, et al: Breast carcinoma in situ: A retrospective review of 112 cases with a minimum 10-year follow-up. Am J Surg 150:44, 1985.

[5]Data from Von Rueden DG, Wilson RE: Intraductal carcinoma of the breast. Surg Gynecol Obstet 158:105, 1984.

[6]Data from Ashikari R, Hajdu SI, Robbins GF: Intraductal carcinoma of the breast (1960–1969). Cancer 28:1182, 1971.

[7]Data from Schuh ME, Nemoto T, Penetrante R, et al: Intraductal carcinoma: Analysis of presentation, pathologic findings, and outcome of disease. Arch Surg 121:1303, 1986.

[8]Data from Kinne DW, Petrek JA, Osborne MP, et al: Breast carcinoma in situ. Arch Surg 124:33, 1989.

[9]Data from Lagios MD, Westdahl PR, Margolin FR, et al: Duct carcinoma in situ: Relationship of extent of noninvasive disease to the frequency of occult invasion, multicentricity, lymph node metastases, and short-term treatment failures. Cancer 50:1309, 1982.

[10]Data from Fisher ER, Sass R, Fisher B, et al: Pathologic findings from the National Surgical Adjuvant Breast Project (protocol 6), I: Intraductal carcinoma (DCIS). Cancer 57:197, 1986.

[11]Data from Arnesson LG, Smeds S, Fagerberg G, et al: Follow-up of two treatment modalities for ductal cancer in situ of the breast. Br J Surg 76:672, 1989.

[12]Data from Ward BA, McKhann CF, Ravikumar TS: Ten-year follow-up of breast carcinoma in situ in Connecticut. Arch Surg 127:1392, 1992.

[13]Data from Silverstein MJ (ed): Ductal Carcinoma in Situ of the Breast. Baltimore, Williams & Wilkins, 1997, p 443.

are rare and are suggestive of malignant transformation of residual glandular tissue. Metastatic recurrences are suggestive of either a histologically unrecognized invasive carcinoma in the mastectomy specimen or the development of a contralateral primary.

There are no prospective, randomized trials comparing the efficacy of mastectomy to breast conservation. For patients choosing preservation of the breast, the efficacy of treatment is measured as (1) the risk of a recurrence in the conserved breast, (2) the risk of an invasive breast cancer recurrence, (3) the risk of dying from a recurrent breast cancer, and (4) the physical side effects of surgery combined with radiation versus the avoidance of those associated with a mastectomy. For women choosing mastectomy for DCIS, reconstruction is an attractive option.

Mastectomy in DCIS

Mastectomy for DCIS is usually a "simple mastectomy" or total mastectomy without removal of ipsilateral axillary nodes. Historically, the rationale for total mastectomy included concern for the risk of occult multicentric disease. When occult multicentric disease is sought in mastectomy specimens from women undergoing the procedure for DCIS, rates of distant disease in the same breast range from 2% to as high as 78%, depending on the diligence of examination. Schwartz and colleagues examined four random sections from each remote quadrant and from under the areola and found occult intraductal carcinoma in 37% of the breasts examined. In contrast, in a meticulous radiologic and pathologic assessment of 82 mastectomy specimens by Holland, only one case of multicentricity was found. The risk of multicentric disease depends on the size and pathologic extent of the primary cancer and on the histologic type of intraductal tumor. In a study by Lagios and associates, disease was found in other quadrants of the breast in 2 (8%) of 24 tumors less than 2 cm, in 2 (12.5%) of 16 tumors between 2 and 5 cm, and in all 13 tumors larger than 5 cm. Patchefsky and colleagues examined multicentricity as a function of histology of the primary tumor. Micropapillary histology was associated with the highest rate of multicentricity (80%). An intermediate number of papillary and comedo carcinomas were associated with remote disease, and the solid and cribriform types were lowest.

In current practice, reasons to select total mastectomy for treatment of DCIS include (1) mammographically identified multicentric disease, (2) diffuse suspicious mammographic calcifications suggestive of extensive in-breast disease, (3) persistent positive margins after reexcision(s), (4) unacceptable cosmesis to obtain negative margins, and (5) a patient not motivated to preserve her breast. Contraindications to breast radiation include (1) prior radiation to the breast region, (2) the presence of collagen vascular disease (scleroderma or active lupus), and (3) first- or second-trimester pregnancy.

Breast Conservation in DCIS

For patients choosing breast conservation, factors that reduce the risk of local recurrence include excising the tumor to an adequate margin, the use of postexcision radiation, and the use of tamoxifen in patients with estrogen receptor–positive disease. Tables 32-14 and 32-15 summarize local failure rates for patients who have undergone breast conservation with and without postoperative radiation. Local recurrence after excision of intraductal carcinoma is reduced by 50% by the use of radiation to the ipsilateral breast.

There are three peer-reviewed, prospective, randomized trials evaluating the efficacy of breast-conserving surgery (referred to as BCS in this paragraph) with and without radiation for treatment of DCIS. In 1971, the NSABP B-06 prospectively randomized 1855 women with

invasive breast cancer to mastectomy versus BCS with radiation versus BCS alone. During subsequent pathology review, 76 specimens were identified as having DCIS only, without an invasive breast cancer component. With 10 years of reported follow-up, the local recurrence rate was 0% (0/28) in those who underwent mastectomy, 7% (2/27) in those who underwent BCS with radiation, and 43% (9/21) for those who underwent BCS alone.

In 1985, the NSABP prospectively randomized 818 women with DCIS to lumpectomy alone versus lumpectomy plus 50 Gy of postoperative radiation. The 12-year actuarial recurrence rates of the B-17 trial were published in 2001. The addition of radiation decreased the ipsilateral recurrence rate from 30.8% for patients undergoing excision alone, to 14.9% for patients undergoing excision with radiation ($P < .000005$). This decrease was seen in the incidence of invasive breast cancer occurrence (16.4% vs. 7.1%, $P < .00001$), with a smaller decrease in the incidence of in situ recurrence (14.1% vs. 7.8%, $P < .001$).

In 1986, the EORTC prospectively randomized 1010 women with DCIS to lumpectomy alone versus lumpectomy plus 50 Gy of postoperative radiation. The 4.25-year actuarial recurrence rates of the EORTC-10853 trial were published in 2000. The addition of radiation decreased the ipsilateral recurrence rate from 16% for patients undergoing excision alone, to 9% for patients undergoing excision with radiation ($P < .005$). This decrease was statistically significant in the reduction of invasive breast cancer occurrence (8% vs. 4%, $P < .04$), and was not statistically significant in the reduction of an in-situ recurrence (8% vs. 4%, $P < .06$).

Pathologic findings from the NSABP B-17 study were published in 1995. Of nine tumor characteristics evaluated, the two predictors of an ipsilateral breast tumor

TABLE 32-14. Treatment of Intraductal Carcinoma by Excision with Radiation Therapy

Study	No. of Patients	Median Follow-up (mo)	Total No. of Recurrences (%)	No. of Invasive Recurrences (%)
Solin[1]	270	124	45 (17)	24 (53)
Bornstein[2]	38	81	8 (21)	5 (13)
FONCAM[3]	37	66*	2 (5)	2 (5)
Silverstein[4]	185	90	30 (16)	16 (9)
Cutuli[5]	34	56	3 (9)	1 (3)
NSABP[6]	411	90	47 (11)	17 (4)
Hiramatsu[7]	76	74	7 (9)	4 (5)

[1]Data from Solin LJ, Kurtz J, Fourquet A, et al: Fifteen-year results of breast-conserving surgery and definitive breast irradiation for the treatment of ductal carcinoma in situ of the breast. J Clin Oncol 14:754, 1996.
[2]Data from Bornstein BA, Recht A, Connolly JL, et al: Results of treating ductal carcinoma in situ of the breast with conservative surgery and radiation therapy. Cancer 67:7, 1991.
[3]Data from Ciatto S, Bonardi R, Cataliotti L, et al: Review of a multicenter series of 350 cases. Coordinating Center and Writing Committee of FONCAM (National Task Force for Breast Cancer), Italy. Tumori 76:552, 1990.
[4]Data from Silverstein MJ (ed): Ductal Carcinoma in Situ of the Breast. Baltimore, Williams & Wilkins, 1997.
[5]Data from Cutuli B, Teissier E, Piat JM, et al: Radical surgery and conservative treatment of ductal carcinoma in situ of the breast. Eur J Cancer 28:649, 1992.
[6]Data from Fisher B, Dignam J, Wolmark N, et al: Lumpectomy and radiation therapy for the treatment of intraductal breast cancer: Findings from National Surgical Adjuvant Breast and Bowel Project B-17. J Clin Oncol 16:441, 1998.
[7]Data from Hiramatsu H, Bornstein BA, Recht A, et al: Local recurrence after conservative surgery and radiation therapy for ductal carcinoma in situ. Cancer J Sci Am 1:55, 1995.
*Mean follow-up (months).

TABLE 32-15.   Local Recurrence after Conservative Surgery and Radiation Therapy

Study (Year)	No. of Patients	Median Follow-up (yr)	Ipsilateral Local Recurrence (%)
Retrospective			
Amichetti (1997)[1]	139	6.8	9
McCormick (1991)[2]	54	3.0	18
Fourquet (1992)[3]	67	8.7	10
Vicini (2001)[4]	146	7.2	12 (10-yr. actuarial)
Solin (1996)[5]	268	10.3	17
Mammographically Detected			
Fowble (1997)[6]	110	5.3	
Hiramatsu (1995)[7]	54	6.2	7
White (1995)[8]	52	5.7	6 (5- & 8-yr. actuarial)
Solin (2001)[9]	418	9.4	11
Kestin (2000)[10]	146	7.2	9 (10-yr. actuarial)
Vicini (1997)[11]	105	6.5	9 (5-yr.), 10 (10-yr. actuarial)
Prospective, Randomized			
Fisher (NSABP B-06, 1991)[12]	27	6.9 (mean)	7
Fisher (NSABP B-17, 1998)[13]	411	7.5 (mean)	12
Julien (EORTC, 2000)[14]	502	4.25	9
Houghton (2002)[15]	522	4.38	8

[1]Data from Amichetti M, Caffo O, Richetti A, et al: Ten-year results of treatment of ductal carcinoma in situ (DCIS) of the breast with conservative surgery and radiotherapy. Eur J Cancer 33(10):1559, 1997.

[2]Data from McCormick B, Rosen PP, Kinne D, et al: Duct carcinoma in situ of the breast: an analysis of local control after conservation surgery and radiotherapy. Int J Radiat Oncol Biol Phys 21(2):289, 1991.

[3]Data from Fourquet A, Zafrani B, Campana F, et al: Breast-conserving treatment of ductal carcinoma in situ. Semin Radiat Oncol 2:116, 1992.

[4]Data from Vicini FA, Kestin LL, Goldstein NS, et al: Relationship between excision volume, margin status, and tumor size with the development of local recurrence in patients with ductal carcinoma in situ treated with breast-conserving therapy. J Surg Oncol 76:245, 2001.

[5]Data from Solin LJ, Kurtz J, Fourquet A, et al: Fifteen-year results of breast-conserving surgery and definitive breast irradiation for the treatment of ductal carcinoma in situ of the breast. J Clin Oncol 14:754, 1996.

[6]Data from Fowble B, Hanlon AL, Fein DA, et al: Results of conservative surgery and radiation for mammographically detected ductal carcinoma in situ (DCIS). Int J Radiat Oncol Biol Phys 38:949, 1997.

[7]Data from Hiramatsu H, Bornstein BA, Recht A, et al: Local recurrence after conservative surgery and radiation therapy for ductal carcinoma in situ. Cancer J Sci Am 1:55, 1995.

[8]Data from White J, Levine A, Gustafson G, et al: Outcome and prognostic factors for local recurrence in mammographically detected ductal carcinoma in situ of the breast treated with conservative surgery and radiation therapy. Int J Radiat Oncol Biol Phys 31:791, 1995.

[9]Data from Solin LJ, Fourquet A, Vicini FA, et al: Mammographically detected ductal carcinoma in situ of the breast treated with breast-conserving surgery and definitive breast irradiation: Long-term outcome and prognostic significance of patient age and margin status. Int J Radiat Oncol Biol Phys 50:991, 2001.

[10]Data from Kestin LL, Goldstein NS, Martinez AA, et al: Mammographically detected ductal carcinoma in situ treated with conservative surgery with or without radiation therapy: Patterns of failure and 10-year results. Ann Surg 231: 235, 2000.

[11]Data from Vicini FA, Lacerna MD, Goldstein NS, et al: Ductal carcinoma in situ detected in the mammographic era: An analysis of clinical, pathologic, and treatment-related factors affecting outcome with breast-conserving therapy. Int J Radiat Oncol Biol Phys 39:627, 1997.

[12]Data from Fisher ER, Leeming R, Anderson S, et al: Conservative management of intraductal carcinoma (DCIS) of the breast. J Surg Oncol 47:139, 1991.

[13]Data from Fisher B, Dignam J, Wolmark N, et al: Lumpectomy and radiation therapy for the treatment of intraductal breast cancer: Findings from National Surgical Adjuvant Breast and Bowel Project B-17. J Clin Oncol 16:441, 1998.

[14]Data from Julien JP, Bijker N, Fentiman IS, et al: Radiotherapy in breast-conserving treatment for ductal carcinoma in situ: First results of the EORTC randomised phase III trial 10853. EORTC Breast Cancer Cooperative Group and EORTC Radiotherapy Group. Lancet 355:528, 2000.

[15]Data from Silverstein MJ (ed): Ductal Carcinoma in Situ of the Breast. Philadelphia, Lippincott Williams & Wilkins, 2002, p 453.

recurrence were the presence of uncertain or involved specimen margins and the presence of comedo necrosis. Uncertain or involved margins were present in 101 (17.6%) of the 573 cases reviewed. For this study, margins were regarded as free "when the tumor was not transected." In 2001, 4.25-year follow-up analysis of the pathologic predictors of local recurrence in the EORTC-10853 study, involved surgical margins and solid and cribiform histology were identified as factors increasing the risk of local recurrence. Solin and colleagues in 1996 reported on 15-year results of DCIS treatment with surgical excision and radiation. With 5 years of follow-up, only 2% of the noncomedo lesions had an in-breast recurrence, as compared with 11% of comedo lesions. With 15 years of follow-up, in-breast recurrence for noncomedo lesions was 15% and for comedo lesions was 17%. These data suggest that histologic subtype impacts on short-term recurrences but does not have an impact with extended follow-up. Thus, in addition to postexcision radiation, adequate surgical margins, often defined as 3 mm or greater, is another modifiable factor that has long-term implications of the success of breast-conserving surgery.

These three prospective and other retrospective studies demonstrate that radiation decreases the chance of local recurrence after breast-conserving surgery by 50%. Furthermore, if an ipsilateral breast tumor recurs, in half of patients it recurs as DCIS and in the other half it recurs as an invasive cancer. Of those patients whose recurrences are an invasive tumor, a proportion of these patients are found to have positive axillary nodes, and a smaller proportion develop metastatic disease. The chance of developing metastatic disease when breast conservation is chosen for treatment of DCIS is estimated as between 0% and 3%.

Role of Axillary Dissection and Sentinel Node Biopsy in DCIS

DCIS, by definition, represents breast cancer contained within an intact basement membrane and without access to lymphatic or vascular channels. However, when axillary dissection is performed during mastectomy for intraductal disease, positive nodes can be seen in up to 3.6% of the cases, as identified in a review of more than 10,000 patients in the National Cancer Database. These probably represent cases in which microinvasion was present but not detected pathologically. Indeed, in a series of 227 patients reported by Silverstein with intraductal carcinoma selected for the absence of microscopic invasion, 163 axillary dissections were performed and all were negative.

Lagios and associates used careful specimen radiography and demanding pathologic processing to examine 111 specimens of intraductal carcinoma. For lesions 45 mm or less ($N = 80$), there were no cases of microscopic invasion. For DCIS measuring 46 to 55 mm ($N = 6$), 17% harbored occult microscopic disease. In 25 patients whose DCIS measured 56 mm or greater, 12 (48%) had evidence of microscopic invasion and 2 of these patients had cancer in axillary nodes. The extent of the primary tumor in these two patients was 68 and 160 mm. Therefore, for patients with small mammographically detected in situ tumors, axillary dissection is not recommended. For women with larger tumors, particularly if mastectomy is required, sentinel node mapping or a level I axillary dissection to evaluate the lymph nodes should be considered.

In addition, when a patient is proceeding directly from a core needle biopsy diagnosis of DCIS to mastectomy, sentinel node mapping should be considered. The possibility of an invasive breast cancer being identified in the mastectomy specimen is inversely proportional to the diameter of the core needle used to obtain the biopsy specimen and directly proportional to the size and grade of DCIS. At the Brigham and Women's Hospital, when the diagnosis of DCIS is made by core needle biopsy, at the time of excisional biopsy, an invasive breast cancer was identified in 19% of patients who underwent 14-gauge core needle biopsy, in 17% who underwent 14-gauge directional vacuum-assisted (DVA) biopsy, and in 12% who underwent 11-gauge DVA biopsy. Furthermore, the likelihood of an invasive breast cancer being diagnosed at the time of surgical excision increases with the grade of DCIS seen in the core biopsy specimen: low grade, 0 of 26 contained invasive disease; intermediate, 2 (6%) of 31 cases contained invasive cancer; and high, 10 (28%) of 36 cases were upstaged. These conversions of DCIS to invasive breast cancer could prompt the need for a second axillary procedure. Should a patient choose to proceed from core needle biopsy to mastectomy, consideration of sentinel node mapping or axillary sampling at the time of mastectomy should occur.

Some investigators are evaluating the role of sentinel node biopsy in patients with DCIS undergoing breast-conserving surgery, but this is still investigational. Importantly, particularly for patients in whom an invasive breast cancer is not identified but in whom a micrometastatic sentinel node has been identified, there is controversy as to the role of adjuvant therapy.

Role of Tamoxifen in DCIS

In 1991, the NSABP B-24 protocol was initiated to evaluate the benefit of tamoxifen for women with DCIS undergoing lumpectomy and radiation. Endpoints included the incidence of invasive and in situ breast cancers in the ipsilateral and contralateral breasts. In this prospective randomized, placebo-controlled, double-blinded trial, 1804 women with DCIS who underwent lumpectomy and radiation were randomized to either 5 years of tamoxifen 20 mg daily or placebo. Seven-year (82-month mean) follow-up results were reported in 2001. Of the 362 patients who experienced a recurrent breast cancer in the ipsilateral or contralateral breast, axillary nodes, chest wall, or distant sites, 156 were randomized to tamoxifen and 206 to placebo. The addition of tamoxifen to lumpectomy and radiation decreased the incidence of ipsilateral breast cancer by 31% (risk reduction predominantly for invasive cancer recurrence—47%). Subsequent contralateral breast cancer was reduced by 47% (with reduction seen predominantly with in situ cancer—68%), and of cancer on either side by 37% (Table 32-16). Thus, as calculated using the 5-year follow-up data, for every 19 women given tamoxifen, one event was avoided. At 7 years of follow-up, the characteristics associated with an increased occurrence of post-treatment ipsilateral invasive and in situ breast cancer include the presence of positive margins, comedo necrosis, a mass on physical examination, and a patient 50 years of age and older.

The question has been raised as to whether the benefit of tamoxifen is restricted to women with estrogen receptor–positive lesions. Receptor status was not a prerequisite for enrollment in this trial. To determine the relationship between estrogen receptor status and response to tamoxifen in DCIS, a retrospective analysis of a subset of 676 (344 placebo- and 332 tamoxifen-treated) patients from NSABP B-24 was performed and recently presented in abstract. More than 75% of DCIS lesions tested estrogen receptor positive. With a median follow-up of 8.7 years, those who were estrogen receptor positive experienced a 59% reduction of first events if taking tamoxifen compared with placebo (RR, 0.41; $P = 0.0002$). For those whose lesions were estrogen receptor negative, a statistically significant difference in event rates was not observed between the two groups, though the number of events were small (RR, 0.80; 95% CI, 0.41 to 1.56; $P = 0.51$; number of events = 36).

Selection criteria for trial enrollment in NSABP B-24 were liberal. Patients with involved surgical margins made up one third of enrolled patients. Mammography inclusion criteria suggest that patients with more than one area of DCIS may have been included. The study does not specifically address the benefit that tamoxifen would yield for patients with a single focus of DCIS excised with wide margins and without mammographic evidence of potential additional foci.

Fisher presented the combined 7-year follow-up results of NSABP B-17 and B-24 in 2001 (see Table 32-16). With 7 years of follow-up, ipsilateral and contralateral breast cancer recurrence for patients undergoing excision alone was 30%; for patients undergoing excision with radiation, 17%; and for patients treated with excision, radiation, and tamoxifen, 10%. Thus, when compared with those in B-17 treated with lumpectomy alone, the addition of radiation and tamoxifen in NSABP B-24 provided a 66% lower cumulative incidence of all breast cancer events at 7 years. On a cautionary note, the definition of negative margins may be considered too lenient by some and was simply no tumor touching the ink used to stain the outside margin, as described earlier. For a patient with estrogen receptor–positive DCIS treated with lumpectomy, radiation, and tamoxifen, the risk of an ipsilateral recurrence is about 7%. Importantly for complete understanding of these studies, mortality differences between any of these assigned groups have not been confirmed. If half of the recurrences are invasive cancer, this would be a 3.5% rate of invasive disease. Particularly for women with estrogen receptor–positive DCIS, the absolute improvement in the risk of developing an invasive breast cancer by adding tamoxifen to radiation therapy for estrogen receptor–positive DCIS may be substantial.

Treatment of Locally Advanced and Inflammatory Breast Cancer

Locally advanced breast cancer is difficult to precisely define but generally refers to patients with large primary tumors (>5 cm, T3), chest wall extension (T4a), skin ulceration or satellite skin nodules (t4b), inflammatory carcinoma (t4d), fixed axillary nodes (N2a), or clinically apparent internal mammary nodes (N2b) or periclavicular nodes (N3). Such cancers span stages IIb, IIIa, and IIIb disease. Central to the concept is the notion that the disease is advanced on the chest wall (T3 or T4 tumor) and/or in regional lymph nodes (N1 to N3 in the 2003 TNM system) and not metastatic to distant sites (M0).

The treatment of locally advanced breast cancer has been changing. The disease is heterogeneous and defies a uniform treatment approach. Prior to the 1970s, treatment included surgery and radiation, with little effect on survival. When surgery is used alone, local relapse rates in the range of 30% to 50% can be anticipated and the long-term cure rates rarely exceed 30%. Similar results are reported when radiation therapy is the sole modality of treatment. These poor results suggest that locally advanced disease is actually metastatic in most patients, emphasizing the role of chemotherapy in these patients. A trimodality approach with the addition of chemotherapy improved both disease-free and overall survivals.

Neoadjuvant Chemotherapy

Seven prospective, randomized trials have evaluated the efficacy of chemotherapy administered in the neoadjuvant setting prior to breast surgery versus administered in the adjuvant setting after surgery. Although two of these trials reported improvement in disease-free survival with the use of neoadjuvant chemotherapy, none have demonstrated improvement in overall survival. Consistently, patients treated with chemotherapy in the neoadjuvant setting were more likely to be treated surgically with breast conservation. Such treatment produces a 50% to 80% partial or complete clinical response. Thus, neoadjuvant chemotherapy can be pursued in those patients who would be candidates for breast conservation, if their primary tumor size could be reduced prior to surgery.

From a practical perspective, prior to initiating chemotherapy in the neoadjuvant setting, under image guidance, a metallic clip is placed into the tumor. Should a complete clinical and radiologic tumor response occur, preoperative stereotactic wire placement alongside the clip will facilitate excision of the tumor site. If histology demonstrates a localized tumor with negative margins, radiation can commence and the breast preserved. For a diffuse tumor with satellite lesions, consideration of re-excision prior to radiation should be given, even if margins are technically cleared. For a diffuse tumor with many satellite foci and positive margins, mastectomy may be required.

For the patient with a clinically negative axilla and a primary breast cancer larger than 5 cm, approximately 25% have pathologically negative lymph nodes. In the context of neoadjuvant chemotherapy for tumor downstaging prior to breast-conserving surgery, sentinel node biopsy at the time of breast surgery is appealing. In a compilation of 11 studies totaling 724 patients, in 99 (14%)

Table 32-16. Combining National Surgical Adjuvant Breast and Bowel Project B-17 and B-24: Seven-Year Follow-up		
	All Breast Cancer Events (Ipsilateral + Contralateral) (%)	
	B-17	B-24
Lumpectomy	30.3	—
Lumpectomy + XRT	18.0	16.9
Lumpectomy + XRT + Tam	—	10.3

XRT, radiation therapy; Tam, tamoxifen.

Adapted from Fisher B, Land S, Mamounas E, et al: Prevention of invasive breast cancer in women with ductal carcinoma in situ: An update of the National Surgical Adjuvant Breast and Bowel Project experience. Semin Oncol 28:400, 2001.

patients the sentinel node could not be identified and in 66 (9%) the sentinel node was falsely negative with remaining axillary nodes harboring metastatic disease. Thus, sentinel node biopsy is recommended prior to neoadjuvant chemotherapy. If the sentinel node is negative, after chemotherapy and at the time of definitive breast surgery, no further surgery of the axilla is performed. If the sentinel node is positive, a completion Level I and II axillary dissection may be performed following chemotherapy and at the time of breast surgery. In a trial by Rouzier, 152 patients with fine-needle aspiration confirmed positive nodal disease received neoadjuvant cyclophosphamide, doxorubicin (Adriamycin), and fluorouracil (CAF) chemotherapy. In multivariate analysis, parameters associated with improved distant disease-free survival included age older than 40 years, absence of residual nodal disease, and S-phase fraction less than 4%. Other studies have demonstrated surgical node staging after neoadjuvant chemotherapy retains prognostic significance, and disease-free and overall survival are improved for the node-negative patient.

Inflammatory Breast Cancer

In 1986, the AJCC specifically defined inflammatory carcinoma according to clinical criteria and assigned a new T code, T4d, which falls under stage IIIb disease. This designation is maintained in the 2002 AJCC staging. Inflammatory breast cancer presents clinically with extensive erythema, edema, and warmth of the breast, most pronounced in the dependent position. These findings may exist independently of a palpable breast mass or any mammographic abnormality beyond skin thickening. The pathologic hallmark is the presence of tumor cells within the dermal lymphatic. Diffuse invasion of lymphatic channels within the breast unifies the clinical picture. *Peau d'orange* is a term used to describe the orange peel appearance of the skin. The dermal lymphatics are congested with tumor cells, precluding draining of lymphatic fluid from the breast. The lymphatic fluid congests the skin, resulting in edema. Axillary nodal metastases are commonly present and distant disease should be sought using radiographic modalities such as bone scan and computed tomography.

Inflammatory breast cancer was once a uniformly fatal disease that claimed its victims after a median survival of 9 to 12 months. Current approaches emphasize aggressive use of combined modality treatment, which includes chemotherapy, mastectomy, and radiation therapy. Newer treatment protocols use intensive chemotherapy as the first modality. Objective response rates are in the range of 60% to 80%, and most patients are rendered free of disease after mastectomy and nodal dissection. A reasonable approach practiced in many North American centers uses a sequence of chemotherapy, mastectomy, and radiation therapy to treat inflammatory breast cancer. For instance, results of combining these three treatment modalities produced a relapse-free survival of 50% at 5 years. In a single institution, this result compared favorably to historical series of patients who received less treatment (7% at 5 years).

Treatment of Special Conditions

Paget's Disease[37]

Paget's disease of the breast clinically presents as nipple erythema and mild eczematous scaling and flaking, progressing to nipple crusting, skin erosions, and ulceration. The condition spreads outward off the nipple and onto the areola and surrounding skin of the breast.

Pathologically, the Paget's cell is a large, pale-staining cell with round or oval nuclei and large nucleoli. The cells are between the normal keratinocytes of the nipple epidermis. They spread into the lactiferous sinuses under the nipple and upward to invade the overlying epidermis of the nipple. Serous fluid can seep through the disrupted keratinocyte layer, resulting in crusting and scaling of the nipple skin. Paget's cells do not invade through the dermal basement membrane and therefore are a form of carcinoma in situ.

The clinical differential diagnosis of scaling skin and erythema of the nipple-areolar complex includes eczema, contact dermatitis, postradiation dermatitis, and Paget's disease. A skin specimen containing Paget's cells and a lactiferous duct secures the diagnosis and can be obtained by nipple-scrape cytology or biopsy.

More than 97% of patients with Paget's disease have an underlying breast carcinoma. Paget's may present with (54%) or without (46%) a mass. Invasive breast cancer coexists with Paget's disease in 93% of patients with a mass and in 38% of patients without a mass.

For patients considering breast preservation, presurgical evaluation should include evaluation for occult multicentric disease with mammography with retroareolar spot compression views. Some advocate breast MRI. For patients with Paget's disease confined clinically and radiologically to the nipple-areolar complex, surgery may include excision of the nipple-areolar complex with at least a 2-cm cone of retroareolar tissue, encompassing all radiographic abnormalities. Alternatively, simple mastectomy with or without an axillary node procedure is probably the most common way Paget's disease is treated in the United States. Nodal evaluation may be based on identification of an invasive component preoperatively or if invasive cancer is strongly suggested.

Male Breast Cancer[2,37,38]

Breast cancer occurring in the mammary gland of men is infrequent, accounting for 0.8% of all breast cancers, less than 1% of all newly diagnosed male cancers, and 0.2% of male cancer deaths. Annually in the United States, there are 1500 new cases and 400 deaths. The median age at diagnosis is 68, 5 years older than for women.

Risk factors include age (exponential increase with age) and those that may be related to abnormalities in estrogen and androgen balance, including testicular disease (undescended testes, congenital inguinal hernia, orchiectomy, orchitis, testicular injury), infertility, obesity, and cirrhosis. Other factors include benign breast conditions (nipple discharge, breast cysts, breast trauma) and radiation exposure. Risk factors related to a genetic predisposition include Klinefelter's syndrome (47,XXY karyotype), family history, and Jewish ancestry. *BRCA2* mutations predispose men to breast cancer and account for 4% of male breast cancers in the absence of a family history, 40% of cases in Iceland where a founder mutation exists, and between 60% and 76% of cases in which a male and female relative have breast cancer. Gynecomastia is not a risk factor: Its rate in men with breast cancer is not higher than in men without.

Histologically, 90% of male breast cancers are invasive, with most being ductal carcinomas. Approximately 80% are estrogen receptor positive, 75% progesterone receptor positive, and 35% over express *HER2/neu*. The remaining 10% are in situ of the ductal type with 75% of these being of the papillary subtype. Given the absence of terminal lobules in the normal male breast, lobular carcinoma, both invasive and in situ, is rarely seen

The majority of men with breast cancer (50% to 97%) present with a breast mass, with the differential diagnosis including gynecomastia, primary breast carcinoma, metastatic carcinoma to the breast, sarcoma, and breast abscess. In addition to local pain and axillary adenopathy, other presenting symptoms include those of the nipple (retraction, ulceration, bleeding, and discharge). Evaluation includes breast imaging studies and, when there is uncertainty of a diagnosis of gynecomastia, needle or surgical biopsy.

The negative prognostic factors for breast cancer in men are the same as in women and include nodal involvement, tumor size, histologic grade, and hormone receptor status. When matched for age and stage, survival is similar to that in women.

The treatment of carcinoma in the male breast depends on the stage and local extent of the tumor. The rarity of male breast cancer has precluded large randomized trials, and thus treatment choices frequently use the same guidelines for women. Small tumors, movable across the chest wall, may be treated by local excision and radiation, if preferred and technically feasible, or by mastectomy. Nodal evaluation by sentinel node biopsy or axillary dissection is governed by the presence of invasive disease. Breast tumors in men more commonly involve the pectoralis major muscle, probably because breast tissue in men is scant. If the underlying pectoral muscle is involved, modified radical mastectomy with excision of the involved portion of muscle is adequate treatment and may be combined with postoperative radiation therapy.

There is little experience with adjuvant chemotherapy or hormonal therapy in male breast cancer. Because most of these tumors are hormone sensitive, the use of adjuvant tamoxifen for node-positive and high-risk node-negative patients seems logical. For men at substantial risk for metastatic disease, adjuvant chemotherapy can be offered.

Angiosarcoma[37]

Malignant sarcomas originating from either lymphatic (lymphangiosarcoma) or capillary endothelium (hemangiosarcoma) are termed *angiosarcomas*. Angiosarcomas are exceedingly malignant tumors, with an annual incidence rate for white females of 1.6/100,000, with 44% of these originating in the breast and 25% in the upper extremity.

Angiosarcoma of the breast or arm is viewed as either primary or secondary based on the absence or presence of a previous breast cancer diagnosis. The interval between breast cancer diagnosis and subsequent upper extremity angiosarcoma is 5 to 10 years. Post-treatment sarcomas can occur in an arm afflicted by lymphedema after radical mastectomy (Stewart-Treves syndrome), in the chest wall following mastectomy and radiation, and in the breast following breast-conserving surgery and radiation. In a case-control study by Cozen using the Los Angeles County Cancer Registry, the incidence of angiosarcoma following treatment for invasive breast cancer was increased when compared to the incidence of angiosarcoma in those without a previous breast cancer diagnosis. The adjusted ORs were 59.3 for upper extremity angiosarcoma, 11.6 for angiosarcoma of the chest and breast, and 3.3 for nonvascular breast sarcomas. Risk factors for the development of soft tissue sarcomas following breast cancer include postmastectomy lymphedema. Using the Swedish Cancer Registry in a population-based study by Karlson, 67 of 122,991 women with breast cancer were subsequently diagnosed with a soft tissue sarcoma of the breast region or arm. In a case-control analysis of the Swedish data, the development of angiosarcoma correlated with lymphedema (OR, 9.5). This analysis also demonstrated that radiation was not a risk factor for the development of angiosarcoma but is a risk factor for the development of nonangiosarcoma sarcomas. Sarcomas of other types correlated with radiation by dose-response, with an OR of 2.4 for an energy of 50 J.

Most commonly, the initial presentation of angiosarcoma is that of a cutaneous or subcutaneous bluish nodule that rapidly becomes multiple in number and converges within edematous skin. Rarely, the lesion may present as erythema within edematous skin and is frequently painful. Finally, it may present within the breast parenchyma, mimicking a hematoma-filled cyst. Metastasis to regional nodes is extraordinarily rare; the usual mode of spread is hematogenous, most commonly to the lungs and bone, and less commonly to abdominal viscera, brain, and even the contralateral breast.

Mammography is unrevealing in one third of cases. Skin-punch biopsy of a single nodular lesion may be insufficient to secure a diagnosis, and a second, larger biopsy may be needed. Histologically, the lesion is composed of numerous slitlike, irregularly dilated vascular channels dissecting between the collagen bundles lined by atypical endothelial cells (described earlier).

In the absence of metastatic disease at presentation, surgery to negative margins, most commonly involving a simple or radical mastectomy, frequently with a split-thickness skin graft or myocutaneous flap is required to secure negative skin margins. In the past, radical surgery offered the only hope of cure. Axillary dissection is neither necessary nor helpful, with the exception of the rare patient with concomitant axillary adenopathy. With the appreciation that all vascular changes in the irradiated skin are at risk and may be part of an evolving spectrum of disease, more conservative approaches involving the use of systemic therapy may be more appropriate for some patients.

Because radiation therapy is of benefit in the treatment of related sarcomas in other body sites, some authors recommend postoperative radiation therapy to the chest wall for the treatment of primary angiosarcoma. For those patients with secondary angiosarcoma where their breast cancer treatment included radiation, additional radiation is offered selectively to regions outside the original radiation port.

Chemotherapy can be considered prior to surgery in efforts to facilitate resection and limit its scope. After surgery, chemotherapy is usually reserved for palliation. The experience with adjuvant therapy is anecdotal, and thus its place is uncertain. Most regimens that are reported to have activity in this tumor contain either dactinomycin or doxorubicin. Treatment principles are changing, and the disease may be increasing in prevalence with the increased use of breast-conserving surgery and radiation. At the Dana-Farber Cancer Institute in Boston, neoadjuvant chemotherapy is used more frequently. Liposomal-formulated, doxorubicin-based chemotherapy has been used with some success and is relatively well tolerated by many women.

After diagnosis, local progression in skin and distant progression most frequently to the lungs and bones occurs rapidly. Within 2 years, there is a 90% mortality. Prognosis is dependent on the histologic grade (I to III) and size of the tumor. High-grade lesions (grade 3) are said to be the most lethal of all primary breast cancers. In contrast, low-grade lesions are more likely to be cured after total mastectomy. For those free of metastatic disease at presentation, after mastectomy, the median time to recurrence is 8 months and the median survival is 2 years. Practitioners should be aware of this disease, and the index of suspicion should be kept high for patients who have been previously irradiated for breast cancer.

Phyllodes Tumor (Cystosarcoma Phyllodes)[39]

Phyllodes tumor and its cousin, the fibroadenoma, are the most common neoplasms of nonepithelial origin in the breast. Phyllodes tumors comprise less than 1% of all breast neoplasms and are unique in their occurrence exclusively in the female breast and appearance in no other site in the body. The term *phyllodes* comes from the Greek word *phyllon,* which means "leaf." This descriptive terminology refers to a bulky tumor whose cut surface is embossed with a leaflike appearance. The term *cystosarcoma* refers to the microscopic cystlike spaces lined with a low epithelium reminiscent of fibroadenoma. The inclusion of sarcoma in the terminology is to reflect the "fleshy" consistency of the tumor, though this may be confusing because the majority of these lesions are considered to be benign. For this reason, the World Health Organization classification of breast tumors uses the term *phyllodes tumor,* which carries no implication of biologic potential. A phyllodes tumor is differentiated from the fibroadenoma by the presence of stromal overgrowth and its diagnosis

is qualified by indication of its malignancy (25%), of its benignity (60%), or whether it has indeterminate characteristics, a so-called borderline lesion (15%), with this differentiation made based on the lesion's stromal characteristics. The clinical behavior of this tumor is difficult to predict with accuracy. Metastases occur in 20% of "malignant" lesions and in less than 5% of "benign" lesions.

The majority of tumors are sharply demarcated and freely mobile with a smooth contour. These tumors can be any size but are frequently large, with a median size of 4 to 5 cm. They can occur in patients at any age, with a median age being 45—20 years later than the average age of patients being seen with fibroadenomas. Thus, particularly for women aged 35 and older who present with a clinically benign but rapidly enlarging breast mass, the differential diagnosis includes phyllodes tumor. Mammographically, these lesions present as round densities with smooth borders and are indistinguishable from fibroadenomas. Ultrasound may reveal a discrete structure with cystic spaces. The diagnosis is suggested by the larger size, a history of rapid growth, and the occurrence in older patients. Cytology is unreliable in differentiating a low-grade phyllodes tumor from a fibroadenoma. In one series of core needle biopsy, the correct diagnosis was rendered in only 50% of cases. Thus, the diagnosis is usually made by excisional biopsy followed by careful pathologic review.

For benign lesions that had been enucleated, 5-year local recurrence rates up to 4% have been reported. Thus, excision with a 1-cm minimum negative margin is advocated. For malignant tumors, if adequate margins are achieved with breast-conserving surgery, mastectomy is not required. In a review of seven series reporting 332 patients, axillary metastases were present in 3 (0.9%) of the patients. Formal axillary dissection seems to be unnecessary, but removal of low axillary lymph nodes cannot be criticized, particularly if patients have palpable adenopathy.

Local recurrences are usually seen within the first few years of surgery, at the site of the original excision, and are inversely correlated with the width of the negative resection margin. There is an unacceptable local recurrence rate, regardless of histologic type or tumor size, if the lesion is enucleated. There are multiple reports of the recurrence being of more aggressive histology than the primary, a condition termed *malignant transformation.* Most patients with a local recurrence are treated with total mastectomy.

Most metastatic phyllodes tumors have spread hematogenously, with common sites including lung, bone, abdominal viscera, and mediastinum, and histologically may contain only the stromal elements. There are no reports of long-term survivors. In multivariate analysis, distant recurrence rates were related to histologic type in one study and stromal type plus the presence of necrosis in a second study and were not related to tumor size or margin status. The optimal palliative treatment of metastatic phyllodes tumors has not been found. Most authors have used cyclophosphamide- or doxorubicin-containing combinations, and several have used cisplatin and etoposide combination chemotherapy. Radiation to symptomatic metastases may be helpful. The majority of the tumors contain either estrogen or progesterone receptors, although palliation with hormone manipulation has not been extensively explored.

CHEMOTHERAPY AND HORMONE THERAPY FOR BREAST CANCER

As radical local surgery gave way to less invasive surgical procedures, the concept of cancer as spreading sequentially from primary site to more and more distant sites was challenged by newer theories of cancer metastasis. Surgical trials of local therapies were at the forefront of this changing concept, as reviewed earlier. Current thinking places the metastatic event early in the progression of breast cancer, probably before the finding of a mass for the majority of patients. This explains the insensitivity of outcome to local treatments for patients in whom metastasis has already occurred. This concept also argues for a systemic approach to breast cancer, administered in concert with local treatment. This missing link is the ability to accurately detect the metastatic disease and select the appropriate patients to receive systemic treatment.

Metastatic disease is the principal cause of death due to breast cancer. Patients who benefit from chemotherapy or hormonal therapy do so because metastasis is prevented, cured, or delayed. The first prospective trials of systemic treatment combined oophorectomy, depriving patients of estrogens, with radical mastectomy. Since these early trials, hundreds of prospective studies have involved thousands of women. The literature on systemic adjuvant treatment of breast cancer is now more than 25 years old. A comprehensive analysis of systemic therapy after surgery for early-stage breast cancer is updated continuously by the EBCTCG. Centered in England, the EBCTCG has conducted meta-analyses of randomized clinical trials for nearly 20 years. For instance, the 1998 update on adjuvant chemotherapy (the latest report) included 75,000 women enrolled worldwide on randomized trials of surgery with or without systemic therapy and was estimated to include 90% of those ever randomized. Interpreting the results of these studies requires a basic knowledge of descriptive and analytical statistics.

Interpreting Results of Clinical Trials

Survival curves are the most familiar way to compare groups of patients in randomized trials of different therapies. To estimate the survival curve for any group of people, investigators use the life-table method (also called the *actuarial method*). Kaplan and Meier proposed a popular modification of these general methods that suit clinical trials, and the resulting curves are often called *Kaplan-Meier curves*. This method tabulates the number of patients surviving as a proportion of the total number of patients reaching the interval of time in question after entering the trial. Plotting data for each time interval generates the familiar curves. Survival or death is only one outcome that can be expressed in actuarial terms. Disease-free survival, event-free survival, and freedom from local failure (just to list a few) all can be expressed in actuarial terms.

Comparisons between groups (e.g., treated vs. control) can be described in several ways, each of which has limitations and ambiguities. As shown in Figure 32-16, the simplest way is to measure the absolute difference between the curves at any specified interval of time during follow-up, shown by the vertical dashed lines between the Kaplan-Meier curves. Alternatively, for any specific proportion of patients, there is a different time until relapse or death between the two curves, shown by the horizontal dashed line in Figure 32-16. For instance, the median survival time is the length of survival free of relapse or death for 50% of the patients. Differences in median survival times between treated and control patients may be significant, even though absolute differences are small. For most treatment comparisons, there are three groups

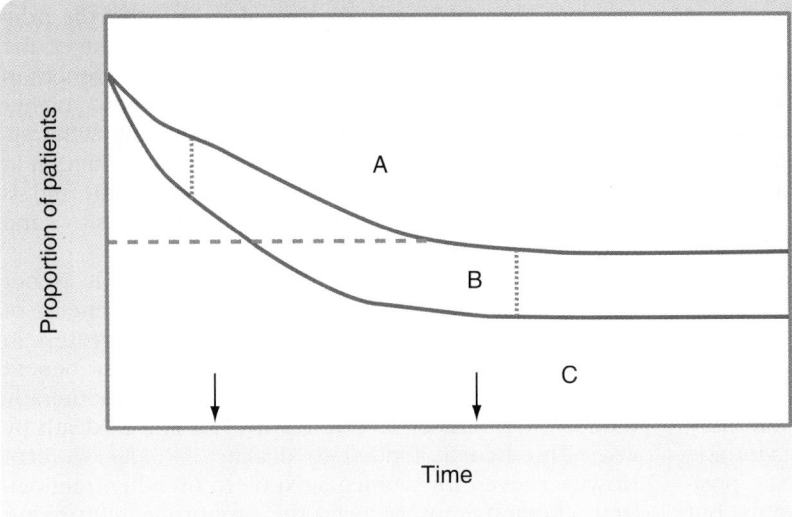

FIGURE 32-16. Interpretation of actuarial curves used in clinical trials comparing two groups of patients. The reader should refer to the text for an explanation of the annotations.

to consider. There are those patients that will remain free of recurrence or death with the control treatment, shown as the area under the lower curve (C). There are patients who are destined to fail both the experimental and control treatments, shown as the area above the experimental (upper curve [A]). It is only the patients falling between the two curves (B) that benefit (or are harmed) by the experimental treatment. The concept of proportional benefit is important when evaluating adjuvant chemotherapy or hormonal therapy for breast cancer; only a small proportion of treated patients benefit from receiving postoperative adjuvant treatments.

A popular way to express the difference between control and experimental groups is to cite the proportional reduction in treatment failures. For instance, the proportional reduction in mortality is the difference in survival between the two groups at an interval divided by the percentage of patients dead in the control group in the same interval. For the same proportional reduction in mortality, the absolute difference in survival varies greatly and is generally larger for groups of patients with higher risks of dying (node-positive vs. node-negative patients). The proportional increase in survival divides the absolute difference between the control and experimental curves in a specified interval by the total surviving in the experimental group (assuming it is larger). For groups with poor survival, small absolute differences lead to larger estimates of the percentage increase in survival.

Adjuvant Chemotherapy for Operable Breast Cancer[37]

The first trials of prolonged postoperative chemotherapy in operable breast cancer were started by the NSABP in 1972 and by the NCI of Italy (NCI-Milan) in 1973. Only patients with positive axillary nodes were chosen for study. The NSABP B-05 compared oral L-phenylalanine mustard (L-PAM, melphalan) with a placebo in patients receiving radical mastectomy. The NCI-Milan trial studied a combination of cyclophosphamide, methotrexate, and 5-fluorouracil (CMF) versus no treatment after either radical mastectomy or extended radical mastectomy. Neither study allowed the use of postoperative radiation therapy or antiestrogen therapy. Both studies stratified patients into a group younger than 50 years of age (commonly denoted premenopausal) and a group older than age 50 years. Nodal involvement was used in both studies to further divide patients into either a group with one to three positive nodes and a group with four or more positive nodes.

The results from these two trials are similar and convincingly positive for women undergoing chemotherapy who are younger than 50 years of age. In both studies, the magnitude of difference in this subgroup was relatively large and statistically significant. In contrast to the positive effect of chemotherapy in younger patients, women older than 50 years of age did not significantly benefit, as a whole, from the use of adjuvant cytotoxic chemotherapy. Subsequent studies show that postmenopausal women also benefit from chemotherapy, but to a lesser extent. Significantly, the 20-year follow-up of

the initial NCI-Milan CMF combination has shown few complications.

Meta-Analysis of Adjuvant Chemotherapy for Breast Cancer[40]

Although clinically worthwhile, the benefits of adjuvant systemic therapy for operable breast cancer are modest and in the range of a 20% to 30% reduction in the odds of recurrence or death. Detection of these small differences requires large trials with a high degree of statistical power; therefore, it is helpful to combine results of randomized clinical trials and ask simple questions that average large numbers of heterogeneous patients. Thus, an international collaboration was begun in 1985 that sought primary data from any randomized trial of adjuvant systemic therapy of breast cancer begun before that same year. Data from more than 75,000 patients were first published in 1995 and were most recently updated in 1998, concerning the benefits of adjuvant chemotherapy, ovarian ablation, immunotherapy, and tamoxifen.

With respect to adjuvant chemotherapy, information from 30,000 women in 69 trials was collected. These patients were involved in randomization between polychemotherapy versus no treatment (18,000), longer versus shorter polychemotherapy (6000), or anthracycline-containing regimens versus CMF (6000). Overall, results for all treated versus all untreated patients indicate a proportional reduction in recurrence of 23.5% and a proportional reduction in death (from any cause) of 15.3%. Subgroup analysis is possible in an overview, as long as the data are present and the groups are uniform. In the first division by subgroup, the overview considered the benefit of adjuvant chemotherapy according to nodal status: those with positive nodes and those with negative nodes. Absolute benefits appear greater for node-positive patients than for node-negative patients. However, the reduction in annual odds of recurrence is similar (28% to 34% for node-negative patients and 33% to 42% for node-positive women). Reduction in the odds of death from any cause is also similar for node-positive and node-negative patients. This relationship is a good example of the principle, discussed earlier, that a constant reduction of the odds of recurrence or death leads to larger differences in absolute benefits for groups with an inherently higher event rate. In summary, adjuvant chemotherapy with multiple drugs produces a statistically significant reduction in the odds of breast cancer recurrence or death and is thought to be proportionately similar in node-positive and node-negative patients.

The rule of a constant proportional benefit is not entirely true. Illustrated in Figure 32-17, the benefits of adjuvant polychemotherapy appeared to be greatest in younger women, with an inverse relationship of benefit to age. For women younger than 40, polychemotherapy reduced the odds of recurrence by 37% and of death by 28%. This benefit tended to decline in older women. However, even for women aged 60 to 69 when randomized, chemotherapy reduced the proportion with recurrence by 18% and the proportion dying by 9%. Women

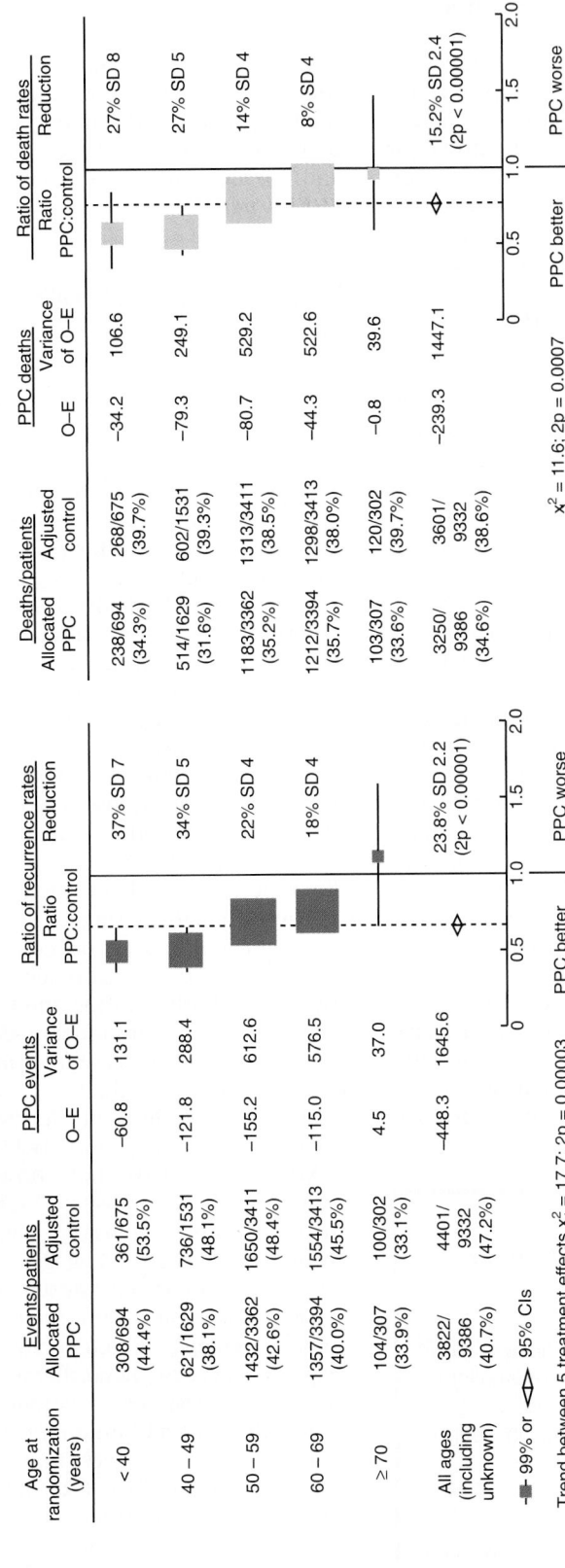

FIGURE 32-17. Risk reductions in the international overview of adjuvant chemotherapy following surgery for operable breast cancer. The position of the *squares* relative to the center line represents the proportion of event rates for chemotherapy treated groups compared to control groups. The *lines* show 95% confidence intervals, and the *area of each square* represents the amount of information available for each age group; *larger squares* mean more women are randomized. This figure shows the influence of age on the effect of chemotherapy; in general, younger women show larger reductions in recurrence rates after taking chemotherapy compared with younger women who did not receive adjuvant treatment. Older women receive somewhat less overall benefit, but statistically important benefits remain even for women older than 60 years. (From Polychemotherapy for early breast cancer: An overview of the randomized trials. Early Breast Cancer Trialists' Collaborative Group. Lancet 352:930-942, 1998.)

older than 70 years did not appear to benefit from the addition of adjuvant polychemotherapy, although the numbers in this group were small ($n = 609$). A significant interaction of chemotherapy and estrogen receptor status was also seen with estrogen receptor–poor disease receiving more benefit than estrogen receptor–unknown or estrogen receptor–positive disease, particularly in postmenopausal women. A small advantage of anthracycline-containing regimens (RR reduction of 12% compared with other polychemotherapy) was also seen in this large analysis.

The overview analysis from the EBCTCG provides useful answers to questions about adjuvant chemotherapy for patients of different ages with dissimilar diseases. Major findings are shown in Box 32-4 from the 1998 Overview. The meta-analysis conducted by the EBCTCG provides principles about adjuvant chemotherapy but recognizes that treatment decisions involve consideration of the benefit and the adverse side effects of treatments. These decisions are more difficult when the likelihood of recurrence is low or when the toxicity of treatment is high. Consider women with small, node-negative breast cancers. Rosen and associates reviewed survival statistics from Memorial Sloan-Kettering Cancer Center for patients undergoing operation alone between 1964 and 1970, allowing a long follow-up. For node-negative patients with tumors 1 cm or less, the likelihood of remaining free of disease at 10 years was 92% (only 8% of these women suffer recurrence). Imagine a woman older than 50 years of age with a 1-cm, estrogen receptor–positive cancer. The proportional benefit of chemotherapy (reduction in the odds of recurrence), although present, is small and in the range of 20%. The absolute benefit is 20% of the odds of recurrence (0.2×0.8), or between 1% and 2%.

In contrast, for node-negative tumors between 1.1 and 2.0 cm, the chance of remaining free of disease decreased to 78%. For young women, with estrogen receptor–negative disease, the proportional reduction in recurrence and mortality is significant (40% and 35%, respectively). In this situation, a 40% reduction in the risk of recurrence

produces a large absolute benefit and may seem sensible. Other groups of node-negative patients may suffer even higher relapse rates, and poor prognostic signs include (1) tumor size greater than 2 cm, (2) poor histologic and nuclear grade, (3) absent hormone receptors, (4) high proliferative fraction (S-phase), (5) aneuploid DNA content, and (6) content of certain oncogenes such as *erbB-2 (HER2/neu)*.

Newer Approaches in Chemotherapy for Breast Cancer[41-43]

Dose Intensity

In the analysis of the Milan CMF trial, the question of chemotherapy dose was investigated as a determinant of effectiveness. The outcome of patients receiving greater than 85% of their calculated chemotherapy dose was significantly better than for patients who received less than 65% of their scheduled dose. This and other analyses have led to the hypothesis that dose intensity of chemotherapy is important in patient outcome. Dose intensity is defined as the amount of drug given over an interval of time (milligrams of delivered dose/m^2/unit of time); more intense regimens give a higher dose in a shorter interval than less intense regimens.

The hypothesis that dose intensity is an important determinant of response has been tested in national cooperative trials by the Cancer and Leukemia Group B (CALGB) and NSABP. The first was a randomized trial of different dose levels of chemotherapy given to women with node-positive (stage II) breast cancer after curative surgery (mastectomy or conservation with radiation). Three arms in this study received escalating dose intensity (by varying both duration and total dose) of CAF. Women given either high- or moderate-dose intense CAF had a significantly longer disease-free and better overall survival rate compared with the low-dose (and low-intensity) arm. Subsequent studies of further increasing doses of cyclophosphamide (NSABP B-22 and B-25) or doxorubicin (CALGB 9344) have not shown additional benefit for patients with node-positive breast cancer. There may be an optimal dose intensity, which must be reached for a given drug, but exceeding that level does not add benefit. The concept of an ideal dose is supported by Skipper and Schabel's work from the Southern Research Institute in animal models, which demonstrates that the dose-response curve of chemotherapy drugs is sigmoid shaped. In this dose-response relationship, very low doses and very high doses add little incremental benefit.

The benefit of very high-dose chemotherapy was addressed in a CALGB trial 9082. In this study, women with 10 or more positive lymph nodes received standard doxorubicin-based chemotherapy followed by a randomization to high-dose chemotherapy with bone marrow transplantation versus moderate-dose chemotherapy. To date, this trial shows a modest disease-free survival advantage, but no overall survival advantage, to high-dose therapy. Even though these results may improve with time, data from other randomized trials currently do not

---

Box 32-4. Overview of Adjuvant Chemotherapy from Early Breast Cancer Trialists' Collaborative Group

1. Benefit is similar for node-positive and node-negative patients, although absolute differences are smaller for patients at lower risk for recurrence or death.
2. All ages (up to 70 years) benefit, although younger patients receive more benefit.
3. Three to six months of adjuvant treatment is similar to longer durations.
4. Anthracycline-containing regimens are slightly more effective.
5. For young women, those with both estrogen receptor–negative and estrogen receptor–positive tumors benefit; for older women, there is more benefit for those with estrogen receptor–negative cancers.

support the use of high-dose chemotherapy, generally given with infusions of hematopoietic cells, outside of a clinical trial.

Most recently, the concept of dose density has been tested in women with positive axillary lymph nodes as an adjuvant to surgery in a national study reported in 2003 by Citron and associates. In this study, patients were randomly assigned to multiple schedules of three chemotherapy drugs (doxorubicin, cyclophosphamide, and paclitaxel). Although it was a complicated study, the women receiving compressed schedules of the three drugs at higher doses were better off during follow-up than their counterparts, that received "less dense" treatment (disease-free survival at 4 years was 82% for the dose-dense group compared to 75% for the other groups). In practice, the duration of adjuvant treatment for breast cancer may shorten to even less than the usual 4 to 6 months.

New Agents[43]

Addition of the novel class of drugs, the taxanes, to the doxorubicin-containing regimens in CALGB 9344 resulted in an improved disease-free and overall survival outlook. The results of this trial in node-positive patients led to U.S. Food and Drug Administration approval of paclitaxel for the adjuvant treatment of breast cancer. Thus, it appears that the addition of an agent, which is "non-cross resistant," can kill additional cancer cells when an increased dose of the same drug may be unable to do so. Further studies, which evaluate optimal timing and duration of taxane therapy, are currently under way within U.S. cooperative treatment groups.

Trastuzumab (Herceptin) is a humanized murine monoclonal antibody raised against the erbB-2 or HER2 surface receptor. This receptor, related to *erbB-1* or the epidermal growth factor receptor (EGFr), is the target of gene amplification and high-level overexpression in about 20% of human breast cancers. Overexpression of the protein product of the *erbB-2* gene is measured by immunohistochemistry and usually quantitatively expressed from zero to 3+. Gene amplification is measured by fluorescent in situ hybridization (FISH). Those cancers with 3+ expression or amplification by FISH may respond to trastuzumab. In fact, the addition of trastuzumab to conventional chemotherapy has improved survival in metastatic breast cancer patients, and some patients have experienced dramatic regression of cancer.

These exciting results are leading to trials of chemotherapy plus trastuzumab in high-risk patients receiving adjuvant chemotherapy, generally whose tumors highly express the *HER2* receptor protein, or contain gene amplification by FISH. Limitations to this approach are the relatively small number of patients with *HER2*-positive tumors and the additive adverse effects of trastuzumab and anthracyclines on cardiac function. On a positive note, biological agents (such as designer drugs and antibodies) that target specific carcinogenic pathways in the cancer (such as growth, apoptosis, or angiogenesis) are being developed and tested with increasing frequency. It is hoped that trastuzumab is the first in a line of new agents that target specific biochemical pathways, leading to less toxic side effects and more potency for cancers reliant on those pathways for their growth and progression.

Neoadjuvant Chemotherapy for Operable Breast Cancer

Neoadjuvant chemotherapy refers to chemotherapy (systemic therapy), given in addition to surgery or radiation (local therapies), which precedes local treatments. Neoadjuvant therapy can achieve high response rates and may permit conservative surgery in more advanced breast cancer, as noted earlier. There are reasons to apply this treatment to earlier stages of disease. For lower tumor burdens, the probability of drug-resistant cells is theoretically less. The absolute number of tumor cells left after treating a small tumor burden may be below a threshold, above which regrowth will occur. For these and other concerns, investigators have treated earlier stage patients with preoperative chemotherapy. The largest randomized trial was conducted through the NSABP and assessed the timing of chemotherapy in operable breast cancer. This trial, which included 1523 patients, demonstrated no survival detriment for patients who received preoperative chemotherapy compared with the same regimen delivered postoperatively. Six percent of participants judged ineligible for lumpectomy before chemotherapy were able to undergo conservative surgery after chemotherapy.

Whereas the preoperative approach may not offer survival advantage, it provides an in vivo assessment of tumor response. The magnitude of this response has independent prognostic significance and may guide subsequent systemic therapy. For patients who do not respond adequately, therapists might consider additional treatment in the form of non–cross-resistant drugs. Perhaps more enticing is the possibility of dictating therapy based on molecular markers measured in the primary tumor. In this setting, response might be measured not only by tumor response but also by changes in molecular characteristics, which could be used to dictate further biologically based therapy. The ability to treat breast cancer, assess response, and measure properties in the target cancer cells makes continued investigation of preoperative therapy worthwhile.

Hormonal Therapy for Breast Cancer[37]

The effect of steroid hormones on sensitive tissues has been the subject of important basic and clinical efforts. Beatson, surgeon to the Glasgow Cancer Hospital, was the first to demonstrate that bilateral oophorectomy can lead to regression of metastatic breast cancer. Surgically induced menopause became the first effective means to control advanced breast cancer, producing a beneficial regression in 25% to 40% of premenopausal patients. Huggins re-emphasized oophorectomy and demonstrated the effectiveness of adrenalectomy in the treatment of postmenopausal metastatic breast cancer patients. Endocrine organ ablation has been replaced by antiestrogen therapy in most patients. The drug tamoxifen is an estrogen agonist-antagonist and currently the first-line treatment for estrogen-sensitive breast cancer. However, there has been a renaissance in the development and use of hormonally active drugs; many new agents and treatment approaches will be tested in the coming years. The molecular basis for hormonal treatment is yielding to investigation, and scientists are learning that the traditional model of the estrogen receptor, its ligand, and its DNA target is an oversimplification. Multiple signal transduction pathways intersect, modify, and are modified by the estrogen receptor.

Steroid Hormone Receptors[2,37]

Reproductive and certain other sensitive tissues possess high-affinity protein receptors for estrogen and progesterone. Specific receptors for both hormones may be present in tumor tissue of mammary origin. These receptor proteins are activated when occupied by their specific hormone ligand. Activation of estrogen receptor leads to the induction of numerous cellular genes, including those that may encode critical enzymes and secrete peptide growth factors (Fig. 32-18). Clinically, the most important protein induced by estrogen receptor is the receptor for progesterone. Therefore, progesterone may serve as an indicator for the presence of a functional estrogen receptor, which may explain why progesterone-positive breast cancers display intermediate responsiveness to hormonal treatments, even if the measured value of estrogen receptor is very low or absent.

Newer assay formats for estrogen and progesterone receptors are based on immunohistochemistry and have virtually replaced the more cumbersome hormone-binding assays, which required fresh tissue. These slide-based assays may be done on either frozen or paraffin-embedded tumor sections. In general, if greater than 10% of tumor cells stain positive for the nuclear receptor, the assay is reported as "positive" and a response to hormonal treatment is likely. The majority of human breast tumors contain detectable amounts of either estrogen receptor or progesterone or both, and the likelihood that a patient's tumor is hormone sensitive increases with increasing age at diagnosis, shown in Table 32-17. Male breast cancer is almost always estrogen receptor positive. In contrast, the relationship between age and progesterone is not as significant.

The presence of estrogen receptor predicts clinical response to all types of endocrine therapies, both additive and ablative. Furthermore, because progesterone expression is induced by estrogen binding to its receptor, the presence of progesterone correlates with response to endocrine therapy. The presence of both receptors in a tumor is associated with almost an 80% chance of favorably responding to hormone addition or blockade (Table 32-18).

Hormonal manipulation for the treatment of breast cancer has been simplified by the introduction of tamoxifen and related compounds. Tamoxifen is a weak estrogen agonist. In molar excess, tamoxifen acts like a

TABLE 32-17. Distribution of Steroid Receptors in Tumor Biopsy Specimens According to Patient Endocrine Status*

Receptor Status of Tumor Biopsy Specimen	Endocrine Status of Patient	
	Premenopausal (%)	Postmenopausal (%)
ER⁺, PgR⁺	222 (45)	520 (63)
ER⁺, PgR⁻	58 (12)	128 (15)
ER⁻, PgR⁻	136 (28)	137 (17)
ER⁻, PgR⁺	72 (15)	41 (5)
Total	488 (44)	826 (44)

*Fifty-five years of age was chosen as an age at which virtually every woman may be considered postmenopausal.

From Wittlift JL: Steroid hormone receptors in breast cancer. Cancer 53(3 Suppl):630-643, 1984.

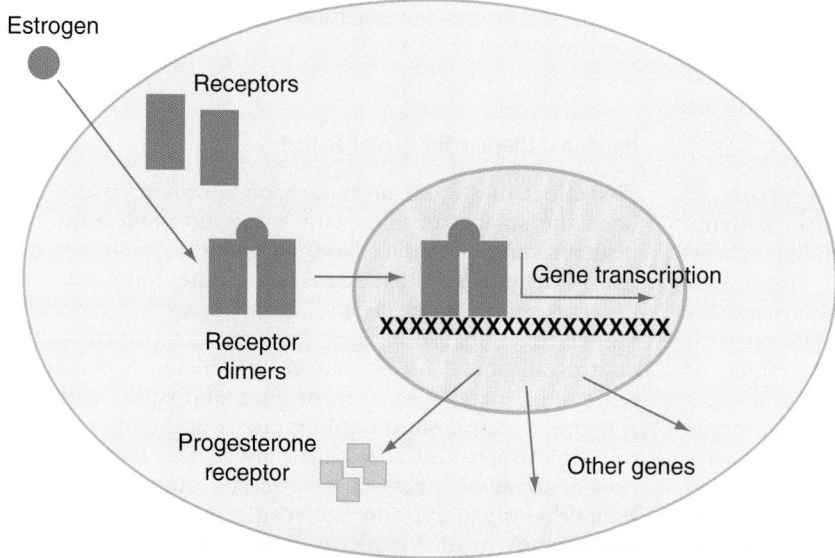

FIGURE 32-18. Physiology of estrogen and the estrogen receptor, shown schematically. Estrogen binds to estrogen receptors, either in the cytoplasm or nucleus, and the ligand-activated receptor interacts with promoter elements in target genes. This interaction results in gene transcription of estrogen-response genes, such as the progesterone receptor. Other genes induced directly or indirectly by the estrogen receptor influence cell growth and differentiation.

TABLE 32-18. Relationship Between Steroid Receptor Status of Breast Tumor and Patients' Objective Response to Endocrine Therapy

Steroid Receptor Status*			
ER⁺, PgR⁺	ER⁺, PgR⁻	ER⁻, PgR⁻	ER⁻, PgR⁺
137/174 (78%)	55/164 (34%)	17/165 (10%)	5/11 (45%)

*Number of patients responding to treatment/number of women with receptor status designated.
Based on the collective paper presented at the National Institutes of Health (NIH) Consensus Development Conference on Steroid Receptors in Breast Cancer (Proceedings of the NIH Consensus Development Conference, 1980). From Donegan WL, Spratt JS (eds): Cancer of the Breast. Philadelphia, WB Saunders, 1988.
ER, estrogen receptor; PgR, progesterone receptor.

competitive antagonist of estrogen activity in the breast but not in other estrogen-sensitive tissues. Both the beneficial and unfavorable actions of tamoxifen in tissues other than the breast are due to its estrogen-like actions. Tamoxifen can replace oophorectomy in premenopausal women with estrogen receptor–positive metastatic cancer, and it is considered the drug of first choice in both premenopausal and postmenopausal patients with estrogen receptor–positive or progesterone receptor–positive cancers. As noted in Table 32-18, response rates in metastatic disease are high when the tumor is estrogen receptor positive or progesterone receptor positive and decrease to 10% for receptor-negative tumors. Tamoxifen has been tested as an adjuvant after surgery or radiation therapy for primary breast cancer, and clinical trials have evaluated the use of tamoxifen to prevent breast cancer in certain high-risk women.

New Hormonal Agents for Breast Cancer[44,45]

Targeting the estrogen/estrogen receptor pathway is both selective for breast cancer cells that overexpress estrogen receptor and relatively nontoxic (compared to many cytotoxic agents and regimens). Novel drugs developed in the last 2 decades target both the production of estrogen, its interaction with estrogen receptor, and the receptor itself. These drugs fall into several new classes, and each class of compounds or mechanisms of action has several competing new agents available for clinical use. The selective estrogen receptor modulators (SERMs) are exemplified by tamoxifen. These agents are agonist-antagonists with differing spectra of activity in different tissues. The newer SERMS include raloxifene, idoxifene, GW5638, and others. The ideal SERM blocks the estrogen receptor in breast cancer tissue; is neutral or inhibitory in the endometrium; lacks the procoagulant activity of estrogen and tamoxifene; and acts like estrogen in the skeletal, cardiovascular, and central nervous systems. SERMs act at the level of the interaction of estrogen with estrogen receptor and influence the recruitment of transcriptional coactivators and repressors to the DNA-bound estrogen receptor dimer.

The aromatase inhibitors are agents that block the conversion of androstenedione to estrone. This is the last step in steroid conversion to active hormones, and it does not interfere with production of corticosteroids or mineralocorticoids. The first inhibitor and prototype of this class is aminoglutethimide. However, this compound does inhibit several upstream enzymes and interferes with the synthesis of cortisone. Therefore, selective aromatase inhibitors (SAIs) were developed that only inhibit the last enzymatic step in the formation of estrone. These include the nonsteroidal compounds that are reversible inhibitors (letrozole and anastrozole) and the steroid-based compounds that are irreversible (suicide) inhibitors (exemestane and formestane) of aromatase.

The SAI group of drugs is used in postmenopausal women and completely suppresses production of estrogen from extragonadal, nonovarian peripheral sites (principally in adipose tissue). Clinically, their usefulness will be second-line agents in postmenopausal women failing tamoxifen, as first-line hormonal agents in postmenopausal women with estrogen receptor–positive breast cancer, and even as alternative drugs to tamoxifen in healthy postmenopausal women as preventives. In premenopausal women, SAIs cause reflex pituitary release of gonadotropins and development of polycystic ovaries and excessive androgen production. However, these drugs may find application in premenopausal patients when combined with luteinizing hormone–releasing hormone agonists (LHRH-As) (see later).

As noted earlier, the SERMs are agents with both agonist and antagonist activity. Pure antiestrogens have been developed. The first of these agents in clinical use is fulvestrant (Faslodex). Fulvestrant is a steroid that binds with high affinity to the estrogen receptor and blocks estrogen receptor dimerization and DNA binding; it also leads to rapid degradation of the receptor protein. This compound has reached phase III testing in postmenopausal women with estrogen receptor–negative metastatic breast cancer who have progressed after tamoxifen treatment. Fulvestrant is probably as effective as the SAI group of drugs in these women. This compound is given at a single intramuscular injection every month, making it a convenient agent to use.

Although not new, estrogen levels can be reduced in premenopausal women, with functioning ovaries, by use of LHRH-As. The LHRH-As are superagonists that cause an early, massive release of pituitary gonadotropins, followed by paralysis of the pituitary and resistance to normal LHRH. Gonadotropin levels fall and result in rapidly declining estrogen levels and suppression of ovarian hormonal function. LHRH-As are peptide analogues of the normal releasing hormone that are 50 to 100 times as potent. Two are in clinical use for the treatment of breast cancer (goserelin and leuprolide).

Adjuvant Hormonal Therapy for Operable Breast Cancer

Early trials of endocrine manipulation after breast cancer operation used ovarian irradiation or surgical oophorectomy. The first modern trial of adjuvant tamoxifen was begun in Copenhagen in 1975. In 1977, the Nolvadex

Adjuvant Trial Organization (NATO) enrolled 1285 patients age 75 years or younger into a two-arm study of tamoxifen versus observation after surgery for operable breast cancer. Premenopausal women with positive axillary nodes and postmenopausal women with or without positive nodes were eligible. Treatment with tamoxifen was continued for 2 years or until relapse resulted in withdrawal from study. Nearly one half (49%) of tumors were assayed for estrogen receptor content. Overall, 34% fewer fatalities were observed in the treatment arm compared with the control group. Similar findings were reported at 5 years from the Cancer Research Campaign in England. This study treated stages I and II breast cancer patients with 20 mg of tamoxifen daily for 2 years.

The second major trial of adjuvant tamoxifen in operable breast cancer was conducted in Scotland and began in 1978, 1 year after the NATO trial opened. The Scottish trial randomized 1312 patients 80 years of age or younger who had negative lymph nodes or who were postmenopausal and had positive axillary nodes. The trial differed from the NATO study by using 5 years of adjuvant tamoxifen and by treatment of first relapses in the control arm with tamoxifen. More tumors (57%) were analyzed for their estrogen receptor content in the Scottish trial. When assessing survival data, it is necessary to note that 93% of patients suffering relapse in the control arm were treated with therapeutic tamoxifen. Therefore, survival prolongation by use of adjuvant tamoxifen in the treatment arm is compared with a policy of delayed tamoxifen therapy after first relapse.

Moderate reduction in both recurrence and fatality rates was observed in the tamoxifen-treated patients. In the control arm, 38% of patients suffered a recurrence and 23% had died by 1987. In the tamoxifen-treated arm, there were recurrences in 24% of patients and 18% died of disease. The results of these trials in the United Kingdom have been confirmed by 24 other randomized comparisons of adjuvant tamoxifen to a no-treatment control arm. In all but one of these trials, tamoxifen has improved disease-free survival, and most trials show a survival benefit. These results have been combined into a large meta-analysis, which confirms the benefits of adjuvant tamoxifen.

Meta-Analysis of Adjuvant Tamoxifen for Breast Cancer[21,46]

The overview from the EBCTCG looked at 42,000 women participating in 63 randomized trials in which tamoxifen was compared with placebo or no treatment. Statistically significant benefits for both node-positive and node-negative women were discovered, as shown in Figure 32-19. The benefits gained by taking tamoxifen for 1 to 5 years were observed after treatment had ceased. For recurrence, the curves are parallel past 5 years. For survival, the benefits gained during years of treatment continued to grow steadily after treatment was stopped. In addition, the benefit of tamoxifen increased with longer duration of use, to a maximum of 5 years in which a 47% ± 3% reduction in the annual hazard rate of recurrence (reduction in the odds of recurrence) was seen. The corresponding

mortality rate reduction was 26% ± 4%. Remarkably, these proportional reductions were largely unaffected by age, menopausal status, nodal status, or concomitant treatment. The only significant predictor was estrogen receptor status, which clearly showed the benefit from tamoxifen was limited to estrogen receptor–positive patients and higher estrogen receptor values correlated with increased benefit.

Adjuvant Ovarian Ablation[46]

One surprising result of the overview process was to rekindle interest in ovarian ablation as an effective adjuvant for operable breast cancer in premenopausal women. Ten trials were reviewed that accomplished ovarian ablation by oophorectomy, ovarian irradiation, and certain drugs (other than tamoxifen). Results were strikingly positive for premenopausal women younger than 50 years of age. Overall survival rate was improved by 25% in women younger than 50 years who received ovarian ablative therapy. Consideration of node-negative women younger than 50 years who died of breast cancer, excluding other causes of death, left an odds reduction of 47% in breast cancer deaths for women whose ovaries were removed or ablated. These data suggest that oophorectomy is as effective as chemotherapy for premenopausal, estrogen receptor–positive patients.

Aromatase Inhibitors as Adjuvant Therapy[47,48]

Several clinical trials are introducing SAIs into adjuvant therapy and comparing these agents against tamoxifen, the current standard for adjuvant therapy of estrogen receptor–positive breast cancer after local treatment. One of the oldest and largest trials directly compares 5 years of tamoxifen with 5 years of the SAI anastrozole, and adds a third arm that combines tamoxifen with anastrozole. The so-called ATAC Trial is a large, multinational, prospective, double-blinded study that accrued 9,366 women from 381 centers in 21 countries. Postmenopausal women with invasive breast cancer were eligible after surgical treatment, or following completion of chemotherapy. Women with estrogen receptor–positive, estrogen receptor–negative or unknown receptor status were eligible, and these subsets were analyzed individually after unmasking the randomization and analyzing results.

After 33 months of follow-up, the first published results of ATAC appeared. Disease-free survival was slightly better with the use of anastrozole as a single agent, compared to both tamoxifen alone and the combination of tamoxifen plus anastrozole (89.4% disease-free survival for anastrozole compared to 87.4% for tamoxifen and 87.2% for tamoxifen alone). The hazard ratio for disease-free survival was 0.83 (0.71 to 0.96; $P = 0.013$) comparing tamoxifen to anastrozole as single agents. The combination of drugs was no better than tamoxifen alone and inferior to anastrozole alone. As expected, the treatment differential was seen in women with estrogen receptor–positive breast cancers. It is likely with longer follow-up in ATAC, and with more adjuvant studies of aromatase inhibitors (at

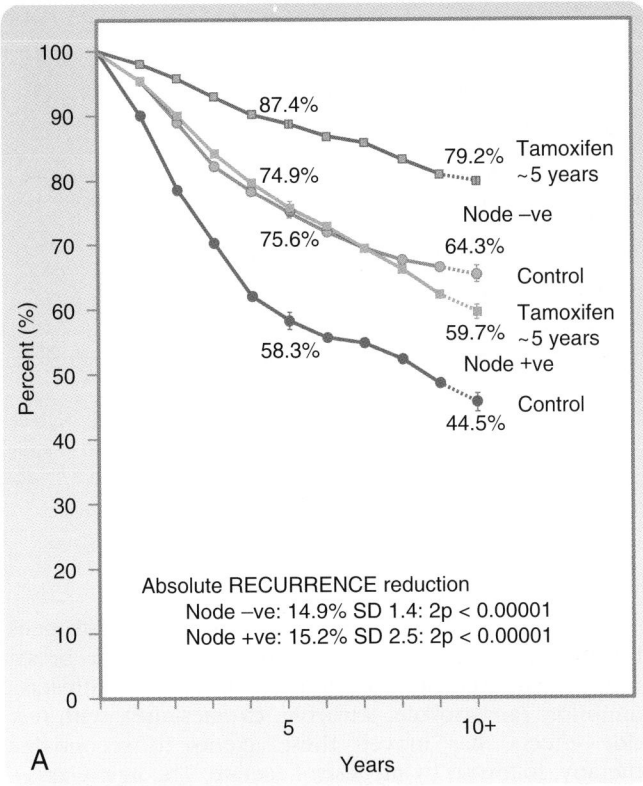
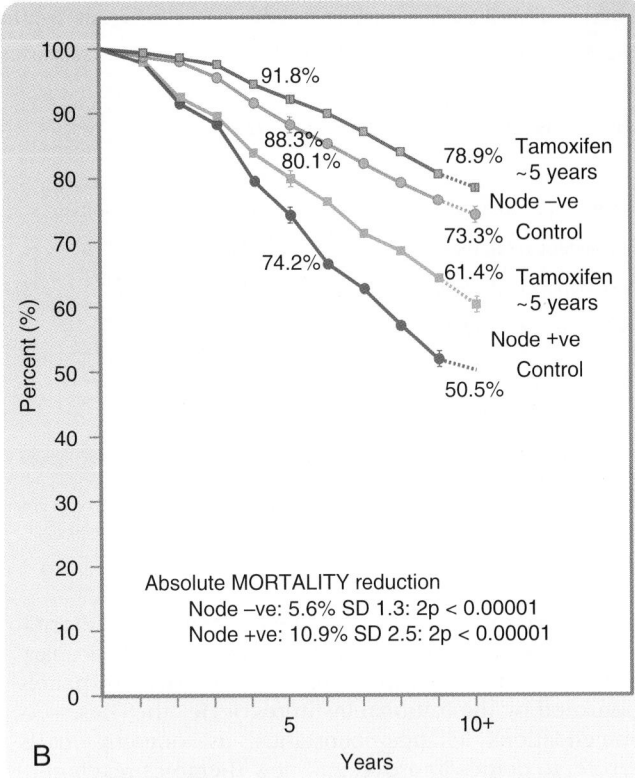

FIGURE 32-19. Results of the international overview of randomized trials comparing tamoxifen-treated patients to control subjects after either mastectomy or breast-conserving surgery for operable breast cancer. **A** shows recurrence-free survival and **B** shows overall survival rates (death from any cause). The s*quares* plot the results of women receiving adjuvant tamoxifen, and the *circles* represent untreated, control women. The *open squares* and *circles* plot the results of axillary node–negative women and the *closed squares* and *circles* plot the results of axillary node–positive women. The absolute differences between treatment and control groups at 10 years of follow-up are shown below the lines. (**A** and **B**, From Tamoxifen for early breast cancer: An overview of the randomized trials. Early Breast Cancer Trialists' Collaborative Group. Lancet 351:1451-1467, 1998.)

least six trials have opened with various strategies), aromatase inhibitors will find a place in the first-line adjuvant treatment of postmenopausal women with estrogen receptor-positive breast cancer. As noted earlier, the SAI group of drugs are not appropriate as single agents in premenopausal women.

Summary of Adjuvant Therapy for Operable Breast Cancer[49]

Guidelines for adjuvant therapy after primary treatment of breast cancer have evolved toward extending treatment recommendations to more patients. In fact, it has been difficult to identify a group of women who do not benefit from some form of adjuvant systemic treatment. Therefore adjuvant chemotherapy is likely to benefit nearly all patients with invasive breast cancers, and hormonal adjuvants probably benefit all breast cancer patients with estrogen receptor-positive or progesterone receptor-positive cancers. A risk-benefit ratio must be estimated for each patient, in which the reduction in risk of recurrence is weighed against the morbidity of treatment. Some form

of adjuvant therapy should be considered for nearly all patients with invasive breast cancer. Exception is made for patients with very favorable tumors (<1 cm in size or tumors with good histologies up to 2 or 3 cm, e.g., tubular or mucinous cancers), in whom side effects of cytotoxic treatment may outweigh benefits. For older patients, the benefits of chemotherapy are generally less and the ability to deliver optimal therapy is made more difficult by the presence of other impairments. For elderly patients, the decision to administer adjuvant chemotherapy should be made on an individual basis.

Adjuvant tamoxifen is recommended for estrogen receptor-positive or progesterone receptor-positive cancers and treatment is continued for 5 years. Although remarkably free of toxicity, a slightly increased incidence of endometrial cancer and venous thrombosis are the major complications of tamoxifen. Therapy in excess of 5 years, or doses larger than 20 mg per day are not recommended outside clinical trials. Tamoxifen should not be routinely recommended for receptor-negative tumors. Aromatase inhibitors may play a role in the adjuvant treatment of breast cancer, but the current standard remains tamoxifen. These recommendations are

TABLE 32-19.   Recommendations for Adjuvant Treatment of Operable Breast Cancer, Stratified by Patient Categories and by Risk of Recurrence

Patient Category	Treatment Stratified by Risk Profile		
	Low	Intermediate	High
Premenopausal, receptor +*	± Hormone†	Hormone, ± chemotherapy	Chemotherapy + hormone
Premenopausal, receptor −	No recommendations	± Chemotherapy	Chemotherapy
Postmenopausal, receptor +	± Hormone	Hormone, ± chemotherapy	Hormone
Postmenopausal, receptor −	± Chemotherapy	± Chemotherapy	± Chemotherapy
Elderly + comorbidities	± Hormone	± Hormone	± Hormone

Risk Definitions:
  Low risk: T ≤ 1 cm; ER or PR +; age ≥ 35 (has all factors)
  Intermediate risk: T = 1–2 cm; ER or PR +, grade 1-2 (has all factors)
  High risk: T ≥ 2 cm; ER and PR −; grade 2-3; age ≤ 35 (has at least one factor)
*Either ER or PR is positive
†Hormone generally refers to tamoxifen for five years, although the use of an aromatase inhibitor in place of, or sequentially, is under investigation. Adapted from multiple sources.

summarized in Table 32-19, adapted from a recent international consensus panel on the treatment of primary breast cancer and from a series of consensus panels sponsored by the National Institutes of Health. These recommendations change constantly as ongoing trials mature, toxicities improve, and new therapies reach clinical application.

Treatment of Metastatic Disease[37,50]

When breast cancer recurs, it is generally thought to be incurable, with a median life expectancy between 18 and 24 months. There are exceptions, including patients with regional lymph node recurrence or women with ipsilateral breast recurrence after wide excision and radiation. In these circumstances, cure rates after local therapy may exceed 30%. Despite aggressive approaches, such as high-dose chemotherapy, distant metastatic disease is probably not curable. Nonetheless, breast cancer is often sensitive to both chemotherapy and hormonal therapy, offering disease control for many patients. Subsets of women live for many years with metastatic disease; in these women, breast cancer can be a chronic disease. In other women, systemic therapy can extend life and improve quality of life during the metastatic phase of breast cancer. This is particularly true for hormone-sensitive metastatic breast cancer. Response rates to endocrine treatment in metastatic disease for patients whose tumors harbor hormone receptors are in excess of 50%. These rates for endocrine therapy are at least as good as those achieved with cytotoxic chemotherapy. Because the time required for response is longer for hormone treatment than for chemotherapy, some estrogen receptor–positive patients with a heavy disease burden or aggressive disease are first treated with chemotherapy. Hormonal agents can be used later in the course of disease. This manipulation of the disease by skilled medical oncologists can prolong quality life in patients with otherwise incurable disease.

Tamoxifen is the first choice among the antiestrogens for patients with metastatic, hormone-sensitive breast cancer. The recent development of newer aromatase inhibitors (anastrozole, letrozole, exemestane), with few side effects, has moved these agents to second-line therapy, followed by megestrol acetate. The new class of pure antiestrogens, exemplified by fulvestrant, is probably equally effective as aromatase inhibitors in the treatment of metastatic breast cancer progressing after prior hormone treatments.

At some point in the treatment of most patients with metastatic breast cancer, chemotherapy is indicated. Although more toxic than hormonal therapy, several trials have indicated that chemotherapy improves quality of life. Response rates for the initial use of chemotherapy range between 50% and 70%. In general, cyclophosphamide and doxorubicin are first-line agents, although many patients receive these drugs as adjuvant treatment. The taxanes (paclitaxel, docetaxel) have essentially replaced other drugs as second-line therapy for most patients, because of their considerable single-agent activity and toxicity profiles. Vinorelbine, oral 5-fluorouracil preparations, and gemcitabine are commonly used third-line agents in patients failing taxanes.

Agents that target specific molecular pathways have been developed for few cancer types. One exciting discovery is the monoclonal antibody against the *HER-2 (erbB-2)* receptor protein, trastuzumab, which has recently been approved for use in metastatic breast cancer. Based on a multi-institution clinical trial looking at therapy for patients with metastatic disease that expressed the *HER-2* receptor, the addition of trastuzumab to paclitaxel tripled the time to progression and extended survival time by 4 to 6 months. This development is an example of targeting a specific oncogenic pathway with a nontoxic biological agent. Furthermore, this agent has remarkable activity against some breast cancers. Other agents, such as inhibitors of signal transduction pathways, inhibitors of angiogenesis, and immune modulators, are in the foreseeable future.

Selected References

Claus EB, Risch N, Thompson WD: Autosomal dominant inheritance of early-onset breast cancer: Implications for risk. Cancer 73:643-651, 1994.

> The "Claus model" is an empiric risk model that predicts a woman's chance of developing breast cancer based on her family history. This model considers the number of affected relatives in both the maternal and paternal lineages (up to 2), their relationship to the patient (whether they are first- or second-degree relatives) and the age of onset of breast cancer in each relative. It does not factor in ethnic background, whether the cancer was bilateral, or a family history of ovarian cancer.

Early Breast Cancer Trialists' Collaborative Group: Polychemotherapy for early breast cancer: An overview of the randomised trials. Lancet 352:930-942, 1998.

> This paper is one in a series of overview analyses (meta-analyses) from the Early Breast Cancer Trialists' Collaborative Group (EBCTCG). This compilation and analysis combines results from 47 worldwide trials of chemotherapy given to early breast cancer patients following surgical treatment. The manuscript provides the modern rationale for prescribing adjuvant chemotherapy to patients and uses the concept of proportional reduction in the chance of adverse events (recurrence and death). Reading past publications, and watching for periodic updates from this group, is recommended as well.

Early Breast Cancer Trialists' Collaborative Group: Tamoxifen for early breast cancer: An overview of the randomized trials. Lancet 351:1451-1467, 1998.

> Similar in scope to the EBCTCG report on polychemotherapy given as adjuvant treatment, this work summarizes the results of 55 worldwide trials using tamoxifen for treatment of early breast cancer after surgical treatment. Concepts and methods of analysis are similar to the previously cited report on chemotherapy, and the results of the overview summarize the current practice for tamoxifen in estrogen receptor-positive breast cancer. As recommended in the previous citation, previous work from the EBCTCG is worth reading, and future analysis will be of interest to practitioners of breast surgery.

Fisher B, Anderson S, Bryant J, et al: Twenty-year follow-up of a randomized trial comparing total mastectomy, lumpectomy, and lumpectomy plus irradiation for the treatment of invasive breast cancer. N Engl J Med 347:1233-1241, 2002.

> A prospective three-arm trial of more than 1800 women with breast cancer and clinically negative axillary lymph nodes, randomized to total mastectomy versus lumpectomy with or without radiation. With 20 years of follow-up, overall and disease free survival rates were equivalent between the three arms. However, local failure in the conserved breast was unacceptably high in the arm receiving only lumpectomy, without postoperative radiation. This 20-year experience is valuable for its comprehensive summary of modern surgery for breast cancer.

Fisher B, Jeong J-H, Anderson S, et al: Twenty-five-year follow-up of a randomized trial comparing radical mastectomy, total mastectomy, and total mastectomy followed by irradiation. N Engl J Med 347:567-575, 2002.

> This is the 25-year summary of a prospective trial of more than 1079 women with breast cancer and both clinically negative and positive axillary nodes. Node-negative patients were randomized to radical mastectomy, simple mastectomy, or simple mastectomy with radiation to the axilla. Node-positive patients were randomized to radical mastectomy or to simple mastectomy, leaving involved nodes, and giving radiation to the nodes. With 25 years of follow-up, overall and disease-free survival rates were equivalent between node-negative patients randomized to three different treatments and node-positive patients randomized to two treatment arms. Published accounts of NSABP B-04 provide a sound basis for understanding the principles behind the surgical approach to the axillary nodes in patients with breast cancer. B-04 also can be studied for the insights it provides into the mechanism and timing of breast cancer metastasis.

Gail MH, Brinton LA, Byar DP, et al: Projecting individualized probabilities of developing breast cancer for white females who are being examined annually. J Natl Cancer Inst 81:1879-1886, 1989.

> The "Gail model" calculates actuarial estimates of future breast cancer risk based on race, age, reproductive risk factors, maternal family history, and previous breast biopsy status. However, the Gail model may underestimate the risk for those with a strong paternal family history of breast cancer, a history of breast and ovarian cancer, and those who carry a *BRCA1* or *BRCA2* mutation.

Hartmann LC, Schaid DJ, Woods JE, et al: Efficacy of bilateral prophylactic mastectomy in women with a family history of breast cancer. N Engl J Med 340:77, 1999.

> In this retrospective, 639 women with a family history of breast cancer underwent prophylactic mastectomy. Based on family pedigrees, the women were divided into high (*n* = 214) and moderate (*n* = 425) risk groups, with high-risk patients defined as those with a family history suggestive of an autosomal dominant predisposition to breast cancer. For women of moderate risk, the number of expected breast cancers was calculated using the Gail model and yielded an incidence risk reduction of 89%. For women in the high-risk cohort, the expected number of breast cancers was calculated using three different statistical models, yielding an incident risk reduction of at least 90%.

Rossouw JE, Anderson GL, Prentice RL, et al: Risks and benefits of estrogen plus progestin in healthy postmenopausal women: Principal results from the Women's Health Initiative randomized controlled trial. JAMA 288:321-333, 2002.

> This prospective, randomized control trial from the Women's Health Initiative (WHI) enrolled 16,608 healthy postmenopausal women ages 50 to 79. The study assessed the benefits and risks of hormone replacement therapy, low-fat diet, and calcium and vitamin D supplementation on rates of cancer, cardiovascular disease, and osteoporosis-related fractures. Results from the WHI will be announced and published in the coming years and will certainly influence thinking about hormone replacement, diet and vitamin supplements.

References

1. Bennett S, Kaelin CM: Benign breast disease. *In* Branch WT (ed): Office Practice of Medicine, 4th ed. Philadelphia, WB Saunders, 2003, pp 545.

2. Donegan WL, Spratt JS: Cancer of the Breast, 5th ed. Philadelphia, WB Saunders, 2002.

3. Haagensen CD: Diseases of the Breast, 3rd ed. Philadelphia, WB Saunders, 1986.

4. Rossouw JE, Anderson GL, Prentice RL, et al: Risks and benefits of estrogen plus progestin in healthy postmenopausal women: Principal results from the Women's Health Initiative randomized controlled trial. JAMA 288:321-333, 2002.

5. Love SM, Gelman RS, Silen W: Sounding board: Fibrocystic "disease" of the breast—a nondisease? N Engl J Med 307:1010-1014, 1982.

6. Controlled Risk Insurance Company of Vermont, Inc: CRICO Risk Management Guidelines. Cambridge, Risk Management Foundation of the Harvard Medical Institutions, 2002.

7. Lewin JM, D'Orsi CJ, Hendrick RE, et al: Clinical comparison of full-field digital mammography and screen-film mammography for detection of breast cancer. AJR Am J Roentgenol 179:671-677, 2002.

8. Meyer JE, Smith DN, Lester SC, et al: Large-core needle biopsy of nonpalpable breast lesions. JAMA 281:1638-1641, 1999.

9. US Preventive Task Force: Screening for breast cancer: Recommendations and rationale. Ann Intern Med 137:344-346, 2002.

10. Humphrey LL, Helfand M, Chan BK, et al: Breast cancer screening: A summary of the evidence for the US Preventive Services Task Force. Ann Intern Med 137:347-360, 2002.

11. Liberman L, Abramson AF, Squires FB, et al: The breast imaging reporting and data system: Positive predictive value of mammographic features and final assessment categories. AJR Am J Roentgenol 171:35-40, 1998.

12. Liberman L, Menell JH: Breast imaging reporting and data system (BI-RADS). Radiol Clin North Am 40:409-430, 2002.

13. Darling ML, Smith DN, Lester SC, et al: Atypical ductal hyperplasia and ductal carcinoma in situ as revealed by large-core needle breast biopsy: Results of surgical excision. AJR Am J Roentgenol 175:1341-1346, 2000.

14. Fisher B, Costantino JP, Wickerham DL, et al: Tamoxifen for prevention of breast cancer: Report of the National Surgical Adjuvant Breast and Bowel Project P-1 Study. J Natl Cancer Inst 90:1371-1388, 1998.

15. National Comprehensive Cancer Network. Retrieved 2002, from *www.nccn.com*.

16. Powels TJ: Anti-oestrogenic prevention of breast cancer—the make- or break-point. Natl Rev Cancer 2:787-794, 2002.

17. Dupont WD, Page DL: Risk factors for breast cancer in women with proliferative breast disease. N Engl J Med 312:146-151, 1985.

18. Claus EB, Risch N, Thompson WD: Autosomal dominant inheritance of early-onset breast cancer: Implications for risk prediction. Cancer 73:643-651, 1994.

19. Gail MH, Brinton LA, Byar DP, et al: Projecting individualized probabilities of developing breast cancer for white females who are being examined annually. J Natl Cancer Inst 81:1879-1886, 1989.

20. National Comprehensive Cancer Network Breast Cancer Risk Reduction. Retrieved 2002, from *www.nci.nih.gov http://brca.nci.gov/brc*.

21. Early Breast Cancer Trialists' Collaborative Group: Tamoxifen for early breast cancer: An overview of the randomised trials. Lancet 351:1451-1467, 1998.

22. Hartmann LC, Schaid DJ, Woods JE, et al: Efficacy of bilateral prophylactic mastectomy in women with a family history of breast cancer. N Engl J Med 340:77-84, 1999.

23. Elston CW, Ellis IO: Systemic Pathology: The Breast, 3rd ed. Edinburgh, Churchill Livingstone, 1998.

24. Rosen PR: Rosen's Breast Pathology, 2nd ed. Philadelphia, Lippincott Williams & Wilkins, 2001.

25. Green FL, Page DL, Fleming ID, et al: AJCC Cancer Staging Manual, 6th ed. Heudekberg, Springer, 2002.

26. Jemal A, Murray T, Samuels A, et al: Cancer statistics, 2003. CA Cancer J Clin 53:5-26, 2003.

27. Fisher B, Jeong JH, Anderson S, et al: Twenty-five-year follow-up of a randomized trial comparing radical mastectomy, total mastectomy, and total mastectomy followed by irradiation. N Engl J Med 347:567-575, 2002.

28. Arriagada R, Le MG, Rochard F, et al: Conservative treatment versus mastectomy in early breast cancer: Patterns of failure with 15 years of follow-up data. Institut Gustave-Roussy Breast Cancer Group. J Clin Oncol 14:1558-1564, 1996.

29. Fisher B, Anderson S, Bryant J, et al: Twenty-year follow-up of a randomized trial comparing total mastectomy, lumpectomy, and lumpectomy plus irradiation for the treatment of invasive breast cancer. N Engl J Med 347:1233-1241, 2002.

30. van Dongen JA, Voogd AC, Fentiman IS, et al: Long-term results of a randomized trial comparing breast-conserving therapy with mastectomy: European Organization for Research and Treatment of Cancer 10801 trial. J Natl Cancer Inst 92:1143-1150, 2000.

31. Veronesi U, Cascinelli N, Mariani L, et al: Twenty-year follow-up of a randomized study comparing breast-conserving surgery with radical mastectomy for early breast cancer. N Engl J Med 347:1227-1232, 2002.

32. Early Breast Cancer Trialists' Collaborative Group: Favourable and unfavourable effects on long-term survival of radiotherapy for early breast cancer: An overview of the randomised trials. Lancet 355:1757-1770, 2000.

33. Chao C, McMasters K: The current status of sentinel lymph node biopsy for breast cancer. Adv Surg 36:167-192, 2002.

34. Schwartz GF, Giuliano AE, Veronesi U: Proceedings of the consensus conference on the role of sentinel lymph node biopsy in carcinoma of the breast, April 19-22, 2001, Philadelphia, Pennsylvania. Cancer 94:2542-2551, 2002.

35. Fisher B, Dignam J, Wolmark N, et al: Tamoxifen in treatment of intraductal breast cancer: National Surgical Adjuvant Breast and Bowel Project B-24 randomised controlled trial. Lancet 353:1993-2000, 1999.

36. Fisher B, Land S, Mamounas E, et al: Prevention of invasive breast cancer in women with ductal carcinoma in situ: An update of the national surgical adjuvant breast and bowel project experience. Semin Oncol 28:400-418, 2001.

37. Harris JR, Lippman ME, Morrow M, et al: Diseases of the Breast, 2nd ed. Philadelphia, Lippincott Williams & Wilkins, 2000.

38. Giordano SH, Buzdar AU, Hortobagyi GN: Breast cancer in men. Ann Intern Med 137:678-687, 2002.

39. Parker SJ, Harries SA: Phyllodes tumours. Postgrad Med J 77:428-435, 2001.

40. Early Breast Cancer Trialists' Collaborative Group: Polychemotherapy for early breast cancer: An overview of the randomised trials. Lancet 352:930-942, 1998.

41. Citron ML, Berry DA, Cirrincione C, et al: Randomized trial of dose-dense versus conventionally scheduled and sequential versus concurrent combination chemotherapy as postoperative adjuvant treatment of node-positive primary breast cancer: First report of Intergroup Trial C9741/Cancer and Leukemia Group B Trial 9741. J Clin Oncol 21:1431-1439, 2003.

42. Harris L, Swain SM: The role of primary chemotherapy in early breast cancer. Semin Oncol 23:31-42, 1996.

43. Perez EA, Hortobagyi GN: Ongoing and planned adjuvant trials with trastuzumab. Semin Oncol 27:26-32; 92-100, 2000.

44. Goss PE, Strasser K: Aromatase inhibitors in the treatment and prevention of breast cancer. J Clin Oncol 19:881-894, 2001.

45. Howell A, Robertson JF, Quaresma Albano J, et al: Fulvestrant, formerly ICI 182,780, is as effective as anastrozole in postmenopausal women with advanced breast cancer progressing after prior endocrine treatment. J Clin Oncol 20:3396-3403, 2002.

46. Early Breast Cancer Trialists' Collaborative Group: Systemic treatment of early breast cancer by hormonal, cytotoxic, or immune therapy: 133 randomised trials involving 31,000 recurrences and 24,000 deaths among 75,000 women. Lancet 339:1-15, 1992.

47. Baum M, Budzar AU, Cuzick J, et al: Anastrozole alone or in combination with tamoxifen versus tamoxifen alone for adjuvant treatment of postmenopausal women with early breast cancer: First results of the ATAC randomised trial. Lancet 359:2131-2139, 2002.

48. Winer EP, Hudis C, Burstein HJ, et al: American Society of Clinical Oncology technology assessment on the use of aromatase inhibitors as adjuvant therapy for women with hormone receptor–positive breast cancer: Status report 2002. J Clin Oncol 20:3317-3327, 2002.

49. Goldhirsch A, Glick JH, Gelber RD, et al: Meeting highlights: International Consensus Panel on the Treatment of Primary Breast Cancer. J Natl Cancer Inst 90:1601-1608, 1998.

50. Slamon DJ, Leyland-Jones B, Shak S, et al: Use of chemotherapy plus a monoclonal antibody against *HER2* for metastatic breast cancer that overexpresses *HER2*. N Engl J Med 344:783-792, 2001.

CHAPTER 33

BREAST RECONSTRUCTION

Bradon J. Wilhelmi, M.D., and **Linda G. Phillips, M.D.**

THE ROLE OF THE GENERAL SURGEON IN BREAST RECONSTRUCTION

Breast cancer is an extremely emotional topic by virtue of its anatomic location and the importance of the female breast in today's society. Therefore, it is imperative for surgeons performing breast surgery to have a basic understanding of which patients are candidates for breast reconstruction and what the reconstructive options are. Most patients start their inquiry about breast reconstruction with the surgeon who will be performing the mastectomy. They may ask, "What will it look like when you are done?" or "Will I have to live without a breast?" It is at this point that general surgeons greatly influence a woman's decision to pursue breast reconstruction. Although the reconstructive surgeon goes into detail about the surgical options, risk, and expected outcomes, ablative surgeons must be prepared for at least a basic discussion with patients. Whether breast implants versus autogenous tissue will be used, where the scars will be, and how long the recovery will take are all questions that most patients want answered. Whether they receive breast reconstruction or not can be influenced by the bias of the ablative surgeons. Oncologic surgeons are trained to place priority on ablation of the tumor; however, care standards now dictate that we also be sensitive to the resulting deformity. Only through a close alliance between the surgical oncologist and reconstructive surgeon can the patient's emotional, physical, and oncologic needs be addressed.

HISTORY

In the late 1800s, breast cancer prognosis was poor. Such notable surgeons as Volkmann, Czerny, and Billroth reported local recurrence rates ranging from 52% to 85%.[1] Within two decades of these reports, William Halsted presented his successful treatment of breast cancer with only a 6% recurrence rate. The halstedian theory of breast cancer treatment would remain the mainstay of breast cancer surgery for the next 60 years. He believed: "The slightest inattention to detail and or attempts to hasten convalescence by such plastic operations as are feasible only when a restricted amount of skin is removed may sacrifice his patient to the disease." So, concerned with the possibility of inadequate skin excision, Halsted went on to say: "To attempt to close the breast wound more or less regularly by any plastic method is hazardous, and in my opinion, to be vigorously discounted." Therefore, true attempts at breast reconstruction would have to wait for almost 50 years.[1]

Despite Halsted's condemnation of reconstructive procedures, it was recognized that the sizable defects left after this radical surgery did need to be closed. Although primary closure was often used, skin grafting of larger wounds was acceptable. Although plastic procedures had been reported by Legueu and Graeve of France and J. Collins Warren of the United States, these were merely chest wall closure techniques and not true breast mound reconstructions.[2]

The first attempt at a true breast reconstruction was in 1895, when Vincent Czerny transplanted a large lipoma from his patient's flank to the mastectomy site.[3] In a recount of this case by Dr. Robert Goldwyn, it was noted that 1 year after surgery the patient was doing well and had good breast symmetry. In this particular case, the mastectomy was for fibrocystic disease and not cancer. Tansini described the first use of the latissimus dorsi myocutaneous flap in 1906.[4] Unfortunately, this remarkable operation would not gain acceptance for another 70 years.

In 1942, Sir Harold Gillies of England started using a tubed pedicle technique of breast reconstruction. In this operation, he would "waltz" a flap from the abdomen to the chest to reconstruct the breast. Although this was very successful, the multiple procedures and prolonged treatment course precluded its widespread application.[5]

Since about 1970, many advances in reconstructive surgery have occurred and have been applied to breast reconstruction. The development of breast implants was the first of these revolutions. In 1963, the silicone breast implant was introduced for breast augmentation and was quickly adopted for breast reconstruction. In 1963, Cronin and Gerow presented a series of patients who had implants used to reconstruct mastectomy defects.[6] For the first time, the plastic surgeon had a procedure that could simulate the missing breast without the need for multiple procedures and a prolonged treatment course. In many ways, it was the simplicity and the safety of breast implants that ignited an interest in breast reconstruction. By the later 1970s, reconstruction was being performed immediately after breast ablation.[7-9]

The development of muscle, musculocutaneous, and fasciocutaneous flaps and microsurgical transplantation has had a tremendous impact on breast reconstruction. The ideal material to reconstruct any defect is like tissue. Up until the early 1970s, this was available only in limited quantities for breast reconstruction. The landmark work by Manchot[10] on vascular territories of the body was rediscovered, and surgeons were then able to exploit this basic knowledge to design flaps based on the axial patterns of named blood vessels. These technical developments allowed surgeons to reliably rearrange tissues and more precisely reconstruct all types of defects, including those of the breast.[11]

PATIENT SELECTION

Opinions as to which patients should receive breast reconstruction are as varied as the surgeons who perform the procedures. In general, young healthy patients with early-stage disease are the best candidates for reconstruction, and, consequently, older patients with advanced disease are poorer candidates. However, because of the multitude of different reconstructive options available, all women should at least be presented with the options before being excluded.[12]

With the increasing popularity of autogenous breast reconstruction, more stringent guidelines may be needed in the selection of potential reconstructive candidates. Compared with mastectomy alone, the greater surgical trauma, increased operative time, increased blood loss,

and prolonged recovery mandate that all patients, regardless of their desire for reconstruction, be thoroughly evaluated both physically and psychologically.

Although designed to help select candidates for transverse rectus abdominis myocutaneous (TRAM) flap reconstruction, the risk factor severity score by Carl Hartrampf can be applied to most patients, regardless of technique used. Each risk is given a numerical weight. The total is added and given a numerical score. Any patient with a score greater than 5 or with three or more risk factors is a poor candidate for TRAM reconstruction but may also be a poor candidate for the other procedures. Those with two risk factors are considered marginal candidates (Table 33-1). Of those risk factors listed, advanced age, obesity, smoking, concomitant disease, and patient psychological/emotional state are the most important to consider (Box 33-1).

TIMING

The timing of breast reconstruction after mastectomy has been advanced from delayed to immediate because of advances and refinements in breast reconstructive techniques and recognition of beneficial psychological

TABLE 33-1. Operative Risk Factors for Breast Reconstruction With the TRAM Flap

Obesity

Moderate: <25% above ideal body weight	1
Severe: >25% over ideal body weight	5

Small-Vessel Disease

Light-to-moderate smoking (1+ pack/day for 2-10 yr)	1
Chronic heavy smoking (10-20 packs/yr)	2
Chronic heavy smoking (20-30 packs/yr)	5
Autoimmune disease (e.g., scleroderma, Raynaud's)	8
Diabetes mellitus: non–insulin dependent	5
Diabetes mellitus: insulin dependent	10

Psychosocial Problems

Unstable emotional state (life crisis)	2
Personality disorder	3
Substance abuse	5

Abdominal Scars

If "planned out" of flap design	0.5
Disruption of vascular perforators: transection of superior epigastric vessels (e.g., Chevron incision, abdominoplasty)	10

Patient's Attitude

Patient unwilling or unable to invest time required for healing or objects to abdominal scar	10

Surgeon's Inexperience

<10 TRAM flaps	1

Major System Disease Process

Chronic lung disease	10
Severe cardiovascular disease	10

TRAM, transverse rectus abdominis myocutaneous.
Adapted from Hartrampf CR Jr: The transverse abdominal island flap for breast reconstruction: A 7-year experience. Clin Plast Surg 15:703-716, 1988.

effects.[13-15] Because studies have shown with immediate breast reconstruction a psychological benefit, cost effectiveness, cosmetic advantage, and no increased risk for complications or oncologic risk, immediate breast reconstruction has become the preferred time for reconstruc-

tion. In 1990, the American Society of Plastic and Reconstructive Surgeons reported that members performed 38% immediate versus 62% delayed reconstructions.[16] In a more recent study, 75% of reconstructions were performed immediately.[17]

Physician support for immediate reconstruction is based on the absence of medical contraindications and the anticipation of significant benefits to the woman. Early reconstruction after mastectomy reduces the emotional impact of mastectomy. Patients who underwent immediate breast reconstruction did not experience the loss of femininity, self-esteem, body image, and sexuality as patients did who had a delay in reconstruction.[18] Another study confirmed that patients who underwent immediate breast reconstruction experienced less depression than those who underwent reconstruction later.[19]

Immediate reconstruction is more cost effective, requiring only one major operation, anesthetic, and hospitalization. Delayed breast reconstruction is 62% more expensive.[20] Moreover, immediate breast reconstruction less frequently results in the need for secondary symmetry procedure.[21] Interruption of lifestyle occurs once, not twice.

Better breast symmetry can be achieved with immediate breast reconstruction because the skin flaps are pliable and not contracted to the chest wall. This improved symmetry with immediate reconstruction was confirmed by a recent study in which 67% (462/689) of delayed reconstructions required a symmetry procedure versus only 22% (155/705) of immediate reconstructions.[22] With immediate breast reconstruction using autologous tissue more of the original breast skin that is sensate can be preserved, whereas with delayed breast reconstruction much of the reconstructed breast skin is insensate. The skin-sparing mastectomy technique can be used with immediate breast reconstruction, which maximizes the sensate breast skin and confines the scar to around the areola (Fig. 33-1). With immediate reconstruction, it is easier to

Box 33-1. Factors Affecting Choice of Reconstruction Procedures

Patient Factors

Age
Medical conditions
 Previous abdominal or thoracic surgeries
 Coronary artery disease
 Chronic obstructive pulmonary disease
 Medications
 Chronic corticosteroid use
 Obesity
Body morphology
Occupation
Social activities
Financial resources
Support systems
Expectations/desires

Disease Factors

Stage of disease
Type of tumor
Need for adjuvant therapy

Miscellaneous Factors

Experience of the surgeon
Availability of equipment (e.g., microscope)
Religious beliefs regarding blood transfusions
Blood banking facilities

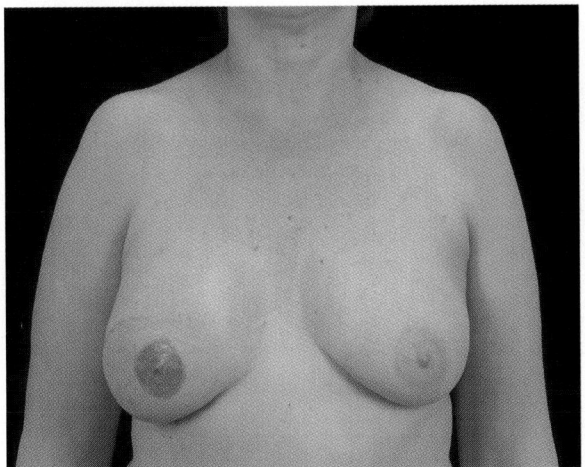 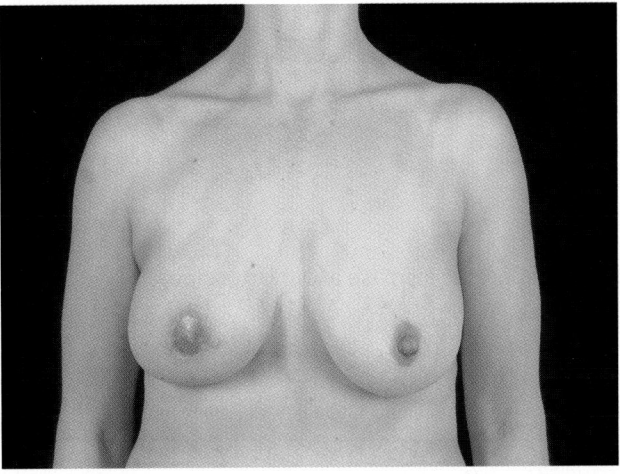

A   B

FIGURE 33-1. **A,** Represents a patient who underwent immediate breast reconstruction of skin-sparing mastectomy with pedicled TRAM flap and nipple areolar reconstruction, later. **B,** This patient underwent delayed breast reconstruction 5 years after modified radical mastectomy. A pedicled TRAM flap was used for her breast reconstruction. Notice the much larger skin paddle on the delayed breast reconstruction versus the skin paddle confined to the areola in the immediate reconstruction.

preserve the inframammary crease than to reestablish it at a later date.[23]

Studies have demonstrated no statistically significant difference in complication rates after intermediate versus delayed breast reconstruction.[24] Furthermore, there is no increased oncologic risk for immediate breast reconstruction. Clinical trials have shown there is no increased risk of cancer recurrence and no increased difficulty with surveillance for breast cancer recurrence with immediate reconstruction.[19,24,25] Because breast cancer recurrence in reconstructed breasts is usually in skin or subcutaneous tissues, the diagnosis is generally not delayed by immediate reconstruction. When breast cancer recurs in the chest wall it is highly associated with metastatic disease and the survival rate is not likely to have been influenced by earlier detection.[26] Studies have shown that immediate breast reconstruction does not delay postoperative administration of chemotherapy and radiotherapy.[27]

SURGICAL PLANNING

For the ideal breast reconstruction, the patient's native chest skin is preserved, leaving the reconstructive surgeon to merely fill a skin brassiere. Unfortunately, this is not always possible, but ablative surgical planning as early as the breast biopsy can improve the reconstructive outcome. In most patients, the surgical approach for the biopsy or the insertion site for the needle core biopsy can be made in or very near the nipple-areola complex. If the scars are placed around the areolar-cutaneous junction, the most favorable scar can be achieved. If the results of the biopsy are positive for cancer, re-excision of the first scar with a limited amount of skin prepares the patient for the most favorable reconstruction.

Contrary to previous teachings, large amounts of skin do not need to be removed to effectively treat breast cancer. Therefore, skin-sparing mastectomy can be performed whenever feasible. The skin-sparing mastectomy spares the breast skin by removing the breast tissue through a small opening only around the areola. Depending on the size and the location of the lesion, only the nipple-areola complex may need to be excised.[28] Additional incisions can be added to help with the dissection, such as a lateral extension of the periareolar incision for access to a large mammary gland or a separate incision in the axillary crease for the lymphadenectomy (Fig. 33-2).

The nipple and areola are removed because of the oncologic risk of involvement, which has been shown to be around 10.6%.[29] The skin-sparing mastectomy can provide superior aesthetic results, by confining the scar to the area around the skin paddle of the flap, which will ultimately be camouflaged as the rim around the reconstructed nipple-areolar complex. The skin-sparing mastectomy is oncologically safe. Studies have demonstrated no increased risk for local recurrence and no increased risk for distant metastasis or spread of cancer, and the disease-free survival for skin-sparing mastectomy is the same as for traditional mastectomy.[30-34]

A skin-sparing mastectomy with the skin flaps shaved too thin leads to tissue necrosis of the mastectomy flap skin over the viable flap. It is critical that the mastectomy skin not be too thin because this compromises blood flow to this skin. The perfusion of this skin can be assessed with a fluorescein test. If the mastectomy skin has questionable viability, it can be discarded and the skin paddle on the flap made larger or alternatively the reconstruction may have to be delayed. Care should be taken to avoid disrupting the inframammary crease. Although a small amount of breast tissue is present below the level of this

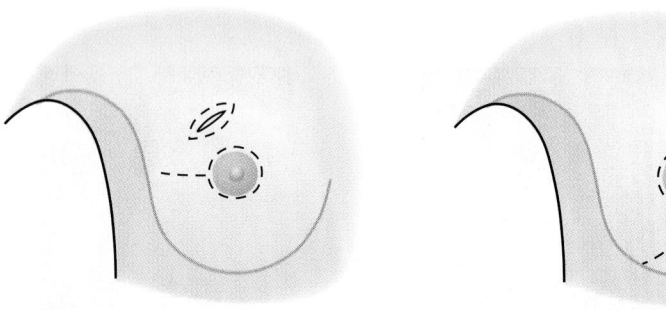

Lateral extension can increase axillary exposure

Wise pattern

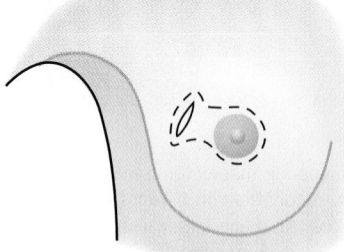

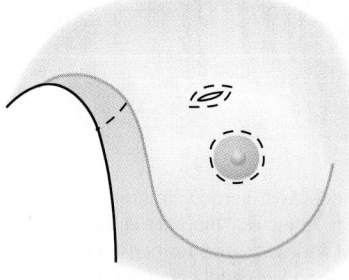

FIGURE 33-2.   Diagrams of options for incision placement in patients undergoing skin-sparing mastectomy. The more native chest skin that can be spared, the more natural the reconstructions tend to be. If possible, the biopsy incision should be placed periareolar to avoid using multiple incisions or increasing the amount of tissue excised from the breast.

crease, it usually does not need to be excised in a standard mastectomy. Preoperative marking of the inframammary crease helps remind the surgeon to avoid releasing this important surface landmark.[35] With the patient supine, the breast can be lifted. The natural crease is evident by the indentation made by the dermal fascial attachments. The crease can be marked with methylene blue, a permanent marker, or staples. Other surgeons have advocated placing sutures at the inframammary crease that are palpable during dissection of the inferior breast tissue.

In large or very ptotic breasts with lesions in the middle or lower third of the breast mound, alternative skin incisions can be planned with the reconstructive surgeon. A breast reduction type of skin incision using the keyhole type pattern provides the ablative surgeon with excellent exposure of the breast mound and adequate exposure for the axillary dissection (Fig. 33-3). If the patient is undergoing a contralateral breast reduction or mastopexy, the standard elliptical mastectomy incision provides less symmetry. The keyhole (pattern of Wise) incision design affords skin excision in the horizontal and vertical planes, resulting in a less ptotic, more conical, breast mound that is easier to shape.

SURGICAL OPTIONS

Breast reconstruction is a process that involves more than just creation of a mound on a woman's chest. Even the most perfectly shaped breast will leave a patient unhappy if it is not matched to the other side. It is often said that asymmetry is worse than ugliness and symmetry is ultimately more important to a successful outcome than anything else. Therefore, the reconstructive plan must accommodate not only the size and shape of the opposite breast but also the position on the chest wall; the location of the inframammary crease; the height, size, and color of the nipple-areolar complex; and the amount of breast ptosis.[36]

Reconstructive options can be divided into two main types: those that utilize autogenous tissue and those that require alloplastic material.[37] In general, autogenous tissue will usually provide better symmetry than an implant. Only 35% of TRAM flap reconstructions required a symmetry procedure versus 55% of implant reconstruction in one study.[38] The choice of procedure for a given patient is affected by her age, her health, her contralateral breast size and shape, her personal preference, and the expertise of the reconstructive surgeon (Box 33-2).

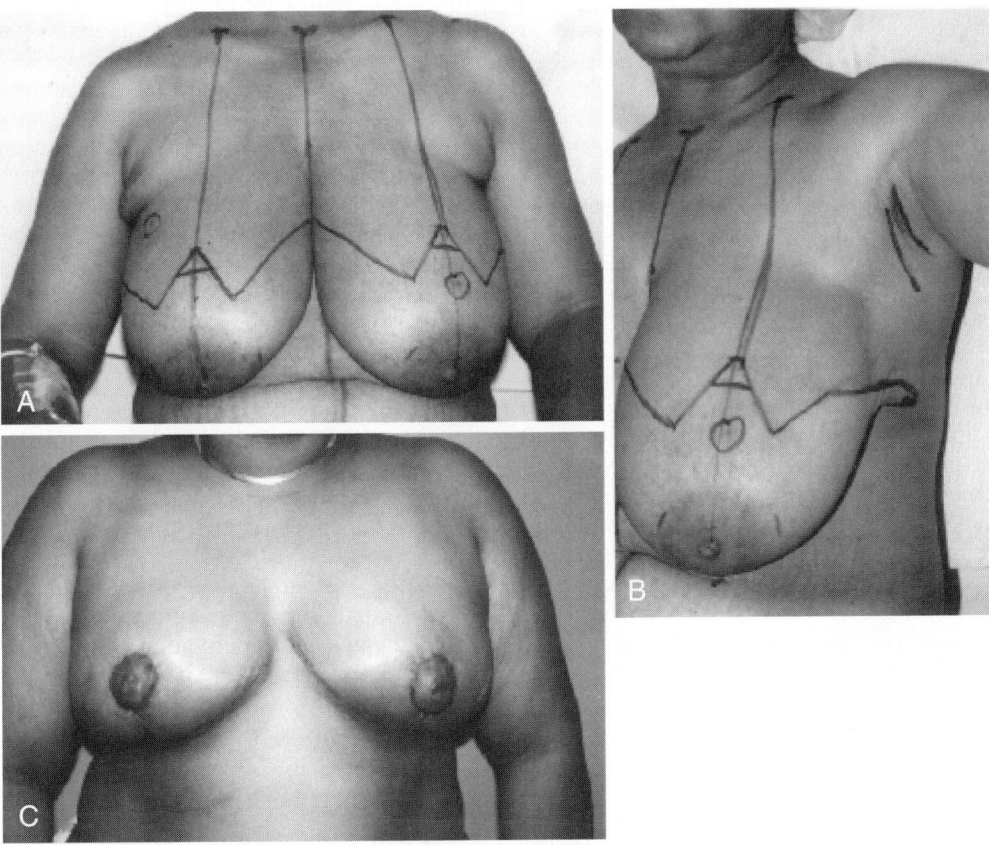

FIGURE 33-3.   A, View of a patient marked with a Wise pattern breast reduction incision. *Circles* show previous biopsy sites. Left breast biopsy result was positive for carcinoma. Patient was otherwise a candidate for lumpectomy but requested breast reduction in conjunction with ablative surgery. Right breast biopsy and subsequent pathology failed to demonstrate carcinoma. **B,** Marking for breast reduction as well as separate axillary incision for axillary node sampling. **C,** Photograph demonstrates postoperative results after breast reduction. The patient started adjunct therapy 5 weeks after surgery.

Box 33-2. Options for Breast Reconstruction

Autogenous
  Abdominal-based flaps
  TRAM
    Single pedicle
    Double pedicle
    Free flap*
    Deep inferior epigastric perforator flap*
  Upper abdominal horizontal flap
  Vertical abdominal flap
  Tubed abdominal flap
Latissimus dorsi musculocutaneous flap
Gluteal flap*
  Superior-based
  Inferior-based
Rubens flap*
Thoracoepigastric flap
Lateral thigh flap*
Breast-splitting procedure†
Alloplastic
  Silicone gel implant
  Silicone implant with saline fill
    Smooth wall
    Textured wall
    Round shaped
    Anatomic shaped
  Silicone injection†
Combination procedures
  Latissimus dorsi flap with implant
  TRAM flap with implant

TRAM, transverse rectus abdominis myocutaneous.
*Require microsurgical procedure.
†Historical note only.

Complications can occur with any type of breast reconstruction. The most significant effect is delay of initiation of adjuvant therapy. Partial or complete flap loss, wound breakdown, and infection are all reasons why chemotherapy or radiation therapy would be delayed. Complication rates are higher for patients who require radiotherapy postoperatively. In patients who required postoperative radiotherapy, TRAM reconstructions can provide better cosmetic outcomes and lower complication rates than implant reconstructions.[39] Because postoperative radiotherapy has been identified to worsen the outcome of an immediate TRAM reconstruction there has been a movement to delay reconstruction in patients who are expected to need postoperative radiotherapy.[40] However, the just-stated advantages to immediate reconstruction outweigh the risk of late complications seen with irradiated immediate TRAM reconstructions. Although survival in patients who have undergone reconstruction is no different than that in patients who have undergone mastectomy alone, the anxiety associated with delays in treatment can be significant to patients and waiting oncologists.[25,41,42]

Another concern to patients is blood loss. The average blood loss from reconstructive procedures ranges from 300 to 575 mL, depending on the pedicle technique used. It may be advisable for patients to autodonate 2 units of blood before surgery to minimize the need for allotransfusion.

Breast Reconstruction with Implants

Of the several methods of breast reconstruction available, breast implants can provide a technically simple means of achieving breast symmetry and pose minimal risk in properly selected patients. This approach to breast reconstruction is appropriate for patients requiring bilateral breast reconstruction. Through the use of bilateral, identical implants, excellent symmetry can be achieved (Fig. 33-4). Unilateral mastectomy patients with small breasts and minimal ptosis can also benefit from this technique. Although initially popularized for breast augmentation, use of the silicone implant was extended to breast reconstruction after mastectomy procedures.[6,43] In the original description, the implant was inserted in the subcutaneous breast wound. The use of saline implants precludes subcutaneous placement because these implants visibly ripple the skin. Placement of the implant in a submuscular plane beneath the pectoralis major, superior portion of rectus abdominis, and serratus anterior muscles provides better protection against implant extrusion as well as a decreased risk for capsular contracture and implant displacement (Fig. 33-5).[44] In approximating the pectoralis major to the serratus anterior muscles, preservation of the clavipectoral fascia, when possible, facilitates prevention of the suture pulling through muscle and ripping muscle fibers.[45,46]

In women with a large contralateral breast, a larger implant may be required for symmetrical reconstruction than can be placed submuscularly in the immediate setting. For these patients, permanent or temporary tissue expanders are utilized (Fig. 33-6). These are silicone envelopes with an integrated or remote port for episodic injection of saline in the outpatient setting.[47,48] Most surgeons overinflate past the desired size. This affords a larger skin envelope that gives some ptosis to the end result. Waiting at least 6 weeks from last expansion to implant exchange is believed to limit the rapid shrinking of expanded skin. At a secondary procedure, the expander is exchanged for a permanent implant. In women with very large breasts a Wise pattern incision can be used for the mastectomy. The complication of implant exposure through the inverted-T wound separation can be avoided by preserving and de-epithelializing the inferior breast skin and repairing the cephalic edge of this de-epithelialized inferior breast skin to the pectoralis major muscle caudal edge to protect the implant (Fig. 33-7).[49]

An alternative technique involves use of a permanent Becker silicone/saline implant expander with a remote port. This implant expander is filled to the desired breast size over several weeks, postoperatively. Later, the port can be taken out as an outpatient procedure.

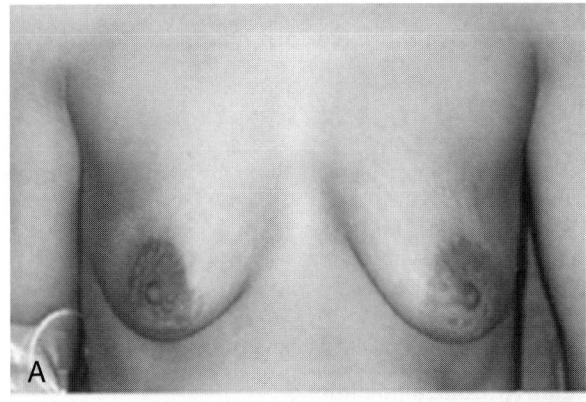
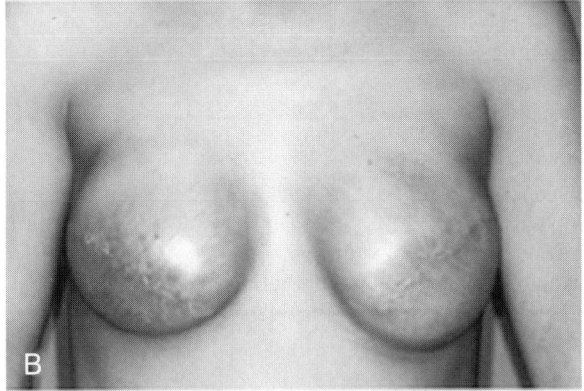
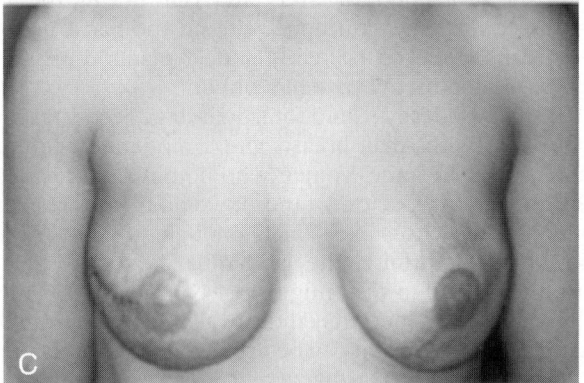

FIGURE 33-4. **A,** A 37-year-old woman with right breast carcinoma and a significant family history of breast cancer elected bilateral mastectomies and implant reconstruction. **B,** First stage of reconstruction with bilateral implants in place after mastectomies. **C,** Completed reconstruction, including secondary nipple reconstruction with local flaps and areola reconstruction with tattooed pigment.

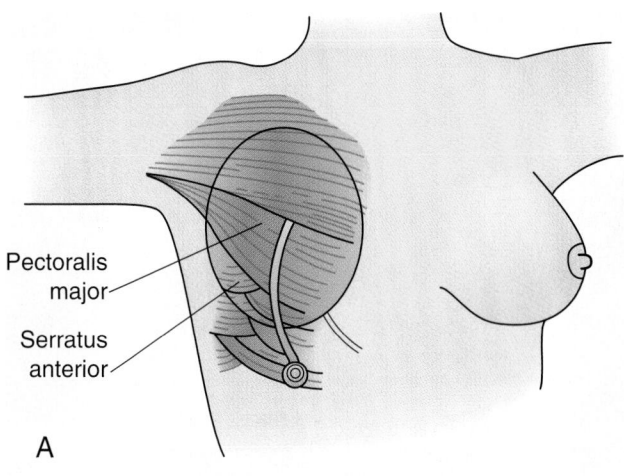
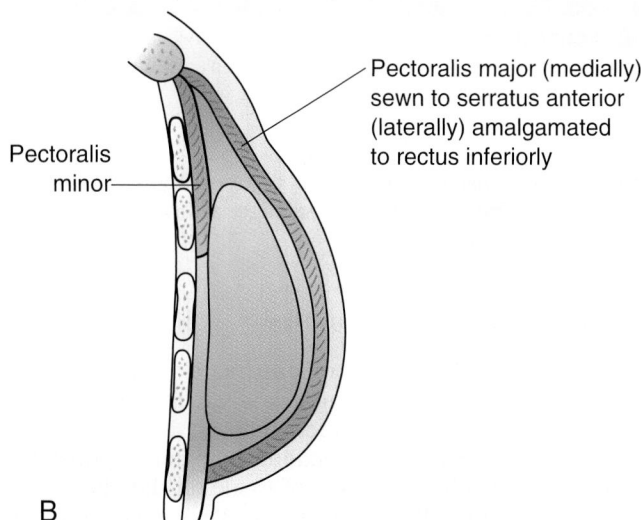

FIGURE 33-5. **A,** Proper placement of tissue expander underneath the pectoralis major/serratus anterior muscle. **B,** Sagittal cut demonstrates pectoralis major/serratus anterior muscle anteriorly, creating a complete muscular pocket to protect the implant from exposure through the thin remaining mastectomy flaps; this is also used to help re-create the inframammary fold.

Complications associated with the use of breast implants can occur in the immediate perioperative period or years later.[50] These complications include exposure, extrusion, or infection of the implants.[51,52] Careful attention when closing the submuscular pocket and skin can help avoid these problems. Longer-term problems also include asymmetry, capsular contracture, and malposition of the implant, rupture, and pain.[53-55]

Additionally, the breast implant may be used for thin patients who have inadequate abdominal and back soft

tissue for use with the TRAM or latissimus dorsi myocutaneous flaps. The breast implant may also be employed in conjunction with a myocutaneous flap to provide coverage and protection. Certain abdominal (subcostal and transverse) or chest (lateral thoracotomy) scars represent previous transection of flap muscle and blood supply and serve as absolute contraindications to the use of modes of autogenous reconstruction, thus requiring the use of the breast implant for reconstruction of the breast. Women expected to receive radiotherapy have a relative contraindication to reconstruction with implants because of increased risk for capsular contracture and inelastic skin impeding tissue expansion (Box 33-3). In those patients who unexpectedly require postoperative radiation

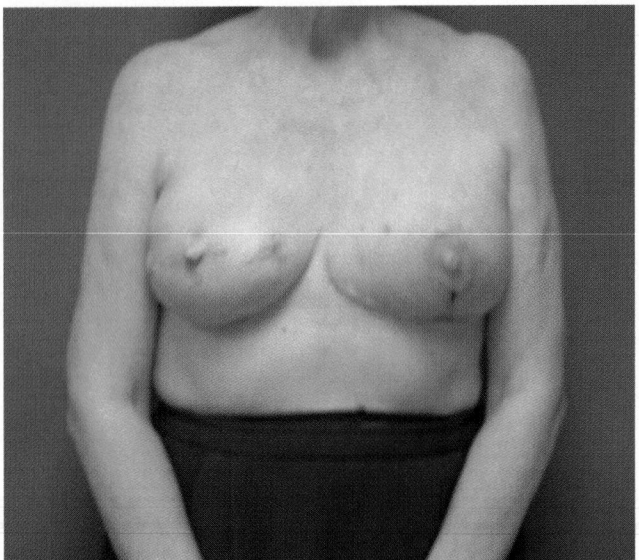

FIGURE 33-6. This patient underwent immediate breast reconstruction with expander that was later replaced with a permanent breast implant.

Box 33-3. Implant Reconstruction

Indications

Bilateral reconstruction
Patient requesting augmentation in addition to reconstruction
Patient not suited for long surgery
Lack of adequate abdominal tissue
Patient unwilling to have additional scars on either back or abdomen
Small breast mound with minimal ptosis

Relative Contraindications

Young age (may need implant replaced multiple times)
Patient unwilling to follow up
Very large breast
Very ptotic breast

Contraindications

Silicon allergy
Implant fear
Previous failed implants
Need for adjuvant radiation therapy

therapy, reconstruction with a myocutaneous flap technique may be required to salvage a firm, contracted implant reconstruction.[56]

Latissimus Dorsi Myocutaneous Flap

By the early 1970s, breast reconstruction with implants was widely accepted as a simple and safe means of reconstruction, but there were some significant limitations. One of the main problems plaguing implant reconstruction was, and still is, the lack of tissue on the chest wall after mastectomy. If a moderate- to large-sized breast is matched or if there is any degree of breast ptosis, then there is never enough skin to cover the needed implant. In an effort to improve outcome, plastic surgeons worked toward developing single-stage operations for breast reconstruction that would supply the necessary additional skin to the chest wall and provide bulk to create a larger breast mound. The latissimus dorsi myocutaneous flap was the first to be widely applied in breast reconstruction.

Although first described by Professor Iginio Tansini for chest wall coverage in 1906, the latissimus dorsi myocutaneous flap was not commonly used until the 1970s.[4,57] The latissimus dorsi is a flat, triangular muscle that originates from the spines of the lumbar and sacral vertebrae and inserts into the intertubular groove of the humerus. Its blood supply comes from the thoracodorsal artery and from multiple segmental perforators off the lumbar intercostal arteries.[58,59] These arteries provide musculocutaneous perforating vessels that penetrate the subcutaneous tissue to supply a territory of skin directly overlying the muscle (Fig. 33-8). This flap is so hardy that it can be safely elevated even if the thoracodorsal artery is cut, receiving retrograde blood flow from a branch to the serratus anterior muscle. Nevertheless, if this flap is the planned method of reconstruction, care should be taken not to injure the thoracodorsal artery and vein during the axillary dissection. The skin donor site on the back, in most cases, can be closed primarily and, if planned properly, will be hidden by the patient's bra line.

This flap is ideally suited for single-stage reconstruction for women with small breasts and a moderate degree of breast ptosis. In some women who do not require a modified radical mastectomy and in whom the resultant segmental resection excision is enough to cause significant breast deformity, the latissimus dorsi flap can be extremely useful in restoring breast contour. If the breast volume requirements exceed the available tissue from this region, a breast implant can be used to augment the reconstruction (Fig. 33-9). However, if a large or very ptotic breast is needed, this technique would be discouraged in favor of the TRAM flap to provide a larger and bulkier skin envelope.

Despite the popularity of the latissimus dorsi flap in breast reconstruction, not all patients are candidates (Box 33-4). Women with large breast volume requirements are not ideal candidates. Patients who have had previous surgery in the back or the axilla (lateral thoracotomies) usually have had their latissimus muscle divided and should be discouraged from undergoing this form of reconstruction. In women with a history of radiation therapy to the axilla, the resultant fibrosis and arteritis may impair the blood supply to this flap, and the use of the latissimus dorsi flap is prohibited.

One of the disadvantages of this technique is that simultaneous harvesting of the flap while the mastectomy is being performed is not possible. Although the mastectomy can be performed with the patient in the lateral decubitus position, inset of the flap necessitates the repositioning of the patient before breast shaping and closure.

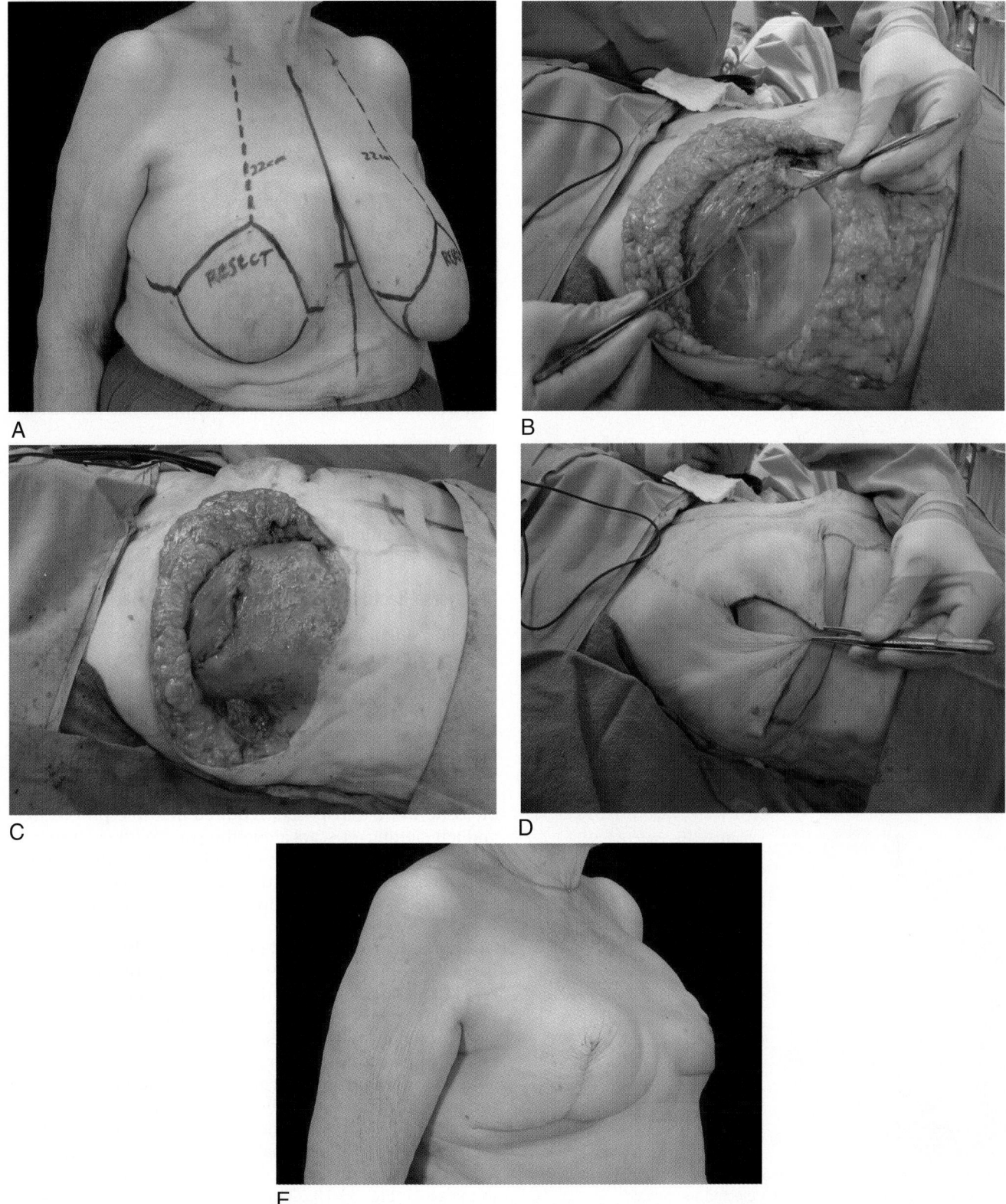

■ FIGURE 33-7. This patient underwent immediate breast reconstruction with implants through a Wise pattern breast reduction incision protected by de-epithelialized inferior skin flap. This inferior-based skin flap is repaired to the lower edge of the pectoralis major muscle to fully cover the implant should the Wise pattern skin incision break down.

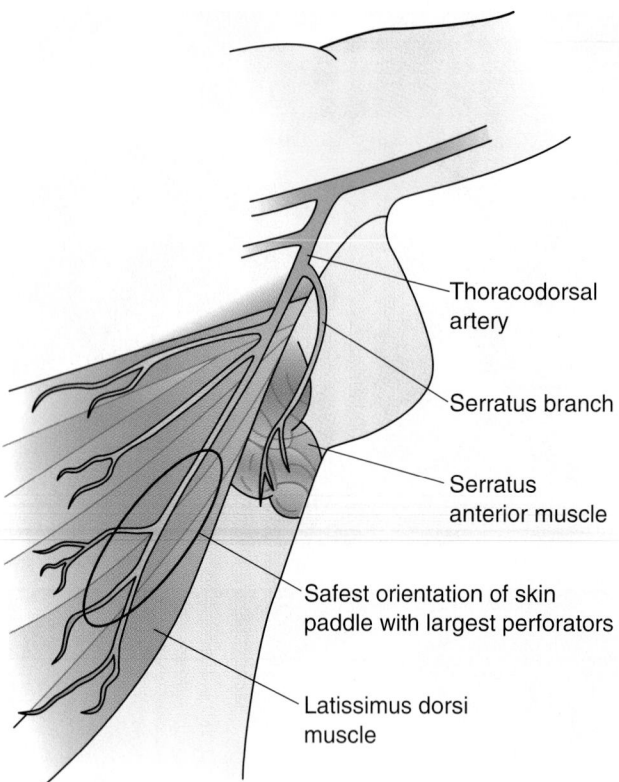

FIGURE 33-8. Pertinent anatomy in latissimus dorsi muscle reconstruction, including the latissimus dorsi muscle subscapular axis with thoracodorsal vessels, as well as communication with serratus anterior muscle via the serratus anterior communicating branch.

Labels in figure:
- Thoracodorsal artery
- Serratus branch
- Serratus anterior muscle
- Safest orientation of skin paddle with largest perforators
- Latissimus dorsi muscle

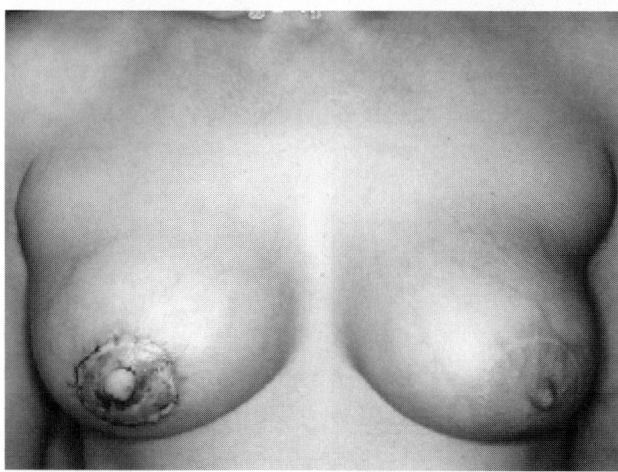

FIGURE 33-9. Woman undergoing right-sided simple mastectomy for chronic mastitis who elected to undergo latissimus dorsi reconstruction with an implant on the right with immediate nipple-areola reconstruction and left mastopexy augmentation. She is seen 3 weeks after her single-stage surgery.

Box 33-4. Latissimus Dorsi Reconstruction

Indications

Small breast
Minor breast ptosis
Abdominal donor site unavailable (e.g., scars, lack of tissue)
Salvage of previous breast reconstruction

Relative Contraindications

Planned postoperative radiation therapy
Bilateral reconstruction
Significant breast ptosis

Contraindications

Previous lateral thoracotomy
Very large breast in patient who does not desire reduction

This results in mild inconvenience to the operating staff, delays the operation, and raises the theoretical consideration of contamination and increased rates of infection.

Transverse Rectus Abdominis Myocutaneous Flap

The TRAM flap is the most commonly performed autogenous reconstructive procedure. The abdomen has always been seen as a potential source of donor tissue, especially for breast reconstruction. The skin and adipose composition between the breast and abdomen are very similar. Sir Harold Gillies[60] reported the initial use of tubed pedicle flaps of abdominal tissue more than 50 years ago. Unfortunately, his operation allowed for only a limited amount of tissue to be transposed, required multiple procedures, and left significant scars along the way. With each step of the transfer, more fat necrosed, which left a firm scar and a smaller flap volume. Further use of this technique was abandoned with the growing application of axial pattern flaps.

Although first suggested in 1979 by Robbins, the TRAM flap was popularized in 1982 by Hartrampf and coworkers.[61] In its original description, an ellipse of skin from the upper abdomen was used. This skin paddle design was later modified to be placed over the lower abdomen to take advantage of the larger amount of adipose tissue available, the more favorable scar location, and longer pedicle for ease in transposition (Box 33-5). Anatomic studies by Moon and Taylor[62] confirmed the rich supply of perforating vessels of the abdominal wall. The flap is divided into four regions on the basis of the entrance of the perforating vessels (Fig. 33-10). The most reliable zones are either directly over the muscle (zone I) or directly adjacent to this zone (zones II, III). Zone IV is the contralateral tissue farthest away from the musculocutaneous perforators and, in most cases, must be discarded, especially in obese patients and those who are smokers.

One of the advantages of this technique over other forms of breast reconstruction is the diversity of configu-

Box 33-5. Transverse Rectus Abdominis Muscle Flap Reconstruction

Indications

Breasts of all sizes
Breast ptosis

Relative Contraindications

Smoking
Abdominal liposuction
Previous abdominal surgery
Pulmonary disease
Obesity

Contraindications

Previous abdominoplasty
Patient unable to tolerate 4- to 6-week recovery period
Patient unable to tolerate longer procedure

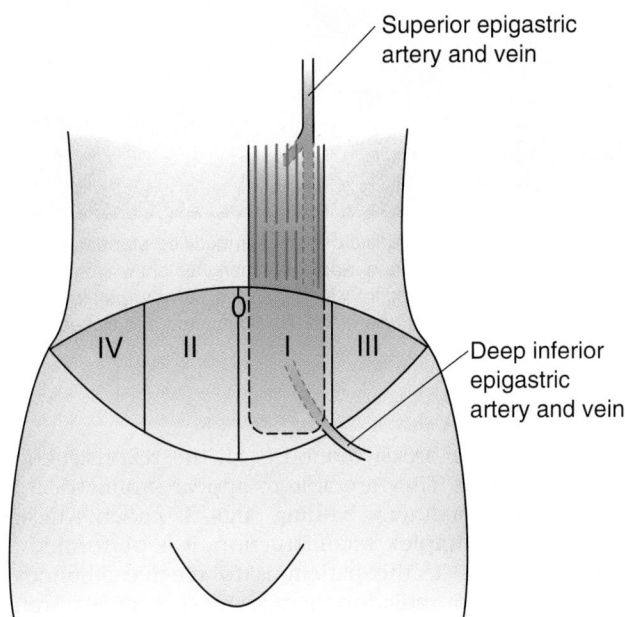

FIGURE 33-10. Vascular territories of the abdominal wall provided by unilateral transverse rectus abdominis myocutaneous (TRAM) flap. Studies by Moon and Taylor show the most reliable cutaneous portion directly overlying the muscle (zone I), followed by zones III, II, and IV, respectively.

rations available to the surgeon. This flap can be harvested as a single- or double-pedicle flap,[63] utilizing the deep superior epigastric blood supply.[64,65] It may also be harvested as a free flap based on the deep inferior epigastric vessels anastomosed to the thoracodorsal or internal mammary artery and vein.[66] The inferior epigastric artery is the dominant blood supply to the abdominal skin. In patients who are obese, needing larger tissue requirements, or with a history of upper abdominal scars, use of the free inferiorly based TRAM flap is considered more reliable. The free TRAM is also advocated for patients who

smoke because the relatively increased blood supply through the deep inferior epigastric artery protects against the nicotine-induced vasospasm that these patients have. Preparation of the artery for the microanastomosis results in stripping of the sympathetic nerves in the adventitia, protecting against vasospasm. Recently, the free flap has been harvested based only on perforators from the deep inferior epigastric artery with preservation of the entire rectus abdominis muscle. The disadvantage to the perforator TRAM flap is the reported increased risk of fat necrosis from less reliable blood supply.[67]

Complications may occur at either the breast or the abdominal donor sites. Donor site complications can include abdominal wall laxity (as opposed to true anatomic hernias), diastasis, abdominal skin necrosis, umbilical malposition, seroma, and severe pain.[68] The incidence of abdominal wall laxity has been reported to be as high as 20%. Although postoperative abdominal function is considered to be best in patients undergoing free TRAM reconstruction, most patients have a greater than 95% preoperative abdominal wall function within 1 year of surgery.[69-71]

Many surgeons use mesh to close the abdominal wall defect caused by the elevation of the muscle flap. Others close the defect by approximating the fascia. For subsequent abdominal procedures, it is helpful to obtain a plastic surgery consultation, perhaps for even opening and closing the abdominal surgery.

Breast complications include partial or complete flap loss. Most large series report less than a 4% flap failure rate and up to a 20% partial flap loss. Although the total flap loss rate is greater with free TRAMs (8%), partial loss is greatest with pedicle flaps (13% to 20%). There is an indication that the ipsilateral pedicled TRAM may have a lower rate of partial necrosis than the contralateral design.[72] Fat necrosis is a late complication affecting about 7% of pedicled TRAMs and 1% to 2% of free TRAMs.[73] Frequently, patients and oncologists are concerned about a firm nodule in the reconstructed breast. Biopsy may be needed to make the final diagnosis and to satisfy both the patient and the oncologist.

Other Options for Autologous Breast Reconstructions

When autologous breast reconstruction is desired but the TRAM and latissimus flaps are not available, other flaps have been described for postmastectomy reconstruction. The free gluteal flap has been used for breast reconstruction as a myocutaneous flap based on either the inferior or the superior vessels (Fig. 33-11).[74,75] Because of the technical complexity of the procedure and complications, including sciatica, seroma, unfavorable scar location, and asymmetrical buttock contour, this option is a secondary choice for breast reconstruction. The vascular pedicle is quite short, requiring either vein interposition or removal of costochondral cartilage to permit anastomosis to the internal mammary vessels.

The Rubens flap is based on the circumflex iliac vessels.[44,76] This option is most applicable for women who have an excess of soft tissue over the hips, as accentuated in women painted by Rubens during the Renaissance. The

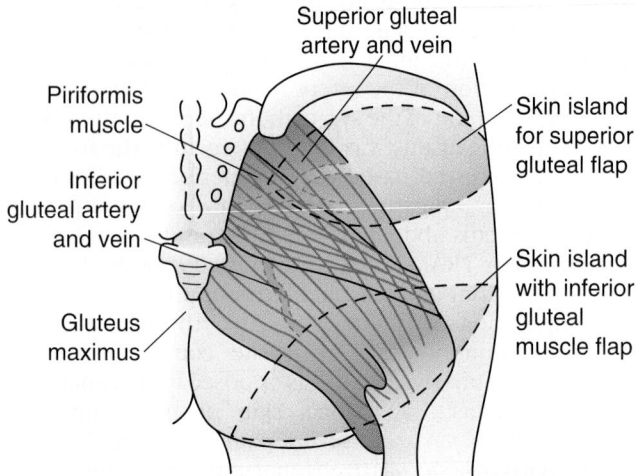

FIGURE 33-11. Pertinent anatomy and outline for free gluteal flap. Either superior- or inferior-based skin paddle can be designed on the respective inferior/superior gluteal artery and vein. Cosmesis is considered good and is best suited in patients with slight buttock ptosis.

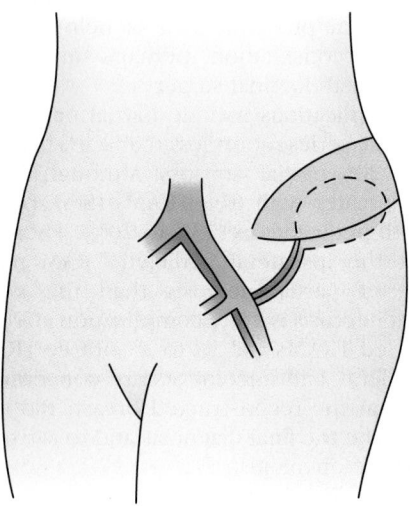

FIGURE 33-12. Diagram of the Rubens flap as described by Hartrampf and coworkers[76] in 1994. This flap is based on the circumflex iliac artery and is best suited in women who are not candidates for TRAM flaps and have adequate soft tissue in their hip region. Symmetry procedures usually need to be performed with excision of a similar amount of tissue from the contralateral hip.

flap is elevated with a full thickness of tissue over the hip and underlying musculature, including the oblique and transverse muscles (Fig. 33-12). Because this reconstructive procedure is limited in bulk and skin envelope and often requires a balancing procedure on the contralateral hip, it is not usually considered as a first option.

Nipple Areola Reconstruction

The first stage of breast reconstruction centers solely on reconstruction of the breast mound. For some patients,

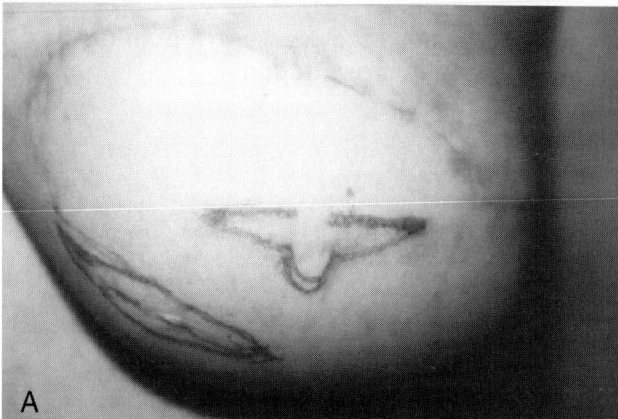

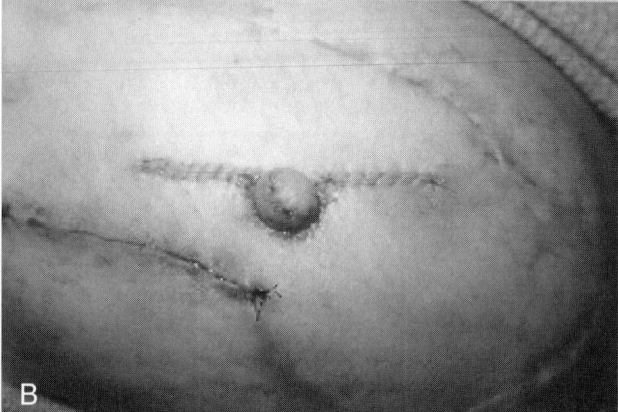

FIGURE 33-13.   A, Basic design of a modified star flap on a left breast before elevation. Additional markings show area of minor revision. This procedure was performed with the patient under local anesthesia in the office. **B,** Completed and closed nipple reconstruction.

merely having a breast mound is all the reconstruction that they desire. They are able to appear symmetrical in their clothes, including bathing suits. If patients desire nipple-areola complex reconstruction, it is performed as a second stage. If the patient is to receive adjunctive chemotherapy or radiation therapy, most surgeons prefer to wait until after that is completed. Changes in breast mound shape and position on the chest wall are expected after surgery and in response to radiation. Therefore, proper position of the nipple may not be able to be determined until 2 to 3 months after the initial surgery.

The nipple is created from local flaps on the breast mound.[77] Numerous different techniques have been described, but all have similar limitations.[78-83] Within 12 months, most undergo at least a 50% reduction in projection. Therefore, at the initial surgery, the nipple should be made larger than desired (Fig. 33-13). The pigmented areola was originally reconstructed with split-thickness skin grafts from the hyperpigmented upper medial thigh, labia majora, or retroauricular regions. This has been replaced with medical tattooing. Pigment is matched to the native nipple areola from the other side. Tattooing is performed 3 to 6 weeks after nipple creation. In most cases, the pigment fades over time and should be tattooed darker than desired.[84,85] Because of areolar tattoo fading and nipple flap flattening, others have attempted cryopreservation of the nipple, which has only produced mediocre results, owing to injury to the tissues with the freezing process.[86] Also, as mentioned earlier, preservation of the nipple-areolar complex poses an oncologic risk.

OUTCOME

In the past, the concerns of immediate breast reconstruction have been possible compromise of the ablative procedure, increased risks of surgery, altered survival, and impaired detection of locally recurrent disease. Therefore, surgeons have been reluctant to suggest reconstruction to their patients. One of the main concerns expressed by surgeons who perform mastectomies is whether a reconstructed breast can be adequately monitored for recurrence. These concerns are only increased as more and more surgeons are performing skin-sparing mastectomies in conjunction with immediate reconstruction. To date, no study has been able to demonstrate any difference in survival between patients undergoing breast reconstruction and those with mastectomy alone. Even in cases of advanced disease, reconstruction has not adversely affected outcomes. Some studies have even stated that complications of seroma and mastectomy skin flap necrosis are significantly decreased. Therefore, based on oncologic concerns alone, breast reconstruction should not be excluded from the treatment of breast cancer.

MANAGEMENT OF THE CONTRALATERAL BREAST

The challenge of breast reconstruction requires not only creating a natural-appearing breast but also achieving breast symmetry. Accordingly, on occasion, breast reconstruction requires an additional procedure on the contralateral breast. Occasionally, the mastectomy affords the patient the opportunity to obtain breast size or shape modification she had long desired previously. In reconstructing postmastectomy breasts, matching preexisting ptosis and larger contralateral breast size are difficult tasks. In the absence of medical contraindications, a reduction mammoplasty, mastopexy, or implant insertion may be required to optimize the breast reconstruction to achieve optimal symmetry (Fig. 33-14).[87] Although the risk of developing cancer in the contralateral breast is low (approximately 4%), in reconstructing the contralateral breast, results are best if done with the same reconstructive option.[88]

SURVEILLANCE

Reconstructed breasts can be followed clinically for evidence of recurrence. If the patient develops a firm subcutaneous mass or cobblestoning of the skin, a fine-needle biopsy or core biopsy should be performed.[89] This firm mass is usually fat necrosis, which is very common after radiotherapy. Routine mammographic screening of the

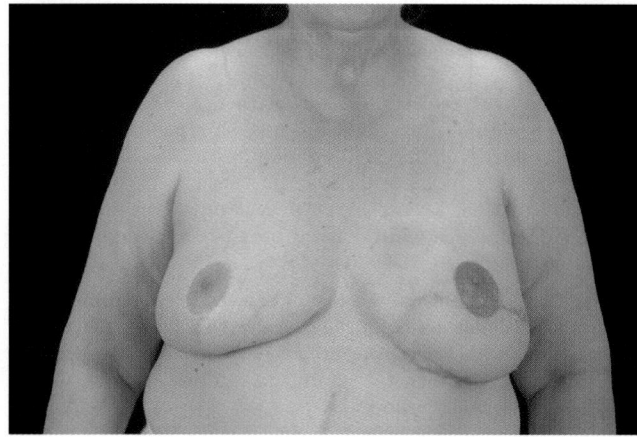

FIGURE 33-14.   This patient underwent delayed breast reconstruction with a pedicled TRAM flap of her left breast and a breast reduction symmetry procedure on the right breast.

TRAM flap breast reconstruction for surveillance is not recommended. Several other tools have been used to evaluate for recurrent breast cancer, including ultrasound, magnetic resonance imaging, computed tomography, and scintimammography. Overall, the most reliable means of diagnosing recurrent breast cancer after TRAM flap reconstruction has been the fine-needle, core, or open biopsy when indicated.[89]

CONCLUSION

Breast reconstruction may be one of the most significant female surgeries of this era and may reverse the dread that has been associated with the loss of one's breast. Breast reconstruction may even lessen the fear that contributes to a women's avoidance of medical evaluation of breast problems. Immediate breast reconstruction is favored because studies have demonstrated no increased oncologic risk, no delay for adjuvant therapy, better aesthetic outcomes, less depression, and more cost effectiveness. Skin-sparing mastectomy can provide a better outcome at no increased risk for local recurrence, distant spread, or disease-free survival. The planning and options for breast reconstruction must be individualized for each patient to minimize the risk for complications. The use of autogenous tissue can provide superior results but at a cost of a donor site. With the advent of tissue engineering some day it may be possible to reconstruct the patient's breast with her own cultured adipocytes harvested by liposuction with minimal risk of donor site complications.[90]

Selected References

Grotting JC, Urist MM, Maddox WA, Vasconez LO: Conventional TRAM flap versus free microsurgical TRAM flap for immediate breast reconstruction. Plast Reconstr Surg 83:828-844, 1989.

The authors described use of the lower abdomen skin paddle and rectus abdominis muscle as a free flap for microvascular tissue transfer in breast reconstruction with several advantages over the pedicle TRAM.

Hartrampf CR, Scheflan M, Black PW: Breast reconstruction with a transverse abdominal island flap. Plast Reconstr Surg 69:216-225, 1982.

> The authors re-described reconstruction of mastectomy defects with a transversely oriented skin paddle based on perforators from the rectus abdominis muscle.

Khoo A, Kross SS, Reece GP, et al: A comparison of resource costs of immediate and delayed breast reconstruction. Plast Reconstr Surg 101:964-970, 1998.

> The report evaluated the cost of delayed versus immediate breast reconstruction in 276 patients, concluding that mastectomy with immediate breast reconstruction is significantly less expensive than mastectomy followed by delayed reconstruction.

Noguchi M, Fukushima W, Ohta N, et al: Oncological aspect of immediate breast reconstruction in mastectomy patients. J Surg Oncol 50:241-246, 1992.

> In this study, multivariate analysis revealed no increased risk for recurrence in 83 patients stratified by menopausal status or axillary lymph node metastases, concluding that immediate breast reconstruction did not compromise survival.

Shaw WW: Breast reconstruction by superior gluteal microvascular free flaps without silicone implants. Plast Reconstr Surg 72:490-501, 1983.

> The author described his successful experience in reconstructing mastectomy defects with the free superior gluteal flap in 10 patients.

Singletary SE: Skin-sparing mastectomy with immediate breast reconstruction: The M.D. Anderson Cancer Center experience. Ann Surg Oncol 3:411-416, 1996.

> This report on 545 patients undergoing skin-sparing mastectomies and immediate breast reconstruction demonstrated a low regional recurrence rate of 2.6%. This recurrence was found to be a function of the tumor biology and disease stage, not use of immediate breast reconstruction or skin-sparing mastectomy.

Slavin SA, Love SM, Goldwyn RM: Recurrent breast cancer following immediate reconstruction with myocutaneous flaps. Plast Reconstr Surg 93:1191-1207, 1994.

> This study of 161 patients who underwent immediate breast reconstruction with myocutaneous flaps did not show concealment by the flap of any recurrent tumor.

Stevens LA, McGrath MH, Druss GD, et al: The psychological impact of immediate breast reconstruction for women with early breast cancer. Plast Reconstr Surg 73:619-628, 1984.

> This prospective study evaluated the psychological effects of immediate versus delayed breast reconstruction. Patients' mood, body image, sexuality, femininity, and social and occupational functioning were found superior in the group who underwent immediate breast reconstruction.

References

1. Halstead WS: Surgical Papers, 2. Baltimore, Johns Hopkins Press, 1924.
2. Rodman WL: Diseases of the Breast With Special Reference to Cancer. Philadelphia, P Blakiston's Sons, 1908.
3. Goldwyn RM: Vincenz Czerny and the beginnings of breast reconstruction. Plast Reconstr Surg 61:673-681, 1978.
4. Bostwick J III, Scheflan M: The latissimus dorsi musculocutaneous flap: A one-stage breast reconstruction. Clin Plast Surg 7:71-78, 1980.
5. Mendelson BC: The evolution of breast reconstruction. Med J Aust 1:7-8, 1982.
6. Cronin TD, Gerow FJ: Augmentation mammaplasty: A new natural feel prosthesis. In: Transactions of the Third International Congress of Plastic Surgery. Amsterdam, Excerpta Medica Foundation, 1963.
7. Mandel MA: Subcutaneous mastectomy with immediate reconstruction of the large breast. Surg Gynecol Obstet 146:90-92, 1978.
8. Pontes R: Single stage reconstruction of the missing breast. Br J Plast Surg 26:377-380, 1973.
9. Snyderman RK, Guthrie RH: Reconstruction of the female breast following radical mastectomy. Plast Reconstr Surg 47:565-567, 1971.
10. Manchot C: Die Hautarterien des Menschlichen Korpers. Leipzig, Vogel, 1889.
11. Ryan JJ: A lower thoracic advancement flap in breast reconstruction after mastectomy. Plast Reconstr Surg 70:153-160, 1982.
12. Dowden RV: Selection criteria for successful immediate breast reconstruction. Plast Reconstr Surg 88:628-634, 1991.
13. Brandberg Y, Malm M, Blomqvist L: A prospective and randomized study, "SVEA," comparing effects of three methods for delayed breast reconstruction on quality of life, patient-defined problem areas of life, and cosmetic result. Plast Reconstr Surg 105:66-76, 2000.
14. Schain WS, Wellisch DK, Pasnau RO, et al: The sooner the better: A study of psychological factors in women undergoing immediate versus delayed breast reconstruction. Am J Psychiatry 142:40-46, 1985.
15. Schain WS, Jacobs E, Wellisch DK: Psychosocial issues in breast reconstruction: Intrapsychic, interpersonal, and practical concerns. Clin Plast Surg 11:237-251, 1984.
16. Rowland JH: Psychological impact of treatments for breast cancer. In Spear SL (ed): Surgery of the Breast: Principles and Art. Philadelphia, Lippincott-Raven, 1998, pp 295-313.
17. Rowland J, Meyerowitz B, Ganz PA, et al: Body image and sexual functioning following reconstructive surgery in breast cancer survivors. Proc ASCO 15:124, 1996.
18. Stevens LA, McGrath MH, Druss RG, et al: The psychological impact of immediate breast reconstruction for women with early breast cancer. Plast Reconstr Surg 73:619-628, 1984.
19. Wellisch DK, Schain WS, Noone RB, et al: Psychosocial correlates of immediate versus delayed reconstruction of the breast. Plast Reconstr Surg 76:713-718, 1985.
20. Khoo A, Kroll SS, Reece GP, et al: A comparison of resource costs of immediate and delayed breast reconstruction. Plast Reconstr Surg 101:964-970, 1998.
21. Losken A, Carlson GW, Bostwick J III, et al: Trends in unilateral breast reconstruction and management of the contralateral breast: The Emory experience. Plast Reconstr Surg 110:89-97, 2002.
22. Losken A, Elwood ET, Styblo TM, et al: The role of reduction mammaplasty in reconstructing partial mastectomy defects. Plast Reconstr Surg 109:968-977, 2002.
23. English JM, Tittle BJ, Barton FE: Breast cancer, cancer prophylaxis and breast reconstruction: Selected readings. Plast Surg 7:11, 1994.

24. Trabulsy PP, Anthony JP, Mathes SJ: Changing trends in post-mastectomy breast reconstruction: A 13-year experience. Plast Reconstr Surg 93:1418-1427, 1994.

25. Slavin SA, Love SM, Goldwyn RM: Recurrent breast cancer following immediate reconstruction with myocutaneous flaps. Plast Reconstr Surg 93:1191-1207, 1994.

26. Langstein HN, Cheng MH, Singletary SE, et al: Breast cancer recurrence after immediate reconstruction: Patterns and significance. Plast Reconstr Surg 111:712-722, 2003.

27. Allweis TM, Boisvert ME, Otero SE, et al: Immediate reconstruction after mastectomy for breast cancer does not prolong the time to starting adjuvant chemotherapy. Am J Surg 183:218-221, 2002.

28. Singletary SE: Skin-sparing mastectomy with immediate breast reconstruction: The M. D. Anderson Cancer Center experience. Ann Surg Oncol 3:411-416, 1996.

29. Simmons RM, Brennan M, Christos P, et al: Analysis of nipple/areolar involvement with mastectomy: Can the areola be preserved? Ann Surg Oncol 9:165-168, 2002.

30. Kroll SS, Ames F, Singletary SE, et al: The oncologic risks of skin preservation at mastectomy when combined with immediate reconstruction of the breast. Surg Gynecol Obstet 172:17-20, 1991.

31. Kroll SS, Schusterman MA, Tadjalli HE, et al: Risk of recurrence after treatment of early breast cancer with skin-sparing mastectomy. Ann Surg Oncol 4:193-197, 1997.

32. Spiegel AJ, Butler CE: Recurrence following treatment of ductal carcinoma in situ with skin-sparing mastectomy and immediate breast reconstruction. Plast Reconstr Surg 111:706-711, 2003.

33. Foster RD, Esserman LJ, Anthony JP, et al: Skin-sparing mastectomy and immediate breast reconstruction: A prospective cohort study for the treatment of advanced stages of breast carcinoma. Ann Surg Oncol 9:462-466, 2002.

34. Gherardini G, Thomas R, Basoccu G, et al: Immediate breast reconstruction with the transverse rectus abdominis musculocutaneous flap after skin-sparing mastectomy. Int Surg 86:246-251, 2001.

35. Pennisi VR: Making a definite inframammary fold under a reconstructed breast. Plast Reconstr Surg 60:523-525, 1977.

36. Birnbaum L: Reconstruction of the aesthetically pleasing breast. Plast Reconstr Surg 67:745-752, 1981.

37. Elliott LF: Options for donor sites for autogenous tissue breast reconstruction. Clin Plast Surg 21:177-189, 1994.

38. Giacalone PL, Bricout N, Dantas MJ, et al: Achieving symmetry in unilateral breast reconstruction: 17 years experience with 683 patients. Aesthetic Plast Surg 26:299-302, 2002.

39. Chawla AK, Kachnic LA, Taghian AG, et al: Radiotherapy and breast reconstruction: Complications and cosmesis with TRAM versus tissue expander/implant. Int J Radiat Oncol Biol Phys 54:520-526, 2002.

40. Tran NV, Chang DW, Gupta A, et al: Comparison of immediate and delayed free TRAM flap breast reconstruction in patients receiving postmastectomy radiation therapy. Plast Reconstr Surg 108:78-82, 2001.

41. Fajardo LL, Roberts CC, Hunt KR: Mammographic surveillance of breast cancer patients: Should the mastectomy site be imaged? AJR Am J Roentgenol 161:953-955, 1993.

42. Noguchi M, Fukushima W, Ohta N, et al: Oncological aspect of immediate breast reconstruction in mastectomy patients. J Surg Oncol 50:241-246, 1992.

43. Freeman BS: Subcutaneous mastectomy for benign breast lesions with immediate or delayed prosthetic replacement. Plast Reconstr Surg 30:6, 1962.

44. Gruber RP, Kahn RA, Lash H, et al: Breast reconstruction following mastectomy: A comparison of submuscular and sub-cutaneous techniques. Plast Reconstr Surg 67:312-317, 1981.

45. Bostwick J III: Plastic and Reconstructive Breast Surgery. St. Louis, Quality Medical, 1990.

46. McShane RH, Omotunde O, Weatherly-White RC: Individualized muscle coverage of implants in breast reconstruction. Plast Reconstr Surg 67:318-327, 1981.

47. Gibney J: Use of a permanent tissue expander for breast reconstruction. Plast Reconstr Surg 84:607-620, 1989.

48. Radovan C: Breast reconstruction after mastectomy using the temporary expander. Plast Reconstr Surg 69:195-208, 1982.

49. Hammond DC, Capraro PA, Ozolins EB, et al: Use of a skin-sparing reduction pattern to create a combination skin-muscle flap pocket in immediate breast reconstruction. Plast Reconstr Surg 110:206-211, 2002.

50. Bailey MH, Smith JW, Casas L, et al: Immediate breast reconstruction: Reducing the risks. Plast Reconstr Surg 83:845-851, 1989.

51. Armstrong RW, Berkowitz RL, Bolding F: Infection following breast reconstruction. Ann Plast Surg 23:284-288, 1989.

52. Schlenker JD, Bueno RA, Ricketson G, et al: Loss of silicone implants after subcutaneous mastectomy and reconstruction. Plast Reconstr Surg 62:853-861, 1978.

53. Asplund O: Capsular contracture in silicone gel and saline-filled breast implants after reconstruction. Plast Reconstr Surg 73:270-275, 1984.

54. Gylbert L, Asplund O, Jurell G: Capsular contracture after breast reconstruction with silicone-gel and saline-filled implants: A 6-year follow-up. Plast Reconstr Surg 85:373-377, 1990.

55. Holmes JD: Capsular contracture after breast reconstruction with tissue expansion. Br J Plast Surg 42:591-594, 1989.

56. Spear SL, Onyewu C: Staged breast reconstruction with saline-filled implants in the irradiated breast: Recent trends and therapeutic implications. Plast Reconstr Surg 105:930-942, 2000.

57. Biggs TM, Cronin ED: Technical aspects of the latissimus dorsi myocutaneous flap in breast reconstruction. Ann Plast Surg 6:381-388, 1981.

58. Cohen BE, Cronin ED: Breast reconstruction with the latissimus dorsi musculocutaneous flap. Clin Plast Surg 11:287-302, 1984.

59. Maxwell GP, McGibbon BM, Hoopes JE: Vascular considerations in the use of a latissimus dorsi myocutaneous flap after a mastectomy with an axillary dissection. Plast Reconstr Surg 64:771-780, 1979.

60. Gillies HD: Design of direct pedicle flaps. BMJ 2:1008, 1932.

61. Hartrampf CR, Scheflan M, Black PW: Breast reconstruction with a transverse abdominal island flap. Plast Reconstr Surg 69:216-225, 1982.

62. Moon HK, Taylor GI: The vascular anatomy of rectus abdominis musculocutaneous flaps based on the deep superior epigastric system. Plast Reconstr Surg 82:815-832, 1988.

63. Wagner DS, Michelow BJ, Hartrampf CR Jr: Double-pedicle TRAM flap for unilateral breast reconstruction. Plast Reconstr Surg 88:987-997, 1991.

64. Scheflan M, Dinner MI: The transverse abdominal island flap: I. Indications, contraindications, results, and complications. Ann Plast Surg 10:24-35, 1983.

65. Scheflan M, Dinner MI: The transverse abdominal island flap: II. Surgical technique. Ann Plast Surg 10:120-129, 1983.

66. Serafin D, Voci VE, Georgiade NG: Microsurgical composite tissue transplantation: Indications and technical considerations in breast reconstruction following mastectomy. Plast Reconstr Surg 70:24-36, 1982.

67. Kroll SS: Fat necrosis in free transverse rectus abdominis myocutaneous and deep inferior epigastric perforator flaps. Plast Reconstr Surg 106:576-583, 2000.

68. Kroll SS, Netscher DT: Complications of TRAM flap breast reconstruction in obese patients. Plast Reconstr Surg 84:886-892, 1989.

69. Grotting JC, Urist MM, Maddox WA, et al: Conventional TRAM flap versus free microsurgical TRAM flap for immediate breast reconstruction. Plast Reconstr Surg 83:828-844, 1989.

70. Hartrampf CR Jr: Abdominal wall competence in transverse abdominal island flap operations. Ann Plast Surg 12:139-146, 1984.

71. Lejour M, Dome M: Abdominal wall function after rectus abdominis transfer. Plast Reconstr Surg 87:1054-1068, 1991.

72. Clugston PA, Gingrass MK, Azurin D, et al: Ipsilateral pedicled TRAM flaps: The safer alternative? Plast Reconstr Surg 105:77-82, 2000.

73. Baldwin BJ, Schusterman MA, Miller MJ, et al: Bilateral breast reconstruction: Conventional versus free TRAM. Plast Reconstr Surg 93:1410-1417, 1994.

74. Paletta CE, Bostwick J III, Nahai F: The inferior gluteal free flap in breast reconstruction. Plast Reconstr Surg 84:875-885, 1989.

75. Shaw WW: Breast reconstruction by superior gluteal microvascular free flaps without silicone implants. Plast Reconstr Surg 72:490-501, 1983.

76. Hartrampf CR Jr, Noel RT, Drazan L, et al: Rubens' fat pad for breast reconstruction: A peri-iliac soft-tissue free flap. Plast Reconstr Surg 93:402-407, 1994.

77. Little JW III, Munasifi T, McCulloch DT: One-stage reconstruction of a projecting nipple: The quadrapod flap. Plast Reconstr Surg 71:126-133, 1983.

78. Brent B, Bostwick J: Nipple-areola reconstruction with auricular tissues. Plast Reconstr Surg 60:353-361, 1977.

79. Chang BW, Slezak S, Goldberg NH: Technical modifications for on-site nipple-areola reconstruction. Ann Plast Surg 28:277-280, 1992.

80. Gruber RP: Nipple-areola reconstruction: A review of techniques. Clin Plast Surg 6:71-83, 1979.

81. Hallock GG, Altobelli JA: Cylindrical nipple reconstruction using an H flap. Ann Plast Surg 30:23-26, 1993.

82. Kroll SS, Hamilton S: Nipple reconstruction with the double-opposing-tab flap. Plast Reconstr Surg 84:520-525, 1989.

83. Little JW III: Nipple-areola reconstruction. Clin Plast Surg 11:351-364, 1984.

84. Becker H: The use of intradermal tattoo to enhance the final result of nipple-areola reconstruction. Plast Reconstr Surg 77:673-676, 1986.

85. Brent B: Nipple-areola reconstruction following mastectomy: An alternative to the use of labial and contralateral nipple-areolar tissues. Clin Plast Surg 6:85-92, 1979.

86. Nakagawa T, Yano K, Hosokawa K: Cryopreserved autologous nipple-areola complex transfer to the reconstructed breast. Plast Reconstr Surg 111:141-149, 2003.

87. Herrmann JB: Management of the contralateral breast after mastectomy for unilateral carcinoma. Surg Gynecol Obstet 136:777-779, 1973.

88. Chang DW, Kroll SS, Dackiw A, et al: Reconstructive management of contralateral breast cancer in patients who previously underwent unilateral breast reconstruction. Plast Reconstr Surg 108:352-360, 2001.

89. Shaikh N, LaTrenta G, Swistel A, et al: Detection of recurrent breast cancer after TRAM flap reconstruction. Ann Plast Surg 47:602-607, 2001.

90. Shenaq SM, Yuksel E: New research in breast reconstruction: Adipose tissue engineering. Clin Plast Surg 29:111-125, vi, 2002.

ENDOCRINE

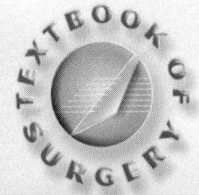

CHAPTER 34

THYROID

John B. Hanks, M.D.

HISTORICAL PERSPECTIVE

The name *thyroid* is derived from the Greek description of a shield-shaped gland in the anterior neck ("thyreoides"). Classical anatomic descriptions of the thyroid were available in the 16th and 17th centuries, but the function of the gland was not well understood. By the 19th century, pathologic enlargement of the thyroid, or goiter, was described. Medical treatment of this condition was described, using what was most likely iodine-rich seaweed. Direct surgical approaches of thyroid masses had frighteningly high complication and mortality rates.

In the late 19th century, two surgeon-physiologists revolutionized treatment of thyroid diseases. Theodor Billroth and Emil Theodor Kocher established large clinics in Europe and, through development of skilled surgical techniques combined with newer anesthetic and antiseptic principles, provided surgical results that proved the safety and efficacy of thyroid surgery for benign and malignant problems. As a result of his pioneering developments in the understanding of thyroid physiology, Kocher received the Nobel Prize in 1909.

The 20th century started with the contributions of Kocher and Billroth. In rapid succession, the understanding of altered physiology, including hypothyroidism and hyperthyroidism, thyroid cancer, advances in imaging, epidemiology, and most recently, minimally invasive diagnostic and surgical techniques have taken place. These advances have allowed the diagnosis and treatment of thyroid diseases to become rapid, cost-effective, low-morbidity procedures.

THYROID EMBRYOLOGY AND ANATOMY

Embryology

The tissue bud that ultimately becomes the thyroid gland arises initially as a midline diverticulum in the floor of the pharynx. This tissue originates in the primitive alimentary tract and consists of cells of endodermal origin. The main portion of this cellular structure descends into the neck and develops into a bilobar solid organ. The original attachment in the pharynx is in the buccal cavity at the foramen cecum, and this becomes the thyroglossal duct, which after 6 weeks of age is usually reabsorbed. The very distal end of this remnant may occasionally be retained and mature as a pyramidal lobe in the adult thyroid.

Microscopic thyroid follicles are first apparent as the lateral lobes develop. When the embryo is about 6 cm in length, these follicles can begin to develop colloid. In the 3rd month, the follicular cells first demonstrate iodine trapping, and thyroid hormone secretion initially begins. Calcitonin-producing C cells arise from the fourth pharyngeal pouch and migrate from the neural crest into the lateral lobes of the thyroid. These cells migrate into the lateral and posterior upper two thirds of the thyroid lobes and are distributed among the follicles. In adults, they remain limited to the upper and middle areas of the gland, usually in the posterior and medial aspects. These C cells are the only component of the adult gland not of endodermal origin.[1]

Knowledge of basic embryology is essential for understanding certain embryologic congenital malformations.

These include the thyroglossal duct cysts and fistulas, which result from retained tissue along the thyroglossal duct. Most thyroglossal duct cysts are found immediately beneath the hyoid bone and are noted in early childhood or infancy. These cysts are almost always in the midline and can be found from the base of the tongue to the suprasternal notch. They usually occur as a mass found in the midline on physical examination or when a localized infection occurs within that mass. A chronically infected or draining thyroglossal duct cyst can lead to a chronic draining fistula. For this reason, all thyroglossal duct cysts, on diagnosis, should be treated surgically and excised because of the potential for infection. Exposure should be made from the foramen cecum through the hyoid bone and as far distally as appropriate. The thyroglossal duct commonly passes through the center of the hyoid bone, requiring removal of the central portion of the structure. Occasionally, papillary cancer can occur in the thyroid tissue within the thyroglossal duct cyst, which requires complete removal of the tract.

When the median thyroid anlage does not descend in a normal fashion, a lingual thyroid can result. In most of these cases, this may be the only thyroid tissue that remains. Enlargement of a lingual thyroid can cause airway obstruction, dysphagia, or bleeding. Most lingual thyroid glands can be suppressed with thyroid hormone administration. In particularly resistant lingual thyroids, radioactive iodine treatment may represent another alternative.

Ectopic thyroid tissue can be found in unusual circumstances contained in the central compartment of the neck. Small amounts of ectopic tissue may be found under the lower poles of normal thyroid and occasionally in the anterior mediastinum. Historically, thyroid tissue described in lateral neck compartments was known as *lateral aberrant thyroid tissue* and was explained as an embryologic variation. This concept has essentially been disproved, and it is thought that any thyroid tissue found in the lateral neck, including around the vascular structures of the neck, may represent metastatic deposits from well-differentiated thyroid carcinoma.

Anatomic Considerations

The normally developed thyroid is a bilobed structure that lies immediately next to the thyroid cartilage in a position anterior and lateral to the junction of the larynx and trachea. In this position, the thyroid encircles about 75% of the diameter of the junction of the larynx and the upper trachea. The two lateral lobes are joined at the midline by an isthmus, which is situated in a directly anterior position at or below the cricoid cartilage. The pyramidal lobe represents the most distal portion of the thyroglossal duct and in the adult may be a prominent structure, which may extend from the midline of the isthmus as far cephalad as the hyoid bone.

A thin layer of connective tissue surrounds the thyroid in this normal anatomic position. This tissue is part of the fascial layer, which invests the trachea. This fascia is different from the thyroid capsule, and during surgery it can be separated easily from the capsule, whereas the true capsule of the thyroid cannot. This fascia coalesces with the thyroid capsule posteriorly and laterally to form a suspensory ligament, known as the *ligament of Berry*. The ligament of Berry is closely attached to the cricoid cartilage and has important surgical implications because of its relation to the recurrent laryngeal nerve.

Recurrent Laryngeal Nerve

The recurrent laryngeal nerves ascend on either side of the trachea, and each lies just lateral to the ligament of Berry as they enter the larynx. There are a number of important variations. In about 25% of patients, the recurrent laryngeal nerve is contained within the ligament as it enters the larynx. On the right side, the recurrent laryngeal nerve separates from the vagus as it crosses the subclavian artery, passing posteriorly and ascending in a lateral position to the trachea along the tracheoesophageal groove. The right recurrent laryngeal nerve can usually be found no further than 1 cm lateral to or within the tracheoesophageal groove at the level of the lower border of the thyroid. As it ascends to the midportion of the thyroid, however, the nerve assumes its position within the tracheoesophageal groove. At this location, the nerve might divide into one, two, or more branches as it enters into the first or second ring of the trachea, with the most important branch disappearing beneath the inferior border of the cricothyroid muscle. The nerve can usually be found immediately anterior or posterior to a main arterial trunk of the inferior thyroid artery at this level. Unusually, a nonrecurrent right laryngeal nerve can arise directly from the vagus and course directly medially into the larynx. This nonrecurrent anatomy is found in 0.5% to 1.5% of patients. Even more infrequently, patients may have both a recurrent and a nonrecurrent laryngeal nerve on the right. These two nerves usually join in a position beneath the lower border of the thyroid.[2]

On the left side, the recurrent laryngeal nerve separates from the vagus as that nerve traverses over the arch of the aorta. The left recurrent laryngeal nerve then passes inferiorly and medially to the aorta and begins to ascend toward the larynx, finding its way into the tracheoesophageal groove as it ascends to the level of the lower lobe of the thyroid. Both recurrent laryngeal nerves are consistently found within the tracheoesophageal groove when they are within 2.5 cm of their entrance into the larynx. These nerves pass either inferiorly or posteriorly to an arterial branch of the inferior thyroid artery and eventually enter the larynx at the level of the cricothyroid articulation on the caudal border of the cricothyroid muscle. Here the nerve is immediately adjacent to the superior parathyroid, the inferior thyroid artery, and the most posterior aspect of the thyroid. Great care is needed in surgical dissection in this area because the nerve is essentially tethered as it dives beneath the cricothyroid muscle and can be placed on stretch by overly vigorous dissection (Fig. 34-1).

The motor function of the recurrent laryngeal nerve is abduction of the vocal cords from the midline. Damage to a recurrent laryngeal nerve results in paralysis of the vocal cord on the side affected. Such damage might result in a

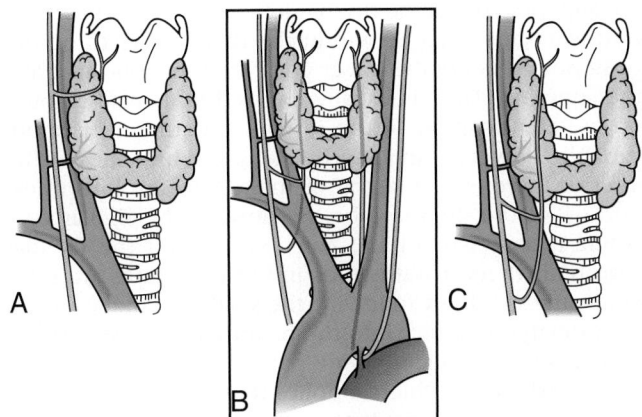

FIGURE 34-1. Anomalous variations in the course of the right recurrent laryngeal nerve. **A,** A nonrecurrent laryngeal nerve arises from the vagus. **B,** The normal course of the recurrent laryngeal nerve arises from the vagus after it passes beneath the subclavian artery. **C,** The unusual nonrecurrent nerve and recurrent laryngeal nerve join to form a common distal nerve. (A to C, From Greenfield LJ [ed]: Surgery: Scientific Principles and Practice, 2nd ed. Philadelphia, Lippincott-Raven, 1997, p 1165.)

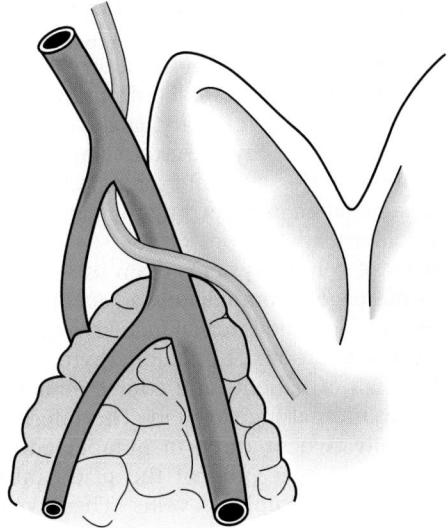

FIGURE 34-2. The relationship between the external branch of the superior laryngeal nerve (black) and the superior thyroid artery. The nerve can course inferiorly and medially and may run partly along with or around the artery or the branches of the artery as they enter the superior lobe of the thyroid. (From Duh QY: Surgical anatomy and embryology of the thyroid and parathyroid glands and recurrent and external laryngeal nerves. In Clark OH, Duh QY [eds]: Textbook of Endocrine Surgery. Philadelphia, WB Saunders, 1997, p 11.)

cord that remains in a medial position or just lateral to the midline. A normal voice, albeit weakened, can occur if the remaining functioning contralateral cord is able to approximate the paralyzed cord. If the vocal cord remains paralyzed in an abducted position and closure cannot occur, a severely impaired voice and ineffective cough can be the result. If recurrent laryngeal nerves are damaged bilaterally, complete loss of voice or airway obstruction requiring emergency intubation and tracheostomy may be necessary. Occasionally, bilateral damage can result in cords taking an abducted position, which, although allowing airway movement, may result in upper respiratory infection due to ineffective cough.

Superior Laryngeal Nerve

The superior laryngeal nerve separates from the vagus nerve at the base of the skull and descends toward the superior pole of the thyroid along the internal carotid artery. At the level of the hyoid cornu, it divides into two branches: The larger internal branch has sensory function and enters the thyrohyoid membrane, where it innervates the larynx. The smaller external branch continues to travel along the lateral surface of the inferior pharyngeal constrictor muscle and usually descends anteriorly and medially along with the superior thyroid artery. Within 1 cm of the superior thyroid artery's entrance into the thyroid capsule, the nerve usually takes a medial course and enters into the cricothyroid muscle (Fig. 34-2). This is an extremely important relation because, during the performance of a thyroid lobectomy, the external branch is not usually visualized because it has already entered the inferior pharyngeal muscle fascia. This nerve is at risk of being severed or entrapped, however, if superior pole vessels are ligated at too great a distance above the superior pole of the thyroid.[3] Damage to the external branch can result in a severe loss in quality of voice or voice

strength. Although this may not be as clinically devastating as recurrent laryngeal nerve damage, it is extremely bothersome to patients whose occupation demands good voice quality.

Blood Supply

The arterial supply to the thyroid gland is supplied by four main arteries, two superior and two inferior. The superior thyroid artery is the first branch of the external carotid artery and separates from that structure immediately above the bifurcation of the common carotid artery. The superior thyroid artery then drops medially onto the surface of the inferior pharyngeal constrictor muscle and enters the substance of the superior pole of the thyroid at its apex. The superior thyroid artery courses medially with the external branch of the superior laryngeal nerve, and this structure must be separated from it when gaining control of the artery.

The inferior thyroid artery takes its origin from the thyrocervical trunk. This artery ascends into the neck on either side behind the carotid sheath and then arches medially and enters the thyroid gland posteriorly. There is no direct arterial supply to the thyroid at the inferior boundaries because most of these vascular structures are venous. An occasional inferior arterial supply may occur from a thyroidea ima artery that occurs in the absence of a well-defined inferior arterial supply. The thyroidea ima arteries occur in less than 5% of patients and usually arise directly from the innominate artery or from the aorta.

The inferior thyroid artery has important anatomic relationships. The recurrent laryngeal nerve is usually directly adjacent (in either an anterior or posterior position) to the inferior thyroid artery within 1 cm of its entrance into the larynx. Careful dissection of the artery in this case is mandatory and cannot be completed until knowledge of the position of the recurrent laryngeal nerve is gained. Additionally, the inferior thyroid artery almost always supplies both the superior and inferior parathyroid glands, and care must be taken in evaluating the parathyroids after inferior thyroid artery division.

Three pairs of venous systems drain the thyroid. Superior venous drainage is immediately adjacent to the superior arteries and joins the internal jugular vein at the level of the carotid bifurcation. The middle thyroid veins exist in more than half of patients and course immediately laterally into the internal jugular vein. The inferior thyroid veins are usually two or three in number and descend directly from the lower pole of the gland into the innominate and brachiocephalic veins. These veins often descend into the tail of the thymus gland.[4]

Lymphatic System

The relationship of the thyroid gland to its lymphatic drainage is most important when considering surgical treatment of thyroid carcinoma. The thyroid gland and its neighboring structures have a rich lymphatic supply that drains the thyroid in almost every direction. Within the gland, lymphatic channels occur immediately beneath the capsule and communicate between lobes through the isthmus. This drainage connects to structures immediately adjacent to the thyroid with numerous lymphatic channels into the regional lymph nodes. These regional lymph nodes exist in a pretracheal position immediately superior to the isthmus; paratracheal nodes; tracheoesophageal groove lymph nodes; mediastinal nodes in the anterior and superior position; jugular lymph nodes in the upper, middle, and lower distribution; and retropharyngeal and esophageal lymph nodes. Laterally, cervical lymph nodes within the posterior triangle may be involved in patients with widespread thyroid cancers. Additionally, lymph nodes within the submaxillary triangle may be involved with metastatic activity.

Papillary carcinoma of the thyroid is commonly associated with adjacent nodal metastasis. Medullary carcinoma has a strong predilection for metastatic lymphatic involvement, usually within the central compartment (the space between the internal jugular veins). For this reason, central-compartment lymph node dissection is indicated at the time of total thyroidectomy for medullary carcinoma.

Parathyroid Glands

The thyroid sheath encases the lateral and posterior portion of each thyroid lobe and, as such, frequently provides a covering substance to the superior parathyroid gland. When the superior portion of the thyroid lobe is dissected and rolled medially, an area containing fat beneath this fascia is apparent. The superior parathyroid gland almost always lies within the fat beneath the thyroid sheath in this location in a posterior position relative to the superior part of the thyroid lobe. The inferior parathyroid gland may also be within the thyroid sheath on the posterior aspect of the lower portion of the lobe and, like the superior gland, is usually encased in a small amount of fat. The position of the inferior parathyroid is more variable, however, and can be along the branches of the inferior thyroid vein lateral or inferior to the lowermost portion of the thyroid lobe. Because of the similar consistency and color of the parathyroids and the fat that surrounds them, parathyroids in both positions are most efficiently sought by following the smaller branches of the inferior thyroid artery into the parathyroid substance.[1]

The superior and inferior parathyroid glands have a single end artery, which supplies them medially from the inferior thyroid artery. If the main trunk of the inferior thyroid artery is sacrificed for dissection, both parathyroids on that side can be devascularized because there is no collateral blood supply to maintain viability. Careful dissection should attempt to divide only the branches of the inferior thyroid entering the thyroid capsule during excision. Using careful technique, it is possible to maintain good vascular supply to the superior and inferior parathyroid even when a total thyroidectomy is performed.

PHYSIOLOGY OF THE THYROID GLAND

The thyroid gland is responsible for the production of two families of metabolic hormones: the thyroid hormones thyroxine (T_4) and triiodothyronine (T_3) and the hormone calcitonin. The thyroid follicular unit is the important site of thyroid hormone production. The thyroid follicle is made up of a single layer of cuboidal follicular cells that encompass a central depository filled with the protein substance colloid, which is part of the storage mechanism. Each follicle is surrounded by a rich network of capillaries, which interdigitate among the multiple follicular units contained within normal thyroid matrix. The thyroid follicle is the major production unit as well as a storage place for thyroid hormones.[5]

Cells derived from the neural crest are called *C cells* and migrate into the thyroid during embryologic development. These cells come to rest in a parafollicular position predominantly in the upper lobe of each thyroid. C cells are responsible for production of the hormone calcitonin, which has important calcium metabolism regulatory properties.

Iodine Metabolism

Iodine can be efficiently absorbed from the gastrointestinal tract in the form of inorganic iodide and rapidly enters the extracellular iodide pool. The thyroid gland is responsible for storing 90% of the total-body iodide at any given time, leaving less than 10% existing in the extracellular pool. The extracellular pool consists of freshly absorbed iodide as well as the total derived from the breakdown of previously formed thyroid hormone. Within the thyroid, iodide is stored either as preformed thyroid hormone or as iodinated amino acids.

Iodide is taken up into the follicular cells by an active transport process from the extracellular space. Iodide can be lost from the extracellular space through renal excretion and through the skin, saliva, or respiration. Iodide transport into the follicular cells is regulated by thyroid-stimulating hormone (TSH) as well as by the follicular content of iodide. The active transport of iodide into the follicular cells results in a significant iodide gradient across the cell. Although the process of iodide transport is not completely understood, it appears to be linked to a sodium-potassium adenosine triphosphatase system.

The relationship between iodine ingestion and thyroid disease has been known for more than 100 years. At the turn of the 20th century, the practice of iodine supplementation of food and water came as the result of careful study in areas where iodine insufficiency was demonstrated and linked to endemic goiter. Significant iodine deficiency still occurs in various undeveloped parts of the world. Iodine deficiency can result in nodular goiter, hypothyroidism and cretinism, and possibly, the development of follicular thyroid carcinoma. The World Health Organization has been involved with using iodine dietary supplementation to treat entire populations in such undeveloped areas of the world. In situations in which iodine excess occurs, disease processes such as Graves' disease and Hashimoto's thyroiditis can occur.[6]

Thyroid Hormone Synthesis

On entrance into the follicular cell, inorganic iodide is efficiently oxidized and coupled with tyrosine moieties to form iodotyrosines in either a single conformation (monoiodotyrosine [MIT]) or in a coupled conformation (diiodotyrosine [DIT]) (Fig. 34-3). These forms are contained within the follicle as the storage protein thyroglobulin. The formation of DIT and MIT is dependent on an important intracellular catalytic agent, thyroid peroxidase, which has been well characterized and is an integral part of the initial process of organification and storage of the inorganic iodide.[7] This enzyme is localized to the apical part of the follicular cell, where it reacts at the cell-colloid interface.

MIT and DIT are biologically inert. The coupling of these two residues gives rise to the two biologically active thyroid hormones. T_4 is formed by the coupling of two molecules of DIT; T_3 is formed by coupling a molecule of MIT with a molecule of DIT. In normal circumstances, the formation of T_4 is the major pathway. Both T_3 and T_4 are bound to thyroglobulin and stored within the colloid in the center of the follicular unit. This rapid and metabolically active process results in the storage of about 2 weeks' worth of thyroid hormone within the organism under normal circumstances.[8]

Release of T_4 and T_3 is regulated by the apical membrane of the follicular cell, which results in lysosomal hydrolysis of the colloid that contains the thyroglobulin-bound hormones. The apical membrane of the thyroid cell forms multiple pseudopodia and incorporates thyroglobulin into small vesicles that are then brought within the cell apparatus. Within the vesicles, lysosomal hydrolysis results in the reduction of disulfide bonds, and both T_3 and T_4 are then free to pass through the basement mem-

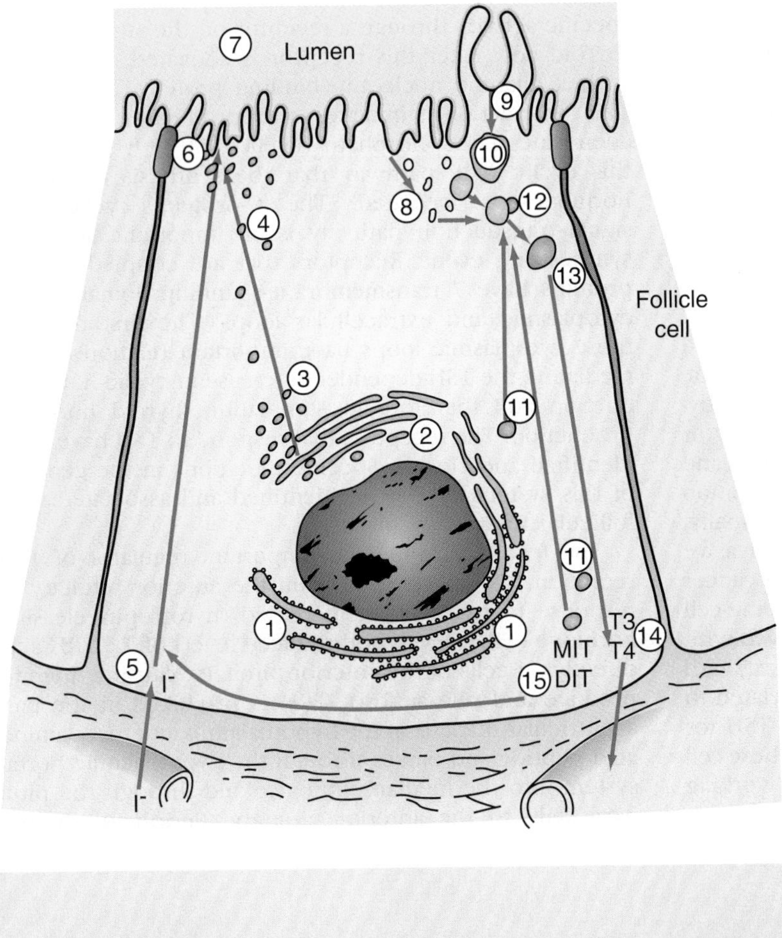

FIGURE 34-3. Diagrammatic scheme of thyroid hormone formation and secretion. 1, Thyroglobulin and protein synthesis in the rough endoplasmic reticulum. 2, Coupling of the thyroglobulin carbohydrate units in the smooth endoplasmic reticulum and Golgi apparatus. 3, Formation of exocytotic vesicles. 4, Transport of exocytotic vesicles with noniodinated thyroglobulin to the apical surface of the follicle cell and into the follicular lumen. 5, Iodide transport at the basal cell membrane. 6, Iodide oxidation, thyroglobulin iodination, and coupling of iodotyrosyl to iodothyronyl residues. 7, Storage of iodinated thyroglobulin in the follicular lumen. 8, Endocytosis by micropinocytosis. 9, Endocytosis by macropinocytosis (pseudopods). 10, Colloid droplets. 11, Lysosome migrating to the apical pole. 12, Fusion of lysosomes with colloid droplets. 13, Phagolysosomes with thyroglobulin hydrolysis. 14, Triiodothyronine (T_3) and thyroxine (T_4) secretion. 15, Monoiodotyrosine (MIT) and diiodotyrosine (DIT) deiodination.

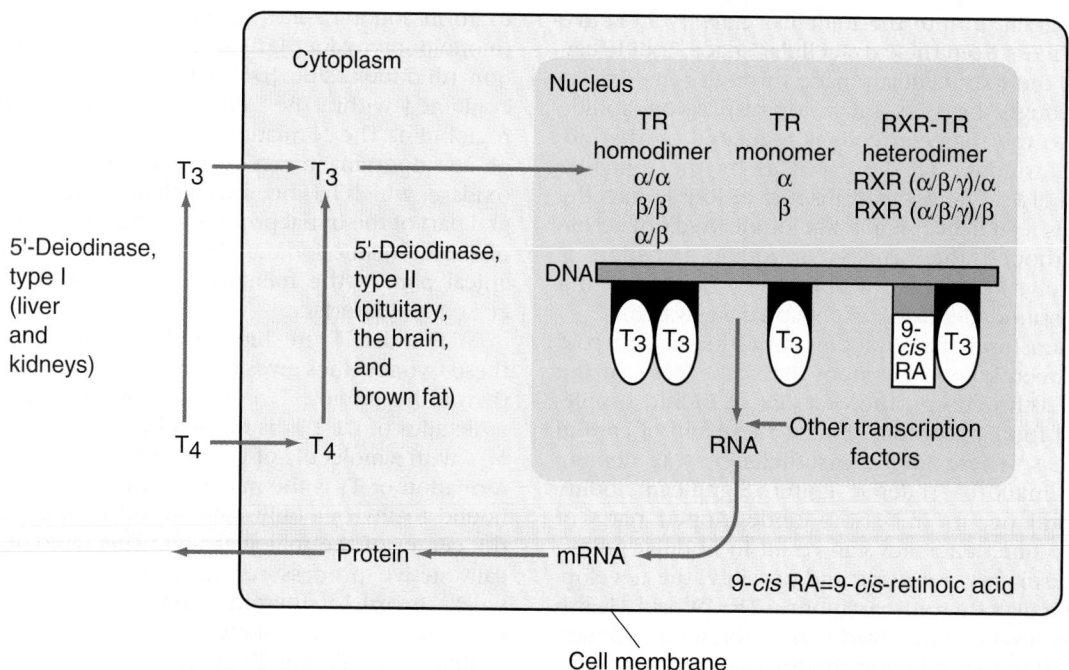

FIGURE 34-4.   Cellular and molecular events involved in thyroid hormone function. Thyroxine (T_4) is converted in the periphery and in the cytoplasm of the cell into triiodothyronine (T_3). T_3 travels to the nucleus, where it binds to the thyroid hormone receptor, either homodimer, monomer, or heterodimer. Thyroid hormone receptor binding leads to RNA transcription in association with other transcription factors, with expression of messenger RNA that is then translated into protein.

brane and absorbed into the circulation. This metabolic process is efficient in releasing T_3 and T_4 while maintaining the storage components of thyroglobulin and colloid within the follicular apparatus. Although sensitive assays of peripheral blood can measure thyroglobulin, peripheral thyroglobulin represents an extremely small fraction of total-body stores. Residual iodotyrosines undergo peripheral breakdown, deiodination, and recycling and then can be added to the recently absorbed iodide stores and become available for new thyroid hormone synthesis (Fig. 34-4).[8]

Regulation of Thyroid Hormone Secretion

Triiodothyronine and Thyroxine

The hypothalamic-pituitary-thyroid axis regulates thyroid hormone production and release in a classic endocrine feedback system. The major regulator of thyroid gland activity is the glycoprotein TSH. TSH is a major growth factor for the thyroid. TSH stimulates thyroid cell growth and differentiation as well as iodine uptake and organification and release of T_3 and T_4 from thyroglobulin. Additionally, TSH has been shown to stimulate the growth and invasive characteristics of some well-differentiated thyroid cancer cell lines in vitro. Ironically, there are other intriguing cell culture data demonstrating that TSH may be involved with suppressing other human thyroid cell lines or, at least, with making them less aggressive. Certain cell lines related to anaplastic human thyroid are not dependent on TSH for growth, and it appears that TSH administration to these cell lines in vitro may slow their growth, perhaps working through suppression of TSH receptor genes.[9,10]

TSH is a glycoprotein weighing 28,000 daltons that is secreted by the anterior pituitary gland. It is composed of two components, an alpha subunit and a beta subunit, of which the alpha subunit is common to a family of glycoproteins secreted by the anterior pituitary. TSH has specific activity through a receptor on the surface of the thyroid cell. After this receptor is activated, it interacts with a guanine nucleotide-binding protein (G protein). This interaction stimulates the production of cyclic adenosine monophosphate (cyclic AMP). It is through this cyclic AMP pathway that the synthesis of thyroid hormones is mediated. The G-protein, cyclic AMP signal–transduction pathway is an important hormone-synthesizing event. Receptors that are coupled with G proteins have 7 transmembrane-spanning domains with cytoplasmic and extracellular loops. The first three of these cytoplasmic loops have important relationships in mediating the TSH-dependent increase in cyclic AMP production and therefore in stimulating thyroid hormone production. The receptors that respond to TSH have been identified and cloned. Specific mutations in the genetics of this system have been identified and associated with follicular thyroid neoplasms.[10]

The feedback loop is an important regulator of TSH secretion. TSH is released from the anterior pituitary in response to two events, increased thyrotropin-releasing hormone (TRH) levels and reduced levels of T_3. TRH acts directly on cells of the anterior pituitary, causing them to produce and release TSH. TRH is produced in the paraventricular nucleus of the hypothalamus as a three-amino acid peptide and passes through the hypothalamic portal system into the median eminence and through the pituitary stalk to the anterior pituitary. Peripheral thyroid hormone levels may, in addition to stimulating TSH release from the anterior pituitary, enhance TRH secretion.

Negative feedback through increased peripheral levels of T_3 and T_4 can affect TSH secretion. Peripheral T_4 is locally deiodinated in the pituitary and converted to T_3, which then directly inhibits release and synthesis of TSH. It may be that T_3 results in this process by decreased TRH receptor numbers on the surface of anterior pituitary cells, therefore decreasing local responsiveness to TRH. Other metabolic events appear to affect the synthesis of thyroid hormone secretion. Catecholamines, especially epinephrine, may have a direct stimulatory effect on thyroid hormone release and production. Human chorionic gonadotropin stimulates thyroid hormone production and results in increased synthesis during pregnancy. Occasional gynecologic malignancies, including hydatidiform moles with resultant elevated human chorionic gonadotropin levels, may result in elevated thyroid hormone levels. Glucocorticoids suppress thyroid hormone production through suppression of pituitary TSH secretions. A wide variety of disorders that include a nonspecific yet drastically severe illness lead to reduced levels of peripheral thyroid hormone without a resultant rise in TSH (sick euthyroid syndrome). Chronic hyperthermia and chronic starvation are associated with markedly reduced levels of both T_4 and T_3 with or without compensatory elevations in TSH.[11]

Intrinsic autoregulatory mechanisms are another way that the thyroid can control intraglandular stores of thyroid hormones. In areas where dietary iodide is excessive, the thyroid gland has an autoregulated process that inhibits iodide uptake into the follicular cells. The reverse is true in iodide deficiency. Excessively large doses of iodide have interesting and complex effects, including an initial increase in organification followed by suppressive effects, a syndrome known as the *Wolff-Chaikoff effect*.

Thyroglobulin

Thyroglobulin is a glycoprotein weighing 660,000 daltons and is the primary component of the colloid matrix contained within the follicle. Thyroglobulin facilitates the conversion of MIT and DIT into T_3 and T_4. This process is accompanied by thyroglobulin escape into the peripheral bloodstream, where it can be assayed. TSH enhances the whole process of endocytosis, proteolysis, and release through an adenylate cyclase system. Excess peripheral levels of iodine inhibit further release by enhancing thyroglobulin resistance to proteolysis.

Peripheral thyroglobulin can be measured to evaluate benign or malignant thyroid neoplasms. The measurement of peripheral thyroglobulin has predictive value for recurrence of well-differentiated thyroid carcinoma either locally or in metastatic deposits after initial total thyroidectomy.[12]

Calcitonin

Calcitonin is a 32-amino acid polypeptide and is secreted by the C cells, which are parafollicular cells located superolaterally in each thyroid lobe. Calcitonin acts principally to inhibit calcium absorption by osteoclasts and thereby to lower peripheral serum calcium levels. Increased peripheral levels of serum calcium stimulate calcitonin secretion. Calcitonin secretion can be stimulated clinically by infusion of calcium, pentagastrin, and alcohol.

The specific action of calcitonin is on the surface receptors of osteoclasts. Calcitonin receptors have also been found in renal tubular epithelium and in lymphocytes. Calcitonin has a direct action on osteoclasts, which may or may not result in a marked decrease in calcium levels. In fact, patients with clinical calcitonin excess syndromes, such as medullary carcinoma of the thyroid (MCT), have little alteration in peripheral calcium metabolism. Basal or stimulated calcitonin levels are sensitive markers for primary or recurrent MCT. Whether calcitonin should be evaluated routinely for all thyroid masses in an attempt to discover the unusual sporadic medullary carcinoma is not universally agreed on.

Peripheral Action of Thyroid Hormones

In the periphery, T_4 is relatively inactive compared with T_3. T_4 has a low affinity for peripheral nuclear thyroid hormone receptors (TRs) compared with T_3, most likely because T_4 is converted to the active form of T_3 to gain the most efficient use of thyroid hormone release. As a result, the action of thyroid hormones in the periphery is essentially T_3 interaction with the nuclear TR, which then binds to regulatory regions in various gene-regulated processes. TR belongs to the steroid hormone receptor family. Two genes regulate TR production and activity, the alpha and beta forms, which are located on chromosomes 17 and 3. The receptors modulate specific patterns of expression with regard to the tissue that contains them. The beta form of TR is contained within the liver; the central nervous system contains predominantly an alpha form of TR. Expression of TR may be regulated by peripheral thyroid hormone concentrations; low peripheral serum thyroid hormone concentrations appear to result in an increase in TR numbers as a compensatory response. The TR is directly responsible for the clinical manifestation of hormone action. The clinical result of thyroid hormone action is regulated through TR and its effect on various genes, the expressions of which are then regulated in the nucleus, resulting in polypeptide production. For example, T_3 acts on the pituitary by regulating transcription of the genes for both the alpha and beta subunits of TSH, which results in TSH secretion. T_3 affects cardiac contractility by regulating the transcription of myosin heavy-chain production in cardiac muscle.[5]

In the periphery T_3 and T_4 are principally bound to thyroxine-binding globulin. Additionally, T_4 is bound to a prealbumin thyroxine-binding protein and albumin. Thyroxine-binding globulin is the major transport vehicle for about 80% of circulating peripheral thyroid hormone. In pregnancy and other clinical situations with elevated estrogen levels, thyroxine-binding globulin levels are significantly increased, resulting in higher levels of bound T_4 in the periphery. Such states are clinically euthyroid, however, because *free* T_4 levels are not altered.

Most T_3 and T_4 are bound to the extent that free thyroxine constitutes less than 1% of peripheral hormone.

The bound form of thyroid hormones is unable to pass from the extracellular space and must be in the free form to diffuse into the extracellular tissues to affect major metabolic activity. T_3 is especially important in this regard. The process whereby T_3 and T_4 dissociate from binding protein and diffuse into the extracellular tissues is an efficient process, which allows tight control of peripheral metabolic activities. Most T_3 is peripherally derived from conversion from T_4. This conversion occurs by a deiodination, which takes place largely in the plasma and liver. Other deiodination processes are found in the central nervous system, especially the pituitary gland and brain tissues, as well as in brown adipose tissue. Peripheral conversion of T_4 to T_3 can be impaired in many clinical circumstances, such as overwhelming sepsis and malnutrition, and massive steroid therapy can result in functional hypothyroidism.[11]

The half-life of T_3 is about 8 to 12 hours, and free levels disappear rapidly from the peripheral circulation. In adults, the half-life of T_4 is about 7 days because of the efficient and significant degree of binding to carrier proteins. Therefore, thyroid hormones generally have a slow turnover time in the peripheral circulation, and the body is assured of at least a 7- to 10-day supply of T_4 availability for peripheral metabolism.

Inhibition of Thyroid Synthesis

Drugs

Drug therapy for treatment of thyroid excess states is often the first choice from a variety of treatment options. The thioamide class of antithyroid drugs includes propylthiouracil (PTU) and methimazole (Tapazole). This class of drugs acts by inhibiting the organification and oxidation of inorganic iodine as well as by inhibiting the linking of the initial iodotyrosine molecules MIT and DIT. In addition to these effects, PTU inhibits the peripheral conversion of T_4 to T_3. Because of this added capability, PTU is a popular choice for a rapid treatment of hyperthyroid conditions. Methimazole has longer activity and requires a single daily dose; however, it has the capability of crossing the placenta and can affect fetal development in pregnant patients. Both drugs have an effect on peripheral white blood cell development and can cause agranulocytosis; this occurs in less than 1% of cases. Other side effects include rash, arthralgias, neuritis, and liver dysfunction.

Iodine

Inorganic iodine given in large doses can inhibit thyroid hormone release by altering the organic binding process (Wolff-Chaikoff effect). The effect is transient; however, the use of iodine supplementation can be used as a treatment for hyperactivity of the gland in preparation for surgery.

Steroids

Exogenous glucocorticoids can effectively suppress the pituitary-thyroid axis. They can act in the periphery to inhibit peripheral conversion of T_4 to T_3. This effectively lowers serum T_3 levels, allowing steroids to be used as a rapid inhibitory agent in hyperthyroid conditions. Steroids can also lower serum TSH. The rapid action of steroids makes them a potentially important primary treatment for severe, previously untreated or resistant hyperthyroidism.

β Blockers

Patients with thyrotoxicosis have increased sensitivity to catecholamine secretion. Adrenergic antagonists, although not inhibiting thyroid hormone synthesis per se, are valuable in controlling peripheral sensitivity to catecholamines by blocking their effects. Therefore, cardiovascular symptoms such as pulse rate, tremor, and anxiousness can be improved, but the hypermetabolic state can remain or progress.

Tests of Thyroid Function

Evaluation of the Pituitary-Thyroid Feedback Loop

Evaluation of serum TSH is an important screening test for the diagnosis of thyroid status. TSH is measured by an ultrasensitive radioimmunometric assay that has greatly improved clinical diagnosis. This assay is especially important in the delineation of hypothyroid from euthyroid states. Additionally, clinically euthyroid patients may have suppressed TSH values, demonstrating hyperthyroidism before it becomes clinically manifest. The sensitivity of the TSH assay is also less affected by nonthyroid disease processes and remains unaffected by changes in the thyroid hormone–binding proteins.

More elaborate tests of the functional status of the hypothalamic-pituitary axis may require the use of a TRH stimulation test. An intravenous dose of TRH is given, for which a normal response should be an elevation in TSH that peaks within 15 to 35 minutes. Pituitary insufficiency then demonstrates a subnormal response to TRH, whereas patients with primary hypothyroidism demonstrate an enhanced TSH release from the anterior pituitary.

The use of the T_3 suppression tests evaluates the autonomous function of the gland because T_3 suppresses TSH release from the pituitary. An 8- to 10-day course of T_3 is administered, and a radioactive iodine uptake is then performed. The normal response should be a suppression of radioactive iodine uptake to less than 50% of initial values. An autonomously hyperfunctioning thyroid gland demonstrates a lack of suppression of the radioactive iodine uptake.

Serum Triiodothyronine and Thyroxine Levels

Thyroid production is initially screened by measuring serum total T_4 and free T_4 index. Total T_4 can be affected by changes in hormone production or hormone binding to serum proteins; therefore, an accurate evaluation of thyroid function requires measurement of free T_4 levels. The total T_4 assay measures both the free and the protein-bound hormones. Measurement of serum free T_4 is difficult, however, and indirect methods usually suffice. In this regard, the T_3 resin uptake test is one of the most common indirect measurements of the proportion of T_4 that is not protein bound. This test involves radiolabeled T_3, which is added to the individual patient serum. The mixture is incubated with an ion exchange resin, which allows competition for the serum-binding proteins for thyroid hormone. At higher levels of free T_4, the availability of unoccupied binding sites diminishes, and a greater percentage of the radiolabeled T_3 is attached to the resin. If the absolute concentration of free T_4 is low, more radiolabeled T_3 is bound, and the resin uptake is therefore low. The percentage of tracer bound varies inversely with the concentration and the affinity of unoccupied binding sites on the serum T_4-binding proteins. The product of the percentage of uptake and the total serum T_4 concentration is used to calculate the free T_4 index. This value reflects the absolute concentration of serum T_4. These measures are not usually involved with routine screening but are helpful in the diagnosis of T_3 thyrotoxicosis.

Calcitonin

The parafollicular cells, or C cells, of the thyroid elaborate a 32-amino acid polypeptide, calcitonin. The important physiologic consequence of calcitonin is to decrease peripheral levels of calcium. Malignancies that involve calcitonin excess include MCT, although the physiologic action of calcitonin does not appear to be manifest; hypocalcemia is not a problem in these patients. In patients with thyroid masses and in whom multiple endocrine neoplasia (MEN) type 2 syndrome is suspected, a baseline calcitonin level can be drawn. If there is doubt about the diagnosis, a pentagastrin- or calcium-stimulated calcitonin evaluation can be performed employing a 4- to 5-hour test. Additionally, calcitonin can be used as a screening test in families with MEN type 2 syndrome in documenting clinically inapparent disease. Use of calcitonin screening in patients with a thyroid mass, however, is most likely not cost efficient.

Radioactive Iodine Uptake

The radioactive iodine uptake test is becoming less widely used because of the more precise biochemical measurements of T_3, T_4, and TSH. This test has in the past used oral administration of iodine 123 (^{123}I) and calculated uptake using radioscintigraphy. The normal values should show 15% to 30% uptake of the radionuclide after about 24 hours. The use of ^{123}I is preferable because of shorter half-life and lesser radiation exposure compared with ^{131}I, which is used to radioablate thyroid neoplasms.

Thyroid Autoantibody Levels

Thyroid antigens are produced with autoimmune thyroid disorders, including Graves' disease and Hashimoto's thyroiditis. The detection of autoantibodies to the autoimmune disorders is extremely useful diagnostically. About 95% of patients with Hashimoto's thyroiditis and 80% with Graves' disease have detectable antimicrosomal antibodies. In Graves' disease, circulating antibodies have high affinity to a TSH receptor on thyroid follicular cells. These antibodies detected by older assays were given the name *long-acting thyroid stimulators*. Newer assays have a greater sensitivity and may allow earlier detection of Graves' disease while monitoring the success of thyroid medication treatment.

Radiologic Evaluation of The Thyroid

Thyroid Scintigraphy

The use of radionuclide agents has been helpful in delineating the presence, size, and function of thyroid nodules. Two radioactive iodine isotopes have been employed in clinical use. Scanning with ^{123}I has as its advantage low-dose radiation (30 mrad) and a short half-life (12 to 14 hours). This compares favorably with the use of ^{131}I, which has a higher dose of radiation (500 mrad) and a longer half-life (8 to 10 days). Scanning with ^{123}I is usually used for patients with a suspected lingual thyroid or substernal goiter, whereas ^{131}I is used in patients with well-differentiated thyroid carcinoma to screen for distant metastasis. Thyroid cancers should have little uptake of the radionuclide; however, this deficient area on scanning could be masked by overlying normally functioning tissue. Malignancy has been shown to occur in 15% to 20% of "cold" nodules and, additionally, in 5% to 9% of nodules with uptake that is "warm" or "hot," mandating continued aggressive approach to clinically suspicious nodules even if they are not "cold."[13]

Technetium-pertechnetate 99m (^{99m}Tc) is also used for evaluation of thyroid nodules. This substance is trapped by the thyroid but not organified, and it has a short half-life and low radiation dose. Screening with ^{99m}Tc also shows uptake in salivary glands and major vascular structures and, therefore, requires a higher sophistication of interpretation.

Thyroid Ultrasound

The use of directed cervical ultrasound has, as its advantages, increased portability, cost effectiveness, and lack of ionizing radiation. Although ultrasound may add little to the diagnosis of a diffusely enlarged gland, it has become increasingly important in the work-up of discrete nodules. Ultrasound is sensitive to delineating solid compared with cystic characteristics, diameter, and multicentricity of nodules. Additionally, enlarged cervical lymph nodes can be assessed for staging of malignancy. B-mode ultrasonography can be used preoperatively or intraoperatively, usually before and sometimes in conjunction with fine-needle aspiration (FNA).[14,15]

DISORDERS OF THYROID METABOLISM—BENIGN THYROID DISEASE

Hypothyroidism

A delicate balance between central production and peripheral action of T_3 and T_4 is required for a euthyroid state in the periphery. Clinical hypothyroidism is usually associated with decreased production in the thyroid gland, although states of limited activity in the periphery can also occur. In many underdeveloped countries, lack of sufficient iodine intake explains a large percentage of hypothyroid conditions. In more developed countries, most cases of adult hypothyroidism are caused by Hashimoto's thyroiditis, overaggressive radioactive iodine therapy, or surgical ablation. Other causes of hypothyroidism are becoming increasingly relevant, including drug-related altered thyroid function, particularly in the case of the cardiac antiarrhythmic drug amiodarone.[9] Other rarer causes of hypothyroidism include inherited defects in thyroid hormone synthesis, which include defects in thyroid peroxidase and thyroglobulin production. Additionally, congenital aberrant thyroid development can occur in children, which includes thyroid agenesis or thyroid hypoplasia. Central nervous system abnormalities resulting in either anterior pituitary gland disease or hypothalamic disorders can result in a centrally based hypothyroidism resulting from the lack of either TSH or TRH secretion. Finally, a peripheral tissue resistance to thyroid hormone action, possibly through an altered receptor mechanism, has been described.[16]

Endemic Goiter

Iodine deficiency can result in a completely preventable disease referred to as *endemic goiter*, which in its severest form results in endemic cretinism. It may be that as many as one third of the world's population, specifically in underdeveloped countries, are at risk for iodine deficiency, and about 12 million people may suffer from endemic cretinism. Although countries in Southeast Asia, including India, Indonesia, and China, account for most of the total population of the world at risk for iodine deficiency, mild to moderate iodine deficiency can still be seen in a number of European countries, including Italy, Spain, Hungary, Poland, and Yugoslavia. In areas with the most severe iodine deficiency, clinical signs and symptoms of goiter appear at an earlier age. The prevalence increases dramatically in the later childhood years, attaining a peak at puberty. The appearance of goiter decreases during adulthood, remaining slightly greater in women.[17]

Metabolic Consequences of Iodine Deficiency

The chronic physiologic changes that result from a lifetime of iodine deficiency involve anatomic and metabolic alterations of varying significance. As a result of chronic deficient iodine intake, decreased T_4 and T_3 production occurs. This results in gradually increasing thyroid clearance of iodine and decreased renal excretion. Chronic preferential production of T_3 rather than T_4 occurs as well as enhanced peripheral conversion of T_4 to T_3. By making production of T_3 and clearance of the metabolically active hormone as efficient as possible, clinical hypothyroidism is largely avoided by a biochemical pattern of low serum T_4 with elevated TSH and normal or above-normal levels of T_3. In the severest cases, serum T_3 and T_4 concentrations are low, and serum TSH elevations occur. In these situations, endemic cretinism is often found. Accompanying the physiologic changes in response to iodine deficiency, a diffuse enlargement in the thyroid gland often occurs. The thyroid follicles demonstrate a hypertrophic response with reduction in follicular spaces. As the iodine deficiency becomes more severe, follicles can become inactive and then become distended with colloid. Focal areas of nodular hyperplasia may develop and form nodules, some of which may become hot nodules and have autonomous function. Others become inactive and inert. Necrosis, scarring, and hemorrhage can occur, resulting in a fibrous ingrowth; all these disorders include marked enlargement of the gland, often in an asymmetrical pattern.[17]

Postirradiation Hypothyroidism

Planned clinical hypothyroidism can be the result of treatment of certain disorders with ^{131}I. This treatment has become increasingly popular for patients with hyperthyroid conditions, including Graves' disease. Between 50% and 70% of patients who receive greater than 10 mCi can be predicted to become clinically hypothyroid. For patients undergoing this type of treatment, continued thyroid monitoring is necessary on an annual basis.

External-beam irradiation of patients with lymphomatous disease of the mediastinum or head and neck cancers is associated with subclinical hypothyroidism. This becomes particularly important in patients who have had previous thyroid resection for either benign or malignant disease processes.[18]

Postsurgical Hypothyroidism

In the event that ^{131}I therapy is not available for patients with hyperthyroidism or Graves' disease, surgical ablation is an effective way to induce permanent hypothyroidism. Subtotal or total thyroidectomy effectively produces postoperative hypothyroidism. The incidence of postoperative permanent hypothyroidism varies with the skill of the operating surgeon and the amount of thyroid that is truly ablated. The rate of complications, however, such as recurrent laryngeal nerve damage and hypocalcemia, is increased with more aggressive surgical ablation. Other factors affecting postoperative occurrence of hypothyroidism include antithyroid drug administration, dietary iodine availability, and lymphocytic infiltration of the remaining tissue.

Pharmacologic Hypothyroidism

Cytokines. The effects of cytokines in thyroiditis may well be responsible for the generation and aggravation of the disease process. The exact nature of the cytokine effects in the development of Hashimoto's thyroiditis is unclear. It is known that patients undergoing treatment with interferon-alfa or interleukin-2 treatment for certain malignant diseases can develop hypothyroidism, which is reversible on discontinuation of these drugs. This point is particularly important in patients with underlying Hashimoto's thyroiditis, and a careful history should be taken from these patients.

Lithium. Certain psychiatric disorders, including manic depressive disorders, rely on lithium for treatment. Lithium has the capability of inhibiting the cyclic AMP-dependent pathway of hormone formation and may, by this mechanism, inhibit thyroid hormone formation. Hypothyroidism in patients taking lithium is usually seen more frequently in those with underlying Hashimoto's thyroiditis, although it can occur in patients with normal thyroid function.[19]

Amiodarone. Amiodarone is an antiarrhythmic drug that is efficacious in treating ventricular arrhythmias. This drug contains a significant amount of iodine, of which a standard dosage can aggravate thyroid dysfunction. Prolonged administration can result in thyroiditis and resultant hyperthyroidism followed by transient hypothyroidism. This thyroiditis is often associated with an increase in serum interleukin-6 levels, suggesting a cytokine inflammatory response. Severe thyroid dysfunction can occur in patients taking amiodarone, especially those with previously documented Hashimoto's thyroiditis.[20]

Antithyroid Drugs. Common antithyroid drugs (carbimazole, methimazole, and PTU) can, if given in sufficient quantity, result in hypothyroidism. Careful monitoring of patients taking these drugs and understanding the disease process for which they are given are mandatory in following these patients.

Peripheral Tissue Hormone Resistance

A rare familial disorder resulting in generalized thyroid hormone resistance may be caused by thyroid receptor (TR) abnormalities. Malfunction of the TR results in clinically apparent hypothyroidism in the setting of elevated serum thyroid hormone levels.[16] Two separate TRs, TR-α and TR-β, are coded by separate genes on chromosomes 17 and 3, respectively, in the human genome. Mutations in TR-β appear to be responsible for the rare familial disorder of thyroid hormone resistance. TR-α appears to be unaffected and uninvolved with such mutations.

Clinical Presentation and Diagnosis of Hypothyroidism

The developing fetus and newborn are usually protected from hypothyroidism by the transplacental passage of T_4. After birth, the failure of thyroid function, if prolonged, can result in significant and sometimes irreversible changes in development resulting in poor growth, mental retardation, and dwarfism. This syndrome is referred to as *cretinism.* During later childhood years, hypothyroidism can result in decreased intellectual capacity but not necessarily mental retardation. Physical signs such as rectal prolapse, abdominal distention, and umbilical hernia may be present. During adolescence, this situation is known as *juvenile hypothyroidism.*

In adults, spontaneous hypothyroidism is usually manifested in females (80%) and is a more insidious process associated with a slow, progressive failure of function. In the majority of cases, this process is due to a lymphocytic thyroiditis. The classic symptoms are fatigue, headache, weight gain, dry skin, brittle hair, and muscle cramps. Severe progression of disease can result in cardiovascular symptoms including hypertension, pericardial effusions, and pleural effusions. Abdominal distension and constipation are signs of severe hypothyroidism. Anemia may occur in 12% of cases.

Diagnosis. In the work-up of the patient with subjective symptoms of fatigue or constipation, or in the work-up of cardiac abnormalities, the evaluation of thyroid function cannot be forgotten. Classic hypothyroid laboratory evaluation demonstrates decreased T_4 and T_3 values with increased TSH and cholesterol levels.

Treatment. L-Thyroxine is a safe and effective treatment, once the diagnosis is made. An oral dose of 100 μg is effective over a wide range of adult body weight and body mass index. Patients with severe clinical hypothyroidism should be monitored closely and gradually started on increasing doses due to sensitivity to the hormone as a result of chronic depletion of catecholamines in the myocardium.

Thyroiditis

Acute Suppurative Thyroiditis

Acute suppurative thyroiditis infection of the thyroid is extremely rare and is usually the result of a severe pyogenic infection of the upper airway. The process results in severe localized pain and is usually unilateral. Abscess drainage followed by antibiotics is effective and minimal long-term effect on thyroid function results.

Hashimoto's Thyroiditis

One of the major causes of hypothyroidism in the adult population is Hashimoto's thyroiditis. A complex immunologic phenomenon results in the formation of immune complex and complement in the basement membrane of the follicular cells. Complement fixation results in thyroid cell function alterations that impair T_3 and T_4 production. A cascade of cytokine production can result in an exacerbation of immune response that directly interferes with thyroid function. These cellular reactions ultimately result in an infiltration of lymphocytes and a resultant fibrosis, which decreases the number and efficiency of individual follicles.[21] As this immune phenomenon continues, the presence of TSH-blocking antibodies can be detected. Thyroid microsomal antibodies are produced that are most likely key mediators in the initial complement-fixation process. As the immune process continues, changes in thyroid function can be altered by levels of these antibodies. Ultimately, a hypothyroid clinical state can occur in patients with persistent TSH-blocking antibodies.[22]

Subacute Thyroiditis

Subacute thyroiditis occurs in females (2:1) in the United States, England, and Japan. The mean age is in the 40s in most series. The exact cause is not known, although it is not thought to be due to a viral or autoimmune origin. Patients present with a diffuse swelling in the cervical area and a sudden increase in pain. Approximately two thirds of patients have fever, weight loss, and severe fatigue. An FNA can be diagnostic if it demonstrates the giant cells of an epithelioid foreign body type, which characterizes the lesion. Microscopic pathology shows large follicles infiltrated by mononuclear cells, neutrophils, and lymphocytes.

Treatment with steroids and adrenocorticotropic hormone are effective in relieving symptoms. However, the disease process usually continues, unaffected by these medications.

Riedel's Struma

Riedel's thyroiditis (struma) is a rare entity that is a firm, chronic inflammatory process involving the entire thyroid. Symptoms of severe discomfort due to extension into the trachea, esophagus, and laryngeal nerve can occur. As a result, patients may present with impending airway obstruction or dysphagia. Unilateral involvement of symptoms may suggest a malignancy, leading to surgical intervention. The findings at surgery can also be impressive, because the process can extend into the trachea and esophagus with obliteration of the anatomic planes and landmarks. Surgical pathology reveals a dense fibrous tissue and nearly total obliteration of normal follicle architecture. Grossly, direct involvement of the process can result in severe tracheal and esophageal obstruction.

Treatment with thyroid hormone replacement is effective. Immediate tracheal or esophageal obstruction may require a surgical approach to relieve symptoms. Such surgery should be performed by an experienced thyroid surgeon and remove only the constricting portion of the thyroid.

Hyperthyroidism

The disease processes associated with increased thyroid secretion result in a predictable hypermetabolic state. Increased thyroid secretion can be caused by primary alterations within the gland (Graves' disease, toxic nodular goiter, toxic thyroid adenoma) or central nervous system disorders and increased TSH-produced stimulation of the thyroid. Most hyperthyroid states occur because of primary malfunction. Even more unusual hyperthyroid states can result from mismanaged exogenous thyroid ingestion, molar pregnancy with increased release of human chorionic gonadotropin, and, unusually, thyroid malignancy with overproduction of thyroid hormone.

Graves' Disease

Most hyperthyroid states are caused by Graves' disease (diffuse toxic goiter). This disease entity was originally described by an Irish physician, Dr. Robert Graves, in 1835. Most patients are women between the ages of 20 and 40 years. Around 1960, the pathogenesis of Graves' disease was thought to be due to the long-acting thyroid-stimulating antibody, which resulted in exaggerated

thyroid hormone secretion. More recently, it has been demonstrated that a wide variety of antibodies result in a thyroid-stimulating process that incorporates the TSH receptor on follicular cells. Thyroid-stimulating immunoglobulins may stimulate TSH receptors at the same time that certain other immunoglobulins may block TSH binding in the same family of receptors. Although there are several theories about the stimulus that initiates production of these antibodies, there is no universal agreement about the etiology of the process. Genetic susceptibility to this disease is possible. Descriptions of increased probability of Graves' disease in identical and fraternal twins have been described.

Pathology. Patients with Graves' disease have an enlarged nodular gland with increased vascularity. The size may be diffuse or asymmetrical, resulting in significant enlargement that is grossly visible and that can result in cosmetic deformity and significant tracheal deviation or compression. On microscopic examination, the follicles are small, with hyperplastic columnar epithelium. Hyperplasia of these cells is exhibited by rapidly dividing nuclei and papillary projections of the follicular epithelium within the central follicles. Increased lymphoid tissue deposition is also demonstrable in many patients with Graves' disease.

Clinical Presentation. The patient with classic Graves' disease usually has a visibly enlarged neck mass consistent with a goiter. Accompanying clinical thyrotoxicosis and exophthalmos complete the classic triad of the disease. Hair loss, myxedema, gynecomastia, and splenomegaly can accompany the clinical presentation. Physical examination is remarkable for an enlarged palpable thyroid with bilateral and central enlargement. With increased vascularity, a bruit is often heard. Tracheal compression can result in airway obstructive symptoms, although acute compression with respiratory distress is exceedingly rare.

The ocular consequences of prolonged and untreated thyrotoxicosis can be severe. Exophthalmos is thought to be due to the stimulation of fatty fibrous tissue behind the orbit causing outward pressure. Proptosis and supraorbital and infraorbital swelling can result. Conjunctival swelling with accompanying congestion and edema are advanced signs of exophthalmos. In its most severe form, spasm of the upper eyelid resulting in retraction and visualization of a larger amount of sclera than normal can lead to a lid lag and exacerbation of the already swollen conjunctiva. All of these pressure-related phenomena can progress to decreased oculomuscular movements, ophthalmoplegia, and diplopia. Optic nerve damage and blindness can be a long-term result if the underlying condition is not corrected. Sustained hyperthyroidism should be aggressively treated to remove the stimulus to the retro-orbital tissues.

Clinical presentation of hyperthyroidism also includes the protean manifestations of an increased hypermetabolic state. The classic presentation of patients with long-term thyrotoxicosis includes sweating, weight loss, heat intolerance, and thirst. The menstrual cycle can be altered to the point of amenorrhea. Cardiovascular stress can be demonstrated by high-output cardiac failure and congestive heart failure with peripheral edema. Arrhythmias include ventricular tachycardia or atrial fibrillation. Gastrointestinal signs may include increased bowel frequency to the point of diarrhea and electrolyte wasting. Psychiatric signs may include altered sleep patterns, emotional mood swings, fatigue, excitability, and agitation.

Diagnosis. An enlarged smooth thyroid mass and signs and symptoms of thyrotoxicosis suggest the diagnosis. A cost-effective work-up can include an extensive history, physical examination, and thyroid function tests. In addition to elevated levels of T_3 and T_4, a decreased or undetectable level of TSH should be demonstrated. Thyroid antibodies are usually detected in elevated quantities. Extensive use of imaging studies may or may not be required, given the clinical suspicion. A ^{123}I radionuclide scan should demonstrate diffuse uptake throughout an enlarged gland. An ultrasound or computed tomography (CT) scan of the neck may be used to evaluate clinical landmarks (Fig. 34-5). However, the absolute requirement of the latter two images for preoperative assessment is not universally agreed on.[23,24]

Treatment. When a diagnosis of Graves' disease has been made, rapid initiation of therapy should be undertaken. This is particularly crucial for the patients with vision-threatened exophthalmos. There have been three classic methods to treat Graves' disease: radioiodine ablation, surgery, and antithyroid medication. As recently as the 1980s, surgery was the most commonly employed method of treatment; however, advances in the understanding of radionuclide application and efficacy of thyroid medication have made nonsurgical options more prevalent, particularly in the United States. In fact, only a minority of patients with Graves' disease require surgery. Clearly, patients with Graves' disease need to be educated regarding appropriate choices, the risks of each treatment, and the expectation of complete success.

Radionuclide Therapy. The use of radioactive iodine therapy is offered to and chosen by most patients with Graves' disease in the United States. The most commonly employed radionuclide is ^{131}I. Pretreatment establishment of a euthyroid state should be accomplished by using antithyroid medication for 3 to 4 weeks before treatment. The drug therapy should then be terminated to allow efficient uptake of the isotope. A pretreatment screening radionuclide scan should then be done to allow calculation of the appropriate dosage of ^{131}I, which can be ingested orally in a typical dose of 8 to 12 mCi. After ingestion of between 10 to 15 mCi, the overall cure rate should be in the range of 90%. If the initial dosage is successful, most patients are expected to demonstrate normal thyroid function tests without medication in 8 to 12 weeks. A 10% to 15% incidence of hypothyroidism may occur within 12 months, with as much as a 3% increase in each succeeding year. It is important to monitor patients after ^{131}I treatment by carefully measuring circulating hormones and TSH levels.[23,25]

The ideal application of radioactive iodine therapy would be for those patients with small to moderate enlargement of the gland and those in whom antithyroid drugs have clearly not worked. Additional candidates would include patients who desire not to have surgery or for whom surgery is contraindicated. Another group includes those who have recurrence after surgical or medical therapy. Radioactive iodine is probably not the most efficacious in younger patients, including adolescents, or in patients with larger goiters. It is obviously contraindicated in pregnant or lactating patients. There are no absolute contraindications to the use of radioactive iodine therapy in women of child-producing age.

The advantages of ^{131}I therapy include avoidance of surgery and the associated risks for recurrent laryngeal nerve damage, hypothyroidism, or postsurgical recurrence. It may be that ^{131}I therapy is more cost effective in the long run; however, the financial advantage is not as clear if repeated ^{131}I therapy is needed. Disadvantages include a 10% initial incidence, with an increasing long-term incidence of hypothyroidism requiring thyroid replacement therapy and a higher relapse rate after primary treatment requiring further ^{131}I dosage. Additional disadvantages include exacerbation of cardiac arrhythmias, particularly in elderly patients, possible fetal damage in pregnant women, worsening ophthalmic problems, and rare but possibly life-threatening thyroid storm.

Antithyroid Medication. The main antithyroid action of the drugs PTU, methimazole, and carbimazole is through the inhibition of the organification of intrathyroid iodine as well as inhibition of the coupling of iodotyrosine molecules to form T_3 and T_4. It may be that PTU has the additive effect of blocking peripheral conversion of T_4 to T_3. Peripheral excess of T_3 and T_4 has multiple hyperdynamic and hypermetabolic effects. Drugs that block the peripheral conversion of T_4 to T_3 can effectively modulate peripheral effects of thyrotoxicosis. Additionally, peripheral adrenergic effects of thyrotoxicosis can be modulated by the use of β-blocking agents such as propranolol. In the acute circumstance, steroids and β blockers combine both effects to gain rapid control of the hypermetabolic effects of increased peripheral T_4 and T_3.

Medical treatment of patients with severe thyrotoxicosis initially starts with β blockers such as propranolol,

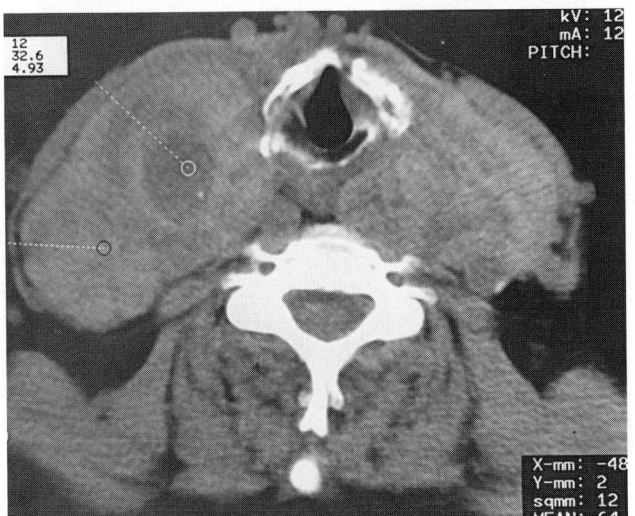

FIGURE 34-5. CT scan at the level of the larynx demonstrates this heterogeneous, large thyroid mass that has involved both lobes of the thyroid and has displaced the larynx. This patient ultimately proved to have a large multinodular goiter.

which is specifically effective in treating tachycardia. Propylthiouracil, carbimazole, or methimazole may then be added, with close monitoring of T_4 and TSH levels. If, after several weeks, clinical or chemical hypothyroidism has occurred, thyroid replacement should be carefully given. Antithyroid medication is effective in gaining rapid control of thyrotoxicosis; however, the relapse rate after discontinuation of medication may approach 50% 12 to 18 months after cessation. Additionally, patients need to be monitored for side effects of the drugs, particularly PTU. These drugs can have major hematologic disorders, which include agranulocytopenia and, in rare instances, aplastic anemia. Other side effects include fever, polyarteritis, and skin rashes.[25]

Thyroid Resection. The advantages of surgical ablation of the thyroid include rapid, effective treatment of thyrotoxicosis without necessity for medications and accompanying side effects. The amount of residual tissue is a subject of debate.[26] Complete ablation of thyroid tissue requires a total thyroidectomy, which is associated with the highest rates of hypoparathyroidism and recurrent laryngeal nerve damage. Some groups have reported that total thyroidectomy is the most effective way to treat patients with severe Graves' disease because it offers the lowest rate of relapse. It may be that patients, particularly those with ophthalmopathy, are stabilized most successfully by total thyroidectomy. Removal of the entire antigenic focus may be the most likely explanation for this observation. Other subtotal resections include near-total thyroidectomy or subtotal thyroidectomy, in which one would do a complete lobectomy on one side, leaving a rim of tissue on the contralateral side (near-total thyroidectomy) or leaving a rim of tissue on both sides (subtotal thyroidectomy). One to 2 g of thyroid tissue can be left at the discretion of the surgeon, thereby minimizing risk of damage to the recurrent laryngeal nerve but exposing the patient to some risk of recurrence within this remaining tissue.[23]

Patients should be considered for surgery who have had obvious failure of medication or radioiodine treatment. Additionally, younger patients, particularly adolescents, pregnant patients, and patients with suspicious masses contained within the large thyroid, should undergo surgical resection. Patients with severe cosmetic deformities or tracheal compression causing discomfort should also be candidates for resection. Before surgery, it is important to counsel the patient on the risks and options of the surgery, including hypoparathyroidism and recurrent laryngeal nerve damage, as well as on the possibility of relapse if less than a total thyroidectomy is contemplated. The patient should be rendered euthyroid before surgery by use of antithyroid medication and, occasionally, β-blocker medication. The use of Lugol's solution has been recommended for about 7 days before surgery to decrease the vascularity of the thyroid parenchyma.

Careful documentation of euthyroid status before surgery in all hyperthyroid patients is mandatory. If the patient is not properly treated preoperatively, thyroid storm can be life threatening. Fortunately, this circumstance is rarely encountered if appropriately anticipated.

Thyroid storm is manifested by severe tachycardia, fever, confusion, vomiting to the point of dehydration, and adrenergic overstimulation to the point of mania and coma after thyroid resection in an uncontrolled hyperthyroid patient. The best way to treat thyroid storm is preoperative anticipation and preparation. Additionally, all patients undergoing general anesthesia should be checked for undiagnosed hyperthyroidism, if clinically suspected. Treatment of the patient with overt thyroid storm should include rapid fluid replacement and rapid institution of antithyroid drugs, β blockers, iodine solutions, and steroids. In life-threatening circumstances, peritoneal dialysis or hemodialysis may be effective in lowering T_4 and T_3 levels.

Toxic Nodular Goiter-Toxic Adenoma

Toxic nodular goiter, also known as *Plummer's disease*, refers to a nodule contained within an otherwise goitrous thyroid gland that has autonomous function. This usually occurs in the setting of a patient with endemic goiter. Increased thyroid hormone production occurs independent of TSH control. Such patients usually have a milder course and are older than patients with Graves' disease. The thyroid in such patients may be diffusely enlarged or associated with retrosternal goiters. Presenting symptoms are mild, peripheral thyroid hormone levels are elevated, and TSH levels are suppressed. Antithyroid antibody levels are usually decreased. The diagnosis is usually confirmed after clinical suspicion, and an ^{131}I radionuclide scan is performed that localizes one or two autonomous areas of function while the rest of the gland shows decreased activity (Fig. 34-6).[23] Treatment of toxic nodular goiter is most effectively performed by resection of the area, usually by

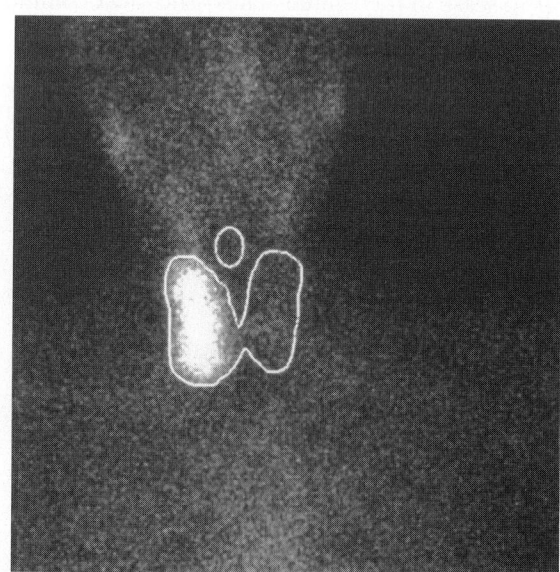

FIGURE 34-6. An ^{131}I scan demonstrates an area of increased uptake in the right lobe of a 32-year-old woman with increased thyroid function tests and a palpable nodule. This scan is consistent with a toxic or hyperfunctioning nodule.

lobectomy or near-total thyroidectomy, particularly when clinical symptoms are pronounced. In the case of the single, hyperfunctioning adenoma, a lobectomy is usually curative. Antithyroid medication can control symptoms, but relapse is common. Radioiodine therapy is not as effective as in patients with Graves' disease.

Nontoxic Goiter

Multinodular Goiter

Multinodular goiter describes an enlarged, diffusely heterogeneous thyroid gland. Initial presentation may include diffuse enlargement, but the mass often develops asymmetrical nodularity. The cause of this mass is usually iodine deficiency. Initially, the mass is euthyroid; however, with increasing size, elevations in T_3 and T_4 can occur and progress gradually into clinical hyperthyroidism. Work-up and diagnosis include evaluation of thyroid function tests. Ultrasound and radioisotopic scanning demonstrate heterogeneous thyroid substance. Nodules with poor uptake can present as lesions suspicious for malignancy. The incidence of carcinoma in multinodular goiter has been reported as 5% to 10%. Therefore, FNA for diagnosis and resection for suspicious lesions should be considered.[27]

Substernal Goiter

Substernal goiter is an unusual presentation of an intrathoracic extension of an enlarged thyroid, usually as a result of multinodular goiter. Most intrathoracic or substernal goiters are labeled "secondary" because they are enlargements or extensions of multinodular goiters, based on the inferior thyroid vasculature. They expand downward into the anterior mediastinum. The extremely rare (~1%) "primary" substernal goiter arises as aberrant thyroid tissue within the anterior or posterior mediastinum and is based on intrathoracic vasculature and not supplied by the inferior thyroid artery.

Most substernal goiters can be approached through a cervical incision. The requirement for a mediastinal approach by sternotomy is unusual, although it provides excellent exposure. Complications of surgery include intrathoracic bleeding, recurrence in unresected tissue, and recurrent laryngeal nerve damage, although in experienced hands the complication rate should be less than 5%.[28,29]

Special Considerations for the Patient With Goiter

Patients with an enlarged thyroid mass (>5 cm) can present with a spectrum of symptoms ranging from none to severe dysphagia, choking, and pain. Occasionally, the diagnosis is suggested by findings of an anterior mediastinal mass on chest radiograph. In 10% to 20% of cases, an asymptomatic patient may have no palpable abnormality in the cervical area and a completely intrathoracic lesion.

CT is the preferred imaging study that should include all regions from the mandible to the upper abdomen. The lesion itself should be scrutinized. Benign goiters have rounded, smooth borders. Thyroid malignancies usually have more ill-defined borders. CT also allows evaluations of regional lymph nodes and metastasis. If the patient has a history of pain and night sweats, a diagnosis of a lymphoma should be considered. The use of FNA with CT guidance is important to secure a tissue diagnosis. Magnetic resonance imaging (MRI) does not usually add significant information to a well-performed CT scan. For the patient with an intrathoracic lesion and a history of cough, preoperative bronchoscopy can give important information about vocal cord status and possible luminal invasion by a malignancy.

The initial surgical approach for almost all goiters and other thyroid masses is through a cervical incision. Goiters are usually easily mobilized, even when they are substernal. Blood supply is usually based on the inferior thyroid artery that is in its normal position, allowing even large substernal masses to be gently mobilized into the neck. Careful attention must be given to the location of the esophagus, trachea, and recurrent laryngeal nerve. The esophagus can be injured by overaggressive manipulation of the thyroid mass. The recurrent laryngeal nerve is usually displaced posteriorly and inferiorly; however, it can be draped anteriorly over the mass and damaged in that position. Great care must be used in mobilization of the mass until the nerve is identified. Extension of the cervical incision to a median sternotomy should be employed if there is significant bleeding from the anterior mediastinum, or if the anatomy and location of the recurrent laryngeal nerve are in doubt or if the mass cannot be mobilized through the surgical field.

WORK-UP AND DIAGNOSIS OF THE SOLITARY THYROID NODULE

The management and ultimate decision for surgical intervention after the finding of a solitary nodule depend on the knowledge of a cost-effective work-up and prognosis (Fig. 34-7). Most patients presenting with a solitary thyroid nodule most likely have a benign lesion; however, thyroid cancer is a definite possibility in all patients. Deciding between conservative management or surgical therapy relies on the careful analysis of the presentation, image assessment, and interventional diagnostic methods.[24]

Presentation

The frequency of the appearance of a thyroid nodule increases with age. Solitary palpable nodules are about four times more prevalent in women than in men. Exposure to radiation, especially during childhood, is associated with an increased prevalence of thyroid nodules, and malignancy, particularly between the late teenage years and early 20s. Rapid recent growth of the mass and signs

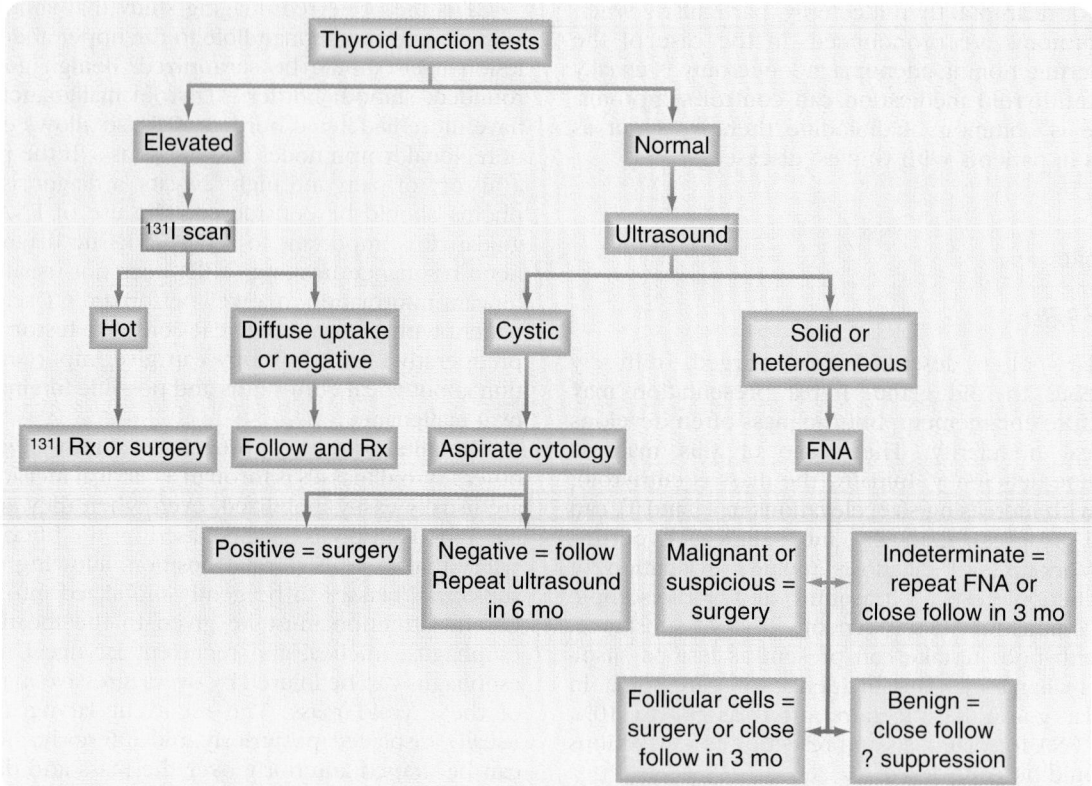

FIGURE 34-7.   The work-up of a solitary thyroid nodule. FNA, fine-needle aspiration; Rx, therapy.

of possible invasion, such as pain or hoarseness, are most suggestive but not conclusive for malignancy (Figs. 34-8 and 34-9).[24,30]

Diagnostic Evaluation

The work-up of the patient with a solitary nodule begins with a careful history and physical examination. The possibility of a thyroid nodule being cancer is greatest in men older than 50 years of age. A careful history should also include exposure to radiation either through occupational sources or through radiographs to the head or neck, particularly earlier in life. Additionally, a thorough history for specific endocrine disorders, including medullary carcinoma, MEN type 2, or papillary thyroid cancer, or of familial polyposis, including Gardner's syndrome, is warranted.[31]

On physical examination, it is important to include a thorough palpation of the thyroid as well as the anterior and posterior cervical triangles. Determining the size and consistency of the nodule is important. Multiple nodules or diffuse nodularity are associated with more benign diagnosis. A firm solitary nodule, particularly in older men, is suspicious for a malignant diagnosis. The use of ultrasound in the office setting to supplement the physical examination is becoming increasingly useful. Ultrasound is extremely useful in evaluating whether the nodule is cystic or solid, multicentricity, and lateral lymph node status. It is important to realize that specific exceptions to the rules exist. Papillary carcinoma can take the form of a cystic lesion. In addition, a firm or solid lesion that is filled

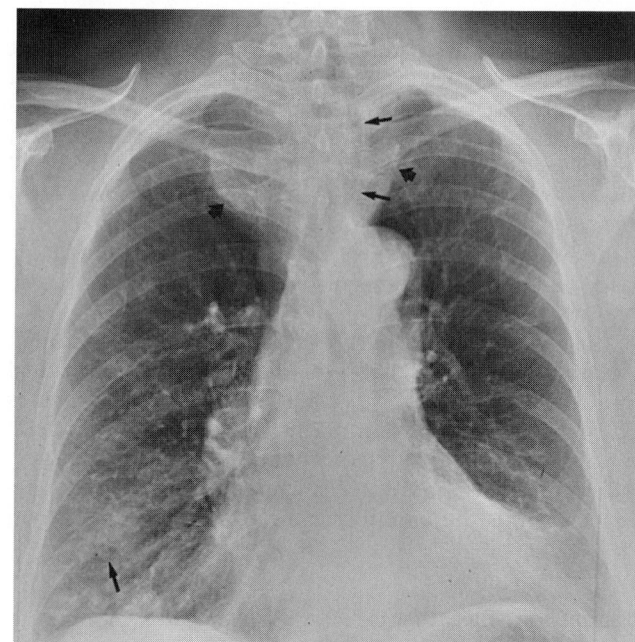

FIGURE 34-8.   An elderly woman presented with an anterior mediastinal mass (*thick arrows*) and tracheal deviation (*thin arrows* at top). Work-up demonstrated pulmonary masses that had squamous cell components (*thin arrow* in right lower lung field). A biopsy of this anterior mediastinal mass was performed and demonstrated anaplastic carcinoma of the thyroid.

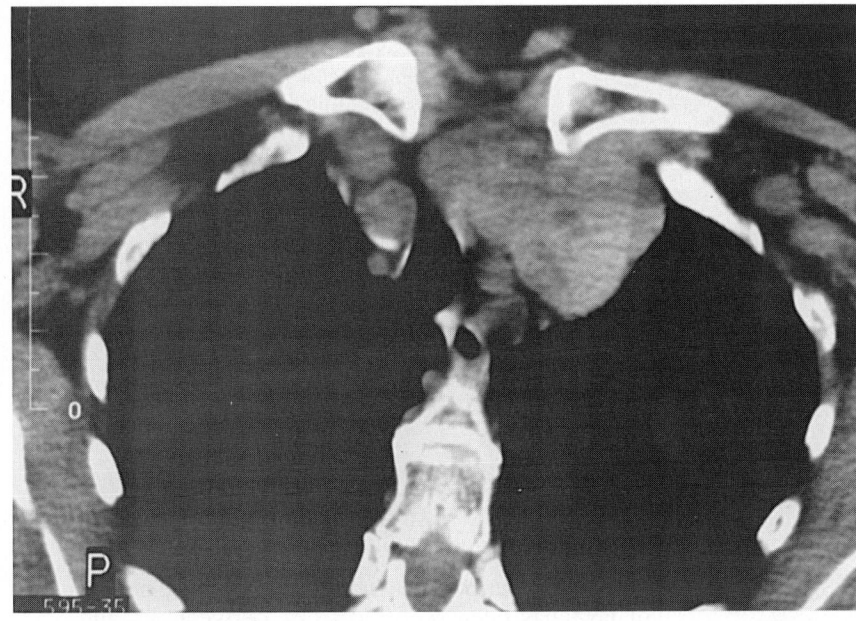

FIGURE 34-9. CT scan of an ill-defined 4-cm mass in the anterior mediastinum immediately beneath the clavicular head in a patient with a mass that proved at biopsy to be anaplastic carcinoma of the thyroid.

with calcified hemorrhage, although suspicious to palpation, is usually benign.

Laboratory Evaluation

The use of a complete blood count, including hematocrit and white blood cell count, in addition to the standard laboratory electrolyte evaluation is usually unhelpful in the work-up of a patient with a thyroid nodule. Thyroid function tests, including measures of T_4 and T_3 resin uptake, and TSH should identify patients with unsuspected hyperthyroid states and dictate appropriate work-up (see Fig. 34-7). Therefore, the use of a standard screening thyroid function test panel is warranted. Serum thyroglobulin has been reported as useful in predicting a well-differentiated carcinoma; however, its standard use is not universally agreed on. When there is clinical suspicion of medullary carcinoma, either by family history or by FNA biopsy, serum calcitonin level can be measured. The routine use of serum calcitonin measurement for thyroid masses is not likely to be helpful.[30]

Radiologic Evaluation

Ultrasound is helpful in determining the volume of a nodule, its multicentricity, and whether it is solid or cystic. Additionally, ultrasound is extremely useful in those patients who are managed conservatively for follow-up of possible increased volume of a suspicious lesion. The use of ultrasound has expanded into the office setting and is also available for intraoperative evaluation. Ultrasound has proven highly effective in determining location and characteristics (cystic vs. solid) of nodules but is unable to accurately predict the diagnosis of solid nodules (Fig. 34-10). The finding of a cystic lesion may be reassuring, but these represent a small minority of thyroid nodules (1% to 5%). Additionally, well-differentiated

thyroid cancers had cystic components in as many as 25% of cases in one series.[32]

The use of radionuclide scanning has decreased as other modalities, such as FNA, have improved. The determination of increased (hot) or poor (cold) uptake in a thyroid nodule does not have acceptable accuracy to warrant its exclusive use for diagnostic decision making. A large series has shown that 16% of patients with cold nodules and 4% of patients with hot nodules had thyroid cancer documented by surgical resection.[33] It may be that the most useful current application for radionuclide scanning is in the setting of the work-up for apparent Graves' disease. The finding of a cold nodule in such a setting should warrant strong consideration of surgery instead of radionuclide therapy or antithyroid medication.

Fine-Needle Aspiration

The use of a small-gauge needle for aspiration biopsy of the thyroid has become increasingly popular and has now become one of the initial diagnostic modalities in patients with thyroid nodules. The use of the smaller-gauge needle has allowed a marked drop in the complication rate from the use of large-bore or core needle biopsies while maintaining diagnostic accuracy. A series of 561 FNA biopsy results reported an 86% sensitivity rate at 91% specificity.[34] The accurate diagnosis of a benign lesion has significantly decreased surgery rates on patients with thyroid nodules. Additionally, preoperative FNA is replacing the use of intraoperative frozen-section analysis of pathology.[34] Despite the widespread use of ultrasound-guided FNA, this modality is also associated with a significant rate of initial nondiagnostic cytology approaching 20% to 25%.[15] The finding of a malignant diagnosis on FNA is associated with a high accuracy rate, approaching 100%. Certain discrete cytologic characteristics of papillary carcinoma allow the use of FNA to be extremely accurate in its diagnosis.

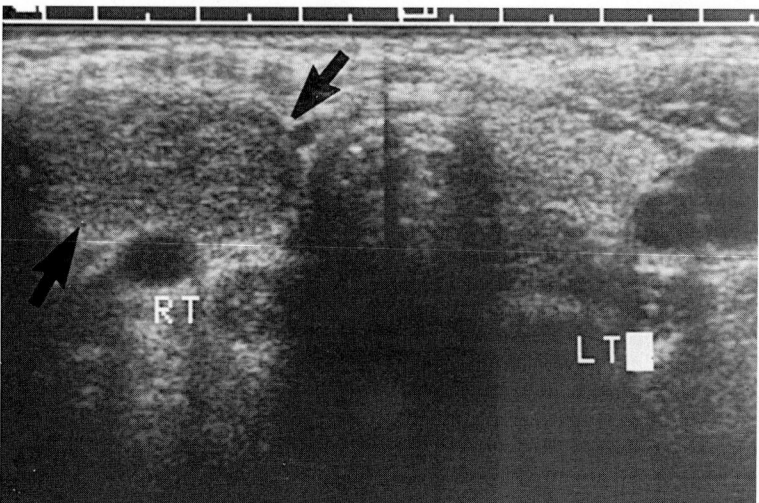

FIGURE 34-10.   Preoperative ultrasound of a patient with a 4 × 2-cm homogeneous right thyroid (RT) mass (*arrows*). Resection demonstrated a follicular adenoma. LT, left thyroid.

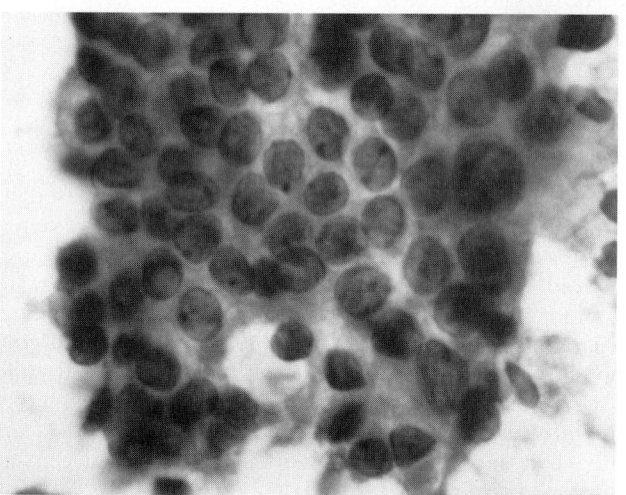

FIGURE 34-11.   Fine-needle aspiration of a thyroid mass allows determination of individual cellular morphology. Cells in this aspirate demonstrate intranuclear grooving as well as "ground-glass" cytoplasm ("Orphan Annie eyes"). These cellular features are consistent with a diagnosis of papillary carcinoma of the thyroid.

The diagnosis of follicular carcinoma cannot be made with FNA. The FNA diagnosis of medullary or anaplastic carcinoma is somewhat more difficult but can be made by experienced cytopathologists (Fig. 34-11). When FNA reveals "follicular cells," an important decision must be made. Although most of these cases are benign (follicular adenoma), this diagnosis cannot be secure and ultimately depends on complete microscopic examination of the resected specimen. Large series show malignancy in 6% to 20% of thyroid lesions with follicular cells demonstrated on FNA.[35]

The diagnosis of a benign lesion is strongly suggested by the findings of colloid and macrophage within the aspirated cytology. In this circumstance, a safe diagnosis of a colloid nodule or benign process can be made. The patient must understand, however, that this diagnosis depends only on the aspirated material. Tissue immediately adjacent to or contained within another part of the

nodule may harbor malignant cells. The false-negative rate of FNA has been reported to be between 1% and 6%.[30] Therefore, benign nodules diagnosed by FNA should be followed sequentially with ultrasound to make sure the characteristics do not change. If FNA leads to a diagnosis that is "suspicious but not confirmatory," an aggressive work-up should continue for the possibility of malignancy. Certain series state that more than half of such FNA results are associated with malignant cells. If an FNA is indeterminate, either a repeat aspiration or close conservative follow-up of the nodule should be undertaken.[24]

FNA can also be used for lesions that are determined to be cystic by ultrasound. A larger-bore needle can be used to aspirate the cyst fluid. Examination of most cystic fluid results in benign cytologic findings; however, an occasional papillary carcinoma can present as a cyst and be diagnosed through cytologic examination of cystic fluid.

Decision Making and Treatment (Table 34-1)

Decision making about thyroid nodules depends on interpretation and the judicious use of thyroid function tests, imaging, and FNA. All patients with a thyroid nodule should have thyroid function tests (including T_4, TSH, and T_3 resin uptake). If these are elevated, the patient should undergo a technetium scan that should confirm a "hot" nodule. If this is confirmed the patient should undergo careful monitoring with thyroid suppression and be seen again after 6 months to confirm successful suppression and re-evaluation. If suppressive therapy fails, surgery (usually lobectomy) is highly effective but usually not required (see Toxic Nodular Goiter-Toxic Adenoma).

For the patient with a thyroid nodule and normal thyroid function tests, an ultrasound should be performed. Cystic lesions on ultrasound are usually benign; however, cystic papillary carcinomas, although rare, do occur. Cystic lesions should be aspirated (bloody or suspicious aspirations can be sent for cytology). After aspiration, these patients should be placed on suppression and seen again in 6 months. Patients with recurrent cysts should be considered surgical candidates.

TABLE 34-1. Thyroid Nodules

Diagnosis	Factors Associated With Diagnosis	Factors that Confirm Diagnosis	Factors Associated With Worse Prognosis
BENIGN			
Colloid	Multinodular goiter FNA shows colloid and macrophages	Surgery	—
Hyperfunctioning nodule	Hyperthyroidism	Iodine 131 scan	—
MALIGNANT			
Papillary carcinoma	Radiation exposure Previous surgery for papillary carcinoma	FNA or surgery	Male gender, age >40 yr, size >3 cm, tall cell variant
Follicular carcinoma	"Follicular cells" by FNA	Permanent section pathology	Male gender, age >40 yr, size >3 cm, poorly differentiated cell type
Medullary carcinoma	MEN types 2a and 2b Elevated calcitonin level	Surgery, FNA Calcitonin levels *ret* oncogene	MEN type 2b and sporadic
Anaplastic carcinoma	Rapid progression of tumor mass Pain, hoarseness	FNA Surgery	Diagnosis

FNA, fine-needle aspiration; MEN, multiple endocrine neoplasia.

For patients whose nodules are solid or of mixed solid-cystic components, decision making depends on additional information. Patients who are male, older than 40 years of age, or who have a history of radiation exposure have an increased likelihood of having a malignancy in a thyroid nodule. These patients should be informed about such factors and counseled to consider a surgical option. In the remainder of the patients, the option of FNA exists. FNA can diagnose papillary cancer and strongly suggest medullary cancer or anaplastic cancer. It cannot confirm follicular cancer, nor can it confirm a completely benign diagnosis. Patients with follicular cells seen on FNA have a 6% to 20% incidence of malignancy. Therefore, the factors just discussed (age, sex, history of radiation) should be considered in advising patients with a solid nodule for whom the diagnosis is not secure with FNA. Colloid nodules are usually suggested by a mixed solid-cystic appearance on ultrasound and FNA shows colloid and macrophages. If not otherwise suspicious, these lesions can be followed by properly informed patients. There is no uniform agreement that thyroid suppression is superior to observation in such patients. The use of thyroid suppression must be carefully monitored, particularly in postmenopausal women, because elevated thyroid hormone levels are a significant risk factor for osteoporosis. Such nodules should be re-evaluated, at least with ultrasound, on a 6-month basis to establish stability of nodule size. Thyroid function tests should document appropriate response to suppression. Alterations in either should be an indication for surgery.[24]

THYROID MALIGNANCIES

Thyroid cancer represents less than 1% of all malignancies in the United States, occurring in about 40 per 1 million people per year. Six deaths per 1 million people occur annually. Ninety percent to 95% of thyroid cancer cases are categorized as well-differentiated tumors arising from follicular cell origin. These include papillary, follicular, and Hürthle cell carcinomas. Medullary thyroid cancer (MCT) accounts for about 6% of thyroid cancers (of which ~ 20% to 30% are on a familial basis MEN types 2A and 2B). Anaplastic carcinoma is an aggressive malignancy and is responsible for less than 1% of thyroid carcinomas in the United States. These cases occur primarily in iodine-deficient areas.

Thyroid Oncogenesis

A gene that contributes directly to tumorigenesis is referred to as an *oncogene*. A *protooncogene* is a gene that can give rise to an oncogene after genetic alteration or through modification of the genetic proteins, which are expressed. After modification, these oncogenes may encode for an altered or mutated receptor on the cell membrane. Such altered receptor activity may result in abnormal growth and development signals transmitted to the nucleus and thus in overexpression or altered expression. As a result, normal growth and differentiation of any cell line may be transformed into a malignant phenotype.[9]

The most recent understanding of a genetic model that leads to thyroid neoplasia includes two important processes: mutated protooncogenes, which result in altered protein production and thus in acceleration in growth, and alterations in growth suppression genes that, when altered, allow unregulated cell growth. There are several examples of each of these groups.[36]

Oncogene Activators

ras *Gene Family.* The *ras* gene family encodes signal-transduction G proteins. Mutational activation of this oncogene results in the production of an inactive form of an enzyme (guanosine triphosphatase), which is ineffective in inactivating protein degradation. Thus, a continued activation of protein accumulation is allowed because of a failed enzymatic process. It appears that as many as 40% of thyroid tumors may have one of the three *ras* gene point mutations (H-*ras*, K-*ras*, or N-*ras*). Additionally, *ras* mutations may occur in benign and malignant neoplasms. Patients who live in iodine-deficient areas may have a slightly decreased incidence of *ras* mutations compared with patients in iodine-sufficient areas. K-*ras* mutations appear more frequently in radiation-induced papillary cancers. As knowledge is gained about this particular oncogene family, it appears that tumor oncogenesis may be related not only to the prevalence of certain mutations but also to other genetic factors as well as environmental factors such as iodine availability.[36]

RET Protooncogene. The *RET* protooncogene encodes for a tyrosine kinase receptor on the cell membrane. This protooncogene may well be involved in the differentiation of neuronal cells. Cells of neural crest origin appear to have increased expression of this oncogene because it has been found in neuroblastoma, pheochromocytoma, and medullary thyroid cancer tissue. Alterations in this system have been shown to result in developmental abnormalities in a number of other neuronal tissues, including gastrointestinal nervous system in Hirschsprung's disease. Expression of the *RET* oncogene is predominantly found only in malignant tissue. It has not been found to any substantial degree in nonmalignant thyroid disease processes. The activation of the *RET* oncogene has been demonstrated in the development of papillary thyroid cancer. It may also be that patients with the oncogene may have a predilection for distant metastasis. In addition, it may be that the expression of *RET* varies markedly in different geographic areas. Japan is associated with a low incidence of *RET* expression in papillary carcinoma of the thyroid (3% to 5%), whereas patients in Italy have a much higher rate (33% to 36%).[37] There also appears to be an increased prevalence in children and adults who have had radiation exposure. These data suggest that the *RET* oncogene may well be a specific genetic event for papillary carcinoma of the thyroid but may, like the *ras* gene, vary greatly geographically or depending on environmental exposure. The *RET* protooncogene is also associated with a high frequency of missense mutations in patients with MEN type 2A. Genetic analysis for this mutation allows a secure diagnosis of children before the clinical appearance of MCT.

Thyroid-Stimulating Hormone Receptor. The thyroid-stimulating hormone receptor (TSH-R) is a member of the G-protein–coupled receptor family. This receptor controls the function and growth of thyroid cells by activation of the adenylate cyclase and phospholipase C pathways. Genetic alterations allowing mutations in the TSH-R gene have been shown in patients with toxic thyroid hyperplasia. Presently, despite a thorough search for mutations in the TSH-R genetic apparatus, there are no associated definite mutations that cause specific malignancies. All the mutations that have been found have resulted in hyperplastic, but benign, nodule formation.[38]

Tyrosine Kinase Receptors. As many as 50 different tyrosine kinase proteins can be categorized as oncoproteins, making the thyroxine kinase group the largest family of oncoproteins. Activation of tyrosine kinase receptors results in a cascade of events, which through phosphorylation activate downstream signaling pathways with multiple metabolic results. Three different tyrosine kinase receptor groups (*RET*, *trk*, and *met*) have been implicated in the development of thyroid cancer. *RET* and *trk* represent activated protooncogene events, and *met* is an overexpressed gene event.[36]

Tumor Suppressor Genes: p53

Mutations in the tumor suppressor gene *p53* are some of the most common genetic alterations and have been found in as many as 50 types of human tumor cell lines. This gene encodes a phosphoprotein that inhibits several genes responsible for normal cell growth and differentiation. Mutations of *p53* are generally found in tumor tissue representing the late stage of tumor growth and spread and in the more poorly differentiated anaplastic thyroid cancer.[36]

Papillary Carcinoma

Papillary carcinoma is the most common of the thyroid neoplasms and is usually associated with an excellent prognosis. This is particularly true in female patients younger than 40 years of age. About 70% to 80% of patients in the United States who are newly diagnosed with thyroid carcinoma have papillary carcinoma. Several studies have shown that the incidence of well-differentiated thyroid carcinoma has increased perhaps as much as 50% since 1990. Whether this is due to increased sophistication in screening and diagnostic techniques or the possible exposure to environmental factors such as radiation or environmental mutagenic chemicals is not clear (Figs. 34-12 and 34-13).

The association of irradiation and thyroid cancer has been known for years. The use of external-beam irradiation in children and young adults in the 1950s and 1960s for acne and tonsillitis has been shown to result in an increased incidence of well-differentiated carcinoma (usually papillary) at any time, usually 5 years after exposure. Additionally, patients who have received external

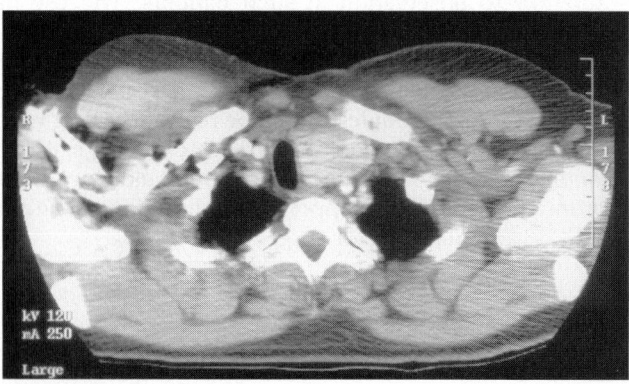

FIGURE 34-12. CT findings of a 4-cm mass in the left lobe of a 40-year-old man suggest an infraclavicular or substernal location. The mass ultimately proved to be a papillary carcinoma.

irradiation for soft tissue malignancy, such as Hodgkin's lymphoma, have an increased incidence of thyroid nodules and cancer (as many as 30% to 35% of those exposed).[39] Areas near known nuclear fallout contamination, such as Chernobyl in the former Soviet Union and in areas of the Southwest United States, have increased incidence rates of well-differentiated thyroid carcinoma.[40]

Pathologic Classification

The pathologic diagnosis of papillary carcinoma depends on the cytologic findings of well-recognized papillary cytomorphology. The neoplasm may form well-defined follicles with only minimal papillary architecture. The latter group can be classified as the follicular variant of papillary carcinoma. Classic papillary carcinoma and the follicular variant of papillary carcinoma have much the same prognostic implications. Individual cellular morphology may

be used to make the diagnosis of papillary carcinoma. Intranuclear inclusion bodies and cellular "grooving" allow the diagnosis of papillary carcinoma on inspection of individual cellular components of an FNA. This allows an important diagnostic capability with a minimally invasive technique (see Fig. 34-11). Additionally, the finding of calcified clumps of cells, most likely from sloughed papillary projections, known as *psammoma bodies*, is diagnostic for papillary cancer.

Other subtypes of papillary carcinoma are more unpredictably aggressive in their biologic behavior. Insular, columnar, and tall cell carcinomas represent these forms of papillary carcinoma. Although these subtypes are rare, they tend to occur in older patients, and the prognosis is predictably worse for these groups. These latter groups represent perhaps less than 1% of all papillary carcinomas (Fig. 34-14).[41]

Clinical Presentation (Table 34-2)

Thyroid masses may occur in either males or females at almost any age. Solitary masses that are painless and firm should be regarded with particular suspicion. Occasionally, a mass in the lateral neck presents as a painless entity and an FNA biopsy confirms a metastatic thyroid malignancy, even in the case of a normal thyroid examination. Thorough head and neck examination often aided by office-based ultrasound allows characterization of the mass.

Most patients with papillary carcinoma can expect an excellent prognosis, approaching a 95% 10-year survival rate for the most favorable stages. Various factors included in clinical presentation and pathologic staging, however, may alter the excellent prognosis. In 1979, Cady and others[42] first evaluated a clinical scoring system and reported a 30-year study of a group of patients in an attempt to place them into risk stratification groups. These studies described the AMES Clinical Scoring System and are based on *a*ge, distant *m*etastasis, *e*xtent of primary tumor, and *s*ize of the primary tumor. Hay[43] reported the

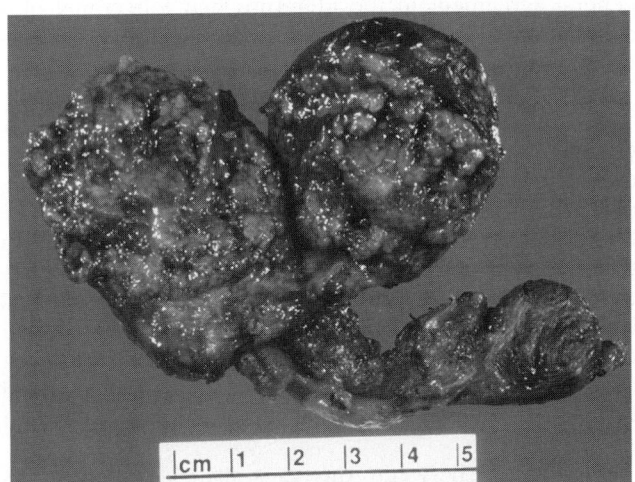

FIGURE 34-13. This 4 × 5-cm right lobe mass was removed as part of a total thyroidectomy. Permanent section pathology revealed papillary carcinoma.

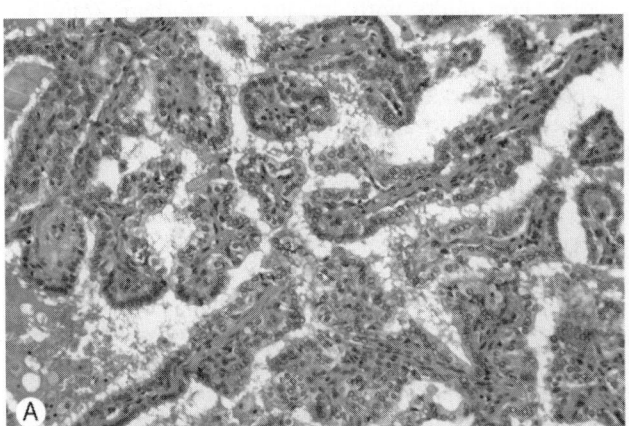
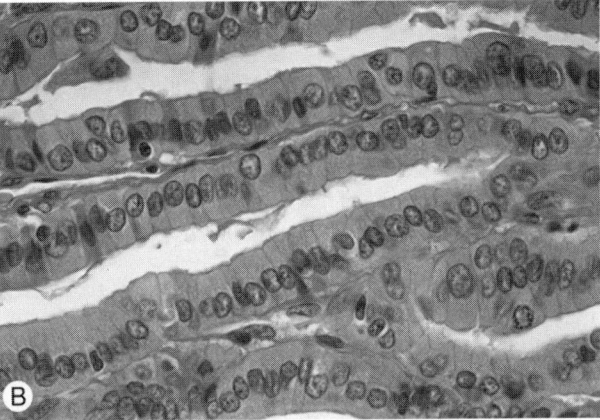

FIGURE 34-14. **A,** Hematoxylin and eosin (H&E) staining of a thyroid mass reveals papillary projections consistent with papillary carcinoma. **B,** H&E staining of a papillary carcinoma shows cells with increased height-to-width ratio in a single row of cells. This is the "tall-cell" variant of papillary carcinoma, which is associated with a poorer prognosis than that of well-differentiated papillary cancer.

TABLE 34-2.   Prognostic Risk Classification for Patients with Well-Differentiated Thyroid Cancer (AMES or AGES*)

	Low Risk	High Risk
Age	<40 years	>40 years
Sex	Female	Male
Extent	No local extension, intrathyroidal, no capsular invasion	Capsular invasion, extrathyroidal extension
Metastasis	None	Regional or distant
Size	<2 cm	>4 cm
Grade	Well differentiated	Poorly differentiated

*For explanation of AMES and AGES, see text.

Mayo Clinic experience and developed his own scoring scale, the AGES Clinical Scoring System. This was based on *a*ge, pathologic *g*rade of tumor, and *e*xtent and *s*ize of the primary tumor. Both the AMES and the AGES Clinical Scoring Systems have proved beneficial in predicting the prognosis of patients. Age at diagnosis turns out to be the most important clinical prognosis; diagnosis at age younger than 40 years is an important prognostic factor of long-term survival. Women may well extend this age cutoff to 50 years. Absence of distant metastasis at the time of initial treatment and size less than 4 cm are likewise important positive predictors. Tumor size greater than 4 cm and extension of the primary tumor through the capsule of the lesion likewise increase the risk for mortality. The AGES system describes a scoring system for presence or absence of these factors. A score of less than 4 is associated with a 20-year mortality rate of less than 1%. The more advanced stages have 5-year survival rates approaching 50%.

The study of DNA ploidy has been used to evaluate clinical prognosis. Increased nuclear DNA (aneuploidy) has been thought to increase the risk for mortality. Universal agreement about this concept does not exist. The overall value in obtaining DNA ploidy information may have some implication for prognosis but has had no definite impact on therapeutics.

Papillary carcinoma may be found incidentally in a thyroid sample resected for a benign process. These carcinomas are usually less than 5 mm in size and are not usually associated with clinically apparent cervical or distant metastatic activity. They may be considered appropriately treated if they are contained within a lobectomy and isthmectomy.

Presentation of a solitary palpable mass (1 to 2 cm) strongly suggests a malignant diagnosis. Confirmation of the diagnosis may be initiated by ultrasound, which can evaluate multinodularity and whether the nodule is solid or cystic. FNA of a palpable solid lesion is the next step. Papillary carcinoma of the thyroid can be diagnosed by this technique because individual cellular architecture can be evaluated and a secure diagnosis made. Multicentricity can be anticipated in as many as 70% of patients with

the diagnosis of papillary cancer. Additionally, cervical lymph node metastasis must be anticipated. Palpable lymphadenopathy should lead to FNA of suspected lesions. Intraoperative evaluation of any suspicious lymph nodes must also be performed by resection or by frozen-section evaluation. Younger patients have been shown to have a high rate of lymph node metastasis; however, this does not appreciably affect mortality. The presence of lymph node metastasis in patients with completely contained intrathyroidal primary papillary carcinoma also does not affect long-term survival. If the final pathology demonstrates extension of a primary papillary carcinoma through the thyroid capsule, a poor prognosis and possibly a higher rate of lymph node metastasis may be anticipated.[44,45]

Treatment

The main treatment of papillary carcinoma of the thyroid is surgical ablation. For lesions smaller than 1 cm, there is general agreement in the literature that lobectomy plus isthmectomy is the appropriate treatment. This is particularly true for incidentally found papillary carcinomas.

Several factors enter into surgical decision making. Younger patients, particularly those 15 years of age or younger, have a high rate of cervical metastasis to the extent that perhaps 90% of children with papillary carcinoma may have documented metastatic activity within the lymph nodes. Therefore, there is a strong consideration that patients in this age group undergo total thyroidectomy and lymph node dissection if palpable cervical lymph nodes occur. Additionally, in older patients with a history of neck irradiation, a more aggressive approach may be taken, including total thyroidectomy and modified neck dissection in the presence of palpable cervical lymph nodes.

In patients between the ages of 15 and 40 years with lesions smaller than 2 cm, surgical treatment is more controversial. Some surgeons perform total thyroidectomy in any event; however, there is sufficient literature that shows that lobectomy and isthmectomy may well suffice when the lesion clearly involves only one lobe. For adults with lesions larger than 2 cm, a total or near-total thyroidectomy is favored by most surgeons. In patients of any age in whom there is palpable adenopathy, a modified radical neck dissection on the side affected should be performed in concert with a total thyroidectomy.

Controversy exists about the use of total thyroidectomy versus lobectomy and isthmectomy in adults with a 1- to 2-cm papillary thyroid carcinoma. The advantages of a total thyroidectomy include the efficient use of radioiodine postoperative treatment. Clearly, if residual thyroid exists, radioablation is much less effective and requires a larger dosage. The advantages of the lesser procedure are the decreased rates of bilateral recurrent laryngeal nerve damage and hypoparathyroidism.

If the papillary carcinoma presents as a palpable lesion larger than 2 cm, a more aggressive surgical resection, including a total thyroidectomy, should be considered. Diligent search for multicentricity within the thyroid as well as regional lymph node metastasis may be employed by the use of ultrasound or neck CT scanning. Distant metastatic activity may be evaluated through chest radiographs, radionuclide scanning, CT, and other techniques as guided by clinical suspicion. In patients with total thyroidectomy, postoperative thyroglobulin levels may be followed to monitor recurrence.[45]

For patients with lower-stage disease (by AMES or AGES), surgical resection should result in an excellent 5- to 10-year survival rate exceeding 90%. For larger lesions, survival numbers may decrease, especially in older men. For larger lesions, postoperative ^{131}I therapy has been advocated.[46,47] Recurrence in local or regional lymph nodes after initial surgery should be treated with completion thyroidectomy, if residual tissue exists, plus regional lymph node dissection. Radioiodine therapy should be used as adjunctive therapy. Distant metastases are rare but have a poor prognosis (Fig. 34-15).

Follicular Carcinoma

Follicular thyroid cancer (FTC) is the second category of well-differentiated thyroid cancers. All types of papillary, follicular, and mixed papillary-follicular cancers account for about 90% of all thyroid cancers. Pure FTC represents the minority of these, constituting about 10% of all thyroid malignancies. FTC is a disease of an older population, often 50 years of age or older. It has a predilection for women, with a ratio of about 3:1. The subtype of FTC, which consists of oxyphilic cells, is known as *Hürthle cells,* and these tend to occur in older patients, usually 60 to 75 years of age.[41,45] There appears to be an increased incidence of FTC in geographic distributions associated with iodine deficiency.

Pathologic Classification

FTC is a malignant neoplasm of the thyroid epithelium, which can present as a wide spectrum of microscopic changes anywhere from virtually normal follicular architecture and function to severely altered cellular architecture. In large series, FTC represents 10% to 15% of patients with thyroid cancer.[45] The histologic diagnosis of FTC depends on the demonstration of what would appear to be normal follicular cells occupying abnormal positions, including capsular, lymphatic, or vascular invasion (Fig. 34-16). If well-differentiated follicular cells are not demonstrated to involve these structures, a diagnosis of a benign follicular adenoma is made. Using these criteria, two types of follicular carcinoma are usually described: minimally invasive and widely invasive.[41] Thorough microscopic examination is required for the former, whereas the latter is usually grossly obvious and clearly different from a well-encapsulated lesion. In both cases, lymph node involvement is unusual, occurring in less than 10% of cases. This is in contradistinction to papillary carcinoma, with which a higher rate of lymph node involvement at the time of presentation occurs. With widely invasive FTC, distant spread is more common, often involving lung, bone, and other solid organs.[48]

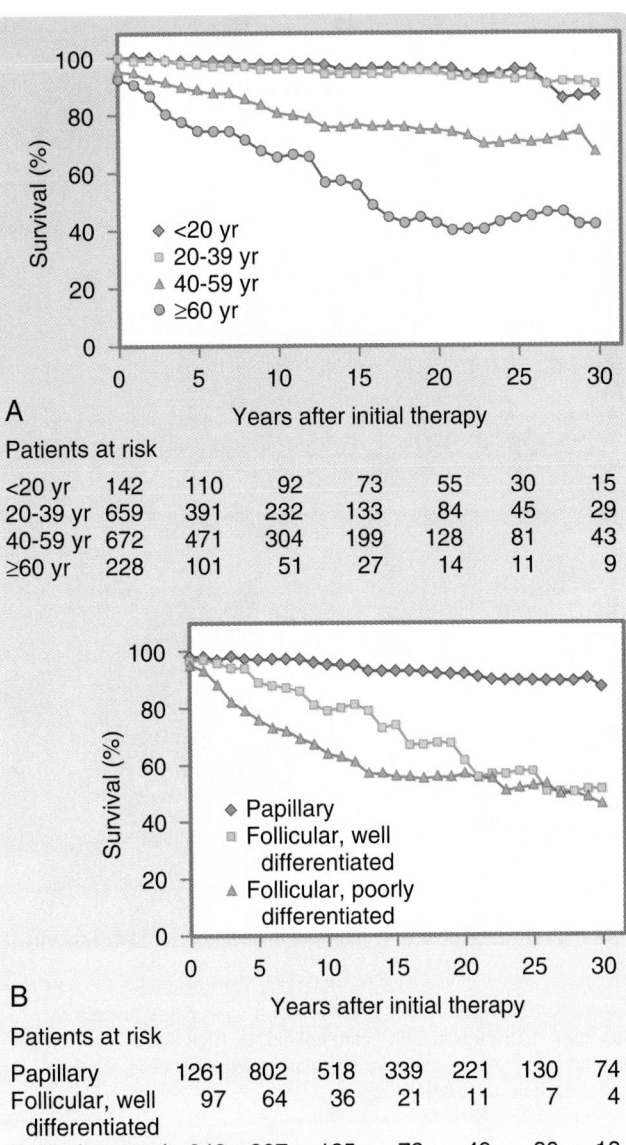

Patients at risk							
<20 yr	142	110	92	73	55	30	15
20-39 yr	659	391	232	133	84	45	29
40-59 yr	672	471	304	199	128	81	43
≥60 yr	228	101	51	27	14	11	9

Patients at risk							
Papillary	1261	802	518	339	221	130	74
Follicular, well differentiated	97	64	36	21	11	7	4
Follicular, poorly differentiated	343	207	125	72	49	30	18

FIGURE 34-15. Survival rates of 1701 patients with papillary or follicular carcinoma (no distant metastasis at time of diagnosis). Overall survival rates were 82% at 10 years, 72% at 20 years, and 60% at 30 years. Patients were followed at Institut Gustav-Roussy in France. **A,** Effect of age at diagnosis on mortality for combined groups. **B,** Survival rate according to histologic subtype. (**A** and **B,** From Schlumberger ML: Medical progress: Papillary and follicular thyroid carcinoma. N Engl J Med 338:300, 1998. Copyright © 1998 Massachusetts Medical Society. All rights reserved.)

Clinical Presentation

FTC, like papillary cancer, classically presents as a painless thyroid mass. Although most patients have a benign mass, the existence of FTC in a patient with multinodular goiter can occur in as many as 10% of cases. The coexistence of lymph node involvement is extremely rare and cervical adenopathy even less so, perhaps occurring in less than 5% of patients. Although the findings of hoarseness and firm fixation of the mass on clinical presentation

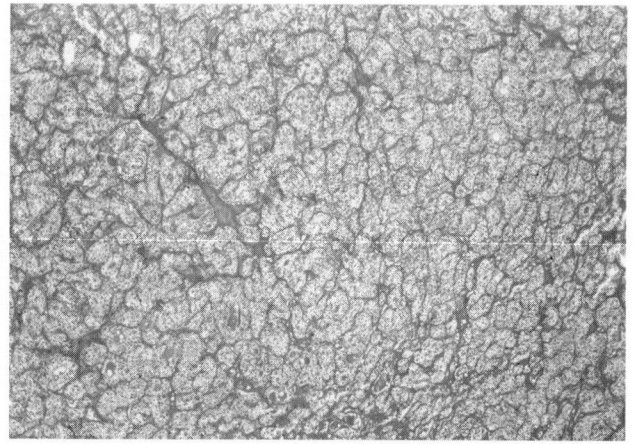

A

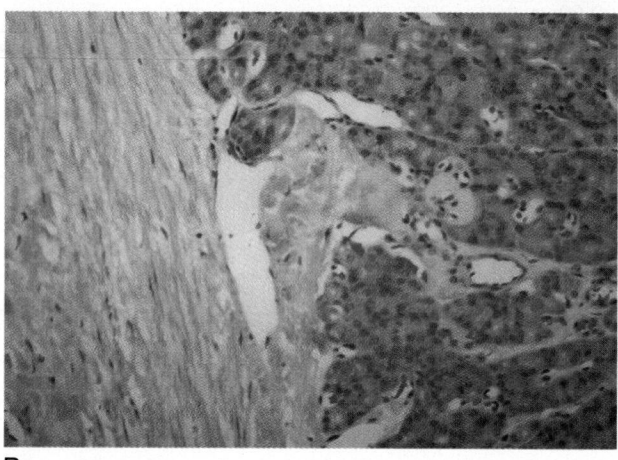

B

FIGURE 34-16.   **A,** H & E stain of a solid mass reveals a microfollicular pattern with scant colloid. **B,** High power examination reveals capsular invasion of follicular cells allowing the diagnosis of follicular cancer.

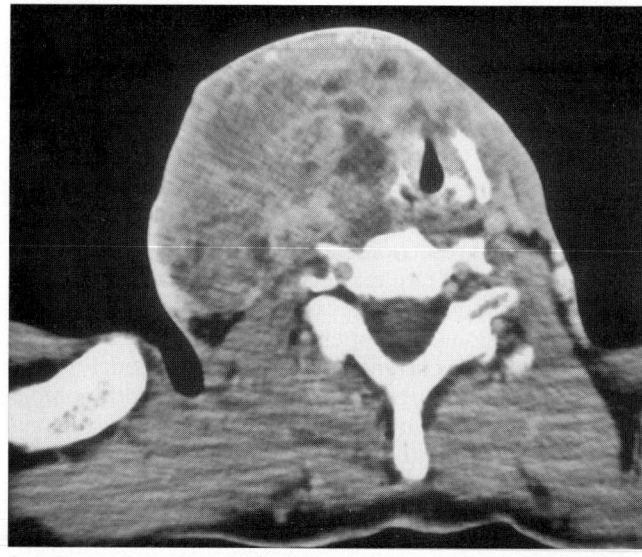

A

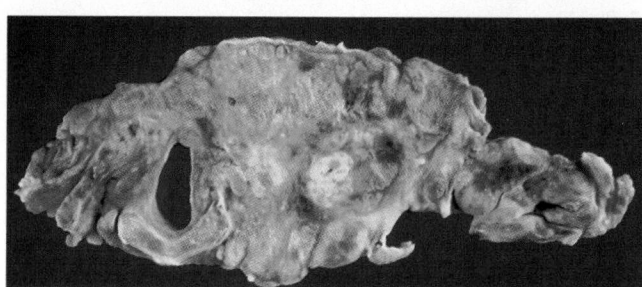

B

FIGURE 34-17.   A 70-year-old man presented with a rapidly enlarging thyroid mass. **A,** CT demonstrates displacement of the larynx and lateral involvement of both jugular veins. This patient died within 6 months of a rapidly progressing follicular cancer. **B,** Autopsy evaluation of the anterior neck compartment demonstrates infiltration of the larynx, clot within the jugular veins, and lateral lymph node involvement.

suggest advanced disease and a poor prognosis, these circumstances are again in the minority of cases. In these cases, diligent search for aggressive extension into the trachea and distant metastasis, particularly in older patients, should be carried out by use of CT or MRI evaluation of the neck and chest (Fig. 34-17).[44]

Laboratory work-up usually reveals a euthyroid state. Thyroid malignancies are almost never associated with hyperfunctioning or hypofunctioning tissue. The incidence of thyrotoxicosis in association with a thyroid malignancy, including FTC, has been reported to approach 2%. Preoperative imaging may be of some assistance to assess the extent of a palpable mass. Ultrasound can determine the size and multicentricity; however, FTC usually presents as a solitary mass. Radionuclide scanning can determine whether a mass has function or is cold, although a minority of cold nodules actually prove to be malignant.

The use of FNA cytology has been of immense help in arriving at a cytologic diagnosis before surgery. In the case of FTC, however, FNA is of limited value. The diagnosis of FTC requires the demonstration of cellular invasion of the capsule or of vascular or lymphatic channels. This cannot be determined through the use of preoperative FNA. Additionally, intraoperative frozen section has been notoriously ineffective in making a definitive diagnosis of FTC.[34,35]

Treatment

The treatment of follicular carcinoma is primarily surgical. The presentation often takes the form of a preoperative FNA or an intraoperative frozen-section diagnosis of a "follicular lesion." The surgeon is left to make the choice as to the most efficacious treatment of a follicular lesion, which, lacking obvious gross characteristics of malignancy and widely invasive FTC, is most likely a benign lesion. If the lesion is 2 cm or smaller and well contained within one thyroid lobe, an argument may be made for thyroid lobectomy and isthmectomy. If the lesion is larger than 2 cm, the surgeon may well proceed with total thyroidectomy. If the follicular lesion is larger than 4 cm, the risk for cancer is greater than 50%; therefore, total thyroidectomy is an obvious choice. Lymph node dissection is not necessary in the absence of palpable lymph nodes and adds nothing to survival data unless obviously involved.[48]

Prognosis after treatment for FTC is dependent on age. Patients younger than 40 years of age have the best prognosis, approaching 95% at 5 and 10 years. Series that compare follicular carcinoma with papillary carcinoma have shown poorer prognosis for FTC, although this disparity is more prominent after 10 to 15 years. Poorly differentiated FTC and well-differentiated FTC have 60% and 80% 10-year survival rates, respectively (see Fig. 34-15).[44]

A particularly vexing problem occurs when a thyroid lobectomy has been performed for a presumed thyroid adenoma but the final pathologic diagnosis is follicular carcinoma. Two considerations must then take place. After determining an AMES or AGES score, a decision needs to be made regarding whether the lesion is low risk (small lesion in younger patient), in which case the patient might be watched closely with ultrasound evaluations every 6 months. Alternatively, the lesion might be higher risk (>2 cm in a patient older than 60 years of age) and require radioablation. This circumstance requires reoperation and completion thyroidectomy, albeit with increased technical difficulty and possibility of complications. The best way to prevent the dilemma is to review any intraoperative frozen-section analyses carefully and to perform the initial surgery keeping the circumstance in mind. The safety of performing more extensive surgery initially rather than completion of surgery at a later time should be considered. As stated previously, intraoperative decision making cannot rely exclusively on the diagnosis being made by frozen section.

Postoperative treatment with T_4 is based on the assumption that TSH suppression minimizes its growth-promoting influence on thyroid cancer. The literature does not completely agree about the efficacy of thyroid suppression. In fact, more recent studies have demonstrated that overaggressive treatment with T_4 may have unproved effects on FTC recurrence and significant enhancement of osteoporotic side effects.[46]

Radioiodine treatment is likewise controversial. There is no substantial benefit to patients with completely resected lesions and more favorable stages. Obviously, radioiodine treatment is most efficacious in patients who have undergone total thyroidectomy. In patients who have undergone subtotal thyroidectomy or lobectomy and isthmectomy, higher doses of radioiodine are needed for remnant ablation. Although there are mixed results in the literature, the use of postoperative radioiodine ablation appears to be warranted in more advanced-stage FTC patients. Additionally, ^{131}I treatment may be given in older patients (≥75 years of age) or in patients whose thyroglobulin levels have increased later than 3 months after surgery.

Hürthle Cell Carcinoma

Hürthle cell carcinoma is a subtype of follicular carcinoma that closely resembles FTC both grossly and on microscopic examination. The tumor contains an abundance of oxyphilic cells, or oncocytes. These cells are derived from follicular cells and have abundant granular acidophilic cytoplasm. Some studies have suggested that Hürthle cell carcinoma may have a worse clinical prognosis than standard FTC; however, there is no uniform agreement on these findings. It does appear that Hürthle cell carcinoma may have a higher rate of recurrence, particularly in regional lymph nodes.[49] Most studies consider Hürthle cell carcinoma to be clinically and prognostically equivalent to FTC.

Prognosis and Treatment

Hürthle cell carcinoma presents in much the same fashion as follicular cell neoplasms. The use of preoperative FNA raises many of the same issues, the finding of Hürthle cells leaving open the question of invasiveness and the diagnosis of malignancy. The treatment is surgical, following the same principles as the work-up of the follicular neoplasm.[49,50]

Medullary Carcinoma

MCT accounts for 5% to 10% of thyroid malignancies. The malignancy involves the parafollicular cell, or C cell, derived from the neural crest. MCT is associated with the secretion of a biological marker, calcitonin. The excess secretion of calcitonin has been demonstrated to be an effective marker for the existence of MCT. The calcitonin excess is *not* associated with hypocalcemia.

Medullary carcinoma can occur in a sporadic form or as part of MEN type 2A or 2B. The MEN syndromes are covered in more detail elsewhere in this text. MEN type 2A usually has a more favorable long-term outcome than MEN type 2B or sporadic MCT.[51]

Presentation

The patient with a sporadic medullary carcinoma may present in either of two ways: with a palpable mass for which a diagnosis can be made through FNA or with the finding of an elevated calcitonin level. In sporadic MCT, the tumors are usually single and unilateral and have no familial predisposition. The presence of both a mass and an elevated calcitonin level is certainly diagnostic of MCT, whereas the finding of an elevated basal calcitonin level in the absence of a thyroid mass might require a further work-up, including repeat basal calcitonin measurement and the completion of a calcium-stimulated or gastrin-stimulated test. The work-up of these patients should include a detailed and in-depth family history inquiring for characteristics of MEN type 2 in the patient and family members (Fig. 34-18). Screening for pheochromocytoma with 24-hour urinary catecholamines is mandatory in any patient whose thyroid mass is suspected as being MCT.

Treatment

The surgical approach to sporadic medullary carcinoma involves at least a total thyroidectomy with or without

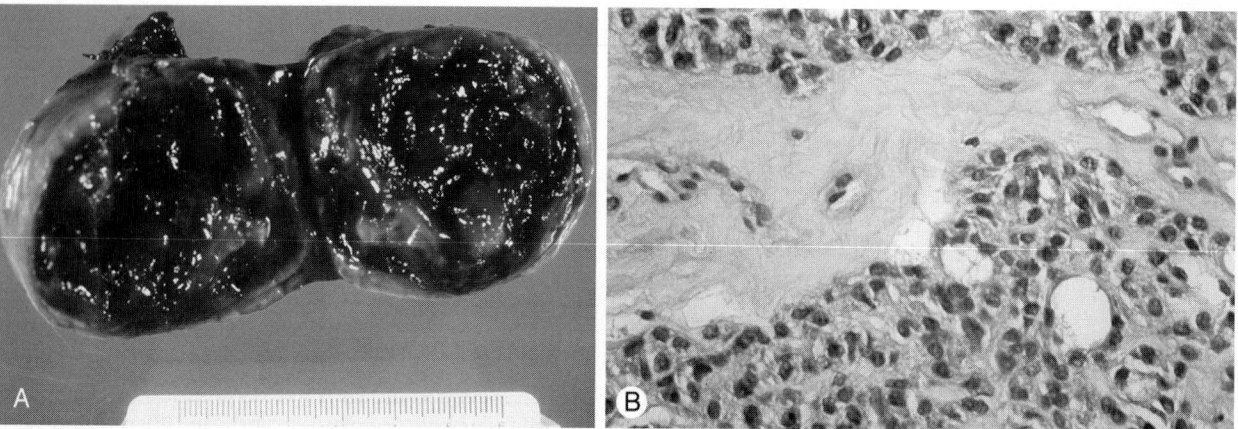

FIGURE 34-18. **A,** This 4-cm solitary mass in a thyroid lobe was removed by total thyroidectomy. H&E staining revealed sporadic medullary carcinoma. **B,** H&E staining of this mass demonstrated cells consistent with medullary carcinoma with amyloid infiltrate.

central lymph node dissection. The total thyroidectomy allows complete removal of the gland and search for multicentricity. In sporadic MCT, the lesion is usually contained within one lobe, whereas MEN involves the upper halves of both lobes. Central lymph node compartment dissection allows appropriate staging of this process. Any palpable lymph nodes in lateral areas require a modified radical neck dissection. A successful operation with good prognosis is predicted for patients with smaller masses and for whom calcitonin levels are undetectable after surgery. Radioactive scanning may be used to ablate any residual thyroid. The literature has described some uses of basal and stimulated calcitonin tests to follow recurrence because the stimulated calcitonin values may rise before the basal calcitonin levels. Unfortunately, documentation by biochemical means of recurrent MCT is often associated with unresectable recurrence in distant metastatic locations, including lung and liver.[51]

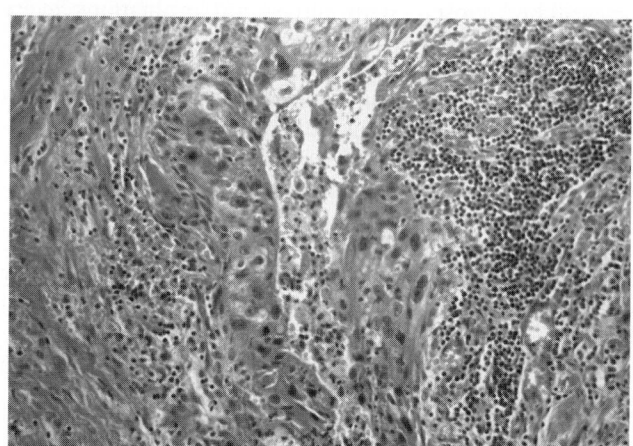

FIGURE 34-19. H&E staining of a thyroid mass reveals a lymphocytic infiltrate into a mass with poorly differentiated cells, many of which are multinucleated. This is consistent with anaplastic carcinoma of the thyroid.

Anaplastic Thyroid Cancer

Anaplastic thyroid carcinoma represents less than 1% of all thyroid malignancies. It is the most aggressive form of thyroid cancer. A typical presentation is in an older patient who presents with dysphagia, cervical tenderness, and a painful neck mass. Superior vena cava syndrome can also be part of the presentation. The clinical situation deteriorates rapidly into tracheal obstruction and rapid local invasion of surrounding structures.

Pathology

Grossly, the tumor is locally invasive, with a firm, whitish appearance. On microscopic evaluation, giant cells with intranuclear cytoplasmic invaginations can be seen. There is a wide variety of cell types, ranging from moderately differentiated to extremely poorly differentiated cell types (Fig. 34-19). Occasionally, squamous cell elements or islands of more recognizable differentiated thyroid carcinoma, such as papillary carcinoma, can be identified within the locus of the tumor. This has led to the specu-

lation that anaplastic carcinoma might arise from more well-differentiated carcinoma; however, there has been no solid proof of this theory.[52]

Treatment

The results of any surgical treatment of anaplastic thyroid carcinoma are tempered by the rapidly progressive clinical course. Most reports with resection are not optimistic. Junor and colleagues[53] reported that less than one third of 91 cases in their series with anaplastic carcinoma were resectable. Two thirds of their patients had biopsy confirmation and no further surgical therapy. Postoperative external-beam irradiation or adjunctive chemotherapy adds little to the overall prognosis. Overall survival in this series was dismal. There was a 50% mortality rate within 6 months and an 11% 3-year survival rate. An interesting recent report discusses the rare findings of "incidental" anaplastic carcinomas in resected specimens that had, not surprisingly, a better prognosis.[54]

It appears that if anaplastic carcinoma initially presents with a resectable mass, some small improvement in survival may be made. The finding of distant metastasis or invasion into locally unresectable structures, such as the trachea or vasculature of the anterior mediastinum, should lead to a more conservative surgical approach, such as tracheostomy.

Lymphoma

Primary thyroid lymphoma, although rare, is being recognized more often. This diagnosis should be considered in patients who present with a goiter, especially one that has apparently grown significantly in a short period. Other presenting symptoms include hoarseness, dysphagia, and fever. There is also an increased association between lymphoma and Hashimoto's thyroiditis. There has been no correlation seen in thyroid lymphoma with neck irradiation or with human immunodeficiency virus infection.

Work-Up and Diagnosis

Because these patients present rarely, the standard work-up for thyroid mass or goiter has usually been completed. There is evidence that ultrasound may have a classic "pseudocystic pattern." The use of FNA can be diagnostic in this situation. The use of flow cytometry for monoclonality can confirm the diagnosis. In some series, FNA is associated with an accurate diagnosis in as many as 78% of cases.[55] If FNA is nondiagnostic, the use of core needle biopsy or open biopsy can be considered. If the diagnosis is either confirmed or highly suspicious, additional preoperative evaluation should include neck, chest, and abdominal CT or MRI evaluation to assess extrathyroidal spread.

Treatment

Treatment philosophies differ with regard to preoperative chemotherapy or surgical ablation. The use of the CHOP regimen (cyclophosphamide, doxorubicin [Adriamycin], vincristine, and prednisolone) has been associated with excellent survival. The use of surgical resection, including a near-total or a total thyroidectomy, is thought to enhance these results. Thyroidectomy, especially the near-total or total procedures, is daunting in these cases. There can be a significant amount of pericapsular edema and swelling with loss of normal tissue planes. Bleeding, parathyroid damage, and recurrent laryngeal nerve damage can occur with increased predictability in such cases.

SURGICAL APPROACHES TO THE THYROID GLAND AND ADJACENT STRUCTURES (Table 34-3)

Cervical Approach

The cervical approach to the thyroid can be used in most benign and malignant processes. A transverse incision is made about two fingerbreadths above the clavicular heads. The incision should be placed in a way that allows a direct approach to the thyroid gland and its adjacent structures while allowing optimal postoperative cosmetic results. It is important that the incision be slightly curved and symmetrical. If possible, the incision should incorporate normal skin lines because this aids in optimal cosmetic healing. The lateral borders of the incision can approach the medial borders of the sternocleidomastoid muscle but can be lengthened if the lateral neck is to be investigated. The skin incision should be carried through subcutaneous fat and the platysmal muscle and superior and inferior flaps dissected medially beneath the platysmal layer. At this layer, anterior jugular veins are identified, and any of those crossing or running along the midline can be divided (Fig. 34-20).

The midline raphe should then be identified between sternohyoid muscles, and this raphe should be divided in a bloodless plane from the thyroid cartilage superiorly to the sternal notch inferiorly. As one enters the plane immediately beneath the sternohyoid muscles, one encounters the isthmus of the thyroid in the midline and each of the lobes laterally. Above and below the isthmus are the cartilaginous rings of the trachea. Blunt finger dissection can separate the sternohyoid muscle from the thyroid capsule medially and identify the sternothyroid muscles in a deep and lateral position. The sternothyroid muscles do not meet in the midline and must be separated off the thyroid capsule to gain lateral exposure of the thyroid. In patients who have had previous FNAs, it may be that the planes under the sternothyroid muscle are obliterated by recent hemorrhage or scarring. If the patient had previous thyroid surgery, these muscle groups will be densely adherent to the trachea and perhaps the tracheoesophageal groove. Great care must be used in this circumstance in identifying the parathyroids and recurrent laryngeal nerve.

On the left side, the tracheoesophageal groove is usually more easily palpated, especially if an esophageal stethoscope is in place. When the recurrent laryngeal nerve has been identified on either side, it is mandatory to track it through any scar tissue or thyroid carcinoma. Every effort should be made to avoid sacrificing the nerve, particularly in patients who are known to have preoperative normal vocal cord function and anatomy. In rare situations, such as anaplastic thyroid carcinoma, aggressive well-differentiated carcinoma, or obvious involvement with other head and neck tumors, the nerve may be sacrificed. If a recurrent laryngeal nerve is seen to have been injured during the course of an otherwise uncomplicated operation, every attempt should be made to repair it initially with microscope-aided visualization and microvascular technique (8-0 or 9-0 monofilament sutures).

The extent of thyroid resection has been shown to affect the rate of complications. Newman and coworkers[56] have reported the incidence of permanent hypocalcemia to be 4% with lobectomy and 17% with total thyroidectomy for resection of thyroid cancer in children. Temporary hypocalcemia occurred in 46% of patients with total thyroidectomy in this series. Although recurrent laryngeal nerve damage occurred with more extensive resections in

TABLE 34-3.   Indications for Interventional Procedures

Procedure	Advantage	Disadvantage or Complications	Indication
Fine-needle aspiration (FNA)	Accurate diagnosis for malignancy	Cannot confirm benign diagnosis Capsular hemorrhage	Tissue diagnosis of ultrasound-determined solid nodule Previous "nondiagnostic" result
Open biopsy	Direct visualization	Requires operating room, possibly general anesthesia	Complex case where FNA has failed to give diagnosis
"Nodulectomy" (less than a lobectomy)	None	Difficult second operation to complete lobectomy if cancer diagnosis is made	None
Lobectomy (with isthmectomy)	Lower rates of hypocalcemia and nerve damage	May require completion thyroidectomy if cancer diagnosis is made	Strong suspicion of benign disease Well-differentiated cancer <1 cm
Near-total thyroidectomy	Lower rates of hypocalcemia and nerve damage	Possible recurrence in residual thyroid tissue	Benign multinodular disease <2-cm nodule on the complete lobectomy side Hyperthyroidism
Total thyroidectomy	Use of postoperative ^{131}I is most efficacious Use of post-thyroglobulin levels for recurrence	Higher rate of hypocalcemia and nerve damage	Extensive multinodular disease Hyperthyroidism >2-cm thyroid cancer (nonpalpable lymph nodes)
Modified radical lymph node dissection	Decreased rate of recurrence	Cranial nerve XII damage Loss of sensation over ear and lateral cervical area (Left) thoracic duct leak and lymphocele Horner's syndrome	Palpable adenopathy with diagnosis of papillary, follicular, or medullary cancer
Median sternotomy	Exposure of mediastinal contents	Bleeding Nonunion of sternum (if complete sternotomy) Increased hospital stay	Extension of malignancy into anterior mediastinum Inability to mobilize large substernal goiter
Central lymph node dissection	Decreased risk of recurrence	Increased risk of hypocalcemia and nerve damage	Medullary carcinoma requires removal of lymph nodes in central cervical compartment (medial to jugular veins)

this study, it is still advisable to employ careful technique for such cases.

Dissection between the sternohyoid and the sternothyroid muscles gains exposure to the lateral and deeper structures. Exposure of these lateral structures is enhanced by placing medial traction on the thyroid lobes on either side. Care must be used to divide the middle thyroid vein before it is placed on excessive traction by this maneuver. With lateral retraction of the muscles and medial retraction of the thyroid lobe, the common carotid is quickly defined. On the left side, the esophagus is more prominent because of its more lateral position at this level in the neck. The tracheoesophageal groove is particularly prominent on the left because of this position of the esophagus. The definition of this area can be enhanced by placement of an esophageal stethoscope, which allows easier palpation of the esophagus (Figs. 34-21 to 34-23).

In the case of complicated lateral thyroid masses, lymphadenopathy, or previous surgery, it may be necessary to gain exposure laterally by dividing the sternohyoid and sternothyroid muscles. It is rarely necessary to employ division of these two muscles because lateral traction usually provides good exposure. If transection of the sternohyoid or sternothyroid muscle is necessary, this should be done superiorly to minimize denervation because both of these muscle groups are innervated from a caudal direction through the ansa hypoglossi nerves.

By gaining access to the plane immediately above the thyroid sheath and lateral traction on the strap muscles of the neck, the operating surgeon should be able to visualize the entirety of the anterior surface of the thyroid. Traction of the thyroid lobes in a medial direction should help identify a dissection plane gaining access to the superior pole vessels (Figs. 34-24 and 34-25). To skeletonize the superior pole vessels, one should have good exposure laterally between the common carotid artery and the superior aspect of the ipsilateral thyroid lobe. One can then enter behind or posterior to the superior thyroid pole adjacent to the cricothyroid muscle. Careful dissection of this area avoids injury to the external laryngeal nerve. Most patients (75% to 80%) have external laryngeal nerves that run on the cricothyroid muscle and are separate from the superior vessels; however, this leaves a significant number of patients in whom the nerve runs in close proximity to the superior pole vessels and can be divided if care is not

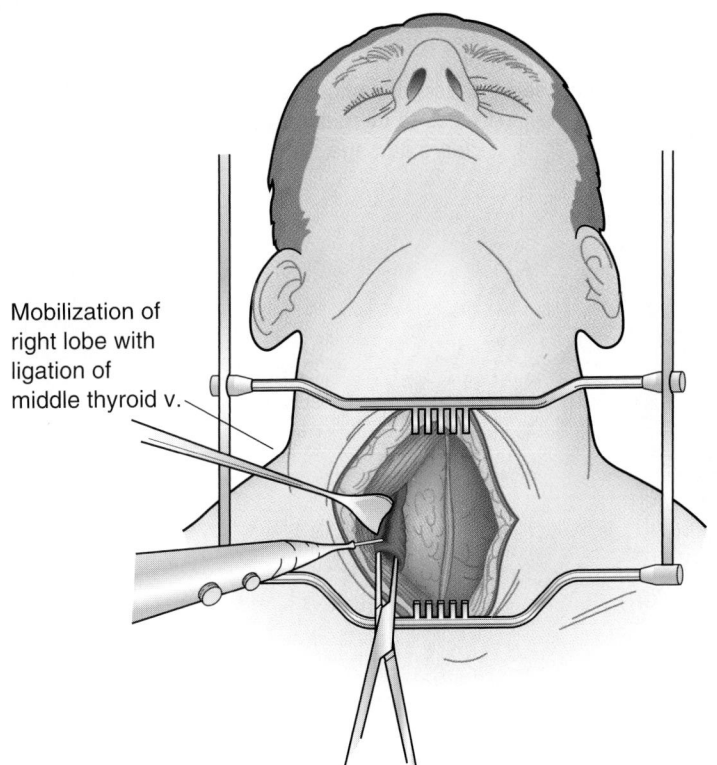

Mobilization of
right lobe with
ligation of
middle thyroid v.

FIGURE 34-20. A Mahorner retractor is inserted, and towels (not shown) are placed so that only the incision is exposed. The strap muscles (sternohyoid and sternothyroid) are then separated by dividing the tissues in the avascular midline plane from the thyroid cartilage to the suprasternal notch. The thyroid lobe is exposed by mobilizing the strap muscles away from the lobe by means of lateral retraction on the muscles and blunt dissection of a Kuettner peanut dissector. The middle vein is exposed, divided, and ligated. (From Sabiston DC Jr [ed]: Atlas of General Surgery. Philadelphia, WB Saunders, 1995.)

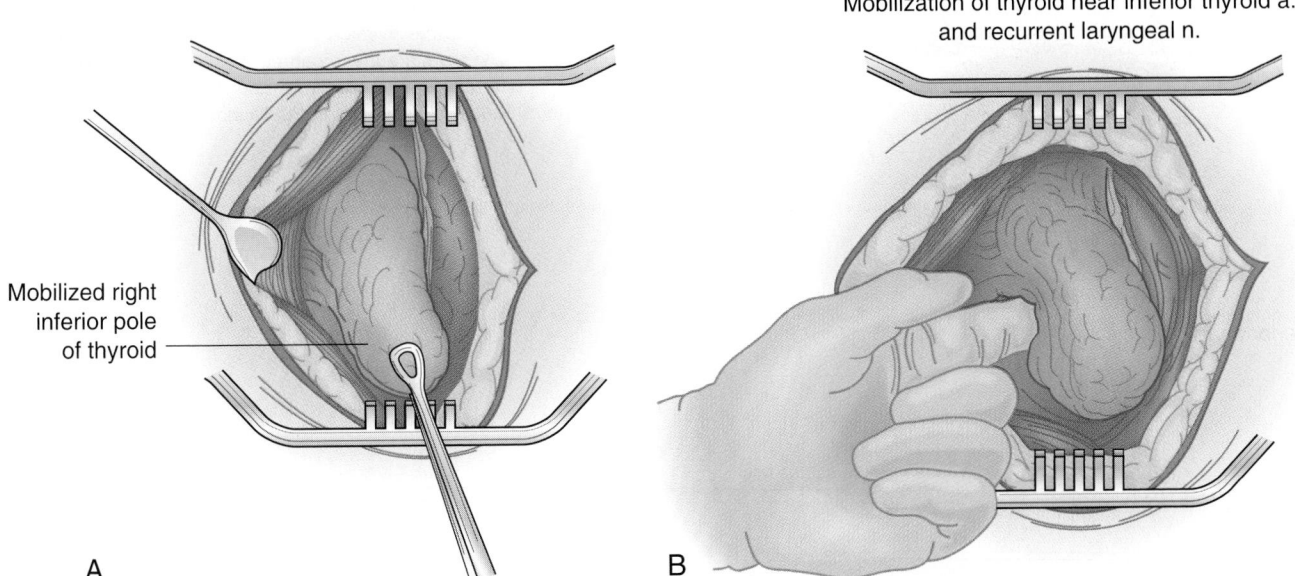

Mobilization of thyroid near inferior thyroid a.
and recurrent laryngeal n.

Mobilized right
inferior pole
of thyroid

A

B

FIGURE 34-21. **A** and **B**, Babcock clamps are applied to inferior and superior (not shown) aspects of the thyroid lobe to facilitate medial retraction on the gland. This exposes the area where the parathyroid glands and recurrent laryngeal nerve are located. (**A** and **B**, From Sabiston DC Jr [ed]: Atlas of General Surgery. Philadelphia, WB Saunders, 1995.)

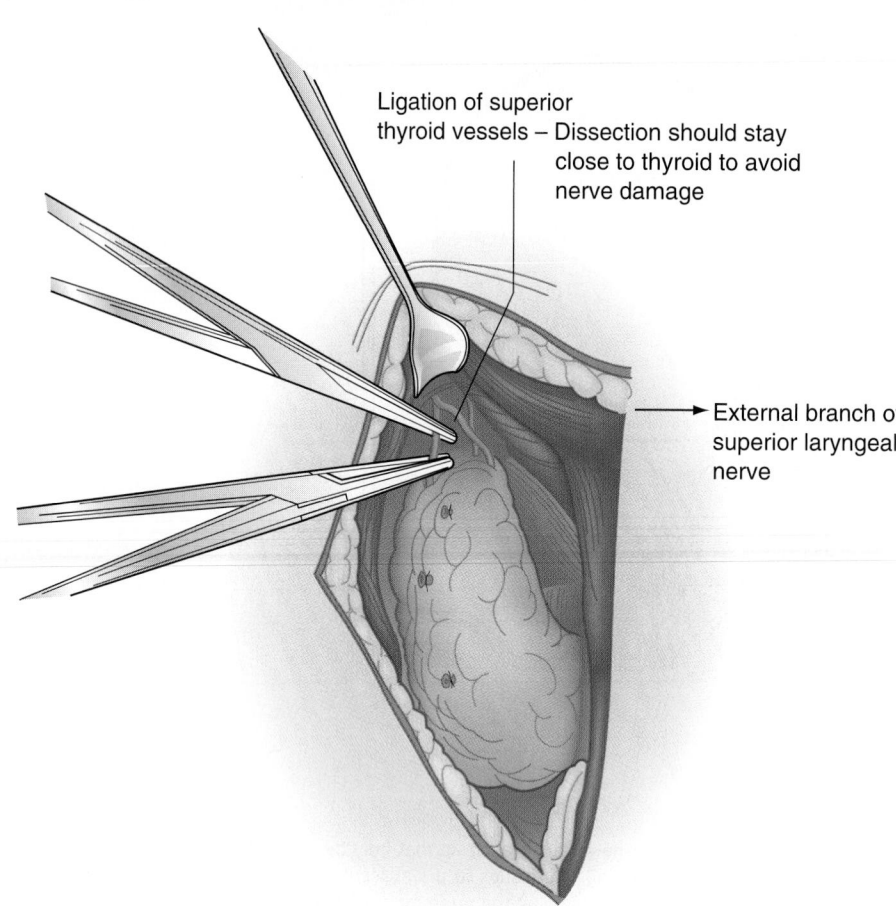

Ligation of superior thyroid vessels – Dissection should stay close to thyroid to avoid nerve damage

External branch of superior laryngeal nerve

FIGURE 34-22. Downward traction on the superior Babcock clamp exposes the superior pole vessels, including the branches of the superior thyroid artery. The external laryngeal nerve courses along the cricothyroid muscle just medial to the superior pole vessels. To avoid injury to this nerve, which controls tension of the vocal cords, the superior pole vessels are divided individually as close as possible to the point where they enter the thyroid gland. (From Sabiston DC Jr [ed]: Atlas of General Surgery. Philadelphia, WB Saunders, 1995.)

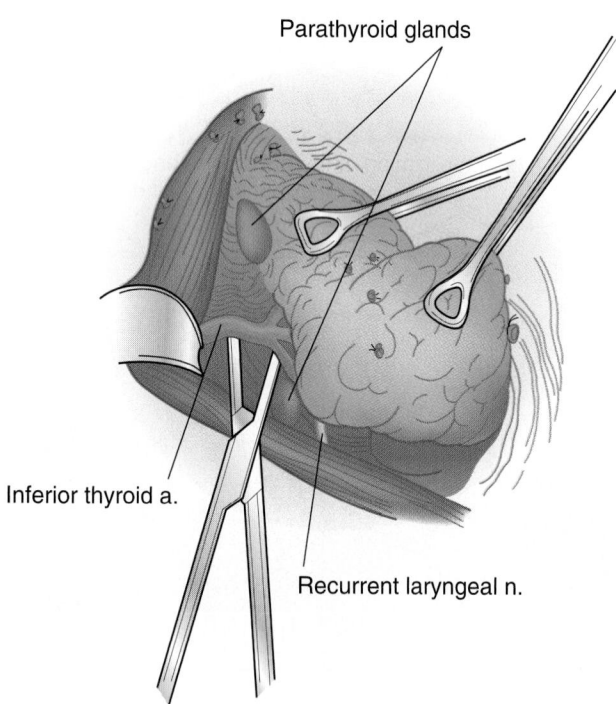

Parathyroid glands

Inferior thyroid a.

Recurrent laryngeal n.

FIGURE 34-23. As the thyroid is retracted medially, gentle dissection with a Hoyt clamp is used to expose the parathyroid glands, inferior thyroid artery, and recurrent laryngeal nerve. The recurrent nerve usually passes behind the inferior thyroid but occasionally lies anterior to it. It is best found by careful dissection just inferior to the artery. The nerve can then be traced upward, and its position in relation to the thyroid can be determined. Parathyroid glands that lie on the thyroid surface can be mobilized with their vascular supply and thus preserved. (From Sabiston DC Jr [ed]: Atlas of General Surgery. Philadelphia, WB Saunders, 1995.)

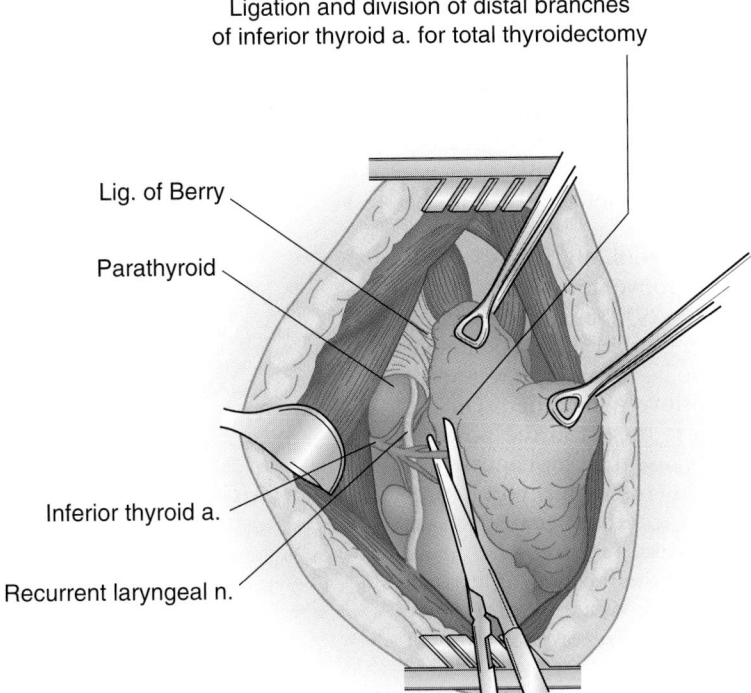

Ligation and division of distal branches
of inferior thyroid a. for total thyroidectomy

Lig. of Berry

Parathyroid

Inferior thyroid a.

Recurrent laryngeal n.

FIGURE 34-24. To perform total lobectomy, the branches of the inferior thyroid artery are divided at the surface of the thyroid gland. The inferior thyroid veins can now be ligated and divided. Superiorly, the connective tissue (ligament of Berry), which binds the thyroid to the tracheal rings, is carefully divided. There are usually several small accompanying vessels, and the recurrent nerve is closest to the thyroid and most vulnerable at this point. Division of the ligament allows the thyroid to be mobilized medially. (From Sabiston DC Jr [ed]: Atlas of General Surgery. Philadelphia, WB Saunders, 1995.)

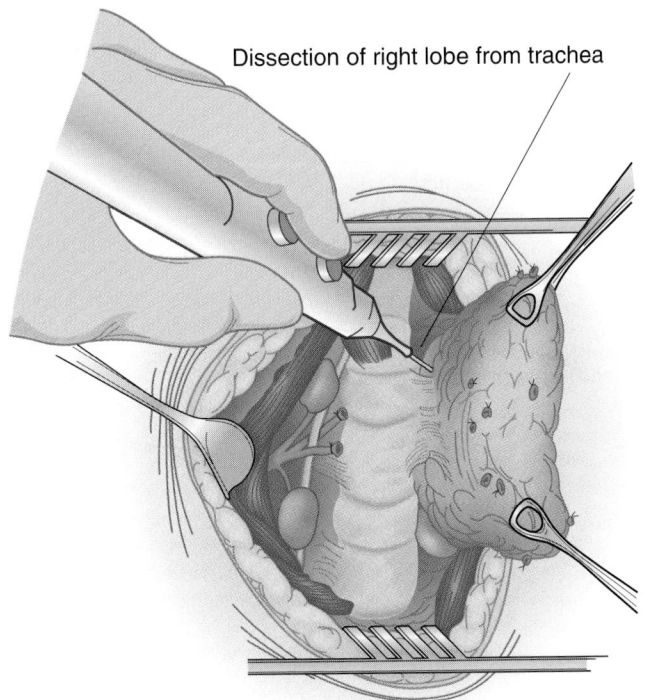

Dissection of right lobe from trachea

FIGURE 34-25. The dissection of the thyroid from the trachea can be performed with the cautery by division of the loose connective tissue between these structures. Dissection is extended under the isthmus, and the specimen is divided so that the isthmus is included with the resected lobe. The pyramidal lobe also should be included if present. (From Sabiston DC Jr [ed]: Atlas of General Surgery. Philadelphia, WB Saunders, 1995.)

used. After the superior pole vessels are carefully dissected and identified, they can be double-ligated adjacent to their entrance into the thyroid lobe. After the superior thyroid vessels and middle thyroid veins have been divided, continued medial retraction of the thyroid lobe allows the posterior aspect of the thyroid lobe to be visualized. It is in this area that the superior parathyroids are usually found lying within small deposits of fat within the thyroid sheath.

Further mobilization of the thyroid lobe allows exposure of the tracheoesophageal groove and the recurrent laryngeal nerve (Figs. 34-26 to 34-29). Minimal dissection of the lower vessels entering the thyroid should be undertaken, and no division should be done until the recurrent laryngeal nerve is seen and positively identified. On the right side, care should be used to dissect in the posterolateral aspects of the trachea because the esophagus is not well palpated in this area. In patients with thyroid reoperations, this area is extremely treacherous because of scar tissue. It is usually advisable, if the recurrent laryngeal nerve is not immediately visible at the level of the thyroid lobe, to proceed lower in the neck tissue in previously undissected areas to gain access to the recurrent laryngeal nerve.

After the recurrent laryngeal nerve is seen on either side, the pace of the operation may be increased; the inferior vessels may be divided while the course of the recurrent laryngeal nerve is directly visualized. Continued medial traction of the lobe then identifies the cephalad course of the nerve to where it disappears under the ligament of Berry or into its final destination, the caudal border of the cricothyroid muscle. The ligament of Berry

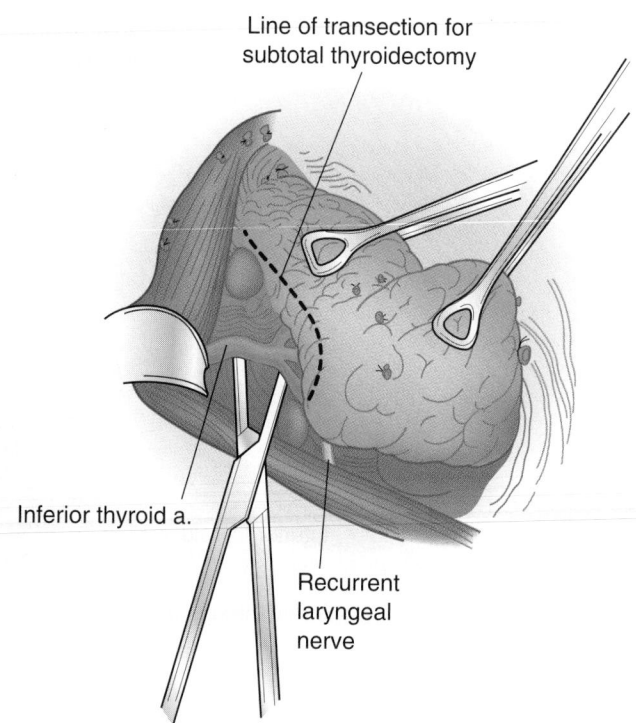

FIGURE 34-26.   Subtotal lobectomy necessitates identification of the parathyroid glands, inferior thyroid artery, and recurrent laryngeal nerve, as previously described. The line of resection is selected to preserve the parathyroid glands and their blood supply and to protect the recurrent laryngeal nerve. It should be based on the inferior thyroid artery or its major branches. (From Sabiston DC Jr [ed]: Atlas of General Surgery. Philadelphia, WB Saunders, 1995.)

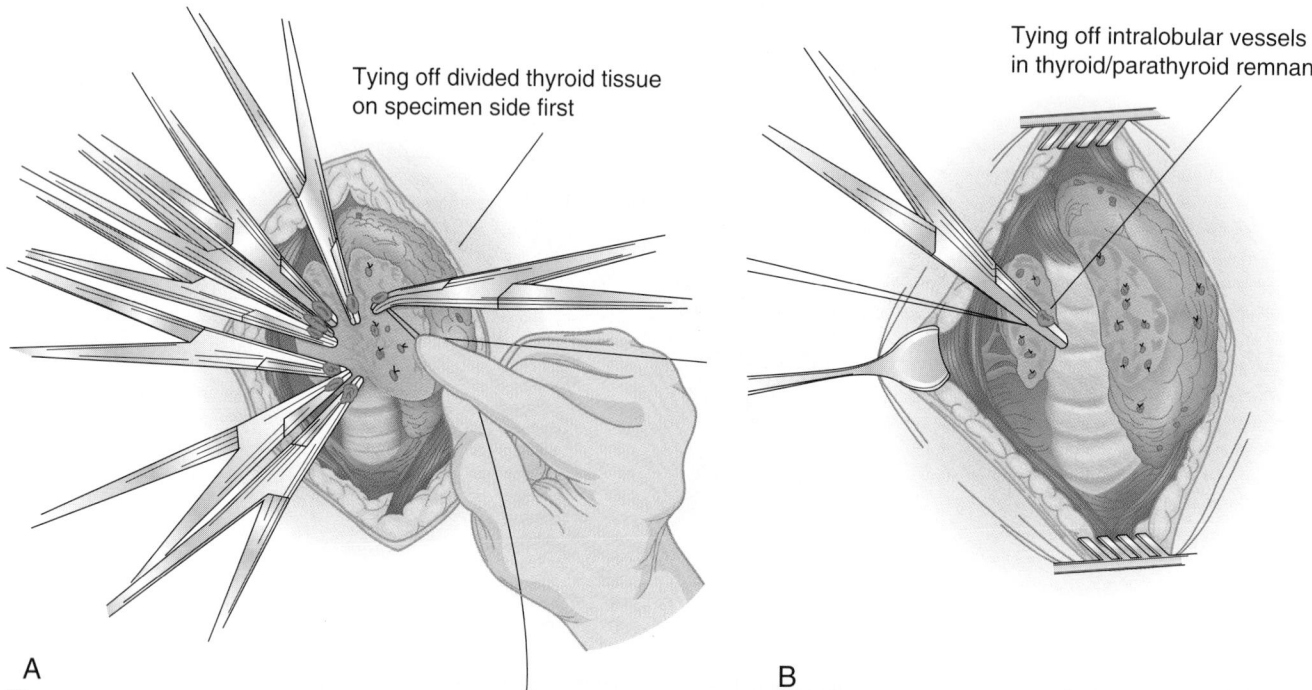

FIGURE 34-27.   **A** and **B,** Clamps are placed along the line of resection and the thyroid gland is divided. The divided tissue is ligated or suture-ligated with 3-0 silk sutures. The dissection is extended to the trachea. (**A** and **B,** From Sabiston DC Jr [ed]: Atlas of General Surgery. Philadelphia, WB Saunders, 1995.)

is in a position just anterior and slightly medial to the nerve's entrance underneath the cricothyroid muscle, and this structure, with a small rim of thyroid tissue, can be ligated using 3-0 silk suture. After division of the ligament of Berry, the attachment of the thyroid medially on the trachea can be divided using low-energy Bovie dissection (see Fig. 34-26).

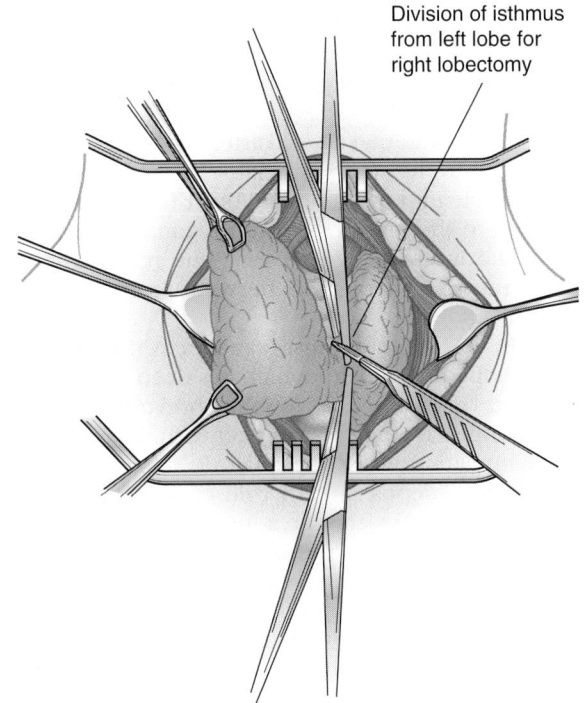

FIGURE 34-28. The thyroid can now be divided so that the isthmus is included in the specimen. A running 2-0 silk suture is used to secure the line of division along the remaining thyroid lobe. (From Sabiston DC Jr [ed]: Atlas of General Surgery. Philadelphia, WB Saunders, 1995.)

Terminology for thyroid surgery is inconsistent in the literature. A total thyroidectomy involves division of all thyroid tissue between the entrance of the recurrent laryngeal nerves bilaterally by the ligament of Berry, resulting in complete removal of virtually all visible thyroid tissue. A near-total thyroidectomy should involve complete dissection on one side while leaving a remnant of thyroid tissue laterally on the contralateral side, which should incorporate the parathyroids. A subtotal thyroidectomy leaves a rim of thyroid tissue bilaterally, ensuring parathyroid viability and avoiding entrance of the recurrent laryngeal nerves into the larynx (see Figs. 34-24 to 34-28).

Central lymph node dissection can be carried out under direct vision, removing all lymph nodes immediately adjacent to the thyroid, especially in the tracheoesophageal groove in those patients with well-differentiated carcinomas. This dissection should proceed laterally to and including lymph nodes within the carotid sheath. If a patient has palpable lymph nodes in the lateral neck, a more complete modified radical neck dissection should be done.[4]

Postoperative monitoring of the thyroid and parathyroid function is extremely important. The surgeon is obligated to evaluate both glands and inform the patient and referring physician of the details of the resection and their expected impact on postoperative function. Calcium determination should be made within 24 hours of surgery. If there are no signs of hypocalcemia, particularly if the surgeon has visualized the glands during surgery, no calcium supplementation may be necessary. If symptoms occur, or if the surgeon is concerned about parathyroid status, the patient may be started on 1500 to 3000 mg of elemental calcium daily supplements.

If the patient was euthyroid prior to surgery, it is reasonable to expect at least 10 days before replacement may need to be started, even for a total thyroidectomy. This allows time for complete specimen evaluation by pathol-

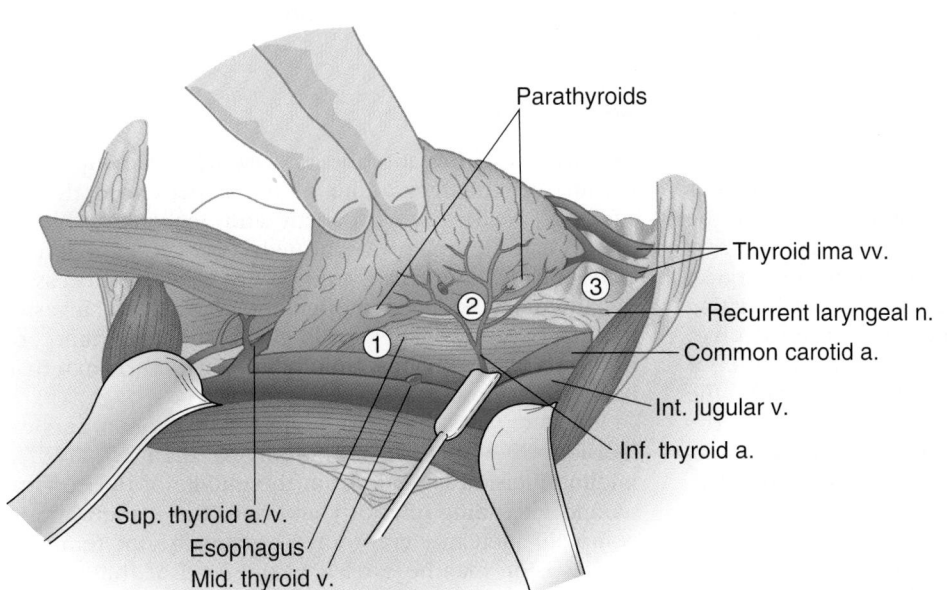

FIGURE 34-29. During thyroidectomy, the recurrent laryngeal nerve is at greatest risk for injury (1) at the ligament of Berry, (2) during ligation of branches of the inferior thyroid artery, and (3) at the thoracic inlet. (From Kahky MP, Weber RS: Intraoperative problems: Complications of surgery of the thyroid and parathyroid glands. Surg Clin North Am 73:307, 1993.)

ogy. Thyroid replacement usually requires a daily dose of 100 μg of levothyroxine (Synthroid) for a person of normal weight. Most endocrinologists believe that levothyroxine dose should be adjusted to keep TSH levels at low normal values after resection for a cancer or suppressive therapy.

Modified Radical Neck Dissection

Although there is some controversy about when to perform a modified radical neck dissection for thyroid carcinoma, it is safe to say that this operation is most widely employed in patients with documented disease in whom obvious and palpable lymphadenopathy lateral to the carotid sheath exists at the time of the original diagnosis or occurs after preceding thyroid surgery. There appear to be limited data on the use of prophylactic neck dissection in patients with well-differentiated thyroid carcinoma who do not have palpable lymph nodes.

In the case of papillary carcinoma, concern about multicentricity and microscopic lymph node involvement appears to fuel this controversy. For larger tumors and palpable nodes in this area, most authors advocate total thyroidectomy and, at least, a central lymph node dissection. In the case of microscopic lymph node involvement in the absence of palpable lateral lymph nodes, the use of radioactive iodine before proceeding with prophylactic lateral lymph node dissection has been advocated but not overwhelmingly accepted. Radioactive iodine appears to be beneficial in this circumstance but is much less effective in ablating palpable regional metastatic lymph node involvement. The use of selected removal of palpable nodes in the lateral compartment ("cherry-picking") has been largely abandoned. Therefore, the use of modified radical neck dissection is primarily reserved for patients with thyroid carcinoma and clinically palpable cervical lymph node metastases. This can be accomplished using an en bloc dissection that removes all the lymphatic and adipose tissue in the lateral neck compartment while avoiding the cosmetic or functional abnormality of removal of muscle groups employed in the classic radical neck dissection. The sternocleidomastoid muscle and spinal accessory nerve are spared.[57]

The operation employs the cervical skin incision, which is standard for most thyroid operations. This is extended laterally and superiorly along the border of the sternocleidomastoid muscle. Occasionally, it is necessary to make a higher parallel incision to the previous surgical incision if higher lymph nodes are palpable. In initiating the neck dissection, the surgeon must gain access deep to the sternocleidomastoid muscle and remain anterior to the carotid sheath above the clavicle. Laterally, the phrenic nerve is identified and preserved in the prevertebral fascia on the anterior scalene muscle. On the left side, the phrenic nerve is immediately adjacent to the thoracic duct at the level of the internal jugular vein junction with the subclavian vein. The dissection should begin just above the clavicle in this area. The goal of the dissection should be the removal of all tissues between the superficial and the prevertebral fascia except for the carotid

artery, jugular vein, vagus, and phrenic and spinal accessory nerves. Additionally, the sympathetic chain and the sternocleidomastoid muscle must be preserved. Dissection should continue in the cephalad direction, where the spinal accessory nerve is identified at the deep and lateral surface of the sternocleidomastoid muscle. The nerve runs inferiorly in the lateral aspect of the posterior triangle of the neck. The nerve can be traced as it gives a branch to the sternocleidomastoid muscle at this level and then passes adjacent and posterior to the digastric muscle.

As the dissection proceeds in a more cephalad direction, the hypoglossal nerve is encountered, which crosses anteriorly to the internal carotid artery and internal jugular vein yet deep to the anterior facial vein. It follows the stylohyoid muscle into the submandibular triangle as it gives innervation to the muscles of the tongue. If one chooses to ligate the internal jugular vein, one must be careful not to injure the hypoglossal nerve as it crosses at this area.

Medially, the surgeon must take care not to injure the cervical sympathetic chain, which lies deep to the carotid sheath and just anterior to the prevertebral fascia. Retropharyngeal lymphatics connect with the cervical and jugular lymphatics across the chain in this area and may have metastatic deposits of thyroid cancer. Injury to the sympathetic chain in this area results in Horner's syndrome, which includes ptosis, miosis, anhidrosis, and increased skin temperature on the involved side.

On completion of the modified radical dissection, a triangle of fibrofatty tissue, which may or may not include the internal jugular vein, is dissected free and oriented for pathology. It is usually not necessary to extend dissection into the suprahyoid area unless there is extensive lymph node involvement, which occurs in only a few patients with well-differentiated thyroid carcinoma (<1%). Great care should be used to dissect structures in the lateral neck, including the sympathetic chain and recurrent laryngeal and spinal accessory nerves, unless they are obviously and grossly involved with tumor.[4]

Median Sternotomy

Exploration of the anterior mediastinal space should be within the armamentarium of the experienced thyroid surgeon. Nearly every benign and malignant thyroid tumor can be removed through cervical exploration. Occasionally, a median sternotomy may be necessary in patients who need reoperation, have large invasive tumors, have low-lying thyroid glands and large tumor, or have received previous radioiodine ablation or external-beam irradiation.

Initial exploration usually always involves a cervical incision. If a median sternotomy is then required, a midline incision is made from the middle of the cervical wound extending inferiorly and onto the manubrium. A complete median sternotomy is generally not required. The incision may be carried to the level of the third or fourth intercostal space and then carried out laterally. Before dividing the sternum, access should be gained on the superior border of the manubrium and all tissues deep to the sternum swept away bluntly with cotton sponges or finger dissection. The midline inferior sternal incision is employed using a saw or splitting device and carried to the level of the second, third, or fourth intercostal space as needed. A lateral T incision is then taken out into the appropriate intercostal space. At this time, injury to the internal mammary arteries can occur if care is not taken to anticipate their course about 1 to 2 cm lateral to the sternal edge.

A sternal separating retractor (Finochietto) can then provide good exposure to the anterior mediastinum. Substernal thyroid masses, including goiters, or extension of malignancies as well as ectopic parathyroid adenomatous tissue can be approached through this incision. The anteromedial fat pad and thymus can be dissected to gain visualization of the pericardium superiorly. As one proceeds laterally in this dissection, one must be careful to avoid injuring the pleura and the phrenic nerves. The innominate vein is deep to the thymus. Virtually all low-lying thyroid masses can be approached through this incision.[4,28]

Complications of Surgery

The advantage of complete removal of disease-bearing tissue and efficient subsequent application of postprocedure radioiodine ablation after total thyroidectomy must be weighed against lesser procedures such as lobectomy in terms of surgical complications. The most important complications are postprocedure hypocalcemia due to devascularization of parathyroid and significant hoarseness due to recurrent laryngeal nerve injury, either traction induced or division.

Hypocalcemia

The rates of postprocedure hypocalcemia should be about 5%, which resolves in 80% of these cases in about 12 months.[58,59] Therefore, every effort should be made to evaluate parathyroid tissue intraoperatively. For those glands that appear to be devascularized, the use of immediate parathyroid autotransplantation of 1-mm fragments of saline-chilled tissue into pockets made in sternocleidomastoid muscle tissue is extremely effective in avoiding hypocalcemia.

Recurrent Laryngeal Nerve Injury

Permanent hoarseness as a result of injury to the recurrent laryngeal nerve should be less than 3% after total thyroidectomy and less for lesser procedures. Great care in dissection around the tracheoesophageal groove should be taken as even small amounts of traction or electrocautery near the nerve is associated with transient hoarseness.

Bleeding

Other complications such as bleeding and wound hematomas may require immediate re-exploration, which should be done in the operating room unless airway compromise dictates otherwise. This can be avoided by meticulous hemostasis at closing, which should result in less than 1% occurrence.

Complication rates appear to be affected by surgeon's experience. A study in Maryland of 5860 patients reported the lowest complication rates in patients of surgeons who performed more than 100 neck explorations annually.[29]

Selected References

Work-up of Thyroid Nodules

Burman KD, Ringel MP, Wartofsky L: Unusual types of thyroid nodules. Endocrinol Metab Clin North Am 25:49-68, 1996.

An excellent discussion of unusual thyroid neoplasms, including tall cell variant of papillary cancer, insular cancer, squamous cell cancer, and lymphoma, among others. Good review of a small literature on the subject.

Hermus AR, Huysmans DA: Treatment of benign nodular thyroid disease. N Engl J Med 338:1438-1447, 1998.

An excellent update on diagnosis and treatment of solitary nodules, multinodular goiter, and nontoxic and toxic nodules. This paper has 77 references and is based on the author's extensive experience in the field.

Mazzaferri EL: Management of a solitary thyroid nodule. N Engl J Med 328:553-559, 1993.

An older article, but still a classic by a prominent endocrinologist. Excellent discussion, with 62 references.

Sabel MS, Staren ED, Gianakakis LM, et al: Use of fine-needle aspiration biopsy and frozen section in the management of the solitary thyroid nodule. Surgery 122:1021-1027, 1997.

This study was presented at the American Association of Endocrine Surgeons in 1997. It reviews fine-needle aspiration and frozen section in 561 patients and assessed the accuracy, sensitivity, and specificity of both procedures, documenting the clinical usefulness of fine-needle aspiration.

Wong CKM, Wheeler MH: Thyroid nodules: Rational management. World J Surg 24:934-941, 2000.

A good review and discussion of work-up and management strategies from an internationally known surgical group from Wales, United Kingdom.

Thyroid Malignancy

Hundahl SA, Cady B, Cunningham MP, et al: Initial results from a prospective cohort study of 5583 cases of thyroid carcinoma treated in the United States during 1996. Cancer 89:202-217, 2000.

An excellent update of the U.S. experience compiled by the Commission on Cancer of the American College of Surgeons.

Schlumberger MJ: Papillary and follicular thyroid cancer. N Engl J Med 338:297-306, 1998.

An excellent update on the topic, with 93 references. Modern controversies and classic observations are well discussed and presented. The author's experience with 1700 patients is included in the discussion.

Surgical Techniques

Attie JN: Modified neck dissection in treatment of thyroid cancer: A safe procedure. Eur J Cancer Clin Oncol 24:315-324, 1998.

A good discussion of the use and applicability of a technique that is not often employed in thyroid cancer but should be understood by surgeons who perform the operation. This series of 313 neck dissections is the author's 35-year experience.

References

1. Henry JF: Surgical anatomy and embryology of the thyroid and parathyroid glands and recurrent and external laryngeal nerves. *In* Clark OH, Duh QY (eds): Textbook of Endocrine Surgery. Philadelphia, WB Saunders, 1997, pp 8-14.
2. Henry JF, Audiffret J, Denizot A, et al: The nonrecurrent inferior laryngeal nerve: Review of 33 cases, including two on the left side. Surgery 104:977-984, 1988.
3. Lennquist S, Cahlin C, Smeds S: The superior laryngeal nerve in thyroid surgery. Surgery 102:999-1008, 1987.
4. Clark OH: Surgical anatomy. *In* Braverman LE, Utiger RE (eds): Werner and Ingbar's The Thyroid, 7th ed. Philadelphia, Lippincott-Raven, 1996, pp 462-468.
5. Brent GA: The molecular basis of thyroid hormone action. N Engl J Med 331:847-853, 1994.
6. Braverman LE: Iodine and the thyroid: 33 years of study. Thyroid 4:351-356, 1994.
7. McLachlan SM, Rapoport B: The molecular biology of thyroid peroxidase: Cloning, expression, and role as autoantigen in autoimmune thyroid disease. Endocr Rev 13:192-206, 1992.
8. Chopra IJ: Nature, source, and relative significance of circulating thyroid hormones. *In* Braverman LE, Utiger RE (eds): Werner and Ingbar's The Thyroid, 7th ed. Philadelphia, Lippincott-Raven, 1996, pp 111-124.
9. Duh QY, Grossman RF: Thyroid growth factors, signal transduction pathways, and oncogenes. Surg Clin North Am 75:421-437, 1995.
10. Parma J, Duprez L, Van Sande J, et al: Somatic mutations in the thyrotropin receptor gene cause hyperfunctioning thyroid adenomas. Nature 365:649-651, 1993.
11. Delbridge LW: Thyroid physiology. *In* Clark OH, Duh QY (eds): Textbook of Endocrine Surgery. Philadelphia, WB Saunders, 1997, pp 3-7.
12. Harvey RD, Matheson NA, Grabowski PS, et al: Measurement of serum thyroglobulin is of value in detecting tumour recurrence following treatment of differentiated thyroid carcinoma by lobectomy. Br J Surg 77:324-326, 1990.
13. Price DC: Radioisotopic evaluation of the thyroid and the parathyroids. Radiol Clin North Am 31:991-1015, 1993.
14. Gooding GA: Sonography of the thyroid and parathyroid. Radiol Clin North Am 31:967-989, 1993.
15. Alexander EK, Heering JP, Benson CB, et al: Assessment of nondiagnostic ultrasound-guided fine-needle aspirations of thyroid nodules. J Clin Endocrinol Metab 87:4924-4927, 2002.
16. Refetoff S: Resistance to thyroid hormone: An historical overview. Thyroid 4:345-349, 1994.
17. Cheung P: Medical and surgical treatment of endemic goiter. *In* Clark OH, Duh QY (eds): Textbook of Endocrine Surgery. Philadelphia, WB Saunders, 1997, pp 15-21.
18. Barsano CP: Other forms of primary hypothyroidism. *In* Braverman LE, Utiger RE (eds): The Thyroid, 6th ed. Philadelphia, JB Lippincott, 1992, p 956.
19. Urabe M, Hershman JM, Pang XP, et al: Effect of lithium on function and growth of thyroid cells in vitro. Endocrinology 129:807-814, 1991.
20. Franklyn JA, Sheppard MC: Amiodarone and thyroid dysfunction. Trends Endocrinol Metab 4:128, 1993.
21. Knecht H, Saremaslani P, Hedinger C: Immunohistological findings in Hashimoto's thyroiditis, focal lymphocytic thyroiditis, and thyroiditis de Quervain: Comparative study. Virchows Arch A Pathol Anat Histol 393:215-231, 1981.
22. Sato K, Yamazaki K, Shizume K, et al: Pathogenesis of autoimmune hypothyroidism induced by lymphokine-activated killer (LAK) cell therapy: In vitro inhibition of human thyroid function by interleukin-2 in the presence of autologous intrathyroidal lymphocytes. Thyroid 3:179-188, 1993.
23. Harada T, Katagiri M, Ito K: Hyperthyroidism: Graves' disease and toxic nodular goiter. *In* Clark OH, Duh QY (eds): Textbook of Endocrine Surgery. Philadelphia, WB Saunders, 1997, pp 47-53.
24. Wong CKM, Wheeler MH: Thyroid nodules: Rational management. World J Surg 24:934-941, 2000.
25. Torring O, Tallstedt L, Wallin G, et al: Graves' hyperthyroidism: Treatment with antithyroid drugs, surgery, or radioiodine—a prospective, randomized study. Thyroid Study Group. J Clin Endocrinol Metab 81:2986-2993, 1996.
26. Menegaux F, Ruprecht T, Chigot JP: The surgical treatment of Graves' disease. Surg Gynecol Obstet 176:277-282, 1993.
27. Hermus AR, Huysmans DA: Treatment of benign nodular thyroid disease. N Engl J Med 338:1438-1447, 1998.
28. Mack E: Management of patients with substernal goiters. Surg Clin North Am 75:377-394, 1995.
29. Sosa JA, Bowman HM, Tielsch JM, et al: The importance of surgeon experience for clinical and economic outcomes from thyroidectomy. Ann Surg 228:320-330, 1998.
30. Mazzaferri EL: Management of a solitary thyroid nodule. N Engl J Med 328:553-559, 1993.
31. Woeber KA: Cost-effective evaluation of the patient with a thyroid nodule. Surg Clin North Am 75:357-363, 1995.
32. Burch HB: Evaluation and management of the solid thyroid nodule. Endocrinol Metab Clin North Am 24:663-710, 1995.
33. Ashcraft MW, Van Herle AJ: Management of thyroid nodules: II. Scanning techniques, thyroid suppressive therapy, and fine-needle aspiration. Head Neck Surg 3:297-322, 1981.
34. Sabel MS, Staren ED, Gianakakis LM, et al: User of fine-needle aspiration biopsy and frozen section in the management of the solitary thyroid nodule. Surgery 122:1021-1027, 1997.
35. Boyd LA, Earnhardt RC, Dunn JT, et al: Preoperative evaluation and predictive value of fine-needle aspiration and frozen section of thyroid nodules. J Am Coll Surg 187:494-502, 1998.
36. Jossart GH, Grossman RF: Tumor oncogenesis. *In* Clark OH, Duh QY (eds): Textbook of Endocrine Surgery. Philadelphia, WB Saunders, 1997, pp 237-242.
37. Jhiang SM, Mazzaferri EL: The *ret/PTC* oncogene in papillary thyroid carcinoma. J Lab Clin Med 123:331-337, 1994.
38. Said S, Schlumberger M, Suarez HG: Oncogenes and anti-oncogenes in human epithelial thyroid tumors. J Endocrinol Invest 17:371-379, 1994.
39. Fraker DL: Radiation exposure and other factors that predispose to human thyroid neoplasia. Surg Clin North Am 75:365-375, 1995.

40. Pacini F, Vorontsova T, Demidchik EP, et al: Post-Chernobyl thyroid carcinoma in Belarus children and adolescents: Comparison with naturally occurring thyroid carcinoma in Italy and France. J Clin Endocrinol Metab 82:3563-3569, 1997.

41. Schneider AB, Ron E: Carcinoma of the follicular epithelium. *In* Braverman LE, Utiger RE (eds): Werner and Ingbar's The Thyroid. Philadelphia, Lippincott-Raven, 1995, pp 902-943.

42. Cady B, Sedgwick CE, Meissner WA, et al: Risk factor analysis in differentiated thyroid cancer. Cancer 43:810-820, 1979.

43. Hay ID: Prognostic factors in thyroid carcinoma. Thyroid Today 12:1-9, 1989.

44. Schlumberger MJ: Papillary and follicular thyroid carcinoma. N Engl J Med 338:297-306, 1998.

45. Hundahl SA, Cady B, Cunningham MP, et al: Initial results from a prospective cohort study of 5583 cases of thyroid carcinoma treated in the United States during 1996: U.S. and German Thyroid Cancer Study Group. An American College of Surgeons Commission on Cancer Patient Care Evaluation study. Cancer 89:202-217, 2000.

46. Mazzaferri EL, Jhiang SM: Long-term impact of initial surgical and medical therapy on papillary and follicular thyroid cancer. Am J Med 97:418-428, 1994.

47. Patwardhan N, Cataldo T, Braverman LE: Surgical management of the patient with papillary cancer. Surg Clin North Am 75:449-464, 1995.

48. Grebe SKG, Hay ID: Follicular thyroid cancer. Endocrinol Metab Clin North Am 24:761-801, 1995.

49. Stojadinovic A, Ghossein RA, Hoos A, et al: Hurthle cell carcinoma: A critical histopathologic appraisal. J Clin Oncol 19:2616-2625, 2001.

50. Grant CS: Operative and postoperative management of the patient with follicular and Hurthle cell carcinoma: Do they differ? Surg Clin North Am 75:395-403, 1995.

51. Moley JF: Medullary thyroid cancer. Surg Clin North Am 75:405-420, 1995.

52. Burman KD, Ringel MD, Wartofsky L: Unusual types of thyroid neoplasms. Endocrinol Metab Clin North Am 25:49-68, 1996.

53. Junor EJ, Paul J, Reed NS: Anaplastic thyroid carcinoma: 91 patients treated by surgery and radiotherapy. Eur J Surg Oncol 18:83-88, 1992.

54. Sugino K, Ito K, Mimura T, et al: The important role of operations in the management of anaplastic thyroid carcinoma. Surgery 131:245-248, 2002.

55. Matsuzuka F, Miyauchi A, Katayama S, et al: Clinical aspects of primary thyroid lymphoma: diagnosis and treatment based on our experience of 119 cases. Thyroid 3:93-99, 1993.

56. Newman KD, Black T, Heller G, et al: Differentiated thyroid cancer: Determinants of disease progression in patients < 21 years of age at diagnosis: A report from the Surgical Discipline Committee of the Children's Cancer Group. Ann Surg 227:533-541, 1998.

57. Attie JN: Modified neck dissection in treatment of thyroid cancer: A safe procedure. Eur J Cancer Clin Oncol 24:315-324, 1988.

58. Mazzaferri EL, Kloos RT: Clinical review 128: Current approaches to primary therapy for papillary and follicular thyroid cancer. J Clin Endocrinol Metab 86:1447-1463, 2001.

59. Pattou F, Combemale F, Fabre S, et al: Hypocalcemia following thyroid surgery: Incidence and prediction of outcome. World J Surg 22:718-724, 1998.

CHAPTER 35

PARATHYROID GLAND

PAUL G. GAUGER, M.D.   and   GERARD M. DOHERTY, M.D.

Historical Aspects	**Parathyroid Pathophysiology**
Embryology and Anatomy	**Surgical Management of Hyperparathyroidism**
Normal Parathyroid Physiology	

The treatment of parathyroid disease is fascinating and rewarding on many levels. To best serve patients, a broad appreciation of clinical issues as well as excellent technical skills and intraoperative judgment are required.

HISTORICAL ASPECTS

The parathyroid gland was first discovered during a post-mortem dissection of an Indian rhinoceros in 1850. Later, a Swedish student, Ivar Sandstrom, described the gross and histologic appearance of the parathyroid glands in several animals and in humans.[1] Early clinical observations led to the prevailing thought that parathyroid tumors arose to compensate for osseous abnormalities. The converse theory eventually considered that parathyroid tumors were primary and were responsible for secondary changes in the skeleton.[2] Mandl confirmed this hypothesis 10 years later when he excised an enlarged parathyroid gland from a patient with hypercalcemia, hypercalciuria, and severe bone disease.[3] Human parathyroid hormone (PTH) was isolated and purified in 1959.[4,5] The first radioimmunoassay for PTH was described in 1963.[6]

EMBRYOLOGY AND ANATOMY

Embryology

The superior parathyroid glands arise from branchial pouch IV and the inferior parathyroids arise from III. The glands are intimately associated with the derivatives of their respective pouches—the inferior glands with the thymus and the superior glands with the lateral thyroid component (later to become the tubercle of Zuckerkandl). As the thymus descends, the inferior glands also migrate caudally and settle near the lower pole of the thyroid. Migration is variable. At one extreme, the ectopic glands may be found high in the carotid sheath, or at the other, they may be found deep in the mediastinum (Fig. 35-1). The inferior glands are more likely to be found in an ectopic location than the superior glands. Rarely, a parathyroid becomes completely enclosed within the thyroid parenchyma (typically an inferior gland).

Anatomy

Normally, there are four parathyroid glands. Åkerström performed autopsy studies on 503 cadavers and found four parathyroid glands in all but 18 cadavers (3%).[7] In 421 cases there were four glands; however, more than four glands were detected in 64 cases (13%).[7] Most often, the supernumerary gland was located in the thymus. The distribution of superior and inferior parathyroid glands in this study is shown in Figure 35-2. The vascular supply to the parathyroid glands is usually from the inferior thyroid artery, but it can arise from the superior thyroid artery, or from anastomoses between these vessels. The inferior, middle, and superior thyroid veins drain the parathyroid glands. The superior parathyroid glands are usually embedded in fat and located on the posterior surface of the upper portion of the thyroid lobe within a 2-cm circumscribed area cranial to the point where the recurrent laryngeal nerve (RLN) intersects the course of the inferior thyroid artery. The lower parathyroid glands are more ventral, usually close to the lower pole of the thyroid gland and the thyrothymic ligament.

Normal glands tend to be flat and ovoid, but on enlargement they become globular. Normally, they measure 5 to 7 × 3 to 4 × 0.5 to 2 mm. The combined weight of the glands is 90 to 200 mg, and the upper glands

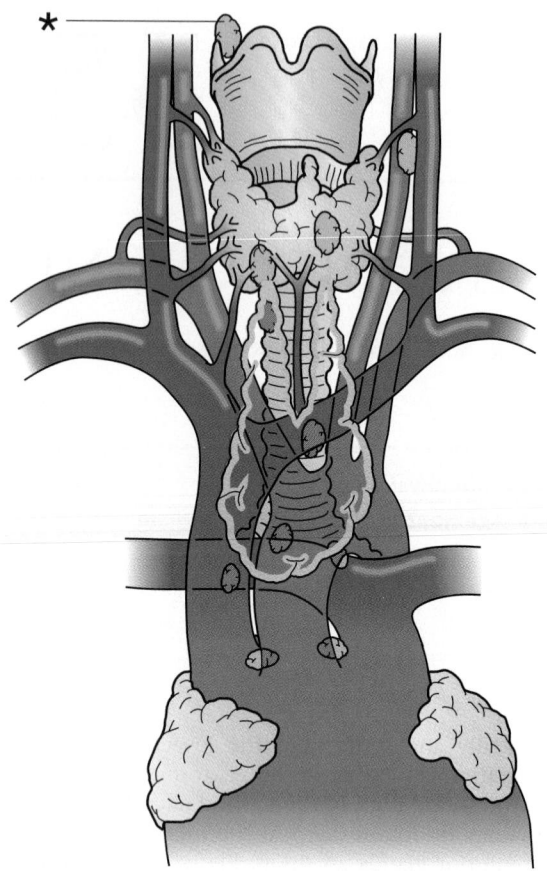

FIGURE 35-1.   Many possible locations of ectopic parathyroid adenomas. Indicated gland locations apply to ectopic inferior parathyroid glands, with the exception of the uppermost gland in the illustration (*), which indicates the position of the rare undescended superior parathyroid gland in the wall of the pharynx. (From Gauger PG, Thompson NW: Persistent or recurrent hyperparathyroidism. *In* Cameron JL [ed]: Current Surgical Therapy, 7th ed. St. Louis, Mosby, 2001, p 670.)

are generally smaller than the lower. In adults, the glands are red-brown to yellow in color. The parathyroid glands consist of a parenchyma containing chief and oxyphil cells and a stroma composed primarily of adipocytes. Less common are the polygonal water-clear cells, which are glycogen-laden chief cells with little visible cytoplasm. Acidophilic, mitochondria-rich oxyphil cells appear near puberty and increase in number with age. The functional significance of the various cell types remains unclear.

NORMAL PARATHYROID PHYSIOLOGY

Mineral Metabolism

Plasma calcium exists in an ionized and a protein-bound phase. Normally, about 1 g of calcium, in the inorganic form, is absorbed daily in the upper small intestine. Extracellular calcium is constantly being exchanged with that in the bone, intracellular fluid, and the glomerular filtrate (99% of which is reabsorbed by the normal kidney). The adult body contains about 700 g of phosphate, most being

located in the bones and teeth. The plasma levels of calcium and phosphate vary inversely with one another. The primary agents responsible for calcium metabolism are PTH, vitamin D, and calcitonin. Their major actions are summarized in Table 35-1.

Parathyroid Hormone

Parathormone (PTH) is synthesized within the parathyroid as pre-proparathormone, which is cleaved first to proparathormone and then to the 84-amino acid PTH. PTH is metabolized in the liver into the active N-terminal and inactive C-terminal fragments. The intact molecule and N-terminal fragment have half-lives of minutes, whereas the C-terminal fragment has a half-life of hours. Normally, PTH secretion is inversely related to levels of serum ionized calcium and 1,25-dihydroxyvitamin D. It has direct effects on the kidney and skeleton and indirect effects on the gastrointestinal tract through vitamin D hydroxylation. In the skeleton, PTH promotes a release of calcium by both an active transport process and by the influence of lysosomal and hydrolytic enzymes. PTH inhibits osteoblasts and stimulates osteoclasts. In the kidney, PTH causes a decrease in calcium clearance. PTH also causes increased renal excretion of phosphate by inhibiting its reabsorption in the tubule. PTH stimulates hydroxylation of 25-hydroxyvitamin D to 1,25-dihydroxyvitamin D in the kidney. It is the latter which causes enhanced absorption of calcium in the intestine.

Vitamin D

The major D vitamins are D_2 and D_3. The most important is vitamin D_3, which is derived from ultraviolet activation of 7-dehydrocholesterol in the skin. The bulk of commercially prepared vitamin D is vitamin D_2. It is derived from ergosterol and is the major form of vitamin D used clinically.

Calcitonin

Calcitonin inhibits bone resorption and produces hypocalcemia when administered to experimental animals. Although it can be used therapeutically, calcitonin is not normally important in the control of serum calcium in humans.

PARATHYROID PATHOPHYSIOLOGY

Hypoparathyroidism

The most common cause of hypoparathyroidism is damage to the parathyroid glands during total thyroidectomy, but it can also occur following parathyroid exploration. A temporary postoperative drop in the serum calcium level is common—likely from compromise of the blood supply to the parathyroids. In patients with significant bone disease, there may be remarkable postoperative

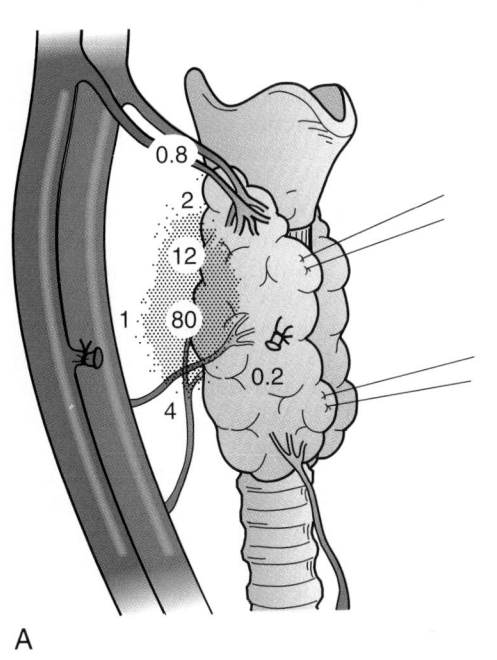

A

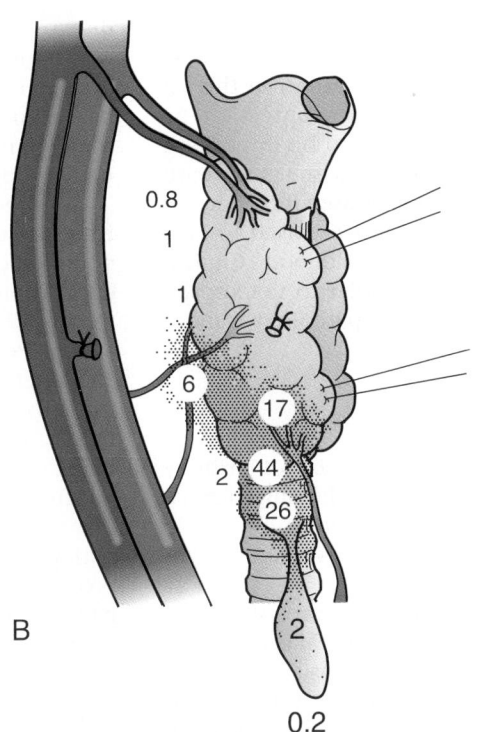

B

0.2

FIGURE 35-2.

Locations of the superior (**A**) and inferior (**B**) parathyroid glands. The more common locations are indicated by the darker shading. The numbers represent the percentages of glands found at the different locations. (*A* and *B*, Adapted from Åkerström G, Malmaeus J, Bergström R: Surgical anatomy of human parathyroid glands. Surgery 95:14-21, 1984.)

TABLE 35-1.   Actions of Major Calcium-Regulating Hormones

	Bone	Kidney	Intestine
Parathyroid hormone	Stimulates resorption of calcium and phosphate	Stimulates reabsorption of calcium and conversion of 25(OH)D₃ to 1,25(OH)₂D₃; inhibits reabsorption of phosphate and bicarbonate	No direct effects
Vitamin D	Stimulates transport of calcium	Inhibits reabsorption of calcium	Stimulates absorption of calcium and phosphate
Calcitonin	Inhibits resorption of calcium and phosphate	Inhibits reabsorption of calcium and phosphate	No direct effects

---

skeletal calcium deposition (bone hunger). The major signs and symptoms of hypocalcemia are attributable to increased neuromuscular excitability from reduced plasma ionized calcium. The earliest manifestations are numbness and tingling in the circumoral area and the fingers. Mental symptoms such as anxiety or confusion can occur. Tetany may develop, characterized by carpopedal spasms, convulsions, or laryngospasm—which can be fatal. On examination, contraction of the facial muscles is elicited by tapping on the facial nerve anterior to the ear (Chvostek's sign). This sign is present in a small number of normal individuals. Acute symptomatic hypocalcemia is treated with intravenous calcium gluconate. Oral calcium and vitamin D analogues are used for long-term management. If there is concomitant hypomagnesemia, it is difficult to correct the hypocalcemia until the magnesium level has been corrected. A far less common cause of hypoparathyroidism is idiopathic lack of function. Neonatal hypoparathyroidism can follow prenatal suppression of fetal parathyroid glands by the hyperparathyroid mother.

Primary Hyperparathyroidism

The incidence of primary hyperparathyroidism (HPT) is approximately 25 per 100,000 in the general population, and approximately 50,000 new cases occur annually in the United States. The incidence increases with age and it is especially common in postmenopausal women.

Etiology

The cause of primary HPT is unknown and probably varies with the specific pathologic condition. Single-gland disease is consistent with a mechanism involving spontaneous growth and hyperfunction, whereas multiglandular disease suggests the presence of some exogenous stimulus or underlying genetic defect. An alteration in the set point (the sensitivity of the glands to suppression by serum or intracellular calcium) appears to be important. Loss of renal function with age is associated with increased plasma levels of PTH. An increased incidence of primary HPT has been noted in patients exposed to low-dose ionizing irradiation—usually in childhood. Clinical presentations of these patients are similar to unexposed patients, although synchronous thyroid pathology is more frequent (57% vs. 7%).[8]

Clinical Presentation (Signs and Symptoms)

In the last century, the typical presentation of primary HPT has changed from a severe, debilitating disease toward a disease with subtle symptoms and physiologic derangements. Some common symptoms are delineated in Table 35-2.[9]

Renal Complications. Renal complications are often the most severe manifestations of primary HPT. Many patients have only frequency, nocturia, and polydipsia, but symptoms related to nephrolithiasis occur in a significant number of patients. Conversely, a small fraction of previously unscreened patients presenting with nephrolithiasis have primary HPT. Renal calculi are usually composed of calcium phosphate or calcium oxalate. Nephrocalcinosis (calcification within the renal parenchyma) occurs in only 5% to 10% of patients with primary HPT.

Hypertension. Hypertension is frequently present in patients with primary HPT. Various mechanisms have been proposed to explain this relationship. It appears to be most closely correlated with the degree of renal impairment. Despite this, one study found that parathyroidectomy led to a substantial fall in both systolic and diastolic pressures in 54% of hypertensive subjects that was unrelated to improvement in renal function.[10]

Bone Disease. With the use of dual-energy x-ray absorption scanning, subtle derangements in bone density can be detected. In modern series, the incidence of overt bone

disease in patients with primary HPT is 5% to 15%. Although the significance of subtle bone loss has been questioned, an increased prevalence of vertebral fractures has been demonstrated in patients undergoing parathyroidectomy compared with a matched control group undergoing cholecystectomy.[11]

Neurologic, Psychiatric, and Neuromuscular Manifestations. Patients with hypercalcemia of any cause may develop neurologic or psychiatric disturbances ranging from depression or anxiety to psychosis or coma. Most of the mental derangements associated with primary HPT are subtle. Petersen performed psychiatric examinations on 54 patients with primary HPT and detected mental disturbances in more than 50%.[12] Many patients who have undergone parathyroidectomy experience a sense of well-being and relief from fatigue and dullness that often was not fully appreciated before surgery. It is well recognized that muscular weakness and fatigue may occur in patients with primary HPT. Most commonly, the weakness is in the proximal muscle groups. In one study, 14 (87.5%) of 16 patients with primary HPT demonstrated weakness, easy fatigability, and muscle atrophy.[13]

Laboratory Diagnosis

The diagnosis of primary HPT is typically made on documentation of an elevated serum calcium concentration, usually in conjunction with an elevated serum intact PTH. The ionized calcium is the active fraction (rather than the protein bound portion), although the reliability and reproducibility of the measurement technique can be limiting. Ionized calcium is useful in defining biochemically subtle disease. The finding of an elevated plasma level of PTH does not in itself establish the diagnosis of HPT. One must evaluate the PTH level as a function of the serum calcium concentration. Subjects with increased serum concentrations of both calcium and PTH generally have HPT.

Approximately half of patients with primary HPT have hypophosphatemia. However, in the presence of significant renal impairment, serum phosphate levels may be elevated. Because of the effect of PTH on bicarbonate excretion in the kidney, patients with primary HPT often have a hyperchloremic metabolic acidosis. Ten to 40% of patients with HPT have increased levels of alkaline phosphatase, which indicates some degree of bone disease. Dual-energy x-ray absorption scanning of the lumbar spine, hip, and forearm has become the standard method for assessing bone density to diagnose osteoporosis in the setting of primary HPT. The demonstration of osteopenia may help establish the importance of primary HPT in the patient's overall health and may document the need for intervention in patients who are otherwise asymptomatic.

Hyperparathyroidism in Pregnancy

Primary HPT in pregnancy is rare and is associated with neonatal tetany, stillbirth, and spontaneous abortion. The risk of fetal complications appears to be higher if it is left untreated. When the diagnosis is made, the mother should undergo operation, if possible, during the second trimester.

TABLE 35-2. Presenting Symptoms in 100 Patients with Primary Hyperparathyroidism

Symptom	Percentage of Population
Nephrolithiasis	30
Bone disease	2
Peptic ulcer disease	12
Psychiatric disorders	15
Muscle weakness	70
Constipation	32
Polyuria	28
Pancreatitis	1
Myalgia	54
Arthralgia	54

Neonatal Primary Hyperparathyroidism and Familial Hypocalciuric Hypercalcemia

Neonatal primary HPT and familial hypocalciuric hypercalcemia (FHH) are caused by a defect in the gene coding for the calcium-sensing receptor.[14] Homozygote infants present with hypotonia, poor feeding, constipation, and respiratory distress (neonatal severe HPT). The 1-year survival in symptomatic untreated patients is less than 50%. Total parathyroidectomy with autotransplantation is the treatment of choice. Heterozygotes for calcium-sensing receptor gene defects have FHH. This benign condition manifests later in life as an elevation in the calcium set point, causing an elevated serum calcium level and mildly elevated serum PTH level without complications of primary HPT. This disease can be distinguished from primary HPT by a low 24-hour urine calcium measurement.

Hyperparathyroid Crisis

Most patients presenting with primary HPT are mildly, chronically ill with symptoms referable to the kidneys or the skeleton. The earliest complaints, such as muscle weakness, anorexia, nausea, constipation, polyuria, and polydipsia, occasionally cause the patient to seek medical advice. Often the examining physician does not suspect primary HPT. Rarely, however, patients may become acutely ill, which is termed *acute HPT* and *hyperparathyroid crisis*. The onset is usually characterized by rapidly developing muscular weakness, nausea and vomiting, weight loss, fatigue, drowsiness, and confusion. The serum calcium concentration is almost always remarkably elevated (16 to 20 mg/dL). Hypercalcemic crisis can also occur due to malignancy (typically multiple myeloma, some lymphomas or leukemias, and breast, lung, or pancreatic carcinoma). In hyperparathyroid crisis, the offending parathyroid gland is usually large, and in about one third of the patients, a tumor is palpable in the neck before surgery. The genesis of the condition involves uncontrolled PTH secretion followed by hypercalcemia, polyuria, dehydration, and reduced renal function, which worsens the hypercalcemia.

The management of severe hypercalcemia addresses four main goals: (1) to correct dehydration, (2) to enhance renal excretion of calcium, (3) to inhibit bone resorption, and (4) to treat the underlying disorder. Although the definitive therapy is resection of the hyperfunctioning parathyroid tissue, it is unwise to proceed with neck exploration until the calcium concentration is lowered. Resuscitation with 0.9% NaCl is instituted to maintain urinary output above 100 mL/hr (typically an extra 2 to 4 L/day or more if tolerated), and subsequent diuresis with loop diuretics (furosemide) increases the renal excretion of sodium and calcium. If the serum calcium level remains elevated despite this, other agents that can lower the serum calcium concentration should be administered (e.g., bisphosphonates, calcitonin). Their use is summarized in Table 35-3.

Secondary and Tertiary Hyperparathyroidism

In contrast to the intrinsic feedback inhibition defect of primary HPT, secondary HPT is caused by chronic extrinsic overstimulation of otherwise normal parathyroid glands—almost always in the setting of chronic renal failure. Secondary HPT develops as a complex sequence of interactions. As glomerular filtration rate falls, the renal production of 1,25-dihydroxyvitamin D_3 decreases, which then reduces intestinal calcium absorption to create a negative calcium balance. A compensatory increase in PTH secretion keeps serum calcium near normal by mobilizing calcium from bone. PTH secretion is further stimulated by hyperphosphatemia (via a phosphorus-specific receptor) and a decrease in ionized calcium (from reduced solubility caused by hyperphosphatemia). Intact PTH levels of 500 to 1500 pg/mL are common (normal, 10 to 65 pg/mL). Long-standing hyperparathormonemia contributes to alteration of the set point of the parathyroid cells to feedback inhibition from ionized calcium. Tertiary HPT follows long-standing secondary HPT when the chronically stimulated parathyroid glands act independently of the serum calcium concentration. Autonomous hypersecretion of PTH may persist despite correction of the underlying condition (such as renal transplantation) or can manifest itself as new refractory hypercalcemia following previously stable secondary HPT. The distinction between secondary and tertiary HPT is not important because the indications and rationale for surgical therapy are the same.

Parathyroid Carcinoma

Parathyroid carcinoma is present in 0.5% or less of patients with primary HPT, but this figure varies with

---

TABLE 35-3. Agents Used in the Treatment of Severe Hypercalcemia

Agent	Dosing	Comment
Calcitonin	4–8 IU/kg subcutaneous q 6–12 hr for 2–3 days	Onset rapid but effect is short lived; nausea and flushing are side effects
Bisphosphonates	Pamidronate 45–90 mg IV	Onset 1–2 days; can be repeated after 7 days

referral patterns and specific diagnostic criteria. In contrast with benign primary HPT, patients are often younger at diagnosis and gender distribution is equal. The symptoms and biochemical perturbations are often, but not always, profound at diagnosis. Many patients have nausea, vomiting, dehydration, polyuria, generalized weakness, and weight loss. In about 50% of patients with parathyroid carcinoma, the involved parathyroid gland is palpable, a finding rarely observed in patients with benign primary HPT. In one series, the mean calcium level at diagnosis was 13.7 mg/dL.[15] Elevated serum alkaline phosphatase level is common.

SURGICAL MANAGEMENT OF HYPERPARATHYROIDISM

Primary Hyperparathyroidism: Operative Versus Nonoperative Management

Serum calcium level is commonly measured, and thus the diagnosis of primary HPT is often made in asymptomatic patients. There is general agreement that most *symptomatic* patients should undergo parathyroidectomy. However, some physicians have proposed that *asymptomatic* patients be followed without operative intervention. A National Institutes of Health Consensus Development Conference reviewed the available data on this subject in 1990.[16] A second conference took place in 2002 to review and revise the recommendations.[17] The panel again agreed that parathyroidectomy is indicated for all patients with symptoms. The indications for operation in asymptomatic patients were outlined as follows:

1. Significant hypercalcemia (serum calcium = 1 mg/dL above the upper limit of normal reference range)

2. Significant hypercalciuria (24-hour urinary calcium excretion ≥ 400 mg)
3. Creatinine clearance reduced by 30% compared to age-matched subjects
4. Decreased bone density at the lumbar spine, hip, or distal radius (as determined by dual-energy x-ray absorptiometry) that is more than 2.5 SDs below peak bone mass (*t*-score <−2.5)
5. Age younger than 50 years
6. Patients for whom medical surveillance is either not desirable or not possible

If patients are to be managed without operation, they must have serum calcium measurements every 6 months and bone mineral densitometry on a yearly basis. Surgical indications are outlined in Box 35-1.

Operative Approaches for Primary Hyperparathyroidism: Standards and Developments

Parathyroidectomy without preoperative localization studies enjoys a high success rate (>95%) and low complication rate (<2%). Despite this, the specific operative approach continues to evolve through the influence of a number of synergistic factors, including (1) improvements

---

> **Box 35-1. Indications for Operative Treatment of Asymptomatic Patients with Primary Hyperparathyroidism**
>
> On initial evaluation of a patient with a known complication of primary hyperparathyroidism such as
>   Overtly symptomatic hypercalcemia
>   Nephrolithiasis
>   Neuromuscular symptoms
>   Neuropsychological symptoms
>   Bone disease
>   Pancreatitis
>   Peptic ulcer disease
> Patients who request operative intervention
> During monitoring of an asymptomatic patient with
>   Significant hypercalcemia (≥1 mg/dL above the upper limit of reference range)
>   Significant hypercalciuria (24-hour calcium excretion ≥400 mg/day)
>   Creatinine clearance reduced 30% from age-matched subjects
>   Decreased bone mineral density at lumbar spine, hip, or distal radius >2.5 SDs below peak bone mass (*t*-score <−2.5)
>   Age <50 years
>   Factors that make ongoing close surveillance difficult

---

in ^{99m}Tc-sestamibi scintigraphy and high-resolution cervical ultrasound; (2) rapid intraoperative PTH measurement; and (3) adjunctive surgical technologies such as hand-held gamma detection probes and small videoscopic equipment. A confusing plethora of options exists, but all rely on accurate preoperative localization. Although these studies occasionally localize an adenoma that would have been relatively more difficult to find during standard exploration, the net result is to influence patient selection so that "easy" explorations become even easier. However, difficult explorations will remain difficult. Therefore, any surgeon performing parathyroidectomy must be completely facile and comfortable with standard four-gland parathyroid exploration, or else parathyroidectomy will lose its standing as a successful, low-morbidity procedure.

Conventional Exploration

General or locoregional anesthesia is used, and the neck is opened through a 2.5 to 4.0-cm transverse cervical incision (Fig. 35-3). Subplatysmal flaps are developed to the level of the thyroid cartilage above and the sternal notch below and onto the sternocleidomastoid muscles laterally (Fig. 35-4). After the strap muscles are separated in the midline (Fig. 35-5), a lobe of the thyroid gland is elevated and rotated medially. The initial critical maneuver is complete division of connective tissue between the thyroid and carotid sheath to widely open the prevertebral space (Fig. 35-6). The tissues inferior to the thyroid lobe are cleaned down to the trachea to locate the RLN and the inferior thyroid artery. In most patients, the RLN lies in the

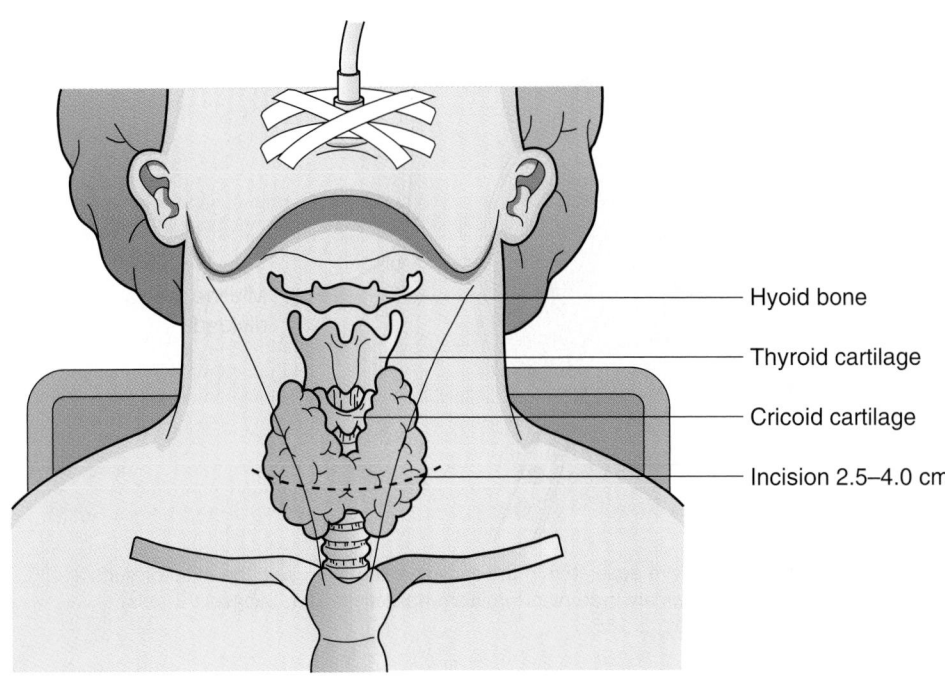

FIGURE 35-3. The incision is placed over the isthmus of the thyroid gland, which lies about 1 cm caudal to the palpable cricoid cartilage. The entire central compartment of the neck can be explored through the small incision, although it cannot all be seen at one time. (From Yim JH, Doherty GM: Operative strategies in primary hyperparathyroidism. *In* Doherty GM, Skogseid B [eds]: Surgical Endocrinology. Philadelphia, Lippincott Williams & Wilkins, 2001, p 164.)

Hyoid bone

Thyroid cartilage

Cricoid cartilage

Incision 2.5–4.0 cm

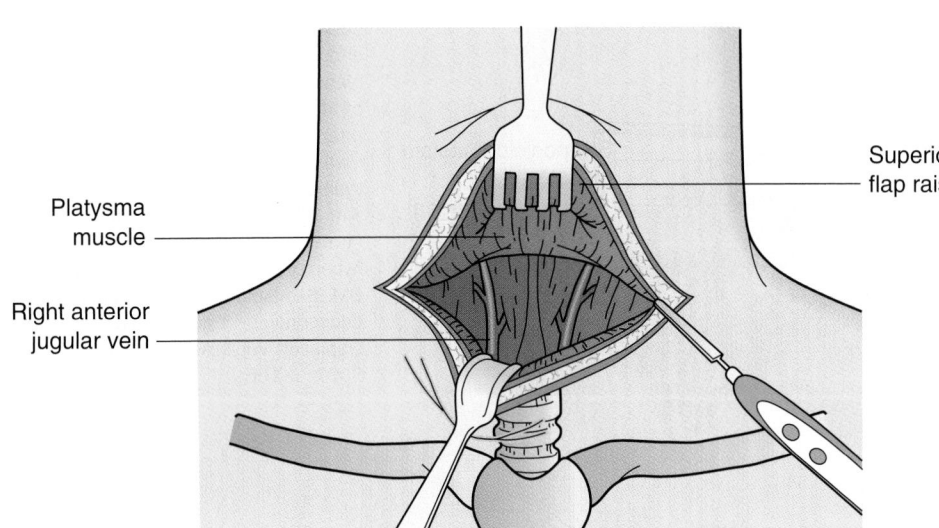

FIGURE 35-4. Flaps are raised deep to the platysma and superficial to the anterior jugular veins. The wide flaps can compensate for a smaller skin incision and can be retracted to expose the various sites in the neck to be explored. (From Yim JH, Doherty GM: Operative strategies in primary hyperparathyroidism. *In* Doherty GM, Skogseid B [eds]: Surgical Endocrinology. Philadelphia, Lippincott Williams & Wilkins, 2001, p 164.)

Superior flap raised

Platysma muscle

Right anterior jugular vein

tracheoesophageal groove; less commonly, it is lateral to the trachea; and rarely, it is anterolateral to the trachea, where it is especially vulnerable to injury. To be certain that one has identified parathyroid tissue, a small biopsy of the suspicious tissue may be necessary but is not routine. The glands must be handled with great care because their blood supply is easily damaged. Although the pathologist can readily distinguish parathyroid from other tissue on frozen section, it is usually not possible to discriminate between parathyroid *adenoma* and *hyperplasia*. Because of the possibility of multiple-gland involvement, every effort must be made to identify all four parathyroids. Complete exploration requires great patience.

The typical anatomic distribution of parathyroid glands was delineated earlier, but even more important is the understanding of atypical locations for normal glands and typical locations for abnormal glands. The most common distribution of superior parathyroid adenomas (normally and ectopically located) is shown in Figure 35-7, and the distribution of inferior parathyroid adenomas is shown in Figure 35-8. When a parathyroid cannot be located during thorough exploration, the surgeon must re-evaluate the findings de novo while remembering basic embryologic and anatomic principles. Critical in determining the next sequence of maneuvers is the inference of which gland is missing—the superior or the inferior—based on proper identification of normal glands already found. Because the RLN obliquely bisects the lateral view of the trachea and esophagus, the inferior gland should generally be located anterior and caudal to this plane (Fig. 35-9). The superior

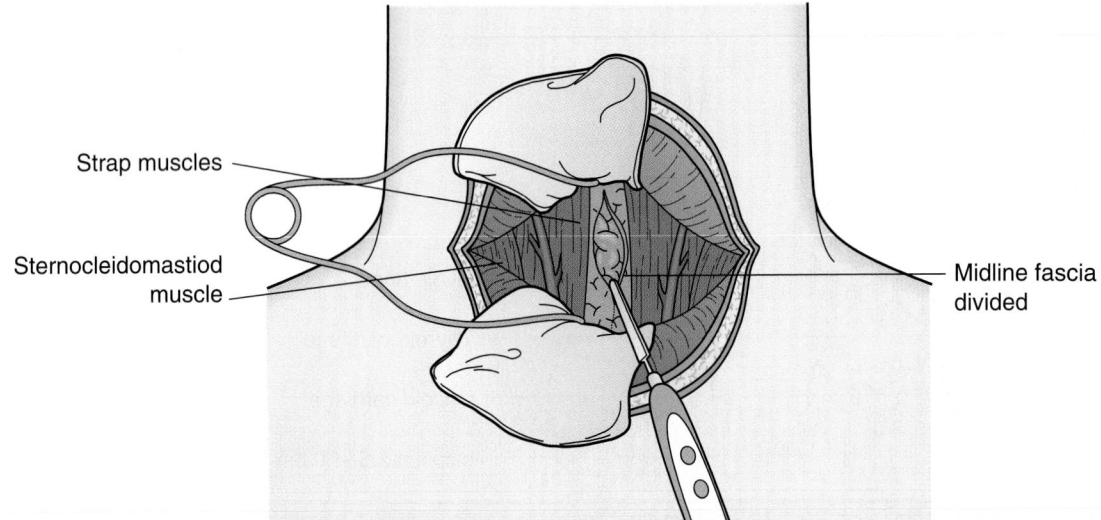

Strap muscles

Sternocleidomastiod
muscle

Midline fascia
divided

FIGURE 35-5.   The paired sternohyoid and sternothyroid muscles are separated in the midline raphe to expose the anterior surface of the thyroid gland. (From Yim JH, Doherty GM: Operative strategies in primary hyperparathyroidism. *In* Doherty GM, Skogseid B [eds]: Surgical Endocrinology. Philadelphia, Lippincott Williams & Wilkins, 2001, p 165.)

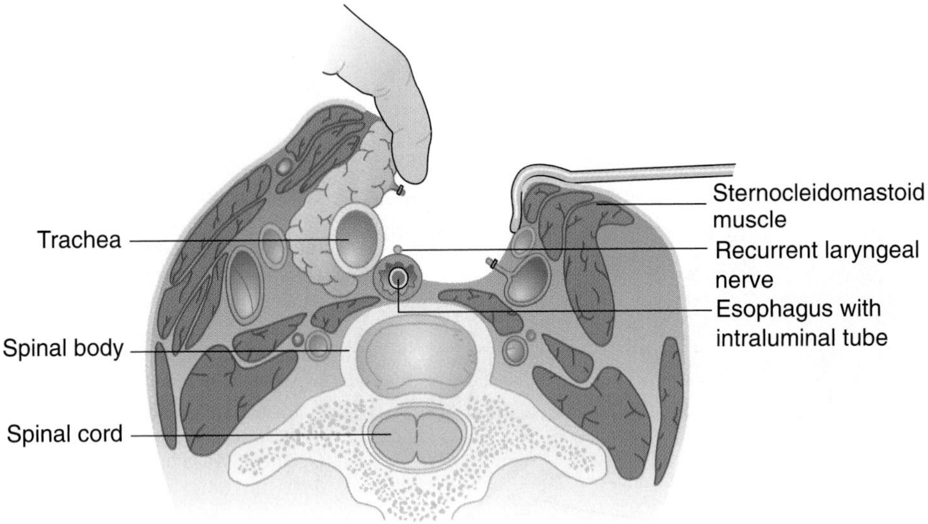

FIGURE 35-6.   The prevertebral plane is found at the posterior aspect of the pharynx and esophagus. Entry into this plane allows for medial retraction of all tissue medial to the carotid artery to assist in visual and manual inspection of the tracheoesophageal groove. (From Yim JH, Doherty GM: Operative strategies in primary hyperparathyroidism. *In* Doherty GM, Skogseid B [eds]: Surgical Endocrinology. Philadelphia, Lippincott Williams & Wilkins, 2001, p 166.)

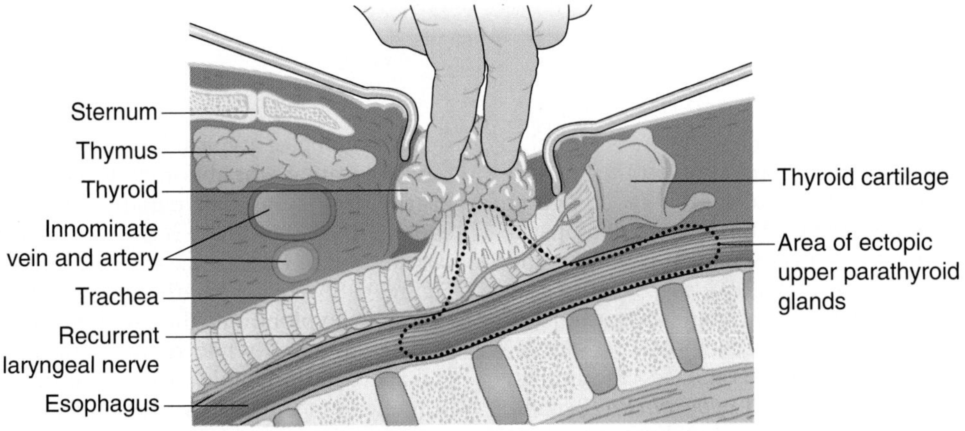

Trachea

Spinal body

Spinal cord

Sternocleidomastoid muscle

Recurrent laryngeal nerve

Esophagus with intraluminal tube

Sternum

Thymus

Thyroid

Innominate vein and artery

Trachea

Recurrent laryngeal nerve

Esophagus

Thyroid cartilage

Area of ectopic upper parathyroid glands

FIGURE 35-7.   The upper parathyroid glands are generally located as shown in Figure 35-2. They can be ectopic, particularly if enlarged. The vascular supply and the tip of the gland may remain in the usual position, but the bulk of the gland may be displaced caudad and posteriorly with growth (acquired ectopia). The shaded area shows the common locations for the upper parathyroid glands. (From Yim JH, Doherty GM: Operative strategies in primary hyperparathyroidism. *In* Doherty GM, Skogseid B [eds]: Surgical Endocrinology. Philadelphia, Lippincott Williams & Wilkins, 2001, p 168.)

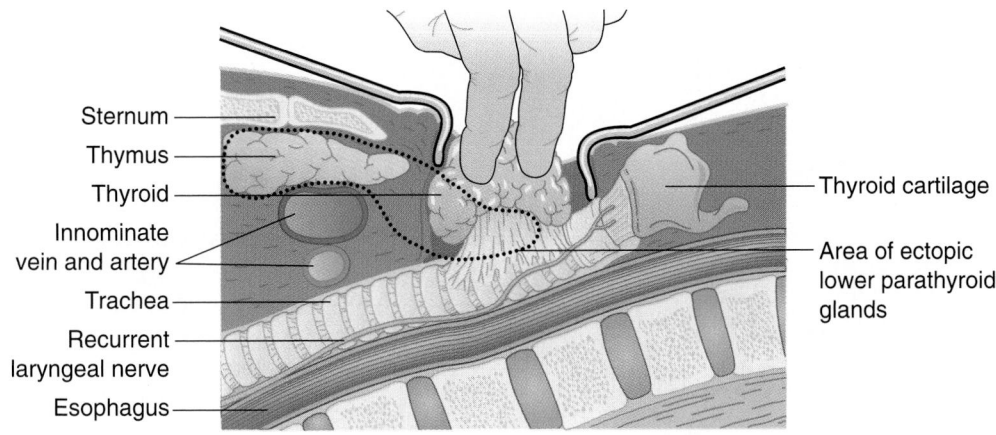

FIGURE 35-8. The lower parathyroid glands can be intimately associated with the thyroid gland and may be difficult to identify in patients with nodular thyroid glands. They may be displaced downward into the mediastinum, as shown in the shaded area, but usually remain anterior to the recurrent laryngeal nerve. (From Yim JH, Doherty GM: Operative strategies in primary hyperparathyroidism. *In* Doherty GM, Skogseid B [eds]: Surgical Endocrinology. Philadelphia, Lippincott Williams & Wilkins, 2001, p 169.)

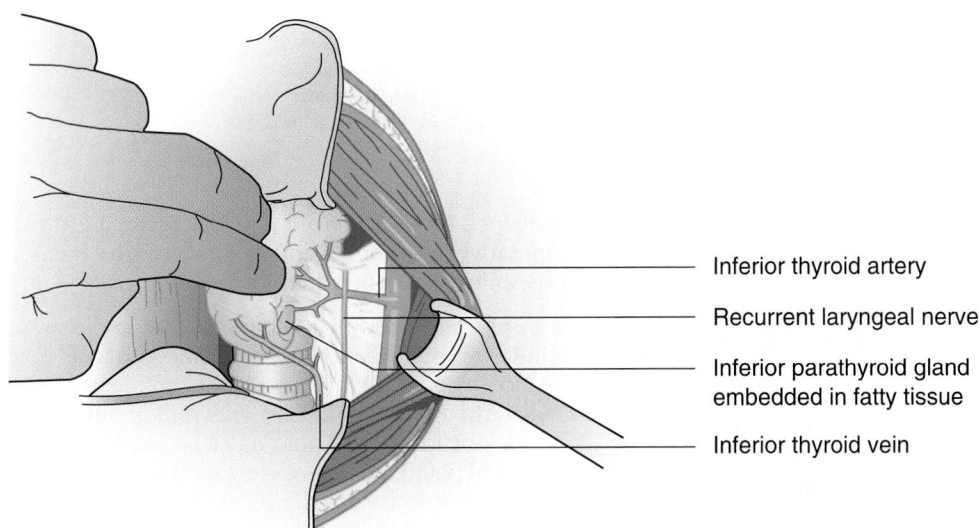

FIGURE 35-9. To expose the lower parathyroid gland, the inferior pole of the thyroid gland is retracted in the direction of the contralateral ear. The soft tissue immediately caudal to the inferior pole of the thyroid gland and anterior to the recurrent laryngeal nerve nearly always contains the parathyroid gland. (From Yim JH, Doherty GM: Operative strategies in primary hyperparathyroidism. *In* Doherty GM, Skogseid B [eds]: Surgical Endocrinology. Philadelphia, Lippincott Williams & Wilkins, 2001, p 167.)

parathyroid gland should be located posterior and cranial to this plane (Fig. 35-10). There is often close association with the tubercle of Zuckerkandl because they share similar embryologic migration.[18] There is contralateral symmetry of superior glands in approximately 80% of patients (inferior in 70%), so the location of a gland on one side can lead to discovery of a difficult-to-find gland on the other. True ectopia of a superior gland is rare. Only 2% to 4% of *normal* superior glands are caudal to the inferior thyroid artery in the tracheoesophageal groove or more cephalad along the superior pole of the thyroid—compressed within its sheath.[7] Less than 1% are even more cephalad in close relationship with the posterior pharyngeal wall.[19] Even so, abnormal superior parathyroid glands often descend to positions of "acquired ectopia" or "pseudoectopia." By far, the most common location is into a paraesophageal or retroesophageal position descending toward the posterior mediastinum; and it is here that

the adenoma is often obvious to the palpating finger of the surgeon before it is visible. A truly intrathyroidal superior parathyroid gland rarely exists, and thyroid lobectomy is not routinely indicated for a missing superior adenoma.

True ectopia (based on embryologic influences) is much more common with inferior parathyroids. Approximately 80% of inferior glands are located within 2 cm of the inferior thyroid pole due to their common migration with the thymus that persists as the nearby *thyrothymic tract.*[20] About 15% are located within the true sheath of the thymic cord.[20] If no parathyroid tissue is found after thymectomy, the surgeon should mobilize, examine, and palpate the ipsilateral lobe of the thyroid gland because occasionally (1% to 4%) an inferior parathyroid is completely encapsulated within the thyroid parenchyma.[21] Intraoperative ultrasound may assist with this assessment. Removal of a thyroid lobe on the side where an inferior

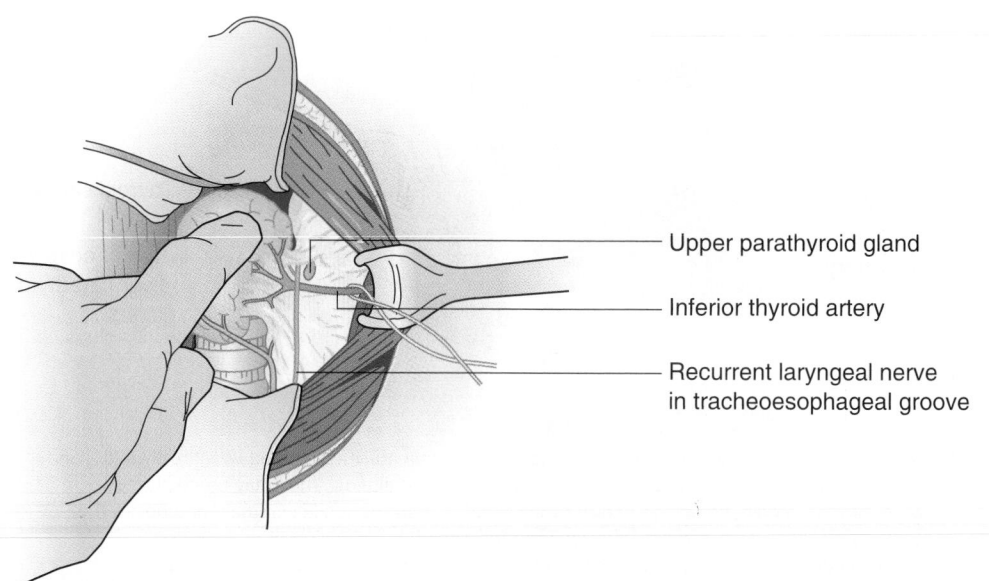

Upper parathyroid gland

Inferior thyroid artery

Recurrent laryngeal nerve
in tracheoesophageal groove

FIGURE 35-10.   To expose the upper parathyroid gland, the thyroid lobe is retracted in the direction of the contralateral shoulder. The recurrent laryngeal nerve is identified in the tracheoesophageal groove. Often, when the nerve is identified, the parathyroid gland is identified also, lying over the nerve near the inferior thyroid artery. The superior parathyroid gland is often found within the confines of an imaginary 2-cm circle located craniad to the intersection of the recurrent laryngeal nerve and the inferior thyroid artery. (From Yim JH, Doherty GM: Operative strategies in primary hyperparathyroidism. *In* Doherty GM, Skogseid B [eds]: Surgical Endocrinology. Philadelphia, Lippincott Williams & Wilkins, 2001, p 166.)

gland is not found is occasionally indicated as a last resort but must not substitute for a meticulous search for parathyroid tissue.

The definitive operative management depends on the number of enlarged parathyroid glands. In fact, the definition of multiglandular disease is a current controversy that considers both gross morphologic features and functional information gained from intraoperative PTH monitoring. While the definition of multiglandular disease is under debate, it is useful to consider that approximately 80% to 90% of patients with HPT undergoing parathyroidectomy are likely to have their disease caused by a single enlarged gland. If one gland is large and the remaining three are of normal size, resection of the enlarged gland is curative in nearly all patients. However, sometimes it is possible to locate three normal parathyroid glands while the adenoma causing the disease is not evident. With this information, an algorithm can be developed to guide the "failing" exploration to make certain that every possibility of curing the patient is provided at the initial operation.

If the missing adenoma is an inferior gland, the next regions to be explored include medially on the anterior tracheal surface, laterally toward the carotid sheath and inferiorly to expose the cervical thymic horn. If the inferior adenoma is not found, a sequence of the following three maneuvers is undertaken:

1. A full cervical thymectomy is performed.
2. The ipsilateral carotid sheath is opened to visually and manually explore the contents to at least the level of the arterial bifurcation.

3. The ipsilateral inferior thyroid pole is interrogated with intraoperative ultrasound and/or resected to include the possibility of an intrathyroidal gland.

If it is a superior gland that is missing, the exploration must include the region encompassing the superior pole of the thyroid. Specifically, the posterolateral aspect, the most cranial tip of the pole and the region medial to the posterior portion of the pole must be explored. The retropharyngeal plane must be widely mobilized for visual and manual inspection from the level of the hyoid bone to the posterior mediastinum. A superior gland may be "undescended" and be found above the level of the thyroid associated with some residual thymic tissue. The tracheoesophageal groove along the RLN should be explored. Rarely, a gland is discovered in the lateral neck associated with the scalene fat pad.

If, despite the maneuvers described earlier, the causative parathyroid adenoma is still not found, it is wise to gently perform small biopsies of each identified parathyroid gland to confirm the surgeon's assessment of which glands are accounted for. Under no circumstances should morphologically normal parathyroid glands be removed in an attempt to decrease PTH levels. Along these lines, it is critical that a detailed operative report is created that explains the specific anatomic locations of the normal glands as well as the specific exploratory maneuvers undertaken. Depending on the biochemical and clinical severity of the persistent disease, the patient will eventually need to undergo a number of localization studies before another exploration is undertaken. These are explained later.

In the event that two or three parathyroid glands are enlarged, most surgeons resect them, leaving the normal-sized glands undisturbed. The question of whether these represent multiple adenomas or primary hyperplasia has not been resolved. Of 76 patients treated in this manner and followed for up to 140 months, 8 (10.5%) had recurrent hypercalcemia.[22] This recurrent disease tended to be mild, and it was concluded that this management is generally acceptable.

In patients with generalized (glandular) enlargement or parathyroid hyperplasia, the surgical management is more difficult and the postoperative results are less satisfactory. Parathyroid hyperplasia occurs in two forms: water-clear cell hyperplasia and chief cell hyperplasia. Clinically, the forms are indistinguishable, but the gross appearance at operation can be quite suggestive. In the former, all four glands are diffusely enlarged and dark brown, with uneven surfaces and numerous pseudopods. In the latter, there may be a great difference in the size of the glands, with the superior frequently being larger than the inferior. Chief cell hyperplasia is the pathologic entity most commonly associated with familial HPT, particularly multiple endocrine neoplasia (MEN) type 1.

The standard therapy for patients with HPT and generalized parathyroid enlargement has been subtotal ($3\frac{1}{2}$-gland) parathyroidectomy. In patients with sporadic parathyroid hyperplasia, the reported incidence of recurrent hypercalcemia is 0 to 16%. The incidence of permanent hypoparathyroidism is 4% to 5%. However, patients with MEN type 1 have a recurrent hypercalcemia rate of 26% to 36% with long-term follow-up. One institution with a lower reported rate of recurrence also reports a high rate of permanent hypoparathyroidism (25%).[23] Because of the relatively increased incidence of postoperative hypoparathyroidism and HPT in patients with *familial parathyroid hyperplasia*, many surgeons have elected to treat these patients by total parathyroidectomy and heterotopic autotransplantation. In humans, normal and abnormal parathyroid glands eventually function as autografts when they are immediately implanted into muscle. The autograft tissue is sliced into 20 to 25 very small pieces for subsequent implantation into a muscle bed. This increases surface area of the graft tissue that is angiogenic. This operation has the advantage of allowing re-exploration for recurrent HPT to take place in the nondominant forearm rather than the neck. In either operation, parathyroid tissue should be cryopreserved. Tissue can be viably frozen in dimethyl sulfoxide and in autologous serum for more than 12 to 18 months. This capability offers the surgeon great versatility because when there is uncertainty about the amount of parathyroid tissue in a patient undergoing reoperation, a portion can be viably frozen to await the postoperative course. If the patient becomes hypocalcemic, parts of the frozen autologous parathyroid tissue can be reimplanted.

Targeted Exploration

Currently, there is a profusion of different "minimally invasive parathyroidectomy" procedures in practice. Whether conventional instruments, intraoperative radioguidance,

or videoscopic technology is employed is not the central issue. The essential change from conventional management is more strategic than it is procedural and can be summarized in two cardinal issues: (1) reliance on preoperative localization of the adenoma by sestamibi scintigraphy or high-resolution ultrasound, and (2) intraoperative indication of cure that does not require morphologic assessment of uninvolved normal glands (e.g., intraoperative PTH monitoring). The main advantages of this "concise" strategy are that it easily allows the use of local anesthesia and sedation to facilitate same-day discharge and greatly decreases the role of frozen section. The main objections are that it increases preoperative costs and that it fails to identify some patients with multigland disease. A fascinating observation that has emerged from this recent experience is that the defined prevalence of multiglandular disease may be lower if the determination is made by functional means (PTH monitoring) versus morphologic means (surgeon inspection).[24,25]

Intraoperative PTH monitoring is predicated on the fact that intact PTH has an extremely short half life (2.5 to 4.5 minutes) and that large decrements can be measured in 10 to 15 minutes. The most commonly used criterion to define cure is a 50% fall from the baseline level by 10 minutes following gland resection. It is important that the baseline level used to index the values in each patient be remeasured immediately before adenoma removal. The baseline can be prematurely lowered by aggressive dissection and or falsely elevated by even gentle manipulation of the gland.

Persistent or Recurrent Hyperparathyroidism

Biochemical HPT evident within the first 6 months after exploration is termed *persistent*. It is usually caused by failure to find the causative adenoma or a second adenoma, or failure to recognize and aggressively treat hyperplasia. *Recurrent* disease occurs after 6 months and is often caused by growth of hyperplastic tissue knowingly or unknowingly left behind at the initial operation. It can also result from autotransplanted tissue or parathyromatosis (diffuse soft tissue implants from spontaneous or iatrogenic tumor rupture). Metachronous second adenomas are rarely the cause. The diagnosis of HPT must be reconfirmed before re-exploration, and urinary calcium level should be measured to rule out FHH if PTH levels are within 15% of the upper limit of normal. Patients should have clear indications for surgical management of their disease such as significant hypercalcemia, nephrolithiasis, or osteopenia. The site of missed disease is often discernible from careful scrutiny of the sequence of operative decisions and events during the original operation.

In contrast to initial operation, surgeons agree that localization studies must be performed before re-exploration. This necessity is reflected in the fact that the likelihood of cure in the best hands may only approach 50% to 60% if the tumor is not localized preoperatively, but should be 90% if preoperative localization is successful. A wise practice is to offer reoperation when two localization studies are in agreement. Noninvasive studies such

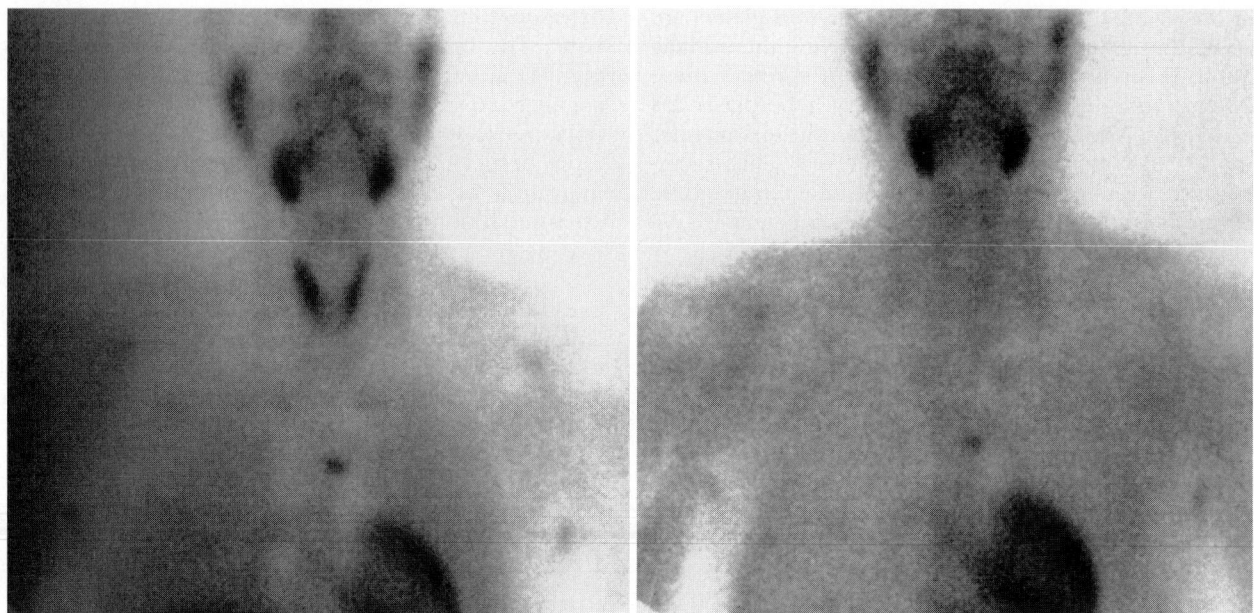

FIGURE 35-11.   Dual-phase ^{99m}Tc-sestamibi scintigraphy in a 22-year-old man with persistent hyperparathyroidism following a cervical exploration during which no inferior parathyroid glands were identified. Anteroposterior views are shown (early on left, delayed on right). Note the persistent focus of activity in the mediastinum that corresponded to an ectopic inferior parathyroid gland within the thymus.

as ^{99m}Tc-sestamibi scintigraphy or cervical ultrasound are usually pursued first (Fig. 35-11). Some centers aspirate the potential occult adenoma under ultrasound guidance to confirm high levels of PTH in the target tissue. Computed tomographic and magnetic resonance images are of limited use for occult disease in the neck near the thyroid. However, either technique can be valuable in detecting the ectopic occult adenoma in the thoracic inlet or mediastinum. Invasive studies are often required to corroborate imaging studies. Selective venous sampling for PTH requires multilevel sampling in bilateral internal jugular veins, innominate veins, and the superior vena cava. Superselective catheterization of the superior thyroid veins, thymic veins, and supreme intercostal veins can add additional information. A step-up in PTH concentration in the specified venous effluent is able to regionally localize approximately 80% of tumors (Fig. 35-12). Selective arteriography of the superior and inferior thyroid arteries and thymic arteries may demonstrate an occult adenoma in up to 60% of patients—especially within the mediastinum. In a patient not suited for operation, therapeutic embolization is possible.

Reoperation for an occult cervical adenoma usually utilizes the previous incision. If a superior gland is suspected, the lateral approach is ideal to establish a less distorted route of access. The plane lateral to the strap muscles and medial to the sternocleidomastoid is developed (Fig. 35-13). The contents of the carotid sheath are gently retracted laterally and the area adjacent to the thyroid and the tracheoesophageal axis is exposed. This approach emphasizes early identification of the RLN and is consequently quite safe.[26] If an inferior parathyroid gland is the target of re-exploration, a low anterior approach reopening the midline raphe exposes the lower thyroid lobes,

trachea, and cervical thymus. Inferior thyroid pole resection is easily performed for the intrathyroidal adenoma. This approach provides access for cervical thymectomy. Blunt dissection and firm, consistent traction on the cervical thymus allows delivery of the entire gland and any contained adenoma. In the past, mediastinal adenomas were estimated to account for 20% of persistent or recurrent disease. However, that definition was made in relation to the clavicles. As most of these tumors are accessible through routine cervical exploration, true deep mediastinal adenomas are present in no more than 2% of patients.

With the exception of patients with hyperparathyroid crisis in whom thorough cervical exploration fails to uncover the abnormal parathyroid gland, mediastinotomy is best deferred until the diagnostic and localizing tests discussed earlier are completed. For mediastinal exploration, a vertical incision is made from the center of the cervical incision. The sternum is either partially divided past the manubrium or completely divided to the xyphoid, and a spreading retractor is inserted. The remaining thymus tissue is first isolated and examined for adenomatous tissue. If the anterior mediastinal exploration is negative, the posterior mediastinum is next examined, especially posterior and lateral to the trachea.

Secondary and Tertiary Hyperparathyroidism

Careful medical management prevents most patients (>90%) from requiring surgical intervention. Oral calcium and 1,25-D_3 supplementation are instituted as renal function worsens. Vitamin D_2 supplements are not effective because the failing kidney cannot convert the vitamin

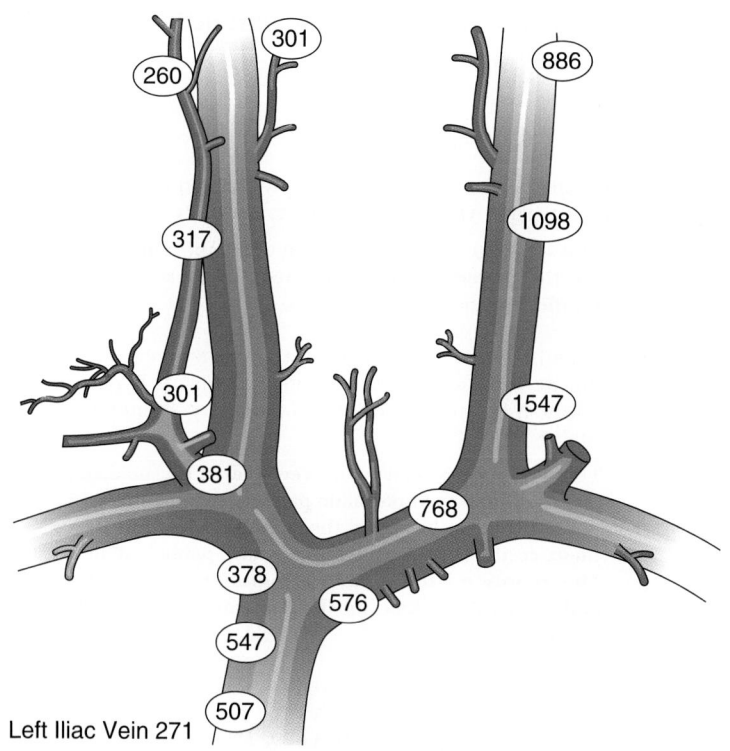

FIGURE 35-12. Example of data obtained from selective venous sampling study in a patient with persistent primary hyperparathyroidism. The step-up was located in the region of the left internal jugular vein, which indicated the presence of an adenoma high in the left neck. This was confirmed at reoperation to be an undescended inferior parathyroid adenoma in the carotid sheath near the arterial bifurcation.

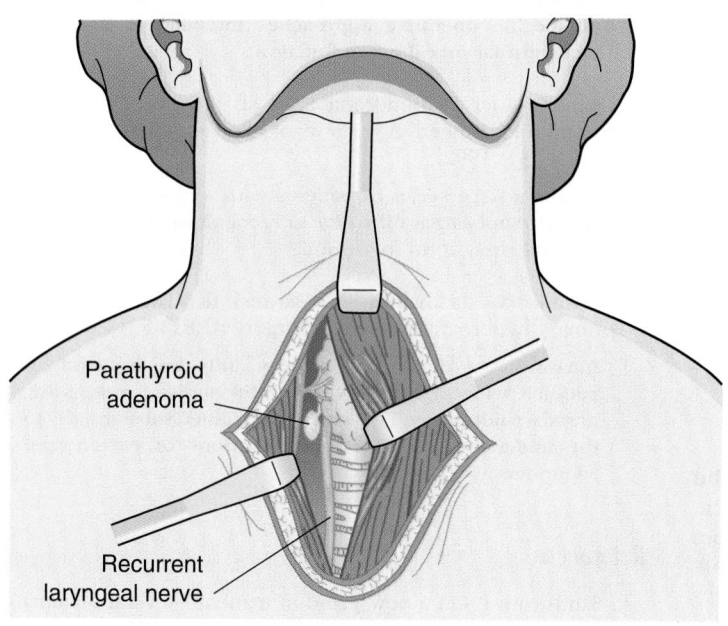

FIGURE 35-13. The lateral approach during reoperation may provide unimpeded access to a superior parathyroid adenoma while allowing safe identification of the recurrent laryngeal nerve. (From Gauger PG, Thompson NW: Persistent or recurrent hyperparathyroidism. *In* Cameron JL [ed]: Current Surgical Therapy, 7th ed. St. Louis, Mosby, 2001, p 669.)

to active form. Oral phosphate binders (e.g., calcium acetate) and dietary adjustments are used to control hyperphosphatemia. Parathyroidectomy is indicated when medical management fails to prevent or control significant morbidity. Indications include musculoskeletal complications such as bone and joint pain, generalized muscular weakness, decreasing bone density under serial measurement, and pathologic fractures. Symptomatic soft tissue

calcification and severe pruritus may occur. Open skin lesions mandate urgent skin biopsy to establish the diagnosis of calciphylaxis (medial arterial calcification), which requires urgent parathyroidectomy. The development of significant hypercalcemia during treatment for secondary HPT—especially after cessation of calcium and 1,25-D_3—indicates development of tertiary HPT and the need for operation.

Preoperative localization studies are an unnecessary expense and do not obviate the need for thorough bilateral exploration. There are two accepted operations for these conditions: (1) subtotal parathyroidectomy and (2) total parathyroidectomy with heterotopic (nondominant forearm) autotransplantation. A randomized, prospective trial has been reported for patients with secondary HPT comparing these two surgical options.[27] Because of the improved clinical parameters (less pruritus and muscle weakness), the improved radiologic parameters, and no need for reoperation compared with up to 20% who have indications for reoperation after subtotal resection, total parathyroidectomy with autotransplantation was preferred. Subtotal parathyroidectomy requires less costly and intense postoperative medical care because the degree of hypocalcemia (albeit temporary) is not as severe. Additionally, reoperation rates with this approach have been comparably low in many hands. Many surgeons prefer this option, especially if the patient does not appear to have tertiary HPT and anticipates renal transplantation within the next 2 to 3 years. Most other patients appear best served by total parathyroidectomy and autotransplantation.

A complete bilateral neck exploration is undertaken for either procedure. All four enlarged parathyroid glands are located as discussed for standard treatment of primary HPT. Complete cervical thymectomy is mandatory since a supernumerary gland is present in 15% to 20% of patients. For total parathyroidectomy, a 75-mg portion of resected parathyroid is transplanted into individual muscle pockets in the manner described earlier for treatment of parathyroid hyperplasia. For subtotal parathyroidectomy, a similar-sized remnant is preserved on the vascular pedicle, preferably an inferior gland. A metallic clip is used both to facilitate hemostatic division of the parathyroid gland as well as to mark the position of the remnant. The viability of the remnant is ensured under observation before the remainder of the parathyroid glands are completely resected.

Parathyroid Carcinoma

It is important to recognize parathyroid carcinoma at the initial neck exploration because radical resection of the malignant parathyroid gland, the ipsilateral thyroid lobe, and involved adjacent soft tissue offers the only possibility for cure. Unfortunately, the diagnosis is not always made intraoperatively. Nineteen percent of patients did not have parathyroid carcinoma recognized at operation in one series.[28] Histologic diagnosis can be difficult. Some factors such as capsular and/or vascular invasion can clearly support the diagnosis, whereas others such as fibrosis, nuclear atypia, and mitotic figures can be seen in equivocal cases as well. Currently, there is no completely reliable molecular marker for diagnosis, but assessment of the proliferative activity of the tumor with immunostaining for Ki-67 can be quite valuable.[29] The long-term prognosis is poor; the opportunity for survival depends on complete initial resection.[30] If disease recurs, reoperation is indicated (including resection of pulmonary and liver metastases) because patients, if untreated, die of uncontrolled hypercalcemia.

Selected References

Åkerström G, Malmaeus J, Bergström R: Surgical anatomy of human parathyroid glands. Surgery 95:14-21, 1984.

This is a large autopsy study that was important in increasing the understanding of the many typical and atypical locations of parathyroid glands.

Bilezikian JP, Potts JT Jr, Fuleihan EH, et al: Summary statement from a workshop on asymptomatic primary hyperparathyroidism: A perspective for the 21st century. J Clin Endocrinol Metab 87:5353-5361, 2002.

This is a recent review and revision of the management principles for asymptomatic patients with primary hyperparathyroidism based on the original consensus development conference findings that were published in 1991. This represents the combined opinions of many medical and surgical leaders in the treatment of parathyroid disease.

Moley JF, Lairmore TC, Doherty GM, et al: Preservation of the recurrent laryngeal nerves in thyroid and parathyroid reoperations. Surgery 125:673-679, 1999.

This is a large series of 132 patients undergoing thyroid or parathyroid reoperations. It provides useful descriptions of specific operative approaches intended to preserve recurrent laryngeal nerve function.

Sandelin K, Auer G, Bondeson L, et al: Prognostic factors in parathyroid cancer: A review of 95 cases. World J Surg 16:724-731, 1992.

This is a large series of patients with a rare cancer. This report emphasizes difficulty in recognition and the need for close long-term follow-up.

Thompson NW, Eckhauser FE, Harness JK: The anatomy of primary hyperparathyroidism. Surgery 92:814-821, 1982.

In contrast to Åkerström's autopsy study, this is a study of patients with primary hyperparathyroidism undergoing parathyroidectomy. This study contributed substantially to the understanding of ectopic locations of parathyroid adenomas.

References

1. Sandstrom I: On a new gland in man and several mammals (glandulae parathyroideae). Ups Lak Foren Forh 15:441, 1879.
2. Schlagenhaufer F: Zwei faller von parathyreoideatumoren. Wien Klin Wochenschr 28:1362, 1915.
3. Mandl F: Therapeutischer versuch bein einem falle von ostitis fibrosa generalisata mittels exstirpation eines epithelkorperchen tumors. Zentrabl Chir 5:260, 1926.
4. Rasmussen H, Craig LC: Purification of the parathyroid hormone by use of countercurrent distribution. J Am Chem Soc 81:5003, 1959.
5. Aurbach GD: Isolation of parathyroid hormone after extraction with phenol. J Biol Chem 234:3179, 1959.
6. Berson SA, Yalow RS, Aurbach GD, et al: Immunoassay of bovine and human parathyroid glands. Surgery 95:14-21, 1963.

7. Åkerström G, Malmaeus J, Bergström R: Surgical anatomy of human parathyroid glands. Surgery 95:14-21, 1984.

8. Tezelman S, Rodriguez JM, Shen W, et al: Primary hyperparathyroidism in patients who have received radiation therapy and in patients who have not received radiation therapy. J Am Coll Surg 180:81-87, 1995.

9. Wells SA, Leight GF, Ross A: Primary hyperparathyroidism. Curr Probl Surg 17:398, 1980.

10. Diamond TW, Both JR, Wing J, et al: Parathyroid hypertension: A reversible disorder. Arch Intern Med 146:1709-1712, 1986.

11. Kochersberger G, Buckley NJ, Leight GS, et al: What is the clinical significance of bone loss in primary hyperparathyroidism? Arch Intern Med 147:1951-1953, 1987.

12. Petersen P: Psychiatric disorders in primary hyperparathyroidism. J Clin Endocrinol Metab 28:1491-1495, 1968.

13. Patten BM, Bilezikian JP, Mallette LE, et al: Neuromuscular disease and primary hyperparathyroidism. Ann Intern Med 80:182-193, 1974.

14. Pollack MR, Brown EM, Chou YHW, et al: Mutations in the human Ca-sensing receptor gene causing familial hypocalciuric hypercalcemia and neonatal severe hyperparathyroidism. Cell 75:1297-1303, 1993.

15. Kebebew E, Arici C, Duh QY, et al: Localization and reoperation results for persistent and recurrent parathyroid carcinoma. Arch Surg 136:878-885, 2001.

16. NIH Conference: Diagnosis and Management of Asymptomatic Primary Hyperparathyroidism: Consensus Development Conference Statement. Ann Intern Med 114:593-597, 1991.

17. Bilezikian JP, Potts JT Jr, Fuleihan EH, et al: Summary Statement from a Workshop on Asymptomatic Primary Hyperparathyroidism: A Perspective for the 21st Century. J Clin Endocrinol Metab 87:5353-5361, 2002.

18. Gauger PG, Delbridge LW, Thompson NW, et al: The incidence and importance of the tubercle of Zuckerkandl in thyroid surgery. Eur J Surg 167:249-254, 2001.

19. Simeone DM, Sandelin K, Thompson NW: Undescended superior parathyroid gland: A potential cause of failed cervical exploration for hyperparathyroidism. Surgery 118:949-956, 1995.

20. Thompson NW, Eckhauser FE, Harness JK: The anatomy of primary hyperparathyroidism. Surgery 92:814-821, 1982.

21. Wheeler MH, Williams ED, Wade JSH: The hyperfunctioning intrathyroidal parathyroid gland: A potential pitfall in parathyroid surgery. World J Surg 11:110-114, 1987.

22. Wells SA Jr, Leight GF, Hensley M, et al: Hyperparathyroidism associated with the enlargement of two or three parathyroid glands. Ann Surg 202:533-538, 1985.

23. van Heerden JA, Kent RB III, Sizemore GW, et al: Primary hyperparathyroidism in patients with multiple endocrine neoplasia syndromes: Surgical experience. Arch Surg 118:533-536, 1983.

24. Molinari AS, Irvin GL III, Deriso GT, et al: Incidence of multiglandular disease in primary hyperparathyroidism determined by parathyroid hormone secretion. Surgery 120:934-936, 1996.

25. Gauger PG, Agarwal G, England BG, et al: Intraoperative parathyroid hormone monitoring fails to detect double parathyroid adenomas: A two-institution experience. Surgery 130:1005-1010, 2001.

26. Moley JF, Lairmore TC, Doherty GM, et al: Preservation of the recurrent laryngeal nerves in thyroid and parathyroid reoperations. Surgery 125:673-679, 1999.

27. Rothmund M, Wagner PK, Schark C: Subtotal parathyroidectomy versus total parathyroidectomy and autotransplantation in secondary hyperparathyroidism: A randomized trial. World J Surg 15:745-750, 1991.

28. Sandelin K, Auer G, Bondeson L, et al: Prognostic factors in parathyroid cancer: A review of 95 cases. World J Surg 16:724-731, 1992.

29. Abbona GC, Papotti M, Gasparri G, et al: Proliferative activity in parathyroid tumors as detected by Ki-67 immunostaining. Hum Pathol 26:135-138, 1995.

30. Wang CA, Gaz RD: Natural history of parathyroid carcinoma: Diagnosis, treatment, and results. Am J Surg 149:522-527, 1985.

CHAPTER 36

ENDOCRINE PANCREAS

James C. Thompson, M.D. and **Courtney M. Townsend, Jr., M.D.**

History	Islet Cell Tumors
Embryology	Medical Therapy for Islet Cell Tumors
Histomorphology of Islets	What's Next?
Endocrine Physiology	

HISTORY

Endocrine cells are diffusely scattered in small clumps throughout the pancreas. While a medical student in 1869, Paul Langerhans described collections of pale-staining cells within the pancreas, the islets that now bear his name. In 1889, Minkowski, after learning that the urine of a pancreatectomized dog attracted flies, analyzed the urine and found glycosuria. Eugene Opie found hyaline changes in the islets of diabetic patients in 1901 and is generally credited with establishing the association between diabetes and islet pathology. In 1908, A. G. Nichols[1] reported a patient with a simple adenoma of islet tissue. Frederick Banting, an orthopedist, and Charles Best, a medical student in Toronto, discovered insulin in 1922, and soon thereafter, insulin became available for the treatment of diabetes. The relationship between hyper-insulinism and an unresectable pancreatic islet cell carcinoma was established by W. J. Mayo, and the first surgical cure of the insulinoma syndrome was achieved by Roscoe Graham in Toronto in 1929. In 1935, Whipple and Frantz[23] described a diagnostic triad for insulinoma: symptoms of hypoglycemia, low concentrations of blood glucose, and relief of symptoms by administration of glucose.

Endocrine cells of the pancreas reside in islets, and the adult human pancreatic islet contains multiple types (Table 36-1): the A (alpha) cell secretes glucagon, the B (beta) cell secretes insulin, the D (delta) cell secretes somatostatin, the D_2 (delta-2) cell secretes vasoactive intestinal peptide (VIP), and the PP (or F) cell secretes pancreatic polypeptide (PP). Enterochromaffin cells are quite rare. Gastrin cells are present normally only in the fetal pancreas. Ectopic gastrin cells may give rise to gastrinomas in the pancreas, duodenum, or adjacent structures. Tumors of any of these cells may in fact secrete

multiple peptides, serially or simultaneously. The syndromes produced are named for the peptide whose symptoms predominate. Thus, the endocrine pancreas may produce insulinomas, glucagonomas, somatostatinomas, VIPomas, PPomas, or gastrinomas. The characteristics of each islet cell tumor syndrome are summarized in Table 36-1.

In 1955, Robert M. Zollinger and Edwin H. Ellison[44] at the Ohio State University Hospital reported on two patients on whom they had operated, both of whom had a fulminant peptic ulcer diathesis, massive acid hyper-secretion, and a non-beta islet cell tumor of the pancreas. Mort Grossman and Rod Gregory determined that the secretagogue was gastrin, and we know that gastrinomas cause Zollinger-Ellison syndrome (ZES).

In 1958, J. V. Verner and A. B. Morrison[59] reported two patients who died of watery diarrhea and hypokalemia, both of whom had been found at autopsy to have benign islet cell tumors. Bloom and colleagues[5] measured high levels of circulating VIP in patients with this watery diarrhea, hypokalemia, and achlorhydria syndrome and proposed VIP to be the responsible agent. In 1942, Becker and colleagues[6] reported on a patient with a severe dermatitis (later determined to be necrolytic migratory erythema), anemia, and diabetes. She was found to have an islet cell carcinoma of the pancreas, but it was not until 1966 that McGavran and associates[7] identified glucagon from an alpha cell carcinoma of the pancreas as the responsible agent. In 1977, two patients with somatostatin-producing islet cell tumors were described in separate reports.[8,9] The syndrome produced is not specific but is usually characterized by diabetes, gallstones, steatorrhea, and hypochlorhydria. The tumor is often discovered at cholecystectomy, and preoperative diagnosis is extraordinarily rare. Many endocrine tumors produce PP,

TABLE 36-1.   Endocrine Cells of Pancreas and Tumor Syndromes

Cells	Content	% Islet Cells	Secretory Granule Size (nm)	Tumor Syndromes	Clinical Features	Diagnostic Hormone Levels	% Malignant	% Multiple	MEN 1	At Operation: % Identified/% Resectable
A	**Glucagon,** glicentin (TRH, CCK, endorphin, PYY, pancreastatin)	15	225	Glucagonoma	Necrolytic migratory erythema, diabetes, anemia	Normal = <150 pg/mL Tumor = 200–2000 pg/mL	Nearly all	Rare	Few	98/35
B	**Insulin** (TRH, CGRP, amylin, pancreastatin, prolactin)	65	300	Insulinoma	Hypoglycemic symptoms (catecholamine release) plus mental confusion	>5 µU/mL in face of hypoglycemia	10	10	10%	80–100/ >90
D	**Somatostatin** (met-encephalon)	5	200–235	Somatostatinoma	Diabetes, gallstones, steatorrhea	Normal = 10–25 pg/mL Tumor = 100–400 pg/mL	Nearly all	0	—	100/60
D₂	VIP	<1	120	VIPoma (watery diarrhea, hypokalemia, achlorhydria [WDHA] [Verner-Morrison])	High-volume secretory diarrhea, hypokalemia, metabolic acidosis, hypochlorhydria	Normal = <200 pg/mL Tumor = 225–2000 pg/mL	50	Rare	Few	100/70
EC	**Substance P** and **serotonin**	<1	325	?	—	—	—	—	—	—
G*	**Gastrin** (ACTH-related peptides)	—	300	Gastrinoma (Zollinger-Ellison syndrome)	Abdominal pain with ulcer disease, massive gastric hypersecretion, secretory diarrhea that can be halted by nasogastric aspiration	Normal = <100 pg/mL Tumor = 100–1000 pg/mL Suspicious = >1000 pg/mL With secretin test, ↑ >200 pg/mL diagnostic	70	—	25%	50–85/79 Of the 70%: pancreatic, <20 duodenal, all ectopic, 80
PP (F)	**Pancreatic polypeptide** (met-encephalon, PHI)	15	140	Tumors (PPomas) are without endocrine symptoms	—	—	—	—	Frequent	—

*Gastrin is present in fetal but not in normal adult pancreatic islets.

TRH, thyrotropin-releasing hormone; CCK, cholecystokinin; PYY, peptide YY; CGRP, calcitonin gene–related peptide; VIP, vasoactive intestinal peptide; ACTH, adrenocorticotropic hormone; MEN 1, multiple endocrine neoplasia type 1; PHI, peptide histidine isoleucine.

Modified from Bonner-Weir S: Anatomy of the islet of Langerhans. *In* Samols E (ed): The Endocrine Pancreas. New York, Raven Press, 1991, p 16; and Marx M, Newman JB, Guice KS, et al: Clinical significance of gastrointestinal hormones. *In* Thompson JC, Greeley GH Jr, Rayford PL, Townsend CM Jr (eds): Gastrointestinal Endocrinology. New York, McGraw-Hill, 1987, p 416.

and its chief usefulness is that of a marker for endocrine tumors of the pancreas; coelevations of PP and of Ca²⁺ signal multiple endocrine neoplasia (MEN) type 1 syndrome. Pancreatic islet tumors have been found on rare occasions to produce growth hormone–releasing factor (GRF), adrenocorticotropic hormone (ACTH), and parathyroid hormone–related peptide. Development of radioimmunoassay by Berson and associates in 1956[10] allowed measurements of circulating concentrations of peptides in picograms per milliliter and has greatly facilitated the diagnosis of the islet cell tumor syndromes. The efficacy of various imaging and sampling techniques for

localization of islet cell tumors of the pancreas and duodenum is shown in Table 36-2.

Surgical management of these tumors has undergone serial evolution. All pancreatic endocrine tumors are rare (estimated at about 5 cases per 1 million population per year), so time is required for evolution of logical strategies for treatment. We attempt briefly to cover the major points the reader would like to know about the endocrine pancreas, and we focus on clinical identification of the tumors, their preoperative localization, their operative management, the usefulness of palliation, and the outcomes that can be expected.

TABLE 36-2. Efficacy of Localization of Endocrine Tumors of the Pancreas and Duodenum

Modality	True Positives (%)
Noninvasive	
Ultrasonography	23
Octreotide radioimaging (SRS)*	86
CT	43
MRI	26
Invasive	
Endoscopic ultrasonography	82
Selective angiography	56
Portal venous sampling	76
Provocative angiography†	65

*Rarely for melanoma.
†Calcium for insulinoma; secretin for gastrinoma.
SRS, somatostatin receptor scintigraphy.
Modified from Norton JA: Neuroendocrine tumors of the pancreas and duodenum. Curr Probl Surg 31:97, 1994.

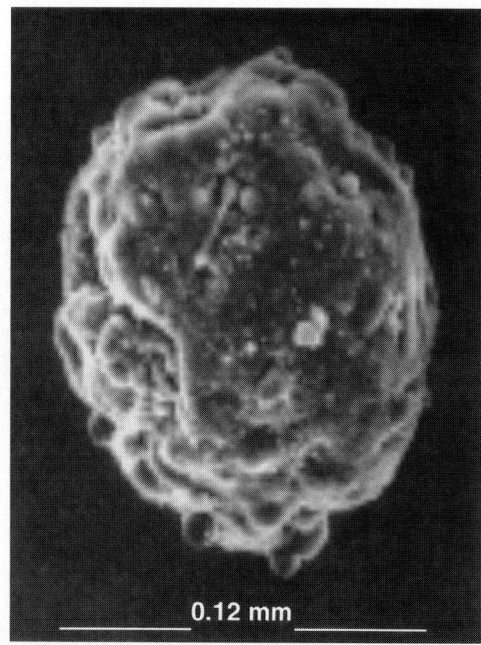

FIGURE 36-1. Scanning electron micrograph of an isolated islet of Langerhans. (From Orci L: Macro- and micro-domains in the endocrine pancreas. Diabetes 31:563, 1982.)

EMBRYOLOGY

The pancreas originates from two diverticular buds of the foregut that give rise to a ventral and a dorsal pancreas. With rotation of the foregut, the two masses fuse in human embryos during the 5th and 6th weeks of fetal development. In humans, the first islets of endocrine tissue appear in the early fetal period (~10 weeks); islets appear initially and in greater number in the tail of the pancreas. The *origin* of the endocrine cells of the pancreas has been a subject of hot debate.[11] Pearse[12] strongly supported an embryologic origin from the fetal neural crest and noted that all neural crest cells have the capacity of *a*mine *p*recursor *u*ptake *d*ecarboxylation (the so-called APUD theory). Falin[13] reported that the islets of Langerhans first appear in the human fetus in the 10th to 11th week of development, arising from epithelium of small ducts and later from centroacinar cells. Gittes and Rutter[14] studied the patterns of genetic expression of hormonal messenger RNA and concluded that both endocrine and exocrine cells of the pancreas arise from embryonic foregut endoderm (not from the neural crest), a view now generally accepted.

Development of human fetal islets has been divided into three stages[15]: in the first phase (weeks 14 to 16), the islet cells bud off of ductules; in the second phase (weeks 17 to 20), beta cells appear in the center of the islets with non-beta cells on the periphery; in phase three (weeks 21 to 26), beta and non-beta cells become positioned throughout the islet. Some exceptions to this orderly arrangement persist: 10% of total islet cells consist of beta cells outside discrete pancreatic islets. In rat embryos, specific insulin, glucagon, and cholecystokinin (CCK) cells can be identified at the beginning of the second half of gestation (day 12), and somatostatin cells appear 3 to 4 days later. Glucagon cells have been found in human embryos at 3 weeks. An example of the genetic mechanisms controlling the appearance of peptide hormones is that the upstream promoter element of the glucagon gene, *G1,* has been shown to restrict glucagon gene expression

to alpha cells[16]; although widely expressed at several embryonic stages, expression of the insulin gene in adults is restricted to islet beta cells.[17]

HISTOMORPHOLOGY OF ISLETS

Islets account for less than 2% of the adult pancreatic mass and thus in humans weigh about 1 g. In the fetus, islets comprise nearly one third of the pancreatic mass, but after birth, this percentage is greatly diluted by the accelerated growth of exocrine tissue. The adult human pancreas contains about 10^6 islets scattered throughout the parenchyma. The average adult human islet contains about 3000 cells, but islets vary greatly in size (40 to 400 µm in diameter). A scanning electromicrograph of an isolated islet is shown in Figure 36-1. Most islets are small, but the largest 15% of islets make up 60% of total islet volume. Adult islets are composed of four major cell types (A, B, D, and PP) and two or more minor types (see Table 36-1). Location of cells within the islet itself is tightly regulated: beta cells occupy the center, and the peripheral mantle is composed of A, D, and PP cells. A cells are columnar and well supplied with granules measuring 200 to 250 nm in diameter. B cells are polyhedral, truncated pyramids with secretory granules 250 to 300 nm (Fig. 36-2). D cells are smaller than A and B cells and are often dendritic. PP cells are the most variable: in humans the granules are elongated, electron dense, and 120 to 160 nm, whereas in other species they are spherical and much larger. Any single cell may secrete more than one peptide; for example, the A cell may secrete CCK, and the B cell may secrete thyrotropin-releasing hormone and amylin (see Table 36-1). Glucagon-producing A cells and

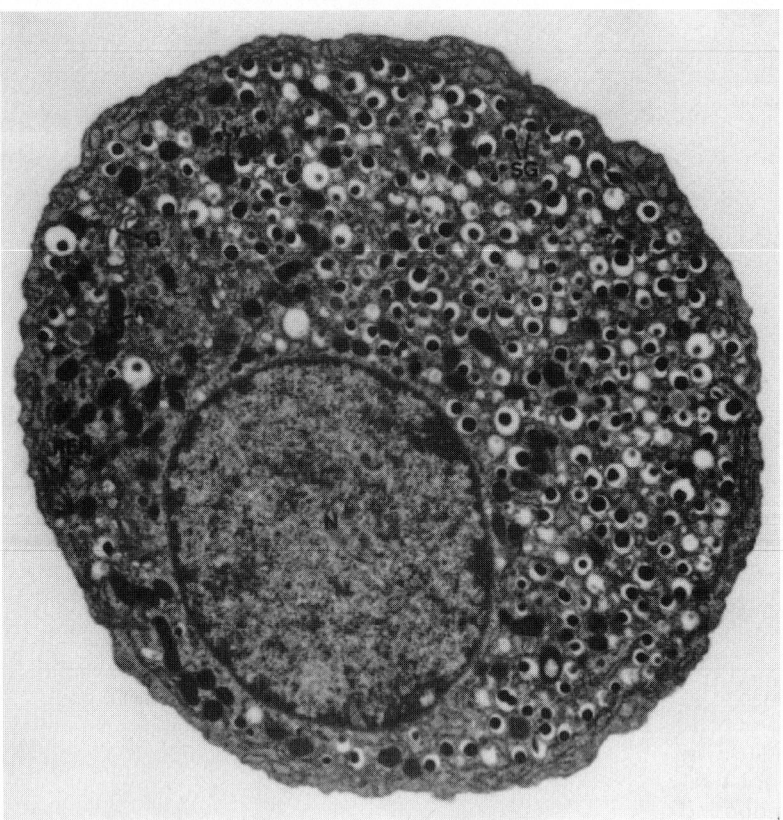

FIGURE 36-2. Electron micrograph of an isolated beta cell that allows identification of the three main membrane compartments characterizing a polypeptide-secreting cell: the rough endoplasmic reticulum (RER), Golgi apparatus (G), and secretory granules (SG). The nucleus (N), the mitochondria (m) and lysosomes (Ly) are also shown. ×10,000. (From Orci L: Macro- and micro-domains in the endocrine pancreas. Diabetes 31:539, 1982.)

PP-producing PP cells have mutually exclusive domains that follow a regional distribution: islets in the head and uncinate process are rich in PP cells but poor in A cells, whereas islets in the body and tail show the opposite predominance; B and D cells are evenly distributed. The physiologic significance of these quirks of distribution is unknown but sometimes important; for example, a Whipple resection removes nearly all PP cells but spares most all glucagon-producing A cells.

Great interest has been focused on the microcirculation of islets and its putative significance in endocrine-to-endocrine cell signaling. A popular concept holds that arterioles pierce the islet through short discontinuities of the mantle of non-beta cells, entering directly into the B cell core.[18,19] Efferent capillaries coalesce at the edge of the islets and pass through the mantle of non-beta cells (Fig. 36-3). This has given rise to the concept that there is a simple B to A to D cell order of cellular perfusion, with resultant control of glucagon secretion, for example, depending on insulin output. This concept has been challenged in a study on rat islet microcirculation that found the supplying arteriole to deliver blood first to capillaries in the mantle of the islet and then to the core, suggesting a more complex pattern and casting doubt on the circulating progression from B to A to D cells.[20] This is not a matter solely of academic interest, because the core-to-mantle interislet portal microcirculation has been held responsible for major abnormalities in glucagon secretion in diabetes.[19]

Studies on a possible portovenous connection between endocrine islets and exocrine acini have been reviewed[21]; insulin stimulates exocrine pancreatic secretion, transport of amino acids, and synthesis of proteins and enzymes. Glucagon inhibits pancreatic secretion and enzyme synthesis. Insulin and glucagon act antagonistically on the exocrine pancreas, but the role of somatostatin is controversial; it may act via its inhibitory effect on islet B cells, although acinar cells themselves possess receptors for somatostatin.

ENDOCRINE PHYSIOLOGY

The chief physiologic function of the endocrine pancreas might be starkly summarized as the regulation of body energy—a role largely achieved by hormonal control of carbohydrate metabolism. Simply stated, insulin is the hormone of energy storage and glucagon the hormone of energy release. Insulin stores energy by decreasing blood glucose level, increasing protein synthesis, decreasing glycogenolysis, decreasing lipolysis, and increasing glucose transport into cells (except beta cells, hepatocytes, and central nervous system cells). Glucagon releases energy by increasing blood glucose level via stimulation of glycogenolysis and stimulating gluconeogenesis and lipolysis. Chief attention in this chapter is directed to the physiology of insulin and glucagon and their interactions with somatostatin.

Insulin

The insulin molecule contains 56 amino acids and is arranged into A and B chains connected by two disulfide

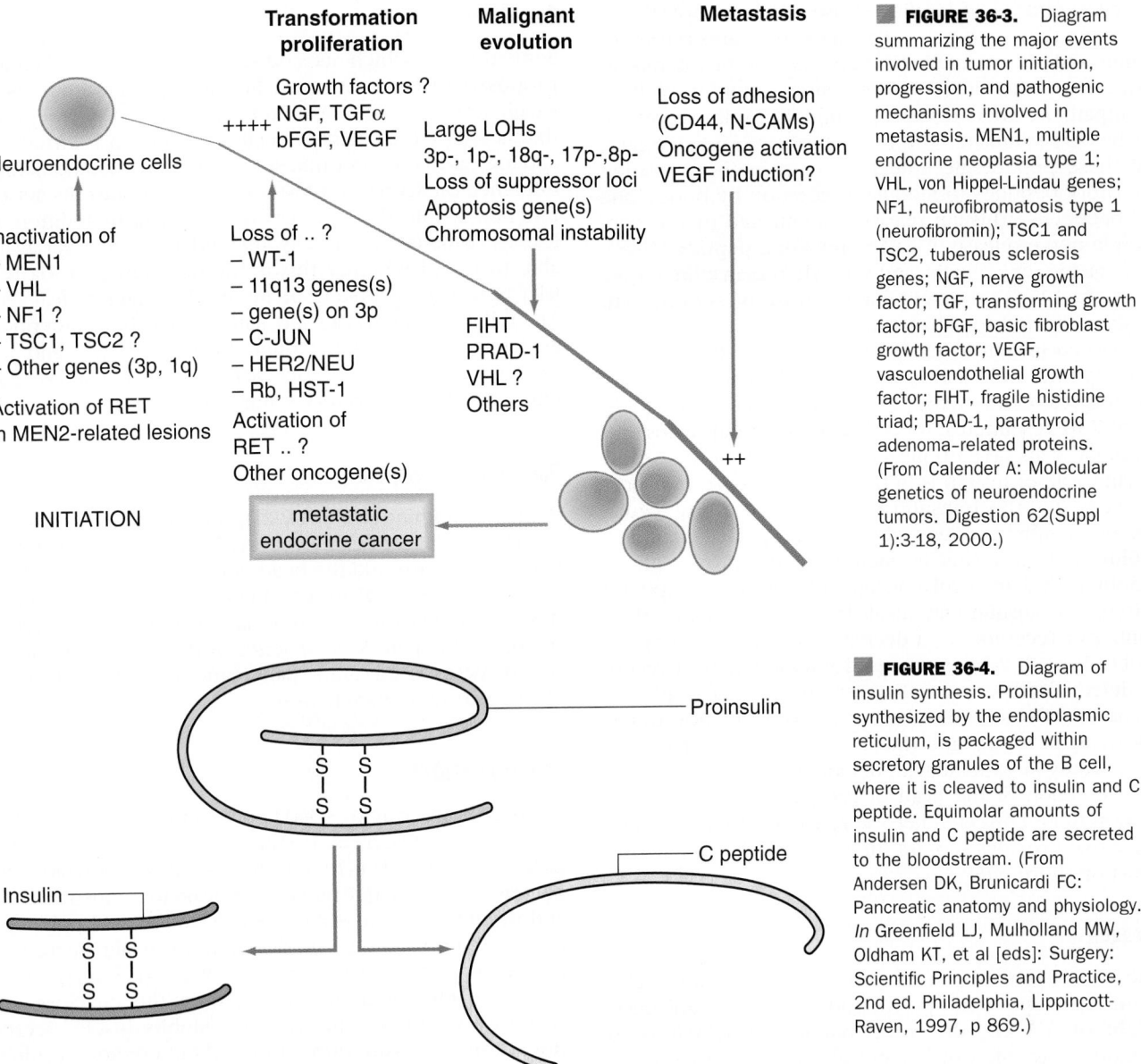

Transformation proliferation

Malignant evolution

Metastasis

Neuroendocrine cells

Growth factors ?
NGF, TGFα
bFGF, VEGF
++++

Large LOHs
3p-, 1p-, 18q-, 17p-,8p-
Loss of suppressor loci
Apoptosis gene(s)
Chromosomal instability

Loss of adhesion
(CD44, N-CAMs)
Oncogene activation
VEGF induction?

Inactivation of
– MEN1
– VHL
– NF1 ?
– TSC1, TSC2 ?
– Other genes (3p, 1q)

Activation of RET
in MEN2-related lesions

Loss of .. ?
– WT-1
– 11q13 genes(s)
– gene(s) on 3p
– C-JUN
– HER2/NEU
– Rb, HST-1

Activation of
RET .. ?

Other oncogene(s)

FIHT
PRAD-1
VHL ?
Others

++

INITIATION

metastatic
endocrine cancer

FIGURE 36-3. Diagram summarizing the major events involved in tumor initiation, progression, and pathogenic mechanisms involved in metastasis. MEN1, multiple endocrine neoplasia type 1; VHL, von Hippel-Lindau genes; NF1, neurofibromatosis type 1 (neurofibromin); TSC1 and TSC2, tuberous sclerosis genes; NGF, nerve growth factor; TGF, transforming growth factor; bFGF, basic fibroblast growth factor; VEGF, vasculoendothelial growth factor; FIHT, fragile histidine triad; PRAD-1, parathyroid adenoma–related proteins. (From Calender A: Molecular genetics of neuroendocrine tumors. Digestion 62(Suppl 1):3-18, 2000.)

Proinsulin

C peptide

Insulin

S—S
S—S

S—S
S—S

FIGURE 36-4. Diagram of insulin synthesis. Proinsulin, synthesized by the endoplasmic reticulum, is packaged within secretory granules of the B cell, where it is cleaved to insulin and C peptide. Equimolar amounts of insulin and C peptide are secreted to the bloodstream. (From Andersen DK, Brunicardi FC: Pancreatic anatomy and physiology. *In* Greenfield LJ, Mulholland MW, Oldham KT, et al [eds]: Surgery: Scientific Principles and Practice, 2nd ed. Philadelphia, Lippincott-Raven, 1997, p 869.)

bridges. In newly synthesized insulin, these chains are joined by means of a connecting (C) peptide (Fig. 36-4). This proinsulin, which is synthesized in the endoplasmic reticulum, travels on stimulation to the Golgi complex of the beta cell, where the C peptide is cleaved, and insulin is moved via microtubules into secretory granules to be released into the bloodstream by extrusion of the 6-kD polypeptide through the cell membrane (exocytosis). Patients with type I (insulin-dependent) diabetes have undergone loss of beta cells and have an absolute insulin deficiency. In common with structures that are truly vital, there is a great back-up supply of beta cells: Development of diabetes requires destruction of more than 80% of the beta cells. Insulin secretion is regulated by circulating levels of glucose and by humoral and neural factors. The glucose-sensing mechanism of the beta cell is highly alert, and on detecting high blood glucose level, reacts with an immediate output of stored insulin that lasts about 5 minutes, followed by a longer sustained secretion, which appears to be newly synthesized insulin.

Oral ingestion of glucose in humans and other species has been shown repeatedly to cause a release of pancreatic insulin in an amount that is greater than the insulin response to an identical dose of glucose given intravenously, even though blood levels of glucose may be the same. Several peptides released from the proximal gut by a normal meal have the capacity to augment nutrient-induced release of insulin. These insulinotropic factors apparently act directly on beta cells and are called *incretins*. Gastric inhibitory peptide is by far the best candidate for a physiologic incretin action, with CCK a distant second. Humoral inhibitors of insulin release include somatostatin, pancreastatin, amylin, and the fatty tissue hormone leptin.

Neural control of insulin release can be simplistically summarized by stating that the vagus stimulates release of insulin and the sympathetic nervous system inhibits it. However, further study shows a more complex picture: α-sympathetic fibers do strongly inhibit insulin secretion, but β-fibers stimulate. The nerve fibers release peptides, and these peptidergic influences react with circulating regulatory peptides to modulate secretion by both alpha and beta cells.[22] Insulin release is stimulated by the peptidergic nerve release of gastrin-releasing peptide (GRP), CCK, gastrin, enkephalin, and VIP, whereas insulin release is inhibited by peptidergic nerve release of neurotensin, substance P, and somatostatin.

Secreted insulin is transported rapidly to the portovenous system, and slightly more than half is cleared by hepatocytes on first transit of the liver; insulin has a half-life of 7 to 10 minutes. All cells except cerebrocytes and red blood cells take up insulin. Renal excretion is scant. A major role of insulin is in promoting glucose transport into cells, and this transport may be enhanced by regulation of membrane-bound glucose transporter peptides. Insulin binds to a specific membrane receptor, a glycoprotein with a molecular weight of 300 kD. Peripheral resistance to insulin may result from either a diminished number of receptors or a decreased receptor affinity for insulin. Type II diabetes is caused at least in part by receptor defects leading to insulin resistance. The complexity of control of insulin metabolism has been demonstrated repeatedly in normal individuals and in diabetic patients. In one study in patients with hepatic resistance to insulin after resection of the head of the pancreas for trauma, infusion of PP corrected hepatic resistance to insulin, evidence that provides support for a role for PP as a glucose-regulatory hormone.[4]

Glucagon

Glucagon, secreted by the A cells of the islet, is a straight-chain, 29-amino acid polypeptide, with a molecular weight of 3.5 kD, the main function of which is to promote conversion of hepatic glycogen to glucose. As with insulin, glucagon secretion is controlled by a complex interaction of neural, hormonal, and nutrient factors. As with insulin, the primary regulator of glucagon release is circulating glucose, high levels of which inhibit glucagon secretion. Glucagon and insulin exercise a yin-yang reciprocal control of carbohydrate metabolism. Failure of glucagon secretion can cause hypoglycemia, and excess glucagon may bring about hyperglycemia. Insulin and somatostatin suppress glucagon release, probably via the islet portovenous system. Neural control of glucagon output is similar to that of insulin,[22] but sympathetic neural transmitters and the neural hormone epinephrine stimulate the A cell, whereas they inhibit the B cell. The putative hormone-hormone interrelation (B to A to D) among islet cells as mediated by the portovenous islet flow has been discussed in the section on insulin. Another item of uncertainty is whether the hormone-hormone interrelations all are carried out via the interislet circulation or whether some may be simply cell-to-cell paracrine effects.

Somatostatin

Somatostatin, which its codiscoverer, Roger Guillemin, proposed to be a universal hormonal "off-switch," is a small, straight-chain, 14-amino acid (1.6-kD) polypeptide that is secreted by acinar D cells. Although it is attractive and logical to consider that somatostatin has a modulating influence on secretion of other islet hormones, its actual function within the pancreas is unknown. In addition, if it does influence other cells, techniques are not yet available to reveal whether this is through transport via the islet portovenous system or by simple paracrine leakage. The full molecule has a short half-life, but the octapeptide analogue octreotide has a longer life in circulation and has been used to treat secretory diarrhea, bowel fistulas, and endocrine hypersecretory syndromes.

Pancreatic Polypeptide

PP is a 36-amino acid, 4.2-kD, straight-chain molecule secreted by PP (or F) cells that are located primarily in the uncinate process and the head of the pancreas. The physiologic actions of PP are unknown, and its clinical usefulness is limited to its role as a marker for other endocrine tumors of the pancreas. Absence of PP may play a role in the diabetes seen after pancreatic resection or after chronic atrophic pancreatitis.[4]

OTHER PEPTIDES

VIP is a 28-amino acid, 3.3-kD polypeptide secreted by the D_2 cell of the pancreas. It stimulates insulin and inhibits gastric secretion. It is found throughout the gastrointestinal tract, and its major function appears to be vasodilation and bronchodilation. Amylin is a 36-amino acid polypeptide secreted by the B cell that inhibits insulin secretion and uptake. Pancreastatin is part of a larger ubiquitous molecule, chromogranin A, found in the envelope of secretory granules. Pancreastatin inhibits insulin secretion. Gastrin cells are present in fetal but not normal adult islets. Other peptides (glicentin, thyrotropin-releasing hormone, CCK, endorphin, peptideYY [PYY]), GRF, calcitonin gene–related peptide [CGRP], prolactin, metenkephalin, ACTH, peptide histidine isoleucine [PHI], and parathyroid hormone–related peptide) have been reported in normal islets and in islet cell tumors.

ISLET CELL TUMORS

In 1935, Whipple and Frantz[23] reported the association of hyperinsulinism with adenomas of pancreatic islet cells, establishing a functional connection between islet cell tumors and endocrine syndromes. Later, syndromes were described for islet tumors producing gastrin, glucagon, somatostatin, VIP, and other peptides. To repeat, these tumors are rare. The annual incidence in this country has been estimated between 5 and 10 cases per 1 million population per year. The autopsy rate is said to be 1%, or, expressed another way, these tumors are 1000 to 2000 times more common in autopsy statistics than in annual clinical incidence; most are clearly nonfunctional and benign.

The incidence of malignancy in these tumors varies greatly, from about 10% in insulinomas to nearly all glucagonomas and somatostatinomas (see Table 36-1). In a manner reminiscent of stage-by-stage progression of normal gut epithelium to eventual malignancy, tumorigenesis of neuroendocrine cells appears to involve multiple genetic events (mutational activation or inactivation of oncogenes or tumor suppressor genes) (see Fig. 36-3).[24] For these tumors, the criterion of malignancy is simple: if they metastasize, they are malignant. On hematoxylin and eosin stains, all pancreatic endocrine tumors (including carcinoid tumors of the bowel) look alike. Immunostaining using antibodies to specific hormones allows identification of the endocrine content of cells. By light microscopy, there are no characteristics that separate benign from malignant tumors. Some large aggressive tumors may invade adjacent structures and by such action proclaim their malignancy, but most tumors larger than 2 cm are malignant anyway. Mixed exocrine-endocrine tumors are rare; when present, the endocrine cells are inactive, except in pancreaticoblastomas.

Endocrine tumors of the pancreas vary greatly in mode of onset and severity of symptoms, location, and malignant potential. With time, they may vary greatly in secretion and biologic aggressiveness. So great is the variation even within specific tumor syndromes that any generalization may not apply to a particular patient. One accurate generalization is that even though multiple hormones may be produced by a single tumor (or even by a single cell within that tumor), the syndrome is recognized and named by the clinical signs of the predominant endocrine agent. As many as 40% of patients with islet cell neoplasms may have elevated levels of multiple hormones, not all of which produce symptoms. We treated a young woman several years ago with ZES who did well after total gastrectomy until she developed a virulent syndrome of hypertension, muscle weakness, and anorexia. She was found to have high levels of ACTH and died in steroid crisis as we were preparing her for adrenalectomy. Her ACTH levels were more than 200 times normal, and she was asymptomatic from remaining gastrinoma tissue (the tumor cell line was established in nude mice[25,26]). Moertel[27] wondered whether this phenomenon represents multiple clones of tumor cells or a common stem cell with multiple potentials for hormone production. We followed a man for several years after an operation for gastrinoma, watching his extraordinarily high serum gastrin levels and watching his hepatic metastatic tumor grow. When he died, the hepatic metastases contained, to our surprise, huge amounts of somatostatin with scant residual gastrin.

Although the tumor syndromes are classically ascribed to *pancreatic* islet tumors, tumors are often in extrapancreatic locations, especially in the duodenum and in the peripancreatic areas above, below, and to the right of the duodenum. Nearly all insulinomas, glucagonomas, and VIPomas occur within the pancreas itself, whereas most gastrinomas occur in the duodenum, with the pancreas a close second. Somatostatinomas are equally divided between the pancreas and the proximal small bowel. Patients with von Recklinghausen's disease may have somatostatinomas or gastrinomas in the duodenum.[28]

Tumors may show an anatomic preference for bimodal distribution. An analysis of several reported series suggests that gastrinomas, PPomas, and somatostatinomas show a 75% preference to an anatomic location to the right of the superior mesenteric arteries in peripancreatic tissue, in the duodenum, and in the head of the pancreas. By contrast, about 75% of insulinomas and glucagonomas were located in the body and tail of the pancreas to the left of the superior mesenteric artery.[29] Further review of these findings suggested that the distribution of glucagonomas, insulinomas, and PPomas corresponded to the normal distribution of these endocrine cell types within the pancreas.

Pancreatic endocrine tumors may occur sporadically or in conjunction with the MEN 1 syndrome. MEN 1 is characterized by tumors of the parathyroid, pituitary, and pancreas and occasionally the adrenal. MEN 1 is associated genetically with a defect on chromosome 11 and is inherited in an autosomal dominant fashion. Because islet cell tumors in MEN 1 patients are always multiple, preoperative recognition of the MEN 1 status is necessary. About 25% of patients with gastrinomas, 10% of those with insulinomas, and lesser percentages of those with glucagonomas and VIPomas have MEN syndrome. Of all MEN 1 patients, more than half have gastrinomas, and one in five has an insulinoma. Most (70% to 90%) MEN 1 patients manifest hyperparathyroidism, usually caused by hyperplasia of all four glands. Any patient with a pancreatic endocrine tumor syndrome should have a measurement of calcium level, and if that is elevated, the parathyroids and the pituitary should be studied. A general principle is that in MEN 1 patients with islet tumors, the hyperparathyroidism should be surgically managed first, preferably by removing all four glands with immediate autograft.

From a clinical viewpoint, the most important aspects of dealing with patients with endocrine tumors of the pancreas are the means of localization and the proper operative treatment. In a meta-analysis of a dozen individual reports, the efficacy of true positive tumor localization has been summarized (see Table 36-2). Techniques of both localization and of surgical excision have undergone radical changes in the past decade and are still in the process of evolution. The following sections offer a brief review of current methods of diagnosis, localization, and surgical techniques. Each is discussed in detail under the appropriate tumor heading.

Insulinoma

Insulinoma is the most common functioning tumor of the pancreas, and affected patients present a tableau of symptoms referable to hypoglycemia (symptoms of catecholamine release), mental confusion and obtundation, or both. Many patients have symptoms for years. Some have been greatly troubled by emotional instability and fits of rage, often followed by somnolence. A review of the world literature from 1914 to 1957 reported 356 cases of hyperinsulinism due to benign islet cell adenomas.[30]

Clinical Features and Diagnosis

The diagnostic hallmark of the syndrome is the so-called Whipple triad, namely, symptoms of hypoglycemia (catecholamine release), low blood glucose level (40 to 50 mg/dL), and relief of symptoms after intravenous administration of glucose. The triad is not entirely diagnostic, because it may be emulated by factitious administration of hypoglycemic agents, by rare soft tissue tumors, or occasionally by reactive hypoglycemia. The clinical syndrome of hyperinsulinism may follow one of two patterns or sometimes a combination of both. The symptom complex may be due to autonomic nervous overactivity, expressed by fatigue, weakness, fearfulness, hunger, tremor, sweating, and tachycardia, or alternatively, a central nervous system disturbance with apathy (or irritability or anxiety), confusion, excitement, loss of orientation, blurring of vision, delirium, stupor, coma, or convulsions. The pathognomonic finding is an inappropriately high (>5 µU/mL) level of serum insulin during symptomatic hypoglycemia. A diagnostic ratio of blood insulin (in microunits per milliliter) to glucose (in milligrams per deciliter) of greater than 0.4 has proved valuable in diagnosis. The best way to induce hypoglycemia is with fasting: two thirds of patients will experience hypoglycemic symptoms in 24 hours, and nearly all other patients experience symptoms by 72 hours of fasting. Provocative tests, usually involving tolbutamide or glucagon, have been used, but these may cause dangerously profound hypoglycemia and are usually not necessary. Because cerebrocytes metabolize only glucose, prolonged profound hypoglycemia may cause permanent brain damage. Clinicians need to be alert to this when attempting to induce hypoglycemia by fasting. Most important, preoperative NPO orders *must* be accompanied by intravenous administration of glucose.

A particularly troubling cause of the clinical picture of hyperinsulinemia is brought about by factitious administration of insulin or a hypoglycemic agent such as sulfonylurea. Individuals so involved are usually workers in health care who have access to insulin or other hypoglycemic agents. Their motives are obscure but are clearly aimed at securing attention. Self-administration of insulin can be detected because these patients do not have the usual consonant concentrations of C-peptide or proinsulin (see Fig. 36-4); sulfonylurea may be detected, with difficulty, in blood (and more important, insulin levels are not inappropriately high).

As soon as a patient with insulinoma is identified, care must be taken to prevent severe hypoglycemia with possible loss of cerebrocytes. Diet should be modified to include frequent meals, even awakening at night to eat. The standard drug is diazoxide, which is helpful in about two out of three patients but should be discontinued at least a week before operation because it may cause intraoperative hypotension. The long-acting somatostatin analogue octreotide, although helpful in children with nesidioblastosis, has been effective only rarely in adults.

Localization

Insulinomas are small (usually <1.5 cm), usually single (only 10% are multiple and those are usually associated with MEN 1 syndrome), usually benign (only 5% to 10% are malignant), and usually hard to find. Success in localization often parallels the degree of invasiveness of the study (see Table 36-2). Plain abdominal radiographic and ultrasound studies are rarely helpful, but contrast-augmented computed tomography (CT) and magnetic resonance imaging (MRI) locate 50% to 60% of tumors. Since few insulinomas have many somatostatin receptors, somatostatin receptor scintigraphy (SRS) is not highly successful. Success in localization by selective arteriography varies with the size of the tumor; rates of 90% accuracy have been reported with insulinomas. Demonstration of islet tumors by enhanced CT (Fig. 36-5),[31] enhanced MRI, or arteriography depends, of course, on the relatively rich blood supply to islet tumors compared with the rest of the pancreatic parenchyma. Also helpful has been selective portovenous sampling for measurement of insulin levels in pancreatic venous tributaries (Fig. 36-6), a method that does not absolutely localize the site of the tumor, but in about 75% of cases does provide accurate information on the region of the pancreas from which high levels of insulin are released. The method has a relatively high incidence of problems with bleeding into the peritoneal cavity or biliary tree. It is expensive and requires skill.

Calcium is known to release insulin, and, taking a page from the intra-arterial secretin test for gastrinoma,[32] a highly promising test has been developed for localizing insulinomas by means of selective intra-arterial injection of calcium (into the gastroduodenal, superior mesentery, right hepatic, or splenic arteries), obtaining samples for radioimmunoassay of insulin from the right hepatic vein.[33] (The dose of calcium is 0.025 mEq calcium per kilogram.) A study from the National Institutes of Health (NIH) has compared the accuracy of several techniques in the localization of insulinoma in 36 patients: the accuracy of CT was 24%; MRI, 45%; SRS, 17%; abdominal ultrasound, 13%; selective angiogram, 43%; and intra-arterial calcium stimulation, 94%. By combinations of these studies, all tumors were identified before surgery; a surgeon unaware of the preoperative localization study was successful in identifying the tumor by intraoperative ultrasound in 12 (86%) of 14 patients.[34]

Operation

Treatment for insulinoma is surgical. At operation, the incision is dictated by operator preference, either a midline incision from the xiphoid to below the umbilicus or a bilateral subcostal incision. Exposure should be generous, and mechanical ring retractors are an asset. The entire abdomen should be explored, with particular attention being paid to possible liver metastases. Next, the pancreas should be mobilized by dividing the gastrocolic ligament from left to right, by incising the posterior lining of the lesser sac along the inferior and superior margins of the pancreas, and by performing a generous medial

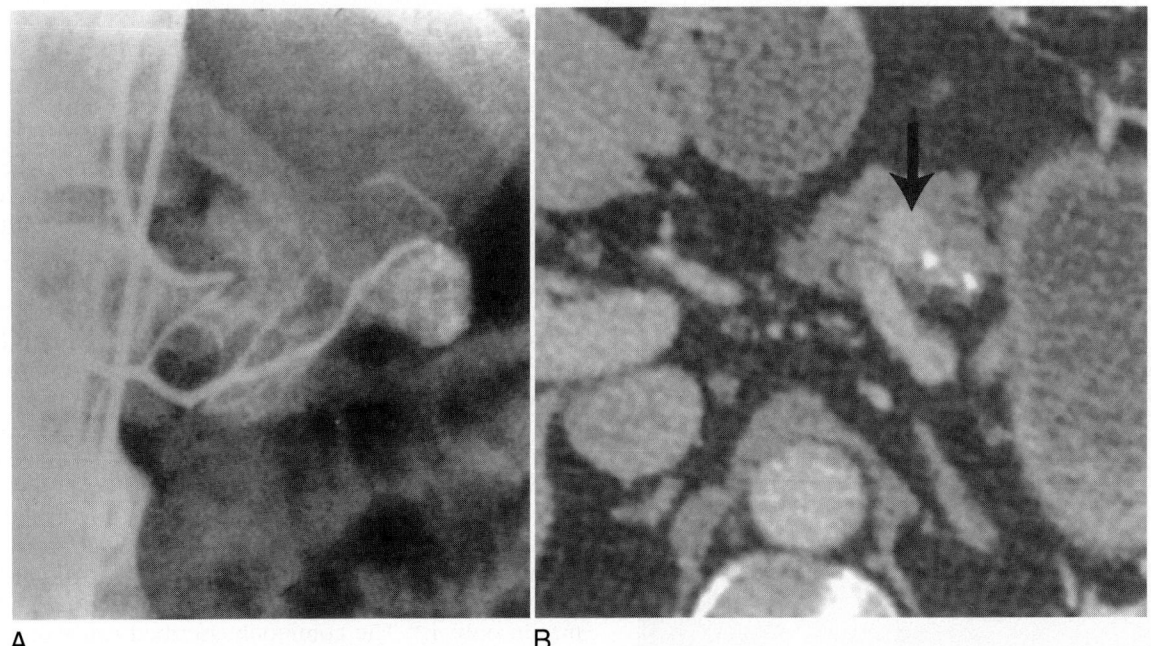

A   B

FIGURE 36-5. Arteriographic demonstration of an insulinoma. **A,** Selective injection into the specific dorsal pancreatic artery demonstrates the tumor precisely. **B,** Insulinoma with triphasic enhancement on CT. The mass in pancreatic body (*arrow*) demonstrates early and prolonged enhancement with wash-out during the portal venous phase; note the maximal difference in enhancement between tumor and normal pancreas occurs during pancreatic phase (shown). (**A,** From Edis AJ, McIlrath DC, Van Heerden JA, et al: Insulinoma: Current diagnosis and surgical management. Curr Probl Surg 13:1-45, 1976; **B,** From Ros PR, Mortele KJ: Imaging features of pancreatic neoplasms. Jbr-Btr 84:239-249, 2001.)

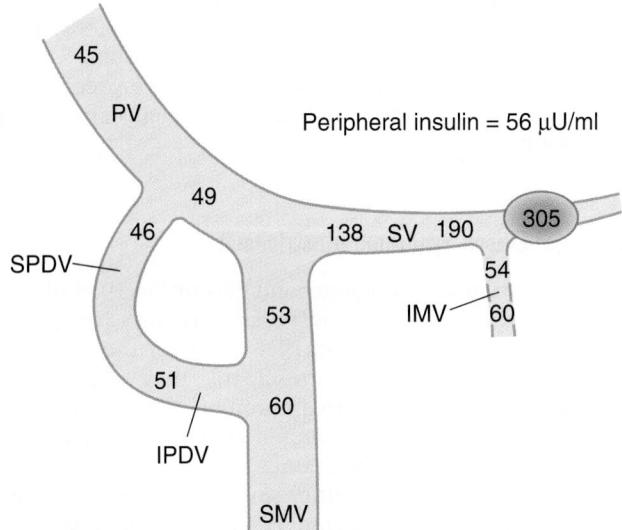

FIGURE 36-6. Transhepatic selective venous sampling of the portal vein and its tributaries for insulin. Venous insulin levels are greatly elevated in the distal splenic vein (*shaded circle*). Intraoperative ultrasound and palpation of the pancreas failed to reveal an insulinoma. A distal pancreatectomy was performed on the basis of the portovenous sampling gradient shown here, and the pathologists confirmed the presence of a 1-cm insulinoma. IMV, inferior mesenteric vein; IPDV, inferior pancreatic duodenal vein; PV, portal vein; SMV, superior mesenteric vein; SPDV, superior pancreatic duodenal vein; SV, splenic vein. Insulin concentrations are given in microunits per milliliter. (From Norton JA, Shawker TH, Doppman JL, et al: Localization and surgical treatment of occult insulinomas. Ann Surg 212:615-620, 1990.)

mobilization of the C-loop of the duodenum, incising the peritoneum along the right border (Kocher maneuver). The head of the pancreas should be palpated carefully and examined anteriorly and posteriorly; the body and tail of the pancreas should be palpated, dividing any ligamentous attachments to the spleen, delivering the spleen into the wound, and rotating the tail anteriorly to allow palpation and visualization.

Anyone operating on patients with islet adenomas should be familiar with techniques for, and limitations of, intraoperative ultrasonography. The higher-resolution (7.5- to 10-MHz) transducers are used in the pancreas; because of its greater depth of penetration, a 5-MHz transducer is better for the liver. Islet tumors are detected as sonolucent masses, usually of uniform consistency. Several reports attest to the high degree of accuracy of intraoperative ultrasound.[35,36] Figure 36-7 shows a pancreatic insulinoma detected by intraoperative ultrasonography. The color-Doppler attachment allows detection of adjacent vessels and aids in identification of the pancreatic ductal system, which shows up as a lucent tube without flow. A fair conclusion is that intra-arterial calcium infusion is the most sensitive study for preoperative localization of insulinomas and that intraoperative ultrasound is essential for their intraoperative detection.[37]

Careful review of current literature leads to the almost startling conclusion that nearly all syndromes of hyperinsulinism are due to insulinomas and that nearly all insulinomas can now be detected before or during surgery. If this experience holds true, the former bête noire of the

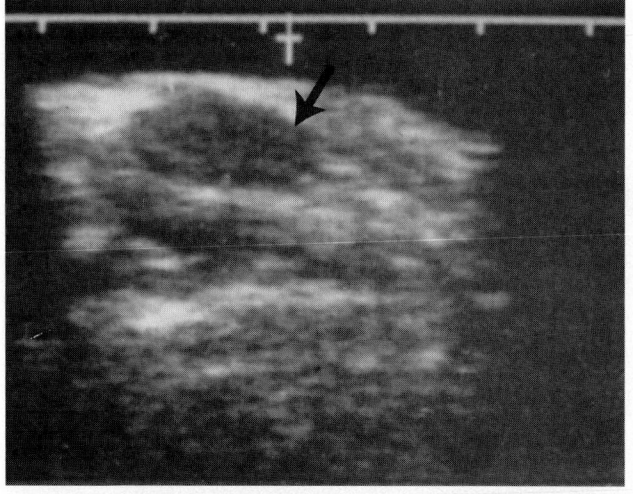

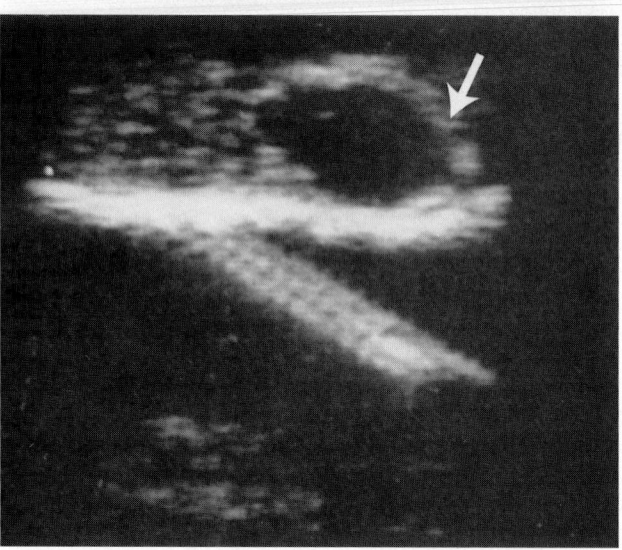

FIGURE 36-7. **A** and **B**, Intraoperative ultrasonographic demonstration of insulinoma using 7.5-MHz probe. Tumor of the midbody of the pancreas *(arrows)* is clearly shown in both panels; the *horizontal (white) line* beneath the tumor is the surgeon's glove. (**A** and **B**, Courtesy of W. H. Nealon, M.D.)

endocrine surgeon, namely, exploring a patient with known hyperinsulinism and not finding the tumor, will have been vanquished, and, in being vanquished, taking with it the idea that B cell hyperplasia, or some form of adult nesidioblastosis, is to blame when the operating surgeon is unable to locate an insulinoma. Having said this, there appears to be scant justification for an empirical ("blind") partial pancreatectomy except in patients with insulinoma plus MEN 1; this previously stated decision has received support.[38]

Most insulinomas are benign and can be enucleated. Nutrient vessels in the bed of the adenoma should be cauterized. Care should be taken in enucleation to avoid injury to ductal structures, and if a duct is injured, it should be sutured and drained. If malignant, the tumor should be resected in a cancer-type operation, and if metastatic, it is worthwhile to attempt to remove all primary and metastatic tumor tissue in an attempt to minimize persistent hyperinsulinism.

The 10% of patients with hyperinsulinism who have MEN 1 syndrome have multiple islet tumors, one of which is usually dominant and responsible for the excessive insulin output. These are probably best managed by resecting the area of the pancreas that shows the highest insulin output on selective portovenous sampling or on selective intra-arterial calcium challenge.[39]

Persistent hyperinsulinemia after operation for metastatic islet cell tumor may be managed by diazoxide[40] or by streptozotocin plus fluorouracil.[41] The usual dose of diazoxide is 100 mg three times a day; side effects are rare and are chiefly fluid retention and hirsutism. The usual dose of streptozotocin is 500 mg/m^2 of body surface daily for 5 consecutive days plus fluorouracil 400 mg/m^2 daily over 5 days. White blood cell and platelet counts must be monitored carefully.

Insulinomas are rare in infants; a review of 160 patients with neonatal and infantile hyperinsulinism found adenomas in only 4.[42] The commonly ascribed cause of hyperinsulinism in the very young is nesidioblastosis, literally a nestlike increase in islet cells. The problem with this concept is that nesidioblastosis appears to be a normal phase of fetal islet development rather than a pathologic entity. The best explanation for hyperinsulinism appears to be a regulatory defect in insulin synthesis, storage, or release. The problem is serious because prolonged hypoglycemia leads to mental retardation in many, perhaps most, of these children. A near-total (95% to 98%) pancreatectomy appears to offer the best results,[43] with octreotide therapy reserved for preoperative preparation and those few children not rendered euglycemic after operation.

Zollinger-Ellison Syndrome (Gastrinoma)

The initial report by Zollinger and Ellison[44] in 1955 of two patients with a virulent ulcer diathesis, massive gastric acid hypersecretion, and an islet tumor of the pancreas introduced a new disease. Presciently, they ascribed the acid secretory symptoms to a hormone elaborated by the tumor. This hormone was shown later to be gastrin, and we now know that a gastrinoma is the hallmark of ZES. In the less than half a century since the original description of ZES, gradual accumulation of experience has changed and greatly improved diagnostic and therapeutic approaches.[45] All interested parties have witnessed the disease in evolution, and we describe it here as it is best known in the early years of this century. Gastrinoma is the second most common islet cell tumor and is the most common symptomatic, malignant endocrine tumor of the pancreas. Having said that, current information is that about half of gastrinomas arise in the duodenum. Rare pulmonary, acoustic neuroma, and colon tumors may produce gastrin without causing hypergastrinemia, but outside the area of the pancreas and duodenum, only ovarian cancers can process progastrin to gastrin to bring about ZES.

Clinical Features and Diagnosis

In 75% of patients with ZES, the gastrinoma is sporadic, whereas 25% have an associated MEN 1 syndrome. In the sporadic form, there is a slight (60%) male predominance; the average age of onset is 50 years. With MEN 1, onset is usually 5 to 10 years earlier. The main symptoms are those caused by peptic acid hypersecretion, with abdominal pain the chief complaint in about 75% of patients. Nearly two thirds of patients have diarrhea, and 10% to 20% of patients present with diarrhea alone. A unique characteristic of this diarrhea is that it is halted by nasogastric aspiration of gastric secretion, a feature that separates it from *all other* secretory diarrheas. Most patients have peptic ulcers; duodenal are the most common, but jejunal ulceration may be found (both patients in the original report by Zollinger and Ellison had jejunal ulcers). The most common complications of peptic ulcer are nausea and vomiting in 30%, bleeding in 10%, and perforation in 7%. About one third of patients present with signs and symptoms of gastroesophageal reflux disease, and this number appears to be increasing.

Of all MEN 1 patients, the organ most commonly involved is the parathyroid, and 70% to 95% of patients show hypercalcemia (albumin corrected). The next most common syndrome is ZES (54%), followed by insulinoma (21%), glucagonoma (3%), and VIPoma (1%). Nonfunctioning PPoma occurs in more than 80%.[46] Pituitary adenomas are common, most of which are nonfunctioning, with prolactinomas being the next most common.

As is true with any new disease, the most flagrant examples are those seen first, and with time, early and less severe cases become evident. Thus, all early reports of ZES were concerned with the startling virulence of the ulcer diathesis, with massive acid hypersecretion, severe unrelenting diarrhea, intractable abdominal pain, and frequent episodes of bleeding and perforation. Patients with ulcer symptoms are currently likely to have a gastrin measurement early, and those who have ZES are recognized and their hypersecretion managed with antisecretory drugs before evolving into grave clinical states.

ZES must be excluded in all patients with intractable peptic ulcer, severe esophagitis, or persistent secretory diarrhea. The diagnosis depends on the presence of hypergastrinemia in the face of increased secretion of gastric acid. Most laboratories have an upper limit of normal of 100 pg/mL for fasting levels of gastrin. Levels of 100 to 1000 pg/mL are occasionally seen in non-ZES patients, and levels higher than 1000 are nearly diagnostic for ZES, provided that the patient makes gastric acid (some pernicious anemia patients have very high gastrin levels but make no gastric acid; the same is true to a lesser degree in patients taking proton-pump inhibitors [e.g., omeprazole]). The upper limit of normal for basal acid output is 5 mEq/hour; most ZES patients secrete more than 15 mEq/hour or, if postgastrectomy, more than 5 mEq/hour. Measurement of gastric juice pH shows a value of less than 2; a pH of greater than 2.5 in a nasogastric aspirate virtually rules out ZES. Other causes of hypergas-

trinemia must be ruled out (Box 36-1). If the diagnosis is in doubt, the secretin provocative test is highly useful. In this test, fasting gastrin level is measured before intravenous secretin (2 CU/kg) is administered, and further samples for gastrin determination are obtained at 2, 5, 10, and 20 minutes after secretin administration. An increase in the gastrin value of more than 200 pg/mL after secretin administration is found in 87% of patients, with no false-positive results. The false-negative results may be due to *Helicobacter pylori*.

Current clinical clues to patients with ZES are the following:

- A virulent peptic ulcer or gastroesophageal reflux disease diathesis
- Absence of *H. pylori* or failure of the peptic ulcer to heal after either anti-*H. pylori* therapy or H₂ blockade
- A secretory diarrhea that persists (especially if the diarrhea is halted by nasogastric suction)
- Signs or symptoms of MEN 1 syndrome (elevated serum calcium and parathyroid hormone levels, pituitary tumor)

Once the diagnosis is established, acid secretion should be controlled to prevent complications and to afford symptomatic relief. The best results are achieved with the proton-pump inhibitor drugs, which should be given in an appropriate dose (60 to 120 mg/day; usual dose, 80 mg/day). These drugs have proven safe and effective, and enough should be given so as to curtail gastric acid output to less than 5 mEq/hour.

Box 36-1. Causes of Hypergastrinemia

↑ Stimulation of Gastrin Release

Zollinger-Ellison syndrome (gastrinoma)
Antral G cell hyperplasia ± pheochromocytoma
Pyloric obstruction

↓ Inhibition of Gastrin Release

Hypochlorhydria or achlorhydria
    Atrophic gastritis
    Pernicious anemia
    Gastric carcinoma
    Vitiligo
    Most important: antisecretory drugs (H₂-receptor antagonist and especially proton-pump inhibitors)
Antral exclusion operation
Vagotomy

↓ Catabolism

Chronic renal failure

Unknown

Rheumatoid arthritis
Small bowel resection (temporary)

Adapted from Townsend CM Jr, Thompson JC: Up-to-date treatment of the patient with hypergastrinemia. Adv Surg 20:161, 1987.

Pathology

Gastrinomas were originally assumed to arise in the pancreas, but most subsequent series have shown that at least half originate in the duodenum. Sixty to 90% are found in the so-called gastrinoma triangle,[47] an area in the upper abdomen with its superior point at the junction of the cystic and common bile ducts, its inferior point at the junction or the inferior margin of the second and third parts of the duodenum, and its left lateral point at the junction of the head and neck of the pancreas (Fig. 36-8). The duodenum is the site of gastrinomas in 45% to 60% of patients, and there is a pronounced proximal-to-distal gradient within the duodenum (i.e., most are in the first part, none in the fourth). Gastrinomas have been reported in the renal capsule and in ovarian cancers. Histologic criteria for malignancy are either absent or unreliable. Again, if the tumors metastasize, they are malignant. In early series, 60% to 90% of tumors were malignant, whereas most subsequent studies report that only about one third are malignant, which suggests that with time, all tumors may become malignant. The cell of origin is certainly not clear, because the normal postembryonic pancreas and duodenum contain no gastrin cells. Candidates would be a nest of embryonal cells or an undifferentiated line of pancreatic stem cells. Gastrinomas in the duodenum and pancreas may have a different embryologic origin; that is, gastrinomas in the duodenum and pancreatic head may arise from the ventral pancreatic anlage, and tumors of the body and tail may arise from the dorsal anlage. ZES patients with the MEN 1 syndrome have multiple tumors, often microadenomas, scattered throughout the pancreas and duodenum. Sixty to 80% of these MEN 1 patients have duodenal gastrinomas, which usually metastasize to local nodes (85% have lymph node metastases). In general, metastases to the liver occur from large (>3-cm) sporadic pancreatic tumors, whereas lymph node metastases do not appear to be dependent on size or location of the primary tumor (duodenal and pancreatic gastrinomas appear to be equally malignant, with about 50% of the metastases going to lymph nodes). Whether all of these lymph nodes containing gastrinoma tissue are true metastases is questionable because long-standing cures have, on occasion, resulted from their excision.[48,49] More sporadic cases of ZES present initially with liver metastases than do those with ZES plus MEN 1 syndrome, but survival without metastases (95% vs. 96% at 5 years) is not different. Because of these early liver metastases, the sporadic form of ZES is more virulent than ZES plus MEN 1. An NIH study with a mean follow-up of 12.5 years of patients with sporadic ZES showed liver metastases to be the dominant factor in survival; for instance, the 10-year survival for patients with hepatic metastases was 30%, and that for patients without hepatic metastases was 90%. Surprisingly, the presence or absence of lymph node metastases did not affect survival.[50] All of this suggests that there is an initial biological division into either a benign or a malignant clinical syndrome (Table 36-3).

Gastrinomas are usually slow growing, and some patients may live for years with metastatic disease. Zollinger and Ellison's[44] second patient (JM) was found to have lymph node metastases at the time of her total gastrectomy in 1954. Forty years later, she had a parathyroidectomy and was alive and well in 1999 (C. Ellison, personal communication, 1999). Patients with unresectable liver metastases have a 5-year survival of 20% to 40% and a 10-year survival of between 0 and 30%. A 10-year prospective study of 73 ZES patients who had no radiographic evidence of liver metastases showed that long-term survival was excellent compared with survival of patients with distant spread, even when no tumor was found and even when resection was not curative (Fig. 36-9).

Gastrin is a potent growth factor for parietal cells, and ZES patients have greatly increased numbers of parietal cells (from a normal population of 1×10^9 to approximately 5×10^9 parietal cells in ZES patients). In addition to the physiologically active G17 and G34 forms, gastrinomas release smaller and larger forms of gastrin, fragments of gastrin, and glycine-extended forms. All ZES patients have an elevated level of chromogranin A (present in the wall of the secretory granule).

Localization

Attempts to localize gastrinomas by means of ultrasonography, arteriography, and enhanced CT and MRI have been only partly successful. The highly invasive technique of selective portovenous sampling has proved to be less helpful with gastrinomas than with insulinomas. An improvement was achieved by selective intra-arterial injection of secretin with sampling from the right hepatic vein.[32] If, for example, venous gastrin levels spiked after secretin injection into, say, the dorsal pancreatic artery, the gastrinoma would presumably reside within the distribution of that artery. The most promising current method is SRS, which involves radionuclide scanning after injection of radiolabeled octreotide.[51,52] Because more than 90% of gastrinomas have receptors for somatostatin,

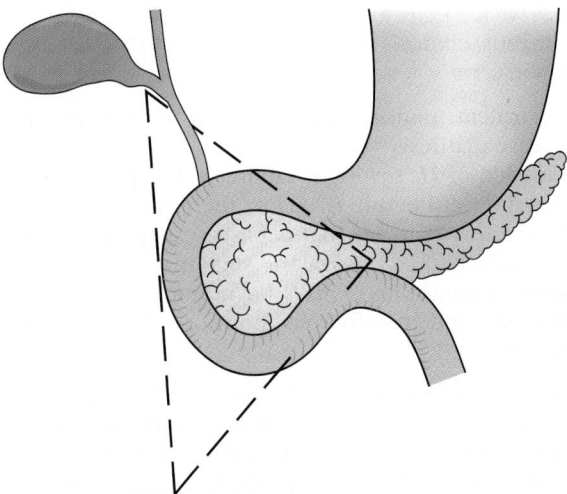

FIGURE 36-8.   The anatomic triangle in which approximately 90% of gastrinomas are found. (From Stabile BE, Morrow DJ, Passaro E Jr: The gastrinoma triangle: Operative implications. Am J Surg 147:25-31, 1984.)

TABLE 36-3. Comparison of Clinical and Laboratory Characteristics of Patients with a Benign or Malignant Clinical Course with Gastrinoma

Characteristics*	Clinical Course (% all patients)	
	Benign† (n =140)	Malignant† (n = 45)
Percentage of patients	76	24
Present with liver metastases	0	19
Develop liver metastases	0	5
Gender	Predominantly male (68)	Predominantly female (67)
MEN 1 at initial evaluation	21	Uncommon (6)
Time from onset to diagnosis	Long (mean 5.9 yr)	Short (mean 2.7 yr)
Serum gastrin level‡	Moderately elevated (mean, 1711 pg/mL)	Very elevated (mean, 5157 pg/mL)
Size of primary tumor	Small (≤1 cm)	Large (>3 cm)
Location of primary tumor	Primarily duodenum (66)	Primarily pancreatic (92)
Survival at 10 yr	Excellent (96)	Poor (30)
Flow cytometry of tumor	Low S phase (mean 3.3) High percentage of nontetraploid aneuploid (32) Multiple stem line aneuploid rare	High S phase (mean 5.1) Low percentage of nontetraploid aneuploid Multiple stem line aneuploid frequent (25)

*All characteristics were significantly different (P <0.0001) between the two groups.
†The benign or nonaggressive course was not associated with the development of liver metastases (n = 140), whereas patients in whom the gastrinoma pursued a malignant or aggressive course had liver metastases either at the initial evaluation (n = 36) or developed liver metastases (n = 9) during follow-up.
‡Normal serum gastrin level <100 pg/mL.
MEN 1, multiple endocrine neoplasia type 1.
From Jensen RT: Gastrin-producing tumors. Cancer Treat Res 89:304, 1997.

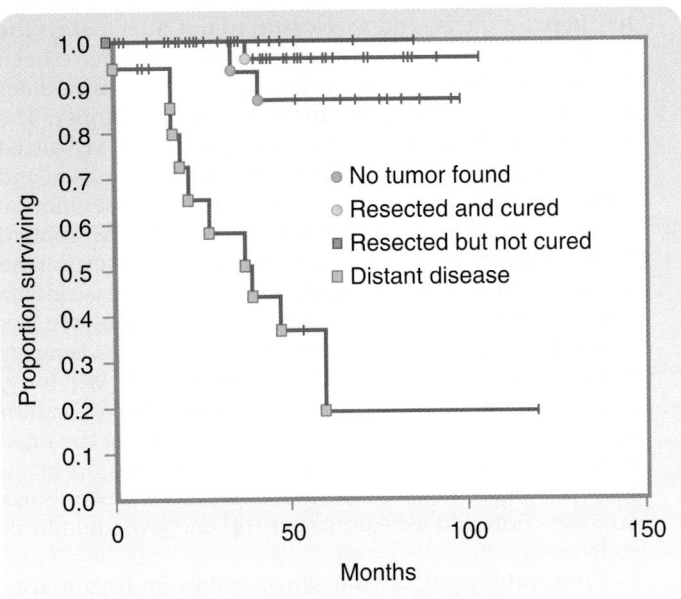

FIGURE 36-9. Proportion of patients surviving with Zollinger-Ellison syndrome from day of diagnosis. Patients were divided into four groups on the basis of preoperative evaluation, operative findings, and initial postoperative evaluation: 18 patients who had distant metastatic disease at diagnosis (included as controls), patients who had no tumor found at surgery (n = 16), patients who had tumor resected and were disease free (cured) (n = 42), and patients who had all of the tumor resected but who were not disease free (n = 15). There were no differences among the three groups with localized gastrinoma, but the group with distant disease had a significantly shorter survival time (P < .001). (From Norton JA, Doppman JL, Jensen RT: Curative resection in Zollinger-Ellison syndrome: Results of a 10-year prospective study. Ann Surg 215:8-18, 1992.)

SRS is particularly sensitive in imaging both primary and metastatic gastrinoma tissue. In this technique, 6 mCi of ^{111}In-labeled octreotide is given intravenously, and body images are obtained with a gamma camera at 4 and 24 hours (Fig. 36-10). A study from NIH compared tumor localization in 80 ZES patients by use of ultrasonography, CT, MRI, selective angiography, and bone scanning with SRS and found SRS to be the most sensitive method for either primary or metastatic liver gastrinomas.[53] The authors concluded that because of its sensitivity, simplicity, and cost-effectiveness, SRS should be the first imaging method used for gastrinoma localization in ZES patients. Detection depends on size; a later study reported that SRS detected only 30% of lesions that were 1.1 cm or less and that SRS failed to increase the disease-free rate.[51] Duodenal gastrinomas are usually small and are the most resistant to preoperative localization. Direct endoscopy and endoscopic ultrasonography are probably the most effective

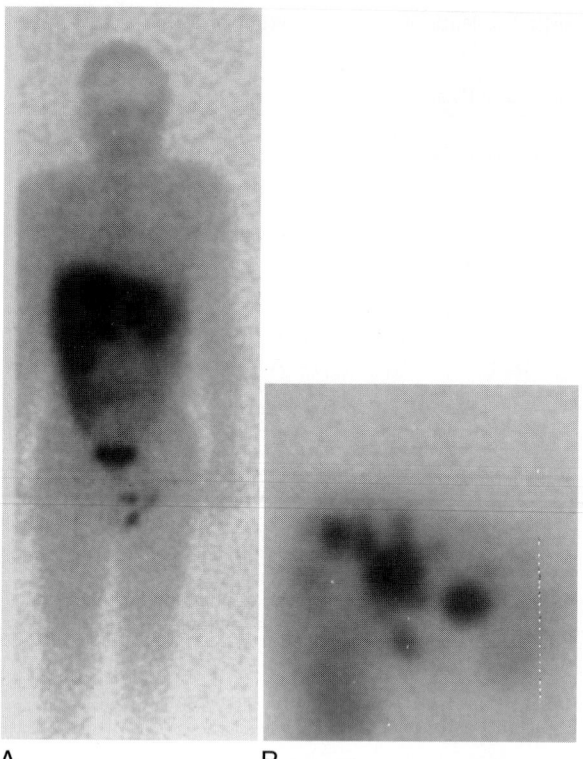

FIGURE 36-10. Somatostatin receptor scintigram of a patient with metastatic gastrinoma. **A,** Whole-body scan at 24 hours after injection of ^{111}In octreotide shows metastatic tumor in the liver with primary tumor in the head of the pancreas. **B,** Detail of hepatic metastases with pancreatic primary.

preoperative studies for detection of duodenal gastrinomas. All localizing studies have overlapping sensitivities, and most patients with gastrinomas, either primary or metastatic, will have undergone two, three, or more of the available localization techniques (ultrasound, enhanced CT and MRI, arteriography, selective portovenous sampling, selective intra-arterial secretin with hepatic vein sampling, endoscopic ultrasonography, and SRS) (see Table 36-2). The percentage of patients with a positive diagnosis but with a nonlocalized tumor has steadily decreased, but it is not yet always possible to localize the tumor before operation. Because of the complications associated with the procedure and because of often equivocal results, one study concluded that portal venous sampling for gastrin is no longer indicated[39]; we agree.

Great progress has been made in localizing tumors, but the number of true cures is still disappointing. Improvement must await the development of techniques for earlier detection or more extensive surgical procedures.

Operation

Pharmacologic control of acid secretion has rendered total gastrectomy unnecessary. The role of lesser acid-reducing surgical procedures (e.g., selective proximal vagotomy) in patients with unresectable gastrinomas is unclear but doubtful. Omeprazole therapy is so effective that we now operate only for tumor removal, and every ZES patient is a candidate for tumor-removal operation until proved otherwise because of systemic illness or widespread metastases. Although gastrinomas have a high rate of malignancy, they are more apt to be cured than is cancer of any other abdominal viscera. Efforts at surgical cure are clearly justified.

Every attempt is made to localize the tumor before surgery, and CT and MRI are effective with larger tumors and especially with hepatic metastases. Gastric secretion should be controlled during the perioperative period, and because parenteral forms of proton-pump inhibitors are not yet available, this control depends on parenteral administration of H$_2$ antagonists, the dose of which should be adjusted so as to secure a gastric acid output of 5 mEq/hour or less. Acid secretion fluctuates and must be tested often (at least three times a day).

The abdominal incision should be either a vertical midline or a bilateral subcostal, and exposure should be generous. Exploration should include the entire abdomen, from the undersurface of the diaphragm to the pelvic floor, with particular attention being paid to the liver, to the right subhepatic and paraduodenal area, and to the pelvic cul-de-sac and ovaries. The entire small bowel and colon should be examined with care, with the surgeon looking for lymph nodes in the mesentery or attached to the wall of the bowel.

We have found small primary gastrinomas free in the small bowel mesentery, adjacent to the duodenum, in the wall of the stomach, above the confluence of the right and left hepatic ducts, and as a cystic tumor attached to the lesser curvature of the stomach.[48] Gastrinomas have been reported in the ovary and colon. Any suspicious nodules should be excised and sent for frozen section biopsy. The liver should be mobilized freely and carefully visualized and palpated. Any superficial mass should be excised and should undergo biopsy; specimens of deep masses may be obtained by fine needle. When asked why he robbed banks, Willie Sutton said, "That's where the money is": the highest yield in search for gastrinomas is in the gastrinoma triangle, especially the pancreas and duodenum (see Fig. 36-8). The pancreas should be mobilized by incising its retroperitoneal attachments superiorly and inferiorly, mobilizing the spleen to allow visualization and palpation of the back of the tail of the pancreas, mobilizing the head with a wide Kocher maneuver, and taking care to maintain hemostasis in all efforts at mobilization. Gastrinomas are often firm, reddish-tan masses (others have said bluish red).

We carefully palpate the pancreas time and again, fore and aft, as well as possible, and then flood the abdomen with saline to facilitate intraoperative ultrasonography. Higher-resolution transducers (7.5 to 10 MHz) should be used for the pancreas and a 5-MHz transducer for the liver. Intraoperative ultrasonography plus palpation is effective in localizing 90% to 98% of pancreatic gastrinomas.

Finding tumors in the pancreas may be difficult, but finding duodenal tumors is more difficult. Intraoperative endoscopy with transillumination of the duodenal wall facilitates visualization of many duodenal tumors (Fig. 36-11). Some are large enough to be seen directly through

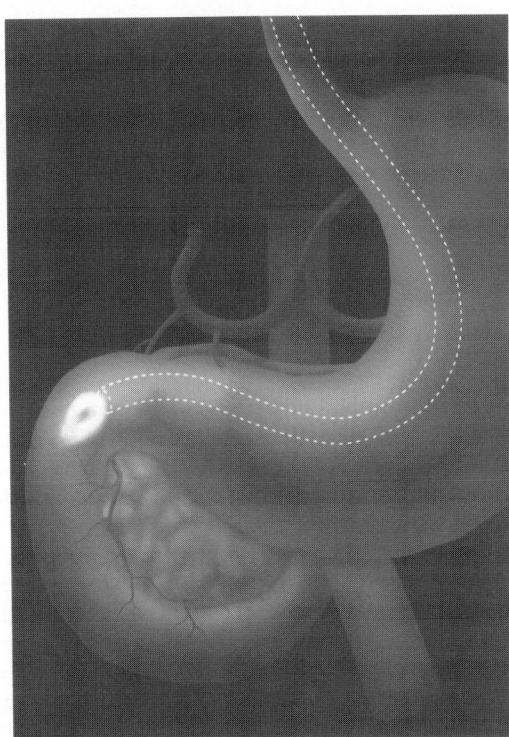

FIGURE 36-11. Duodenal gastrinoma is demonstrated by transmural endoscopic illumination. Operating room lights must be turned off to see these small tumors, which are the most common in the first part of the duodenum. (Modified from Thompson JC: Atlas of Surgery of the Stomach, Duodenum, and Small Bowel. St. Louis, Mosby–Year Book, 1992, p 301.)

the endoscope itself. Palpation occasionally localizes the larger tumors, but duodenotomy is essential for identification of duodenal gastrinomas, which are much more common proximally than distally (70% are in the first portion, 20% in the second, 10% in the third, and none in the fourth). Transillumination allows placement of the duodenotomy incision so as to avoid tumor tissue; the duodenotomy should also avoid injury to the papilla. Tumors should be excised with a full-thickness elliptical incision, and again, the papilla should be protected. If a paraduodenal lymph node shows tumor on frozen section, the primary lesion is almost always within the duodenum.

Tumors within the pancreas should be enucleated if at all possible. If they are adjacent to a duct, care must be taken not to injure the duct, but if the duct is injured, it should be fine-sutured and a drain placed. Large tumors located distally can be excised by distal pancreatectomy. Tumors within the head should be enucleated if at all possible. Because the mortality for Whipple resection has diminished greatly in the past decade, there are several reports of such successful removal of gastrinomas of the head of the pancreas that were otherwise not susceptible to enucleation. Tumors to the left of the superior mesenteric artery have a higher incidence of hepatic metastases and show more aggressive tumor behavior.[54] If all apparent tumor is removed, immediate cure rates now approach 90%. Unfortunately, with long follow-up, nearly half of the patients initially free of disease show

symptomatic or biochemical (i.e., a positive secretin test result) recurrence by 5 years. An abnormal secretin test antedates recurrent symptoms. Early reports show that with careful exploration of the duodenum, mortality greatly diminishes. Routine addition of duodenotomy yields improved detection of tumors.

The treatment of metastatic disease has undergone serial changes but is still unsatisfactory.[65] Radiation and chemotherapy are largely ineffective. The combination of doxorubicin, streptozotocin, and 5-fluorouracil has a low, temporary response rate but is highly toxic and has no impact on survival. Similarly, octreotide and interferon-alfa have few temporary and partial responses. Surgical treatment of distant metastases by cytoreduction procedures (debulking) appears useful, and some patients with solitary localized metastatic disease have prolonged postoperative disease-free survival. In patients with unresectable metastases, the question of whether to resect the primary tumor is not settled.

No consensus has yet been achieved in the treatment of patients with ZES and MEN 1, who often have multiple pancreatic and duodenal islet cell tumors.[45] A study from the Mayo Clinic suggested that because no patients were cured and few tumors are malignant, surgery was not indicated.[55] Some surgical reports of short-term cures contradict this wait-and-see attitude,[39,56] but in one small, tightly controlled series, a biochemical cure (i.e., a negative secretin test) was not achieved in any of 10 patients.[57] One review concluded that because the interval required to pronounce a patient cured is long and variable, this argument will not be settled for years.[52] Certainly, all ZES/MEN 1 patients with hyperparathyroidism should undergo parathyroidectomy. Because missed duodenal wall gastrinomas may account for the previous inability to cure patients with combined MEN 1 and ZES, we believe that in the absence of widespread disease, laparotomy is indicated to delay progress of these gastrin-producing tumors.

In a report of 151 patients operated on between 1981 and 1998, 123 of whom had sporadic gastrinomas and 28 of whom had ZES/MEN 1, gastrinomas were found in 93% of patients and in 100% of the last 81 patients operated on.[58] Gastrinomas were located in the duodenum in 49% of patients, in the pancreas in 24%, in lymph nodes in 11%, and in other locations in 9% of patients, with 16% having unknown primaries. The overall 10-year survival rate was 94%, and 34% of patients with sporadic gastrinomas were free of disease at 10 years, whereas none of the ZES/MEN 1 patients were free of disease. The authors of this NIH series concluded that all patients with the sporadic form of the ZES without metastatic disease should be offered surgical exploration. The role of surgery in patients with the ZES/MEN 1 syndrome remains unclear.

Verner-Morrison Syndrome (VIPoma)

VIPomas are endocrine tumors usually arising from pancreatic islets that secrete VIP and cause a syndrome of profound watery diarrhea, hypokalemia, and achlorhydria. The diarrhea persists despite fasting (which qualifies it as a secretory diarrhea) and despite nasogastric aspiration (which differentiates it from the diarrhea of ZES). The condition was first described in 1958 in a report of two fatal cases, both of which at autopsy revealed a pancreatic islet cell adenoma.[59] The etiologic agent was found to be a VIP-producing tumor in 1973,[5] and a later report indicated that some VIPomas may be ectopic.[60] There is actually some argument about whether VIP is a normal islet hormone: some ascribe it to the D_2 cell, and others state that, like gastrin, it occurs only in islet tumors. Verner-Morrison syndrome is highly variable. Constant features are diarrhea, hypovolemia, hypokalemia, and acidosis; variable features are achlorhydria or hypochlorhydria, hypercalcemia, hyperglycemia, and flushing with rash.[1]

The diagnostic triad in Verner-Morrison syndrome is a secretory diarrhea, high levels of circulating VIP, and a pancreatic tumor. Diarrhea volumes are often massive, 3 to 5 L/day, and the diagnosis of VIPoma is unlikely if stool volume is less than 700 mL/day. The conditions to be considered in the differential diagnosis are laxative abuse, bacterial and parasitic diarrhea, carcinoid syndrome (which shows an elevated level of 5-hydroxyindole acetic acid in the urine), and ZES (which shows an elevated serum gastrin level). Of these, VIPomas alone show elevated levels of VIP; normal levels are higher than 200 pg/mL, and VIPoma patients have levels ranging from 225 to 2000 pg/mL.

Most tumors are large by the time the syndrome is manifest, and localization is often achieved with enhanced CT, MRI, or arteriography. About 50% of patients have metastatic spread by the time of diagnosis. If abdominal studies fail to locate the tumor, a thoracic CT should be performed because as many as 10% of the tumors are intrathoracic. As soon as the diagnosis is established, treatment with the long-acting somatostatin analogue octreotide should be used to control fluid loss.

Surgical removal of VIPoma should be attempted in all VIPoma patients. Most VIPomas can be excised by distal pancreatectomy. The adrenals and retroperitoneal tissues should be carefully examined if no pancreatic tumor is found. In the 50% of patients with metastatic disease, local excision of as much tumor as can be safely removed (debulking) is indicated. Partial pancreatectomy and resection of liver metastases have been reported to bring about resolution of recurrent Verner-Morrison syndrome. In patients with nonresectable tumors, chemotherapy is rarely effective, but octreotide is helpful in the control of diarrhea.

Glucagonoma

A tumor of islet alpha cells, a glucagonoma causes a syndrome of a characteristic skin rash, diabetes mellitus, anemia, weight loss, and elevated circulating levels of glucagon. The syndrome was first described in 1942 by dermatologists who noted the relationship between a pancreatic tumor and a severe, unrelenting dermatitis.[6] The characteristic skin lesion, a necrolytic migrating erythema (Fig. 36-12), was reported to be associated with the glucagon-secreting alpha cell carcinoma of the pancreas.[7] The syndrome is rare (the largest single series reported until 1995 was 18 patients), and most patients are initially recognized by their skin lesions and referred to surgeons by dermatologists. Glucagonoma was found to be associated with a low level of amino acids, and parenteral administration of amino acid was found to bring about the disappearance of the skin lesions.[61] Diabetes is usually mild.

A pseudoglucagonoma syndrome has been described in patients who have necrolytic migratory erythema without pancreatic tumor; the cause is unknown, but the condition is associated with several chronic illnesses, and only a few patients show elevated levels of glucagon.[62]

The diagnosis is made from the characteristic skin lesion, elevated levels of glucagon (whose release can be

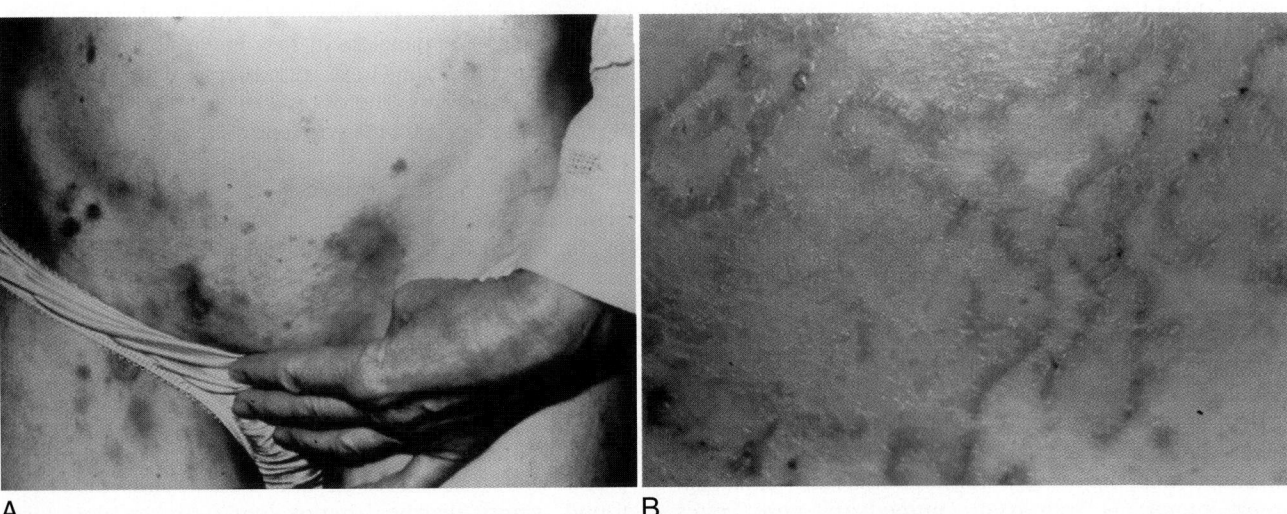

A   B

FIGURE 36-12.   The characteristic necrolytic migrating erythematous dermatitis of the glucagonoma syndrome. **A,** Confluent patches with superficial necrosis. **B,** Close-up shows serpiginous margins. (**A** and **B,** Courtesy of Hugo V. Villar, M.D.)

provoked by secretin, if necessary), and a pancreatic tumor. The upper limit of normal for glucagon is 150 to 190 pg/mL; glucagonoma patients have levels of 200 to 2000 pg/mL. The islet tumor may be demonstrated by enhanced CT or MRI or by selective angiography.

Once the diagnosis is made, the patient should be prepared by administration of total parenteral nutrition containing amino acids, with simultaneous octreotide for symptomatic relief. Because one third of these patients have been reported to have thrombotic complications after surgery, perioperative heparin is indicated.

Treatment is surgical excision of the tumor, which usually lies in the body or tail of the pancreas. Nearly all glucagonomas are malignant, but an aggressive approach to removal of the primary and metastatic tumor is warranted. Even so, the cure rate appears to be only 30%, and long-term chemotherapy has proved disappointing for metastatic disease. Symptomatic relief can be achieved with octreotide.

Somatostatinoma

All endocrine tumors of the pancreas are rare; somatostatinomas are exceedingly rare, and fewer than 60 cases have been reported. The tumor syndrome was first described in 1977 in separate reports on two individuals,[8,9] and the full syndrome (steatorrhea, diabetes mellitus, hypochlorhydria, and gallstones) was characterized 2 years later.[63] The features of the syndrome are variable and do not always coincide with predictable effects of high circulating levels of somatostatin. Most patients present with mild diabetes, but 10% have symptoms of hypoglycemia. This illustrates the unpredictability of hormone-hormone interactions: In the case of diabetes, the suppressive effect of somatostatin on insulin release predominates; in hypoglycemic patients, the predominant inhibition affects glucagon.

The clinical presentation is unpredictable; some patients have developed obstructive jaundice caused by tumor pressure on the common bile duct, whereas presenting complaints in other patients have been diarrhea and gallstones. Some duodenal somatostatinomas have been associated with von Recklinghausen's neurofibromatosis.[28] Tumors can be localized by CT, MRI, arteriography, and even SRS because somatostatinomas do possess functioning somatostatin receptors.

Treatment is surgical. Seventy to 90% of tumors have been reported to be malignant. Most tumors are in the tail of the pancreas, and caudal pancreatectomy is indicated. Localization is rarely a problem because the tumors are usually large. Hepatic metastases are common, and debulking of metastatic tumor tissue is indicated. The large size and frequency of malignancy dictate resection rather than enucleation of the pancreatic tumor. Metastases should, of course, be excluded before consideration is given to Whipple's resection of the head of the pancreas. Small duodenal tumors can be treated by local excision. At operation, cholecystectomy should be performed whether or not the patient has gallstones because if they are not present, they will likely occur.

Still-Rarer Tumors

Various functional tumors of the endocrine pancreas have been reported, some secreting GRF, some secreting neurotensin, some parathyroid hormone–related peptide, some PP, and some ACTHs, with the appropriate resultant endocrine syndrome. GRFomas are invariably associated with MEN 1 syndrome: 30% of GRF tumors originate in the pancreas, 50% in the lung, and 10% in the small bowel. Forty percent of GRFoma patients have ZES, and 40% have Cushing's syndrome. Patients with ACTH-secreting tumors usually have other endocrine syndromes, most frequently ZES. They have classic symptoms of Cushing's syndrome (which occurs in 5% of all ZES patients and in 20% of patients with both ZES and MEN 1). Neurotensinomas cause hypokalemia, weight loss, hypotension, cyanosis, flushing, and diabetes. They are usually malignant. PPomas are associated with high circulating PP levels and no characteristic symptoms, although patients with PPomas have been reported with watery diarrhea and with skin rash. PPomas are almost always large and, except when associated with MEN 1 syndrome, are usually solitary and in the head of the pancreas. Elevated levels of PP are often seen with other islet cell tumor syndromes.

Nonfunctioning Endocrine Tumors

Patients with nonfunctioning islet tumors are late in seeking help and do so finally because of symptoms of tumor progression. Most such tumors are malignant and have metastasized by the time of diagnosis. Abdominal pain and jaundice are common initial complaints that result from mechanical or mass effects of the tumor. Surgical resection should be attempted for cure when possible. More than 60% of tumors are metastatic at the time of diagnosis, but most appear to grow slowly, and prolonged survival is possible even with incurable disease (44% at 5 years).

MEDICAL THERAPY FOR ISLET CELL TUMORS

The best agent for pharmacologic control of hyperinsulinemia is diazoxide, which is widely used in preparing patients for operation and in maintenance therapy for patients with unresectable metastatic insulinoma. Octreotide therapy has also been effective, although its response rate compared with diazoxide is not yet clear. Streptozocin combined with fluorouracil has proved effective in the treatment of advanced islet cell carcinoma, both functioning and nonfunctioning, with some long-term, symptom-free intervals.[41]

In ZES patients, the achievement of pharmacologic control of gastric acid secretion, first partially with H_2-receptor antagonists and then more effectively with proton-pump inhibitors, revolutionized therapy. By defusing the risk of hypersecretory catastrophes, these drugs have virtually eliminated most of the urgent problems (bleeding, perforation, diarrhea, and fluid imbalance).

The proton-pump inhibitors have been particularly effective and have proved to be safe, despite early concerns about the potential risk of causing gastric carcinoids or other enterochromaffin cell tumors. There is a question of whether persistent hypergastrinemia in patients with MEN 1 will lead to the development of gastric carcinoids that could become malignant. The dosage should be adjusted to achieve a gastric acid secretion of less than 10 mEq/hour for the hour before the next dose of drug (in patients with severe gastroesophageal reflux disease, the reduction in acid secretion to <1 mEq/hour may be required).[45] In patients with unresectable metastatic disease, long-term antisecretory therapy with proton-pump inhibitor drugs has proved more effective and more reliable than treatment with H_2-receptor antagonists or with octreotide, the long-acting somatostatin analogue.

Long-term use of octreotide has its greatest success in the long-term treatment of VIPoma symptoms, especially diarrhea. Several attempts have been made to demonstrate an antitumor effect, but significant decreases were found only in rare patients with VIPoma or GRFoma.[64]

When metastatic disease is contained within lymph nodes and the liver, various chemotherapeutic regimens, cytoreduction (debulking) surgery, hepatic artery embolization, or combinations of these are useful. However, when metastases to bone occur, only chemotherapy, interferon treatment, or use of octreotide may be helpful. Since these tumors are rare and chemotherapeutic success unusual, accurate assessment of the role of chemotherapy will await multi-institutional trials.[65]

All islet cell tumors except insulinomas (10%) and GRFomas (30%) have a malignancy rate of greater than 60%.[66] Responses to chemotherapy have been variable: In a review of more than 700 patients with metastatic islet tumors, responses to various agents (streptozocin, chlorozotocin, 5-fluorouracil, interferon-alfa, doxorubicin, and octreotide, alone and in combination) yielded objective responses in from 0 to 26% of patients. In control studies, cytoreductive operations appear to be effective. Hepatic artery embolization is recommended for patients with hepatic metastases without extensive extrahepatic disease and may be a valuable palliative procedure, but it does not seem to prolong life.

WHAT'S NEXT?

Immunotherapy and Transplantation

Future advances in immune therapy, molecular biology, and genetics offer great hope in the management of pancreatic endocrinopathies.

The immune treatment of diabetes is underway, and patients with early-onset type I diabetes appear to respond to cyclosporine. Immunization with selected T-cell receptor peptides may lead to the generation of antibodies against clones of T cells reacting to beta cells.[67] The current best hope for surgical treatment of diabetes, of course, is to transplant islet tissue by means of either pancreatic organ transplantation or embolization of isolated islets (usually into the portal vein). The first pancreas transplantation was performed in 1966 by Kelly and colleagues.[68] By the end of 1989, nearly 2300 transplants had been performed worldwide, and the actuarial survival between 1985 and 1989 was 87% for patients and 56% for grafts. There are several problems: Where should the pancreatic duct be drained, what type of venous anastomosis (portal or systemic) should be used, how should rejection be detected, and most important, what are the life-threatening consequences of leaks and rejection?

Transplantation of isolated islets has been performed in animals since 1972 and in humans since 1980. In most of these, islets are isolated by collagenase digestion of the cadaveric pancreas. They are selected for viability by means of vital staining, and the viable islets are injected into the portal circulation (other sites, e.g., the spleen and the kidney, have been used). Between 200,000 and 500,000 islets are required to achieve euglycemia, which in most instances has been transient. A few moderately long-term successes are enticing.[69] The use of fetal tissue for islet transplantation appears to offer promise. Whole-organ transplantation is cumbersome and complicated and carries a significant risk, but it has a success rate that is considerably higher than that of isolated islet grafts. Current experimental efforts are in progress to modify xenogenic (pig, cow) islets to genetically engineer human/nonhuman insulin-producing cells that will be suitable for grafting within special immunoisolation barrier membranes.[70]

Experimental Oncology and Molecular Genetics

Experimental oncology is one of the richest fields in all of biomedical research, and we cover here only a few examples that may prove clinically useful in patients with endocrine tumors of the pancreas. Recent genomic studies have accelerated studies in the molecular genetics of these tumors. Genetic studies of endocrine tumors of the pancreas have suggested novel loci for tumor suppressor genes *3p25*, *3p27*, and *11p13*, among others. Loss of alleles in these regions may serve as markers for malignant endocrine tumors of the pancreas. The cyclin-dependent kinase inhibitor, $p27^{kip1}$, was found to be abundant in well-differentiated tumors and to be low or absent in aggressive tumors.[71]

More than 90% of these tumors show a silencing of the tumor suppressor gene *p16/MTS1*. p53 protein is prominent in exocrine tumors of the pancreas but appears to be surprisingly absent in endocrine tumors. Chromosome 3 is often deleted in sporadic malignant endocrine tumors of the pancreas and studies suggest that chromosome 3q27-qter may contain a tumor suppressor gene.[72] Evers and colleagues[73] have shown that gastrinomas amplify the protooncogene HER-2/*neu* but not *p53* or *ras*. Others report an increase in HER-2/*neu* only in aggressive tumors.[74] Studies of insulinomas have shown that the G protein $G_{s\alpha}$ has a threefold greater expression in insulinoma than in normal islet cells, suggesting that it may be involved in unregulated insulin secretion or in tumorigenesis. The progression of malignant insulinomas has been shown to be accompanied by progressive accumulation of multiple genetic lesions; activation of *myc*, transforming growth factor-α, and *ras* genes may be early events in insulinoma development. Loss of sex chromosome (X in women and Y in men) is frequent in endocrine tumors of the pancreas and appears to be associated with metastases and local invasion.[75] Cytometry of benign and malignant endocrine tumors of the pancreas has shown that hypertriploid tumors have a statistically worse prognosis than do diploid, triploid, and hypotriploid tumors.

Selected References

Doherty GM, Doppman JL, Shawker TH, et al: Results of a prospective strategy to diagnose, localize, and resect insulinomas. Surgery 110:989-997, 1991.

> **This report from the National Institutes of Health provided clear evidence that transhepatic selective portal venous sampling for insulin was the best single method for localizing insulinomas, and the authors found that intraoperative ultrasound located tumors in seven patients who did not have a palpable lesion.**

Gibril F, Reynolds JC, Doppman JL, et al: Somatostatin receptor scintigraphy: Its sensitivity compared with that of other imaging methods in detecting primary and metastatic gastrinomas: A prospective study. Ann Intern Med 125:26-34, 1996.

> **In 80 consecutive patients with Zollinger-Ellison syndrome (ZES), these National Institutes of Health authors compared conventional tumor localization methods with somatostatin receptor scintigraphy (SRS) and found SRS to be the single most sensitive method for localizing either primary gastrinomas or metastatic liver lesions. The authors concluded that because of its sensitivity, simplicity, and cost-effectiveness, SRS should be the first imaging method used in patients with ZES.**

Jensen RT: Gastrin-producing tumors. Cancer Treat Res 89:293-334, 1997.

> **In 41 tightly packed pages, Jensen provides a scholarly précis of whatever was known about gastrinoma up to 1997. He discusses growth factors, oncogenes, and tumor suppressor genes as they affect growth of gastrinoma. Particularly helpful are the discussions on pathology (especially of duodenal gastrinoma), tumor biology, and techniques of localization, as well as a plan for patients with Zollinger-Ellison syndrome (ZES) and multiple endocrine neoplasia type 1. The concept of two separate clinical forms of ZES, one benign and one malignant, is strongly substantiated.**

Norton JA: Neuroendocrine tumors of the pancreas and duodenum. Curr Probl Surg 31:77-156, 1994.

> **This review of the immense National Institutes of Health experience with surgical management of endocrine tumors of the pancreas and duodenum provides a vade mecum for the student of these syndromes. Especially helpful are discussions of localization methods for insulinomas and gastrinomas and the variabilities brought about by multiple endocrine neoplasia type 1 syndrome. Norton concludes that nearly all of these tumors can be located and that aggressive surgical management is highly beneficial. Localizing and removing duodenal gastrinomas are of paramount import in achieving improved rates of cure of Zollinger-Ellison syndrome.**

Norton JA, Fraker DL, Alexander HR, et al: Surgery to cure the Zollinger-Ellison syndrome. N Engl J Med 341:635-644, 1999.

> **This report of 151 consecutive patients operated on at the National Institutes of Health between 1981 and 1998 reported an overall rate of localization of 93% (actually 100% in the last 81 patients to undergo operation). In patients with sporadic gastrinoma, 34% were free of disease at 10 years compared with none with Zollinger-Ellison syndrome/multiple endocrine neoplasia type 1 (ZES/MEN 1) syndrome. The overall 10-year survival was 94%. The role of surgery in patients with ZES/MEN 1 remained unclear.**

Orci L: Macro- and micro-domains in the endocrine pancreas. Diabetes 31:538-565, 1982.

> **In this 1981 Banting lecture, Orci summarizes two decades of his work on the histomorphology and cytomorphology of islets, in which he details the subcellular organization of the beta cell in the biosynthesis and release of insulin, the cellular environment of beta cells, and the cross-talk between beta and neighboring islet cells. The illustrations alone invite the reader into a new world, with electron micrographs showing freeze-fracture replicas across the Golgi apparatus of a B cell, and other gifts.**

Stabile BE, Morrow DJ, Passaro E Jr: The gastrinoma triangle: Operative implications. Am J Surg 147:25-31, 1984.

> **Early efforts at operative localization of gastrinomas involved random searches of the pancreas, the subhepatic space, the retrogastric area, and the liver. Stabile and colleagues provide us with a treasure map showing where gastrinomas are likely found. The duodenum, which is one wall of that triangle, has been shown to contain about half of all gastrinomas.**

Zollinger RM, Ellison EH: Primary peptic ulcerations of the jejunum associated with islet cell tumors of the pancreas. Ann Surg 142:709-723, 1955.

> **At the 1955 meeting of the American Surgical Association in Philadelphia, Zollinger and Ellison discussed their experience with two patients, and that discussion led to the introduction of the entire clinical field of gastrointestinal endocrinopathies. Isolated observations of endocrine tumors in patients with gut dysfunction had been made, but Zollinger and Ellison made the prescient observation that the pancreatic tumor elaborated a secretagogue that caused the ulcer diathesis. Citation indices reveal that thousands of papers have recounted the experience of other scholars with Zollinger-Ellison syndrome. This paper was the "can opener" for that vast picnic.**

References

1. Nichols AG: Simple adenoma of the pancreas arising from an islet of Langerhans. J Med Res 8:385-395, 1908.
1a. Krejs GJ: VIPoma syndrome. Am J Med 82:37-48, 1987.
2. Solorzano CC, Lee JE, Pisters PW, et al: Nonfunctioning islet cell carcinoma of the pancreas: Survival results in a contemporary series of 163 patients. Surgery 130:1078-1085, 2001.
3. Srivastava A, Alexander J, Lomakin I, et al: Immunohistochemical expression of transforming growth factor-α and epidermal growth factor receptor in pancreatic endocrine tumors. Hum Pathol 32:1184-1189, 2001.

4. Seymour NE, Brunicardi FC, Chaiken RL, et al: Reversal of abnormal glucose production after pancreatic resection by pancreatic polypeptide administration in man. Surgery 104:119-129, 1988.

5. Bloom SR, Polak JM, Pearse AG: Vasoactive intestinal peptide and watery-diarrhoea syndrome. Lancet 2:14-16, 1973.

6. Becker SW, Kahn D, Rothman S: Cutaneous manifestations of internal malignant tumors. Arch Dermatol Syphilol 45:1069-1080, 1942.

7. McGavran MH, Unger RH, Recant L, et al: A glucagon-secreting alpha-cell carcinoma of the pancreas. N Engl J Med 274:1408-1413, 1966.

8. Ganda OP, Weir GC, Soeldner JS, et al: "Somatostatinoma": A somatostatin-containing tumor of the endocrine pancreas. N Engl J Med 296:963-967, 1977.

9. Larsson LI, Hirsch MA, Holst JJ, et al: Pancreatic somatostatinoma. Clinical features and physiological implications. Lancet 1:666-668, 1977.

10. Berson SA, Yalow RS, Bauman A, et al: Insulin-I^{131} metabolism in human subject: Demonstration of insulin-binding globulin in the circulation of insulin treated subjects. J Clin Invest 35:170, 1956.

11. Debas HT: Molecular insights into the development of the pancreas. Am J Surg 174:227-231, 1997.

12. Pearse AGE: The cytochemistry and ultrastructure of polypeptide hormone–producing cells of the APUD series and the embryologic, physiologic, and pathologic implications of the concept. J Histochem Cytochem 17:303-313, 1969.

13. Falin LI: The development and cytodifferentiation of the islets of Langerhans in human embryos and foetuses. Acta Anat (Basel) 68:147-168, 1967.

14. Gittes GK, Rutter WJ: Onset of cell-specific gene expression in the developing mouse pancreas. Proc Natl Acad Sci U S A 89:1128-1132, 1992.

15. Hahn von Dorsche H, Reiher H, Hahn HJ: Phases in the early development of the human islet organ. Anat Anz 166:69-76, 1988.

16. Morel C, Cordier-Bussat M, Philippe J: The upstream promoter element of the glucagon gene, G1, confers pancreatic alpha cell–specific expression. J Biol Chem 270:3046-3055, 1995.

17. Dumonteil E, Philippe J: Insulin gene: organisation, expression, and regulation. Diabetes Metab 22:164-173, 1996.

18. Bonner-Weir S, Orci L: New perspectives on the microvasculature of the islets of Langerhans in the rat. Diabetes 31:883-889, 1982.

19. Samols E, Stagner JI: Intraislet and islet-acinar portal systems and their significance. In Samols E (ed): The Endocrine Pancreas. New York, Raven, 1991, pp 93-124.

20. Liu YM, Guth PH, Kaneko K, et al: Dynamic in vivo observation of rat islet microcirculation. Pancreas 8:15-21, 1993.

21. vön Schonfeld J, Goebell H, Müller MK: The islet-acinar axis of the pancreas. Int J Pancreatol 16:131-140, 1994.

22. Havel PJ, Taborsky GJ Jr: The contribution of the autonomic nervous system to changes of glucagon and insulin secretion during hypoglycemic stress. Endocr Rev 10:332-350, 1989.

23. Whipple AO, Frantz VK: Adenoma of islet cells with hyperinsulinism: A review. Ann Surg 101:1299-1335, 1935.

24. Calender A: Molecular genetics of neuroendocrine tumors. Digestion 62(Suppl 1):3-18, 2000.

25. Evers BM, Townsend CM Jr, Thompson JC: Zollinger-Ellison syndrome. Probl Gen Surg 14:119-131, 1997.

26. Upp JR Jr, Trudel JL, Townsend CM Jr, et al: Establishment of a human gastrinoma in nude mice. Surgery 104:1037-1045, 1988.

27. Moertel CG: Karnofsky Memorial Lecture. An odyssey in the land of small tumors. J Clin Oncol 5:1502-1522, 1987.

28. Green BT, Rockey DC: Duodenal somatostatinoma presenting with complete somatostatinoma syndrome. J Clin Gastroenterol 33:415-417, 2001.

29. Howard TJ, Stabile BE, Zinner MJ, et al: Anatomic distribution of pancreatic endocrine tumors. Am J Surg 159:258-264, 1990.

30. Moss NH, Rhoads JE: Hyperinsulinism and islet cell tumors of the pancreas. In Howard JM, Jordon GL Jr (eds): Surgical Diseases of the Pancreas. Philadelphia, JB Lippincott, 1960, pp 321-370.

31. Ros PR, Mortele KJ: Imaging features of pancreatic neoplasms. Jbr-Btr 84:239-249, 2001.

32. Imamura M, Takahashi K, Adachi H, et al: Usefulness of selective arterial secretin injection test for localization of gastrinoma in the Zollinger-Ellison syndrome. Ann Surg 205:230-239, 1987.

33. Doppman JL, Miller DL, Chang R, et al: Insulinomas: localization with selective intraarterial injection of calcium. Radiology 178:237-241, 1991.

34. Brown CK, Bartlett DL, Doppman JL, et al: Intraarterial calcium stimulation and intraoperative ultrasonography in the localization and resection of insulinomas. Surgery 122:1189-1194, 1997.

35. Huai JC, Zhang W, Niu HO, et al: Localization and surgical treatment of pancreatic insulinomas guided by intraoperative ultrasound. Am J Surg 175:18-21, 1998.

36. Norton JA, Cromack DT, Shawker TH, et al: Intraoperative ultrasonographic localization of islet cell tumors: A prospective comparison to palpation. Ann Surg 207:160-168, 1988.

37. Doherty GM, Doppman JL, Shawker TH, et al: Results of a prospective strategy to diagnose, localize, and resect insulinomas. Surgery 110:989-997, 1991.

38. Hirshberg B, Libutti SK, Alexander HR, et al: Blind distal pancreatectomy for occult insulinoma, an inadvisable procedure. J Am Coll Surg 194:761-764, 2002.

39. Norton JA: Neuroendocrine tumors of the pancreas and duodenum. Curr Probl Surg 31:77-156, 1994.

40. Gill GV, Rauf O, MacFarlane IA: Diazoxide treatment for insulinoma: a national UK survey. Postgrad Med J 73:640-641, 1997.

41. Moertel CG, Hanley JA, Johnson LA: Streptozocin alone compared with streptozocin plus fluorouracil in the treatment of advanced islet-cell carcinoma. N Engl J Med 303:1189-1194, 1980.

42. Thomas CG Jr, Cuenca RE, Azizkhan RG, et al: Changing concepts of islet cell dysplasia in neonatal and infantile hyperinsulinism. World J Surg 12:598-609, 1988.

43. Martin LW, Ryckman FC, Sheldon CA: Experience with 95% pancreatectomy and splenic salvage for neonatal nesidioblastosis. Ann Surg 200:355-362, 1984.

44. Zollinger RM, Ellison EH: Primary peptic ulcerations of the jejunum associated with islet cell tumors of the pancreas. Ann Surg 142:709-723, 1955.

45. Jensen RT: Gastrin-producing tumors. Cancer Treat Res 89:293-334, 1997.

46. Beauchamp RD, Thompson JC: Endocrine tumors of the pancreas. In Zinner MJ, Schwartz SI, Ellis H, et al (eds): Maingot's Abdominal Operations. Stamford, CT, Appleton & Lange, 1997, pp 1961-1976.

47. Stabile BE, Morrow DJ, Passaro E Jr: The gastrinoma triangle: operative implications. Am J Surg 147:25-31, 1984.

48. Thompson JC, Lewis BG, Wiener I, et al: The role of surgery in the Zollinger-Ellison syndrome. Ann Surg 197:594-607, 1983.

49. Thompson JC, Reeder DD, Villar HV, et al: Natural history and experience with diagnosis and treatment of the Zollinger-Ellison syndrome. Surg Gynecol Obstet 140:721-739, 1975.

50. Weber HC, Venzon DJ, Lin JT, et al: Determinants of metastatic rate and survival in patients with Zollinger-Ellison syndrome: A prospective long-term study. Gastroenterology 108:1637-1649, 1995.

51. Alexander HR, Fraker DL, Norton JA, et al: Prospective study of somatostatin receptor scintigraphy and its effect on operative outcome in patients with Zollinger-Ellison syndrome. Ann Surg 228:228-238, 1998.

52. Jensen RT: Management of the Zollinger-Ellison syndrome in patients with multiple endocrine neoplasia type 1. J Intern Med 243:477-488, 1998.

53. Gibril F, Reynolds JC, Doppman JL, et al: Somatostatin receptor scintigraphy: Its sensitivity compared with that of other imaging methods in detecting primary and metastatic gastrinomas: A prospective study. Ann Intern Med 125:26-34, 1996.

54. Howard TJ, Sawicki MP, Stabile BE, et al: Biologic behavior of sporadic gastrinoma located to the right and left of the superior mesenteric artery. Am J Surg 165:101-106, 1993.

55. Malagelada JR, Edis AJ, Adson MA, et al: Medical and surgical options in the management of patients with gastrinoma. Gastroenterology 84:1524-1532, 1983.

56. Thompson NW, Pasieka J, Fukuuchi A: Duodenal gastrinomas, duodenotomy, and duodenal exploration in the surgical management of Zollinger-Ellison syndrome. World J Surg 17:455-462, 1993.

57. MacFarlane MP, Fraker DL, Alexander HR, et al: Prospective study of surgical resection of duodenal and pancreatic gastrinomas in multiple endocrine neoplasia type 1. Surgery 118:973-980, 1995.

58. Norton JA, Fraker DL, Alexander HR, et al: Surgery to cure the Zollinger-Ellison syndrome. N Engl J Med 341:635-644, 1999.

59. Verner JV, Morrison AB: Islet cell tumor and a syndrome of refractory watery diarrhea and hypokalemia. Am J Med 25:374-380, 1958.

60. Said SI, Faloona GR: Elevated plasma and tissue levels of vasoactive intestinal polypeptide in the watery-diarrhea syndrome due to pancreatic, bronchogenic, and other tumors. N Engl J Med 293:155-160, 1975.

61. Norton JA, Kahn CR, Schiebinger R, et al: Amino acid deficiency and the skin rash associated with glucagonoma. Ann Intern Med 91:213-215, 1979.

62. Schwartz RA: Glucagonoma and pseudoglucagonoma syndromes. Int J Dermatol 36:81-89, 1997.

63. Krejs GJ, Orci L, Conlon JM, et al: Somatostatinoma syndrome. Biochemical, morphologic, and clinical features. N Engl J Med 301:285-292, 1979.

64. Maton PN: The use of the long-acting somatostatin analogue, octreotide acetate, in patients with islet cell tumors. Gastroenterol Clin North Am 18:897-922, 1989.

65. Townsend CM Jr, Thompson JC: Up-to-date treatment of the patient with hypergastrinemia. Adv Surg 20:155-181, 1987.

66. Gibril F, Doppman JL, Jensen RT: Recent advances in the treatment of metastatic pancreatic endocrine tumors. Semin Gastrointest Dis 6:114-121, 1995.

67. Eisenbarth GS: Type I diabetes mellitus. A chronic autoimmune disease. N Engl J Med 314:1360-1368, 1986.

68. Kelly WD, Lillehei RC, Merkel FK, et al: Allotransplantation of the pancreas and duodenum along with the kidney in diabetic nephropathy. Surgery 61:827-837, 1967.

69. Shapiro AM, Lakey JR, Ryan EA, et al: Islet transplantation in seven patients with type 1 diabetes mellitus using a glucocorticoid-free immunosuppressive regimen. N Engl J Med 343:230-238, 2000.

70. Calafiore R: Perspectives in pancreatic and islet cell transplantation for the therapy of IDDM. Diabetes Care 20:889-896, 1997.

71. Canavese G, Azzoni C, Pizzi S, et al: p27: A potential main inhibitor of cell proliferation in digestive endocrine tumors but not a marker of benign behavior. Hum Pathol 32:1094-1101, 2001.

72. Guo SS, Arora C, Shimoide AT, et al: Frequent deletion of chromosome 3 in malignant sporadic pancreatic endocrine tumors. Mol Cell Endocrinol 190:109-114, 2002.

73. Evers BM, Rady PL, Sandoval K, et al: Gastrinomas demonstrate amplification of the HER-2/*neu* proto-oncogene. Ann Surg 219:596-604, 1994.

74. Goebel SU, Iwamoto M, Raffeld M, et al: HER-2/*neu* expression and gene amplification in gastrinomas: Correlations with tumor biology, growth, and aggressiveness. Cancer Res 62:3702-3710, 2002.

75. Missiaglia E, Moore PS, Williamson J, et al: Sex chromosome anomalies in pancreatic endocrine tumors. Int J Cancer 98:532-538, 2002.

CHAPTER 37

THE PITUITARY AND ADRENAL GLANDS

L. Michael Brunt, M.D. and **Jeffrey Moley, M.D.**

Pituitary Gland	Adrenal Gland

PITUITARY GLAND

Anatomy/Embryology

The pituitary is composed of two parts: an anterior lobe or adenohypophysis and the neurohypophysis, which consists of the posterior lobe, neural stalk, and infundibulum (Fig. 37-1). The anterior pituitary arises from embryonic ectoderm (Rathke's pouch) and includes the pars distalis, pars intermedia (vestigial in humans), and pars tuberalis. The pars distalis is the largest and functionally most important portion of the anterior pituitary. The neural portion of the gland arises from the diencephalon and includes the neural stalk, infundibulum, and posterior lobe. Embryonic defects in invagination and obliteration of the pharyngeal extent of Rathke's pouch may lead to craniopharyngiomas or hormonally active ectopic pituitary adenomas.

The average adult pituitary measures $10 \times 15 \times 5$ mm and weighs between 0.4 and 0.9 g. The gland is oval, bilaterally symmetrical, and brownish red. The pituitary is approximately 20% larger in females than in males and it enlarges about 10% in females during pregnancy. The adenohypophysis makes up 80% of the gland and, together with the posterior lobe, fills approximately three fourths of the sellar space. The pituitary resides within the sella turcica *(Turkish saddle)*, which is bordered anteriorly, posteriorly, and inferiorly by the sphenoid bone and laterally by the cavernous sinus (Fig. 37-2). The floor of the sella forms the roof of the sphenoidal sinus. The carotid arteries and cranial nerves III, IV, and VI traverse the cavernous sinus lateral to the sella. Nearby structures also include the optic nerves and chiasm, the maxillary body, and the median eminence of the hypothalamus, which gives rise to the pituitary stalk. The diaphragma sellae, a thick reflection of dura mater, covers the roof of the sella and closely encircles the pituitary stalk in 50% of individuals. In remaining individuals, the diaphragma sellae incompletely surrounds the stalk and may permit superior extension of pituitary tumors.

The arterial supply to the hypothalamic-pituitary region is complex and arises from three sources. The inferior hypophyseal artery, a branch of the carotid artery, supplies the posterior pituitary. The superior hypophyseal arteries branch from the circle of Willis to supply the median eminence. The middle hypophyseal arteries are of variable origin and supply the pituitary stalk. Capillary portions of the superior hypophyseal arteries drain from the hypothalamus, the median eminence, and the superior portions of the pituitary stalk into the hypophyseal portal system, which forms a secondary venous plexus in the anterior pituitary and ultimately empties into the cavernous sinus. This portal venous system constitutes the principal blood supply to the anterior pituitary and serves as the medium through which releasing hormones from the hypothalamus reach the pituitary.

Histology

Cell types of the anterior pituitary are classified by their secretory products: lactotrophs produce prolactin (PRL), somatotrophs produce growth hormone (GH), adrenocorticotrophs produce adrenocorticotropic hormone (ACTH), thyrotrophs produce thyroid-stimulating hormone (TSH), and gonadotrophs produce follicle-stimulating hormone (FSH) and luteinizing hormone (LH). Pituitary cells may, however, have plurihormonal potential, and some pituitary tumors secrete several hormones concurrently. The five pituitary cell types are regionally distributed within the gland. Lactotrophs and

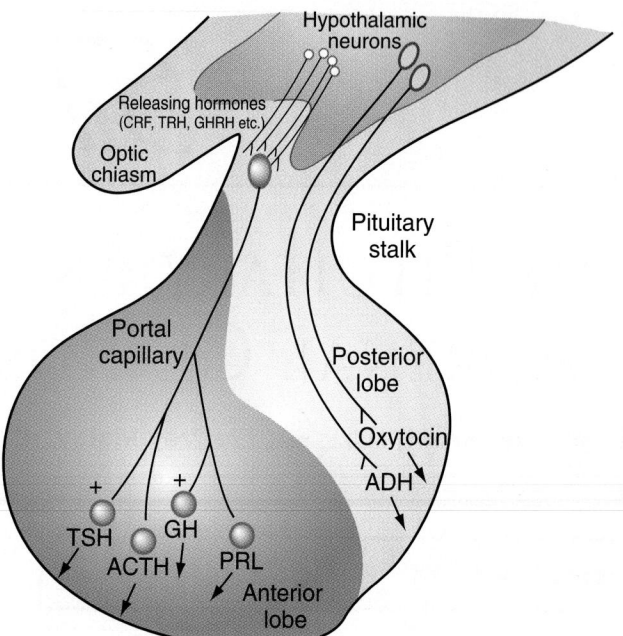

FIGURE 37-1.   Schematic representation of hypothalamic-pituitary region. Releasing hormones synthesized by hypothalamic neurons reach the adenohypophysis via the hypothalamic-pituitary portal blood system. Cells of the anterior lobe include lactotrophs, which produce prolactin (PRL); somatotrophs, which produce growth hormone (GH); corticotrophs, which produce adrenocorticotropin (ACTH); thyrotrophs, which produce thyroid-stimulating hormone (TSH); and gonadotrophs, which produce follicle-stimulating hormone (FSH) and luteinizing hormone (LH). The neurohypophysis contains antidiuretic hormone (ADH) and oxytocin synthesized by neurons of the hypothalamus.

gonadotrophs are widely distributed, somatotrophs reside peripherally within two lateral wings of the gland, thyrotrophs are anteromedially located, and corticotrophs are found within a central median wedge.

The neurohypophysis, or posterior pituitary, includes the posterior lobe, the pituitary stalk, and the median eminence. Antidiuretic hormone (ADH) and oxytocin are synthesized in the supraoptic and paraventricular nuclei of the hypothalamus and are transported through axons from these nuclei to the posterior pituitary where the active hormones are released into the capillary circulation.

Physiology

Anterior pituitary hormone secretion is controlled by the hypothalamus. Axons from the arcuate and other anterior hypothalamic nuclei terminate in the median eminence next to portal capillaries, where they release hormones into the hypothalamic-pituitary portal circulation to inhibit or stimulate cells of the anterior pituitary (Table 37-1).

The anterior pituitary secretes three groups of hormones: (1) pro-opiomelanocortin (POMC)-derived ACTH and β-lipotropin (β-LPH); (2) the related hormones GH and PRL; and (3) the glycoprotein hormones LH, FSH, and TSH. ACTH controls glucocorticoid production by the adrenal cortex; GH regulates growth and intermediary metabolism; PRL is necessary for lactation; TSH regulates the thyroid; and LH and FSH together control the gonads in males and females. Target gland hormones, in turn, participate in feedback control of the pituitary and hypothalamus.

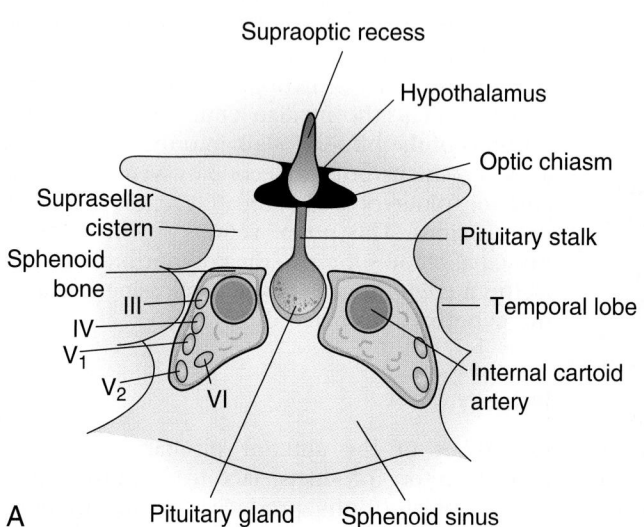

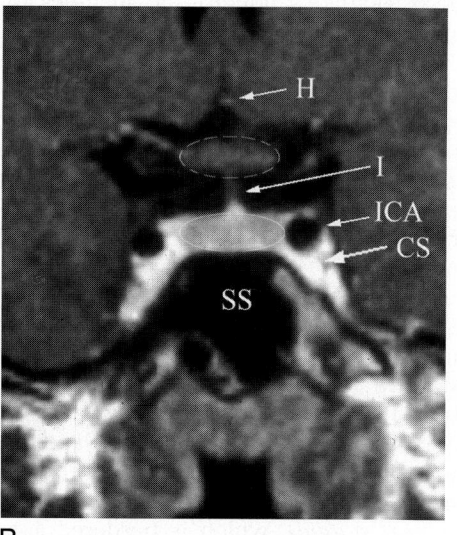

FIGURE 37-2.   Magnetic resonance (MR) image and schematic diagram of the pituitary fossa. **A,** The pituitary is bordered laterally by the cavernous sinus, which contains the internal carotid artery and cranial nerves III, IV, and VI. The optic chiasm lies immediately above the pituitary stalk. **B,** Enhanced coronal MR image. The pituitary is identified by the solid ellipse and the optic chiasm by the dotted one. Other structures seen are the hypothalamus (H), infundibulum (I) or pituitary stalk, internal carotid artery (ICA), cavernous sinus (CS), and sphenoidal sinus (SS).
(**A,** From Lechan RM: Neuroendocrinology of pituitary hormone regulation. Endocrinol Metab Clin North Am 16:475, 1987; **B,** Courtesy of FJ Wippold, MD, Mallinckrodt Institute of Radiology, Washington University School of Medicine, St. Louis, Missouri).

TABLE 37-1.   Hypothalamic and Pituitary Hormones and Their Actions

Hypothalamic Hormone	Hormone or Organ Affected	Ultimate Peripheral Action
Corticotropin-releasing hormone (CRH)	Adrenocorticotropic hormone (ACTH)	Stimulates adrenal secretion of cortisol and androgens
Thyrotropin-releasing hormone (TRH)	Thyroid-stimulating hormone (TSH)	Stimulates thyroid hormone secretion
Prolactin-releasing hormone	Prolactin (PRL)	Stimulates lactation
Gonadotropin-releasing hormone (GNRH)	Follicle-stimulating hormone (FSH), luteinizing hormone (LH)	Stimulates estradiol and progesterone secretion, folliculogenesis, and ovulation in women; stimulates testosterone secretion and sperm production in men
Growth hormone–releasing hormone (GHRH)	Growth hormone (GH)	Stimulates insulin-like growth factor-1 production
Vasopressin	Kidney	Stimulates free-water reabsorption in renal collecting ducts
Oxytocin	Uterus, breast	Stimulates uterine contraction and milk ejection
Dopamine	Prolactin	Inhibits release
Somatostatin	Growth hormone	Inhibits release

Adapted from Vance ML: Hypopituitarism. N Engl J Med 330:1651, 1994. Copyright 1994. Massachusetts Medical Society. All rights reserved.

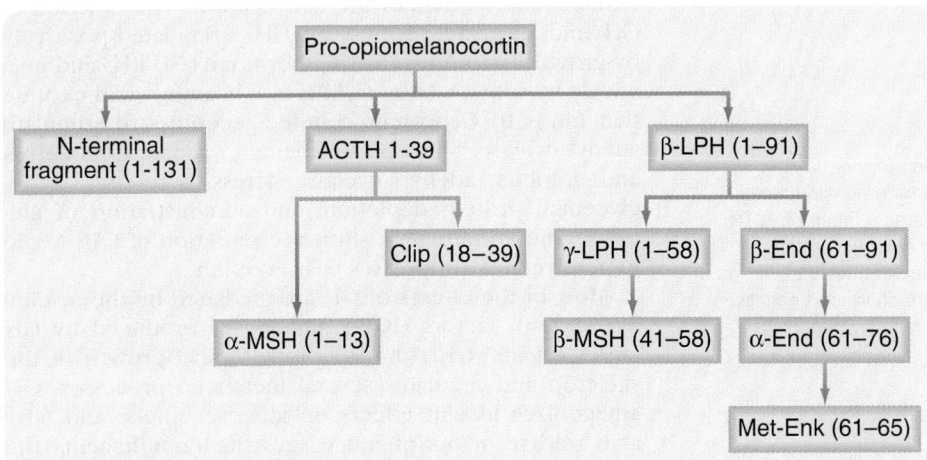

FIGURE 37-3.   High-molecular-weight precursor of ACTH and several other peptides secreted by the anterior pituitary. Clip, Clip peptide; MSH, melanocyte-stimulating hormone; LPH, lipotropin; End, endorphin; Met-Enk, met-enkephalin.

Adrenocorticotropic Hormone

ACTH is produced by corticotrophs of the anterior pituitary. This 39-amino acid peptide is part of the 241-amino acid precursor POMC. Tissue-specific processing of POMC occurs at the post-translational level to form several biologically active polypeptides, including ACTH, β-LPH, a joining peptide, and an NH2-terminal peptide (Fig. 37-3). The biologic activity of ACTH resides in its initial 18-amino acid sequence, and a stable synthetic ACTH (1-24 amino acids; Cortrosyn) is available for diagnostic use. ACTH and β-LPH have melanocyte-stimulating activity, which may explain the increased skin pigmentation seen with corticotroph hyperactivity in patients with Addison's disease and Nelson's syndrome.

Corticotropin-releasing hormone (CRH) regulates ACTH release through receptor-mediated cyclic adenosine monophosphate production in corticotrophs. Stress of major surgery, burns, fever, or hypoglycemia may elicit large (2-fold to 10-fold) increases in ACTH and cortisol secretion. ACTH stimulates cortisol production by the adrenal gland. Secretion of both hormones is normally pulsatile and follows a circadian rhythm. Plasma ACTH and serum cortisol levels are lowest between 10 PM and 2 AM and are highest at approximately 8 AM. Glucocorticoids exert negative feedback at several levels, including hypothalamic CRH release, POMC transcription and processing, and CRH-stimulated ACTH release (Fig. 37-4). In addition, ACTH exerts *short loop* negative feedback to hypothalamic CRH release.

Opioids

Cleavage of the β-LPH sequence of POMC releases the endogenous opioids β-endorphin and met-enkephalin.

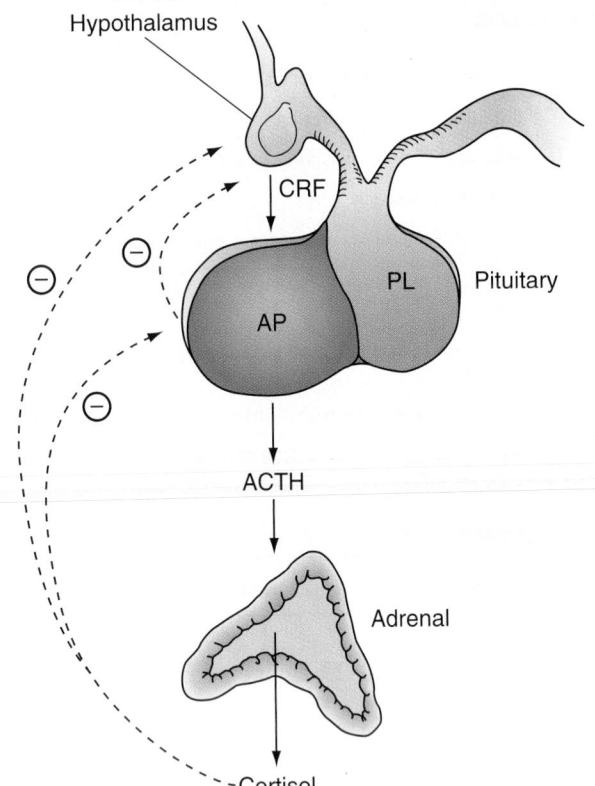

FIGURE 37-4. Schematic representation of the hypothalamic-pituitary-adrenal axis. Corticotropin-releasing factor (CRF) produced by the hypothalamus stimulates release of ACTH from the pituitary, which in turn stimulates cortisol secretion by the adrenal. Cortisol exerts negative feedback at both the hypothalamus and pituitary. ACTH also exerts short loop negative feedback of hypothalamic CRF release. AP, anterior pituitary; PL, posterior lobe.

Opioids stimulate opiate receptors in the brain and spinal cord to produce analgesia. The endogenous opioids are released from many central nervous system sites during periods of stress, shock, or hypoglycemia.

Prolactin and Growth Hormone Family

Prolactin, human GH, and human placental lactogen (hPL) make up a related family of hormones sharing a common ancestral gene. Within the human PRL-GH family, a single PRL gene is present on chromosome 6 and five GH-related genes are located on chromosome 17. Only PRL and GH seem relevant to pituitary function.

PROLACTIN

PRL circulates as a 23,000-molecular-weight monomeric polypeptide, and normal baseline levels are less than 20 µg/L in women and less than 10 µg/L in men. Synthesis and release of PRL by lactotrophs are under tonic inhibition by hypothalamic dopamine. Suckling of the breast is the principal physiologic stimulus for PRL release under normal conditions and causes a 10- to 100-fold increase in PRL within 30 minutes of stimulation. Prolactin is secreted by lactotrophs, which constitute 10% to 30% of the cells of the normal pituitary and 70% of cells in females during pregnancy. Prolactin-releasing peptide is a potent stimulator of prolactin release. Thyrotropin-releasing hormone (TRH) also has PRL releasing effects.

PRL binds to specific receptors in the breast to initiate and sustain lactation. Physiologic hyperprolactinemia suppresses gonadotropin-releasing hormone (GnRH) and transiently depresses the hypothalamic-pituitary-gonadal axis during lactation. This effect may explain the often observed, although unreliable, phenomenon of decreased fertility in lactating women. Dopamine, L-dopa, and the ergot alkaloid bromocriptine inhibit PRL release and lactation. Metoclopramide, haloperidol, chlorpromazine, and reserpine can interfere with release of dopamine into the pituitary portal circulation, enhance PRL secretion, and cause galactorrhea.

GROWTH HORMONE

Growth hormone is a 191-amino acid peptide that circulates bound to a GH-binding protein that is identical to the extracellular domain of the GH receptor. The function of GH-binding protein is unclear. GH is regulated positively by growth hormone-releasing hormone (GH-RH) and negatively by somatostatin. GH-RH is a 44-amino acid peptide that binds to G protein–coupled receptors to stimulate adenyl cyclase. Somatostatin binds to separate receptors and inhibits adenyl cyclase. Stress, exercise, hypoglycemia, protein depletion, and administration of glucagon and arginine can stimulate secretion of GH. Acute hyperglycemia suppresses GH secretion.

Most of the effects of GH are mediated by the insulin-like growth factors (IGF-1 and IGF-2) produced by GH target organs. GH stimulates longitudinal growth of the skeleton and regulates several metabolic processes. GH antagonizes insulin effects on glucose uptake and fatty acid release in peripheral tissues but complements the anabolic effect of insulin on amino acid uptake. GH also stimulates insulin secretion by the pancreas and stimulates hepatocyte growth and adipocyte metabolism. GH promotes anabolism in burn patients and has been shown to prevent corticosteroid-induced catabolism.

Glycoprotein Hormones

TSH, FSH, and LH are glycoprotein hormones of the anterior pituitary. Each is composed of two subunits: A 92-amino acid alpha subunit is encoded by a gene on chromosome 6 and is identical among these three hormones. The beta subunit is unique for each hormone and confers specificity.

THYROID-STIMULATING HORMONE

TSH is a 28,000-molecular-weight glycoprotein whose alpha subunit is encoded by a gene on chromosome 1. TSH secretion follows a pulsatile circadian pattern in response to stimulation by the hypothalamic tripeptide TRH. TSH binds to receptors on thyroid epithelium, stimulates iodide transport and thyroglobulin proteolysis, and stimulates thyroid hormone release, which activates adenyl cyclase. TSH also increases the size and vascularity of the thyroid gland. The thyroid hormones, triiodothyronine (T_3) and thyroxine (T_4), exert negative feedback on TSH release by the pituitary. TSH also inhibits hypothalamic release of TRH by a short-loop negative feedback (Fig. 37-5). Somatostatin, dopamine, and glucocorticoids also decrease TSH release.

LUTEINIZING HORMONE AND FOLLICLE-STIMULATING HORMONE

In males, LH stimulates Leydig cells to produce testosterone, whereas FSH binds to receptors on the Sertoli cells to promote spermatogenesis. Testosterone and the gonadotropins influence both the rate and numbers of germ cells that ultimately differentiate into mature sperm. Testosterone and its metabolite dihydrotestosterone stimulate growth of the penis and scrotum, promote development of facial, axillary, and pubic hair, and influence states of libido and aggressiveness.

In females, LH and FSH regulate cyclic ovarian function. FSH stimulates maturation of the graafian follicle and its production of estradiol. A mid-cycle surge of LH causes follicular rupture, ovulation, and establishment of the corpus luteum. LH maintains luteal function until either pregnancy or luteolysis. In general, sex steroids exert negative feedback on release of LH and FSH by the pituitary. Over a 24- to 36-hour interval before ovulation, however, estradiol and progesterone transiently stimulate LH secretion and, to a lesser extent, FSH secretion. A gradual increase in plasma estradiol to levels above 300 pg/mL for a duration of 5 to 7 days followed by a rise in plasma progesterone from 0.5 to 1.5 ng/mL enhances release of LH and FSH and leads to ovulation. Gonadotropin-releasing hormone (GnRH) stimulates gonadotropin secretion from the pituitary. Androgens suppress GnRH from the hypothalamus, whereas estradiol, converted from testosterone in peripheral tissues, inhibits GnRH-induced LH release from the pituitary. Sertoli cells release the peptide inhibin, which suppresses release of FSH but not LH.

Neurohypophyseal Hormones

Antidiuretic hormone (ADH, also known as vasopressin) and oxytocin are the two principal hormones secreted by the posterior pituitary. These hormones both contain nine amino acids and are derived from a common ancestral hormone, vasotocin.

ANTIDIURETIC HORMONE

ADH is synthesized by the pituitary and is released into the circulation in conjunction with the carrier protein neurophysin II. ADH circulates to the kidney, where it stimulates sodium and chloride reabsorption by epithelial cells of the medullary thick ascending loop of Henle. In addition, ADH enhances permeability to water within the collecting ducts of the medulla. Release of ADH is stimulated by a rise in plasma osmolality above 285 mOsm or a decrease in circulating blood volume by 5% or more. ADH is also secreted in response to catecholamines, angiotensin, opiates, and other analgesic or anesthetic agents. Drugs such as phenytoin, alcohol, and lithium suppress release of ADH.

OXYTOCIN

Oxytocin and its carrier protein neurophysin I are released by neural pathways during distention of the vagina or uterus or by suckling of the nipples. Oxytocin stimulates uterine contraction during labor and elicits milk ejection by myoepithelial cells of the mammary ducts during lactation.

Pituitary Tumors

Pituitary tumors are the most common intracranial neoplasm and account for 10% to 15% of all intracranial tumors. The incidence increases with advancing age and prevalence rates in autopsy series have been as high as 20%.[1] The clinical disease prevalence rate, however, is approximately 1000-fold less. Pituitary tumors are classified both according to their hormone content and by their size. Pituitary microadenomas are defined as less than 10 mm in diameter and are located completely within the

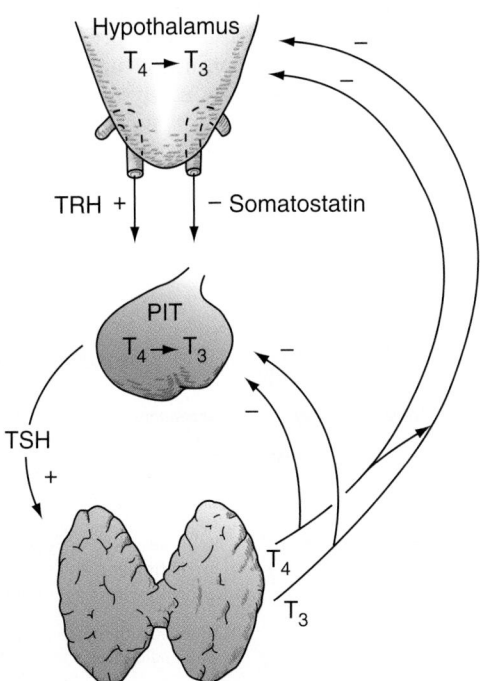

FIGURE 37-5. Schematic representation of hypothalamic-pituitary-thyroid gland axis. Hypothalamic thyrotropin-releasing hormone (TRH) regulates secretion of thyrotropin-stimulating hormone (TSH) by the pituitary (PIT), which in turn stimulates thyroid production of thyroid hormones triiodothyronine (T_3) and thyroxine (T_4). Thyroid hormones feed back to inhibit TRH and TSH in the hypothalamus and pituitary, respectively. In addition, there is a "short loop" by which TSH feeds back at the hypothalamic level to inhibit TRH.
(From Wilson JD, Foster DW [eds]: Williams Textbook of Endocrinology, 8th ed. Philadelphia, WB Saunders, 1992, p 169.)

sella, whereas macroadenomas are more than 10 mm in size and are often associated with extrasellar extension. Prolactinomas and GH-producing adenomas are the most frequent pituitary tumor types. ACTH-producing adenomas and gonadotroph adenomas are less common, and TSH-producing adenomas are rare. Other sellar or parasellar tumors include craniopharyngiomas, germ cell tumors, and metastatic lesions.

Pathogenesis

X chromosomal inactivation studies have shown that the majority of pituitary tumors are clonal in origin.[2] This observation and the absence of associated hyperplasia in most pituitary adenomas suggest that a molecular defect is the basis for the pathogenesis of pituitary tumors.[1] However, hormonal and other promoting factors are also likely important in tumor development, because autopsy studies show a much higher prevalence of these tumors than is apparent clinically.[3] Mutations in the G protein signaling system have been identified in a subset of GH-secreting pituitary tumors. These point mutations occur in the alpha chain of the guanosine triphosphate–binding protein G_s (gsp mutations), which is the adenylate cyclase–stimulating G protein associated with the GH-RH receptor.[4] Constitutive activation of this pathway leads to elevated cyclic adenosine monophosphate in these cells, which in turn results in GH hypersecretion. These gsp mutations have been found in approximately 40% of GH-secreting tumors as well as in a small percentage of nonfunctioning and ACTH-secreting pituitary adenomas.[3]

Clinical Presentation

The frequency of various functioning pituitary tumors and their clinical presentation are given in Table 37-2. Prolactinomas cause galactorrhea and hypogonadism (e.g., amenorrhea and infertility in women and impotence in men). GH-secreting tumors cause gigantism in children and acromegaly in adults. ACTH-producing tumors produce signs and symptoms of hypercortisolism (Cushing's syndrome). Glycoprotein hormone (LH, FSH, and TSH)–producing adenomas cause infertility and sexual dysfunction. Pituitary tumors may also cause deficiency of one or more hormones or may even result in panhypopituitarism.

Pituitary tumors may also cause symptoms from local mass effects. Headaches may occur as well as signs and symptoms related to compression of nearby cranial nerves. Headache from pituitary tumors is variable, and its pathogenesis is unknown. Pituitary neoplasms enlarge superiorly toward the optic chiasm and may produce visual field changes. The classic defect, bitemporal hemianopsia, is variable, and other visual defects occur. Extraocular muscle movements can be limited secondary to compression of cranial nerves III, IV, and VI in the cavernous sinus. Fundoscopic examination may reveal pallor of the optic disc, yet papilledema is unusual. Spontaneous cerebrospinal fluid (CSF) rhinorrhea occurs rarely (0.5% of patients), but a pituitary tumor is the most common cause of this symptom. Despite the presence of local extension in some patients, pituitary tumors are usually considered benign because they rarely metastasize.

TABLE 37-2.   Classification and Treatment of Pituitary Tumors

Tumor	Frequency	Primary Clinical Manifestations	Primary Therapy	Secondary Therapy
Prolactinoma	30%-50%	Females: galactorrhea, amenorrhea Males: mass effects	Dopamine agonists	Surgical resection
Growth hormone–producing adenoma	20%	Adults: acromegaly Children: gigantism	Surgical resection	Somatostatin analogue, radiation therapy, ?growth hormone receptor antagonists
Corticotropin-producing adenoma	10%-15%	Cushing's syndrome	Surgical resection	Radiation therapy, bilateral adrenalectomy, ketoconazole
Gonadotropin-producing adenoma	10%-15%	Mass effects, hypopituitarism Females: ovarian hyperstimulation* Males: ↑ testosterone, ↑ libido	Surgical resection	Radiation therapy
Thyrotropin-producing adenoma	1%-2.8%	Hyperthyroidism/goiter	Surgical resection	Somatostatin analogue
Nonfunctioning adenoma	5%-10%	Mass effect/hypopituitarism	Microadenomas: observation Macroadenomas: surgical resection	Radiation therapy

*Ovarian hyperstimulation: multiple ovarian cysts, endometrial hyperplasia.

Diagnostic Evaluation

In the past, patients with pituitary tumors often presented with classic endocrine and neuro-ophthalmologic abnormalities caused by an advanced tumor. Today, most pituitary tumors are diagnosed earlier with symptoms of endocrine hypersecretion only. The symptomatic patient with features of a pituitary lesion should undergo a complete neurologic examination with formal visual field evaluation. Bedside testing with confrontation may detect gross field cuts only. Neuro-ophthalmologic examination with visual field testing and evaluation of acuity, contrast, and color vision is necessary to detect subtle field defects and should be performed in patients before and after treatment for macroadenomas. A complete endocrinologic battery should be considered, including PRL, GH, TSH, FSH, LH, and fasting early morning cortisol level.

Biochemical assessment of anterior pituitary function includes measurement of basal plasma levels of a hormone under standard conditions as outlined in Table 37-3. Dynamic testing of pituitary reserve using individual provocative or suppression tests may occasionally be required when basal levels are equivocal. Careful consideration of time of day and stress factors must be made because even the discomfort associated with blood drawing may stimulate pituitary hormone secretion. Further details of the biochemical evaluation for each specific tumor type are given later in this chapter.

Diagnostic Imaging and Localization

Dynamic high-resolution magnetic resonance imaging (MRI) with intravenous gadolinium contrast medium enhancement is the diagnostic imaging modality of choice for patients with suspected pituitary disease.[5] MRI visualizes the optic chiasm, pituitary gland, pituitary stalk, cavernous portion of the internal carotid, and cavernous sinus with excellent detail (Figs. 37-6 through 37-8). It detects pituitary adenomas over 5 mm with a sensitivity approaching 100%, although very small microadenomas, as in Cushing's disease, may be missed.[6] MRI also reliably identifies macroadenomas and pituitary apoplexy (hemorrhage into a macroadenoma), as well as most other pituitary pathology. MRI is superior to computed tomography (CT) in assessing the dimensions of the sella turcica and in identifying pathologic processes in juxtasellar regions. In patients who are unable to undergo MRI, fine-section (1 mm) coronal CT with intravenous contrast medium enhancement may also be used to image pituitary adenomas and to demonstrate the relationship of the sella to surrounding structures. About 50% of microadenomas, however, are isodense with surrounding tissues or are not large enough to be resolved with present CT scanning techniques.

Inferior petrosal sinus (IPS) sampling and venous sampling of the cavernous sinus assist in the evaluation of patients with acromegaly or Cushing's syndrome by localizing GH- or ACTH-secreting pituitary tumors that are undetectable by MRI or CT. Measurement of basal and corticotropin-releasing hormone (CRH)-stimulated ACTH levels reliably differentiates pituitary from adrenal and ectopic causes of Cushing's syndrome. IPS may, however, be associated with serious complications, including venous thrombosis, pulmonary embolus, and vascular damage to the brain stem. Catheter angiography, particularly when performed with digital subtraction techniques, can detect abnormal carotid siphon anatomy, identify the positions of segments of the circle of Willis, and detect aneurysms or vascular malformations but is not often indicated.

TABLE 37-3.   Pituitary Hormone Evaluation

Pituitary Hormone	Basal Test	Dynamic Test	
		Hyperfunction	**Hypofunction**
Prolactin	AM serum prolactin	None	TRH stimulation
Growth hormone	Serum IGF-1 and growth hormone	Glucose suppression of growth hormone	Insulin-induced hypoglycemia, ?GHRH stimulation
ACTH	Urine free cortisol* Plasma ACTH	Low-dose DST* High-dose DST† IPS-CRH†	ACTH stimulation
Gonadotropins	Fasting prolactin, luteinizing hormone, FSH, TSH, IGF-1, glycoprotein α subunit, estradiol, testosterone	TRH stimulation of TSH, luteinizing hormone, gonadotropins, and subunits	TRH stimulation
TSH	Serum T$_4$, serum TSH	None	TRH stimulation

TRH, thyrotropin-releasing hormone; ACTH, adrenocorticotropic hormone; FSH, follicle-stimulating hormone; TSH, thyroid-stimulating hormone; DST, dexamethasone suppression test; IPS-CRH, inferior petrosal sinus sampling—corticotropin-releasing hormone test; GHRH, growth hormone–releasing hormone; IGF-1, insulin-like growth factor-1; T$_4$, thyroxine.
*Establishes hypercortisolism (Cushing's syndrome).
†Localizes cause of hypercortisolism to the pituitary (Cushing's disease).
See text for details of testing.

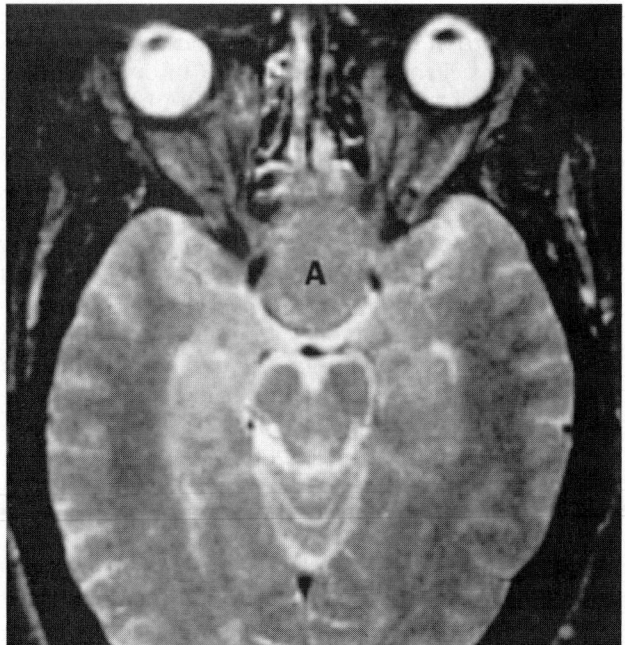

FIGURE 37-6.   Axial spin-echo T2-weighted MR image of a large pituitary adenoma (A) that occupies the suprasellar cistern. (Courtesy of F. J. Wippold, M.D., Mallinckrodt Institute of Radiology, Washington University School of Medicine, St. Louis, Missouri.)

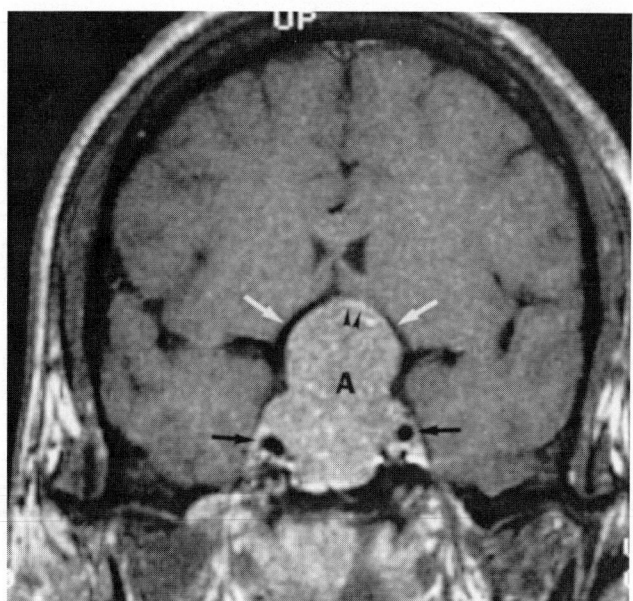

FIGURE 37-8.   Coronal spin-echo T1-weighted MR image of a pituitary adenoma after Gd-DTPA enhancement. The adenoma (A) enhances, therefore increasing its signal. The tumor displaces the carotid arteries laterally *(black arrows)*. Note that the A1 segments of the anterior cerebral arteries *(white arrows)* and the chiasm *(arrowheads)* drape over the mass. (Courtesy of F. J. Wippold, M.D., Mallinckrodt Institute of Radiology, Washington University School of Medicine, St. Louis, Missouri.)

General Approach to Management of Pituitary Disorders

MEDICAL THERAPY

Medical management of pituitary disease serves two purposes: primary or adjuvant treatment for select functioning tumors and hormone replacement for hypopituitarism. Three classes of agents are available for the treatment of hormone excess due to pituitary tumors: (1) dopamine agonists; (2) somatostatin analogues; and (3) hormone receptor antagonists. Both the dopamine antagonists and somatostatin analogues exist in short- and long-acting preparations. Primary medical treatment of functioning pituitary tumors is generally limited to dopamine receptor agonists (bromocriptine or cabergoline) for the treatment of prolactinomas. Further details regarding medical management options are given below under the specific tumor types and in the section on hypopituitarism.

SURGICAL THERAPY

Surgical resection is the primary therapy for pituitary adenomas other than prolactinoma and for pituitary apoplexy unresponsive to medical therapy. A transsphenoidal approach is appropriate for over 95% of pituitary lesions. Either an endoscopic transnasal or a sublabial transsphenoidal approach may be used (Fig. 37-9), but the transnasal procedure is generally preferred.[7] In this approach, the sphenoidal sinus and floor of the sella are exposed using an endoscope inserted into one nostril. The pituitary lesion is then removed using standard microsurgical

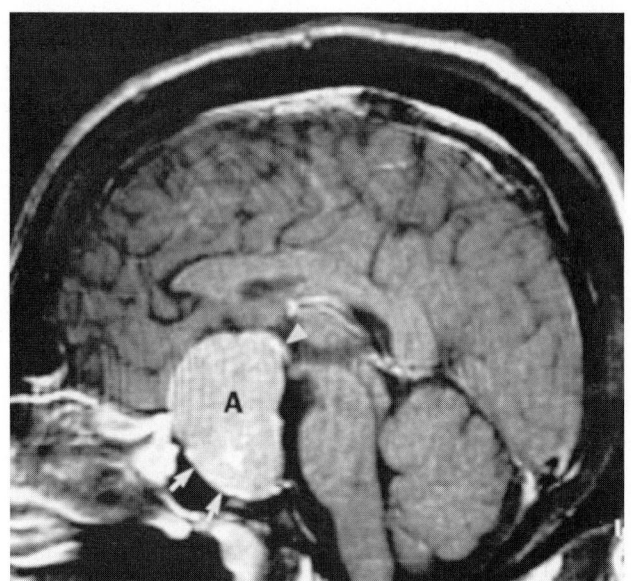

FIGURE 37-7.   Sagittal spin-echo T1-weighted MR image of a pituitary adenoma after Gd-DTPA enhancement. The enhancing adenoma (A) fills an expanded sella turcica *(white arrows)* and extends into the suprasellar cistern. The mass indents the third ventricle *(white arrowhead)*. (Courtesy of F. J. Wippold, M.D., Mallinckrodt Institute of Radiology, Washington University School of Medicine, St. Louis, Missouri.)

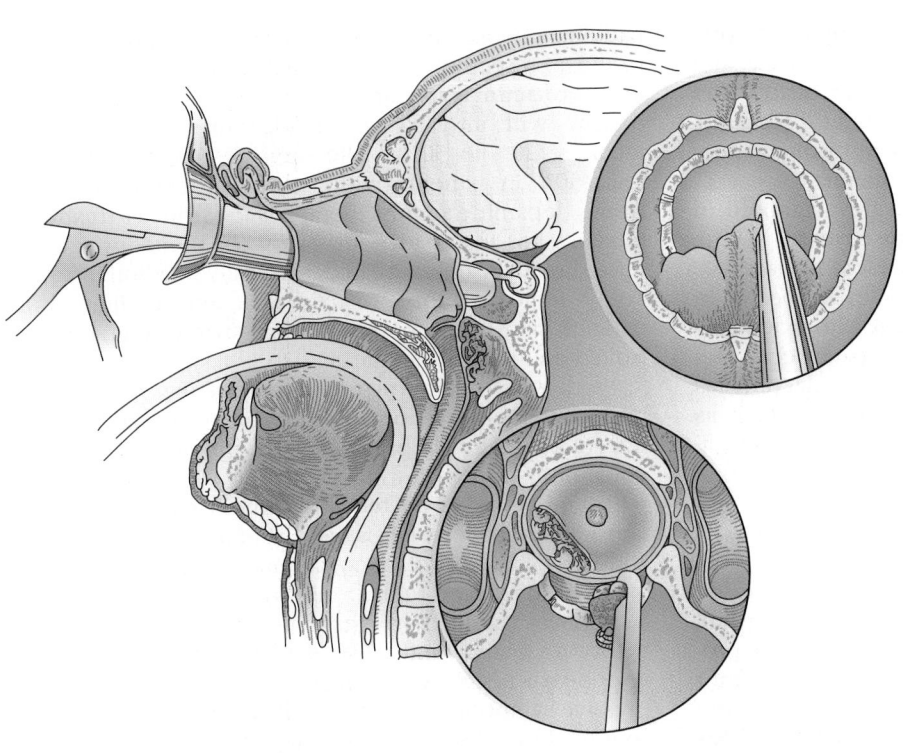

FIGURE 37-9. Endonasal transsphenoidal resection of a pituitary tumor. **Top Inset,** Removal of the sella floor with small rongeurs. **Bottom Inset,** Exposed inferior aspect of a pituitary adenoma. (Reproduced from Tindall GT, Barrow DL: Disorders of the Pituitary. St. Louis, CV Mosby, 1986, with permission.)

techniques.[8] This approach can be converted to a sublabial incision if wider exposure is needed. In some cases, a transfrontal craniotomy approach is necessary to remove larger pituitary tumors that have grown into the subarachnoid space, suprasellar cistern, or cavernous sinus with compression of neural and vascular structures. The results of transsphenoidal pituitary surgery reflect the expertise of the surgeon, the size of the tumor, and previous therapy.[9,10] Transsphenoidal resection of microadenomas results in remission rates of 70% to 90%.[8] Recurrence rates over 10-year follow-up ranged from 8% to 16% in one series and were highest in patients with clinically nonfunctioning tumors.[8] Transsphenoidal resection of macroadenomas is curative in only 40% to 50% of cases, although visual field abnormalities are improved in 70% to 80% of patients.[8,11]

Complication rates for transsphenoidal pituitary surgery are low, and current mortality rates are less than 0.5%. Major complications such as CSF rhinorrhea, cranial nerve palsy, and vision loss occur in 1.5% of patients.[8] Panhypopituitarism is observed in approximately 3% of operations performed for microadenoma and in a somewhat higher percentage of operations for macroadenoma. Diabetes insipidus occurs in 5% to 30% of cases and is usually transient.[8,11]

RADIATION THERAPY

Radiation therapy is reserved for patients with incompletely resected tumors, with recurrent symptoms after surgery, and for those who refuse surgery or who are a prohibitive surgical risk. Options include conventional external-beam radiotherapy or stereotactic radiosurgery (gamma knife). Conventional radiotherapy is usually given as 45 to 50 Gy over a 5- to 6-week period. In properly selected cases, external-beam radiotherapy results in a 70% response rate; however, the onset of effect is slow and panhypopituitarism occurs in up to 50% of cases. Other complications of this technique include damage to the optic pathways and development of a second brain tumor (estimated risk up to 16 times that of the general population).[12] Stereotactic (gamma knife) radiosurgery delivers radiation with high precision to the target with a low dose to surrounding tissue. Done under local anesthesia in an outpatient setting, a single dose of 20 to 30 Gy is delivered to the tumor using stereotactic MRI guidance.[13] Complications of optic neuropathy are infrequent, but pituitary insufficiency may still develop. The principal role of this technique is largely adjunctive, after incomplete or failed resection, or for unresectable tumors with extrasellar extension into the cavernous sinus.[12,13]

Diagnosis and Management of Specific Pituitary Tumors

PROLACTINOMA

Prolactinomas are the most common functioning pituitary tumors, representing 30% to 50% of all pituitary neoplasms,[14] and they are the most common cause of nonphysiologic hyperprolactinemia. The causes of hyperprolactinemia are numerous and include (1) medications such as tricyclic antidepressants, monoamine oxidase inhibitors, metoclopramide, verapamil, opiates, and cocaine; (2) hypothalamic disorders (tumors, irradiation, inflammatory processes); (3) medical conditions such as cirrhosis, renal insufficiency, hypothyroidism, adrenal insufficiency, and pregnancy; (4) pituitary stalk compression by tumors; and (5) rarely ectopic PRL production.[14,15] Oral estrogens may cause galactorrhea, but prolactinoma should be suspected if amenorrhea and galactorrhea persist more than 6 months after discontinuing oral contraceptive use. A pregnancy test is mandatory in all female patients with hyperprolactinemia.

Most pituitary prolactinomas (85%) are diagnosed in women, two thirds of which are discovered in the microadenoma stage. Galactorrhea is present in over 75% of women with prolactinoma, and amenorrhea occurs in up to 50%. Men are more likely to present with macroadenomas and experience symptoms of a space-occupying lesion of the sella. A minority of men with prolactinomas present with symptoms of hyperprolactinemia, such as impotence, infertility, decreased libido, or galactorrhea. Prolonged hyperprolactinemia may result in hypogonadism, which can lead to osteopenia in both males and females. Prolactinomas occur in up to 40% of individuals with multiple endocrine neoplasia (MEN) type 1.

A serum PRL level greater than 200 ng/mL is diagnostic of a prolactinoma, and levels between 100 and 200 ng/mL in a nonpregnant patient are usually caused by a prolactinoma.[11] Moderately elevated levels (25 to 100 ng/mL) should be repeated to exclude stress-induced hyperprolactinemia. The degree of hyperprolactinemia correlates roughly with tumor size. Basal PRL levels above 250 ng/mL in males and in nonpregnant females are almost invariably due to a macroprolactinoma.[15] Prolactin levels between 100 and 200 ng/mL suggest either a microprolactinoma or pituitary stalk compression by an adenoma with disruption of dopamine transport to the anterior pituitary (pseudoprolactinoma). Most medications do not cause plasma PRL levels above 100 ng/mL.

Most asymptomatic microprolactinomas, found during screening of patients with MEN 1, remain stable over time and require only observation. Treatment is necessary for symptomatic prolactinomas with the goal of correction of the endocrinopathy and relief of symptoms due to a sellar mass. Medical therapy with one of the dopamine agonists is highly effective for both microprolactinomas and macroprolactinomas. These agents act by binding to the dopamine receptors on the surface of PRL cells and act to inhibit synthesis and secretion of prolactin. The currently used dopamine agonists include bromocriptine, pergolide, and cabergoline. Cabergoline is a newer agent that has the advantages of a longer half-life and less frequent dosing.[15] In patients with microprolactinomas, normalization of PRL levels occurs within several weeks of therapy in 80% to 90% of patients.[16] Demonstrable tumor shrinkage is seen in 60% to 70% of microprolactinomas within 3 to 6 months of medical treatment, and 30% to 40% have no tumor that can be visualized after medical therapy. The duration of therapy is controversial but should be at least 5 to 6 years and may be lifelong.

Transsphenoidal resection is indicated in patients who fail medical therapy or who are intolerant to it. In patients with microprolactinomas, restoration of prolactin levels to normal occurs in 85% to 90% of patients, with recurrence rates less than 10% at 10-year follow-up.[16,17] Because treatment with dopamine agonists is costly, is of long term, and may be associated with significant side effects, some patients choose operation as primary therapy.[18,19] The results of resection are less favorable for macroprolactinomas. Prolactin levels are normalized in 60% to 70% of patients with intrasellar macroadenomas, but recurrence rates are 20% to 50%.[20] The surgical success rate is less than 50% in patients with extrasellar extension. As a result, dopamine agonist therapy is the primary treatment modality for macroadenomas as well. Pseudoprolactinomas should also be treated surgically. Radiotherapy is rarely indicated for prolactinomas and is limited to patients with symptomatic tumors that cannot be controlled medically or surgically.

Fertility is usually restored within a few weeks once prolactin levels are normalized. Women should use contraception to avoid pregnancy to minimize the use of dopamine agonists during pregnancy. Pregnant patients with known or suspected prolactinomas require special consideration because less than 5% of microprolactinomas and 15% of macroprolactinomas enlarge during pregnancy and produce symptoms.[21] All women with macroprolactinomas should have quantitative visual field testing before pregnancy and must be observed closely. Bromocriptine has been used during pregnancy to suppress compressive symptoms and has not been associated with fetal abnormalities.[16] Surgical debulking of the tumor should be considered in women who have had minimal tumor shrinkage during medical therapy and who wish to become pregnant, to minimize the risk of tumor expansion during pregnancy.[11]

GROWTH HORMONE–PRODUCING ADENOMA

GH–producing adenomas are the second most common pituitary adenoma, accounting for 20% of functional pituitary tumors.[11] These tumors cause acromegaly, a disease of bone and soft tissue overgrowth. The peak incidence is in the fourth to fifth decades, and the diagnosis is often delayed 5 to 10 years or more, owing to the slow progression of symptoms and physical changes. In children, these tumors may cause gigantism when GH excess occurs before epiphyseal plate closure. Over 98% of cases of acromegaly are due to a primary pituitary adenoma.[22]

The clinical features of acromegaly are listed in Table 37-4. These characteristic physical changes cause disfigurement and pain. Overproduction of the GH-dependent factor IGF-1, also known as somatomedin C, is responsible for most of the symptoms and complications of acromegaly.[11] GH–induced insulin resistance and glucose intolerance are frequent, yet only 10% to 20% of patients with acromegaly are overtly diabetic. Amenorrhea is common in women with GH-producing adenomas and may be caused by tumor compression of normal surrounding pituitary tissue with hyposecretion of FSH and LH. About 30% of patients have hyperprolactinemia as a result of compression of the pituitary stalk or tumor cosecretion of GH and PRL.[11] Patients with untreated acromegaly experience chronic, debilitating symptoms and often die prematurely of cardiovascular and respiratory sequelae of GH excess.

The diagnosis of a GH-producing tumor relies on measurement of serum GH and IGF-1 concentrations and an

TABLE 37-4. Clinical Features of Acromegaly	
Features	Prevalence (%)
Acral enlargement	98
Hyperhidrosis	70
Menstrual disturbance	69
Headache	59
Weakness	59
Glucose intolerance	40
Skin tags	38
Impotence	34
Visual field abnormality	28
Goiter	25
Hypertension	23

Modified from Melmed S, Brannstein GD, Chang RJ, Becker DP: UCLA Conference: Pituitary tumors secreting growth hormone and prolactin. Ann Intern Med 105:245, 1986.

oral glucose tolerance test with measurement of glucose suppression of GH release.[23] Random GH levels less than 0.4 µg/L with a normal IGF-1 and a GH nadir of less than 1 µg/L during an oral glucose tolerance test effectively exclude the diagnosis of acromegaly. GH concentration at 60 and 120 minutes after oral administration of 100 g of glucose should be greater than 2 µg/L (frequently over 10 µg/L) in patients with acromegaly. Positive biochemical testing should prompt MRI of the sella. If the pituitary MRI is negative, plasma GHRH levels should be measured to exclude the rare (<1%) ectopic GHRH-secreting tumors.[24] Localization of suspected ectopic GH or GHRH-secreting tumors consists of abdominal and chest CT, although these tumors may also be localized with ^{111}In-diethylenetriamine pentetic acid (DTPA)-octreotide scintigraphy (Octreoscan).

Treatment goals in acromegaly include normalization of serum GH levels, alleviation of mass effects (headache, vision abnormalities), and preservation of anterior pituitary function. Transsphenoidal resection of the adenoma is the preferred treatment but may be technically difficult because of the greater distance from the patient's lip to the sphenoidal sinus.[9] Preoperative treatment with a somatostatin analogue may be advisable to improve diabetes, hypertension, or congestive heart failure. Criteria for cure after surgery include normalization of IGF-1 levels and serum GH levels less than 1 µg/L after oral glucose challenge.[24] The cure rate after surgery is approximately 80% for microadenomas but falls to less than 50% for macroadenomas. Radiation may be used in patients with incompletely resected tumors and controls tumor growth in up to 70% to 80% of patients.[11] The main long-term complication of radiation is hypopituitarism.

The use of somatostatin analogues has significantly advanced the medical management of acromegaly. GH and IGF-1 levels are lowered in 80% to 90% of patients[22] with acromegaly and normalized in 50% to 60%.[11] Some groups have used octreotide to shrink large tumors preoperatively,[25] but whether this approach improves outcomes is unclear. Octreotide may be used in conjunction with a dopamine agonist in selected cases.[26] Alternate medical therapies to octreotide such as GH receptor antagonists are under evaluation.[27]

CORTICOTROPIN-PRODUCING ADENOMA

Corticotropin-producing pituitary adenomas (Cushing's disease) constitute 10% to 15% of functional pituitary adenomas. They cause up to 60% to 75% of cases of Cushing's syndrome and are diagnosed in the microadenoma stage in 90% of cases. The clinical presentation and diagnostic evaluation of Cushing's syndrome are described in detail in the adrenal section.

Once the biochemical diagnosis of ACTH-dependent Cushing's syndrome has been established, pituitary MRI should be done to look for a pituitary adenoma. Pituitary MRI identifies 60% to 70% of Cushing's adenomas,[11] although many patients have microadenomas less than 5 mm that may not be detected by this modality.[28,29] Bilateral inferior petrosal sinus (IPS) sampling with CRH stimulation is indicated in patients with negative or equivocal MRI findings.[30] Simultaneous bilateral sampling of both inferior petrosal sinuses should be carried out with CRH administration. An IPS:peripheral ACTH ratio of 3.0 or larger indicates a pituitary source, whereas patients with ectopic ACTH should have an IPS:peripheral ratio of 2.0 or less.[31] Comparison of right and left inferior petrosal sinus ratios may also lateralize the adenoma.[9] The sensitivity and specificity of this procedure are between 80% and 90% or even higher in experienced hands.[31,32]

Surgical resection is the preferred management of corticotroph microadenomas causing Cushing's disease. The surgical approach is similar to that for other pituitary tumors and is successful in 75% to 90% of cases, although recurrence rates may be as high as 10% to 20%.[29] Transsphenoidal resection of macroadenomas is less successful, and recurrence is more common. Hypopituitarism occurs infrequently after transsphenoidal resection if the tumor has not replaced the entire sella. Patients with persistent or recurrent ACTH hypersecretion after pituitary surgery require adjuvant radiation therapy. Up to 90% of patients so treated experience remission.[33] Increasingly, these patients are being treated with stereotactic radiosurgery. Because remission may be delayed for several months after radiation, the hypercortisolemic state should be managed medically until a response has occurred. All patients undergoing pituitary resection for Cushing's disease require administration of stress-dose corticosteroids both perioperatively and chronically until the hypothalamic-pituitary-adrenal axis returns to normal.

Agents used in the medical treatment of Cushing's disease act to reduce ACTH secretion by the pituitary (bromocriptine, octreotide), at the adrenal level to inhibit cortisol synthesis (ketoconazole, metyrapone, aminoglutethimide), or at the peripheral level to block cortisol receptors (RU486). Octreotide is not effective for pituitary Cushing's but may inhibit ectopic ACTH production. Ketoconazole inhibits the cytochrome p450 enzymes involved in steroid hormone synthesis and is the primary medical agent used. Medical treatment is reserved for short-term reduction of serum cortisol before surgery or if surgical therapy fails. These drugs have numerous side effects and are not indicated as primary therapy in Cushing's disease.

Bilateral adrenalectomy is occasionally indicated for patients who fail treatment with both pituitary surgery and pituitary radiation. Adrenalectomy may also be warranted in patients with severe forms of the disease as the surest means of reducing cortisol production. Patients with invasive corticotropin-producing tumors may experience enhancement of tumor growth after bilateral adrenalectomy (Nelson's syndrome).[34] The predominant manifestations of Nelson's syndrome are skin hyperpigmentation and headaches and visual changes from tumor enlargement.[11] These tumors may be locally invasive and have been associated with the development of pituitary apoplexy. Pituitary radiation may lower the incidence of Nelson's syndrome.[35] This complication is no longer as common because of the low frequency with which bilateral adrenalectomy is now performed in patients with Cushing's disease.

GONADOTROPIN-PRODUCING ADENOMA

Gonadotropin-cell adenomas constitute 10% to 15% of all pituitary tumors.[11,14] Because these tumors typically secrete minimal or inefficient amounts of FSH or LH, most are clinically silent hormonally.[36] As a result, these tumors are usually large (>10 mm) at the time of diagnosis and may have extrasellar extension. The most common presenting features are visual symptoms (bitemporal hemianopsia, fifth or sixth cranial nerve palsies), headaches, and hypopituitarism. Increased LH production may result in increased testosterone concentrations and increased libido in males and ovarian hyperstimulation with increased estradiol levels, multiple ovarian cysts, and endometrial hyperplasia in females.[11] Patients are more likely to present with partial or panhypopituitarism, however, because of the large tumor size and they should undergo thorough biochemical assessment of pituitary endocrine function. Diagnostic evaluation for gonadotropin hypersecretion consists of determination of intact FSH and LH and measurement of the LH alpha subunit after TRH stimulation.[37] Transsphenoidal resection is the primary treatment. Patients with large tumors that traverse the diaphragma sellae and who present with visual impairment may require transfrontal resection.

THYROTROPIN-PRODUCING ADENOMA

These tumors are the rarest pituitary adenomas (1% to 2.8%)[11,14] and produce symptoms of an enlarging sellar mass as well as hyperthyroidism secondary to elevated TSH levels. Over 90% of patients have macroadenomas at presentation, with an average tumor size of 23 mm.[38,39] Most patients with TSH-producing adenomas have mild hyperthyroidism and a goiter. The diagnosis is established by measurement of serum T_3, T_4, TSH, and the alpha subunit of TSH. Serum PRL and GH levels should be measured as well because of the potential for mixed hormone secretion.[38] Thyroid hormone resistance should be considered in the differential diagnosis if the pituitary MRI is negative.[14] Dynamic testing with TRH stimulation should be done to differentiate these two disorders: TSH levels should not rise after TRH in patients with TSH-secreting tumors, whereas the TSH response to TRH is intact in patients with thyroid hormone resistance. The treatment of thyrotroph adenomas is transsphenoidal resection. Octreotide may control persistent TSH hypersecretion in 80% to 90% of incompletely resected tumors but has limited effects on tumor growth.[40]

NONFUNCTIONING OR INCIDENTALLY DISCOVERED PITUITARY ADENOMAS

Nonfunctioning or null cell tumors account for 5% to 10% of pituitary adenomas.[11] These tumors usually present because of mass effects or some degree of hypopituitarism. Treatment of symptomatic patients is surgical resection. Patients with pituitary adenomas discovered incidentally on MRI done for other reasons should undergo biochemical screening for PRL and other pituitary hormones as clinically indicated.[41] Visual field testing is recommended for patients with macroadenomas. Microadenomas should be followed annually with MRI. Surgical resection should be considered for macroadenomas because up to 20% enlarge or cause pituitary apoplexy during follow-up.[42]

Other Pituitary Disorders

Posterior Pituitary Disorders

The syndrome of inappropriate antidiuretic hormone secretion (SIADH) is characterized by euvolemic hyponatremia with an inappropriately concentrated urine. SIADH is generally a diagnosis of exclusion after other causes of euvolemic hyponatremia, including hypothyroidism and adrenal insufficiency, have been excluded. Ectopic production of ADH is the most common cause of SIADH and is most often due to small cell lung carcinoma.

Deficiency of antidiuretic hormone (diabetes insipidus) is suggested by prolonged polyuria and polydipsia, and it is confirmed by a combination of high plasma osmolality (>285 mOsm) and low urine osmolality (<200 mOsm) after water deprivation. Correction of diabetes insipidus after exogenously administered ADH differentiates central versus nephrogenic diabetes insipidus. Partial diabetes insipidus may be treated with unrestricted free water access. Patients with more severe diabetes insipidus should be treated with intranasally or parenterally administered desmopressin (DDAVP, 1-deamino-8-D-arginine vasopressin).

Hypopituitarism

Hypopituitarism may be either selective (partial hypopituitarism) or complete (panhypopituitarism) and may be caused by untreated pituitary adenomas, pituitary radiation or surgery, or head injury. Hypopituitarism in patients with large pituitary tumors may result from increased intrasellar pressure with compression of portal vessels and the pituitary stalk,[43] from ischemia, necrosis, hemorrhage, or a combination thereof. It is usually a slow, gradual process that develops over months to years. Although variation occurs, the progressive loss of pituitary function typically occurs in the following order: LH/FSH, GH, TSH, then ACTH. The most common symptoms, sexual dysfunction in men and amenorrhea and infertility in women, are caused by hypogonadotropic hypogonadism. GH deficiency causes growth retardation in children; adults with GH deficiency may have increased body fat, reduced skeletal and cardiac muscle mass, decreased bone density, reduced energy levels, and a sense of social isolation.[44] TSH deficiency causes secondary hypothyroidism with weight gain, fatigue, depression, and cold intolerance. ACTH deficiency leads to symptoms of adrenal insufficiency, although mineralocorticoid production is spared and hyperpigmentation is not observed. The goal of replacement therapy for partial or panhypopituitarism is to restore circulating hormone levels within the normal range. Adrenal insufficiency is treated with twice-daily hydrocortisone, hypothyroidism with once-daily thyroxine, and hypogonadism with oral or transdermal estrogen and progesterone in women and parenteral or transdermal testosterone biweekly in men. GH replacement is critical in children and is probably beneficial in adults as well.

Pituitary Apoplexy

Pituitary apoplexy follows acute hemorrhage into or infarction of a pituitary tumor. Symptoms occur suddenly owing to expansion of blood within the sella and include severe headache, stiff neck, loss of vision, and extraocular nerve palsies. Secondary adrenal insufficiency may lead to hypotension and shock. Pituitary apoplexy most often occurs in an undiagnosed pituitary tumor but can appear during radiation therapy for pituitary tumors, during anticoagulation, or after closed-head trauma.[45] Mild forms of pituitary apoplexy may be treated conservatively with glucocorticoid therapy.[46] Patients with severe symptoms or persistent neural deficits require urgent transsphenoidal decompression of the sella.

Sheehan's Syndrome

Pituitary necrosis may occur rarely after postpartum hemorrhage and hypovolemia. The degree of subsequent hypopituitarism reflects the extent of pituitary necrosis and may include adrenal insufficiency, hypothyroidism, and amenorrhea. An inability to breast feed postpartum due to destruction of oxytocin-containing neurons of the posterior pituitary is an early clue to this diagnosis.

Empty Sella Syndrome

An empty sella turcica results from arachnoid herniation through an incomplete diaphragma sellae. This syndrome may occur in the absence of a recognized pituitary tumor and is either primary due to a congenital diaphragmatic defect or secondary due to an injury to the diaphragm by pituitary surgery, radiation, or infarction.[45] Primary empty sella syndrome typically occurs in obese, multiparous, hypertensive women who experience headaches but have no underlying neurologic disorders. Pituitary function is usually normal, but occasionally PRL is increased and GH reserve is reduced. Secondary empty sella syndrome is observed in patients with otherwise benign CSF hypertension and in patients with a loss of pituitary function due to apoplexy or surgical therapy. Abnormal GH, PRL, or ACTH secretion may persist in such patients. The diagnosis is confirmed with MRI or CT. No treatment is necessary for the primary condition, whereas correction of the underlying cause is necessary for the secondary form.

ADRENAL GLAND

History

The anatomy of the adrenal gland was first described by Eustachius in 1563. In 1855, Addison described clinical features present in patients with adrenal disease identified at autopsy. Cushing described the clinical features of hypercortisolism in 1912, but the role of adrenal tumors in this syndrome was not understood until 1934.[47] Primary hyperaldosteronism was described by Conn in 1955.[48] Pheochromocytoma was first described by Frankel in 1886.

Embryology

Each adrenal is composed of two functionally distinct endocrine units contained within a single capsule. The adrenal cortex and the medulla each have distinct embryologic, anatomic, histologic, and functional characteristics. The adrenal cortex arises from coelomic mesoderm adjacent to the urogenital ridge between the fourth and sixth gestational weeks. The gland then differentiates into a thin outer *definitive cortex* and a thick inner *fetal cortex* by the eighth week. The fetal cortex actively produces fetal steroids during gestation but involutes rapidly after birth. The definitive cortex persists and develops into the functional adrenal cortex, which has distinct zonae glomerulosa and fasciculata at birth. The zona reticularis develops later, during the first year of life. Aberrant adrenocortical tissue may be found near the kidney or in the pelvis along the path of migration of structures arising from the urogenital ridge. Adrenocortical tissue may also be found in locations that are not explained by normal patterns of migration of fetal tissues (Fig. 37-10).

The adrenal medulla and sympathetic nervous system develop together. During the fifth gestational week, neural crest cells migrate to the para-aortic and paravertebral regions and along the adrenal vein toward the medial aspect of the developing adrenal fetal cortex. Most extra-adrenal chromaffin cells regress. However, some cells remain and form the organ of Zuckerkandl, which is located generally to the left of the aortic bifurcation near the origin of the inferior mesenteric artery. Extra-adrenal chromaffin tissue may persist anywhere along the path of neural crest cell migration (see Fig. 37-10).

Anatomy

The adrenal glands are bilateral retroperitoneal organs located on the superomedial aspect of the upper pole of each kidney (Fig. 37-11). Each gland weighs approximately 4 g. The pyramid-shaped right adrenal lies close to the inferior vena cava and frequently abuts the right diaphragmatic crus and the bare area of the liver. The left adrenal is larger and flatter and is found between the kidney and aorta near the tail of the pancreas and the

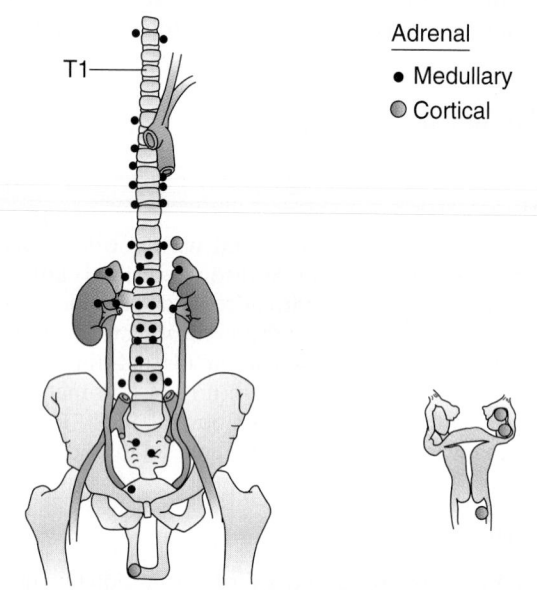

FIGURE 37-10.   Sites of extra-adrenal cortical and medullary tissues.

splenic artery. The adrenal glands are often not visible on direct inspection of the retroperitoneum and are found after dissection and mobilization of adjacent structures. The normal adrenal cortex is bright yellow and thicker than the red-brown medulla.

The adrenal glands derive their blood supply from branches of the inferior phrenic artery superiorly, the aorta medially, and the renal artery inferiorly (see Fig. 37-11). The primary blood supply of the right adrenal comes from the superior and inferior adrenal arteries, whereas the left adrenal is supplied primarily by the middle and inferior adrenal arteries. Additionally, numerous small arterial branches enter the perimeter of the gland. Microvasculature within each adrenal integrates function of the cortex and medulla. Cortisol-rich venous effluent flows from the cortex to the medulla where cortisol stimulates the synthesis and activity of phenylethanolamine-N-methyl transferase (PMNT), leading to the conversion of norepinephrine to epinephrine. Extra-adrenal chromaffin tissues lack this regulatory mechanism and, thus, secrete predominantly norepinephrine.

The right adrenal vein drains to the inferior vena cava through a wide but short central vein. The left adrenal vein empties primarily into the left renal vein but may occasionally drain directly to the vena cava. Lymphatic plexuses drain to para-aortic and renal lymph nodes. The adrenal cortex has no known direct innervation, although the adrenal medulla is richly supplied by preganglionic sympathetic nerves. Parasympathetic nerves to the medulla have not been identified.

Histologically, the adult adrenal cortex is composed of three zones: an outer zona glomerulosa, a middle zona fasciculata, and an inner zona reticularis. Cells of the zona fasciculata are large, appear foamy secondary to

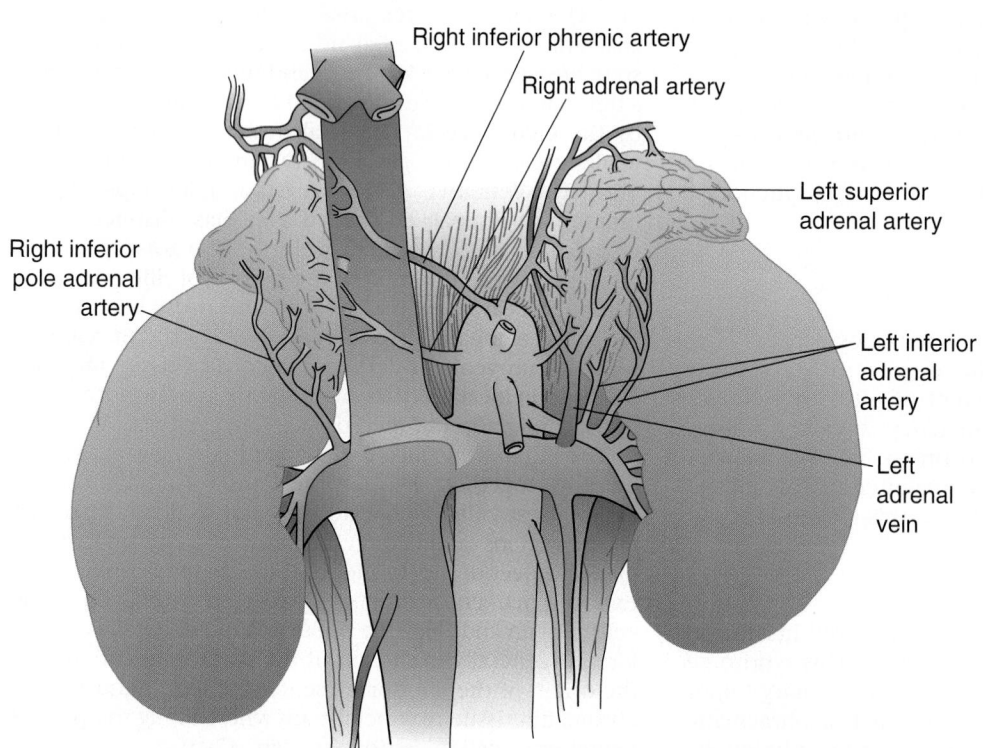

FIGURE 37-11.   Anatomy of the adrenal glands. (Reprinted with permission from Brunt LM: Laparoscopic adrenalectomy. *In* Eubanks WS, Swanstrom LL, Soper NJ [eds]: Mastery of Endoscopic and Laparoscopic Surgery. Philadelphia, Lippincott Williams & Wilkins, 2000, p 321.)

many lipid inclusions, and constitute 75% of the cortex. Cells of the zona reticularis have compact cytoplasm and few lipid inclusions. ACTH stimulation causes cells of these two inner zones to enlarge, owing to increased storage of lipid and proliferation of mitochondria and endoplasmic reticulum. Cells of the zona glomerulosa are small, have an intermediate number of lipid inclusions, and constitute about 15% of the cortex.

The adrenal medulla is smaller than the cortex and contributes approximately 10% of the total gland weight. Adrenal medullary cells are polyhedral, are arranged in cords, and contain catecholamines that precipitate chromium salts (thus the name chromaffin cells). Core vesicles containing epinephrine and norepinephrine are apparent on electron microscopy.

Adrenal Steroid Biochemistry and Physiology

Three major biosynthetic pathways lead to the production of glucocorticoids, mineralocorticoids, and adrenal androgens. These pathways are compartmentalized within the adrenal gland and reflect the enzymatic capabilities of each zone. Mineralocorticoids are synthesized in the zona glomerulosa, whereas glucocorticoids and adrenal androgens are synthesized in the zonae fasciculata and reticularis. All adrenal steroids share a common 17-carbon structure composed of three hexane rings and a single pentane ring. The androgenic C-19 steroids have methyl groups at positions 18 and 19 on the basic structure. Glucocorticoids and mineralocorticoids have an additional two-carbon side chain (C-20, 21) attached at position 17.

Adrenocortical hormones are synthesized from cholesterol that is either extracted from plasma or synthesized within the adrenal cortex. Cholesterol is cleaved within the mitochondria to form Δ5-pregnenolone, the common precursor for glucocorticoids, mineralocorticoids, and androgenic steroids. After leaving the mitochondrion, pregnenolone enters the smooth endoplasmic reticulum, where it is shunted to divergent biosynthetic pathways (Fig. 37-12). The zona glomerulosa and zona reticularis contain the enzyme 17α-hydroxylase, which oxidizes pregnenolone and progesterone at C-17. From these, cortisol and sex steroids are synthesized sequentially. Mineralocorticoid biosynthesis follows a parallel pathway in the zona glomerulosa but does not undergo initial hydroxylation at C-17, owing to absence of 17α-hydroxylase activity in this zone. Congenital absence of enzymes involved in any one of these pathways shunts pregnenolone derivatives through unaffected pathways and causes specific clinical syndromes.

Glucocorticoids

Adrenal cortisol production is regulated by pituitary-derived ACTH under most conditions. The amount of cortisol production is a function of body size (12 mg/m^2 of body surface area). A normal adult secretes 10 to 30 mg of cortisol each day.

In plasma, 75% of cortisol is bound to corticosteroid-binding globulin (transcortin), 15% is bound to albumin, and 10% to 15% is unbound and active. Plasma transcortin levels increase during pregnancy and in response to pharmacologic doses of estrogen. Alterations in transcortin or albumin concentrations in plasma can alter total plasma cortisol concentration without affecting its free concentration. On the other hand, excessive cortisol production may exceed transcortin- and albumin-binding capabilities and lead to sharp increases in free cortisol.

The plasma half-life of cortisol is approximately 90 minutes. In the liver, cortisol is transformed to the inactive metabolites dihydrocortisol and tetrahydrocortisol. These metabolites are conjugated to glucuronate and excreted in the urine, where they may be measured as 17-hydroxycorticosteroids. A small fraction of unmetabolized cortisol can be measured in the urine.

Steroid hormones exert their effects by binding to specific soluble intracellular cytosolic receptors. The activated steroid-receptor complex then moves to the nucleus, binds to DNA, and activates transcription of target genes. The diverse physiologic actions of glucocorticoids center on intermediary metabolism, immune modulation, and regulation of intravascular volume.

Cortisol regulates the intermediary metabolism of carbohydrates, proteins, and lipids. Cortisol stimulates release of glucagon, and together these substances raise blood glucose by antagonizing insulin-stimulated glucose uptake by peripheral tissues and also by stimulating hepatic gluconeogenesis. Cortisol also decreases peripheral protein synthesis and amino acid uptake, thereby increasing glycogenic amino acid delivery to the liver, and it stimulates peripheral lipolysis. Thus, glucocorticoids function anabolically in vital tissues such as liver and brain but catabolically in skin, muscle, lymphoid tissues, and adipocytes. Cortisol maintains intravascular volume by retarding entry of free water into cells, by decreasing capillary permeability to water, and by a weak mineralocorticoid effect. Cortisol also maintains blood pressure through stimulation of angiotensinogen release and by inhibition of prostaglandin I$_2$, a potent vasodilator.

Prolonged exposure to high levels of endogenous corticosteroids leads to a catabolic state with negative nitrogen balance, proximal muscle weakness, and insulin-resistant diabetes mellitus. Additionally, a redistribution of body fat occurs that results in truncal obesity and peripheral depletion. Glucocorticoids retard wound healing by impairing collagen formation and fibroblast activity, produce osteopenia by inhibiting osteoblast bone formation, and promote early closure of epiphyseal plates in children and adolescents. Other effects of chronic corticosteroid excess include emotional and psychologic disturbances, cataracts, and corneal ulcers.

Glucocorticoids possess profound anti-inflammatory and immunosuppressive properties.[49] These steroids suppress interleukin-2 production and inhibit lymphocyte activation and both monocyte and neutrophil migration to areas of inflammation. Cortisol inhibits histamine release and histamine-induced lysosomal degranulation by mast cells. Corticosteroids also modulate humoral immunity by regulating T-cell activation of B cells and, at high doses, by directly inhibiting B-cell activation and proliferation.

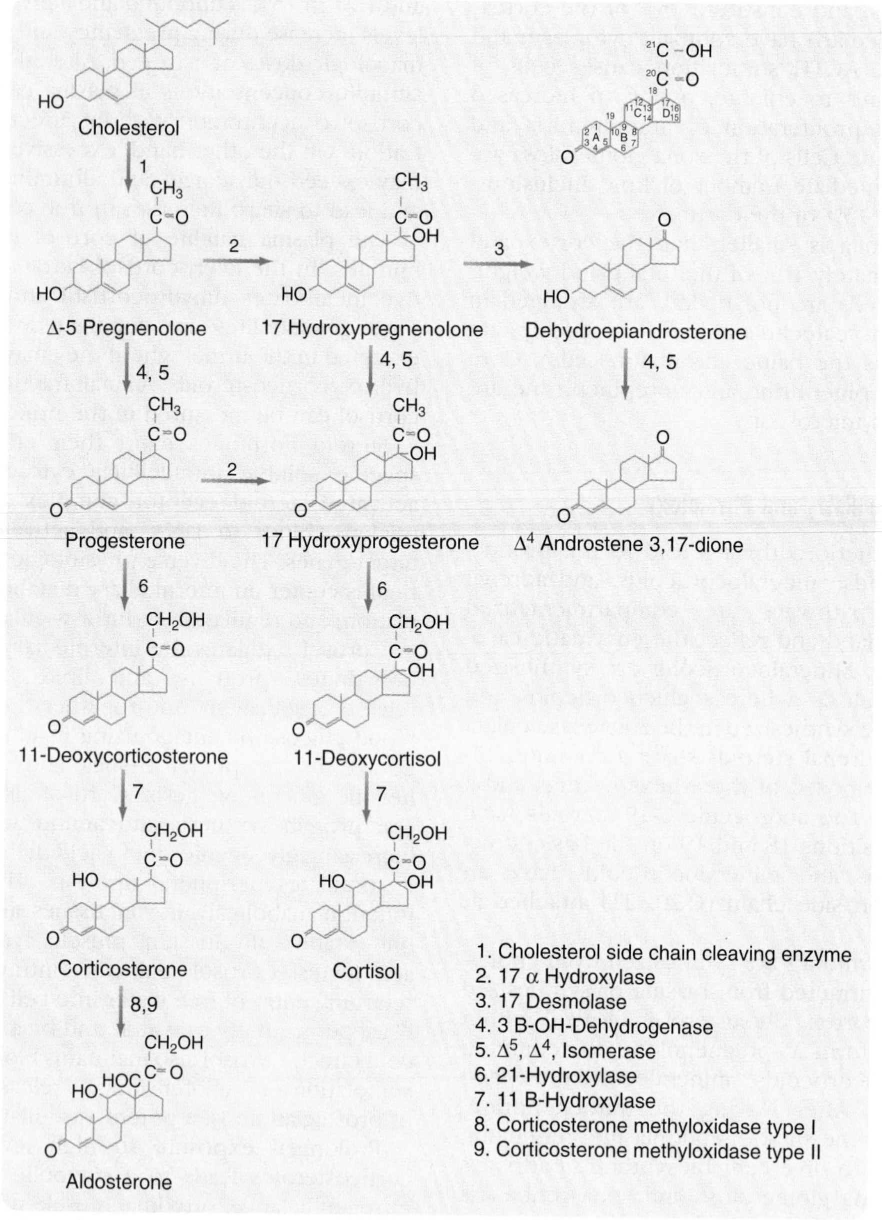

FIGURE 37-12. Biosynthetic pathways of adrenal corticosteroids.

Mineralocorticoids

Aldosterone is the major mineralocorticoid in humans. From 100 to 150 mg of aldosterone is secreted from the zona glomerulosa into the bloodstream each day, where it is bound to transcortin (20%) and albumin (40%), with the remainder circulating free. The plasma half-life of aldosterone is approximately 15 minutes, and 90% is cleared from the plasma after a single pass through the liver. Metabolic degradation of aldosterone occurs in the liver by enzymatic reduction and conjugation with glucuronic acid before excretion by the kidney. Only minute amounts of free aldosterone are excreted in the urine.

Aldosterone regulates fluid and electrolyte balance by stimulating sodium retention and potassium and hydrogen ion secretion by the distal convoluted tubule of the kidney. Aldosterone also promotes sodium absorption by

a variety of epithelia, including sweat glands, gastrointestinal mucosa, and salivary glands. High levels of circulating mineralocorticoid thus tend to expand intravascular volume.

The renin-angiotensin system and plasma potassium concentration are the principal regulators of aldosterone secretion. ACTH, plasma sodium, and POMC-derived peptides and others are minor contributors.[50] Activation of the renin-angiotensin system begins with release of renin from juxtaglomerular cells of the kidney in response to a decrease in renal blood flow, to sympathetic nervous system stimulation, or to a decrease in plasma sodium. Renin enzymatically cleaves angiotensinogen to produce the decapeptide angiotensin I, which is then cleaved by angiotensin-converting enzyme (ACE) in the lung to form the active octapeptide angiotensin II. Angiotensin II directly stimulates aldosterone biosynthesis and release from the adrenal through receptor-mediated activation of phospholipase C.[50] Angiotensin II is also a potent vasoconstrictor and directly elicits a marked increase in arterial blood pressure. Factors that decrease renal arterial blood flow such as hemorrhage, dehydration, upright posture, or renal artery stenosis stimulate the renin-angiotensin system. Restoration of blood volume and pressure, as well as high levels of aldosterone, inhibit release of renin and angiotensin.

Aldosterone secretion is exquisitely sensitive to changes in serum potassium levels. An increase of serum potassium level by as little as 0.1 mEq/L increases aldosterone secretion by 35%, whereas a fall in serum potassium by 0.3 mEq/L decreases aldosterone secretion by 50%. Hypokalemia blunts the aldosterone response that would otherwise be observed in a number of clinical settings, and restoration of the serum potassium level restores this response.

ACTH plays a comparatively minor role in aldosterone regulation. In fact, the zona glomerulosa does not atrophy after hypophysectomy, unlike the zona reticularis and zona fasciculata. ACTH may acutely stimulate aldosterone hypersecretion, although prolonged ACTH exposure ultimately leads to diminished aldosterone response. Other pituitary factors including POMC derivatives and ADH stimulate aldosterone secretion. Sodium intake regulates aldosterone indirectly through changes in renin secretion and through modulation of the sensitivity of the zona glomerulosa to angiotensin II.

Adrenal Sex Steroids

In cells of the zona reticularis, pregnenolone is converted to 17-hydroxypregnenolone and subsequently to dehydroepiandrosterone (DHEA). DHEA is the major C-19 sex steroid produced by the adrenal cortex, although the sulfated derivative of DHEA and Δ4-androstenedione are also formed. DHEA and androstenedione are weak androgens and exert their effect on peripheral tissues after local conversion to testosterone. Only minute amounts of testosterone or estrone are synthesized under normal circumstances, and the gonads are the primary source of these sex steroids. Adrenal androgen release is stimulated by ACTH and not by the gonadotropins.

Adrenal androgens promote development of male secondary sexual characteristics and cause virilization in women. During fetal life, circulating androgens influence development of the male external genitalia, the male ductal structures such as vas deferens, epididymis, and seminal vesicles, and the prostate. Absence of androgens prenatally prompts development of female genitalia and the vagina. Normally, the gonads are the principal source of sex steroids in males and females. During puberty, androgens contribute to growth of the phallus, muscle mass, and body hair in the male. Estrogens promote growth and maturation of the breast, uterus, and vagina in the female. Excessive production of adrenal sex steroids either prenatally or postnatally results in disorders of sexual development.

Diseases of the Adrenal Cortex

Cushing's Syndrome

BACKGROUND

The syndrome named after Harvey Cushing was described by him in 1932.[51] At that time he reported a series of eight patients with central obesity, glucose intolerance, hypertension, plethora, hirsutism, osteoporosis, nephrolithiasis, menstrual irregularity, muscle weakness, and emotional lability. He called the syndrome "pituitary basophilism" because basophilic adenomas of the pituitary were noted in six of these patients. The contribution of hypercortisolism and adrenal cortical hyperplasia was subsequently recognized. To this day Cushing's syndrome refers to the signs and symptoms of hypercortisolism regardless of their cause. "Cushing's disease" refers to the syndrome when caused by a pituitary adenoma.

The incidence of Cushing's syndrome is approximately 10 per million population. The most common cause of this syndrome is exogenous administration of synthetic corticosteroids. Endogenous hypercortisolism in all cases is due to increased adrenal production of cortisol, which may be ACTH dependent or independent. As noted in Box 37-1, endogenous Cushing's syndrome is ACTH dependent in 80% of cases and ACTH independent in 20% of cases. Causes of ACTH-dependent Cushing's syndrome include ACTH-producing pituitary tumors (Cushing's disease) and ectopic ACTH-producing tumors (most commonly bronchial carcinoids and small cell lung cancer). ACTH-dependent Cushing's syndrome is always associated with bilateral adrenal hyperplasia.

Pseudo-Cushing's syndrome occurs in some patients with major depression or alcoholism. These patients may have abnormally high cortisol secretion and appear to have clinical and biochemical features of Cushing's syn-

---

Box 37-1 Causes of Cushing's Syndrome

Diagnosis	Percentage
ACTH Dependent	
Cushing's disease	68
Ectopic ACTH syndrome	12
Ectopic CRH syndrome	<1
ACTH Independent	
Adrenal adenoma	10
Adrenal carcinoma	8
Adrenal cortical hyperplasias	1
Pseudo-Cushing's Syndrome	
Major depression	1
Alcoholism	<1

ACTH, adrenocorticotropic hormone.
Adapted from Orth DN: Cushing's syndrome. N Engl J Med 332:791-803, 1995. Copyright 1995, Massachusetts Medical Society. All rights reserved.

drome. The syndrome rapidly disappears with remission of the primary disorder.

SIGNS AND SYMPTOMS

The clinical signs and symptoms of Cushing's syndrome are listed in Box 37-2.[52] The features of full blown Cushing's syndrome are dramatic and easily recognizable. In contrast, many patients with early or mild Cushing's syndrome have subtle findings. Some of these features, such as obesity and hypertension, are quite prevalent in the population and are not necessarily caused by hypercortisolism. Conversely, the presence of central obesity with prominent supraclavicular fat pads, plethora, wide purple striae on the abdomen and extremities, proximal muscle weakness and inappropriate osteopenia, are relatively specific for Cushing's syndrome and should prompt a work-up for hypercortisolism.

BIOCHEMICAL EVALUATION OF CUSHING'S SYNDROME

The diagnostic evaluation of the patient with suspected Cushing's syndrome is outlined in Figure 37-13. The evaluation should proceed in a stepwise fashion to first determine whether the patient has hypercortisolism. If hypercortisolism is present, then the next step is to deter-

---

Box 37-2 Clinical Features of Cushing's Syndrome

General

*Central obesity**
Proximal muscle weakness
Hypertension
Headaches
Psychiatric disorders

Skin

Wide (>1 cm) purple striae
Spontaneous ecchymoses
Facial plethora
Hyperpigmentation
Acne
Hirsutism
Fungal skin infections

Endocrine and Metabolic Derangements

Hypokalemic alkalosis
Osteopenia
Delayed bone age in children
Menstrual disorders, decreased libido, impotence
Glucose tolerance, diabetes mellitus
Kidney stones
Polyuria
Elevated white blood cell count

*Symptoms and signs in italics indicate relatively specific findings in patients with the syndrome.
Adapted from Meier CA, Biller BMK: Clinical and biochemical evaluation of Cushing's syndrome. Endocrinol Metab Clin North Am 26:741, 1997.

---

mine whether it is due to ACTH-dependent or ACTH-independent causes. Finally, the source of the Cushing's syndrome should be identified by imaging. No single test is absolutely reliable in establishing a diagnosis of Cushing's syndrome, and, therefore, multiple tests are usually performed. The sine qua non of this disorder is the presence of hypercortisolism that is insensitive to suppression by administration of exogenous glucocorticoid.[53] Loss of the normal diurnal variation in cortisol secretion is also characteristic of Cushing's syndrome, but because of variability in levels, random plasma cortisol levels are of little value in making the diagnosis.

Establishing the Presence of Cushing's Syndrome

24-Hour Urinary Free Cortisol. The most useful test in the initial diagnostic evaluation of the patient with suspected Cushing's syndrome is determination of 24-hour urinary free cortisol.[31] Collections should be carefully timed and urinary creatinine should be measured concurrently. Ideally, two sequential 24-hour collections should be done to ensure adequacy of the specimen. This test has a reported sensitivity of 95% to 100% and specificity of 98% for the diagnosis of Cushing's syndrome. However, elevated urinary free cortisol levels have been observed in some patients with pseudo-Cushing's syndrome conditions.

Overnight Low-Dose Dexamethasone Suppression Test. Dexamethasone is a synthetic glucocorticoid that does not cross react in standard cortisol radioimmunoassays. In this test, 1 mg of dexamethasone is administered orally at 11 PM and plasma cortisol is obtained at 8 AM the following day. Plasma cortisol level should be suppressed to less than 3 to 5 µg/dL after dexamethasone in normal individuals but not in patients with Cushing's syndrome. Because of its simplicity, this test may be especially useful in screening patients with adrenal incidentalomas for subclinical Cushing's syndrome. However, false-positive test results occur in 10% to 15% of cases with the overnight test, mainly in patients with obesity, alcoholism, or those taking estrogens or phenytoin. Some patients with mild Cushing's syndrome may still demonstrate sensitivity to dexamethasone. Consequently, some endocrinologists have used stricter criteria for suppression of cortisol to less than 1.8 µg/dL to exclude the diagnosis.[31,54]

Late Night Salivary Cortisol. The concentration of cortisol in the saliva is a good indicator of free biologically active cortisol.[31] Measurement of late night (11 PM) salivary cortisol appears to have high sensitivity as a screening test for Cushing's syndrome.[55] A commercially available saliva collecting kit is used to measure two or three 11 PM cortisol levels. Salivary cortisol levels greater than 6.0 nmol/L are diagnostic for Cushing's syndrome, whereas levels between 3 and 6 nmol/L are indeterminate and require further testing.

CRH/Dexamethasone Suppression Test. This test is useful in patients with borderline screening test results because it identifies partially suppressible pituitary adenomas and nonsuppressible ectopic or adrenal lesions. In this test, 0.5 mg of dexamethasone is given every 6 hours for 48 hours followed by an 8 AM CRH bolus. Plasma cortisol is measured 15 minutes later. A 15-minute cortisol level greater than 1.4 µg/dL is consistent with the presence of Cushing's syndrome.[52]

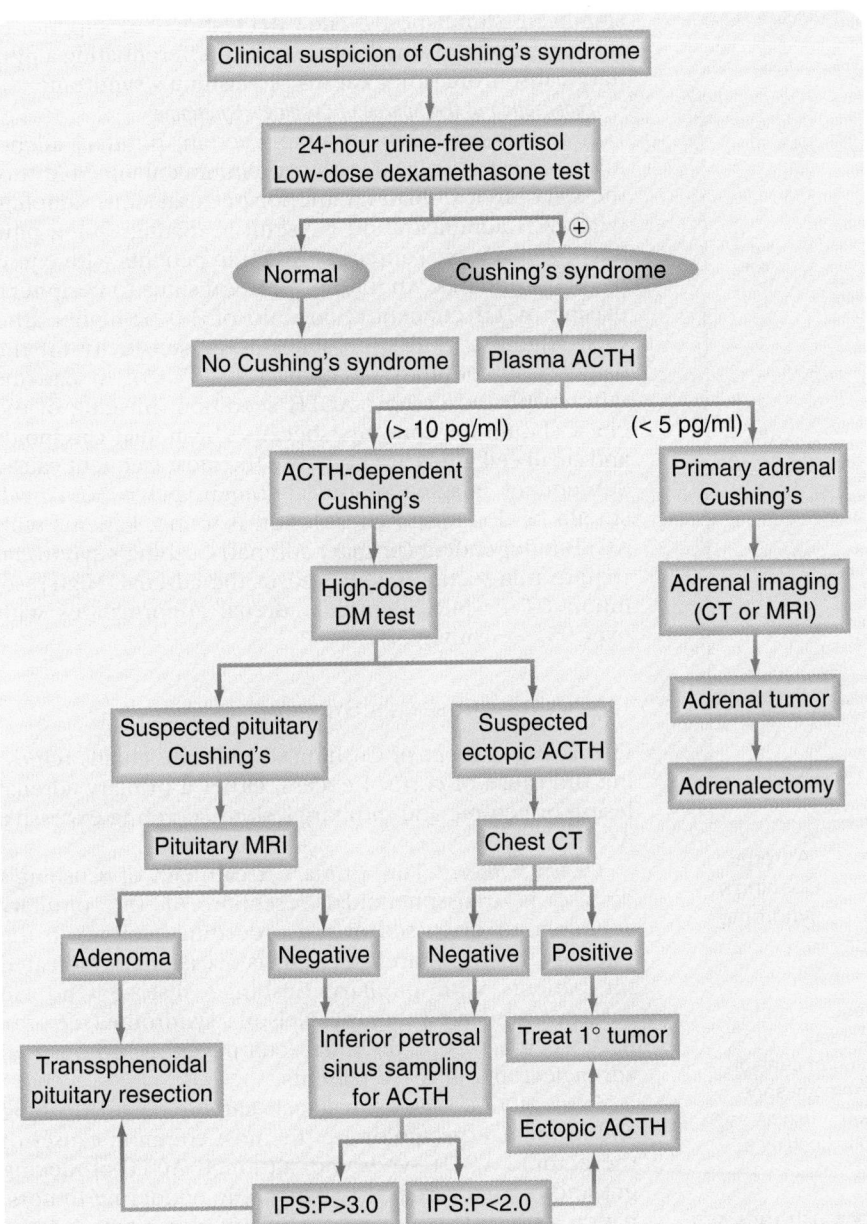

FIGURE 37-13. Diagnostic algorithm for evaluation of Cushing's syndrome. IPS:P; inferior petrosal sinus to peripheral plasma ACTH.

Differentiation of ACTH-Dependent from ACTH-Independent Cushing's Syndrome

Plasma ACTH Level. Measurement of plasma ACTH levels, which is done using a two-site immunometric assay, is the best test to distinguish ACTH-dependent (pituitary or ectopic ACTH) from ACTH-independent (primary adrenal) causes of Cushing's syndrome. Plasma ACTH levels are normally between 10 and 60 pg/mL. Suppression of plasma ACTH to below 5 pg/mL is characteristic of adrenocortical neoplasms,[31] which secrete high levels of cortisol and inhibit ACTH release by the pituitary. Patients with pituitary neoplasms and secondary bilateral adrenocortical hyperplasia have ACTH levels that may range from 15 to 500 pg/mL. Ectopic ACTH production is generally associated with higher plasma ACTH levels than pituitary Cushing's syndrome, although there is overlap in the degree of ACTH elevation between these two disorders.[31]

High-Dose Dexamethasone Suppression Test. In patients with nonsuppressed or elevated ACTH levels, the differential diagnosis is between a pituitary and an ectopic source of ACTH. The high-dose dexamethasone suppression test is based on the principle that hypercortisolism due to ACTH-secreting pituitary adenomas will be suppressed at least partially by high-dose dexamethasone whereas that due to adrenal tumors and ectopic ACTH-producing tumors will not. The standard test employs 2 mg of dexamethasone given orally every 6 hours over 2 days, with a 24-hour urine collection for free cortisol taken basally and again during the second day of dexamethasone administration. Urinary free cortisol is suppressed by more than 90% from baseline in 60% to 70% of patients with pituitary adenomas.[56,57] Failure to suppress urinary free cortisol supports a diagnosis of an ectopic ACTH-producing tumor, an adrenal neoplasm, or primary bilateral adrenal hyperpla-

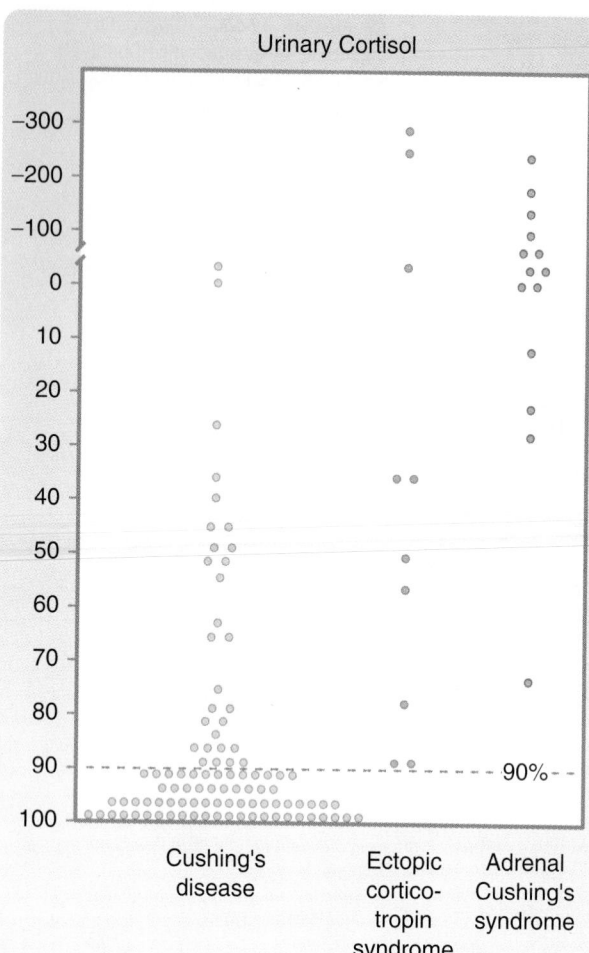

FIGURE 37-14. High-dose dexamethasone test results in patients with Cushing's syndrome. Shown is the percent suppression from baseline of 24-hour urine excretion of cortisol on the second day of treatment with high-dose dexamethasone (2 mg every 6 hours for eight doses) in patients with Cushing's syndrome. (Reprinted with permission from Orth DN: Cushing's syndrome. N Engl J Med 332:797, 1995.)

sia. However, some patients with pituitary Cushing's syndrome may also fail to suppress urinary free cortisol, as shown in Figure 37-14. An overnight high-dose suppression test (8 mg at midnight) is available and has similar diagnostic accuracy.

CRH Test. The CRH stimulation test is based on the principle that pituitary but not adrenal or ectopic ACTH sources of Cushing's syndrome respond to CRH by increasing ACTH levels. This test has been used (1) to evaluate ACTH responsiveness in patients with borderline or low ACTH levels and (2) for differentiating pituitary from ectopic ACTH sources.[52] In this test, ovine CRH (1 μg/kg) is administered intravenously over 30 seconds and plasma ACTH and serum cortisol levels are obtained at 15, 30, and 60 minutes. Patients with primary adrenal Cushing's syndrome have a blunted peak ACTH response (increase of <10 pg/mL over baseline). A rise in plasma ACTH levels of more than 35% to 50% after administration of CRH is highly suggestive of pituitary Cushing's syndrome, whereas patients with ectopic ACTH rarely demonstrate

significant stimulation.[58] The CRH test may be superior to the high-dose dexamethasone test in differentiating a pituitary cause from other causes of Cushing's syndrome.

Localization of the Source of Cushing's Syndrome

As discussed in the pituitary section, pituitary adenomas are best visualized with gadolinium-enhanced MRI of the sella turcica. Bilateral inferior petrosal sinus sampling with CRH administration is useful in distinguishing pituitary from ectopic sources of ACTH in patients with equivocal MRI findings. An inferior petrosal sinus to peripheral plasma ACTH concentration ratio of 3.0 or higher after CRH administration approaches 100% sensitivity for the diagnosis of pituitary adenoma (Fig. 37-15). In patients with suspected ectopic ACTH secretion, imaging of the chest should be done first because bronchial carcinoids and small cell lung carcinoids are the most frequent cause. Subsequent imaging of the abdomen, pelvis, and neck should be done if no chest lesion is found. Patients with ACTH-independent (primary adrenal) Cushing's syndrome require thin-section CT or MRI of the adrenal. High-resolution CT or MRI identifies adrenal abnormalities with over 95% sensitivity.

TREATMENT OF CUSHING'S SYNDROME

Effective treatment of Cushing's syndrome entails removing the cause of cortisol excess, either a primary adrenal lesion or ectopic and pituitary lesions secreting excessive ACTH.

Cushing's Disease The primary treatment of Cushing's disease is transsphenoidal resection of the pituitary adenoma, as discussed in the preceding section on the pituitary. Bilateral adrenalectomy is occasionally indicated for patients with pituitary Cushing's disease who fail surgery or radiation therapy. Nelson's syndrome (see pituitary section) is a potential complication of bilateral adrenalectomy in these patients.

Ectopic ACTH Syndrome Small cell carcinoma of the lung and bronchial carcinoids are the most common causes of the ectopic ACTH syndrome, although ACTH-producing gut and thymic carcinoids, pancreatic endocrine tumors, pancreatic cystadenomas, medullary carcinoma of the thyroid, and pheochromocytomas have all been reported. Ectopic production of CRF is a rare cause of Cushing's syndrome, and described sources include medullary carcinoma of the thyroid and carcinoma of the prostate. Patients with ectopic ACTH syndrome usually appear cushingoid, but they more often present with signs of an advanced malignancy such as weakness and weight loss. These patients often have a severe metabolic alkalosis with hypokalemia. A presumptive diagnosis of ectopic ACTH hypersecretion is made on the basis of (1) increased urinary free cortisol, (2) increased plasma ACTH, and (3) failure to suppress ACTH and hypercortisolism with high-dose dexamethasone.

Treatment of ectopic ACTH syndrome is removal of the primary lesion. Debulking of unresectable primary lesions or recurrences with or without bilateral adrenalectomy may provide palliation in some patients. Medical treatment with ketoconazole, metyrapone, aminoglutethimide, and mitotane has been used to suppress production of corticosteroid in inoperable cases. Bilateral

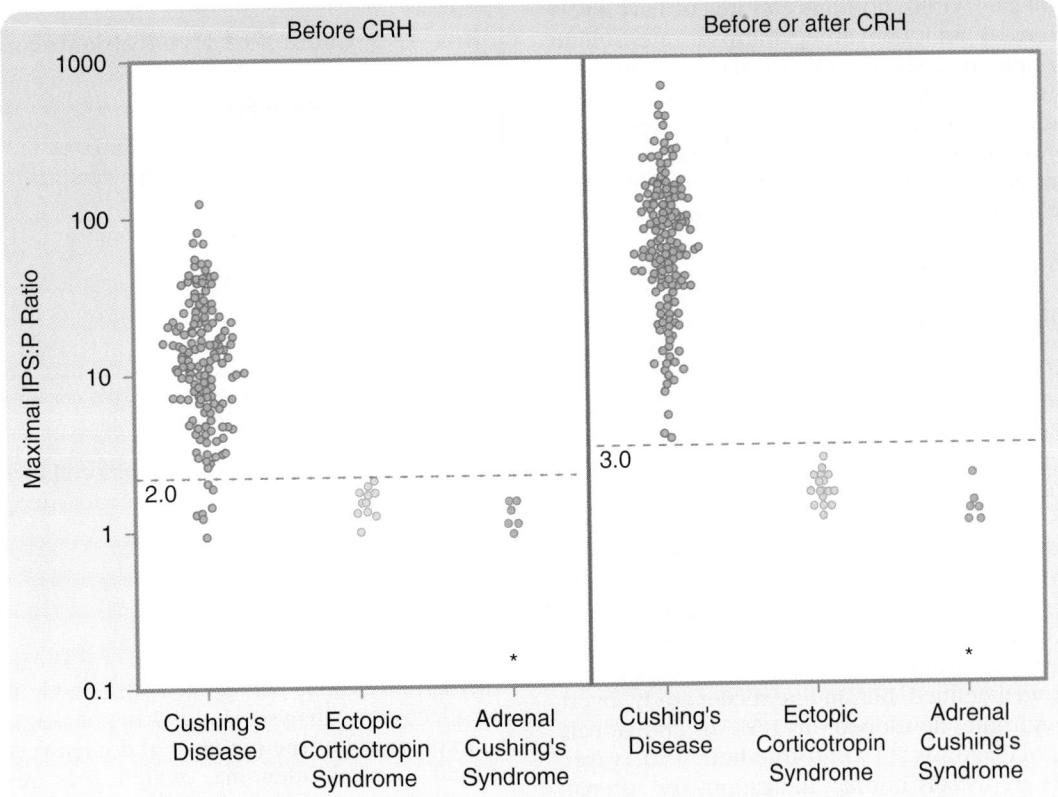

FIGURE 37-15. Results of inferior petrosal sinus sampling in patients with Cushing's syndrome. Shown are the ratios of plasma ACTH concentrations in either the right or left inferior petrosal sinus (IPS) to samples in a peripheral (P) vein either before *(left panel)* or after *(right panel)* administration of ovine corticotropin-releasing hormone (CRH) (1 g/kg). *Dashed lines* indicate the lower limit of values considered to indicate Cushing's disease. (Reprinted with permission from Orth DN: Cushing's syndrome. N Engl J Med 332:799, 1995.)

adrenalectomy may be beneficial in select patients with uncontrollable hypercortisolism or after unsuccessful localization of the ectopic ACTH source.

PRIMARY ADRENAL CUSHING'S SYNDROME

Adrenal Adenoma From 10% to 25% of patients with endogenous Cushing's syndrome have a primary adrenal cause. A solitary adrenal adenoma is present in 80% to 90% of these patients and is often associated with atrophy of both adjacent and contralateral adrenocortical tissue. Adrenal adenomas are cured by adrenalectomy, and prognosis is good after resection. Most lesions less than 6 cm in diameter may be resected laparoscopically. Large or invasive adrenal cortical carcinomas should be removed via an open anterior approach.

All patients who undergo adrenalectomy for primary adrenal causes of Cushing's syndrome require perioperative and postoperative glucocorticoid replacement, since the contralateral gland is suppressed. Replacement therapy with prednisone, at a starting dose of 5 mg in the morning and 2.5 mg in the evening, may be required for 6 to 18 months postoperatively. Adequacy of replacement is monitored clinically. Inadequate replacement results in signs of adrenal insufficiency, whereas overreplacement results in features of Cushing's syndrome. The duration of

replacement therapy can be guided by normalization of the ACTH stimulation test.

Primary Adrenal Hyperplasia A small subset of patients have primary adrenal Cushing's syndrome due to bilateral nodular adrenal hyperplasia, which may occur in two forms: primary pigmented nodular adrenal hyperplasia (PPNAD) and macronodular adrenal hyperplasia. PPNAD is characterized by the presence of multiple, small hyperfunctioning adrenal nodules that vary in size from 1 to 2 mm up to 3 cm.[59] The etiology is unclear, but adrenal stimulating autoantibodies have been demonstrated in many of these patients. About 20% of cases of PPNAD occur in a familial setting in association with multiple other tumors, including cardiac myxomas, pigmented skin lesions, pituitary, testicular, and other tumors (Carney's complex). In macronodular adrenal hyperplasia, the adrenals may be markedly enlarged and weigh up to 500 g. Large bilateral adrenal nodules that range in size from 0.5 to 7 cm are present. Adrenal sensitivity to gastric inhibitory peptide has been implicated in the pathogenesis of some of these cases.[60] The treatment of Cushing's syndrome due to primary adrenal hyperplasia is total bilateral adrenalectomy.

Adrenocortical Carcinoma Patients with this rare but aggressive malignancy may present with Cushing's syndrome. An acute and rapidly progressive course of Cushing's syndrome, weight gain, virilization, and elevated urinary levels of 17-ketosteroids and dehydroepiandrosterone sulfate (DHEAS) strongly suggests adrenocortical carcinoma. This contrasts to the more gradual onset of symptoms experienced by patients with an adrenal adenoma. Adrenocortical carcinoma requires aggressive surgical resection, although cure is infrequent. Details of the management of adrenocortical carcinoma are discussed subsequently.

SUBCLINICAL CUSHING'S SYNDROME

Some patients may have evidence of autonomous glucocorticoid production without the classic clinical signs and symptoms of Cushing's syndrome—termed *preclinical* or *subclinical Cushing's syndrome*.[61] Subclinical Cushing's syndrome has been identified in 5% to 20% of patients with incidentally discovered adrenal masses. These patients have a high incidence of hypertension, obesity, and diabetes mellitus but lack the other clinical features of Cushing's syndrome. Biochemical findings in these patients have included partially autonomous secretion of cortisol, resistance to suppression with dexamethasone, and loss of the normal diurnal variation in cortisol secretion.[62] The natural history of subclinical Cushing's syndrome is not well defined, but, in one recent study, overt Cushing's syndrome developed in 1.5% of individuals within 1 year of diagnosis.[63] Twenty-four-hour urinary free cortisol levels are usually normal. Indications for adrenalectomy in this population include age younger than 50 years and the presence of possible disease-related hypertension, diabetes, obesity, and osteoporosis.[61] Patients with suppression of plasma ACTH levels or elevated urinary free cortisol should also undergo adrenalectomy because of the likely progression to clinically overt Cushing's syndrome. Supplemental glucocorticoids should be administered postoperatively because of suppression of the contralateral normal adrenal.

CUSHING'S SYNDROME IN CHILDREN

Cushing's syndrome is rare in children and affects girls three times as often as boys. As in adults, the most common cause is a pituitary microadenoma. Adrenal neoplasms are more common than ACTH-dependent causes in children younger than age 7 years; in this age group, adrenal cortical carcinomas constitute about 70% of Cushing's-related adrenal tumors.[64] Ectopic ACTH production in children is uncommon. The clinical manifestations of Cushing's syndrome in children differ somewhat from adults in that generalized obesity and growth retardation are the predominant features.[64] Menstrual irregularities, striae, plethora, headaches, hypertension, ecchymoses, and impaired carbohydrate tolerance may also be present. Virilization associated with hirsutism and acne is also a frequent finding. Young children may have premature sexual development and accelerated epiphyseal maturation from increased adrenal androgen production.[65]

Children with Cushing's disease are best managed by transsphenoidal resection of the microadenoma. Pituitary irradiation has been used after failure of pituitary surgery, but some endocrinologists have expressed concern regarding the long-term effects of irradiation in children. Adrenal-

---

Box 37-3 Causes of Hyperaldosteronism

Primary Aldosteronism

Aldosterone-producing adenoma (65-70%)
Idiopathic bilateral adrenal hyperplasia (30%)
Adrenal carcinoma (<1%)
Glucocorticoid-suppressible aldosteronism (<1%)

Secondary Aldosteronism

Renal artery stenosis
Congestive heart failure

Modified from Melby JC: Diagnosis of hyperaldosteronism. Endocrinol Metab Clin North Am 20:248, 1991.

---

ectomy is the treatment of choice for a child with Cushing's syndrome secondary to an adrenocortical neoplasm.

Primary Hyperaldosteronism

BACKGROUND

In 1955, Jerome Conn described a 34-year-old woman with hypertension, generalized weakness, and polyuria. Her electrolyte analysis showed hypokalemia, and surgical exploration of the patient's abdomen revealed a right adrenal cortical adenoma, which was resected. The patient's blood pressure and metabolic abnormalities normalized within 2.5 weeks after operation, which led Conn to hypothesize that these abnormalities were due to secretion of aldosterone by the adenoma.[48]

High levels of circulating plasma aldosterone cause hypokalemia and hypertension. Aldosteronism may be primary, owing to autonomous adrenal hypersecretion of aldosterone with suppressed plasma renin, or may be secondary, as a result of elevated plasma renin (Box 37-3). Primary aldosteronism is twice as common in women as in men, and it usually occurs between the ages of 30 and 50. The incidence of primary aldosteronism was previously thought to be approximately 1%. Recent reports, however, have estimated that primary aldosteronism is more common than previously thought. Gordon and colleagues reported that 8.5% of a series of 199 hypertensive patients with normal serum potassium levels had primary aldosteronism.[66] The most common cause of primary aldosteronism is an aldosterone-producing adrenal adenoma, which accounts for two thirds of cases (see Box 37-3).[67] Idiopathic hyperaldosteronism from bilateral adrenal cortical hyperplasia causes 30% to 40% of cases.[68] Rare causes include aldosterone-producing adrenocortical carcinoma and glucocorticoid-remediable aldosteronism. The latter is an autosomal dominant condition in which ACTH-dependent hyperaldosteronism is corrected by administration of exogenous glucocorticoids. This rare disorder occurs secondary to fusion of the ACTH-responsive 11β-hydroxylase gene promoter to the aldosterone synthase gene.[69] ACTH-induced overexpression of this chimeric gene by cells of the zona fasciculata results in excessive aldosterone production.

Secondary aldosteronism is a physiologic response of the renin-angiotensin system to renal artery stenosis, cirrhosis, congestive heart failure, and normal pregnancy. The adrenal functions normally and secretes aldosterone in response to the elevated plasma renin and angiotensin caused by these conditions. Secondary aldosteronism responds to treatment of the underlying cause.

SIGNS AND SYMPTOMS

Patients with primary aldosteronism have moderate to severe diastolic hypertension that is often resistant to medical treatment.[70] Hypokalemia occurs spontaneously in 80% to 90% of patients with this disorder and can usually be induced in those who have a normal potassium concentration by oral sodium loading.[71] The clinical signs and symptoms associated with primary hyperaldosteronism are nonspecific but may include headache from the hypertension. Peripheral edema is rare despite the volume expansion effects of increased circulating aldosterone. Potassium depletion may cause symptoms of muscle weakness and cramps, fatigue, polyuria, and polydipsia. In addition to hypokalemia, initial laboratory findings may include mild metabolic alkalosis and relative hypernatremia (serum sodium concentration >142mEq/L).[70]

DIAGNOSIS

Primary aldosteronism should be screened for in any hypertensive patient with hypokalemia, even if the patient is on diuretics. Other individuals who should be evaluated for hyperaldosteronism include those with severe hypertension, hypertension refractory to medical therapy, and young age at onset of hypertension.

The goals of diagnostic evaluation of the patient with suspected primary aldosteronism are (1) to establish the presence of hyperaldosteronism biochemically and (2) to distinguish surgically correctable aldosterone-producing adrenal adenoma (aldosteronoma) from medically treatable idiopathic cortical hyperplasia. A diagnostic algorithm for the evaluation of patients suspected to have this diagnosis is shown in Figure 37-16. The biochemical diagnosis of primary aldosteronism requires demonstration of elevated aldosterone levels with suppressed plasma renin activity. The initial screening evaluation, therefore, consists of measurement of upright plasma aldosterone concentration (PAC) and plasma renin activity (PRA). A PAC:PRA ratio of more than 20 to 30 in the setting of a plasma aldosterone level of greater than 15 ng/dL is suggestive of the diagnosis and merits further evaluation to confirm the presence of inappropriate aldosterone secretion.[72] Patients should be off spironolactone for 6 weeks as well as off ACE inhibitors before testing. Calcium-channel blockers, α_1-adrenergic receptor blockers, and β-receptor blockers do not usually affect the accuracy of the results and can be used for hypertensive control.[72]

Patients with an elevated PAC:PRA ratio should be investigated further by measurement of urinary aldosterone excretion while on a high-sodium diet. Patients

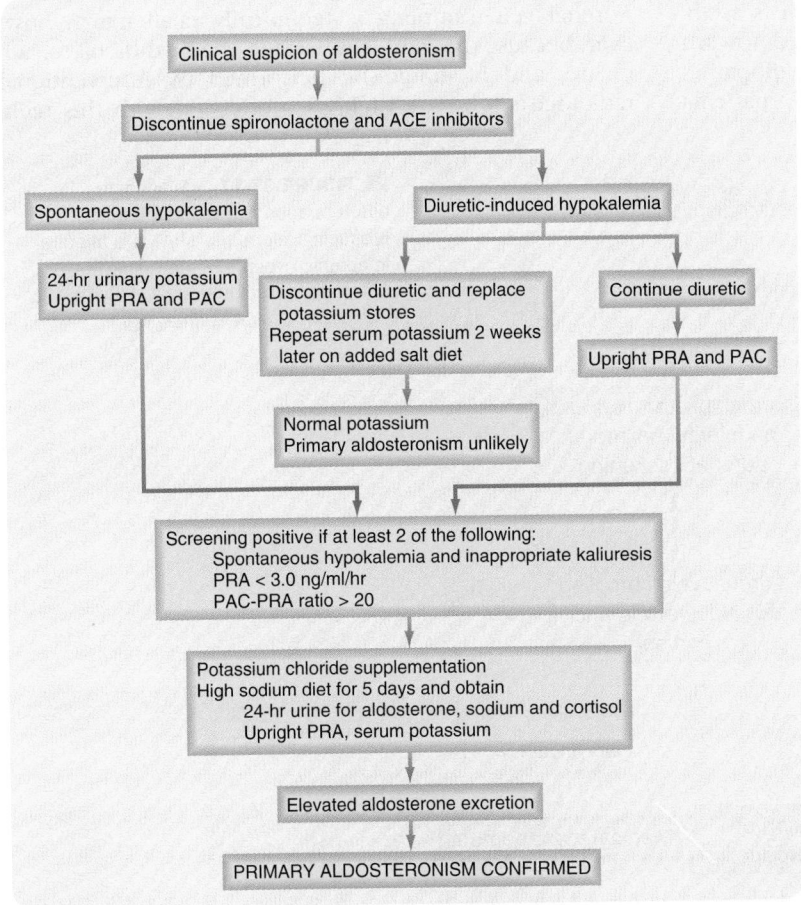

FIGURE 37-16. Screening and diagnostic confirmation of primary aldosteronism. ACE, angiotensin-converting enzyme; PAC, plasma aldosterone concentration; PRA, plasma renin activity. (From Young WF, Hogan MJ, Klee GG, et al: Primary aldosteronism: Diagnosis and treatment. Mayo Clin Proc 65:99, 1990.)

with primary hyperaldosteronism should not exhibit aldosterone suppressibility after salt loading, whereas in other conditions aldosterone secretion should be suppressed by a high sodium intake. It is important that potassium be repleted before testing because the increased sodium intake may lead to increased urinary potassium excretion and exacerbation of hypokalemia. Patients should be on a high-sodium diet for at least 3 days, and a 24-hour urine collection for aldosterone, potassium, and sodium is carried out on the third day. The 24-hour urine sodium excretion rate should be more than 200 mEq to verify adequate sodium intake. In this setting, the urine aldosterone excretion rate in patients with hyperaldosteronism should be more than 12 μg/24 hr.[72] A urinary potassium output of more than 30 mEq/day in the presence of a serum potassium value less than 3.5 mEq/L is also supportive of a diagnosis of primary aldosteronism.

An alternative method for the biochemical confirmation of primary hyperaldosteronism is the intravenous saline infusion test. In this test, patients who have followed a low sodium diet for 3 days are given 2 L of normal saline over 4 hours while supine, and a concurrent 24-hour urine collection for aldosterone and sodium is started. A urine aldosterone excretion rate of less than 14 μg/24 hr excludes primary hyperaldosteronism except for the glucocorticoid-remediable type. Plasma aldosterone may also be measured; a level less than 8.5 ng/dL excludes primary aldosteronism. The intravenous saline test may precipitate congestive heart failure in patients with limited cardiac reserve, however, and should be used judiciously.

Once the diagnosis of primary aldosteronism is established biochemically, further tests are directed toward distinguishing between an aldosteronoma and idiopathic adrenal hyperplasia (Fig. 37-17). In general, patients with aldosteronomas tend to have more pronounced hypokalemia, have higher plasma and urinary aldosterone levels, and are younger in age (<50 years) when compared with those with idiopathic hyperaldosteronism.[72,73] However, these factors do not reliably predict unilateral versus bilateral adrenal disease in any given patient, and adrenal imaging should be carried out as the next step. Adrenal imaging should not be done, however, until the biochemical diagnosis is clear because of the potential to be misled by an unrelated nonfunctional "incidentaloma," as is discussed later.

The preferred imaging modality for suspected aldosteronoma is CT because of the sensitivity of CT for detecting adrenal lesions greater than 0.5 to 1.0 cm in more than 90% of patients.[74] MRI is more costly but may be useful during pregnancy or in situations in which CT is undesirable or contraindicated. The presence of a unilateral adenoma 1 cm or larger on CT with a normal contralateral adrenal is strong evidence for the presence of a unilateral aldosteronoma and further localization before adrenalectomy is probably unnecessary. However, if the CT shows bilateral adrenal nodularity, a unilateral adrenal lesion less than 1 cm, unilateral adrenal thickening, or bilateral normal adrenals, additional testing is indicated to determine whether a unilateral source for increased aldosterone production is present.[75]

Sampling of the adrenal veins for aldosterone and cortisol is the preferred method for differentiating unilateral aldosteronoma from idiopathic hyperaldosteronism in cases in which the radiographic imaging is unclear.[75,76] Adrenal vein sampling is technically challenging, however, because the right adrenal vein can be difficult to cannulate, and it should be performed by interventional radiologists who are highly experienced with this tech-

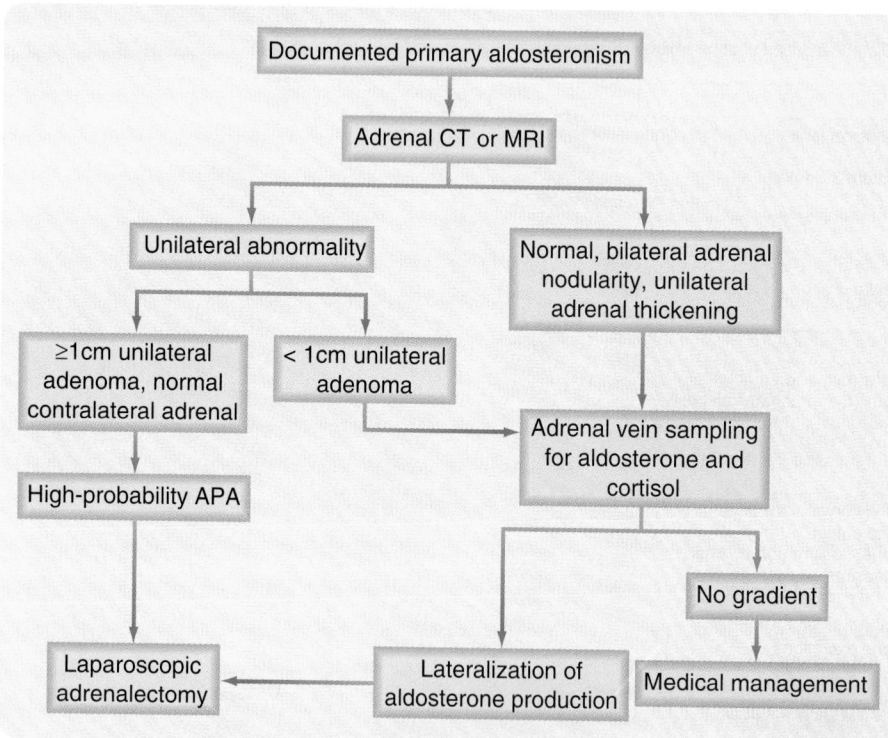

FIGURE 37-17. Diagnostic differentiation between aldosterone-producing adenoma (APA) and bilateral idiopathic hyperaldosteronism (IHA). CT, computed tomography; MRI, magnetic resonance imaging.

nique. In this procedure, percutaneous transfemoral cannulation of both adrenal veins is performed and intravenous ACTH is administered. Blood samples for aldosterone and cortisol are obtained from the inferior vena cava (IVC) and from both adrenal veins. Comparison of cortisol levels from the IVC and adrenal veins is used to confirm adequate placement of catheters; right and left adrenal vein cortisol levels should be similar and should be higher than the IVC level. In a study from Mayo Clinic of 65 patients who underwent bilateral adrenal vein sampling, the mean adrenal to IVC cortisol gradient was 32:1 on the right and 22:1 on the left.[75] The lower left-sided values were believed to be due to the contribution of the inferior phrenic vein to left adrenal vein effluent. Expression of the result as the ratio of aldosterone concentration to cortisol corrects for this dilution factor. An adrenal vein aldosterone to cortisol ratio that is four to five times higher on one side than the other is predictive of an aldosteronoma in greater than 90% of cases.

MANAGEMENT OF PRIMARY ALDOSTERONISM

Adrenal Adenoma Surgical removal of an aldosterone-secreting adenoma results in resolution of hypokalemia in virtually 100% of cases and substantial improvement of hypertension in over 90%.[77] However, long-term cure of hypertension occurs in only 60% to 70%.[72] Preoperative spironolactone and potassium are given to replete potassium stores and correct alkalosis before anesthesia. Blood pressure response to spironolactone in patients with primary hyperaldosteronism also correlates with outcome after operation; a significant fall in blood pressure with spironolactone often predicts a successful outcome after adrenalectomy. Response to adrenalectomy is also influenced by the duration and severity of hypertension and by the presence of histologic changes in the kidney.[72,78] Age older than 50 years, male sex, and the presence of multiple nodules within the adrenal are also associated with a poor response to surgery.[79]

Surgical removal of the affected adrenal gland is appropriate treatment for patients with solitary unilateral aldosteronoma (Fig. 37-18). These tumors are usually small (1 to 2 cm) and, therefore, laparoscopic adrenalectomy is the preferred approach. If an aldosterone-producing carcinoma is suspected (these are extremely rare), an open transabdominal approach should be used so that en bloc resection of the adrenal with adjacent structures (e.g., kidney, liver, pancreas, spleen or colon) may be accomplished if necessary. Bilateral adrenalectomy for adenomas is not recommended because the resulting adrenal insufficiency may be more difficult to manage than the hypertension.[68] Patients do not require perioperative glucocorticoid coverage after unilateral adrenalectomy for aldosteronoma but may require treatment with synthetic mineralocorticoids when oral intake resumes. Selective hypoaldosteronism generally resolves within 3 months of resection of the aldosteronoma.

Idiopathic Adrenal Hyperplasia and Glucocorticoid-Remediable Aldosteronism

Medical management is indicated for patients with idiopathic hyperaldosteronism. Spironolactone is effective

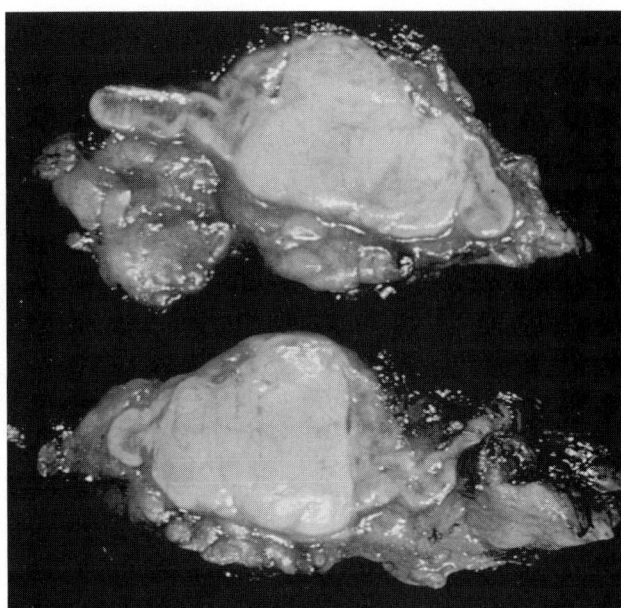

FIGURE 37-18. Bisected right adrenalectomy specimen from a patient with primary aldosteronism. Specimen reveals a 1.5-cm adrenal adenoma with the characteristic yellow-orange color of an aldosteronoma. After resection, the patient's hypertension and hypokalemia corrected.

in controlling hypertension and hypokalemia but may not be well tolerated because of side effects of impotence, decreased libido, and gynecomastia. Other agents that have been used for this problem include amiloride, thiazide diuretics, and calcium-channel blockers. Adrenalectomy may be indicated when symptomatic hypokalemia is refractory to medical therapy.

Glucocorticoid-remediable aldosteronism is important to diagnose and treat because these patients are at increased risk for developing hemorrhagic stroke.[80] Treatment consists of administration of dexamethasone, 0.5 to 1.0 mg/day, to suppress ACTH production. Small doses should be used to avoid Cushing's syndrome. A combination of spironolactone, triamterene, or other potassium-sparing diuretic regimens may be helpful in reducing corticosteroid requirements.

ADRENAL NEOPLASMS ASSOCIATED WITH EXCESS SEX STEROIDS

Virilizing Adrenal Tumors Benign and malignant adrenal cortical tumors may cause virilization by production of excess adrenal androgens, in particular the androgen precursor DHEA. DHEA may be measured directly in plasma or in urine as a 17-ketosteroid. Often, glucocorticoids are concurrently overproduced, which leads to virilization and Cushing's syndrome. Girls prematurely develop clitoral enlargement and pubic hair. Boys prematurely develop hirsutism and macrogenitosomia praecox, but the testes remain small and there may be inhibition of spermatogenesis. Development of an adrenal virilizing tumor in women causes hirsutism and masculinization. Adult males with these tumors may have no signs until primary tumor enlargement or distant metastases cause symptoms. Abdominal CT or MRI is used to localize these lesions.

Resection of tumor and involved adrenal gland is the primary treatment for patients with adrenal virilizing tumors. It is hard to distinguish benign from malignant lesions by histology alone. Invasion of adjacent structures and nodal or distant metastases occur with malignant lesions, but these features may not be obvious until a recurrence has occurred. Tumor recurrence may also manifest itself by return of virilization and by detection of increased 17-ketosteroids in the urine. Aminoglutethimide or mitotane may be useful in controlling signs and symptoms in patients with metastatic disease.

Feminizing Adrenal Tumors

Feminizing adrenal neoplasms are extremely rare. Most of these tumors occur in adult males in the second to fourth decade of life. Impotence is common, and gynecomastia and testicular atrophy are frequent findings. In young males, the association of bilateral gynecomastia, rapid growth, and advanced bone age should suggest a feminizing adrenal tumor. Usually, levels of urinary 17-ketosteroids and estrogens are elevated. Girls with a feminizing adrenal tumor experience precocious puberty with breast enlargement, development of a female escutcheon, and early onset of menses. Approximately 50% of patients have a palpable abdominal mass at the time of diagnosis. Diagnosis depends on biochemical demonstration of elevated urinary levels of estrogens and 17-ketosteroids. Surgical resection is the treatment of choice. Generally, patients with benign adenomas experience a normal survival, whereas the prognosis is poor in patients with adrenocortical carcinoma.

Adrenogenital Syndromes

CONGENITAL ADRENAL HYPERPLASIA

The congenital adrenal hyperplasias are the most common adrenal disorders of infancy and childhood. These syndromes result from inherited defects of one or several of the enzymes necessary for cortisol biosynthesis (Table 37-5). Cortisol deficiency leads to ACTH overproduction and secondary hyperplasia of the adrenal cortex with shunting of cortisol precursors into adrenal androgen pathways. Peripheral tissues convert the excess adrenal androgens to testosterone, which causes virilization of the patient.

Prenatal adrenal virilization in females produces ambiguous external genitalia (female pseudohermaphro-

TABLE 37-5.   Defects of Adrenal Steroidogenesis*

Deficiency	Syndrome	Ambiguous Genitalia	Postnatal Virilization	Salt Metabolism	Steroids Increased	Steroids Decreased	Enzyme	Frequency†
Cholesterol desmolase	Lipoid hyperplasia	Males	No	Salt wasting	None	All	P-450scc	Rare
3β-OH-steroid dehydrogenase	Classic	Males and ?females	Yes	±Salt wasting	DHEA, 17-OH-pregnenolone	Aldosterone, cortisol, testosterone	3β-OH-steroid dehydrogenase	Rare
	Nonclassic	No	Yes	Normal	DHEA, 17-OH-pregnenolone		3β-OH-steroid dehydrogenase	? Frequent
17-Hydroxylase		Males	No	Hypertension	DOC, corticosterone	Cortisol, testosterone	P-450c17	Rare
17,20-Lyase		Males	No	Normal	DHEA, testosterone, androstenedione	P-450c17	Rare	Rare
21-Hydroxylase	Salt wasting	Females	Yes	Salt wasting	17-OHP, androstenedione	Aldosterone, cortisol	P-450c21	1/10,000
	Simple virilizing	Females	Yes	Normal	17-OHP, androstenedione	Cortisol	P-450c21	1/20,000
	Nonclassic	No	Yes	Normal	17-OHP, androstenedione		P-450c21	0.1%-1% (3% in European Jews)
11-Hydroxylase	Classic	Females	Yes	Hypertension	DOC, 11-deoxycortisol	Cortisol, ±aldosterone	P-450c11	1/100,000
	Nonclassic	No	Yes	Normal	11-deoxycortisol, ±DOC		P-450c11	? Frequent
Corticosterone methyloxidase II		No	No	Salt wasting	18-OH-corticosterone	Aldosterone	P-450c11	Rare (except in Iranian Jews)

DHEA, dehydroepiandrosterone; DOC, deoxycorticosterone; 17-OHP, 17-hydroxyprogesterone.
*Deficiency of 17,20-lyase is expressed in the gonads but is included here because it apparently involves the same gene as 17-hydroxylase deficiency.
†"Rare" denotes a syndrome accounting for less than 1% of reported cases of congenital adrenal hyperplasia, which has an overall frequency of about 1 in 5000 births.
"? Frequent" syndromes may occur at frequencies similar to that of nonclassic 21-hydroxylase deficiency, but prevalence data are not available.
Reprinted by permission of The New England Journal of Medicine from White PC, New MI, Dupont B: Congenital adrenal hyperplasia. N Engl J Med 316:1580, 1987. Copyright 1987, Massachusetts Medical Society.

ditism). The müllerian structures (ovaries, fallopian tubes, uterus) are not influenced by androgens and develop normally. Surgical correction of the external anomalies and control of the endocrine defect may allow these females to ultimately bear children.[81]

Postnatal congenital adrenal hyperplasia causes virilization of females and sexual precocity of males. Females develop hirsutism, polycystic ovaries, and irregular menses. Male patients exhibit hypertrophy of the phallus and accelerated growth of body hair and secondary sexual attributes. Fertility is often impaired. Both sexes experience rapid somatic growth, an advanced bone age, early closure of epiphyses, and short stature. Hyperpigmentation may also occur from high levels of circulating pro-opiomelanocortin derivatives.

21-HYDROXYLASE DEFICIENCY

Most cases (>90%) of congenital adrenal hyperplasia are secondary to deficiency of 21-hydroxylase. Mutations of the 21-hydroxylase gene cause the various forms of 21-hydroxylase deficiency.[81] Without 21-hydroxylase, progesterone and 17-hydroxyprogesterone cannot be converted to 11-deoxycortisol and 11-deoxycorticosterone, respectively, and both cortisol and aldosterone are decreased. Two forms of this deficiency are recognized that reflect partial or complete absence of the enzyme. The complete form is characterized by androgen excess at birth, salt wasting in the urine and stool, diarrhea, hypovolemia, hyponatremia, hyperkalemia, and hyperpigmentation. The partial form is characterized by virilization only, which may occur at birth or perhaps not until late childhood or puberty. Increased levels of ACTH may be capable of driving cortisol and aldosterone production into their normal range; therefore, salt wasting, hypovolemia, and hyperpigmentation may be mild or absent.

The laboratory diagnosis of 21-hydroxylase deficiency is straightforward, because elevation of plasma 17-hydroxyprogesterone is the most characteristic abnormality found. Untreated patients with 21-hydroxylase deficiency also have variable deficiencies in both plasma cortisol and 24-hour urinary free cortisol excretion. Comparison of baseline and stimulated levels of 17-hydroxyprogesterone after ACTH stimulation testing can identify complete forms of the disorder.[81]

Treatment of 21-hydroxylase deficiency consists of glucocorticoid and mineralocorticoid replacement. Adequacy of therapy is documented by correction of plasma androgen and 17-hydroxyprogesterone levels. Female patients with ambiguous genitalia require surgical correction, which is best undertaken between age 2 and 18 months. Salient features of the other adrenogenital syndromes are summarized in Table 37-5.

Adrenocortical Carcinoma

BACKGROUND

Adrenocortical carcinoma is a rare tumor that constitutes less than 0.2% of all cancers. These cancers are usually large and advanced when discovered and are rarely curable. The age distribution of adrenocortical carcinoma is bimodal, with peaks in the first and fifth decades. Females are affected more commonly than are males. Most patients (75%) present with stage III or IV disease (Table 37-6).[82,83] Syndromes of adrenal hormone overproduction occur in 36% to 60% of adult patients and may include hypercortisolism, hyperaldosteronism, or virilization. Functional tumors occur more often in females. Nonfunctioning adrenocortical carcinomas present most commonly with abdominal pain, increased abdominal girth, weight loss, weakness, anorexia, and nausea. Approximately 50% of patients have a palpable abdominal mass, and 25% have hepatomegaly. The right adrenal is involved as often as is the left.

DIAGNOSIS

An adrenocortical carcinoma should be suspected in patients with rapidly progressive Cushing's syndrome or in patients with both cushingoid and virilizing features. Large (>6 cm) adrenal masses that extend to nearby structures on CT are more likely to represent carcinomas than are small (<6 cm) adrenal masses. These tumors are as bright as or brighter than liver on T2-weighted MRI.[84] On opposed-phase chemical shift MRI, the signal does not "drop out" in adrenocortical carcinomas as it does in adenomas.[85] In this regard, these tumors appear similar to metastatic lesions or pheochromocytomas. Once the diagnosis of an adrenocortical carcinoma is established, a metastatic evaluation with CT of the chest and bone scan should be done.

The clinical and histologic criteria for malignancy are not well established. Metastasis and invasion of adjacent structures are considered definite evidence of malignancy. Although there are exceptions, adrenal neoplasms weighing more than 100 g or greater than 10 cm in diameter should be considered malignant.[84] Tumor necrosis, hemorrhage, and local invasion are gross pathologic features associated with adrenocortical carcinoma. Histopathologic features of malignancy include the presence of cells

TABLE 37-6. Staging of Adrenocortical Carcinoma

Stage	TNM	Criteria	Percentage of Cases
I	T_1, N_0, M_0	<5 cm; confined to adrenal	2
II	T_2, N_0, M_0	>5 cm; confined to adrenal	19
III	T_3, N_0, M_0	Local invasion or positive nodes	18
	T_1/T_2, N_1, M_0		
IV	T_3/T_4, N_1, M_0	Local invasion and positive nodes, or metastases	61
	Any T/N, M_1		

TNM, tumor-node-metastasis classification; subscript numbers represent the level of malignant involvement.
Modified from Pommier RF, Brennan MF: Management of adrenal neoplasms. Curr Probl Surg 28:684, 1991.

with large hyperchromatic nuclei and more than 20 mitoses per high-power field.

MANAGEMENT

Complete surgical resection of locally confined tumor is the only chance for cure of adrenocortical carcinoma. Wide exposure and a generous incision are needed for several reasons: to allow en bloc resection of tumor and adjacent involved structures; to minimize the risk of rupture of the tumor capsule with spillage; to permit access to the renal veins and vena cava if tumor thrombus is present; and to provide exposure for aortocaval node clearance. A bilateral subcostal incision with midline extension (Mercedes incision) usually provides adequate exposure. Occasionally, a thoracoabdominal incision may be necessary for extremely large right-sided tumors with vena caval involvement. The patient should be rolled up slightly on his or her side to facilitate exposure and retraction of adjacent organs.

In two series, patients with stage I and II disease had a mean survival of 24 and 25 months, with 50% and 10% 5-year survivals after resection, respectively.[86,87] However, spread to local structures including the peritoneum, retroperitoneum, and lymph nodes is evident in 65% of cases and only about 80% of patients are able to undergo attempted resection for cure.[85] Treatment then involves en bloc resection of locally invasive stage III disease. The 5-year survival rate in a series of 113 patients who had a complete primary resection was 55%.[88] Patients with stage I and II tumors had much better 5-year survival (60%) than those with stage III and IV disease (10%). In other series, overall 5-year survival for patients with stage III disease after en bloc resection was 22% to 24%.[85,89]

Common sites for metastases from adrenocortical carcinoma include the lung, lymph nodes, liver, and bone. Surgical debulking of locally advanced or metastatic tumor may provide symptomatic relief from some slow-growing, hormonally productive cancers.[90] Close biochemical and radiologic follow-up is required after resection because locally recurrent or metastatic disease is best treated by reoperation.[82,90]

Mitotane (o, p-DDD) is an adrenal cytotoxic agent with limited effectiveness in some patients with adrenocortical carcinoma. The mechanism of action of mitotane is unknown; however, serious side effects including neurotoxicity, nausea, vomiting, diarrhea, and adrenal insufficiency limit the number of patients who can tolerate this agent. Partial, unsustained responses have been reported in approximately one third or fewer patients, and survival is unchanged.[82,90] Although anecdotal reports of long-term survivors after mitotane treatment exist, no controlled studies have established efficacy of mitotane in this disease.[85] Adjuvant chemotherapy with mitotane after complete resection for adrenocortical carcinoma is controversial, and most oncologists reserve its use for recurrent, unresectable, or metastatic disease.[84] Other chemotherapeutic regimens have been ineffective, and combination regimens of mitotane with other agents have not demonstrated superiority over mitotane alone.[91]

Adrenal Insufficiency

BACKGROUND

In 1855, Thomas Addison described 11 patients with primary adrenal insufficiency, including 5 patients with tuberculous destruction of the adrenal glands.[92] The most common causes of primary adrenal insufficiency are listed in Box 37-4.[93] Although overt adrenal insufficiency is not common, an insidious onset of symptoms and signs of adrenal insufficiency may be present in up to 20% to 30% of patients with bilateral adrenal metastatic lesions detected by CT.[94] These patients are recognized by their weak responses to ACTH stimulation testing. Intra-adrenal hemorrhage and acute adrenal insufficiency may occur in a number of conditions, including trauma, shock, and coagulopathy. Spontaneous adrenal hemorrhage occurring during fulminant meningococcal, gram-negative, or pneumococcal septicemia is known as Waterhouse-Friderichsen syndrome. Exogenous steroid use, surgical resection of cortisol-producing adrenal tumors or ACTH-producing pituitary tumors, and bilateral adrenalectomy are important causes of secondary adrenal insufficiency.

SIGNS AND SYMPTOMS

Acute adrenal insufficiency is a medical emergency and should be suspected in stressed patients with a history of adrenal surgery, adrenal insufficiency, or exogenous steroid use. Signs and symptoms include fever, nausea, vomiting, severe hypotension, and lethargy (Table 37-7). Chronic adrenal insufficiency presents more subtly, and diagnosis is often delayed. Most frequent chronic symptoms include fatigue, weight loss, anorexia, nausea and vomiting, abdominal pain, and diarrhea.

Box 37-4 Causes of Adrenal Insufficiency

Primary Adrenal Insufficiency

Autoimmune conditions: polyglandular autoimmune syndromes I and II

Infections: tuberculosis, fungal infections, cytomegalovirus infection, human immunodeficiency virus-associated infection

Adrenal hemorrhage: Waterhouse-Friderichsen syndrome, coagulopathy

Secondary Adrenal Insufficiency

Exogenous steroid use
Pituitary disease: tumor, hemorrhage
Surgery
    After transsphenoidal removal of a pituitary tumor
    After removal of a functioning adrenal tumor
Metastatic disease: lung, gastric, breast, melanoma, lymphoma
Drugs: mitotane, metyrapone, aminoglutethimide

Modified from Werbel SS, Ober KP: Acute adrenal insufficiency. Endocrinol Metab Clin North Am 22:303, 1993.

TABLE 37-7. Symptoms and Signs in Acute Adrenocortical Insufficiency ("Adrenal Crisis")

Symptoms/Signs (Clinical Deterioration Without Obvious Cause)	Prevalence (%)
Fever	70
Nausea and vomiting	64
Abdominal pain	46
Hypotension	36
Abdominal distention	32
Obtundation/lethargy	26
Hyponatremia	45
Hyperkalemia	25

Modified from May ME, Vaughan ED Jr, Carey RM: Adrenocortical insufficiency: Clinical aspects. *In* Vaughan ED Jr, Carey RM (eds): Adrenal Disorders. New York, Thieme, 1989, p 176.

DIAGNOSIS

The characteristic laboratory findings of adrenal insufficiency include hyponatremia, hyperkalemia, azotemia, and fasting or reactive hypoglycemia. Hypercalcemia may also be present. The peripheral blood smear may demonstrate eosinophilia in 15% to 20% of patients. Adrenal calcifications may be visible on plain abdominal radiographs in 15% of cases.

The rapid ACTH stimulation test is the best test for detection of adrenal insufficiency. Before this test, patients on chronic steroid replacement should be changed to dexamethasone for several days because hydrocortisone acetate is detected by the laboratory assay for cortisol. Synthetic ACTH (250 µg) is administered intravenously, and plasma cortisol levels are measured at 0, 30, and 60 minutes. Normal peak cortisol response should exceed 20 µg/dL. Subnormal stimulation should be confirmed by the standard, prolonged ACTH infusion test. Measurement of ACTH by immunoradiometric assay is then used to distinguish primary from secondary and tertiary adrenal insufficiency. High plasma concentration of ACTH (>200 pg/dL) and low plasma cortisol (<10 mg/dL) are diagnostic of primary adrenal insufficiency in a patient with characteristic symptoms and signs. Low levels of plasma ACTH indicate secondary (pituitary) or tertiary (hypothalamic) causes that can be differentiated by CRH stimulation testing.

MANAGEMENT

Treatment of adrenal insufficiency must be based on clinical suspicion before laboratory confirmation is available. Intravenous volume replacement with normal or hypertonic saline and dextrose is essential, as is immediate intravenous corticosteroid replacement therapy with 4 mg of dexamethasone. Extreme states of hyponatremia should not be corrected too rapidly. Subsequent recognition and treatment of the underlying cause, particularly if it is infectious, usually resolve the crisis.

A rapid ACTH stimulation test is performed to establish the diagnosis of adrenal insufficiency after resuscitation and corticosteroid replacement. Thereafter, 100 mg of hydrocortisone is administered intravenously every 6 to 8 hours and is tapered to standard replacement doses as the patient's condition stabilizes. Mineralocorticoid replacement is not required until intravenous fluids are discontinued and oral intake resumes. Chronic adrenal insufficiency requires corticosteroid and mineralocorticoid replacement. Determination of appropriate replacement doses is imprecise, and follow-up with occasional adjustments is necessary. The average adult requires 12 mg/m² of hydrocortisone, or its equivalent, each day, administered in divided doses along with 0.05 to 0.10 mg of the mineralocorticoid fludrocortisone.

Patients who have known adrenal insufficiency or have received supraphysiologic doses of corticosteroid for more than 1 week in the year preceding surgery should receive perioperative stress-dose corticosteroids. If in doubt, rapid ACTH stimulation testing may be performed during the preoperative evaluation of the patient. Corticosteroid replacement should approximate the known capacity of the normal adrenal to secrete up to 300 mg/day of cortisol under maximal stress. An accepted regimen includes administration of 100 mg of hydrocortisone on the morning of major surgery followed by 100 mg of hydrocortisone every 8 hours during the perioperative 24 hours. If high doses of corticosteroids are administered for less than 72 hours, they can be rapidly tapered to replacement levels as the patient's condition permits. A rapid taper is desirable to minimize corticosteroid-related wound complications and infection.

Physiology of the Adrenal Medulla

The adrenal medulla is derived from the embryonic neural crest. Adrenal medullary or chromaffin cells store and secrete several biologically active amines, including dopamine, norepinephrine, and epinephrine. These catecholamines are also synthesized in the brain and in sympathetic neurons.

The synthesis of catecholamines from tyrosine involves the sequential action of four enzymes: (1) tyrosine hydroxylase, which converts tyrosine to L-dihydroxyphenylalanine (dopa); (2) aromatic L-amino acid decarboxylase, which converts dopa to dopamine; (3) dopamine-β-hydroxylase, which converts dopamine to L-norepinephrine; and (4) phenylethanolamine-N-methyltransferase (PNMT), which converts L-norepinephrine to L-epinephrine. PNMT is localized exclusively in cells of the adrenal medulla and the organ of Zuckerkandl. Thus, with rare exceptions, epinephrine-secreting tumors arise only in these two sites.

Excitation of adrenal chromaffin cells stimulates discharge of catecholamines from intracellular granules into the circulation. The physiologic responses to catecholamines are mediated by α- and β-adrenergic receptors on peripheral tissues. α-Adrenergic receptors have highest affinity for norepinephrine, less for epinephrine, and least for isoproterenol. β-Adrenergic receptors are most responsive to isoproterenol and least to norepinephrine. Specific antagonists recognize each receptor class: α receptors are antagonized by phentolamine and phenoxybenzamine, and β receptors are blocked by propranolol. The β-receptor subtypes have been characterized: β_1 receptors are present in cardiac muscle, adipose tissue, and small intestine, whereas β_2 receptors are found in vascular, tracheal, and uterine smooth muscle, skeletal muscle, and liver. The α receptors have been similarly subdivided: α_1 receptors mediate vasoconstriction, pupillary dilatation, and uterine contraction, whereas α_2 receptors modulate presynaptic norepinephrine release and platelet aggregation. Dopamine receptor activation causes positive inotropic and chronotropic effects on cardiac muscle, induces mild peripheral vasoconstriction, and dilates renal arterioles.

Three pathways govern clearance of catecholamines from the circulation: specific uptake by sympathetic neurons, nonspecific uptake and degradation by peripheral tissues, and excretion in the urine. Catecholamines are metabolized in liver and kidney by two enzymes, monoamine oxidase (MAO) and catechol-O-methyl transferase (COMT). In these tissues, MAO and COMT convert epinephrine or norepinephrine to methoxyhydroxyphenylglycol (MHPG), vanillylmandelic acid (VMA), normetanephrine, and metanephrine (Fig. 37-19). These inactive metabolites are renally cleared and are measurable in the urine either as free compounds or as conjugates of glucuronide or sulfate.

Diseases of the Adrenal Medulla

Pheochromocytoma

BACKGROUND

Pheochromocytomas are catecholamine-secreting adrenal tumors that arise from chromaffin cells of the adrenal medulla. Extra-adrenal pheochromocytomas are also called *functional paragangliomas* and may occur in sympathetic ganglia in the neck, mediastinum, abdomen, pelvis, and organ of Zuckerkandl. The first description of a pheochromocytoma is credited to Frankel, who reported finding bilateral adrenal tumors in an 18-year-old woman who died precipitously in 1886. Roux and Mayo independently reported the first successful resections of pheochromocytomas in 1926 and 1927, respectively.[95,96]

Pheochromocytomas are rare tumors, occurring in 2 to 8 persons per million.[97] These tumors may occur in a sporadic or familial manner and are found with increased frequency in screened hypertensive populations. The peak incidence of pheochromocytoma occurs during the fourth and fifth decades of life, and males and females are affected about equally. The *rule of tens* is a commonly cited and fairly accurate description of pheochromocytomas: tumors are bilateral in 10%, extra-adrenal in 10%, familial in 10%, and malignant in 10% and occur in children in 10% of cases.

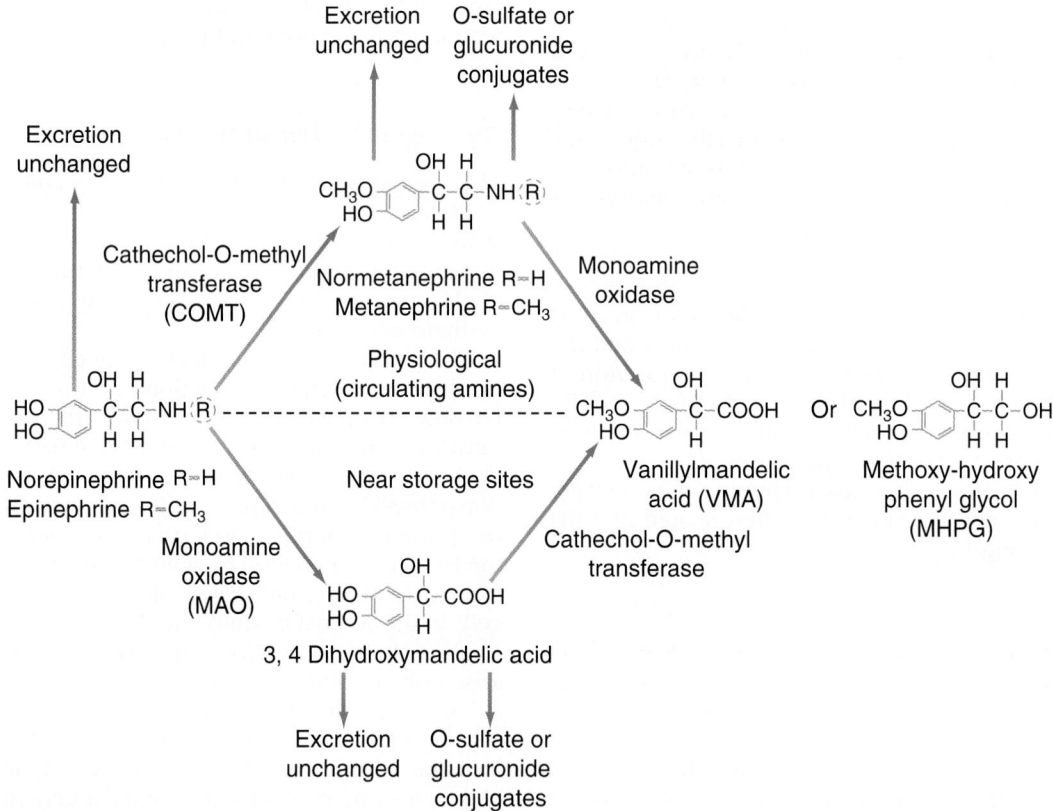

FIGURE 37-19. Biochemical pathways of catecholamine metabolism. (From Melmon KL: Catecholamines and the adrenal medulla. *In* Williams RH [ed]: Textbook of Endocrinology, 6th ed. Philadelphia, WB Saunders, 1981.)

Pheochromocytomas occur in the adrenal medulla in 90% of cases and are more frequent in the right gland than in the left. The organ of Zuckerkandl is the most common extra-adrenal site of pheochromocytoma. Because of the absence of the enzyme PMNT, extra-adrenal pheochromocytomas generally secrete norepinephrine but not epinephrine.

SIGNS AND SYMPTOMS

Pheochromocytomas present with signs and symptoms of catecholamine excess (Table 37-8). Elevation of the blood pressure, which may range from mild hypertension to a dramatic hypertensive crisis, is the most consistent manifestation of this disorder. Hypertension is sustained in roughly one half of patients, is paroxysmal in one third, and is absent in one fifth.[98] Other symptoms include spells that consist of palpitations, anxiety, headache, and flushing. Cardiovascular complications may develop, including myocardial infarction, cardiac dysrhythmias, and stroke. Orthostatic hypotension may occur and results from diminished plasma volume and blunted autonomic reflexes. Gastrointestinal motility may be depressed and results in ileus, obstipation, and sometimes megacolon. Asymptomatic patients with functioning tumors are relatively uncommon, and nonfunctioning tumors are distinctly uncommon. Sudden death has been reported in patients with known or unsuspected pheochromocytomas who have undergone provocative testing, percutaneous biopsy of the tumor, or surgical procedures for other indications.

DIAGNOSIS

Demonstration of increased plasma or urinary levels of catecholamines and their metabolites is the sine qua non for the diagnosis of pheochromocytoma. More than 90% of patients with pheochromocytomas have distinctly elevated 24-hour urine levels of catecholamines, metanephrine, and VMA. Urinary VMA is the least specific test, because false-positive findings may result from ingestion of coffee, tea, raw fruits, or drugs such as α-methyldopa. Recently, the measurement of plasma fractionated metanephrines (metanephrine and normetanephrine) has become available as a screening test for the detection of pheochromocytomas.[99,100] This test is now preferred in many institutions as the initial method of biochemical evaluation because it is highly sensitive for detecting pheochromocytomas and is simple to perform.[101] False-positive results are more common with this test, however, and additional testing is recommended to confirm the diagnosis in positive test cases with measurement of urine catecholamines and metanephrines or of plasma catecholamines and repeat plasma fractionated metanephrines.[101] A comparison of the sensitivity and specificity of these various biochemical tests for the diagnosis of pheochromocytomas is given in Table 37-9.

Provocative testing with glucagon and the clonidine suppression test have been used in the past to aid in the diagnosis in difficult cases but are no longer commonly employed. In one series of 542 patients with normal 24-hour urine studies, not one patient had positive results on provocative testing.[102] Furthermore, the clonidine suppression test may cause hypotension whereas the administration of glucagon can result in severe hypertension.

Up to 98% of pheochromocytomas are found in the abdomen, 2% to 3% in the thorax, and 1% in the neck.[103] CT and MRI are the two radiologic modalities of choice to localize pheochromocytomas. CT readily detects tumors 1 cm and larger, with a reported sensitivity of 87% to 100%.[104] MRI is similarly sensitive, and a T2-weighted image brightness three times greater than liver is highly specific for pheochromocytoma (Fig. 37-20).[105] Adrenal arteriography and venography no longer have a role in the imaging of these patients.

Iodine-131-metaiodobenzylguanidine (^{131}I-MIBG) selectively accumulates in chromaffin tissues and accumulates more rapidly in pheochromocytoma than in normal tissue. Multi-institutional experience with ^{131}I-MIBG imaging for pheochromocytomas demonstrated an overall sensitivity of 77% to 87% and a specificity of 96% to 100%.[104] This test is most useful in localizing extra-adrenal tumors not seen with conventional imaging and in following patients with malignant pheochromocytomas.

TABLE 37-8. Symptoms of Pheochromocytoma		
Symptoms*	Approximate Percentage	
	Paroxysmal (37 Patients)	Persistent (39 Patients)
Headaches (severe)	92	72
Excess sweating (generalized)	65	69
Palpitations ± tachycardia	73	51
Anxiety or nervousness (± fear of impending death; panic)	60	28
Tremulousness	51	26
Pain in chest and/or abdomen (usually epigastric) and/or lumbar regions and/or lower abdomen and/or groin	48	28
Nausea ± vomiting	43	26
Weakness, fatigue, prostration	38	15
Weight loss (severe)	14	15
Dyspnea	11	18
Warmth ± heat intolerance	13	15
Visual disturbances	3	21
"Dizziness" or faintness	11	3
Constipation	0	13
Paresthesias or pain in arms	11	0
Bradycardia (noted by patient)	8	3
Grand mal seizures	5	3

*Symptoms presumably result from excess catecholamines and/or hypertension. From Manger WM, Gifford RW: Pheochromocytoma. New York, Springer-Verlag, 1977, p 89.

TABLE 37-9. Sensitivity and Specificity of Biochemical Tests for Diagnosis of Pheochromocytoma

Biochemical Test	Sensitivity (%)	Specificity (%)	Sensitivity at 100% Specificity (%)
Plasma metanephrine level	99	89	82
Plasma catecholamine level	85	80	38
Urinary catecholamine level	83	88	64
Urinary metanephrine level	76	94	53
Urinary vanillylmandelic acid level	63	94	43

Sensitivity was determined for tests in 151 patients with mainly sporadic pheochromocytoma, and specificity was determined for tests in 349 patients studied at the National Institutes of Health. Reprinted with permission from Pacak K, Linehan WM, Eisenhofer G, et al: Recent advances in genetics, diagnosis, localization, and treatment of pheochromocytoma. Ann Intern Med. 134:318, 2001.

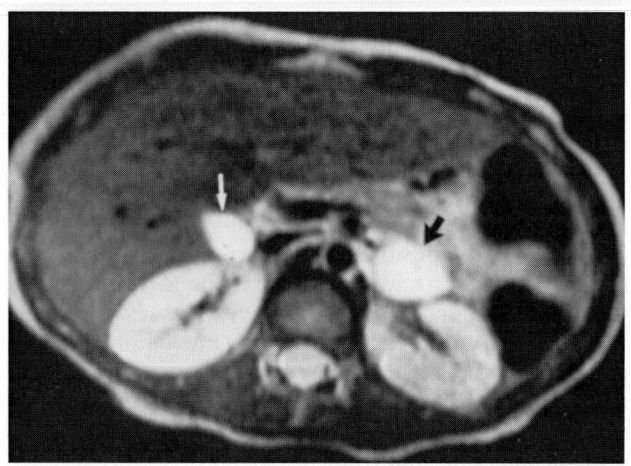

FIGURE 37-20. T2-weighted MR study of a left-sided pheochromocytoma *(black arrow)*. The gallbladder *(white arrow)* has an increased signal intensity because of its high water content. Pheochromocytomas, adrenocortical carcinomas, and metastatic lesions to the adrenal gland demonstrate this high signal intensity, possibly because of their high water content. (Courtesy of J. Heiken, M.D., Mallinckrodt Institute of Radiology, Washington University School of Medicine, St. Louis, Missouri.)

MANAGEMENT

Preoperative management of patients with pheochromocytoma centers on (1) control of hypertension, (2) α blockade to prevent intraoperative hypertensive crisis due to tumor manipulation and release of catecholamines, and (3) fluid resuscitation to prevent circulatory collapse after removal of the catecholamine-secreting tumor. α-Adrenergic blockade is achieved with phenoxybenzamine, starting at a dose of 10 mg twice daily. The dose is increased by 10 to 20 mg/day until hypertension and symptoms are controlled and the patient demonstrates mild postural hypotension. Phenoxybenzamine is usually administered for at least 1 week before operation, and the patient should be hospitalized the last 24 hours before adrenalectomy for observation and administration of intravenous fluids. Patients with marked hypertension and symptoms may require hospitalization for several days

before operation while α blockade is adjusted. Because the patient's volume status may be restricted owing to the increased adrenergic mediated vasoconstriction, fluid volume expansion is important as α blockade progresses to avoid severe postural hypotension and to minimize hemodynamic fluctuations during surgery. Side effects of α blockade include reflex tachycardia, nasal congestion, and an inability to ejaculate.

β-Adrenergic blockade is indicated in patients who develop tachycardia with α blockade or who have tachyarrhythmias or predominately epinephrine-secreting tumors. β Blockers may enhance pressor response to endogenous norepinephrine and thus should not be given until adequate α blockade has been established. β Blockade can also produce profound bradycardia, myocardial depression, and congestive heart failure. Cardiac asystole and death after propranolol administration have been reported in patients with pheochromocytoma. Other agents that may be used to manage hypertension in pheochromocytoma include selective α₁-adrenergic antagonists (terazosin and doxazosin) and calcium-channel blockers.

Patients with pheochromocytoma can be expected to have blood pressure volatility and high fluid volume requirements during and immediately after surgery. All patients should have additional hydration by preoperative intravenous fluid administration for 12 to 24 hours before surgery to avoid cardiovascular collapse after removal of the tumor. An arterial pressure line is indicated for intraoperative monitoring in symptomatic patients.

Anesthetic agents may trigger the release of catecholamines from pheochromocytomas. The anesthetic plane is now considered more important than the choice of agent, and both enflurane and isoflurane have been used successfully. Intraoperative hypertension is best treated with a sodium nitroprusside drip, and cardiac arrhythmias are best managed with short-acting β blockers (e.g., esmolol) or lidocaine. Morphine and phenothiazines may precipitate hypertensive crisis and should be avoided preoperatively.[103]

In the past, an open anterior approach through either a midline or bilateral subcostal incision was used to resect pheochromocytomas. This approach allowed complete abdominal exploration and was necessary to evaluate possible extra-adrenal locations, metastases, and multifocal lesions. Today, CT, MRI, and radionuclide scans permit preoperative localization of tumor in 95% or more of cases, so that the surgical approach may be more directed. In most cases, pheochromocytomas are appropriate for excision using a laparoscopic approach.[106,107] Regardless of the approach, important common principles include minimal handling of the tumor, early isolation of the adrenal vein, and avoidance of capsular rupture.

Immediately after resection of the pheochromocytoma, profound hypotension as a result of vasodilatation may occur. Fluid resuscitation is necessary to expand intravascular volume. Symptomatic patients are usually admitted to an intensive care unit where arterial blood pressure and urine output should be monitored continuously during the first 24 hours after operation. Monitoring of the serum glucose concentration should also be carried out because of the risk of hypoglycemia owing to rebound hyperinsulinemia from catecholamine-induced suppression of insulin secretion.

SPECIAL ISSUES IN PHEOCHROMOCYTOMA

Hereditary Pheochromocytomas Pheochromocytomas may occur as a component of a variety of inherited endocrine tumor syndromes, including multiple endocrine neoplasia (MEN) type 2, von Hippel-Lindau (VHL) disease, and neurofibromatosis type 1 (NF-1). Mutations responsible for development of these hereditary tumors have been identified and include the *RET* proto-oncogene in MEN 2A and 2B, the *VHL* tumor suppressor gene in von Hippel-Lindau disease, and the *NF1* gene in neurofibromatosis type 1. Recently, familial paragangliomas of the neck have been shown to be associated with mutations in the succinate dehydrogenase subunit B *(SDHB)* and succinate dehydrogenase subunit D genes *(SDHD)* that encode mitochondrial enzymes involved in oxidative phosphorylation.[108] It was previously thought that approximately 10% of pheochromocytomas were hereditary. Recent evidence indicates that this number may be higher. Neumann and associates[109] performed genetic testing for germ-line mutations in the genes just mentioned in 271 patients with apparent nonhereditary pheochromocytomas. Mutations were found in 66 cases (24%); 30 had mutations of *VHL*, 13 of *RET*, 11 of *SDHD*, and 12 of *SDHB.*

Multiple Endocrine Neoplasia 2 (MEN 2). The MEN 2 syndromes are hereditary, autosomal dominant predispositions to medullary carcinoma of the thyroid (MTC) and pheochromocytomas. MEN 2A is also associated with parathyroid hyperplasia, whereas MEN 2B patients have multiple mucosal neuromas, ganglioneuromatosis, and a characteristic "marfanoid" body habitus but lack hyperparathyroidism. Nearly all individuals affected with MEN 2 develop medullary carcinoma of the thyroid, whereas only 30% to 40% develop pheochromocytomas.[110-112] It is imperative that patients with medullary carcinoma of the thyroid be screened for pheochromocytoma, especially if there is a family history of either tumor. Approximately 10% of patients with MEN 2A present with symptoms of pheochromocytoma as the initial manifestation of

disease.[110] Relatives of these patients should be screened for associated endocrinopathies even if they are asymptomatic. Screening strategies are more thoroughly discussed in Chapter 38.

The adrenal medullary disease in patients with MEN 2 may be bilateral and is often preceded by the onset of adrenal medullary hyperplasia (Fig. 37-21). Management consists of removal of all grossly identifiable pheochromocytomas by adrenalectomy. A cortical-sparing procedure to preserve adrenal function may be considered in carefully selected patients with bilateral tumors. Patients with unilateral tumors should undergo unilateral adrenalectomy and should be followed closely with annual biochemical screening. The risk of development of a contralateral pheochromocytoma 5 years after unilateral adrenalectomy in this population is approximately 33%.[107]

Von Hippel-Lindau Disease. Patients with von Hippel-Lindau disease may develop bilateral kidney tumors and cysts, cerebellar and spinal hemangioblastomas, retinal angiomas, pancreatic cysts and tumors, epididymal cystadenomas, and inner ear canal tumors as well as pheochromocytomas.[113] Some von Hippel-Lindau families may present with pheochromocytoma as the primary manifestation. It is important to screen patients with bilateral or multifocal pheochromocytomas for mutations in both the *VHL* and *RET* genes.[101]

Neuroectodermal Dysplasias. Von Recklinghausen's neurofibromatosis is diagnosed in 5% to 10% of patients with pheochromocytoma, although less than 1% of patients with von Recklinghausen's disease develop pheochromocytoma. Other neuroectodermal dysplasia syndromes associated with pheochromocytoma include tuberous sclerosis and Sturge-Weber syndrome.

MALIGNANT PHEOCHROMOCYTOMA

The diagnosis of malignant pheochromocytoma is often difficult to make either by preoperative criteria or by

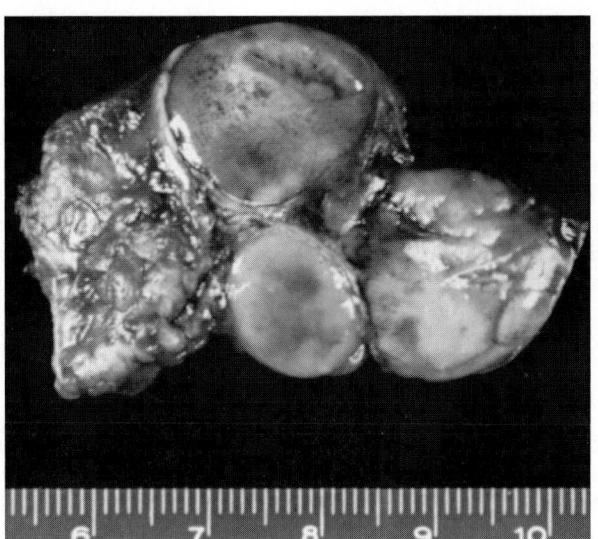

FIGURE 37-21. Multiple pheochromocytomas in a single adrenal gland resected from a patient with multiple endocrine neoplasia type 2A.

inspection of the resected specimen. On gross examination, many benign tumors penetrate the adrenal capsule and may even invade the veins draining the gland. Microscopic examination of both benign and malignant lesions may reveal cellular pleomorphism, mitoses, and atypical nuclei. Therefore, a diagnosis of malignant pheochromocytoma is established only by demonstrating invasion of adjacent structures or by documenting nodal or distant metastases.

Ten to 20 percent of sporadically occurring pheochromocytomas prove to be malignant. Females are three times more likely than males to harbor such a malignancy. It is controversial whether such lesions in children are more or less likely to be malignant than in adults.[114] There is much stronger evidence, however, that pheochromocytomas found in extra-adrenal sites are two to three times as likely to be malignant as those of adrenal origin.[115] Hypertension associated with malignant pheochromocytomas is sustained and is rarely paroxysmal.

Pheochromocytomas may spread to bone, liver, lymph nodes, lungs, and the central nervous system. Less common metastatic sites are the pleura, kidney, omentum, and pancreas. Recurrences usually appear within 5 to 10 years after resection of the primary lesion but may be detected as many as 20 years later. There are no clear differences in secretion rates of the different catecholamines to distinguish benign from malignant lesions.

The treatment of malignant pheochromocytoma includes resection of metastases and medical control of hypertension. Radiation therapy may be helpful to ameliorate pain from bony metastases. Ablative therapy with ^{131}I-MIBG has produced partial responses,[116] and combination chemotherapy with cyclophosphamide, vincristine, and dacarbazine may also be effective.[117,118] Overall 5-year survival is 36% to 60%.[119]

EXTRA-ADRENAL PHEOCHROMOCYTOMA

Extra-adrenal pheochromocytomas, also known as *functional paragangliomas,* can occur at any site in the abdomen where chromaffin tissue is located and have been found in the paravertebral ganglia, the organ of Zuckerkandl, and the urinary bladder (Fig. 37-22). Pheochromocytomas that arise in the organ of Zuckerkandl can become large enough to press on adjacent vascular or genitourinary structures and can be quite vascular and difficult to resect. Pheochromocytomas located in the bladder can cause hypertensive episodes during micturition. Thoracic and cervical pheochromocytomas have also been identified in sympathetic ganglia of the posterior mediastinum, the carotid body *(chemodectomas),* the heart, and the jugular bulb.

PHEOCHROMOCYTOMA IN PREGNANCY

Pheochromocytoma in pregnancy is an extremely dangerous problem that can cause death of both the mother and fetus. Nearly 130 cases of pheochromocytoma requiring management during pregnancy have been reported.[120] Although antenatal diagnosis is made in less than half of the patients, it significantly reduces maternal and fetal mortality at the time of delivery.[120] Pheochromocytoma

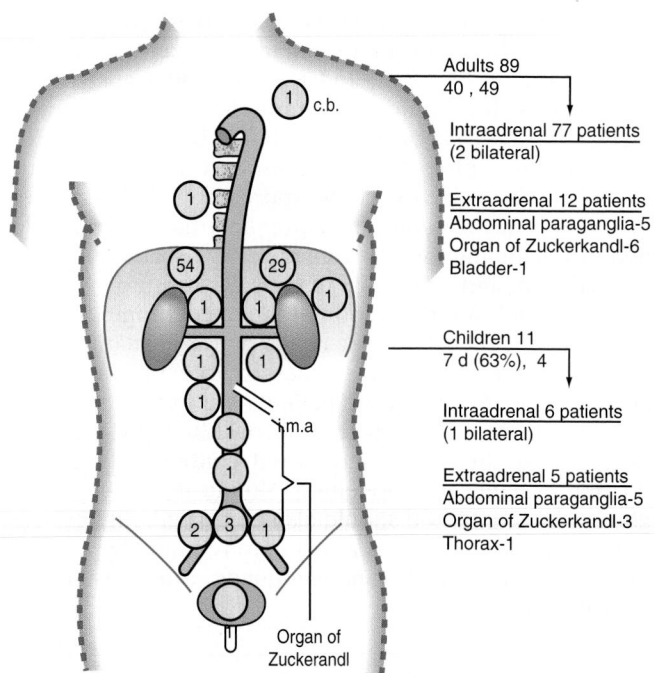

FIGURE 37-22. Locations of 107 pheochromocytomas in 100 patients. c.b., carotid body; i.m.a., inferior mesenteric artery. (From Manger WM, Gifford RW, Melicow MM: Pheochromocytoma. New York, Springer-Verlag, 1977, p 45.)

may be suspected in pregnant women who experience preeclampsia, paroxysmal hypertension, or unexplained hyperpyrexia after delivery. Unfortunately, the diagnosis may not be made until after sudden shock and death of the mother occur at the time of anesthesia and delivery. The period of greatest hazard occurs from the onset of labor until 48 hours post partum.

The timing of surgical intervention in the pregnant patient with a pheochromocytoma should be individualized depending on the degree of medical control of hypertension, tumor size, likelihood of malignancy, and stage of pregnancy.[121] If the diagnosis is made during the second trimester of pregnancy when the risk of spontaneous abortion is low, surgical resection is recommended as soon as pharmacologic α blockade can be established.[122,123] In the first trimester, the patient should be managed medically until the second trimester, at which time adrenalectomy is performed. For patients with pheochromocytomas diagnosed during the third trimester, medical management is preferred until delivery, provided hypertensive control is adequate. However, the mother and fetus must be closely monitored because hypertensive crises can be precipitated by labor, fetal movement, and mechanical pressure from the uterus. The optimal method of childbirth in these patients is controversial. Combined cesarean section and removal of the pheochromocytoma has been advocated by some,[122] but vaginal delivery may be possible in selected cases if the patient is well controlled medically.[123] Adrenalectomy is then carried out after recovery from childbirth. There is no direct evidence that short-term use of phenoxybenzamine is harmful to the fetus, although few patients have been studied and the long-term effects of the drug are unclear. A laparoscopic approach has been used successfully to remove pheochromocytomas in some pregnant patients.[124]

PHEOCHROMOCYTOMA IN CHILDHOOD

Approximately 10% of pheochromocytomas occur in individuals younger than 20 years of age. Childhood pheochromocytomas occur more commonly in familial settings (MEN 2, NF-1). Symptoms are similar to those in adults, but sustained hypertension, sweating, visual symptoms, weight loss, polydipsia, and polyuria are more common.[125] Multiple, bilateral, and extra-adrenal tumors occur in 25% to 40% of pediatric cases.[97]

Incidental Adrenal Mass

The number of incidentally discovered adrenal masses has increased dramatically over the past 2 decades as a result of the widespread use and improved resolution of abdominal imaging modalities. Autopsy data taken from a compilation of 25 series have demonstrated adrenal adenomas in patients without premortem evidence of adrenal disease in 5.9% cases.[126] The prevalence of unsuspected adrenal masses detected in CT series has ranged from 1% to 5%.[127] Adrenal nodules also increase in incidence with advancing age; the incidence before age 30 is only 0.2% compared with 6.9% in individuals older than age 70.[128] Proper evaluation of the patient with an adrenal incidentaloma requires an understanding of the differential diagnosis of adrenal masses, the biochemical profile of hyperfunctioning adrenal tumors, and risk factors for adrenal malignancy.[129] Adrenalectomy is reserved for patients with hyperfunctioning tumors and for potentially malignant lesions. Therefore, the diagnostic evaluation should consist of both a determination of the functional status of the adrenal lesion and an assessment of its malignant potential.

Differential Diagnosis

The differential diagnosis of adrenal incidentalomas and their relative frequency are shown in Table 37-10.[130-135] Nonfunctioning cortical adenomas are the most common lesions, accounting for between 36% and 94% of cases.[136] Hormonally active tumors including pheochromocytomas, cortisol-producing adenomas, and aldosteronomas are much less common. Primary adrenocortical carcinomas are usually apparent from their large size and other radiographic features, as are discussed later. Adrenal metastases are uncommon in patients without a history of malignancy but increase in frequency dramatically in the setting of a known diagnosis of cancer. Myelolipomas, adrenal cysts, and ganglioneuromas are other adrenal lesions that commonly present as incidental findings.

Functioning Tumors

Although most adrenal incidentalomas are nonfunctioning, hormonally active tumors such as pheochromocytomas, cortisol-producing adenomas, and aldosteronomas may occasionally present as asymptomatic, incidentally discovered lesions. Aldosteronoma is the least common functioning adrenal tumor to present as an incidentaloma and should be screened for only in patients who have hypertension or a history of hypokalemia. It is not necessary to test for hyperaldosteronism in patients who are normotensive and normokalemic. Pheochromocytomas have compromised 5% to 7% of incidental adrenal masses in major reported series.[127] The diagnosis of pheochromocytoma should always be excluded before any invasive procedure in a patient with an adrenal mass to avoid precipitating a hypertensive crisis. In one center, 10% of all benign, sporadic adrenal pheochromocytomas actually presented as adrenal incidentalomas.[137] Subclinical hypercortisolism (subclinical Cushing's syndrome) is the most common biochemical abnormality detected in patients with adrenal incidentalomas and has been reported in 5%

TABLE 37-10. Frequency of Various Tumors in Major Series of Adrenal Incidentalomas

Diagnosis	Herrera et al[130]	Kasperlik-Zaluska et al[131]	Barzon et al[132]	*Proye et al[133]	*Favia et al[134]	*Mantero et al[135]	Total
Nonfunctioning adenoma	330	122	121	50	25	138	786 (60%)
Pheochromocytoma	5	19	9	15	4	42	94 (7.2%)
Subclinical Cushing's	2	8	20	—	8	48	86 (6.6%)
Aldosteronoma	—	2	6	5	6	12	31 (2.4%)
Adrenocortical cancer	4	18	23	5	15	47	112 (8.6%)
Metastatic cancer	1	19	7	4	3	7	41 (3.1%)
Myelolipoma	—	10	2	4	1	30	47 (3.6%)
Other†	—	10	14	20	6	56	106 (8.1%)

*Surgical series of operated cases.
†Most commonly includes adrenal cysts and ganglioneuromas.

to 20% of cases.[61] These patients have evidence of autonomous cortisol secretion but lack overt signs and symptoms of Cushing's syndrome, as discussed in detail in the section on Cushing's syndrome.

Nonhypersecretory Tumors

NONFUNCTIONING CORTICAL ADENOMAS

Nonfunctioning adrenocortical adenomas account for the majority of incidentally discovered adrenal masses in patients with no prior history of cancer. Radiographically, these tumors appear as homogeneous lesions with smooth, encapsulated margins. The natural history of nonfunctioning masses has not been clearly shown, but there have been isolated reports of nonfunctioning lesions that later progressed to functional autonomy. In a study of 251 patients at the Mayo Clinic with nonfunctioning masses who were followed for a minimum of 1 year, however, none subsequently developed clinical or biochemical abnormalities.[130]

ADRENOCORTICAL CARCINOMA

Adrenocortical carcinomas are rare tumors that are large (>6 cm) and typically exhibit radiographic features suggestive of malignancy, such as irregular borders, regional lymphadenopathy, or local invasiveness. About half of these tumors are hormonally active. In the Mayo Clinic series,[130] only 4 nonfunctioning adrenocortical carcinomas were identified of 342 incidentalomas evaluated (incidence: 1.2%). Over 90% of reported adrenocortical carcinomas are more than 6 cm in diameter, and the likelihood that an incidentaloma represents a primary adrenal carcinoma increases with increasing size of the lesion. However, small adrenal cancers do occur. In one recent series of 117 patients with adrenal tumors, five adrenocortical cancers (13.5%) were smaller than 5.0 cm.[138] Imaging features were predictive of malignancy in four of these five cases.

ADRENAL METASTASES

The adrenal gland is a common site for metastases, which have been found in 1% to 30% of patients with an adrenal incidentaloma. Cancers that frequently metastasize to the adrenal include breast, lung, and renal cell carcinomas as well as melanoma and lymphoma. Adrenalectomy may be indicated in patients with solitary adrenal metastases who have no evidence of metastatic disease elsewhere. Fine-needle aspiration biopsy (FNA) under CT or ultrasound guidance may be used to confirm the diagnosis but should be done only if the results of biopsy will alter therapy. FNA should never be attempted until biochemical studies have excluded the possibility of a pheochromocytoma.

OTHER ADRENAL LESIONS

Myelolipomas are benign lesions composed of fat and bone marrow elements. They can become quite large and have a typical radiographic appearance with evidence of macroscopic fat and calcification (Fig. 37-23). Adrenalectomy is not indicated for myelolipomas unless they are

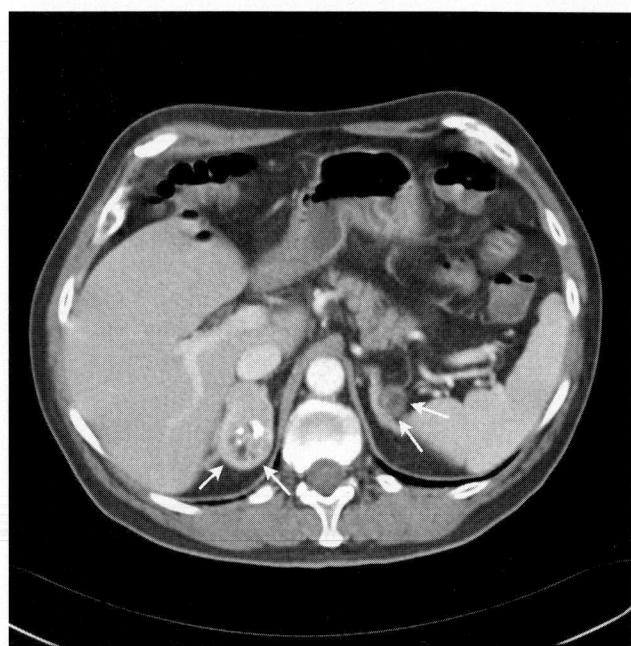

FIGURE 37-23.   CT scan of bilateral adrenal myelolipomas *(arrows).* The characteristic features of a myelolipoma shown here include both macroscopic fat (seen as hypodense areas within the myelolipomas) and calcification in the right-sided lesion.

large and symptomatic. Adrenal cysts are variable in size and also have a characteristic appearance on CT. Adrenal hemorrhage occurs more frequently on the right and is more common in the setting of trauma or anticoagulation.

Biochemical Evaluation

Biochemical screening for pheochromocytoma in the setting of an adrenal incidentaloma should consist of measurement of plasma fractionated metanephrines or a 24-hour urine collection for catecholamines and metanephrines. Screening for hypercortisolism consists of an overnight, single-dose (1 to 3 mg) dexamethasone test. Patients who fail to suppress 8 AM plasma cortisol to less than 3 mg/dL after dexamethasone administration should be suspected of having subclinical Cushing's syndrome and should undergo further testing with measurement of 24-hour urinary free cortisol and plasma ACTH. Screening for hyperaldosteronism should consist of measurement of PAC and PRA. A PAC:PRA of more than 20 in conjunction with a PAC greater than 15 ng/dL is suggestive of the diagnosis.[128] Confirmation should be obtained by measuring 24-hour urinary aldosterone levels.

Radiographic Evaluation

The CT characteristics of adrenal incidentalomas have also been used to help determine the risk of malignancy of these tumors. Cysts, myelolipomas, and adrenal hemorrhage each have specific CT features that are diagnostic and do not require further evaluation. Benign adenomas are usually homogeneous lesions with smooth, regular, encapsulated margins that do not increase in size over time (Fig. 37-24). Primary adrenal carcinomas, in contrast, are typically large tumors with irregular borders and features of inhomogeneity, such as hemorrhage, necrosis, and calcification. They may also have evidence of local invasion or associated lymphadenopathy. Most adenomas are low attenuation lesions (<10 Hounsfield units) on unenhanced CT, whereas carcinomas have much higher attenuation values (>18 Hounsfield units). However, some adenomas have also had attenuation values greater than 10 Hounsfield units.

MRI has been used to further characterize the nature of adrenal masses and to differentiate benign from malignant lesions. It has the advantage of avoiding exposure to ionizing radiation but is more expensive than CT. Adenomas usually exhibit low signal intensity on T2-weighted image sequences, whereas both pheochromocytomas and adrenal metastases have a brighter signal intensity on T2-weighted images. Another useful MRI sequence is that of in phase/opposed phase chemical shift imaging, which is a technique used to differentiate various adrenal neoplasms based on their lipid content.[139] Adrenal lesions with a high lipid content such as adenomas and myelolipomas typically show a loss of signal intensity on opposed phase chemical shift sequences (Fig. 37-25). In contrast, malignant lesions and pheochromocytomas fail to show any appreciable loss of signal intensity on opposed phase MRI.

Biopsy

FNA biopsy is rarely indicated for the evaluation of the patient with an adrenal mass. Because FNA cytology does not reliably differentiate an adenoma from a primary adrenal cancer, this technique should be reserved for the rare patient in whom tissue diagnosis of an adrenal metastasis is necessary to guide therapy. FNA of an adrenal mass is usually done under CT guidance and has associated risks, including bleeding, pneumothorax, pancreatitis, and seeding of the needle tract by tumor. It is imperative that a pheochromocytoma be excluded biochemically before any adrenal biopsy is carried out to avoid precipitating a hypertensive crisis.

Management

An evaluation and management algorithm for patients with adrenal incidentalomas is shown in Figure 37-26. The presence of a hormonally active tumor is an indication for adrenalectomy. In patients with nonfunctional adrenal masses, adrenalectomy should be performed if the tumor is more than 6 cm in diameter or if the imaging features on CT and/or MRI are atypical for an adenoma. Patients with nonfunctioning lesions less than 4 cm may be observed with interval CT or MRI at 3 to 4 months and again at 1 year. A repeat functional assessment should be carried out at 12 and 24 months.[128] Management of nonfunctional lesions between 4 and 6 cm is controversial. Most groups recommend adrenalectomy for lesions greater than 4 to 5 cm, although close follow-up is a reasonable option if the appearance is consistent with an

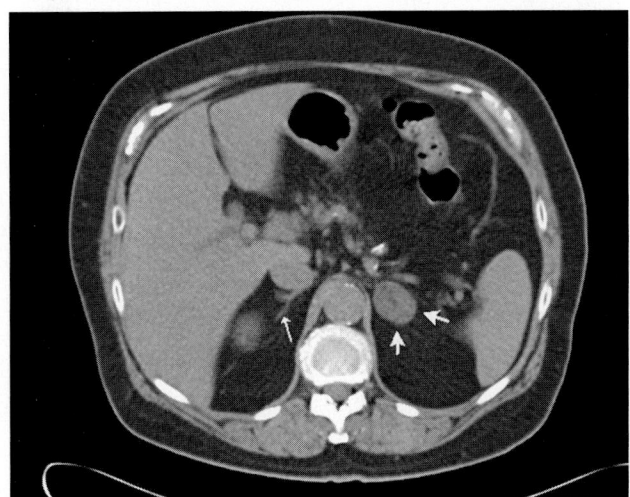

FIGURE 37-24. CT scan of an adrenal adenoma. The adenoma *(arrows)* is well circumscribed and low in attenuation compared with adjacent liver. A normal right adrenal is also seen *(small arrow).*

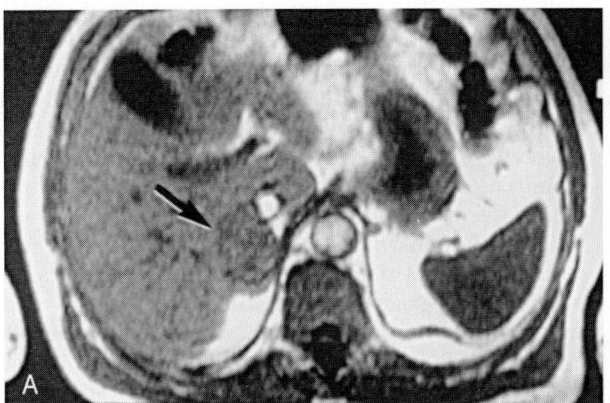 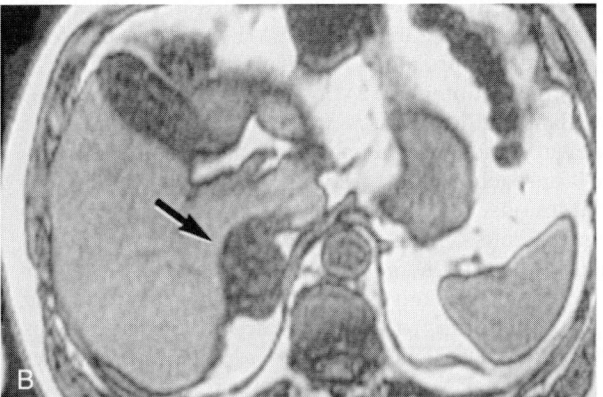

FIGURE 37-25. MR chemical shift imaging sequences of an adrenal adenoma. A right adrenal mass is present *(arrow).* **A,** The in-phase image shows the adrenal mass to be almost isointense compared with the liver. **B,** Opposed-phase imaging shows the adrenal mass to be markedly darker with loss of signal intensity compared with the liver, consistent with an adenoma. (Courtesy of Jeff Brown, M.D., Washington University School of Medicine, St. Louis, Missouri.)

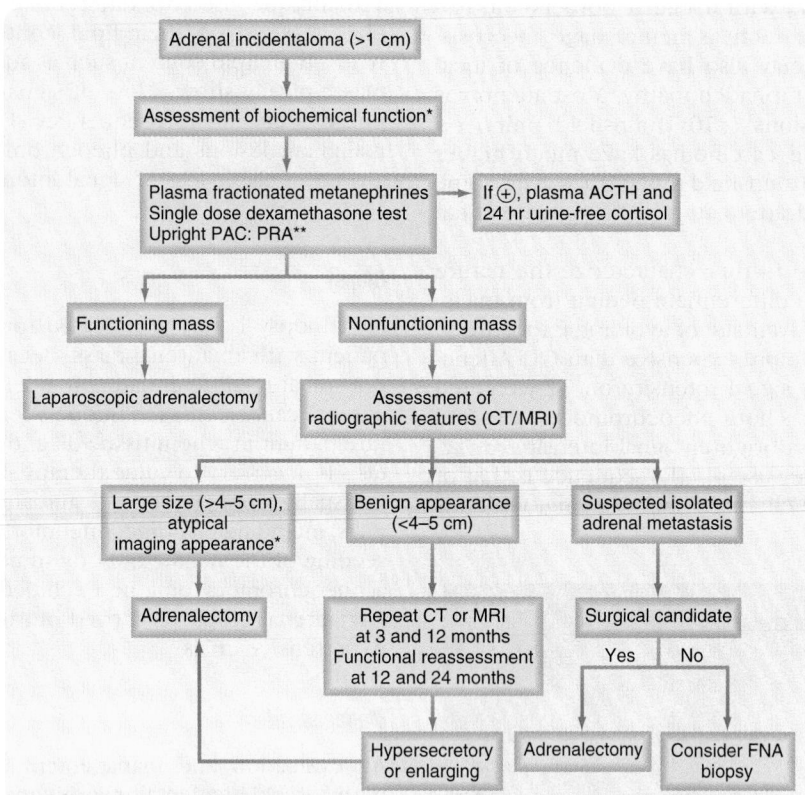

FIGURE 37-26. Evaluation and management algorithm for an incidental adrenal mass. The asterisks indicate details are in the text. Screening for hyperaldosteronism is done only if the patient is hypertensive or hypokalemic. PAC:PRA, plasma aldosterone concentration to plasma renin activity ratio; FNA, fine-needle aspiration.

adenoma. Adrenalectomy should be considered for intermediate-size lesions that enlarge during follow-up or that have imaging findings that are not typical for an adenoma.

Technique of Adrenalectomy

A number of different surgical approaches are available for the removal of the adrenal glands. Historically, the four open surgical approaches that have been used are (1) anterior transabdominal, (2) posterior retroperitoneal, (3) lateral flank, and (4) thoracoabdominal. Over the past decade, laparoscopic adrenalectomy has become the preferred approach in most centers for removal of benign adrenal lesions. The choice of approach in an individual patient depends on the suspected pathology, size of the adrenal lesion, and surgeon experience. Tumors smaller than 6 cm that are likely benign are usually resected using a laparoscopic approach.[140-142] Large adrenal masses (>10 cm) and suspected primary adrenal malignancies larger than 6 cm should generally be resected using an anterior approach to adequately explore the entire abdomen and to ensure resection with negative margins. Very large adrenocortical carcinomas, 10 to 15 cm or larger, that require en bloc resection of involved adjacent structures may necessitate a thoracoabdominal approach.

Open Adrenalectomy

ANTERIOR APPROACH

Open anterior adrenalectomy can be carried out via an upper midline, extended unilateral, or bilateral subcostal incision. This approach provides wide exposure and access to both adrenals and allows staging of adrenal malignancies. The open anterior approach is the preferred route for resection of large, potentially invasive adrenal tumors. In patients with extremely large (>10 to 15 cm) adrenocortical carcinomas, the bilateral subcostal incision can be extended in the upper midline to the xiphoid (Mercedes incision) to allow improved exposure and mobilization of the liver, thereby avoiding the morbidity of a thoracoabdominal approach.

For the open anterior approach, the flank is elevated 30 degrees on a pillow or beanbag. The table is flexed, opening the space between the costal margin and the anterior superior iliac spine. A bilateral subcostal or midline incision is made that allows access to both adrenals and facilitates exploration of the abdomen (Fig. 37-27). The abdomen is opened and explored for evidence of metastatic disease, including biopsy or excision of suspicious lesions. Resection of the right adrenal proceeds with mobilization and anteromedial retraction of the right hepatic lobe by dividing the right triangular ligament. Sub-

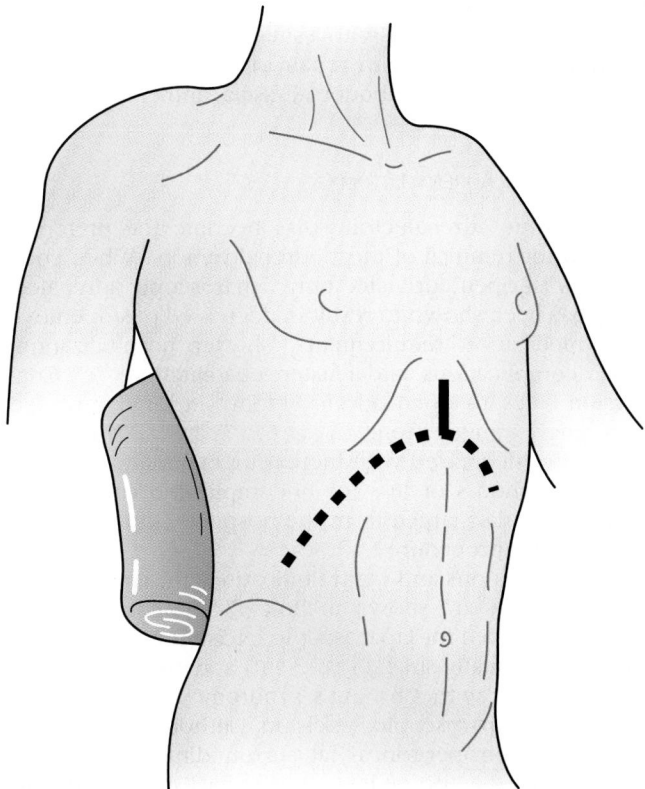

FIGURE 37-27. Patient position and incision for the open anterior approach to adrenalectomy. The patient's side is elevated somewhat to facilitate exposure. The incision may be extended in the midline up to the xiphoid *(solid line)* if necessary to improve exposure and access to larger tumors.

sequently, the hepatic flexure and transverse colon are mobilized and are retracted medially. A Kocher maneuver of the duodenum may be performed to expose the inferior vena cava, the right kidney, and the right adrenal. The retroperitoneal space is entered behind the liver to expose the adrenal. Dissection of the gland proceeds from its superomedial aspect, where small feeding arteries are individually clipped and divided. The vena cava is carefully dissected along its posterolateral border, which allows identification of the right adrenal vein where it drains directly into the inferior vena cava from the medial aspect of the gland. The adrenal vein is ligated with a 2-0 silk tie and divided close to the vena cava. For large pheochromocytomas that require open resection, the adrenal vein is isolated early during the operation to avoid catecholamine surges and blood pressure fluctuations during manipulation of the gland. Once the adrenal vein is ligated, arterial feeding vessels are clipped and divided sequentially, beginning at the superolateral aspect of the gland and continuing medially.

Resection of the left adrenal gland requires mobilization of the spleen and left colon. The left colon is freed from its peritoneal attachments and is reflected inferiorly. The spleen is then delivered from the left upper quadrant medially by dividing the splenorenal ligament. The spleen, stomach, and pancreatic tail are retracted medially en bloc to expose the left kidney and adrenal (Fig. 37-28). The left adrenal vein is isolated, ligated with 2-0 silk tie at its junction with the left renal vein, and divided. The gland is dissected and the arterial vessels are clipped and divided sequentially, beginning at the superolateral aspect of the gland and continuing medially.

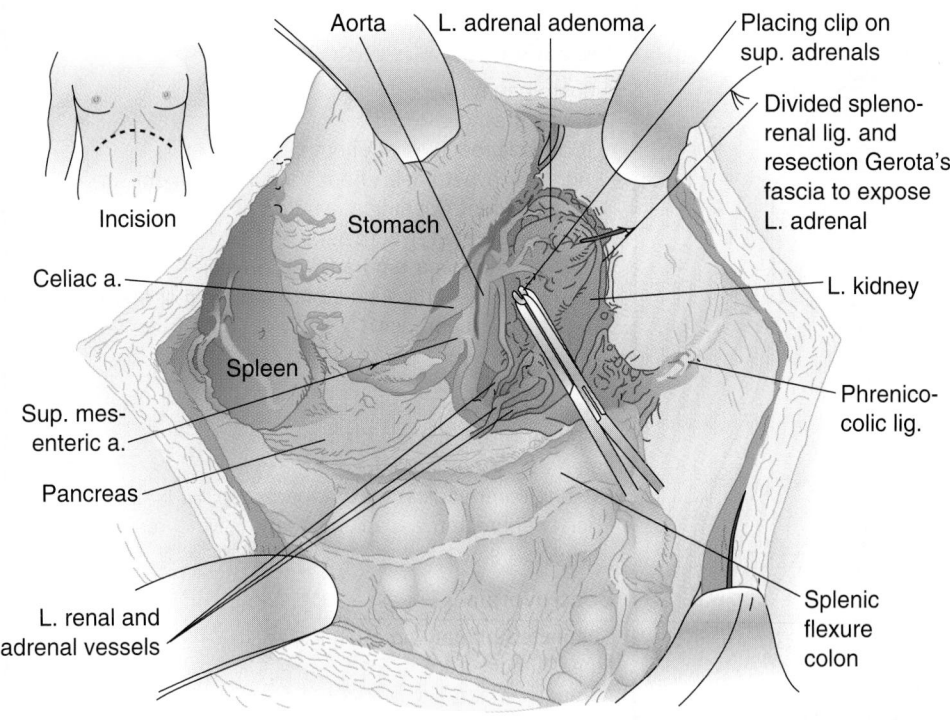

FIGURE 37-28.
Operative approach to the left adrenal gland through an open anterior incision. Exposure is provided by medial visceral rotation of the colon, spleen, and tail of the pancreas.

OPEN POSTERIOR APPROACH

Open posterior adrenalectomy is performed using a hockey stick-type incision in the back with resection of the 12th rib. In the past, this approach was used primarily for patients with small, unilateral tumors or those who had adrenal hyperplasia and required bilateral adrenalectomy. Today, the open posterior approach has been almost completely replaced by laparoscopic adrenalectomy. The only indication currently is the patient with a small (<5 cm) tumor who has contraindications to laparoscopy.

The patient is placed prone on the operating table, and a curvilinear skin incision is made from the midline at the 10th rib extending inferiorly and laterally to the superior border of the posterior iliac crest (Fig. 37-29). The latissimus dorsi muscle is divided, and the lumbodorsal fascia is incised longitudinally. The sacrospinalis muscle is retracted medially, and the 12th rib and vascular bundle are resected as far medially as possible. The 12th intercostal nerve is gently retracted superiorly. The retroperitoneum is entered to expose retroperitoneal fat and Gerota's fascia. The diaphragm is bluntly elevated from Gerota's fascia, the pleura is separated from the diaphragm, and the diaphragm is then divided. Gerota's fascia is incised, and the kidney is retracted inferiorly to expose the adrenal gland. Arterial vessels are clipped, and the adrenal vein, located deep to the arteries, is ligated as it is encountered. The gland is then freed circumferentially from its lateral to medial aspect. The inferior border of the gland is dissected last to maintain attachment to the kidney and inferior retraction of the gland. If the pleura is entered during the operation, it is closed after first evacuating the pleural space with a small suction catheter. The operation concludes with repair of the diaphragm, reapproximation of the lumbodorsal fascia, and closure of the skin.

LAPAROSCOPIC ADRENALECTOMY

Laparoscopic adrenalectomy has become the preferred method for removal of most adrenal tumors. When compared with open adrenalectomy, laparoscopic adrenalectomy has been shown to result in decreased postoperative pain medication requirements, shorter hospitalization, fewer complications, and a faster rehabilitation.[143-146] Conversion rates to open adrenalectomy in large reported series have ranged from 1% to 5%.[140-142,147,148] Operative times have decreased with increasing experience and are typically 2 hours or less for uncomplicated cases. Most patients are discharged from the hospital within 24 to 48 hours of the procedure.

The indications and contraindications for laparoscopic adrenalectomy are shown in Box 37-5. Aldosteronomas are ideally suited for laparoscopic excision because these tumors are usually small (1 to 2 cm) and are rarely malignant. Patients with Cushing's syndrome are also appropriate for laparoscopic excision, although the large amount of retroperitoneal fat surrounding the adrenals may make the procedure somewhat more difficult. Pheochromocytomas may also be more challenging to remove laparoscopically because of their larger size and

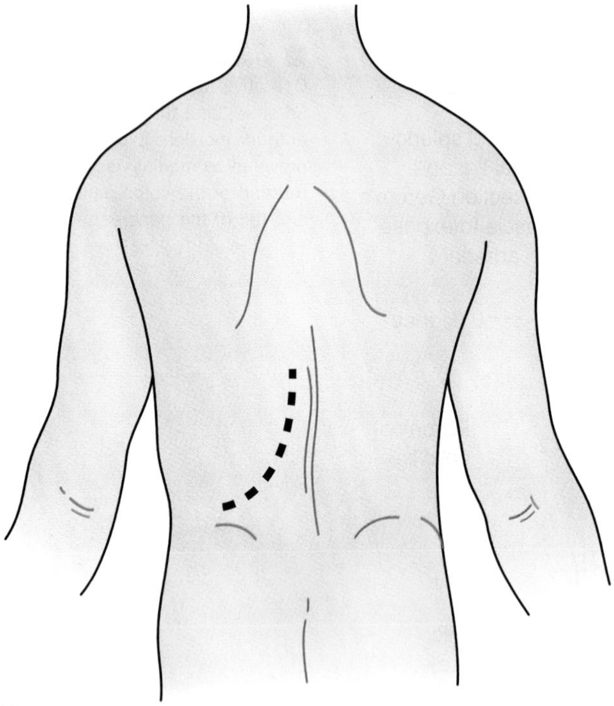

FIGURE 37-29.   Incision location for open posterior approach to adrenalectomy. The incision is extended inferiorly and laterally from the tenth rib to the posterior iliac crest.

Box 37-5 Indications and Contraindications for Laparoscopic Adrenalectomy

Indications

Aldosteronoma
Cushing's syndrome
  Cortisol-producing adenoma
    Adrenal hyperplasia from failed treatment of ACTH-dependent Cushing's syndrome
  Primary adrenal hyperplasia
Pheochromocytoma (sporadic or familial)
Nonfunctioning cortical adenoma (>4-5 cm or atypical radiographic appearance)

Contraindications

Any locally invasive adrenal tumor
Regional lymph node metastases
Large adrenocortical cancer
Existing contraindication to laparoscopic surgery
Prior nephrectomy, splenectomy, liver resection on affected side*

Controversial

Suspected primary adrenal malignancy
Large tumor size
Adrenal metastasis

* Relative contraindication

increased vascularity. Laparoscopic bilateral adrenalectomy has been carried out for patients with bilateral pheochromocytomas and in patients with ACTH-dependent Cushing's syndrome who have failed treatment of the primary lesion. The only absolute contraindications to laparoscopic adrenalectomy are local tumor invasiveness or the presence of regional lymph node metastases. Relative contraindications include tumor size larger than 10 to 12 cm or primary adrenal malignancy greater than 6 cm. The precise size limit for recommending laparoscopic adrenalectomy is controversial but depends on several factors, including the nature of the underlying adrenal lesion, favorable local conditions, and laparoscopic experience of the surgeon. Prior nephrectomy, splenectomy, or liver resection on the side of the adrenal lesion may also contraindicate a laparoscopic approach.

The two principal laparoscopic approaches to adrenalectomy are the transabdominal lateral flank approach and the retroperitoneal endoscopic approach. The transabdominal lateral approach is the most commonly used laparoscopic technique. In this approach, the patient is placed in a lateral decubitus position as shown in Figure 37-30. Stable patient positioning is facilitated by the use of a padded bean bag mattress. A roll is placed under the chest wall to protect the axilla, and the hips and legs should also be well padded to avoid nerve compression injuries. The arm is suspended, and the patient is secured to the operating table with tape and a safety strap. The operating table is then flexed to open up the space between the costal margin and the anterior superior iliac spine. The anterior and posterior axillary lines serve as useful landmarks for port placement and should be marked before draping the patient.

Initial access to the peritoneal cavity is usually obtained with a closed Veress needle technique; alternatively, direct open insertion of a blunt-tipped cannula can be employed. The first access site is usually in the subcostal region just medial to the anterior axillary line. The other ports are then inserted under direct laparoscopic visualization in a transverse line from the lateral edge of the rectus sheath to the posterior axillary line between the costal margin and iliac crest as shown in Figure 37-31. The ports should be spaced 5 cm or more apart to allow adequate freedom of movement of the instruments both internally and externally. A single 12-mm port is necessary for insertion of a clip applier and for specimen extraction. The other ports used for placement of the laparoscope and dissecting instruments can be 5 mm or smaller. Four ports are necessary for right adrenalectomy, whereas left adrenalectomy can be carried out with either three or four ports. Operating instruments needed for laparoscopic adrenalectomy include an angled (30- or 45-degree) laparoscope, atraumatic grasping forceps, dissecting forceps, hook electrocautery, endoscopic clip applier, ultrasonic coagulator (optional), and an irrigation/suction apparatus.

The principles of adrenal dissection are the same laparoscopically as for open adrenalectomy. The adrenal gland should be well exposed by mobilizing overlying structures and dividing the related ligamentous attachments as described next. The dissection must be extracapsular to the adrenal to prevent bleeding from the adrenal capsule and to avoid fragmentation and implantation of adrenal tissue or tumor. For the same reasons, the adrenal should be handled carefully at all times and should be manipulated by gently pushing or elevating it or grasping periadrenal fat and not the adrenal gland itself.

For laparoscopic right adrenalectomy, the initial step in the dissection is to divide the right triangular ligament of

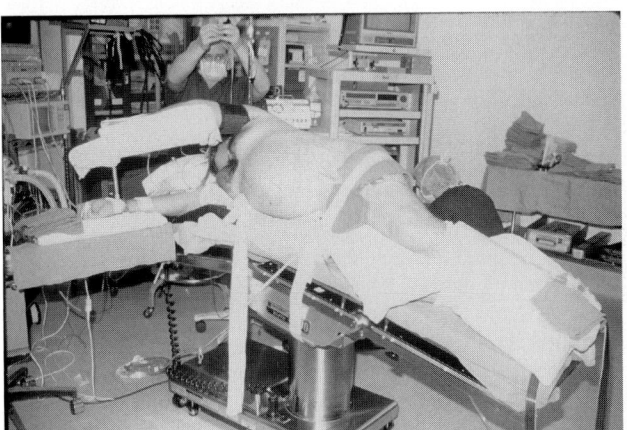

FIGURE 37-30. Patient position for the transabdominal lateral approach to laparoscopic (left) adrenalectomy. The patient is on a padded bean bag mattress and is secured to the operating table with tape and safety straps. The table is flexed at the waist and placed in a reverse Trendelenburg position. The chest wall and other pressure points are well padded to avoid nerve compression injuries.

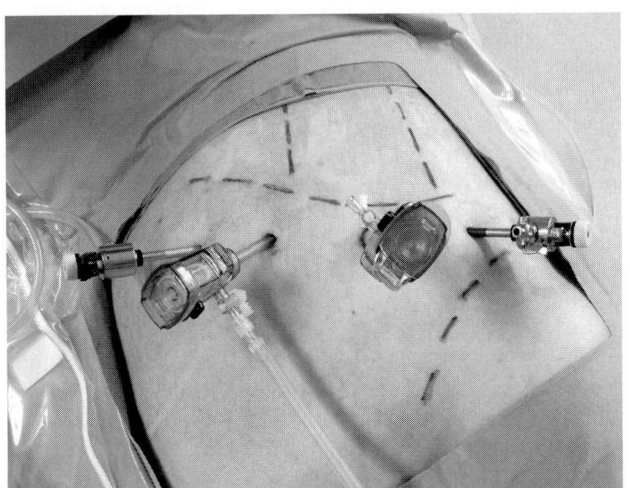

FIGURE 37-31. Port site placement for laparoscopic left adrenalectomy using the transabdominal lateral approach. The anterior and posterior axillary lines, costal margin, and iliac crest are identified by the *dashed lines*. The ports should be spaced at intervals of 5 cm or greater to allow external freedom of movement.

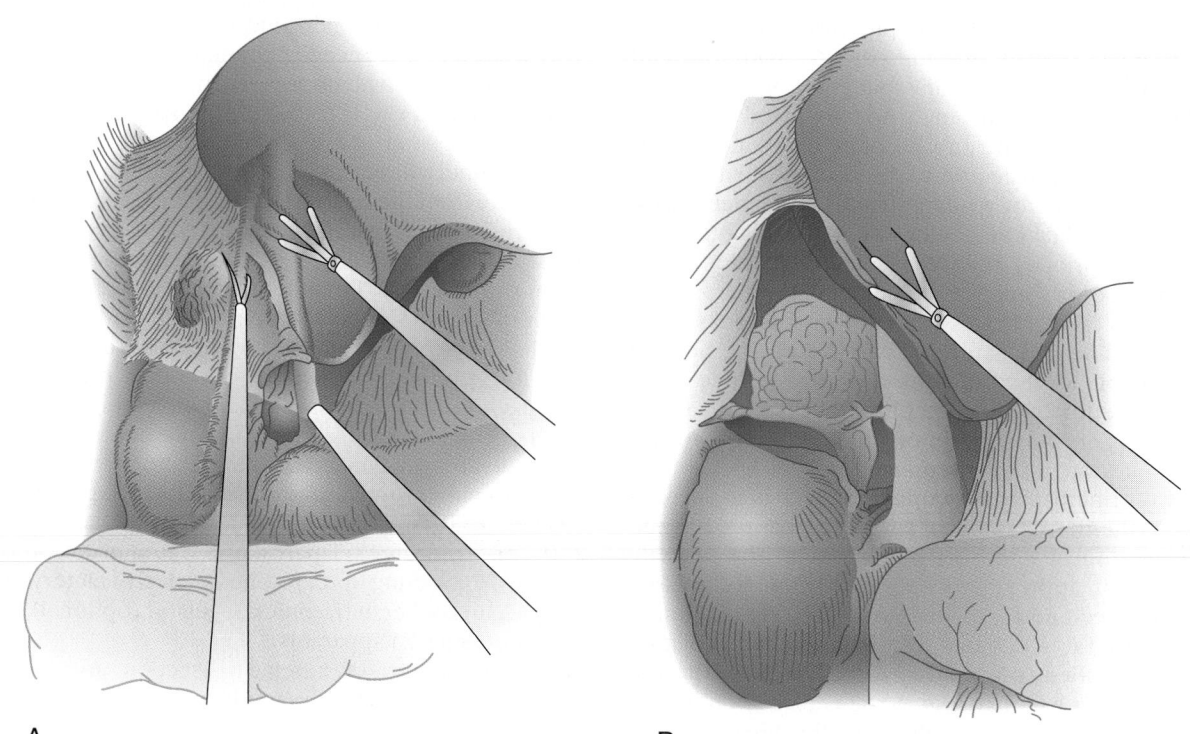

A   B

FIGURE 37-32.   Schematic representation of anatomic relationships as viewed during laparoscopic right adrenalectomy with the transabdominal lateral flank approach. **A,** The right triangular ligament of the liver is divided to allow full medial rotation of the right lobe of the liver. **B,** The medial border of the adrenal has been partially dissected free to expose the inferior vena cava and right adrenal vein. (Reprinted with permission from Brunt LM: Laparoscopic adrenalectomy. *In* Eubanks WS, Swanstrom LL, Soper NJ [eds]: Mastery of Endoscopic and Laparoscopic Surgery. Philadelphia, Lippincott Williams & Wilkins, 2000, p 325.)

the liver from its inferior margin to the diaphragm. This maneuver allows medial rotation of the right hepatic lobe and is the key to safe exposure of the adrenal and inferior vena cava (Fig. 37-32). A flexible or fan-shaped retractor inserted through the most medial port is used to retract the liver. It is not usually necessary to mobilize the hepatic flexure of the colon. The adrenal gland is identifiable posterolateral to the inferior vena cava and superior to the kidney. The connective tissue between the medial border of the adrenal and inferior vena cava is separated with a hook electrocautery (Fig. 37-33), and small vessels entering the adrenal medially are either cauterized or clipped and divided (see Fig. 37-32). The right adrenal vein is encountered early in the dissection and is carefully isolated, doubly clipped, and divided. A second smaller right adrenal vein may sometimes be present superior to the main vein. After division of the adrenal vein, the superior and inferior pole attachments and vessels are divided. Larger arterial branches may either be clipped or divided with an ultrasonic coagulator. The adrenal is then dissected off the superior pole of the kidney and the posterior diaphragm. The specimen is then placed in an endoscopic retrieval bag and is extracted at the 12-mm port site after enlarging the incision somewhat. The adrenal bed is checked for hemostasis, and the retractor, instruments, and videoscope are withdrawn. The operation concludes with closure of the fascia at the 12-mm port site and the skin incisions.

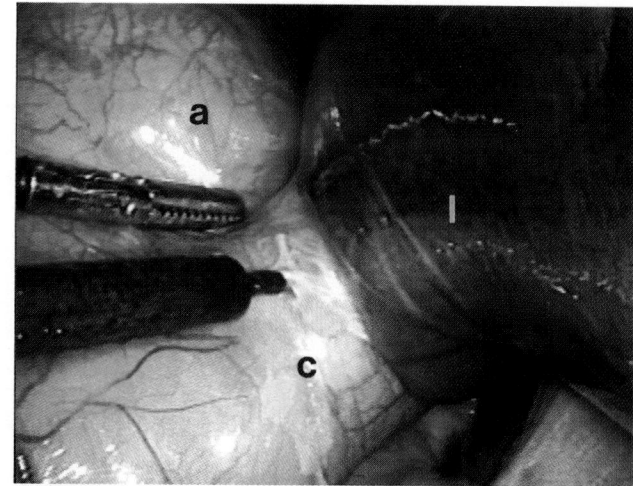

FIGURE 37-33.   View of the right adrenal gland as exposed laparoscopically. The adrenal tumor (a), inferior vena cava (c), and liver (l) are visible. Dissection of the connective tissue plane between the inferior vena cava and adrenal is facilitated with a hook electrocautery.

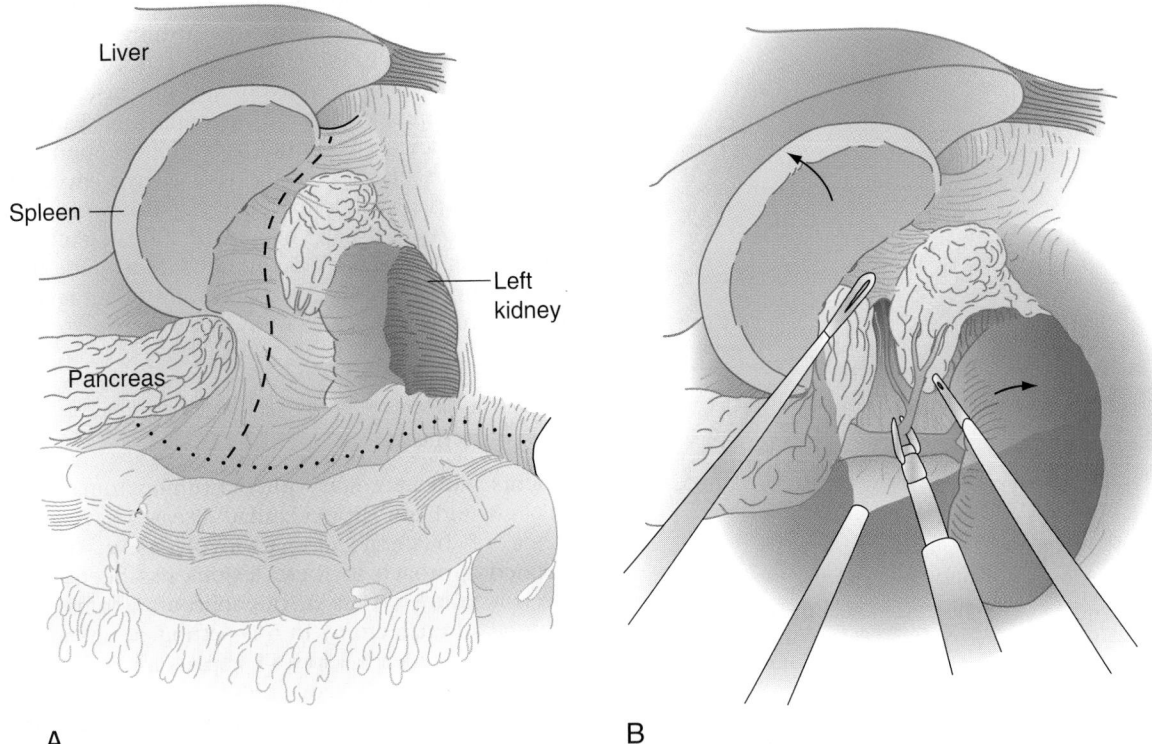

Liver

Spleen

Pancreas

Left kidney

A

B

FIGURE 37-34. Schematic illustration of sequential steps in laparoscopic exposure of the left adrenal gland (lateral flank approach). **A,** The splenocolic ligament is divided first *(dotted line),* followed by complete division of the splenorenal ligament *(dashed line).* **B,** The spleen is rotated medially, and the kidney is retracted laterally. The vein is ligated at the inferomedial border of the adrenal with endoscopic clips. (Reprinted with permission from Brunt LM: Laparoscopic adrenalectomy. *In* Eubanks WS, Swanstrom LL, Soper NJ [eds]: Mastery of Endoscopic and Laparoscopic Surgery. Philadelphia, Lippincott Williams & Wilkins, 2000, pp 326, 327.)

Left adrenalectomy is performed with opposite patient position and port placement. The steps in exposure of the left adrenal are shown in Figure 37-34. The splenic flexure of the colon is first mobilized by dividing the splenocolic ligament. A fourth port may then be safely placed in the posterior axillary line. The splenorenal ligament is next divided from the inferior border of the spleen to the diaphragm to allow the spleen to roll medially. It is important not to mobilize the kidney posteriorly because this will result in the kidney and adrenal falling medially and the dissection of the adrenal gland will be more difficult. The plane between the kidney and tail of the pancreas is then developed, and the pancreas is retracted medially. The adrenal gland is usually visible at this stage in the procedure. Intraoperative ultrasound may be used to find the adrenal in cases in which it is difficult to locate, such as in obese patients or those with Cushing's syndrome. The medial, lateral, and inferior borders of the adrenal are defined by dissection with the cautery or ultrasonic scalpel. The inferior pole of the adrenal should be carefully dissected away from the renal vein to expose the left adrenal vein, which courses somewhat obliquely at the inferomedial border of the adrenal (Fig. 37-35). The inferior phrenic vein frequently joins the adrenal vein just above where the latter empties into the renal vein. The left adrenal is also more closely applied to the kidney than on the right side. Otherwise, the rest

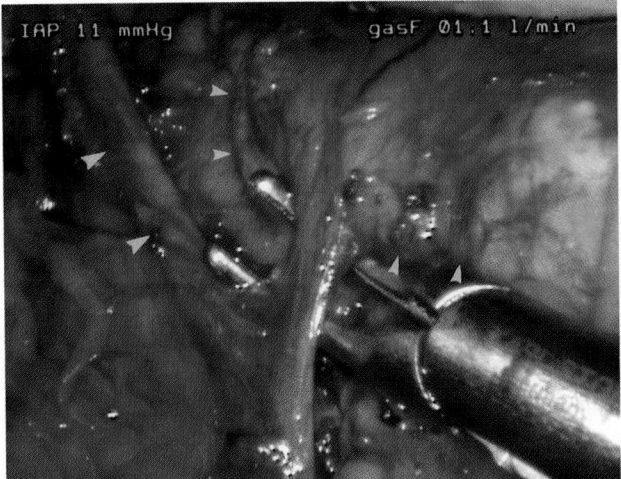

IAP 11 mmHg   gasF 01.1 l/min

FIGURE 37-35. Laparoscopic exposure and ligation of the left adrenal vein. A right angle dissector is elevating the left adrenal vein. The adrenal gland is indicated by the *small arrowheads.* Note the inferior phrenic vein *(larger arrowheads)* entering the left adrenal vein proximal to the latter's entry into the renal vein.

serum potassium value is checked in the first week after adrenalectomy. Patients with Cushing's syndrome or those who undergo bilateral adrenalectomy are given stress steroids perioperatively and are discharged home on a maintenance dose of prednisone. Patients with pheochromocytomas should have glucose monitoring the first 24 hours because of the risk of hypoglycemia from rebound hyperinsulinemia. After laparoscopic adrenalectomy, liquids are usually begun the morning after surgery and the diet is advanced as tolerated. Most patients are discharged home within 24 to 48 hours of surgery without restrictions in physical activity.

Partial Adrenalectomy for Patients With Inherited Pheochromocytomas

Patients with hereditary pheochromocytomas (MEN 2A, MEN 2B, and von Hippel-Lindau disease) have a high incidence of bilateral adrenal involvement. The recommended approach to these lesions has been to perform adrenalectomy when a pheochromocytoma develops. Bilateral adrenalectomy in this setting results in the need for life-long adrenal steroid replacement and the risk of addisonian crisis. For this reason, partial adrenalectomy removing only the tumor-containing portion of the gland has been recommended as an alternative to total adrenalectomy in highly selected patients with hereditary pheochromocytomas.[149-151] This approach may prevent some patients from requiring life-long adrenal corticosteroid replacement and may reduce the threat of lethal addisonian crisis. Partial adrenalectomy has been performed using both open and laparoscopic approaches. Long-term follow-up is not available, and, in the event of recurrence, a difficult open procedure needs to be performed. Partial adrenalectomy for other tumors such as aldosteronomas has been performed but is controversial.[152]

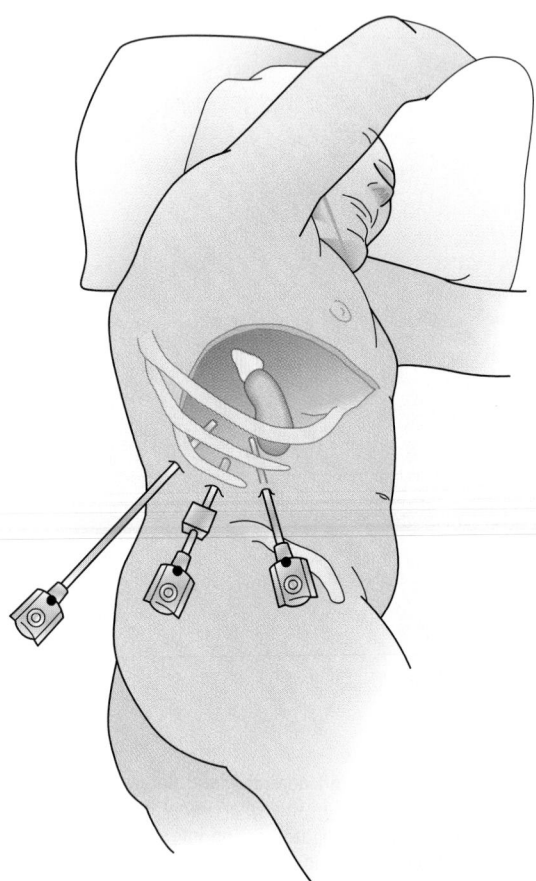

■ FIGURE 37-36. Port site location for the lateral retroperitoneal approach to laparoscopic adrenalectomy. (Reprinted with permission from Brunt LM: Laparoscopic adrenalectomy. *In* MacFadyen BM [ed]: Laparoscopic Surgery of the Abdomen. New York, Springer, 2004, p226.)

of the procedure is similar to laparoscopic right adrenalectomy.

Laparoscopic adrenalectomy can also be performed using a totally retroperitoneal approach. Retroperitoneal endoscopic adrenalectomy may be carried out with the patient in either a semi-jackknife or lateral position (Fig. 37-36). The advantages of the retroperitoneal approach are that the peritoneal cavity does not need to be entered, which may be especially important in the patient with extensive prior upper abdominal surgery; also, the patient may not need to be repositioned for bilateral adrenalectomy. However, this approach is generally more difficult and has a smaller working space, and the orientation can be difficult.

Postoperative Management

Postoperatively, the patient should have close monitoring of vital signs and urine output. A complete blood cell count is obtained on the first postoperative day and electrolytes are monitored as clinically indicated. Patients with hyperaldosteronism are taken off spironolactone, and a

Selected References

Pituitary

Arafah BM, Nasrallah MP: Pituitary tumors: Pathophysiology, clinical manifestation and management. Endocr Relat Cancer 8:287-305, 2001.

> **This review article contains an in-depth summary of the clinical presentation, diagnostic evaluation, and management options for patients with pituitary tumors.**

Lamberts SW, de Herder WW, van der Lely AJ: Pituitary insufficiency. Lancet 352:127-134, 1998.

> **Up-to-date review of the diagnosis and management of hypopituitarism.**

Molitch ME (ed): Advances in the management of pituitary tumors. Endocrinol Metab Clin North Am 28(1), 1999.

> **This monograph contains 11 chapters that cover the current approach to diagnosis and management of pituitary disorders. Each chapter is written by an expert in the field.**

Wilson CB: Extensive personal experience: Surgical management of pituitary tumors. J Clin Endocrinol Metab 82:2381-2385, 1997.

Dr. Wilson has performed over 3000 transsphenoidal procedures over 27 years and shares his experience and approach.

Adrenal

Brunt LM, Moley JF. Adrenal incidentaloma. World J Surg 25:905-913, 2001.

Detailed review of the diagnostic evaluation and management approach to patients with adrenal incidentalomas.

Dackiw AP, Lee JE, et al: Adrenal cortical carcinoma. World J Surg 25:914-926, 2001.

Comprehensive review of the current management of adrenal cortical carcinoma.

Findling JW, Raff H: Diagnosis and differential diagnosis of Cushing's syndrome. Endocrinol Metab Clin North Am 30:729-747, 2001.

This comprehensive review of the diagnostic approach to Cushing's syndrome includes a discussion of some newer diagnostic studies.

Moley JF, Lairmore TC, et al: Hereditary endocrinopathies. Curr Probl Surg 36:653-762, 1999.

Overview of current understanding of familial tumor syndromes.

Pacek K, Linehan WM, Eisenhofer G, et al: Recent advances in genetics, diagnosis, localization, and treatment of pheochromocytoma. Ann Intern Med 134:315-329, 2001.

Up-to-date review of molecular genetics and diagnostic evaluation of pheochromocytoma.

Stewart P: Mineralocorticoid hypertension. Lancet 353:1341-1347, 1999.

Thorough review of the diagnostic approach to hyperaldosteronism.

Young WF: Pheochromocytomas and primary aldosteronism: Diagnostic approaches. Endocrinol Metab Clin North Am 26:801-827, 1997.

Comprehensive discussion by an expert.

References

1. Asa SL, Ezzat S: The cytogenesis and pathogenesis of pituitary adenomas. Endocr Rev 19:798-827, 1998.
2. Herman V, Fagin J, Gonsky R, et al: Clonal origin of pituitary adenomas. J Clin Endocrinol Metab 71:1427-1433, 1990.
3. Faglia G, Spada A: Genesis of pituitary adenomas: State of the art. J Neurooncol 54:95-110, 2001.
4. Landis C, Masters SB, Spada A, et al: GTPase inhibiting mutations activate the alpha chains of Gs and stimulate adenylate cyclase in human pituitary tumours. Nature 340:692-696, 1989.
5. Naidich MJ, Russell EJ: Current approaches to imaging of the sellar region and pituitary. Endocrinol Metab Clin North Am 28:45-79, 1999.
6. Maroldo TV, Dillon WP, Wilson CB: Advances in diagnostic techniques of pituitary tumors and prolactinomas. Curr Opin Oncol 4:105-115, 1992.
7. Liu JK, Weiss MH, Couldwell WT: Surgical approaches to pituitary tumors. Neurosurg Clin North Am 14:93-107, 2003.
8. Laws ER Jr, Thapar K: Pituitary surgery. Endocrinol Metab Clin North Am 28:119-131, 1999.
9. Wilson CB: Extensive personal experience: Surgical management of pituitary tumors. J Clin Endocrinol Metab 82:2381-2385, 1997.
10. Shimon I, Melmed S: Management of pituitary tumors. Ann Intern Med 129:472-483, 1998.
11. Arafah BM, Nasrallah MP: Pituitary tumors: Pathophysiology, clinical manifestations and management. Endocr Relat Cancer 8:287-305, 2001.
12. Jackson IM, Noren G: Role of gamma knife therapy in the management of pituitary tumors. Endocrinol Metab Clin North Am 28:133-142, 1999.
13. Thoren M, Hoybye C, Grenback E, et al: The role of gamma knife radiosurgery in the management of pituitary adenomas. J Neurooncol 54:197-203, 2001.
14. Simard MF: Pituitary tumor endocrinopathies and their endocrine evaluation. Neurosurg Clin North Am 14:41-54, 2003.
15. Molitch ME: Disorders of prolactin secretion. Endocrinol Metab Clin North Am 30:585-609, 2001.
16. Molitch ME, Thorner MO, Wilson CB: Management of prolactinomas: Overview and introduction. J Clin Endocrinol Metab 82:996-1000, 1997.
17. Arafah BM, Brodkey JS, Pearson OH: Gradual recovery of lactroph responsiveness to dynamic stimulation following surgical removal of prolactinomas: Long-term follow-up studies. Metabolism 35:905-912, 1986.
18. Turner HE, Adams CB, Wass J: Transsphenoidal surgery for microprolactinoma: An acceptable alternative to dopamine agonists? Eur J Endocrinol 140:43-47, 1999.
19. Losa M, Mortini P, Barzaghi R, et al: Surgical treatment of prolactin-secreting pituitary adenomas: Early results and long-term outcome. J Clin Endocrinol Metab 87:3180-3186, 2002.
20. Feigenbaum SL, Downey DE, Wilson CB, et al: Extensive personal experience: Transsphenoidal pituitary resection for preoperative diagnosis of prolactin-secreting pituitary adenoma in women: Long-term follow-up. J Clin Endocrinol Metab 81:1711-1719, 1995.
21. Molitch ME: Pregnancy and the hyperprolactinemic woman. N Engl J Med 312:1364-1370, 1985.
22. Melmed S: Acromegaly. N Engl J Med 322:966-977, 1990.
23. Giustina A, Barkan AL, Casanueva F, et al: Criteria for cure of acromegaly: A consensus statement. J Clin Endocrinol Metab 85:526-529, 2000.
24. Ben-Shlomo A, Melmed S: Acromegaly. Endocrinol Metab Clin North Am 30:565-583, 2001.
25. Barkan AL, Lloyd RV, Chandler WF, et al: Preoperative treatment of acromegaly with long-acting somatostatin analog SMS 201-995: Shrinkage of invasive pituitary macroadenomas and improved surgical remission rate. J Clin Endocrinol Metab 67:1040-1048, 1988.
26. Melmed S, Casanueva FF, Cavagnini F, et al: Guidelines for acromegaly management. J Clin Endocrinol Metab 87:4054-4058, 2002.
27. Trainer PJ, Drake WM, Katznelson L, et al: Treatment of acromegaly with the growth hormone receptor antagonist pegvisomant. N Engl J Med 342:1171-1177, 2000.

28. Findling JW, Doppman JL: Biochemical and radiologic diagnosis of Cushing's syndrome. Endocrinol Metab Clin North Am 23:511-537, 1994.

29. Tyrrell JB, Wilson CB: Cushing's disease: Therapy of pituitary adenomas. Endocrinol Metab Clin North Am 23:925-938, 1994.

30. Tsigos C, Chrousos GP: Differential diagnosis and management of Cushing's syndrome. Annu Rev Med 47:443-461, 1996.

31. Findling JW, Raff H: Diagnosis and differential diagnosis of Cushing's syndrome. Endocrinol Metab Clin North Am 30:729-747, 2001.

32. Invitti C, Giraldi FP, Cavagnini F: Inferior petrosal sinus sampling in patients with Cushing's syndrome and contradicting response to dynamic testing. Clin Endocrinol 51:255-257, 1999.

33. Vincenti A, Estrada A, de la Cuerda C, et al: Results of external pituitary irradiation after unsuccessful transsphenoidal surgery in Cushing's disease. Acta Endocrinol 125:470, 1991.

34. Ludecke DK, Flitsch J, Knappe UJ, et al: Cushing's disease: A surgical view. J Neurooncol 54:151-166, 2001.

35. Jenkins PJ, Trainer PJ, Plowman PN, et al: The long-term outcome after adrenalectomy and prophylactic pituitary radiotherapy in adrenocorticotropin-dependent Cushing's syndrome. J Clin Endocrinol Metab 80:165-171, 1995.

36. Freda PU, Wardlaw SL: Clinical review 110: Diagnosis and treatment of pituitary tumors. J Clin Endocrinol Metab 84:3859-3866, 1999.

37. Daneshdoost L, Gennarelli TA, Bashey HM, et al: Recognition of gonadotroph adenomas in women. N Engl J Med 324:589-594, 1991.

38. Beck-Peccoz P, Bruckner-Davis F, Persani L, et al: Thyrotropin-secreting pituitary tumors. Endocr Rev 17:610-638, 1996.

39. Bruckner-Davis F, Oldfield EH, Skarulis MC, et al: Thyrotropin-secreting pituitary tumors: Diagnostic criteria, thyroid hormone sensitivity, and treatment outcome in 25 patients followed at the National Institutes of Health. J Clin Endocrinol Metab 84:476-486, 1999.

40. Caron P, Arlot S, Chanson P, et al: Efficacy of the long-acting octreotide formulation (octreotide-Lar) in patients with thyrotropin-secreting pituitary adenomas. J Clin Endocrinol Metab 86:2849-2853, 2001.

41. King JJ, Justice AC, Aaron D: Management of incidental pituitary microadenomas: A cost-effective analysis. J Clin Endocrinol Metab 82:3625, 1997.

42. Nishizawa S, Ohta S, Yokoyama T, et al: Therapeutic strategy for incidentally found pituitary tumors. Neurosurgery 43:1344-1348, 1998.

43. Arafah BM, Prunty D, Ybarra J, et al: The dominant role of increased intrasellar pressure in the pathogenesis of hypopituitarism, hyperprolactinemia, and headaches in patients with pituitary adenomas. J Clin Endocrinol Metab 85:1789-1793, 2000.

44. Vance ML, Mauras N: Growth hormone therapy in adults and children. N Engl J Med 341:1206-1216, 1999.

45. Vance ML: Hypopituitarism. N Engl J Med 330:1651-1652, 1994.

46. Arafah BM, Ybarra J, Tarr RW, et al: Pituitary tumor apoplexy: Pathophysiology, clinical manifestations, and management. J Intens Care Med 12:123-134, 1997.

47. Walters W, Wilder RM, Kepler EJ: The suprarenal cortical syndrome with presentation of ten cases. Ann Surg 100:670, 1934.

48. Conn JW: Presidential Address: 1) Painting background. 2) Primary aldosteronism. J Lab Clin Med 45:661-664, 1955.

49. McPartland RP: Metabolic and Pharmacologic Actions of Glucocorticoids. Amsterdam, Elsevier, 1986.

50. Quinn SJ: Regulation of aldosterone secretion. Annu Rev Physiol 50:409-426, 1988.

51. Cushing H: The basophil adenomas of the pituitary body and their clinical manifestations (pituitary basophilism). Bull Johns Hopkins Hosp 50:137, 1932.

52. Meier CA, Biller BMK: Clinical and biochemical evaluation of Cushing's syndrome. Endocrinol Metab Clin North Am 26:741-762, 1997.

53. Orth DN: Cushing's syndrome. N Engl J Med 332:701-803, 1995.

54. Wood PJ, Barth JH, Freedman DB, et al: Evidence for the low dose dexamethasone test to screen for Cushing's syndrome—recommendations for a protocol for biochemistry laboratories. Ann Clin Biochem 34:222-229, 1997.

55. Raff H, Raff JL, Findling JW: Late-night salivary cortisol as a screening test for Cushing's syndrome. J Clin Endocrinol Metab 83:2681-2686, 1998.

56. Flack MR, Oldfield EH, Cutler GB Jr, et al: Urine free cortisol in the high dose dexamethasone suppression test for the differential diagnosis of Cushing's syndrome. Ann Intern Med 116:211-217, 1992.

57. Avgerinos PC, Yanovski JA, Oldfield EH, et al: The metyrapone and dexamethasone suppression tests for the differential diagnosis of the adrenocorticotrophic-dependent Cushing's syndrome: A comparison. Ann Intern Med 121:318-327, 1994.

58. Nieman LK, Oldfield EH, Wesley R, et al: A simplified morning ovine corticotropin-releasing hormone stimulation test for the differential diagnosis of adrenocorticotropin-dependent Cushing's syndrome. J Clin Endocrinol Metab 77:1308-1312, 1993.

59. Samuels MH, Loriaux DL: Cushing's syndrome and the nodular adrenal gland. Endocrinol Metab Clin North Am 23:555-568, 1994.

60. Lacroix A, Bolte E, Tremblay J, et al: Gastric inhibitory polypeptide-dependent cortisol hypersecretion—a new cause of Cushing's syndrome. N Engl J Med 327:974-980, 1992.

61. Reincke M: Subclinical Cushing's syndrome. Endocrinol Metab Clin North Am 29:43-56, 2000.

62. Reincke M, Nieke J, Krestin GP, et al: Preclinical Cushing's syndrome in adrenal "incidentalomas": Comparison with adrenal Cushing's syndrome. J Clin Endocrinol Metab 75:826, 1992.

63. Barzon L, Fallo F, Soninoo N, et al: Development of overt Cushing's syndrome in patients with adrenal incidentaloma. Eur J Endocrinol 146:61-66, 2002.

64. Magiakou MA, Chrousos GP: Cushing's syndrome in children and adolescents: Current diagnostic and therapeutic strategies. J Endocrinol Invest 25:181-194, 2002.

65. Magiakou MA, Mastorakos G, Oldfield EH, et al: Cushing's syndrome in children and adolescents: Presentation, diagnosis, therapy. N Engl J Med 331:629-636, 1994.

66. Gordon RD, Stowasser M, Klevin S, et al: High incidence of primary aldosteronism in 199 patients referred with hypertension. Clin Exp Pharmacol Physiol 21:315-318, 1994.

67. Irony I, Kater CE, Biglieri EG: Correctable subsets of primary aldosteronism: Primary adrenal hyperplasia and renin-responsive adenoma. Am J Hypertens 3:576-582, 1990.

68. Bravo EL: Primary aldosteronism: Issues in diagnosis and management. Endocrinol Metab Clin North Am 23:271-283, 1994.

69. Lifton RP, Kluhy RG, Powers M: A chimeric 11-beta-hydroxylase/aldosterone synthase gene causes glucocorticoid-remediable aldosteronism and human hypertension. Nature 355:262-265, 1992.

70. Young WF, Hogan MJ, Klee GG: Primary aldosteronism: Diagnosis and management. Mayo Clin Proc 65:96-110, 1990.

71. Ganguly A: Primary aldosteronism. N Eng J Med 339:1828-1834, 1998.

72. Young WF Jr: Primary aldosteronism: A common and curable form of hypertension. Cardiol Rev 7:207-214, 1999.

73. Blumenfeld JD, Sealey JE, Schlussel Y, et al: Diagnosis and treatment of primary hyperaldosteronism. [Comment]. Ann Intern Med 121:877-885, 1994.

74. Dunnick NR, Leight GS, Roubidoux MA: CT in the diagnosis of primary aldosteronism: Sensitivity in 29 patients. Am J Radiol 160:321-324, 1993.

75. Young WF Jr, Stanson AW, Grant CS: Primary aldosteronism: Adrenal venous sampling. Surgery 120:913-919, 1996.

76. Gordon RD, Stowasser M, Rutherford JC: Primary aldosteronism: Are we diagnosing and operating on too few patients? World J Surg 25:941-947, 2001.

77. Sywak M, Pasieka JL: Long-term follow-up and cost benefit of adrenalectomy in patients with primary hyperaldosteronism. Br J Surg 89:1587-1593, 2002.

78. Sawka AM, Young WF, Thompson GB, et al: Primary aldosteronism: Factors associated with normalization of blood pressure after surgery. Ann Intern Med 135:258-261, 2001.

79. Obara T, Ito Y, Okamoto T: Risk factors associated with postoperative persistent hypertension in patients with primary aldosteronism. Surgery 112:987-993, 1992.

80. Litchfield WR, Anderson BF, Weiss RJ, et al: Intracranial aneurysm and hemorrhagic stroke in glucocorticoid-remediable aldosteronism. Hypertension 31:445-450, 1998.

81. White PC, New MI, Dupont BO: Congenital adrenal hyperplasia. N Engl J Med 316:1519-1524, 1987.

82. Pommier RF, Brennan MF: Management of adrenal neoplasms. Curr Probl Surg 28:659-739, 1991.

83. Zografos GC, Driscoll DL, Karakousis CP: Adrenal adenocarcinoma: A review of 53 cases. J Surg Oncol 55:160-164, 1994.

84. Norton JA, Levin B, Jensen RT: Cancer of the Endocrine System: The Adrenal Gland. Philadelphia, JB Lippincott, 1993.

85. Luton J-P, Cerdas S, Billaud L: Clinical features of adrenocortical carcinoma, prognostic factors, and the effect of mitotane therapy. N Engl J Med 322:1195-1201, 1990.

86. Henley DJ, van Heerden JA, Grant CS, et al: Adrenal cortical carcinoma—a continuing challenge. Surgery 94:926-931, 1983.

87. Bodie B, Novick AC, Pontes JE: The Cleveland Clinic experience with adrenal cortical carcinoma. J Urol 141:257-260, 1989.

88. Schulick RD, Brennan MF: Long-term survival after complete resection and repeat resection in patients with adrenocortical carcinoma. Ann Surg Oncol 6:719-726, 1999.

89. Icard P, Goudet P, Charpenay C, et al: Adrenocortical carcinomas: Surgical trends and results of a 253-patient series from the French Association of Endocrine Surgeons study group. World J Surg 25:891-897, 2001.

90. Jensen JC, Pass HI, Sindelar WF: Recurrent or metastatic disease in select patients with adrenocortical carcinoma: Aggressive resection vs chemotherapy. Arch Surg 126:457-461, 1991.

91. Abraham J, Bakke S, Rutt A, et al: A phase II trial of combination chemotherapy and surgical resection for the treatment of metastatic adrenocortical carcinoma: Continuous infusion doxorubicin, vincristine, and etoposide with daily mitotane as a P-glycoprotein antagonist. Cancer 94:2333-2343, 2002.

92. Addison T: On the Constitutional Effects of Disease of the Suprarenal Capsules. London, Highly, 1885.

93. Werbel SS, Ober KP: Acute adrenal insufficiency. Endocrinol Metab Clin North Am 22:303-328, 1993.

94. Kung AW, Pun KK, Lam K: Addisonian crisis as presenting feature in malignancies. Cancer 65:177-179, 1990.

95. Saegesser F: Cesar Roux (1857-1934) et son epogue. Rev Med Suisse Romande 104:403, 1984.

96. Mayo CH: Paroxysmal hypertension with tumor of retroperitoneal nerve. JAMA 89:1047, 1927.

97. Cryer PE: Pheochromocytoma. Clin Endocrinol Metab 14:203-220, 1985.

98. Bravo EL, Gifford RW Jr: Pheochromocytoma. Endocrinol Metab Clin North Am 22:329-341, 1993.

99. Lenders JW, Keiser HR, Goldstein DS, et al: Plasma metanephrines in the diagnosis of pheochromocytoma. Ann Intern Med 123:101-109, 1995.

100. Eisenhofer G, Lenders JW, Linehan WM, et al: Plasma normetanephrine and metanephrine for detecting pheochromocytoma in von Hippel-Lindau disease and multiple endocrine neoplasia type 2. N Engl J Med 340:1872-1879, 1999.

101. Pacak K, Linehan WM, Eisenhofer G, et al: Recent advances in genetics, diagnosis, localization, and treatment of pheochromocytoma. Ann Intern Med 134:315-329, 2001.

102. Young WF Jr: Pheochromocytoma and primary aldosteronism: Diagnostic approaches. Endocrinol Metab Clin North Am 27:801-827, 1997.

103. Bravo EL: Evolving concepts in the pathophysiology, diagnosis, and treatment of pheochromocytoma. Endocr Rev 15:356, 1994.

104. Velchick MG, Alavi A, Kressel HY: Localization of pheochromocytoma: MIBG, CT and MRI correlation. J Nucl Med 30:328, 1989.

105. Peplinski GR, Norton JA: The predictive value of diagnostic tests for pheochromocytoma. Surgery 116:1101-1110, 1994.

106. Gagner M, Breton G, Pharand D, et al: Is laparoscopic adrenalectomy indicated for pheochromocytomas? Surgery 120:1076-1080, 1996.

107. Brunt LM, Lairmore TC, Doherty GM, et al: Adrenalectomy for familial pheochromocytoma in the laparoscopic era. Ann Surg 235:713-721, 2002.

108. Baysal BE, Ferrell RE, Willett-Brozick JE, et al: Mutations in SDHD, a mitochondrial complex II gene, in hereditary paraganglioma. Science 287:848-851, 2000.

109. Neumann HP, Bausch B, McWhinney SR, et al: Germ-line mutations in nonsyndromic pheochromocytoma. N Engl J Med 346:1459-1466, 2002.

110. Cance WG, Wells SA Jr: Multiple endocrine neoplasia type IIa. Curr Probl Surg 22:1-56, 1985.

111. Howe JR, Norton JA, Wells SA Jr: Prevalence of pheochromocytoma and hyperparathyroidism in multiple endocrine neoplasia type IIa: Results of long-term follow-up. Surgery 114:1070-1077, 1993.

112. Moley JF, Lairmore TC, Phay JE: Hereditary endocrinopathies. Curr Probl Surg 36:653-762, 1999.

113. Linehan WM, Lerman MI, Zbar B: Identification of the von Hippel-Lindau (VHL) gene: Its role in renal cancer. JAMA 273:564-570, 1995.

114. Kaufman BH, Telander RL, van Heerden JA: Pheochromocytoma in pediatric age groups: Current status. J Pediatr Surg 18:879-884, 1983.

115. Remine WH, Chong GC, van Heerden JA: Current management of pheochromocytoma. Ann Surg 179:740-748, 1974.

116. Krempf M, Lumbroso J, Mornex R: Use of ^{131}I-iodobenzylguanidine in the treatment of malignant pheochromocytoma. J Clin Endocrinol Metab 72:455-461, 1991.

117. Keiser HR, Goldstein DS, Wade JL: Treatment of malignant pheochromocytoma with combination chemotherapy. Hypertension 7:1, 1985.

118. Averbach SD, Steakly CS, Young RC: Malignant pheochromocytoma: Effective treatment with a combination of cyclophosphamide, vincristine and dacarbazine. Ann Intern Med 109:267, 1988.

119. van Heerden JA, Steps SG, Hamberger B: Pheochromocytoma: Current status and changing trends. Surgery 91:367-373, 1982.

120. Fudge TL, McKinnon WM, Geary WL: Current surgical management of pheochromocytoma during pregnancy. Arch Surg 115:1224-1225, 1980.

121. Brunt LM: Phaeochromocytoma in pregnancy. Br J Surg 88:481-483, 2001.

122. Freier DT, Thompson NW: Pheochromocytoma and pregnancy: The epitome of high risk. Surgery 114:1148-1152, 1993.

123. Harrington JL, Farley DR, van Heerden JA, et al: Adrenal tumors and pregnancy. World J Surg 23:182-186, 1999.

124. Demeure MJ, Carlsen B, Traul D: Laparoscopic removal of a right adrenal pheochromocytoma in a pregnant woman. J Laparoendosc Adv Surg Tech 8:315-319, 1998.

125. Jones MT, Gillham B: Factors involved in the regulation of adrenocorticotropic hormone/beta-lipotropic hormone. Physiol Rev 68:743-818, 1988.

126. Young WFJ: Management approaches to adrenal incidentalomas: A view from Rochester, Minnesota. Endocrinol Metab Clin North Am 29:159-185, 2000.

127. Mantero F, Arnaldi G: Management approaches to adrenal incidentalomas: A view from Ancona, Italy. Endocrinol Metab Clin North Am 29:107-125, 2000.

128. Thompson GB, Young WF Jr: Adrenal incidentaloma. Curr Opin Oncol 15:84-90, 2003.

129. Brunt LM, Moley JF: Adrenal incidentaloma. World J Surg 25:905-913, 2001.

130. Herrera MF, Grant CS, van Heerden JA, et al: Incidentally discovered adrenal tumors: An institutional perspective. Surgery 110:1014-1021, 1991.

131. Kasperlik-Zaluska AA, Roslonowska E, Slowinska-Srzednicka J, et al: Incidentally discovered adrenal mass (incidentaloma): Investigation and management of 208 patients. Clin Endocrinol 46:29-37, 1997.

132. Barzon L, Scaroni C, Sonino N, et al: Incidentally discovered adrenal tumors: Endocrine and scintigraphic correlates. J Clin Endocrinol Metab 83:55-62, 1998.

133. Proye CAG, Manjili MJ, Combemale FP, et al: Experience gained from operation of 103 adrenal incidentalomas. Langenbeck's Arch Surg 383:330-333, 1998.

134. Favia G, Lumachi F, Basso S, et al: Management of incidentally discovered adrenal masses and risk of malignancy. Surgery 128:918-924, 2000.

135. Mantero F, Terzolo M, Arnaldi G, et al: A survery on adrenal incidentaloma in Italy. J Clin Endocrinol Metab 85:637-644, 2000.

136. Kloos RT, Gross MD, Francis IR, et al: Incidentally discovered adrenal masses. Endocr Rev 16:460-484, 1995.

137. Kudva YC, Young WF Jr, Thompson GB, et al: Adrenal incidentaloma: An important component of the clinical presentation spectrum of benign sporadic adrenal pheochromocytoma. Endocrinologist 9:77-80, 1999.

138. Barnett CC, Varma DG, El-Naggar AK, et al: Limitations of size as a criterion in the evaluation of adrenal tumors. Surgery 128:973-983, 2000.

139. Mitchell DG, Crovello M, Matteuci T, et al: Benign adrenocortical masses: Diagnosis with chemical shift MR imaging. Radiology 185:345-351, 1992.

140. Gagner M, Pomp A, Heniford BT, et al: Laparoscopic adrenalectomy: Lessons learned from 100 consecutive cases. Ann Surg 226:238-247, 1997.

141. Brunt LM, Moley JF, Doherty GM, et al: Outcomes analysis in patients undergoing laparoscopic adrenalectomy for hormonally active adrenal tumors. Surgery 130:629-635, 2001.

142. Lezoche E, Guerrieri M, Paganini AM, et al: Laparoscopic adrenalectomy by the transperitoneal approach. Surg Endosc 14:920-925, 2000.

143. Brunt LM, Doherty GM, Norton JA, et al: Laparoscopic compared to open adrenalectomy for benign adrenal neoplasms. J Am Coll Surg 183:1-10, 1996.

144. Thompson GB, Grant CS, van Heerden JA, et al: Laparoscopic versus open posterior adrenalectomy: A case-control study. Surgery 122:1132-1136, 1997.

145. Imai T, Kikumori T, Phiwa M, et al: A case-controlled study of laparoscopic compared with open lateral adrenalectomy. Am J Surg 178:50-54, 1999.

146. Brunt LM: The positive impact of laparoscopic adrenalectomy on complications of adrenal surgery. Surg Endosc 16:252-257, 2001.

147. Bonjer HJ, Berends FJ, Kazemier G, et al: Endoscopic retroperitoneal adrenalectomy: Lessons learned from 111 consecutive cases. Ann Surg 232:796-803, 2000.

148. Henry J-F, Defechereux T, Raffaelli M, et al: Complications of laparoscopic adrenalectomy: Results of 169 consecutive cases. World J Surg 24:1342-1346, 2000.

149. Lee JE, Curley SA, Gagel RF, et al: Cortical-sparing adrenalectomy for patients with bilateral pheochromocytoma. Surgery 120:1064-1071, 1996.

150. Neumann HPH, Bender BU, Reincke M, et al: Adrenal-sparing surgery for phaeochromocytoma. Br J Surg 86:94-97, 1999.

151. Walther MM, Keiser HR, Choyke PL, et al: Management of hereditary pheochromocytoma in von Hippel-Lindau kindreds with partial adrenalectomy. J Urol 161:395-398, 1999.

152. Walz MK, Peitgen K, Saller B, et al: Subtotal adrenalectomy by the posterior retroperitoneoscopic approach. World J Surg 22:621-627, 1998.

CHAPTER 38

THE MULTIPLE ENDOCRINE NEOPLASIA SYNDROMES

Terry C. Lairmore, M.D., and **Jeffrey F. Moley, M.D.**

Multiple Endocrine Neoplasia Type 1	Multiple Endocrine Neoplasia Type 2 Syndromes

The familial multiple endocrine neoplasia (MEN) syndromes result from genetic changes in both a tumor suppressor gene and a proto-oncogene. These hereditary cancer syndromes are characterized by the predisposition to neoplastic transformation in multiple target endocrine tissues as well as the pathologic involvement of nonendocrine tissues. The associated endocrine tumors may be benign or malignant and may develop either synchronously or metachronously. Within an affected endocrine target tissue, a diffuse preneoplastic hyperplasia typically precedes the development of microscopic invasion or grossly evident multifocal carcinoma. Importantly, the recent discovery of the specific genetic basis for the MEN types 1 and 2 syndromes has allowed the development of strategies for direct genetic testing and early surgical intervention. Early thyroidectomy is indicated for patients with a genetic diagnosis of MEN 2, with the aim of preventing the subsequent development of regional or distant medullary thyroid carcinoma (MTC) metastases. The optimal early surgical intervention to prevent metastatic spread of the potentially malignant neuroendocrine tumors in patients with a genetic diagnosis of MEN 1 is currently more controversial.

The MEN syndromes are characterized by differing patterns of involvement. In its full expression, MEN 1 is characterized by the concurrence of parathyroid hyperplasia, neuroendocrine tumors of the pancreas and duodenum, and adenomas of the anterior pituitary gland. MEN 2A is characterized by the concurrence of MTC, pheochromocytomas, and parathyroid hyperplasia, whereas MEN 2B consists of MTC, pheochromocytomas, mucosal neuromas, and a distinctive marfanoid habitus.

MULTIPLE ENDOCRINE NEOPLASIA TYPE 1

Genetic Studies and Pathogenesis

In 1988, the *MEN1* locus was originally mapped to chromosome 11q13 by a combination of genetic linkage analysis and tumor deletion mapping.[1] The MEN1 disease gene was ultimately identified by positional cloning in 1997.[2] Frequent chromosome deletions involving the *MEN1* locus, termed loss of heterozygosity (LOH), are observed in the deoxyribonucleic acid (DNA) from tumor tissue derived from patients with MEN 1 and from mice with an engineered deletion of one *Men1* allele. This pattern of allelic deletion is consistent with a two-mutational model of oncogenesis,[3] in which *two hits* are required to inactivate both copies of a tumor suppressor gene. The normal protein product of a tumor suppressor gene is presumed to function as a negative influence or brake on cellular growth and proliferation, such that complete elimination of its function would be expected to result in unregulated cell growth or neoplastic transformation. According to this model, the first event is a mutation inherited in the germline that confers susceptibility to neoplastic change in the involved tissues. Elimination of the remaining functional copy of the gene in a single cell through a chance somatic mutational event, or *second hit* (such as a gene deletion), results in clonal expansion and cancer development. The occurrence of individual second hits in several target organ cells explains the multifocal involvement characteristically observed in affected endocrine tissues. Overexpression of menin has been shown to diminish the tumorigenic phenotype of *Ras*-transformed NIH-3T3 cells, consistent with its putative tumor suppressor function.[4] In addition, researchers in one study have suggested a possible role for menin in repressing telomerase activity in somatic cells, perhaps explaining in part its tumor suppressor properties.[5]

The *MEN1* gene consists of 10 exons spanning 9 kb of genomic DNA and encodes a 610 amino acid protein product termed *menin*.[2] The 2.8-kb menin mRNA transcript is ubiquitously expressed in both endocrine and nonendocrine tissues. The menin protein sequence is highly conserved among human, mouse (98%),[6,7] and rat (97%)[8,9] and more distantly among zebrafish (75%)[10,11] and *Drosophila* (47%).[12] However, database analysis of menin protein sequence reveals no significant homology to other known protein families. In the mouse embryo, *Men1* expression appears as early as gestational day 7 and ultimately is detectable at high levels in diverse tissues including testis and the central nervous system. Knockout of both *Men1* alleles in mice results in embryonic lethality.[13] These findings suggest that menin is essential for early development and may have a broader role in the regulation of cell growth that is not limited to the tissues affected in MEN 1. Menin is predominantly a nuclear protein[14] that binds to JunD, a member of the AP-1 transcription factor family, and represses JunD-mediated transcription.[15,16] In addition, menin has been shown to bind physically to a variety of proteins (Smad3, NF-κB, nm23, and others).[17-21] The combination of findings from all current studies has not yielded a clear picture of the mechanisms of menin's tumor suppressor activity or the specific role for menin in endocrine tumorigenesis.

More than 300 independent mutations have been described in the *MEN1* gene.[22] Therefore, there are almost as many unique mutations as there are genetically independent families. The diverse array of *MEN1* mutations that has been reported includes nonsense, missense, frameshift, deletions, and RNA splicing defects.[23-27] The mutations are scattered throughout the coding sequence and intron-exon junctions of the gene. Missense mutations are point mutations in which a DNA base-pair change results in the substitution of an erroneous amino acid for the appropriate amino acid at a specific residue within the protein. Nonsense mutations are base-pair changes that result in a codon that does not specify an amino acid and therefore result in premature termination of translation. Frameshift mutations change the reading frame and therefore usually cause premature termination of translation downstream. Approximately two thirds of the reported mutations in the *MEN1* gene result in premature termination of translation and truncation of the C-terminal portion of the menin protein. No specific genotype-phenotype correlations have been established to date for MEN 1, although phenotypic variants (isolated hyperparathyroidism, frequent prolactinomas) have been described.[28,29]

Genetic testing is available in selected centers with certain limitations. The detection of a disease-associated mutation in a family with a previously defined specific genetic change is straightforward. However, in a novel family for which the specific mutation is not known in advance, a comprehensive search of the coding sequence and intron-exon junctions is necessary to search for all possible mutations. Formal genetic counseling and informed consent, including disclosures relevant to privacy of medical information and the potential impact of the genetic information on treatment, are essential to a comprehensive program of genetic testing.

Clinical Features and Management

The MEN 1 syndrome is characterized by parathyroid hyperplasia, neuroendocrine tumors of the pancreas and duodenum, and adenomas of the anterior pituitary. In addition, bronchial and thymic carcinoids, thyroid nodules, adrenocortical nodular hyperplasia, lipomas, ependymomas, and cutaneous angiofibromas occur with increased frequency in patients with MEN 1.

The clinical expression of MEN 1 most often develops in the third or fourth decade, with the onset of signs or symptoms being rare before age 10 years. Males and females are affected in equal numbers, as predicted by the autosomal dominant inheritance pattern. MEN 1 has been described in many geographic regions and in many ethnic groups, and no racial predilection has been demonstrated.

The MEN 1 trait is transmitted with essentially 100% penetrance but with variable expressivity, such that each affected person may exhibit some but not necessarily all of the components of the syndrome. The most common abnormality in MEN 1 is parathyroid hyperplasia, which eventually develops in 90% to 97% of affected individuals. Duodenopancreatic neuroendocrine tumors (which carry a malignant potential) and pituitary adenomas occur with variable frequency. The clinical manifestation of neuroendocrine tumors of the duodenum and pancreas occurs in 30% to 80% of patients, whereas pituitary tumors become clinically evident in 15% to 50% of affected patients.[30] At autopsy, pathologic involvement in all three endocrine tissues has been described in more than 90% of patients.[31] When compared with sporadic endocrine tumors, the endocrine tumors arising in association with the familial MEN 1 syndrome are characterized by an earlier age at onset, multifocal involvement within a target endocrine tissue, and the development of concurrent neoplasms in multiple endocrine tissues.

The clinical manifestations of patients with MEN 1 depend on the endocrine tissue involved, the overproduction of a specific hormone, or the local mass effect and malignant progression of the neoplasm. Previously, complications related to hormone excess such as severe ulcer disease or hypoglycemia were the most frequent presenting complaints.[32] Currently, the principal cause of mortality in patients with MEN 1 is malignant progression of duodenopancreatic neuroendocrine cancers or bronchial/thymic carcinoids.[33,34]

Parathyroid Glands

The most common endocrine abnormality in MEN 1 is hyperparathyroidism, occurring in more than 95% of patients. Most affected persons exhibit parathyroid hyperplasia with involvement of all four glands. In contrast, fewer than 20% of patients with sporadic primary hyperparathyroidism have multiglandular involvement. Histopathologically, generalized chief cell hyperplasia is seen in the parathyroid glands from patients with MEN 1.

Hypercalcemia is usually the first biochemical abnormality detected in patients with MEN 1 and may precede the clinical onset of a pancreatic neuroendocrine tumor or pituitary neoplasm by several years. The symptoms in the setting of MEN 1 are similar to those of patients with sporadic primary hyperparathyroidism. Asymptomatic hypercalcemia may be present in many patients over a long period of observation. Symptomatic patients may develop renal lithiasis or nephrocalcinosis. Skeletal complications of hyperparathyroidism occur but are uncommon. In general, hyperparathyroidism in patients with MEN 1 has an earlier age at onset and usually causes a milder hypercalcemia than that observed in primary sporadic hyperparathyroidism. The diagnosis is made by measuring serum calcium and parathyroid hormone levels.

The aim of surgical treatment for hyperparathyroidism in patients with MEN 1 is to achieve the lowest incidence of recurrent hypercalcemia while minimizing the complication of permanent hypoparathyroidism. Because patients with MEN 1 develop multiglandular disease, there is a significantly higher rate of recurrent or persistent hyperparathyroidism[35-38] after parathyroidectomy when compared with the results for the treatment of sporadic parathyroid adenoma. The appropriate surgical procedure for patients with MEN 1 is either three-and-one-half gland parathyroidectomy, leaving the parathyroid tissue remnant in situ in the neck, or total four-gland parathyroidectomy with intramuscular autotransplantation of parathyroid tissue into the forearm muscle.[36,39] A potential advantage of the latter technique includes the feasibility of managing recurrent hyperparathyroidism, should it develop, by excision of a portion of the grafted parathyroid tissue under local anesthesia (obviating the morbidity of repeat neck exploration). A transcervical, partial thymectomy should also be performed, owing to the possibility of an ectopic or supernumerary parathyroid gland within the cranial horns of the thymus. In general, preoperative imaging tests are not necessary for patients with MEN 1 undergoing initial neck exploration, because appropriate treatment requires bilateral neck exploration and identification of all four glands. Noninvasive imaging tests, such as sestamibi scanning and ultrasound, may be useful for parathyroid localization before reoperative surgery.

Pancreas and Duodenum

The second most frequent component of MEN 1 is the development of neuroendocrine tumors of the duodenum or pancreas. Depending on the method of study, 30% to 80% of patients with MEN 1 develop these tumors. The pathologic change is typically multifocal, and diffuse islet cell hyperplasia and microadenoma formation may be present in areas of the pancreas distant from grossly evident tumor. Gastrinomas frequently occur within the wall of the duodenum or in extrapancreatic sites. The pancreaticoduodenal tumors in patients with MEN 1 cause symptoms either due to hormone oversecretion or to the mass effects from tumor growth itself and are characterized by a high malignant potential. Pancreatic neuroendocrine tumors that are nonfunctioning or that secrete pancreatic polypeptide are probably the most frequent neuroendocrine tumors that occur in patients with MEN 1.[40]

The most common *functional* neuroendocrine tumor in patients with MEN 1 is gastrinoma. The presenting signs and symptoms in patients with hypergastrinemia, or the Zollinger-Ellison syndrome, may include epigastric pain, reflux esophagitis, secretory diarrhea, and weight loss. Active peptic ulcer disease is present in 70% to 80% of patients at the time of diagnosis. Patients may infrequently present with a severe ulcer diathesis, as well as stricture or perforation of the esophagus due to severe reflux esophagitis. Gastrinomas associated with MEN 1 account for 20% of all cases of the Zollinger-Ellison syndrome.[41] Gastrinoma is diagnosed by the documentation of gastric acid hypersecretion (basal acid output [BAO] >15mEq/hr in patients without operation or >5mEq/hr in patients with prior ulcer surgery), associated with elevated fasting levels of serum gastrin (>100 pg/mL). The diagnosis can be confirmed by an abnormal secretin test. A test result is positive when serum levels of gastrin rise more than 200 pg/mL after the intravenous administration of secretin (2 U/kg).

Gastrinomas that develop in patients with MEN 1 are usually malignant, as indicated by the presence of regional lymph node or distant metastases. Gastrinomas were previously thought to be located predominantly in the head of the pancreas within the *gastrinoma triangle*.[42] More recent data suggest that gastrinomas in patients with MEN 1 occur most frequently within the wall of the duodenum.[43-45] Owing to the small size of these neoplasms, the primary gastrinoma may not be localized preoperatively by computed tomography (CT) or angiography. Endoscopic ultrasound, although dependent on the operator's experience, has been utilized successfully to localize gastrinomas within the wall of the duodenum or head of the pancreas.

The value of surgical resection for intended cure of gastrinoma in patients with MEN 1 is controversial. Although most evidence indicates that patients with Zollinger-Ellison syndrome and MEN 1 are rarely cured by operation,[46-49] localized resection of a potentially malignant neuroendocrine tumor may be indicated in an attempt to control the tumoral process and prevent subsequent malignant dissemination. The recognition that primary gastrinomas occur frequently in the duodenal wall, combined with efforts to perform an extensive regional lymphadenectomy or even pancreaticoduodenectomy, may improve the success rate of surgery for Zollinger-Ellison syndrome in the setting of MEN 1.[50] Total gastrectomy is rarely indicated for patients with gastrinoma, because medical management with high dose H_2-receptor antagonists or proton pump inhibitors effectively prevents most of the symptoms or complications resulting from the acid hypersecretion. Patients with primary hyperparathyroidism should undergo parathyroidectomy, because normalization of the serum calcium level improves the Zollinger-Ellison syndrome.[51]

The second most common clinically evident pancreatic neuroendocrine neoplasm in patients with MEN 1 is insulinoma. These are usually small (<2 cm) and occur with even distribution throughout the pancreas. Patients typically present with recurrent symptoms of neuroglycopenia: sweating, dizziness, confusion, or syncope. The diagnosis of insulinoma is made by documenting symptomatic hypoglycemia in association with inappropriately elevated plasma levels of insulin and C-peptide during a supervised 72-hour fast. Factitious hypoglycemia, the purposeful administration of insulin or hypoglycemic drugs, must be excluded. Insulinomas may be occult and are infrequently localized by conventional preoperative imaging studies such as CT, ultrasound, magnetic resonance imaging (MRI), or angiography.

There is no ideal medical therapy for insulinoma; therefore, the preferred treatment is accurate localization and surgical resection of the functioning tumor to correct life-threatening hyperinsulinemia. Patients with MEN 1 characteristically develop multiple neuroendocrine tumors, a fact that may complicate identification of the specific functional tumor responsible for the hyperinsulinism. Preoperative regional localization of the functioning tumor within the pancreas may be provided by selective catheterization of the arteries supplying the pancreas, followed by injection of an insulin secretagogue (calcium gluconate) and measurement of insulin gradients in the hepatic veins.[52,53] The operative approach includes complete mobilization of the pancreas and careful examination of the gland by inspection and palpation. Intraoperative ultrasound greatly facilitates the identification of small tumors, especially within the pancreatic head or uncinate process.[54-56] Small, benign insulinomas are amenable to enucleation. Partial pancreatectomy may be required for multiple or potentially malignant tumors.[57] In the event the insulinoma is not identified despite an exhaustive intraoperative search, blind subtotal pancreatectomy is not recommended.

Approximately 10% of insulinomas occurring in patients with MEN 1 are malignant. Patients with malignant insulinoma and disseminated metastases may respond to treatment with streptozotocin, and some control of hypoglycemia may be achieved by the administration of either diazoxide or octreotide.

Other functional neuroendocrine tumors of the pancreas, such as glucagonoma, somatostatinoma, and tumors secreting vasoactive intestinal peptide or pancreatic polypeptide, occur rarely in association with MEN 1.

Pituitary Gland

Pituitary neoplasms occur in 15% to 50% of patients. Most of these tumors are prolactin-secreting adenomas. Pituitary tumors cause symptoms either by hypersecretion of hormones or compression of adjacent structures. Large adenomas may cause visual field defects by pressure on the optic chiasm or manifestations of hypopituitarism through compression of the adjacent normal gland. Prolactin-secreting tumors result in amenorrhea and galactorrhea in women or hypogonadism in men. Approximately 30% of MEN 1 patients with pituitary tumors exhibit acromegaly resulting from overproduction of growth hormone.[32] Much less commonly, corticotropin-producing tumors cause Cushing's disease.

Pituitary tumors, either functioning or nonfunctioning, may require surgical ablation or irradiation. Bromocriptine (Parlodel), a dopamine agonist and an inhibitor of prolactin secretion, and cabergoline (Dostinex) have been used to treat prolactinomas medically.

Other Tumors

Bronchial and thymic carcinoids, benign thyroid tumors, benign and malignant adrenocortical tumors, lipomas, ependymomas of the central nervous system, and facial cutaneous angiofibromas and collagenomas[58] occur with increased frequency in patients with MEN 1.

THE MULTIPLE ENDOCRINE NEOPLASIA TYPE 2 SYNDROMES

Epidemiology and Clinical Features

The multiple endocrine neoplasia (MEN) type 2 syndromes include MEN 2A, MEN 2B, and familial, non-MEN medullary thyroid carcinoma (FMTC). These autosomal dominant inherited syndromes are caused by germline mutations in the *RET* gene on chromosome 10.[59] The hallmark of these syndromes is medullary thyroid carcinoma (MTC), which is multifocal, is bilateral, and occurs at a young age. In patients affected by MEN 2A, MEN 2B, or FMTC there is complete penetrance of MTC; all persons who inherit the disease allele develop MTC. Other features of the syndromes are variably expressed, with incomplete penetrance. These features are summarized in Table 38-1.

Twenty-five percent of all MTC cases are familial. In MEN 2A, patients develop multifocal, bilateral MTC, associated with C-cell hyperplasia. Approximately 42% of affected patients develop pheochromocytomas, which may also be multifocal and bilateral and are associated with adrenal medullary hyperplasia. Hyperparathyroidism develops in 10% to 35% of patients and is due to hyperplasia, which may be asymmetrical, with one or more glands becoming enlarged.[39,60] Cutaneous lichen amyloidosis has been described in some patients with MEN 2A. In this entity, macular amyloidosis presents as brownish plaques of multiple tiny papules, usually in the interscapular area.[61] Microscopically, these lesions demonstrate a hyperplastic epidermis, acanthosis, lymphocytic infiltrate, and amyloid goblets. Lastly, Hirschsprung's disease is infrequently associated with MEN 2A.[62-64] This disease is characterized by absence of autonomic ganglion cells within the distal colonic parasympathetic plexus, resulting in obstruction and megacolon.

In MEN 2B, as in MEN 2A, all patients who inherit the disease develop MTC. All MEN 2B individuals have mucosal neuromas, and 40% to 50% of patients develop pheochromocytomas. These patients often have a distinct physical appearance with a prominent mid-upper lip,

TABLE 38-1.   Clinical Features of Sporadic MTC, MEN 2A, MEN 2B, and FMTC

Clinical Setting	Features of MTC	Inheritance Pattern	Associated Abnormalities	Genetic Defect
Sporadic MTC	Unifocal	None	None	Somatic *RET* mutations in >20% of tumors
MEN 2A	Multifocal, bilateral	Autosomal dominant	Pheochromocytomas, hyperparathyroidism	Germline missense mutations in extracellular cysteine codons of *RET*
MEN 2B	Multifocal, bilateral	Autosomal dominant	Pheochromocytomas, mucosal neuromas, megacolon, skeletal abnormalities	Germline missense mutation in tyrosine kinase domain of *RET*
FMTC	Multifocal, bilateral	Autosomal dominant	None	Germline missense mutations in extracellular or intracellular cysteine codons of *RET*

MTC, medullary thyroid carcinoma; MEN, multiple endocrine neoplasia; FMTC, familial medullary thyroid carcinoma.
Reproduced with permission from Moley JF, Lairmore TC, Phay JE: Hereditary endocrinopathies. Curr Probl Surg 36:653-764, 1999.

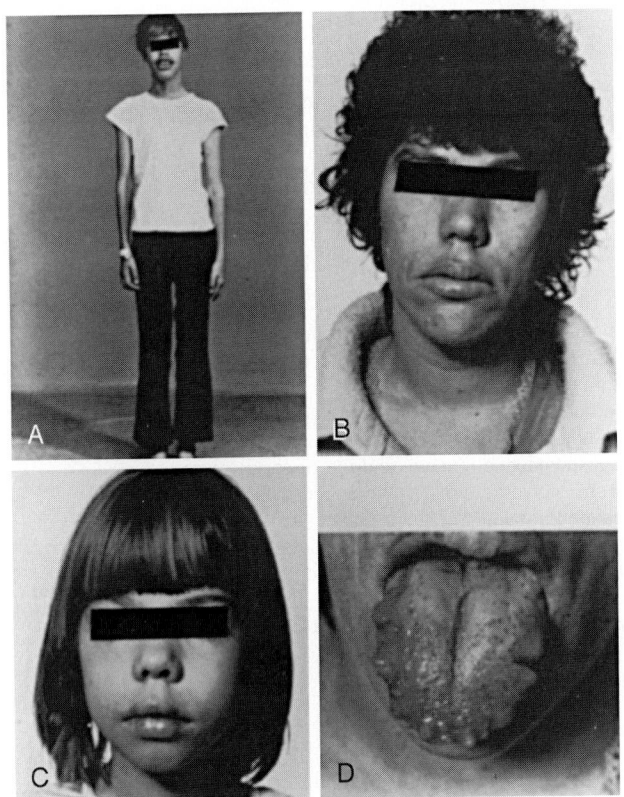

FIGURE 38-1.   A to C, Characteristic phenotypic appearance of three patients with multiple endocrine neoplasia (MEN) 2B. **D,** Multiple neuromas on the tongue and oral mucosa in a patient with MEN 2B.

Familial, non-MEN medullary thyroid carcinoma (FMTC) is characterized by the occurrence of MTC without any other endocrinopathies.[67] MTC in these patients has a later age at onset and a more indolent clinical course than MTC in patients with MEN 2A and MEN 2B. Occasional patients with FMTC will never manifest clinical evidence of MTC (symptoms or a palpable neck mass), although biochemical testing and histologic evaluation of the thyroid always demonstrates MTC.

Medullary Thyroid Carcinoma

MTC originates from the parafollicular cells, or C cells, of the thyroid. These cells comprise 1% of the total thyroid mass and are dispersed throughout the gland, with the highest concentration in the upper poles. The C cells produce, store, and secrete the hormone calcitonin. In the MEN 2 syndromes, MTC is associated with C cell hyperplasia, which is presumed to be a precursor lesion. Histologically, MTC can be identified by calcitonin staining and by the presence of amyloid in the tumors. Hereditary MTC is often multifocal and bilateral. Basal and stimulated serum calcitonin levels correlate with tumor burden and are always elevated in patients with palpable thyroid tumors. MTCs may also secrete other hormones, including carcinoembryonic antigen (CEA).[68] Secretory diarrhea and flushing, most often attributed to elevated calcitonin, are the main paraneoplastic manifestations of advanced MTC.

Early diagnosis in hereditary MTC is critical, because metastases occur in the early stages of disease. Lymph node metastases are rarely present in patients in whom genetic testing established the diagnosis of MEN 2A or FMTC in childhood, when thyroidectomy is performed before the occurrence of a thyroid mass or elevation of calcitonin level.[69,70] In contrast, most cases of sporadic MTC, and cases of hereditary MTC not detected by genetic screening, present as a neck mass detected on physical examination. Diagnosis is made by biopsy (fine-needle aspiration cytology) and measurement of calcitonin levels. Lymph node metastases are usually present in these patients by the time the diagnosis is made.

MTC spreads within the central compartment to perithyroidal and paratracheal lymph nodes (level VI nodes) (Fig.

everted eyebrows, multiple tongue nodules, and "marfanoid" body habitus, with a relatively small torso and long limbs (Fig. 38-1). MEN 2B patients do not develop hyperparathyroidism. MTC in MEN 2B patients presents at a very young age—in infancy—and appears to be the most aggressive form of hereditary MTC, although its aggressiveness may be more related to the extremely early age at onset, rather than to the biologic virulence of the tumor. Once it presents clinically, MTC in patients with MEN 2B is rarely curable.[65,66]

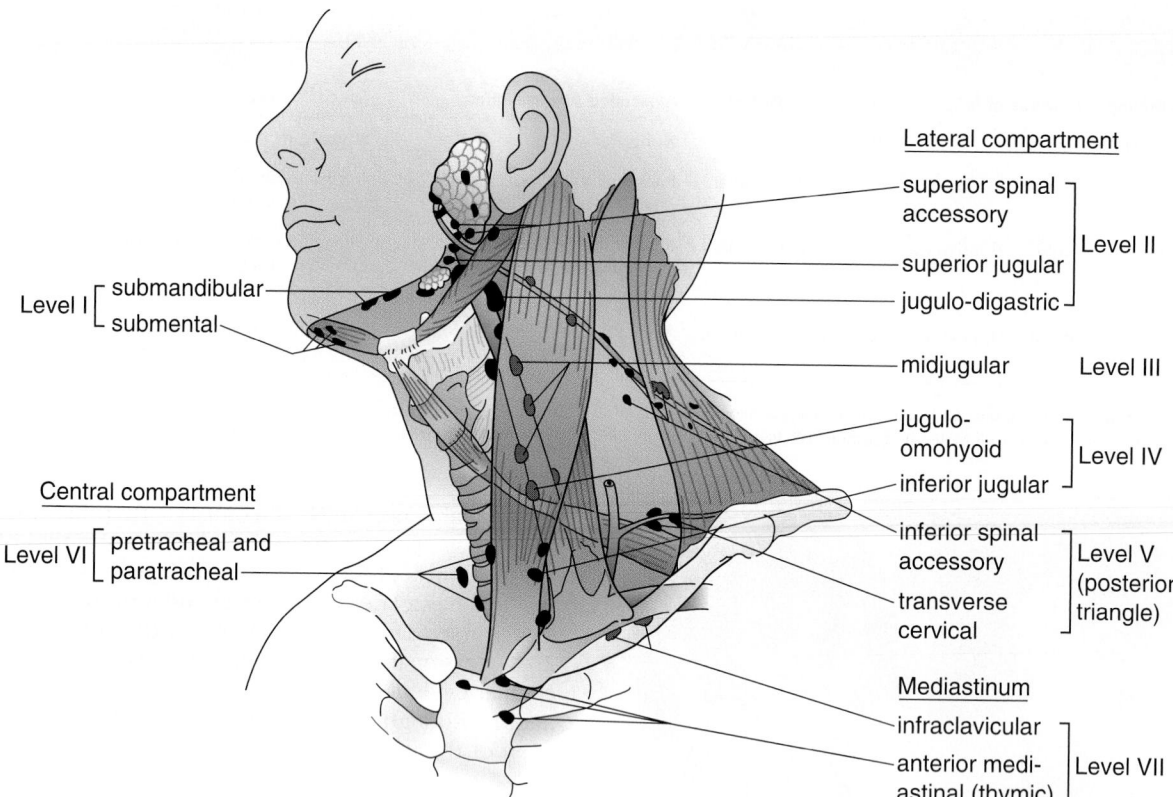

FIGURE 38-2. Schematic representation of the anatomic landmarks and lymph node compartments in the neck and upper mediastinum. The central compartment is delimited inferiorly by the innominate vein, superiorly by the hyoid bone, laterally by the carotid sheaths, and dorsally by the prevertebral fascia. It comprises lymphatic and soft tissues around the esophagus as well as pretracheal and paratracheal lymph nodes that drain the thyroid bed (level VI). The submandibular nodal group (level I) is subsumed in the central compartment by some classifications. The lateral compartments span the area between the carotid sheath, the sternocleidomastoid muscle, and the trapezius muscle. The inferior border is defined by the subclavian vein, and the hypoglossal nerve determines the superior boundary. The lymph node chain adjacent to the jugular vein is divided craniad to caudad in superior jugular nodes (level II), midjugular nodes (level III), and inferior jugular nodes (level IV). Lymph nodes situated in the posterior triangle between the dorsolateral sternocleidomastoid muscle, the trapezius muscle, and the subclavian vein are classified as level V nodes. Mediastinal lymphatic tissue is referred to as level VII lymph nodes. (Reprinted with permission from Musholt TJ, Moley JF: Management of persistent or recurrent medullary thyroid carcinoma. Probl Gen Surg 14:89-109, 1997.)

38-2).[71] The central compartment includes tissue on the trachea, extending laterally to the carotid sheath, and from the hyoid bone superiorly, to the innominate vein inferiorly. Within this compartment, spread is commonly bilateral. Upper mediastinal nodes (level VII nodes) are also frequently involved. Further lymphatic spread can also occur to the lateral neck compartment, including jugular (levels II, III, and IV nodes), posterior triangle (level V nodes), and supraclavicular nodes. The outcome of patients with involvement of lower tracheobronchial lymph nodes is equivalent to that of patients with distant metastases. In one report, a colleague and I analyzed the distribution of nodal metastases in a series of MTCs that presented as a palpable neck mass and in whom central and bilateral cervical nodes were removed and examined histologically. We found that the incidence of central (levels VI and VII) node involvement was extremely high (80%), regardless of the size of the primary tumor. There was also

frequent involvement of ipsilateral (75%) and contralateral (47%) level II, III, and IV nodes (Table 38-2).[71]

MTC may involve adjacent structures by direct invasion or compression. Structures most commonly affected include the trachea, recurrent laryngeal nerve, jugular veins, and carotid arteries. Invasion of these structures may result in stridor, upper airway obstruction, hoarseness, dysphagia, and bleeding or arterial stenosis or occlusion. MTC in the thyroid or in cervical metastases may cause localized pain.

Distant metastases occur in liver, lung, bone, and other soft tissues, including the breast (Fig. 38-3). In a study from a Swedish registry it was noted that MTC patients with a palpable mass in the neck had distant metastatic disease in 20% of cases, regardless of heritability.[72] Occult remote metastases are the likely cause of persistent hypercalcitoninemia after thyroidectomy and extensive lymph node dissection.

TABLE 38-2. Lymph Node Metastases in Palpable Medullary Thyroid Carcinoma

Tumor Size (cm)	No. Patients	Central Metastases	Ipsilateral Metastases	Contralateral Metastases
0-0.9	16	11/16	12/16	5/16
1-1.9	16	13/16	14/16	7/16
2-2.9	13	11/13	7/13	8/13
3-3.9	12	9/12	10/12	8/12
4 cm+	16	14/16	12/16	6/16
Total	73	58/73 (80%)	55/73 (75%)	34/73 (47%)

Reprinted with permission from Moley JF, DeBenedetti MK: Patterns of nodal metastases in palpable medullary thyroid carcinoma: Recommendations for extent of node dissection. Ann Surg 229:880-888, 1999.

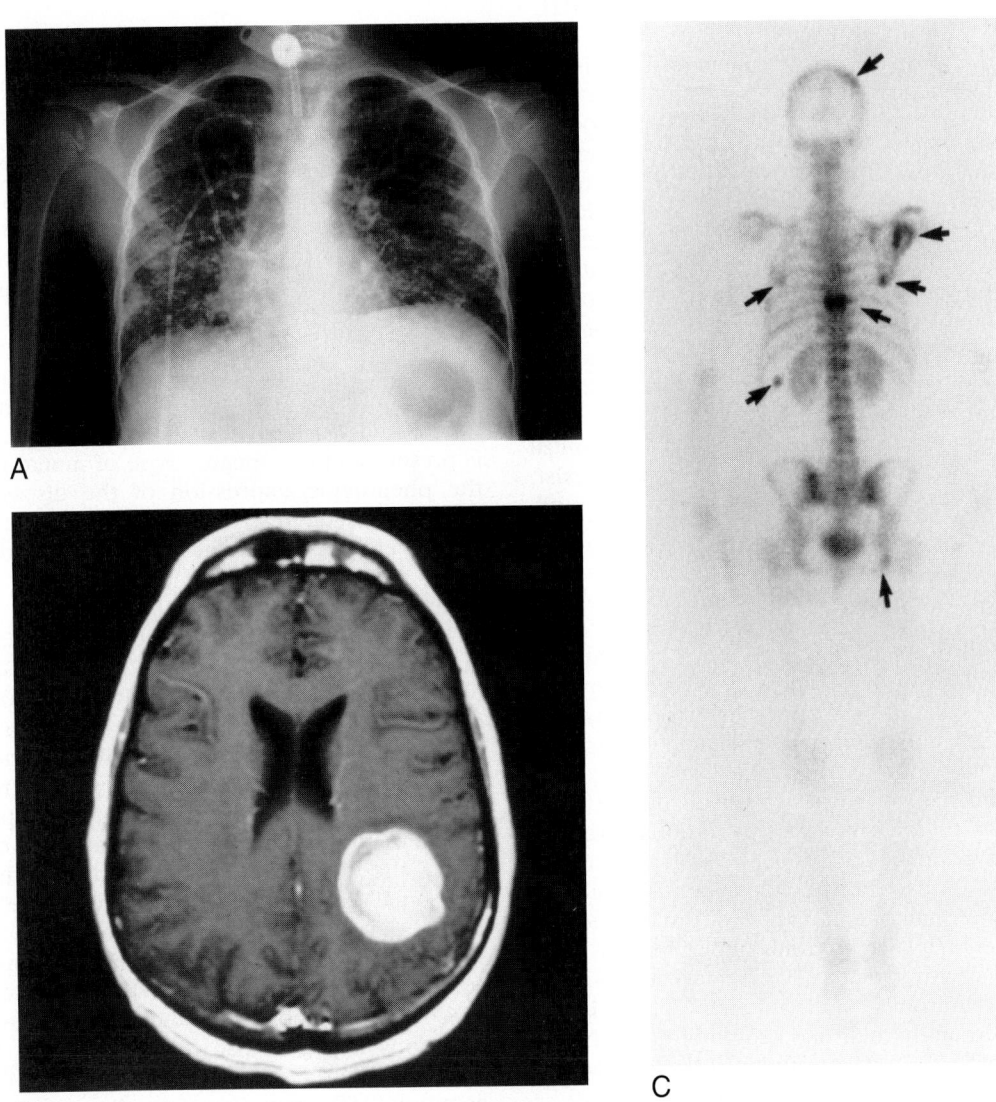

FIGURE 38-3.   Distant metastatic disease in patients with medullary thyroid carcinoma. **A,** Lymphangitic pulmonary spread in child with MEN 2B and MTC. **B,** Solitary brain metastasis in patient with MEN 2A and MTC. **C,** Multiple skeletal metastases *(arrows)* in a patient with sporadic MTC. (Reprinted with permission from Moley JF, Lairmore TC, Phay JE: Hereditary endocrinopathies. Curr Probl Surg 36:653-764, 1999.)

Pheochromocytoma

Pheochromocytomas occur in 40% to 50% of MEN 2A and MEN 2B patients, with the incidence increasing with age. Pheochromocytomas arise in adrenal medullary or chromaffin cells that synthesize, store, and secrete catecholamines. These tumors often present as classic signs and symptoms of excess catechol secretion (i.e., hypertension, headache, heart palpitations, anxiety, and tremulousness). Complications of unrecognized disease include malignant hypertension, stroke, myocardial infarction, and cardiac arrhythmias. There are frequent reports of sudden death in patients with known or unsuspected pheochromocytomas who have undergone unrelated surgical procedures or biopsies or died during childbirth.

Pheochromocytomas rarely precede the development of C-cell abnormalities in MEN 2 syndrome. Approximately 10% of MEN 2 patients present with signs or symptoms of pheochromocytomas that precede those of MTC. As with the thyroid C cells, adrenal medullary cells undergo similar, predictable morphologic changes in the development of a pheochromocytoma. Histologically, the lesion progresses from diffuse hyperplasia to nodular hyperplasia, with nodules greater than 1 cm being defined as pheochromocytomas. In MEN 2, pheochromocytomas are often multifocal, with bilateral tumors occurring in more than half of these patients. As opposed to the sporadic form of the disease, malignant and extra-adrenal pheochromocytomas are very rare within MEN 2 populations. The frequency of development of pheochromocytomas varies among MEN 2 kindreds, with some kindreds displaying the tumor as the dominant characteristic. Pheochromocytomas may be clinically silent in up to 60% of MEN 2 cases, when they are detected by biochemical testing. Multiple biochemical markers for this tumor exist, including epinephrine, norepinephrine, dopamine, vanillylmandelic acid, and metanephrines.

Parathyroid Disease

Hyperparathyroidism occurs in 10% to 35% of patients with MEN 2A.[60] Parathyroid hormone is secreted by the parathyroid glands and is integral in calcium homeostasis. Serum excess of this hormone can lead to hypercalcemia and its associated symptomatology, such as renal stone formation, osteopenia, and mental status changes. Unlike MEN 1, hyperparathyroidism is rarely the initial presenting problem in patients with MEN 2A. Hyperparathyroidism in MEN 2A is characterized by multiglandular hyperplasia. Fewer than one in five patients have a single parathyroid adenoma. Parathyroid hyperplasia is not found in patients with sporadic MTC or in patients with MTC in MEN 2B syndrome. Parathyroid hyperplasia, in the absence of hyperparathyroidism, is common in MEN 2A. Many patients with MEN 2A are found to have enlarged parathyroids at the time of surgery for MTC.

Phenotypic Features of MEN 2B

MEN 2B is distinguished by characteristic physical features (see Fig. 38-1), unlike MEN 2A and FMTC, in which patients have a normal outward appearance. As described earlier, mucosal neuromas and a marfanoid habitus are present. The mucosal neuromas are unencapsulated, thickened proliferation of nerves that occur principally on the lips and tongue but can also be found on the gingiva, buccal mucosa, nasal mucosa, vocal cords, and conjunctiva. MEN 2B patients can also develop ganglioneuromas of the intestine in the submucosal and myenteric plexus. This results in an extremely large colon. Intestinal dysfunction may manifest early in life with poor feeding, failure to thrive, constipation, or pseudo-obstruction.[73] Adults with this disorder may have dysphagia from esophageal dysmotility. Rarely, a patient can present with toxic megacolon. MEN 2B patients do not develop Hirschsprung's disease, however, as do some patients with MEN 2A.

Genetics

MEN 2 is inherited in an autosomal dominant mendelian fashion. Mutations in the *RET* proto-oncogene are responsible for MEN 2A, MEN 2B, and FMTC. This gene encodes a *trans*-membrane protein tyrosine kinase (Fig. 38-4). The mutations that cause the MEN 2 syndromes are activating, gain-of-function mutations that cause constitutive activation of the protein. This is unusual among hereditary cancer syndromes, which are usually caused by loss-of-function mutations in the predisposition gene (e.g., familial polyposis, BRCA 1 and 2, von Hippel-Lindau, and MEN 1). Over 30 missense mutations have been described in patients affected by the MEN 2 syndromes (Table 38-3).[62,74-76] Within an affected kindred, a single *RET* mutation is present and the specific type of mutation is related to the phenotypic expression of the disease within that kindred. The aggressiveness of MTC, and the probability of developing pheochromocytoma and parathyroid disease, is influenced by the specific *RET* mutation in a kindred.

Patients with MEN 2B most commonly have a germline mutation in codon 918 of *RET* (ATG>ACG), which is in the tyrosine kinase domain. Other mutations have been described (codon 883 and 922). In contrast to MEN 2A and FMTC, 50% of mutations in MEN 2B patients arise de novo and are not present in the parents. In almost all of these cases, the mutation occurred in the patient's paternal allele. In offspring of the patients with de novo mutations, the disease is transmitted to offspring in an autosomal dominant fashion. The rate of de novo cases of MEN 2A and FMTC is extremely low.

In MEN 2A, codon 634 and 618 mutations are the most common, although mutations at other codons (see Table 38-3) are also observed and there is overlap in the mutations that give rise to MEN 2A and FMTC. FMTC patients have the most indolent form of MTC. The most common FMTC mutations occur in codons 609, 611, 618, and 620, although mutations of other codons have also been identified (see Table 38-3). Many patients with FMTC are cured by thyroidectomy alone, and those with persistent elevation of calcitonin levels do well for many years. Occasional patients survive into the seventh or

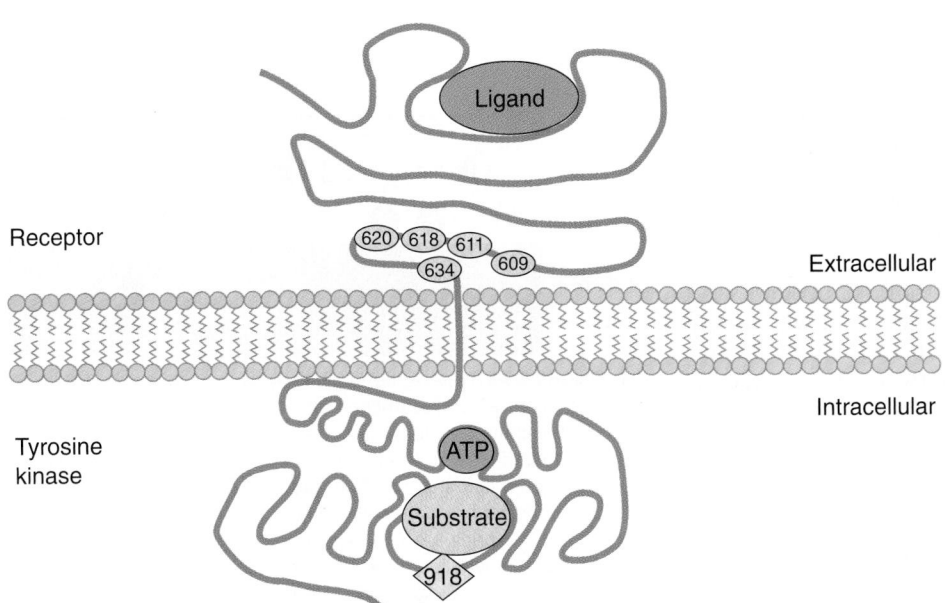

FIGURE 38-4. Schematic representation of the *RET* proto-oncogene structure. The locations of the multiple endocrine neoplasia (MEN) 2A and familial medullary thyroid carcinoma mutations that affect conserved cysteine residues in the portion of the extracellular domain immediately adjacent to the transmembrane segment are indicated by numbers in the *ovals.* The single MEN 2B mutation that replaces methionine with threonine in a critical position within the tyrosine kinase catalytic domain is indicated by the number in the *diamond.* The numbers within the symbols indicate the codon number. ATP, adenosine triphosphate.

TABLE 38-3. *RET* Mutations and Associated Clinical Syndromes

Exon	Affected Codon	Affected Amino Acid	Clinical Syndrome	MEN 2 Mutations (%)
10	609	Cysteine	MEN 2A, FMTC, MEN 2A, and Hirschsprung's disease	0-1
10	611	Cysteine	MEN 2A, FMTC	2-3
10	618	Cysteine	MEN 2A, FMTC	3-5
10	620	Cysteine	MEN 2A, FMTC	6-8
11	634	Cysteine	MEN 2A	80-90
11	635	Thr Ser Cys Ala	MEN 2A	<1
11	637	Cys Arg Thr	MEN 2A	<1
13	768	Glutamine	FMTC	0-1
13	790	Leucine	MEN 2A, FMTC	<1
13	791	Tryptophan	FMTC	0-1
14	804	Valine	FMTC, MEN 2A	<1
15	883	Ala → Phe	MEN 2B	<1
15	891	Ser → Ala	FMTC	<1
16	918	Met → Thr	MEN 2B	3-5
16	922	Ser → Tyr	MEN 2B	<1

FMTC, familial medullary thyroid carcinoma; MEN, multiple endocrine neoplasia.

eighth decade without any treatment for or symptoms of MTC, although pathologic examination of the thyroid reveals MTC or C-cell hyperplasia. It has been suggested that appropriate management of patients with FMTC (particularly those with codon 13 and 14 *RET* mutations) is observation and yearly calcitonin testing, with thyroidectomy only if stimulated calcitonin levels become elevated.[77]

The exon 16 mutation common in MEN 2B patients has also been identified in approximately 40% of sporadic MTC tumors, where it is assumed to be a somatic, rather than an inherited, mutation in the tumor cells only.[62]

Diagnosis

Medullary Thyroid Carcinoma

The age at onset and the aggressiveness of MTC may vary considerably, depending on the clinical situation. Sporadic MTC is unilateral and unifocal in the majority of cases, whereas MTC in the MEN 2 syndromes is usually bilateral and multifocal. MTC in MEN 2A often becomes clinically apparent in late childhood or in the teenage years. In FMTC, the tumors are indolent and appear later in life, whereas MTC in MEN 2B presents in infancy or early childhood, with gross evidence of cancer present in children as young as 6 months of age.

The prognosis of MTC is associated with disease stage at the time of diagnosis. Numerous studies of patients with MEN 2A have shown a direct correlation between early diagnosis and cure of MTC.[69,70] Patients with MEN 2A and FMTC have a completely normal outward appearance. In these patients, the diagnosis of MTC has been made through screening efforts (measurement of calcitonin levels or *RET* gene mutation testing), undertaken because of other affected family members, or by detection of a thyroid nodule on physical examination. Over 50% of patients with MEN 2B have normal parents, and the diagnosis in these de novo cases is not usually made until a mass is discovered in the neck. Very rarely, the diagnosis is made earlier by an astute clinician who notes the characteristic phenotype. Most index cases of MEN 2A, MEN 2B, and FMTC present as a thyroid mass that is identified as MTC by biopsy. Palpable cervical adenopathy is present in over 50% of patients who present with palpable MTC, and lymph node metastases are present histologically in up to 80%. Respiratory complaints, hoarseness, and dysphagia can be seen in about 13% of patients. Approximately 12% of patients with palpable MTC present with evidence of distant metastatic disease.[78] Occasional index cases of MEN 2 present with clinical pheochromocytoma or hyperparathyroidism before the diagnosis of MTC is made.

Approximately 25% of all patients with MTC have MEN 2A, MEN 2B, or FMTC. Because of this, it is believed that genetic testing should be considered in all patients who present with MTC. An in-depth family history with close attention to any relatives with severe hypertension or thyroid and adrenal tumors is essential. A careful review of systems to identify any evidence of symptomatic pheochromocytoma or hyperparathyroidism should be conducted. The caregiver should also note any phenotypic physical characteristics that might suggest MEN 2B. If a *RET* mutation is found on genetic screening, first-degree relatives should be tested for the same mutation (Fig. 38-5). Patients found to have a mutation in the *RET* proto-oncogene should have biochemical testing for pheochromocytoma before thyroidectomy. Failure to identify a pheochromocytoma in a patient who undergoes thyroid surgery can have disastrous consequences, because induction of anesthesia may cause a catechol surge with resultant malignant hypertension.

Thyroid C cells and MTC cells secrete calcitonin, which is an invaluable serum marker for the presence of disease in screening and follow-up settings. Carcinoembryonic antigen level is also elevated in over 50% of patients with MTC.[68] Calcitonin is a more useful tumor marker for MTC than carcinoembryonic antigen, because of its shorter half-life (days compared with months) and because many MTCs do not secrete this antigen. Blood levels of calci-

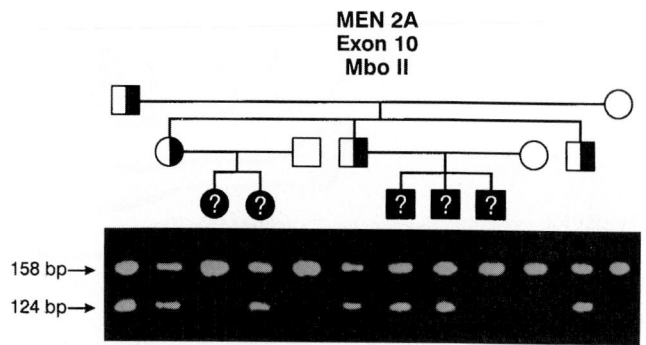

FIGURE 38-5. Pedigree of a family with multiple endocrine neoplasia type 2A and restriction endonuclease digestion of polymerase chain reaction fragments of the *RET* proto-oncogene. The pedigree illustrates three generations of a family affected by MEN 2A. In the oldest generation, the grandfather (square-half-filled in to indicate medullary thyroid carcinoma) is affected. All three of his offspring are affected; and in the third generation, genetic testing identifies three mutation carriers (the granddaughter on the right and the two grandsons on the left). In the restriction digest gel at the bottom of the figure, two bands indicate a mutation carrier and one band indicates no mutation (wild type). (Reprinted with permission from Chi D, Toshima K, Donis-Keller H, Wells SA Jr: Predictive testing for multiple endocrine neoplasia type 2A: Based on the detection of mutations in the *RET* proto-oncogene. Surgery 116:128, 1994.)

tonin may be measured in the basal state or after the administration of the secretagogues calcium and pentagastrin.[79,80] After basal levels have been obtained, intravenous calcium (2 mg/kg/1 min) is infused, followed immediately by pentagastrin (0.5 µg/kg/5 sec), and then blood is drawn for measurement of calcitonin levels at 1, 3, and 5 minutes. Recently, pentagastrin has not been made in the United States; however, European-made pentagastrin has been obtained and approved for use at Washington University in St. Louis (IND #61,205) and at Duke University. The development of immunoradiometric assays has greatly improved the sensitivity and specificity of calcitonin measurements. Calcium-pentagastrin–stimulated calcitonin testing is still useful in patients at risk for MTC and in patients who have normal basal levels of calcitonin after definitive surgery. Elevated stimulated levels of calcitonin indicate the presence of MTC in these patients.

Genetic screening of all individuals in a known MEN 2 kindred is the standard of care. If patients from a kindred with a known mutation are shown not to have inherited the mutation, they need no further follow-up. Controversy exists over the management of patients found to have a *RET* mutation with no clinical or biochemical evidence of disease. At present, in-depth genetic counseling is recommended and prophylactic thyroidectomy is encouraged in childhood for carriers of the mutant gene. The near-complete penetrance of MEN 2 manifesting as MTC, combined with the morbidity and mortality associated with the tumor, warrants surgery before the tumor can be detected biochemically. In a study by Wells and colleagues, seven MEN 2A kindreds were evaluated by genetic screening.[69] Twenty-one patients had *RET* mutations and were offered prophylactic thyroidectomy. Thirteen patients opted for surgery, and all were found to have either C-cell hyperplasia or foci of MTC on pathologic examination. Of these 13 patients, only 7 had abnormal calcium-pentagastrin–stimulated calcitonin testing preoperatively. Recent studies have shown that 10% of patients diagnosed by abnormal biochemical testing had metastatic MTC despite diligent screening.[81]

Pheochromocytoma

Biochemical screening for pheochromocytoma is best done by measurement of plasma or 24-hour urine catecholamines and metanephrines. This test should be done on an annual basis. If testing is negative, no further workup is necessary until the next year. If the test is positive or borderline, imaging is needed to determine if a pheochromocytoma is present. Almost all MEN 2A and MEN 2B patients have some degree of adrenal medullary hyperplasia and may have borderline elevations of urinary catechols and thickening of the adrenals without a definite pheochromocytoma.

Adrenal CT or MRI can detect tumors 1 cm or larger. Opposed phase chemical shift MRI may distinguish a pheochromocytoma from an adrenal adenoma, which may occur in up to 9% of normal patients.[82] ^{131}I-Metaiodobenzylguanidine (^{131}I-MIBG) scanning is useful in detecting extra-adrenal pheochromocytomas, although extra-adrenal tumors are extremely rare in patients with MEN 2A and MEN 2B.

Parathyroid Disease

All known MEN 2A carriers should be screened annually for the presence of hyperparathyroidism by serum calcium measurements. Parathyroid hormone levels should be measured if the serum calcium is high or borderline.

Medical and Surgical Therapy

Medullary Thyroid Carcinoma

Recommended surgical treatment of MTC is influenced by several factors. First, the clinical course of MTC is usually more aggressive than that of differentiated thyroid cancer, with higher recurrence and mortality rates. Second, MTC cells do not take up radioactive iodine, and radiation therapy and chemotherapy are ineffective. Third, MTC is multicentric in 90% of patients with the hereditary forms of the disease. Fourth, in patients with palpable disease, over 70% have nodal metastases. Last, the ability to measure postoperative stimulated calcitonin levels has allowed assessment of the adequacy of surgical extirpation. Screening for pheochromocytoma should be done before performing thyroid surgery. If patients are found to have evidence of pheochromocytoma, adrenal surgery with perioperative α-adrenergic blockade should precede other procedures.

Preventative thyroidectomy is recommended before age six in patients with MEN 2A and FMTC. Patients with MEN 2B should undergo thyroidectomy during infancy because of the aggressiveness and earlier age at onset of MTC in these patients. These procedures are best performed by surgeons experienced in thyroid surgery in children because finding the parathyroids can be extremely difficult owing to their small size and translucent appearance.[59,69]

Thorough surgical extirpation is the only curative treatment for MTC. In patients without a palpable neck mass who are found to be carriers of a *RET* mutation by genetic testing, total thyroidectomy and central node dissection is recommended. At my institution, total parathyroidectomy with autotransplantation is often done at the same time as total thyroidectomy for MTC.[39,69] This is because the blood supply to the parathyroids is closely associated with the posterior capsule of the thyroid and with the perithyroidal lymph nodes. Preservation of the parathyroids is usually not possible if all thyroid tissue and central nodes are removed. Parathyroid glands are therefore removed, sliced into 1×3-mm fragments, and autotransplanted into individual muscle pockets in the muscle of the nondominant forearm (in patients with MEN 2A) or sternocleidomastoid muscle (in patients with FMTC or MEN 2B).[83] Patients are maintained on calcium and vitamin D supplementation for 4 to 8 weeks postoperatively. In a recent series of thyroidectomies performed in 13 patients with hereditary MTC identified by genetic screening, total thyroidectomy and central node dissection with parathyroidectomy and parathyroid autografting was performed in all patients.[69] All patients were normocalcemic after stopping calcium supplementation 8 weeks postoperatively. In other series, the percentage of patients requiring calcium supplementation after parathyroidectomy with parathyroid autografting has ranged from 0% to 18%. Other experts in this field attempt to preserve the glands with vascular supply intact during thyroidectomy for MTC.[84-86] Parathyroidectomy with autotransplantation should be done in all patients with gross parathyroid enlargement or biochemical evidence of parathyroid disease at the time of operation for MTC.

In patients with MTC who present with a palpable thyroid mass, the risk of more extensive nodal metastatic disease is increased. In the past, authors recommended total thyroidectomy with node dissections only if nodes are clinically palpable. This is an effective strategy for differentiated thyroid cancer, where suppression with thyroxine and radioactive iodine ablation are effective adjuncts to surgery, but MTC cells do not respond to these nonsurgical treatments. Surgery is the only effective therapeutic modality for MTC at the present time. Overall, persistent disease, evidenced by elevation of calcitonin levels, is present in over 50% of patients after surgery for MTC. In the absence of effective adjuvant therapy there is a need to better define or predict the extent of spread of these tumors at the time of diagnosis, so that appropriate operative resection can be performed.

Metastatic involvement of cervical lymph nodes is present in over 75% of patients with palpable MTC tumors.[71] Based on this observation, my recommendation for patients who present with palpable MTC is total thyroidectomy, parathyroidectomy with autotransplantation,

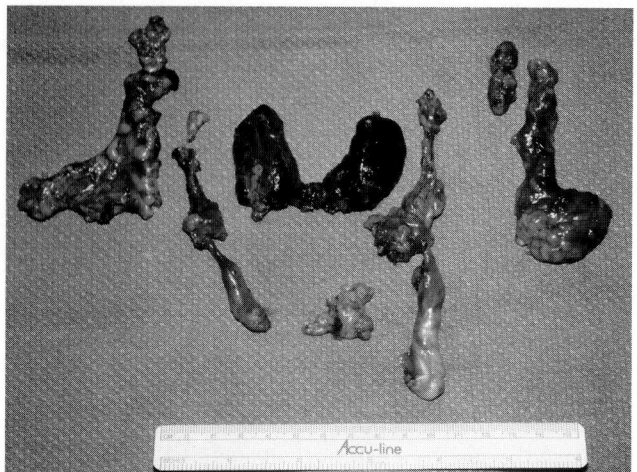

FIGURE 38-6.   Total thyroidectomy and central (levels VI and VII) and bilateral levels II to V node dissections from a thin young male and bilateral palpable medullary thyroid carcinoma (parathyroids not shown). Microscopic metastases were present in all nodal groups. (Reprinted with permission from Moley JF, Lairmore TC, Phay JE: Hereditary endocrinopathies. Curr Probl Surg 36:653-764, 1999.)

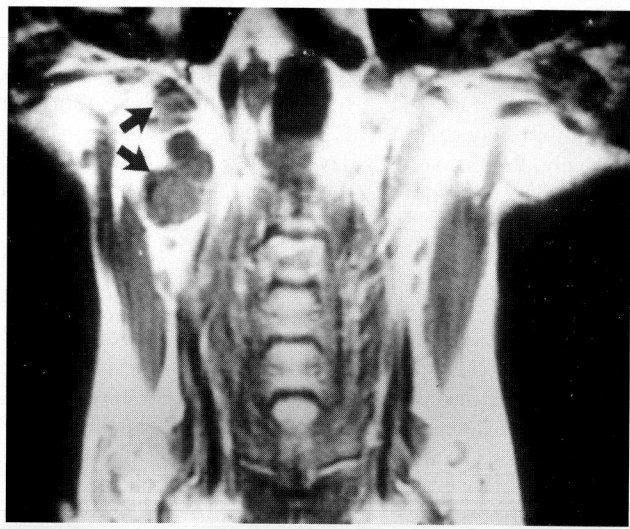

FIGURE 38-7.   Bulky mediastinal adenopathy *(arrows)* in a man with medullary thyroid carcinoma. Note tracheal narrowing and deviation.

central neck dissection (right and left levels VI and VII), and ipsilateral level II through V node dissection. Bilateral level II through V node dissections may be done, depending on the extent of nodal involvement apparent at operation. The central node dissection encompasses all tissue from the level of the hyoid bone superiorly to the innominate vessels inferiorly and laterally to the carotid sheaths (Fig. 38-6). Nodal tissue on the anterior surface of the trachea is removed, exposing the superior surface of the innominate vein behind the sternal notch. Fatty and nodal tissue between the carotid artery and the trachea is removed, including paratracheal nodes along the recurrent nerves. On the right, the junction of the innominate and right carotid arteries is exposed; and on the left, nodal tissue is removed to a comparable level behind the head of the left clavicle. A systematic approach to the removal of all nodal tissue in these patients has been reported to improve recurrence and survival rates when compared retrospectively with procedures where only grossly involved nodes were removed.[87]

Persistent or Recurrent Disease

Patients who present with palpable MTC often have elevated calcitonin levels after primary surgery, indicating residual or recurrent MTC. Currently, there is no defined role for chemotherapy or radiation therapy in these patients. Reoperation for patients with recurrent disease can be done with curative or palliative intent. Evidence of distant metastases is a contraindication to surgery unless some palliative benefit can be identified (Fig. 38-7). Two such indications are to prevent invasion or compression of the airway and to debulk large tumors that cause profuse, intractable diarrhea secondary to hormone secretion. If no evidence of distant metastases is found in a

patient who has not had previous cervical node dissections, re-exploration of the neck with completion of node dissection is an option for patients with persistent or recurrent elevations of calcitonin.[88,89] At my institution, metastatic work-up consists of neck, chest, and abdominal CT or MRI, and diagnostic laparoscopy. I have not found octreotide, technetium/thallium, or fluorodeoxyglucose-positron emission tomography (FDG-PET) to be more sensitive than CT or MRI.[90] If no evidence of metastatic disease is found, surgery with completion node dissections is discussed with the patient as an option. Reoperations in such patients resulted in reduction of calcitonin levels to normal in one third of patients. In patients with elevated calcitonin levels only, and no palpable or radiologically visualized disease, observation is another option.

Diagnostic laparoscopy with direct examination of the liver is extremely useful in detecting distant metastases in these patients before reoperation on the neck (Fig. 38-8). In one series, liver metastases were identified by laparoscopy in 25% of patients with persistent elevation of calcitonin levels despite negative CT or MRI of the liver.[91] If distant metastases are identified, observation of the neck is recommended and neck reoperation is recommended only if the patient develops gross cervical recurrence that threatens the airway. If laparoscopy and imaging studies show no evidence of metastatic disease, re-exploration of the neck is considered to remove residual nodal tissue. The operative strategy in these reoperations is to remove all residual thyroid and nodal tissue in at-risk areas that was not removed at the previous operation, guided by the previous operative records, pathology reports, and imaging studies (Fig. 38-9). Reoperation resulted in normalization of the calcitonin level in one third of patients in a study from my institution. Long-term follow-up of these patients is in progress to determine if these responses are durable.

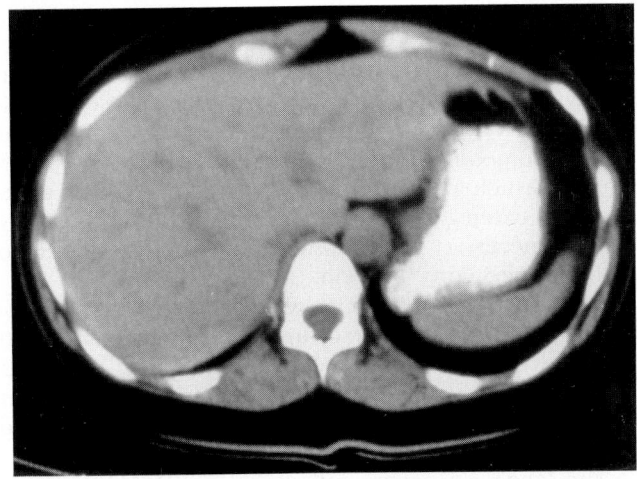

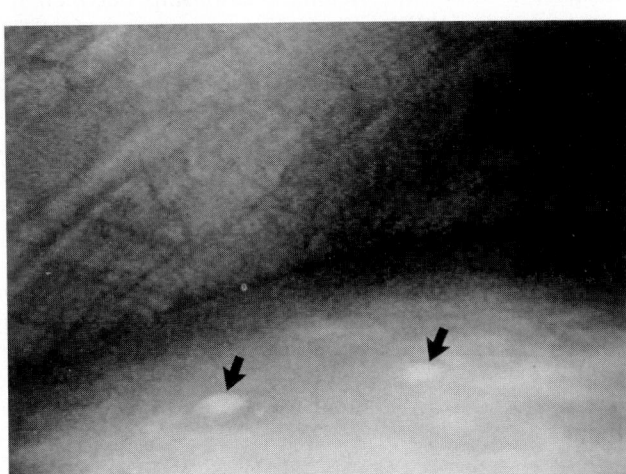

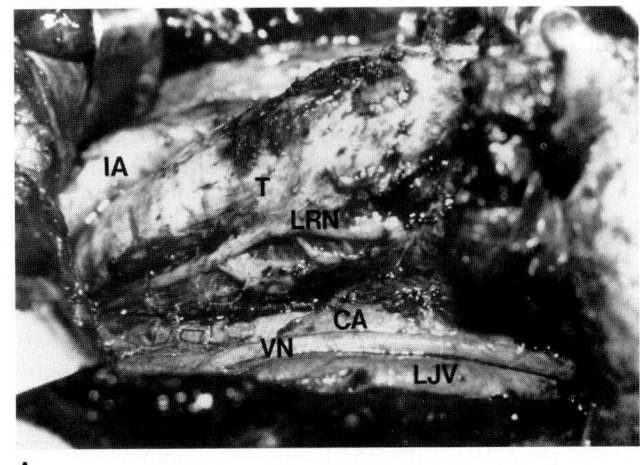

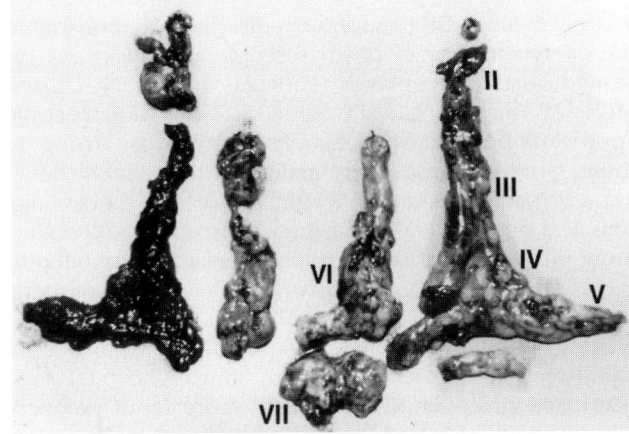

FIGURE 38-8. **A,** CT of liver from patient with MEN 2A, recurrent MTC, and elevated calcitonin levels. There is no evidence of liver metastases on the scan. **B,** Laparoscopic view of liver from the same patient showing multiple small raised whitish lesions on and just beneath the surface of the liver *(arrows),* confirmed to be metastatic MTC by biopsy. These small, multiple metastases are often not seen on routine CT or other imaging modalities, including nuclear scanning. (Reprinted with permission from Tung WS, Vesely TM, Moley JF: Laparoscopic detection of hepatic metastases in patients with residual or recurrent medullary thyroid cancer. Surgery 118:1024-1030, 1995.)

FIGURE 38-9. This patient with MEN 2B had recurrent elevation of calcitonin levels 20 years after total thyroidectomy for MTC. Redo central neck dissection and bilateral functional neck dissections (microdissection) were performed. **A,** View of trachea and dissected central and left paratracheal compartment. The photograph was taken from the patient's left side. Patient's head is to the right and chest is to the left. IA, innominate vein; T, trachea; LRN, left recurrent laryngeal nerve; CA, left carotid artery; VN, left vagus nerve; LJV, left jugular vein. Note markedly enlarged nerves characteristic of MEN 2B. **B,** Surgical specimen from same patient. The photograph shows central and upper mediastinal nodes (level VII), bilateral paratracheal nodes (level VI), and bilateral jugular chain and posterior triangle nodes (levels II, III, IV, and V nodes). Microscopic foci of MTC were found in paratracheal dissection specimens. (Reprinted with permission from Moley JF: Medullary thyroid cancer. *In* Clark OH, Duh QY [eds]: Textbook of Endocrine Surgery. Philadelphia, WB Saunders, 1997.)

Pheochromocytoma

Partial or complete adrenalectomy is recommended in patients with MEN 2A and MEN 2B who are found to have a pheochromocytoma. It is important to medically stabilize the patient before surgery to avoid any perioperative events owing to excessive catechol secretion. Preoperative α-adrenergic blockade is achieved by administration of phenoxybenzamine (40 to 200 mg/day) for 5 days to 2 weeks before surgery. The dose is titrated to the lowest blood pressure tolerated by these patients without symptomatic relative hypotension. Should tachycardia or cardiac arrhythmia result from treatment with phenoxy-

benzamine, a β-adrenergic blocker is added to the treatment regimen. After medical stabilization, the patient is taken for operation. During the procedure, it may be necessary to control intraoperative paroxysmal hypertension with short-acting antihypertensives such as sodium nitroprusside or phentolamine.

Traditionally, controversy has existed as to whether unilateral or bilateral adrenalectomy should be performed for unilateral tumors. In a series at our institution, the results of unilateral and bilateral adrenalectomies were compared.[92] Nearly one fourth of patients undergoing bilateral adrenalectomy experienced at least one episode of acute adrenal insufficiency requiring hospitalization. Two of these patients died of episodes of adrenal insufficiency. Of the patients who had unilateral adrenalectomies, 52% developed contralateral pheochromocytomas after a mean interval of 12 years. Conversely, 48% of patients remained disease free by biochemical and symptomatic standards during a mean interval of 5 years. Based on these results, it is my practice to perform resection of the involved adrenal only and maintain yearly biochemical screening thereafter.

The classic surgical approach for adrenalectomy in MEN 2 patients is through an anterior abdominal midline incision. The first report of successful laparoscopic removal of adrenal tumors was by Gagner and colleagues in 1992.[93] Since then, several studies have demonstrated the safety and efficacy of laparoscopic adrenalectomy for benign adrenal neoplasms. Patients with MEN 2A and MEN 2B may be ideally suited to the laparoscopic approach, because the pheochromocytomas arising in these syndromes are rarely malignant and almost never extra-adrenal. Pheochromocytomas may be successfully removed by unilateral or bilateral laparoscopic adrenalectomy provided the adrenal tumors are small, confined to the adrenal gland(s), and accurately localized preoperatively by high-resolution CT or MRI and the patient is adequately prepared pharmacologically. Laparoscopic adrenalectomy is associated with shorter hospital stay, decreased postoperative pain, and more rapid recovery when compared with open adrenalectomy.[94,95] Contraindications to the laparoscopic approach include large tumors (>8 to 10 cm), malignant pheochromocytomas, and existing contraindications to laparoscopy.

Parathyroid Disease

The need for isolated parathyroidectomy in MEN 2 patients is rare. As discussed earlier, routine total parathyroidectomy with autotransplantation is usually performed at the time of thyroidectomy, regardless of gross appearance of the parathyroid glands.[39,83] Should hyperparathyroidism occur at a later time in these patients with forearm grafts, surgical removal of a portion of the graft can be done under local anesthetic in an outpatient setting. If, at the time of the initial neck exploration, the parathyroids are left in situ, subsequent development of hyperparathyroidism requires re-exploration of the neck with identification and removal of all four glands followed by autotransplantation.

Complications and Postoperative Care

The complications and immediate postoperative care in surgery for the various endocrinopathies in MEN 2 are similar to those described in more detail in the previous chapters dealing with each specific disease. In thyroidec-

tomy for MEN 2–related MTC, the complications include injury to the recurrent laryngeal nerve, hypocalcemia secondary to parathyroid damage, and compromise of the airway secondary to hematoma formation. These complications are very unusual in the hands of an experienced thyroid surgeon.[96] If both recurrent nerves have been injured (which may occur in a patient after multiple operations or extensive tumor involvement), a tracheostomy may be necessary. Fiberoptic laryngoscopy is done to monitor vocal cord function.

After total thyroidectomy with parathyroid autotransplantation, it is necessary to supplement calcium, vitamin D, and thyroid hormone. Calcium and vitamin D supplementation is withdrawn 4 to 8 weeks postoperatively as the parathyroid grafts begin to function. Lifelong thyroid replacement is required.

The long-term postoperative care for MEN 2 patients demands a close and lifelong relationship between the care provider and the patient. Yearly screenings for MTC recurrences and other manifestations of the syndrome must still be conducted. After thyroidectomy for MTC, calcitonin levels should be documented in the immediate postoperative period and should be followed closely. If a patient is found to have persistent or elevated calcitonin level postoperatively, an extensive physical examination and imaging work-up for focal and metastatic disease must be conducted, as outlined in the previous section.

In patients who have undergone adrenalectomy for pheochromocytoma, routine yearly plasma or 24-hour urine screens must be performed to rule out a contralateral tumor.[97] If catecholamines or metanephrines become elevated, MRI or CT should be repeated to localize the tumor.

MEN 2A patients must have lifelong screening for evidence of hyperparathyroidism. Graft-dependent hyperparathyroidism may occur in patients with parathyroid autografts, and in these cases debulking of the parathyroid autografts should be performed. Intraoperative quick parathyroid hormone assays are helpful in determining the adequacy of these procedures.

Prognosis

MTC in the MEN 2 syndromes is usually indolent and slow growing, but it is lethal in most patients with distant metastases. Patients with MEN 2A and FMTC have a better long-term outcome than patients with MEN 2B or sporadic tumors. Within these clinical settings, however, there is variation. In the MEN 2 population, with the relatively recent widespread use of genetic screening modalities and related changes in treatment for patients identified by these methods, long-term prognosis has yet to be established. Before the use of these screening techniques, average life expectancy was 50 years for patients with MEN 2A and 30 years for patients with MEN 2B. As more kindreds are followed by genetic and biochemical screening, the long-term prognosis for MEN 2 patients in the modern era of treatment should become more clear.

Conclusion

The identification of mutations in the *RET* protooncogene associated with MEN 2A, MEN 2B, and FMTC has led to a new paradigm in surgery—the performance of an operation based on the result of a genetic test. Prophylactic thyroidectomy based on direct mutation analysis appears to be curative in MEN 2A and FMTC patients when they are screened at a young age. The application of meticulous reoperative strategies for persistent hypercalcitoninemia combined with more accurate staging studies has led to better patient selection for surgery and improved outcome.

Selected References

Chandrasekharappa SC, Guru SC, Manickamp P, et al: Positional cloning of the gene for multiple endocrine neoplasia-type 1. Science 276:404, 1997.

> Original article reporting the successful positional cloning of the *MEN1* gene.

Larsson C, Skogseid B, Oberg K, et al: Multiple endocrine neoplasia type 1 gene maps to chromosome 11 and is lost in insulinoma. Nature 332:85, 1988.

> This is the original report that maps the *MEN1* gene to chromosome 11 by genetic studies. Important observations of allelic loss on chromosome 11 in tumor DNA from a pair of brothers with MEN 1 and insulinoma also demonstrate that oncogenesis in MEN 1 is consistent with a two-hit model that involves inactivation of both copies of a tumor-suppressor gene.

Donis-Keller H, Dou S, Chi D, et al: Mutations in the *RET* proto-oncogene are associated with MEN 2A and FMTC. Hum Mol Genet 2:851, 1993.

Mulligan LM, Kwok JBJ, Healey CS, et al: Germ-line mutations of the *RET* proto-oncogene in multiple endocrine neoplasia type 2A. Nature 363:458, 1993.

> These papers report the identification of missense germline mutations in the RET proto-oncogene that are associated with MEN 2A. The mutations produce amino acid substitutions affecting one of several conserved cysteine residues in the extracellular ligand-binding domain of RET, a tyrosine kinase receptor. These reports allowed the introduction of direct DNA testing to identify patients who have inherited a mutation for MEN 2A.

Wells SA Jr, Chi D, Toshima K, et al: Predictive DNA testing and prophylactic thyroidectomy in patients at risk for multiple endocrine neoplasia type 2A. Ann Surg 220:237, 1994.

> The investigators used direct DNA testing to identify patients who had inherited a mutation for MEN 2A and performed prophylactic thyroidectomy in 13 patients. C-cell hyperplasia with or without medullary thyroid carcinoma was present in the resected thyroid gland from each patient. There were no metastases to cervical lymph nodes, and postoperative plasma calcitonin levels were normal. This article reports the utilization of preventative surgical treatment based on direct DNA testing for germline mutations in this familial cancer syndrome.

References

1. Larsson C, Skogseid B, Öberg K, et al: Multiple endocrine neoplasia type 1 gene maps to chromosome 11 and is lost in insulinoma. Nature 332:85-87, 1988.
2. Chandrasekharappa SC, Guru SC, Manickam P, et al: Positional cloning of the gene for multiple endocrine neoplasia-type 1. Science 276:404-407, 1997.
3. Knudson AG Jr, Hethcote HW, Brown BW: Mutation and childhood cancer: A probabilistic model for the incidence of retinoblastoma. Proc Natl Acad Sci U S A 72:5116-5120, 1975.
4. Kim YS, Burns AL, Goldsmith PK, et al: Stable overexpression of *MEN1* suppresses tumorigenicity of *RAS*. Oncogene 18:5936-5942, 1999.
5. Elledge SJ, Lin S-Y: Multiple tumor suppressor pathways negatively regulate telomerase. Cell 113:881-889, 2003.
6. Stewart C, Parente F, Piehl F, et al: Characterization of the mouse *Men1* gene and its expression during development. Oncogene 17:2485-2493, 1998.
7. Guru SC, Crabtree JS, Brown KD, et al: Isolation, genomic organization, and expression analysis of Men1, the murine homolog of the *MEN1* gene. Mamm Genome 10:592-596, 1999.
8. Karges W, Maier S, Wissmann A, et al: Primary structure, gene expression and chromosomal mapping of rodent homologs of the *MEN1* tumor suppressor gene. Biochim Biophys Acta 1446:286-294, 1999.
9. Maruyama K, Tsukada T, Hosono T, et al: Structure and distribution of rat menin mRNA. Mol Cell Endocrinol 156:25-33, 1999.
10. Khodaei S, O'Brien KP, Dumanski J, et al: Characterization of the MEN1 ortholog in zebrafish. Biochem Biophys Res Commun 264:404-408, 1999.
11. Manickam P, Vogel AM, Agarwal SK, et al: Isolation, characterization, expression, and functional analysis of the zebrafish ortholog of *MEN1*. Mamm Genome 11:448-454, 2000.
12. Maruyama K, Tsukada T, Honda M, et al: Complementary DNA structure and genomic organization of *Drosophila menini*. Mol Cell Endocrinol 168:135-140, 2000.
13. Crabtree JS, Scacheri PC, Ward JM, et al: A mouse model of multiple endocrine neoplasia, type 1, develops multiple endocrine tumors. Proc Natl Acad Sci U S A 98:1118-1123, 2001.
14. Guru SC, Goldsmith PK, Burns AL, et al: Menin, the product of the *MEN1* gene, is a nuclear protein. Proc Natl Acad Sci U S A 95:1630-1634, 1998.
15. Agarwal SK, Guru SC, Heppner C, et al: Menin interacts with the AP1 transcription factor JunD and represses JunD-activated transcription. Cell 96:143-152, 1999.
16. Gobl AE, Berg M, Lopez-Egido JR, et al: Menin represses JunD-activated transcription by a histone deacetylase-dependent mechanism. Biochim Biophys Acta 1447:51-56, 1999.
17. Kaji H, Canaff L, Lebrun JJ, et al: Inactivation of menin, a Smad3-interacting protein, blocks transforming growth factor type beta signaling. Proc Natl Acad Sci U S A 98:3837-3842, 2001.
18. Heppner C, Bilimoria KY, Agarwal SK, et al: The tumor suppressor protein menin interacts with NF-kappaB proteins and inhibits NF-kappaB-mediated transactivation. Oncogene 20:4917-4925, 2001.
19. Ohkura N, Kishi M, Tsukada T, et al: Menin, a gene product responsible for multiple endocrine neoplasia type 1, inter-

acts with the putative tumor metastasis protein nm23. Biochim Biophys Res Commun 282:1206-1210, 2001.

20. Lemmens IH, Forsberg L, Pannett AA, et al: Menin interacts directly with the homeobox-containing protein Pem. Biochem Biophys Res Commun 286:426-431, 2001.

21. Sukhodolets KE, Hickman AB, Agarwal SK, et al: The 32-kilodalton subunit of replication protein A interacts with menin, the product of the *MEN1* tumor suppressor gene. Mol Cell Biol 23:493-509, 2003.

22. Schussheim DH, Skarulis MC, Agarwal SK, et al: Multiple endocrine neoplasia type 1: New clinical and basic findings. Trends Endocrinol Metab 12:173-178, 2001.

23. Lemmens I, Van de Ven WJM, Kas K, et al: Identification of the multiple endocrine neoplasia type 1 *(MEN1)* gene. Hum Mol Genet 6:1177-1183, 1997.

24. Bassett JHD, Forbes SA, Pannett AAJ, et al: Characterization of mutations in patients with multiple endocrine neoplasia type 1. Am J Hum Genet 62:232-244, 1998.

25. Agarwal SK, Kester MB, Debelenko LV, et al: Germline mutations in the *MEN1* gene in familial multiple endocrine neoplasia type 1 and related states. Hum Mol Genet 6:1169-1175, 1997.

26. Mayr B, Apenberg S, Rothamel T, et al: Menin mutations in patients with multiple endocrine neoplasia. Eur J Endocrinol 137:684-687, 1997.

27. Mutch MG, Dilley WG, Sanjurjo F, et al: Germline mutations in the multiple endocrine neoplasia type 1 gene: Evidence for frequent splicing defects. Hum Mutat 13:175-185, 1999.

28. Olufemi SE, Green JS, Manickam P, et al: Common ancestral mutation in the *MEN1* gene is likely responsible for the pro-lactinoma variant of MEN 1 (MEN1 Burin) in four kindreds from Newfoundland. Hum Mutat 11:264-269, 1998.

29. Kassem M, Kruse TA, Wong FK, et al: Familial isolated hyperparathyroidism as a variant of multiple endocrine neoplasia type 1 in a large Danish pedigree. J Clin Endocrinol Metab 85:165-167, 2000.

30. Brandi M, Marx S, Aurbach A, et al: Familial multiple endocrine neoplasia type 1: A new look at pathophysiology. Endocr Rev 8:391-405, 1987.

31. Majewski JT, Wilson SD: The MEA-I syndrome: An all or none phenomenon. Surgery 86:475-484, 1979.

32. Ballard HS, Frame B, Hartsock RJ: Familial multiple endocrine adenoma-peptic ulcer complex. Medicine 43:481-516, 1964.

33. Wilkinson S, Teh BT, Davey KR, et al: Cause of death in multiple endocrine neoplasia type 1. Arch Surg 128:683, 1993.

34. Doherty GM, Olson JA, Frisella MM, et al: Lethality of multiple endocrine neoplasia type 1. World J Surg 22:581-586, 1997.

35. Rizzoli R, Green J, Marx SJ: Long-term follow-up of serum calcium levels after parathyroidectomy. Am J Med 78:467-473, 1985.

36. Wells SA Jr, Farndon JR, Dale JK, et al: Long-term evaluation of patients with primary parathyroid hyperplasia managed by total parathyroidectomy and heterotopic autotransplantation. Ann Surg 192:451-8, 1980.

37. Kraimps JL, Duh QY, Demeure M, et al: Hyperparathyroidism in multiple endocrine neoplasia syndrome. Surgery 112:1080-1086, 1992.

38. van Heerden JA, Kent RB, Sizemore GW, et al: Primary hyperparathyroidism in patients with multiple endocrine neoplasia syndromes: Surgical experience. Arch Surg 118:533-536, 1983.

39. Herfarth KK-F, Bartsch D, Doherty GM, et al: Surgical management of hyperparathyroidism in patients with multiple endocrine neoplasia type 2A. Surgery 120:966-974, 1996.

40. Mutch MG, Frisella MM, DeBenedetti MK, et al: Pancreatic polypeptide is a useful plasma marker for radiographically evident pancreatic islet cell tumors in patients with multiple endocrine neoplasia type 1. Surgery 122:1012-1020, 1997.

41. Vieto RJ, Hickey RC, Samaan NA: Type 1 multiple endocrine neoplasias. Curr Probl Cancer 7:1-25, 1982.

42. Stabile BE, Morrow DJ, Passaro EJ: The gastrinoma triangle: Operative indications. Am J Surg 147:25-32, 1984.

43. Thompson N, Vinik A, Eckhauser F: Microgastrinomas of the duodenum: A cause of failed operations for the Zollinger-Ellison syndrome. Ann Surg 209:396-404, 1989.

44. Delcore RJ, Cheung LY, Friesen SR: Characteristics of duodenal wall gastrinomas. Am J Surg 160:621-624, 1990.

45. Norton JA, Doppman JL, Jensen RT: Curative resection in Zollinger-Ellison syndrome: Results of a 10-year prospective study. Ann Surg 215:8-18, 1992.

46. Sheppard BC, Norton JA, Doppman JL, et al: Management of islet cell tumors in patients with multiple endocrine neoplasia: A prospective study. Surgery 106:1108-1118, 1989.

47. van Heerden JA, Smith SL, Miller LJ: Management of the Zollinger-Ellison syndrome in patients with multiple endocrine neoplasia type I. Surgery 100:971-977, 1986.

48. Wolfe MM, Jensen RT: Zollinger-Ellison syndrome: Current concepts in diagnosis and management. N Engl J Med 317:1200-1209, 1987.

49. Norton JA, Fraker DL, Alexander R, et al: Surgery to cure the Zollinger-Ellison syndrome. N Engl J Med 341:635-644, 1999.

50. Thompson NW: Current concepts in the surgical management of multiple endocrine neoplasia type 1 pancreatic-duodenal disease: Results in the treatment of 40 patients with Zollinger-Ellison syndrome, hypoglycaemia or both. J Intern Med 243:495-500, 1998.

51. Norton JA, Cornelius MJ, Doppman JL: Effect of parathyroidectomy in patients with hyperparathyroidism and multiple endocrine neoplasia type I. Surgery 102:958-966, 1987.

52. Doppman JL, Miller DL, Chang R, et al: Insulinomas: Localization with selective intraarterial injection of calcium. Radiology 178:237-241, 1991.

53. Cohen MS, Picus D, Lairmore TC, et al: Prospective study of provocative angiograms to localize functional islet cell tumors of the pancreas. Surgery 122:1091-1100, 1997.

54. Grant CS, van Heerden J, Charboneau JW, et al: Insulinoma—the value of intraoperative ultrasonography. Arch Surg 123:843-848, 1988.

55. Norton JA, Cromack DT, Shawker TH, et al: Intraoperative ultrasonographic localization of islet cell tumors. Ann Surg 207:160-168, 1988.

56. Doherty GM, Doppman JL, Shawker TH, et al: Results of a prospective strategy to diagnose, localize, and resect insulinomas. Surgery 110:989-987, 1991.

57. Lairmore TC, Chen VY, DeBenedetti MK, et al: Duodenopancreatic resections in patients with multiple endocrine neoplasia type 1. Ann Surg 231:909-918, 2000.

58. Darling TN, Skarulis MC, Steinberg SM, et al: Multiple facial angiofibromas and collagenomas in patients with multiple endocrine neoplasia type 1. Arch Dermatol 133:853-857, 1997.

59. Moley JF, Lairmore TC, Phay JE: Hereditary endocrinopathies [Review]. Curr Probl Surg 36:653-762, 1999.

60. Howe JR, Norton JA, Wells SAJ: Prevalence of pheochromocytoma and hyperparathyroidism in multiple endocrine neoplasia type 2A: Results of long-term follow-up. Surgery 114:1070-1077, 1993.

61. Robinson MF, Furst EJ, Nunziata V, et al: Characterization of the clinical features of five families with hereditary primary

cutaneous lichen amyloidosis and multiple endocrine neoplasia type 2. Henry Ford Hosp Med J 40:249-252, 1992.

62. Eng C, Mulligan LM: Mutations of the *RET* Proto-oncogene in the multiple endocrine neoplasia type 2 syndromes, related sporadic tumors, and Hirschsprung disease. Hum Mutat 9:97-109, 1997.

63. Edery P, Lyonnet S, Mulligan L, et al: Mutations of the *RET* proto-oncogene in Hirschsprung's disease. Nature 367:378-380, 1994.

64. Romeo G, Ronchetto P, Luo Y, et al: Point mutations affecting the tyrosine kinase domain of the *RET* proto-oncogene in Hirschsprung's disease. Nature 367:377-378, 1994.

65. Norton JA, Froome LC, Farrell RE, et al: Multiple endocrine neoplasia type IIb. Symp Endocr Surg 59:109-118, 1979.

66. O'Riordain DS, O'Brien T, Crotty TB, et al: Multiple endocrine neoplasia type 2B: More than an endocrine disorder. Surgery 118:936-942, 1995.

67. Farndon JR, Leight GS, Dilley WG, et al: Familial medullary thyroid carcinoma without associated endocrinopathies: A distinct clinical entity. Br J Surg 73:278-281, 1986.

68. Wells S, Haagensen D, Linehan W, et al: The detection of elevated plasma levels of carcinoembryonic antigen in patients with suspected or established medullary thyroid carcinoma. Cancer 42:1498, 1978.

69. Wells SA, Chi DD, Toshima K, et al: Predictive DNA testing and prophylactic thyroidectomy in patients at risk for multiple endocrine neoplasia type 2A. Ann Surg 220:237-250, 1994.

70. Gagel RF, Tashjian AHJ, Cummings T, et al: The clinical outcome of prospective screening for multiple endocrine neoplasia type 2A, an 18-year experience. N Engl J Med 318:478-484, 1988.

71. Moley JF, DeBenedetti MK: Patterns of nodal metastases in palpable medullary thyroid carcinoma: Recommendations for extent of node dissection. Ann Surg 229:880-888, 1999.

72. Bergholm U, Adami HO, Bergstrom R, et al: Clinical characteristics in sporadic and familial medullary thyroid carcinoma. Cancer 63:1196-1204, 1989.

73. Cohen MS, Phay JE, Albinson C, et al: Gastrointestinal manifestations of multiple endocrine neoplasia type 2. Ann Surg 235:648-654, 2002.

74. Donis-Keller H, Dou S, Chi D, et al: Mutations in the *RET* proto-oncogene are associated with MEN 2A and FMTC. Hum Mol Genet 2:851-856, 1993.

75. Mulligan L, Kwok J, Healy C: Germ-line mutations of the *RET* protooncogene in multiple endocrine neoplasia type 2A (MEN 2A). Nature 363:458-460, 1993.

76. Mulligan LM, Eng C, Healey CS, et al: Specific mutations of the *RET* proto-oncogene are related to disease phenotype in MEN 2A and FMTC. Nat Genet 6:70-74, 1994.

77. Libroa I: Familial medullary thyroid carcinoma, clinical management. *In* Seventh International Workshop on Multiple Endocrine Neoplasia. Gubbio, Italy, 1999, pp 113-118.

78. Saad MF, Ordonez NG, Rashid RK, et al: Medullary carcinoma of the thyroid: A study of the clinical features and prognostic factors in 161 patients. Medicine 63:319-342, 1984.

79. Wells S, Baylin S, Linehan W, et al: Provocative agents and the diagnosis of medullary carcinoma of the thyroid gland. Ann Surg 188:139-141, 1978.

80. Wells SA, Baylin SB, Gann DS: Medullary thyroid carcinoma: Relationship of method of diagnosis to pathologic staging. Ann Surg 188:377, 1978.

81. Ledger GA, Khosla S, Lindor NM, et al: Genetic testing in the diagnosis and management of multiple endocrine neoplasia type II. Ann Intern Med 122:118-124, 1995.

82. Mitchell DG, Crovello M, Matteucci T, et al: Benign adrenocortical masses: Diagnosis with chemical shift MR imaging. Radiology 185:345, 1992.

83. Olson JA, DeBenedetti MK, Baumann DS, et al: Parathyroid autotransplantation during thyroidectomy: Results of long-term follow-up. Ann Surg 223:472-477, 1996.

84. Lips C, Landsvater R, Hoppener J, et al: Clinical screening as compared with DNA analysis in families with multiple endocrine neoplasia type 2A. N Engl J Med 331:828-835, 1994.

85. Frilling A, Dralle H, Eng C, et al: Presymptomatic DNA screening in families with multiple endocrine neoplasia type 2 and familial medullary thyroid carcinoma. Surgery 118:1099-1104, 1995.

86. Dralle H, Gimm O, Simon D, et al: Prophylactic thyroidectomy in 75 children with hereditary medullary thyroid carcinoma: German and Austrian experience. World J Surg 22:744-751, 1998.

87. Dralle H: Lymph node dissection and medullary thyroid carcinoma. Br J Surg 89:1073-1075, 2002.

88. Tisell L, Hansson G, Jansson S, et al: Reoperation in the treatment of asymptomatic metastasizing medullary thyroid carcinoma. Surgery 99:60-66, 1986.

89. Moley JF, Dilley WG, DeBenedetti MK, et al: Improved results of cervical reoperation for medullary thyroid carcinoma. Ann Surg 225:734-740, 1997.

90. Musholt T, Musholt P, Dehdashti F, et al: Evaluation of FDG-PET scan and its association with glucose transporter expression in medullary thyroid cancer and pheochromocytoma—a clinical and molecular study. Surgery 122:1049-1061, 1997.

91. Tung WS, Vesely TM, Moley JF, et al: Laparoscopic detection of hepatic metastases in patients with residual or recurrent medullary thyroid cancer. Surgery 118:1024-1029, 1995.

92. Lairmore TC, Ball DW, Baylin SB, et al: Management of pheochromocytomas in patients with multiple endocrine neoplasia type 2 syndromes. Ann Surg 217:595-603, 1993.

93. Gagner M, Lacroix A, Prinz RA, et al: Early experience with laparoscopic approach for adrenalectomy. Surgery 114:1120-1125, 1993.

94. Brunt LM, Doherty GM, Norton JA, et al: Laparoscopic adrenalectomy compared to open adrenalectomy for benign adrenal neoplasms. J Am Coll Surg 183:1-10, 1996.

95. Brunt LM, Lairmore TC, Doherty GM, et al: Adrenalectomy for familial pheochromocytoma in the laparoscopic era. Ann Surg 235:713-720, 2002.

96. Moley JF, Lairmore TC, Doherty GM, et al: Preservation of the recurrent laryngeal nerves in thyroid and parathyroid reoperations. Surgery 126:673-679, 1999.

97. Eisenhofer G, Lenders JW, Linehan WM, et al: Plasma normetanephrine and metanephrine for detecting pheochromocytoma in von Hippel-Lindau disease and multiple endocrine neoplasia type 2. N Engl J Med 340:1872-1879, 1999.

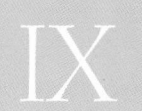
ESOPHAGUS

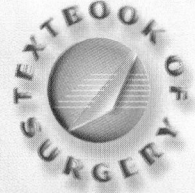

CHAPTER 39

ESOPHAGUS

Joseph B. Zwischenberger, M.D.,   Clare Savage, M.D.,

and   Manoop S. Bhutani, M.D.

| Anatomy | Diseases |
| Physiology | |

ANATOMY

Esophagus

The *embryonic esophagus* forms when paired longitudinal grooves appear on each side of the laryngotracheal diverticulum, grow medially, and fuse to form the tracheoesophageal septum. This septum divides the foregut into the ventral laryngotracheal tube and the dorsal esophagus. Esophageal elongation occurs rapidly, with the final length attained by the seventh gestational week. The striated muscle of the upper esophagus is derived from the caudal branchial arches and is innervated by the vagus nerve. The smooth muscle of the lower esophagus arises from splanchnic mesenchyme and is supplied by a visceral nerve plexus derived from neural crest cells. The position of the vagus nerve on the esophagus results from unequal growth of the greater curve of the stomach relative to the lesser curve, with consequent rotation of the left vagus anteriorly and of the right vagus posteriorly.

The *esophagus* is a hollow tube of muscle 25 to 30 cm long, beginning at C6 (cricoid cartilage level) and ending at T11, that penetrates the diaphragm and joins the cardia of the stomach (Fig. 39-1). The esophagus lies anterior to the vertebral column and longus colli muscles, posterior to the trachea, and adjacent to the descending aorta. It is divided into four segments: pharyngoesophageal, cervical, thoracic, and abdominal. The length between the laryngopharynx and cervical esophagus is the pharyngoesophageal segment. The pharyngeal musculature includes the superior, middle, and inferior constrictors, as well as the stylopharyngeus muscles. The inferior pharyngeal constrictor (thyropharyngeus muscle) passes obliquely and superiorly from its origin on the thyroid cartilage to its posterior insertion in the median raphe. The

esophageal introitus (cricopharyngeus muscle or upper esophageal sphincter) is the most inferior portion of the inferior pharyngeal constrictor and is identifiable by the transverse direction of its fibers. The transition between the oblique fibers of the thyropharyngeus muscle and the transverse fibers of the cricopharyngeus muscle creates a point of potential weakness (Killian's triangle) in the pharyngoesophageal segment (site of origin of a Zenker diverticulum and a common site of perforation during esophagoscopy). The cricopharyngeal sphincter is unique to the gastrointestinal tract because it does not consist of a circular ring of muscle, but rather it is a bow of muscle connecting the two lateral borders of the cricoid cartilage. The cricopharyngeus muscle fibers blend into the longitudinal and circular muscle of the cervical esophagus, a 5- to 6-cm segment that extends to the beginning of the first thoracic vertebra.

Although the cervical esophagus is a midline structure positioned posterior to the trachea, it courses to the left of the trachea and is therefore more easily approached through a left-sided neck incision. The cervical esophagus lies just anterior to the prevertebral fascia and can normally be separated from its loose fibrous posterior attachments by blunt finger dissection of the prevertebral space. On each side of the cervical esophagus lie the carotid sheath and the thyroid gland, with the recurrent laryngeal nerves passing bilaterally in the groove between the esophagus and the trachea.

The thoracic esophagus passes into the posterior mediastinum, behind the aortic arch and great vessels, and curves to the left of the trachea behind the left mainstem bronchus. It then deviates to the right in the subcarinal area for several centimeters and returns to the left of midline and anterior to the thoracic aorta as it proceeds behind the pericardium to the level of the seventh thoracic vertebra. At this point, the esophagus deviates

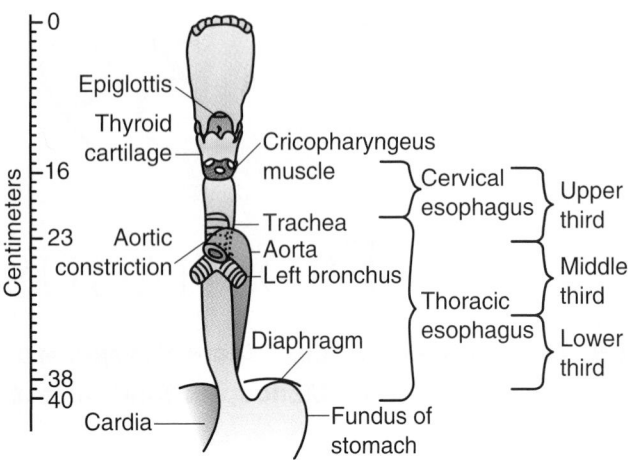

FIGURE 39-1. Normal anatomy of the esophagus.

farther to the left and anteriorly, entering the esophageal diaphragmatic hiatus at the level of the 11th thoracic vertebra. The lateral boundaries of the thoracic esophagus are the right and left parietal pleurae.

The *diaphragmatic esophageal hiatus* is a sling of muscle fibers that arise from the right crus or both the right and left crura. The abdominal esophagus (1 to 2 cm long) extends from the esophageal hiatus to the cardia of the stomach to form the *esophagogastric junction.* The location of the esophagogastric junction has been defined in different ways: (1) the junction of esophageal squamous and gastric columnar epithelium; (2) the point at which the tubular esophagus joins the gastric pouch; and (3) the junction of the esophageal circular muscle layer with the oblique sling fibers of the stomach (loop of Willis or collar of Helvetius). Clinically, the squamocolumnar epithelial junction (ora serrata or Z line), as identified endoscopically, is the most practical definition of the gastroesophageal junction, provided the patient does not have a columnar-lined lower esophagus. The *phrenoesophageal membrane* is a fibroelastic sheet of tissue that extends circumferentially from the muscular margins of the diaphragmatic hiatus to the esophagus. The majority of the phrenoesophageal membrane arises from the endoabdominal fascia and inserts into the esophagus for 2 to 3 cm above the hiatus and 3 to 5 cm above the mucosal junction. Fibrous strands from the upper surface of the diaphragm (fascia of Laimer) contribute to the phrenoesophageal membrane. The functional significance of the phrenoesophageal membrane is unknown; however, this tissue lacks sufficient strength to reliably anchor the esophagogastric junction in the abdomen during an antireflux operation.

The esophagus has three distinct areas of anatomic narrowing. The *cervical constriction* occurs at the level of the cricopharyngeal sphincter, the narrowest point of the gastrointestinal tract (14 mm in diameter). The *bronchoaortic constriction* (15 to 17 mm) is located at the level of the fourth thoracic vertebra behind the tracheal bifurcation where the left mainstem bronchus and the aortic arch abut the esophagus. The *diaphragmatic constriction* (16 to 19 mm) occurs where the esophagus trav-

erses the diaphragm. Between these areas of constriction, the esophagus has a wider caliber, termed the *superior* and *inferior dilatations.* The normal adult thoracic esophagus has a maximum diameter of approximately 2.5 cm on barium swallow examination.

The esophagus is a mucosal-lined muscular tube that lacks a serosa and is surrounded by a layer of loose fibroalveolar adventitia. Beneath the adventitia is a layer of longitudinal muscle overlying an inner layer of circular muscle. Between the two muscular layers is a thin intramuscular septum of connective tissue that contains fine blood vessels and ganglion cells (Auerbach plexus). Both the longitudinal and the circular muscle layers of the upper third of the esophagus are striated, whereas the layers of the lower two thirds are smooth. The fatty and relatively thick submucosa permits considerable mobility of the esophageal mucosa. The submucosa contains the mucous glands, blood vessels, the Meissner neural plexus, and an extensive lymphatic network. The esophageal mucosa consists of squamous epithelium except for the distal 1 to 2 cm, which is junctional columnar epithelium. Occasionally, ectopic gastric mucosa may be found throughout the length of the esophagus.

The esophagus is nourished by numerous segmental arteries, all of which contribute to the extensive capillary network (Fig. 39-2). The cervical esophagus receives blood from the superior thyroid artery as well as the inferior thyroid artery of the thyrocervical trunk, with both sides communicating through collateral vessels. The major blood supply of the thoracic esophagus is from four to six aortic esophageal arteries, supplemented by collateral vessels from the inferior thyroid, intercostal and

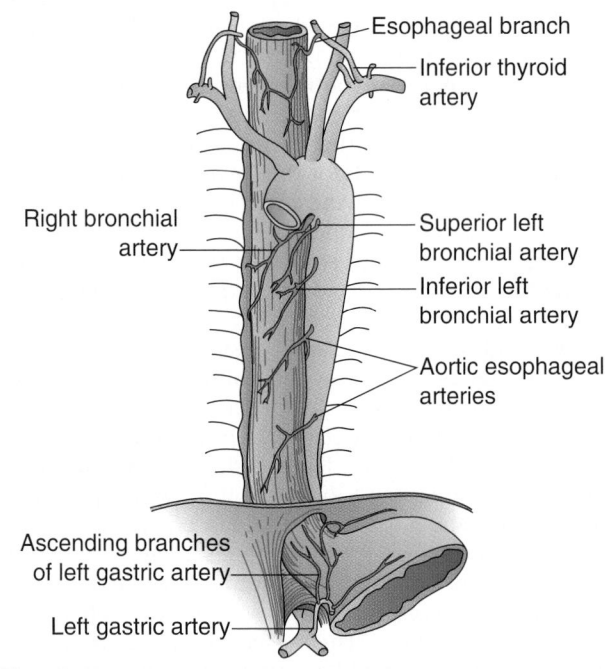

FIGURE 39-2. Arterial blood supply of the esophagus. (Adapted from Hagen JA, DeMeester TR: Anatomy of the esophagus. *In* Shields TW, LoCicero J III, Ponn RB [eds]: General Thoracic Surgery, 5th ed, vol 2. Philadelphia, Lippincott Williams & Wilkins, 2000, p 1599.)

bronchial, inferior phrenic, and left gastric arteries. The aortic esophageal arteries terminate in fine capillary networks before they actually penetrate the esophageal muscle layer. After penetrating and supplying the muscle layers of the esophagus, the esophageal capillary network runs longitudinally in the submucosa. The extensive venous drainage of the esophagus includes the hypopharyngeal, azygous, hemiazygous, intercostal, and gastric veins (Fig. 39-3).

The esophagus has both sympathetic and parasympathetic innervation (Fig. 39-4). In the neck, the superior laryngeal nerves arise from the vagus nerve and divide into the external and internal laryngeal branches. The external laryngeal nerve innervates the cricothyroid muscle and also, in part, the inferior pharyngeal constrictor. The internal laryngeal nerve is the sensory nerve of the pharyngeal surface of the larynx and the base of the tongue. The recurrent laryngeal branches of the vagus nerve provide parasympathetic innervation to the cervical esophagus as well as innervation to the upper esophageal sphincter. Injury to the recurrent laryngeal nerve may result in hoarseness as well as upper esophageal sphincter dysfunction, with secondary aspiration on swallowing. In the thorax, the vagus nerve sends fibers to the striated muscle as well as parasympathetic preganglionic fibers to the smooth muscle. Sympathetic innervation consists of fibers to the cervical esophagus from the superior and inferior cervical sympathetic ganglia, to the thoracic esophagus from the upper thoracic and splanchnic nerves, and to the intra-abdominal esophagus from the celiac ganglion. The Meissner and Auerbach plexuses provide an intrinsic autonomic nervous system within the esophageal wall. The

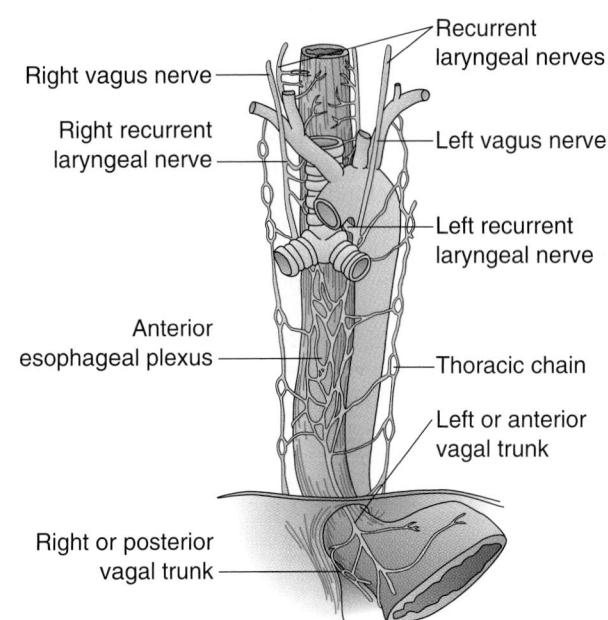

FIGURE 39-4. Innervation of the esophagus. (Adapted from Hagen JA, DeMeester TR: Anatomy of the esophagus. *In* Shields TW, LoCicero J III, Ponn RB [eds]: General Thoracic Surgery, 5th ed, vol 2. Philadelphia, Lippincott Williams & Wilkins, 2000, p 1599.)

Meissner plexus of nerves is located in the submucosa, whereas the Auerbach plexus is in the connective tissue between the circular and longitudinal muscle layers. The two major branches of the vagus nerve lie along either side of the thoracic esophagus and form two large nerve plexuses supplying the esophagus and the lungs. The esophageal vagus plexuses coalesce and become single trunks, 2 to 6 cm above the esophageal hiatus. The left branch of the vagus nerve lies anterior to the esophagus, and the right branch is posterior, at the diaphragmatic hiatus.

The esophagus has an extensive lymphatic drainage that consists of two lymphatic plexuses, one arising in the mucosa and the other in the muscular layer. Mucosal lymphatic capillaries pierce the muscular layer and drain to regional lymph nodes. These lymphatic capillaries run longitudinally in the esophageal wall before they exit through muscle into adjacent lymph nodes. The flow of lymphatics of the upper two thirds of the esophagus tends to be upward, whereas the distal third tends to be downward; however, all lymphatics intercommunicate. Therefore, esophageal carcinomas may spread directly to internal jugular nodes in the neck, paratracheal nodes in the superior mediastinum, subcarinal nodes in the middle chest, paraesophageal nodes in the lower mediastinum, and inferior pulmonary ligament, perigastric, and left gastric artery lymph nodes.

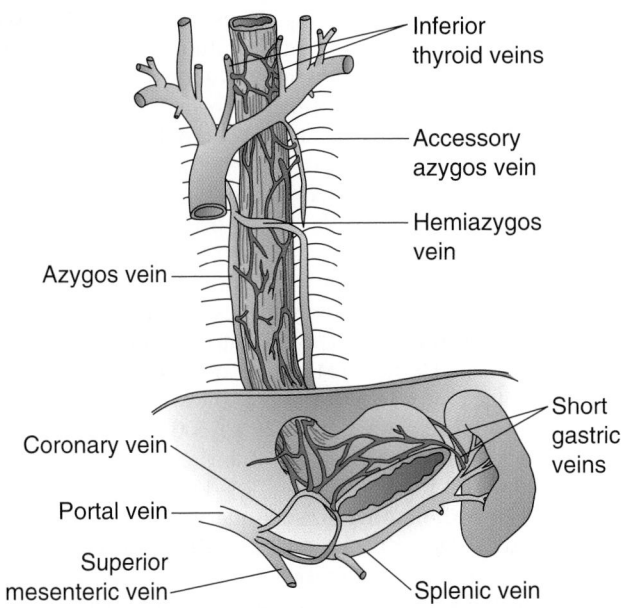

FIGURE 39-3. Venous drainage of the esophagus. (Adapted from Hagen JA, DeMeester TR: Anatomy of the esophagus. *In* Shields TW, LoCicero J III, Ponn RB [eds]: General Thoracic Surgery, 5th ed, vol 2. Philadelphia, Lippincott Williams & Wilkins, 2000, p 1599.)

Thoracic Duct

The proximity of the thoracic duct to the esophagus makes it vulnerable to injury during esophageal surgery.

The *thoracic duct* forms at the confluence of the cisterna chyli at a level between the T12 and L2 vertebrae and to the right side of the abdominal aorta. The duct enters the posterior mediastinum through the aortic hiatus at the level of T10 to T12 and continues cephalad on the anterior surface of the vertebral column between the aorta and the azygos vein and behind the esophagus. At T4 to T5, the duct crosses to the left of the spine, passes under the aortic arch, and continues along the left side of the esophagus, to ascend into the neck posterior to the left subclavian artery. In the neck, the duct lies anterior to the vertebral artery and vein, thyrocervical trunk, and phrenic nerve, and it enters the venous system at the junction of the left subclavian and left internal jugular veins. Operations on the thoracic esophagus, particularly after previous surgery or radiation therapy with consequent periesophageal fibrosis, may result in chylothorax from thoracic duct injury.

PHYSIOLOGY

The basic function of the esophagus is to transport swallowed material from the pharynx into the stomach. Secondarily, gastric reflux into the esophagus is prevented by the lower esophageal sphincter (LES). The entry of air into the esophagus with each inspiration is prevented by the upper esophageal sphincter (UES), which normally remains closed as a result of tonic contraction of the cricopharyngeus muscle. Intraesophageal pressures, including the amplitude and length of the UES and LES, the extent and duration of relaxation of these sphincters with swallowing, and the characteristics of peristaltic activity in the body of the esophagus, can be measured with a multilumen motility catheter (Fig. 39-5). Micropressure transducers, fastened directly along recording catheters, are extremely accurate and are more sensitive to pressure changes within the esophagus than water-perfused systems. Although esophageal motility studies have become a basic diagnostic tool in evaluating disorders of esophageal motor function such as dysphagia, chest pain of undetermined origin, and gastroesophageal reflux, many factors affect the pressures recorded from patient to patient and from one laboratory to another. These variables include catheter size, the character of the swallowed bolus (e.g., hot vs. cold liquid, dry vs. wet swallow), and resting time between swallows.[1] The quantitative values obtained from esophageal manometry are not absolute, and this study provides but one additional bit of corroborative information to be used along with the patient's medical history, results of barium swallow, and endoscopic findings in the assessment of esophageal function.

Swallowing is a complex, rapid series of events that has been divided radiologically into six phases.[2] The rapidity of these events causes difficulty in measuring pharyngeal function precisely.[3] The UES is 2.5 to 4.5 cm in length and has a basal resting pressure ranging from 16 to 118 mm Hg (mean, 42 mm Hg) and a duration of relaxation with swallowing of 0.5 to 1.2 seconds. Contraction of the UES after the relaxation phase produces intraluminal pressures that are often twice as high as resting pres-

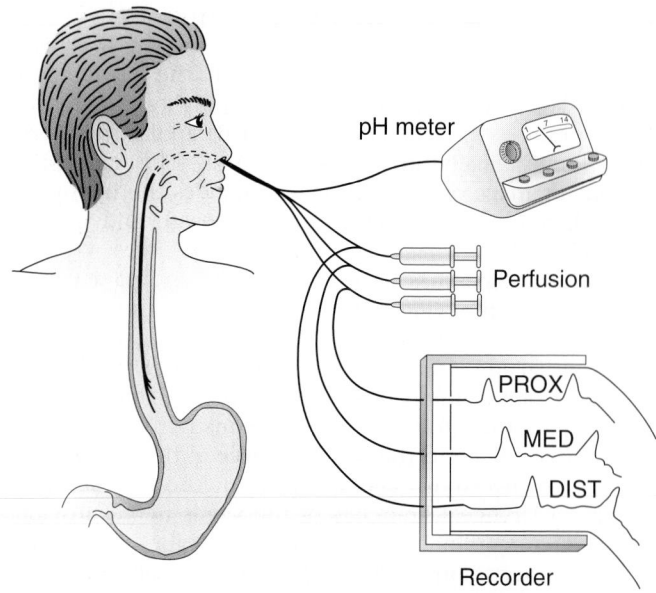

FIGURE 39-5.   Combined manometric-pH recording system used in the evaluation of esophageal function. The triple-lumen perfused recording catheter measures intraluminal pressures from three levels in the esophagus. Measurements are made in terms of centimeters from the nostrils to the proximal opening of the recording catheter (PROX). The medial catheter (MED) records pressures 5 cm distal to the proximal opening, and the distal catheter (DIST) 5 cm below this. The intraesophageal pH electrode is used to document gastroesophageal reflux.

sures and last 2 to 4 seconds. Three types of contractions are seen in the esophageal body. *Primary peristalsis* is progressive and is triggered by voluntary swallowing. *Secondary peristalsis* is also progressive, but it is generated by distention or irritation, not by voluntary swallowing. *Tertiary contractions* are nonprogressive (simultaneous) contractions that may occur either after voluntary swallowing or spontaneously between swallows. As the swallowed bolus enters the esophagus from the pharynx, a primary peristaltic wave is activated that traverses the esophageal body at a speed of 2 to 5 cm/sec and propels the swallowed material from the pharynx into the stomach in 4 to 8 seconds in an orderly, progressive manner (Fig. 39-6). Normally, a progressive peristaltic contraction (primary wave) follows 97% of all wet swallows.[4]

Pressure within the body of the esophagus is a reflection of negative intrathoracic pressure, being maximally negative (−5 to −10 mm Hg) during deep inspiration and highest (0 to 5 mm Hg) during expiration. Esophageal peristaltic pressure ranges from 20 to 100 mm Hg, with a duration of contraction between 2 and 4 seconds.[4] If the entire swallowed bolus of food does not empty from the esophagus into the stomach, secondary peristaltic waves are initiated. These contractions, like the primary waves, are progressive and sequential, but they begin in the smooth muscle segment of the esophagus (near the level of the aortic arch) and continue until retained intraesophageal contents are emptied into the stomach. Thus, unlike the primary wave, the secondary contraction is not initiated by a voluntary swallow but by local distention of the esophagus. Tertiary contractions are simul-

Progressive Peristalsis

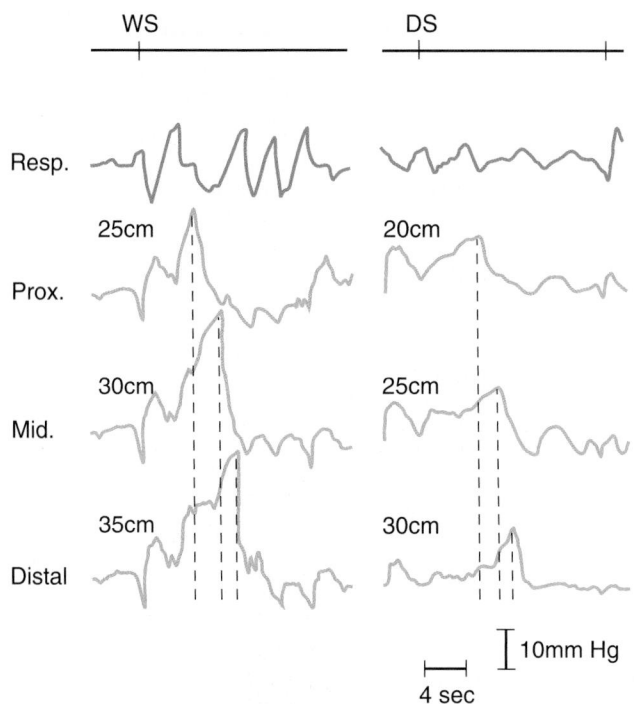

Normal HPZ

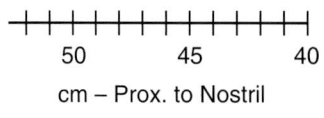

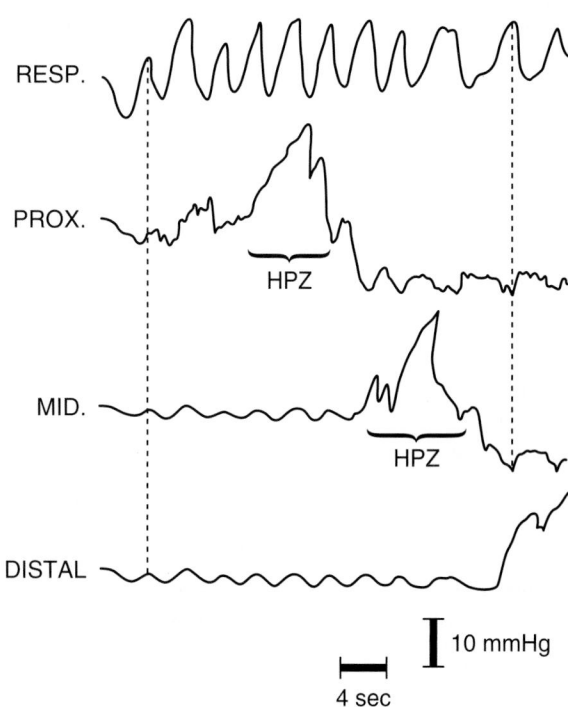

FIGURE 39-6. Motility tracing shows normal peristalsis. With each swallow, a progressive esophageal contraction is generated, passing first by the proximal recording port (PROX.), then the middle (MID.), and finally the distal port. DS, dry swallow; RESP., respiration; WS, wet swallow.

FIGURE 39-7. Motility tracing shows normal distal sphincter mechanism or high-pressure zone (HPZ). As the recording catheter is withdrawn from the stomach into the esophagus, the HPZ is identified sequentially in each catheter. Mean basal pressure within the thoracic esophagus is lower than that within the stomach (below the diaphragm). Below the diaphragm, within the stomach, a positive deflection is seen during respiratory excursions at the peak of inspiration (when diaphragm is lowest). Conversely, in the esophagus, at the peak of inspiration, intrathoracic pressure is maximally negative and a negative deflection during inspiration is observed (*dotted lines*). MID., middle; PROX., proximal; RESP., respiration.

taneous, nonprogressive, nonperistaltic, monophasic, or multiphasic waves that can occur throughout the esophagus and represent uncoordinated contractions of the smooth muscle that are responsible for the classic "corkscrew" appearance of esophageal spasm on barium swallow examination.

The term *lower esophageal sphincter* implies an anatomic sphincter such as the pylorus. Although no such *anatomic* LES is present, manometry has defined an elevated distal esophageal resting pressure that is 3 to 5 cm in length, which serves as the barrier against abnormal gastroesophageal reflux and represents a *functional* sphincter (Fig. 39-7). Thus, the LES is more accurately referred to as the *LES mechanism* or the *distal esophageal high-pressure zone* (HPZ). The factors responsible for maintaining competence of the LES are poorly understood. Most antireflux procedures rely on an intra-abdominal segment of esophagus to prevent reflux.

Normal resting pressure within the HPZ ranges from 10 to 20 mm Hg, but no absolute value predicts competence or incompetence of the LES mechanism. Patients with no gastroesophageal reflux may have an extremely low HPZ amplitude on manometric recordings, whereas others with massive reflux may have seemingly high distal pressures. This inconsistency is a reflection of both HPZ variation from individual body habitus and the radial asymmetry of the LES that results in varied readings during pull-

through determinations, depending on the orientation of the catheter recording port. Mean HPZ pressures less than 6 mm Hg and overall sphincter length less than 2 cm are likely to be associated with incompetence of the LES and gastroesophageal reflux.

The distal HPZ is located in the region of the diaphragmatic hiatus. The distal portion of the sphincter demonstrates respiratory variations like those in the abdomen —increased pressure with inspiration and decreased pressure with expiration. In the proximal portion of the HPZ, however, one notes an intrathoracic pattern of respiratory variation, namely, negative pressure with inspiration and positive pressure with expiration. The terms *point of respiratory reversal* and *pressure inversion point* are used to designate the site at which this transition in respiratory pattern occurs on manometric tracings. In patients who lack a distal HPZ, the pressure inversion

Relaxation of HPZ with Swallowing

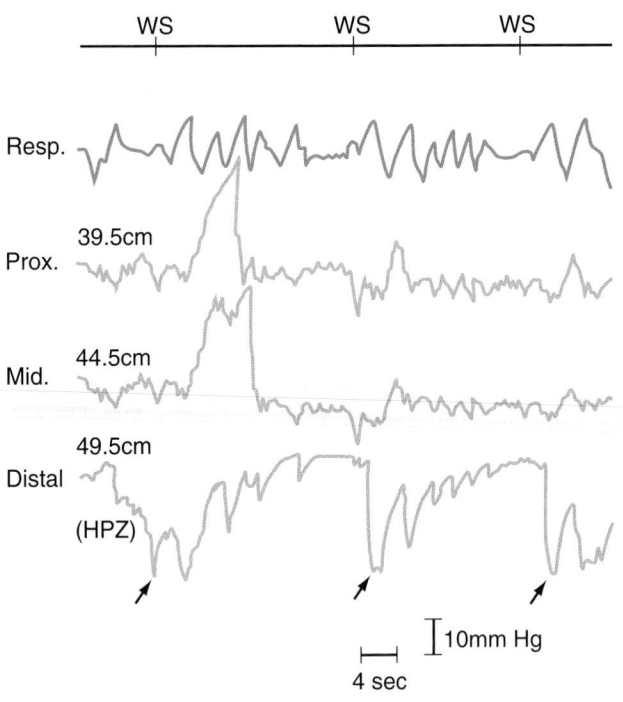

FIGURE 39-8. Motility tracing shows normal relaxation of the distal high-pressure zone (HPZ) with swallowing. The distal recording port is within the HPZ (49.5 cm from the nostrils). Each swallow normally results in relaxation of the HPZ *(arrows)*, followed by a sustained postdeglutitive contraction, after which pressure again returns to basal levels. MID., middle; PROX., proximal; RESP., respiration; WS, wet swallow.

point is used as a reference point indicative of the cardia, 5 cm above which the pH electrode can be positioned for acid reflux testing. Within 1.5 to 2.5 seconds after a swallow is initiated, distal HPZ relaxation occurs and lasts 4 to 6 seconds (Fig. 39-8). A post-deglutitive contraction then occurs that generates pressures of 25 to 35 mm Hg for 7 to 10 seconds, after which HPZ tone returns to resting levels. Distal HPZ pressure varies continually in everyone and is influenced by a host of neural, hormonal, myogenic, mechanical, and environmental factors (Table 39-1).

DISEASES

Vascular Rings

Vascular rings usually become apparent during early adult life as esophageal obstruction. Barium swallow or endoscopy reveals a typical constriction of the esophagus at the aortic arch and great vessels, and angiography or magnetic resonance imaging (MRI) usually shows which vessels are involved. The definitive treatment, if dysphagia is persistent or progressive, is to divide the vascular ring by a transthoracic procedure. The anatomy and repair

TABLE 39-1.   Factors Affecting Distal High-Pressure Zone Tone

Factors	Increased Tone	Decreased Tone
Hormonal	Gastrin	Vasoactive intestinal polypeptide
	Motilin	Secretin
	Prostaglandin F_{2a}	Cholecystokinin
	Bombesin	Glucagon
	Substance P	Progesterone
	Histamine	Estrogen
		Prostaglandins E_1, E_2, A_1
Drug-related	Caffeine	α-Adrenergic blockers
	α-Adrenergic agents	Phentolamine
	Norepinephrine	Anticholinergics
	Phenylephrine	Atropine
	Anticholinesterase	Theophylline
	Edrophonium	β-Adrenergic blockers
	Cholinergic agents	Isoproterenol
	Bethanechol	Meperidine
	Methacholine	H_2-Blocker
	Betazole	Calcium-channel blockers
	Metoclopramide	Dopamine
		Ethanol
		Epinephrine
		Nicotine
		Nitroglycerin
Food-related	Protein meal	Fatty meal
		Ethanol
		Chocolate
Myogenic	Normal resting muscle tone	?Aging
		?Diabetes mellitus
Mechanical	Antireflux operation	Hiatal hernia
		Abnormal phrenoesophageal ligament insertion
		Short or absent intra-abdominal distal esophageal segment
		Nasogastric tube
Miscellaneous	Gastric alkalinization	Gastric acidification
	Gastric distention	Gastrectomy
		Hypoglycemia
		Hypothyroidism
		Amyloidosis
		Pernicious anemia
		Epidermolysis bullosa

Adapted from Hurwitz AL, Haddad JK: Disorders of Esophageal Motility. Philadelphia, WB Saunders, 1979, p 120

can be complex because the abnormality often involves aberrant great vessels.

Esophageal Webs

Upper Esophageal Webs (Plummer-Vinson Syndrome)

Plummer-Vinson syndrome *(sideropenic dysphagia)* refers to the development of cervical dysphagia in patients with chronic iron-deficiency anemia. These patients are usually edentulous, malnourished women older than 40 years of age with atrophic oral mucosa, glossitis, and brittle, spoon-shaped fingernails *(koilonychia).* The cause of dysphagia is usually a cervical esophageal web, but abnormal pharyngeal and esophageal motility may also play a role. Treatment consists of esophageal dilatation and correction of the nutritional deficiency. This syndrome is regarded as a premalignant lesion because approximately 10% of patients develop squamous cell carcinoma of the hypopharynx, oral cavity, or esophagus.[5]

Lower Esophageal Webs (Schatzki's Ring)

Distal esophageal webs, or a *Schatzki ring,* occur at the squamocolumnar epithelial junction and are seen radiographically on a barium swallow because the squamocolumnar junction is above the diaphragm due to a hiatal hernia (Fig. 39-9 [also see Fig. 39-19]). The presence of a ring does not predict either gastroesophageal reflux or esophagitis. These lesions appear as annular strictures that project into the esophageal lumen at a right angle to the long axis of the lower esophagus. Most patients are asymptomatic, although intermittent dysphagia may occur when the ring diameter is less than 20 mm (the critical ring diameter at which dysphagia invariably occurs is less than 13 mm). The web involves only the mucosa and submucosa, not the esophageal muscle. Histologically, one sees only a slight amount of increased submucosal fibrosis beneath the squamocolumnar epithelium.[6]

Many patients with dysphagia have no reflux symptoms and respond to intermittent esophageal bougienage. Others, especially with dysphagia and reflux, require periodic dilatations and antireflux medical therapy. In those with refractory dysphagia or gastroesophageal reflux disease (GERD) that fails to respond to medical therapy, intraoperative dilatation with an antireflux procedure is indicated. Resection of the ring alone, without repair of the associated hiatal hernia, will fail because the inciting cause of reflux is not addressed.

Congenital Webs

Congenital esophageal webs are rare lesions that usually present as inability to feed with regurgitation during infancy, although some remain asymptomatic until adulthood. Symptomatic webs may be successfully disrupted by endoscopic or oral dilatation. Rarely, dense webs within the body of the esophagus require transthoracic resection.

Esophageal Cysts and Duplications

Esophageal congenital cysts form during the embryonic process of separation of the pulmonary tree and the esophagus from their common origin. These cysts are theoretically separable into three categories: duplications, bronchogenic cysts, and neurenteric cysts. Because of the difficulty in distinguishing one type of cyst from another, these can be considered collectively as *duplication cysts.* Cysts can be found at any location, but those associated with the intrathoracic esophagus are the most common. Cyst size, shape, and degree of connection to the esophagus are all highly variable, although communication with the true lumen is uncommon. In adults, most cysts are asymptomatic and are found incidentally when a posterior mediastinal mass is identified on a chest radiograph.[7] However, duplications can cause dysphagia when they are large enough, become infected, perforate, or bleed if they contain gastric mucosa. In infants, pulmonary compromise can be caused by airway compression.

The natural history of esophageal cysts is variable. Malignant degeneration has been reported, but because the incidence appears extremely low, duplication cysts are considered benign. The possibilities of enlargement, infection, and bleeding warrant removal for most patients. Open thoracotomy and video-assisted thoracoscopic (VATS) techniques can be used similar to leiomyoma excision (see Fig. 39-28). If the wall of the cyst cannot be separated from the common esophageal wall, it may be left behind, but the mucosa of the cyst should be stripped away to prevent cyst recurrence. Marsupialization of the cyst with internal drainage and cauterization of the mucosa are alternative methods of management. The long-term results of resection are excellent, and recurrence is rare if the initial excision is complete. Alternatively, endoscopic ultrasound (EUS) or computed tomography (CT)-guided aspiration, cytologic evaluation, and follow-up have been used successfully.[8]

Disorders of Esophageal Motility

Disorders of esophageal motility are *functional* disorders that interfere with swallowing or produce dysphagia without any intraluminal organic obstruction or

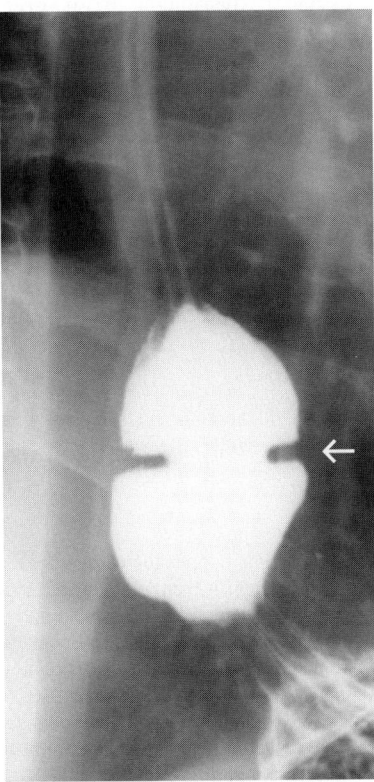

FIGURE 39-9. Esophagogram shows a distal esophageal (Schatzki) ring *(arrow)*. (Courtesy of Ronelle A. Dubrow, M.D., MD Anderson Cancer Center, Houston, TX.)

extrinsic compression. Barium swallow examination, esophagoscopy, and esophageal function tests, including manometry and intraesophageal pH reflux testing, constitute the basic evaluation for suspected esophageal motility disorders.

Upper Esophageal Sphincter Dysfunction

The terms *oropharyngeal dysphagia* and *cricopharyngeal dysfunction* describe the symptom complex that occurs when patients have difficulty swallowing liquid or solid food from the oropharynx into the upper esophagus. The causes of this difficulty include abnormalities of the central and peripheral nervous system, metabolic and inflammatory myopathy, gastroesophageal reflux, and complications of neck or thoracic surgery. Anatomically related causes of upper esophageal dysphagia, such as carcinoma, caustic stricture, cervical vertebral bone spurs, thyromegaly, and trauma, should be excluded. A purely psychological cause of a complaint of cervical dysphagia, *globus hystericus*, is a diagnosis of exclusion made only after ruling out primary esophageal disease.

Despite the variety of neurogenic and myogenic conditions involving the pharyngoesophageal junction, the resulting oropharyngeal dysphagia has a consistent clinical presentation.[9] The dysphagia is localized between the thyroid cartilage and the suprasternal notch as a lump in the throat or as occasional pain radiating to the jaw and ears. Expectoration of excessive saliva is common in patients who are unable to swallow the 1 to 1.5 L of saliva produced daily. Hoarseness often occurs with cricopharyngeal dysfunction. Weight loss secondary to impaired caloric intake completes the diagnostic symptom complex of cricopharyngeal dysfunction. Symptoms of gastroesophageal reflux occur in 30% to 90% of patients with cricopharyngeal dysfunction.[10]

DIAGNOSIS

Studies to evaluate cricopharyngeal dysfunction include barium swallow, manometry, and acid reflux testing. The barium swallow may be normal, particularly in patients with intermittent symptoms, or may demonstrate a spectrum of hypertonicity of the UES, a posterior cricopharyngeal bar, or a pharyngoesophageal (Zenker's) diverticulum. A complete barium swallow should exclude other significant esophageal disease, particularly a hiatal hernia with gastroesophageal reflux or a distal tumor, which may produce symptoms referred to the cervical esophagus. Esophagoscopy may rule out neoplasm and reflux esophagitis, both of which can result in cervical dysphagia. Esophageal function studies (manometry and acid reflux testing) should also be performed. Abnormalities of thoracic esophageal peristalsis may be found in one third of patients with cricopharyngeal dysfunction, suggesting that cervical esophageal complaints are a manifestation of more generalized disordered esophageal motor function.

TREATMENT

In the presence of persistent cervical dysphagia or aspiration and a radiographically or manometrically documented abnormal UES, a cervical esophagomyotomy is a low-risk operation with high benefit. Patients with an incompetent LES may respond to medical antireflux therapy.[11] Finally, surgical treatment of severe or intractable gastroesophageal reflux may eliminate secondary cervical esophageal symptoms. Intermittent outpatient esophageal bougienage to 54 to 56 French may produce dramatic temporary relief of incapacitating cervical dysphagia in patients with polymyositis, Parkinson's disease, or the residua of a midbrain (basilar artery) cerebrovascular accident.

A cervical esophagomyotomy for cricopharyngeal dysfunction is performed through a 5- to 8-cm oblique left-sided cervical incision centered at the level of the cricoid cartilage and paralleling the anterior border of the sternocleidomastoid muscle (Fig. 39-10). The sternocleidomastoid muscle and carotid sheath and its contents are retracted laterally while the trachea is retracted medially (one should avoid placement of retractors on the tracheoesophageal groove with subsequent injury to the recurrent laryngeal nerve). The dissection proceeds posteriorly through the cervical fascial layers to the prevertebral fascia to mobilize the esophagus. The esophagus is *not* encircled. With a 40-French bougie in the esophagus, the cervical esophagomyotomy is performed on the posterolateral esophageal wall. The incision (7 to 10 cm long) extends from the level of the tip of the superior cornu of the thyroid cartilage inferiorly to 1 to 2 cm behind the clavicle. This "extended" cervical esophagomyotomy is recommended to ensure division of all uncoordinated UES muscle fibers. A cervical esophagomyotomy is successful in relieving cervical dysphagia from cricopharyngeal

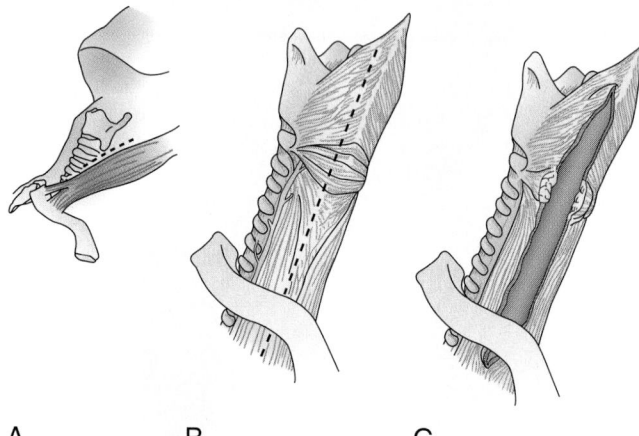

A   **B**   **C**

■ **FIGURE 39-10.**   Cervical esophagomyotomy for cricopharyngeal dysfunction. **A,** A 5-cm oblique skin incision is made anterior to the sternocleidomastoid muscle and centered over the cricoid cartilage. **B,** With a 40-French bougie within the esophagus, the esophagomyotomy is performed on the left posterolateral aspect of the esophagus to avoid injury to the recurrent laryngeal nerve, seen in the tracheoesophageal groove. **C,** Completed esophagomyotomy extends from the level of the superior cornu of the thyroid cartilage inferiorly to 1 to 2 cm behind the clavicle. (**A** to **C,** Adapted from Orringer MB: Extended cervical esophagomyotomy for cricopharyngeal dysfunction. J Thorac Cardiovasc Surg 80:669-678, 1980.)

motor dysfunction in 65% to 85% of patients undergoing the operation.[11]

Motor Disorders of the Body of the Esophagus

Esophageal motor disorders are best viewed as a continuum, with hypomotility (*achalasia*) at one extreme and hypermotility (*diffuse esophageal spasm* [DES]) at the other. Between these extremes is *vigorous achalasia,* which has elements of both achalasia and DES, as well as less clearly characterized examples of neuromotor dysfunction. Primary motor disturbances often present as mixed components and symptoms ranging from the severe crushing retrosternal pain of esophageal spasm (often mimicking a myocardial infarction) to the heavy fullness of retained food from achalasia.

Nonspecific neuromotor esophageal dysfunction, manifested by progressive peristalsis and simultaneous, weak-to-absent esophageal contractions after swallowing, is seen in numerous conditions, such as peripheral neuropathy (diabetes, alcoholism), collagen vascular diseases (scleroderma, dermatomyositis), myasthenia gravis, multiple sclerosis, and amyotrophic lateral sclerosis. In these conditions, patients have an alteration of normal sequential peristaltic contractions with swallowing. In the presence of distal obstruction from either a tumor or a benign stricture, tertiary esophageal contractions may be seen in the body of the esophagus during barium swallow and motility studies.

ACHALASIA

The term *achalasia* is of Greek derivation and literally means "failure or lack of relaxation." Achalasia is the most common functional disorder of the esophageal body and LES, usually occurring during middle age, with equal incidence for either sex. The classic triad of presenting symptoms includes dysphagia, regurgitation, and weight loss. In the early stages of achalasia, the patient notes a sticking sensation, usually at the level of the xiphoid, after ingestion of liquids, especially cold liquids, and later after ingestion of solids. Patients with achalasia eat slowly, use large volumes of water to wash food into the stomach, and may twist the upper torso, elevate the chin and extend the neck, or walk in an effort to aid esophageal emptying. As more water is swallowed, the weight of the fluid column in the esophagus increases, along with the sensation of retrosternal fullness, until the LES is forced open, with sudden relief as the esophagus empties. Dysphagia progresses slowly and is well tolerated for many years. Therefore, patients with achalasia often do not seek medical attention until progressive dysphagia interferes with their lifestyle. Regurgitation of undigested food is common as the disease progresses, and aspiration becomes life threatening. Effortless regurgitation occurs after eating, particularly on bending forward or reclining. As the esophagus dilates, regurgitation of foul-smelling, stagnant intraesophageal contents occurs. Achalasia often results in recurrent respiratory symptoms related to aspiration, such as pneumonia, lung abscess, bronchiectasis, hemoptysis, or bronchospasm. Marked distention of the dilated esophagus may produce dyspnea from compression of the mainstem bronchi and hilum.

The dysfunctional or absent esophageal peristaltic waves, impaired relaxation of the LES on receipt of the food bolus, and the increased LES resting pressure result from loss of the ganglion cells in the intermyenteric (Auerbach's) plexus. The etiology of these neuronal changes is unknown; however, the characteristic clinical, radiographic, and manometric findings have resulted from various situations, including severe emotional stress, major physical trauma, drastic weight reduction, and Chagas' disease in South America. Chagas' disease, a parasitic infection by the leishmanial forms of *Trypanosoma cruzi,* is characterized by destruction of the smooth muscle ganglion cells of the Auerbach myenteric plexus, with resulting motor dysfunction and progressive dilation not only of the esophagus but also of the colon, ureters, and other viscera. In achalasia, the parasympathetic ganglion cells within the myenteric plexus, between the longitudinal and circular muscle layers of the esophagus, are markedly reduced in number. At autopsy, a decrease in the dorsal motor nucleus of the vagus has been found. Likewise, injury to the esophageal myenteric plexus by cold, heat, chemicals, or excision also leads to the characteristic manometric signs of the disease.

Achalasia is a premalignant esophageal lesion, with a prevalence of carcinoma in 2% to 8% of patients with known achalasia followed an average of 15 to 28 years, with squamous cell carcinoma the most common type.[12,13] Long-standing mucosal irritation from retention esophagitis appears to induce the metaplasia. Esophageal carcinoma in achalasia tends to arise in the middle third of the esophagus, below the air-fluid level, where the mucosal irritation is most pronounced.

Diagnosis The radiographic appearance of achalasia varies with progression of the disease. The characteristic appearance on a standard chest radiograph is an air-fluid level within a dilated esophagus. Barium swallow shows uniform esophageal dilatation with a distal tapering ("beak") secondary to failure of the LES to relax. Later stages demonstrate massive dilatation, tortuosity, and a sigmoid-shaped esophagus, often termed a *megaesophagus.* Retained intraesophageal food contents are typically seen (Fig. 39-11).[14] The manometric criteria of achalasia are failure of the LES to relax reflexively with swallowing and lack of progressive peristalsis throughout the length of the esophagus. In the early stages of achalasia, contractions after swallowing may be of normal amplitude, synchronous, and simultaneous. Later, contractions are either weak or totally absent. The distal esophageal HPZ pressure is generally normal or elevated, but the marked hypertonicity of DES is not seen. Administration of a mild vagomimetic agent (i.e., bethanechol [Urecholine]) produces marked elevation of intraesophageal pressure and increased amplitude and frequency of simultaneous esophageal contractions that correspond with the patient's complaint of chest pain. This response does not occur in scleroderma, but it is common both in DES and achalasia.

In achalasia, esophagoscopy is indicated to evaluate the severity of esophagitis, the possibility of associated

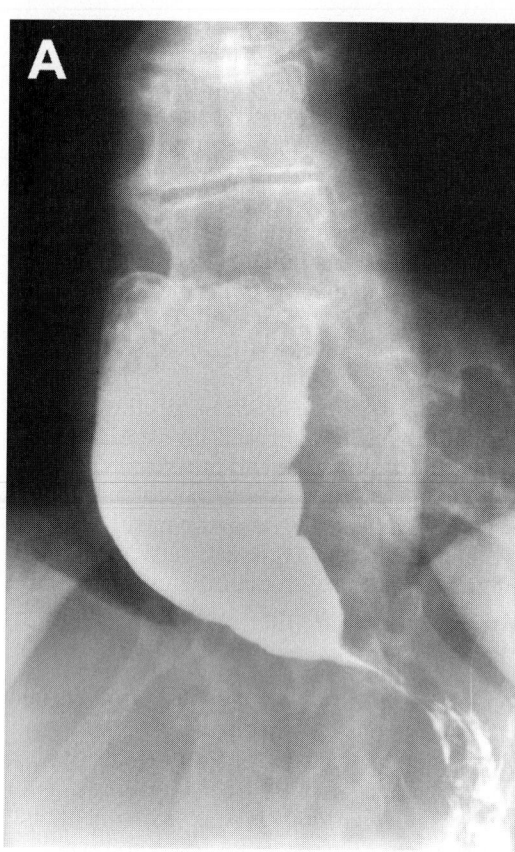

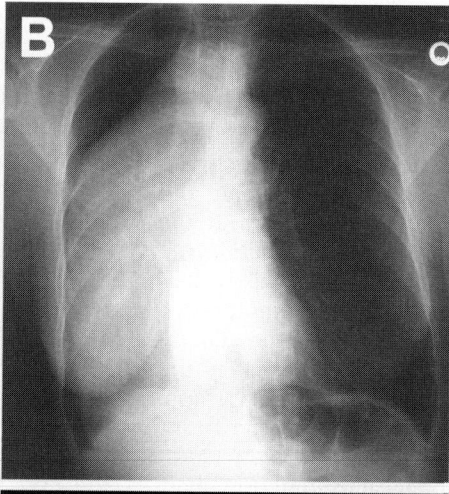

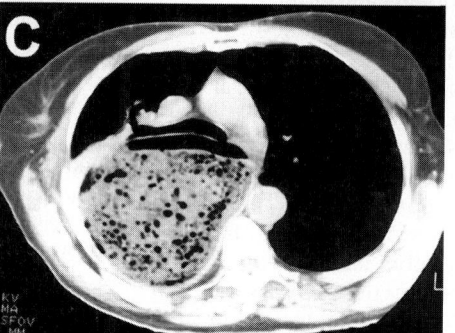

FIGURE 39-11.
A, Esophagogram shows a dilated esophagus, an air-fluid level, and a distal tapering typical of achalasia. **B,** A sigmoid-shaped esophagus is evident on a chest radiograph in a patient with long-standing achalasia and megaesophagus with retained intraesophageal food. **C,** CT scan of megaesophagus. (**A,** Courtesy of Ronelle A. Dubrow, M.D., MD Anderson Cancer Center, Houston, TX; **B** and **C** from Zwischenberger JB, Savage C: Megaesophagus from a 26-year history of achalasia. Ann Thorac Surg 69:1597, 2000.)

carcinoma, a distal esophageal stricture from reflux esophagitis, or a tumor of the cardia mimicking achalasia *(pseudoachalasia).* Retention esophagitis in advanced achalasia is different endoscopically from reflux esophagitis. When the patient has prolonged retention esophagitis from achalasia, the irritating effects of putrefying food on the esophageal mucosa may induce severe edema, with reddish purple discoloration and marked friability. The presence of retained fluid and food in the dilated esophagus, even after an overnight fast, may complicate esophagoscopy, and cricoid pressure to protect the airway is indicated.

Secondary achalasia or pseudoachalasia, caused by a tumor at or near the gastroesophageal junction, is also best detected by endoscopy and biopsy. The precise imaging of EUS can be used when endoscopic examination alone fails to confirm the diagnosis of secondary or primary achalasia. EUS may identify subepithelial tumor infiltration in secondary achalasia when results of biopsies of the cardia or gastroesophageal junction are negative.

Treatment Because the derangement in esophageal motor function does not return to normal, the treatment of achalasia is purely palliative. Both nonsurgical and surgical treatments of achalasia are directed toward relieving the obstruction caused by the nonrelaxing LES.

In the early stages of the disease, before the esophagus dilates, use of sublingual nitroglycerin before or during meals, long-acting nitrates, and calcium-channel blocking agents may improve swallowing. Passage of mercury-weighted bougies, 48 to 54 French, may relieve the dysphagia for several days or weeks, but it is seldom a satisfactory long-term solution. The definitive treatment of achalasia requires disruption of the circular layer of smooth muscle within the LES area. The two most widely used and analyzed methods of therapy for achalasia are forceful dilatation, either pneumatic or hydrostatic, and esophagomyotomy.[12] Results were considered excellent or good in 65% of patients with dilatation and 85% of those after esophagomyotomy. The perforation (4% vs. 1%) and mortality rates (0.5% vs. 0.2%) were reported to be higher with dilatation than with esophagomyotomy. However, the advent of volume-limited pressure-controlled balloons (Gruntzig-type) has decreased the perforation rate and mortality of balloon dilatation. A Gruntzig-type balloon is positioned under fluoroscopic control within the LES. The balloon is rapidly inflated to a pressure of 300 mm Hg for 15 seconds. Results from dilatation show that approximately 60% of patients receive complete relief of symptoms after one treatment and that an additional 10% respond to a second treatment. Most patients referred for myotomy have had at least one failed balloon dilatation.

The proposed mechanism of failure of the LES to relax in achalasia is the selective loss of inhibitory neurons in the myenteric plexus, which results in unopposed excitation of the smooth muscle by acetylcholine. Injections of botulinum toxin (Botox), a protein produced by *Clostridium botulinum,* into the LES during endoscopy, blocks acetylcholine release, providing symptomatic relief. Encouraging early results, with initial improvement in 70% of patients, have been reported. Longer follow-up, however, has been disappointing, with symptomatic relief lasting only 6 to 9 months. Fortunately, success is most often seen in higher-risk elderly patients.[15,16] Experimental techniques such as EUS-guided injections have been proposed to maximize delivery of botulinum toxin to the esophageal smooth muscle, increasing the efficacy of treatment.[16] Pneumatic dilatation was compared with Botox treatment in a double-blind, randomized study showing remission of symptoms in 38% with Botox versus 89% with pneumatic dilatation at 1 year.[17] In summary, Botox injections and pneumodilatation have almost equal short-term results; however, the long-term efficacy of pneumodilatation is considered superior.[12]

Surgical treatment, either open or video-assisted, with division of the circular muscle of the lower end of the esophagus, offers precise and less traumatic division of the circular muscle layer than that achieved by forceful dilatation. Results appear superior to those of balloon dilatation, and mortality is low. Major disadvantages include the need for hospitalization and thoracic access, and an incidence of 5% to 10% of reflux postoperative esophagitis. Excellent results with laparoscopic esophagomyotomy in the treatment of achalasia have been reported.[18] This approach is clearly superior to transthoracic video-assisted esophagomyotomy and appears to increase referrals for surgical management.[19]

The traditional transthoracic distal esophagomyotomy for achalasia is performed through a left thoracotomy in the sixth or seventh intercostal space. The pleural reflection is incised and the distal esophagus is mobilized, with careful preservation of the vagus nerve. In addition, the esophagogastric junction is mobilized from the esophageal hiatus to allow visualization of 1 to 2 cm of stomach. A linear incision (7 to 10 cm) is made through the longitudinal and circular muscle layer, from the level of the inferior pulmonary vein across the lower sphincter inferiorly for complete division of circular muscle fibers (Fig. 39-12). Separation of the muscularis from the submucosa at the margin of the incision is important to ensure that the divided layers do not reapproximate as healing occurs.[20]

Unresolved technical questions concern the distal extent of the esophagomyotomy and the need for a concomitant antireflux procedure.[21] Some surgeons advocate a short esophagomyotomy carried onto the stomach only far enough to ensure complete division of the distal esophageal musculature but not far enough to induce incompetence of the LES mechanism. With this approach, several surgeons reported a late incidence of postoperative gastroesophageal reflux of about 8%.[22] Many surgeons believe that complete relief of the obstruction caused by the uncoordinated LES can be achieved only by rendering the LES incompetent and, therefore, carrying the esophagomyotomy onto the stomach for 1 to 2 cm.[23] Many esophageal surgeons perform a complete esophagocardiomyotomy for achalasia with some type of fundoplication to prevent the subsequent development of gastroesophageal reflux. A 360-degree loose fundoplasty, in which the stomach is wrapped around the lower esophagus, has the potential disadvantage of offering too much

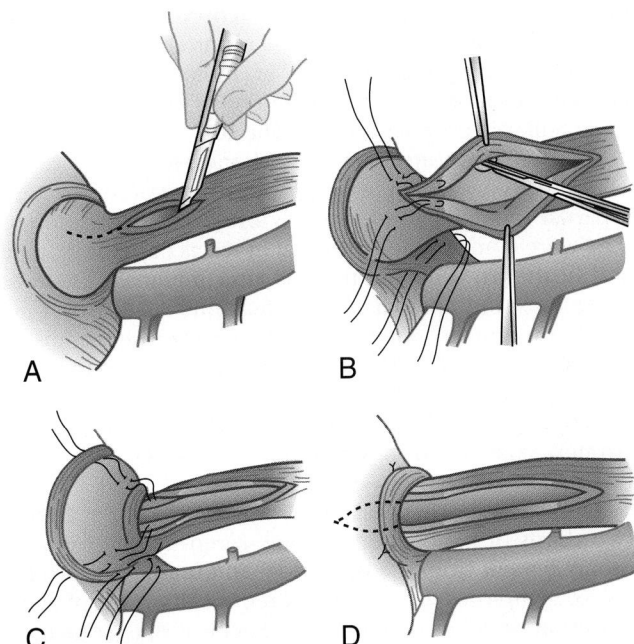

FIGURE 39-12. **A,** Esophageal body myotomy extends from the inferior pulmonary vein to include the lower esophageal sphincter and 1 to 1.5 cm of the gastric wall muscle. **B,** The mucosa is mobilized over 50% of the esophageal circumference to allow pouting of the mucosa between the transected pieces of muscle. A partial fundoplication is often added to protect the esophagus from reflux disease. Two stitches approximate the esophageal muscle layer and the gastric fundus. This modified Belsey fundoplication omits the third suture, which normally would lie at the site of the myotomy. **C,** A second row of sutures approximates esophageal muscle and gastric fundus. These same sutures are then passed through the diaphragm and tied on the thoracic side of the hiatus. This maneuver both reduces the fundoplication into the abdomen and anchors it beneath the hiatus. **D,** Operative appearance after repair. (**A** to **D,** Adapted from Duranceau A: Esophageal dysmotility. *In* Baue AE, Geha AS, Hammond GL, et al [eds]: Glenn's Thoracic and Cardiovascular Surgery, 6th ed, vol 1. Norwalk, CT, Appleton & Lange, 1996, p 848. With permission of the McGraw-Hill Companies.)

resistance to the passage of food. Recent reports suggest a longer (3-cm) myotomy may more completely obliterate the LES than reflux controlled with a Toupet (270-degree) fundoplication.[24] With any technique, however, gradual deterioration of esophageal function over time and the late development of gastroesophageal reflux and esophagitis jeopardize the long-term outcome.[25]

Minimally invasive video-assisted techniques to accomplish an esophagomyotomy have yielded comparable results to the open approach with less postoperative pain and a shorter hospital stay.[26,27] Most surgeons prefer a laparoscopic (transabdominal) approach with a partial fundoplication to avoid postoperative reflux. The laparoscopic myotomy has advantages over the thoracoscopic technique. First, anesthesia is easier to administer because a double-lumen tube is not needed. Second, the myotomy can be performed more easily through the abdomen. Last, the absence of a chest tube may decrease postoperative pain. A large series of 168 patients undergoing minimally invasive esophagomyotomy (thoracoscopic, 35; laparoscopic, 133) over an 8-year period reported good or excellent relief of dysphagia in 90%.[18] Even those with a dilated, end-stage esophagus had excellent relief of dysphagia, and none required esophagectomy. The authors originally performed the myotomy through a thoracoscopic approach but now prefer the laparoscopic approach combined with a partial fundoplication. A study of 62 patients reported 92% were comparable to normal in terms of quality of life and heartburn score 19 months after minimally invasive myotomy and partial fundoplication.[28] Laparoscopic myotomy appears safe and effective even after unsuccessful treatment with botulinum toxin[29] or when the esophagus is dilated.[30]

Esophagectomy for end-stage achalasia should be strongly considered in symptomatic patients with tortuous megaesophagus (see Fig. 39-11B and C), failure of prior myotomy, or undilatable reflux stricture.[31,31a] Only two thirds of patients undergoing a repeat esophagomyotomy benefit from the operation, and fundoplication for reflux symptoms has even poorer results.[32] Esophageal resection provides definitive treatment of the esophageal abnormality and eliminates the late risk of carcinoma. Transhiatal resection is recommended with increased frequency in patients with failed prior operations for achalasia or in those with a megaesophagus that may fail to empty adequately after an esophagomyotomy.[33] Banbury and associates[34] reported that 32 patients underwent esophagectomy with gastric transposition during a 10-year period with excellent functional results. Eighty-three percent had no or only mild dysphagia, and most had no dietary restrictions. In 93 patients undergoing transhiatal esophagectomy for achalasia, 95% were eating well at an average 3-year follow-up.[31a]

DIFFUSE ESOPHAGEAL SPASM AND RELATED HYPERMOTILITY DISORDERS

DES is a poorly understood hypermotility disorder in which patients experience chest pain and/or dysphagia as a result of repetitive, simultaneous, high-amplitude esophageal contractions. The origin of DES is unknown. The patient with DES is typically anxious and complains of chest pain inconsistently related to eating, exertion, and position. The character of the chest pain may mimic that of angina pectoris, often described as squeezing, oppressive, retrosternal pressure that has variable intensity and radiates toward the jaw, down the arms, and frequently to the intrascapular region of the back. Symptoms are often greatest during periods of emotional stress, but the lack of association with exercise and the occasional association of dysphagia with the chest pain suggests an esophageal rather than a cardiac abnormality. Obstructive symptoms are unusual. Many patients experience regurgitation of retained intraesophageal saliva during bouts of DES. Ingestion of cold liquids or foods may aggravate DES, as can gastroesophageal reflux, but most patients with DES do not have reflux. A history of irritable bowel syndrome, pylorospasm, or other functional gastrointestinal complaints is common. Gallstones, peptic ulcer disease, and pancreatitis can all trigger DES.

Diagnosis The initial evaluation of the patient with DES is the same as that of the patient with chest pain of undetermined origin. A careful history is essential to elucidate causative intra-abdominal disease (e.g., gallstones, gastritis, or peptic ulcer disease). On barium swallow examination, DES is frustratingly variable. Classic curling or a corkscrew esophagus caused by segmental contractions of the circular muscle may be apparent (Fig. 39-13); however, findings range from a distal beaklike taper (suggesting early achalasia) to normal-appearing peristalsis. An esophageal pulsion diverticulum, particularly in a patient with angina-like symptoms, implicates DES. Esophagoscopy should be performed to rule out an infiltrating tumor, esophageal fibrosis, or esophagitis causing radiographic distal esophageal narrowing. Unfortunately, some of the radiographic and manometric criteria of DES are seen in asymptomatic patients. Unless the patient is experiencing spasm at the time of the manometric study, just as with the barium esophagogram, the results may be entirely normal.

The issue is further confounded by the inclusion of a variety of related hypermotility disorders, such as nutcracker esophagus, hypertensive LES, nonspecific esophageal motility disorders, and vigorous achalasia under the generic heading of DES (Table 39-2). These conditions, however, are best defined by manometric criteria (Box 39-1). The classic manometric criteria of DES are simultaneous, multiphasic, repetitive, often high-

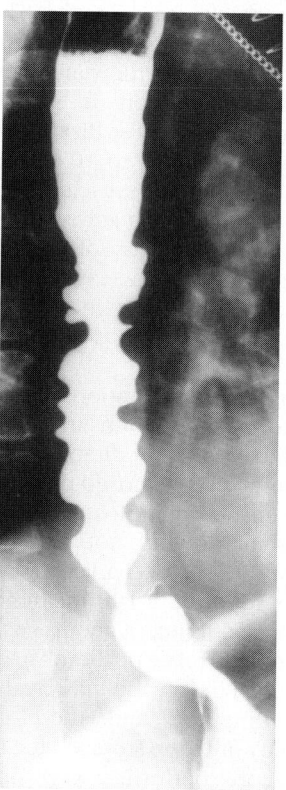

FIGURE 39-13. Barium swallow of diffuse esophageal spasm showing the classic corkscrew appearance secondary to segmental contractions of the circular muscle. (Courtesy of Ronelle A. Dubrow, M.D., MD Anderson Cancer Center, Houston, TX.)

TABLE 39-2. Differential Characteristics of Achalasia and Primary Spasm

Characteristic	Achalasia	Vigorous Achalasia	Diffuse Esophageal Spasm	Nutcracker Esophagus
Dysphagia	Common	Common	Rare	Common
Pain	Rare	Common	Common	Common
Barium esophagogram	Abnormal: dilated esophagus, bird-beak taper	Abnormal	Normal caliber "corkscrew" esophagus	Normal contraction progression
Endoscopy	Normal	Normal	Normal	Normal
Motility	Nonrelaxing LES, absent or weak simultaneous contraction after swallowing	Nonrelaxing LES + hypertonic simultaneous, multiphasic contractions after swallowing	Hypertonic simultaneous, multiphasic contractions after swallowing	Normal peristalsis present, very high amplitude and duration of contractions

LES, lower esophageal sphincter.

Box 39-1 Manometric criteria of primary esophageal motility disorders

NORMAL

LES pressure 15-25 mm Hg (never > 45 mm Hg) with normal relaxation with swallowing

Mean amplitude of distal esophageal peristaltic wave 30-100 mm Hg (never > 180 mm Hg)

Simultaneous contractions occurring after < 10% of wet swallows

Monophasic waveforms (with no more than two peaks)

Duration of distal esophageal peristaltic wave: 2-6 sec

No repetitive contractions

PRIMARY MOTILITY DISORDERS

Achalasia

Aperistalsis in esophageal body

Partial or absent LES relaxation with swallowing

LES pressure normal or > 45 mm Hg

Intraesophageal basal pressure higher than intragastric

Diffuse esophageal spasm

Simultaneous (nonperistaltic) contractions

Repetitive (≥3 wk)

Increased duration (>6 sec)

Spontaneous contractions

Intermittent normal peristalsis

Contractions possibly of increased amplitude

Nutcracker esophagus

Mean peristaltic amplitude (10 wet swallows) in distal esophagus > 180 mm Hg

Increased duration of contractions (>6 sec) frequent

Normal peristaltic sequences

Hypertensive LES

LES pressures > 45 mm Hg but with normal relaxation

Normal esophageal peristalsis

NONSPECIFIC ESOPHAGEAL MOTILITY DISORDERS

No or decreased amplitude of peristalsis
 Normal LES pressure
 Normal LES relaxation

Abnormal peristalsis, including any of the following:
 Abnormal waveforms
 Isolated simultaneous contractions
 Isolated spontaneous contractions
 Normal peristalsis sequence maintained
 LES normal

VIGOROUS ACHALASIA

Repetitive simultaneous contractions in body of esophagus
 (as with diffuse esophageal spasm)

Partial or absent LES relaxation (as with achalasia)

LES, lower esophageal sphincter.
Adapted from Khan AA, Castell DO: Primary diffuse esophageal spasm and related disorders. *In* Jamieson GG (ed): Surgery of the Oesophagus. Edinburgh, Churchill Livingstone, 1988, pp 483-488.

---

amplitude contractions that occur after a swallow and spontaneously in the smooth muscle portion of the esophagus. The diagnostic hallmark of DES is the correlation of subjective complaints with objective evidence of spasm (inducible by a vagomimetic drug, bethanechol [Urecholine]) on manometric tracings.

Treatment The treatment of DES is far from satisfactory. Documented psychiatric disorders, including depression, psychosomatic complaints, and anxiety, have been reported in more than 80% of patients with esophageal manometric contraction abnormalities.[35] For many patients with DES, simply establishing an esophageal cause of their previously unexplained chest pain and providing reassurance are therapeutic. Patients who complain of dysphagia should avoid stress during meals as well as "trigger" foods or drinks. If gastroesophageal reflux is symptomatic or documented with esophageal function tests, medical treatment of reflux should be initiated.

Antispasmodics and calcium-channel blockers are occasionally helpful. The response of DES to nitrates is variable but may be dramatic. Esophageal dilation with Hurst-Maloney bougies (50 to 60 French) may relieve dysphagia and chest pain.

Although thoracic esophagomyotomy has been advocated in the treatment of DES,[36] results are much less favorable than in achalasia, with success in only 50% to 60%. Despite improvement in manometric and radiographic indicators of DES after esophagomyotomy, patients may continue to complain of chest pain and slow emptying. Therefore, only when a patient with DES is incapacitated by chest pain or dysphagia, or in the presence of a pulsion diverticulum of the intrathoracic esophagus, should one perform a long esophagomyotomy in which the muscular layers of the esophagus are split from the esophagogastric junction to above the aortic arch. Controversy exists about whether the LES should be divided in this procedure and whether an antireflux procedure should be included, but obstructive symptoms may not be relieved unless *all* circular esophageal muscle fibers in this area are transected.

The *nutcracker* or *super-squeeze esophagus* is a hypermotility disorder characterized by extremely high-amplitude (as high as 225 to 430 mm Hg) progressive peristaltic contractions, often of prolonged duration. Symptoms of chest pain, dysphagia, and odynophagia are like those of DES, and treatment considerations are similar.

Esophageal motor disturbances occur in several collagen vascular diseases, such as dermatomyositis, polymyositis, and lupus erythematosus, but particularly scleroderma. Disruption of normal esophageal peristalsis is so common in scleroderma that it is a major diagnostic sign of the disease. Normal, progressive peristalsis gives way to weak, simultaneous, nonpropulsive contractions with severe gastroesophageal reflux. Use of the combined Collis gastroplasty-fundoplication (Figs. 39-14 to 39-16) has particular merit in the patient with scleroderma, who typically has severe esophagitis, esophageal shortening, stricture formation, fibrinoid degeneration, and atrophy of distal esophageal smooth muscle that jeopardize the long-term success of the traditional operations.

Obstructive symptoms due to a competent lower esophageal sphincter mechanism in a patient with an atonic esophagus, however, may require postoperative dilatation therapy. Advanced esophageal scleroderma, manifested by either severe dilatation or reflux stricture (refractory to dilatation and medical therapy), may require esophagectomy with a cervical esophagogastric anastomosis to eliminate reflux esophagitis and to restore the ability to swallow.[37]

Esophageal Diverticula

Esophageal diverticula are epithelial-lined mucosal pouches that protrude from the esophageal lumen. Almost all are acquired and are classified according to their site of occurrence, wall thickness, and mechanism of formation. Diverticula commonly occur at three distinct sites: (1) *pharyngoesophageal* (Zenker's) diverticula occur at the junction of the pharynx and esophagus, (2)

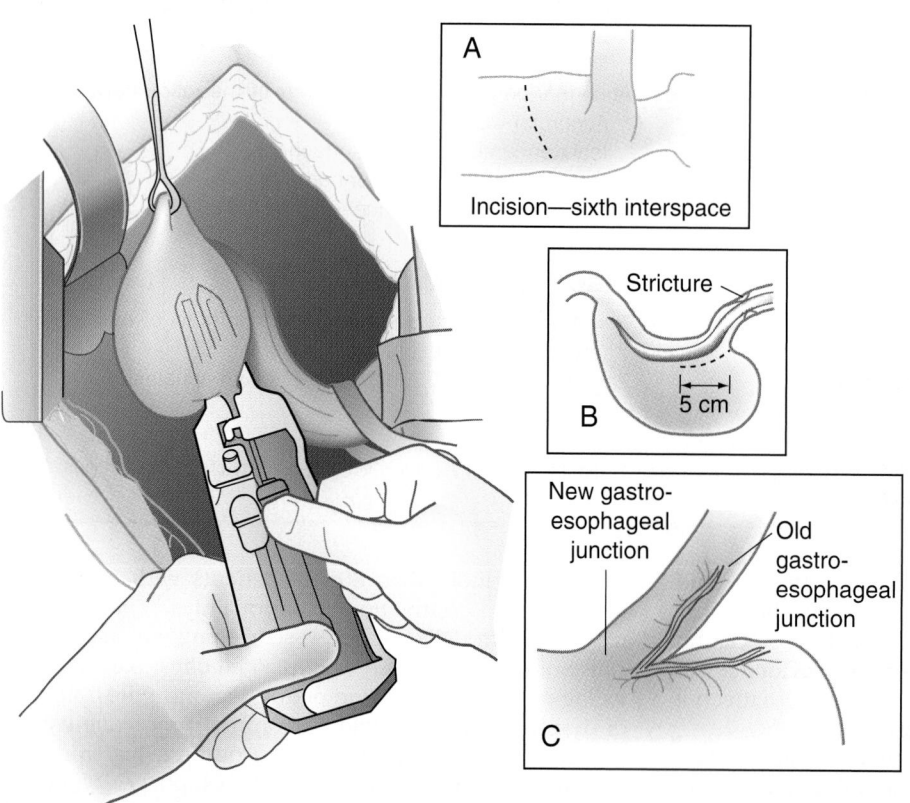

FIGURE 39-14. Construction of the Collis gastroplasty tube with the GIA surgical stapler. **A,** Mobilization of the esophagus and gastric fundus is performed through a lateral thoracotomy in the sixth or seventh left intercostal space. **B,** A 54- or 56-French Maloney dilator is passed through the esophagogastric junction and is displaced against the lesser curvature of the stomach, and the stapler is applied. The knife assembly is advanced *(main illustration),* and the stapler is removed. The staple suture line is oversewn with a running 4-0 Prolene Lembert stitch. **C,** The result is a 5-cm long gastric tube extension into the esophagus. (**A** to **C,** Adapted from Orringer MB, Sloan H: Collis-Belsey reconstruction of the esophagogastric junction: Indications, physiology, and technical considerations. J Thorac Cardiovasc Surg 71:295-303, 1976.)

Figure labels: Incision—sixth interspace; Stricture; 5 cm; B; New gastroesophageal junction; Old gastroesophageal junction; C; A

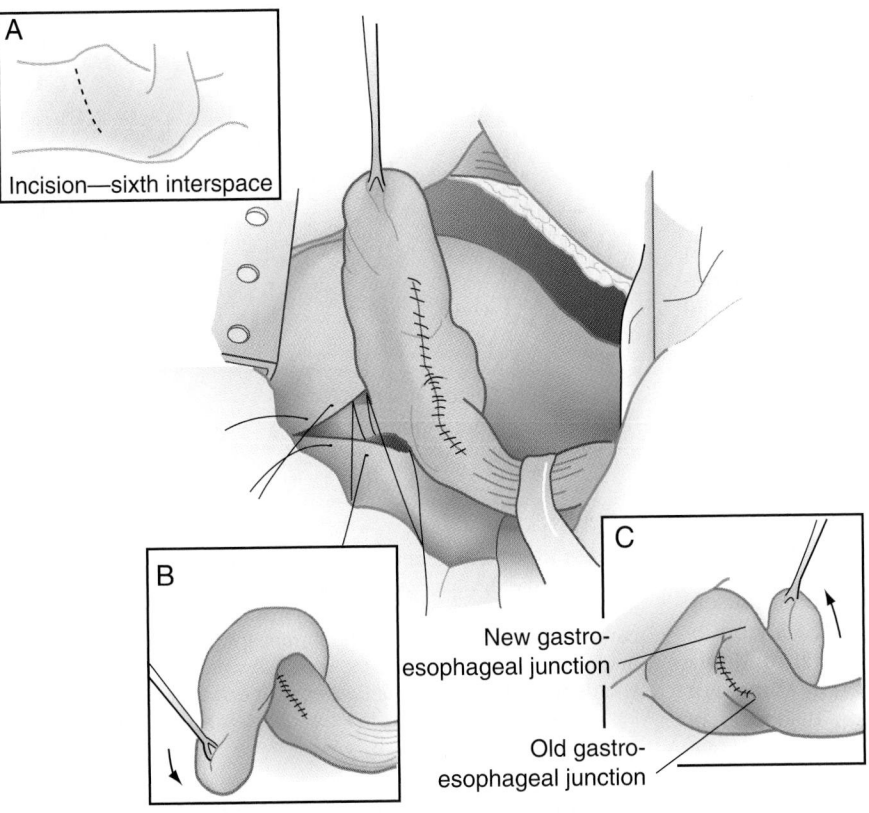

FIGURE 39-15. The combined Collis-Nissen reconstruction of the esophagogastric junction. The *main drawing* illustrates the elongated, narrowed gastric fundus available for fundoplication after completion of the Collis procedure. **A,** Placement of the left thoracotomy. **B** and **C,** The gastric fundus is wrapped around the gastroplasty tube and adjacent stomach. The posterior crural sutures are placed but left untied until the fundoplication is reduced below the diaphragm. (**A** to **C,** Adapted from Orringer MB, Sloan H: Collis-Nissen reconstruction of the esophagogastric junction. Ann Thorac Surg 22:120-130, 1976. Adapted with permission from the Society of Thoracic Surgeons.)

New gastro-esophageal junction

Old gastro-esophageal junction

Incision—sixth interspace

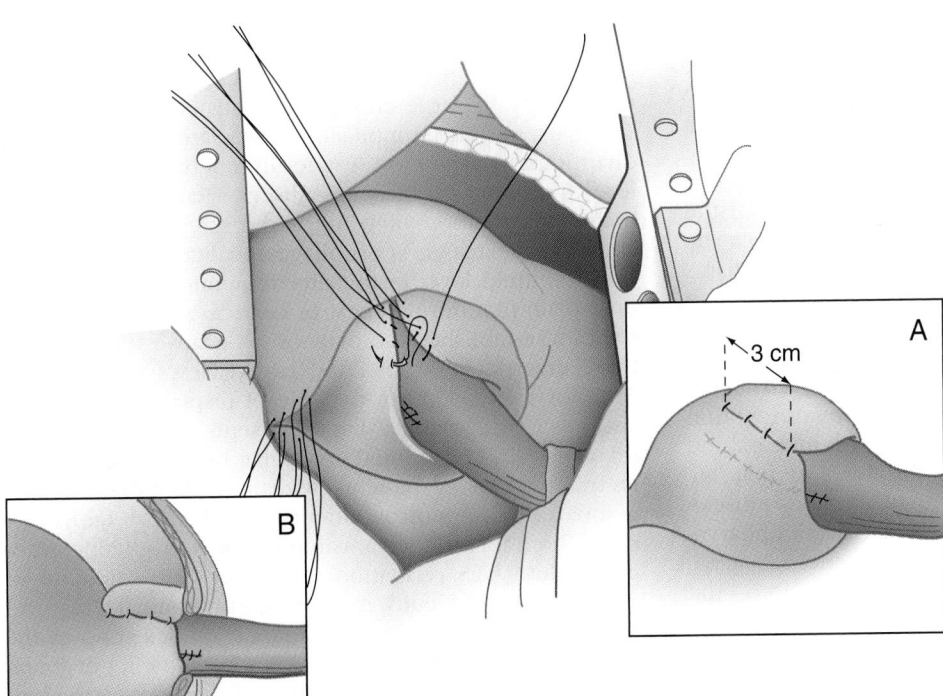

FIGURE 39-16. Completion of the combined Collis-Nissen procedure, with fundoplication limited to 3 cm in length. **A,** Four seromuscular 2-0 silk sutures placed 1 cm apart *(main illustration)* are used to construct the fundoplication around the gastroplasty tube. **B,** The fundoplication is reduced beneath the diaphragm. In scleroderma patients who have impaired esophageal motility, the fundoplication must be performed loosely to minimize postoperative obstructive symptoms. (**A** and **B,** Adapted from Stirling MC, Orringer MB: The combined Collis-Nissen operation for esophageal reflux strictures. Ann Thorac Surg 45:148-157, 1988.)

3 cm

parabronchial (midesophageal) diverticula occur near the tracheal bifurcation, and (3) *epiphrenic* (supradiaphragmatic) diverticula arise from the distal 10 cm of esophagus. A *true* diverticulum contains all layers of the normal esophageal wall, including mucosa, submucosa, and muscle, whereas a false diverticulum consists primarily of mucosa and submucosa. *Pulsion diverticula* (pharyngoesophageal and epiphrenic) are false diverticula that arise because elevated intraluminal pressure forces the mucosa and submucosa to herniate through the esophageal musculature. Abnormally elevated intraluminal pressure, secondary to an esophageal motility disorder or distal obstruction, is responsible for the mucosal herniation through the muscle of the esophagus. Traction diverticula (parabronchial) are true diverticula that result from external inflammatory reactions in adjacent mediastinal lymph nodes that adhere to the esophagus and pull the entire wall toward these lesions as they heal and contract. The overall decreased incidence of tuberculosis in the West has almost eliminated tuberculous mediastinal lymphadenitis and traction diverticula of the midesophagus. Therefore, almost all diverticula of the body of the esophagus are pulsion diverticula caused by an underlying motility abnormality.[38] Symptoms are a result of the primary motility disturbance, retained food within the diverticulum, or aspiration.

Treatment of patients with diverticula is designed to relieve dysphagia, palliate chest pain, and protect against pulmonary soilage caused by chronic aspiration of regurgitated esophageal contents. Surgical therapy must address the esophageal motility disorder; therefore, esophagomyotomy of the abnormally functioning muscle is essential. If the myotomy crosses the LES, a nonobstructive antireflux procedure such as a partial fundoplication to prevent iatrogenic reflux is favored by some. For a complete discussion, see the section on disorders of esophageal motility.

Pharyngoesophageal (Zenker's) Diverticula

The pharyngoesophageal diverticulum (Zenker's diverticulum) is the most common esophageal diverticulum. Zenker's diverticulum usually presents in patients older than 60 years, which is thought to be due to loss of tissue elasticity and decreased muscle tone.[39] The diverticulum characteristically arises from the dorsal wall of the hypopharynx between the oblique fibers of the posterior pharyngeal constrictors and the transverse fibers of the cricopharyngeus muscle of the UES (Fig. 39-17). The transition in direction of these muscle fibers (Killian's triangle) represents a point of potential weakness in the posterior pharynx. Zenker's diverticulum is a pulsion diverticulum resulting from a transient incomplete opening in the UES,[40] also referred to as *cricopharyngeal achalasia*.[41] The swallowed bolus exerts pressure within the pharynx above the UES and causes the mucosa and submucosa eventually to herniate through the anatomically weak area proximal to the cricopharyngeus muscle. The diverticulum enlarges, drapes over the cricopharyngeus, and dissects inferiorly in the prevertebral space behind the esophagus, occasionally well into the mediastinum.

DIAGNOSIS

Zenker's diverticula are usually asymptomatic initially and are discovered during a routine radiographic evaluation. Symptomatic patients may complain of a vague sensation or sticking in the throat, intermittent cough, excessive salivation, and intermittent dysphagia (particularly with solid foods). When the sac enlarges, especially in elderly persons, more severe symptoms develop, including cervical dysphagia, gurgling sounds during swallowing,

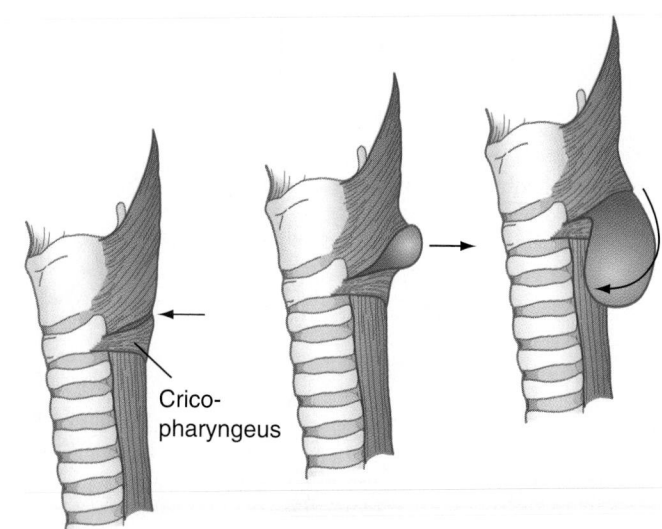

FIGURE 39-17.   Formation of pharyngoesophageal (Zenker's) diverticulum. **Left,** Herniation of the pharyngeal mucosa and submucosa occurs at the point of transition *(arrow)* between the oblique fibers of the thyropharyngeus muscle and the more horizontal fibers of the cricopharyngeus muscle. **Center** and **right,** As the diverticulum enlarges, it dissects toward the left side and downward into the superior mediastinum in the prevertebral space.

regurgitation of food (ingested several hours earlier), halitosis, voice change, retrosternal pain, and respiratory obstruction. To aid in swallowing, patients often develop various "maneuvers," including clearing the throat, coughing, or placing pressure on the neck. In rare cases, the pouch may be large enough to obstruct the esophagus. The most serious complication associated with Zenker's diverticula is aspiration, especially nocturnal, which can lead to pneumonia or a lung abscess. Rare complications include perforation, bleeding, and carcinoma. Weight loss and dysphagia suggest esophageal malignancy.

An air-fluid level in the diverticulum can be detected on a plain film during chest or cervical studies. A barium swallow establishes the diagnosis. Because the origin of these diverticula is posterior, lateral views are essential. Anterior views confirm the side of displacement. A persistent cricopharyngeal bar represents the incompletely relaxed or hypertrophied cricopharyngeal muscle. Manometric tracings of patients with a Zenker diverticulum compared with control patients (matched for age) show no difference, a finding casting doubt on the concept of incomplete UES relaxation in Zenker's diverticulum or reflecting the difficulty measuring intraluminal pressures during deglutition effects. Histologic studies support the concept of diminished UES opening by showing degenerative changes. Manometric testing of the cricopharyngeal area is generally not necessary in evaluating patients with Zenker's diverticulum.[42]

Endoscopic assessment and biopsy are necessary when mass defects or ulcers are seen on a barium swallow. When the endoscope tip enters a diverticulum, the endoscopist may feel a typical "give" as the scope passes distal to the cricopharyngeus and enters the proximal esophagus; however, within a few centimeters, no lumen is found distally. An association exists between the Zenker's diverticulum-cricopharyngeal bar complex and GERD. Assessment of associated GERD with esophagoscopy and manometry may be best performed after surgical correction of the diverticulum because the operative risk of Zenker's diverticulectomy myotomy is so low.

TREATMENT

Zenker's diverticulum can be treated surgically or endoscopically. In general, surgical therapy consists of esophagomyotomy with (diverticulectomy) or without resection of the diverticulum (diverticulotomy) or invagination of the diverticulum (diverticuloplexy). Treatment of symptomatic patients is indicated, regardless of size of the pouch. The degree of cricopharyngeal muscle dysfunction, not the absolute size of the diverticulum, determines the severity of cervical dysphagia. Therefore, the proper treatment of Zenker's diverticulum, like that of every pulsion diverticulum, is directed toward the underlying motor abnormality responsible for formation of the pouch.

A commonly used surgical approach is cervical esophagomyotomy and resection of the diverticulum performed through an oblique left cervical incision that parallels the anterior border of the sternocleidomastoid muscle or a transverse cervical incision centered over the cricoid cartilage.[11] The sternocleidomastoid muscle and carotid sheath and its contents are retracted laterally, and the thyroid and the trachea are retracted medially. The diverticulum is located beneath the inferior thyroid artery, which is identified and divided. With a 40-French bougie within the esophagus, the pouch is dissected to its base and an extramucosal esophagomyotomy is performed in both directions from the base of the pouch (7 to 10 cm) to ensure that all cricopharyngeal muscle fibers are divided (Fig. 39-18). Because most pouches between 1 and 2 cm in diameter blend into the exposed mucosa and submucosa after the cervical esophagomyotomy, some surgeons terminate the operation at this point without

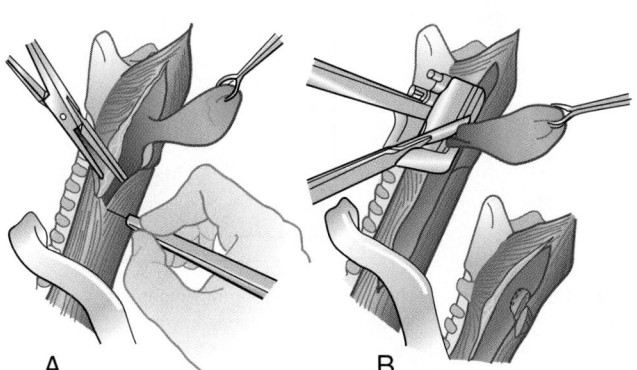

FIGURE 39-18. Cervical esophagomyotomy and concomitant resection of a pharyngoesophageal diverticulum. **A,** After mobilization of the diverticulum, the esophagomyotomy is performed in either direction from the base of the pouch. **B,** After the esophagomyotomy is completed, the base of the diverticulum is crossed with a TA-30 stapler and amputated. (**A** and **B,** Adapted from Orringer MB: Extended cervical esophagomyotomy for cricopharyngeal dysfunction. J Thorac Cardiovasc Surg 80:669-678, 1980.)

resecting the diverticulum.[39,43] Most surgeons advocate excising larger pouches by using a surgical stapler. Alternatively, diverticulopexy (mobilizing the pouch and suspending it from adjacent tissues so the mouth is dependent) combined with a cricopharyngeal myotomy may be used and has been shown to have both shorter hospital stays and fasting periods compared with myotomy and diverticulectomy.[44,45] Endoscopic division of the common wall between the diverticulum and the esophagus (internal pharyngoesophagotomy, the Dohlman procedure) using a laser or stapler has also been successful. A comparison of endoscopic versus surgical treatment, however, showed a significantly higher percentage overall of patients asymptomatic after surgery.[45-47] For diverticula smaller than 3 cm, the percentage of patients with excellent or good post-procedural symptom control was significantly higher for those who had surgical rather than endoscopic treatment. For diverticula larger than 3 cm, there was no significant difference between surgery and endoscopy in patients reporting excellent to good symptom control. For this reason, some advocate endoscopic resection only for large diverticula.

Resection of the pouch without myotomy predisposes to the development of a cervical fistula and to long-term recurrence of the pouch.[45,48] Patients with known incompetence of the lower sphincter must be postured upright postoperatively after a cricopharyngeal myotomy is performed that renders the upper sphincter incompetent. Regardless of the surgical approach, recurrence is rare, and results are excellent.

Midesophageal Diverticula

Patients with midesophageal diverticula may be asymptomatic; however, dysphagia, retrosternal pain, regurgitation, belching, epigastric pain, heartburn, and weight loss are noted. Although rare, complications include spontaneous rupture, aspiration, esophagobronchial fistula, carcinoma, and exsanguination. A barium swallow is the most effective imaging study for midesophageal diverticula. Midesophageal diverticula are often wide mouthed, are more common on the right side, and are usually singular. Most are less than 5 cm long; and as they enlarge, food may become trapped.

In the past, these diverticula were caused by traction in patients with mediastinal fibrosis and/or chronic lymphadenopathy from pulmonary tuberculosis or histoplasmosis. More recent studies emphasize pulsion forces from motility disorders as the cause of these diverticula. Manometrically, these patients may have achalasia, DES, or other nonspecific esophageal motor disorders. The dysmotility can be classified as normal, achalasia-like, scleroderma-like, or nonspecific. Endoscopy is often required to pass the manometry catheter into the stomach, particularly if an epiphrenic diverticulum is also present.

Epiphrenic Diverticula

Epiphrenic (supradiaphragmatic) diverticula are pulsion diverticula that appear in the distal third of the esophagus, within 10 cm of the gastroesophageal junction. As with midesophageal diverticula, they are more common on the right side. Epiphrenic diverticula are occasionally asymptomatic, but most patients have a motility disorder and present with dysphagia, regurgitation, vomiting, chest and epigastric pain, anorexia, weight loss, cough, halitosis, or noisy swallowing. No predictable relationship exists between symptoms and the size of the diverticulum.

DIAGNOSIS

Barium swallow best detects the presence of epiphrenic diverticula and often characterizes the underlying motility disorder (Fig. 39-19). In addition to fixed, relatively wide-mouthed diverticula, transient outpouchings may occur proximally in segments where peristalsis is absent. Although epiphrenic diverticula are readily detected with a barium swallow, motility studies are necessary to rule out an underlying motor disorder.[49] A distal esophageal stricture or tumor can also lead to abnormally elevated intraesophageal pressure with a resultant pouch. Rarely, epiphrenic diverticula may be congenital (Ehlers-Danlos syndrome) or may result from trauma.

TREATMENT

Minimally symptomatic patients with pouches smaller than 3 cm often require no treatment, whereas those with severe dysphagia, chest pain, or a pouch greater than 3 cm are candidates for esophagomyotomy and resection of the diverticula. Surgery is performed through a left

thoracotomy (or VATS) for resection of the diverticulum and a long extramucosal thoracic esophagomyotomy from beneath the aortic arch to the esophagogastric junction (Fig. 39-20). An associated hiatal hernia or incompetent LES should also be repaired during the operation. When an esophagomyotomy for motor disturbances is performed, the question of how far the incision should extend onto the stomach arises and whether a concomitant antireflux operation is necessary. Ellis and colleagues[50] reported

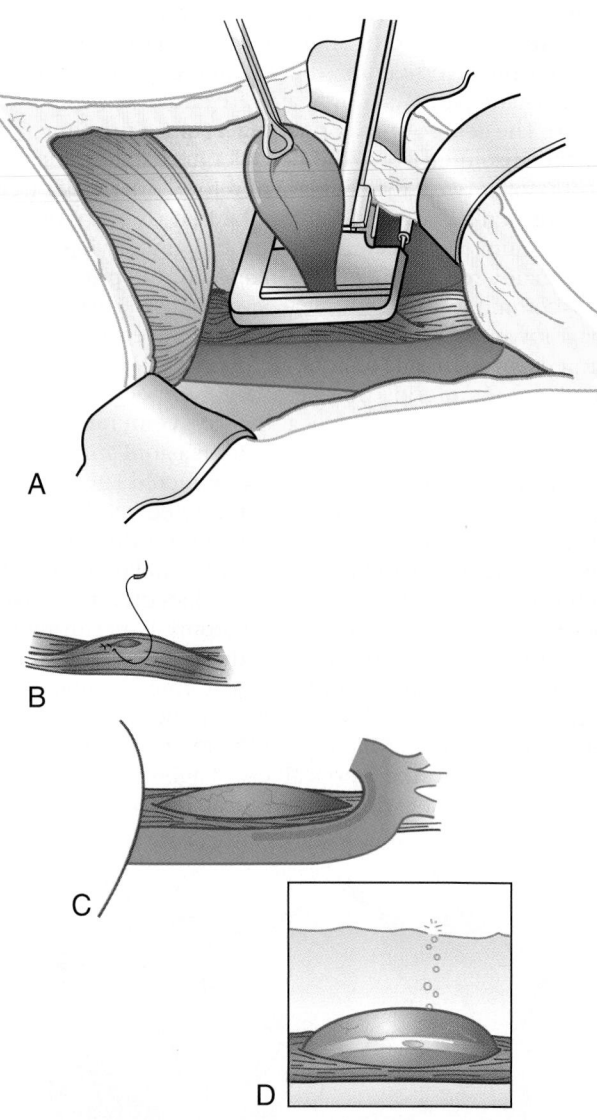

A

B

C

D

FIGURE 39-20.   Technique of resection of epiphrenic diverticulum and concomitant thoracic esophagomyotomy. **A,** After the diverticulum is mobilized to its base, it is amputated with a TA-30 surgical stapler. **B,** The staple suture line is oversewn by approximating adjacent muscle. **C,** A long esophagomyotomy from the esophagogastric junction to the aortic arch is performed on the opposite wall of the esophagus. **D,** Air is insufflated through an intraesophageal nasogastric tube with the esophagus immersed under saline solution so that any disruption of the mucosa can be identified and repaired. (**A** to **D,** Adapted from Orringer MB: Complications of esophageal surgery and trauma. *In* Greenfield LJ [ed]: Complications of Surgery and Trauma, 2nd ed. Philadelphia, JB Lippincott, 1990, pp 302-325.)

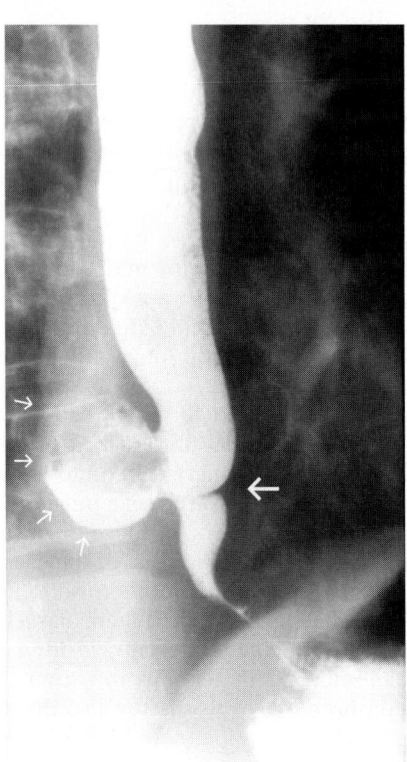

FIGURE 39-19.   Barium swallow showing an epiphrenic diverticulum *(multiple small arrows)* just proximal to a Schatzki ring *(arrow)*. (Courtesy of Ronelle A. Dubrow, M.D., MD Anderson Cancer Center, Houston, TX.)

that the LES should not be disturbed if preoperative esophageal function tests are normal. Belsey emphasized the need to eliminate the distal esophageal obstruction completely and routinely divided the LES by carrying the muscle incision 1.5 cm onto the stomach. If reflux is a major component of the symptoms, an antireflux procedure in addition to the esophageal myotomy will be necessary. In these circumstances, a partial fundoplication (Belsey type), rather than a 360-degree Nissen fundoplication, is less likely to produce functional obstruction on long-term follow-up.[44] Although thought of as procedures with relatively low morbidity and mortality, diverticulectomy and esophagomyotomy have been associated with a 9% operative mortality.[51] As a result, operative intervention for asymptomatic or minimally symptomatic epiphrenic diverticulum is discouraged.

Caustic Injury

The severity and site of caustic esophageal injury depend on the substance ingested (alkali vs. acid, solid vs. liquid, and concentration), quantity ingested, residual food in the stomach, and duration of tissue contact. Alkali causes liquefactive necrosis, resulting in a deep burn, whereas acids cause coagulative necrosis, forming an eschar that limits tissue penetration.[52] Solid alkali tends to adhere to and burn the oropharynx, whereas liquid alkali is rapidly swallowed, causing less oropharyngeal but more esophageal and/or gastric injury.[53,54] Sites susceptible to injury because of a relative delay in transit include the upper esophagus in the area of the cricopharyngeus, the mid-esophagus where the aorta and left mainstem bronchus impinge, and the distal esophagus proximal to the lower esophageal sphincter (LES).

Caustic injury also results in a hypotensive LES with reflux and prolonged exposure of the distal esophagus.[55] Alkali ingestion results in pylorospasm, with regurgitation of caustic agent into the esophagus, followed by cricopharyngeal muscle spasm and propulsion back into the stomach, aggravating both the esophageal and gastric burns. With acid ingestion, the esophagus may escape injury because of relative tolerance by the squamous epithelium. However, in the stomach, acid induces immediate pylorospasm, pooling the acid in the distal antrum and producing severe gastritis that may progress within 24 to 48 hours to full-thickness necrosis and perforation.

Symptoms of caustic ingestion include oral pain, hematemesis, drooling, and inability or refusal to swallow. Hoarseness, stridor, and dyspnea suggest laryngeal edema or epiglottic injury, prompting a thorough airway evaluation with bronchoscopy and laryngoscopy and possible intubation or tracheostomy to maintain airway patency. Corticosteroids may be administered to relieve airway obstruction due to mucosal edema and bronchospasm. Substernal, back, or abdominal pain may signify mediastinal or peritoneal perforation. Absence of symptoms or evidence of oropharyngeal burns does not exclude esophageal injury.[53,54,56,57] A report of caustic ingestion in 85 pediatric patients, however, showed absence of symptoms was always associated with no or minimal injury, whereas hematemesis, respiratory distress, or presence of

at least three symptoms was consistently associated with severe injury.[58]

Management of caustic ingestion involves immediate verification of the etiologic agent, followed by chest and abdominal radiographs and then esophagoscopy. Esophagoscopy is recommended 12 to 24 hours after injury to allow gastric emptying and stabilization of the patient,[52-54,56,57,59,60] unless esophageal or gastric perforation is suspected (Fig. 39-21). The severity of esophageal injury is classified as first degree (hyperemia and edema), second degree (ulceration), or third degree (massive edema and eschar formation with or without full-thickness necrosis). Esophagoscopy, which usually requires general anesthesia in children, may not be necessary in asymptomatic pediatric patients. Instead, some advocate close observation.[58,61] A prospective study by Millar and coworkers[61] of 22 patients showed a 100% negative predictive value for detection of caustic esophageal injury with radiolabeled sucralfate. The authors suggest screening children with suspected caustic ingestion with radiolabeled sucralfate before esophagoscopy. Treatment of first-degree esophageal burns, which do not perforate or form strictures, is usually observation for up to 48 hours.[53,54,56,62,63] Patients with second- or third-degree esophageal burns without evidence of perforation are placed in the intensive care unit (ICU), kept *nil per os* (NPO), and given intravenous fluids and antibiotics to decrease the risk of aspiration and bacterial contamination of the mediastinum through the injured esophageal wall.[53] Because acid reflux may increase stricture formation, prophylactic H blockers, proton-pump inhibitors, or antacids are recommended.[58,64] A large retrospective case series[63] indicated that corticosteroids are efficacious in preventing stricture formation; however, they may mask signs of peritonitis, especially at higher doses (e.g., 1.5 to 2 mg/kg/day of prednisone).[62] The endoscope is advanced to the area of the first severe burn to avoid iatrogenic perforation, often precluding full assessment of the esophagus and stomach. In addition, assessment of the depth of burn is difficult during esophagoscopy.[53,57] An alternative approach, advocated by Estrera and associates,[56] is exploratory laparotomy for all patients with second- or third-degree burns seen during esophagoscopy. With this approach, all burns with full-thickness necrosis undergo radical esophagogastrectomy, cervical esophagostomy, and jejunostomy for feeding. Those with second-degree and third-degree burns without full-thickness esophagogastric necrosis have an intraluminal stent placed for at least 21 days to prevent obliteration of the esophageal lumen and provide a template for epithelial ingrowth.[56] Estrera and coworkers reported four of four patients with second-degree burns and three of five patients with limited third-degree burns treated with a stent did not develop strictures.[56]

Patients with second- or third-degree injuries are monitored for evidence of perforation with serial chest and abdominal radiographs plus a barium swallow performed at 24 hours. Treatment alternatives include, first, an elective gastrostomy for feeding with passage of a nasogastric string for retrograde dilatation of strictures, which is commonly used in pediatric patients.[57,62] A second alternative

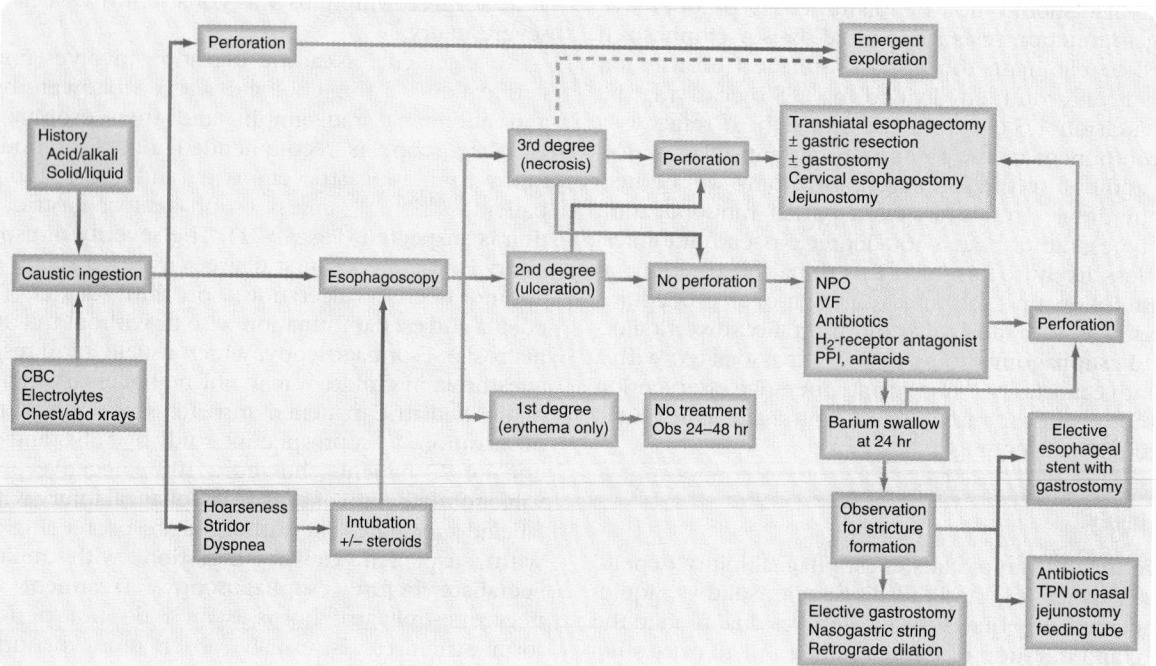

FIGURE 39-21.   Algorithm for treatment of caustic ingestion. CBC, Complete blood count; Abd, abdomen; NPO, nil per os; IVF, intravenous fluids; PPI, proton-pump inhibitor; TPN, total parenteral nutrition. (Modified from Zwischenberger JB, Savage C, Bidani A: Surgical aspects of esophageal disease. Am J Respir Crit Care Med 164:1037-1040, 2001.)

is intraluminal stent placement for prevention of strictures plus gastrostomy, as discussed previously.[56] The third option is to continue antibiotics and initiate feeding via a Dobhoff tube or total parenteral nutrition. All patients are kept NPO until they can swallow their saliva without pain, after which the diet is advanced as tolerated. Esophagogastroduodenoscopy is performed at 3 weeks for full evaluation. The esophagus and stomach are also evaluated with a barium swallow performed at 3 weeks, 3 months, and 6 months to rule out stricture formation, gastric outlet obstruction, or the development of either an hourglass or *linitis plastica*–like appearance.[65,66]

If the physical examination and chest or abdominal radiographs indicate a perforation has occurred, abdominal exploration is mandatory with resection of all injured organs to prevent extension of the injury.[60] Caustic esophageal perforations are best treated by esophagectomy, with the transhiatal route preferred.[67] Extensive fullthickness esophageal and gastric necrosis is treated with urgent radical total esophagogastrectomy with delayed (6 months) reconstruction. All patients receive a cervical esophagostomy and feeding jejunostomy.

The most frequent complication of second- or thirddegree esophageal burns is stricture formation, which usually develops between 3 and 8 weeks after initial injury.[62,63] Some lesions are mild and respond to dilatation without recurrence. Bougienage for early treatment of caustic esophageal burns is performed daily for several weeks, then every other day for 2 to 3 weeks, and finally once a week for months. Dilatations should not be initiated until esophageal re-epithelialization is complete, generally not sooner than 6 weeks after injury. For localized strictures extending beyond 1.5 cm and failing to respond to bougienage alone, local injection of corticosteroids

visualized through an esophagoscope, followed by bougienage, may be beneficial.[68]

Other complications include tracheoesophageal fistula, hiatal hernia, reflux, and esophageal carcinoma. Diagnosis of a tracheoesophageal fistula is suggested by progressive pneumonia, choking, coughing with feedings, or bilestained mucus in the airway with confirmation by a contrast study using barium. Hiatal hernia and reflux can develop years after injury, causing late esophagitis and peptic stricture. An acquired form of achalasia has also been reported as a consequence of extensive intramural fibrosis. The incidence of esophageal carcinoma in patients with caustic injury is 1000-fold greater than in the general population; therefore, any change in symptoms warrants immediate radiographic and endoscopic examination.

In summary, management of caustic ingestion requires radiologic and endoscopic evaluation to assess the injury. First-degree burns are observed, whereas second- and third-degree burns without perforation are managed by supportive care, with or without stent placement or gastrostomy, and with surveillance for late strictures. Caustic perforation requires immediate esophageal and/or gastric resection.

Perforation of the Esophagus

Esophageal perforation presents as an emergency because treatment delay reduces survival. Iatrogenic perforation, spontaneous perforation, and trauma account for a large majority of esophageal perforations.[69-72] Endoscopic procedures are the most common cause of iatrogenic esophageal perforation, with the cricopharyngeal area most commonly injured.[69] Mid- and distal esophageal perforations usually result from biopsies to document malignancy or from dilatations. Infrequent causes of iatrogenic esophageal perforation include difficult endotracheal intubation, blind insertion of a minitracheostomy, resection of lung cancer, blind dissection of the abdominal esophagus, operations on the cervical spine, thyroidectomy, and palliative intubation, stenting, or laser treatment of esophageal tumors. Boerhaave's syndrome, esophageal rupture induced by straining, is the most common type of spontaneous perforation. Ruptures usually occur in the left posterior aspect of the lower esophagus and are five times more frequent in males.[69] Severe reflux, caustic ingestion, and candidal, herpetic, and immunodeficiency infections also cause pathologic perforations. Destruction of the esophageal wall by carcinoma may cause mediastinal or pleural perforations. Esophageal perforations from penetrating or blunt trauma are frequently overshadowed by associated injuries and have a poor prognosis if unrecognized.[69,73,74]

Diagnosis

Symptoms and signs (pain, vomiting, hematemesis, dysphagia, tachypnea, tachycardia, fever, subcutaneous emphysema, mediastinal crunch, chest hypersonarity, or dullness) of esophageal perforation vary with cause, location (cervical, thoracic, or abdominal) and pathway of soilage (Fig. 39-22). Pain is the most common symptom, present in 70% to 90% of patients, usually referring directly to the site of perforation.[75] Cervical perforation is characterized by neck ache and stiffness due to esophageal attachment to the prevertebral fascia limiting spread of oropharyngeal soilage.[69] In the abdomen, subxiphoid pain is present with anterior perforations, and dull epigastric pain radiating to the back may occur if the perforation is posterior and communicates with the lesser sac. Severe retrosternal or chest pain lateralizing to the side of perforation is seen with thoracic perforation. Severe chest pain after straining and hematemesis occur with postemetic ruptures. Tachycardia and tachypnea are documented in most patients with perforation. Hypotension and shock are present when sepsis or significant inflammatory third spacing have occurred. Subcutaneous emphysema is seen frequently with cervical perforations but less often with thoracic or abdominal perforations. The Mallory-Weiss syndrome refers to a mucosal laceration (single or multiple) at the esophagogastric junction with hematemesis following retching or vomiting, but is not associated with pain. Dysphagia appears late and is usually related to a thoracic perforation.

Chest radiography is suggestive in 90% of patients but may be normal immediately after perforation. Pneumomediastinum, subcutaneous emphysema, mediastinal widening, or a mediastinal air-fluid level prompt investigation to rule out esophageal perforation. Hydropneumothorax on the left is seen in patients with distal third esophageal perforations. Esophagogram using barium should be used for esophageal perforations that are not expected to communicate with the peritoneal cavity to reveal the primary area of leakage. Water-soluble contrast (such as Gastrografin) should be used for esophageal perforations expected to communicate with the peri-

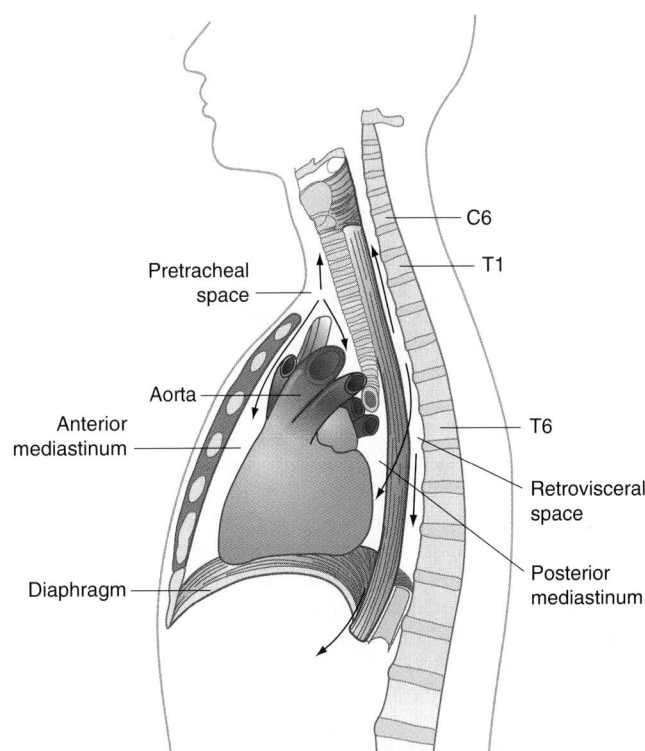

FIGURE 39-22. Diagram showing pathways for spread of infection to mediastinum and pleural cavities after cervical or thoracic esophageal perforation. (From Fell SC: Esophageal perforation. *In* Pearson FG, Cooper JD, Deslauriers J, et al [eds]: Esophageal Surgery, 2nd ed. Philadelphia, Churchill Livingstone, 2002, p 617.)

toneal cavity. In summary, barium is inert in the chest, whereas aspirated Gastrografin causes pneumonitis. However, barium in the peritoneal cavity causes peritonitis, while Gastrografin in the peritoneal cavity is inert. Unfortunately, the rate of false-negative esophagograms may be as high as 10%.[76] Chest CT often shows mediastinal fluid and air at the site of perforation. If a perforation is suspected during an endoscopic procedure, careful inspection of the esophagus without air insufflation is warranted. Based on our experience, esophagoscopy can miss a perforation hidden in a mucosal fold or aggravate soilage by air insufflation and is not recommended as a primary diagnostic study for esophageal perforation.

Treatment

Etiology, location, and delay between rupture and treatment affect prognosis and management of esophageal perforation. Lapse of time before drainage or repair of the perforation, regardless of cause and location, is the most significant influence on outcome.[75,77] Postemetic perforation is the most morbid, with decreased survival from massive contamination and delayed diagnosis. Morbidity and mortality increase as the perforation extends into the thorax.[78] Iatrogenic perforation, often noted immediately during endoscopic instrumentation, results in less morbidity and mortality. Patients with perforations of the cervical esophagus have a 94% survival, those with perforations of the thoracic esophagus have a 66% survival, and those with perforations of the abdominal esophagus have a 71% survival.[69]

Nonoperative management of esophageal perforations has been associated with a 20% to 38% mortality[79,80]; however, in carefully selected patients, mortality can approach zero.[71,81] The difficulty with nonoperative management is prospective determination of which perforation will remain contained and which will cause ongoing contamination with subsequent uncontrolled infection. Criteria for nonoperative management proposed by Cameron and associates[81] include a well-contained leak in a stable patient without evidence of sepsis or communication with the pleural or peritoneal cavity. The perforation must easily drain back into the esophagus, although this may be difficult to determine on an esophagogram. Signs and symptoms of sepsis during nonoperative management warrant immediate surgical treatment. Pneumothorax, mediastinal emphysema, and respiratory failure are also indications for surgical interventions.

Surgery, with primary repair reinforced with vascularized tissue, is the mainstay for esophageal perforation treatment (Fig. 39-23).[69-72,82,83] Preoperative preparation includes nasogastric intubation for gastric decompression, broad-spectrum antibiotics for oropharyngeal contamination, and intravenous fluid resuscitation. Cervical perforations are treated by primary closure and drainage of the neck. Thoracic esophageal perforations require a right thoracotomy for exposure of the upper two thirds and left thoracotomy for the lower third. Lesions at the esophagogastric junction are approached by left thoracotomy or upper midline celiotomy, with repairs often reinforced by fundoplication. Perforations require wide mediastinal drainage by opening the parietal pleura the entire length of the esophagus. Nonviable and grossly contaminated

tissue in the mediastinum and the parietal pleura is débrided. The esophagus and often the esophagogastric junction must be dissected completely to identify the site of perforation and mobilize the esophagus for a tension-free repair. Esophagomyotomy (an incision through the longitudinal and circular muscle layers, exposing the submucosa) is often necessary to visualize the mucosal injury. Primary repair is accomplished with closure of the mucosal defect over a bougie and reapproximation of the muscle.[83] The technique of repair may be a single-layer or a double-layer suture closure, but recent experience with the three-layered stapled ENDO-GIA repair has produced gratifying results even after long periods of delay in diagnosis. Compared with an unreinforced primary repair (39% fistula formation, 25% mortality), reinforcement with vascularized tissue may decrease fistula formation (13%) and mortality (6%).[75] Esophageal repairs are then drained by a large-bore chest tube. A mobilized gastric fundus provides the best protection as a partial or total fundoplication around perforations of the distal esophagus (Fig. 39-24A). A fundic (Thal) patch may be used if the perforation extends above the diaphragm (see Fig. 39-24B). Protection of thoracic esophageal perforation repairs can be added by an autologous pleural flap[84] (see Fig. 39-24C) or by pedicled muscle flaps from the intercostal muscles, chest wall musculature, the diaphragm, or a mobilized pedicle of omentum (Fig. 39-25).[85]

Late perforations can usually still be repaired primarily, then reinforced by muscle or pleura.[75,83,86] If repair is not possible or if severe mediastinitis is present, options include esophageal resection or exclusion and diversion. Most favor esophageal resection, cervical esophagostomy, and enteral feeding tube with plans for late (6 months) reconstruction. Perforations encountered late may initially be treated by wide drainage of the mediastinum by

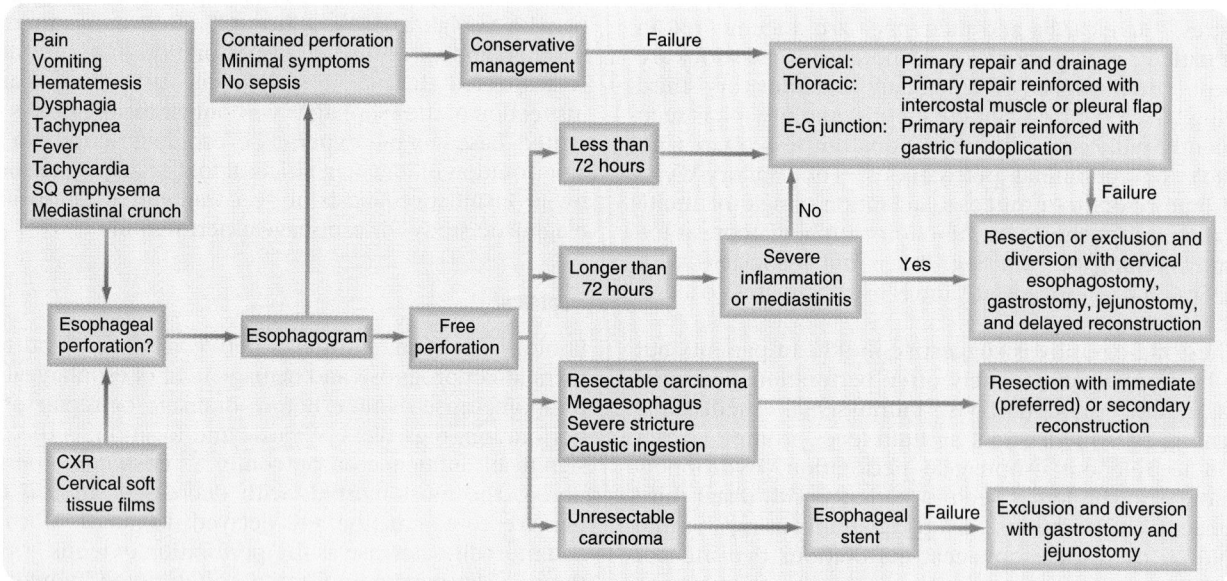

FIGURE 39-23. Algorithm for treatment of esophageal perforation. SQ, subcutaneous; CXR, chest radiograph; E-G, esophagogastric. (Modified from Zwischenberger JB, Savage C, Bidani A: Surgical aspects of esophageal disease. Perforation and caustic injury. Am J Respir Crit Care Med 164:1037-1040, 2001.)

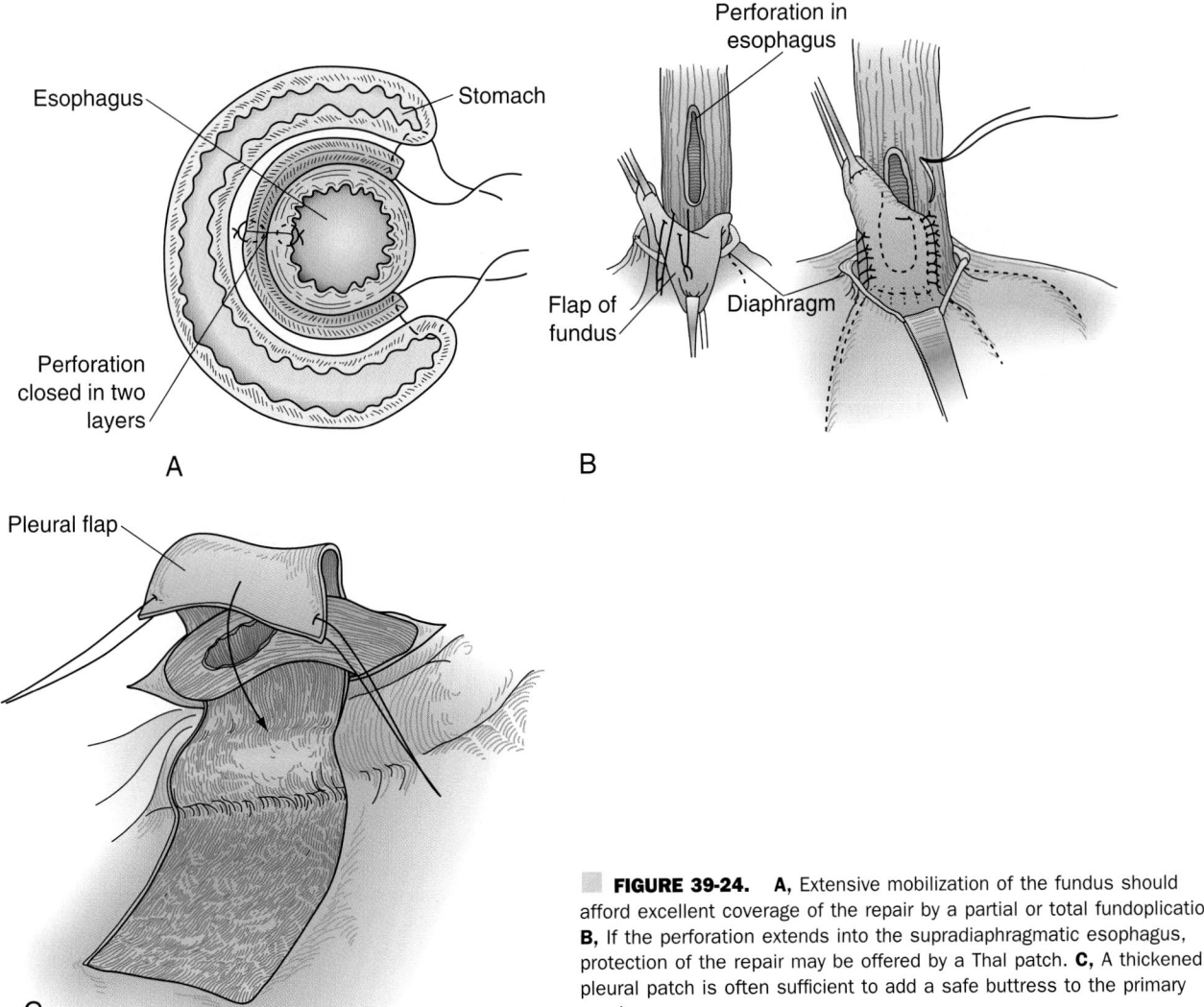

FIGURE 39-24.   **A,** Extensive mobilization of the fundus should afford excellent coverage of the repair by a partial or total fundoplication. **B,** If the perforation extends into the supradiaphragmatic esophagus, protection of the repair may be offered by a Thal patch. **C,** A thickened pleural patch is often sufficient to add a safe buttress to the primary repair.

opening the parietal pleura the entire length of the esophagus (not just a chest tube). Patients with complex perforations should preferably be treated with jejunostomy enteral nutrition or parenteral hyperalimentation because gastrostomy should be avoided for later reconstruction. Broad-spectrum antibiotics should be continued for at least 10 days. If the site is grossly inflamed, diversion and drainage may allow survival with later resection or reconstruction. Exclusion and diversion entail cervical esophagostomy (diversion of the cervical esophagus, creating a salivary fistula), gastric decompression with a gastrostomy, and jejunostomy with delayed (6 months) reconstruction (Fig. 39-26A). An alternative to exclusion and diversion is T-tube drainage of the perforation, creating a controlled esophagocutaneous fistula (see Fig. 39-26B).[71,87] T-tube placement can be used in high-risk patients, but continued leakage can progress to sepsis and is often not recommended as a routine procedure.[71,75,87]

Esophageal resection, with or without immediate reconstruction, should be considered a first-line procedure for perforations in patients with megaesophagus, carcinoma, caustic ingestion or stenosis, or severe undilatable reflux strictures.[70,72,82,83] If the underlying pathologic process is esophageal carcinoma, resection and immediate reconstruction are indicated if the lesion is otherwise resectable. If perforation has occurred during palliative treatment of unresectable esophageal carcinoma, a covered metallic stent, which closely follows the contours of the esophagus, usually prevents leakage.[88] Treatment of a spontaneous perforation with a flexible covered stent has also been reported.[89]

Early primary repair still has significant morbidity and mortality ranging from 33% to 43% in patients with a postemetic rupture, even if the condition is diagnosed and treated less than 24 hours after perforation,[69] to as low as 5% in some reports.[83] Principles of repair include a local esophagomyotomy proximal and distal to the tear to expose the mucosal defect and normal mucosa beyond débridement of the mucosal defect, closure over a bougie, and reapproximation of the muscle. Reinforcement with vascularized tissue and wide drainage reportedly decreases the incidence of fistulas (13%) and mortality (6%) compared with treatment by a simple primary repair (fistula, 39%; mortality, 25%).[90]

Postoperative care includes nasogastric tube decompression of the stomach until resolution of the postoperative

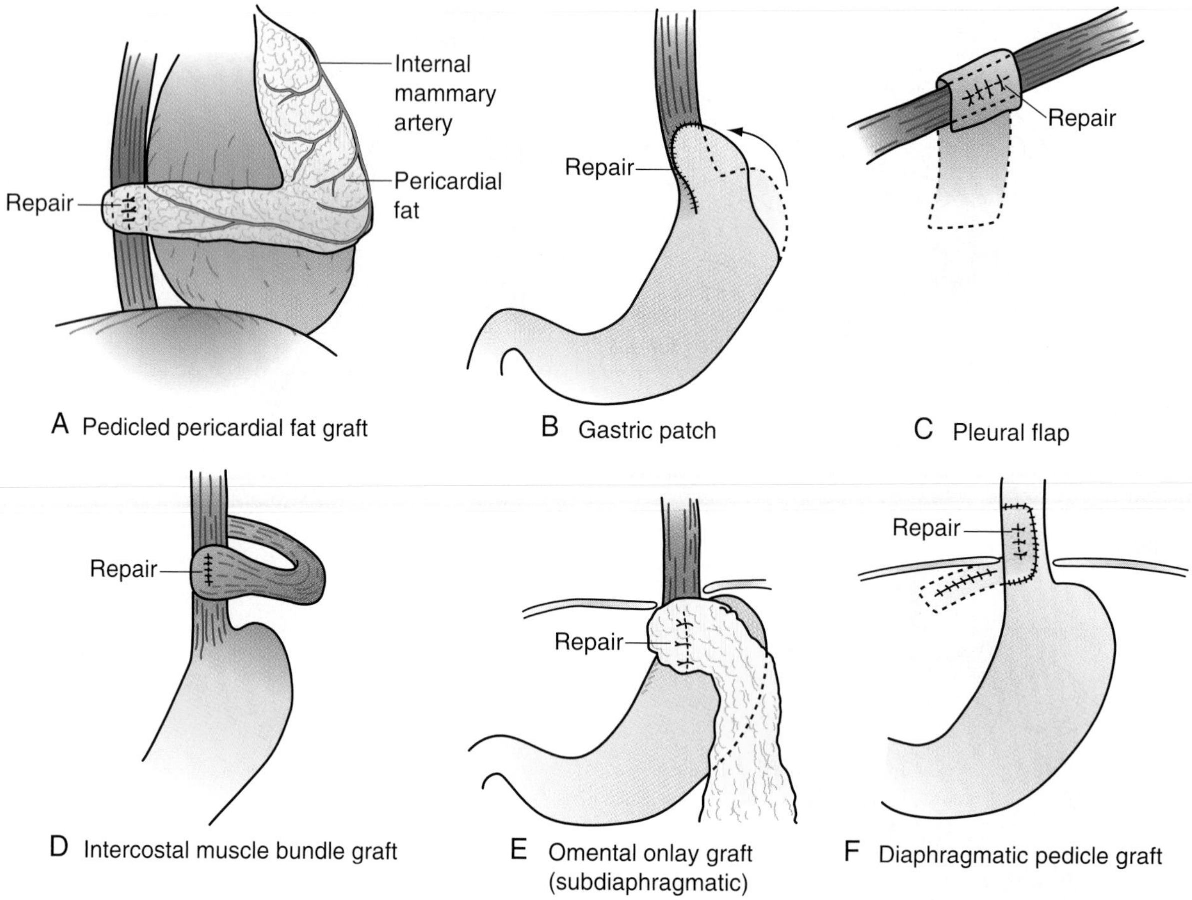

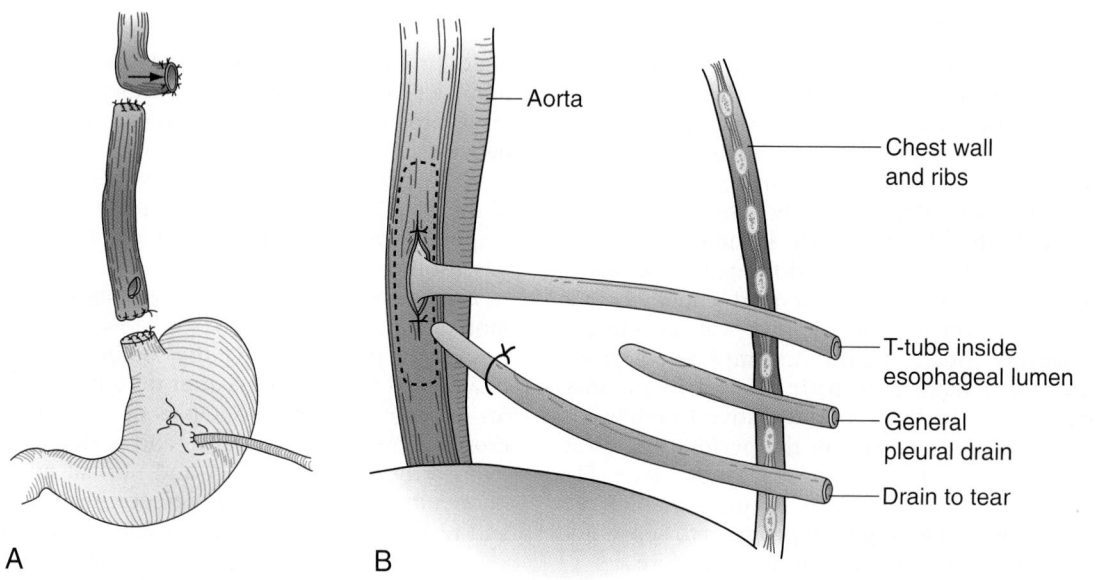

A Pedicled pericardial fat graft

Internal mammary artery

Pericardial fat

Repair

B Gastric patch

Repair

C Pleural flap

Repair

D Intercostal muscle bundle graft

Repair

E Omental onlay graft (subdiaphragmatic)

Repair

F Diaphragmatic pedicle graft

Repair

FIGURE 39-25.   **A to F,** Techniques of buttressing the primary repair of esophageal perforation. (**A** to **F,** Adapted from Brewer LA III, Carter R, Mulder GA, Stiles QR: Options in the management of perforations of the esophagus. Am J Surg 152:62-69, 1986, with permission from Excerpta Medica Inc.)

Aorta

Chest wall and ribs

T-tube inside esophageal lumen

General pleural drain

Drain to tear

A

B

FIGURE 39-26.   **A,** Exclusion of the perforated esophagus by closure or division at the cardia and into the neck. **B,** T-tube drainage of the esophageal perforation with pleural drainage.

ileus, after which enteral feeding is slowly advanced through a jejunostomy or Dobhoff tube. An esophagogram is obtained 3 to 7 days postoperatively to document absence of a leak and allow oral intake. Long-term surveillance for stricture formation, reflux, or carcinoma is also recommended.

In summary, treatment of an esophageal perforation requires fluid resuscitation, control of sepsis, operative drainage of the mediastinum and pleural cavity, primary repair of the esophagus, and reinforcement with vascularized tissue. Although delayed diagnosis increases the complexity because of friable tissue at the site of perforation, primary repair may still be possible. In cases with severe inflammation, either resection or exclusion with diversion is recommended. Primary resection is indicated for undilatable strictures, megaesophagus, carcinoma, or caustic stenosis or ingestion.

tracheostomy. Long-term intubation, however, still accounts for the majority of acquired, nonmalignant TEFs because of either overinflation of the cuff or placement of a small tracheostomy tube necessitating overinflation of the cuff to provide airway sealing. Associated risk factors increasing the likelihood of TEF include excessive motion of the tracheostomy tube, infections, hypotension, corticosteroid use, and diabetes. Diagnosis is by bronchoscopy and esophagoscopy.

Operative closure of a TEF is necessary because spontaneous closure is rare. Before undertaking the operation, it is best if patients are weaned from the ventilator because positive-pressure ventilation after tracheal repair increases the risk of dehiscence. Various surgical options are available for repair of a TEF; however, postintubation TEF is best treated with tracheal resection and anastomosis with the primary esophageal closure buttressed by a pedicled strap muscle flap.[91,92]

Tracheoesophageal Fistula (Acquired)

The widespread use of high-volume low-pressure cuffs has reduced the incidence of cuff-related *tracheoesophageal fistulas* (TEFs) to 0.5% in patients undergoing

Benign Esophageal Tumors

Benign tumors of the esophagus are rare, constituting only 0.5% to 0.8% of all esophageal neoplasms.[93] A useful classification is listed in (Table 39-3).[94] Approximately 60%

TABLE 39-3. Human Esophagus and Histogenetic Classification of Benign Esophageal Tumors

Esophageal Wall Tissue of Origin	Tumor Type	Tissue Type
Mucosa		
Epithelial lining		
Normal stratified squamous epithelium	Squamous cell papilloma	Epithelial
Acquired metaplastic columnar epithelium	True adenoma (rare) or adenomatous hyperplasia	Epithelial
Lamina propria		
Simple esophageal cardiac mucous gland	Mucus retention cyst	Epithelial
	True adenoma (rare)	Epithelial
Epithelial lining plus lamina propria	Inflammatory pseudotumor	Mesenchymal
	Fibrovascular polyp	Mesenchymal
Muscularis mucosae	Leiomyoma	Nonepithelial
Inflamed gastric mucosal fold at gastroesophageal junction	Inflammatory reflux polyp	Reflux polyp-fold complex
Submucosa		
Esophageal mucous gland proper	Mucus retention cyst	Epithelial
	Adenoma	Epithelial
Vascular connective tissue	Fibrovascular polyp (fibrolipoma, fibromyxoma)	Mesenchymal
Blood vessel	Hemangioma	Mesenchymal
Schwann cell	Granular cell tumor	Mesenchymal
	Neurilemoma	Mesenchymal
Muscularis Propria		
Striated muscle (upper one third)	Rhabdomyoma	Mesenchymal
Smooth muscle (lower two thirds)	Leiomyoma	Mesenchymal
Nerve fiber	Neurofibroma	Mesenchymal
Schwann cell	Granular cell tumor	Mesenchymal
	Neurilemoma	
Tunica Adventitia		
Connective tissue	Fibroma	Mesenchymal
Nerve plexus	Schwannoma (neurilemoma)	Mesenchymal
Ectopic Tissues		
Sebaceous gland	Adenoma	Epithelial
Tracheobronchial rests	Choristoma	Mixed tissues

From Shamji F, Todd TRJ: Benign tumors. *In* Pearson FG, Cooper JD, Deslauriers J, et al (eds): Esophageal Surgery, 2nd ed. Philadelphia, Churchill Livingstone, 2002, p 639.

of benign esophageal neoplasms are leiomyomas, 20% are cysts, and 5% are polyps.

Leiomyomas

Leiomyomas, leiomyosarcomas, and leiomyoblastomas were originally named for their histologic resemblance to smooth muscle cells. Recent studies show the cell of origin is actually mesenchymal, making the more appropriate term *gastrointestinal stromal tumors* (GISTs). GISTs are the most common mesenchymal tumors of the gastrointestinal tract and may be benign, malignant, or of intermediate malignant potential. Virtually all GISTs occur from mutations of the c-*KIT* oncogene, exhibiting consistent expression of c-*KIT (CD117),* which is considered the most specific criterion for diagnosis.[94a] True leiomyomas (c-*KIT* negative) are less frequent than previously described. These tumors, when benign, do not infiltrate surrounding tissue, so the overlying mucosa is rarely, if ever, invaded.[95]

These intramural tumors typically occur between 20 and 50 years of age, have no clear-cut gender preponderance, and are multiple in 3% to 10% of patients. More than 80% of these tumors occur in the middle and lower thirds of the esophagus, rarely in the cervical region.

DIAGNOSIS

Despite infringement into the lumen by the tumor, symptoms of dysphagia and vague retrosternal pressure or pain are produced only by large tumors (usually larger than 5 cm) because of the distensibility of the uninvolved esophagus. Most are found incidentally at autopsy and are asymptomatic. Esophageal symptoms prompt performance of a barium swallow and/or an endoscopic examination. The barium swallow appearance (Fig. 39-27) is distinctive because the well-localized mass has a smooth surface with distinct margins and is not circumferential. Most frequently, a leiomyoma is seen on a chest radiograph as a posterior mediastinal mass or is found unexpectedly during endoscopic examination. During endoscopy, the mucosa is intact and the extrinsic mass narrows the lumen but can easily be displaced and passed with the esophagoscope. Endoscopic biopsy should be avoided because adherence of the tumor to the mucosal biopsy site may complicate subsequent surgical resection. EUS confirms the diagnosis of leiomyoma as a hypoechoic lesion arising in the submucosa or muscularis propria.

TREATMENT

Excision of symptomatic leiomyomas or those larger than 5 cm is advised (Fig. 39-28). Asymptomatic or smaller tumors discovered incidentally can be observed and followed. Although excision of the esophageal tumor provides the only absolute proof that it is benign, leiomyomas have such a characteristic radiographic appearance, slow growth rate, and low risk of malignant degeneration that periodic follow-up of these lesions is reasonable. The malignant variant of leiomyosarcoma is extremely rare.

When resection is indicated, benign tumors of the middle third of the esophagus are approached through a

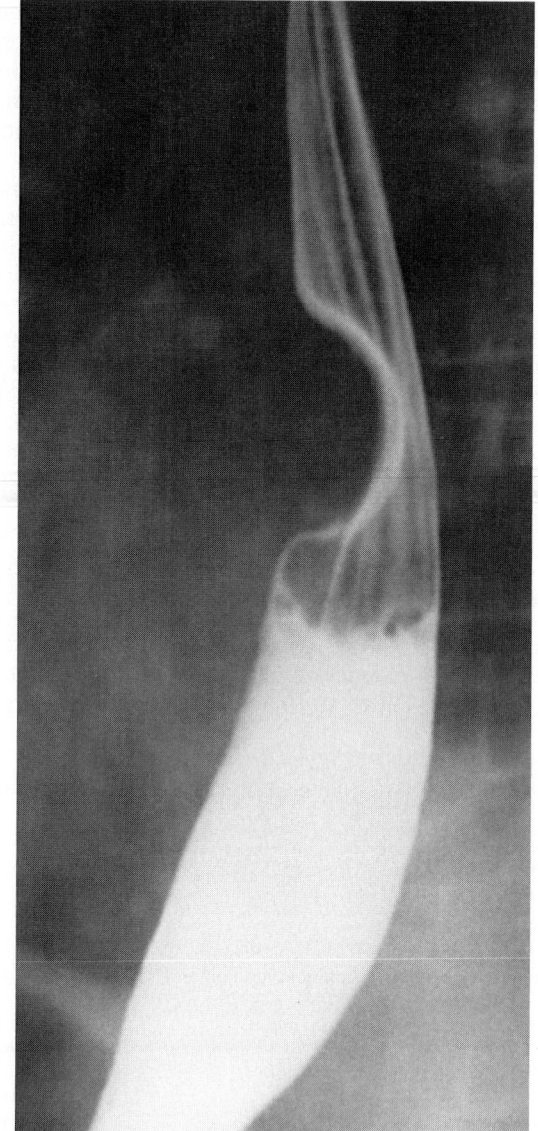

FIGURE 39-27. Esophagogram shows a typical leiomyoma.

right thoracotomy; those in the distal third are approached through a left thoracotomy. The tumor is located, and the overlying longitudinal esophageal muscle is split in the direction of its fibers, to reveal the mass. The tumor is then gently dissected away from contiguous tissues and the underlying submucosa. Once the tumor has been enucleated, the longitudinal muscle should be reapproximated if possible. Esophageal resection may be required for either giant leiomyomas of the cardia that involve the adjacent stomach or for diffuse esophageal leiomyomatosis, although multiple enucleations may be performed.

Using minimally invasive surgical techniques, the surgeon approaches the lesion from the left side of the patient's chest, which allows access to the distal esophagus. The right side of the chest is preferable for access to lesions of the middle and upper esophagus, in which the

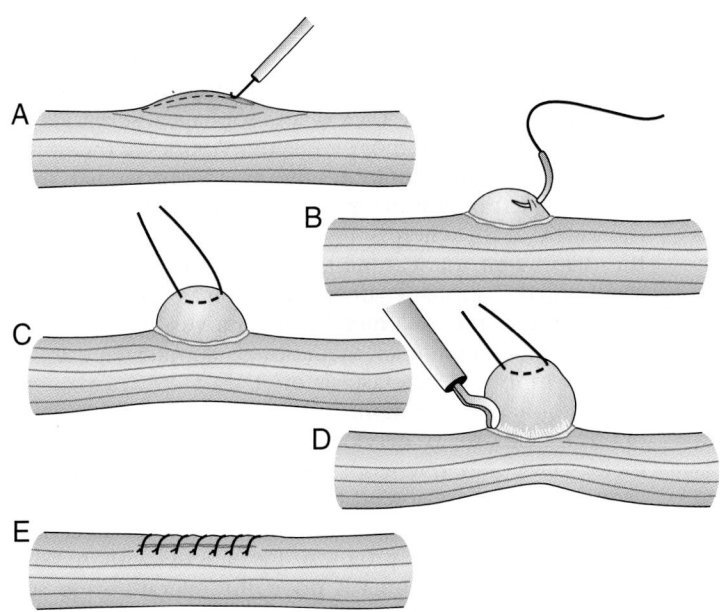

FIGURE 39-28. Operation for leiomyoma of the esophagus. **A,** Incision of the muscle wall. **B,** Dissection of the muscle wall. **C,** A traction stitch placed through the tumor. **D,** Separation of the tumor from the mucosa. **E,** Closure of the myotomy. (**A** to **E,** Adapted from Lerut T: Thoracoscopic esophageal surgery. *In* Baue AE, Geha AS, Hammond GL, et al [eds]: Glenn's Thoracic and Cardiovascular Surgery, 6th ed, vol 1. Norwalk, CT, Appleton & Lange, 1996, p 867. With permission of the McGraw-Hill Companies.)

aorta interferes with left-sided approaches. The patient is placed in the lateral decubitus thoracotomy position, with the operating table flexed to maximize the intercostal distances. Ventilation of the contralateral lung is continued through a double-lumen endotracheal tube, and the ipsilateral lung is allowed to collapse. Thoracoports are arrayed, and the lung is retracted anteriorly to expose the posterior mediastinum. Retraction can be accomplished with a fan-shaped retractor or by grasping and elevating the lung. Exposure is further facilitated by tilting the operating table to lean the patient forward.

The parietal pleura overlying the esophagus is grasped, elevated, and incised to gain entry into the posterior mediastinum. The azygos vein is divided between hemoclips or with an endoscopic gastrointestinal anastomosis stapling device, if necessary, for exposure of the upper esophagus. Further, blunt and sharp dissection suffices to separate the esophagus from the mediastinal fat. To provide countertraction, it is safer to push gently on the esophagus with a blunt-tipped instrument than to grasp the easily torn muscle. Enlarging a trocar site can be useful in allowing the placement of a long standard instrument to facilitate dissection. When the dissection is between the esophagus and the aorta, the esophageal arteries need to be either clipped or controlled with a Harmonic scalpel. If the operation is performed for a cyst or a leiomyoma, only enough dissection to expose the lesion is necessary.

After exposure has been gained and the esophagus mobilized, the benign tumor is dissected from the muscle and mucosa. The tumor can be either grasped directly or lifted by a suspension suture that transfixes the tumor. Invasion of or attachment to the muscle or mucosa is rare, so the tumor can be easily separated. Electrocautery should not be used for fear of injuring the mucosa. A small

muscle defect can be covered by suturing the muscle layers in a transverse orientation. If the muscle gap is large, an onlay patch of parietal pleura or adjacent vascularized tissue is an option (see Fig. 39-25).

Polyps of the cervical esophagus (20% of benign tumors) are intraluminal lesions that may cause dysphagia or may be regurgitated into the larynx with the potential for asphyxiation. They are composed of a fibroelastic core and usually are covered with normal epithelium. The preferred approach for resection is through a lateral cervical esophagomyotomy, thereby delivering the polyp to allow resection of the mucosal origin of the pedicle under direct vision. Esophageal polyps have also been removed endoscopically by electrocoagulating the pedicle. Lipomas, vascular tumors, and neurofibromas are extremely rare, but they must be removed to control symptoms or to exclude malignancy.

Esophageal Cancer

Esophageal cancer is the sixth most common malignancy worldwide and represents 4% of newly diagnosed cancers in North America. Unfortunately, most North American patients still present with locally advanced (stage T3 and/or N1) disease. Variations in incidence occur among countries or even within regions in a given country, especially among the male population. Besides these geographic patterns, a major shift in the histologic type of tumors has occurred. Traditionally, esophageal cancer has been squamous cell in patients with the usual risk factors for other aerodigestive tract carcinomas, specifically smoking (5-fold) and alcohol (5-fold) abuse. Heavy smoking and heavy drinking combine to increase the risk

25- to 100-fold. African-Americans are five times more likely to develop squamous cell carcinoma than other socioeconomic groups; and males are affected four to six times more often than females.[97] Within North America and Europe, the incidence of adenocarcinoma rose 100% in the 1990s, strongly correlated with reflux, Barrett's metaplasia, and dietary factors (a diet high in fat).[98]

Although the origin of this shift remains unknown, carcinoma of the esophagus now appears to affect younger, healthier patients. Nutritional factors and potential carcinogens have been incriminated, including alcohol, tobacco, zinc, nitrosamines, malnutrition, vitamin deficiencies, anemia, poor oral hygiene and dental caries, previous gastric surgery, and long-term ingestion of hot foods or beverages. An increased incidence of esophageal carcinoma is noted in patients with familial keratosis palmaris et plantaris (*tylosis*), which is inherited as an autosomal dominant trait. Some esophageal lesions increase the incidence of cancer, including achalasia, reflux esophagitis, Barrett's (columnar epithelial-lined) esophagus,[99] radiation esophagitis,[100] caustic burns, Plummer-Vinson syndrome, leukoplakia, esophageal diverticula, and ectopic gastric mucosa. The rising prevalence of adenocarcinoma associated with Barrett's esophagus suggests a possible link to untreated or silent gastroesophageal reflux. This observation potentially defines high-risk patients who may potentially benefit from surveillance to achieve earlier detection of dysplasia or malignancy.

Esophageal cancer is notorious for its aggressive biologic behavior; it infiltrates locally, involves adjacent lymph nodes (Fig. 39-29), and metastasizes widely by hematogenous spread. Lack of an esophageal serosal layer tends to favor local tumor extension. Tumors of the upper and middle thirds infiltrate the tracheobronchial tree, aorta, and left recurrent laryngeal nerve as it loops around the aortic arch, whereas lower-third tumors may invade the diaphragm, pericardium, or stomach. The extensive mediastinal lymphatic drainage, which communicates with cervical and abdominal collateral vessels, is responsible for the finding of mediastinal, supraclavicular, or celiac lymph node metastasis in at least 75% of patients with esophageal carcinoma. Cervical esophageal cancers drain to the deep cervical, paraesophageal, posterior mediastinal, and tracheobronchial lymph nodes. Lower esophageal tumors spread to paraesophageal, celiac, and splenic hilar lymph nodes. Distant spread to liver and lungs is common. The prognosis for patients with invasive squamous cell carcinoma is poor; the overall 5-year survival for patients with treated tumors is 5% to 12%. Extraesophageal tumor extension is present in 70% of cases at the time of diagnosis, and the 5-year survival is only 3% when lymph node metastases are present, compared with 42% when no lymph node spread has occurred.

Histologically, approximately 95% of esophageal cancers worldwide are squamous cell carcinomas. In areas of China where the disease is endemic and mass

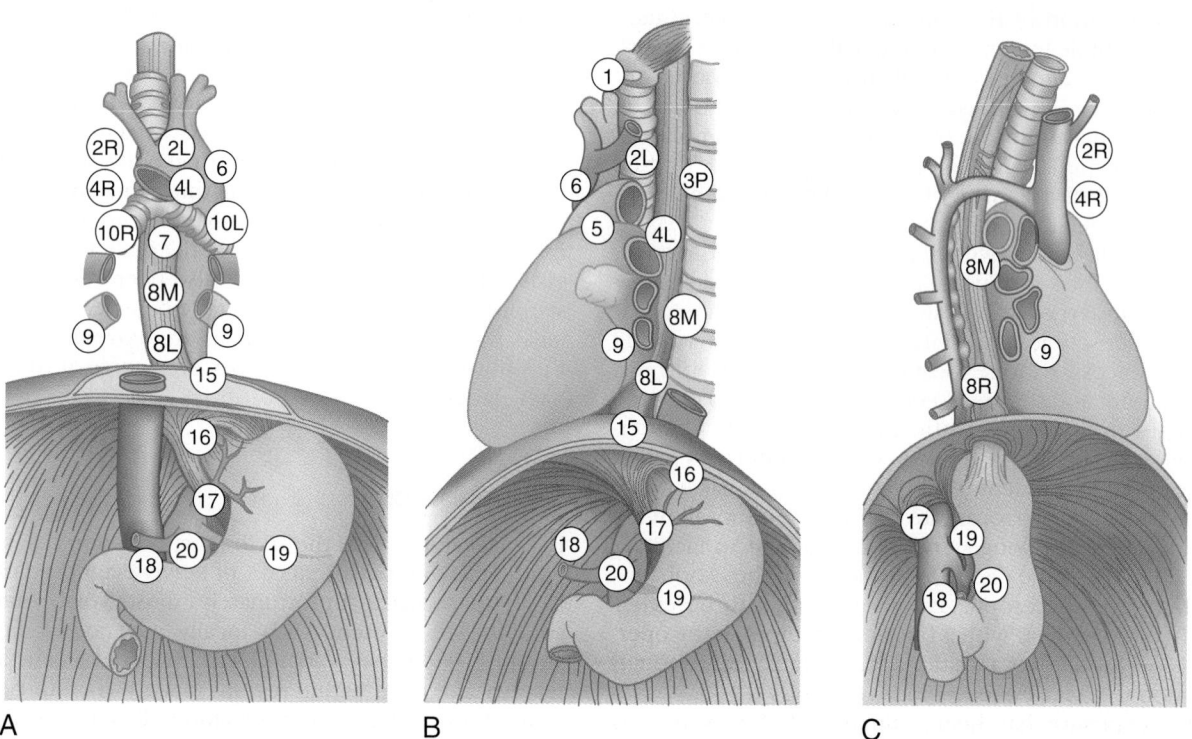

FIGURE 39-29.   Lymph node map for esophageal cancer. **A,** Anterior view. **B,** Left lateral view. **C,** Right lateral view. Lymph node stations: 1, supraclavicular; 2R, right paratracheal; 2L, left paratracheal; 3P, posterior mediastinal; 4R, right tracheobronchial angle; 4L, left tracheobronchial; 5, aortopulmonary; 6, anterior mediastinal; 7, subcarinal; 8M, middle paraesophageal; 8L, lower paraesophageal; 9, inferior pulmonary ligament; 10, hilar; 15, diaphragmatic; 16, paracardial; 17, left gastric; 18, common hepatic; 19, splenic; 20, celiac. (From Rice TW: Esophageal carcinoma: Diagnosis and staging of esophageal carcinoma. *In* Pearson FG, Cooper JD, Deslauriers J, et al [eds]: Esophageal Surgery, 2nd ed. Philadelphia, Churchill Livingstone, 2002, p 688.)

screening using esophageal brush cytology for detection of early carcinomas is economically and medically justifiable, several macroscopic varieties of early esophageal cancer have been defined. These early forms of esophageal cancer have been variously termed *carcinoma in situ, superficial spreading carcinoma,* and *intramucosal carcinoma.* They constitute fewer than 5% of all resected cases, are asymptomatic, and may take 3 to 4 years to progress to invasive squamous cell carcinoma. Endoscopically, carcinoma in situ most often presents as a slightly raised, granular, reddish, plaquelike lesion, although superficial erosions or papillary lesions smaller than 3 cm in diameter may also be seen. Endoscopic surveillance by staining with supravital dyes has been suggested as a form of chemoendoscopy to increase identification of dysplastic areas in high-risk patients. However, the utility of this technique is not uniformly reproducible in various studies and the routine use of chemoendoscopy remains controversial.[101,102]

Squamous cell carcinoma arises from the mucosa of the esophagus. Histologically, it is characterized by invasive sheets of cells that run together and are polygonal, oval, or spindle-shaped with a distinct or ragged stromal-epithelial interface. Located mainly in the thoracic esophagus, approximately 60% of these tumors are found in the middle third and about 30% in the distal third. Squamous cell neoplasms have four major gross pathologic presentations: (1) fungating—predominantly intraluminal growth with surface ulceration and extreme friability that frequently invades mediastinal structures; (2) ulcerating—flat-based ulcer with slightly raised edges; hemorrhagic, friable with surrounding induration; (3) infiltrating—a dense, firm, longitudinal and circumferential intramural growth pattern; and (4) polypoid—intraluminal polypoid growth with a smooth surface on a narrow stalk (fewer than 5% of cases).[103] A 5-year survival of 70% is associated with the polypoid tumor compared with a 5-year survival of less than 15% for all other types.[104]

Adenocarcinoma is now the most common cell type of esophageal cancer in the United States. It arises from the superficial and deep glands of the esophagus, mainly in the lower third of the esophagus, especially near the gastroesophageal junction (Fig. 39-30). Whites are at four times greater risk than blacks, and men have an 8-fold higher risk than women. Esophageal adenocarcinoma may have one of three origins: (1) the esophageal submucosal glands; (2) heterotopic islands of columnar epithelium; or (3) malignant degeneration of metaplastic columnar epithelium (Barrett's mucosa). Gastric adenocarcinoma may also involve the esophagus secondarily. Unlike the mucin-secreting cells of origin, adenocarcinoma cytologically has a reduced cytoplasmic-nuclear ratio. A loss of cellular polarity demonstrates variable atypia and nuclear size, enlarged nucleoli, and increased mitoses. Gastroesophageal junction tumors arise initially as flat or raised patches of mucosa that may subsequently ulcerate and become large (up to 5 cm) nodular masses. Tumor size is related to prognosis. For tumors smaller than 5 cm, 40% are localized, 25% have spread beyond the esophagus, and 35% have metastasized or are unresectable. For tumors that are more than 5 cm in length, 10% are localized, 15%

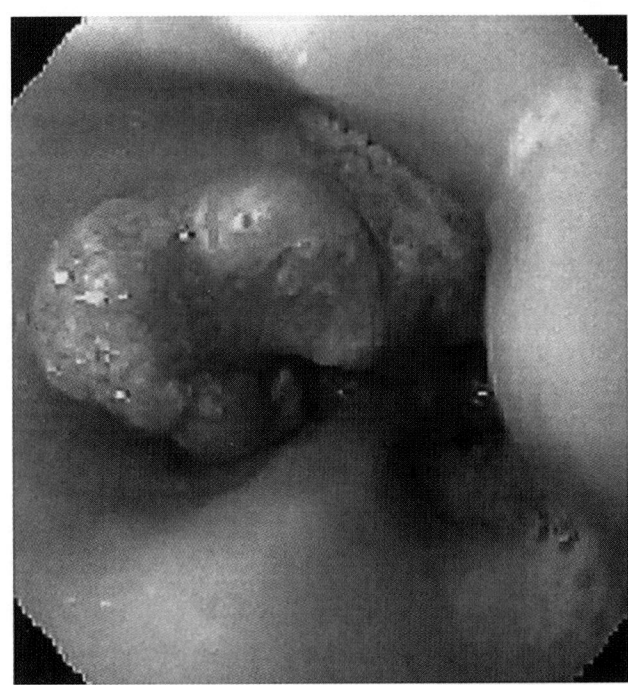

FIGURE 39-30. Adenocarcinoma of the esophagogastric junction. (From Rice TW, Zuccaro G Jr: Flexible esophagoscopy. *In* Pearson FG, Cooper JD, Deslauriers J, et al [eds]: Esophageal Surgery, 2nd ed. Philadelphia, Churchill Livingstone, 2002, p 153.)

have invaded mediastinal structures, and 75% have metastasized.[105]

As with squamous cell carcinoma, adenocarcinoma of the esophagus exhibits aggressive behavior with frequent transmural invasion and lymphatic spread. Because many of these tumors arise in the distal esophagus, spread to paraesophageal, celiac axis, and splenic hilar lymph nodes is common. Metastases to the lung and liver are frequent.

Seven percent of the U.S. population suffers from symptomatic GERD, and 2% to 15% of those patients with chronic reflux disease develop Barrett's esophagus (metaplastic columnar epithelium replaces the distal squamous mucosa attributable to prolonged exposure of the distal esophageal mucosa to gastroesophageal reflux).[98,98a] Barrett's esophagus is of clinical importance because adenocarcinoma occurs in patients with Barrett's esophagus at a rate 30 to 40 times greater than that of the general population. Although the true incidence of Barrett's esophagus in the general population is unknown, adenocarcinoma arises in 8% to 15% of patients with a columnar-lined esophagus.[99] The finding of dysplasia in Barrett's mucosa is a prognostic sign of potential malignant degeneration,[106] with 30% of patients with severe dysplasia developing adenocarcinoma (see Barrett's Esophagus, later in this chapter).

Diagnosis

Symptoms of esophageal carcinoma are usually insidious, beginning as nonspecific retrosternal discomfort or indigestion, followed by the common symptoms of dysphagia and weight loss (Table 39-4). Because of the elasticity of the esophagus, two thirds of the lumen must be obstructed to produce dysphagia. Patients complain of food "getting stuck," often directly at the location of the lesion. Pain can be caused by spasm or contractions proximal to an obstruction, tumor invasion, or interference with swallowing, or it may be related to metastases into the surrounding esophageal lymph nodes. Because dysphagia is the presenting complaint in 80% to 90% of patients with esophageal carcinoma,[111] any adult who complains of dysphagia (usually progressive) warrants esophagoscopy to rule out carcinoma. Likewise, esophagoscopy and biopsy are mandatory in every patient with an esophageal stenosis. Less frequent symptoms are coughing or hoarseness associated with tumors of the cervical esophagus. As the tumor enlarges, esophageal obstruction results in progressive weight loss, regurgitation, and aspiration, which, together with tobacco and alcohol abuse, result in poor general physical condition. All these factors have a negative impact on morbidity and mortality, whatever therapeutic regimen is chosen.

Although various imaging modalities (chest radiography, barium swallow, CT and positron emission tomography [PET]) assist in determining the presence and extent of disease, diagnosis of esophageal cancer is based on esophageal biopsy. Plain chest radiography is abnormal in only 50% of patients with esophageal cancer, with findings such as an air-fluid level in the obstructed esophagus, a dilated esophagus, abnormal mediastinal soft tissue representing adenopathy, or tracheal deviation. The chest radiograph, however, may be deceivingly normal even in patients with advanced disease. Double-contrast barium swallow shows the presence of obstruction or fistulas, as well as the tumor length and location. Advanced cancers manifest as luminal narrowing, ulceration, and strictures with an abrupt shelflike (shouldered) proximal border on barium swallow (Fig. 39-31). CT or EUS can determine the anatomic location and enlargement of the mediastinal, perigastric, or celiac lymph nodes. Esophagoscopy is required to establish a tissue diagnosis and determine the extent of longitudinal intramural tumor spread. The entire esophagus is visualized, and brush cytology plus biopsy tissue samples are obtained for histologic analysis. The accuracy of brush cytology alone is 85% to 97%, and that of biopsy alone ranges from 83% to 90%. The accuracy of

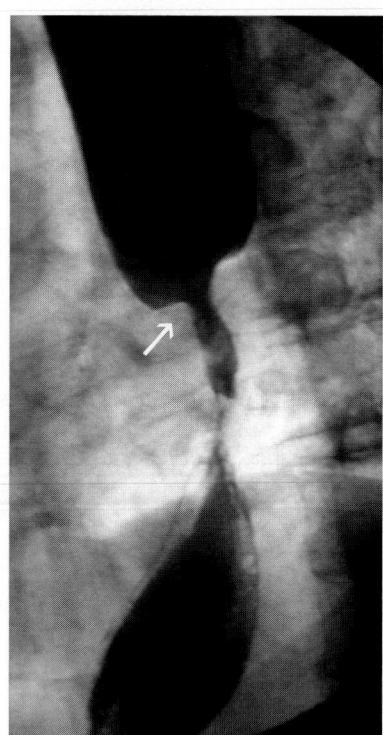

FIGURE 39-31.   Double-contrast barium swallow shows abrupt shouldered narrowing (*arrow*) at the transition between normal-appearing esophagus and the esophageal cancer.

the combination of brush cytology and biopsy is more than 97%.[107] If the lesion remains undiagnosed by biopsy or brush cytology because of the depth of the tumor, EUS-guided fine-needle aspiration (FNA) will further increase the diagnostic yield. Unfortunately, programs for early detection of esophageal carcinoma using mass screening of patients with barium swallow, flexible fiberoptic esophagoscopy, or exfoliative cytology are not cost effective in Western cultures, where the incidence of this disease is still relatively low.

Staging

Once the diagnosis of esophageal carcinoma has been histologically established after esophagoscopy and biopsy, staging of the tumor is the next step in determining which therapeutic option is appropriate (Fig. 39-32). The stage of a tumor is classified most frequently by the staging system devised by the American Joint Committee on Cancer. This system is a TNM-based system. The "T" (*tumor*) indicates the progressive degree (1 to 4) of invasion of the tumor into the esophageal wall (Fig. 39-33). "N" stands for *nodal involvement*, and "M" represents distant *metastasis* (Table 39-5).

Appropriate staging is important because survival is closely correlated with the T and N stage and with the presence of celiac node involvement.[112] T4 cancers, which do not benefit from surgery, can be reliably identified by EUS. Five-year survivals for esophageal cancer are as follows: stage I, 50% to 94%; stage II, 15% to 65%; stage III, 6% to 23%; and stage IV, less than 5%, although

TABLE 39-4.   Clinical Features of Esophageal Cancer

Sign or Symptom	Patients with Symptom (%)
Dysphagia	87-95
Weight loss	42-71
Vomiting or regurgitation	29-45
Pain	20-46
Cough or hoarseness	7-26
Dyspnea	5

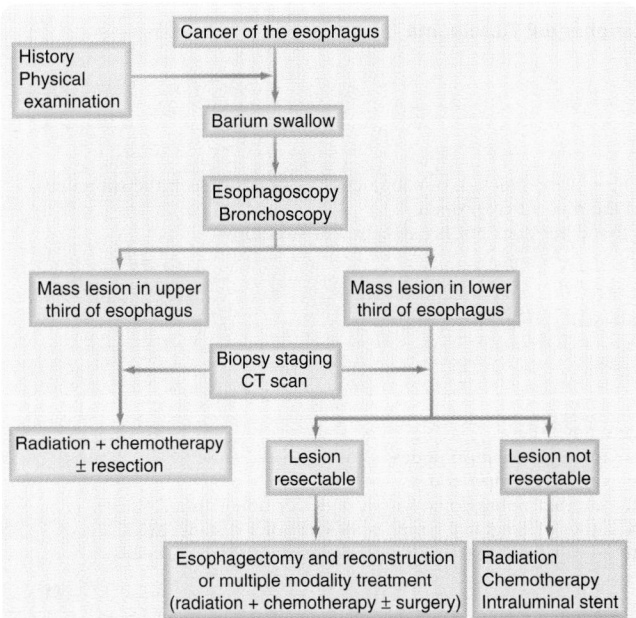

FIGURE 39-32. Management algorithm for cancer of the esophagus. CT, computed tomography.

some have reported stage IV survival as high as 27% (Table 39-6).[22,113]

LYMPH NODES (N STAGE)

Until recently, surgical exploration with lymph node sampling had been standard for definitive staging of esophageal cancer. As described in the anatomy section, esophageal lymphatics are extensive and form a continuous network from the neck to the abdomen (Fig. 39-34). Advances in imaging technology have greatly changed the preoperative staging schema. Lymph node involvement may be assessed by EUS, CT, PET, MRI, or video-assisted thoracoscopy and laparoscopy (Table 39-7). Lymph nodes are considered malignant by EUS when larger than 1-cm and hypoechoic with distinct margins and a round shape.[114] CT and EUS imaging rely on the anatomic size of the node as a predictor of malignancy but cannot differentiate between hyperplastic nodes and nodes enlarged because of metastasis. Therefore, EUS and CT can be used for image-directed FNA of mediastinal or celiac nodes. EUS has the advantage of "real-time" imaging during FNA. Histologic examination of lymph nodes is currently the standard for evaluating N stage disease, yet patients with negative nodal involvement often have recurrent disease. To decrease this error, immunohistochemical analysis to

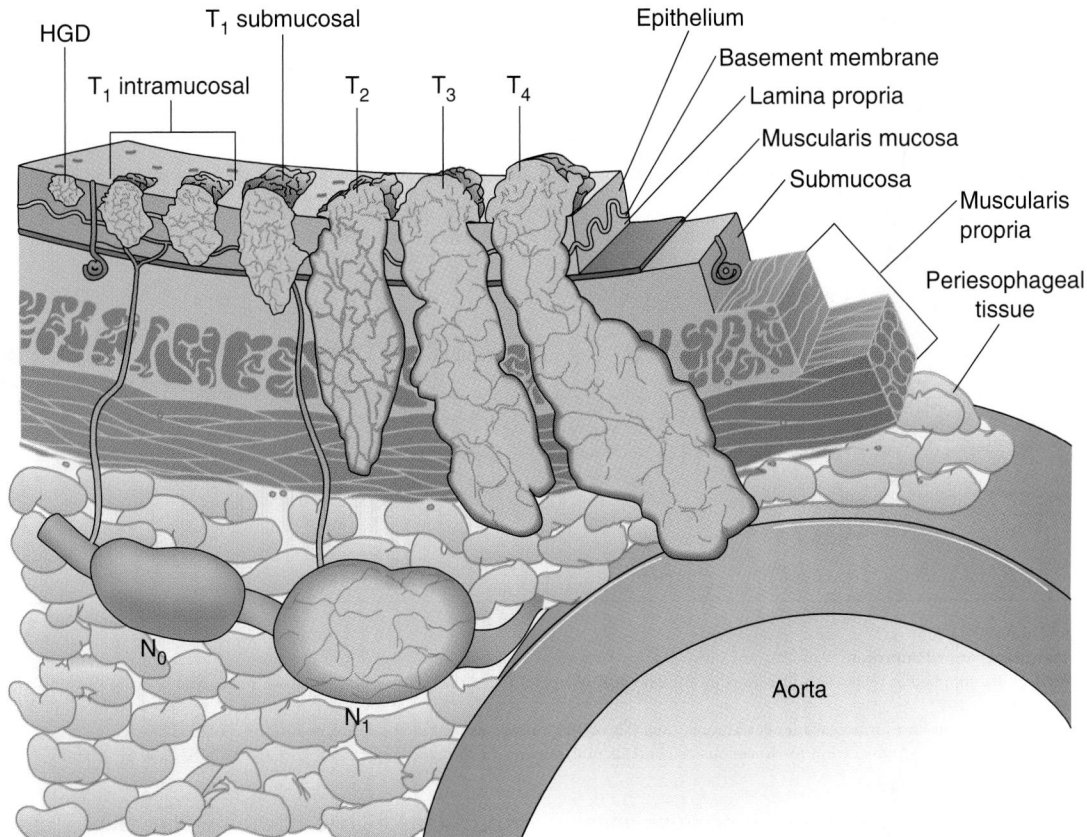

FIGURE 39-33. Primary tumor status (T) is defined by depth of tumor invasion. Regional lymph node (N) status is defined by the absence (N0) or presence (N1) of regional nodal metastases. HGD, high-grade dysplasia. (From Rice TW: Esophageal carcinoma: Diagnosis and staging of esophageal carcinoma. *In* Pearson FG, Cooper JD, Deslauriers J, et al [eds]: Esophageal Surgery, 2nd ed. Philadelphia, Churchill Livingstone, 2002, p 687.)

TABLE 39-5.   Tumor-Node-Metastasis (TNM) Staging of Esophageal Carcinoma

T: Primary Tumor

TX	Tumor cannot be assessed
T0	No evidence of tumor
Tis	High-grade dysplasia
T1	Tumor invades the lamina propria, muscularis mucosa, or submucosa; does not breach the submucosa
T2	Tumor invades into but not beyond the muscularis propria
T3	Tumor invades the paraesophageal tissue but does not invade adjacent structures
T4	Tumor invades adjacent structures

N: Regional Lymph Nodes

NX	Regional lymph nodes cannot be assessed
N0	No regional lymph node metastases
N1	Regional lymph node metastases

M: Distant Metastases

MX	Distant metastases cannot be assessed
M1a	Upper thoracic esophagus metastatic to cervical lymph nodes
	Lower thoracic esophagus metastatic to celiac lymph nodes
M1b	Upper thoracic esophagus metastatic to other nonregional lymph nodes or other distant sites
	Midthoracic esophagus metastatic to either nonregional lymph nodes or other distant sites
	Lower thoracic esophagus metastatic to other nonregional lymph nodes or other distant sites

Stage Groupings	T	N	M
Stage 0	Tis	N0	M0
Stage I	T1	N0	M0
Stage IIA	T2	N0	M0
	T3	N0	M0
Stage IIB	T1	N1	M0
	T2	N1	M0
Stage III	T3	N1	M0
	T4	Any N	M0
Stage IVA	Any T	Any N	M1a
Stage IVB	Any T	Any N	M1b

From Rice TW: Esophageal carcinoma: Diagnosis and staging of esophageal carcinoma. *In* Pearson FG, Cooper JD, Deslauriers J, et al (eds): Esophageal Surgery, 2nd ed. Philadelphia, Churchill Livingstone, 2002, p 686.

TABLE 39-6.   Esophageal Cancer Survival Rates

Stage	Skinner et al, 1986*	Ellis et al, 1993	Roder et al, 1994	Killinger et al, 1996†	Ellis et al, 1997‡	Hagen et al, 2001§	Altorki et al, 2002¶
I	55%	50.8%	18%	50%	50.3%	94%	88%
IIA	15%	37.5%	14%	38%	22.5%	65%	84%
IIB	27%	16.2%	6%		22.5%	65%	
III	6%	13.6%	4%	10%	16.7%	23%	54%
IV		0%	2%		0%	27%	25%

*En bloc surgical resection.
†Thoracotomy or transhiatal surgical approach.
‡The first four references are supplied in full in Ellis FHJ, Heatley GJ, Balogh K: Proposal for improved staging criteria for carcinoma of the esophagus and cardia. Eur J Cardiothorac Surg 12:361-364, 1997.
§Hagen JA, et al: Curative resection for esophageal adenocarcinoma: Analysis of 100 en bloc esophagectomies. Ann Surg 234:520-531, 2001.
¶Altorki N, et al: Three-field lymph node dissection for squamous cell and adenocarcinoma of the esophagus. Ann Surg 236:177-183, 2002.

predict tumor occurrence in patients with negative nodal involvement by histologic criteria is under investigation using multiple different tumor markers. A study of node-negative esophageal cancer patients showed significant prognostic value of certain tumor markers (low-level P-gp expression, high-level expression of p53, and low-level expression of transforming growth factor-α) in predicting outcomes after esophagectomy.[115] VATS coupled with laparoscopy has been found to be an accurate, although invasive, lymph node staging technique (90% to 94%).

DISTANT METASTASIS (M STAGE)

Cross-sectional imaging techniques used to assess metastatic disease are EUS, CT, and MRI. EUS is especially suited to visualize lymph nodes around the celiac axis and the left liver lobe (both considered distant metastases) but cannot fully assess the extent of metastatic disease. CT and

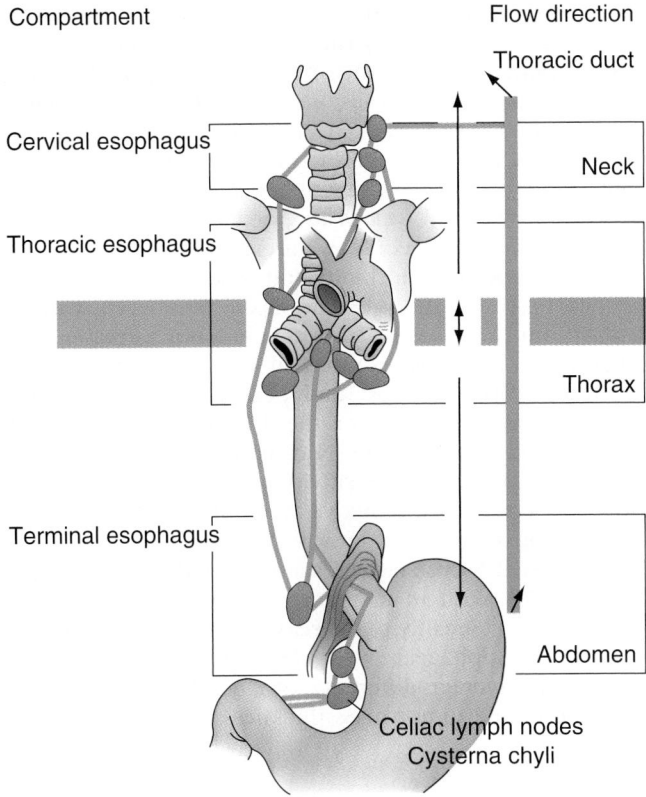

Compartment

Flow direction

Thoracic duct

Cervical esophagus

Neck

Thoracic esophagus

Thorax

Terminal esophagus

Abdomen

Celiac lymph nodes
Cysterna chyli

FIGURE 39-34. Concept of lymphatic pathways. Owing to the embryonic development of the lymphatic pathways from two sources, the branchiogenic and the body mesenchyme, lymph drains toward two different directions. There is bidirectional flow at the tracheal bifurcation, which is the area of embryologic tissue transition. This feature is consistent with clinical observations. The knowledge of lymph flow and the corresponding lymph node distribution is essential in understanding potential spread of malignancy. (From Liebermann-Meffert D: Anatomy, embryology, and histology. *In* Pearson FG, Cooper JD, Deslauriers J, et al [eds]: Esophageal Surgery, 2nd ed. Philadelphia, Churchill Livingstone, 2002, p 17.

MRI can detect mediastinal lymphadenopathy, mediastinal invasion, and distant metastases,[116] but evaluation with FNA or transbronchial biopsy is necessary for the determination of malignancy. Bronchoscopy is required for patients with tumors of the upper and middle third of the esophagus to view the pharynx, larynx, and tracheobronchial tree for synchronous and metachronous malignancies. If a patient complains of bone pain, a nuclear medicine bone scan should be performed.[117]

COMPUTED TOMOGRAPHY

CT of the chest and abdomen is standard for staging of esophageal cancer and permits evaluation of esophageal wall thickness, direct mediastinal invasion by the tumor, presence of regional and distant lymphadenopathy, and distant metastasis (including pulmonary, liver, and adrenal). CT enables detection of distant metastases (M stage), especially in the liver,[118,119] and evaluation of adjacent organ (T4) invasion, especially tracheobronchial.[119] Regional adenopathy immediately adjacent to the esophagus (that can be resected) does not preclude esophagectomy. However, histologically documented distant metastatic (stage IV) esophageal carcinoma (e.g., liver, pulmonary, or supraclavicular lymph node) contraindicates esophagectomy, because the survival is only 6 to 12 months. Esophagectomy in the presence of celiac lymph node metastasis (stage IV, M1a disease) has advocates because select series show a survival rate similar to local lymph node involvement.[113]

Although CT signs of mediastinal invasion have been well described, including obliteration of periesophageal fat planes, mass effect on adjacent structures (such as the aorta, heart, or tracheobronchial tree), as well as the presence of a tracheoesophageal fistula, accuracy is too low for definitive staging. Many esophageal carcinomas deemed unresectable by CT because of the proximity of the esophagus to vital mediastinal structures are found to be resectable at surgery.[120] The accuracy for N stage ranges from 39% to 74% and from 33% to 57% for T staging alone[121,122]; therefore, the only absolute confirmation of unresectability is FNA histology or operative exploration.

ENDOSCOPIC ULTRASOUND

EUS is the most accurate method for assessing locoregional disease including depth of tumor invasion, length of tumor and degree of luminal stenosis, regional nodal

TABLE 39-7.   Accuracy of Staging Techniques

Modality	T Accuracy (%)	N Accuracy (%)	M Accuracy (%)
Computed tomography	49-60	39-74	85-90
Endoscopic ultrasound	76-92	50-88	66-86
Magnetic resonance imaging	96	56-74	
Positron emission tomography		48-76	71-91
Thoracoscopy or laparoscopy		90-94	

disease, and involvement of adjacent structures. EUS has an 85% accuracy for T stage and 75% for N stage.[123] For patients in whom the probe can be positioned within the esophageal lumen involved by tumor, EUS has an 86% accuracy in defining involved mediastinal lymph nodes.[124] Up to 30% of advanced esophageal cancers present as stricture and are more likely to have celiac node involvement. For accurate staging, the echoendoscope can be safely passed beyond a stricture following dilation (up to 14-16 mm diameter).[25] However, not all endoscopists agree on this approach because it increases the rate of esophageal perforation. Ultrasonic miniprobes enable safe passage through high-grade malignant strictures and achieve higher accuracy rates for T staging but similar rates for N staging.[125a,125b] Similarly, 91% of patients with an obstructing tumor precluding passage of an endoscope have stage III to IV disease.[126]

Early esophageal tumors involve either the mucosa (T1m) or submucosa (T1sm). T1m tumors are associated with less than 5% lymph node involvement compared with 30% to 40% in T1sm tumors.[127,128] Overall, T1 tumors have a 90% five-year survival. Early tumors involving the mucosa (T1m) can be resected endoscopically in patients who are not surgical candidates or refuse esophagectomy. Ideal candidates for endoscopic mucosal resection include intramucosal cancers that are limited in size (<2 cm, <three-fourths circumferential involvement) with less than four areas of tumor involvement.[129,130] High-frequency ultrasound probe sonography can better differentiate T1m from T1sm compared with standard EUS. These probes can be introduced through the lumen of a gastroscope during routine upper endoscopy, thus obviating the need for two examinations. A significant error

associated with EUS T staging is to overstage 7% to 11% of early disease.[127-130] Diagnostic accuracy ranges from 84% to 92%, with increasing accuracy directly correlated with increasing T stage[127,129-131] (about 85% accuracy for T1 to more than 95% for T4 disease).

A learning curve is involved with using EUS to stage esophageal tumors (Fig. 39-35). Rice and associates[132] reported an overall T-staging accuracy of 59% (first 28 patients) with an increase to 81% (following 52 patients). T1 lesions are limited to the mucosa or submucosa. T2 lesions penetrate into the muscularis propria but not beyond (Fig. 39-36). T3 lesions penetrate the muscularis propria and invade the adventitia. T4 lesions invade locally into an adjacent structure such as the aorta.[131] Reported high accuracies of T4 detection occur with EUS when compared with CT analysis. Accurately detecting T4 disease prevents unnecessary surgical intervention while reducing associated morbidity and costs. In a prospective multi-institutional study by the Japan Esophageal Oncology Group[133] to assess the accuracy of preoperative staging of resectable esophageal cancer, using barium swallow, esophagoscopy, and percutaneous and endoscopic ultrasonography, for the T category, the overall accuracy was 80%. For the N category, the overall accuracy was 72%, with a sensitivity of 78%, a specificity of 60%, and a positive predictive value of 78%. Overall, the accuracy of stage grouping was 56%.

Whereas EUS overstages T status, it tends to understage lymph nodes, with an accuracy ranging from 50% to 88% for N stage.[122] Sensitivity decreases as distance increases from the esophageal wall. Brugge and colleagues[97] reported an average difference of 2.8 ± 1.0 mm between EUS-determined tumor mass thickness and the histologic

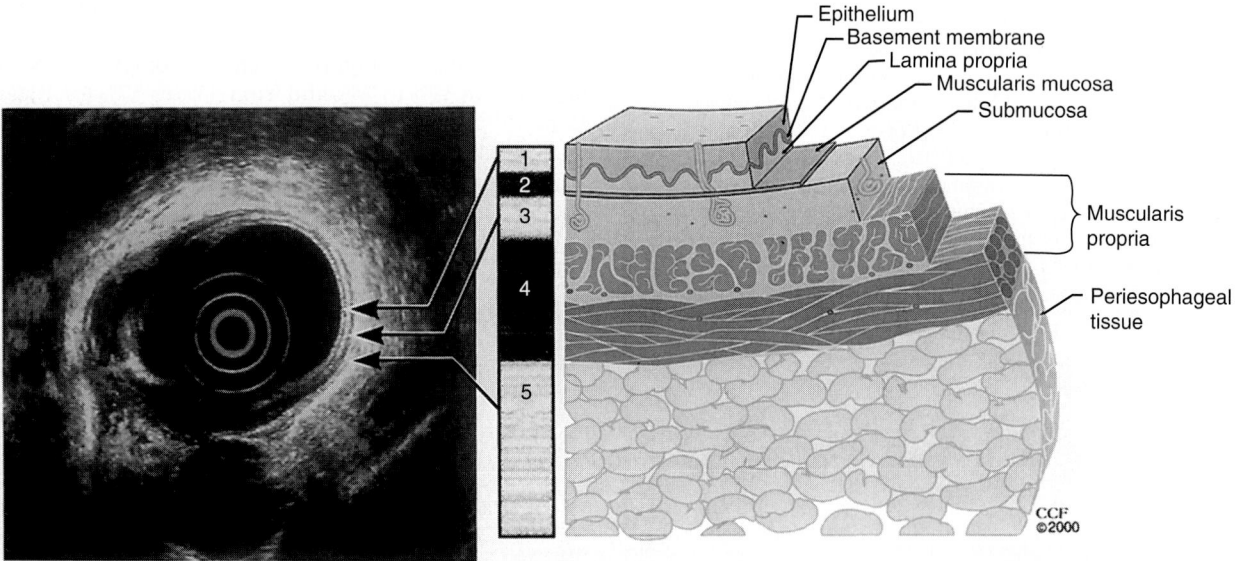

FIGURE 39-35.   Comparison of endoscopic ultrasonographic image with layers of gut wall. The first layer, hyperechoic, represents the interface between the endoscope and superficial mucosa. The second layer, hypoechoic, represents the lamina propria and muscularis mucosae. The third layer, hyperechoic, represents submucosa and the interface between submucosa and muscularis propria. The fourth layer, hypoechoic, represents the muscularis propria. The fifth layer, hyperechoic, represents the interface between serosa and surrounding tissues. (From Rice TW, Zuccaro G Jr: Endoscopic esophageal ultrasound. In Pearson FG, Cooper JD, Deslauriers J, et al [eds]: Esophageal Surgery, 2nd ed. Philadelphia, Churchill Livingstone, 2002, p 124.)

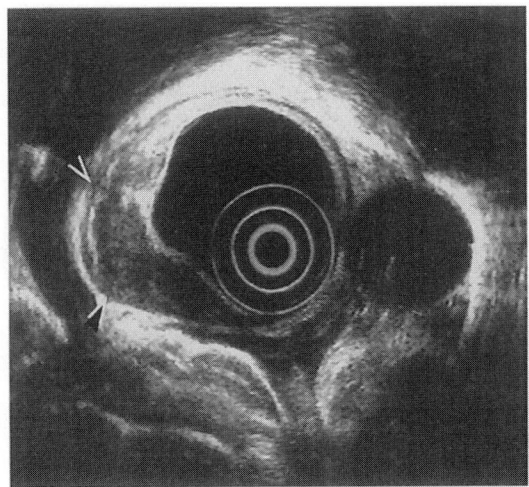

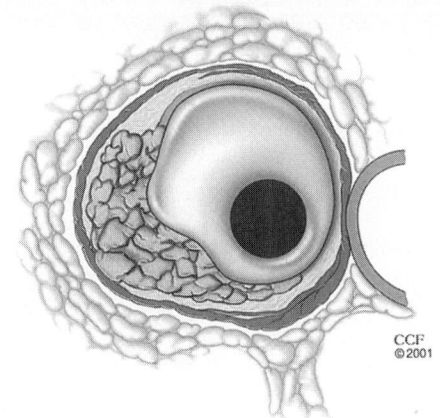

FIGURE 39-36.   A T2 esophageal carcinoma. **Top,** A T2 tumor as seen by endoscopic ultrasound. The hypoechoic *(black)* tumor invades the hypoechoic *(black)* fourth ultrasound layer (muscularis propria) but does not breach the boundary between fourth and fifth ultrasound layers *(arrows).* **Bottom,** A T2 tumor invades but does not breach the muscularis propria. (From Rice TW, Zuccaro G Jr: Endoscopic esophageal ultrasound. *In* Pearson FG, Cooper JD, Deslauriers J, et al [eds]: Esophageal Surgery, 2nd ed. Philadelphia, Churchill Livingstone, 2002, p 688.)

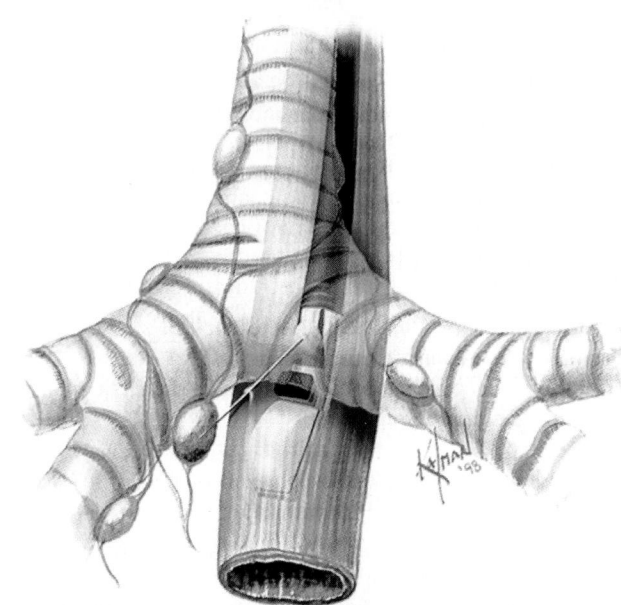

FIGURE 39-37.   Use of endoscopic ultrasound allows real-time imaging of lymph nodes within 5 cm of the esophagus, including subcarinal nodes, providing direct access for fine-needle aspiration.

specimen. The rising incidence in distal and gastro-esophageal junction adenocarcinoma increases the need for accurately staging celiac lymph nodes.[119] The sensitivity and specificity of EUS for determining the presence or absence of malignant celiac nodes are 72% and 97%, respectively, with a decrease in sensitivity for nodal metastases smaller than 1 cm in diameter.

Advances in endoscopically guided FNA allow direct cytologic evaluation of lymph nodes or masses within 5 cm of the esophagus (Fig. 39-37). Sensitivity, specificity, and accuracy rates of 85% to 93% have been reported with EUS and FNA, with little to no increase in morbidity and cost.[119] However, data on the negative predictive value are lacking.[134] Certain EUS image characteristics may increase the probability of a lymph node being malignant. These features include (1) homogenous and hypoechoic appearance, (2) sharp borders, (3) round shape, and (4) size larger than 10 mm.[135] If all four features are present, then the chance of malignancy is close to 90%. However, only a small percentage of malignant lymph nodes have all four sonographic features suggesting malignant invasion. EUS-guided FNA can access lymph nodes in the periesophageal, periaortic, subcarinal, aortopulmonary window, and celiac axis locations in the esophageal cancer.[16,135-138] A disadvantage of EUS-guided FNA is the inability to biopsy lymph nodes directly adjacent to the primary tumor that require traversing the primary tumor with the needle, resulting in a false-positive result.[138a]

POSITRON EMISSION TOMOGRAPHY

The role of PET in esophageal cancer staging continues to be a topic of debate. [18]Fluorodeoxyglucose (FDG)-PET increases recognition of distant metastasis, with increased emission in areas of increased glucose metabolism (including cancer) but with poor overall anatomic detail.[30] The main characteristic of PET is that it does not rely on anatomic or structural distortion for detecting malignancy. PET produces whole-body images in three dimensions, but without anatomic resolution, to assess both metastatic spread and primary disease. While the sensitivity and specificity are comparable to or exceed those of CT, they remain low for definitive staging. The sensitivity of PET in evaluating distant metastases ranges from 67% to 88%, compared with 61% to 83% for CT. The specificity of PET ranges from 92% to 93%, compared with 71% to 75% for CT.[30,139,140] PET results in upstaging of approximately 20% of patients who have no distant metastases detected with conventional staging. PET has a 71% to 72% sensitivity, 82% to 86% specificity, and 48% to 76% accuracy in detecting nodal involvement.[139-141] A recent meta-analysis shows the detection of hepatic metastases using PET has a 90% specificity compared with 76% for MR and 72% for CT.[142] The disadvantage of PET is that cellular FDG uptake is not specific for tumors and that areas of inflammation often predispose to false-positive results. Moreover, because PET is an emission technique based on increased cellular metabolism and not on anatomic changes, the level of tumor invasion (T stage) cannot be determined and periesophageal lymph nodes directly adjacent to the tumor are difficult to distinguish from the primary tumor. Although PET is more reliable than CT alone for identifying metastatic disease, the functional advantages of PET can be combined with the anatomic superiority of CT to enhance the detection rate for metastasis to 80% to 90% accuracy (Fig. 39-38).

MAGNETIC RESONANCE IMAGING

Additional studies such as MRI to evaluate mediastinal structures, bone and brain scans to detect metastatic disease, and staging mediastinoscopy are not performed routinely unless these tests are indicated by specific symptoms or findings. MRI can accurately detect T4 and metastatic disease, especially disease involving the liver; however, MRI tends to overstage lymph node involvement and T disease.[143,144] MRI has a 56% to 74% accuracy in detecting lymph node metastases.[145] When CT is compared with MRI, the sensitivity and specificity for metastatic detection are almost equal; however, CT costs less and is more readily available than MRI.

THORACOSCOPY AND MINIMALLY INVASIVE STAGING

The use of VATS to stage esophageal cancer has been shown to be highly accurate, although invasive, in evaluating nodal status. Thoracoscopy allows visualization of the entire thoracic cavity and esophagus, from the thoracic inlet to the diaphragmatic hiatus, for biopsy of lymph nodes as well as visualization of the extent of local involvement.[144] Thoracoscopy can also visualize metastatic disease involving nearby or adjacent structures, such as the trachea, azygos vein, aorta, pericardium, and diaphragm. Krasna and colleagues[146] reported the sensitivity, specificity, and positive and negative predictive value to be 80%, 100%, 100%, and 88%, respectively, with an accuracy of 93% for the detection of thoracic lymph nodes involving primary esophageal tumors. A right-sided thoracoscopy is most commonly performed so the esophagus can be viewed and manipulated without interference from the aorta. A left-sided thoracoscopy is used when the patient has suspicious left-sided nodal findings, especially aortopulmonary window nodes, from prior radiologic imaging.[147]

Akiyama and associates[148] identified and mapped the most common areas of lymph node metastases from primary esophageal tumors (Fig. 39-39). These metastases were then correlated with the location of the primary tumor to see whether certain primary tumors had tendencies to spread to specific lymph node regions. Distant nodal metastases were common regardless of the location of the primary tumor. One of the most common sites of

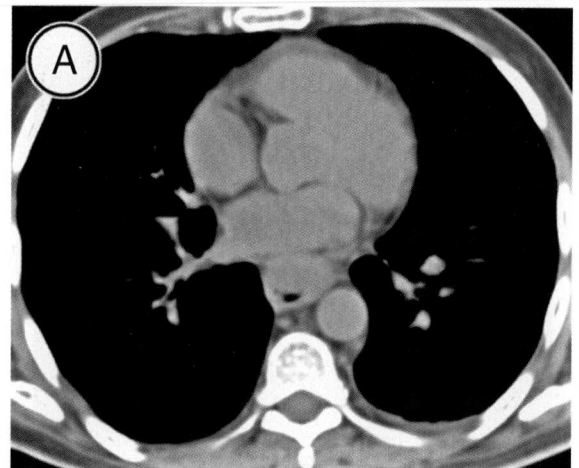

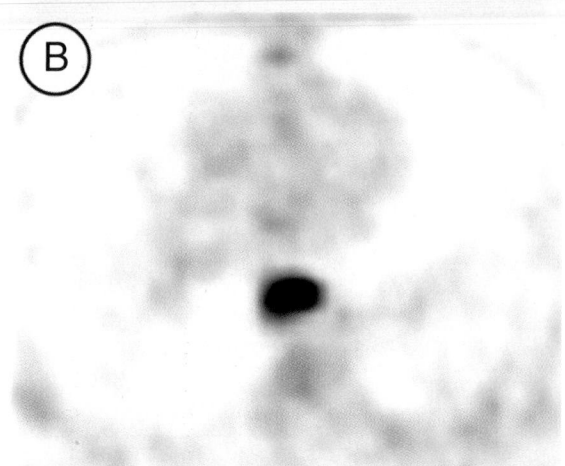

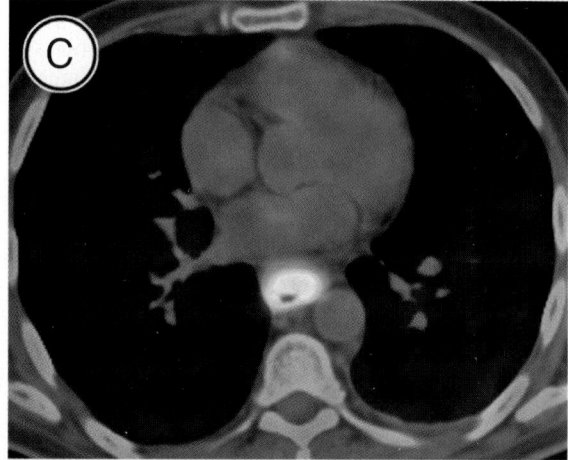

FIGURE 39-38.   A, CT shows diffuse esophageal thickening *(arrow).* **B,** FDG-PET shows increased emission in the region of the esophagus. **C,** CT-PET fusion images show precise anatomic location of the lesion. (Courtesy of Jeremy J. Erasmus, M.D., MD Anderson Cancer Center, Houston, TX.)

spread was the celiac axis, an area not visualized by minimally invasive thoracoscopy.

Laparoscopy is useful in evaluation and biopsy of the celiac axis, the surface of the peritoneal cavity, the esophagogastric junction, and the liver.[149] Laparoscopy

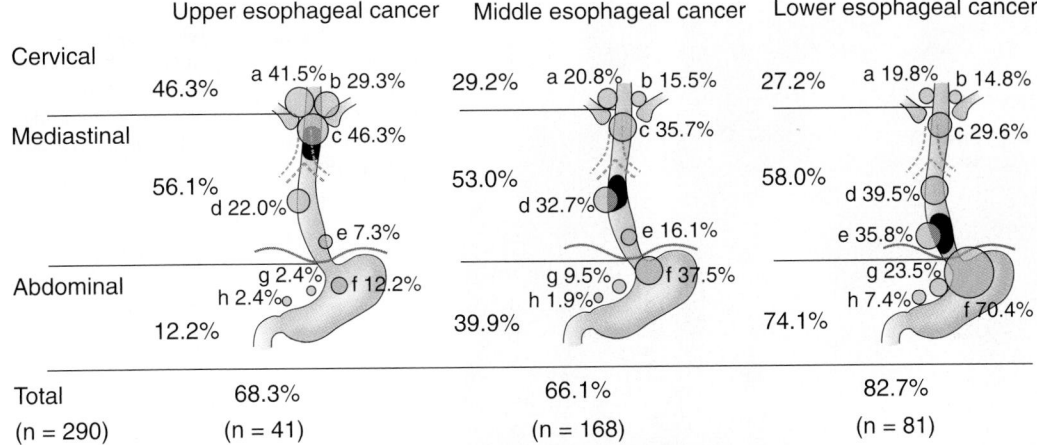

FIGURE 39-39. Ratio of positive lymph nodes per number of resected cases. Letters a to h refer to the lymph node groups listed in Box 39-2. (Adapted from Akiyama H, Tsurumaru M, Udagawa H, Kajiyama Y: Radical lymph node dissection for cancer of the thoracic esophagus. Ann Surg 220:364-373, 1994.)

Treatment

Treatment includes surgery, chemotherapy, radiation, or a combination of these techniques; however, despite multitudes of clinical trials and retrospective reviews, no treatment modality has proved superior. In the absence of metastatic disease, an esophagectomy can be performed in patients who are able to tolerate the procedure. A gastric pull-up is the preferred technique of reconstruction unless the stomach is extensively involved with tumor, precluding adequate tumor-free margin, or previous disease or surgery has compromised gastric length or blood supply.

Current trials have focused on radiation and chemotherapy with or without resection. Therapy for esophageal carcinoma is influenced by the knowledge that in most of these patients, local tumor invasion or distant metastatic disease precludes cure. In fact, 85% to 95% of patients have lymph node involvement at the time of surgical resection. Fewer than 10% of patients with lymph node involvement survive for 5 years.[127] In the past, palliative techniques were advocated because of the poor long-term survival rates of patients with esophageal carcinoma. Palliation affords the patient the ability to swallow (at least saliva) and perhaps to resume a normal life for 9 to 12 months. After the initial evaluation for staging, the physician can assess whether palliative or curative approaches are indicated.

complements thoracoscopy to provide a method for accurate minimally invasive staging. Laparoscopic ultrasound can visualize nodes as small as 3 mm in diameter with resolution comparable to that of EUS to potentially improve overall TNM staging accuracy.

PALLIATIVE TREATMENT

Palliation is appropriate when patients are too debilitated to undergo resection or have a tumor that is unresectable because of extensive invasion of vital structures, recurrence of resected or irradiated tumor, and/or metastases. Most of these patients have complete or partial obstruction of the esophagus resulting from the tumor, and swallowing is painful or impossible. The goal of palliation is to use the most effective and least invasive means possible to relieve dysphagia and discomfort, to support nutrition, and to limit hospitalization. Depending on the perceived life expectancy, palliation includes dilatation, intubation, photodynamic therapy, radiotherapy with or without chemotherapy, surgical bypass, and/or laser therapy. None of these methods has proven superior.

Dilatation/Stenting Dilatation of malignant strictures to palliate dysphagia and to allow EUS evaluation is associated with a 2% to 3% risk of esophageal wall rupture or bleeding. Unfortunately, relief is measured only in weeks. Patients with high-grade malignant strictures more likely present with advanced disease. The purpose of a stent is to bridge the obstruction in the esophagus to allow luminal patency primarily for control of saliva and secondarily for nutrition (Fig. 39-40). Flexible, self-expanding stents are constructed of two layers of superalloy monofilament wire with a layer of silicon between them. The silicon sandwiched between the layers delays tumor ingrowth through the holes in the wire mesh. After administration of local or general anesthesia, the stricture is dilated to 42 to 45 French, the lesion is identified, and the expandable covered stent is inserted under fluoroscopic or endoscopic control. Once the stent is inserted and expanded, the ends flange out to anchor to the wall of the esophagus. Patients note chest discomfort initially

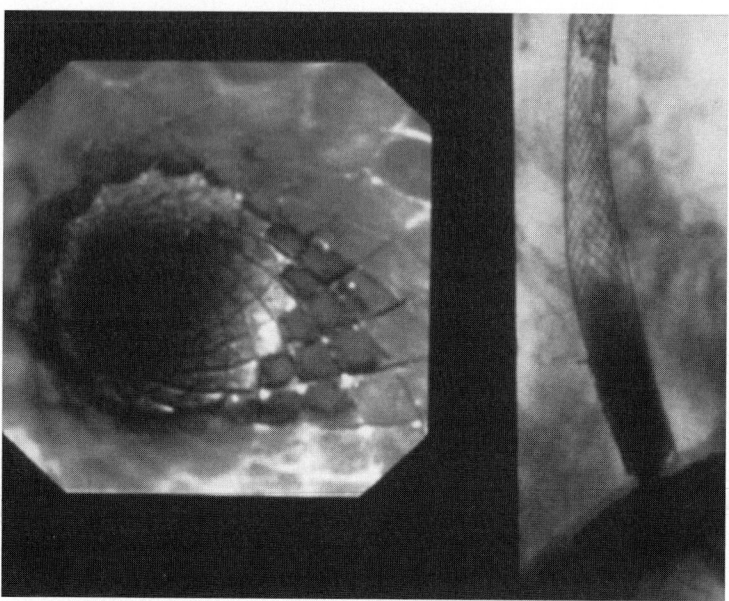

FIGURE 39-40.   Endoscopic view of covered wallstent after stenting (**left**) shows patency of the stent on contrast agent study (**right**). (Adapted from Chan ACW, Chung SCS: Interventional esophagoscopy. *In* Yim APC, Hazelrigg SR, Izzat MB, et al [eds]: Minimal Access Cardiothoracic Surgery. Philadelphia, WB Saunders, 2000, p 385.)

because of the stretching of the stricture. The insertion of self-expanding metal stents does not preclude further treatment with chemotherapy or radiation.

Although the ability of the patient to handle saliva is improved, oral intake must be restricted to foods able to pass through the rigid, indwelling esophageal stent. The average survival after palliative stent placement for esophageal carcinoma is less than 6 months. This method of therapy is also suited to patients with malignant tracheoesophageal fistula, in whom an intraesophageal stent may both occlude the fistula and permit oral alimentation for several months.

Photodynamic Therapy For photodynamic therapy, a photosensitizer such as dihematoporphyrin ether is given intravenously and after 24 to 72 hours is retained in the tumor in a much higher concentration than in healthy tissue. A low-power red laser is delivered to the tumor via flexible endoscope. The photosensitizer absorbs the red light and produces oxygen radicals to destroy the tumor. Two to 3 days after photodynamic therapy, esophagoscopy is repeated, and necrotic tumor tissue is débrided, often monthly. Complications include development of fistulas and aspiration. Edema of the hands and face and photosensitivity after this therapy are common complaints.[150] Photodynamic therapy has high 5-year survival rates in limited disease with a complete response in some stage I tumors. At present, photodynamic therapy in early stage disease is reserved for patients considered unsuitable for surgery.[151] For patients with advanced disease, treatment with photodynamic therapy can provide relief from dysphagia, with a reported mean survival of 9.5 months.[151] This form of therapy can be used in conjunction with chemotherapy and can be repeated indefinitely.

Radiation Therapy External-beam radiation relieves dysphagia in approximately 80% of the patients. In half of the patients, tumor regrowth occurs 6 months after radiation therapy has been completed.[152] An example of a curative effort would be a total dose of 6000 to 6400 cGy in 180-to 200-cGy daily fractions, 5 days a week for 6 to 7 weeks. Conversely, pain relief may be more rapidly attained by increasing the daily dose per fraction. For example, a total dosage of 4000 to 4500 cGy in 220- to 260-cGy daily fractions, or 3000 cGy in 300-cGy/day fractions.

Intracavitary radiation minimizes exposure to radiosensitive adjacent structures such as the lungs and spinal cord that may be affected with external-beam therapy, especially in patients who have had the maximum tolerable safe dose of external-beam radiation.[153] A type of intracavitary radiation, brachytherapy, has been used as primary therapy for palliation or as a boost after external beam radiation or combined modality treatment.[154] A major limitation of brachytherapy is the effective treatment distance of the primary isotope iridium-192. Tumor more than 1 cm from the source will receive a suboptimal radiation dose.[155] In the palliative setting, intraluminal brachytherapy decreases dysphagia.[156]

Laser Therapy Endoscopic laser therapy similarly improves dysphagia, but multiple treatments are required and long-term benefit is seldom achieved. The goal is to produce necrosis of the tumor. A neodymium:yttrium-aluminum-garnet (Nd:YAG) laser is set at high-power (80 to 120 watts) and short-power durations of 1 to 2 seconds with the tip of the laser probe 5 to 10 mm from the tissue. The laser is directed in retrograde fashion when possible to avoid an obstructive accumulation of necrotic tissue and to reduce the likelihood of esophageal perforation. When the tumor is completely obstructing, laser therapy is administered in antegrade fashion. Treatments to reestablish luminal patency are required every 3 to 10 weeks. Morbidity and mortality risks with laser therapy are relatively low (less than 5%). Complications include esophageal perforation, bacterial infection, abdominal distention, hemorrhage, and fistula formation.

Surgical Palliation. Before effective dilatation, stenting, radiation, laser, or ablative techniques were available, when a tumor was unresectable, a palliative surgical bypass with interposed stomach or colon was advocated in patients with severe dysphagia or a TEF. The operative mortality was a prohibitive 11% to 40%, and mortality was much higher in patients with cervical fistulas or TEFs.[157] Most (75%) were able to eat a full diet,[158] but postoperative mean survival was only 3 to 6 months.[157]

A more recent palliative surgical bypass technique is an endothoracic endoesophageal pull-through operation, which consists of stripping the esophagus of its mucosal layer and tumor and using the muscular tube of the esophagus as a sleeve through which the stomach is pulled. Normal swallowing and normal diet are achieved in almost 80% of the patients. Operative mortality rates are still approximately 15%, and morbidity rates approach 25%. Complications include anastomotic and respiratory conditions.[159]

CURATIVE TREATMENT

Factors such as general debility, malnutrition, cardiac risk, multisystem dysfunction, liver failure, infection, invasion of a vital structure, or metastatic disease limit the patient's health and chances of tolerating a curative surgical procedure.[160] At best, only 50% of patients are eligible for a curative resection at presentation.[161] The lymphatic drainage of the esophagus is extensive, both within the esophageal wall and in the surrounding mediastinal tissues. As a result, longitudinal spread of the esophageal carcinoma may be extensive and tumors may be multicentric. Tumor recurs at the resection margin in 10% of patients who have had a 6- to 8-cm margin of normal esophagus removed.

There are four types of esophagectomy (transthoracic, en bloc, transhiatal, and video-assisted), with none shown to have a relative survival advantage. Transthoracic esophagectomy entails a midline celiotomy for mobilization of the stomach and a right thoracotomy for proximal esophageal lesions or a left thoracotomy for distal lesions. En bloc esophagectomy involves complete resection of the thoracic esophagus with a two- (chest and abdomen) or three-field (chest, abdomen, and neck) lymph node dissection using a midline celiotomy, right thoracotomy, and a cervical incision for the proximal anastomosis of the stomach tube to the cervical esophageal remnant. Transhiatal esophagectomy requires a cervical incision to mobilize the esophagus and perform the proximal anastomosis then a midline celiotomy to mobilize the esophagus and stomach. Video-assisted esophagectomy uses laparoscopy to mobilize the stomach, VATS to mobilize the esophagus, and a cervical incision for the anastomosis of the stomach tube to the cervical esophageal remnant.

Regardless of technique, surgeons generally agree on the desirability of a so-called R0 resection (i.e., a complete macroscopic and microscopic removal of tumor). Great controversy remains on the extent of the resection and the type of surgical access (i.e., transthoracic, left- or right-sided, or transhiatal resection best suited to achieve an R0 resection for a given stage and tumor location). Some reports, especially from Japanese groups, focus on the value of extended lymphadenectomy both in the mediastinum and in the superior abdominal compartment

(two-field lymphadenectomy). Many surgeons think that adding bilateral cervical lymphadenectomy (three-field lymphadenectomy) is essential, especially in patients with supracarinal tumors. As expected, these extensive resections and reconstructions adversely affect surgical morbidity and mortality. Some evidence indicates that extensive lymphadenectomy improves prolonged disease-free survival times and cure rates through better control of local and regional recurrence, which may result in better control of distant metastases. As a result, even in patients with advanced stage III disease, 5-year survival rates of around 20% can be obtained after an R0 resection. Extended lymphadenectomy obviously adds to improved pathologic staging.

Since 1970, the reported 5-year survival rates for patients undergoing esophagectomy have risen from an average of 10% to 15% to a high of 35% secondary to refinements in surgical technique and risk management, improved anesthesia and critical care management, and an emphasis on nutrition by enteral and/or parenteral routes.[161a] Despite these improvements in surgical outcome, the overall survival rate for carcinoma of the esophagus has changed little. Katlic and colleagues[162] noted only an 11% five-year survival rate in patients with locally advanced N1 disease (stages IIB or III) who were treated in the 1990s.

Transhiatal Esophagectomy Transhiatal esophagectomy without thoracotomy was developed because of the pulmonary and intrathoracic leak complications associated with the thoracotomy required for transthoracic and en bloc esophagectomies. For transhiatal esophagectomy, the entire thoracic esophagus is resected through a widened hiatus and reconstructed with the stomach anastomosed to the remaining cervical esophagus above the level of the clavicles (Fig. 39-41). The overall in-hospital mortality for transhiatal esophagectomy is 5.7% versus 9.2% for transthoracic esophagectomy, with no significant difference in 3- and 5-year survival.[163] Advocates of transhiatal esophagectomy report a low operative mortality of 2% to 8% and a low anastomotic leak rate of 5% to 7.9%.[164-169] Orringer and coauthors[169] reviewed their 22-year experience with transhiatal esophagectomy in 1085 patients. They reported a hospital mortality rate of 4% and an average blood loss of less than 700 mL. Anastomotic leak occurred in 13% of patients. A modified technique of reconstituting the gastrointestinal tract by switching to a side-to-side stapled esophagogastric anastomosis has reduced the leak rate to less than 3%.[170]

In performing a transhiatal esophagectomy, the surgeon removes accessible cervical, intrathoracic, and intra-abdominal lymph nodes for staging, but a complete en bloc resection of adjacent lymph node-bearing tissue is not accomplished. The advantages of this approach include (1) a thoracotomy is avoided; (2) an intrathoracic esophageal anastomosis is avoided (if a cervical esophagogastric anastomotic leak does occur, it is easily drained and rarely causes mediastinitis or fatal complications); and (3) no intra-abdominal or intrathoracic gastrointestinal suture lines are present.[168a]

The transhiatal esophagectomy is performed through an upper-midline abdominal and cervical incision without thoracotomy; therefore, the thoracic esophagus is resected through the widened diaphragmatic hiatus and the neck. The stomach is mobilized by dividing the left gastric and left gastroepiploic vessels, and the right gastric and the right gastroepiploic arcades are preserved (Fig. 39-42). Pyloromyotomy and feeding jejunostomy are performed routinely. The entire thoracic esophagus from the level of the clavicles to the cardia is resected, while one carefully monitors intra-arterial blood pressure to avoid prolonged hypotension from cardiac displacement during the transhiatal esophageal dissection (Fig. 39-43). The sur-

gical stapler is used to fashion a gastric tube from the greater curvature of the stomach (Fig. 39-44) while still preserving the entire length. The stomach is mobilized through the posterior mediastinum in the original esophageal bed (Fig. 39-45) and is anastomosed (hand sewn or stapled) to the cervical esophagus (Fig. 39-46). The normal stomach, properly mobilized, reaches to the neck in every patient. For distal-third esophageal tumors localized to the cardia, the high lesser curvature of the stomach is resected 4 to 6 cm beyond the gross tumor, while preserving the point on the high greater curvature

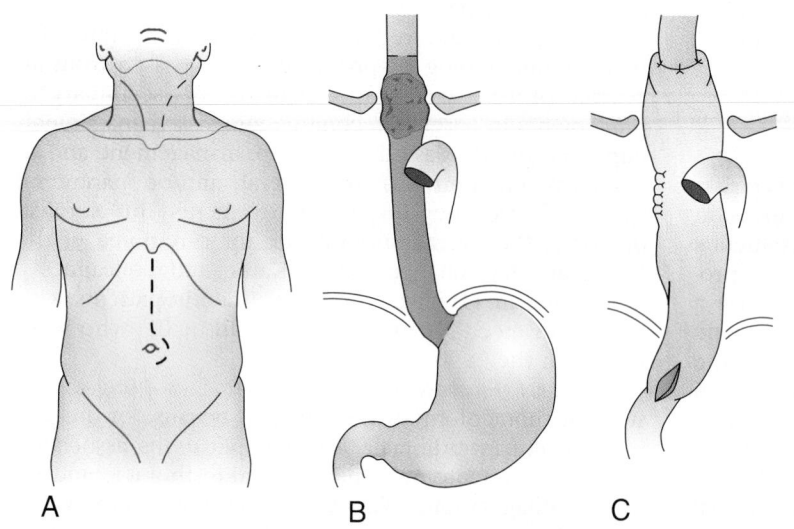

A   **B**   **C**

FIGURE 39-41.   A to **C,** Overview of transhiatal esophagectomy with gastric mobilization and gastric pull-up for cervical-esophagogastric anastomosis. (**A** to **C,** Adapted from Ellis FH Jr: Esophagogastrectomy for carcinoma: Technical considerations based on anatomic location of lesion. Surg Clin North Am 60:275, 1980.)

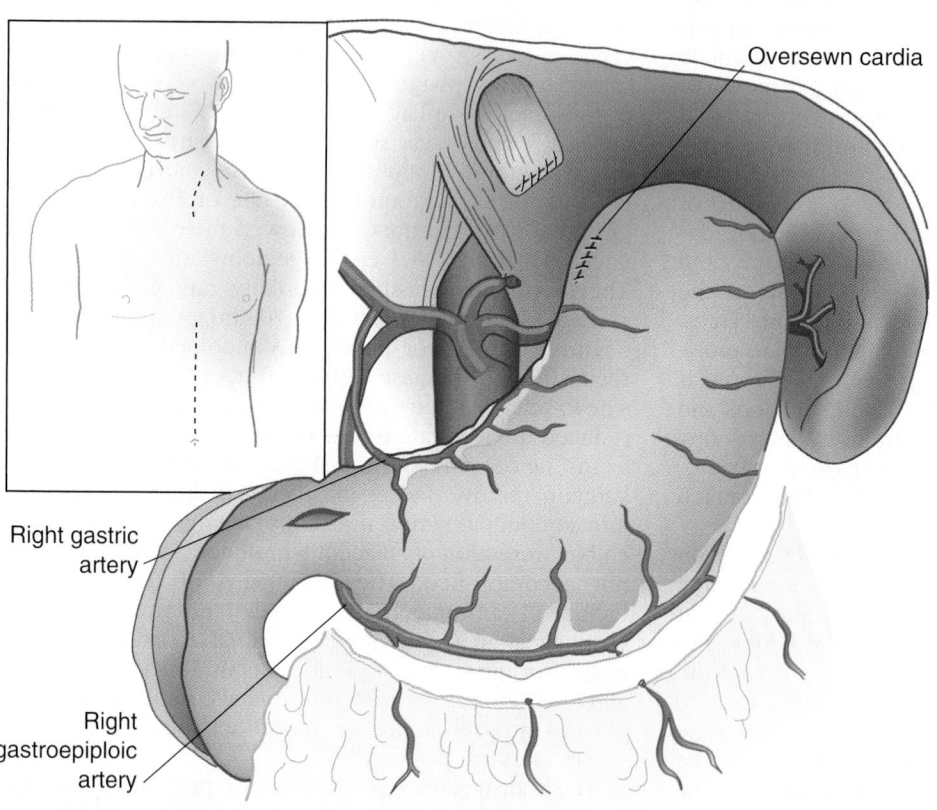

Oversewn cardia

Right gastric artery

Right gastroepiploic artery

FIGURE 39-42.   Mobilization of the stomach for either substernal gastric bypass or esophageal replacement after transhiatal esophagectomy. The gastric and right gastroepiploic vessels are preserved, a Kocher maneuver and pyloromyotomy are performed, and the divided cardia is stapled and oversewn. (Adapted from Orringer MB, Sloan H: Substernal gastric bypass of the excluded thoracic esophagus for palliation of esophageal carcinoma. J Thorac Cardiovasc Surg 70:836-851, 1975.)

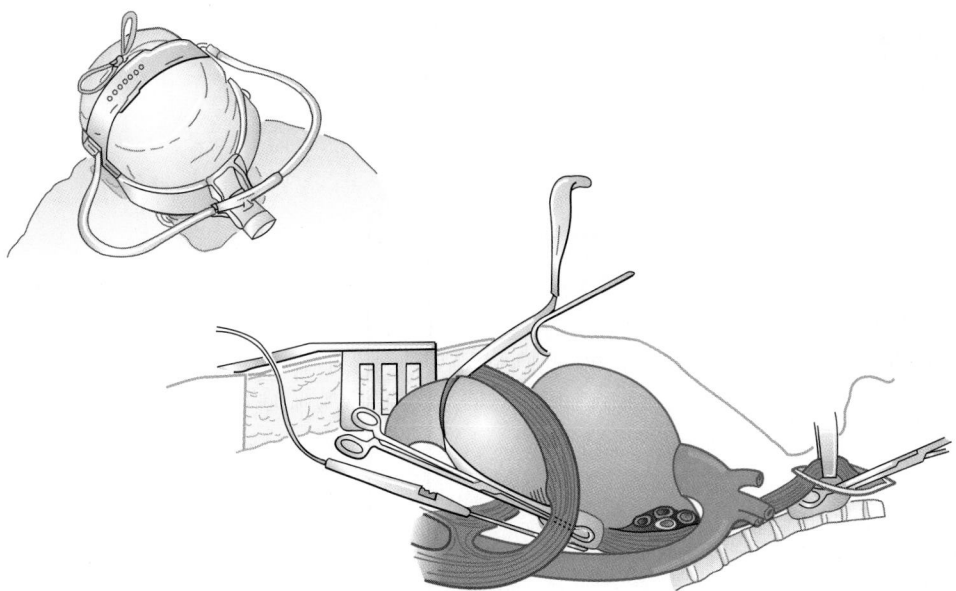

FIGURE 39-43.
Esophageal mobilization during transhiatal esophagectomy under direct vision is aided by enlargement of the diaphragmatic hiatus and anterior retraction of the middle mediastinal structures. (Adapted from Zwischenberger JB, Sankar AB: Transhiatal esophagectomy. Chest Surg Clin North Am 5:527-542, 1995.)

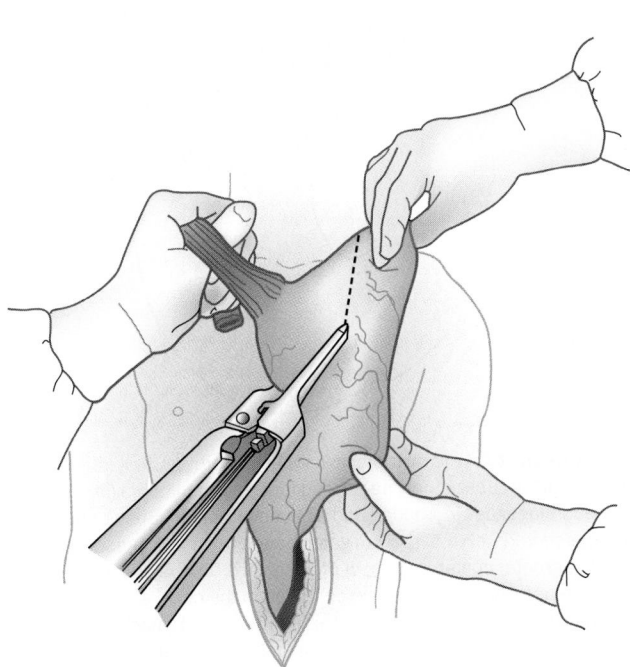

FIGURE 39-44. After completing the transhiatal esophagectomy for a localized distal third carcinoma, the surgical stapler is used to fashion a gastric tube from the greater curvature, resecting as much stomach as possible distal to gross tumor. The remaining stomach is then positioned in the posterior mediastinum in the original esophageal bed and is anastomosed to the cervical esophagus. (Adapted from Orringer MB, Sloan H: Esophageal replacement after blunt esophagectomy. *In* Nyhus LM, Baker RJ [eds]: Mastery of Surgery. Boston, Little, Brown, 1984.)

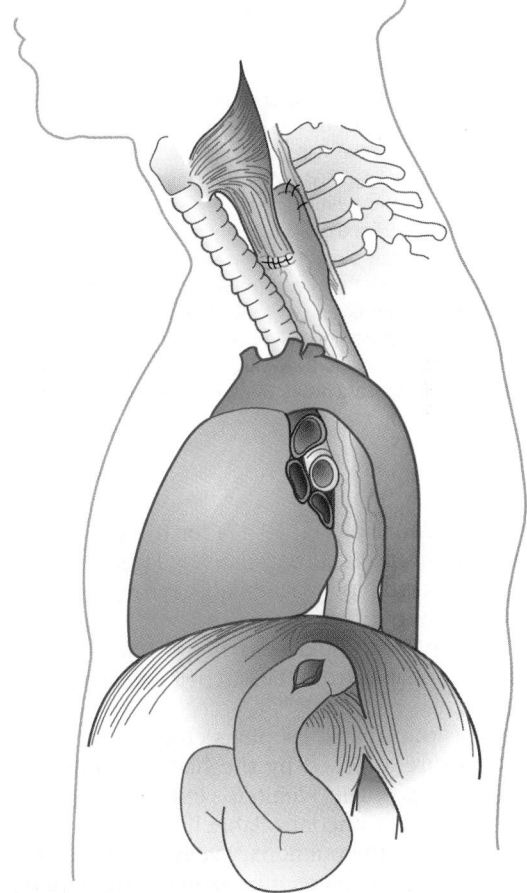

FIGURE 39-45. After transhiatal esophagectomy and pyloromyotomy, the stomach is mobilized through the posterior mediastinum, the fundus is sutured to the cervical prevertebral fascia, and an end-to-side esophagogastrotomy is performed. (Adapted from Orringer MB, Sloan H: Esophagectomy without thoracotomy. J Thorac Cardiovasc Surg 76:643-654, 1978.)

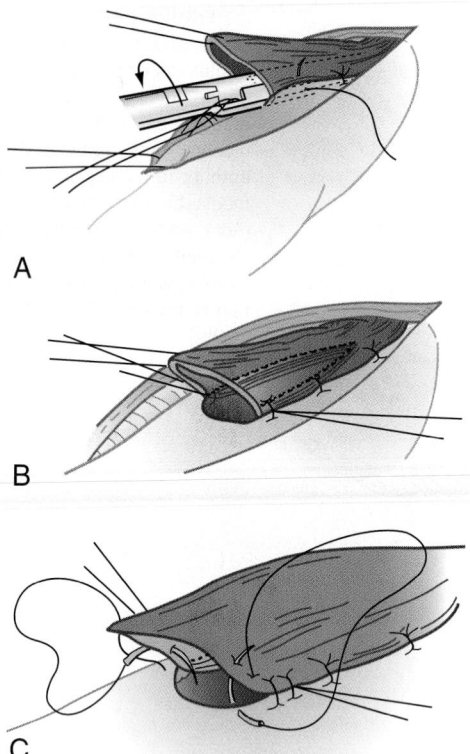

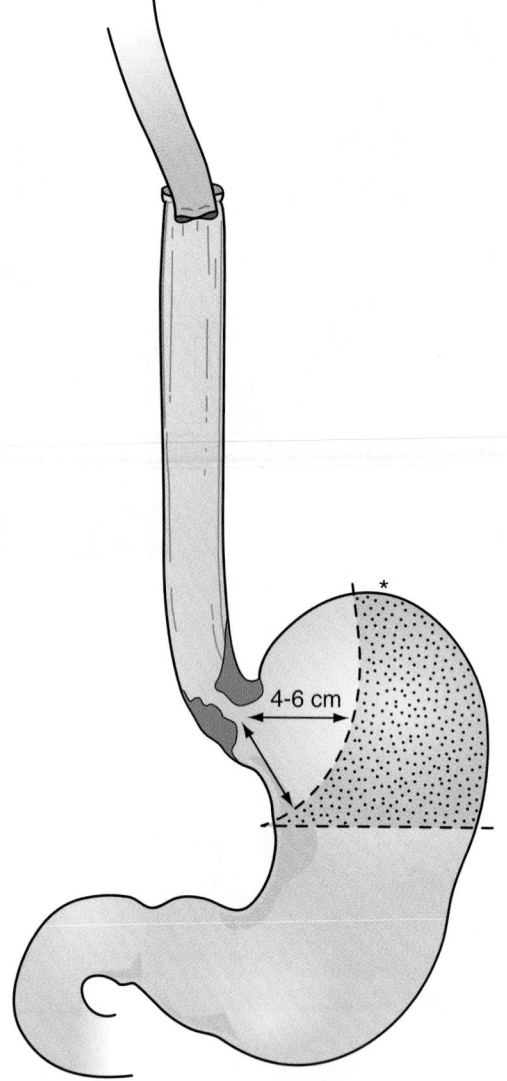

FIGURE 39-46. **A,** The stapler is closed, thereby approximating the jaws; but before firing it, two suspension sutures are placed on either side between the anterior stomach and the adjacent esophagus. **B,** When the knife assembly of the stapler is advanced, the "common wall" between the esophagus and the stomach is cut and a 3-cm-long side-to-side anastomosis is created. Corner sutures are then placed at either side of the gastrotomy. **C,** The gastrotomy and remaining open esophagus are approximated in two layers. (**A** to **C,** Adapted from Orringer MB, Marshall B, Iannettoni MD: Eliminating the cervical esophagogastric anastomotic leak with a side-to-side stapled anastomosis. J Thorac Cardiovasc Surg 119:277-288, 2000.)

FIGURE 39-47. Total thoracic esophagectomy and proximal partial gastrectomy performed for adenocarcinoma limited to the esophagogastric junction and adjacent stomach. Such tumors may be resected with a 4- to 6-cm gastric margin, thereby preserving the entire greater curvature aspect of the gastric fundus and that point *(asterisk)* that reaches most cephalad to the neck. A proximal hemigastrectomy for such a tumor wastes valuable stomach *(stippled area)* that can be used for esophageal replacement and contributes little to the "cancer operation." (Adapted from Orringer MB, Sloan H: Esophagectomy without thoracotomy. J Thorac Cardiovasc Surg 76:643-654, 1978.)

that reaches cephalad (Fig. 39-47) for the cervical esophagogastric anastomosis. Even relatively large intrathoracic esophageal carcinomas are resectable through an enlarged hiatus. For tumors of the upper-thoracic esophagus, the addition of a partial upper sternal split facilitates dissection of the esophagus from the trachea under direct vision (Fig. 39-48).[170]

Critics of transhiatal esophagectomy object to the limited exposure afforded by the hiatus to the intrathoracic esophagus. The limited exposure potentially increases the risk of uncontrollable hemorrhage by injury to the azygos vein, the pulmonary veins, or the aortic arch and precludes a complete mediastinal lymph node dissection for purposes of staging and potential cure. A review of the literature with a meta-analysis, however, has shown that operative blood loss is significantly less during transhiatal esophagectomy compared with transthoracic esophagectomy.[163] In addition to the contraindications of performing any esophagectomy, contraindications to the

transhiatal approach include evidence of tumor invasion of the pericardium, aorta, and/or tracheobronchial tree.[167] No esophagectomy (transthoracic, transhiatal, or radical) technique has demonstrated superiority in survival or local tumor control.

Transthoracic resections, which involve a posterolateral thoracotomy, have a higher incidence of pulmonary complications compared with the transhiatal approach. The transhiatal cervical anastomosis predisposes to a higher rate of leaks (13.6% for transhiatal vs. 7.2% for transthoracic); however, the majority are detected by

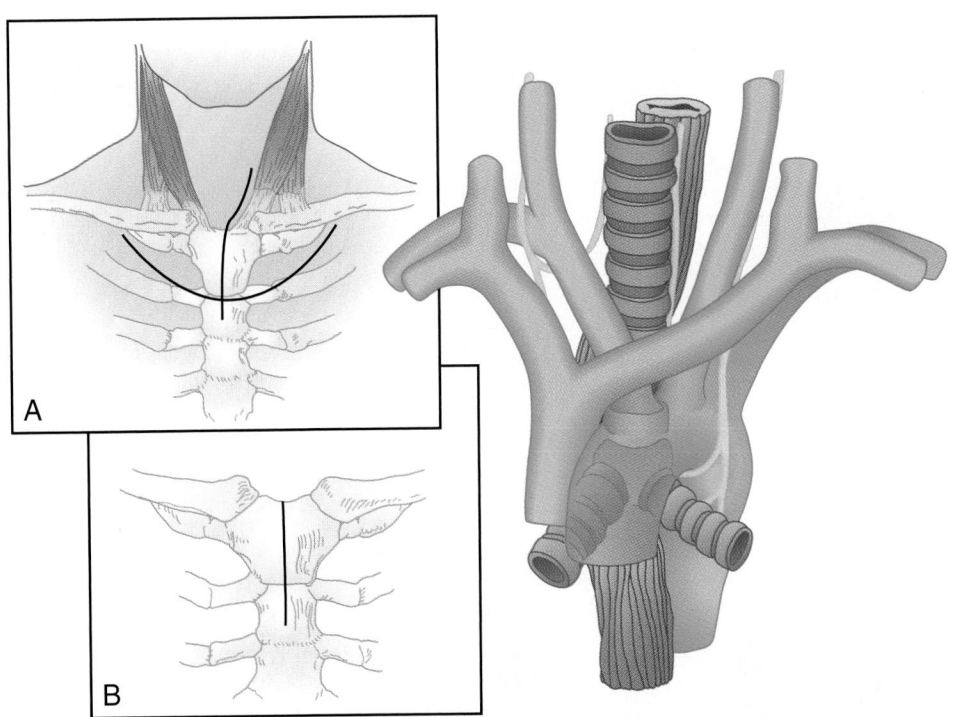

FIGURE 39-48. Exposure of the upper thoracic esophagus through a partial upper sternal split. The course of the left recurrent laryngeal nerve beneath the aortic arch and then in the tracheoesophageal groove is demonstrated. **A,** The usual left cervical incision extended onto the anterior chest in the midline and the alternative curved anterior thoracic skin incision avoid a scar on the lower anterior neck. **B,** The sternotomy incision extends from the suprasternal notch through the manubrium and across the angle of Louis. (**A** and **B,** Adapted from Orringer MB: Anterior approach to the upper thoracic esophagus. J Thorac Cardiovasc Surg 87:124-129, 1984.)

routine postoperative barium swallows and resolve spontaneously.[163] If drainage is required, the cervical incision can be reopened to create a fistula, which will close over the following weeks. Performance of the cervical esophagogastric anastomoses with a side-to-side staple technique has reduced the leak rate to less than 3%. Likewise, techniques to decrease traction on the recurrent laryngeal nerve have decreased the incidence of hoarseness. Additional early and late complications associated with the transhiatal approach are wound infection, pneumothorax, esophageal stricture, and delayed gastric emptying. Intensive care is minimized as the reported average total length of hospital stay is now 7 days.

While some advocate performance of transhiatal esophagectomy regardless of tumor level, others have suggested that surgical outcomes may be optimized by tailoring the surgical approach to the tumor location.[171] These advocates propose using transthoracic esophagectomy for mid and upper esophageal tumors to ensure safe dissection, reserving the transhiatal approach for lesions arising in the lower one third of the esophagus.

Transthoracic Esophagectomy While transhiatal esophagectomy focuses on decreasing postoperative morbidity by avoiding a thoracotomy, transthoracic esophagectomy allows complete lymph node dissection under direct vision, complete resection of tumor mass and adjacent tissue, and complete staging of the tumor with possibly higher perioperative morbidity. The esophagus lies in the right side of the mediastinum, except for the most distal third, which bends to the left. Moreover, the aortic arch overlies the left side of the upper esophagus and obscures visibility during resection of a tumor in the middle to upper third. The traditional surgical approach to distal esophageal carcinoma has been a left-sided thoracoab-

dominal incision (Fig. 39-49). The distal esophagus, proximal stomach, and adjacent lymph node-bearing tissues are resected, and an intrathoracic esophagogastric anastomosis is performed. For higher thoracic esophageal tumors, a right thoracoabdominal incision or separate right thoracic and abdominal incisions are used, and a high intrathoracic esophagogastric anastomosis is performed (Fig. 39-50) as proposed by Ivor Lewis in 1946. In either case, a gastric drainage procedure (pyloromyotomy or pyloroplasty) is recommended to prevent subsequent postvagotomy gastric outlet obstruction from pylorospasm.

Unfortunately, a combined thoracic and abdominal operation in a debilitated patient may lead to respiratory insufficiency, resulting from postoperative incisional pain and an inability to breathe deeply, that requires prolonged mechanical ventilatory assistance and increases mortality.[172,173] In addition, although disruption of an intrathoracic esophageal anastomosis is reported less frequently than a cervical anastomotic leak from a transhiatal esophagectomy, the consequences, including mediastinitis and sepsis, are fatal in up to 40% of patients. An additional disadvantage of the intrathoracic esophageal anastomosis is inadequate long-term relief of dysphagia either because of anastomotic suture-line tumor recurrence or because of the development of reflux esophagitis above the anastomosis, which follows disruption of the LES mechanism. The operative mortality varies significantly, ranging from as high as 14%[35] to as low as 2.2%.[50]

The posterior lateral thoracotomy incision is made on the right at the fifth intercostal space, and on the left at the sixth or seventh. An upper midline laparotomy is performed if the tumor is in the upper third of the esophagus. A left neck incision ensures exposure of the cervical

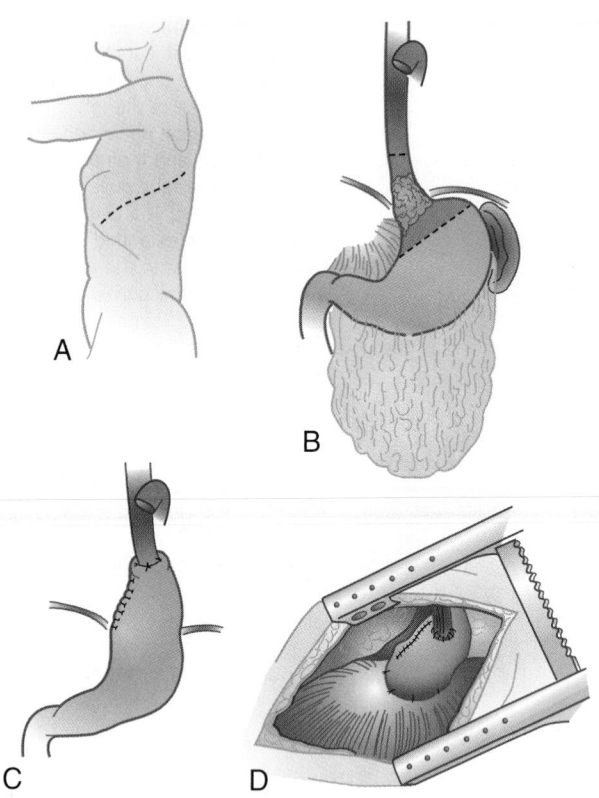

FIGURE 39-49. Overview of left thoracotomy (**A**) and esophageal mobilization with gastric pull-up (**B**) for intrathoracic anastomosis (**C**). **D,** The completed low intrathoracic esophagogastric anastomosis is shown. The remaining distal stomach has been mobilized into the chest through the diaphragmatic hiatus and the stomach suspended from the prevertebral fascia with several sutures. The anastomosis is constructed away from the suture line of the gastric transection. The edge of the diaphragmatic hiatus has been sutured to the stomach to prevent herniation of abdominal viscera. The diaphragmatic incision is closed with everting horizontal mattress sutures followed by a running whipstitch of nonabsorbable suture. (**A** to **C,** Adapted from Ellis FH Jr, Shahian DM: Tumors of the esophagus. *In* Glenn WWL, Baue AE, Geha AS, et al [eds]: Thoracic and Cardiovascular Surgery, 4th ed. Norwalk, CT, Appleton & Lange, 1983, p 566, with permission of the McGraw-Hill Companies. **D,** Adapted from Orringer MB: Surgical options for esophageal resection and reconstruction with stomach. *In* Baue AE, Geha AS, Hammond GL [eds]: Glenn's Thoracic and Cardiovascular Surgery, 5th ed. Norwalk, CT, Appleton & Lange, 1991, p 793, with permission of the McGraw-Hill Companies.)

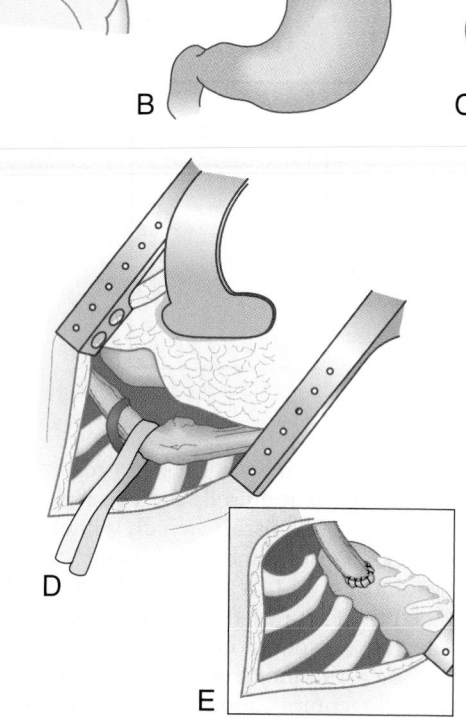

FIGURE 39-50. Overview of right thoracotomy (**A**) with esophageal resection, gastric mobilization (**B**), and intrathoracic anastomosis (**C**) for midesophageal tumor. **D,** The azygos vein has been divided and the esophagus encircled and dissected away from the posterior membranous trachea. **E,** Completed high intrathoracic esophagogastric anastomosis at the apex of the right chest is shown. The gastric fundus has been suspended from the prevertebral fascia. (**A** to **C,** Adapted from Ellis FH Jr: Esophagogastrectomy for carcinoma: Technical considerations based on anatomic location of lesion. Surg Clin North Am 60:273, 1980; **D** and **E,** Adapted from Orringer MB: Surgical options for esophageal resection and reconstruction with stomach. *In* Baue AE, Geha AS, Hammond GL [eds]: Glenn's Thoracic and Cardiovascular Surgery, 5th ed. Norwalk, CT, Appleton & Lange, 1991, p 794.)

esophagus and cricopharyngeus to obtain a tumor-free margin. The lung and pleural space are examined for any evidence of metastatic disease. The inferior pulmonary ligament is divided to the inferior pulmonary vein. The tumor area is examined for evidence of direct invasion of vital mediastinal structures. The esophagus, periesophageal lymphatics, and adjacent pleura are resected, preferably en bloc. The paratracheal lymph nodes are removed along with the primary specimen. Taking great care to avoid damage to or retraction of the recurrent laryngeal nerve decreases the incidence of hoarseness. The azygos vein and thoracic duct are resected along with the primary specimen. The opposing pleura is not resected unless it appears to be invaded with tumor. The esophagus is mobilized from the anterior longitudinal ligament of the spine. The esophagus is then transected 5 to 8 cm from the UES, yet a sufficient distance away from the primary tumor (at least 5 cm but usually 10 cm) to avoid skip metastases or longitudinal lymphatic spread.

The most direct route for the conduit of reconstruction (stomach, colon, roux-en-Y loop of jejunum) is the posterior mediastinum in the prevertebral space created by the resected esophagus. Some investigators have advocated placing the neoesophagus in a substernal position to reduce the likelihood of a local recurrence that causes obstruction.[174] For distal-third tumors that are located at the esophageal hiatus and the diaphragm, a left thoracotomy alone allows sufficient exposure of the esophagus and diaphragm to be resected with the specimen to achieve a negative margin. A cephalad transection site is then chosen approximately 10 cm above the most superior portion of the esophageal tumor. The gastric margin is at least 5 cm from the lowest portion. The remaining stomach is then pulled up into the posterior mediastinum, and an anastomosis is performed (end-to-end or end-to-side anastomosis) using either a single-layer or a two-layered hand-sewn anastomosis or stapling devices.[175,176]

A total thoracic esophagectomy is similar but includes removal of the entire esophagus to maximize the resection margin. This procedure begins with a laparotomy, to mobilize the conduit of choice. A right-sided thoracotomy is performed, and the esophagus is resected from a 5-cm gastric margin at the cardia to within 2 to 3 cm of the UES. The conduit, whether it be stomach or colon, is placed either retrosternally or in the original esophageal bed, and a cervical anastomosis is performed.

En Bloc Esophagectomy Because many patients present with metastases to regional lymph nodes as well as to the surrounding tissue and organs, a more radical resection, the *en bloc esophagectomy,* has been advocated by a few thoracic surgeons. An envelope of normal tissue is removed along with the spleen, celiac nodes, posterior pericardium, azygos vein, thoracic duct, and adjacent diaphragm (Fig. 39-51 and Box 39-2). With this aggressive surgery, operative mortality ranges from 5.1% to 11%, higher but not significantly different from other approaches.[176a] The two major complications are similar to transhiatal and transthoracic esophagectomy: anastomotic leak and respiratory complications. With the en bloc technique, 5-year survival rate is 40% to 55% overall.[176b] In adenocarcinoma, increased incidence of regional lymph node metastases has been reported with increasing depth of invasion of the primary tumor. Lymph nodes are involved in 80% of patients with muscular invasion.[9] Forty-four patients with transmural adenocarcinoma who underwent en bloc esophagectomy had an overall 5-year actuarial survival of 26%, with the presence and number of lymph node metastases the most important predictors of survival.[177] Some surgeons advocate a three-field dissection (bilateral cervical, mediastinal, and abdominal) followed by esophagectomy for patients with locally advanced carcinoma of the thoracic esophagus in the presence of lymph node metastasis; overall 5-year survival is 56% and >60% in patients Stage I or II.[177a]

Thoracoscopic Esophagectomy Several authors have reported the use of video-assisted thoracoscopy or laparoscopy in performing esophagectomy.[28,79,178-182] Techniques described include a standard laparotomy with thoracoscopic mobilization of the esophagus, a totally laparo-

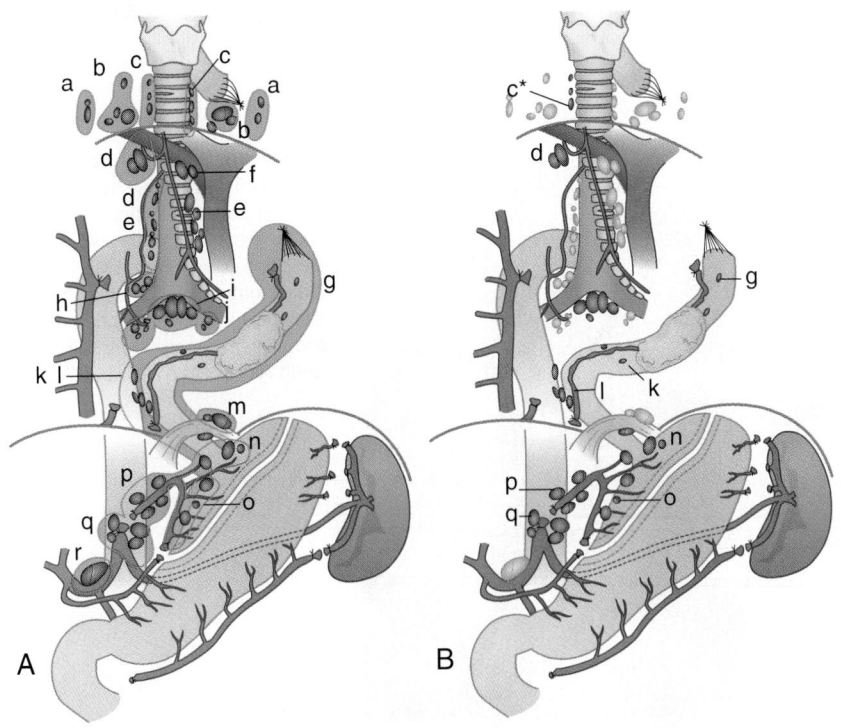

FIGURE 39-51. **A,** Extent of resection and lymph node dissection routinely carried out for cancer of the thoracic esophagus. The mediastinal part is the lateral view. The right main bronchus is retracted anteriorly. Letters a to r represent the lymph node groups shown in Box 39-2. **B,** Less extensive dissection for cancer of the thoracic esophagus. Letters c to q represent the lymph node groups shown in Box 39-2. c* represents the lowest nodes in the right recurrent nerve chain in the neck and can be removed via a thoracotomy. (**A** and **B,** Adapted from Akiyama H: Squamous cell carcinoma of the thoracic esophagus. *In* Surgery for Cancer of the Esophagus. Baltimore, Williams & Wilkins, 1990, p 23.)

A

B

Box 39-2 Classification of lymph nodes

Cervical Lymph Nodes

Deep lateral nodes (a) (spinal accessory lymphatic chain)
Deep external nodes (b)
Deep internal nodes (c) (recurrent nerve lymphatic chain)

Superior Mediastinal Lymph Nodes

Recurrent nerve lymphatic chain (d)
Paratracheal nodes* (e)
Brachiocephalic artery nodes (f)
Paraesophageal nodes (g)
Infra-aortic arch nodes (h)

Middle Mediastinal Lymph Nodes

Tracheal bifurcation nodes (i)
Pulmonary hilar nodes (j)
Paraesophageal nodes (k)

Lower Mediastinal Lymph Nodes

Paraesophageal nodes (l)
Diaphragmatic nodes (hiatal part) (m)

Superior Gastric Lymph Nodes

Paracardiac nodes (n)
Lesser curvature nodes (o)
Left gastric artery nodes (p)

Celiac Trunk Lymph Nodes (Q)

Common Hepatic Artery Lymph Nodes (R)

*The left paratracheal nodes are regarded as the left recurrent nerve lymphatic chain.

Adapted from Akiyama H: Squamous cell carcinoma of the thoracic esophagus. *In* Surgery for Cancer of the Esophagus. Baltimore, Williams & Wilkins, 1990, p 22.

scopic transhiatal technique, laparoscopic gastric mobilization with a right mini-thoracotomy, and the combined laparoscopic and thoracoscopic technique with thoracoscopic mobilization of the esophagus, followed by laparoscopic gastric mobilization.[28,182] Thoracoscopic esophagectomy has three stages. The first is the thoracoscopic dissection of the thoracic esophagus (Fig. 39-52). The second is the laparoscopic mobilization of the intended gastric conduit (Fig. 39-53), and the third is the cervical anastomosis.

Studies reporting on thoracoscopic esophagectomy have indicated an operative mortality between 0% and 13.5%.[28] The morbidity has been reported to be 27% to 55%. Major causes of complications include respiratory disorders, anastomotic leak, chylothorax, and laryngeal nerve injury.[28,90] Although technically feasible, the success of thoracoscopic esophagectomy is highly dependent on the experience of the surgeon, with no current technique considered standard. Thoracoscopic esophagectomy has not been shown to reduce the length of hospitalization or complications relative to open surgical procedures. Randomized trials with longer follow-up are required to fully evaluate the procedure.

Reconstruction After Esophagectomy After a portion of the esophagus is removed, or after complete esophagectomy, a conduit must be established for alimentary continuity. The stomach, colon, and jejunum have all been successfully used as esophageal substitutes[183-185] (Fig. 39-54) most often utilizing the posterior mediastinum or retrosternal routes (Fig. 39-55).[174] The stomach is the conduit of choice because of ease in mobilization and ample vascular supply (Fig. 39-56). A higher incidence of mortality is noted with the use of the colon because of the necessity for three anastomoses (coloesophagostomy, colojejunostomy, and colocolostomy). The colon is used if the patient has undergone a partial or total gastrectomy previously or if tumor involves the stomach to preclude a 5-cm margin

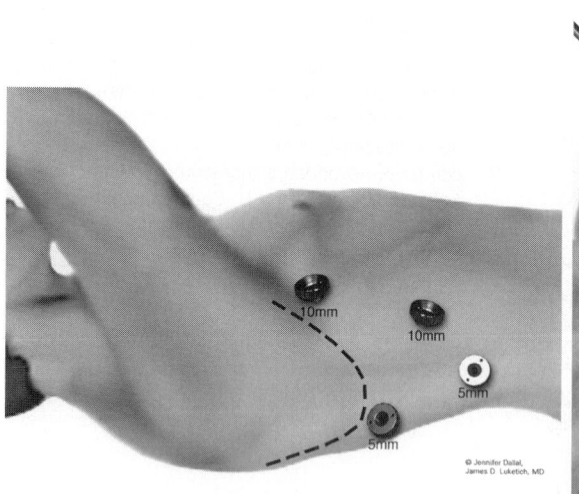

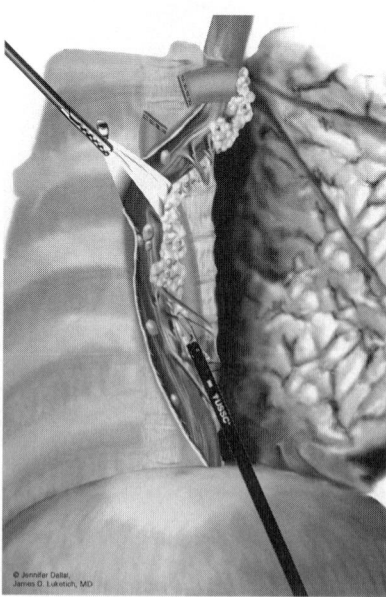

FIGURE 39-52. **Left,** Video-assisted thoracoscopic surgical port sites. **Right,** Thoracoscopic mobilization of the esophagus. (From Litle VR, Buenaventura PO, Luketich JD: Minimally invasive resection of esophageal cancer. Surg Clin North Am 82:711-728, 2002.)

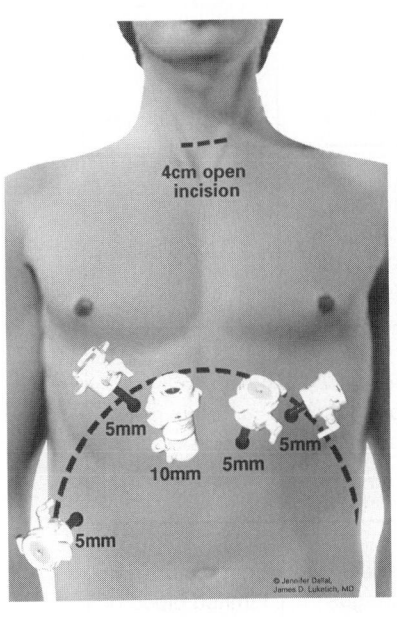

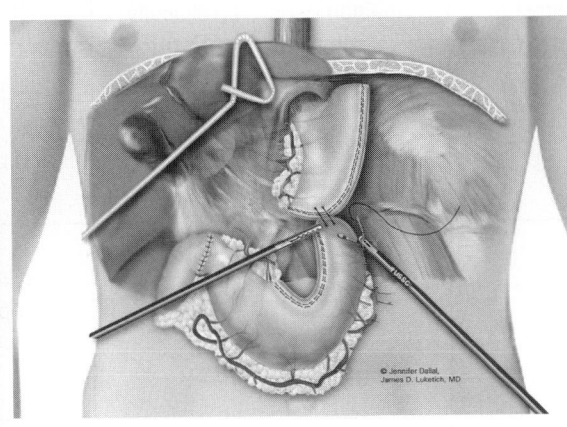

FIGURE 39-53. **Right,** Laparoscopic pyloroplasty and gastric tubularization preceding esophageal removal. **Left,** Abdominal port sites for laparoscopy and position of the neck incision. (From Litle VR, Buenaventura PO, Luketich JD: Minimally invasive resection for esophageal cancer. Surg Clin North Am 82:711-728, 2002.)

(Fig. 39-57). Jejunal loops can also be used, but their limited vascular supply restricts mobility and length (Fig. 39-58).

Anastomosis can be performed in the chest just below the arch of the aorta (intrathoracic anastomosis), or a cervical anastomosis can be made in the neck, depending on the choice of reconstruction. Mechanical staplers continue to improve, and leak rates are decreasing. Leakage is more likely to occur in patients who are malnourished, who have had preoperative radiation therapy, and who have tension at the anastomosis. A leak most frequently occurs within 10 days of the surgical procedures. Patients with a leak may also present with signs of sepsis or increased drainage output from previously placed chest tubes and drains. For a cervical anastomotic leak, the drainage can be controlled by opening the cervical incision to create a cervical fistula.[170] With adequate drainage, the leak usually spontaneously closes within 1 to 2 weeks and mortality is rare. Nutritional support is maintained by an enteral feeding tube. Approximately half of the patients who have an anastomotic leak develop a stricture relieved by serial esophageal dilatation. For small leaks that readily drain into the lumen, the patient may be managed with antibiotics, nutritional support, and close observation.

Leaks from an anastomosis in the mediastinum are significantly more serious, with mortality rates of 20% to 40%. For an intrathoracic anastomotic leak, in most cases, reoperation should be performed. If repair of the anastomosis seems feasible, it may be attempted with primary repair and reinforcement with vascularized tissue, as discussed for primary perforation. Often, the safest option is to take down the anastomosis and mobilize the remaining esophagus out of the chest through a cervical incision for construction of an anterior thoracic end-esophagostomy (Fig. 39-59). Devitalized stomach is resected, and the remaining stomach is returned to the abdominal cavity. A decompressing gastrostomy is performed. The pleural cavity and mediastinum should be débrided, thoroughly irrigated, and adequately drained. Future reconstruction

with a colon interposition is the goal at 6 to 12 months, following complete recovery.

Carcinomas involving the cervicothoracic esophagus (and frequently the larynx), either primarily or secondarily, pose unique problems for esophageal reconstruction after laryngopharyngectomy. Concomitant radical neck dissection is often required because of regional lymph node involvement. Resection of tumors that involve the high retrosternal trachea is facilitated by removal of the anterior breast plate and construction of a mediastinal tracheostomy.[186,187] Although replacement of the pharynx and cervical esophagus is possible with skin tubes, myocutaneous flaps, and isolated segments of jejunum anastomosed to a cervical arterial and venous blood supply using microvascular technique, these operations are frequently multistaged, prolonged, and technically difficult.[188-190] Laryngopharyngectomy for cervicothoracic tumors and concomitant transhiatal esophagectomy without thoracotomy provide the maximum distal esophageal margin beyond the tumor and permit restoration of continuity of the alimentary tract. However, a colon interposition is often recommended for restoring alimentary continuity in this situation, because regurgitation after a pharyngogastric anastomosis gives a less satisfactory functional result.

Preoperative Preparation for Esophagectomy If the esophageal obstruction precludes adequate fluid or caloric intake, endoscopic dilatation of the malignant stricture and insertion of a nasogastric feeding tube or an intraluminal stent for enteral nutrition are performed to achieve an intake of approximately 2000 calories per day. Intravenous hyperalimentation is seldom indicated, because of the associated septic and metabolic complications. Oral hygiene is often neglected, and abscessed or severely carious teeth should be removed or repaired preoperatively to minimize the severity of an infection that may result from anastomotic disruption and swallowed oral bacteria. If the patient has a history of prior gastric operations that may preclude the use of the entire stomach as an esophageal substitute, a barium enema or colonoscopy should be

Organ	Technique	Number of anastomoses	Inherent morbidity difficulty	Upper level of usefulness	Disadvantages
Stomach	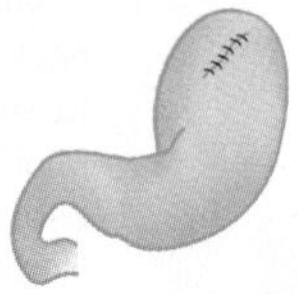	1	+	Cervical esophagus and pharynx	Bulky Reflux risk
Greater curvature tube	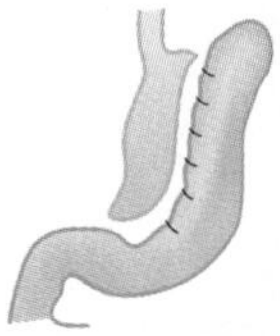	1	+	Cervical esophagus and pharynx	Reflux risk
Reversed gastric tube	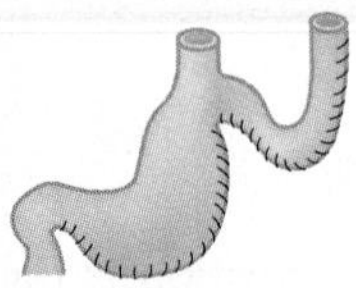	1	+++	Cervical esophagus and pharynx	Long suture line Limited blood supply
Nonreversed gastric tube	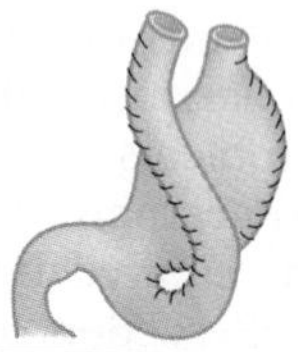	1	++	Lower cervical esophagus	Long suture line
Right colon	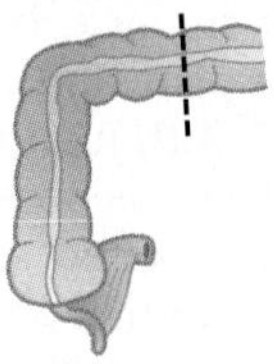	3	+++	Lower cervical esophagus	Thin-walled Bulky Short pedicle
Left colon	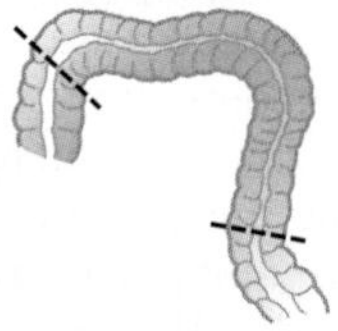	3	++++	Most versatile organ for use at any level Lower third to pharynx	Extensive operation Redundancy over time
Jejunum	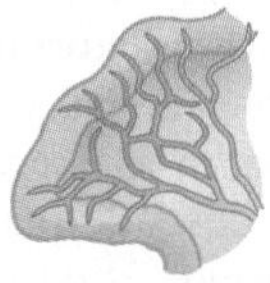	2 (Roux loop) 3 (Interposition)	++	Lower third	Limited graft length without revision of pedicle or bowel
Free graft	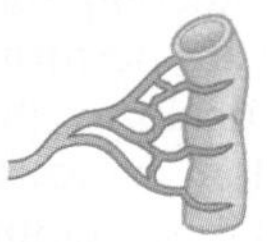	5 (2 micro-vascular)	+++++	Pharynx and cervical esophagus	Microvascular anastomoses required

FIGURE 39-54.   Options for esophageal substitution. (Adapted from Hiebert CA, Bredenberg CE: Selection and placement of conduits. *In* Pearson FG, Deslauriers J, Ginsberg RJ, et al [eds]: Esophageal Surgery. New York, Churchill Livingstone, 1995, p 652.)

Route	Procedure	Advantages	Disadvantages
Subcutaneous	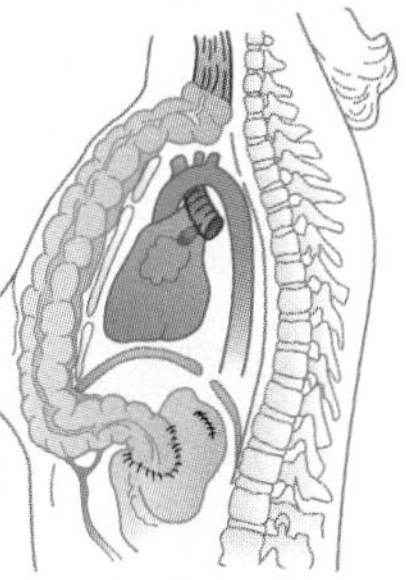	Ease of construction Avoids encroachment on heart or lungs Facilitates early detection of graft failure	Cosmetically far from ideal Longest course of any route
Substernal	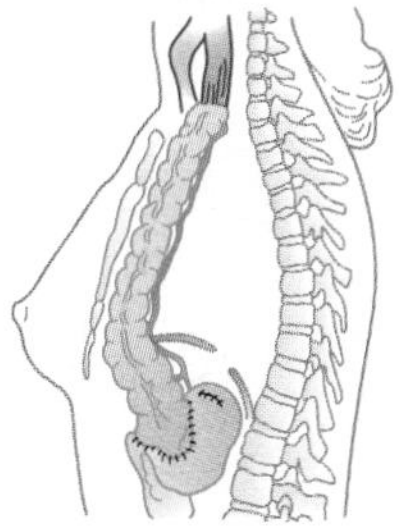	Ease of construction Useful when mediastinum is unavailable	Long route Graft angulation Cardiac surgery concerns (past or proposed)
Transpleural	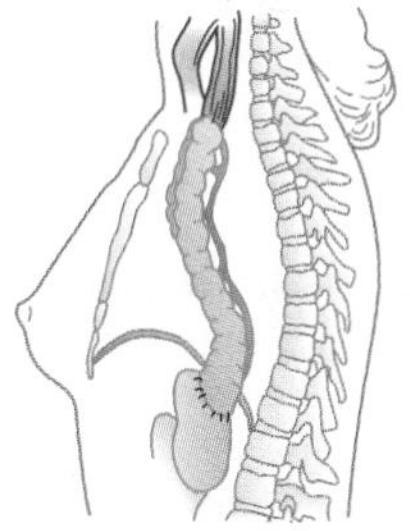	Convenient from left thoracic approach	Displaces lung
Posterior mediastinal	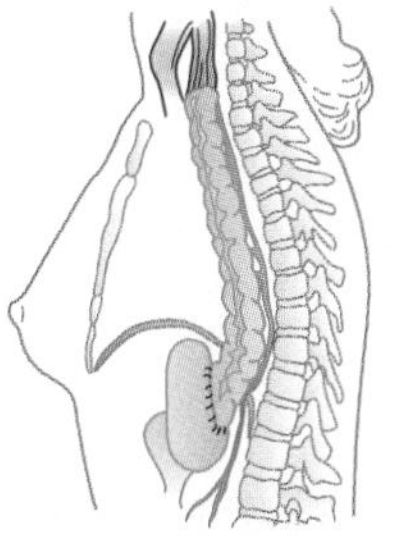	Short and direct	Mediastinum may be unavailable if inflamed, scarred, or involved with cancer
Endo-esophageal	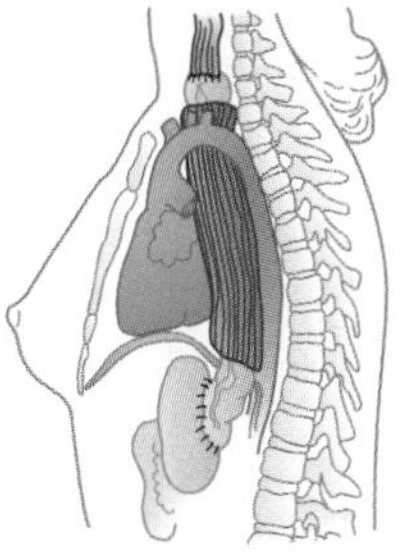	Lessened risk of bleeding Short and direct Promotes a straight lie of the viscus	? Compromise of cancer operation ? Possibility for constriction

FIGURE 39-55.   Options for esophageal substitution. (Adapted from Hiebert CA, Bredenberg CE: Selection and placement of conduits. *In* Pearson FG, Deslauriers J, Ginsberg RJ, et al [eds]: Esophageal Surgery. New York, Churchill Livingstone, 1995, p 654.)

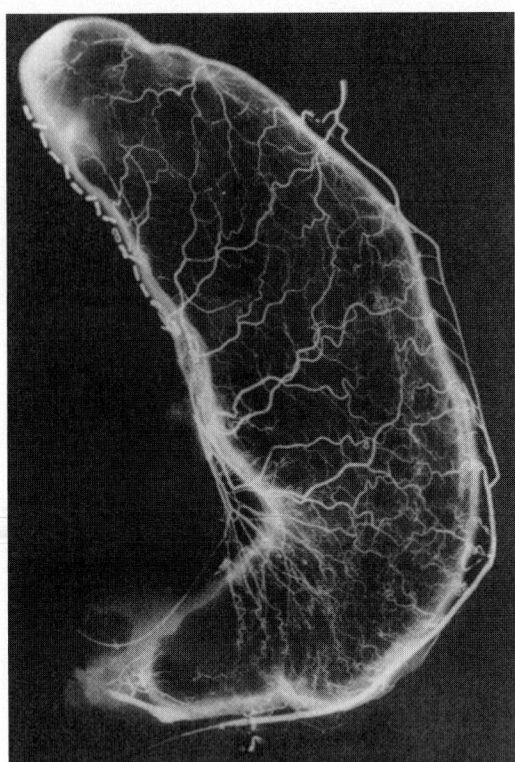

FIGURE 39-56. Arteriogram of the stomach after preparation for esophageal substitute. The intramural arterial network is sufficiently seen, even after resection of the cardia and the left gastric area of the lesser curvature. (Adapted from Akiyama H, Miyazono H, Tsurumaru M, et al: Use of the stomach as an esophageal substitute. Ann Surg 188:606-610, 1978.)

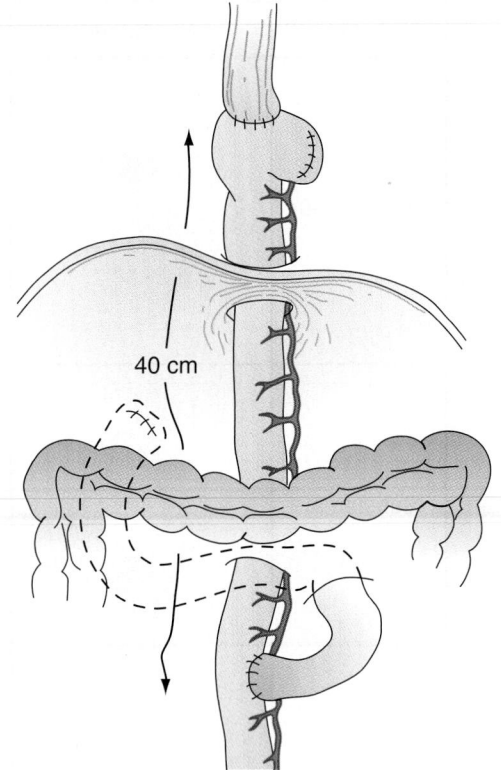

FIGURE 39-58. Roux-en-Y reconstruction of the distal esophagus after distal esophagectomy and total gastrectomy for tumor involving the cardia of the stomach. (Adapted from Akiyama H: Total gastrectomy and roux-en-Y reconstruction. *In* Pearson FG, Deslauriers J, Ginsberg RJ, et al [eds]: Esophageal Surgery. New York, Churchill Livingstone, 1995, p 736.)

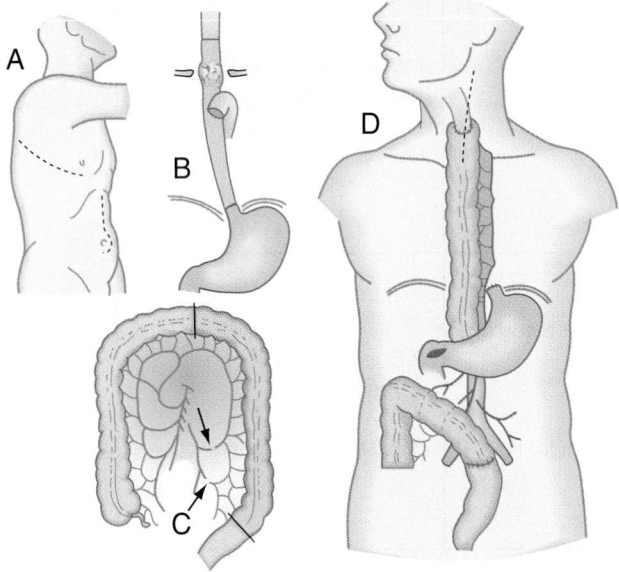

FIGURE 39-57. Esophagectomy with interposition of antiperistaltic segment of left colon. **A,** Incisions used in performance of esophagectomy, cervical esophagostomy, pyloromyotomy, and gastrostomy. **B,** Extent of esophageal resection *(shaded area).* **C,** Preparation of segment of left colon *(shaded area)* for interposition based on middle colic artery (note sites of vascular interruption, which maintain the integrity of the vascular arcade). **D,** Completed operation. (**A** to **D,** Adapted from Ellis FH Jr: Esophagogastrectomy for carcinoma: Technical considerations based on anatomic location of lesion. Surg Clin North Am 60:265-279, 1980.)

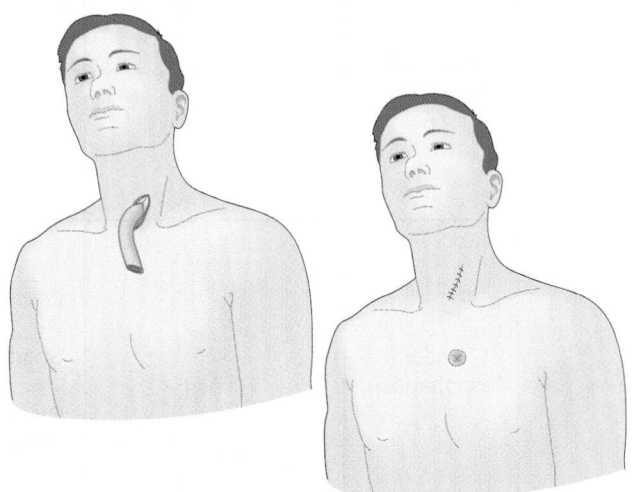

FIGURE 39-59. Construction of anterior thoracic esophagostomy after esophagectomy for esophageal disruption. Rather than discarding viable esophagus that has been mobilized through the cervical incision (**A**), the remaining esophagus is tunneled subcutaneously and a stoma is constructed on the upper anterior thorax (**B**). (**A** and **B**, from Orringer MB, Stirling MC: Esophagectomy for esophageal disruption. Ann Thorac Surg 49:35-43, 1990.)

done to assess the suitability of the colon for esophageal replacement, and the colon then prepared in the event that a colonic interposition is required.

Radiation Therapy The goal of radiation therapy is to destroy the tumor, its microscopic extensions, and other local sites of metastases without crossing the radiation threshold of normal adjacent cells. Patients who undergo external-beam radiation therapy, used alone in the treatment of esophageal carcinoma, have only a 0% to 10% five-year survival, so this therapy is not considered curative. In general, radiation therapy alone should be reserved for palliation or for patients who are medically unable to tolerate chemotherapy.[154] Radiation therapy has low morbidity and can improve esophageal obstruction in most patients in 4 to 7 days. Relief of dysphagia, however, is short lived and recurrence is seen usually within 6 months.[152] The field includes a 5-cm margin on either side of the tumor and adjacent lymph node stations. The supraclavicular or celiac lymph nodes are targets if the tumor is in the upper or lower esophagus, respectively. In the chest, the vulnerable structures are the lung, heart, spinal cord, and bone marrow; therefore, specific oblique fields utilize custom-molded casts or cradles to achieve immobilization and reproducibility. Treatment can be given by hyperfractionation (small fractions two to three times a day), accelerated fractionation (normal-sized fractions given more than once a day), or conventionally (normal-sized fractions [180 to 250 cGy] once a day). The range is from 50 Gy in 20 treatments over 4 weeks to 66 Gy in 33 treatments over 7 weeks. Some of the complications seen are pneumonitis, pericarditis, myocarditis, stricture (40%), fistula formation, and spinal cord damage.[191] Radiation therapy is contraindicated in the presence of a tracheoesophageal fistula. Radiation necrosis of the tumor promotes fistula formation when the tumor has penetrated the trachea or bronchus.

Preoperative radiation therapy is designed to reduce the tumor size, to control the amount of local spread of the tumor before surgery, and to reduce the risk of tumor spread at the time of surgical manipulation. Randomized trials of preoperative radiation therapy for clinically resectable disease show no increase in resectability or survival. Likewise, a recent meta-analysis from the Esophageal Cancer Collaborative group showed no survival advantage with preoperative radiation.[191a] The goal of postoperative radiation therapy is to destroy residual malignant cells after surgical resection, especially if positive tumor margins are discovered after resection. Randomized trials limited to patients treated with postoperative radiation therapy also failed to show improved survival. A recent prospective randomized study comparing surgery alone to surgery plus postoperative radiotherapy (50 to 60 Gy) showed significantly improved survival in stage III patients.[192]

Chemotherapy Chemotherapy as a single modality in the treatment of esophageal cancer is the least effective strategy. Although radiographic improvement is reported in up to one half of patients, two or three cycles (6 to 12 weeks) of chemotherapy are required, relief of dysphagia is slow and/or incomplete, and no survival improvement is observed. Chemotherapy is most often used preoperatively alone or in combination with radiation therapy to treat micrometastases and reduce the tumor size to improve resectability. If surgery is not indicated, chemotherapy is combined with radiation therapy for primary treatment to achieve palliation and possibly improve survival. Chemotherapy is typically given in a combination of two or more drugs, with cisplatin and 5-fluorouracil the most frequently used agents. Other agents with activity in esophageal cancer include paclitaxel, camptothecin, irinotecan, and vinorelbine. Combination therapy has shown promise, with response rates between 50% and 70% for cisplatin-based doublets. Adding a third agent has only fractionally improved response while almost universally worsening toxicity.

Neoadjuvant (preoperative) therapy and combined modality therapy have become focuses of interest in the effort to prolong survival and to reduce recurrence rates. The proposed benefits of preoperative chemotherapy are the preoperative elimination of systemic micrometastases in local, regional, and locally advanced tumors, potentially lowering the stage of the primary tumor. Such a regimen should increase the complete (R0) resection rate in patients with locally advanced tumors, reduce the rate of local and distant recurrences, and increase the chances for long-term survival.

To date, preoperative (neoadjuvant) chemotherapy for resectable esophageal cancer has had mixed results, with no definite improvement in survival for either squamous cell or adenocarcinoma of the esophagus. Few trials have separated chemotherapeutic and radiation responses of squamous cell from adenocarcinoma, which may be a factor in the mixed efficacy reported in various large esophageal cancer studies. A series from Walsh and associates randomized 113 patients with adenocarcinoma of the mid- or distal esophagus (including the cardia) to two cycles of 5-fluorouracil/cisplatin plus preoperative radiation versus surgery alone.[193] There was a significant improvement in both median survival (16 vs. 11 months) and 3-year survival (32% vs. 6%). A criticism of this study is the high operative mortality of 9% and the low 3-year survival (6%) in the surgical control arm, which is below that of historic controls, potentially contributing to the statistical significance. Overall, response rates to chemotherapy are approximately 20%, with few complete pathologic responses.[180,194] Most studies focusing on neoadjuvant chemotherapy are based on combinations that contain cisplatin, which seems to be well tolerated without increasing the postoperative mortality or morbidity rates. A recent large randomized controlled trial comparing preoperative cisplatin and fluorouracil to surgery alone showed a significant improvement in median survival (16.8 months) in the chemotherapy/surgery group compared with surgery alone (13.3 months).[195] In the Intergroup study (INT 0123), patients were randomly assigned to receive either standard (50.4 Gy) or high-dose (64.8 Gy) radiation therapy in addition to chemotherapy. The study consisted of 236 patients, and preliminary results demonstrate no survival difference between the two treatment arms.[196] In the largest multi-institutional randomized study (440 patients) comparing preoperative chemotherapy followed by surgery with surgery alone for patients with local and operable esophageal cancer, Kelsen and associates[197] noted no significant difference between groups in median, 1-year, or 2-year survival rates. There are several active trials to assess the potential benefits of combined modality therapy in the treatment of resectable carcinoma of the esophagus. Details of these studies can be found on CancerNet, the National Cancer Institute website.[198] In addition to neoadjuvant therapy, a recent large trial studying the effects of surgery with or without postoperative (adjuvant) chemotherapy in adenocarcinoma of the stomach or gastroesophageal junction showed improved survival in the chemotherapy group (36 months) versus surgery alone (27 months).[199]

Neoadjuvant therapy that adds radiation to the chemotherapeutic regimen may be more efficacious than radiation or chemotherapy alone. A meta-analysis of 26 phase II and III preoperative chemoradiation therapy trials has demonstrated that increasing the dose of preoperative radiation therapy produces a higher rate of complete pathologic response.[199a] In addition, higher doses of either fluorouracil or cisplatin are also associated with a higher response rate.[200] Randomized trials comparing preoperative radiation therapy and chemotherapy plus surgery to surgery alone have been disappointing with no significant differences in median survival in most studies.[193,201-204]

Given the substantial limitations and criticisms of the previous randomized trials, the Intergroup developed a randomized trial (CALGB C9781) of preoperative combined modality therapy. Unfortunately, the trial was closed prematurely due to lack of accrual. The impression of both physicians and patients that preoperative therapy is superior has made accrual of patients to randomized trials comparing preoperative treatment with surgery alone difficult. Despite lack of convincing data to support its use, the combined use of chemotherapy and radiation therapy followed by surgical resection is perceived as standard treatment in most centers for all but the earliest of esophageal tumors. After resection, a complete histologic response rate of 25% to 30% is observed. As seen with other trials involving radiation therapy and chemotherapy, survival rates are dramatically increased when no residual cancer is found in the tumor specimen. Five-year survival rates approach 60% when this occurs. Unfortunately, no reliable method exists to identify "responders" before therapy is begun.

Another major focus of research is on the development of molecular markers to allow better selection of patients for chemotherapy regimens. In the future, molecular markers may facilitate more stratified therapy and may identify patients better suited for multiple modality therapy including chemotherapy, radiation therapy, and/or surgery.

Barrett's Esophagus

Injured squamous cells in the distal esophagus can be replaced either by more squamous cells or, through the process of metaplasia, by columnar cells (Barrett's esophagus). Chronic gastroesophageal reflux both injures the squamous epithelium and provides the abnormal esophageal environment that stimulates repair through columnar cell metaplasia. Up to three different types of columnar epithelia can be found in Barrett's esophagus: (1) specialized intestinal metaplasia, which has a villiform surface and intestinal-type crypts lined by mucus-secreting columnar cells and goblet cells; (2) gastric fundic-type epithelium; and (3) junctional-type epithelium. Specialized intestinal metaplasia is the most common, and dysplasia and carcinoma in Barrett's esophagus are almost invariably associated with specialized intestinal metaplasia.

Diagnosis

Barrett's esophagus is more common in men than in women, with a 3:1 male predominance (the average age at diagnosis is 55 years). Barrett's esophagus and severe GERD are uncommon in blacks. The prevalence of Barrett's esophagus increases with age up to 70 years. Barrett's esophagus often remains stable, and no conclusive evidence indicates that either ongoing severe reflux or effective treatment of reflux alters the progression of Barrett's esophagus despite the association with cancer. The extent of intestinal metaplasia is related to the status of the LES and the degree of esophageal acid exposure.[205] Barrett's esophagus can be found in 10% to 15% of patients who have endoscopic examinations for symptoms of GERD. Most patients with Barrett's esophagus do not seek medical attention for esophageal symptoms and may have no symptoms of GERD. GERD associated with Barrett's esophagus, however, often is severe, with esophageal ulceration, stricture, and hemorrhage. Barrett's esophagus has been identified in approximately 1 in 10 persons with erosive esophagitis and 1 in 3 persons with a peptic esophageal stricture. In one study, small areas of specialized columnar epithelium with intestinal metaplasia were identified histologically in the region of the gastroesophageal junction in 18% of patients undergoing endoscopy. This finding indicates that "short segment Barrett's esophagus" may be common in the general population. Whether short-segment Barrett's esophagus represents a substantial risk factor for esophageal adenocarcinoma is not yet clear.

Cancer registries in the United States document that the rate of increase in the frequency of adenocarcinoma of the distal esophagus and gastric cardia exceeds that for any other type of cancer. Most of these tumors arise from Barrett's epithelium, a finding suggesting that the prevalence of specialized intestinal metaplasia that predisposes to adenocarcinoma is far more common in the general population than had been appreciated. Carcinogenesis in Barrett's esophagus may involve activation of proto-oncogenes, dysfunction of tumor suppressor genes, or both. Molecular studies have shown that genomic abnormalities in Barrett's esophagus result in the loss of heterozygosity in a variety of tumor suppressor genes including 17P (encoding p53), 5Q (APC, MCC), 18Q (DCC), and 13Q (RBI). Tumor suppressor genes (p53, P16), oncogenes (c-erbB-2, H-ras, K-ras, cyclin D1, and src), and growth factors or receptors (transforming growth factor-α, epidermal growth factor receptor) are implicated in the malignant transformation of Barrett's esophagus and may soon serve as prognostic indicators. Notably, the degree of angiogenesis is not a significant prognostic indicator of esophageal cancer. Flow cytometry has also been used to detect aneuploidy in Barrett's esophagus.

True dysplasia in Barrett's esophagus represents a neoplastic alteration of the columnar epithelium and is widely regarded as the precursor of invasive malignancy. Unfortunately, dysplasia is not an ideal biomarker of malignant potential in Barrett's epithelium for several reasons. The histologic interpretation of dysplasia is largely subjective, and the natural history of dysplasia is not clear. Dysplastic Barrett's mucosa often is indistinguishable from nondysplastic mucosa, and small foci of dysplasia can be easily missed. Despite limitations, dysplasia remains the best biomarker for evaluating malignancy in Barrett's esophagus. Approximately one third of patients with high-grade dysplasia in Barrett's esophagus either already have or will develop invasive cancer within several years. The prevalence of adenocarcinoma at the time of diagnosis of Barrett's esophagus is approximately 8%. The high incidence of esophageal adenocarcinoma has led to the recommendation that all patients with Barrett's esophagus undergo prospective screening for the development of dysplasia and carcinoma. Although this approach seems reasonable, the benefits of screening in Barrett's esophagus have not been proven by a prospective clinical trial.

A number of optical biopsy and light fluorescence or scattering techniques are being investigated for early detection of dysplasia and improve surveillance of Barrett's. The newest to most promising of these techniques is optical coherence tomography (OCT). OCT is an optical biopsy technique that uses infrared light, allowing high resolution imaging of the gastrointestinal wall, including the esophagus. The OCT probe can be passed through the biopsy channels of conventional endoscopes for application during routine endoscopy, with a resolution of 10 mm. A number of trials investigating the utility of OCT in Barrett's esophagus have been initiated; however, OCT remains investigational.[206]

Treatment

Although some severe dysplastic lesions remain stable, most physicians advocate prophylactic esophagectomy in this patient population.[107-110] No medical or surgical treatment, other than resection of the esophagus with dysplastic mucosa, has been demonstrated to produce regression or to prevent malignancy from developing in patients with Barrett's esophagus. The Collis-Nissen gastroplasty controls reflux symptoms and the associated mucosal damage. It restores the LES gradient but increases the resistance to bolus transit; however, no regression of the abnormal mucosa occurs despite reflux control.[207] Given all the uncertainties about the meaning of dysplasia, whether esophageal resection, with its substantial attendant risks, should be recommended for all affected patients is not clear. Hence, endoscopic surveillance is the current recommended approach to management (Fig. 39-60).

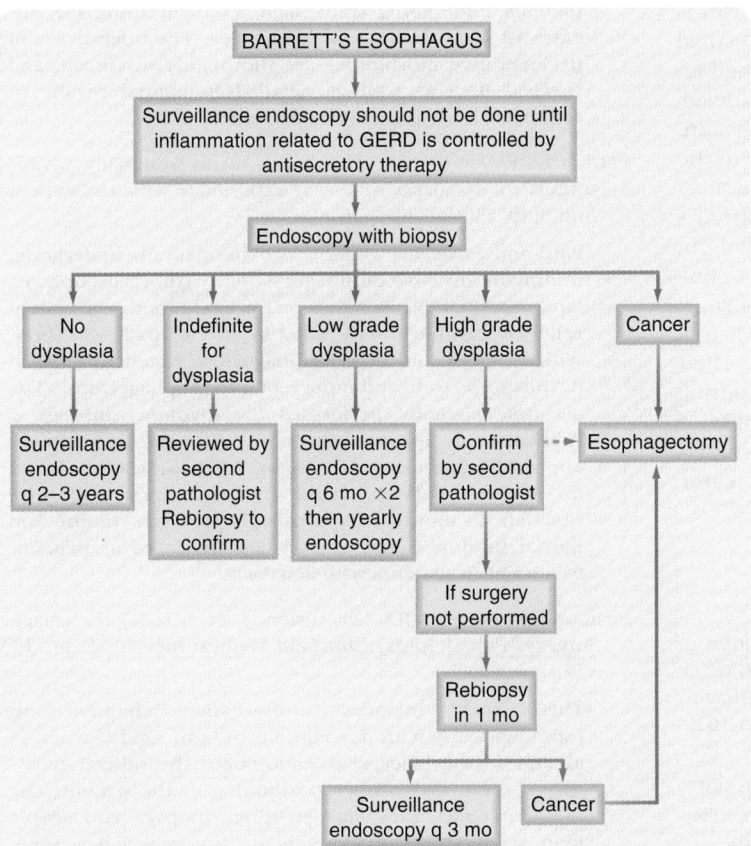

FIGURE 39-60. Management algorithm for Barrett's esophagus.

Patients undergoing surgery for carcinoma in situ or confirmed high-grade dysplasia should have an esophagectomy that includes the entire columnar-lined esophageal segment. The reasons for this recommendation are twofold. First, Barrett's esophagus is a premalignant condition, and high-grade dysplasia or carcinoma may develop subsequently in any columnar-lined tissue that remains after surgery. Second, some studies have reported that as many as 50% of patients who undergo esophagectomy for high-grade dysplasia have an unrecognized adenocarcinoma in the surgical specimen. Multicentric cancers are common, occurring in 13% to 37% of resection specimens for Barrett's esophageal adenocarcinoma.

Laser ablation of Barrett's epithelium has been described but is an experimental therapy, the safety and efficacy of which remain to be established. Photodynamic therapy is a local, endoscopically controlled therapeutic technique based on the sensitization of malignant and precancerous lesions before light-induced tissue destruction. High-grade dysplasia appears to be eradicated in patients, and mucosal cancer is destroyed in 75%. Mucosectomy uses endoscopic snare resections of the mucosa to remove dysplastic areas. Endoscopic argon plasma coagulation may offer patients with small early Barrett's esophageal carcinoma an effective, minimally invasive alternative to mucosectomy or photodynamic therapy. Other clinicians have noted that endoscopic examination with systematic biopsy cannot reliably exclude the presence of occult adenocarcinoma in Barrett's esophagus with invasion beyond the muscularis mucosa, and these investigators caution against the use of mucosal ablative procedures.

After ablation of Barrett's epithelium, the neoplasm is squamous in nature; however, islands of residual intestinal metaplasia may still be present beneath the neoepithelium regardless of ablation technique. Cancer can and has developed in these residual intestinal metaplasia islands that are inaccessible to routine endoscopic surveillance due to the overlying new squamous mucosa that may be normal.[208,209] Because of these concerns, routine ablation of Barrett's epithelium without dysplasia is not recommended. In select high surgical risk patients, ablation may be of clinical benefit for high-grade dysplasia or early carcinoma.

Cyclooxygenase-2 (COX-2) inhibitors may play a role in the chemoprevention of Barrett's esophagus. Their expression is increased in Barrett's esophagus during metaplasia, dysplasia, and carcinoma. COX-2 inhibitor drugs may provide chemoprevention and avert progression of dysplasia or development of esophageal carcinoma. Studies remain investigational.

Selected References

Duranceau A, Ferraro P: Physiology and physiologic studies of the esophagus. *In* Shields TW, LoCicero J III, Ponn RB (eds): General Thoracic Surgery, 5th ed, Vol 2, The Esophagus. Philadelphia, Lippincott Williams & Wilkins, 2000, pp 1619-1634.

This is an authoritative discussion of esophageal physiology that contains clear and understandable manometric tracings of sphincter relaxation and peristaltic activity.

Ellis FH Jr: Standard resection for cancer of the esophagus and cardia. Surg Oncol Clin North Am 8:279-294, 1999.

Standard techniques of esophagectomy as currently performed for cancer of the esophagus and cardia are described. A review of the literature discloses a wide difference in findings and postoperative results. A review of his personal findings and results in 505 operations for cancer of the esophagus on one surgical service from January 1, 1970, to January 1, 1997, reveals a resectability rate of 90%, a hospital mortality rate of 3.3%, a postoperative complication rate of 33.9%, and an adjusted actuarial 5-year survival rate of 24.7%.

Lagergren J, Bergstrom R, Lindgren A, Nyren O: Symptomatic gastroesophageal reflux as a risk factor for esophageal adenocarcinoma. N Engl J Med 340:825-831, 1999.

A nationwide, population-based, case-control study in Sweden that demonstrates a strong and probably causal relation between gastroesophageal reflux and esophageal adenocarcinoma.

Lerut T, Coosemans W, De Leyn P, et al: Treatment of esophageal carcinoma. Chest 116:463S-465S, 1999.

DeCamp MM Jr, Swanson SJ, Jaklitsch MT: Esophagectomy after induction chemoradiation. Chest 116:466S-469S, 1999.

These two excellent overviews illustrate the current controversies regarding surgery alone versus neoadjuvant treatment modalities.

Orringer MB, Marshall B, Iannettoni MD: Transhiatal esophagectomy (THE): Clinical experience and refinements. Ann Surg 230:392-400, 1999.

This is the latest University of Michigan report of 1085 patients undergoing transhiatal esophagectomy for diseases of the intrathoracic esophagus. The operative and perioperative morbidities are thoroughly discussed, and survival data as well as detailed functional results of esophageal substitution are presented.

Patti MG, Pellegrini CA, Horgan S, et al: Minimally invasive surgery for achalasia: An 8-year experience with 168 patients. Ann Surg 230:587-594, 1999.

Patti and associates reported on 168 patients undergoing minimally invasive esophagomyotomy (thoracoscopic 35, laparoscopic 133) over an 8-year period. Good or excellent relief of dysphagia was noted in 90% of patients. Those with a dilated, end-stage esophagus had excellent relief of dysphagia as well, and none required esophagectomy. The authors originally performed the myotomy through a thoracoscopic approach but now prefer the laparoscopic approach combined with a partial fundoplication. Based on these excellent results and long-term follow-up (median 28 months), laparoscopic Heller myotomy and partial fundoplication should be considered as primary treatment in patients with achalasia.

Pearson FG, Cooper JD, Deslauriers J, et al (eds): Esophageal Surgery. Philadelphia, Churchill Livingstone, 2002, pp 133-157.

This work includes authoritative chapters on esophagoscopy with descriptions of both rigid (Savary, et al) and flexible (Rice, et al) endoscopes, the indications for use of each, and proper positioning of the patient. The methodologies for vital staining, biopsy, endoscopic hemostasis, and photodynamic therapy are well described.

Pearson FG, Cooper JD, Deslauriers J, et al (eds): Esophageal Surgery. Philadelphia, Churchill Livingstone, 2002, pp 515-550.

> This authoritative textbook contains outstanding chapters on primary esophageal motor disorders (pp. 515-535) and Chagas' disease (pp. 536-550). In the former, Wood and associates present radiographic and manometric depictions of the various esophageal motor disorders and schematic illustrations of the operative approaches. The chapter by the Brazilian surgeon Ximenes-Netto is based on his vast personal experience with Chagas' disease and provides a unique perspective for those who are unfamiliar with this infectious cause of achalasia.

Reed CE, Mishra G, Sahai AV, et al: Esophageal cancer staging: Improved accuracy by endoscopic ultrasound of celiac lymph nodes. Ann Thorac Surg 67:319-322, 1999.

> With the rising incidence of distal and gastroesophageal junction adenocarcinomas, assessment of the celiac axis lymph nodes becomes important because it is a common nodal drainage basin. EUS permits evaluation of these lymph nodes and biopsy by FNA. EUS with FNA is emerging as an important tool in guiding treatment for patients with distal adenocarcinoma and in documenting disease before neoadjuvant therapy.

Rice TW: Esophageal diverticula. Semin Thorac Cardiovasc Surg 11:325-367, 1999.

> Comprehensive seminar on current evaluation and surgical techniques, including minimally invasive surgery.

References

1. Meyer GW, Castell DO: In support of the clinical usefulness of lower esophageal sphincter pressure determination. Dig Dis Sci 26:1028-1031, 1981.
2. Donner MW, Bosma JF, Robertson DL: Anatomy and physiology of the pharynx. Gastrointest Radiol 10:196-212, 1985.
3. Kahrilas PJ, Logemann JA, Lin S, et al: Pharyngeal clearance during swallowing: A combined manometric and videofluoroscopic study. Gastroenterology 103:128-136, 1992.
4. Duranceau AC, Devroede G, LaFontaine E, et al: Esophageal motility in asymptomatic volunteers. Surg Clin North Am 63:777-786, 1983.
5. Wynder EL, Hultberg S, Jacobsson F, et al: Environmental factors in cancer of the upper alimentary tract; a Swedish study with special reference to Plummer-Vinson (Paterson-Kelly) syndrome. Cancer 10:470-487, 1957.
6. Wilkins EW Jr: Rings and webs. In Pearson FG, Cooper JD, Deslauriers J, et al (eds): Esophageal Surgery. Philadelphia, Churchill Livingstone, 2002, pp 297-305.
7. Salo JA, Ala-Kulju KV: Congenital esophageal cysts in adults. Ann Thorac Surg 44:135-138, 1987.
8. Van Dam J, Rice TW, Sivak MV Jr: Endoscopic ultrasonography and endoscopically guided needle aspiration for the diagnosis of upper gastrointestinal tract foregut cysts. Am J Gastroenterol 87:762-765, 1992.
9. Nigro JJ, Hagen JA, DeMeester TR, et al: Prevalence and location of nodal metastases in distal esophageal adenocarcinoma confined to the wall: Implications for therapy. J Thorac Cardiovasc Surg 117:16-25, 1999.
10. Henderson RD: Disorders of the pharyngoesophageal junction. In Henderson RD (ed): Esophagus: Reflux and Primary Motor Disorders. Baltimore, Williams & Wilkins, 1980, pp 223-247.
11. Orringer MB: Extended cervical esophagomyotomy for cricopharyngeal dysfunction. J Thorac Cardiovasc Surg 80:669-678, 1980.
12. St Peter SD, Swain JM: Achalasia: A comprehensive review. Surg Laparosc Endosc Percutan Tech 13:227-240, 2003.
13. Streitz JM Jr, Ellis FH Jr, Gibb SP, et al: Achalasia and squamous cell carcinoma of the esophagus: Analysis of 241 patients. Ann Thorac Surg 59:1604-1609, 1995.
14. Zwischenberger JB, Savage C: Megaesophagus from a 26-year history of achalasia. Ann Thorac Surg 69:1597, 2000.
15. Neubrand M, Scheurlen C, Schepke M, et al: Long-term results and prognostic factors in the treatment of achalasia with botulinum toxin. Endoscopy 34:519-523, 2002.
16. Bhutani MS: Gastrointestinal uses of botulinum toxin. Am J Gastroenterol 92:929-933, 1997.
17. Bansal R, Nostrant TT, Scheiman JM, et al: Intrasphincteric botulinum toxin versus pneumatic balloon dilation for treatment of primary achalasia. J Clin Gastroenterol 36:209-214, 2003.
18. Patti MG, Pellegrini CA, Horgan S, et al: Minimally invasive surgery for achalasia: An 8-year experience with 168 patients. Ann Surg 230:587-594, 1999.
19. Patti MG, Fisichella PM, Perretta S, et al: Impact of minimally invasive surgery on the treatment of esophageal achalasia: A decade of change. J Am Coll Surg 196:698-705, 2003.
20. Chen LQ, Chughtai T, Sideris L, et al: Long-term effects of myotomy and partial fundoplication for esophageal achalasia. Dis Esophagus 15:171-179, 2002.
21. Ferguson MK: Achalasia: Current evaluation and therapy. Ann Thorac Surg 52:336-342, 1991.
22. Ellis FH Jr: Treatment of carcinoma of the esophagus or cardia. Mayo Clin Proc 64:945-955, 1989.
23. Castrini G, Pappalardo G: Our experience in the surgical treatment of achalasia. In DeMeester TR, Skinner DB (eds): Esophageal Disorders: Pathophysiology and Therapy. New York, Raven Press, 1985, pp 423-426.
24. Oelschlager BK, Chang L, Pellegrini CA: Improved outcome after extended gastric myotomy for achalasia. Arch Surg 138:490-497, 2003.
25. Malthaner RA, Tood TR, Miller L, et al: Long-term results in surgically managed esophageal achalasia. Ann Thorac Surg 58:1343-1347, 1994.
26. Wiechmann RJ, Ferguson MK, Naunheim KS, et al: Video-assisted surgical management of achalasia of the esophagus. J Thorac Cardiovasc Surg 118:916-923, 1999.
27. Sharp KW, Khaitan L, Scholz S, et al: 100 consecutive minimally invasive Heller myotomies: Lessons learned. Ann Surg 235:631-639, 2002.
28. Luketich JD, Schauer PR, Christie NA, et al: Minimally invasive esophagectomy. Ann Thorac Surg 70:906-912, 2000.
29. Horgan S, Hudda K, Eubanks T, et al: Does botulinum toxin injection make esophagomyotomy a more difficult operation? Surg Endosc 13:576-579, 1999.
30. Luketich JD, Schauer PR, Meltzer CC, et al: Role of positron emission tomography in staging esophageal cancer. Ann Thorac Surg 64:765-769, 1997.
31. Orringer MB, Stirling MC: Esophageal resection for achalasia: Indications and results. Ann Thorac Surg 47:340-345, 1989.
31a. Devaney EJ, Iannettoni MD, Orringer MB, et al: Esophagectomy for achalasia: Patient selection and clinical experience. Ann Thorac Surg 72:854-858, 2001.

32. Ellis FH Jr, Watkins E Jr, Gibb SP, et al: Ten to 20-year clinical results after short esophagomyotomy without an antireflux procedure (modified Heller operation) for esophageal achalasia. Eur J Cardiothorac Surg 6:86-90, 1992.

33. Orringer MB, Marshall B, Iannettoni MD: Transhiatal esophagectomy: Clinical experience and refinements. Ann Surg 230:392-403, 1999.

34. Banbury MK, Rice TW, Goldblum JR, et al: Esophagectomy with gastric reconstruction for achalasia. J Thorac Cardiovasc Surg 117:1077-1084, 1999.

35. Clouse RE, Lustman PJ: Psychiatric illness and contraction abnormalities of the esophagus. N Engl J Med 309:1337-1342, 1983.

36. Vantrappen G, Hellemans J: Treatment of achalasia and related motor disorders. Gastroenterology 79:144-154, 1980.

37. Orringer MB: Transhiatal esophagectomy for benign disease. J Thorac Cardiovasc Surg 90:649-655, 1985.

38. Evander A, Little AG, Ferguson MK, et al: Diverticula of the mid- and lower esophagus: pathogenesis and surgical management. World J Surg 10:820-828, 1986.

39. van Overbeek JJ: Pathogenesis and methods of treatment of Zenker's diverticulum. Ann Otol Rhinol Laryngol 112:583-593, 2003.

40. Cook IJ, Gabb M, Panagopoulos V, et al: Pharyngeal (Zenker's) diverticulum is a disorder of upper esophageal sphincter opening. Gastroenterology 103:1229-1235, 1992.

41. Sutherland HD: Cricopharyngeal achalasia. J Thorac Cardiovasc Surg 43:114-126, 1962.

42. Fulp SR, Castell DO: Manometric aspects of Zenker's diverticulum. Hepatogastroenterology 39:123-126, 1992.

43. Payne WS: The treatment of pharyngoesophageal diverticulum: The simple and complex. Hepatogastroenterology 39:109-114, 1992.

44. Duranceau A, Rheault MJ, Jamieson GG: Physiologic response to cricopharyngeal myotomy and diverticulum suspension. Surgery 94:655-662, 1983.

45. Gutschow CA, Hamoir M, Rombaux P, et al: Management of pharyngoesophageal (Zenker's) diverticulum: Which technique? Ann Thorac Surg 74:1677-1683, 2002.

46. Dohlman G, Mattsson O: The endoscopic operation for hypopharyngeal diverticula: A roentgen cinematographic study. Arch Otolaryngol 71:744-752, 1960.

47. Peracchia A, Bonavina L, Narne S, et al: Minimally invasive surgery for Zenker diverticulum: Analysis of results in 95 consecutive patients. Arch Surg 133:695-700, 1998.

48. Colombo-Benkmann M, Unruh V, Krieglstein C, et al: Cricopharyngeal myotomy in the treatment of Zenker's diverticulum. J Am Coll Surg 196:370-378, 2003.

49. Falk GW: Regurgitation in a patient with an esophageal diverticulum. Cleve Clin J Med 61:409-411, 1994.

50. Ellis FH Jr, Crozier RE, Gibb SP: Reoperative achalasia surgery. J Thorac Cardiovasc Surg 92:859-865, 1986.

51. Benacci JC, Deschamps C, Trastek VF, et al: Epiphrenic diverticulum: Results of surgical treatment. Ann Thorac Surg 55:1109-1114, 1993.

52. DiPalma JA: Esophageal disorders. In Civetta JM, Taylor RW, Kirby RR (eds): Critical Care. Philadelphia, Lippincott-Raven, 1997, pp 2071-2077.

53. Kirsh MM, Ritter F: Caustic ingestion and subsequent damage to the oropharyngeal and digestive passages. Ann Thorac Surg 21:74-82, 1976.

54. Greenberg RE, Bank S, Blumstein M, et al: Common gastrointestinal disorders in the intensive care unit. In Bone RC (ed): Pulmonary and Critical Care Medicine. Chicago, Mosby, 1993, pp 1-27.

55. Spitz L, Lakhoo K: Caustic ingestion. Arch Dis Child 68:157-158, 1993.

56. Estrera A, Taylor W, Mills LJ, et al: Corrosive burns of the esophagus and stomach: A recommendation for an aggressive surgical approach. Ann Thorac Surg 41:276-283, 1986.

57. Symbas PN, Vlasis SE, Hatcher CR Jr: Esophagitis secondary to ingestion of caustic material. Ann Thorac Surg 36:73-77, 1983.

58. Lamireau T, Rebouissoux L, Denis D, et al: Accidental caustic ingestion in children: Is endoscopy always mandatory? J Pediatr Gastroenterol Nutr 33:81-84, 2001.

59. Anderson KD: Corrosive injury. In Pearson FG, Deslauriers J, Ginsberg RJ, et al (eds): Esophageal Surgery/Trauma. New York, Churchill Livingstone, 1995, pp 465-478.

60. Cattan P, Munoz-Bongrand N, Berney T, et al: Extensive abdominal surgery after caustic ingestion. Ann Surg 231:519-523, 2000.

61. Millar AJ, Numanoglu A, Mann M, et al: Detection of caustic oesophageal injury with technetium 99m-labelled sucralfate. J Pediatr Surg 36:262-265, 2001.

62. Anderson KD, Rouse TM, Randolph JG: A controlled trial of corticosteroids in children with corrosive injury of the esophagus. N Engl J Med 323:637-640, 1990.

63. Mamede RC, De Mello Filho FV: Treatment of caustic ingestion: An analysis of 239 cases. Dis Esophagus 15:210-213, 2002.

64. Gunnarsson M: Local corticosteroid treatment of caustic injuries of the esophagus: A preliminary report. Ann Otol Rhinol Laryngol 108:1088-1090, 1999.

65. Goldman LP, Weigert JM: Corrosive substance ingestion: A review. Am J Gastroenterol 79:85-90, 1984.

66. Kikendall JW: Caustic ingestion injuries. Gastroenterol Clin North Am 20:847-857, 1991.

67. Hwang TL, Shen-Chen SM, Chen MF: Nonthoracotomy esophagectomy for corrosive esophagitis with gastric perforation. Surg Gynecol Obstet 164:537-540, 1987.

68. Gandhi RP, Cooper A, Barlow BA: Successful management of esophageal strictures without resection or replacement. J Pediatr Surg 24:745-749, 1989.

69. Jones WG II, Ginsberg RJ: Esophageal perforation: A continuing challenge. Ann Thorac Surg 53:534-543, 1992.

70. Altorjay A, Kiss J, Voros A, et al: The role of esophagectomy in the management of esophageal perforations. Ann Thorac Surg 65:1433-1436, 1998.

71. Bufkin BL, Miller JI Jr, Mansour KA: Esophageal perforation: Emphasis on management. Ann Thorac Surg 61:1447-1451, 1996.

72. Iannettoni MD, Vlessis AA, Whyte RI, et al: Functional outcome after surgical treatment of esophageal perforation. Ann Thorac Surg 64:1606-1609, 1997.

73. English GM, Hsu SF, Edgar R, et al: Oesophageal trauma in patients with spinal cord injury. Paraplegia 30:903-912, 1992.

74. Pass LJ, LeNarz LA, Schreiber JT, et al: Management of esophageal gunshot wounds. Ann Thorac Surg 44:253-256, 1987.

75. Gouge TH, Depan HJ, Spencer FC: Experience with the Grillo pleural wrap procedure in 18 patients with perforation of the thoracic esophagus. Ann Surg 209:612-617, 1989.

76. Sarr MG, Pemberton JH, Payne WS: Management of instrumental perforations of the esophagus. J Thorac Cardiovasc Surg 84:211-218, 1982.

77. White RK, Morris DM: Diagnosis and management of esophageal perforations. Am Surg 58:112-119, 1992.

78. Dolgin SR, Wykoff TW, Kumar NR, et al: Conservative medical management of traumatic pharyngoesophageal perforations. Ann Otol Rhinol Laryngol 101:209-215, 1992.

79. Jagot P, Sauvanet A, Berthoux L, et al: Laparoscopic mobilization of the stomach for oesophageal replacement. Br J Surg 83:540-542, 1996.

80. Altorjay A, Kiss J, Voros A, et al: Nonoperative management of esophageal perforations. Is it justified? Ann Surg 225:415-421, 1997.

81. Cameron JL, Kieffer RF, Hendrix TR, et al: Selective nonoperative management of contained intrathoracic esophageal disruptions. Ann Thorac Surg 27:404-408, 1979.

82. Orringer MB, Stirling MC: Esophagectomy for esophageal disruption. Ann Thorac Surg 49:35-42, 1990.

83. Whyte RI, Iannettoni MD, Orringer MB: Intrathoracic esophageal perforation: The merit of primary repair. J Thorac Cardiovasc Surg 109:140-144, 1995.

84. Grillo HC, Wilkins EW Jr: Esophageal repair following late diagnosis of intrathoracic perforation. Ann Thorac Surg 20:387-399, 1975.

85. Richardson JD, Martin LF, Borzotta AP, et al: Unifying concepts in treatment of esophageal leaks. Am J Surg 149:157-162, 1985.

86. Wright CD, Mathisen DJ, Wain JC, et al: Reinforced primary repair of thoracic esophageal perforation. Ann Thorac Surg 60:245-248, 1995.

87. Shields TW: Esophageal trauma. In Shields TW (ed): General Thoracic Surgery. Philadelphia, Lippincott Williams & Wilkins, 2000, pp 1769-1782.

88. Morgan RA, Ellul JP, Denton ER, et al: Malignant esophageal fistulas and perforations: Management with plastic-covered metallic endoprostheses. Radiology 204:527-532, 1997.

89. Davies AP, Vaughan R: Expanding mesh stent in the emergency treatment of Boerhaave's syndrome. Ann Thorac Surg 67:1482-1483, 1999.

90. Lawrence DR, Ohri SK, Moxon RE, et al: Primary esophageal repair for Boerhaave's syndrome. Ann Thorac Surg 67:818-820, 1999.

91. Reed MF, Mathisen DJ: Tracheoesophageal fistula. Chest Surg Clin North Am 13:271-289, 2003.

92. Macchiarini P, Verhoye JP, Chapelier A, et al: Evaluation and outcome of different surgical techniques for postintubation tracheoesophageal fistulas. J Thorac Cardiovasc Surg 119:268-276, 2000.

93. Postlethwait RW, Lowe JE: Benign tumors and cysts of the esophagus. In Orringer MB, Zuidema GD (eds): Shackelford's Surgery of the Alimentary Tract. Philadelphia, WB Saunders, 1996.

94. Shamji F, Todd TR: Benign tumors. In Pearson FG, Cooper JD, Deslauriers J, et al (eds): Esophageal Surgery. Philadelphia, Churchill Livingstone, 2002, pp 636-648.

94a. Logrono R, Jones DV, Faruqi S, Bhutani MS: Recent advances in cell biology, diagnosis, and therapy of gastrointestinal stromal tumor (GIST). Cancer Biol Ther 3(3), 2004.

95. Seremetis MG, Lyons WS, deGuzman VC, et al: Leiomyomata of the esophagus: An analysis of 838 cases. Cancer 38:2166-2177, 1976.

96. Lewis RJ, Caccavale RJ, Sisler GE: Imaged thoracoscopic surgery: A new thoracic technique for resection of mediastinal cysts. Ann Thorac Surg 53:318-320, 1992.

97. Brugge WR, Lee MJ, Carey RW, et al: Endoscopic ultrasound staging criteria for esophageal cancer. Gastrointest Endosc 45:147-152, 1997.

98. Lagergren J, Bergstrom R, Lindgren A, et al: Symptomatic gastroesophageal reflux as a risk factor for esophageal adenocarcinoma. N Engl J Med 340:825-831, 1999.

98a. Koop H: Gastroesophageal reflux disease and Barrett's esophagus. Endoscopy 36(2):103-109, 2004.

99. Sarr MG, Hamilton SR, Marrone GC, et al: Barrett's esophagus: Its prevalence and association with adenocarcinoma in patients with symptoms of gastroesophageal reflux. Am J Surg 149:187-193, 1985.

100. Sherrill DJ, Grishkin BA, Galal FS, et al: Radiation-associated malignancies of the esophagus. Cancer 54:726-728, 1984.

101. Wong RK, Horwhat JD, Maydonovitch CL: Sky blue or murky waters: The diagnostic utility of methylene blue. Gastrointest Endosc 54:409-413, 2001.

102. Canto MI, Setrakian S, Willis J, et al: Methylene blue-directed biopsies improve detection of intestinal metaplasia and dysplasia in Barrett's esophagus. Gastrointest Endosc 51:560-568, 2000.

103. Glickman JN: Section II: Pathology and pathologic staging of esophageal cancer. Semin Thorac Cardiovasc Surg 15(2):167-179, 2003.

104. Sasajima K, Takai A, Taniguchi Y, et al: Polypoid squamous cell carcinoma of the esophagus. Cancer 64:94-97, 1989.

105. Takagi I, Karasawa K: Growth of squamous cell esophageal carcinoma observed by serial esophagographies. J Surg Oncol 21:57-60, 1982.

106. Riddel RH: Dysplasia and regression in Barrett's epithelium. In Spechler SJ, Goyal RK (eds): Barrett's Esophagus: Pathophysiology, Diagnosis, and Management. New York, Elsevier, 1985, pp 143-153.

107. Lin OS, Mannava S, Hwang KL, et al: Reasons for current practices in managing Barrett's esophagus. Dis Esophagus 15:39-45, 2002.

108. Hameeteman W, Tytgat GN, Houthoff HJ, et al: Barrett's esophagus: Development of dysplasia and adenocarcinoma. Gastroenterology 96:1249-1256, 1989.

109. Miros M, Kerlin P, Walker N: Only patients with dysplasia progress to adenocarcinoma in Barrett's oesophagus. Gut 32:1441-1446, 1991.

110. Reid BJ, Weinstein WM, Lewin KJ, et al: Endoscopic biopsy can detect high-grade dysplasia or early adenocarcinoma in Barrett's esophagus without grossly recognizable neoplastic lesions. Gastroenterology 94:81-90, 1988.

111. Ferguson MK, Skinner DB: Carcinoma of the esophagus and cardia. In Orringer MG, Zuidema GD (eds): Shackelford's Surgery of the Alimentary Tract. Philadelphia, WB Saunders, 1990, pp 305-332.

112. Pfau PR, Ginsberg GG, Lew RJ, et al: EUS predictors of long-term survival in esophageal carcinoma. Gastrointest Endosc 53:463-469, 2001.

113. Hagen JA, DeMeester SR, Peters JH, et al: Curative resection for esophageal adenocarcinoma: Analysis of 100 en bloc esophagectomies. Ann Surg 234:520-531, 2001.

114. Parmar KS, Zwischenberger JB, Reeves AL, et al: Clinical impact of endoscopic ultrasound-guided fine needle aspiration of celiac axis lymph nodes (M1a disease) in esophageal cancer. Ann Thorac Surg 73:916-921, 2002.

115. Aloia TA, Harpole DH Jr, Reed CE, et al: Tumor marker expression is predictive of survival in patients with esophageal cancer. Ann Thorac Surg 72:859-866, 2001.

116. Kumbasar B: Carcinoma of esophagus: Radiologic diagnosis and staging. Eur J Radiol 42:170-180, 2002.

117. Halvorsen RA Jr, Thompson WM: Primary neoplasms of the hollow organs of the gastrointestinal tract: Staging and follow-up. Cancer 67:1181-1188, 1991.

118. Koch J, Halvorsen RA Jr: Staging of esophageal cancer: Computed tomography, magnetic resonance imaging, and endoscopic ultrasound. Semin Roentgenol 29:364-372, 1994.

119. Reed CE, Mishra G, Sahai AV, et al: Esophageal cancer staging: Improved accuracy by endoscopic ultrasound of celiac lymph nodes. Ann Thorac Surg 67:319-322, 1999.

120. Quint LE, Glazer GM, Orringer MB, et al: Esophageal carcinoma: CT findings. Radiology 155:171-175, 1985.

121. Tio TL, Cohen P, Coene PP, et al: Endosonography and computed tomography of esophageal carcinoma: Preoperative classification compared to the new (1987) TNM system. Gastroenterology 96:1478-1486, 1989.

122. Vilgrain V, Mompoint D, Palazzo L, et al: Staging of esophageal carcinoma: Comparison of results with endoscopic sonography and CT. AJR Am J Roentgenol 155:277-281, 1990.

123. Botet JF, Lightdale CJ, Zauber AG, et al: Preoperative staging of esophageal cancer: Comparison of endoscopic US and dynamic CT. Radiology 181:419-425, 1991.

124. Murata Y, Muroi M, Yoshida M, et al: Endoscopic ultrasonography in the diagnosis of esophageal carcinoma. Surg Endosc 1:11-16, 1987.

125. Pfau PR, Ginsberg GG, Lew RJ, et al: Esophageal dilation for endosonographic evaluation of malignant esophageal strictures is safe and effective. Am J Gastroenterol 95:2813-2815, 2000.

125a. Menzel J, Hoepffner N, Nottberg H, et al: Preoperative staging of esophageal carcinoma: Miniprobe sonography versus conventional endoscopic ultrasound in a prospective histopathologically verified study. Endoscopy 31(4):291-297, 1999.

125b. Hunerbein M, Ulmer C, Handke T, Schlag PM: Endosonography of upper gastrointestinal tract cancer on demand using miniprobes or endoscopic ultrasound. Surg Endosc 17(4):615-619, 2003.

126. Van Dam J, Rice TW, Catalano MF, et al: High-grade malignant stricture is predictive of esophageal tumor stage: Risks of endosonographic evaluation. Cancer 71:2910-2917, 1993.

127. Siewert JR, Holscher AH, Dittler HJ: Preoperative staging and risk analysis in esophageal carcinoma. Hepatogastroenterology 37:382-387, 1990.

128. Van Dam J: Endosonographic evaluation of the patient with esophageal cancer. Chest 112:184S-190S, 1997.

129. Ell C, May A, Gossner L, et al: Endoscopic mucosal resection of early cancer and high-grade dysplasia in Barrett's esophagus. Gastroenterology 118:670-677, 2000.

130. Nijhawan PK, Wang KK: Endoscopic mucosal resection for lesions with endoscopic features suggestive of malignancy and high-grade dysplasia within Barrett's esophagus. Gastrointest Endosc 52:328-332, 2000.

131. Vickers J: Role of endoscopic ultrasound in the preoperative assessment of patients with oesophageal cancer. Ann R Coll Surg Engl 80:233-239, 1998.

132. Rice TW, Boyce GA, Sivak MV: Esophageal ultrasound and the preoperative staging of carcinoma of the esophagus. J Thorac Cardiovasc Surg 101:536-544, 1991.

133. Nishimaki T, Tanaka O, Ando N, et al: Evaluation of the accuracy of preoperative staging in thoracic esophageal cancer. Ann Thorac Surg 68:2059-2064, 1999.

134. Penman ID, Williams DB, Sahai AV, et al: Ability of EUS with fine-needle aspiration to document nodal staging and response to neoadjuvant chemoradiotherapy in locally advanced esophageal cancer: A case report. Gastrointest Endosc 49:783-786, 1999.

135. Bhutani MS, Hawes RH, Hoffman BJ: A comparison of the accuracy of echo features during endoscopic ultrasound (EUS) and EUS-guided fine-needle aspiration for diagnosis of malignant lymph node invasion. Gastrointest Endosc 45:474-479, 1997.

136. Bhutani MS: Interventional Endoscopic Ultrasound. Amsterdam, Harwood Academic Publishers, 1999.

137. Bhutani MS: Interventional endoscopic ultrasonography: State of the art at the new millennium. Endoscopy 32:62-71, 2000.

138. Slater MS, Holland J, Faigel DO, et al: Does neoadjuvant chemoradiation downstage esophageal carcinoma? Am J Surg 181:440-444, 2001.

138a. Bhutani MS: Emerging indications for interventional ultrasonography. Endoscopy 35(8):S45-S48, 2003.

139. Flanagan FL, Dehdashti F, Siegel BA, et al: Staging of esophageal cancer with ^{18}F-fluorodeoxyglucose positron emission tomography. AJR Am J Roentgenol 168:417-424, 1997.

140. Wren SM, Stijns P, Srinivas S: Positron emission tomography in the initial staging of esophageal cancer. Arch Surg 137:1001-1007, 2002.

141. Luketich JD, Schauer P, Landreneau R, et al: Minimally invasive surgical staging is superior to endoscopic ultrasound in detecting lymph node metastases in esophageal cancer. J Thorac Cardiovasc Surg 114:817-823, 1997.

142. Kinkel K, Lu Y, Both M, et al: Detection of hepatic metastases from cancers of the gastrointestinal tract by using noninvasive imaging methods (US, CT, MR imaging, PET): A meta-analysis. Radiology 224:748-756, 2002.

143. Krasna MJ, McLaughlin JS: Thoracoscopic lymph node staging for esophageal cancer. Ann Thorac Surg 56:671-674, 1993.

144. Krasna MJ, Reed CE, Jaklitsch MT, et al: Thoracoscopic staging of esophageal cancer: A prospective, multiinstitutional trial. Cancer and Leukemia Group B Thoracic Surgeons. Ann Thorac Surg 60:1337-1340, 1995.

145. Petrillo R, Balzarini L, Bidoli P, et al: Esophageal squamous cell carcinoma: MRI evaluation of mediastinum. Gastrointest Radiol 15:275-278, 1990.

146. Krasna MJ, Reed CE, Nedzwiecki D, et al: CALGB 9380: A prospective trial of the feasibility of thoracoscopy/laparoscopy in staging esophageal cancer. Ann Thorac Surg 71:1073-1079, 2001.

147. Krasna MJ: Minimally invasive staging for esophageal cancer. Chest 112:191S-194S, 1997.

148. Akiyama H, Tsurumaru M, Udagawa H, et al: Radical lymph node dissection for cancer of the thoracic esophagus. Ann Surg 220:364-372; discussion 372-373, 1994.

149. Krasna MJ: The role of thoracoscopic lymph node staging in esophageal cancer. Int Surg 82:7-11, 1997.

150. McCaughan JS Jr, Ellison EC, Guy JT, et al: Photodynamic therapy for esophageal malignancy: A prospective twelve-year study. Ann Thorac Surg 62:1005-1010, 1996.

151. Moghissi K, Dixon K: Photodynamic therapy (PDT) in esophageal cancer: A surgical view of its indications based on 14 years experience. Technol Cancer Res Treat 2:319-326, 2003.

152. Hishikawa Y, Kurisu K, Taniguchi M, et al: High-dose-rate intraluminal brachytherapy (HDRIBT) for esophageal cancer. Int J Radiat Oncol Biol Phys 21:1133-1135, 1991.

153. Fleischman EH, Kagan AR, Bellotti JE, et al: Effective palliation for inoperable esophageal cancer using intensive intracavitary radiation. J Surg Oncol 44:234-237, 1990.

154. Minsky BD: Combined modality therapy for esophageal cancer. Semin Oncol 30:46-55, 2003.

155. Sur M, Sur R, Cooper K, et al: Morphologic alterations in esophageal squamous cell carcinoma after preoperative high dose rate intraluminal brachytherapy. Cancer 77:2200-2205, 1996.

156. Sur RK, Levin CV, Donde B, et al: Prospective randomized trial of HDR brachytherapy as a sole modality in palliation of advanced esophageal carcinoma—an International Atomic Energy Agency study. Int J Radiat Oncol Biol Phys 53:127-133, 2002.

157. Meunier B, Spiliopoulos Y, Stasik C, et al: Retrosternal bypass operation for unresectable squamous cell cancer of the esophagus. Ann Thorac Surg 62:373-377, 1996.

158. Conlan AA, Nicolaou N, Hammond CA, et al: Retrosternal gastric bypass for inoperable esophageal cancer: A report of 71 patients. Ann Thorac Surg 36:396-401, 1983.

159. Saidi F, Abbassi A, Shadmehr MB, et al: Endothoracic endoesophageal pull-through operation: A new approach to cancers of the esophagus and proximal stomach. J Thorac Cardiovasc Surg 102:43-50, 1991.

160. Orringer MB, Forastiere AA, Perez-Tamayo C, et al: Chemotherapy and radiation therapy before transhiatal esophagectomy for esophageal carcinoma. Ann Thorac Surg 49:348-355, 1990.

161. Ajani JA: Current status of new drugs and multidisciplinary approaches in patients with carcinoma of the esophagus. Chest 113:112S-119S, 1998.

161a. Naunheim KS, Hanosh J, Zwischenberger JB, et al: Esophagectomy in the septuagenarian. Ann Thorac Surg 56:880-884, 1993.

162. Katlic MR, Wilkins EW Jr, Grillo HC: Three decades of treatment of esophageal squamous carcinoma at the Massachusetts General Hospital. J Thorac Cardiovasc Surg 99:929-938, 1990.

163. Hulscher JB, Tijssen JG, Obertop H, et al: Transthoracic versus transhiatal resection for carcinoma of the esophagus: A meta-analysis. Ann Thorac Surg 72:306-313, 2001.

164. Goldfaden D, Orringer MB, Appelman HD, et al: Adenocarcinoma of the distal esophagus and gastric cardia: Comparison of results of transhiatal esophagectomy and thoracoabdominal esophagogastrectomy. J Thorac Cardiovasc Surg 91:242-247, 1986.

165. Hankins JR, Attar S, Coughlin TR Jr, et al: Carcinoma of the esophagus: A comparison of the results of transhiatal versus transthoracic resection. Ann Thorac Surg 47:700-705, 1989.

165a. Zwischenberger JB, Sankar AB: Transhiatal esophagectomy. Chest Surg Clin North Am 5:527-542, 1995.

166. Millikan KW, Silverstein J, Hart V, et al: A 15-year review of esophagectomy for carcinoma of the esophagus and cardia. Arch Surg 130:617-624, 1995.

167. Pac M, Basoglu A, Kocak H, et al: Transhiatal versus transthoracic esophagectomy for esophageal cancer. J Thorac Cardiovasc Surg 106:205-209, 1993.

168. Vigneswaran WT, Trastek VF, Pairolero PC, et al: Transhiatal esophagectomy for carcinoma of the esophagus. Ann Thorac Surg 56:838-846, 1993.

168a. Zwischenberger JB, Sankar AB: Transhiatal esophagectomy. Chest Surg Clin North Am 5:527-542, 1995.

169. Orringer MB, Marshall B, Iannettoni MD: Transhiatal esophagectomy (THE): Clinical experience and refinements. Ann Surg 230:392-400, 1999.

170. Orringer MB, Marshall B, Iannettoni MD: Eliminating the cervical esophagogastric anastomotic leak with a side-to-side stapled anastomosis. J Thorac Cardiovasc Surg 119:277-288, 2000.

170a. Orringer MB: Partial median sternotomy: Anterior approach to the upper thoracic esophagus. J Thorac Cardiovasc Surg 87:124-129, 1984.

171. Bousamra M II, Haasler GB, Parviz M: A decade of experience with transthoracic and transhiatal esophagectomy. Am J Surg 183:162-167, 2002.

172. Fok M, Law SY, Wong J: Operable esophageal carcinoma: current results from Hong Kong. World J Surg 18:355-360, 1994.

173. Savage C, McQuitty C, Wang D, et al: Post-thoracotomy pain management. Chest Surg Clin North Am 12:251-263, 2002.

174. Kirk RM: A trial of total gastrectomy, combined with total thoracic oesophagectomy without formal thoracotomy, for carcinoma at or near the cardia of the stomach. Br J Surg 68:577-579, 1981.

175. Akiyama H, Hiyama M, Hashimoto C: Resection and reconstruction for carcinoma of the thoracic oesophagus. Br J Surg 63:206-209, 1976.

176a. Hulscher JB, van Sandick JW, de Boer AG, et al: Extended transthoracic resection compared with limited transhiatal resection for adenocarcinoma of the esophagus. N Engl J Med 347:1662-1669, 2002.

176b. Altorki N, Skinner D: Should en bloc esophagectomy be the standard of care for esophageal carcinoma. Ann Surgery 234:581-587, 2001.

177. Nigro JJ, DeMeester SR, Hagen JA, et al: Node status in transmural esophageal adenocarcinoma and outcome after en bloc esophagectomy. J Thorac Cardiovasc Surg 117:960-968, 1999.

177a. Nakagawa S, Kanda T, Kosugi S, et al: Recurrence pattern of squamous cell carcinoma of the thoracic esophagus after extended radical esophagectomy with three-field lymphadenectomy. J Am Coll Surg 198:205-211, 2004.

178. Luketich JD, Schauer PR, Christie NA, et al: Minimally invasive esophagectomy. Ann Thorac Surg 70:906-911; discussion 911-912, 2000.

179. Dexter SP, Martin IG, McMahon MJ: Radical thoracoscopic esophagectomy for cancer. Surg Endosc 10:147-151, 1996.

180. Law S, Fok M, Chu KM, et al: Thoracoscopic esophagectomy for esophageal cancer. Surgery 122:8-14, 1997.

181. Robertson GS, Lloyd DM, Wicks AC, et al: No obvious advantages for thoracoscopic two-stage oesophagectomy. Br J Surg 83:675-678, 1996.

182. Nguyen NT, Schauer PR, Luketich JD: Combined laparoscopic and thoracoscopic approach to esophagectomy. J Am Coll Surg 188:328-332, 1999.

183. Ikeda Y, Tobari S, Niimi M, et al: Reliable cervical anastomosis through the retrosternal route with stepwise gastric tube. J Thorac Cardiovasc Surg 125:1306-1312, 2003.

184. Davis PA, Law S, Wong J: Colonic interposition after esophagectomy for cancer. Arch Surg 138:303-308, 2003.

185. Young MM, Deschamps C, Trastek VF, et al: Esophageal reconstruction for benign disease: Early morbidity, mortality, and functional results. Ann Thorac Surg 70:1651-1655, 2000.

186. Orringer MB: As originally published in 1992: Anterior mediastinal tracheostomy with and without cervical exenteration. Updated in 1998. Ann Thorac Surg 67:591, 1999.

187. Grillo HC, Mathisen DJ: Cervical exenteration. Ann Thorac Surg 49:401-409, 1990.

188. Chen HC, Kuo YR, Hwang TL, et al: Microvascular prefabricated free skin flaps for esophageal reconstruction in difficult patients. Ann Thorac Surg 67:911-916, 1999.

189. Spriano G, Pellini R, Roselli R: Pectoralis major myocutaneous flap for hypopharyngeal reconstruction. Plast Reconstr Surg 110:1408-1413; discussion 1414-1416, 2002.

190. Wadsworth JT, Futran N, Eubanks TR: Laparoscopic harvest of the jejunal free flap for reconstruction of hypopharyngeal and cervical esophageal defects. Arch Otolaryngol Head Neck Surg 128:1384-1387, 2002.

191. O'Rourke IC, Tiver K, Bull C, et al: Swallowing performance after radiation therapy for carcinoma of the esophagus. Cancer 61:2022-2026, 1988.

191a. Arnott SJ, Duncan W, Gignoux M, et al: Preoperative radiotherapy in esophageal carcinoma: A meta-analysis using individual patient data (oesophageal cancer collaborative group). Int J Radiat Oncol Biol Phys 41:579-583, 1998.

192. Xiao ZF, Yang ZY, Liang J, et al: Value of radiotherapy after radical surgery for esophageal carcinoma: A report of 495 patients. Ann Thorac Surg 75:331-336, 2003.

193. Walsh TN, Noonan N, Hollywood D, et al: A comparison of multimodal therapy and surgery for esophageal adenocarcinoma. N Engl J Med 335:462-467, 1996.

194. Schlag PM: Randomized trial of preoperative chemotherapy for squamous cell cancer of the esophagus. The Chirurgische Arbeitsgemeinschaft für Onkologie der Deutschen Gesellschaft für Chirurgie Study Group. Arch Surg 127:1446-1450, 1992.

195. Medical Research Council Oesophageal Cancer Working Party and Girling DJ: Surgical resection with or without preoperative chemotherapy in oesophageal cancer: A randomised controlled trial. Lancet 359:1727-1733, 2002.

196. Minsky BD, Pajak TF, Ginsberg RJ, et al: INT 0123 (Radiation Therapy Oncology Group 94-05) phase III trial of combined-modality therapy for esophageal cancer: High-dose versus standard-dose radiation therapy. J Clin Oncol 20:1167-1174, 2002.

197. Kelsen DP, Ginsberg R, Pajak TF, et al: Chemotherapy followed by surgery compared with surgery alone for localized esophageal cancer. N Engl J Med 339:1979-1984, 1998.

198. Entwistle JW III, Goldberg M: Multimodality therapy for resectable cancer of the thoracic esophagus. Ann Thorac Surg 73:1009-1015, 2002.

199. Macdonald JS, Smalley SR, Benedetti J, et al: Chemoradiotherapy after surgery compared with surgery alone for adenocarcinoma of the stomach or gastroesophageal junction. N Engl J Med 345:725-730, 2001.

199a. Geh JI, Bond SJ, Bentzen SM, Glynne-Jones R: Preoperative chemoradiotherapy in esophageal cancer: evidence of dose response. Proc ASCO 19:247a, 2000.

200. Geh JI, Bond SJ, Bentzen SM, et al: Preoperative chemoradiotherapy in esophageal cancer: Evidence of dose response. Proc ASCO 247a, 2000.

201. Bosset JF, Gignoux M, Triboulet JP, et al: Chemoradiotherapy followed by surgery compared with surgery alone in squamous cell cancer of the esophagus. N Engl J Med 337:161-167, 1997.

202. Burmeister BH, Smithers BM, Fitzgerald L, et al: Randomized phase III trial of preoperative chemoradiation followed by surgery (CR-S) versus surgery alone (S) for localized resectable cancer of the esophagus. Proc Am Soc Clin Oncol 19:305-313, 2001.

203. Urba SG, Orringer MB, Turrisi A, et al: Randomized trial of preoperative chemoradiation versus surgery alone in patients with locoregional esophageal carcinoma. J Clin Oncol 19:305-313, 2001.

204. Law S, Fok M, Chow S, et al: Preoperative chemotherapy versus surgical therapy alone for squamous cell carcinoma of the esophagus: a prospective randomized trial. J Thorac Cardiovasc Surg 114:210-217, 1997.

205. Oberg S, DeMeester TR, Peters JH, et al: The extent of Barrett's esophagus depends on the status of the lower esophageal sphincter and the degree of esophageal acid exposure. J Thorac Cardiovasc Surg 117:572-580, 1999.

206. Poneros JM, Brand S, Bouma BE, et al: Diagnosis of specialized intestinal metaplasia by optical coherence tomography. Gastroenterology 120:7-12, 2001.

206a. Corey KE, Schmitz SM, Shaheen NJ: Does a surgical antireflux procedure decrease the incidence of esophageal adenocarcinoma in Barrett's esophagus? A metaanalysis. Am J Gastroenterol 98(11):2390-2394, 2003.

207. Csendes A, Braghetto I, Burdiles P, et al: Comparison of forceful dilatation and esophagomyotomy in patients with achalasia of the esophagus. Hepatogastroenterology 38:502-505, 1991.

208. Bonavina L, Ceriani C, Carazzone A, et al: Endoscopic laser ablation of nondysplastic Barrett's epithelium: Is it worthwhile? J Gastrointest Surg 3:194-199, 1999.

209. Van Laethem JL, Peny MO, Salmon I, et al: Intramucosal adenocarcinoma arising under squamous re-epithelialisation of Barrett's oesophagus. Gut 46:574-577, 2000.

CHAPTER 40

HIATAL HERNIA AND GASTROESOPHAGEAL REFLUX DISEASE

Brant K. Oelschlager, M.D., **Thomas R. Eubanks**, D.O.

and **Carlos A. Pellegrini**, M.D.

Gastroesophageal Reflux Disease
Paraesophageal Hernias

Summary

The role of operative treatment for hiatal hernias changed dramatically during the 1990s. Once a relatively uncommon event, antireflux operations are now performed in large numbers at many institutions around the world. The driving force behind increased surgical referral for treatment was the popularity of minimally invasive surgery. Although the techniques of antireflux operations have not changed, the approach to the surgery has become more palatable to the patient and the referring physician. More and more surgeons are called on to treat gastroesophageal reflux disease (GERD) and paraesophageal hernias. Thus, the surgeon must be familiar with all aspects of evaluating and treating both entities, because he or she is ultimately responsible for the successful outcome of the patient.

GASTROESOPHAGEAL REFLUX DISEASE

Pathophysiology

The lower esophageal sphincter (LES) has the primary role of preventing reflux of the gastric contents into the esophagus. The sphincter is a unique physiologic entity, as opposed to an anatomic structure, that is located just cephalad to the gastroesophageal junction and is clearly identifiable as a zone of high pressure during manometric evaluation as the sensing device passes from the stomach into the esophagus. Several factors contribute to the high-pressure zone. The first is the intrinsic musculature of the distal esophagus. These muscle fibers differ from those in other areas of the esophagus in that they are in a state of tonic contraction. They normally relax with initiation of a swallow and then return to a state of tonic contraction. The second contributing factor to LES pressure is the sling fibers of the cardia. These fibers are at the same anatomic depth of the circular muscle fibers of the esophagus but are oriented in a different direction. They run diagonally from the cardia-fundus junction to the lesser curve (Fig. 40-1). These fibers are responsible for a significant percentage of the lower esophageal high-pressure zone.[1] The third contributing factor to the maintenance of the high-pressure zone in the distal esophagus is the diaphragm.[2] As the esophagus passes from the chest to the abdomen, it is surrounded by the crura of the diaphragm. During inspiration, the anteroposterior diameter of the crural opening is decreased, compressing the esophagus and increasing the measured pressure at the LES. This concept is particularly important for the interpretation of esophageal manometry tracings. By convention, the LES pressure should be assessed at mid or end expiration, thereby providing reliable, reproducible pressure measurements. The last component of the pressure generated at the lower esophageal high-pressure zone is the transmitted pressure of the abdominal cavity. The abdominal compartment has a relatively higher pressure than does the thoracic cavity. A gastroesophageal junction that is firmly anchored in the abdominal cavity will be exposed to a greater transmural pressure than one that is in the posterior mediastinum.

Gastroesophageal reflux may occur when the high-pressure zone in the distal esophagus is too low to prevent gastric contents from entering the esophagus or when a

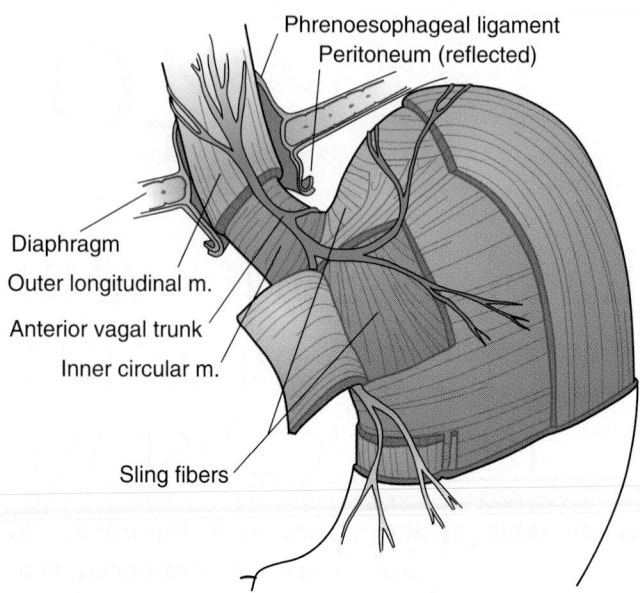

FIGURE 40-1. Schematic drawing of the muscle layers of the esophagogastric region. The intrinsic muscle of the esophagus, the diaphragm, and the sling fibers contribute to the lower esophageal sphincter pressure. The circular muscle fibers of the esophagus are at the same depth as the sling fibers of the cardia.

sphincter with normal pressure undergoes spontaneous relaxation, not associated with a peristaltic wave in the body of the esophagus.[3,4] Although both conditions may lead to abnormal amounts of reflux, some degree of reflux is present in most individuals. Thus, the distinction between GERD and gastroesophageal reflux must be made by considering all aspects of the patient's presentation and evaluation.

GERD is often associated with a hiatal hernia. Although any type of hiatal hernia may give rise to the classic symptoms of reflux, the most common is the type I hernia (Fig. 40-2A), also called a *sliding hiatal hernia*. A type I hernia is present when the gastroesophageal junction is not maintained in the abdominal cavity by the phreno-esophageal ligament (membrane). Thus, the cardia is allowed to migrate back and forth between the posterior mediastinum and the peritoneal cavity. The phreno-esophageal ligament is a continuation of the endoabdominal fascia, which reflects onto the esophagus at the hiatus. It lies just superficial to the peritoneal reflection at the hiatus and continues into the mediastinum (Fig. 40-3).[5] Although the presence of a small sliding hernia does not necessarily imply an incompetent cardia, the larger its size, the greater the risk of abnormal gastroesophageal reflux.[6] A type II hernia (see Fig. 40-2B), also called a *rolling* or *paraesophageal hernia*, occurs when the gastroesophageal junction is anchored in the abdomen but the hiatal defect, which is usually large, provides space for viscera to migrate into the mediastinum. The relatively negative pressure in the thorax facilitates visceral migration. Most commonly, the fundus of the stomach migrates into the mediastinum; however, the colon and spleen are also occasionally identified. This is discussed in

more detail in the second part of this chapter in the discussion of paraesophageal hernias. A type III hernia (see Fig. 40-2C) is a combination of the first two, in which the gastroesophageal junction and the fundus (or other viscera) are free to move into the mediastinum.

A hiatal hernia is neither necessary nor sufficient to make the diagnosis of GERD, and the presence of such a hernia does not constitute an indication for operative correction. The theoretical implications of a type I and type III hiatal hernia being present is that the cardia and distal esophagus have the potential to be exposed to the negative pressure of the thoracic cavity. This would have the effect of lowering the pressure at the LES, thereby allowing reflux to occur more readily. Many patients with hiatal hernias do not have symptoms and do not require treatment.

Symptoms

The most common presentation of patients with GERD includes a long-standing history of heartburn and a shorter history of regurgitation. Heartburn, when typical, is a very reliable symptom. Heartburn should be confined to the epigastric and retrosternal areas. It should be identified as a caustic or stinging sensation. It does not radiate to the back and is not characteristically described as a pressure sensation. It is best to ask the patient to describe in detail the sensation he or she is experiencing. Sometimes the symptoms will be more characteristic of peptic ulcer disease, cholelithiasis, or coronary artery disease.

The presence of regurgitation indicates progression of the disease. Some patients will be unable to bend over without experiencing the unpleasant event. A distinction between regurgitation of undigested and digested food should be made. Undigested food in the regurgitant is indicative of a different pathologic process, such as an esophageal diverticulum or achalasia.

In addition to heartburn and regurgitation, dysphagia is an important symptom to elicit. Most commonly, dysphagia represents a mechanical obstruction and is more pronounced with solid food ingestion than with liquids. If dysphagia for both liquids and solids occurs at the same time and is present with the same intensity, a neuromuscular disorder should be suspected. When a patient is found to have dysphagia, peptic stricture of the distal esophagus is most likely to be the cause. However, tumor, diverticula, and motor disorders should be excluded because this determination will affect the operative approach.

Other symptoms may be present in patients with gastroesophageal reflux. Most of them arise from the gastrointestinal tract; however, many patients will have symptoms involving the respiratory tract as well. These are called *extraesophageal* (or *supraesophageal*) *symptoms*. The frequency of symptoms in more than 1000 patients evaluated at the gastrointestinal function laboratory of the University of Washington is shown in Table 40-1. Although many patients with gastrointestinal symptoms will complain of extraesophageal symptoms as well, it is less common for a patient to present with only respiratory symptoms. This is discussed in detail at the end of this section.

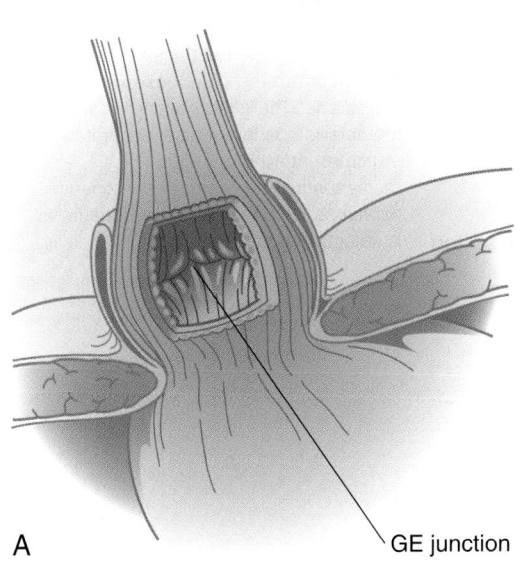

A — GE junction

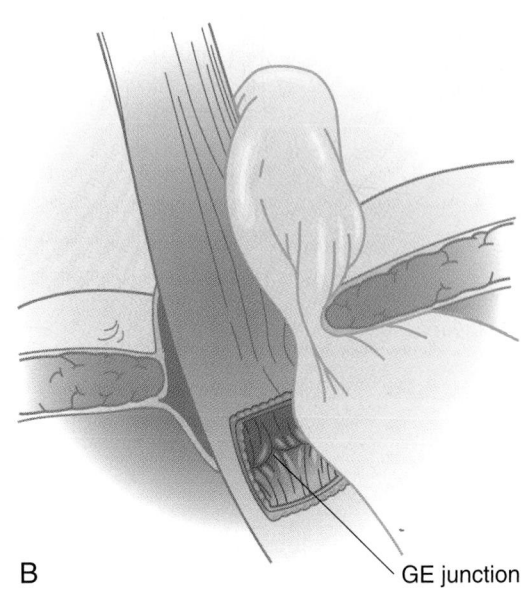

B — GE junction

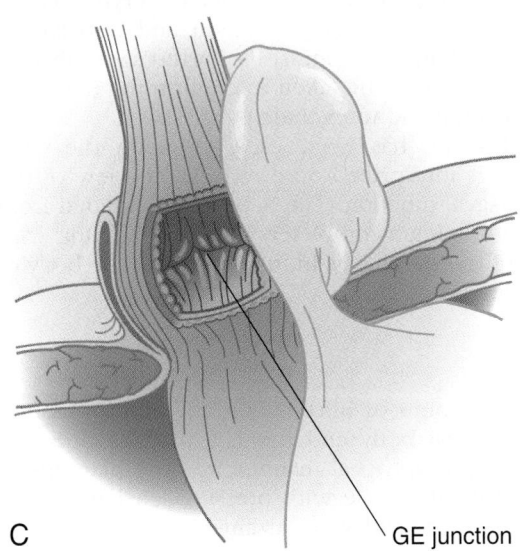

C — GE junction

FIGURE 40-2. The three types of hiatal hernia. **A,** Type I is also called a sliding hernia. **B,** Type II is known as a rolling hernia. **C,** Type III is referred to as a mixed hernia. GE, gastroesophageal.

Physical Examination

The physical examination of patients with GERD rarely contributes to confirmation of the diagnosis. In patients with advanced disease, several observations may help identify the source of the patient's discomfort. A patient who constantly drinks water during the interview is facilitating esophageal clearance, which may be indicative of continual reflux or distal obstruction. Other patients with advanced disease will sit leaning forward and carry out the interview with their lungs inflated to near vital capacity. This is an attempt to keep the diaphragm flattened, the anteroposterior diameter of hiatus narrowed, and, thus, the LES pressure elevated. Patients who have severe proximal reflux with regurgitation of gastric contents into their mouth may have erosion of their dentition (revealing yellow teeth due to the loss of dentin), injected oropharyngeal mucosa, or signs of chronic sinusitis.

The physical examination may be helpful in determining the presence of other pathologic entities. The presence of abnormal supraclavicular lymph nodes in a patient with heartburn and dysphagia may suggest esophageal or gastric cancer. If the patient's retrosternal pain is reproducible with palpation, then a somatic cause is likely.

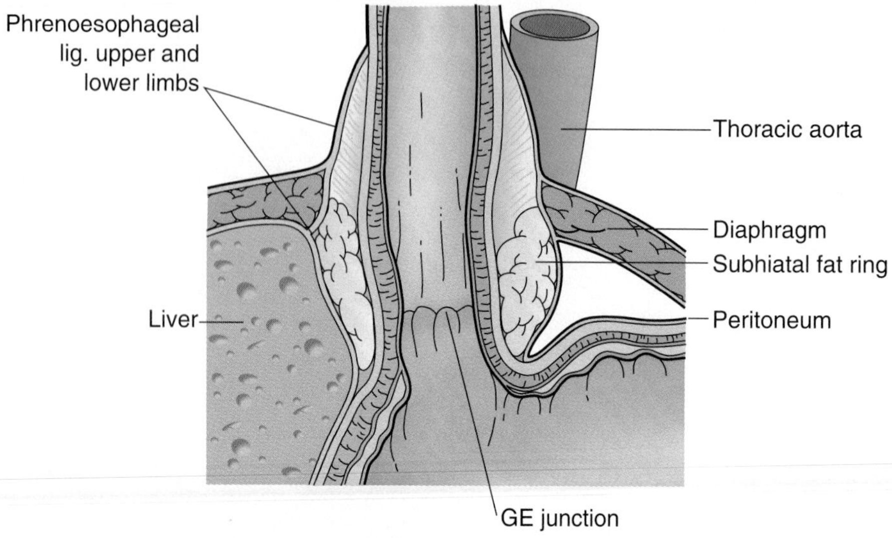

Phrenoesophageal lig. upper and lower limbs

Thoracic aorta

Diaphragm

Subhiatal fat ring

Liver

Peritoneum

GE junction

FIGURE 40-3. Section of the gastroesophageal (GE) junction demonstrates the relationship of the peritoneum to the phrenoesophageal membrane. The phrenoesophageal membrane continues as a separate structure into the posterior mediastinum. The parietal peritoneum continues as the visceral peritoneum as it reflects onto the stomach.

TABLE 40-1.   Prevalence of Symptoms in 1000 Patients Evaluated for Gastroesophageal Reflux Disease*

Symptom	Predominance (%)
Heartburn	80
Regurgitation	54
Abdominal pain	29
Cough	27
Dysphagia for solids	23
Hoarseness	21
Belching	15
Bloating	15
Aspiration	14
Wheezing	7
Globus	4

*Symptoms reported occurred more frequently than once a week.

Short of these extreme presentations, the physical examination is generally not helpful in confirming or excluding gastroesophageal reflux as a pathologic entity.

Preoperative Evaluation

The preoperative work-up in a patient being considered for operative treatment will help confirm the diagnosis, exclude other pathologic entities, and direct the operative intervention.

Endoscopy

Endoscopy is an essential step in the evaluation of patients with GERD who are being considered for operative intervention. The value of the study is in its ability to exclude other diseases, especially a tumor, and to document the

presence of peptic esophageal injury. The degree of injury can be measured using a scoring system such as the Savary-Miller interpretation (1 indicates erythema; 2, linear ulceration; 3, confluent ulceration; and 4, stricture). The extreme of mucosal injury is Barrett's esophagus. Biopsy samples should be taken to confirm the metaplastic transformation and to exclude dysplasia.

The endoscope has been used to grade the "flap valve."[7] This is interpreted on a retroflexed view of the gastroesophageal junction. The flap valve is graded from 1 to 4, with 4 being a completely patulous junction with the lumen of the esophagus in full view from the body of the stomach.

Manometry

A significant amount of information about the function of the esophageal body and the LES may be obtained from stationary esophageal manometry. The manometry catheter is a flexible tube with pressure-sensing devices (water perfused or solid state) arranged at 5-cm intervals (Fig. 40-4). The upper esophageal sphincter is notoriously difficult to analyze because it migrates during the cervical phase of swallowing. Fortunately, the characteristics of the upper esophageal sphincter are infrequently relevant to clinical practice. The pertinent information to be gained from the manometry tracings concerns the function of the LES and the esophageal body.

The LES is analyzed for mean resting pressure. This may be determined in two ways: a station pull-through and a rapid pull-through. The majority of laboratories report the values recorded from the station pull-through. With this method, the pressures are measured while the catheter is stagnant with the radial ports at the high-pressure zone of the LES. Rapid pull-through measurements are obtained while the catheter is being pulled across the high-pressure zone at a rate of 1 cm/second. The latter measurements are usually higher than the station pull-through measurements, owing to the artifact of catheter movement. Normal pressures for a station pull-through at the LES range between 12 and 30 mm Hg. The sphincter should

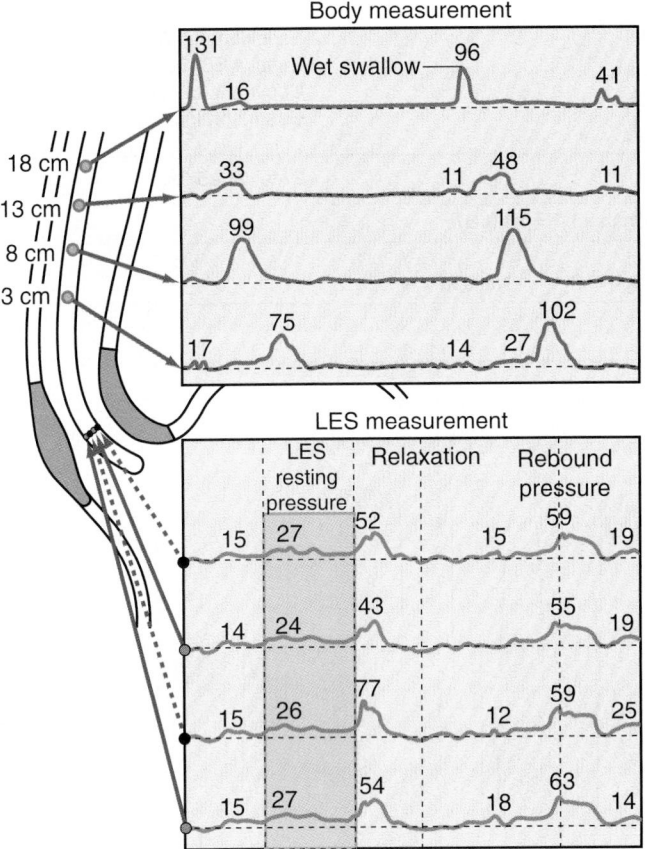

Body measurement

Wet swallow

LES measurement

	LES resting pressure	Relaxation		Rebound pressure	

FIGURE 40-4. Representative tracings from the body of the esophagus and the lower esophageal sphincter (LES) show the relative positions of the pressure-sensing channels during the study. Peristalsis is seen after a wet swallow in the body, whereas the LES is seen to relax to gastric baseline levels during the same interval.

relax to the pressure of the gastric baseline for several seconds when a swallow is initiated. Other information to be gained from the LES is the total length, the intra-abdominal length, and the location of the sphincter relative to the nares. The longer the length of the high-pressure zone and the longer the intra-abdominal component, the greater the barrier to reflux of gastric contents.[8]

The esophageal body is assessed to determine the effectiveness of peristalsis. With the four channels located at 3, 8, 13, and 18 cm above the LES, the patient is given a series (at least 10) of 5-mL aliquots of water to swallow. The peristaltic activity is reported as the percentage of initiated swallows that are transmitted to each channel successfully. Normally, a patient should have greater than 80% peristalsis. The second characteristic of clinical importance is the amplitude of the peristaltic wave. The amplitude is simply the average of the pressures generated in the distal esophagus during effectively transmitted peristaltic waves. Ineffective esophageal motility (IEM) is defined as less than 60% peristalsis or distal esophageal amplitudes of less than 30 mm Hg and is often associated with significant GERD. It was traditionally thought that a 360-degree fundoplication is likely to cause an insurmountable obstruction to swallowing and to result in dys-

phagia, but this idea has been challenged recently. This is discussed further in the section on surgical therapy.

pH Monitoring

The gold standard for diagnosing and quantifying acid reflux is the 24-hour pH test.[9] The study is performed by placing a thin catheter containing one or more solid-state electrodes in the esophagus. The electrodes are spaced 5 to 10 cm apart and are capable of sensing fluctuations in the pH between 2 and 7. The electrodes are connected to a data recorder that the patient wears for the period of observation. There is a digital clock displayed on the recorder. When the patient has an event (e.g., heartburn, chest pain, eructation), he or she is to record the event in a diary, noting the time on the recorder (Fig. 40-5).

A large amount of information may be gleaned from the study: total number of reflux episodes (pH <4), longest episode of reflux, number of episodes lasting longer than 5 minutes, extent of reflux in the upright position, and extent of reflux in the supine position. An overall score is obtained with the use of a formula that assigns a weight to each item according to its capacity to cause esophageal injury. This value, known as the *DeMeester score*, should be less than 14.7. A simpler way to determine whether abnormal reflux is occurring is to estimate the total percent of time the pH is below 4 in the proximal and distal channel.[10] The total percent time is calculated by dividing the time the pH was less than 4 by the total time of the study and multiplying by 100. In the proximal esophagus (15 cm above the LES), acid exposure normally occurs less than 1% of the time; in the distal esophagus (5 cm above the LES), it normally occurs less than 4%.

The patient's symptom diary should be correlated with episodes of reflux. The correlation of heartburn or chest pain with a drop in the pH has significant clinical value because it helps to confirm a cause-and-effect relationship. When interpreting these studies, one should keep in mind that patients often do not proceed with their normal activities and eating patterns when they have the catheter in place. Thus, their symptoms may not be as prevalent during the study period. If there is symptom correlation with low pH measurements, the suspicion of reflux-induced disease may be confirmed, even if the total acid exposure is normal.

Esophagogram

The esophagogram provides valuable information in the evaluation of patients with symptoms of GERD when an operation is contemplated or when the symptoms do not respond as expected. Often, spontaneous reflux during the examination will be demonstrated. Although reflux may be induced in patients who do not have the disease, the occurrence of spontaneous reflux lends support to the diagnosis of abnormal gastroesophageal reflux. The true value of the study is to determine the external anatomy of the esophagus and the proximal stomach. The presence and size of a hiatal hernia may be characterized (Fig. 40-6). Although this neither confirms nor refutes the presence of disease, it is extremely beneficial in planning the

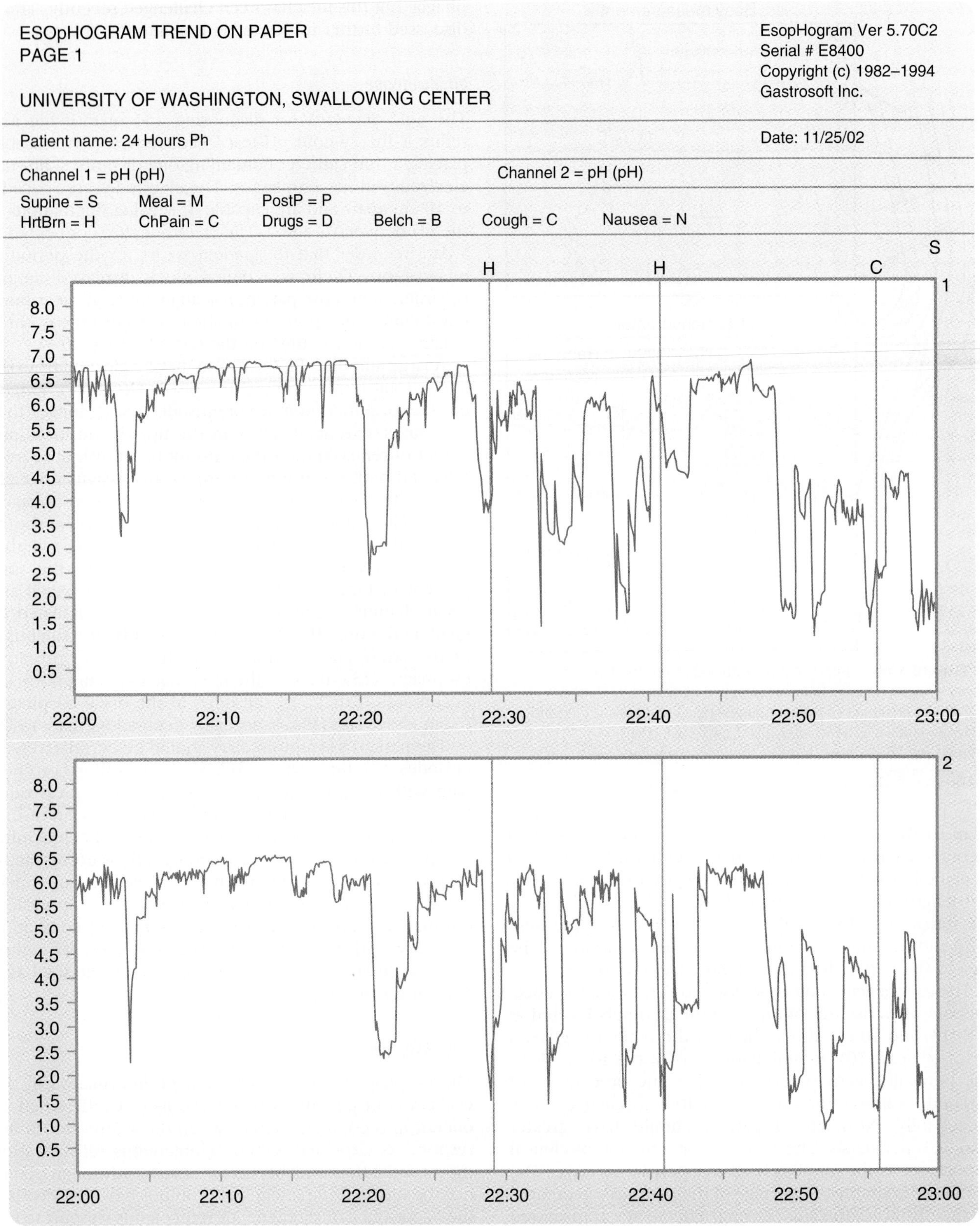
ESOpHOGRAM TREND ON PAPER
PAGE 1
UNIVERSITY OF WASHINGTON, SWALLOWING CENTER
EsopHogram Ver 5.70C2
Serial # E8400
Copyright (c) 1982–1994
Gastrosoft Inc.
Patient name: 24 Hours Ph
Date: 11/25/02
Channel 1 = pH (pH)
Channel 2 = pH (pH)
Supine = S
Meal = M
PostP = P
HrtBrn = H
ChPain = C
Drugs = D
Belch = B
Cough = C
Nausea = N
H
H
C
S
1
8.0
7.5
7.0
6.5
6.0
5.5
5.0
4.5
4.0
3.5
3.0
2.5
2.0
1.5
1.0
0.5
22:00
22:10
22:20
22:30
22:40
22:50
23:00
2
8.0
7.5
7.0
6.5
6.0
5.5
5.0
4.5
4.0
3.5
3.0
2.5
2.0
1.5
1.0
0.5
22:00
22:10
22:20
22:30
22:40
22:50
23:00

FIGURE 40-5. Compressed tracing of a 24-hour pH study. Time is marked on the x-axis, and pH is marked on the y-axis. Symptom events are marked along the top of the tracing (H, heartburn; B, belching; S, supine position; and so on, as noted along the top). (Courtesy of the University of Washington Swallowing Center.)

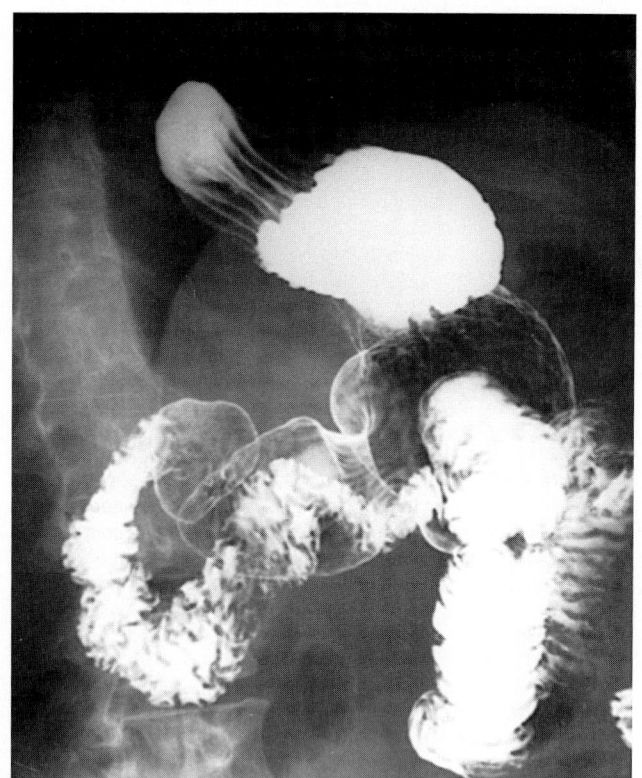

FIGURE 40-6. Upper gastrointestinal contrast material study shows a large hiatal hernia with the rugal folds of the stomach clearly transgressing the shadow of the left hemidiaphragm.

operation. A mediastinal gastroesophageal junction that does not reduce into the peritoneal cavity during the study is a predictor of a more difficult operation that may require an esophageal lengthening procedure. Peptic esophageal strictures may also be found on an esophageal contrast study. The presence of a stricture will taint the interpretation of the 24-hour pH study, especially if it is tight enough to prevent reflux. Other anatomic abnormalities, such as diverticula, tumors, and unexpected paraesophageal hernias, will be discovered during an esophagogram.

Other Tests

In unique circumstances, other diagnostic tests may be valuable. Occasionally, a patient will not be able to tolerate nasoesophageal intubation. A scintigraphic study to evaluate esophageal clearance and reflux may provide evidence of motility disorder and gastroesophageal reflux.[11] Gastric distention resulting from delayed emptying may also be diagnosed with a scintigraphic study. Although this condition may contribute to reflux, it is not clear whether a gastric emptying procedure (pyloroplasty) should be added to an antireflux procedure in a patient with delayed gastric emptying.

Some patients will have laryngeal symptoms of gastroesophageal reflux. Laryngoscopy and stroboscopic examinations will help provide objective evidence of extraesophageal reflux; findings include inflammation of laryngeal mucosa, muscle tension abnormalities, and, in severe cases, subglottic stenosis.

Treatment

Most people will experience symptoms of reflux during their life. A smaller percent will proceed with self-treatment. Those with persistent symptoms will seek help from a physician, and a fraction of them will eventually be referred to a surgeon for evaluation. The surgeon sees a preselected group of patients with this disease, but it is imperative to ensure that each individual has had an appropriate trial of less aggressive therapy. Lifestyle modifications are certainly helpful in avoiding gastroesophageal reflux. Cessation of smoking, decreased caffeine intake, and avoidance of large meals before lying down will help decrease transient episodes of LES relaxation. Elevation of the head of the bed and avoidance of constricting clothing will help prevent unfavorable pressure gradients across the gastroesophageal junction.

Medical Management

When a patient is first seen, a lengthy work-up is not necessary if the history and examination are consistent with GERD. It would be prudent to check for chronic anemia in such a patient and to prescribe a 6-week course of acid suppression therapy. Most authors agree that a double dose of a proton pump inhibitor should be the initial approach to medical management. Given in this manner, the use of medical therapy becomes in itself a diagnostic tool.[12] If the symptoms persist after a trial of medical therapy, a more extensive evaluation, as described earlier, would be indicated.[13] The medications available to treat acid reflux include antacids, motility agents, H_2 blockers, and proton pump inhibitors. Although lifestyle modification has been advocated before or as an adjunct to medical therapy, the efficacy of such changes in the treatment of esophagitis has not been proved.[14]

Pharmacologic treatment of GERD has been revolutionized by the advent of proton pump inhibitors. These drugs act by irreversibly binding the proton pump in the parietal cells of the stomach, thus effectively stopping gastric acid production. The maximal effect occurs after approximately 4 days of therapy, and the effects will linger for the life of the parietal cell. Thus, the acid suppression will persist for 4 to 5 days after therapy has ended. For this reason, the patient should be off therapy for 1 week before being evaluated with pH monitoring.

Compared with H_2 blockers, proton pump inhibitors are more effective at healing esophageal ulceration secondary to acid exposure.[15] The medications are relatively expensive but are well tolerated. The side effects may include headache, abdominal pain, and diarrhea. Long-term therapy appears to be safe even though it has been linked to gastric polyp formation.[16] The polyps are usually hyperplastic and do not appear to be premalignant.

Surgical Therapy

The indications for surgical therapy have changed somewhat with the advent of proton pump inhibitors. Certainly, patients with evidence of severe esophageal injury (ulcer, stricture, or Barrett mucosa) and incomplete resolution of symptoms or relapses while on medical therapy are appropriate to consider for operative intervention. Other patients with a long duration of symptoms or those in whom symptoms persist at a young age should be considered for operative treatment initially. In these patients, operative therapy should be considered an alternative to medical therapy rather than a treatment of last resort.

There are some patients who have absolutely no response of their symptoms to the use of proton pump inhibitors. They should be scrutinized further before offering surgical treatment, as opposed to being considered medical failures who need operative treatment. Because the proton pump inhibitors are so effective at decreasing the acid production of the stomach, the diagnosis of GERD in such patients should be questioned and must be demonstrated with objective testing.

Since the application of minimally invasive techniques to the treatment of GERD, the cost of the operative treatment has decreased. This has changed the way in which surgical treatment is viewed. Considering the cost of proton pump inhibitor use and the cost of operative treatment with its accepted success rate, the length of time required for medical therapy to become more expensive than the operation is about 10 years.[17,18] This assumes the patient uses the lowest dose of the medication. Therefore, in patients who have more than 10 years of life expectancy and are in need of lifelong therapy due to a mechanically defective sphincter, surgical therapy may be considered as the treatment of choice.

360-DEGREE WRAP (LEFT CRUS APPROACH)

The technique described here is the left crus approach to a 360-degree wrap (*Nissen fundoplication*), which should be the procedure of choice for the majority of patients. The left crus approach provides the advantage of a direct and early view of the short gastric vessels and the spleen. Once this obstacle is negotiated, there is little chance of injuring the spleen during the remainder of the procedure.

The patient is placed in a low lithotomy position. The surgeon stands between the patient's legs, with the assistant on the left side of the patient. The five trocars are placed so that two equilateral triangles sharing a common medial angle are created (Fig. 40-7). The surgeon operates through the two most cephalad ports. The assistant operates through the two closest caudad ports. The right-sided, caudad port is used for the liver retractor.

With the assistant first retracting the greater curve and then the omentum, the left crus and the greater curve are dissected by the surgeon. The short gastric vessels are taken early to mobilize the fundus (Fig. 40-8). With the fundus mobilized, the phrenoesophageal membrane over the left crus may be dissected until the crural fibers are identified. The entire length of the left crus is mobilized at this time (Fig. 40-9).

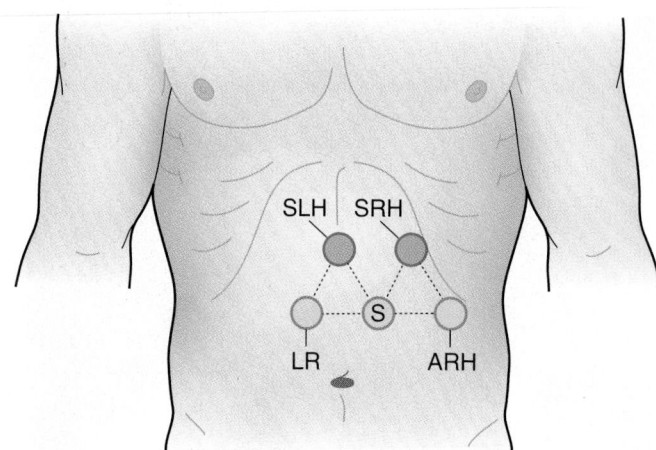

FIGURE 40-7.   Port placement for a laparoscopic approach to hiatus. The apices of the two triangles denote the surgeon's right (SRH) and left (SLH) hand working ports. The base port sites of the two triangles are for the liver retractor (LR), the videoendoscope (S), and the assistant's right hand (ARH).

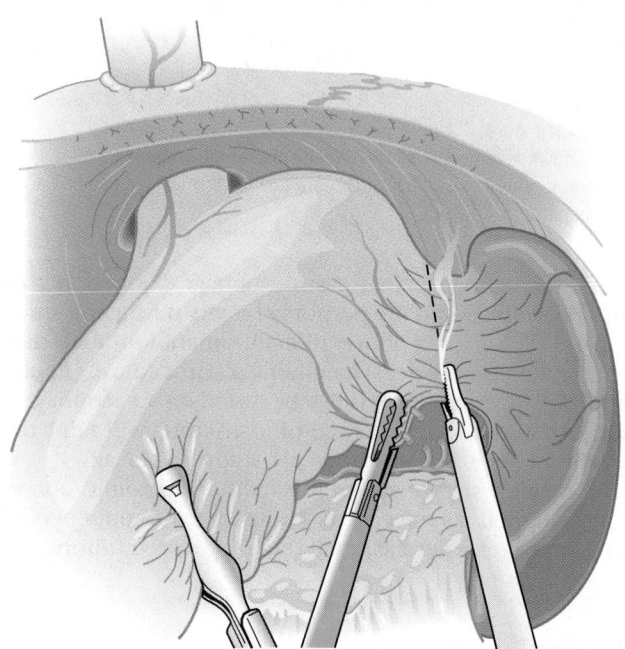

FIGURE 40-8.   Left crus approach shows early mobilization of the fundus of the stomach. The spleen is in plain view during dissection, which helps to prevent injury.

Right crural dissection is then performed by opening the lesser omentum and mobilizing this to the phrenoesophageal membrane on the right. Anterior and posterior dissection of the right crus will reveal the previously dissected left crus. Care should be taken to preserve the anterior and posterior vagi during this mobilization (Fig. 40-10). Both will be contained by the wrap. A Penrose drain is placed around the esophagus to facilitate more proximal dissection and to assist with creation of the wrap.

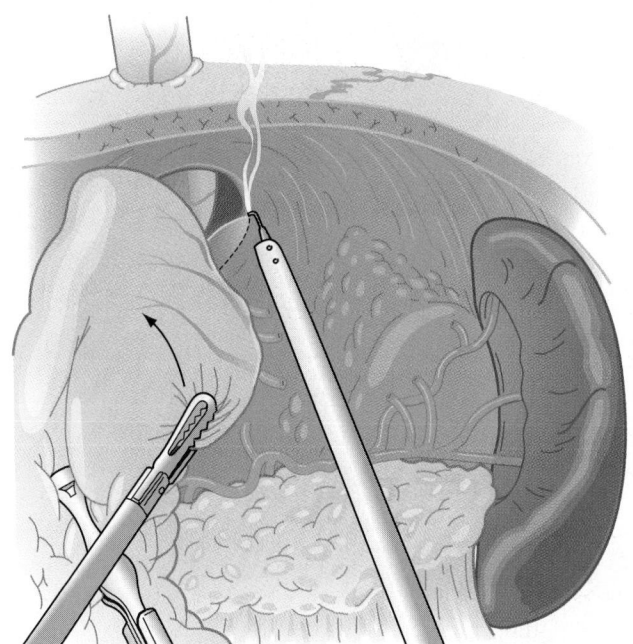

FIGURE 40-9. After the fundus has been mobilized, the peritoneal reflection at the hiatus and the phrenoesophageal membrane are incised anterior to the left crus to avoid injury to the esophagus and posterior vagus.

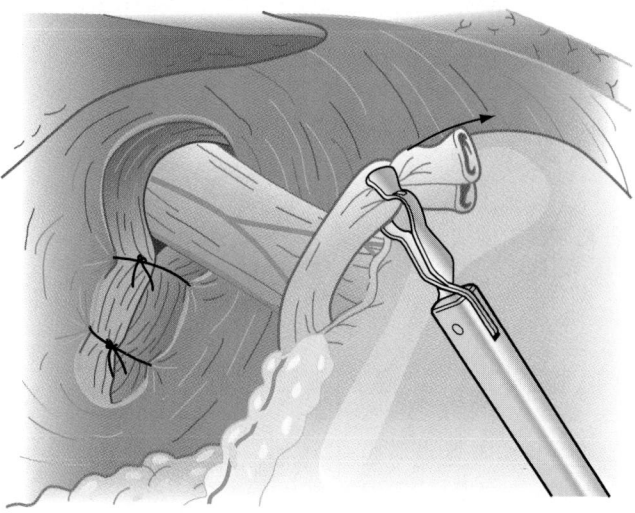

FIGURE 40-11. Posterior crural closure is performed with heavy permanent suture. Note how the peritoneum and, thus, the phrenoesophageal membrane are incorporated into the closure. The exposure is facilitated by displacement of the esophagus to the left and anterior.

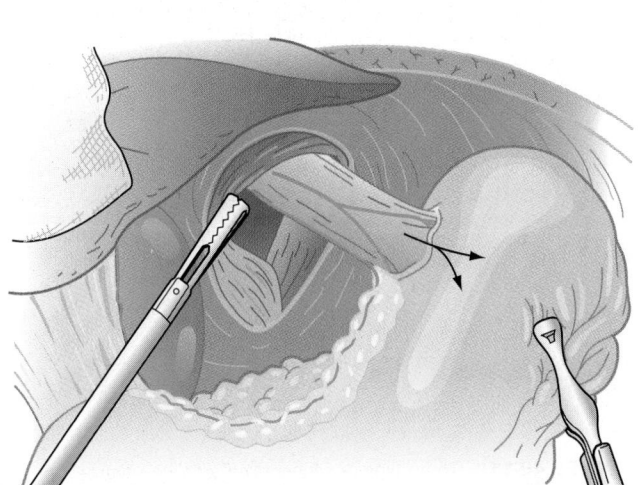

FIGURE 40-10. A similar dissection of the right crus will complete the posterior and lateral exposure of the hiatus. As long as the dissection is performed along the crura, the likelihood of injury to adjacent structures is minimal.

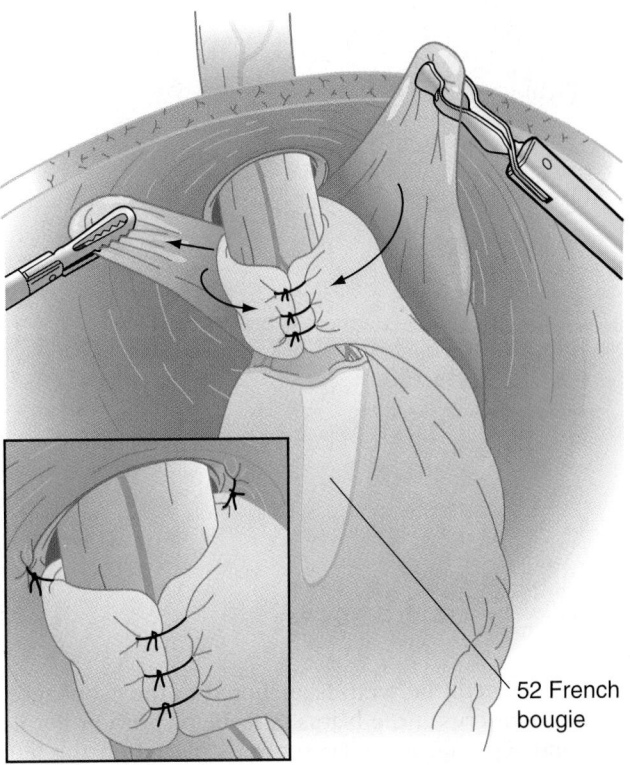

52 French bougie

FIGURE 40-12. The wrap is fashioned with fundus over a length of 2.5 to 3 cm. The bougie is placed after the first suture of wrap is secured to ensure a "floppy" fundoplication. The wrap is secured to the diaphragm with right and left coronal sutures (inset).

Once the esophagus is mobilized, the crura are reapproximated posteriorly with heavy permanent sutures to allow the easy passage of a 52-French bougie (Fig. 40-11). The posterior aspect of the fundus is then passed behind the esophagus from left to right. The wrap is created over a length of 2.5 to 3 cm with three or four interrupted permanent sutures. This repair should also allow the easy passage of a 52-French bougie (Fig. 40-12). With the

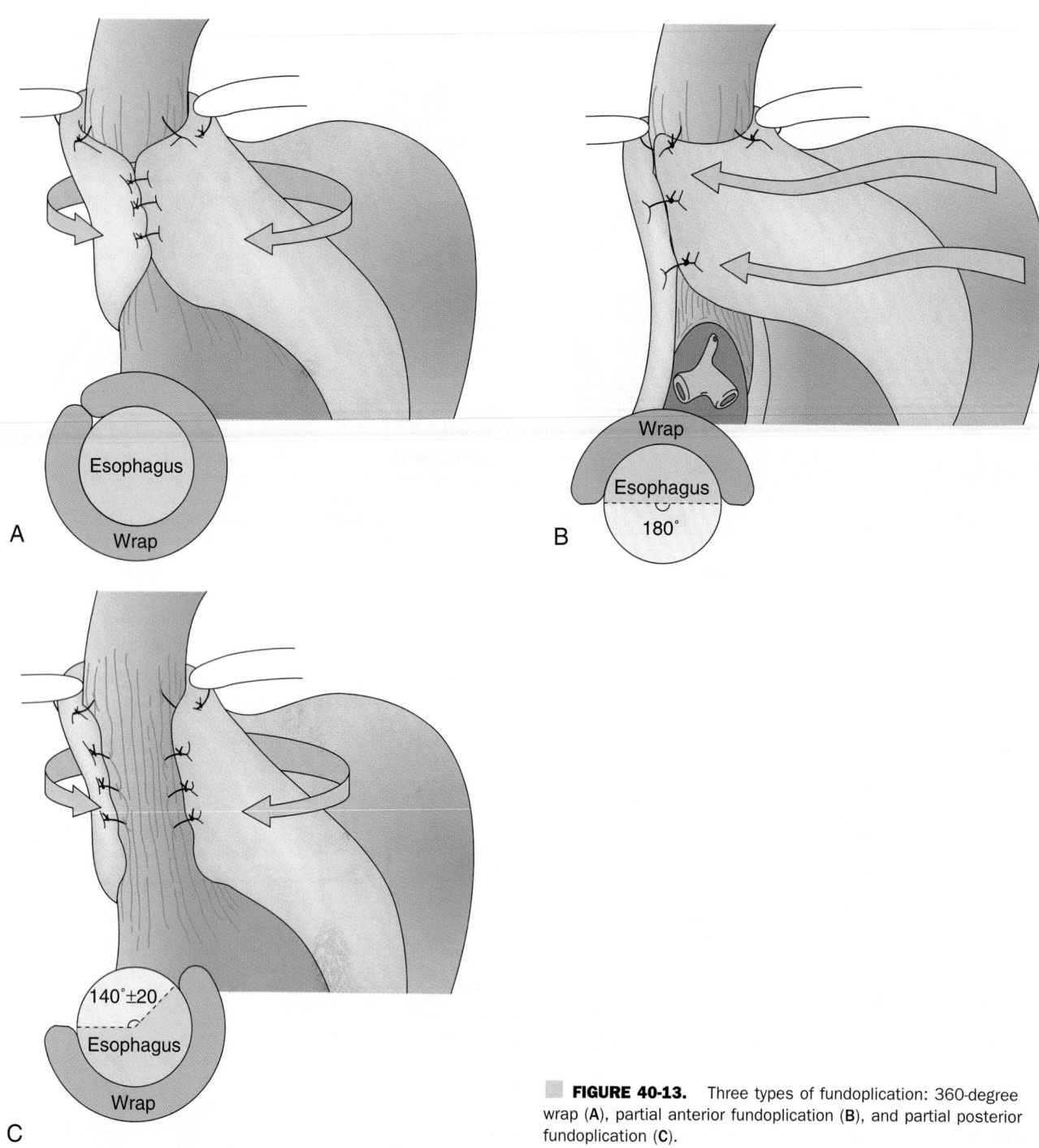

FIGURE 40-13. Three types of fundoplication: 360-degree wrap (**A**), partial anterior fundoplication (**B**), and partial posterior fundoplication (**C**).

bougie removed, the wrap is anchored to the esophagus and the right crus at the hiatus. This helps prevent herniation and slipping. A similar suture is placed on the left (see Fig. 40-12, *inset*). The wrap is anchored anteriorly and posteriorly to the crura with two additional sutures.

The wrap is inspected. The suture line should lie just to the right of the middle of the esophagus. The posterior aspect of the wrap should not have redundant stomach, which would imply the wrap was made too far inferior, possibly with the body instead of the fundus. There should be a gentle sweeping of the wrap toward the greater curvature (Fig. 40-13*A*). If it is angulated abruptly,

there may be too much tension on the fundus. When all of these steps are completed, the wrap is completed. All trocar sites of more than 5 mm should have fascial closure.

PARTIAL FUNDOPLICATION

When esophageal motility is poor, then a partial fundoplication may be considered to prevent obstruction to bolus propagation in the esophagus. While this was thought mandatory in all patients with IEM (peristalsis <60% or distal esophageal amplitudes <30 mm Hg), this practice has been questioned in recent years. Our experience is that a total fundoplication can be performed in most patients with IEM (except perhaps those patients with absent peristalsis), without an increase in development of dysphagia.[19] In fact, effective control of reflux with a total fundoplication usually improves premorbid dysphagia and often improves the esophageal motility. When needed, there are many types of partial fundoplications. Regardless of the type used, the initial dissection of the esophagus is the same.

If an anterior wrap (Thal, Dor) is to be performed, there is no need to disrupt the posterior attachments of the esophagus (see Fig. 40-13B). The Dor and Thal fundoplications are created with the fundus folded over the anterior aspect of the esophagus. They are anchored to the hiatus and esophagus as in the 360-degree wrap. The experience with these repairs is limited in patients being treated for gastroesophageal reflux. They are more commonly used in patients with achalasia after an anterior myotomy has been performed.

If a posterior wrap (Toupet) is to be performed, the entire esophageal dissection is the same as for a 360-degree wrap, and the crura are reapproximated as well. The reconstruction of the posterior fundoplication is initiated by passing the posterior fundus behind the esophagus from left to right. The fundoplication is created by anchoring the posterior fundus to the crura and the esophagus. The most cephalad sutures of the wrap incorporate all three structures (fundus, crus, esophagus). The wrap is anchored posteriorly to the crura with two or three sutures. The fundus is then sutured to the esophagus along the anterolateral aspects, creating a 220- to 250-degree wrap (see Fig. 40-13C).

Endoscopic Therapy

Recently several endoscopic techniques have been developed for the treatment of GERD. These procedures have sparked significant interest, because they each promise a mechanical treatment for reflux with less invasion than a fundoplication. These techniques attempt to augment the LES by suturing (EndoCinch, Bard), radiofrequency energy (Stretta, Curon Medical), Plexiglas injection (polymethylmethacrylate), or biocompatiable polymer injection (Enteryx, Boston Scientific).

The first technique developed is an endoscopic suturing device that attempts to re-create a fundoplication by placing sutures to augment the cardiac flap valve. Initial results revealed a decrease in patient symptoms, with only modest improvement in reflux by pH monitoring.[20] There is a suggestion of decreased efficacy with time, and durability of this procedure must be confirmed with longer follow-up.[21]

The second device to be approved for clinical use is the Stretta procedure. By applying radiofrequency energy to the gastroesophageal junction, collagen is deposited, thus augmenting the reflux barrier. Like the suturing device, this technique results in symptom improvement and modest objective changes in esophageal pH.[22] The other devices are still completing clinical trials and no data are yet available. At the time of this writing each of these approaches should be considered experimental

and longer follow-up is needed before recommending their widespread use.

Outcome

The results of operative intervention may be measured by relief of symptoms, improvement in acid exposure, complications, and failures.

Symptomatic and Objective Results

Success after the operation may be measured by the patient's relief of symptoms and by the quantitative analysis on postoperative physiologic testing. Unfortunately, postoperative testing is difficult to obtain owing to the cost and the patient's reluctance to undergo repeated nasoesophageal intubation, especially when he or she has no symptoms.

Symptom response to the operative treatment of GERD is excellent. Most authors report response rates of 90% to 94%.[23-26] Long-term follow-up is still not available because the laparoscopic technique was introduced in the early 1990s. It appears as though the results are similar to those experienced with the open approach.

Two randomized trials with long-term follow-up are available comparing medical and surgical therapy for GERD. Spechler and colleagues found that surgical therapy conferred good symptom control after 10-year follow-up.[27] Interestingly, 62% of patients in the surgical group were taking antisecretory medications at this time, although not necessarily for GERD because reflux symptoms did not change significantly when these patients stopped taking medications. In a separate study, surgical therapy was associated with far fewer treatment failures than medical therapy with long-term follow-up.[28] Although more long-term follow-up studies are needed, antireflux procedures seem to provide an excellent alternative to medical therapy with fairly durable results.

Complications

In general, complications have been reported in 3% to 10% of patients.[23,25,29,30] Many of the complications are minor and are related to surgical intervention in general (urinary retention, wound infection, venous thrombosis, and ileus). Others are related specifically to the procedure or the approach (splenic injury, hollow viscus perforation, dysphagia, and pneumothorax). All complications in patients at the University of Washington are shown in Table 40-2. The complications may be divided into those that are identified at the time of the procedure and those that are identified in the postoperative period.

OPERATIVE

Pneumothorax is one of the most common intraoperative complications, occurring in 5% to 8% of patients. The actual incidence of pneumothorax is unknown, because routine postoperative chest radiographs are generally not performed. Because the pneumothorax results from a violation of the pleural space by carbon dioxide, there is

TABLE 40-2. Complications in 400 Laparoscopic Antireflux Procedures

Complication	No. (%)
Postoperative ileus	28 (7)
Pneumothorax	13 (3)
Urinary retention	9 (2)
Dysphagia	9 (2)
Other minor complications	8 (2)
Liver trauma	2 (0.5)
Acute herniation	1 (0.25)
Perforated viscus	1 (0.25)
Death	1 (0.25)
Total	72 (17.25)

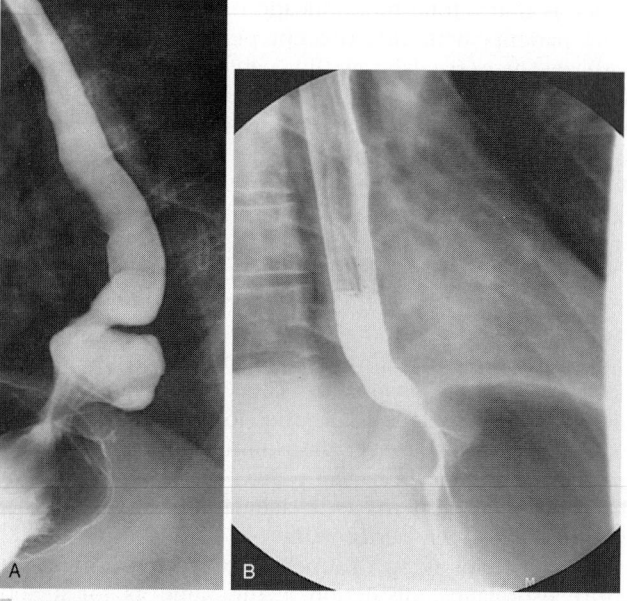

FIGURE 40-14. Contrast material studies are invaluable in the assessment of persistent or recurrent postoperative symptoms. **A,** Patient with a herniated (into mediastinum) and slipped (wraparound stomach) 360-degree fundoplication. **B,** Normal anatomic appearance of 360-degree wrap. Note the smooth tapering of the distal esophagus, the fluid level in the distal esophagus, and the air in the distended fundus above the wrap.

no need to evacuate the gas. Because carbon dioxide is absorbed rapidly and no underlying lung injury exists, the lung will reexpand without incident. If a pneumothorax is identified, the patient is maintained on oxygen therapy and the chest radiograph is repeated 2 hours after the operation. The pneumothorax should be resolved by this time.

Gastric and esophageal injuries are far less common and usually result from overaggressive tissue manipulation or from passage of the bougie. Although usually reported as less than 1%,[31] population-based studies suggest the incidence may be as high as 1.7% in inexperienced hands.[32] The injuries may be repaired with suture or an automatic stapler without sequelae if identified at the time of operation. If the injury is not seen at surgery, then the patient will likely need a second operation to repair the viscus, unless the leak is small and contained.

Major liver injury is reported rarely, and the incidence of splenic injury is about 2.3% in population-based studies.[32] Careful retraction of the left lobe of the liver will prevent significant lacerations and subcapsular hematomas. The use of a fixed retractor decreases the likelihood of liver injury. Splenic injury may result from dissection of the fundus and greater curve. Excessive traction on the lienogastric ligament should be avoided. In over 1000 laparoscopic antireflux operations performed at the University of Washington, splenectomy has not occurred.

Postoperative

Early postoperative complaints of bloating may occur in up to 30% of patients; however, fewer than 4% of patients have the symptom after 2 months.[24] There are at least three reasons for bloating. First, the patient may have more difficulty belching owing to the wrap. Second, vagal trauma may contribute to delayed gastric emptying.[33] Third, the patients will still have a tendency to swallow saliva (an unconscious effort to relieve symptoms of reflux) and with it a significant amount of air. Few patients require nasogastric tube decompression after surgery.

Postoperative dysphagia may occur in up to 20% of patients initially. A smaller percentage of patients require dilation for this problem.[24,34] Because the dissection of the hiatus and handling of the esophagus will cause some edema, dysphagia due to this will be short lived. When placing the wrap sutures, hematomas of the stomach or esophageal wall may result, resulting in dysphagia. If the wrap is too tight, the dysphagia is unlikely to resolve without dilation. The use of a graduated diet over the course of 4 to 6 weeks after the operation will limit the amount of dysphagia from the first two causes.

Death is uncommon with this operation and is less than 0.5% in our experience. Mortality does increase when age reaches 60, and patients over 80 have a 8.3% mortality.[32] This must be considered with the severity of GERD when deciding to perform an antireflux procedure.

Failures

Operative failures are patients who have persistent symptoms and physiologic evidence of continued acid exposure. The incidence is about 5%. The majority of these patients may be treated with acid suppression therapy with good results. All patients who present with recurrent or persistent symptoms should be evaluated with manometry and pH studies. If acid exposure is documented or if symptoms are severe, an esophagogram should be obtained. The presence of an anatomic abnormality of the wrap, particularly a sizable herniation, is almost always best treated with surgery (Fig. 40-14A). If the esophagogram reveals good location of the wrap and the absence of a recurrent hernia, then an attempt may be made to treat the patient medically (see Fig. 40-14B). We have found, however, that in some instances reoperation will relieve symptoms even in patients with normal-appearing wraps on esophagogram.

Special Cases

Within the purview of GERD there are several entities that have received special attention. The surgeon should be aware of these variations and the considerations that arise from them.

Strictures

Strictures pose a serious problem for the patient with GERD, although with better medical therapy this is a fairly rare complication today. Dysphagia, a most troublesome symptom, often results from stricture formation. Furthermore, strictures are a manifestation of acute and chronic inflammation, which not only decreases the diameter of the esophagus but also shortens the esophagus, making operative intervention more difficult. The evaluation of these patients may be more difficult, because the presence of a tight stricture may prevent reflux on the 24-hour pH study. The study would be ideally performed after dilation. Other causes of stricture (tumor or caustic injury) must be excluded before operative intervention. Strictures resulting from GERD are indicative of long-standing disease and may be associated with a shortened esophagus or Barrett's esophagus.

The most effective therapy for peptic stricture of the esophagus is an antireflux procedure. Although there is evidence to support effective symptom control with endoscopic dilation and proton pump inhibitor maintenance therapy, operative treatment results in fewer dilations per patient. Of 27 patients treated at the University of Washington for refractory peptic stricture, 21 proceeded with operative control of reflux. In these patients, the average number of dilations per patient was 2.8 preoperatively and 0.33 postoperatively. This compares favorably with the 6 patients who continued on medical therapy; they required an average of 9 dilations per patient throughout the course of treatment.

Barrett's Esophagus

In some patients, prolonged acid and perhaps alkaline injury leads to a change in the esophageal mucosa from its usual squamous epithelium to a columnar configuration (*Barrett's esophagus*). The cells almost always extend proximally from the squamocolumnar junction in a contiguous pattern. If Barrett's esophagus is found, multiple biopsies are necessary to exclude dysplasia, which may indicate a tendency toward the development of adenocarcinoma. Although the incidence of adenocarcinoma in patients with Barrett's esophagus is about 40 times greater than that in the general population (Barrett's studies with increased incidence), the incidence of cancer in these patients is still very low.

Because Barrett's esophagus arises from gastroesophageal reflux injury (of acid or bile), an antireflux procedure might be expected to decrease the rate of dysplasia and cancer. This issue is not resolved; the evidence in the literature is not conclusive.[35] Two recent series report the regression of intestinal metaplasia in 14% to 42% of patients after antireflux surgery.[36,37] Our own experience at the University of Washington supports this, having seen regression in 57% of patients with short segment Barrett's esophagus (<3 cm). Regardless of the impact of an antireflux procedure on the evolution of Barrett's esophagus, the patients should still be examined endoscopically for surveillance of metaplasia after the operation is performed.

Short Esophagus

As a result of repeated injury, the esophagus narrows (*stricture*) and shortens. The real challenge in these patients comes in the operative approach.

By mobilizing the esophagus well into the mediastinum, a 2- to 3-cm segment of esophagus can usually be placed into the abdomen without tension. However, if this cannot be accomplished, a Collis gastroplasty may be performed. A double-staple technique may be used to create the neoesophagus (Fig. 40-15) once the dissection has been performed.

Unfortunately, the postoperative physiologic testing on these patients reveals an abnormal acid exposure in 50% of patients.[38] One reason for this is because the lengthening procedure often leaves parietal cells in the neoesophagus above the wrap.

Extraesophageal Symptoms

A relatively new area of study in GERD is the involvement of the respiratory tract. Symptoms of hoarseness, laryngitis, cough, wheezing, and aspiration may occur when patients have high proximal reflux. Pulmonary fibrosis has also been associated with high gastroesophageal reflux.[39]

About 30% of patients with typical symptoms of reflux will have some type of extraesophageal symptom; however, about 10% of patients will have only extraesophageal symptoms when they present for evaluation. Of the patients who present with primary laryngeal symptoms, fewer than half will have typical manifestations of heartburn or regurgitation.[40] Unfortunately, standard diagnostic testing for GERD has diminished sensitivity and specificity in this group of patients. Often, the initial pH study will show abnormal acid exposure in the upper esophagus,[41,42] but this is not necessary for the diagnosis.[43] The detection of acid in the pharynx on pH monitoring improves the diagnostic rates of laryngeal reflux.[44] Furthermore, pharyngeal reflux is a better predictor of response to medical[45] and surgical therapy[46] than standard esophageal measurements. Still, the measurement of pharyngeal reflux has poor sensitivity, likely because the mechanism of extraesophageal disease is via vagal stimulation from esophageal acid exposure. The diagnosis may also be supported by a stroboscopic examination of the vocal cords showing evidence of inflammation and

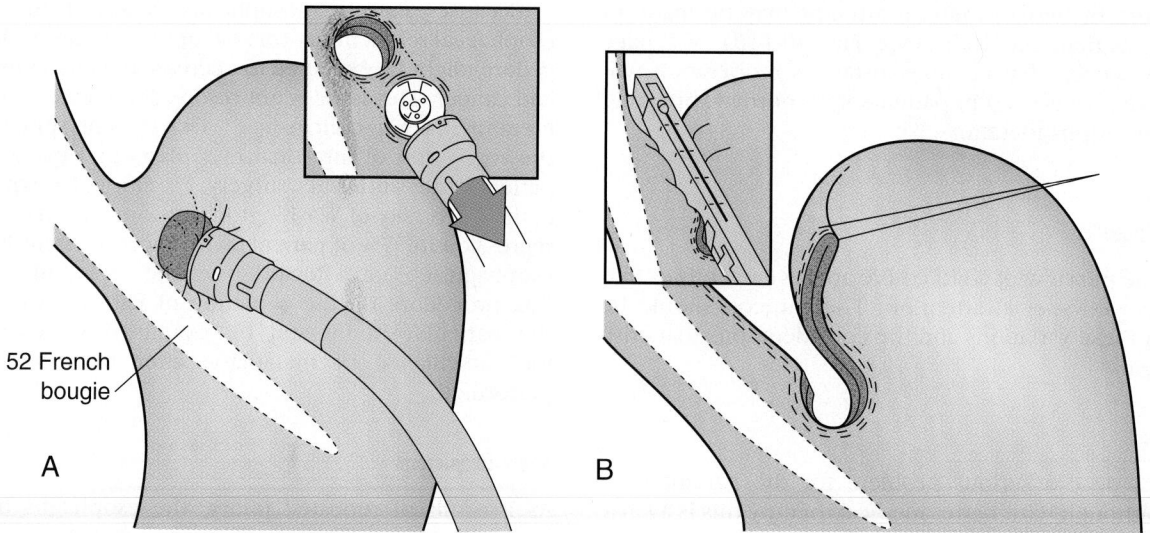

FIGURE 40-15.   Double-staple technique for esophageal lengthening. **A,** A circular stapling and cutting device is used to create a through-and-through opening of the cardia-fundus junction. **B,** A linear stapling and cutting device is then used to transect the remaining stomach toward the gastroesophageal junction.

injury,[31] although these findings are too nonspecific by themselves to reliably diagnose reflux as the culprit.

Both medical and surgical therapies have been used to treat the extraesophageal manifestations of GERD. The resolution of symptoms, increased exercise, and cessation of corticosteroid use have all been observed. The rate of symptom response to therapy is less than that of heartburn and regurgitation (75% to 80%).[47,48] The reason for this may be due to the selection of patients. With further evaluation of this unique group of patients, selection criteria may improve the results of both medical and operative intervention.

PARAESOPHAGEAL HERNIAS

Paraesophageal hernias, type II or type III (see Fig. 40-2B and C), are less commonly encountered in surgical practice than GERD. The operative approach has varied considerably for several decades. The central issues have remained the same in the era of videoendoscopic surgery: the need to operate on asymptomatic patients, whether to add an antireflux procedure, whether to anchor the stomach to the abdominal wall, and the need to remove the hernia sac. The repair of a paraesophageal hernia is another procedure that is ideally suited for a laparoscopic approach.

Pathophysiology

The most common structure to herniate through the esophageal hiatus is the fundus of the stomach. Occasionally, the fundus of the stomach will rotate toward the right pleural cavity along the organoaxial axis defined by the phrenoesophageal membrane at the hiatus and the retroperitoneal attachment of the first portion of the duodenum. This results in what has been referred to as an *upside-down stomach.* Other structures that may be

located in the hernia sac include the spleen, colon, and omentum. After repeated episodes of the viscera entering the hernia sac, adhesions between the wall of the sac and the structures may form, thus preventing the structures from returning to their position in the peritoneal cavity. The natural history of these large hernias is a matter of debate. Rarely, the herniated contents will become strangulated, causing an emergent condition that requires immediate operative intervention. Because of these risks and early reports of Belsey and Hill,[49,50] most for decades have recommended repair of these hernias when detected regardless of symptoms. Recent evidence, however, suggests that the risk of acute strangulation is around 1% per year.[22] Therefore we, and many others, recommend surgical intervention only for younger patients (<60 years) and those with significant symptoms.

Symptoms

The most common symptoms include intermittent dysphagia for solids that result from episodes of acute gastric or esophageal obstruction, abdominal and chest pain secondary to visceral torsion, gastrointestinal bleeding from mucosal ischemia, and heartburn. This profile varies considerably from that of GERD. The symptoms are often nonspecific and do not lead the clinician to the diagnosis. Often, a diagnosis of paraesophageal hernia is made only after a contrast study or endoscopy is performed for proximal gastrointestinal tract complaints.

In the series of patients at the University of Washington, symptoms of heartburn were present in 50% of patients. Episodic attacks of abdominal pain and dysphagia were also present in 50% of patients. Other symptoms occurred with varying frequency (Table 40-3). Regurgitation is likely to occur in patients with large hiatal defects and a type III hernia, which allows the gastroesophageal junction to migrate into the chest, thus promoting a pres-

TABLE 40-3.   Symptoms in 42 Patients Presenting With Paraesophageal Hernias*

Symptom	Predominance (%)
Heartburn	50
Dysphagia	43
Chest pain	37
Gastrointestinal blood loss	34
Regurgitation	31
Bloating	31
Abdominal pain	27
Cough	23

*Symptoms reported occurred more frequently than once a week.

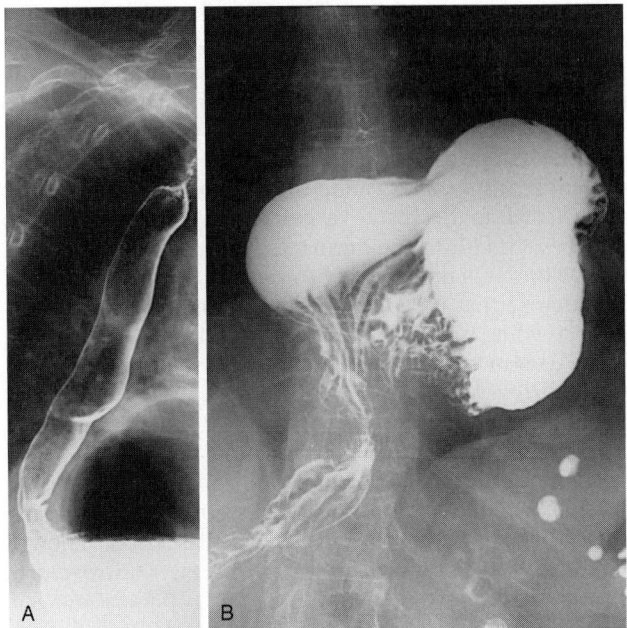

FIGURE 40-16.   Upper gastrointestinal contrast material study is essential in the evaluation of a paraesophageal hernia. **A,** Oblique view shows the stomach with an air-fluid level anterior to the esophagus and well into the mediastinum. **B,** An anteroposterior view of a patient with complete organoaxial volvulus, with the entire stomach in the mediastinum and the pylorus at the hiatus.

sure gradient and encouraging reflux. Episodic attacks of pain are thought to arise from transient distention and ischemia of the hernia contents. Spontaneous reduction provides relief. Dysphagia will occur if the gastroesophageal junction is angled such that a food bolus may not enter the stomach after a swallow is initiated. Gastrointestinal bleeding is caused by ulceration of the mucosa at an area where the stomach folds back onto itself. Thirty-four percent of patients presenting to the University of Washington were found to have a gastrointestinal source of blood loss.

Preoperative Evaluation

The evaluation of patients with paraesophageal hernias is similar to that of patients undergoing work-up for GERD. A contrast esophagogram, however, in these patients is the most important diagnostic test (Fig. 40-16). Endoscopy helps to identify mucosal erosions as a source of gastrointestinal blood loss. Manometry is needed to determine the motor function of the esophageal body. The pH testing can be avoided if an antireflux procedure is performed as part of the operative repair. However, if an antireflux procedure is not planned, the extent of gastroesophageal reflux should be evaluated.

In patients with large paraesophageal hernias, it may be very difficult to complete the manometry, and pH studies can be difficult. When the fundus of the stomach is angled such that the distal esophagus and gastroesophageal junction may not be negotiated with the catheters, the studies may be incomplete. It is important to obtain some idea of the degree of peristalsis in the body of the esophagus before proceeding with the operation. This can be accomplished even if the stomach and distal esophagus cannot be cannulated.

Treatment

After the introduction of laparoscopic techniques for the treatment of sliding hiatal hernias, the use in the repair of paraesophageal hernias naturally followed. Although technically more difficult, laparoscopic paraesophageal hernia repair is safe, feasible, and generally associated with less perioperative morbidity than open approaches. However, there are recent reports suggesting recurrence rates as high as 30% to 40% (although recurrence rates are likely 15% to 20% with open approaches).[51,52] Although most of these recurrences are asymptomatic and found only on barium studies, it is of concern, and techniques to reduce recurrences are needed. Unfortunately, synthetic mesh, which is used for most other hernia repairs, is associated with occasional esophageal erosion, limiting its practical use.[53]

The operative approach via laparoscopy, our preferred approach, is similar to that of gastroesophageal reflux procedures described previously with respect to patient positioning and port placement. Several variations in the technique must be made to accommodate the unique operative findings in paraesophageal hernias.

The initial dissection for paraesophageal hernias begins with mobilization of the greater curve and fundus. Because the left crus is usually obscured by the lienogastric ligament and the short gastric vessels, crural dissection may be hazardous at the beginning of the operation. By mobilizing the fundus and dividing the short gastric vessels with ultrasonic transection, the left crus may be exposed safely.[54]

Once the crural fibers are exposed on the left, the hernia sac will, by necessity, have been divided. At this point, the peritoneal sac may be divided anteriorly with minimal risk. Further dissection of the sac from its mediastinal attachments will free the stomach and allow it to be delivered into the peritoneal cavity. Once the hernia contents are returned to the peritoneal cavity, the hernia sac must be transected circumferentially at the hiatus. The technically challenging aspect of the dissection is encountered during the posterior sac dissection. The esophagus and the anterior vagus nerve are intimately associated with the sac posteriorly. Often, a lighted bougie is useful to identify the exact location of the esophagus. Once the sac is freed at the hiatus, a concerted effort is made to remove as much of the hernia sac from the mediastinum as possible. It is unnecessary to remove all of the sac, and considering that the pleura, esophagus, and inferior pulmonary veins may be injured during the dissection, the desire to remove the entire sac must be tempered by the possible injury to vital structures.

After the dissection is completed, the crura are reapproximated with interrupted nonabsorbable suture, as with any antireflux procedure. An antireflux procedure should be added to the procedure to prevent postoperative reflux after the extensive hiatal dissection. Though the need for an antireflux procedure is controversial, approximately 60% of patients with paraesophageal hernias have abnormal reflux and a hypotensive LES; thus we consider a fundoplication appropriate.[55] The fundoplication will also act to seal the hiatus, preventing access by other viscera. As with fundoplication for GERD, the type of wrap is dictated by the preoperative manometry. Postoperative management of the patient is the same as for operations performed for type I hernias and GERD.

Outcome

Operative treatment of paraesophageal hernias is effective in the control of symptoms in 90% to 100% of patients.[56-59] Of 42 patients operated laparoscopically for paraesophageal hernia at the University of Washington, all had resolution of their primary symptoms.[24] Anemia, which was found in 36% of patients preoperatively, resolved after the surgery. The average operative time was 3.3 hours, and the average hospital stay was 4 days (range, 2 to 8 days).

Five patients had postoperative 24-hour pH studies performed. Four had normal results, with a mean acid exposure time of 0.8%. One patient had abnormal acid exposure (total percent time, 16.6%) but had no symptoms. One patient had a recurrent hernia but is currently asymptomatic.

Complication rates were similar to those for GERD. The pneumothorax rate was higher (7%) because the mediastinal dissection is more extensive. During the postoperative course, 20 patients (48%) had subcutaneous emphysema in the cervical region that resolved spontaneously. This is due to the extensive mediastinal dissection that is carried out during the operation. One patient died of portal venous thrombosis 7 days after the operation.

Strangulation of Hernia Contents

The clinical finding of persistent thoracic or epigastric pain, fever, or sepsis in a patient known to have a para-esophageal hernia is a surgical emergency. The mortality rate for ischemic stomach in the mediastinum is high. Although the consequences of this clinical situation are grave, it is a relatively rare occurrence in patients with paraesophageal hernias. In 31 patients with complicated paraesophageal hernias, only 2 were found to have gastric necrosis and perforation.[60] Of the initial 42 patients operated on at the University of Washington, only 1 required an emergent repair. Interestingly, 11 patients were found to have gastric volvulus at the time of the operation. Thus, 25% of the patients had the potential to develop vascular compromise, and only 1 (2%) did. Emergent reduction of a paraesophageal hernia may be approached laparoscopically, but a low threshold for conversion should be maintained.

SUMMARY

Operative treatment of GERD and paraesophageal hernias has become more common in the era of laparoscopic procedures. Careful patient selection based on symptom assessment, response to medical therapy, and preoperative testing will optimize chances for successful surgical treatment. Scrupulous operative technique will allow for resolution of symptoms in almost all patients. Complications of the laparoscopic approach to these diseases are uncommon.

Selected References

Branton SA, Hinder RA, Floch NR, et al: Surgical treatment of gastroesophageal reflux disease. *In* Castell DO, Richter JE (eds): The Esophagus, 3rd ed. Philadelphia, Lippincott Williams & Wilkens, 1999, pp 511-525.

> **An excellent review of pathophysiology, work-up, and surgical treatment of GERD. Excellent diagrams and technical explanations.**

Duranceau A, Ferraro P, Jamieson GG: Evidence-based investigation for reflux disease. Chest Surg Clin North Am 11:495-506, 2001.

> **A comprehensive review of the work-up of GERD, which is the cornerstone of treating the disease appropriately.**

Oelschlager BK, Pellegrini CA: Paraesophageal hernias: Open, laparoscopic, or thoracic repair? Chest Surg Clin North Am 11:589-603, 2001.

> **This review covers the presentation, management, and controversies surrounding the repair of paraesophageal hernias.**

References

1. Clemente G, D'Ugo D, Granone P, et al: Intraoperative esophageal manometry in surgical treatment of achalasia: A reappraisal. Hepatogastroenterology 43:1532-1536, 1996.
2. Mittal RK, Balaban DH: The esophagogastric junction. N Engl J Med 336:924-932, 1997.
3. Galmiche JP, Janssens J: The pathophysiology of gastro-oesophageal reflux disease: An overview. Scand J Gastroenterol Suppl 211:7-18, 1995.

4. Katzka DA, Sidhu M, Castell DO: Hypertensive lower esophageal sphincter pressures and gastroesophageal reflux: An apparent paradox that is not unusual. Am J Gastroenterol 90:280-284, 1995.

5. Friedland GW: Progress in radiology: Historical review of the changing concepts of lower esophageal anatomy: 430 B.C.-1977. AJR Am J Roentgenol 131:373-378, 1978.

6. Patti MG, Goldberg HI, Arcerito M, et al: Hiatal hernia size affects lower esophageal sphincter function, esophageal acid exposure, and the degree of mucosal injury. Am J Surg 171:182-186, 1996.

7. Hill LD, Kozarek RA, Kraemer SJ, et al: The gastroesophageal flap valve: In vitro and in vivo observations. Gastrointest Endosc 44:541-547, 1996.

8. Stein HJ, DeMeester TR: Who benefits from antireflux surgery? World J Surg 16:313-319, 1992.

9. Demeester TR, Johnson LF, Joseph GJ, et al: Patterns of gastroesophageal reflux in health and disease. Ann Surg 184:459-470, 1976.

10. Grande L, Culell P, Ros E, et al: Comparison of stationary vs ambulatory 24-hour pH monitoring systems in diagnosis of gastroesophageal reflux disease. Dig Dis Sci 38:213-219, 1993.

11. Stacher G, Bergmann H: Scintigraphic quantitation of gastrointestinal motor activity and transport: Oesophagus and stomach. Eur J Nucl Med 19:815-823, 1992.

12. Schenk BE, Kuipers EJ, Klinkenberg-Knol EC, et al: Omeprazole as a diagnostic tool in gastroesophageal reflux disease. Am J Gastroenterol 92:1997-2000, 1997.

13. Richter JE: Typical and atypical presentations of gastroesophageal reflux disease: The role of esophageal testing in diagnosis and management. Gastroenterol Clin North Am 25:75-102, 1996.

14. Dent J: Long-term aims of treatment of reflux disease, and the role of non-drug measures. Digestion 51(Suppl 1):30-34, 1992.

15. Skoutakis VA, Joe RH, Hara DS: Comparative role of omeprazole in the treatment of gastroesophageal reflux disease. Ann Pharmacother 29:1252-1262, 1995.

16. Freston JW: Long-term acid control and proton pump inhibitors: Interactions and safety issues in perspective. Am J Gastroenterol 92:51S-57S, 1997.

17. Heudebert GR, Marks R, Wilcox CM, et al: Choice of long-term strategy for the management of patients with severe esophagitis: A cost-utility analysis. Gastroenterology 112: 1078-1086, 1997.

18. Vaezi MF, Schroeder PL, Richter JE: Reproducibility of proximal probe pH parameters in 24-hour ambulatory esophageal pH monitoring. Am J Gastroenterol 92:825-829, 1997.

19. Oleynikov D, Eubanks TR, Oelschlager BK, et al: Total fundoplication is the operation of choice for patients with gastroesophageal reflux and defective peristalsis. Surg Endosc 16:909-913, 2002.

20. Filipi CJ, Lehman GA, Rothstein RI, et al: Transoral, flexible endoscopic suturing for treatment of GERD: A multicenter trial. Gastrointest Endosc 53:416-422, 2001.

21. Rothstein RI, Pohl H, Grove M, et al: Endoscopic gastric plication for the treatment of GERD: Two year follow-up results. Am J Gastroenterol 96(Suppl 1):S35, 2001.

22. Stylopoulos N, Gazelle GS, Rattner DW: Paraesophageal hernias: Operation or observation? Ann Surg 236:492-501, 2002.

23. Cadiere GB, Himpens J, Rajan A, et al: Laparoscopic Nissen fundoplication: Laparoscopic dissection technique and results. Hepatogastroenterology 44:4-10, 1997.

24. Horgan S, Pellegrini CA: Surgical treatment of gastroesophageal reflux disease. Surg Clin North Am 77:1063-1082, 1997.

25. Peracchia A, Rosati R, Bona S, et al: Laparoscopic treatment of functional diseases of the esophagus. Int Surg 80:336-340, 1995.

26. Peters JH, DeMeester TR: Indications, benefits and outcome of laparoscopic Nissen fundoplication. Dig Dis 14:169-179, 1996.

27. Spechler SJ, Lee E, Ahnen D, et al: Long-term outcome of medical and surgical therapies for gastroesophageal reflux disease: Follow-up of a randomized controlled trial. JAMA 285:2331-2338, 2001.

28. Lundell L, Miettinen P, Myrvold HE, et al: Continued (5-year) followup of a randomized clinical study comparing antireflux surgery and omeprazole in gastroesophageal reflux disease. J Am Coll Surg 192:172-181, 2001.

29. Anvari M, Allen C, Borm A: Laparoscopic Nissen fundoplication is a satisfactory alternative to long-term omeprazole therapy. Br J Surg 82:938-942, 1995.

30. Cadiere GB, Houben JJ, Bruyns J, et al: Laparoscopic Nissen fundoplication: Technique and preliminary results. Br J Surg 81:400-403, 1994.

31. Oelschlager BK, Eubanks TR, Maronian N, et al: Laryngoscopy and pharyngeal pH are complementary in the diagnosis of gastroesophageal-laryngeal reflux. J Gastrointest Surg 6:189-194, 2002.

32. Flum DR, Koepsell T, Heagerty P, et al: The nationwide frequency of major adverse outcomes in antireflux surgery and the role of surgeon experience, 1992-1997. J Am Coll Surg 195:611-618, 2002.

33. Hunter RJ, Metz DC, Morris JB, et al: Gastroparesis: A potential pitfall of laparoscopic Nissen fundoplication. Am J Gastroenterol 91:2617-2618, 1996.

34. Zaninotto G, Anselmino M, Costantini M, et al: Laparoscopic treatment of gastro-esophageal reflux disease: Indications and results. Int Surg 80:380-385, 1995.

35. DeMeester SR, Campos GM, DeMeester TR, et al: The impact of an antireflux procedure on intestinal metaplasia of the cardia. Ann Surg 228:547-556, 1998.

36. Hofstetter WL, Peters JH, DeMeester TR, et al: Long-term outcome of antireflux surgery in patients with Barrett's esophagus. Ann Surg 234:532-539, 2001.

37. Bowers SP, Mattar SG, Smith CD, et al: Clinical and histologic follow-up after antireflux surgery for Barrett's esophagus. J Gastrointest Surg 6:532-539, 2002.

38. Jobe BA, Horvath KD, Swanstrom LL: Postoperative function following laparoscopic collis gastroplasty for shortened esophagus. Arch Surg 133:867-874, 1998.

39. Mays EE, Dubois JJ, Hamilton GB: Pulmonary fibrosis associated with tracheobronchial aspiration: A study of the frequency of hiatal hernia and gastroesophageal reflux in interstitial pulmonary fibrosis of obscure etiology. Chest 69:512-515, 1976.

40. Koufman JA: The otolaryngologic manifestations of gastroesophageal reflux disease (GERD): A clinical investigation of 225 patients using ambulatory 24-hour pH monitoring and an experimental investigation of the role of acid and pepsin in the development of laryngeal injury. Laryngoscope 101:1-78, 1991.

41. Patti MG, Debas HT, Pellegrini CA: Clinical and functional characterization of high gastroesophageal reflux. Am J Surg 165:163-168, 1993.

42. Patti MG, Debas HT, Pellegrini CA: Esophageal manometry and 24-hour pH monitoring in the diagnosis of pulmonary aspiration secondary to gastroesophageal reflux. Am J Surg 163:401-406, 1992.

43. Triadafilopoulos G, DiBaise JK, Nostrant TT, et al: The Stretta procedure for the treatment of GERD: 6 and 12 month follow-up of the U.S. open label trial. Gastrointest Endosc 55:149-156, 2002.

44. Cote DN, Miller RH: The association of gastroesophageal reflux and otolaryngologic disorders. Compr Ther 21:80-84, 1995.

45. Eubanks TR, Omelanczuk P, Hillel A, et al: Pharyngeal pH measurements in patients with respiratory symptoms before and during proton pump inhibitor therapy. Am J Surg 181:466-470, 2001.

46. Oelschlager BK, Eubanks TR, Oleynikov D, et al: Symptomatic and physiologic outcomes after operative treatment for extraesophageal reflux. Surg Endosc 16:1032-1036, 2002.

47. Hunter JG, Trus TL, Branum GD, et al: A physiologic approach to laparoscopic fundoplication for gastroesophageal reflux disease. Ann Surg 223:673-687, 1996.

48. Johnson WE, Hagen JA, DeMeester TR, et al: Outcome of respiratory symptoms after antireflux surgery on patients with gastroesophageal reflux disease. Arch Surg 131:489-492, 1996.

49. Hill LD: Incarcerated paraesophageal hernia: A surgical emergency. Am J Surg 126:286-291, 1973.

50. Skinner DB, Belsey RH: Surgical management of esophageal reflux and hiatus hernia: Long-term results with 1,030 patients. J Thorac Cardiovasc Surg 53:33-54, 1967.

51. Hashemi M, Peters JH, DeMeester TR, et al: Laparoscopic repair of large type III hiatal hernia: objective followup reveals high recurrence rate. J Am Coll Surg 190:553-561, 2000.

52. Mattar SG, Bowers SP, Galloway KD, et al: Long-term outcome of laparoscopic repair of paraesophageal hernia. Surg Endosc 16:745-749, 2002.

53. Carlson MA, Condon RE, Ludwig KA, et al: Management of intrathoracic stomach with polypropylene mesh prosthesis reinforced transabdominal hiatus hernia repair. J Am Coll Surg 187:227-230, 1998.

54. Horgan S, Eubanks TR, Jacobsen G, et al: Repair of paraesophageal hernias. Am J Surg 177:354-358, 1999.

55. Walther B, DeMeester TR, Lafontaine E, et al: Effect of paraesophageal hernia on sphincter function and its implication on surgical therapy. Am J Surg 147:111-116, 1984.

56. Casabella F, Sinanan M, Horgan S, et al: Systematic use of gastric fundoplication in laparoscopic repair of paraesophageal hernias. Am J Surg 171:485-489, 1996.

57. Hawasli A, Zonca S: Laparoscopic repair of paraesophageal hiatal hernia. Am Surg 64:703-710, 1998.

58. Krahenbuhl L, Schafer M, Farhadi J, et al: Laparoscopic treatment of large paraesophageal hernia with totally intrathoracic stomach. J Am Coll Surg 187:231-237, 1998.

59. Perdikis G, Hinder RA, Filipi CJ, et al: Laparoscopic paraesophageal hernia repair. Arch Surg 132:586-591, 1997.

60. Ozdemir IA, Burke WA, Ikins PM: Paraesophageal hernia: A life-threatening disease. Ann Thorac Surg 16:547-554, 1973.

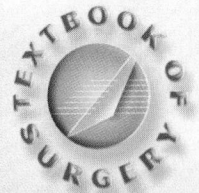

CHAPTER 41

ABDOMINAL WALL, UMBILICUS, PERITONEUM, MESENTERIES, OMENTUM, AND RETROPERITONEUM

Richard H. Turnage, M.D.,   Benjamin D. L. Li, M.D.
and   John C. McDonald, M.D.

Abdominal Wall and Umbilicus	**Mesentery and Omentum**
Peritoneum and Peritoneal Cavity	**Retroperitoneum**

ABDOMINAL WALL AND UMBILICUS

Embryology

The abdominal wall begins to develop in the earliest stages of embryonic differentiation from the lateral plate of the intraembryonic mesoderm. At this stage, the embryo consists of three principal layers: an outer protective layer termed *ectoderm,* an inner nutritive layer termed *endoderm,* and the *mesoderm.* The intraembryonic mesoderm becomes segmented into mesodermal somites or myotomes from which proliferating cells grow into the developing abdominal wall or somatopleure. The developing mesoderm of the future anterolateral abdominal wall splits into three layers that ultimately give rise to the transversus abdominis and the internal and external oblique muscles.

At this early stage, the lining of the coelomic cavity communicates broadly with the lining outside the body cavity. As the embryo enlarges and the abdominal wall components grow toward one another, the ventral open area, bounded by the edge of the amnion, becomes smaller. This results in the development of the umbilical cord as a tubular structure containing the yolk stalk (omphalomesenteric duct), allantois, and the fetal blood vessels, which pass to and from the placenta.

By the end of the third month of gestation the body walls have closed, except at the umbilical ring. Because the alimentary tract increases in length more rapidly than the coelomic cavity increases in volume, much of the developing gut protrudes through the umbilical ring to lie within the umbilical cord. As the coelomic cavity enlarges enough to accommodate the intestine, the latter returns to the developing peritoneal cavity such that only the omphalomesenteric duct, the allantois, and the fetal blood vessels pass through the shrinking umbilical ring. At birth, blood no longer courses through the umbilical vessels and the omphalomesenteric duct has been reduced to a fibrous cord and no longer communicates with the intestine. After division of the umbilical cord, the umbilical ring heals rapidly by scarring.

Anatomy

There are nine layers to the abdominal wall: skin, subcutaneous tissue, superficial fascia, external oblique muscle, internal oblique muscle, transversus abdominis muscle, endoabdominal or transversalis fascia, extraperitoneal or preperitoneal adipose and areolar tissue, and peritoneum (Fig. 41-1).

Subcutaneous Tissues

The subcutaneous tissue consists of Camper's and Scarpa's fascia. Camper's fascia is the superficial layer that

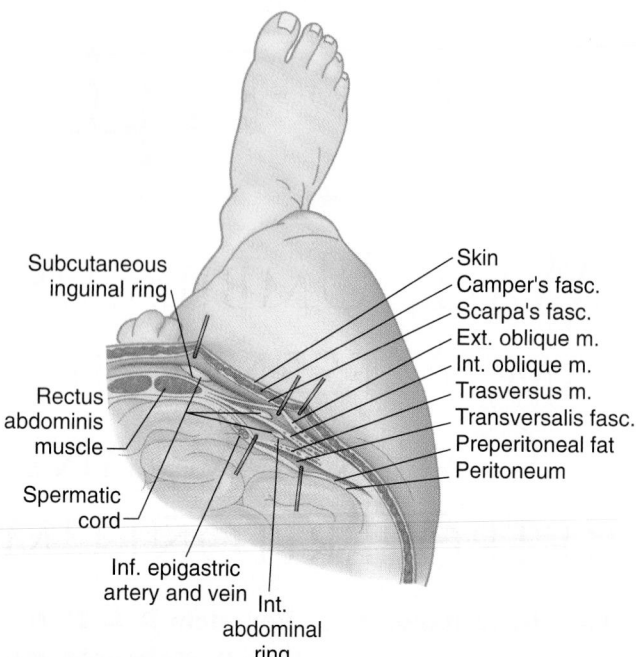

FIGURE 41-1. The nine layers of the anterolateral abdominal wall. (From Thorek P: Anatomy in Surgery, 2nd ed. Philadelphia, JB Lippincott, 1962, p 358.)

contains the bulk of the subcutaneous fat; Scarpa's fascia is a denser layer of fibrous connective tissue contiguous with the fascia lata of the thigh. Approximation of Scarpa's fascia aids in the alignment of the skin after surgical incisions.

Muscle and Investing Fascias

The muscles of the anterolateral abdominal wall include the external and internal oblique and the transversus abdominis. These flat muscles enclose much of the circumference of the torso and give rise anteriorly to a broad, flat aponeurosis investing the rectus abdominis muscles (i.e., rectus sheath). The external abdominal oblique muscles are the largest and the thickest of the flat abdominal wall muscles. They originate from the lower seven ribs and course in a superolateral to inferomedial direction. The most posterior of the fibers run vertically downward to insert into the anterior half of the iliac crest. At the midclavicular line, the muscle fibers give rise to a flat, strong aponeurosis that passes anteriorly to the rectus sheath to insert medially into the linea alba (Fig. 41-2). The lower portion of the external oblique aponeurosis is rolled

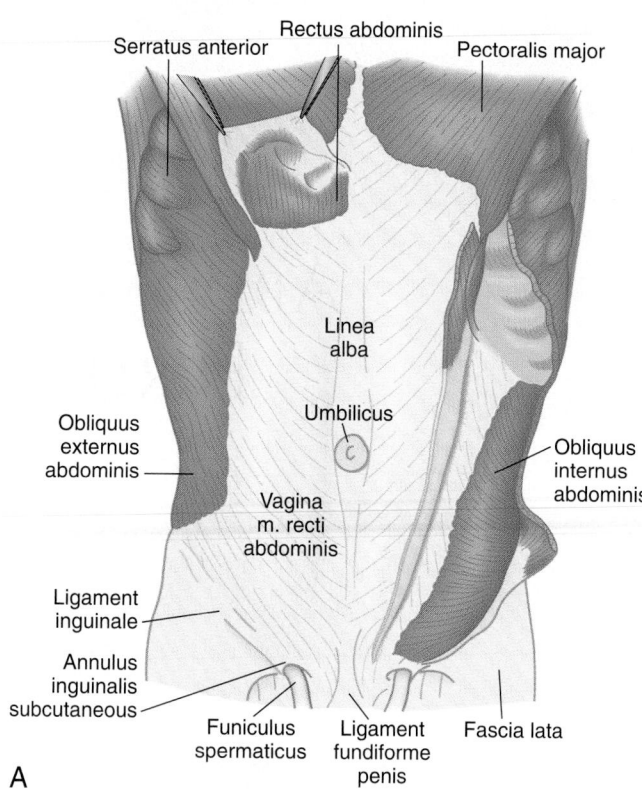

A

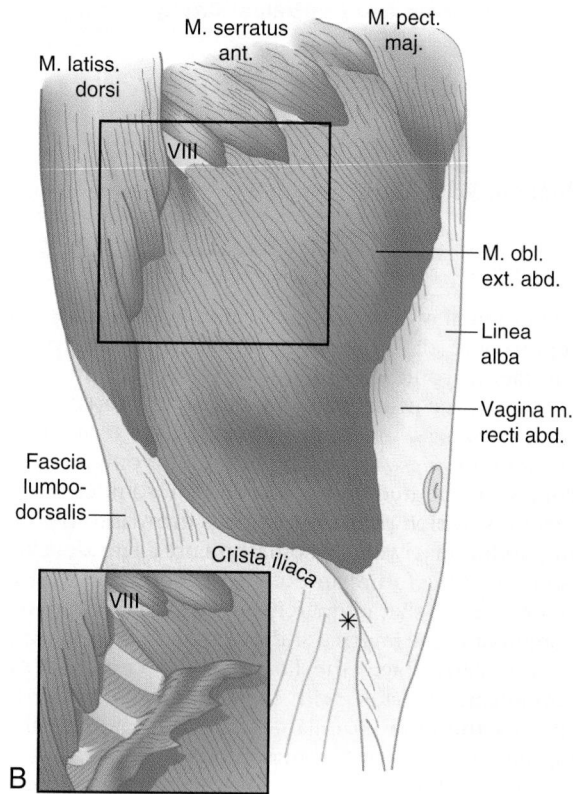

B

FIGURE 41-2. **A,** The external oblique, internal oblique, and rectus abdominis muscles and the anterior rectus sheath. **B,** A lateral view of the external oblique muscle and its aponeurosis as it enters the anterior rectus sheath. The inset shows the origin of the external oblique muscle fibers from the lower ribs and their costal cartilages. (From McVay C: Anson and McVay's Surgical Anatomy, 6th ed. Philadelphia, WB Saunders, 1984, pp 477 and 478.)

posteriorly and superiorly on itself to form a groove on which the spermatic cord lies. This portion of the external oblique aponeurosis extends from the anterior superior iliac spine to the pubic tubercle and is termed the *inguinal* or *Poupart's ligament.* The inguinal ligament is the lower, free edge of the external oblique aponeurosis under which pass the femoral artery, vein, and nerve and the iliacus, psoas major, and pectineus muscles. A femoral hernia passes posterior to the inguinal ligament, whereas an inguinal hernia passes anterior and superior to this ligament. The shelving edge of the inguinal ligament is utilized in various repairs of inguinal hernia, including the Bassini and the Lichtenstein tension-free repair (see Chapter 42).

The internal abdominal oblique muscle originates from the iliopsoas fascia beneath the lateral half of the inguinal ligament, from the anterior two thirds of the iliac crest and the lumbodorsal fascia. Its fibers course in a direction opposite to those of the external oblique (i.e., inferolateral to superomedial). The uppermost fibers insert into the lower five ribs and their cartilages (Figs. 41-2 and 41-3). The central fibers form an aponeurosis at the semilu-

nar line, which, above the semicircular line (of Douglas), is divided into anterior and posterior lamellae that envelop the rectus abdominis muscle. Below the semicircular line, the aponeurosis of the internal oblique muscle courses anteriorly to the rectus abdominis muscle as a part of the anterior rectus sheath. The lowermost fibers of the internal oblique muscle pursue an inferomedial course paralleling that of the spermatic cord to insert into the pubis between the symphysis and the pubic tubercle. Some of the lower muscle fascicles accompany the spermatic cord into the scrotum as the cremasteric muscle.

The transversus abdominis muscle is the smallest of the muscles of the anterolateral abdominal wall. It arises from the lower six costal cartilages, the spines of the lumbar vertebra (where it forms a portion of the lumbodorsal fascia), the iliac crest, and the iliopsoas fascia beneath the lateral third of the inguinal ligament. The fibers course transversely to give rise to a flat aponeurotic sheet that passes posterior to the rectus abdominis muscle above the semicircular line and anterior to this muscle below it (Fig. 41-4). The inferiormost fibers of the transversus abdominis originating from the iliopsoas fascia pass inferomedially along with the lower fibers of the internal oblique muscle. These fibers form the aponeurotic arch of the transversus abdominis muscle, which lies superiorly to Hesselbach's triangle and is an important anatomic landmark in the repair of inguinal hernias, particularly Bassini's operation and Cooper's ligament repair. Hesselbach's triangle is the site of direct inguinal hernias and is bordered by the inguinal ligament inferiorly, the lateral margin of the rectus sheath medially, and the inferior epigastric vessels laterally. The floor of this triangle is composed of transversalis fascia (see Chapter 42).

The transversalis fascia covers the deep surface of the transversus abdominis muscle and with its various extensions forms a complete fascial envelope around the abdominal cavity (Fig. 41-5). This fascial layer is regionally named for the muscles that it covers (e.g., the iliopsoas fascia, obturator fascia, and the inferior fascia of the respiratory diaphragm). The transversalis fascia binds together the muscle and aponeurotic fascicles into a continuous layer and reinforces weak areas where the aponeurotic fibers are sparse. This layer is responsible for the structural integrity of the abdominal wall, and, by definition, a hernia results from a defect in the transversalis fascia.

The rectus abdominis muscles are paired muscles that appear as long, flat triangular ribbons that are wider at their origin on the anterior surfaces of the fifth, sixth, and seventh costal cartilages and the xiphoid process than at their insertion on the pubic crest and pubic symphysis. Each muscle is composed of long, parallel fascicles interrupted by three to five tendinous inscriptions (see Fig. 41-5). These irregular tendinous intersections provide attachments of the rectus abdominis muscle to the anterior rectus sheath. There is no similar attachment to the posterior rectus sheath. These muscles lie adjacent to each other, being separated only by the linea alba. In addition to supporting the abdominal wall and protecting its contents, contraction of these powerful muscles flexes the vertebral column.

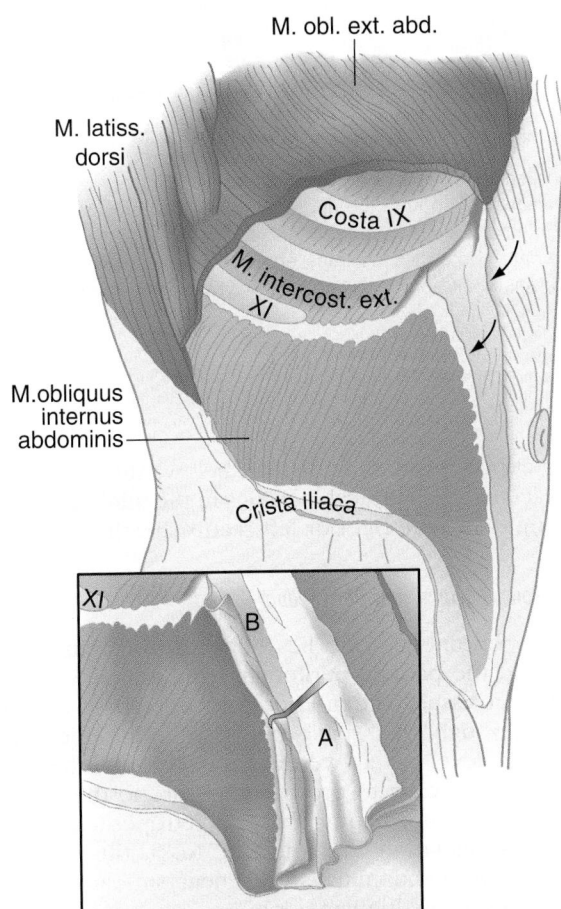

FIGURE 41-3. A lateral view of the internal oblique muscle. The external oblique muscle has been removed to show the underlying internal oblique muscle originating from the lower ribs and costal cartilages. (From McVay C: Anson and McVay's Surgical Anatomy, 6th ed. Philadelphia, WB Saunders, 1984, p 479.)

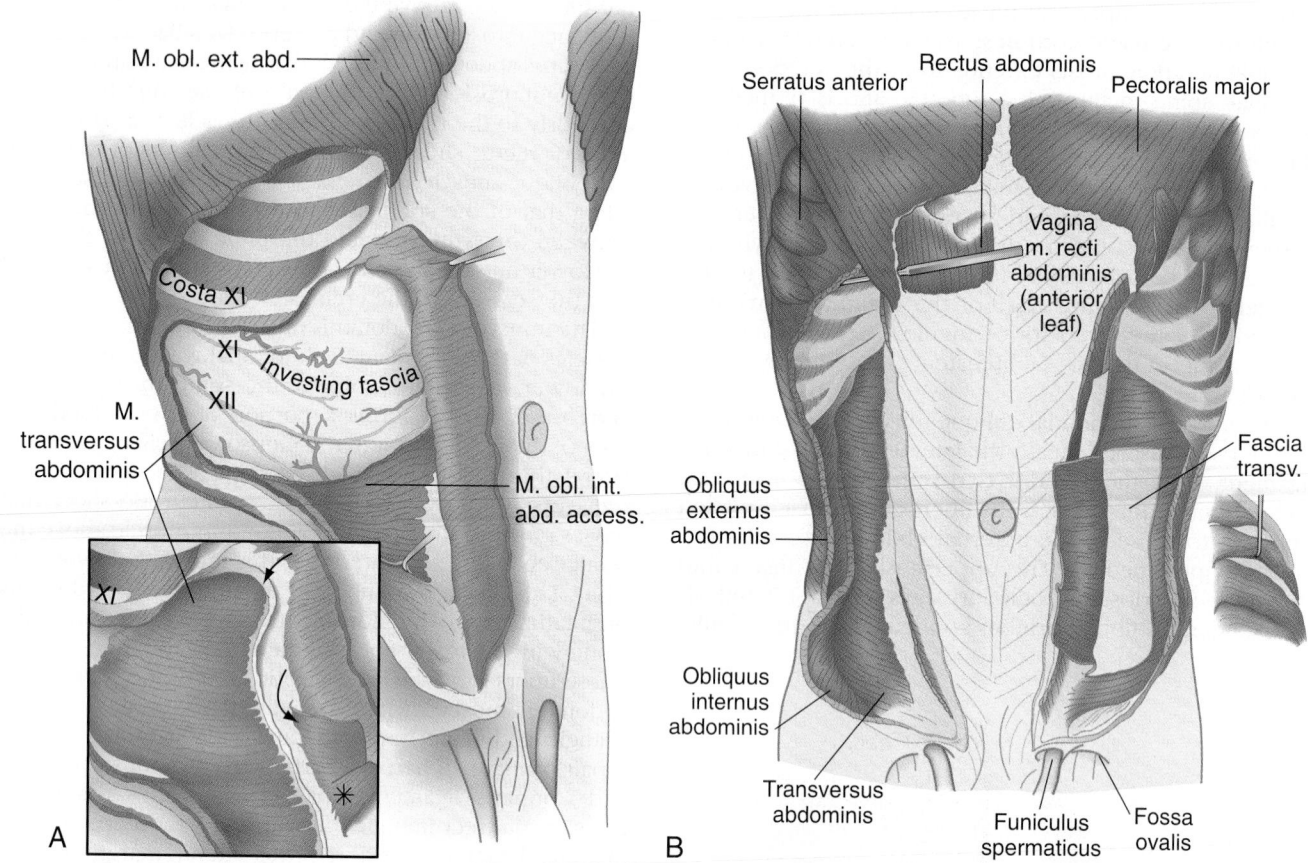

FIGURE 41-4.   A, An anterolateral view of the investing fascia of the transversus abdominis muscle and the muscle itself with the fascia removed (inset). The external and internal oblique muscles have been removed. Also note the appearance of the intercostal nerves lying between the fascia of the transversus abdominis muscle and the internal oblique muscle. **B,** An anterior view of the transversus abdominis muscle *(on the left)* and the transversalis fascia *(on the right)*. Note that the transversalis fascia is shown by reflecting the overlying transversus abdominis muscle medially. (From McVay C: Anson and McVay's Surgical Anatomy, 6th ed. Philadelphia, WB Saunders, 1984, pp 480 and 481.)

The rectus abdominis muscles are contained within a fascial sheath, the rectus sheath, which is derived from the aponeuroses of the three flat abdominal muscles. Superior to the semicircular line of Douglas, the fascial sheath completely envelops the rectus abdominis muscle with the external oblique and the anterior lamellae of the internal oblique aponeuroses passing anterior to the rectus abdominis and the aponeuroses from the posterior lamellae of the internal oblique muscle, the transversus abdominis muscle, and the transversalis fascia passing posterior to the rectus muscle. Below the semicircular line, all of these fascial layers pass anteriorly to the rectus abdominis except for the transversalis fascia. In this location the posterior aspect of the rectus abdominis is covered only by transversalis fascia, preperitoneal areolar tissue, and peritoneum.

The rectus abdominis muscles are held closely in apposition near the anterior midline by the linea alba. The linea alba consists of a band of dense, crisscross fibers of the aponeuroses of the broad abdominal muscles. It extends from the xiphoid to the pubic symphysis and is much wider above the umbilicus than below, thus facilitating the placement of surgical incisions in the midline without entering either the right or left rectus sheath.

Preperitoneal Space and Peritoneum

The preperitoneal space lies between the transversalis fascia and the parietal peritoneum and contains adipose and areolar tissue. The inferior epigastric artery and vein course through this space before entering the rectus sheath at a level just above the hypogastrium. This space is utilized surgically to provide exposure to the inguinal region for herniorrhaphy and the retroperitoneum for renal transplantation into the iliac fossa, the extraperitoneal repair of abdominal aortic aneurysms, and anterior approaches to the lumbar spine.

This space also contains the remnants of three fetal structures that are apparent during laparotomy or laparoscopy. These include (1) the medial umbilical ligaments, which are the vestiges of the fetal umbilical arteries arising from the superior vesical arteries to course

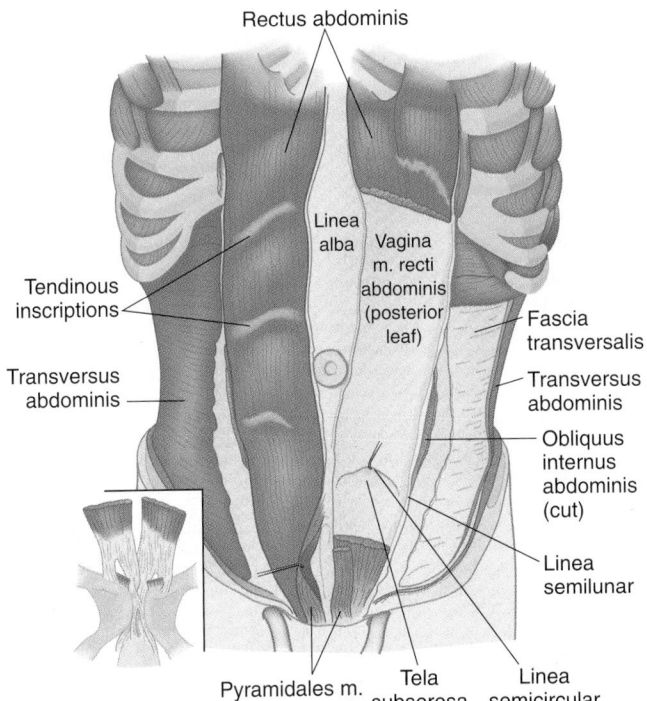

FIGURE 41-5. The rectus abdominis muscle and the contents of the rectus sheath. Note the semicircular line below which the posterior rectus sheath is absent and the rectus abdominis muscle overlies the transversalis fascia, preperitoneal areolar tissue, and peritoneum. (From McVay C: Anson and McVay's Surgical Anatomy, 6th ed. Philadelphia, WB Saunders, 1984, p 482.)

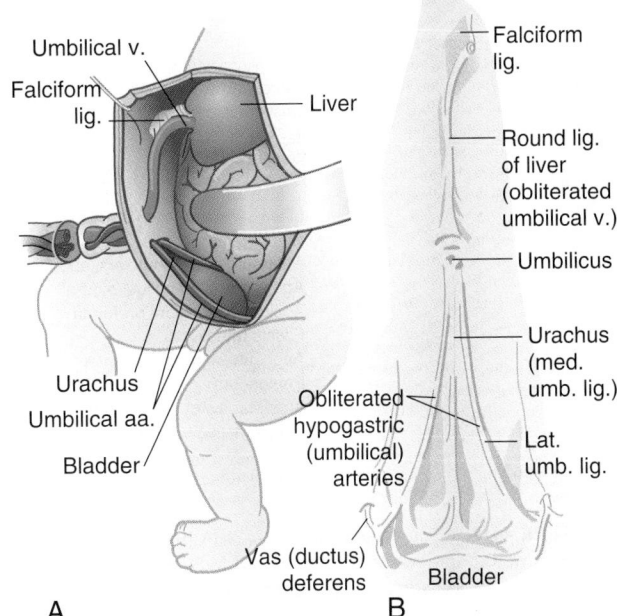

FIGURE 41-6. The umbilicus. **A,** In the fetus, the umbilical vein superiorly and the two umbilical arteries and urachus inferiorly radiate from the umbilicus. **B,** A view of the umbilicus from within the peritoneal cavity showing the round ligament of the liver (derived from the obliterated umbilical vein) superiorly and the median umbilical ligament (derived from the obliterated urachus) and medial umbilical ligaments (also called the lateral umbilical ligaments, derived from the obliterated umbilical arteries). (From Thorek P: Anatomy in Surgery, 2nd ed. Philadelphia, JB Lippincott, 1962, p 375.)

superiorly to the umbilicus; (2) the median umbilical ligament, which is a midline fibrous cord representing the remnant of the fetal allantoic stalk (or urachus) passing from the apex of the bladder to the umbilicus; and (3) the falciform ligament of the liver, which is a peritoneum-covered projection of extraperitoneal adipose tissue extending from the umbilicus to the liver. The round ligament or ligamentum teres is contained within the free margin of the falciform ligament and represents the obliterated umbilical vein coursing from the umbilicus to the left branch of the portal vein (Fig. 41-6).

The parietal peritoneum is the innermost layer of the abdominal wall. It consists of a thin layer of dense, irregular connective tissue covered on its inner surface by a single layer of squamous mesothelium.

Vessels and Nerves of the Abdominal Wall

VASCULAR SUPPLY

The anterolateral abdominal wall receives its arterial supply from the last six intercostals and four lumbar arteries, the superior and inferior epigastric arteries, and the deep circumflex iliac arteries (Fig. 41-7). The trunks of the intercostal and lumbar arteries, together with the inter-

costal, iliohypogastric, and ilioinguinal nerves, course between the transversus abdominis and the internal oblique muscles. The most distal extensions of these vessels pierce the lateral margins of the rectus sheath at various levels and anastomose freely with branches of the superior and inferior epigastric arteries. The superior epigastric artery, one of the terminal branches of the internal mammary artery, reaches the posterior surface of the rectus abdominis muscle through the costoxiphoid space in the diaphragm. It descends within the rectus sheath to anastomose with branches of the inferior epigastric artery. The inferior epigastric artery derived from the external iliac artery just proximal to the inguinal ligament courses through the preperitoneal areolar tissue to enter the lateral rectus sheath at the semilunar line of Douglas. The deep circumflex iliac artery, arising from the lateral aspect of the external iliac artery near the origin of the inferior epigastric artery, gives rise to an ascending branch that penetrates the abdominal wall musculature just above the iliac crest, near the anterior superior iliac spine.

The venous drainage of the anterior abdominal wall follows a relatively simple pattern in which the superficial veins above the umbilicus empty into the superior vena cava by way of the internal mammary, intercostal, and long thoracic veins. The veins inferior to the umbilicus (i.e., the superficial epigastric, circumflex iliac, and the

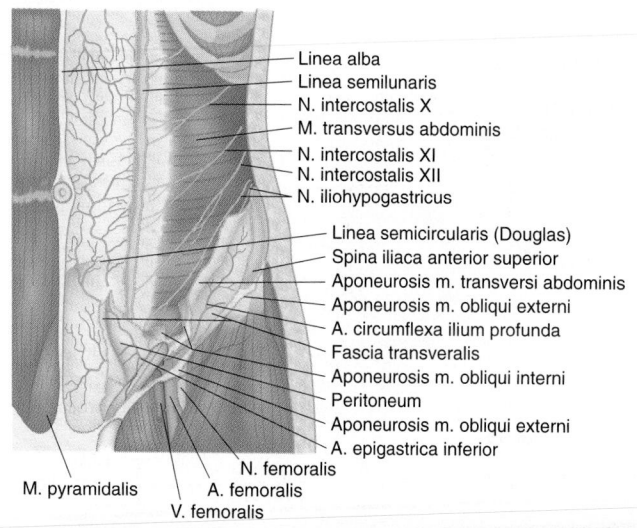

FIGURE 41-7.   The arteries and nerves of the anterolateral abdominal wall. (From McVay C: Anson and McVay's Surgical Anatomy, 6th ed. Philadelphia, WB Saunders, 1984, p 501.)

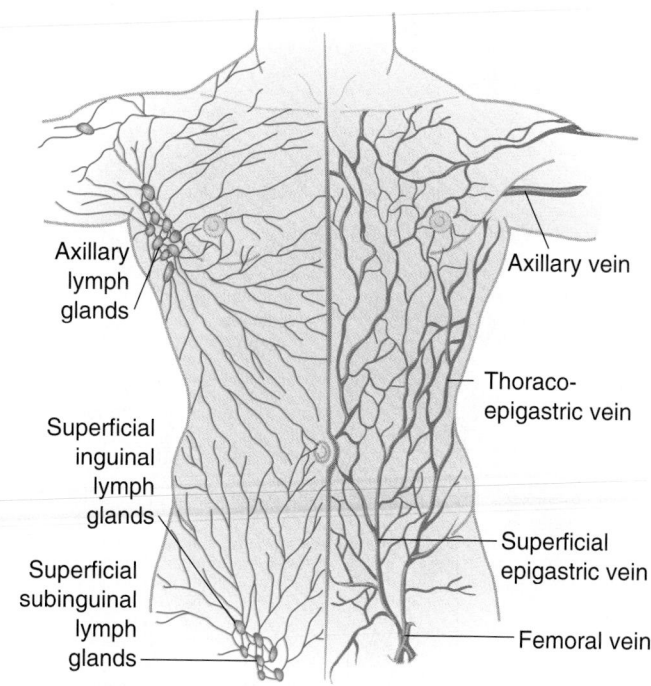

FIGURE 41-8.   The venous and lymphatic drainage of the anterolateral abdominal wall. (From Thorek P: Anatomy in Surgery, 2nd ed. Philadelphia, JB Lippincott, 1962, p 345.)

pudendal veins) converge toward the saphenous opening in the groin to enter the saphenous vein and become tributary to the inferior vena cava (Fig. 41-8). The numerous anastomoses between the infraumbilical and supraumbilical venous systems provide collateral pathways by which venous return to the heart may bypass an obstruction of either the superior or inferior vena cava. The paraumbilical vein, which passes from the left branch of the portal vein along the ligamentum teres to the umbilicus, provides important communication between the veins of the superficial abdominal wall and the portal system in patients with prehepatic or intrahepatic portal venous obstruction. In this setting, portal blood flow is diverted away from the higher pressure portal system through the paraumbilical veins to the lower pressure veins of the anterior abdominal wall. The dilated superficial paraumbilical veins in this setting are termed *caput medusae.*

The lymphatic supply of the abdominal wall follows a pattern similar to the venous drainage. Those lymphatic vessels arising from the supraumbilical region drain into the axillary lymph nodes whereas those arising from the infraumbilical region drain toward the superficial inguinal lymph nodes. The lymphatic vessels from the liver course along the ligamentum teres to the umbilicus to communicate with the lymphatics of the anterior abdominal wall. It is from this pathway that carcinoma in the liver may spread to involve the anterior abdominal wall at the umbilicus (Sister Mary Joseph node).

INNERVATION

The anterior rami of the thoracic nerves follow a curvilinear course forward in the intercostal spaces toward the midline of the body (see Fig. 41-7). The upper six thoracic nerves end near the sternum as anterior cutaneous sensory branches. Thoracic nerves 7 through 12 pass behind the costal cartilages and lower ribs to enter a plane between the internal oblique muscle and the transversus abdominis. The 7th and 8th nerves course slightly upward or horizontally to reach the epigastrium, whereas the lower nerves have an increasingly caudal trajectory. As these nerves course medially they provide motor branches to the abdominal wall musculature. Medially, they perforate the rectus sheath to provide sensory innervation to the anterior abdominal wall. The anterior ramus of the 10th thoracic nerve reaches the skin at the level of the umbilicus, and the 12th thoracic nerve innervates the skin of the hypogastrium.

The ilioinguinal and iliohypogastric nerves often arise in common from the anterior rami of the 12th thoracic and 1st lumbar nerves to provide sensory innervation to the hypogastrium and lower abdominal wall. The iliohypogastric nerve runs parallel to the 12th thoracic nerve to pierce the transversus abdominis muscle near the iliac crest. After coursing between the transversus abdominis muscle and the internal oblique for a short distance, the nerve pierces the latter to travel under the external oblique fascia toward the external inguinal ring. It emerges through the superior crus of the external inguinal ring to provide sensory innervation to the anterior abdominal wall in the hypogastrium.

The ilioinguinal nerve courses parallel to the iliohypogastric but closer to the inguinal ligament. Unlike the iliohypogastric, the ilioinguinal nerve courses with the spermatic cord to emerge from the external inguinal ring, with its terminal branches providing sensory innervation to the skin of the inguinal region and the scrotum or labium. The ilioinguinal, iliohypogastric, and genital branch of the genitofemoral nerves are commonly encountered during the performance of inguinal herniorrhaphy.

Congenital Abnormalities

Umbilical Hernias

Umbilical hernias may be classified into three distinct forms: (1) omphalocele, (2) infantile umbilical hernia, and (3) acquired umbilical hernia.

OMPHALOCELE

An omphalocele is a funnel-shaped defect in the central abdomen through which the viscera protrude into the base of the umbilical cord. It is caused by failure of the abdominal wall musculature to unite in the midline during fetal development. The umbilical vessels may be splayed over the viscera or pushed to one side. In larger defects, the liver and spleen may lie within the cord along with a major portion of the bowel. These large hernias are covered by peritoneum and, more superficially, amnion. There is no skin covering these defects. These lesions are associated with a high incidence of concomitant congenital anomalies.

Gastroschisis is another defect of the abdominal wall presenting at birth in which the umbilical membrane has ruptured, allowing the intestine to herniate outside the abdominal cavity. The defect is nearly always to the right of the umbilical cord, and the intestine is not covered with skin or amnion. Concomitant congenital anomalies occur in only about 10% of patients. Both omphalocele and gastroschisis are discussed in greater detail in Chapter 70.

INFANTILE UMBILICAL HERNIA

Infantile umbilical hernias appear within a few days or weeks after the stump of the umbilical cord has sloughed. It is caused by a weakness in the adhesion between the scarred remains of the umbilical cord and the umbilical ring. In contrast to omphalocele, the infantile umbilical hernia is covered by skin. Generally, these small hernias occur in the superior margin of the umbilical ring. They are easily reducible and become prominent when the infant cries. Most of these hernias resolve within the first 24 months of life, and complications such as strangulation are rare. Operative repair is indicated for those patients in whom the hernia has persisted beyond the age of 3 or 4 years. This condition and its management are further discussed in Chapters 42 and 70.

ACQUIRED UMBILICAL HERNIA

In this condition, an umbilical hernia develops at a time remote from closure of the umbilical ring. This hernia occurs most commonly at the upper margin of the umbilicus and results from weakening of the cicatricial tissue that normally closes the umbilical ring. This may be due to excessive stretching of the abdominal wall such as occurs with pregnancy, vigorous labor, or ascites. In contrast to infantile umbilical hernias, acquired umbilical hernias do not spontaneously resolve but instead gradually increase in size. The dense fibrous hernia ring at the neck of this hernia makes strangulation of herniated intestine or omentum an important complication.

Abnormalities Resulting from Persistence of the Omphalomesenteric Duct

During fetal development, the midgut communicates widely with the yolk sac. As the abdominal wall components approximate one another, the omphalomesenteric duct narrows and comes to lie within the umbilical cord. Over time, communication between the yolk sac and the intestine becomes obliterated and the intestine resides free within the peritoneal cavity. Persistence of part or all of the omphalomesenteric duct results in a variety of abnormalities related to the intestine and abdominal wall (Fig. 41-9).

Persistence of the intestinal end of the omphalomesenteric duct results in an abnormality known as Meckel's diverticulum. These congenital diverticula arise from the antimesenteric border of the small intestine, most often, the ileum. They are found in about 2% of the population and may be associated with inflammation, perforation, hemorrhage, or obstruction. Gastrointestinal bleeding is caused by peptic ulceration of adjacent intestinal mucosa from hydrochloric acid secreted by ectopic parietal cells within the diverticulum. Intestinal obstruction associated with Meckel's diverticulum is usually due to intussusception or to volvulus around an abnormal fibrous connection between the diverticulum and the posterior aspect of the umbilicus. These lesions are discussed in Chapter 46.

The omphalomesenteric duct may remain patent throughout its course, producing an enterocutaneous fistula between the distal small intestine and the umbilicus. This condition presents as the passage of meconium and mucus from the umbilicus in the first days of life. Because of the risk of mesenteric volvulus around a persistent omphalomesenteric duct, these lesions should be promptly treated with laparotomy and excision of the fistulous tract. Persistence of the distal end of the omphalomesenteric duct results in an umbilical polyp, which is a small excrescence of omphalomesenteric ductal mucosa at the umbilicus. Such polyps resemble umbilical granulomas except that they do not disappear after silver nitrate cauterization. They suggest the presence of a persistent omphalomesenteric duct or umbilical sinus and are most appropriately treated by excision of the mucosal remnant and underlying omphalomesenteric duct or umbilical sinus if present. Umbilical sinuses result from the persistence of the distal omphalomesenteric duct. The morphology of the sinus tract may be readily delineated by a sinogram. Treatment involves excision of the sinus. Lastly, the accumulation of mucus in a portion of a persistent omphalomesenteric duct may result in the formation of a cyst, which may be associated with either the intestine or the umbilicus by a fibrous band. Treat-

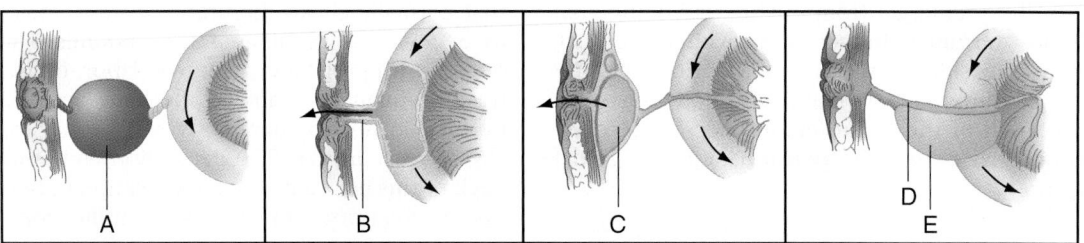

FIGURE 41-9.   Abnormalities resulting from persistence of the omphalomesenteric duct.
A, Omphalomesenteric duct cyst. **B,** Persistent omphalomesenteric duct with an enterocutaneous fistula.
C, Omphalomesenteric duct cyst and sinus. **D,** Fibrous cord between the small intestine and the posterior
surface of the umbilicus. **E,** Meckel's diverticulum. (From McVay C: Anson and McVay's Surgical Anatomy, 6th ed.
Philadelphia, WB Saunders, 1984, p 576.)

ment consists of excision of the cyst and the associated persistent omphalomesenteric duct.

Abnormalities Resulting from Persistence of the Allantois

The allantois is the most cranial component of the embryologic ventral cloaca. The intra-abdominal portion of the allantois is termed the *urachus* and connects the urinary bladder with the umbilicus, whereas the extra-abdominal part of the allantois is contained within the umbilical cord. At the end of gestation, the urachus is converted into a fibrous cord that courses between the extraperitoneal urinary bladder and the umbilicus as the median umbilical ligament. Persistence of a part or all of the urachus may result in the formation of a vesicocutaneous fistula with the appearance of urine at the umbilicus, an extraperitoneal urachal cyst presenting as a lower abdominal mass, or a urachal sinus with the drainage of a small amount of mucus. Proper treatment is excision of the urachal remnant with closure of the bladder, if necessary.

Acquired Abnormalities of the Abdominal Wall

Diastasis Recti

Diastasis recti refers to a thinning of the linea alba in the epigastrium and is manifested by a midline protrusion of the anterior abdominal wall. The transversalis fascia is intact, and hence this is not a hernia. There are no identifiable fascial margins and there is no risk of intestinal strangulation. The presence of diastasis recti may be particularly noticeable to the patient on straining or on lifting the head from the pillow. Appropriate management consists of reassurance of the patient and the family regarding the innocuous nature of this condition.

Anterior Abdominal Wall Hernias

Epigastric hernias occur at sites through which vessels and nerves perforate the linea alba to course into the subcutaneum. Through these openings extraperitoneal areolar tissue and, at times, peritoneum may herniate into the subcutaneous tissue. Although these hernias are often small, they may produce significant localized pain and tenderness owing to direct pressure of the hernia sac and its contents on the nerves emerging through the same fascial opening.

Spigellian hernias occur through the fascia in the region of the semilunar line and present as localized pain and tenderness and rarely as a palpable mass. The hernia sac is often small, tends to remain beneath the external oblique aponeurosis, and is only rarely palpable. Ultrasonography of the abdominal wall or computed tomography (CT) with thin cuts through the abdomen, after careful marking of the suspected site, may be diagnostic. Treatment consists of simple operative closure of the fascial defect. These hernias are discussed in Chapter 42.

Rectus Sheath Hematoma

Bleeding into the rectus sheath may result from blunt or penetrating injuries to the abdominal wall, including needle punctures during paracentesis or injections, violent contraction or stretching of the rectus muscle during sneezing or coughing, or, less commonly, spontaneously in patients receiving anticoagulants. Rectus sheath hematomas occur more commonly in women than men and have been reported at all ages. The most common cause in young women is pregnancy, and the most common cause in young men is trauma or muscular exertion. In older patients, anticoagulation, particularly if poorly controlled, is an important causative factor in the development of rectus sheath hematomas.

Superior to the semicircular line, the dissection of blood along the length of the rectus sheath is limited by the nondistensible nature of the rectus sheath and the tendinous inscriptions of the rectus muscle that bind the muscle to the anterior rectus sheath. Above the semicircular line, the rectus sheath tamponades the bleeding, thus limiting expansion of the hematoma. In this instance, localized abdominal pain and tenderness are relatively early findings. Below the semicircular line, the posterior rectus muscle is covered only by the transversalis fascia and the readily distensible preperitoneal layer of fatty areolar tissue. This allows expansion of the hematoma to a much larger size before the occurrence of symptoms. Most rectus sheath hematomas occur in the lower abdomen.

Abdominal pain is the most common symptom associated with rectus sheath hematomas. It is often severe and exacerbated by movements that require muscular contraction of the abdominal wall. Physical examination will demonstrate tenderness over the rectus sheath, often with voluntary guarding. A diffuse mass, or fullness, may be noted in thin patients; however, in others this will not be seen. The pain and tenderness associated with this process may be severe enough to suggest peritonitis. Ecchymosis is present only if there is a several-day delay from the onset of symptoms to presentation. In those cases in which the hematoma expands into the perivesical and preperitoneal space, the hematocrit may fall, although hemodynamic instability is uncommon.

Ultrasonography or CT will confirm the presence of the hematoma and localize it to the abdominal wall in nearly all cases. The management of patients with rectus sheath hematomas depends on the etiology and the nature of the hematoma, that is, whether there is evidence of continued hemorrhage or the hematoma is stable. In general, coagulopathy should be corrected, but continued anticoagulation of selected patients may be prudent depending on the indications for anticoagulation and the seriousness of the hemorrhage. For patients in whom the hematoma is stable, pain medication and avoidance of abdominal wall muscular strain is usually sufficient. Progression of the hematoma necessitates operative evacuation and hemostasis. In the lower abdomen, special attention should be given to the inferior epigastric vessels, which, if injured, require ligation above and below the site of bleeding.

Malignancies of the Abdominal Wall

The two most common primary malignancies of the abdominal wall are desmoid tumors and sarcomas. Although the abdominal wall may also be the site of metastatic disease, this is usually a late occurrence in the natural history of that disease. One exception is the transperitoneal seeding of the abdominal wall by intra-abdominal malignancies complicating transabdominal biopsies or operative procedures.

Desmoid Tumor

Desmoid tumor, sometimes referred to as aggressive fibromatosis, is an uncommon neoplasm that occurs sporadically or as part of an inherited syndrome, most notably, familial adenomatous polyposis (FAP). The tumor may arise from fascia or muscle and has been classified as superficial (fascial) or deep (musculoaponeurotic). The superficial disease, also known as Dupuytren's fibromatosis, is slow growing, is small, and rarely involves deeper structures. Deep fibromatosis has a relatively rapid growth rate, often attains a large size, has a high rate of local recurrence, and involves the musculature of the trunk and extremities. Desmoid tumors are also classified as extraabdominal (e.g., shoulder girdle), abdominal wall, and intra-abdominal (mesenteric and pelvic desmoid). Most spontaneous desmoid tumors occur at the shoulder girdle or the abdominal wall, whereas intra-abdominal desmoids, especially mesenteric desmoids, are more common in patients with FAP.[1-3]

In the general population, desmoid tumors occur with a frequency of 2.4 to 4.3 cases per million people[4]; this risk is increased 1000-fold in patients with FAP.[3] Typically, abdominal wall desmoid tumors occur in young women during gestation or, more frequently, within a year of childbirth. Oral contraceptive use has also been associated with the occurrence of these tumors.[5] These associations, combined with the detection of estrogen receptors within the substance of the tumor, suggest a regulatory role for estrogen in this disease. There is also often a temporal association between the development of this neoplasm and an antecedent history of abdominal trauma or operation.[4]

Patients with desmoid tumors present with a painless enlarging mass. Local symptoms may arise from compression of adjacent organs or neurovascular structures. Magnetic resonance imaging (MRI) provides information regarding the extent of the disease and its relationship to intra-abdominal organs. These tumors appear homogeneous and isointense to muscle on T1-weighted images; T2-weighted images demonstrate greater heterogeneity with a signal slightly less intense than fat. After MRI, an incisional biopsy or a core needle biopsy should be performed. This will demonstrate a tumor composed of interwoven bundles of spindle cells with variable amounts of collagen. The core of the tumor is often acellular, whereas the periphery has diffuse cellularity, suggesting a low-grade fibrosarcoma. Unlike sarcoma, the fibroblasts are highly differentiated and lack mitotic activity. Despite this benign histologic appearance, desmoids are diffusely infiltrative and tend to recur locally, even after complete resection.

The treatment of abdominal wall desmoids is complete resection with a tumor-free margin. Even with tumor-free margins the local recurrence rate approaches 40%. Although multiple local recurrences are unfortunately common, systemic metastases are extremely rare.[1] The role for radiation therapy in the management of desmoid tumors either as an adjunct to surgery or as primary treatment is evolving. In a review of 22 publications, Nuyttens and colleagues reported local control rates of 61% for surgery alone and 75% for surgery plus radiation therapy. More importantly, the combination of radiation therapy and resection improved local failure rates in patients after incomplete resection, particularly for those patients with close or microscopically positive margins, from 50% to 60% to 80% to 90%.[6] Although reports of radiation therapy alone for the treatment of desmoid tumor exist in the literature, this is generally reserved for those patients with tumors deemed unresectable.

Antiproliferative agents and cytotoxic chemotherapy have been used to palliate the aggressive nature of desmoid tumors with variable results.[4,7] The two most widely used groups of noncytotoxic drugs are nonsteroidal anti-inflammatory drugs (NSAIDs) and antiestrogens. The objective response rate for each of these agents is about 50%.[7,8] Chemotherapy has generally been reserved for unresectable, symptomatic, and clinically aggressive disease. Partial responses have been observed after treatment with doxorubicin, dactinomycin, dacarbazine, or carboplatin, although toxicity has been relatively high.[4]

Abdominal Wall Sarcoma

Truncal sarcomas (including both chest and abdominal wall) account for about 10% of sarcomas. Histologic subtypes include liposarcoma, fibrosarcoma, rhabdomyosarcoma, leiomyosarcoma, and malignant fibrous histiocytoma. The clinical behavior of these tumors is determined more by anatomic site, grade, and size than by specific histologic pattern. Similar to desmoid tumors, abdominal wall sarcomas present as a painless mass. The differential diagnosis includes many common lesions, such as ventral hernias, benign soft tissue tumors such as lipoma, and inflammatory processes, such as needle site granulomas in diabetics. Clinical characteristics that suggest an abdominal wall malignancy are (1) nonreducible lesions arising from below the superficial fascia, (2) size greater than 5 cm, (3) recent increase in size, (4) fixation to the abdominal wall, and (5) fixation to organs in the abdomen.

MRI will provide information regarding the location and extent of these neoplasms as well as involvement of contiguous structures. But definitive diagnosis requires biopsy, which may be performed with a core needle or by incision. If an incisional biopsy is performed, the incision should be placed in the same plane as the underlying muscle to minimize unnecessary tissue loss at the definitive procedure and ease reconstructive efforts. No attempt should be made to develop tissue flaps around the lesion, and hemostasis should be meticulous to avoid dissemination of the tumor along the tissue planes by a postoperative hematoma. The treatment of these malignancies is resection with a tumor-free margin. Reconstruction of the abdominal wall defect may be accomplished primarily, with myocutaneous flaps, or with prosthetic meshes, depending on the site and extent of resection.

Symptoms of Intra-abdominal Diseases Referred to the Abdominal Wall

Abdominal pain may be categorized as visceral, somatoparietal, and referred. Visceral pain is caused by stimulation of visceral nociceptors by inflammation, distention, or ischemia. The pain is dull and poorly localized to the epigastrium, periumbilical regions, or hypogastrium, depending on the embryonic origin of the organ involved. Inflammation of the stomach, duodenum, and biliary tract (derivatives of the embryonic foregut) localizes visceral pain to the epigastrium. Stimulation of nociceptors in midgut-derived organs (i.e., small intestine, appendix, and right colon) causes the sensation of pain in the periumbilical region, whereas inflammation or distention of hindgut-derived organs (left colon and rectum) causes hypogastric pain. The pain is felt in the midline because these organs transmit sympathetic sensory afferents to both sides of the spinal cord. The pain is poorly localized because the innervation of most viscera is multisegmental and contains fewer nerve receptors than highly sensitive organs such as the skin. The pain is often characterized as cramping, burning, or gnawing and may be accompanied by secondary autonomic effects, such as sweating, restlessness, nausea, vomiting, perspiration, and pallor.

Somatoparietal pain arises from inflammation of the parietal peritoneum and is more intense and more precisely localized than visceral pain. The nerve impulses mediating parietal pain travel within the somatic sensory spinal nerves and reach the spinal cord in the peripheral nerves corresponding to the cutaneous dermatomes from the sixth thoracic to the first lumbar region. Lateralization of parietal pain is possible because only one side of the nervous system innervates a given part of the parietal peritoneum.

The difference between visceral and somatoparietal pain is well illustrated by the pain associated with acute appendicitis in which the early vague periumbilical visceral pain is followed by the localized somatoparietal pain at McBurney's point. The visceral pain is produced by distention and inflammation of the appendix, whereas the localized somatoparietal pain in the right lower quadrant of the abdomen is caused by extension of the inflammation to the parietal peritoneum.

Referred pain is felt in anatomic regions remote from the diseased organ. This phenomenon is caused by convergence of visceral afferent neurons innervating an injured or inflamed organ with somatic afferent fibers arising from a specific anatomic region at the level of second-order neurons in the spinal cord. Well-known examples of referred pain include shoulder pain on irritation of the diaphragm, scapular pain associated with acute biliary tract disease, or testicular or labial pain caused by retroperitoneal inflammation.

PERITONEUM AND PERITONEAL CAVITY

Embryology

The first indication of the intraembryonic coelom occurs during the initial stages of somite differentiation when a midline cavity forms in the mesoderm. The mesoderm becomes divided by clefts on each side of the lateral plate that ultimately develop into somatic and splanchnic layers. The somatic layer was discussed earlier because it contributes to the development of the abdominal wall as the somatopleure. The splanchnic layer with its underlying endoderm becomes the splanchnopleure, which ultimately contributes to the formation of the viscera by differentiating into muscle, blood vessels, lymphatics, and connective tissues of the alimentary tract. Growth of the somatopleure results in the development of an inverted U-shaped tube that in its early stages communicates freely with the extraembryonic coelom, thus allowing the free movement of fluid into the interior of the embryo at this stage of development. As the mesodermal and ectodermal elements of the primordial somatopleure meet in the ventral midline the peritoneal cavity becomes sealed.

Anatomy

The peritoneum consists of a single sheet of simple squamous epithelium of mesodermal origin, termed *mesothelium,* lying on a thin connective tissue stroma. The surface area is 1.0 to 1.7 m², approximately that of the total body surface area. In males, the peritoneal cavity is sealed, whereas in females it is open to the exterior via the ostia of the fallopian tubes. The peritoneal membrane is divided into parietal and visceral components. The parietal peritoneum covers the anterior, lateral, and posterior abdominal wall surfaces as well as the inferior surface of the diaphragm and the pelvis. The visceral peritoneum covers most of the surface of the intraperitoneal organs (i.e., the stomach, jejunum, ileum, transverse colon, liver, and spleen) and the anterior aspect of the retroperitoneal organs (i.e., the duodenum, left and right colon, pancreas, kidneys, and adrenal glands).

The peritoneal cavity is subdivided into interconnected compartments or spaces by 11 ligaments and mesenteries. The peritoneal ligaments or mesenteries include the coronary, gastrohepatic, hepatoduodenal, falciform, gastrocolic, duodenocolic, gastrosplenic, splenorenal, and phrenicocolic ligaments and the transverse mesocolon and small bowel mesentery (Fig. 41-10). These structures partition the abdomen into nine potential spaces: right and left subphrenic, subhepatic, supramesenteric and inframesenteric, right and left paracolic gutters, pelvis, and lesser space. These ligaments, mesenteries, and peritoneal spaces direct the circulation of fluid in the peritoneal cavity and thus may be useful in predicting the route of spread of infectious and malignant diseases. For example, perforation of the duodenum from peptic ulcer disease may result in the movement of fluid (and the development of abscesses) in the subhepatic space, the right paracolic gutter, and the pelvis. The blood supply to the visceral peritoneum is derived from the splanchnic blood vessels, whereas the parietal peritoneum is supplied by branches of the intercostals, subcostal, lumbar, and iliac vessels. The innervation of the visceral and parietal peritoneum was discussed earlier.

Physiology

The peritoneum is a bidirectional, semipermeable membrane that controls the amount of fluid within the peritoneal cavity, promotes the sequestration and removal of bacteria from the peritoneal cavity, and facilitates the migration of inflammatory cells from the microvasculature into the peritoneal cavity. Normally the peritoneal cavity contains less than 100 mL of sterile serous fluid. Microvilli on the apical surface of the peritoneal mesothelium markedly increase the surface area and promote the rapid absorption of fluid from the peritoneal cavity into the lymphatics and the portal and systemic circulation. The amount of fluid within the peritoneal cavity may increase to many liters in various diseases, such as cirrhosis, nephrotic syndrome, and peritoneal carcinomatosis.

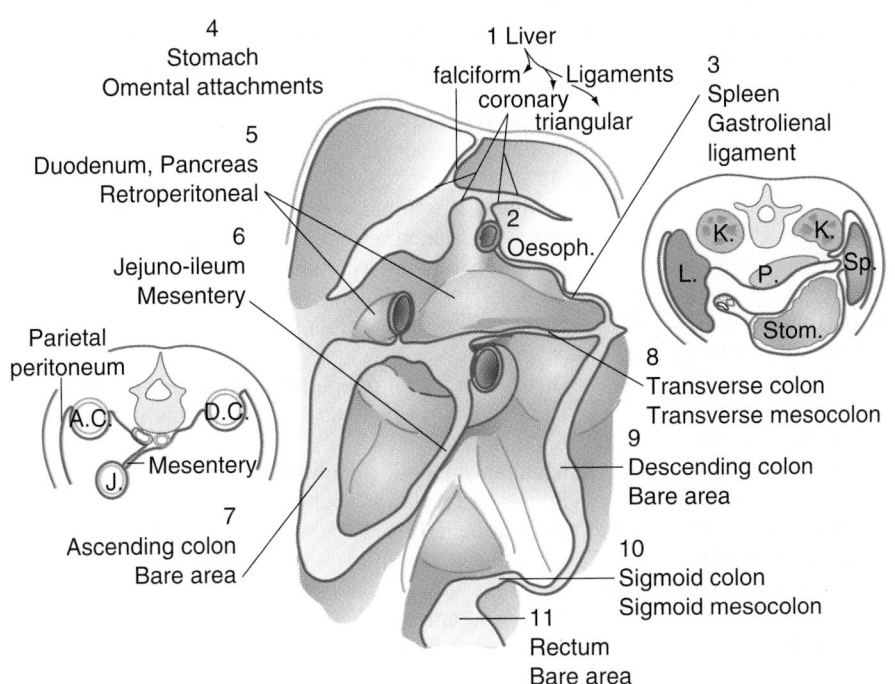

4
Stomach
Omental attachments

1 Liver
falciform   Ligaments
coronary
triangular

3
Spleen
Gastrolienal
ligament

5
Duodenum, Pancreas
Retroperitoneal

2
Oesoph.

6
Jejuno-ileum
Mesentery

Parietal
peritoneum

A.C.   D.C.

Mesentery

J.

7
Ascending colon
Bare area

K.   K.

L.   P.   Sp.

Stom.

8
Transverse colon
Transverse mesocolon

9
Descending colon
Bare area

10
Sigmoid colon
Sigmoid mesocolon

11
Rectum
Bare area

FIGURE 41-10. Peritoneal ligaments and mesenteric reflections in the adult. These attachments partition the abdomen into nine potential spaces: right and left subphrenic, subhepatic, supramesenteric and inframesenteric spaces, right and left paracolic gutters, pelvis, and omental bursa (shown in inset on right side of illustration). (From McVay C: Anson and McVay's Surgical Anatomy, 6th ed. Philadelphia, WB Saunders, 1984, p 589.)

The circulation of fluid within the peritoneal cavity is driven in part by the movement of the diaphragm. Intercellular pores in the peritoneum covering the inferior surface of the diaphragm were first described by von Recklinghausen in 1863. These intercellular pores (termed *stomata*) communicate with lymphatic pools within the diaphragm. Lymph flows from these diaphragmatic lymphatic channels via subpleural lymphatics to the regional lymph nodes and, ultimately, the thoracic duct. Relaxation of the diaphragm during exhalation opens the stomata, and the negative intrathoracic pressure draws fluid and particles, including bacteria, into the stomata. Contraction of the diaphragm during inhalation propels the lymph through the mediastinal lymphatic channels into the thoracic duct. It is postulated that this "diaphragmatic pump" drives the movement of peritoneal fluid in a cephalad direction toward the diaphragm and into the thoracic lymphatic vessels.[9,10] This circulatory pattern of peritoneal fluid toward the diaphragm and into the central lymphatic channels is consistent with the rapid appearance of sepsis in patients with generalized intra-abdominal infections as well as the perihepatitis of the Fitz-Hugh–Curtis syndrome in patients with acute salpingitis.

The peritoneum and peritoneal cavity responds to infection in five ways: (1) bacteria are rapidly removed from the peritoneal cavity via the diaphragmatic stomata and lymphatics, as described in the preceding paragraph; (2) peritoneal macrophages release proinflammatory mediators that promote the migration of leukocytes into the peritoneal cavity from the surrounding microvasculature; (3) degranulation of peritoneal mast cells releases histamine and other vasoactive products causing local vasodilation and the extravasation of protein-rich fluid containing complement and immunoglobulins into the peritoneal space; (4) protein within the peritoneal fluid opsonizes bacteria that, along with activation of the complement cascade, promote neutrophil- and macrophage-mediated bacterial phagocytosis and destruction; and (5) bacteria become sequestered within fibrin matrices, thereby promoting abscess formation and limiting the generalized spread of the infection.

Ascites

Pathophysiology and Etiology

Ascites is the pathologic accumulation of fluid within the peritoneal cavity. The principal causes of ascites formation and their pathophysiologic basis are listed in Box 41-1. Cirrhosis is an important cause of ascites in the United States. Two pathophysiologic processes contribute to the pathogenesis of ascites formation in cirrhotics: (1) hepatic fibrosis increases resistance to portal venous flow with resulting portal hypertension, and (2) nitric oxide release causes vasodilation and the systemic release of vasoconstrictors and sodium-retentive hormones, which produce a physiologic state consistent with intravascular volume depletion despite total body volume expansion.

BOX 41-1. Principal causes of ascites formation categorized according to their underlying pathophysiology

Portal Hypertension

Cirrhosis
Noncirrhotic
    Prehepatic portal venous obstruction
        Chronic mesenteric venous thrombosis
        Multiple hepatic metastases
    Posthepatic venous obstruction
        Budd-Chiari syndrome

Cardiac

Congestive heart failure
Chronic pericardial tamponade
Constrictive pericarditis

Malignancy

Peritoneal carcinomatosis
    Primary peritoneal malignancies
        Primary peritoneal mesothelioma
        Serous carcinoma
    Metastatic carcinoma
        Gastrointestinal carcinomas (e.g., gastric, colonic, and pancreatic cancer)
        Genitourinary carcinomas (e.g., ovarian cancer)
Retroperitoneal obstruction of lymphatic channels
    Lymphoma
    Lymph node metastases (e.g., testicular cancer, melanoma)
    Obstruction of the lymphatic channels at the base of the mesentery
    Gastrointestinal carcinoid tumors

Miscellaneous

Bile ascites
    Iatrogenic after operations on the liver and/or biliary tract
    Traumatic after injuries to the liver and/or biliary tract
Pancreatic ascites
    Acute pancreatitis
    Pancreatic pseudocyst
Chylous ascites
    Disruptions of retroperitoneal lymphatic channels
        Iatrogenic during retroperitoneal dissections
            Retroperitoneal lymphadenectomy
            Abdominal aortic aneurysmorrhaphy
        Blunt or penetrating trauma
    Malignancy
        Obstruction of retroperitoneal lymphatic channels
        Obstruction of lymphatic channels at the base of the mesentery
    Congenital lymphatic abnormalities
        Primary lymphatic hypoplasia
Peritoneal Infections
    Tuberculous peritonitis
Myxedema
Nephrotic syndrome
Serositis in connective tissue disease

Ascites occurs in the absence of cirrhosis in 15% to 20% of patients. Increased portal venous pressure due to obstruction of the portal venous system in the absence of cirrhosis causes the transudation of fluid across the mesenteric and intestinal wall into the peritoneal cavity. A similar pressure-based mechanism is operative in instances of cardiac failure, although in the latter cases there is also profound sodium and water retention owing to the release of vasopressin and activation of the renin-aldosterone and sympathetic nervous systems (similar to that of patients with cirrhosis). Patients with malignancies develop ascites by one of three mechanisms: (1) multiple hepatic metastases cause stenosis or occlusion of the branches of the portal vein with resultant portal hypertension; (2) multiple foci of malignant cells scattered throughout the peritoneal cavity release protein-rich fluid into the peritoneal cavity; and (3) obstruction of retroperitoneal lymphatics by malignant disease, such as lymphoma, leads to rupture of the major lymphatic channels and the leakage of chyle into the peritoneal cavity. Lastly, ascites may result from the leakage of pancreatic juice or bile into the peritoneal cavity after disruption or injury of a major pancreatic or bile duct.

Clinical Presentation

The diagnosis of ascites is made on the basis of the medical history and the appearance of the abdomen. Risk factors for hepatitis or cirrhosis should be carefully sought by questioning patients about alcohol or intravenous drug use, blood transfusions, sex with a member of the same sex, acupuncture, tattoos, or ear or body piercing. Long-standing obesity is associated with nonalcoholic steatohepatitis, an important cause of cirrhosis in the United States. Also, patients with a history of cirrhosis who suddenly develop ascites should be suspected of having hepatocellular carcinoma. Lastly, pancreatic ascites may occur in those patients with a history of pancreatitis or a pancreatic pseudocyst.

A full, bulging abdomen with dullness of the flanks on percussion is consistent with the presence of ascites. Cattau and colleagues found that about 1.5 L of fluid must be present before dullness can be detected by percussion.[11] Physical evidence of cirrhosis should be sought, including palmar erythema, large dilated abdominal wall collateral veins, and multiple spider angiomata. Patients with cardiac ascites should have impressive jugular venous distention and other evidence of congestive heart failure.

Ascitic Fluid Analysis

Paracentesis with ascitic fluid analysis is the most rapid and cost-effective method of determining the etiology of ascites. Paracentesis should be performed and ascitic fluid analyzed in all patients with new onset of ascites. The occurrence of symptoms, signs, or laboratory evidence of infection (e.g., abdominal pain or tenderness, fever, encephalopathy, hypotension, renal failure, acidosis, or leukocytosis) in patients with ascites should also prompt paracentesis with ascitic fluid analysis.

Abdominal paracentesis can be performed safely in most patients, including those with cirrhosis and mild coagulopathy. Runyon[12] suggests that only ongoing disseminated intravascular coagulation and clinically evident fibrinolysis are contraindications to paracentesis in patients with ascites. He reported no cases of hemoperitoneum, deaths, or infections in more than 229 paracenteses performed on 125 cirrhotics; abdominal hematomas occurred in 2% of cases, with only half of these requiring blood transfusion. Paracentesis is performed most commonly in the lower abdomen, with the left lower quadrant preferred over the right. Ultrasound guidance may be particularly useful in obese patients and in those with laparotomy scars and potential intra-abdominal adhesions. Consideration should be given to avoid the inferior epigastric vessels.

Examination of the ascitic fluid begins with its gross appearance. Normal ascitic fluid is slightly yellow and transparent. If the ascitic fluid contains more than 5000 neutrophils/mm^3 it will be cloudy, whereas ascitic fluid specimens with a neutrophil count less than 1000 cells/mm^3 is nearly clear. Blood within the ascitic fluid may be due to a traumatic tap, in which case the fluid may be blood-streaked and will often clot unless immediately transferred to an anticoagulant tube. Nontraumatic blood-tinged ascitic fluid does not clot because the required factors have been depleted by previous clotting with clot lysis within the peritoneal cavity. Lipid within the ascitic fluid will cause it to appear opalescent, ranging from cloudy to completely opaque and chylous. If placed in the refrigerator for 48 to 72 hours the lipids will usually layer out.

The most valuable laboratory tests on ascitic fluid include the cell count and differential and the ascitic fluid albumin and total protein concentrations. The leukocyte count in uncomplicated cirrhotic ascites is usually less than 500 cells/mm^3, with about half of these cells being neutrophils. More than 250 neutrophils/mm^3 of ascitic fluid suggests an acute inflammatory process, the most common of which is spontaneous bacterial peritonitis. In this instance, both the total white blood cell count and the absolute neutrophil count are elevated and neutrophils usually account for more than 70% of the total cell count.

The serum-ascites albumin gradient (SAAG) is the most reliable method to categorize the various causes of ascites. The SAAG is calculated by measuring the albumin concentration of serum and ascitic fluid specimens and subtracting the ascitic fluid value from the serum value. If the SAAG is greater than or equal to 1.1 g/dL, the patient has portal hypertension; a SAAG less than 1.1 g/dL is consistent with the absence of portal hypertension. Examples of high and low gradient causes of ascites are shown in Table 41-1. The accuracy of this measurement in predicting the presence or absence of portal hypertension is about 97%.[13]

Management of Ascites in Cirrhotics

For those patients in whom alcohol is an important factor in the pathogenesis of their cirrhosis, it is important to

TABLE 41-1.   Classification of Ascites by Serum–Ascites Albumin Gradient

High Gradient (≥1.1 g/dL)	Low Gradient (<1.1 g/dL)
Cirrhosis	Peritoneal carcinomatosis
Alcoholic hepatitis	Tuberculous peritonitis
Cardiac ascites	Pancreatic ascites
Massive liver metastases	Biliary ascites
Fulminant hepatic failure	Nephrotic syndrome
Budd-Chiari syndrome	Postoperative lymphatic leak
Portal vein thrombosis	Serositis in connective tissue diseases
Myxedema	

From Runyon B: Ascites and spontaneous bacterial peritonitis. *In* Sleisenger and Fordtran's Gastrointestinal and Liver Disease: Pathophysiology/Diagnosis/Management, 7th ed. Philadelphia, WB Saunders, p 1523.

convince the patient to stop drinking alcohol. Over a period of months, abstinence can allow healing of the reversible component of their liver disease and the ascites may resolve or become more responsive to medical management. The mainstays of medical management of ascites are dietary sodium restriction and diuretics. A reasonable dietary sodium restriction for most cirrhotic patients with ascites is 2 g/day. Patient compliance with this regimen may be assessed by measuring the 24-hour urinary sodium excretion. Patients compliant with their dietary restriction and who excrete more than 78 mmol/day of sodium in their urine should lose weight. If the weight is increasing despite urinary sodium losses greater than 78 mmol/day, one can assume that the patient is consuming more sodium than is prescribed. Spironolactone and furosemide, when given in a dosing ratio of 100:40, will promote natriuresis while maintaining normokalemia. In general, spironolactone (100 mg/day) and furosemide (40 mg/day) is begun initially. If this regimen is ineffective in both increasing urinary sodium and decreasing body weight, the doses of these drugs may be increased simultaneously while maintaining the 100:40 ratio.

Management of Refractory Ascites in Cirrhotics

Refractory ascites refers to that which is unresponsive to sodium restriction and high-dose diuretic treatment, a situation occurring in less than 10% of patients with ascites due to cirrhosis.[14] Current therapeutic options for these patients include liver transplantation, serial therapeutic paracentesis, transjugular intrahepatic portosystemic stent shunt, and peritoneovenous shunts. These modalities are discussed in Chapter 51.

Chylous Ascites

Chylous ascites is the collection of chyle in the peritoneal cavity and may result from one of three principal mechanisms: (1) obstruction of the major lymphatic channels at the base of the mesentery or the cisterna chyli with exudation of chyle from dilated mesenteric lymphatics; (2) direct leakage of chyle through a lymphoperitoneal fistula due to abnormal or injured retroperitoneal lymphatic vessels; and (3) exudation of chyle through the walls of retroperitoneal megalymphatics without a visible fistula or thoracic duct obstruction.

In adults, the most common cause of chylous ascites is an intra-abdominal malignancy producing obstruction of the lymphatic channels at the base of the mesentery or in the retroperitoneum. Lymphoma is the most common malignancy associated with chylous ascites, although chylous ascites has also been associated with ovarian, colon, renal, prostate, pancreatic, and gastric malignancies. Gastrointestinal carcinoids may be associated with chylous ascites owing to obstruction of the lymphatics at the base of the mesentery by invasion and the dense fibrosis characteristic of this neoplasm. In children, chylous ascites is most often caused by congenital lymphatic abnormalities, such as primary lymphatic hypoplasia, resulting in lower extremity lymphedema, chylothorax, and chylous ascites. Chylous ascites may also result from division or injury of the retroperitoneal lymphatics during operative procedures such as aortic procedures and retroperitoneal lymph node dissections. Lastly, blunt and penetrating traumatic injuries are also important causes of chylous ascites, particularly in children.

Patients with chylous ascites most often present with painless abdominal distention. Malnutrition and dyspnea occur in about 50% of cases. Paracentesis yields a characteristic milky-appearing ascitic fluid with a high protein and fat content. The serum-ascites albumin gradient will be less than 1.1 mg/dL, and the triglyceride level will be greater than that of plasma, often two to eight times that of plasma. CT, lymphoscintigraphy, and lymphangiography may provide information regarding the site of obstruction, although the latter two modalities are rarely used or available.

Management of patients with chylous ascites includes the maintenance or improvement of nutrition, reduction in the rate of chyle formation, and correction of the underlying disease process. Nutrition may be improved by enteral or parenteral formulations. In one series, a low-fat, medium-chain triglyceride diet combined with diuretics allowed the successful nonoperative management of 9 of 18 patients with chylous ascites complicating retroperitoneal lymph node dissection for testicular cancer.[15] Paracentesis may be used to temporarily relieve the dyspnea and abdominal discomfort associated with chylous ascites; however, repeated paracentesis leads to hypoproteinemia and malnutrition. Experience with peritoneovenous shunts to treat chylous ascites has generally been disappointing, owing to a variety of complications, not the least of which is rapid shunt occlusion by the highly viscous chyle. Surgical exploration of the abdomen and the retroperitoneum is recommended for those patients failing to improve with nonoperative management, an occurrence in as many as 50% to 66% of patients. Exploration of a previous operative site may identify a discrete lymphatic channel leaking chyle that may be ligated.

Peritonitis

Peritonitis is inflammation of the peritoneum and peritoneal cavity and is most commonly due to a localized or generalized infection. Primary peritonitis results from bacterial, chlamydial, fungal, or mycobacterial infection in the absence of a perforation of the gastrointestinal tract, whereas secondary peritonitis occurs in the setting of gastrointestinal perforation. Frequent causes of secondary bacterial peritonitis include perforated peptic ulcer disease, acute perforated appendicitis, perforated colonic diverticulum, and pelvic inflammatory disease.

Spontaneous Bacterial Peritonitis

Spontaneous bacterial peritonitis (SBP) is defined as a bacterial infection of ascitic fluid in the absence of an intra-abdominal, surgically treatable source of infection. Although most commonly associated with cirrhosis, SBP may also occur in patients with nephrotic syndrome and, less commonly, congestive heart failure. It is extremely rare for patients in whom the ascitic fluid has a high protein concentration to develop SBP, such as those with peritoneal carcinomatosis.[16] The most common pathogens in adults with SBP are the aerobic enteric flora *E. coli* and *Klebsiella pneumoniae*. In children with nephrogenic or hepatogenic ascites, group A *Streptococcus, Staphylococcus aureus,* and *Streptococcus pneumoniae* are common isolates. The pathogenesis of SBP remains unclear; however, several lines of evidence suggest that bacterial translocation from the gastrointestinal tract plays an important role in the development of this infection. It is postulated that local and systemic immune deficiencies in cirrhotics prevent effective opsonization, phagocytosis, and killing of translocated bacteria. Gomez and associates reported impaired Fc gamma receptors on the surface of macrophages of cirrhotics that may prevent effective phagocytosis.[17] Others have suggested that a low ascitic fluid opsonic activity also prevents effective uptake and killing of bacteria by both macrophages and neutrophils. These investigators have demonstrated both in vivo and in vitro a correlation between the total protein and C3 concentration of ascitic fluid, the capacity to kill bacteria, and the frequency of SBP.[18-20]

The diagnosis of SBP is made initially by demonstrating greater than or equal to 250 neutrophils/mm³ of ascitic fluid in a clinical setting consistent with this diagnosis (i.e., abdominal pain, fever, and/or peripheral leukocytosis in a patient with low-protein ascites).[16] It is very unusual to document bacterascites on Gram stain of ascitic fluid, and delay of appropriate antibiotic management until the ascitic fluid cultures grow bacterial isolates risks the development of overwhelming infection and death.

Broad-spectrum antibiotics, such as a third-generation cephalosporin, should be started immediately in patients suspected of having ascitic fluid infection. These agents cover about 95% of the flora most commonly associated with SBP. The spectrum of the antibiotic coverage may be narrowed once the results of antibiotic sensitivity tests are known. Repeat paracentesis with ascitic fluid analysis is not needed in the usual case in which there is rapid improvement in response to antibiotic therapy. If the setting, symptoms, ascitic fluid analysis, or response to therapy is atypical, repeat paracentesis may be helpful in detecting secondary peritonitis. Multiple bacterial isolates, particularly of gram-negative enteric organisms, combined with a poor response to antibiotic therapy, suggests the presence of secondary peritonitis. In the setting of perforation of the gastrointestinal tract, an upright abdominal or chest radiograph will often demonstrate pneumoperitoneum, the presence of which necessitates emergent laparotomy. In those instances in which pneumoperitoneum is not present on plain radiograph, CT with parenteral and enteral contrast medium enhancement may demonstrate evidence of intra-abdominal inflammation such as that associated with acute appendicitis, acute cholecystitis, or diverticulitis.

The immediate mortality risk due to SBP is low, particularly if the disease is recognized and treated expeditiously. However, the development of other complications of hepatic failure, including gastrointestinal hemorrhage or hepatorenal syndrome, contributes to the death of many of these patients during the hospitalization in which SBP is detected. The occurrence of SBP is an important landmark in the natural history of cirrhosis, with 1- and 2-year survival rates about 30% and 20%, respectively.[16]

Tuberculous Peritonitis

Tuberculosis is common in impoverished areas of the world. In the United States, tuberculosis and tuberculous peritonitis were quite common in the first half of the 20th century; however, between 1953 and 1985 the number of cases of tuberculosis declined by about 5% per year. Since 1985, the number of cases of tuberculosis has increased dramatically, especially in Hispanics, African Americans, immigrants, refugees, and individuals with acquired immunodeficiency syndrome (AIDS). The peritoneum is the sixth most common site of extrapulmonary tuberculosis after lymphatic, genitourinary, bone and joint, miliary, and meningeal sites. Most cases of tuberculous peritonitis result from reactivation of latent peritoneal disease that had been previously established hematogenously from a primary pulmonary focus. About one sixth of cases are associated with active pulmonary disease.

The illness often presents insidiously with patients having had symptoms for several weeks to months at the time of presentation. Abdominal swelling due to ascites formation is the most common symptom, occurring in more that 80% of instances. Fever, weight loss, and abdominal pain are also commonly reported. Only about half of these patients will have an abnormal chest radiograph. The tuberculin skin test is positive in most cases. The ascitic fluid SAAG is less than 1.1 g/dL. Microscopic examination of the ascitic fluid will show erythrocytes and an increased number of leukocytes, most of which are lymphocytes.

The diagnosis is best made by laparoscopy with directed biopsy of the peritoneum. This will provide a presumptive diagnosis in nearly 90% of cases. Laparotomy or laparoscopy will demonstrate multiple whitish nodules (<5 mm) scattered over the visceral and parietal peritoneum. Histologic examination will demonstrate caseating granulomas in nearly 90% of cases. Multiple adhesions between the abdominal organs and the parietal peritoneum are another common feature. Blind percutaneous peritoneal biopsy has a much lower yield than directed biopsy. Laparotomy with peritoneal biopsy is reserved for those instances in which laparoscopy has been nondiagnostic. Microscopic examination of ascitic fluid for acid-fast bacilli will identify the organism in less than 3% of cases. Similarly, the frequency of positive ascites culture for *Mycobacterium tuberculosis* occurs in less than 20% of instances. Furthermore, it may take up to 8 weeks for the culture to yield definitive information, thus limiting its diagnostic usefulness. Lastly, determination of ascitic fluid adenosine deaminase activity has been shown to have a very high accuracy for diagnosing tuberculous peritonitis. Adenosine deaminase is an enzyme involved in the catabolism of purine bases, and levels are increased in tuberculous peritonitis as a result of stimulation of T lymphocytes by mycobacterial antigens.

The treatment of peritoneal tuberculosis is antituberculous drugs. Drug regimens useful in treating pulmonary tuberculosis are also effective for peritoneal disease, with isoniazid and rifampin daily for 9 months being a commonly used and effective regimen.

Peritonitis Associated with Chronic Ambulatory Peritoneal Dialysis (CAPD)

In the United States, about 8% of patients with chronic renal failure undergo peritoneal dialysis. Peritonitis is one of the most common complications of CAPD, occurring with an incidence of approximately one episode every 1 to 3 years. Patients present with abdominal pain, fever, and cloudy peritoneal dialysate containing more than 100 leukocytes/mm^3, with more than 50% of the cells being neutrophils. Gram stain will detect organisms in only 10% to 40% of cases. About 75% of infections are due to gram-positive organisms, with *Staphylococcus epidermidis* accounting for 50% of cases. *Staphylococcus aureus*, gram-negative enteric organisms, and fungal species are also important causes of peritonitis associated with CAPD.

Peritonitis associated with CAPD is treated by the intraperitoneal administration of antibiotics with an appropriate antibacterial spectrum (e.g., first-generation cephalosporins). Ultimately, the most appropriate regimen must be based on the antibiotic sensitivities of the specific causative agents. Recurrent or persistent peritonitis requires removal of the dialysis catheter and resumption of hemodialysis.

Malignant Neoplasms of the Peritoneum

Malignant neoplasms of the peritoneum may be classified as primary or secondary, depending on the site of origin of the tumor. Primary malignancies of the peritoneum are rare and include malignant mesothelioma and its subtypes, serous tumors, malignant tumors of other müllerian types, desmoplastic small round cell tumor, and sarcomas. Most malignancies of the peritoneum are transperitoneal metastases from a carcinoma of the gastrointestinal tract (especially the stomach, colon, and pancreas), the genitourinary tract (most commonly, ovarian), or, more rarely, an extra-abdominal site (e.g., breast). In its advanced stage, where metastatic cancer deposits diffusely coat the visceral and parietal peritoneum, these peritoneal metastases are referred to as carcinomatosis.

Malignant Peritoneal Mesothelioma

The most common primary malignant peritoneal neoplasm is malignant mesothelioma. The median survival rate for patients with this rare tumor is 4 to 12 months. At least in part, this poor prognosis is due to the very advanced stage of the disease at the time of presentation. Patients present with abdominal pain, ascites, and weight loss. Fifty to 70 percent of patients will have a history of asbestos exposure.[21] The omentum may be diffusely involved with tumor and present as an epigastric mass. CT will demonstrate mesenteric thickening, peritoneal studding, hemorrhage within the tumor, and ascites. At laparotomy the ascitic fluid ranges from a serous transudate to a viscous fluid rich in mucopolysaccharides. The neoplasm tends to involve all peritoneal surfaces producing large masses of tumor. In contrast to pseudomyxoma peritonei, local invasion of intra-abdominal organs, such as the liver, intestine, bladder, and abdominal wall, is the rule.

It may be difficult to differentiate a malignant peritoneal mesothelioma from diffuse peritoneal carcinomatosis arising from an intra-abdominal organ such as the stomach, pancreas, colon, or ovary. Careful intra-operative examination of the pattern of spread and a generous biopsy for histologic evaluation will often allow this distinction to be made. Furthermore, malignant peritoneal mesothelioma generally remains confined to the abdomen whereas advanced-stage intra-abdominal carcinomas frequently have pulmonary and other extra-abdominal metastases. Extension of the mesothelioma into one or both pleural cavities is more likely than hematogenous dissemination.

Complete surgical resection is rarely possible, and most commonly operative intervention is used to provide palliation for intestinal obstruction. Radiation therapy alone, whether using open field techniques, intraperitoneal instillation of radioactive agents, or external-beam radiation therapy, has had very limited success and significant associated morbidity. Intraperitoneal chemotherapy, including the use of cisplatin and mitomycin C, have been reported, but with very limited success.[22] Even in those patients with complete response, relapse is generally rapid.[23] Combined modality approaches hint of a brighter future. In one retrospective review of 15 patients treated with cytoreductive surgery and chemotherapy, Eltabbakh and associates reported a median survival of 29 months.[24] Park and colleagues reported that cytoreductive surgery, followed by hyperthermic peritoneal perfusion with cisplatin, led to a median progression-free survival of 26 months with an overall 2-year survival of 80%.[25] Similarly, Loggie and coworkers combined cytoreductive surgery with intraperitoneal heated chemotherapy perfusion of mitomycin-C in 12 patients for whom the median survival was 34.2 months with follow-up to 45 months.[21]

Pseudomyxoma Peritonei

Pseudomyxoma peritonei is a rare malignant process of the peritoneal cavity that characteristically arises from a ruptured ovarian or appendiceal adenocarcinoma. In this disease, the peritoneum becomes coated with a mucus-secreting tumor that fills the peritoneal cavity with tenacious, semisolid mucus. Large loculated cystic masses may also form within the abdomen.

Pseudomyxoma peritonei is most prevalent in women between 50 and 70 years of age. It is often asymptomatic until very late in its course, and patients often experience a global deterioration in their health long before the diagnosis of pseudomyxoma peritonei is made. Symptoms include abdominal pain and distention as well as numerous nonspecific symptoms. Physical examination reveals a distended abdomen with nonshifting dullness. On occasion, a palpable abdominal mass may be present, especially in tumors of appendiceal origin. CT may demonstrate posterior displacement of the small intestine, loculated collections of fluid density material, and scalloping of intra-abdominal organs due to extrinsic pressure of adjacent peritoneal implants. At laparotomy, liters of yellowish gray mucoid material are present on the omental and peritoneal surfaces.

The management of these patients includes drainage of the mucus and intraperitoneal fluid and cytoreduction of the primary and secondary tumor implants, including peritonectomy and omentectomy. For those tumors originating from an appendiceal adenocarcinoma, a right colectomy should also be performed. Ovarian malignancies should be treated with total abdominal hysterectomy and bilateral salpingo-opherectomy as well as cytoreduction. In the setting of an indeterminant site of origin, a right colectomy and resection of the omentum along with bilateral oophorectomy and cytoreduction surgery should be performed. Postoperative adjuvant therapy has included the use of intraperitoneal 5-fluorouracil, mitomycin-C, and cisplatin[26] as well as intraperitoneal mucolytics, such as dextran sulfate and plasminogen activator (urokinase).[27] Although the tumor will recur in approximately two thirds of patients, the slow progression of the disease results in 5- and 10-year survival rates of 50% and 20%, respectively.[28] In one report, aggressive cytoreductive surgery combined with intraperitoneal 5-fluorouracil and mitomycin-C resulted in a 10-year survival rate of 80%.[26,29]

MESENTERY AND OMENTUM

Embryology and Anatomy

The greater and lesser omenta are complex peritoneal folds that pass from the stomach to the liver, transverse colon, spleen, bile duct, pancreas, and diaphragm. They originate from the dorsal and ventral midline mesenteries of the embryonic gut. In the very early stages of development, the alimentary canal traverses the future coelomic cavity as a straight tube suspended posteriorly by an uninterrupted dorsal mesentery and anteriorly by a ventral mesentery in the cranial portion of its extent. The embryonic stomach appears as a fusiform swelling in the proximal alimentary tube that rotates 90 degrees on its longitudinal axis such that the lesser curvature faces to the right and the greater curvature to the left. Much of the embryonic ventral mesentery is resorbed; however, the portion extending from the fissure of the ligamentum venosum and the porta hepatis to the proximal duodenum, the lesser curvature of the stomach (gastrohepatic ligament), persists as the lesser omentum. The right border is a free edge at which the two continuous layers form the anterior border of the opening into the lesser sac termed the *foramen of Winslow.* Between the layers of the lesser omentum and at its right border are the common hepatic duct, the portal vein, and the hepatic artery.

The embryonic dorsal mesogastrium grows as a sheet of peritoneum extending from the greater curvature of the stomach over the anterior surface of the small intestine. After passing inferiorly almost to the pelvis, the peritoneal membrane turns upon itself to pass upward to a line of attachment on the transverse colon slightly above that of the transverse mesocolon. Fat is laid down in this omental apron and provides an insulating layer of protection of the abdominal viscera.

In the early stages of development, the embryonic small intestine elongates to form an anteriorly oriented intestinal loop that then rotates counterclockwise, such that the cecum and the future ascending colon move to the right side of the peritoneal cavity and the descending colon assumes a vertical position on the left wall of the peritoneal cavity. The jejunum and ileum are supported by a peritoneum-covered dorsal mesentery carrying the mesenteric blood vessels and lymphatics. The posterior line of attachment extends obliquely from the duodenojejunal junction at the left side of the second lumbar vertebra toward the right iliac fossa to terminate anterior to the sacroiliac articulation.

Physiology

The omentum and the intestinal mesentery are rich in lymphatics and blood vessels. The omentum contains areas with high concentrations of macrophages that may aid in the removal of foreign material and bacteria. Furthermore, the omentum becomes densely adherent to intraperitoneal sites of inflammation, often preventing free peritonitis during instances of intestinal gangrene or perforation (e.g., acute diverticulitis or acute appendicitis).

Diseases of the Omentum

Omental Cysts

Omental cysts are unilocular or multilocular cysts containing serous fluid that are thought to arise from congenital or acquired obstruction of omental lymphatic channels. They are lined by a lymphatic endothelium similar to that of cystic lymphangiomas. Most commonly omental cysts are discovered in children or young adults. Small cysts are often asymptomatic and discovered at the time of laparotomy for an unrelated problem, whereas larger cysts may present as a palpable abdominal mass. Uncomplicated cysts usually lie in the lower mid abdomen and are freely movable, smooth, and nontender. Complications are more common in children and include torsion, infection, or rupture.

Plain radiographs of the abdomen may show a well-circumscribed soft tissue density in the mid abdomen, and contrast studies of the intestine may show displacement of intestinal loops and extrinsic compression on adjacent bowel. Ultrasound or CT will show a fluid-filled mass with internal septations, the differential diagnosis of which includes cysts and solid tumors of the mesentery, peritoneum, and retroperitoneum, including desmoid tumors. Ultimately, the diagnosis is made by excision of the cyst and histologic examination of the wall. Local excision is curative.

Omental Torsion and Infarction

Torsion of the greater omentum is defined as the axial twisting of the omentum along its long axis, causing ischemia. This condition requires the omentum to be fixed in one point with the remainder of the structure redundant and free within the peritoneal cavity. If the twist is tight enough (or the venous obstruction is of sufficient duration), arterial inflow will become compromised leading to infarction and necrosis. Omental torsion is classified as primary when no coexisting causative condition is identified or as secondary when the torsion occurs in association with a causative condition such as a hernia, tumor, or adhesion. Secondary omental torsion is more common than primary torsion and occurs when the central portion of the omentum twists between the two fixed points. Primary omental torsion most frequently involves the right side of the omentum; it is postulated that the greater weight and relative freedom of the right omentum makes torsion more likely on the right that the left.

Omental torsion occurs twice as often in men as women and is most frequent in patients in their fourth or fifth decades of life. Patients present with the acute onset of severe abdominal pain, which is localized to the right side of the abdomen in 80% of patients. Nausea and vomiting may be present but is not a predominant finding. There may be a moderate leukocytosis, and the patient's temperature is often normal or only slightly elevated. Physical examination demonstrates localized abdominal tenderness, with guarding suggesting peritonitis. A mass may be palpable if the involved omentum is sufficiently large.

The differential diagnosis includes any disease associated with right-sided abdominal pain and tenderness, most notably acute appendicitis, acute cholecystitis, and torsion of an ovarian cyst. CT may demonstrate an omental mass and may suggest the presence of inflammation but is generally not adequately specific to make the diagnosis. Often the patient's clinical presentation will justify laparotomy, at which time free serosanguineous fluid, a congested and inflamed portion of the omentum, and the absence of another pathologic condition will suggest the occurrence of omental torsion. Treatment consists of resection of the involved omentum and correction of any related condition.

Omental Neoplasms

Primary malignancies of the omentum are extremely rare events, and when they do occur they are most commonly of soft tissue origin. A more common scenario is involvement of the omentum by metastatic tumor spread transperitoneally from an intra-abdominal carcinoma. In an advanced stage, the omentum becomes replaced by the metastatic tumor, resulting in the descriptive term *omental cake.*

Omental Grafts and Transpositions

The arterial and venous blood supply to the greater omentum is derived from omental branches of the right and left gastroepiploic arteries, which course along the greater curvature of the stomach. Division of the right or left gastroepiploic artery and the vasa recta along the greater curvature of the stomach with mobilization of the omentum from the transverse colon allows the development of a vascularized omental pedicle flap. This graft may be used to cover chest and mediastinal wounds after chest wall resections and to prevent the small intestine from entering the pelvis after abdominal perineal resection (thus preventing radiation enteritis during radiation therapy for rectal carcinoma). Lastly, the formation of dense adhesions between the omentum and sites of perforation or inflammation facilitates its use as a patch for perforations of the duodenum (Graham patch [Fig. 41-11]) or for buttressing anastomoses.

Diseases of the Mesentery

Mesenteric Cysts

The most common non-neoplastic mesenteric cysts are termed *mesothelial cysts* based on the ultrastructure of the cells lining the cyst. The cysts contain either chyle or a clear serous fluid and may occur in the mesentery of either the small intestine (60%) or the colon (40%). These cysts occur most commonly in adults, with a mean age of 45 years, and are twice as common in women as in men. Depending on the size of the cyst, patients may present with complaints of abdominal pain, fever, and emesis. A mid-abdominal mass may be palpable on examination of the abdomen. The diagnosis can usually be made preoperatively with ultrasonography or CT. Enucleation of the cyst at laparotomy is curative and can usually be accomplished because the mesenteric blood vessels and the intestinal wall are usually not adherent to the cyst wall.

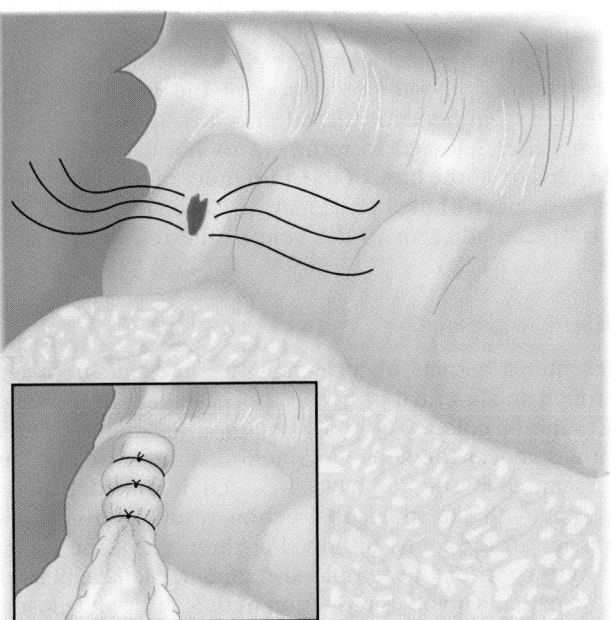

FIGURE 41-11.   Closure of a perforated duodenal ulcer with an omental (Graham) patch. (From Graham: Surg Gynecol Obstet 64:235-238, 1937.)

Internal drainage of the cyst into the peritoneal cavity has also been successfully employed in the management of very large cysts. Aspiration alone has a very high rate of cyst recurrence. In those instances in which the cyst is not completely excised, the contents of the cyst and the internal architecture of the cyst wall must be carefully inspected and the cyst wall examined histologically to ensure a non-neoplastic etiology.

Acute Mesenteric Lymphadenitis

Acute mesenteric lymphadenitis is a syndrome of acute right lower quadrant abdominal pain associated with mesenteric lymph node enlargement and a normal appendix. Generally, the diagnosis is made on exploration of the abdomen of a patient suspected of having acute appendicitis, at which time a normal appendix and enlarged mesenteric lymph nodes are discovered. This syndrome occurs most commonly in children and young adults and with equal frequency in males and females.

Numerous causative agents have been implicated in the pathobiology of acute mesenteric lymphadenitis, including viral, bacterial, parasitic, and fungal infections. *Yersinia enterocolitica* in particular has been associated with this syndrome in children. Culture and histologic examination of the enlarged lymph nodes, stool culture, and antibody titers have been used to identify causative agents but are not routinely employed in the management of these patients.

The symptom-complex associated with acute mesenteric lymphadenitis is similar to acute appendicitis and includes the acute onset of periumbilical pain, which shifts to the right lower quadrant over time. Physical examination demonstrates right lower quadrant tenderness with abdominal wall muscular rigidity and rebound tenderness. Nausea, vomiting, and anorexia may also be present but are not dominant features. Generally, the patient's temperature and white blood cell count are normal or only slightly elevated.

The diagnosis is made at the time of operation for presumed acute appendicitis, at which time a normal-appearing appendix is found with enlarged mesenteric lymph nodes. Excision of an enlarged lymph node with culture and nodal histology may provide information regarding the etiology but is not routinely employed.

Mesenteric Panniculitis

Mesenteric panniculitis is an inflammatory disease of the adipose tissue of the mesentery. It is also referred to as mesenteritis, isolated lipodystrophy, retroperitoneal xanthogranuloma, sclerosing lipogranulomatosis, and lipogranuloma of the mesentery. The small bowel mesentery is most frequently involved, although the mesocolon may also be affected. Grossly, the disease is characterized by a thickened, hard, rubbery, or nodular mesentery or by multiple mesenteric masses of this consistency. The process most often involves the root of the small bowel mesentery and frequently encompasses the mesenteric vessels. In advanced cases, mesenteric venous and lymphatic obstruction may be present. Irregular areas of discoloration, ranging from gray to reddish brown to pale yellow, suggesting fat necrosis are scattered throughout the mesentery. In some patients there is foreshortening and scarring of the mesentery with distortion of the bowel. Histologic findings include abnormal fat cells with foamy cytoplasm and infiltration by mononuclear inflammatory cells. Lipid-laden macrophages are invariably present and foreign body giant cells, fatty necrosis, calcification, and collagenous replacement may also be present in advanced cases.

Mesenteric panniculitis occurs most commonly in the fifth decade of life, but it has been reported in persons of nearly all ages. The disease is twice as common in males as females. The majority of patients present with abdominal pain; vomiting and abdominal swelling occur less commonly. Other complaints include anorexia, weight loss, constipation, diarrhea, and rectal bleeding. An abdominal mass is palpable in about half of patients; abdominal tenderness and/or distention, fever, and evidence of peritoneal irritation are present in a small number of cases.

Laboratory studies are usually normal except that the erythrocyte sedimentation rate may be elevated. Barium contrast studies of the intestine and colon may reveal extrinsic displacement of intestinal loops, fixed, dilated loops of small intestine, and a spiculated or serrated mucosal appearance suggestive of extrinsic inflammation. Laparotomy or laparoscopy with biopsy of the involved mesentery remains necessary for definitive diagnosis.

Mesenteric panniculitis requires treatment only infrequently. Resection or bypass is necessary only in those instances associated with bowel obstruction. The prognosis in mesenteric panniculitis is good, with lethal disease reported only rarely. In general, abdominal pain continues or recurs in about 25% of patients after diagnosis.

Intra-abdominal (Internal) Hernias

Internal Hernias Due to Developmental Defects

There are three general mechanisms by which developmental abnormalities cause the formation of internal hernias: (1) abnormal retroperitoneal fixation of the intestinal mesentery resulting in anomalous positioning of the intestine (i.e., mesocolic or paraduodenal hernias); (2) abnormally large internal foramina or fossa (i.e., foramen of Winslow and supravesical hernias); and (3) incomplete mesenteric surfaces with the presence of an abnormal opening or orifice through which the intestine herniates (i.e., mesenteric hernias).

MESOCOLIC (OR PARADUODENAL) HERNIAS

Mesocolic hernias are unusual congenital hernias in which the small intestine herniates behind the mesocolon. They result from abnormal rotation of the midgut and have been categorized as either right or left. A right mesocolic hernia occurs when the prearterial limb of the midgut loop fails to rotate around the superior mesenteric artery. This results in the majority of the small intestine remaining to the right of the superior mesenteric artery. Normal counterclockwise rotation of the cecum and proximal colon into the right side of the abdomen and its fixation to the posterolateral peritoneum causes the small intestine to become trapped behind the mesentery of the right side of the colon. The ileocolic, right colic, and middle colic vessels lie within the anterior wall of the sac, and the superior mesenteric artery courses along the medial border of the neck of the hernia (Fig. 41-12A).

It is postulated that the left mesocolic hernia occurs as a consequence of in utero herniation of the small intestine between the inferior mesenteric vein and the posterior parietal attachments of the descending mesocolon to the retroperitoneum. The inferior mesenteric artery and vein are integral components of the hernia sac (see Fig. 41-12B). About 75% of mesocolic hernias occur on the left side.

The most common clinical presentation is that of small intestinal obstruction, in which patients may present with symptoms of either acute or chronic small bowel obstruction. Barium radiographs will demonstrate displacement of the small intestine to the left or the right side of the abdomen. CT with intravenous contrast medium enhancement may demonstrate displacement of the mesenteric vessels.

The operative management of patients with a right mesocolic hernia involves incision of the lateral peritoneal reflections along the right colon with reflection of the right colon and cecum to the left. The entire gut then assumes a position simulating that of nonrotation of both the prearterial and postarterial segments of the midgut. Opening the neck of the hernia will injure the superior mesenteric vessels and fail to free the herniated bowel (see Fig. 41-12C).

The operative management of patients with a left mesocolic hernia consists of incision of the peritoneal attachments and adhesions along the right side of the inferior mesenteric vein with reduction of the herniated small intestine from beneath the inferior mesenteric vein. The vein is then allowed to return to its normal position on the left side of the base of the mesentery of the small intestine. The neck of the hernia may be closed by suturing the peritoneum adjacent to the vein to the retroperitoneum (see Fig. 41-12D).

MESENTERIC HERNIAS

Mesenteric hernias occur when the intestine herniates through an abnormal orifice in the mesentery of the small intestine or colon. The most common location for these hernias is near the ileocolic junction, although defects in the sigmoid mesocolon have also been described. Patients present with intestinal obstruction resulting from compression of the loops of bowel at the neck of the hernia or by torsion of the herniated segment. Management of these patients involves reduction of the hernia and closure of the mesenteric defect.

Acquired Internal Hernias

Acquired internal hernias result from the creation of abnormal mesenteric defects after operative procedures or trauma. Most commonly these result from inadequate closure (or dehiscence) of mesenteric defects created during the performance of gastrojejunostomy, colostomy, ileostomy, or bowel resection. The creation of a small space allows the herniation of the small intestine through the mesenteric rent and the development of intestinal obstruction. The treatment of these patients is operative with reduction of the hernia and closure of the peritoneal defect.

Malignancies of the Mesentery

Similar to the situation in the peritoneum and omentum, the most common neoplasm involving the mesentery is metastatic disease from an intra-abdominal adenocarcinoma. This may result from the direct invasion of the primary tumor (or its lymphatic metastases) into the mesentery or from the transperitoneal spread of the malignancy into the mesentery. Distortion and fixation of the mesentery by the tumor itself or by the resultant desmoplastic reaction may cause intestinal obstruction. The most common primary malignancy of the mesentery is a desmoid tumor.

Mesenteric Desmoid

Mesenteric desmoid accounts for less than 10% of sporadic desmoid tumors; however, it is a particularly common tumor in patients with FAP. In this group of patients, 70% of the desmoid tumors are intra-abdominal and one half to three fourths of these involve the mesentery.[2-4] The association between desmoid tumor and FAP is particularly strong in that subset of patients with

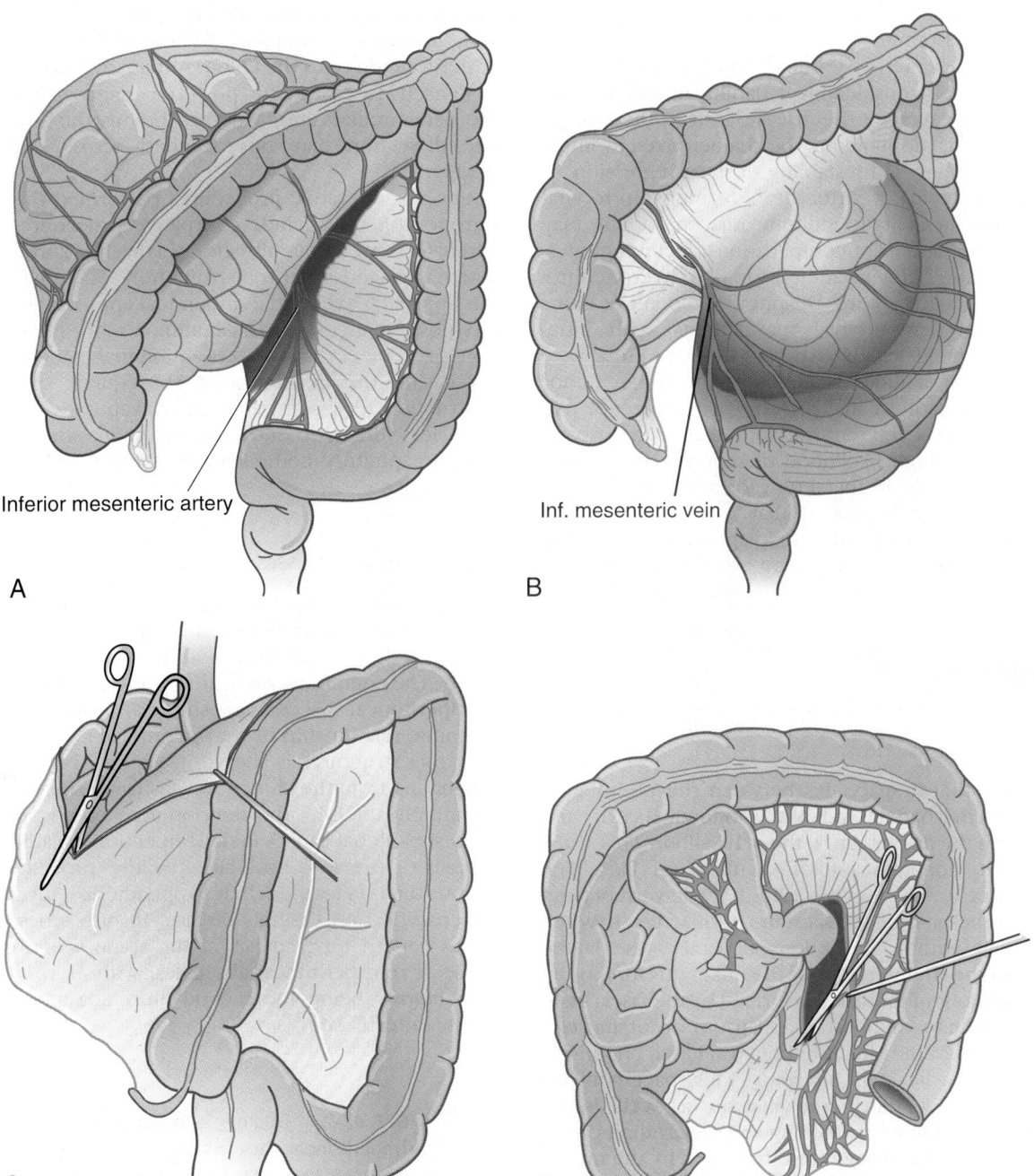

Inferior mesenteric artery

A

Inf. mesenteric vein

B

C

D

FIGURE 41-12.   A, Right mesocolic (paraduodenal) hernia. Note that the anterior wall of a right mesocolic hernia is the ascending mesocolon. The hernia orifice lies to the right of the midline and the superior mesenteric artery and ileocolic artery course along the anterior border of the hernia neck. **B,** Left mesocolic (paraduodenal) hernia. The hernia orifice is to the left of the midline and the herniated intestine lies behind the anterior wall of the descending mesocolon. **C,** A right mesocolic hernia is repaired by division of the lateral peritoneal attachments of the ascending colon, reflecting it toward the left side of the abdomen. The small and large intestine then assumes a position simulating that of nonrotation of both the pre-arterial and postarterial segments of the midgut. Opening the neck of the hernia will injure the superior mesenteric vessels and fail to free the herniated bowel. **D,** A left mesocolic hernia is reduced by incising the hernia sac along an avascular plane immediately to the right of the inferior mesenteric vessels. (**A** and **B,** From Brigham R, d'Avis JC: Paraduodenal hernia. *In* Nyhus LM, Condon RE [eds]: Hernia, 3rd ed. Philadelphia, JB Lippincott, 1989, pp 484 and 485; **C** and **D,** from Brigham R, et al: Paraduodenal hernia: Diagnosis and surgical management. Surgery 96:498, 1984.)

Gardner's syndrome. Patients with FAP and a family history of desmoid tumors have a 25% chance of developing a desmoid tumor.[3]

Although mesenteric desmoid tumors tend to be aggressive, there is considerable variability in their growth rate during the course of the disease. In fact, the biology of intra-abdominal desmoid may be characterized by initial rapid growth followed by stability or even regression.[5,30] Mesenteric desmoid, by virtue of its relationship to vital structures and its ability to infiltrate adjacent organs, may however cause significant complications, including intestinal obstruction, ischemia and perforation, hydronephrosis, and even aortic rupture. Despite these complications the overall 10-year survival for patients with intra-abdominal desmoids can be as high as 60% to 70%.[4,30]

The treatment of choice is complete resection of tumor with margins free of the malignancy. The recurrence rate after resection has been reported to be between 60% and 85%.[4] Given the high likelihood of recurrence and prolonged survival even in the setting of advanced disease, some authors have suggested that a trial of watchful waiting along with minimally toxic agents such as sulindac and antiestrogen therapy may be the best strategy, particularly in patients with minimal symptoms.[5,30]

RETROPERITONEUM

Anatomy

The retroperitoneal space lies between the peritoneum and the posterior parietal wall of the abdominal cavity and extends from the diaphragm to the pelvic floor. This space contains two contiguous fossa: lumbar and iliac. The lumbar fossa extends from the 12th thoracic vertebra and 12th rib to the base of the sacrum and iliac crest. When viewed from within the abdominal cavity, the lateral margin is to the lateral border of the quadratus lumborum muscle. The floor of the space is formed by the fascia overlying the quadratus lumborum and psoas major muscles and extends from the lateral lumbocostal arch superiorly to the iliolumbar ligament inferiorly. This space contains varying amounts of fatty areolar tissue as well as the adrenal glands, kidneys, ascending and descending colon, and duodenum. This space is also traversed by the ureter, renal vessels, gonadal vessels, the inferior vena cava, and aorta. The iliac fossa is continuous with that of the lumbar region above, the lateral and anterior preperitoneal spaces of the abdominal wall, and the pelvis inferiorly. The iliacus muscle with its investing fascia represents the floor of the iliac fossa. The iliac fossa contains the iliac vessels, ureter, genitofemoral nerve, spermatic or ovarian vessels, and the iliac lymph nodes.

Retroperitoneal Operative Approaches

The aorta, vena cava, iliac vessels, kidneys, and adrenal glands may be approached operatively through the retroperitoneal space. The extent of dissection is limited in the posterior midline by the major visceral branches of the aorta. Superiorly, dissection is limited by fusion of the peritoneum to the undersurface of the diaphragm; and, inferiorly, dissection is limited by the reflection of peritoneum onto the colon. Anteriorly, the peritoneum is densely fused to the posterior rectus sheath above the semicircular line, whereas below the semicircular line dissection may be extended across the midline readily.

Specific operative procedures performed through the retroperitoneum include extirpative procedures such as adrenalectomy and nephrectomy as well as aortic aneurysmorrhaphy and renal transplantation. The advantages to this approach over a transabdominal approach include (1) less postoperative ileus facilitating a more rapid resumption of a diet; (2) no intra-abdominal adhesions, thus decreasing the likelihood of subsequent small bowel obstruction; (3) less intraoperative evaporative fluid losses with less dramatic intravascular fluid shifts; and (4) fewer respiratory complications such as atelectasis and pneumonia.

Retroperitoneal Abscesses

Retroperitoneal abscesses may be classified as primary if the infection results from hematogenous spread or secondary if they are related to an infection in an adjacent organ. The conditions associated with the development of retroperitoneal abscesses are shown in Table 41-2, and the anatomic relationship of retroperitoneal abscesses to surrounding structures is shown in Figure 41-13. Infections originating from the kidney and gastrointestinal tract most commonly underlie the development of retroperitoneal abscesses. Renal causes include infections related to renal lithiasis or previous urologic operative procedures. Gastrointestinal causes include appendicitis, diverticulitis, pancreatitis, and Crohn's disease. In one series from an urban center, tuberculosis of the spine was a common cause of retroperitoneal abscesses, with *Mycobacterium tuberculosis* being the second most common bacterial isolate, after *E. coli*.[31]

TABLE 41-2. Etiology and Relative Frequency of Retroperitoneal Abscesses	
Etiology	**Frequency (%)**
Renal diseases	47
Gastrointestinal diseases, including diverticulitis, appendicitis, and Crohn's disease	16
Hematogenous spread from remote infections	11
Abscesses complicating operative procedures	8
Bone infections, including tuberculosis of the spine	7
Trauma	4.5
Malignancies	4
Miscellaneous causes	3

These data were compiled from three retrospective reviews[31-33] of 134 patients treated between 1971 and 2001.

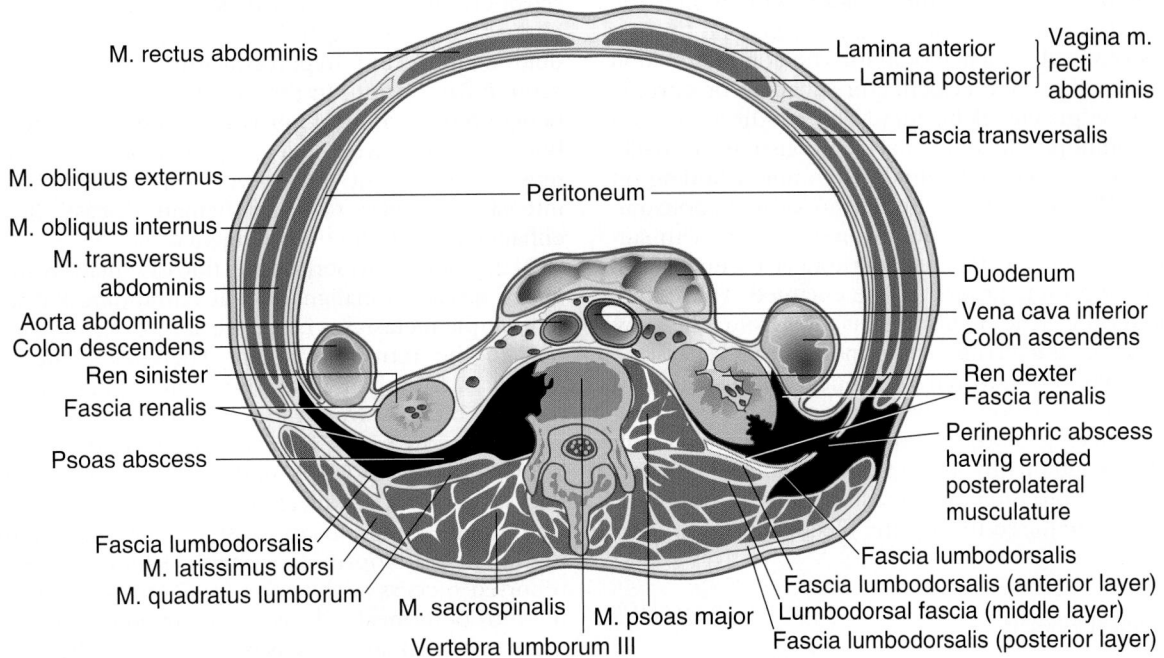

FIGURE 41-13. The anatomic relationships of retroperitoneal abscesses to surrounding structures. A psoas abscess is shown on the left side of the image, and a perinephric abscess is shown to the right. (From McVay C: Anson and McVay's Surgical Anatomy, 6th ed. Philadelphia, WB Saunders, 1984, p 735.)

The bacteriology of retroperitoneal abscesses is related to the etiology. Infections originating from the kidney are often monomicrobial and involve gram-negative rods such as *Proteus mirabilis* and *E. coli*. Retroperitoneal abscesses associated with diseases of the gastrointestinal tract involve *E. coli*, *Enterobacter* species, enterococcus, as well as anaerobic species such as *Bacteroides*. These infections often involve numerous bacterial species, including gram-negative bacilli, enterococcus, and anaerobic species. Infections from hematogenous spread are most commonly monomicrobial and related to staphylococcal species. Tuberculosis of the spine is an important cause of retroperitoneal abscesses in immunocompromised individuals and those emigrating from underdeveloped countries.

The most common symptoms include abdominal or flank pain (60% to 75%), fever and chills (30% to 90%), malaise (10% to 22%), and weight loss (12%).[32,33] Patients with psoas abscesses may have referred pain to the hip, groin, or knee. The duration of symptoms is often greater than 1 week. Patients with retroperitoneal abscesses frequently have concurrent, chronic illnesses such as renal lithiasis, diabetes mellitus, human immunodeficiency virus infection, or malignancies.

CT will demonstrate a low density mass within the retroperitoneum with surrounding inflammation. Gas may be present in as many as a third of these lesions.[31] CT will provide important information regarding the exact location of the abscess as well as its relationship to contiguous organs, hence likely sources of the infection.

Treatment of retroperitoneal abscesses includes appropriate antibiotics and adequate drainage. Many reports have demonstrated the efficacy of CT-guided drainage in managing this aspect of the treatment.[31,33] In one recent study, 86% of abscesses resolved with this approach.[33] Operative drainage through a retroperitoneal approach is indicated for those lesions not amenable to percutaneous drainage or those lesions that fail percutaneous drainage.

The mortality rate for patients with retroperitoneal abscesses is related, at least in part, to the presence of significant medical comorbidities. In one study in which 72% of their patients had significant concurrent medical problems the overall mortality rate was 26% and the major complication rate was 50%.[32] In another recent study, in which many fewer patients had diabetes or other systemic illnesses, the mortality rate was only 1.6%.[33]

Retroperitoneal Hematomas

Retroperitoneal hematomas most commonly occur after blunt or penetrating injuries, in the setting of abdominal aortic or visceral artery aneurysms, or after acute or chronic anticoagulation or fibrinolytic therapy. The diagnosis and management of retroperitoneal hematomas occurring in the setting of trauma or aneurysmal rupture are considered in detail in Chapters 20, 64, and 66. Bleeding into the retroperitoneum also may complicate anticoagulant therapy, including low molecular weight heparin for medical conditions such as atrial fibrillation or deep venous thrombosis. Retroperitoneal hematomas have also been described in patients undergoing fibrinolytic therapy for peripheral or coronary arterial thrombosis as well as in patients with bleeding diatheses such as hemophilia.

Patients present with abdominal or flank pain that may radiate into the groin, labia, or scrotum. Clinical evidence of acute blood loss may be present depending on the volume of blood lost and the rapidity with which the patient bled. A palpable abdominal mass may be present as well as physical evidence of ileus. The complete blood cell count may provide evidence of subacute or chronic blood loss or platelet deficiency. The prothrombin and partial thromboplastin times may demonstrate a coagulopathy. Microscopic hematuria is a common finding on urinalysis. CT will establish the diagnosis by demonstrating a high density mass in the retroperitoneum with surrounding stranding in the retroperitoneal tissue planes. The involved muscle group may be enlarged. These findings should be readily distinguishable from the low density mass characteristic of retroperitoneal abscesses.

Patients who develop retroperitoneal hematomas as a result of anticoagulation are best managed by the restoration of circulating blood volume and correction of the underlying coagulopathy. In rare circumstances, arteriography with embolization of a bleeding artery or operative exploration is required to stop the bleeding.

Retroperitoneal Fibrosis

Retroperitoneal fibrosis is an uncommon inflammatory condition characterized by the proliferation of fibrous tissue in the retroperitoneum. Seventy percent of cases are idiopathic (termed *Ormand's disease*), whereas 30% are associated with various drugs (most notably, ergot alkaloids or dopaminergic agonists), infections, trauma, retroperitoneal hemorrhage or retroperitoneal operations, radiation therapy, or primary or metastatic neoplasms. Many of the idiopathic cases are associated with inflammatory abdominal aortic aneurysms or vasculitis syndromes. The fibrosis is usually confined to the central and paravertebral spaces between the renal arteries and sacrum and tends to encase the aorta, inferior vena cava, and ureters. The process usually begins at the level of the aortic bifurcation and spreads cephalad. In 15% of instances, the fibrotic process extends outside the retroperitoneum to also involve the peripancreatic and periduodenal spaces, the pelvis, and the mediastinum.

Patients present with a vague constellation of symptoms, including abdominal or flank pain, weight loss, malaise, and hypertension. Scrotal or leg edema caused by lymphatic obstruction may also be present. Laboratory tests will often provide evidence of renal insufficiency and anemia. Other laboratory abnormalities include an elevated erythrocyte sedimentation rate and an elevated C-reactive protein. The diagnosis is based on the patient's history and intravenous urography demonstrating hydronephrosis and hydroureter associated with delayed excretion and medial deviation of the ureters. Most commonly the disease is bilateral, although unilateral cases do occur. CT without intravenous contrast medium enhancement will show a fibrous plaque that is usually isodense or slightly hyperdense compared with surrounding muscle. In early lesions, intravenous instillation of contrast medium will cause enhancement of the fibrous plaques owing to the greater vascularity of lesions at this stage, whereas at later stages of disease the avascular fibrotic plaque shows no enhancement. MRI of early benign retroperitoneal fibrosis may show areas of high signal intensity on T2-weighted images owing to the abundant fluid content and hypercellularity associated with the acute inflammation. In the mature and quiescent stage of benign retroperitoneal fibrosis, the low signal intensity on both T1- and T2-weighted images is similar to that of psoas muscle. Malignant retroperitoneal fibrosis has signal intensities similar to early benign disease (i.e., early enhancement with contrast agent).

Malignant retroperitoneal fibrosis may result from direct spread of malignant cells entrapping the ureter or to multiple metastases causing a severe desmoplastic reaction in the retroperitoneum. Therefore, differentiating malignant from benign fibrosis is important and requires multiple biopsies from the retroperitoneal fibrotic tissue. Katz and coworkers have reported good success with Tru-Cut needle biopsies under CT guidance.[34] Primary, idiopathic retroperitoneal fibrosis is treated with ureteral stenting and immunosuppression, including methylprednisolone, azathioprine, or penicillamine. Others have reported success with tamoxifen.[35] Most secondary cases of retroperitoneal fibrosis are treated with midline transperitoneal ureterolysis with wrapping the ureter with an omental flap or lateral retroperitoneal ureteral transposition. In one report of 14 patients undergoing ureterolysis with an omental flap, 12 had relief of ureteral obstruction evident on follow-up intravenous urograms.[34]

Retroperitoneal Malignancies

Malignancies in the retroperitoneum may result from (1) extracapsular growth of a primary neoplasm of a retroperitoneal organ such as the kidney, adrenal, colon, or pancreas; (2) development of a primary germ cell neoplasm from embryonic rest cells; (3) development of a primary malignancy of the retroperitoneal lymphatic system (e.g., lymphoma); (4) metastases from a remote primary malignancy into a retroperitoneal lymph node (e.g., testicular cancer); and (5) development of a malignancy of the soft tissue of the retroperitoneum, including sarcomas and desmoid tumors. The most common primary malignancy of the retroperitoneum is a sarcoma.

Retroperitoneal Sarcoma

About 15% of all soft tissue sarcomas occur in the retroperitoneum and about 8300 new cases of retroperitoneal sarcomas present in the United States each year.[36,37] Patients with von Recklinghausen's disease and Li-Fraumeni syndrome have an increased incidence of sarcoma. Furthermore, patients with mutations of the *p53* and *RB1* genes also appear to have a predilection for the development of sarcoma, suggesting that these genes may play an important regulatory role in the malignant transformation to sarcoma.

Most patients with retroperitoneal sarcomas present with an asymptomatic abdominal mass, often after the primary tumor has reached a considerable size. Abdominal pain is present in half of patients and less common symptoms, depending on the location of the tumor and the specific organs involved, include gastrointestinal hemorrhage, early satiety, nausea and vomiting, weight loss, and lower extremity swelling. Symptoms related to nerve compression by the tumor, such as lower extremity paresthesia and paresis, have also been associated with retroperitoneal sarcoma. CT and MRI will provide important information regarding the size and precise location of the primary tumor and its relationship to major vascular structures as well as the presence or absence of metastatic disease. Preoperative imaging studies will provide important clues to the diagnosis, and hence a histologic diagnosis of sarcoma by CT-guided core biopsy is usually reserved for those lesions with a significant likelihood to be lymphoma or germ cell tumor. The CT and gross appearance of a large retrohepatic sarcoma is shown in Figure 41-14. In general, the diagnosis can be confirmed at the time of definitive resection by simple incisional or core needle biopsy.

The goal of sarcoma treatment is the complete en bloc resection of the tumor and any involved adjacent organs. Lymph node metastasis by sarcoma is rare (<5%), and hence radical lymphadenectomy is not indicated unless there is gross evidence of lymph node involvement at the time of resection. The most important prognostic variable is the ability to resect the neoplasm with a tumor-free resection margin. Table 41-3 summarizes the results from several large series of patients with retroperitoneal sarcoma. Rates of resectability of the primary retroperitoneal sarcoma vary widely, based on the extent of disease at presentation, surgeon's experience, and the institution's referral pattern. Local recurrence after complete resection of retroperitoneal sarcoma is common, occurring in 40% to 80% of cases.[38,39] There is no difference in the rate of local recurrence when comparing high-grade and low-grade sarcomas; however, the median time to recurrence is much shorter in high-grade than in low-grade sarcoma (15 months vs. 42 months).[40] Patients with high-grade sarcoma also have a higher risk for systemic disease and death than do those patients with low-grade sarcoma.[38,39]

In patients with recurrent disease, complete resection of recurrent sarcoma is beneficial. In a report by Lewis and colleagues at the Memorial Sloan-Kettering Cancer Center, of the 61 patients with recurrent sarcoma, 35 underwent complete resection. This group of patients had a significantly higher survival rate than those undergoing incomplete resection (60% vs. 18% 5-year disease-specific

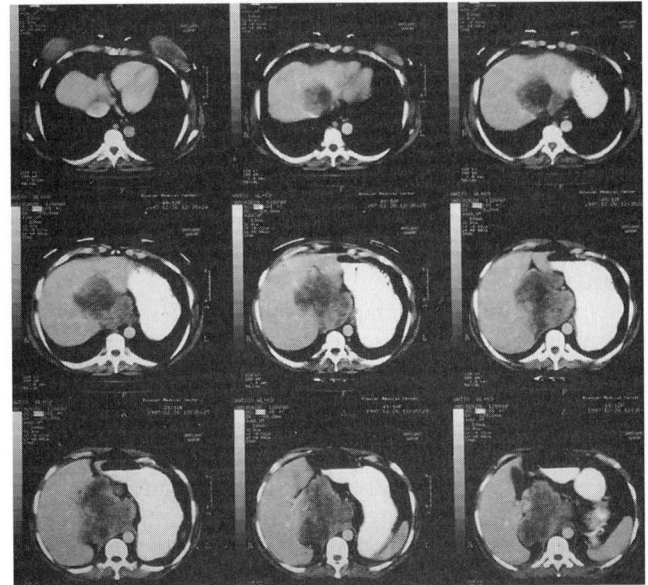

A

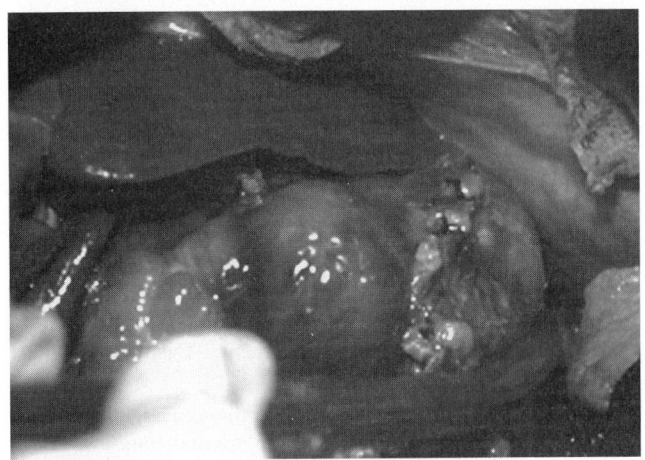

B

FIGURE 41-14. **A,** CT scan of the upper abdomen of a patient with a large sarcoma originating from the upper retroperitoneum. **B,** Intraoperative photograph of this tumor presenting in the subhepatic space.

TABLE 41-3. Outcomes in the Primary Resection of Retroperitoneal Sarcoma

Study	No. of Patients	Resectability (%)	Local Recurrence at 5 Yr (%)	Survival at 5 Yr (%)	Median Survival (mo)
Lewis et al., 1998[38]	278	83	41	NR	72
Alvarenga et al., 1991[48]	120	25	80	29	NR
Singer et al., 1995[39]	83	NR	NR	54*	NR
Karakousis et al., 1996[46]	57	100	42	66	NR

NR, not reported.
*Reported at 12 years.

survival).[38] Unlike extremity sarcoma, the role for external-beam radiation therapy for local control after surgical resection is limited by the low tolerance for radiation injury of the surrounding normal tissue. External-beam radiation therapy[41,42] as well as combined intraoperative brachytherapy plus external-beam irradiation[43,44] have been used for local control of these malignancies. Unfortunately, the potential benefits of radiation therapy after complete resection have been offset by the early and late radiation toxicity.[45,46]

As with radiation therapy, most of the literature on the use of chemotherapy has been on extremity sarcoma. Specific retrospective studies on the efficacy of postoperative chemotherapy for retroperitoneal sarcoma have not shown significant benefits.[39,46] Limited experience with preoperative chemotherapy and radiation therapy for sarcoma has also been disappointing.[47] As such, adjuvant therapy (chemotherapy and radiation therapy) in retroperitoneal sarcoma should be offered in the context of a clinical trial. These may also play a role in the palliation of symptomatic inoperable disease.

Selected References

McVay C (ed): Anson and McVay's Surgical Anatomy, 6th ed. Philadelphia, WB Saunders, 1984.

Thorek P: Anatomy in Surgery, 2nd ed. Philadelphia, JB Lippincott, 1962.

> Thorek's Anatomy in Surgery and Anson and McVay's Surgical Anatomy are classic texts of anatomy, beautifully illustrated and written from a surgeon's perspective.

Guarner C, Runyon BA: Spontaneous bacterial peritonitis: Pathogenesis, diagnosis and management. Gastroenterologist 3:311-328, 1995.

> This is an outstanding review of the causes, diagnosis, and management of patients with spontaneous bacterial peritonitis.

Runyon BA, Montano AA, Akrividadis EA, et al: The serum-ascites albumin gradient is superior to the exudates-transudate concept in the differential diagnosis of ascites. Ann Intern Med 117:215-220, 1992.

> This very well-written paper describes and defends the use of the serum-ascites albumin gradient in the elucidation of the pathophysiology of ascites formation.

Willwerth BM, Zollinger RM, Izant RJ: Congenital mesocolic (paraduodenal) hernia: Embryologic basis of repair. Am J Surg 128:358-361, 1974.

> This is a classic description of right and left mesocolic hernias. The authors suggest an embryologic basis for the occurrence of these hernias as well as a clear description on their management.

References

1. Biermann JS: Desmoid tumors. Curr Treat Options Oncol 1:262-266, 2000.
2. Anthony T, Rodriguez-Bigas MA, Weber TK, Petrelli NJ: Desmoid tumors. J Am Coll Surg 182: 369-377, 1996.
3. Gurbuz AK, Giardiello FM, Peterson GM, et al: Desmoid tumours in familial adenomatous polyposis. Gut 35:377-381, 1994.
4. Kulaylat MN, Karakousis CP, Keaney CM, et al: Desmoid tumour: A pleomorphic lesion. Eur J Surg Oncol 25:487-497, 1999.
5. Burke AP, Sobin LH, Shekitka KM, et al: Intra-abdominal fibromatosis: A pathologic analysis of 130 tumors with comparison of clinical subgroups. Am J Surg Pathol 14:335-341, 1990.
6. Nuyttens JJ, Rust PF, Thomas CT, Turrisi AT: Surgery versus radiation therapy for patients with aggressive fibromatosis or desmoid tumors: A comparative review of 22 articles. Cancer 88:1517-1523, 2000.
7. Klein WA, Miller HH, Anderson M: The use of indomethacin, sulindac, and tamoxifen for the treatment of desmoid tumours associated with familial polyposis. Cancer 60:2863-2868, 1987.
8. Kinzbrunner B, Ritter S, Domingo J, Rosenthal CJ: Remission of rapidly growing desmoid tumors after tamoxifen therapy. Cancer 52:2201-2204, 1983.
9. Abu-Hijleh MF, Habbal OA, Moqattash ST: The role of the diaphragm in lymphatic absorption from the peritoneal cavity. J Anat 186:453-467, 1995.
10. Last M, Kurtz L, Stein TA, Wise L: Effect of PEEP on the rate of thoracic duct lymph flow and clearance of bacteria from the peritoneal cavity. Am J Surg 145:126-130, 1983.
11. Cattau E, Benjamin SB, Knuff TE, Castell DO: The accuracy of the physical exam in the diagnosis of suspected ascites. JAMA 247:1164-1166, 1982.
12. Runyon BA: Paracentesis of ascitic fluid: A safe procedure. Arch Intern Med 146:2259-2261, 1986.
13. Runyon BA, Montano AA, Akrividadis EA, et al: The serum-ascites albumin gradient is superior to the exudates-transudate concept in the differential diagnosis of ascites. Ann Intern Med 117:215-220, 1992.
14. Stanley MM, Ochi S, Lee KK, et al: Peritoneovenous shunting as compared with medical management in patients with alcoholic cirrhosis and massive ascites. N Engl J Med 321:1632-1638, 1989.
15. Baniel J, Rowland R: Management of chylous ascites after retroperitoneal lymph node dissection for testicular cancer. J Urol 150:1422-1424, 1993.
16. Guarner C, Runyon BA: Spontaneous bacterial peritonitis: Pathogenesis, diagnosis and management. Gastroenterologist 3:311-328, 1995.
17. Gomez P, Ruiz P, Schreiber AD: Impaired function of macrophage FC-gamma receptors and bacterial infection in alcoholic cirrhotics. N Engl J Med 331:1122-1128, 1994.
18. Runyon BA: Low-protein-concentration ascitic fluid is predisposed to spontaneous bacterial peritonitis. Gastroenterology 91:1343-1346, 1986.
19. Such J, Guarner C, Enriquez J: Low C3 in ascitic fluid predisposes to spontaneous bacterial peritonitis. J Hepatol 6:80-84, 1988.
20. Runyon BA: Patients with deficient ascitic fluid opsonic activity are predisposed to spontaneous bacterial peritonitis. Hepatology 8:632-635, 1988.
21. Loggie BW, Fleming RA, McQuellon RP, et al: Prospective trial for the treatment of malignant peritoneal mesothelioma. Am Surg 67:999-1003, 2001.
22. Hayashi T, Nasu Y, Aramaki K, et al: A case of peritoneal malignant mesothelioma with disappearance of ascites: Results of intraperitoneal instillation of mitomycin C and oral administration of UFT. Gan To Kagaku Ryoho 16:2449-2452, 1989.

23. Howell SB, Pfeifle CL, Wung WE, et al: Intraperitoneal cisplatin with systemic thiosulfate protection. Ann Intern Med 97:845-851, 1982.

24. Eltabbakh GH, Piver MS, Hempling RE, et al: Clinical picture, response to therapy, and survival of woman with diffuse malignant peritoneal mesothelioma. J Surg Oncol 70:6-12, 1999.

25. Park BJ, Alexander HR, Libutti SK: Treatment of primary peritoneal mesothelioma by continuous hyperthermic peritoneal perfusion (CHPP). Ann Surg Oncol 6:582-590, 1999.

26. Sugarbaker PH, Fernandez-Trigo V, Shamsa F: Clinical determinants of treatment failure in patients with pseudomyxoma peritonei. Cancer Treat Res 81:121-132, 1996.

27. Beller FK, Zimmerman RE, Nienhaus H: Biochemical identification of mucus of pseudo-myxoma peritonei as the basis of mucolytic treatment. Am J Obstet Gynecol 155:970-973, 1986.

28. Jivan S, Bahal V: Pseudomyxoma peritonei. Postgrad Med J 78:170-172, 2002.

29. Sugarbaker PH: Pseudomyxoma peritonei. Cancer Treat Res 81:105-119, 1996.

30. Smith AJ, Lewis JJ, Merchant NB, et al: Surgical management of intra-abdominal desmoid tumours. Br J Surg 87:608-613, 2000.

31. Paley M, Sidhu PS, Evans RA, Karani JB: Retroperitoneal collections—aetiology and radiological implications. Clin Radiol 52:290-294, 1997.

32. Crepps JT, Welch JP, Orlando R: Management and outcome of retroperitoneal abscesses. Ann Surg 205:276-281, 1987.

33. Manjon CC, Sanchez AT, Lara JD, et al: Retroperitoneal abscesses. Scand J Nephrol 37:139-144, 2003.

34. Katz R, Golijanin D, Pode D, Shapiro A: Primary and postoperative retroperitoneal fibrosis—experience with 18 cases. Urology 60:780-783, 2002.

35. Owens LV, Cance WG, Huth JF: Retroperitoneal fibrosis treated with tamoxifen. Am J Surg 61:842-844, 1995.

36. Fieg BW: Retroperitoneal sarcomas. Surg Oncol Clin North Am 12:369-377, 2003.

37. Jemal A, Murray T, Samuels A, et al: Cancer Statistics, 2003. CA Cancer J Clin 53:5-26, 2003.

38. Lewis JJ, Leung D, Woodruff JM, Brennan ME: Retroperitoneal sarcoma: Analysis of 500 patients treated and followed at a single institution. Ann Surg 228:355-365, 1998.

39. Singer S, Corson JM, Demnetri GD: Prognostic factors predictive of survival for truncal and retroperitoneal soft tissue sarcoma. Ann Surg 222:185-195, 1995.

40. Jacques D, Coit D, Hajdu S, Brennan M: Management of primary and recurrent soft tissue sarcoma of the retroperitoneum. Ann Surg 212:51-59, 1990.

41. Catton C, O'Sullivan B, Kotwall C, et al: Outcome and prognosis in retroperitoneal soft tissue sarcoma. Int J Radiat Oncol Biol Phys 29:1005-1010, 1994.

42. Fein D, Corn B, Lanciano R, et al: Management of retroperitoneal sarcomas: Does dose escalation impact on locoregional control? Int J Radiat Oncol Biol Phys 31:129-134, 1995.

43. Tepper JE, Suit HD, Wood WC: Radiation therapy of retroperitoneal soft tissue sarcomas. Int J Radiat Oncol Biol Phys 10:825-830, 1984.

44. Sindelar WF, Kinsella TJ, Chen PW: Intraoperative electron beam radiotherapy in retroperitoneal sarcomas: Results of a prospective randomized clinical trial. Arch Surg 128:402-407, 1993.

45. Glenn J, Sindelar WF, Kinsella T: Results of multi-modality therapy of resectable soft tissue sarcomas of the retroperitoneum. Surgery 97:316-325, 1985.

46. Karakousis CP, Velez AF, Gerstenbluth R: Resectability and survival in retroperitoneal sarcomas. Ann Surg Oncol 3:150-158, 1996.

47. Sondak VK, Robertson JM, Sussman JJ, et al: Preoperative idoxuridine and radiation for large soft tissue sarcomas: Clinical results with five-year follow-up. Ann Surg Oncol 5:106-112, 1998.

48. Alvaranga JC, Ball AB, Fisher C: Limitations of surgery in the treatment of retroperitoneal sarcoma. Br J Surg 78:912-916, 1991.

CHAPTER 42

HERNIAS

Mark A. Malangoni, M.D. and **Raymond J. Gagliardi, M.D.**

Incidence	Special Problems
Anatomy	Umbilical Hernias
Classification	Epigastric Hernias
Diagnosis	Incisional and Ventral Hernias
Nonoperative Management	Unusual Hernias
Operative Repair	Complications
Femoral Hernias	Quality of Life

More than 600,000 hernias are repaired annually in the United States, making hernia repair one of the most common operations performed by general surgeons. Despite the frequency of this procedure, no surgeon has ideal results, and complications such as postoperative pain, nerve injury, infection, and recurrence continue to challenge surgeons.

"Hernia" is derived from the Latin word for rupture. A hernia is defined as an abnormal protrusion of an organ or tissue through a defect in its surrounding walls. Although a hernia can occur at various sites of the body, these defects most commonly involve the abdominal wall, particularly the inguinal region. Abdominal wall hernias occur only at sites when the aponeurosis and fascia are not covered by striated muscle (Box 42-1). These sites most commonly include the inguinal, femoral, and umbilical areas, the linea alba, the lower portion of the semilunar line, and sites of prior incisions (Fig. 42-1). The "neck" or orifice of a hernia is located at the innermost musculoaponeurotic layer whereas the hernia sac is lined by peritoneum and protrudes from the neck. There is no consistent relationship between the area of a hernia defect and the size of a hernia sac.

A hernia is *reducible* when its contents can be replaced within the surrounding musculature, and it is *irreducible* or *incarcerated* when it cannot be reduced. A *strangulated* hernia has compromised blood supply to its contents, which is a serious and potentially fatal complication. Strangulation occurs more often in large hernias that have small orifices. In this situation, the small neck of the hernia obstructs arterial blood flow, venous drainage, or both to the contents of the hernia sac. Adhesions between the contents of the hernia and the peritoneal lining of the sac can provide a tethering point that entraps the hernia contents and predisposes to intestinal obstruction and strangulation. A more unusual type of strangulation is a Richter's hernia. In a Richter's hernia, a small portion of the antimesenteric wall of the intestine is trapped within the hernia and strangulation can occur without the presence of intestinal obstruction.

An *external* hernia protrudes through all layers of the abdominal wall, whereas an *internal* hernia is a protrusion of intestine through a defect within the peritoneal cavity. An *interparietal* hernia occurs when the hernia sac is contained within a musculoaponeurotic layer of the abdominal wall.

Inguinal hernias are classified as either *direct* or *indirect*. The sac of an indirect inguinal hernia passes from the internal inguinal ring obliquely toward the external inguinal ring and ultimately into the scrotum. In contrast, the sac of a direct inguinal hernia protrudes outward and forward and is medial to the internal inguinal ring and inferior epigastric vessels. Although it sometimes can be difficult to distinguish between an indirect and a direct inguinal hernia, this distinction is of little importance because the operative repair of these types of hernias is similar.

INCIDENCE

Hernias are a common problem; however, their true incidence is unknown. It is estimated that 5% of the population will develop an abdominal wall hernia, but the

Box 42-1. Abdominal Wall Hernias

Groin

Inguinal
  Indirect
  Direct
  Combined
Femoral

Anterior

Umbilical
Epigastric
Spigelian

Pelvic

Obturator
Sciatic
Perineal

Posterior

Lumbar
  Superior triangle
  Inferior triangle

prevalence may be even higher. Approximately 75% of all hernias occur in the inguinal region. Two thirds of these are indirect, and the remainder are direct inguinal hernias. Based on national operative statistics, incisional hernias account for 15% to 20% of all abdominal wall hernias, umbilical and epigastric hernias constitute 10% of hernias, femoral hernias for about 5%, and unusual hernias for the remainder.

Men are 25 times more likely to have a groin hernia than women. An indirect inguinal hernia is the most common hernia, regardless of gender. In men, indirect hernias predominate over direct hernias at a ratio of 2 to 1. Direct hernias are very uncommon in women. There is a female dominance in femoral and umbilical hernias of approximately 10 to 1 and 2 to 1, respectively. Although

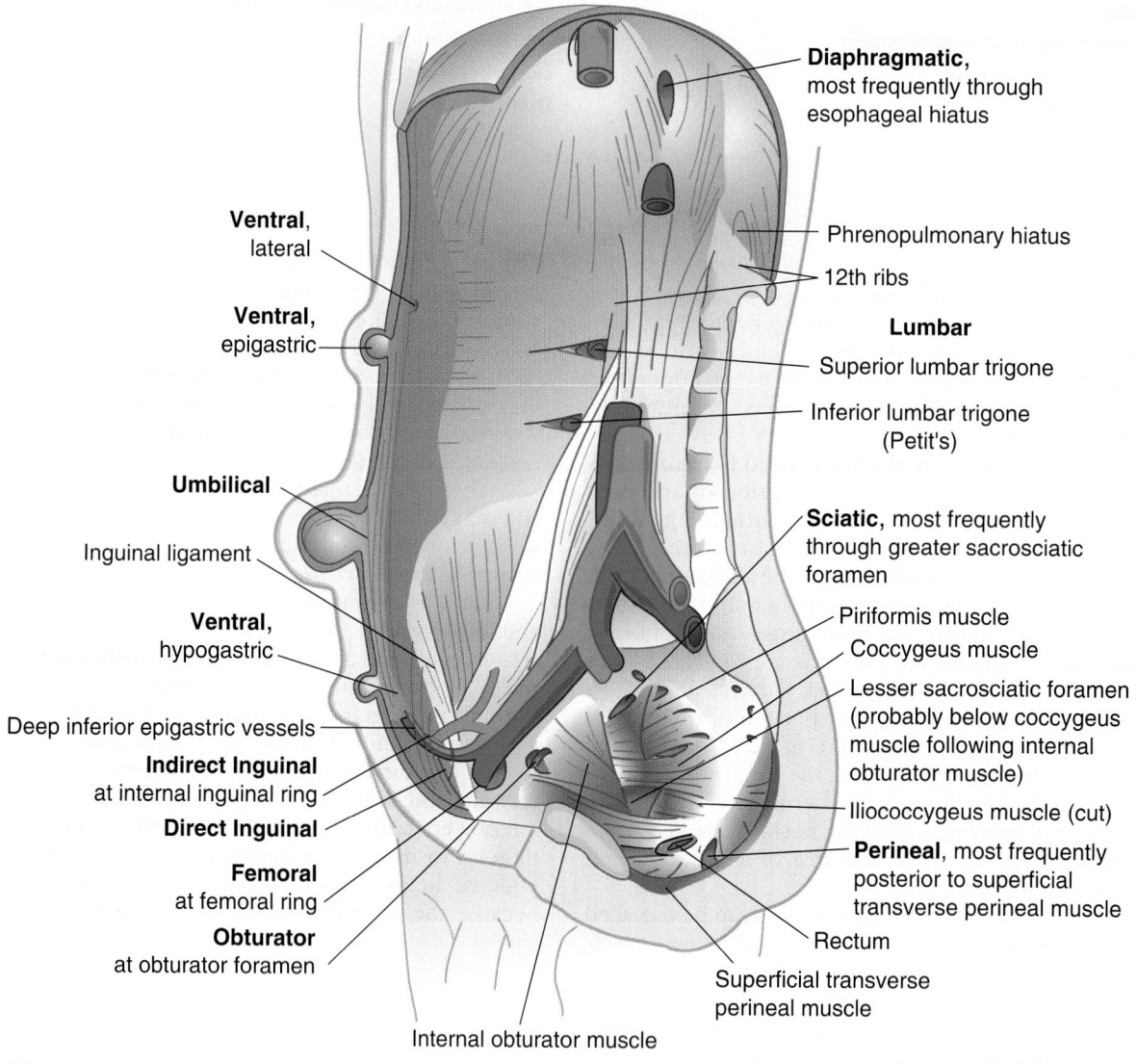

FIGURE 42-1. Types of abdominal wall hernias. (From Dorland's Illustrated Medical Dictionary, 26th ed, Philadelphia, WB Saunders, 1985, plate XXI.)

femoral hernias occur more frequently in women than in men, inguinal hernias remain the most common hernia in women. Femoral hernias are rare in men. Ten percent of women and 50% of men who have a femoral hernia either have or will develop an inguinal hernia. Incisional hernias are twice as common in women as in men.

Both indirect inguinal and femoral hernias occur more commonly on the right side. This is attributed to a delay in atrophy of the processus vaginalis following the normal slower descent of the right testis to the scrotum during fetal development.[1] The predominance of right-sided femoral hernias is thought to be due to the tamponading effect of the sigmoid colon on the left femoral canal.

The prevalence of hernias increases with age, particularly for inguinal, umbilical, and femoral hernias. The likelihood of strangulation and need for hospitalization also increases with aging. Strangulation, the most common serious complication of a hernia, occurs in only 1% to 3% of groin hernias and is more common at the extremes of life. Most strangulated hernias are indirect inguinal hernias; however, femoral hernias have the highest rate of strangulation (15% to 20%) of all hernias, and for this

reason it is recommended that all femoral hernias be repaired at the time of discovery.

ANATOMY

Anatomy of the Groin

The surgeon must have a comprehensive understanding of the anatomy of the groin to properly select and utilize various options for hernia repair.[1-3] In addition, the relationships of muscles, aponeuroses, fascia, nerves, blood vessels, and spermatic cord structures in the inguinal region must be mastered to obtain the lowest incidence of recurrence and to avoid complications. These anatomic considerations must be understood from both the anterior and posterior approaches, because both approaches are useful in different situations (Figs. 42-2 and 42-3).

Because most hernias are repaired through an anterior approach, it is essential to understand the anatomy from the skin surface to the preperitoneal space. Beneath the skin and subcutaneous tissues are the superficial circumflex iliac, superficial epigastric, and external pudendal

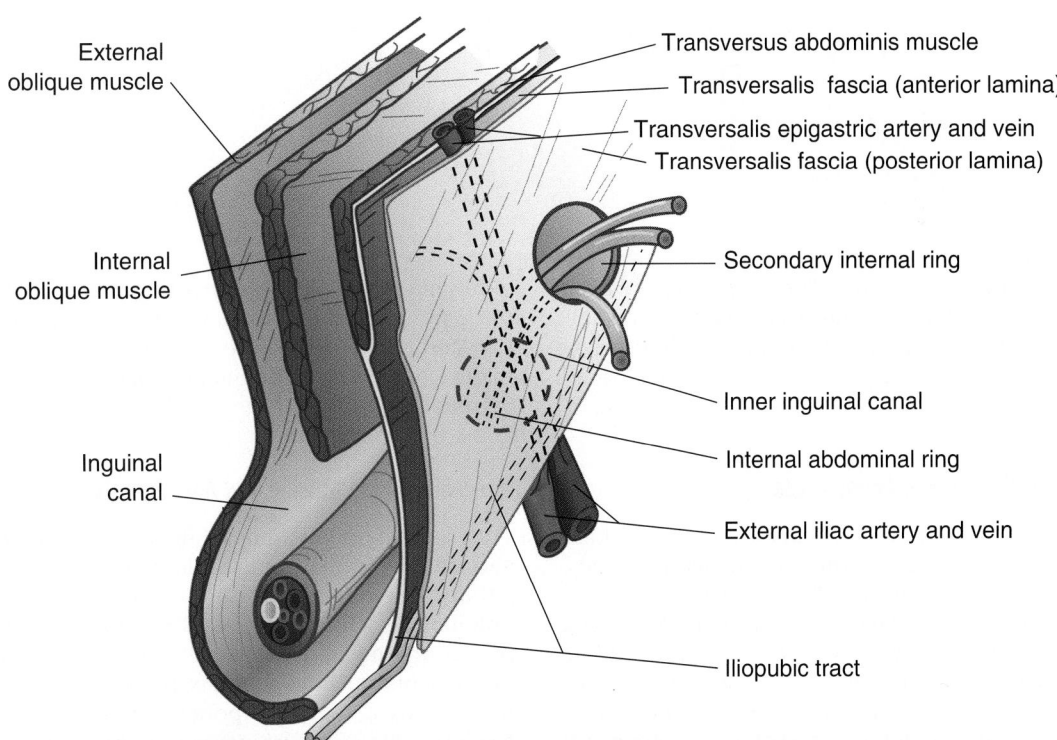

FIGURE 42-2. Nyhus' classic parasagittal diagram of the right midinguinal region illustrating the muscular aponeurotic layers separated into anterior and posterior walls. The posterior laminae of the transversalis fascia has been added, with the inferior epigastric vessels coursing through the abdominal wall medially to the inner inguinal canal (From Read RC: The transversalis and preperitoneal fasciae—a re-evaluation. *In* Nyhus LM, Condon RE [eds]: Hernia, 4th ed, Philadelphia, JB Lippincott, 1995, pp 57-63.)

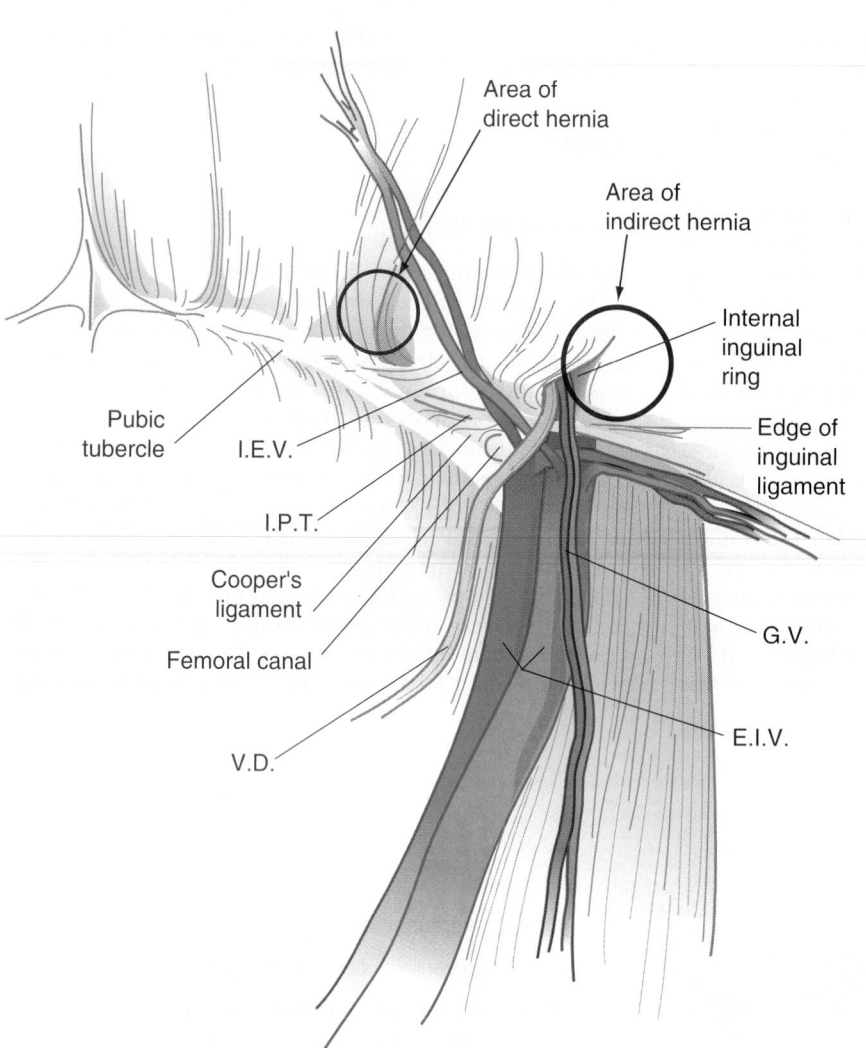

Area of
direct hernia

Area of
indirect hernia

Internal
inguinal
ring

Pubic
tubercle

I.E.V.

Edge of
inguinal
ligament

I.P.T.

Cooper's
ligament

Femoral canal

G.V.

V.D.

E.I.V.

FIGURE 42-3. Anatomy of the important preperitoneal structures in the right inguinal space. IEV, inferior epigastric vessels; IPT, iliopubic tract; VD, vas deferens; GV, gonadal vessels; EIV, external iliac vessels. (From Talamini MA, Are C: Laparoscopic hernia repair. *In* Zuidema GD, Yeo CJ [eds]: Shackelford's Surgery of the Alimentary Tract, 5th ed. Philadelphia, WB Saunders, 2002, vol 5, p 140.)

arteries and accompanying veins. These vessels arise from and drain to the proximal femoral artery and vein, respectively, and are directed superiorly. If encountered during operation, these vessels can be retracted or even divided when necessary.

External Oblique Muscle and Aponeurosis

The external oblique muscle fibers are directed inferiorly and medially and lie deep to the subcutaneous tissues. The aponeurosis of the external oblique muscle is formed by a superficial and deep layer. This aponeurosis, along with the bilaminar aponeuroses of the internal oblique and transversus abdominis, forms the anterior rectus sheath and, finally, the linea alba by linear decussation. The external oblique aponeurosis serves as the superficial boundary of the inguinal canal. The inguinal ligament (Poupart's ligament) is the inferior edge of the external oblique aponeurosis and extends from the anterior superior iliac spine to the pubic tubercle, turning posteriorly to form a shelving edge. The lacunar ligament is formed by the insertion of the inguinal ligament to the pubis. The

external (superficial) inguinal ring is an ovoid opening of the external oblique aponeurosis that is positioned superior and slightly lateral to the pubic tubercle. The spermatic cord exits the inguinal canal through the external inguinal ring.

Internal Oblique Muscle and Aponeurosis

The internal oblique muscle fibers are directed superiorly and laterally in the upper abdomen; however, they run in a transverse direction in the inguinal region. The internal oblique muscle serves as the cephalad (or superior) border of the inguinal canal. The medial aspect of the internal oblique aponeurosis fuses with fibers from the transversus abdominis aponeurosis to form a conjoined tendon. This structure actually is present in only 5% to 10% of patients and is most evident at the insertion of these muscles on the pubic tubercle. The cremasteric muscle fibers arise from the internal oblique and encompass the spermatic cord. These muscle fibers are essential to the cremasteric reflex but have little relevance to hernia repairs.

Transversus Abdominis Muscle and Aponeurosis and Transversalis Fascia

The transversus abdominis muscle layer is oriented transversely throughout most of its area; in the inguinal region these fibers course in a slightly oblique downward direction. The strength and continuity of this muscle and aponeurosis are important for the prevention of inguinal hernia.

The aponeurosis of the transversus abdominis covers both anterior and posterior surfaces. The lower margin of the transversus abdominis arches along with the internal oblique muscle over the internal inguinal ring to form the *transversus abdominis aponeurotic arch*. The transversalis fascia is the connective tissue layer that underlies the abdominal wall musculature. The transversalis fascia, sometimes referred to as the endoabdominal fascia, is a component of the inguinal floor. It tends to be more dense in this area but still remains relatively thin.

The iliopubic tract is a continuation of the transverse abdominis aponeurosis and fascia at the upper border of the femoral sheath. The iliopubic tract also forms the inferior crus of the deep inguinal ring. The superior crus of the deep ring is formed by the transversus abdominis aponeurotic arch. The iliopubic tract is located posterior to the inguinal ligament, and it crosses over the femoral vessels and inserts on the anterior superior iliac spine and inner lip of the wing of the ilium.

The iliopubic tract is an extremely important structure in the repair of hernias from both the anterior and posterior approaches.[4] It comprises the inferior margin for most anterior repairs. The portion of the iliopubic tract lateral to the internal inguinal ring serves as the inferior border below which staples or tacks should not be placed during a laparoscopic inguinal hernia repair because the lateral femoral cutaneous and genitofemoral nerves are located inferior to the iliopubic tract.

Cooper's Ligament

Cooper's ligament is formed by the periosteum and fascia along the superior ramus of the pubis. This structure is posterior to the iliopubic tract and forms the posterior border of the femoral canal.

Inguinal Canal

The inguinal canal is approximately 4 cm in length and is located 2 to 4 cm cephalad to the inguinal ligament. The canal extends between the internal (deep) inguinal and the external (superficial) inguinal rings. The inguinal canal contains the spermatic cord and the round ligament of the uterus.

The spermatic cord is composed of cremasteric muscle fibers, the testicular artery and accompanying veins, the genital branch of the genitofemoral nerve, the vas deferens, the cremasteric vessels, the lymphatics, and the processus vaginalis. The cremaster muscle arises from the lowermost fibers of the internal oblique muscle and encompasses the spermatic cord in the inguinal canal. The cremasteric vessels are branches of the inferior epigastric vessels and pass through the posterior wall of the inguinal canal through their own foramen. These vessels supply the cremaster muscle and can be divided to expose the floor of the inguinal canal during hernia repair without damaging the testis.

The inguinal canal is bounded superficially by the external oblique aponeurosis. The internal oblique and transversus abdominis musculoaponeurosis form the cephalad wall of the inguinal canal. The inferior wall of the inguinal canal is formed by the inguinal ligament and lacunar ligament. The posterior wall or floor of the inguinal canal is formed by the transversalis fascia and the aponeurosis of the transversus abdominis muscle.

The *Hesselbach triangle* refers to the margins of the floor of the inguinal canal. The inferior epigastric vessels serve as its superolateral border, the rectus sheath as medial border, and the inguinal ligament as the inferior border. Direct hernias occur within the Hesselbach triangle, whereas indirect inguinal hernias arise lateral to the triangle. It is not uncommon, however, for medium and large indirect inguinal hernias to involve the floor of the inguinal canal as they enlarge.

The iliohypogastric and ilioinguinal nerves and the genital branch of the genitofemoral nerve are the important nerves in the groin area (Fig. 42-4). The iliohypogastric and ilioinguinal nerves provide sensation to the skin of the groin, the base of the penis, and the ipsilateral upper medial thigh. The iliohypogastric and ilioinguinal nerves lie beneath the internal oblique muscle to a point just medially and superior to the anterior superior iliac spine, where they penetrate the internal oblique muscle and lie beneath the external oblique aponeurosis. The main trunk of the iliohypogastric nerve runs on the anterior surface of the internal oblique muscle and aponeurosis medial and superior to the internal ring. The iliohypogastric nerve may provide an inguinal branch that joins the ilioinguinal nerve. The ilioinguinal nerve runs anterior to the spermatic cord in the inguinal canal and branches at the superficial inguinal ring. The genital nerve innervates the cremaster muscle and the skin on the lateral side of the scrotum and labia. This nerve lies on the iliopubic tract and accompanies the cremaster vessels to form a neurovascular bundle.

Preperitoneal Space

The preperitoneal space contains adipose tissue, lymphatics, blood vessels, and nerves. The nerves of the preperitoneal space of specific concern to the surgeon include the lateral femoral cutaneous nerve and the genitofemoral nerve. The lateral femoral cutaneous nerve originates as a root of L2 and L3 and is occasionally a direct branch of the femoral nerve. This nerve courses along the anterior surface of the iliac muscle beneath the iliac fascia and passes either under or through the lateral attachment of the inguinal ligament at the anterior superior iliac spine. This nerve runs beneath or occasionally through the iliopubic tract lateral to the internal inguinal ring.

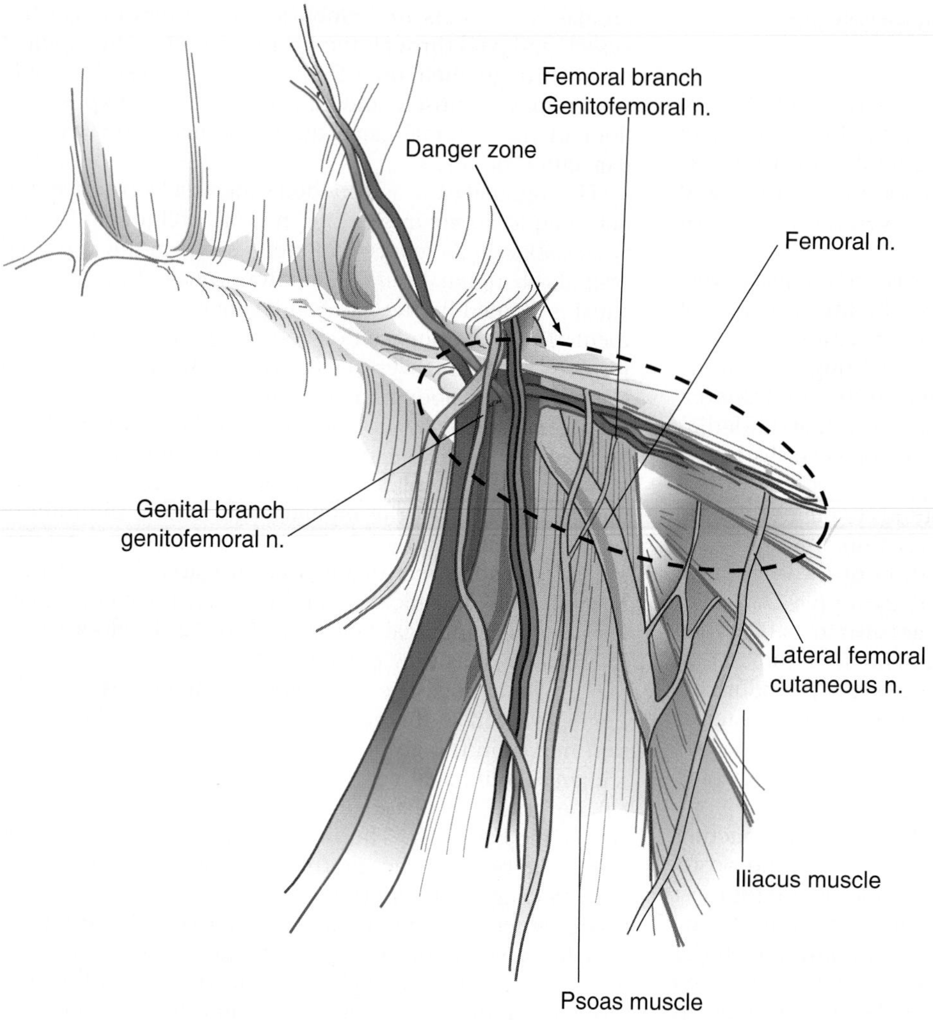

FIGURE 42-4. Important nerves and their relationship to inguinal structures (right side is illustrated). (From Talamini MA, Are C: Laparoscopic hernia repair. *In* Zuidema GD, Yeo CJ [eds]: Shackelford's Surgery of the Alimentary Tract, 5th ed, Philadelphia, WB Saunders, 2002, vol 5, p 140.)

The genitofemoral nerve usually arises from the L2 or the L1 and L2 nerve roots. It divides into genital and femoral branches on the anterior surface of the psoas muscle. The genital branch enters the inguinal canal through the deep ring, whereas the femoral branch enters the femoral sheath lateral to the artery.

The inferior epigastric artery and vein are branches of the external iliac vessels and are important landmarks for laparoscopic hernia repair. These vessels course medial to the internal inguinal ring and eventually lie beneath the rectus abdominis muscle immediately beneath the transversalis fascia. The inferior epigastric vessels serve to define the types of inguinal hernia. Indirect inguinal hernias occur lateral to the inferior epigastric vessels, whereas direct hernias occur medial to these vessels.

The vas deferens courses through the preperitoneal space from caudad to cephalad and medial to lateral to join the spermatic cord at the deep inguinal ring.

Femoral Canal

The boundaries of the femoral canal are the iliopubic tract anteriorly, Cooper's ligament posteriorly, and the femoral vein laterally. The pubic tubercle forms the apex of the femoral canal triangle. A femoral hernia occurs through this space and is medial to the femoral vessels.

Anatomy of the Anterior Abdominal Wall

The anatomy of the anterior abdominal wall is straightforward and considerably easier to grasp than the anatomy of the inguinal area. The lateral musculature is composed of three layers, with the fascicles of each directed obliquely at different angles to create a strong envelope for the abdominal contents. Each of these muscles forms an aponeurosis that inserts into the linea alba, a midline structure joining both sides of the abdominal wall. The external oblique muscle is the most superficial muscle of the lateral abdominal wall. Deep to the external oblique lies the internal oblique muscle. The fibers of the external oblique course inferomedially (as "hands in pockets"), whereas those of the internal oblique muscle run deep to and in the opposite direction of the external oblique. The deepest muscular layer of the abdominal wall is the transversus abdominis muscle. These three lateral muscles give rise to aponeurotic layers lateral to the rectus, which contribute to the anterior and posterior layers of the rectus sheath.[5]

ities may play a greater role in diagnosis of more unusual hernias of the abdominal wall.

NONOPERATIVE MANAGEMENT

Most surgeons recommend operation on discovery of an inguinal hernia because the natural history of a groin hernia is that of progressive enlargement and weakening, with the potential for incarceration and strangulation. Patients with a short life expectancy or significant comorbid illnesses with minimal symptoms are the exception. There is no direct comparison between operation and observation, particularly in asymptomatic patients, although one such study is in progress.[8]

Trusses can provide symptomatic relief of hernias and are used more commonly in Europe.[9] Correct measurement and fitting are important. Hernia control has been reported in approximately 30% of patients. Complications associated with the use of a truss include testicular atrophy, ilioinguinal or femoral neuritis, and hernia incarceration. It is generally agreed that nonoperative management should not be used for femoral hernias because of the high incidence of associated complications, particularly strangulation.

OPERATIVE REPAIR

Anterior Repairs

Anterior repairs are the most common operative approach for inguinal hernias. Tension-free repairs are now standard, and there are a variety of different types. Older types of repair are indicated for small hernias.

There are some technical aspects of operation common to all anterior repairs. Open hernia repair is begun by making a transversely oriented, linear, or slightly curvilinear incision 2 to 3 cm above and parallel to the inguinal ligament. Dissection is continued through the subcutaneous tissues and Scarpa's fascia. The external oblique fascia and external inguinal ring should be identified. The external oblique fascia is incised through the superficial inguinal ring to expose the inguinal canal. The ilioinguinal and iliohypogastric nerves should be identified and mobilized to avoid transection and entrapment. The spermatic cord is mobilized at the pubic tubercle by a combination of blunt and sharp dissection. Improper mobilization of the spermatic cord too lateral to the pubic tubercle can cause confusion in the identification of tissue planes and essential structures and may result in disruption of the floor of the inguinal canal.

The cremasteric muscle fibers of the mobilized spermatic cord are divided and separated from the underlying cord structures. The cremasteric artery and vein, which join the cremaster muscle near the inguinal ring, are usually cauterized or ligated and divided.

When an indirect hernia is present, the hernia sac is located deep to the cremaster muscle and anterior and superior to the spermatic cord structures. Incising the cremaster muscle in a longitudinal direction and dividing it circumferentially near the internal inguinal ring helps expose the indirect hernia sac. The hernia sac is carefully dissected from adjacent cord structures and dissected to the level of the internal inguinal ring. The sac should be opened and examined for visceral contents if it is large; however, this step is unnecessary in small hernias. The neck of the sac is ligated at the level of the internal ring, and any excess sac is excised. If a large hernia sac is present, it can be divided using the electrocautery to facilitate ligation. It is not necessary to excise the distal portion of the sac. If the sac is broad based, it may be easier to displace it into the peritoneal cavity rather than to ligate it. Direct hernia sacs protrude through the floor of the inguinal canal and can be reduced below the transversalis fascia before repair. A "lipoma of the cord" represents retroperitoneal fat that has herniated through the deep inguinal ring and should be suture ligated and removed.

A sliding hernia presents a special challenge in handling the hernia sac. With a sliding hernia, a portion of the sac is composed of visceral peritoneum covering part of a retroperitoneal organ, usually the colon or bladder. In this situation, the grossly redundant portion of the sac (if present) should be excised and the peritoneum re-closed. The organ and sac then can be reduced below the transversalis fascia similar to a direct hernia.

Iliopubic Tract Repair

The iliopubic tract has been identified by Condon as an essential component of anatomic hernia repairs.[3] This structure is contiguous with the transversus abdominis aponeurotic arch in normal groin anatomy but separates from the transversus abdominis when the inguinal floor weakens. The iliopubic tract repair approximates the transversus abdominis aponeurotic arch to the iliopubic tract with the use of interrupted sutures (Fig. 42-6). The repair begins at the pubic tubercle and extends laterally past the internal inguinal ring. This repair was initially described using a relaxing incision (see later); however, many surgeons who use this repair do not perform a relaxing incision.

Shouldice Repair

The Shouldice repair emphasizes a multilayer imbricated repair of the posterior wall of the inguinal canal with a continuous running suture technique. After completion of the dissection, the posterior wall of the inguinal canal is reconstructed by superimposing running suture lines progressing from deep to more superficial layers. The initial suture line secures the transversus abdominis aponeurotic arch to the iliopubic tract. Next, the internal oblique and transversus abdominis muscles and aponeuroses are sutured to the inguinal ligament. The Shouldice repair is associated with a very low recurrence rate and a high degree of patient satisfaction. The original description of the Shouldice repair used running stainless steel wire repair, although most who practice this technique now use other types of permanent suture.

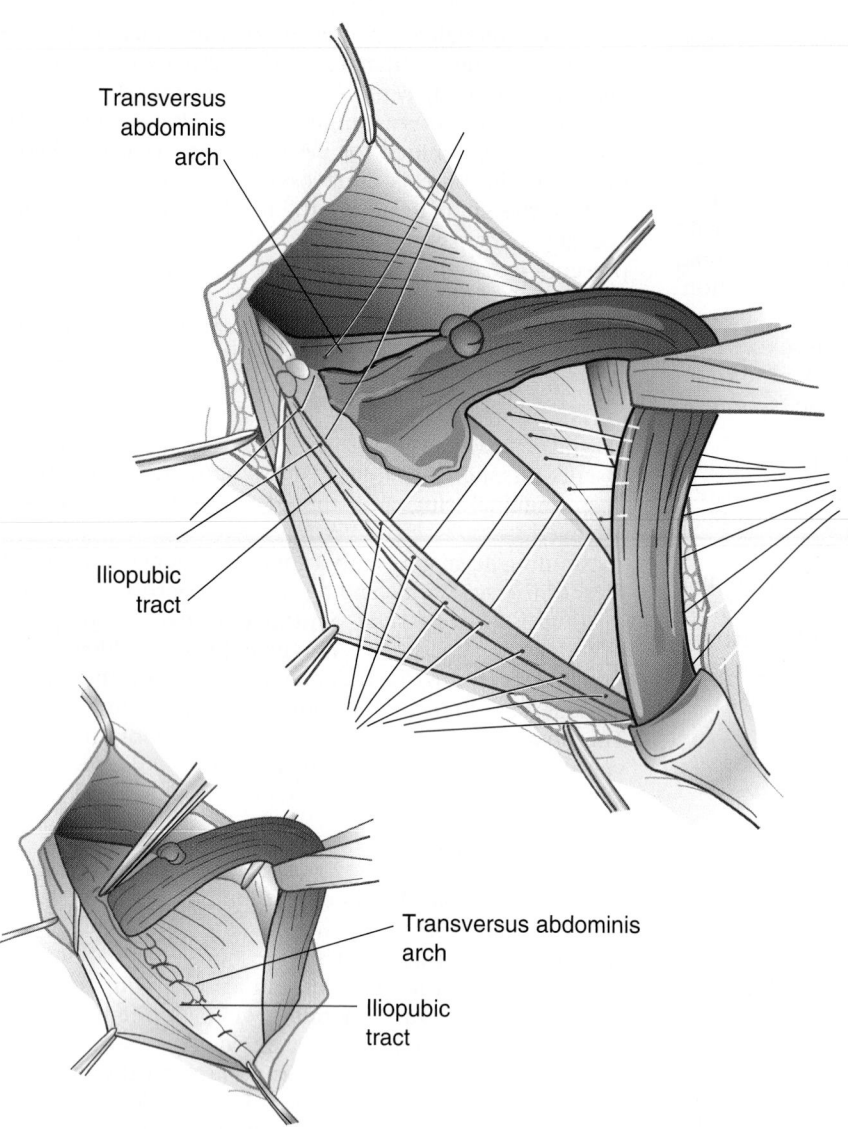

Transversus
abdominis
arch

Iliopubic
tract

Transversus abdominis
arch

Iliopubic
tract

FIGURE 42-6.   Iliopubic tract repair.
Top, Sutures lateral to the cord complete
reconstruction of the deep inguinal ring. These
sutures encompass the transversus abdominis
arch above and the cremaster origin and
iliopubic tract below. **Bottom,** The complete
repair is ready for wound closure. The
reconstruction of the deep ring should be snug
but also loose enough to admit the tip of a
hemostat. (From Condon RE: Anterior iliopubic
tract repair. *In* Nyhus LM, Condon RE [eds]:
Hernia, 2nd ed. Philadelphia, JB Lippincott,
1974, p 204.)

Bassini Repair

The Bassini repair is performed by suturing the transversus abdominis and internal oblique musculoaponeurotic arches or conjoined tendon (when present) to the inguinal ligament. This once popular technique is the basic approach to nonanatomic hernia repairs and was the most popular type of repair done before the advent of tension-free repairs.

Cooper Ligament (McVay) Repair

The Cooper ligament repair has traditionally been popular for the correction of direct inguinal hernias, large indirect hernias, recurrent inguinal hernias, and femoral hernias. The repair begins at the pubic tubercle. Interrupted, nonabsorbable sutures are used to approximate the edge of the transversus abdominis aponeurosis to Cooper's ligament. When the medial aspect of the femoral canal is reached, a transition suture is placed to incorporate Cooper's ligament and the iliopubic tract. Lateral to this

transition stitch, the transversus abdominis aponeurosis is secured to the iliopubic tract.

An important principle of this repair is the need for a relaxing incision. The relaxing incision is made by reflecting the external oblique aponeurosis cephalad and medial to expose the anterior rectus sheath. An incision is then made in a curvilinear direction beginning 1 cm above the pubic tubercle throughout the extent of the anterior sheath to near its lateral border. This relieves tension on suture line and results in decreased postoperative pain and hernia recurrence. The fascial defect is covered by the body of the rectus muscle, which prevents herniation at the relaxing incision site.

The "tension-free" repair has become the dominant method of inguinal hernia repair (Fig. 42-7). Recognizing that tension in a repair is the principal cause of recurrence, current practices in hernia management employ a synthetic mesh prosthesis to bridge the defect, a concept first popularized by Lichtenstein.[10] In the Lichtenstein repair, a piece of prosthetic nonabsorbable mesh is fashioned to fit the canal. A slit is cut into the distal, lateral

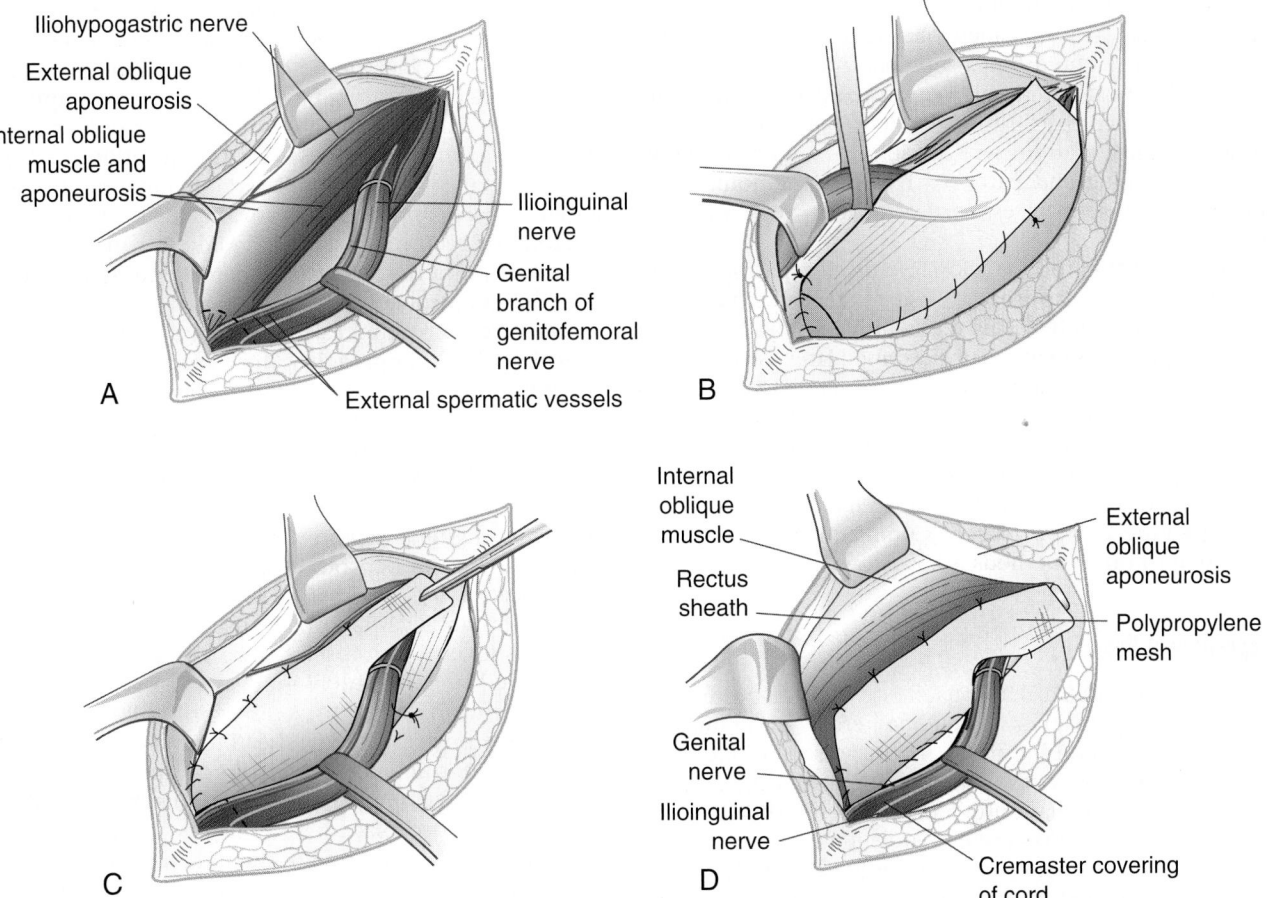

FIGURE 42-7. The Lichtenstein tension-free hernia repair. **A,** This procedure is performed by careful dissection of the inguinal canal. High ligation of an indirect hernia sac is performed, and the spermatic cord structures are retraced inferiorly. The external oblique aponeurosis is separated from the underlying internal oblique muscle high enough to accommodate a 6- to 8-cm wide mesh patch. Overlap of the internal oblique muscle edge by 2 to 3 cm is necessary. An 8 × 16-cm sheet of Marlex mesh is fashioned to fit the inguinal canal. A slit is made in the lateral aspect of the mesh, and the spermatic cord is placed between the two tails of the mesh. **B,** The spermatic cord is retracted in the cephalad direction. The medial aspect of the mesh overlaps the pubic bone by approximately 2 cm. The mesh is secured to the aponeurotic tissue overlying the pubic tubercle using a running suture of nonabsorbable monofilament material. The suture is continued laterally by suturing the inferior edge of the mesh to the shelving edge of the inguinal ligament to a point just lateral to the internal inguinal ring. **C,** A second monofilament suture is placed at the level of the pubic tubercle and continued laterally by suturing the mesh to the internal oblique aponeurosis or muscle approximately 2 cm from the aponeurotic edge. **D,** The lower edges of the two tails are sutured to the shelving edge of the inguinal ligament to create a new internal ring made of mesh. The spermatic cord structures are placed within the inguinal canal overlying the mesh. The external oblique aponeurosis is closed over the spermatic cord. (Reproduced from Arregui ME, Nagan RD [eds]: Inguinal Hernia: Advances or Controversies? Oxford, England, Radcliffe Medical, 1994.)

edge of the mesh to accommodate the spermatic cord. There are preformed commercially available prostheses available for use. Monofilament, nonabsorbable suture is used in a continuous fashion beginning at the pubic tubercle and running a length of suture in both directions toward the superior aspect above the internal inguinal ring to the level of the "tails" of the mesh. The mesh is sutured to the aponeurotic tissue overlying the pubic bone medially, continuing superiorly along the transversus abdominis or conjoined tendon. The inferolateral edge of the mesh is sutured to the iliopubic tract or the shelving edge of the inguinal (Poupart's) ligament to a point lateral to the internal inguinal ring. At this point, the tails created by the slit are sutured together around the sper-

matic cord snugly forming a "new" internal inguinal ring. The ilioinguinal nerve and genital branch of the genitofemoral nerve are placed with the cord structures and are passed through this newly fashioned internal inguinal ring.

The "tension-free" mesh repair has been modified from the original Lichtenstein repair. Gilbert reported using a cone-shaped "plug" of polypropylene mesh that when inserted into the internal inguinal ring would deploy like an upside-down umbrella and occlude the hernia.[11] This plug is sewn to the surrounding tissues and held in place by an additional overlying mesh patch. This patch may not need to be secured by sutures; however, to do so requires dissection to create a sufficient space between the external and internal oblique for the patch to lie flat over the inguinal canal. This so-called plug and patch repair, an extension of Lichtenstein's original mesh repair, has become the most commonly performed primary anterior inguinal hernia repair. Although this repair can be done without suture fixation by experienced surgeons, many secure both plug and patch with several monofilament nonabsorbable sutures, especially for very weak inguinal floors.

Another option for a tension-free mesh repair involves a preperitoneal approach using a self-expanding polypropylene patch.[12] This technique employs the principles for preperitoneal repair described later. A pocket is created in the preperitoneal space by blunt dissection, and then a preformed mesh patch is inserted into the hernia defect that expands to cover the direct, indirect, and femoral spaces. The patch lies parallel to the inguinal ligament. It can remain without suture fixation, or a small tacking suture can be placed. Comparative data of this technique to other methods are lacking.

Preperitoneal Repair

The open preperitoneal approach is useful for the repair of recurrent inguinal hernias, sliding hernias, strangulated hernias, and femoral hernias.[13] A transverse skin incision is made 2 cm above the internal inguinal ring and is directed to the medial border of the rectus sheath. The muscles of the anterior abdominal wall are incised transversely, and the preperitoneal space is identified. If further exposure is needed, the anterior rectus sheath can be incised and the rectus muscle retracted medially. The preperitoneal tissues are retracted cephalad to visualize the posterior inguinal wall and the site of herniation. The inferior epigastric artery and veins are generally beneath the midportion of the posterior rectus sheath and usually do not need to be divided. The posterior approach avoids mobilization of the spermatic cord and injury to the sensory nerves of the inguinal canal, which is particularly important for hernias previously repaired through an anterior approach. If the peritoneum is incised, it should be sutured close to avoid evisceration of intraperitoneal contents into the operative field. The transversalis fascia and transversus abdominis aponeurosis are identified and sutured to the iliopubic tract. Femoral hernias repaired by this approach require closure of the femoral canal by securing the repair to Cooper's ligament. A mesh prosthesis is frequently used to reinforce the closure of the femoral canal, particularly with large hernias.

Laparoscopic Management

The application of minimally invasive surgical techniques to inguinal hernia repair has added to the ongoing debate over the "best" inguinal hernia repair. Laparoscopic inguinal hernia repair is another method of tension-free mesh repair, based on a preperitoneal approach. Proponents tout quicker recovery, less pain, better visualization of anatomy, utility in fixing all inguinal hernia defects, and decreased surgical site infections. Critics emphasize longer operative times, technical challenges, and increased cost. There are over 700 publications of laparoscopic inguinal hernia repair. Most report a complication rate of less than 10% and a recurrence rate of 0% to 3%.[8,14] Although controversy exists about the utility of laparoscopic repair of primary unilateral inguinal hernias, most agree that this approach has advantages for patients with bilateral or recurrent hernias.[15] Adopting practice guidelines for the performance of laparoscopic hernia repairs may help control costs.

Early reports emphasized a transabdominal preperitoneal (TAPP) approach. More recently, the totally extraperitoneal approach (TEP) repair has become more popular. Both techniques are similar in actual repair but differ in the manner by which the preperitoneal space is accessed. The TAPP repair uses traditional intraperitoneal trocars and the creation of a peritoneal flap to expose the posterior inguinal region. The TEP approach provides access to the preperitoneal space without entering the peritoneal cavity.[16]

An infraumbilical incision is used. The anterior rectus sheath is incised, the ipsilateral rectus abdominis muscle is retracted laterally, and blunt dissection is used to create a space beneath the rectus. A dissecting balloon is inserted deep to the posterior rectus sheath, advanced to the pubic symphysis, and inflated under direct laparoscopic vision (Fig. 42-8). Once opened, the space is insufflated and additional trocars are placed. A 30-degree laparoscope provides the best visualization of the inguinal region (see Fig. 42-3). The inferior epigastric vessels are identified along the lower portion of the rectus muscle and retracted anteriorly. Cooper's ligament must be cleared from the pubic symphysis medially to the level of the external iliac vein. The iliopubic tract is also identified. Care must be taken to avoid injury to the femoral branch of the genitofemoral nerve and the lateral femoral cutaneous nerve, which are located lateral and below the iliopubic tract (see Fig. 42-4). Lateral dissection is carried out to the anterior superior iliac spine. Finally, the spermatic cord is skeletonized.

A direct hernia sac and associated preperitoneal fat is gently reduced by traction if it has not already been reduced by balloon expansion of the peritoneal space. A small indirect hernia sac is mobilized from the cord structures and reduced into the peritoneal cavity. A large sac may be difficult to reduce. In this case, the sac is divided with cautery near the internal inguinal ring, leaving the distal sac in situ. The proximal peritoneal sac should be closed with a loop ligature to prevent pneumoperitoneum from occurring. Once any hernias are reduced, a 10 × 15-cm piece of polypropylene mesh is inserted through a trocar and unfolded. It should cover the direct, indirect, and femoral spaces and rest over the cord structures. The mesh is carefully secured with a tacking stapler to Cooper's ligament from the pubic tubercle to the external iliac vein, anteriorly to the posterior rectus musculature and transversus abdominis aponeurotic arch at least 2 cm above the hernia defect, and laterally to the iliopubic tract. The mesh should extend beyond the pubic symphysis and below the spermatic cord and peritoneum (Fig.

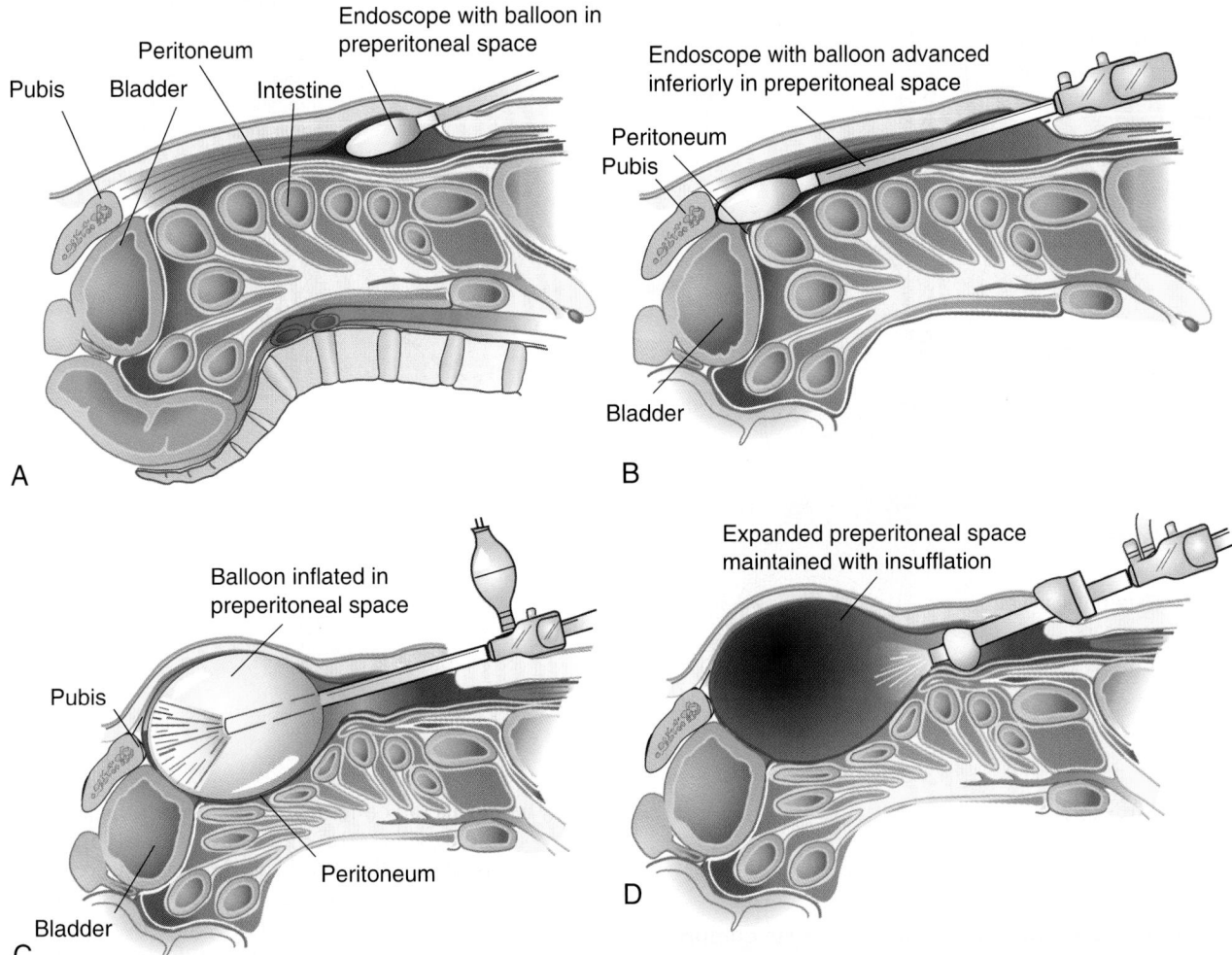

FIGURE 42-8. The total extraperitoneal (TEP) laparoscopic hernia repair. **A,** The TEP approach for laparoscopic hernia repair is demonstrated. Access to the posterior rectus sheath is gained in the periumbilical region. A balloon dissector is placed on the anterior surface of the posterior rectus sheath. **B,** The balloon dissector is advanced to the posterior surface of the pubis in the preperitoneal space. **C,** The balloon is inflated, thereby creating an optical cavity. **D,** The optical cavity is insufflated by carbon dioxide, and the posterior surface of the inguinal floor is dissected. (From Shadduck PP, Schwartz LB, Eubanks WS: Laparoscopic inguinal herniorrhaphy. *In* Pappas TN, Schwartz LB, Eubanks WE [eds]: Atlas of Laparoscopic Surgery. Philadelphia, Current Medicine, 1996. Copyright 1996 by Current Medicine. Reproduced by permission of the publisher.)

42-9). The mesh should not be fixed in this area, and tacks should not be placed inferior to the iliopubic tract beyond the external iliac artery. Staples placed in this area may injure the femoral branch of the genitofemoral nerve or the lateral femoral cutaneous nerve. Staples should also be avoided in the "triangle of doom" bounded by the ductus deferens medially and the spermatic vessels laterally to avoid injury to the external iliac vessels and femoral nerve.

FEMORAL HERNIAS

A femoral hernia occurs through the femoral canal that is bounded superiorly by the iliopubic tract, inferiorly by Cooper's ligament, laterally by the femoral vein, and medially by the junction of the iliopubic tract and Cooper's lig-

ament. A femoral hernia produces a mass or bulge below the inguinal ligament. On occasion, some femoral hernias will present over the inguinal canal. In this situation, the femoral hernia sac still exits inferior to the inguinal ligament through the femoral canal but ascends in a cephalad direction.

A femoral hernia can be repaired using the standard Cooper ligament repair, a preperitoneal approach, or a laparoscopic approach. The essential elements of femoral hernia repair include dissection and removal of the hernia sac and obliteration of the defect in the femoral canal, either by approximation of the iliopubic tract to Cooper's ligament or by placement of prosthetic mesh to obliterate the defect. The incidence of strangulation in femoral hernias is high; therefore, incarcerated femoral hernias should have the hernia sac contents examined for viability.

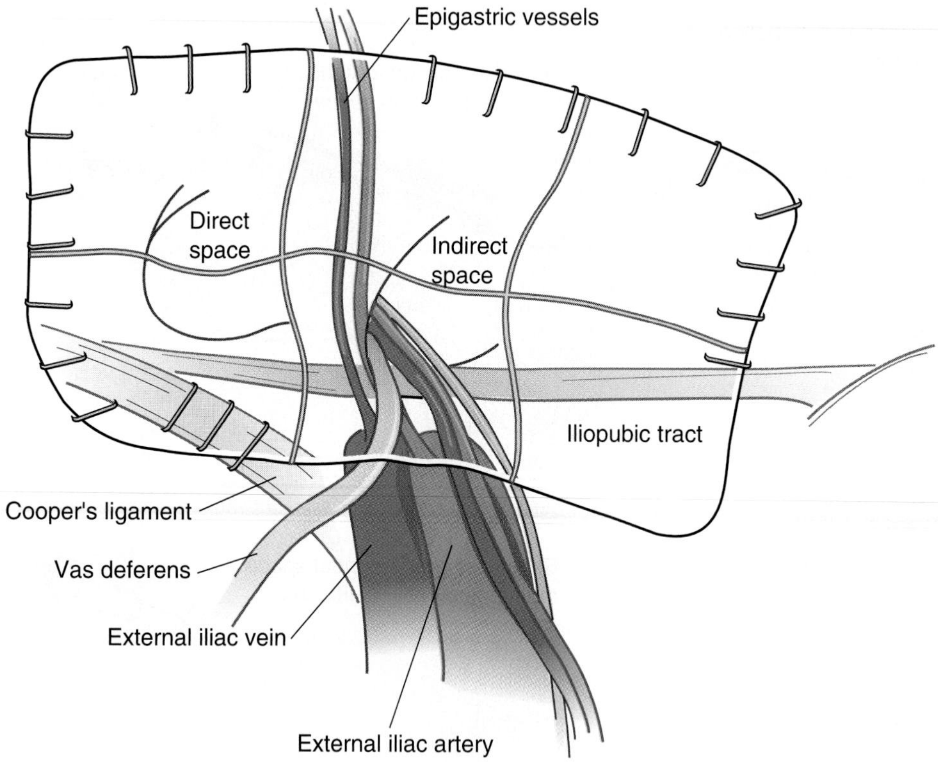

Epigastric vessels

Direct space

Indirect space

Iliopubic tract

Cooper's ligament

Vas deferens

External iliac vein

External iliac artery

FIGURE 42-9. Illustration of prosthetic mesh placement for the total extraperitoneal (TEP) hernia repair. (From Corbitt J: Laparoscopic transabdominal transperitoneal patch hernia repair. *In* Ballantyne GH [ed]: Atlas of Laparoscopic Surgery. Philadelphia, WB Saunders, 2000, p 511.)

SPECIAL PROBLEMS

Sliding Hernia

A sliding hernia occurs when an internal organ comprises a portion of the wall of the hernia sac. The most common viscus involved is the colon or urinary bladder. Most sliding hernias are a variant of indirect inguinal hernias, although femoral and direct sliding hernias can occur. The primary danger associated with a sliding hernia is the failure to recognize the visceral component of the hernia sac before injury to the bowel or bladder. The sliding hernia contents are reduced into the peritoneal cavity, and any excess hernia sac should be ligated and divided. After reduction of the hernia, one of the aforementioned techniques can be used for repair of the inguinal hernia.

Recurrent Hernias

The repair of recurrent inguinal hernias is challenging, and results are associated with a higher incidence of secondary recurrence. Recurrent hernias almost always require placement of a prosthesis for successful repair. Recurrences after anterior hernia repair using mesh are best managed by a posterior approach and placement of a second prosthesis.

Strangulated Hernias

Repair of a suspected strangulated hernia is most easily done using a preperitoneal approach.[17] With this expo-

sure, the hernia sac contents can be directly visualized and their viability assessed through a single incision. The constricting ring is identified and can be incised to reduce the entrapped viscus with minimal danger to the surrounding organs, blood vessels, and nerves. If it is necessary to resect strangulated intestine, the peritoneum can be opened and resection done without the need for a second incision.

Bilateral Hernias

The approach to repair of bilateral inguinal hernias is based on the extent of the hernia defect. Simultaneous repair of bilateral hernias has traditionally been associated with a recurrence rate approximately twice that of unilateral hernia repair. The use of a giant prosthetic reinforcement of the visceral sac (Stoppa repair)[18] or the TEP laparoscopic repair are appropriate techniques for simultaneous repair of bilateral inguinal hernias, although bilateral anterior repair through separate incisions can be used.

UMBILICAL HERNIA

The umbilicus is formed by the umbilical ring of the linea alba and is a common site of hernia. Intra-abdominally, the round ligament (ligamentum teres) and the paraumbilical veins join into the umbilicus superiorly and the median umbilical ligament (obliterated urachus) enters inferiorly. Umbilical hernias in infants are congenital and are quite common. They close spontaneously in the vast majority of cases by the age of 2 years. Those that persist after the age of 5 years are frequently repaired surgically, although complications related to these hernias in children are unusual. There is a strong predisposition toward the development of these hernias in individuals of African descent. In the United States, the incidence is eight times higher in African American than in white infants.[19]

Umbilical hernias in adults are largely acquired. These hernias occur more frequently in women and in patients with conditions that result in increased intra-abdominal pressure, such as pregnancy, obesity, ascites, or abdominal distention. Umbilical hernia is more common among individuals who have only a single midline aponeurotic decussation compared with the normal triple decussation of fibers.[20] Strangulation is unusual, but strangulation and rupture of the hernia can occur in chronic ascitic conditions. Small asymptomatic umbilical hernias barely detectable on examination need not be repaired. Adults who have symptoms, a large hernia, incarceration, thinning of the overlying skin, or uncontrollable ascites should have hernia repair. Spontaneous rupture of umbilical hernias in patients with ascites can result in peritonitis and death.[21]

Classically, repair was done using the vest-over-pants repair proposed by Mayo.[22] This technique employs imbrication of superior and inferior fascial edges, although, because of increased tension on the repair, it is rarely performed today. Instead, small defects are closed primarily after separation of the sac from the overlying umbilicus. Larger defects (greater than 3 to 4 cm) should be closed using prosthetic mesh either to bridge the defect or as a reinforcement with suture repair, because some data suggest that the recurrence rate may be reduced with prosthetic repair.[23] Large umbilical hernias also can be repaired by a laparoscopic approach with intra-abdominal mesh placement. This technique should be reserved for unusually large umbilical defects, where it can provide a decreased recurrence rate and potentially fewer complications.[24]

EPIGASTRIC HERNIAS

Epigastric hernias are two to three times more common in men. These hernias are located between the xiphoid process and umbilicus and are usually within 5 to 6 cm above the umbilicus. Like umbilical hernias, epigastric hernias are more common in individuals with a single aponeurotic decussation.[20] The defects are small and often produce pain out of proportion to their size owing to incarceration of preperitoneal fat. They are multiple in up to 20% of patients. Repair is often accomplished by simple closure of the fascial defect similar to umbilical hernias.

INCISIONAL AND VENTRAL HERNIAS

Of all hernias encountered, incisional (ventral) hernias can be the most frustrating and difficult to treat. Incisional hernias occur as a result of excessive tension and inadequate healing of a previous incision, which is often associated with surgical site infections. These hernias enlarge over time, leading to pain, bowel obstruction, incarceration, and strangulation. Obesity, advanced age, malnutrition, ascites, pregnancy, and conditions that increase intra-abdominal pressure are predisposed factors to the development of an incisional hernia. Obesity can cause an incisional hernia to occur, owing to increased tension on the abdominal wall provided by the excessive bulk of a thick pannus and large omental mass. Chronic pulmonary disease and diabetes mellitus have also been recognized as risk factors for the development of incisional hernia. Medications such as corticosteroids and chemotherapeutic agents and surgical site infection can contribute to poor wound healing and increase the risk of developing an incisional hernia. Incisional hernias have been reported to occur in up to 10% of laparotomies.[25]

Large ventral hernias can result in loss of abdominal domain, which occurs when the abdominal contents no longer reside in the abdominal cavity. These large abdominal wall defects also can result from the inability to close the abdomen primarily because of bowel edema, abdominal packing, peritonitis, and repeat laparotomy. With loss of domain, the natural rigidity of the abdominal wall becomes compromised and the abdominal musculature is often retracted. Respiratory dysfunction can occur because these large ventral defects cause paradoxical respiratory abdominal motion. Loss of abdominal domain also can result in bowel edema, stasis of the splanchnic venous system, urinary retention, and constipation. Return of displaced viscera to the abdominal cavity during repair may lead to increased abdominal pressure, abdominal compartment syndrome, and acute respiratory failure.

Primary repair of incisional hernias can be done when the defect is small (<4 cm) and there is viable surrounding tissue. Larger defects (>4 cm in diameter) have a high recurrence rate if closed primarily and should be repaired with a prosthesis. Recurrence rates vary between 10% and 50% and are generally lower with prosthetic mesh repairs.[25] Prosthetic material may be placed as an onlay patch to buttress a tissue repair, interposed between the fascial defect, or sandwiched between tissue planes.

A variety of synthetic mesh products are available. Polypropylene mesh has been used extensively and allows for ingrowth of native fibroplasts and incorporation into the surrounding fascia. It is semi-rigid, somewhat flexible, and porous. It is preferable to interpose omentum between this mesh and the intestine to minimize the occurrence of enterocutaneous fistula. Expanded polytetrafluoroethylene (PTFE) can also be used for ventral hernia repair. This product differs from other synthetic meshes in that it is flexible, is smooth, and contains microscopic pores. Fibroblast proliferation occurs through the pores, but PTFE is impermeable to fluid. Unlike polypropylene, PTFE is not incorporated into the native tissue. Encapsulation occurs slowly and infection can occur during the encapsulation process. When infected, PTFE almost always must be removed. Composite mesh is a newer product that combines attributes of both polypropylene and PTFE by layering the two substances on top of one another. The PTFE surface serves as a protective interface against the bowel, and the polypropylene side faces superficially to be incorporated into the native fascial tissue. The newest development in prosthesis for ventral hernia repair is "nonsynthetic" or natural tissue mesh. Porcine intestinal submucosa and human-derived acellular tissue matrix from cadaveric dermis are available for repair of ventral abdominal defects. There are no data comparing the effectiveness of these natural tissue alternatives to synthetic mesh repairs.

The use of laparoscopic ventral hernia repair has been increasing, particularly for large defects. Trocars are placed lateral to the hernia defect. In general, scope placement and trocar location is not consistent and depends on the size and location of the hernia. The hernia contents are reduced, and adhesions are lysed. The surface area of the defect is measured, and a piece of mesh several centimeters larger than the defect is cut to size. The mesh is rolled, placed into the abdomen, and deployed. It is secured to the anterior abdominal wall with pre-placed mattress sutures that are passed through separate incisions, and tacking staples are placed between these sutures to secure the mesh several centimeters beyond the defect. The advantages of this approach are quicker recovery time and less postoperative pain. Complications are similar to those of open ventral hernia repair.[26]

Massive ventral hernias can present a particular challenge. Originally, methods to gradually stretch the abdominal wall were used to allow for restoration of abdominal domain and closure. This was accomplished by insufflation of air into the abdominal cavity to create a progressive pneumoperitoneum. Repeated administrations of increasing volumes of air over 1 to 3 weeks allowed the muscles of the abdominal wall to become lax enough for primary closure of the defect. This technique is usually unnecessary with prosthetic repairs.

Mesh reinforcement of the abdominal cavity was initially described by Stoppa for bilateral inguinal hernia repair.[27] The inguinal hernia defects were not closed, but instead a large piece of nonabsorbable mesh was inserted into the preperitoneal space to reinforce the lower abdominal wall. This procedure is referred to as giant prosthetic reinforcement of the visceral sac (GPRVS). This technique also has been used for massive ventral hernias, in which a large piece of mesh is placed in the retromuscular space on top of either the posterior rectus sheath or peritoneum. This space must be dissected laterally on both sides of the linea alba (for midline defects) to a distance of 8 to 10 cm beyond the defect. The prosthetic mesh should expand 5 to 6 cm beyond the superior and inferior borders of the defect. It does not need to be sutured because it is held in place by intra-abdominal pressure (Pascal's principle), allowing eventual incorporation into the surrounding tissues. Lateral fixation sutures can be used to hold the mesh in place when the aponeurotic defect cannot be closed.

Another recent development in the repair of complex or large ventral defects is the components separation technique. This involves separating the lateral muscular layers of the abdominal wall to allow their advancement. Primary fascial closure at the midline is often possible, eliminating the need for mesh insertion. Relaxing incisions are made on the lateral external oblique aponeurosis to allow its advancement, and additional relaxing incisions may be needed on the aponeurotic layers of the internal oblique and transversus abdominis. This technique is very useful in patients who have had damage-control laparotomies performed or in other situations in which large hernia defects exist.[28]

UNUSUAL HERNIAS

Spigelian Hernia

A spigelian hernia occurs through the spigelian fascia, which is composed of the aponeurotic layer between the rectus muscle medially and the semilunar line laterally. Nearly all spigelian hernias occur at or below the arcuate line. The absence of posterior rectus fascia may contribute to an inherent weakness in this area. These hernias are often interparietal, with the hernia sac dissecting posterior to the external oblique aponeurosis.

Most spigelian hernias are small (1 to 2 cm in diameter) and develop during the fourth to seventh decades of life. Patients often present with localized pain in the area without a bulge because the hernia lies beneath the intact external oblique aponeurosis. Ultrasound or CT of the abdomen can be useful to establish the diagnosis.

A spigelian hernia should be repaired because of the risk of incarceration associated with its relatively narrow neck. The hernia site should be marked before operation. A transverse incision is made over the defect and carried through the external oblique aponeurosis. The hernia sac is opened and dissected free of the neck of the hernia and either excised or inverted. The defect is closed transversely by simple suture repair of the transversus abdominis and internal oblique muscles, followed by closure of the external oblique aponeurosis. Larger defects should be repaired using a mesh prosthesis. Recurrence is uncommon.

Obturator Hernia

The obturator canal is formed by the union of the pubic bone and ischium. This canal is covered by a membrane pierced by the obturator nerve and vessels. Weakening of the obturator membrane may result in enlargement of the canal and formation of a hernia sac, which can lead to intestinal incarceration and strangulation. The patient can present with evidence of compression of the obturator nerve, which causes pain in the medial aspect of the thigh (Howship-Romberg sign). Nearly one half of patients with obturator hernia present with complete or partial bowel obstruction. An abdominal CT can establish the diagnosis if necessary.

A posterior approach, either open or laparoscopic, is preferred. This approach provides direct access to the hernia. Patients with compromised bowel should have a preperitoneal open repair. After reduction of the hernia sac and contents, any preperitoneal fat within the obturator canal should be reduced. The obturator nerve can be manipulated gently with a blunt nerve hook to facilitate reduction of the fat pad. The obturator foramen is repaired with sutures or a small piece of prosthetic mesh, with care to avoid injury to the obturator nerve and vessels.

Lumbar Hernia

Lumbar hernias can be either congenital or acquired and occur in the lumbar region of the posterior abdominal wall. Hernias through the superior lumbar triangle (Grynfeltt's triangle) are more common. The superior lumbar triangle is bounded by the 12th rib, paraspinal muscles, and internal oblique muscle. Less common are hernias through the inferior lumbar triangle (Petit's triangle), which is bounded by the iliac crest, latissimus dorsi muscle, and external oblique muscle. Weakness of the lumbodorsal fascia through either of these areas results in progressive protrusion of extraperitoneal fat and a hernia sac. Lumbar hernias are not prone to incarceration.

Satisfactory suture repair is difficult because of the immobile bony margins of these defects. Repair is best done by placement of prosthetic mesh, which can be sutured to the margins of the hernia. There is usually sufficient fascia over the bone to anchor the mesh.

Interparietal Hernia

Interparietal hernias are rare and occur when the hernia sac lies between layers of the abdominal wall. Interparietal hernias most frequently occur in previous incisions. Spigelian hernias are nearly always interparietal.

The correct preoperative diagnosis of interparietal hernia can be difficult. Many patients with complicated interparietal hernias present with intestinal obstruction. Abdominal CT can assist in the diagnosis. Large interparietal hernias usually require placement of prosthetic mesh for closure. When this cannot be done, the separation of components technique may be useful to provide natural tissues to obliterate the defect.

Sciatic Hernia

The greater sciatic foramen can be a site of hernia formation. These hernias are extremely unusual and difficult to diagnose and frequently are asymptomatic until intestinal obstruction occurs. The most common symptoms are the presence of an uncomfortable or slowly enlarging mass in the gluteal or intragluteal area. Sciatic nerve pain can occur, but sciatic hernia is a rare cause of sciatic neuralgia.

A transperitoneal approach is preferred if bowel obstruction or strangulation is suspected. Hernia contents can usually be reduced with gentle traction. Prosthetic mesh repair is usually preferred. A transgluteal approach can be used if the diagnosis is certain and the hernia is reducible. With the patient prone, an incision is made from the posterior edge of the greater trochanter across the hernia mass. The gluteus maximus muscle is opened, and the sac is visualized. The muscle edges of the defect are either reapproximated with interrupted sutures or the defect is obliterated with mesh.

Perineal Hernia

Perineal hernias are caused by congenital or acquired defects and are very uncommon. These hernias also may occur after abdominoperineal resection or perineal prostatectomy. The hernia sac protrudes through the pelvic diaphragm. Primary perineal hernias are rare, occur most commonly in older, multiparous women, and can be quite large. Symptoms are usually related to protrusion of a mass through the defect that is worsened by sitting or standing. A bulge is frequently detected on bimanual rectal-vaginal examination.

Perineal hernias are generally repaired through a transabdominal approach or combined transabdominal and perineal approaches. After the sac contents are reduced, small defects may be closed with nonabsorbable suture whereas large defects should be repaired with prosthetic mesh.

COMPLICATIONS

There are a myriad of complications related to hernia repair (Tables 42-1 and 42-2). Some are general complications that are related to underlying diseases and the effects of anesthesia. These will vary by patient population and risk. In addition, there are technical complications that are directly related to the repair. Technical complications are affected by the experience of the surgeon and are more frequent after repair of recurrent hernias. There is increased scarring and disturbed anatomy with hernia recurrence that can result in an inability to identify important structures at operation. This is the principal reason why we recommend using a different approach for recurrent hernia.

Although the overall complication rate from hernia repair has been estimated to be about 10%, many of these complications are transient and can be addressed easily. More serious complications from a large experience are listed in Table 42-1.

Surgical Site Infection

The risk of surgical site (wound) infection is estimated to be 1% to 2% after open inguinal hernia repair and less with

TABLE 42-1. Complications After 4114 Shouldice Hernia Repairs		
Complication	No. Patients	%
Wound infection	24	0.58
Hematoma	18	0.43
Pulmonary embolus	3	0.07
Hemorrhage	1	0.02
Ischemic orchitis	25	0.61
Testicular atrophy	14	0.34

From Wantz GE: The Canadian repair of inguinal hernia. *In* Nyhus LM, Condon RE (eds): Hernia, 3rd ed. Philadelphia, JB Lippincott, 1989, pp 236-248.

TABLE 42-2.   Complications After 867 Laparoscopic Hernia Repairs

Complication	No. (%)
Transient groin pain	30 (3.5)
Persistent groin pain	14 (1.6)
Transient leg pain	29 (3.3)
Persistent leg pain	11 (1.3)
Seroma/no aspiration	21 (2.4)
Seroma/aspiration	9 (1.0)
Hematoma	13 (1.5)
Transient testicular pain	8 (0.9)
Persistent testicular pain	5 (0.6)
Orchitis/epididymitis	8 (0.9)
Hydrocele	8 (0.9)
Incisional infection	2 (0.2)
Prosthesis infection	1 (0.1)
Transection vas deferens	1 (0.1)
Total	160 in 148 hernias (17.1)

From Fitzgibbons RJ Jr, Camps J, Cornet DA, et al: Laparoscopic inguinal herniorrhaphy: Results of a multicenter trial. Ann Surg 221:3-13, 1995.

laparoscopic repairs. These are clean operations, and the risk of infection is primarily influenced by associated patient diseases. Most would agree that there is no need to use routine antimicrobial prophylaxis for hernia repair.[29] Patients who have significant underlying disease, as reflected by an American Society of Anesthesiology (ASA) score greater than or equal to 3, should receive perioperative prophylaxis with cefazolin, 1 to 2 g, given intravenously within 30 to 60 minutes before the incision. Either clindamycin, 600 mg intravenously, or erythromycin, 250 mg intravenously, can be used for patients allergic to penicillin. Only a single dose of antibiotic is necessary. The placement of prosthetic mesh does not increase the risk of infection and should not affect the use of prophylaxis. The risk of infection can be decreased by using proper operative technique, preoperative antiseptic skin preparation, and appropriate hair removal. There is an increased risk of infection for patients who have had prior hernia incision infections, chronic skin infections, or an infection at a distant site.[30] These infections should be treated before elective operation.

Nerve Injuries

Nerve injuries are an infrequent complication of inguinal hernia repair. Injury can occur from traction, electrocautery, transection, and entrapment. The use of prosthetic mesh can result in dysesthesias from an inflammatory response.

The nerves most commonly affected during open hernia repair are the ilioinguinal, genital branch of the genitofemoral, and iliohypogastric.[31] During laparoscopic repair, the lateral femoral cutaneous and genitofemoral nerves are most often affected.[32] Rarely, the main trunk of the femoral nerve can be injured during either open or laparoscopic inguinal hernia repair.

Transient neuralgias can occur and are usually self-limited and resolve within a few weeks after operation. Persistent neuralgias usually result in pain and hyperesthesia in the area of distribution. Symptoms are often reproduced by palpation over the point of entrapment. Transection of a sensory nerve usually results in an area of numbness corresponding to the distribution of the involved nerve.

Various approaches to management of residual neuralgia have been described. These include analgesics, local anesthetic nerve blocks, transcutaneous electrical stimulation, and various medications. Patients presenting with nerve entrapment syndromes are usually best treated by repeat exploration with neurectomy. Mesh removal is usually needed as well.[33]

Laparoscopic nerve injuries are minimized by not placing any tacks or staples below the lateral portion of the iliopubic tract. If nerve entrapment occurs, patients should be reoperated to remove the offending tack or staple.

Ischemic Orchitis

Ischemic orchitis occurs from thrombosis of the small veins of the pampiniform plexus within the spermatic cord. This results in venous congestion of the testis, which becomes swollen and tender 2 to 5 days after operation. The process continues for an additional 6 to 12 weeks and usually results in testicular atrophy. Orchiectomy is rarely necessary.

The incidence of ischemic orchitis can be minimized by avoiding unnecessary dissection within the spermatic cord. The incidence can increase with dissection of the distal portion of a large hernia sac and among patients who have anterior operations for hernia recurrence or for spermatic cord pathology. In these situations, the use of a posterior approach is preferred.

Injury to the Vas Deferens and Viscera

Injury to the vas deferens and the intra-abdominal viscera is unusual. Most of these injuries occur in patients with sliding inguinal hernias when there is failure to recognize the presence of intra-abdominal viscera in the hernia sac. With large hernias, the vas deferens can be displaced in an enlarged inguinal ring before its entry into the spermatic cord. In this situation, the vas deferens should be identified and protected.

Hernia Recurrence

Hernia recurrence rates are variable but can be as low as 1% to 3% over a 10-year period of follow-up. Most hernias recur within the first 2 years after repair. In general, recurrences are lowest with tension-free repairs and higher with anatomic repairs.[10,14,24,32,34-39]

Hernia recurrences are usually due to technical factors, such as excessive tension on the repair, missed hernias, failure to include an adequate musculoaponeurotic margin in the repair, and improper mesh size and placement.[40] Recurrence also can result from failure to close a patulous internal inguinal ring, the size of which should always be assessed at the conclusion of the primary operation. Other factors that can cause hernia recurrence are chronically elevated intra-abdominal pressure, a chronic cough, deep incisional infections, and poor collagen formation in the wound. Recurrences are more common among patients with direct hernias and usually involve the floor of the inguinal canal near the pubic tubercle, where suture line tension is greatest. The use of a relaxing incision when there is excessive tension at the time of primary hernia repair is helpful to reduce recurrence.

Most recurrent hernias will require use of prosthetic mesh for successful repair.[13,41-44] Choosing a different approach (usually posterior) avoids dissection through scar tissue, improves visualization of the defect and reduction of the hernia, and decreases the incidence of complications, particularly ischemic orchitis and injury to the ilioinguinal nerve. Recurrences after initial prosthetic mesh repairs can be due to displaced prostheses or the use of a prosthetic of inadequate size. Recurrences are best managed by placing a second prosthesis through a different approach.

The Shouldice repair has been demonstrated to have a recurrence rate of less than 2%, which is the lowest rate of recurrence among repairs that do not use a tension-free approach.[45] A recent meta-analysis of 58 reports comparing synthetic mesh techniques to non-mesh repairs has shown a nearly 60% reduction in recurrence with the use of mesh.[46] This same report concluded that there was no difference in the rate of hernia recurrence between laparoscopic and open approaches that used mesh.

Recurrence is even more common after repair of recurrent hernias and is directly related to the number of previous attempts at repair. Large population-based studies report a re-recurrence rate of 4% to 5% overall.[44] Tension-free and mesh-based repairs have the lowest rates of reoperation after recurrence and provide a reduction in recurrence of approximately 60% compared with more traditional repairs.[41-43]

QUALITY OF LIFE

The major quality indicators that have been assessed for hernia repair are postoperative pain and return to work. Tension-free and laparoscopic mesh-based approaches have been demonstrated to be less painful than non-mesh repairs.[8] Laparoscopic repairs have the least amount of postoperative pain and have been shown to provide a marginal advantage in reducing time off work.[8,15]

Selected References

Anson BJ, McVay CB: Inguinal hernia: The anatomy of the region. Surg Gynecol Obstet 66:186, 1938.

Condon RE: Surgical anatomy of the transversus abdominis and transversalis fascia. Ann Surg 173:1, 1971.

Nyhus LM: An anatomic reappraisal of the posterior inguinal wall, with special consideration of the iliopubic tract and its relation to groin hernias. Surg Clin North Am 44:1305, 1960.

These three references are classic descriptions of the anatomy of the groin. All are well illustrated.

Anthony T, Bergen PC, Kim LT, et al: Factors affecting recurrence following incisional herniorrhaphy. World J Surg 24:95-100, 2000.

Excellent report comparing primary and mesh repairs for incisional hernia in a Veterans Administration hospital.

EU Hernia Trialists Collaboration: Repair of groin hernia with synthetic mesh. Meta-analysis of randomized controlled trials. Ann Surg 235:322-332, 2002.

Excellent meta-analysis of tension-free repairs compared with other methods. It demonstrates a 60% reduction in recurrence among mesh repairs.

Gilbert AI: Sutureless repair of inguinal hernia. Am J Surg 163:331, 1992.

This report describes the "plug and patch" tension-free inguinal hernia repair.

Lichtenstein IL, Shulman AG, Amid PK, et al: The tension-free hernioplasty. Am J Surg 157:188, 1989.

This article reports excellent results of a large number of tension-free hernia repairs.

Lowham AS, Filipi CJ, Fitzgibbons RJ Jr: Mechanisms of hernia recurrence after preperitoneal mesh repair: Traditional and laparoscopic. Ann Surg 225:422-431, 1997.

This article outlines the important causes for inguinal hernia recurrence. These principles also apply to other hernias.

Stoppa RE: The treatment of complicated groin and incisional hernias. World J Surg 13:545, 1989.

Reference describing the giant prosthetic reinforcement of the visceral sac (Stoppa) repair and its indications.

References

1. Skandalakis J, Colborn G, Androulakis J: Embryologic and anatomic basis of inguinal herniorrhaphy. Surg Clin North Am 74:799-836, 1993.
2. Anson BJ, McVay CB: Inguinal hernia: The anatomy of the region. Surg Gynecol Obstet 66:186, 1938.
3. Condon RE: Surgical anatomy of the transversus abdominis and transversalis fascia. Ann Surg 173:1, 1971.
4. Nyhus LM: An anatomic reappraisal of the posterior inguinal wall, with special consideration of the iliopubic tract and its relation to groin hernias. Surg Clin North Am 44:1305, 1960.
5. Netter FH: Atlas of Human Anatomy. Summit, NJ, Ciba-Geigy Corp, 1993.

6. Bradley M, Morgan D, Pentlow B, et al: The groin hernia—an ultrasound diagnosis? Ann R Coll Surg Engl 85:178-180, 2003.

7. Della Santa V, Groebli Y: Diagnosis of non-hernia groin masses. Ann Chir 125:179-183, 2000.

8. Neumayer L, Jonasson O, Fitzgibbons R Jr: Tension-free inguinal hernia repair: The design of a trial to compare open and laparoscopic surgical techniques. J Am Coll Surg 196:743-752, 2003.

9. Cheek CM, Williams MH, Farndon JR: Trusses in the management of hernia today. Br J Surg 82:1611-1613, 1995.

10. Lichtenstein IL, Shulman AG, Amid PK, et al: The tension-free hernioplasty. Am J Surg 157:188, 1989.

11. Gilbert AI: Sutureless repair of inguinal hernia. Am J Surg 163:331, 1992.

12. Kugel RD: Minimally invasive, nonlaparoscopic, preperitoneal, and sutureless, inguinal herniorrhaphy. Am J Surg 178:298-302, 1999.

13. Nyhus LM, Pollak R, Bombeck CT, et al: The preperitoneal approach and prosthetic buttress repair for recurrent hernia. Ann Surg 208:733, 1988.

14. Swanstrom LL: Laparoscopic hernia repairs: The importance of cost as an outcome measurement at the century's end. Surg Clin North Am 80:1341-1351, 2000.

15. Voyles CR, Hamilton BJ, Johnson WD, et al: Meta-analysis of laparoscopic inguinal hernia trials favors open hernia repair with preperitoneal mesh prosthesis. Am J Surg 184:6-10, 2002.

16. Memon MA, Fitzgibbons RJ: Laparoscopic inguinal hernia repair: Transabdominal preperitoneal (TAPP) and totally extraperitoneal (TEP). In Scott-Connor CEH (ed): The Sages Manual. New York, Springer, 1999.

17. Malangoni MA, Condon RE: Preperitoneal repair of acute incarcerated and strangulated hernias of the groin. Surg Gynecol Obstet 162:65-67, 1986.

18. Stoppa RE: The treatment of complicated groin and incisional hernias. World J Surg 13:545, 1989.

19. Radhakris H, Nan J: Umbilical hernia. In Nyhus LM, Condon RE (eds): Hernia, 4th ed. Philadelphia, JB Lippincott, 1995.

20. Askar OM: Aponeurotic hernias: Recent observations upon paraumbilical and epigastric hernias. Surg Clin North Am 64:315, 1984.

21. Lemmer JH, Strodel WE, Knol JA, et al: Management of spontaneous umbilical hernia disruption in the cirrhotic patient. Ann Surg 181:85, 1983.

22. Mayo WJ: Radical cure of umbilical hernia. JAMA 48:1842, 1907.

23. Arroyo A, et al: Randomized clinical trial comparing suture and mesh repair of umbilical hernia in adults. Br J Surg 88:1321-1323, 2001.

24. Wright BE, et al: Is laparoscopic umbilical hernia repair with mesh a reasonable alternative to conventional repair? Am J Surg 184:505-508, 2002.

25. Anthony T, Bergen PC, Kim LT, et al: Factors affecting recurrence following incisional herniorrhaphy. World J Surg 24:95-100, 2000.

26. Parker HH III, Nottingham JM, Bynoe RP, et al: Laparoscopic repair of large incisional hernias. Am Surg 68:530-533, 2002.

27. Stoppa RE, Rives JL, Warlaumont CR, et al: The use of Dacron in the repair of hernias of the groin. Surg Clin North Am 64:269-285, 1984.

28. Ewart CJ, Lankford AB, Gamboa MG: Successful closure of abdominal wall hernias using the components separation technique. Ann Plast Surg 50:269-273, 2003.

29. Taylor EW, Byrne DJ, Leaper DJ, et al: Antibiotic prophylaxis and open groin hernia repair. World J Surg 21:811-815, 1997.

30. Cramer SO, Malangoni MA, Schulte WJ, Condon RE: Inguinal hernia repair before and after prostatic resection. Surgery 94:627-630, 1983.

31. Starling JR, Harms BA, Schroeder ME, et al: Diagnosis and treatment of genitofemoral and ilioinguinal entrapment neuralgia. Surgery 102:581-586, 1987.

32. Fitzgibbons RJ Jr, Camps J, Cornet DA, et al: Laparoscopic inguinal herniorrhaphy: Results of a multicenter trial. Ann Surg 221:3-13, 1995.

33. Heise CP, Starling JR: Mesh inguinodynia: A new clinical syndrome after inguinal herniorrhaphy? J Am Coll Surg 187:514, 1998.

34. Johansson B, Hallerback B, Glise H, et al: Laparoscopic mesh versus open preperitoneal mesh versus conventional technique for inguinal hernia repair: A randomized multicenter trial (SCUR Hernia Repair Study). Ann Surg 230:225-231, 1999.

35. Juul P, Christensen K: Randomized clinical trial of laparoscopic versus open inguinal hernia repair. Br J Surg 86:316-319, 1999.

36. MacFadyen BV, Mathis CR: Inguinal herniorrhaphy: Complications and recurrence. Semin Laparosc Surg 1:128, 1994.

37. Millikan KW, Kosik ML, Doolas A: A prospective comparison of transabdominal preperitoneal laparoscopic hernia repair versus traditional open hernia repair in a university setting. Surg Laparosc Endosc 4:247, 1994.

38. Paganini A, Lezoche E, Carle F, et al: A randomized, controlled clinical study of laparoscopic vs open tension-free inguinal hernia repair. Surg Endosc 12:979-986, 1998.

39. Liem MS, van Duyn EB, van der Graaf Y, et al: Recurrences after conventional anterior and laparoscopic inguinal hernia repair. A randomized comparison. Ann Surg 237:136-141, 2003.

40. Lowham AS, Filipi CJ, Fitzgibbons RJ Jr: Mechanisms of hernia recurrence after preperitoneal mesh repair: Traditional and laparoscopic. Ann Surg 225:422-431, 1997.

41. Shulman AG, Amid PK, Lichtenstein IL: The "plug" repair of 1402 recurrent inguinal hernias: 20-year experience. Arch Surg 125:265-267, 1990.

42. Rutkow IM, Robbins AW: The mesh plug technique for recurrent groin herniorrhaphy: A nine-year experience of 407 repairs. Surgery 124:844-847, 1998.

43. Janu PG, Sellers KD, Mangiante EC: Recurrent inguinal hernia: Preferred operative approach. Am Surg 64:569-573, 1998.

44. Haapaniemi S, Gunnarsson U, Nordin P, et al: Reoperation after recurrent groin hernia repair. Ann Surg 234:122-126, 2001.

45. Simons MP, Kleijnen J, van Geldere D, et al: Role of Shouldice technique in inguinal hernia repair: a systematic review of controlled trials and a meta-analysis. Br J Surg 83:734-738, 1996.

46. The EU Hernia Trialists Collaboration: Repair of groin hernia with synthetic mesh: Meta-analysis of randomized controlled trials. Ann Surg 235:322-332, 2002.

CHAPTER 43

ACUTE ABDOMEN

R. Scott Jones, M.D. **and Jeffrey A. Claridge,** M.D.

The term *acute abdomen* designates symptoms and signs of intra-abdominal disease usually treated best by surgical operation. Many diseases, some of which do not require surgical treatment, produce abdominal pain, so the evaluation of patients with abdominal pain must be methodical and careful. The proper management of patients with acute abdominal pain requires a timely decision about the need for surgical operation. This decision requires evaluation of the patient's history and physical findings, laboratory data, and imaging tests. The syndrome of acute abdominal pain generates a large number of hospital visits and may affect the very young, the very old, either sex, and all socioeconomic groups.[1-4] All patients with abdominal pain should undergo evaluation to establish a diagnosis so that timely treatment can minimize morbidity and mortality.

Abdominal pain accounts for 5% to 10% of all emergency department visits or 5 to 10 million patient encounters in the United States annually.[5] Another study demonstrated that 25% of patients presenting to the emergency department complained of abdominal pain.[6] Diagnoses vary according to age group: pediatric, geriatric, and everyone else. Chapter 70 deals with abdominal pain in children. Appendicitis is more common in children, whereas biliary disease, colonic diverticulitis, and intestinal infarction occur more commonly in the elderly. Hospitalized patients may develop abdominal pain during the course of their illness, making diagnosis and treatment more difficult.

ANATOMY AND PHYSIOLOGY

Developmental Anatomy

The developmental anatomy of the abdominal cavity and of its viscera determines normal structure and influences the pathogenesis and clinical manifestations of most abdominal diseases.[7] Peritoneal attachments and visceral sensory innervation are particularly important to the evaluation of acute abdominal disease. After the 3rd week of fetal development, the primitive gut divides into foregut, midgut, and hindgut. The superior mesenteric artery supplies the midgut (the fourth portion of the duodenum to the midtransverse colon). The foregut includes the pharynx, the esophagus, the stomach, and the proximal duodenum, whereas the hindgut comprises the distal colon and the rectum. The afferent fibers accompanying the vascular supply provide sensory innervation to the bowel and associated visceral peritoneum.

Thus, disease in the proximal duodenum (foregut) stimulates celiac axis afferents to produce epigastric pain. Stimuli in the cecum or appendix (midgut) activate afferent nerves accompanying the superior mesenteric artery to cause periumbilical pain, and distal colon disease induces inferior mesenteric artery afferent fibers to cause suprapubic pain. The phrenic nerve and afferent fibers in C3, C4, and C5 dermatomes accompanying the phrenic arteries innervate the diaphragmatic musculature and the peritoneum on its undersurface. Stimuli to the diaphragm therefore cause referred shoulder pain. The parietal peritoneum, abdominal wall, and retroperitoneal soft tissue receive somatic innervation corresponding to the segmental nerve roots (Fig. 43-1).

The richly innervated parietal peritoneum is particularly sensitive. Parietal peritoneal surfaces sharply localize painful stimuli to the site of the stimulus. When visceral inflammation irritates the parietal peritoneal surface, localization of pain occurs. Maneuvers that exacerbate this irritation then intensify the pain. The many "peritoneal signs" useful in the clinical diagnosis of the acute abdomen originate in this fashion. Dual-sensory innervation of the abdominal cavity by both visceral

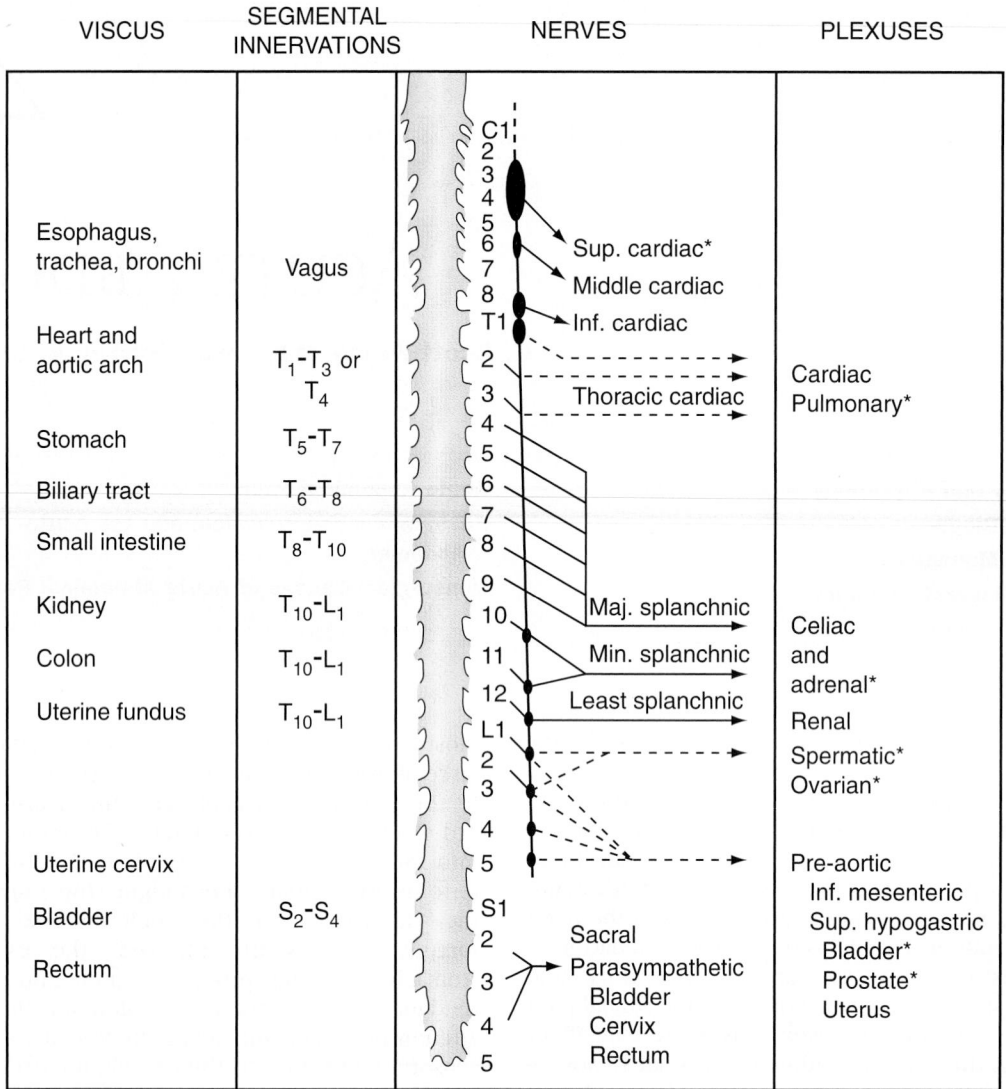

VISCUS	SEGMENTAL INNERVATIONS	NERVES	PLEXUSES
Esophagus, trachea, bronchi	Vagus	Sup. cardiac* Middle cardiac Inf. cardiac	
Heart and aortic arch	T_1-T_3 or T_4	Thoracic cardiac	Cardiac Pulmonary*
Stomach	T_5-T_7		
Biliary tract	T_6-T_8		
Small intestine	T_8-T_{10}		
Kidney	T_{10}-L_1	Maj. splanchnic	Celiac and adrenal*
Colon	T_{10}-L_1	Min. splanchnic	Renal
Uterine fundus	T_{10}-L_1	Least splanchnic	Spermatic* Ovarian*
Uterine cervix			Pre-aortic Inf. mesenteric Sup. hypogastric
Bladder	S_2-S_4	Sacral Parasympathetic Bladder Cervix Rectum	Bladder* Prostate* Uterus
Rectum			

* No known sensory fibers in sympathetic rami.

FIGURE 43-1.   Sensory innervation of the viscera. (From White JC, Sweet WH: Pain and the Neurosurgeon. Springfield, IL, Charles C Thomas, 1969, p 526.)

afferents and somatic nerves produces clinical pain patterns that aid in diagnosis. For example, the pain of acute appendicitis originates with poorly localized periumbilical pain progressing to sharply localized right lower quadrant pain when the inflammation involves the parietal peritoneal surface.

Peripheral nerves mediate sharp, sudden, well-localized pain. Sensory afferents involved with intraperitoneal abdominal pain transmit dull, sickening, poorly localized pain of more gradual onset and protracted duration. The vagus nerve does not transmit pain from the gut. Small, unnamed sympathetic afferent nerves transmit pain from the esophagus to the spinal cord. Afferent nerves from the liver capsule, the hepatic ligaments, the central portion of the diaphragm, the splenic capsule, and the pericardium enter the central nervous system from C3 to C5. The spinal cord from T6 to T9 receives pain fibers from the

periphery of the diaphragm, the gallbladder and the stomach, the pancreas, and the small intestine. Pain fibers from the colon, appendix, and pelvis viscera enter the central nervous system at the 10th and 11th thoracic segments. The sigmoid colon, rectum, renal pelvis and capsule, ureter, and testes pain fibers enter the central nervous system at T11 and L1. The bladder and the rectosigmoid colon send afferent nerves to the spinal cord from S2 to S4.[8,9]

Cutting, tearing, crushing, or burning usually does not produce pain in the abdominal viscera. However, stretching or distention of the peritoneum produces pain. Bacterial or chemical peritoneal inflammation produces visceral pain, as does ischemia. Cancer can cause intra-abdominal pain by invading sensory nerves. Abdominal pain may be visceral, parietal, or referred. *Visceral pain* is dull and poorly localized, usually in the epigastrium, periumbilical region, or suprapubic region, and it usually does not lateralize well. Patients with visceral pain may also experience sweating, restlessness, and nausea. The *parietal* or *somatic pain* associated with intra-abdominal disorders may be more intense and precisely localized. *Referred pain* is perceived at a site distant from the source of stimulus. For example, irritation of the diaphragm may produce pain in the shoulder. Disease in the bile duct or gallbladder may produce shoulder pain. Distention of the small bowel can produce pain referred to the back.

During the 5th week of fetal development, the bowel outgrows the peritoneal cavity, protrudes through the base of the umbilical cord, and undergoes a 180-degree counterclockwise rotation. During this process, the bowel remains outside the peritoneal cavity until approximately the 10th week, when it returns to the abdomen, and an additional 90-degree counterclockwise rotation occurs. This embryologic rotation places the viscera in their adult positions, and subsequent fusion of the portions of the colonic and duodenal mesenteries with the mesothelium of the posterior abdomen forms the normal ultimate peritoneal attachments. Knowledge of these attachments is clinically important during the evaluation of patients with the acute abdomen because of variation in the exact position of the viscera (e.g., pelvic or retrocecal appendix) and the compartmentalization of the abdomen by mesenteric attachments.[10] The latter, for example, may channel duodenal or gastric contents from the site of a perforated ulcer to the right lower quadrant.

Peritoneal Pathophysiology

Mesothelial cells cover the visceral and parietal peritoneal surfaces. Openings into radially arranged lymphatics penetrate the diaphragmatic peritoneal surface. Introduction of bacteria into the peritoneal cavity can cause an outpouring of fluid from the peritoneal membrane. This loss of fluid from the circulation may lead to dehydration and may produce the clinical signs of resting or orthostatic hypotension and tachycardia. Diaphragmatic lymphatics are the major route for the clearance of bacteria and cellular debris from the abdominal cavity. This process leads to an intraperitoneal circulation of fluid toward the subdiaphragmatic regions bilaterally. Fluid not cleared in this fashion tends to accumulate in the deep end of the pelvis. Thus, subdiaphragmatic, subhepatic, paracolic, or pelvic fluid collections can accompany visceral perforation. The peritoneal surfaces localize bacteria and the products of inflammation. The peritoneum responds to inflammation by increased blood flow, increased permeability, and the formation of a fibrinous exudate on its surface. The bowel also responds to inflammation with localized or generalized paralysis. The fibrinous surface thus created, aided by decreased intestinal movement, causes adherence between bowel and omentum and effectively walls off inflammation. An abscess may produce sharply localized pain with normal bowel sounds and gastrointestinal function, whereas a disseminated process, such as a perforated ulcer, produces generalized abdominal pain

with a quiet abdomen. Peritonitis may affect the entire abdominal cavity or a portion of the visceral or parietal peritoneum. Transudation can produce an increase in the peritoneal fluid, which is rich in protein and leukocytes that facilitate the formation of fibrin on peritoneal surfaces.

Peritonitis denotes peritoneal inflammation from any cause. Primary or spontaneous peritonitis can occur as a diffuse bacterial infection without an obvious intra-abdominal source of contamination. Primary peritonitis, most commonly caused by *Pneumococcus* or hemolytic *Streptococcus,* occurs more commonly in children than in adults. However, adults with ascites and cirrhosis are susceptible to spontaneous peritonitis resulting from *Escherichia coli* and *Klebsiella.*[11]

The more common secondary peritonitis results from perforation, infection, or gangrene of an intra-abdominal organ, usually of the gastrointestinal tract. Gastrointestinal secretions, pancreatic secretions, bile, blood, urine, and meconium cause chemical peritonitis when in contact with the peritoneum. A common form of chemical peritonitis follows perforation of a peptic ulcer. Bile peritonitis may result from perforation of the gallbladder or leakage from the bile ducts. Ordinarily, slow bleeding into the abdominal cavity produces relatively few signs of inflammation; the addition of bacteria to blood produces suppuration (Box 43-1). The sickest postoperative patients may have tertiary peritonitis that kills 30% to 64% of affected patients. The syndrome of poorly localized intra-abdominal infection, an altered microbial flora, progressive organ dysfunction, and high mortality define tertiary peritonitis.[12,13]

Peritonitis causes abdominal pain, either generalized or localized, depending on the disease. Appendicitis usually causes localized pain. Perforated peptic ulcer usually produces generalized abdominal pain. Acute cholecystitis causes right upper quadrant pain referred to the right scapula or shoulder. Physical findings of patients with peritonitis are abdominal tenderness, guarding, and rebound tenderness.

Box 43-1. Causes of Hemoperitoneum

Gastrointestinal
 Traumatic laceration of liver, spleen, pancreas, mesentery, bowel
Gynecologic
 Ruptured ectopic pregnancy
 Ruptured graafian follicle
 Ruptured uterus
Vascular
 Ruptured aneurysm: aortoiliac, hepatic, renal, and splenic artery
Urologic
 Ruptured bladder
Hematologic
 Ruptured spleen

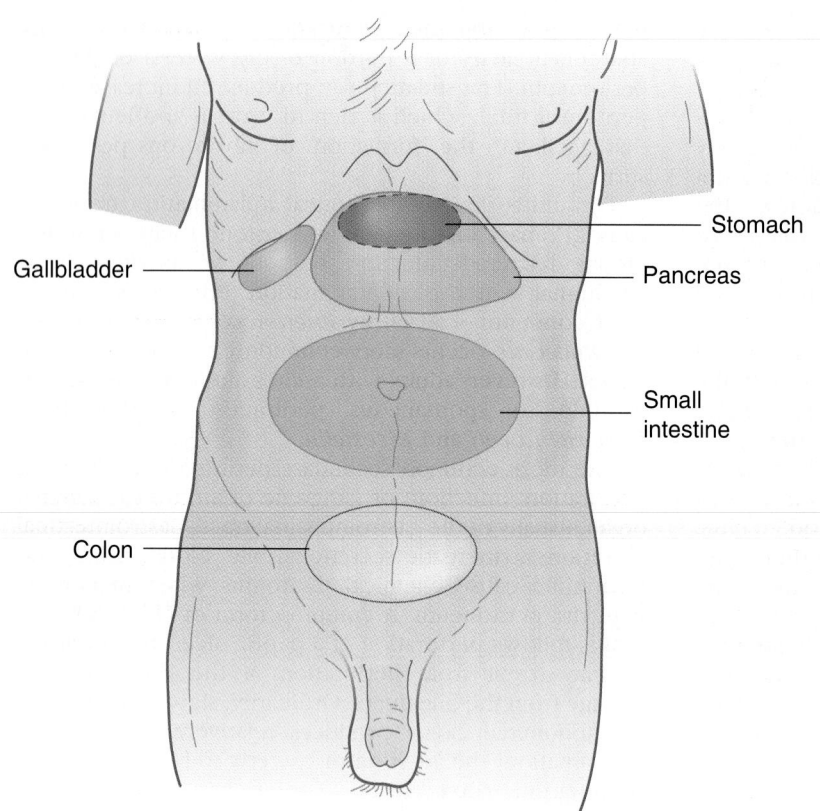

FIGURE 43-2.   Pain from intra-abdominal viscera.

Gallbladder

Stomach

Pancreas

Small intestine

Colon

CLINICAL DIAGNOSIS

History and Present Illness

Pain is the focal issue in the evaluation of the patient suspected of having an acute abdomen.[8,9,14] The history should therefore characterize and document the pain as precisely as possible. The duration of the pain is important, but the location, mode of onset, and character of the pain help in making a diagnosis. Abdominal pain that persists for 6 hours or more with severe intensity increases the likelihood that surgical operation will be required. If the pain ebbs after a few hours, however, the probability of surgical disease decreases, but not to zero. Visceral pain caused by distention, inflammation, or ischemia usually feels dull and poorly localized in the midabdomen. Depending on the organ involved, the pain may be felt in the epigastrium, the periumbilical area, or the lower abdomen (Fig. 43-2). Diseases of the kidneys or ureters produce pain in the flanks. Parietal pain, however, is sharper and better localized. Localized parietal peritonitis can produce pain confined to one of the four quadrants of the abdomen.

In an evaluation of the location of the pain, the concept of referred pain becomes important. Subdiaphragmatic disorders can produce pain referred to the shoulder. Blood or pus beneath the left diaphragm can cause left shoulder pain. Biliary disease can cause referred pain in the right shoulder or the back. Diseases above the diaphragm such as basal pneumonia can cause pain referred to the neck or shoulder in the C4 distribution. Upper abdominal pain suggests peptic ulcer, acute cholecystitis, or pancreatitis. Conversely, ovarian cysts, diverticulitis, and ruptured tubo-ovarian abscesses produce lower abdominal pain. Small bowel obstruction usually causes midabdominal pain sometimes referred to the back (Fig. 43-3).

Migratory pain shifting from one place to another can give insight into the diagnosis. For example, pain that moves from the epigastrium to the periumbilical area to the right lower quadrant suggests acute appendicitis. Distention and inflammation of the appendix produce visceral pain perceived in the periumbilical area.[15] When the inflammation spreads and produces parietal peritonitis, the pain localizes in the right lower quadrant of the abdomen. Another example of moving or migratory pain occurs with perforated duodenal ulcer. The leakage of duodenal contents from a perforated ulcer causes intense and localized epigastric pain. However, if the leaked duodenal content gravitates down the right paracolic gutter into the right lower quadrant, the patient may also experience right lower quadrant pain. Although the location of abdominal pain may be helpful, particularly early in the course of the disease, it may not be typical in all patients. Late in many cases, the pain may become generalized because of diffuse peritonitis.

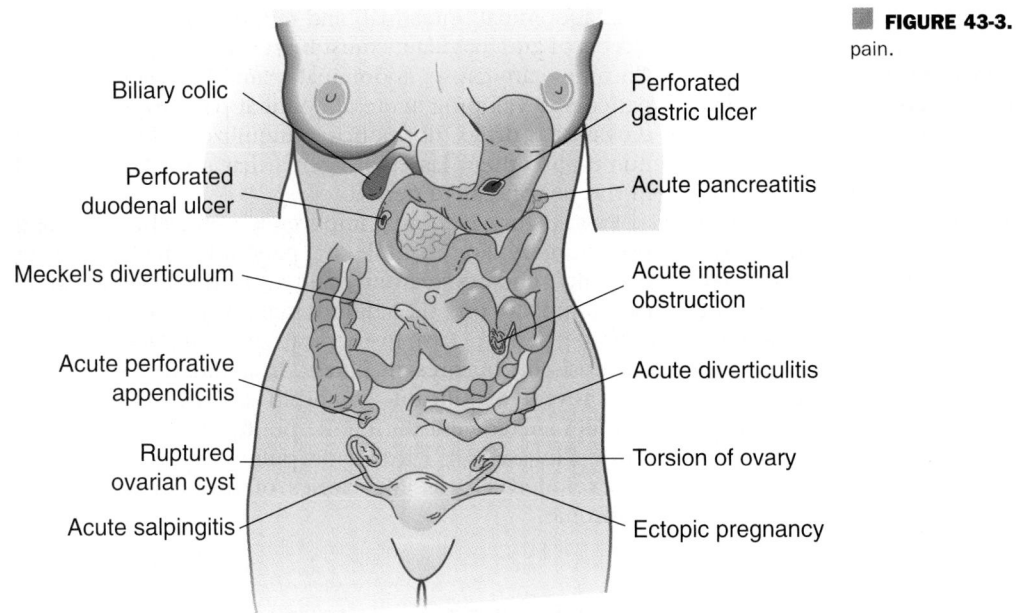

FIGURE 43-3. Common causes of abdominal pain.

Biliary colic

Perforated gastric ulcer

Perforated duodenal ulcer

Acute pancreatitis

Meckel's diverticulum

Acute intestinal obstruction

Acute perforative appendicitis

Acute diverticulitis

Ruptured ovarian cyst

Torsion of ovary

Acute salpingitis

Ectopic pregnancy

Box 43-2. Abdominal Pain Secondary to Inflammatory Lesions of the Gastrointestinal Subsystem

Stomach
  Gastric ulcer
  Duodenal ulcer
Biliary tract
  Acute cholecystitis with or without choledocholithiasis
Pancreas
  Acute, recurrent, or chronic pancreatitis
Small intestine
  Crohn's disease
  Meckel's diverticulum
Large intestine
  Appendicitis
  Diverticulitis

Box 43-3. Abdominal Pain Secondary to Obstructing Lesions of the Gastrointestinal Tract

Jejunum
  Malignancy
  Volvulus
  Adhesions
  Intussusception
Ileum
  Malignancy
  Volvulus
  Adhesions
  Intussusception
Colon
  Malignancy
  Volvulus: cecal or sigmoid
  Diverticulitis

The initial manifestations of the acute abdomen and the evolution of the pain syndrome may give some insight into the cause of the pain. The pain can start suddenly or instantly with no prior symptoms. Sudden or explosive onset of severe abdominal pain suggests free perforation of a viscus such as the duodenum or acute intestinal ischemia from a visceral artery embolus. This type of pain onset can awaken patients from sleep or can incapacitate them during work or play. Sudden, generalized, excruciating pain suggests an intra-abdominal catastrophe that may produce shock requiring resuscitation and prompt operation. In other conditions, the pain comes on with progressively increasing intensity over 1 to 2 hours. This progressive pain represents the usual manifestation of the diseases that commonly produce the acute abdomen such as acute cholecystitis, acute pancreatitis, and proximal small bowel obstruction. Some illness begins with vague general abdominal discomfort that progresses to abdominal pain over a few hours. The pain becomes more intense and subsequently localizes. This group of illnesses generally includes acute appendicitis, incarcerated hernia, distal small bowel obstruction, colon obstruction, diverticulitis, and contained or walled-off visceral perforation (Box 43-2).

The quality, severity, and periodicity of the pain may provide clues to the diagnosis. Steady, sharp pain accompanies perforated duodenal ulcer or perforated appendix. The early pain of small bowel obstruction is vague and deep seated. This pain then assumes a crescendo-decrescendo character described as *colicky pain* (Box 43-3). However, if obstruction produces intestinal infarction, then the pain becomes dull and constant. The pain of ureteral obstruction is extremely severe and intense.

Patients with kidney stones appear restless, agitated, or hyperactive and tend to move about, in contrast to patients with peritoneal inflammation, who prefer to lie quietly and remain undisturbed. Sudden, excruciating pain in the upper abdomen or the lower chest or interscapular region suggests aortic dissection.

Radiation of pain or referral of pain may help in diagnosis. Radiation of pain around the right costal margin to the right shoulder and scapula suggests acute cholecystitis. Pancreatitis usually produces epigastric pain that may radiate along the costal margins to the back or straight through to the back. Kidney stones may cause pain radiating to the groin or the perineal area.

Vomiting may occur from the severity of the pain or because of disease in the gastrointestinal tract. Generally, patients with abdominal pain requiring surgical treatment experience the pain before vomiting occurs. Vomiting frequently precedes the pain in patients with medical conditions. Patients with appendicitis usually have pain and anorexia for a while before vomiting, and patients with gastroenteritis experience vomiting before abdominal pain. Vomiting frequently occurs in patients with acute cholecystitis, acute gastritis, acute pancreatitis, and bowel obstruction. Proximal small bowel obstruction produces more vomiting than distal small bowel obstruction. Vomiting occurs uncommonly in patients with colon obstruction. Small bowel obstruction of longer duration can cause feculent vomiting. Obstruction distal to the ampulla of Vater causes bile-stained vomitus, whereas obstruction proximal to the ampulla causes clear vomitus. Most patients with acute abdominal pain have no desire to eat. Anorexia may precede the pain of acute appendicitis.

Bowel function, including a history of constipation, diarrhea, or a recent change in bowel habits, can be important. Watery diarrhea associated with abdominal pain suggests gastroenteritis. Immunosuppressed patients can contract cytomegalovirus (CMV) infection, salmonellosis, or cryptosporidiosis, which may produce diarrhea. A past history of diarrhea raises the suspicion of inflammatory bowel disease, either Crohn's disease or ulcerative colitis. Failure to pass gas or bowel movements suggests mechanical intestinal obstruction. A history of jaundice, hematemesis, hematochezia, or hematuria is important in the evaluation of acute abdominal pain.

A careful menstrual history is important in women with abdominal pain. Ovulation can produce significant abdominal pain. Furthermore, abdominal pain in a woman with a missed menstrual period or irregular menstrual periods can be related to complications of an undiagnosed pregnancy or an ectopic pregnancy.

The drug history is important in managing patients with acute abdominal pain. Corticosteroids predispose to gastroduodenal ulceration and the possibility of perforation. Corticosteroids also immunosuppress patients and obscure the manifestations of acute intra-abdominal disease. Furthermore, patients who have taken steroids for long periods require perioperative steroid supplementation. Patients who take diuretics need evaluation of their fluid and electrolyte status. Anticoagulants can cause intra-abdominal, intestinal, and mesenteric bleeding. The effects of anticoagulants must be reversed preoperatively. Cocaine can cause abdominal pain. Of course, many patients developing acute abdominal pain are taking cardiovascular drugs, hormones, tranquilizers, diuretics, and numerous other classes of agents that must be managed in the perioperative period.

Past history becomes important, especially regarding prior surgery. For example, if a patient has had an appendectomy, cholecystectomy, and so forth, it has a significant impact on the differential diagnosis of acute abdominal pain. Past history can also give clues to the diagnosis of the present illness. In addition, past history may reveal significant comorbid conditions requiring careful management during the perioperative period. Systemic illnesses or cardiac or pulmonary disease must be excluded as possible causes of the abdominal pain syndrome.

Physical Examination

The physical examination usually provides important information that helps in the diagnosis and management of patients with acute abdominal pain.[8,14] The patient's overall appearance, ability to communicate, habitus, and signs of pain should be noted. Does the patient lie quietly in bed or actively move about? Does the patient lie on his or her side with knees and hips flexed? Does the patient appear dehydrated with dry mucous membranes? An apprehensive patient lying quietly in bed, avoiding motion, and complaining of abdominal pain probably has serious intra-abdominal disease. The physical examination continues with the evaluation of the vital signs. Low fever often accompanies diverticulitis, appendicitis, and acute cholecystitis. High fever more often occurs in pneumonia, urinary tract infection, septic cholangitis, or gynecologic infection. Rapid heart rate and hypotension may mean advanced complicated disease with peritonitis. Peritonitis causes hypovolemia as plasma volume leaves the intravascular space. The general appearance of the patient and the vital signs determine the urgency of the diagnostic work-up and implementation of therapy.

Examination of the abdomen always begins with inspection, with particular attention to scars, hernias, masses, or abdominal wall defects. Hernias incarcerated in the groin, umbilicus, or incisions of obese patients can be difficult to detect. The examiner should observe whether the contour of the abdomen appears scaphoid, flat, or distended. Abdominal distention can mean intestinal obstruction, ileus, or fluid including ascites, blood, or bile.

Palpation is a crucial step in evaluating the patient with acute abdominal pain. For this examination, the patient and the examiner should be positioned comfortably to conduct gentle palpation. The examiner should assess the patient's facial expression for signs of pain or discomfort during the examination. Careful palpation for tenderness is important. This must be done gently to avoid hurting the patient and should begin in an area away from the pain site if possible. The finding and the description of tenderness are the most important steps in palpation of the abdomen of patients with acute abdominal pain. Localized tenderness over the McBurney point suggests appendicitis. Tenderness in the right upper quadrant suggests an inflamed gallbladder. Diverticulitis produces tenderness in the left lower quadrant. Tenderness throughout the abdomen may reflect diffuse peritonitis.

The detection of increased abdominal muscle tone during palpation is called *guarding.* Guarding may be voluntary, involuntary, localized, or generalized. To detect guarding, the examiner should press gently but slowly and firmly on the patient's abdomen. Using two hands works best. The detection of muscle spasm denotes guarding. If, after asking the patient to relax and breathe deeply, the patient's muscles relax, it denotes voluntary guarding. If the muscles remain rigid or tense, it indicates involuntary guarding, which means underlying peritonitis. Guarding may be localized or generalized. Generalized intense guarding produces the boardlike abdomen characteristic of perforated duodenal ulcer. Careful deep palpation can detect abdominal masses. Acute cholecystitis, acute pancreatitis, abdominal aortic aneurysm, and diverticulitis can produce abdominal masses. Severe guarding can interfere with the detection of abdominal masses by palpation.

Rebound tenderness is also a sign of peritonitis. To detect rebound tenderness, the examiner presses deep into the patient's abdomen with flattened fingers. Sudden withdrawal of that hand may cause an increase in the abdominal pain, and this symptom indicates peritonitis. Rebound tenderness can be elicited directly over the site of the abdominal pain. Pressing and releasing the abdomen away from the site of pain can exacerbate the pain at the original site. Careful, deep palpation can detect abdominal masses. Severe guarding can interfere with the detection of abdominal masses by palpation. In acute cholecystitis, palpation in the right subcostal area during deep inspiration by the patient may elicit pain. This finding is called a positive *Murphy's sign.* This sign can be detected either with the patient sitting or supine. The gallbladder may be palpated during this maneuver. Direct compression by the probe may cause pain during ultrasound examination.

Auscultation of the abdomen should give information about the presence or absence of bowel sounds. A quiet abdomen indicates ileus. Hyperactive bowel sounds may occur in gastroenteritis. Periods of quiet interrupted by the onset of high-pitched hyperactive bowel sounds characterize the peristaltic rushes of mechanical small bowel obstruction. Evaluation of bowel sounds requires careful auscultation for several minutes. During auscultation of the abdomen, the examiner can effectively evaluate tenderness and guarding further by palpating gently with the stethoscope. The examiner should also note the presence or absence of bruits in the abdomen.

Percussion is an important part of the abdominal examination. When percussion elicits tenderness, it indicates inflammation and has the same implication as rebound tenderness. Hyper-resonance or tympany to percussion of the abdomen means gaseous distention of the intestine or

> ### Box 43-4. Abdominal Pain Secondary to Lesions of the Gynecologic Subsystem
>
> **Ovary**
>   Ruptured graafian follicle
>   Torsion of ovary
> **Fallopian tube**
>   Ectopic pregnancy
>   Acute salpingitis
>   Pyosalpinx
> **Uterus**
>   Uterine rupture
>   Endometritis

stomach. Resonance to percussion over the liver suggests free intra-abdominal gas.

Other tests or maneuvers can aid in the assessment of patients with abdominal pain. Pain during gentle tapping of a fist or deep palpation at the costovertebral angles may suggest pyelonephritis. An inflamed retrocecal appendix or a psoas abscess can produce pain or tenderness on motion of the psoas muscle. If passively extending the hip or actively flexing the hip against resistance causes pain, this is called a positive *iliopsoas sign.* If internal or external rotation of the flexed hip causes pain, it is referred to as a positive *obturator sign.*

During the bimanual pelvic examination, the physician should seek evidence of uterine or adnexal masses or tenderness. Acute salpingitis, tubo-ovarian abscess, or torsion of an ovarian cyst can cause acute abdominal pain (Box 43-4). The speculum examination allows inspection of the cervix for discharge. Rectal examination should include tests for occult blood, and the examiner should note the presence of masses or tenderness. An inflamed pelvic appendix or a pelvic abscess can cause tenderness detected by rectal examination.

Laboratory Testing

Laboratory investigation of most patients with acute abdominal pain usually includes a complete blood count. Intra-abdominal inflammation can produce elevation in the white blood cell count, although this is not always true. One study demonstrated a poor correlation between the white blood cell count and the degree of intra-abdominal inflammation in patients operated on because of acute abdominal pain.[16] If a patient with unequivocal and persistent abdominal pain has a normal or low white blood cell count, a differential count may disclose a marked left shift, which can be more significant than finding an elevation in the white blood cell count. If patients have obvious dehydration, a history of vomiting or diarrhea, or if they have been taking medications such as diuretics that may influence their serum electrolyte values, one should measure the concentrations of serum sodium, potassium, blood urea nitrogen, creatinine, glucose, chloride, and carbon dioxide. In addition, these laboratory tests enable one to detect diabetes, renal failure, or other systemic diseases. Measurements of serum amylase and lipase may help in the evaluation of upper abdominal pain by giving evidence of pancreatitis. Although elevated serum amylase accompanies pancreatitis, other diseases such as perforated duodenal ulcer and small bowel infarction can also cause increased serum amylase concentrations. Patients with right upper quadrant abdominal pain should have measurements of serum bilirubin, alkaline phosphatase, and serum transaminase because of the possibility of obstructive jaundice or acute hepatitis. Urinalysis can detect evidence of urinary tract infection, hematuria, proteinuria, or hemoconcentration. Women of childbearing age who have acute abdominal pain or hypotension should have measurement of the serum or urine β-human chorionic gonadotropin concentration.

Diagnostic Imaging

History and physical examination are the most important and useful steps in the evaluation of patients with abdominal pain. However, advances in imaging of the abdomen have improved the diagnostic accuracy and the overall management of patients experiencing acute abdominal pain. Before the widespread availability of ultrasonography and computed tomography (CT), surgeons performed a careful history and physical examination, obtained laboratory tests, and reviewed plain films of the abdomen and chest. With that information, a decision to operate or not was made usually on the basis that the patient probably had some disease best treated surgically. The laparotomy was considered diagnostic as well as therapeutic. Historically, before modern imaging tests, as many as 20% of patients operated on for acute appendicitis did not have it.

Plain films still have usefulness in several circumstances. A radiograph centered on the diaphragm detects pneumoperitoneum better than other radiographic techniques. An upright chest radiograph can detect under the diaphragm as little as 1 mL of air injected into the peritoneal cavity.[17] For the occasional patient who cannot stand up, a lateral decubitus radiograph of the abdomen can also detect pneumoperitoneum effectively. A cross-table lateral radiograph with the patient in the left lateral position can detect 5 to 10 mL of gas under the lateral abdominal wall. Free air in the peritoneal cavity indicates a perforation of the gastrointestinal tract. Perforated duodenal ulcers usually allow small amounts of air to escape into the peritoneal cavity. About 75% of patients with perforated duodenal ulcers have radiographically detectable pneumoperitoneum. Perforations of the stomach and the colon can cause extensive pneumoperitoneum. The amount of pneumoperitoneum can also depend on the duration of the leak from the perforation. Plain films of the abdomen can show extensive pneumoperitoneum. If the film defines both the serosal and the related mucosal walls of the bowel, it means free air is at that serosal surface. In addition, free air can delineate the falciform ligament on plain abdominal films. An extensive hydro-

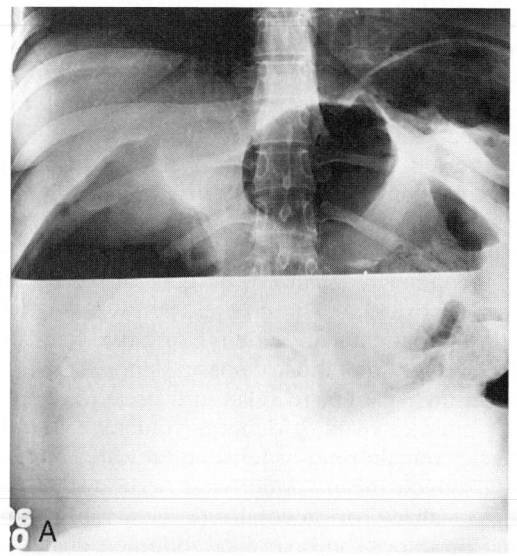

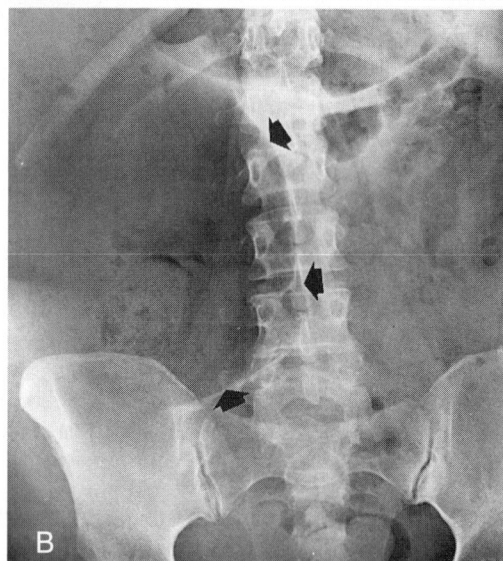

FIGURE 43-4.   Plain film findings in hydropneumoperitoneum. **A,** Upright view shows fluid level too long to be within a loop of bowel. **B,** In the supine position, the free air is well defined by the interface with the fluid in the peritoneal cavity *(arrows).*

pneumoperitoneum appears as an extremely long air-fluid level on an upright film. A supine film can show a large air collection beneath the abdominal wall that does not conform to any bowel loop (Fig. 43-4).

Plain films show abnormal calcifications. About 10% of gallstones and 90% of kidney stones contain sufficient calcium to be radiopaque. Appendicoliths can calcify and appear radiographically in 5% of patients with appendicitis. Pancreatic calcifications characteristic of chronic pancreatitis show on plain films, and vascular calcifications can aid in the evaluation of abdominal aortic aneurysms, visceral artery aneurysms, and atherosclerosis of visceral vessels.

Supine and erect plain films of the abdomen show gastric outlet obstruction; proximal, mid, and distal small bowel obstruction; and colon obstruction. The characteristics of small bowel obstruction include multiple air-fluid levels in dilated, centrally located loops of intestine with visible valvulae conniventes and an absence or paucity of colon gas. Obstructed colon usually appears as peripherally located distended bowel with haustral markings. If the ileocecal valve is incompetent, colon obstruction will cause distention of the distal small bowel.

Some patients with an acute abdomen have plain abdominal films that show a bowel pattern suggesting mechanical obstruction when no obstruction exists. Paralytic ileus can produce distended bowel with multiple air-fluid levels. Plain radiographs show paralytic ileus resulting from intra-abdominal or retroperitoneal inflammation. The radiographic findings of paralytic ileus include excessive distention and fluid with gas distributed from stomach to rectum.

Plain films of the abdomen may also detect gas in the portal or mesenteric venous system, intramural gas in the gastrointestinal tract, gas in the biliary ducts or gallbladder, and gas in the urinary tract or retroperitoneal areas. When plain films show gas in the portal or mesenteric veins, it usually means advanced and serious disease. CT can show small amounts of gas in veins and also may delineate the cause of the abnormality. If the patient's history suggests renal colic, an intravenous pyelogram may confirm the diagnosis of a kidney stone.

CT scanning has provided definite improvements in diagnostic accuracy in evaluating patients with abdominal pain and also reveals anatomic and pathologic detail not possible with plain radiographs (Fig. 43-5).[18] Therefore, CT and ultrasonography now occupy the central imaging role in this situation. Although history and physical examination provide essential information in evaluating patients with the acute abdomen, modern imaging techniques, including ultrasound and CT, can lead to an anatomic diagnosis in most cases. One prospective study of 40 patients with acute abdominal pain revealed that CT significantly improved the diagnostic accuracy of clinical evaluation plus plain radiographs.[19] Clinical examination and plain films were 50% correct, but CT scanning was 95% correct. CT scans accurately detected the specific anatomic lesion in 57.5% of cases compared with 17.5% with clinical examination and plain films. This study included no patients with appendicitis, the most common cause of the acute abdomen, because the surgeons did not refer any cases of suspected appendicitis for inclusion in the study. However, other investigators evaluated the role of CT in the diagnosis of acute appendicitis in 100 consecutive patients studied prospectively.[20] The CT interpretation had 98% sensitivity, 98% specificity, 98% positive predictive value, 98% negative predictive value, and 98% overall accuracy for diagnosing or ruling out appendicitis. According to the authors' calculations, these 100 CT scans produced a net savings of $44,731 in the care of the study patients because of improved diagnostic accuracy. CT scans can add important value to the diagnosis of acute appendicitis. However, focused specialists using excellent equipment in an environment of inquiry conducted this study, and the results may not be reproducible in all hospitals.[20] Other workers questioned the value of CT scanning in the diagnosis of acute appendicitis.[21]

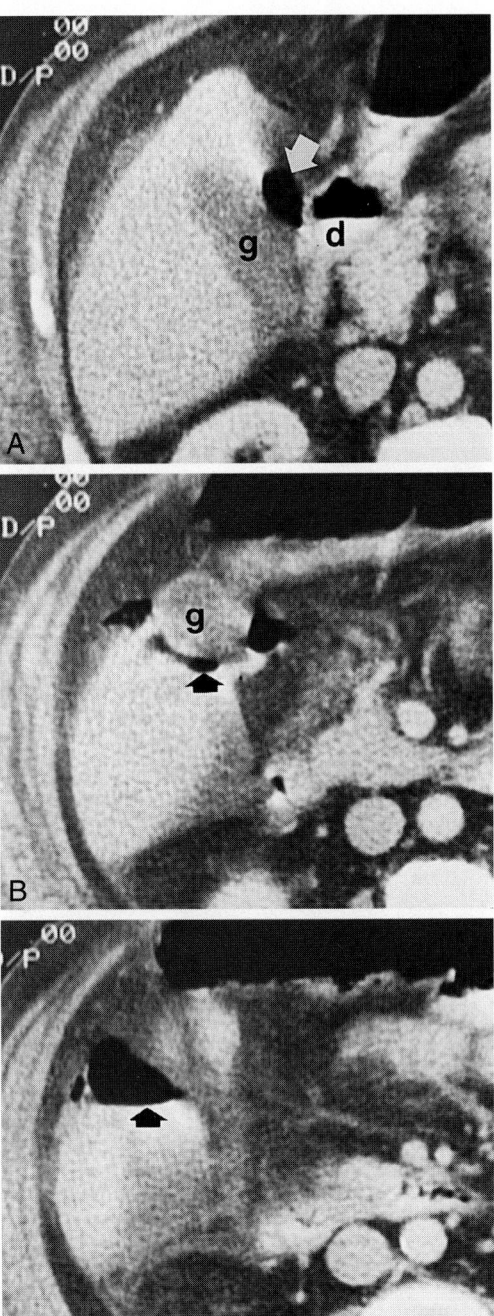

FIGURE 43-5. Unsuspected perforated duodenal ulcer. **A,** Small amount of extraluminal gas *(arrow)* lies lateral to duodenal bulb (d). g, gallbladder. **B,** At 3 cm caudad, gas *(arrow)* tracks behind the gallbladder (g) laterally. **C,** The air-fluid level *(arrow)* identifies the loculated extravasated duodenal contents. Inflammatory changes are present in the surrounding mesenteric fat.

Ultrasonography is useful for patients with acute abdominal pain because it provides rapid, safe, low-cost evaluation of the liver, gallbladder (Fig. 43-6), bile ducts, spleen, pancreas, appendix, kidneys, ovaries, adnexa, and uterus. Transabdominal and intravaginal ultrasonography can aid in the evaluation of the ovaries, adnexa, and uterus. Ultrasonography also detects and characterizes the

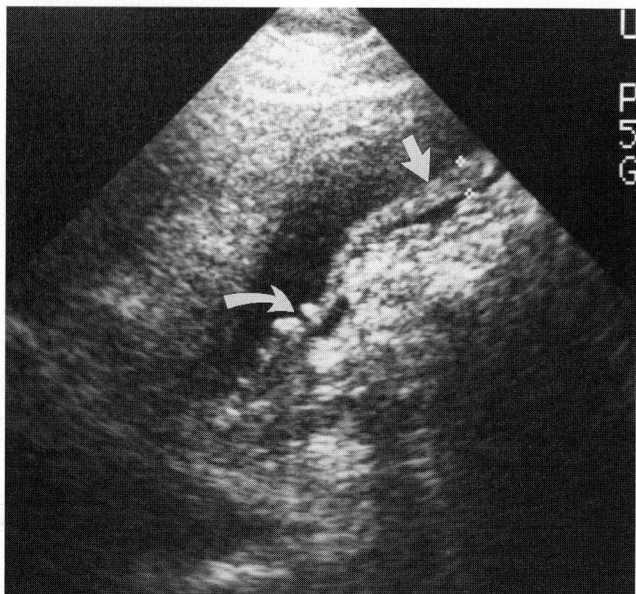

FIGURE 43-6.   Acute cholecystitis. Ultrasound evaluation shows two small stones *(curved arrow)* present in the neck of the gallbladder. The wall of the gallbladder in the fundus *(straight arrow)* is thickened, and pericholecystic fluid is present.

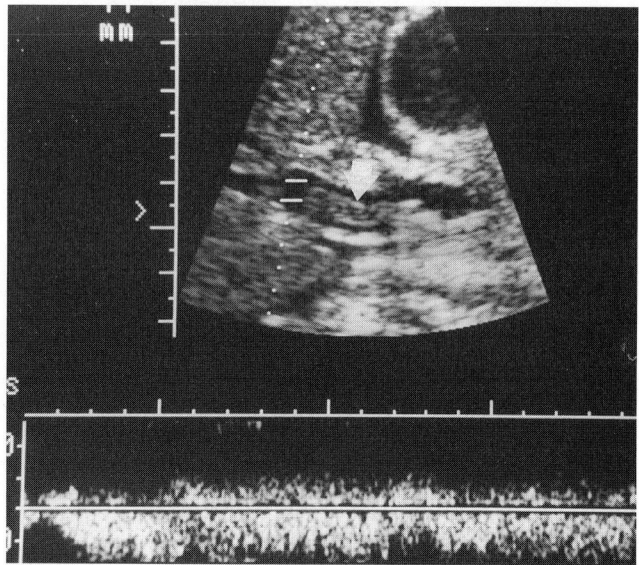

FIGURE 43-7.   Thrombus in portal vein evident on pulsed Doppler ultrasonography. An echogenic thrombus *(arrow)* is within the lumen of the portal vein. The Doppler tracing indicates flow within the portal vein.

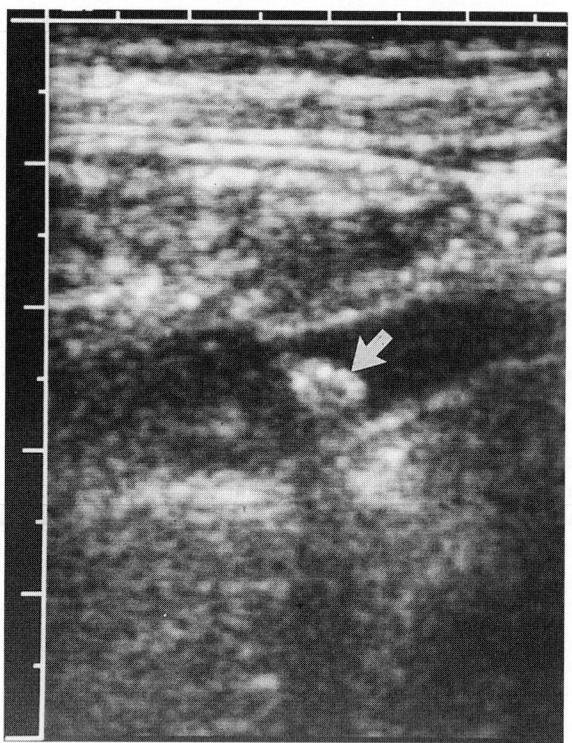

FIGURE 43-8.   Acute appendicitis. On ultrasonography, a radiographically nonopaque appendicolith *(arrow)* is evident within a thick-walled, distended appendix (longitudinal view).

distribution of intra-abdominal fluid. Color-Doppler ultrasonography allows evaluation of the intra-abdominal and retroperitoneal blood vessels. Aortic and visceral artery aneurysms, venous thrombosis, arteriovenous fistulas, and vascular anomalies can be evaluated with ultrasound (Fig. 43-7). Unfortunately, patients with acute abdominal disease frequently have excessive abdominal gas that interferes with careful and detailed sonographic evaluation of the abdominal organs, but overlying gas, bone, and

fat do not impair imaging with CT. Therefore, CT has become important for evaluating causes of the acute abdomen.

Appendicitis, the most common cause of the acute surgical abdomen in North America, can be difficult to diagnose.[1,2] Plain films and barium enema studies generally add little to the diagnosis. However, in patients with uncomplicated appendicitis, ultrasonography can detect appendicoliths, demonstrate a distended or thick-walled appendix, or detect periappendiceal and pericecal inflammatory changes (Fig. 43-8). Ultrasound is reliable and sensitive for the detection of appendicoliths and the demonstration of an abnormally distended or thick-walled appendix.[22] Conversely, CT detects acute appendicitis and defines the changes of complicated appendicitis (Fig. 43-9). CT scans can enable the examiner to differentiate diffuse periappendiceal inflammation from an abscess. In addition, CT scans detect many of the diseases included in the differential diagnosis of acute appendicitis.

CT detects blood and other fluids in the abdominal cavity. Intramural intestinal hemorrhage is readily detected by CT (Fig. 43-10). CT scans accurately reveal mesenteric venous thrombosis (Fig. 43-11). CT scans can delineate diverticulitis and its complications, such as abscess and even pyelophlebitis (Fig. 43-12). CT is especially helpful in evaluating pancreatitis by revealing minimal edema, extensive edema, fluid collections, hemorrhage, and necrosis; in addition, it effectively evaluates the complications of pancreatitis such as abscess or

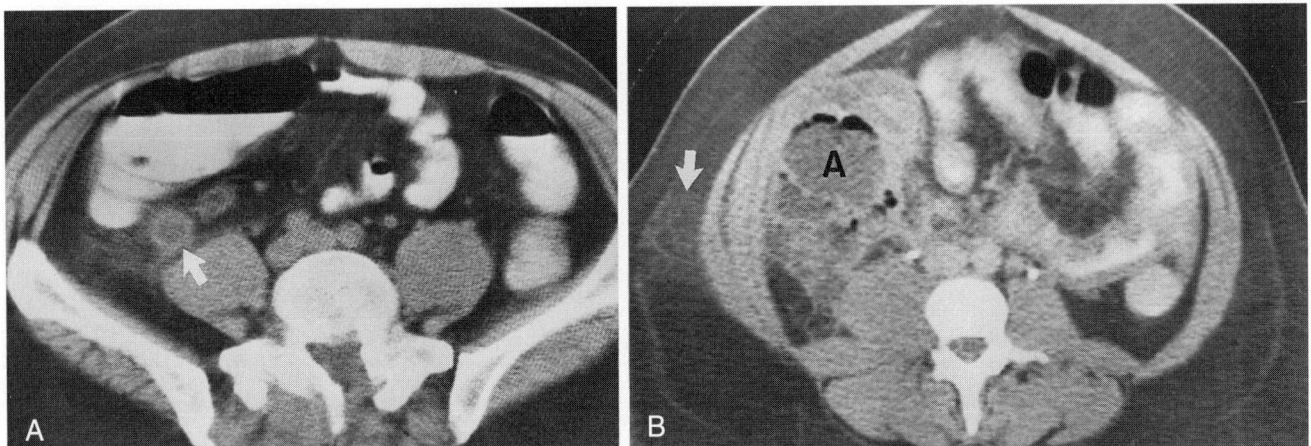

FIGURE 43-9. Appendicitis. **A,** CT scan of uncomplicated appendicitis. A thick-walled, distended, retrocecal appendix *(arrow)* is seen with inflammatory change in the surrounding fat. **B,** CT scan of complicated appendicitis. A retrocecal appendiceal abscess (A) with an associated phlegmon posteriorly was found in a 3-week-postpartum, obese woman. Inflammatory change extends through the flank musculature into the subcutaneous fat *(arrow)*.

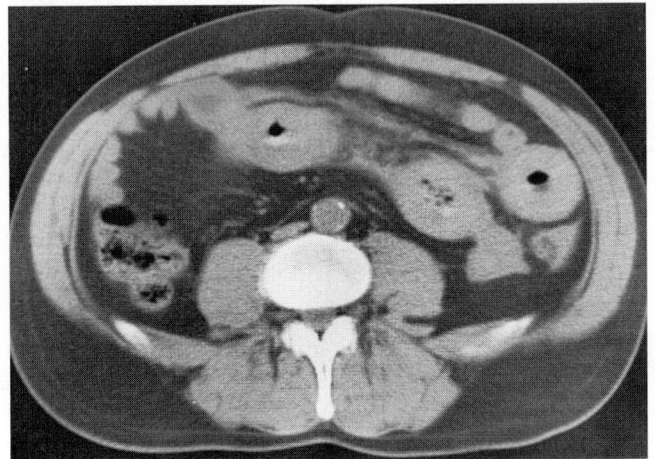

FIGURE 43-10. Intramural hematoma of small bowel. Uniform, concentric, high-density thickening of the wall of jejunal loops is characteristic.

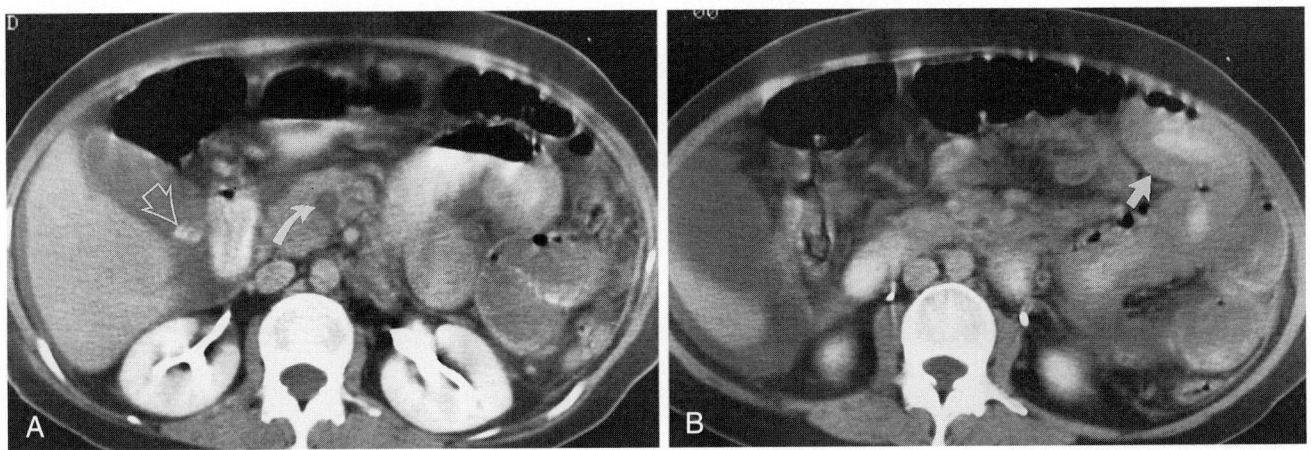

FIGURE 43-11. Small bowel infarction associated with mesenteric venous thrombosis. **A,** Note the low-density thrombosed superior mesenteric vein *(solid arrow)* and incidental gallstones *(open arrow)*. **B,** Thickening of proximal small bowel wall *(arrow)* coincided with several feet of infarcting small bowel at time of surgery.

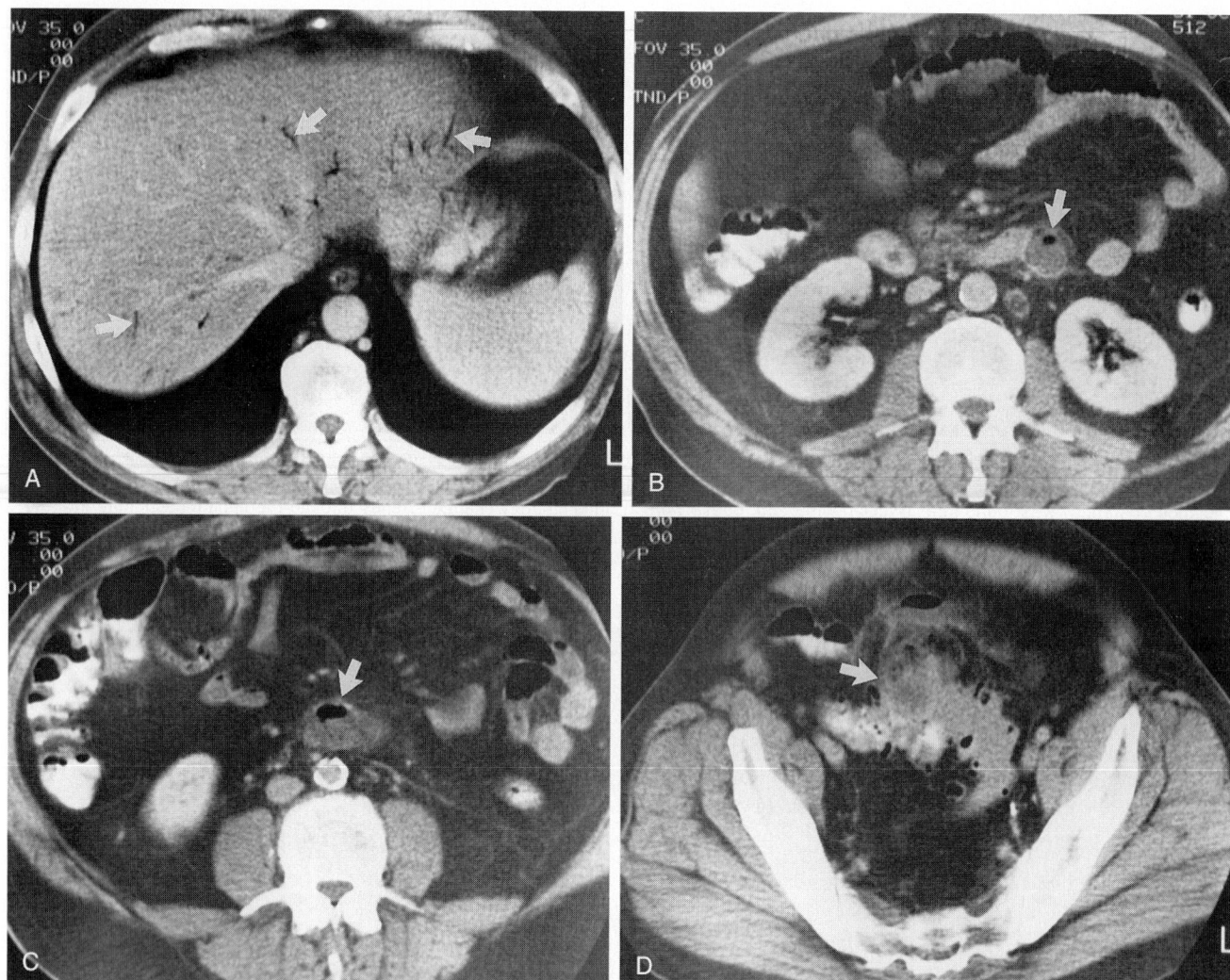

FIGURE 43-12.   Acute pyelophlebitis resulting from diverticulitis with abscess. **A,** Minute quantities of gas *(arrows)* within peripheral branches of the portal venous system were not visible on a plain radiograph. **B,** A gas-containing thrombus *(arrow)* is visible in the inferior mesenteric vein at its junction with the splenic vein. **C,** A chain of abscesses *(arrow)* extended along the course of the thrombosed inferior mesenteric vein. **D,** The septic thrombus led directly to a pericolonic abscess *(arrow)* caused by diverticulitis of the sigmoid colon.

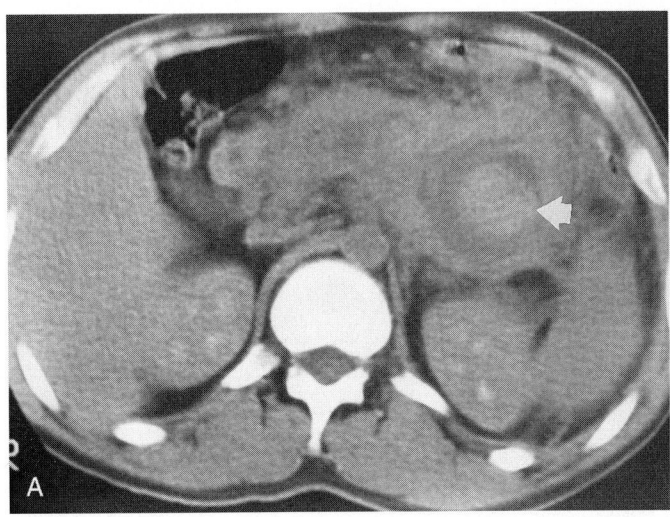

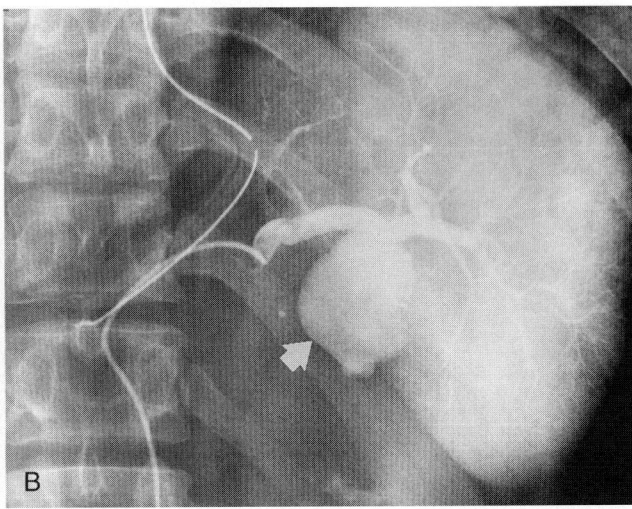

FIGURE 43-13.   Hemorrhage and false aneurysm complicating pancreatitis. **A,** Intraparenchymal hemorrhage enlarges the body and tail of the pancreas. The lumen of the false aneurysm *(arrow)* is shown as an area of increased density resulting from the enhancement of the flowing blood. **B,** Selective splenic arteriogram. A false aneurysm *(arrow)* arises from a branch of the splenic artery and was successfully treated with transcatheter embolization.

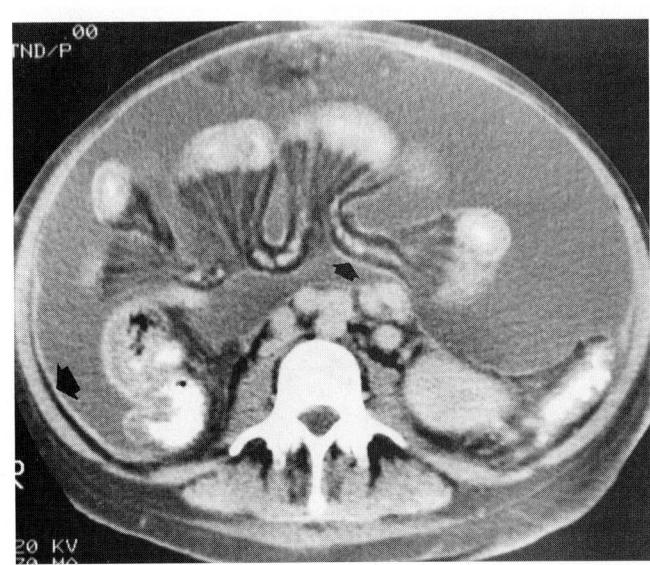

FIGURE 43-14.   Peritonitis. CT scan shows inflammatory thickening of the parietal *(large arrow)* and visceral *(small arrow)* peritoneum. The ascitic fluid is of high density, characteristic of peritonitis.

pseudocyst (Fig. 43-13). CT scans show the signs of advanced peritonitis (Fig. 43-14). With this technique, one can also evaluate the complications of colon perforation (Fig. 43-15) and of small bowel disease such as intussusception (Fig. 43-16). Although history and physical examination provide essential information in evaluating patients with the acute abdomen, modern imaging techniques, including ultrasound and CT, can lead to an anatomic diagnosis in the majority of cases.

CLINICAL MANAGEMENT

Differential Diagnosis

Information from the patient's history, physical examination, laboratory tests, and imaging studies usually permits a diagnosis, but uncertainty can still remain (see Fig. 43-3). Because appendicitis is a common disease, it must remain in the differential diagnosis of any patient with persistent abdominal pain, particularly right lower quadrant pain.[3,4] The diagnosis of appendicitis is easy to miss, and perforation substantially increases morbidity and mortality from the disease.[1,2] Delay in diagnosis is the principal reason for unfavorable outcomes in appendicitis. Appendicitis is the most common cause of the acute abdomen in childhood; however, in older patients, acute cholecystitis, bowel obstruction, cancer, and acute vascular conditions assume importance in addition to appendicitis. The differential diagnosis in young women can be difficult because they can have salpingitis, dysmenorrhea, ovarian lesions, and urinary tract infections as well as complications of pregnancy, which can confound the evaluation of abdominal pain. Of course, the medical causes of abdominal pain must be considered, but patients with medical disease generally lack specific localized tenderness and guarding. The other problem is that about one third of patients who present with acute abdominal pain have nonspecific abdominal pain, and no clear diagnosis is ever established.

Decision to Operate

These difficulties notwithstanding, the surgeon must make a decision to operate or not. Certain indications for surgical treatment exist. For example, definite signs of

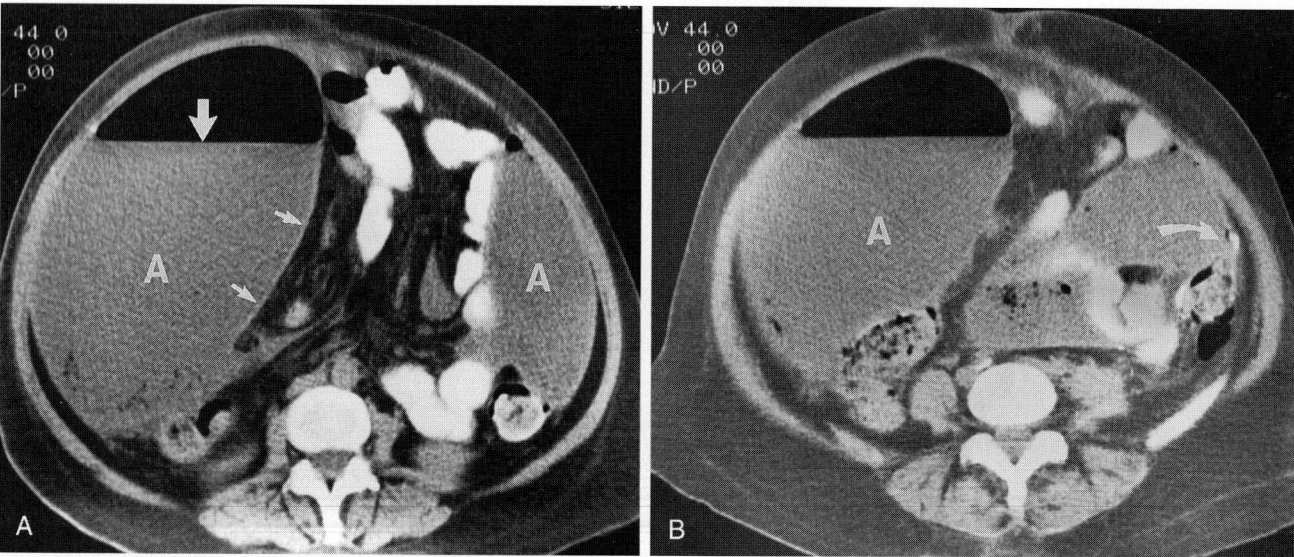

FIGURE 43-15.   Pyopneumoperitoneum secondary to a perforated descending colon. **A,** Pyopneumoperitoneum interface *(large arrow)* and inflammatory thickening of visceral peritoneum *(small arrows)* are shown. Seven liters of grossly infected ascitic fluid (A) were drained percutaneously. **B,** A trail of small gas bubbles in the left flank led to a point of discrete perforation of the descending colon *(arrow)*, which was confirmed by contrast material enema and was surgically repaired.

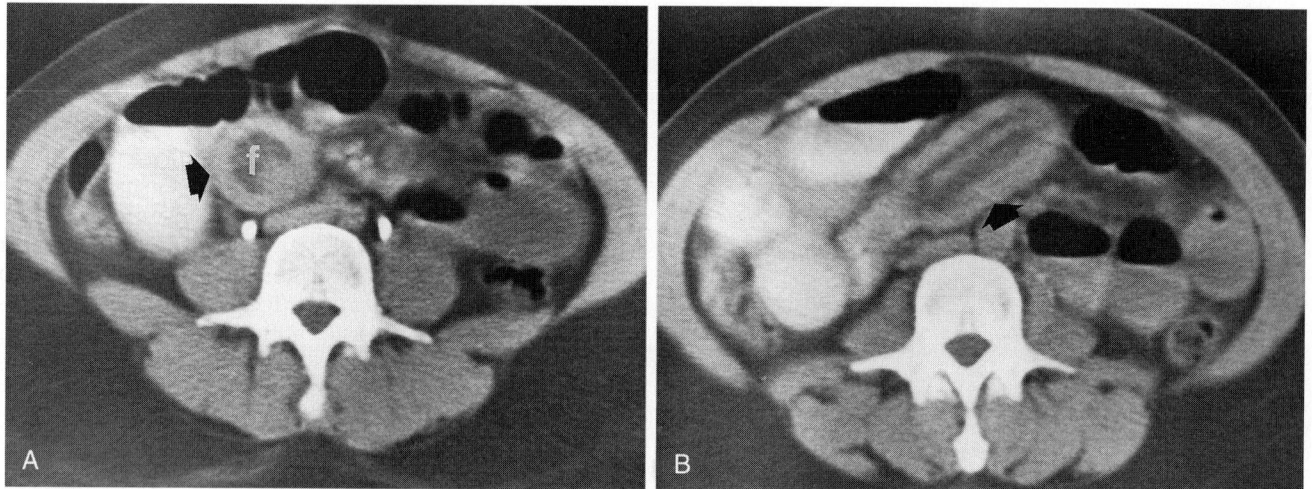

FIGURE 43-16.   Acute small bowel intussusception. The patient had a sudden onset of severe mid-abdominal pain with nonspecific plain film findings. Cross-sectional (**A**) and longitudinal (**B**) CT scans showed a small bowel intussusception *(arrows)*. Mesenteric fat (f) accompanies the intussusceptum. A benign spindle cell tumor was the cause.

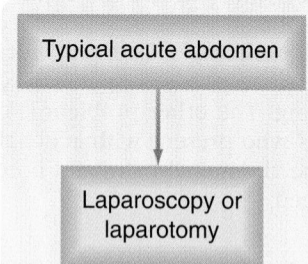

FIGURE 43-17.   Patients with unrelenting abdominal pain, tenderness, guarding, and rebound should undergo laparoscopy or laparotomy following suitable resuscitation and preparation.

peritonitis such as tenderness, guarding, and rebound tenderness support the decision to operate (Fig. 43-17). Likewise, severe or increasing localized abdominal tenderness should prompt an operation. Patients with abdominal pain and signs of sepsis that cannot be explained by any other finding should undergo operation. Those patients suspected of having acute intestinal ischemia should be operated on after complete evaluation. Certain radiographic findings confidently predict the need for operation. These findings include pneumoperitoneum and radiologic evidence of gastrointestinal perforation. Patients presenting with abdominal pain and free intra-abdominal gas seen on radiograph warrant operation with limited exceptions (Fig. 43-18). Observation with serial examinations may be

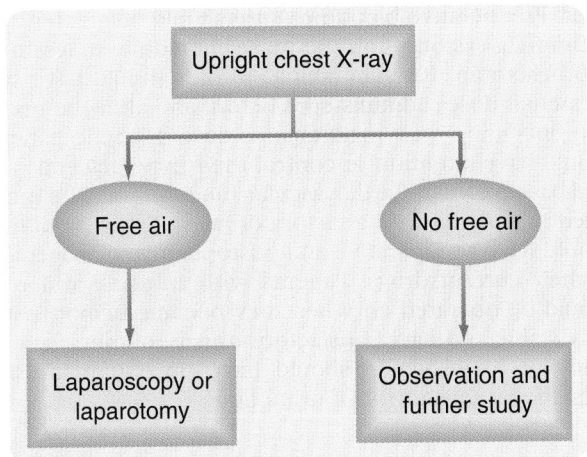

FIGURE 43-18. Most patients with free air in the peritoneal cavity should undergo laparoscopy or laparotomy following suitable resuscitation and preparation.

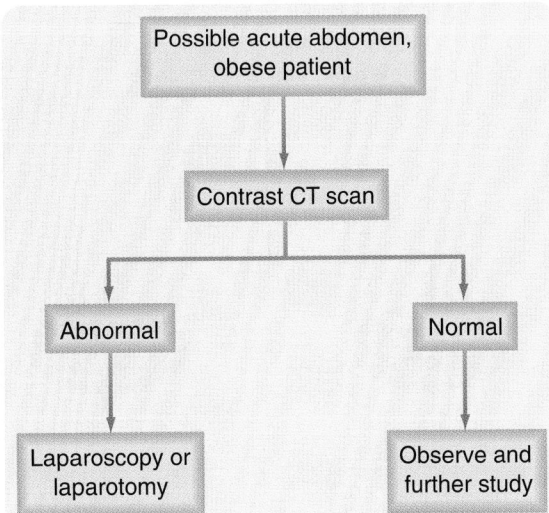

FIGURE 43-20. When obesity impairs physical examination, CT scan of the abdomen can aid in the evaluation of abdominal pain.

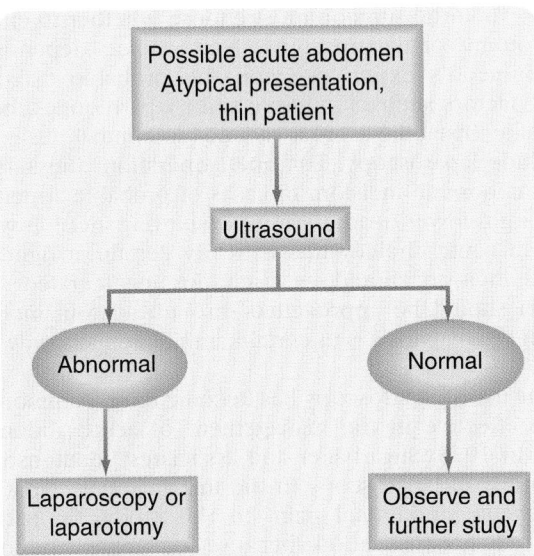

FIGURE 43-19. Patients with abdominal pain and doubtful findings for an acute abdomen should undergo imaging tests beginning with abdominal ultrasound.

appropriate for a patient with free gas after a colonoscopy.[23] Intra-abdominal gas can persist for a day or two following celiotomy. Imaging tests can reveal signs of vascular occlusion requiring operation.

After careful examination and evaluation, diagnostic uncertainty can remain. Some patients may have equivocal physical findings (Figs. 43-19 and 43-20). When this occurs and the diagnosis is unclear and the patient's wellness is unclear, it may be advisable to defer operation and to re-examine the patient carefully after several hours.[24] This is best done in a short-stay unit in the hospital, in a special unit in the emergency department, or if necessary, by regular hospital admission. In a period of hours, vague pain with minimal physical findings may proceed to defi-

nite localized pain with tenderness, guarding, and rebound tenderness; if that occurs, operation should follow. After several hours, the patient's symptoms and signs may also resolve. When that happens, the patient can be dismissed, although the patient should have a follow-up appointment scheduled within a day or so to permit re-examination to be certain that an important diagnosis was not missed. Certain patients are difficult to evaluate because of special characteristics. For example, patients who are neurologically impaired as a result of a stroke or a spinal cord injury may be difficult to evaluate.[25] Patients who are under the influence of drugs or alcohol may require special or subsequent examination. Patients who take steroids or are otherwise immunosuppressed deserve special mention because steroids and immunosuppression mask the intensity of abdominal pain and the physical findings of severe, life-threatening intra-abdominal disease. Patients in this category who have persistent, unequivocal abdominal pain and even minimal findings should be considered for surgical operation.

Some patients with clear findings of the acute abdomen may be treated without surgical operation. For example, patients with perforated duodenal ulcer who seek attention late in the course of their disease after they have been sick for several days may be treated best by careful supportive care including nasogastric suction, intravenous fluids, and pain relief. Certain patients with empyema of the gallbladder, especially those with other serious concomitant illnesses, can be treated by percutaneous drainage of the infected gallbladder and careful supportive care rather than with cholecystectomy. Some patients who have acute appendicitis may not seek attention until several days into the course of the illness, at which time they may have walled off the perforation and may have an appendiceal abscess. These patients have right lower quadrant pain, tenderness, and perhaps guarding, but if they have an appendiceal abscess, this is usually best managed by percutaneous drainage of the abscess and

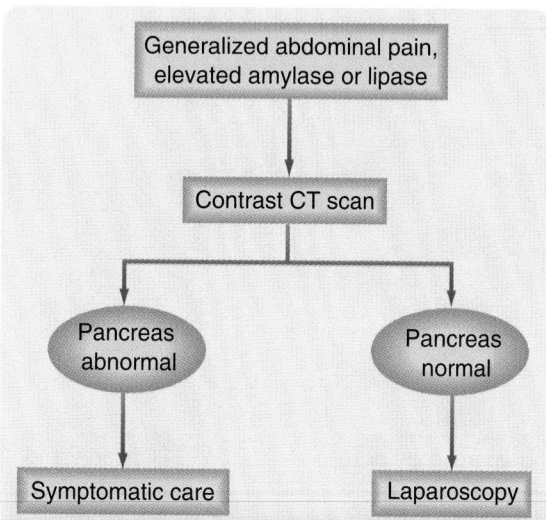

FIGURE 43-21.   Pancreatitis can produce the acute abdomen. Acute pancreatitis should be managed with supportive care. Complications of acute pancreatitis may require operation.

avoidance of appendectomy at that time. Acute diverticulitis is usually best managed nonsurgically. If a patient with diverticular disease has a diverticular abscess, percutaneous drainage and supportive care will suffice, and the diverticular disease may be removed electively later. Most patients with acute pancreatitis should be managed without operation unless they have a specific indication for operation (Fig. 43-21). Indications for operation include the development of an abscess.

Preoperative Preparation

In a stable, otherwise healthy patient, preoperative procedures should include insertion of a nasogastric tube, establishment of access for intravenous fluid administration, insertion of a Foley catheter in the urinary bladder to record urinary output, and pain relief. Once a decision has been made to perform an operation, the patient should be given a narcotic or other suitable analgesic unless he or she is being taken immediately to the operating room. Most patients with an acute abdomen requiring an operation have conditions in which infection is either present or likely. For that reason, antibiotics should be administered preoperatively.

Unstable patients must have more careful evaluation and resuscitation before one proceeds to surgical intervention. These patients also require a nasogastric tube, a Foley catheter, intravenous fluids, and antibiotics, but if patients have hypotension, tachycardia, or oliguria and evidence of dehydration, they will need a period of supportive care and intravenous fluids before they undergo general anesthesia and operation. After evaluation of their fluid and electrolyte status and degree of dehydration, these patients should receive sufficient quantities of intravenous fluid to establish urinary output of 0.5 mL/kg per hour. Preoperative blood pressure should be greater than 100 mm Hg systolic, and the pulse should fall to less than 100 beats/min. Patients taking steroids should have supplemental doses administered before and after the operation, including their maintenance dose. Diabetic patients should have attention to control their hyperglycemia and acid-base balance. Cardiovascular function must be monitored in patients with a history of heart disease, and they should have preoperative and postoperative management of their current drugs. Patients with an acute abdomen should be operated on when they become hemodynamically stable and have satisfactory urinary output. Patients who are hypokalemic should have potassium infusion after the establishment of urine flow.

Operation

After concluding that a patient with abdominal pain needs an operation, the surgeon must plan the surgical approach. General inhalation anesthesia administered through an endotracheal tube should be used in most cases. Then the surgeon must choose whether to employ laparotomy or laparoscopy. That choice depends on the surgeon's experience and the probable diagnosis. Some factors such as multiple prior laparotomies, hemodynamic instability, or advanced abdominal distention preclude laparoscopy. For open operation, the surgeon must choose an incision. In cases of probable appendicitis, a right lower quadrant muscle-splitting incision works well. If acute cholecystitis is nearly certain, a right subcostal incision should be used. An incarcerated groin hernia should be approached through a groin incision. When the diagnosis is uncertain, a midline incision works well.

The use of laparoscopy has become more common and more effective in the management of acute abdominal pain. In 1975, Sugarbaker and associates[26] demonstrated the utility of laparoscopy in the management of patients with acute abdominal pain. In this study, 56 patients required hospitalization because of acute abdominal pain. Twenty-seven of these patients had a "definite" clinical diagnosis and underwent laparotomy. Six, or 22%, of these patients had a negative laparotomy, whereas 21 patients had diseases managed best by laparotomy. Twenty-nine patients without an "exact" diagnosis underwent laparoscopy. Eighteen of those patients had, at laparoscopy, a definitive diagnosis of a disease that did not require laparotomy, and 11 patients required laparotomy after laparoscopy. Laparoscopy required 20 minutes on average and incurred no complications. The patients in the laparoscopy group had shorter hospital stays and lower hospital charges. Since 1975, of course, laparoscopic surgical skills and technology have improved dramatically, and the usefulness of laparoscopy in managing patients with acute abdominal pain is generally recognized and accepted.

Laparoscopy has become an important technique in the management of patients with acute abdominal pain. In a study of 255 patients with acute abdomen, laparoscopy proved helpful.[27] In this set of patients, laparoscopy provided a definitive diagnosis in 93%, and the remaining 7% required laparotomy for diagnosis. The treatment of the acute abdominal pain was exclusively laparoscopic in 73% of the patients, whereas 23% were treated by conventional surgery. Four percent had a combined procedure of conventional surgery assisted by laparoscopy. Eight patients died from the natural course of their disease, five from nonresectable intestinal infarctions, and three from disseminated peritoneal malignant disease. Excluding these patients, the operative mortality was 2%, that is, 5 of 247 cases. One 80-year-old patient had a fatal stroke, an 89-year-old patient who was operated on for a large intestinal obstruction had multiple organ failure, an 82-year-old patient had an intraoperative complication resulting in massive blood loss and died on the 48th postoperative day, and an 89-year-old patient died of a thoracic empyema.

More recently, several authors reported favorable experiences using laparoscopy in the diagnosis and treatment of patients with acute abdominal pain.[28-33] The diagnostic accuracy of laparoscopy varied from 93% to 100%. Laparoscopic techniques accomplished definitive treatment of the underlying disease in 44% to 73% of cases. From 10% to 38% of patients required laparotomy for definitive treatment. In 20% to 38% of patients, laparoscopy revealed either no abnormality or discovered a disease requiring no surgery for proper treatment. The morbidity rates ranged from 0 to 20%, and the mortality rates ranged from 0 to 5%.

Diagnostic and therapeutic laparoscopic techniques have an important place in the management of patients with acute abdominal pain. The diagnostic accuracy spares many patients an unnecessary laparotomy and also allows definitive laparoscopic therapy that prevents additional patients from undergoing unnecessary laparotomy. Evidence suggests that diagnostic laparoscopy reduces the cost of managing patients with acute abdominal pain. Whether diagnostic laparoscopy and therapeutic laparoscopy reduce the cost remains unclear. Most patients with acute abdominal pain should be suitable candidates for laparoscopy. Laparoscopy should be avoided in hemodynamically unstable patients and in patients with extensive gaseous distention of the abdomen. Whether pregnant women with the acute abdomen should undergo laparoscopy is a practical question. One study suggested that laparoscopy in this setting was safe and effective.[34]

Outcomes

It is difficult to know the mortality rate for patients with the acute abdomen. A study from the United Kingdom of patients hospitalized with abdominal pain revealed a mortality rate for all patients of 3.0% and an operative mortality of 7.7%.[35] Another study of 300 consecutive patients undergoing laparotomy within 6 hours of consultation for gastrointestinal perforation, intestinal infarction, or hemorrhage demonstrated a mortality rate of 20%.[36] This study included mostly critically ill patients. Other studies revealed a 16% to 40% mortality rate for emergency in older patients.[35]

ACUTE VISCERAL ISCHEMIA

Although patients experiencing acute visceral ischemia account for a small percentage of the population seeking medical attention for acute abdominal pain, this topic deserves special attention because of extreme difficulty in establishing a correct and timely diagnosis and because the condition has a high mortality rate. Acute arterial disease may be either occlusive or nonocclusive, and venous disease can also produce the syndrome. Arterial occlusion may be either embolic or thrombotic. Generally, acute superior mesenteric artery embolism causes a sudden onset of extremely severe abdominal pain. This ischemic pain persists for a long time before the development of intestinal necrosis. Because the pain results from ischemia and not from peritonitis, these patients have no abdominal tenderness, guarding, or rebound. Therefore, abdominal pain out of proportion to the abdominal physical findings should raise a question about this diagnosis. Because ischemia stops bowel motility promptly, the abdomen may be quiet to auscultation, depending on the amount of ischemic bowel. The heart is the most likely source of a superior mesenteric artery embolus. Therefore, any patient with cardiac arrhythmias, particularly atrial fibrillation, a known mural thrombus, or a recent myocardial infarction who develops acute abdominal pain should have acute superior mesenteric artery embolism high in the differential diagnosis. Patients with atherosclerosis can develop thrombosis at a superior mesenteric artery stenosis. Patients with acute visceral ischemia usually have marked leukocytosis and acidosis. Because cardiovascular disease is important in the development of acute visceral ischemia, most patients with that condition are persons who are middle aged or older.

Conversely, venous thrombosis can cause visceral ischemia, and those patients can be younger. Birth control pills have been implicated in venous thrombosis in young women. Patients suspected of having acute visceral ischemia should undergo arteriography. Although duplex scanning can provide information about the visceral circulation, arteriography provides better images for planning arterial reconstruction or embolectomy. However, arteriography may not help in venous disease. CT scans or magnetic resonance imaging studies can reveal and delineate clots in visceral veins. Most patients with acute visceral ischemia should undergo laparotomy. Some patients develop visceral ischemia because of poor perfusion resulting from decreased cardiac output. Patients usually develop nonocclusive visceral ischemia while they are in the hospital, particularly in an intensive care setting. Improving cardiac output to restore intestinal perfusion is an important step in managing this problem. Arteriography may be required for complete evaluation and allows direct infusion of vasodilators for therapy.

ACUTE ABDOMINAL PAIN

During Pregnancy

The development of acute abdominal pain during pregnancy presents a diagnostic challenge because of the enlarged uterus and the difficulty in evaluating the abdomen.[34] Appendicitis occurs once in 1500 pregnancies, evenly distributed in the trimesters. The diagnosis may be particularly difficult because the pregnant uterus can push the cecum and appendix into the right upper quadrant. Cholecystitis also occurs during pregnancy. Cholecystectomy has been performed in 3% to 8% of 10,000 pregnancies. Other conditions, such as acute pancreatitis and perforated ulcer, occur less frequently. Preeclamptic patients may experience spontaneous rupture of the liver. This is a serious and difficult complication to manage. Other causes of abdominal pain during pregnancy include placental abruption, ruptured uterus, torsion of the ovary, urinary tract infection, and pulmonary embolus.

The pregnant patient with right-sided abdominal pain, tenderness, and guarding should be strongly suspected of having appendicitis. Ultrasound examination may help to detect evidence of appendicitis. In this setting, the patient should undergo operation, probably laparoscopy. The patient and the fetus are likely to face more risk from a ruptured appendix than from the procedure. If possible, surgical treatment of symptomatic cholelithiasis should be avoided during pregnancy. Patients with infrequent, mild, self-limited attacks of right upper quadrant pain should delay the operation until after delivery. If biliary colic becomes disabling but not an emergency, operation should be delayed and performed in the second trimester. Procedures are safer during the second trimester of pregnancy. Procedures during the first trimester pose a risk to the fetus, whereas procedures during the third trimester carry the risk of premature labor. If a pregnant patient with cholelithiasis develops unrelenting right upper quadrant abdominal pain, tenderness, guarding, and fever, she should undergo operation, probably laparoscopic cholecystectomy. Hemodynamic monitoring, perhaps including an arterial line, should be used. When laparoscopy is used, intra-abdominal pressures up to 15 mm Hg should be safe. Carbon dioxide values should be monitored. Fetal heart tones should be monitored, and exsufflation should follow any sign of fetal distress.

The Patient in the Medical Intensive Care Unit

Patients in the medical intensive care unit (MICU) who develop abdominal pain while undergoing treatment for another primary condition pose a common and difficult management challenge. Gajic and associates[37] studied a cohort of 77 abdominal catastrophe patients from 6000 MICU admissions (1.3%). The conditions producing the acute abdomen in that cohort included peptic ulcer, ischemic bowel, cholecystitis, bowel obstruction, and bowel inflammation. The APACHE III score on admission to the MICU predicted a mortality rate of 31% in this group of patients who experienced an actual mortality rate of 63%. The development of an acute abdomen in this setting doubled the mortality risk. All of the 26 patients not undergoing operation died, while 23 of the 51 patients undergoing operation died postoperatively. In the unoperated group some patients were judged too ill for surgery, 2 died during resuscitation, and 3 cases were only diagnosed at autopsy. For the patients undergoing operation significant predictors of mortality included delay in surgical evaluation, delay in surgical intervention, admission APACHE III scores, renal insufficiency, and ischemic bowel. Surgical delay occurred in patients with altered mental state, absence of peritoneal signs, opioid analgesia, antibiotics, and mechanical ventilation. It is noteworthy that in this cohort 84% of patients had abdominal pain, 95% had abdominal tenderness, 73% had abdominal distention, and 33% had free intra-abdominal air on radiograph or CT.

MICU intensivists should maintain a low threshold for obtaining surgical consultation for patients with abdominal pain. The surgeon will approach such patients with high clinical suspicion. Repeated abdominal examinations, radiologic and sonographic investigations, and abdominal paracentesis must be evaluated carefully. Laparoscopy may help in this setting. Gagne and colleagues[38] reported using bedside minilaparoscopy to evaluate abdominal pain in ICU patients. Minilaparoscopy can be performed with a 3.3-mm laparoscope and instruments using local anesthesia and intravenous sedation. In any case, early surgical intervention remains crucial to survival of patients developing the acute abdomen in the MICU.

AIDS, IMMUNOSUPPRESSION, AND THE ACUTE ABDOMEN

The diagnosis and treatment of acute abdominal pain in patients with immunodeficiency pose special problems.[39,40] One must recognize the immunosuppressed patient and determine the degree of immunosuppression.[41] Mild to moderate immunodeficiency occurs in the elderly, the malnourished, the diabetic, the uremic, and patients with malignancy. In addition transplant patients on maintenance immunosuppression therapy and acquired immunodeficiency syndrome (AIDS) patients with $CD4^+$ counts greater than 200/mm^3 fall in this category. Patients in this mild to moderate immunodeficient category have the same kinds of diagnoses and surgical problems as other patients except they present in later or more advanced stages of the acute abdominal disease. Severe immunodeficiency includes AIDS patients with $CD4^+$ counts less than 200/mm^3, transplant patients taking high doses or potent immunosuppressants, and cancer patients taking chemotherapy especially if neutropenic. Severe immunodeficient patients with the acute abdomen have unusual diseases and seek medical attention late in the course of their disease. Their symptoms are vague, and they are unlikely to have fever, abdominal tenderness, or guarding. Immunodeficient patients have particular susceptibility to unusual infections caused by fungi, mycobacteria, viruses, and infestations by parasites. They are also prone to develop unusual malignant tumors.

Parente and coworkers[42] studied 458 AIDS patients hospitalized 752 times over 4 years. Seventy-one of the patients had an episode of abdominal pain severe enough to require surgical consultation. Forty-two of those patients had a premortem diagnosis of the condition causing the pain. Twenty-three patients had the cause of the abdominal pain explained by postmortem examination. The most common causative disorders in decreasing order included gastrointestinal non-Hodgkin's lymphoma, acute pancreatitis, CMV colitis/enteritis, *Mycobacterium avium-intracellulare* colitis/enteritis, sclerosing cholangitis, CMV gastritis, cryptosporidial infection, acute cholecystitis, and gastrointestinal Kaposi's sarcoma. Ten patients underwent emergency laparotomy: six for perforated viscus or peritonitis, two for intestinal obstruction, one for toxic megacolon, and one for hemoperitoneum. The postoperative survival was 40% at 1 month, 30% at 3 months, and 10% at 6 months. The median survival of the abdominal pain patients was 180 days from the diagnosis of AIDS, significantly lower than the median survival rate of the patients without abdominal pain, which was 540 days.

Patients with advanced AIDS are debilitated, malnourished, and catabolic. In addition to being particularly susceptible to unusual bacterial, viral, and fungal agents, these patients are also at risk for the common causes of the acute abdomen. Patients with AIDS are particularly prone to CMV infections, and these infections commonly invade the gastrointestinal tract and produce mucosal ulceration, bleeding, and even perforation. One should avoid surgery in patients with CMV infection unless perforation occurs. If the diagnostic work-up indicates that a patient with AIDS has an acute abdomen from a common AIDS-unrelated disease, he or she should have conventional treatment without delay.

Patients who have received organ transplants, particularly patients taking high doses of steroids, are at risk of developing the same diseases as those that occur in AIDS patients.[8,43] Because immunosuppression obscures the signs and symptoms of intra-abdominal infections and perforation, physicians caring for organ transplant recipients must have a heightened awareness of the serious significance of acute abdominal pain in their patients. Transplant recipients with intestinal perforation, appendicitis, and so forth should be operated on as soon as possible.

Any new complaint of abdominal pain expressed by an immunocompromised patient requires professional attention. Internists and family physicians should consult surgeons promptly in this situation. The surgeon should obtain a careful description of the nature of the pain and its onset. Immunocompromised patients may harbor advanced intra-abdominal disease yet exhibit minimal physical findings including fever, abdominal tenderness, guarding, and rebound. Imaging tests may help with the decision to operate. Although establishing strict criteria or guidelines for operating remains difficult, severely immunocompromised patients with unrelenting abdominal pain should undergo laparoscopy or laparotomy. In such cases the risks of intervention remain far less than the risks of untreated potentially catastrophic disease.

Box 43-5. Nonsurgical Causes of Abdominal Pain

Cardiac
  Myocardial infarction
  Acute pericarditis
Pulmonary
  Pneumonia
  Pulmonary infarction
Gastrointestinal
  Acute pancreatitis
  Gastroenteritis
  Acute hepatitis
Endocrine
  Diabetic ketoacidosis
  Acute adrenal insufficiency
Metabolic
  Acute porphyria
  Familial Mediterranean fever
  Hyperlipidemia
Musculoskeletal
  Rectus muscle hematoma
Central and peripheral nervous system
  Tabes dorsalis
  Nerve root compression
Genitourinary
  Pyelonephritis
  Acute salpingitis
Hematologic
  Sickle cell crisis

NONSURGICAL CAUSES OF ACUTE ABDOMINAL PAIN

Many diseases produce acute abdominal pain and may be treated best by means other than surgery.[44] Certain nonsurgical conditions can cause acute abdominal pain, such as spontaneous bacterial peritonitis, as mentioned earlier (Box 43-5). Sickle cell anemia may produce an attack of severe abdominal pain, referred to as *sickle cell crisis,* and this condition may result from a splenic infarction. These patients also may have attacks of bone and joint pain. Gastroenteritis may produce severe abdominal pain. Patients who develop abdominal pain and who have had a recent exposure to antibiotic therapy may have *Clostridium difficile* colitis or pseudomembranous colitis, which can mimic the acute abdomen. This diagnosis can usually be clarified by a careful history, and sigmoidoscopy reveals the pseudomembrane, which is virtually pathognomonic for the condition. Other diseases, such as lead poisoning, acute porphyria, and familial Mediterranean fever, may also cause abdominal pain. Pneumonia can produce abdominal pain, and of course, acute myocardial infarction may produce epigastric pain and can mimic acute pancreatitis or perforated ulcer. Hepatitis may produce abdominal pain. Acute adrenal insufficiency may cause abdominal pain, and patients with hyperlipidemia may have acute abdominal pain with or without acute pancreatitis.

To manage patients with abdominal pain effectively, the surgeon must always remember that many nonsurgical diseases cause abdominal pain and may mimic the acute abdomen. Surgical and nonsurgical causes of abdominal pain are not mutually exclusive. Patients with sickle cell disease can develop acute cholecystitis or appendicitis. After performing a careful history, physical examination, and imaging tests, the surgeon must evaluate the strength of the evidence that the patient actually has a nonsurgical disease versus the strength of the evidence for an acute surgical abdomen. Diagnostic laparoscopy should find liberal application in this situation.

Selected References

Jeffrey RB Jr: CT and Sonography of the Acute Abdomen. New York, Raven, 1989.

> This textbook provides complete discussion and illustration of the use of CT and sonography in the evaluation of patients with acute abdominal pain.

Lee JKT, Sagel SS, Stanley RJ: Computed Body Tomography with MRI Correlation, 2nd ed. New York, Raven, 1989.

> This textbook is an important source of information on the use of CT and MRI in the diagnosis of abdominal pain.

Rao PM, Rhea JT, Novelline RA, et al: Effect of computed tomography of the appendix on treatment of patients and use of hospital resources. N Engl J Med 338:141-146, 1998.

> This careful prospective study determined the sensitivity and specificity of CT imaging in the diagnosis of acute appendicitis. The authors also evaluated the role of CT in patient outcome.

Salky BA, Edye MB: The role of laparoscopy in the diagnosis and treatment of abdominal pain syndromes. Surg Endosc 12:911-914, 1998.

> The authors reviewed their experiences with 121 patients with acute abdominal pain who underwent laparoscopy for diagnosis and treatment. They discussed the role of laparoscopy for acute abdominal pain.

Silen W: Copes' Early Diagnosis of the Acute Abdomen, 19th ed. New York, Oxford University Press, 1995.

> All surgical residents and all surgeons who treat patients for acute abdominal pain should review this classic book.

References

1. Brewer BJ, Golden GT, Hitch DC, et al: Abdominal pain: An analysis of 1,000 consecutive cases in a University Hospital emergency room. Am J Surg 131:219-223, 1976.
2. Lewis FR, Holcroft JW, Boey J, et al: Appendicitis: A critical review of diagnosis and treatment in 1,000 cases. Arch Surg 110:677, 1975.
3. Owens BJ, Hamit HF: Appendicitis in the elderly. Ann Surg 187:392-396, 1978.
4. Yusuf MF, Dunn E: Appendicitis in the elderly: Learn to discern the untypical picture. Geriatrics 34:73-79, 1979.
5. Graff LG, Robinson D: Abdominal pain and emergency department evaluation. Emerg Med Clin North Am 19:123-136, 2001.
6. Cordell WH, Keene KK, Giles BK, et al: The high prevalence of pain in emergency medical care. Am J Emerg Med 20:165-169, 2002.
7. Gray SW, Skandalakis JE: Embryology for Surgeons: The Embryological Basis for the Treatment of Congenital Defects. Philadelphia, WB Saunders, 1972.
8. Diethelm AG, Stanley RJ, Robbin ML: The acute abdomen. In Sabiston DC (ed): Textbook of Surgery: The Biological Basis of Modern Surgical Practice, 15th ed. Philadelphia, WB Saunders, 1997, pp 825-846.
9. Way LW: Abdominal pain. In Sleisenger MH, Fordtran JS (eds): Gastrointestinal Disease, 2nd ed. Philadelphia, WB Saunders, 1978, pp 207-221.
10. Buschard K, Kjaeldgaard A: Investigation and analysis of the position, fixation, length, and embryology of the vermiform appendix. Acta Chir Scand 139:293-298, 1973.
11. Gilbert JA, Kamath PS: Spontaneous bacterial peritonitis: An update. Mayo Clin Proc 70:365-370, 1995.
12. Nathens AB, Rotstein OD, Marshall JC: Tertiary peritonitis: Clinical features of a complex nosocomial infection. World J Surg 22:158-163, 1998.
13. Rotstein OD, Meakins JL: Diagnostic and therapeutic challenges of intra-abdominal infections. World J Surg 14:159-166, 1990.
14. Boey JH: Acute abdomen. In Way LW (ed): Current Surgical Diagnosis and Treatment, Vol 21, 10th ed. Norwalk, CT, Appleton & Lange, 1994, pp 441-452.
15. Van Zwalenburg C: The relation of mechanical distension to the etiology of appendicitis. Ann Surg 41:437, 1905.
16. Blennerhassett L, Hall JL, Hall JC: White blood cell counts in patients undergoing abdominal surgery. Aust N Z J Surg 66:369-371, 1996.
17. Miller RE, Nelson SW: The roentgenologic demonstration of tiny amounts of free intraperitoneal gas: Experimental and clinical studies. Am J Roentgenol Radium Ther Nucl Med 112:574-585, 1971.
18. Siewert B, Raptopoulos V, Mueller MF, et al: Impact of CT on diagnosis and management of acute abdomen in patients initially treated without surgery. AJR Am J Roentgenol 168:173-178, 1997.
19. Taourel P, Baron MP, Pradel J, et al: Acute abdomen of unknown origin: Impact of CT on diagnosis and management. Gastrointest Radiol 17:287-291, 1992.
20. Rao PM, Rhea JT, Novelline RA, et al: Effect of computed tomography of the appendix on treatment of patients and use of hospital resources. N Engl J Med 338:141-146, 1998.
21. Morris KT, Kavanagh M, Hansen P, et al: The rational use of computed tomography scans in the diagnosis of appendicitis. Am J Surg 183:547-550, 2002.
22. Jeffrey RB Jr, Laing FC, Townsend RR: Acute appendicitis: Sonographic criteria based on 250 cases. Radiology 167:327-329, 1988.
23. Araghizadeh FY, Timmcke AE, Opelka FG, et al: Colonoscopic perforations. Dis Colon Rectum 44:713-716, 2001.
24. White JJ, Santillana M, Haller JA Jr: Intensive in-hospital observation: A safe way to decrease unnecessary appendectomy. Am Surg 41:793-798, 1975.
25. Bar-On Z, Ohry A: The acute abdomen in spinal cord injury individuals. Paraplegia 33:704-706, 1995.
26. Sugarbaker PH, Sanders JH, Bloom BS, et al: Preoperative laparoscopy in diagnosis of acute abdominal pain. Lancet 1:442-445, 1975.
27. Navez B, d'Udekem Y, Cambier E, et al: Laparoscopy for management of nontraumatic acute abdomen. World J Surg 19:382-387, 1995.
28. Chung RS, Diaz JJ, Chari V: Efficacy of routine laparoscopy for the acute abdomen. Surg Endosc 12:219-222, 1998.

29. Kaiser AM, Katkhouda N: Laparoscopic management of the perforated viscus. Semin Laparosc Surg 9:46-53, 2002.

30. Paterson-Brown S: Emergency laparoscopic surgery. Br J Surg 80:279-283, 1993.

31. Salky BA, Edye MB: The role of laparoscopy in the diagnosis and treatment of abdominal pain syndromes. Surg Endosc 12:911-914, 1998.

32. Sanna A, Adani GL, Anania G, et al: The role of laparoscopy in patients with suspected peritonitis: Experience of a single institution. J Laparoendosc Adv Surg Tech A 13:17-19, 2003.

33. Vander Velpen GC, Shimi SM, Cuschieri A: Diagnostic yield and management benefit of laparoscopy: A prospective audit. Gut 35:1617-1621, 1994.

34. Gurbuz AT, Peetz ME: The acute abdomen in the pregnant patient: Is there a role for laparoscopy? Surg Endosc 11:98-102, 1997.

35. Hawthorn IE: Abdominal pain as a cause of acute admission to hospital. J R Coll Surg Edinb 37:389-393, 1992.

36. Rozycki GS, Tremblay L, Feliciano DV, et al: Three hundred consecutive emergent celiotomies in general surgery patients: Influence of advanced diagnostic imaging techniques and procedures on diagnosis. Ann Surg 235:681-689, 2002.

37. Gajic O, Urrutia LE, Sewani H, et al: Acute abdomen in the medical intensive care unit. Crit Care Med 30:1187-1190, 2002.

38. Gagne DJ, Malay MB, Hogle NJ, et al: Bedside diagnostic minilaparoscopy in the intensive care patient. Surgery 131:491-496, 2002.

39. Bizer LS, Pettorino R, Ashikari A: Emergency abdominal operations in the patient with acquired immunodeficiency syndrome. J Am Coll Surg 180:205-209, 1995.

40. Jeffrey RB Jr: Abdominal imaging in the immunocompromised patient. Radiol Clin North Am 30:579-596, 1992.

41. Scott-Conner CE, Fabrega AJ: Gastrointestinal problems in the immunocompromised host: A review for surgeons. Surg Endosc 10:959-964, 1996.

42. Parente F, Cernuschi M, Antinori S, et al: Severe abdominal pain in patients with AIDS: Frequency, clinical aspects, causes, and outcome. Scand J Gastroenterol 29:511-515, 1994.

43. Meyers WC, Harris N, Stein S, et al: Alimentary tract complications after renal transplantation. Ann Surg 190:535-542, 1979.

44. Steinheber FU: Medical conditions mimicking the acute surgical abdomen. Med Clin North Am 57:1559-1567, 1973.

CHAPTER 44

ACUTE GASTROINTESTINAL HEMORRHAGE

Barbara Lee Bass, M.D. and Douglas J. Turner, M.D.

Initial Evaluation and Treatment of Patients With Acute Gastrointestinal Hemorrhage	**Acute Gastrointestinal Hemorrhage From an Obscure Source**
Acute Upper Gastrointestinal Hemorrhage	**Rare Causes of Gastrointestinal Hemorrhage From an Obscure Source**
Acute Lower Gastrointestinal Hemorrhage	

Hemorrhage from the gastrointestinal tract is a common and serious clinical problem. In the United States, 1% to 2% of acute hospital admissions are for patients requiring evaluation and treatment of gastrointestinal hemorrhage. With an incidence of 170 per 100,000 adults per year, gastrointestinal hemorrhage is a leading diagnosis in patients admitted to intensive care units (ICUs).[1] Although the overall mortality rate for these patients ranges from 5% to 12%, the mortality rate in patients with persistent or recurring hemorrhage approaches 40%. Mortality is linked not only to the degree of hemorrhage but also, more importantly, to the coexisting medical conditions in the patient with hemorrhage.[2] Up to 85% of bleeding episodes cease spontaneously, allowing a less urgent approach to identify the source of bleeding and to provide definitive therapy; however, 15% of patients present with major, ongoing bleeding that requires aggressive emergency diagnosis and management to allow successful clinical outcomes. These high-risk patients are most likely to require surgical intervention and to have poor outcomes.[3]

Hemorrhage can arise in any area of the gastrointestinal tract: the esophagus, stomach and duodenum, small bowel, and colon as well as organs that empty secretions into the gastrointestinal tract, such as the liver through the biliary system and the pancreas through the pancreatic duct. Although the spectrum of conditions giving rise to acute hemorrhage are legion, more than 85% of major bleeding episodes can be linked to one of four diagnoses: peptic ulcer disease, variceal hemorrhage, colonic diverticulosis, or angiodysplasia. Other sources of hemorrhage are distinctly less common. Gastrointestinal hemorrhage spans the socioeconomic strata and is equally common in

urban and rural environments. Only advancing age appears to be a risk factor for hemorrhage that applies across the full spectrum of bleeding conditions of the intestinal tract. Up to half of patients with acute gastrointestinal hemorrhage are older than 60 years of age.

Numerous advances in medical technology during the 1990s, particularly the improved availability and application of diagnostic and therapeutic endoscopy, have been instrumental in the evaluation and successful treatment of patients with major bleeding. Although surgery is required for control of hemorrhage in only 5% to 10% of patients hospitalized with gastrointestinal hemorrhage, it remains an essential emergency intervention for those patients with severe or recurrent hemorrhage from both the upper and lower gastrointestinal tract. Successful collaboration between the surgeon and the gastroenterologist is essential for optimal management of these complicated patients.

In all patients, regardless of bleeding source, successful initial management requires that the treating physician be mindful of the potential severity of gastrointestinal hemorrhage. Appropriate resuscitation to restore volume and red blood cell deficits is critical in patients with major hemorrhage. This resuscitation phase must be followed by rapid diagnosis of the source of bleeding. Thereafter, institution of appropriate specific therapies may be offered to effect successful management.

This chapter focuses on diagnosis and treatment of the two major categories of gastrointestinal hemorrhage: upper gastrointestinal hemorrhage, bleeding originating in the gastrointestinal tract proximal to the ligament of Treitz; and lower gastrointestinal hemorrhage, bleeding arising in the bowel distal to the ligament. Upper gastrointestinal hemorrhage is present in 85% of patients with acute gastrointestinal bleeding; lower gastrointestinal bleeding occurs in 10% to 15% of patients, with the small bowel as the source in only 1% to 5% of patients. Hemorrhage from small bowel sources may be difficult to diagnose and is frequently referred to as *hemorrhage of obscure origin*. The introduction of video capsule endoscopy 3 years ago has enhanced the diagnosis and treatment of the uncommon small bowel lesion.

INITIAL EVALUATION AND TREATMENT OF PATIENTS WITH ACUTE GASTROINTESTINAL HEMORRHAGE

Initial management of a patient with acute gastrointestinal hemorrhage has four primary goals: (1) comprehensive patient assessment, with attention to hemodynamic status and identification of significant medical comorbidities; (2) institution of appropriate resuscitation and monitoring; (3) identification of the major source of gastrointestinal bleeding; and (4) institution of specific therapeutic interventions to stop or control the bleeding. When the level of severity of the bleeding is clarified and initial assessment and resuscitation are complete, the patient may be triaged to the appropriate level unit of care.

Goal 1: Initial Patient Assessment

Most patients with acute gastrointestinal hemorrhage present for initial assessment in the emergency department. One quarter of patients develop gastrointestinal hemorrhage during hospitalization for a concurrent illness; this group is particularly high risk for subsequent mortality.[4] Initial assessment in either case calls for a focused history and physical examination, with attention to risk factors for gastrointestinal hemorrhage and laboratory evaluation.

History

Except for patients in hemorrhagic shock, revealing information can be obtained from the patient's history. The essential elements to be ascertained are the characteristics of the bleeding; the onset and duration of bleeding (hours or days antecedent); the associated symptoms; the use of concurrent medications; and previous significant medical conditions, particularly liver disease.

Characteristics of Bleeding

Acute gastrointestinal hemorrhage can present with hematemesis (vomiting of blood or bloody gastric contents), melena (passage of dark tarry or maroon stool), or hematochezia (passage of bright red blood from the rectum). On initial evaluation of a patient with acute gastrointestinal hemorrhage, it is important to determine whether the patient has experienced hematemesis, melena, or hematochezia. Gastrointestinal bleeding that is slow or intermittent is usually not evident to the patient; hence, the

term *occult* is associated with this pattern of blood loss. Such patients present to primary care venues with secondary signs of slow blood loss, such as anemia or fatigue.

Hematemesis is diagnostic of upper gastrointestinal bleeding, that is, bleeding from the esophagus, stomach, or duodenum. Rarely, hematemesis may result from brisk hemorrhage from the nasal passages or pharynx when the patient swallows large volumes of blood. Melena can be indicative of either upper or lower gastrointestinal hemorrhage. Dark, tarry stools are most commonly a sign of an upper gastrointestinal source in which the blood has traversed the small bowel and colon. Gastric acid degrades hemoglobin to hematin, and the actions of digestive enzymes and luminal bacteria further contribute to the appearance of melena. Melena may also represent bleeding from lesions in the small bowel or right colon. Hematochezia is the characteristic sign of colonic hemorrhage and reflects rapid elimination of blood from the bowel. Ten percent of patients with very rapid upper gastrointestinal hemorrhage may also have a history of hematochezia and syncope. It is essential to determine the onset of bleeding and the frequency of episodes of hematemesis, melena, or hematochezia and to make a rough estimate of volume.

Associated Symptoms

Inquiry regarding associated symptoms is also of value. A history of orthostatic dizziness or syncope indicates rapid and profound blood loss. Antecedent dyspepsia is suggestive of peptic ulcer disease; crampy abdominal pain is more consistent with upper gastrointestinal bleeding, whereas hematochezia is usually painless. Antecedent vomiting may suggest Mallory-Weiss tears; weight loss raises the possibility of malignancy.

Medications

The risk for gastrointestinal ulceration and hemorrhage is elevated in patients taking salicylates or nonsteroidal anti-inflammatory drugs (NSAIDs). Use of these medications is linked not only to gastritis and gastric and duodenal ulcers but also to much less commonly seen ulcerated lesions of the colon and small bowel. Further, salicylates and NSAIDs impair platelet function and may contribute to poor coagulation in patients who develop the complication of hemorrhage. These agents are widely used by middle-aged and elderly patients; up to half of patients older than 50 years of age may use NSAIDs over the course of a given 30-day period. Use of other medications that predispose to hemorrhage, such as warfarin and low-molecular-weight heparin, should be elicited. All medications should be reviewed, particularly those for cardiovascular disorders, including β blockers, calcium-channel blockers, and antihypertensives, because these agents alter the normal physiologic signs of hypovolemia.

Past Medical History

The past medical history should identify previous episodes of gastrointestinal bleeding or past history of conditions associated with acute hemorrhage. A history of dysphagia or reflux esophagitis, recent gastrointestinal distress with vomiting, peptic ulceration, *Helicobacter pylori* infection, liver disease, alcohol abuse, inflammatory bowel disease, intestinal polyps, diverticulosis, or malignancy may point to the source of bleeding. Equally important is identification of comorbid medical conditions that alter the patient's ability to respond to hemorrhage. Complications and mortality are much more likely to occur in patients with a history of renal insufficiency, atherosclerotic cardiovascular disease, congestive heart failure, chronic respiratory conditions, preexisting liver disease, or central nervous system disability.[5]

Physical Examination

The major initial objective of the physical examination is to determine the degree of blood loss and volume depletion. Patients in shock with hypotension (systolic blood pressure <90 mm Hg in the supine position), tachycardia, and cold extremities can be assumed to have a deficit of at least 40% of blood volume. Patients with less severe but substantial blood loss of 20% to 40% show hypotension in the upright position. Orthostatic vital signs should be checked in all patients not in shock by allowing the patient to sit up with the legs dangling for a period of 5 minutes. An elevation in pulse of more than 20 beats/min or a fall in blood pressure of more than 10 mm Hg is a positive sign, indicative of at least a 20% blood volume loss. Signs of peripheral hypoperfusion, such as clammy, cool, pale extremities, also reflect a volume loss of at least 20%. These signs are less reliable in elderly patients, who may show exaggerated postural changes or blunted changes in heart rate, or are more likely to be using β-blocker medication. All patients showing a volume deficit of greater than 20% of blood volume require prompt and aggressive resuscitation.

The physical examination generally offers few specific signs relative to the source of gastrointestinal hemorrhage. The oropharynx and nose should be examined to exclude the rare unrecognized nasopharyngeal source of bleeding. Although epigastric tenderness may be elicited in patients with peptic ulcer conditions, this is not a reliable sign. Patients with hematemesis and cirrhosis may show jaundice, abdominal distention with ascites, palmar erythema, and caput medusae, suggesting bleeding related to portal hypertension; even these signs, however, are not sufficient to forego complete diagnostic evaluation for the actual bleeding source. A rectal examination, noting the quality of the stool (i.e., brown, melena, or hematochezia) should also be completed. Peutz-Jeghers syndrome, a rare heritable condition, is characterized by small intestinal polyposis and may be identified by melanin spots on the lips, oral mucosa, and digits; patients with Osler-Weber-Rendu syndrome may have cutaneous telangiectasias.

Initial Laboratory Assessment

All patients with gastrointestinal hemorrhage should have basic laboratory testing, including hemoglobin and hematocrit, coagulation profile, liver function tests, serum electrolytes, and renal function. The initial hematocrit may not reflect the actual degree of hemorrhage because intravascular volume repletion from extracellular fluids may not have occurred.[6] The finding of initial hemoglobin of less than 10 g/100 mL is associated with an increased risk for morbidity and mortality. A specimen should also be sent to the blood bank for type and crossmatching.

Goal 2: Resuscitation

Based on the estimated volume deficit, rapid restoration of intravascular volume is indicated. All patients with gastrointestinal hemorrhage should have two large-bore intravenous lines for administration of lactated Ringer's solution. Patients in shock should receive prompt transfusion of packed red blood cells if immediate response to electrolyte solutions is not evident. Patients with major hemorrhage, elderly patients, and patients with significant comorbidities (including cardiac, pulmonary, hepatic, or renal insufficiency) should be monitored with central venous or pulmonary artery catheters. Urine output should be monitored with a Foley catheter.

Ongoing hemorrhage requires continuous resuscitation with saline and red blood cell transfusion. Coagulation defects should be corrected with component therapy or fresh frozen plasma and platelets. These measures should be instituted in the hospital environment that can best support these rapid maneuvers. In some hospitals, this is the emergency department; in others, this resuscitation is best accomplished in an ICU. Patients with massive hematemesis and mental obtundation are at high risk for pulmonary aspiration. These and hemodynamically unstable patients should have endotracheal intubation performed to protect the airway.

Despite general improvements in management of critically ill patients, the mortality rate for patients with major gastrointestinal hemorrhage, particularly upper gastrointestinal hemorrhage related to peptic ulceration, has remained unchanged at 5% to 12%. In fact, elderly patients with defined comorbid risk factors, including impaired cardiac, renal, and pulmonary function, may have mortality rates for major upper gastrointestinal hemorrhage in excess of 60%. These patients rarely die of hemorrhage, however. Rather, they die of multisystem organ failure precipitated by episodes of shock due to initial or recurrent episodes of hemorrhage or as a consequence of pneumonia or cardiac events. Hence, appropriate management on initial presentation is essential to salvage these patients.

Goal 3: Identification of Source of Bleeding

Successful management of a patient with acute gastrointestinal hemorrhage requires knowledge of the site of bleeding. The specific aspects of diagnostic testing are considered in the detailed sections that follow. The general considerations are reviewed here.

Patients with hematemesis, melena, or hematochezia require emergency upper endoscopy by an endoscopist capable of therapeutic intervention. Preparatory to this examination, a large-caliber orogastric tube should be placed to lavage the gastric lumen to enhance visual examination. Airway protection may require endotracheal intubation. Active volume resuscitation must continue during the examination. If patients are hemodynamically stable and show no signs of ongoing hemorrhage, endoscopic examination may be deferred to an urgent status (within 12 hours) provided the patient can be carefully observed in the interim.

Patients presenting with melena and hematochezia without a history of hematemesis should have a nasogastric tube inserted to examine the gastric contents. Findings of blood-tinged secretions, "coffee grounds," or guaiac-positive fluid should prompt upper endoscopy. Patients with melena and hematochezia with hemodynamic instability should have initial emergency upper endoscopy. Bleeding peptic lesions in the duodenum can elicit pyloric spasm precluding reflux of sufficient amounts of blood into the gastric lake to cause hematemesis. Endoscopy is essential to examine the duodenum in these patients. Even in stable patients, this examination should be performed within 24 hours of the bleeding episode to optimize outcome.[7]

Hemodynamically stable patients with hematochezia and patients with melena with a negative upper gastrointestinal examination may be presumed to have acute lower gastrointestinal hemorrhage. For these patients, the choice of initial diagnostic test remains controversial. Mesenteric arteriography, colonoscopy, and labeled red blood cell scintigraphy are potentially valuable based on the clinical presentation. Diagnostic approaches are considered later in the section on lower gastrointestinal hemorrhage.

Goal 4: Institution of Specific Therapy

After resuscitation and identification of the source of bleeding, specific therapy can be instituted. For the 15% of patients with ongoing gastrointestinal hemorrhage and hemodynamic instability, the time interval until this intervention should be less than 2 hours, and all measures to provide ongoing support to avoid shock should be employed during the interval. Fortunately, bleeding stops spontaneously in most patients, allowing a more deliberate evaluation. After the source of bleeding has been identified, specific intervention can be provided. An algorithm for diagnosis of acute upper gastrointestinal bleeding is shown in Figure 44-1.

Interventions for specific conditions are reviewed in the following sections.

ACUTE UPPER GASTROINTESTINAL HEMORRHAGE

Definition and Incidence

Upper gastrointestinal bleeding is defined as bleeding from a source proximal to the ligament of Treitz. Acute upper gastrointestinal hemorrhage is a common and potentially deadly condition accounting for approximately 85% of hospital admissions for gastrointestinal bleeding. Despite the availability of effective antiulcer medications and an improved understanding of the pathogenesis of ulcer disease, gastroduodenal ulcer disease remains the most common cause, responsible for half of bleeding episodes. In urban environments, hemorrhage from esophageal and gastric varices secondary to portal hypertension of alcoholic cirrhosis constitutes the next most frequent source, identified in 10% to 20% of patients.[8] Acute mucosal lesions, broadly characterized as gastritis or duodenitis, are observed in 15% to 30% of patients with hemorrhage in both urban and nonurban settings. Other causes have remained relatively stable in frequency since the early 1970s, including Mallory-Weiss mucosal tears at the gastroesophageal junction (8% to 10%), esophagitis (3% to 5%), malignancy (3%), Dieulafoy's lesion (1% to 3%), and more recently, "watermelon" stomach (1% to 2%). A differential diagnosis for acute upper gastrointestinal hemorrhage is shown in Box 44-1.

Clinical Presentations

Hematemesis and melena are the most frequent clinical findings in significant upper gastrointestinal bleeding. However, massive bleeding from an upper source may be associated with hematochezia. Even in instances where a lower gastrointestinal bleeding source is suspected, the passage of a nasogastric tube is required to interrogate for the presence of blood in the stomach. Although all sources of gastrointestinal bleeding have high associated morbidities, upper gastrointestinal bleeding has the highest risk for life-threatening hemorrhage.

Etiology

Although the conditions described earlier (see Box 44-1) share similar clinical presentations and initial assessment and resuscitation protocols are similar, definitive endoscopic evaluation is essential to correctly determine the cause of bleeding. Each condition has unique features of management that can be appropriately applied only with timely definitive diagnosis. Diagnostic endoscopy is the mandatory initial diagnostic test. However, endoscopy in the setting of acute hemorrhage carries specific risks compared with elective endoscopy. Complication rates of 0.9%, most of which are cardiopulmonary in nature, are reported for patients undergoing emergency endoscopy for hemorrhage, as compared with rates of 0.1% to 0.3% in the elective setting. Arterial desaturation during the procedure occurs four times as frequently in patients undergoing emergency compared with elective upper endoscopy. Patients with hypotension have a decreased level of consciousness and are at increased risk for pulmonary aspiration. The gastric lumen may contain large amounts of blood or clot; thorough evacuation of the lumen with a large-bore orogastric tube may not only facilitate visualization but also help prevent aspiration. Elderly patients with these and other comorbid conditions are most likely to have these risks. Careful airway protection is mandatory, and elective orotracheal intubation is often

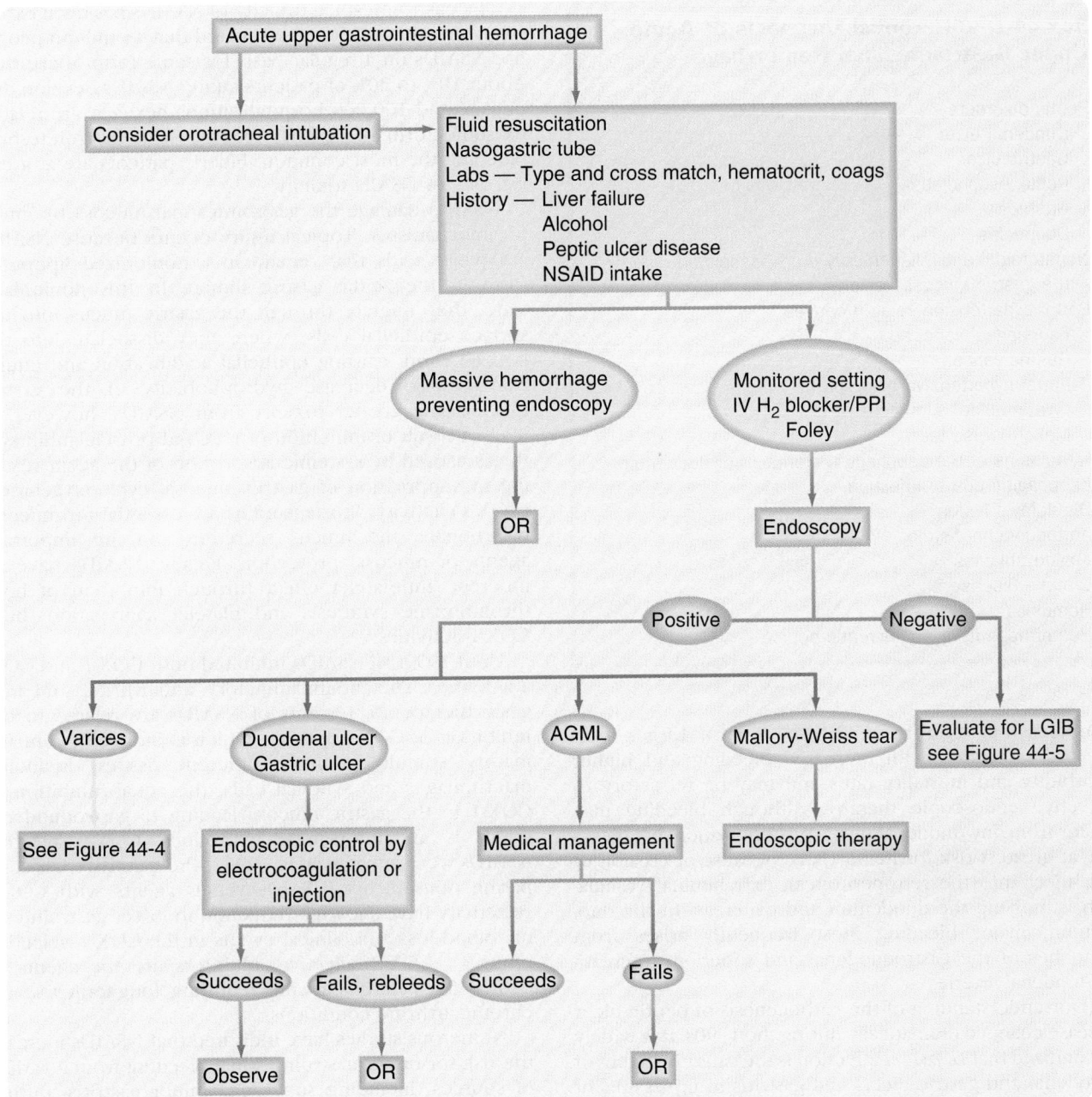

FIGURE 44-1. Algorithm for the management of upper gastrointestinal bleeding. NSAID, nonsteroidal anti-inflammatory drug; PPI, proton-pump inhibitor; LGIB, lower gastrointestinal bleeding; AGML, acute gastric mucosal lesions; OR, operating room.

appropriate for these patients. Despite the risks, endoscopy is essential.

Bleeding Peptic Ulcer

Peptic gastric and duodenal ulcers are the most common cause of acute hemorrhage in the upper gastrointestinal tract, each accounting for about 25% of cases. Despite improved understanding of the pathogenesis of ulcer disease and improved therapies to manage bleeding with nonsurgical endoscopic therapies, only a few recent studies have indicated that surgical and mortality rates for this condition may have declined slightly since about

1995. About 5% of patients with peptic ulcer disease have hemorrhage as the initial manifestation of the condition, and up to 20% of patients with peptic ulcers develop bleeding at least once. Hemorrhage remains the most lethal form of complicated ulcer disease; 80% of ulcer deaths in the elderly occur as a consequence of an episode of acute hemorrhage.

Pathogenesis

Bleeding ulcer is caused by acid-peptic erosion into the submucosal or extraluminal vessels. In the stomach, the vessel is typically a small submucosal artery with a mean

> ### Box 44-1. Differential Diagnosis of Acute Upper Gastrointestinal Hemorrhage
>
> Peptic disorders
>   Duodenal ulcer
>   Gastric ulcer
>   Reflux esophagitis
>   Gastritis
>   Duodenitis
> Nonsteroidal anti-inflammatory drug–associated disorders
> Acute gastric mucosal lesions
> Portal hypertension–related causes
>   Esophageal varices
>   Gastric varices
>   Portal hypertensive gastropathy
>   "Watermelon" stomach
>   Mallory-Weiss tear
> Neoplasms of the esophagus, stomach, or duodenum
> Esophagitis due to infection
> Dieulafoy's lesion
> Aortoduodenal fistula
> Angiodysplasias
> Crohn's disease
> Hemobilia
> Hemorrhage from a pancreatic source

diameter of 0.7 mm (range, 0.1 to 1.8 mm).[9] Larger arteries are associated with increased bleeding and higher morbidity and mortality rates and may be refractory to effective endoscopic therapy. Although bleeding may occur from any duodenal ulcer, posterior duodenal ulcers are at greatest risk for hemorrhage because of erosion of the ulcer into the retroperitoneal, extraluminal vasculature supplying the duodenum and pancreas. In the duodenum, major bleeding most frequently arises from branches of the gastroduodenal and superior pancreaticoduodenal arteries.

Our understanding of the pathogenesis of peptic ulcer disease changed dramatically during the 1990s. It is widely recognized that *H. pylori* infection is the causative agent of duodenal and gastric ulcers and gastritis in up to 80% of patients not taking NSAIDs. *H. pylori*–associated ulcers represent 40% to 50% of cases of peptic disease. NSAIDs are responsible for the remaining cases, and up to 30% of these patients may also have *H. pylori* infection. *H. pylori* is not uniformly identifiable in non-NSAID–using patients with bleeding peptic ulcer. In some series, only 40% to 60% of patients with bleeding ulcer were found to have *H. pylori* infection. Hence, the role of "physiologic" acid hypersecretion in patients with complicated ulcer disease is being reappraised. Patients using NSAIDs have a 15% to 20% greater risk for bleeding ulcer than patients with *H. pylori* infection, and NSAID use may be an independent indicator of adverse outcome. Only 1% to 2% of patients with ulcer disease develop the condition as a result of acid hypersecretion caused by gastrin-secreting endocrine tumors of the gastrointestinal tract (Zollinger-Ellison syndrome).

The gastrointestinal toxicity of NSAIDs has been extensively investigated.[10] It is estimated that 13 million people use NSAIDs on a regular basis for some form of arthritis. About 10% to 20% of patients taking NSAIDs develop dyspepsia, and 100,000 hospitalizations per year are related to some form of NSAID toxicity, with gastrointestinal bleeding the most common. Elderly patients are at greatest risk for NSAID toxicity.

NSAIDs damage the gastrointestinal mucosa by multiple mechanisms. Topical injury occurs because NSAIDs are weak acids that remain in a nonionized lipophilic form in the acidic gastric lumen. In this nonionized state, they migrate through the gastric mucus into the surface epithelial cells, where they dissociate into the ionized form, causing epithelial acidification and injury. NSAIDs also decrease hydrophobicity of the gastric mucus. The greater toxicity from NSAIDs, however, is likely a result of inhibition of mucosal prostaglandin synthesis caused by systemic absorption of the agent resulting in suppression of gastric mucosal cyclooxygenase-1 (COX-1) activity. Prostaglandins are essential for mucosal bicarbonate and mucus secretion and are important agents of mucosal protection. Finally, NSAIDs have an inherent antiplatelet effect through inhibition of both thromboxane synthesis and platelet aggregation, both COX-1 activities.[11]

Until 1999, all NSAIDs inhibited both COX-1 and COX-2 activities. The anti-inflammatory, antiarthritic, and analgesic therapeutic benefits of NSAIDs are related to the inhibition of COX-2 activity, which is induced by inflammatory stimuli in many different tissues, including macrophages and synovial cells; the equal inhibition of COX-1 in the gastric mucosa leading to gastroduodenal injury is an unfortunate byproduct. COX-2–selective NSAIDs were introduced in 1999.[12] Prospective trials comparing nonselective NSAIDs versus agents with COX-2 selectivity have shown a reduction in lower gastrointestinal blood loss and clinical events in the COX-2–selective group.[6,11] COX-2–selective inhibitors are the agents of choice for elderly patients requiring long-term use for chronic arthritic conditions.

Numerous studies have indicated that NSAIDs increase the risk for upper gastrointestinal bleeding from a variety of sources, including superficial minor gastritis, diffuse gastritis, and gastric and duodenal ulcer. Bleeding may be related not only to gastrointestinal toxicity but also to platelet dysfunction as a result of NSAID use. In 160 consecutive patients with upper gastrointestinal hemorrhage, 19% of the patients had a prolonged skin bleeding time on initial presentation. Excluding those patients with chronic liver disease, the bleeding time was significantly higher in patients using NSAIDs than in patients not taking NSAIDs. Although acid suppression is recommended for patients who must continue to use NSAIDs after an episode of bleeding, there is no prospective trial that has proved the ability of proton-pump inhibitors, type 2 histamine (H₂) receptor antagonists, or misoprostol to prevent rebleeding. Rather, NSAIDs should be discontinued and alternative therapy provided for the original condition whenever possible.

TABLE 44-1. Mortality Associated With Underlying Medical Illnesses and Gastrointestinal Bleeding

Condition	Mortality Rate (%)
Renal disease	29
Acute renal failure	63
Liver disease	25
Jaundice	42
Pulmonary disease	23
Respiratory failure	57
Cardiac disease	13
Congestive heart failure	28

From Lieberman D: Gastrointestinal bleeding: Initial management in gastrointestinal bleeding. Gastroenterol Clin North Am 22:723, 1993.

Clinical Prognostic Features

Many reviews have identified clinical features associated with poor clinical outcomes (Table 44-1). Organ-specific complications, need for emergency surgery, and death are the primary factors cited as adverse outcomes after acute upper gastroduodenal hemorrhage. The primary factors associated with poor outcome are severe magnitude (rate and volume) of the initial hemorrhage; persistence or recurrence of major hemorrhage during the hospitalization for the acute hemorrhage; advanced age, generally older than 60 years of age; and presence of medical comorbid conditions.

Several risk assessment measures have been developed. The BLEED risk classification schema predicts risk on initial presentation based on five criteria: ongoing bleeding; low systolic blood pressure (i.e., <100 mm Hg, excluding orthostatic measures); elevated prothrombin time (i.e., >1.2 times the control value); altered mental status; and presence of an unstable comorbid disease (defined as any ongoing organ system abnormality that ordinarily would require ICU admission, e.g., myocardial ischemia, hepatic dysfunction).[13] The presence of any one of these factors places a patient at a roughly threefold increased risk for in-hospital complications of recurrent gastrointestinal hemorrhage, need for surgical intervention, or death. This risk tool can be applied independently of findings at endoscopy and may allow appropriate triage to the ICU or other levels of care. Similar estimates of mortality can be made based on age, systolic blood pressure on presentation, appearance of initial nasogastric aspirate, and transfusion requirement, as shown in Table 44-2.

Prognostic Findings at Endoscopy

The actual appearance of the ulcer at endoscopy is the most important predictor of rebleeding. Ulcers generally have one of five appearances: a clean ulcer base; a flat, pigmented spot, which may be purple, brown, or black, on the ulcer surface; an adherent clot; a visible vessel, which appears as a smooth surfaced or tubular protuberance on the smooth ulcer surface; or active bleeding with either spurting blood, continuous oozing, or oozing around an adherent clot. The latter four appearances are

TABLE 44-2. Prognostic Indicators for Mortality From Peptic Ulcer Hemorrhage

Clinical Parameter	Mortality Rate (%)
Overall	5-8
Age	
≥60 years	10-15
≥80 years	25-30
Systolic blood pressure on presentation	
80-90 mm Hg	12-15
<80 mm Hg	30-35
Nasogastric aspirate on presentation	
Coffee-ground appearance	6-10
Red blood	18-20
Transfusion requirement	
≥10 units	28-34

From Dudnick R, Martin P, Friedman LS: Management of bleeding ulcers. Med Clin North Am 75:948, 1991.

considered to be stigmata of hemorrhage.[14] The probability of rebleeding can be estimated based on this endoscopic appearance: a clean ulcer base rarely bleeds; a flat, pigmented spot ulcer bleeds again in about 10% of patients; an adherent, nonbleeding clot carries a rebleeding risk of about 20%; and a visible vessel carries a rebleeding risk of 40% to 80%.

Descriptive identification of the ulcer characteristics has also been reported as the Forrest classification system, wherein FI ulcers show active bleeding, FIIa represents an ulcer with a visible vessel or pigmented protuberance, FIIb represents an ulcer with an adherent clot, FIIc represents an ulcer with a pigmented spot, and FIII shows a clean ulcer base without stigmata of bleeding. Rebleeding rates increase with ulcer size; ulcers greater than 2 cm in diameter are high risk. As discussed later, endoscopic therapy is appropriate for ulcers with stigmata of bleeding. In contrast, active bleeding not controlled with endoscopic measures mandates immediate surgical intervention.

The transendoscopic Doppler device has been evaluated to assess blood flow beneath the ulcer surface.[14] A positive Doppler study indicating a blood vessel beneath the ulcer was a strong predictor of rebleeding, although the value of this method of evaluation to predict rebleeding is yet to be demonstrated in a large cohort.

Therapeutic Interventions

Medical Management. Therapy is based on clinical presentation and endoscopic findings. A patient with minimal bleeding and a clean ulcer base on endoscopy is at very low risk for recurrent hemorrhage. Young patients may be discharged with specific antiulcer therapy: an antisecretory agent (either an H_2-receptor antagonist or proton-pump inhibitor), cessation of NSAIDs if applicable, and *H. pylori* eradication with antibiotics if *H. pylori* positive.[15] Older patients with this clinical presentation should be admitted for a brief period of in-hospital observation before discharge on a similar regimen. Follow-up endoscopy is indicated at 6 weeks for patients with gastric ulcer to ensure healing and exclude malignancy but not for patients with duodenal ulcer.

Patients with more significant hemorrhage and findings on endoscopy with stigmata for lesions at increased risk for rebleeding should be admitted to the hospital. Patients with clinical risk factors for adverse outcome should be admitted to the ICU.

Recent evidence has focused on the ability of antisecretory therapy to decrease the incidence of rebleeding following endoscopic therapy. Several recent large clinical trials have been reported demonstrating reduced rates of recurrent bleeding with the use of intravenous proton-pump inhibitors.[16,17] An additional recent study also showed favorable rebleeding results with oral proton-pump inhibitor therapy versus placebo.[18] All the trials demonstrating benefit for proton-pump inhibitor therapy have been completed in patients with significant hemorrhage who have also had a therapeutic endoscopy and were not treated solely with medication. Hence, the proton-pump inhibitors were used as adjuncts to endoscopic therapy.

Endoscopic Therapy. Endoscopic therapy can be used to arrest active ulcer bleeding and to prevent rebleeding in patients with ulcers at high risk for rebleeding (FI, FIIa, and FIIb ulcers). Several endoscopic devices can deliver the thermal energy required to achieve coagulation. Transendoscopic bipolar electrocoagulation and heater probe therapy can decrease rebleeding rates and the need for surgical intervention by up to 50%. In skilled hands, light amplification by stimulated emission of radiation (LASER) coagulation offers similar results, although the risk for perforation is higher; LASER is generally not used as the initial therapeutic modality in most institutions. Each of these modalities can result in activation of bleeding or transmural bowel injury with consequent perforation, although these are rare, with reported incidence rates of less than 0.5%.

Injection therapy is an equally effective nonthermal method to secure hemostasis. Available sclerosing or vasoconstricting agents include absolute alcohol, epinephrine, fibrin glue, and polidocanol. The choice of method and agent is the preference of the endoscopist and equipment availability. Sclerosants are injected around the ulcer perimeter or visible vessel. Rebleeding rates are reduced by half, relative to those ulcers with similar characteristics not subjected to endoscopic therapy.

Irrespective of the method of endoscopic hemostasis, endoscopy is highly successful in stopping initial active bleeding, with initial success rates in more than 95% of cases in ulcers that are actively bleeding or with non-bleeding visible vessels.[19] Nevertheless, bleeding recurs in about 20% of patients, and 97% of this rebleeding occurs within 96 hours of the initial endoscopy.[20]

Individual studies have not shown a significant decrease in mortality in patients subjected to endoscopic therapies for hemorrhage; however, two meta-analyses have suggested this benefit. Overall reduction in mortality rate is roughly 40% in patients subjected to endoscopic interventions relative to those patients not subjected to endoscopic treatments.[21]

Endoscopic therapy fails in about 20% of patients, manifest as either failure to control hemorrhage on initial presentation or as early recurrent hemorrhage. In the recent past, rebleeding patients were treated surgically, but more recent experience suggests that repeat endoscopy may be a safe and effective alternative for these patients. Repeat endoscopy may be able to salvage half of these patients; however, morbidity and mortality are high in this subset of patients,[22] with high risk of perforation and overall worse outcomes when surgery was required. Optimal management strategies for this high-risk group remain controversial. Before embarking on repeat endoscopy to control recurrent hemorrhage, surgical options should be considered, particularly in patients who are at high risk for rebleeding and in elderly patients who are at high risk for multisystem organ dysfunction and death from recurrent episodes of hypotension and stress.

Surgical Therapy. Surgery is ultimately required in roughly 10% of patients with bleeding ulcer. Surgery is indicated for patients with active hemorrhage not responsive to endoscopic measures, significant recurrent hemorrhage after endoscopic treatment, an ongoing transfusion requirement, or transfusion requirements exceeding 6 units of packed red blood cells in a 24-hour interval. Given the now extensive successful experience with endoscopic therapy, surgery is generally reserved for those patients in whom endoscopic measures have failed as the primary intervention, assuming expert endoscopy is readily available. There are surgical reports to support early elective operation after initial endoscopic hemostasis in elderly patients with lesions at high risk for rebleeding (FI and FIIa ulcers); however, this practice has not been uniformly embraced by gastrointestinal surgeons.[23] Before improved success with endoscopic methods, the presence of a visible vessel was considered an absolute indication for surgery. Now, the decision for surgery is balanced by endoscopic expertise, patient characteristics, and transfusion requirements. In contrast, expertise in interventional endoscopy may not be available in some communities; thus, surgery becomes an important treatment modality earlier in the course of disease in patients in these locations.

A number of studies have attempted to clarify the group of patients that can benefit from early definitive surgical therapy.[24] Unfortunately, no study series with a sizable cohort has been collected since the advent of effective endoscopic therapy. Earlier, pre-endoscopy series support a role for early surgery for patients with clear evidence of ongoing hemorrhage (>4 units of packed red blood cells), presence of shock, history of previous hemorrhage, endoscopic evidence of high risk for rebleeding (FI or FIIa lesions), and age older than 65 years. A retrospective review of 66 patients managed with early definitive surgery accrued from an urban hospital between 1986 and 1990 showed that these patients were successfully managed without a death. Unlike more recent surgical series, however, the average age of the patients in this study was 53 years, in contrast to the current average age of 63 years in patients with acute upper gastrointestinal hemorrhage. Moreover, it is likely that many patients were treated surgically who by today's standards would not have required surgical therapy.

Clinical judgment is essential in deciding who will benefit from surgical intervention at what time. Early definitive surgical intervention is clearly indicated for patients in whom primary endoscopic therapies fail. It is also clear that elderly patients with lesions at highest risk for rebleeding fair better with early definitive operation than with episodes of recurrent hemorrhage as a result of failed repeated efforts at hemostasis. Whether early elective operation should be provided to elderly patients after initial successful endoscopic therapy for a high-risk FI or FII lesion has not been definitively settled. Such a decision needs to take into consideration local technical expertise, critical care support, and ongoing advances in endoscopic intervention.

Choice of Operation. The goal of surgical intervention in bleeding peptic ulcer is to control hemorrhage. This may be achieved by either direct suture ligation of the bleeding vessel or, in the case of gastric ulcer, with gastric resection or ulcer excision. The role for a definitive acid-reducing procedure is a secondary, but important, objective of the surgical procedure.

Bleeding Duodenal Ulcer. Operative intervention for bleeding duodenal ulcer requires direct exposure of the ulcer in the duodenum by way of duodenotomy or duodenopyloromyotomy. Because these ulcers are typically located on the posterior duodenal wall, direct suture ligation with a nonabsorbable suture suffices in most patients to arrest bleeding. Occasionally, direct suture ligation fails to stop bleeding, so that four-quadrant suture ligation around the perimeter of the bleeding ulcer may be necessary to control bleeding. Rarely, these two measures fail, and ligation of the gastroduodenal artery cephalad and inferior to the duodenum may be necessary.

Provided the patient is stable and free of life-threatening, preoperative comorbid conditions, a definitive antisecretory procedure is indicated (Fig. 44-2). Truncal vagotomy is the least time-consuming and a highly effective procedure to decrease acid secretion. Alternatively, the parietal cell vagotomy has been advocated by some surgeons. In this procedure, a limited duodenotomy is performed for ulcer ligation, preserving normal gastric emptying in conjunction with the parietal cell vagotomy. Because the typical patient undergoing emergency or urgent surgery for bleeding ulcer is at high risk for adverse outcome, careful consideration should be used before proceeding with this more time-consuming operation. The patient should be well resuscitated and hemodynamically stable. In actual practice, parietal cell vagotomy with limited duodenotomy is rarely applied in this setting today, given the typical clinical features of patients with refractory bleeding ulcer. Although technically feasible, similar concerns have limited the use of the laparoscopic approach to patients with actively bleeding ulcer. Gastric resection is generally not indicated in the management of duodenal ulcer hemorrhage.

Suture ligation of bleeding duodenal ulcer with pyloroplasty and truncal vagotomy is successful in acutely controlling hemorrhage in 90% of patients. Up to 10% of patients may develop early rebleeding. Repeat surgical intervention is rarely required for these patients, however, because bleeding frequently ceases with supportive measures. Reported operative mortality rates range from less than 1% to 50% based on the patient's comorbid conditions.

Bleeding Gastric Ulcer. Again, the primary goal of surgical intervention for bleeding gastric ulcer disease is to stop

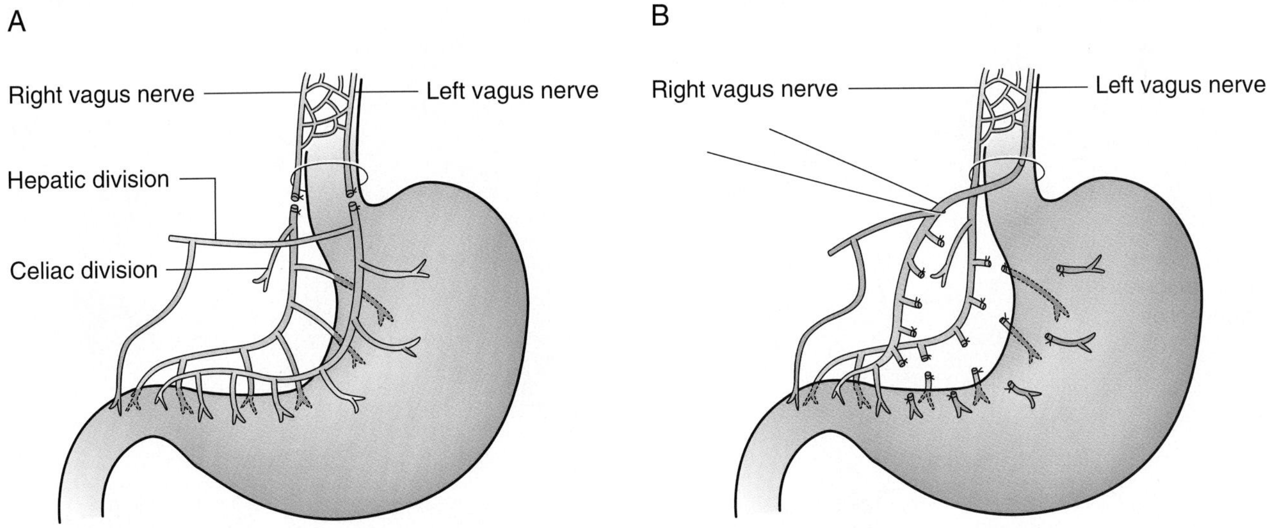

FIGURE 44-2. Truncal vagotomy and parietal cell vagotomy. **A,** During truncal vagotomy, both vagal trunks are divided at the esophageal hiatus. The vagal branches to the gastric cardia, fundus, antrum, and pylorus are divided, as are the hepatic and celiac branches. A gastric-emptying procedure, either pyloroplasty or gastrojejunostomy, is required because pyloric opening is impaired. **B,** Parietal cell vagotomy denervates only the parietal cell mass. Innervation of the antropyloric region and the hepatic and celiac branches is preserved. Parietal cell vagotomy preserves normal gastric emptying, but the procedure requires considerably longer operative time and should be used only in stable patients who do not have significant risk factors for poor outcome. (**A** and **B,** From Mulholland MW: Duodenal ulcer. *In* Greenfield LJ, Mulholland MW, Oldham KT [eds]: Surgery: Scientific Principles and Practice, 2nd ed. Philadelphia, Lippincott-Raven, 1997, p 766.)

hemorrhage. Unlike duodenal ulcer, there is a chance that a gastric ulcer may be malignant; up to 10% of gastric ulcers prove to be a gastric adenocarcinoma or lymphoma. Additionally, rebleeding rates for gastric ulcer treated with simple ligation approach 30%. Ideally, therefore, the surgical procedure should include ulcer excision.

Ulcers of the incisura, antrum, and distal body of the stomach should be managed with distal gastrectomy and Billroth I or II reconstruction (Fig. 44-3). Truncal vagotomy is indicated in the setting of hemorrhage in stable patients and those free of life-threatening comorbid conditions. Fortunately, most bleeding gastric ulcers arise in these regions of the stomach, reflecting the distribution of gastric ulcers. Fewer than 10% of gastric ulcers are located high on the lesser curvature. Ulcers in this position can be managed with either subtotal or near-total gastrectomy or with local ulcer excision and distal gastrectomy without vagotomy. Aggressive proximal gastric resections carry high morbidity and mortality rates, however, particularly in the setting of hemorrhage, and the need for such resections is infrequent.

Ulcer Surgery in Patients with H. pylori Infection. A role for definitive antisecretory ulcer surgery is clear in the setting of hemorrhage from peptic ulcer in patients taking NSAIDs who must continue this therapy. Some gastroenterologists and surgeons have questioned the need for definitive antiulcer surgery in patients with *H. pylori*-associated ulcer disease. A definitive judgment cannot be made at this time. A role for excluding a definite antisecretory procedure in perforated duodenal ulcer is supported by a recent study showing that in *H.*

pylori-infected patients with perforated duodenal ulcers, those treated with *H. pylori* therapy after closure alone had significantly less ulcer recurrence than those treated with closure and omeprazole alone.[15] Eradication of *H. pylori* can decrease the incidence of rebleeding in patients with *H. pylori*-related ulcer disease with bleeding, as shown in another recent study. However, this may be true only of patients with relatively minor bleeding, not those with significant hemorrhage of a magnitude to warrant transfer or surgery.[25] Gastrointestinal surgeons who have cared for many of these critically ill patients with severe bleeding will note that only 10% of patients with *H. pylori* infection develop ulcer disease related to their infection, and of those 10%, only 1 in 5 develops hemorrhage as a complication. Of that 2%, only 1 in 10 ultimately requires surgery to control bleeding; that is, 0.2% of all *H. pylori*-infected patients eventually face surgery for bleeding peptic ulcer disease. Moreover, recent evidence also suggests that patients requiring surgical intervention for bleeding peptic ulcer had an *H. pylori* infection rate that was far lower than that commonly seen in other populations with ulcer disease.[25] Extrapolation of the data from uncomplicated patients has led to the postulation that simple oversewing of the bleeding ulcer and *H. pylori* treatment would be sufficient surgical therapy; however, recent evidence demonstrates that more than 50% of these patients would be at high risk for recurrent hemorrhage. Hence, using the long-standing effective modality of acid-reducing surgery as definitive management of ulcer diathesis in these patients seems prudent at this time.

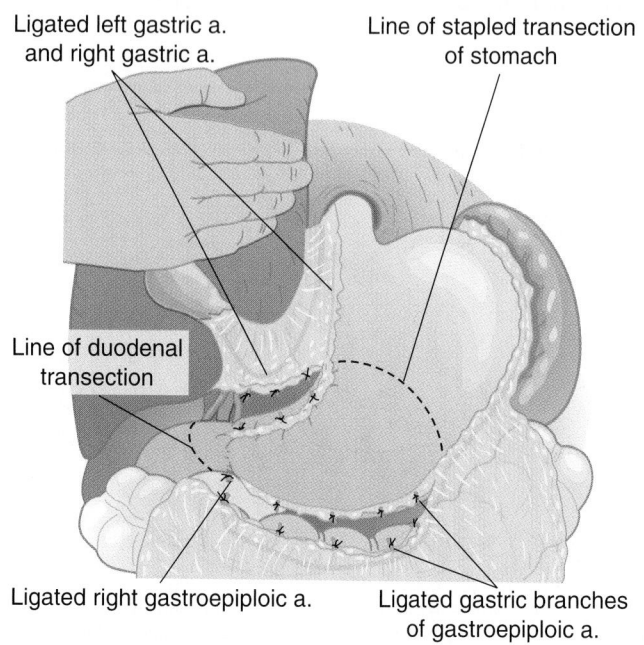

Ligated left gastric a. and right gastric a.

Line of stapled transection of stomach

Line of duodenal transection

Ligated right gastroepiploic a.

Ligated gastric branches of gastroepiploic a.

A

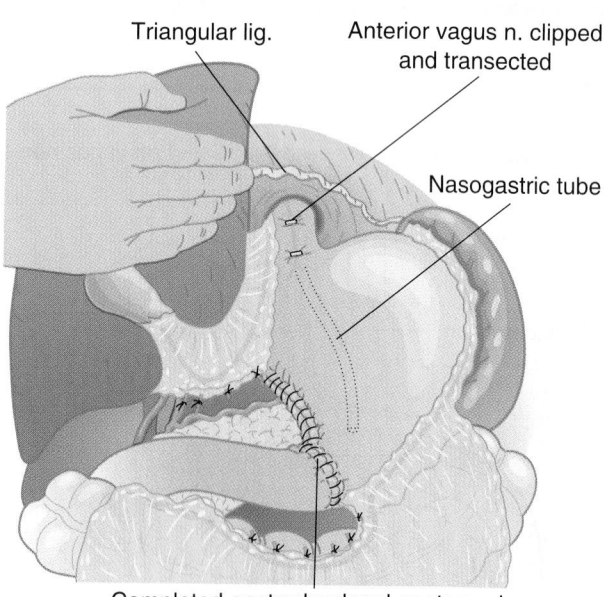

Triangular lig.

Anterior vagus n. clipped and transected

Nasogastric tube

Completed gastroduodenal anatomosis

B

FIGURE 44-3.   **A,** Lines mark limits of gastric resection for antrectomy. For patients with more proximal gastric ulcers, the proximal line of resection can be extended or tailored to include the ulcer in the resection. **B,** Billroth I reconstruction with gastroduodenostomy. Note that truncal vagotomy is included in the procedure. (**A** and **B,** From Sabiston DC Jr: Atlas of General Surgery. Philadelphia, WB Saunders, 1994, pp 271-272.)

Bleeding Caused by Portal Hypertension

For completeness we briefly discuss bleeding related to portal hypertension, a frequent cause of upper gastrointestinal bleeding. This is more extensively covered in Chapter 51.

Bleeding from esophagogastric varices is responsible for one third of all deaths in patients with cirrhosis and portal hypertension. As many as 90% of cirrhotic patients develop esophageal varices, and 25% to 30% of these develop hemorrhage. The mortality risk from each episode of hemorrhage approaches 25%. After bleeding has occurred, repeated hemorrhage develops in 70% of patients.

Esophageal varices are dilated submucosal veins that communicate with the portocollateral circulation and the systemic venous system. Varices range in size from small (1- to 2-mm) irregular protuberances to large (1- to 2-cm) serpentine structures that abut into the esophageal lumen. Most varices are initially restricted to the distal esophagus, although with time gastric varices along the cardia and high greater curvature of the stomach are evident in most patients.

Treatment of Acute Variceal Hemorrhage

Hemorrhage from varices in cirrhotic patients is a potentially highly lethal event. The clinical presentation includes massive hematemesis, melena, and occasionally hematochezia. Hemodynamic instability is common. Initial management calls for prompt resuscitation with particular attention to correction of volume deficit, coagulopathy, and airway management. Patients with poor liver function as reflected by Child's classification system are at high risk for mortality. Treatment in an ICU is imperative.

Emergency endoscopy is required to evaluate the source of bleeding. Although varices may be suspected based on clinical stigmata of cirrhosis, bleeding is equally likely to be caused by gastritis, ulcer disease, or portal hypertensive gastropathy in patients without a prior history of bleeding varices. About 70% of patients with prior episodes of variceal hemorrhage are bleeding from varices.

An algorithm for the management of bleeding resulting from portal hypertension is shown in Figure 44-4.

Endoscopy is necessary both to confirm the source of bleeding and to allow endoscopic therapy. Both variceal sclerotherapy and rubber band ligation are effective endoscopic measures. Sclerotherapy can be completed with a variety of sclerosants, and both intravariceal and paravariceal injections are equally effective. Complications of sclerotherapy include esophageal ulceration, bleeding perforation, mediastinitis, pleural effusion, and pulmonary edema. Late stricture has also been observed. Esophageal variceal rubber band ligation is comparable to sclerotherapy, although complications may be less common than with sclerotherapy, particularly those related to mediastinal and pulmonary inflammation. Gastric varices are not effectively treated by sclerotherapy. In good-risk patients with bleeding gastric varices, prompt surgical decompression should be considered.

Concomitant treatment with vasoactive drugs is indicated. The somatostatin analogue octreotide, given by continuous intravenous infusion, offers the best efficacy and safety profile. Somatostatin decreases splanchnic blood flow, thereby decreasing portal and variceal pressure without eliciting coronary vasoconstriction. Vasopressin alone and vasopressin plus nitroglycerin by continuous systemic intravenous infusion are also of benefit in decreasing splanchnic blood flow and decreasing variceal bleeding. One of these agents should be started as soon as the diagnosis of variceal hemorrhage is established. In patients with a known history of variceal hemorrhage, the infusions should begin empirically in the emergency department on presentation with hematemesis.

Endoscopic therapy and somatostatin infusions are effective in arresting hemorrhage in 80% to 90% of cases. Sclerotherapy may be repeated up to two times in the initial 48 hours if initial efforts fail. If sclerotherapy is successful, attention must be directed toward future prevention of rebleeding, which occurs in more than 70% of patients with portal hypertension who have bled from esophageal varices. If sclerotherapy is ineffective, a Sengstaken-Blakemore tube should be inserted. This device has a large gastric balloon and an esophageal balloon that can be passed through the mouth into the stomach. Careful positioning is required to avoid esophageal perforation. When in position, the gastric balloon is inflated, and traction is applied to the tube, placing pressure on the esophagogastric junction venous plexus. This results in cessation of bleeding in most patients. In the few that continue to bleed, the esophageal balloon should be inflated. With this intraluminal control, resuscitation, correction of coagulopathy, and definitive management plans can be pursued. Failure to control bleeding with these measures carries a mortality rate in excess of 70% in patients with Child's class C liver dysfunction.

The patient with acute variceal hemorrhage who continues to bleed after endoscopic and medical therapies have been applied can be considered for transjugular intrahepatic shunt (TIPS) or emergency surgical decompression of the portal circulation. The TIPS procedure involves placement of a transvenous intrahepatic portosystemic stent to decompress the portal circulation. Results have varied widely in different institutions. Clinical expertise and aggressive medical management are required for a successful outcome, particularly in high-risk candidates, those with ongoing bleeding and poor liver function. Child's class A and B patients have a 30-day mortality rate of 10%, whereas Child's class C patients have a reported 30-day mortality rate in excess of 50%. Rebleeding is also likely and occurs in 22% of patients within the first month, usually a result of TIPS thrombosis.

In most reported series, emergency decompressive surgery for patients (procedures discussed in Chapter 51) with uncontrolled hemorrhage carries an operative mortality rate in excess of 50%. This reflects the fact that ongoing hemorrhage is more likely to occur in patients with poor liver function (Child's class C).

The risks for early and late mortality after variceal hemorrhage are largely determined by the patient's liver

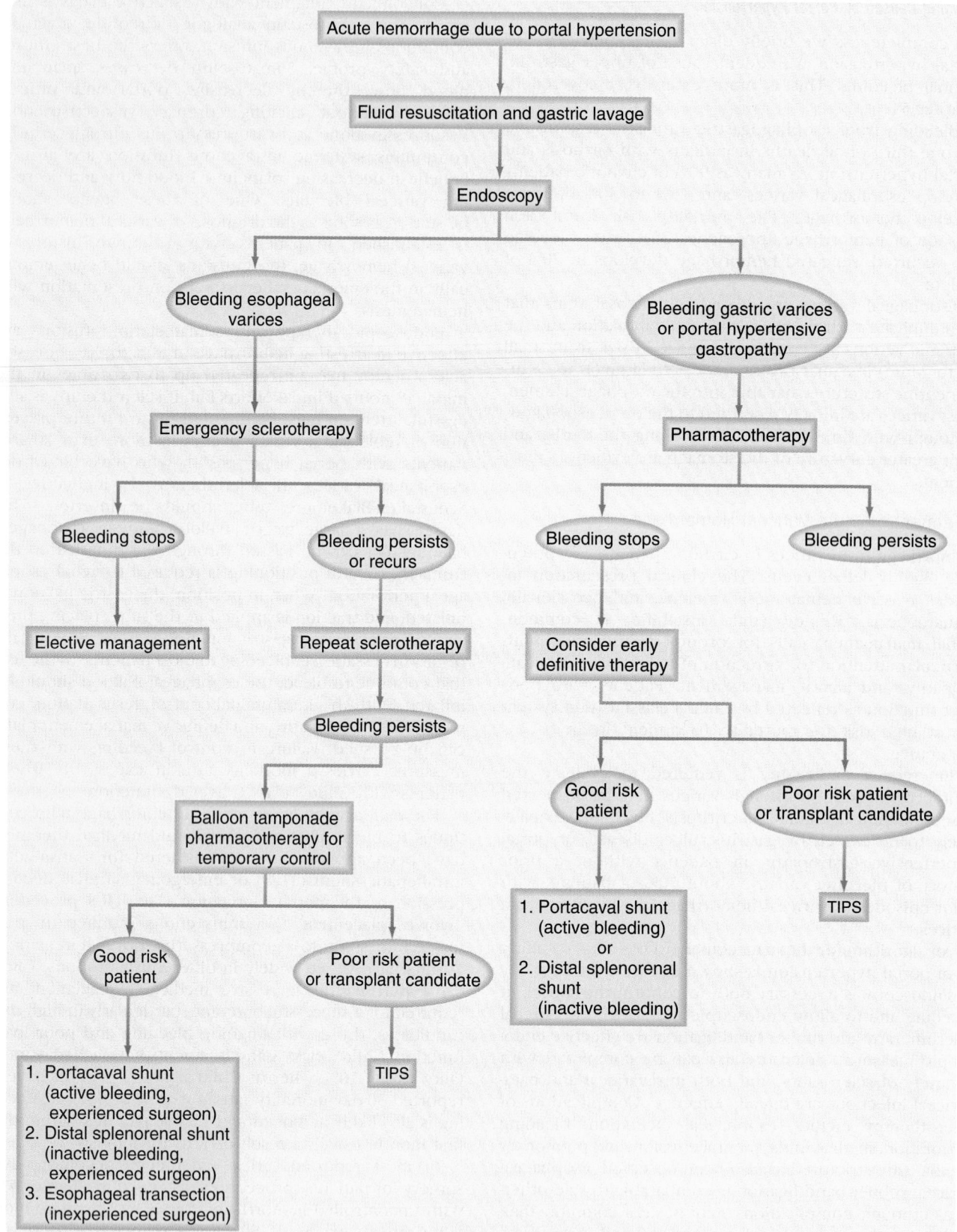

■ **FIGURE 44-4.** Algorithm for the management of acute hemorrhage due to portal hypertension. TIPS, transjugular intrahepatic portosystemic shunt. (From Rikkers LF: Portal hypertension. *In* Levine BA, Copeland E, Howard R, et al [eds]: Current Practice of Surgery, Vol. 3. New York, Churchill Livingstone, 1995.)

TABLE 44-3.   Child's Criteria for Hepatic Functional Reserve

Measure	A: Minimal	B: Moderate	C: Advanced
Serum bilirubin (mg/100 mL)	<2.0	2–3	>3
Serum albumin (g/100 mL)	>3.5	3–3.5	<3
Ascites	None	Easily controlled	Poorly controlled
Encephalopathy	None	Minimal	Advanced, "coma"
Nutrition	Excellent	Good	Poor, "wasting"

From Boyer TD: Portal hypertension and its complications: Bleeding esophageal varices, ascites, and spontaneous bacterial peritonitis. *In* Zakim D, Boyer TD (eds): Hepatology: A Textbook of Liver Disease. Philadelphia, WB Saunders, 1982, pp 464-499.

function at the time of hemorrhage. Several classification schemes have been developed to predict the degree of liver dysfunction, but the most durable has been based on the original assessment presented by Child. Simply stated, assessment of the degree of encephalopathy, hyperbilirubinemia, ascites, albumin, and prolongation of the prothrombin time can provide a good estimate of 30-day mortality. Table 44-3 shows Child's classification parameters. Predicted 30-day mortality rates after an episode of variceal hemorrhage are as follows: Child's class A, less than 10%; Child's class B, 30%; and Child's class C, 50%. Mortality rates increase at the 1-year interval to Child's class A, 24%; Child's class B, 45%; and Child's class C, 85%, overall.

Acute Gastric Mucosal Lesions

Acute gastric mucosal lesions (AGMLs) include a broad category of acute erosive mucosal conditions that develop in critically ill patients. Also known as *stress gastritis, acute mucosal ischemia, erosive gastritis,* or *stress ulceration,* these conditions share a common epidemiology and clinical presentation. They are characterized by stigmata of mucosal injury evidenced by mucosal pallor, petechiae, and erosions. The lesions can be distributed throughout the gastric mucosa but are predominantly identified in the body of the stomach. Bleeding is the clinical presenting sign in critically ill patients. The bleeding may be massive and life threatening. Prompt correction of the factors leading to the critical illness is the most important priority in management. Lesions resembling AGMLs are also observed in patients on chronic NSAID therapy. Up to 40% of patients using NSAIDs for a chronic condition may have endoscopic evidence of gastritis, but evolution of the lesions to AGMLs with stigmata of bleeding is unusual. Significant bleeding from AGMLs is seen in fewer than 1% of all NSAID users. Hence, the NSAID-associated mucosal erosions are clinicopathologically distinct from the AGMLs of critical illness.

Patients at risk for non-NSAID–associated AGML include virtually all critically ill patients in medical and surgical ICUs. Particular risk factors include sepsis, respiratory failure, hemodynamic instability, coma following head injury or intracranial operation, burns covering more than 35% of body surface area, multiple trauma, cardiopulmonary bypass, and coagulopathy. The condition is particularly lethal in postoperative cardiovascular patients and in patients with sepsis and multiorgan failure.

The pathogenesis of AGML is related to a combination of both gastric acid and activated pepsin injuring the gastric mucosa and is exacerbated by mucosal ischemia secondary to hypoperfusion. Activated pepsin is a proteolytic enzyme that directly digests the mucosal lining and is inactivated at a pH of approximately 4.5. This understanding has led to broad application of prophylaxis against stress ulceration in critical care practice. In fact, such prophylaxis has greatly diminished the incidence of major bleeding from this condition; thus, surgical intervention for control of bleeding is now a rare procedure.

Prophylaxis

AGML can be prevented by any of several strategies. The most widely applied methods involve neutralization of the contents in the gastric lake. Administration of antacids to maintain the intragastric pH above 4.0 is effective provided that dosing is at a frequency and volume sufficient to maintain the desired pH range. Antisecretory therapy with either H_2-receptor antagonists (multiple trials) and proton-pump inhibitor therapy (limited trials) is also efficacious, administered by either a continuous intravenous infusion or bolus dosing.[26] Again, pH monitoring is required to ensure efficacy because acid hypersecretion may be present in these patients, rendering conventional dosing inadequate.

Despite the proven efficacy of gastric pH neutralization at reducing clinically significant bleeding, many intensivists have questioned whether this normalization contributes to nosocomial pneumonia by allowing bacterial colonization of the gastric lake. Although early trials appeared to confirm this fear, a more recent large comparative trial showed no increased incidence in pneumonia in patients receiving H_2-receptor therapy rather than sucralfate (while clinically important bleeding episodes were significantly decreased).[27] With these observations, the current recommendation regarding stress ulceration calls for gastric neutralization with either H_2-receptor antagonists or proton-pump inhibitors.

DIAGNOSIS AND TREATMENT

AGMLs in hospitalized patients are heralded by gastrointestinal bleeding evidenced by hematemesis, nasogastric aspiration of blood or coffee ground–like material, or an unexplainable drop in hematocrit. The magnitude of bleeding may be slight or massive; both forms tend to cease spontaneously with appropriate management, which includes resuscitation, transfusion, and correction of coagulopathy. Emergency evaluation with upper endoscopy, a procedure that should be completed in the ICU, is indicated. Careful attention to prevent aspiration and hypovolemia during the procedure is mandatory.

Findings at endoscopy are characterized by diffuse petechiae, superficial erosions, and mucosal pallor. If a solitary site of bleeding is identified, endoscopic therapy, such as thermal or bipolar electrocoagulation, fibrin glue application, or injection therapy, is appropriate. Frequently, however, bleeding is too diffuse to allow endoscopic therapy. In this case, aggressive medical management with transfusion and component therapy to correct coagulation defects and anemia is indicated. Measures to correct hypoperfusion, hypovolemia, and gastric acid neutralization are also important elements of management.

The role of angiography in stress ulceration is limited to diffuse, unremitting hemorrhage. Selective celiac catheterization may allow identification of the bleeding arteries of origin. Embolization with coils or collagen gel or selective intra-arterial infusion of vasopressin may arrest bleeding in up to 80% of patients provided that selective bleeding vessels can be identified.[28] Recurrent bleeding is common, however, and the mortality of patients with this degree of hemorrhage is in excess of 50%. Death ensues from multisystem failure precipitated by ongoing hemorrhage and recurrent shock.

Surgery is rarely used to treat AGML. Only those patients who have failed aggressive medical management and endoscopic therapy and who have treatable critical illness are candidates for surgery. These are particularly challenging patients because they are critically ill with preexisting multisystem failure, sepsis, or other highly lethal conditions. Frequently, noncorrectable coagulopathy secondary to sepsis or hepatic failure is present. In the few patients that do come to surgery, the goal of surgery is hemostasis. At laparotomy, a generous gastrotomy is made to evaluate the sites of hemorrhage. In the unlikely finding of a single bleeding site or bleeding from only a few small sites, oversewing of these sites and truncal vagotomy and drainage are appropriate. Unfortunately, multiple sites are usually found, leaving only subtotal or near-total gastrectomy, with Roux-en-Y gastrojejunostomy as the only viable option. Regardless of surgical procedure, the postoperative mortality rate is high, in excess of 50%. Death is usually from multisystem organ failure.

Mallory-Weiss Tears

About 10% of cases of upper gastrointestinal hemorrhage are caused by Mallory-Weiss tears. The lesion is characterized by a tear in the proximal gastric mucosa near the esophagogastric junction. The clinical presentation is typified by an antecedent history of vomiting, retching, or coughing followed by hematemesis. The mean age for patients with this condition is older than 60 years; 80% are men. Alcoholism, disease-related bleeding diatheses, hiatal hernia, and NSAID use are frequently observed. Up to 10% of patients may have bleeding of sufficient magnitude to have hematochezia and hypotension as presenting signs. Up to 90% of these lesions stop bleeding spontaneously without specific intervention. Patients with cirrhosis and portal hypertension with coagulopathy are at greatest risk for morality, which overall averages 3%.[29] Initial assessment and treatment should include prompt history and physical examination, resuscitation, and endoscopic evaluation. The tear is typically located on the lesser curvature and measures 15 to 20 mm in length and 2 to 3 mm in width. Findings at initial endoscopy may reveal active bleeding or oozing, stigmata of recent bleeding, or a clean-based tear. Endoscopic therapy by either injection or thermal energy is efficacious in patients with active bleeding.

Transfusion of packed red blood cells is required in 40% to 70% of patients. Patients with active bleeding at initial endoscopy and those with coagulation disorders are at greatest risk for rebleeding; roughly 30% bleed again within the first 24 hours. Rebleeding is rare in patients without coagulation disorders. Medical therapy includes acid reduction with antisecretory agents. Although this is not an acid-peptic condition, findings of associated gastritis are common in these patients.

Surgery is rarely required for control of hemorrhage. If bleeding fails to stop after endoscopic therapy, laparotomy for oversewing of the mucosal tear through a high gastrotomy is appropriate. An acid-reducing procedure is not required. Rebleeding is most likely related to ongoing, or uncorrectable, coagulopathy; thus, aggressive, ongoing efforts to maintain a normal coagulation profile are needed.

Unusual Causes of Acute Upper Gastrointestinal Hemorrhage

Esophageal Sources

The esophagus is the source of major hemorrhage in fewer than 3% of patients admitted for evaluation of acute upper gastrointestinal hemorrhage. The most common causes are infectious esophagitis, gastroesophageal reflux disease, Barrett's epithelium, malignancy (including adenocarcinomas and squamous carcinomas), medication-induced erosions, Crohn's disease, and radiation. Patients with human immunodeficiency virus (HIV) infection and other immunocompromised patients are at particular risk for infectious esophagitis, including erosive esophagitis caused by *Candida albicans*, other fungi, herpes simplex virus, cytomegalovirus, and mycobacterial infection. Bleeding may be massive, although episodes of less severe hemorrhage are typical.

Therapy is targeted to the cause of bleeding. If active hemorrhage is identified, endoscopic electrocoagulation or heater probe therapy is usually effective in stopping hemorrhage, at least temporarily while definitive management is planned. Specific therapy is targeted to the etiology and includes appropriate antibiotics for infectious causes, proton-pump inhibitors for reflux-associated conditions, and definitive multimodality cancer therapies for malignant tumors. Sucralfate is a useful adjunct to specific therapies in patients with acute inflammatory conditions of the esophagus. Emergency surgery to control hemorrhage is rarely required. Treatment with definitive surgical management, resection for tumors, or antireflux therapy for patients with reflux-induced esophagitis is dictated by the specific cause of the hemorrhage.

Dieulafoy's Lesion

Dieulafoy's vascular malformations are rare causes of acute upper gastrointestinal hemorrhage. The lesions are unusually large submucosal or mucosal vessels found in the gastric mucosa, most commonly along the lesser curvature in the mid-stomach. The lesion is most frequently diagnosed in middle life and is not associated with identifiable factors for mucosal injury, vascular disease, or medical conditions.

Bleeding occurs when superficial erosion into the vessel occurs, resulting in brisk, voluminous hemorrhage that ceases spontaneously. Endoscopic diagnosis is difficult because the lesion is rarely associated with an obvious ulcerated lesion. Rather, reliable diagnosis depends on fortuitous timely endoscopy during hemorrhage to allow visualization of bleeding from a pinpoint mucosal defect. Occasionally, the endoscopist may appreciate a vessel wall at the site of bleeding. If a lesion is definitively identified, the site should be marked endoscopically with India ink injection to allow precise surgical resection.

Recurrent hemorrhage is common; often, several episodes occur before accurate diagnosis. Efforts at endoscopic ablation with sclerotherapy and electrocoagulation have not proved effective in the few reported series. Rather, appropriate definitive management calls for wedge resection of the gastric wall. Precise endoscopic localization of the lesion allows this limited resection in lieu of more extended blind gastric resection. Because the condition is not associated with peptic mucosal injury, vagotomy is not indicated.

Aortoenteric Fistula

Aortoenteric fistula is an uncommon condition in which an inflammatory tract develops between the aorta and the gastrointestinal tract. The fistula may develop as a primary process resulting from infectious aortitis, or inflammatory aortic aneurysm, or as a secondary process following aortic replacement with a synthetic graft for treatment of abdominal aortic aneurysm. The secondary aortoenteric fistulas are by far the more common cause, and this complication may develop in up to 1% of patients after aortic aneurysm repair. The fistulas characteristically develop between the proximal anastomosis and the overlying small bowel (duodenum or jejunum), although communication to the colon has also been noted. It is thought that a low-grade infection at the site of contact between the anastomosis and the bowel leads to the fistula formation. This diagnosis must be considered in any patient with acute gastrointestinal hemorrhage and a history of aortic surgery. The "herald" bleed, an episode of acute hemorrhage that ceases spontaneously, occurs hours to days prior to the inevitable exsanguinating hemorrhage that will ensue if the condition is not recognized and treated.

Emergency upper endoscopy is mandatory for all patients with suspected aortoenteric fistula. If endoscopy is negative, computed tomography (CT) to look for evidence of inflammation at the aortic anastomosis is indicated. Others advocate emergency angiography, including lateral views, to identify the small mycotic aneurysm that is frequently present. Angiography should be pursued in all patients with negative CT scans.

In patients with exsanguinating hemorrhage, emergency laparotomy with control of the proximal aorta is indicated. Effective surgical management calls for removal of the aortic graft and extra-anatomic vascular bypass to restore distal aortic flow.

ACUTE LOWER GASTROINTESTINAL HEMORRHAGE

Definition and Incidence

Acute lower gastrointestinal bleeding is hemorrhage arising distal to the ligament of Treitz. The colon is the source of hemorrhage in more than 95% to 97% of cases, with the remaining 3% to 5% arising in small bowel sites. Lower gastrointestinal bleeding accounts for about 15% of major episodes of gastrointestinal hemorrhage and hence is much less common than upper gastrointestinal bleeding. The incidence of lower gastrointestinal bleeding increases with age, reflecting the parallel increase in acquired lesions responsible for colonic bleeding: diverticulosis and angiodysplasias. The differential diagnosis of acute lower gastrointestinal hemorrhage is shown in Box 44-2.

Clinical Presentation

The hallmark of acute lower gastrointestinal hemorrhage is hematochezia; passage of bloody stool, blood, or blood clots per rectum. If bleeding is slower and of lesser volume, melena may also be a presenting sign, although this is more characteristic of an upper gastrointestinal source. Similarly, up to 15% of patients with massive hemorrhage from an upper gastrointestinal source may present with hematochezia, which is indicative of at least 1000 mL of hemorrhage over a short interval from an upper gastrointestinal source.

Roughly half of patients present with both a decrease in hemoglobin and hematocrit and hemodynamic instability; 30% have orthostatic changes, 10% syncope, and 19% shock. Although lower gastrointestinal hemorrhage represents a genuine emergency, it is generally less life-threatening than upper gastrointestinal hemorrhage. Patients are less likely to present in shock, more likely to cease bleeding spontaneously, and usually have a lower transfusion requirement.

Box 44-2. Differential Diagnosis of Lower Gastrointestinal Hemorrhage

Diverticulosis
Angiodysplasia
Neoplasm
Polyps
Meckel's diverticulum
    Inflammatory disorders
    Ulcerative colitis
    Crohn's disease
    Infectious colitis
    Radiation-induced disorders
Nonsteroidal anti-inflammatory drug–associated disorder
Hemorrhoids
Varices
Dieulafoy's lesions
Osler-Weber-Rendu syndrome
Aortoenteric fistula
Vasculitis
Mesenteric ischemia

Etiology

Unlike upper gastrointestinal hemorrhage, in which endo-scopic findings can accurately identify mucosal lesions responsible for acute hemorrhage, validating the source of an episode of hemorrhage from the colon is more problem-atic. First, lower gastrointestinal hemorrhage is character-ized by episodes of intermittent hemorrhage; bleeding may well have ceased by the time the diagnostic procedure is obtained. Second, up to 42% of patients are found to have multiple potential bleeding sources at the time of diagnostic evaluation. It is therefore important to have a clear under-standing of the significance of findings on diagnostic evalu-ation and to keep in mind the limited certainty that may accompany some of these findings. The direct observation of a bleeding lesion or findings of stigmata of recent hemor-rhage at endoscopy are required to establish a definitive diagnosis.[30] Understanding the degree of certainty of a bleeding source is of great importance when contemplating surgical resection to treat hemorrhage.

Diverticulosis

Colonic diverticulosis represents the most common source of lower gastrointestinal hemorrhage, responsible for 40% to 55% of cases of hemorrhage in most series. Colonic diverticula are common acquired lesions of the abdominal colon. Although 40% of patients in the 5th decade of life have diverticula, this incidence rises to 80% by the 9th decade. Hemorrhage complicates 3% to 5% of patients with diverticulosis. The anatomic basis for bleed-ing is thought to be asymmetrical rupture of intramural branches (the vasa recta) of the marginal artery at the dome of the diverticulum or at its antimesenteric margin. It appears likely that luminal traumatic factors, including impacted fecaliths with abrasion of the vessels, lead to hemorrhage. Hemorrhage is rarely associated with the inflammation of clinical diverticulitis.

Diverticular hemorrhage ceases spontaneously in up to 90% of patients. Transfusion of greater than 4 units of packed red blood cells is rare. Although left colon diver-ticula are more common, bleeding tends to be more common from right colon diverticular sources. Hemor-rhage from right colon lesions may also be of greater rate and volume than that from left-sided diverticula. After an initial episode of hemorrhage, rebleeding is likely to occur in 10% of patients in the first year; thereafter, the risk for rebleeding increases to 25% at 4 years.

Given the prevalence of colonic diverticulosis, and the fact that most episodes of hemorrhage tend to cease spon-taneously, many episodes of lower intestinal hemorrhage are attributed to colonic diverticulosis as a presumptive rather than a definitive diagnosis.

Angiodysplasia

Angiodysplasias are responsible for 3% to 20% of cases of acute lower intestinal bleeding. Angiodysplasias, also referred to as *arteriovenous malformations*, are small ectatic blood vessels in the submucosa of the gastroin-testinal tract. The overlying mucosa is often thin, and superficial erosion at the site of an angiodysplasia has been observed on histologic examination of surgical or autopsy specimens. Angiodysplasias are identified in 1% to 2% of autopsy evaluations and increase in frequency with the age of the patient. Angiodysplasias may occur throughout the gastrointestinal tract and represent the most common cause of hemorrhage from the small bowel in patients older than 50 years of age.

Angiodysplasias are evident on colonoscopy as red, flat lesions about 2 to 10 mm in diameter. Lesions may appear stellate, oval, sharp, or indistinct. Colonoscopy is the most sensitive method to identify angiodysplasias, although angiography is also able to identify these lesions. The use of meperidine during colonoscopy may decrease the ability to identify angiodysplasias because of a reduction in mucosal blood flow. Another study has identified that the use of a narcotic antagonist may increase the size of angiodysplasias and enhance the detection rate. On angiography, angiodysplasias appear as ectatic, slowly emptying veins or as arteriovenous malformations with brisk, early venous filling.

More than half of angiodysplasias are localized to the right colon, and bleeding from angiodysplasia correlates with this distribution. Angiodysplasias may be associated with many medical conditions, including end-stage renal disease, aortic stenosis, von Willebrand's disease, and others. It is not clear whether this association reflects the greater tendency of angiodysplasias to bleed in these con-ditions or whether, in fact, angiodysplasias are more common structural findings in them.

Neoplasia

Colonic neoplasms, including adenomatous polyps, juvenile polyps, and carcinomas, present in a variety of manners. Typically, bleeding from these lesions is slow, characterized by occult bleeding and secondary anemia. These neoplasms can bleed briskly, however, and in some series, up to 20% of cases of acute hemorrhage are ultimately found to arise from colonic polyps or cancers. Juvenile polyps are the second most common cause of hemorrhage in patients younger than the age of 20 years.

Inflammatory Conditions

A wide variety of inflammatory conditions can cause acute lower gastrointestinal hemorrhage. Hemorrhage is rarely the presenting sign; rather, it develops in the course of the disease, and the cause is suspected based on the patient's history. Up to 20% of cases of acute lower gastrointestinal hemorrhage may be due to one of these inflammatory conditions. Most episodes of bleeding cease spontaneously or with specific therapy directed at the cause.

Hemorrhage complicates the course of ulcerative colitis in up to 15% of cases. Emergency colectomy for persistent hemorrhage accounts for 6% to 10% of emergency surgical colectomies in patients with this disease. Crohn's disease is less likely to cause massive colonic hemorrhage and occurs in roughly 1% of patients with this condition. Infectious causes include *Escherichia coli*, typhoid, cytomegalovirus, and *Clostridium difficile*. Radiation injury is most common in the rectum after pelvic radiotherapy for prostate or gynecologic malignancies. Bleeding is most common 1 year after radiation treatments but may occur up to 4 years later. Patients with immunosuppression or acquired immunodeficiency syndrome (AIDS) are at risk for acute lower intestinal hemorrhage from a unique set of causes. Cytomegalovirus is the most common cause; Kaposi's sarcoma, histoplasmosis, and perianal fistulas and fissures are also problematic and are more likely to hemorrhage in patients with AIDS-induced thrombocytopenia.

Vascular Causes

Vascular causes of acute lower intestinal hemorrhage include the vasculitides (polyarteritis nodosa, Wegener's granulomatosis, rheumatoid arthritis, and others), which are associated with punctate ulceration of the colon and small bowel. Colonic ischemia with mucosal ulceration and friability may also result in acute hemorrhage, often in the setting of acute abdominal pain and sepsis. Acute mesenteric ischemia may be heralded by an episode of hematochezia in the context of severe abdominal pain, preexisting vascular disease, arterial embolism risk, or hypercoagulability. Although hemorrhage is an element in the clinical management of these patients, only rarely does the control of hemorrhage become the major focus of therapy. Rather, restoration of visceral perfusion is the primary therapeutic objective.

Hemorrhoids

Hemorrhoids are usually noted on physical examination in more than half of patients with lower gastrointestinal hemorrhage. In fewer than 2% can the hemorrhage be attributed to these lesions, however. Unless unequivocal signs of bleeding are evident on anoscopy, investigation of the patient for another source of lower intestinal bleeding should be pursued. Patients with portal hypertension may develop massive hemorrhage from hemorrhoids, as can patients with HIV-associated thrombocytopenia with hemorrhoids.

Uncommon Causes

Rare causes of lower gastrointestinal hemorrhage include solitary rectal ulcer, Dieulafoy's lesion of the colon, portal colopathy, NSAIDs, intussusception, or bleeding following colonoscopic biopsy or polypectomy.

Initial Assessment

The initial history and physical examination are directed to determining the potential source of the hemorrhage and the severity of initial hemorrhage. Most cases eventually are determined to result from angiodysplasia or diverticulosis, both of which are usually asymptomatic before initial hemorrhage. Nonetheless, the initial history should exclude other, less common causes of the bleeding. Specific inquiry should be made regarding use of NSAIDs or anticoagulants. Abdominal pain or recent diarrhea and fever may point to colitis, either infectious or ischemic. Patients with prior aortic surgery should be considered to have an aortoenteric fistula until proved to the contrary. Prior radiation therapy for pelvic malignancy may indicate radiation proctitis. Recent colonoscopy may suggest bleeding from a biopsy or polypectomy site. The cause of previous episodes of bleeding should be elicited, as should the possibility of a history of inflammatory bowel disease. Family history of polyposis syndromes or colonic malignancy may also be pertinent. Young patients—those less than 30 years of age—are at greatest risk for bleeding from Meckel's diverticula or intestinal polyps.

Physical examination should include measurement of orthostatic vital signs in patients without overt shock. All patients should be resuscitated, as outlined in the previous section. Pertinent findings on physical examination may include scars from previous abdominal incisions, the presence of abdominal masses, or skin and oral lesions suggestive of polyposis syndromes. Stigmata of cirrhosis suggestive of bleeding from hemorrhoids or varices secondary to portal hypertension should be considered. The rectal examination is important to identify any anorectal pathology, including tumors, ulcers, or polyps. The color of the rectal contents and the presence of formed stool or blood clot should also be noted. Anoscopic examination to exclude hemorrhage from hemorrhoids should be completed. A nasogastric tube should be inserted to look for blood or coffee ground–like material to exclude an upper gastrointestinal source. In patients with hematochezia and hemodynamic instability, emergency upper endoscopy is required.

Diagnosis

Emergency surgical intervention for ongoing massive hemorrhage is rarely necessary before attempts are made to localize the precise source of bleeding. This allows an orderly approach to identification of the bleeding site, which is essential for appropriate therapy. After the patient has been resuscitated and stabilized, diagnostic testing should begin. The choice of initial investigation remains controversial and is dependent to some degree on local availability of procedures and expertise. The three options for primary diagnostic testing are colonoscopy, selective visceral angiography, and technetium 99m (^{99m}Tc)-labeled red blood cell scintigraphy. An algorithm for diagnosis of acute lower gastrointestinal bleeding is shown in Figure 44-5.

Colonoscopy

Recognition that most episodes of hemorrhage cease spontaneously and that stigmata of bleeding are subtle has led to efforts to perform colonoscopy as early as possible in the course of evaluation. Urgent colonoscopy, completed within 12 hours of admission, is indicated in patients who have ceased to have ongoing significant hemorrhage and in whom resuscitation and hemodynamic stability have been achieved. In this setting, colonoscopy can be completed after colonic purging.[31] Positive findings on colonoscopy include identification of an active bleeding site, identification of a nonbleeding visible vessel, clot adherent to a diverticular ulcerated orifice, clot adherent to a discrete focus of mucosa, or fresh blood localized to a colonic segment. Similarly, the finding of fresh blood

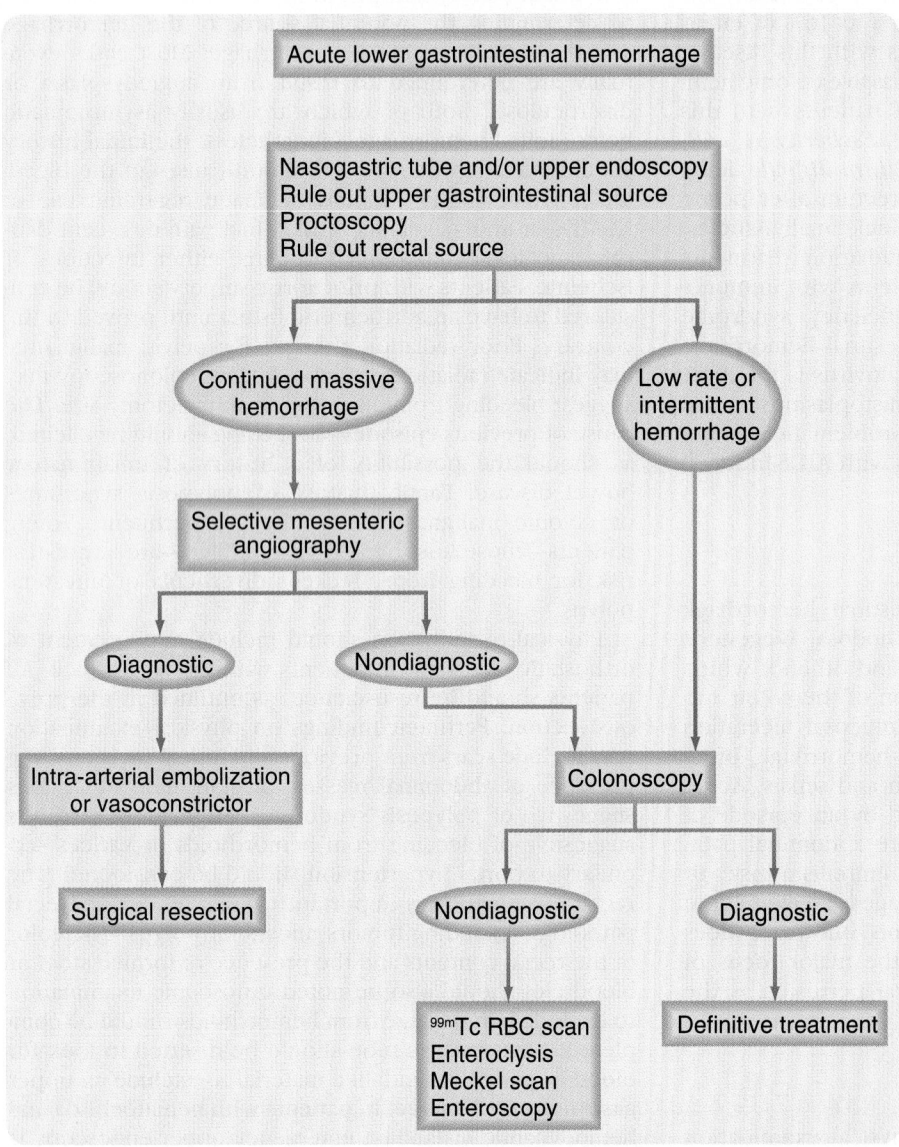

FIGURE 44-5. Diagnostic steps in the evaluation of acute lower gastrointestinal hemorrhage. RBC, red blood cell; UGI, upper gastrointestinal. (Modified from Turnage RH: Acute gastrointestinal hemorrhage. *In* Greenfield LJ, Mulholland MW, Oldham KT [eds]: Surgery: Scientific Principles and Practice. Philadelphia, Lippincott-Raven, 1997, p 1158.)

only in the terminal ileum after a negative upper endoscopy strongly suggests the small bowel as a bleeding source. It is important that incidental lesions, such as blood clots in multiple diverticular orifices, nonbleeding arteriovenous malformation, nonbleeding polyps, and nonbleeding diverticula, are not concluded to be the site of recent hemorrhage. Hemorrhage can be attributed only to lesions with clear stigmata of bleeding.

Patients presenting with massive lower gastrointestinal hemorrhage are poor candidates for emergency colonoscopy. The procedure is technically difficult because of the inability to clear the mucosal surfaces of old or new hemorrhage. Finding a discrete, actively bleeding vessel in the unprepared bowel is difficult even for the most experienced endoscopist. Second, patients with massive hemorrhage have hemodynamic instability, precluding the use of sedation and increasing the risk for hypoxemia and complication. Further, resuscitation may be compromised during the procedure.

Hence, colonoscopy is most appropriately used as the initial diagnostic procedure in patients presenting with acute hemorrhage that has ceased or in patients with a more moderate degree of bleeding. Colonoscopy is the procedure of choice in patients who develop hemorrhage after colonoscopic polypectomy.

Selective Visceral Angiography

Mesenteric arteriography has been widely used in the evaluation and treatment of patients with lower gastrointestinal hemorrhage. Selective injection of radiographic contrast into the superior mesenteric or inferior mesenteric arteries identifies hemorrhage in patients bleeding at a rate of 0.5 mL/min or greater. The study can accurately identify arterial hemorrhage in 45% to 75% of patients if they are actively bleeding at the time of contrast injection. Given the characteristic intermittent bleeding seen in lower gastrointestinal hemorrhage associated with diverticulosis, arteriovenous malformations, and other causes, bleeding may have ceased by the time of the study. Some radiologists have advocated evocative testing, including intra-arterial vasodilators, heparin, and fibrinolytic agents, in an effort to identify a bleeding source accurately. This approach does not appear to be warranted except in patients with refractory intermittent episodes of hemorrhage in a fully staffed suite. Because 90% of cases of hemorrhage cease spontaneously, and only 10% rebleed, such evocative testing is inappropriate for most patients.

About 10% of patients develop a complication of angiography. Major complications include stroke, renal failure, femoral artery thrombosis, lower extremity immobilization, and hematoma formation. Given that most patients with lower gastrointestinal hemorrhage are older than 60 years of age, medical comorbidities, including vascular disease and renal insufficiency, may place these patients at high risk for the procedure. Hence, angiography is reserved for patients with evidence of significant ongoing hemorrhage.

Technetium 99m-Red Blood Cell Scintigraphy

[99m]Tc-red blood cell scintigraphy has met with mixed success in the diagnosis of lower gastrointestinal hemorrhage. In this noninvasive nuclear medicine imaging procedure, the patient's red blood cells are labeled with a technetium isotope and reintroduced into the circulation. With each bleeding episode, labeled blood is shed into the colonic lumen, creating an isotopic focus that can be imaged with whole abdominal scintigraphy. Rates of bleeding as low as 0.1 mL/min can be detected. Images are obtained at distinct intervals after injection, within the first 2 hours, and thereafter at 4- to 6-hour intervals, or at the time of clinical evidence of rebleeding.[29] After extravasation into the lumen, the blood moves through the colonic lumen, generally from the right colon to the left, but occasionally in retrograde fashion because of colonic contractions.

If bleeding is present at the time of injection and initial imaging, ^{99m}Tc-red blood cell scans can accurately identify a source of bleeding in up to 85% of cases.[32] If bleeding is not active at the time of the initial study, or if delayed bleeding occurs, subsequent imaging to detect the luminal isotope can be inaccurate because of the sporadic movement of the tracer in the gut lumen.[33] The study is accurate in only 40% to 60% of patients, little better than a 50:50 ratio, to isolate bleeding to the left or right colon. Hence, patients in whom a surgical resection is anticipated to control recurrent or persistent hemorrhage should have the bleeding confirmed with either a positive angiogram or a positive colonoscopy. The red blood cell scans serve primarily to target the subsequent confirmatory study.

Treatment

Endoscopic Treatment

Endoscopic therapy includes the use of the same modalities available for upper gastrointestinal hemorrhage. Thermal heater probes, electrocoagulation, and sclerotherapy have been used. Reports suggest that electrocoagulation can be successfully applied for bleeding colonic diverticula, although this approach has not been widely embraced. Efforts at endoscopic control of diverticular hemorrhage may precipitate more significant bleeding. In contrast, angiodysplasias are readily treated with endoscopic measures. Acute bleeding can be controlled in up to 80% of patients with bleeding angiodysplasias, although rebleeding may develop in up to 15%. Care must be taken to avoid precipitating massive hemorrhage when treating angiodysplasias. Many endoscopists recommend approaching the lesion from the perimeter, obliterating feeder vessels before cauterization of the central vessel. Endoscopic therapy is also appropriate for patients with bleeding from a recent snare polypectomy site. Bleeding develops in 1% to 2% of patients after polypectomy and may occur up to 2 weeks after polypectomy. An endoscopic approach is recommended for these lesions.

Angiographic Treatment

In patients whose bleeding source is identified by angiography, a trial of angiographic therapy may be appropriate as a perioperative temporizing measure or as a definitive measure for high-risk surgical candidates.[34] Provided selective catheterization of a mesenteric vessel leading directly to the bleeding site can be completed, intra-arterial vasoconstrictor therapy with vasopressin can temporarily achieve control of bleeding in up to 80% of patients. Rebleeding is common, however, after discontinuing the therapy. Complications are frequent and serious and include myocardial ischemia, pulmonary edema, mesenteric thrombosis, and hyponatremia. Transarterial vasopressin should not be used in patients with coronary artery disease or other vascular disease. The primary role of this therapy is to achieve temporary control of bleeding before emergency definitive surgical resection.

Transcatheter embolization of massive bleeding may also be used for patients who are poor candidates for surgical resection. Embolization of gelatin sponges or microcoils can achieve temporary control of bleeding from angiodysplasias and diverticula. Given the lack of collateral blood supply to the colonic wall, these procedures may be complicated by colonic infarction heralded by abdominal pain, fever, and sepsis. Hence, like vasoconstrictive therapy, this procedure should be restricted to patients who cannot tolerate surgery or as a temporizing measure in massive hemorrhage in patients for whom a definitive surgical resection is imminent.

Surgery

Surgery is indicated for patients with ongoing or recurrent hemorrhage. Transfusion of more than 6 units of packed red blood cells, ongoing transfusion requirement, or persistent hemodynamic instability is an indication for colectomy in acute hemorrhage. Patients who develop recurrent lower gastrointestinal hemorrhage are also appropriately treated with colectomy because the risk for subsequent hemorrhage increases with time. Segmental colectomy is indicated in patients with persistent or recurrent colonic hemorrhage. Every effort should be made to localize the source of bleeding so that a hemicolectomy can be performed rather than a blind subtotal abdominal colectomy. Certainty of the site of bleeding is important; operation based on a positive ^{99m}Tc-red blood cell scan alone can result in recurrent hemorrhage in up to 35% of patients. "Blind" total abdominal colectomy carries significantly higher perioperative morbidity, and associated mortality rates approach 25% in some series. Diarrhea and rapid transit after total abdominal colectomy can also be debilitating conditions for elderly patients. There is no indication for a blind segmental colectomy, for which rebleeding rates as high as 75% are seen.

Mortality after colectomy for acute lower gastrointestinal hemorrhage overall is less than 5%. As in upper gastrointestinal hemorrhage, bleeding is not the cause of death; rather, pneumonia, cardiovascular events, and renal failure lead to poor outcomes, primarily in elderly patients with recurrent hemorrhage. Thoughtful timely management can lead to a successful outcome in most patients.

ACUTE GASTROINTESTINAL HEMORRHAGE FROM AN OBSCURE SOURCE

Definition and Incidence

The small bowel is a rare source of acute hemorrhage. Only 2% to 5% of patients with acute gastrointestinal hemorrhage are ultimately determined to have bled from a small intestinal source. This low frequency is fortunate because the small bowel is a difficult organ to visualize and precise detection of the bleeding lesion is characteristically delayed.

Clinical Presentation

The clinical presentation of patients with acute small bowel hemorrhage is similar to that of acute lower gastrointestinal hemorrhage from a colonic source. Small bowel hemorrhage is frequently episodic, characterized by recurrent brisk hemorrhage, which ceases spontaneously only to recur weeks or months later. Most patients are evaluated on multiple occasions after multiple bouts of hemorrhage before a correct diagnosis is made and effective definitive therapy completed.[35] Szold and associates[36] reported that the typical patient referred with acute gastrointestinal hemorrhage of obscure origin had intermittent episodes of hemorrhage during a 26-month period, had undergone 1 to 20 diagnostic tests, and had received an average of 20 units of packed red blood cells before diagnosis.

Etiology

The causes of hemorrhage identified in the 71 patients as studied by Szold and associates are shown in Table 44-4. In adults the most common source of bleeding from the small bowel is angiodysplasia, responsible for 50% to 75% of cases in older patients, and 30% to 40% of those in younger patients. These acquired lesions are most common in the right colon but can be found throughout the gastrointestinal tract.[37] The telangiectasias of Osler-Weber-Rendu syndrome are distinct from angiodysplasias. Most patients with this hereditary disorder present with skin and oral lesions in youth and acquire gastrointestinal lesions with bleeding in the 4th decade of life, or later. These telangiectasias are diffuse, and surgical intervention is not appropriate. Small bowel tumors are the second most common source of bleeding (25%) and include collectively gastrointestinal stromal tumors, lymphomas, adenocarcinomas, carcinoids, and metastatic melanomas. Less common possibilities include Meckel's diverticulum (more common in children), small bowel diverticula, Crohn's disease, radiation enteritis, ulcers due to NSAIDs, celiac sprue, and other rare findings.

TABLE 44-4. Sources of Obscure Gastrointestinal Bleeding: Findings in 71 Patients Treated with Surgery

Diagnosis	Patients (%)
Arteriovenous malformation	40
Small bowel leiomyoma	11
Small bowel adenocarcinoma	7
Small bowel lymphoma	6
Crohn's disease	6
"Watermelon" stomach	4
Meckel's diverticulum	4
Small bowel leiomyosarcoma	3
Metastatic colon carcinoma to small bowel	3
Small bowel varices	3
Small bowel melanoma	3
Others	10
Total	100

From Szold A, Katz L, Lewis B: Surgical approach to occult gastrointestinal bleeding. Am J Surg 163:90-93, 1992.

Initial Assessment

Initial priorities in management are resuscitation followed by prompt diagnostic testing as described for patients with lower gastrointestinal bleeding. Emergency upper endoscopy is indicated in hemodynamically unstable patients with hematochezia; patients with melena should have nasogastric aspiration to check for blood in the gastric contents. If negative, selective visceral angiography or emergency colonoscopy should be completed based on the clinical assessment of the rate and degree of bleeding. The role of ^{99m}Tc-red blood cell scintigraphy remains controversial, as in lower gastrointestinal hemorrhage.

In the rare patient with significant, ongoing small bowel bleeding at the time of these initial evaluations, a positive small intestinal source may be identified. Colonoscopy may reveal hemorrhage coming through the ileocecal valve or pooling in the terminal ileum, whereas selective mesenteric angiography may reveal the bleeding source from any of many possible small bowel sources. Obviously, it is critical not only to identify the small bowel as the source of hemorrhage but also to identify the precise site within the small bowel, so that a limited bowel resection can be completed.

In most patients, however, bleeding has ceased before the time these studies are completed, and only aggressive subsequent evaluation allows definitive diagnosis and treatment. Primary surgical exploration without investigation is to be condemned because the surgeon is rarely able to identify the actual source of small intestinal bleeding by visual inspection or palpation. Undirected exploration has a high risk of failure and should not be pursued except in patients with acute exsanguinating hemorrhage.

Diagnosis

The diagnostic evaluation of a patient with suspected bleeding from a small bowel source can be laborious and frustrating. Most of these patients have already undergone many of the more common and previously described modalities without success. The choice of diagnostic test varies depending on the particular presentation of the patient.

Spiral Computed Tomography

CT scanning with intravenous and oral contrast medium is a noninvasive diagnostic tool that is particularly useful if there is concomitant abdominal pain or symptoms of obstruction. CT images can identify areas of bowel thickening, mass lesions, or extraintestinal lesions that may be contributing to the patient's overall symptoms. These structural changes may be diagnostic of tumor, inflammatory conditions, or diverticula.

Enteroclysis

Enteroclysis is a small bowel contrast imaging study that can correctly identify mass lesions and structural mucosal processes, such as inflammatory or ulcerated lesions, in up to 80% of cases. It is unable, however, to identify angiodysplasias, the most common source of bleeding in these patients. Though still popular at some institutions, enteroclysis is poorly tolerated by patients and many centers have abandoned its use. When used strictly to evaluate the source of occult small intestinal bleeding, enteroclysis has a reported yield of only 10% to 21%. The ordinary small bowel follow-through contrast study is not adequate to evaluate these patients and should not be used, with a reported diagnostic yield of only 0 to 5.6%.[38]

Meckel's Scans

Meckel's diverticula may contain ectopic acid-secreting gastric mucosa that can lead to ulceration of the adjacent small bowel mucosa. The parietal cells in the gastric mucosa take up ^{99m}Tc pertechnetate, allowing imaging by a gamma camera. Congenital duplications of the intestinal tract may also contain ectopic gastric mucosa and be imaged with this test. This procedure should be the initial evaluation in young patients (those <30 years of age), in whom Meckel's diverticulum is the most common cause of small intestinal bleeding.

Small Bowel Endoscopy

Small bowel endoscopy, enteroscopy, has historically been completed by two methods. However, the recent introduction of video capsule endoscopy has greatly diminished the use of these technically challenging procedures. "Push" small bowel endoscopy uses a pediatric colonoscope to visualize the proximal small bowel directly.[39] The procedure is of limited value because only the proximal jejunum and duodenum can be visualized, even by skilled endoscopists. The Sonde (pull) enteroscopy has been abandoned in the United States. In this interesting historical method, a small fiberoptic imaging scope was "pulled" through the small bowel lumen by peristalsis to the ileocecal valve. Several hours later, the enteroscope was slowly pulled back through the intestine, and a careful inspection of the mucosa was completed through the 120-degree vision angle lens.[35] Although fine mucosal lesions and angiodysplasias could be identified with this technique, localization and therapy could not be accomplished.

Video Capsule Endoscopy

The Given wireless video capsule endoscope is an 11 × 26-mm capsule containing a miniature video camera, light source, battery, and transmitter.[40] It transmits video images to a torso-mounted recorder system at a rate of two images per second, up to 50,000 images overall, after being swallowed by the patient. The lens yields an 8-to-1 magnification, and the capsular coating prevents intestinal contents from interfering with the images. Relative contraindications include obstructive symptoms, motility disorders, and pacemakers. The major complication is capsule retention, which can occur at a stricture and has been reported in 5% of cases, although less than 1% of all mandated surgical retrieval.[41] Although it has not been available for long, in preliminary reports it has proven far superior to push endoscopy in diagnosis, and is tolerated much better as well. It does not have the capacity for therapeutic interventions as yet, nor can precise localizations within the bowel be achieved. It is, however, valuable in identifying diffuse disease that would not be amenable to surgical exploration and for identifying lesions for surgical or medical treatment. It is also an appropriate test to identify potential small bowel lesions prior to intraoperative endoscopy.

Intraoperative Endoscopy

A combined surgical and endoscopic procedure to evaluate and treat the small bowel sources of bleeding offers the best strategy for success. During exploratory laparotomy, small bowel enteroscopy is completed by an endoscopist. The operating surgeon carefully plicates the small bowel over the enteroscope while the lumen is visualized. The operating room lights are dimmed to image angiodysplasia better by transillumination. Identification of a mucosal ulcerated lesion or a single or multiple angiodysplasia allows definitive surgical treatment with small bowel resection. This combined approach may identify a bleeding source in up to 70% of patients; in patients with prior findings noted on video capsule endoscopy or angiography, the precise site of the abnormality can be identified to allow limited small bowel resection.

Treatment

The most common cause of small bowel bleeding, angiodysplasia, should be treated with endoscopic sclerotherapy or coagulation, if the lesion is within reach of the endoscope. For those in whom endoscopic measures

fail, surgical segmental resection of the small bowel is indicated. Because angiodysplasias are acquired with age, up to 25% of patients develop new hemorrhage from other angiodysplasias in subsequent years; thus, long-term follow-up is required. With both these and with telangiectasias some success with conjugated estrogen therapy to decrease the frequency and degree of hemorrhage has been reported.

Neoplasms are the second most common cause of small intestinal hemorrhage. Most are benign, although malignant tumors may also bleed. Therapy is surgical resection. Bleeding Meckel's diverticulum and small bowel diverticula are also appropriately treated with resection as well.

RARE CAUSES OF GASTROINTESTINAL HEMORRHAGE FROM AN OBSCURE SOURCE

Acute gastrointestinal hemorrhage from an obscure source has been reported to occur from a variety of conditions. These include radiation enteritis, small intestinal varices, Crohn's disease, tuberculosis, syphilis, typhoid, histoplasmosis, vasculitis, small bowel ulcerated lesions in patients with gastrin-secreting tumors, and Dieulafoy's lesions. Medical treatment is appropriate for most infectious causes and in patients with Zollinger-Ellison syndrome. Enterectomy is required in the other conditions.

Disorders of the pancreas can cause acute gastrointestinal hemorrhage as blood is delivered into the duodenum through the pancreatic duct. Such bleeding has been reported in the setting of acute pseudoaneurysms after pancreatectomy and in pancreatic tumors. Bleeding is a rare complication of these disorders. Angiography may confirm the presence of a pseudoaneurysm and allow angiographic embolization for acute hemorrhage control. Pancreatic resection may be appropriate, depending on the clinical condition.

The liver may also be the source of presumed acute gastrointestinal hemorrhage. Bleeding into the hepatic duct presents as gastrointestinal hemorrhage as blood enters the duodenum from the common bile duct, a condition known as *hemobilia*. Hemobilia has been reported to occur secondary to hepatic trauma with intrahepatic hematoma, hepatic aneurysms or other vascular malformations, hepatic tumors, hepatic abscess, or after hepatic resection or percutaneous liver biopsy. This diagnosis is usually considered when endoscopic visualization during acute hemorrhage shows blood entering the duodenum at the ampulla of Vater, depending on the clinical scenario. Selective visceral angiography is usually required to define the source and often allows definitive management by intra-arterial embolization.

Selected References

Church NI, Palmer KR: Ulcers and nonvariceal bleeding. Endoscopy 35:22-26, 2003.

> This review article details the current strategies for managing patients with bleeding peptic ulcer based on a detailed analysis of the reported clinical experience. The cited references are excellent.

Kollef MH, Canfield DA, Zuckerman G: Triage considerations for patients with acute gastrointestinal hemorrhage admitted to a medical intensive care unit. Crit Care Med 23:1048-1054, 1995.

> **This important paper identifies clinical parameters, independent of endoscopic findings, to predict adverse outcome for patients with acute gastrointestinal hemorrhage and provides an algorithm for triage considerations.**

Rikkers LF: The changing spectrum of treatment for variceal bleeding. Ann Surg 228:536-546, 1998.

> **This paper, which will become a classic, details a single surgeon's experience in managing patients with acute gastrointestinal hemorrhage secondary to portal hypertension. The author's contributions have defined the approach to the management of these patients during the past 4 decades, and the evolution of his current treatment strategy is presented.**

Vernava AM, Moore BA, Longo WE, et al: Lower gastrointestinal bleeding. Dis Colon Rectum 40:846-858, 1997.

> **This paper offers a complete summary of evaluation and work-up for lower gastrointestinal bleeding.**

Wara P: Endoscopic prediction of major rebleeding: A prospective study of stigmata of hemorrhage in bleeding ulcer. Gastroenterology 88:1209-1214, 1985.

> **This classic paper describes the now widely embraced classification system for endoscopic stigmata that predict the risk for recurrent hemorrhage in patients with bleeding peptic ulcer.**

Wolfe MM, Lichtenstein DR, Singh G: Gastrointestinal toxicity of nonsteroidal anti-inflammatory drugs. N Engl J Med 340:1888-1899, 1999.

> **This review summarizes the pathogenesis on nonsteroidal anti-inflammatory drug–induced gastrointestinal complications.**

Zuckerman GR, Prakash C, Askin MP, et al: AGA technical review on the evaluation and management of occult and obscure gastrointestinal bleeding. Gastroenterology 118:201-221, 2000.

> **This paper provides a great summary of evaluation protocols in these patients.**

References

1. Peura DA, Lanza FL, Gostout CJ, et al: The American College of Gastroenterology Bleeding Registry: Preliminary findings. Am J Gastroenterol 92:924-928, 1997.
2. Bass B, Wolpert S: Management of the complications of peptic ulcer disease. Probl Gen Surg 14:54-68, 1997.
3. Bulut OB, Rasmussen C, Fischer A: Acute surgical treatment of complicated peptic ulcers with special reference to the elderly. World J Surg 20:574-577, 1996.
4. Bhatti N, Amoateng-Adjepong Y, Qamar A, et al: Myocardial infarction in critically ill patients presenting with gastrointestinal hemorrhage: Retrospective analysis of risks and outcomes. Chest 114:1137-1142, 1998.
5. Valentine RJ, Hagino RT, Jackson MR, et al: Gastrointestinal complications after aortic surgery. J Vasc Surg 28:404-412, 1998.
6. Hunt RH, Bowen B, Mortensen ER, et al: A randomized trial measuring fecal blood loss after treatment with rofecoxib, ibuprofen, or placebo in healthy subjects. Am J Med 109:201-206, 2000.
7. Cooper GS, Chak A, Way LE, et al: Early endoscopy in upper gastrointestinal hemorrhage: Associations with recurrent bleeding, surgery, and length of hospital stay. Gastrointest Endosc 49:145-152, 1999.
8. Wilcox CM, Clark WS: Causes and outcome of upper and lower gastrointestinal bleeding: The Grady Hospital experience. South Med J 92:44-50, 1999.
9. Laine L, Peterson WL: Bleeding peptic ulcer. N Engl J Med 331:717-727, 1994.
10. Wolfe MM, Lichtenstein DR, Singh G: Gastrointestinal toxicity of nonsteroidal anti-inflammatory drugs. N Engl J Med 340:1888-1899, 1999.
11. Laine L, Connors LG, Reicin A, et al: Serious lower gastrointestinal clinical events with nonselective NSAID or coxib use. Gastroenterology 124:288-292, 2003.
12. Pennisi E: Building a better aspirin. Science 280:1191-1192, 1998.
13. Kollef MH, O'Brien JD, Zuckerman GR, et al: BLEED: A classification tool to predict outcomes in patients with acute upper and lower gastrointestinal hemorrhage. Crit Care Med 25:1125-1132, 1997.
14. Kohler B, Maier M, Benz C, et al: Acute ulcer bleeding: A prospective randomized trial to compare Doppler and Forrest classifications in endoscopic diagnosis and therapy. Dig Dis Sci 42:1370-1374, 1997.
15. Ng EKW, Lam YH, Sung JJ, et al: Eradication of *Helicobacter pylori* prevents recurrence of ulcer after simple closure of duodenal ulcer perforation: Randomized controlled trial. Ann Surg 231:153-158, 2000.
16. Lau JYW, Sung JJY, Lee KK, et al: Effect of intravenous omeprazole on recurrent bleeding after endoscopic treatment of bleeding peptic ulcers. N Engl J Med 343:310-316, 2000.
17. Zed PJ, Loewen PS, Slavik RS, et al: Meta-analysis of proton pump inhibitors in treatment of bleeding peptic ulcers. Ann Pharmacother 35:1528-1534, 2001.
18. Javid G, Masoodi I, Zargar SA, et al: Omeprazole as adjuvant therapy to endoscopic combination injection sclerotherapy for treating bleeding peptic ulcer. Am J Med 111:280-284, 2001.
19. Church NI, Palmer KR: Ulcers and nonvariceal bleeding. Endoscopy 35:22-26, 2003.
20. Jiranek GC, Kozarek RA: A cost-effective approach to the patient with peptic ulcer bleeding. Surg Clin North Am 76:83-103, 1996.
21. Cook DJ, Guyatt GH, Salena BJ, et al: Endoscopic therapy for acute nonvariceal upper gastrointestinal hemorrhage: A meta-analysis. Gastroenterology 102:139-148, 1992.
22. Lau JY, Sung JJ, Lam YH, et al: Endoscopic retreatment compared with surgery in patients with recurrent bleeding after initial endoscopic control of bleeding ulcers. N Engl J Med 340:751-756, 1999.
23. Rockall TA: Management and outcome of patients undergoing surgery after acute upper gastrointestinal haemorrhage. Steering Group for the National Audit of Acute Upper Gastrointestinal Haemorrhage. J R Soc Med 91:518-523, 1998.
24. Imhof M, Schroders C, Ohmann C, et al: Impact of early operation on the mortality from bleeding peptic ulcer—ten years' experience. Dig Surg 15:308-314, 1998.
25. Callicutt CS, Behrman SW: Incidence of *Helicobacter pylori* in operatively managed acute nonvariceal upper gastrointestinal bleeding. J Gastrointest Surg 5:614-619, 2001.
26. Cook DJ, Reeve BK, Guyatt GH, et al: Stress ulcer prophylaxis in critically ill patients: Resolving discordant meta-analyses. JAMA 275:308-314, 1996.

27. Cook D, Guyatt G, Marshall J, et al: A comparison of sucralfate and ranitidine for the prevention of upper gastrointestinal bleeding in patients requiring mechanical ventilation. Canadian Critical Care Trials Group. N Engl J Med 338:791-797, 1998.

28. Walsh RM, Anain P, Geisinger M, et al: Role of angiography and embolization for massive gastroduodenal hemorrhage. J Gastrointest Surg 3:61-66, 1999.

29. Bharucha AE, Gostout CJ, Balm RK: Clinical and endoscopic risk factors in the Mallory-Weiss syndrome. Am J Gastroenterol 92:805-808, 1997.

30. Zuckerman GR, Prakash C: Acute lower intestinal bleeding: II. Etiology, therapy, and outcomes. Gastrointest Endosc 49:228-238, 1999.

31. Chaudhry V, Hyser MJ, Gracias VH, et al: Colonoscopy: The initial test for acute lower gastrointestinal bleeding. Am Surg 64:723-728, 1998.

32. Gunderman R, Leef J, Ong K, et al: Scintigraphic screening prior to visceral arteriography in acute lower gastrointestinal bleeding. J Nucl Med 39:1081-1083, 1998.

33. Vernava AM III, Moore BA, Longo WE, et al: Lower gastrointestinal bleeding. Dis Colon Rectum 40:846-858, 1997.

34. Gordon RL, Ahl KL, Kerlan RK, et al: Selective arterial embolization for the control of lower gastrointestinal bleeding. Am J Surg 174:24-28, 1997.

35. Lewis BS: Small intestinal bleeding. Gastroenterol Clin North Am 23:67-91, 1994.

36. Szold A, Katz LB, Lewis BS: Surgical approach to occult gastrointestinal bleeding. Am J Surg 163:90-93, 1992.

37. Vu H, Adams CZ Jr, Hoover EL: Jejunal angiodysplasia presenting as acute lower gastrointestinal bleeding. Am Surg 56:302-304, 1990.

38. Zuckerman GR, Prakash C, Askin MP, et al: AGA technical review on the evaluation and management of occult and obscure gastrointestinal bleeding. Gastroenterology 118:201-221, 2000.

39. Waye JD: Small bowel endoscopy. Endoscopy 35:15-21, 2003.

40. Appleyard M, Glukhovsky A, Swain P: Wireless-capsule diagnostic endoscopy for recurrent small-bowel bleeding. N Engl J Med 344:232-233, 2001.

41. Cave DR: Wireless video capsule endoscopy. Clin Perspect Gastroenterol 5:203-207, 2002.

CHAPTER 45

STOMACH

David W. Mercer, M.D. and **Emily K. Robinson, M.D.**

Anatomy	Stress Gastritis
Physiology	Gastric Neoplasia
Peptic Ulcer Disease	Other Gastric Lesions

ANATOMY

Gross Anatomy

Divisions

Wallace P. Ritchie, Jr., called the stomach an elegant organ, once thought to be the seat of the soul, always handy to bring to the dinner table, and a recognized source of ecstasy and grief. It originates as a dilation in the tubular embryonic foregut during the 5th week of gestation. By the 7th week, it descends, rotates, and further dilates with a disproportionate elongation of the greater curvature into its normal anatomic shape and position. Following birth, it is the most proximal abdominal organ of the alimentary tract (Fig. 45-1). The most proximal region of the stomach is called the *cardia*, and it attaches to the esophagus. Immediately proximal to the cardia is a physiologically competent lower esophageal sphincter. Distally, the pylorus connects the distal stomach (antrum) to the proximal duodenum. Although the stomach is fixed at the gastroesophageal (GE) junction and the pylorus, its large mid portion is mobile. The fundus represents the superior-most part of the stomach and is floppy and distensible. It is bounded superiorly by the diaphragm and laterally by the spleen. The body of the stomach represents the largest portion and is also referred to as the *corpus*. The body also contains most of the parietal cells and is bounded on the right by the relatively straight lesser curvature and on the left by the longer greater curvature. At the angularis incisura, the lesser curvature abruptly angles to the right. It is at this point that the body of the stomach ends and the antrum begins. Another important anatomic angle (angle of His) is that which the fundus forms with the left margin of the esophagus.

Most of the stomach resides within the left upper quadrant of the abdomen. The left lateral segment of the liver usually covers a large portion of the stomach anteriorly. The diaphragm, chest, and abdominal wall bound the remainder of the stomach. Inferiorly, the stomach is attached to the transverse colon, spleen, caudate lobe of the liver, diaphragmatic crura, and retroperitoneal nerves and vessels. Superiorly, the GE junction is found about 2 to 3 cm below the diaphragmatic esophageal hiatus in the horizontal plane of the seventh chondrosternal articulation, a plane only slightly cephalad to that containing the pylorus. The gastrosplenic ligament attaches the proximal greater curvature to the spleen.

Blood Supply

As shown in Figure 45-2, most of the blood supply to the stomach is from the celiac artery. There are four main arteries: the left and right gastric arteries along the lesser curvature and the left and right gastroepiploic arteries along the greater curvature. In addition, a substantial quantity of blood may be supplied to the proximal stomach by the inferior phrenic arteries and by the short gastric arteries from the spleen. The largest artery to the stomach is the left gastric artery, and it is not uncommon (15% to 20%) for an aberrant left hepatic artery to originate from it. Consequently, proximal ligation of the left gastric artery may result in acute left-sided hepatic ischemia because the aberrant left hepatic artery occasionally represents the only arterial flow to the left hepatic lobe. The right gastric artery arises from the hepatic artery (or the gastroduodenal artery). The left gastroepiploic artery originates from the splenic artery, and the right gastroepiploic originates from the gastroduodenal artery. The extensive anastomotic connection between these major vessels ensures that, in most cases, the stomach will survive if three of four arteries are ligated, provided that the arcades along the greater and lesser curvatures are not disturbed. In general, the veins of the stomach parallel the arteries. The left gastric (coronary) and right gastric veins usually drain into the portal vein. The right

gastroepiploic vein drains into the superior mesenteric vein, and the left gastroepiploic vein drains into the splenic vein.

Lymphatic Drainage

Generally, the lymphatic drainage of the stomach parallels the vasculature and essentially drains into four zones of lymph nodes as depicted in Figure 45-3. The superior gastric group drains lymph from the upper lesser curvature into the left gastric and paracardial nodes. The suprapyloric group of nodes drains the antral segment on the lesser curvature of the stomach into the right suprapancreatic nodes. The pancreaticolienal group of nodes drains lymph high on the greater curvature into the left gastroepiploic and splenic nodes. The inferior gastric/subpyloric group of nodes drains lymph along the right gastroepiploic vascular pedicle. All four zones of lymph nodes drain into the celiac group and into the thoracic duct. Although the aforementioned lymph nodes drain different areas of the stomach, it remains widely recognized that gastric cancers may metastasize to any of the four nodal groups regardless of the cancer location. In addition, the extensive submucosal plexus of lymphatics accounts for the fact that there is frequently microscopic evidence of malignant cells several centimeters from the resection margin of gross disease.

FIGURE 45-1. Divisions of the stomach. (From Zuidema G: Shackelford's Surgery of the Alimentary Tract, 4th ed. Philadelphia, WB Saunders, 1995.)

FIGURE 45-2. Blood supply to the stomach and duodenum with anatomical relationships to the spleen and pancreas. The stomach is reflected cephalad. (From Zuidema G: Shackelford's Surgery of the Alimentary Tract, 4th ed. Philadelphia, WB Saunders, 1995.)

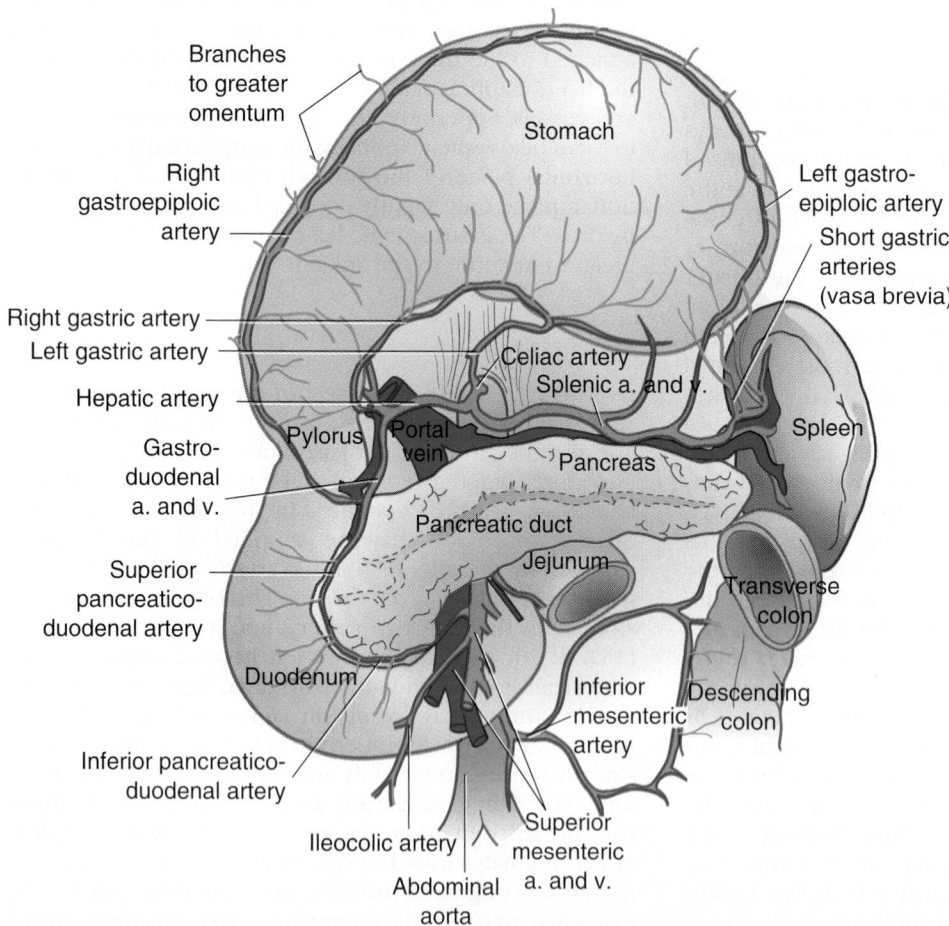

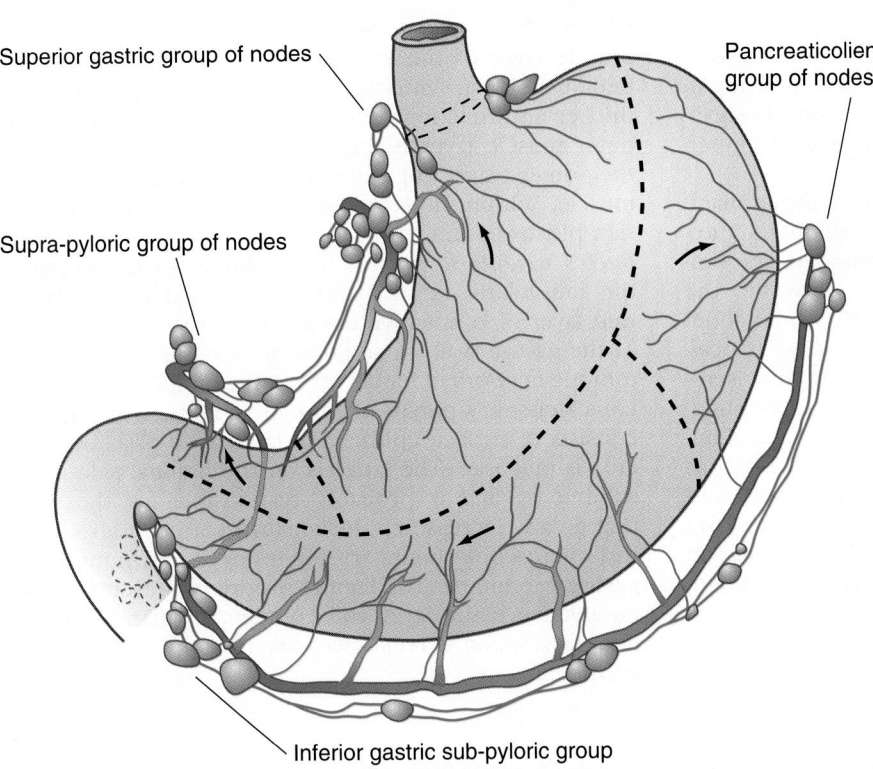

Superior gastric group of nodes

Supra-pyloric group of nodes

Pancreaticolienal group of nodes

Inferior gastric sub-pyloric group

FIGURE 45-3. Lymphatic drainage of the stomach. (From Moody F, McGreevy J, Miller T: Stomach. In Schwartz SI, Shires GT [eds]: Principles of Surgery, 5th ed. New York, McGraw-Hill, 1989.)

Innervation

As shown in Figure 45-4, the extrinsic innervation of the stomach is both parasympathetic through the vagus and sympathetic through the celiac plexus. The vagus nerve originates in the vagal nucleus in the floor of the fourth ventricle and traverses the neck in the carotid sheath to enter the mediastinum, where it divides into several branches around the esophagus. These branches coalesce above the esophageal hiatus to form the left and right vagus nerves. However, it is not uncommon to find more than two vagal trunks at the distal esophagus.[1] At the GE junction, the left vagus is anterior, and the right vagus is posterior (L-A-R-P, mnemonic). As shown in Figure 45-4, the left vagus gives off the hepatic branch to the liver and then continues along the lesser curvature as the anterior nerve of Latarjet. Although not shown, the "criminal" nerve of Grassi is the first branch of the right or posterior vagus nerve and is recognized as a potential etiology of recurrent ulcers when left undivided. The right nerve also gives a branch off to the celiac plexus and then continues posteriorly along the lesser curvature. As depicted, a truncal vagotomy is performed above the celiac and hepatic branches of the vagi, whereas a selective vagotomy is performed below. A highly selective vagotomy is performed by dividing the crow's feet to the proximal stomach while preserving the innervation of the antral and pyloric parts of the stomach. Most (>90%) of the vagal fibers are afferent, carrying stimuli from the gut to the brain. Efferent vagal fibers originate in the dorsal nucleus of the medulla and synapse with neurons in the myenteric and submucosal plexuses. These neurons utilize acetyl-

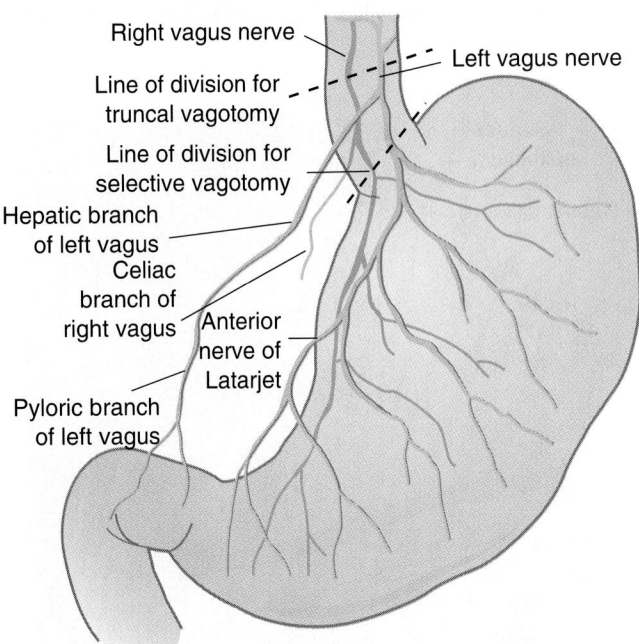

Right vagus nerve

Left vagus nerve

Line of division for truncal vagotomy

Line of division for selective vagotomy

Hepatic branch of left vagus

Celiac branch of right vagus

Anterior nerve of Latarjet

Pyloric branch of left vagus

FIGURE 45-4. Vagal innervation of the stomach. The line of division for truncal vagotomy is shown and is above the hepatic and celiac branches of the left and right vagus nerves, respectively. The line of division for selective vagotomy is shown and occurs below the hepatic and celiac branches. (From Mercer D, Liu T: Open truncal vagotomy. In Operative Techniques in General Surgery 5:8-85, 2003.)

choline as their neurotransmitter and influence gastric motor function and gastric secretion. In contrast, the sympathetic nerve supply comes from T5 to T10, traveling in the splanchnic nerve to the celiac ganglion. Postganglionic fibers then travel with the arterial system to innervate the stomach.

The intrinsic or enteric nervous system of the stomach consists of neurons in Auerbach's and Meissner's autonomic plexuses. In these locations, cholinergic, serotonergic, and peptidergic neurons are present. However, the function of these neurons remains poorly understood. Nevertheless, a number of neuropeptides have been localized to these neurons and include acetylcholine, serotonin, substance P, calcitonin gene–related peptide, bombesin, cholecystokinin (CCK), and somatostatin. Consequently, it is oversimplified to think of the stomach as only containing parasympathetic (cholinergic input) and sympathetic (adrenergic input) supply. Moreover, the parasympathetic nervous system contains adrenergic neurons, and the sympathetic system also contains cholinergic neurons.

Gastric Morphology

Except for a small posterior area at the proximal cardia and distal pyloric antrum, the stomach is covered by peritoneum. The peritoneum forms the outer serosa of the stomach. Below it is the thicker, muscularis propria, or muscularis externa, which is made up of three layers of smooth muscles (Fig. 45-5). The middle layer

of smooth muscle is circular and is the only complete muscle layer of the stomach wall. At the pylorus, this middle circular muscle layer becomes progressively thicker and functions as a true anatomic sphincter. The outer muscle layer is longitudinal and continuous with the outer layer of longitudinal esophageal smooth muscle. Within the layers of the muscularis externa, is a rich plexus of autonomic nerves and ganglia called *Auerbach's myenteric plexus*. The submucosa lies between the muscularis externa and mucosa and is a collagen-rich layer of connective tissue that is the strongest layer of the gastric wall. In addition, it contains the rich anastomotic network of blood vessels and lymphatics and contains Meissner's plexus of autonomic nerves. The mucosa consists of surface epithelium, lamina propria, and muscularis mucosae. The latter is on the luminal side of the submucosa and is probably responsible for the rugae that greatly increase epithelial surface area. It also marks the microscopic boundary for invasive and noninvasive gastric carcinoma. The lamina propria represents a small connective tissue layer and contains capillaries, vessels, lymphatics, and nerves necessary to support the surface epithelium.

Gastric Glandular Organization

Gastric mucosa consists of columnar glandular epithelia. The functions of the glands and the cells lining the glands vary according to the region of the stomach in which they are found (Table 45-1). The endocrine cells such as the gastrin (G) cells or somatostatin (D) cells can be either open or closed. Open-type endocrine cells have their microvilli on the apical membranes, which allows direct contact with gastric contents. The microvilli likely possess chemical and pH sensors that signal the cell to secrete their prestored peptides. In contrast, closed-type endocrine cells do not have microvilli in contact with the gastric lumen. In the antrum, there are G cells and D cells that are of the open-type variety. In contrast, the D cells located in the fundus/body of the stomach are of the closed-type variety and are in direct contact with the acid-secreting parietal cells. In the cardia, the mucosae are arranged in branched glands that primarily secrete mucus, and the pits are short. In the fundus and body, the glands are more tubular and the pits longer. In the antrum, the glands are more branched. The luminal ends of the gastric glands and pits are lined with mucus-secreting surface epithelial cells, which extend down into the necks of the glands for variable distances. In the cardia, the glands are predominantly mucus secreting. In the body, the glands are lined from the neck to the base mostly with parietal and chief cells (Fig. 45-6). There are a few parietal cells in the fundus and proximal antrum, but none in the cardia or prepyloric antrum. Biopsy specimens taken from the stomach have demonstrated that parietal cells account for 13% of epithelial cells, whereas chief cells account for 44%; mucus cells account for 40%; and endocrine cells account for 3%.

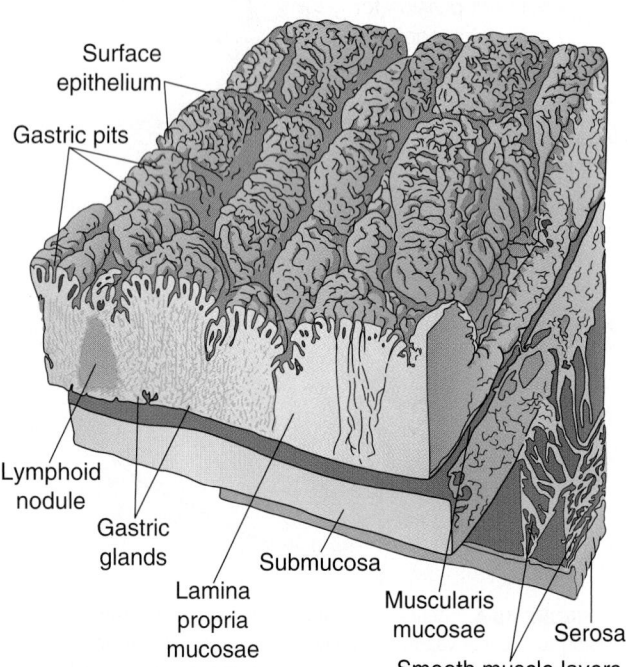

Surface epithelium

Gastric pits

Lymphoid nodule

Gastric glands

Lamina propria mucosae

Submucosa

Muscularis mucosae

Serosa

Smooth muscle layers

FIGURE 45-5. Gastric mucosa surface. The normal distribution of gastric glands is depicted on the left. The glands are gray and the gastric pits are black (×17). (From Zuidema G: Shackelford's Surgery of the Alimentary Tract, 4th ed. Philadelphia, WB Saunders, 1995.)

TABLE 45-1 Gastric Cell Types, Location, and Function

Cells	Location	Function
Parietal	Body	Secretion of acid and intrinsic factor
Mucus	Body, antrum	Mucus
Chief	Body	Pepsin
Surface epithelial	Diffuse	Mucus, bicarbonate, prostaglandins (?)
ECL	Body	Histamine
G	Antrum	Gastrin
D	Body, antrum	Somatostatin
Gastric mucosal interneurons	Body, antrum	Gastrin-releasing peptide
Enteric neurons	Diffuse	CGRP, others

ECL, enterochromaffin-like; CGRP, calcitonin gene–related peptide.

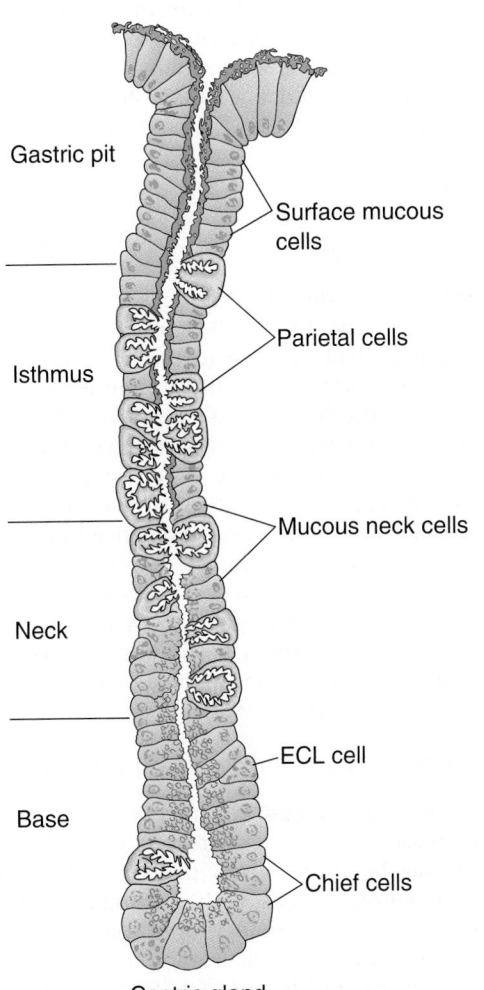

Gastric pit

Surface mucous cells

Parietal cells

Isthmus

Mucous neck cells

Neck

ECL cell

Base

Chief cells

Gastric gland

FIGURE 45-6. Cells residing within a gastric gland. (From Zuidema G: Shackelford's Surgery of the Alimentary Tract, 4th ed. Philadelphia, WB Saunders, 1995.)

PHYSIOLOGY

General Considerations

The principal function of the stomach is to prepare ingested food for digestion and absorption as it is propulsed into and through the small intestine. The initial period of digestion requires that solid components of a meal be stored for several hours while they undergo a reduction in size and breakdown into their basic metabolic constituents.

Receptive relaxation of the proximal stomach enables the stomach to function as a storage organ. *Receptive relaxation* refers to the process whereby the proximal portion of the stomach relaxes in anticipation of food intake. This relaxation enables liquids to pass easily from the stomach along the lesser curvature, whereas the solid food settles along the greater curvature of the fundus. In contrast to liquids, emptying of solid food is facilitated by the antrum, which pumps solid food components into and through the pylorus. The antrum and pylorus function in a coordinated fashion allowing entry of food components into the duodenum and also returning material to the proximal stomach until it is appropriate for delivery into the duodenum.

In addition to storing food, the stomach participates in digestion of a meal. For example, starches undergo enzymatic breakdown through the activity of salivary amylase, although the pH within the center of the gastric bolus needs to be greater than pH 5. Peptic digestion metabolizes a meal into fats, proteins, and carbohydrates by breaking down cell walls. Although the duodenum and proximal small intestine are primarily responsible for digestion of a meal, the stomach clearly facilitates this process.

Regulation of Gastric Function

Gastric function is under both neural and hormonal control, and both systems interact to provide additional regulation. Hormonal mediators of gastric function are usually peptides or amines that interact with their target cells in one of three ways: endocrine, paracrine, or neurocrine. Endocrine cells release peptides from their basolateral membranes into the bloodstream that circulate, arrive at target cells, and exert their hormonal effects. In contrast, paracrine cells release their peptides locally, arriving at target cells by diffusion across the interstitial space. Finally, neurocrine mediators are released from nerve endings that diffuse across the synapse with a target cell and bind to a receptor. Some peptides such as somatostatin can act as either endocrine or paracrine mediators of gastric function depending on the circumstances. Moreover, the precise state of any target cell depends on the relative balance of endocrine, paracrine, and neurocrine mediators acting on it.

Gastric Peptides

Gastrin

SYNTHESIS AND ACTION

Gastrin is produced by G cells located in the gastric antrum (see Table 45-1). It is synthesized as a pre-propeptide and undergoes post-translational processing to produce biologic reactive gastrin peptides. Several molecular forms of gastrin exist. G-34 (big gastrin), G-17 (little gastrin), and G-14 (mini gastrin) all have been identified. However, 90% of antral gastrin is released as the 17-amino acid peptide, although G-34 predominates in the circulation because its metabolic half-life is longer than that of G-17.[2] The pentapeptide sequence contained at the carboxyl terminus of gastrin is the biologically active component and is identical to that found on another gut peptide, CCK. CCK and gastrin differ by tyrosine sulfation sites.[3] The release of gastrin is stimulated by food components contained within a meal, especially protein digestion products. Luminal acid inhibits the release of gastrin. Somatostatin (see later) has paracrine actions on antral G cells and acts to inhibit gastrin release. In the antral location, somatostatin and gastrin release are functionally linked, and an inverse reciprocal relationship exists between these two peptides.[4] Moreover, somatostatin exerts a tonic inhibitory effect on gastrin release and likely mediates the inhibitory effects of luminal acid on gastrin release.

Gastrin is the major hormonal regulator of the gastric phase of acid secretion following a meal. Although parietal cells possess receptors to gastrin and exogenous gastrin elicits gastric acid secretion, it is likely that histamine, released from enterochromaffin-like (ECL) cells, is the principal mediator of this action. Evidence supporting this concept is the finding that gastrin-stimulated gastric acid secretion is significantly blunted following administration of H₂-receptor antagonists.[5] Both exogenous gastrin and endogenous gastrin have been shown to prevent gastric injury from luminal irritants, suggesting that gastrin also plays a role in the intrinsic gastric mucosal defense system.[6] Gastrin also has considerable trophic

effects on the parietal cells and the gastric ECL cells. In fact, prolonged hypergastrinemia from any cause leads to mucosal hyperplasia as well as an increase in the number of ECL cells and, under some circumstances, is associated with the development of gastric carcinoid tumors.[7]

HYPERGASTRINEMIA

Hypergastrinemia can result from a variety of causes. Hypergastrinemia that results from administration of antisecretory agents is an appropriate response caused by loss of feedback inhibition of gastrin release by luminal acid. Lack of acid causes a reduction in somatostatin release, which in turn causes increased release of gastrin from antral G cells. Hypergastrinemia can also occur in the setting of pernicious anemia or uremia or following surgical procedures such as vagotomy or retained gastric antrum after gastrectomy. In contrast, gastrin levels increase inappropriately in patients with gastrinoma (Zollinger-Ellison syndrome). These gastrin-secreting tumors are not located in the antrum and secrete gastrin autonomously. The clinical triad of Zollinger-Ellison syndrome is the finding of gastric acid hypersecretion, severe peptic ulcer disease, and a non-beta islet cell tumor of the pancreas (see later).

Somatostatin

SYNTHESIS AND ACTION

Somatostatin is produced by D cells and exists endogenously as either the 14- or 28-amino acid peptide.[8] The predominant molecular form in the stomach is somatostatin 14. It is produced by diffuse neuroendocrine cells located in both the fundus and the antrum. In these locations, their cytoplasmic extensions have direct contact with the parietal cells and the G cells, where it presumably exerts its actions through paracrine effects on acid secretion and gastrin release.[9] Somatostatin is able to directly inhibit parietal cell acid secretion but can also indirectly inhibit acid secretion through inhibition of gastrin release and downregulation of histamine release from ECL cells. The principal stimulus for somatostatin release is antral acidification, whereas acetylcholine from vagal fibers inhibits its release.

EFFECTS OF *HELICOBACTER PYLORI* ON SOMATOSTATIN

Basal and stimulated gastrin concentrations are significantly increased in patients infected with *Helicobacter pylori*. It has been proposed that *H. pylori* causes a decrease in antral D cells with a resultant decrease in somatostatin levels. The reduction in somatostatin causes disinhibition of antral G cells leading to increased gastrin release.[9] Eradication of *H. pylori* restores the antral D-cell population, causing an increase in antral somatostatin with a resultant decrease in gastrin levels.[9] These data suggest that infection with *H. pylori* decreases antral D cells and somatostatin levels to cause an increase in gastrin release, which in turn leads to an increase in gastric acid secretion. However, while *H. pylori* infected patients with duodenal ulcer disease usually have enhanced acid secretion, there are a number of *H. pylori*–positive healthy volunteers with no peptic ulcer disease who have little or no increase in acid secretion when compared to *H. pylori*–negative volunteers. Nevertheless, cure of the infection in patients with duodenal ulcer has been demonstrated by some, but not all, investigators to diminish acid secretion.[9]

Gastrin-Releasing Peptide

Bombesin was discovered 20 years ago, from an extract prepared from skin of the amphibian *Bombina bombina.* Its mammalian counterpart is gastrin-releasing peptide (GRP). GRP-staining immunoreactivity is particularly prominent in nerves ending in the acid secreting and the gastrin-secreting portions of the stomach and is found in the circular muscular layer.[10] In the antral mucosa, GRP stimulates gastrin and somatostatin release by binding to receptors located on the G and D cells, respectively. It is rapidly cleared from the circulation by a neutral endopeptidase and has a half-life of around 1.4 minutes.[10] Peripheral administration of exogenous GRP stimulates gastric acid secretion, whereas central administration in the ventricles inhibits acid secretion.[10] This inhibitory pathway is not mediated by a humoral factor, is unaffected by vagotomy, and appears to involve the sympathetic nervous system.

Histamine

Histamine plays a prominent role in parietal cell stimulation. Administration of H_2-receptor antagonists almost completely abolishes gastric acid secretion in response to both gastrin and acetylcholine.[5] These data suggest that histamine may be a necessary intermediary of gastrin- and acetylcholine-stimulated acid secretion. Histamine is stored in the acidic granules of ECL cells as well as in resident mast cells. Its release is stimulated by gastrin, acetylcholine, and epinephrine following receptor-ligand interactions on ECL cells. In contrast, somatostatin inhibits gastrin-stimulated histamine release through interactions with somatostatin receptors located on the ECL cell. Thus, the ECL cell plays an essential role in parietal cell activation that possesses both stimulatory and inhibitory feedback pathways that modulate the release of histamine and therefore acid secretion.

Gastric Acid Secretion

Gastric acid secretion by the parietal cell is regulated by three local stimuli: acetylcholine, gastrin, and histamine. These three stimuli account for basal and stimulated gastric acid secretion. Acetylcholine is the principal neurotransmitter modulating acid secretion and is released from the vagus and parasympathetic ganglion cells. Vagal fibers innervate not only parietal cells but also G and ECL cells to modulate release of their peptides. Gastrin has hormonal effects on the parietal cell and stimulates histamine release. Histamine has paracrine-like effects on the parietal cell and, as shown in Figure 45-7, plays a central role

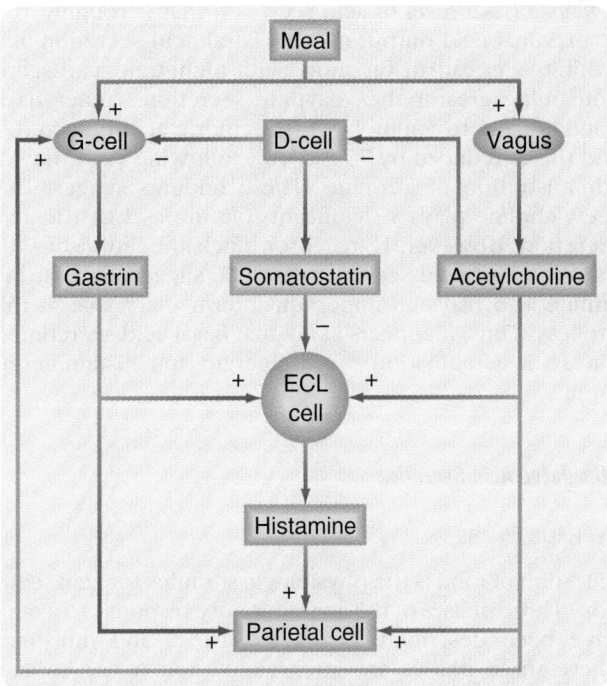

FIGURE 45-7.   The central role of the enterochromaffin-like (ECL) cell in regulation of acid secretion by the parietal cell is shown. As demonstrated, ingestion of a meal stimulates vagal fibers to release acetylcholine (cephalic phase). Binding of acetylcholine to M_3 receptors located on the ECL cell, parietal cell, and G cell results in the release of histamine, hydrochloric acid, and gastrin, respectively. Binding of acetylcholine to M_3 receptors on D cells results in the inhibition of somatostatin release. Following a meal, G cells are also stimulated to release gastrin, which interacts with receptors located on ECL cells and parietal cells to cause the release of histamines and hydrochloric acid (gastric phase). Release of somatostatin from D cells decreases histamine release and gastrin release from ECL cells and G cells, respectively. In addition, somatostatin inhibits parietal cell acid secretion (not shown). The principal stimulus for activation of D cells is antral luminal acidification (not shown). (From Zuidema G: Shackelford's Surgery of the Alimentary Tract, 4th ed. Philadelphia, WB Saunders, 1995.)

in the regulation of acid secretion by the parietal cell following its release from ECL cells. As depicted, somatostatin exerts inhibitory actions on gastric acid secretion. Release of somatostatin from antral D cells is stimulated in the presence of intraluminal acid (i.e., pH of ≤ 3). Following its release, somatostatin inhibits gastrin release through paracrine effects and also modifies histamine release from ECL cells.[11] In some patients with peptic ulcer disease, this negative feedback response is defective.[12] Consequently, the precise state of acid secretion by the parietal cell is dependent on the overall influence of the positive and negative stimuli.

Basal Acid Secretion

In the absence of food, the precise secretory status of the parietal cell varies among species. In humans, there is always a basal level of acid secretion that is roughly 10% of maximal acid output (MAO). Basal acid secretion also exhibits a circadian variation, with night-time acid secretion being greater than daytime secretion. Under basal conditions, 1 to 5 mmol of hydrochloric acid is secreted, and this is reduced by 75% to 90% following vagotomy or administration of atropine. These findings suggest that acetylcholine plays a significant role in basal gastric acid secretion. However, H_2-receptor blockade diminishes the magnitude of acid secretion by 90%, suggesting that histamine also plays an important intermediary role in this process. Thus, it appears likely that basal acid secretion is due to a combination of cholinergic and histaminergic input.

Stimulated Acid Secretion

CEPHALIC PHASE

Ingestion of food is the physiologic stimulus for acid secretion. Three phases of the acid secretory response to a meal have been described: cephalic, gastric, and intestinal. These three phases are inter-related and occur concurrently, not consecutively.

The cephalic phase originates with the sight, smell, thought, or taste of food, which stimulates neural centers in the cortex and hypothalamus. Although the exact mechanisms by which senses stimulate acid secretion remain to be fully elucidated, it is hypothesized that several sites are stimulated in the brain. These sensitive sites include, but are not limited to, the dorsal vagal complex, nucleus tract solitarius, and dorsal motor nucleus and may involve release of thyrotropin-releasing hormone.[13] These higher centers transmit signals to the stomach by the vagus nerves, which release acetylcholine that in turn activates muscarinic receptors located on target cells. Acetylcholine directly increases acid secretion by the parietal cell and can both inhibit and stimulate gastrin release, the net effect being a slight increase in gastrin levels.[14] Vagal stimulation by sham feeding (chew and spit) to humans increases acid secretion to roughly 50% of the maximal acid response to exogenous gastrin or histamine. Although the intensity of the acid secretory response in the cephalic phase surpasses that of the other phases, it accounts for only 20% to 30% of the total volume of gastric acid produced in response to a meal in humans because of the short duration of the cephalic phase.

GASTRIC PHASE

The gastric phase of acid secretion begins when food enters the gastric lumen. Digestion products of ingested food interact with microvilli of antral G cells to stimulate gastrin release. Protein components and amino acids are particularly effective at stimulating gastrin release, with the aromatic amino acids phenylalanine and tryptophan being the most potent. Food stimulates acid secretion by causing mechanical distention of the stomach. Gastric distention activates stretch receptors in the stomach to elicit the long vagovagal reflex arc. It is abolished by proximal gastric vagotomy and is, at least in part, independent of changes in serum gastrin levels. However, antral distention also causes gastrin release in humans, and this reflex has been called the *pyloro-oxyntic reflex*.[15] In humans, mechanical distention of the stomach accounts for about 30% to 40% of the maximal acid secretory response to a peptone meal, with the remainder due to gastrin release. The entire gastric phase accounts for most (60% to 70%) of meal-stimulated acid output, because it lasts until the stomach is empty.

INTESTINAL PHASE

The intestinal phase of gastric secretion remains poorly understood but appears to be initiated by entry of chyme into the small intestine. It occurs after gastric emptying and lasts as long as partially digested food components remain within the proximal small bowel.[16] It accounts for only 10% of the acid secretory response to a meal and does not appear to be mediated by serum gastrin levels. It is hypothesized that a distinct acid-stimulatory peptide hormone (entero-oxyntin), which is released from small bowel mucosa, may mediate the intestinal phase of acid secretion.

Cellular Basis of Acid Secretion

GASTRIN RECEPTORS

Gastrin initiates its biologic actions by activation of surface membrane receptors. These receptors are members of the classic G-protein–coupled 7-transmembrane-spanning receptor family and are classified as either type A or type B CCK receptors. The gastrin or CCK-B receptor has high affinity for both gastrin and CCK, whereas the type A CCK receptors have affinity for sulfated CCK analogues and a low affinity for gastrin.[6] Binding of gastrin to the CCK-B receptor is coupled to the calcium signaling pathway.[17]

MUSCARINIC RECEPTORS

Acetylcholine exerts its effect on the parietal cell through interactions with the M_3 subtype of the muscarinic receptor family. This receptor is coupled to increased levels of intracellular calcium, mediated by phospholipase-induced production of inositol trisphosphate.[17]

HISTAMINE RECEPTORS

Histamine receptors are members of the family of G-protein–coupled 7-transmembrane-spanning receptors. On the parietal cell, the H_2 subtype binds histamine to activate adenylate cyclase, which in turn leads to an increase in intracellular cyclic adenosine monophosphate (AMP) levels.

SOMATOSTATIN RECEPTORS

Somatostatin receptors are also 7-transmembrane-spanning receptors; there are at least five different types. Binding of somatostatin with its receptors is coupled to one or more inhibitory guanine nucleotide–binding proteins. The different somatostatin receptors also appear to have divergent pharmacologic effects, since one somatostatin receptor may associate with an inhibitory G protein whereas another may not.[8] Parietal cell somatostatin receptors appear to be a single subunit of glycoproteins, having a molecular weight of 99 kD with equal affinity for somatostatin 14 and somatostatin 28.[8] Somatostatin can inhibit parietal cell secretion via both G-protein–dependent and G-protein–independent mechanisms. However, the ability of somatostatin to exert its inhibitory actions on cellular function is primarily thought to be mediated via inhibition of adenylate cyclase with a resultant reduction in cyclic AMP levels.

SECOND MESSENGERS

The two second messengers principally involved in stimulation of acid secretion by parietal cells are intracellular cyclic AMP and calcium. Synthesis of these two messengers in turn activates a variety of protein kinases and phosphorylation cascades. Although these protein kinases become activated and phosphorylate a variety of parietal cell proteins, little is known about the precise phosphorylation pathways that result in activation of the proton pump that is ultimately responsible for acid secretion. Nevertheless, the intracellular events following ligand binding to receptors on the parietal cell are demonstrated in Figure 45-8. As depicted, histamine causes an increase in intracellular cyclic AMP, which activates protein kinases to initiate a cascade of phosphorylation events that culminate in activation of the H/K-adenosine triphosphatase (ATPase). In contrast, acetylcholine and gastrin stimulate phospholipase C, which converts membrane-bound phospholipids into inositol triphosphate (IP_3) to mobilize calcium from intracellular stores. Increased intracellular calcium activates other protein kinases that likewise ultimately activate the H/K-ATPase to initiate secretion of hydrochloric acid.

Activation and Secretion by the Parietal Cell

The H/K-ATPase is the final common pathway for gastric acid secretion by the parietal cell. It is composed of two subunits: an alpha catalytic (100-kD) subunit and a glycoprotein beta (60-kD) subunit. During the resting or nonsecreting state, gastric parietal cells store the H/K-ATPase within intracellular tubulovesicular elements. Cellular relocation of the proton-pump subunits through cytoskeletal rearrangements must occur for acid secretion to increase in response to stimulatory factors. The subsequent insertion and heterodimer assembly of the H/K-ATPase subunits into the microvilli of the secretory canaliculus causes an increase in gastric acid secretion.[17] A KCl efflux pathway must exist to supply potassium to the extracytoplasmic side of the pump. Cytosolic hydrogen is secreted by the H/K-ATPase in exchange for extracytoplasmic potassium (see Fig. 45-8) which is an electroneutral exchange and therefore does not contribute to the transmembrane potential difference across the parietal cell. Secretion of chloride is accomplished through a chloride channel, moving chloride from the parietal cell cytoplasm to the gastric lumen. The secre-

tion/exchange of hydrogen for potassium, however, does require energy in the form of ATP because hydrogen is being secreted against a gradient of more than 1 million-fold. Because of this large energy requirement, the parietal cell also has the largest mitochondrial content of any mammalian cell, with a mitochondrial compartment representing 34% of its cell volume. In response to a secretagogue, the parietal cell undergoes a conformational change and a several-fold increase in the canalicular surface area occurs (Fig. 45-9). In contrast to stimulated acid secretion, cessation of acid secretion requires endocytosis of the H/K-ATPase with regeneration of cytoplasmic tubulovesicles containing the subunits, and this occurs through a tyrosine-based signal.[18] The tyrosine-containing sequence is located on the cytoplasmic tail of the beta subunit and is highly homologous to the motif responsible for internalization of the transferrin receptor.

More than 1 billion parietal cells are found within the normal human stomach and are responsible for secreting about 20 mmol of hydrochloric acid per hour in response to a proton meal. Each individual parietal cell secretes 3.3 billion hydrogen ions per second, and there is a linear relationship between MAO and parietal cell number. However, gastric acid secretory rates may be altered in patients with upper gastrointestinal diseases. For example, gastric acid is often increased in patients with duodenal ulcer or gastrinoma, whereas it is decreased in patients with pernicious anemia, gastric atrophy, gastric ulcer, or gastric cancer. The lower secretory rates observed in gastric ulcer patients are typically for proximal gastric ulcers, whereas distal, antral, or prepyloric ulcers are associated with acid secretory rates similar to those obtained in duodenal ulcer patients.

Pharmacologic Regulation of Gastric Acid Secretion

Site-specific receptor antagonists for histamine, gastrin, and acetylcholine inhibit gastric acid secretion by competitive inhibition of the receptor. The best known site-specific antagonists are the group collectively known as the *H₂-receptor antagonists*. The most potent of the H₂-receptor antagonists is famotidine followed by ranitidine, nizatidine, and cimetidine. The half-life is 3 hours for famotidine and approximately 1.5 hours for the others. All undergo hepatic metabolism, are excreted by the kidney, and do not differ much in bioavailability. The newest class of antisecretory agents is the substituted benzimidazoles, of which omeprazole is a prime example. These agents inhibit acid secretion more completely because they irreversibly inhibit the proton pump. These proton-pump inhibitors are weak acids with a pKa of 4.0 and therefore become selectively localized in the secretory canaliculus of the parietal cell, which is the only structure in the body with a pH less than 4. Following oral administration, these agents are absorbed into the bloodstream as prodrugs and then selectively concentrate in the secretory canaliculus. At low pH, they become ionized and activated with formation of an active sulfur group. Because the proton pump is located on the luminal surface, the transmembrane pump proteins are also exposed to acid or low pH. The cysteine residues on the alpha subunit form a cova-

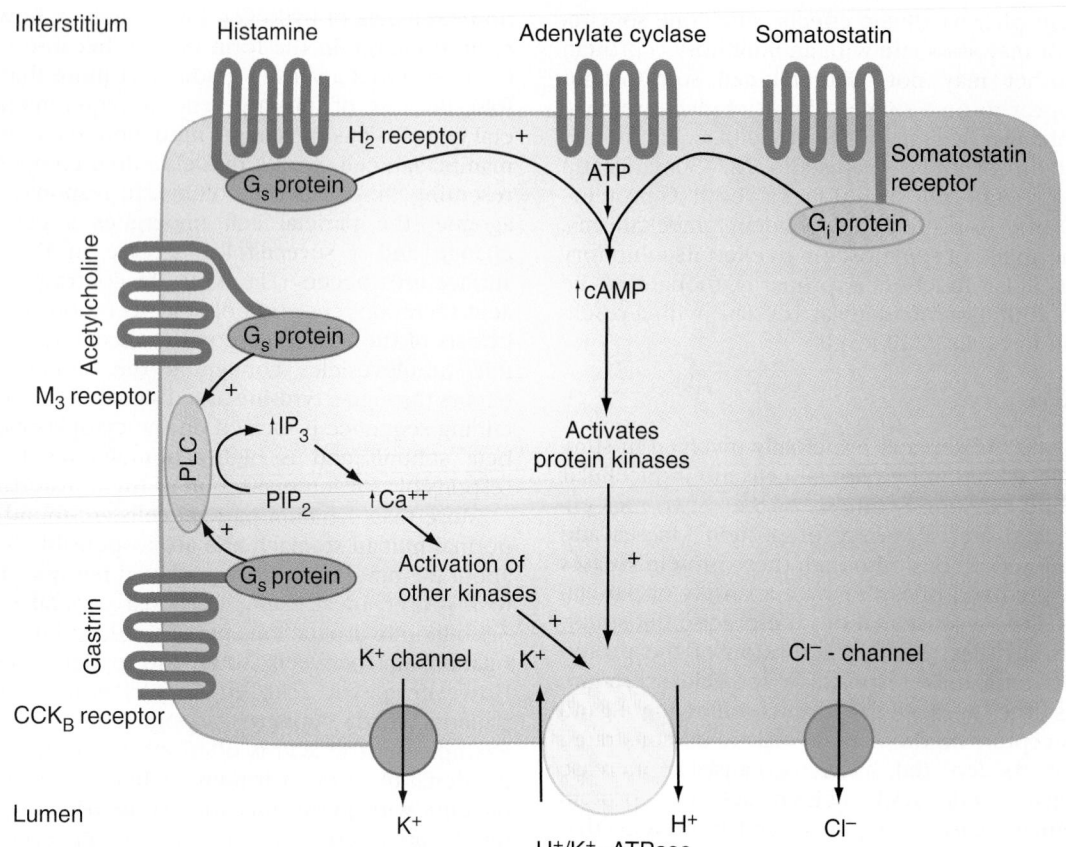

FIGURE 45-8. Intracellular signaling events within parietal cell are depicted. As shown, histamine binds to H₂ receptors, stimulating adenylate cyclase through a G-protein–linked mechanism. Adenylate cyclase activation causes an increase in intracellular cyclic AMP levels, which in turn activates protein kinases. Activated protein kinases stimulate a phosphorylation cascade with a resultant increase in levels of phosphoproteins that activate the proton pump. Activation of the proton pump leads to extrusion of cytosolic hydrogen in exchange for extracytoplasmic potassium. In addition, chloride is secreted through a chloride channel located on the luminal side of the membrane. Gastrin binds to type B cholecystokinin receptors and acetylcholine binds to M₃ receptors. Following the interaction of gastrin or acetylcholine with their receptors, phospholipase C is stimulated through a G-protein–linked mechanism to convert membrane-bound phospholipids into inositol triphosphate (IP₃). IP₃ stimulates the release of calcium from intracellular calcium stores, leading to an increase in intracellular calcium that in turn activates protein kinases, which activate the H/K-ATPase. ATP, adenosine triphosphate; ATPase, adenosine triphosphatase; cAMP, cyclic adenosine monophosphate; Gₛ protein, stimulatory guanine nucleotide protein; Gᵢ, inhibitory guanine nucleotide protein; PLC, phospholipase C; PIP₂, phosphatidylinositol 4,5 diphosphate. (From Zuidema G: Shackelford's Surgery of the Alimentary Tract, 4th ed. Philadelphia, WB Saunders, 1995.)

lent disulfate bond with activated benzimidazoles that irreversibly inhibits the proton pump. Because of the covalent nature of this bond, these proton-pump inhibitors have more prolonged inhibition of gastric acid secretion than H₂ blockers. For recovery of acid secretion to occur, new proton pumps need to be synthesized. As a result, these agents have a longer duration of action than the plasma half-life for these agents, with intragastric pH being maintained higher than 3 for 18 hours or more.

One notable side effect for the proton-pump inhibitors is that an elevation of serum gastrin levels occurs, an effect also found in response to the other antisecretory agents. However, 24-hour plasma gastrin levels are greater following proton-pump inhibitors than with H₂-receptor antagonists, and this effect is accompanied by hyperplasia of G cells and ECL cells when these agents are adminis-

tered chronically. Chronic administration of omeprazole was in fact found to cause ECL hyperplasia that could progress to carcinoid tumors in rats.[7] These tumors were more common in women than in men and occurred only when the rats were at the end of their natural life span. This sequence of events, however, was not specific for omeprazole and was reproduced by other agents that caused prolonged inhibition of acid secretion and resultant hypergastrinemia. The effects of these agents on gastric acidity are reversed following discontinuation of these agents and gastric acidity returns to normal levels.

Functions of Gastric Acid

Gastric acid plays a critical role in digestion of a meal. It is required to convert pepsinogen (see later) into pepsin,

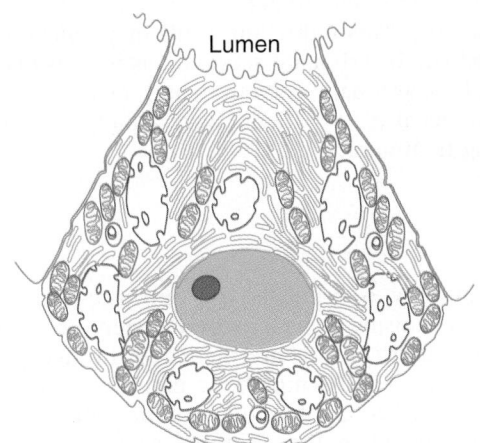

Lumen

Nonsecreting parietal cell

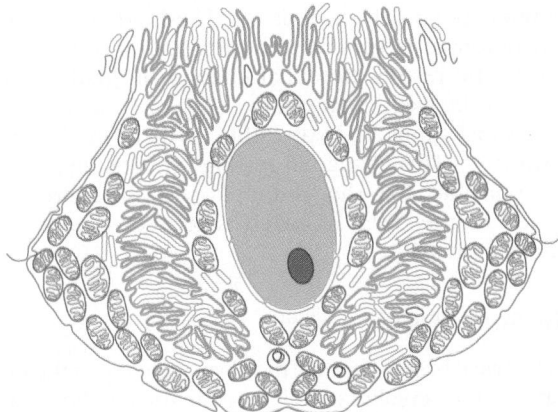

Acid-secreting parietal cell

FIGURE 45-9. Diagrammatic representation of resting and stimulated parietal cell. Note the morphologic transformation between the nonsecreting parietal cell and the stimulated parietal cell with increases in secretory canalicular membrane surface area. (From Mulholland MW: Anatomy and physiology. In Greenfield LJ, Mulholland MW [eds]: Surgery: Scientific Principles and Practice. Philadelphia, JB Lippincott, 1993.)

which is necessary for hydrolysis of proteins into polypeptides. Gastric acid also elicits the release of secretin from the duodenum, which results in pancreatic bicarbonate secretion. In addition, gastric acid functions to limit colonization of the upper gastrointestinal tract with bacteria. Colonization of the stomach and duodenum is known to occur in patients with achlorhydria or in patients receiving antisecretory agents. There is evidence for causation between gastric colonization and the subsequent development of nosocomial pneumonias in the intensive care unit (ICU).[19] Gastric luminal alkalinization attenuates the natural bactericidal effect of gastric acid, creating an environment conducive to bacterial overgrowth. It is noteworthy that the pathogens involved in nosocomial pneumonia, the principal infection of patients with multiple organ dysfunction syndrome in the ICU, are frequently found in gastric aspirates and appear to tem-

porarily colonize the stomach prior to the development of clinical pneumonia.[20] However, some studies challenge the importance of increased gastric colonization with bacterial pathogens on subsequent nosocomial pneumonia development.[21]

Gastric Analysis

There are numerous ways to assess acid secretion in the stomach. Aspiration of gastric contents via a nasogastric tube is probably the most accurate. The study requires complete emptying of gastric contents followed by instillation and recovery of 50 mL of saline. The stomach is then aspirated every 5 minutes for 1 hour and the aspirates pooled in 15-minute aliquots. At the end of 1 hour, the stomach is stimulated to secrete acid by intravenous administration of a secretagogue such as histamine (2 µg/kg) or pentagastrin (6 µg/kg). Aspiration of the stomach continues with four 15-minute collections obtained over a 1-hour period. The volume of collections is measured and each aliquot is titrated electrometrically to determine the amount of hydrogen ions present. The rate of secretion is expressed as the number of milliequivalents produced per hour during the basal or unstimulated state and during maximal and peak acid output. MAO is obtained by averaging the output of the two final 15-minute periods. Peak acid output is the highest rate of secretion obtained during a 15-minute period following secretagogue stimulation. Basal acid output (BAO) is generally around 2 to 3 mEq/hour and MAO is in the range of 10 to 15 mEq/hour.

Other Gastric Secretory Products

GASTRIC JUICE

Gastric juice is the result of secretion by the parietal cells, chief cells, and mucus cells, in addition to swallowed saliva and duodenal refluxate. The electrolyte composition of parietal and nonparietal gastric secretion varies with the rate of gastric secretion. Parietal cells secrete an electrolyte solution that is isotonic with plasma and contains 160 mmol/L. The pH of this solution is 0.8. The lowest intraluminal pH commonly measured in the stomach is 2, due to dilution of the parietal cell secretion by other gastric secretions that also contain sodium, potassium, and bicarbonate.

INTRINSIC FACTOR

Intrinsic factor is a 60,000-dalton mucoprotein secreted by the parietal cell that is essential for the absorption of vitamin B_{12} in the terminal ileum. It is secreted in amounts that far exceed that which is necessary for vitamin B_{12} absorption. In general, its secretion parallels that of gastric acid secretion, yet the secretory response is not necessarily linked to acid secretion. For example, proton-pump inhibitors do not block intrinsic factor secretion in humans, nor do they alter absorption of labeled vitamin B_{12}.[22] Intrinsic factor deficiency can develop in the setting of pernicious anemia or in patients undergoing total gastrectomy and both groups of patients require vitamin B$_{12}$ supplementation.

PEPSINOGEN

Pepsinogens are proteolytic proenzymes with a molecular weight of 42 kD that are secreted by the glands of the gastroduodenal mucosa. Two types of pepsinogens are secreted. Group 1 pepsinogens are secreted by chief cells and by mucus neck cells located in the glands of the acid-secreting portion of the stomach. Group 2 pepsinogens are produced by surface epithelial cells throughout the acid-secreting portion of the stomach as well as the antrum and the proximal duodenum. Consequently, group 1 pepsinogens are secreted by the same glands that secrete acid, whereas group 2 pepsinogens are secreted by acid-secreting and gastrin-secreting mucosa. In the presence of acid, both forms of pepsinogen are converted to pepsin by removal of a short amino-terminal peptide. Pepsins become inactivated at a pH greater than 5, although group 2 pepsinogens are active over a wider range of pH values than the group 1 pepsinogens.[23] As a result, group 2 pepsinogens may be involved in peptic digestion in the setting of increased gastric pH, which commonly occurs in the setting of stress or in patients with gastric ulcer.

MUCUS AND BICARBONATE

Mucus and bicarbonate combine to neutralize gastric acid at the gastric mucosal surface. They are secreted by the surface mucus cells and by mucus neck cells located in the acid-secreting and antral portions of the stomach. Mucus is a viscoelastic gel that contains approximately 85% water and 15% glycoproteins. It provides a mechanical barrier to injury by contributing to the unstirred layer of water found at the luminal surface of the gastric mucosa. It also provides an impediment to ion movement from the lumen to the apical cell membrane and is relatively impermeable to pepsins. Mucus is in a constant state of flux because it is secreted continuously by mucosal cells on one hand and solubilized by luminal pepsin on the other. Mucus production is stimulated by vagal stimulation, cholinergic agonists, prostaglandins, and some bacterial toxins. In contrast, anticholinergic drugs and nonsteroidal anti-inflammatory drugs (NSAIDs) inhibit its secretion. *H. pylori,* on the other hand, secretes various proteases and lipases that break down mucin, which impairs the protective function of the mucus layer.[24]

In the acid-secreting portion of the stomach, bicarbonate secretion is an active process, whereas in the antrum, both active and passive secretion of bicarbonate occur. The magnitude of bicarbonate secretion, however, is considerably less than acid secretion. Yet, although the luminal pH is 2, the pH observed at the surface epithelial cell is usually 7.[25] The pH gradient found at the epithelial surface is due to the aforementioned unstirred layer of water contained within the mucus gel and to the continuous secretion of bicarbonate by the surface epithelial cells. In fact, gastric cell surface pH remains greater than 5 until the luminal pH is less than 1.4. However, the luminal pH in duodenal ulcer patients is frequently less than 1.4, so the cell surface is exposed to lower pH in these patients. This reduction in pH may reflect a reduction in gastric bicarbonate secretion as well as decreased duodenal bicarbonate secretion and may explain why some duodenal ulcer patients have a higher relapse rate following treatment.[26]

Motility

Gastric motility is regulated by extrinsic and intrinsic neural mechanisms as well as by myogenic control. The extrinsic neural controls are mediated through parasympathetic (vagus) and sympathetic pathways, whereas the intrinsic controls involve the enteric nervous system already discussed in the Anatomy section. In contrast, myogenic control resides within the excitatory membranes of the gastric smooth muscle cells. When the cell membrane potential exceeds its threshold potential, an action potential is generated and results in muscle contraction. The resting potential changes in gradient from −48 mV in the gastric pacemaker cells of Cajal, located in the proximal stomach, to a resting gradient of −75 mV in the pylorus.[27] This change in resting potential may in part be responsible for the reduced rate of contractions observed in the distal stomach when compared to the proximal stomach.

Fasting Gastric Motility

The electrical basis of gastric motility begins with the depolarization of pacemaker cells located in the mid-body of the stomach along the greater curvature. Once initiated, slow waves travel at 3 cycles/minute in a circumferential and antegrade fashion toward the pylorus.[28] In addition to these slow waves, gastric smooth muscle cells are capable of producing action potentials, which are associated with larger changes in membrane potential than slow waves. In comparison to slow waves, which are not associated with gastric contractions, action potentials are associated with actual muscle contractions. During fasting, the stomach goes through a cyclical pattern of electrical activity composed of slow waves and electrical spikes, which has been termed the *myoelectric migrating complex* (MMC). Each cycle of MMC lasts 90 to 120 minutes and is made up of four phases of electrical activity.[29] *Phase I* of the MMC is the quiescent phase, where slow waves are present without action potentials, therefore resulting in an increase in gastric tone but no gastric contraction. In *phase II* of the MMC, the motor spikes are associated with slow waves and occasional gastric contractions. During *phase III*, motor spike activity is associated with each slow wave, resulting in forceful gastric contractions every 15 to 20 seconds. The net effect of phase III MMC activity is clearance of large undigestible food substances contained within the stomach. *Phase IV* activity is characterized as a brief period of recovery prior to the next MMC cycle. The net effects of the MMC are frequent clearance of gastric contents during periods of fasting. The exact regulatory mechanisms of MMC activities are unknown, but these activities remain intact following vagal denervation.

Postprandial Gastric Motility

Ingestion of a meal results in a decrease in the resting tone of the proximal stomach and fundus, referred to as *receptive relaxation* and *gastric accommodation*. Because these reflexes are mediated by the vagus nerves, interruption of vagal innervation to the proximal stomach, such as by truncal vagotomy or proximal gastric vagotomy, can eliminate these reflexes with resultant early satiety and rapid emptying of ingested liquids.[30] In addition to its storage function, the stomach is responsible for the mixing and grinding of ingested solid food particles. This activity involves repetitive forceful contractions of the mid-portion and antral portions of the stomach, causing food particles to be propelled against a closed pylorus with subsequent retropulsion of solids and liquids. The net effect is a thorough mixing of solids and liquids and sequential shearing of solid food particles to less than 1 mm in size.

The emptying of gastric contents is under the influence of well-coordinated neural and hormonal mediators. Systemic factors such as anxiety, fear, depression, and exercise can affect the rate of gastric motility and emptying. Additionally, the chemical and mechanical properties, and temperature of the intraluminal contents can influence the rate of gastric emptying. In general, liquids empty more rapidly than solids, and carbohydrates empty more readily than fats. Increases in the concentration and/or acidity of liquid meals cause a delay in gastric emptying. In addition, hot and cold liquids tend to empty at a slower rate than ambient temperature fluids. These responses to luminal stimuli are regulated by the enteric nervous system. Osmoreceptors and pH-sensitive receptors in the proximal small bowel have also been shown to be involved in the activation of feedback inhibition of gastric emptying. Inhibitory peptides, proposed to be active in this setting, include CCK, glucagon, vasoactive intestinal peptide, and gastric inhibitory polypeptide.

Abnormal Gastric Motility

Symptoms of abnormal gastric motility are nausea, fullness, early satiety, abdominal pain, and discomfort. Although mechanical obstruction can and should be ruled out with upper endoscopy and/or radiographic contrast studies, objective evaluation of a patient with a suspected motility disorder can be accomplished with gamma scintigraphy, real-time ultrasound, and magnetic resonance imaging. Gastric motility disorders that are most commonly encountered in clinical practice are gastric dysmotility following vagotomy, delayed gastric emptying associated with diabetes mellitus, and gastric motility dysfunction related to *H. pylori* infection. Vagotomy results in loss of receptive relaxation and gastric accommodation in response to meal ingestion with resultant early satiety, postprandial bloating, accelerated emptying of liquids, and a delay in emptying of solids. Clinical manifestations of diabetic gastropathy, which can occur in insulin-dependent or -independent patients, closely resemble the clinical picture of postvagotomy gastroparesis. Furthermore, structural changes have been identified in the vagus

nerves of patients with diabetes, suggesting that a diabetic autonomic neuropathy may be responsible. However, the metabolic effects of diabetes have also been implicated. Specifically, hyperglycemia has been shown to cause a decrease in contractility of the gastric antrum, an increase in pyloric contractility, and a suppression of phase III activity of the MMC.[31] Suppression of phase III MMC activity is thought to be responsible for the accumulation of gastric bezoars seen in some diabetic patients. In contrast, hyperinsulinemia, which is often associated with non-insulin-dependent diabetics, may play a role in the gastroparesis seen in non-insulin-dependent diabetics since it also leads to suppression of phase III MMC activity.[32]

H. pylori–infected patients with nonulcer dyspepsia have also been demonstrated to have impaired gastric emptying that is accompanied by a reduction in gastric compliance.[33] In rats, lipopolysaccharide derived from *H. pylori* causes a reduction in gastric emptying of a liquid meal for up to 12 hours by an unknown mechanism. Regardless of the etiology of gastroparesis, treatment consists of prokinetic agents, such as metoclopramide and erythromycin, that have been shown to have some benefit, although the evidence is more compelling in diabetic patients.[34]

Gastric-Emptying Studies

There are a number of ways to assess gastric emptying. The saline load test is perhaps the simplest and is accomplished by instilling a known volume of saline into the stomach and aspirating the amount remaining at a certain time. For example, some recommend instillation of 750 mL and then aspirating at 30 minutes. If the return is less than 200 mL, this indicates normal gastric function. In contrast, gastric dysfunction is usually present if there is more than 400 mL of saline present at the end of 30 minutes. Alternatively, fluoroscopic procedures can also provide information on gastric emptying and may reveal mechanical causes that could contribute to a delay such as gastric outlet obstruction. However, the computed radionucleotide scans are more commonly used to assess gastric emptying. This can be done with radiolabeled liquids or with a radiolabeled solid meal. Once a mechanical obstruction has been ruled out, gastric-emptying studies utilizing these radionucleotide scans can be particularly helpful in patients with gastric atony from associated illness such as diabetes or in postgastrectomy patients.

Gastric Barrier Function

Gastric barrier function depends on a number of physiologic and anatomic factors. These include but are not limited to cell membranes, tight junctions, cell renewal processes, mucus secretion, alkaline secretion, and arterial pH. Blood flow also plays a role in gastric mucosal defense by providing nutrients and delivering oxygen to ensure that those intracellular processes that underlie mucosal resistance to injury can proceed unabated. Decreased gastric mucosal blood flow has minimal effects on lesion production until it approaches 50% of normal. When blood flow is reduced by more than 75%, marked mucosal injury results, and this is exacerbated in the presence of a luminal acid. Once damage does occur, injured surface epithelial cells are replaced rapidly by migration of surface mucus cells located along the basement membranes. This process is referred to as *restitution* or *reconstitution*.[35] It occurs within minutes and does not require cell division.

Exposure of the stomach to noxious agents causes a reduction in the potential difference across the gastric mucosa. In normal gastric mucosa, the potential difference across the mucosa is –30 to –50 mV and results from the active transport of chloride into the lumen and sodium into the blood whose gradients are maintained by the activity of the Na/K-ATPase.[36] Damage disrupts the tight junctions between mucosal cells causing the epithelium to become leaky to ions (i.e., Na^+ and Cl^-) and a resultant loss of the high transepithelial electrical resistance normally found in gastric mucosa. In addition, damaging agents like NSAIDs or aspirin possess carboxyl groups that are nonionized at low intragastric pH because they are weak acids. Consequently, they readily enter the cell membranes of gastric mucosal cells because they are now lipid soluble, whereas they will not penetrate the cell membranes at neutral pH because they are ionized. On entry into the neutral pH environment found within the cystosol, they become reionized, will not exit the cell membrane, and are toxic to the mucosal cells.

Peptic ulcers are caused by increased aggressive factors and/or decreased defense factors.[37] This, in turn, leads to mucosal damage and subsequent ulceration. Protective or (defensive) factors include mucosal bicarbonate secretion, mucus production, blood flow, growth factors, cell renewal, and endogenous prostaglandins. Damaging or (aggressive) factors include hydrochloric acid secretion, pepsins, ethanol ingestion, smoking, duodenal reflux of bile, ischemia, NSAIDs, hypoxia, and, most notably, *H. pylori*.

PEPTIC ULCER DISEASE

Epidemiology

Peptic ulcer disease remains one of the most prevalent and costly gastrointestinal diseases. The annual incidence of active ulcer (gastric ulcer and duodenal ulcer) in the United States is about 1.8% or roughly 500,000 new cases per year. In addition, there are approximately 4 million ulcer recurrences yearly.[38] Because peptic ulcer disease is a chronic and recurrent disease, the prevalence is always considerably higher than the incidence of new cases. During the past couple of decades, elective admissions have decreased dramatically while admissions for complications related to ulcer disease have shown little change.[39] It is estimated that 3 million to 4 million patients are seen by a physician each year for diagnosis and treatment of peptic ulcer disease, and an additional 3 to 4 million patients are self-medicating. Moreover, it is estimated that

more than 130,000 operations for peptic ulcer disease are performed yearly, and approximately 9000 patients die from complications of their peptic ulcer disease yearly. Hospitalization rates have decreased for duodenal ulcer but have remained stable for gastric ulcer.[38,40] Although the decreasing hospitalization rate for duodenal ulcer may represent a true decrease in incidence, it is more likely a change in hospitalization patterns, with a lower rate of elective hospitalizations. In contrast, gastric ulcer is also more likely to occur in elderly patients, and admissions for bleeding gastric ulcers have increased over the last several years.[38,41] The increase in gastric ulcer complicated by hemorrhage is also associated with an increase in NSAID ingestion. Peptic ulcer disease in the United States has decreased in men and increased in women.[38] Although the reason for the decrease in men is unknown, it may reflect the decrease in smoking among men over the last 2 decades. It is speculated that the increase in women with peptic ulcer disease is in part due to an increase in smoking and an increase in NSAID ingestion.

H. pylori may represent the most drastic change in our understanding of peptic ulcer disease and has led many experts to conclude that peptic ulcer disease is in reality an infectious disease. Human gastric bacteria were first discovered in the early 1900s. In the 1920s, urease was erroneously thought to be produced by humans and to be protective. Thirty years later, in the 1950s, these previously observed bacteria were dismissed as contaminants. However, in the 1970s, gastric bacteria were rediscovered and found to be associated with inflammation. Twelve years later, the first successful culture of the organism was accomplished by Marshall and Warren, who named it *Campylobacter pyloridis*. Then, in 1987, it was reported that eradication of the organism reduced duodenal ulcer recurrence. Following reclassification of the organism to *H. pylori* in 1989, the National Institutes of Health (NIH) convened a consensus panel that issued guidelines for management of ulcer disease, taking *H. pylori* into account. Consequently, any treatment plan for peptic ulcer disease, both medical and surgical, requires that *H. pylori* be taken into account. The association between *H. pylori* and peptic ulcer disease is discussed in more detail in the section on pathophysiology.

Despite advances in medical therapy to inhibit acid secretion and to eradicate *H. pylori*, surgery remains important in managing these patients. Over the last 2 decades, there has been an increase in emergency operations performed for complications of peptic ulcers while the number of operations for elective indications has decreased markedly. Moreover, there is a high recurrence rate for peptic ulcerations following discontinuation of medical therapy. Thus, there is a renewed interest in operative management of patients suffering from peptic ulcer disease. Although the indications for surgery have not changed dramatically over the last several decades (i.e., bleeding, perforation, obstruction), the type of operation performed has changed in the *H. pylori* era.[42-44] The earliest surgical procedures usually employed subtotal gastrectomy, with removal of the parietal cell secreting mass as the role of the vagus nerve in secretory stimulation was not completely understood. Later, based on important contributions from Dr. Lester Dragsteadt regarding the functional significance of vagal innervation in acid secretion, vagotomy, and its use in the treatment of peptic ulcer disease evolved. Then, in the late 1960s, proximal gastric vagotomy came into favor as the role of the vagus in modulating gastric emptying became better understood. As a result, proximal vagotomy became the procedure of choice in elective surgery for peptic disease, and this procedure became even more attractive when it was discovered that it could be performed laparoscopically. However, recent studies indicate that vagotomy may not even be necessary in some situations such as perforation of the duodenum, provided that *H. pylori* is eradicated.[44]

Location and Type of Ulcer

Peptic ulcer disease can be divided into gastric and duodenal ulcers. Both types tend to occur near mucosal junctions. For example, duodenal ulcers usually occur at the duodenal pyloric junction, whereas gastric ulcers tend to occur at the oxyntic-antral junction, the antral-pyloric junction, or the esophagogastric junction. An ulcer by definition extends through the muscularis mucosa in contrast to an erosion, which is superficial to the muscularis mucosa. Duodenal ulcer disease is a disease of multiple etiologies.[37] The only absolute requirements are secretion of acid and pepsin in conjunction with either *H. pylori* infection or ingestion of NSAIDs. In comparison, gastric ulcer may present in four forms. Type 1 gastric ulcers are most common, accounting for about 60% to 70% of the total. Typically, they are located on the lesser curvature at or proximal to the incisura, near the junction of the oxyntic and antral mucosa. Most are associated with diffuse antral gastritis or multifocal atrophic gastritis. Type 2 gastric ulcers (~15%) occur in the same location as the type 1 lesion but are associated with either active or chronic duodenal ulcer disease. Type 3 gastric ulcers (20%) are typically located within 2 cm of the pylorus (pyloric channel ulcer). The fourth type of gastric ulcer is located in the proximal stomach or in the gastric cardia and is rare in the United States and Europe but common in Latin America. Types 2 and 3 gastric ulcers appear to behave more like duodenal ulcers and are associated with excess acid, whereas types 1 and 4 gastric ulcers are not. Moreover, gastric cancers may ulcerate and resemble gastric ulcers. Furthermore, ulcers may be caused by nonacid or other peptic disorders such as Crohn's disease, pancreatic rests, syphilis, *Candida* infection, or malignant diseases such as Kaposi's sarcoma, lymphoma, carcinoma, or pancreatic carcinoma.

Pathogenesis

Helicobacter pylori *Infection*

It is now believed that 90% of duodenal ulcers and roughly 75% of gastric ulcers are associated with *H. pylori* infection. If this organism is eradicated as part of ulcer treatment, ulcer recurrence is extremely rare. Warren and Marshall were the first to identify and isolate the organism.[45] They were also the first to note its close relationship with the inflammatory gastritis that occurred in the stomach. The organism was found to be a spiral or helical gram-negative rod with 4 to 6 flagella that resided in gastric-type epithelium within or beneath the mucus layer, which protected it from both acid and antibiotics. Its shape and flagella aided its movement through the mucus layer, and it was also found to produce a variety of enzymes that helped it adapt to a hostile environment. Most notably, it is one of the most potent producers of urease of any bacteria yet described. This enzyme is capable of splitting urea into ammonia and bicarbonate, creating an alkaline microenvironment in the setting of an acidic gastric milieu. However, the presence of urease also helps greatly in establishing a diagnosis of this organism through utilization of various laboratory tests. The organism is microaerophilic, and the optimal temperature for isolation is 35°C to 37°C, with growth occurring after 2 to 5 days. *H. pylori* can live only in gastric epithelium because only gastric epithelium expresses specific adherence receptors in vivo that can be recognized by the organism. Thus, it can also be found in heterotopic gastric mucosa in proximal esophagus, Barrett's esophagus, gastric metaplasia in the duodenum, Meckel's diverticulum, and heterotopic gastric mucosa in the rectum.

The mechanisms responsible for *H. pylori*–induced gastrointestinal injury remain to be fully elucidated. Three potential mechanisms for *H. pylori*–induced gastrointestinal injury have been proposed: (1) production of toxic products to cause local tissue injury; (2) induction of a local mucosal immune response; or (3) increased gastrin levels with a resultant increase in acid secretion. Some of the locally produced toxic mediators include breakdown products from urease activity (i.e., ammonia); cytotoxins; a mucinase that degrades mucus and glycoproteins; phospholipases that damage epithelial cells and mucus cells; and platelet-activating factor, which is known to cause mucosal injury and thrombosis in the microcirculation. In contrast, *H. pylori*–induced mucosal immune responses may also contribute to gastrointestinal injury. *H. pylori* is known to cause a local inflammatory reaction in the gastric mucosa and to produce chemotactic factors that attract neutrophils and monocytes. Activated monocytes and neutrophils in turn produce a number of proinflammatory cytokines and reactive oxygen metabolites. *H. pylori* appears to directly induce production of interleukin 8 by gastric epithelial cells, which is known to be proinflammatory. Subsequent stimulation of $CD4^+$ T cells also leads to the production of a variety of cytokines. These cells can further stimulate B cells to differentiate into specific antibody-producing cells, and IgM, IgG, and secretory IgA production follows. In addition, *H. pylori* causes a gastric mucosal neutrophil and mononuclear cell infiltration that leads to epithelial damage and lymphoid follicle formation, which is not normally present in the gastric mucosa.

The increased levels of serum gastrin associated with duodenal ulcer disease appear to be secondary to *H. pylori* infection. In patients with *H. pylori* infection, basal and stimulated gastrin levels are significantly increased. It appears that the mechanism for this increase is secondary to a reduction in antral D cells caused by infection with

H. pylori. The reduction in antral D cells leads to a reduction in somatostatin levels, which as previously discussed leads to an increase in serum gastrin levels due to disinhibition of the G cells with a resultant increase in serum gastrin and antral gastrin levels. Eradication of *H. pylori* leads to an increase in antral D cells and somatostatin with a consequent decrease in gastrin levels.[9] However, the association of acid secretion with *H. pylori* is not as straightforward. Although *H. pylori*–positive healthy volunteers have a small increase or no increase in acid secretion as compared to *H. pylori*–negative volunteers, *H. pylori*–infected patients with duodenal ulcers do have a marked increase in acid secretion.[46] In one study, basal plasma gastrin, BAO, and GRP-stimulated plasma gastrin and acid output were measured in volunteers and in patients with duodenal ulcers before and 1 month following completion of *H. pylori* therapy. In that study, acid secretion was significantly higher in *H. pylori*–positive patients with ulcers than in *H. pylori*–positive volunteers. Significant decreases were documented in all four measurements after cure of the infection.[47] In other words, both basal and GRP-stimulated gastrin and acid secretion returned to normal after *H. pylori* eradication. However, in another study examining the effects of *H. pylori* on MAO, it was found that compared with *H. pylori*–negative healthy volunteers, BAO was significantly higher in *H. pylori*–positive healthy volunteers ($P < 0.05$), *H. pylori*–positive patients with duodenal ulcer ($P < 0.0001$), and patients with duodenal ulcers 1 month posteradication ($P < 0.01$). *H. pylori* had the same significant effects on GRP-stimulated acid output in these patients. Gastrin 17 was also used to stimulate MAO in subjects from the various groups in whom maximal GRP-stimulated responses were observed. Duodenal ulcer patients were examined before and 1 year after *H. pylori* eradication. In this study, it was found that MAO, which is related to parietal cell mass, was higher in *H. pylori*–positive patients with duodenal ulcer than in healthy volunteers with and without *H. pylori* and was unchanged 1 year after *H. pylori* had been eradicated. This suggested that increased parietal cell mass was independent of, not related to, *H. pylori*.[48]

Peptic ulcers are also strongly associated with antral gastritis. A multitude of studies before the *H. pylori* era demonstrated that almost all peptic ulcer patients had histologic evidence of antral gastritis. McDonald, in 1973, found that the only patients with gastric ulcers and no gastritis were those ingesting aspirin.[49] It is now recognized that most cases of histologic gastritis are due to *H. pylori* infection. Even those patients with an NSAID-associated ulcer had evidence of a histologic antral gastritis in 25% of the patients as opposed to 95% in non-NSAID–associated ulcers. In most cases, the infection tends to be confined initially to the antrum and results in antral inflammation. Other evidence supporting a causal role for *H. pylori* in histologic gastritis comes from two separate volunteer physicians who ingested inocula of *H. pylori* after first confirming normal gross and microscopic gastric mucosa. Both men developed gastric *H. pylori* infection. Acute inflammation was observed histologically on days 5 and 10. By 2 weeks, it had been replaced by chronic inflammation with evidence of a mononuclear cell infiltration. These two reports provide documentation that *H. pylori* can cause histologic gastritis. Furthermore, eradication of *H. pylori* improves gastric histology. However, histologic gastritis does not necessarily equate with symptoms of dyspepsia.[50]

H. pylori represents a chronic infection found worldwide. Once a person is infected, usually in childhood, it is probably for life because spontaneous remission is rare. There tends to be an inverse relationship between infection and socioeconomic status. The reasons for this remain poorly understood but may be due to factors such as sanitary conditions, familial clustering, and crowding. In fact, one study documented familial clustering of *H. pylori* infection, demonstrating that *H. pylori* in one household member is associated with a greater chance of infection in other members.[51] In this study, other family members of a child with *H. pylori* infection had exceptionally high rates of seropositivity since more than 75% had evidence of infection. This would suggest a person-to-person transmission of *H. pylori* such as via the fecal-oral or oral-oral route, although acquisition of the infection from a common source is also possible. The same study found that children in North America are infrequently infected with *H. pylori* and that even adult patients have a low prevalence of *H. pylori* infection (24% in this study). In another study evaluating 150 African Americans and Hispanics between 19 and 49 years of age, the current *H. pylori* rate of infection was studied in relation to a variety of factors, including childhood crowding and socioeconomic status at 8 years of age and at the time of study. *H. pylori* infection was most common in the lowest socioeconomic class (85%), intermediate in the middle class (52%), and the lowest in the highest class (11%). The odds ratio for *H. pylori* infection comparing the highest childhood crowding index with the lowest crowding was 4.5 (95% confidence interval of 3.3 to 5.7) indicating a marked and significant effect of childhood crowding on *H. pylori* infection. Again, data such as these combined with the evidence of familial clustering of *H. pylori* infection provide strong evidence that the infection is transmitted by a person-to-person route and that the infection is commonly acquired early in life.[52]

Developing countries have a higher rate of *H. pylori* infection, and this is especially true in children. Multiple studies have demonstrated what appears to be a steady, linear increase in acquisition of *H. pylori* infection with age, especially in the United States and Northern European nations. In these countries, *H. pylori* infection is relatively uncommon in childhood and increases to approximately 40% to 50% after 50 years of age. It appears that childhood is the period of major risk for acquiring *H. pylori* infection in developed countries. In comparison, in developing countries with evidence of low socioeconomic status, crowding, or poor sanitary conditions, approximately 80% of people have *H. pylori* infection by the time they reach adulthood. *H. pylori* prevalence also varies with racial and ethnic groups, which is true even in the United States. Whites tend to have the lowest rates of infection, whereas in a study from Houston, African American rates of infection at each age approximately doubled that of whites.[53] This difference in prevalence among different racial/ethnic groups is probably related to lower socioeconomic status and to poorer living conditions during childhood in the nonwhite subjects.

H. pylori infection is associated with a number of common upper gastrointestinal disorders. In the United States, normal blood donors have an overall prevalence of about 20% to about 55% with variations by age and ethnicity of the population. *H. pylori* infection is virtually always present in the setting of active chronic gastritis and is present in the majority of duodenal (>90%) and gastric (60% to 90%) ulcer patients. Noninfected gastric ulcer patients tend to be NSAID users. There is a less strong association with nonulcer dyspepsia that is probably in the range of about 50%. In addition, a vast majority of gastric cancer patients show evidence of past *H. pylori* infection. However, although the association is strong, no causal relationship has been proven. There is also a strong association between mucosa-associated lymphoid tissue (MALT) lymphoma and *H. pylori* infection. Regression of these lymphomas has been demonstrated following eradication of the organism; therefore, *H. pylori* eradication should be attempted before chemotherapy. Again, *H. pylori* infection is present in almost all patients with duodenal ulcers and most patients with gastric ulcers. Furthermore, virtually all cases of ulcer disease without *H. pylori* infection are related to utilization of NSAIDs. Because NSAIDs cause gastric ulcers more frequently than duodenal ulcers, it may explain the greater frequency of *H. pylori*–negative gastric ulcers.

Limited data are available to estimate the lifetime risk of developing an ulcer in patients with *H. pylori* infection. However, a study by Cullen and associates was performed as a serologic study from Australia with a mean period of evaluation of 18 years. During this time frame, 15% of *H. pylori*–positive subjects developed verified duodenal ulcer as compared to 3% of seronegative individuals.[54] Another study by Sipponen and colleagues evaluated patients after 10 years in Scandinavia. This study was related to the presence or absence of histologic gastritis at the time of their initial assessments. Because *H. pylori* causes most cases of histologic gastritis, this observation was used as a marker for *H. pylori* infection. In this study, 11% of the patients with histologic gastritis developed peptic ulcer disease over a 10-year period as compared with only 1% of those without gastritis.[55] The incidence of ulcers in these two studies may have been underestimated because many patients with asymptomatic or minimally symptomatic ulcers may not have presented for medical evaluation. However, another factor implicating a causative role for *H. pylori* and ulcer formation is that eradication of *H. pylori* dramatically reduces ulcer recurrence. Although ulcers are easily cured using a variety of medications, they tend to recur if maintenance medical therapy or acid-lowering surgery is not used. Furthermore, even in the study of maintenance medical therapy, a significant number (25%) will have an ulcer recurrence. However, a large number of prospective trials now document that patients with *H. pylori* infection and ulcer disease who have documented eradication of the organism virtually never (<2%) develop recurrent ulcers. In those patients who do develop recurrent ulcers, they are usually associated with NSAID utilization.

NSAIDs

After *H. pylori* infection, ingestion of NSAIDs is the most common cause of peptic ulcer disease. As previously mentioned, hospitalizations for bleeding upper gastrointestinal lesions are increasing along with increased NSAID use. Most of the increased NSAID utilization has occurred in women older than 50 years of age, which is also the group with the increase in bleeding gastric ulcers.[56] The increased risk of bleeding has been documented in placebo-controlled trials with chronic aspirin utilization for prevention of recurrent heart attack or stroke.[57] Furthermore, the increased risk of bleeding and ulcerations is proportional to the daily dosage of NSAID. Consequently, the ingestion of NSAIDs remains an important factor in ulcer pathogenesis, especially in relationship to the development of complications and death.[58] The role of NSAIDs in peptic ulcer disease becomes even more meaningful if one considers the fact that roughly 3 million people in the United States take daily NSAIDs and about 1 in 10 patients taking daily NSAIDs have an acute ulcer. In addition, 2% to 4% of NSAID users have gastrointestinal complications each year, and more than 3000 deaths and more than 25,000 hospitalizations per year are attributable to NSAID-induced gastrointestinal complications. Moreover, when compared to the general population, NSAIDs increase the risk of gastrointestinal complications approximately 2- to 10-fold.

NSAID ingestion not only causes acute gastroduodenal injury but is also associated with chronic gastroduodenal injury.[58] This risk of mucosal injury and or ulceration is roughly proportional to the anti-inflammatory effect associated with each NSAID.[58] Although acute epigastric pain is common during the acute phase, it does not necessarily correlate with mucosal lesions. However, the presence of chronic epigastric pain is more suggestive of ulceration. The acute gastroduodenal lesions typically appear within 1 to 2 weeks of ingestion of the NSAIDs and range from mucosal hyperemia to superficial gastric erosions. In contrast, chronic injury typically occurs after 1 month and may be seen in the stomach as erosions or ulcerations in the gastric antrum or in the duodenum. Again, ulcer risk is dose related, and the acute mucosal response does not necessarily predict subsequent ulcer risk. In comparison to *H. pylori* ulcers, which are more frequently found in the duodenum, NSAID-induced ulcers are more frequently found in the stomach. *H. pylori* ulcers are also nearly always associated with chronic active gastritis, whereas gastritis is not frequently found with an NSAID-induced ulcer, occurring about 25% of the time. In addition, when NSAID use is discontinued, the ulcers usually do not recur, whereas with *H. pylori*–related ulcers, there is a 50% to 80% recurrence rate in 1 year unless the organism is eradicated with therapy.

Acid

There is a linear relationship between MAO and parietal cell number. However, gastric acid secretory rates are altered in patients with upper gastrointestinal diseases. Basal acid secretion is normally in the 1- to 8-mmol/hour rate, and the response to pentagastrin ranges from 6 to 40 mmol/hour. In diseases such as pernicious anemia, gastric atrophy, types 1 and 4 gastric ulcers, and gastric cancer, both basal and pentagastrin-stimulated acid output are decreased. In contrast, gastric secretory rates are increased in patients with duodenal ulcer and gastrinoma. In fact, an adequate level of acid secretion is a prerequisite for duodenal ulcers, and their presence is rare in patients who have an MAO of less than 12 to 15 mmol/hour. For types 1 and 4 gastric ulcers, which are not associated with excessive acid secretion, acid acts as an important cofactor, exacerbating the underlying ulcer damage and attenuating the ability of the stomach to heal. For patients with type 2 or 3 gastric ulcers, gastric acid hypersecretion does seem to be more common, and consequently they behave more like duodenal ulcers than the type 1 or 4 gastric ulcers.

Duodenal Ulcer Pathophysiology

Duodenal ulcer is a disease of multiple etiologies. The only relatively absolute requirements are acid and pepsin secretion in combination with either infection with *H. pylori* or ingestion of NSAIDs. Many secretory abnormalities are found in patients with duodenal ulcer disease, and clearly not every patient has the same secretory abnormalities (Box 45-1).[59] The more common secretory abnormalities relate to decreased bicarbonate secretion, increased nocturnal acid secretion, increased duodenal acid load, and increased daytime acid secretion. Less frequently found secretory abnormalities include increased pentagastrin-stimulated MAO, increased sensitivity to gastrin, increased basal levels of gastrin, increased gastric emptying, decreased inhibition of gastrin release, and increased postprandial gastrin release. As previously mentioned, there is a strong correlation between parietal cell number and MAO. Mean parietal cell number is increased in duodenal ulcer patients but not in gastric ulcer patients.[60] However, at least two thirds of duodenal ulcer patients and gastric ulcer patients fall within the normal range. Additionally, there is marked overlap in gastric acid secretion between duodenal ulcer patients and normal patients without ulcer disease. Although MAOs are greater in patients with duodenal ulcers than when compared with normal subjects, about 70% of duodenal ulcers still fall within the normal range. Because the overlap between duodenal ulcer patients and normal subjects is so great, acid secretory testing is of little value in establishing a diagnosis of duodenal ulcer. Nevertheless, subjects with maximal acid secretion of less than 10 mmol/hour are unlikely to develop or have duodenal ulcer disease.

Gastric Ulcer Pathophysiology

Gastric ulcers can occur anywhere in the stomach, although they usually present on the lesser curvature near the incisura angularis as shown in Figure 45-10. Approximately 60% of ulcers are located in this location and are classified as type 1 gastric ulcers. These ulcers generally are not associated with excessive acid secretion and may, in fact, have low-to-normal acid output. Most occur within 1.5 cm of the histologic transition zone between the fundic and antral mucosa and are not associated with duodenal, pyloric, or prepyloric mucosal abnormalities. In contrast, type 2 gastric ulcers are located in the body of the stomach in combination with a duodenal ulcer. These types of ulcers usually are associated with excess acid secretion. Type 3 gastric ulcers are prepyloric ulcers and account for about 20% of the lesions. These ulcers also behave like duodenal ulcers and are associated with hypersecretion of gastric acid. Type 4 gastric ulcers occur high on the lesser curvature near the GE junction. The incidence of type 4 gastric ulcers is less than 10%, and they are not associated with excessive acid secretion. Finally, some ulcers may appear on the greater curvature of the stomach, but the incidence is less than 5%.

Gastric ulcers rarely develop before 40 years of age, and the peak incidence occurs between 55 and 65 years of age. They are more likely to occur in lower than higher social economic classes and are slightly more common in the nonwhite than the white population. The exact pathogenesis of a benign gastric ulcer remains unknown. Some conditions that may predispose to gastric ulceration are age older than 40 years, sex (female:male, 2:1), ingestion of barrier-breaking drugs such as aspirin or NSAIDs, abnormalities in acid and pepsin secretion, gastric stasis through delayed gastric emptying, coexisting duodenal ulcer, duodenal gastric reflux of bile, gastritis, and infection with *H. pylori*. Some clinical conditions that may predispose to gastric ulceration include chronic alcohol intake, smoking, long-term corticosteroid therapy, infection, and intra-arterial therapy. With regard to acid and pepsin secretion, the presence of acid appears to be essential to the production of gastric ulcer; however, the total secretory output appears to be less important. Rapid healing follows acid reduction therapy, even when the lesion-bearing portion of the stomach is left intact because in the presence of gastric mucosal damage, acid is ulcerogenic even when present in normal or less than normal amounts.

Box 45-1. Frequency of secretory abnormalities in duodenal ulcer patients

Decreased duodenal bicarbonate secretion: 70%
Increased nocturnal acid secretion: 70%
Increased duodenal acid load: 65%
Increased daytime acid secretion: 50%
Increased pentagastrin-stimulated MAO: 40%
Increased sensitivity to gastrin: 35%
Increased basal gastrin: 35%
Increased gastric emptying: 30%
Decreased pH inhibition of gastrin release: 25%
Increased postprandial gastrin release: 25%

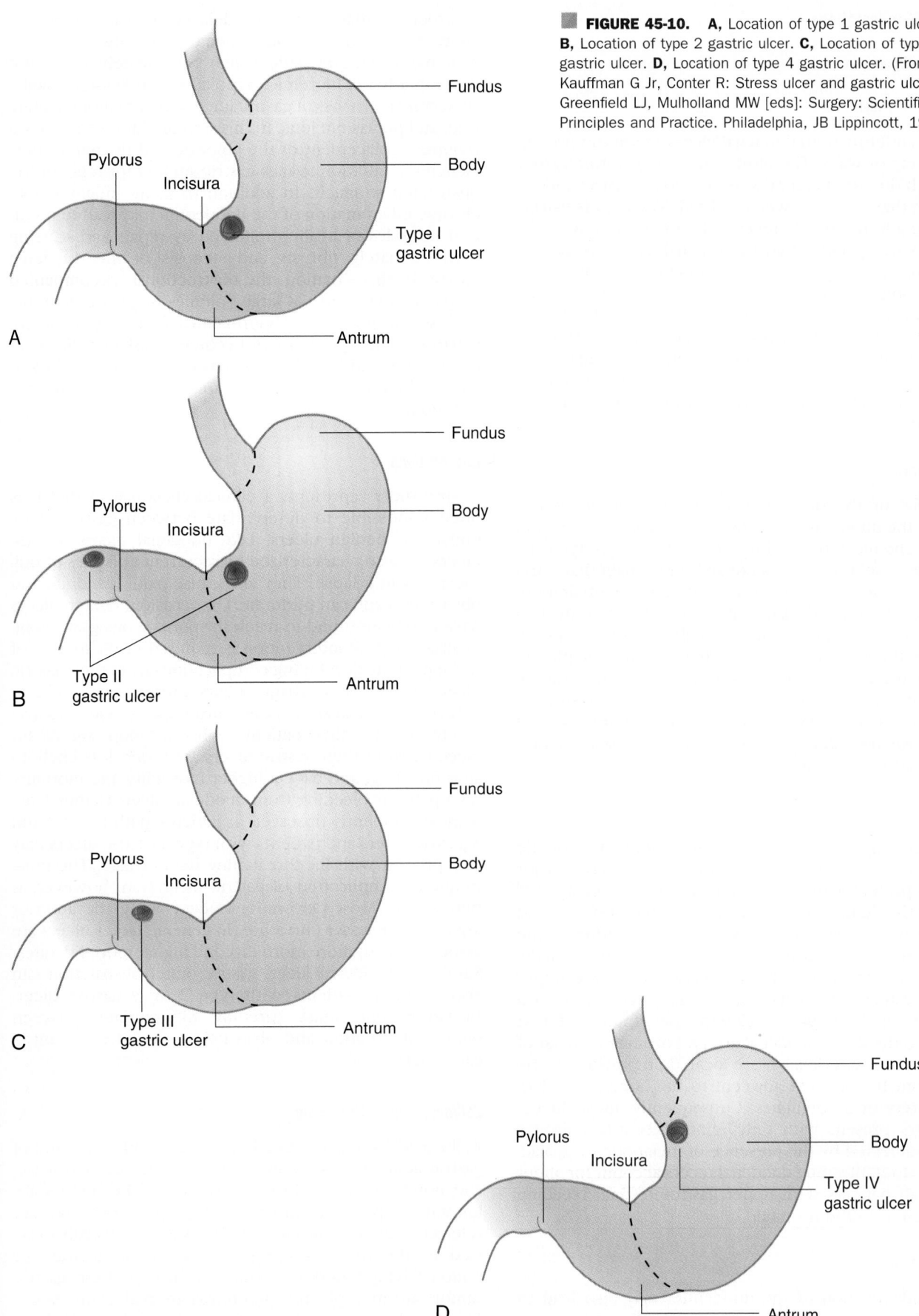

FIGURE 45-10. **A,** Location of type 1 gastric ulcer. **B,** Location of type 2 gastric ulcer. **C,** Location of type 3 gastric ulcer. **D,** Location of type 4 gastric ulcer. (From Kauffman G Jr, Conter R: Stress ulcer and gastric ulcer. In Greenfield LJ, Mulholland MW [eds]: Surgery: Scientific Principles and Practice. Philadelphia, JB Lippincott, 1993.)

Clinical Manifestations

Duodenal Ulcer

ABDOMINAL PAIN

Patients suffering from duodenal ulcer disease can present in a variety of ways. The most common symptom associated with duodenal ulcer disease is mid-epigastric abdominal pain that is usually well localized. The pain is usually tolerable and frequently relieved by food. Moreover, the pain may be episodic, may be seasonal in the spring and fall, or may relapse during periods of emotional stress. For these reasons and because it is relieved, many patients do not seek medical attention until they have had the disease for many years. When the pain becomes constant, this suggests that there is deeper penetration of the ulcer, and referral of pain to the back is usually a sign of penetration into the pancreas. Diffuse peritoneal irritation is usually a sign of free perforation.

PERFORATION

About 5% of the time, a penetrating ulcer penetrates through the duodenum into the free peritoneal cavity and elicit a chemical peritonitis. The patient can typically recall the exact time of onset of abdominal pain that is frequently accompanied by fever, tachycardia, dehydration, and ileus. Abdominal examination reveals exquisite tenderness, rigidity, and rebound. A hallmark of free perforation is the demonstration of free air underneath the diaphragm on an upright chest radiograph. This complication of duodenal ulcer disease represents a surgical emergency. Once the diagnosis is made, operation should be performed in an expeditious fashion following appropriate fluid resuscitation.

BLEEDING

The most common cause of death in patients with peptic ulcer disease is bleeding in patients who have major medical problems or are older than 65 years of age.[61,62] Because the duodenum has an abundant blood supply and the gastroduodenal artery lies directly posterior to the duodenum bulb, gastrointestinal bleeding from a duodenal ulcer is fairly common. Most cases of massive upper gastrointestinal hemorrhage are in fact secondary to a bleeding duodenal ulcer following penetration of that ulcer into the gastroduodenal artery. Fortunately, most of the ulcers are superficial or are located on portions of the duodenum that are not adjacent to the large gastroduodenal artery or its branches. Consequently, most duodenal ulcers present with only minor bleeding episodes that are detected by the presence of melanotic or guaiac-positive stool. Bleeding duodenal ulcers account for about 25% of all patients with upper gastrointestinal bleeding who present to the hospital.

OBSTRUCTION

Acute inflammation of the duodenum may also lead to mechanical obstruction with a functional gastric outlet obstruction manifested by delayed gastric emptying, anorexia, or nausea accompanied by vomiting. In cases of prolonged vomiting, patients may become dehydrated and develop a hypochloremic, hypokalemic metabolic alkalosis secondary to loss of gastric juice rich in hydrogen, chloride, and potassium ions. In this setting, fluid resuscitation requires replacement of the chloride and potassium deficiencies in addition to nasogastric suction for relief of the obstructed stomach. In addition to acute inflammation, chronic inflammation of the duodenum may lead to recurrent episodes of healing followed by repair and scarring with ultimately fibrosis and stenosis of the duodenal lumen. In this situation, the obstruction is accompanied by painless vomiting of large volumes of gastric contents with similar metabolic abnormalities as seen in the acute situation. The stomach can become massively dilated in this setting, and it rapidly loses its muscular tone. Marked weight loss and malnutrition are also common in this situation.

Gastric Ulcer

Gastric ulcer represents a clinical challenge in that it is often impossible to differentiate between gastric carcinoma and benign ulcers. Like duodenal ulcers, gastric ulcers are also characterized by recurrent episodes of quiescence and relapse. They also cause pain, bleeding, and obstruction and can perforate. On occasion, benign ulcers have also been found to result in spontaneous gastrocolic fistulas. Surgical intervention is required in 8% to 20% of those patients developing complications from their gastric ulcer disease. Hemorrhage occurs approximately 35% to 40% of the time at some point during the course of gastric ulceration. Usually, patients who develop significant bleeding from their gastric ulcers are older, less likely to stop bleeding, and have a higher morbidity and mortality than patients bleeding from duodenal ulcer. Hemorrhage is most frequently observed in patients with types 2 and 3 gastric ulcers and patients with type 4 gastric ulcers may also present with life-threatening hemorrhage. The most frequent complication of gastric ulceration, however, is perforation. Most perforations occur along the anterior aspect of the lesser curvature. In general, larger ulcers are associated with more morbidity and higher mortality rates. Similar to duodenal ulcer, gastric outlet obstruction can also occur in patients with type 2 or 3 gastric ulcer. However, one must carefully differentiate between benign obstruction and obstruction secondary to antral carcinoma.

Zollinger-Ellison Syndrome

Zollinger-Ellison syndrome is a clinical triad consisting of gastric acid hypersecretion, severe peptic ulcer disease, and non-beta islet cell of the pancreas. The tumors are known to produce gastrin (G-17 and G-34) and are referred to as *gastrinomas*. These tumors are usually localized to the head of the pancreas, duodenal wall, or regional lymph nodes. About one half of these gastric tumors are multiple and two thirds are malignant. About one fourth have multiple endocrine neoplasia (MEN) 1 syndrome, with tumors of the parathyroid, pituitary, and pancreatic islet cells being present. Pathophysiologic features of Zollinger-Ellison syndrome that distinguish it from duodenal ulcer are present and all are explained either by the actions of gastrin to stimulate gastric acid secretion and mucosal growth or by association with production of other hormones in MEN 1 syndrome. In general, Zollinger-Ellison syndrome is accompanied by diarrhea secondary to increased gastric acid secretion as well as weight loss and steatorrhea secondary to decreased duodenal/jejunal pH and inactivation of lipase. Large gastric folds are often found, and this is thought to be secondary to the tropic effects of gastrin. The large amounts of gastric acid secretion are also due to the excessive secretion of gastrin. In those patients with MEN 1, there is frequently a family history of endocrine tumors or hypercalcemia. In addition, intractable or postsurgical recurrences of ulcer disease are frequently encountered in patients with Zollinger-Ellison syndrome secondary to acid hypersecretion as a result of the gastrin-secreting tumor. Provocative tests are rarely needed for establishing the diagnosis of a gastrinoma because fasting and stimulated plasma gastrin levels are usually elevated and provide a sensitive and specific method to diagnosis Zollinger-Ellison syndrome. The secretin test is probably the most sensitive and specific provocative test and produces few adverse effects. Treatment of Zollinger-Ellison syndrome is based on clinical findings. If an isolated duodenal wall tumor is present on computed tomography (CT) and/or visceral angiography, surgical resection followed by measurement of gastric acid secretion is performed. If there is no evidence of tumor or evidence of metastatic tumor, proton-pump inhibitors or H_2-receptor antagonists to suppress fasting acid output to less than 10 mmol/hour is effective. However, drug efficacy needs to be checked regularly at 3-month intervals. Total gastrectomy is generally obsolete.

Diagnosis

History and physical examination are probably of limited value in distinguishing between gastric and duodenal ulceration. Routine laboratory studies include a complete blood count, liver chemistries, serum creatinine, and calcium levels. A serum gastrin level should also be obtained in patients with ulcers that are refractory to medical therapy or require surgery. An upright chest radiograph is usually performed when ruling out perforation. The two principal means of diagnosing peptic ulcers are upper gastrointestinal radiographs and fiberoptic endoscopy. Contrast radiography is less expensive and most (90%) can be diagnosed accurately. However, about 5% of ulcers that appear radiographically benign are malignant. *H. pylori* testing (see later) should also be done in all patients with suspected peptic ulcer disease.

Helicobacter pylori *Testing*

Diagnostic tests for *H. pylori* are divided between tests that do or do not require a sample of gastric mucosa. The noninvasive tests available are serology and the carbon-labeled urea breath test. The invasive tests available are the rapid urease test, histology, and culture. Noninvasive tests do not require endoscopy, whereas invasive tests do.

SEROLOGY

Because *H. pylori* infection elicits a local as well as a systemic IgG-mediated immune response, serology can be used to diagnose *H. pylori*. There are a variety of ELISA laboratory-based tests available as well as some rapid office-based immunoassays. Serology is the diagnostic test of choice when endoscopy is not indicated and has about 90% sensitivity and specificity associated with it. Serology testing, however, is not without its limitations as antibody titers can remain high for a year or more and consequently this test cannot be used to assess eradication following therapy. The current estimated cost for the office serology test is about $15.00 whereas the laboratory test is approximately $75.00.

UREA BREATH TEST

Another noninvasive test used for diagnosing *H. pylori* is the carbon-labeled urea breath test. This test is based on the ability of *H. pylori* to hydrolyze urea. Its sensitivity and specificity are both greater than 95%. The test is performed by having the patient ingest a carbon isotope–labeled urea using either C14 or C13. If C13 is used, mass spectrometry is required, whereas C14 does not but is associated with a low level of radiation exposure. Following ingestion of the carbon isotope, urea will be metabolized to ammonia and labeled bicarbonate if *H. pylori* infection is present. The labeled bicarbonate is excreted in the breath as labeled carbon dioxide, which is then quantified. The urea breath test is less expensive than endoscopy and samples the entire stomach. False-negative results can occur if the test is done too soon after treatment, so it is usually best to test 4 weeks after therapy is finished. The urea breath test currently costs about $200 and is the method of choice to document eradication.

RAPID UREASE ASSAY

The method of choice to diagnosis *H. pylori* if endoscopy is employed is the rapid urease test. This is another test based on the ability of *H. pylori* to hydrolyze urea. The enzyme urease catalyzes degradation of urea to ammonia and bicarbonate, creating an alkaline environment that can be detected by a pH indicator. Consequently, endoscopy is performed and gastric mucosal tissue biopsied. Mucosal biopsies are placed into a liquid or solid medium containing urea and a pH indicator. Sensitivity is approximately 90% and specificity is 98%, and the results are available within hours. It currently costs about $10, which is negligible with respect to the cost of endoscopy.

HISTOLOGY

Endoscopy can also be performed with biopsy samples of gastric mucosa followed by histologic visualization of *H. pylori*. Histologic visualization of *H. pylori* is still the gold standard of diagnostic tests. *H. pylori* is identified by its appearance and colonization sites with routine hematoxylin and eosin stains or with special stains such as silver, Giemsa, or Genta for improved visibility. Sensitivity is about 95% and specificity is 99%. This test is widely available and affords the clinician the ability to assess the severity of gastritis as well as to confirm the presence or absence of the organism. Histology costs approximately $150 to perform, plus the cost of endoscopy.

CULTURE

Culturing of gastric mucosa obtained at endoscopy can also be performed to diagnose *H. pylori*. The sensitivity is approximately 80% and specificity is 100%. However, it requires laboratory expertise, it is not widely available, it is relatively expensive ($150), and diagnosis requires up to 3 to 5 days. Nevertheless, it does provide the opportunity to perform antibiotic sensitivity testing on isolates should the need arise.

HELICOBACTER PYLORI TESTING SUMMARY

In summary, it is not necessary to perform endoscopy to diagnose *H. pylori*. Serology is the test of choice for initial diagnosis when endoscopy is not required. If, however, endoscopy is to be performed, the rapid urease assay or histology are both excellent options, but the cost advantage lies with the rapid urease assay. After treatment (only if necessary) the urea breath test is the method of choice but again should not be performed until 4 weeks after therapy ends. If the breath test is unavailable, endoscopy may be performed in selected patients such as those with bleeding ulcers or other complications of their peptic ulcer disease.

Upper Gastrointestinal Radiography

Diagnosis of peptic ulcer by upper gastrointestinal radiography requires the demonstration of barium within the ulcer crater, which is usually round or oval and that may or may not be surrounded by edema. This study is useful to determine the location and the depth of penetration of the ulcer as well as the extent of deformation from chronic fibrosis. A characteristic barium radiograph of a peptic ulcer is demonstrated in Figure 45-11. The ability to detect ulcers on radiography does require the technical skills and abilities of the radiologist but is also dependent on the size and location of the ulcer. With single-contrast radiographic techniques, as many as 50% of duodenal ulcers may be missed, whereas with double-contrast studies 80% to 90% of ulcer craters can be detected. The location of a gastric ulcer is of little predictive value in establishing malignancy as benign, and malignant ulcers can occur anywhere in the stomach. However, the size of the gastric ulcer may have some predictive value in that larger lesions are more likely to be malignant than smaller ones. In addition, the finding of an ulcer with an associated mass, interrupted, fused, or nodular mucosal folds approaching the margin of the crater, or an ulcer with irregular filling defects in the ulcer crater is suggestive of a malignancy.

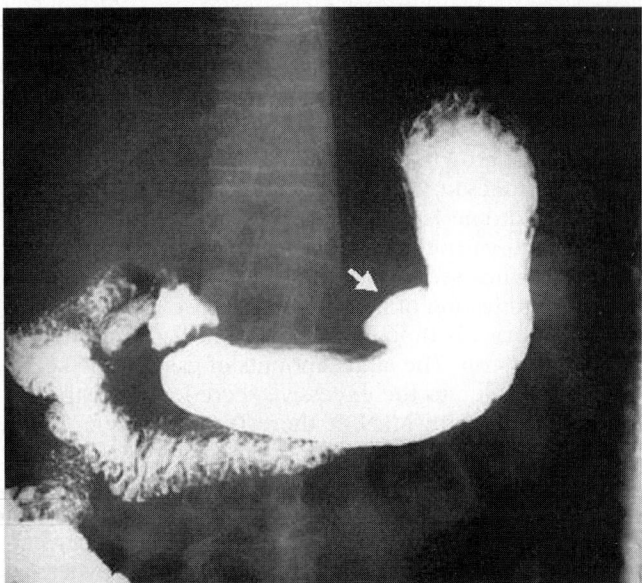

FIGURE 45-11.   There is a large benign-appearing gastric ulcer protruding medially from the lesser curvature of the stomach (arrow) just above the gastric incisura. (Courtesy of Agnes Guthrie, M.D., Department of Radiology, University of Texas Medical School–Houston.)

Fiberoptic Endoscopy

Endoscopy is the most reliable method of diagnosing a gastric ulcer, with an accuracy higher than 97%. In addition, if multiple biopsies and brushings for cytology are performed, the probability of diagnosing a malignancy is also in excess of 97%. In general, benign ulcers have smoother, more regular, rounded edges with a flat, smooth ulcer base. Malignancy is more often associated with a mass that may protrude into the lumen or have folds surrounding the ulcer crater that are nodular, clubbed, fused, or stop short of the ulcer margin. Again, however, multiple biopsy specimens are necessary for any of these ulcers because ruling out a malignancy is mandatory. Clinical symptoms or signs that may prompt early endoscopic evaluation include major weight loss, symptoms of gastric outlet obstruction, a palpable abdominal mass, guaiac-positive stool, or blood loss anemia. In addition to providing diagnostic abilities, endoscopy provides the ability to sample tissue for *H. pylori* testing and may also be used for therapeutic purposes in the setting of gastrointestinal bleeding (see treatment of bleeding later) or in the therapy of obstruction (see the following section).

Treatment

Medical Management

Drugs may heal ulcers by a variety of mechanisms. Some of the mechanisms by which medications may be used include eradication of *H. pylori* infection, neutralization of acid secretion, or by other mechanisms. Lifestyle modifications are also in order. Cigarette smoking has clearly been shown to retard ulcer healing and should be avoided. Discontinuation of aspirin or NSAIDs should also be undertaken if possible. If the patient is unable to discontinue NSAIDs, consideration should be given to utilization of some of the newer, more selective cyclooxygenase (COX)-2 inhibitors, which are associated with fewer gastrointestinal side effects. Because coffee strongly stimulates acid secretion and because alcohol may damage the mucosa, their ingestion should be moderate at most.

Most of the agents designed to treat ulcers medically are designed to either inhibit or neutralize acid secretion or are aimed at eradicating *H. pylori*. Parietal cell secretion is regulated by site-specific agonists and antagonists. Histamine, gastrin, and acetylcholine all stimulate parietal cell secretion through activation of receptors located on the basolateral membrane of the parietal cell. Prostaglandins inhibit acid secretion by interacting with another specific receptor. Histamine stimulates production of cyclic AMP and prostaglandins inhibit this stimulation. In contrast, gastrin and acetylcholine stimulate calcium and protein kinase C pathways. The H/K-ATPase is located on the apical surface of the parietal cell, and its function can be inhibited through administration of a proton-pump inhibitor. Acid secretion can be inhibited by blocking the histamine, gastrin, or acetylcholine receptors, by activation of the prostaglandin receptor, or by antagonizing the hydrogen-potassium pump.

ANTACIDS

Antacids are the oldest form of therapy for peptic ulcer disease. Antacids reduce gastric acidity by reacting with hydrochloric acid, forming a salt and water to inhibit peptic activity by raising pH. Antacids differ greatly in their buffering ability, absorption, taste, and side effects. They are most effective when ingested 1 hour after a meal. If taken on an empty stomach, the antacids are emptied rapidly and have only a transient buffering effect. However, if taken after meals, they are retained in the stomach and exert their buffering action for a longer period. The minimum dose of antacids required to produce optimal healing rates represents only a few tablets or liquid doses of antacids per day, usually in doses of 200 to 1000 mmol/day. This dosage level produces minimal side effects and results in approximately 80% ulcer healing at 1 month. The mechanism for ulcer healing at lower doses is not clear because gastric acidity is only neutralized for brief periods. Magnesium antacids tend to be the best buffers but can cause significant diarrhea by a cathartic action. In contrast, aluminum acids precipitate with phosphorous and can occasionally result in hypophosphatemia and sometimes constipation. Consequently, although antacids may heal duodenal ulcers with an efficacy comparable to that observed with H$_2$-receptor antagonists, many patients have found large, frequent doses to be unacceptable.

H$_2$-RECEPTOR ANTAGONISTS

The H$_2$-receptor antagonists are structurally similar to histamine. Variations in the ring structure and the side chains cause differences in potency and side effects. Currently available H$_2$-receptor antagonists differ in their potency but only modestly in half-life and bioavailability. All undergo hepatic metabolism and are excreted by the kidney. Famotidine is probably the most potent and cimetidine is the least potent. Continuous intravenous infusion of H$_2$-receptor antagonists has been shown to produce more uniform acid inhibition than intermittent administration. The fluctuating effects of intermittently administered H$_2$-receptor antagonists are probably caused by the relatively short half-life of these agents, which ranges from 1.5 to 3 hours. Many randomized, controlled trials indicate that all H$_2$-receptor antagonists result in duodenal ulcer healing rates from 70% to 80% after 4 weeks and from 80% to 90% after 8 weeks of therapy. Split-dose, evening, and night-time therapy all are effective, but again continuous intravenous infusion produces the most uniform acid inhibition.

PROTON-PUMP INHIBITORS

The most potent class of antisecretory agents is the class of inhibitors known as the proton-pump inhibitors, otherwise as the substituted benzimidazoles. These enzymes covalently bond to the catalytic subunit of the proton pump and, once bound, acid secretion can recommence only by synthesis of new proton pumps. Because the pump is the final step in acid secretion, proton-pump inhibitors negate all types of acid secretion from all types of secretagogues. Not surprisingly, proton-pump inhibitors provide more complete inhibition of acid secretion than the H$_2$-receptor antagonists. Inhibition of acid secretion is more prolonged than with H$_2$-receptor antagonists because of the irreversible inhibition of the enzyme caused by the covalent bond to the proton pump. In general, the action lasts for approximately 18 hours. Proton-pump inhibitors suppress not only basal acid secretion but also meal-stimulated gastric acid secretion and acid secretion in response to exogenously administered secretagogues. Both H$_2$-receptor antagonists and H/K-ATPase inhibitors are effective at night, but the H/K-ATPase inhibitor is more effective during the day.[63] Twenty-four-hour plasma gastrin levels are also greater following inhibition of acid secretion with proton-pump inhibitors than with H$_2$-receptor antagonists. Proton-pump inhibitors also produce more rapid healing of ulcers than standard H$_2$-receptor antagonists. In fact, data from eight trials revealed that a 20-mg dose of omeprazole had a 14% advantage at 2 weeks and a 9% advantage at 4 weeks when compared to a 300-mg dose of cimetidine. Proton-pump inhibitors have a healing rate of 85% at 4 weeks and 96% at 8 weeks. In addition, proton-pump inhibitors require an acidic environment within the gastric lumen to become activated and bind to the proton pump at the secretory canaliculus. Thus, utilization of antacids or H$_2$-receptor antagonists in combination with proton-pump inhibitors could have deleterious effects by promoting an alkaline environment and thereby preventing activation of the proton-pump inhibitor. Consequently, antacids and H$_2$-receptor antagonists should not be used in combination with proton-pump inhibitors.

SUCRALFATE

Sucralfate is structurally related to heparin but does not have any anticoagulant effects. It has been shown to be quite effective in the treatment of ulcer disease, although its exact mechanism of action is not entirely understood. It is an aluminum salt of sulfated sucrose that disassociates under the acidic conditions in the stomach. It is speculated that the sucrose polymerizes and binds to protein in the ulcer crater to produce a kind of protective coating that can last as long as 6 hours. It has also been suggested that it may bind and concentrate endogenous basic fibroblast growth factor, which appears to be important in mucosal healing. Duodenal ulcer healing after 4 to 6 weeks of treatment with sucralfate (1 g four times daily) is superior to placebo and comparable to H_2-receptor antagonists such as cimetidine. Similar healing rates have been reported with twice-daily dosing (2 g twice daily 30 minutes before breakfast and at bedtime).

TREATMENT OF HELICOBACTER PYLORI INFECTION

The clinician has three major goals when faced with a patient with ulcer disease: (1) symptoms need to be relieved; (2) the ulcer needs to be healed; and (3) recurrence must be prevented. Antisecretory agents with acid suppression have traditionally achieved the first two goals. With NSAID-related ulcers, discontinuation of NSAIDs achieves the third goal. However, in the setting of non-NSAID ulcers, which are usually secondary to *H. pylori*, eradication of *H. pylori* can also almost completely prevent recurrence of ulcers. For duodenal ulcers, the recurrence rate following successful healing is roughly 72% if no additional therapy is employed. If H_2-receptor antagonists are used as maintenance therapy, patients still have a 25% recurrence rate. However, if *H. pylori* is eradicated, only 2% of the patients have an ulcer recurrence. The gold standard in the past for eradicating *H. pylori* was triple therapy in combination with a bismuth-based therapy for 2 weeks. This regimen was considered more effective with tetracycline, with eradication rates up to 95%. A standard 2-week bismuth-based therapy comprised Pepto-Bismol (2 tablets four times daily) in combination with metronidazole (500 mg four times daily) and tetracycline (500 mg four times daily). For acute ulcers, H_2-receptor antagonists or proton-pump inhibitors were used for 2 additional weeks after completion of the standard bismuth-based therapy (i.e., 4 weeks total). However, various triple regimens for *H. pylori* eradication have emerged. Most of these employ a proton-pump inhibitor in combination with antibiotics such as metronidazole, chlorythromycin, or amoxicillin. These regimens are 1 to 2 weeks in duration, have the advantage of not containing bismuth, and are given only twice a day. Some of these triple regimens are currently available in a packet such as Helidac and are taken anywhere from 7 to 10 days to 2 weeks. Eradication rates for these new triple regimens range from 80% to 95%. For acute ulcers, all three drugs are given for 1 week, then 2 additional weeks with a proton-pump inhibitor alone or 4 to 6 weeks' treatment with a full-dose H_2-receptor antagonist.

In February 1994, the NIH convened a consensus conference on *H. pylori* in peptic ulcer disease. At this conference, the following recommendations were made. All patients with gastric or duodenal ulcers who were infected with *H. pylori*, regardless of whether first presentation or recurrence, should be treated. *H. pylori*–infected ulcer patients receiving maintenance treatment or with a history of complicated or refractory disease should also be treated. They added that there was no reason to consider routine detection or treatment in the absence of ulcers and concluded that NSAID use should not alter treatment. The NSAID should be discontinued if possible, but if *H. pylori* is present, *H. pylori* should be treated. For patients with complications such as bleeding or perforation, documentation of eradication was imperative. Again, this is most easily performed with a urea breath test. Although not recommended by the NIH, it is not inappropriate to treat *H. pylori*–positive patients with MALT lymphoma for the previously mentioned reasons. Nevertheless, some controversial treatment issues still exist. In nonulcer dyspepsia, the infected patient who insists on eradication of *H. pylori* needs to be advised of the benefits or lack of benefits *H. pylori* eradication might have because it is unlikely that eradication will improve symptoms and it is possible that it will contribute to the emergence of antibiotic resistance. The success of therapy for *H. pylori* depends on the correct use of the regimens. One cannot substitute ampicillin for amoxicillin and one cannot substitute doxycycline for tetracycline. Appropriate dosages need to be used, the recommended frequency of administration adhered to, and the duration of drug therapy enforced.

For treatment of active NSAID ulcers, it is best to discontinue the NSAID if at all possible while the ulcer is being treated. If not, an attempt should be made to switch to the selective COX-2 inhibitors. Testing should be performed for *H. pylori* and, if present, treatment administered. For patients with gastric ulcers, proton-pump inhibitors have been shown to be more effective that H_2-receptor antagonists in patients taking NSAIDs. Again, if patients cannot discontinue their NSAIDs, then switching to selective COX-2 inhibitors should be considered or, alternatively, cotherapy with misoprostol, a prostaglandin analogue, might be of benefit.

Approach to the Patient Bleeding from Peptic Ulcer Disease

Approximately 80% of upper gastrointestinal bleeds are self-limited. The overall mortality of 8% to 10% for those who continue to bleed or in whom bleeding recurs has not changed dramatically over the last several decades despite an older and probably sicker patient population. The initial step in management of patients with acute upper gastrointestinal hemorrhage is adequate initial and ongoing resuscitation. Following resuscitation, endoscopy is performed to assess the cause and severity of the bleed, which will dictate the required intensity of therapy and predict the risk of further bleeding and/or death. Several factors are associated with continued or recurrent bleeding and increase the risk of mortality. Most studies have demonstrated that mortality increases with age, such as the American Society for Gastrointestinal Endoscopy (ASGE) study that found a mortality of 8.7% for patients 60 years old or younger and 13.4% for those older than 60 years of age.[64] The severity of the initial bleed is also an adverse prognostic factor, and this might include the presence of shock, a high transfusion requirement, or bright red blood in the nasogastric tube or in the stool. Recurrent bleeding increased the mortality rate from 8% to 30% in one study and from 7% to 44% in another. The onset of bleeding in a hospital was also associated with a higher mortality rate (33%) compared to those who bled outside of the hospital or prior to admission (7%). In the ASGE study, eight disease categories were looked at to assess their contribution to the mortality rate in patients with upper gastrointestinal bleeding. These disease states included cardiac, central nervous system, gastrointestinal, hepatic, neoplastic, pulmonary, renal, and stress. In the absence of any concomitant disease, the mortality rate was 2.5%. However, if there were three concomitant diseases, the mortality rate rose to 14.6%. With six concomitant diseases, the mortality rate rose to 66.7%. Stigmata of recent hemorrhage from peptic ulcers also predict an adverse prognostic sign. These stigmata included a visible vessel on endoscopy, oozing of bright red blood, and fresh or old blood clot at the base of the ulcer. When a visible vessel was seen, it was associated with a 50% rebleeding rate, whereas other signs were associated with a lower rebleeding rate of about 8%. In the ASGE study, pumping or oozing lesions had a significantly greater mortality (16%) and need for surgery (24%) when compared to those with clot or no blood (mortality 6.7%, surgery 11%). In addition, patients undergoing emergency surgery had a 30% mortality rate compared to 10% for those undergoing elective surgery.[64] Mortality also rises with increased severity of bleeding, which correlates with transfusion requirement. If no units are transfused, the mortality rate is approximately 2%; for 1 to 3 units, approximately 5%; for 4 to 6 units, approximately 12%; for 7 to 9 units, approximately 15%; and when more than 10 units are used, the mortality rate rises to approximately 35%. A pumping or oozing lesion in the ASGE study was associated with a transfusion requirement greater than 5 units (37.6%), which was significantly different when compared to patients who had a clot or no blood on the lesion. In the latter group, only 20% required more than 5 units of blood. Pumping lesions were seen in only 5.5% of the cases in the ASGE study as compared to the 24.2% frequency of oozing lesions. The risk of rebleeding in a patient with no active bleeding and overlying clot varies from 8% to 30%. The visible vessel is regarded as the one stigma of recent hemorrhage that is associated with the highest incidence of rebleeding. In patients with a visible vessel, rebleeding has occurred in 56% of patients in one study compared to 8% of those with oozing and 0% of those with no stigmata of recent hemorrhage. Mortality was also limited to those patients with visible vessels.

Endoscopy remains the investigation of choice for patients with upper gastrointestinal bleeding from peptic ulcer disease. As previously mentioned, endoscopy provides the opportunity not only for diagnosis but also therapy. Hemostatic methods currently employed include thermotherapy (heater probe, multipolar or bipolar electrocoagulation), as well as injection of ethanol or epinephrine solutions. When the bleeding is controlled, long-term medical therapy includes antisecretory agents usually in the form of a proton-pump inhibitor plus testing for *H. pylori,* with treatment if positive. If *H. pylori* is present, documentation of eradication should be performed following therapy. If the bleeding continues or recurs, surgery may be indicated (discussed under Duodenal and Gastric Ulcer Disease individually).

Surgical Procedures for Peptic Ulcer Disease

The four classic indications for surgery on peptic ulcers are intractability, hemorrhage, perforation, and obstruction. Elective surgery for intractability is becoming rarer as medical therapy becomes more effective. The recognition of *H. pylori* and its eradication suggest that the intractability indication for surgery may apply only to patients in whom the organism cannot be eradicated or who cannot be taken off NSAIDs. In contrast to uncomplicated ulcers, the incidence of ulcers with complications requiring surgery does not seem to have diminished, and therefore familiarity with the various methods for treating bleeding, perforation, and obstruction is essential.

One goal of ulcer surgery is to prevent gastric acid secretion. As previously mentioned, subtotal gastrectomy was considered optimal management for duodenal and gastric ulcers until Dragstedt's description of vagotomy and its impact on ulcer healing and recurrence. As described later, there are three levels of vagotomy that can be performed, and these are shown in Figures 45-4 and 45-13. Vagotomy decreases peak acid output by approximately 50%, whereas vagotomy plus antrectomy, which removes the gastrin-secreting portion of the stomach, decreases peak acid output by approximately 85%.

TRUNCAL VAGOTOMY

As shown in Figure 45-4, truncal vagotomy is performed by division of the left and right vagus nerves above the hepatic and celiac branches just above the GE junction. Truncal vagotomy is probably the most common operation performed for duodenal ulcer disease. Most surgeons employ some form of drainage procedure in association with truncal vagotomy. The classic truncal vagotomy in combination with a Heineke-Mikulicz pyloroplasty is shown in Figure 45-12. When the duodenal bulb is scarred, a Finney pyloroplasty or Jaboulay gastroduodenostomy may be useful alternatives. In general, there is little difference in the side effects associated with the type of drainage procedure performed, although bile reflux may be more common after gastroenterostomy and diarrhea is more common after pyloroplasty. The incidence of dumping is about the same for both. From a technical standpoint, truncal vagotomy with pyloroplasty represents an uncomplicated procedure that can be performed quickly, making it especially attractive for patients who are hemodynamically unstable from bleeding ulcers.

HIGHLY SELECTIVE VAGOTOMY (PARIETAL CELL VAGOTOMY)

The highly selective vagotomy is also called the *parietal cell vagotomy* or the *proximal gastric vagotomy.* This procedure was developed after recognition that truncal vagotomy in combination with a drainage procedure or

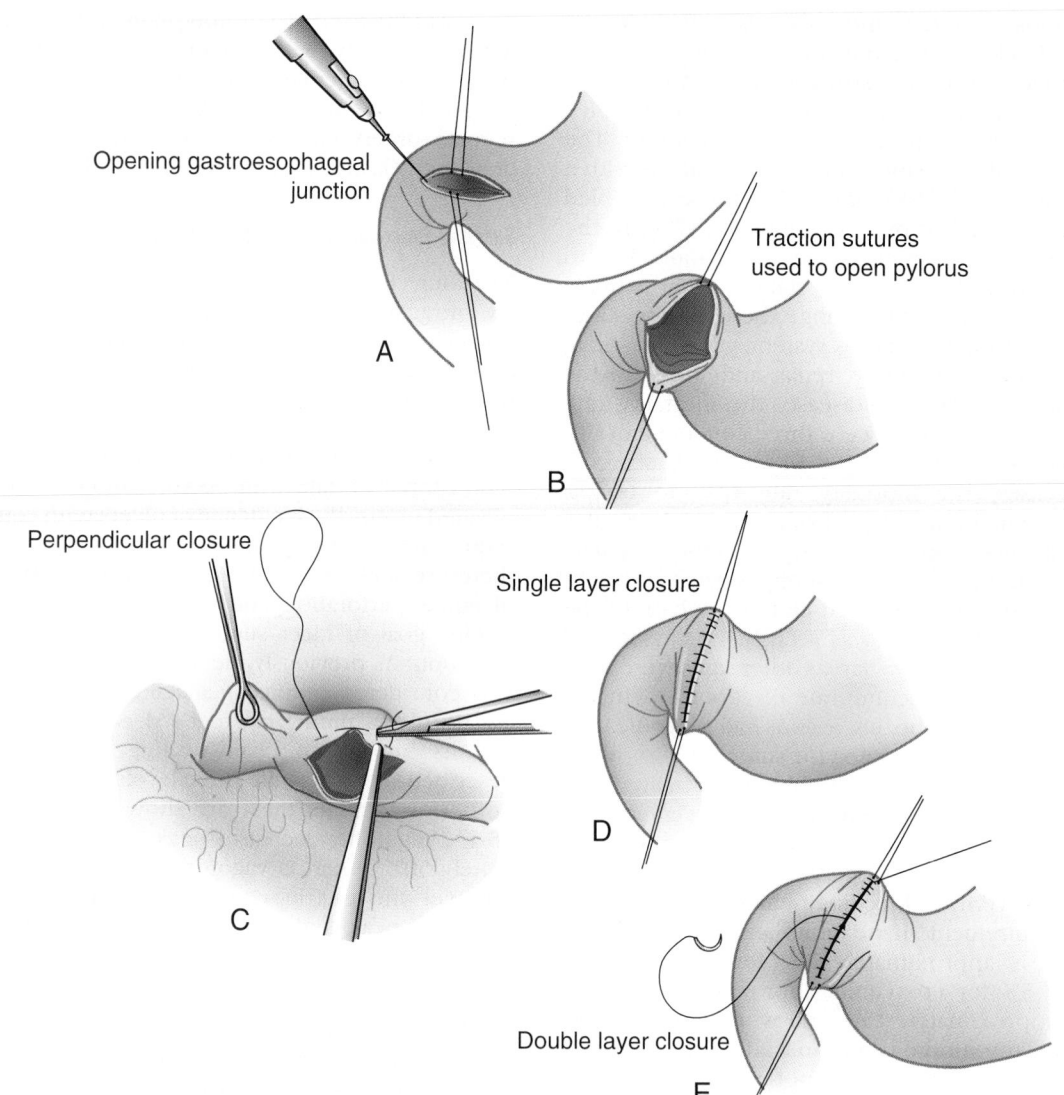

FIGURE 45-12. **A** to **E,** Heineke-Mikulicz pyloroplasty. (**A–E,** From Soreide JA, Soreide A: Pyloroplasty. Operative Techniques in General Surgery 5:65-72, 2003.)

gastric resection adversely affected the pyloral-antral pump function. This procedure divides only the vagus nerves supplying the acid-producing portion of the stomach and preserves the vagal innervation of the gastric antrum so that there is no need for routine drainage procedures. Consequently, there are fewer postoperative complications. In general, the nerves of Latarjet are identified anteriorly and posteriorly, and the crow's feet innervating the fundus and body of the stomach are divided. These nerves are divided up to a point approximately 7 cm proximal to the pylorus or the area in the vicinity of the gastric antrum. Superiorly, division of these nerves is carried to a point at least 5 cm proximal to the GE junction on the esophagus that is shown in Figure 45-13. Ideally, two or three branches to the antrum and pylorus should be preserved. The "criminal nerve of Grassi" represents a very proximal branch of the posterior trunk of

the vagus, and great attention needs to be taken to avoid missing this branch in the division process because it is frequently cited as a predisposition for ulcer recurrence if left intact.

The recurrence rates following highly selective vagotomy are variable and depend on the skill of the operator and the duration of follow-up. Lengthy longitudinal follow-up is necessary to evaluate the results of this procedure because of the consistently reported rise in recurrent ulceration with time. Recurrence rates of 10% to 15% are reported for this procedure when performed by skilled surgeons. These compare very favorably or even slightly higher than those reported after truncal vagotomy in combination with pyloroplasty. However, truncal vagotomy with pyloroplasty is more commonly associated with postvagotomy dumping syndrome and postvagotomy diarrhea. The moderate ulcer recurrence rate with highly

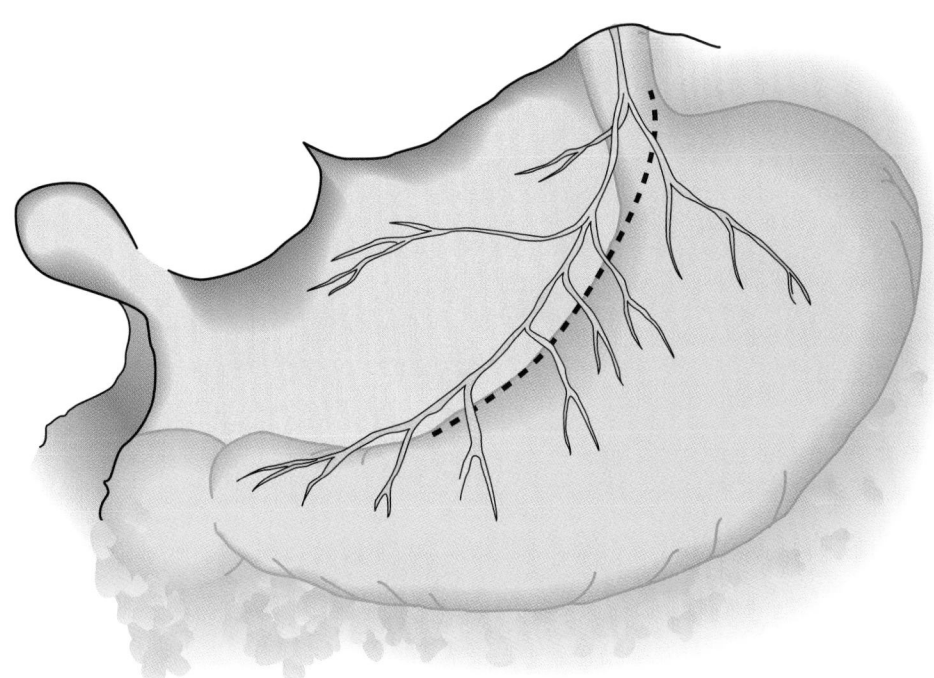

FIGURE 45-13.   Anterior view of the stomach and the anterior nerve of Latarjet. The dotted line represents the line of dissection for parietal cell or highly selective vagotomy. Note that the last major branches of the nerve are left intact and that the dissection begins 7 cm from the pylorus. At the gastroesophageal junction, the dissection is well away from the origin of the hepatic branches of the left vagus. (From Kelly KA, Teotia SS: Proximal gastric vagotomy. In Baker RJ, Fischer JE (eds): Mastery of Surgery. Philadelphia, Lippincott, Williams and Wilkins, 2001.)

selective vagotomy is considered acceptable by many surgeons because recurrences in this scenario are usually responsive to medical therapy with proton-pump inhibitors. When the results of this procedure are broken down by the preoperative ulcer site, there appears to be strong data suggesting that prepyloric ulcers are more likely to be associated with recurrence than duodenal ulcers for unclear reasons. As a result, it may not be the procedure of choice for prepyloric ulcers.

TRUNCAL VAGOTOMY AND ANTRECTOMY

The most common indications for antrectomy or distal gastrectomy are duodenal ulcer disease, gastric ulcer, and large benign gastric tumors. Relative contraindications include cirrhosis, extensive scarring of the proximal duodenum that leaves a difficult or tenuous duodenal closure, and previous operations on the proximal duodenum such as choledochoduodenostomy. When done in combination with truncal vagotomy, it is far more effective in reducing acid secretion and recurrence than either truncal vagotomy in combination with a drainage procedure or highly selective vagotomy. In fact, the recurrence rate for ulceration after truncal vagotomy and antrectomy is approximately 0 to 2% and probably represents the gold standard with regard to recurrence rates. However, this low recurrence rate needs to be balanced against postgastrectomy and postvagotomy syndromes (see later) that rarely occur following highly selective vagotomy but appear in 20% of the patients undergoing this procedure. Distal gastrectomy or antrectomy requires reconstruction of gastrointestinal continuity that can be accomplished by either a gastroduodenostomy (Billroth I) (Fig. 45-14) or gastrojejunostomy (Billroth II) (See Fig. 45-20B). For benign diseases, gastroduodenostomy is usually favored because it avoids the problem of retained-antrum

syndrome, duodenal stump leak, and afferent loop obstruction associated with gastrojejunostomy following resection. If the duodenum is significantly scarred, gastroduodenostomy may be technically more difficult, necessitating gastrojejunostomy. If a gastrojejunostomy is performed, the loop of jejunum chosen for anastomosis is usually brought through the transverse mesocolon in a retrocolic fashion rather than in front of the transverse colon in an antecolic fashion. The retrocolic anastomosis minimizes the length of the afferent limb and decreases the likelihood of twisting or kinking that could potentially lead to afferent loop obstruction and predispose to the devastating complication of a duodenal stump leak. Although vagotomy and antrectomy are clearly effective at managing ulcerations, they are used infrequently in the treatment of patients with peptic ulcer disease, as described later. In general, operations of lesser magnitude are performed more frequently in the *H. pylori* era. The overall mortality rate for antrectomy is about 2% but obviously is higher in patients with comorbid conditions such as insulin-dependent diabetes or immunosuppression. Approximately 20% of patients develop some form of postgastrectomy and/or postvagotomy complications and these are described in the following sections.

SUBTOTAL GASTRECTOMY

Subtotal gastrectomy is rarely performed for treatment of patients with peptic ulcer disease. It is usually reserved for patients with underlying malignancies or patients who have developed recurrent ulcerations following truncal vagotomy and antrectomy. The latter scenario assumes that medical therapy has been unable to heal the recurrent ulcer and that Zollinger-Ellison syndrome has been ruled out. Following subtotal gastrectomy, restoration of gastrointestinal continuity can be accomplished with

■ **FIGURE 45-14.**   Hemigastrectomy with Billroth 1 (gastroduodenal) anastomosis. (From Dempsey D, Pathak A: Antrectomy. Operative Techniques in General Surgery 5:86-100, 2003.)

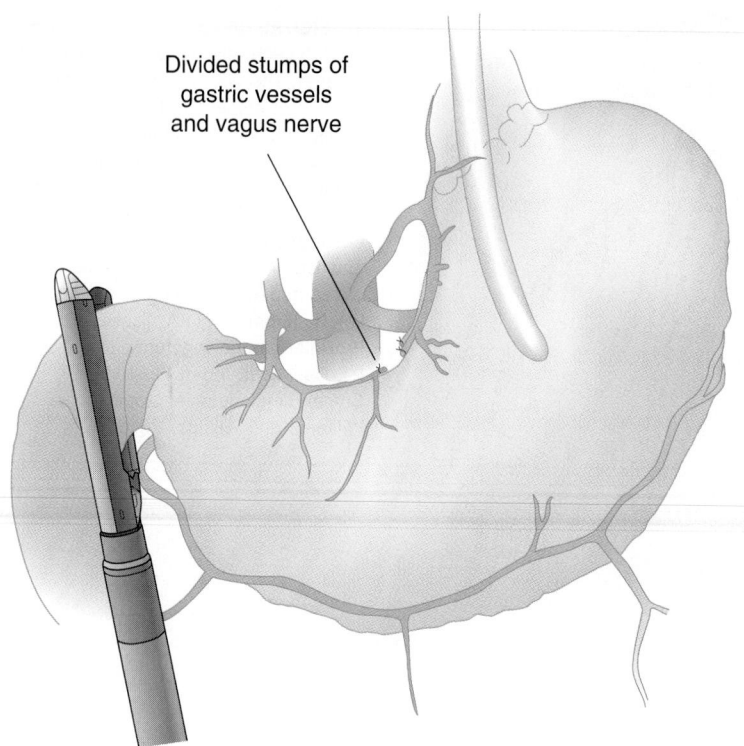

Divided stumps of
gastric vessels
and vagus nerve

A

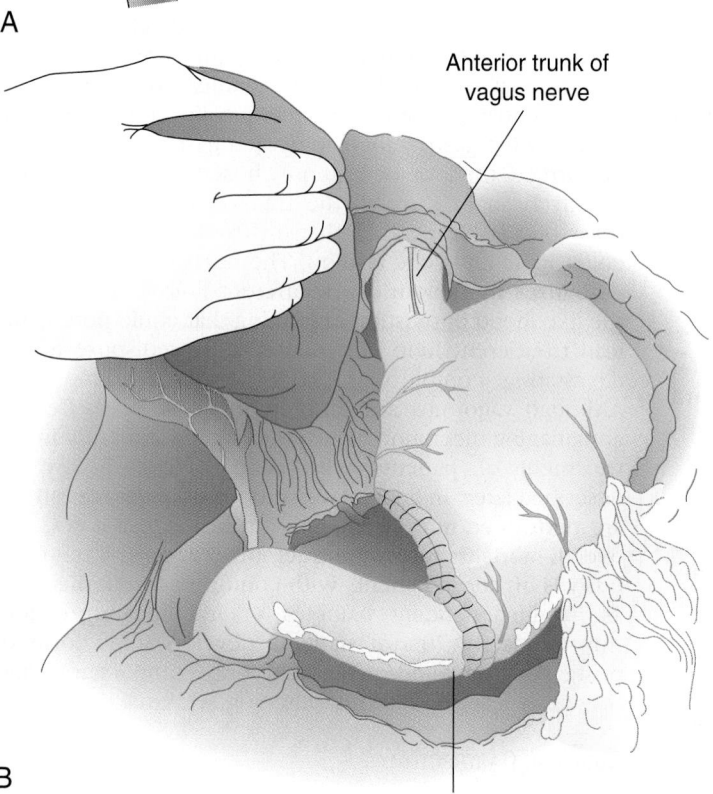

Anterior trunk of
vagus nerve

B

Billroth I gastroduodenal
anastomosis completed

either a Billroth II anastomosis or via a Roux-en-Y gastrojejunostomy.

LAPAROSCOPIC PROCEDURES

Not surprisingly, since the advent of laparoscopic cholecystectomy, many surgeons have applied minimally invasive surgical approaches to gastric surgery. Both parietal cell vagotomy and posterior truncal vagotomy with anterior seromyotomy (Taylor procedure) can be accomplished laparoscopically and represent effective antiulcer operations. However, long-term results are still unavailable to compare with those of the openly performed procedures. Dumping syndrome and postvagotomy diarrhea are similar in incidences to that observed after open highly selective vagotomy. Major concerns regarding this operation relate primarily to its efficacy and prevention of recurrent ulcers. Because incomplete innervation predisposes patients to recurrent ulcerations following highly selective vagotomy, anterior seromyotomy might place patients at risk for recurrence due to failure to completely denervate the parietal cell mass. Laparoscopic approaches can also be used for repair of simple perforations and offer clear advantages as opposed to the formal laparotomy required in open procedures.

Surgical Indications

Surgical therapy serves several purposes. It salvages patients from life-threatening complications associated with perforation, hemorrhage, and gastric outlet obstruction. It provides cure for the disease in the form of protection from recurrence, and it rules out the potential for malignancy in the case of gastric ulcerations. The indications for surgery are intractable abdominal pain, bleeding, perforation, and obstruction. For all ulcers being considered for elective surgery, antisecretory agents should probably be discontinued for about 72 hours prior to operation to allow gastric acidity to return to normal values, which minimizes bacterial overgrowth and the extent of contamination.

Intractable Duodenal Ulcer

Intractability is loosely defined as failure of an ulcer to heal after an initial trial of 8 to 12 weeks of therapy or if patients relapse once therapy has been discontinued. This is unusual for duodenal ulcer disease in the *H. pylori* era; however, it still exists for benign gastric ulcers in which malignancy needs to be ruled out. Although rarely seen today, intractable duodenal ulcer should be treated by parietal cell vagotomy. Although this can be performed openly, many prefer a laparoscopic approach. The current laparoscopic technology allows performance of parietal cell vagotomy in exactly the same way it is performed openly and probably provides better visualization. Proximal gastric vagotomy is associated with a morbidity of less than 1% and a mortality of less than 0.5%. Unfortunately, the recurrence rate is roughly 5% to 25%. Some surgeons prefer a Taylor procedure in which the posterior truncal vagotomy is performed laparoscopically and then an endoscopic gastrointestinal stapler is used to perform a seromyotomy across the anterior portion of the stomach to divide all the vagal fibers coursing through the seromuscular layer. Although some surgeons are concerned about dividing vagal innervation to the celiac ganglion and to the rest of the viscera, there is considerable evidence that preserving vagal innervation of the celiac axis and small bowel does little to reduce the side effects of vagotomy. Thus, the Taylor procedure appears to be equivalent to parietal cell vagotomy and the side effects are not any greater. Taylor has published data suggesting that anterior lesser curve seromyotomy and posterior truncal vagotomy result in acid suppression that is similar in magnitude to that achieved following highly selective vagotomy or truncal vagotomy with drainage. Gastric emptying following the Taylor procedure is also similar to that of highly selective vagotomy (increased emptying of liquids and normal emptying of solids), and dumping and diarrhea are less than those observed following truncal vagotomy and drainage.

Intractable Gastric Ulcer

TYPE 1 GASTRIC ULCER

For type 1 gastric ulcers, malignancy remains a major concern and excision of the ulcer is necessary. Consequently, the distal gastrectomy is probably the best operation in this clinical situation. Re-establishment of intestinal continuity can be performed with a Billroth I or Billroth II, but, again, a Billroth I is the preferred choice, providing malignancy has been ruled out. The morbidity associated with a distal gastrectomy without vagotomy and Billroth I reconstruction is approximately 3% to 5% for elective treatment of type 1 gastric ulcers. Mortality ranges from 1% to 2% and is associated with recurrence rate of less than 2%. It is important to remember, however, that the presentation of a nonhealing gastric ulcer in the *H. pylori* era should raise serious concerns about the presence of underlying malignancy. If malignancy is encountered, a subtotal gastrectomy with a Billroth II gastrojejunostomy or Roux-en-Y gastrojejunostomy should be performed. Vagotomy usually is not necessary for the type 1 gastric ulcer because it is not dependent on gastric acid. Although technically more difficult, a parietal cell vagotomy with wedge excision of the ulcer could also be performed. Because intractable peptic ulcer disease is so uncommon, it is important to ensure that adequate time has elapsed and appropriate therapy has been administered to allow healing of the ulcer to occur. This includes confirmation that *H. pylori* has been eradicated and that NSAIDs have been eliminated as a potential cause. Most patients with a type 1 gastric ulcer should in fact heal following appropriate medical therapy, as described in the medical therapy section.

TYPE 2 OR 3 GASTRIC ULCERS

Assuming that patients have had adequate time to heal their type 2 or 3 gastric ulcer and *H. pylori* has been eradicated, a distal gastrectomy in combination with vagotomy should be performed. Several studies have demonstrated that patients undergoing highly selective vagotomy for type 2 or 3 gastric ulcers have a poorer outcome than those undergoing resection. The type of vagotomy performed in combination with the resection could be either a selective or truncal vagotomy. However, there are still some who advocate performing a laparoscopic parietal cell vagotomy and reserve resection for those who develop ulcer recurrence. Management of type 4 gastric ulcers is discussed separately.

Bleeding Duodenal Ulcers

As a result of aggressive endoscopic management, there has been a significant reduction in the number of patients with bleeding duodenal ulcers who require surgery to control their bleeding. The patients who come to surgery are usually sicker, more elderly, and more likely to have complications. Laine and Peterson demonstrated that you can treat at least one recurrence of bleeding by endoscopic management with no increase in mortality and morbidity and have long-term control of hemorrhage in approximately half of the patients.[65] However, these patients need to be observed closely, and treatment with endoscopy needs to be prompt and as aggressive as possible. Provided that the gastroenterologist or surgical endoscopist can stop the bleeding and is confident that it can be managed by endoscopy, the patient still needs to be treated with a proton-pump inhibitor and undergo therapy for *H. pylori* after testing. For those patients who continue to bleed or who are referred by the endoscopist, the duodenal bleeding is usually controlled by opening the duodenum and oversewing the ulcer with a U stitch from the vessel, which is usually the pancreaticoduodenal artery or gastroduodenal artery. As most of these patients are elderly, have bled a significant amount, and have some degree of hypotension, the more time-consuming parietal cell vagotomy is usually not performed. Instead, a truncal vagotomy with pyloroplasty is performed. Although not proven, there are some who advocate opening the duodenum, ligating the gastroduodenal vessel, closing the duodenum, and then eradicating *H. pylori*. The clear exception to this would be if the patient had received therapy in the past for *H. pylori* and failed or if the patient was known to be *H. pylori* negative. In this situation, an acid-reducing procedure is clearly indicated. Most surgeons would not perform any form of gastrectomy for a bleeding duodenal ulcer.

Bleeding Gastric Ulcers

For bleeding type 1 gastric ulcers, a distal gastrectomy with Billroth I anastomosis is usually performed. Some have advocated adding vagotomy for patients who remain on NSAIDs, although the data on this are likewise unclear. However, if patients still require NSAIDs, they should be given misoprostol, a prostaglandin analogue, since it has been found to have a 40% reduction in serious gastrointestinal complications in those patients who have to stay on NSAIDs.[66] Alternatively, the use of selective COX-2 inhibitors is also an option. For types 2 and 3 gastric ulcers, distal gastrectomy in combination with vagotomy is indicated.

Perforated Duodenal Ulcers

The available evidence suggests that simple patching of a perforated duodenal ulcer followed by treatment with *H. pylori* is all that is necessary for patients who present with a perforated duodenum secondary to peptic ulcer disease. However, this assumes that the patient is *H. pylori* positive and will be compliant with therapy to eradicate *H. pylori*. If the patient is known to be *H. pylori* negative, then an acid-reducing procedure (i.e., truncal vagotomy with pyloroplasty) should be performed.[44] Patch closure of the duodenum can be performed by either a laparoscopic or open procedure.[67] In some cases, patients present with a sealed perforation. One of the first studies assessing this group of patients came out of Hong Kong, where a series of patients were treated prospectively and successfully with nonoperative management.[68] These patients were hemodynamically stable and without signs of toxicity. Unfortunately, the patients who failed were the ones where it would be most desirable to use nonoperative management (i.e., the elderly and the very ill). In this situation, upper gastrointestinal radiography needs to demonstrate that the ulcer is indeed sealed, as suggested by Berne and Donovan.[69] Nonoperative therapy in this situation would include treatment for *H. pylori* and acid suppression. For all perforated duodenal ulcer patients who are *H. pylori* positive, documentation of *H. pylori* eradication with a urea breath test is mandatory, and it is paramount that the patients are compliant with their medications to treat *H. pylori* regardless of whether they are managed surgically or nonoperatively.

Perforated Gastric Ulcer

For perforated type 1 gastric ulcers that occur in hemodynamically stable patients, distal gastrectomy with Billroth I reanastomosis is usually performed. However, simple patching of the gastric ulcer, testing for *H. pylori*, and treatment if positive can also be considered. However, the risk of malignancy needs to be ruled out; therefore, biopsy of the ulcer bed also needs to be performed. In addition, even if initial biopsies are negative, documentation of healing needs to be undertaken at a later date with repeat endoscopy and rebiopsy of the ulcer if it has not healed. Adding vagotomy for perforated type 1 gastric ulcers is unlikely to be of any value. Types 2 and 3 gastric ulcers, because they behave like duodenal ulcers, can be simply treated with patch closure followed by treatment for *H. pylori*. Again, this assumes that patients are *H. pylori* positive.

Gastric Outlet Obstruction

Gastric outlet obstruction is more common with duodenal and type 3 gastric ulcers but can occur in patients with a type 2 ulcer. Obstruction is an unusual presentation for type 1 gastric ulcers, and its presence should suggest an occult malignancy. All patients with gastric outlet obstruction require preoperative nasogastric decompression for several days, correction of fluid and electrolyte imbalances, antisecretory therapy, and endoscopy with biopsies prior to surgical intervention. The first principle is to categorize the patient as either acutely or chronically obstructed. If the patient is acutely obstructed, the patient should be treated nonoperatively with nasogastric decompression, intravenous fluid, nutritional support as needed, and acid-suppressive therapy. *H. pylori* should be tested for and treated. On the other hand, if the patient has chronic gastric outlet obstruction, as might be the case with a chronic duodenal ulcer with fibrosis, operative therapy is usually indicated to open up the gastric outlet. In addition, an acid-reducing procedure is necessary. Gastrectomy can be done if technically feasible. Alternatively, gastrojejunostomy with truncal vagotomy is also an option. The only randomized trial examining the management of operation for gastric outlet obstructions was done by Csendes and associates.[70] They found that gastroduodenostomy in conjunction with a highly selective vagotomy yielded the poorest results in terms of symptomatic relief of the three operations, the other two being selective vagotomy with antrectomy and highly selective vagotomy with gastroenterostomy. Endoscopic balloon dilation has also been tried in this situation, although those who benefit from this procedure are likely those with acute gastric outlet obstruction and not those with chronic gastric outlet obstruction.[71] The preferred procedure for those patients presenting with a gastric outlet obstruction is parietal cell vagotomy with a gastrojejunostomy. In addition, these patients require therapy for *H. pylori*. The physiologic argument for doing the parietal cell vagotomy with a gastrojejunostomy as opposed to truncal vagotomy is that it maintains innervation to the chronically obstructed antrum. As a result, the patient may have fewer chronic emptying problems compared with truncal vagotomy.

Type 4 Gastric Ulcers

The type 4 gastric ulcer presents a difficult management problem.[72] The surgical treatment depends on the ulcer size, the distance from the GE junction, and the degree of surrounding inflammation. Whenever possible, the ulcer should be excised. The most aggressive approach would be to perform a distal gastrectomy including a small portion of the esophageal wall and ulcer with a Roux-en-Y esophagogastrojejunostomy to restore intestinal continuity. For type 4 gastric ulcers that are located 2 to 5 cm from the GE junction, a distal gastrectomy can be performed with a vertical extension of the resection to include the lesser curvature with the ulcer. After resection, bowel continuity is restored with an end-to-end gastroduodenostomy. Some have even advocated leaving the ulcer in place or locally excising it in conjunction with the truncal vagotomy and pyloroplasty.

Giant Gastric Ulcers

Giant gastric ulcers are defined as ulcers with a diameter of 3 cm or greater. They are usually found on the lesser curvature; only 4% occur along the greater curvature. It is not uncommon for these ulcers to penetrate into contiguous structures such as the spleen, pancreas, liver, or transverse colon and be falsely diagnosed as unresectable malignancy, despite normal biopsy results. The incidence of malignancy ranges from 6% to 30% and increases with the size of the ulcer. Giant gastric ulcers have a high likelihood of developing complications (i.e., perforation, bleeding) and therefore early operation is thought to be the treatment of choice. The operation of choice is resection including the ulcer bed, with vagotomy reserved for types 2 and 3 gastric ulcers. In the high-risk patient with significant underlying comorbid conditions, a local excision combined with vagotomy and pyloroplasty may be considered; otherwise, resection has the highest chance for successful outcome.

Postgastrectomy Syndromes

Postoperative Complications for Peptic Ulcer Disease

The overall mortality rate for vagotomy and pyloroplasty or a vagotomy with antrectomy is about 1% or less, whereas for highly selective vagotomy it is around 0.05%. Postoperative complications include bleeding, infection, and delayed gastric emptying, which can occur in roughly 5% of patients following vagotomy and pyloroplasty or vagotomy and antrectomy. Highly selective vagotomy has the lowest rate of associated complications, which occur in only about 1% of patients. In addition to these early complications, gastric surgery results in a number of physiologic derangements due to loss of reservoir function, interruption of the pyloric sphincter mechanism, the type of gastric reconstruction, and vagal nerve transection.

These disorders are collectively referred to as *postgastrectomy syndromes*. Although the physiologic derangements account for most of the symptoms, there are also some psychological elements associated with the disease process that remain poorly understood. Approximately 25% of the patients who undergo surgery for peptic ulcer disease subsequently develop some degree of postgastrectomy syndrome, although this frequency is much lower in highly selective vagotomy. Fortunately, only about 1% of them become permanently disabled from their symptoms. When these postgastrectomy symptoms develop, it has become more apparent that every attempt should be made to avoid reoperation since many of these patients lack a clearly mechanical or physiologic defect and because many of the problems persist despite reoperation. If reoperation is attempted, it should not be performed until an adequate trial of conservative therapy has been administered and for an adequate period of time.

Postgastrectomy Syndromes Secondary to Gastric Resection

DUMPING SYNDROME

Dumping syndrome refers to a symptom complex that occurs following ingestion of a meal when a portion of the stomach has been removed or the normal pyloric sphincter mechanism has become disrupted. Dumping syndrome exists in either a late or an early form, with the early form occurring more frequently.

EARLY DUMPING

The early form of dumping syndrome usually occurs within 20 to 30 minutes following ingestion of a meal and is accompanied by both gastrointestinal and cardiovascular symptoms. The gastrointestinal symptoms include nausea and vomiting, a sense of epigastric fullness, eructations, cramping abdominal pain, and often explosive diarrhea. The cardiovascular symptoms include palpitations, tachycardia, diaphoresis, fainting, dizziness, flushing, and occasionally blurred vision. The symptoms characteristically occur while the patient is seated at the table eating or shortly after eating. This symptom complex can develop after any operation on the stomach. However, it is more common after partial gastrectomy with the Billroth II reconstruction, in which as many as 50% to 60% of patients may develop this complication, especially if more that two thirds of the stomach has been removed. It is far less commonly observed following the Billroth I gastrectomy or in patients following vagotomy and drainage procedures. Usually, the gastrointestinal symptoms are more common and only rarely does the full-blown symptom complex occur with the cardiovascular and vasomotor aberrations noted earlier.

Although the exact sequence of events responsible for this syndrome remains to be fully defined, it is generally agreed that it occurs because of the rapid passage of food of high osmolarity from the stomach into the small intestine. This occurs because gastrectomy or interruption of the pyloric sphincteric mechanism prevents the stomach from preparing its contents and delivering them to the proximal bowel in the form of small particles in isotonic solution. The resultant hypertonic food bolus passes into the small intestine, which induces a rapid shift of extracellular fluid into the intestinal lumen to achieve isotonicity. Following this shift of extracellular fluid, luminal distention occurs and induces the autonomic responses listed earlier.

The symptoms associated with early dumping syndrome appear to be secondary to the release of several humoral agents such as serotonin, bradykinin-like substances, neurotensin, and enteroglucagon. Usually, the symptoms of dumping are sufficiently obvious that the diagnosis can be made on this basis alone. However, if there is doubt, gastric-emptying scans can be obtained that demonstrate rapid gastric emptying. Alternatively, a provocative test can also be done in the form of a 200-mL meal of 50% glucose solution and water. Patients with early dumping syndrome have symptoms following ingestion of this glucose solution.

The majority of patients subjected to gastric surgery complain of some dumping-like symptoms following surgery. Most, however, experience spontaneous relief and require no specific therapy. In those situations where symptoms are prolonged, dietary measures are usually sufficient to manage these patients. These dietary measures include avoiding foods containing large amounts of sugar, frequent feeding of small meals rich in protein and fat, and separating liquids from solids during a meal. In the past, serotonin antagonists were given to these patients with marginal benefit. Recently, however, the long-acting somatostatin analogue octreotide acetate (Sandostatin) has been shown to be highly effective in preventing the development of symptoms, both vasomotor and gastrointestinal. This synthetic analogue has been shown to inhibit the hormonal responses associated with this syndrome and to completely abolish the associated diarrhea. This peptide not only inhibits gastric emptying but also induces a fasting or interdigestive small bowel motility pattern in patients with dumping syndrome such that intestinal transit of the ingested meal is prolonged. The side effects associated with administration of this synthetic peptide are relatively benign; however, the agent is somewhat expensive.

In the less than 1% of patients who fail to respond to the conservative measures mentioned earlier, operative intervention may become necessary. The physiologic rationale for surgery is to improve the gastric reservoir function, decrease rapid gastric emptying, or, ideally, accomplish both goals. Although a variety of surgical procedures have been used to manage early dumping, the use of isoperistaltic or antiperistaltic jejunal segments has had the greatest success in dealing with this problem in most centers. This procedure is done by utilizing a 10- to 20-cm loop of jejunum and interposing it between the stomach and small intestine in an isoperistaltic fashion. This loop dilates over time and therefore promotes the reservoir function. In the antiperistaltic approach, a jejunal segment 10 cm in length is used, and the jejunum is twisted on its mesentery so that its distal end is anastomosed to the stomach and its proximal end to the small intestine. This reversal in peristalsis permits the loop to act as a substitute pylorus and delay the rate of gastric emptying. Another technique is the creation of a long-limb Roux-en-Y anastomosis to delay gastric emptying. Whether this approach is superior to the use of isoperistaltic or antiperistaltic jejunal segments has yet to be determined.

LATE DUMPING

The syndrome of late dumping appears 2 to 3 hours after a meal and is far less common than early dumping. The basic defect in this disorder is also rapid gastric emptying; however, it is related specifically to carbohydrates being delivered rapidly into the proximal intestine. When carbohydrates are delivered to the small intestine, they are quickly absorbed, resulting in hyperglycemia that triggers the release of large amounts of insulin to control the rising blood sugar. This results in an actual "overshooting" such that a profound hypoglycemia occurs in response to the insulin. This activates the adrenal gland to release catecholamines, which results in diaphoresis, tremulousness, lightheadedness, tachycardia, and confusion. The symptom complex is indistinguishable from insulin or hypoglycemic shock.

These patients should be advised to ingest frequent small meals and to reduce their carbohydrate intake. Some patients have found benefit with pectin, either alone or in combination with acarbose, an α-glucoside hydrolase inhibitor that delays carbohydrate absorption through impairment of intraluminal starch and sucrose digestion. If conservative measures fail, the use of an antiperistaltic loop of jejunum between the residual gastric pouch and intestine has been shown to effectively manage this problem. The antiperistaltic limb accomplishes a delay in gastric emptying and also results in flattening of the glucose tolerance curve to alleviate the hypoglycemic symptomatology.

METABOLIC DISTURBANCES

A number of metabolic consequences arise following gastric procedures but are more common and serious after partial gastrectomy than after vagotomy. The incidence following gastrectomy is also much greater if a Billroth II as opposed to a Billroth I is used for reconstruction. As for dumping, the severity of these disturbances is directly related to the extent of gastric resection.

The most common metabolic defect appearing following gastrectomy is anemia. Two types have been identified: One is related to a deficiency in iron and the other is related to an impairment in vitamin B_{12} metabolism. Iron deficiency anemia is more common than vitamin B_{12} deficiency anemia. More than 30% of patients undergoing gastrectomy suffer from iron deficiency anemia. The exact cause remains to be fully understood but appears to be related to a combination of decreased iron intake, impaired iron absorption, and chronic subclinical blood loss secondary to the hyperemic, friable gastric mucosa primarily involving the margins of the stoma where the stomach connects to the small intestine. In general, the addition of iron supplements to the patient's diet corrects this metabolic problem.

Megaloblastic anemia can also occur following gastrectomy, especially when more than 50% of the stomach is removed, such as that occurring during subtotal gastrectomy. Megaloblastic anemia from vitamin B_{12} deficiency only rarely develops following partial gastrectomy such as that seen with antrectomy. Vitamin B_{12} deficiency occurs secondary to poor absorption of the substance due to lack of intrinsic factor secretion in the gastric juice. If a patient develops a macrocytic anemia, serum vitamin B_{12} levels should be obtained. If the vitamin B_{12} level is abnormal, the patient should be treated with intramuscular injections of cyanocobalamin every 3 to 4 months indefinitely since its administration orally is not reliable. The other cause of macrocytic anemia is folate deficiency, which is rare following gastric resection but may coexist with either an iron or vitamin B_{12} deficiency. Folate deficiency can usually be corrected by dietary supplementation.

Another common metabolic disturbance following gastric resection is impaired absorption of fat. On occasion, steatorrhea may be seen after gastrectomy and Billroth II reconstruction as a result of inadequate mixing of bile salts and pancreatic lipase with ingested fat because of the duodenal bypass. If this occurs, a deficiency in uptake of fat-soluble vitamins may also occur. In the setting of steatorrhea, pancreatic replacement enzymes are often effective in decreasing fat loss.

Both osteoporosis and osteomalacia have also been observed following gastric resection and appear to be caused by deficiencies in calcium. If fat malabsorption is also present, the calcium malabsorption is further aggravated as fatty acids bind calcium. The incidence of this problem also increases with the extent of gastric resection and is usually associated with a Billroth II gastrectomy. Development of bone disease generally occurs approximately 4 to 5 years after surgery. Treatment of this disorder usually requires calcium supplements (1 to 2 g/day) in conjunction with vitamin D (500 to 5000 units daily).

Postgastrectomy Syndromes Related to Gastric Reconstruction

A number of disorders can develop following gastric resection as a result of the technique used to re-establish gastrointestinal continuity. Patients undergoing Billroth II gastrectomy are more likely to encounter these problems than those undergoing other types of reconstruction. The afferent loop and retained-antrum syndromes occur only in patients with this type of gastrectomy.

AFFERENT LOOP SYNDROME

Afferent loop syndrome occurs as a result of partial obstruction of the afferent limb that is unable then to empty its contents. As shown in Figure 45-15, afferent loop syndrome can occur from a variety of causes. It can arise secondary to kinking and angulation of the afferent limb, internal herniation behind the efferent limb, stenosis of the gastrojejunal anastomosis, a redundant twisting of the afferent limb with a resultant volvulus, or secondary to adhesions involving the afferent limb. The syn-

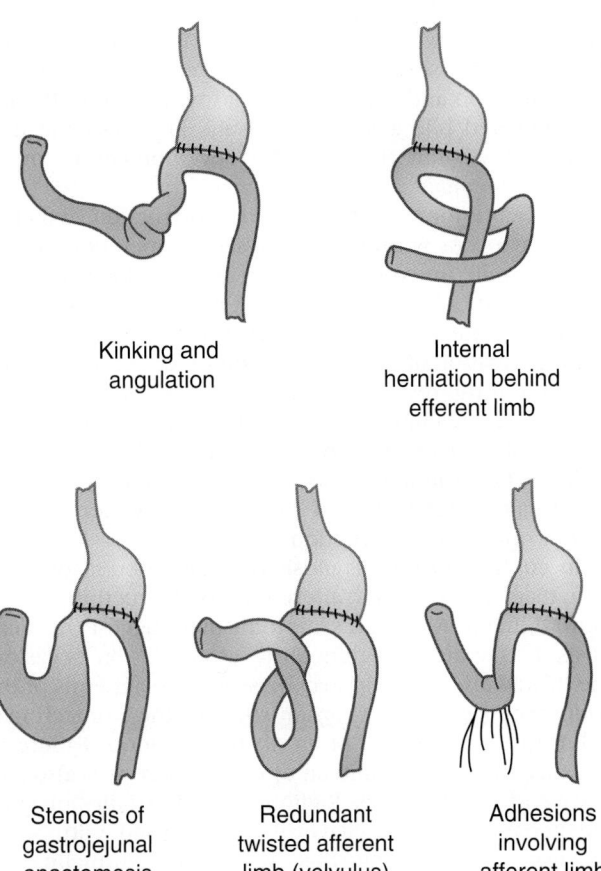

Kinking and
angulation

Internal
herniation behind
efferent limb

Stenosis of
gastrojejunal
anastomosis

Redundant
twisted afferent
limb (volvulus)

Adhesions
involving
afferent limb

FIGURE 45-15. Causes of afferent loop syndrome.

drome usually occurs when the afferent limb is longer than 30 to 40 cm and has been anastomosed to the gastric remnant in an antecolic fashion. Although acute afferent loop syndrome can occur, it is usually found chronically.

Following obstruction of the afferent limb, there is an accumulation of pancreatic and hepatobiliary secretion within the limb, resulting in its distention. Pancreatic and hepatobiliary secretion occur in response to ingestion of food in the gastric remnant or passage of food into the efferent loop. Accumulation of these secretions results in distention, which causes epigastric discomfort and cramping. In the setting of partial obstruction, the intraluminal pressure increases to forcefully empty its contents into the stomach, resulting in bilious vomiting that is often projectile but offers immediate relief of symptoms. There is no food contained within the vomitus since the ingested meal has already passed into the efferent limb. In the setting of complete obstruction, necrosis and perforation of the loop can occur because the obstruction is a closed loop due to the fact that the duodenum proximally has already been closed during the Billroth II gastrectomy. In this situation, constant abdominal pain is noted and may be more pronounced in the right upper quadrant, with radiation into the interscapular area. Like any complete bowel obstruction, this is a surgical emergency and requires immediate attention. In most patients with afferent loop syndrome, the obstruction is only partial. Whether or not a patient seeks medical attention depends on the degree of afferent loop obstruction present. If the obstruction has been present for a long period, it can also be aggravated by the development of the blind loop syndrome. In this situation, bacterial overgrowth occurs in the static loop and the bacteria bind with vitamin B_{12} and deconjugated bile acids. This results in a systemic deficiency of vitamin B_{12} with the development of megaloblastic anemia.

The acute form of afferent loop obstruction, which is rare, may occur within a few days after operation or may develop quite unexpectedly years after the Billroth II gastrectomy. In both circumstances it is caused by the acute blockage of the afferent limb such as that seen with volvulus or herniation of the afferent loop posterior to the efferent limb. If the resulting obstruction is of the closed-loop type, it requires immediate operative intervention. A palpable abdominal mass may be present in about one third of patients, although the associated pain and tenderness are usually severe enough to indicate the necessity of urgent operative intervention.

In contrast to the diagnosis of acute afferent obstruction, diagnosing chronic afferent loop obstruction may be more difficult. Although symptoms may suggest this diagnosis, it is sometimes difficult to establish. On occasion, the dilated afferent loop may be seen on plain films of the abdomen or a contrast barium study of the stomach may delineate the presence of an obstructed loop. Failure to visualize the afferent limb on upper endoscopy is also suggestive of the diagnosis. Radionucleotide studies imaging the hepatobiliary tree have also been used with some success in diagnosing this syndrome. Normally, the radionucleotide should pass into the stomach or distal small bowel after being excreted into the afferent limb. If

there is failure to do so, the possibility of an afferent loop obstruction should be considered. The medical usefulness of radionucleotide studies remains to be determined.

For both forms of afferent loop syndrome, acute and chronic, operation is indicated because it is a mechanical problem, not a functional problem. A long afferent limb is usually the underlying problem, and treatment therefore involves the elimination of this loop. Some have advocated converting the Billroth II construction into a Billroth I anastomosis, whereas others have advocated an enteroenterostomy below the stoma or the use of a Roux-en-Y anastomosis. However, if a Roux-en-Y anastomosis is performed, a concomitant vagotomy should also be performed to prevent marginal ulceration from the diversion of duodenal contents from the gastroenteric stoma.

EFFERENT LOOP OBSTRUCTION

Obstruction of the efferent limb is usually quite rare. The most common cause of efferent loop obstruction is herniation of the limb behind the anastomosis in a right-to-left fashion. This can occur with both antecolic and retrocolic gastrojejunostomies. The preference for herniation in the right-to-left direction is probably a result of the fact that gastrojejunostomies lie to the left of the main mass of the small intestine, making it mechanically easier for herniation to occur from right to left. With this type of herniation, obstruction of the efferent limb is usually all that occurs; however, it may also compress the mesentery of the afferent limb, compromising its blood supply or obstructing the afferent limb as well. Efferent loop obstruction may occur anytime following surgery; however, more than 50% of the patients become obstructed within the first postoperative month. Establishing a diagnosis is difficult, although initial complaints may include left upper quadrant abdominal pain that is colicky in nature, bilious vomiting, and abdominal distention. The diagnosis is usually established on a contrast barium study of the stomach with failure of barium to enter the efferent limb. Operative intervention is almost always necessary and consists of reducing the retroanastomotic hernia and closing the retroanastomotic space to prevent recurrence of this condition.

ALKALINE REFLUX GASTRITIS

Following gastrectomy, reflux of bile is fairly common. In a small percentage of patients, this reflux is associated with severe epigastric abdominal pain accompanied by bilious vomiting and weight loss. It is usually not relieved by food or antacids. The vomiting may occur anytime during the day or night and can even awaken patients from sleep. Although the diagnosis can be made by taking a careful history, HIDA scans are usually diagnostic, demonstrating biliary secretion into the stomach and even into the esophagus in severe cases. Upper endoscopy can also be performed, with multiple biopsies taken away from the stoma, and the gastric fluid can be analyzed for bile acid concentrations. On endoscopy, the mucosa is frequently friable and beefy red and superficial mucosal ulcerations may be apparent on microscopy. Iron deficiency anemia and weight loss are also common.

Most patients suffering from alkaline reflux gastritis have had gastric resection performed with a Billroth II anastomosis. Symptoms may occur at any time following the operation. Although bile reflux appears to be the inciting event, a number of issues remain unanswered with respect to the role of bile in its pathogenesis. For example, many patients have reflux of bile into their stomach following gastrectomy without any symptoms. Moreover, there is no clear correlation between the volume of bile or its composition and the subsequent development of alkaline reflux gastritis. Although it is clear that the syndrome does exist, caution needs to be exercised to be sure that it is not overdiagnosed. Once a diagnosis is made, therapy is directed at relief of symptoms. Unfortunately, most of the medical therapies that have been tried to treat alkaline reflux gastritis have not shown any consistent benefit. Thus, for those patients with intractable symptoms, surgery is recommended. The surgical procedure of choice usually means converting the Billroth II anastomosis into a Roux-en-Y gastrojejunostomy in which the Roux limb has been lengthened to 41 to 46 cm.

RETAINED-ANTRUM SYNDROME

Because the antral mucosa may extend 0.5 cm past the pyloric muscle, the syndrome of retained gastric antrum may occur following partial gastrectomy even if the resection is carried beyond the pyloric sphincter. A Billroth II anastomosis can therefore result in the development of retained-antrum syndrome if residual antrum is left in the duodenal stump. In this situation, the retained antrum is continually bathed in alkaline pH from the duodenal, pancreatic, and biliary secretions, which in turn stimulate the release of large amounts of gastrin with a resultant increase in acid secretion. This highly ulcerogenic circumstance is responsible for approximately 9% of recurrent ulcers following previous surgery for peptic ulcer disease and is associated with an incidence of recurrent ulceration as high as 80%. It can be eliminated if biopsy confirmation of duodenal mucosa is obtained following resection of the proximal duodenum at the time of the Billroth II gastrectomy.

In patients who develop a recurrent ulcer following previous gastrectomy for ulcer disease in which a Billroth II anastomosis was performed, a technetium scan may prove helpful in diagnosing retained antrum. In patients with a retained antrum, this scan demonstrates a "hot spot" that is adjacent to the area where normal uptake of technetium by the gastric mucosa of the remaining stomach occurs. If a retained antrum is diagnosed, H_2-receptor blockade or proton-pump inhibitors may prove helpful in controlling acid hypersecretion. If this is ineffective, either conversion of the Billroth II to a Billroth I reconstruction or excision of the retained antral tissue in the duodenal stump is indicated.

Postvagotomy Syndromes

POSTVAGOTOMY DIARRHEA

Approximately 30% or more of patients suffer from diarrhea after gastric surgery. For most patients, it is not severe and usually disappears within the first 3 to 4 months. For some patients, the diarrhea is part of the dumping syndrome previously described. However, vagotomy is also associated with alterations in stool frequency. Truncal vagotomy has been reported to result in increased frequency of daily bowel movements in 30% to 70% of patients. In some, the diarrhea may occur two or three times weekly or manifest itself once or twice a month. In others, it may be more explosive and result in soiled clothing. Most patients with postvagotomy diarrhea have their symptoms resolve over time. In those patients who fail to resolve their symptoms, cholestyramine, an anionic exchange resin that absorbs bile salts and renders them unabsorbable and inactive, can significantly diminish the severity of diarrhea. However, because postvagotomy diarrhea is usually self-limited, treatment should be symptomatic. Treatment with cholestyramine should show signs of improvement within 1 to 4 weeks of initiation of treatment. Four grams of cholestyramine with meals three times daily followed by an adjustment to a maintenance dosage should decrease bowel movements to once or twice a day. Only in rare cases is operative therapy necessary for postvagotomy diarrhea. When diarrhea has remained incapacitating for at least 1 year following initial gastric surgery, the diarrhea fails to respond to cholestyramine therapy, and other causes have been ruled out, surgery is indicated. This should involve no more than 1% of all patients undergoing vagotomy. The operative procedure of choice is to interpose a 10-cm segment of reverse jejunum 70 to 100 cm from the ligament of Treitz. This has led to sustained relief from diarrhea in most patients subjected to this operation.

POSTVAGOTOMY GASTRIC ATONY

Following vagotomy, gastric emptying is delayed. This is true for both truncal and selective vagotomies but not in the case of highly selective or parietal cell vagotomy. With selective or truncal vagotomy, patients lose antral pump function and therefore they have a reduction in their ability to empty solids. In contrast, emptying of liquids is accelerated because of loss of receptive relaxation in the proximal stomach that regulates liquid emptying. Although most patients undergoing vagotomy and a drainage procedure manage to adequately empty their stomach, some patients have persistent gastric stasis that results in retention of food within the stomach for several hours. This may be accompanied by a feeling of fullness and occasionally by abdominal pain. In still rarer cases, it may be associated with a functional gastric outlet obstruction. The diagnosis of gastroparesis is confirmed on scintigraphic assessment of gastric emptying. However, other causes of delayed gastric emptying such as diabetes mellitus, electrolyte imbalance, drug toxicity, and neuromuscular disorders must also be excluded. In addition, a mechanical cause of gastric outlet obstruction such as postoperative adhesions, afferent or efferent loop obstruction, and internal herniations must be ruled out. Endoscopic examination of the stomach also needs to be performed to rule out any anastomotic obstructions. In those patients with a functional gastric outlet obstruction and documented gastroparesis, pharmacotherapy is usually employed. The agents most commonly utilized are prokinetic agents such as metoclopramide and/or erythromycin. Metoclopramide exerts its prokinetic effects by acting as a dopamine antagonist and by cholinergic-enhancing effects as a result of facilitation of acetylcholine release from enteric cholinergic neurons. In contrast, erythromycin markedly accelerates gastric emptying by binding to motilin receptors on gastrointestinal smooth muscle cells, where it acts as a motilin agonist. One of these two agents usually is sufficient to enhance gastric tone and improve gastric emptying.

INCOMPLETE VAGAL TRANSECTION

When performing vagotomy, it is important to denervate the acid secretion portion of the stomach. If not performed properly, it predisposes the patient to the possible development of recurrent ulcer formation. The type of vagotomy performed influences the likelihood of this problem. In highly selective vagotomy, incomplete vagotomy is rarely a problem because of the meticulous dissection required during this procedure. In contrast, truncal vagotomy may be associated with incomplete transection because of the variability in size of the two trunks and their anatomic position. Either vagus nerve may be incompletely transected during truncal vagotomy, although the right vagus nerve is more frequently transected inadequately than the left. In contrast to the left vagus nerve, which usually hugs the anterior esophageal surface, the right vagus nerve is frequently buried in the periesophageal tissue, potentially leading to incomplete transection. Histologic confirmation of vagal transection decreases the incidence of incomplete vagotomy.

STRESS GASTRITIS

Stress gastritis has been referred to as *stress ulcerations, stress erosive gastritis,* and *hemorrhagic gastritis.* These lesions may lead to life-threatening gastric bleeding and by definition occur after physical trauma, shock, sepsis, hemorrhage, respiratory failure, or severe burns. They are characterized by multiple, superficial (nonulcerating) erosions that begin in the proximal or acid-secreting portion of the stomach and progress distally. They may also occur in the setting of central nervous system disease such as that seen with a Cushing ulcer or as a result of thermal burn injury involving more than 30% of the body surface area (Curling ulcer).

Stress gastritis lesions typically change with time. They may be detected within hours following injury and are considered early if they appear within the first 24 hours. These early lesions are typically multiple, shallow, and discrete areas of erythema along with focal hemorrhage or an adherent clot. If the lesion erodes into the submucosa that contains the blood supply, frank bleeding may result. On microscopy, these lesions appear as wedge-shaped mucosal hemorrhages with coagulation necrosis of the superficial mucosal cells. They are almost always seen in the fundus of the stomach and only rarely in the distal stomach. Acute stress gastritis can be classified as late if

there is a tissue reaction, organization around a clot, or an inflammatory exudate. This picture may be seen by microscopy 24 to 72 hours after injury. Late lesions appear identical to those of regenerating mucosa around a healing gastric ulcer. Both types of lesions can be seen endoscopically.

Pathophysiology

Although the precise mechanisms responsible for the development of stress gastritis remain to be fully elucidated, current evidence suggest a multifactorial etiology. These stress-induced gastric lesions appear to require the presence of acid. Other factors that may predispose to the development of these lesions include impaired mucosal defense mechanisms against luminal acid such as a reduction in blood flow, a reduction in mucus, a reduction in bicarbonate secretion by mucosal cells, or a reduction in endogenous prostaglandins. All of these factors render the stomach more susceptible to damage from luminal acid with the resultant hemorrhagic gastritis. "Stress" is considered present when hypoxia, sepsis, or organ failure occurs. When stress is present, mucosal ischemia is thought to be the main factor responsible for the breakdown of these normal defense mechanisms. In this setting, luminal acid is then able to damage the compromised mucosa. There is little evidence to suggest that increased gastric acid secretion occurs in this situation. However, the presence of luminal acid appears to be a prerequisite for this form of gastritis to evolve. Moreover, complete neutralization of luminal acid or antisecretory therapy precludes the development of experimental stress gastritis.

The frequency of life-threatening hemorrhage from stress gastritis appears to be diminishing and may be related to improvements in our ability to manage critically ill patients. Consequently, there are few well-designed prospective, randomized control trials to identify risk factors for patients at risk for developing this disease process. With the studies that have been performed with a limited number of patients, other risk factors or predisposing clinical conditions have been identified. These include the presence of adult respiratory syndrome, multiple trauma, major burn over 35% of body surface area, oliguric renal failure, large transfusion requirements, hepatic dysfunction, hypotension, prolonged surgical procedures, and sepsis from any source. A direct correlation has also been identified between acute upper gastrointestinal hemorrhage and the severity of the underlying critical illness.

Most studies probably underestimate the true incidence of stress gastritis unless endoscopy is performed because at least one study has shown that gastric erosions are present in almost every patient with a life-threatening injury. The major predisposing condition appears to be sepsis. Major thermal burns also significantly increase the risk for development of stress gastritis. In severely burned patients, one study demonstrated that gastric erosions are present in 93% of these patients on endoscopy but that the occurrence of severe acute upper gastrointestinal hemorrhage was around 25% to 50%.

Presentation and Diagnosis

More than 50% of patients develop their stress gastritis within 1 to 2 days following a traumatic event. The only clinical sign may be painless upper gastrointestinal bleeding that may be delayed at onset. The bleeding is usually slow and intermittent and may be detected by only a few flecks of blood in the nasogastric tube or an unexplained drop in the hemoglobin. On occasion, there may be profound upper gastrointestinal hemorrhage that is accompanied by hypotension and hematemesis. The stool is frequently guaiac positive, although melena and hematochezia are rare. Endoscopy is required to confirm the diagnosis and to differentiate stress gastritis from other sources of gastrointestinal hemorrhage. Usually, the bleeding source is correctly identified in more than 90% of cases, as previously discussed in the approach to patients with upper gastrointestinal hemorrhage.

Therapy

Any patient with upper gastrointestinal bleeding requires prompt and definitive fluid resuscitation with correction of any coagulation or platelet abnormalities. If blood is required, then it should be administered without delay, and if there are specific clotting abnormalities or platelet deficiencies, fresh frozen plasma and platelets should likewise be administered. In patients being treated for sepsis, broad-spectrum antibiotics in conjunction with source control of the infection needs to be undertaken. Treatment of the underlying sepsis plays a major role in treating the underlying gastric erosions. Saline lavage of the stomach through a nasogastric tube helps remove any pooled blood and prevents gastric distention that stimulates gastrin release. Nasogastric decompression also removes noxious substances such as bile and pancreatic juice that could potentially further compromise the stomach. More than 80% of patients who present with upper gastrointestinal hemorrhage stop bleeding using this approach. Once the nasogastric tube aspirate is clear, indicating that bleeding has ceased, intraluminal gastric pH should be maintained at greater than 5.0 with antisecretory agents. Usually this involves the utilization of proton-pump inhibitors or, alternatively, H_2-receptor antagonists with or without combination antacid therapy. There is little evidence to suggest that endoscopy with electrocautery or heater probe coagulation has any benefit in the therapy of bleeding from acute stress gastritis. However, some studies suggest that acute bleeding can be effectively controlled by selective infusion of vasopressin into the splanchnic circulation via the left gastric artery. Vasopressin is administered by continuous infusion through the catheter at a rate of 0.2 to 0.4 IU/min for a maximum of 48 to 72 hours. If the patient has underlying cardiac disease or liver disease, vasopressin should not be used. Although vasopressin may decrease blood loss, it has not been shown to result in improved survival. Other angiographic techniques that can be employed include embolization of the left gastric artery if bleeding is identified on angiography. However, the extensive plexus of submucosal arterial vessels within the stomach makes this approach less appealing and not as successful.

Bleeding that recurs or persists requiring more than 6 units of blood (3000 mL) is an indication for operation. Because most of the lesions are in the proximal stomach or fundus, a long anterior gastrotomy should be made in this area. The gastric lumen is cleared of blood, and the mucosal surface is inspected for bleeding points. Bleeding areas are oversewn with figure-of-eight stitches taken deep within the gastric wall. Each actively bleeding site needs to be secured in this way. Most of the superficial erosions are not actively bleeding and therefore do not require ligature unless a blood vessel is seen at its base. The operation is completed by closing the anterior gastrotomy and then performing a truncal vagotomy and pyloroplasty to reduce acid secretion. The incidence of rebleeding is less than 5% if bleeding points are carefully looked for and secured. In contrast, other surgeons prefer a partial gastrectomy in combination with vagotomy. Rarely, and only in patients with life-threatening hemorrhage refractory to other forms of therapy, total gastrectomy may be the only alternative.

Prophylaxis

Because of the high mortality in patients with acute stress gastritis who develop massive upper gastrointestinal hemorrhage, high-risk patients should be treated prophylactically. Because mucosal ischemia may alter a number of mucosal defense mechanisms that then enable the stomach to withstand luminal irritants and protect itself from injury, every effort should be made to correct any perfusion deficits from shock. Sepsis needs to be controlled with antibiotics and source control; ventilatory support needs to be optimized in addition to correcting any systemic acid-base abnormalities or electrolyte abnormalities; and patients require adequate nutrition preferably via the enteral route, which is associated with fewer infectious complications. In addition to optimizing patient care, several medical therapies are available for prophylaxis, and most are aimed at neutralizing or preventing acid secretion. The patients at risk for stress gastritis in the ICU setting appear to be patients with respiratory failure and who have underlying coagulopathy. For patients who do not have coagulopathy or require mechanical ventilation for less than 48 hours, one study suggested that prophylaxis for stress gastritis was unnecessary.[73]

Antacids can be administered as prophylaxis for stress gastritis and have an efficacy of 96%. This usually requires hourly administration of antacids (30 to 60 mL) by nasogastric tube to maintain the intraluminal gastric pH above 3.5. If the pH can be maintained above 5.0, more than 99.9% of acid will be neutralized and pepsin will be inactive. In a review of data collected from 16 prospective trials (2133 patients), 3.7% of patients given antacids had evidence of blood loss versus 17.4% given cimetidine for prophylaxis against stress gastritis and 27.3% for those given placebo. Thus, there appears to be no significant advantage of H_2 blockers over antacids. In fact, most studies have demonstrated that it is easier to maintain a pH greater than 5 with antacids than with standard intermittent doses of H_2-receptor antagonist. However, recent data suggest that continuous infusions of the H_2-receptor antagonists provide more consistent maintenance of intraluminal gastric pH than do standard intermittent infusions. Whether continuous infusion of H_2-receptor antagonists has a better clinical outcome or improves drug safety has yet to be determined. Nevertheless, H_2-receptor antagonists have about a 97% efficacy when used as medical prophylaxis for stress gastritis.

Sucralfate has also been used for prophylaxis against stress gastritis, and, like antacids and H_2-receptor antagonists, is extremely efficacious in the 90% to 97% range. Sucralfate, given 1 g every 6 hours, appears to be just as effective as antacids or cimetidine. This form of prophylaxis has the added effect of allowing the stomach to maintain its normal pH and thus prevent bacterial overgrowth. This latter effect may be beneficial because several studies have suggested that gastric luminal alkalinization predisposes the stomach to bacterial overgrowth and subsequent nosocomial pneumonia. Exogenous prostaglandins have also been utilized as stress gastritis prophylaxis agents, although their efficacy appears to be much less than that of the other agents.

GASTRIC NEOPLASIA

Benign Tumors

Gastric Polyps

Gastric polyps are usually an incidental finding on endoscopy, detected in 2% to 3% of gastroscopic evaluations. Fundic gland polyps constitute 47% of all gastric polyps and have no malignant potential. Typically, they present as multiple 2- to 3-mm sessile lesions in the body and fundus, most commonly in healthy gastric mucosa. Most cases are sporadic but can occur in 53% of patients with familial adenomatous polyposis or Gardner's syndrome. Although the polyps themselves are non-neoplastic, retrospective studies have reported colorectal neoplasms in up to 60% of patients with gastric fundic gland polyps.[74]

Hyperplastic polyps are among the most frequently observed polyps and compose 28% to 75% of all gastric polyps. The lesions are typically less than 1.5 cm in size and arise in a setting of chronic atrophic gastritis 40% to 75% of the time. Most commonly, the chronic atrophic gastritis is secondary to *H. pylori* infection, the treatment of which may result in polyp regression. Although the hyperplastic polyp itself is non-neoplastic, dysplastic changes may occasionally develop in the polyp. Frank adenocarcinoma is detected in 2% of hyperplastic polyps. When detected, endoscopic polypectomy is indicated for histologic examination.

Adenomatous polyps have a distinct risk for malignancy. They account for 10% of all gastric polyps and most commonly are antral, sessile, solitary, and eroded. The adenomas can present as tubular, tubulovillous, or villous. Gastric adenocarcinoma may be found in 21% of cases, with increased risk with larger size and villous histology. Polyps larger than 4 cm in diameter may harbor carcinoma 40% of the time. Focal carcinomas were found in 6% of flat tubular adenomas and 33% of villous and tubulovillous adenomas.[75] Additionally, the presence of gastric adenomas is a marker for increased risk of developing adenocarcinoma in another part of the stomach. Coincident carcinomas have been reported in 8% to 59% of cases.[76] Endoscopic polypectomy is sufficient treatment if the entire polyp is removed and there is no invasive cancer in the specimen. Operative excision is recommended for sessile lesions larger than 2 cm, polyps found to have areas of invasive tumors, or polyps that are symptomatic secondary to pain or bleeding. Due to the increased risk of coincident gastric carcinoma, these patients should be followed closely by serial endoscopies.

Ectopic Pancreas

Ectopic pancreatic tissue arises during embryonal development during the fusion of the dorsal and ventral pancreatic buds. The ectopic pancreatic tissue is implanted in the bowel wall and carried to its final location. The incidence of ectopic pancreatic tissue is 1% to 2% in autopsy series, with 70% of cases occurring in the stomach, duodenum, and jejunum.[77] Most patients with gastric ectopic pancreatic tissue are asymptomatic, whereas others present with symptoms similar to those of peptic ulcer disease. The most common presenting symptoms are abdominal pain (45%), epigastric discomfort (12%), nausea and vomiting (10%), and bleeding (8%). The mass can be visualized on upper gastrointestinal endoscopy; however, tissue diagnosis can be difficult due to the submucosal location of the rests. Endoscopic ultrasonography (EUS) can be a useful adjunct for diagnosis as well as for guided biopsy. Pancreatic rests that cause symptoms are treated by surgical excision.

Malignant Tumors

Adenocarcinoma

EPIDEMIOLOGY

Gastric carcinoma was the most common cancer worldwide in the 1980s and is now surpassed only by lung cancer in incidence. There is substantial geographic variation in the incidence of gastric carcinoma internationally, with higher rates in Japan and some parts of South America and lower rates in Western Europe and the United States.

Gastric cancer is the 10th most common cancer in the United States, the incidence of which has been decreasing over the last 70 years. It is estimated that 22,000 patients will develop the disease each year and 13,000 of those will die. Gastric cancer in the United States is twice as common in men as it is in women (11 cases per 100,000 vs. 5 cases per 100,000, respectively), and the incidence is higher among U.S. black men than white men (17.5 vs. 10 cases, respectively, per 100,000).[78] The incidence also increases with age, peaking in the 7th decade. Studies of migrant populations from areas of high incidence to areas of low incidence suggest that environmental exposure as well as other cultural or genetic factors influences the predisposition to gastric cancer. The risk of gastric cancer in individuals who migrated from the highest risk areas in Japan persisted even when they adopted a Western diet. However, offspring who adopted a Western-style diet had a markedly decreased risk.

There has been a noticeable shift in the site of gastric cancer from the distal stomach to the more proximal stomach over the past several decades. The incidence of adenocarcinoma of the gastric cardia has increased steadily while the incidence of cancer in other anatomic subsites has decreased. The increase was most noticeable for white men and is possibly linked to a history of smoking or heavy alcohol use.

RISK FACTORS

Most epidemiologic studies investigating the role of diet in relation to the development of gastric cancer associate diets low in animal protein and fat, high in complex carbohydrates, high in salted meats and fish, and high in nitrates or *H. pylori* in drinking water with an increased risk for gastric cancer. It appears the long-term ingestion of nitrates in dried, smoked, and salted food contributes to this increased risk. Nitrates are converted to carcinogenic nitrites by bacteria. Such bacteria may be introduced through consumption of partially decayed foods, a practice that is more common in the lower social economic strata worldwide. Conversely, the consumption of raw vegetables, citrus fruits, and high-fiber breads is associated with a lower risk for gastric cancer. The ascorbic acid and β carotene found in fruits and vegetables act as antioxidants, whereas ascorbic acid can also prevent the conversion of nitrates to nitrites (Box 45-2).

Other factors associated with an increased risk of gastric cancer include low socioeconomic status (except in Japan), cigarette smoking, male gender, and *H. pylori* infection. The presence of IgG antibodies to *H. pylori* in a given population correlates with the local incidence and mortality rates of gastric cancer. Different strains of this organism elicit different levels of antibody response. For example, infection with the *cagA* strain elicits more mucosal inflammation than *cagA*-negative strains and also confers a greater risk for developing gastric cancer.[79] Host genetic factors also tend to play a role in which individuals with *H. pylori* infection will eventually develop gastric cancer. Interleukin-1 gene cluster polymorphisms, which enhance the production of interleukin-1β, are associated with an increased risk of hypochlorhydria induced by *H. pylori* and thus gastric cancer.[80] Therefore, the familial clustering of *H. pylori* infection associated with inherited genetic polymorphisms linked to hypochlorhydria may explain the increase in cancer risk in individuals with a family history of gastric cancer.

Balfour first reported a correlation between prior gastric surgery for benign disease and the subsequent

---

Box 45-2. Factors associated with increased risk of developing stomach cancer

Nutritional

Low fat or protein consumption
Salted meat or fish
High nitrate consumption
High complex-carbohydrate consumption

Environmental

Poor food preparation (smoked, salted)
Lack of refrigeration
Poor drinking water (well water)
Smoking

Social

Low social class

Medical

Prior gastric surgery
Helicobacter pylori infection
Gastric atrophy and gastritis
Adenomatous polyps
Male gender

---

development of gastric cancer in 1922. Subsequent meta-analyses support the conclusion that there is an increased risk for gastric remnant cancer in patients with prior partial gastrectomy. However, the risk is observed only after a latency of 15 years and is increased in patients operated on for gastric but not duodenal ulcers.

Patients with pernicious anemia are also at increased risk for developing gastric cancer. Pernicious anemia is an autoimmune gastritis of the oxyntic mucosa and increases the risk of gastric cancer, as do other types of chronic inflammation. Achlorhydria is the defining feature of this condition because the autoimmune reaction destroys chief and parietal cells. The mucosa becomes very atrophic and develops antral and intestinal metaplasia. The relative risk for a patient with pernicious anemia developing gastric cancer is approximately 2.1 to 5.6.[81]

The presence of gastric polyps can increase a patient's risk of gastric cancer. Hyperplastic polyps, the most common histologic type, are benign. However, their presence is associated with an increased risk of gastric cancer because they form in stomachs with established gastritis, a known risk factor for carcinoma.

Adenomatous polyps carry a distinct risk for the development of malignancy in the polyp. Mucosal atypia is frequent, and progression from dysplasia to carcinoma in situ has been observed. The risk for the development of carcinoma is approximately 10% to 20% and increases with increasing size of the polyp. Endoscopic removal is indicated for pedunculated lesions and is sufficient if the polyp is completely removed and there are no foci of invasive cancer on histologic examination. If the polyp is larger than 2 cm or sessile or has a proven focus of invasive carcinoma, then operative excision is warranted.

Recently, several genetic alterations have been identified that are associated with gastric adenocarcinoma. These changes can be classified as the activation of oncogenes, the inactivation of tumor suppressor genes, the reduction of cellular adhesion, the reactivation of telomerase, and the presence of microsatellite instability. The c-*met* protooncogene is the receptor for the hepatocyte growth factor and is frequently overexpressed in gastric cancer as are the k-*sam* and c-*erbB2* oncogenes. The inactivation of the tumor suppressor genes *p53* and *p16* have been reported in both diffuse and intestinal-type cancers, whereas adenomatous polyposis coli (*APC*) gene mutations tend to be more frequent in intestinal type gastric cancers. Additionally, a reduction or loss in the cell adhesion molecule E-cadherin can be found in approximately 50% of diffuse-type gastric cancers.[82] Microsatellite instability can be found in approximately 20% to 30% of intestinal-type gastric cancer. Microsatellites are lengths of DNA in which a short (1- to 5-nucleotide) motif is repeated several times. Microsatellite instability reflects a gain or loss of repeat units in a germline microsatellite allele, indicating the clonal expansion that is typical of a neoplasm.

PATHOLOGY

Ninety-five percent of all malignant gastric neoplasms are adenocarcinomas. Other histologic types include squamous cell carcinoma, adenoacanthoma, carcinoid tumors, gastrointestinal stromal tumors (GISTs), and lymphoma. Numerous pathologic classification schemes of gastric cancer have been proposed. The Borrmann classification system was developed in 1926 and remains useful today for the description of endoscopic findings. The Borrmann system divides gastric carcinoma into five types depending on the lesion's macroscopic appearance. Borrmann type I represents polypoid or fungating lesions; type II ulcerating lesions surrounded by elevated borders; type III represents ulcerating lesions with infiltration into the gastric wall; type IV are diffusely infiltrating lesions; and type V are lesions that do not fit into any of the other categories (Fig. 45-16). *Linitis plastica* is the term to describe type IV carcinoma when it involves the entire stomach. The original histologic classification system was developed by Borders in 1942. Borders classified gastric carcinomas according to the degree of cellular differentiation, independent of morphology, and ranged from 1 (well differentiated) to 4 (anaplastic). Many other classification systems have been proposed; however, the most useful and widely used system remains the one proposed by Lauren in 1965. The Lauren system separates gastric adenocarcinoma into intestinal or diffuse types based on histology. This schema characterizes two varieties of gastric adenocarcinoma that manifest different pathology, epidemiology, pathogenesis, and prognosis (Table 45-2). The intestinal variant typically arises in the setting of a recognizable precancerous condition such as gastric atrophy or intestinal metaplasia. Men are more commonly affected than women, and the incidence of the intestinal type gastric adenocarcinoma increases with age. The intestinal type is also the dominant histology in areas

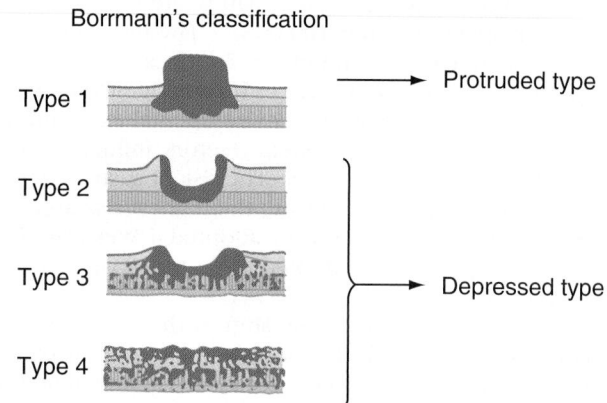

Borrmann's classification

FIGURE 45-16. Borrmann's pathologic classification of gastric cancer based on gross appearance. (From Iriyama K, Asakawa T, Koike H, et al: Is extensive lymphadenectomy necessary for surgical treatment of intramucosal carcinoma of the stomach? Arch Surg 124:309, 1989.)

TABLE 45-2.   Lauren Classification System

Intestinal	Diffuse

Environmental
    Gastric atrophy, intestinal
    metaplasia
	Familial
	    Blood type A

Men > women
    Increasing incidence with age
	Women > men
	    Younger age group

Gland formation	Poorly differentiated, signet ring cells
Hematogenous spread	Transmural/lymphatic spread
Microsatellite instability	Decreased E-cadherin
APC gene mutations	
p53, *p16* inactivation	*p53*, *p16* inactivation

APC, adenomatous polyposis coli.

in which gastric cancer is epidemic, suggesting an environmental etiology. Correa and colleagues proposed a model for the pathogenesis of the intestinal type that is based on progression from gastritis to carcinoma over the course of several decades (Fig. 45-17). The intestinal variety is well differentiated with a tendency to form glands. Metastatic spread is generally hematogenous to distant organs.

The diffuse form of gastric adenocarcinoma is poorly differentiated, lacks gland formation, and is composed of signet ring cells. The diffuse variant consists of tiny clusters of small uniform cells, tends to spread submucosally, has less inflammatory infiltration, and metastasizes early. The route of spread is generally by transmural extension and through lymphatic invasion. The diffuse form does not generally arise in the setting of prior gastritis, is more common in women and affects a slightly younger age group. The diffuse form also has an association with blood type A and familial occurrences, suggesting a genetic eti-

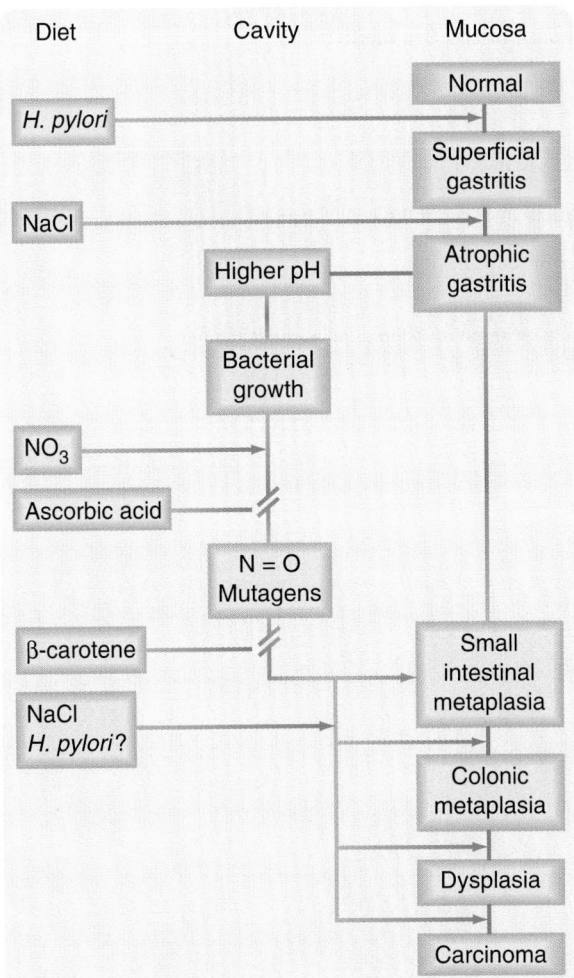

Diet	Cavity	Mucosa
		Normal
H. pylori		Superficial gastritis
NaCl		Atrophic gastritis
	Higher pH	
	Bacterial growth	
NO₃		
Ascorbic acid		
	N = O Mutagens	
β-carotene		Small intestinal metaplasia
NaCl H. pylori?		Colonic metaplasia
		Dysplasia
		Carcinoma

FIGURE 45-17. Correa mode of the pathogenesis of human gastric adenocarcinoma. (From Corrrea P: Human gastric carcinogenesis: A multistep and multifactoral process—First Cancer Society Award Lecture on Cancer Epidemiology and Prevention. Cancer Res 52:6735, 1992.)

ology. Intraperitoneal metastases are frequent, and in general the prognosis is less favorable for patients with diffuse-subtype histology.

In 1990, the World Health Organization (WHO) recommended another classification system for gastric cancers that is based on morphologic features.[83] In the WHO system, gastric cancer is divided into five main categories: adenocarcinoma, adenosquamous cell carcinoma, squamous cell carcinoma, undifferentiated carcinoma, and unclassified carcinoma. Adenocarcinomas are further subdivided into four types according to their growth pattern: papillary, tubular, mucinous, and signet ring. Each type is further subdivided by degree of differentiation. Although widely used, the WHO classification system offers little in terms of patient management, and there are a significant number of gastric cancers that do not fit into these categories. There is little evidence that any of the classification systems mentioned earlier can add to the prognostic information provided by the American Joint Commission on Cancer (AJCC) tumor node metastases (TNM) staging system (Table 45-3).

CLINICAL PRESENTATION

Gastric adenocarcinoma lacks specific symptoms early in the course of the disease. Patients often ignore early vague epigastric discomfort and indigestion, which are often mistaken for gastritis, leading to symptomatic treatment for 6 to 12 months before diagnostic studies are ordered. The epigastric pain is similar to pain caused by benign ulcers and similarly may mimic angina. Typically, however, the pain is constant, nonradiating, and unrelieved by food ingestion. More advanced disease may present with weight loss, anorexia, fatigue, or vomiting. Symptoms often reflect the site of origin of the tumor. Proximal tumors involving the GE junction often present with dysphagia, whereas distal antral tumors may present as gastric outlet obstruction. Diffuse mural involvement by tumor, as occurs in linitis plastica, leads to decreased distensibility of the stomach and complaints of early satiety. Clinically significant gastrointestinal bleeding is rare, but as many as 15% of patients may develop hematemesis and 40% of patients are anemic. Very large tumors may erode through the stomach and into the transverse colon, presenting as large bowel obstruction.

Physical signs develop late in the course of the disease and are most commonly associated with locally advanced or metastatic disease. Patients may present with a palpable abdominal mass, a palpable supraclavicular (Virchow's) or periumbilical (Sister Mary Joseph's) lymph node, peritoneal metastasis palpable by rectal examination (Blumer's shelf), or a palpable ovarian mass (Krukenberg's tumor). As the disease progresses, patients may develop hepatomegaly secondary to metastasis, jaundice, ascites, and cachexia.

PREOPERATIVE EVALUATION

Once gastric cancer is suspected based on history and physical examination, flexible upper endoscopy is the diagnostic modality of choice. Although double-contrast barium upper gastrointestinal radiology is cost effective with 90% diagnostic accuracy, the inability to distinguish benign from malignant gastric ulcers makes endoscopy preferable. During endoscopy, multiple biopsies (seven or more) should be obtained around the ulcer crater to facilitate histologic diagnosis. Biopsy of the ulcer crater itself may reveal only necrotic debris. If multiple biopsies are taken, the diagnostic accuracy of the procedure approaches 98%. The addition of direct-brush cytology to multiple biopsies may increase the diagnostic accuracy of the study. Additionally, the size, location, and morphology of the tumor should be noted, and other mucosal abnormalities should be carefully evaluated. In select patients with advanced disease, esophagogastroduodenoscopy provides a means for palliation through the use of laser ablation, dilation, or tumor stenting. Although EUS is not included in the National Comprehensive Cancer Network guidelines for the evaluation of gastric adenocarcinoma, some centers are using this procedure to assist in the staging of this disease. EUS can gauge the extent of gastric wall invasion as well as evaluate local nodal status. However, EUS cannot reliably distinguish tumor from fibrosis; therefore, it is not a good modality for evaluating

TABLE 45-3.   TNM Classification of Carcinoma of the Stomach

Category	Criteria
PRIMARY TUMOR (T)	
TX	Primary tumor cannot be assessed
T0	No evidence of primary tumor
Tis	Carcinoma in situ: intraepithelial tumor without invasion of the lamina propria
T1	Tumor invades lamina propria or submucosa
T2	Tumor invades muscularis propria or subserosa
T2a	Tumor invades muscularis propria
T2b	Tumor invades subserosa
T3	Tumor penetrates serosa (visceral peritoneum) without invasion of adjacent structures
T4	Tumor invades adjacent structures
REGIONAL LYMPH NODES (N)	
NX	Regional lymph node(s) cannot be assessed
N0	No regional lymph node metastasis
N1	Metastasis in 1 to 6 regional lymph nodes
N2	Metastasis in 7 to 15 regional lymph nodes
N3	Metastasis in more than 15 regional lymph nodes
DISTANT METASTASIS (M)	
MX	Distant metastasis cannot be assessed
M0	No distant metastasis
M1	Distant metastasis

STAGE GROUPING

Stage 0	Tis	N0	M0
Stage 1A	T1	N0	M0
Stage IB	T1	N1	M0
	T2a/b	N0	M0
Stage II	T1	N2	M0
	T2a/b	N1	M0
	T3	N0	M0
Stage IIIA	T2a/b	N2	M0
	T3	N1	M0
	T4	N0	M0
Stage IIIB	T3	N2	M0
Stage IV	T4	N1–3	M0
	T1–3	N3	M0
	Any T	Any N	M1

From AJCC Cancer Staging Manual, 6th ed. New York, Springer-Verlag, 2001.

response to therapy. Overall, staging accuracy with EUS is about 75%. Correct assignment of tumor stage by EUS is poor for AJCC (see Table 45-3) T2 lesions (38%) but better for T1 (80%) and T3 (90%) lesions. Overall accuracy of nodal staging is 77%.[84] Although the accuracy of nodal staging can be improved by fine-needle aspiration biopsy, the application of this technique is limited by technical challenges. Because of these limitations, the use of EUS in the evaluation of gastric cancer is largely confined to regional referral centers.

Once the diagnosis of gastric cancer is confirmed, further studies should include a complete blood count, serum chemistries to include liver function tests, coagulation studies, chest radiograph, and CT scan of the abdomen. In women, a pelvic CT scan or ultrasound is also recommended. CT of the chest may be needed for proximal gastric cancers. CT can readily detect the presence of visceral metastatic disease as well as malignant ascites. The major limitations of CT are in the evaluation of early gastric primaries and in the detection of small (<5 mm) metastases in the liver or on peritoneal surfaces.

The reported accuracy for CT staging of lymph node metastasis ranges from 25% to 86%.[85,86]

Due to the inaccuracy of CT and other modalities for the detection of 5 mm or smaller macrometastases on the peritoneal surface or liver, laparoscopy is recommended as the next step in the evaluation of patients with locoregional disease. Laparoscopy can detect metastatic disease in 23% to 37% of patients judged to be eligible for potentially curative resection by current-generation CT scanning.[87,88] In a combined series between M. D. Anderson Cancer Center and Memorial Sloan-Kettering Cancer Center of 40 patients with distant disease detected by staging laparoscopy, only one patient later presented in need of a palliative procedure. Therefore, given the infrequent occurrence of life-threatening hemorrhage or complete gastric outlet obstruction in the presence of stage IV gastric cancer, laparoscopy improves palliation by avoiding nontherapeutic laparotomy in approximately one fourth of patients presumed to have localized gastric cancer. The addition of laparoscopic ultrasonography may increase the sensitivity of laparoscopic staging in gastric cancer as it has in other abdominal malignancies. However, given the limitations of the available data and the operator-dependent nature of the technique, further investigation is required to define its role in the staging of gastric cancer.

Cytologic analysis of peritoneal fluid or of fluid obtained by peritoneal lavage may reveal the presence of free intraperitoneal gastric cancer cells, identifying patients with otherwise occult carcinomatosis. Patients with positive findings on peritoneal cytology have a poor prognosis, similar to that of patients with macroscopic stage IV disease. However, false-positive results can be obtained, and not all studies confirm the prognostic significance of positive findings. More sensitive methods of detecting free intraperitoneal gastric cancer cells such as immunostaining and reverse-transcriptase polymerase chain reaction for carcinoembryonic antigen messenger RNA are under investigation.

STAGING

Many staging systems have been proposed for gastric adenocarcinoma. A basic understanding of the older systems is necessary to understand the literature. The pathologic staging system currently in use worldwide is the AJCC TNM staging system (see Table 45-3). T, N, and M stand for tumor, nodes, and metastasis, respectively, and are based on depth of primary tumor invasion through the gastric wall (Fig. 45-18), the number of involved lymph nodes, and the presence or absence of distant metastasis. The TNM system can adequately stratify patients into distinct groups with different risks for tumor-related death. A major revision occurred in the AJCC staging system for gastric cancer in 1997 when nodal status stratification was changed from location of nodes to number of positive

nodes. In the current staging system, a minimum of 15 nodes must be evaluated for accurate staging. Nodal staging is then determined by the number of positive nodes, with pN1 reflecting 1 to 6 positive nodes, pN2 7 to 15 positive nodes, and pN3 more than 15 positive nodes. Some data suggest location of the primary (cardia compared to distal tumors) may independently predict survival. However, the current AJCC staging system does not reflect the poorer prognosis for proximal gastric tumors seen in some studies.

The term *R status* was first described by Hermanek in 1994 and is used to describe the tumor status after resection. The term *R0* describes a microscopically margin negative resection, in which no gross or microscopic tumor remains in the tumor bed. *R1* indicates removal of all macroscopic disease but microscopic margins are positive for tumor. *R2* indicates gross residual disease. As the extent of resection can influence survival, some authors include this R designation to complement the TNM system. Long-term survival can be expected only after an R0 resection; therefore, a significant effort should be made to avoid R1 or R2 resections. Knowledge of the older staging systems and the Japanese system is crucial to the understanding of the debate regarding lymphadenectomies for gastric cancer. In the previous edition of Union Internationale Contre le Cancer (UICC) TNM system, N categories were defined by the location of lymph node metastases relative to the primary. In 1982, UICC and AJCC agreed to define pN1 as 3 cm or less from the primary and pN2 as greater than 3 cm from the primary or nodal metastases along named blood vessels. The Japanese Classification for Gastric Carcinoma (JCGC) staging system was designed to describe the anatomic locations of nodes removed during gastrectomy. Sixteen distinct anatomic locations of lymph nodes are described (Fig.

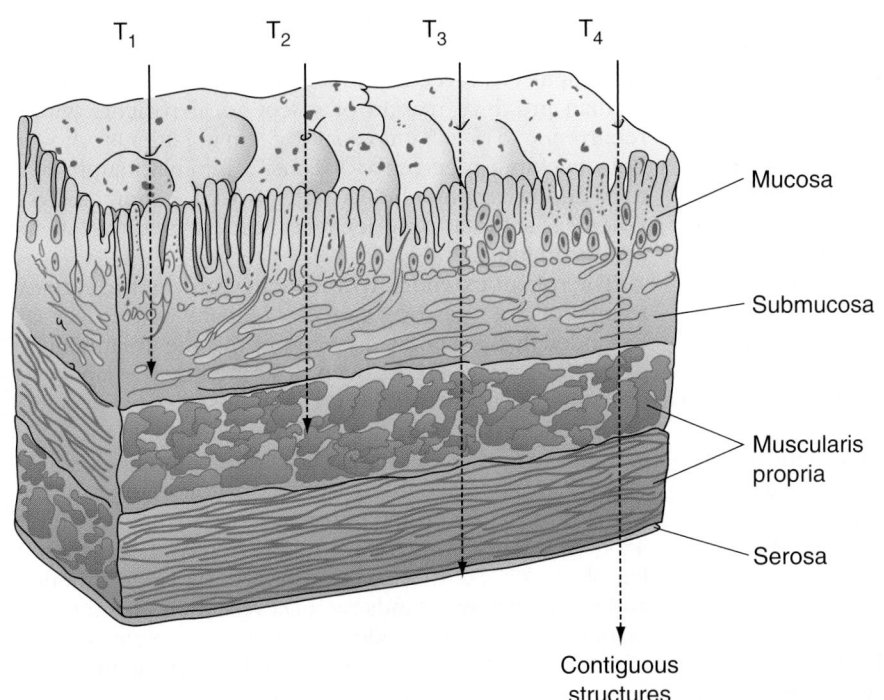

FIGURE 45-18. T stage as defined by depth of penetration into the gastric wall. (From Alexander HR, Kelsen DG, Tepper JC: Cancer of the stomach. In De Vita VT, Hellman S, Rosenberg SA [eds]: Cancer: Principles and Practice of Oncology, 5th ed. Philadelphia, Lippincott-Raven, 1997.)

Mucosa

Submucosa

Muscularis propria

Serosa

Contiguous structures

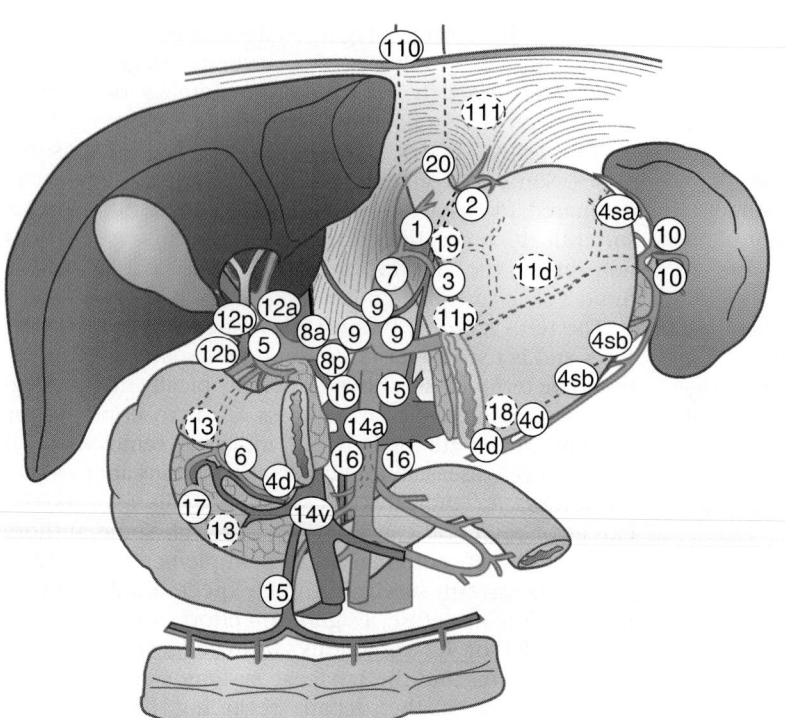

FIGURE 45-19. Lymph node station numbers as defined by the Japanese Gastric Cancer Association. (From Japanese Gastric Cancer Association: Japanese Classification of Gastric Carcinoma—2nd English Edition. Gastric Cancer 1:10-24, 1998.)

45-19), with the recommendation for nodal basin dissection dependent on the location of the primary. The lymph node stations or "echelons" are numbered and then further classified into groups of echelons that correspond to the location of the primary and reflect the likelihood of harboring metastases (Table 45-4). The presence of metastasis to each lymph node group then determines the N classification. For example, metastases to any of the group 1 lymph nodes in the absence of disease in more distant lymph node groups are classified as N1.

SURGICAL TREATMENT

The optimal surgical management of gastric cancer must be tailored to the extent and location of disease. In the absence of distant metastatic spread, aggressive surgical resection of the gastric tumor is justified. The extent of gastric resection is determined by the need to obtain a resection margin free of microscopic disease. Because gastric tumors are characterized by extensive intramural spread, a line of resection at least 6 cm from the tumor mass is necessary to ensure a low rate of anastomotic recurrence. The appropriate surgical procedure should be determined by the location of the tumor and the known pattern of spread.

Tumors of the cardia and proximal stomach account for 35% to 50% of all gastric adenocarcinomas. In general, proximal tumors are more advanced on presentation than more distant tumors, so curative resections are rare. For proximal lesions, either total gastrectomy (Fig. 45-20A) or proximal gastric resection is necessary to remove the tumor. Although there is no evidence that one operation is better than the other for tumor removal, there is abundant evidence that proximal gastric resection results in higher morbidity and mortality than total gastrectomy. In a series by Buhl and colleagues, patients with a proximal

gastric resection had higher incidences of dumping, heartburn, and reduced appetite than patients treated with distal or total gastrectomy.[89] In the Norwegian Stomach Cancer Trial, the incidence of morbidity and mortality following proximal gastric resections was 52% and 16%, respectively, compared to 38% and 8% for total gastrectomy.[90] Thus, total gastrectomy should be considered the procedure of choice for proximal gastric lesions. Distal tumors account for approximately 35% of all gastric cancers. Since recent studies have indicated no difference in 5-year survival between patients undergoing potentially curative subtotal versus total gastrectomy, subtotal gastrectomy is appropriate for patients in whom a negative margin resection can be performed (Fig. 45-20B). Studies on patients with recurrent gastric cancer have noted the median proximal margin of resection in patients with a recurrence to be 3.5 cm versus 6.5 cm in patients who did not develop a recurrence.[91] Thus, a luminal margin of 5 to 6 cm is recommended with frozen-section analysis when a subtotal gastric resection is performed for adenocarcinoma.

The role of extended lymphadenectomy in the surgical treatment of gastric cancer remains controversial. Extended lymph node dissections for the treatment of gastric cancer have best been described by the Japanese, and subsequently the JCGC D categories are used to define the extent of lymphatic dissection performed. In the JCGC system, lymph node basins are numbered and subsequently grouped according to the location of the primary. The groupings according to primary site are listed in Table 45-4. A *D1* resection refers to the removal of group 1 lymph nodes, *D2* to dissection of groups 1 and 2 nodes, and a *D3* resection stands for a D2 resection plus removal of para-aortic lymph nodes. To effect complete removal of station 10 (parasplenic) and station 11 (parapancreatic) nodes, Japanese surgeons perform splenectomy and

TABLE 45-4. Grouping of Regional Lymph Nodes (Groups 1–3) by Location of Primary Tumor According to the Japanese Classification of Gastric Carcinoma[11]

Lymph Node Station (No.)	Description	Location of Primary Tumor in Stomach		
		Upper Third	Middle Third	Lower Third
1	Rt. paracardial	1	1	2
2	Lt. paracardial	1	3	M
3	Lesser curvature	1	1	1
4sa	Short gastric	1	3	M
4sb	Lt. gastroepiploic	1	1	3
4d	Rt. gastroepiploic	2	1	1
5	Suprapyloric	3	1	1
6	Infrapyloric	3	1	1
7	Lt. gastric artery	2	2	2
8a	Ant. comm. hepatic	2	2	2
8p	Post. comm. hepatic	3	3	3
9	Celiac artery	2	2	2
10	Splenic hilum	2	3	M
11p	Proximal splenic	2	2	2
11d	Distal splenic	2	3	M
12a	Lt. hepatoduodenal	3	2	2
12b,p	Post. hepatoduodenal	3	3	3
13	Retropancreatic	M	3	3
14v	Sup. mesenteric v.	M	3	2
14a	Sup. mesenteric a.	M	M	M
15	Middle colic	M	M	M
16a1	Aortic hiatus	M	M	M
16a2,b1	Para-aortic, middle	3	3	3
16b2	Para-aortic, caudal	M	M	M

a., artery; ant., anterior; lt., left; M, lymph nodes regarded as distant metastasis; post., posterior; rt., right; sup., superior; v., vein.

partial pancreatectomy during D2 resections for primaries whose drainage includes these echelons. Because of the increased morbidity in the patients receiving these adjunctive resections, Western surgeons do not typically resect the spleen or pancreas unless it is involved by direct extension from a T4 tumor.

Splenectomy is no longer advocated as a routine adjunctive procedure to gastrectomy for cancer. The purpose of splenectomy in gastric cancer, aside from managing direct tumor extension, is for removal of lymph nodes at the splenic hilus (station 10) as a part of an extended lymph node resection (D2) for proximal gastric cancer. However, multivariate analysis in the Dutch trial comparing D1 versus D2 resections for gastric cancer indicated that splenectomy carried a major risk for hospital death (hazard ratio 2.16) and overall complications (hazard ratio 2.13).[92] It is clear that any extended resection is accompanied by an increase in morbidity and mortality without an improvement in survival. Thus, local

organ resection, especially of the spleen, pancreas, or transverse colon, should be performed only when needed to accomplish an R0 resection.

Extended D2 lymph node dissections are routinely performed in Japan and have been demonstrated in studies performed in that country to provide a survival benefit over more limited D1 dissections. The first evidence of a survival benefit for an extended dissection was in 1981 by Kodama and associates, who reported a 39% 5-year survival rate after a D2 dissection compared to 18% for D1.[93] Many other Japanese studies have confirmed these findings. However, randomized controlled trials in the West of D2 versus D1 dissections for gastric cancer have failed to demonstrate a survival benefit for the extended dissections. The British trial reported an elevated postoperative morbidity (28% for D1 and 46% for D2) and mortality (6.5% for D1 and 13% for D2) in the D2 arm without any difference in 5-year survival (35% for D1 and 32% for D2).[94] Similarly, the Dutch trial also observed

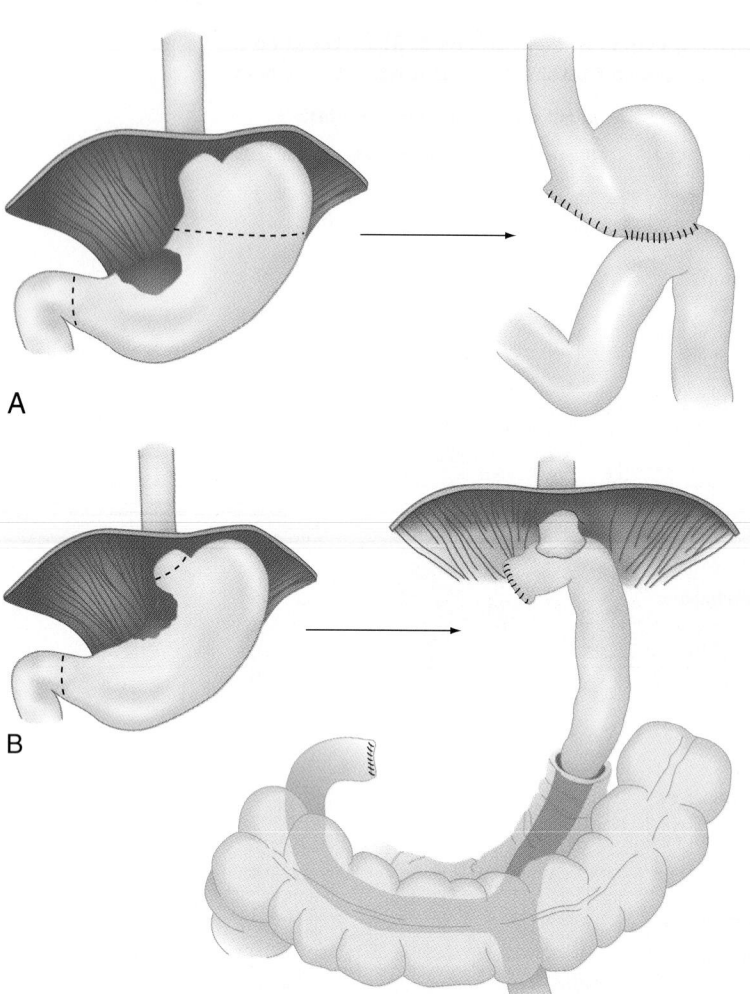

increased morbidity (25% for D1 and 43% for D2) and mortality (6.5% for D1 and 13% for D2) with no survival benefit associated with the extended resection.[92] Extended lymph node dissections for gastric cancer remain an investigational treatment option and should be performed at specialized centers in the context of a clinical trial.

PALLIATIVE TREATMENT

Because 20% to 30% of gastric cancer patients present with stage IV disease, clinicians must be familiar with different methods of palliative treatment. The goal of palliative treatment is the relief of symptoms with minimal morbidity. Surgical palliation of advanced gastric cancer may include resection or bypass alone or in conjunction with percutaneous, endoscopic, or radiotherapeutic techniques. Complete staging is necessary to determine the appropriate method of palliation for individual patients. In the presence of peritoneal disease, hepatic metastases, diffuse nodal metastases, or ascites, palliation of bleeding or proximal gastric obstruction would preferably be obtained nonoperatively. Nonoperative therapies include laser recanalization and endoscopic dilation, with or without stent placement. Patients who undergo stent placement for gastric outlet obstruction are frequently able to tolerate solid foods and may not require additional interventions.

ADJUVANT THERAPY

In a 1999 review of the National Cancer Database by Hundahl and colleagues, it was reported that only 29% of patients undergoing gastrectomy for gastric adenocarcinoma received some type of adjuvant treatment, whereas 71% were treated by surgery alone.[95] These practice trends reflected the lack of convincing data to support the use of chemotherapy or radiation therapy in the management of gastric adenocarcinoma. However, many investigators believe the standard of care has changed on the basis of the Southwest Cancer Oncology Group trial (INT-00116). This trial evaluated two cycles of 5-fluorouracil and leucovorin with subsequent concurrent chemotherapy and radiation therapy, using the same chemotherapeutic agents, as adjuncts following an R0 resection of gastric adenocarcinoma. The median survival for the surgery-only arm was 27 months compared to 36 months ($P = 0.005$) for the chemotherapy and radiation therapy group. The three-year survival rates were 41% in the surgery-only group compared to 50% in the chemotherapy and radiation therapy group ($P = 0.005$).[96] These data would support the addition of postoperative chemoradiation to the treatment of patients with resectable gastric adenocarcinoma.

Neoadjuvant chemotherapy is currently under investigation and has yielded some promising results. A few studies have demonstrated acceptable toxicities, with an increased number of patients completing all planned therapy and undergoing R0 resections compared to historical controls.

OUTCOMES

Overall, 5-year survival after the diagnosis of gastric cancer is 10% to 21%. Stage-stratified 5-year survival rates for all patients and those undergoing surgical excision are depicted in Figures 45-21 and 45-22. Patients who undergo a potentially curative resection have a better prognosis, with a 5-year survival rate of 24% to 57%.

Recurrence rates after gastrectomy remain high, ranging from 40% to 80%, depending on the series. Most recurrences occur within the first 3 years. The locoregional failure rate ranges from 38% to 45%, whereas peritoneal dissemination as a component of failure occurs in 54% of patients in several series. Isolated distant metastases are uncommon, because most patients with distant failure also have locoregional recurrence as well. The most common sites of locoregional recurrence are the gastric remnant at the anastomosis and in the gastric bed

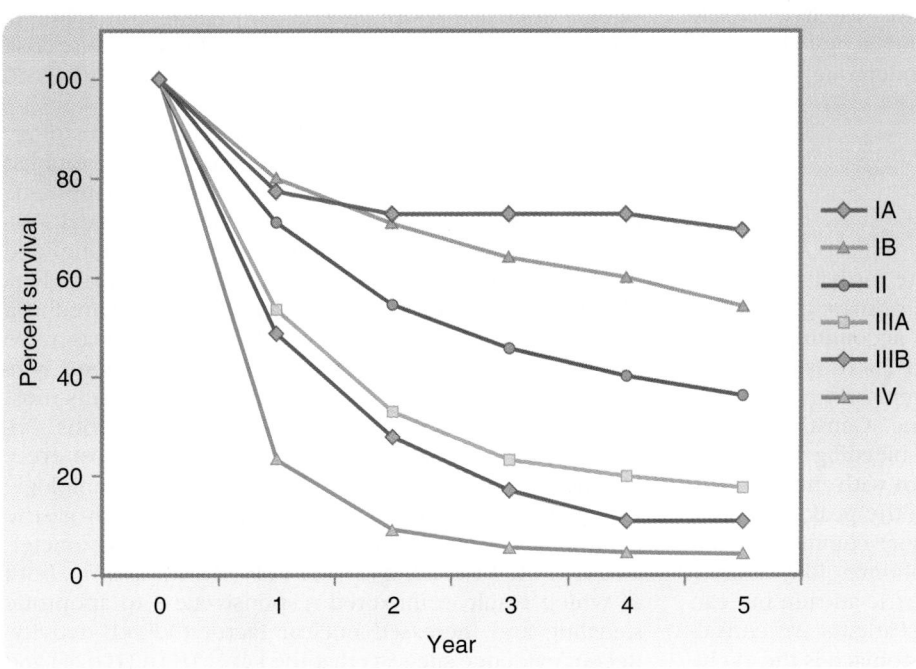

FIGURE 45-21. Survival rates for all patients with gastric carcinoma stratified by combined American Joint Committee on Cancer (AJCC), 5th edition, stage.

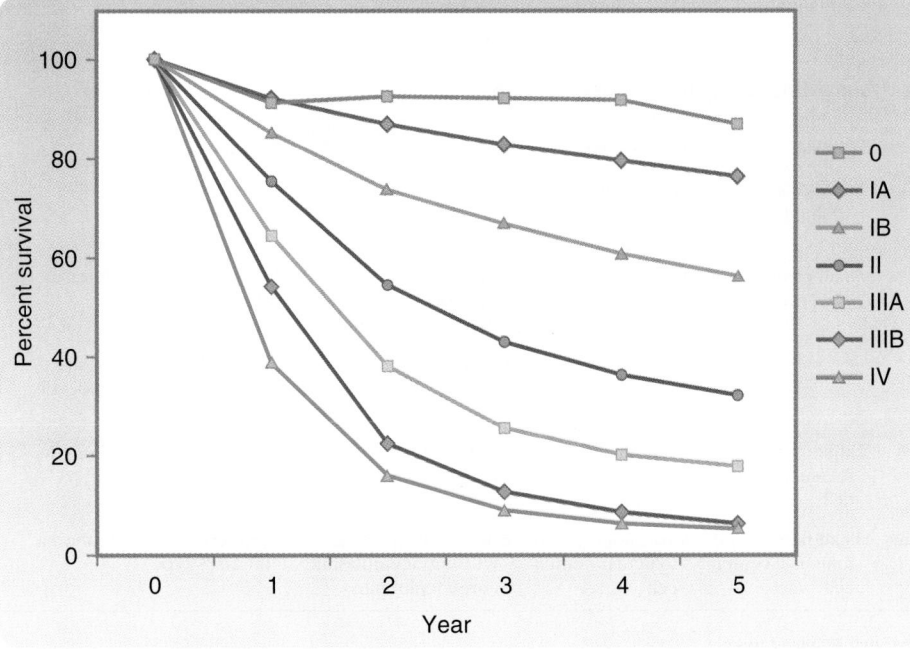

FIGURE 45-22. Survival rates for gastric cancer patients undergoing gastrectomy as stratified by combined American Joint Committee on Cancer (AJCC), 5th edition, stage.

and the regional nodes. Hematogenous spread occurs to the liver, lung, and bone.

SURVEILLANCE

All patients should be followed up systematically. Because most recurrences occur within the first 3 years, surveillance examinations are more frequent in the first several years. Follow-up should include a complete history and physical examination every 4 months for 1 year, then every 6 months for 2 years and then annually thereafter. Laboratory examinations including complete blood counts and liver function tests should be obtained as clinically indicated. Many clinicians obtain chest radiographs as well as CT scans of the abdomen and pelvis routinely, whereas others obtain studies only when clinically suspicious of a recurrence. Yearly endoscopy should be considered in patients who have undergone a subtotal gastrectomy.

Gastric Lymphoma

EPIDEMIOLOGY

The stomach is the most common site for lymphomas in the gastrointestinal system. However, primary gastric lymphoma is still relatively uncommon, accounting for less than 15% of gastric malignancies and 2% of lymphomas. Patients often present with vague symptoms, namely epigastric pain, early satiety, and fatigue. Constitutional B symptoms are rare. Although overt bleeding is uncommon, more than half of patients present with anemia. Lymphomas occur in older patients, with the peak incidence in the 6th and 7th decades, and are more common in men (male:female ratio, 2:1). Gastric lymphomas, like carcinomas, most commonly occur in the gastric antrum but can arise from any part of the stomach. Patients are considered to have gastric lymphoma if the stomach is the exclusive or predominant site of disease.

PATHOLOGY

In the management of gastric lymphomas, as in the management of nodal lymphomas, it is important to determine not only the stage of disease but also the subtype of lymphoma. There are multiple classification systems for lymphomas (Table 45-5). The most common gastric lymphoma is diffuse large B-cell lymphoma (55%) followed by extranodal marginal cell lymphoma (MALT) (40%), Burkitt's lymphoma (3%), and mantle cell and follicular lymphomas (each < 1%).

Diffuse large B-cell lymphomas most commonly are primary lesions; however, they may also occur from progression of less aggressive lymphomas such as chronic lymphocytic leukemia/small lymphocytic lymphoma, follicular lymphoma, or MALT lymphoma. Immunodeficiencies as well as H. pylori infection are risk factors for the development of primary diffuse large B-cell lymphoma.

In 1983, Isaacson and Wright noted that the histology of primary low-grade gastric B-cell lymphoma resembled that of MALT.[97] Subsequently, the MALT lymphoma concept was extended to include other extranodal low-grade B-cell lymphomas of the salivary gland, lung, and thyroid. These organs lack native lymphoid tissue; the lymphomas at these sites arise from the MALT acquired as a result of chronic inflammation. MALT lymphomas were recently reclassified as "extranodal marginal zone lymphomas of MALT type." Gastric MALT lymphoma is most commonly preceded by H. pylori–associated gastritis. Evidence of H. pylori infection can be found in almost every instance of gastric MALT lymphoma. Epidemiologic studies have also linked H. pylori infection with gastric lymphomas. Genetically, MALT lymphoma is characterized by t (1; 14)(p22; q32) and t (11; 18)(q21; q21), both of which result in impaired responsiveness to apoptotic signaling and increased nuclear factor (NF)-κB activity. Recent evidence suggests that the t (11; 18)(q21; q21) and B-cell lymphoma/leukemia 10 (Bcl-10) nuclear expression

---

TABLE 45-5.   Comparison of Gastrointestinal Lymphoma Classifications

WHO Classification	REAL	Working	Lukes-Collins	Kiel	Rappaport
Extranodal marginal zone lymphoma (MALT lymphoma)	—	Small cleaved cell type	Small cleaved cell type	Immunocytoma	Well-differentiated lymphocytic
Follicular lymphoma	Follicular center lymphoma	Small cleaved cell type	Small cleaved cell type	Centroblastic/ centrocytic, follicular and diffuse	Nodular, poorly differentiated lymphocytic
Mantle cell lymphoma	—	—	—	Centrocytic	Intermediately or poorly differentiated lymphocytic, diffuse or nodular
Diffuse large B-cell lymphoma	Diffuse large B-cell lymphoma	Large cleaved follicular center cell	Large cleaved follicular center cell	Centroblastic, B-immunoblastic	Diffuse mixed lymphocytic and histiocytic
Burkitt's lymphoma	Burkitt's lymphoma	Small noncleaved follicular center cell	Small noncleaved follicular center cell	Burkitt's lymphoma with intracytoplasmic immunoglobulin	Undifferentiated lymphoma, Burkitt's type

WHO, World Health Organization; MALT, mucosa-associated lymphoid tissue.

may predict for nonresponsiveness to treatment by *H. pylori* eradication and lymphoma regression.[98]

Burkitt's lymphomas of the stomach are associated with Epstein-Barr virus infections, as they are in other sites. Burkitt's lymphoma is highly aggressive and tends to affect a younger aged population than other types of gastric lymphomas. Burkitt's is most commonly found in the cardia or body of the stomach as opposed to the antrum.

EVALUATION

Endoscopy generally reveals nonspecific gastritis or gastric ulcerations, with mass lesions being unusual. Occasionally, a submucosal growth pattern renders endoscopic biopsies nondiagnostic. EUS is useful to determine the depth of gastric wall invasion, specifically to identify patients at risk for perforation secondary to full-thickness involvement of the gastric wall. Evidence of distant disease should be sought through upper airway examination, bone marrow biopsy, and CT of the chest and abdomen to detect lymphadenopathy. Any enlarged lymph nodes should undergo biopsy. *H. pylori* testing should be performed by histology and, if negative, confirmed by serology.

STAGING

The best staging system remains controversial. When possible, the TNM staging system should be used (with the criteria proposed for gastric carcinoma). Several other staging systems for primary gastric non-Hodgkin's lymphoma are available (Table 45-6).

TREATMENT

Most centers employ a multimodality treatment program for patients with gastric lymphoma. The role of resection in gastric lymphoma remains controversial, and many patients are now being treated with chemotherapy plus radiation therapy alone. The risk of perforation in patients treated with chemotherapy has been overstated in the past and approaches 5%. The most common chemothera-peutic combination is CHOP (cyclophosphamide, hydroxy-daunomycin, Oncovin, prednisone). A prospective, non-randomized study evaluating patients with early-stage (stage IE, IIE) disease demonstrated similar disease-free 5-year survival rates in patients treated with surgery, chemotherapy, and radiation therapy versus chemotherapy and radiation therapy alone (82% vs. 84.4%; NS).[99] Radiation therapy is limited in usefulness for larger tumors, with local control rates dropping from 100% for tumors 3 cm or less to 60% to 70% for tumors larger than 6 cm.[100] Late complications of radiation therapy such as stricture, enteritis, and secondary tumor formation can be significant. The overall risk of severe radiation complications after treatment to 30 Gy for gastrointestinal tumors can approach 30% at 10 years. Thus, treatment should be individualized, with careful consideration given to treating a younger patient with high-dose gastrointestinal radiation.

Patients who present with late-stage disease are not amenable to surgical cure and should be referred for chemotherapy. The diagnosis of lymphoma discovered unexpectedly at operation can be confirmed by frozen section. Additionally, fresh tissue should be sent for fluorescence-activated cell sorting, immunohistochemistry, and genetic analysis. Consideration should be given to performing a bone marrow aspiration at the time of surgery. If isolated stage IE or IIE lymphoma is encountered, surgical removal of all gross disease is ideal. Patients with disseminated lymphoma cannot be cured surgically, and the operation should focus on obtaining enough tissue for diagnosis and repairing perforations.

Recent evidence suggests that early-stage MALT lymphomas as well as some patients with very limited diffuse large B-cell lymphoma may be effectively treated by *H. pylori* eradication alone. Successful eradication resulted in remission in more than 75% of cases. However, careful follow-up is necessary, with repeat endoscopy in 2 months to document clearance of the infection as well as biannual endoscopy for 3 years to document regression. Some patients will continue to demonstrate the lymphoma clone after *H. pylori* eradication, suggesting the lymphoma became dormant rather than disappearing.

TABLE 45-6. Staging Systems for Primary Gastrointestinal Non-Hodgkin's Lymphoma

Ann Arbor*	Rao et al†	Musshoff†	Description	Relative Incidence (%)
IE	IE	IE	Tumor confined to gastrointestinal tract	26
IIE	IIE	IIE	Tumor with spread to regional lymph nodes	26
IIE	IIIE	IIE	Tumor with nodal involvement beyond regional lymph nodes (para-aortic, iliac)	17
IIIE-IV	IVE	IIIE-IV	Tumor with spread to other intra-abdominal organs (liver, spleen) or beyond abdomen (chest, bone marrow)	31

*Carbone PP, Kaplan HS, Musshoff K, et al: Report of the Committee on Hodgkin's Disease Staging Classification. Cancer Res 31:1860-1861, 1971.
†Rao AR, Kagan AR, Kagan AR, et al: Management of gastrointestinal lymphoma. Am J Clin Oncol 7:213-219, 1984.
‡Musshoff K: [Clinical staging classification of non-Hodgkin's lymphomas (author's trans, German)]. Strahlentherapie 153:218-221, 1977.
From Bozzetti F, Audisio RA, Giardini R, Gennari L: Role of surgery in patients with primary non-Hodgkin's lymphoma of the stomach: An old problem revised. Br J Surg 80:1102, 1993.

The presence of transmural tumor extension, nodal involvement, transformation into a large cell phenotype, transformation t (11; 18), or nuclear Bcl-10 expression all predict for failure after *H. pylori* eradication alone. Additionally, a small subset of MALT lymphoma patients will be *H. pylori* negative. In these patients, consideration should be given to surgical resection, radiation therapy, and chemotherapy. Five-year disease-free survival with multimodality treatment is greater than 95% in stage IE and 75% in stage IIE disease.

Gastric Sarcomas

EPIDEMIOLOGY

Gastric sarcomas arise from mesenchymal components of the gastric wall and constitute about 3% of all gastric malignancies. GISTs are the most common mesenchymal tumor of the gastrointestinal tract and are most frequently located in the stomach (60% to 70%). Patients usually present after the 4th decade, with the mean age of 60 years at diagnosis.

PATHOLOGY

Initially thought to arise from smooth muscle cells, GISTs were previously classified as leiomyomas or leiomyosarcomas. Histologically, they appear to arise from the muscularis propria and most likely originate from the cells of Cajal, autonomic nerve–related gastrointestinal pacemaker cells that regulate intestinal motility. GISTs are defined as cellular, spindle cell, or occasionally pleomorphic mesenchymal tumors located in the gastrointestinal tract and express the Kit (CD117, stem cell factor receptor) protein. Kit is a transmembrane tyrosine kinase receptor, the ligand for which is stem cell factor. The Kit protein is detected by immunohistochemistry and can reliably distinguish GISTs from true smooth muscle neoplasms. Most GISTs (70% to 80%) also are positive for CD34, a hematopoietic progenitor cell antigen. Recently, a new activating mutation has been detected in GISTs. A subset of GISTs lack c-*kit* mutations and have intragenic activation mutations in a related tyrosine kinase receptor, platelet-derived growth factor-α.

STAGING

No current staging system exists for GISTs; however, several factors have been identified that correlate with clinical behavior. Tumors that show low mitotic frequency (≤5 mitoses per 50 high-powered fields [HPF]) usually have a benign behavior. Tumors with mitotic counts more than 5 per 50 HPF are considered malignant, and tumors with more than 50 mitoses per 50 HPF are classified as high-grade malignant. Malignancy is also associated with tumors greater than 5 cm in size, cellular atypia, necrosis, or local invasion. C-*kit* mutations occur predominantly in malignant GISTs and are an unfavorable prognostic marker. Most c-*kit* mutations occur in exon 11 and result in activation of c-*kit*. More than 80% of gastric GISTs are classified as benign according to these criteria.

However, many histologically malignant-appearing lesions never metastasize, whereas, rarely, benign-appearing lesions do. Benign gastric GISTs occur more frequently than malignant ones (3 to 5:1). Since GISTs with a low mitotic count and malignant behavior are generally larger, this has led to the designation "uncertain malignant potential" to a significant number of GISTs.

CLINICAL MANIFESTATION/EVALUATION

The most common presentations of gastric GISTs are gastrointestinal bleeding and pain/dyspepsia. Endoscopy may be the first diagnostic test if patients present with bleeding; however, since the neoplasm grows intramurally, the true extent of the tumor can best be assessed with CT. Double-contrast upper gastrointestinal series may show a smooth-edged filling defect. Endoscopic biopsy is diagnostic in approximately 50% of the cases. Percutaneous or endoscopic biopsy should be performed only if the results would obviate the need for surgery.

TREATMENT

The goal of surgery is a margin-negative resection to include en-bloc resection of adjacent organs if involved by direct extension. If at the time of surgical resection the histology is uncertain, a frozen section should be performed because the diagnosis of adenocarcinoma or lymphoma would change the surgical management. Rupture of the tumor should be avoided to prevent inoculation of the peritoneal cavity with tumor cells. Because lymph node metastases are rare (<10%), there is no known added benefit of extended lymphadenectomy. Most recurrences are in the first 2 years, presenting as local disease frequently associated with liver metastases. Other common patterns of failure include peritoneal recurrences. Salvage surgery to resect recurrent disease has not been demonstrated to improve survival. Overall, 5-year survival for gastric GISTs is 48% (19% to 56%), with survival after complete surgical resection ranging from 32% to 63%. Indices that independently predict recurrence include mitotic rate of more than 15 mitoses per 30 HPF, mixed cytomorphology (spindle cell and epithelioid), presence of deletion/insertion c-*kit* exon 11 mutations, and male sex.

Until recently there was no good adjuvant therapy for GISTs. Radiation therapy has not been proven to be effective in their management, and only 5% of tumors respond to doxorubicin-based cytotoxic chemotherapy. Imatinib mesylate (formerly ST1517, now Glivic/Gleevec) is a competitive inhibitor of certain tyrosine kinases, including the kinases associated with the transmembrane receptor Kit and platelet-derived growth factor receptors. Initial studies showed encouraging results, with 54% of patients exhibiting at least a partial response.[101] Imatinib mesylate is approved for use in CD117-positive unresectable and/or metastatic GISTs. Further studies are ongoing, and patients with a diagnosis of GIST should be considered for enrollment in one of the many active clinical trials.

OTHER GASTRIC LESIONS

Hypertrophic Gastritis (Ménétrier's Disease)

Ménétrier's disease (hypoproteinemic hypertrophic gastropathy) is a rare, acquired, premalignant disease characterized by massive gastric folds in the fundus and corpus of the stomach, giving the mucosa a cobblestone or cerebriform appearance. Histologic examination reveals foveolar hyperplasia (expansion of surface mucous cells) with absent parietal cells. The condition is associated with protein loss from the stomach, excessive mucus production as well as hypochlorhydria or achlorhydria. The cause of Ménétrier's disease is unknown but has been associated with cytomegalovirus infection in children and *H. pylori* infection in adults. Additionally, increased transforming growth factor-α has been noted in the gastric mucosa of patients with the disease.[102] Patients often present with epigastric pain, vomiting, weight loss, anorexia, and peripheral edema. Typical gastric mucosal changes can be detected by radiographic or endoscopic examination. Biopsy should be performed to rule out gastric carcinoma or lymphoma. Twenty-four-hour pH monitoring reveals hypochlorhydria or achlorhydria, whereas a chromium-labeled albumin test reveals increased gastrointestinal protein loss. Medical treatment has yielded inconsistent results; however, some benefit has been shown through the use of anticholinergic drugs, acid suppression, octreotide, and *H. pylori* eradication. Total gastrectomy should be performed on patients who continue to have massive protein loss despite optimal medical therapy or if dysplasia or carcinoma develops.

Mallory-Weiss Tear

Mallory-Weiss tears are related to forceful vomiting, retching, coughing, or straining that results in disruption of the gastric mucosa high on the lesser curve at the GE junction. They account for 15% of acute upper gastrointestinal hemorrhages and are rarely associated with massive bleeding. The overall mortality for the lesion is 3% to 4%, with the greatest risk of massive hemorrhage in alcoholic patients with preexisting portal hypertension. Most patients with active bleeding can be managed by endoscopic methods such as multipolar electric coagulation, epinephrine injection, endoscopic band ligation, or endoscopic hemoclipping. Angiographic intra-arterial infusion of vasopressin or transcatheter embolization may be of use in very selective high-risk cases. The need for operative intervention is rare. If surgery is required, the lesion at the GE junction is approached through an anterior gastrotomy and the bleeding site is oversewn with several deep 2-0 silk ligatures to reapproximate the gastric mucosa in an anatomic fashion.

Dieulafoy's Gastric Lesion

Dieulafoy's lesions account for 0.3% to 7% of nonvariceal upper gastrointestinal hemorrhages. Bleeding from a gastric Dieulafoy's lesion is caused by an abnormally large (1 to 3 mm), tortuous artery coursing through the submucosa. Erosion of the superficial mucosa overlying the artery occurs secondary to the pulsations of the large submucosal vessel. The artery is then exposed to the gastric contents, and further erosion and bleeding occur. Generally, the mucosal defect is 2 to 5 mm in size and is surrounded by normal-appearing gastric mucosa. The lesions generally occur 6 to 10 cm from the GE junction, generally in the fundus near the cardia. In one series, 67% were located high in the body of the stomach, with 25% in the gastric fundus. Dieulafoy's lesions are more common in men (2:1) with the peak incidence in the 5th decade. Most patients present with hematemesis. The classic presentation of a patient with a Dieulafoy's lesion is sudden onset of massive, painless, recurrent hematemesis with hypotension. Detection and identification of the Dieulafoy's lesion can be difficult. Esophagogastroduodenoscopy is the diagnostic modality of choice, correctly identifying the lesion in 80% of patients. Because of the intermittent nature of the bleeding, repeated endoscopies may be needed to correctly identify the lesion. If the lesion can be identified endoscopically, attempts should be made to stop the bleeding using endoscopic modalities such as multipolar electrocoagulation, heater probe, noncontact laser photocoagulation, injection sclerotherapy, band ligation, or endoscopic hemoclipping. Angiography can be useful in cases where endoscopy could not definitely identify the source. Angiographic findings may include a tortuous, ectatic artery in the distribution of the left gastric artery with accompanied contrast extravasation in the setting of acute bleeding. Gelfoam embolization has been reported to successfully control bleeding in patients with Dieulafoy's lesion, though the reported experience is limited.

Surgery was once the only therapy for a Dieulafoy's lesion but is now reserved for patients in whom other modalities have failed. The surgical management consists of gastric wedge resection to include the offending vessel. The difficulty at the time of surgery is locating the lesion unless it is actively bleeding. The surgical procedure can be greatly facilitated by asking the endoscopist to tattoo the stomach when the lesion is identified. The traditional surgical approach has been through laparotomy with wide gastrotomy to identify the lesion with subsequent wide wedge resection. The lesion can also be approached laparoscopically, combined with intraoperative endoscopy. A wedge resection is performed with a linear stapling device using endoscopic transillumination to determine the resection margin.

Gastric Varices

Gastric varices are broadly classified by Sarin and Kumar into two types: gastroesophageal varices and isolated gastric varices.[103] Isolated gastric varices are subclassified into type 1 (varices located in the fundus of the stomach) and type 2 (isolated ectopic varices located anywhere in the stomach).

Gastric varices can develop secondary to portal hypertension, in conjunction with esophageal varices, or secondary to sinistral hypertension from splenic vein thrombosis. In generalized portal hypertension, the increased portal pressure is transmitted by the left gastric vein to esophageal varices and by the short and posterior gastric veins to the fundic plexus and cardia veins. Isolated gastric varices tend to occur secondary to splenic vein thrombosis. Splenic blood flows retrograde through the short and posterior gastric veins into the varices, then hepatopetally through the coronary vein into the portal vein. Left-to-right retrograde flow through the gastroepiploic vein to the superior mesenteric vein can explain the development of ectopic varices in the stomach.

The incidence of bleeding from gastric varices has been reported to be between 3% and 30%, but in most series it is less than 10%. However, the incidence of bleeding can be as high as 78% in patients with splenic vein thrombosis and fundic varices. There are limited data on risk factors associated with hemorrhage in patients with gastric varices, though increasing size of the varices or, worse, Child's status increases the risk of bleeding.

Gastric varices in the setting of splenic vein thrombosis are readily treated by splenectomy. Patients with bleeding gastric varices should have an abdominal ultrasound to document splenic vein thrombosis prior to surgical intervention, because gastric varices are most often associated with generalized portal hypertension.

Gastric varices in the setting of portal hypertension should be managed like esophageal varices. The patient should be volume resuscitated, with attention paid to correction of abnormal coagulation profiles. Temporary tamponade can be attempted with a Sengstaken-Blakemore tube. Endoscopy serves as a diagnostic as well as a therapeutic tool. Successful eradication of the esophageal varices through banding or sclerotherapy often results in obliteration of the gastric varices. Because gastric varices arise in the submucosa, a common complication associated with gastric variceal sclerotherapy is ulceration. A major problem with gastric varices is rebleeding, 50% of which is secondary to ulcers. Endoscopic variceal band ligation can achieve hemostasis in approximately 89% of patients[104]; however, concerns over gastric perforations with this technique have tempered its use. Transjugular intrahepatic portosystemic shunting (TIPS) can be effective in controlling gastric variceal hemorrhage, with rebleeding rates around 30%. A gastrorenal shunt between gastric varices and the left renal vein is present in 85% of patients with gastric varices.[105] This spontaneous shunt decompresses the portal system and lessens the efficacy of TIPS. A balloon catheter can be inserted into the gastrorenal shunt through the left renal vein and the shunt occluded by inflating the balloon. A sclerosant (ethanolamine oleate) is then injected and left to remain until clots have formed in the varices. Balloon-occluded retrograde transvenous obliteration has been reported to have a high success rate (100%) with a low recurrence rate (0 to 5%).[106] The major complication of this procedure is aggravation of esophageal varices secondary to a rise in portal pressure as a consequence of occluding the gastrorenal shunt. Additionally, ethanolamine oleate can cause hemolysis (treated by haptoglobin administration) with subsequent renal damage.

Gastric Volvulus

Gastric volvulus is an uncommon condition. Torsion occurs along the stomach's longitudinal axis (organoaxial) in approximately two thirds of cases and along the vertical axis (mesenteroaxial) in one third of cases (Fig. 45-23). Most commonly, organoaxial gastric volvulus occurs acutely and is associated with a diaphragmatic defect, whereas mesenteroaxial volvulus is partial (<180 degrees) and recurrent and is not associated with a diaphragmatic defect. In adults, the diaphragmatic defects are most commonly traumatic or paraesophageal hernias, whereas in children congenital defects such as the foramen of Bochdalek or eventration are involved. The major symptoms at presentation are abdominal pain that is acute in onset, distention, vomiting, and upper gastrointestinal hemorrhage. The sudden onset of constant and severe upper abdominal pain, recurrent retching with production of little vomitus, and the inability to pass a nasogastric tube constitute Borchardt's triad. Plain films of the abdomen reveal a gas-filled viscus in the chest or upper abdomen. The diagnosis can be confirmed by barium contrast study or upper gastrointestinal endoscopy. Acute volvulus is a surgical emergency. Through a transabdominal approach

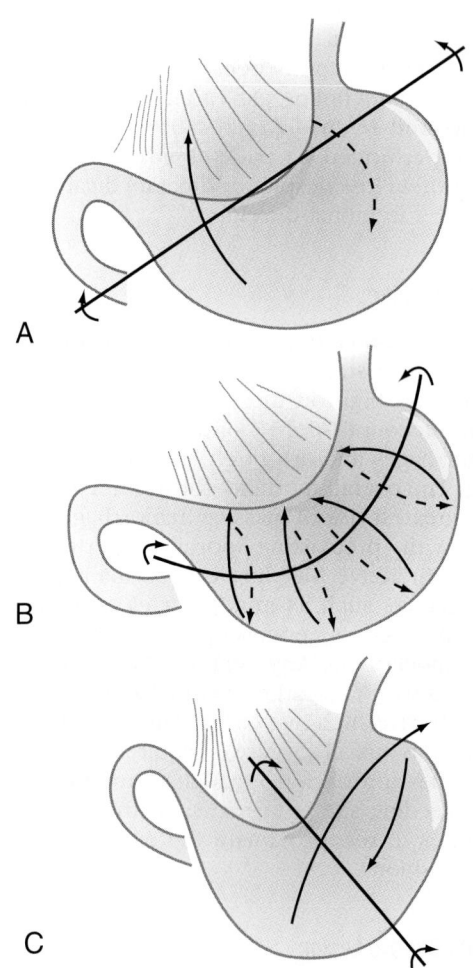

FIGURE 45-23. Torsion of the stomach along the longitudinal axis (organoaxial) (**A** and **B**) and along the vertical axis (mesoaxial) (**C**). (**A-C**, From Dalgaard JG: Acta Chir Scand 103:131, 1952.)

the stomach is reduced and uncoiled. The diaphragmatic defect is repaired with consideration given to a fundoplication in the setting of a paraesophageal hernia. In the unusual case where strangulation has occurred (5% to 28%), the compromised segment of stomach is resected. Spontaneous volvulus, without an associated diaphragmatic defect, is treated by detorsion and fixation of the stomach by gastropexy or tube gastrostomy.

Bezoars

Bezoars are collections of nondigestible materials, usually of vegetable origin (phytobezoar) but also of hair (trichobezoar). Phytobezoars are most commonly found in patients who have undergone surgery of the stomach and have impaired gastric emptying. Diabetic patients with autonomic neuropathy are also at risk. The symptoms of gastric bezoars include early satiety, nausea, pain, vomiting, and weight loss. A large mass may be palpable on physical examination, and the diagnosis is confirmed by a barium examination or endoscopy. Dan and coworkers in 1959 were the first to suggest enzymatic therapy to attempt dissolution of the bezoar. Papain, found in Adolph's Meat Tenderizer (AMT), is given in a dose of 1 tsp in 150 to 300 mL of water several times daily. The sodium concentration in AMT is high, so hypernatremia may result if large quantities are administered. Alternative enzymes such as cellulase have been used with some success. Generally, enzymatic débridement is followed by aggressive Ewald tube lavage or endoscopic fragmentation. Failure of these therapies would necessitate surgical removal.

Trichobezoars are concretions of hair, generally found in long-haired girls or women who often deny eating their own hair (trichophagy). Symptoms include pain from gastric ulceration, fullness from gastric outlet obstruction with occasional gastric perforation, and small bowel obstruction. Trichobezoars tend to form a cast of the stomach, with strands of hair having been observed as far distally as the transverse colon. Small trichobezoars may respond to endoscopic fragmentation, vigorous lavage, or enzymatic therapy. However, these techniques are of limited usefulness, and larger trichobezoars require surgical removal. The small bowel should be examined to be certain additional bezoars are not present. The trichophagy requires psychiatric care, because recurrent bezoar formation is common.

Annotated References

Aoki T: Current status of and problems in the treatment of gastric and duodenal ulcer disease: Introduction. World J Surg 24:249-327, 2000.

This is an excellent symposium on the management of gastric and duodenal ulcers in the modern era. Surgical as well as medical management of bleeding and perforated ulcers is discussed.

Bonenkamp JJ, Hermans J, Sasako M, van de Velde CJ: Extended lymph-node dissection for gastric cancer. Dutch Gastric Cancer Group. N Engl J Med 340:908-914, 1999.

Prospective, randomized trial in 80 Dutch hospitals comparing D1 with D2 lymph node dissection for gastric cancer in terms of morbidity. The results in Dutch patients do not support the routine use of D2 lymph node dissection in patients with gastric cancer.

Cook DJ, Fuller HD, Guyatt GH, et al: Risk factors for gastrointestinal bleeding in critically ill patients. Canadian Critical Care Trials Group. N Engl J Med 330:377-381, 1994.

A prospective, multicenter cohort study evaluating the potential risk factors for stress ulceration in patients admitted to intensive care units and the occurrence of clinically important gastrointestinal bleeding (defined as overt bleeding in association with hemodynamic compromise or the need for blood transfusion). Few critically ill patients had clinically important gastrointestinal bleeding; therefore, prophylaxis against stress ulcers can be safely withheld from critically ill patients unless they have coagulopathy or require mechanical ventilation.

Cuschieri A, Weeden S, Fielding J, et al: Patient survival after D1 and D2 resections for gastric cancer: Long-term results of the MRC randomized surgical trial. Surgical Co-operative Group. Br J Cancer 79:1522-1530, 1999.

In this prospective trial, D1 resection (removal of regional perigastric nodes) was compared with D2 resection (extended lymphadenectomy to include levels 1 and 2 regional nodes). In a multivariate analysis, clinical stages II and III, old age, male sex, and removal of spleen and pancreas were independently associated with poor survival. These findings indicate that the classic Japanese D2 resection offers no survival advantage over D1 surgery. However, the possibility that D2 resection without pancreaticosplenectomy may be better than standard D1 resection cannot be dismissed by the results of this trial.

Demetri GD, von Mehren M, Blanke CD, et al: Efficacy and safety of imatinib mesylate in advanced gastrointestinal stromal tumors. N Engl J Med 347:472-480, 2002.

Prospective, open-label, randomized, multicenter trial to evaluate the activity of imatinib in patients with advanced gastrointestinal stromal tumor. Imatinib induced a sustained objective response in more than half of patients with an advanced unresectable or metastatic gastrointestinal stromal tumor.

Driks MR, Craven DE, Celli BR, et al: Nosocomial pneumonia in intubated patients given sucralfate as compared with antacids or histamine type 2 blockers: The role of gastric colonization. N Engl J Med 317:1376-1382, 1987.

A prospective, randomized trial evaluating the rate of nosocomial pneumonia among 130 patients given mechanical ventilation in an intensive care unit who were receiving as prophylaxis for stress ulcer either sucralfate (n = 61), which does not raise gastric pH, or conventional treatment with antacids, H2 blockers, or both (n = 69). The rate of pneumonia was twice as high in the antacid-H2 group as in the sucralfate group (95% confidence interval, 0.89 to 4.58; P = 0.11). In patients receiving mechanical ventilation, the use of a prophylactic agent against stress ulcer bleeding that preserves the natural gastric acid barrier against bacterial overgrowth may be preferable to antacids and H2 blockers.

Fries JF, Miller SR, Spitz PW, et al: Toward an epidemiology of gastropathy associated with nonsteroidal antiinflammatory drug use. Gastroenterology 96:647-655, 1989.

> The thesis of this paper is that gastropathy associated with nonsteroidal anti-inflammatory drugs (NSAIDs) is the most frequent and, in aggregate, the most severe drug side effect in the United States. Patients on NSAIDs had a hazard ratio for gastrointestinal hospitalization that was 6.45 times that of patients not on NSAIDs. The syndrome of NSAID-associated gastropathy can be estimated to account for at least 2600 deaths and 20,000 hospitalizations each year in patients with rheumatoid arthritis alone.

Hundahl SA, Phillips JL, Menck HR, et al: The National Cancer Data Base Report on poor survival of U.S. gastric carcinoma patients treated with gastrectomy: Fifth Edition American Joint Committee on Cancer staging, proximal disease, and the "different disease" hypothesis. Cancer 88:921-932, 2000.

> A review of the management of gastric cancer patients in the United States diagnosed during the years 1985-1996 and treated with gastrectomy. Based on a review of the National Cancer Data Base Reports.

Koch P, del Valle F, Berdel WE, et al: Primary gastrointestinal non-Hodgkin's lymphoma: II. Combined surgical and conservative or conservative management only in localized gastric lymphoma—results of the prospective German Multicenter Study GIT NHL 01/92. J Clin Oncol 19:3874-3883, 2001.

> Prospective nonrandomized, multicenter trial of patients with primary gastrointestinal non-Hodgkin's lymphomas undergoing combined surgical and conservative treatment versus conservative treatment alone for primary gastric lymphoma in localized stages. The study showed no survival benefit through the addition of surgery. Although the study was not randomized, a stomach-conserving approach may be favored.

Koniaris LG, Drugas G, Katzman PJ, Salloum R: Management of gastrointestinal lymphoma. J Am Coll Surg 197:127-141, 2003.

> Excellent review of gastrointestinal lymphomas and their management.

Macdonald JS, Smalley SR, Benedetti J, et al: Chemoradiotherapy after surgery compared with surgery alone for adenocarcinoma of the stomach or gastroesophageal junction. N Engl J Med 345:725-730, 2001.

> First study to show adjuvant chemoradiotherapy to be of benefit in patients with gastric adenocarcinoma. Postoperative chemoradiotherapy should be considered for all patients at high risk for recurrence of adenocarcinoma of the stomach or gastroesophageal junction who have undergone curative resection.

Ng EK, Lam YH, Sung JJ, et al: Eradication of *Helicobacter pylori* prevents recurrence of ulcer after simple closure of duodenal ulcer perforation: Randomized controlled trial. Ann Surg 231:153-158, 2000.

> A randomized trial to determine whether eradication of *Helicobacter pylori* could reduce the risk of ulcer recurrence after simple closure of perforated duodenal ulcer. The data suggest that eradication of *H. pylori* prevents ulcer recurrence in patients with *H. pylori*–associated perforated duodenal ulcers. Immediate acid-reducing surgery in the presence of generalized peritonitis is unnecessary.

References

1. Gray SW, Skandalakis DA: Atlas of Surgical Anatomy for General Surgeons. Baltimore, Williams & Wilkins, 1985.
2. Berson SA, Yalow RS: Nature of immunoreactive gastrin extracted from tissues of gastrointestinal tract. Gastroenterology 60:215-222, 1971.
3. Liddle RA: Cholecystokinin. New York, Raven Press, 1994.
4. Saffouri B, Weir GC, Bitar KN, et al: Gastrin and somatostatin secretion by perfused rat stomach: Functional linkage of antral peptides. Am J Physiol 238:G495-G501, 1980.
5. Berglindh T: The mammalian gastric parietal cell in vitro. Annu Rev Physiol 46:377-392, 1984.
6. Mercer DW, Cross JM, Smith GS, et al: Protective action of gastrin-17 against alcohol-induced gastric injury in the rat: Role in mucosal defense. Am J Physiol 273:G365-G373, 1997.
7. Carney JA, Go VL, Fairbanks VF, et al: The syndrome of gastric argyrophil carcinoid tumors and nonantral gastric atrophy. Ann Intern Med 99:761-766, 1983.
8. Chiba T, Yamada T: Gut somatostatins. *In* Walsh JH, Docray JG (eds): Gut Peptides: Biochemistry and Physiology. New York, Raven Press, 1994, pp 123-145.
9. Queiroz DM, Mendes EN, Rocha GA, et al: Effect of *Helicobacter pylori* eradication on antral gastrin- and somatostatin-immunoreactive cell density and gastrin and somatostatin concentrations. Scand J Gastroenterol 28:858-864, 1993.
10. Bunnett N: Gastrin-releasing peptide. *In* Walsh JH, Docray JG (eds): Gut Peptides: Biochemistry and Physiology. New York, Raven Press, 1994, pp 423-445.
11. Schubert ML, Edwards NF, Makhlouf GM: Regulation of gastric somatostatin secretion in the mouse by luminal acidity: A local feedback mechanism. Gastroenterology 94:317-322, 1988.
12. Walsh JH, Richardson CT, Fordtran JS: pH dependence of acid secretion and gastrin release in normal and ulcer subjects. J Clin Invest 55:462-468, 1975.
13. Tache Y: Central nervous system regulation of gastric acid secretion. *In* Johnson LR (ed): Physiology of the Gastrointestinal Tract, 2nd ed. New York, Raven Press, 1987, p 911.
14. Lucey MR, Wass JA, Fairclough P, et al: Autonomic regulation of postprandial plasma somatostatin, gastrin, and insulin. Gut 26:683-688, 1985.
15. Debas HT, Konturek SJ, Walsh JH, et al: Proof of a pylorooxyntic reflex for stimulation of acid secretion in the dog. Gastroenterology 66:526, 1947.
16. Konturek SJ, Radecki T, Kwiecien N: Stimuli for intestinal phase of gastric secretion in dogs. Am J Physiol 234:E64-E69, 1978.
17. Sach G: Regulation and structure/function of the acid pump of the stomach. *In* Johnson LR (ed): Physiology of the Gastrointestinal Tract, 3rd ed. New York, Raven Press, 1994, pp 1119-1138.
18. Courtois-Coutry N, Roush D, Rajendran V, et al: A tyrosine-based signal targets H/K-ATPase to a regulated compartment and is required for the cessation of gastric acid secretion. Cell 90:501-510, 1997.
19. Heyland D, Mandell LA: Gastric colonization by gram-negative bacilli and nosocomial pneumonia in the intensive care unit patient: Evidence for causation. Chest 101:187-193, 1992.
20. Driks MR, Craven DE, Celli BR, et al: Nosocomial pneumonia in intubated patients given sucralfate as compared with antacids or histamine type 2 blockers: The

role of gastric colonization. N Engl J Med 317:1376-1382, 1987.

21. Tryba M, Zevounou F, Torok M, et al: Prevention of acute stress bleeding with sucralfate, antacids, or cimetidine: A controlled study with pirenzepine as a basic medication. Am J Med 79:55-61, 1985.

22. Kittang E, Aadland E, Schjonsby H: Effect of omeprazole on the secretion of intrinsic factor, gastric acid, and pepsin in man. Gut 26:594-598, 1985.

23. Samloff IM: Peptic ulcer: The many proteinases of aggression. Gastroenterology 96:586-595, 1989.

24. Dunn BE: Pathogenic mechanisms of *Helicobacter pylori*. Gastroenterol Clin North Am 22:43-57, 1993.

25. Kivilaakso E, Flemstrom G: Surface pH gradient in gastroduodenal mucosa. Scand J Gastroenterol Suppl 105:50-52, 1984.

26. Quigley EM, Turnberg LA: pH of the microclimate lining human gastric and duodenal mucosa in vivo: Studies in control subjects and in duodenal ulcer patients. Gastroenterology 92:1876-1884, 1987.

27. el-Sharkawy TY, Morgan KG, Szurszewski JH: Intracellular electrical activity of canine and human gastric smooth muscle. J Physiol 279:291-307, 1978.

28. Hinder RA, Kelly KA: Human gastric pacesetter potential: Site of origin, spread, and response to gastric transection and proximal gastric vagotomy. Am J Surg 133:29-33, 1977.

29. Code CF, Marlett JA: The interdigestive myo-electric complex of the stomach and small bowel of dogs. J Physiol 246:289-309, 1975.

30. Azpiroz F, Malagelada JR: Gastric tone measured by an electronic barostat in health and postsurgical gastroparesis. Gastroenterology 92:934-943, 1987.

31. Barnett JL, Owyang C: Serum glucose concentration as a modulator of interdigestive gastric motility. Gastroenterology 94:739-744, 1988.

32. Abrahamsson H: Gastrointestinal motility disorders in patients with diabetes mellitus. J Intern Med 237:403-409, 1995.

33. Saslow SB, Thumshirn M, Camilleri M, et al: Influence of *H. pylori* infection on gastric motor and sensory function in asymptomatic volunteers. Dig Dis Sci 43:258-264, 1998.

34. Peeters TL: Erythromycin and other macrolides as prokinetic agents. Gastroenterology 105:1886-1899, 1993.

35. Silen W, Ito S: Mechanisms for rapid re-epithelialization of the gastric mucosal surface. Annu Rev Physiol 47:217-229, 1985.

36. Sernka TJ, Hogben CA: Active ion transport by isolated gastric mucosae of rat and guinea pig. Am J Physiol 217:1419-1424, 1969.

37. Soll AH: Pathogenesis of peptic ulcer and implications for therapy. N Engl J Med 322:909-916, 1990.

38. Kurata JH: Ulcer epidemiology: an overview and proposed research framework. Gastroenterology 96:569-580, 1989.

39. Sonnenberg A: Costs of medical and surgical treatment of duodenal ulcer. Gastroenterology 96:1445-1452, 1989.

40. Sonnenberg A: Changes in physician visits for gastric and duodenal ulcer in the United States during 1958–1984 as shown by National Disease and Therapeutic Index (NDTI). Dig Dis Sci 32:1-7, 1987.

41. Armstrong CP, Blower AL: Non-steroidal anti-inflammatory drugs and life-threatening complications of peptic ulceration. Gut 28:527-532, 1987.

42. Tytgat GN: Treatments that impact favourably upon the eradication of *Helicobacter pylori* and ulcer recurrence. Aliment Pharmacol Ther 8:359-368, 1994.

43. Dempsey D, Ashley S, Mercer DW, et al: Peptic ulcer surgery in the *H. pylori* era: II. Indications for operation. Contemp Surg 57:433-441, 2001.

44. Ng EK, Lam YH, Sung JJ, et al: Eradication of *Helicobacter pylori* prevents recurrence of ulcer after simple closure of duodenal ulcer perforation: Randomized controlled trial. Ann Surg 231:153-158, 2000.

45. Warren JR: Unidentified curved bacilli on gastric epithelium in active chronic gastritis [Letter]. Lancet 1:1273, 1983.

46. Peterson WL, Barnett CC, Evans DJ Jr, et al: Acid secretion and serum gastrin in normal subjects and patients with duodenal ulcer: The role of *Helicobacter pylori*. Am J Gastroenterol 88:2038-2043, 1993.

47. El-Omar EM, Oien K, El-Nujumi A, et al: *Helicobacter pylori* infection and chronic gastric acid hyposecretion. Gastroenterology 113:15-24, 1997.

48. Valenzuela M, Martin-Ruiz JL, Cahallero-Plasencia AM, et al: Parietal cell hyperactivity is not due to *Helicobacter pylori* infection in patients with duodenal ulcer. Am J Gastroenterol 91:2114-2119, 1996.

49. MacDonald WC: Correlation of mucosal histology and aspirin intake in chronic gastric ulcer. Gastroenterology 65:381-389, 1973.

50. Rauws EA, Langenberg W, Houthoff HJ, et al: *Campylobacter pyloridis*–associated chronic active antral gastritis: A prospective study of its prevalence and the effects of antibacterial and antiulcer treatment. Gastroenterology 94:33-40, 1988.

51. Drumm B, Perez-Perez GI, Blaser MJ, et al: Intrafamilial clustering of *Helicobacter pylori* infection. N Engl J Med 322:359-363, 1990.

52. Dooley CP, Cohen H, Fitzgibbons PL, et al: Prevalence of *Helicobacter pylori* infection and histologic gastritis in asymptomatic persons. N Engl J Med 321:1562-1566, 1989.

53. Smoak BL, Kelley PW, Taylor DN: Seroprevalence of *Helicobacter pylori* infections in a cohort of U.S. Army recruits. Am J Epidemiol 139:513-519, 1994.

54. Cullen DJE, Collins BJ, Christiansen KJ, et al: Long-term risk of peptic ulcer disease in people with *H. pylori* infection—a community-based study. Gastroenterology 104:A60, 1993.

55. Sipponen P, Varis K, Fraki O, et al: Cumulative 10-year risk of symptomatic duodenal and gastric ulcer in patients with or without chronic gastritis: A clinical follow-up study of 454 outpatients. Scand J Gastroenterol 25:966-973, 1990.

56. Somerville K, Faulkner G, Langman M: Non-steroidal anti-inflammatory drugs and bleeding peptic ulcer. Lancet 1:462-464, 1986.

57. Kurata JH, Abbey DE: The effect of chronic aspirin use on duodenal and gastric ulcer hospitalizations. J Clin Gastroenterol 12:260-266, 1990.

58. Fries JF, Miller SR, Spitz PW, et al: Toward an epidemiology of gastropathy associated with nonsteroidal antiinflammatory drug use. Gastroenterology 96:647-655, 1989.

59. Lam SK: Pathogenesis and pathophysiology of duodenal ulcer. Clin Gastroenterol 13:447-472, 1984.

60. Cox AJ: Stomach size and its relation to chronic peptic ulcer. Arch Pathol 54:407-422, 1952.

61. Kurata JH, Elashoff JD, Haile BM, et al: A reappraisal of time trends in ulcer disease: Factors related to changes in ulcer hospitalization and mortality rates. Am J Public Health 73:1066-1072, 1983.

62. Susser M: Period effects, generation effects, and age effects in peptic ulcer mortality. J Chronic Dis 35:29-40, 1982.

63. Fimmel CJ, Etienne A, Cilluffo T, et al: Long-term ambulatory gastric pH monitoring: Validation of a new method and effect of H_2 antagonists. Gastroenterology 88:1842-1851, 1985.

64. Silverstein FE, Gilbert DA, Tedesco FJ, et al: The national ASGE survey on upper gastrointestinal bleeding: I. Study design and baseline data. Gastrointest Endosc 27:73-79, 1981.

65. Laine L, Peterson WL: Bleeding peptic ulcer. N Engl J Med 331:717-727, 1994.

66. Silverstein FE, Graham DY, Senior JR, et al: Misoprostol reduces serious gastrointestinal complications in patients with rheumatoid arthritis receiving nonsteroidal anti-inflammatory drugs: A randomized, double-blind, placebo-controlled trial. Ann Intern Med 123:241-249, 1995.

67. Stabile BE: Redefining the role of surgery for perforated duodenal ulcer in the *Helicobacter pylori* era. Ann Surg 231:159-160, 2000.

68. Crofts TJ, Park KG, Steele RJ, et al: A randomized trial of nonoperative treatment for perforated peptic ulcer. N Engl J Med 320:970-973, 1989.

69. Berne TV, Donovan AJ: Nonoperative treatment of perforated duodenal ulcer. Arch Surg 124:830-832, 1989.

70. Csendes A, Maluenda F, Braghetto I, et al: Prospective randomized study comparing three surgical techniques for the treatment of gastric outlet obstruction secondary to duodenal ulcer. Am J Surg 166:45-49, 1993.

71. Lau JY, Chung SC, Sung JJ, et al: Through-the-scope balloon dilation for pyloric stenosis: Long-term results. Gastrointest Endosc 43:98-101, 1996.

72. Aoki T: Current status of and problems in the treatment of gastric and duodenal ulcer disease: Introduction. World J Surg 24:249, 2000.

73. Cook DJ, Fuller HD, Guyatt GH, et al: Risk factors for gastrointestinal bleeding in critically ill patients. Canadian Critical Care Trials Group. N Engl J Med 330:377-381, 1994.

74. Eidt S, Stolte M: Gastric glandular cysts—investigations into their genesis and relationship to colorectal epithelial tumors. Z Gastroenterol 27:212-217, 1989.

75. Nakamura T, Nakano G: Histopathological classification and malignant change in gastric polyps. J Clin Pathol 38:754-764, 1985.

76. Oberhuber G, Stolte M: Gastric polyps: An update of their pathology and biological significance. Virchows Arch 437:581-590, 2000.

77. Harold KL, Sturdevant M, Matthews BD, et al: Ectopic pancreatic tissue presenting as submucosal gastric mass. J Laparoendosc Adv Surg Tech A 12:333-338, 2002.

78. Group UScSW: United States Cancer Statistics: 1999 Incidence. Atlanta, GA, Department of Health and Human Services, Centers for Disease Control and Prevention and National Cancer Institute, 2002.

79. Israel DA, Peek RM: Pathogenesis of *Helicobacter pylori*-induced gastric inflammation. Aliment Pharmacol Ther 15:1271-1290, 2001.

80. Figueiredo C, Machado JC, Pharoah P, et al: *Helicobacter pylori* and interleukin-1 genotyping: An opportunity to identify high-risk individuals for gastric carcinoma. J Natl Cancer Inst 94:1680-1687, 2002.

81. Stemmermann GN, Fenoglio-Preiser C: Gastric carcinoma distal to the cardia: A review of the epidemiological pathology of the precursors to a preventable cancer. Pathology 34:494-503, 2002.

82. Becker KF, Atkinson MJ, Reich U, et al: E-cadherin gene mutations provide clues to diffuse-type gastric carcinomas. Cancer Res 54:3845-3852, 1994.

83. Borchard F: Classification of gastric carcinoma. Hepatogastroenterology 37:223-232, 1990.

84. Willis S, Truong S, Gribnitz S, et al: Endoscopic ultrasonography in the preoperative staging of gastric cancer: Accuracy and impact on surgical therapy. Surg Endosc 14:951-954, 2000.

85. Mani NB, Suri S, Gupta S, et al: Two-phase dynamic contrast-enhanced computed tomography with water-filling method for staging of gastric carcinoma. Clin Imaging 25:38-43, 2001.

86. Davies J, Chalmers AG, Sue-Ling HM, et al: Spiral computed tomography and operative staging of gastric carcinoma: A comparison with histopathological staging. Gut 41:314-319, 1997.

87. Lowy AM, Mansfield PF, Leach SD, et al: Laparoscopic staging for gastric cancer. Surgery 119:611-614, 1996.

88. Burke EC, Karpeh MS, Conlon KC, et al: Laparoscopy in the management of gastric adenocarcinoma. Ann Surg 225:262-267, 1997.

89. Buhl K, Schlag P, Herfarth C: Quality of life and functional results following different types of resection for gastric carcinoma. Eur J Surg Oncol 16:404-409, 1990.

90. Viste A, Haugstvedt T, Eide GE, et al: Postoperative complications and mortality after surgery for gastric cancer. Ann Surg 207:7-13, 1988.

91. Papachristou DN, Fortner JG: Local recurrence of gastric adenocarcinomas after gastrectomy. J Surg Oncol 18:47-53, 1981.

92. Bonenkamp JJ, Hermans J, Sasako M, et al: Extended lymph-node dissection for gastric cancer. Dutch Gastric Cancer Group. N Engl J Med 340:908-914, 1999.

93. Kodama Y, Sugimachi K, Soejima K, et al: Evaluation of extensive lymph node dissection for carcinoma of the stomach. World J Surg 5:241-248, 1981.

94. Cuschieri A, Weeden S, Fielding J, et al: Patient survival after D1 and D2 resections for gastric cancer: Long-term results of the MRC randomized surgical trial. Surgical Cooperative Group. Br J Cancer 79:1522-1530, 1999.

95. Hundahl SA, Phillips JL, Menck HR: The National Cancer Data Base Report on poor survival of U.S. gastric carcinoma patients treated with gastrectomy: Fifth Edition American Joint Committee on Cancer staging, proximal disease, and the "different disease" hypothesis. Cancer 88:921-932, 2000.

96. Macdonald JS, Smalley SR, Benedetti J, et al: Chemoradiotherapy after surgery compared with surgery alone for adenocarcinoma of the stomach or gastroesophageal junction. N Engl J Med 345:725-730, 2001.

97. Isaacson P, Wright DH: Malignant lymphoma of mucosa-associated lymphoid tissue: A distinctive type of B-cell lymphoma. Cancer 52:1410-1416, 1983.

98. Wundisch T, Kim TD, Thiede C, et al: Etiology and therapy of *Helicobacter pylori*-associated gastric lymphomas. Ann Hematol 82:535-545, 2003.

99. Koch P, del Valle F, Berdel WE, et al: Primary gastrointestinal non-Hodgkin's lymphoma: II. Combined surgical and conservative or conservative management only in localized gastric lymphoma—results of the prospective German Multicenter Study GIT NHL 01/92. J Clin Oncol 19:3874-3883, 2001.

100. Koniaris LG, Drugas G, Katzman PJ, et al: Management of gastrointestinal lymphoma. J Am Coll Surg 197:127-141, 2003.

101. Demetri GD, von Mehren M, Blanke CD, et al: Efficacy and

safety of imatinib mesylate in advanced gastrointestinal stromal tumors. N Engl J Med 347:472-480, 2002.

102. Dempsey PJ, Goldenring JR, Soroka CJ, et al: Possible role of transforming growth factor alpha in the pathogenesis of Ménétrier's disease: Supportive evidence from humans and transgenic mice. Gastroenterology 103:1950-1963, 1992.

103. Sarin SK, Kumar A: Gastric varices: Profile, classification, and management. Am J Gastroenterol 84:1244-1249, 1989.

104. Shiha G, El-Sayed SS: Gastric variceal ligation: A new technique. Gastrointest Endosc 49:437-441, 1999.

105. Watanabe K, Kimura K, Matsutani S, et al: Portal hemodynamics in patients with gastric varices: A study in 230 patients with esophageal and/or gastric varices using portal vein catheterization. Gastroenterology 95:434-440, 1988.

106. Sarin SK, Agarwal SR: Gastric varices and portal hypertensive gastropathy. Clin Liver Dis 5:727-767, 2001.

CHAPTER 46

SMALL INTESTINE

B. Mark Evers, M.D.

Embryology	**Obstruction**
Anatomy	**Inflammatory Diseases**
Physiology	**Neoplasms**
Motility	**Diverticular Disease**
Endocrine Function	**Miscellaneous Problems**
Immune Function	

The small intestine is a marvel of complexity and efficiency. The primary role of the small intestine is the digestion and absorption of dietary components once they leave the stomach. This process depends on a multitude of structural, physiologic, endocrine, and chemical factors. Exocrine secretions from the liver and pancreas enable complete digestion of the foodstuffs. The enlarged surface area of the small intestinal mucosa then absorbs these nutrients. In addition to its role in digestion and absorption, the small bowel is the largest endocrine organ in the body and is one of the most important organs of immune function. Given its essential role and complexity, it is amazing that diseases of the small bowel are not more frequent. In this chapter, the normal anatomy and physiology of the small intestine are described, as well as disease processes involving the small bowel, which include obstruction, inflammatory diseases, neoplasms, diverticular disease, and various miscellaneous problems.

EMBRYOLOGY

The primitive gut is formed during the fourth week of fetal human gestation.[1,2] The endodermal layer gives rise to the epithelial lining of the digestive tract, and the splanchnic mesoderm surrounding the endoderm gives rise to the muscular connective tissue and all of the other layers of the intestine. Except for the duodenum, which is a primitive foregut structure, the small intestine is derived from the midgut. During the fifth week of fetal development, when the intestinal length is rapidly increasing, herniation of the midgut occurs through the umbilicus (Fig. 46-1). This midgut loop has both a cranial and caudal limb, with the cranial limb developing into the distal duodenum, jejunum, and proximal ilium and the caudal limb becoming the distal ilium and proximal two thirds of the transverse colon. The juncture of the cranial and caudal limbs is where the vitelline duct joins to the yolk sac. This duct structure normally becomes obliterated before birth; however, it can persist as a Meckel diverticulum in approximately 2% of the population. This midgut herniation persists until approximately 10 weeks of fetal gestation, when the intestine returns to the abdominal cavity. After completing a 270-degree rotation from its initial starting point, the proximal jejunum reenters the abdomen and occupies the left side of the abdomen with subsequent loops lying more to the right. The cecum enters last and is located temporarily in the right upper quadrant; however, with time, it descends to its normal position in the right lower quadrant. Congenital anomalies of gut malrotation and fixation can occur during this process.

The primitive small bowel is lined by a sheet of cuboidal cells until about the ninth week of gestation, when villi begin to form in the proximal intestine and then proceed in a caudal fashion until the entire small bowel and even the colon, for a period of time, are lined by these finger-like projections. Crypt formation begins in the 10th to 12th weeks of gestation. The crypt

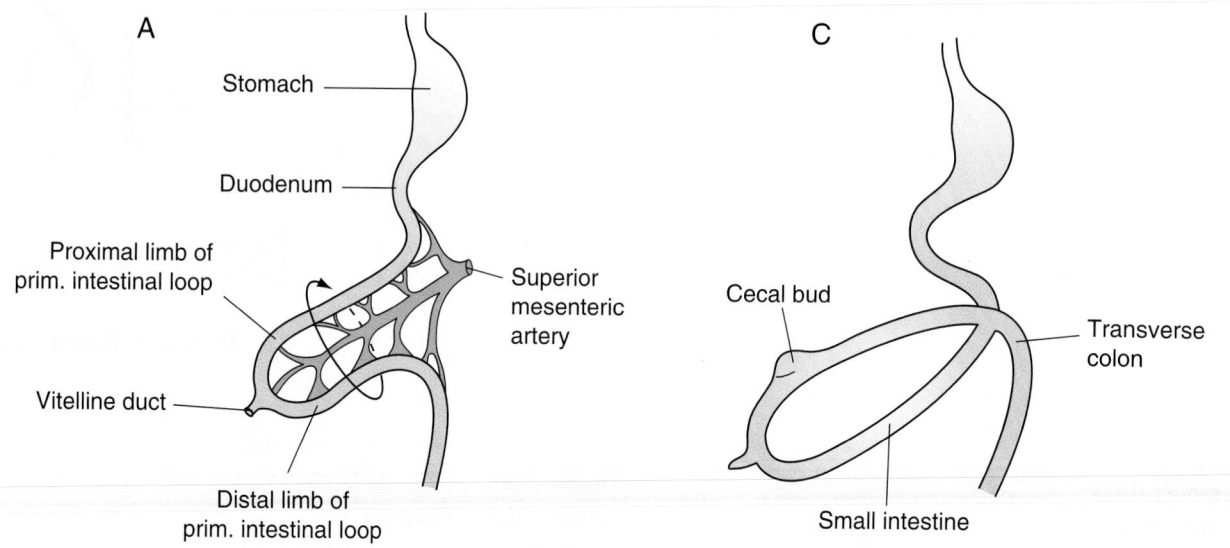

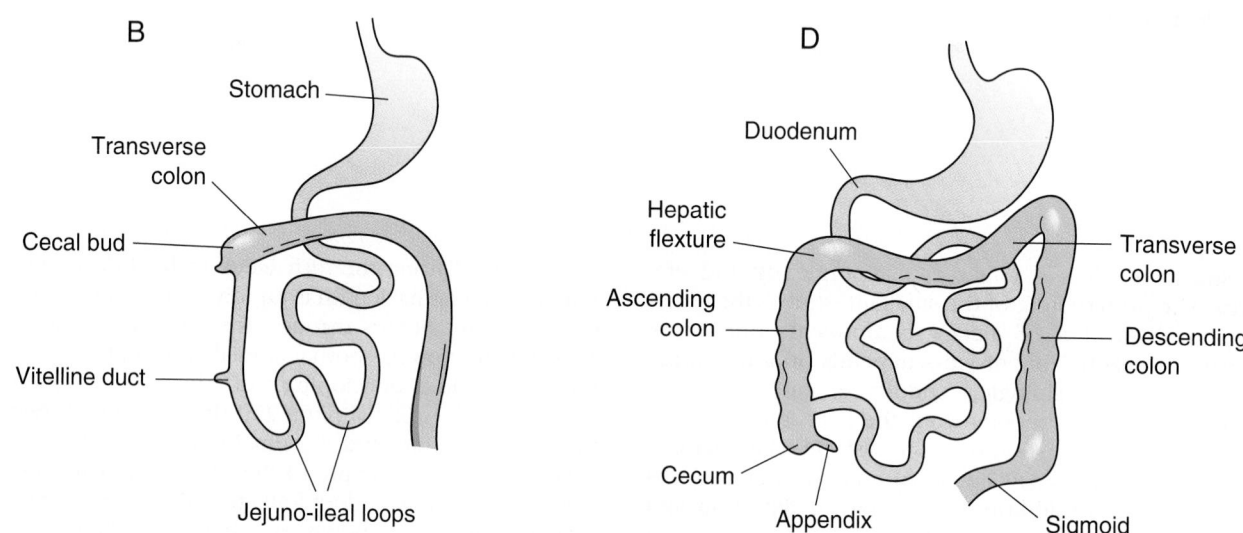

FIGURE 46-1.   Rotation of the intestine. **A,** The intestine after a 90-degree rotation around the axis of the superior mesenteric artery, the proximal loop on the right, and the distal loop on the left. **B,** The intestinal loop after a further 180-degree rotation. The transverse colon passes in front of the duodenum. **C,** Position of the intestinal loops after reentry into the abdominal cavity. Note the elongation of the small intestine, with formation of the small intestine loops. **D,** Final position of the intestines after descent of the cecum into the right iliac fossa. (From Podolsky DK, Babyatshy MW: Growth and development of the gastrointestinal tract. *In* Yamada T [ed]: Textbook of Gastroenterology. Philadelphia, JB Lippincott, 1995, vol 2, chap 23, with permission. Adapted from Sadler TW [ed]: Langman's Medical Embryology, 5th ed. Baltimore, Williams & Wilkins, 1985).

layer of the small bowel is the site of continual cell renewal and proliferation. As the cells ascend the crypt-villus axis, proliferation ceases and cells differentiate into one of the four main cell types: *absorptive enterocytes*, which compose approximately 95% of the intestinal cell population; *goblet cells*; *Paneth cells*; and *enteroendocrine cells*.[3,4] Cells are eventually extruded into the intestinal lumen. Amazingly, this entire process of complete renewal of the intestinal lining occurs in less than 1 week in humans.

ANATOMY

Gross Anatomy

General Description

The entire small intestine, which extends from the pylorus to the cecum, measures 270 to 290 cm, with duodenal length estimated at approximately 20 cm, jejunal length at 100 to 110 cm, and ileal length at 150 to 160 cm.[5] The jejunum begins at the duodenojejunal angle, which is

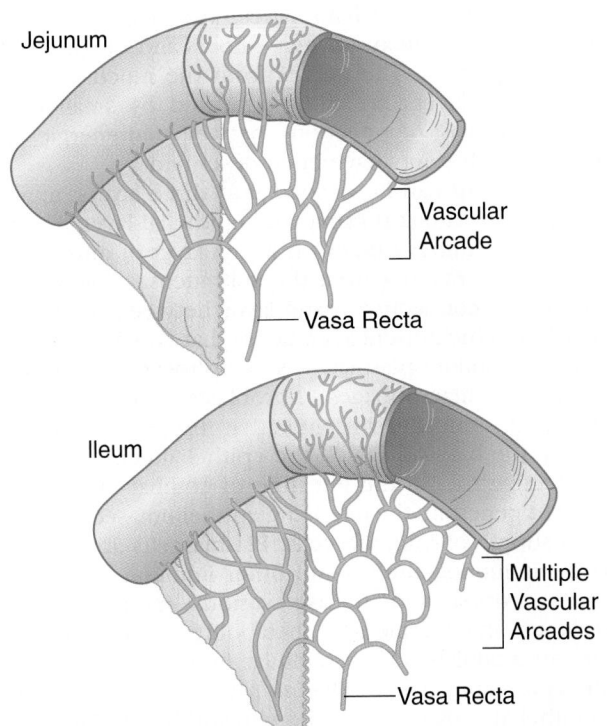

FIGURE 46-2. The jejunal mucosa is relatively thick with prominent plicae circulares; the mesenteric vessels form only one or two arcades with long vasa recta. The ileum is smaller in circumference and has thinner walls; the mesenteric vessels form multiple vascular arcades with short vasa recta. (Adapted from Thompson JC: Atlas of Surgery of the Stomach, Duodenum, and Small Bowel. St. Louis, Mosby–Year Book, 1992, p 263.)

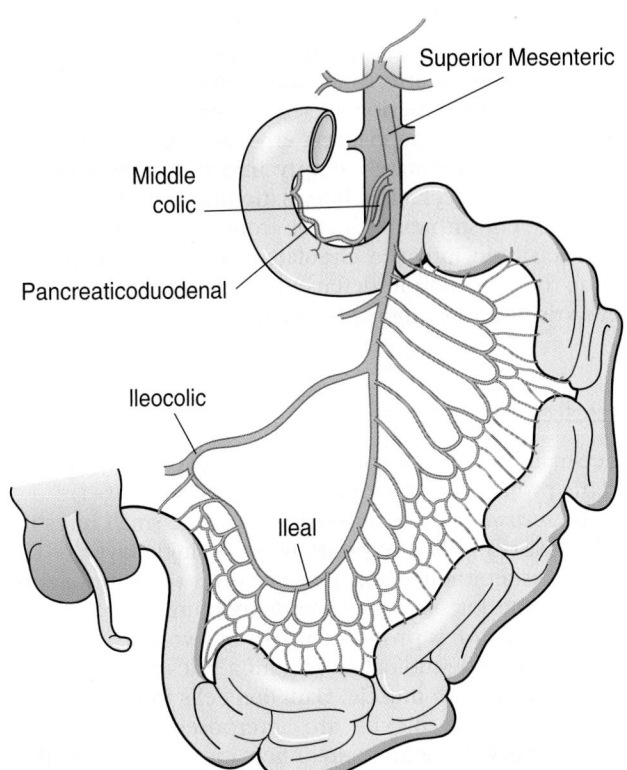

FIGURE 46-3. Blood supply to the jejunoileum and distal duodenum is entirely from the superior mesenteric artery, which courses anterior to the third portion of the duodenum. The celiac artery supplies the proximal duodenum. (Adapted from Thompson JC: Atlas of Surgery of the Stomach, Duodenum, and Small Bowel. St. Louis, Mosby–Year Book, 1992, p 265.)

supported by a peritoneal fold known as the *ligament of Treitz*. There is no obvious line of demarcation between the jejunum and the ileum; however, the jejunum is commonly considered to make up the proximal two fifths of the small intestine and the ileum takes up the remaining three fifths. The jejunum has a somewhat larger circumference, is thicker than the ileum, and can be identified at surgery by examining mesenteric vessels (Fig. 46-2). In the jejunum, only one or two arcades send out long, straight vasa recta to the mesenteric border, whereas the blood supply to the ileum may have four or five separate arcades with shorter vasa recta. The mucosa of the small bowel is characterized by transverse folds (*plicae circulares*), which are prominent in the distal duodenum and jejunum.

Neurovascular-Lymphatic Supply

The small intestine is served by rich vascular, neural, and lymphatic supplies, all traversing through the mesentery. The base of the mesentery attaches to the posterior abdominal wall to the left of the second lumbar vertebra and passes obliquely to the right and inferiorly to the right sacroiliac joint. The blood supply of the small bowel, except for the proximal duodenum that is supplied by branches of the celiac axis, comes entirely from the superior mesenteric artery (Fig. 46-3). The superior mesenteric artery courses anterior to the uncinate process of the pan-

creas and the third portion of the duodenum, where it divides to supply the pancreas, distal duodenum, the entire small intestine, and the ascending and transverse colon. There is an abundant collateral blood supply to the small bowel provided by vascular arcades coursing in the mesentery. Venous drainage of the small bowel parallels the arterial supply, with blood draining into the superior mesenteric vein, which joins the splenic vein behind the neck of the pancreas to form the portal vein.

The innervation of the small bowel is provided by both parasympathetic and sympathetic divisions of the autonomic nervous system, which in turn provide the efferent nerves to the small intestine. Parasympathetic fibers are derived from the vagus, and they traverse the celiac ganglion and affect secretion, motility, and probably all phases of bowel activity. Vagal afferent fibers are present but apparently do not carry pain impulses. The sympathetic fibers come from three sets of splanchnic nerves and have their ganglion cells usually in a plexus around the base of the superior mesenteric artery. Motor impulses affect blood vessel motility and probably gut secretion and motility. Pain from the intestine is mediated through general visceral afferent fibers in the sympathetic system.

The lymphatics of the small intestine are noted in major deposits of lymphatic tissue, particularly in the Peyer patches of the distal small bowel. Lymphatic drainage proceeds from the mucosa through the wall of the bowel to a set of nodes adjacent to the bowel in the mesentery. Drainage continues to a group of regional nodes adjacent to the mesenteric arterial arcades and then to a group at the base of the superior mesentery vessels. From there, lymph flows into the cisterna chyli and then up the thoracic ducts to ultimately empty into the venous system located in the neck. The lymphatic drainage of the small intestine constitutes a major route for transport of absorbed lipid into the circulation and likewise plays a major role in immune defense and also in the spread of cells arising from cancers of the gut.

Microscopic Anatomy

The small bowel wall consists of four layers: serosa, muscularis propria, submucosa, and mucosa (Fig. 46-4).

The *serosa* is the outermost layer of the small intestine and consists of visceral peritoneum, a single layer of flattened mesoepithelial cells that encircles the jejunoileum, and the anterior surface of the duodenum.

The *muscularis* propria consists of two muscle layers, a thin outer longitudinal layer, and a thicker inner circular layer of smooth muscle. Ganglion cells from the myenteric (Auerbach) plexus are interposed between the muscle layers and send neural fibers into both layers, thus providing electrical continuity between the smooth muscle cells and permitting conduction through the muscle layer.

The *submucosa* consists of a layer of fibroelastic connective tissue containing blood vessels and nerves. It is the strongest component of the intestinal wall and therefore must be included in anastomotic sutures. It contains

elaborate networks of lymphatics, arterials, and venules and an extensive plexus of nerve fibers and ganglion cells (Meissner plexus). The nerves from the mucosa/submucosa muscle layers are interconnected by small nerve fibers, and cross connections between adrenergic and cholinergic elements have been described.

The *mucosa* can be divided into three layers: muscularis mucosa, lamina propria, and epithelial layer (Fig. 46-5). The *muscularis mucosa* is a thin layer of muscle that separates the mucosa from the submucosa. The *lamina propria* is a connective tissue layer between the epithelial cells and the muscularis mucosa that contains a variety of cells, including plasma cells, lymphocytes, mast cells, eosinophils, macrophages, fibroblasts, smooth muscle cells, and noncellular connective tissue. The lamina propria, the base on which the epithelial cells lie, serves a protective role in the intestine to combat microorganisms that penetrate the overlying epithelium, secondary to a rich supply of immune cells. Plasma cells actively synthesize immunoglobulins and other immune cells in the lamina propria and release various mediators (e.g., cytokines, arachidonic acid metabolites, and histamines) that can modulate various cellular functions of the overlying epithelium. The *epithelial layer* is a continual sheet of epithelial cells covering the villi and lining the crypts. The main functions of the crypt epithelium are cell renewal and exocrine, endocrine, water, and ion secretion; the main functions of the villus epithelium are digestion and absorption. Four main cell types are contained in the mucosal layer: (1) goblet cells, which secrete mucus; (2) Paneth cells, which secrete lysozyme, tumor necrosis factor (TNF), and the cryptidins, which are homologues of leukocyte defensins and thought to be related to the

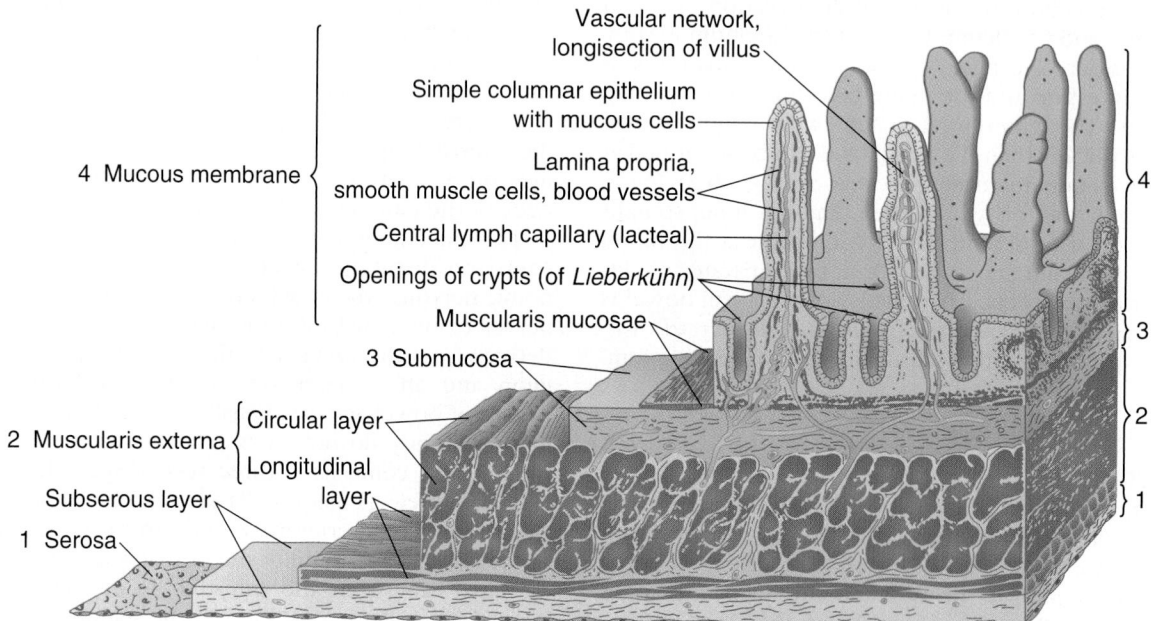

FIGURE 46-4.   Layers of the small intestine. A large surface is provided by villi for the absorption of required nutriments. The solitary lymph follicles in the lamina propria of the mucous membrane are not labeled. In the stroma of both sectioned villi are shown the central chyle (lacteal) vessels or the villous capillaries. (From Sobotta J, Figge FHJ, Hild WJ: Atlas of Human Anatomy. New York, Hafner, 1974, with permission.)

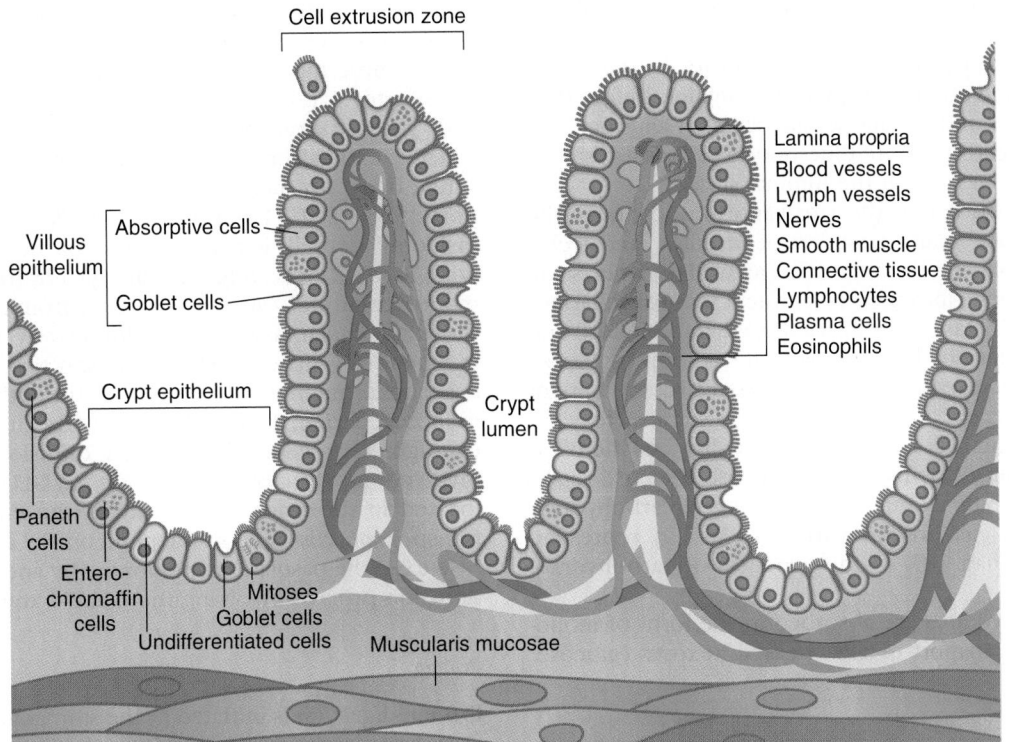

FIGURE 46-5. Schematic diagram of the histologic organization of the small intestinal mucosa. (Adapted from Keljo DJ, Gariepy CE: Anatomy, histology, embryology, and developmental anomalies of the small and large intestine. *In* Feldman M, Scharschmidt BF, Sleisenger MH [eds]: Sleisenger & Fordtran's Gastrointestinal and Liver Disease: Pathology/Diagnosis/Management. Philadelphia, WB Saunders, 2002, p 1646.)

host mucosal defense system; (3) absorptive enterocytes; and (4) enteroendocrine cells, of which there are more than 10 distinct populations that produce the gastrointestinal hormones.

Microscopically, the mucosa is designed for maximal absorptive surface area with villi protruding into the lumen.[2,6] Villi are the tallest in the distal duodenum and proximal jejunum and shortest in the distal ileum. Absorptive enterocytes represent the main cell type in the mucosa and are responsible for digestion and absorption. Their luminal surface is covered by microvilli that rest on a terminal web. The microvilli increase the absorptive capacity by 30-fold. To further increase absorption, the microvilli are covered by a fuzzy coat of glycoprotein, the *glycocalyx*.

PHYSIOLOGY

Digestion and Absorption

The complex process of digestion and eventual absorption of nutrients, water, electrolytes, and minerals is the main role of the small intestine.[7] Liters of water and hundreds of grams of food are delivered to the small intestine daily; and, with remarkable efficiency, nearly all food is absorbed, except for indigestible cellulose. The stomach initiates the process of digestion with the breakdown of solids to particles 1 mm or smaller, which are then delivered to the duodenum, where pancreatic enzymes, bile, and brush border enzymes continue the process of digestion and eventual absorption through the small intestinal wall.[8] The small bowel is primarily responsible for absorption of the dietary components (carbohydrates, proteins, and fats), as well as ions, vitamins, and water.

Carbohydrates

An adult consuming a normal Western diet will ingest 300 to 350 g of carbohydrates a day, with approximately 50% consumed as starch, 30% as sucrose, 6% as lactose, and the remainder as maltose, trehalose, glucose, fructose, sorbitol, cellulose, and pectins.[8-11] Dietary starch is a polysaccharide consisting of long chains of glucose molecules (Fig. 46-6). Amylose makes up approximately 20% of starch in the diet and is broken down at the α-1,4 bonds by salivary (i.e., ptyalin) and pancreatic amylases that convert amylose to maltotriose and maltose. Amylopectin, making up approximately 80% of dietary starch, has branching points every 25 molecules along the straight glucose chains; the α-1,6 glucose linkages in amylopectin produce the end products of amylase digestion: maltose, maltotriose, and the residual branch saccharides, the dextrins. In general, the starches are almost totally converted into maltose and other small glucose polymers before they have passed beyond the duodenum or upper jejunum. The remainder of carbohydrate digestion occurs as a result of brush border enzymes of the luminal surface.

The brush border of the small intestine contains the enzymes lactase, maltase, sucrase-isomaltase, and trehalase, which split the disaccharides, as well as other small glucose polymers, into their constituent monosaccharides (Table 46-1). Lactase hydrolyzes lactose into glucose and galactose. Maltase hydrolyzes maltose to produce glucose monomers. Sucrase-isomaltase possesses two subunits of the same molecule; sucrase hydrolyzes sucrose to yield glucose and fructose, and isomaltase hydrolyzes the α-1,6 bonds in α-limit dextrins to yield glucose. Glucose represents more than 80% of the final products of carbohydrate digestion with galactose and fructose, usually representing no more than 10% of the products of carbohydrate digestion.

The carbohydrates are absorbed in the form of monosaccharides. Transport of the released hexoses (glucose, galactose, and fructose) is carried by specific mechanisms involving active transport. The major routes of absorption are by three membrane carrier systems, sodium glucose transporter 1 (SGLT-1), glucose transporter 5 (GLUT-5), and glucose transporter 2 (GLUT-2) (Fig. 46-7).[8,9,11] Glucose and galactose are absorbed by a carrier-mediated active transport mechanism, which involves the cotransport of Na^+ (SGLT-1 transporter). As Na^+ diffuses into the inside of the cell, it pulls the glucose or galactose along with it, thus providing the energy for transport of the monosaccharide. The exit of glucose from the cytosol into the intracellular space is predominantly due to a Na^+-independent carrier (GLUT-2 transporter) located at the basolateral membrane. Fructose, the other significant monosaccharide, is absorbed from the intestinal lumen through a process of facilitated diffusion. The carrier involved for fructose absorption is GLUT-5, which is located in the apical membrane of the enterocyte. This transport process does not depend on Na^+ or energy. Fructose exits the basolateral membrane by another facilitated diffusion process involving the GLUT-2 transporter.

Protein

Protein digestion is initiated in the stomach, where gastric acid denatures proteins.[8-10,12] Digestion is continued in the small intestine, where the protein comes in contact with pancreatic proteases. Pancreatic trypsinogen is secreted in the intestine by the pancreas in an inactive form but becomes activated by the enzyme enterokinase, a brush border enzyme in the duodenum. Activated trypsin then activates the other pancreatic proteolytic enzyme precursors. The endopeptidases, which include trypsin, chymotrypsin, and elastase, act on peptide bonds at the interior of the protein molecule, producing peptides that are substrates for the exopeptidases (carboxypeptidases), which serially remove a single amino acid from the carboxyl end of the peptide (Table 46-2). This results in splitting the complex proteins into dipeptides, triglycerides, and some larger proteins, which are absorbed

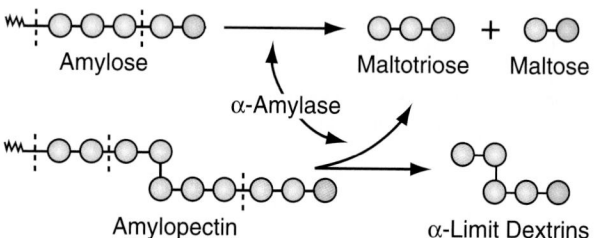

FIGURE 46-6. Action of pancreatic α-amylase on linear (amylose) and branched (amylopectin) forms of starch to produce the breakdown products maltotriose, maltose, and dextrins. (Adapted from Alpers DH: Digestion and absorption of carbohydrates and proteins. *In* Johnson LR, Alpers DH, Christensen J, et al [eds]: Physiology of the Gastrointestinal Tract, 3rd ed. New York, Raven, 1994, vol 2, p 1727.)

TABLE 46-1.   Characteristics of Brush Border Membrane Carbohydrases

Enzyme	Substrate	Products
Lactase	Lactose	Glucose Galactose
Maltase (glucoamylase)	α-1,4-linked oligosaccharides up to nine residues	Glucose
Sucrase-isomaltase (sucrose-α-dextrinase)		
Sucrase	Sucrose	Glucose Fructose
Isomaltase	α-Limit dextrin	Glucose
Both enzymes	α-Limit dextrin α-1,4 link at nonreducing end	Glucose
Trehalase	Trehalose	Glucose

From Marsh MN, Riley SA: Digestion and absorption of nutrients and vitamins. *In* Feldman M, Sleisenger MH, Scharschmidt BF (eds): Sleisenger & Fordtran's Gastrointestinal and Liver Disease. Pathophysiology/Diagnosis/Management. Philadelphia, WB Saunders, 1998, vol 2, p 1480.

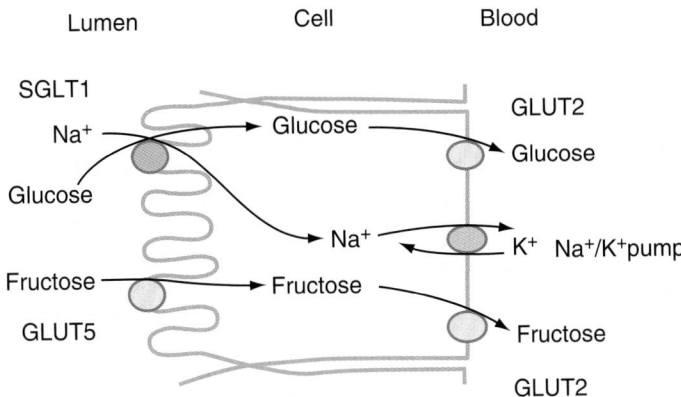

FIGURE 46-7. Model for glucose, galactose, and fructose transport across the intestinal epithelium. Glucose and galactose are transported into the enterocyte across the brush border membrane by the Na⁺/glucose cotransporter (SGLT-1) and then transported out across the basolateral membrane down their concentration gradients by GLUT-2. The low intracellular Na⁺ driving uphill sugar transport across the brush border is maintained by the Na⁺/K⁺ pump on the basolateral membrane. Glucose and galactose therefore stimulate Na⁺ absorption across the epithelium. Fructose is transported across the cell down the concentration gradient across the brush border and basolateral membranes. GLUT-5 is the brush border fructose transporter, whereas GLUT-2 handles fructose transport across the basolateral membrane. (From Wright EM, Hirayama BA, Loo DDF, et al: Intestinal sugar transport. *In* Johnson LR, Alpers DH, Christensen J, et al [eds]: Physiology of the Gastrointestinal Tract, 3rd ed. New York, Raven Press, 1994, p 1752, with permission.)

TABLE 46-2. Principal Pancreatic Proteases

Enzyme	Primary Action
Endopeptidases	Hydrolyze interior peptide bonds of polypeptides and proteins
Trypsin	Attacks peptide bonds involving basic amino acids; yields products with basic amino acids at carboxyl-terminal end
Chymotrypsin	Attacks peptide bonds involving aromatic amino acids, leucine, glutamine, and methionine; yields peptide products with these amino acids at carboxyl-terminal end
Elastase	Attacks peptide bonds involving neutral aliphatic amino acids; yields products with neutral amino acids at carboxyl-terminal end
Exopeptidases	Hydrolyze external peptide bonds of polypeptides and protein
Carboxypeptidase A	Attacks peptides with aromatic and neutral aliphatic amino acids at carboxyl-terminal end
Carboxypeptidase B	Attacks peptides with basic amino acids at carboxyl-terminal end

From Castro GA: Digestion and absorption. *In* Johnson LR (ed): Gastrointestinal Physiology. St. Louis, CV Mosby, 1991, pp 108-130, with permission.

from the intestinal lumen by a Na⁺-mediated active transport mechanism and digested further by enzymes in the brush border and in the cytoplasm of the enterocytes (Fig. 46-8). These peptidase enzymes include amino peptidases and several dipeptidases, which split the remaining larger polypeptides into tripeptides and dipeptides and some amino acids. The amino acids, dipeptides, and tripeptides are easily transported through the microvilli into the epithelial cells, where, in the cytosol, additional peptidases hydrolyze the dipeptides and tripeptides into single amino acids, which then pass through the epithelial cell membrane into the portal venous system. In normal humans, digestion and absorption of protein are usually 80% to 90% completed in the jejunum.

Fats

Emulsification of Fats

Most adults in North America consume 60 to 100 g/day of fat. Triglycerides, the most abundant fats, are composed of a glycerol, nucleus, and three fatty acids; small quantities of phospholipids, cholesterol, and cholesterol esters also are found in the normal diet. Essentially all fat digestion occurs in the small intestine, where the first step is the breakdown of fat globules into smaller sizes so as to facilitate further breakdown by water-soluble digestive enzymes, a process called emulsification.[8-10,13] This process is facilitated by bile from the liver that contains bile salts and the phospholipid lecithin. The polar parts of

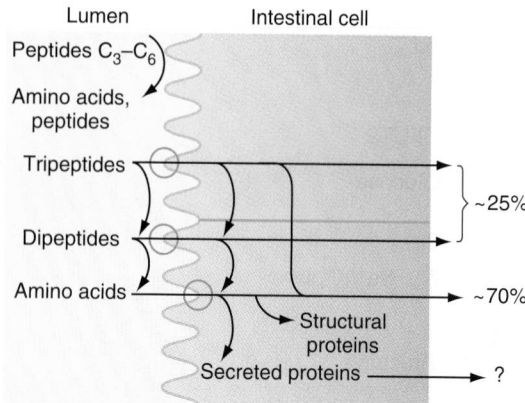

FIGURE 46-8. Digestion and absorption of proteins. (Adapted from Alpers DH: Digestion and absorption of carbohydrates and proteins. *In* Johnson LR, Alpers DH, Christensen J, et al [eds]: Physiology of the Gastrointestinal Tract, 3rd ed. New York, Raven Press, 1994, vol 2, p 1733.)

the bile salts and lecithin molecules are soluble in water, whereas the remaining portions are soluble in fat. Therefore, the fat-soluble portions dissolve in the surface layer of the fat globules and the polar portions, projecting outward, are soluble in the surrounding aqueous fluids. This arrangement renders the fat globules more accessible to fragmentation by agitation in the small intestine. Therefore, a major function of bile salts, and especially lecithin in the bile, is to allow the fat globules to be readily fragmented by agitation in the intestinal lumen. With the increase in surface area of the fat globules resulting from the action of the bile salts and lecithin, the fats can now be readily attacked by pancreatic lipase, the most crucial enzyme in the digestion of triglycerides, which splits triglycerides into free fatty acids and 2-monoglycerides.

Micelle Formation

Fat digestion is further accelerated by bile salts, which, secondary to their amphipathic nature, can form micelles.[9,14] Micelles are small spherical globules composed of 20 to 40 molecules of bile salts with a sterol nucleus that is highly fat soluble and a hydrophilic polar group that projects outward. The mixed micelles thus formed are arrayed so that the insoluble lipid is surrounded by the bile salts oriented with their hydrophilic ends facing outward. Therefore, as quickly as the monoglycerides and free fatty acids are formed from lipolysis, they become dissolved in the central hydrophobic portion of the micelles, which then act to carry these products of fat hydrolysis to the brush borders of the epithelial cells, where absorption occurs.

Intracellular Processing

The monoglycerides and free fatty acids, which are dissolved in the central lipid portion of the bile acid micelles, are absorbed through the brush border due to their highly lipid-soluble nature and simply diffuse into the interior of the cell.[8,9,13] After disaggregation of the micelle, bile salts remain within the intestinal lumen to enter into the for-

mation of new micelles and act to carry more monoglycerides and fatty acids to the epithelial cells. The released fatty acids and monoglycerides in the cell re-form into new triglycerides. This re-formation of a triglyceride occurs in the cell through the interactions of intracellular enzymes that are associated with the endoplasmic reticulum. The major pathway for resynthesis involves synthesis of triglycerides from 2-monoglycerides and coenzyme A (CoA)-activated fatty acids. Microsomal acyl-CoA lipase is necessary to synthesize acyl-CoA from the fatty acid before esterification. These reconstituted triglycerides then combine with cholesterol, phospholipids, and apoproteins to form chylomicrons that consist of an inner core containing triglycerides and a membranous outer core of phospholipids and apoproteins. The chylomicrons pass from the epithelial cells into the lacteals, where they pass through the lymphatics into the venous system. Eighty to 90 percent of all fat absorbed from the gut is absorbed in this manner and transported to the blood by way of the thoracic lymph in the form of chylomicrons. Small quantities of short- to medium-chain fatty acids may be absorbed directly into the portal blood rather than being converted into triglycerides and absorbed into the lymphatics. These shorter-chain fatty acids are more water soluble, which allows for the direct diffusion into the bloodstream. Figure 46-8 summarizes the process of fat digestion and absorption.

Enterohepatic Circulation

The proximal intestine absorbs most of the dietary fat. Although the unconjugated bile acids are absorbed into the jejunum by passive diffusion, the conjugated bile acids that form micelles are absorbed in the ileum by active transport and are reabsorbed from the distal ileum. The bile acids then pass via the portal venous system to the liver for resection as bile. The total bile salt pool in humans is 2 to 3 g, and it recirculates about six times every 24 hours (the enterohepatic circulation of bile salts).[9,10,13] Almost all of the bile salts are absorbed, with only approximately 0.5 g lost in the stool every day; this is replaced by resynthesis from cholesterol.

Water, Electrolytes, and Vitamins

Eight to 10 L of water per day enter the small intestine. Much of this is absorbed, with only approximately 500 mL or less leaving the ileum and entering the colon[8,9] (Fig. 46-9). Water may be absorbed by the process of simple diffusion. In addition, water may be drawn in and out of the cell through a process of osmotic pressure, resulting from active transport of sodium, glucose, or amino acids into cells.

Electrolytes can be absorbed in the small bowel by active transport or by coupling to organic solute.[8,9,15,16] Na^+ is absorbed by active transport through the basolateral membranes. Cl^- is absorbed in the upper part of the small intestine by a process of passive diffusion. Large quantities of HCO_3^- must be reabsorbed, and this is accomplished in an indirect fashion. As the Na^+ is absorbed, H^+ is secreted into the lumen of the intestine. It then com-

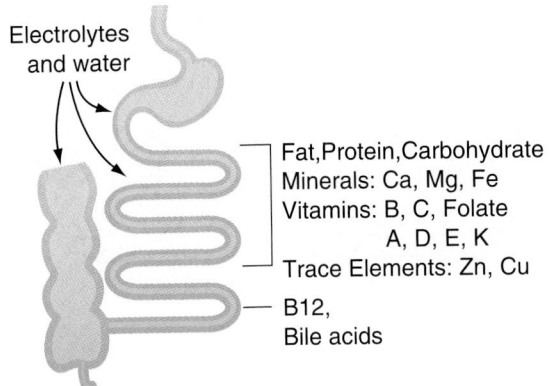

Electrolytes
and water

Fat, Protein, Carbohydrate
Minerals: Ca, Mg, Fe
Vitamins: B, C, Folate
           A, D, E, K
Trace Elements: Zn, Cu

B12,
Bile acids

FIGURE 46-9. Absorption of water and electrolytes in the small bowel and colon. (Adapted from Westergaard H: Short bowel syndrome. *In* Feldman M, Scharschmidt BF, Sleisenger MH [eds]: Gastrointestinal and Liver Disease: Pathophysiology, Diagnosis, Management. Philadelphia, WB Saunders, 1998, p 1549.)

bines with HCO_3^- to form carbonic acid, which then dissociates to form water and carbon dioxide. The water remains in the chyme, but the carbon dioxide is readily absorbed in the blood and subsequently expired. Calcium is absorbed, particularly in the proximal intestine (duodenum and jejunum), by a process of active transport; absorption appears to be facilitated by an acid environment and is enhanced by vitamin D and parathyroid hormone. Iron is absorbed as either a heme or nonheme component in the duodenum by an active process. Iron then is either deposited within the cell as ferritin or is transferred to the plasma bound to transferrin. The total absorption of iron is dependent on body stores of iron and the rate of erythropoiesis; any increase in erythropoiesis increases iron absorption. Potassium, magnesium, phosphate, and other ions also can be actively absorbed throughout the mucosa.

Vitamins are either fat soluble (e.g., A, D, E, and K) or water soluble (e.g., ascorbic acid [vitamin C], biotin, nicotinic acid, folic acid, riboflavin, thiamine, pyridoxine [vitamin B_6], and cobalamin [vitamin B_{12}]).[9,10,16] The fat-soluble vitamins are carried in mixed micelles and transported in chylomicrons of lymph to the thoracic duct and into the venous system. The absorption of water-soluble vitamins appears to be more complex than originally thought. Vitamin C is absorbed by an active transport process that incorporates a sodium-coupled mechanism as well as a specific carrier system. Vitamin B_6 appears to be rapidly absorbed by simple diffusion into the proximal intestine. Thiamine (vitamin B_1) is rapidly absorbed in the jejunum by an active process similar to the sodium-coupled transport system for vitamin C. Riboflavin (vitamin B_2) is absorbed in the upper intestine by facilitated transport. The absorption of vitamin B_{12} occurs primarily in the terminal ileum. Vitamin B_{12} is derived from cobalamin, which is freed in the duodenum by pancreatic proteases. The cobalamin binds to intrinsic factor, which is secreted by the stomach, and is protected from prote-

olytic digestion. Specific receptors in the terminal ileum take up the cobalamin-intrinsic factor complex, probably by translocation. In the ileal enterocyte, free vitamin B_{12} is bound to an ileal pool of transcobalamin II, which transports it into the portal circulation.

MOTILITY

Food particles are propelled through the small bowel by a complex series of muscular contractions.[8,9,17,18] Peristalsis consists of intestinal contractions passing aborally at a rate of 1 to 2 cm/sec. The major function of peristalsis is the movement of intestinal chyme through the intestine. Motility patterns in the small bowel vary greatly between the fed and fasted states. Pacesetter potentials, which are thought to originate in the duodenum, initiate a series of contractions in the fed state that propel food through the small bowel. During the interdigestive (fasting) period between meals, the bowel is regularly swept by cyclical contractions that move aborally along the intestine every 75 to 90 minutes. These contractions are initiated by the migrating myoelectric complex (MMC), which is under the control of both neural and humoral pathways. Extrinsic nerves to the small bowel are vagal and sympathetic. The vagal fibers have two functionally different effects: one is cholinergic and excitatory, and the other is peptidergic and probably inhibitory. Sympathetic activity inhibits motor function, whereas parasympathetic activity stimulates it. Although intestinal hormones are known to affect small intestinal motility, the one peptide that has been clearly shown to function in this regard is motilin, which is found at its peak plasma level during phase III (intense bursts of myoelectrical activities resulting in regular, high-amplitude contractions) of MMCs.

ENDOCRINE FUNCTION

Gastrointestinal Hormones

The gastrointestinal hormones are distributed along the length of the small bowel in a spatial-specific pattern. In fact, the small bowel is the largest endocrine organ in the body.[19,20] Although often classified as hormones, these agents do not always function in a truly endocrine fashion (i.e., discharged into the bloodstream, where an action is produced at some distant site) (Fig. 46-10). Sometimes, these peptides are discharged and act locally in a paracrine or an autocrine manner. In addition, these peptides may serve as neurotransmitters (e.g., vasoactive intestinal peptide). The gastrointestinal hormones play a major role in pancreaticobiliary and intestinal secretion and motility. In addition, certain gastrointestinal hormones exert a trophic effect on both normal and neoplastic intestinal mucosa and pancreas.[21-23] The location, major stimulants of release, and primary effects of the more important gastrointestinal hormones are summarized in Table 46-3. In addition, the diagnostic and therapeutic uses of gastrointestinal hormones are listed in Table

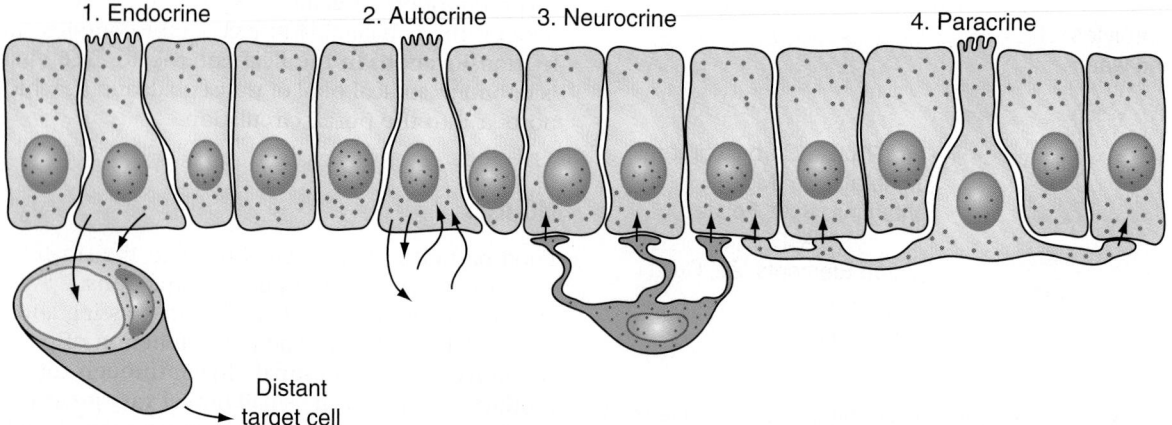

FIGURE 46-10.   Actions of intestinal hormones may be via endocrine, autocrine, neurocrine, or paracrine effects. (Adapted from Miller LJ: Gastrointestinal hormones and receptors. *In* Yamada T, Alpers DH, Laine L, et al [eds]: Textbook of Gastroenterology, 3rd ed. Philadelphia, Lippincott Williams & Wilkins, 1999, vol 1, p 37.)

46-4. (For a more in-depth discussion of the structure, molecular biology, physiologic functions, and uses of these hormones, the reader is referred to references 20 and 22 to 25.)

Receptors

The gastrointestinal hormones interact with their cell surface receptors to initiate a cascade of signaling events that eventually culminate in their physiologic effects. These hormones primarily signal through G protein–coupled receptors that traverse the plasma membrane seven times and represent the largest group of receptors found in the body.[26] The heterotrimeric G proteins, which are composed of α, β, and γ subunits, are the molecular switches for signal transduction. Agonist binding to the seven-transmembrane domain receptor is thought to cause a conformational change in the receptor that allows it to interact with the G proteins. Intracellular second messengers that can then be activated include cyclic adenosine monophosphate, Ca^{2+}, cyclic guanosine monophosphate, and inositol phosphate.

In addition to the gastrointestinal hormones, a number of other peptides and growth factors are located in the gastrointestinal mucosa, including epidermal growth factor, transforming growth factors-α and -β, insulin-like growth factor, fibroblast growth factor, and platelet-derived growth factor.[27] These peptides play a role in cell growth and differentiation and act through tyrosine kinase receptors, which have a single membrane-spanning domain.

A third class of surface receptors, the ion channel-linked receptors, are found most commonly in cells of neuronal lineage and usually bind specific neurotransmitters.[27] Examples include receptors for excitatory (acetylcholine and serotonin) and inhibitory (γ-aminobutyric acid, glycine) neurotransmitters. These receptors undergo a conformational change on binding of the mediator, which allows passage of ions across the cell membrane and results in changes in voltage potential.

IMMUNE FUNCTION

During the course of a normal day, we ingest a number of bacteria, parasites, and viruses. The large surface areas of the small bowel mucosa represent a potential major portal of entry for these pathogens; the small intestine serves as a major immunologic barrier in addition to its important role in digestion and endocrine function. As a result of constant antigenic exposure, the intestine possesses abundant lymphoid cells (i.e., B and T lymphocytes) and myeloid cells (macrophages, neutrophils, eosinophils, and mast cells).[28,29] To deal with the constant barrage of potential toxins and antigens, the gut has evolved into a highly organized and efficient mechanism for antigen processing, humoral immunity, and cellular immunity. The gut-associated lymphoid tissue is localized in three areas: Peyer patches, lamina propria lymphoid cells, and intraepithelial lymphocytes.

The Peyer patches are unencapsulated lymphoid nodules that constitute an afferent limb of the gut-associated lymphoid tissue that recognizes antigens through the specialized sampling mechanism of the microfold (M) cells contained within the follicle-associated epithelium (Fig. 46-11). Antigens that gain access to the Peyer patches activate and prime B and T cells in that site. The M cells cover the lymphoid follicles in the gastrointestinal tract and provide a site for the selective sampling of intraluminal antigens. Activated lymphocytes from intestinal lymphoid follicles then leave the intestinal tract and migrate into afferent lymphatics that drain into mesenteric lymph nodes. Furthermore, these cells migrate into the lamina propria. The B lymphocytes become surface immunoglobulin (Ig) A-bearing lymphoblasts, which serve a critically important role in mucosal immunity.

B lymphocytes and plasma cells, T lymphocytes, macrophages, dendritic cells, eosinophils, and mast cells are scattered throughout the connective tissue of the lamina propria. Approximately 60% of the lymphoid cells are T cells. These T lymphocytes are a heterogeneous group of cells and can differentiate into one of several types of T-effector cells. Cytotoxic T-effector cells directly

TABLE 46-3. Gastrointestinal Hormones

Hormone	Location	Major Stimulants of Peptide Secretion	Primary Effects
Gastrin	Antrum, duodenum (G cells)	Peptides, amino acids, antral distention, vagal and adrenergic stimulation, gastrin-releasing peptide (bombesin)	Stimulates gastric acid and pepsinogen secretion Stimulates gastric mucosal growth
Cholecystokinin	Duodenum, jejunum (I cells)	Fats, peptides, amino acids	Stimulates pancreatic enzyme secretion Stimulates gallbladder contraction Relaxes sphincter of Oddi Inhibits gastric emptying
Secretin	Duodenum, jejunum (S cells)	Fatty acids, luminal acidity, bile salts	Stimulates release of water and bicarbonate from pancreatic ductal cells Stimulates flow and alkalinity of bile Inhibits gastric acid secretion and motility and inhibits gastrin release
Somatostatin	Pancreatic islets (D cells), antrum, duodenum	Gut: fat, protein, acid, other hormones (e.g., gastrin, cholecystokinin) Pancreas: glucose, amino acids, cholecystokinin	Universal "off" switch: Inhibits release of gastrointestinal hormones Inhibits gastric acid secretion Inhibits small bowel water and electrolyte secretion Inhibits secretion of pancreatic hormones
Gastrin-releasing peptide (mammalian equivalent of bombesin)	Small bowel	Vagal stimulation	Universal "on" switch: Stimulates release of all gastrointestinal hormones (except secretin) Stimulates gastrointestinal secretion and motility Stimulates gastric acid secretion and release of antral gastrin Stimulates growth of intestinal mucosa and pancreas
Gastric inhibitory polypeptide	Duodenum, jejunum (K cells)	Glucose, fat, protein adrenergic stimulation	Inhibits gastric acid and pepsin secretion Stimulates pancreatic insulin release in response to hyperglycemia
Motilin	Duodenum, jejunum	Gastric distention, fat	Stimulates upper gastrointestinal tract motility May initiate the migrating motor complex
Vasoactive intestinal peptide	Neurons throughout the gastrointestinal tract	Vagal stimulation	Primarily functions as a neuropeptide Potent vasodilator Stimulates pancreatic and intestinal secretion Inhibits gastric acid secretion
Neurotensin	Small bowel (N cells)	Fat	Stimulates growth of small and large bowel mucosa
Enteroglucagon	Small bowel (L cells)	Glucose, fat	Glucagon-like peptide-1 Stimulates insulin release Inhibits pancreatic glucagon release Glucagon-like peptide-2 Potent enterotrophic factor
Peptide YY	Distal small bowel, colon	Fatty acids, cholecystokinin	Inhibits gastric and pancreatic secretion Inhibits gallbladder contraction

damage the target cells. T-helper cells are effector cells that help mediate induction of other T cells or the induction of B cells to produce humoral antibodies. T-suppressor cells perform just the opposite function. Approximately 40% of the lymphoid cells in the lamina propria are B cells, which are primarily derived from precursors in Peyer patches. These B cells and their progeny, plasma cells, are predominantly focused on IgA synthesis and, to a lesser extent, on IgM, IgG, and IgE synthesis.

The intraepithelial lymphocytes are located in the space between the epithelial cells that line the mucosal surface and lie close to the basement membrane. It is suspected that most of the intraepithelial lymphocytes are T cells. On activation, the intraepithelial lymphocytes may acquire cytolytic functions that can contribute to epithelial cell death through apoptosis. These cells may be important in the immunosurveillance against abnormal epithelial cells.

As already stated, one of the major protective immune mechanisms for the intestinal tract is the synthesis and secretion of IgA. The intestine contains more than 70% of the IgA-producing cells in the body. IgA is produced by plasma cells in the lamina propria and is secreted into the intestine where it can bind antigens at the mucosal surface. The IgA antibody traverses the epithelial cell to the lumen by means of a protein carrier (the secretory component) that not only transports the IgA but also protects it against the intracellular lysosomes. IgA does not activate complement and does not enhance cell-mediated opsonization or destruction of infectious organisms or antigens, which sharply contrasts to the role of other immunoglobulins. Secretory IgA inhibits the adherence of bacteria to epithelial cells and prevents their colonization and multiplication. In addition, secretory IgA neutralizes bacterial toxins and viral activity and blocks the absorption of antigens from the gut.

OBSTRUCTION

The description of patients presenting with small bowel obstruction dates back to the third or fourth century, when Praxagoras created an enterocutaneous fistula to relieve a bowel obstruction. Despite this success with operative therapy, the nonoperative management of these patients with attempted reduction of hernias, laxatives, ingestion of heavy metals (e.g., lead or mercury), and leeches to remove toxic agents from the blood was the rule until the late 1800s, when antisepsis and aseptic surgical techniques made operative intervention safer and more acceptable. A better understanding of the pathophysiology of bowel obstruction and the use of isotonic fluid resuscitation, intestinal tube decompression, and antibiotics have greatly reduced the mortality rate for patients with mechanical bowel obstruction.[30,31] However, patients with a bowel obstruction still represent

TABLE 46-4.   Diagnostic and Therapeutic Uses of Gastrointestinal Hormones

Hormone	Diagnostic/Therapeutic Uses
Gastrin	Pentagastrin (gastrin analogue) used to measure maximal gastric acid secretion
Cholecystokinin	Biliary imaging of gallbladder contraction
Secretin	Provocative test for gastrinoma Measurement of maximal pancreatic secretion
Glucagon	Suppresses bowel motility for endocrine spasm Relieves sphincter of Oddi spasm Provocative test for insulin, catecholamine, and growth hormone release
Somatostatin analogues	Treatment of carcinoid diarrhea and flushing Decrease secretion from pancreatic and intestinal fistulas Ameliorate symptoms associated with hormone-overproducing endocrine tumors Treatment of esophageal variceal bleeding

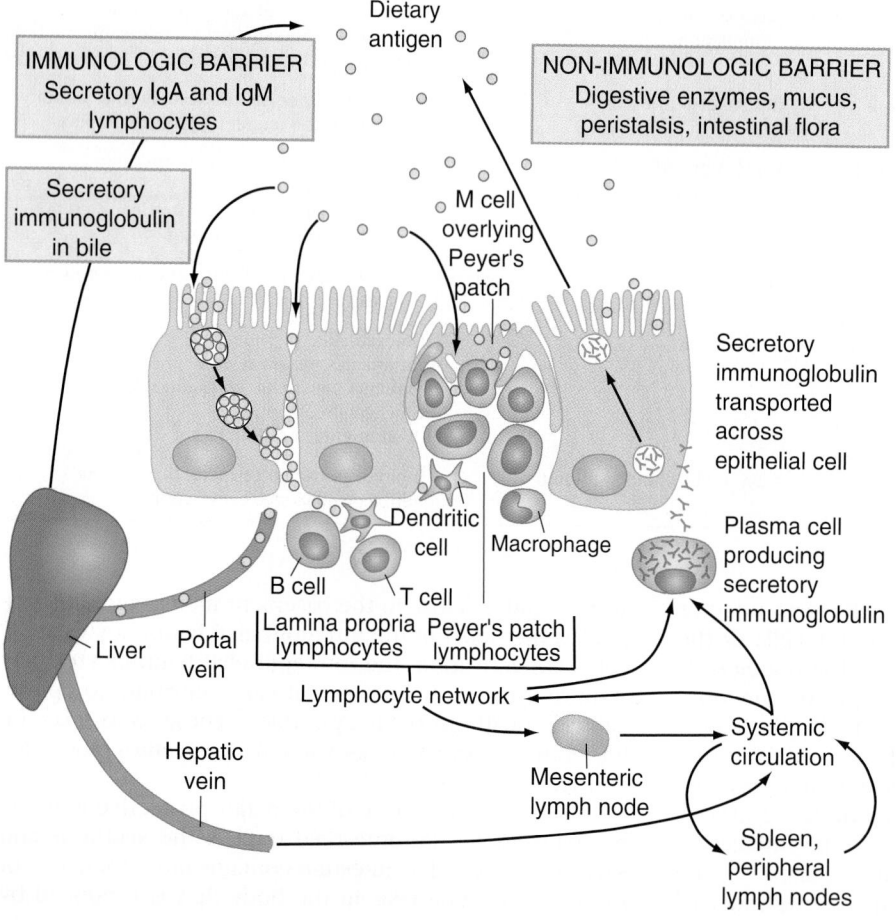

FIGURE 46-11.   The mucosal barrier of the gut. Antigens contact specialized microfold (M) cells overlying Peyer's patches, which then process and present the antigen to the immune system. When B lymphocytes are stimulated by antigenic material, the cells develop into antibody-forming cells that secrete various types of immunoglobulins (Igs), the most important of which is IgA. (Adapted from Duerr RH, Shanahan F: Food allergy. *In* Targan SR, Shanahan F [eds]: Immunology and Immunopathology of the Liver and Gastrointestinal Tract. New York, Igaku-Shoin, 1990, p 510.)

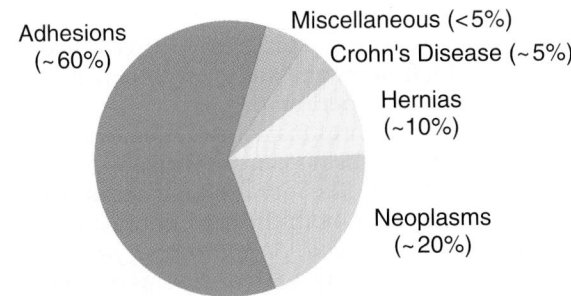

FIGURE 46-12. Common causes of small bowel obstruction in industrialized countries.

some of the most difficult and vexing problems that surgeons face with regard to the correct diagnosis, the optimal timing of therapy, and the appropriate treatment. Ultimate clinical decisions regarding the management of these patients dictates a thorough history and work-up and a heightened awareness of potential complications.

Etiology

The causes of a small bowel obstruction can be divided into three categories: (1) obstruction arising from extraluminal causes such as adhesions, hernias, carcinomas, and abscesses; (2) obstruction intrinsic to the bowel wall (e.g., primary tumors); and (3) intraluminal obturator obstruction (e.g., gallstones, enteroliths, foreign bodies, and bezoars) (Box 46-1). The cause of small bowel obstruction has changed dramatically during the past century.[32] At the turn of the 20th century, hernias accounted for more than half of mechanical intestinal obstructions. With the routine elective repair of hernias, this cause has dropped to the third most common cause of small bowel obstruction in industrialized countries. Adhesions secondary to previous surgery are by far the most common cause of small bowel obstruction (Fig. 46-12).

Adhesions, particularly after pelvic operations (e.g., gynecologic procedures, appendectomy, and colorectal resection), are responsible for more than 60% of all causes of bowel obstruction in the United States.[33,34] This preponderance of lower abdominal procedures to produce adhesions that result in obstruction is thought to be due to the fact that the bowel is more mobile in the pelvis and more tethered in the upper abdomen.

Malignant tumors account for approximately 20% of the cases of small bowel obstruction. The majority of these tumors are metastatic lesions that obstruct the intestine secondary to peritoneal implants that have spread from an intra-abdominal primary tumor such as ovarian, pancreatic, gastric, or colonic. Less often, malignant cells from distant sites, such as breast, lung, and melanoma, may metastasize hematogenously and account for peritoneal implants and result in an obstruction. Large intra-abdominal tumors may also cause small bowel obstruction through extrinsic compression of the bowel lumen. Primary colonic cancers (particularly those arising from

the cecum and ascending colon) may present as a small bowel obstruction. Primary small bowel tumors can cause obstruction but are exceedingly rare.

Hernias are the third leading cause of intestinal obstruction and account for approximately 10% of all cases. Most commonly, these represent ventral or inguinal hernias. Internal hernias, usually related to prior abdominal surgery, can also result in small bowel obstruction. Less common hernias can also produce obstruction, such as femoral, obturator, lumbar, and sciatic hernias.

Box 46-1. Causes of Mechanical Small Intestinal Obstruction in Adults

Lesions Extrinsic to the Intestinal Wall

Adhesions (usually postoperative)
Hernia
    External (e.g., inguinal, femoral, umbilical, or ventral hernias)
    Internal (e.g., congenital defects such as paraduodenal, foramen of Winslow, and diaphragmatic hernias or postoperative secondary to mesenteric defects)
Neoplastic
    Carcinomatosis
    Extraintestinal neoplasms
Intra-abdominal abscess

Lesions Intrinsic to the Intestinal Wall

Congenital
    Malrotation
    Duplications/cysts
Inflammatory
    Crohn's disease
    Infections
        Tuberculosis
        Actinomycosis
        Diverticulitis
Neoplastic
    Primary neoplasms
    Metastatic neoplasms
Traumatic
    Hematoma
    Ischemic stricture
Miscellaneous
    Intussusception
    Endometriosis
    Radiation enteropathy/stricture

Intraluminal/Obturator Obstruction

Gallstone
Enterolith
Bezoar
Foreign body

Adapted from Tito WA, Sarr MG: Intestinal obstruction. In Zuidema GD (ed): Surgery of the Alimentary Tract. Philadelphia, WB Saunders, 1996, pp 375-416.

Crohn's disease is the fourth leading cause of small bowel obstruction and accounts for approximately 5% of all cases. Obstruction can result from acute inflammation and edema, which may resolve with conservative management. In patients with long-standing Crohn's disease, strictures can develop that may require resection and reanastomosis or strictureplasty.

An important cause of small bowel obstruction that is not routinely considered is obstruction associated with an intra-abdominal abscess, commonly from a ruptured appendix, diverticulum, or dehiscence of an intestinal anastomosis. The obstruction may occur as a result of a local ileus in the small bowel adjacent to the abscess. In addition, the small bowel can form a portion of the wall of the abscess cavity and become obstructed by kinking of the bowel at this point.

Miscellaneous causes of bowel obstruction account for 2% to 3% of all cases but should be considered in the differential diagnosis. These include intussusception of the bowel, which in the adult is usually secondary to a pathologic lead point such as a polyp or tumor; gallstones, which can enter the intestinal lumen by a cholecystenteric fistula and cause obstruction; enteroliths originating from jejunal diverticula; foreign bodies; and phytobezoars.

Pathophysiology

Early in the course of an obstruction, intestinal motility and contractile activity increase in an effort to propel luminal contents past the obstructing point. The increase in peristalsis that occurs early in the course of bowel obstruction is present both above and below the point of obstruction, thus accounting for the finding of diarrhea that may accompany partial or even complete small bowel obstruction in the early period. Later in the course of obstruction, the intestine becomes fatigued and dilates, with contractions becoming less frequent and less intense.

As the bowel dilates, water and electrolytes accumulate both intraluminally and in the bowel wall itself. This massive third-space fluid loss accounts for the dehydration and hypovolemia. The metabolic effects of fluid loss depend on the site and duration of the obstruction. With a proximal obstruction, dehydration may be accompanied by hypochloremia, hypokalemia, and metabolic alkalosis associated with increased vomiting. Distal obstruction of the small bowel may result in large quantities of intestinal fluid into the bowel; however, abnormalities in serum electrolytes are usually less dramatic. Oliguria, azotemia, and hemoconcentration can accompany the dehydration. Hypotension and shock can ensue. Other consequences of bowel obstruction include increased intra-abdominal pressure, decreased venous return, and elevation of the diaphragm, compromising ventilation. These factors can serve to further potentiate the effects of hypovolemia.

As the intraluminal pressure increases in the bowel, a decrease in mucosal blood flow can occur. These alterations are particularly noted in patients with a closed-loop obstruction in which greater intraluminal pressures are attained. A closed-loop obstruction, produced commonly by a twist of the bowel, can progress to arterial occlusion and ischemia if left untreated and may potentially lead to bowel perforation and peritonitis.

In the absence of intestinal obstruction, the jejunum and proximal ileum of the human are virtually sterile. With obstruction, however, the flora of the small intestine changes dramatically, in both the type of organism (most commonly *Escherichia coli*, *Streptococcus faecalis*, and *Klebsiella*) and the quantity, with organisms reaching concentrations of 10^9 to 10^{10}/mL. Studies have shown an increase in the number of indigenous bacteria translocating to mesenteric lymph nodes and even systemic organs.[35] However, the overall importance of this bacterial translocation on the clinical course has not been entirely defined.

Clinical Manifestations and Diagnosis

A thorough history and physical examination are critical to establishing the diagnosis and treatment of the patient with an intestinal obstruction. In the majority of patients, a meticulous history and physical examination complemented by plain abdominal radiographs are all required to establish the diagnosis and to devise a treatment plan. More sophisticated radiographic studies may be necessary in certain patients in whom the diagnosis and cause are uncertain. However, a computed tomographic (CT) scan of the abdomen should not be the starting point in the work-up of a patient with intestinal obstruction.

History

The cardinal symptoms of intestinal obstruction include colicky abdominal pain, nausea, vomiting, abdominal distention, and a failure to pass flatus and feces (i.e., obstipation). These symptoms may vary with the site and duration of obstruction. The typical crampy abdominal pain associated with intestinal obstruction occurs in paroxysms at 4- to 5-minute intervals and occurs less frequently with distal obstruction. Nausea and vomiting are more common with a higher obstruction and may be the only symptoms in patients with gastric outlet or high intestinal obstruction. An obstruction located distally is associated with less emesis, and the initial and most prominent symptom is the cramping abdominal pain. Abdominal distention occurs as the obstruction progresses, and the proximal intestine becomes increasingly dilated. Obstipation is a later development, and it must be reiterated that patients, particularly in the early stages of bowel obstruction, may relate a history of diarrhea that is secondary to increased peristalsis. Therefore, the important point to remember is that a complete bowel obstruction cannot be ruled out based on a history of loose bowel movements. The character of the vomitus is also important to obtain in the history. As the obstruction becomes more complete with bacterial overgrowth, the vomitus becomes more feculent, indicating a late and established intestinal obstruction.

Physical Examination

The patient with intestinal obstruction may present with tachycardia and hypotension, demonstrating the severe dehydration that is present. Fever suggests the possibility of strangulation. Abdominal examination demonstrates a distended abdomen, with the amount of distention somewhat dependent on the level of obstruction. Previous surgical scars should be noted. Early in the course of bowel obstruction, peristaltic waves can be observed, particularly in thin patients, and auscultation of the abdomen may demonstrate hyperactive bowel sounds with audible rushes associated with vigorous peristalsis (i.e., borborygmi). Late in the obstructive course, minimal or no bowel sounds are noted. Mild abdominal tenderness may be present with or without a palpable mass; however, localized tenderness, rebound, and guarding suggest peritonitis and the likelihood of strangulation. A careful examination must be performed to rule out incarcerated hernias in the groin, the femoral triangle, and the obturator foramen. A rectal examination should be performed to assess for intraluminal masses and to examine the stool for occult blood, which may be an indication of malignancy, intussusception, or infarction.

Radiologic and Laboratory Examinations

The diagnosis of intestinal obstruction is often immediately evident after a thorough history and physical examination. Therefore, plain radiographs usually confirm the clinical suspicion and define more accurately the site of obstruction. The accuracy of diagnosis of the small intestinal obstruction on plain abdominal radiographs is estimated to be approximately 60%, with an equivocal or a nonspecific diagnosis obtained in the remainder of cases. Characteristic findings on supine radiographs are dilated loops of small intestine without evidence of colonic distention. Upright radiographs demonstrate multiple air-fluid levels, which often layer in a stepwise pattern (Fig. 46-13). Plain abdominal films may also demonstrate the cause of the obstruction (e.g., foreign bodies or gallstones) (Fig. 46-14). In uncertain cases or when one is unable to differentiate partial from complete obstruction, further diagnostic evaluations may be required.

In the more complex patient in whom the diagnosis is not readily apparent, CT has proved to be beneficial (Fig. 46-15).[36] A CT is particularly sensitive for diagnosing complete or high-grade obstruction of the small bowel and for determining the location and cause of obstruction. The CT examination is less sensitive, however, in patients with partial small bowel obstruction.[37,38] In addition, CT is helpful if an extrinsic cause of bowel obstruction (e.g., abdominal tumors, inflammatory disease, or abscess) is suggested (Fig. 46-16). CT has also been described as useful in determining bowel strangulation. Unfortunately, CT findings associated with strangulation are those of irreversible ischemia and necrosis.

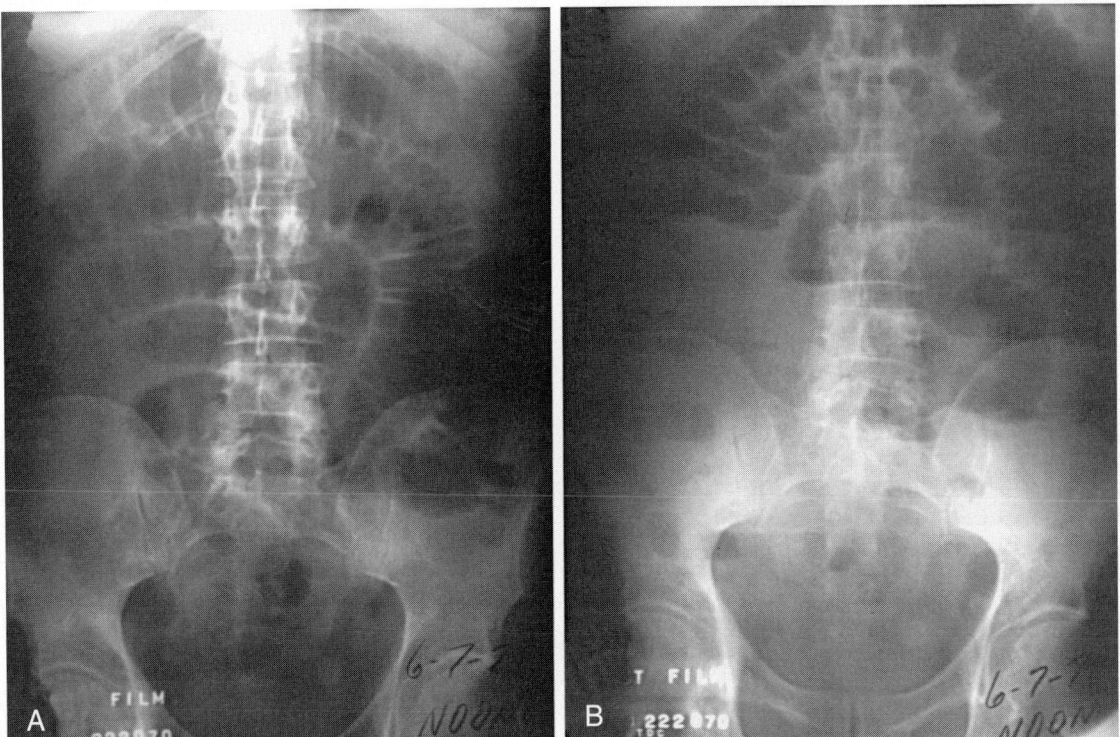

FIGURE 46-13.   Plain abdominal radiographs of a patient with a complete small bowel obstruction. **A,** Supine film shows dilated loops of small bowel in an orderly arrangement, without evidence of colonic gas. **B,** Upright film shows multiple, short, air-fluid levels arranged in a stepwise pattern. (Courtesy of Melvyn H. Schreiber, M.D., The University of Texas Medical Branch.)

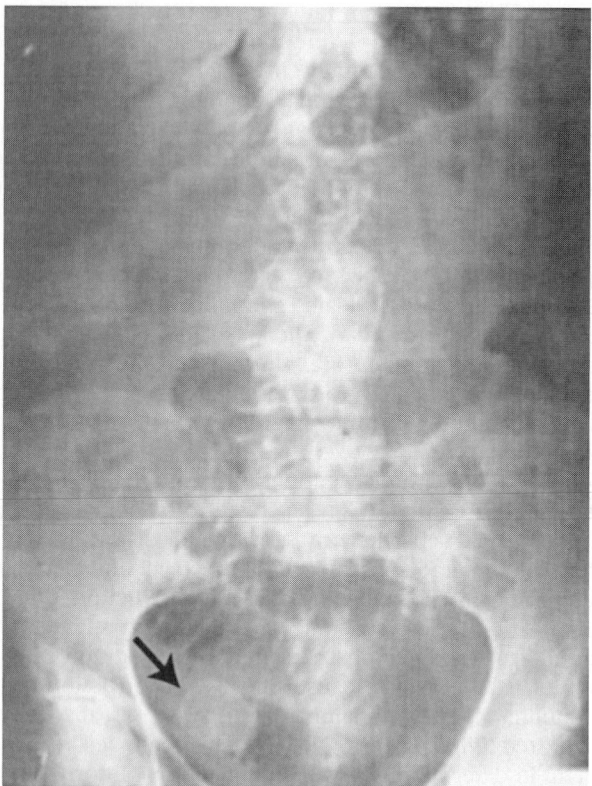

FIGURE 46-14. Plain abdominal film shows complete bowel obstruction caused by a large radiopaque gallstone *(arrow)* obstructing the distal ileum.

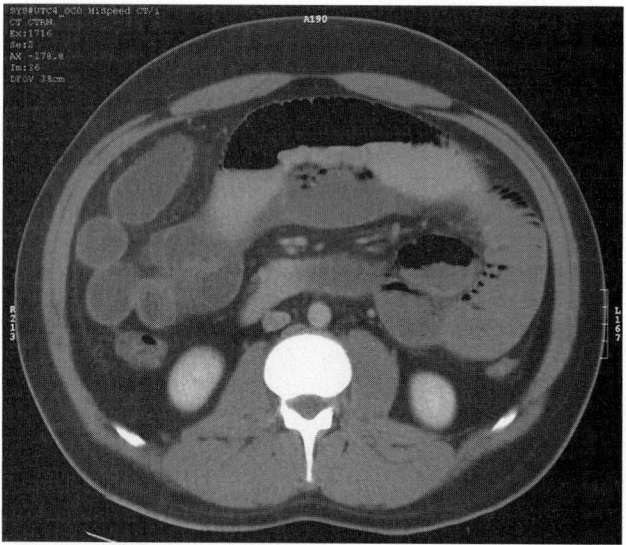

FIGURE 46-15. CT scan through the mid abdomen shows dilated small bowel loops filled with fluid and decompressed ascending and descending colon. These are typical CT findings in small bowel obstruction. (Courtesy of Eric Walser, M.D., The University of Texas Medical Branch.)

Barium studies have been a useful adjunct in certain patients with a presumed obstruction. In particular, enteroclysis, which involves the oral insertion of a tube into the duodenum to instill air and barium directly into the small intestine and to follow the movement fluoroscopi-

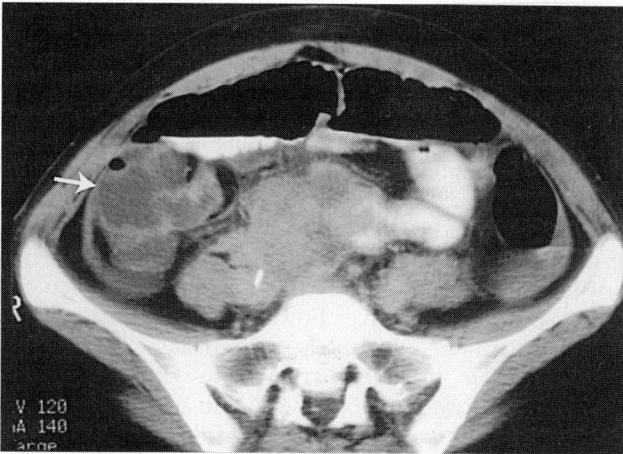

FIGURE 46-16. CT scan of the abdomen of a patient with a mechanical bowel obstruction secondary to an abscess in the right lower quadrant *(arrow)*. Multiple dilated and fluid-filled loops of small bowel are noted. (Courtesy of Melvyn H. Schreiber, M.D., The University of Texas Medical Branch.)

cally, has been helpful in the assessment of obstruction.[36,39] Enteroclysis has been advocated as the definitive study in patients in whom the diagnosis of low-grade, intermittent small bowel obstruction is clinically uncertain. In addition, barium studies can precisely demonstrate the level of the obstruction as well as the cause of the obstruction in certain instances (Fig. 46-17). The main disadvantages of enteroclysis are the need for nasoenteric intubation, the slow transit of contrast material in patients with a fluid-filled hypotonic small bowel, and the enhanced expertise required by the radiologist to perform this procedure.

Ultrasound has been reported to be useful in pregnant patients where radiation exposure is a concern. Magnetic resonance imaging (MRI) has been described in patients with obstruction; however, it appears to be no better diagnostically than CT.

To summarize, plain abdominal radiographs are usually diagnostic of bowel obstruction in more than 60% of the cases, but further evaluation (possibly by CT or barium radiography) may be necessary in 20% to 30% of cases. CT examination is particularly useful in patients with a history of abdominal malignancy, in postsurgical patients, and in patients who have no history of abdominal surgery and present with symptoms of bowel obstruction. Barium studies are recommended in patients with a history of recurring obstruction or low-grade mechanical obstruction to precisely define the obstructed segment and degree of obstruction.

Laboratory examinations are not helpful in the actual diagnosis of patients with small bowel obstruction but are extremely important in assessing the degree of dehydration. Patients with a bowel obstruction should routinely have laboratory measurements of serum sodium, chloride, potassium, bicarbonate, and creatinine. The serial determination of serum electrolytes should be performed to assess the adequacy of fluid resuscitation. Dehydration may result in hemoconcentration, as noted by an elevated

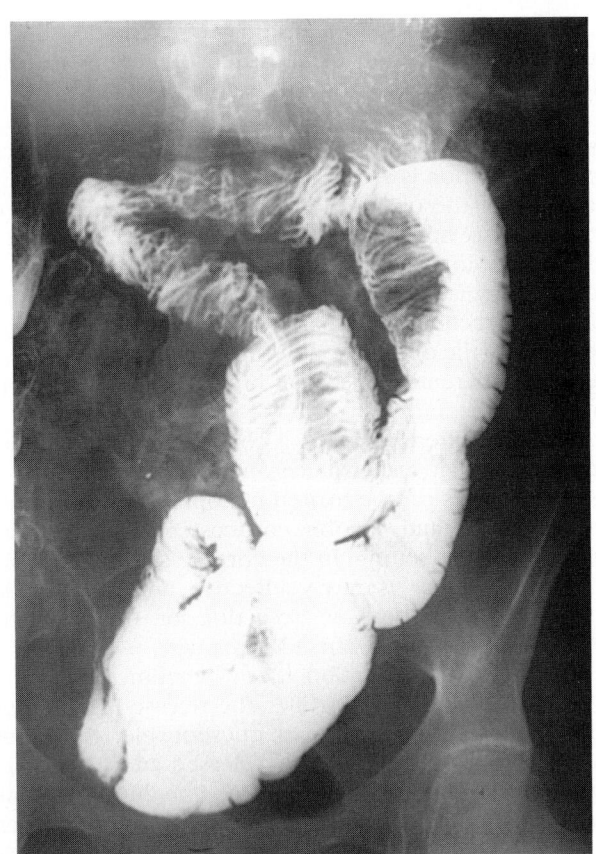

FIGURE 46-17. Barium study demonstrates jejunojejunal intussusception. (Courtesy of Melvyn H. Schreiber, M.D., The University of Texas Medical Branch.)

hematocrit. This value should be monitored because fluid resuscitation results in a decrease in the hematocrit and some patients (e.g., those with intestinal malignancies) may require blood transfusions before surgery. In addition, the white blood cell count should be assessed. Leukocytosis may be found in patients with strangulation; however, an elevated white blood cell count does not necessarily denote strangulation. Conversely, the absence of leukocytosis does not eliminate strangulation as a possibility.

Simple Versus Strangulating Obstruction

The majority of patients with small bowel obstruction are classified as having simple obstructions that involve mechanical blockage of the flow of luminal contents without compromised viability of the intestinal wall. In contrast, strangulation obstruction, which usually involves a closed-loop obstruction in which the vascular supply to a segment of intestine is compromised, can lead to intestinal infarction. Strangulation obstruction is associated with an increased morbidity and mortality risk, and therefore recognition of early strangulation is important in differentiating from simple intestinal obstruction. "Classic" signs of strangulation have been described and include tachycardia, fever, leukocytosis, and a constant, noncramping abdominal pain. However, a number of

studies have convincingly shown that no clinical parameters or laboratory measurements can accurately detect or exclude the presence of strangulation in all cases.[40]

CT examination is useful only in detecting the late stages of irreversible ischemia. Various serum determinations, including lactate dehydrogenase, amylase, alkaline phosphatase, and ammonia levels, have been assessed with no real benefit. Initial reports have described some limited success in discriminating strangulation by measuring serum D-lactate, creatine phosphokinase isoenzyme (particularly the BB isoenzyme), or intestinal fatty acid binding protein; however, these are only investigational and cannot be widely applied to patients with obstruction. Finally, noninvasive determinations of mesenteric ischemia were described by Richards and associates[41] using a superconducting quantum interference device (SQUID) magnetometer to noninvasively detect mesenteric ischemia. Intestinal ischemia is associated with changes in the basic electric rhythm of the small intestine. Clinical assessment of this technique is under way.

To reiterate, it is important to remember that bowel ischemia and strangulation cannot be reliably diagnosed or excluded preoperatively in all cases by any known clinical parameter, combination of parameters, or current laboratory and radiographic examinations.

Treatment

Fluid Resuscitation and Antibiotics

Patients with intestinal obstruction are usually dehydrated and depleted of sodium, chloride, and potassium, requiring aggressive intravenous replacement with an isotonic saline solution such as lactated Ringer's. Urine output should be monitored by the placement of a Foley catheter. After the patient has formed adequate urine, potassium chloride should be added to the infusion if needed. Serial electrolyte measurements, as well as hematocrit and white blood cell count, are performed to assess the adequacy of fluid repletion. Because of large fluid requirements, patients, particularly the elderly, may require central venous assessment and, in some cases, the placement of a Swan-Ganz catheter. Broad-spectrum antibiotics are given prophylactically by some surgeons based on the reported findings of bacterial translocation occurring even in simple mechanical obstructions. In addition, antibiotics are administered as a prophylaxis for possible resection or inadvertent enterotomy at surgery.

Tube Decompression

In addition to intravenous fluid resuscitation, another important adjunct to the supportive care of patients with intestinal obstruction is nasogastric suction. Nasogastric suction with a Levin tube empties the stomach, reducing the hazard of pulmonary aspiration of vomitus and minimizing further intestinal distention from preoperatively swallowed air. The use of long intestinal tubes (e.g., Cantor or Baker tubes) has been advocated by some groups. However, prospective randomized trials demonstrated no significant differences with regard to the decompression achieved, the success of nonoperative treatment, or the morbidity rate after surgical intervention compared with the use of nasogastric tubes.[42] Furthermore, the use of these long tubes has been associated with a significantly longer hospital stay, duration of postoperative ileus, and postoperative complications in some series. Therefore, it appears that long intestinal tubes offer no benefit in the preoperative setting over nasogastric tubes.

Patients with a partial intestinal obstruction may be treated conservatively with resuscitation and tube decompression alone. Resolution of symptoms and discharge without the need for surgery have been reported in 60% to 85% of patients with a partial obstruction.[32] Enteroclysis can assist in determining the degree of obstruction, with higher-grade partial obstructions requiring earlier operative intervention. Although an initial trial of nonoperative management of most patients with partial small bowel obstruction is warranted, it should be emphasized that clinical deterioration of the patient or increasing small bowel distention on abdominal radiographs during tube decompression warrants prompt operative intervention. The decision to continue to treat a patient nonoperatively with a presumed bowel obstruction is based on clinical judgment and requires constant vigilance to ensure that the clinical course has not changed.

Operative Management

In general, the patient with a complete small bowel obstruction requires operative intervention. A nonoperative approach to selected patients with complete small intestinal obstruction has been proposed by some, who argue that prolonged intubation is safe in these patients provided that no fever, tachycardia, tenderness, or leukocytosis is noted. Nevertheless, one must realize that nonoperative management of these patients is undertaken at a calculated risk of overlooking an underlying strangulation obstruction and delaying the treatment of intestinal strangulation until after the injury becomes irreversible. Retrospective studies report that a 12- to 24-hour delay of surgery in these patients is safe but that the incidence of strangulation and other complications increases significantly after this time period.[43]

The nature of the problem dictates the approach to management of the obstructed patient. Patients with intestinal obstruction secondary to an adhesive band may be treated with lysis of adhesions. Great care should be used in the gentle handling of the bowel to reduce serosal trauma and avoid unnecessary dissection and inadvertent enterotomies. Incarcerated hernias can be managed by manual reduction of the herniated segment of bowel and closure of the defect.

The treatment of patients with an obstruction and a history of malignant tumors can be particularly challenging. In the terminal patient with widespread metastasis, nonoperative management, if successful, is usually the best course; however, only a small percentage of cases of complete obstruction can be successfully managed nonoperatively. In this case, a simple bypass of the obstruct-

ing lesion, by whatever means, may offer the best option rather than a long and complicated operation that may entail bowel resection.

Patients with an obstruction secondary to Crohn's disease will often resolve with conservative management if the obstruction is acute. If a chronic fibrotic stricture is the cause of the obstruction, then a bowel resection or strictureplasty may be required.

Patients with an intra-abdominal abscess can present in a manner indistinguishable from those with mechanical bowel obstruction. CT is particularly useful in diagnosing the cause of the obstruction in these patients; drainage of the abscess percutaneously may be sufficient to relieve the obstruction.

Radiation enteropathy, as a complication of radiation therapy for pelvic malignancies, may cause bowel obstruction. Most cases can be treated nonoperatively with tube decompression and possibly corticosteroids, particularly during the acute setting. In the chronic setting, nonoperative management is rarely effective and will require laparotomy with possible resection of the irradiated bowel or bypass of the affected area.

At the time of exploration, it can sometimes be difficult to evaluate bowel viability after the release of a strangulation. If intestinal viability is questionable, the bowel segment should be completely released and placed in a warm, saline-moistened sponge for 15 to 20 minutes and then reexamined. If normal color has returned and peristalsis is evident, it is safe to retain the bowel. A prospective controlled trial comparing clinical judgment with the use of a Doppler probe or the administration of fluorescein for the intraoperative discrimination of viability found that the Doppler flow probe added little to the conventional clinical judgment of the surgeon.[44] In difficult borderline cases, fluorescein fluorescence may supplement clinical judgment. Another approach to the assessment of bowel viability is the "second look" laparotomy 18 to 24 hours after the initial procedure. This decision should be made at the time of the initial operation. A second-look laparotomy is clearly indicated in a patient whose condition deteriorates after the initial operation.

Some groups have evaluated the efficacy of laparoscopic management of acute small bowel obstruction.[45,46] The laparoscopic treatment of small bowel obstruction appears to be effective and leads to a shorter hospital stay in a highly selected group of patients. Patients fitting the criteria for consideration of laparoscopic management include those with (1) mild abdominal distention allowing adequate visualization, (2) a proximal obstruction, (3) a partial obstruction, and (4) an anticipated single-band obstruction. Currently, patients who have advanced, complete, or distal small bowel obstructions are not candidates for laparoscopic treatment. Unfortunately, the majority of patients with obstruction are in this group. Similarly, patients with matted adhesions or carcinomatosis or those who remain distended after nasogastric intubation should be managed with conventional laparotomy. Therefore, the future role of laparoscopic procedures in the treatment of these patients remains to be defined.

Management of Specific Problems

Recurrent Intestinal Obstruction

All surgeons can readily (and most often painfully) remember the complicated patient with multiple previous abdominal operations and a "frozen" abdomen who presents with yet another bowel obstruction. An initial nonoperative trial is usually desirable and often safe. In those patients who do not respond conservatively, reoperation is required. This can often be a long and arduous procedure with great care taken to prevent enterotomies. In these difficult patients, various surgical procedures and pharmacologic agents have been tried in an effort to prevent recurrent adhesions and obstruction.

External plication procedures have been described in which the small intestine or its mesentery is sutured in large, gently curving loops.[47,48] Common complications have included the development of fistulas, gross leakage, peritonitis, and death. For this reason, and because of the low overall success rate, these procedures have largely been abandoned. Several series have reported moderate success with internal fixation or stenting procedures using a long intestinal tube inserted via the nose, a gastrostomy, or even a jejunostomy and left in place for 2 weeks or longer.[49,50] Complications associated with these tubes include prolonged drainage of bowel contents from the tube insertion site, intussusception, and difficult removal of the tube, which may require surgical reexploration.

Pharmacologic agents, including corticosteroids and other anti-inflammatory agents, cytotoxic drugs, and antihistamines, have been used with limited success. The use of anticoagulants, such as heparin, dextran solutions, dicumarol, and sodium citrate, has modified the extent of adhesion formation, but their side effects far outweigh their efficacy. Intraperitoneal instillation of various proteinases (e.g., trypsin, papain, and pepsin), which cause enzymatic digestion of the extracellular protein matrix, has been unsuccessful. Hyaluronidase has been of questionable value, and conflicting results have been obtained with fibrinolytic agents such as streptokinase, urokinase, and fibrinolytic snake venoms. In a prospective, multicenter trial, Becker and colleagues[51] reported that the use of a hyaluronate-based, bioresorbable membrane reduced the incidence and severity of postoperative adhesion formation. Another study by Vrijland and associates found that placement of this membrane reduced the severity, but not the incidence, of postoperative adhesion in patients undergoing a Hartmann procedure.[52] This could represent a significant advance if the long-term incidence of obstruction is likewise shown to be reduced.

To date, the most effective means of limiting the number of adhesions is a good surgical technique, which includes the gentle handling of the bowel to reduce serosal trauma, avoidance of unnecessary dissection, exclusion of foreign material from the peritoneal cavity (the use of absorbable suture material when possible, the avoidance of excessive use of gauze sponges, and the removal of starch from gloves), adequate irrigation and removal of infectious and ischemic debris, and preservation and use of the omentum around the site of surgery or in the denuded pelvis.[53]

Acute Postoperative Obstruction

Small bowel obstruction that occurs in the immediate postoperative period presents a challenge in both the diagnosis and treatment. Diagnosis is often difficult because the primary symptoms of abdominal pain and nausea or emesis may be attributed to a postoperative ileus. Electrolyte deficiencies, particularly hypokalemia, can be a cause of ileus and should be corrected. Plain abdominal films are usually not helpful in distinguishing an ileus from obstruction. CT may be useful in this regard and, in particular, enteroclysis studies may be quite helpful in determining if an obstruction exists and, if so, then the level of the obstruction. Conservative management should be attempted for a partial obstruction. Complete obstruction requires reoperation and correction of the underlying problem.

Ileus

An ileus is defined as intestinal distention and the slowing or absence of passage of luminal contents without a demonstrable mechanical obstruction. An ileus can result from a number of causes, including drug induced, metabolic, neurogenic, and infectious (Box 46-2).

Pharmacologic agents that can produce an ileus include anticholinergic drugs, autonomic blockers, antihistamines, and various psychotropic agents, such as haloperidol and tricyclic antidepressants. One of the more common causes of drug-induced ileus in the operative patient is the use of opiates, such as morphine or meperidine. Metabolic causes of ileus are common and include hypokalemia, hyponatremia, and hypomagnesemia. Other metabolic causes include uremia, diabetic coma, and hypoparathyroidism. Neurogenic causes of an ileus include postoperative ileus, which occurs after abdominal operations. Spinal injury, retroperitoneal irritation, and

---

Box 46-2. Causes of Ileus

Post laparotomy
Metabolic and electrolyte derangements (e.g., hypokalemia, hyponatremia, hypomagnesemia, uremia, diabetic coma)
Drugs (e.g., opiates, psychotropic agents, anticholinergic agents)
Intra-abdominal inflammation
Retroperitoneal hemorrhage or inflammation
Intestinal ischemia
Systemic sepsis

Adapted from Turnage RH, Bergen PC: Intestinal obstruction and ileus. *In* Feldman M, Scharschmidt FG, Sleisenger MH (eds): Gastrointestinal and Liver Disease. Pathophysiology/Diagnosis/Management. Philadelphia, WB Saunders, 1998, pp 1799-1810.

orthopedic procedures on the spine or pelvis can result in an ileus. Finally, a number of infectious causes can result in an ileus; common infectious causes include pneumonia, peritonitis, and generalized sepsis from a nonabdominal source.

Patients often present in a manner similar to those with a mechanical small bowel obstruction. Abdominal distention, usually without the colicky abdominal pain, is the typical and most notable finding. Nausea and vomiting may occur but may also be absent. Patients with an ileus may continue to pass flatus and diarrhea, and this may help distinguish these patients from those with a mechanical small bowel obstruction.

Radiologic studies may help to distinguish ileus from small bowel obstruction. Plain abdominal radiographs may reveal distended small bowel as well as large bowel loops. In cases that are difficult to differentiate from obstruction, barium studies may be beneficial.

The treatment of an ileus is entirely supportive with nasogastric decompression and intravenous fluids. The most effective treatment to correct the underlying condition may be aggressive treatment of the sepsis, correction of any metabolic or electrolyte abnormalities, and discontinuation of medications that may produce an ileus. Pharmacologic agents have been used but for the most part have been ineffective. Drugs that block sympathetic input (e.g., guanethidine) or stimulate parasympathetic activity (e.g., bethanechol or neostigmine) have been tried. In addition, hormonal manipulation, using cholecystokinin or motilin, has been evaluated, but the results have been inconsistent. Intravenous erythromycin has been ineffective, and cisapride, although apparently beneficial in stimulating gastric motility, does not appear to alter intestinal ileus.

INFLAMMATORY DISEASES

Crohn's Disease

Crohn's disease is a chronic, transmural inflammatory disease of the gastrointestinal tract of unknown cause. Crohn's disease can involve any part of the alimentary tract from the mouth to the anus but most commonly affects the small intestine and colon. The most common clinical manifestations are abdominal pain, diarrhea, and weight loss. Crohn's disease can be complicated by intestinal obstruction or localized perforation with fistula formation. Both medical and surgical treatments are palliative; however, operative therapy can provide effective symptomatic relief for those patients with complications from Crohn's disease and produces a reasonable long-term benefit.

History

The first documented case of Crohn's disease was described by Morgagni in 1761. In 1913, the Scottish surgeon Dalziel described nine cases of intestinal inflammatory disease.[54] However, it is the landmark paper by Crohn, Ginzburg, and Oppenheimer in 1932 that provided, in eloquent detail, the pathologic and clinical findings of this inflammatory disease in young adults.[55] This classic paper crystallized the description of this inflammatory condition. Although many different (and sometimes misleading) terms have been used to describe this disease process, *Crohn's disease* has been universally accepted as its name.

Incidence and Epidemiology

Crohn's disease is the most common primary surgical disease of the small bowel, with an annual incidence of 3 to 7 cases per 100,000 of the general population; the incidence is highest in North America and Northern Europe.[56] Crohn's disease primarily attacks young adults in the second and third decades of life. However, a bimodal distribution is apparent with a second smaller peak occurring in the sixth decade of life. Crohn's disease is more common in urban dwellers, and although earlier reports suggested a somewhat higher female predominance, the two genders are affected equally. The risk of developing Crohn's disease is about two times higher in smokers than that in nonsmokers. Several studies have indicated an increased incidence of Crohn's disease in women using oral contraceptives; however, more recent studies have shown no differences. Although Crohn's disease is uncommon in African blacks, blacks in the United States have rates similar to whites. Certain ethnic groups, particularly Jews, have a greater incidence of Crohn's disease than do age- and gender-matched control subjects. There is a strong familial association, with the risk of developing Crohn's disease increased approximately 30-fold in siblings and 14- to 15-fold for all first-degree relatives. Other analyses supporting a genetic role for Crohn's disease show a concordance rate of 67% in monozygotic twins for Crohn's disease.

Etiology

The cause of Crohn's disease remains unknown. A number of potential causes have been proposed, with the most likely possibilities being infectious, immunologic, and genetic.[56,57] Other possibilities that have met with various levels of enthusiasm include environmental and dietary factors, smoking, and psychosocial factors. Although these latter factors may contribute in the overall disease process, it is unlikely that they represent the primary etiologic mechanism for Crohn's disease.

Infectious Agents

Although a number of infectious agents have been proposed as potential causes of Crohn's disease, the two that have received the most attention include mycobacterial infections, particularly *Mycobacterium paratuberculosis*, and the measles virus. The existence of atypical mycobacteria as a cause for Crohn's disease was proposed by Dalziel in 1913.[54] Subsequent studies using polymerase chain reaction (PCR) techniques have confirmed the presence of mycobacteria in intestinal samples of patients with

Crohn's disease. Transplantation of tissue from patients with Crohn's disease has resulted in ileitis,[58] but antimicrobial therapy directed against mycobacteria has not been effective in ameliorating the disease process.

Immunologic Factors

Immunologic abnormalities that have been demonstrated in patients with Crohn's disease have included humoral as well as cell-mediated immune reactions directed against intestinal cells, suggesting an autoimmune phenomenon. Attention has focused on the role of cytokines, such as interleukin (IL)-1, IL-2, IL-8, and TNF-α, as contributing factors in the intestinal inflammatory response. The role of the immune response remains controversial in Crohn's disease and may represent an effect of the disease process rather than an actual cause.

Genetic Factors

Genetic factors play an important role in the pathogenesis of Crohn's disease because the single strongest risk factor for developing disease is having a relative with Crohn's disease. European and American studies reported the presence of a locus on chromosome 16q (called the *IBD1* locus).[59,60] Independent investigative groups identified the *IBD1* locus as the *NOD2* gene, a member of the CED4/APAF1 superfamily of apoptosis regulatory proteins, which mediates the innate immune response to microbial pathogens, leading to NF-κB activation.[60,61] Individuals with allelic variants of *NOD2* have a 40-fold relative risk of Crohn's disease compared with the general population; the *IBD1* locus appears to be relatively specific for Crohn's disease and not ulcerative colitis. Other inflammatory bowel disease genomic regions include *IBD2* on chromosome 12q (observed more in ulcerative colitis) and *IBD3*, containing the major histocompatibility complex region located on chromosome 6p. Putative *IBD* loci have been identified on chromosomes 5q, 19p, 7q and 3p.[60,61]

Even with strong evidence for a genetic link to Crohn's disease, it is worth reiterating that there is a substantially less than 100% concordance rate between monozygotic twins, suggesting that simple mendelian inheritance cannot account for the pattern of occurrence. Therefore, it is likely that multiple causes (e.g., environmental factors) contribute to the etiology and pathogenesis of this disease.

Pathology

The most common sites of occurrence of Crohn's disease are the small intestine and colon. The involvement of both large and small intestine has been noted in approximately 55% of patients. Thirty percent of patients present with small bowel disease alone, and in 15% the disease appears limited to the large intestine. The disease process is discontinuous and segmental. In patients with colonic disease, rectal sparing is characteristic of Crohn's disease and helps to distinguish it from ulcerative colitis. Perirectal and perianal involvement occurs in about one third of patients with Crohn's disease, particularly those with

colonic involvement. Crohn's disease can also involve the mouth, esophagus, stomach, duodenum, and appendix. Involvement of these sites can accompany disease in the small or large intestine, but in only rare cases have these locations been the only apparent sites of involvement.

Gross Pathologic Features

At exploration, thickened grayish-pink or dull purple-red loops of bowel are noted, with areas of thick gray-white exudate or fibrosis of the serosa. Areas of diseased bowel separated by areas of grossly appearing normal bowel called "skip areas" are commonly encountered. A striking finding of Crohn's disease is extensive fat wrapping caused by the circumferential growth of the mesenteric fat around the bowel wall (Fig. 46-18). As the disease progresses, the bowel wall becomes increasingly thickened, firm, rubbery, and virtually incompressible. The uninvolved proximal bowel may be dilated secondary to obstruction of the diseased segment. Involved segments often are adherent to adjacent intestinal loops or other viscera with internal fistulas common in these areas. The mesentery of the involved segment is usually thickened, with enlarged lymph nodes often noted.

On opening the bowel, the earliest gross pathologic lesion is a superficial aphthous ulcer noted in the mucosa. As the disease progresses, the ulceration becomes pronounced and complete transmural inflammation results. The ulcers are characteristically linear and may coalesce to produce transverse sinuses with islands of normal mucosa in between, thus giving the characteristic cobblestone appearance.

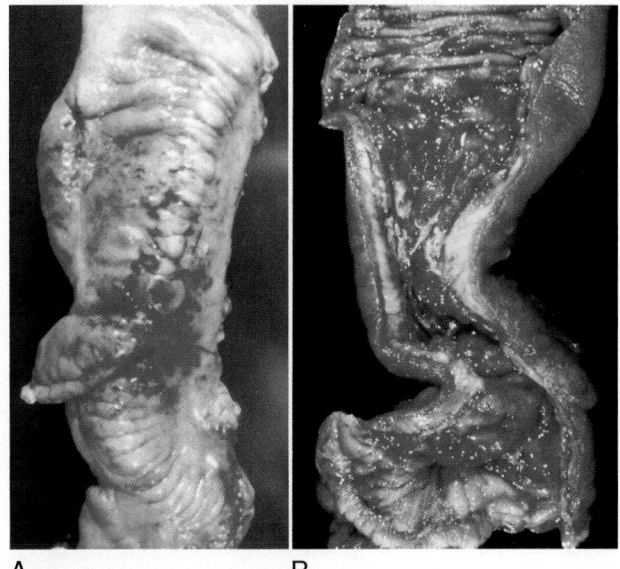

A   B

FIGURE 46-18. Gross pathologic features of Crohn's disease. **A,** Serosal surface demonstrates extensive "fat wrapping" and inflammation. **B,** Resected specimen demonstrates marked fibrosis of the intestinal wall, stricture, and segmental mucosal inflammation. (Courtesy of Mary R. Schwartz, M.D., Baylor College of Medicine.)

Microscopic Features

Mucosal and submucosal edema may be noted microscopically before any gross changes.[62] A chronic inflammatory infiltrate appears in the mucosa and submucosa and extends transmurally. This inflammatory reaction is characterized by extensive edema, hyperemia, lymphangiectasia, an intense infiltration of mononuclear cells, and lymphoid hyperplasia. Characteristic histologic lesions of Crohn's disease are noncaseating granulomas with Langer-

hans' giant cells. Granulomas appear later in the course and are found in the wall of the bowel or in regional lymph nodes in 60% to 70% of patients (Fig. 46-19).

Clinical Manifestations

Crohn's disease can occur at any age, but the typical patient is the young adult in the second or third decade of life. The onset of disease is often insidious, with a slow

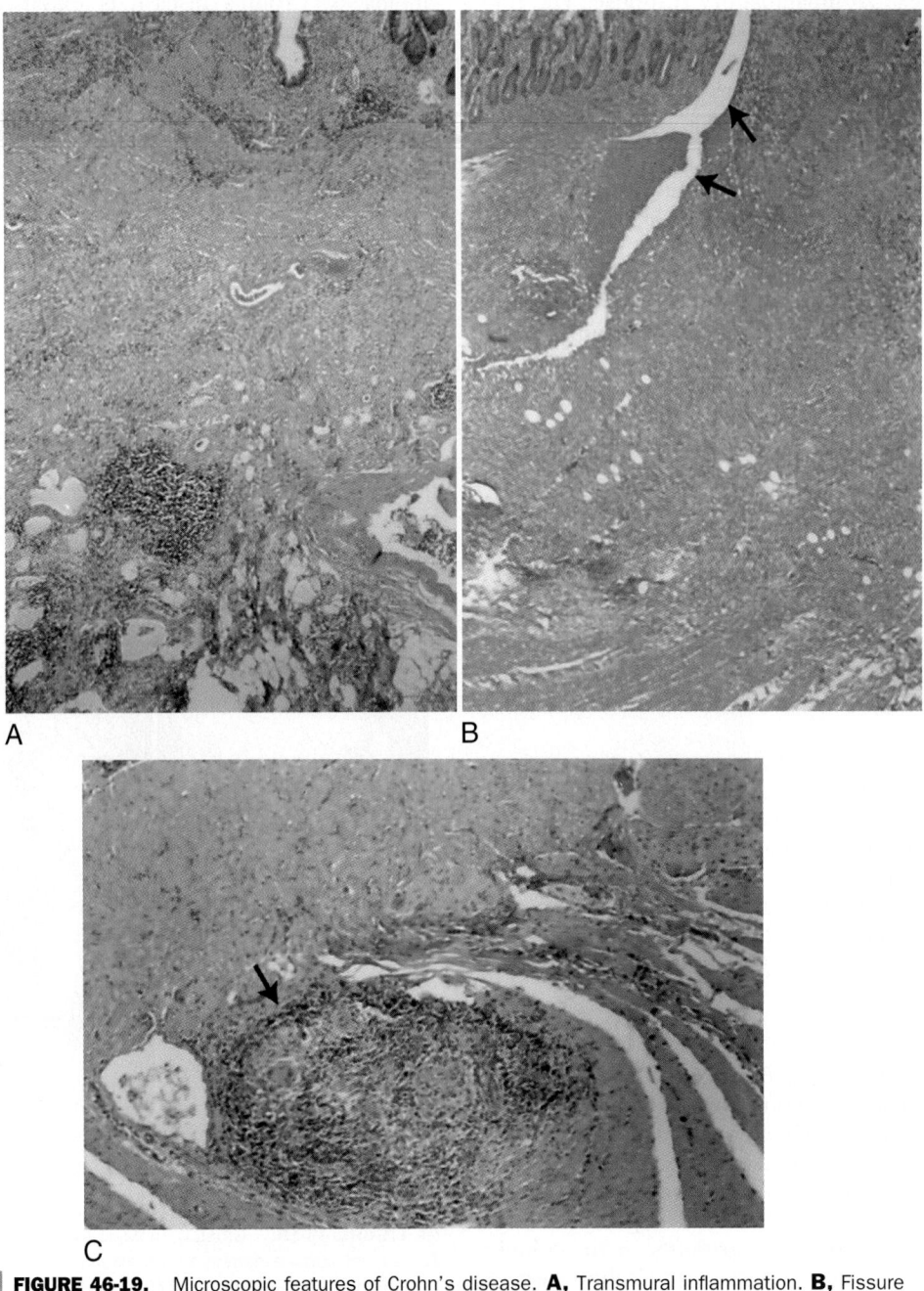

A

B

C

■ **FIGURE 46-19.**   Microscopic features of Crohn's disease. **A,** Transmural inflammation. **B,** Fissure ulcer *(arrows)*. **C,** Noncaseating granuloma located in the muscular layer of the small bowel *(arrow)*. (Courtesy of Mary R. Schwartz, M.D., Baylor College of Medicine.)

and protracted course. Characteristically, there are symptomatic periods of abdominal pain and diarrhea interspersed with asymptomatic periods of varying lengths. With time, the symptomatic periods gradually become more frequent, more severe, and longer lasting. The most common symptom is intermittent and colicky abdominal pain, most commonly noted in the lower abdomen. The pain, however, may be more severe and localized and may mimic the signs and symptoms of acute appendicitis. Diarrhea is the next most frequent symptom and is present, at least intermittently, in approximately 85% of patients. In contrast to ulcerative colitis, patients with Crohn's disease typically have fewer bowel movements and the stools rarely contain mucus, pus, or blood. Systemic nonspecific symptoms include a low-grade fever (present in about one third of the patients), weight loss, loss of strength, and malaise.

The main intestinal complications of Crohn's disease include obstruction and perforation. Obstruction occurs as a result of chronic fibrosing lesions, which eventually narrow the lumen of the bowel, producing partial or near-complete obstruction. Free perforations into the peritoneal cavity leading to a generalized peritonitis can occur in patients with Crohn's disease, but this presentation is rare. More commonly, fistulas occur between the sites of perforation and adjacent organs, such as loops of small and large intestine, the urinary bladder, the vagina, the stomach, and sometimes the skin, usually at the site of a previous laparotomy. Localized abscesses can occur near the sites of perforation. Patients with Crohn's colitis may develop toxic megacolon and present with a marked colonic dilatation, abdominal tenderness, fever, and leukocytosis.

Long-standing Crohn's disease predisposes to cancer of both the small intestine and colon.[63,64] The relative risk for adenocarcinoma of the small bowel in Crohn's disease is at least 100-fold greater than in matched control subjects. These carcinomas typically arise at sites of chronic disease and more commonly occur in the ileum. Most are not detected until the advanced stages and prognosis is poor. Although this relative risk of small bowel cancer in Crohn's disease is quite high, the absolute risk is still small. Of greater concern is the development of colorectal cancer in patients with colonic involvement and a long duration of disease. Although the cancer risk is lower in Crohn's disease than in patients with extensive ulcerative colitis, recent evidence indicates that with the same duration and anatomic extent of disease, the risk of cancer in Crohn's disease of the colon is at least as great as that in ulcerative colitis. Dysplasia is the putative precursor lesion for Crohn's-associated cancer. Although the dysplasia-carcinoma sequence has not been as extensively studied in Crohn's disease compared with ulcerative colitis, patients with long-standing Crohn's disease should have an equally aggressive colonoscopic surveillance regimen as in patients with extensive ulcerative colitis. Extraintestinal cancer, such as squamous cell carcinoma of the vulva and anal canal and Hodgkin's and non-Hodgkin's lymphomas, may be more frequent in patients with Crohn's disease.

Perianal disease (fissure, fistula, stricture, or abscess) is common and occurs in 25% of patients with Crohn's disease limited to the small intestine, 41% of patients with ileocolitis, and 48% of patients with colonic involvement alone. Perianal disease may be the sole presenting feature in 5% of patients and may precede the onset of intestinal disease by months or even years. Crohn's disease should be suspected in any patient with multiple, chronic perianal fistulas.

Extraintestinal manifestations of Crohn's disease may be present in 30% of patients (Box 46-3). The most common symptoms are skin lesions, which include erythema nodosum and pyoderma gangrenosum, arthritis and arthralgias, uveitis and iritis, hepatitis and pericholangitis, and aphthous stomatitis. In addition, amyloidosis, pancreatitis, and nephrotic syndrome may occur in these patients. These symptoms may precede, accompany, or appear independent of the underlying bowel disease.

Diagnosis

A diagnosis of Crohn's disease should be considered in patients with chronic, recurring episodes of abdominal pain, diarrhea, and weight loss. Typically, the diagnostic modalities most commonly used include barium contrast studies and endoscopy.[65,66] Barium radiographic studies of the small bowel reveal a number of characteristic findings, including a cobblestone appearance of the mucosa composed of linear ulcers, transverse sinuses, and clefts. Long lengths of narrowed terminal ileum (Kantor string sign) may be present in long-standing disease (Fig. 46-20). Segmental and irregular patterns of bowel involvement may

---

Box 46-3. Extraintestinal Manifestations of Crohn's Disease

Skin

Erythema multiforme
Erythema nodosum
Pyoderma gangrenosum

Eyes

Iritis
Uveitis
Conjunctivitis

Joints

Peripheral arthritis
Ankylosing spondylitis

Blood

Anemia
Thrombocytosis
Phlebothrombosis
Arterial thrombosis

Liver

Nonspecific triaditis
Sclerosing cholangitis

Kidney

Nephrotic syndrome
Amyloidosis

Pancreas

Pancreatitis

General

Amyloidosis

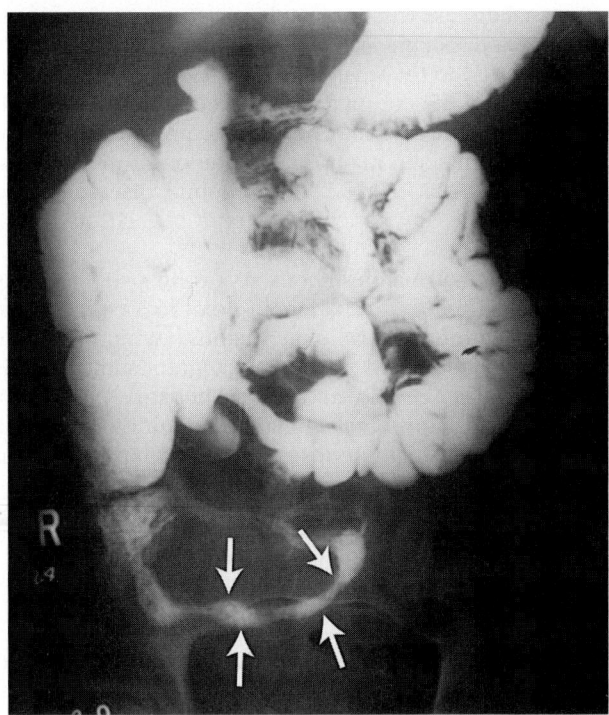

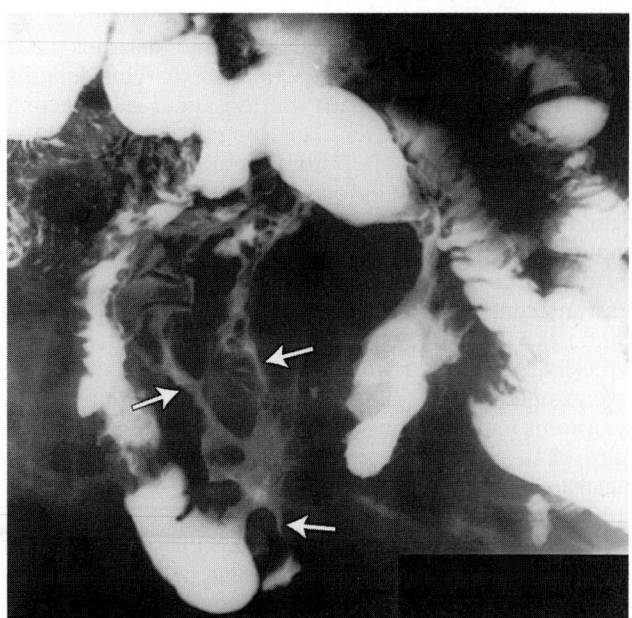

FIGURE 46-20.   Small bowel series in a patient with Crohn's disease demonstrates a narrowed distal ileum *(arrows)* secondary to chronic inflammation and fibrosis. (Courtesy of Melvyn H. Schreiber, M.D., The University of Texas Medical Branch.)

FIGURE 46-21.   Crohn's disease with multiple short fistulous tracks communicating between the distal loops of ileum and the proximal colon *(arrows)*. (Courtesy of Melvyn H. Schreiber, M.D., The University of Texas Medical Branch; adapted from Evers BM, Townsend CM Jr, Thompson JC: Small intestine. *In* Schwartz SI [ed]: Principles of Surgery, 7th ed. New York, McGraw-Hill, 1999, p 1233, with permission of The McGraw-Hill Companies.)

be noted. Fistulas between adjacent bowel loops and organs may be apparent (Fig. 46-21). CT may be useful in demonstrating the marked transmural thickening, and it can also greatly aid in diagnosing extramural complications of Crohn's disease (Fig. 46-22). Ultrasonography has limited value in the evaluation of patients with Crohn's disease, but it is useful in the assessment of undiagnosed right lower quadrant pain. When the colon is involved, sigmoidoscopy or colonoscopy may reveal characteristic aphthous ulcers with granularity and a normal-appearing surrounding mucosa. With more progressive and severe disease, the ulcerations involve more and more of the bowel lumen and may be difficult to distinguish from ulcerative colitis. However, the presence of discrete ulcers and cobblestoning, as well as the discontinuous segments of involved bowel, favors a diagnosis of Crohn's disease. Intubation of the ileocecal valve during colonoscopy allows examination and biopsy of the terminal ileum. Serologic markers may also be useful in the diagnosis of Crohn's disease. In particular, perinuclear antineutrophil cytoplasmic antibody (pANCA) and anti-*Saccharomyces cerevisiae* (ASCA) are two autoantibodies associated with inflammatory bowel disease. A large cohort study reported a specificity of 92% for Crohn's disease in patients who were ASCA positive/pANCA negative and 98% for ulcerative colitis in patients who were ASCA negative/pANCA positive.[62,67]

The differential diagnosis of Crohn's disease includes both specific and nonspecific causes of intestinal inflammation. Bacterial inflammation, such as that caused by

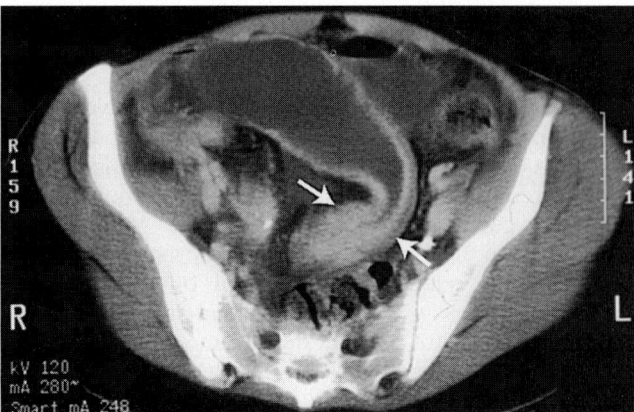

FIGURE 46-22.   CT scan of a patient with Crohn's disease demonstrates marked thickening of the bowel *(arrows)* with a high-grade partial small bowel obstruction and dilated proximal intestine. (Courtesy of Melvyn H. Schreiber, M.D., The University of Texas Medical Branch; adapted from Evers BM, Townsend CM Jr, Thompson JC: Small intestine. *In* Schwartz SI [ed]: Principles of Surgery, 7th ed. New York, McGraw-Hill, 1999, p 1233, with permission of The McGraw-Hill Companies.)

Salmonella and *Shigella*; intestinal tuberculosis; and protozoan infections, such as amebiasis, may present as an ileitis. In the immunocompromised host, rare infections, particularly mycobacterial and cytomegaloviral, have become more common and may cause ileitis. Acute distal ileitis may be a manifestation of early Crohn's disease, but it also may be unrelated such as when it is caused by a bacteriologic agent (e.g., *Campylobacter* or *Yersinia*). Patients usually present in a similar fashion as those presenting with acute appendicitis with a sudden onset of right lower quadrant pain, nausea, vomiting, and fever. These entities normally resolve spontaneously; and when noted during surgery, no biopsy or resection should be performed.

In most instances, Crohn's disease of the colon can be readily distinguished from ulcerative colitis; however, in 5% to 10% of patients, the delineation between Crohn's and ulcerative colitis may be difficult, if not impossible, to make (Table 46-5). Ulcerative colitis nearly always involves the rectum most severely, with lessening inflammation from the rectum to the ileocolic area. In contrast, Crohn's disease may be worse on the right side of the colon than on the left side and sometimes the rectum is spared. Ulcerative colitis also demonstrates continuous involvement from rectum from proximal segments, whereas Crohn's disease is segmental. Although ulcerative colitis involves the mucosa of the large intestine, it does not extend deep into the wall of the bowel, as does Crohn's disease. Bleeding is a more common symptom in ulcerative colitis. Perianal involvement and rectovaginal fistulas are unusual in ulcerative colitis but are more common in Crohn's disease. Other endoscopic features of Crohn's disease are "skip" lesions, asymmetrical involvement of bowel, and the cobblestone appearance that results from ulcerations interspersed with islands of edematous mucosa.

Management

Medical Therapy

There is no cure for Crohn's disease, so both medical and surgical therapy is mainly palliative and directed toward relieving acute exacerbations or complications of the disease.[68] Drugs that have demonstrated efficacy in the induction and maintenance of remission include aminosalicylates (e.g., sulfasalazine, mesalamine), corticosteroids, immunosuppressive agents (e.g., azathioprine, 6-mercaptopurine, and methotrexate), antibiotics, and infliximab (an anti-TNF-α antibody). Other innovative therapies based on selective molecular targets are currently being analyzed.

Aminosalicylate Sulfasalazine (Azulfidine), an aminosalicylate, is the most commonly prescribed drug for Crohn's disease. The active moiety of sulfasalazine is 5-aminosalicylic acid. Sulfasalazine is taken orally and has been shown in randomized, controlled trials to be efficacious in patients with Crohn's disease. A clear benefit is noted in patients with colitis and ileocolitis, whereas the effectiveness of sulfasalazine alone in the treatment of Crohn's disease limited to the small bowel is controversial. In contrast to its use in ulcerative colitis, sulfasalazine has not been conclusively proved to maintain remission in Crohn's disease or to prevent recurrence after surgery. Newer sulfasalazine-like drugs (e.g., mesalamine) that provide for a slow release of 5-aminosalicylic acid during their passage through the small bowel and the colon are being evaluated.[68,69] Clinical trials have demonstrated efficacy of mesalamine at a dosage of 4 g/day without an increase in side effects. Studies are being conducted to evaluate even higher dosages. Mesalamine is considered first-line therapy for Crohn's disease.[68]

Corticosteroids Corticosteroids, particularly prednisone, have been beneficial in the induction of remission in active Crohn's disease. However, they are ineffective in maintaining remission in Crohn's disease. Newer corticosteroids have been evaluated, of which budesonide has been found to be the most promising.[70] In one study, high-dose budesonide was more effective than placebo in achieving remission in patients with active Crohn's

TABLE 46-5. Diagnosis of Crohn's Colitis Versus Ulcerative Colitis		
	Crohn's Colitis	**Ulcerative Colitis**
Symptoms and Signs		
Diarrhea	Common	Common
Rectal bleeding	Less common	Almost always
Abdominal pain (cramps)	Moderate to severe	Mild to moderate
Palpable mass	At times	No (unless large cancer)
Anal complaints	Frequent (>50%)	Infrequent (<20%)
Radiologic Findings		
Ileal disease	Common	Rare (backwash ileitis)
Nodularity, fuzziness	No	Yes
Distribution	Skip areas	Rectum extending upward and continuously
Ulcers	Linear, cobblestone, fissures	Collar-button
Toxic dilatation	Rare	Uncommon
Proctoscopic Findings		
Anal fissure, fistula, abscess	Common	Rare
Rectal sparing	Common (50%)	Rare (5%)
Granular mucosa	No	Yes
Ulceration	Linear, deep, scattered	Superficial, universal

disease. Although the combination of sulfasalazine and corticosteroids may be used to maintain patients for short periods after resolution of an acute inflammatory exacerbation, the long-term use of these compounds, either alone or in combination, has not been shown to be of benefit in preventing recurrence of disease. Given a relatively good response to mesalamine and its relative safety, budesonide may be considered an alternative to mesalamine as first-line therapy for patients with active Crohn's disease.

Antibiotics Certain antibiotics have also been found to be effective in the primary therapy of Crohn's disease. The antibiotic used most is metronidazole, which has been shown in some studies to result in significant improvement in disease activity. Other antibiotics that have been used with varying success include ciprofloxacin, tetracycline, ampicillin, and clindamycin. The mechanism of action of antibiotics in Crohn's disease is unclear, and side effects of these antibiotics preclude their long-term use. Therefore, antibiotics may play an adjunctive role in the treatment of Crohn's disease and, in selected patients, may be useful in treating perianal disease, enterocutaneous fistulas, or active colonic disease.

Immunosuppressive Agents The immunosuppressive agents azathioprine and 6-mercaptopurine are effective in the treatment of Crohn's disease. Despite the potential toxicity, these drugs have proved to be relatively safe in these patients, with the most common side effects including pancreatitis, hepatitis, fever, and rash. The most disconcerting implications of these immunosuppressants are bone marrow suppression and the potential for malignancy. Other immunosuppressive agents that have been used with some effectiveness include methotrexate, cyclosporine, and tacrolimus (FK-506). Tacrolimus inhibits the production of IL-2 by T-helper cells and, in a recent randomized multicenter trial, was found to be effective for fistula improvement, but not fistula remission, in patients with perianal Crohn's disease.[71]

Anticytokine and Cytokine Therapies Perhaps the most promising therapy to emerge in recent years is the introduction of immunomodulatory treatments using cytokines and anticytokines.[72] Monoclonal antibodies to TNF-α have shown promise, with clinical trials demonstrating a rapid control of active Crohn's disease, tissue healing, and potential remission.[73] A randomized controlled trial demonstrated that infliximab, a chimeric monoclonal antibody to TNF-α, is both efficacious and safe in the treatment of moderate-to-severe Crohn's disease and resulted in fistula closure in 46% of patients compared with only 13% of patients receiving placebo.[74] Although highly effective in certain Crohn's patients with fistulas, not every patient responds to infliximab. Also, there is an increased risk of tuberculosis reactivation, invasive fungal and other opportunistic infections, demyelinating central nervous system lesions, activation of latent multiple sclerosis, and exacerbating congestive heart disease. Promising results have also been obtained using the anti-inflammatory cytokine IL-10.[75] A multicenter randomized trial found that IL-10 demonstrated significant improvement in the clinical status in 46% of patients with Crohn's disease compared with 19% of placebo control subjects.

Novel Therapies Other therapeutic agents under investigation include IL-1 receptor antagonists, anti–IL-12, anti–IL-18, and anti–interferon-γ antibodies, anti-adhesion molecule antibodies, and growth factors. Compounds are also being evaluated that block certain signaling pathways (e.g., NF-κB, MAP kinases, and PPARγ); in limited studies, some of these compounds have shown clinical improvements.[76] A recent trial has also been reported using natalizumab, a recombinant humanized monoclonal antibody against α₄ integrin, with efficacy in reducing signs and symptoms of Crohn's disease that was at least similar to that of infliximab.[77]

Nutritional Therapy

Nutritional therapy in patients with Crohn's disease has been used with varying success. The use of chemically defined elemental diets has been shown in some studies to reduce disease activity, particularly in patients with disease localized to the small bowel.[78,79] Liquid polymeric diets may be as effective as elemental feedings and are more acceptable to patients. With few exceptions, standard elemental diets have not been effective in the maintenance of remission in Crohn's disease. Total parenteral nutrition (TPN) has also been shown to be of use in patients with active Crohn's disease; however, complication rates exceed those for enteral nutrition. Although the primary role of nutritional therapy is questionable in patients with inflammatory bowel disease, there is definitely a secondary role for nutritional supplementation to replenish depleted nutrient stores, allowing intestinal protein synthesis and healing, and for preparing patients for operation.

Surgical Treatment

Although medical management is indicated during acute exacerbations of disease, the majority of patients with chronic Crohn's disease will require surgery some time during the course of their illness. In patients with more than 20 years of disease, the National Cooperative Crohn's Disease Study reported that the cumulative probability of surgery was 78%.[80] The indications for operation are limited to complications that include intestinal obstruction, intestinal perforation with fistula formation or abscess, free perforation, gastrointestinal bleeding, urologic complications, cancer, and perianal disease.[81] Children with Crohn's disease and resulting systemic symptoms, such as growth retardation, may benefit from resection. The extraintestinal complication of Crohn's disease, although not a primary indication for operation, often subsides after resection of involved bowel with the exception of ankylosing spondylitis and hepatic complications.

Operative therapy in patients with Crohn's disease should be specifically directed to the complication, and only the segment of bowel involved in the complicating process should be resected.[82] Even if adjacent areas of bowel are clearly diseased, they should be ignored. Early in the history of the surgical therapy of Crohn's disease, surgeons tended to perform wider resections with the hope of cure or significant remission. However, repeated wide resections resulted in no greater remissions or cure and led to the short bowel syndrome, which is a devastating surgical complication. Frozen sections to determine microscopic disease are unreliable and are not recommended. *Therefore, operative treatment of a complication should be limited to that segment of bowel involved with the complication and no attempt should be made to resect more bowel even though grossly evident disease may be apparent.*

The role of laparoscopic surgery for patients with Crohn's disease has not been clearly defined. In appropriately selected patients, for example those with localized abscesses, simple intra-abdominal fistulas, and perianastomotic recurrent disease, this technique appears feasible and safe.[83,84] However, the advantage of laparoscopic surgery over conventional open surgery in this disease has not been established. Randomized clinical trials are required to assess the potential future role of laparoscopic surgery in the management of patients with Crohn's disease.

Management of Specific Problems

Acute Ileitis

Patients can present with acute abdominal pain localized to the right lower quadrant and signs and symptoms consistent with a diagnosis of acute appendicitis. At exploration, the appendix is found to be normal, but the terminal ileum is edematous and beefy red, with a thickened mesentery and enlarged lymph nodes. This condition, known as *acute ileitis*, is a self-limited disease. Acute ileitis may be a manifestation of early Crohn's disease but is most often unrelated. Bacteriologic agents such as *Campylobacter* or *Yersinia* may result in acute ileitis. Intestinal resection should not be performed. Although in the past the management of the appendix was controversial, it is clear now that in the absence of acute inflammatory involvement of the appendix or the cecum, appendectomy should be performed. This eliminates the appendix as a source of abdominal pain in the future.

Obstruction

Intestinal obstruction is the most common indication for surgical therapy in patients with Crohn's disease. Obstruction in these patients is often partial, and nonoperative management is indicated initially. Operative intervention is required in instances of complete obstruction and in patients with partial obstruction whose condition does not resolve with nonoperative management. The treatment of choice of intestinal obstruction in patients with Crohn's disease is segmental resection of the involved segment with primary reanastomosis. This may involve segmental resection and primary anastomosis of a short segment of ileum if this is the site of the complication. More commonly, the cecum is involved contiguously with

the terminal ileum, in which case resection of the involved terminal ileum and colon is required and the ileum is anastomosed to the ascending or transverse colon (Fig. 46-23).

In selected patients with obstruction caused by strictures (either single or multiple), one option is to perform a strictureplasty that effectively widens the lumen but avoids intestinal resection.[85] Strictureplasty is performed by making a longitudinal incision through the narrowed area of the intestine followed by closure in a transverse fashion in a manner similar to a Heineke-Mikulicz pyloroplasty (Fig. 46-24A). For longer diseased segments (>10 cm), the strictureplasty can be performed similar to a Finney pyloroplasty (see Fig. 46-24B) or a side-to-side isoperistaltic strictureplasty.[86] Strictureplasty has the most application in those patients in whom multiple short areas of narrowing are present over long segments of intestine, in those patients who have already had several previous resections of the small intestine, and when the areas of narrowing are due to fibrous obstruction rather than acute inflammation. This procedure preserves intestine and is associated with complication and recurrence rates comparable to resection and reanastomosis.

In the past, bypass procedures were commonly used. Currently, bypass with exclusion is used only in elderly, poor-risk patients; patients who have had several prior resections and cannot afford to lose any more bowel; and patients in whom resection would necessitate entering an abscess or endangering normal structures.

Fistula

Fistulas in patients with Crohn's disease are relatively common and are usually to adjacent small bowel, colon, or other surrounding viscera (e.g., bladder). The presence of a radiographically demonstrable enteroenteral fistula without any signs of sepsis or other complications is not in itself an indication for surgery. However, many of these

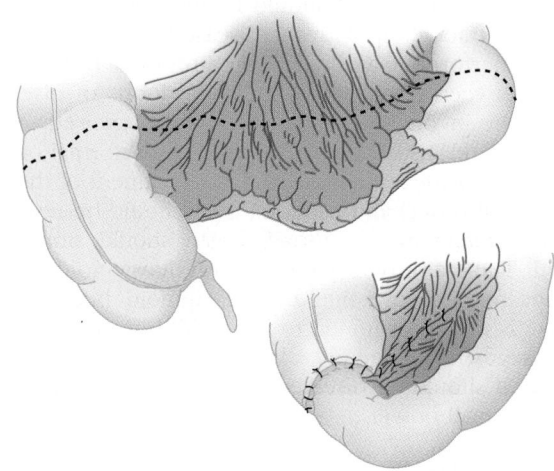

FIGURE 46-23. Resection of the ileum, ileocecal valve, cecum, and ascending colon for Crohn's disease of the ileum. Intestinal continuity is restored by end-to-end anastomosis.

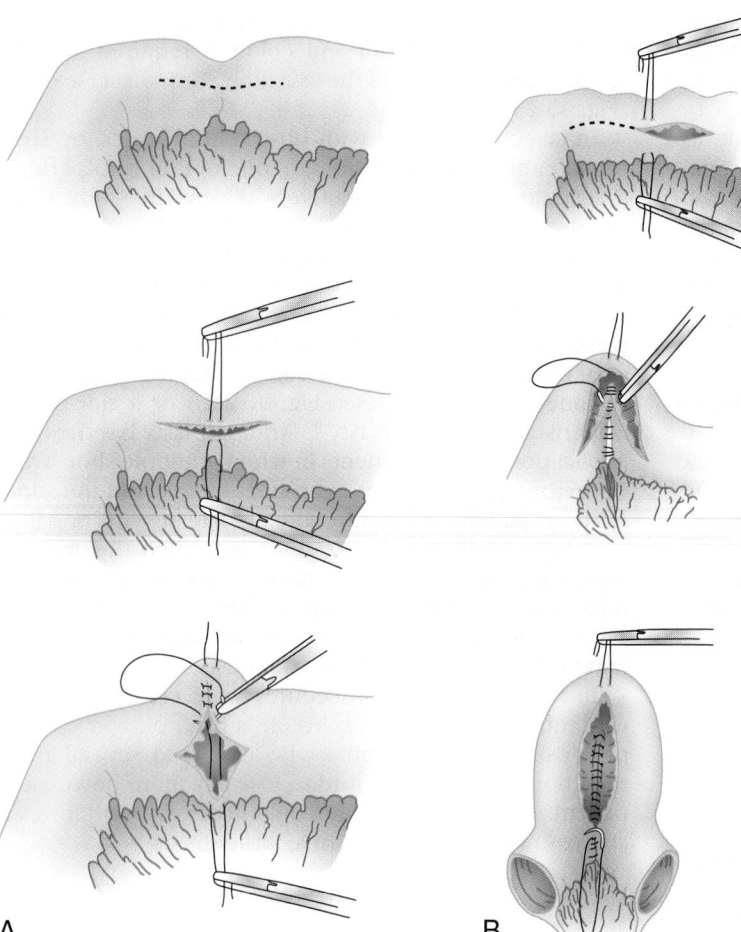

A

B

FIGURE 46-24.   **A,** Technique of short strictureplasty in the manner of a Heineke-Mikulicz pyloroplasty. **B,** For longer diseased segments, strictureplasty may be performed in a manner similar to Finney pyloroplasty. (Adapted with permission from Alexander-Williams J, Haynes IG: Up-to-date management of small-bowel Crohn's disease. *In* Advances in Surgery. St. Louis, Mosby, 1987, pp 245-264.)

patients will require eventual resection as the disease progresses and the patients have progressively worsening abdominal pain. Enterocutaneous fistulas may develop but are rarely spontaneous and are more likely to follow resection or drainage of intra-abdominal abscesses. Ideally, enterocutaneous fistulas should be managed by excising the fistula tract along with the diseased segment of intestine and performing a primary reanastomosis. If the fistula forms between two or more adjacent loops of diseased bowel, the involved segments should be excised. Alternatively, if the fistula involves an adjacent normal organ, such as the bladder or colon, only the segment of the diseased small bowel and fistulous tract should be resected and the defect in the normal organ should simply be closed. The majority of patients with ileosigmoid fistulas do not require resection of the sigmoid because the disease is usually confined to the small bowel. However, if the segment of sigmoid is also found to have Crohn's disease, it should be resected along with the segment of diseased small bowel.

Free Perforation

Perforation into the free peritoneal cavity occurs occasionally but is not common in patients with Crohn's disease. When this occurs, the segment of involved bowel should be resected and, in the presence of minimal contamination, a primary anastomosis should be performed. If generalized peritonitis is present, a safer option may be to perform enterostomies until the intra-abdominal sepsis is controlled and then return for restoration of intestinal continuity.

Gastrointestinal Bleeding

Although anemia from chronic blood loss is common in patients with Crohn's disease, life-threatening gastrointestinal hemorrhage is rare. The incidence of hemorrhage is more common in patients with Crohn's disease involving the colon rather than the small bowel. As with the other complications, the segment involved should be resected and intestinal continuity restored. Arteriography may be useful to localize the bleeding before surgery.

Urologic Complications

Genitourinary complications occur in 4% to 35% of patients with Crohn's disease.[87] The most common urologic complication is ureteral obstruction, which is usually secondary to ileocolic disease with retroperitoneal abscess. Surgical treatment of the primary intestinal disease is adequate in most patients. In a few instances of long-standing inflammatory disease, periureteric fibrosis may be present and require ureterolysis.

Cancer

Patients with long-standing Crohn's disease of the small bowel and, in particular, the colon have an increased incidence of cancer. The management of these patients is the same as any patient (i.e., resection of the cancer with appropriate margins and regional lymph nodes). Patients with cancer associated with Crohn's disease commonly have a worse prognosis than those who do not have Crohn's, based largely on the fact that the diagnosis in these patients is delayed.

Colorectal Disease

The same principle applies to patients with Crohn's disease limited to the colon as those with disease to the small bowel; that is, surgical resection should be limited to the segment producing the complications.[88] Indications for surgery include a lack of response to medical management or complications of Crohn's colitis, which include obstruction, hemorrhage, perforation, and toxic megacolon. Depending on the diseased segments, operations commonly include segmental colectomy with colocolonic anastomosis, subtotal colectomy with ileoproctostomy, and in patients with extensive perianal and rectal disease, total proctocolectomy with Brooke ileostomy. Patients with toxic megacolon should undergo colectomy, closure of the proximal rectum, and end ileostomy.

A particularly troubling problem after proctocolectomy in patients with Crohn's disease is delayed healing of the perineal wound. Several series have reported that 25% to 60% of perineal wounds are open 6 months after surgery. Persistent nonhealing wounds require excision with secondary closure. Large cavities or sinuses may be filled using well-vascularized pedicles of muscle (gracilis, semimembranosus, rectus abdominis) or omentum or by using an inferior gluteal myocutaneous graft.[88]

Although controversial, continence-preserving operations, such as ileoanal pouch anastomoses or continent ileostomies (Kock pouch) that have been used in patients with ulcerative colitis, are not recommended for patients with Crohn's colitis because of the high rate of recurrence of Crohn's disease in the pouch, fistulas to the anastomosis, and peripouch abscesses.

Perianal Disease

Diseases involving the perianal region include fissures and fistulas and are quite common in patients with Crohn's disease, particularly those with colonic involvement. The treatment of perianal disease should be conservative.[89,90] Antibiotics and immunosuppressive agents (e.g., azathioprine and 6-mercaptopurine) have been used with varying success. Encouraging reports have been obtained using the TNF-α antibody infliximab and tacrolimus.[71,74] Wide excision of abscesses or fistulas is not indicated, but more conservative interventions, including the liberal placement of drainage catheters and noncutting setons, are preferable.[91] Definitive fistulotomy is indicated in the majority of patients with superficial, low transsphincteric, and low intersphincteric fistulas, although one must recognize that some degree of anal stenosis may occur as a result of chronic inflammation. High transsphincteric, suprasphincteric, and extrasphincteric fistulas are usually treated with noncutting setons. Fissures usually are lateral, relatively painless, large, and indolent and usually respond to conservative management. Abscesses should be drained, but large excisions of tissue should not be performed. Advancement flap closure of perineal fistulas may be required in certain instances. Selective construction of diverting stomas has good results when combined with optimal medical therapy to induce remission of inflammation. Proctectomy may be infrequently required in a subset of patients who have persistent and unremitting disease despite conservative medical and surgical therapy.

Duodenal Disease

Crohn's disease of the duodenum occurs in 2% to 4% of patients with Crohn's disease. Operative intervention is uncommon. The primary indication for surgery in these patients is duodenal obstruction that does not respond to medical therapy. The use of gastrojejunostomy to bypass the disease rather than duodenal resection is the procedure of choice. Strictureplasties have been performed with success in selected patients.

Prognosis

Operations directed at Crohn's disease are not curative. They provide patients with often significant symptomatic relief. Rates of recurrence are reported as high in most series.[92,93] It is important, however, to note how recurrence is defined in these studies. Endoscopic evidence of recurrence is detected in approximately 70% of patients within 1 year of surgery and in 85% by 3 years. Most of these recurrences are asymptomatic. If defined exclusively by the need for reoperation, however, recurrence rates are only 25% to 30% at 5 years and 40% to 50% at 20 years. To put this in perspective, after a first resection for Crohn's disease, approximately 45% of patients will ultimately require a second operation, of whom only 25% will require a third operation. Overall, nearly 90% of people undergoing operation for Crohn's disease will never require more than one additional operation. Despite the risk of recurrence, many patients who have had surgery for Crohn's disease wish that they had had their operation sooner. Performed for proper indications, surgery almost invariably rehabilitates those disabled by Crohn's disease. The overwhelming majority of such patients report relief of symptoms after surgery, restoration of a feeling of well-being and the ability to eat normally, and a reduction in the need for medical therapy.[94]

Standardized mortality rates in patients with Crohn's disease are increased in those patients whose disease began before the age of 20 and in those who have had disease present for longer than 13 years. Long-term survival studies have suggested that patients with Crohn's disease have a death rate that is approximately two to three times higher than that in the general population. Gastrointestinal cancer remains the leading cause of disease-related death in patients with Crohn's disease; other causes of disease-related deaths include sepsis, thromboembolic complications, and electrolyte disorders.

Typhoid Enteritis

Typhoid fever remains a significant problem in developing countries, most commonly in areas with contaminated water supplies and inadequate waste disposal. Children and young adults are most often affected. Improvements in sanitation have decreased the incidence of typhoid fever in industrialized countries; however, approximately 500 cases per year are still reported in the United States.

Typhoid enteritis is an acute systemic infection of several weeks' duration caused primarily by *Salmonella typhosa*. The pathologic events of typhoid fever are initiated in the intestinal tract after oral ingestion of the typhoid bacillus. These organisms penetrate the small bowel mucosa, making their way rapidly to the lymphatics and then systemically. Hyperplasia of the reticuloendothelial system, including lymph nodes, liver, and spleen, is characteristic of typhoid fever. Peyer patches in the small bowel become hyperplastic and may subsequently ulcerate with complications of hemorrhage or perforation.

The diagnosis of typhoid fever is confirmed by isolating the organism from blood (positive in 90% of the patients during the first week of the illness), bone marrow, and stool cultures. In addition, the finding of high titers of agglutinins against the O and H antigens is strongly suggestive of typhoid fever. Assays for the diagnosis of *S. typhosa* using PCR have been developed but are still experimental.

Treatment of typhoid fever and uncomplicated typhoid enteritis is accomplished by antibiotic administration. Chloramphenicol, ampicillin, amoxicillin, and trimethoprim-sulfamethoxazole have all been used as therapy with good results. In addition, short courses of third-generation cephalosporins have been used successfully to treat typhoid fever.

Complications requiring potential surgical intervention include hemorrhage and perforation.[95] The incidence of hemorrhage was reported to be as high as 20% in some series, but with the availability of antibiotic treatment this figure has decreased. When hemorrhage occurs, transfusion is indicated and usually suffices. Rarely, laparotomy must be performed for uncontrollable, life-threatening hemorrhage. Intestinal perforation through an ulcerated Peyer patch occurs in approximately 2% of cases. Typically, it is a single perforation in the terminal ileum, and simple closure of the perforation is the treatment of choice. With multiple perforations, which occur in about one fourth of the patients, resection with primary anastomosis or exteriorization of the intestinal loops may be required.

Enteritis in the Immunocompromised Host

The AIDS epidemic, as well as the widespread use of immunosuppressive agents after organ transplantation, has resulted in a number of rare and exotic pathogens infecting the gastrointestinal tract.[96] Almost all patients with AIDS have gastrointestinal symptoms during their illness, the most common of which is diarrhea.[97] However, the surgeon may be asked to evaluate the immunocompromised patient with abdominal pain, an obvious acute abdomen, or gastrointestinal bleeding; a number of protozoal, bacterial, viral, and fungal organisms may be responsible.

Protozoa

Protozoa (e.g., *Cryptosporidium*, *Isospora*, and *Microsporidium*) are the most frequent class of pathogens causing diarrhea in patients with AIDS. The small bowel is the most common site of infection. Diagnosis is established most often by acid-fast stain of the stool or duodenal secretions. Symptoms are most commonly related to diarrhea, which may be at times intractable. Current treatment regimens have not been entirely effective.

Bacteria

Infections by enteric bacteria are more frequent and more virulent in human immunodeficiency virus (HIV)-infected individuals than in healthy hosts. *Salmonella*, *Shigella*, and *Campylobacter* are associated with higher rates of both bacteremia and antibiotic resistance in the immunocompromised patient. The diagnosis of *Shigella* or *Salmonella* may be established by stool cultures. The diagnosis of *Campylobacter*, however, may be more difficult, with stool cultures often negative. These enteric infections manifest clinically with high fever, abdominal pain, and diarrhea that may be bloody. Abdominal pain may mimic an acute abdomen. Bacteremia should be treated by administration of parenteral antibiotics; ciprofloxacin is an attractive choice if the organisms are multiply resistant.

Diarrhea caused by *Clostridium difficile* is more common among patients with AIDS owing to the increased antibiotic use in this population compared with healthy hosts. Diagnosis is by standard assays of stool for *C. difficile* enterotoxin. Treatment with metronidazole or vancomycin is usually effective.

Mycobacteria

Mycobacterial infection is a frequent cause of intestinal disease in immunocompromised hosts. This can be either secondary to *Mycobacterium tuberculosis* or *Mycobacterium avium* complex (MAC), which is an atypical mycobacterium related to the type that causes cervical adenitis (scrofula). The usual route of infection is by swallowed organisms that directly penetrate the intestinal mucosa. The luminal gastrointestinal tract is involved by MAC, with massive thickening of the proximal small intestine often noted (Fig. 46-25). Clinically, patients with MAC present with diarrhea, fever, anorexia, and progressive wasting.

The most frequent site of intestinal involvement of *M. tuberculosis* is the distal ileum and cecum, with 85% to 90% of patients demonstrating disease at this site.[98] The gross appearance can be ulcerative, hypertrophic, or ulcerohypertrophic. The bowel wall appears thickened, and often an inflammatory mass surrounds the ileocecal region. Acute inflammation is apparent, as well as strictures and even fistula formation. The serosal surface is normally covered with multiple tubercles, and mesenteric lymph nodes are frequently enlarged and thickened; on sectioning, caseous necrosis is noted. The mucosa is hyperemic, edematous, and, in some cases, ulcerated. Histologically, the distinguishing lesion is a granuloma, with caseating granulomas found most commonly in the lymph nodes. Most patients complain of chronic abdominal pain, which may be nonspecific, weight loss, fever, and diarrhea.

The diagnosis of mycobacterial infection is made by identification of the organism in tissue, either by direct visualization with an acid-fast stain, by culture of the excised tissue, or by PCR techniques. Radiographic examinations usually reveal a thickened mucosa with distorted mucosal folds and ulcerations. CT may be useful and shows a thickening of the ileocecal valve and cecum.

The treatment of *M. tuberculosis* is similar in the immunocompromised or nonimmunocompromised host. The organism is usually responsive to multidrug, antimicrobial therapy. The therapy for MAC infection is evolving; drugs that have been successfully used in vivo and in vitro include amikacin, ciprofloxacin, cycloserine, and ethionamide. Clarithromycin has also been successfully used in combination with other agents. Surgical intervention may be required for intestinal tuberculosis, particularly *M. tuberculosis*. Obstruction and fistula formation are the leading indications for surgery; however, with modern treatment, most fistulas now respond to medical management. Regarding ulcerative complications, surgery may be necessary when free perforation, perforation with abscess, or massive hemorrhage occurs. The treatment is usually resection with anastomosis.

Viruses

Cytomegalovirus (CMV) is the most common viral cause of diarrhea in immunocompromised patients. Clinical manifestations include intermittent diarrhea accompanied by fever, weight loss, and abdominal pain. The manifestations of enteric CMV infection result from mucosal ischemic ulcerations, which account for the high rate of perforations noted with CMV. As a result of the diffuse, ulcerating involvement of the intestine, patients may present with abdominal pain, peritonitis, or hematochezia. Diagnosis of CMV is made by demonstrating viral inclusions. The most characteristic form is an intranuclear inclusion, which is often surrounded by a halo, producing an "owl's-eye" appearance. There may also be cytoplasmic inclusions (Fig. 46-26). Cultures for CMV are usually positive when inclusion bodies are present, but these cultures are less sensitive and specific than histopathologic identification. Once diagnosed, the treatment for CMV is usually affected by ganciclovir. An alternative to ganciclovir is foscarnet, a pyrophosphate analogue that inhibits viral replication. Other less common viral infections have been reported and include adenovirus, rotavirus, and novel enteric viruses such as astrovirus and picornavirus.

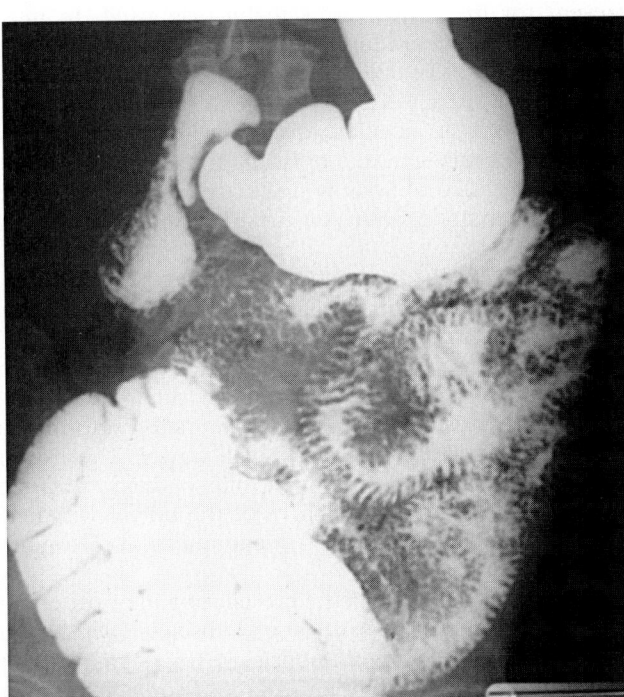

FIGURE 46-25. Barium radiograph of a patient with AIDS shows thickened intestinal folds consistent with enteritis secondary to atypical mycobacterium. (Courtesy of Melvyn H. Schreiber, M.D., The University of Texas Medical Branch.)

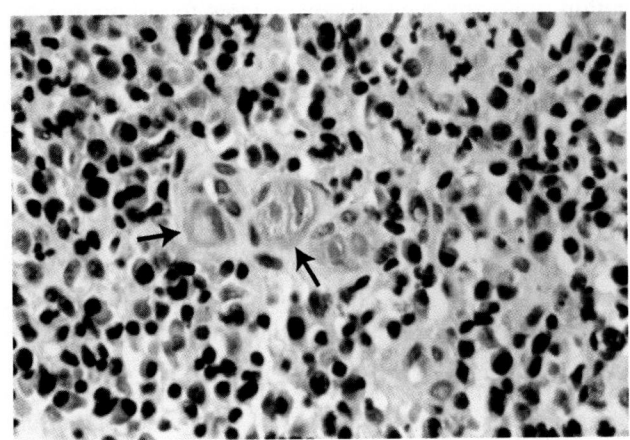

FIGURE 46-26. Microscopic section of small bowel in a patient with AIDS who has cytomegalovirus enteritis. Multiple large cells with both intranuclear and intracytoplasmic inclusions typical of cytomegalovirus are demonstrated (*arrows*). (Courtesy of Mary R. Schwartz, M.D., Baylor College of Medicine.)

Fungi

Fungal infections of the intestinal tract have been recognized in patients with AIDS. Gastrointestinal histoplasmosis occurs in the setting of systemic infection, often in association with pulmonary and hepatic disease. Diagnosis is made by fungal smear and culture of infected tissue or blood. The infection is most commonly treated by the administration of amphotericin B. Coccidioidomycosis of the intestinal tract is rare and, like histoplasmosis, occurs in the context of systemic infection.

NEOPLASMS

General Considerations

Small bowel neoplasms are exceedingly rare despite the fact that the small bowel constitutes approximately 80% of the total length of the gastrointestinal tract and makes up more than 90% of the mucosal surface area.[99-101] Only 5% of all gastrointestinal neoplasms and only 1% to 2% of all malignant tumors of the gastrointestinal tract occur in the small bowel. Approximately 5300 new cases of primary small intestinal cancer occurred in the United States in 2003 (equally distributed between men and women) with 1100 estimated cancer deaths.[102] The reasons for this decreased incidence in cancer despite the rapidly proliferating mucosa are entirely speculative but may include such factors as the rapid transit of luminal contents; the high turnover rate of small bowel epithelial cells, which may minimize carcinogenic exposure; the alkalinity of small intestinal contents; the high level of IgA in the intestinal wall; and the low bacterial count of small intestinal luminal contents.

The mean age at onset is approximately 59 years; the mean age of the presentation is 62 years for benign tumors and approximately 57 years for malignant lesions. Similar to other cancers, there appears to be a geographic distribution, with the highest cancer rates found among the Maori of New Zealand and ethnic Hawaiians.[103] The incidence of small bowel cancer is particularly low in India, Romania, and other parts of Eastern Europe. Although as previously stated, the incidence of small bowel cancer is exceedingly small, there appears to be a disturbing trend of increased rates since the mid 1980s, possibly reflecting the spread of AIDS and the increase in neoplasms, such as lymphomas, that occur in the immunocompromised host.

The incidence of small bowel neoplasia varies considerably, with benign lesions identified more often in autopsy series. In contrast, malignant neoplasms account for 75% of symptomatic lesions that lead to surgery. This reflects the fact that the majority of benign neoplasms are asymptomatic and therefore are not found unless as an incidental finding. Leiomyomas and adenomas are the most frequent of the benign tumors. Benign lesions appear to be more common in the distal small bowel, but these numbers may be somewhat misleading, owing to the relatively short length of the duodenum. In fact, per

unit area, duodenal tumors are most frequent. Depending on the series, either adenocarcinoma or carcinoid tumor is the most common malignant neoplasm. Adenocarcinomas are more numerous in the proximal small bowel, whereas the other malignant lesions are more common in the distal intestine. Patients with Crohn's disease and familial adenomatous polyposis are at a higher risk for small bowel neoplasms than the general population. Although the molecular genetics of small bowel neoplasms have not been entirely characterized, similar to colorectal cancers, mutations of the K-ras gene are commonly found.[104] Allelic losses, particularly involving tumor suppressor genes at chromosome locations 5q (the APC gene), 17q (the p53 gene), and 18q (the DCC [Deleted in Colon Cancer] and DPC4 [SMAD4] genes) have been noted in some small bowel cancers.[105]

Numerous risk factors and associated conditions have been described with relation to neoplasia of the small bowel. These include patients with familial adenomatous polyposis, hereditary nonpolyposis colorectal cancer (HNPCC), Peutz-Jeghers syndrome, Crohn's disease, gluten-sensitive enteropathy (i.e., celiac sprue), and biliary diversion (e.g., previous cholecystectomy). Controversial factors that may contribute to small bowel cancers include smoking, heavy alcohol consumption ($\geq$ 80 g/day of ethanol), and consumption of red meat or salt-cured foods.[105]

Diagnosis

Owing to the insidious nature of many of the small bowel neoplasms, a high index of suspicion must be present for these neoplasms to be diagnosed. In most series, a correct preoperative diagnosis is made in only 20% to 50% of symptomatic patients. An upper gastrointestinal tract series with small intestinal follow-through yields an accurate diagnosis in 50% to 70% of patients with malignant neoplasms of the small intestine (Fig. 46-27). Enteroclysis appears to be an even more sensitive technique, with a diagnostic accuracy of approximately 90%.

Flexible endoscopy may be useful, particularly in diagnosing duodenal lesions, and often the colonoscope can be advanced into the terminal ileum for visualization and biopsy of ileal neoplasms. Push enteroscopy has not been used routinely to evaluate lesions in the small bowel because this test may take up to 8 hours to perform and it may not visualize the entire small bowel. The use of swallowed radiotelemetry capsules (e.g., capsule endoscopy) that transmit images of the bowel wall may be of diagnostic value as this technique becomes more widely available.[106]

Plain films may confirm the presence of an obstruction; however, for the most part, they are useless in making a diagnosis of small bowel neoplasms. Angiography is of value in diagnosing and localizing tumors of vascular origin. CT of the abdomen can prove particularly useful in detecting extraluminal tumors such as gastrointestinal stromal tumors (GISTs) and can provide helpful information regarding staging of malignant cancers (Fig. 46-28).[107] Ultrasonography has not proved to be effective in making the preoperative diagnosis of small bowel neoplasm. Despite the sophisticated imaging and diagnostic modalities, diagnosis of a small bowel tumor is often achieved only at the time of surgical exploration, performed either as an elective procedure or as an emergency procedure.

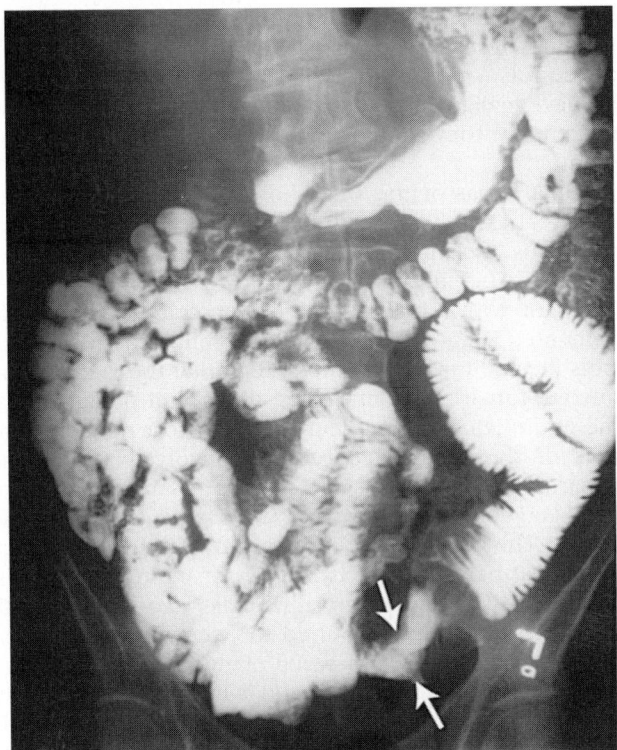

FIGURE 46-27. Barium radiograph demonstrates a typical "apple-core" lesion *(arrows)* caused by adenocarcinoma of the small bowel, producing a partial obstruction with dilated proximal bowel. (Courtesy of Melvyn H. Schreiber, M.D., The University of Texas Medical Branch.)

Benign Neoplasms

The most common benign neoplasms include benign GISTs, adenomas, and lipomas. Adenomas are the most common benign tumors reported in autopsy series, but GISTs are the most common benign small bowel lesions that produce symptoms.

Clinical Manifestations

Symptoms associated with small bowel neoplasms are often vague and nonspecific and may include dyspepsia, anorexia, malaise, and dull abdominal pain (often intermittent and colicky). These symptoms may be present for months or years before surgery. The majority of patients with benign neoplasms remain asymptomatic, and the neoplasms are only discovered at autopsy or as incidental findings at laparotomy or upper gastrointestinal radiologic studies. Of the remainder, pain, most often related to obstruction, is the most frequent complaint. Most frequently, obstruction is the result of intussusception, and benign small tumors are the most common cause of this condition in adults. Hemorrhage is the next most common symptom. Bleeding is usually occult; hematochezia or hematemesis may occur, although life-threatening hemorrhage is uncommon.

Treatment

Surgical treatment of benign tumors is nearly always indicated because of the risk of subsequent complications and because the diagnosis of benign disease cannot be made without microscopic evaluation. The complications of benign neoplasms that most often require treatment include bleeding and obstruction. Segmental resection and primary anastomosis are most commonly used except for very small lesions, which may be excised by enterotomy. The entire small bowel should be searched for other lesions because they are often multiple.

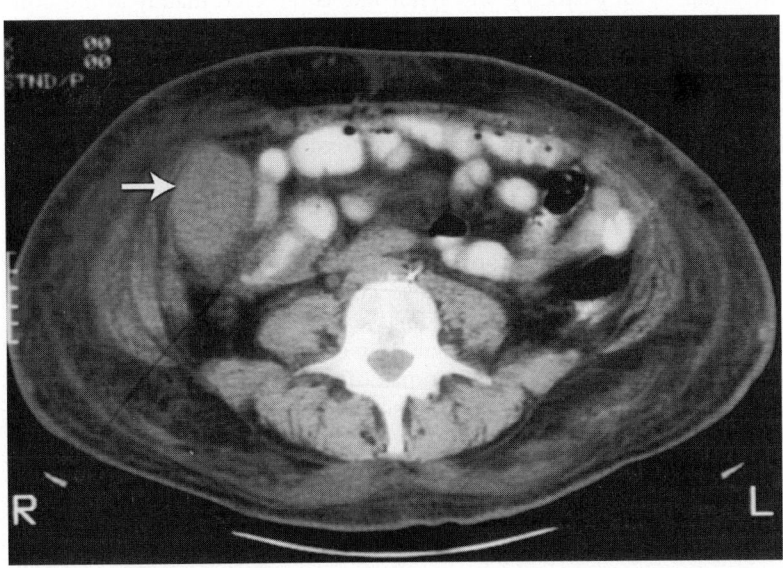

FIGURE 46-28. CT scan of abdomen demonstrates a small bowel neoplasm *(arrow).* (Courtesy of Melvyn H. Schreiber, M.D., The University of Texas Medical Branch.)

Pathology

Leiomyomas, benign tumors of smooth muscle origin, are the most common symptomatic benign neoplasms of the small bowel. In recent years as the origin of these tumors has become more clear, pathologists have begun to shift from designations such as leiomyoma or leiomyosarcoma to the term *stromal tumors* (i.e., GISTs).[108,109] Currently, these tumors are thought to arise from the interstitial cell of Cajal, an intestinal pacemaker cell of mesodermal descent. These tumors are made up of spindle (70%) and epithelioid (30%) cells, and benign GISTs are three to four times more common than malignant GISTs. The majority (>90%) of GISTs express CD117, the c-*kit* protooncogene protein that is a transmembrane receptor for the stem cell growth factor, and 70% to 80% express CD34, the human progenitor cell antigen; less frequently these tumors stain positive for actin and desmin.[105,110] The incidence is equal in men and in women, and they are most frequently diagnosed in the fifth decade of life. Grossly, they are firm, gray-white lesions with a whorled appearance noted on cut surface; microscopic examination demonstrates well-differentiated smooth muscle cells. These tumors may grow intramurally and cause obstruction. Alternatively, the tumors demonstrate intramural and extramural growth, sometimes achieving considerable size and eventually outgrowing their blood supply and resulting in bleeding manifestations, which is the most common indication for surgery in patients with benign stromal tumors. Surgical resection is necessary for appropriate treatment. Mitotic counts higher than 2 per 50 high-powered fields imply an increased risk of local recurrence.[111,112]

Adenomas account for approximately 15% of all benign small bowel tumors and are of three primary types: true adenomas, villous adenomas, and Brunner gland adenomas. Twenty percent of adenomas are found in the duodenum, 30% are found in the jejunum, and 50% are found in the ileum. The majority of these lesions are asymptomatic, with most occurring singly and found incidentally at autopsy. The most common presenting symptoms are bleeding and obstruction. Villous adenomas of the small bowel are rare but do occur, are most commonly found in the duodenum, and may be associated with the familial polyposis syndrome. These lesions have a propensity for malignant degeneration and may be of relatively large size (>5 cm) in diameter. They are usually noted secondary to abdominal pain or bleeding; obstruction may also occur. The malignant potential of these lesions is reportedly between 35% and 55%. The treatment of choice is segmental resection, although, in the duodenum, polypectomy may be performed if the tumor is histologically benign. Invasive changes necessitate more extensive resection, such as a pancreaticoduodenectomy. Brunner gland adenomas represent benign hyperplastic lesions arising from the Brunner glands of the proximal duodenum. These adenomas may produce symptoms mimicking those of peptic ulcer disease. Diagnosis can usually be accomplished by endoscopy and biopsy, and symptomatic lesions in an accessible region should be resected by simple excision. There is no malignant potential for Brunner gland adenomas, and a radical resection should not be used.

Lipomas, which are also included in the category of stromal tumors, are most common in the ileum and present as single intramural lesions located in the submucosa. They occur most commonly in the sixth and seventh decades of life and are more frequent in men. Less than one third of these tumors are symptomatic; and of these, the most common manifestations are obstruction and bleeding from superficial ulcerations. The treatment of choice for symptomatic lesions is excision. Lipomas do not have malignant potential, and, therefore, when found incidentally, they should be removed only if the resection is simple.

Hamartomas of the small bowel occur as part of the Peutz-Jeghers syndrome, an inherited syndrome of mucocutaneous melanotic pigmentation and gastrointestinal polyps.[113] The pattern of inheritance is simple mendelian dominant with a high degree of penetrance. The classic pigmented lesions are small, 1- to 2-mm, brown or black spots located in the circumoral region of the face, buccal mucosa, forearms, palms, soles, digits, and perianal area. The entire jejunum and ileum are the most frequent portions of the gastrointestinal tract involved with these hamartomas; however, 50% of patients may also have rectal and colonic lesions and 25% of patients have gastric lesions. The most common symptom is recurrent colicky abdominal pain, usually as a result of intermittent intussusception. Lower abdominal pain associated with a palpable mass has been reported to occur in one third of patients. Hemorrhage as a result of autoamputation of the polyps occurs less frequently and is most commonly manifested by anemia. Acute life-threatening hemorrhage is uncommon but may occur. Although once considered as a purely benign disease, adenomatous changes have been reported in 3% to 6% of hamartomas. Extracolonic cancers are common, occurring in 50% to 90% of patients (small intestine, stomach, pancreas, ovary, lung, uterus, and breast). The small intestine represents the most frequent site for cancer, with a relative risk of 520 compared with the general population.[105] The treatment of complications of Peutz-Jeghers syndrome is directed mainly at the complication of obstruction or persistent bleeding. Resection should be limited to the segment of bowel that is producing complications and most often involves a limited resection. Because of the widespread nature of intestinal involvement, cure is not possible and extensive resections are not indicated.

Hemangiomas are developmental malformations consisting of submucosal proliferation of blood vessels. They can occur at any level of the gastrointestinal tract, and the jejunum is the most commonly affected small bowel segment. Hemangiomas account for 3% to 4% of all benign tumors of the small bowel and are multiple in 60% of patients. Hemangiomas of the small bowel may occur as part of an inherited disorder known as Rendu-Osler-Weber disease. In addition to the small bowel, hemangiomas may also be present in the lung, liver, and mucus membranes. Patients with Turner's syndrome are likely also to have cavernous hemangiomas of the intestine. The most common symptom of small bowel hemangiomas is intestinal bleeding. Angiography and ^{99m}Tc-red blood cell scanning are the most useful diagnostic studies. If a hemangioma is localized preoperatively, resection of the involved segment of intestine is warranted. If not identified, intraoperative transillumination and palpation can be helpful.

Malignant Neoplasms

The most common malignant neoplasms of the small bowel in the approximate order of frequency are adenocarcinomas, carcinoid tumors, malignant GISTs, and lymphomas. Because of differences in clinical presentation, diagnosis, and treatment, carcinoid tumors are considered separately.

Clinical Manifestations

In contrast to benign lesions, malignant neoplasms almost always produce symptoms, the most common of which include pain and weight loss. Obstruction develops in 15% to 35% of patients and, in contrast to the intussusception produced by benign lesions, is usually the result of tumor infiltration and adhesions. Diarrhea with tenesmus and passage of large amounts of mucus may occur. Adenocarcinomas may produce the typical constricting apple-core lesions similar to those observed in the colon. Gastrointestinal bleeding, manifested by anemia and guaiac-positive stools or occasionally by melena or hematochezia, occurs to varying degrees with malignant lesions and is more common with leiomyosarcomas. A palpable mass may be felt in 10% to 20% of patients, and perforations develop in approximately 10%, usually secondary to lymphomas and sarcomas.

Pathology

Adenocarcinomas constitute approximately 50% of the malignant tumors of the small bowel in most reported series.[114] The peak incidence is in the seventh decade of life, and most series show a slight male predominance. The majority of these tumors are located in the duodenum and proximal jejunum (Fig. 46-29). Those arising in association with Crohn's disease tend to occur at a somewhat younger age, and more than 70% arise in the ileum. Tumors of the duodenum tend to present somewhat earlier than those occurring in the most distal intestine, with symptoms of jaundice and chronic bleeding. Adenocarcinomas of the jejunum and ileum usually produce symptoms that may be more nonspecific and include vague abdominal pain and weight loss. Intestinal obstruction and chronic bleeding can also occur. Perforation is uncommon. As with adenocarcinomas in other organs, survival of patients with small bowel adenocarcinomas is related to the stage of disease at the time of diagnosis. Unfortunately, diagnosis is often delayed and the disease is advanced at the time of surgery, secondary to a number of factors (e.g., the vagueness of symptoms, absence of physical findings, and lack of clinical suspicion owing to the rarity of these lesions).

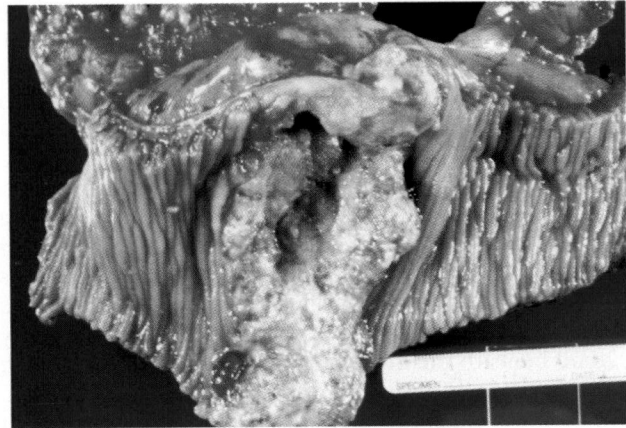

FIGURE 46-29. Large circumferential mucinous adenocarcinoma of the jejunum. (Courtesy of Mary R. Schwartz, M.D., Baylor College of Medicine.)

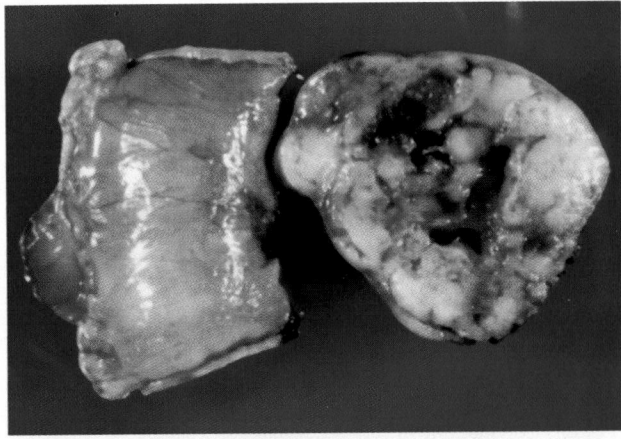

FIGURE 46-30. Small bowel leiomyosarcoma (malignant gastrointestinal stromal tumor) with hemorrhagic necrosis. (Courtesy of Mary R. Schwartz, M.D., Baylor College of Medicine.)

Malignant GISTs, which arise from mesenchymal tissue, constitute approximately 20% of malignant neoplasms of the small bowel (Fig. 46-30). These tumors are more common in the jejunum and ileum, typically are diagnosed in the fifth and sixth decades of life, and occur with a somewhat more male preponderance. Malignant GISTs are greater than 5 cm at the time of diagnosis in 80% of patients. GISTs mostly arise from the muscularis propria and generally grow extramurally. Most common indications for surgery include bleeding and obstruction, although free perforation may occur as a result of hemorrhagic necrosis in large tumor masses. Typically, GISTs tend to invade locally and spread by direct extension into adjacent tissues and hematogenously to the liver, lungs, and bone; lymphatic metastases are unusual. The most useful indicators of survival and the risk of metastasis include the size of the tumor at presentation, the mitotic index, and evidence of tumor invasion into the lamina propria.

Malignant lymphomas involve the small bowel primarily or as a manifestation of systemic disease. Primary gastrointestinal lymphomas, of which approximately one third occur in the small bowel, account for 5% of all lymphomas. Lymphomas constitute 7% to 25% of small bowel malignant tumors in the adult; in children younger than age 10 years, they are the most common intestinal neoplasm. Lymphomas are most commonly found in the ileum, where there is the greatest concentration of gut-associated lymphoid tissue. Increased risk of developing primary small bowel lymphomas has been reported in patients with celiac disease and immunodeficiency states (e.g., AIDS). Grossly, small intestine lymphomas are usually large, with the majority larger than 5 cm; they may extend beneath the mucosa (Fig. 46-31). Microscopically, there is often diffuse infiltration of the intestinal wall. Symptoms of small bowel lymphoma include pain, weight loss, nausea, vomiting, and change in bowel habits. Perforation may occur in up to 25% of the patients (Fig. 46-32). Fever is uncommon and suggests systemic involvement.

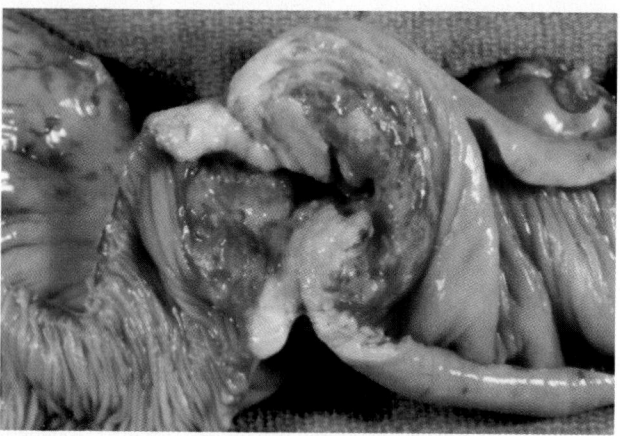

FIGURE 46-31.   Gross photograph of primary lymphoma of the ileum shows replacement of all layers of the bowel wall with tumor. (Courtesy of Mary R. Schwartz, M.D., Baylor College of Medicine.)

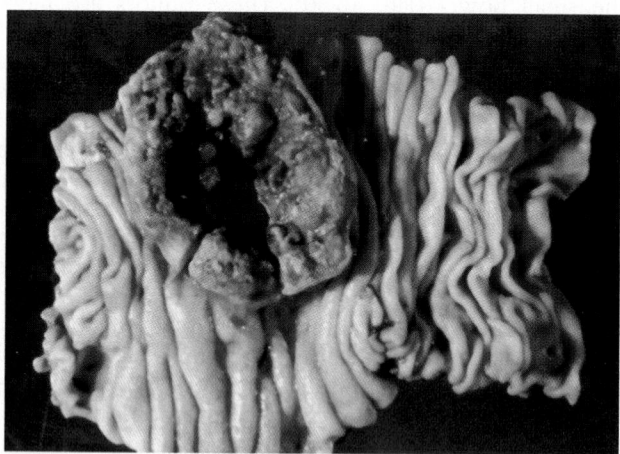

FIGURE 46-32.   Small bowel lymphoma presents as perforation and peritonitis. (Courtesy of Mary R. Schwartz, M.D., Baylor College of Medicine.)

Treatment

The treatment of adenocarcinomas and lymphomas of the small bowel is wide resection including regional lymph nodes (Fig. 46-33). This may require pancreaticoduodenectomy (Whipple operation) for duodenal lesions. Often, surgical resection for cure is not possible. Therefore, palliative resection should be performed to prevent further complications of bleeding, obstruction, and perforation. If this is not possible, bypass of the involved segment may provide relief of symptoms. For GISTs, segmented bowel resection is required; wide margins and extensive lymph node dissection are not necessary. Resection of organ segments that have been invaded with tumor and of hepatic metastases appear to confer an improvement in survival.

Adjuvant radiation and chemotherapy have little role in the treatment of patients with adenocarcinomas of the small bowel. Radiotherapy and chemotherapy combined with surgical excision provide the best survival rates for patients with lymphomas. The adjuvant treatment of GISTs may be favorably impacted by recent reports demonstrating an effect on GIST tumor progression using the tyrosine kinase inhibitor imatinib mesylate (Gleevec; formerly referred to as STI571), which blocks the unregulated mutant *c-kit* (CD117) tyrosine kinase.[115] Imatinib also inhibits the Bcr-Abl and platelet-derived growth factor (PDGF) receptor tyrosine kinases. Mutations in *c-kit* are thought to represent the primary cause of the proliferative capacity and malignant potential of GIST. Clinical trials are underway using imatinib for metastatic and primary GIST, and the preliminary results appear encouraging.[116,117]

Prognosis

Only half of the patients operated on for malignant tumors of the small intestine have lesions amenable to curative

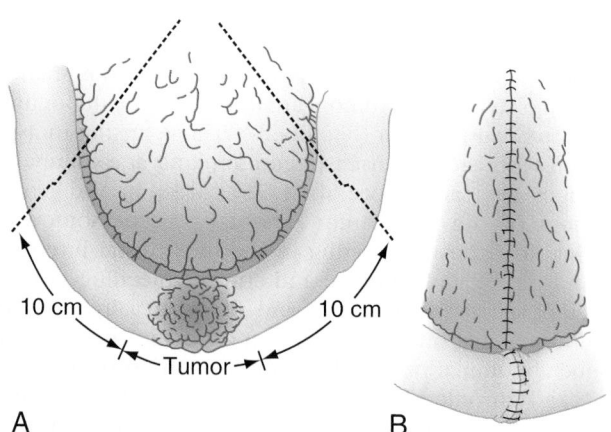

FIGURE 46-33.   Surgical management of carcinoma of the small bowel. **A,** Malignant tumors should be resected with a wide margin of normal bowel and a wedge of mesentery to remove the immediate draining lymph nodes. **B,** End-to-end anastomosis of the small bowel and repair of the mesentery. (Adapted from Thompson JC: Atlas of Surgery of the Stomach, Duodenum and Small Bowel. St. Louis, Mosby–Year Book, 1992, p 299.)

resection.[118] One third have a distant metastasis at the time of initial surgery, and the overall 5-year survival rate after surgical treatment of malignant tumors is only 25%. Adenocarcinoma has the poorest prognosis, with an overall survival rate of 15% to 20%. Overall 5-year survival rates for GISTs are variable, ranging from 7% to 56%.

Carcinoid Tumors

Carcinoids of the small bowel arise from enterochromaffin cells (Kulchitsky cells) found in the crypts of Lieberkühn.[119,120] These cells are also known as argentaffin cells because of their staining by silver compounds. These tumors were first described by Lubarsch in 1888; and in 1907, Oberndorfer coined the term *Karzinoide* to indicate the carcinoma-like appearance and the presumed lack of malignant potential. Carcinoid tumors have been reported in a number of organs including, most commonly, the lungs, bronchi, and gastrointestinal tract. Most patients with small bowel carcinoids are in the fifth decade of life.

Carcinoids may be classified by the embryologic site of origin and secretory product.[121] Carcinoid tumors may be derived from the foregut (respiratory tract, thymus), midgut (jejunum, ileum and right colon, stomach, and proximal duodenum), and hindgut (distal colon and rectum). Foregut carcinoids characteristically produce low levels of serotonin (5-hydroxytryptamine) but may secrete 5-hydroxytryptophan or adrenocorticotrophic hormone. Midgut carcinoids are characterized by having high serotonin production. Hindgut carcinoids rarely produce serotonin but may produce other hormones, such as somatostatin and peptide YY. The gastrointestinal tract is the most common site for carcinoid tumors. After the appendix, the small intestine is the second most frequently affected site in the gastrointestinal tract. In the small intestine, carcinoids almost always occur within the last 2 feet of the ileum. Carcinoid tumors have a variable malignant potential and are composed of multipotential cells with the ability to secrete numerous humoral agents, the most prominent of which are serotonin and substance P (Table 46-6). In addition to these substances, carcinoid tumors have been found to secrete corticotropin, histamine, dopamine, neurotensin, prostaglandins, kinins, gastrin, somatostatin, pancreatic polypeptide, calcitonin, and neuron-specific enolase.

The primary importance of carcinoid tumors is the malignant potential of the tumors themselves. Although the carcinoid syndrome, which is characterized by episodic attacks of cutaneous flushing, bronchospasm, diarrhea, and vasomotor collapse, can occur and is quite dramatic in its most florid form, it occurs in only a small percentage of patients with malignant carcinoids.

Pathology

Carcinoid tumors may arise in organs derived from the foregut, midgut, and hindgut. Seventy to 80 percent of carcinoids are asymptomatic and found incidentally at the time of surgery.[122] In the gastrointestinal tract, more than 90% of carcinoids are found in three sites: the appendix (45%), the ileum (28%), and the rectum (16%) (Table 46-7). The malignant potential (ability to metastasize) is related to location, size, depth of invasion, and growth pattern. Only approximately 3% of appendiceal carcinoids metastasize, but approximately 35% of ileal carcinoids are associated with metastasis. The majority (~75%) of gastrointestinal carcinoids are less than 1 cm in diameter, and approximately 2% of these are associated with metastasis. In contrast, carcinoid tumors 1 to 2 cm in diameter and over 2 cm are associated with metastasis in 50% and 80% to 90% of cases, respectively.

Grossly, these tumors are small, firm submucosal nodules that are usually yellow on cut surface (Fig. 46-34). They tend to grow very slowly, but after invasion of the serosa there often is an intense desmoplastic reaction producing mesenteric fibrosis, intestinal kinking, and intermittent obstruction. Small bowel carcinoids are multicentric in 20% to 30% of patients.[119] This tendency to multicentricity exceeds that of any other malignant neoplasm of the gastrointestinal tract. Another unusual observation is the frequent coexistence of a second primary malignant neoplasm of a different histologic type.[123] This usually is a synchronous adenocarcinoma (most commonly in the large intestine) that can occur in 10% to 20%

TABLE 46-6. Secretory Products of Carcinoid Tumors			
Amines	**Tachykinins**	**Peptides**	**Other**
5-HT	Kallikrein	Pancreatic polypeptide (40%)	Prostaglandins
5-HIAA (88%)	Substance P (32%)	Chromogranins (100%)	
5-HTP	Neuropeptide K (67%)	Neurotensin (19%)	
Histamine		HCGα (28%)	
Dopamine		HCGβ	
		Motilin (14%)	

HCG, human chorionic gonadotropin; 5-HIAA, 5-hydroxyindoleacetic acid; 5-HT, 5-hydroxytryptamine; 5-HTP, 5-hydroxytryptophan.
Values in parentheses represent percentage frequency.

TABLE 46-7. Distribution of Gastrointestinal Carcinoids: Incidence of Metastases and of Carcinoid Syndrome

Site	Cases	Average Metastasis (%)	Cases of Carcinoid Syndrome
Esophagus	1		0
Stomach	93 (2%)	23	8
Duodenum	135 (4%)	20	4
Jejunoileum	1032 (28%)	34	91
Meckel's diverticulum	42 (1%)	19	3
Appendix	1686 (45%)	2	6
Colon	91 (2%)	60	5
Rectum	592 (16%)	18	1
Ovary	34	6	17
Biliary tract	10	30	0
Pancreas	2		1
Total	3718		136

Adapted from Cheek RC, Wilson H: Carcinoid tumors. Curr Probl Surg (November):4-31, 1970.

of patients with carcinoid tumors. Carcinoid tumors are associated with multiple endocrine neoplasia type 1 in approximately 10% of cases.

Clinical Manifestations

Carcinoid Tumors In the absence of carcinoid syndrome, symptoms of patients with carcinoid tumors of the small bowel are similar to those with small bowel tumors of other histologic types. The most common symptoms include abdominal pain, which is variably associated with partial or complete small intestinal obstruction. Obstructive symptoms are often caused by intussusception but may occur secondary to a local desmoplastic reaction, apparently produced by humoral agents elaborated by the tumor. Diarrhea and weight loss may also occur. The diarrhea is a result of a partial bowel obstruction rather than a secretory diarrhea that is noted in patients with the malignant carcinoid syndrome.

Malignant Carcinoid Syndrome The malignant carcinoid syndrome is a relatively rare disease, occurring in fewer than 10% of patients with carcinoid tumors. The syndrome is most commonly associated with carcinoid tumors of the gastrointestinal tract, particularly from the small bowel, but carcinoids in other locations, such as the bronchus, pancreas, ovary, and testes, have also been described in association with the syndrome. The classic description of the carcinoid syndrome typically includes vasomotor, cardiac, and gastrointestinal manifestations.[124] A number of humoral factors are produced by carcinoid tumors, but those considered to contribute to the carcinoid syndrome include serotonin, 5-hydroxytryptophan (a precursor of serotonin synthesis), histamine, dopamine, kallikrein, substance P, prostaglandin, and neuropeptide K. The major-

ity of patients who exhibit malignant carcinoid syndrome have massive hepatic replacement by metastatic disease. However, tumors that bypass the liver, specifically ovarian and retroperitoneal carcinoids, may produce the syndrome in the absence of liver metastasis.

Common symptoms and signs include cutaneous flushing (80%); diarrhea (76%); hepatomegaly (71%); cardiac lesions, most commonly right heart valvular disease (41% to 70%); and asthma (25%). Cutaneous flushing in the carcinoid syndrome may be of four varieties: diffuse erythematosus, which is short lived and normally affects the face, neck, and upper chest; violaceous, which is similar to diffuse erythematosus flush except that the attacks may be longer and patients may develop a permanent cyanotic flush with watery eyes and injected conjunctiva; prolonged flushes, which may last up to 2 to 3 days and involve the entire body and be associated with profuse lacrimation, hypotension, and facial edema; and a bright-red patchy flushing, which is typically seen with gastric carcinoids. The diarrhea associated with carcinoid syndrome is episodic (usually occurring after meals), watery, and often explosive. Increased circulating serotonin levels are thought to be the cause of the diarrhea because the serotonin antagonist methysergide effectively controls the symptom. Cardiac lesions and carcinoid tumors mainly involve the right side of the heart and are usually limited to the tricuspid and pulmonary valves. The three most common cardiac lesions are pulmonary stenosis (90%), tricuspid insufficiency (47%), and tricuspid stenosis (42%).[124] Asthmatic attacks are usually observed during the flushing symptom, and both serotonin and bradykinin have been implicated in this symptom. Malabsorption and pellagra (dementia, dermatitis, and diarrhea) are occasionally present and are thought to be caused by excessive diversion of dietary tryptophan.

Diagnosis

The elevation of various humoral factors forms the basis for diagnostic tests in patients with carcinoid tumors and the carcinoid syndrome. Carcinoid tumors produce serotonin, which is then metabolized in the liver and the lung to the pharmacologically inactive 5-hydroxyindoleacetic acid. Elevated urinary levels of 5-hydroxyindoleacetic acid measured over 24 hours with high-performance liquid chromatography are highly specific. A potentially useful marker of neuroendocrine tumors is plasma concentrations of chromogranin A, a protein made in the secretory granules, which is elevated in more than 80% of patients with carcinoid tumors. Plasma serotonin, substance P, neurotensin, neurokinin A, and neuropeptide K can be measured, but these peptides may not be elevated in all patients. Provocative tests using pentagastrin, calcium, or epinephrine may be used to reproduce the symptoms of carcinoid tumors. The administration of pentagastrin is the safest and most reliable and the most frequently used; however, with the accuracy of current diagnostic tests, there are relatively few indications today for provocative tests.

Carcinoid tumors of the small intestine are rarely diagnosed preoperatively. Barium radiographic studies of the

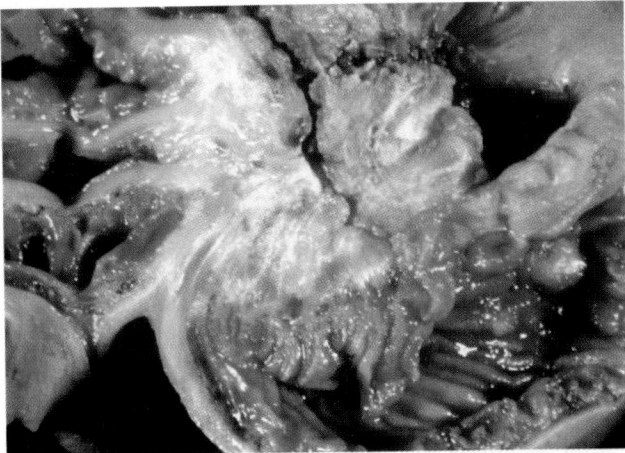

A

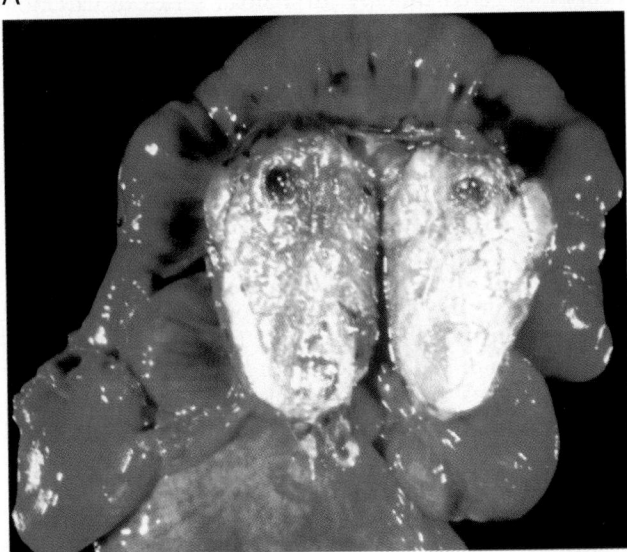

B

FIGURE 46-34. Gross pathologic characteristics of carcinoid tumor. **A,** Carcinoid tumor of the distal ileum demonstrates the intense desmoplastic reaction and fibrosis of the bowel wall. **B,** Mesenteric metastases from a carcinoid tumor of the small bowel. (Adapted from Evers BM, Townsend CM Jr, Thompson JC: Small intestine. In Schwartz SI [ed]: Principles of Surgery, 7th ed. New York, McGraw-Hill, 1999, p 1245, with permission of The McGraw-Hill Companies.)

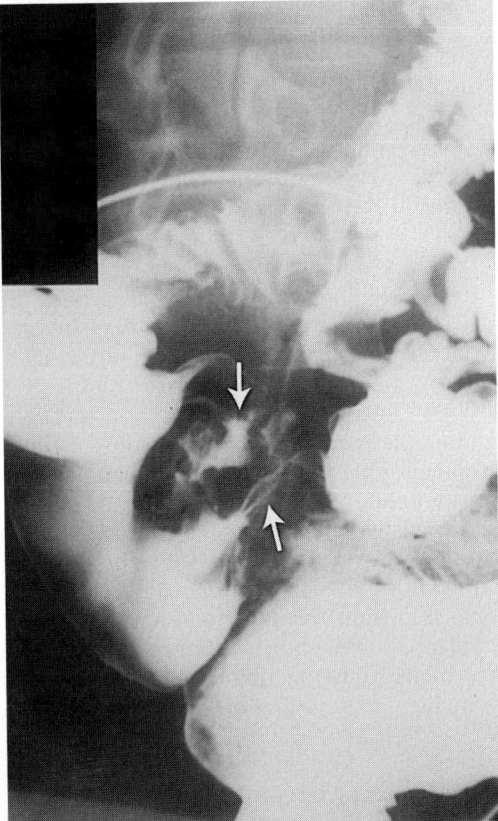

FIGURE 46-35. Barium radiograph of a carcinoid tumor of the terminal ileum demonstrates fibrosis with multiple filling defects and high-grade partial obstruction *(arrows).* (Courtesy of Melvyn H. Schreiber, M.D., The University of Texas Medical Branch.)

small bowel may exhibit multiple filling defects as a result of kinking and fibrosis of the bowel (Fig. 46-35). There are a number of imaging techniques used to diagnose the extent and spread of carcinoid tumors. Angiography and high-resolution ultrasonography can provide information on mesenteric involvement as well as hepatic involvement. Angiography may show an abnormal arrangement of mesenteric arteries and narrowing of branches associated with poor accumulation of contrast medium and poor venous drainage of the tumor area. In addition, encasement and pseudoaneurysm formation, typical of a malignant process in the mesentery, may be noted. CT is useful in detecting hepatic and lymph node metastases and the extent of bowel wall and mesenteric involvement.

A novel imaging study that takes advantage of the fact that many of these tumors possess somatostatin receptors is somatostatin receptor scintigraphy using ^{111}In-labeled pentetreotide.[125,126] This scintigraphic localization study has shown encouraging results with a higher reported sensitivity than conventional imaging techniques, such as CT, in delineating and localizing carcinoid tumors.

Treatment

The treatment of patients with small bowel carcinoid tumors is based on tumor size and site and presence or absence of metastatic disease.[127,128] For primary tumors of less than 1 cm in diameter without evidence of regional lymph node metastasis, a segmental intestinal resection is adequate. For patients with lesions of more than 1 cm, with multiple tumors or with regional lymph node metastasis, regardless of the size of the primary tumor, wide excision of bowel and mesentery is required. Lesions of the terminal ileum are best treated by right hemicolectomy. Small duodenal tumors can be excised locally; however, more extensive lesions may require pancreaticoduodenectomy. In addition to treatment of the primary tumor, it is important that the abdomen be thoroughly explored for multicentric lesions.

Caution should be exerted in the anesthetic management of patients with carcinoid tumors because anesthesia may precipitate a carcinoid crisis characterized by hypotension, bronchospasm, flushing, and tachycardia predisposing to arrhythmias. The treatment of carcinoid crisis is intravenous octreotide given as a bolus of 50 to 100 µg, which may be continued as an infusion at 50 µg/hr. In addition, intravenous antihistamine and hydrocortisone may be of some benefit.

In patients with carcinoid tumors and widespread metastatic disease, surgery is still indicated. In contrast to metastases from other tumors, there is a definite role for surgical debulking, which, in many series, provides beneficial symptomatic relief.[121] This may involve hepatic resection by either wedge resection or formal hepatic lobectomy. In the case of widespread multiple hepatic metastases, hepatic artery ligation or percutaneous embolization has produced good results. Others have reported regression of tumors when hepatic artery occlusion was combined with chemotherapy, concluding that combined modality therapy should be further evaluated. The role of liver transplantation in the treatment of metastatic carcinoid tumors is unclear, and the number of patients in whom this has been attempted has been small. A recent multicenter study reported a 5-year survival rate of 69% among highly selected patients who underwent liver transplantation for metastatic carcinoid tumors.[129]

Medical therapy for patients with malignant carcinoid syndrome is primarily directed toward the relief of symptoms caused by the excess production of humoral factors.[130] Various long-acting analogues of somatostatin, such as octreotide (Sandostatin), relieve symptoms (diarrhea and flushing) of the carcinoid syndrome in a majority of patients.[131] Kvols and associates[132,133] reported not only dramatic relief of symptoms using octreotide but also tumor regression in 17% of patients. There is no doubt of the important role of somatostatin analogues in the control of symptoms; however, their potential role in tumor inhibition has not been resolved. Results using newer somatostatin analogues with a slow-release formulation (e.g., Sandostatin LAR) in patients with carcinoid tumors are pending. Interferon-α has also been shown to provide symptomatic relief in patients with carcinoid syndrome.[134] A clinical trial that evaluated the use of interferon-α in more than 100 patients with carcinoid syndrome identified decreases in urinary 5-hydroxyindoleacetic acid in 42% of patients and tumor regression in 15%. However, the increased incidence of side effects (e.g., fever, fatigue, anorexia, and weight loss) precludes the widespread use of this drug.

Serotonin receptor antagonists have been used with limited success. Methysergide is no longer used owing to the incidence of retroperitoneal fibrosis. Ketanserin and cyproheptadine have been shown to provide some control of symptoms, and other antagonists, such as ondansetron, may be even more effective and more extensive clinical trials are underway.[135]

Cytotoxic chemotherapy has had only limited success.[127] The role of chemotherapy is confined predominantly to patients with metastatic disease who are symptomatic and unresponsive to other therapies. The most frequent combination used is streptozotocin and 5-fluorouracil or cyclophosphamide, which may result in some tumor regression in up to one third of the patients. The duration of response, however, is short lived. The use of cisplatin and etoposide has shown some promise only in patients with well-differentiated carcinoids. Results using dacarbazine (DTIC) are conflicting.

In summary, the treatment of carcinoid tumors requires a multidisciplinary approach, and combined modalities may be the best option, including surgical debulking, hepatic artery embolization or chemoembolization, and medical therapy. In addition, newer therapies are being developed that may be useful in the future.[125,126,134] The expression of neuroendocrine peptide receptors on carcinoid tumors and their avid uptake of ^{111}In-octreotide and ^{123}I-labeled metaiodobenzylguanidine (MIBG) for scintigraphic scanning have led to the development of novel receptor-targeted therapy. In a small series of carcinoid tumors, this therapy resulted in decreased size and reduced 5-hydroxyindoleacetic acid output with repeated high-dose ^{111}In-octreotide. Studies with ^{131}I-MIBG therapy have shown up to a 60% response in patients. Most recently, ^{90}Y–labeled octreotide has been reported to be of therapeutic benefit in a limited group of patients; controlled trials are planned for the future.

Prognosis

Carcinoid tumors have the best prognosis of all small bowel tumors, whether the disease is localized or metastatic. Resection of a carcinoid tumor localized to its primary site approaches a 100% survival rate. Five-year survival rates are approximately 65% among patients with regional disease and 25% to 35% among those with distant metastasis. When widespread metastatic disease precludes cure, extensive resection for palliation is indicated. In fact, long-term palliation often can be obtained because these tumors are relatively slow growing. A number of factors have been evaluated in an attempt to identify patients with carcinoid tumors who have a poor prognosis. Probably the most useful factor identified is an elevated level of chromogranin A, which was found to be an independent predictor of an adverse prognosis.

Metastatic Neoplasms

Metastatic tumors involving the small bowel are much more common than primary neoplasms. The most common metastases to the small intestine are those arising from other intra-abdominal organs, including the uterine cervix, ovaries, kidneys, stomach, colon, and pancreas. Small intestinal involvement is by either direct extension or implantation of tumor cells. Metastases from extra-abdominal tumors are rare but may be found in patients with adenocarcinoma of the breast and carcinoma of the lung. Cutaneous melanoma is the most common extra-abdominal source to involve the small intestine, with involvement of the small intestine noted in more than half of patients dying of malignant melanoma (Fig. 46-36). Common symptoms include anorexia, weight loss, anemia, bleeding, and partial bowel obstruction. Treatment is palliative resection to relieve symptoms or, occa-

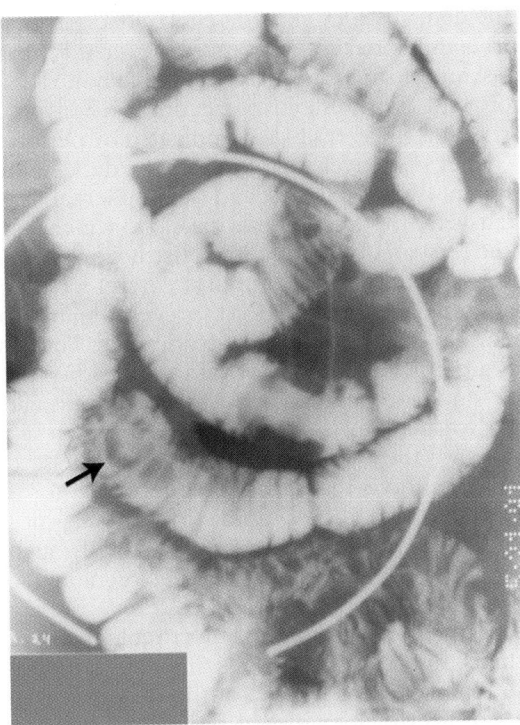

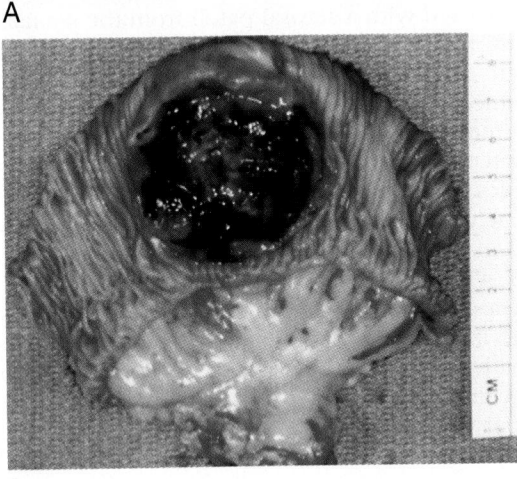

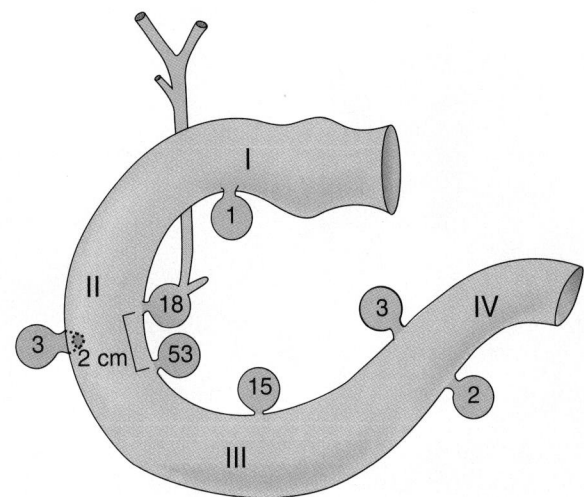

FIGURE 46-37. Distribution of 95 duodenal diverticula within the four portions of the duodenum. (From Eggert A, Teichmann W, Wittmann DH: The pathologic implication of duodenal diverticula. Surg Gynecol Obstet 154:62-64, 1982, with permission.)

FIGURE 46-36. **A,** Barium radiograph shows "target lesions" consistent with metastatic melanoma of the small bowel (arrow). **B,** Gross specimen demonstrating metastatic melanoma to the small bowel. (**A,** Courtesy of Melvyn H. Schreiber, M.D., The University of Texas Medical Branch. **B,** Courtesy of Mary R. Schwartz, M.D., Baylor College of Medicine.)

sionally, bypass if the metastatic tumor is extensive and not amenable to resection.

DIVERTICULAR DISEASE

Diverticular disease of the small intestine is relatively common. It may present as either true or false diverticula. A true diverticulum contains all layers of the intestinal wall and is usually congenital. False diverticula consist of mucosa and submucosa protruding through a defect in the

muscle coat and are usually acquired defects. Small bowel diverticula may occur in any portion of the small intestine. Duodenal diverticula are the most common acquired diverticula of the small bowel, and Meckel's diverticulum is the most common true congenital diverticulum of the small bowel.

Duodenal Diverticula

Incidence and Etiology

First described by Chomel, a French pathologist, in 1710,[136] diverticula of the duodenum are relatively common, representing the second most common site for diverticulum formation after the colon. The incidence of duodenal diverticula is varied depending on the age of the patient and the method of diagnosis. Upper gastrointestinal radiographic studies identify duodenal diverticula in 1% to 5% of all studies, whereas some autopsy series report the incidence as being as high as 15% to 20%. Duodenal diverticula occur twice as often in women as in men and are rare in patients younger than age 40 years. They have been classified as congenital or acquired, true or false, and intraluminal or extraluminal. Two thirds to three fourths of duodenal diverticula are found in the periampullary region (within a 2-cm radius of the ampulla) and project from the medial wall of the duodenum (Fig. 46-37).

Clinical Manifestations

The important thing to remember is that the overwhelming majority of duodenal diverticula are asymptomatic and are usually noted incidentally by an upper gastrointestinal series for an unrelated problem (Fig. 46-38). Diagnosis may also be obtained by upper gastrointestinal endoscopy or suggested by plain abdominal films showing an atypi-

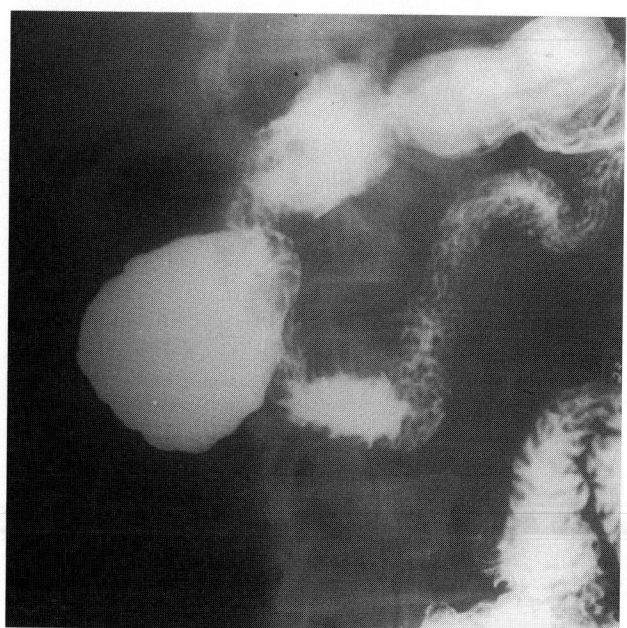

FIGURE 46-38.   Large diverticulum arises from the second portion of the duodenum. (Courtesy of Melvyn H. Schreiber, M.D., The University of Texas Medical Branch.)

cal gas bubble; CT can identify large diverticula. Less than 5% of duodenal diverticula will require surgery because of a complication of the diverticulum itself. Major complications of duodenal diverticula include obstruction of the biliary or pancreatic ducts that may contribute to cholangitis and pancreatitis, respectively; hemorrhage; perforation; and rarely, "blind loop" syndrome.

Only those diverticula associated with the ampulla of Vater are significantly related to complications of cholangitis and pancreatitis.[137] In these patients, the ampulla most often enters the duodenum at the superior margin of the diverticulum rather than through the diverticulum itself. The mechanism proposed for the increased incidence of complications of the biliary tract is the location of the perivaterian diverticula that may produce mechanical distortion of the common bile duct as it enters the duodenum, resulting in partial obstruction and stasis. Hemorrhage can be caused by inflammation, leading to erosion of a branch of the superior mesenteric artery.[138] Perforation of duodenal diverticula has been described but is rare. Finally, stasis of intestinal contents within a distended diverticulum can result in bacterial overgrowth, malabsorption, steatorrhea, and megaloblastic anemia (i.e., blind loop syndrome). Symptoms related to duodenal diverticula in the absence of any other demonstrable disease usually are nonspecific epigastric complaints that can be treated conservatively and may actually prove to be the result of another problem not related to the diverticulum itself.

Treatment

As stated previously, the vast majority of duodenal diverticula are asymptomatic and benign; and when they are

found incidentally, they should be left alone. Several operative procedures have been described for the treatment of the symptomatic duodenal diverticulum. The most common and most effective treatment is diverticulectomy, which is most easily accomplished by performing a wide Kocher maneuver that exposes the duodenum. The diverticulum is then excised, and the duodenum is closed in a transverse or longitudinal fashion, whichever produces the least amount of luminal obstruction. Because of the close proximity of the ampulla, careful identification of the ampulla is essential to prevent injury to the common bile duct and the pancreatic duct. For diverticula that are embedded deep within the head of the pancreas, a duodenotomy is performed with invagination of the diverticulum into the lumen, which is then excised, and the wall is closed (Fig. 46-39A to C). Alternative methods that have been described for duodenal diverticula associated with the ampulla of Vater include an extended sphincteroplasty through the common wall of the ampulla in the diverticulum (see Fig. 46-39D to F).

The treatment of a perforated diverticulum may require procedures similar to those described in patients with massive trauma-related defects of the duodenal wall. The perforated diverticulum should be excised and the duodenum closed with a serosal patch from the jejunal loop. If the surrounding inflammation is severe, it may be necessary to divert the enteric flow away from the site of the perforation with a gastrojejunostomy or duodenojejunostomy. Interruption of duodenal continuity proximal to the perforated diverticulum may be accomplished with a row of staples. Great care should be taken if the perforation is adjacent to the papilla of Vater. Intraluminal duodenal diverticula have been described but are highly uncommon and, if symptomatic, can be completely excised if they arise at a site distant from the ampulla. However, if a symptomatic intraluminal diverticulum is encountered associated with the ampulla of Vater, subtotal resection of the diverticulum should be carried out to protect the entry of the biliary-pancreatic ducts.

Jejunal and Ileal Diverticula

Incidence/Etiology

Diverticula of the small bowel are much less common than duodenal diverticula, with an incidence ranging from 0.1% to 1.4% noted in autopsy series and 0.1% to 1.5% noted in upper gastrointestinal studies.[139] Jejunal diverticula are more common and are larger than those in the ileum. These are false diverticula, occurring mainly in an older age group (after the sixth decade of life). These diverticula are multiple, usually protrude from the mesenteric border of the bowel, and may be overlooked at surgery because they are embedded within the small bowel mesentery (Fig. 46-40). The cause of jejunoileal diverticulosis is thought to be a motor dysfunction of the smooth muscle or the myenteric plexus, resulting in disordered contractions of the small bowel, generating increased intraluminal pressure, and resulting in herniation of the

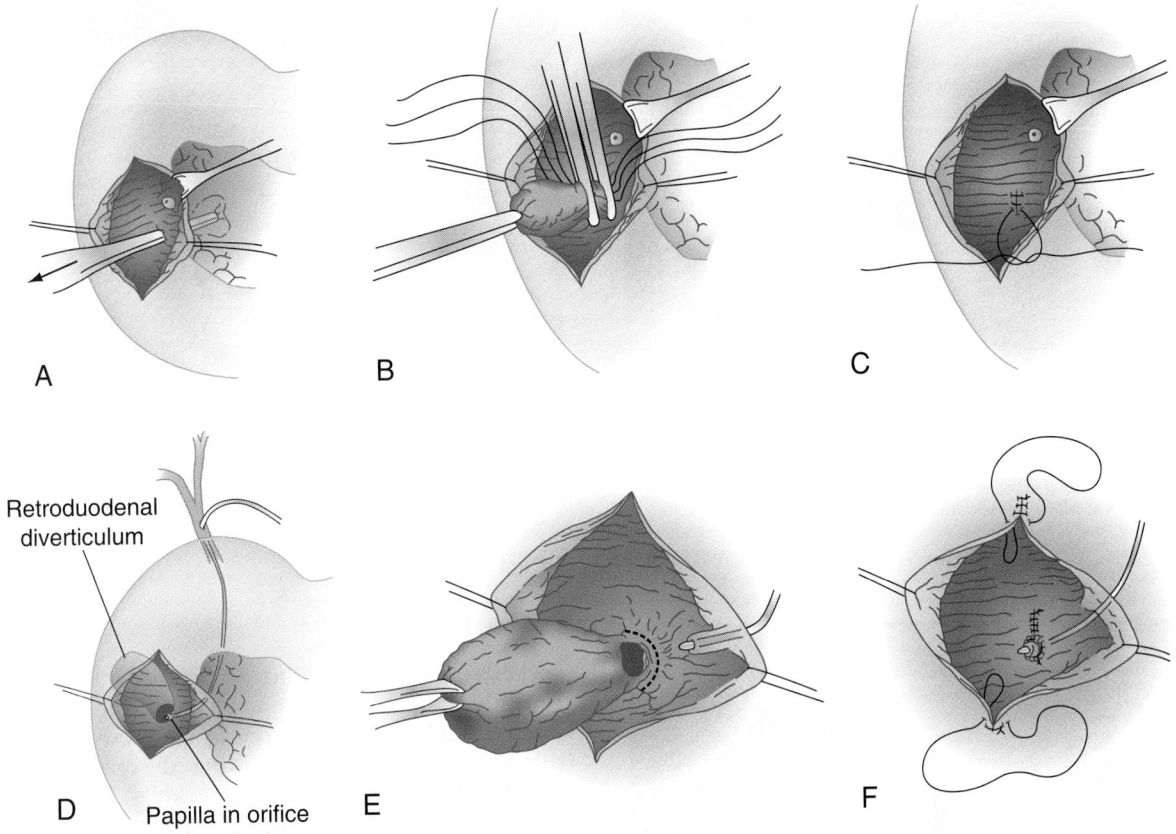

FIGURE 46-39. **A** to **C,** Treatment of a diverticulum protruding into the head of the pancreas. The duodenum is opened vertically. A clamp is used to invert the diverticulum into the lumen, where it is excised and the posterior wall defect is closed. **D** to **F,** Management of the unusual duodenal diverticula that arise in the periampullary location. A tube stent should be placed into the common bile duct and passed distally into the duodenum to facilitate identification and later dissection of the sphincter of Oddi. The diverticulum is inverted into the lumen of the duodenum. The round opening in the wall of the base of the diverticulum is the site at which the ampullary structures were freed by a circumferential incision. The *heavy broken line* in **E** shows the line of division of the base of the diverticulum, which is accomplished by free-hand dissection. After the diverticulum has been removed, the stent and enveloping papilla are protruded into the defect left by the division of the base of the diverticulum. The mucosa and muscle wall of the papilla are then sewn circumferentially to the wall of the duodenum. (Adapted from Thompson JC: Atlas of Surgery of the Stomach, Duodenum and Small Bowel. St. Louis, Mosby–Year Book, 1992, pp 209-213.)

mucosa and submucosa through the weakest portion of the bowel (i.e., the mesenteric side).

Clinical Manifestations

Jejunoileal diverticula are usually found incidentally at laparotomy or during the performance of an upper gastrointestinal study (Fig. 46-41); the great majority remain asymptomatic. Acute complications such as intestinal obstruction, hemorrhage, or perforation can occur but are rare.[140] Chronic symptomatology includes vague chronic abdominal pain, malabsorption, functional pseudo-obstruction, and chronic low-grade gastrointestinal hemorrhage. Acute complications are diverticulitis, with or without abscess or perforation; gastrointestinal hemorrhage; and intestinal obstruction. Stasis of intestinal flow with bacterial overgrowth (i.e., blind loop syndrome),

owing to the jejunal dyskinesia, may lead to deconjugation of bowel salts and uptake of vitamin B_{12} by the bacterial flora, resulting in steatorrhea and megaloblastic anemia, with or without neuropathy.

Treatment

For incidentally noted, asymptomatic jejunoileal diverticula, no treatment is required. Treatment of complications of obstruction, bleeding, and perforation is usually by intestinal resection and end-to-end anastomosis. Patients presenting with malabsorption secondary to the blind loop syndrome and bacterial overgrowth within the diverticulum can usually be given antibiotics. Obstruction may be caused by enteroliths that form in a jejunal diverticulum and are subsequently dislodged and obstruct the distal intestine. This condition may be treated by enterotomy

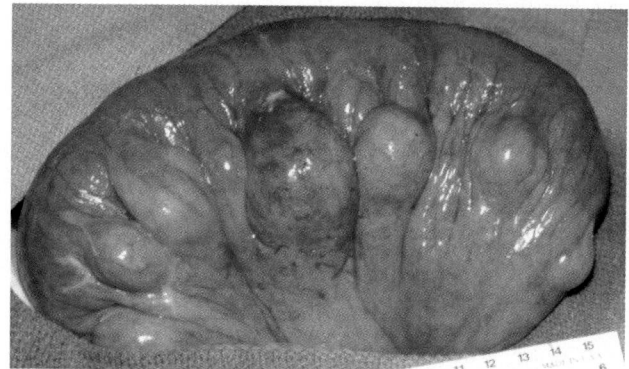

FIGURE 46-40. Multiple large jejunal diverticula located in the mesentery in an elderly patient presenting with obstruction secondary to an enterolith. (Adapted from Evers BM, Townsend CM Jr, Thompson JC: Small intestine. *In* Schwartz SI [ed]: Principles of Surgery, 7th ed. New York, McGraw-Hill, 1999, p 1248, with permission of The McGraw-Hill Companies.)

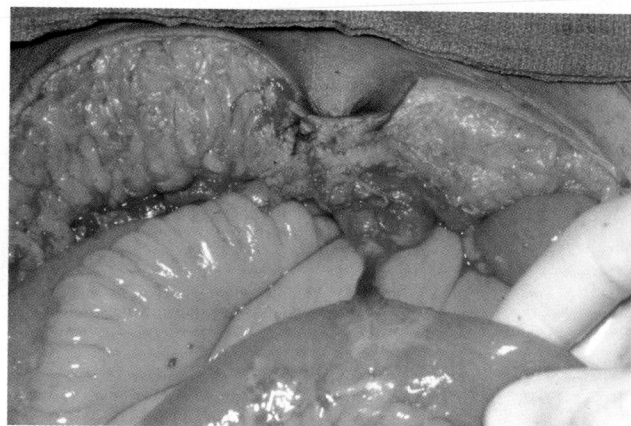

FIGURE 46-42. Omphalomesenteric remnant persisting as a fibrous cord from the ileum to the umbilicus.

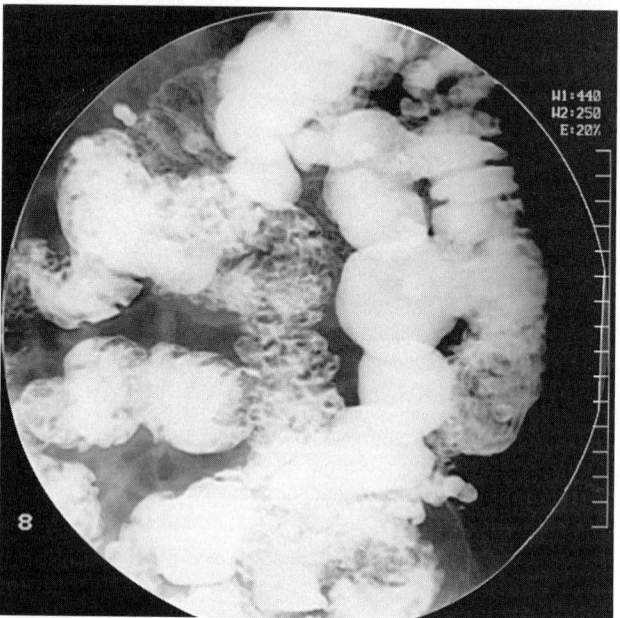

FIGURE 46-41. Multiple jejunal diverticula demonstrated by a barium contrast upper gastrointestinal study. (Courtesy of Melvyn H. Schreiber, M.D., The University of Texas Medical Branch.)

and removal of the enterolith, or sometimes the enterolith can be milked distally into the cecum. When the enterolith causes obstruction at the level of the diverticulum, bowel resection is necessary. When a perforation of a jejunoileal diverticulum is encountered, resection with reanastomosis is required, because lesser procedures such as simple closure, excision, or invagination are associated with greater mortality and morbidity rates. In extreme cases, such as diffuse peritonitis, enterostomies may be required if judgment dictates that reanastomosis may be risky.

Meckel's Diverticulum

Incidence/Etiology

Meckel's diverticulum is the most commonly encountered congenital anomaly of the small intestine, occurring in approximately 2% of the population.[141] It was reported initially in 1598 by Hildanus and then described in detail by Johann Meckel in 1809.[142] Meckel's diverticulum is located on the antimesenteric border of the ileum 45 to 60 cm proximal to the ileocecal valve and results from incomplete closure of the omphalomesenteric, or vitelline, duct. An equal incidence is found among men and women. The Meckel diverticulum may exist in different forms, ranging from a small "bump" that may be easily missed to a long projection that communicates with the umbilicus by a persistent fibrous cord (Fig. 46-42) or, much less commonly, a patent fistula. The usual manifestation is a relatively wide-mouth diverticulum measuring approximately 5 cm in length, with a diameter of up to 2 cm (Fig. 46-43). Cells lining the vitelline duct are pluripotent; therefore, it is not uncommon to find heterotopic tissue within the Meckel diverticulum, the most common of which is gastric mucosa (present in 50% of all Meckel's diverticula). Pancreatic mucosa is encountered in approximately 5% of diverticula; less commonly, these diverticula may harbor colonic mucosa.

Clinical Manifestations

The vast majority of Meckel's diverticula are entirely benign and are incidentally discovered during autopsy, laparotomy, or barium studies (Fig. 46-44). The most common clinical presentation of a Meckel diverticulum is gastrointestinal bleeding, which occurs in 25% to 50% of patients who present with complications; hemorrhage is the most common symptomatic presentation in children aged 2 years or younger. This complication may present as acute massive hemorrhage, as anemia secondary to chronic bleeding, or as a self-limiting recurrent episodic event. The usual source of the bleeding is a chronic acid-

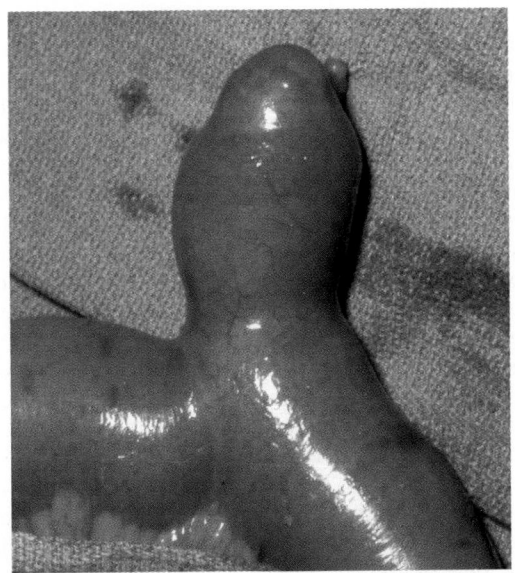

FIGURE 46-43. Common presentation of a Meckel diverticulum projecting from the antimesenteric border of the ileum.

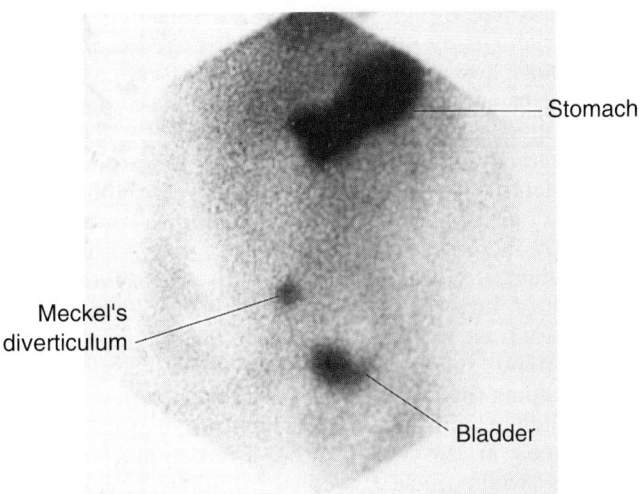

FIGURE 46-45. ^{99m}Tc pertechnetate scintigraphy in a child demonstrates a Meckel diverticulum clearly differentiated from the stomach and bladder. (Courtesy of Melvyn H. Schreiber, M.D., The University of Texas Medical Branch.)

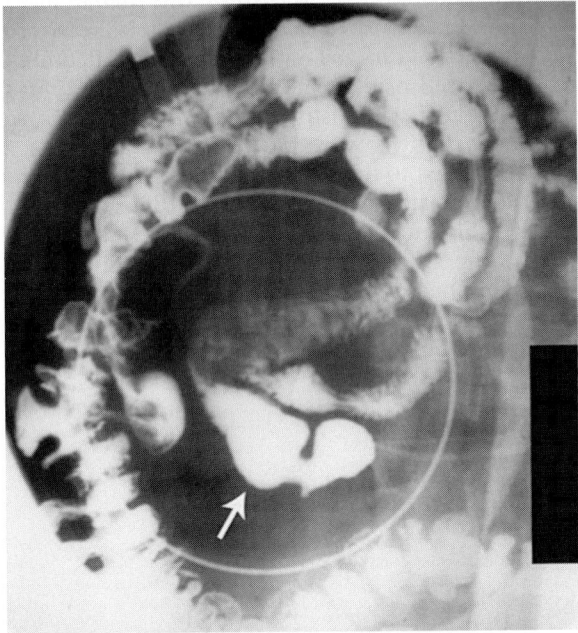

FIGURE 46-44. Barium radiograph demonstrates an asymptomatic Meckel diverticulum *(arrow)*. (Courtesy of Melvyn H. Schreiber, M.D., The University of Texas Medical Branch.)

induced ulcer in the ileum adjacent to a Meckel diverticulum that contains gastric mucosa.

Another common presenting symptom of Meckel's diverticulum is intestinal obstruction, which may occur as a result of a volvulus of the small bowel around a diverticulum associated with a fibrotic band attached to the abdominal wall, intussusception, or, rarely, incarceration of the diverticulum in an inguinal hernia (Littre's hernia). Volvulus is usually an acute event and, if allowed to progress, may result in strangulation of the involved bowel. In intussusception, a broad-based diverticulum invaginates and then is carried forward by peristalsis. This may be ileoileal or ileocolic and present as acute obstruction associated with an urge to defecate, early vomiting, and, occasionally, the passage of the classic currant-jelly stool. A palpable mass may be present. Although reduction of an intussusception secondary to a Meckel diverticulum can sometimes be performed by barium enema, the patient should still undergo resection of the diverticulum to negate subsequent recurrence of the condition.

Diverticulitis accounts for 10% to 20% of symptomatic presentations. This complication is more common in adult patients. Meckel's diverticulitis, which is clinically indistinguishable from appendicitis, should be considered in the differential diagnosis of a patient with right lower quadrant pain. Progression of the diverticulitis may lead to perforation and peritonitis. It is important to remember that when the appendix is found to be normal during exploration for suspected appendicitis, the distal ileum should be inspected for the presence of an inflamed Meckel diverticulum. Finally, much rarer complications of Meckel's diverticula include neoplasms, with the most common benign tumors reported as leiomyomas, angiomas, and lipomas. Malignant neoplasms include adenocarcinomas, which commonly originate from the gastric mucosa, sarcoma, and carcinoid tumor.

Diagnostic Studies

The diagnosis of Meckel's diverticulum may be difficult. Plain abdominal radiographs, CT, and ultrasonography are rarely helpful. In children, the single most accurate diagnostic test for Meckel's diverticula is scintigraphy with sodium ^{99m}Tc-pertechnetate.[143] The ^{99m}Tc-pertechnetate is preferentially taken up by the mucus-secreting cells of gastric mucosa and ectopic gastric tissue in the diverticulum (Fig. 46-45). The diagnostic sensitivity of this scan has been reported as high as 85%, with a specificity of 95% and an accuracy of 90% in the pediatric age group.

In adults, however, ^{99m}Tc-pertechnetate scanning is less accurate because of the reduced prevalence of ectopic gastric mucosa within the diverticulum. The sensitivity and specificity can be improved by the use of pharmacologic agents such as pentagastrin and glucagon or H$_2$-receptor antagonists (e.g., cimetidine). Pentagastrin indirectly increases the metabolism of mucus-producing cells, whereas glucagon inhibits peristaltic dilution and washout of intraluminal radionuclide. Cimetidine may be used to increase the sensitivity of scintigraphy by decreasing the peptic secretion, but not the radionuclide uptake, and retarding the release of pertechnetate from the diverticular lumen, thus resulting in higher radionuclide concentrations in the wall of the diverticulum. In adult patients, when nuclear medicine findings are normal, barium studies should be performed. In patients with acute hemorrhage, angiography is sometimes useful.

Treatment

The treatment of a symptomatic Meckel diverticulum should be prompt surgical intervention with resection of the diverticulum or resection of the segment of ileum bearing the diverticulum. Segmental intestinal resection is required for treatment of patients with bleeding because the bleeding site usually is in the ileum adjacent to the diverticulum. Resection of the diverticulum for nonbleeding Meckel's diverticula can be performed using either a hand-sewn technique or stapling across the base of the diverticulum in a diagonal or transverse line so as to minimize the risk of subsequent stenosis. Reports have demonstrated the feasibility and safety of laparoscopic diverticulectomy.[144] Long-term outcomes with this procedure, however, are lacking.

Although the treatment for a complicated Meckel diverticulum is straightforward, controversy still exists regarding the optimal treatment of a Meckel diverticulum noted as an incidental finding. It is generally recommended that asymptomatic diverticula found in children during laparotomy be resected. The treatment of Meckel's diverticula encountered in the adult patient, however, remains controversial.[145,146] In a landmark paper by Soltero and Bill,[147] which formed the basis of the surgical management of asymptomatic Meckel's diverticula in adults for a number of years, the likelihood of a Meckel diverticulum becoming symptomatic in the adult patient was estimated as 2% or less; morbidity rates from incidental removal, which was reported to be as high as 12% in some studies, far exceeded the potential for prevention of disease. This study was criticized, however, because it was not a population-based analysis. An epidemiologic population-based study by Cullen and associates[148] challenged the practice of ignoring an incidentally found Meckel's diverticulum. A 6.4% rate of development of complications from the Meckel diverticulum was calculated to occur over a lifetime. This incidence of complications does not appear to peak during childhood as originally thought. Therefore, the recommendation from this study was that an incidentally found Meckel's diverticulum should be removed at any age up to 80 years as long as no additional conditions (e.g., peritonitis) made removal hazardous. The rates of short- and long-term postoperative complications from prophylactic removal were low (approximately 2%), and death was related to the primary operation or the general health of the patient and not to the diverticulectomy. Therefore, this study, as well as other recent studies, suggests that the issue of prophylactic diverticulectomy in adults should be reevaluated and that in selected patients diverticulectomy in the asymptomatic patient may be beneficial and safer than originally reported.

TABLE 46-8.	Causes of Small Intestine Ulceration
Infections	Tuberculosis, syphilis, cytomegalovirus, typhoid, parasites, *Strongyloides* hyperinfection, *Campylobacter*, *Yersiniosis*
Inflammatory	Crohn's disease, systemic lupus erythematosus, celiac disease, ulcerative enteritis
Ischemia	Mesenteric insufficiency
Idiopathic	Primary ulcer, Behçet's syndrome
Drug induced	Potassium, indomethacin, phenylbutazone, salicylates, antimetabolites
Radiation	Therapeutic, accidental
Vascular	Vasculitis, giant cell arteritis, amyloidosis (ischemit lesion), angiocentric lymphoma
Metabolic	Uremia
Hyperacidity	Zollinger-Ellison syndrome, Meckel's diverticulum, stomal ulceration
Neoplastic	Lymphoma, adenocarcinoma, melanoma
Toxic	Acute jejunitis (β-toxin-producing *Clostridium perfringens*), arsenic
Mucosal lesions	Lymphocytic enterocolitis

Adapted from Rai R, Bayless TM: Isolated and diffuse ulcers of the small intestine. *In* Feldman M, Scharschmidt BF, Sletsenger MH (eds): Gastrointestinal and Liver Disease: Pathophysiology/Diagnosis/Management. Philadelphia, WB Saunders, 1998, pp 1771-1778.

MISCELLANEOUS PROBLEMS

Small Bowel Ulcerations

Ulcerations of the small bowel are relatively uncommon and may be attributed to Crohn's disease, typhoid fever, tuberculosis, lymphoma, and ulcers associated with gastrinoma (Table 46-8). Drug-induced ulcerations can occur and have been, in the past, attributed to enteric-coated potassium chloride tablets and corticosteroids. In addition, ulcerations of the small intestine in which no causative agent can be identified have been described. Reports suggest that small bowel complications from nonsteroidal anti-inflammatory drugs (NSAIDs) may be more common than originally considered.[149] NSAID-induced ulcers occur more commonly in the ileum, with single or multiple ulcerations noted. Complications necessitating operative intervention include bleeding, perforation, and obstruction. In addition to ulcerations, NSAIDs are known to induce an enteropathy characterized by increased intestinal permeability leading to protein loss and hypoalbuminemia, malabsorption, and anemia. Kessler and coworkers[149] identified NSAID use and complications as responsible for at least 4% of all small bowel resections performed during a 3-year period. Often, this cause is unrecognized, and the diagnosis is delayed in patients who present with bleeding. Treatment of complications from small bowel ulcerations is segmental resection and intestinal reanastomosis.

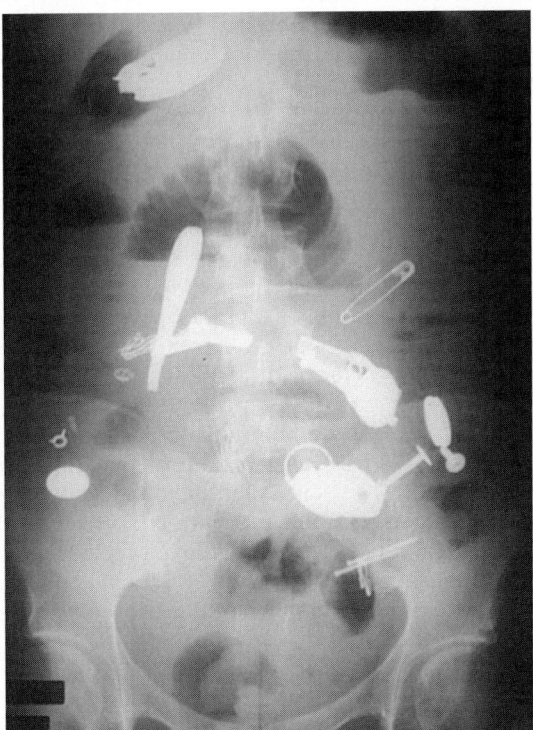

FIGURE 46-46. Plain abdominal film demonstrates a number of ingested foreign bodies in a patient presenting with a small bowel obstruction. (Courtesy of Melvyn H. Schreiber, M.D., The University of Texas Medical Branch.)

Ingested Foreign Bodies

Ingestion of foreign bodies that could lead to subsequent perforation or obstruction of the gastrointestinal tract are swallowed, usually accidentally, by children or adults. These include glass and metal fragments, pins, needles, toothpicks, fish bones, coins, whistles, toys, and broken razor blades, among others (Fig. 46-46). Intentional ingestion of foreign bodies is sometimes seen in the incarcerated and the mentally deranged. For the vast majority of patients, treatment is observation, which allows the safe passage of these objects through the intestinal tract.[150] If the object is radiopaque, progress can be followed by serial abdominal films. Cathartic agents are contraindicated. Sharp, pointed objects such as needles, razor blades, or fish bones may penetrate the bowel wall. If abdominal pain, tenderness, fever, or leukocytosis occurs, immediate laparotomy and surgical removal of the offending object are indicated. Laparotomy is also required for intestinal obstruction.

Small Bowel Fistulas

Enterocutaneous fistulas are most commonly iatrogenic, usually the result of a surgical misadventure (e.g., anastomotic leakage, injury of the bowel or blood supply, laceration of the bowel by wire mesh, or retention suture).[151] In addition, fistulas may result from erosion by suction catheters, adjacent abscesses, or trauma. Contributing factors in some patients may include previous radiation therapy, intestinal obstruction, inflammatory bowel disease, mesenteric vascular disease, or intra-abdominal sepsis. Less than 2% of enterocutaneous fistulas occur spontaneously, and they are usually the result of Crohn's disease.

Recognition of enterocutaneous fistulas is usually not difficult. The typical clinical presentation is that of a febrile, postoperative patient with an erythematous wound. When a few skin sutures are removed, a purulent or bloody discharge is noted; leakage of enteric contents then occurs, sometimes immediately, but often within 1 or 2 days. If the diagnosis is in doubt, confirmation can be obtained by oral administration of a nonabsorbable marker, such as charcoal or Congo red, or by injection of water-soluble contrast medium into the fistula. This is the most common presentation of a small bowel fistula in which the process is more or less walled off in the immediate area of damage to the small bowel. Less commonly, small bowel fistulas may present as generalized peritonitis.

Enterocutaneous fistulas are classified according to their location and volume of daily output. These factors dictate both treatment and morbidity/mortality rates. In general, the more proximal the fistula in the intestine, the more serious the problem, with greater fluid and electrolyte loss. The drainage has a greater digestive capacity, and the distal segment is not available for absorption of nutrients. High-output fistulas are those that discharge 500 mL or more per 24 hours. Factors that prevent the spontaneous closure of fistulas are shown in Box 46-4.

Radiographic investigation of the fistula by injection of water-soluble contrast material through the fistula tract should be carried out early to delineate the presence and

Box 46-4.   Factors Preventing Spontaneous Fistula Closure

High output (>500 mL/24 hr)
Severe disruption of intestinal continuity (>50% of bowel circumference)
Active inflammatory bowel disease of bowel segment
Cancer
Radiation enteritis
Distal obstruction
Undrained abscess cavity
Foreign body in the fistula tract
Fistula tract <2.5 cm in length
Epithelialization of fistula tract

extent of any abscess cavities; to obtain information about the length of the tract, the extent of bowel wall disruption, and the location of the fistula; and to determine whether a distal obstruction is present. CT is helpful in determining if underlying collections of fluid or pus are present. Often these collections can be drained percutaneously.

The major complications associated with small bowel fistulas include sepsis, fluid and electrolyte depletion, necrosis of the skin at the site of external drainage, and malnutrition. Mortality rates for patients with enterocutaneous fistulas remain high, with some series reporting a 15% to 20% mortality rate.

Treatment

Successful management of patients with intestinal fistulas requires establishment of controlled drainage, usually using a sump suction apparatus, management of sepsis, prevention of fluid and electrolyte depletion, protection of the skin, and provision of adequate nutrition.[152,153] The control of fistula output is most easily accomplished by intubation of the fistula tract with a drain. Protection of the skin around the fistulous opening is important to prevent excoriation and destruction of the skin. This is most easily accomplished by using Stomahesive appliances with applications of zinc oxide, aluminum paste ointment, or karaya powder. The suction catheter can be brought out through the end of the Stomahesive bag, which is cut to just fit the fistulous opening. This will allow for collection and accurate measurement of the output. The use of TPN has been an important advance in the management of patients with enterocutaneous fistulas and significantly prevents the problems of malnutrition.

The volume depletion that occurs from a proximal small bowel fistula may present a formidable problem. Agents that inhibit gut motility, such as codeine or diphenoxylate, are generally not helpful. The long-acting somatostatin analogue octreotide has been used in patients with enterocutaneous fistulas with a successful decrease in the volume of output.[154] Some series have reported that octreotide significantly improved the rate of fistula closure, whereas other studies have failed to document this increased closure rate. However, there is no

doubt that octreotide greatly ameliorates the problems associated with a massive volume loss and allows better control of the fistula tract.

When sepsis has been controlled and nutritional therapy has been instituted, a course of conservative management should be followed. Some have advocated conservative management for up to 3 months to allow for spontaneous closure. However, Reber and associates[155] showed that after sepsis was controlled, more than 90% of small intestinal fistulas that closed did so within 1 month. Fewer than 10% of the fistulas closed after 2 months, and none closed spontaneously after 3 months. Therefore, a reasonable management plan would be to follow a conservative course for 4 to 6 weeks, at which time, if closure has not been obtained, surgical management should be considered. This period of conservative management not only allows those fistulas to heal spontaneously but also allows for optimization of nutritional status and control of the wound and fistula sites. Also, a reasonable delay permits the peritoneal reaction and inflammation to subside, thus making a second operation easier and safer.

Surgery is most easily accomplished by entering the previous abdominal wound, with great care taken to avoid further damage to adherent bowel. The preferred operation is fistula tract excision and segmental resection of the involved segment of intestine and reanastomosis. Simple closure of the fistula after removing the fistula tract almost always results in a recurrence of the fistula. If an unexpected abscess is encountered or if the bowel wall is rigid and distended over a long distance, thus making primary anastomosis unsafe, exteriorization of both ends of the intestine should be accomplished. Various bypass procedures have also been described as part of a staged approach in which exclusion of the segment containing the fistula is accomplished in the first reoperation and then another operation is required for resection of the involved segment and the fistula tract. Although this may be necessary in extreme circumstances, this is certainly not the preferred surgical management.

In summary, enterocutaneous fistulas occur most commonly as a result of a previous operative procedure. Once identified, radiologic studies must be performed to define the precise location as well as other factors, such as a surrounding abscess cavity or disruption of the bowel wall. This is most directly accomplished by a fistulogram, although CT may also be helpful in certain patients. The key elements to treating an enterocutaneous fistula include the control of sepsis, fluid and electrolyte depletion, skin necrosis, and malnutrition. A majority of these fistulas will heal spontaneously within 4 to 6 weeks of conservative management. If closure is not accomplished after this time, surgery is indicated.

Pneumatosis Intestinalis

Pneumatosis intestinalis is an uncommon condition presenting as multiple gas-filled cysts of the gastrointestinal tract. The cysts may be located in the subserosa, submucosa, and, rarely, muscularis layer and vary in size from microscopic to several centimeters in diameter. They can occur anywhere along the gastrointestinal tract, from the esophagus to the rectum; however, they are most common in the jejunum, followed by the ileocecal region and the colon. Extraintestinal structures such as mesentery, peritoneum, and the falciform ligament may also be involved. There is an equal incidence among males and females, and this condition most commonly occurs in the fourth to seventh decades of life. Pneumatosis in neonates is usually associated with necrotizing enterocolitis. The cause of pneumatosis intestinalis has not been completely delineated. A number of theories have been proposed, of which the mechanical, mucosal damage, bacterial, and pulmonary theories appear to be the most promising.

The majority of cases of pneumatosis intestinalis are associated with chronic obstructive pulmonary disease or the immunocompromised state (e.g., AIDS; post transplantation; in association with leukemia, lymphoma, vasculitis, or collagen vascular disease; and in those patients taking chemotherapy or corticosteroids).[156] Other associated conditions include inflammatory, obstructive, or infectious conditions of the intestine; iatrogenic conditions such as endoscopy and jejunostomy placement; ischemia; and extraintestinal diseases such as diabetes. Pneumatosis not associated with other lesions is referred to as *primary pneumatosis*.

Grossly, the cysts resemble cystic lymphangiomas or hydatid cysts. On histologic section, the involved portion has a honeycomb appearance. The cysts are thin walled and break easily. Spontaneous rupture gives rise to pneumoperitoneum. Symptoms are nonspecific, and in pneumatosis associated with other disorders, the symptoms may be those of the associated disease. Symptoms in primary pneumatosis intestinalis, when present, include most commonly diarrhea, abdominal pain, abdominal distention, nausea, vomiting, weight loss, and mucus in stools. Hematochezia and constipation have also been described. Complications associated with pneumatosis intestinalis occur in approximately 3% of cases and include volvulus, intestinal obstruction, hemorrhage, and intestinal perforation. Most commonly, pneumoperitoneum occurs in these patients, usually in association with small bowel rather than large bowel pneumatosis. Peritonitis is unusual. In fact, pneumatosis intestinalis represents one of the few cases of sterile pneumoperitoneum and should be considered in the patient with free abdominal air but no evidence of peritonitis.

The diagnosis is usually made radiographically by plain abdominal or barium studies. On plain films, pneumatosis intestinalis appears as radiolucent areas within the bowel wall, which must be differentiated from luminal intestinal gas (Fig. 46-47). The radiolucency may be linear or curvilinear or appear as grapelike clusters or tiny bubbles. Alternatively, barium contrast or CT studies can be used to confirm the diagnosis. Visualization of intestinal cysts has also been described by ultrasound.

No treatment is necessary unless one of the very rare complications supervenes, such as rectal bleeding, cyst-induced volvulus, or tension pneumoperitoneum. Prognosis in most patients is that of the underlying disease. The important point is to recognize that pneumatosis

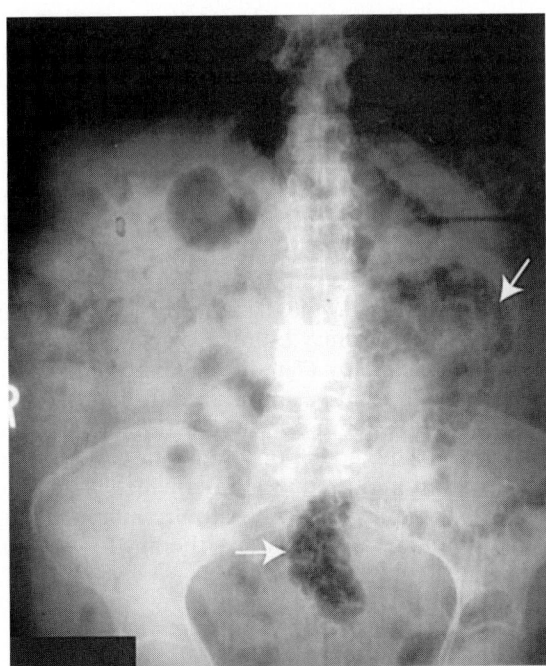

FIGURE 46-47. Plain abdominal film demonstrates pneumatosis intestinalis *(arrows)*. (Courtesy of Melvyn H. Schreiber, M.D., The University of Texas Medical Branch.)

intestinalis is a benign cause of pneumoperitoneum. Treatment should be directed at the underlying cause of the pneumatosis, and surgical intervention should be predicated on the clinical course of the patient.

Blind Loop Syndrome

This is a rare condition manifested by diarrhea, steatorrhea, megaloblastic anemia, weight loss, abdominal pain, and deficiencies of the fat-soluble vitamins (A, D, E, and K), as well as neurologic disorders. The underlying cause of this syndrome is bacterial overgrowth in stagnant areas of the small bowel produced by stricture, stenosis, fistulas, or diverticula (e.g., jejunoileal or Meckel's diverticulum). Under normal circumstances the upper gastrointestinal tract contains fewer than 10^5 bacteria/mL, mostly gram-positive aerobes and facultative anaerobes. However, with stasis, the number of bacteria increases with excessive proliferation of aerobic and anaerobic bacteria (bacteroides, anaerobic lactobacilli, coliforms, and enterococci are likely to be present in varying numbers). The bacteria compete for vitamin B_{12}, producing systemic deficiency of vitamin B_{12} and megaloblastic anemia.

The syndrome can be confirmed by a series of laboratory investigations. Bacterial overgrowth can be diagnosed with cultures obtained through an intestinal tube or by indirect tests such as the ^{14}C-xylose or ^{14}C-cholylglycine breath tests. Excessive bacterial use of ^{14}C substrate leads to an increase in $^{14}CO_2$. Once bacterial overgrowth and steatorrhea are confirmed, a Schilling test (^{57}Co-labeled vitamin B_{12} absorption) may be performed next, which should reveal a pattern of urinary excretion of vitamin B_{12} resembling that of pernicious anemia (a urinary loss of 0%

to 6% of vitamin B_{12} compared with the normal of 7% to 25%). In patients with a blind loop syndrome, vitamin B_{12} excretion is not altered by the addition of intrinsic factor, but a course of a broad-spectrum antibiotic (e.g., tetracycline) should return vitamin B_{12} absorption to normal.

Treatment of patients with the blind loop syndrome is parenteral vitamin B_{12} therapy and a broad-spectrum antibiotic, most commonly tetracycline or amoxicillin/clavulanate potassium (Augmentin). An alternative choice is the combination of a cephalosporin (e.g., cephalexin [Keflex]) and metronidazole. If these agents are not effective, chloramphenicol may be used. For most patients, a single course of therapy (7 to 10 days) is sufficient, and the patient may remain symptom free for months. Prokinetic agents have been used without real success. Surgical correction of the condition producing stagnation and blind loop syndrome produces a permanent cure and is indicated in those patients who require multiple rounds of antibiotics or are on continuous therapy.

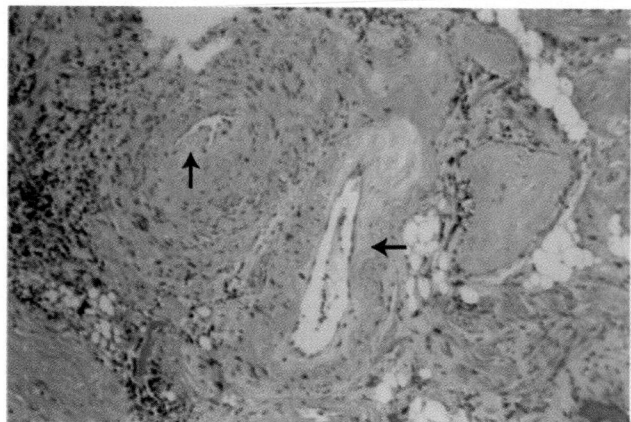

FIGURE 46-48. Photomicrograph of the ileum of a patient with ulceration and stricture secondary to radiation enteritis. Note the obliterative arteritis, thickened arterial walls, and submucosal fibrosis (arrows), which are characteristic findings of chronic radiation injury. (Courtesy of Mary R. Schwartz, M.D., Baylor College of Medicine.)

Radiation Enteritis

Radiation therapy is commonly used as adjuvant therapy for various abdominal and pelvic cancers. In addition to tumor cells, however, other rapidly dividing cells in normal tissues may be affected by radiation. Surrounding normal tissue such as the small intestinal epithelium may sustain severe, acute, and chronic deleterious effects.[157,158] The amount of radiation appears to correlate with the probability of developing radiation enteritis. Serious late complications are unusual if the total radiation dosage is less than 4000 cGy; morbidity risk increases with dosages exceeding 5000 cGy.[159] Other factors, including previous abdominal operations, preexisting vascular disease, hypertension, diabetes, and adjuvant treatment with certain chemotherapeutic agents such as 5-fluorouracil, doxorubicin, dactinomycin, and methotrexate, contribute to the development of enteritis after radiation treatments. A previous history of laparotomy increases the risk of enteritis, presumably owing to adhesions that fix portions of the small bowel into the irradiated field. Radiation damage tends to be acute and self-limiting, with symptoms consisting mainly of diarrhea, abdominal pain, and malabsorption. The late effects of radiation injury are the result of damage to the small submucosal blood vessels with a progressive obliterative arteritis and submucosal fibrosis, resulting eventually in thrombosis and vascular insufficiency (Fig. 46-48).[160] This injury may produce necrosis and perforation of the involved intestine, but more commonly it leads to stricture formation with symptoms of obstruction or small bowel fistulas.

Radiation enteritis may be minimized by adjusting ports and dosages of radiation to deliver optimal treatment specifically to the tumor and not to surrounding tissues. Placement of radiopaque markers, such as titanium clips, at the time of the original operation facilitates better targeting of the radiation treatment. Methods designed to exclude the small bowel from the irradiated field include reperitonealization, omental transposition, and placement of absorbable mesh slings.[161]

Numerous pharmacologic interventions have also been described to reduce the side effects of radiation enteritis.[162] Sucralfate has been shown to be of value in preventing the diarrhea associated with abdominal radiation. Superoxide dismutase, a free radical scavenger, has been used successfully to reduce complications. Other compounds that have been evaluated include glutathione, antioxidants (e.g., vitamin A, vitamin E, β-carotene), and histamine antagonists. The most effective radioprotectant agent appears to be amifostine (WR-2721), a sulfhydryl compound that is converted intracellularly to an active metabolite, WR-1065, which in turn binds to free radicals and protects the cell from radiation injury. Other agents that may prove useful in the prevention of the acute symptoms of acute radiation enteritis include glutamine-enriched enteral formulas and the hormones bombesin, growth hormone, glucagon-like peptide 2, and insulin-like growth factor-I, which have demonstrated effectiveness in experimental studies in preventing or reducing symptoms associated with radiation enteritis.[163,164]

The treatment of acute radiation enteritis is directed at controlling symptoms. Antispasmodics and analgesics may alleviate abdominal pain and cramping, and diarrhea usually responds to opiates or other antidiarrheal agents. The use of corticosteroids for acute radiation enteritis is of uncertain value. Dietary manipulation, including oral elemental diets, has also been advocated to ameliorate the acute effects of radiation enteritis; however, results are conflicting.

Operative intervention may be required in a subgroup of patients with the chronic effects of radiation enteritis. This subgroup of patients represents only a small percentage (2% to 3%) of the total number of patients who have received abdominal or pelvic irradiation. Indications for operation include obstruction, fistula formation, perforation, and bleeding, with obstruction being the most common presentation. Operative procedures include a bypass or resection with reanastomosis.[165] Advocates for bypass procedures contend that this procedure is safer and controls the symptoms better than resection. Advocates of resection contend that the high morbidity and mortality rates previously reported with resection and reanastomosis reflect inadequate resection and anastomosis of diseased intestine. In patients presenting with obstruction, extensive lysis of adhesions should be avoided. Obstruction due to rigid, fixed intestinal loops in the pelvis is best bypassed. If resection and reanastomosis are planned, at least one end of the anastomosis should be from intestine outside the irradiated field. An incidence as high as 50% of anastomotic breakdown has been reported after resection and anastomosis involving diseased segments of bowel, owing to the poor healing qualities of the irradiated tissue. Macroscopic findings may not be accurate in evaluating the full extent of radiation damage. Frozen sections and laser Doppler flowmetry have been used to assist resection and anastomosis. However, reports of the clinical usefulness of these techniques are conflicting. Perforation of the intestine should be treated with resection and anastomosis. When reanastomosis is thought to be unsafe, the ends should be exteriorized.

Radiation enteritis can be a relentless disease process. Almost half of patients who survive their first laparotomy for radiation bowel injury require further surgery for ongoing bowel damage. Up to 25% of these patients die of radiation enteritis and complications from its management.

Short Bowel Syndrome

The short bowel syndrome results from a total small bowel length that is inadequate to support nutrition. Seventy-five percent of cases of short bowel syndrome occur from massive intestinal resection.[166] In the adult, mesenteric occlusion, midgut volvulus, and traumatic disruption of the superior mesenteric vessels are the most frequent causes. Multiple sequential resections, most commonly associated with recurrent Crohn's disease, account for 25% of patients. In neonates, the most common cause of short bowel syndrome is bowel resection secondary to necrotizing enterocolitis. The clinical hallmarks of the short bowel syndrome include diarrhea, fluid and electrolyte deficiency, and malnutrition. Other complications include an increased incidence of gallstones due to disruption of the enterohepatic circulation and of nephrolithiasis from hyperoxaluria. Specific nutrient deficiencies must be prevented, and levels must be monitored closely; these nutrients include iron, magnesium, zinc, copper, and vitamins. The likelihood that a patient with short bowel syndrome will be permanently dependent on TPN is thought to be primarily influenced by the length, location, and the health of the remaining intestine. In patients with short bowel syndrome, postabsorptive levels of plasma citrulline, a nonprotein amino acid produced by intestinal mucosa, may provide an indicator to differentiate transient from permanent intestinal failure.[167]

The bowel has a remarkable capacity to adapt after small bowel resection; and in many instances, this process of intestinal adaptation, called adaptive hyperplasia, effectively prevents severe complications resulting from the markedly decreased surface area that is available for absorption and digestion.[168] However, any adaptive mechanism can be overwhelmed, and adaptation can be inadequate if too much small bowel is lost. Although there is considerable individual variation, resection of up to 70% of the small bowel usually can be tolerated if the terminal ileum and ileocecal valve are preserved. Length alone, however, is not the only determining factor of complications related to small bowel resection. For example, if the distal two thirds of the ileum, including the ileocecal valve, is resected, significant abnormalities of absorption of bile salts and vitamin B_{12} may occur, resulting in diarrhea and anemia, although only 25% of the total length of the small bowel has been removed. Proximal bowel resection is tolerated much better than distal resection because the ileum can adapt and increase its absorptive capacity more efficiently than the jejunum.

Treatment

The most important aspect to remember about short bowel syndrome is prevention. In patients with Crohn's disease, resections limited to the particular complication should be performed. In addition, during surgery for problems related to intestinal ischemia, the smallest possible resection should be performed, and, if necessary, second-look operations should be carried out to allow the ischemic bowel to demarcate, thus potentially preventing unnecessary extensive resection of the bowel.

After massive small bowel resection, the treatment course may be divided into early and late phases. In its early phase, treatment is primarily directed at the control of diarrhea, replacement of fluid and electrolytes, and prompt institution of TPN.[169] Volume losses may exceed 5 L/day, and vigorous monitoring of intake and output with adequate replacement must be carried out. Diarrhea in this early phase can be caused by a multitude of sources. For example, hypergastrinemia and gastric hypersecretion occur after massive small bowel resection and greatly contribute to diarrhea after a massive small bowel resection. Acid hypersecretion can be managed by H_2-receptor antagonists or proton pump blockers, such as omeprazole. Diarrhea may also be caused by ileal resection, resulting in disruption of the enterohepatic circulation and excessive amounts of bile salts entering the colon. Cholestyramine may be beneficial when diarrhea is related to the cathartic effects of unabsorbed bile salts in the colon. In addition, the judicious use of agents that inhibit gut motility (e.g., codeine and diphenoxylate) may be helpful. The long-acting somatostatin analogue octreotide also appears to reduce the amount of diarrhea during the early phase of short bowel syndrome.[170] Some studies suggest that octreotide may inhibit gut adaptation; other studies, however, have not confirmed this deleterious effect of octreotide.

As soon as the patient has recovered from the acute phase, enteral nutrition should begin so intestinal adaptation may be started early and proceed successfully.[171] The most common types of enteral diets are elemental

(Vivonex, Flexical) or polymeric (Isocal, Ensure). Controversy exists regarding the optimal diet for these patients. Initially, a high-carbohydrate, high-protein diet is appropriate to maximize absorption. Milk products should be avoided, and diet should be begun at iso-osmolar concentrations and with small amounts. As the gut adapts, the osmolality, volume, and caloric content can be increased. The provision of nutrients in their simplest forms is an important part of the treatment. Simple sugars, dipeptides, and tripeptides are rapidly absorbed from the intestinal tract. Reduction in dietary fat has long been considered to be important in the treatment of patients with short bowel syndrome. Supplementation of the diet with 100 g or more of fat, however, should be carried out, often requiring the use of medium-chain triglycerides, which are absorbed in the proximal bowel. Vitamins, especially fat-soluble vitamins, as well as calcium, magnesium, and zinc supplementation, should be provided. The roles of hormones administered systemically and glutamine administered enterally are being evaluated. The hormones neurotensin, bombesin, and glucagon-like peptide 2 (GLP-2) have demonstrated marked mucosal growth in various experimental studies and have been shown to prevent the gut atrophy associated with TPN in experimental studies; combination therapy appears more efficacious than single-agent administration.[172,173] In addition, limited clinical studies using GLP-2 show improved intestinal absorption and nutritional status in patients with short bowel syndrome.[172,174]

Two other hormones not derived from the gut that have been evaluated extensively in various experimental and limited clinical trials include growth hormone and insulin-like growth factor-I. In an uncontrolled clinical trial, Byrne and colleagues[175] used a combination of growth hormone, glutamine, and a modified diet and demonstrated a reduction in or elimination of TPN requirements in some refractory patients with severe short bowel syndrome and TPN dependence. However, in a double-blind, placebo-controlled randomized study, Scolapio and associates[176] demonstrated only modest improvements in electrolyte absorption but no improvements in small bowel morphology, stool losses, or macronutrient absorption using the combination of glutamine and growth hormone. In contrast, a study by Seguy and colleagues[177] suggested that a 3-week course of low-dose growth hormone significantly improved intestinal absorption in TPN-dependent patients. Given the conflicting results in these studies, the potential efficacy of this treatment in TPN-dependent patients remains to be defined. The combination of various trophic hormones with glutamine and a modified diet may prove more efficacious in this difficult group of patients.[178]

A number of surgical strategies have been attempted in patients who are chronically TPN dependent with limited success; these include procedures to delay intestinal transit time, methods to increase absorptive area, and small bowel transplantation.[179] Methods to delay intestinal transit time include the construction of various valves and sphincters, with inconsistent results reported. Antiperistaltic segments of small intestine have been constructed to slow the transit, thus allowing additional contact time for nutrient and fluid absorption. Moderate successes have been described with this technique. Other procedures, including colonic interposition, recirculating loops of small bowel, and retrograde electrical pacing, have been tried but were found to be unsuccessful in humans and were largely abandoned. Surgical procedures to increase absorptive area include the intestinal tapering and lengthening procedure originally described by Bianchi.[180] This procedure improves intestinal function by correcting the dilatation and ineffective peristalsis of the remaining intestine, as well as by doubling the intestinal length while preserving the mucosal surface area. Although beneficial in selected patients, potential complications can include necrosis of divided segments and anastomotic leaks.

Intestinal transplantation has improved with the introduction of the new immunosuppressive agent tacrolimus (FK506).[181] More than 200 intestinal transplantations have been performed worldwide in humans during the 1990s. These have included primarily isolated small intestinal grafts and combined liver/small intestinal grafts with a few more extensive cluster grafts in a large series reported from the International Intestinal Transplant Registry. Under tacrolimus treatment, 1-year graft and patient survival rates were 65% and 83%, respectively, for isolated bowel transplantation and 65% and 68% for liver/small bowel transplantation. Seventy-eight of the 86 survivors in this series had stopped TPN and were receiving oral nutrition. The largest experience in the United States has been at the University of Pittsburgh, where the reported patient survival rate has been 72% at 1 year, 53% at 2 years, and 42% at 3 years. Currently, liver/small intestine transplantation has a survival rate similar to that for kidney and heart transplantation. The challenges of small bowel transplantation continue to be the need for better immunosuppression and earlier detection of rejection. An alternative to intestinal transplantation is mucosal stem cell transplantation, which involves transplanting enterocytes onto a biomatrix and achieving regeneration of intestinal mucosa. This procedure is, at best, preliminary but has shown some promise in experimental studies.

Vascular Compression of the Duodenum

Vascular compression of the duodenum, also known as superior mesenteric artery syndrome or Wilkie's syndrome, is a rare condition characterized by compression of the third portion of the duodenum by the superior mesenteric artery as it passes over this portion of the duodenum.[182] Symptoms include profound nausea and vomiting, abdominal distention, weight loss, and postprandial epigastric pain, which varies from intermittent to constant depending on the severity of the duodenal obstruction. Weight loss usually occurs before the onset of symptoms and contributes to the syndrome.

This syndrome is most commonly seen in young asthenic individuals, with women being more commonly affected than men. Predisposing factors for vascular compression of the duodenum, aside from weight loss, include supine immobilization, scoliosis, and the placement of a body cast (sometimes called the cast syndrome). An asso-

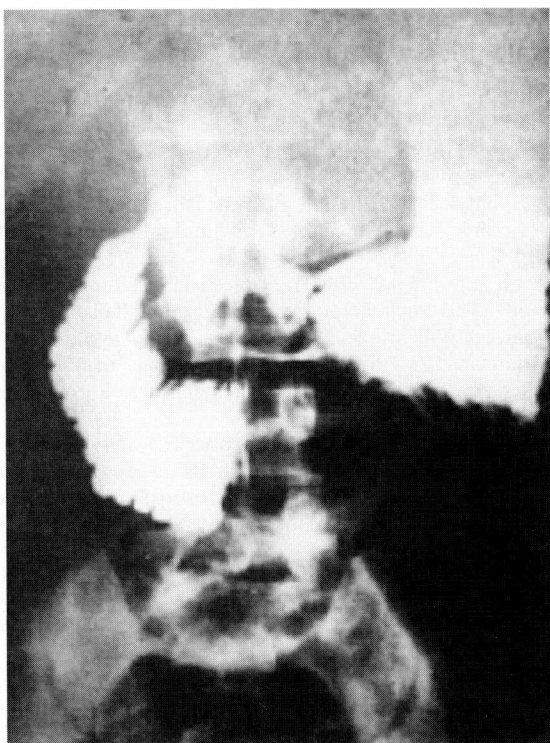

FIGURE 46-49. Barium radiograph demonstrates obstruction of the third portion of the duodenum secondary to superior mesenteric artery compression as a consequence of burn injury. (Adapted from Reckler JM, Bruck HM, Munster AM, et al: Superior mesenteric artery syndrome as a consequence of burn injury. J Trauma 12:979-985, 1972.)

ciation between vascular compression of the duodenum and peptic ulcer has been observed. Vascular compression of the duodenum has been reported in association with anorexia nervosa and after proctocolectomy and J-pouch anal anastomosis, resection of an arterial venous malformation of the cervical cord, abdominal aortic aneurysm repair, and orthopedic procedures, usually spinal surgery. One report in the literature describes a family with a preponderance of vascular compression of the duodenum.

Diagnosis of this condition is made by barium upper gastrointestinal series (Fig. 46-49) or hypotonic duodenography, which demonstrates abrupt or near-total cessation of flow of barium from the duodenum to the jejunum.[183] CT has been useful in certain instances. Treatment of this syndrome varies. Conservative measures are tried initially and have been increasingly successful as definitive treatment. The operative treatment of choice for vascular compression of the duodenum is duodenojejunostomy.[184]

Selected References

Bonen DK, Cho JH: The genetics of inflammatory bowel disease. Gastroenterology 124:521-536, 2003.

> This review nicely summarizes recent findings regarding the genetic changes that may contribute to the development of Crohn's disease.

Crohn BB, Ginzburg L, Oppenheimer GD: Regional ileitis: A pathologic and clinical entity. JAMA 99:1323-1329, 1932.

> This landmark paper succinctly crystallizes the clinical course, differential diagnosis, and pathologic findings of regional ileitis in young adults. Although other terms have been applied to this disease process, based on the descriptions in this classic paper, Crohn's disease has been universally accepted as the name.

Cullen JJ, Kelly KA, Moir CR, et al: Surgical management of Meckel's diverticulum: An epidemiologic, population-based study. Ann Surg 220:564-569, 1994.

> This study, which was a carefully performed, epidemiologic, population-based analysis, challenges the prior dogma of selective resection of incidentally discovered Meckel's diverticula in the adult patient.

DeCosse JJ, Rhodes RS, Wentz WB, et al: The natural history and management of radiation induced injury of the gastrointestinal tract. Ann Surg 170:369-384, 1969.

> This report, presented at the annual meeting of the American Surgical Association in 1969, is a landmark article that clearly delineates the clinical features, complications, and management of patients with radiation enteritis.

Fazio VW, Marchetti F: Recurrent Crohn's disease and resection margins: Bigger is not better. Adv Surg 32:135-168, 1999.

> This review summarizes the surgical principles of treating complications of Crohn's disease, that is, bigger resection margins are not associated with fewer recurrence rates.

Hartwell JA, Hoguet JP: Experimental intestinal obstruction in dogs with special reference to the cause of death and the treatment by large amounts of normal saline solution. JAMA 59:82, 1912.

> This experimental study emphasizes the importance of fluid loss in intestinal obstruction and demonstrates that the administration of saline solutions prevented death from a high intestinal obstruction in dogs. The observations are as timely today as they were in 1912.

Joensuu H, Roberts PJ, Sarlomo-Rikala M, et al: Effect of the tyrosine kinase inhibitor STI571 in a patient with a metastatic gastrointestinal stromal tumor. N Engl J Med 344:1052-1056, 2001.

> This is the first study to demonstrate the clinical effectiveness of imatinib (Gleevec) for the treatment of malignant gastrointestinal stromal tumor. This further highlights the fact that agents that selectively target molecular pathways may provide important adjuvant therapies for certain cancers.

Johnson LR (ed): Gastrointestinal Physiology, 6th ed. St. Louis, Mosby, 2001.

> This is a current, concise and nicely illustrated mini-text on gastrointestinal physiology.

Moertel CG, Sauer WG, Dockerty MB, Baggenstoss AH: Life history of the carcinoid tumor of the small intestine. Cancer 14:901-912, 1961.

> This carefully performed study from the Mayo Clinic includes a total of 209 cases of carcinoid tumors of the small bowel.

Present DH, Rutgeerts P, Targan S, et al: Infliximab for the treatment of fistulas in patients with Crohn's disease. N Engl J Med 340:1398-1405, 1999.

> This article represents the first randomized, multicenter, double-blind trial demonstrating significant improvement in patients with enterocutaneous fistulas due to Crohn's disease using infliximab, an antibody to tumor necrosis factor-α. Further studies have demonstrated the effectiveness of this treatment in selected patients.

Thomas RP, Hellmich MR, Townsend CM Jr, Evers BM: Role of gastrointestinal hormones in the proliferation of normal and neoplastic tissues. Endocr Rev 24:571-599, 2003.

> This review summarizes the effects of various gastrointestinal hormones on the growth of normal tissues and gastrointestinal cancers; possible treatment options are discussed.

Thompson JC, Marx M: Gastrointestinal hormones. Curr Probl Surg 21:1-80, 1984.

> This authoritative treatise provides a succinct summary of the function and clinical significance of the gastrointestinal hormones. This monograph is easy to read and should serve as a nice introduction to the field.

Thorson A, Biorck G, Bjorkman G, Waldenstrom J: Malignant carcinoid of the small intestine with metastases to the liver, valvular disease of the right side of the heart (pulmonary stenosis and tricuspid regurgitation without septal defects), peripheral vasomotor symptoms, bronchoconstriction, and an unusual type of cyanosis: A clinical and pathologic syndrome. Am Heart J 47:795-817, 1954.

> This report nicely describes the clinical manifestations of the carcinoid syndrome with an emphasis on right-sided heart disease. The role of 5-hydroxytryptamine, which was known to be produced by carcinoid tumors of the intestine, was postulated as the causative factor for right-sided valvular disease.

Vanderhoof JA, Langnas AN: Short-bowel syndrome in children and adults. Gastroenterology 113:1767-1778, 1997.

> This review article describes management strategies, both medical and surgical, in patients with small bowel syndrome. The role for transplantation in these patients is discussed.

References

1. Moore KL, Persaud TVN: The digestive system. *In* The Developing Human: Clinically Oriented Embryology. Philadelphia, WB Saunders, 1998, pp 271-302.
2. Keljo DJ, Gariepy CE: Anatomy, histology, embryology, and developmental anomalies of the small and large intestine. *In* Feldman M, Friedman LS, Sleisenger MH (eds): Sleisenger and Fordtran's Gastrointestinal and Liver Disease: Pathology/Diagnosis/Management. Philadelphia, WB Saunders, 2002, pp 1643-1664.
3. Cheng H, Leblond CP: Origin, differentiation and renewal of the four main epithelial cell types in the mouse small intestine: V. Unitarian theory of the origin of the four epithelial cell types. Am J Anat 141:537-561, 1974.
4. Simon TC, Gordon JI: Intestinal epithelial cell differentiation: New insights from mice, flies and nematodes. Curr Opin Genet Dev 5:577-586, 1995.
5. Hirsch J, Ahrens EH Jr: Measurement of the human intestinal length in vivo and some causes of variation. Gastroenterology 31:274-284, 1956.
6. Madara JL, Trier JS: The functional morphology of the mucosa of the small intestine. *In* Johnson LR (ed): Physiology of the Gastrointestinal Tract. New York, Raven Press, 1994, pp 1577-1622.
7. Davenport HW: Physiology of the Digestive Tract: An Introductory Text. Chicago, Year Book Medical Publishers, 1982.
8. Chung DH, Evers BM: The Digestive System. *In* O'Leary JP (ed): The Physiologic Basis of Surgery. Philadelphia, Lippincott Williams & Wilkins, 2002, pp 457-490.
9. Johnson LR: Digestion and absorption. *In* Johnson LR, Gerwin TA (eds): Gastrointestinal Physiology. St. Louis, Mosby, 2001, pp 119-140.
10. Farrell JJ: Digestion and absorption of nutrients and vitamins. *In* Feldman M, Friedman LS, Sleisenger MH (eds): Sleisenger & Fordtran's Gastrointestinal and Liver Disease: Pathology/Diagnosis/Management. Philadelphia, WB Saunders, 2002, pp 1715-1743.
11. Traber PG: Carbohydrate assimilation. *In* Yamada T, Alpers DH, Kaplowitz N, et al (eds): Textbook of Gastroenterology. Philadelphia, Lippincott Williams & Wilkins, 2003, pp 389-412.
12. Ganapathy V, Ganapathy ME, Leibach FH: Protein digestion and assimilation. *In* Yamada T, Alpers DH, Kaplowitz N, et al (eds): Textbook of Gastroenterology. Philadelphia, Lippincott Williams & Wilkins, 2003, pp 438-448.
13. Davidson NO: Intestinal lipid absorption. *In* Yamada T, Alpers DH, Kaplowitz N, et al (eds): Textbook of Gastroenterology. Philadelphia, Lippincott Williams & Wilkins, 2003, pp 413-437.
14. Guyton AC, Hall JE: Digestion and absorption in the gastrointestinal tract. *In* Textbook of Medical Physiology. Philadelphia, WB Saunders, 2000, pp 754-763.
15. Sellin JH: Intestinal electrolyte absorption and secretion. *In* Feldman M, Friedman LS, Sleisenger MH (eds): Sleisenger and Fordtran's Gastrointestinal and Liver Disease: Pathology/Diagnosis/Management. Philadelphia, WB Saunders, 2002, pp 1693-1714.
16. Halsted CH, Lonnerdal BL: Vitamin and mineral absorption. *In* Yamada T, Alpers DH, Kaplowitz N, et al (eds): Textbook of Gastroenterology. Philadelphia, Lippincott Williams & Wilkins, 2003, pp 449-471.
17. Hasler WL: Motility of the small intestine and colon. *In* Yamada T, Alpers DH, Kaplowitz N, et al (eds): Textbook of Gastroenterology. Philadelphia, Lippincott Williams & Wilkins, 2003, pp 220-247.
18. Andrews JM, Dent J: Small intestinal motor physiology. *In* Feldman M, Friedman LS, Sleisenger MH (eds): Sleisenger & Fordtran's Gastrointestinal and Liver Disease: Pathology/Diagnosis/Management. Philadelphia, WB Saunders, 2002, pp 1665-1678.
19. Thompson JC, Marx M: Gastrointestinal hormones. Curr Probl Surg 21:1-80, 1984.
20. Greeley GH Jr: Gastrointestinal Endocrinology. Totowa, NY, Humana Press, 1999.
21. Johnson LR: Regulation: Peptides of the gastrointestinal tract. *In* Johnson LR, Gerwin TA (eds): Gastrointestinal Physiology. St. Louis, Mosby, 2001, pp 1-16.
22. Reubi JC: Peptide receptors as molecular targets for cancer diagnosis and therapy. Endocr Rev 24:389-427, 2003.
23. Thomas RP, Hellmich MR, Townsend CM Jr, et al: Role of gastrointestinal hormones in the proliferation of normal and neoplastic tissues. Endocr Rev 24:571-599, 2003.

24. Dockray GJ, Varro A, Dimaline R: Gastric endocrine cells: Gene expression, processing, and targeting of active products. Physiol Rev 76:767-798, 1996.

25. Merchant JL, Dickinson CJ, Yamada T: Molecular biology of the gut: Model of gastrointestinal hormones. In Johnson LR, Alpers DH, Christensen J, et al (eds): Physiology of the Gastrointestinal Tract. New York, Raven Press, 1994, pp 295-350.

26. Thompson JC, Cooper CW, Rayford PL, et al: Gastrointestinal Endocrinology: Receptors and Post-receptor Mechanisms. San Diego, Academic Press, 1990.

27. Shetzline MA, Liddle RA: Gastrointestinal hormones and neurotransmitters. In Feldman M, Friedman LS, Sleisenger MH (eds): Sleisenger & Fordtran's Gastrointestinal and Liver Disease: Pathology/Diagnosis/Management. Philadelphia, WB Saunders, 2002, pp 3-20.

28. Sartor RB: Mucosal immunology and mechanisms of gastrointestinal inflammation. In Feldman M, Friedman LS, Sleisenger MH (eds): Sleisenger and Fordtran's Gastrointestinal and Liver Disease: Pathology/Diagnosis/Management. Philadelphia, WB Saunders, 2002, pp 21-52.

29. Blumberg RS, Stenson WF: The immune system and gastrointestinal inflammation. In Yamada T, Alpers DH, Kaplowitz N, et al (eds): Textbook of Gastroenterology. Philadelphia, Lippincott Williams & Wilkins, 2003, pp 117-150.

30. Hartwell JA, Hoguet JP: Experimental intestinal obstruction in dogs with special reference to the cause of death and the treatment by large amounts of normal saline solution. JAMA 59:82-87, 1912.

31. Wangensteen OH: Historical aspects of the management of acute intestinal obstruction. Surgery 65:363-383, 1969.

32. Bass KN, Jones B, Bulkley GB: Current management of small-bowel obstruction. Adv Surg 31:1-34, 1997.

33. Ellis H, Moran BJ, Thompson JN, et al: Adhesion-related hospital readmissions after abdominal and pelvic surgery: A retrospective cohort study. Lancet 353:1476-1480, 1999.

34. Miller G, Boman J, Shrier I, et al: Natural history of patients with adhesive small bowel obstruction. Br J Surg 87:1240-1247, 2000.

35. Sagar PM, MacFie J, Sedman P, et al: Intestinal obstruction promotes gut translocation of bacteria. Dis Colon Rectum 38:640-644, 1995.

36. Maglinte DD, Heitkamp DE, Howard TJ, et al: Current concepts in imaging of small bowel obstruction. Radiol Clin North Am 41:263-283, vi, 2003.

37. Furukawa A, Yamasaki M, Furuichi K, et al: Helical CT in the diagnosis of small bowel obstruction. Radiographics 21:341-355, 2001.

38. Burkill G, Bell J, Healy J: Small bowel obstruction: The role of computed tomography in its diagnosis and management with reference to other imaging modalities. Eur Radiol 11:1405-1422, 2001.

39. Blackmon S, Lucius C, Wilson JP, et al: The use of water-soluble contrast in evaluating clinically equivocal small bowel obstruction. Am Surg 66:238-244, 2000.

40. Sarr MG, Bulkley GB, Zuidema GD: Preoperative recognition of intestinal strangulation obstruction: Prospective evaluation of diagnostic capability. Am J Surg 145:176-182, 1983.

41. Richards WO, Garrard CL, Allos SH, et al: Noninvasive diagnosis of mesenteric ischemia using a SQUID magnetometer. Ann Surg 221:696-705, 1995.

42. Richards WO, Williams LF Jr: Obstruction of the large and small intestine. Surg Clin North Am 68:355-376, 1988.

43. Sosa J, Gardner B: Management of patients diagnosed as acute intestinal obstruction secondary to adhesions. Am Surg 59:125-128, 1993.

44. Bulkley GB, Zuidema GD, Hamilton SR, et al: Intraoperative determination of small intestinal viability following ischemic injury: A prospective, controlled trial of two adjuvant methods (Doppler and fluorescein) compared with standard clinical judgment. Ann Surg 193:628-637, 1981.

45. Leon EL, Metzger A, Tsiotos GG, et al: Laparoscopic management of small bowel obstruction: Indications and outcome. J Gastrointest Surg 2:132-140, 1998.

46. Fischer CP, Doherty D: Laparoscopic approach to small bowel obstruction. Semin Laparosc Surg 9:40-45, 2002.

47. Childs WA, Phillips RB: Experience with intestinal plication and a proposed modification. Ann Surg 152:258-265, 1960.

48. Noble TB Jr: Plication of small intestine as prophylaxis against adhesions. Am J Surg 35:41-44, 1937.

49. Rodriguez-Ruesga R, Meagher AP, Wolff BG: Twelve-year experience with the long intestinal tube. World J Surg 19:627-631, 1995.

50. Sprouse LR II, Arnold CI, Thow GB, et al: Twelve-year experience with the Thow long intestinal tube: A means of preventing postoperative bowel obstruction. Am Surg 67:357-360, 2001.

51. Becker JM, Dayton MT, Fazio VW, et al: Prevention of postoperative abdominal adhesions by a sodium hyaluronate-based bioresorbable membrane: A prospective, randomized, double-blind multicenter study. J Am Coll Surg 183:297-306, 1996.

52. Vrijland WW, Tseng LN, Eijkman HJ, et al: Fewer intraperitoneal adhesions with use of hyaluronic acid-carboxymethylcellulose membrane: A randomized clinical trial. Ann Surg 235:193-199, 2002.

53. Liakakos T, Thomakos N, Fine PM, et al: Peritoneal adhesions: Etiology, pathophysiology, and clinical significance: Recent advances in prevention and management. Dig Surg 18:260-273, 2001.

54. Dalziel TK: Chronic interstitial enteritis. BMJ 2:1068-1070, 1913.

55. Crohn BB: Regional ileitis: A pathologic and clinical entity. JAMA 99:1323-1329, 1932.

56. Sartor RB: Current concepts of the etiology and pathogenesis of ulcerative colitis and Crohn's disease. Gastroenterol Clin North Am 24:475-507, 1995.

57. Hodgson HJ: Pathogenesis of Crohn's disease. Baillieres Clin Gastroenterol 12:1-17, 1998.

58. Van Kruiningen HJ, Ruiz B, Gumprecht L: Experimental disease in young chickens induced by a Mycobacterium paratuberculosis isolate from a patient with Crohn's disease. Can J Vet Res 55:199-202, 1991.

59. Hugot JP, Laurent-Puig P, Gower-Rousseau C, et al: Mapping of a susceptibility locus for Crohn's disease on chromosome 16. Nature 379:821-823, 1996.

60. Bonen DK, Cho JH: The genetics of inflammatory bowel disease. Gastroenterology 124:521-536, 2003.

61. Satsangi J, Morecroft J, Shah NB, et al: Genetics of inflammatory bowel disease: Scientific and clinical implications. Best Pract Res Clin Gastroenterol 17:3-18, 2003.

62. Finkelstein SD, Sasatomi E, Regueiro M: Pathologic features of early inflammatory bowel disease. Gastroenterol Clin North Am 31:133-145, 2002.

63. Itzkowitz SH: Inflammatory bowel disease and cancer. Gastroenterol Clin North Am 26:129-139, 1997.

64. Solomon MJ, Schnitzler M: Cancer and inflammatory bowel disease: Bias, epidemiology, surveillance, and treatment. World J Surg 22:352-358, 1998.

65. Carucci LR, Levine MS: Radiographic imaging of inflammatory bowel disease. Gastroenterol Clin North Am 31:93-117, ix, 2002.

66. Rubesin SE, Scotiniotis I, Birnbaum BA, et al: Radiologic and endoscopic diagnosis of Crohn's disease. Surg Clin North Am 81:39-70, viii, 2001.

67. Abreau MT, Vasiliauskas EA, Kam LY, et al: Use of serologic tests in Crohn's disease. Clin Perspect Gastroenterol May/June:155-164, 2001.

68. Hanauer SB, Present DH: The state of the art in the management of inflammatory bowel disease. Rev Gastroenterol Disord 3:81-92, 2003.

69. Lochs H, Mayer M, Fleig WE, et al: Prophylaxis of postoperative relapse in Crohn's disease with mesalamine: European Cooperative Crohn's Disease Study VI. Gastroenterology 118:264-273, 2000.

70. Thomsen OO, Cortot A, Jewell D, et al: A comparison of budesonide and mesalamine for active Crohn's disease. International Budesonide-Mesalamine Study Group. N Engl J Med 339:370-374, 1998.

71. Sandborn WJ, Present DH, Isaacs KL, et al: Tacrolimus for the treatment of fistulas in patients with Crohn's disease: A randomized, placebo-controlled trial. Gastroenterology 125:380-388, 2003.

72. Van Deventer SJ: Immunotherapy of Crohn's disease. Scand J Immunol 51:18-22, 2000.

73. Hanauer SB, Cohen RD, Becker RV III, et al: Advances in the management of Crohn's disease: Economic and clinical potential of infliximab. Clin Ther 20:1009-1028, 1998.

74. Present DH, Rutgeerts P, Targan S, et al: Infliximab for the treatment of fistulas in patients with Crohn's disease. N Engl J Med 340:1398-1405, 1999.

75. Narula SK, Cutler D, Grint P: Immunomodulation of Crohn's disease by interleukin-10. Agents Actions Suppl 49:57-65, 1998.

76. van Deventer SJ: New biological therapies in inflammatory bowel disease. Best Pract Res Clin Gastroenterol 17:119-130, 2003.

77. Ghosh S, Goldin E, Gordon FH, et al: Natalizumab for active Crohn's disease. N Engl J Med 348:24-32, 2003.

78. Graham TO, Kandil HM: Nutritional factors in inflammatory bowel disease. Gastroenterol Clin North Am 31:203-218, 2002.

79. Song HK, Buzby GP: Nutritional support for Crohn's disease. Surg Clin North Am 81:103-115, viii, 2001.

80. Singleton JW, Law DH, Kelley ML Jr, et al: National Cooperative Crohn's Disease Study: Adverse reactions to study drugs. Gastroenterology 77:870-882, 1979.

81. Delaney CP, Fazio VW: Crohn's disease of the small bowel. Surg Clin North Am 81:137-158, ix, 2001.

82. Fazio VW, Marchetti F: Recurrent Crohn's disease and resection margins: bigger is not better. Adv Surg 32:135-168, 1999.

83. Aleali M, Milsom JW: Laparoscopic surgery in Crohn's disease. Surg Clin North Am 81:217-230, x, 2001.

84. Ogunbiyi OA, Fleshman JW: Place of laparoscopic surgery in Crohn's disease. Baillieres Clin Gastroenterol 12:157-165, 1998.

85. Spencer MP, Nelson H, Wolff BG, et al: Strictureplasty for obstructive Crohn's disease: The Mayo experience. Mayo Clin Proc 69:33-36, 1994.

86. Michelassi F, Hurst RD, Melis M, et al: Side-to-side isoperistaltic strictureplasty in extensive Crohn's disease: A prospective longitudinal study. Ann Surg 232:401-408, 2000.

87. Manganiotis AN, Banner MP, Malkowicz SB: Urologic complications of Crohn's disease. Surg Clin North Am 81:197-215, x, 2001.

88. Fazio VW, Wu JS: Surgical therapy for Crohn's disease of the colon and rectum. Surg Clin North Am 77:197-210, 1997.

89. Schwartz DA, Pemberton JH, Sandborn WJ: Diagnosis and treatment of perianal fistulas in Crohn disease. Ann Intern Med 135:906-918, 2001.

90. McClane SJ, Rombeau JL: Anorectal Crohn's disease. Surg Clin North Am 81:169-183, ix, 2001.

91. Kosinski L, Welton ML: Surgical options in the management of perianal Crohn's disease. Semin Gastrointest Dis 9:15-20, 1998.

92. Wolff BG: Factors determining recurrence following surgery for Crohn's disease. World J Surg 22:364-369, 1998.

93. Rutgeerts P: Strategies in the prevention of postoperative recurrence in Crohn's disease. Best Pract Res Clin Gastroenterol 17:63-73, 2003.

94. Krupnick AS, Morris JB: The long-term results of resection and multiple resections in Crohn's disease. Semin Gastrointest Dis 11:41-51, 2000.

95. Meier DE, Tarpley JL: Typhoid intestinal perforations in Nigerian children. World J Surg 22:319-323, 1998.

96. Baden LR, Maguire JH: Gastrointestinal infections in the immunocompromised host. Infect Dis Clin North Am 15:639-670, xi, 2001.

97. Craig RM, Carlson S, Ehrenpreis E: Acquired immunodeficiency syndrome enteropathy: A perspective. Compr Ther 21:184-188, 1995.

98. al Karawi MA, Mohamed AE, Yasawy MI, et al: Protean manifestation of gastrointestinal tuberculosis: Report on 130 patients. J Clin Gastroenterol 20:225-232, 1995.

99. North JH, Pack MS: Malignant tumors of the small intestine: A review of 144 cases. Am Surg 66:46-51, 2000.

100. Gill SS, Heuman DM, Mihas AA: Small intestinal neoplasms. J Clin Gastroenterol 33:267-282, 2001.

101. Blanchard DK, Budde JM, Hatch GF III, et al: Tumors of the small intestine. World J Surg 24:421-429, 2000.

102. Jemal A, Murray T, Samuels A, et al: Cancer statistics, 2003. CA Cancer J Clin 53:5-26, 2003.

103. Neugut AI, Jacobson JS, Suh S, et al: The epidemiology of cancer of the small bowel. Cancer Epidemiol Biomarkers Prev 7:243-251, 1998.

104. Arber N, Neugut AI, Weinstein IB, et al: Molecular genetics of small bowel cancer. Cancer Epidemiol Biomarkers Prev 6:745-748, 1997.

105. Bresalier RS, Ben-Menachem T: Tumors of the small intestine. In Alpers DH, Kaplowitz N, Laine L, et al (eds): Textbook of Gastroenterology. Philadelphia, Lippincott Williams & Wilkins, 2003, pp 1643-1662.

106. Iddan G, Meron G, Glukhovsky A, et al: Wireless capsule endoscopy. Nature 405:417, 2000.

107. Buckley JA, Jones B, Fishman EK: Small bowel cancer: Imaging features and staging. Radiol Clin North Am 35:381-402, 1997.

108. Berman J, O'Leary TJ: Gastrointestinal stromal tumor workshop. Hum Pathol 32:578-582, 2001.

109. Pidhorecky I, Cheney RT, Kraybill WG, et al: Gastrointestinal stromal tumors: Current diagnosis, biologic behavior, and management. Ann Surg Oncol 7:705-712, 2000.

110. DeMatteo RP: The GIST of targeted cancer therapy: A tumor (gastrointestinal stromal tumor), a mutated gene (c-kit), and a molecular inhibitor (STI571). Ann Surg Oncol 9:831-839, 2002.

111. Kim CJ, Day S, Yeh KA: Gastrointestinal stromal tumors: Analysis of clinical and pathologic factors. Am Surg 67:135-137, 2001.

112. Yao KA, Talamonti MS, Langella RL, et al: Primary gastrointestinal sarcomas: Analysis of prognostic factors and results of surgical management. Surgery 128:604-612, 2000.

113. Jeghers H, McKusick VA, Katz KH: Generalized intestinal polyposis and melanin spots on the oral mucosa, lips, and digits: Syndrome of diagnostic significance. N Engl J Med 241:993-1005, 1949.

114. Neugut AI, Marvin MR, Rella VA, et al: An overview of adenocarcinoma of the small intestine. Oncology (Huntingt) 11:529-550, 1997.

115. Joensuu H, Roberts PJ, Sarlomo-Rikala M, et al: Effect of the tyrosine kinase inhibitor STI571 in a patient with a metastatic gastrointestinal stromal tumor. N Engl J Med 344:1052-1056, 2001.

116. Blanke CD, von Mehren M, Joensuu H: Evaluation of the molecularly targeted therapy STI571 in patients with unresectable or metastatic gastrointestinal stromal tumors expressing KIT. Proc Am Soc Clin Oncol 20:2. Available at: http://virtualmeeting.asco.org/vm2001/interest_areas/special_sessions/plenary.htm. Accessed: October 2003.

117. van Oosterom AT, Judson I, Verweij J, et al: Safety and efficacy of imatinib (STI571) in metastatic gastrointestinal stromal tumours: A phase I study. Lancet 358:1421-1423, 2001.

118. Cunningham JD, Aleali R, Aleali M, et al: Malignant small bowel neoplasms: Histopathologic determinants of recurrence and survival. Ann Surg 225:300-306, 1997.

119. Moertel CG, Sauer WG, Dockerty MB, et al: Life history of the carcinoid tumor of the small intestine. Cancer 14:901-912, 1961.

120. Pearse AG, Takor TT: Neuroendocrine embryology and the APUD concept. Clin Endocrinol (Oxf) 5(Suppl):229S-244S, 1976.

121. Kulke MH, Mayer RJ: Carcinoid tumors. N Engl J Med 340:858-868, 1999.

122. Soga J: Carcinoids of the small intestine: A statistical evaluation of 1102 cases collected from the literature. J Exp Clin Cancer Res 16:353-363, 1997.

123. Gerstle JT, Kauffman GL Jr, Koltun WA: The incidence, management, and outcome of patients with gastrointestinal carcinoids and second primary malignancies. J Am Coll Surg 180:427-432, 1995.

124. Thorson A, Biorck G, Bjorkman G, et al: Malignant carcinoid of the small intestine with metastases to the liver, valvular disease of the right side of the heart (pulmonary stenosis and tricuspid regurgitation without septal defects), peripheral vasomotor symptoms, bronchoconstriction, and an unusual type of cyanosis: A clinical and pathologic syndrome. Am Heart J 47:795-817, 1954.

125. Benevento A, Dominioni L, Carcano G, et al: Intraoperative localization of gut endocrine tumors with radiolabeled somatostatin analogs and a gamma-detecting probe. Semin Surg Oncol 15:239-244, 1998.

126. Pelley RJ, Bukowski RM: Recent advances in diagnosis and therapy of neuroendocrine tumors of the gastrointestinal tract. Curr Opin Oncol 9:68-74, 1997.

127. Memon MA, Nelson H: Gastrointestinal carcinoid tumors: Current management strategies. Dis Colon Rectum 40:1101-1118, 1997.

128. Stinner B, Kisker O, Zielke A, et al: Surgical management for carcinoid tumors of small bowel, appendix, colon, and rectum. World J Surg 20:183-188, 1996.

129. Le Treut YP, Delpero JR, Dousset B, et al: Results of liver transplantation in the treatment of metastatic neuroendocrine tumors: A 31-case French multicentric report. Ann Surg 225:355-364, 1997.

130. Arnold R: Medical treatment of metastasizing carcinoid tumors. World J Surg 20:203-207, 1996.

131. Anthony L, Johnson D, Hande K, et al: Somatostatin analogue phase I trials in neuroendocrine neoplasms. Acta Oncol 32:217-223, 1993.

132. Kvols LK: Therapy of the malignant carcinoid syndrome. Endocrinol Metab Clin North Am 18:557-568, 1989.

133. Kvols LK, Reubi JC, Horisberger U, et al: The presence of somatostatin receptors in malignant neuroendocrine tumor tissue predicts responsiveness to octreotide. Yale J Biol Med 65:505-536, 1992.

134. Oberg K: Advances in chemotherapy and biotherapy of endocrine tumors. Curr Opin Oncol 10:58-65, 1998.

135. Wilde MI, Markham A: Ondansetron: A review of its pharmacology and preliminary clinical findings in novel applications. Drugs 52:773-794, 1996.

136. Chomel JBL: Diverse observations anatomiques. In Histoire de L'Academie Royale des Sciences. Paris, Institute de France, 1710, pp 37-39.

137. Mackenzie ME, Davies WT, Farnell MB, et al: Risk of recurrent biliary tract disease after cholecystectomy in patients with duodenal diverticula. Arch Surg 131:1083-1085, 1996.

138. Mosimann F, Bronnimann B: The duodenal diverticulum: An exceptional site of massive bleeding. Hepatogastroenterology 45:603-605, 1998.

139. Akhrass R, Yaffe MB, Fischer C, et al: Small-bowel diverticulosis: Perceptions and reality. J Am Coll Surg 184:383-388, 1997.

140. de Bree E, Grammatikakis J, Christodoulakis M, et al: The clinical significance of acquired jejunoileal diverticula. Am J Gastroenterol 93:2523-2528, 1998.

141. Yahchouchy EK, Marano AF, Etienne JC, et al: Meckel's diverticulum. J Am Coll Surg 192:658-662, 2001.

142. Meckel JF: Ueber die Divertikel am Darmkanal. Arch Physiol 9:421-453, 1809.

143. Rossi P, Gourtsoyiannis N, Bezzi M, et al: Meckel's diverticulum: Imaging diagnosis. AJR Am J Roentgenol 166:567-573, 1996.

144. Sanders LE: Laparoscopic treatment of Meckel's diverticulum: Obstruction and bleeding managed with minimal morbidity. Surg Endosc 9:724-727, 1995.

145. Pinero A, Martinez-Barba E, Canteras M, et al: Surgical management and complications of Meckel's diverticulum in 90 patients. Eur J Surg 168:8-12, 2002.

146. Groebli Y, Bertin D, Morel P: Meckel's diverticulum in adults: Retrospective analysis of 119 cases and historical review. Eur J Surg 167:518-524, 2001.

147. Soltero MJ, Bill AH: The natural history of Meckel's diverticulum and its relation to incidental removal: A study of 202 cases of diseased Meckel's diverticulum found in King County, Washington, over a fifteen-year period. Am J Surg 132:168-173, 1976.

148. Cullen JJ, Kelly KA, Moir CR, et al: Surgical management of Meckel's diverticulum: An epidemiologic, population-based study. Ann Surg 220:564-569, 1994.

149. Kessler WF, Shires GT III, Fahey TJ III: Surgical complications of nonsteroidal antiinflammatory drug-induced small bowel ulceration. J Am Coll Surg 185:250-254, 1997.

150. Webb WA: Management of foreign bodies of the upper gastrointestinal tract: Update. Gastrointest Endosc 41:39-51, 1995.

151. Tassiopoulos AK, Baum G, Halverson JD: Small bowel fistulas. Surg Clin North Am 76:1175-1181, 1996.

152. Tulsyan N, Abkin AD, Storch KJ: Enterocutaneous fistulas. Nutr Clin Pract 16:74-77, 2001.

153. Hwang RF, Schwartz RW: Enterocutaneous fistulas: Current diagnosis and management. Curr Surg 57:443-445, 2000.

154. Sancho JJ, di Costanzo J, Nubiola P, et al: Randomized double-blind placebo-controlled trial of early octreotide in patients with postoperative enterocutaneous fistula. Br J Surg 82:638-641, 1995.

155. Reber HA, Roberts C, Way LW, et al: Management of external gastrointestinal fistulas. Ann Surg 188:460-467, 1978.

156. Pear BL: Pneumatosis intestinalis: A review. Radiology 207:13-19, 1998.

157. Quastler H: The nature of intestinal radiation death. Radiat Res 4:303, 1956.

158. Vanagunas A: Radiation-induced gastrointestinal disease. Clin Perspect Gastroenterol, Mar/Apr:69-75, 2001.

159. Warren SL, Whipple GH: Roentgen ray intoxication: I. Unit dose over thorax negative–over abdomen lethal: Epithelium of small intestine-sensitive to x-rays. J Exp Med 35:187-203, 1922.

160. DeCosse JJ, Rhodes RS, Wentz WB, et al: The natural history and management of radiation-induced injury of the gastrointestinal tract. Ann Surg 170:369-384, 1969.

161. Deutsch AA, Stern HS: Technique of insertion of pelvic Vicryl mesh sling to avoid postradiation enteritis. Dis Colon Rectum 32:628-630, 1989.

162. Waddell BE, Rodriguez-Bigas MA, Lee RJ, et al: Prevention of chronic radiation enteritis. J Am Coll Surg 189:611-624, 1999.

163. Alexandrides T, Spiliotis J, Mylonas P, et al: Effects of growth hormone and insulin-like growth factor-I on radiation enteritis: A comparative study. Eur Surg Res 30:305-311, 1998.

164. Klimberg VS, Souba WW, Dolson DJ, et al: Prophylactic glutamine protects the intestinal mucosa from radiation injury. Cancer 66:62-68, 1990.

165. Nakashima H, Ueo H, Shibuta K, et al: Surgical management of patients with radiation enteritis. Int Surg 81:415-418, 1996.

166. Scolapio JS, Fleming CR: Short bowel syndrome. Gastroenterol Clin North Am 27:467-479, viii, 1998.

167. Crenn P, Coudray-Lucas C, Thuillier F, et al: Postabsorptive plasma citrulline concentration is a marker of absorptive enterocyte mass and intestinal failure in humans. Gastroenterology 119:1496-1505, 2000.

168. Dowling RH, Booth CC: Functional compensation after small-bowel resection in man: Demonstration by direct measurement. Lancet 2:146-147, 1966.

169. Vanderhoof JA, Langnas AN: Short-bowel syndrome in children and adults. Gastroenterology 113:1767-1778, 1997.

170. Thompson JS: Management of the short bowel syndrome. Gastroenterol Clin North Am 23:403-420, 1994.

171. Sundaram A, Koutkia P, Apovian CM: Nutritional management of short bowel syndrome in adults. J Clin Gastroenterol 34:207-220, 2002.

172. Drucker DJ: Biological actions and therapeutic potential of the glucagon-like peptides. Gastroenterology 122:531-544, 2002.

173. Izukura M, Evers BM, Parekh D, et al: Neurotensin augments intestinal regeneration after small bowel resection in rats. Ann Surg 215:520-527, 1992.

174. Jeppesen PB, Hartmann B, Thulesen J, et al: Glucagon-like peptide 2 improves nutrient absorption and nutritional status in short-bowel patients with no colon. Gastroenterology 120:806-815, 2001.

175. Byrne TA, Persinger RL, Young LS, et al: A new treatment for patients with short-bowel syndrome: Growth hormone, glutamine, and a modified diet. Ann Surg 222:243-255, 1995.

176. Scolapio JS, Camilleri M, Fleming CR, et al: Effect of growth hormone, glutamine, and diet on adaptation in short-bowel syndrome: A randomized, controlled study. Gastroenterology 113:1074-1081, 1997.

177. Seguy D, Vahedi K, Kapel N, et al: Low-dose growth hormone in adult home parenteral nutrition-dependent short bowel syndrome patients: A positive study. Gastroenterology 124:293-302, 2003.

178. Wilmore DW, Byrne TA, Persinger RL: Short bowel syndrome: New therapeutic approaches. Curr Probl Surg 34:389-444, 1997.

179. Thompson JS, Langnas AN, Pinch LW, et al: Surgical approach to short-bowel syndrome: Experience in a population of 160 patients. Ann Surg 222:600-607, 1995.

180. Bianchi A: Intestinal loop lengthening—a technique for increasing small intestinal length. J Pediatr Surg 15:145-151, 1980.

181. Gilroy R, Sudan D: Liver and small bowel transplantation: Therapeutic alternatives for the treatment of liver disease and intestinal failure. Semin Liver Dis 20:437-450, 2000.

182. Jones SA, Carter R, Smith LL, et al: Arteriomesenteric duodenal compression. Am J Surg 100:262-277, 1960.

183. Reckler JM, Bruck HM, Munster AM, et al: Superior mesenteric artery syndrome as a consequence of burn injury. J Trauma 12:979-985, 1972.

184. Gustafsson L, Falk A, Lukes PJ, et al: Diagnosis and treatment of superior mesenteric artery syndrome. Br J Surg 71:499-501, 1984.

CHAPTER 47

APPENDIX

Kevin P. Lally, M.D., Charles S. Cox, Jr., M.D., and Richard J. Andrassy, M.D.

Anatomy and Embryology	**Neoplasms**
Appendicitis	**Miscellaneous Conditions**

ANATOMY AND EMBRYOLOGY

The appendix is a derivative of the midgut along with the ileum and ascending colon. The cecum is first visible during the 5th week of gestation, with the appendix first appearing around the 8th week of gestation as an outpouching of the cecum.[1] The appendix initially projects from the apex of the cecum, but the base gradually rotates in a more medial location toward the ileocecal valve. During development, the gut undergoes a series of rotations, with the cecum ending fixed in the right lower quadrant. Because the appendiceal orifice is always at the confluence of the cecal taenia, the final location of the appendix is determined by the location of the cecum.

The appendiceal artery, a branch of the ileocolic artery, supplies the appendix. Histologic examination of the appendix shows a number of lymphoid follicles in the submucosa. Lymphoid nodules first appear in the 7th month of gestation. There is a gradual increase in lymphoid tissue through adolescence and then a decrease over time. The lumen of the appendix is often obliterated in elderly persons.[1] As with the rest of the colon, there are mucus-producing goblet cells throughout the mucosa.

The appendix in the adult can vary widely in length from 2 to 22 cm but averages about 9 cm in length. Although the base of the appendix is consistently found at the confluence of the taenia at the base of the cecum, the tip can be located in a variety of locations (Fig. 47-1). The "normal" location of the appendix is retrocecal but within the peritoneal cavity, because the most inferior portion of the cecum is within the peritoneal cavity. This situation occurs approximately 65% of the time. It is pelvic in location in 30% and retroperitoneal in 2% of the population. The tip of the appendix can also be found in a preileal or postileal location. The varying location of the tip of the appendix explains the myriad of symptoms that can be found in patients with appendicitis.

APPENDICITIS

History

Although appendicitis has been a common problem for centuries, it was not until the early 19th century that the appendix was recognized as an organ capable of causing disease. There was continued debate through the mid 1800s about the cause of right lower quadrant inflammation, with terms such as *perityphlitis* and *paratyphlitis* commonly used. In 1827, Melier described several autopsy cases of appendicitis and clearly stated the opinion that the appendix was the likely cause, including the presumed pathophysiology that is accepted today. However, a strongly opposing position by Dupuytren, the most eminent surgeon of the time, caused Melier's views not to gain widespread acceptance. Continued work in Britain and Germany pointed to the appendix as a potential source of disease, and indeed, the number of publications on diseases of the appendix began to increase significantly. By 1880, both Matterstock in Germany and With in Norway published papers that clearly suggest the appendix as a significant cause of iliac fossa inflammation. In 1886, Reginald Fitz of Boston made a landmark contribution by discussing the appendix as the primary cause of right lower quadrant inflammation.[2] He coined the term *appendicitis* and, importantly, recommended early surgical treatment of the disease. By 1886, the widespread availability of anesthesia and the growing acceptance of antisepsis set the stage for the rapid application of these recommendations, with several U.S. surgeons making important contributions.

Before 1886, a number of cases of intervention for appendicitis had been reported. However, most of these patients had operative intervention well after the disease was established, with the primary goal to drain the infection. Several papers of note were published in the ensuing

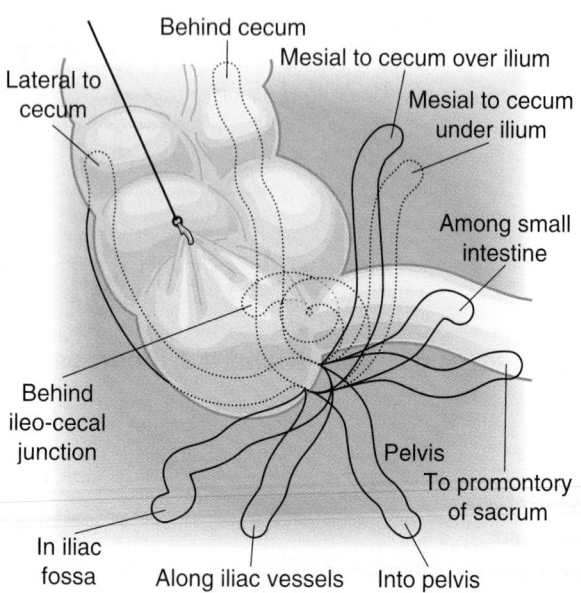

FIGURE 47-1. Various locations in which the tip on the appendix can be found. (From Kelly HA, Hurdon E: The Vermiform Appendix and Its Diseases. Philadelphia, WB Saunders, 1905.)

years. In 1889, Chester McBurney described the migratory pain as well as the finger point localization of pain between 1.5 and 2 inches from the anterior iliac spine on an oblique line to the umbilicus. He incorrectly stated that this was an almost constant finding in patients with appendicitis.[3] McBurney in New York and McArthur in Chicago described a right lower quadrant muscle splitting incision for surgical treatment in 1894. It is interesting to note that McBurney kept his patients on bed rest for at least 4 weeks after surgery! In 1905, Murphy clearly described the appropriate sequence of symptoms of pain followed by nausea and vomiting with fever and exaggerated local tenderness in the position occupied by the appendix.[4] There continued to be significant improvements in survival, so by the time penicillin became routinely available in the late 1940s, the mortality rate for appendicitis was less than

2%. Further advances in the management of appendicitis have included the recognition of the polymicrobial flora, improved diagnostic studies, and interventional radiologic procedures for treatment of abscesses. Currently, the mortality rate is 0.25% if all ages are considered (Fig. 47-2).[5,6]

Appendicitis occurs infrequently in very young children and elderly persons. The disease has a maximal incidence in patients in their late teens and 20s. There is a slight increased prevalence in males versus females.

Pathophysiology

It is widely accepted that the inciting event in most instances of appendicitis is obstruction of the appendiceal lumen. This may be due to lymphoid hyperplasia, inspissated stool (a fecalith), or some other foreign body. Given the correlation with the incidence of appendicitis by age and the size and distribution of the lymphoid tissue, it is likely that lymphoid obstruction or partial obstruction of the lumen is a common cause. Obstruction of the lumen leads to bacterial overgrowth as well as continued mucus secretion. This causes distention of the lumen, and the intraluminal pressure increases. This may lead to lymphatic and then venous obstruction. With bacterial overgrowth and edema, an acute inflammatory response ensues. The appendix then becomes more edematous and ischemic. Necrosis of the appendiceal wall subsequently occurs along with translocation of bacteria through the ischemic wall. This is gangrenous appendicitis. Without intervention, the gangrenous appendix will perforate, with spillage of the appendiceal contents into the peritoneal cavity. If this sequence of events occurs slowly, the appendix is contained by the inflammatory response and the omentum, leading to localized peritonitis and eventually an appendiceal abscess. If the body does not wall off the process, the patient may develop diffuse peritonitis.

Bacteriology

The flora in the noninflamed appendix is similar to the colon with a variety of facultative aerobic and anaerobic

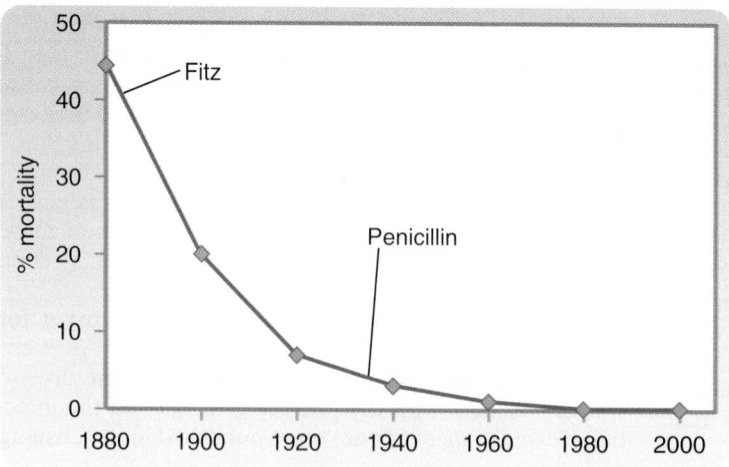

FIGURE 47-2. Mortality rates from appendicitis since 1880. The landmark paper by Fitz was published in 1886. Penicillin became widely available in the late 1940s.

bacteria found; hence, the bacteria involved in appendicitis are the same as for other colonic diseases. The incidence of obtaining positive cultures from the peritoneal cavity depends on the stage of appendicitis found. In patients with acute, nonperforated appendicitis, peritoneal fluid cultures bacteria in fewer than half of the patients.[7] However, peritoneal cultures are positive in more than 85% of patients with gangrenous or perforated appendicitis.[8] The number of bacterial species that can be cultured depends on how vigorously the investigators attempt to isolate them, with some investigators showing an average of more than nine different species. In 1938, Altemeier demonstrated the polymicrobial nature of perforated appendicitis, and for practical purposes, little has changed.[9] The most common facultative aerobic and anaerobic bacteria that are isolated are outlined in Box 47-1.

The usefulness of routine peritoneal cultures in patients with perforated appendicitis has been questioned.[10] The flora are generally known, the results are not available for several days, and many times, no change in treatment plan is made despite culture results. It appears reasonable to avoid routine cultures and to obtain them only in patients with persisting infection or surgical site infection.

Diagnosis

Clinical

The diagnosis of acute appendicitis is made primarily on the basis of the history and the physical findings, with additional assistance from laboratory and radiographic examinations. The typical history is onset of generalized abdominal pain followed by anorexia and nausea. The pain then becomes most prominent in the epigastrium and gradually moves toward the umbilicus, finally localizing in the right lower quadrant. Vomiting may occur during this time. Examination of the abdomen usually shows diminished bowel sounds, with direct tenderness and muscle spasm in the right lower quadrant. As the process continues, the amount of spasm increases, with the appearance of rebound tenderness. The temperature is often mildly elevated (~38°C) and usually rises to higher levels in the event of perforation, although this is highly variable. Direct tenderness is usually present in the right lower quadrant and may involve other parts of the abdomen, particularly if perforation has occurred. The appendix is often situated at or around McBurney's point. However, it must be emphasized that the exact anatomic location of the appendix can be at any point on a 360-degree circle surrounding the base of the cecum. This is the site at which the pain and tenderness are usually maximal, and the exact site can vary from patient to patient.

Rovsing's sign, which is elicited when pressure applied in the left lower quadrant reflects pain in the right lower quadrant, is often present but is not specific. The psoas sign may be positive and is elicited by extension of the right thigh with the patient lying on the left side. As the examiner extends the right thigh with stretching of the muscle, pain suggests the presence of an inflamed appendix overlying the psoas muscle. The obturator sign can be elicited with the patient in the supine position with passive rotation of the flexed right hip. Pain with this maneuver indicates a positive sign. Rectal examination is of little value in establishing the diagnosis of acute appendicitis but can be useful to determine the presence or absence of a mass.[11] If the appendix ruptures, abdominal pain becomes intense and more diffuse, the muscular spasm increases, and there is a simultaneous increase in the heart rate, with a rise in temperature to 39°C to 40°C. At this time, the patient appears quite ill, and it becomes obvious that the clinical situation has deteriorated. Infrequently, there may be a slight diminishing of pain with rupture, presumably due to the decreased distention of the appendix, but a true pain-free interval is uncommon.

Box 47-1. Bacteria Frequently Isolated From Perforated Appendicitis

Aerobic and Facultative

Escherichia coli
Viridans streptococci
Pseudomonas aeruginosa
Group D streptococci
Enterococcus species

Anaerobic

Bacteroides fragilis
Other *Bacteroides* species
Peptostreptococcus micros
Bilophila species
Lactobacillus species
Fusobacterium species

Radiographic

ABDOMINAL RADIOGRAPHS

Abdominal radiographs obtained in the evaluation of patients with acute abdominal pain typically include the flat and upright abdominal radiograph, as well as a chest radiograph. This sequence of studies may be useful in patients with atypical presenting symptoms and physical signs. However, plain abdominal radiographs should not be considered "routine" or "mandatory" components of the evaluation of patients with acute abdominal pain. Pneumoperitoneum on an upright abdominal radiograph suggests a diagnosis other than appendicitis. Rarely does a perforated appendix present with pneumoperitoneum (1% to 2%). Abdominal radiographs may demonstrate a fecalith, localized ileus, or loss of the peritoneal fat stripe. Gas in the appendix is not a sign specific for appendicitis and should not mandate laparotomy for appendicitis.[12]

Ultrasound

Ultrasonography is often used as the initial diagnostic imaging study in the majority of patients in whom the clinical diagnosis of appendicitis is equivocal. Ultrasound is noninvasive and rapidly available and avoids radiation exposure. Most studies of graded compression ultrasound demonstrate a sensitivity of more than 85% and a specificity of more than 90%.[13,14] In experienced hands, ultrasound has been reported to significantly lower the negative exploration rate.[15] However, the sonogram for appendicitis is a highly operator-dependent study. Sonographic criteria for the diagnosis of acute appendicitis are the demonstration of a noncompressible appendix of 7 mm or greater in anteroposterior diameter, the presence of an appendicolith, interruption of the continuity of the echogenic submucosa, and periappendiceal fluid or mass (Fig. 47-3A). A fecalith in combination with localized right lower quadrant pain is highly diagnostic of appendicitis.[16] False-positive studies can be due to secondary inflammation of the appendix as a result of inflammatory bowel disease, salpingitis, or other causes. False-negative sonograms are usually due to nonvisualization of a retrocecal appendix and a gas-filled cecum, which prevents visualization of the appendix. In addition, perforation significantly decreases the diagnostic accuracy of graded compression of the appendix. Thus, the ultrasonographic diagnosis of perforated appendicitis depends on the secondary findings on periappendiceal fluid, mass, and loss of the integrity of the submucosa layer (Fig. 47-3B). Gaseous distention of the right lower quadrant bowel loops or prolonged symptoms suggesting perforation should make computed tomography (CT) the preferred imaging study for improved accuracy and potential utility in planning intervention for appendiceal abscess or phlegmon.

Computed Tomography

Improved image resolution to the 0.5- to 1.0-cm range has improved the accuracy of CT scanning.[17,18] Typically, CT has been reserved for patients with an equivocal history and physical and laboratory findings. CT is useful in patients with an observed inflammatory abdominal process, and the presentation is atypical for appendicitis. The accuracy of CT is greatest when a deliberate effort is made to visualize the appendix. Although some reports discount the use of intravenous contrast agent and use limited enteric contrast agent, the optimal technique requires complete small bowel opacification.[19] The terminal ileum and cecum must be filled with contrast agent to improve the recognition of the normal or abnormal appendix and to avoid confusing unopacified ileal loops with the appendix. Unless contraindicated, intravenous contrast agent should be used as well. Specific, fine (5-mm)-image intervals should be obtained in the region of the appendix.

In general, CT findings of appendicitis increase with the severity of the disease. The normal appendix appears as a thin tubular structure in the right lower quadrant that may or may not opacify with contrast agent. Appendicoliths appear as ringlike homogeneous calcifications and are

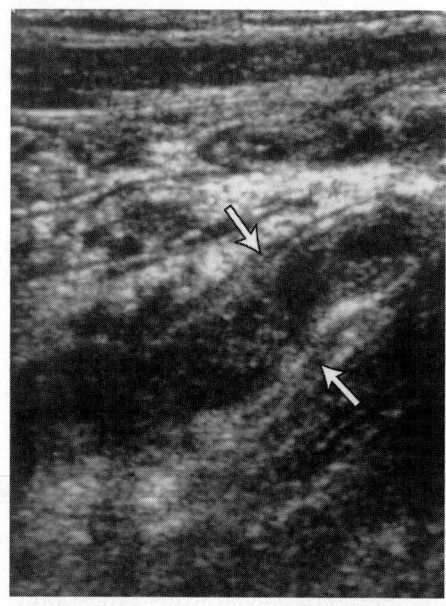

A

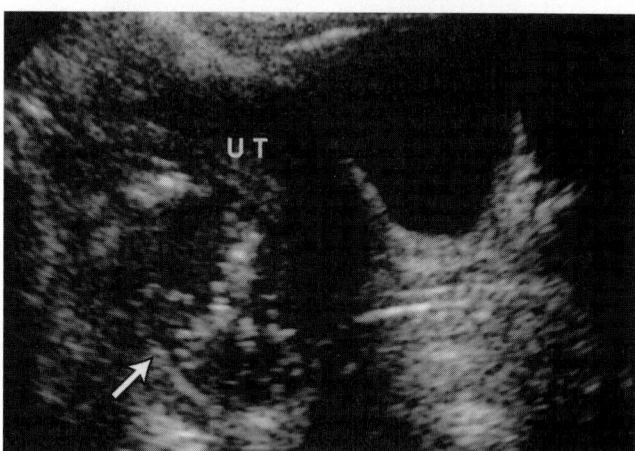

B

FIGURE 47-3. **A,** Ultrasonogram of the right lower quadrant demonstrates acute appendicitis with a thickened appendiceal wall and increased diameter *(arrows).* **B,** Ultrasonogram of perforated appendicitis with a complex abscess cavity in the right lower quadrant. UT, uterus; *arrow,* fluid collection.

seen in approximately 25% of the population. Classically, a CT diagnosis of acute appendicitis includes an abnormal appendix with periappendiceal inflammation (Fig. 47-4A). The appendix is considered abnormal when it is distended or thickened and greater than approximately 5 to 7 mm in diameter. The wall of the inflamed appendix is circumferentially thickened and may appear as a "halo" or "target." CT findings of periappendiceal inflammation suggest appendicitis; these include periappendiceal abscess, fluid collections, edema, and phlegmon.[20] Periappendiceal inflammation or edema is visualized as clouding of the mesenteric fat ("dirty fat"), local fascial thickening, and ill-defined right lower quadrant soft tissue densities. Intravenous contrast agent–enhanced studies help to define the

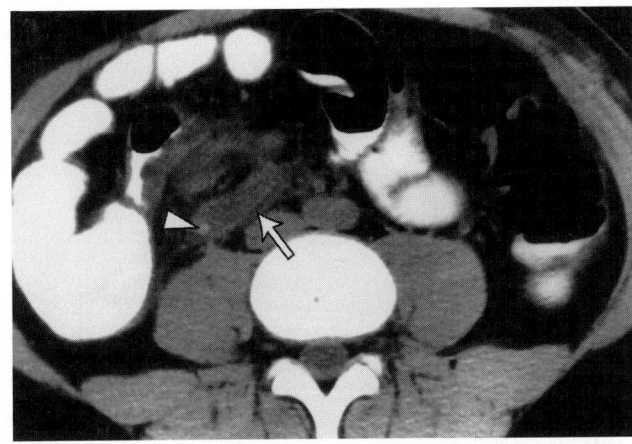

A

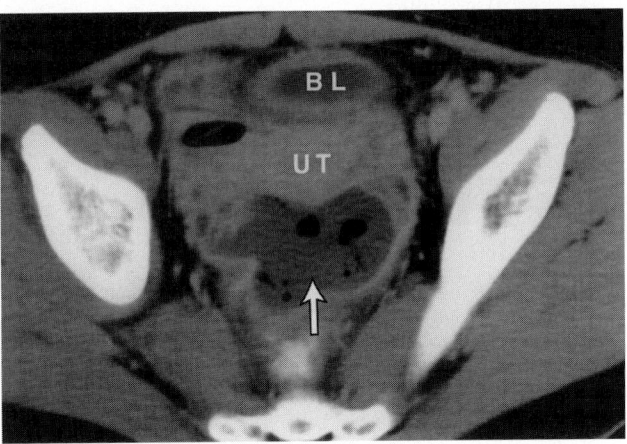

B

FIGURE 47-4. **A,** CT scan of the abdomen demonstrates an edematous, thickened appendix *(arrow)* with obstructing appendicolith *(arrowhead).* **B,** CT scan of abdomen demonstrates a perforated appendix with a complex abscess and pelvic fluid collection *(arrow).* BL, bladder; UT, uterus.

inflamed appendiceal and periappendiceal tissue. CT is especially useful in distinguishing those patients presenting late in their clinical course (48 to 72 hours) who may have developed a phlegmon or abscess, thus altering potential therapy (Fig. 47-4*B*).

The true sensitivity of CT in diagnosing acute appendicitis is unknown.[21,22] Retrospective studies, studies of consecutive patients, and studies with debatable inclusion criteria have made the application of CT to individual patients with a truly equivocal presentation (those who have undergone nondiagnostic ultrasonography, evaluation by an experienced surgeon, and a brief period of repetitive examination) problematic.[23] Use of CT has increased significantly since its introduction.[24] A reasonable estimate is that CT is 90% sensitive to the detection of intra-abdominal inflammation, with an 80% to 90% positive predictive value.

Our use of imaging studies, shown in Figure 47-5, is currently similar to that described by Wilson and associates.[24] CT is used in conjunction with repetitive examina-

tion and clinical observation in patients with equivocal findings, high-risk populations for false-positive examinations (negative appendectomies) and a high suspicion of late or complicated disease that may prompt treatment of percutaneous drainage and antibiotics. Using this approach, the frequency of negative explorations has been significantly reduced.[25,26]

NUCLEAR MEDICINE

Nuclear medicine studies can be used to evaluate patients with suspected appendicitis.[27] Two types of imaging studies have been used: radiolabeled white blood cells (Tc 99m WBC) and immunoglobulin G (Tc 99 IgG).[28,29] The studies take 1 to 3 hours to perform, not including white blood cell labeling time and incubation period after injection. These techniques rely on the localization of the leukocyte or IgG at the site of appendiceal inflammation; with the use of scintigraphy, the inflamed tissue is observed in the right lower quadrant. The sensitivity, specificity, and accuracy of these studies in populations similar to those studied to evaluate the usefulness of ultrasonography and CT scanning are not superior to the aforementioned imaging studies. Moreover, although noninvasive, the studies are not promptly available. The true potential value of these studies may be in patients with persistent symptoms and negative ultrasonography and CT studies. To date, the accuracy of these studies in these diagnostically challenging patients is unknown.

Laboratory

The majority of patients undergoing evaluation for acute abdominal pain have a complete blood count as a component of the evaluation. The leukocyte count is usually elevated to the range of 12,000 to 18,000 mm^3.[30] In addition, an increase in the percentage of neutrophils (the "left shift") with a normal total white blood cell count supports the clinical diagnosis of appendicitis. A completely normal leukocyte count and differential is uncommon in patients with appendicitis but can be seen. Other laboratory indices of inflammation have been studied as adjuncts to diagnosis of appendicitis. C-reactive protein has been studied and correlated with the clinical and pathologic findings.[31,32] In general, this is not a clinically useful laboratory study because it is nonspecific.

A urinalysis is often obtained in the evaluation of patients with abdominal pain to determine whether genitourinary tract inflammation is present. The urinalysis may show a mild pyuria with appendicitis owing to the proximity of the ureter to the inflamed appendix. The increased specific gravity of the urine adds to the clinical diagnosis of hypovolemia. Proteinuria can also be an adjunct to the diagnosis of spontaneous bacterial peritonitis as a complication of nephrotic syndrome in children evaluated for acute abdominal pain.

Diagnoses

Appendicitis should be considered in the differential diagnosis of almost all patients with abdominal pain, but there

DIAGNOSTIC EVALUATION FOR SUSPECTED APPENDICITIS

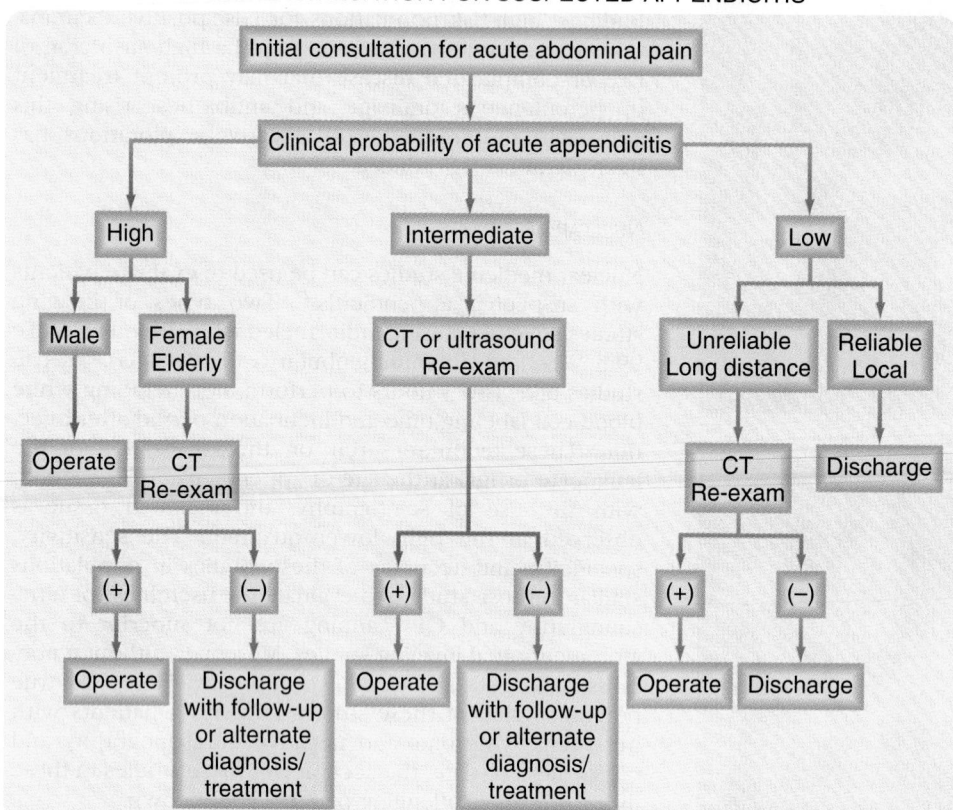

FIGURE 47-5. Algorithm for the evaluation and consultation for acute abdominal pain.

are other problems that are most frequently confused with appendicitis and should be excluded. The large majority of these problems can be excluded on the basis of a thorough history and physical examination and limited laboratory tests.

Diagnostic laparoscopy may be useful in some patients in whom the diagnosis cannot be ruled out. The most common patients that would be in this group are women between 15 and 45 years of age. Laparoscopy can be useful to rule out other disorders as well. There is some controversy about whether to remove a normal appearing appendix at laparoscopy. Although this can be achieved with low morbidity, some surgeons think that if the appendix is normal, it should be left in place.[33] There is no consensus on this in the literature, and we will routinely remove the appendix in these patients. However, with current diagnostic modalities, the need for laparoscopy for diagnosis is quite low. As with other causes of abdominal pain, it is important to consider the patient's age and sex because the differential diagnosis may be quite different.

DIFFERENTIAL DIAGNOSES

The differential diagnosis of appendicitis can incorporate almost all causes of abdominal pain. Cope's textbook on the diagnosis of the acute abdomen[33a] remains a classic reference for the myriad of conditions that can mimic appendicitis. There are, however, some common diagnoses that can be confused with appendicitis. These will vary some by gender and age.

Preschool Children. In the preschool child, the diagnoses to consider include intussusception, Meckel's diverticulitis, and acute gastroenteritis. Intussusception with colicky-type pain is more common in children younger than 3 years of age. The child may have a mass, but true peritonitis is not common. Meckel's diverticulitis is much less common than appendicitis. The pain may be similar but will localize to the periumbilical area. Diagnostic studies may show an inflammatory mass in the mid-abdomen. Although accurate preoperative diagnosis may be difficult, the surgical therapy is the same. Perhaps the most difficult diagnosis to differentiate is acute gastroenteritis.[34] Patients with gastroenteritis will have diarrhea and nausea. There are often leukocytes in the stool. Vomiting is frequent, but peritoneal signs are absent. Many young children with acute appendicitis have been initially diagnosed incorrectly as having gastroenteritis.

School-Age Children. Gastroenteritis remains a common differential diagnosis. Functional pain is common. These children may complain of abdominal pain, but supportive laboratory findings such as a leukocytosis or left shift are absent. True signs of peritonitis are also absent. Constipation can be a cause of significant abdominal pain in children. However, systemic findings such as fever and peritoneal irritation are absent. Clearly, to establish this diagnosis, there must be a history of infrequent stools and supportive findings on rectal examination. Appending a diagnosis of constipation or gastroenteritis implies the diagnostic criteria for these have been met. Otherwise, it is better to call the pain "undiagnosed" or "unclear." Omental infarction can also be seen in children, and the symptoms can mimic those of appendicitis.[35] These patients often have a palpable mass and the pain does not migrate.

Adolescent Boys and Young Adult Men. The differential diagnoses shift again. Diseases to be considered in this age patient include Crohn's disease (discussed elsewhere), ulcerative colitis, and epididymitis. Physical examination of the scrotum helps diagnose epididymitis: The patient has clear tenderness over the epididymis on examination.

Adolescent Girls and Young Adult Women. The differential diagnoses in young women are quite broad and encompass a number of gynecologic conditions. Despite this, an accurate diagnosis can be established in most patients. Pelvic inflammatory disease has a history of onset in the lower abdomen. The pain is usually bilateral and exacerbated on pelvic examination. Although the patients often have a fever and leukocytosis, a good history and examination usually establishes the diagnosis. Ovarian cysts are also common. The physical findings of a ruptured cyst or ovarian torsion can mimic appendicitis exactly. However, the history is one of acute onset in the right lower quadrant. There is no migration or changing symptoms. The absence of a clear-cut history and physical examination in this age woman should prompt other diagnostic studies. Urinary tract infections are also quite common in women of this age group. A good history and findings on urinalysis and examination differentiate the large majority of these patients.

Elderly Age Group. Appendicitis in the elderly can be difficult to diagnose preoperatively. The differential includes malignancies of the gastrointestinal tract and reproductive system. Other diagnoses to consider include diverticulitis, perforated ulcers, and cholecystitis. Malignancies are often seen on a CT scan. The history may be atypical for appendicitis, and symptoms are often more than a few hours in duration. Diverticulitis, especially right sided, can be extremely difficult to differentiate since both are right-sided inflammatory processes. Age and a previous history may help. The history for patients with a perforated ulcer is usually one of an acute onset and not a migratory pain. The pain is rarely in the right lower quadrant. Laboratory findings do not help differentiate many of these conditions, but a CT scan can be quite useful.

Types of Treatment

The treatment of appendicitis varies somewhat depending on the stage of the disease. In general, patients should receive fluid resuscitation before surgery. This may require only 1 or 2 hours in patients with nonperforated disease but may take substantially longer in patients with perforated appendicitis.

Acute

MEDICAL

Patients with acute, nonperforated appendicitis should undergo urgent appendectomy. There have been few studies examining the role of antibiotic therapy alone for appendicitis. Eriksson and Granstrom performed a randomized trial of antibiotic therapy versus surgical therapy for patients with appendicitis.[36] In a small number of patients, the initial success with medical therapy was 85%, but there was a recurrence rate of 35% with short follow-up. Antibiotics alone have been used in rare situations such as with sailors on long submarine tours.[37] Owing to the high recurrence rate, the current standard is operative treatment for acute appendicitis. There is a general consensus that prophylactic antibiotics should be administered before the start of the operation, but in acute disease, we use only a single dose.[38] There are a number of antibiotics that can be used as long as they provide activity against enteric anaerobic and gram-negative bacteria.[39] We use a single dose of cefoxitin or cefotetan for prophylaxis.

In the past, the incidence of removing a normal appendix was acceptable if it was 20%. However, much lower rates than this have been quoted.[6] An overall negative exploration rate of 20% should not be viewed as a gold standard with the availability of ultrasound- and CT-assisted diagnosis. The negative exploration rate in women is still higher than that in men owing to the confusion with diseases of the fallopian tubes and ovaries.

SURGICAL

There are two approaches to removal of the nonperforated appendix: One through an open incision, usually a transverse right lower quadrant skin incision (Davis-Rockey) or an oblique version (McArthur-McBurney) with separation of the muscles in the direction of their fibers, or a paramedian incision (not routinely done). The incision is centered on the midclavicular line (Fig. 47-6).

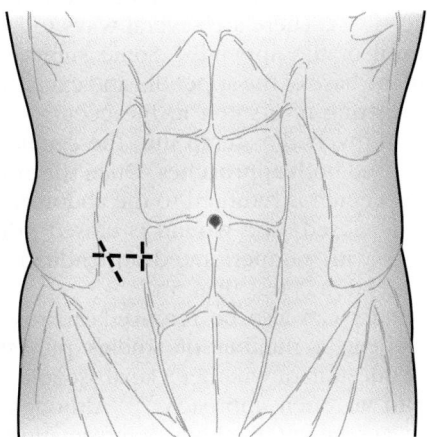

FIGURE 47-6. Location for the common incisions used for an appendectomy. (From Ortega JM, Ricardo AE: Surgery of the appendix and colon. *In* Moody FG [ed]: Atlas of Ambulatory Surgery. Philadelphia, WB Saunders, 1999.)

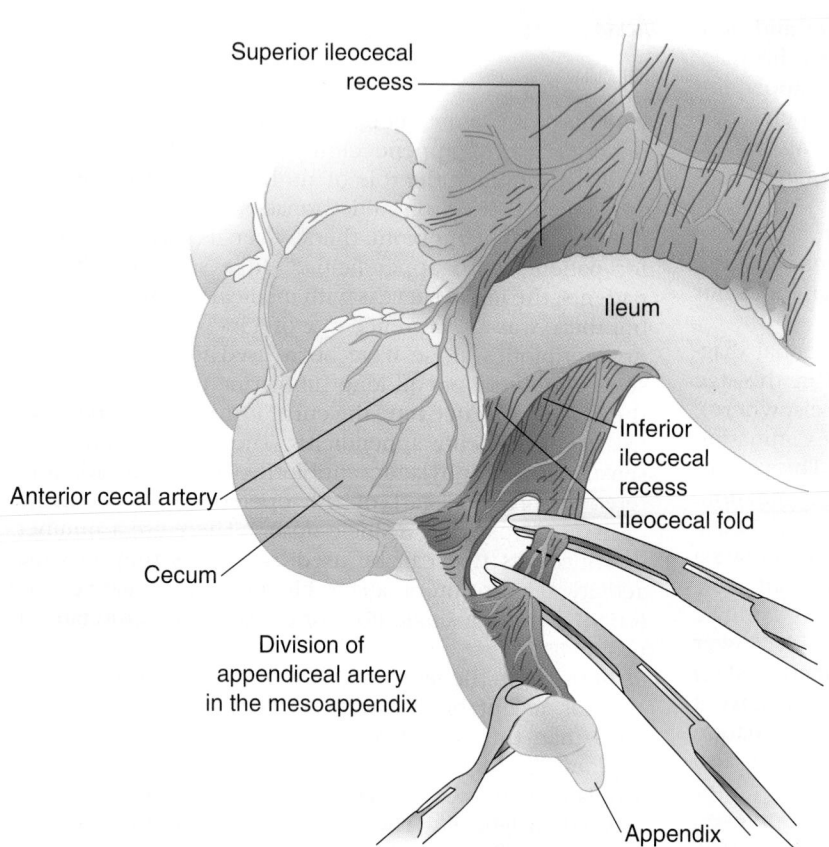

Superior ileocecal
recess

Ileum

Anterior cecal artery

Inferior
ileocecal
recess

Ileocecal fold

Cecum

Division of
appendiceal artery
in the mesoappendix

Appendix

FIGURE 47-7. Division of the mesoappendix during an open appendectomy. (From Ortega JM, Ricardo AE: Surgery of the appendix and colon. *In* Moody FG [ed]: Atlas of Ambulatory Surgery. Philadelphia, WB Saunders, 1999.)

Occasionally, where the diagnosis is uncertain, a periumbilical midline incision can be used. Once the peritoneum is entered, the appendix is delivered into the field. This can usually be accomplished with careful digital manipulation of the appendix and cecum. It is important to avoid too extensive of a blind dissection. In difficult cases, extending the incision 1 to 2 cm can greatly simplify the procedure. Once the appendix is delivered into the wound, the mesoappendix is sacrificed between clamps and ties (Fig. 47-7). There are several ways to handle the actual removal of the appendix. Some surgeons simply suture ligate the base of the appendix and excise it. Others place a pursestring or Z-stitch in the cecum, excise the appendix, and invert the stump into the cecum (Fig. 47-8). We have used both approaches. Once the appendix is removed, the cecum is returned to the abdomen, and the peritoneum is closed. The wound is closed primarily in most patients with nonperforated appendicitis because the risk of infection is less than 5%.

The appendix can also be removed laparoscopically. There have been a number of studies published that examine the question of whether a laparoscopic approach is superior to an open approach.[40,41] Although there is not universal agreement, the body of information suggests that in the adult, although operative costs are higher due to a longer procedure and more equipment needed with laparoscopy, the overall costs may be lower because the pain is less and patients can return to work sooner.[42] It is

more difficult to demonstrate these benefits in small children. Most authors report using three ports to remove the appendix: an umbilical port and two others. The location of the two other ports may vary depending on the surgeon and the patient's body habitus (Fig. 47-9). The appendix can be removed using endoloops or an endoscopic stapling device (Fig. 47-10). The total charges can vary significantly if disposable ports and a stapler are used. The appendiceal stump is not buried when it is removed laparoscopically, and the appendix is removed through one of the port sites (Fig. 47-11). The fascia at the 10-mm port sites is usually closed, as is the skin. Many patients can be discharged within 24 hours of operation.

Perforated Appendicitis

The management of perforated or gangrenous appendicitis varies somewhat from that of acute nonperforated disease. In these patients, the appendix has already perforated, so the need for urgent intervention is less obvious. Patients with perforated appendicitis will often have a longer duration of symptoms, high fever, and a higher white blood cell count. Most of these patients are volume depleted and require several hours or more of fluid resuscitation before operative intervention. It is important to ensure that the patient has been adequately resuscitated before undertaking an operation. Patients with perforated disease have established peritonitis and

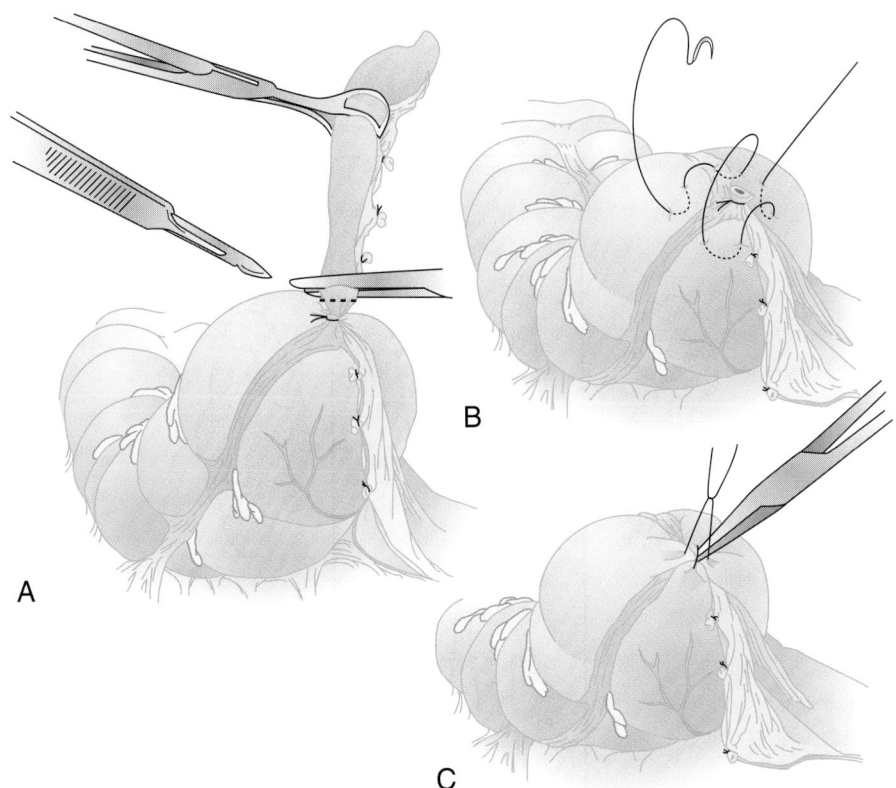

FIGURE 47-8. Steps in an open appendectomy. **A,** The appendix is divided after ligation. **B,** A Z- or pursestring stitch is placed in the cecum. **C,** Inversion of the appendiceal stump. (**A** to **C,** From Ortega JM, Ricardo AE: Surgery of the appendix and colon. *In* Moody FG [ed]: Atlas of Ambulatory Surgery. Philadelphia, WB Saunders, 1999.)

should receive appropriate broad-spectrum intravenous antibiotic therapy targeted against gram-negative aerobes and anaerobes, which should start as soon as the diagnosis is established. The duration of therapy is controversial. Some authors recommend an empiric time of treatment such as 7 or 10 days. Others suggest treatment until the patient is afebrile with a normal white blood cell count.[43]

Some studies in adults and children have now shown that early operative intervention in cases of perforated appendicitis may be associated with more postoperative complications compared to antibiotic therapy followed by interval appendectomy.[44] Experience has shown that patients with perforated appendicitis and evidence of an associated small bowel obstruction may be prone to failure of this approach, but others suggest it is a better approach.[43,45] Our approach to perforated/complicated appendicitis is outlined in Figure 47-12.

If an operative approach is planned, there are two possible approaches: an open laparotomy or laparoscopy. There is some controversy about the use of laparoscopy in patients with advanced disease because the incidence of postoperative intra-abdominal abscess formation in some series has been markedly higher with laparoscopy than with an open approach.[46,47]

Late Presentation With or Without a Mass

Two to 5% of patients with appendicitis present with a palpable right lower quadrant mass.[48] This can represent either a discrete abscess or phlegmon. The management of these patients has been controversial. Historically, this has been fueled by equivocal imaging studies that could not reliably corroborate the physical findings and an inability to reliably drain an abscess percutaneously. There also has been a bias toward early removal of the perforated appendix/appendiceal abscess to "control intra-abdominal sepsis." The preferred approach to the management of the appendiceal mass is percutaneous drainage, which is performed under image guidance (ultrasound or CT) and intravenous antibiotics directed against aerobic gram-negative and anaerobic organisms.[38] Numerous studies have documented the safety and efficacy of this approach.[49,50] In late, complicated appendicitis, appendectomy can be a hazardous procedure. Surgery at this stage can serve to disseminate a localized inflammatory process; to injure surrounding inflamed or edematous bowel, resulting in fistulas; or to require more extensive procedures, such as cecectomy or right hemicolectomy.

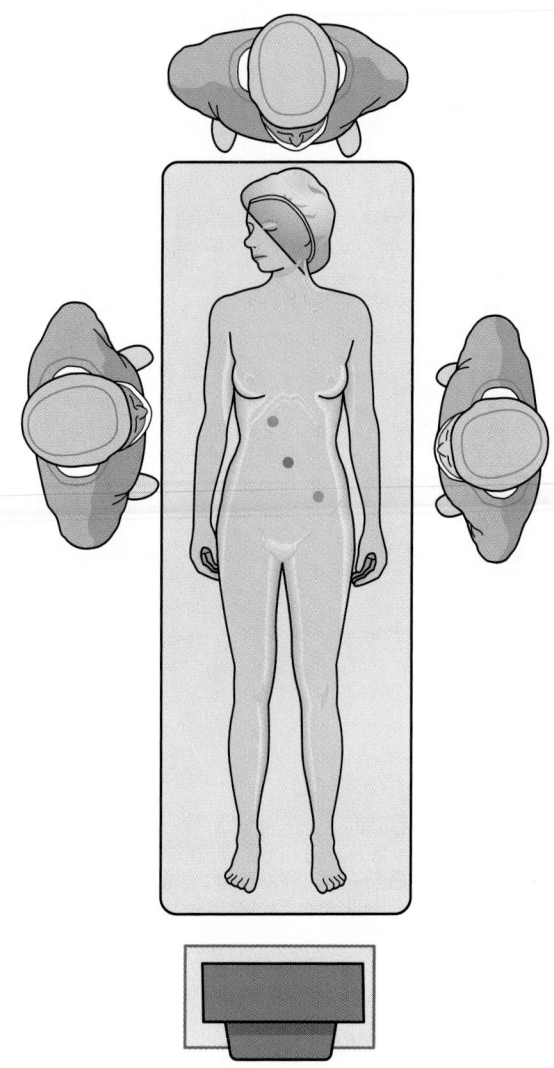

- 5-mm camera port
- 5-mm instrument port
- 12-mm umbilical port

FIGURE 47-9.   Location of the port sites for laparoscopic appendectomy. (From Ortega JM, Ricardo AE: Surgery of the appendix and colon. *In* Moody FG [ed]: Atlas of Ambulatory Surgery. Philadelphia, WB Saunders, 1999.)

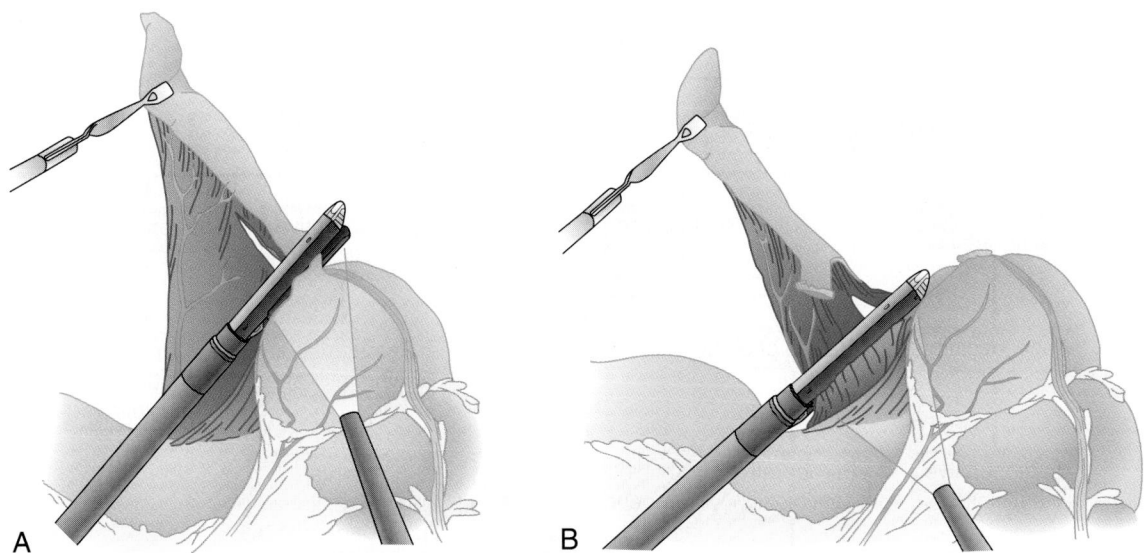

FIGURE 47-10.   **A,** Division of the appendix using an endostapler. **B,** Division of the mesoappendix with an endostapler (sometimes both can be divided at the same time). (**A** and **B,** From Ortega JM, Ricardo AE: Surgery of the appendix and colon. *In* Moody FG [ed]: Atlas of Ambulatory Surgery. Philadelphia, WB Saunders, 1999.)

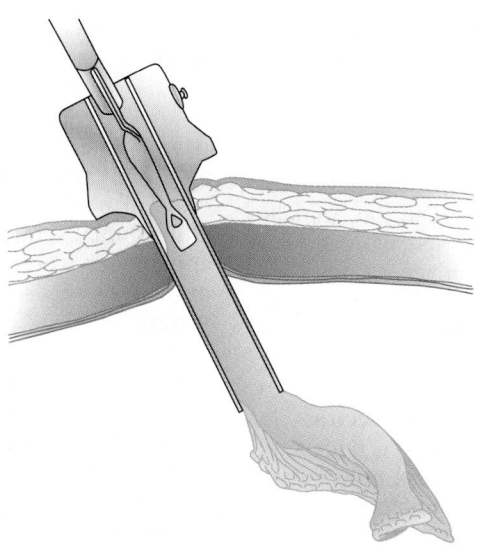

FIGURE 47-11.   Removal of the appendix through one of the ports. (From Ortega JM, Ricardo AE: Surgery of the appendix and colon. *In* Moody FG [ed]: Atlas of Ambulatory Surgery. Philadelphia, WB Saunders, 1999.)

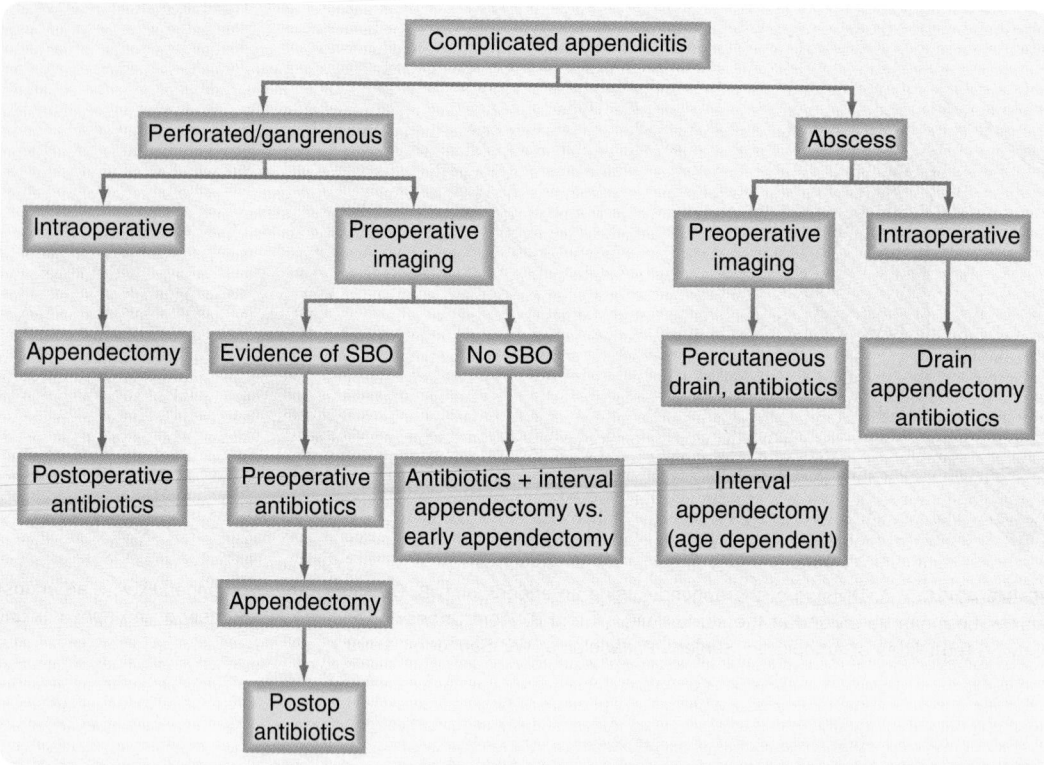

FIGURE 47-12. Algorithm for the management of complicated appendicitis. Complicated appendicitis antibiotic management protocol includes gentamicin 7 mg/kg body weight IV every 24 hours and metronidazole 500 mg IV every 6 hours (adult dose); Administer first doses 1 hour preoperatively and continue until white blood cell count and differential are normal and the patient is afebrile for 24 hours. If there is minimal to no clinical response in 72 hours after initiating treatment, then consider changing antibiotics to imipenem. Complicated appendicitis wound management protocol includes leaving the wound open with consideration of delayed primary closure on postoperative day 3 to 5. SBO, small bowel obstruction.

Interval Appendectomy

There is general consensus that a localized appendiceal abscess from perforated appendicitis can be initially managed with CT-guided percutaneous drainage or limited surgical drainage. When the drainage is combined with adequate antibiotic and fluid administration, most patients will respond to this conservative management and can be discharged without fever or abdominal pain. Controversy exists, however, as to whether interval appendectomy (performing an elective appendectomy in the "interval" between bouts of appendicitis) is necessary to prevent recurrent bouts of appendicitis. In one study that compared early with delayed appendectomy after appendiceal mass formation, 15% of the patients in the delayed group had a recurrent acute episode during the waiting period. The authors concluded that despite a slightly higher incidence of wound infection in the early appendectomy group, it appeared safe and cost effective to remove the appendix early rather than waiting 6 to 10 weeks.[51]

A review of the histopathology in patients who underwent interval appendectomy revealed one patient with appendiceal duplication, three patients with granulomatous appendicitis, and two with persistent acute appendicitis. All appendices at interval appendectomy had patent lumens, and 15 of 17 were patent to the tip. Several authors support the role of interval appendectomy in cases of perforated appendicitis treated conservatively.[52] Others might interpret this study to suggest that the appendices were mostly normal and that appendectomy only for persistent or recurrent disease might be warranted.

In one long-term follow-up of patients with an appendiceal mass treated nonoperatively, only 1 of 10 patients required appendectomy. The rest remained asymptomatic with their appendix intact.[36] The risk of recurrent appendicitis must be balanced against the risk of interval appendectomy. In general, the younger the patient, the higher the lifetime risk of recurrent appendicitis and the lower the operative risk. Although many pediatric surgeons (including ourselves) perform interval appendectomy routinely at 8 to 12 weeks in children, the risk in patients older than 30 to 40 years of age probably would not support this policy.

Chronic or Recurrent Type of Appendicitis

The occurrence of chronic or recurrent appendicitis is controversial, and although rare, its existence is plausible. Intermittent bouts of obstruction of the appendiceal

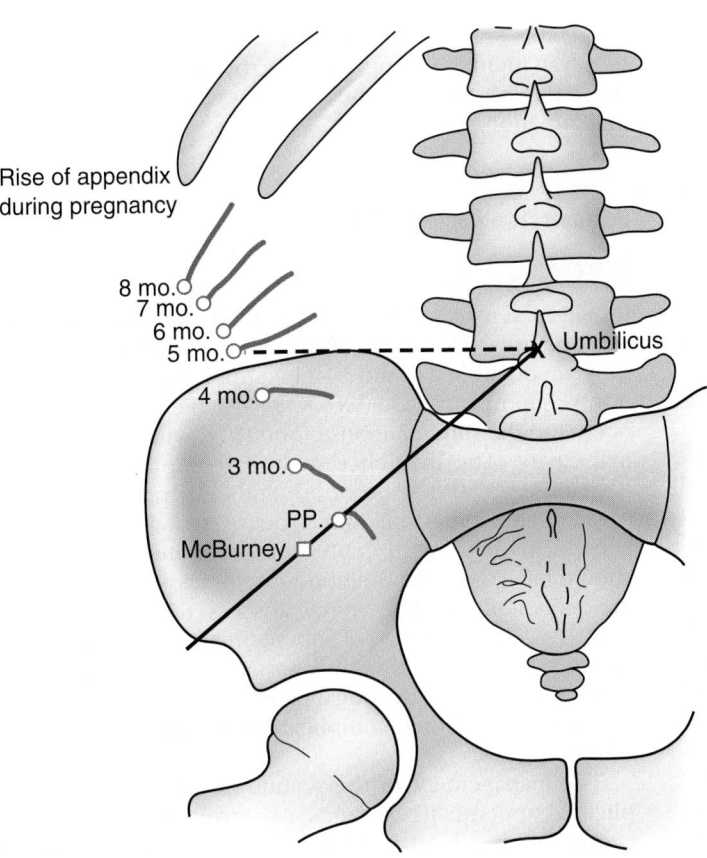

Rise of appendix
during pregnancy

8 mo.
7 mo.
6 mo.
5 mo.
4 mo.
3 mo.
PP.
McBurney

Umbilicus

FIGURE 47-13.   Changes in the location of the appendix during pregnancy. PP, postpartum. (From Baer JL, Reis RA, Arens RA: Appendicitis in pregnancy. JAMA 98:1359, 1932.)

lumen with spontaneous remission may be the cause. Mild local inflammation after a resolving attack of acute appendicitis may result in chronic right lower quadrant discomfort.

The CT appearance of the appendix in patients with recurrent or chronic appendicitis reportedly demonstrates findings similar to acute appendicitis.[53] Patients undergoing appendectomy for chronic lower abdominal pain frequently demonstrate abnormal histology of the appendix and are relieved of their symptoms. In one report, 92% of the removed appendices revealed histologic abnormalities, and 95% of these patients were completely cured.[54]

Appendiceal colic has been reported in children secondary to partial luminal obstruction of the appendix without inflammation.[55] The diagnosis was made if the following three criteria were met: a history of longer than 1 month with three or more recurrent attacks of right lower quadrant abdominal pain; localized tenderness in the right lower abdomen without signs of peritoneal irritation or inflammation; or radiologic findings at barium examination consisting of irregular filling of the appendix, nonfilling or partial filling of the appendix after 24 hours, or nonemptying of the appendix after 72 hours. Twenty-six children diagnosed by the criteria above underwent appendectomy and of these, 23 (88.5%) experienced pain relief in the immediate postoperative period. The remaining three children had pain relief within 4 months after appendectomy.

Appendicitis During Pregnancy

Appendicitis and cholecystitis are the most frequent causes of abdominal pain during pregnancy. Abdominal tenderness is the most important finding in appendicitis, but the location of point tenderness varies during gestation. After the 5th month of gestation, the appendiceal position is shifted superiorly above the iliac crest, and the appendix tip is rotated medially by the gravid uterus (Fig. 47-13). The white blood cell count may not be helpful because it is frequently elevated during pregnancy. Common symptoms such as nausea, vomiting, or anorexia are also common during pregnancy and thus of limited diagnostic value. Ultrasound may be of help if a thickened or dilated appendix is identified.

Suspicion of appendicitis should lead to early surgical intervention in all trimesters. Negative laparotomy results in minimal fetal loss,[56] whereas a delay in diagnosis and perforation may result in a high incidence of fetal death and a relatively high incidence of maternal death.[57] A laparoscopic approach has been used and does not appear to increase maternal or fetal morbidity or mortality rates.

Occasionally, patients will have had a walled-off gangrenous or ruptured appendix that presents with acute abdominal pain immediately after delivery. The contraction and return toward normal size of the uterus may disrupt the walling-off process and lead to a generalized peritonitis.

Special Considerations

INTRAOPERATIVE MANAGEMENT OF THE NONINFLAMED APPENDIX

Despite competent clinical evaluation, including laboratory and imaging studies, abdominal exploration may reveal a noninflamed appendix. Typically, the exploration is accomplished via a right lower quadrant incision, laparoscopy, or occasionally a midline incision. In cases of a normal appendix without succus entericus or purulent peritoneal fluid, there is a low probability of an occult surgical disease process. At that point, a standard evaluation includes inspection of the terminal ileum and ascending colon for evidence of inflammatory bowel disease or mesenteric adenitis and more proximally for the presence of Meckel's diverticulitis. The gallbladder may be palpated and/or visualized in thin patients, and ovarian inspection can be accomplished in women. Occasionally, sigmoid diverticulitis can be palpated and/or visualized as well. In children with turbid abdominal fluid and no anatomically identifiable lesion, the fluid should undergo Gram's stain and culture to evaluate specifically for diplococci. Primary peritonitis complicating nephrotic syndrome may present in this manner. Pancreatitis, occult abdominal trauma with a perforated hollow viscus, or perforated peptic ulcer may occasionally mimic appendicitis, and each case is usually associated with abnormal peritoneal fluid. The omentum should be evaluated for infarction or torsion. These diagnoses often require closure of the right lower quadrant incision and a new vertical midline incision to adequately diagnose and treat these problems. There is an advantage in these patients to a laparoscopic exploration.

As mentioned previously, management of the normal-appearing appendix at exploration once other problems have been ruled out is controversial. Many surgeons are of the opinion that the appendix should be removed since the complication rate is quite low in this setting. We routinely remove the appendix in this setting unless the procedure would prove difficult. Other disease processes found should be managed appropriately and are discussed in the appropriate chapters.

CROHN'S DISEASE

Patients who undergo exploration for presumed appendicitis and have evidence of Crohn's disease should undergo appendectomy. Although there is theoretical concern for the development of an enterocutaneous fistula, this is extremely rare. Moreover, appendectomy prevents future diagnostic confusion.

Appendectomy in those patients with significant cecal inflammation can be difficult and if the appendix appears normal, good judgment would support leaving the appendix in place. There are some reports of an increased risk of Crohn's disease in patients who had an appendectomy for appendicitis.[58]

MECKEL'S DIVERTICULUM

Exploration may reveal an incidental finding of a Meckel's diverticulum. In most cases, we do not think that removal is warranted. Circumstances that would require removal include young age, narrow neck diverticulum, presence of gastric mucosa, or evidence of previous inflammation.

Postoperative Complications

Infection

Infection remains the most common complication after the operative treatment of appendicitis. Although infection can occur in a number of locations, surgical site infection predominates. The two sites at which infections can occur are the subcutaneous wound and within the abdominal cavity. The incidence of both complications varies depending on the stage of appendicitis, patient age and physiologic condition, and type of wound closure. In general, patients with acute, nonperforated appendicitis should have a wound infection rate of less than 5% and an incidence of intra-abdominal abscess formation of less than 1%.[6] The incidence of subcutaneous wound infection appears to be lower with laparoscopic appendectomy. Our approach to evaluating a patient with a potential postoperative infectious complication is shown in Figure 47-14.

The management of the wound in patients with complicated appendicitis remains a controversial issue. Some centers with a high incidence of advanced appendicitis favor a delayed primary wound closure. Other studies have shown no increased risk for wound infection when a subcuticular wound closure is performed with the proper use of antibiotics.[59] One literature review that examined cost-utility found a significant cost saving with primary closure compared with delayed primary closure or secondary closure.[60] Care must be taken in evaluating these studies. The expected incidence in children should be lower than that in adults, and many studies do not stratify the patients by risk. It appears reasonable that in low-risk patients with complicated appendicitis, primary wound closure can be performed.

The incidence of wound infection and intra-abdominal sepsis in patients with complicated appendicitis is higher than that in patients with nonperforated appendicitis. There have been several reports of a much higher incidence of abscess formation in patients with complicated appendicitis who have undergone laparoscopic appendectomy. The mechanism is unclear at this time, and other studies argue against this. The treatment of intra-abdominal abscess is usually percutaneous drainage and intravenous antibiotics with good results.

Bowel Obstruction

Intestinal obstruction can occur after laparotomy for appendicitis. The true long-term incidence is unknown, but it is likely similar to the risk of patients undergoing laparotomy for other reasons. The incidence in one large series was approximately 1% and 1.3% in another, with most patients presenting in the first 6 months after operation.[6,61]

MANAGEMENT OF POST-OPERATIVE INFECTIOUS COMPLICATIONS OF APPENDICITIS

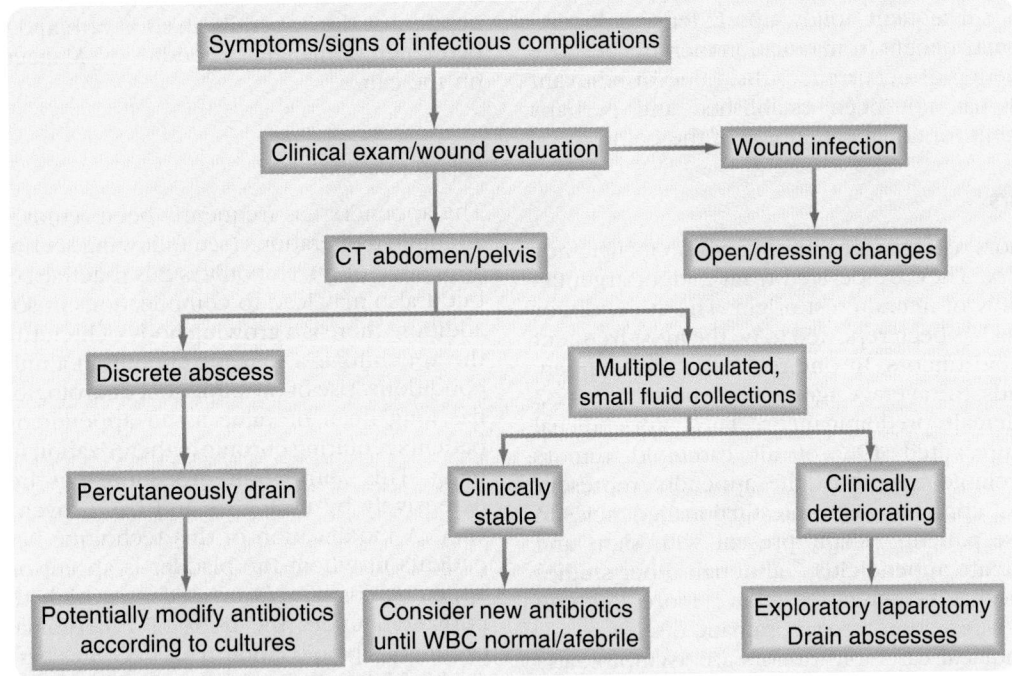

FIGURE 47-14.   Management of postoperative infectious complications of appendicitis. WBC, white blood cell count.

Infertility

The risk of tubal infertility in female patients after appendicitis is unclear.[62,63] In one large study, there was no increased risk of infertility in patients with nonperforated appendicitis but a severalfold increase in infertility in patients with perforated appendicitis.[64] However, another study by Puri and colleagues[65] showed no difference in either group. Regardless, the risk appears to be sufficiently low that patients who have had appendicitis do not require routine evaluations unless there is a proven problem with fertility.

Miscellaneous

As with any operation, a number of other problems may occur. Urinary tract infections, pneumonia, and other complications of hospitalization can occur in patients with appendicitis. Elderly patients have a higher rate of complications.[66] Occasionally, a patient may develop a fecal fistula after operation. This almost always occurs in patients with perforated appendicitis. The majority will close, but in a few patients, surgical closure may be required.

NEOPLASMS

Adenocarcinoma

Appendiceal neoplasms are extremely rare and are infrequently diagnosed preoperatively.[67] Carcinoids are the most common appendiceal neoplasm. Adenocarcinoma of the appendix constitutes less than 0.5% of all gastrointestinal neoplasms. In one review of 94 patients with primary adenocarcinoma of the appendix, 52 (55%) had the mucinous variety, of whom 22 had pseudomyxoma peritonei; the other 45% had the colonic and adenocarcinoid types of tumor. The most common presentation was that of acute appendicitis, and no patient had the diagnosis made preoperatively. The 5-year survival rate for appendiceal carcinoma is 55% and varies with the stage of the tumor. Patients with the mucinous type have a better prognosis than do those with the colonic type. The survival rate is superior after right hemicolectomy versus appendectomy alone (58% vs. 20%). A second primary malignancy occurred in 33 patients (35%), of which 17 were located in the gastrointestinal tract.[68]

In general, mucinous carcinoma or adenocarcinoma of the appendix is seen in older patients thought to have acute appendicitis. Occasionally, the diagnosis is recognized intraoperatively but frequently not until the specimen is reviewed histologically. Right hemicolectomy is indicated for (1) invasive adenocarcinoma, (2) tumors close to the cecum, (3) mucin-producing tumors, (4) invasion of lymphatics, serosa, or mesoappendix, and (5) cellular pleomorphism with a high mitotic rate. Adenocarcinoid tumors of the appendix presenting as a unilateral or bilateral Krukenberg tumor have been reported, and appendectomy is recommended in all patients with Krukenberg tumors when another primary site cannot be identified at the time of surgery.

In summary, these rare tumors generally present as acute appendicitis in older patients. Treatment either primarily or at re-exploration generally requires right hemicolectomy. Synchronous or metachronous secondary tumors are frequent and should be looked for at exploration and in subsequent follow-up. Extensive locoregional disease may benefit from radiation therapy. Because of the infrequency of occurrence, the value of adjuvant chemotherapy has not been established and perhaps mimics treatment for adenocarcinoma of the colon.

Carcinoid Tumors

Carcinoid tumors represent the most common malignancy of the appendix. They are derived from midgut argentaffin cells, possibly of neural crest origin. The appendix or the small bowel has been reported to be the most frequent site for carcinoid tumors. In one review of 1570 appendiceal carcinoids, the average age at presentation was 42.2 years, with a female predominance.[69] These appendiceal carcinoids represented 19% of all carcinoid tumors reviewed. Carcinoid tumors of the appendix represent one of the most common gastrointestinal malignancies in children. These patients usually present with signs and symptoms of acute appendicitis,[70] although other studies have suggested that incidental resection is more common in children than resection for symptomatic disease.

Most appendiceal carcinoid tumors are asymptomatic or found incidentally and are less than 1 cm. Simple appendectomy is adequate treatment. Treatment for tumors between 1 and 2 cm is decided best by location. If the tumor is located at the base of the appendix or invading the mesentery, a right hemicolectomy is recommended. If the tumor can be resected by appendectomy alone, this should be adequate therapy because distant metastases are rare for tumors less than 1.5 to 2 cm. Lesions greater than 2 cm have a higher incidence of distant metastases and should be treated by right hemicolectomy with the hope of decreasing locoregional recurrence.[71] At the time of diagnosis, 35% are nonlocalized. The current overall 5-year survival rate is 94% for localized lesions, 85% for regional invasion, and 34% for distant metastases. Almost 15% of patients have synchronous noncarcinoid tumors at other sites as well.

Sporadic cases of distant metastases from small appendiceal carcinoids have been reported but are extremely rare. The goblet cell carcinoid variant has been reported to be more aggressive, with a higher incidence of peritoneal spread and an increased morbidity rate. More aggressive surgery and multimodal therapy have been recommended, although the value of this recommendation has not been confirmed.

MISCELLANEOUS CONDITIONS

Intussusception

Intussusception of the appendix or appendiceal stump after appendectomy is a rare condition that is difficult to diagnose because symptoms are nonspecific and findings are limited.[72] Intussusception of the appendiceal stump after inversion appendectomy usually presents within 2 weeks after appendectomy. Abdominal pain, vomiting,

blood per rectum, or a palpable mass may be found. Diagnosis can be made with barium enema or CT. Intussusception of the appendix itself is rare and may be caused by benign or malignant conditions. Management depends on the cause.

Appendicostomy

The appendix has frequently been removed during other abdominal operations (see following section on incidental appendectomy). Not only is this practice seldom indicated but it also may lead to complications in some patients. In addition, there is a growing body of literature showing that the appendix is a valuable conduit in a number of clinical conditions. Use of the appendix in urologic reconstruction has long been of value as an appendicovesicostomy in patients requiring chronic catheterization for bladder emptying. This Mitrofanoff procedure has been used fairly extensively by urologists and has proven long-term efficacy. A modification of this technique has been used in patients in whom the bladder is absent or too small. An appendicolostomy is created by which the appendix is implanted under the tenia of a detubularized patch of cecum or sigmoid colon. This becomes part of a continent neobladder or is attached to the bladder itself.

It has been recognized that the appendix can be an excellent conduit in the construction of a hepatoportoappendicostomy. A vascularized appendix can be interposed between the biliary tree and the duodenum after resection of a choledochal cyst. Early experience with this technique has demonstrated excellent bile flow and no episodes of ascending cholangitis. Use of the appendix as a tube conduit for decompression after colon surgery or for the chronic administration of medications or enema has also been reported with good functional characteristics.[72,73]

Incidental Appendectomy

The practice of incidental appendectomy is controversial and, even if safe, probably unnecessary in most patients. Selective incidental appendectomy in patients at high risk for appendicitis or right lower quadrant pain may have a role.

Incidental appendectomy during hysterectomy or cholecystectomy has not resulted in increased complications but probably is not cost effective if there is an increased surgical charge.[74] Because most cases of appendicitis occur in younger patients and most incidental appendectomies are performed in older patients, routine incidental appendectomy may not lead to a significant reduction in hospitalization for appendicitis.

Although incidental appendectomy is contraindicated in certain conditions, the selective use in young patients (i.e., 10 to 30 years) in good health, but at risk for appendicitis, may be of benefit and cost effective.[75] Young female patients who have recurrent pelvic pathology or pain may benefit from incidental appendectomy. We have frequently performed incidental appendectomy when a right lower quadrant incision has been used for operations such as the reduction of an intussusception. This is generally thought to decrease confusion if right lower quadrant pain occurs at some future time. No clinical trials to support this approach have been conducted. Incidental appendectomy during certain procedures such as retroperitoneal lymphadenectomy for testis cancer or vascular grafts may be associated with higher infectious complications and should be avoided. In one study of 455 incidental appendectomies performed on 1910 children undergoing nephrectomy for Wilms' tumor, there was no increase in infectious complications or postoperative intestinal obstructions in the group undergoing incidental appendectomy.[76] Only 3 of the 1455 children who did not have an incidental appendectomy had appendicitis at 2, 7, and 10 months after nephrectomy. Other indications for incidental appendectomy may include acute or chronic right lower quadrant pain where a normal appendix is found at exploration. In addition, patients found to have Crohn's disease at exploration for right lower quadrant abdominal pain and tenderness generally undergo appendectomy to prevent future diagnostic dilemmas.

Selected References

Altemeier WA: The bacterial flora of acute perforated appendicitis with peritonitis. Ann Surg 107:517-528, 1938.

> This is a classic article on the bacteriology of appendicitis. The author studied the bacterial flora in patients with perforated appendicitis over a 2.5-year period. He showed clearly that most patients had multiple bacteria present. He also highlighted the extremely high incidence of anaerobic bacteria in this setting. This study changed the thinking about peritonitis and the bacteriology from one of single organisms to multiple bacteria and helped propel the field of surgical bacteriology.

Garbutt JM, Soper NJ, Shannon WD, et al: Meta-analysis of randomized controlled trials comparing laparoscopic and open appendectomy. Surg Laparosc Endosc 9:17-26, 1999.

> This paper is a good summary of the randomized trials that have been performed comparing laparoscopic to open appendectomy.

Helmer KS, Robinson EK, Lally KP, et al: Standardized patient care guidelines reduce infectious morbidity in appendectomy patients. Am J Surg 183:608-616, 2002.

> This study shows a clear benefit to following a standardized protocol in the management of appendicitis. The antibiotics used may vary, but the important part is to establish a standard, hospital-wide approach.

Mazuski JE, Sawyer RE, Nathens AB, et al: The Surgical Infection Society Guidelines on Antimicrobial Therapy for Intra-Abdominal Infections: An Executive Summary. Surg Infect 3:161-233, 2002.

> This is an excellent discussion of different antibiotics and their appropriate uses. The report outlines indications for both short and prolonged courses of therapy. Also presented are a number of the age-available and potential combinations. Recommended agents for different clinical situations are given. These recommendations represent the consensus of the Surgical Infection Society.

Sandor A, Modlin IM: A retrospective analysis of 1570 appendiceal carcinoids. Am J Gastroenterol 93:422-428, 1998.

> A review of 1570 appendiceal carcinoid tumors demonstrated that this cohort composed 18.9% of all carcinoid tumors and exhibited a marked female predominance. Appendiceal carcinoids presented earlier than other gastrointestinal carcinoids. At the time of diagnosis, 35.4% were nonlocalized. The overall 5-year survival rate was 94% for localized lesions, 84.6% for regional invasion, and 33.7% for distant metastases. The 5-year survival rate for appendiceal carcinoids (85.9%) was the highest among all types of carcinoid tumors.

Silen W: Cope's Early Diagnosis of the Acute Abdomen, 20th ed. New York, Oxford University Press, 2000.

> This is the classic reference for the diagnosis of the acute abdomen. The book is short and easy to read, and reading this book should be part of most clinicians' training.

References

1. Skandalakis JE, Gray SW, Ricketts R: The colon and rectum. *In* Skandalakis JE, Gray SW (eds): Embryology for Surgeons. Baltimore, Williams & Wilkins, 1994, pp 242-281.
2. Fitz RH: Perforating inflammation of the vermiform appendix: With special reference to its early diagnosis and treatment. Trans Assoc Am Phys 1:107-143, 1886.
3. McBurney C: Experience with early operative interference in cases of disease of the vermiform appendix. N Y State Med J 50:676-684, 1889.
4. Murphy JB: Appendicitis with original report histories and analysis of one hundred and forty-one laparotomies for that disease under personal observation. JAMA 22:302-304, 1894.
5. Blomqvist PG, Andersson REB, Granath F, et al: Mortality after appendectomy in Sweden, 1987-1996. Ann Surg 233:455-460, 2001.
6. Hale DA, Molloy M, Pearl RH, et al: Appendectomy: A contemporary appraisal. Ann Surg 225:252-261, 1997.
7. Baron EJ, Bennion R, Thompson J, et al: A microbiological comparison between acute and complicated appendicitis. Clin Infect Dis 14:227-231, 1992.
8. Bennion RS, Baron EJ, Thompson JE, et al: The bacteriology of gangrenous and perforated appendicitis revisited. Ann Surg 211:165-171, 1980.
9. Altemeier WA: The bacterial flora of acute perforated appendicitis with peritonitis. Ann Surg 107:517-528, 1938.
10. Bilik R, Burnweit C, Shandling B: Is abdominal cavity culture of any value in appendicitis? Am J Surg 175:267-270, 1998.
11. Dunning PG, Goldman MD: The incidence and value of rectal examination in children with suspected appendicitis. Ann R Coll Surg Engl 73:233-234, 1991.
12. Shaffer HA, Harrison RB: Gas in the appendix: A sometimes significant but nonspecific diagnostic sign. Arch Surg 114:587-589, 1979.
13. Chen SC, Chem KM, Wong SM, et al: Abdominal sonography screening of clinically diagnosed suspected appendicitis before surgery. World J Surg 22:449-452, 1998.
14. Puylaert JBCM: Acute appendicitis: US evaluation using graded compression. Radiology 158:355-360, 1986.
15. Puig S, Hormann M, Rebhandl W, et al: US as a primary diagnostic tool in relation to negative appendectomy: Six years' experience. Radiology 226:101-104, 2003.

16. Jeffrey RB, Fainig FC, Townsend RC: Acute appendicitis: Sonographic criteria based on 250 cases. Radiology 163:11-14, 1987.

17. Fuchs JR, Schlamberg JS, Shortsleeve MJ, et al: Impact of abdominal CT imaging on the management of appendicitis: An update. J Surg Res 106:131-136, 2002.

18. Rao PM, Rhea JT, Rattner DW, et al: Introduction of appendiceal CT: Impact on negative appendectomy and appendiceal perforation rates. Am J Surg 229:344-349, 1999.

19. Rao PM, Rhea JT, Novelline RA, et al: Helical computed tomography combined with contrast material administered only through the colon for imaging of suspected appendicitis. AJR Am J Roentgenol 169:1275-1280, 1997.

20. Urban BA, Fishman EK: Targeted helical CT of the acute abdomen: Appendicitis, diverticulitis, and small bowel obstruction. Semin Ultrasound CT MR 21:20-39, 2000.

21. Balthazar EJ, Rofsky NM, Zucker R: Appendicitis: The impact of computed tomography imaging on negative appendectomy and perforation rates. Am J Gastroenterol 93:768-771, 1998.

22. Weyrant MJ, Eachempati SR, Maluccio MN, et al: The use of computed tomography for the diagnosis of acute appendicitis in children does not influence the overall rate of negative appendectomy or perforation. Surg Infect 2:19-23, 2001.

23. Raptopoulos V, Katsou G, Rosen MP, et al: Acute appendicitis: Effect of increased use of CT on selecting patients earlier. Radiology 226:521-526, 2003.

24. Wilson EB, Cole JC, Nipper ML, et al: Computed tomography and ultrasonography in the diagnosis of appendicitis. Arch Surg 136:670-675, 2001.

25. Bendeck SE, Nino-Murcia M, Berry GJ, et al: Imaging for suspected appendicitis: Negative appendectomy and perforation rates. Radiology 225:131-136, 2002.

26. Naoum JJ, Mileski WJ, Daller JA, et al: The use of abdominal computed tomography scan decreases the frequency of misdiagnosis in cases of suspected appendicitis. Am J Surg 184:587-590, 2002.

27. Kipper SL, Rypins EB, Evans DG, et al: Neutrophil-specific ^{99m}Tc-labeled anti-CD15 monoclonal antibody imaging for diagnosis of equivocal appendicitis. J Nucl Med 41:449-455, 2000.

28. Typins EB, Kipper SL: ^{99m}Tc-hexamethylpropyleneaurine scan for diagnosing acute appendicitis in children. Ann Surg 63:878-881, 1997.

29. Wong DW, Vasinrapec P, Spieth ME, et al: Rapid detection of acute appendicitis with ^{99m}Tc-labeled intact polyvalent human immune globulin. J Am Coll Surg 185:534-543, 1997.

30. Bongard F, Landers DV, Lewis F: Differential diagnosis of appendicitis and pelvic inflammatory disease: A prospective analysis. Am J Surg 150:90-96, 1985.

31. Albu E, Miller BM, Choi Y, et al: Diagnostic value of C-reactive protein in acute appendicitis. Dis Colon Rectum 37:49-51, 1994.

32. Eriksson S, Granstron L, Olander B, et al: Sensitivity of interleukin-6 and C-reactive protein concentrations in the diagnosis of acute appendicitis. Eur J Surg 161:41-45, 1995.

33. van den Broek WT, Bijnen AB, de Ruiter P, et al: A normal appendix found during diagnostic laparoscopy should not be removed. Br J Surg 88:251-254, 2001.

33a. Silen W: Cope's Early Diagnosis of the Acute Abdomen, 20th ed. New York, Oxford University Press, 2000.

34. Horwitz JR, Gursoy MF, Jaksic T, et al: Importance of diarrhea as a presenting symptom of appendicitis in very young children. Am J Surg 173:80-82, 1997.

35. Grattan-Smith JD, Blews DE, Brand T: Omental infarction in pediatric patients: Sonographic and CT findings. AJR Am J Roentgenol 178:1537-1539, 2002.

36. Eriksson S, Granstrom L: Randomized controlled trial of appendicectomy versus antibiotic therapy for acute appendicitis. Br J Surg 82:166-169, 1995.

37. Adams ML: The medical management of acute appendicitis in a nonsurgical environment: A retrospective case review. Mil Med 155:345-347, 1990.

38. Helmer KS, Robinson EK, Lally KP, et al: Standardized patient care guidelines reduce infectious morbidity in appendectomy patients. Am J Surg 183:608-613, 2002.

39. Mazuski JE, Sawyer RG. Nathens AB, et al: The Surgical Infection Society Guidelines on Antimicrobial Therapy for Intra-Abdominal Infections: An Executive Summary. Surg Infect 3:161-233, 2002.

40. Panton ON, Samson C, Segal J, et al: A four-year experience with laparoscopy in the management of appendicitis. Am J Surg 171:538-541, 1996.

41. Vallina VL, Velasco JM, McCulloch CS: Laparoscopic versus conventional appendectomy. Ann Surg 218:685-692, 1993.

42. Garbutt JM, Soper NJ, Shannon WD, et al: Meta-analysis of randomized controlled trials comparing laparoscopic and open appendectomy. Surg Laparosc Endosc 9:17-26, 1999.

43. Keller MS, McBride WJ, Vane DW: Management of complicated appendicitis: A rational approach based on clinical course. Arch Surg 131:261-264, 1996.

44. Oliak D, Yamin D, Udani VM, et al: Nonoperative management of perforated appendicitis without periappendicial mass. Am J Surg 179:177-181, 2000.

45. So JBY, Chiong EC, Chiong E, et al: Laparoscopic appendectomy for perforated appendicitis. World J Surg 26:1485-1488, 2002.

46. Horwitz JR, Custer D, Mehall J, et al: Should laparoscopic appendectomy be avoided for complicated appendicitis in children? J Pediatr Surg 32:1601-1603, 1997.

47. Krischer SL, Browne A, Dibbins A, et al: Intra-abdominal abscess after laparoscopic appendectomy for perforated appendicitis. Arch Surg 136:438-441, 2001.

48. Jordan JS, Kovalcik PJ, Schwab CW: Appendicitis with a palpable mass. Ann Surg 193:227-229, 1981.

49. Gillick J, Velayudham M, Puri P: Conservative management of appendix mass in children. Br J Surg 88:1539-1542, 2001.

50. Nitecki S, Assalia A, Schein M: Contemporary management of the appendiceal mass. Br J Surg 80:18-20, 1993.

51. Marya SK, Garg P, Singh M, et al: Is long delay necessary before appendectomy after appendiceal formation? Can J Surg 36:268-270, 1993.

52. Gahukamble DB, Gahukamble LD: Surgical and pathological basis for interval appendicectomy after resolution of appendicular mass in children. J Pediatr Surg 35:424-427, 2000.

53. Rao PM, Rhea JT, Novelline RA, et al: The computed tomography appearance of recurrent and chronic appendicitis. Am J Emerg Med 15:26-33, 1998.

54. Fayez JA, Toy NJ, Flanagan TM: The appendix as the cause of chronic lower abdominal pain. Am J Obstet Gynecol 172:122-123, 1995.

55. Gorenstin A, Serour F, Katz R, et al: Appendiceal colic in children: A true clinical entity. J Am Coll Surg 182:246-250, 1996.

56. Halvorsen AC, Brandt B, Andreasen JJ: Acute appendicitis in pregnancy: Complication and subsequent management. Eur J Surg 158:603-606, 1992.

57. Al-Mulhim AA: Acute appendicitis in pregnancy: A review of 52 cases. Int Surg 81:295-297, 1996.

58. Andersson RE, Olaison G, Tysk C, Ekbom A: Appendectomy is followed by increased risk of Crohn's disease. Gastroenterology 124:40-46, 2003.

59. Serour F, Efrati Y, Klin B, et al: Subcuticular skin closure as a standard approach to emergency appendectomy in children: Prospective clinical trial. World J Surg 20:38-42, 1996.

60. Brasel KJ, Burgstrom DC, Weigelt JA: Cost-utility analysis of contaminated appendectomy wounds. J Am Coll Surg 184:23-30, 1997.

61. Andersson REB: Small bowel obstruction after appendicectomy. Br J Surg 88:1387-1391, 2001.

62. Andersson R, Lambe M, Bergstrom R: Fertility patterns after appendicectomy: Historical cohort study. BMJ 318:963-967, 1999.

63. Urbach DR, Cohen MM: Is perforation of the appendix a risk factor for tubal infertility and ectopic pregnancy? An appraisal of the evidence. Can J Surg 42:101-108, 1999.

64. Mueller BA, Daling JR, Moore DE, et al: Appendectomy and the risk of tubal infertility. N Engl J Med 315:1506-1508, 1986.

65. Puri P, McGuinness EP, Guiney EJ: Fertility following perforated appendicitis in girls. J Pediatr Surg 24:547-549, 1989.

66. Hui TT, Major KM, Avital I, et al: Outcome of elderly patients with appendicitis: Effect of computed tomography and laparoscopy. Arch Surg 137:995-1000, 2002.

67. McCusker ME, Cote TR, Clegg LX, et al: Primary malignant neoplasms of the appendix. Cancer 94:3307-3312, 2002.

68. Nitechi SS, Wolff BG, Schlinkert R, et al: The natural history of surgically treated primary adenocarcinoma of the appendix. Ann Surg 219:51-57, 1996.

69. Sandor A, Modlin IM: A retrospective analysis of 1570 appendiceal carcinoids. Am J Gastroenterol 93:422-428, 1998.

70. Corpron CA, Black CT, Herzog CE, et al: A half century of experience with carcinoid tumors in children. Am J Surg 170:606-608, 1995.

71. Kulke MH, Meyer RJ: Carcinoid tumors. N Engl J Med 340:858-868, 1999.

72. La Salle AJ, Andrassy RJ, Page CP, et al: Intussusception of the appendiceal stump. Clin Pediatr 19:432-435, 1980.

73. Aksnes G, Diseth TH, Helseth A, et al: Appendicostomy for antegrade enema: Effects on somatic and psychosocial functioning in children with myelomeningocele. Pediatrics 109:484-489, 2002.

74. Sugimoto T, Edwards D: Incidence and costs of incidental appendectomy as a preventive measure. Am J Public Health 77:471-475, 1987.

75. Wang HT, Sax HC: Incidental appendectomy in the era of managed care and laparoscopy. J Am Coll Surg 192:182-188, 2001.

76. Ritchey ML, Haase GM, Shochat SJ, et al: Incidental appendectomy during nephrectomy for Wilms' tumor. Surg Gynecol Obstet 176:423-426, 1993.

CHAPTER 48

COLON AND RECTUM

Najjia Mahmoud, M.D.,   **John Rombeau**, M.D.,   **Howard M. Ross**, M.D.,
and   **Robert D. Fry**, M.D.

EMBRYOLOGY OF THE COLON AND RECTUM

No comprehensive discussion of colorectal anatomy is complete without a thorough understanding of the genesis of the gastrointestinal tract. Knowledge of the developmental anatomy of the foregut, midgut, and hindgut establish a context in which to consider mature structural and functional anatomic relationships.

The endodermal roof of the yolk sac gives rise to the primitive gut tube. At the beginning of the third week of development, the gut tube is divided into three regions: the midgut, which opens ventrally, is positioned between the foregut in the headfold and the hindgut in the tailfold. Development progresses through the stages of "physiologic herniation," "return to the abdomen," and "fixation." The acquisition of length and formation of dedicated blood and lymphatic supplies takes place during this time (Fig. 48-1).

Foregut-derived structures end at the second portion of the duodenum and rely on the celiac artery for blood supply. The midgut, extending from the duodenal ampulla to the distal transverse colon, is based on the superior mesenteric artery. The distal third of the transverse colon, the descending colon, and the rectum evolve from the hindgut fold and are supplied by the inferior mesenteric artery. Venous and lymphatic channels mirror their arterial counterparts and follow the same embryologic divisions. At the dentate line endoderm-derived tissues fuse with the ectoderm-derived "proctodeum," or ingrowth from the anal pit.

Distal rectal development is complex. The cloaca is a specialized area of the primitive distal rectum composed of both endoderm- and ectoderm-derived tissues. This area is incorporated into the anal transition zone, which surrounds the dentate line in the adult. The cloaca exists in a continuum with the hindgut, but at approximately the sixth week it begins to divide and differentiate into anterior urogenital and posterior anal and sphincter elements. Simultaneously, the urogenital and gastrointestinal tracts are separated by caudal migration of the urogenital septum. During the 10th week of development, the external anal sphincter is formed from the posterior cloaca as the descent of the urogenital septum becomes complete. The internal anal sphincter is formed by the 12th week from enlarged circular muscle layers of the rectum.

ANATOMY OF THE COLON, RECTUM, AND PELVIC FLOOR

The colon and rectum consist of a tube of variable diameter approximately 150 cm in length. The terminal ileum empties into the cecum via a thickened, nipple-shaped invagination, the ileocecal valve. The cecum is a capacious sac-like segment of the proximal colon with an average diameter of 7.5 cm and length of 10 cm. Although it is quite distensible, acute dilatation of the cecum to a diameter of greater than 12 cm, an event that can be measured by a plain abdominal radiograph, can result in ischemic necrosis and perforation of the bowel wall. Surgical intervention may be required when this degree of cecal distention is caused by obstruction or pseudo-obstruction (Fig. 48-2).

The appendix extends from the cecum approximately 3 cm below the ileocecal valve as a blind-ending

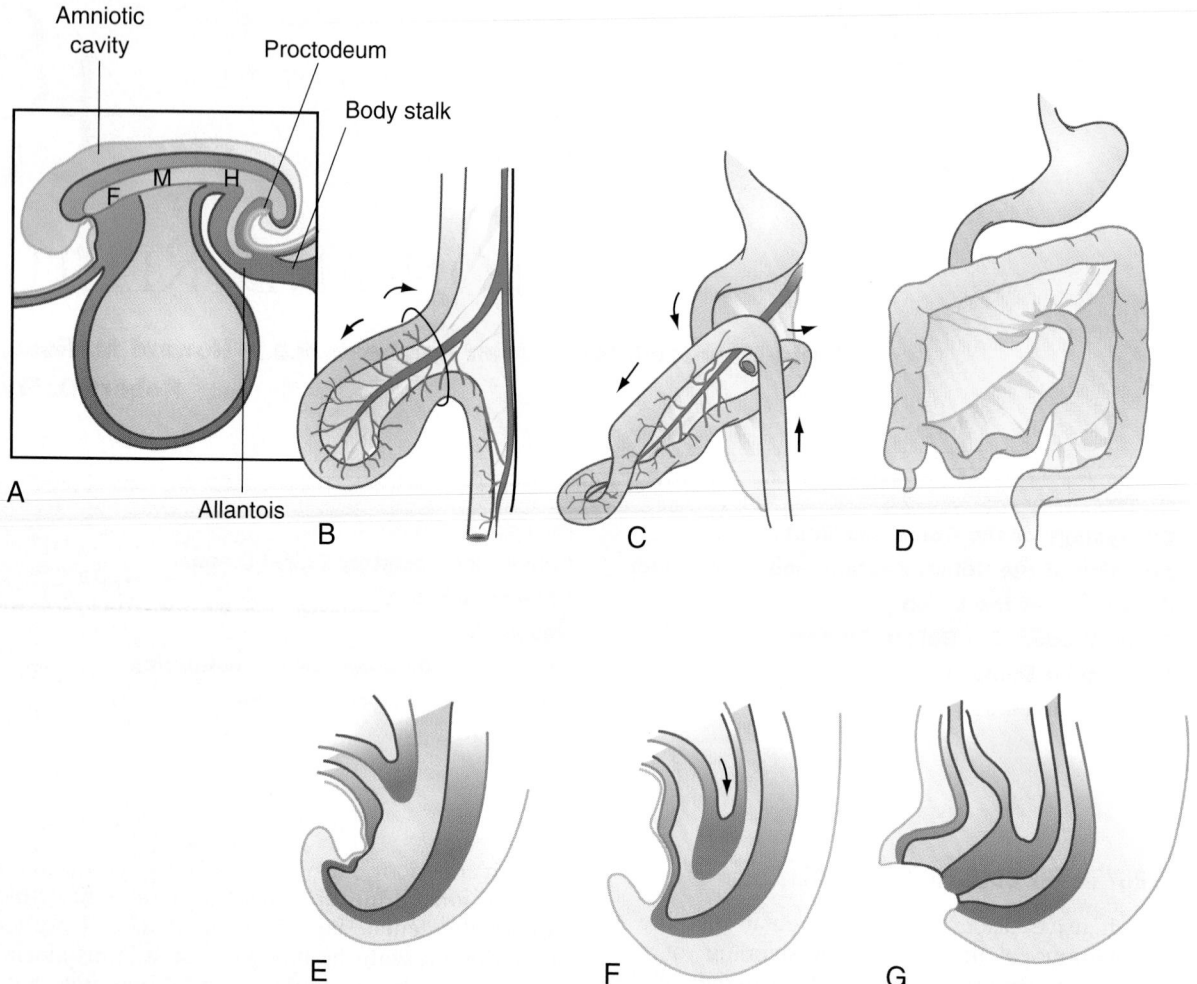

FIGURE 48-1. **A,** At the third week of development, the primitive tube can be divided into three regions: the foregut in the head fold, the hindgut with its ventral allantoic outgrowth in the smaller tail fold, and the midgut between these two portions. Stages of development of the midgut: physiologic herniation (**B**), return to the abdomen (**C**), fixation (**D**). At the sixth week, the urogenital septum migrates caudally (**E**) and separates the intestinal and urogenital tracts (**F, G**). (From Corman ML [ed]: Colon & Rectal Surgery, 4th ed. Philadelphia, Lippincott-Raven, 1998, p 2.)

elongated tube 8 to 10 cm in length. The proximal appendix is fairly constant in location, whereas the end can be located in a wide variety of positions relative to the cecum and terminal ileum. Most commonly, it is retrocecal (65%), followed by pelvic (31%), subcecal (2.3%), pre-ileal (1.0%), and retro-ileal (0.4%). Clinically, the appendix is found at the convergence of the teniae coli. Another clinical aid useful in detecting the location of the appendix through a small abdominal incision is the identification of the fold of Treves, the only antimesenteric epiploic appendage normally found on the small intestine, marking the junction of the ileum and cecum.

The ascending colon, approximately 15 cm in length, runs upward toward the liver on the right side; like the descending colon, the posterior surface is fixed against the retroperitoneum, whereas the lateral and anterior surfaces are true intraperitoneal structures. The "white line of Toldt" represents the fusion of the mesentery with the posterior peritoneum. This subtle peritoneal landmark serves the surgeon as a guide for mobilizing the colon and mesentery from the retroperitoneum.

The transverse colon is approximately 45 cm in length. Hanging between fixed positions at the hepatic and splenic flexures, it is completely invested in visceral peritoneum. The nephrocolic ligament secures the hepatic flexure and directly overlies the right kidney, duodenum, and porta hepatis. The phrenocolic ligament lies ventral to the spleen and fixes the splenic flexure in the left upper quadrant. The angle of the splenic flexure is higher, more acute, and more deeply situated than that of the hepatic flexure. The splenic flexure is typically approached by dissecting the descending colon along the line of Toldt from below and then entering the lesser sac by reflecting the omentum from the transverse colon. This maneuver allows mobilization of the flexure to be achieved with minimal traction required for exposure. Attached to the superior aspect of the transverse colon is the greater omentum, a fused double layer of visceral and parietal peritoneum (four total layers) that contains variable amounts of stored fat. Clinically, it is quite useful in preventing adhesions between surgical abdominal wounds and underlying bowel and is often used to "cover"

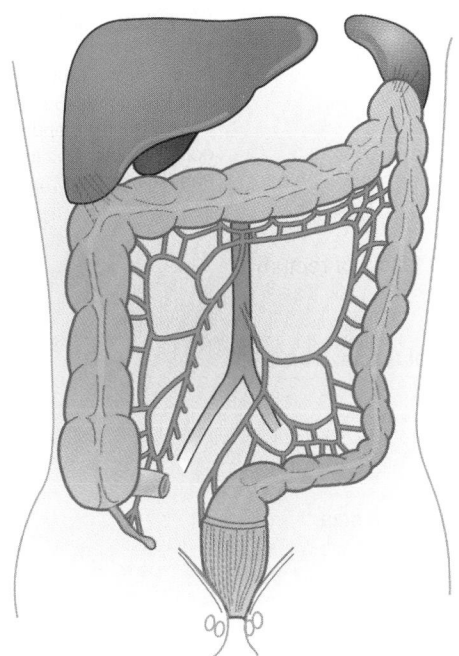

FIGURE 48-2.   Anatomy of the colon and rectum: coronal view. The diameter of the right colon is larger than the diameter of the left side. Note the higher location of the splenic flexure, compared with the hepatic flexure, and the extraperitoneal location of the rectum.

intraperitoneal contents as incisions are closed. The omentum can be mobilized and placed between the rectum and vagina after repair of a high rectovaginal fistula or used to fill the pelvic and perineal space left after excision of the rectum. The living tissue of the greater omentum makes a good "patch" in difficult situations such as treatment of a perforated duodenum, where closure of inflamed and friable tissues is impossible or ill advised.

The descending colon lies ventral to the left kidney and extends downward from the splenic flexure for approximately 25 cm. It is smaller in diameter than the ascending colon. At the level of the pelvic brim there is a transition between the relatively thin-walled, fixed, descending colon and the thicker, mobile sigmoid colon. The sigmoid colon varies in length from 15 to 50 cm (average 38 cm) and is very mobile. It is a small-diameter, muscular tube on a long, floppy mesentery that often forms an "omega" loop in the pelvis. The mesosigmoid is frequently attached to the left pelvic sidewall, producing a small recess in the mesentery known as the intersigmoid fossa. This mesenteric fold is a surgical landmark for the underlying left ureter.

The rectum, along with the sigmoid colon, serves as a fecal reservoir. There is some controversy in the definition of the proximal and distal extent of the rectum. Some consider the rectosigmoid junction to be at the level of the sacral promontory, whereas others consider it to be at the point at which the teniae converge. Anatomists consider the dentate line the distal extent of the rectum, whereas surgeons typically view this union of columnar and squamous epithelium as existing within the anal canal and consider the end of the rectum to be the proximal

border of the anal sphincter complex. The rectum is 12 to 15 cm in length and lacks teniae coli or appendices epiploicae. It occupies the curve of the sacrum in the true pelvis, and the posterior surface is almost completely extraperitoneal in that it is adherent to presacral soft tissues and thus is outside the peritoneal cavity. The anterior surface of the proximal third of the rectum is covered by visceral peritoneum. The peritoneal reflection is 7 to 9 cm from the anal verge in men and 5 to 7.5 cm in women. This anterior peritonealized space is called the pouch of Douglas or the pelvic cul-de-sac, and it may serve as the site of "drop" metastases from visceral tumors. These peritoneal metastases can form a mass in the cul-de-sac ("Bloomer's shelf") that can be detected by a digital rectal examination.

The rectum possesses three involutions or curves known as the valves of Houston. The middle valve folds to the left and the proximal and distal to the right. These "valves" are more properly called folds, for they have no specific function as impediments to flow. They are lost following full surgical mobilization of the rectum, a maneuver that may provide approximately 5 cm of additional length to the rectum, a process that greatly facilitates the surgeon's ability to fashion an anastomosis deep in the pelvis.

The posterior aspect of the rectum is invested with a thick, closely applied mesorectum. A thin layer of investing fascia (fascia propria) coats the mesorectum and represents a distinct layer from the presacral fascia against which it lies. In the course of proctectomy for rectal cancer, mobilization of the rectum entails developing the potential space between the presacral fascia and the fascia propria. Total mesorectal excision is a well-described oncologic maneuver that makes good use of the tissue planes investing the rectum to achieve a relatively bloodless rectal and mesorectal dissection. The lymphatics are contained within the mesorectum, and total mesorectal excision adheres to the basic surgical oncologic principle of removal of the cancer in continuity with its blood and lymphatic supply. Resection of the rectum using this technique based on a thorough understanding of anatomy has been shown to markedly reduce the incidence of subsequent local recurrence of rectal cancer.

Pararectal Fascia

The endopelvic fascia is a thick layer of parietal peritoneum that lines the walls and floor of the pelvis. The portion that is closely applied to the periosteum of the anterior sacrum is the presacral fascia. The fascia propria of the rectum is a thin condensation of the endopelvic fascia that forms an envelope around the mesorectum and continues distally to help form the lateral rectal stalks. The lateral rectal stalks or "ligaments" are actually anterolateral structures containing the middle rectal artery. The stalks reside in close proximity to the mixed autonomic nerves (containing both sympathetic and parasympathetic nerves), and division of these structures close to the pelvic sidewall may result in injury to these nerves, resulting in impotence and bladder dysfunction (Fig. 48-3).

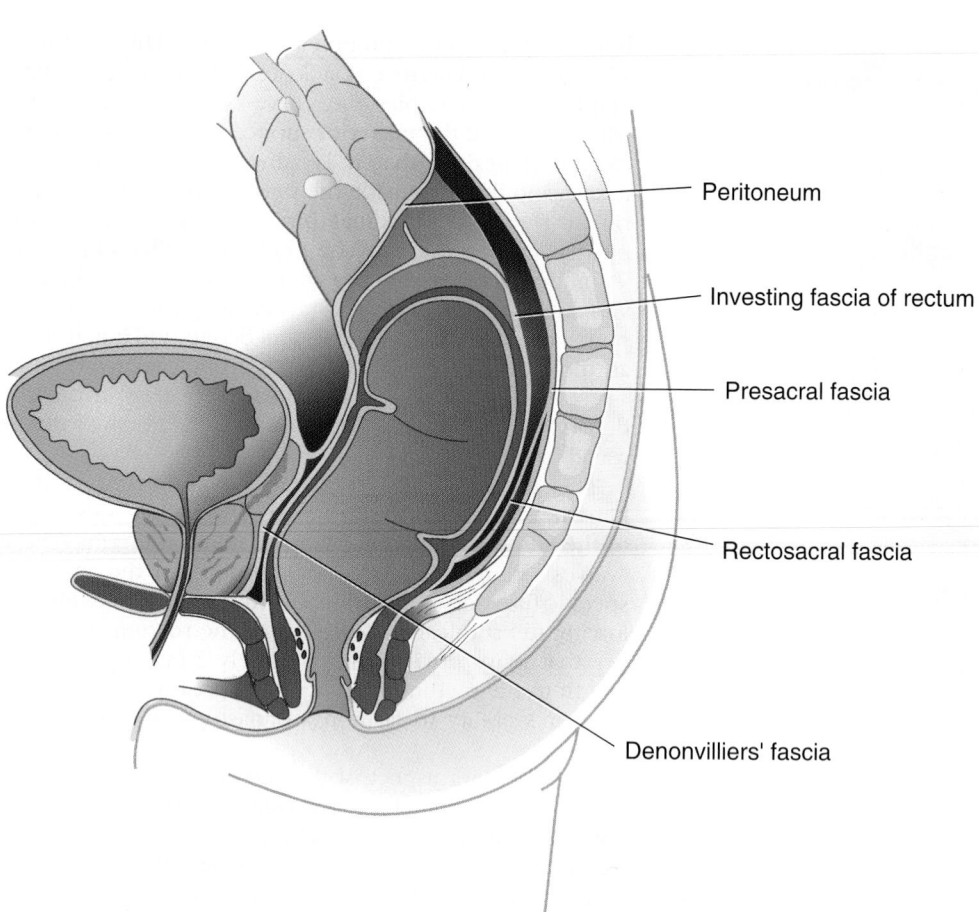

FIGURE 48-3.   Endopelvic fascia. (From Gordon PH, Nivatvongs S [eds]: Principles and Practice of Surgery for the Colon, Rectum, and Anus, 2nd ed. St. Louis, Quality Medical Publishing, 1999, p 10.)

Peritoneum

Investing fascia of rectum

Presacral fascia

Rectosacral fascia

Denonvilliers' fascia

The rectosacral fascia, or Waldeyer's fascia, is a thick condensation of endopelvic fascia connecting the presacral fascia to the fascia propria at the level of S4 and extends to the anorectal ring. Waldeyer's fascia is an important surgical landmark, and its division during dissection from an abdominal approach provides entry to the deep retrorectal pelvis. Dissection between the fascia propria and the presacral fascia follows the principles of surgical oncology and minimizes the risk of vascular or neural injuries. Disruption of the presacral fascia may lead to injury of the basivertebral venous plexus, resulting in massive hemorrhage. Disrupting the fascia propria during an operation for rectal cancer significantly increases the incidence of subsequent recurrence of cancer in the pelvis.

The Pelvic Floor

The muscles of the pelvic floor, like those of the anal sphincter mechanism, arise from the primitive cloaca. The pelvic floor or diaphragm consists of the pubococcygeus, iliococcygeus, and puborectalis, a group of muscles that together form the levator ani. The pelvic diaphragm resides between the sacrum, obturator fascia, ischial spines, and pubis. It forms a strong floor that supports the pelvic organs and, together with the external anal sphincter, regulates defecation. The "levator hiatus" is an opening between the decussating fibers of the pubococcygeus that allows egress of the anal canal, urethra, and dorsal vein in men and the anal canal, urethra, and vagina in women. The puborectalis is a strong U-shaped sling of striated muscle coursing around the rectum just above the level of the anal sphincters. Relaxation of the puborectalis straightens the anorectal angle and permits descent of feces; contraction produces the opposite effect. The puborectalis is in a state of continual contraction, a factor vital to the maintenance of continence. Puborectalis dysfunction is an important cause of defecation disorders. The pubococcygeus and iliococcygeus most likely participate in continence by applying lateral pressure to narrow the levator hiatus (Figs. 48-4 and 48-5).

Arterial Supply and Venous and Lymphatic Drainage

Knowledge of the embryologic development of the intestinal tract provides an excellent foundation for understanding the anatomic blood supply. The foregut is supplied by the celiac artery, the midgut by the superior mesenteric artery (SMA), and the hindgut by the inferior

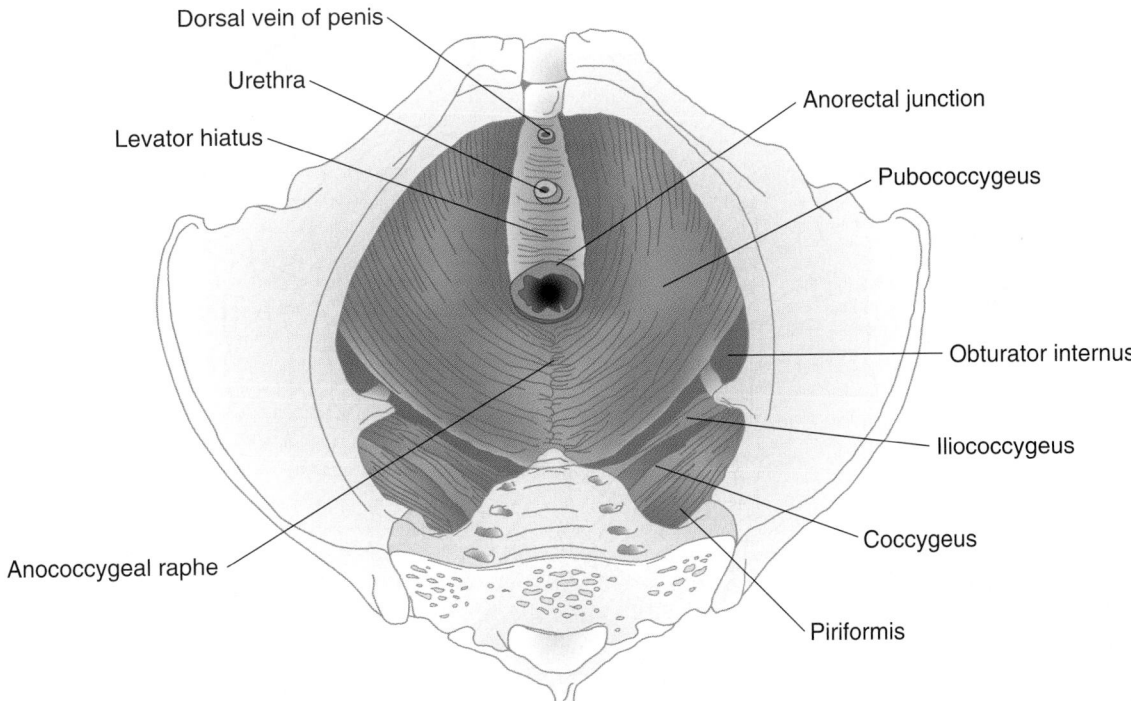

FIGURE 48-4.   Levator muscles. (From Gordon PH, Nivatvongs S [eds]: Principles and Practice of Surgery for the Colon, Rectum, and Anus, 2nd ed. St. Louis, Quality Medical Publishing, 1999, p 18.)

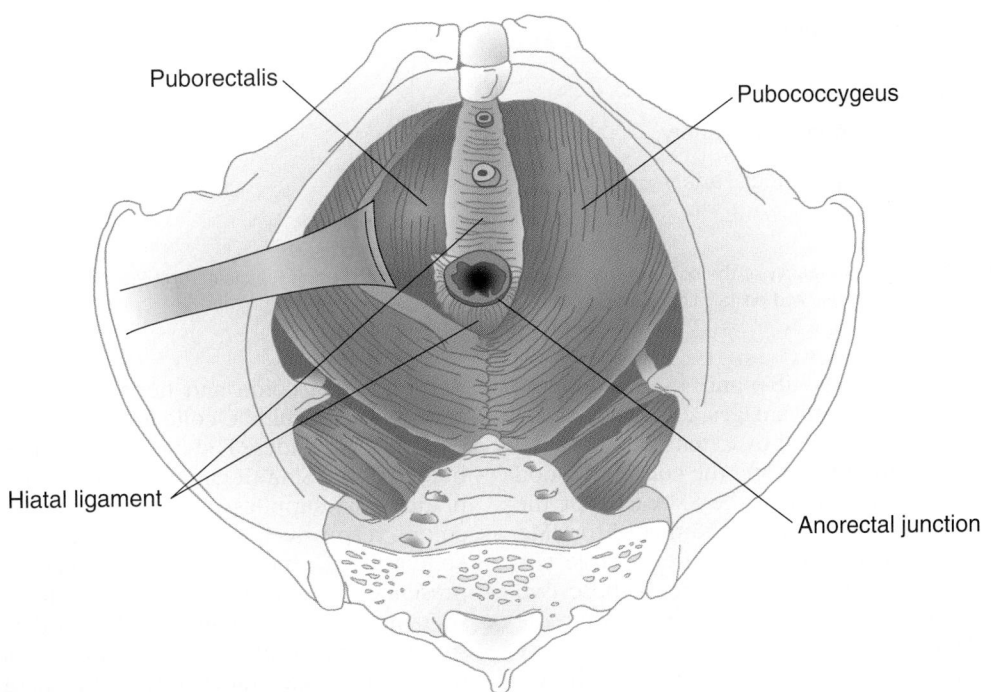

FIGURE 48-5.   Hiatal ligament. (From Gordon PH, Nivatvongs S [eds]: Principles and Practice of Surgery for the Colon, Rectum, and Anus, 2nd ed. St. Louis, Quality Medical Publishing, 1999, p 18.)

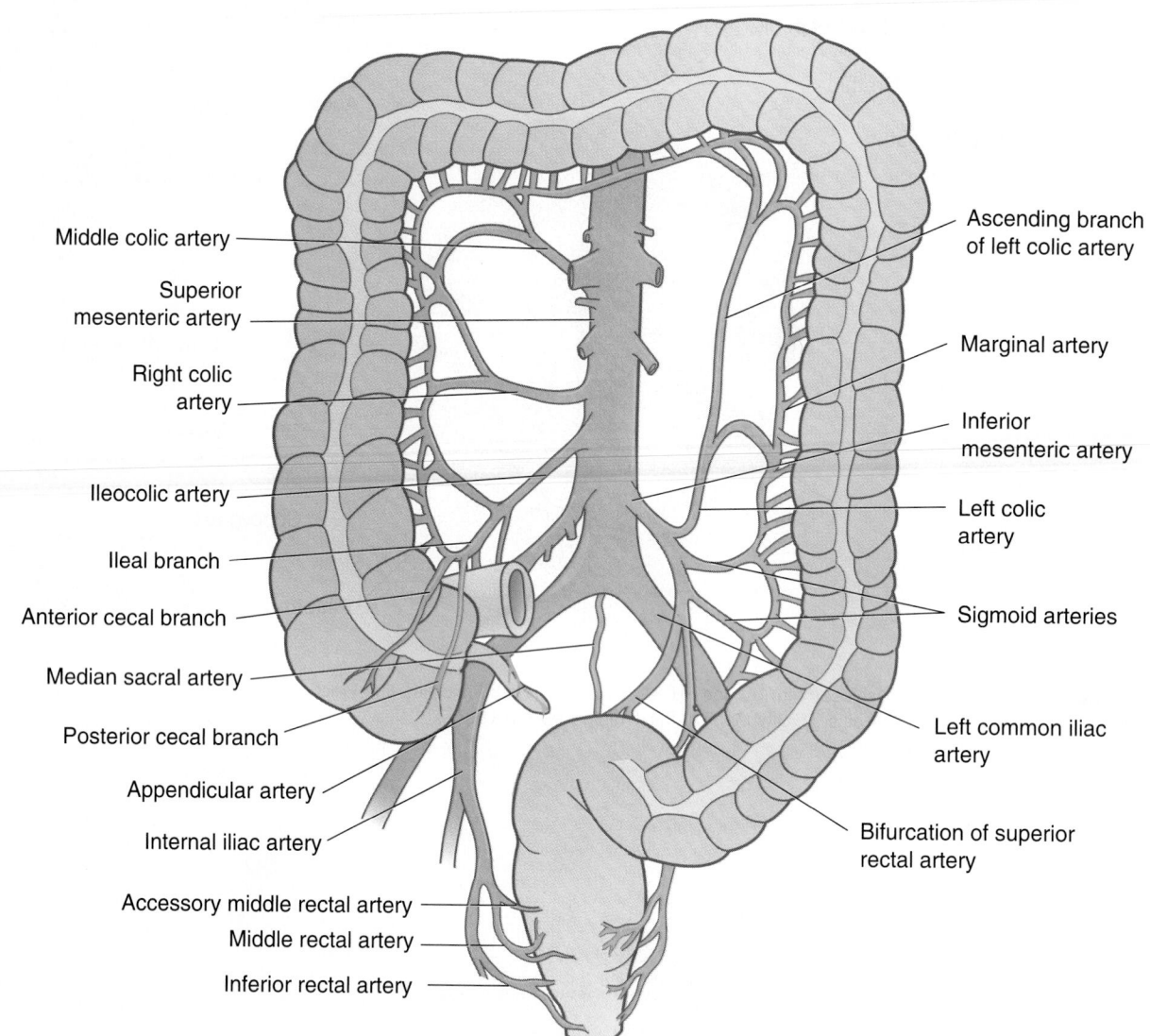

FIGURE 48-6.   Arterial supply of the colon. (From Gordon PH, Nivatvongs S [eds]: Principles and Practice of Surgery for the Colon, Rectum and Anus, 2nd ed. St. Louis, Quality Medical Publishing, 1999, p 23.)

mesenteric artery (IMA) (Figs. 48-6 and 48-7). Anatomic redundancy confers survival advantages, and in the intestinal tract this feature is provided by extensive communication between the major arteries and the collateral blood supply (Fig. 48-8). The territory of the SMA ends at the distal portion of the transverse colon and that of the IMA begins in the region of the splenic flexure. A large collateral vessel, the "marginal artery," connects these two circulations and forms a continuous arcade along the mesenteric border of the colon. Vasa recta from this artery branch off at short intervals and directly supply the bowel wall (Fig. 48-9). The SMA supplies the entire small bowel, giving off 12 to 20 jejunal and ileal branches to the left and up to 3 main colonic branches to the right. The ileocolic artery is the most constant of these branches and supplies the terminal ileum, cecum, and appendix. The right colic artery is absent in 2% to 18% of specimens; when present it may arise directly from the SMA, or as a branch of the ileocolic or middle colic artery. It supplies

the ascending colon and hepatic flexure and communicates with the middle colic artery through collateral marginal artery arcades. The middle colic artery is a proximal branch of the SMA. It generally divides into a right and left branch that supplies the proximal and distal transverse colon, respectively. Anatomic variations of the middle colic artery include complete absence in 4% to 20% and presence of an accessory middle colic artery in 10% of specimens. The left branch of the middle colic artery may supply territory also supplied by the left colic artery through the collateral channel of the marginal artery. This collateral circulation in the area of the splenic flexure is the most inconstant of the entire colon and has been referred to as a "watershed" area, vulnerable to ischemia in the presence of hypotension. In some studies, up to 50% of specimens lack clearly identified arteries in a small segment of colon at the confluence of the blood supplies of the midgut and hindgut. These individuals rely on adjacent vasa recta in this area for arterial supply to the bowel

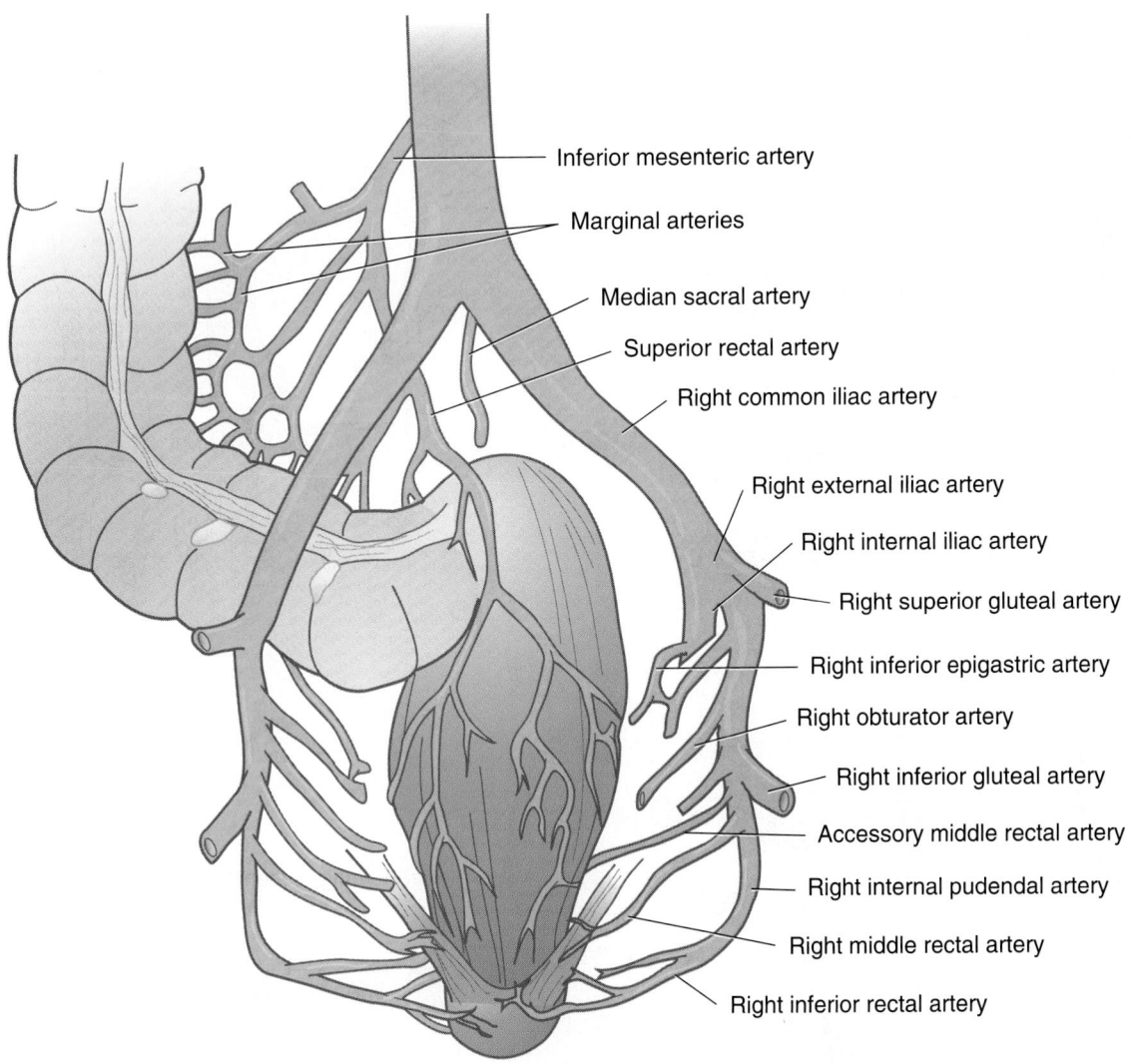

Inferior mesenteric artery

Marginal arteries

Median sacral artery

Superior rectal artery

Right common iliac artery

Right external iliac artery

Right internal iliac artery

Right superior gluteal artery

Right inferior epigastric artery

Right obturator artery

Right inferior gluteal artery

Accessory middle rectal artery

Right internal pudendal artery

Right middle rectal artery

Right inferior rectal artery

FIGURE 48-7. Arterial supply of the rectum. (From Gordon PH, Nivatvongs S [eds]: Principles and Practice of Surgery for the Colon, Rectum, and Anus, 2nd ed. St. Louis, Quality Medical Publishing, 1999, p 24.)

wall. In practice, surgeons avoid making anastomoses in the region of the splenic flexure for fear that the blood supply will not be sufficient to permit healing of the anastomosis, a situation that could lead to anastomotic leak and sepsis.

The IMA originates from the aorta at the level of L2-3, approximately 3 cm above the aortic bifurcation. The left colic artery is the most proximal branch, supplying the distal transverse colon, splenic flexure, and descending colon. Two to six sigmoid branches collateralize with the left colic artery and form arcades that supply the sigmoid colon and contribute to the marginal artery.

The arc of Riolan is a collateral artery first described by Jean Riolan (1580-1657) that directly connects the proximal SMA with the proximal IMA and may serve as a vital conduit when one or the other of these arteries is occluded. It is also known as the meandering mesenteric artery and is highly variable in size. Flow can be either forward (IMA stenosis) or retrograde (SMA stenosis) depending on the site of obstruction. Such obstruction results in increased size and tortuosity of this meandering

artery that may be detected by arteriography; the presence of a large arc of Riolan thus suggests occlusion of one of the major mesenteric arteries (Figs. 48-8 and 48-10).

The IMA terminates in the superior rectal (superior hemorrhoidal) artery that courses behind the rectum in the mesorectum, branching and then entering the rectal submucosa. Here, the capillaries form a submucosal plexus in the distal rectum at the level of the anal columns. The anal canal also receives arterial blood from the middle rectal (hemorrhoidal) and inferior rectal (hemorrhoidal) arteries. The middle rectal artery is a branch of the internal iliac artery. It is variable in size and enters the rectum anterolaterally, passing alongside and slightly anterior to the lateral rectal stalks. It has been reported to be absent in 40% to 80% of specimens studied. The inferior rectal artery is a branch of the pudendal artery that itself is a more distal branch of the internal iliac. From the obturator canal, it traverses the obturator fascia, ischiorectal fossa, and external anal sphincter to reach the anal canal. This vessel is encountered during the perineal dissection of an abdominoperineal resection.

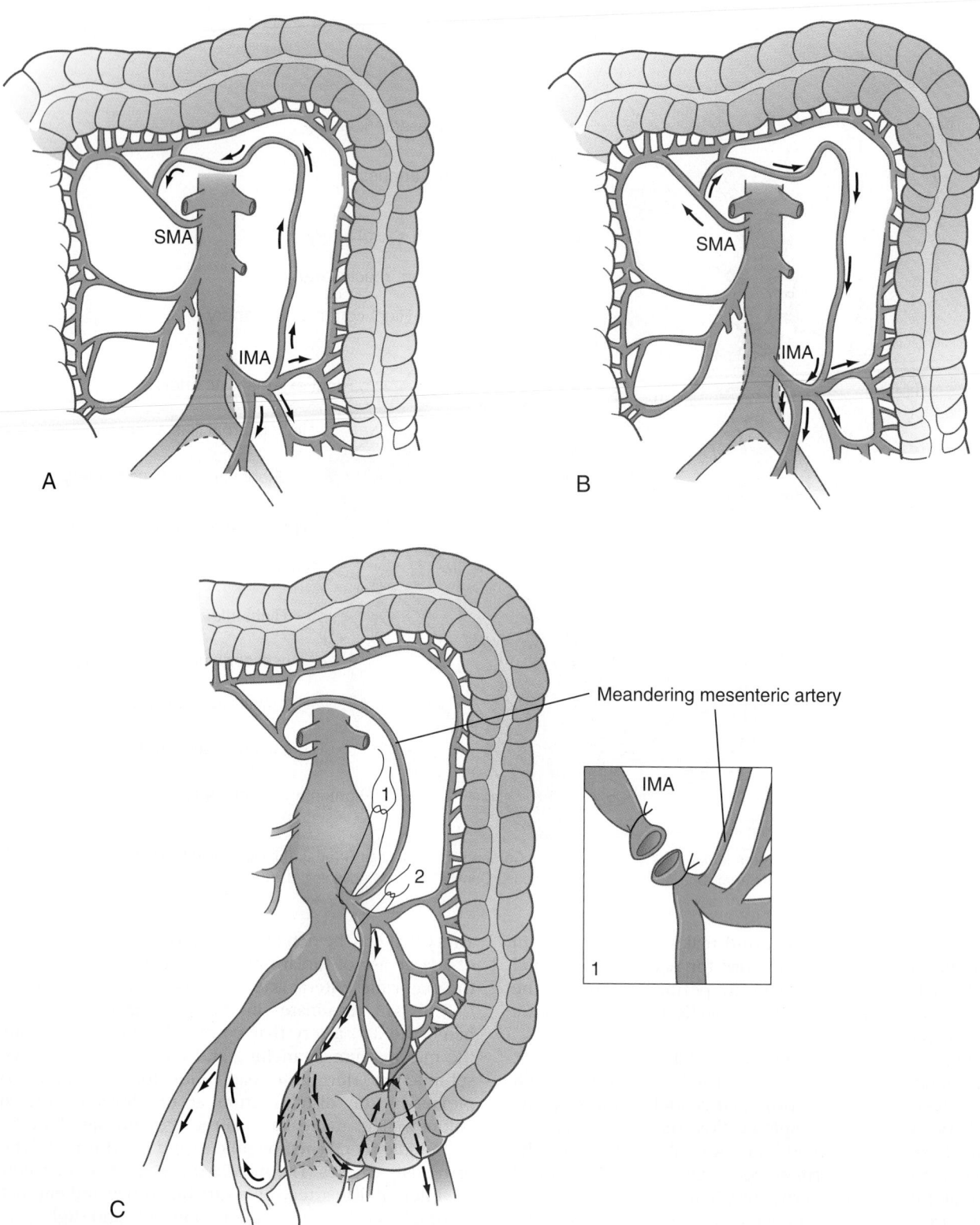

FIGURE 48-8. Pathologic anatomy and occlusion of the superior mesenteric artery (SMA) and the inferior mesenteric artery (IMA). **A,** Occlusion of SMA. **B,** Occlusion of IMA. **C,** Location for ligating IMA: 1, correct location of ligation (see inset); 2, incorrect location of ligation. (From Gordon PH, Nivatvongs S [eds]: Principles and Practice of Surgery for the Colon, Rectum, and Anus, 2nd ed. St. Louis, Quality Medical Publishing, 1999, p 28.)

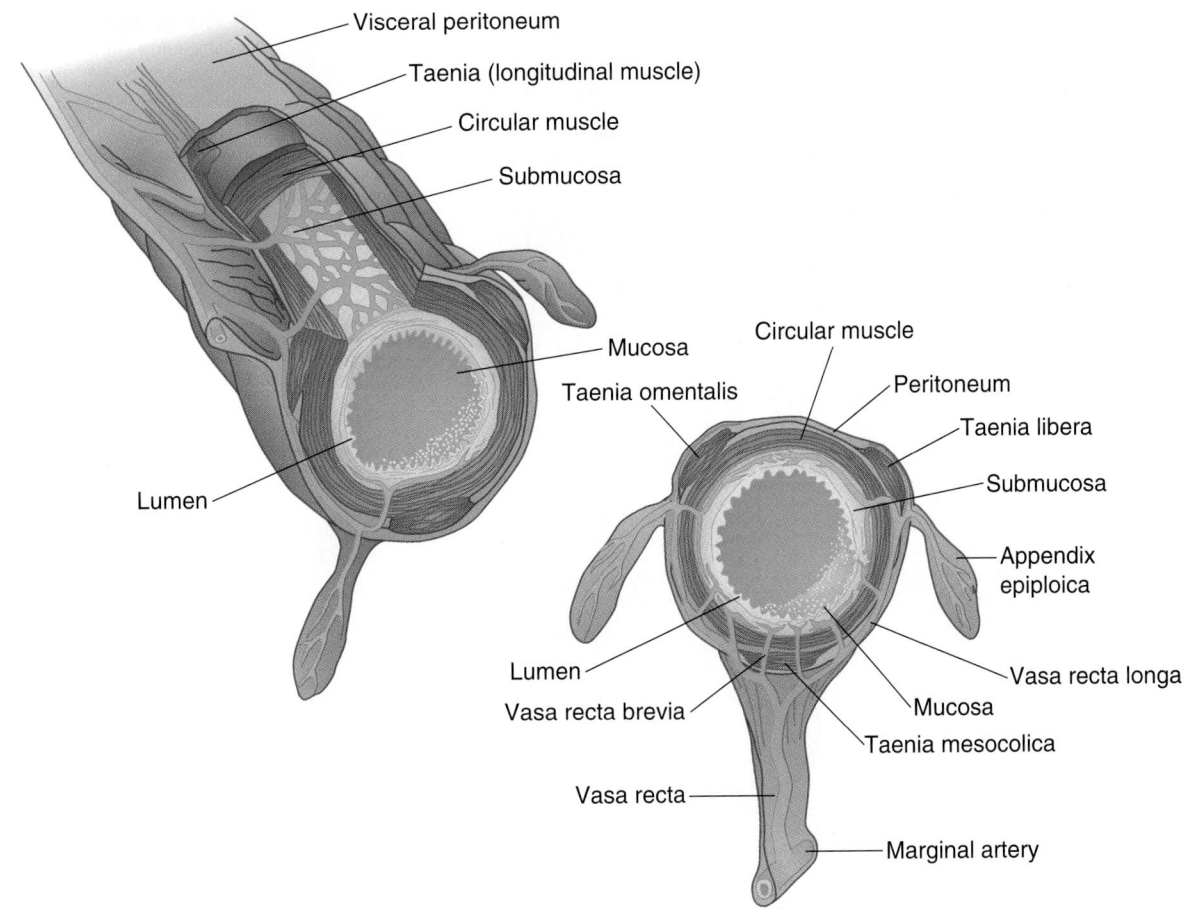

FIGURE 48-9. Cross sectional anatomy of the colon, with vasa brevia and vasa recta. (From Gordon PH, Nivatvongs S [eds]: Principles and Practice of Surgery for the Colon, Rectum, and Anus, 2nd ed. St. Louis, Quality Medical Publishing, 1999, p 26.)

The venous drainage of the colon and rectum mirrors the arterial blood supply. Venous drainage from the right and proximal transverse colon empties into the superior mesenteric vein, which coalesces with the splenic vein to become the portal vein. The distal transverse colon, descending colon, sigmoid, and most of the rectum drain into the inferior mesenteric vein, which empties into the splenic vein to the left of the aorta. The anal canal is drained by the middle and inferior rectal veins into the internal iliac vein and subsequently the inferior vena cava. The bidirectional venous drainage of the anal canal accounts for differences in patterns of metastasis from tumors arising in this region (Fig. 48-11).

Lymphatic drainage also follows the arterial anatomy. The wall of the large bowel is supplied with a rich network of lymphatic capillaries that drain to extramural channels paralleling the arterial supply. Lymphatics from the colon and proximal two thirds of the rectum ultimately drain into the paraortic nodal chain that empties into the cisterna chyli. Lymphatics draining the distal rectum and anal canal may drain either to the paraortic nodes or laterally, via the internal iliac system, to the superficial inguinal nodal basin. Although the dentate line roughly marks the level where lymphatic drainage diverges, classic studies by Block and Enquist using dye injection demonstrate that spread through lymphatic channels to adjacent pelvic organs such as the vagina and broad ligament occurs when injections are administered as high as 10 cm proximal to the dentate line (Figs. 48-12 and 48-13).

Lymph nodes are commonly grouped into "levels" depending on their location. Epicolic nodes are located along the bowel wall and in the epiploicae. Nodes adjacent to the marginal artery are paracolic. Intermediate nodes are located along the main branches of the large blood vessels; primary nodes are located on the SMA or IMA. Lymph node invasion by metastatic cancer is an important prognostic factor for patients with colorectal cancer. Accurate pathologic assessment of lymph nodes is essential for accurate staging, which serves as a determinant for treatment of patients with colorectal cancer.

Nerves

Preganglionic sympathetic nerves from T6 to T12 synapse in preaortic ganglia. Postsympathetic fibers then course along blood vessels to reach the right and transverse colon. The right and transverse colon parasympathetic

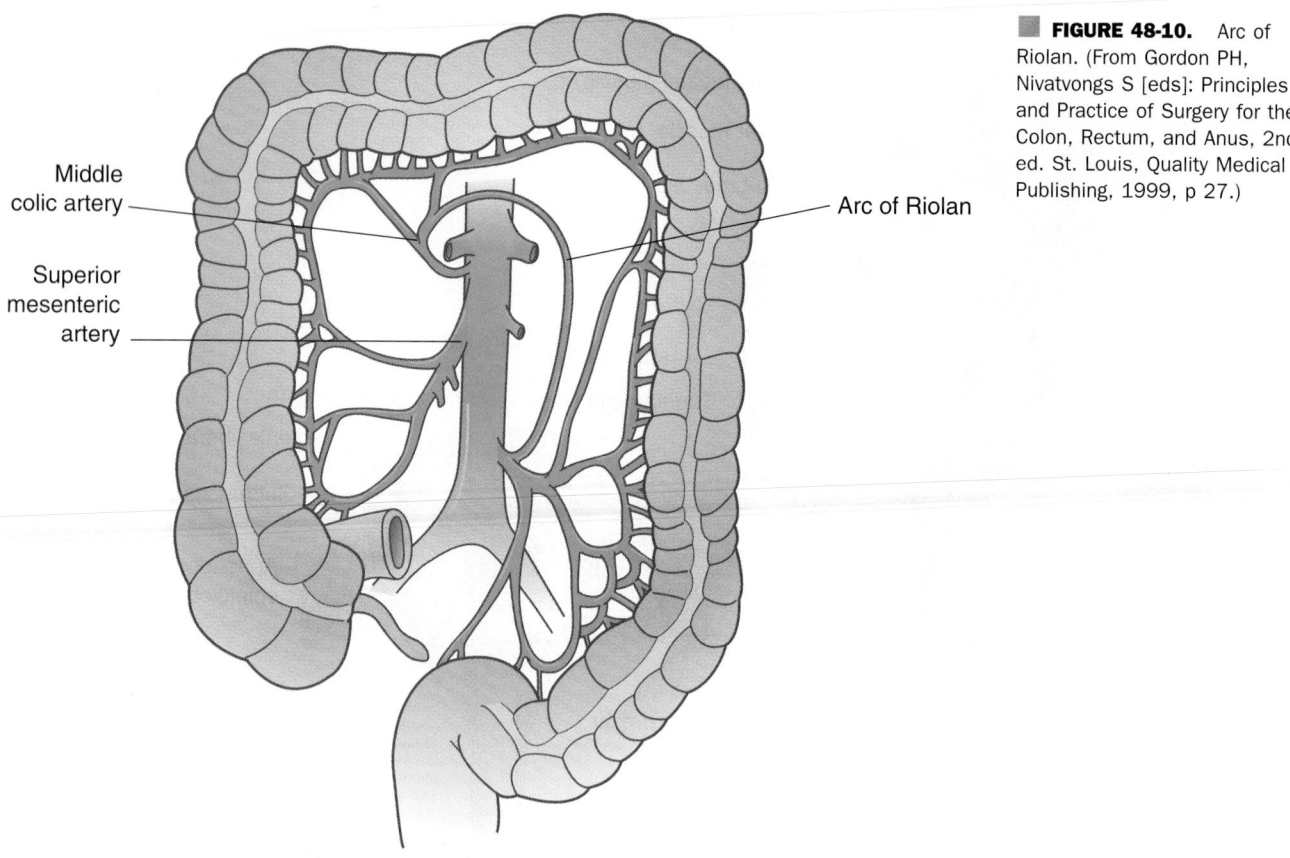

FIGURE 48-10. Arc of Riolan. (From Gordon PH, Nivatvongs S [eds]: Principles and Practice of Surgery for the Colon, Rectum, and Anus, 2nd ed. St. Louis, Quality Medical Publishing, 1999, p 27.)

Middle colic artery

Superior mesenteric artery

Arc of Riolan

supply comes from the right vagus nerve. Parasympathetic fibers follow branches of the SMA to synapse in the wall of the bowel. The left colon and rectum receive sympathetic supply from the preganglionic lumbar splanchnics of L1 to L3. These synapse in the preaortic plexus located above the aortic bifurcation, and the postganglionic elements follow the branches of the IMA and superior rectal artery to the left colon, sigmoid, and rectum. The lower rectum, pelvic floor, and anal canal receive postganglionic sympathetics from the pelvic plexus. The pelvic plexus is adherent to the pelvic sidewalls and is adjacent to the lateral stalks. It receives sympathetic branches from the presacral plexus, which condense at the sacral promontory into the left and right hypogastric nerves. These sympathetic nerves, which descend into the pelvis dorsal to the superior rectal artery, are responsible for delivery of semen to the posterior prostatic urethra. Failure to preserve at least one of the hypogastric nerves during rectal dissection results in ejaculatory dysfunction in males.

The pelvic parasympathetic nerves, or nervi erigentes, arise from S2 to S4. Preganglionic parasympathetic nerves merge with postganglionic sympathetics after the latter emerge from the sacral foramina. These nerve fibers, via the pelvic plexus, surround and innervate the prostate, urethra, seminal vesicles, urinary bladder, and muscles of the pelvic floor. Rectal dissection may disrupt the pelvic plexus and its subdivisions, resulting in neurogenic bladder and sexual dysfunction. Rates of bladder and erectile dysfunction after rectal surgery are as high as 45%. Degree and type of dysfunction is affected by the level of

the neurologic injury. A high IMA ligation severing the hypogastric nerves near the sacral promontory results in sympathetic dysfunction characterized by retrograde ejaculation and bladder dysfunction. Injury to the mixed parasympathetic and sympathetic periprostatic plexus results in impotence and atonic bladder.

PHYSIOLOGY OF THE COLON*

In a broad sense, the function of the colon is the recycling of nutrients, whereas the function of the rectum is the elimination of stool.[1] The recycling of nutrients depends on the metabolic activity of the colonic flora, on colonic motility, and on mucosal absorption and secretion. Stool elimination involves dehydration of colonic contents and defecation.

Recycling of Nutrients

During the digestive process, ingested nutrients are diluted within the intestinal lumen by biliopancreatic and gastrointestinal (GI) secretions. The small intestine absorbs the great majority of ingested nutrients, as well as some of the fluid and bile salts secreted into the lumen. However, the ileal effluent is still rich in water,

---

* Portions of this section previously appeared in the chapter by Dr. Rolando H. Rolandellia, which was published in the 16th edition of this work, pages 932 to 934.

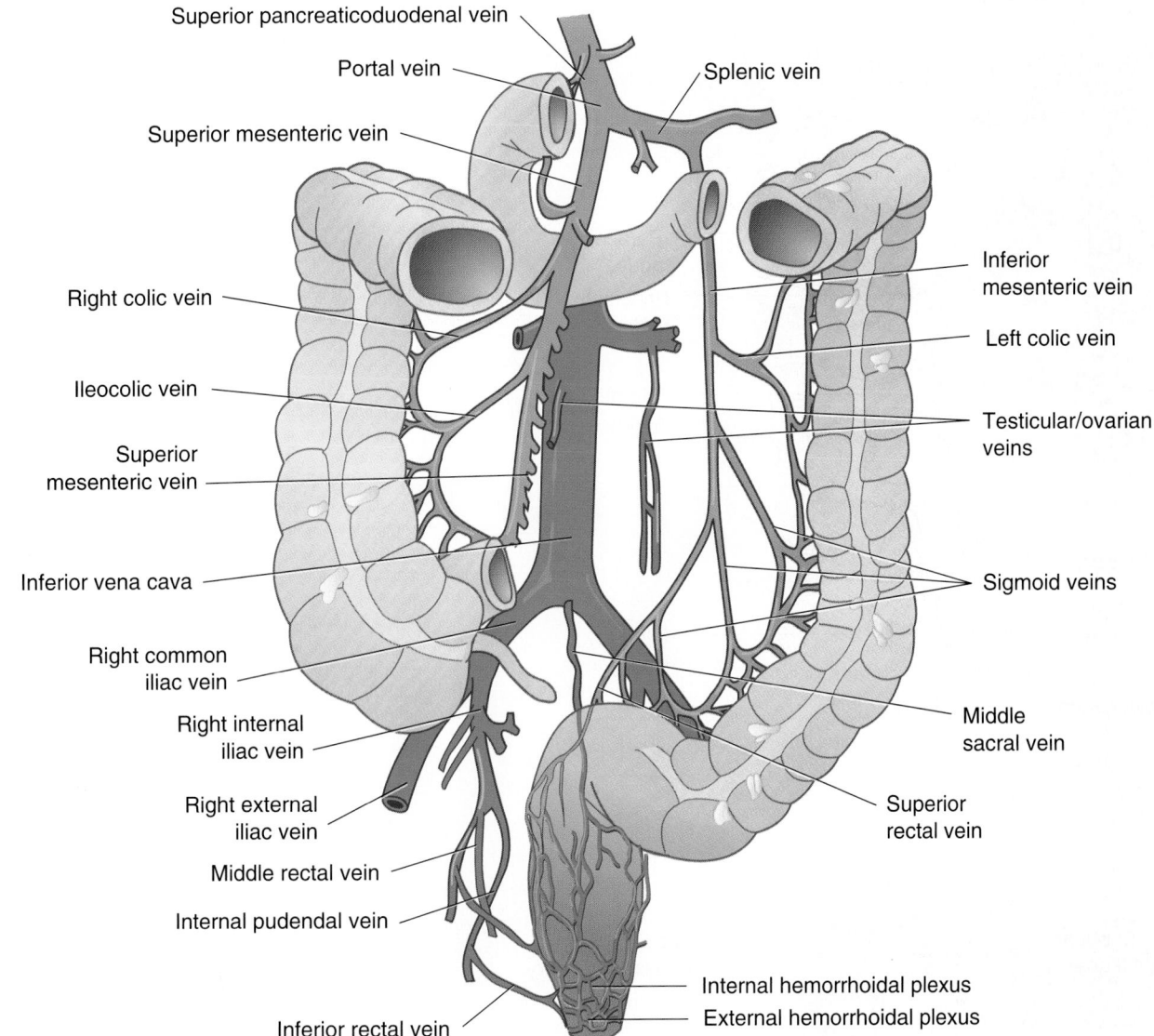

FIGURE 48-11. Venous drainage of the colon and rectum. (From Gordon PH, Nivatvongs S [eds]: Principles and Practice of Surgery for the Colon, Rectum, and Anus, 2nd ed. St. Louis, Quality Medical Publishing, 1999, p 30.)

electrolytes, and nutrients that resist digestion. The colon has the functions to recover these substances and to avoid unnecessary losses of fluids, electrolytes, nitrogen, and energy. To accomplish this, the colon depends highly on its bacterial flora.

Colonic Flora

The colonic microbiota plays an important role in several areas of human physiology.[2] This complex congregate of microorganisms confers great metabolic potential on the colon, primarily through its degradative abilities. Many hundreds of different types of bacteria, varying widely in physiology and biochemistry, exist in the various micro-habitats of the colon: the lumen, the mucin layer, and the mucosal surface. Cultures from colonoscopic biopsies

reveal aerobic counts (aerobes and facultative organisms) ranging from 2.4×10^3 to 1.3×10^6 colony-forming units (cfu)/sample biopsy (5.6 mg) and total anaerobic counts 10 to 10^2 times higher at 1.4×10^5 to $\times 10^7$ cfu/sample.[3] *Bacteroides* species predominate throughout the colon (range, 8.6×10^4 to 1.4×10^7 cfu/sample), composing 66% of total counts from proximal colon and 68.5% from rectum.

Fermentation

Both microbiota and host obtain clear benefits from this association. Although the host provides energy substrates from diet and desquamated cellular debris, together with a relatively stable environment for bacteria to proliferate, bacteria supply the host with *butyrate,* a bacterial

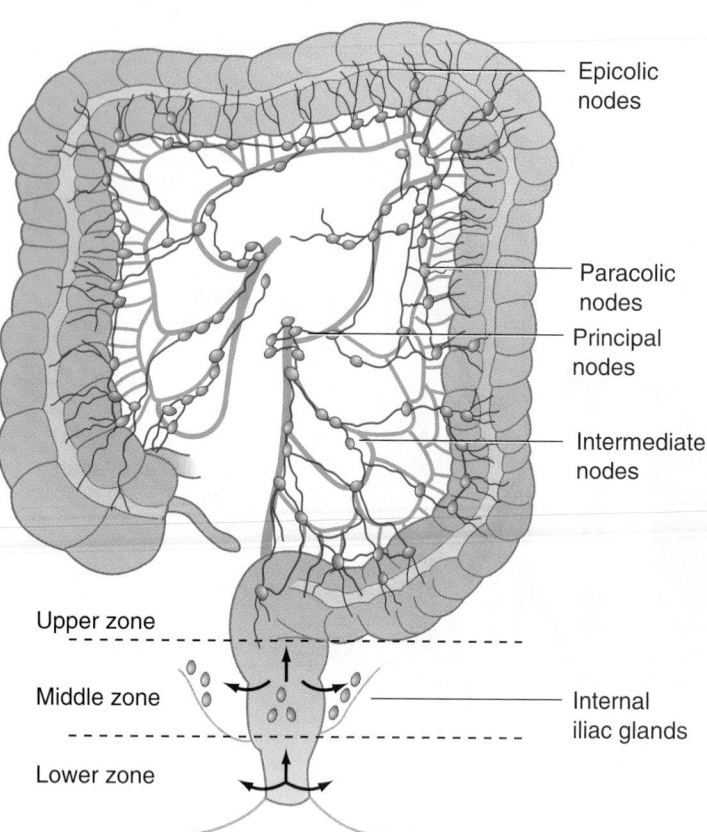

Epicolic nodes

Paracolic nodes

Principal nodes

Intermediate nodes

Upper zone

Middle zone

Lower zone

Internal iliac glands

FIGURE 48-12.   Lymphatic drainage of the colon. (From Corman ML [ed]: Colon & Rectal Surgery, 4th ed. Philadelphia, Lippincott-Raven, 1998, p 21.)

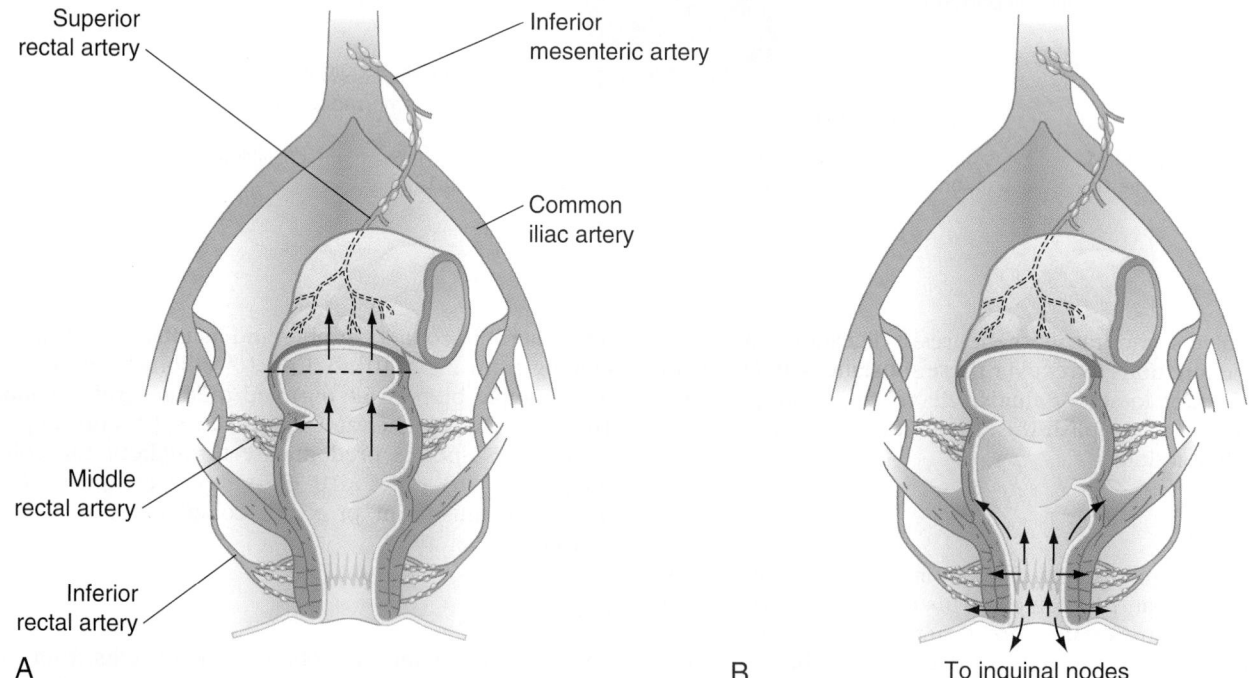

Superior rectal artery

Inferior mesenteric artery

Common iliac artery

Middle rectal artery

Inferior rectal artery

A

B

To inguinal nodes

FIGURE 48-13.   Lymphatic drainage of the rectum (**A**) and anal canal (**B**). (From Gordon PH, Nivatvongs S [eds]: Principles and Practice of Surgery for the Colon, Rectum, and Anus, 2nd ed. St. Louis, Quality Medical Publishing, 1999, p 32.)

fermentation product that has become the main fuel for colonic epithelial cells. Furthermore, bacterial fermentation products are also absorbed and used systemically as a source of energy.[4] One patient population who may benefit from colonic absorption of energy is that of patients with short bowel syndrome.[5] Preservation of the colon in these patients can provide as much as 0.8 MJ (megajoule) per day and reduce carbohydrate excretion by fivefold.[6]

The main sources of energy for intestinal bacteria are complex carbohydrates: starches and nonstarch polysaccharides (NSPs), also known as *dietary fiber.* Carbohydrate metabolism is of great importance in the colon because generically, and in terms of absolute numbers, the vast majority of cultivable microorganisms are saccharolytic. However, the most complex carbohydrates are degraded in a multistep process by a consortium of bacteria rather than by one specific bacterial species.[7] Although NSPs are the main substrate for bacterial fermentation in the colon, not all types of NSPs are equally fermented.[8] *Lignin* is a noncarbohydrate component of plants that is not fermented by human colonic flora and attracts water, thus producing bulk. *Celluloses,* which are primarily found in leafy vegetables, are only partially fermented, whereas *fruit pectins* are completely fermented by colonic bacteria. Colonic transit time and bulking of stool depend on the fermentability of the various NSPs ingested. Poorly fermented NSPs increase luminal bulk and accelerate transit time. Highly fermentable NSPs provide minimal bulk and slow transit time. Consequently, the type of NSP has an impact on both the cause and the treatment of colonic diseases. Constipation, diverticulosis, and colon cancer are uncommon in populations with a high intake of roughage (i.e., water-insoluble NSPs). Thus, water-insoluble fibers are used for the treatment of constipation. Conversely, water-soluble NSPs are easily fermented by colonic bacteria, yielding short-chain fatty acids (SCFAs). Because the absence of SCFAs in the colonic lumen has been linked to impaired absorption, water-soluble NSPs, such as pectin, are used to treat diarrhea.

In addition to NSPs, colonic bacteria ferment malabsorbed starch and protein. The fraction of starch that is not well digested and absorbed in the upper GI tract is known as resistant starch (RS). In this manner, the caloric content of malabsorbed starch and proteins is transferred to SCFAs, which can then be absorbed by the colon and thereby recovered as a calorie supply. It is estimated that approximately 10% of the daily energy expenditure of a normal subject is obtained from the absorption of SCFAs by the colon. Several approaches have been taken to study the significance of RS in colonic physiology. One of these approaches is to measure the amount of starch excreted in the ileal effluent in patients with an ileostomy.[9] When placed in an in vitro fermentation system, the ileal effluent containing RS produces more butyrate and less ammonia than when starch is absent in the ileal effluent. In subjects with an intact colon who receive a diet supplemented with RS, there also is an increase in total fecal output and daily excretion of butyrate and acetate. The fecal excretion of NSPs also increases, suggesting that the

presence of RS in the colon may affect the fermentation of NSPs.[10] Another approach used to assess the degree of fermentation of RS is to measure breath hydrogen and blood levels of SCFAs.[11] Hydrogen, a byproduct of carbohydrate fermentation, diffuses into the venous outflow of the intestine and then into alveoli for elimination in breath.[12] In subjects fed a diet high in RS, breath hydrogen and serum SCFAs are increased compared with subjects fed a diet low in RS. Other gases produced by bacterial fermentation are CO_2, methane (CH_4), and nitrogen (N_2), as well as odoriferous sulfur-containing gases. Gases produced by bacterial fermentation compose approximately 74% of flatus.[13] Excessive gas production from a high consumption of fermentable fiber can produce a feeling of bloating, although bloating is usually more a sign of irritable bowel syndrome than of excessive fiber fermentation.[14]

The amounts and types of fermentation products formed by colonic bacteria depend on the relative amounts of each available substrate, their chemical structures and compositions, and the fermentation strategies (biochemical characteristics and catabolite regulatory mechanisms) of bacteria. Protein fermentation, or *putrefaction,* results in the formation of a number of potentially toxic metabolites, including phenols, indoles, and amines. The production of these substances is inhibited or repressed in many intestinal microorganisms by a fermentable source of carbohydrate.[15] Due to the anatomy and physiology of the colon, putrefactive processes become quantitatively more important in the distal colon, where carbohydrate is more limiting. The more distal location of colon cancer is probably due to the greater exposure to carcinogens formed by protein putrefaction. Although carbohydrates and proteins entering the colon can be salvaged by bacteria and recycled to the benefit of the host, bacterial metabolism of malabsorbed lipids can be harmful to the host. It has been proposed that lipidic bacterial metabolites can act as detergents in the colon, leading to mucosal injury and reactive hyperproliferation, which in turn can promote tumor development.[16]

Short-Chain Fatty Acids

SCFAs constitute approximately two thirds of the colonic anion concentration (70 to 130 mmol/L), mainly as acetate, propionate, and butyrate.[17] Besides their action on gut morphology and function, SCFAs influence GI motility.[18] SCFAs are involved in the so-called ileocolonic brake (i.e., the inhibition of gastric emptying by nutrients reaching the ileocolonic junction). They may involve hormonal messengers, such as peptide YY, and neural pathways, as well as local reflexes and myogenic responses.[19]

Butyrate exerts trophic effects on normal colonocytes both in vitro and in vivo. In contrast, butyrate arrests the growth of neoplastic colonocytes and inhibits the preneoplastic hyperproliferation induced by some tumor promoters in vitro. Its selective effects on G protein activation[20] explain this paradox of the effects of butyrate in normal versus neoplastic colonocytes. Human colonic carcinoma cells exposed to butyrate accumulate simultaneously in G_0 to G_1 and G_2 to M of the cell cycle. During this transition from G_0 to G_1 to G_2 to M arrest, mitochondrial electron transport is enhanced. This change in mitochondrial activity is followed by changes in membrane potential and cellular growth arrest.[21] Butyrate also regulates the expression of molecules involved in colonocyte adhesion. Butyrate-stimulated differentiation inhibits cell proliferation across collagen I, collagen IV, and laminin and decreases β_1-, α_1-, and α_2-integrin subunit surface expression.[22]

Urea Recycling

For many years, urea was thought to be the end product of nitrogen metabolism in humans. This is true in the sense that humans, and mammals in general, do not produce urease. However, colonic bacteria are rich in urease. If urea is labeled with a tracer (radioisotope or heavy isotope) and injected intravenously, 10% of the urea nitrogen is not recovered in urine but rather is incorporated into body protein. Bacteria firmly adherent to the colonic epithelium mediate this process of urea recycling, which produces urease. A low-protein and high-fiber diet such as that of the Papua New Guinea highlanders further increases urea recycling. These individuals ingest only 10 mg of protein per kilogram per day and have normal health with normal muscle mass and serum proteins. Adaptation to this low-protein diet has made the colon very efficient in recycling nitrogen to the point that it may even absorb some essential amino acids (lysine). Urea recycling has been exploited as a therapy for renal failure by excluding nonessential amino acids from the diet to promote maximal urea recycling and diminish the need for dialysis. The one pathologic condition in which urea recycling is not beneficial is liver failure. When the liver cannot reuse the urea nitrogen absorbed by the colon, ammonia enters the blood-brain barrier and produces false neurotransmitters, which result in hepatic coma.

Absorption

The total absorptive area of the colon is estimated to be approximately 900 cm^2. Between 1000 and 1500 mL of fluid is poured into the cecum by the daily ileal effluent. The total volume of water in stool is only 100 to 150 mL/day. This 10-fold reduction in water across the colon represents the most efficient site of absorption in the GI tract per surface area. The net absorption of sodium is even higher: Although the ileal effluent contains 200 mEq/L of sodium, stool contains only 25 to 50 mEq/L. One major difference between sodium and water absorption in the colon is that although water is absorbed passively, sodium requires active transport. Sodium is transported against chemical and electrical gradient at the expense of energy consumption.

The colonic epithelium can use various fuels; however, n-butyrate is oxidized in preference to glutamine, glucose, or ketone bodies. Because mammalian cells do not produce n-butyrate, the colonic epithelium relies on luminal bacteria to produce it through the fermentation of dietary fiber. The lack of n-butyrate, such as that

resulting from the inhibition of fermentation by broad-spectrum antibiotics, leads to less sodium and water absorption and, thus, diarrhea. Conversely, the perfusion of the colonic lumen with n-butyrate stimulates sodium and water absorption. n-Butyrate, acetate, and propionate are SCFAs produced through bacterial fermentation; these constitute the main anions in stool. Other physiologic effects of SCFAs on the colon include stimulation of blood flow, mucosal cell renewal, and regulation of intraluminal pH for homeostasis of the bacterial flora.

In addition to recovering sodium and water, the colonic mucosa absorbs bile acids. The colon absorbs bile acids that escape absorption by the terminal ileum, thus making the colon part of the enterohepatic circulation. Bile acids are passively transported across the colonic epithelium by nonionic diffusion. When the colonic absorptive capacity is exceeded, colonic bacteria deconjugate bile acids. Deconjugated bile acids can then interfere with sodium and water absorption, leading to secretory, or choleretic, diarrhea. Choleretic diarrhea is seen early after right hemicolectomy as a transient phenomenon and more permanently after extensive ileal resection.

Secretion

The physiologic role of colon secretion is demonstrated in patients with chronic renal failure. Uremic patients can remain normokalemic while ingesting a normal amount of potassium before requiring dialysis. This phenomenon is associated with a compensatory increase in colonic secretion and fecal excretion of potassium. This effect is blocked by spironolactone, which illustrates the effect of aldosterone on colonic potassium secretion. Potassium secretion requires both Na^+, K^+ ATPase and Na^+, K^+ 2Cl cotransport on the basolateral membrane and an apical potassium channel.

Many forms of colitis are associated with increased potassium secretion, such as inflammatory bowel disease (IBD), cholera, and shigellosis. In addition, some forms of colitis impair colonic absorption or produce secretion of chloride; examples are collagenous and microscopic colitis and congenital chloridorrhea. Chloride is secreted by colonic epithelium at a basal rate, which is increased in pathologic conditions such as cystic fibrosis and secretory diarrhea. Secretion of chloride also requires the coupling of Na^+, K^+ ATPase and Na^+, K^+ 2Cl cotransport to exit passively through the apical membrane. Calcium and cyclic adenosine monophosphate both stimulate chloride secretion, whereas bicarbonate and SCFAs inhibit chloride secretion.

Colonic secretion of H^+ and bicarbonate is coupled to the absorption of Na^+ and Cl^-, respectively. It is through these exchangers that the colon is linked to systemic acid-base metabolism.[23] The supply of H^+ and bicarbonate for these exchangers is maintained by the hydration of CO catalyzed by colonic carbonic anhydrase. Changes in systemic pH induce changes in the activity of carbonic anhydrase eliciting elimination of H^+ or bicarbonate as needed to bring systemic pH back to normal.

Motility

Fermentation in the colon is made possible by its distinctive morphology. The colon can be divided into three anatomic segments: the right colon, the left colon, and the rectum. The right colon is the fermentation chamber of the human GI tract, with the cecum being the colonic segment where bacteria are most metabolically active. The left colon is a site of storage and dehydration of stool. Colonic transit rate is a determinant of stool SCFA concentration, including butyrate and distal colonic pH. This may explain the interrelations among colonic cancer, dietary fiber intake, stool elimination, and stool pH.[24] Transit through the colon is controlled by the autonomic nervous system. Parasympathetic nervous fibers supply the colon via the vagi and the pelvic nerves. Nerve fibers reaching the colon arrange themselves in several plexuses: the subserosal, myenteric (Auerbach), submucosal (Meissner), and mucosal plexuses. The neurons of the myenteric plexus concentrate along the taeniae but sparsely between them, where the longitudinal muscle layer is thin. Sympathetic nerve fibers originate in the superior and inferior mesenteric ganglia and reach the colon by way of perivascular plexuses.

The motility pattern is different in the three anatomic segments. In the right colon, antiperistaltic, or retropulsive, waves generate retrograde flow of colonic contents back to the cecum. In the left colon, contents are propelled caudad by tonic contractions, separating them into a series of globular masses. A third type of contraction, called *mass peristalsis,* is interspersed with the propulsive and retropulsive contractions and occurs at varying intervals, more frequently after meals. Each mass peristaltic contraction is able to advance a column of colonic contents through one third of the colonic length.

The colon responds to the ingestion of a meal with an increase in the number of migrating and nonmigrating long spike bursts of potentials peaking at 15 minutes after the meal.[25] This increase in electrical activity is followed by an increase in colonic tone.[26] The increased postprandial contractility is greater in the sigmoid than in the transverse colon. The effects of a meal on colonic motility are commonly called the *gastrocolic reflex.*

Formation of Stool

The frequency of defecation is just as variable among individuals as is their perception of abnormal stool frequency.[27] An individual who passes more than three loose stools per day is considered as having diarrhea, whereas fewer than three weekly stools is considered constipation. Any frequency within that range is considered normal, although many individuals will still seek medical attention for what they perceive as either diarrhea or constipation. Many factors influence colonic transit rate. Colonic transit is longer in women than in men and longer in premenopausal women than postmenopausal women. Conversely, colonic transit is shortened in smokers.[28] In normal subjects, supplementation with NSPs does not shorten colonic transit time, although it does increase fecal weight.[29,30] In patients with idiopathic constipation,

however, NSPs, in the form of psyllium seeds, shorten colonic transit and increase stool weight.[31]

Defecation

Normal defecation requires adequate colonic transit time, stool consistency, and fecal continence. Fecal continence implies deferment of stool elimination; discrimination among gas, liquid, and solid stool; and selective elimination of gas without stool. There is some controversy regarding the actual role of the rectum under resting conditions. Some propose that the rectum is simply a conduit, which under resting conditions should be empty. If stool arrives at the rectum, the anorectal inhibitory reflex is triggered, forcing the subject to hold defecation by voluntary contraction of the external sphincter. However, any surgeon who performs routine rigid proctosigmoidoscopies in the office is well aware that a patient can have a rectum full of stool without any awareness. This leads to the opposing view, which regards the rectum as a reservoir. Just as stool triggers the anorectal inhibitory reflex, it also triggers a rectocolic reflex. This reflex allows continuous filling of the rectum with fecal material until the colon is emptied.[32]

The mechanisms involved in fecal continence are not fully understood. A certain reservoir capacity is needed to achieve fecal continence. A stiff, nondistensible rectum such as in radiation proctitis may produce incontinence even when the sphincter muscles are competent. Part of the internal and external sphincter muscle fibers are necessary for adequate continence, although many patients have part of the sphincter severed during a fistulotomy and are still continent. Probably, the only factor certainly needed for fecal continence is innervation of the sphincter. Not only the motor nerve fibers, which produce contraction of the sphincter fibers, but also all of the sensory innervation is important to adequately empty the rectum.

BOWEL PREPARATION BEFORE SURGERY

Purging the feces and reducing the concentration of colonic intraluminal bacteria before operations on the colon have long been basic tenets of surgery. The normal, or autochthonous, microbial organisms in the colon constitute up to 90% of the dry weight of feces, reaching concentrations up to 10^9 organism/mL of feces. The anaerobic *Bacteroides* is the most common colonic microbe, whereas *Escherichia coli* is the most common aerobe. *Pseudomonas* species, *Enterococcus, Proteus* species, *Klebsiella,* and *Streptococcus* species are also present in large numbers.

The process of preparing the colon for an elective operation has traditionally involved two factors: purging the fecal contents ("mechanical preparation") and administration of antibiotics effective against colonic bacteria. Tradition has held that an "unprepared" colon, one which contains intraluminal feces, poses an unacceptably high rate of failure of the anastomosis to heal. However, recent experience with primary repair of colonic injuries by trauma surgeons, and reports from European surgeons describing elective operations conducted safely without the use of preoperative purging, have caused reconsideration concerning the true value of purging the colon before colonic surgery. Because the colonocytes receive nutrition from intraluminal free fatty acids produced by fermentation from colonic bacteria, there are concerns that purging may actually be detrimental to the healing of a colonic anastomosis. However, in the United States at the present time, the colon is generally cleansed in preparation for colonic operations.[33] Effective cleansing is mandatory for adequate colonoscopy or contrast enema.

Although the use of preoperative parenteral antibiotics is well accepted and validated, the related issue of preoperative oral antibiotic use is controversial. A multiplicity of bowel preparation regimens and antibiotic combinations are in current use. A clear superiority of one above another is not present; however, for some patients, certain bowel preparations may have adverse physiologic consequences. Knowledge of the history of bowel preparation practices, current controversies, and data is useful.

Mechanical bowel cleansing methods are used for both colonoscopy and elective surgery. Complete bowel obstruction and free perforation are absolute contraindications to bowel preparation. For colonoscopy, properties of various preparations are judged by safety, patient tolerance, and efficacy or preparation quality. In the past, 4 to 5 days of clear liquids along with laxatives such as senna, castor oil, and bisacodyl; whole bowel nasogastric irrigation; mannitol irrigation; and repeated enemas were among the regimens used. Patient tolerance of these methods is poor and associated with dehydration, electrolyte abnormalities, and severe abdominal cramping and generally not well tolerated by elderly or infirm patients. In the 1980s, polyethylene glycol solution (PEG), a nonabsorbed sodium sulfate-based liquid, was developed as an oral mechanical bowel preparation. Patients are required to drink at least 2 to 4 L of the solution along with additional fluids. Abdominal cramping, nausea, and vomiting are common side effects of the preparation, and prophylactic antiemetics are often routinely administered. Sodium phosphate solution (Fleet's Phospho-soda) was developed in response to patient dissatisfaction with the large fluid volume required for PEG preparation and has been found in most trials to be a more tolerable preparation with higher rates of patient satisfaction and compliance. The smaller volume (45 mL taken twice) seems to be the main benefit, because the side effects are similar. Sodium phosphate pills (Visicol) were recently introduced as an alternative to liquids. The regimen consists of ingesting a total of 40 pills, with 3 pills taken every 15 minutes with 8 oz of fluid. Sodium phosphate, whether in liquid or pill form, has been linked more frequently than PEG to rare, but serious, electrolyte imbalances. In patients with impaired renal function, hyperphosphatemia, hypernatremia, hypokalemia, and hypocalcemia can occur. For this reason, PEG is the recommended bowel preparation in patients with renal insufficiency, cirrhosis, ascites, or congestive heart failure. Recent investigation comparing efficacy of mechanical bowel preparation has focused on comparisons between PEG and sodium phosphate solutions. Cohen and coworkers demonstrated a 90%

"excellent" or "good" bowel preparation with sodium phosphate versus 70% with 4 L of PEG.[34] Frommer and colleagues found that sodium phosphate results in a "cleaner" bowel than PEG with no difference in infectious complications.[35] On the other hand, Poon and associates in 2002 found that there was no difference in bowel cleanliness when the volume of PEG was reduced to 2 L and compared with 90 mL of sodium phosphate and that the reduced volume enhanced patient compliance.[36] In a Canadian study, the use of sodium phosphate was associated with increased patient compliance and an eightfold cost reduction when compared with PEG.[37] Ultimately, patient comfort and economic factors may determine mechanical bowel preparation practices if efficacy is similar.

For patients undergoing colonoscopy, the quality of the bowel preparation is essential for obtaining an accurate examination. For segmental resections, however, the necessity of mechanical bowel preparation has come under scrutiny. A report by Miettinen and colleagues comparing infectious complications in mechanically prepared bowel (PEG solution) versus unprepared bowel in patients undergoing segmental resection failed to reveal differences in any type of infectious complication.[38] Both groups received parenteral antibiotics. Zmora and associates looked at left-sided anastomoses only and found that there was no significant difference between overall infection rates in unprepared (13.2%) versus prepared bowel (12.5%).[39] The wound infection rates in this study did not significantly differ either at 6.6% in the prepared group and 10% in the unprepared group. Although studies of this type have been relatively small and significantly underpowered, they point to the future possibility of avoiding the discomfort of bowel preparation and the small attendant risk of electrolyte irregularities and dehydration.

Antibiotic use in colorectal surgery is a well-established practice that reduces infectious complications. Elective colorectal cases are classified as "clean contaminated" and, as such, benefit from routine single dose administration of parenteral antibiotics 30 minutes before incision. There is evidence to show that when operative times are prolonged, additional doses at 4-hour intervals reduce wound infection. Once the operation is complete, postoperative administration of antibiotics for a clean-contaminated case such as a routine segmental resection does not further reduce infectious complications and may promote *Clostridium difficile* colitis, *Candida* infection, and the emergence of bacterial antibiotic resistance. Polk and Lopez-Mayor showed a reduction in postoperative infection rates from 30% to 8% with the routine use of preoperative parenteral antibiotics.[40] Gomez-Alonso and associates repeated these results, showing a drop from 39% to 9%.[41] Antibiotics active against both aerobes and anaerobes are ideal—second- or third-generation cephalosporins alone or combinations of a fluoroquinolone plus metronidazole or clindamycin are typical. The use of additional oral antibiotics to theoretically further reduce the bacterial lode is widely accepted but not as well validated. In a survey of colon and rectal surgeons in 1990, 87% indicated that both oral and parenteral antibiotic usage is part of their routine preparation for elective colon operations.[42] A preparation often used consists of erythromycin base (1 g) and neomycin (1 g) given in three preoperative doses the day before surgery. However, this regimen is associated with a high incidence of nausea and abdominal cramps, and some surgeons prefer to prescribe oral ciprofloxacin or metronidazole.

In studies comparing oral to parenteral antibiotics, a decrease in wound infection rate from 36% to 6.5% was seen with intravenous administration, whereas others comparing a combination of oral plus parenteral versus oral alone found that the addition of intravenous antibiotics reduced infectious complications by half (from 22% to 11%). It is notable that there have been no prospective randomized trials examining this issue and that most retrospective reviews are poorly powered. While it is clear that preoperative parenteral antibiotics reduce wound infection rates, oral antibiotics do not clearly benefit the patient either by reducing wound infection or by decreasing intra-abdominal abscess or leaks. Perhaps the rate of intra-abdominal abscess formation is more dependent on technical factors affecting anastomotic integrity than on antibiotic prophylaxis.

DIVERTICULAR DISEASE

A diverticulum is an abnormal sac or pouch protruding from the wall of a hollow organ, which is, for the purposes of this discussion, the colon. A *true diverticulum* is composed of all layers of the intestinal wall, whereas a *false diverticulum,* or *pseudodiverticulum,* lacks a portion of the normal bowel wall. The diverticula that commonly occur in the human colon are protrusions of mucosa through the muscular layers of the intestine. Because these mucosal herniations are devoid of the normal muscular layers, they are pseudodiverticula (Fig. 48-14).

Diverticulosis or *diverticular disease* are terms used to indicate the presence of colonic diverticula. Diverticulosis is a common condition of Western society and seems to be an unfortunate product of the Industrial Revolution. It is interesting that there seem to be no specimens of colonic diverticulosis in anatomic or medical museums in Europe that were archived before the Industrial Revolution. The process of roller-milling wheat flour was introduced in Europe approximately a quarter of a century earlier than the appearance of diverticulosis, which was initially observed in the first decade of the 20th century. It has been postulated that the decreased consumption of unprocessed cereals along with the increased consumption of sugar and meat by the general population are factors largely responsible for the appearance of diverticulosis. Over the past 75 years the amount of fiber consumed by individuals in North America and Western Europe has decreased while the prevalence of diverticulosis has increased significantly. The formation of diverticula is also related to aging. Diverticula are rare in individuals younger than the age of 30 years, but at least two thirds of Americans will have developed colonic diverticula by the age of 80.

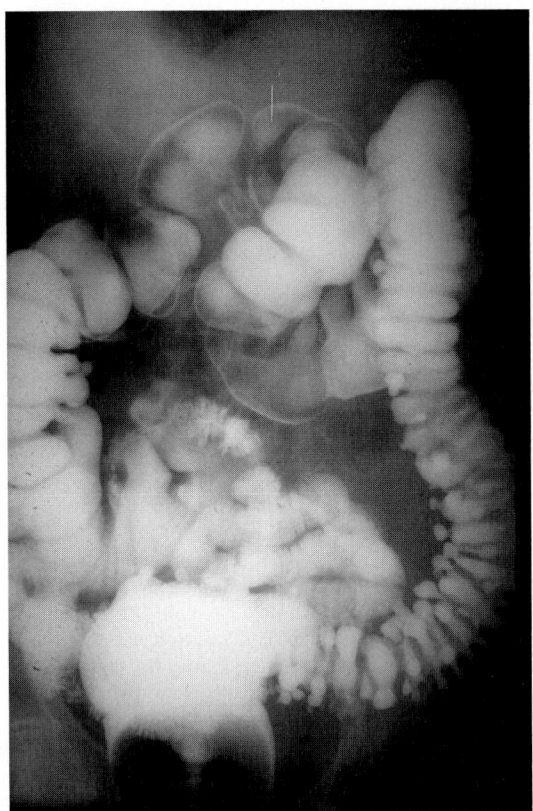

FIGURE 48-14.   Barium enema with extensive sigmoid diverticulosis.

Further evidence that a diet low in fiber and high in carbohydrates and meat contributes to the incidence of diverticulosis is the observation that diverticulosis is rare in sub-Saharan African blacks, who consume a high-fiber diet; however, blacks in Johannesburg who consume a low-fiber diet have the same incidence of diverticulosis as South African whites.

Pathogenesis

Diverticula are actually herniations of mucosa through the colon at sites of penetration of the muscular wall by arterioles. These sites are on the mesenteric side of the antimesenteric teniae. In some cases the arteriole penetrating the wall can be displaced over the dome of the diverticulum. This close relationship between the artery and diverticulum is responsible for the massive hemorrhage that occasionally can complicate diverticulosis (Fig. 48-15).

There is often a striking hypertrophy of the muscular layers of the colonic wall associated with diverticulosis. This thickening of the colonic wall, most commonly affecting the sigmoid colon, may precede the appearance of diverticula. Diverticula most commonly affect the sigmoid colon and are confined to the sigmoid in about half of patients with diverticulosis. The next most common area involved is the descending colon (about 40% of affected individuals), and the entire colon will

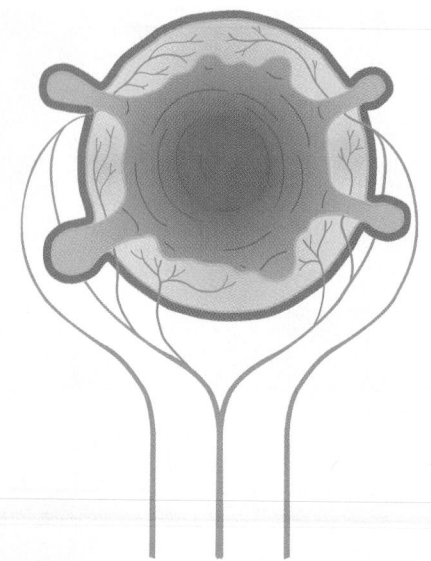

FIGURE 48-15. Pathogenesis of diverticular disease. Diverticula are herniations of the mucosa through the points of entry of blood vessels across the muscular wall. Because the diverticula are formed only by the mucosa rather than by the entire wall of the intestine, they are called false diverticula. Note that the diverticula form only between the mesenteric taeniae and each of the two lateral taeniae. Because there are no perforating vessels, diverticula do not form on the antimesenteric side of the colon.

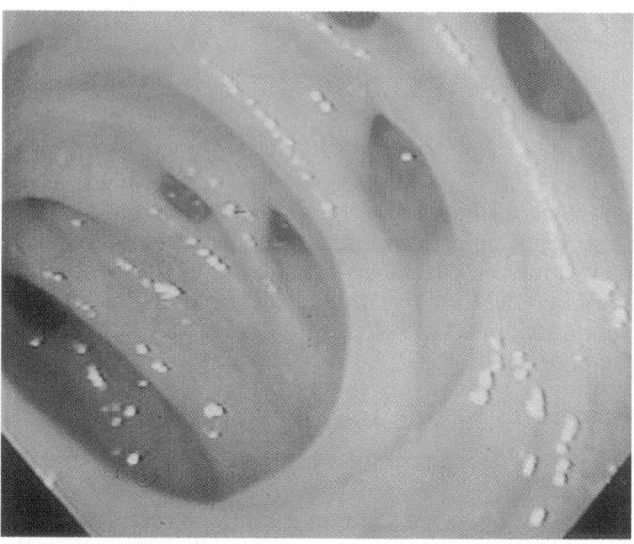

FIGURE 48-16. Colonoscopic view of diverticula.

have diverticula in 5% to 10% of patients with diverticulosis. Even in patients with diverticula involving the entire colon, the muscular thickening characteristic of the disease is usually confined to the sigmoid (Fig. 48-16).

The sigmoid colon, the most common site of diverticula formation, is also the segment of colon with the smallest luminal diameter. If the colonic lumen contains a large volume of fiber, the contractile pressure required to propel the feces forward is low. In such circumstances the colonic pressure in the sigmoid is only slightly above atmospheric pressure. However, with the decreased

amount of fiber typically provided by today's typical dietary regimens, there is decreased colonic luminal content, requiring generation of increased colonic pressures to propel the feces forward. Colonic pressures as high as 90 mm Hg can be generated by contraction of the narrow sigmoid colon. These high intraluminal pressures are thought to be responsible for the herniations of mucosa through the anatomically weak points in the colonic wall.

Diverticulitis

Diverticulitis is the result of a perforation of a colonic diverticulum. The term is somewhat of a misnomer because the disease is actually an extraluminal pericolic infection caused by the extravasation of feces through the perforated diverticulum. *Peridiverticulitis* would actually be the term to more appropriately describe the infectious process. Recognition that the infection is actually caused by a perforation of the colon, an event that is often controlled by the body's natural defenses, provides a basis for understanding the signs and symptoms of the disease as well as the rationale for determining appropriate diagnostic tests and treatment.

The sigmoid colon is the segment of large bowel with the highest incidence of diverticula, and it is by far the most frequent site for involvement with diverticulitis. Patients with diverticulitis usually complain of left lower quadrant abdominal pain that may radiate to the suprapubic area, left groin, or back. Alteration in bowel habit is a very common complaint, and fever, chills, and urinary urgency are common. This is an infectious, inflammatory process, and rectal bleeding is not usually associated with an attack of diverticulitis.

The physical findings are dependent on the site of perforation, the amount of contamination, and the presence or absence of secondary infection of adjacent organs. The most common physical finding is tenderness of the left lower abdomen. There may be voluntary guarding of the left abdominal musculature, and a tender mass in the left lower abdomen is suggestive of a phlegmon or abscess. Abdominal wall distention may be detected if there is associated ileus or small bowel obstruction secondary to the inflammatory process. A rectal or vaginal examination may reveal a tender fluctuant mass typical of a pelvic abscess.

Sigmoid diverticulitis should be distinguished from cancer of the rectosigmoid, although it is seldom necessary to establish the distinction on an emergency basis. However, the surgical approach to diverticulitis is significantly different than that required for a perforated sigmoid cancer, and if urgent operation is indicated an effort should be taken to exclude the diagnosis of cancer. A limited sigmoidoscopic examination may at times be helpful in such circumstances. However, air should not be insufflated through the endoscope because of distention of the colon and the possibility that increased colonic pressure could force more bacteria through the perforation into the peritoneal cavity. The sigmoidoscope can seldom be advanced beyond 12 cm in a patient with diverticulitis, and the examination is usually only useful to exclude a cancer of the rectum as a cause of the symptoms.

The diagnosis of diverticulitis can often be presumed with a fair degree of reliability by a careful history and physical examination, and it is reasonable to begin treatment with antibiotics on this evidence alone. However, if the diagnosis is in doubt, four diagnostic tests can be considered: computed tomography (CT) of the abdomen, magnetic resonance imaging (MRI), abdominal ultrasound, and water-soluble contrast enema. The CT and MRI provide essentially the same information and advantages. There has been more experience with CT, and this is considered by most surgeons to be the preferred test to confirm the suspected diagnosis of diverticulitis. It reliably reveals the location of the infection, the extent of the inflammatory process, the presence and location of an abscess, and the sympathetic involvement of other organs, with secondary complications such as ureteral obstruction or a fistula to the bladder. In addition, an abscess detected by CT may often be drained by a percutaneous approach with the aid of CT guidance.

Ultrasound of the abdomen offers many of the advantages of CT, including the possibility of percutaneous drainage of an abscess with ultrasound guidance. The selection between CT, MRI, and ultrasound examinations varies considerably among institutions, but all have been shown to be useful in establishing the diagnosis of diverticulitis, especially when an abscess has complicated the disease.

The use of a contrast enema in the evaluation of a patient suspected of having diverticulitis has diminished considerably because of the advantages offered by the noninvasive tests described earlier. An enema carries the risk of increasing the colonic pressure and causing further extravasation of feces through the perforated diverticulum. Some studies have shown an advantage of the contrast enema in distinguishing acute diverticulitis from perforated cancer, but many surgeons feel the risk associated with a contrast enema outweighs the potential gain. If a contrast enema is used, the contrast agent should be water soluble. Water-soluble contrast enemas do not carry the risk of barium-fecal peritonitis, but there is still a considerable risk of extravasation of contrast material from the colon that may aggravate the infection and spread the extent of the peritonitis.

Diverticulitis obviously presents in a variety of ways with a broad spectrum of severity, from a single episode of mild self-limited disease to repeated episodes that respond to antibiotics to fulminant complicated disease characterized by life-threatening sepsis. Hinchey and colleagues[43] have described a practical classification system that provides some organization of the broad clinical spectrum of the disease:

Stage I: Pericolic or mesenteric abscess
Stage II: Walled-off pelvic abscess
Stage III: Generalized purulent peritonitis
Stage IV: Generalized fecal peritonitis

Appropriate treatment obviously must be individualized based on the severity of the disease.

Uncomplicated Diverticulitis

Uncomplicated diverticulitis (disease not associated with free intraperitoneal perforation, fistula formation, or obstruction) can often be treated with antibiotics on an outpatient basis. If the patient has significant pain characteristic of localized peritonitis, hospitalization and intravenous antibiotics are indicated. The use of morphine should be avoided because of the increased intracolonic pressure associated with that drug; meperidine has been reported to decrease intraluminal pressure and is a more appropriate analgesic.

Patients with uncomplicated diverticulitis usually respond promptly to antibiotic treatment, with marked improvement in symptoms within 48 hours. After the symptoms have subsided for at least 3 weeks, investigative studies should be conducted to establish the presence of diverticula and to exclude cancer, which can mimic diverticulitis. The preferred test is a colonoscopic examination, which can directly visualize the colonic lumen even in the presence of numerous diverticula. A barium enema can demonstrate the extent of the diverticular disease, but a sigmoid cancer may be hidden by the numerous contrast-filled diverticula of the sigmoid colon, a fact that considerably diminishes the value of the contrast enema in the evaluation of the patient with diverticulosis (Fig. 48-17).

A first attack of uncomplicated diverticulitis that responds to antibiotic therapy is generally treated nonoperatively, with the introduction of a high-fiber diet. The chances of a second attack of diverticulitis are relatively low, less than 25%. The management of patients younger than 45 years of age affected by an attack of uncomplicated diverticulitis is somewhat controversial. Many

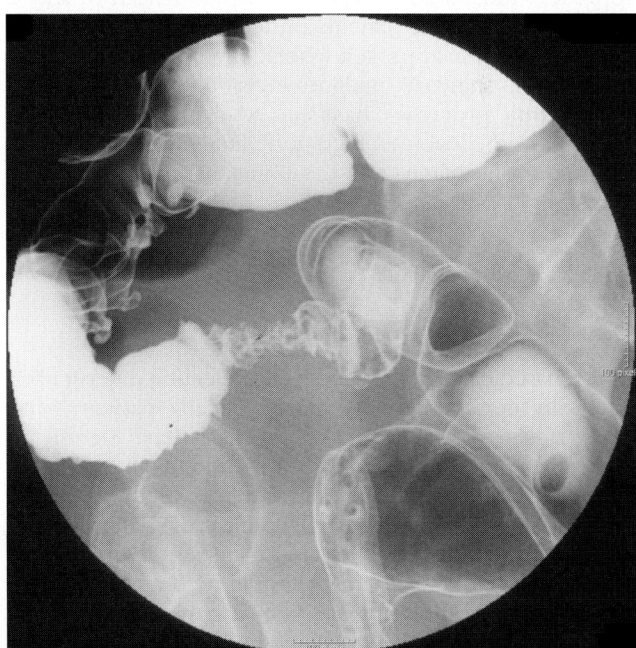

FIGURE 48-17. Barium enema in a patient with a previous attack of diverticulitis. Note stricture in sigmoid colon. Colonoscopy was necessary to exclude cancer.

surgeons have recommended an elective sigmoidectomy after recovery in young patients because the natural history of diverticulitis in the young is not well understood and there may be a high risk of recurrence of the disease over the expected long life span. However, Vignati and coworkers studied 40 patients younger than 50 years of age who were hospitalized with diverticulitis and followed for up to 9 years.[44] Two thirds of these patients did not require surgery during the follow-up period. These results are similar to the expectations for patients older than the age of 50, and the authors concluded that younger patients should be treated in the same manner as patients whose first attack of diverticulitis occurs after the age of 50.

If a patient suffers recurrent attacks of diverticulitis, surgical treatment should be considered. The chance of a third episode after a second bout of diverticulitis is greater than 50%, and the risk increases with each subsequent attack. Each uncomplicated attack of diverticulitis is treated with antibiotics to allow resolution of the acute infection. After the inflammation has resolved, usually 4 to 6 weeks after the episode, elective resection of the involved colon should be done.

Diverticulitis in the immunocompromised host represents a special challenge for the surgeon. We believe that elective sigmoidectomy after a single attack of diverticulitis should be considered in such patients because of their diminished ability to combat an infectious insult. There is some suggestion that medical therapy is less effective in these patients, resulting in an increased incidence of emergent surgery. Unfortunately, mortality rates after surgery are higher when compared with patients whose immune system is not compromised.

A growing trend in elective surgery for diverticular disease has been the utilization of a laparoscopic approach. Most studies reveal a hospital length of stay 2 to 3 days shorter for patients undergoing sigmoidectomy by a laparoscopic approach when compared with patients receiving a standard midline incision. A hand-assisted laparoscopic procedure has been advocated by some surgeons, who believe this technique facilitates the division of fused tissue planes and the blunt disruption of fistula tracts.

Complicated Diverticulitis

Abscess

As discussed earlier, an abscess complicating diverticulitis is usually confined to the pelvis. Usually patients with pelvic abscesses caused by diverticulitis have significant pain, fever, and leukocytosis. The abdominal, pelvic, or rectal examinations may detect a tender, fluctuant mass, and CT, MRI, or ultrasound will confirm the diagnosis and location of the abscess. Unless the abscess is quite small (less than 2 cm in diameter) it should be drained, and the preferred method of drainage is by a percutaneous route guided by CT or ultrasound. Occasionally, a pelvic abscess can be drained into the rectum through a transanal approach. These methods of drainage are highly preferable to a transabdominal approach by laparotomy, which

risks spreading the contents of the abscess throughout the peritoneal cavity (Fig. 48-18).

Adequate drainage of the abscess, accompanied by administration of intravenous antibiotics, usually results in a rapid clinical improvement. Although a fistula may result from the sigmoid colon to the insertion site of the percutaneous catheter that provided drainage, this can be easily handled at the time of elective surgery when the intense intra-abdominal infection has subsided.

Elective surgery should be offered after the patient has completely recovered from the infection, usually about 6 weeks following the drainage of the abscess. At that time it is usually feasible to excise the diseased sigmoid colon and fashion an anastomosis between the descending colon and rectum, thus avoiding a colostomy. It is essential to remove all of the colon that is abnormally thickened and to incorporate rectum that is not inflamed or thickened into the distal component of the anastomosis. A major cause of recurrent diverticulitis after sigmoidectomy is failure to completely remove the entire abnormally thickened bowel that is associated with this disease. If the distal sigmoid colon is not resected, the rate of recurrent diverticulitis is unnecessarily elevated. Benn and colleagues found the rate of recurrent diverticulitis to be 12% if the distal sigmoid was not resected, compared with 6% if the anastomosis was to the top of the rectum.[45] It is seldom necessary to mobilize the rectum farther than 2 cm below the sacral promontory to obtain normal bowel for a satisfactory anastomosis. Although diverticula may be present throughout the colon, it is not necessary to excise the entire colon in such circumstances; only the colon that is thickened and brittle (usually the entire sigmoid) need be resected.

Fistula

A fistula between the sigmoid colon and the skin (which may result from percutaneous drainage of an abscess),

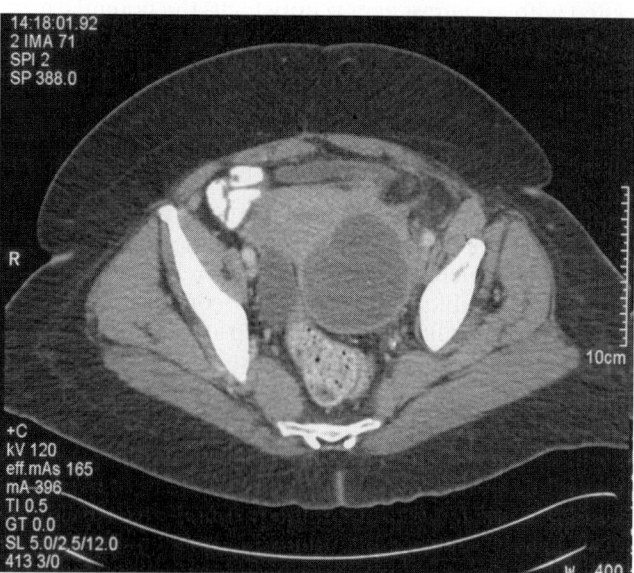

FIGURE 48-18. CT scan of pelvis shows diverticulitis with abscess.

bladder, vagina, or small bowel is a relatively frequent complication of diverticulitis. Such a fistula commonly forms when an abscess is either drained or involves an adjacent organ or the skin. The source of the infection (the perforated diverticulum) continues to supply the fistula, and cure will not be achieved until the source is eradicated by excising the diseased sigmoid colon. Diverticulitis is a more common cause of a fistula between the colon and bladder than is Crohn's disease or cancer. Sigmoid vesical fistulas are more common in men than women, because the uterus prevents the sigmoid from adhering to the bladder in women. Women with sigmoid fistulas have usually had a prior hysterectomy.

Symptoms of a sigmoid-vesical fistula include pneumaturia (with the passage of air from the urethra classically noted at the end of micturition), fecaluria, and recurring urinary tract infections. The fistula may cause significant urosepsis in men, with prostatic hypertrophy causing a relative obstruction of the distal urinary tract. The most reliable test to confirm the suspicion of a fistula between the intestine and the bladder is CT, which may demonstrate air in the bladder (Fig. 48-19). A barium enema will fail to reveal a fistula half of the time, and an intravenous pyelogram is even less accurate. Cystoscopy usually reveals cystitis and bullous edema at the site of the fistula, but the test is helpful to exclude cancer (colon or bladder) as the cause of the fistula.

Initial treatment of any fistula caused by diverticulitis is to control the infection and reduce the associated inflammation. A fistula arising from the colon is rarely a cause for emergency surgery; in fact, the patient's condition is often improved when the drainage of an abscess results in the formation of a fistula. Antibiotics should be administered to reduce the adjacent cellulitis, and diagnostic steps should be taken to confirm the cause of the fistula before a definitive operation is undertaken. A colonoscopy should be done to examine the sigmoid mucosa and exclude colon cancer (or Crohn's disease) as the cause of the fistula. Every effort should be made to rule out cancer, because the operation for a sigmoid-vesical fistula secondary to sigmoid cancer requires en bloc excision of the involved organs, a more extensive operation than is required to interrupt the nonmalignant fistula and excise the diseased (but benign) sigmoid colon.

Fistulas caused by diverticulitis can usually be treated by a one-stage operation, taking down the fistula and excising the sigmoid colon, then fashioning an anastomosis between the descending colon and the rectum. The secondary organs involved (usually the bladder) will heal once the source of the infection, the sigmoid colon, is removed. The bladder defect is usually so small that no closure is necessary, and healing will occur if the bladder is drained with a Foley catheter or suprapubic cystostomy for 7 days after the operation. Larger bladder openings may require suture closure with absorbable (chromic) sutures combined with drainage. If there is significant inflammation in the abdomen and pelvis, despite a "cooling off" period, the use of ureteral stents placed preoperatively can facilitate identification of the ureters and minimize inadvertent ureteral injury. A technique of early identification of the ureter and proximal to distal dissection of the sigmoid colon facilitates the resection when a phlegmon caused by diverticulitis obliterates the normal anatomy.

Generalized Peritonitis

Generalized peritonitis caused by diverticulitis can be caused in two ways: (1) a diverticulum may perforate into the peritoneal cavity and the perforation is not sealed by the body's normal defenses or (2) an abscess that is initially localized expands and suddenly bursts into the unprotected peritoneal cavity. In the former instance the peritoneal cavity is contaminated with feces; in the latter, contamination is from pus containing enteric bacteria. In either situation, the result is an overwhelming infection that requires immediate operative intervention. Fortunately, both of these circumstances are relatively rare.

Patients with generalized peritonitis caused by a perforated diverticulum exhibit diffuse abdominal tenderness, with voluntary and involuntary guarding over the entire abdomen. Abdominal radiographs or CT scans may reveal intraperitoneal free air, but the absence of extraintestinal air does not exclude the diagnosis. Signs of generalized sepsis include an elevated white blood cell count, fever, tachycardia, and hypotension. Immediate celiotomy is mandatory to identify and excise the segment of colon containing the perforation. Under such circumstances it is not safe to restore intestinal continuity because of the high likelihood that an intestinal anastomosis will not heal when fashioned in such a hostile infectious environment. The proper operation in this situation is to resect the diseased sigmoid colon, construct a colostomy using noninflamed descending colon, and suture the divided end of the rectum closed. This procedure is called *Hartmann's operation,* after Henri Hartmann, the French surgeon who described this technique in 1921. Hartmann's operation, although initially described for the treatment of cancer, is the most common technique for emergency operations required for control of infection secondary to diverticulitis.

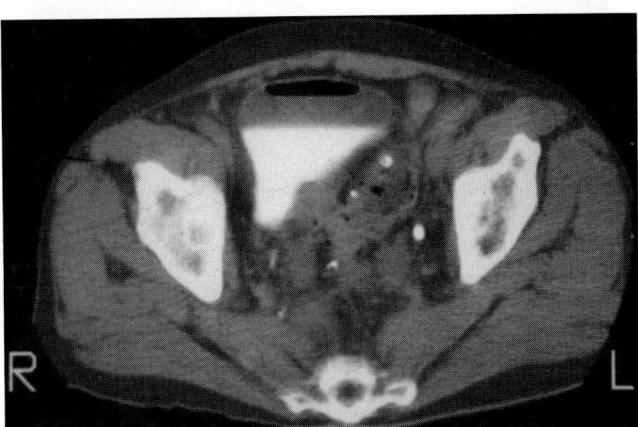

FIGURE 48-19. CT scan of pelvis. The patient has diverticulitis, and air in the bladder indicates a fistula between the sigmoid and the bladder.

Eliminating the source of infection by excising the perforated sigmoid colon, establishing diversion of the feces with a colostomy, and controlling the peritoneal infection by irrigating the peritoneal cavity and administering intravenous antibiotics, along with appropriate generalized and nutritional support, should result in resolution of the infection. When the patient has recovered completely from the illness, usually after a period of at least 10 weeks, taking down the colostomy and fashioning an anastomosis between the descending colon and the rectum will restore intestinal continuity.

COLONIC VOLVULUS

Volvulus describes the condition in which the bowel becomes twisted on its mesenteric axis, a situation that results in partial or complete obstruction of the bowel lumen and a variable degree of impairment of its blood supply. The condition most commonly affects the colon. Although colonic volvulus is relatively rare in the United States, ranking behind cancer and diverticulitis, it is responsible for approximately 5% of cases of large bowel obstruction. However, in Russia volvulus accounts for approximately half of all causes of colonic obstruction, and it is a common cause of colonic obstruction in Iran, India, and some parts of Africa.

Any portion of the large bowel can torse if that segment is attached to a long and floppy mesentery that is fixed to the retroperitoneum by a narrow base of origin. However, the mesenteric anatomy is such that volvulus is most common in the sigmoid colon, with less frequent occurrences involving the right colon and terminal ileum (usually referred to as cecal volvulus), the cecum alone (the condition permitted by a highly mobile cecum, called a cecal bascule, that is mobile in a caudad to cephalad direction), and, most rarely, the transverse colon.

Sigmoid volvulus accounts for two thirds to three fourths of all cases of colonic volvulus. The condition is permitted by an elongated segment of bowel accompanied by a lengthy mesentery with a very narrow parietal attachment, a situation that allows the two ends of the mobile segment to come close together and twist about the narrow mesenteric base. Associated factors include chronic constipation and aging, with the average age at presentation being in the seventh to eighth decade of life. There is an increased incidence of the condition in institutionalized patients afflicted with neuropsychiatric conditions and treated with psychotropic drugs. These medications may predispose to volvulus by affecting intestinal motility. The increased incidence of volvulus in third world countries has been attributed to a diet high in fiber and vegetables.

Patients with sigmoid volvulus may present as acute or subacute intestinal obstruction with signs and symptoms indistinguishable from those caused by cancer of the distal colon. There is usually a sudden onset of severe abdominal pain, vomiting, and obstipation. The abdomen is usually markedly distended and tympanitic, with the distention often more dramatic than would be associated with other causes of obstruction. There is always the

possibility that the condition can be associated with ischemia caused either by mural ischemia associated with the increased tension of the distended bowel wall or by arterial occlusion caused by torsion of the mesenteric arterial supply; therefore, severe abdominal pain, rebound tenderness, and tachycardia are ominous signs.

There may be a history of previous episodes of acute volvulus that spontaneously resolved, and in such circumstances marked abdominal distention may occur with minimal tenderness.

The radiographic findings are often dramatic and enable prompt diagnosis and treatment (Fig. 48-20). They usually reveal a markedly dilated sigmoid colon with the appearance of a "bent inner tube" with its apex in the right upper quadrant. An air-fluid level may be seen in the dilated loop of colon, and gas is usually absent from the rectum. CT reveals a characteristic mesenteric whirl, although the diagnosis can usually be established on the basis of the clinical presentation and the plain film of the abdomen (Fig. 48-21). A contrast enema typically demonstrates the point of obstruction with the pathognomonic "bird's beak" deformity revealing the obstructing twist that obstructs the sigmoid lumen (Fig. 48-22).

Treatment of the sigmoid volvulus begins with appropriate resuscitation, and in most cases involves nonoperative decompression. Decompression relieves the acute problem and allows resection as an elective procedure that can be accomplished with reduced morbidity and mortality. Patients with signs of colonic necrosis are not eligible for nonoperative decompression.

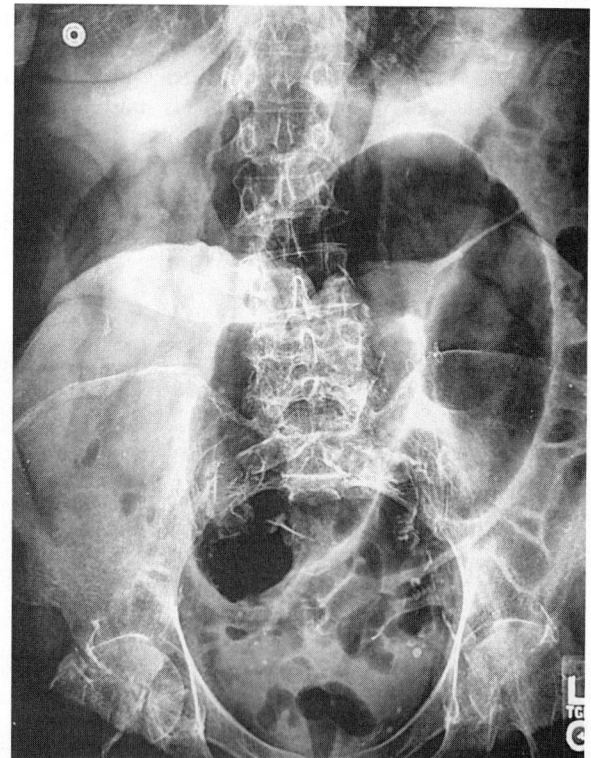

FIGURE 48-20.   Plain film of sigmoid volvulus. Note appearance of "bent inner tube." (Courtesy of Dina F. Caroline, M.D., Ph.D., Temple University Hospital.)

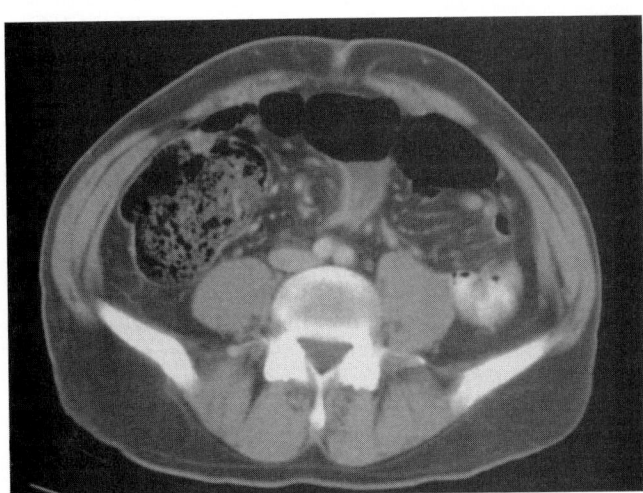

FIGURE 48-21. CT of abdomen in patient with sigmoid volvulus. Note characteristic whirl in mesentery.

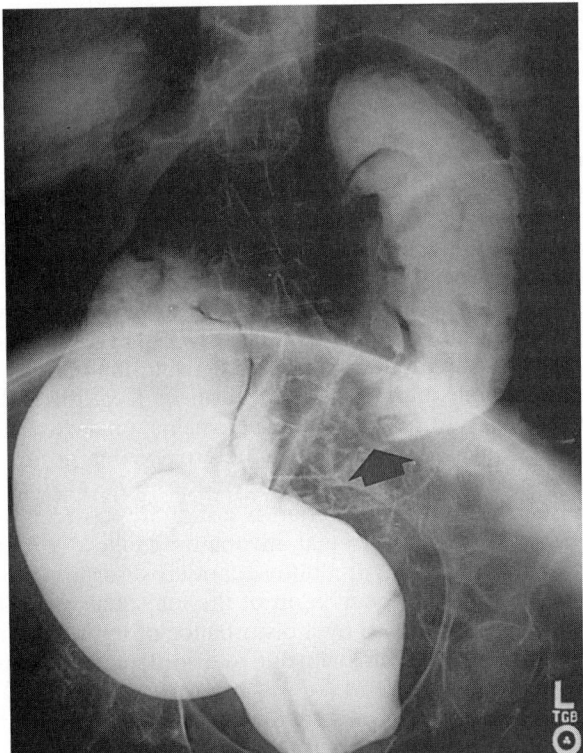

FIGURE 48-22. Barium enema of sigmoid volvulus. Contrast agent and air fills rectum and distal sigmoid colon. The contrast agent stops abruptly at the point of torsion. (Courtesy of Dina F. Caroline, M.D., Ph.D., Temple University Hospital.)

Decompression can occur with placement of a rectal tube through a proctoscope or with the use of a colonoscope. Often, a soft rectal tube can be inserted under direct vision through the twist of the volvulus while the patient is in the emergency department. Decompression results in a sudden gush of gas and fluid, with a decrease in the abdominal distention. The reduction should be

confirmed with an abdominal radiograph. The rectal tube should be taped to the thigh and left in place for 1 or 2 days to allow continued decompression and to prevent immediate recurrence of the volvulus. The bowel can then be cleansed with cathartics and a complete colonoscopic examination performed. If a rectal tube cannot be passed as described, detorsion of the volvulus with the colonoscope should be attempted. If detorsion of the volvulus cannot be accomplished with either a rectal tube or colonoscope, laparotomy with resection of the sigmoid colon (Hartmann's operation) is required.

Even if detorsion of the sigmoid is successful, elective sigmoid resection is indicated in most cases because of the extremely high recurrence rate (which approaches 50%). The operation can be conducted through a small left lower quadrant incision or by a laparoscopic approach. Because the elongated colon and mesentery require virtually no mobilization, resection with primary anastomosis is easily accomplished. Colonoscopy should be performed before elective resection to exclude an associated neoplasm.

Although the term *cecal volvulus* is ingrained in the literature, true volvulus of the cecum probably never occurs. There is a well-recognized condition in which the cecum folds in a cephalad direction anteriorly over a fixed ascending colon. Although gangrene may develop, this is exceedingly rare because there is not major vessel obstruction. This "cecal bascule" commonly causes intermittent bouts of abdominal pain as the mobile cecum permits intermittent episodes of isolated cecal obstruction that are spontaneously relieved as the cecum falls back into its normal position.

The condition commonly referred to as cecal volvulus is actually a cecocolic volvulus and consists of an axial rotation of the terminal ileum, cecum, and ascending colon with concomitant twisting of the associated mesentery. This is a relatively rare condition, accounting for less than 2% of all cases of adult intestinal obstruction and approximately a fourth of all cases of colonic volvulus in the United States. Cecocolic volvulus is possible because of a lack of fixation of the cecum to the retroperitoneum. Studies on cadavers have shown that between 11% and 22% of people have a right colon that is sufficiently mobile to allow a volvulus to occur. Factors that have been implicated in causing a cecal volvulus include previous surgery, pregnancy, malrotation, and obstructing lesions of the left colon. Cecocolic volvulus is somewhat more common in women, whereas sigmoid volvulus occurs with equal frequency in both sexes. Cecocolic volvulus affects a younger age group (most common in the late 50s) compared with sigmoid volvulus.

The typical presentation of patients with cecocolic volvulus is the sudden onset of abdominal pain and distention. In the early phases of a cecocolic volvulus, the pain is mild or moderate in intensity. If the condition is not relieved and ischemia occurs, the pain increases significantly. Physical examination my reveal asymmetrical distention of the abdomen, with a tympanitic mass palpable in either the left upper quadrant or mid abdomen. Plain radiographs of the abdomen reveal a dilated cecum that is usually displaced to the left side of the abdomen.

The distended cecum usually assumes a gas-filled "comma" shape, the concavity of which faces inferiorly and to the right. Occasionally the distended cecum will appear as a circular shape with a narrow, triangular density pointing superiorly and to the right. Haustral markings in the distended loop indicate that the dilated bowel is colon. The torsion results in obstruction of the small bowel, and the radiographic pattern of dilated small intestine can cause diagnostic difficulty.

Although there have been reports of detorsion of ceco-colic volvulus with a colonoscope, most cases will require operation to correct the volvulus and prevent ischemia. If ischemia has already occurred, immediate operation is obviously required. Contrast enema is helpful to confirm the diagnosis and to exclude a carcinoma of the distal bowel as a precipitating cause of the volvulus (Fig. 48-23).

Right colectomy is the procedure of choice. Primary anastomosis is usually preferred unless the volvulus has resulted in frankly gangrenous bowel, when resection of the gangrenous bowel with ileostomy is a safer approach. There have been many reports of correcting cecocolic volvulus with cecopexy, which should avoid the complication associated with an anastomosis. However, the operation to provide fixation of the cecum is actually quite extensive, entailing elevating and attaching a flap of peritoneum over the surface of the cecum and ascending colon. The recurrence rates are high with cecopexy, and

right colectomy remains the procedure of choice for most surgeons.

Volvulus of the transverse colon is extremely rare and tends to be associated with other abnormalities, such as congenital bands, distal obstructing lesions, and pregnancy. Clinical features are indistinguishable from other causes of large bowel obstruction. Radiologic examination is not particularly useful, because many cases are misdiagnosed as sigmoid volvulus. A contrast study may show a "bird's beak" deformity indicating a volvulus. In such cases colonoscopic reduction may result in detorsion and relief of obstruction. Elective resection should follow to prevent recurrence.

PSEUDO-OBSTRUCTION

Pseudo-obstruction of the colon (also called Ogilvie's syndrome, after its description by Sir William Heneage Ogilvie in 1948) describes the condition of distention of the colon, with signs and symptoms of colonic obstruction, in the absence of an actual physical cause of the obstruction. Ogilvie described two patients with clinical features of colonic obstruction despite a normal barium enema. Both patients underwent laparotomy for the condition, neither had mechanical obstruction, but both had unsuspected malignant disease involving the area of the celiac axis and semilunar ganglion. The cause of the dilatation was attributed to the malignant infiltration of the sympathetic ganglia. Subsequently there have been numerous descriptions of cases of colonic distention in the absence of mechanical obstruction and without malignant involvement of the visceral autonomic nerves. Very few cases of pseudo-obstruction have malignant infiltration of the autonomic nerves as the cause; in fact, the exact pathogenesis of the syndrome remains unknown and it has been associated with a heterogeneous group of conditions.

Primary pseudo-obstruction is a motility disorder that is either a familial visceral myopathy (hollow visceral myopathy syndrome) or a diffuse motility disorder involving the autonomic innervation of the intestinal wall. The latter may be modified by a disturbance of intestinal hormones or may be principally due to disordered autonomic innervation.

Secondary pseudo-obstruction is more common and has been associated with neuroleptic medications, opiates, severe metabolic illness, myxedema, diabetes mellitus, uremia, hyperparathyroidism, lupus, scleroderma, Parkinson's disease, and traumatic retroperitoneal hematomas. One mechanism thought to play a role in the pathogenesis is sympathetic overactivity overriding the parasympathetic system. Indirect support for this theory has been derived from the success in treating the syndrome with neostigmine, a parasympathomimetic agent. Further support comes from reports of immediate resolution of the syndrome after administration of an epidural anesthetic that provides sympathetic blockade.

Pseudo-obstruction may present in acute or chronic forms. The acute variety most commonly affects patients with chronic renal, respiratory, cerebral, or cardiovascu-

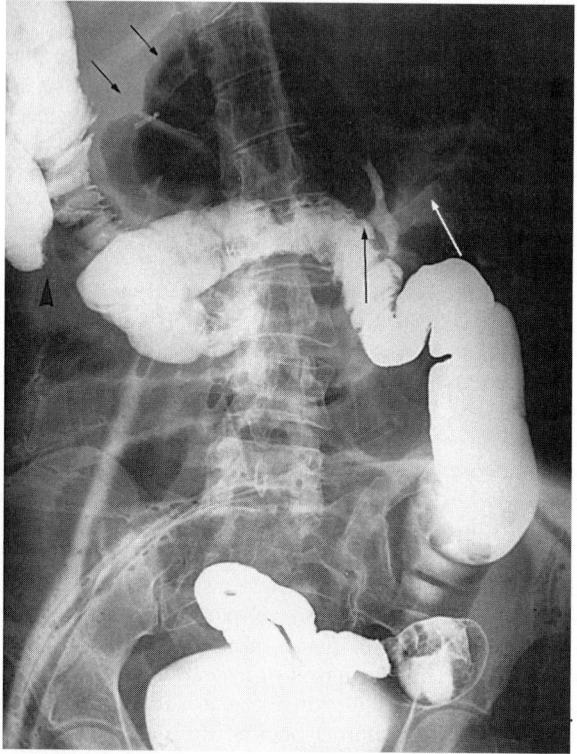

FIGURE 48-23.   Barium enema in patient with cecal volvulus. The contrast stops abruptly at the proximal end of the hepatic flexure *(arrowhead)*. The dilated, air-filled cecum crosses the midline of the abdomen toward the left upper quadrant *(arrows)*. (Courtesy of Dina F. Caroline, M.D., Ph.D., Temple University Hospital.)

lar disease. It usually involves only the colon, whereas the chronic form affects other parts of the gastrointestinal tract, usually presents as bouts of subacute and partial intestinal obstruction, and tends to periodically recur.

Acute colonic pseudo-obstruction should be suspected when a medically ill patient suddenly develops abdominal distention. The abdomen is tympanitic and usually nontender, and bowel sounds are usually present. Plain abdominal radiographs reveal a distended colon, with the right and transverse segments tending to be most dramatically affected. The radiologic appearance is one of large bowel obstruction.

The most useful investigation is a water-soluble contrast enema that should be performed in all patients in whom the diagnosis is suspected, provided their condition is stable enough to warrant the procedure. The contrast enema can reliably differentiate between mechanical obstruction and pseudo-obstruction, a differentiation that is essential to guide appropriate therapy.

Colonoscopy is the alternative diagnostic investigation for pseudo-obstruction and has the attractive advantage that it can be used for treatment. However, at the present time the water-soluble contrast enema is generally the preferred initial test.

Once the diagnosis of acute pseudo-obstruction is suspected, treatment should accompany the diagnostic evaluation. Initial treatment includes nasogastric decompression, replacement of extracellular fluid deficits, and correction of electrolyte abnormalities. All medications that inhibit bowel motility, such as opiates, should be discontinued. Patient response is monitored by serial abdominal examinations and radiographs. Most patients will improve with this regimen. Until the mid-1990s the treatment usually utilized when the colonic distention failed to resolve with supportive measures was colonoscopic decompression. While this approach was generally successful, it required skilled personnel and equipment and carried the risk of colonic perforation from both instrument trauma and insufflation. In addition, the procedure often had to be repeated because of recurrence of the colonic distention.

At the present time the trend has been to treat the condition with neostigmine, a parasympathomimetic agent. It is obviously imperative that mechanical obstruction be excluded (either by water-soluble contrast enema or colonoscopy) before the administration of neostigmine, or the subsequent high pressures generated in the colon against a distal obstruction could cause colonic perforation.

Neostigmine enhances parasympathetic activity by competing with acetylcholine for acetylcholinesterase-binding sites. In the treatment of colonic pseudo-obstruction, 2.5 mg of neostigmine is given intravenously over 3 minutes. The resolution of the condition is indicated within less than 10 minutes of administration of the drug, by the passage of stool and flatus by the patient. The recurrence rates after the administration of neostigmine appear to be far lower than those associated with colonoscopic decompression. Satisfactory decompression of large-bowel distention was achieved in 11 of 12 patients in a study reported in 1995.[46] A study by Trevisani and colleagues in 2000 reported success with a single administration of neostigmine in 26 of 28 patients.[47]

A significant side effect of neostigmine is bradycardia, and all patients must be monitored by telemetry during administration of the drug. Atropine must be immediately available, and patients with significant cardiac disease are not candidates for this treatment.

COLONIC INFLAMMATORY BOWEL DISEASE

Inflammatory bowel disease (IBD) is the term used to describe the two enigmatic disease processes of ulcerative colitis and Crohn's disease. The diseases are related by virtue of having an unknown etiology, common clinical symptoms, and overlapping histologic features. The medical and surgical management of the two entities is quite different, and hence they will be discussed separately.

Ulcerative Colitis

Ulcerative colitis (UC) is a nonspecific inflammatory disease involving the mucosa of the colon and rectum. There is no specific medical cure, and approximately one third of patients with UC undergo operative treatment. This is caused by increasing intractability, disease complications, and the premalignant nature of the disease. Removal of the colon and rectum cures ulcerative colitis, thus all medical treatments should be compared with surgery. Additionally, surgery prevents the possibility for developing colorectal malignancy, which increases with the duration of disease. Moreover, surgery eliminates the chronic need for anti-inflammatory drugs such as corticosteroids and immunosuppressives with adverse effects often exceeding surgical complications. Finally, regardless of whether a permanent ileostomy or a sphincter-saving operation is performed, a satisfactory or good result is observed in approximately 90% of patients.[48]

Epidemiology, Etiology, and Pathogenesis

The incidence of UC varies throughout the world and is more common in developed countries when compared with developing countries. The reasons for this are unclear but are thought to be related, in part, to differences in dietary intake. The incidence of UC has remained relatively constant during the past two decades. In the United States, it occurs in 5 to 6/100,000 population, with a prevalence between 50 and 70 cases/100,000/yr. There is a relatively equal distribution between genders, and it occurs at all ages with peak onsets between the second and fourth decades. UC is more common in Jewish than in non-Jewish people and in whites than in nonwhites.

The specific cause of UC is unknown. Current hypotheses suggest that it probably results from a combination of factors, leading to dysfunctional immunoregulation in the intestinal wall. These factors include dietary intake, genetic predisposition, and an imbalance between the normally controlled states of regulated inflammation in the intestinal wall.[49] Factors that have been hypothesized to predispose to IBD include a low-fiber diet, food allergies, food additives, infectious agents, and shortened duration of breast feedings. Surprisingly, smokers, but not former smokers, have approximately half the risk of developing UC than nonsmokers. In contrast, smokers have approximately a twofold increased risk of developing Crohn's disease 5 to 15 years after the initiation of smoking than nonsmokers.[50] Family history is the most consistent risk factor for IBD. Parent-child and sibling relationships are far more common than relationships involving more distant relatives. Ulcerative colitis probands tend to have more relatives diagnosed with UC, and Crohn's disease probands have more relatives with Crohn's disease. The genetic predisposition for UC is not inherited in a classic mendelian pattern and is probably influenced by additional social factors as discussed previously.

Two genetic abnormalities found to be associated with UC are variations in DNA repair genes and class II major histocompatibility complex genes. Patients with UC display specific alleles of group HLA and DR2 (gene HLA-DRB1). There is an association between certain alleles and the clinical form of the disease. The DR1501 allele is associated with a more benign course, whereas the DR1502 is associated with severe forms of the disease.

The earliest recognizable abnormality that appears to initiate the symptoms associated with UC is the influx of neutrophils into the lamina propria. Seventy-five percent of UC patients exhibit perinuclear antineutrophil cytoplasmic antibodies (p-ANCA); however, the presence of p-ANCA does not correlate with the activity or extent of colitis and is most likely an epiphenomenon. The presence of p-ANCA has been used as a diagnostic test to help differentiate UC from Crohn's disease.

Patients with UC often have elevated levels of interleukin (IL)-4, IL-5, IL-6, IL-10, and IL-13, an observation that supports the inflammatory etiology of the disease. Inflammatory mechanisms such as cytokine mediation do not appear to be unique to IBD. Moreover, extensive immunologic reviews emphasize that UC is not an autoimmune disease. Despite these observations, the immune system remains an important mediator of inflammation in chronic UC. Clinically, the severity of the disease correlates with the presence of immune cells in the inflamed intestine. Additionally, extraintestinal manifestations resemble immune complex disorders. Finally, immunosuppressive drugs that inhibit the release of soluble activation factors are often effective in controlling the disease.

Pathologic Features

There are distinct gross and microscopic features that are characteristic of UC. Whereas some of these features may be found in Crohn's disease, they are more prevalent in UC.

Gross Appearance

The most common disease pattern in UC is inflammation of the rectal mucosa that extends to a variable distance into the more proximal colon. Characteristically, the disease is more severe in the rectum than in more proximal segments of the colon. An exception to this is patients who have been treated with corticosteroid enemas, which have a greater beneficial effect on the rectum than on the more proximal colon. The typical gross appearance is a granular, swollen, and friable mucosa (Fig. 48-24). In extensive disease there may be patchy full-thickness ulcerations of the mucosa. In long-standing active colitis the mucosa may be severely denuded. Additionally, endoscopic examination may reveal multiple polyps that are manifestations of regeneration of inflamed mucosa. These lesions are known as "pseudo-polyps" or "inflammatory polyps" (Fig. 48-25).

UC, as mentioned earlier, always involves the rectum but is often limited to the left colon; there is frequently a

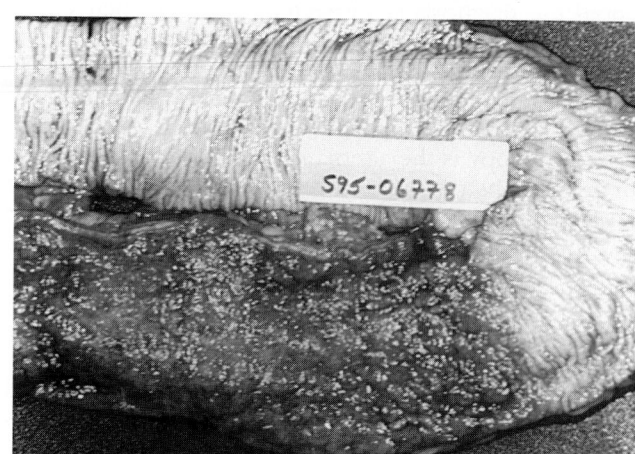

FIGURE 48-24. Ulcerative colitis, macroscopic appearance of left-sided colitis. The left side of the colon displays continuous disease manifested as erythema and granularity of the mucosal surface, whereas the right colon appears normal. (Courtesy of M. Markowitz Haber, M.D., Hahnemann University Hospital.)

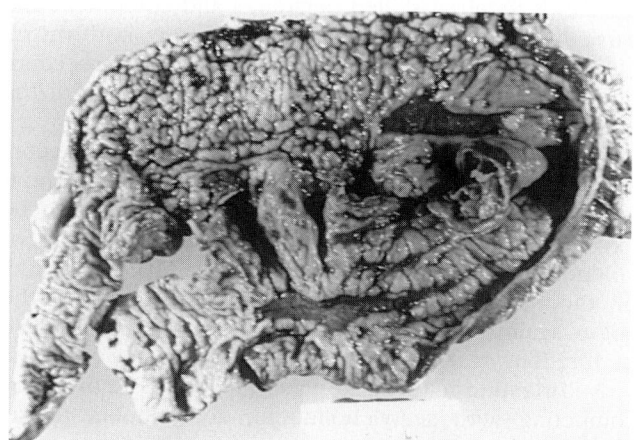

FIGURE 48-25. Ulcerative colitis, macroscopic appearance of pancolitis. Because the entire colon is involved with inflammatory changes, this specimen represents a case of universal colitis or pancolitis. The distal colon shows a large longitudinal ulcer with heaped-up adjacent mucosa. In the midportion of the colon, the mucosa is relatively flat and featureless. In the right side of the colon, there are multiple projections, or pseudopolyps, creating a cobblestone appearance. The ileocecal valve is edematous and irregular, whereas the terminal ileum is spared. (Courtesy of M. Markowitz Haber, M.D., Hahnemann University Hospital.)

demarcation of the proximal margin at the splenic flexure. In more extensive disease, patients may have complete involvement of the colon or pancolitis. Regardless of the extent of involvement, a diagnostic characteristic of UC is the continuous, uninterrupted inflammation of the mucosa beginning at the distal rectum and extending proximally to a variable distance. This is distinctively different from Crohn's colitis, which often involves distinct and separate segments of colonic inflammation. A normal segment of colon interspersed between inflamed segments (skipped area) is characteristic of Crohn's disease and is an important diagnostic aid in distinguishing UC from Crohn's disease.

Strictures occur in 5% to 12% of patients with long-standing UC. Benign strictures are usually caused by hypertrophy of the muscularis mucosa. A common clinical dictum is that a stricture in the presence of UC is malignant until proved otherwise. Three important features are more diagnostic of malignant strictures when compared with benign strictures: (1) appearance late in the course of the disease (60% after 20 years of disease vs. 0% before 10 years of disease), (2) location proximal to the splenic flexure (86%), and (3) cause of large bowel obstruction (much more commonly associated with malignancy) (Fig. 48-26).

Microscopic Features

Inflammation in UC is confined to the mucosal and submucosal layers of the colon. This is an important contrast to Crohn's disease, which is characterized by transmural inflammation of the intestine (Table 48-1). An important

TABLE 48-1. Comparisons of Ulcerative Colitis and Crohn's Colitis

	Ulcerative Colitis	Crohn's Colitis
Gross Appearance		
Thickened wall	0	4+
Thickened mesentery	0	3+
Serosal "fat wrapping"	0	4+
Segmental disease	0	4+
Microscopic Appearance		
Transmural	0	4+
Lymphoid aggregates	0	4+
Granulomas	0	3+
Clinical Features		
Bleeding per rectum	3+	1+
Diarrhea	3+	3+
Obstructive symptoms	1+	3+
Anal/perianal disease	Rare	4+
Risk of cancer	2+	3+
Small bowel disease	0	4+
Colonoscopic Features		
Distribution	Continuous	Discontinuous
Rectal disease	4+	1+
Friability	4+	1+
Aphthous ulcers	0	4+
Deep longitudinal ulcers	0	4+
Cobblestoning	0	4+
Pseudopolyps	2+	2+
Operative Treatment		
Total proctocolectomy	Curative	Combined disease: colon + rectum
Segmental resection	Rare	Absence of anorectal disease
Ileal pouch	Preferred by most patients	Contraindicated
Complications		
Postoperative recurrence	0	4+
Fistulas	Rare	4+
Sclerosing cholangitis	1+	Rare
Cholelithiasis	0	2+
Nephrolithiasis	0	2+

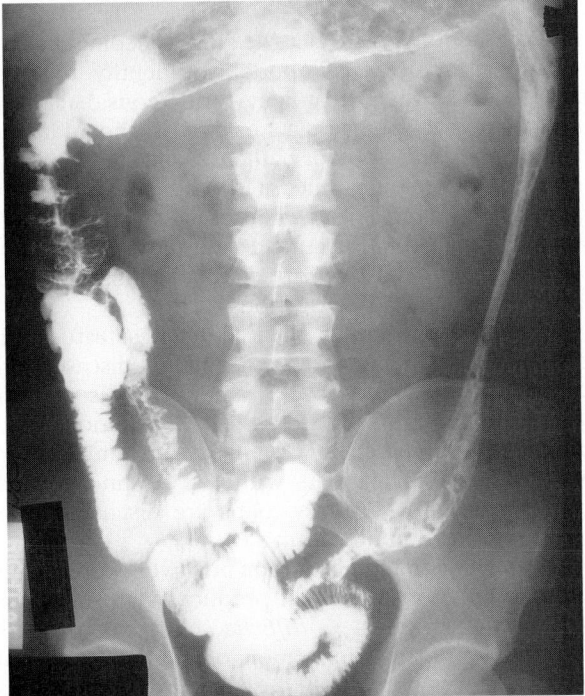

FIGURE 48-26. Stricture in chronic ulcerative colitis. Colonoscopy revealed chronic inflammation but no dysplasia or cancer.

microscopic feature of UC is the infiltration of polymorphonucleocytes and round cells into the crypts of Lieberkühn at the base of the mucosa with multiple crypt abscesses (Fig. 48-27). The marked vascular engorgement accounts for the propensity for rectal bleeding. The number of goblet cells in the crypts is diminished. With more advanced disease there is a coalescence of crypt abscesses and desquamation of overlying cells to form an ulcer that is limited to the mucosa and submucosa. These findings are not exclusive to UC and may be seen in infectious colitis; therefore, it is important to rule out infectious colitis when making the diagnosis of UC.

Confinement of the inflammation to the inner layers of the bowel wall is an important characteristic of UC. However, with the extensive inflammation characteristic of toxic megacolon the full thickness of the bowel wall may be involved, and the process may progress to necrosis and perforation of the colon.

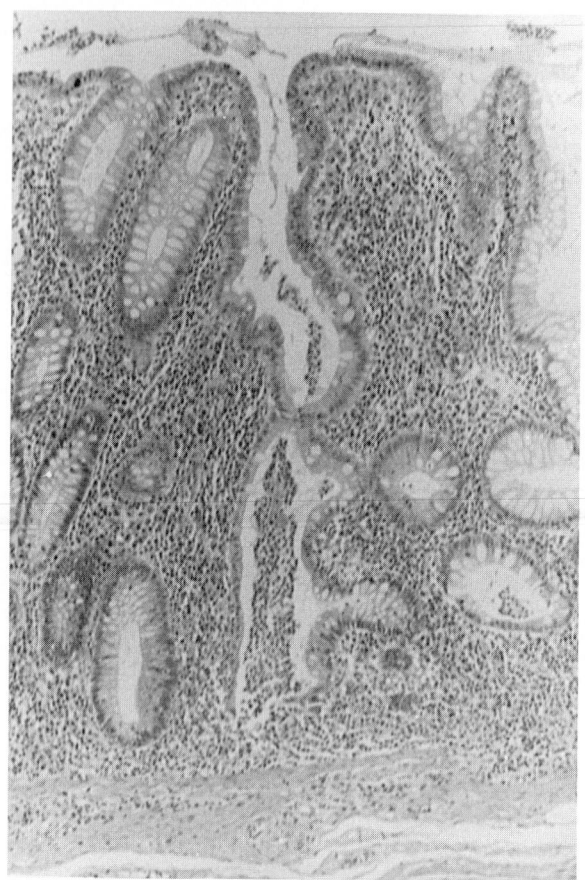

FIGURE 48-27. Active ulcerative colitis. The glands are irregular with branching, and, focally, the long axis of the gland is horizontal rather than perpendicular. A central crypt abscess is present. There are increased numbers of chronic inflammatory cells throughout the lamina propria. (Courtesy of M. Markowitz Haber, M.D., Hahnemann University Hospital.)

Clinical Findings

Diarrhea and rectal bleeding are the most common symptoms of UC. The extent of diarrhea is frequently associated with the severity of the disease and may occur hourly. Nocturnal diarrhea is an ominous symptom and is frequently due to significant disease. There is often an increased frequency of small, mucoid bowel movements with blood. The presence of only blood and mucus per rectum indicates severe disease. Loss of body weight and anemia are frequent findings in patients with chronic UC. Massive bleeding with hypovolemic shock is unusual.

Physical findings reflect the severity of the disease. Abdominal tenderness, particularly on the left side, is common. Abdominal distention, combined with fever, tachycardia, and leukocytosis, are suggestive of toxic megacolon. Urgency, tenesmus, and fecal incontinence may be present in patients with severe and advanced ulcerative proctosigmoiditis.

Extraintestinal Manifestations

Peripheral arthritis and ankylosing spondylitis are the most common extraintestinal manifestations of UC and usually improve or resolve after colectomy. Peripheral arthritis occurs in 15% to 20% of patients with UC and occurs most frequently in knees and ankles. Sacroiliitis may also occur.

Primary sclerosing cholangitis (PSC) is the most serious extraintestinal manifestation of UC and does not resolve with colectomy. The activity of the diseased mucosa is more severe in patients with combined UC and PSC, and the risk of colonic cancer is five times greater when compared with UC alone. Cancer occurs more on the right side of the colon in patients with PSC and UC when compared with patients with UC alone. In some patients, PSC precedes clinical findings of UC.

Diagnosis

Colonoscopy is the best modality for the diagnosis of UC. Proctoscopy or flexible sigmoidoscopy may be sufficient for establishing the diagnosis during the acute phase of the disease because the rectum is almost always involved in UC, and complete colonoscopy increases the risk for perforation. Mucosal appearance varies with disease activity from granular with minimal friability and edema in the milder stage, to frank ulceration with marked edema and bleeding in the acute stage. Multiple biopsies should be performed from sequential sites in patients with chronic UC to identify dysplasia or cancer. This is especially important in patients who have had the disease for at least 10 years. All patients with the new presumed diagnosis of UC should have either an upper gastrointestinal radiograph with small bowel follow-through, or colonoscopic intubation of the ileum, to rule out Crohn's disease.

Differential Diagnosis

Several conditions cause diarrhea and bleeding and may be mistaken for UC. It is important to identify these conditions because their treatment varies considerably. All patients with a suspected diagnosis of UC should have an examination of the stool for pathogenic bacteria, ova, and parasites. The colonic mucosa should be sampled and examined, despite a normal endoscopic appearance. Conditions that may be mistakenly confused with UC include Crohn's disease, *Clostridium difficile* colitis, infectious colitis, amebiasis, and collagenous colitis.

UC involving primarily the rectum has features that are similar to and different from Crohn's disease of the rectum. The presence of perianal disease is far more common in Crohn's colitis than in UC. Additionally, the rectum is often spared in Crohn's colitis and is almost always inflamed in patients with UC. Distinctive endoscopic features for Crohn's colitis are discussed subsequently (see section on Crohn's colitis).

Clostridium difficile is a gram-positive, spore-forming anaerobic microorganism that produces watery diarrhea, fever, and leukocytosis. *C. difficile* colitis has been associated with prior administration of antibiotics. Initially clindamycin was noted to be associated with the disease, but virtually every antibiotic has been reported as a causative agent. Rectal bleeding is usually not present. *C. difficile* colitis may produce abdominal distention and mimic toxic megacolon. The latex agglutination test provides a rapid identification of *C. difficile* antigens in the stool within minutes. If the diagnosis is unclear, proctoscopy or flexible sigmoidoscopy should be performed. Macroscopically, the mucosa appears to be normal or demonstrates mild inflammation. Occasionally, there is a yellowish plaquelike membrane on the inflamed mucosa, which has led to the descriptive term *pseudomembranous colitis.* Colonic involvement is often patchy or segmental. Additional infectious colitides include *Salmonella* enterocolitis, *Campylobacter* enteritis, and amebiasis. These are diagnosed with stool cultures and treated with the appropriate antibiotics or antiamebic drugs. Collagenous colitis is a rare form of idiopathic colitis that is more prevalent in women (80%). It generally occurs in those older than the age of 50 years and has been associated with autoimmune and rheumatologic conditions. Patients with collagenous colitis often present with watery diarrhea. The diagnosis is made by endoscopic biopsy demonstrating the pathognomonic finding of thickening of the subepithelial collagen layer (mean 15.0 μm versus normal 2.5 μm). The surface epithelium usually shows a variable patchy lymphocytic infiltrate, and the crypts may contain intraepithelial lymphocytes but have no degenerative changes. Most patients with collagenous colitis respond to antidiarrheal medication.

Risk of Carcinoma

Dysplasia and cancer are the most serious sequelae of UC. These findings can occur even when patients are asymptomatic. The estimate of carcinoma risk associated with different patterns of dysplasia is low-grade dysplasia (10%), high-grade dysplasia (30% to 40%), and dysplasia associated with a lesion or mass (DALM) (50% or more).[51] Factors predisposing to cancer are the duration of disease, age at onset, and extent of involvement of the colon. Neoplastic lesions in the colon of patients with UC can develop with a precursor DALM lesion or as coincidental adenomas.[52] The risk of carcinoma in pancolitis is directly related to the duration of the disease: 0% to 3% risk at 5 to 10 years and 50% and 75% risk after 30 and 40 years of disease, respectively (Figs. 48-28 to 48-30).

Colonoscopic Surveillance

The optimal method of colonoscopic surveillance has yet to be established. Systematic strategy for colonoscopic follow-up of patients with long-standing UC is a mandatory component of their management. The American Cancer Society guidelines recommend surveillance colonoscopy every 1 to 2 years beginning 8 years after the start of pancolitis and 12 to 15 years after the start of left-sided colitis.[53] This strategy is based on the premise that a dysplastic lesion can be detected endoscopically before invasive cancer has developed. Detailed pathologic studies have confirmed the patchy nature of dysplasia and have recommended as many as 33 colonoscopic biopsies to provide a 90% chance of detecting dysplasia. Approximately 25% of carcinomas diagnosed in patients with UC are not associated with dysplasia elsewhere in the colon.[54]

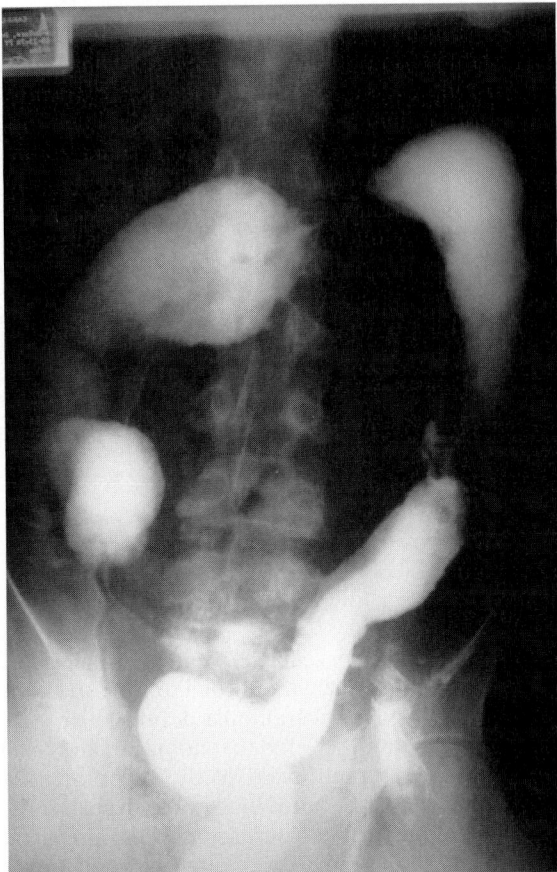

FIGURE 48-28. Barium enema demonstrating stricture in transverse colon of patient with ulcerative colitis of 15 years' duration.

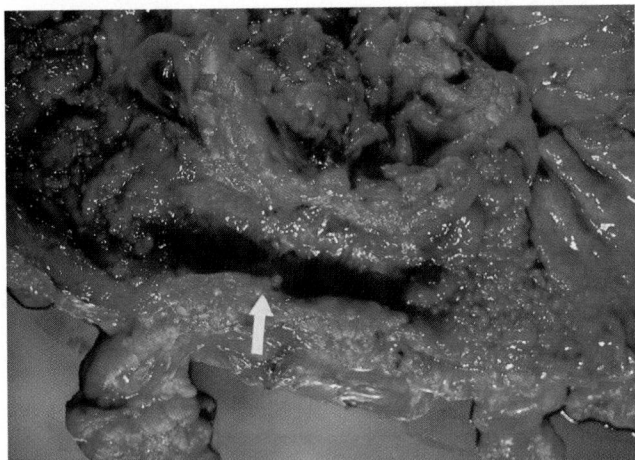

FIGURE 48-29. Photograph of resected colon from patient in Figure 48-28, revealing the stricture (*arrow*) to be invasive cancer. The patient had liver metastases.

Dysplasia is often difficult to diagnose, particularly when it is determined to be of low grade. Even in specialist centers a second opinion by an experienced pathologist should be sought before a diagnosis of low-grade dysplasia is confirmed. An analysis of 10 prospective

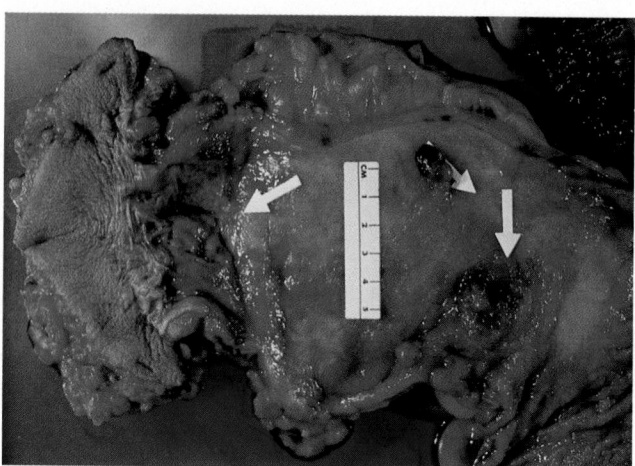

FIGURE 48-30. Resected rectum from patient in Figure 48-28 shows invasive cancers in rectum *(arrows)*.

studies of dysplasia surveillance, with a total of 1225 patients, has shown that when colectomy is performed for high-grade dysplasia, carcinoma is present in 42% of patients.[55] Of major concern is that approximately half of these carcinomas are advanced. If the recommendation for colectomy is delayed until high-grade dysplasia develops, it may be too late for a surgical cure. Approximately 8% of patients undergoing colectomy with low-grade or indefinite dysplasia have cancer, although the data in this category are insufficient to be conclusive.[56]

Despite the absence of prospective randomized controlled trials to confirm specific guidelines for surveillance, the clinician is still required to make diagnostic and therapeutic decisions. The following recommendations have been proposed to improve the accuracy of dysplasia surveillance. When high-grade dysplasia is discovered, the findings should be confirmed by a second experienced pathologist. If the findings are reconfirmed, a colectomy should be performed. If low-grade dysplasia is confirmed by a second experienced pathologist, strong consideration should be given to colectomy.

With the increasing growth of UC genetics, it is hoped that molecular tumor markers may improve the sensitivity of surveillance colonoscopy. Specifically, mutations of the p53 tumor suppressor gene *(TP53)*, aneuploidy, and mucin-associated sialosyl-Tn expression appear to be promising.[57] Although encouraging, these approaches have not yielded a validated reliable cancer marker of high predictive value.

Genetic Changes—Neoplasms and Ulcerative Colitis

There are differences between genetic changes in cells becoming dysplastic and neoplastic cells in patients with UC when compared with patients with sporadic colorectal cancers. For example, only 6% of UC-associated dysplasia and cancer have mutations at the *APC* genes whereas 74% of patients with sporadic cancer have *APC* gene mutations.[58]

Indications for Operations

As mentioned previously, removal of the entire colon and rectum cures UC; thus, it may be argued that surgical treatment is the gold standard to which all treatment should be compared. Most patients referred to surgeons for treatment of UC have received extensive medical regimens to which the disease has become refractory. Indications for surgical treatment of patients with UC include intractability, dysplasia-carcinoma, massive bleeding, and toxic megacolon (Box 48-1).

Intractability

Intractability, or colitis that is refractory to medical management, is the most common indication for operative treatment. The availability of the ileal-anal pouch procedure and avoidance of a permanent stoma has encouraged more patients with refractory UC to choose operation. Most patients with refractory UC have been on long-term medical regimens. In some instances the symptoms persist, whereas in other instances, patients and their clinicians become concerned because of the major side effects of medical treatment. Occasionally, individuals develop attacks of fulminant colitis characterized by significant diarrhea, intolerable abdominal pain, and clinical deterioration. Early operative treatment is recommended if this condition persists for longer than 4 days despite optimal intense nonoperative treatment.

Dysplasia-Carcinoma

High-grade dysplasia is an absolute indication for colectomy (Fig. 48-31). Many clinicians now recommend colectomy for low-grade dysplasia, although this remains controversial. The diagnosis of dysplasia is difficult to establish in the presence of active inflammation, and most authorities recommend that the diagnosis should be confirmed independently by two experienced pathologists. The presence of cancer in the colon does not exclude the possibility of performing an ileal-anal pouch, particularly for T2 and T3 lesions. Patients with T4 lesions are perhaps best treated with a subtotal colectomy, Hartmann's closure of the rectum, and end-ileostomy.

Massive Colonic Bleeding

Massive colonic bleeding is an infrequent indication for operation for UC because most patients respond to conservative management. Massive hemorrhage accounts for less than 5% of all urgent colectomies for UC.

Box 48-1 Ulcerative Colitis—Indications for Surgery

Intractability
Dysplasia-carcinoma
Massive colonic bleeding
Toxic megacolon

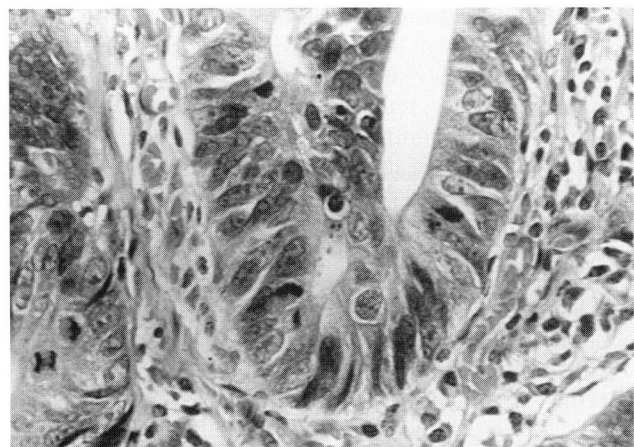

FIGURE 48-31. High-grade colonic dysplasia in ulcerative colitis. Nuclei are large, pleomorphic, hyperchromatic, and crowded. Cells have a high nucleus-to-cytoplasm ratio. Mitotic figures are easily identified. Note that the tubular lumen is irregular with a row of cells seen centrally, suggesting a transition to intramucosal carcinoma. (Courtesy of M. Markowitz Haber, M.D., Hahnemann University Hospital.)

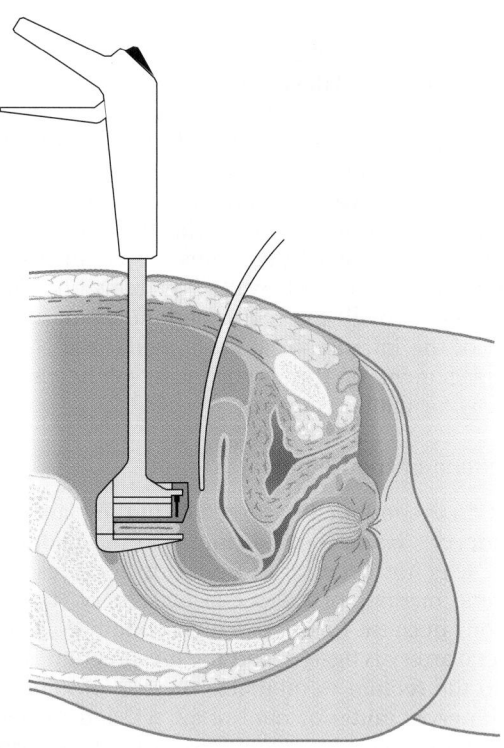

FIGURE 48-32. Closure of rectal stump after resection of abdominal colon.

TOXIC MEGACOLON

Toxic megacolon is a clinical term indicating acute colitis accompanied by significant dilatation of the colon. Patients suffering from toxic megacolon are extremely ill with a high fever, severe abdominal pain, tenderness, tachycardia, and leukocytosis. The characteristic finding is abdominal distention caused by marked colonic dilatation that may predispose to colonic perforation. Vigorous intravenous fluid and pharmacologic resuscitation is required. Transient toxic dilatation in the colon is not an indication for operation, but significant clinical deterioration that does not respond to intensive supporting treatment including intravenous fluids, broad-spectrum antibiotics, corticosteroids, and immunosuppressives is an indication for urgent operation. Most surgeons believe that the appropriate operation for toxic megacolon is abdominal colectomy with ileostomy. The proximal end of the divided rectum is exteriorized as a mucous fistula or closed with sutures or staples (a variant of Hartmann's operation) (Fig. 48-32). Removal of the dilated colon permits the patient to recover from the fulminant effects of the colitis. After adequate recovery (usually several months), the rectum can be removed, the ileostomy taken down, and continuity restored with an ileal-pouch anal anastomosis.

Proctectomy in the presence of toxic megacolon increases the operative time and the risk of pelvic sepsis in a depleted patient, and a subsequent operation to create an ileal-pouch anal anastomosis is much more technically difficult if the proctectomy has been done at an earlier date.

If it is not possible to vent the proximal rectum as a mucous fistula, a drain should be placed into the rectum through the anus in the early postoperative period to prevent distention of the rectum and intraperitoneal perforation through the rectal suture line.

Operations

Preoperative Preparation

Patients in need of major colonic operations require preoperative preparation. Although controversial, most surgeons prescribe some form of bowel preparation before surgery. Despite the absence of prospective controlled data to support this practice, the performance of major colonic surgery in a decompressed colon, versus one full of stool, is technically easier and is more aesthetically pleasing to everyone in the operating room. Patients are given intravenous antibiotics immediately before the skin incision. After endotracheal intubation the patient is placed in the lithotomy position with the lower extremities supported by noncompressing stirrups. A Foley catheter is placed before initiating the operation and remains in place for 3 to 4 days after the operation. A nasogastric catheter decompresses the stomach during the operation and is removed in the recovery room or on the first postoperative day.

Total Proctocolectomy With End-Ileostomy

Total proctocolectomy with end-ileostomy removes all of the colon, rectum, and anus. It is performed in one stage and avoids certain problems associated with staged resections and the restorative ileal-pouch procedure. Disadvantages include a permanent stoma and potential problems with healing of the perineal wound. The problems associated with an unhealed perineal wound can be lessened if an intersphincteric (endoanal) proctectomy is performed (see later). Total proctocolectomy with end-ileostomy is indicated for patients who are poor candidates for restorative proctocolectomy; these include elderly and incontinent patients.

All patients are marked for an ileostomy preoperatively while awake in the sitting and supine positions to prevent improper placement of the stoma at the site of a skin crease on the abdominal wall. Preferably the stoma is brought out through the rectus abdominis muscle at the summit of the infraumbilical fat mound. Care is taken to avoid placement of the stoma next to the iliac crest, umbilicus, or midline incision.

Mobilization of the Rectum

Dissection is continued retrorectally in the plane anterior to Waldeyer's fascia to avoid injury to the middle sacral vessels. It is not necessary to perform total resection of the lateral margins of the rectal mesentery (total meso-resection) because this is a benign condition. The superior rectal artery is ligated, and the mesorectum is divided close to the rectum to minimize the risk of injury to the erectile nerves (anterior rami of S2, S3, and S4 nervi erigentes). Care is taken to avoid injury to the posterior wall of the vagina or the seminal vesicles. The anterior dissection is performed in a plane external to the fascia of Denonvilliers. When the dissection is carried to the level of the levator floor, the proctectomy can be completed by a perineal approach (see later).

An alternative approach is to transect the rectum at the level of the levators and complete the abdominal portion of the operation with primary maturation of the ileostomy, to be followed by the endoanal proctectomy. The ileostomy incision is then made at the previously marked site, and the transected ileum is drawn through the site. The abdominal wall and skin are closed, and the ileostomy is matured primarily with absorbable sutures.

Intersphincteric (Endoanal) Proctectomy

The Lone-Star Retractor (Lone Star Medical Products, Houston, TX) is used to efface the anus and provide adequate visualization of the distal rectum. The intersphincteric space is identified and injected with 1:200,000 epinephrine solution. The circumference of the rectum is dissected sharply or with electrocautery. As a result of the previously transected margin of the low rectum being left open, the index finger of the operator can be inserted transanally into the retrorectal space to facilitate the perineal intersphincteric dissection in the previously identified posterior rectal plane.

Colectomy With Hartmann's Closure of the Rectum or Mucous Fistula

Total abdominal colectomy with either Hartmann's closure of the rectum or distal mucous fistula removes the abdominal colon to the level of the upper rectum or distal sigmoid colon. This operation avoids a long operating time and pelvic dissection, both of which can be deleterious in an acutely ill patient. Disadvantages include retention of the severely diseased rectum and perhaps distal sigmoid. Moreover, rectal bleeding may continue despite the absence of the intra-abdominal colon. This operation is usually performed in acutely ill patients such as those with fulminant colitis or toxic megacolon. Additional indications for this operation include preoperative conditions in which it is difficult to differentiate between Crohn's colitis and UC.

It is important to transect the rectum at a high level to facilitate the next operative stage. The Hartmann, or blind, closure of the rectum is usually done with staples. Long marking sutures of nonabsorbable material are placed at the site of the transected rectum to aid in its identification at the time of reoperation. Usually there is insufficient length of retained sigmoid colon to fashion a mucous fistula; however, when sufficient length is present, creation of a mucous fistula facilitates identification of the rectum at the next operation.

Total Proctocolectomy With Ileal Pouch-Anal Anastomosis

Total proctocolectomy with ileal pouch-anal anastomosis (IPAA) is the gold standard of operative treatment for most patients with UC. This procedure avoids a permanent stoma and permits bowel movements per rectum. Disadvantages include a high percentage of complications related to the pouch and low anastomosis (see ensuing discussion). Indications for this operation are the same as discussed previously, with the requirement of good anorectal function and sphincter tone. Generally this procedure is performed in individuals younger than 65 years of age.

Controversies

Controversies include whether this operation should be performed in one (without ileostomy) or two (with ileostomy) stages and whether all of the rectal mucosa (mucosectomy) should be removed or a short rectal cuff used for a stapled (double-stapled) anastomosis. The one-stage operation includes performing the total abdominal proctocolectomy with IPAA without a temporary diverting ileostomy. The approach has the advantages of a single operation that avoids complications that may accompany an ileostomy. Disadvantages include an increased risk of pelvic sepsis, as well as symptomatic leak of the pouch or ileal-anal suture line.[59] The two-stage procedure includes a temporary diverting ileostomy. Most surgeons routinely perform the two-stage operation in high-risk patients, particularly those on large doses of corticosteroids.

An additional controversy is whether the complete rectal mucosa should be removed (mucosectomy) versus retention of a short segment of retained rectum and a double-stapled mucosa-to-mucosa anastomosis. The advantages of the mucosectomy include complete removal of potentially malignant tissue. Disadvantages include increased nocturnal staining of stool per anus and slight reduction in anal sphincter function. The mucosectomy is also technically more difficult than the double-stapled operation. The major indication for mucosectomy is dysplasia of the rectum.

Operative Technique

The operation must be conducted in a manner to mobilize the ileal mesentery from the retroperitoneum in a fashion that will permit the ileum to reach the anal canal. The mesentery is mobilized to the level of the duodenum, and it may be necessary to divide the ileocolic artery to gain adequate mesenteric length. If the decision is made to perform a double-stapled anastomosis, the rectum is transected with the aid of a stapling instrument at the level of the levator muscles. An ileal pouch is fashioned from the distal 30 cm of ileum, usually with the aid of stapling instruments (Fig. 48-33). An estimate is made of the mobility of the pouch mesentery to ensure a tension-free pouch-anal anastomosis. In the event there is perceived tension of the IPAA, additional mesenteric vessels may need to be ligated and transected. Care is taken to perform this procedure carefully to avoid undue injury to the vascular supply to the pouch. The intraoperative Doppler may be used to identify which mesenteric vessels can be ligated safely. A stapled anastomosis is constructed between the apex of the ileal pouch and the anus (Fig. 48-34). The integrity of the anastomosis is confirmed with the finding of two circumferential tissue margins in the stapler after its removal. In addition, air is insufflated into the pouch through a proctoscope inserted through the anus. Any defects in the anastomosis will be revealed by bubbles rising through saline placed in the pelvis. A loop ileostomy is then placed at the previously marked site. In obese patients, it may be technically impossible to perform a concomitant ileostomy due to insufficient length of the small bowel mesentery and increased distance to the abdominal wall. In these situations, a one-stage procedure without ileostomy may be the best approach.

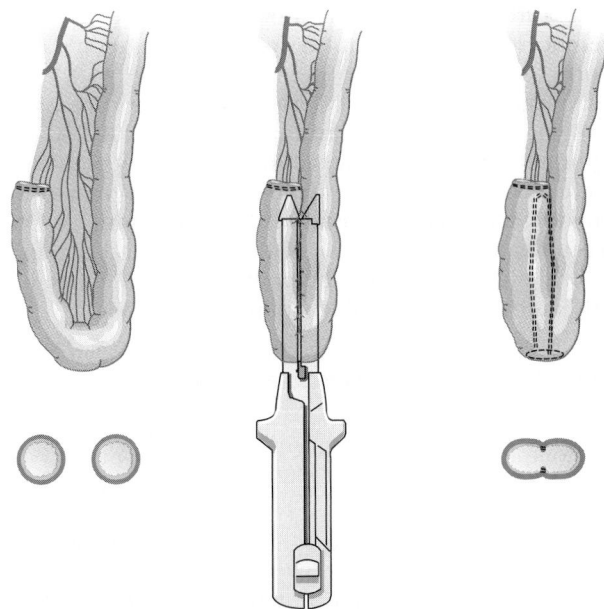

FIGURE 48-33.   Creation of an ileal J pouch using a cutting linear stapler. For replacement of the rectum, a reservoir is created from the distal ileum. The stapler joins two limbs of intestine with staples while dividing the intervening wall. The diameter of the pouch so created is twice as large as the original diameter of the ileum.

Anorectal Mucosectomy With Hand-Sewn Anastomosis

As mentioned, mucosectomy provides the removal of the complete anorectal mucosa, thus theoretically eliminating all potentially premalignant tissue. Disadvantages include impaired continence and increased nocturnal staining. In addition, there have been reported cases of carcinoma arising from the anastomosis of patients treated in this fashion. It has been hypothesized that stripping the

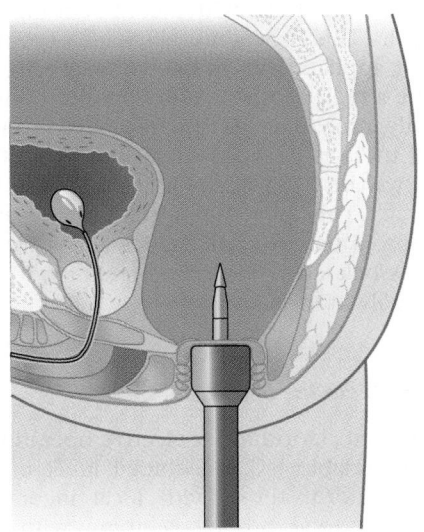
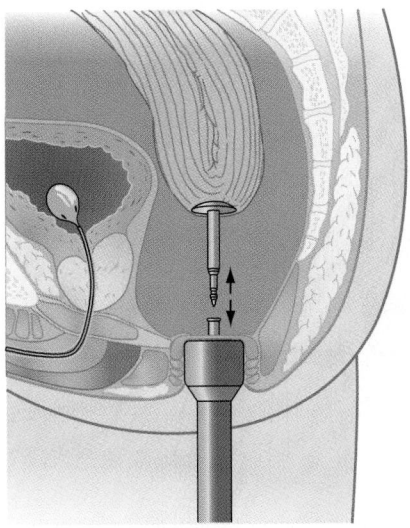

FIGURE 48-34.   Fashioning of stapled ileal pouch anal anastomosis.

mucosa from the muscularis does not remove all of the precancerous epithelium, despite the surgeon's best efforts.

Exposure during the mucosectomy is improved with the Lone-Star Retractor and injection of 1:200,000 epinephrine solution into the submucosa. After completion of the anal mucosectomy the pouch is delivered to the denuded anorectal cuff using a Babcock clamp. A 1-cm incision is made in the base of the pouch, and the anastomosis is made between the pouch and the dentate line with interrupted absorbable sutures (Fig. 48-35).

Complications of Restorative Proctocolectomy

The pouch procedure is associated with many early and late complications. Bowel obstruction is the major postoperative morbidity that occurs after either the initial operation or closure of the ileostomy. In many instances this is a mechanical obstruction due to dietary indiscretion with consumption of inordinate amounts of roughage. This condition usually resolves with bowel rest and a clear liquid diet. Approximately 5% of patients require reoperation for a mechanical small bowel obstruction. Late complications include pouchitis, stricture, fistulas, obstruction, and incomplete evacuation.

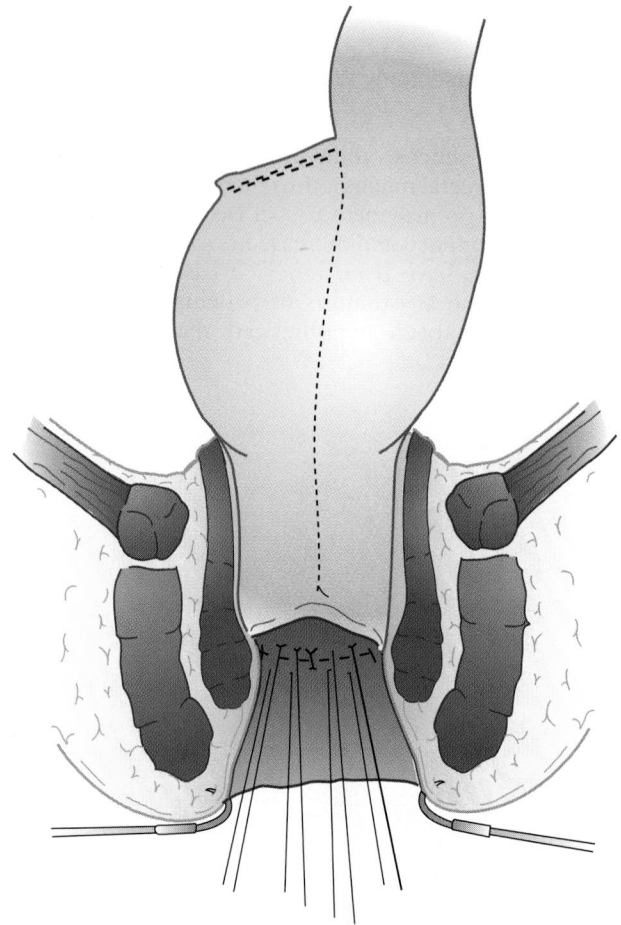

FIGURE 48-35. Hand-sewn ileal pouch anal anastomosis following anorectal mucosectomy.

Pouchitis is acute and/or chronic inflammation of the ileal pouch. It occurs in up to 50% of patients. The risk of pouchitis is highest during the first 2 years after intestinal continuity is restored. There is a significantly higher incidence of pouchitis in patients with extraintestinal manifestations before colectomy. Symptoms include frequent bowel movements, urgency, rectal bleeding, incontinence, and abdominal pain. Additionally, extraintestinal manifestations of IBD may occur during active pouchitis. The most accurate diagnosis is based on combined clinical, endoscopic, and histologic examination of the pouch. The etiology of pouchitis is unknown but it is probably due in part to bacterial proliferation, bacterial stasis, and by-products of bacterial breakdown such as release of endotoxin. Most patients respond readily to broad-spectrum antibiotics such as metronidazole. Clinical improvement usually occurs within 24 to 48 hours of antibiotic therapy.

Anal stricture occurs frequently in patients with ileal pouch-anal anastomoses. In most instances, this does not become problematic; however, up to 15% of patients may have symptoms secondary to this problem. Incomplete evacuation is the most common symptom. In some instances patients can self-dilate strictures with improvement. A stricture of 5 mm or less should be dilated with the aid of an anesthetic.

Laparoscopic Total Abdominal Colectomy With Ileal Pouch-Anal Anastomosis

Recent successes have been reported with the laparoscopic, hand-assisted construction of the ileal pouch-anal anastomosis. Similar to other laparoscopic operations, the advantages of this procedure over open surgery include improved cosmesis, shortened hospital stay, less pronounced immunosuppression and inflammatory response, and lower consumption of analgesia.[60] Disadvantages include increased operative time.

Total Proctocolectomy With Continent Reservoir

Total proctocolectomy with continent reservoir includes removal of all of the colon, rectum, and anus and creation of a skin level stoma with a continent nipple valve in the reservoir. This procedure eliminates the need for a permanent appliance on the abdominal wall. Disadvantages include a high percentage of complications and the need for daily intubations of the abdominal reservoir. Additionally, if there is injury to or malfunction of the reservoir, there may be a considerable loss of small bowel with its removal.[61] This operation is seldom indicated because of the more satisfactory aesthetics and lower complication rate associated with the technique of restorative proctocolectomy.

Summary of Elective Operations

A suggested algorithm for elective operations for patients with intractable UC is included in Figure 48-36. Older patients and/or those with fecal incontinence should undergo a total proctocolectomy with end-ileostomy. Younger individuals with endoscopically confirmed severe proctitis and/or dysplasia should have an IPAA, anal mucosectomy, and hand-sewn anastomosis with a diverting ileostomy. Patients without proctitis or dysplasia and deemed good operative risks are candidates for an IPAA with double-stapled anastomosis and diverting ileostomy. If the patient is a poor operative risk, a total abdominal colectomy with either an ileal-rectal anastomosis or a very low Hartmann closure with ileostomy should be performed.

Postoperative Care

Postoperative care after total proctocolectomies with IPAA is similar to other abdominal operations. Nasogastric tubes are usually discontinued in the recovery room or the morning after surgery. Epidural catheters are left in place 48 to 72 hours. A liquid diet is begun approximately 48 hours postoperatively and rapidly advanced to a low-residue diet. The pelvic drain is generally removed in 48 hours. Foley catheters are often left in place for 3 days, depending on the difficulty of the pelvic dissection. The patient is ambulated rapidly after surgery. Most patients are discharged to home on the fifth to sixth postoperative day. A soluble contrast radiograph is performed on the pouch (pouchgram) at approximately 10 weeks after the initial operation. If the pouchgram is satisfactory, the ileostomy is closed shortly thereafter. If there is evidence of a small leak from the pouch, the radiograph is repeated in approximately 6 weeks. Approximately 95% of pouch leakages seal in the absence of chronic pelvic sepsis.

Patient Satisfaction

The IPAA is characterized by a unique association of a high percentage of complications with a very high level of patient satisfaction, which is seldom observed in postoperative patients. Most large series report a greater than 80% rate of patient satisfaction even in older patients. This is in spite of patients having an average of six to seven bowel movements daily and a 20% rate of perianal seepage. These results are probably due in part to a high motivation level among the patients and the resolution of the primary disease regardless of the operative intervention.

Crohn's Colitis

Crohn's disease is an inflammatory disease that may affect any segment of the gastrointestinal tract. Disease limited exclusively to the colon occurs in approximately 15% of patients with Crohn's disease. The disease may diffusely involve the entire colon, or, in contrast to ulcerative

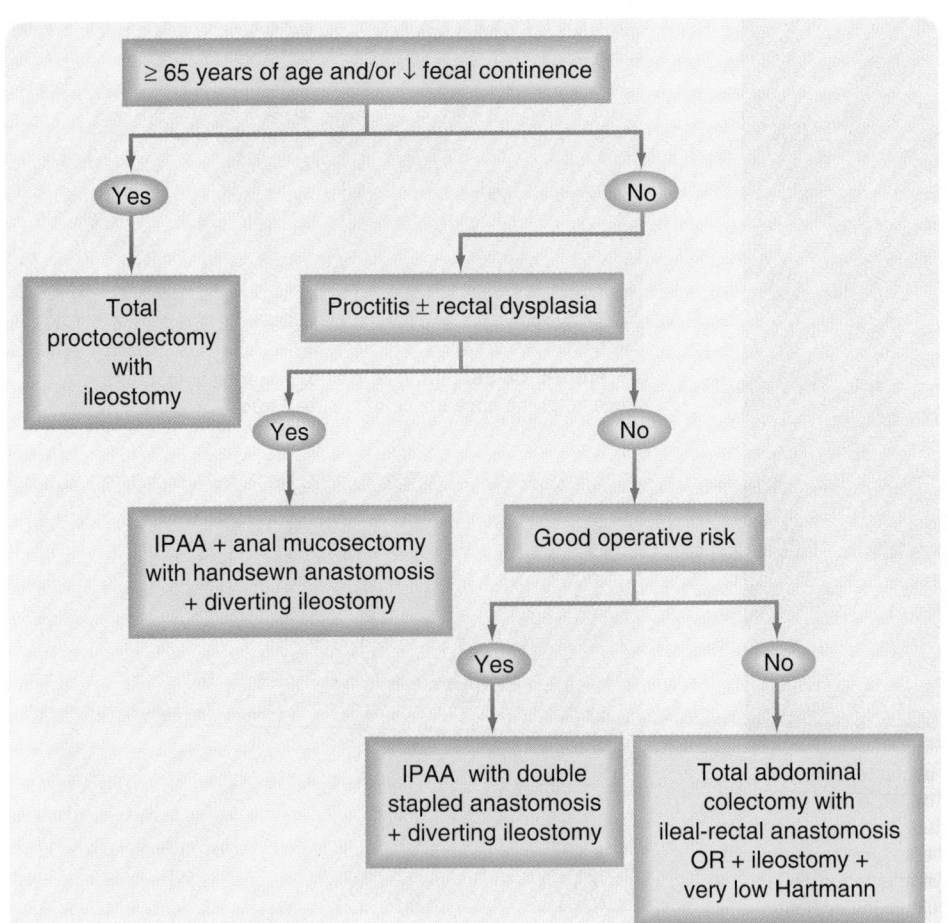

FIGURE 48-36.   Elective operations for ulcerative colitis. IPAA, ileal pouch-anal anastomosis.

colitis, there may be segmental involvement of the colon (Fig. 48-37). This discussion is limited to Crohn's colitis. Additional discussions of Crohn's disease of the remaining intestinal tract are provided in other sections of this text.

Epidemiology, Etiology, and Pathogenesis

The incidence of Crohn's disease continues to increase, albeit slowly. This may be due in part to improved diagnostic modalities. The incidence ranges from 1 to 6/100,000 population depending on geographic area. The highest rates are in Scandinavian countries and Scotland, followed by England and North America. There is a bimodal age distribution with a peak onset between 15 and 30 years and a second smaller peak between 55 and 80 years. It occurs equally between genders and is more common among Jewish people and urban residents.

After intestinal resection, the risk of clinical, endoscopic, and postoperative recurrence is significantly increased in smokers when compared with nonsmokers. Additionally, there is increased association between oral contraceptives and Crohn's disease.

The etiology of Crohn's disease is unknown; the most accepted theories suggest that it is probably due to a combination of events. These include a specific infectious agent, a defective mucosal barrier resulting in increased exposure to antigens, and an abnormal host response to intestinal contents.[62] Chromosome 16 and the HLA region

of chromosome 6 have been implicated in susceptibility to disease. Alleles on specific long-range HLA haplotypes determine overall susceptibility. Additionally, there are novel genetic associations with susceptibility, location, and behavior of Crohn's disease.[63]

Pathologic Features

Crohn's colitis is grossly characterized by a thickened colonic wall and a mucosal appearance of deep, indolent, linear ulcers, cobblestoning, friability, stricturing, and aphthoid ulceration. Single or multiple strictures may be present in both the colon and small bowel. Long linear mucosal ulcers may subsequently become "railroad track" or "bear claw" in appearance (Fig. 48-38).

Microscopic features include transmural inflammation, submucosal edema, lymphoid aggregation, granulomas (Fig. 48-39), and ultimately fibrosis. A pathognomonic microscopic feature of Crohn's disease is the noncaseating granuloma; this is a localized, well-formed aggregate of epithelioid histocytes surrounded by lymphocytes and giant cells. Two thirds of patients with Crohn's disease have granulomas, but they are rarely identified by colonoscopic biopsy.

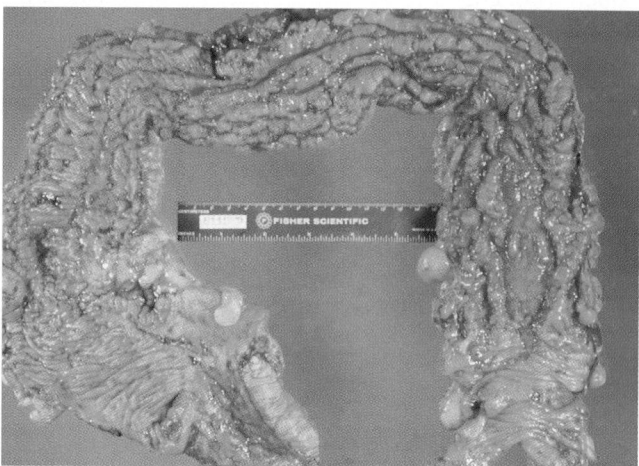

FIGURE 48-38. Crohn's colitis. Linear ulceration of the mucosa, giving appearance of "railroad track" or "bear claw ulcers."

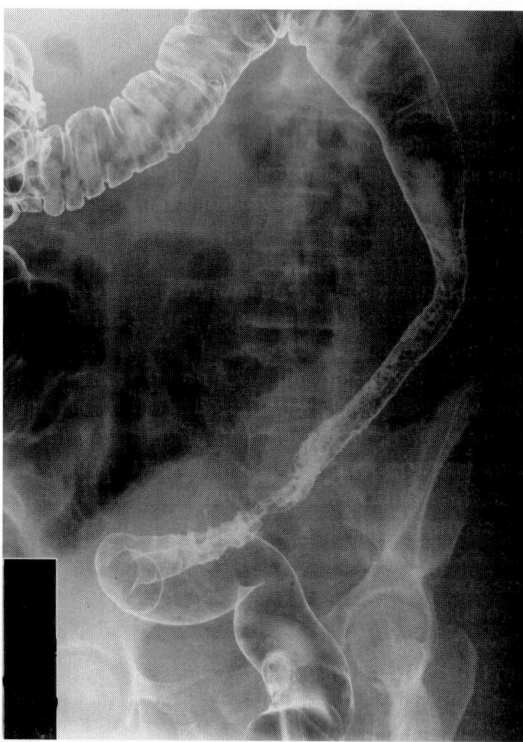

FIGURE 48-37. Crohn's colitis. This barium enema demonstrates segmental inflammation of the left colon, characteristic of Crohn's disease. The rectum is spared, a clinical finding that is useful in distinguishing Crohn's colitis from ulcerative colitis. The rectal mucosa is virtually always affected in patients with ulcerative colitis, whereas the pattern of colonic inflammation is variable in Crohn's colitis.

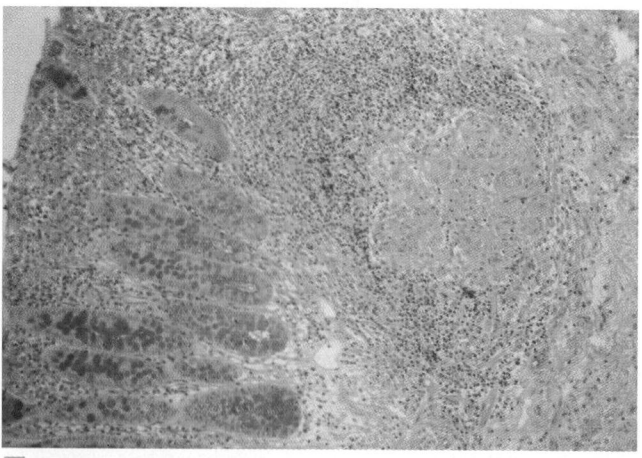

FIGURE 48-39. Crohn's colitis with noncaseating granuloma.

Clinical Characteristics

The onset of Crohn's colitis is often insidious, and symptoms are subtle; thus, early diagnosis is seldom made. The combination of abdominal cramps and diarrhea is often mistaken for viral gastroenteritis or irritable bowel syndrome. Most patients seek further evaluation as symptoms progress and weight loss occurs. Patients with familial Crohn's disease have an earlier age at onset and usually more extensive disease. Of patients who have Crohn's colitis, two thirds have total involvement of the colon and 50% to 75% have rectal disease. This contrasts to UC in which virtually 100% of patients have inflammation of the rectum.

There is also a striking increased incidence of anal disease in patients with Crohn's disease, compared with patients with ulcerative colitis. The anal disease, manifested by fistulas, fissures, edematous skin tags, and erosion of the anoderm, affects approximately 30% of patients with ileocolic Crohn's disease, with a significantly higher incidence occurring in patients with extensive colonic disease. It is an interesting observation that Crohn's disease may spare the rectum but frequently is accompanied by anal disease, whereas ulcerative colitis virtually always involves the rectum but seldom is accompanied by anal disease.

Diagnosis

Most patients are not referred to surgeons until the diagnosis of Crohn's disease is already confirmed. The diagnosis of Crohn's colitis is made through combined investigative studies, including colonoscopy, radiography, and pathology. Colonoscopy is the most sensitive test to diagnose Crohn's colitis, particularly in mild and early disease that is not easily detected with radiographs. The disease is usually patchy in distribution, and aphthous ulcers and edema of the mucosa are early features. Fibrotic strictures are often present in chronic disease. In some instances it is extremely difficult to differentiate Crohn's disease from UC, particularly when inflammation of the rectum is extensive. Biopsies are usually nondiagnostic unless a granuloma is detected.

An upper gastrointestinal examination should be performed in all patients with suspected Crohn's colitis or UC. Concomitant involvement of the small bowel strongly supports the diagnosis of Crohn's disease (Fig. 48-40). Longitudinal and transverse ulcers and a cobblestone-like mucosal pattern are radiographic characteristics, as are skip lesions—areas of normal bowel separating segments of inflamed intestine. An abdominal CT scan is often helpful in evaluating the extent of Crohn's colitis and extraintestinal involvement.

Differential Diagnosis

Differential diagnosis of Crohn's colitis includes infectious colitis and UC. All patients should have a stool culture for enteric organisms and examination for ova and parasites. Organisms that may mimic Crohn's disease in appearance include *Yersinia, Campylobacter, Shigella,* and *Salmonella.*

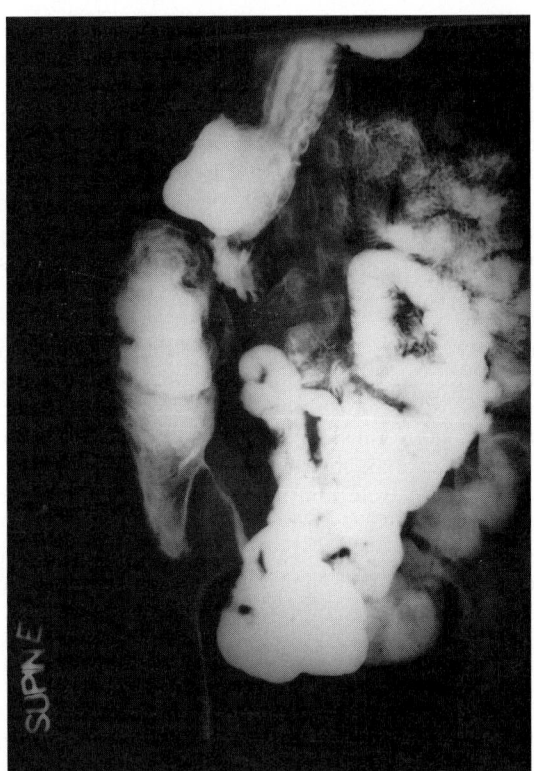

FIGURE 48-40. Small bowel contrast study demonstrating "string sign" caused by inflammation and narrowing of the terminal ileum.

Box 48-2. Crohn's Colitis—Indications for Surgery

Intractability
Intestinal obstruction
Intra-abdominal abscess
Fistulas
Fulminant colitis
Toxic megacolon
Massive bleeding
Cancer
Growth retardation

Indications for Operation (Box 48-2)

In contrast to UC, operative treatment of Crohn's disease is only palliative. Thus, the goals are relief of symptoms, correction of complications, and prevention of cancer.

The timing of operative treatment for Crohn's disease is controversial. The proponents for early operation cite the dramatic relief of symptoms and significant improvement of quality of life. Additional rationale for not delaying operations is the potential for the severity of disease to increase with ensuing adverse sequelae, including perforation, abscesses, obstruction, and enteric fistulas. Moreover, normal segments of intestine may become markedly adherent to diseased bowel, thus making operative resection of the primary disease more difficult and often leading to inadvertent loss of normal intestine. Critics of operative treatment emphasize the high recurrence rate (up to 50% during 15 years of follow-up). Frequently, the final decision for surgery is based on the personal wishes of the patient and his or her referring physician. An important principle in preoperative decision making is to ensure that the patient has received the best available medical therapy before considering surgery. Additionally, it is important not to wait until the disease has become so severe that serious complications may occur.

Indications for surgery in 166 patients with Crohn's colitis were reviewed by the Cleveland Clinic. Internal fistulas and abscess constituted 25% of patients; perianal disease, 23%; chronically ill health, 21%; toxic megacolon, 19%; and intestinal obstruction, 12%.[64] These data may reflect, in part, referral patterns to a major specialty center. Indications for surgery for Crohn's colitis include intractability, intestinal obstruction, intra-abdominal abscess, fistulas, fulminant colitis, toxic megacolon, massive bleeding, cancer, and growth retardation.

Intractability—Refractoriness to Medical Treatment

Similar to UC, the most common indication for operative treatment of Crohn's disease in most institutions is failure to adequately respond to optimal medical management. Clearly, this indication varies as to the symptomatic tolerance of the patient and the experience of the treating physician.

Intestinal Obstruction

Intestinal obstruction is a common reason for operation for Crohn's disease. The most common anatomic pattern is disease of the terminal ileum, which often extends to the cecum. Close attention should be given to antecedent dietary history. In many instances, the ingestion of large amounts of fiber or roughage leads to an obturation type of obstruction at the site of disease. An obturation obstruction frequently resolves when the patient is placed on bowel rest or when dietary intake is restricted to clear liquids. Additional causes of obstruction include adhesions, intra-abdominal abscesses and phlegmons, and occult malignancy. If the obstruction is at the site of a chronically strictured anastomosis attempts at balloon dilation may be performed. If the patient is acutely obstructed, preoperative management consists of aggressive replacement of intravenous fluids and bowel rest.

Intra-abdominal Abscess

Intra-abdominal abscess may occur at any location within the abdominal cavity and is usually the result of a sealed perforation of the bowel. Most of these patients can be treated initially with CT-guided percutaneous drainage and antibiotics. If the patient fails to respond to this regimen or if the abscess is not amenable to percutaneous drainage, exploratory celiotomy is recommended with possible bowel resection. In some instances it is more prudent to perform a diverting ileostomy and intraoperative drainage in preparation for a definitive elective resection several months later.

Fistulas

Internal Fistula

Approximately one third of patients with Crohn's disease develop an internal fistula, and most of these are due to Crohn's disease of the small intestine. Uncomplicated enteroenteric or enterocolic fistulas do not usually require operative treatment. Occasionally, patients with ileal-sigmoid fistulas will develop increased diarrhea and require resection of the diseased terminal ileum. Whether the segment of involved sigmoid needs to be resected depends on the extent of the inflammation. With minimal inflammation the sigmoid defect can be simply closed, as long as the primary site of the fistula (the ileum) is resected.

Colocutaneous and Enterocutaneous Fistula

Most spontaneous fistulas eroding through the abdominal wall and skin are due to terminal ileal disease, rather than colonic Crohn's disease. Ileal-cutaneous and colocutaneous fistulas may be due to early postoperative anastomotic breakdown. Most of these patients can be treated nonoperatively with bowel rest. If high output (>500 mL/day) fistulas occur, total parenteral nutrition may hasten nonoperative closure. In the event the fistula has not healed after 4 to 6 weeks of parenteral nutrition, it is unlikely that it will heal nonoperatively.

Colovesical and Colovaginal Fistula

These fistulas generally are treated by resection of the diseased bowel, with débridement and/or closure of bladder and/or vagina and interposition of omentum between the enteric suture line and contiguous organ.

Fulminant Colitis

Fulminant colitis is initially treated with aggressive intravenous fluids, antibiotics, and close metabolic monitoring in an intensive care unit. Urgent operation is recommended if the patient fails to respond to this treatment regimen within 1 to 5 days. A total abdominal colectomy with ileostomy and mucous fistula or Hartmann's closure of the rectum is the preferred operation.

Toxic Megacolon

Similar to UC, Crohn's disease may cause toxic megacolon. Operative treatment of this serious condition has been discussed previously. It is of interest that because of the stenosing fibrotic nature of Crohn's disease, patients with fulminant colitis may not display the typical dilation that characterizes toxic megacolon. However, the toxicity of these patients is no less threatening than with UC, and colectomy may be required for the nondilated toxic colon characteristic of this disease. (See earlier discussion of toxic megacolon.)

Massive Bleeding

Although significantly less common than UC, massive bleeding may occur in a small percentage of patients with

Crohn's disease. Similar to all patients with intestinal bleeding, an inclusive work-up and aggressive medical treatment should be performed before operative intervention. The most likely site of bleeding is similar to the general distribution of Crohn's disease, with the terminal ileum being the most common site. If the bleeding does not respond to medical treatment and the site cannot be located, proctoscopy should be performed to rule out a rectal site of bleeding. Operative treatment consists of a subtotal colectomy with either end-ileostomy and Hartmann's closure or an ileal-rectal anastomosis.

Cancer Prevention

Patients with chronic, active Crohn's colitis require periodic surveillance through colonoscopy and biopsy similar to UC; however, prophylactic operation is not recommended to prevent cancer. Similar to UC, the presence of high-grade dysplasia is an indication for colectomy. A stricture in long-standing Crohn's disease is a possible sign of cancer. Additionally, a bypassed segment of Crohn's disease should be resected if possible.

Cancer

As mentioned, cancer of the colon is increased in patients with Crohn's colitis. The prognosis is directly related to the stage of the disease at the time of operation.

Extracolonic Manifestations

Many extracolonic manifestations of Crohn's disease will resolve after the diseased bowel has been removed. Exceptions to this include primary sclerosing cholangitis, cirrhosis, and ankylosing spondylitis.

Growth Retardation

Prepubertal resection of severely diseased segments of Crohn's disease, in turn, will eliminate growth retardation and premature closure of epiphyses. Perioperative nutritional support is an important component of the total care of these patients.

Operations

Operative treatment for Crohn's disease is strictly palliative. The most important principle is conservatism to include removal of as little bowel as possible to ameliorate symptoms. A randomized prospective trial of 131 patients requiring surgery for Crohn's disease at the Cleveland Clinic concluded that an operative margin 2 cm from gross disease was sufficient to relieve symptoms and improve outcome.[65] Frozen sections on the margins of resection were not predictive of increased rates of postoperative recurrence. As a result of the high reoperative rate for Crohn's disease, every effort should be made to use medical management before considering surgery.

Ileal-Cecal Resection

Ileal-cecal resection is the most commonly performed operation for patients with Crohn's disease. This operation removes the severely diseased terminal ileum (usually 6 to 12 inches) with concomitant removal of the cecum; anastomosis is then performed between the ileum and the ascending colon. Advantages of ileal-cecal resection include relief of symptoms often resulting from obstruction or perforation. Disadvantages include the high propensity for reoperation and the potential for anastomotic complications. Indications for ileal-cecal resection include patients with obstruction or perforation of the terminal ileum. Because the disease almost always extends to the cecum, it is usually removed concomitantly.

The operation is usually performed through a lower midline incision. Transverse abdominal incisions should be avoided in patients with Crohn's disease because of the elimination of potential sites for stomal placement due to incisional scars, which, in turn, impair adherence of ostomy appliances. In the event a lower abdominal or pelvic mass is identified by preoperative CT, a right ureteral stent is placed at the time of surgery. The terminal ileum is transected 2 to 3 cm proximal to the grossly apparent disease. The technique of feeling for a sharp mesenteric-bowel margin correlates well with the intraluminal disease and prevents removing inordinate amounts of relatively grossly normal small bowel (Fig. 48-41).

Ileal-cecectomy may be performed laparoscopically with efficacy similar to open operations.

Total Proctocolectomy With Ileostomy

This operation removes all of the abdominal colon, rectum, and anus. Its advantages are the complete removal of the diseased colon and rectum. Disadvantages include potential problems with healing of the perineal wound. The technique is essentially the same as described in the operative section under UC. Endoanal or intersphincteric proctectomy should be performed to minimize the size and duration of healing of the perineal wound. Opening and draining of perianal fistulas and abscesses should be performed concomitantly.

Total Abdominal Colectomy With Ileal-Rectal Anastomosis

This operation removes the entire diseased colon to the level of the rectum. Its advantage is the preservation of bowel movements through the rectum. Disadvantages include increased frequency of bowel movements and the high likelihood of future removal of the rectum and anus. This operation is associated with a 3% mortality and a 5% to 10% risk of anastomotic leakage. Ileal-rectal anastomosis is associated with a clinical recurrence rate of 50% to 70% at 5 and 10 years, respectively. Approximately two thirds of patients will require reoperation and permanent ileostomy.

Subtotal Colectomy With Hartmann's Closure of Rectum and Ileostomy or Mucous Fistula

This operation removes the entire colon and preserves the rectum. It is indicated in the acutely ill, high-risk patient in need of surgery for severe Crohn's colitis and proctitis. It has the advantage of elimination of the perineal wound

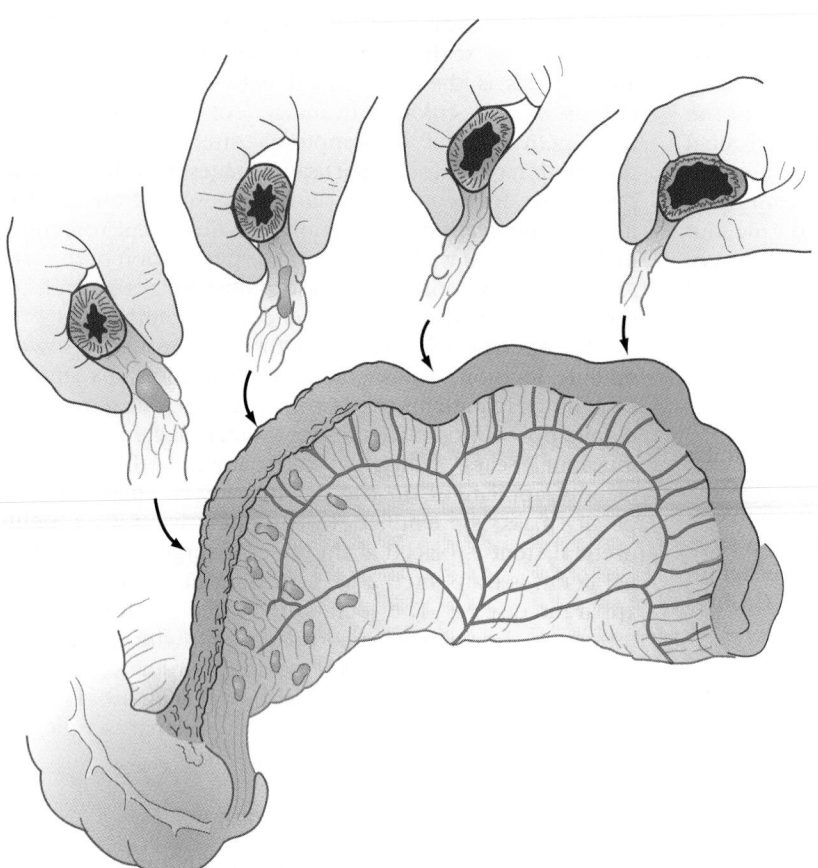

FIGURE 48-41. Method to identify ileal margin free of significant intraluminal disease for ileal-cecal resection of Crohn's disease. A sharp mesenteric-bowel margin correlates with significant absence of intraluminal disease. (From Strong SA: Crohn's disease. *In* Nicholls RJ, Dozois RR [eds]: Surgery of the Colon & Rectum. Edinburgh, Churchill Livingstone, 1997, p 622.)

and is shorter in duration than total proctocolectomy with permanent ileostomy. Disadvantages include residual inflammation and sequelae in the retained rectum and potential ileostomy complications.

Segmental Colectomy With Colocolic Anastomosis

Crohn's disease is limited to a segment of the colon in 10% to 20% of patients with Crohn's colitis. Segmental colectomy provides a stoma-free postoperative period and, despite the potential for adverse sequelae, is particularly appealing to young patients. It is indicated for patients with limited segmental disease in the colon and associated stricture or obstruction. Segmental colectomy is associated with a 30% to 50% recurrence rate within 5 years and a reoperative rate of 45% within 5 years and 60% within 10 years. It is contraindicated in patients with severe rectal or perianal disease. Disadvantages include a very high rate of disease recurrence, which in turn requires reoperation. If the transection of the colon is near the rectum, the anastomosis may be performed transanally with the stapler or as a hand-sewn end-to-end anastomosis. This operation is also performed laparoscopically with excellent results.

Total Proctocolectomy With Ileal Pouch-Anal Anastomosis in Patients With Unsuspected Crohn's Disease

Total proctocolectomy with IPAA is contraindicated in patients with Crohn's disease; however, in some instances, it may be extremely difficult to differentiate between UC and Crohn's colitis. If the pouch procedure is performed in patients who ultimately are proved to have Crohn's disease, the pouch may still function in a satisfactory manner in a small percentage of patients. The majority of patients ultimately have problems with the pouch such as fistulas, fissures, and increased frequency of bowel movements. Most of these patients undergo removal of the pouch.

Summary of Elective Operations—Intractable Disease

A suggested algorithm for elective operations for patients with intractable Crohn's colitis is included in Figure 48-42. Patients with concomitant rectal or perineal disease, such as fistulas, fissures, and recurrent abscesses, should be assessed for their operative risk. Good risk patients should have a total colectomy with intersphincteric proctectomy and ileostomy. Poor risk patients should undergo a total colectomy with low Hartmann's closure and ileostomy. Patients without perianal or rectal disease should be endoscopically assessed for the extent of colonic disease. If disease occurs in greater than 50% of the colon, a total colectomy with ileal-sigmoid or ileal-rectal anastomosis can be performed. Patients without extensive colonic disease are candidates for a segmental colectomy with colocolic or colorectal anastomosis.

Postoperative Recurrence

The reoperative rate for patients with Crohn's disease is 4% to 5% per year. Many factors are associated with

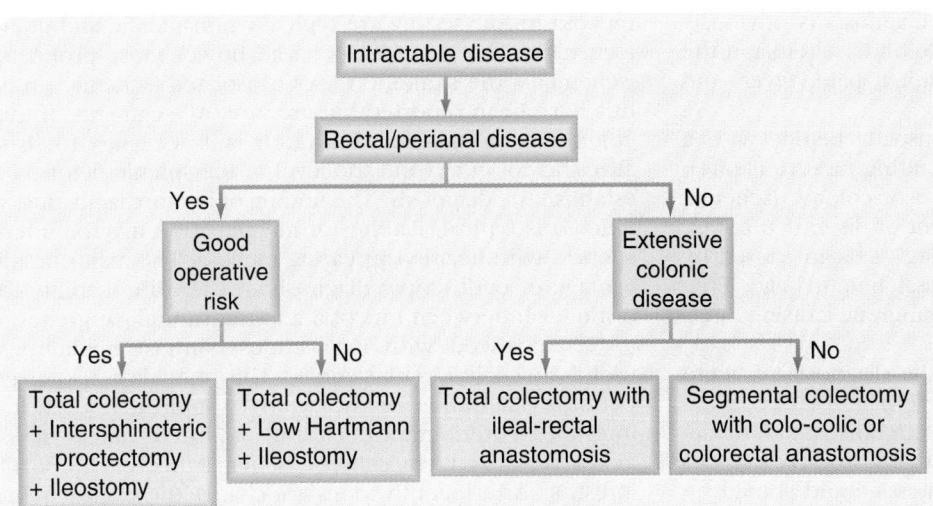

FIGURE 48-42. Elective operations for Crohn's colitis.

increased postoperative recurrence. The presence of perianal disease is associated with a greater risk of recurrence. Total proctocolectomy with ileostomy has a lower rate of recurrence (15% in 5 years), and all operations with anastomosis have an increased risk of recurrence when compared with total proctocolectomy.

Maintaining postoperative remission in patients with Crohn's disease continues to be investigated. The results of a meta-analysis of more than 30 clinical trials in maintenance therapy in Crohn's disease were reported recently.[66] Four trials demonstrated statistically significant reduction in anastomotic recurrence when 5-acetylsalicylic compounds were used when compared with placebo. Not all authors have found similar findings. Salomon[67] reported a meta-analysis of 12 placebo-controlled trials, examining the effect of induction and maintenance therapy in Crohn's disease. There were nearly identical rates of relapse with sulfasalazine, prednisolone, and azathioprine, which revealed a 90% maintenance remission at 3 months; however, this had decreased to 25% at 36 months. Efficacy with maintenance therapy has been noted more frequently in patients with ileal and ileal-colic disease than with colonic disease alone. Recent evidence has confirmed that mesalamine (Procter and Gamble, Cincinnati, OH) at higher doses may be an effective agent to prevent remission.[68] In a carefully performed double-blinded placebo-controlled trial, 750 mg four times a day of mesalamine for 4 years decreased the remission rate to 25% in the treatment group compared with 36% in the placebo group.

COLONIC ISCHEMIA

Colonic ischemia (CI) is the most common form of intestinal ischemia. Most attacks are transient and resolve spontaneously; thus the entity is often misdiagnosed or unrecognized. While the etiology of many cases of CI is obscure, aortic surgery, arteriosclerotic disease, and conditions causing transient hypotension have been implicated. Other factors associated with the disease include the use of oral contraceptives, cocaine abuse, hereditary coagulopathies, long-distance running, and certain bacterial pathogens, including cytomegalovirus and *E. coli* O157:H7.[69]

As described previously, the colon is supplied with arterial blood from the SMA and IMA. There are collateral channels that may develop between these major mesenteric arteries; it is not unusual for the marginal artery or the arc of Riolan to provide collateral circulation adequate to sustain the left colon if the IMA has been gradually occluded by atherosclerosis. Indeed, the IMA is frequently occluded in conditions requiring aortic surgery, and in such circumstances transection of the IMA does not require reimplantation. However, in this situation the left colon is dependent on collateral blood supply, and transient hypotension at the time of the vascular procedure or immediately postoperatively may result in ischemic injury to the vulnerable colonic mucosa.

The spectrum of CI includes transient ischemia, chronic ischemia, and gangrene. The disease is usually segmental. If the ischemia is limited to the most vulnerable layer of the intestine, the mucosa, the disease may be transient, and recovery may be complete. More significant ischemia involving the muscularis may result in scarring and a chronic stricture. Ischemia affecting the full thickness of the bowel wall may result in gangrene with perforation and fecal peritonitis.

The signs and symptoms of colonic ischemia include abdominal pain, hematochezia, and fever. These symptoms vary considerably depending on the severity of the ischemia and the length as well as the thickness of the colon that is affected. Ischemia limited to a small segment of mucosa may cause cramping abdominal pain and passage of a small amount of blood; more significant mucosal ischemia may result in more severe abdominal pain and tenderness over the affected segment of colon, bacterial translocation, fever, leukocytosis, and acidosis; compromise of blood supply to the full thickness of the colonic wall will result in severe abdominal pain, fever, leukocytosis, acidosis, and signs of peritonitis.

Rapid and accurate diagnosis permits institution of supportive measures or withdrawal of offending medications (i.e., oral contraceptives) that may halt the progression of the disease and prevent mucosal ischemia from progressing to transmural gangrene. Early diagnosis is obviously facilitated by a high suspicion for colonic ischemia in the setting of mild to moderate abdominal pain, fever, and bloody diarrhea.

Radiologic investigation of CI usually begins with a plain film of the abdomen. The resulting picture is often nonspecific, but findings suggestive of colonic ischemia include an ileus, an isolated segment of distended colon, or, more specifically, "thumbprinting"—a sign caused by intestinal wall edema or submucosal hemorrhage. Free intraperitoneal air can result from gangrene causing intestinal perforation.

The use of barium enema for the diagnosis of acute colonic ischemia has become obsolete. The risk of perforation and barium peritonitis in this circumstance is unacceptable. Water-soluble contrast studies also carry a risk of perforation of the compromised intestine and should be avoided in the acute setting. However, contrast enemas are quite useful and acceptable for the detection and evaluation of a stricture that may have developed because of ischemia.

Flexible sigmoidoscopy or colonoscopy provides the advantage of direct visualization of the colonic mucosa. Bacterial or viral cultures may be obtained, and biopsy specimens may be taken. Unfortunately, biopsies of the mucosa in this setting are typically nonspecific and uninformative. The segment of large bowel most prone to ischemia is the sigmoid. Cases of isolated ischemic proctitis have been reported but are rare. All segments of the colon may be involved, but rarely is it necessary to visualize the colon beyond the level of the splenic flexure to establish the diagnosis. The finding of hemorrhagic, dusky mucosa is typical. Patches of inflammation may be interspersed with healthy-appearing mucosa. The major disadvantage of endoscopic diagnosis of CI is the inability to distinguish between mucosal and transmural gangrene.

CT enhanced with intravenous contrast medium is useful in such circumstances. This modality also may permit visualization of the arterial supply to the entire intestine. Arteriography is not indicated unless it is believed that acute mesenteric ischemia involves the small intestine. Arteriography does not change the management or outcome of clinically apparent colonic ischemia.

Treatment of CI depends on the presentation and severity of signs and symptoms (Fig. 48-43). Hospital admission, intravenous fluids, bowel rest, and general supportive measures until the patient is pain free usually are adequate treatment for mucosal ischemia. Because loss of integrity of the mucosa may result in bacterial translocation, broad-

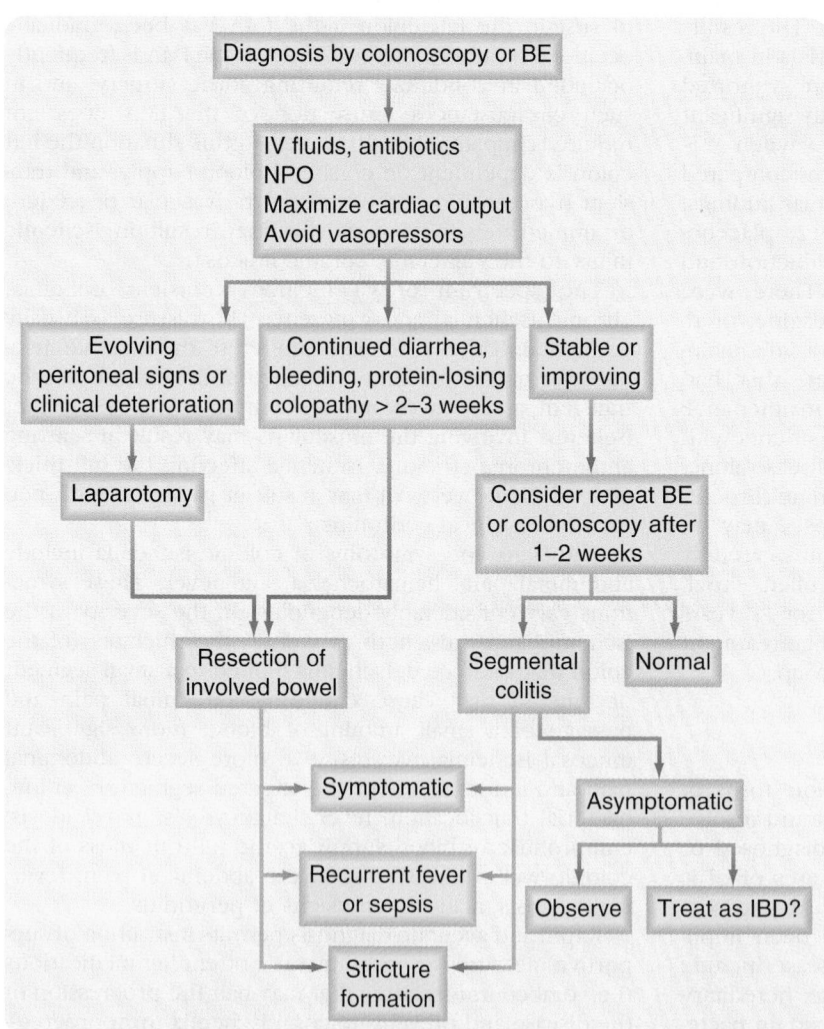

FIGURE 48-43. Management of colonic ischemia. BE, barium enema; IV, intravenous; NPO, nil per os; IBD, inflammatory bowel disease.

spectrum antibiotics are generally advocated for the treatment of CI. Level 1 evidence for antibiotic treatment in humans is nonexistent, but antibiotics are associated with increased survival in rat models of CI.

There is a recognized risk of CI after abdominal aortic operations, and the diagnosis must be considered when abdominal pain, fever, leukocytosis, or acidosis occur after this type of operation. Flexible sigmoidoscopy is indicated to establish the diagnosis. Monitoring of the patient includes serial abdominal examinations and frequent recording of vital signs, urine output, blood pH, and white blood cells. Supportive measures are provided as described earlier. If transmural gangrene is suspected, immediate operation is indicated.

Although surgical intervention for CI is relatively uncommon, when it is indicated, the procedure of choice is partial or total colectomy with or without an end stoma (Box 48-3). Unlike mesenteric ischemia involving the small bowel, revascularization procedures to establish blood flow to the colon are not indicated. Indications for operation in CI are fairly straightforward. Colonic perforation is a clear indication for laparotomy and resection of the ischemic segment with end ileostomy or colostomy. Total colonic ischemia is rare, but cases have been reported to mimic fulminant colitis or toxic megacolon. Such cases require treatment by total colectomy and end ileostomy. Although quite rare, massive bleeding in the setting of acute ischemic colitis is a serious and life-threatening occurrence. Subtotal colectomy with an end ileostomy is usually indicated in this situation unless the specifically involved segment of colon can be accurately identified and resected.[70]

Indications for surgery in subacute situations are uncommon. However, patients who remain symptomatic, with pain, bleeding, diarrhea, or recurrent bouts of sepsis for 2 to 3 weeks after presentation with no improvement may require operation. Whether to fashion an anastomosis in this setting is unclear. The nature of this disease and the potential for serious septic complications argues for creation of a stoma.

Chronic sequelae of CI include stricture formation as well as chronic segmental colitis. Strictures can be symptomatic depending on their location and diameter. The condition most commonly affects the sigmoid colon. Indications for treatment include obstructive symptoms, diagnostic uncertainty (suspicion of cancer as a cause of stricture), and impediment to endoscopic examination of suspected colonic lesions in the colon proximal to the stricture. Ischemic strictures have been successfully dilated by endoscopic techniques and stents. However, resection of the strictured segment with primary anastomosis is generally advocated for relatively healthy patients.

Patients with chronic segmental colitis typically have intermittent symptoms of pain and bleeding. Endoscopic examination reveals inflammation limited to a segment of colon (usually descending or sigmoid). Biopsies of the friable tissue are unrevealing but can rule out infectious causes. Frequently, colonoscopic examination of patients after a bout of CI reveals completely normal mucosa, testifying to the transient, intermittent nature of the attacks. It is extremely rare that attacks recur in an intermittent fashion that requires surgical intervention.

NEOPLASIA

Adenocarcinoma of the colon and rectum is the third most common site of new cancer cases and deaths in both men and women in the United States. The estimated incidence of new cases in 2002 is 148,300, with 56,600 deaths from the disease. The lifetime risk of developing colorectal cancer in the United States is 6%, with over 90% of cases occurring after the age of 50. The death rate from colorectal cancer decreased by 1.8% per year from 1992 to 1998.[71]

Colorectal cancer occurs in hereditary, sporadic, or familial forms. Hereditary forms of colorectal cancer have been extensively described and are characterized by family history, young age at onset, and the presence of other specific tumors and defects. Familial adenomatous polyposis (FAP) and hereditary nonpolyposis colorectal cancer (HNPCC) have been the subject of many recent investigations that have provided significant insights into the pathogenesis of colorectal cancer.

Sporadic colorectal cancer occurs in the absence of family history, generally affects an older population (60 to 80 years of age), and usually presents as an isolated colon or rectal lesion. Genetic mutations associated with the cancer are limited to the tumor itself, unlike hereditary disease where the specific mutation is present in all cells of the affected individual. Nevertheless, the genetics of colorectal cancer initiation and progression proceed along very similar pathways in both hereditary and sporadic forms of the disease. Studies of the relatively rare inherited models of the disease have greatly enhanced the understanding of the genetics of the far more common sporadic form of the cancer.

The concept of "familial" colorectal cancer is relatively new. Lifetime risk of colorectal cancer increases for members in families in which the index case is young (younger than 50 years of age) and the relative is close

---

Box 48-3. Colonic Ischemia—Indications for Surgery

Acute Indications

Peritoneal signs
Massive bleeding
Universal fulminant colitis with or without toxic megacolon

Subacute Indications

Failure of an acute segmental ischemic colitis to respond within 2 to 3 weeks with continued symptoms or a protein-losing colopathy
Apparent healing but with recurrent bouts of sepsis

Chronic Indications

Symptomatic colon stricture
Symptomatic segmental ischemic colitis

TABLE 48-2.   Familial Risk and Colon Cancer

Familial Setting	Approximate Lifetime Risk of Colon Cancer
General U.S. population	6%
One first-degree relative* with colon cancer	Two- to 3-fold increased
Two first-degree relatives* with colon cancer	Three- to 4-fold increased
First-degree relative* with colon cancer diagnosed ≤50 yr	Three- to 4-fold increased
One second- or third-degree relative†‡ with colon cancer	1.5-fold increased
Two second- or third-degree relatives†‡ with colon cancer	Two- to 3-fold increased
One first-degree relative* with adenomatous polyp	Two-fold increased

*First-degree relatives include parents, siblings, and children.
†Second-degree relatives include grandparents, aunts, and uncles.
‡Third-degree relatives include great-grandparents and cousins.
From Burt RW: Colon cancer screening. Gastroenterology 119:837-853, 2000, with permission.

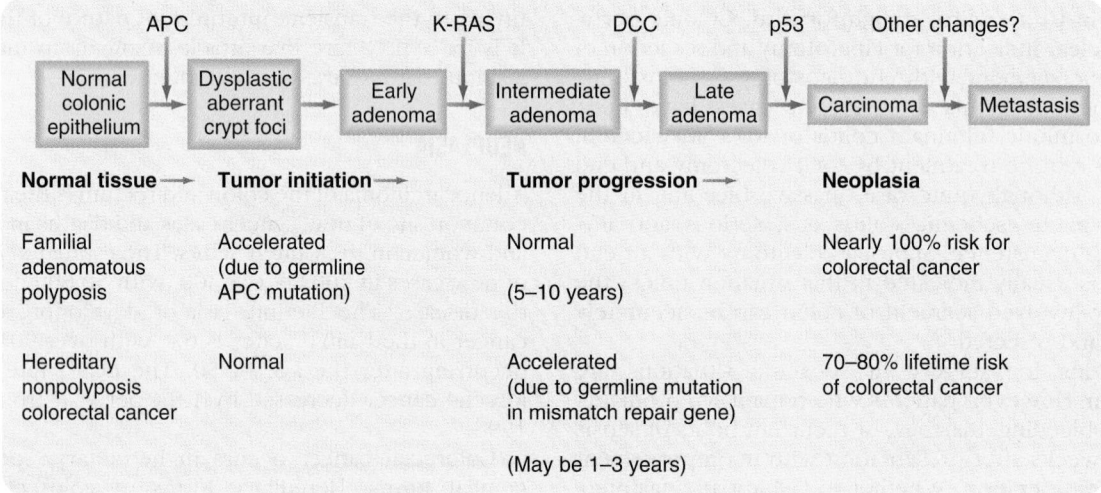

FIGURE 48-44.   The adenoma-carcinoma sequence in sporadic and hereditary colorectal cancer. (From Ivanovich JL, Read TE, Ciske DJ, et al: A practical approach to familial and hereditary colorectal cancer. Am J Med 107:68-77, 1999.)

(first degree). The risk increases as the number of family members with colorectal cancer rises (Table 48-2). An individual who is a first-degree relative of a patient diagnosed with colorectal cancer at an age younger than 50 is twice as likely as the general population to develop the cancer. This more subtle form of inheritance is currently the subject of much investigation. Genetic polymorphisms, gene modifiers, and defects in tyrosine kinases have all been implicated in various forms of familial colorectal cancer.

Colorectal Cancer Genetics

The field of colorectal cancer genetics was revolutionized in 1988 by the description of the genetic changes involved in the progression of a benign adenomatous polyp to invasive carcinoma.[72] Since then, there has been an explosion of additional information about the molecular and genetic pathways resulting in colorectal cancer. Tumor suppressor genes, DNA mismatch repair genes, and protooncogenes all contribute to colorectal neoplasia, both in the sporadic

and inherited forms. The Fearon-Vogelstein "adenoma-carcinoma" multistep model of colorectal neoplasia represents one of the best-known models of carcinogenesis (Fig. 48-44).[73] This sequence of tumor progression involves damage to protooncogenes and tumor suppressor genes. The multistep carcinogenesis model can serve as a template to illustrate how certain early mutations produce accumulated defects resulting in neoplasia. The specific contributing mutations in genes such as *APC* have been intensely studied. It is important to view this model and others as progressive and in flux as interconnected cell cycle control pathways and new functions for well-known genes are becoming recognized (Table 48-3).

Specific Mutations

Tumor Suppressor Genes

Tumor suppressor genes produce proteins that inhibit tumor formation by regulating mitotic activity and pro-

TABLE 48-3. Gene Mutations That Cause Colon Cancer

Mutation Type	Genes Involved	Type of Disease Caused
Germline	*APC*	Familial adenomatous polyposis
	MMR	HNPCC (Lynch syndrome)
Somatic	Oncogenes:	Sporadic disease
	myc	
	ras	
	src	
	erbB2	
	Tumor suppressor genes:	
	TP53	
	DCC	
	APC	
	MMR genes:	
	hMSH2	
	hMLH1	
	hPMS1	
	hPMS2	
	hMSH6	
	hMSH3	
Genetic polymorphism	*APC*	Familial colon cancer in Ashkenazi Jewish persons

DCC, deleted in colorectal carcinoma; HNPCC, hereditary nonpolyposis colorectal cancer; MMR, mismatch repair.

viding inhibitory cell cycle control. Tumor formation occurs when these inhibitory controls are deregulated by mutation. Point mutations, loss of heterozygosity (LOH), frame shift mutations, and promoter hypermethylation are all types of genetic changes that can cause failure of a tumor suppressor gene. These genes are often referred to as "gatekeeper" genes because they provide cell cycle inhibition and regulatory control at specific checkpoints in cell division. The failure of regulation of normal cellular function by tumor suppressor genes is appropriately described by the term *loss of function.* Both alleles of the gene must be nonfunctional to initiate tumor formation.

The adenomatous polyposis coli *(APC)* gene is a tumor suppressor gene located on chromosome 5q21. Its product is 2843 amino acids in length and forms a cytoplasmic complex with GSK-3β (a serine-threonine kinase), β-catenin, and axin. β-Catenin, a multifunctional protein, is a structural component of the epithelial cell adherens junctions and the actin cytoskeleton; it also binds in the cytoplasm to Tcf/LEF and is then transported into the nucleus where it activates transcription of genes like c-*myc* and others that regulate cellular growth and proliferation. *APC* therefore participates in cell cycle control by regulating the intracytoplasmic pool of β-catenin.

The *Wnt* signaling proteins are closely associated with the *APC*/β-catenin pathway. *APC* also influences cell cycle proliferation by regulating *Wnt* expression. *Wnt* gene products are extracellular signaling molecules that help regulate tissue development throughout the organism. The *Wnt* signaling proteins are closely associated with the *APC*/β-catenin pathway. Under normal conditions, reduced intracytoplasmic β-catenin levels inhibit *Wnt* expression. When *APC* is mutated however, β-catenin levels rise and *Wnt* is activated. Overexpression of *Wnt* leads to activation of *Wnt* target genes such as *cyclin*

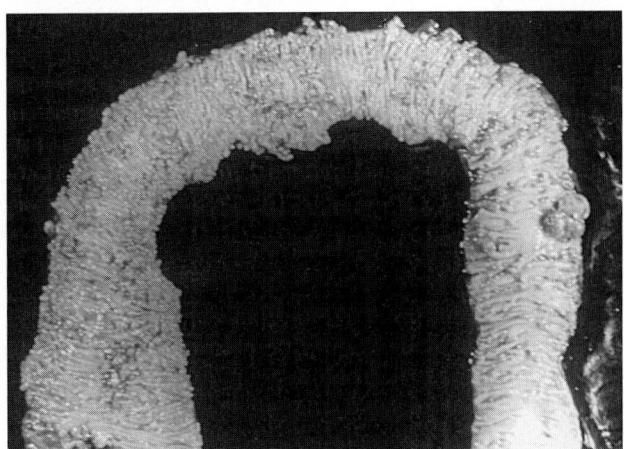

FIGURE 48-45. Familial adenomatous polyposis, macroscopic appearance. The colon has been opened longitudinally, exposing the mucosa. Thousands of small polyps are seen throughout the colon (note the large one on the left side). (Courtesy of M. Markowitz Haber, M.D., Hahnemann University Hospital.)

D1 and *MYC,* which drive cell proliferation and tumor formation.[74]

The earliest mutations in the adenoma-carcinoma sequence occur in the *APC* gene. The earliest phenotypic change present is known as "aberrant crypt formation," and the most consistent genetic aberrations within these cells are abnormally short proteins known as *APC* truncations. Most clinically relevant derangements in *APC* are truncation mutations created by inappropriate transcription of premature termination codons.[75]

A germline *APC* truncation mutation is responsible for the autosomal dominant inherited disease, familial adenomatous polyposis (FAP). Thirty percent of cases of FAP are de novo germline mutations, and thus patients present without a family history of the disease. FAP is rare, with an estimated incidence of 1/8000 in the United States, occurring without gender predilection. It is classically characterized by greater than 100 adenomatous polyps being present in the colon and rectum. These polyps often number in the thousands and are almost always manifest by the late second or early third decade of life (Fig. 48-45). Because some of these polyps proceed through the adenoma-carcinoma sequence, most patients with FAP will die of colon cancer by the fifth decade of life in the absence of surgical intervention. FAP is of great interest to those studying sporadic colorectal cancer because *APC* truncation mutations similar to those found in *APC* patients occur in 85% of sporadic colorectal cancers.

Most *APC* truncation mutations occur in the "mutational cluster region" of the gene, an area responsible for β-catenin binding. However, genotype-phenotype correlations exist with mutations in other regions of the gene. For example, mutations close to the 5′ end of the gene produce a very short truncated protein that causes the syndrome known as "attenuated FAP" or AFAP. These patients usually have far less than the hundreds of polyps usually associated with FAP, and the disease has a tendency to spare the rectum. "Classic" FAP is characterized by truncation mutations occurring in the gene from codon 1250 to codon 1464. Mutations occurring farther along the gene toward the 3′ end are quite rare and most likely result in either a much attenuated phenotype or no detectable abnormality at all (Fig. 48-46).

The variability of the FAP phenotype is also expressed by the presence or absence of extraintestinal manifestations of disease. In the past, the term *Gardner's syndrome* was used to describe the coexpression of profuse colonic adenomatous polyps along with osteomas of the mandible and skull, desmoid tumors of the mesentery, and periampullary neoplasms. Many other associated disorders have been subsequently described, including thyroid papillary tumors, medulloblastomas, hypertrophic gastric fundic polyps, and congenital hypertrophy of the pigmented retinal epithelium of the iris (CHRPE). The expression of extraintestinal manifestations of FAP is dependent on mutation location, with the vast majority of these signs seen only when the truncation occurs in a very small area of the mutational cluster region.

Another *APC* mutation implicated in about 25% of colorectal cancers afflicting Ashkenazi Jewish descendants is the I1307 point mutation caused by substitution of a lysine for isoleucine at codon 1307. This was initially believed to be a genetic polymorphism—a substitution that does not affect the protein structure. However, it is now recognized as probably the most important cause of familial colorectal cancer in this population.

The most frequently mutated tumor suppressor gene in human neoplasia is *p53 (TP53)*, located on chromosome 17p. Mutations in *p53* are present in 75% of colorectal cancers and occur rather late in the adenoma-carcinoma sequence. Under normal conditions, *p53* acts by inducing apoptosis in response to cellular damage or by causing G1 cell-cycle arrest allowing DNA repair mechanisms to

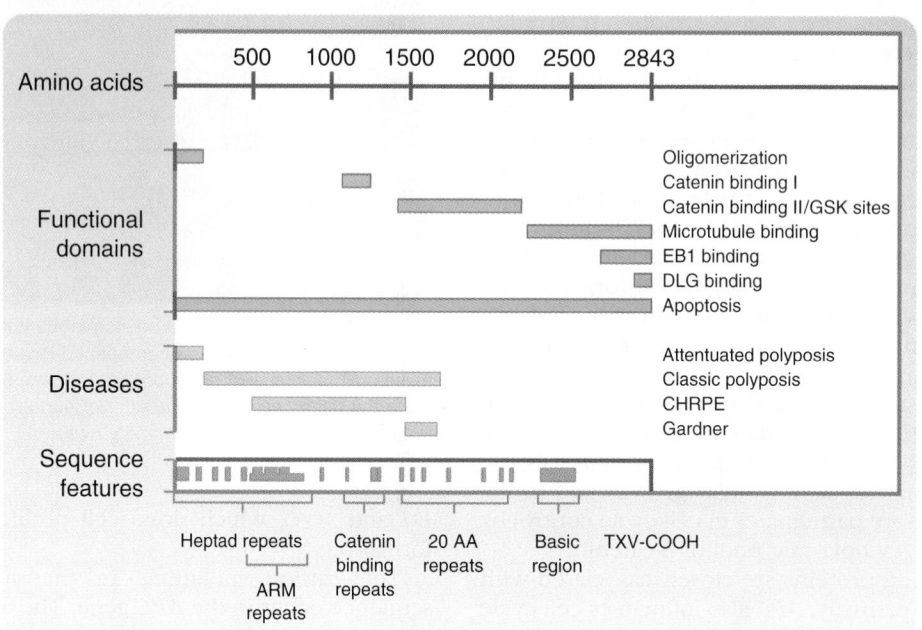

FIGURE 48-46. Functional and pathogenic properties of *APC*. APC is a protein heterodimer 2843 amino acids in length. The figure depicts the functional domains of APC schematically as blue bars where regional mutations result in loss of protein binding as described in the column on the right side of the figure. Mutations in these regions result in truncations that may affect cellular structure and cell signaling, such as the inability to bind catenins and interference with microtubule binding. Cellular processes such as apoptosis are affected by mutations occurring at many sites along the gene. Some mutational affects are unknown, such as those preventing EB1 and DLG binding (proteins with unclear functions). Diseases are similarly represented by gold bars. Mutations within the regions depicted result in the disease phenotypes described in the right column, including attenuated polyposis, classic polyposis, CHRPE, and Gardner's syndrome (extraintestinal manifestations of familial adenomatous polyposis). (From Kinzler KW, Vogelstein B: Lessons from hereditary colorectal cancer. Cell 87:159-170, 1996.)

occur. One of the features of mutated *p53* is that it is unable to activate the *BAX* gene to induce apoptosis. For its role in regulating apoptosis, *p53* is known as the "guardian of the genome." The minority of colon cancer patients who have intact *p53* in their tumors may possess a survival advantage. Several recent studies have indicated that prognostic significance may be related to tumor *p53* status.[76]

A number of genes on chromosome 18q are implicated in colorectal cancer, including *SMAD2, SMAD4,* and *DCC.* SMAD proteins are involved in the TGFβ signal transduction pathway. *SMAD2* and *SMAD4* are mutated in 5% to 10% of sporadic colorectal cancer. DCC is encoded by a large gene and is involved in cell-cell or cell-matrix interactions. It is not clear how DCC is directly involved in colorectal neoplasia. *DPC4* is a gene adjacent to *DCC* and may be the tumor suppressor gene deleted in 18q mutations.[76]

Mismatch Repair Genes

Mismatch repair genes (MMR) are called "caretaker" genes because of their important role in policing the integrity of the genome and correcting DNA replication errors. MMR genes that undergo a loss of function contribute to carcinogenesis by accelerating tumor progression. Mutations in MMR genes (including *hMLH1, hMSH2, hMSH3, hPMS1, hPMS2,* and *hMSH6*) result in the syndrome hereditary nonpolyposis colorectal cancer (HNPCC). Approximately 3% of colorectal cancers in the United States are caused by HNPCC. Mutations in MMR genes produce microsatellite instability. Microsatellites are repetitive sequences of DNA that seem to be randomly distributed throughout the genome. Stability of these sequences is a good measure of the general integrity of the genome. MMR gene mutations result in errors in S phase when DNA is newly synthesized and copied. Microsatellite instability exists in 10% to 15% of sporadic tumors and in 95% of tumors in patients with HNPCC. Even so, only 50% of patients diagnosed with HNPCC have readily identifiable MMR mutations.[75]

Oncogenes

Protooncogenes are genes that produce proteins that promote cellular growth and proliferation. Mutations in protooncogenes typically produce a "gain-of-function" and can be caused by mutation in only one of the two alleles. After mutation, the gene is called an "oncogene." Overexpression of these growth-oriented genes contributes to the uncontrolled proliferation of cells associated with cancer. The products of oncogenes can be divided into categories. For example, growth factors (TGFβ, EGF, insulin-like growth factor); growth factor receptors *(erbB2),* signal transducers *(SRC, ABL, RAS);* and nuclear protooncogenes and transcription factors *(MYC)* are all oncogene products that appear to have a role in the development of colorectal neoplasia. The *RAS* protooncogene is located on chromosome 12, and mutations are believed to occur very early in the adenoma-carcinoma sequence. Mutated *RAS* has been found to be present in aberrant crypt foci as well as adenomatous polyps. Activated *RAS* leads to constitutive activity of the protein that stimulates cellular growth. Fifty percent of sporadic colon cancers possess *RAS* mutations, and current trials of farnesyl transferase inhibitors, which block a step in *RAS* post-translational modification, may hold therapeutic promise.[74]

The Adenoma-Carcinoma Sequence

The adenoma-carcinoma sequence is now recognized as the process through which most colorectal carcinomas develop. Clinical and epidemiologic observations have long been cited to support the hypothesis that colorectal carcinomas evolve through a progression of benign polyps to invasive carcinoma, and the elucidation of the genetic pathways to cancer described earlier has confirmed the validity of this hypothesis. However, before the molecular genesis of colorectal cancer was appreciated, there was considerable controversy as to whether colorectal cancer arose de novo or evolved from a polyp that was initially a benign precursor. Although there have been a few documented instances of tiny colonic cancers arising de novo from normal mucosa, these instances are rare, and the validity of the adenoma-carcinoma sequence is now accepted by virtually all authorities. The historical observations that led to the hypothesis are of interest because of the therapeutic implications implicit in an understanding of the adenoma-carcinoma sequence. Observations that provided support for the hypothesis include the following:

- Larger adenomas are found to harbor cancers more often than smaller ones, and the larger the polyp, the higher the risk of cancer. While the cellular characteristics of the polyp are important, with villous adenomas carrying a higher risk than tubular adenomas, the size of either polyp is also important. The risk of cancer in a tubular adenoma smaller than 1 cm in diameter is less than 5%, whereas the risk of cancer in a tubular adenoma larger than 2 cm is 35%. A villous adenoma larger than 2 cm carries a 50% chance of containing a cancer.
- Residual benign adenomatous tissue is found in the majority of invasive colorectal cancers, suggesting progression of the cancer from the remaining benign cells to the predominant malignant ones.
- Benign polyps have been observed to develop into cancers. There have been reports of the direct observation of benign polyps that were not removed progressing over time into malignancies.
- Colonic adenomas occur more frequently in patients who have colorectal cancer. Nearly a third of all patients with colorectal cancer will also have a benign colorectal polyp.
- Patients who develop adenomas have an increased lifetime risk of developing colorectal cancer.
- Removal of polyps decreases the incidence of cancer. Patients with small adenomas have a 2.3 times increased risk of cancer after the polyp is removed, compared with an 8-fold increased incidence of

colorectal cancer in patients with polyps who do not undergo polypectomy.

- Populations with a high risk of colorectal cancer also have a high prevalence of colorectal polyps.
- Patients with familial adenomatous polyposis will develop colorectal cancer virtually 100% of the time in the absence of surgical intervention. The adenomas that characterize this syndrome are histologically the same as sporadic adenomas.
- The peak incidence for the discovery of benign colorectal polyps is 50 years of age. The peak incidence for the development of colorectal cancer is 60 years of age. This suggests a 10-year time span for the progression of an adenomatous polyp to a cancer. It has been estimated that a polyp larger than 1 cm has a cancer risk of 2.5% in 5 years, 8% in 10 years, and 24% in 20 years.

These observations and the studies by molecular biologists document that colonic mucosa progresses through stages to the eventual development of an invasive cancer. Colonic epithelial cells lose the normal progression to maturity and cell death and begin proliferating in a more and more uncontrolled manner. With this uncontrolled proliferation the cells accumulate on the surface of the bowel lumen as a polyp. With more proliferation and increasing cellular disorganization the cells extend though the muscularis mucosae to become invasive carcinoma. Even at this advanced stage, the process of colorectal carcinogenesis generally follows an orderly sequence of invasion of the muscularis mucosae, pericolic tissue, lymph nodes, and, finally, distant metastasis (Figs. 48-47 and 48-48).

Colorectal Polyps

A colorectal polyp is any mass projecting into the lumen of the bowel above the surface of the intestinal epithelium. Polyps arising from the intestinal mucosa are generally classified by their gross appearance as pedunculated (with a stalk) (Fig. 48-49) or sessile (flat, without a stalk) (Fig. 48-50). They are further classified by their histologic appearance as tubular adenoma (with branched tubular glands), villous adenoma (with long finger-like projections of the surface epithelium) (Fig. 48-51), or tubulovillous adenoma (with elements of both cellular patterns). The most common benign polyp is the tubular adenoma, composing 65% to 80% of all polyps removed. Ten to 25% of polyps are tubulovillous, and 5% to 10% are villous adenomas. Tubular adenomas are most often pedunculated, and villous adenomas are more commonly sessile. The degree of cellular atypia is variable across the span of polyps, but there is generally less atypia in tubular adenomas, and severe atypia or dysplasia (precancerous cellular change) is found more often in villous adenomas. The incidence of invasive carcinoma being found in a polyp is dependent on the size and histologic type of the polyp. As mentioned previously, there is less than a 5% incidence of carcinoma in an adenomatous polyp less than 1 cm in size, whereas there is a 50% chance that a villous adenoma greater than 2 cm will contain a cancer.

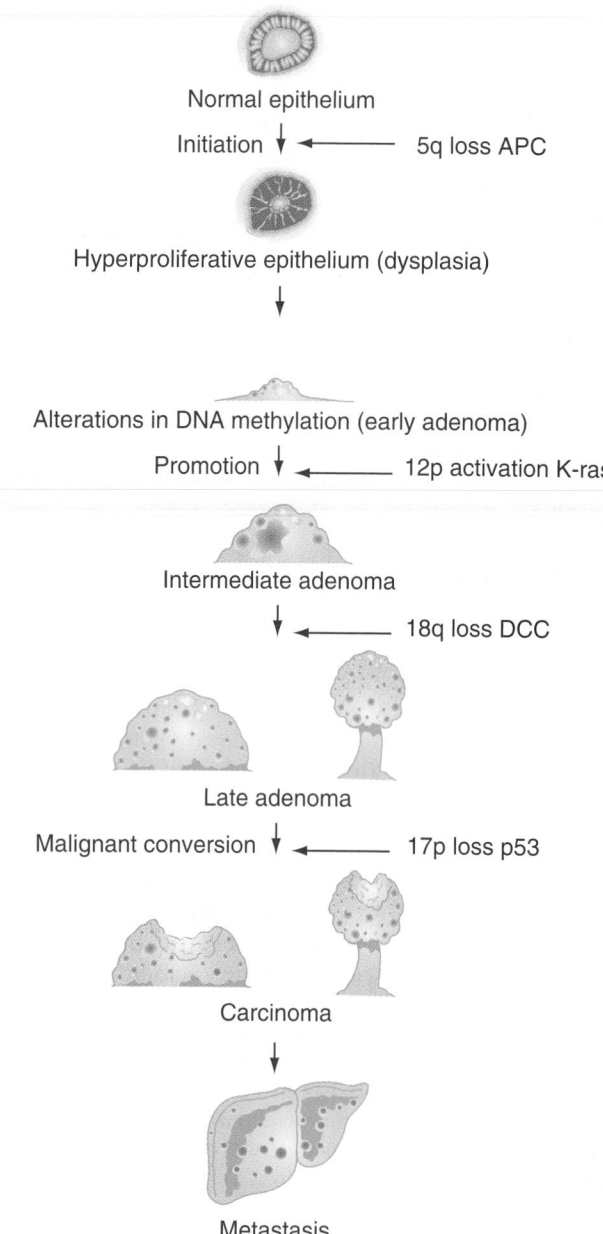

FIGURE 48-47.   Model of colorectal carcinogenesis. (Modified from Corman ML [ed]: Colon & Rectal Surgery, 4th ed. Philadelphia, Lippincott-Raven, 1998, p 593; after Fearon ER, Vogelstein B: A genetic model of colorectal cancer tumorigenesis. Cell 61:759, 1990. With permission.)

The treatment of an adenomatous or villous polyp is removal, usually by colonoscopy. The presence of any polypoid lesion is an indication for a complete colonoscopy and polypectomy, if feasible. Polyps on a stalk are often removed by a snare passed through the colonoscope, whereas sessile (flat) polyps present technical problems with this technique because of danger of perforation associated with the snare technique. Although it may be feasible to elevate the sessile polyp from the underlying muscularis with saline injection, permitting subsequent endoscopic excision, sessile lesions will often

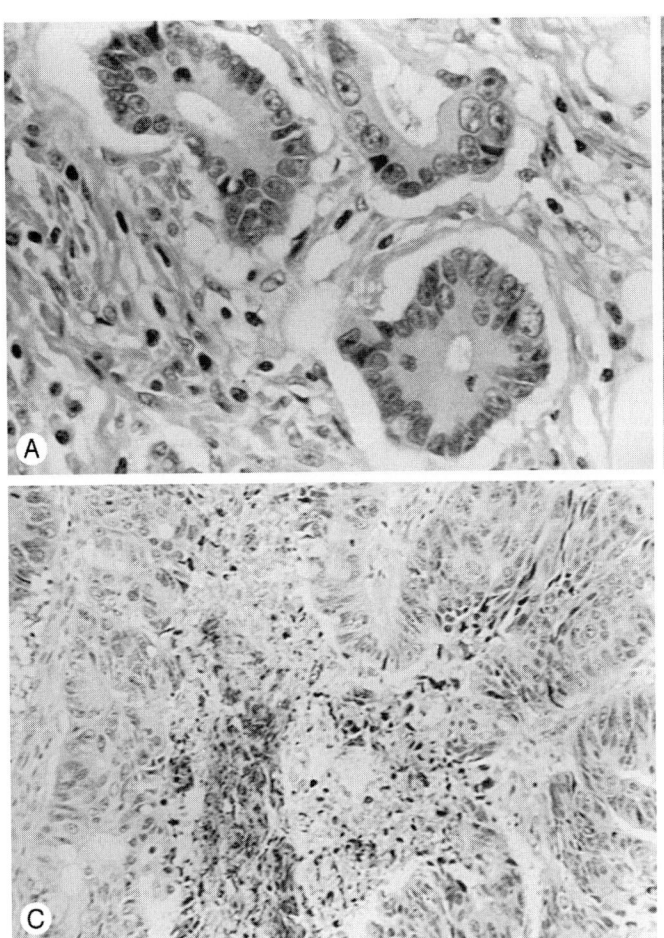

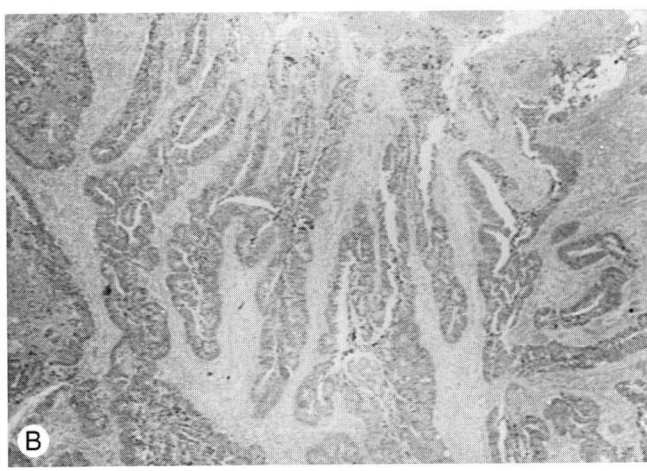

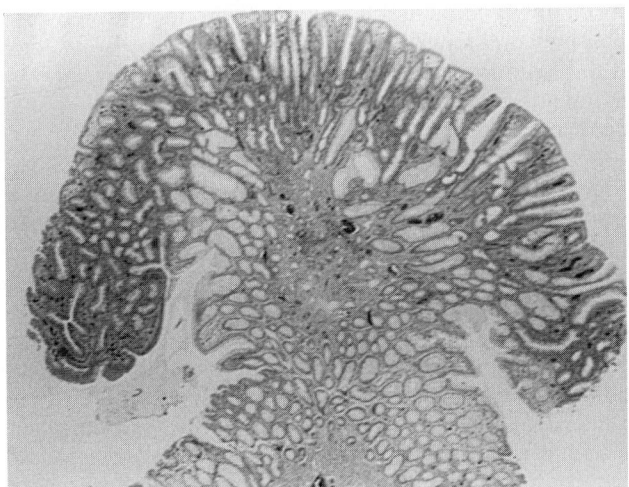

FIGURE 48-48. Colon carcinoma, microscopic appearance. **A,** Neoplastic glands present within desmoplastic stroma. **B,** Neoplastic glands in region of ulcerated surface. **C,** Neoplastic glands with extensive central necrosis present within desmoplastic stroma. (**A** to **C,** Courtesy of M. Markowitz Haber, M.D., Hahnemann University Hospital.)

FIGURE 48-49. Pedunculated adenomatous polyp, microscopic appearance at low-power magnification. The head of the polyp is lined with dysplastic epithelium, whereas the stalk is lined with nondysplastic epithelium. (Courtesy of M. Markowitz Haber, M.D., Hahnemann University Hospital.)

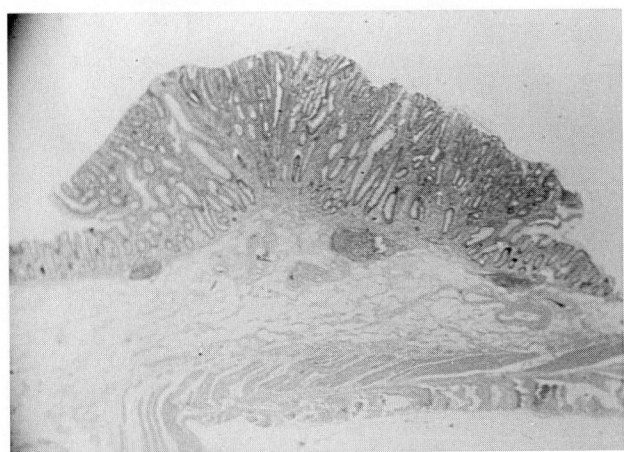

FIGURE 48-50. Sessile adenomatous polyp, microscopic appearance at low-power magnification. This small tubular adenoma is called sessile because of its broad base, the preservation of the muscularis mucosa underneath, and the absence of a stalk. (Courtesy of M. Markowitz Haber, M.D., Hahnemann University Hospital.)

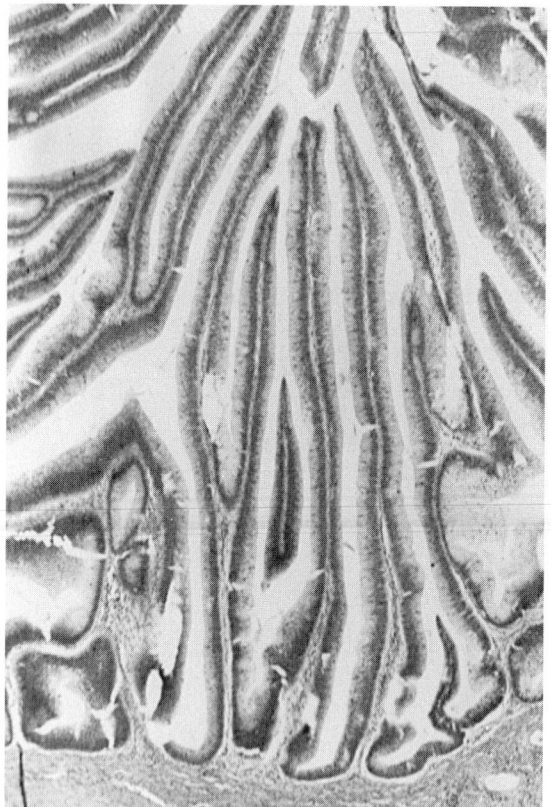

FIGURE 48-51.   Villous adenoma. This photomicrograph reveals the finger-like projections that give the appearance of villi. (Courtesy of M. Markowitz Haber, M.D., Hahnemann University Hospital.)

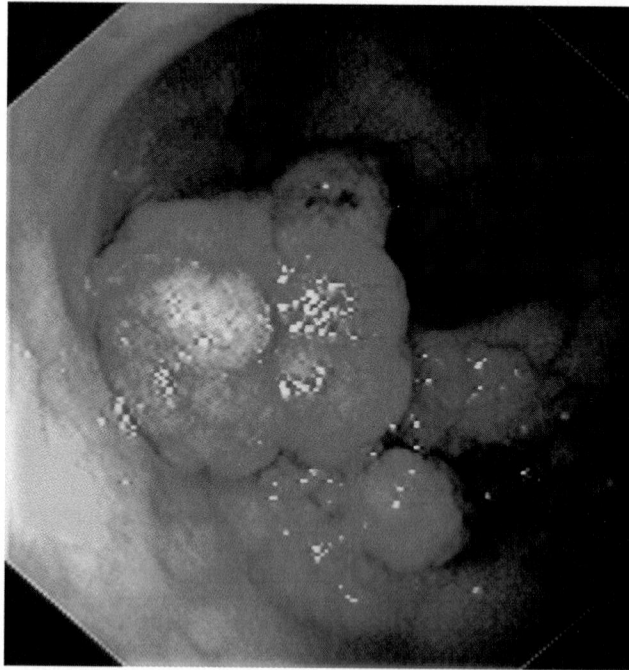

FIGURE 48-52.   Colonoscopic view of sessile polyp. This polyp proved to be a carcinoma after it was removed by segmental resection.

require segmental colectomy for complete removal (Fig. 48-52).

As described earlier, adenomatous polyps should be considered precursors of cancer; and when cancer arises in a polyp careful consideration needs to be given to ensure the adequacy of treatment. "Invasive carcinoma" describes the situation in which malignant cells have extended through the muscularis mucosae of the polyp, whether it is a lesion on a stalk or a sessile lesion. Carcinoma confined to the muscularis mucosae does not metastasize, and the cellular abnormalities should be described as "atypia." Complete excision of this type of polyp is adequate treatment.

If invasive carcinoma penetrates the muscularis mucosae, consideration of the risk of lymph node metastasis and local recurrence is required to determine whether a more extensive resection is required. In 1985, Haggit and associates[77] proposed a classification for polyps containing cancer according to the depth of invasion as follows (Fig. 48-53):

Level 0: Carcinoma does not invade the muscularis mucosae (carcinoma-in-situ or intramucosal carcinoma).
Level 1: Carcinoma invades through the muscularis mucosae into the submucosa but is limited to the head of the polyp.
Level 2: Carcinoma invades the level of the neck of the polyp (junction between the head and the stalk).
Level 3: Carcinoma invades any part of the stalk.
Level 4: Carcinoma invades into the submucosa of the bowel wall below the stalk of the polyp but above the muscularis propria.

By definition, all sessile polyps with invasive carcinoma are level 4 by Haggitt's criteria.

If a polyp contains a histologically poorly differentiated invasive carcinoma, or if there are cancer cells observed in the lymphovascular spaces, there is a greater than 10% chance of metastases and these lesions should be treated aggressively.

A pedunculated polyp with invasion to levels 1, 2, and 3 has a low risk of lymph node metastasis or local recurrence, and complete excision of the polyp is adequate if the above mentioned poor prognostic factors are not present. A sessile polyp containing invasive cancer has at least a 10% chance of metastasis to regional lymph nodes, but if the lesion is well or moderately differentiated and there is no lymphovascular invasion noted, and the lesion can be completely excised, the depth of invasion by the cancer may provide useful prognostic information. There is a high risk of lymph node and distant metastasis associated with sessile cancers in the rectum, and these lesions should be treated aggressively.

Hyperplastic polyps are the most common colonic polyps, but they are usually quite small and composed of cells showing dysmaturation and hyperplasia. The small diminutive polyps have been regarded as benign in nature with no neoplastic potential. The histologic appearance of these polyps is serrated (saw-toothed) (Fig. 48-54). Ninety percent of these polyps are less than 3 mm, and these diminutive lesions are generally considered to have

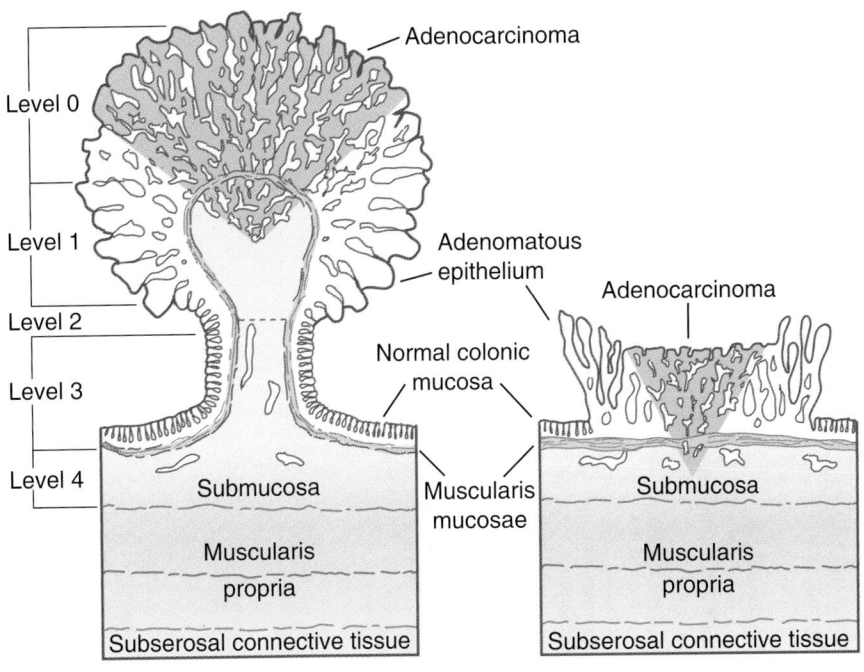

FIGURE 48-53. Anatomic landmarks of pedunculated and sessile adenomas. (From Haggitt RC, Glotzbach RE, Soffer EE, et al: Prognostic factors in colorectal carcinomas arising in adenomas: Implications for lesions removed by endoscopic polypectomy. Gastroenterology 89:328-336, 1985.)

Pedunculated adenoma Sessile adenoma

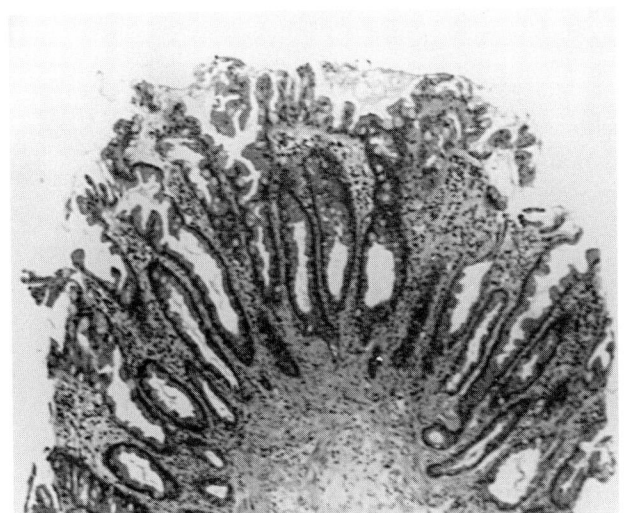

FIGURE 48-54. Hyperplastic polyp. Elongated tubular glands are lined by epithelium with abundant pink cytoplasm and a tufted appearance, seen predominantly at the surface and at the luminal portion of the gland. This gives the glands a serrated, or saw-toothed, appearance. (Courtesy of M. Markowitz Haber, M.D., Hahnemann University Hospital.)

no malignant potential. However, adenomatous changes can be found in hyperplastic polyps, and for this reason the polyps should be excised for histologic examination. Recently, these serrated adenomas have been observed to be associated with development of cancers that predominate in the right side of the colon more frequently in elderly women and smokers. These serrated adenomas appear to be associated with the microsatellite instability characteristic of defects in DNA repair mechanisms.[78]

Hereditary Cancer Syndromes (Table 48-4)

Peutz-Jeghers syndrome is an autosomal dominant syndrome characterized by the combination of hamartomatous polyps of the intestinal tract and hyperpigmentation of the buccal mucosa, lips, and digits. Germline defects in the tumor suppressor serine/threonine kinase 11 (STK11) gene are implicated in this rare autosomal dominant inherited disease. Although the syndrome was first described by Hutchinson in 1896, later separate descriptions by Peutz and then Jeghers in the 1940s brought recognition of the condition. The syndrome is associated with an increased (2% to 10%) risk of cancer of the intestinal tract, with cancers reported throughout the intestinal tract, from the stomach to the rectum. There is also an increased risk of extraintestinal malignancies, including cancer of the breast, ovary, cervix, fallopian tubes, thyroid, lung, gallbladder, bile ducts, pancreas, and testes.

The polyps may cause bleeding or intestinal obstruction (from intussusception). If surgery is required for these symptoms, an attempt should be made to remove as many polyps as possible with the aid of intraoperative endoscopy and polypectomy. Any polyp that is larger than 1.5 cm should be removed if possible. It is reasonable to survey the colon endoscopically every 2 years, and patients should be screened periodically for malignancies of the breast, cervix, ovary, testis, stomach, and pancreas.

Juvenile polyps are benign polyps composed of cystic dilatations of glandular structures within the fibroblastic stroma of the lamina propria. They are relatively uncommon, yet may cause bleeding or intussusception. For these reasons the polyps should be treated by endoscopic removal.

Multiple polyposis coli is an autosomal dominant syndrome with high penetrance that carries an increased risk of both gastrointestinal and extraintestinal cancer. The

TABLE 48-4. Hereditary Cancer Syndromes

	Hereditary Nonpolyposis Colon Cancer	Hereditary Adenomatous Polyposis Syndromes		Hereditary Hamartomatous Polyposis Syndromes			
		Familial Adenomatous Polyposis/Gardner's Syndrome	Turcot's Syndrome	Cowden's Disease	Familial Juvenile Polyposis	Peutz-Jeghers Syndrome	Ruvalcaba-Myhre-Smith Syndrome (Bannayan-Zonana Syndrome)
GI Features	Small number of colorectal polyps	Hundreds to thousands of colorectal polyps; duodenal adenomas and gastric polyps, usually fundic gland	Colorectal polyps, which may be few or resemble classic familial adenomatous polyposis	Polyps most commonly of colon and stomach	Juvenile polyps mostly in the colon but throughout GI tract Defined by ≥ 10 juvenile polyps	Small number of polyps throughout GI tract but most common in small intestine	Hamartomatous GI polyps, usually lipomas, hemangiomas, or lymphangiomas
Other Clinical Features	Muir-Torre variant: sebaceous adenomas, keratoacanthomas, sebaceous epitheliomas, and basal cell epitheliomas	Osteomas, desmoid tumors, epidermoid cysts, and congenital hypertrophy of retinal epithelium	Brain tumors, including cerebellar medulloblastoma and glioblastomas	Mucocutaneous lesions, thyroid adenomas and goiter, fibroadenomas and fibrocystic disease of the breast, uterine leiomyomas, and macrocephaly	Congenital abnormalities in at least 20%, including malrotation, hydrocephalus, cardiac lesions, Meckel's diverticulum, and mesenteric lymphangioma	Pigmented lesions of skin; benign and malignant genital tumors	Dysmorphic facial features, macrocephaly, seizures, intellectual impairment, and pigmented macules of shaft and glans of penis
Malignancy Risk	70%–80% lifetime risk of colorectal cancer; 30%–60% lifetime risk of endometrial cancer; ↑ risk of ovarian cancer, gastric carcinoma, transitional cell carcinoma of the ureters and renal pelvis, small bowel cancer, and sebaceous carcinomas	Colorectal cancer risk approaches 100%; ↑ risk of periampullary malignancy, thyroid carcinoma, central nervous system tumors, and hepatoblastoma	Colorectal carcinoma and brain tumors	10% risk of thyroid cancer and up to 50% risk of adenocarcinoma of breast in affected women	9% to 25% risk of colorectal cancer; ↑ risk of gastric, duodenal, and pancreatic cancer	↑ Risk of GI malignancy and pancreatic cancer and adenoma malignum of cervix; unknown risk of breast cancer	Malignant GI tumors identified but lifetime risk for malignancy unknown

Screening Recommendations	Colonoscopy at age 20-25 yr; repeat every 1-3 yr Transvaginal ultrasound or endometrial aspirate at age 20-25 yr; repeat annually (expert opinion only)	Flexible proctosigmoidoscopy at age 10-12 yr; repeat every 1-2 yr until age 35; after age 35 repeat every 3 yr Upper GI endoscopy every 1-3 yr starting when polyps first identified	Same as for familial adenomatous polyposis Also consider imaging of the brain	Annual physical exam with special attention to thyroid Mammography at age 30 or 5 yr before earliest breast cancer case in the family Routine colon cancer surveillance (expert opinion only)	Screening by age 12yr if symptoms have not yet arisen Colonoscopy with multiple random biopsies every several years (expert opinion only)	Upper GI endoscopy, small bowel radiography, and colonoscopy every 2 yr; pancreatic ultrasound and hemoglobin levels annually; gynecologic examination, cervical smear, and pelvic ultrasound annually; clinical breast exam and mammography at age 25 yr; clinical testicular exam and testicular ultrasound in males with feminizing features (expert opinion only)	No known published recommendations
Genetic Basis	AD *MLH1* (chromosome 3p) *MSH2* (chromosome 2p) *MSH6/GTMP* (chromosome 2p) *PMS1* (chromosome 2q) *PMS2* (chromosome 7q)	AD *APC* (chromosome 5q)	AD *APC* mutations identified predominantly in families with cerebellar medulloblastoma *MLH1, PMS2* mutations identified in families with predominance of glioblastomas	AD *PTEN* (chromosome 10q)	AD inheritance in some families Subset of families with mutation in *SMAD4 (DRC4)* (chromosome 10q)	AD *STK11* (chromosome 19p)	AD *PTEN* (chromosome 10q) in some families
Genetic Testing	Clinical testing of *MLH1* and *MSH2* genes available	Clinical testing of *APC* gene available	Clinical testing of *APC* and *MLH1* genes available	Research testing of *PTEN* gene available	Families being collected for research studies only	Research testing of *STK11* gene available	Research testing of *PTEN* gene available

GI, gastrointestinal; AD, autosomal dominant; ↑, increased.

syndrome is usually discovered because of GI bleeding, intussusception, or hypoalbuminemia associated with protein loss through the intestine. The juvenile polyps in this syndrome are predominately hamartomas, but the hamartomas may contain adenomatous elements and adenomatous polyps also are common. There is an increased cancer risk in the afflicted individuals, with a malignant potential of at least 10% in patients with multiple juvenile polyps. Mutations in the tumor suppressor gene *SMAD4* are believed to cause up to 50% of reported cases.

In patients with a relatively small number of juvenile polyps, endoscopic polypectomy should be done. However, patients with numerous polyps should be treated with abdominal colectomy, ileorectal anastomosis, and frequent endoscopic surveillance of the rectum. If the diffuse form of polyposis involves the rectal mucosa, consideration should be given to restorative proctocolectomy with ileal pouch anal anastomosis.

FAP is the prototypical hereditary polyposis syndrome. The discovery of the gene responsible for the transmission of the disease, the *APC* (adenomatosis polyposis coli) gene, located on chromosome 5q21, lagged behind the first descriptions of cases of FAP by an entire century. In 1863, Virchow reported a 15-year-old boy with multiple colonic polyps. In 1882, Cripps described the occurrence of numerous colonic polyps in multiple family members. In 1927, Cockayne demonstrated that FAP was genetically transmitted in an autosomal dominant fashion. Dukes was the first to establish some form of a familial tumor registry, which he reported with Lockhart-Mummery in 1930. Throughout the 20th century many reports described various extraintestinal manifestations associated with FAP. In 1986, Lemuel Herrera demonstrated that the underlying genetic abnormality was a mutation in the *APC* gene.

The common expression of the syndrome is the invariable presence of multiple colonic polyps, the frequent occurrence of gastric, duodenal, and periampullary polyps, and the occasional association of extraintestinal manifestations, including epidermoid cysts, desmoid tumors in the abdomen, osteomas, and brain tumors. Gastric and duodenal polyps will occur in about half of affected individuals. Most of the gastric polyps represent fundic gland hyperplasia, rather than adenomatous polyps, and have limited malignant potential. However, duodenal polyps are adenomatous and should be considered to be premalignant. Patients with FAP have an increased risk of ampullary cancer. Adenomatous polyps and cancer have also been found in the jejunum and ileum of patients with FAP. Rare extraintestinal malignancies in FAP patients include cancers of the extrahepatic bile ducts, gallbladder, pancreas, adrenals, thyroid, and liver. An interesting marker for FAP is congenital hypertrophy of the retinal pigmented epithelium (CHRPE), which can be detected by indirect ophthalmoscopy in about 75% of affected individuals.

The gene is expressed in 100% of patients with the mutation. Autosomal dominance results in expression in 50% of offspring. There is a negative family history in 10% to 20% of affected individuals who apparently acquire the syndrome as the result of a spontaneous mutation. All patients with the defective gene will develop cancer of the colon if left untreated. The average age of discovery of a new patient with FAP is 29 years. The average age of a patient who is newly discovered to have colorectal cancer related to FAP is 39 years. Eponymous polyposis syndromes now recognized to belong to the general disorder of FAP include Gardner's syndrome (colonic polyps, epidermal inclusion cysts, osteomas) and Turcot's syndrome (colonic polyps and brain tumors).

Osteomas usually present as visible and palpable prominences in the skull, mandible, and tibia of individuals with FAP. They are virtually always benign. Radiographs of the maxilla and mandible may reveal bone cysts, supernumerary and impacted molars, or congenitally absent teeth. Desmoid tumors can present in the retroperitoneum and abdominal wall of affected patients, usually after surgery. These tumors seldom metastasize but are often locally invasive, and direct invasion of the mesenteric vessels, ureters, or walls of the small intestine can result in death.

Surgical treatment of patients with FAP is directed at removal of all affected colonic and rectal mucosa. Restorative proctocolectomy with ileal pouch anal anastomosis (IPAA) has become the most commonly recommended operation. The procedure is usually accompanied by a distal rectal mucosectomy to ensure that all premalignant colonic mucosa is removed, and the IPAA is fashioned between the ileal pouch and the dentate line of the anal canal. Patients who undergo this procedure for FAP have a better functional result than patients similarly treated for ulcerative colitis, in that the incidence of inflammation in the ileal pouch (pouchitis) is much lower in patients with FAP than in patients with ulcerative colitis.

An alternative approach, total abdominal colectomy with ileorectal anastomosis, was used extensively before the development of the technique of IPAA, and has certain advantages to be considered. If a FAP patient has relatively few polyps in the rectum, consideration may be given to this option. The abdominal colon is resected, and an anastomosis fashioned between the ileum and rectum. It is technically a simpler operation to perform, and the pelvic dissection is avoided. This eliminates the potential complication of injury to the autonomic nerves that could result in impotence. In addition, there is theoretically less of a risk of anastomotic leak from the relatively simple ileorectal anastomosis fashioned in the peritoneal cavity, compared with the long suture (or staple) lines required to form the ileal pouch and then fashion the anastomosis between the ileal pouch and the anus.

An additional argument in favor of abdominal colectomy and ileorectal anastomosis is the observation that sulindac and celecoxib have been observed to cause the regression of adenomatous polyps in some patients with FAP.[79] The disadvantages are that the rectum remains at high risk for the formation of new precancerous polyps, a proctoscopic examination is required every 6 months to detect and destroy any new polyps, and there is a definite increased risk of cancer arising in the rectum with the passage of time.

It has been suggested that genetic testing may help make a decision between restorative proctocolectomy with IPAA and abdominal colectomy with ileorectal anastomosis. It has been observed that the risk of rectal cancer is almost three times higher in FAP patients with a mutation after codon 1250 than in patients with mutations before this codon. This fact may influence the decision to offer abdominal colectomy with ileorectal anastomosis to patients whose mutation occurs proximal to codon 1250 if proctoscopic examination should reveal no or few polyps in the rectum.[80]

Patients who choose to be treated by abdominal colectomy with ileorectal anastomosis should realize that the risk of developing rectal cancer is real and has been shown to be 4%, 5.6%, 7.9%, and 25% at 5, 10, 15, and 20 years after the operation, respectively.[81] Even though sulindac and celecoxib can produce partial regression of polyps, semiannual surveillance of the rectal mucosa is required, and about one third of patients treated by abdominal colectomy and ileorectal anastomosis will develop florid polyposis of the rectum that will require proctectomy (and either ileostomy or IPAA) within 20 years.

As discussed earlier, polyps of the stomach and duodenum are not uncommon in patients with FAP. The gastric polyps are usually hyperplastic and do not require surgical removal. However, the duodenal and ampullary polyps are usually neoplastic and require attention. A reasonable surveillance program is for upper gastrointestinal surveillance every 2 years after the age of 30 and endoscopic polypectomy, if possible, to remove all large adenomas from the duodenum. If numerous polyps are identified, the endoscopy obviously should be repeated at greater frequency. If an ampullary cancer is discovered at an early stage, pancreatoduodenectomy (Whipple's procedure) is indicated.

The abdominal desmoid tumor can be an especially vexing and difficult extraintestinal manifestation of FAP. After surgical procedures, dense fibrous tissue forms in the mesentery of the small intestine or within the abdominal wall in some patients with FAP. If the mesentery is involved, the intestine can be tethered or invaded directly by the tumor. The locally invasive tumor can also encroach on the vascular supply to the intestine. Small desmoid tumors confined to the abdominal wall are appropriately treated by resection, but the surgical treatment of mesenteric desmoids is dangerous and generally futile. There have been sporadic reports of regression of desmoid tumors after treatment with sulindac, tamoxifen, radiation, and various types of chemotherapy. The initial treatment is usually with sulindac or tamoxifen.[82]

The ability to identify the genetic mutation in most patients with FAP (although the mutation may not be identified in as many as 20% of patients with a well-documented, transmissible FAP syndrome) permits a method of screening family members that are at risk of inheriting the mutation. It is imperative that the *APC* mutation is clearly identified in the DNA of a family member known to have the disease. The DNA of other family members can then be directly analyzed, requiring only a venipuncture. If the analysis demonstrates noninheritance of a mutated *APC* gene, the individual can avoid yearly endoscopic screening and should require only occasional colonoscopy.

HNPCC is the most frequently occurring hereditary colorectal cancer syndrome in the United States and Western Europe. It accounts for approximately 3% of all cases of colorectal cancer and for approximately 15% of such cancers in patients with a family history of colorectal cancer. Dr. Aldred S. Warthin, chairman of pathology at the University of Michigan, initially recognized this hereditary syndrome in 1985. Dr. Warthin's seamstress prophesied that she would die of cancer because of her strong family history of endometrial, gastric, and colon cancer. Dr. Warthin's investigations of her family's medical records revealed a pattern of autosomal dominant transmission of the cancer risk. This family (Family G) has been further studied and characterized by Dr. Henry Lynch, who described the prominent features of the syndrome, including onset of cancer at a relatively young age (mean of 44 years), proximal distribution (70% of cancers located in the right colon), predominance of mucinous or poorly differentiated (signet cell) adenocarcinoma, an increased number of synchronous and metachronous cancers, and, despite all of these poor prognostic indicators, a relatively good outcome after surgery. Two hereditary syndromes were initially described. Lynch I syndrome is characterized by cancer of the proximal colon occurring at a relatively young age, whereas Lynch II syndrome is characterized by families at risk for both colorectal cancer and extracolonic cancers, including cancers of endometrial, ovarian, gastric, small intestinal, pancreatic, and ureteral and renal pelvic origin.

Before the genetic mechanisms underlying the Lynch syndromes were understood, the syndrome was defined by the Amsterdam criteria, which required three criteria for the diagnosis: (1) colorectal cancer in three family members (first-degree relatives), (2) involvement of at least two generations, and (3) at least one affected individual being younger than the age of 50 at the time of diagnosis. These requirements were recognized as being too restrictive, and the modified Amsterdam criteria expanded the cancers to be included to not only colorectal but also endometrial, ovarian, gastric, pancreatic, small intestinal, ureteral, and renal pelvic cancers. Further liberalization for identifying patients with HNPCC occurred with the introduction of the Bethesda criteria (Box 48-4).

Molecular biologists have demonstrated that the increased cancer risk in these syndromes is due to malfunction of the DNA repair mechanism. Specific genes that have been shown to be responsible for the syndrome include *hMSH2* (located on chromosome 2p21), *hMLH1* (3p21), *hMSH6* (2p16-21), and *hPMS2* (7p21). A mutation in *hMSH2* has been shown to be responsible for the cancer prevalence in Cancer Family G. Mutations in *hMSH2* or *hMLH1* account for over 90% of identifiable mutations in patients with HNPCC. The initially reported difference in types of cancers occurring in Lynch I and Lynch II syndromes cannot be accounted for by mutations in specific mismatch repair genes. The cancer family syndrome involving *hMSH6* is characterized by an increased incidence of endometrial carcinoma.

The mainstay of the diagnosis of HNPCC is a detailed family history. Still, it should be remembered that as many as 20% of newly discovered cases of HNPCC are caused

Box 48-4. Clinical Criteria for Hereditary Nonpolyposis Colorectal Cancer (HNPCC)

Amsterdam Criteria

At least three relatives with colon cancer and all of the following:

One affected person is a first-degree relative of the other two affected persons

Two successive generations affected

At least one case of colon cancer diagnosed before age 50 years

Familial adenomatous polyposis excluded

Modified Amsterdam Criteria

Same as the Amsterdam criteria, except that cancer must be associated with HNPCC (colon, endometrium, small bowel, ureter, renal pelvis) instead of specifically colon cancer

Bethesda Criteria

The Amsterdam criteria or one of the following:

Two cases of HNPCC-associated cancer in one patient, including synchronous or metachronous cancer

Colon cancer and a first-degree relative with HNPCC-associated cancer and/or colonic adenoma (one case of cancer diagnosed before age 45 years and adenoma diagnosed before age 40 years)

Colon or endometrial cancer diagnosed before age 45 years

Right-sided colon cancer that has an undifferentiated pattern (solid-cribriform) or signet-cell histopathologic characteristics diagnosed before age 45 years

Adenomas diagnosed before age 40 years

---

by spontaneous germline mutations, so a family history may not accurately reflect the genetic nature of the syndrome. Colorectal cancer, or an HNPCC-related cancer, arising in a person younger than the age of 50 should raise the suspicion of this syndrome. Genetic counseling and genetic testing can be offered. If the individual proves to have HNPCC by identification of a mutation in one of the known mismatch repair genes, then other family members can be tested after obtaining genetic counseling. However, failure to identify a causative mismatch repair gene mutation in a patient with a suggestive history does not exclude the diagnosis of HNPCC. In as many as 50% of patients with a family history that clearly demonstrates HNPCC type transmission of cancer susceptibility, DNA testing will fail to identify the causative gene.

The management of patients with HNPCC is somewhat controversial, but the need for close surveillance in patients known to carry the mutation is obvious. It is usually recommended that a program of surveillance colonoscopy should begin at the age of 20. Colonoscopy is repeated every 2 years until the age of 35 and then annually thereafter. In women, periodic vacuum curettage is begun at age 25, as well as pelvic ultrasound and determination of CA-125 levels. Annual tests for occult blood in the urine should also be obtained, because of the risk of ureteral and renal pelvic cancer (Table 48-5).

It has been shown that annual colonoscopy and removal of polyps when found will decrease the incidence of colon cancer in patients with HNPCC. However, there have been well-documented cases of invasive colon cancers occurring 1 year after a negative colonoscopy. It is obvious that the slow evolution from benign polyp to invasive cancer is not a feature of pathogenesis in HNPCC patients, and this phenomenon of accelerated carcinogenesis mandates frequent (annual) colonoscopic examinations. Even with annual colonoscopic examinations there is a documented risk of colon cancer, but should a

---

TABLE 48-5.   Screening Recommendations for FAP and HNPCC

Lifetime Cancer Risk		Screening Recommendations
Familial Adenomatous Polyposis (FAP)		
Colorectal cancer	100%	Colonoscopy annually, beginning age 10-12
Duodenal or periampullary cancer	5%-10%	Upper GI endoscopy every 1 to 3 yr, beginning age 20-25
Pancreatic cancer	2%	Possible periodic abdominal ultrasound
Thyroid cancer	2%	Annual thyroid examination
Gastric cancer	<1%	Upper GI endoscopy as for duodenal and periampullary
Central nervous system cancer	<1%	Annual physical examination
Hereditary Nonpolyposis Colorectal Cancer (HNPCC)		
Colorectal cancer	80%	Colonoscopy, every 2 yr beginning age 20, annually after age 40 or 10 years younger than earliest case in family
Endometrial cancer	40%-60%	Pelvic exam, transvaginal ultrasound, endometrial aspirate every 1-2 yr, beginning age 25-35
Upper urinary tract cancer	4%-10%	Ultrasound and urinalysis every 1-2 yr; start at age 30 to 35 yr
Gallbladder and biliary cancer	2%-18%	No recommendation
Central nervous system cancer	<5%	No recommendation
Small bowel cancer	<5%	No recommendation

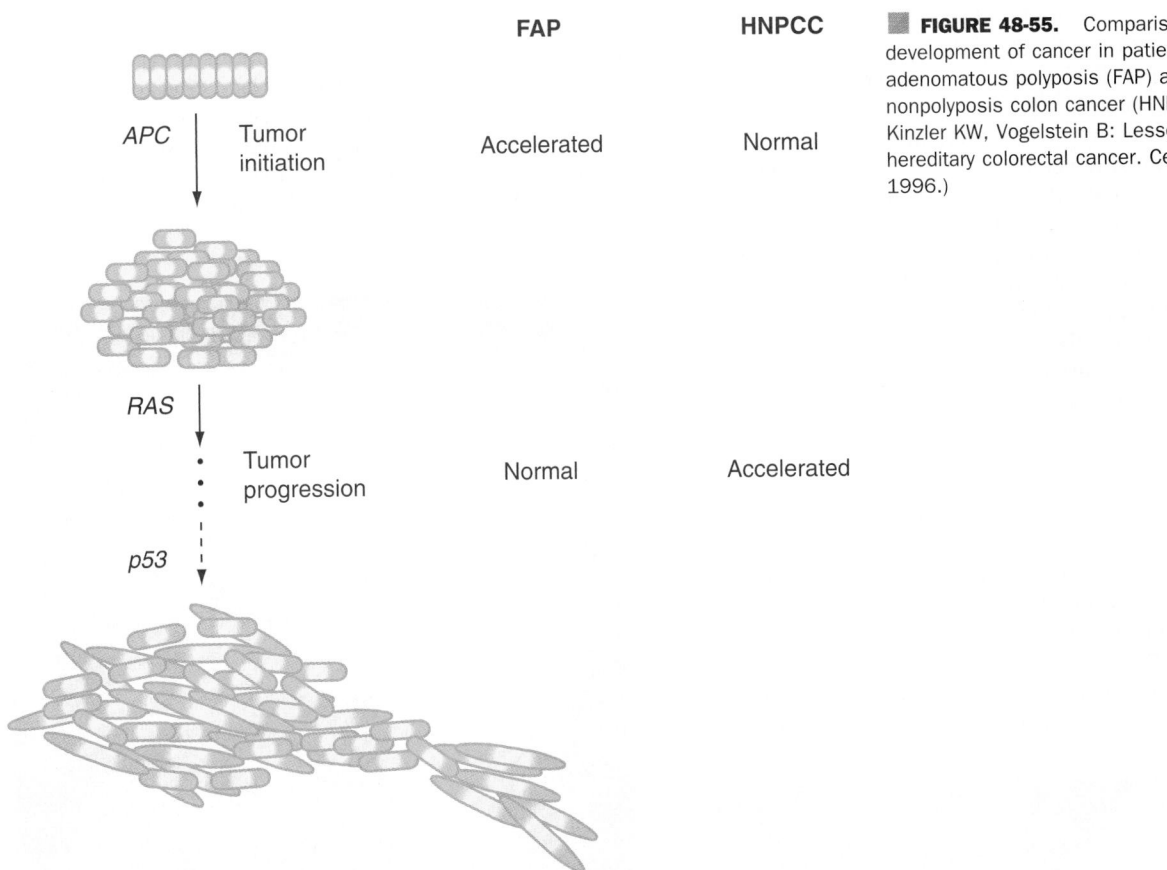

	FAP	HNPCC
APC — Tumor initiation	Accelerated	Normal
RAS — Tumor progression	Normal	Accelerated
p53		

FIGURE 48-55. Comparison of the development of cancer in patients with familial adenomatous polyposis (FAP) and hereditary nonpolyposis colon cancer (HNPCC). (From Kinzler KW, Vogelstein B: Lessons from hereditary colorectal cancer. Cell 87:159-170, 1996.)

cancer arise while the patient is under a vigorous surveillance program the cancer stage is usually favorable (Fig. 48-55).

When a colon cancer is detected in a patient with HNPCC, an abdominal colectomy and ileorectal anastomosis is the procedure of choice. If the patient is a woman with no further plans for childbearing, a prophylactic total abdominal hysterectomy and bilateral salpingo-oophorectomy is recommended. The rectum remains at risk for development of cancer, and annual proctoscopic examinations are mandatory after abdominal colectomy. Other forms of cancer associated with HNPCC are treated according to the same criteria as in nonhereditary cases. The role of prophylactic colectomy for patients with HNPCC has been considered in some instances, but this concept has not received universal acceptance. It is an interesting but well-documented fact that the prognosis is better for cancer patients with HNPCC than for non-HNPCC patients with cancer of the same stage.

Sporadic Colon Cancer

It is important to recognize the increased risk of cancer in patients with hereditary cancer syndromes, but by far the most common form of colorectal cancer is sporadic, without an associated strong family history.

Although the cause and pathogenesis of adenocarcinoma are similar throughout the large bowel, significant differences in the use of diagnostic and therapeutic modalities separate colonic from rectal cancers. This distinction

is largely due to the confinement of the rectum by the bony pelvis. The limited mobility of the rectum allows MRI to generate better images and increases its sensitivity. In addition, the proximity of the rectum to the anus permits easy access of ultrasound probes for more accurate assessment of the extent of penetration of the bowel wall and the involvement of adjacent lymph nodes. The limited accessibility of the rectum, the proximity to the anal sphincter, and the close association with the autonomic nerves supplying the bladder and genitalia require special and unique consideration when planning treatment for cancer of the rectum. Therefore, colon and rectal adenocarcinomas are discussed separately.

The signs and symptoms of colon cancer are varied, nonspecific, and somewhat dependent on the location of the tumor in the colon as well as the extent of constriction of the lumen caused by the cancer. Over the past several decades the incidence of cancer in the right colon has increased in comparison to cancer arising in the left colon and rectum. This is an important consideration, in that at least half of all colon cancers are located proximal to the area that can be visualized by the flexible sigmoidoscope. Colorectal cancers can bleed, causing red blood to appear in the stool (hematochezia). Bleeding from right-sided colon tumors can cause dark, tarry stools (melena). Often the bleeding may be asymptomatic and detected only by anemia discovered by a routine hemoglobin determination. Iron-deficiency anemia in any male or nonmenstruating female should lead to a search for a source of bleeding from the gastrointestinal tract. Bleeding is often associated with colon cancer, but in approximately one third of patients with a proven colon cancer the hemoglobin will be normal and the stool will test negative for occult blood.

Cancers located in the left colon are often constrictive. Patients with left-sided colon cancers may notice a change in bowel habit, most often reported as increasing constipation. Sigmoid cancers can mimic diverticulitis, presenting as pain, fever, and obstructive symptoms. At least 20% of patients with sigmoid cancer will also have diverticular disease, making the correct diagnosis difficult at times. Sigmoid cancers can also cause colovesical or colovaginal fistulas. Such fistulas are more commonly caused by diverticulitis, but it is imperative that the correct diagnosis be established, because the treatment of colon cancer is substantially different than the treatment for diverticulitis.

Cancers in the right colon more often present as melena, fatigue associated with anemia, or, if the tumor is advanced, abdominal pain. Although obstructive symptoms are more commonly associated with cancers of the left colon, any advanced colorectal cancer can cause a change in bowel habits and intestinal obstruction (Figs. 48-56 and 48-57).

Colonoscopy is the gold standard for establishing the diagnosis of colon cancer. It permits biopsy of the tumor

to verify the diagnosis while allowing inspection of the entire colon to exclude metachronous polyps or cancers (the incidence of a metachronous cancer is approximately 3%). Colonoscopy is generally performed even after a cancer is detected by barium enema to obtain a biopsy and to detect (and remove) small polyps that may be missed by the contrast study (Fig. 48-58).

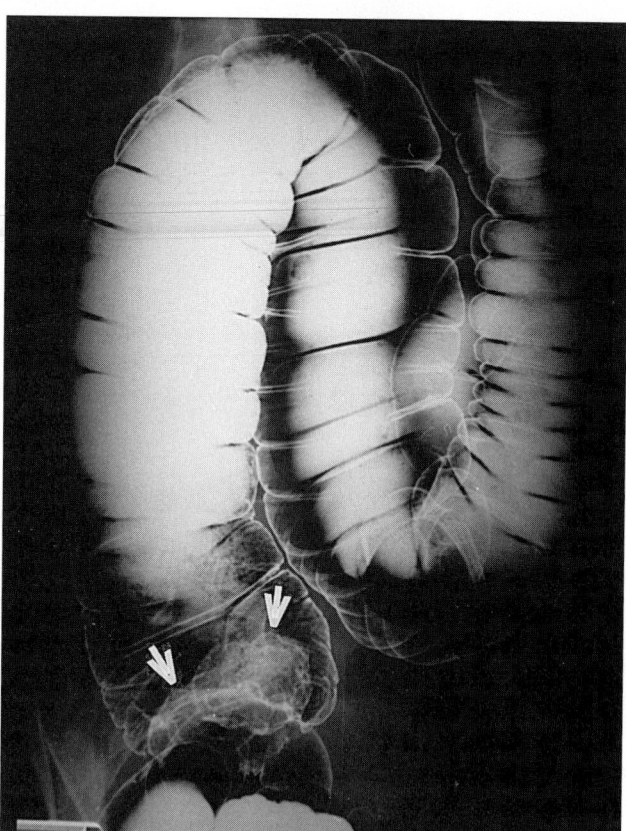

FIGURE 48-57.   Barium enema demonstrating a polypoid carcinoma arising in the cecum of a 35-year-old woman (arrows). (Courtesy of Dina F. Caroline, M.D., Ph.D., Temple University Hospital.)

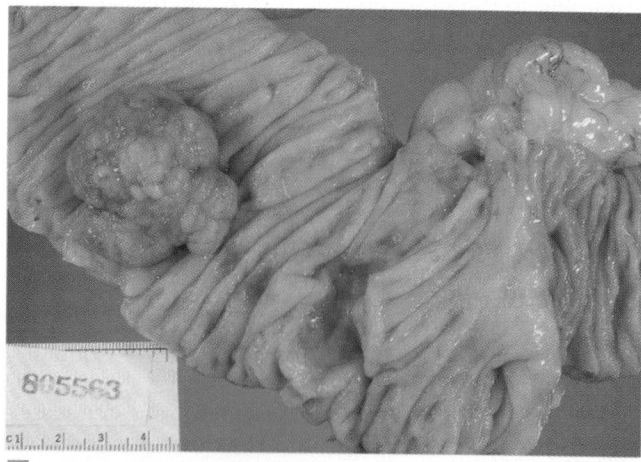

FIGURE 48-58.   Resected right colon containing large benign sessile polyp adjacent to an ulcerated carcinoma.

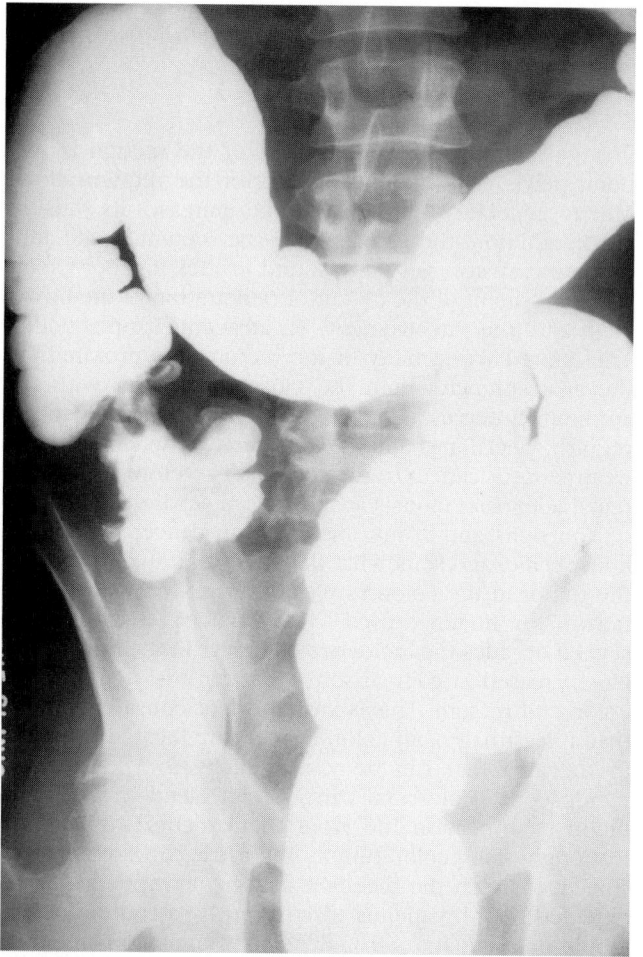

FIGURE 48-56.   Barium enema demonstrating "apple core" or "napkin ring" lesion, caused by a constricting carcinoma.

In patients with tumors causing complete obstruction the diagnosis is most properly established by resection of the tumor without the benefit of preoperative colonoscopy. A water-soluble contrast enema is often useful in such circumstances to establish the anatomic level of the obstruction. Primary anastomosis between the proximal colon and the colon distal to the tumor has been avoided in the past in the presence of obstruction because of a high risk of anastomotic leak associated with such an approach. Thus such patients were usually treated by resection of the segment of colon containing the obstructing cancer, suture closure of the distal sigmoid or rectum, and construction of a colostomy (Hartmann's operation). Intestinal continuity could be reestablished later after the colon had been cleansed with purgatives by taking down the colostomy and fashioning a colorectal anastomosis.

Alternatives to this approach have been to resect the segment of left colon containing the cancer and then cleanse the remaining colon with saline lavage by inserting a catheter through the appendix or ileum into the cecum and irrigating the contents from the colon. A primary anastomosis between the prepared colon and the rectum can then be fashioned without the need for a temporary colostomy. A third approach occasionally used for obstructing cancers of the sigmoid colon is to resect the tumor and the entire colon proximal to the tumor and fashion an anastomosis between the ileum and the distal sigmoid colon (subtotal colectomy and ileosigmoid anastomosis). This approach has the advantage of avoiding a temporary colostomy and eliminating the need to search for synchronous lesions in the colon proximal to the cancer. However, patients treated by this approach may have more frequent bowel movements.

More recently endoscopic techniques have been developed that permit the placement of a stent introduced with the aid of a colonoscope that traverses the obstructed tumor and expands, re-creating a lumen, relieving the obstruction, and permitting a bowel prep and elective operation with primary colorectal anastomosis.[83]

The approaches just discussed concern obstruction of the left colon. Complete obstruction of the right colon or cecum by cancer occurs less frequently. These patients present with signs and symptoms of a small bowel obstruction. If an obstruction of the proximal colon is suspected, a water-soluble contrast study is useful to verify the diagnosis and evaluate the distal colon for the presence of a synchronous lesion. Obstructing cancer of the proximal colon is treated by right colectomy with primary anastomosis between the ileum and the transverse colon.

Patients with tumors that are not obstructing should undergo a thorough evaluation for metastatic disease. This includes a thorough physical examination, chest radiograph, liver function tests, and carcinoembryonic antigen (CEA) level. Most surgeons now order CT or MRI to more thoroughly inspect the liver for metastases and to search for other intra-abdominal pathologic processes.

The presence of hepatic metastatic disease does not preclude the surgical excision of the primary tumor. Unless the hepatic metastatic disease is extensive, excising the primary cancer can provide excellent palliation. Bleeding and obstruction caused by the tumor can be avoided, and if the metastatic disease in the liver is resectable, the patient may yet be cured.

The objective of surgery for colon adenocarcinoma is the removal of the primary cancer with adequate margins, regional lymphadenectomy, and restoration of the continuity of the gastrointestinal tract by anastomosis. The extent of resection is determined by the location of the cancer, its blood supply and draining lymphatic system, and the presence or absence of direct extension into adjacent organs. It is important to resect the lymphatics (which parallel the arterial supply) to the greatest extent possible, to render the abdomen free of lymphatic metastases if possible. Should hepatic metastases subsequently be detected, they may still be resected for cure in some instances if the abdominal disease has been completely eradicated (Fig. 48-59).

To restore the continuity of the gastrointestinal tract, an anastomosis is fashioned with either sutures or staples, joining the ends of the intestine (small or large). It is important that both segments of the intestine used for the anastomosis have excellent blood supply and that there be no tension on the anastomosis. For lesions involving the cecum, ascending colon, and hepatic flexure, a right hemicolectomy is the procedure of choice. This involves removal of the bowel from 4 to 6 cm proximal to the ileocecal valve to the portion of the transverse colon supplied by the right branch of the middle colic artery. An anasto-

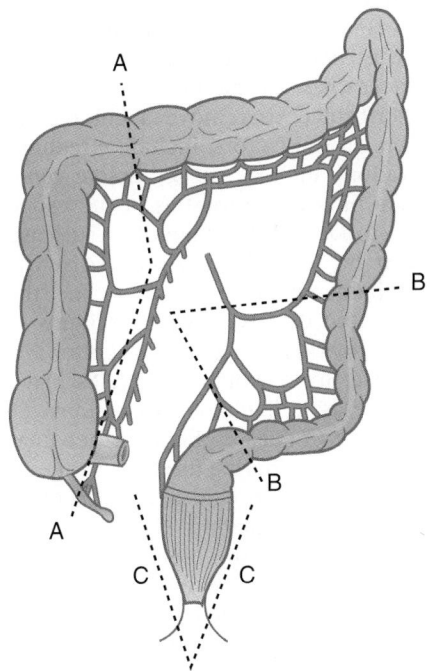

FIGURE 48-59. Operative procedures for right-sided colon cancer, sigmoid diverticulitis, and low-lying rectal cancer. A right hemicolectomy (**A**) involves resection of a few centimeters of terminal ileum and colon up to the division of the middle colic vessels into right and left. A sigmoidectomy (**B**) consists of removing the colon between the partially retroperitoneal descending colon and the rectum. An abdominoperineal resection of the rectum (**C**) is performed in a combined approach through the abdomen and through the perineum for the resection of the entire rectum and anus.

mosis is fashioned between the terminal ileum and the transverse colon. An extended right hemicolectomy is the procedure of choice for most transverse colon lesions and involves division of the right and middle colic arteries at their origin, with removal of the right and transverse colon supplied by these vessels. The anastomosis is fashioned between the terminal ileum and the proximal left colon. A left hemicolectomy (i.e., resection from the splenic flexure to the rectosigmoid junction) is the procedure of choice for tumors of the descending colon, whereas a sigmoidectomy is appropriate for tumors of the sigmoid colon. Most surgeons prefer to avoid incorporating the proximal sigmoid colon into an anastomosis because of the often-tenuous blood supply from the IMA and the frequent involvement of the sigmoid with diverticular disease.

Abdominal colectomy (sometimes called subtotal colectomy or total colectomy) entails removal of the entire colon from the ileum to the rectum, with continuity restored by an ileorectal anastomosis. Owing to loss of the absorptive and storage capacity of the colon, this procedure causes an increase in stool frequency. Patients younger than the age of 60 years generally tolerate this well, with gradual adaptation of the small bowel mucosa, increased water absorption, and an acceptable stool frequency of one to three bowel movements daily. In older individuals, however, abdominal colectomy may result in significant chronic diarrhea. Abdominal colectomy is indicated for patients with multiple primary tumors, for individuals with HNPCC, and occasionally for patients with completely obstructing sigmoid cancers.

The chances that the patient has been cured by an operation performed to remove a colorectal cancer is dependent on several factors, including technical aspects of the operation, such as the complete removal of all tumor, certain biologic properties of the cancer that are poorly understood, and the stage of the disease.

Staging may be defined as the process by which objective data are assembled to try to define the state of progression of the disease.[84] Separate items of data are summated to provide a designated stage for an individual patient's disease, from which inferences may be drawn regarding the relative likelihood of residual disease and hence the chance of cure without further treatment and the advisability of considering further treatment. The ideal staging system would provide one ultimately important and simple item of information: Has the operation cured the patient or will he or she die unless further intervention prevents it? Thus, there would be just two categories: the cured and those destined to die of their disease.[85] Unfortunately, no system extant even remotely approaches that goal. Still, every attempt should be made to accurately assess the extent of the disease to provide guidance for prognosis and the need for further treatment.

At the present time the stage of the tumor is assessed by indicating the depth of penetration of the tumor into the bowel wall (T stage), the extent of lymph node involvement (N stage), and the presence or absence of distant metastases (M stage). For most of the last half century the standard staging system was based on a system developed and modified by Cuthbert Dukes, a pathologist

at St. Mark's Hospital in London.[86] The classification was developed for rectal cancer, but it was generally used to also describe the stage of colon cancer. The Dukes' classification is simple to remember and still frequently used. Dukes' stage A cancer is confined to the bowel wall. Stage B cancer penetrates the bowel wall, and stage C cancer indicates lymph nodal metastases. Kirklin and colleagues, from the Mayo Clinic, established a distinction between tumors that partially penetrated the muscularis propria (B1) and those that fully penetrated this layer (B2). Astler and Coller further separated the tumors that had invaded lymph nodes but did not penetrate the entire bowel wall (C1) from tumors that invaded lymph nodes and did penetrate the entire wall (C2).[87] Turnbull and associates from the Cleveland Clinic added stage D for tumors with distant metastasis. All of these modifications in various combinations are still in use and often called the modified Dukes classifications.

The classification in use by most hospitals in the United States was developed by the American Joint Committee on Cancer (AJCC) and was approved by the International Union Against Cancer (UICC).[88] This classification, known as the TNM (Tumor, Node, Metastasis) system, combines clinical information obtained preoperatively with data obtained during surgery and after histologic examination of the specimen. There have been some modifications in the system since its introduction in 1987. The surgeon is now encouraged to score the completeness of the resection as follows: R0 for complete tumor resection with all margins negative; R1 for incomplete tumor resection with microscopic involvement of a margin, and R2 for incomplete tumor resection with gross residual tumor not resected (Table 48-6).

There are four possible stages of colorectal cancer within the AJCC system. In stage I, there is no lymph node metastasis and the tumor is either T1 or T2 (up to muscularis propria). Patients who undergo appropriate resection of T stage 1 colon cancer have a 5-year survival rate of approximately 90%. Stage II is now subdivided into IIa (if the primary tumor is T3) and IIB (for T4 lesions), with no lymph node metastasis. The 5-year survival rate for patients with stage II colon cancer treated by appropriate surgical resection is approximately 75%. Stage III cancer is characterized by lymph node metastasis and is now subdivided into IIIA (T1 to T2, N1, M0), IIIB (T3 to T4, N1, M0), and IIIC (any T, N2, M0). In the latest version of the staging system (2003) smooth metastatic nodules in the pericolic or perirectal fat are considered lymph node metastasis and should be included in N staging. Irregularly contoured metastatic nodules in the peritumoral fat are considered vascular invasion.[89] The estimated survival for stage III cancer treated by surgery alone is approximately 50%. With the presence of distant metastasis, stage IV, the 5-year survival rate is less than 5%.

The survival rates described above do not reflect the use of adjuvant chemotherapy after curative resection of colon cancer. There is a clearly demonstrated benefit for patients with stage III disease treated postoperatively with 5-fluorouracil/leukovorin (67% 5-year survival). The benefits of adjuvant chemotherapy for patients with stage II colon cancer have not been clearly demonstrated, and

TABLE 48-6. AJCC TNM Staging System for Colorectal Cancer

Primary Tumor (T)

TX	Primary tumor cannot be assessed
T0	No evidence of primary tumor
Tis	Carcinoma in situ: intraepithelial or invasion of lamina propria*
T1	Tumor invades submucosa
T2	Tumor invades muscularis propria
T3	Tumor invades through the muscularis propria into the subserosa, or into nonperitonealized pericolic or perirectal tissues
T4	Tumor directly invades other organs or structures and/or perforates visceral peritoneum†

Regional Lymph Nodes (N)‡

NX	Regional lymph nodes cannot be assessed
N0	No regional lymph node metastasis
N1	Metastasis in 1 to 3 regional lymph nodes
N2	Metastasis in 4 or more regional lymph nodes

Distant Metastasis (M)

MX	Distant metastasis cannot be assessed
M0	No distant metastasis
M1	Distant metastasis

Stage Grouping

Stage	T	N	M	Dukes§	MAC§
0	Tis	N0	M0		
I	T1	N0	M0	A	A
	T2	N0	M0	A	B1
IIA	T3	N0	M0	B	B2
IIB	T4	N0	M0	B	B3
IIIA	T1-T2	N1	M0	C	C1
IIIB	T3-T4	N1	M0	C	C2/C3
IIIC	Any T	N2	M0	C	C1/C2/C3
IV	Any T	Any N	M1		D

Histologic Grade (G)

GX	Grade cannot be assessed
G1	Well differentiated
G2	Moderately differentiated
G3	Poorly differentiated
G4	Undifferentiated

*Tis includes cancer cells confined within the glandular basement membrane (intraepithelial) or lamina propria (intramucosal) with no extension through the muscularis mucosae into the submucosa.

†Direct invasion in T4 includes invasion of other segments of the colorectum by way of the serosa: for example, invasion of the sigmoid colon by a carcinoma of the cecum. Tumor that is adherent to other organs or structures macroscopically is classified T4. However, if no tumor is present in the adhesion microscopically the classification should be pT3. The V and L substaging should be used to identify the presence or absence of vascular or lymphatic invasion.

‡A tumor nodule in the pericolorectal adipose tissue of a primary carcinoma without histologic evidence of residual lymph node in the nodule is classified in the pN category as a regional lymph node metastasis if the nodule has the form and smooth contour of a lymph node. If the nodule has an irregular contour, it should be classified in the T category and also coded as V1 (microscopic venous invasion) or as V2 (if it was grossly evident), because there is a strong likelihood that it represents venous invasion.

§Dukes B is a composite of better (T3N0M0) and worse (T4N0M0) prognostic groups, as is Dukes C (Any TN1M0 and Any TN2M0). MAC is the modified Astler-Coller classification.

Note: The y prefix is to be used for those cancers that are classified after pretreatment, whereas the r prefix is to be used for those cancers that have recurred.

several ongoing clinical trials are now studying the benefit of chemotherapy in this group of patients. There has been no demonstrated efficacy for adjuvant chemotherapy for patients with stage I colon cancer.

Rectal Cancer

The most common symptom of rectal cancer is hematochezia. Unfortunately, this is often attributed to hemorrhoids, and the correct diagnosis is consequently delayed until the cancer has reached an advanced stage. Other symptoms include mucus discharge, tenesmus, and change in bowel habit.

The differential diagnosis of rectal cancer includes ulcerative colitis, Crohn's proctocolitis, radiation proctitis, and procidentia. Occasionally "hidden rectal prolapse" or internal intussusception of the sigmoid into the rectum can produce a solitary rectal ulcer that mimics an ulcerating cancer. It is thought that the chronic trauma from the recurrent intussusception results in ulceration of the rectal mucosa. Instead of a solitary rectal ulcer, this mucosal trauma from intussusception can sometimes produce the entity of *colitis cystica profunda*, a polypoid lesion that is characterized by the presence of benign columnar epithelium and mucous cysts residing deep to the muscularis mucosae. This histologic pattern can be confused with invasive adenocarcinoma, and it is obviously important to recognize this completely benign entity.

The preoperative assessment of patients with rectal cancer is similar to that described for patients with colon cancer, with some significant differences: (1) the requirement for precise characterization of the cancer with respect to proximity to the anal sphincters and (2) the extent of invasion as determined by depth of penetration into the bowel wall and spread to adjacent lymph nodes. The location of the tumor is best determined by examination with a rigid proctosigmoidoscope. Rigid proctosigmoidoscopy should be done even if the tumor has been diagnosed with a colonoscopic examination, because the flexible scope may not accurately measure the exact distance from the tumor to the anal sphincter. The depth of penetration can be estimated by digital rectal examination (superficially invasive tumors are mobile, whereas the lesions become tethered and fixed with increasing depth of penetration), and endorectal ultrasound (EUS) or magnetic resonance imaging (MRI) with endorectal coil can provide fairly accurate assessment of the extent of invasion of the bowel wall (Fig. 48-60).

Treatment

Tumors located in the distal 3 to 5 cm of the rectum present the greatest challenge for the surgeon. Achieving local control of the tumor is more difficult here owing to the confinement of the pelvic anatomy and the proximity of adjacent organs such as the urethra, prostate, seminal vesicles, vagina, cervix, and bladder. For tumors in this location, the challenge for the surgeon is to decide between wide margins of resection and preservation of the anal sphincter. Preoperative radiotherapy, usually

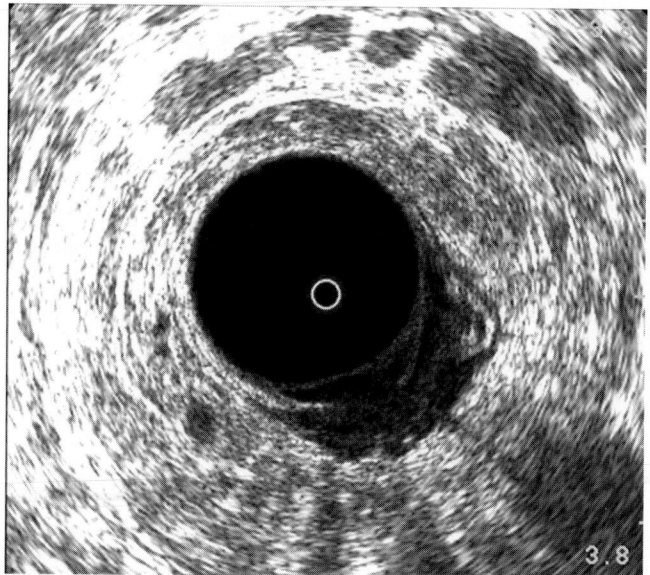

FIGURE 48-60. Endorectal ultrasound of patient with T3N1 rectal cancer. The cancer penetrates through all layers of the rectal wall, and an enlarged lymph node is clearly visible.

combined with chemotherapy, is often recommended to reduce the size of the rectal cancer. In Europe, preoperative radiation usually consists of 2500 cGy of pelvic radiation delivered over the course of 5 days, followed by either low anterior resection or abdominal-perineal resection.[90] In the United States it is becoming increasingly common to treat deeply penetrating (T2 or T3) rectal cancers with preoperative radiation (4500 to 5040 cGy over 5 to 6 weeks) combined with chemotherapy (5-fluorouracil and leucovorin).[91] This treatment program reduces the degree of wall invasion and of lymph node involvement in 70% of patients. There are a variety of advantages for preoperative radiation therapy, including biologic (decreased tumor seeding at the time of surgery and increased radiosensitivity of cells whose oxygenation is not decreased by surgery), physical (no postsurgical small bowel fixation in the pelvis), and functional (ability to change the operation from an abdominal-perineal resection to a sphincter-preserving low anterior resection with a coloanal anastomosis). An additional benefit in patients with locally advanced/unresectable disease is the ability to increase the resectability rate. This reduction in tumor invasiveness by preoperative radiation is known as *downstaging*.

Once the location and stage of the cancer are determined, various options need to be considered for the optimal treatment of the rectal cancer. Other important considerations include the presence or absence of comorbid conditions and the patient's body habitus (an obese male with a narrow pelvis presents technical difficulties different than a thin woman with a wide pelvis). There is no one operation that is appropriate to treat all rectal cancers, and the appropriate operation should be tailored to eradicate the tumor while preserving function to the fullest extent possible. The following procedures all are useful in certain circumstances.

Local Excision

Local excision of a rectal cancer is an excellent operation for a small cancer in the distal rectum that has not penetrated into the muscularis. This is accomplished through a transanal approach and usually involves excision of the full thickness of the rectal wall underlying the tumor. Local excisions do not allow complete removal of lymph nodes in the mesorectum, and therefore operative staging is limited. The operation is indicated for mobile tumors that are less than 4 cm in diameter, that involve less than 40% of the rectal wall circumference, and that are located within 6 cm of the anal verge. These tumors should be stage T1 (limited to the submucosa) or T2 (limited to the muscularis propria), well or moderately differentiated histologically, and with no vascular or lymphatic invasion. There should be no evidence of nodal disease on preoperative ultrasound or MRI. Adherence to these principles results in acceptable local recurrence rates compared with treatment by abdominal-perineal resection. Local excision is also used for palliation of more advanced cancer in patients with severe comorbid disease, in whom extensive surgery carries a high risk of morbidity or mortality. Various technical approaches have been described to achieve transanal local excision, including use of a special proctoscope equipped with a magnifying camera (transanal endoscopic microsurgery), but all approaches require the complete excision of the cancer with adequate margins of normal tissue. Whereas many surgeons suture the rectal defect closed after the local excision, this is not mandatory because the operative site is below the peritoneal reflection. Unfortunately, as experience has accumulated with this approach, it has become clear that close follow-up is mandatory, in that approximately 8% of T1 lesions will recur, and the recurrence rate for T2 lesions has been shown in some series to exceed 20%.[92] Most clinicians believe that local excision is not adequate treatment for a T2 rectal cancer and that further treatment is required, either adjuvant radiation and chemotherapy or radical excision (either low anterior resection or abdominal-perineal resection).

Fulguration

This technique, which eradicates the cancer by using an electrocautery device that destroys the tumor by creating a full-thickness eschar at the tumor site, requires extension of the eschar into the perirectal fat, thus destroying both the tumor and the rectal wall. The procedure can be used only for lesions below the peritoneal reflection. Complications associated with this approach are postoperative fever and significant bleeding that can occur as late as 10 days after the operation. Obviously this technique cannot provide a specimen to assess the pathologic stage, since the tumor and margins are disintegrated by fulguration. The procedure is reserved for patients with a prohibitive operative risk and limited life expectancy.

Abdominal-Perineal Resection

The complete excision of the rectum and anus, by concomitant dissection through the abdomen and perineum, with suture closure of the perineum and creation of a permanent colostomy was first described by Ernest Miles and is thus sometimes referred to as the Miles procedure. The rectum and sigmoid colon are mobilized through an abdominal incision. The pelvic dissection, done through the abdominal incision, mobilizes the mesorectum in continuity with the tumor-bearing rectum. The pelvic dissection is carried to the level of the levator ani muscles. The perineal portion of the operation excises the anus, the anal sphincters, and the distal rectum. The operation may be accomplished sequentially or simultaneously using an abdominal surgeon and a surgeon in the perineal field. An abdominal-perineal resection is indicated when the tumor involves the anal sphincters, when the tumor is too close to the sphincters to obtain adequate margins, or in patients in whom sphincter-preserving surgery is not possible because of unfavorable body habitus or poor preoperative sphincter control.

Low Anterior Resection

Resection of the rectum through an abdominal approach offers the advantage of completely removing the portion of bowel containing the cancer and the mesorectum, which contains the lymphatic channels that drain the tumor bed. The term *anterior resection* (an abbreviation for the more correct term *anterior proctosigmoidectomy with colorectal anastomosis*) indicates resection of the proximal rectum or rectosigmoid above the peritoneal reflection. The term *low anterior resection* indicates that the operation entails resection of the rectum below the peritoneal reflection through an abdominal approach. The sigmoid colon is almost always included with the resected specimen, because diverticulosis often involves the sigmoid and the blood supply to the sigmoid is often not adequate to sustain an anastomosis if the IMA is transected. For cancers involving the lower half of the rectum, the entire mesorectum (which contains the lymph channels draining the tumor bed) should be excised in continuity with the rectum. This technique, *total mesorectal excision,* produces the complete resection of an intact package of the rectum and its adjacent mesorectum, enveloped within the visceral pelvic fascia with uninvolved circumferential margins. The use of the technique of total mesorectal excision has resulted in a significant increase in 5-year survival rates (50% to 75%), decrease in local recurrence rate (from 30% to 5%), and a decrease in the incidence of impotence and bladder dysfunction (from 85% to less than 15%).[93]

Intestinal continuity is reestablished by fashioning an anastomosis between the descending colon and the rectum, a feat that has been greatly facilitated by the introduction of the circular stapling device. After the colorectal anastomosis has been completed, it should be inspected with a proctoscope inserted through the anus. If there is concern about the integrity of the anastomosis, or if the patient has received high-dose preoperative chemoradiation, a temporary proximal colostomy should be made to permit complete healing of the anastomosis. The colostomy can be closed in approximately 10 weeks

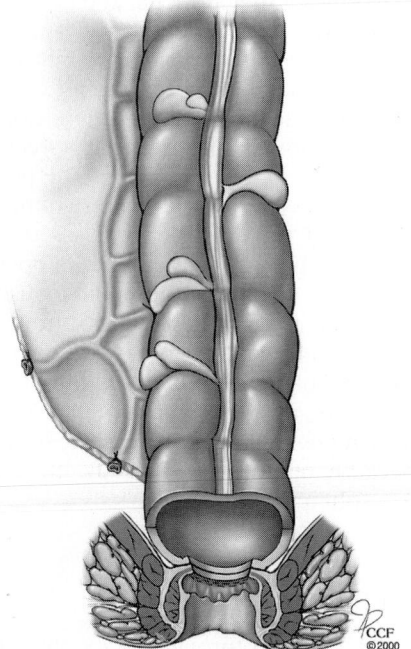

FIGURE 48-61.   Anastomosis between descending colon and anus, following complete resection of the rectum. The absence of the rectum often results in frequent, small bowel movements, a phenomenon known as "clustering" or "low anterior resection syndrome." (From Mantyh CR, Hull TL, Fazio VW: Coloplasty in low colorectal anastomosis: Manometric and functional comparison with straight and colonic J-pouch anastomosis. Dis Colon Rectum 44:37-42, 2001.)

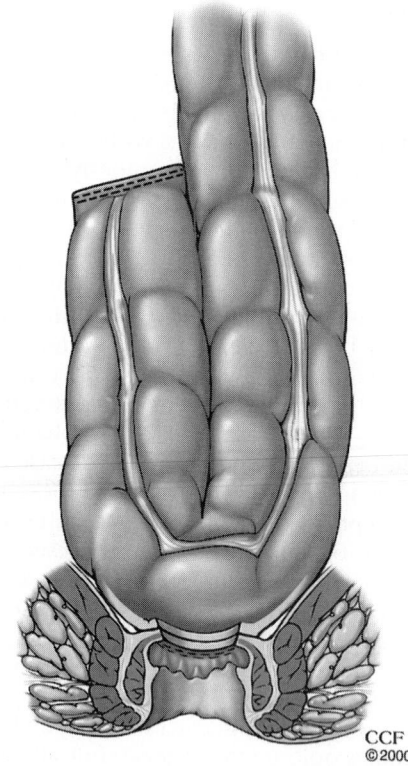

FIGURE 48-62.   J-pouch fashioned from descending colon to form proximal portion of coloanal anastomosis. This increases the "capacitance" to decrease the frequency of bowel movements. (From Mantyh CR, Hull TL, Fazio VW: Coloplasty in low colorectal anastomosis: Manometric and functional comparison with straight and colonic J-pouch anastomosis. Dis Colon Rectum 44:37-42, 2001.)

if proctoscopy and contrast studies verify the integrity of the anastomosis.

An end-to-end anastomosis between the descending colon and the distal rectum or anus may result in significant alteration of bowel habits attributed to the loss of the normal rectal capacity (Fig. 48-61). Patients treated with this operation often experience frequent small bowel movements ("low anterior resection syndrome" or "clustering"). This problem has been addressed by fashioning a colonic J-pouch as the proximal component of the anastomosis (Fig. 48-62). As experience has accumulated with this approach, it appears that improvement in bowel function is significant for cancers located in the distal rectum, but if the anastomosis is created above 9 cm from the anal verge, there is little benefit of a J-pouch compared with an end-to-end anastomosis. The limbs of the J-pouch should be relatively short (6 cm), because patients with larger J-pouches have a significant incidence of difficulty with evacuation.[94]

In obese patients, or patients with a narrow pelvis, it may not be technically feasible to fashion a J-pouch as the proximal component of the low pelvic anastomosis, because the bulk of the pouch simply will not fit into the narrow pelvis. In such circumstances a reservoir can be devised with a "coloplasty." This technique provides a rectal reservoir by making an 8- to 10-cm colotomy 4 to 6 cm from the divided end of the colon. The colotomy is closed transversely to provide increased rectal space and capacitance (Figs. 48-63 and 48-64).[95]

SPHINCTER-SPARING ABDOMINAL-PERINEAL RESECTION WITH COLOANAL ANASTOMOSIS

Abdominal-perineal resection is at times required because a cancer in the distal rectum cannot be resected with adequate margins while preserving the anal sphincter. However, the use of preoperative radiation and chemotherapy has been shown, in some instances, to shrink the tumor to an extent that acceptable margins can be achieved. If the anal sphincters do not need to be sacrificed to achieve adequate margins based on oncologic principles, a permanent stoma may be avoided with a sphincter-sparing abdominal-perineal resection with an anastomosis between the colon and the anal canal. This operation has particular application for young patients with rectal tumors who have a favorable body habitus and good preoperative sphincter function. The operation can be conducted in a variety of ways, but all methods involve mobilizing the sigmoid colon and pelvic rectum through an abdominal approach and dissecting the rectal mucosa from the anal sphincters at the level of the dentate line and completing the resection of the most distal rectum through the anal approach. An anastomosis is then fash-

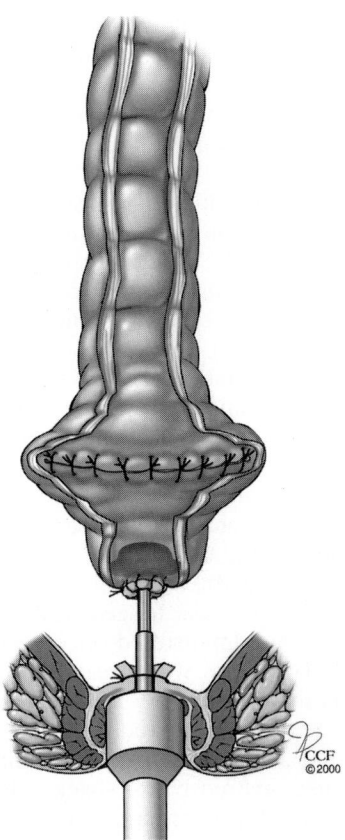

FIGURE 48-63.   A coloplasty is performed by making an 8- to 10-cm colotomy 4 to 6 cm from the cut end of the colon. The longitudinal colotomy is made between the taeniae on the antimesenteric side. It is closed transversely with absorbable sutures. An end-to-end stapled anastomosis then joins the colon to the distal rectum or anus. (From Mantyh CR, Hull TL, Fazio VW: Coloplasty in low colorectal anastomosis: Manometric and functional comparison with straight and colonic J-pouch anastomosis. Dis Colon Rectum 44:37-42, 2001.)

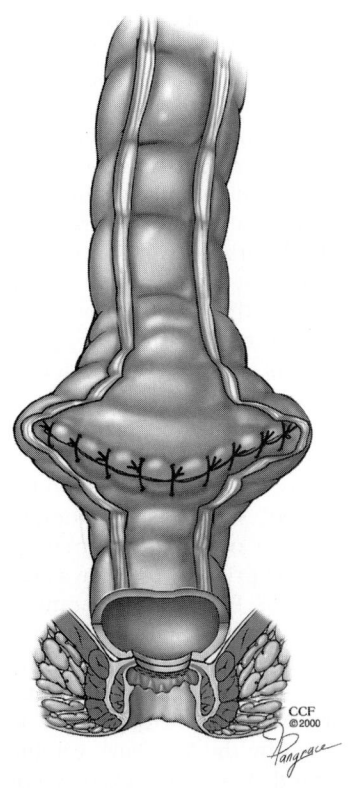

FIGURE 48-64.   The completed stapled coloplasty with anastomosis. (From Mantyh CR, Hull TL, Fazio VW: Coloplasty in low colorectal anastomosis: Manometric and functional comparison with straight and colonic J-pouch anastomosis. Dis Colon Rectum 44:37-42, 2001.)

ioned between the descending colon and the anus, often using a J-pouch or coloplasty procedure described earlier for the low colorectal anastomosis. The anastomosis is made with sutures placed through a transanal approach by the surgeon in the perineal field.

Colorectal Cancer Prevention and Screening

Cancer prevention can be divided into a discussion of primary and secondary prevention. Primary prevention is the identification of environmental factors responsible for cancer and then modifying those factors to reduce risk. Examples of this strategy include dietary modification, avoidance of environmental hazards, and chemoprevention. Secondary prevention involves finding a precursor lesion or cancer at a stage whereby metastasis and death can be prevented. Cancer screening is the cornerstone of secondary prevention. Colorectal cancer is a preventable disease. An understanding of defined risk factors and screening options is essential for every health care practitioner. Our understanding of the natural history of colorectal cancer, precancerous conditions, patient risk

factors, and the efficacy of screening options is currently in flux. Even so, obtaining a basic facility with the current evidence should be the goal.

Colorectal cancer is an ideal candidate for screening strategies: (1) it is a common and serious problem, (2) precursor lesions exist, (3) it is slow growing, and (4) testing is available. In 1993, the National Polyp Study Workgroup published a landmark study documenting a 76% to 90% reduction in colorectal cancer incidence compared with reference populations when adenomatous colon polyps are removed endoscopically.[96] A year prior to this, both Selby[97] and Newcomb[98] and their colleagues independently showed a 60% to 70% rectal cancer mortality reduction after sigmoidoscopy and polypectomy. Clearly, intervention results in mortality reduction.

Far more controversial is the choice of screening method. This area of prevention is rapidly changing, and updated recommendations occur frequently. Patients are risk stratified with frequency and method of screening dictated by category (Table 48-5). By far, most patients (70%) are of average risk: These patients have no personal or family history of colorectal cancer or polyps and no predisposing conditions such as ulcerative colitis or Crohn's disease.

The most difficult risk category to define is the moderate risk group. Recently, the American College of Gastroenterologists stratified it into two groups.[99] Patients with one first-degree relative with colorectal cancer diagnosed after age 60 are twice as likely as an average-risk individual to develop colorectal cancer themselves. Furthermore, their risk of colorectal cancer at age 40 is the same as the general population's risk at age 50. Therefore, these individuals are considered at "moderately" increased risk. Screening recommendations are the same as for average risk patients but should begin at age 40. Patients with a "strong family history" of colorectal cancer include those with multiple first-degree relatives with colorectal cancer or a single first-degree relative with cancer diagnosed when younger than 60 years of age. Overall risk of developing cancer for this cohort is three to four times the average. Patients at "high" risk of developing colorectal cancer are those with a hereditary cancer syndrome such as FAP or HNPCC or those with either ulcerative or Crohn's colitis.

Perhaps the most frequently used, and least well understood, screening tool is fecal occult blood testing (FOBT). It has the advantage of being inexpensive, easy-to-use, and interpretable by primary care physicians. In randomized studies, use of FOBT alone annually with three consecutive stools, produced a colorectal cancer-specific mortality reduction rate of 33%.[100] Unfortunately, the false-negative rate using FOBT alone is unacceptably high. Only 30% to 50% of cancers were detectable in most series. A study conducted by the Veterans Administration Study Group documented that only 24% of colorectal cancers produced a positive result.[101] Only 7.0% of patients with polyps produced positive FOBT (compared with 6.4% of polyp-free patients). In short, FOBT alone is not an adequate test for either polyps or colorectal cancer in any risk group.

For average-risk individuals, combining FOBT with flexible sigmoidoscopy at 5-year intervals is deemed acceptable as a screening option. In 2001, the VA Cooperative Study Group published the results of a large study (2885 patients) comparing FOBT and flexible sigmoidoscopy with colonoscopy.[102] All patients underwent FOBT followed by full colonoscopy. The "flexible sigmoidoscopy" portion of the examination was carefully documented. Although sigmoidoscopy alone identified 70.3% of all cancers, the combination of FOBT and flexible sigmoidoscopy failed to detect 24% of proximal cancers. Flexible sigmoidoscopy is a valuable tool that can be done in an office-based setting by general practitioners without a full bowel preparation. However, poor preparation, patient discomfort, and variable technique may limit the accuracy of the examination. Polyps detected by flexible sigmoidoscopy should prompt full colonoscopic examination. Flexible sigmoidoscopy alone or with FOBT is not an adequate examination for those in either the strong family history or high-risk group.

Double-contrast barium enema (DCBE) was once the diagnostic mainstay for lower gastrointestinal disease. The advent of flexible fiberoptics has largely supplanted its use. Even so, it has retained a place in the screening armamentarium for the average risk patient. In 2000, the National Polyp Study Work Group compared DCBE and colonoscopy in a prospective double-blinded trial in patients with a history of polyps.[103] All 862 study subjects underwent both types of examinations. Colonoscopists were blinded to the results of the antecedent barium enema. Forty-five percent of colonoscopies revealed adenomatous polyps versus only 26% of DCBE. The rate of detection on DCBE is significantly influenced by size. Only 48% of polyps 1.0 cm or greater in size were detected on DCBE.

Colonoscopy is considered the screening gold standard. It is the test of choice for patients with greater-than-average risk and has the advantage of providing a way to intervene in the natural history of colorectal cancer by facilitating endoscopic polypectomy. However, it has several disadvantages. It is the most morbid screening method. Colonic perforation (1/2000 to 1/2500 examinations) as well as significant bleeding (<1% of examinations) can occur. Colonoscopy requires a full bowel preparation accompanied by fasting, sedation, and a skilled endoscopist. Finally, colonoscopy is the most expensive screening test available. Even considering these limitations, the use of colonoscopy has become commonplace. It is among the screening tests recommended for average risk individuals. Indeed, it may be the most cost effective test if administered once every 10 years as recommended. For those with greater-than-average risk, colonoscopy is mandatory both for initial screening and for follow-up. Several good studies have endeavored to establish reliable accuracy statistics for colonoscopy. In 1990, Hixson used paired back-to-back colonoscopies to document a 15% polyp miss rate.[104] Rex, using the same method, had a 24% overall miss rate; however, less than 6% of polyps missed were greater than 1.0 cm.[105] In the National Polyp Study Work Group trial, colonoscopic examination revealed a 20% overall polyp miss rate. However, no polyp greater than 1.0 cm went undetected.[103] Clearly, the "gold standard" could be improved on, particularly for polyps less than 1.0 cm.

PELVIC FLOOR DISORDERS AND CONSTIPATION

Disorders of the pelvic floor can be classified as primarily colorectal, urologic, or gynecologic. Often, problems requiring the attention of multiple specialists present in a synchronous fashion, a condition known as "complex prolapse." Rectal prolapse (procidentia), enterocele, rectocele, and functional disorders of the muscles of the pelvic floor (anismus, levator spasm) are among the pelvic floor disorders that surgeons treat. A "functional disorder" is defined by the concurrent presence of normal anatomy and abnormal function. Surgeons are often consulted concerning functional disorders of the large bowel or pelvic floor. These problems do not usually require operative intervention; in fact, the surgical literature is replete with examples of failed operations to correct these problems. However, the signs and symptoms of these disorders mimic surgical diseases and require proper recognition and treatment. Although chronic constipation is often considered an example of a functional problem, surgery is a consideration in a select number of patients who fail medical management. The surgical evaluation and management of these disorders are discussed in this section.

Testing and Evaluation

Anorectal Physiology Laboratory

Anorectal physiology testing refers to the systematic evaluation of anal canal resting and squeeze pressures, anal reflexes, pudendal nerve conduction velocities, and electromyographic (EMG) muscle fiber recruitment. Measurement of anal canal pressures (manometry) involves the use of water-filled balloons attached to catheters and transducers placed in the anal canal. The measurement of resting and squeeze pressures at various points in the anal canal reflects the strength, tone, and function of the internal and external sphincter. Normal resting and squeeze values are 40 to 80 mm Hg. Resting pressure reflects the function of the internal sphincter, whereas squeeze pressure measures external sphincter (voluntary muscle) contributions. Measurement of anal canal pressures is useful in the evaluation of conditions ranging from incontinence to obstructive defecation. EMG "recruitment" refers to the motor unit potential of the puborectalis muscle and is compared for rest, squeeze, and push (simulated defecation). An increase in the recruitment of fibers during straining is pathognomonic for the syndrome of paradoxic puborectalis, or inappropriate puborectalis contraction. Pudendal nerve terminal motor latency (PNTML) times are measured with a special transducer attached to a glove-like apparatus designed to be worn on the finger and hand. A digital rectal examination is required with application of the finger electrode to the right and left levator ani complex. Values between 1.8 and 2.2 msec are normal. Prolonged values are seen in traumatic injuries of the vagina or anal canal (obstetric in etiology), sacral nerve root damage, or in chronic diseases such as diabetes.

Defecography

Defecography is an extremely useful modality for determining the precise nature of various pelvic floor abnormalities. Barium paste is placed in both the vagina and the rectum after the patient ingests water-soluble contrast to opacify the small bowel. As the patient evacuates the rectal barium paste, abnormalities occurring during the act of defecation can be recorded with fluoroscopic videotaping. A vast amount of both functional and anatomic information can be gathered from this test. The presence of multiple anatomic abnormalities such as rectocele, enterocele, and vaginal vault prolapse can be efficiently evaluated. Functional problems such as paradoxic puborectalis syndrome have very characteristic defecography patterns and can be evaluated in this way. Many contributing anatomic problems can be readily identified.

Rectal Prolapse (Procidentia)

Etiology and Symptoms

Most information regarding how patients develop rectal prolapse is based on observation of the clinical characteristics of those suffering from the problem. The condition was documented in the Hippocratic Corpus, and since then, descriptions of both etiologies and rectifying procedures have been numerous. However, two competing theories of rectal prolapse did evolve. Alexis Moschcowitz proposed in 1912 that a rectal prolapse was caused by a sliding herniation of the pouch of Douglas through the pelvic floor fascia into the anterior aspect of the rectum. His theory was based on the fact that the pelvic floor of prolapse patients is mobile and unsupported and the observation that other adjacent structures can occasionally be seen alongside the rectal component of the prolapse. With the advent of defecography in 1968, however, Broden and Snellman were able to show convincingly that procidentia is basically a full-thickness rectal intussusception starting approximately 3 inches above the dentate line and extending beyond the anal verge. Both explanations take into consideration the weakness of the pelvic floor in rectal prolapse cases, the concept of herniation, and the observation that there are abnormal anatomic features that characterize this condition.[106]

Women aged 50 and older are six times as likely as men to present with rectal prolapse. The peak age of incidence is the seventh decade in women, whereas the relatively few men afflicted with the syndrome may develop prolapse at the age of 40 or less. One striking characteristic of young male patients is their tendency to have psychiatric disorders, and many are institutionalized. Young male patients with procidentia also tend to take constipating medications and report significant symptoms related to bowel function.

Anatomy and Pathophysiology of Prolapse

Patients with prolapse are frequently found to have specific anatomic characteristics. Diastasis of the levator ani, an abnormally deep cul-de-sac, a redundant sigmoid colon, a patulous anal sphincter, and loss of the rectal sacral attachments are commonly described.

Large case reviews aimed at elucidating other predisposing factors support several observations. Chronic or lifelong constipation with a component of straining is present in over 50% of patients. Fifteen percent experience diarrhea. Contrary to the common assumption that rectal prolapse is a consequence of multiparity, 35% of patients with rectal prolapse are nulliparous. Once a prolapse is apparent, fecal incontinence becomes a predominant symptomatic feature, occurring in 50% to 75% of cases. Proximal bilateral pudendal neuropathy is present in incontinent prolapse patients and is responsible for denervation atrophy of the external sphincter musculature. This finding is absent in normal controls. It is speculated that pudendal nerve damage is responsible for pelvic floor and anal sphincter weakening and may be the underlying cause of a spectrum of pelvic floor disorders. Pudendal nerve damage can result from direct trauma (obstetric injury), chronic diseases such as diabetes, and neoplastic processes causing sacral nerve root damage.

Symptoms of prolapse progress as the prolapse develops. Often, the prolapse initially comes down with defecation or straining, only to spontaneously reduce

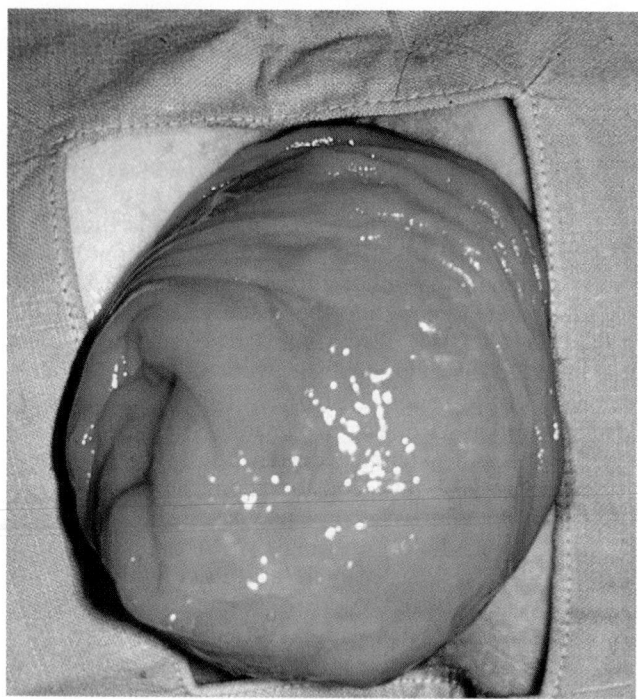

FIGURE 48-65. Procidentia, or rectal prolapse. The entire rectum has protruded through the anal canal.

afterward. Patients describe a "mass" or large "lump" that they may have to push back in after defecation (Fig. 48-65). The presenting complaint may be the concurrent fecal incontinence that results from the prolapse or a sensation of chronic moisture and mucous drainage in the perineal area. Minimal or spontaneously reducible prolapses may progress to chronically prolapsed rectum requiring digital reduction. Chronically prolapsed rectal mucosa may become thickened, ulcerated, and cause significant bleeding. Occasionally, the presentation of rectal prolapse can be quite dramatic when the prolapsed segment becomes incarcerated below the level of the anal sphincter. Emergent operative therapy is indicated in this situation.

Differential Diagnosis and Investigation

A common pitfall in the diagnosis of rectal prolapse is the potential for confusion with prolapsed incarcerated internal hemorrhoids. These conditions may be distinguished by close inspection of the direction of the prolapsed tissue folds. In the case of rectal prolapse, the folds are always concentric, whereas hemorrhoidal tissue develops radial invaginations defining the hemorrhoidal cushions. Prolapsed, incarcerated hemorrhoids produce extreme pain and can be accompanied by fever and urinary retention. Unless incarcerated, rectal prolapse is easily reducible and painless.

Prior to operative intervention, a careful history, physical examination, and colonoscopy should be performed. Thirty-five percent of patients with rectal prolapse complain of urinary incontinence, and another 15% have a significant vaginal vault prolapse. These symptoms will require evaluation and potential multidisciplinary surgical intervention.

If the diagnosis is suspected from the history, but not detected on physical examination, confirmation can be obtained by asking the patient to produce the prolapse by straining while on a toilet. Inspection of the perineum with the patient in the sitting or squatting position is helpful for this purpose. In the event that the prolapse is still elusive, defecography, a technique described earlier, may reveal the problem.

Although uncommon, occasionally, a neoplasm may form the lead point for a rectal intussusception. For this reason, and because these older patients have a significant rist of colorectal neoplasia, a colonoscopy or barium enema should precede an operation. A significant finding on colonoscopic inspection may change the operative approach.

Anal manometry and pudendal nerve terminal motor latencies can be ordered preoperatively to further evaluate symptoms of incontinence. However, rarely do these test results change the operative strategy. A finding of increased nerve conduction periods (nerve damage) may have postoperative prognostic significance for continence, although more studies are required to confirm this. Those patients with evidence of nerve damage may have a higher rate of incontinence after surgical correction of the prolapse. Decreased anal squeeze or resting pressures are expected with this condition and may predate the actual development of the prolapse. Routine manometric studies for obvious prolapse are usually not done.

Operative Repair

The number of procedures described in the literature both historically and in recent times is breathtaking. Over 50 types of repair have been documented, most of historical interest only. Approaches have generally included anal encirclement, mucosal resection, perineal proctosigmoidectomy, anterior resection with or without rectopexy, rectopexy alone, and a host of procedures involving the use of synthetic mesh affixed to the presacral fascia. The apparent enthusiasm and ingenuity of surgeons in their quest to define the ideal prolapse operation only serves to highlight its elusiveness. Two predominant approaches, abdominal and perineal, are considered in the operative repair of rectal prolapse. The surgical approach is dictated by the comorbidities of the patient, the surgeon's preference and experience, and the patient's age. It is generally believed that the perineal approach results in less perioperative morbidity and pain and a reduced length of hospital stay. These advantages have, until recently, been considered to be offset by a higher recurrence rate. Recent data are unclear on this point, however, and a properly executed perineal operation may yield the same good long-term results as abdominal procedures. This point will be clarified by ongoing long-term studies. The advent of laparoscopic options may also provide advantages, but, for now, recurrence data are scant.[107]

The Ripstein repair has many advocates and involves placement of a prosthetic mesh around the mobilized rectum with attachment of the mesh to the presacral fascia below the sacral promontory. Recurrence rates for this procedure range from 2.3% to 5%. The bowel is mechanically prepared for this procedure with a polyethylene glycol or sodium phosphate solution. The procedure involves mobilizing the rectum on both sides posteriorly down to the coccyx. Ripstein described division of the upper portion of the lateral rectal ligaments, but others advocate leaving them wholly intact because the rates of postoperative constipation are fully 50% greater in patients with divided lateral stalks. After mobilization of the rectum, a 5-cm band of rectangular mesh is placed around its anterior aspect at the level of the peritoneal reflection, and both sides of the mesh are sutured with nonabsorbable suture to the presacral fascia, approximately 1 cm from the midline. Sutures are used to secure the mesh to the rectum anteriorly and the rectum is pulled upward and posteriorly. Much controversy has surrounded the choice of mesh. Autologous fascia lata, synthetic nonabsorbable products such as Marlex (Davol, Inc. subsidiary of C.R. Bard, Inc., Cranston, RI), Teflon (E.I. duPont de Nemours & Co., Wilmington, DE), and Ivalon and absorbable prosthetics such as polyglycolic acid have been used. Recurrence rates for all of these techniques are well under 10%, although follow-up times and evaluation criteria between studies have varied and strict comparisons cannot be made. Complications include large bowel obstruction, erosion of the mesh through the bowel, ureteric injury or fibrosis, small bowel obstruction, rectovaginal fistula, and fecal impaction. Postoperative morbidity rates are 20%, but most of these complications are minor. Although mesh rectopexy results in significant improvement in fecal incontinence (50%), no rectal prolapse operation should be advocated as a procedure to restore continence; and patients, especially those with prolapse for more than 2 years, should be warned of the possibility that incontinence could persist.[108]

A significant complication of this operation is the incidence of new-onset or worsened constipation. Fifteen percent of patients experience constipation for the first time after Ripstein rectopexy and at least 50% of those who are constipated preoperatively are made worse. While some of these difficulties are attributed to complications of the procedure such as mesh stricture, obstruction at the level of the repair, or rectal dysfunction after lateral stalk division, a subset of patients will be found to have slow-transit constipation characterizing a global motility disorder. Some authors advocate routine preoperative transit studies to select these patients out, but usually a good bowel habit history will suffice. The etiology of any severe, unremitting postoperative defecation or obstruction problem should be investigated with a barium enema and perhaps with a small bowel study. Strictures, obstructions, adhesions, and fistulas may be identified by the radiograph.

Fiber, fluids, and stool softeners are useful in the management of functional constipation after rectal prolapse repairs of any type. Occasionally, mild laxatives such as milk of magnesia, magnesium citrate, or polyethylene glycol-based therapies (Miralax, Braintree Laboratories, Inc., Braintree, MA) may be necessary for short periods of time. Newer treatments for constipation involve oral administration of 5-HT4 receptor agonists (tegaserod maleate) and may prove invaluable in the short-term treatment of this problem.

The Wells procedure is an alternative mesh technique that reduces the incidence of rectal obstruction by eliminating the anterior placement of the mesh. The mesh is affixed to the posterior aspect of the rectal fascia propria and then to the presacral fascia as previously described. The Ivalon (polyvinyl alcohol) sponge is a method that at one point was very popular among European surgeons but has since fallen out of favor. The sponge is placed posteriorly in the deep pelvis in a manner similar to the Wells technique. In fact, Wells initially described this procedure. Although postoperative recurrence rate results have been as good as those involving synthetic nonabsorbable mesh and reported evacuation disorders have been low, a disturbing feature of the Ivalon sponge is a high rate of pelvic abscess, necessitating sponge removal. Although polyvinyl alcohol is a sarcoma-producing carcinogen in rats, this effect has not been demonstrated in humans.

Resection rectopexy is a technique first described by Frykman and Goldberg in 1969 and popularized in the United States in the past 30 years (Fig. 48-66). Lack of artificial mesh, ease of operation, and reduction of "redundant" sigmoid colon are the principal attractions of the procedure. Recurrence rates are low, ranging from 2% to 5%, and major complication rates range from 0% to 20% and relate either to obstruction or anastomotic leak. Basically, the sigmoid colon and rectum are mobilized to the level of the levators. The lateral ligaments are divided, elevated from the deep pelvis, and sutured to the presacral fascia. The mesentery of the sigmoid colon is then divided, with preservation of the IMA, and a tension-free anastomosis is created. A revised version of this procedure involves preservation of the lateral stalks and unilateral fastening of the rectal mesentery to the sacrum at the level of the sacral promontory. Sigmoid resection is a unique and controversial feature of this procedure. It seems to reduce constipation by 50% in those who complain preoperatively of this symptom in some studies. Others have argued that sigmoidectomy is an inadequate operation for a chronic motility problem that affects the entire bowel, and those patients should be formally evaluated preoperatively and subtotal colectomy recommended if colonic inertia is detected. Interestingly, in patients who complain of incontinence before surgery, this symptom consistently improves in about 35%, even with the sigmoid resection. A variant of this procedure involves forgoing the sigmoid resection in those who report no history of constipation and whose predominant complaint is fecal incontinence.

Perineal proctosigmoidectomy was first introduced by Mikulicz in 1899 and remained the favored treatment for prolapse in Europe for many years. Miles advocated this procedure in the United Kingdom and it was promoted in the United States by Altemeier at the University of Cincinnati. As the abdominal approaches gained favor, principally because of the reduced recurrence rates, the perineal approach was increasingly reserved only for those with the highest operative risk. However, renewed

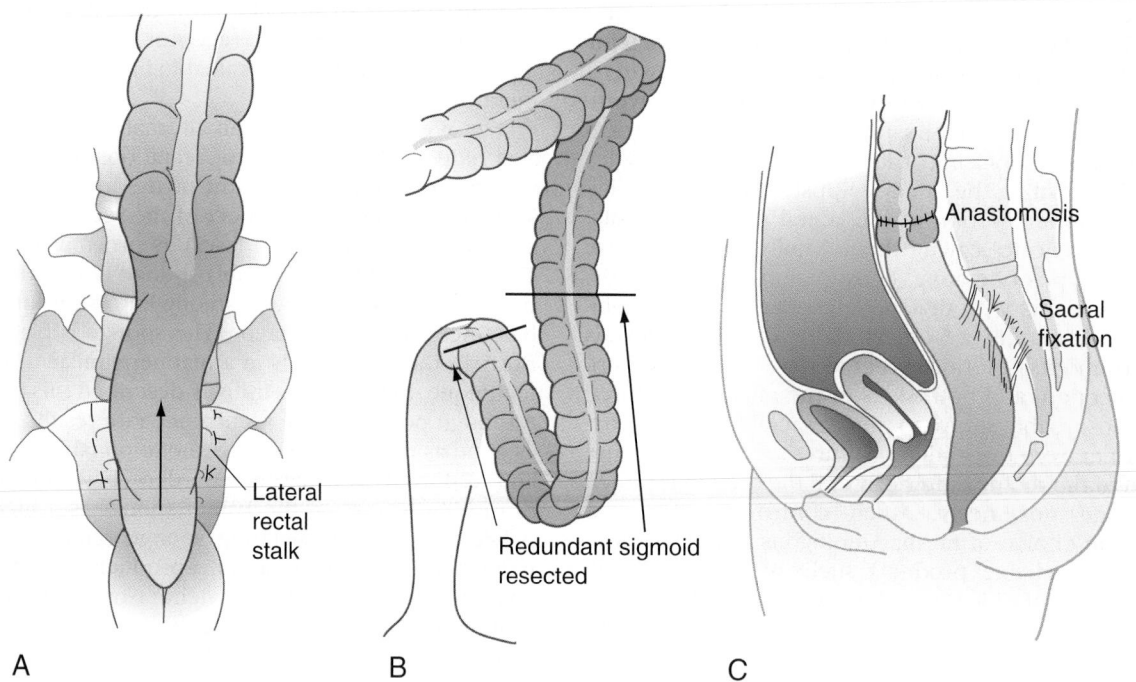

A   B   C

FIGURE 48-66.   Anterior resection with rectopexy, or the Frykman Goldberg procedure, for rectal prolapse.
A, After full mobilization by sharp dissection, the tissues lateral to the rectal wall are swept away laterally.
B, Resection of the redundant sigmoid colon. **C,** Anastomosis completed and rectopexy sutures are placed. (From
Gordon PL, Nivatvongs S [eds]: Principles and Practice of Surgery for the Colon, Rectum, and Anus, 2nd ed. St.
Louis, Quality Medical Publishing, 1999, p 520.)

interest in the technique has accompanied studies
showing recent reduced recurrence rates, and there are a
number of surgeons who believe that strong consideration
should be given to this technique when repairing prolapse
in young men who stand an increased risk of autonomic
nerve injury resulting in impotence.

The Altemeier procedure combines a perineal proctosigmoidectomy with an anterior levatoroplasty (Fig.
48-67). The latter procedure is performed to correct the
levator diastasis commonly associated with this condition.
Theoretically, restoration of fecal continence is enhanced
by this additional maneuver. As always, the large bowel is
mechanically cleansed. The patient is placed in the prone
jackknife position and a Foley catheter is placed. The
rectal mucosa is serially grasped with Babcock or Allis
clamps until a full-thickness prolapse is demonstrated. A
full-thickness circumferential incision is made 1.5 cm
proximal to the dentate line. The low peritoneal reflection
can usually be incised anteriorly and the peritoneal cavity
entered. The mesentery of the rectum and sigmoid colon
is sequentially clamped and tied until no redundant bowel
remains. The colon is transected at this point and an anastomosis fashioned between the colon and the anal canal
with either sutures or staples.

Patients undergoing perineal proctosigmoidectomy are
generally older and with significantly more comorbidities
than those who are considered for abdominal repair. Complication rates are less than 10%, and recurrence rates
have been reported to be as high as 16%, although, as
mentioned, recent series demonstrate significantly lower
recurrence rates. Complications include bleeding from

the staple or suture line, pelvic abscess, and, rarely, dehiscence of the suture line, with perineal evisceration. Lack
of an abdominal incision, reduced pain, and reduced
length of hospitalization make this procedure an attractive
option.[108]

Anal encirclement is one of the oldest surgical techniques for rectal prolapse described. Thiersch described
silver wire anal encirclement in 1891. Since then, it has
been tried with a wide variety of materials, including
stainless steel wire, nonabsorbable mesh, small Silastic
bands, nylon suture, and polypropylene. This technique is
reserved by most surgeons for patients of the highest surgical risk because it can be done under local anesthesia.
With the patient in the prone jackknife or lithotomy position, the anal area is sterilely prepped and draped.
Two small lateral incisions are made, and the wire or
suture is introduced with a curved needle into one and
brought out the other. This is repeated and a knot is tied
and buried laterally. The orifice should be snug but should
easily admit an index finger. Anal encirclement does not
correct the fecal incontinence associated with prolapse
and the recurrence rate is quite high (>30%). In addition,
although the mortality rate is 0%, the morbidity is quite
high. Erosion of the wire into the sphincter, anovaginal
fistula formation, rectal prolapse incarceration, fecal
impaction, and infection can occur. Reoperative rates of
7% to 59% are reported in the literature. The safety of
current anesthetic techniques and the low morbidity and
relative functional success of perineal proctectomy have
made anal encirclement, for the most part, a thing of the
past.[109]

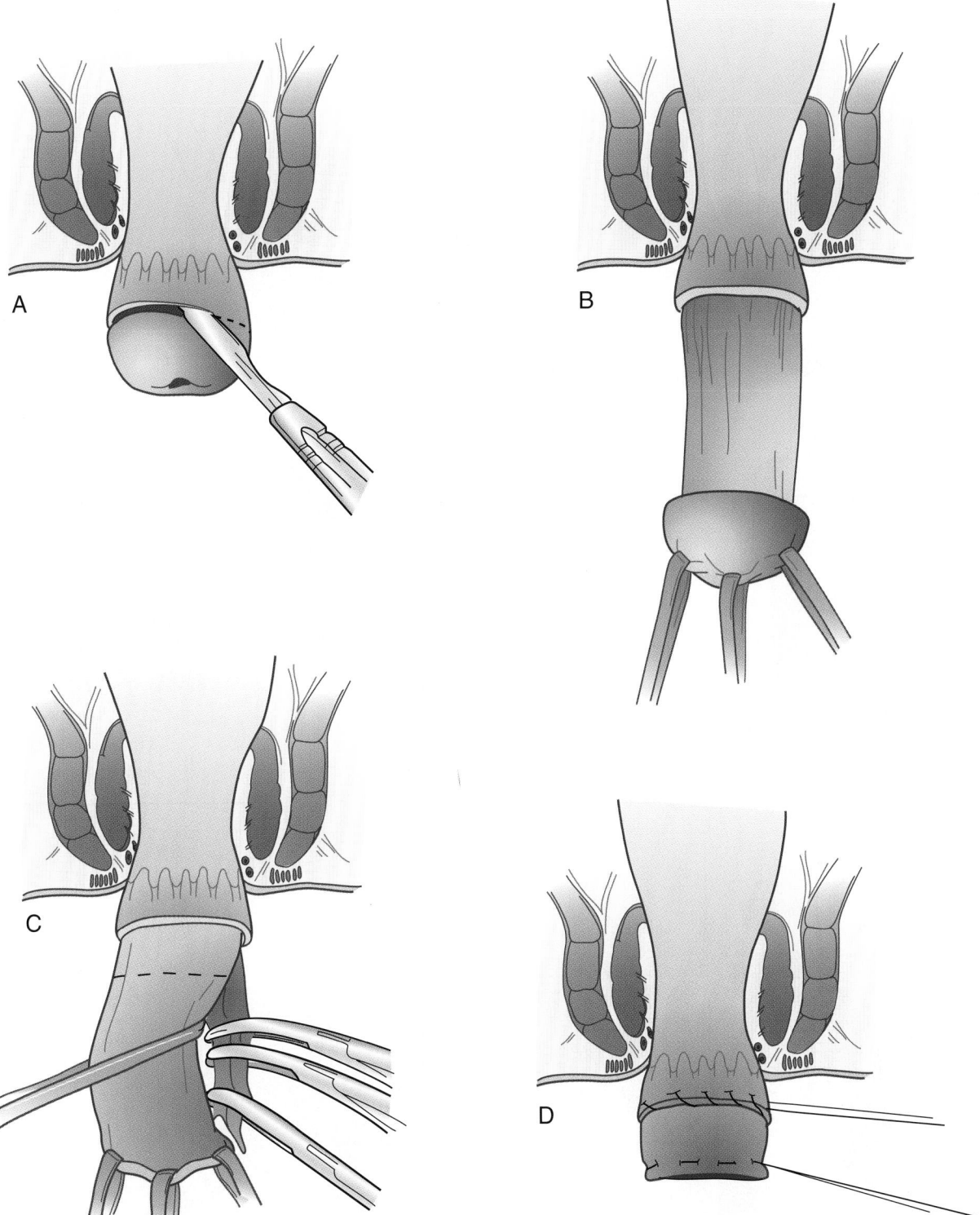

FIGURE 48-67. Altemeier perineal rectosigmoidectomy. **A,** Circumferential incision of rectum proximal to dentate line. **B,** Delivery of redundant rectum and sigmoid colon. **C,** Ligation of blood supply to rectum. **D,** Placement of pursestring suture on proximal bowel and excision of redundant colon and rectum. Whip stitch placed on rectal stump.

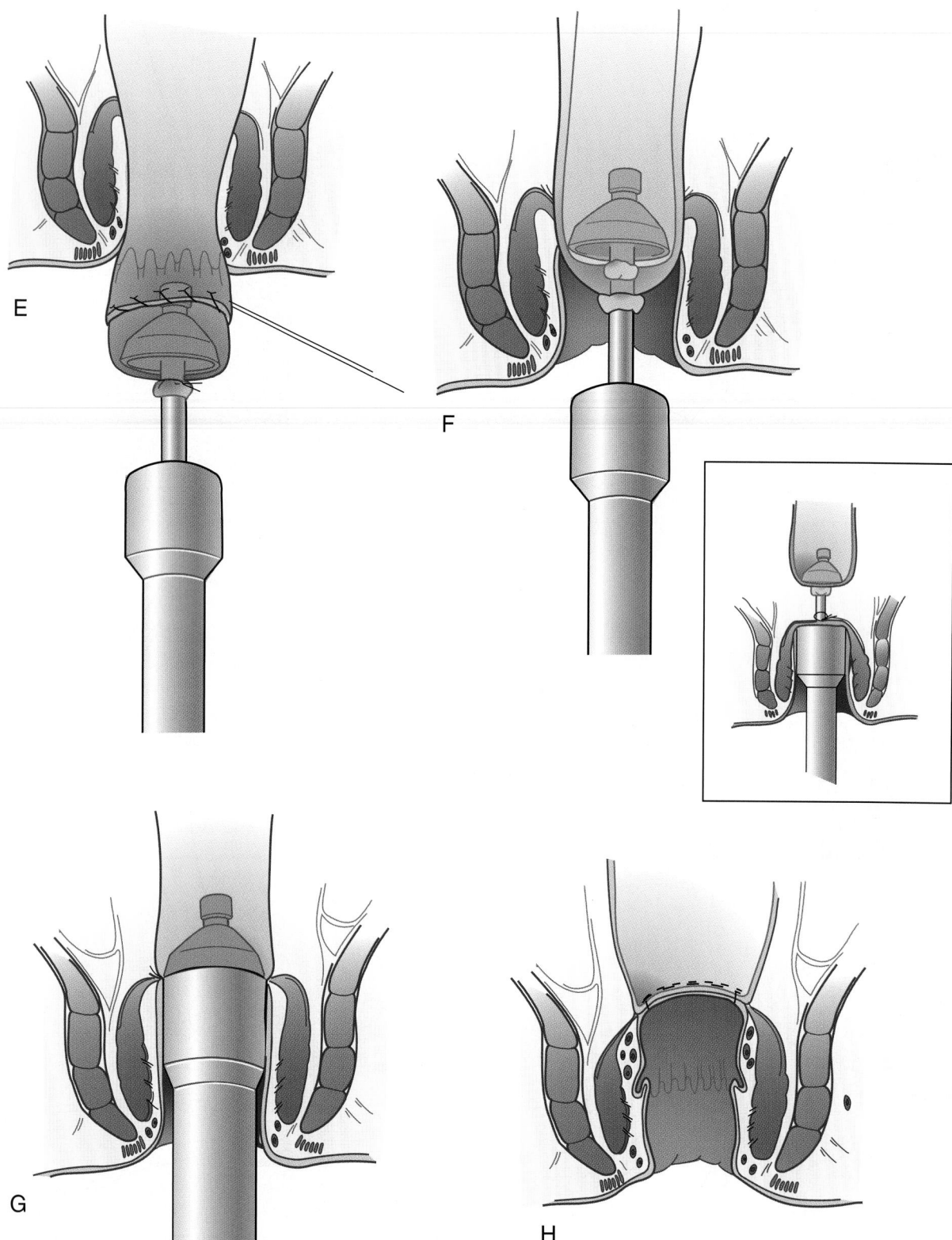

■ **FIGURE 48-67—cont'd.** **E,** Proximal pursestring suture secured around central shaft. **F,** Proximal bowel advanced through anus and distal pursestring tied. **G,** Approximation of anvil to cartridge and activation of stapler. **H,** Completed anastomosis. (From Gordon PL, Nivatvongs S [eds]: Principles and Practice of Surgery for the Colon, Rectum, and Anus, 2nd ed. St. Louis, Quality Medical Publishing, 1999, pp 524-525.)

Internal Prolapse and Solitary Rectal Ulcer Syndrome

Two areas of controversy related to rectal prolapse involve the treatment of solitary rectal ulcer syndrome (SRUS) and internal intussusception of the rectal mucosa. Although it is identified as an "ulcer," the gross pathology of SRUS can range from a typical crater-like ulcer with a fibrinous central depression to a polypoid lesion. It is always located on the anterior aspect of the rectum 4 to 12 cm from the anal verge and is thought to correspond with the location of the puborectalis "sling." It is frequently, though not exclusively, associated with internal intussusception or full-thickness rectal prolapse. Patients are typically young and female, however, with an average age of 25 and a history of straining and difficult evacuation.

The rectal ulcer is usually found on proctoscopy or flexible sigmoidoscopy and commonly presents with rectal bleeding in the setting of straining or constipation. The etiology of SRUS remains somewhat unclear, but speculation centers on chronic ischemia. The fold with the ulcer is thought to form the lead point of an intussusception into the anal canal. Chronic, repeated straining or prolapse of this lead point produces ischemia, tissue breakdown, and ulceration. Possible digital self-disimpaction may also be a contributing factor. Histology reveals a thick layer of fibrosis obliterating the lamina propria and a central fibrinous exudate. Other common pathologic findings include the presence of mucus-filled glands misplaced in the submucosa and lined with normal colonic epithelium (i.e., colitis cystica profunda). Differentiating SRUS from malignancy, infection, or Crohn's disease is important but not difficult. The anterior location in the context of classic symptoms and the pathologic findings are conclusive.

Diagnostic evaluation by defecography is the radiologic procedure of choice and usually reveals the underlying disorder. Full-thickness rectal prolapse, internal prolapse, paradoxic puborectalis syndrome (failure of relaxation of the pelvic floor musculature on straining), and thickened rectal folds are common findings.

Data regarding the treatment of this unusual disorder is retrospective and studies are small, but several common observations have been made. In general, a third of patients with SRUS also suffer from full-thickness rectal prolapse. Abdominal prolapse repairs have resulted in a cure rate of 80% in patients with SRUS and full-thickness rectal prolapse. In the same study, patients treated with the same procedure for mucosal prolapse and SRUS faired far worse—only 25% of patients responded to operative intervention. In most studies, dietary management, pelvic floor retraining (biofeedback), and short-term use of topical anti-inflammatory medications containing mesalamine result in remission for those with either internal prolapse or pelvic muscle dysfunction. Prompt diagnosis of the underlying problem and appropriate treatment can be difficult, but are the keys to cure. Local excision usually results in a larger nonhealing wound and really has no role in management. Very rarely, symptoms of severe bleeding, pain, and spasm may require a temporary diverting sigmoid colostomy.[110]

Internal intussusception was first described in the late 1960s when defecography was first developed and came into widespread use. The condition is also called internal or "hidden" prolapse and is confined to the rectal mucosa and submucosa, which separates from the muscularis mucosae layer and "slides" down the anal canal (Fig. 48-68). Internal intussusception can be identified in 50% of

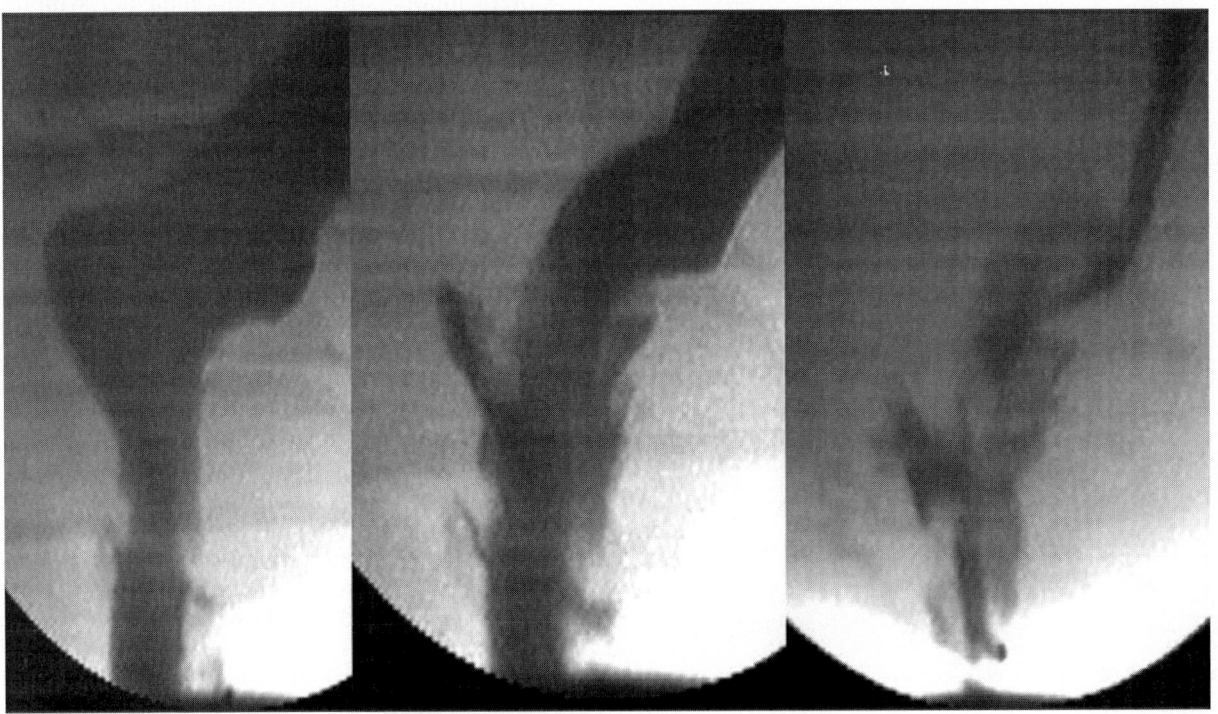

FIGURE 48-68. Defecography showing progression of internal intussusception.

the asymptomatic population and seems to represent a normal variant. However, there are advocates of internal prolapse repair when it is found in patients who complain of dysfunctional defecation. The transanal Delorme mucosal resection procedure involves circumferential removal of redundant anal canal and distal rectal mucosa and imbrication of the muscularis layer with serial vertical sutures. Berman and associates demonstrated improvement in 71% of patients undergoing the Delorme procedure, but these good results were not repeated in studies by other groups.[111]

Abdominal repairs such as the Ripstein have also been advocated as an alternative for symptomatic patients. Unfortunately, the results of these studies are not conclusive. In patients who were repaired via an abdominal approach, only 24% to 38% of patients reported any sort of improvement, whereas a significant number experienced worsening. Like SRUS, the treatment of patients with incomplete or obstructed defecation should be initially evaluated with defecography. Data do not currently support operative intervention for these disorders when internal intussusception alone is present.[112]

Rectocele

A rectocele is an abnormal sac-like projection of the anterior rectum that extends from the distal rectum to the distal anal canal. It usually begins just above the sphincter complex (Figs. 48-69 and 48-70). The etiology of rectoceles is multifactorial. Stretching of the endopelvic fascia from antecedent pelvic floor injury followed by chronic increased intra-abdominal pressure, causes an anterior full-thickness "herniation" of the rectum into the vagina.

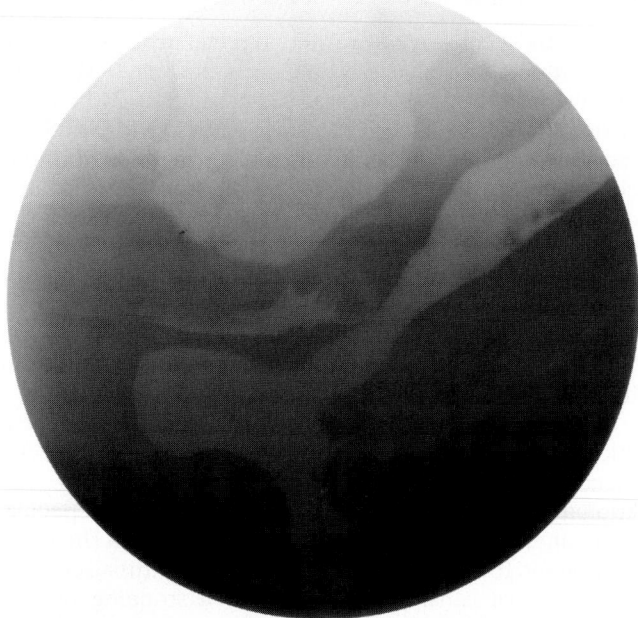

FIGURE 48-70.   Triple contrast radiograph demonstrates large anterior rectocele. Contrast material is also in the vagina and small intestine.

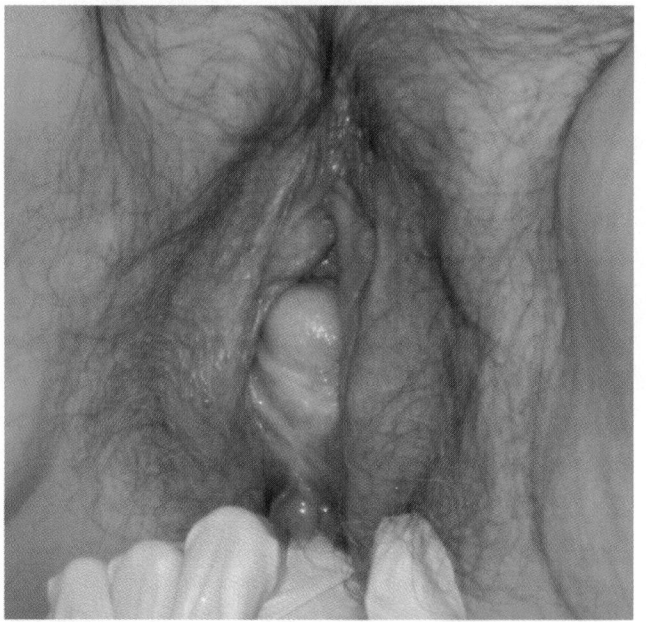

FIGURE 48-69.   Digital anorectal examination demonstrating anterior rectocele protruding from the vaginal introitus.

Rectal pressures are higher than those in the vagina; therefore, pressure tends to push the rectum anteriorly and stretch and shift the rectovaginal septum as well. The major symptom of rectocele is "stool trapping," a form of obstructed defecation. Women commonly describe requiring vaginal pressure to reduce the bulge, effectively stenting the anterior rectum and enabling defecation.

Criteria for operative intervention include symptomatic stool trapping requiring digital evacuation or vaginal support and large protruding rectoceles that push vaginal mucosa beyond the introitus producing dryness, ulceration, and discomfort. Although small rectoceles are common, it is rare that a rectocele less than 2 cm is symptomatic.

There are two major operative approaches to rectoceles: transanal and transvaginal. Although the transvaginal approach has been criticized by surgeons because the repair is done on the "low pressure" side of the rectovaginal septum, it does have certain distinct advantages. The bowel is fully prepped, and the patient is placed in the lithotomy position. After the submucosal injection of lidocaine with 1% epinephrine, a swath of vagina is excised starting at the vaginal introitus and carried to the apex of the vagina. The size of this segment is determined by the depth of the rectocele. The goal is to excise a full-thickness segment of vagina, dissect out and reduce an enterocele if one is found in the rectovaginal septum, and then obliterate the deep cul-de-sac by suturing the cut edges of vagina closed and allow the space to contract by fibrosis.

Alternatively, several approaches for the transanal correction of rectocele have been described. This technique is probably best described by Sullivan who expects 80% of patients to have good to excellent results. An incision is made longitudinally in the rectum over the bulge above the sphincters. The incision's length varies with the size of the rectocele. The underlying vagina is exposed and imbricated to obliterate the sac, and the rectum is separately imbricated and closed over that with absorbable sutures. Unfortunately, direct comparisons in the literature between these techniques are absent. However, the largely unsubstantiated argument is made by surgeons that a repair based in the "high pressure," or rectal side, of the bulge may reduce recurrence. No matter the technique, patient selection and follow-up is crucial. In one study, only 54% of patients who underwent rectocele repair obtained relief from their symptoms of obstructive defecation. Paradoxic puborectalis syndrome was not ruled out and was responsible for continued problems.[113] Postoperative biofeedback therapy is appropriate in these cases. Defecography evaluation is very helpful to distinguish these problems preoperatively.

Constipation

Constipation is a symptom, and it is often used by patients to describe very different problems. It occurs frequently in older populations—in one survey 50% of women and 30% of men older than 65 years of age were affected.[114] Although functional constipation seems to occur most often in the elderly, a small subset of patients present at a very young age with severe unremitting symptoms. These patients are evaluated differently and are discussed in detail later. Although most individuals describe constipation in terms of reduced stool frequency, up to 25% use the term to indicate straining, excessive pushing, or a feeling of incomplete defecation.[115] Normal stool frequencies range from three times per week to three times per day. The causes of constipation are numerous, but the evaluation of constipation is relatively straightforward, and the indications for surgery are few (Fig. 48-71). The initial evaluation of constipation should elicit information regarding acuteness of symptoms, stool frequency, changes in stool form, the presence or absence of blood in the stool, new medications, and any newly diagnosed illnesses. The physical examination should always include a rectal examination and proctoscopy. New-onset constipation can be divided into categories for further diagnostic consideration. These categories are depression or debilitation, new medications, endocrine conditions such as hypothyroidism, and obstructed defecation. For the purposes of this chapter, we will focus on surgically correctable causes, while recognizing that by far, most constipation is chronic and functional and is rectified simply by the addition of fluid and fiber to the diet.

A patient whose symptoms are composed of straining and incomplete defecation with a normal stool frequency should be evaluated for obstructive defecation. The best way to obtain the most information is through physical examination and defecography. Symptomatic rectoceles are those that fail to empty completely on defecography.

Associated anatomic abnormalities (e.g., vaginal vault prolapse and enterocele) can be concurrently corrected. Anal manometry with electromyographic recruitment is an invaluable investigatory tool for the patient with normal anatomy and suspected paradoxic puborectalis syndrome. Biofeedback therapy is indicated in these cases. Occasionally, both surgically correctable rectocele and functional defecatory disorders coexist. In this situation, biofeedback is usually initiated and then rectocele repair is done subsequently.

The primary concern for the physician evaluating new-onset constipation is to rule out large bowel malignancy. A patient who presents with complaints of an acute change in bowel habits should be evaluated by colonoscopy in the absence of obvious causes such as narcotic usage. Suspect medications should be immediately stopped, and reevaluation should take place shortly thereafter. No improvement or a guaiac-positive stool should lead to colonoscopic examination. Barium enema is acceptable as well, but flexible sigmoidoscopy, even combined with stool guaiac testing, fails to detect 25% of right-sided malignancies.[101] A normal colonoscopic examination is reassuring and should lead to trials of dietary therapy. Fluid intake should be increased to 2 L/day at minimum, and fiber therapy should be instituted. Caffeinated beverages should be avoided. There are many other laxative-based strategies for the short-term treatment of functional constipation. Long-term failure to respond to these strategies necessitates further investigation.

Transit Studies

Measurement of colonic transit time is a valuable aid in the establishment of a diagnosis of "slow-transit" constipation or colonic inertia. Although many different techniques exist to assess colonic transit times, two main goals of testing are to establish "whole gut" and "segmental" transit values. A very common and simple test has been devised by Martelli to do both. The patient is asked to refrain from the use of laxatives or constipating medications such as iron supplements for 3 to 4 days before the test. The patient ingests a capsule containing 20 radiopaque markers and an abdominal radiograph is obtained on each subsequent day for a total of 7 days or until the markers are expelled. The capsules are quantified in three areas of the colon: right, left, and rectosigmoid. Normal subjects expel 80% of markers within 5 days after ingestion. Slow-transit constipation is diagnosed in patients who fail to meet these criteria.[116]

Slow-Transit Constipation (Colonic Inertia)

It has been estimated that 2% of the population suffers from chronic, unremitting functional constipation. The majority of patients are female with a mean age younger than 30. Most of these individuals will report that they were constipated as children and that the constipation

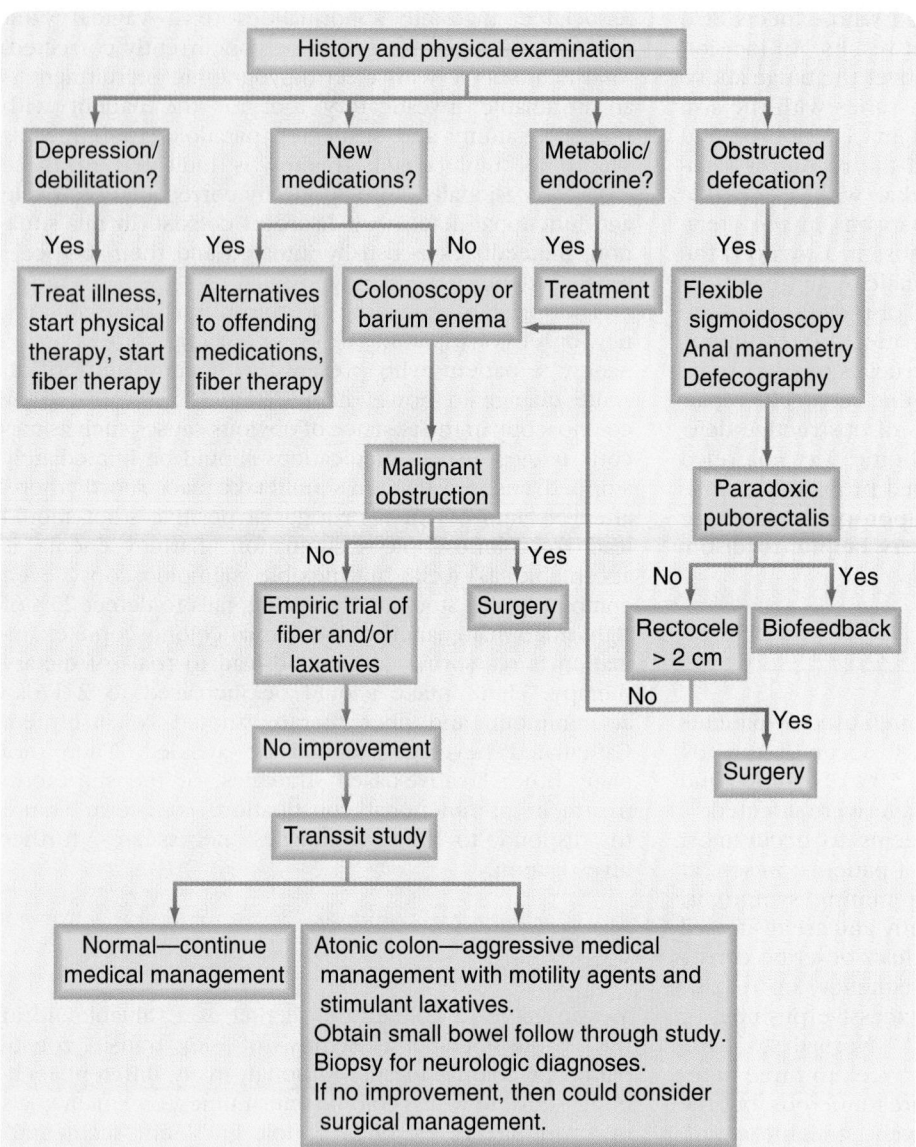

FIGURE 48-71. Algorithm for management of patients with constipation.

worsened during adolescence and early adulthood. Bowel movement frequency is widely variable and ranges from once or twice a week to once every 2 to 3 weeks. Abdominal pain, bloating, and nausea accompany the constipation and make these patients miserable. Frequent use of over-the-counter laxatives and enemas characterize this group, and concurrent psychiatric conditions such as depression are common. Although malignancy in this group is exceedingly rare, it should be ruled out. A barium enema is a useful initial examination: Not only does it screen for large obvious lesions, but the morphology of the colon and the presence of dilation can also be evaluated. A transit study is the next diagnostic step. Biopsies are usually not indicated unless a strong suspicion of neuropathic constipation is harbored. A loss of the argyrophil plexus with a marked increase in Schwann cells indicat-

ing extrinsic damage to the myenteric plexus can be found.[117] This damage is thought to result from chronic laxative abuse. Although the etiology of "idiopathic" or slow-transit constipation is unknown, a study by Schouten and coworkers demonstrated that 29 of 39 patients who had undergone subtotal colectomy for constipation had significantly weaker or absent staining of the myenteric plexus on immunohistochemical staining with a monoclonal antineurofilament antibody.[118] Further study is required to establish this mechanism as causative, but identification of the problem in this manner may lead to more specific therapies. In addition to this, a delay in gastric emptying and small bowel follow-through has been noted in these patients, implying a global motility problem. This motility problem may be responsible for the mixed surgical outcomes noted in the literature.

An aggressive bowel regimen is always the first course of action on diagnosis of slow-transit constipation. A combination of laxatives, fiber, and polyethylene glycol–based solutions can be helpful. A new class of laxative approved for short-term use is 5-HT4 receptor agonists. These may prove beneficial and merit investigation.

Surgery for idiopathic colonic inertia is controversial. The most commonly described procedure is subtotal colectomy with ileorectal anastomosis. Traditionally, only patients with symptoms in the setting of megacolon or megarectum were considered for operative intervention. More and more patients with normal caliber colons and severe refractory constipation have been referred for surgery. The costs and inconvenience associated with medical therapy for severe chronic constipation are not inconsiderable. Intuitively, surgery may seem like an attractive option. However, the data concerning lasting cure are unclear. In most series that include over 20 patients and have more than 2-year follow-up, results range from 33% to 94% success rate (regular defecation without the use of laxatives).[108] The wide range of results is of concern. It has been noted that, often, the symptoms of nausea, bloating, and abdominal pain can persist and can be accompanied by incapacitating diarrhea. In effect, many patients trade one symptom-complex for another. There have been a few small prospective studies exercising strict selection criteria for surgery that includes normal defecography results and diffuse delay on transit study. These patients seem to fair best in follow-up, enjoying a 94% success rate as defined by good or excellent patient satisfaction scores.[119] Subtotal colectomy with ileorectal anastomosis is an option for patients with normal-caliber colonic inertia, but it should not be advocated as a perfect solution. Careful selection criteria applied to motivated, psychologically well-adjusted individuals results in the best long-term surgical results.

Slow-Transit Constipation (Colonic Inertia) With Megacolon

A small, but important, subset of constipation is neurologic in origin. In contrast to colonic inertia with a normal colon, as a group, 50% of these patients are male. Surgical intervention is usually indicated in these cases because medical therapy eventually fails. Among these entities, Chagas' disease, adult Hirschsprung's disease, and neuronal intestinal dysplasia will be considered. Commonly, all of these etiologies will present as slow-transit constipation in the presence of a dilated colon. A dilated rectum is a variable finding and is typically absent in Hirschsprung's disease.

Hirschsprung's disease is occasionally diagnosed in adulthood. These patients are typically young males in their 20s with lifelong evacuation complaints. Commonly, in these cases, a quite short, distal segment of rectum is involved. The remainder of the colon is dilated from chronic distal partial obstruction. Stool is characteristically absent from the distal rectum, similar to the physical finding in children. Barium enema characteristically demonstrates a narrow distal rectum with proximal dilated colon. Anal manometric findings reveal an absent rectoanal inhibitory reflex (RAIR), indicating that the rectum has lost its neurologically mediated ability to relax in response to the presence of a fecal load. Histologic diagnosis is made on biopsy of the distal rectal mucosa at least 3 cm above the dentate line to avoid the normal aganglionic segment in this area. Suction mucosal and superficial punch biopsies are both diagnostic and can be done in the office setting. Acetylcholinesterase staining of the submucosa and lamina propria reveals an increased number of large brown-stained nerve fibers and is considered 99% accurate in establishing the diagnosis. A discussion of surgical interventions for this problem is found in the chapter on pediatric surgery.

Megacolon is the most common complication of intestinal trypanosomiasis. The organism involved is *Trypanosoma cruzi*, a parasite endemic in South America. Nerve damage resulting from trypanosomiasis causes megacolon and -rectum. Fecal impaction and sigmoid volvulus are the most common complications. Subtotal colectomy for this problem results in a residual dyskinetic rectum; therefore, pull-through procedures with excision of the colon and rectum and creation of an ileal reservoir (ileal J-pouch or Park's pouch) are preferable.

Neuronal intestinal dysplasia describes two distinct congenital defects of the intestinal mural ganglia. Type A is seen predominantly in children and consists of hypoplasia of the sympathetic innervation. Type B is present in both children and adults and is characterized by dysplasia of the submucosal plexus resulting in weak forward propulsion of stool. Histologically, hyperplasia and giant ganglia with 7 to 10 nerve cells are present. Acetylcholinesterase staining shows a dense plexus of parasympathetic fibers with increased activity. Laxative therapy in these individuals is usually a short-term strategy and most patients fail treatment. Surgical resection with ileorectal anastomosis is the treatment of choice.

LAPAROSCOPIC COLON RESECTION

The first laparoscopic colon resections were performed in 1991. The experience gained by surgeons performing laparoscopic cholecystectomy provided the impetus to develop the laparoscopic colon resection. Patients undergoing laparoscopic cholecystectomy had smaller incisions, less postoperative pain, shorter hospital stays, and earlier return to work. These benefits were achieved while preserving the time-honored technical aspects of removal of the gallbladder. The goals of laparoscopic colectomy are similar to those of laparoscopic cholecystectomy. The technical requirements and principles of colonic resection cannot be compromised in an effort to avoid the detriment of a standard midline incision. Earlier return to physical activity must be reliably provided. In nearly all studies investigating the implementation of laparoscopic colon resection for various diseases, patients have been discharged 2 to 3 days earlier than patients treated by open colon resection. Laparoscopic colectomy has not been associated with an increased incidence of complications. Data suggest that pulmonary and immune system function is better maintained after laparoscopic operation. Body image satisfaction subsequent to the diminished incision size is well documented. The benefits of laparoscopic colon resection have been found in all age groups, including the elderly.

The accelerated return of bowel function has facilitated earlier discharge from the hospital. The propulsive movement of intestinal content in the nonfed surgical patient is dependent on the migrating motor complex. The migrating motor complex is inhibited by bowel handling, opiate intake, and catecholamine (stress hormone) levels. It is hypothesized that laparoscopic colon resection provides earlier return of bowel function because there is less handling of the bowel and the benefit of the smaller incision includes decreased catecholamine release and decreased narcotic requirement.

Virtually all colon and rectal diseases amenable to surgical treatment are amenable to treatment by a laparoscopic approach. Ileocecectomy for Crohn's disease, right, left, and low anterior colon resection for colon polyps and cancer, ileostomy and colostomy creation and closure, sigmoid resection for diverticulitis, and proctocolectomy with ileoanal J-pouch formation for ulcerative colitis are all performed regularly at centers with colon and rectal surgeons who have advanced laparoscopic training. The indications for surgery are the same, whether the approach is through a standard incision or by laparoscopic technique. The laparoscopic surgeon essentially performs a proven operation by a technique that reduces the length of the abdominal incision.

There are various nuances of the techniques used by laparoscopic surgeons. Laparoscopic techniques of colon resection invariably involve laparoscopic mobilization of the diseased colonic segment(s). The postoperative recovery benefit of laparoscopic colon resection is not altered if hand-assisted techniques are employed or if bowel division and anastomosis are performed intracorporeally or extracorporeally.

There were initially concerns that laparoscopic colon resection for cancer might not achieve cure rates established by standard oncologic operations. These concerns seemed especially pertinent with reports of cancer recurrence at the insertion port sites in the abdominal wall. As experience has accumulated, port site recurrence appears equivalent to recurrence of cancer in the incision of patients treated by conventional operation.

If the operation is conducted correctly, proximal and distal resection margins and lymph node harvest are the same, whether a laparoscopic or conventional incision approach is used. Small prospective randomized trials have revealed at least equivalent survival between laparoscopic and conventional open operations for cancer. The long-term results of large multi-institutional prospective randomized trials, both based in the United States and other countries, have yet to be reported.

Selected References

Corman ML (ed): Colon and Rectal Surgery, 4th ed. Philadelphia, Lippincott-Raven, 1998.

> **Describes colorectal operative procedures in detail with excellent illustrations.**

Gordon PL, Nivatvongs S (eds): Principles and Practice of Surgery for the Colon, Rectum, and Anus, 2nd ed. St. Louis, Quality Medical Publishing, 1999.

> **This text provides excellent anatomic illustrations and detailed descriptions of diverticular disease and common colorectal disorders.**

Kinzler KW, Vogelstein B: Lessons from hereditary colorectal cancer. Cell 87:159-170, 1996.

> **Excellent and thorough description of the genetics of colorectal cancer.**

Pemberton JH, Swash M, Henry MM (eds): The Pelvic Floor, Its Function and Disorders. Philadelphia, WB Saunders, 2002.

> **Excellent in-depth discussion of pelvic floor disorders and colonic motility disorders.**

References

1. Christl SU, Scheppach W: Metabolic consequences of total colectomy. Scand J Gastroenterol Suppl 222:20-24, 1997.
2. Macfarlane GT, Macfarlane S: Human colonic microbiota: Ecology, physiology and metabolic potential of intestinal bacteria. Scand J Gastroenterol Suppl 222:3-9, 1997.
3. Poxton IR, Brown R, Sawyerr A, et al: Mucosa-associated bacterial flora of the human colon. J Med Microbiol 46:85-91, 1997.
4. Nordgaard I, Mortensen PB, Langkilde AM: Small intestinal malabsorption and colonic fermentation of resistant starch and resistant peptides to short-chain fatty acids. Nutrition 11:129-137, 1995.
5. Nordgaard I, Mortensen PB: Digestive processes in the human colon. Nutrition 11:37-45, 1995.
6. Nordgaard I, Hansen BS, Mortensen PB: Importance of colonic support for energy absorption as small-bowel failure proceeds. Am J Clin Nutr 64:222-231, 1996.
7. Rochet V, Bernalier A: Utilization of algal polysaccharides by human colonic bacteria, in axenic culture or in association with hydrogenotrophic microorganisms. Reprod Nutr Dev 37:221-229, 1997.
8. Hillemeier C: An overview of the effects of dietary fiber on gastrointestinal transit. Pediatrics 96:997-999, 1995.
9. Silvester KR, Englyst HN, Cummings JH: Ileal recovery of starch from whole diets containing resistant starch measured in vitro and fermentation of ileal effluent. Am J Clin Nutr 62:403-411, 1995.
10. Phillips J, Muir JG, Birkett A, et al: Effect of resistant starch on fecal bulk and fermentation-dependent events in humans. Am J Clin Nutr 62:121-130, 1995.
11. Muir JG, Lu ZX, Young GP, et al: Resistant starch in the diet increases breath hydrogen and serum acetate in human subjects. Am J Clin Nutr 61:792-799, 1995.
12. Kagaya M, Iwata N, Toda Y, et al: Small bowel transit time and colonic fermentation in young and elderly women. J Gastroenterol 32:453-456, 1997.
13. Suarez F, Furne J, Springfield J, et al: Insights into human colonic physiology obtained from the study of flatus composition. Am J Physiol 272:G1028-1033, 1997.
14. Levitt MD, Furne J, Olsson S: The relation of passage of gas an abdominal bloating to colonic gas production. Ann Intern Med 124:422-424, 1996.
15. Birkett A, Muir J, Phillips J, et al: Resistant starch lowers fecal concentrations of ammonia and phenols in humans. Am J Clin Nutr 63:766-772, 1996.

16. Vonk RJ, Kalivianakis M, Minich DM, et al: The metabolic importance of unabsorbed dietary lipids in the colon. Scand J Gastroenterol Suppl 222:65-67, 1997.

17. Mortensen PB, Clausen MR: Short-chain fatty acids in the human colon: Relation to gastrointestinal health and disease. Scand J Gastroenterol Suppl 216:132-148, 1996.

18. Cherbut C, Aube AC, Blottiere HM, et al: Effects of short-chain fatty acids on gastrointestinal motility. Scand J Gastroenterol Suppl 222:58-61, 1997.

19. Ropert A, Cherbut C, Roze C, et al: Colonic fermentation and proximal gastric tone in humans. Gastroenterology 111:289-296, 1996.

20. Velazquez OC, Lederer HM, Rombeau JL: Butyrate and the colonocyte: Implications for neoplasia. Dig Dis Sci 41:727-739, 1996.

21. Heerdt BG, Houston MA, Augenlicht LH: Short-chain fatty acid-initiated cell cycle arrest and apoptosis of colonic epithelial cells is linked to mitochondrial function. Cell Growth Differ 8:523-532, 1997.

22. Basson MD, Turowski GA, Rashid Z, et al: Regulation of human colonic cell line proliferation and phenotype by sodium butyrate. Dig Dis Sci 41:1989-1993, 1996.

23. Charney AN, Dagher PC: Acid-base effects on colonic electrolyte transport revisited. Gastroenterology 111:1358-1368, 1996.

24. Lewis SJ, Heaton KW: Increasing butyrate concentration in the distal colon by accelerating intestinal transit. Gut 41:245-251, 1997.

25. Medeiros JA, Pontes FA, Mesquita OA: Is colonic electrical activity a similar phenomenon to small-bowel electrical activity? Dis Colon Rectum 40:93-99, 1997.

26. Ford MJ, Camilleri M, Wiste JA, et al: Differences in colonic tone and phasic response to a meal in the transverse and sigmoid human colon. Gut 37:264-269, 1995.

27. Ashraf W, Park F, Lof J, et al: An examination of the reliability of reported stool frequency in the diagnosis of idiopathic constipation. Am J Gastroenterol 91:26-32, 1996.

28. Meier R, Beglinger C, Dederding JP, et al: Influence of age, gender, hormonal status and smoking habits on colonic transit time. Neurogastroenterol Motil 7:235-238, 1995.

29. Haack VS, Chesters JG, Vollendorf NW, et al: Increasing amounts of dietary fiber provided by foods normalizes physiologic response of the large bowel without altering calcium balance or fecal steroid excretion. Am J Clin Nutr 68:615-622, 1998.

30. Stephen AM, Dahl WJ, Sieber GM, et al: Effect of green lentils on colonic function, nitrogen balance, and serum lipids in healthy human subjects. Am J Clin Nutr 62:1261-1267, 1995.

31. Ashraf W, Park F, Lof J, et al: Effects of psyllium therapy on stool characteristics, colon transit and anorectal function in chronic idiopathic constipation. Aliment Pharmacol Ther 9:639-647, 1995.

32. Shafik A: Recto-colic reflex: Role in the defecation mechanism. Int Surg 81:292-294, 1996.

33. Nichols RL, Smith JW, Garcia RY, et al: Current practices of preoperative bowel preparation among North American colorectal surgeons. Clin Infect Dis 24:609-619, 1997.

34. Cohen SM, Wexner SD, Binderow SR, et al: Prospective, randomized, endoscopic-blinded trial comparing precolonoscopy bowel cleansing methods. Dis Colon Rectum 37:689-696, 1994.

35. Frommer D: Cleansing ability and tolerance of three bowel preparations for colonoscopy. Dis Colon Rectum 40:100-104, 1997.

36. Poon CM, Lee DW, Mak SK, et al: Two liters of polyethylene glycol-electrolyte lavage solution versus sodium phosphate as bowel cleansing regimen for colonoscopy: A prospective randomized controlled trial. Endoscopy 34:560-563, 2002.

37. Vanner SJ, MacDonald PH, Paterson WG, et al: A randomized prospective trial comparing oral sodium phosphate with standard polyethylene glycol-based lavage solution (Golytely) in the preparation of patients for colonoscopy. Am J Gastroenterol 85:422-427, 1990.

38. Miettinen RP, Laitinen ST, Makela JT, et al: Bowel preparation with oral polyethylene glycol electrolyte solution vs. no preparation in elective open colorectal surgery: Prospective, randomized study. Dis Colon Rectum 43:669-677, 2000.

39. Zmora O, Pikarsky AJ, Wexner SD: Bowel preparation for colorectal surgery. Dis Colon Rectum 44:1537-1549, 2001.

40. Polk HC Jr, Lopez-Mayor JF: Postoperative wound infection: A prospective study of determinant factors and prevention. Surgery 66:97-103, 1969.

41. Gomez-Alonso A, Lozano F, Perez A, et al: Systemic prophylaxis with gentamicin-metronidazole in appendicectomy and colorectal surgery: A prospective controlled clinical study. Int Surg 69:17-20, 1984.

42. Solla JA, Rothenberger DA: Preoperative bowel preparation: A survey of colon and rectal surgeons. Dis Colon Rectum 33:154-159, 1990.

43. Hinchey EJ, Schaal PG, Richards GK: Treatment of perforated diverticular disease of the colon. Adv Surg 12:85-109, 1978.

44. Vignati PV, Welch JP, Cohen JL: Long-term management of diverticulitis in young patients. Dis Colon Rectum 38:627-629, 1995.

45. Benn PL, Wolff BG, Ilstrup DM: Level of anastomosis and recurrent colonic diverticulitis. Am J Surg 151:269-271, 1986.

46. Stephenson BM, Morgan AR, Salaman JR, et al: Ogilvie's syndrome: A new approach to an old problem. Dis Colon Rectum 38:424-427, 1995.

47. Trevisani GT, Hyman NH, Church JM: Neostigmine: Safe and effective treatment for acute colonic pseudo-obstruction. Dis Colon Rectum 43:599-603, 2000.

48. Karlbom U, Raab Y, Ejerblad S, et al: Factors influencing the functional outcome of restorative proctocolectomy in ulcerative colitis. Br J Surg 87:1401-1408, 2000.

49. Sandborn WJ, Targan SR: Biologic therapy of inflammatory bowel disease. Gastroenterology 122:1592-1608, 2002.

50. Lashner BA: Epidemiology of inflammatory bowel disease. Gastroenterol Clin North Am 24:467-474, 1995.

51. Wexner SD, Rosen L, Lowry A, et al: Practice parameters for the treatment of mucosal ulcerative colitis—supporting documentation. The Standards Practice Task Force. The American Society of Colon and Rectal Surgeons. Dis Colon Rectum 40:1277-1285, 1997.

52. Suzuki K, Muto T, Shinozaki M, et al: Differential diagnosis of dysplasia-associated lesion or mass and coincidental adenoma in ulcerative colitis. Dis Colon Rectum 41:322-327, 1998.

53. Byers T, Levin B, Rothenberger D, et al: American Cancer Society guidelines for screening and surveillance for early detection of colorectal polyps and cancer: Update 1997. American Cancer Society Detection and Treatment Advisory Group on Colorectal Cancer. CA Cancer J Clin 47:154-160, 1997.

54. Mayer R, Wong WD, Rothenberger DA, et al: Colorectal cancer in inflammatory bowel disease: A continuing problem. Dis Colon Rectum 42:343-347, 1999.

55. Bernstein CN, Shanahan F, Weinstein WM: Are we telling patients the truth about surveillance colonoscopy in ulcerative colitis? Lancet 343:71-74, 1994.

56. Befrits R, Ljung T, Jaramillo E, et al: Low-grade dysplasia in extensive, long-standing inflammatory bowel disease: A follow-up study. Dis Colon Rectum 45:615-620, 2002.

57. Cho JH, Nicolae DL, Gold LH, et al: Identification of novel susceptibility loci for inflammatory bowel disease on chromosomes 1p, 3q, and 4q: Evidence for epistasis between 1p and IBD1. Proc Natl Acad Sci U S A 95:7502-7507, 1998.

58. Tarmin L, Yin J, Harpaz N, et al: Adenomatous polyposis coli gene mutations in ulcerative colitis-associated dysplasias and cancers versus sporadic colon neoplasms. Cancer Res 55:2035-2038, 1995.

59. Williamson ME, Lewis WG, Sagar PM, et al: One-stage restorative proctocolectomy without temporary ileostomy for ulcerative colitis: A note of caution. Dis Colon Rectum 40:1019-1022, 1997.

60. Braga M, Vignali A, Zuliani W, et al: Metabolic and functional results after laparoscopic colorectal surgery: A randomized, controlled trial. Dis Colon Rectum 45:1070-1077, 2002.

61. Litle VR, Barbour S, Schrock TR, et al: The continent ileostomy: Long-term durability and patient satisfaction. J Gastrointest Surg 3:625-632, 1999.

62. Sartor RB: Current concepts of the etiology and pathogenesis of ulcerative colitis and Crohn's disease. Gastroenterol Clin North Am 24:475-507, 1995.

63. Ahmad T, Armuzzi A, Bunce M, et al: The molecular classification of the clinical manifestations of Crohn's disease. Gastroenterology 122:854-866, 2002.

64. Fazio VW, Wu JS: Surgical therapy for Crohn's disease of the colon and rectum. Surg Clin North Am 77:197-210, 1997.

65. Fazio VW, Marchetti F: Recurrent Crohn's disease and resection margins: Bigger is not better. Adv Surg 32:135-168, 1999.

66. Stark ME, Tremaine WJ: Maintenance of symptomatic remission in patients with Crohn's disease. Mayo Clin Proc 68:1183-1190, 1993.

67. Salomon P, Kornbluth A, Aisenberg J, et al: How effective are current drugs for Crohn's disease? A meta-analysis. J Clin Gastroenterol 14:211-215, 1992.

68. Sutherland LR, Martin F, Bailey RJ, et al: A randomized, placebo-controlled, double-blind trial of mesalamine in the maintenance of remission of Crohn's disease. The Canadian Mesalamine for Remission of Crohn's Disease Study Group. Gastroenterology 112:1069-1077, 1997.

69. American Gastroenterological Association Medical Position Statement: Guidelines on intestinal ischemia. Gastroenterology 118:951-953, 2000.

70. Brandt LJ, Boley SJ: AGA technical review on intestinal ischemia. American Gastrointestinal Association. Gastroenterology 118:954-968, 2000.

71. Jemal A, Murray T, Samuels A, et al: Cancer statistics, 2003. CA Cancer J Clin 53:5-26, 2003.

72. Vogelstein B, Fearon ER, Hamilton SR, et al: Genetic alterations during colorectal-tumor development. N Engl J Med 319:525-532, 1988.

73. Fearon ER, Vogelstein B: A genetic model for colorectal tumorigenesis. Cell 61:759-767, 1990.

74. Neibergs HL, Hein DW, Spratt JS: Genetic profiling of colon cancer. J Surg Oncol 80:204-213, 2002.

75. Kinzler KW, Vogelstein B: Lessons from hereditary colorectal cancer. Cell 87:159-170, 1996.

76. Calvert PM, Frucht H: The genetics of colorectal cancer. Ann Intern Med 137:603-612, 2002.

77. Haggitt RC, Glotzbach RE, Soffer EE, et al: Prognostic factors in colorectal carcinomas arising in adenomas: Implications for lesions removed by endoscopic polypectomy. Gastroenterology 89:328-336, 1985.

78. Jass JR, Young J, Leggett BA: Evolution of colorectal cancer: Change of pace and change of direction. J Gastroenterol Hepatol 17:17-26, 2002.

79. Steinbach G, Lynch PM, Phillips RK, et al: The effect of celecoxib, a cyclooxygenase-2 inhibitor, in familial adenomatous polyposis. N Engl J Med 342:1946-1952, 2000.

80. Vasen HF, van der Luijt RB, Slors JF, et al: Molecular genetic tests as a guide to surgical management of familial adenomatous polyposis. Lancet 348:433-435, 1996.

81. Heiskanen I, Jarvinen HJ: Fate of the rectal stump after colectomy and ileorectal anastomosis for familial adenomatous polyposis. Int J Colorectal Dis 12:9-13, 1997.

82. Soravia C, Berk T, McLeod RS, et al: Desmoid disease in patients with familial adenomatous polyposis. Dis Colon Rectum 43:363-369, 2000.

83. Dauphine CE, Tan P, Beart RW Jr, et al: Placement of self-expanding metal stents for acute malignant large-bowel obstruction: A collective review. Ann Surg Oncol 9:574-579, 2002.

84. Northover JMA: Staging and management of colorectal cancer. World J Surg 21:672-677, 1997.

85. Jass JR, Love SB, Northover JM: A new prognostic classification of rectal cancer. Lancet 1:1303-1306, 1987.

86. Dukes C: The classification of cancer of the rectum. J Pathol Bacteriol 35:323, 1932.

87. Astler VB, Coller FA: The prognostic significance of direct extension of carcinoma of the colon and rectum. Ann Surg 139:846-852, 1954.

88. Greene FL, Page DL, Fleming ID, et al: AJCC Cancer Staging Manual, 6th ed. New York, Springer-Verlag, 2002.

89. Greene FL, Stewart AK, Norton HJ: A new TNM staging strategy for node-positive (stage III) colon cancer: An analysis of 50,042 patients. Ann Surg 236:416-421, 2002.

90. Swedish Rectal Cancer Trial: Improved survival with preoperative radiotherapy in resectable rectal cancer. N Engl J Med 336:980-987, 1997.

91. Saltz LB, Minsky B: Adjuvant therapy of cancers of the colon and rectum. Surg Clin North Am 82:1035-1058, 2002.

92. Steele GD Jr, Herndon JE, Bleday R, et al: Sphincter-sparing treatment for distal rectal adenocarcinoma. Ann Surg Oncol 6:433-441, 1999.

93. Heald RJ, Moran BJ, Ryall RD, et al: Rectal cancer: The Basingstoke experience of total mesorectal excision, 1978-1997. Arch Surg 133:894-899, 1998.

94. Lazorthes F, Gamagami R, Chiotasso P, et al: Prospective, randomized study comparing clinical results between small and large colonic J-pouch following coloanal anastomosis. Dis Colon Rectum 40:1409-1413, 1997.

95. Mantyh CR, Hull TL, Fazio VW: Coloplasty in low colorectal anastomosis: Manometric and functional comparison with straight and colonic J-pouch anastomosis. Dis Colon Rectum 44:37-42, 2001.

96. Winawer SJ, Zauber AG, Ho MN, et al: Prevention of colorectal cancer by colonoscopic polypectomy. The National Polyp Study Workgroup. N Engl J Med 329:1977-1981, 1993.

97. Selby JV, Friedman GD, Quesenberry CP Jr, et al: A case-control study of screening sigmoidoscopy and mortality from colorectal cancer. N Engl J Med 326:653-657, 1992.

98. Newcomb PA, Norfleet RG, Storer BE, et al: Screening sigmoidoscopy and colorectal cancer mortality. J Natl Cancer Inst 84:1572-1575, 1992.

99. Rex DK, Johnson DA, Lieberman DA, et al: Colorectal cancer prevention 2000: Screening recommendations of the American College of Gastroenterology. American College of Gastroenterology. Am J Gastroenterol 95:868-877, 2000.

100. Mandel JS, Bond JH, Church TR, et al: Reducing mortality from colorectal cancer by screening for fecal occult blood. Minnesota Colon Cancer Control Study. N Engl J Med 328:1365-1371, 1993.

101. Lieberman DA, Weiss DG: One-time screening for colorectal cancer with combined fecal occult-blood testing and examination of the distal colon. Veterans Affairs Cooperative Study Group 380. N Engl J Med 345:555-560, 2001.

102. Lieberman DA, Weiss DG, Bond JH, et al: Use of colonoscopy to screen asymptomatic adults for colorectal cancer. Veterans Affairs Cooperative Study Group 380. N Engl J Med 343:162-168, 2000.

103. Winawer SJ, Stewart ET, Zauber AG, et al: A comparison of colonoscopy and double-contrast barium enema for surveillance after polypectomy. National Polyp Study Work Group. N Engl J Med 342:1766-1772, 2000.

104. Hixson LJ, Fennerty MB, Sampliner RE, et al: Prospective study of the frequency and size distribution of polyps missed by colonoscopy. J Natl Cancer Inst 82:1769-1772, 1990.

105. Rex DK, Rahmani EY, Haseman JH, et al: Relative sensitivity of colonoscopy and barium enema for detection of colorectal cancer in clinical practice. Gastroenterology 112:17-23, 1997.

106. Madoff RD, Mellgren A: One hundred years of rectal prolapse surgery. Dis Colon Rectum 42:441-450, 1999.

107. Kim DS, Tsang CB, Wong WD, et al: Complete rectal prolapse: Evolution of management and results. Dis Colon Rectum 42:460-469, 1999.

108. Gordon PL, Nivatvongs S: Principles and Practice of Surgery for the Colon, Rectum, and Anus, 2nd ed. St. Louis, Quality Medical Publishing, 1999.

109. Fengler SA, Pearl RK: Perineal approaches in the repair of rectal prolapse. Perspect Colon Rectal Surg 9:31-42, 1996.

110. Lawler LP, Fleshman JW: Solitary rectal ulcer, rectocele, hemorrhoids and pelvic pain. In Pemberton JH, Swash M, Henry MM (eds): The Pelvic Floor: Its Function and Disorders. Philadelphia, WB Saunders, 2002, pp 358-384.

111. Berman IR, Harris MS, Rabeler MB: Delorme's transrectal excision for internal rectal prolapse: Patient selection, technique, and three-year follow-up. Dis Colon Rectum 33:573-580, 1990.

112. Fleshman JW, Kodner IJ, Fry RD: Internal intussusception of the rectum: A changing perspective. Neth J Surg 41:145-148, 1989.

113. Arnold MW, Stewart WR, Aguilar PS: Rectocele repair: Four years' experience. Dis Colon Rectum 33:684-687, 1990.

114. Talley NJ, Fleming KC, Evans JM, et al: Constipation in an elderly community: A study of prevalence and potential risk factors. Am J Gastroenterol 91:19-25, 1996.

115. Moore-Gillon V: Constipation: What does the patient mean? J R Soc Med 77:108-110, 1984.

116. Martelli H, Devroede G, Arhan P, et al: Some parameters of large bowel motility in normal man. Gastroenterology 75:612-618, 1978.

117. Preston DM, Butler MG, Smith B, et al: Neuropathology of slow transit constipation. Gut 24:A997, 1983.

118. Schouten WR, ten Kate FJ, de Graaf EJ, et al: Visceral neuropathy in slow transit constipation: An immunohistochemical investigation with monoclonal antibodies against neurofilament. Dis Colon Rectum 36:1112-1117, 1993.

119. Wexner SD, Daniel N, Jagelman DG: Colectomy for constipation: Physiologic investigation is the key to success. Dis Colon Rectum 34:851-856, 1991.

ANUS

Heidi Nelson, M.D.

Disorders of the Anal Canal	**Less Common Benign Anal Disorders**
Pelvic Floor Disorders	**Neoplastic Disorders**
Common Benign Anal Disorders	

DISORDERS OF THE ANAL CANAL

The anal canal can be the site of rare lesions. Most conditions arising in this area, however, are common and benign but may be incapacitating and interfere with the daily quality of life of patients. Moreover, these disorders are often misdiagnosed or maltreated, leading at times to disastrous consequences. A better knowledge of the functional anatomy of this portion of the gastrointestinal tract, as well as recent changes in our understanding of its physiology and that of the pelvic floor, should facilitate diagnosis and management of these ailments and result in more favorable outcomes.

Anatomy

The anal canal, which extends for a distance of about 4 cm from the anorectal ring to the hairy skin of the anal verge, is the most distal portion of the alimentary canal. Its lining, as well as its musculature, has important features that, together with the pelvic floor structures, contribute significantly to the regulation of defecation and continence. Its borders include the coccyx posteriorly, the ischiorectal fossa and its contents bilaterally, and the perineal body and vagina in women and the urethra in men anteriorly.

Anal Canal Lining

The epithelium that lines the anal canal differs at various levels. The characteristically serrated dentate (or pectinate) line made up of anal valves anatomically demarcates the cephalad, pleated mucosa from the caudad, smooth anoderm mucosa. The proximal mucosa is corrugated into a series of 12 to 14 columns of Morgagni with corresponding crypts between each fold. Opening into these crypts are a variable number of anal glands, which traverse

the submucosa to enter the internal sphincter to terminate in the intersphincteric plane.[1] Thus, infection of these cryptoglandular structures may result in fistulas that can be expected to communicate with the dentate line area.

The mucosa of the upper anal canal, like that of the rectum, is pinkish and is lined by columnar epithelium, whereas the mucosa distal to the dentate line is paler and lined by squamous epithelium devoid of hair and glands.[2] The change between the two types of epithelium, however, is not abrupt, and the mucosa of the so-called transitional zone, which lies immediately proximal to the dentate line, consists of layers of cuboidal cells interspersed with tongues of columnar epithelium, which is purplish in color. Differences between the rectal columnar mucosal lining and anal squamous lining have several important clinical implications. For example, diseases affecting the rectal mucosa, such as ulcerative colitis, can extend within the transitional zone area but not distal to the dentate.[3] Cancers proximal to the dentate are typically adenocarcinomas, and those distal are squamous or cloacogenic. At the anal verge, the lining acquires the characteristics of normal skin with its apocrine glands, and this is where infectious complications of the apocrine glands, hidradenitis suppurativa, present. Further, this differentiation also demarcates differences in sensory perception, which influences the surgical approaches to anorectal conditions. For example, internal hemorrhoids can be treated with rubber band ligation without the need for local anesthesia. Excision of external hemorrhoids requires the application of local anesthesia to the sensitive perianal skin.

Anal Canal Musculature

The anal canal musculature with its sphincteric apparatus is the terminal muscular channel of the gastrointestinal

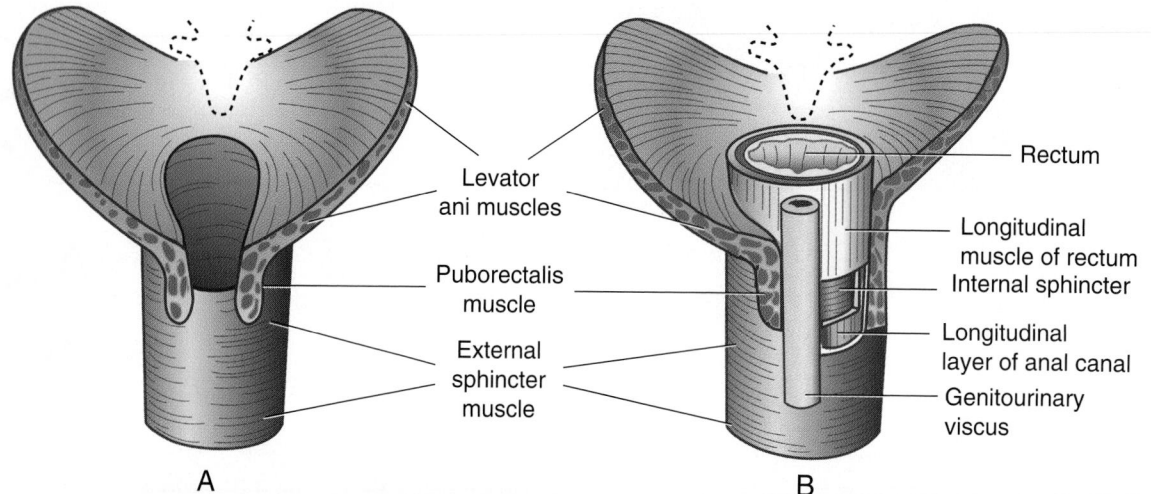

A   B

FIGURE 49-1.   The anal canal mechanism comprises two components, visceral and somatic, each of which is tubular. The visceral tube is enclosed by a skeletal muscle tube by means of which continence is maintained. **A,** Diagrammatic representation of the skeletal muscle component. **B,** Composite arrangement after insertion of a simple visceral component. (**A** and **B,** From Parks AG, Gordon PH, Hardcastle JD: A classification of fistula-in-ano. Br J Surg 63:1-12, 1976.)

tract and can be conceptualized as two tubular structures overlying each other. The inner component is the continuation of the smooth circular layer of the rectum forming the thickened and rounded internal sphincter that ends 1.5 cm below the dentate line slightly cephalad to the external sphincter (intersphincteric groove). The outer component is a continuous sheet of striated muscle constituting the pelvic floor, which comprises the levator ani muscle, the puborectalis muscle, and the external sphincter (Fig. 49-1). The latter is elliptical and engulfs the anal canal and the internal sphincter, beyond which it terminates in a subcutaneous portion. The other two portions, namely the superficial and deep divisions, constitute a single muscular unit,[1] which is continuous superiorly with the puborectalis and levator ani muscles. The external sphincter, bulbospongiosus, and transverse perineal muscles meet together centrally on the perineum to constitute the perineal body. The funnel-shaped configuration of the paired levator ani muscles form the major part of the pelvic floor, and their fibers decussate medially with the contralateral side to fuse with the perineal body around the prostate or vagina.

The internal sphincter, which is innervated by the autonomic nervous system, is independent of voluntary control, whereas the external sphincter, which is supplied by the inferior rectal branch of the internal pudendal nerve and the perineal branch of the fourth sacral nerve, is under voluntary control.[2]

Physiology

The physiology of the anal canal and pelvic floor is complex, but the advent of more sophisticated means to evaluate its functions, such as manometry, defecography, evacuability testing, and electromyography, have improved our understanding of it. The principal function

of the anal canal is the regulation of defecation and maintenance of continence. The ability to control defecation depends on the coordinated functions of the sensory and muscular activities of the anus; the compliance, tone, and evacuability of the rectum; the muscular activities of the pelvic floor; and the consistency, volume, and timing of the colonic fecal movements. Perturbations of any of the critical functions can result in fecal incontinence (Table 49-1).

The anal canal, which has a mean length of 4 cm, lengthens with squeezing of the external sphincter and shortens with straining.[4] *Resting pressure*, or tone, which depends largely on the internal sphincter, averages 90 cm H$_2$O and is lower in women and older patients than in men and younger patients.[5] This high-pressure zone increases resistance to the passage of stool. *Squeeze pressure*, generated by contraction of the external anal sphincter and puborectalis muscle, more than doubles intra–anal canal resting pressure. This maximal increase lasts but for a minute at the most, and consequently, squeeze pressure serves only to prevent leakage on presentation of the rectal content to the proximal anal canal at inappropriate times. The principal mechanism that provides continence is the pressure differential between the rectum (6 cm H$_2$O) and the anal canal (90 cm H$_2$O).[6] The anorectal angle is produced by the anterior pull of the puborectalis muscle as it encircles the rectum at the anorectal ring and contributes to fecal continence. This angle may act as a flap valve[7] or have a sphincter-like function.[8] Maneuvers that sharpen this angle augment continence, whereas those that straighten it favor defecation.

Anorectal sensation allows discrimination of the character of the enteric content (gas, liquids, or solids) and detection of the need to pass that content through sensory receptors located either in the rectal muscular wall or in the pelvic floor musculature.[5] The fact that such sensations persist after proctectomy and ileoanal anastomosis[9]

TABLE 49-1.   Common Causes of Fecal Incontinence

Category	Mechanism	Common Causes
Functional	Fecal impaction; dilated internal anal sphincter	Pelvic floor dyssynergia (difficulty relaxing sphincter when defecating), drug side effect, idiopathic, spinal cord injury
	Diarrhea; rapid transit and/or large volume	Irritable bowel syndrome; infectious and metabolic causes of diarrhea
	Cognitive/psychological; social indifference	Dementia, psychosis, willful soiling
Sphincter weakness	Sphincter muscle injury	Obstetric trauma, motor vehicle accident, foreign body trauma
	Pudendal nerve injury	Obstetric trauma, diabetic peripheral neuropathy, multiple sclerosis, idiopathic
	CNS injury	Spina bifida, traumatic spinal cord injury, cerebrovascular accident, multiple sclerosis
Sensory loss	Afferent nerve injury: unable to detect rectal filling	Diabetic neuropathy, spinal cord injury, multiple sclerosis

CNS, central nervous system.
Adapted from Whitehead WE, Wald A, Norton NJ: Treatment options for fecal incontinence. Dis Colon Rectum 44:134, 2001.

suggests that the receptors are situated in the pelvic floor. For the enteric content to reach the anal canal for discrimination, the internal sphincter must relax while the rectum distends and contracts (rectal anal inhibitory reflex). This reflex involves inhibitory neurons of the myenteric plexus, which innervates the internal sphincter, and intramural nerves and neurotransmitters.[5] Transient relaxation of the internal anal sphincter brings the rectal content into contact with the sensory mucosa of the proximal anal canal so that it can be recognized. Other factors important to continence include rectal compliance, tone, and capacity; rectal filling and emptying; and stool volume and consistency.[5]

Diagnostic Evaluation of the Anus

Systematic evaluation of anorectal disorders includes a careful history and physical examination of the anal canal area before elaborate laboratory testing.

History

Important symptoms include bleeding, pain, discharge (mucoid, purulent, or fecal), and change in bowel habits. It is also paramount to know about associated illnesses, medications, family history, bleeding tendency, and exposure through travel or sexual contacts.

Bleeding is a common presenting symptom of both benign and malignant conditions of the anus and large bowel. Details regarding the type of bleeding can help differentiate between anorectal and large bowel disorders. Inquiry into the type of bleeding should include whether the blood is dark or bright red or associated with clots, whether it is mixed with the stool or separate, and whether it drips into the toilet bowl or only appears on the toilet paper. Blood that drips, is separate from stools, and is bright red is most commonly seen with bleeding internal hemorrhoids. Blood on toilet tissue may be associated with minor hemorrhoidal disease but also with anal fissure. Clots or melena indicate colonic or more proximal bleeding, respectively. Although a careful bleeding history

may suggest a specific etiology, consideration must always be given to proximal bowel evaluation to exclude the possibility of more serious conditions, such as cancer. This is particularly important when examination cannot confirm a bleeding source; when patients are at increased risk for cancer by age or family history; and when bleeding does not resolve promptly after treatment of the presumed source. When there is doubt, evaluate the proximal bowel.

Anorectal pain occurring during or immediately after stooling that is described as severe is usually associated with anal fissure. Pain that may or may not be related to stooling and is throbbing in nature most often is seen with an abscess or poorly draining fistula. Pain totally unrelated to stooling is likely to be associated with proctalgia fugax or levator ani syndrome, a condition characterized by painful episodes of short duration (<20 to 30 minutes) occurring often at night and relieved by walking, warm baths, or other maneuvers. To ascertain change in bowel habits, it is necessary to establish by careful inquiry the previous pattern of bowel habit. Indeed, constipation may mean different conditions to different patients, and it is important to know whether the condition is of recent onset or chronic to determine the course of investigation.

Physical Examination

The left lateral position, with the buttocks projecting slightly beyond the edge of the table, and the prone jackknife position are both suitable for evaluation of anal conditions. Inspection with good lighting should precede any other type of examination. Skin tags, excoriations, scars, or any changes in color or appearance of perianal skin are easily recognized. A patulous anus may indicate incontinence and possibly prolapse. Inspection while straining may help determine the presence of hemorrhoidal or rectal prolapse in multiparous women, and a protruding anus may be an indication of descending perineum syndrome. A careful and systematic digital examination with a well-lubricated index finger gradually inserted into the anal canal helps the examiner to appreciate any mass,

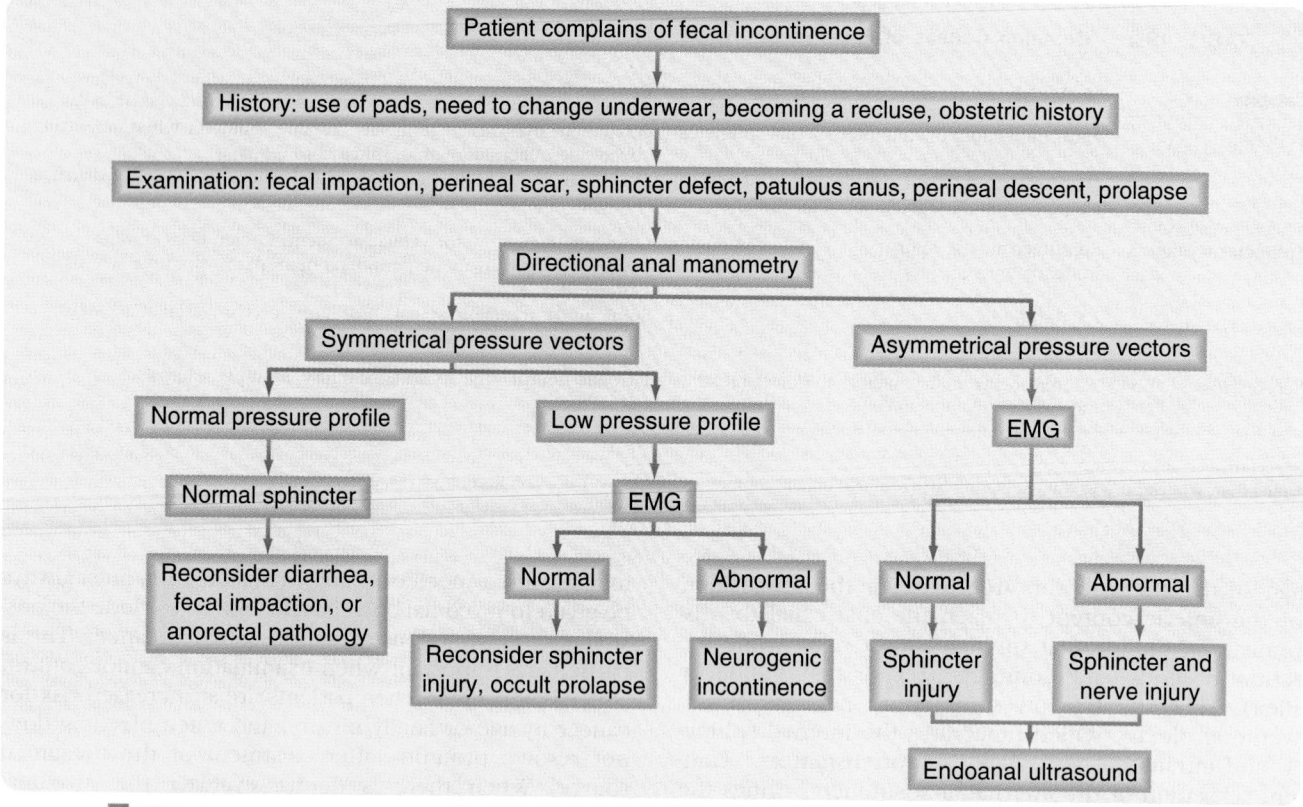

FIGURE 49-2. Investigation of fecal incontinence. EMG, electromyogram. (From Sagar PM, Pemberton JH: Anorectal and pelvic floor function: Relevance to continence, incontinence, and constipation. Gastroenterol Clin North Am 25:173, 1996.)

induration, or stricturing as well as to assess the resting tone and strength of the squeeze pressure of the anal sphincter. In men, the prostate should be palpated; in women, the posterior vaginal wall should be pushed forward to detect rectocele.

After the preliminary evaluation has been completed, proctosigmoidoscopy after enema preparation enables satisfactory visualization of the anorectum. Early signs of mucosal inflammation include the loss of the vascular pattern with erythema, granularity, friability, and even ulcerations. Gross lesions, such as polyps or carcinoma, should be readily identifiable. Any suspicious area or mass should be sampled for biopsy, with the patient's permission, so that a precise histopathologic diagnosis can be established. On withdrawing the scope, the anorectal area can be assessed for mucosal prolapse, hemorrhoids, fissure, polyps, and so forth. The anoscope can also be used for the same purpose; it optimizes the evaluation of lesions confined to the anus.

Other investigations may include barium enema, flexible sigmoidoscopy or colonoscopy, and stool examination, especially if infectious diarrhea or sexually transmitted disease (STD) is suspected. Special studies, such as manometry, defecography, and electromyography, may help in the assessment of anorectal incontinence, constipation, or any other pelvic floor disorders. More recently, ultrasonography and magnetic resonance imaging (MRI) have shown promise in the evaluation of

anorectal suppurative processes. The indications and usefulness of these tests are discussed later under the specific disorders.

PELVIC FLOOR DISORDERS

Incontinence

Clinical Evaluation

Voluntary control of defecation is obviously desirable; fecal incontinence is often a disabling condition. Determining the extent and nature of the problem should start by distinguishing true incontinence, that is, complete loss of solid stools, from minor incontinence, that is, occasional staining from seepage or urgency. Seepage of mucus from prolapsing hemorrhoids or from a large secretory villous polyp, urgency from colitis or proctitis, and overflow incontinence from fecal impaction may be confused with true incontinence. After true incontinence is established, the severity of the disability should be assessed by seeking information on control of flatus, liquid and solid stool, and effect on lifestyle and activities (Fig. 49-2).[10] Fecal incontinence may be multifactorial; hence, details regarding possible causes and associated gastrointestinal disorders should be sought in the patient's history (see Table 49-1).

Defects in the sphincter may be the result of trauma from previous surgical procedures for hemorrhoids, fissures, or fistulas; forceful dilation of the anal canal; impalement injury; or obstetric injuries either directly because of a tear or breakdown of episiotomy repair or indirectly from stretching of the pudendal nerve during labor,[11] which may develop decades later. Other possible causes include radiation damage, primary anal diseases, aging, and neurogenic processes. When associated with other neurologic findings or risk factors, more extensive neurologic evaluations should be performed. Associated gastrointestinal disorders, such as diarrhea, can aggravate disorders of continence.[12] Physical examination should confirm a weak resting tone and squeeze pressure or a patulous anus and the presence of scars, defects, deformities, or keyhole abnormalities. Examination can also exclude the presence of prolapse, hemorrhoids, or other contributory or associated anorectal abnormalities. Endoscopy excludes the diagnoses of proctitis, fecal impaction, rectal polyps, and colitis cystica profunda.

Additional testing can be restricted to a few tests depending on the extent of findings at examination.[12,13] Anal manometry confirms the extent of impairment of the internal and external sphincters by the resting and squeeze pressures, respectively. Manometry can also identify asymmetry, suggesting anatomic defects amenable to repair. Endoanal ultrasound has been recommended to detect occult defects and, in some centers with expertise, is considered more accurate than clinical or conventional methods of evaluation. Finally, electromyography of the pelvic floor can be used to differentiate between anatomic and neurogenic sources of incontinence, and pudendal nerve terminal motor latency testing can predict the likelihood of successful repair.[12-14]

Medical Management

Treatment may be nonoperative, including medications to slow transit or increase stool consistency or diet and sphincter exercises, but in general, results from these approaches have been disappointing, except for cases of mild incontinence.[12] Biofeedback training for strengthening of the anal musculature and improvement of anorectal sensation has been widely applied, particularly in cases of generalized weakness in which repairable anatomic defects are not identified. Variable rates of success have been reported, with typically 75% experiencing at least modest reduction in incontinence frequency and 50% accomplishing complete continence.[12] Biofeedback can also be used before or after surgical repair to optimize results. Another nonsurgical approach is to maximize evacuation regularity; this can be accomplished with the assistance of suppositories or daily tap-water enemas.[12] Accidental eliminations are minimized if the rectum is empty between evacuations.

Surgical Repair

An expanding number of surgical options are available for correction of fecal incontinence, including everything from direct sphincter repair to artificial sphincter implantation and colostomy diversion. For discrete anatomic defects, the most common surgical approach is the direct overlapping sphincteroplasty, in which the separated muscular ends are dissected, reapproximated, and sutured (Fig. 49-3).[15] Fecal diversion is not typically required for these repairs unless there are extenuating circumstances. The overlapping sphincteroplasty is associated with low rates of morbidity and mortality and reasonable rates of success with good to excellent results achieved in 55% to 68% of patients,[12,14] but direct repair of anterior sphincter defects from obstetric injuries can be expected to restore fecal continence in 59% of patients.[11] For nonanatomic defects, postanal repair has been advocated by some authorities as a useful surgical option. Because rates of continence from the postanal repair are reported as low as 35% in specialty-focused centers, it has a rather limited role in the overall management of incontinence.[16]

Anal encirclement, such as with a Thiersch wire or other prosthetic material, is discouraged as a definitive strategy and has largely been replaced by the use of implantable artificial sphincters or the application of neoanal muscular sphincters, or the application of sacral nerve stimulation.[17] Early results from these approaches are encouraging. On rare occasions, a patient may be so disabled from incontinence and refractory to medical and surgical therapies that an end colostomy may be acceptable.

Prolapse of the Rectum

Pathogenesis and Clinical Presentation

Prolapse of the rectum, or procidentia, is an uncommon problem of obscure etiology characterized by full-thickness eversion of the rectal wall through the anus.[18] The exact cause is unclear, but the disorder tends to predominate in women, in those that strain excessively, and in those with chronic mental disorders. Pregnancy and delivery cannot be important because the condition can occur in men and in nulliparous women. Studies would strongly support the concept that rectal prolapse is the result of intussusception or infolding of the rectum or rectosigmoid.[19] As the intussusception progresses caudally, the intussusceptum gradually pulls the upper rectal wall away from its sacral and lateral moorings.[18] With continued straining, the bowel continues to roll inside out until initially the mucocutaneous junction and eventually the rectal wall evert completely. This progressive phenomenon may explain why some patients have occult or hidden prolapse and why the sigmoid mesentery may elongate, the cul-de-sac may deepen, and the pelvic floor musculature may increasingly weaken. Such findings have been implicated as causative, but it is more likely that they are the result of the prolonged process of gradual prolapsing of the rectum.[18]

The symptoms of early prolapse may be vague, including discomfort or a sensation of incomplete evacuation during defecation. A long history of constipation and excessive straining is common. When prolapse is complete, protrusion of the rectum is noted as a mass during

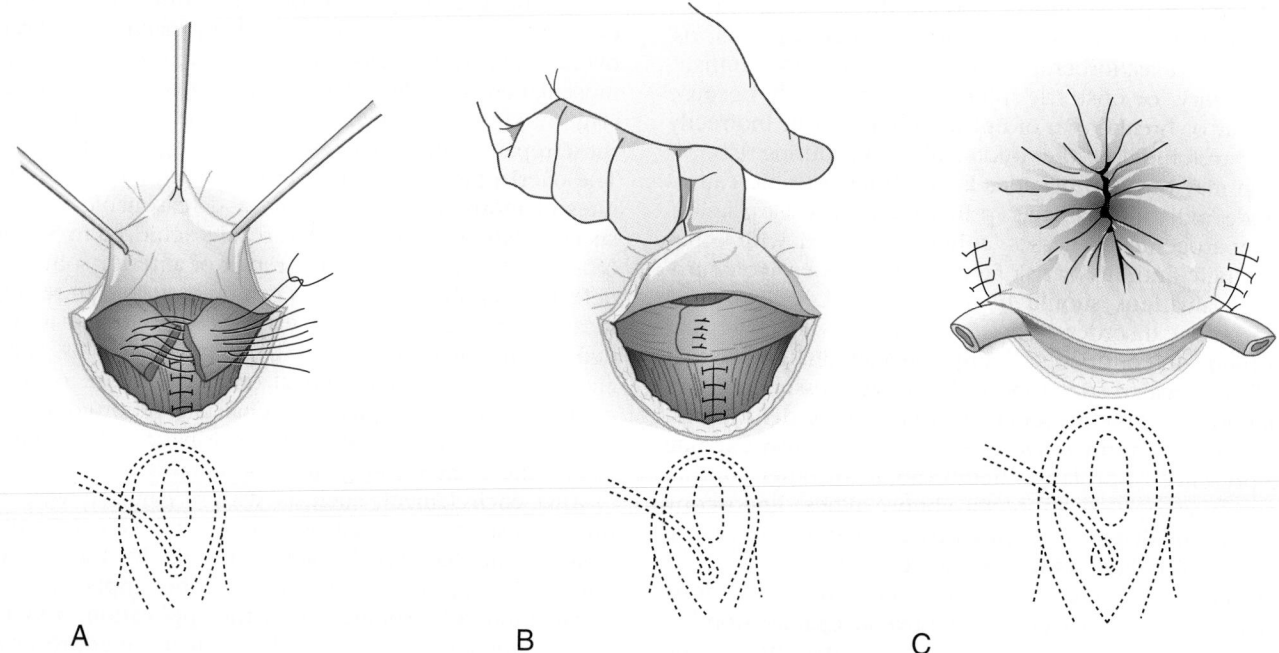

A   B   C

FIGURE 49-3. Overlapping sphincteroplasty. **A,** A curvilinear incision is made midway between the anus and the introitus, limited in its posterolateral extent to avoid pudendal nerve injury. The external sphincter ends are dissected, the scar excised when extensive, and the muscle ends reapproximated using overlapping suture technique. The levator ani muscles are also reapproximated. **B,** Tightness is judged by digital rectal examination. **C,** The wound edges are closed over drains, at times using a Y-configuration to lengthen the perineal body. (**A** to **C,** By permission of Mayo Foundation.)

and after defecation. In patients with occult prolapse, a feeling of pressure and a sensation of incomplete evacuation may be the only symptoms.

Preoperative Evaluation

The preoperative assessment of the patient should focus on establishing the extent of the prolapse; the patient's overall health status; the presence of associated bowel conditions, such as constipation; and complications, such as incontinence. All of these factors influence the operative strategy. At history, nearly half of patients[20] have constipation, and most have fecal incontinence.[21-24] By observing the patient while straining on the commode, the presence and extent of the prolapse can be verified. Complete prolapse demonstrates full-thickness rectal protrusion with concentric rings (Fig. 49-4). Frail elderly patients and those with high-risk comorbid conditions or limited life expectancy are ideally suited for perineal procedures. Young patients, particularly those with constipation or evidence of defecating disorders, are best served with resection and fixation, using open or laparoscopic approaches.

Complete lower gastrointestinal tract evaluations are performed as indicated. On endoscopy, redness of the anterior rectal mucosa or a solitary rectal ulcer 6 to 8 cm anteriorly may be present. A number of additional tests can be ordered but have limited value and are not typically required. Manometry documents the presence of sphincter damage but does not predict recovery. An abnormal pudendal nerve terminal motor latency predicts

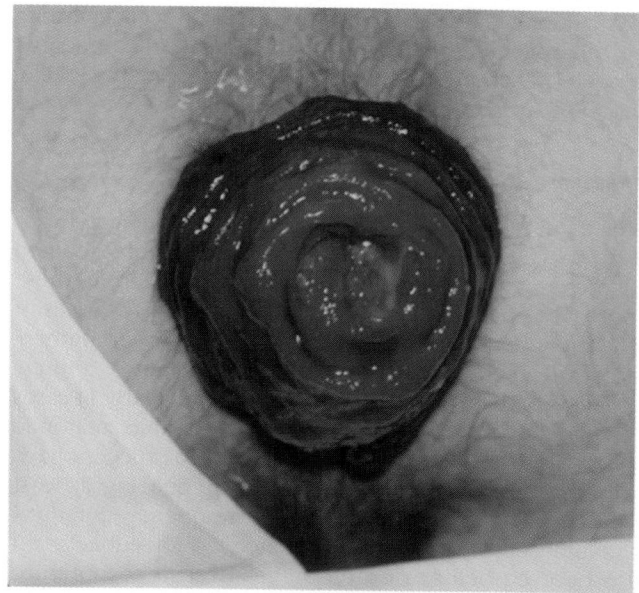

FIGURE 49-4. Complete rectal prolapse. The everted rectal wall appears as a tubular mass made up of several concentric mucosal folds. (By permission of Mayo Foundation.)

a high risk for postoperative anal incontinence but rarely influences the management.[22] Defecography can demonstrate the extent of prolapse and transit studies the extent of constipation. Because a patient with significant prolongation in transit time may respond better to a more

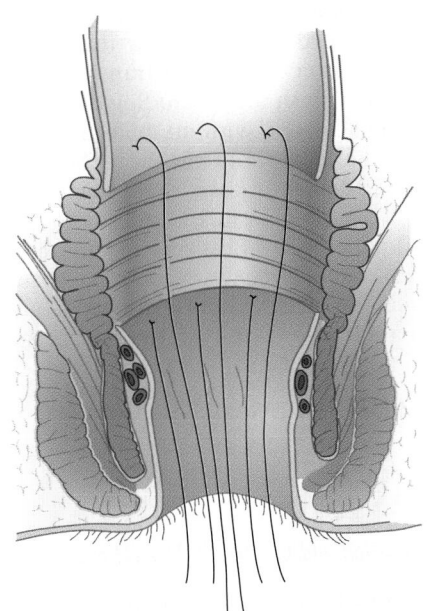

FIGURE 49-5. Schematic representation of Delorme repair of complete rectal prolapse. Mucosal proctectomy is followed by muscular plication, anastomosing the proximal extent of the mucosal resection site to the distal mucosa, just proximal to the dentate. (By permission of Mayo Foundation.)

extensive colonic resection, this may be indicated in select patients with constipation.

Surgical Correction

Two general approaches are used to achieve surgical correction of rectal prolapse: the perineal approach, which includes the Delorme and the Altemeier procedures, and the abdominal approach, which includes but is not limited to anterior resection with or without rectopexy and mesh fixation.[25] The perineal approach is less taxing on the patient and yet has a higher recurrence rate; thus, it is ideally suited for patients with high operative risk and a limited life expectancy. An abdominal approach is preferred for young healthy patients because they can tolerate the procedure with low risk and are less likely to suffer a recurrence requiring reoperation.

Perineal Procedures

The Delorme procedure is essentially a mucosal proctectomy and muscularis plicating procedure (Fig. 49-5). It is ideally applied to patients with up to 3 to 4 cm of prolapse even though the mucosal tube resected can extend for up to 15 cm. Even in frail, elderly patients, the Delorme procedure is associated with low rates of mortality and major morbidity, about 1% and 14%, respectively.[24] Incontinence improves in as many as 69% of patients.[24] Prolapse recurrence is not uncommon and is likely underestimated because this procedure is performed in patients with limited life expectancies and therefore short follow-up.

The Altemeier procedure is similar to the Delorme, but rather than a mucosal resection, a full-thickness rectal resection is performed starting 1 or 2 cm above the dentate. The bowel and attendant mesentery are resected. Because the pelvic cavity is entered, injury to small bowel must be avoided. A full-thickness anastomosis is accomplished after the full extent of resection is completed. For patients with incontinence, a levatorplasty may be added to the resection. Results are similar to those described for the Delorme procedure.[23]

Abdominal Procedures

The abdominal options include bowel resection and rectopexy with or without mesh, performed either alone or together. Complete mobilization of the rectum is required for the abdominal procedures; debate exists about whether the lateral stalks should be preserved.[26] Preservation of the stalks is thought to yield better functional results but a greater risk for recurrence.[20] Although the entire rectum is mobilized to the level of the levators, if resection and anastomosis are being performed, they should be performed high rather than low in the rectum, essentially an anterior resection. This minimizes the risk for anastomotic complications. Rectopexy is performed by securing the rectum to the presacral tissues. Resection with rectopexy is associated with low recurrence rates (0 to 9%)[20,22,27] and can be performed safely, with morbidity and mortality rates commensurate with any large bowel resection. Constipation improves in up to half of patients and incontinence in most patients.[20]

Rectopexy alone with mesh fixation is a well-described procedure, preferred by some centers.[21] The risks of resection and anastomosis are avoided, and recurrence rates are generally low. Complications can result, however, from the presence of a foreign body, and symptoms of constipation are often aggravated. The abdominal procedures can be performed through standard laparotomy or using laparoscopic techniques. Results suggest that postoperative recovery is typically faster after laparoscopic resection with rectopexy. Furthermore, rates of morbidities, mortality, recurrence, and functional improvement are the same with laparoscopic and open techniques.[28]

Incontinence and Biofeedback

Because incontinence resulting from chronic stretching may or may not cause permanent pudendal nerve damage, many patients note improvement in continence after prolapse repair. The role of biofeedback for treating persistent postoperative incontinence[27] or for preventing recurrent prolapse in patients with obvious pelvic floor dysfunction and a tendency toward excessive straining is not well established. That it can be beneficial to some patients and that it is noninvasive encourage its use in select patients.

Rectocele

Clinical Evaluation

Patients with a rectocele present with a bulge or prolapse of the anterior rectal wall into the vagina. Symptoms attributable to a rectocele include the presentation of a vaginal bulge, inability to completely evacuate during defecation, and in most cases the necessity to digitally evacuate through the vagina or through the rectum or perineum. The etiology of rectoceles remains unclear and is probably multifactorial because it is associated with a constellation of a number of pelvic floor disorders, including constipation, paradoxical muscular contraction, and neuropathies or anatomic disorders from childbirth.[29] Rectocele may coexist with other defecation disorders such as slow-transit constipation or pelvic floor dysfunction, including pelvic organ prolapse where factors such as age, parity, obesity, constipation, pelvic surgery, and a number of pulmonary and medical conditions may play a role.[29] Associated disorders must be addressed to achieve resolution of all symptoms. A careful physical examination will reveal the size of the defect where the rectum prolapse extends to the vagina.

Defecography, which can demonstrate dynamic information on the process of rectal emptying, is the only test that is specifically diagnostic for a rectocele.[29] It is probably the most useful test for understanding the relevance of the rectocele in the defecation process even though there is no exact correlation between any single test finding and the results from surgery.[29] Further colorectal evaluations and tests can be ordered as appropriate for other symptoms or coexisting disorders.

Treatment

The optimization of bowel function through proper diet, fiber supplements, and good bowel habits is always appropriate as complementary therapy. Medical therapies, specifically biofeedback, have met with limited success, providing only partial relief in the majority of patients but major relief in only a minority of patients.[30]

Surgical Treatment

Patients with rectoceles should be considered for surgical correction if the rectocele is greater than 2 cm and the patient has to perform digital-assisted defecation.[31]

Although gynecologic surgeons often perform a transvaginal repair, the defect between the vagina and the rectum can be corrected using a transperineal approach (with or without mesh and including a levatorplasty) or using a transanal repair, with an anal mucosa flap and a plication technique without mesh.[31] The repair should extend 7 to 10 cm above the anal canal. Symptomatic improvement can be anticipated in 73% to 79% of properly selected patients.[31,32] Best results can be expected in patients who have a small rectocele, require digital-assisted evacuation, are without evidence of anismus, and who are repaired using a transperineal approach.[31-33]

COMMON BENIGN ANAL DISORDERS

Hemorrhoids

Clinical Presentation and Diagnostic Evaluations

Within the normal anal canal exist specialized, highly vascularized "cushions" forming discrete masses of thick submucosa containing blood vessels, smooth muscle, and elastic and connective tissue.[34] They are located in the left lateral, right anterior, and right posterior quadrants of the canal to aid in anal continence. The term *hemorrhoids* should be restricted to clinical situations in which these "cushions" are abnormal and cause symptoms. The cause of hemorrhoids remains unknown. They may be no more than the downward sliding of anal cushions associated with gravity, straining, and irregular bowel habits. Hemorrhoids can be considered external or internal; the diagnosis is based on the history, physical examination, and endoscopy. External hemorrhoids are covered with anoderm and are distal to the dentate line; they may swell, causing discomfort and difficult hygiene, but cause severe pain only if actually thrombosed. Internal hemorrhoids cause painless, bright red bleeding or prolapse associated with defecation. Internal hemorrhoids are classified according to the extent of prolapse, which influences treatment options (Table 49-2). The patient may report

---

TABLE 49-2.　Internal Hemorrhoids: Grading and Management

Grade	Symptoms and Signs	Management
First degree	Bleeding; no prolapse	Dietary modifications*
Second degree	Prolapse with spontaneous reduction Bleeding, seepage	Rubber band ligation Coagulation Dietary modifications
Third degree	Prolapse requiring digital reduction Bleeding, seepage	Surgical hemorrhoidectomy Rubber band ligation Dietary modifications
Fourth degree	Prolapsed, cannot be reduced Strangulated	Surgical hemorrhoidectomy Urgent hemorrhoidectomy Dietary modifications

*Dietary modifications include increasing consumption of fiber, bran, or psyllium and water. Dietary modifications are always appropriate for the management of hemorrhoids, if not for acute care then for chronic management, and for prevention of recurrence after banding and/or surgery.

dripping or even squirting of blood in the toilet bowl. Chronic occult bleeding leading to anemia is rare, and other causes of anemia must be excluded. Prolapse below the dentate line area can occur, especially with straining, and may lead to mucus and fecal leakage and pruritus. Pain is not usually associated with uncomplicated hemorrhoids but more often with fissure, abscess, or external hemorrhoidal thrombosis.

The physical examination should include inspection during straining, preferably on a commode; digital rectal examination; and anoscopy (Fig. 49-6). Digital examination enables assessment of internal and external hemorrhoidal disease and anal canal tone and exclusion of other lesions, especially low rectal or anal canal neoplasms. Because virtually all anorectal symptoms are ascribed to "hemorrhoids" by patients, it is essential that other anorectal pathologies be considered and excluded. Anoscopy is the definitive examination, but a flexible proctosigmoidoscopy should always be added to exclude proximal inflammation or neoplasia. Colonoscopy or barium enema should be added if the hemorrhoidal disease is unimpressive, the history is somewhat uncharacteristic, or the patient is older than 40 years of age or has risk factors for colon cancer, such as a family history. Depending on degree of disease, treatment falls into two main categories: nonsurgical and hemorrhoidectomy.

Nonoperative Management

In many patients, hemorrhoidal symptoms can be ameliorated or relieved by simple measures, such as better local hygiene, avoidance of excessive straining, and better dietary habits supplemented by medication to keep stools soft, formed, and regular (see Table 49-2). A wide array of fiber supplements are now available over the counter. Symptoms of bleeding but not prolapse can be significantly reduced over a period of 30 to 45 days with the use of fiber supplements.[35] Over-the-counter suppositories and anal salves, although popular, have never been tested for efficacy. Even though all patients should be counseled on dietary and fiber recommendations, patients with prolapse and internal plus external hemorrhoids benefit from additional interventions.

In the absence of symptomatic external hemorrhoids, second- and some third-degree internal hemorrhoids can be treated with office procedures that produce mucosal fixation. Although sclerotherapy, infrared coagulation, heater probe, and bipolar electrocoagulation all have been described, the simplest, most effective,[36] and most widely applied office procedure is rubber band ligation. Rubber band ligation can be performed in the office without sedation through an anoscope using a ligator (Fig. 49-7). Preferably, only one site should be banded each time. Because severe perineal sepsis and even deaths have been reported after rubber band ligation, patients should be instructed to return to the emergency department if delayed or undue pain, inability to void, or a fever develops.[37] With one or more applications, symptoms are alleviated in 79% of patients.[38] Because of the risk for bleeding and sepsis, it is preferable that patients are not taking antiplatelet or blood-thinning medications and that sub-

acute bacterial endocarditis prophylaxis is administered to patients at risk. Rubber band ligation should be avoided in immunodeficient patients.

Surgical Treatment

Hemorrhoidectomy is the best means of curing hemorrhoidal disease and should be considered whenever patients fail to respond satisfactorily to repeated attempts at conservative measures; hemorrhoids are severely prolapsed and require manual reduction; hemorrhoids are complicated by strangulation or associated pathology, such as ulceration, fissure, fistula; or hemorrhoids are associated with symptomatic external hemorrhoids or large anal tags.[39] The choice of anesthesia should be individualized based on the patient's preference, build, and medical status. In most instances, local or regional anesthesia with mild sedation can be used effectively. For simple thrombosed external hemorrhoids, excision in the office is best performed early in the course of the disease, during the period of maximum pain (Fig. 49-8). To remove complex internal and/or external hemorrhoids, an open or closed hemorrhoidectomy can be performed as an outpatient procedure.

Closed hemorrhoidectomy provides simultaneous excision of internal and external hemorrhoids (Fig. 49-9). Preoperative and intraoperative assessment determines the number and location of hemorrhoids requiring excision; typically, three bundles are identified in the right anterior, right posterior, and left lateral positions. The use of a large operative scope retractor, such as the Fansler, ensures that sufficient anoderm is preserved to avoid the long-term complication of anal stenosis. Postoperative complications include fecal impaction, infection, urinary retention, and rarely arterial bleeding. Patients typically recover sufficiently to return to work within 1 to 2 weeks.[39,40] As an alternative to the closed technique, the surgical wounds can be left open to reduce postoperative pain, but at the expense of longer healing times.[14] Early experience with the Harmonic scalpel and the stapled hemorrhoidectomy suggest that newer methods may reduce postoperative pain and recovery times.[39,41]

Anal Fissures

Clinical Presentation and Diagnostic Evaluations

An anal fissure is a linear ulcer of the lower half of the anal canal, usually located in the posterior commissure in the midline (Fig. 49-10). Often misnamed as "rectal fissures," in fact, these lesions truly involve just the anal tissues and are typically best seen by visually inspecting the anal verge with gentle separation of the gluteal cleft. Location may vary, and an anterior midline fissure is seen more often in women, although most fissures in women and men reside in the posterior midline. Characteristic associated findings include a sentinel pile or tag externally and an enlarged anal papilla internally. Fissures away from these two locations should raise the possibility of associated diseases, especially Crohn's disease, hidradenitis suppurativa, or

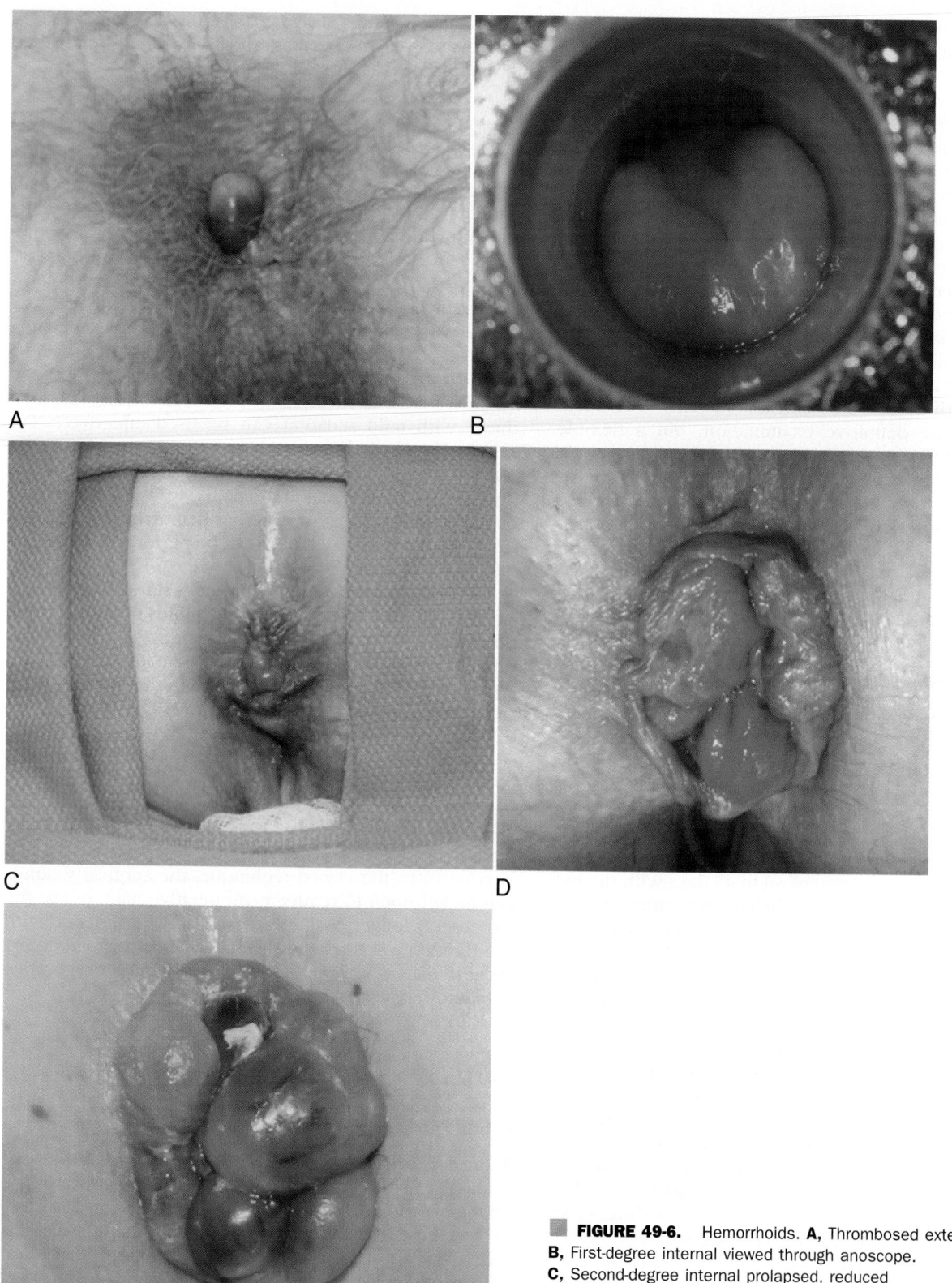

FIGURE 49-6.   Hemorrhoids. **A,** Thrombosed external. **B,** First-degree internal viewed through anoscope. **C,** Second-degree internal prolapsed, reduced spontaneously. **D,** Third-degree internal prolapsed, requiring manual reduction. **E,** Fourth-degree strangulated internal and thrombosed external. (**A,** to **E,** By permission of Mayo Foundation.)

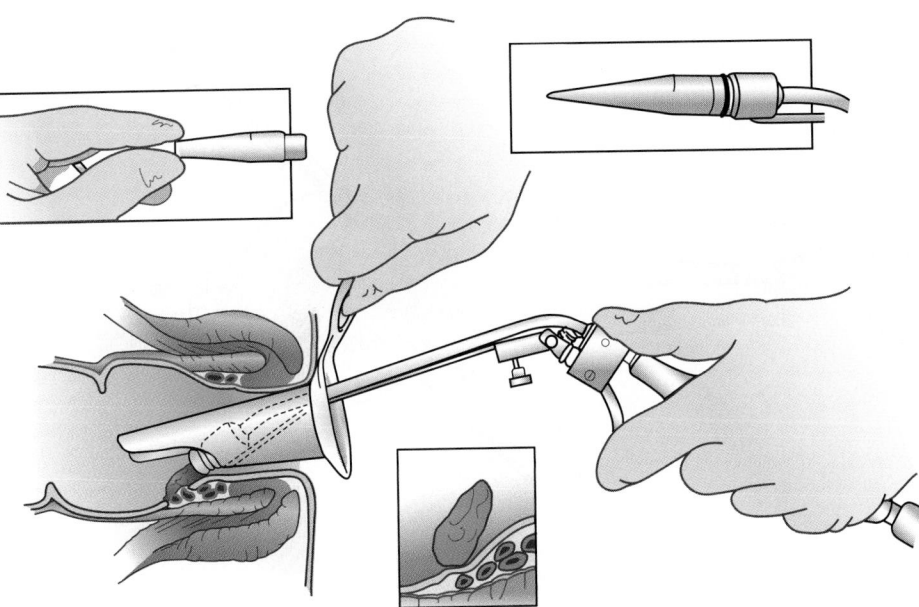

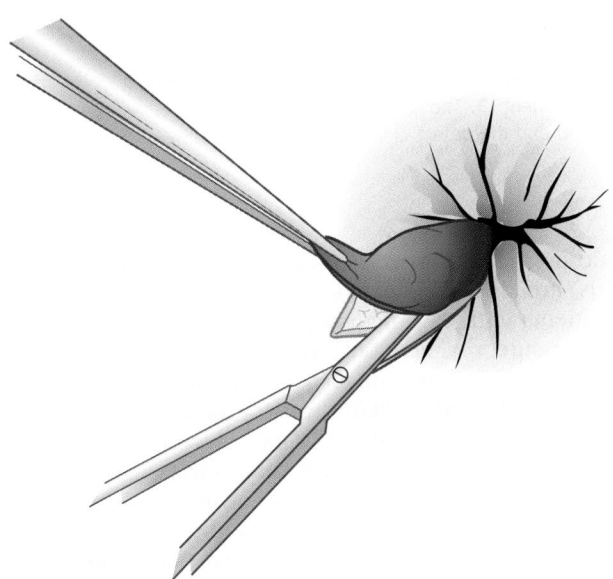

■ **FIGURE 49-8.**   Excision of thrombosed external hemorrhoid. The area is infiltrated with local anesthetic, and the thrombosed hemorrhoid is excised sharply. The wound is left open. (By permission of Mayo Foundation.)

STDs. Because it involves the highly sensitive squamous epithelium, fissure in ano is often a painful condition. With defecation, the ulcer is stretched, causing pain and mild bleeding.

The diagnosis is secured by the typical history of pain and bleeding with defecation, especially if associated with prior constipation and confirmed by inspection after gently parting the posterior anus. Digital as well as proctoscopic examination may trigger severe pain, interfering with the ability to visualize the ulcer. An endoscopic

examination should be performed, but it can be delayed 4 to 6 weeks, until the pain is resolved with medical management or until surgery is performed for those cases refractory to medical therapy.

Pathogenesis

The exact cause of anal fissures is unknown, but many factors appear likely, such as the passage of large, hard stools, which may be the initiating factor; inappropriate diet; previous anal surgery; childbirth; and laxative abuse. Numerous authors have documented higher than normal resting anal canal pressures[42] and reduced anal blood flow in the posterior midline.[43] It is therefore believed that anal fissures are the result of anal sphincter hypertonia and subsequent mucosal ischemia. New information regarding the pathogenesis of anal fissures has led to the introduction of several new medical approaches, including the application of nitric oxide donors, calcium-channel blockers, and botulinum injections, all of which allow for internal sphincter relaxation.

Medical Management

Medical therapies for anal fissures are gaining in popularity, particularly for acute fissures, that is, those presenting within 3 to 6 weeks of symptom onset. The traditional first-line therapy for acute fissures is treatment with warm sitz baths and bran or bulking agents, with rates of fissure healing reported as 87%.[44] Hydrocortisone and lidocaine have been advocated as local topical therapies for acute fissures; however, prospective, randomized evaluations show no benefit over sitz baths and bran.[44] Because improving the dietary and bowel evacuation habits of patients is a good long-term strategy for reducing colon, rectal, and anal problems in general and for reducing the risk of fissures specifically, counseling on proper diet and

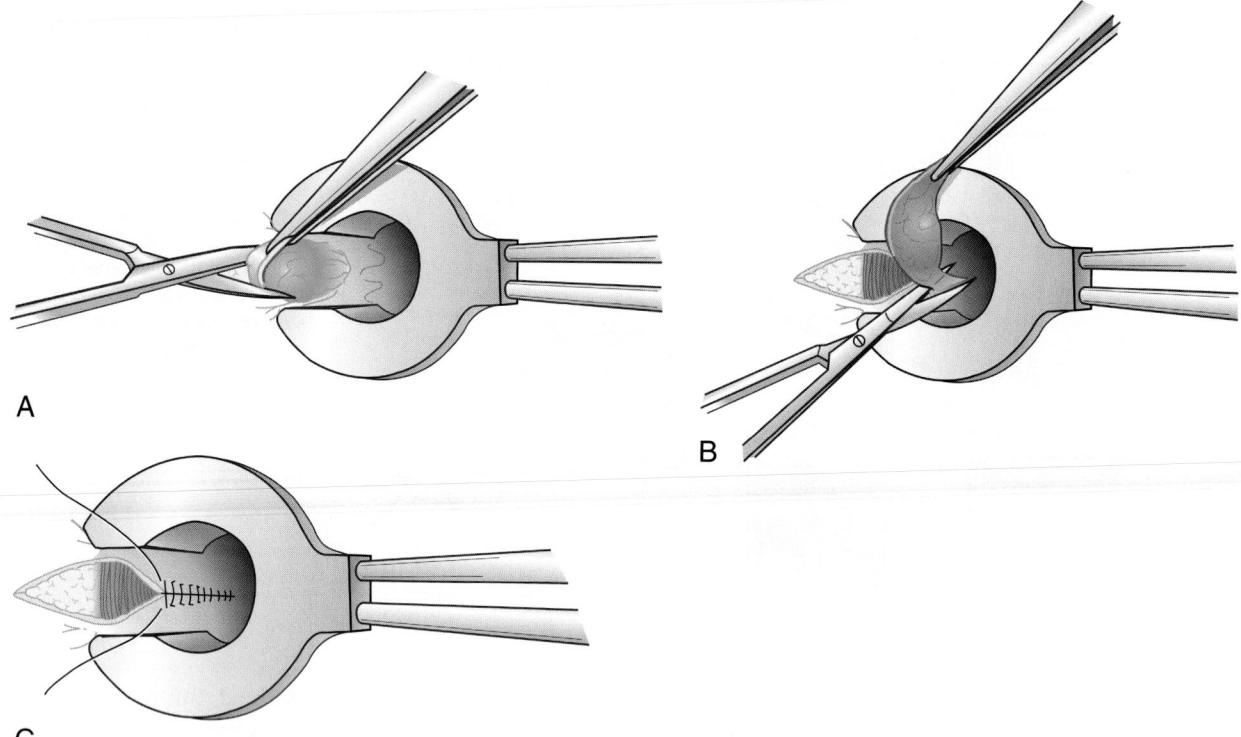

FIGURE 49-9.   Closed hemorrhoidectomy. **A,** Hemorrhoidal tissues are sharply excised starting just beyond the external component and working proximal, finishing with resection of the internal component. **B,** The sphincter muscles are preserved by dissecting only the tissues superficial to them. **C,** The pedicle is transfixed and the defect closed with a running absorbable suture. (**A** to **C,** By permission of Mayo Foundation.)

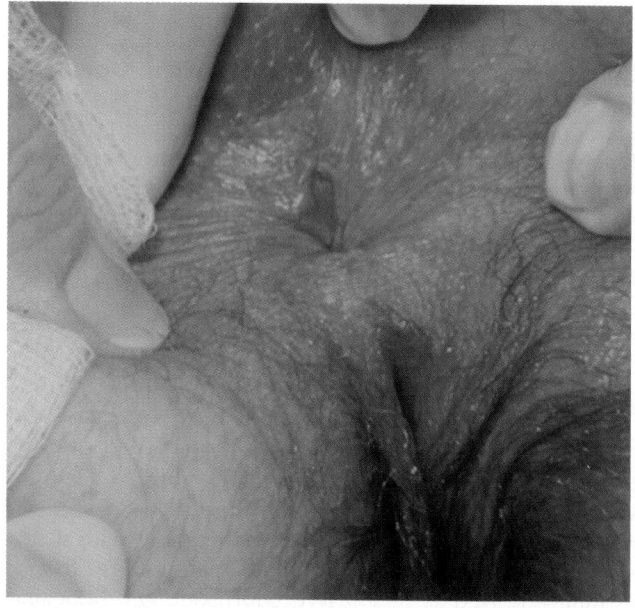

FIGURE 49-10.   Posterior anal fissure. (By permission of Mayo Foundation.)

institution of commercial bulking agents (e.g., psyllium seeds) are always indicated.

Patients with chronic fissures should be started on the acute fissure regimen but are typically also started on other therapies simultaneously, including nitroglycerin or isosorbide dinitrate, theoretically producing "reversible chemical sphincterotomy." For nitroglycerin, the limiting side effects are headaches and tachyphylaxis, which can be reduced by instructing the patient to rest lying down while applying the ointment. The topical application of diltiazem (2%) produces fewer side effects and similar efficacy as nitroglycerin.[45] Fissure healing can be anticipated in about 70% of patients with chronic fissures using nitroglycerin or diltiazem.[45,46] The concept of reversible chemical sphincterotomy has also been applied to the technique of internal sphincter injection of botulinum toxin, a technique that transiently produces striated muscle denervation.[47] Botulinum injections have late recurrence rates as high as 41%; this form of medical therapy is not widely practiced.

Surgical Treatment

Patients with chronic fissures who fail medical therapy either for persistent or recurrent disease and those who develop complications can benefit from surgical therapy. The anal stretch procedure, referred to as the *Lord procedure*, is no longer favored, and the most commonly per-

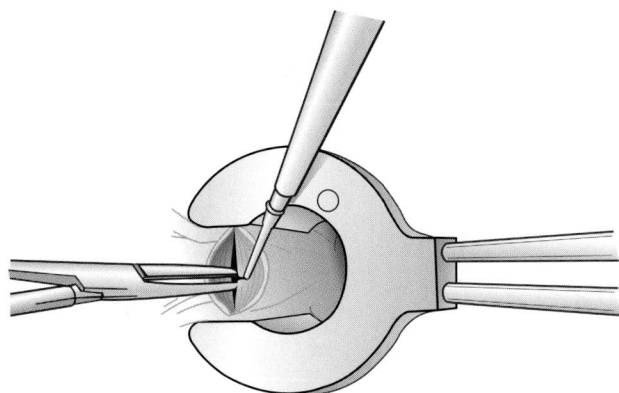

FIGURE 49-11. Partial lateral internal sphincterotomy, closed technique. With an operating scope in place, a small transverse incision is made along the intersphincteric groove. The mucosa is elevated, and the underlying internal sphincter is elevated and divided to release the tight band. (By permission of Mayo Foundation.)

formed procedure is the partial lateral internal sphincterotomy. An alternate surgical approach is the anorectal advancement flap. The flap procedure is particularly attractive for patients with low anal pressures, that is, those who have failed previous sphincterotomy despite a postoperative lowering of anal pressure, and for those with severe anal stenosis. The management of fissures in the setting of Crohn's disease is discussed in the section on perianal Crohn's disease.

Partial lateral internal sphincterotomy can be performed using the closed or open (Fig. 49-11) technique, depending on surgeon preference, training, and experience. Although open sphincterotomy is more appealing from a training standpoint because the internal sphincter can be directly visualized and the extent of transection more readily quantitated, results from the literature do not support better healing rates for the open technique and generally describe a greater frequency of complications.[48] In the past, fissure excision was described as part of the sphincterotomy procedure; it is now accepted that fissure excision is not necessary for achieving complete fissure healing. When open and closed sphincterotomy are considered together, large series confirm high success rates, with rates of fissure nonhealing and recurrence as low as 0 to 10%.[48,49] Early and late complications can occur after lateral internal sphincterotomy, including urinary retention, bleeding, and abscess or fistula formation as well as seepage and, rarely, incontinence.[49]

Anorectal Suppuration

Although anorectal suppuration may have several causes, by far the most common is a nonspecific infection of cryptoglandular origin. Other causes are rare, except for Crohn's disease and hidradenitis suppurativa. The pathogenesis of abscesses and fistulas is usually the same, with the abscess representing the acute phase and the fistula the chronic sequela.

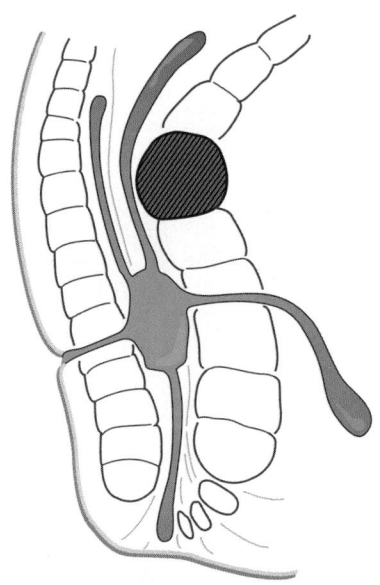

FIGURE 49-12. The various modes of spread from the primary locus in the intersphincteric zone of the mid-anal canal. The puborectalis muscle has been *crosshatched* for easy recognition. (From Parks AG, Gordon PH, Hardcastle JD: A classification of fistula-in-ano. Br J Surg 63:4, 1976.)

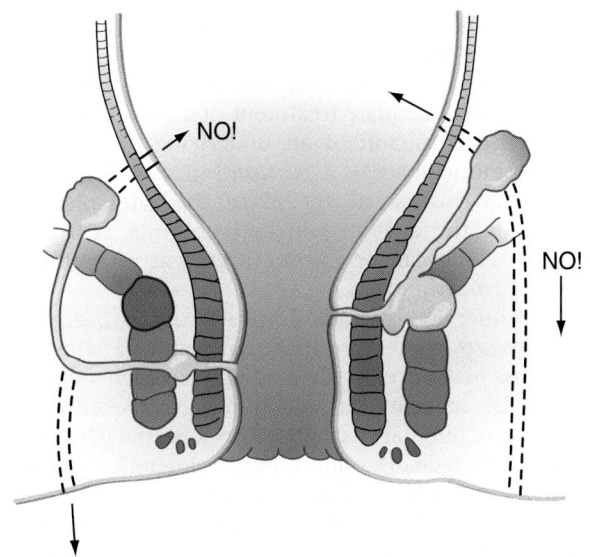

FIGURE 49-13. Diagram demonstrates the two ways in which an acute pararectal abscess can form. It is essential that drainage be carried out in a way appropriate to the type. If incorrectly performed, a different extrasphincteric or suprasphincteric fistula may ensue. (From Parks AG, Gordon PH, Hardcastle JD: A classification of fistula-in-ano. Br J Surg 63:10, 1976.)

Abscess

Infection originates in the intersphincteric plane, most likely in one of the anal glands. This may result in a simple intersphincteric abscess, or it may extend vertically either upward or downward (Fig. 49-12), horizontally (Fig. 49-13), or circumferentially (Fig. 49-14), resulting in a number of clinical presentations.

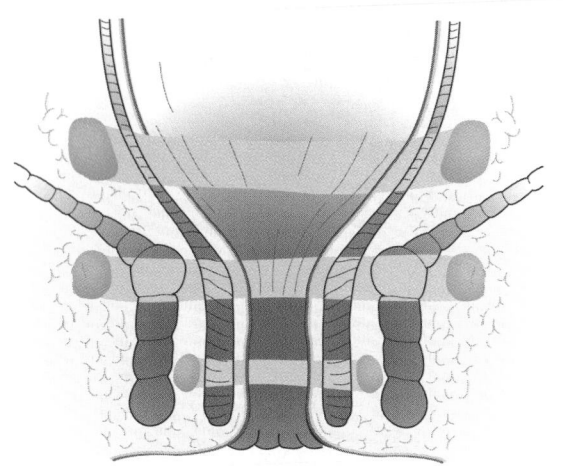

FIGURE 49-14. Diagram illustrates the three planes in which circumferential spread, or "horseshoeing," can occur. (From Parks AG, Gordon PH, Hardcastle JD: A classification of fistula-in-ano. Br J Surg 63:11, 1976.)

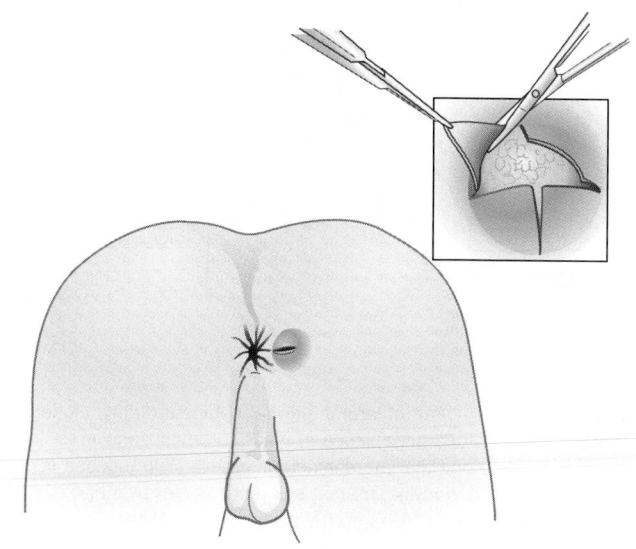

FIGURE 49-15. Incision and drainage of an anorectal abscess. A cruciate incision is made and the wound probed for loculations. The wound edges are kept open to facilitate proper drainage by excising the corners of the cruciate *(inset)* and packing the cavity. (By permission of Mayo Foundation.)

Clinical Presentation: Types of Abscesses

An *intersphincteric abscess* is limited to the primary site of origin and may be asymptomatic or result in severe, throbbing pain that resembles the pain of a fissure. Pain persisting after adequate treatment of a coexisting fissure should raise suspicion of an underlying, unrecognized intersphincteric abscess. A *perianal abscess* results from the vertical downward spread of the intersphincteric infection to the anal margin and presents as a tender swelling, which can be misinterpreted as a thrombosed external hemorrhoid.

If the infection spreads vertically upward, an *intermuscular abscess* within the rectal wall or a *supralevator abscess* may develop, depending on which side of the longitudinal muscle the infection has tracked. These abscesses are difficult to diagnose because the patient may complain of vague discomfort, external manifestations are absent, and the presence of rectal induration and swelling may be clearly established only with the aid of an examination under anesthesia.

Horizontal spread of infection may track across the internal sphincter into the anal canal or in the opposite direction across the external sphincter into the ischiorectal fossa to form an *ischiorectal abscess*. The abscess may be large, especially if neglected or treated only with antibiotics and allowed to expand to the roof of the fossa or even through it into the supralevator space after traversing the levator ani muscle and downward to the perianal skin. The patient may complain of pain and fever before an erythematous mass is detectable. Ultimately, an obvious red, fluctuant mass is visible. The infectious process may spread circumferentially from one side to the other of the intersphincteric space, the supralevator space, or the ischiorectal fossa, producing the complex, horseshoe abscess.

Treatment

Abscesses should be drained when diagnosed. Simple and superficial abscesses can most often be drained under local anesthesia in the office setting in patients who are otherwise healthy. Patients who manifest systemic symptoms; those who are immunocompromised for any reason, including acquired immunodeficiency syndrome (AIDS), diabetes, cancer therapies, or chronic medical immunosuppression; and those with complex, complicated abscesses are best treated in a hospital setting.

An intersphincteric abscess is drained by dividing the internal sphincter at the level of the abscess. For a perianal abscess, a simple skin incision is all that is necessary (Fig. 49-15). Both an intermuscular abscess and a supralevator abscess, so long as it is not an ischiorectal abscess extension, need to be drained into the lower rectum and upper anal canal. An ischiorectal abscess requires immediate, wide local drainage through an appropriate cruciform incision through the skin and subcutaneous tissue overlying the infected space. At times, these abscesses are sufficiently deep that needle localization of the purulent material may be required to guide the surgeon for optimizing the skin incision site. The cavity should be gently digitalized to break down loculations. Neglected abscesses can lead to devastating, necrotizing infections of the perineum that can spread and become lethal. Failure of response to local treatment or recurrent abscesses may suggest inadequate drainage with residual pus, the presence of a fistula, or immunoincompetence. Under these circumstances, antibiotics may be useful, together with examination under anesthesia after preliminary evaluation by computed tomography (CT) of the pelvis and perineum. For horseshoe abscess, the deep postanal space should be drained through a posterior midline incision extending from the subcutaneous portion of the external

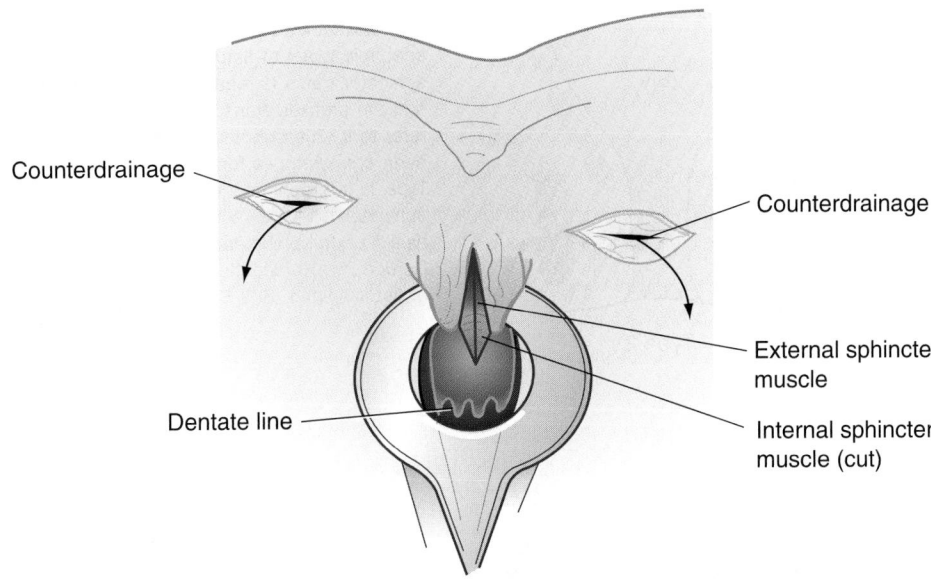

Counterdrainage

Counterdrainage

Dentate line

External sphincter
muscle

Internal sphincter
muscle (cut)

FIGURE 49-16. Modification of Hanley's technique for incision and drainage of a horseshoe abscess. (From Gordon PH: Anorectal abscesses and fistula-in-ano. *In* Gordon PH, Nivatvongs S [eds]: Principles and Practice of Surgery for the Colon, Rectum, and Anus, 2nd ed. St. Louis, Quality Medical, 1992, p 232.)

sphincter over the abscess to the tip of the coccyx, separating the superficial external sphincter and thus unroofing the postanal space and its ischioanal extension (Fig. 49-16). Para-anal incisions can be made and setons placed to drain the anterior extensions of a horseshoe abscess.

Fistula in Ano

Anorectal sepsis can be complicated by a fistula in ano in about 25% of patients during the acute phase of sepsis or within 6 months thereafter.[50] Most fistulas derive from sepsis originating in the anal canal glands at the dentate line. The path of a fistula is determined by the local anatomy; most commonly, they track in the fascial or fatty planes, especially the intersphincteric space between the internal and the external sphincter into the ischiorectal fascia. In such instances, the track passes directly to the perineal skin. In some cases, circumferential spread may also occur in the ischiorectal fossa, with the track passing from one fossa to the contralateral one through the posterior rectum, a fistula known as the *horseshoe fistula*. Fistulas usually fall under four main anatomic categories as described by Parks and colleagues in 1976 (Box 49-1 and Fig. 49-17).[51]

Clinical Presentation: Types of Fistulas

Intersphincteric fistulas are the most common anal fistulas, and in most cases, the infection passes directly downward to the anal margin. However, there are some variants of this type of fistula that are less common and more complex to treat. For instance, the track may travel upward in the rectal wall (higher track), with or without a perineal opening. Rarely, an intersphincteric fistula originates in the pelvis from the colon.[51] In *trans-sphincteric fistulas*, the track traverses the external sphincter to travel through the ischiorectal fossa and end at the perineal skin. If it passes through the muscle at a low level, it is uncom-

---

> **Box 49-1. Classification of Anorectal Fistulas**
>
> *Intersphincteric* (the most common): The fistula track is confined to the intersphincteric plane.
> *Trans-sphincteric:* The fistula connects the intersphincteric plane with the ischiorectal fossa by perforating the external sphincter.
> *Suprasphincteric:* Similar to trans-sphincteric, but the track loops over the external sphincter and perforates the levator ani.
> *Extrasphincteric:* The track passes from the rectum to perineal skin, completely external to the sphincteric complex.

Adapted from classification by Parks AG, Gordon PH, Hardcastle JD: A classification of fistula-in-ano. Br J Surg 63:1, 1976.

---

plicated and readily treatable; if, however, it penetrates the upper portion of the sphincter (high blind track), it constitutes a more difficult therapeutic dilemma. Indeed, it may be felt digitally through the wall of the rectum and may lead the surgeon to create an artificial connection with the rectum by forceful probing, a situation that can be difficult to correct. *Suprasphincteric fistulas* are rare, difficult to treat, and may be hazardous if dealt with by inexperienced surgeons. The track may first travel upward in the intersphincteric plane before taking a lateral direction over the top of the puborectalis and finally downward through the ischiorectal fossa to the perineal skin. Because its trajectory is above all muscles of importance to continence, division of all external muscles results in incontinence. Moreover, the fistula may have an additional extension into the pelvis that runs parallel to the rectum (high blind track). In this instance, an indurated area can be palpated through the rectal wall.

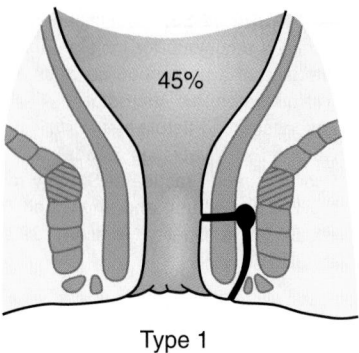

45%

Type 1

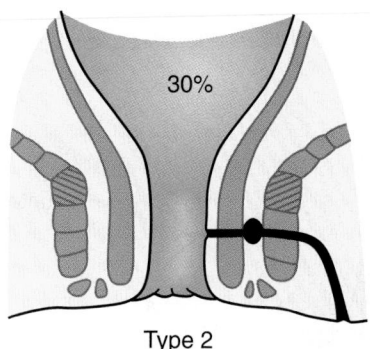

30%

Type 2

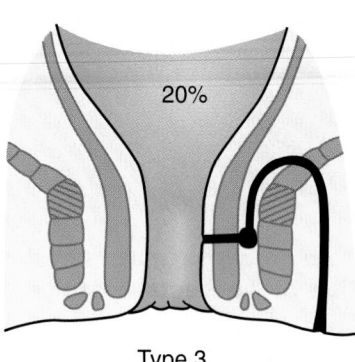

20%

Type 3

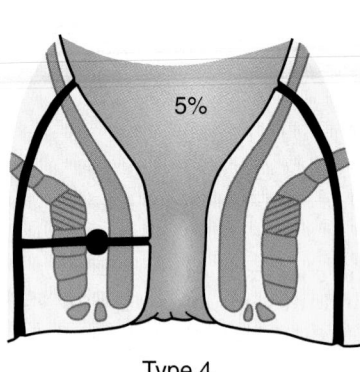

5%

Type 4

FIGURE 49-17. The four main anatomic types of fistulas. The external sphincter mass is regarded as the keystone, and the prefixes *trans*, *supra*, and *extra* refer to it. The puborectalis muscle has been *crosshatched* for easy recognition. Type 1, intersphincteric; type 2, transsphincteric; type 3, suprasphincteric; type 4, extrasphincteric. (From Parks AG, Gordon PH, Hardcastle JD: A classification of fistula-in-ano. Br J Surg 63:5, 1976.)

Finally, *extrasphincteric fistula* is rare and its treatment is also hazardous. It travels from the perineal skin to the rectal wall above the levator ani that it pierces. The track is completely outside the sphincteric apparatus. Causes typically include trauma, either external or internal (e.g., fish bone piercing one wall of rectum), carcinoma, or Crohn's disease. Treatment is difficult, lengthy, and usually involves colostomy.

Treatment

A fistula may first present as an acute abscess or, at times, simply as a draining sinus that may irritate the perineal skin. On examination, subcutaneous induration may be traced from the external opening to the anal canal. Digital examination may reveal a palpable nodule in the wall of the anal canal, an indication of the primary opening. A probe can be eased gently (not forcefully) from the external skin opening to the internal, anal canal opening.

Management of fistula in ano should include the following steps:

1. Under anesthesia, palpation for induration, anoscopy for inspection, and gentle probing along the dentate for internal openings allows accurate definition of the abnormal anatomy. The Goodsall rule (Fig. 49-18) is useful for anticipating the anatomy of simple fistulas. If the internal opening cannot be identified by direct probing, it should be identified by probing the external opening or by injecting a mixture of methylene blue and peroxide into the track using a pediatric feeding tube (Fig. 49-19*A*).

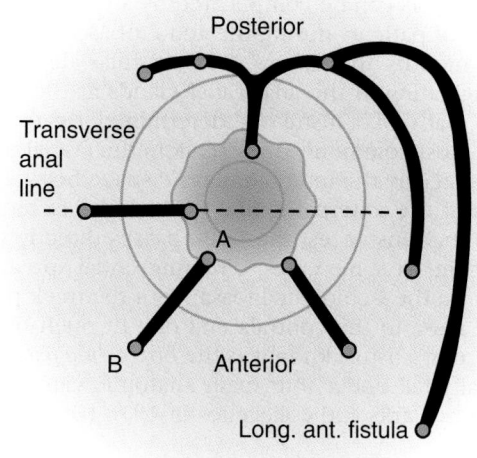

Posterior

Transverse anal line

A

B   Anterior

Long. ant. fistula

FIGURE 49-18. The Goodsall rule. The usual relationship of primary and secondary fistula orifices is diagrammed. The internal (primary orifice) is marked A. The rule predicts that if a line is drawn transversely across the anus, an external opening (B) anterior to this line will lead to a straight radial tract, whereas an external opening that lies posterior to the line will lead to a curved tract and an internal opening in the posterior commissure. The long anterior fistula is an exception to the rule. (From Schrock TR: Benign and malignant disease of the anorectum. *In* Fromm O [ed]: Gastrointestinal Surgery. New York, Churchill Livingstone, 1985, p 612.)

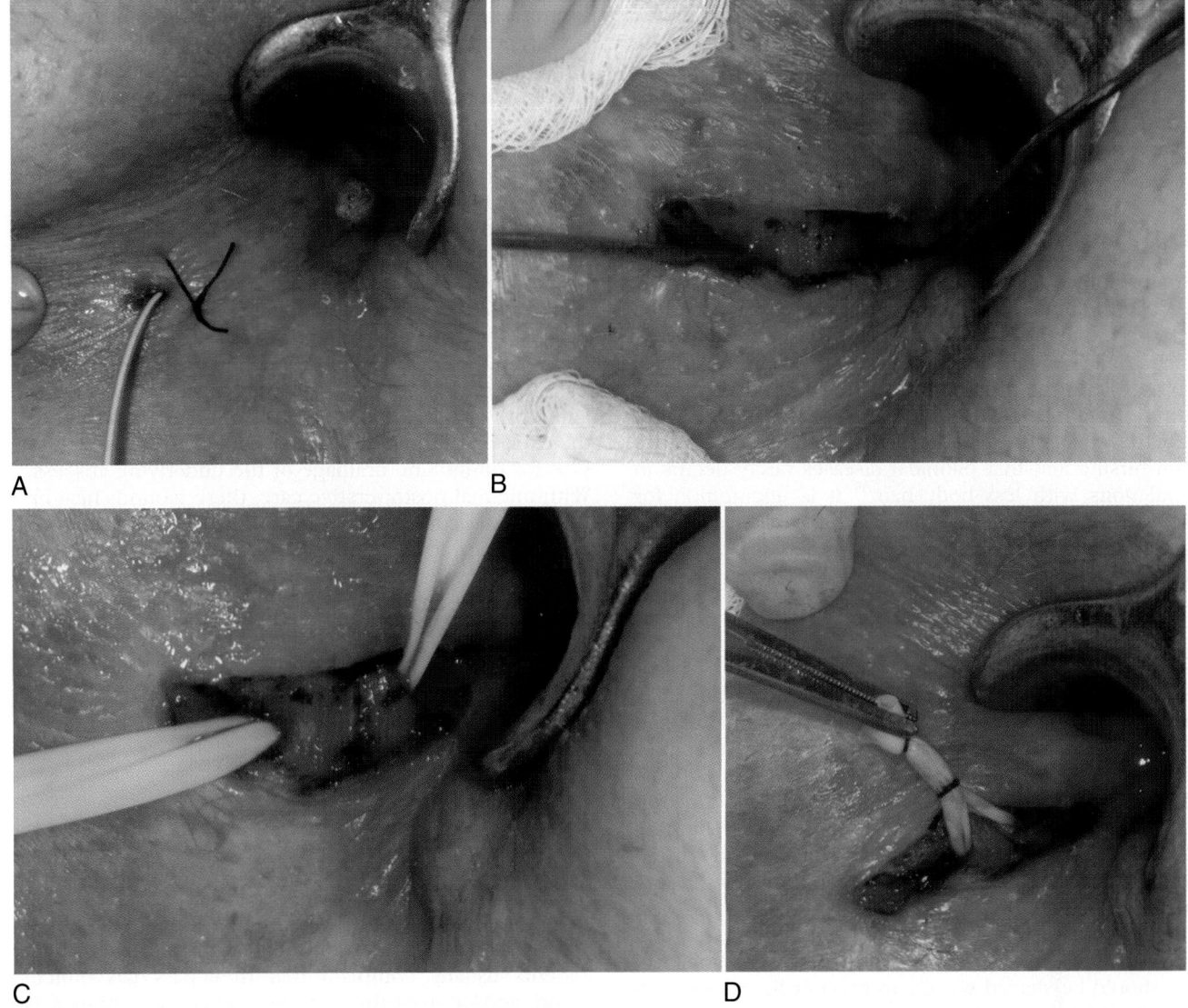

A   B

C   D

FIGURE 49-19.   Seton placement. **A,** If the primary opening cannot be identified by gentle probing along the dentate line, methylene blue plus peroxide injections may better delineate the internal fistula source. **B,** A probe is passed from the primary to the secondary openings, and the skin is incised to reveal the tract and interposed sphincter muscle. **C,** An elastic cutting seton can be placed when generous muscle requires division. **D,** The seton is tightened in the operating room and again once or twice in the office to allow for fibrosis and gradual sphincter transection. (**A** to **D,** By permission of Mayo Foundation.)

2. Drainage of primary intersphincteric infection in all types of fistulas, as well as the primary track across the external sphincter and secondary tracks within the anorectal fossa, is key. For superficial fistulas involving small quantities of sphincter muscle, primary fistulotomy is simple and definitive. For anterior fistulas in women and fistulas involving greater than one fourth to one half the bulk of sphincter muscles, seton placement should be preferred over primary fistulotomy (Fig. 49-19*B to D*). In rare circumstances with complex, deep, or recurrent fistulas, newer alternatives to fistulotomy are preferred to avoid the complication of fecal incontinence. Fibrin glue injections of the track and advancement flap closure of the primary openings can heal 69% of complex fistulas.[52]

3. Close follow-up and careful nursing of the wound by a physician-nurse team involve sitz baths and wound dressing to ensure healing from the depth of the wound to the surface. A seton of monofilament nylon tied loosely around the fistulous track may be used to drain the trans-sphincteric track traveling above the anal valves for a suprasphincteric fistula.[53] The seton may be removed 2 to 3 months later, at which time the track may heal spontaneously. If not, the track may be divided because fibrosis may cause minimal separation of the cut ends. For more straight-forward trans-sphincteric fistulas, a cutting seton can be placed at surgery and tightened in the office. This divides the track gradually over a few weeks and min-imizes the sphincter defect and the risk of significant fecal incontinence.

Difficult and persistent high fistulas can be treated by sliding flap advancement made of mucosa, submucosa, and circular muscle to cover the internal opening.[27] The Goodsall rule (see Fig. 49-18) is of little help in defining the anatomy of complex and recurrent fistulas. Diagnostic tests such as pelvic MRI or endorectal ultrasound and treatment by a specialist may be helpful here.

Pilonidal Disease

Pilonidal infections and chronic pilonidal sinuses typically occur in the midline of the sacrococcygeal skin of young men. Although the exact pathogenesis of pilonidal disease remains elusive and controversial, hair seems to play a central role in the process of infection and in the perpetuation of granulation tissue in sinuses. This is consistent with the clinical observation that pilonidal patients are often hirsute and that pilonidal diseases rarely occurs in populations with less body hair.[54] It is uncommon for pilonidal disease to be confused with clinical disorders such as anal fistulas, skin disorders, underlying malignancies, or true sacrococcygeal sinuses.

Acute Management

Patients presenting acutely with new-onset disease may have a painful fluctuant abscess or a draining infected sinus. Both can be managed with simple office therapies with more definitive procedures reserved for patients who suffer from a recurrence. Abscess can be drained in the office or emergency department using local anesthesia. Typically the fluctuance extends to either side of the midline cleft, and incision and drainage down to the subcutaneous tissues off the midline provides for the best drainage and fastest healing. For both abscesses and sinuses, hair should be removed from the wound and local skin should be shaved weekly to prevent the reintroduction of hair. Laser depilation can also be used to accomplish long-lasting, but temporary, hair removal.[55] Ideally, these patients should be seen weekly in the office for wound care until there is complete healing. Most do not require further care; those who do can be treated as described in the following section.

Operative Management

For those patients who have recurring infections, more definitive operative management is warranted. Numerous procedures have been described in literature ranging from simple incision and drainage to complex plastic flaps for cleft obliteration.[54]

Incision and curettage is advocated by some as the simplest approach to pilonidal disease. After a probe is placed in the sinus, an incision is made over the probe, incising the overlying pits followed by curetting the granulation tissue.[54] Daily care with dry dressings and weekly office visits are required for postoperative management. Wound healing typically requires 4 to 7 weeks, and recurrence rates vary from 1% to 20%.[54] A more common approach is

the simple excision without closure. The entire pilonidal is removed and the wound left to heal by secondary intention, typically requiring 8 to 21 weeks. Recurrence rates are low with this technique, at 2% to 3%.[54] It is appealing to consider excision with immediate closure of the wound because wound healing takes only 2 to 7 weeks; however, recurrences are more likely to occur at rates of 11% to 29%.[54] A technique that is intermediate to the excision with or without closure is that of marsupialization, where the wound edges are approximated to the fibrous base of the pilonidal. Reducing the size of the wound reduces the healing times to under 5 weeks and keeps recurrence rates low at between 1% and 4%.[54]

The majority of other procedures described for pilonidal disease focus on off-midline procedures such as the Bascom[56] or a plastic flap reconstruction like the Limberg[57] or Karydakis.[54] The Bascom procedure involves the excision of the midline pits coupled with a lateral incision for off-midline drainage of the underlying abscess.[56] With minimal postoperative care, these wounds heal in 4 weeks and recurrence rates are as low as 10%.[56] The rhomboid excision and Limberg flap is one example of a flap technique for complete removal of the site of disease and subsequent primary tissue closure.[57] The disadvantage of the flap techniques include the complexity of the procedures; the necessity for inpatient hospitalization, typically less than a week; and the fact that recurrences can still occur in 5% of cases.[57]

LESS COMMON BENIGN ANAL DISORDERS

Rectovaginal Fistula

A rectovaginal fistula is a communication between the epithelial-lined surfaces of the rectum and the vagina. Patients usually complain that they pass gas, mucus, blood, and/or stool through the vagina. Rectovaginal fistulas may be congenital or acquired through trauma, inflammatory bowel disease, irradiation, neoplasia, infection, or other rare causes. For those fistulas associated with a history of trauma, anal manometry and endoanal ultrasound can determine the severity of underlying sphincter and help guide surgical therapies.[58] Rectovaginal fistulas are classified as high or low depending on whether they can be corrected transabdominally or transperineally, respectively.

Surgical Repair

Rectovaginal fistulas need not be corrected immediately, and delay depends on the underlying disease, the size of the fistula, the presence of active inflammation, and the severity of the symptoms. Some fistulas may close spontaneously, whereas others, like those associated with inflammatory bowel disease, may heal with medical therapy alone. High rectovaginal fistulas require a transabdominal approach, whereas low rectovaginal fistulas can be approached transvaginally, transrectally, transperineally, trans-sphincterically, or transanally.

The most common surgical approaches to the low-lying fistula (typically a true anovaginal fistula) are the endorectal advancement flap, sphincteroplasty, and transperineal procedures.[59] An endorectal advancement flap consists of a flap raised of rectal mucosa and underlying internal sphincter that is advanced to cover the primary fistula's opening in the rectum or anus after the fistula's opening has been excised and the underlying muscle reapproximated. The flap is best suited for the first attempt at repair and/or in patients without evidence of an underlying sphincter defect and accordingly associated with a healing rate of 50%.[58] The transperineal repair completely excises the fistula tract and accomplishes a primary reapproximation of the internal, external, and levator muscles in discrete layers. Success rates are as high as 85% to 100% in patients with associated sphincter defects who have already failed other approaches.[59]

For high rectovaginal fistulas, a transabdominal approach is necessary. Whether a portion or the entire rectum is sacrificed depends on the nature and extent of the underlying disease. This approach involves mobilization of the rectovaginal septum, division of the fistula, and a layer closure of the rectal and vaginal defects. In some cases, no rectal resection is necessary, and a live pedicle of tissue may be interposed between the two anastomotic structures to supplement the repair. When rectal tissues are involved by severe irradiation changes, inflammatory bowel disease, or neoplasia, rectal excision is required. Whenever possible, the sphincter apparatus can be preserved using either a low anterior resection or coloanal anastomosis.[59] Whether the outcome of such procedures is favorable or not depends on the underlying disease, selection of patients, and experience and expertise of the surgeon.

In the setting of Crohn's disease, the low anovaginal fistula represents a unique challenge. Primary repair avoids the need for a permanent stoma and can be accomplished in up to 68% of patients using a variety of horizontal, linear, and sleeve advancement flaps.[60]

Condyloma Acuminatum

Condyloma acuminatum is a perineal wart disease caused by the human papillomavirus (HPV); some types are transmitted through sexual contact. Certain types, such as HPV-6 and HPV-11, are found in benign warts, whereas others, such as HPV-16 and HPV-18, are more aggressive and more commonly associated with dysplasia and malignancies. Its incidence has increased considerably since the mid-1960s, and it is the most common STD seen by colorectal surgeons, with a million new cases seen yearly. Most patients with anal condylomata have a history of anal-receptive intercourse, and the occurrence of anal HPV infection is strongly related to human immunodeficiency virus (HIV)-associated immunosuppression.[61]

Clinical Presentation

The usual symptoms include pruritus ani, bleeding, pain, discharge, and wetness. Examination reveals pinkish-

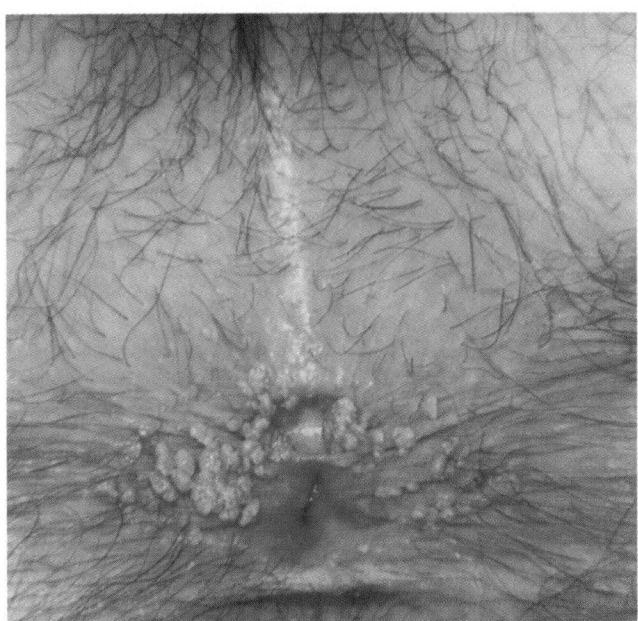

FIGURE 49-20. Perianal condyloma acuminatum. (By permission of Mayo Foundation.)

white warts of varying sizes that may coalesce to form a mass, often foul smelling (Fig. 49-20). Anoscopy may reveal extension in the anal canal. A giant form of the disease has been observed rarely (Buschke-Löwenstein disease). Such lesions can invade, fistulize, and be associated with verrucous carcinoma and squamous cell carcinomas. The diagnosis is based on direct inspection of the perineum and genital organs; anoscopy and proctosigmoidoscopy must be performed because the disease extends intra-anally and a small percentage of patients have only intra-anal disease. The diagnosis is confirmed histologically. Anal warts must be differentiated from condylomata molluscum contagiosum, secondary syphilis, and enlarged anal papillae.

Treatment

Many treatments have been proposed and used, but none offers complete resolution of the disease process. Podophyllin, which is cytotoxic to condylomata but irritating to normal skin, must be applied to the warts. Its use should be limited to minimal disease and extra-anal warts and not repeated because of local complications and potential systemic toxicity. It requires no anesthesia and is inexpensive, but the results are often disappointing. Dichloroacetic acid (bichloracetic acid) can be used to destroy both perianal and intra-anal warts, and it is less irritating than podophyllin. The recurrence rate with both agents is much higher than with surgical excision. Intramuscular or intralesional interferon-β is somewhat effective but may be complicated by systemic symptoms and an influenza-like syndrome.[62]

Electrocauterization with a needle tip is effective and used extensively, often in combination with excision. Local, regional, or general anesthesia is necessary. Carbon dioxide laser can also be effective but is more expensive

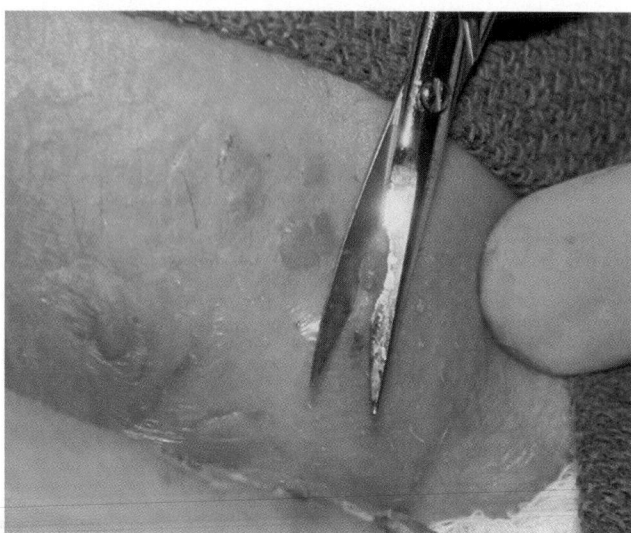

FIGURE 49-21.   Sharp excision of perianal condyloma is facilitated by the raising of the lesion by the injection of a local anesthetic agent. (By permission of Mayo Foundation.)

Box 49-2. Organisms that Cause Sexually Transmitted Diseases

Bacterial

Neisseria gonorrhoeae
Treponema pallidum
Haemophilus ducreyi
Chlamydia species
Shigella flexneri
Campylobacter species

Viral

Herpes simplex
Human papillomavirus
Molluscum contagiosum

Parasitic

Entamoeba histolytica
Giardia lamblia
Cryptococcus species
Isospora belli

and offers no added benefits. With either technique, vapors should be aspirated. Excision with small scissors is preferred because it is precise, provides a tissue diagnosis, minimizes destruction of intervening skin, and can be used on larger lesions (Fig. 49-21). General or regional anesthesia is necessary.

None of the therapeutic options is completely satisfactory; they all are associated with a significant chance of recurrence. Combination of treatments may be valuable. Because recurrence is frequent, close follow-up of patients is recommended.

Sexually Transmitted Diseases and AIDS

STDs, formerly referred to as *venereal diseases,* are exceeded in frequency only by the common cold and influenza. Multiple partners and anal-receptive intercourse increases the risk of STD transmission.[63] STDs can be bacterial, viral, or parasitic in origin (Box 49-2), and a variety of sexual practices may favor their development.

Clinical Presentation

Patients with bacterial STDs may have no symptoms or may have symptoms of pruritus, bloody or mucopurulent rectal discharge, tenesmus, perineal or rectal pain, diarrhea, and fever. Depending on the etiologic agent, proctoscopy may reveal proctitis, discharge (mucopurulent in gonorrhea or *Campylobacter* species infection, bloody in chlamydial infection), anal ulcerations, and abscesses.[64] The diagnosis is based on the clinical signs and physical examination, including endoscopy and cultures of stool or discharge specimens. Treatment is based on the causative agent.

Patients with *viral* STDs may complain of anorectal pain, discharge, bleeding, and pruritus. In molluscum contagiosum, the patient has painless dermal lesions that are flattened, round, and umbilicated.[64] Endoscopy may reveal

vesicles, ulcers, and diffuse friability as in herpes or anal warts in condylomata. The diagnosis is based on cultures, scrapings, or excisional biopsy. Herpes is best treated with acyclovir, whereas the other viral lesions are treated by destruction or excision.[63,64]

Patients with *parasitic* STDs have more systemic symptoms, such as fever, abdominal cramping, and bloody diarrhea. Ulcerations due to *Entamoeba histolytica* are typically hourglass shaped, whereas they are more diffuse when caused by *Giardia lamblia.* Diagnosis is based on biopsy specimens or scrapings and specific stains. *E. histolytica* and *G. lamblia* are treated with metronidazole, and *Isospora belli* is managed with cotrimoxazole.[64]

Acquired Immunodeficiency Syndrome

Anorectal pathology is common in patients who are HIV-positive, affecting about one third of patients at some point in their disease.[65] Anorectal pain, the presence of a mass, and bleeding per rectum are the most frequent presenting complaints.[65] In a consecutive series of 260 HIV-positive patients, the most frequently occurring diseases were condylomata (42%), fistulas (34%), and fissures (32%).[65] For benign noninfectious disorders, fissures and ulcers are the most common presenting problem. This is uniquely different from HIV-negative patients where the primary presenting diagnostics are hemorrhoids and skin tags.[66] In seeing patients with HIV, it is important to distinguish between anal fissures that are amenable to medical therapy and/or lateral internal sphincterotomy and anal ulcers that respond best to operative evaluation, biopsy, viral culture, débridement, and topical antiviral therapy.[66,67] Herpes, cytomegalovirus, and *Chlamydia* are the most typical infectious agents.[65]

Neoplastic disorders in HIV-positive patients include condyloma, anal intraepithelial neoplasia, epidermoid carcinoma, and Kaposi's sarcoma, the incidence of each of these being higher in HIV-positive than HIV-negative patients.[65,66,68] Although therapies for anal condyloma are no different based on HIV status, the recurrence rates seem to be higher for HIV-positive than HIV-negative patients. For the management of in situ and invasive squamous cell carcinoma, it appears that the CD4 count and concomitant treatment with antiretroviral therapy are keys to success with local excision and radiation/chemotherapy, respectively.

Best-practice strategies for anorectal conditions complicating HIV are likely to evolve as we acquire more effective therapies to treat HIV-infected patients.

Hidradenitis Suppurativa

Hidradenitis suppurativa is a chronic inflammatory process affecting the apocrine glands of the perianal region characterized by abscesses and sinus formation. Although recent dermatologic investigations call into question the site of origin of hidradenitis, implicating occluding spongiform infundibulofolliculitis, a follicular disease,[69] hidradenitis has traditionally been considered the result of keratotic debris plugging the apocrine gland. The plugging event is followed by bacterial proliferation, suppurative infection, gland rupture, and spread of inflammation to surrounding subcutaneous tissues. Numerous tracks and pits develop, and the tissues become fibrotic and thickened from the persistent inflammatory response. A number of factors have been implicated in the development and perpetuation of hidradenitis, including the use of depilatories, close shaving, poor personal hygiene, tight-fitting and synthetic clothing, and antiperspirants. The most common bacterial organisms identified include *Streptococcus milleri* and *Staphylococcus aureus, Staphylococcus epidermidis,* and *Staphylococcus hominis.*[70]

Clinical Presentation

Clinically, patients may complain of burning, itching, and hyperhidrosis. Affected patients frequently have seborrheic skin and sometimes have involvement of other areas where apocrine sweat glands are present, such as the axillae and the mammary, inguinal, and genital regions. The affected areas have a purplish appearance with drainage of watery pus. In advanced cases, numerous fistulous tracks are readily identified, and the appearance is classic (Fig. 49-22). When the condition presents early and there are limited fistulous tracks around the anal and perianal tissues, hidradenitis must be differentiated from other types of fistulas, such as those arising from Crohn's disease or infected crypts. Fistulas from hidradenitis arise distal to the dentate in the anal skin, allowing their differentiation from cryptoglandular fistulas, which communicate with the dentate line, and Crohn's disease, which may track to the anorectum proximal to the dentate line (Fig. 49-23).[71] Hidradenitis is more common in women and blacks; however, perianal hidradenitis is more common in men.

Treatment

Perianal hidradenitis can present in one of several states from early acute to late chronic and severe forms and can

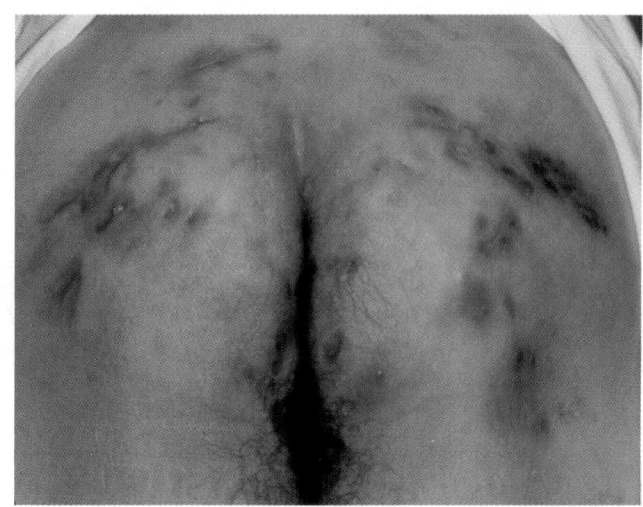

FIGURE 49-22. Hidradenitis suppurativa. (By permission of Mayo Foundation.)

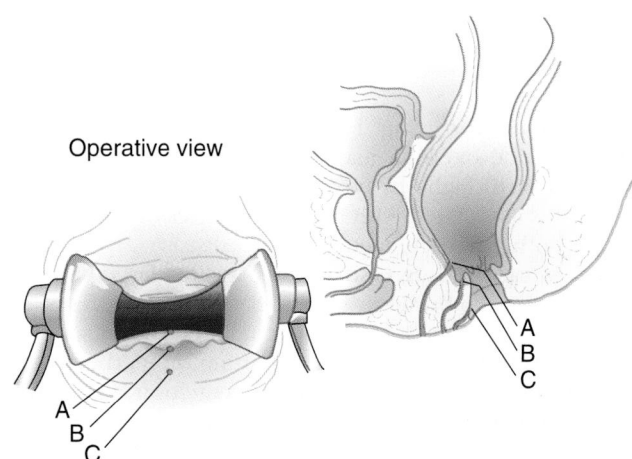

Operative view

FIGURE 49-23. Relationship of fistulous tracks in Crohn's disease, above dentate line (A); cryptoglandular abscess/fistula disease at dentate line (B); and hidradenitis suppurativa, distal to dentate line (C). (From Culp CE: Chronic hidradenitis suppurativa of the anal canal: A surgical skin disease. Dis Colon Rectum 26:669-676, 1983.)

present alone or with associated complications, such as severe anal fibrosis and incontinence, or even copresentation with squamous malignancies.[70] To exclude the possibility of coexisting cancer, biopsies should be performed with liberal indications. For early, limited disease, emphasis should be placed on incision and drainage of infections and prevention of recurrences. The role of oral antibiotic treatment, typically erythromycin, is not established but often recommended. Although not proved, frequent cleansing and warm-water soaking, avoidance of tight-fitting and synthetic clothing, and avoidance of local chemical irritants may help prevent further disease or may reduce the severity of active disease.

When hidradenitis sinus tracks are well established but relatively superficial, they can be unroofed, or laid open.[71] Because these tracks are lined by epithelium, the floor of the track can be preserved; this facilitates rapid healing

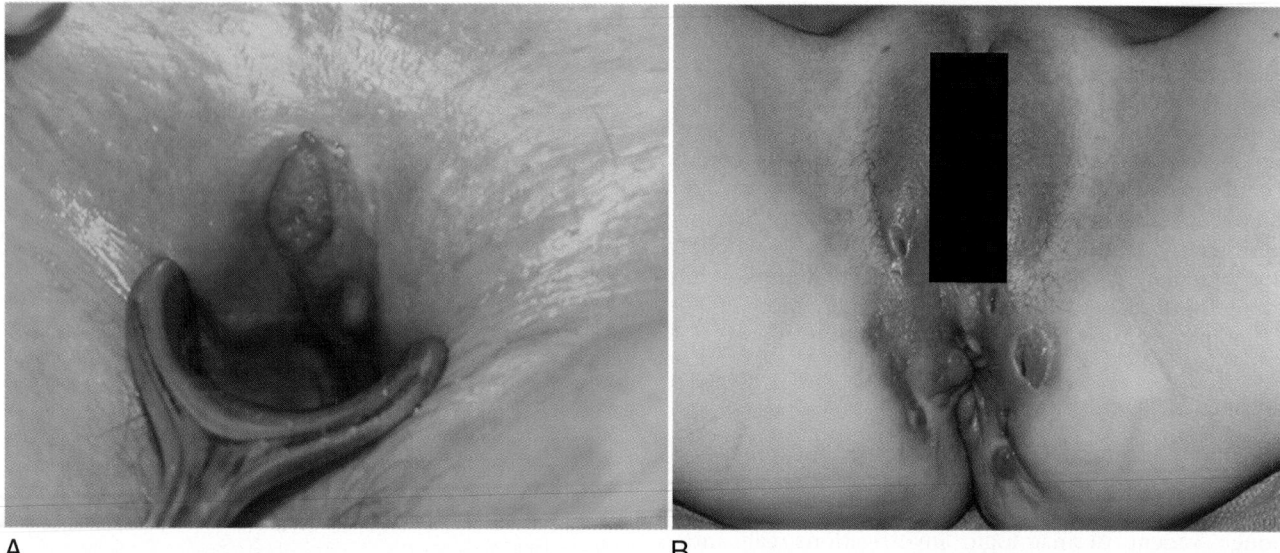

A   B

FIGURE 49-24.   Perineal Crohn's disease. **A,** Characteristic of Crohn's fissures are the shaggy edges, deep ulceration, and granulation tissue. **B,** Uncontrolled perianal Crohn's with multiple fistulas can present as a "watering pot" perineum. (**A** and **B,** By permission of Mayo Foundation.)

and minimizes scarring. For more extensive and deeper disease, wide excision may be required. Although wide excision is thought to be more effective for advanced cases, it is associated with recurrence rates of about 50%, when both same-site and new-site disease are considered.[72] In cases of aggressive wide excision, large wounds can be managed primarily, with delayed healing, flaps, or skin grafts. Wound closure can be tailored to the specific conditions of each patient. Skin grafting offers the advantage of early wound coverage with a reduction in pain and time to complete healing but requires compliance with delicate postoperative wound care. Healing by secondary intention requires less delicate wound care but takes 2 to 3 months for complete healing to be accomplished.[70]

Crohn's Disease of the Anorectum

Clinical Presentation

Anal manifestations of Crohn's disease can be most devastating because of their painful nature and their threat to the patient's continence,[73] and they occur in nearly 20% of patients with Crohn's disease. Patients may suffer from fissures, fistulas, and abscesses. Symptoms and signs of anal Crohn's disease may include pain, swelling, bleeding, soilage or frank incontinence, and fever. Pain may be due to skin excoriation and maceration, hemorrhoids, fissures, or abscess and fistula disease (Fig. 49-24).[73] Edematous, purplish tags are characteristic of the disease. Bleeding may be from distal proctitis, fissures, hemorrhoids, or granulating fistulas. Soilage may result from prolapsing rectal mucosa, seepage of liquid stool, drainage from abscess, or poor continence. Poor continence may result from sphincter damage caused by the disease or aggressive surgery, anoperineal fistulas, rectovaginal fistulas, or loss of rectal compliance.[73]

Evaluation and Treatment

Anorectal examination should include inspection, digital examination, anoscopy, and proctosigmoidoscopy. If the examination cannot be performed satisfactorily because of pain, the patient should be evaluated under anesthesia. The remainder of the gastrointestinal tract should also be assessed. Although conservatism is paramount in importance, patients should not be undertreated if treatment is indicated. Surgery is usually warranted for pain resulting from a poorly draining or undrained abscess. Fissures caused by Crohn's disease are often multiple and located off the midline; they usually respond to conservative measures, such as sitz baths, stool softeners, and oral analgesics. Occasionally, excision of skin tags surrounding deep ulcers to favor better drainage and gentle stretch may be sufficient. Sphincterotomy and fissurectomy should be avoided when perianal Crohn's disease is present. Metronidazole and immunosuppressive drugs, such as steroids, 6-mercaptopurine, azathioprine (Imuran), and cyclosporine have produced mixed results.[73] In some patients, a proctectomy may ultimately be required. The dissection should be done in the intersphincteric plane to favor better perineal healing and help reduce the risk for sexual dysfunction.

Fistulas represent a special challenge in Crohn's disease (Fig 49-25).[74] For patients with superficial fistulas and no active rectal disease, a primary fistulotomy may be indicated. For those patients who have more complex fistulas or who have active proctitis, a combination of surgical management with noncutting setons and medical management is most appropriate. Proctectomy or other definitive surgeries are preserved for those who fail other forms of therapy.

It is now increasingly recognized that patients with Crohn's disease can also present with common anorectal conditions such as fissures, abscesses, and fistulas. In the

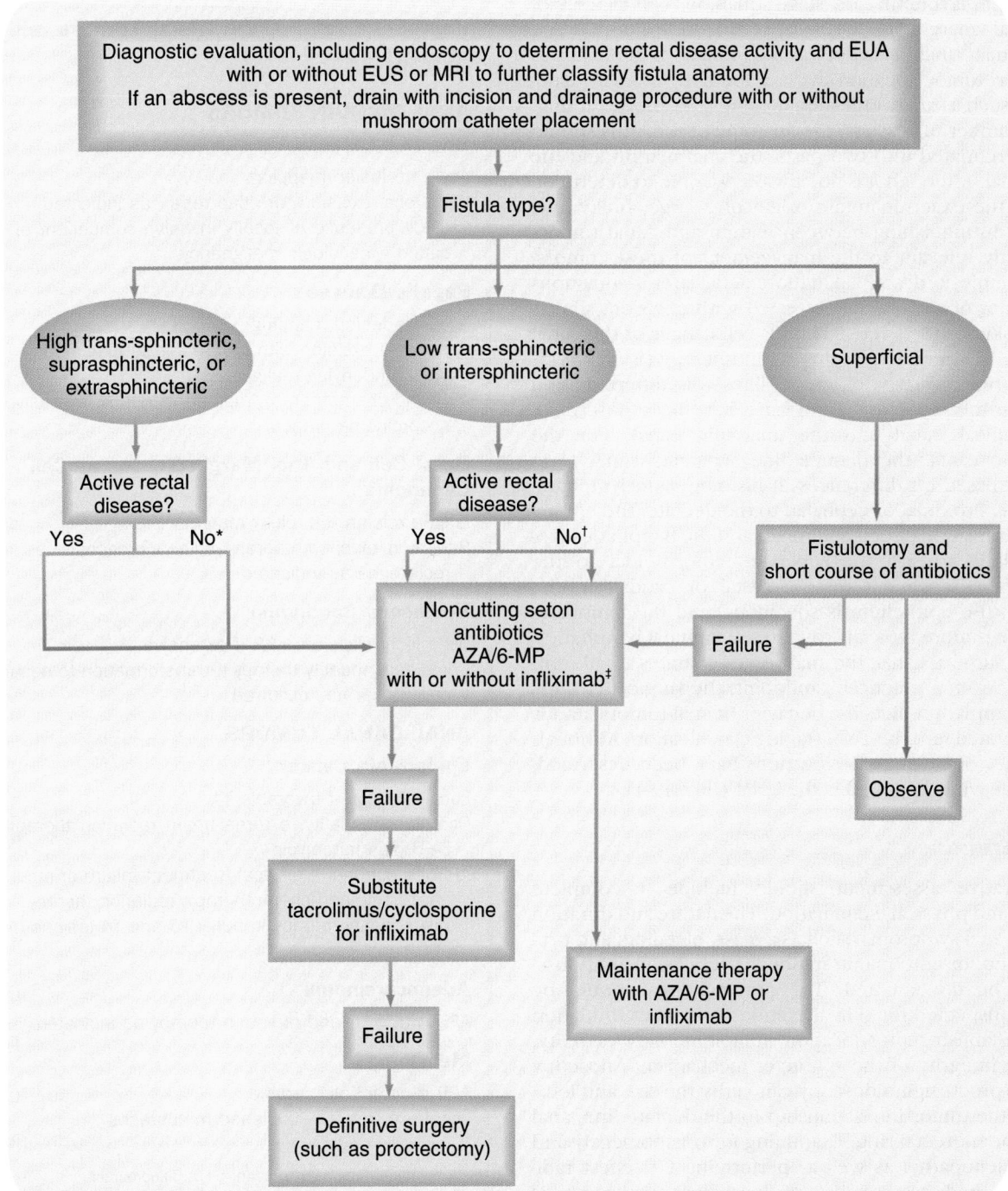

FIGURE 49-25.   Treatment algorithm for perianal Crohn's disease. If the fistula is simple, endorectal advancement flap (*asterisk*) or fistulotomy (*dagger*) can be considered. Use of infliximab should be favored if the fistula is complex, recurrent, or associated with active rectal inflammation (*double dagger*). 6-MP, 6-mercaptopurine; AZA, azathioprine; EUS, endoscopic ultrasonography; MRI, magnetic resonance imaging. (From Schwartz DA, Pemberton JH, Sandborn WJ: Diagnosis and treatment of perianal fistulas in Crohn disease. Ann Intern Med 135:906-918, 2001.)

absence of evidence of rectal or perianal Crohn's, these conditions may be best treated using standard approaches. Although caution is advised against aggressive approaches when treating a Crohn's patient with anorectal problems, undertreatment of symptomatic conditions is also discouraged.

NEOPLASTIC DISORDERS

Neoplasms of the anal area are rare and represent a wide spectrum of benign and malignant tumors. Benign lesions may range from innocuous in situ Bowen's disease to clinically aggressive verrucous lesions; malignant lesions range from favorable early-stage squamous cell cancers of the anal margin to anal canal adenocarcinoma and melanoma.[75] In all instances, it is essential for clinicians to consider tumor location with reference to clear landmarks, such as anal verge, dentate line, and anorectal ring. For a number of reasons, the anatomy of the anus should be differentiated into two parts: the anal margin and the anal canal. Although it is not always possible to determine readily the exact anatomic origin of a large, bulky anal tumor, distinguishing between margin and canal tumors is directly relevant to the management of these tumors. For example, as described in more detail later, a squamous cell tumor of the margin is treated with excision, similar to any skin cancer, yet squamous cell cancer of the canal is treated with radiation plus chemotherapy (Box 49-3).[76]

Historically, two different lines of differentiation between the anal margin and canal have been described: the surgical canal and the anatomic canal. For the anatomic canal, the dentate line separates canal from margin, based on differences in histology and lymphatic drainage. Proximal or cephalad to the dentate, the epithelium is transitional then columnar, and the lymphatics typically drain toward the superior hemorrhoidal to the inferior hemorrhoidal vessels. Distal or caudad to the dentate, the epithelium is squamous, and the lymphatic drainage is more typically toward the inguinal lymphatics. For the surgical canal, the anal verge separates canal from margin. From a practical standpoint, the surgical canal is easy to apply, predicts the behavior of anal tumors, and is incorporated into the TNM staging classification. Although a number of staging classifications have been described, the most widely applied is the TNM (Box 49-4).

Clinical Evaluations

Preoperative assessment should include a complete history and physical examination. The nature and duration of local anal symptoms, such as a mass, bleeding, and pruritus, and distant manifestations, such as weight loss, should be documented. The perianal area should be closely inspected for skin alterations. Digital examination helps establish tumor location, tumor mobility or fixity, and the integrity of the sphincter mechanism. Anoscopy or rigid proctosigmoidoscopy can verify the size and location of the tumor in relationship to the dentate line, anal verge, or anorectal ring. Examining for organomegaly and groin adenopathy, as well as performing CT, chest radiography, and assessments of localizing symptoms, is important when evaluating a malignant lesion.

Anal Margin Tumors

Bowen's Disease

Bowen's disease is an in situ intraepithelial squamous cell carcinoma that rarely (5%) invades or metastasizes.[75] Most patients have no symptoms or have minor complaints, such as burning or pruritus. The perianal skin may be erythematous and thickened with fissuring, brown-red plaques or nodules, or it may be inapparent. Because the appearance of Bowen's disease can be highly variable (Fig.

> **Box 49-3. Summary of Anal Tumors and Management**
>
> **ANAL MARGIN TUMORS**
>
> **Bowen's Disease**
>
> Accurate lesion mapping
> Wide local excision with flap repair as indicated
> Exclude presence of locally invasive component or associated gynecologic malignancy
>
> **Paget's Disease**
>
> Accurate lesion mapping
> Wide local excision with flap repair as indicated
> Exclude underlying malignancy
> APR and chemotherapy/radiation therapy if invasive adenocarcinoma present
>
> **Basal Cell and Anal Margin Squamous Cell Carcinoma**
>
> Local excision with clear margins
> Radiation or chemotherapy in poor-prognosis lesions or recurrence as indicated
>
> **Verrucous Carcinoma**
>
> Wide local excision; APR if extensive
> Combined-modality therapy if transformation to squamous cell cancer has occurred
>
> **ANAL CANAL TUMORS**
>
> **Epidermoid Cancer**
>
> Local excision if favorable T1
> Combined-modality, external-beam radiation therapy plus 5-FU plus mitomycin
> APR if incontinent, or local treatment failure or recurrence after combined chemotherapy/radiation therapy
> Triple-modality therapy in bulky T3 and T4 lesions (role of APR controversial)
>
> **Adenocarcinoma**
>
> APR with 5-FU and radiation therapy as indicated
>
> **Melanoma**
>
> APR if potentially curable
> Local excision if established metastases

APR, abdominal perineal resection; 5-FU, 5-fluorouracil.
Adapted from McMurrick PJ, Nelson H, Goldberg RM, Haddock MG: Cancer of the anal canal. *In* Torosian MH (ed): Integrated Cancer Management. New York, Marcel Dekker, 1999, p 200.

49-26) and even subtle, the differential diagnosis is extensive for a number of dermatologic disorders, including psoriasis, eczema, and leukoplakia, as well as for infections such as monilial infections. Multiple punch biopsies can establish the diagnosis. The concept that Bowen's disease is frequently associated with internal malignancies justifying extensive diagnostic investigations has been challenged and refuted. Having said this, there is evidence

Box 49-4. TNM Staging Classifications for Anal Malignancies

Primary Tumor (T)

Tx   Primary tumor cannot be assessed
T0   No evidence of primary tumor
Tis   Carcinoma in situ
T1   Tumor < 2.0 cm in greatest dimension
T2   Tumor > 2.0 cm but not > 5.0 cm
T3   Tumor > 5.0 cm
T4   Tumor of any size that invades adjacent organ(s)

Regional Lymph Nodes (N)

Nx   Regional lymph nodes cannot be assessed
N0   No regional lymph node metastasis
N1   Metastasis in perirectal lymph node(s)
N2   Metastasis in unilateral internal iliac and/or inguinal lymph node(s)
N3   Metastasis in perirectal and inguinal lymph nodes and/or bilateral internal iliac and/or inguinal lymph nodes

Distant Metastasis (M)

Mx   Distant metastasis cannot be assessed
M0   No distant metastasis
M1   Distant metastasis

Stage Grouping

Stage 0   Tis, N0, M0
Stage I   T1, N0, M0
Stage II   T2, N0, M0
             T3, N0, M0
Stage IIIA   T1, N1, M0
             T2, N1, M0
             T3, N1, M0
             T4, N0, M0
Stage IIIB   T4, N1, M0
             Any T, N2, M0
             Any T, N3, M0
Stage IV   Any T, any N, M1

From AJCC Cancer Staging Manual, 6th ed. New York, Springer-Verlag, 2002.

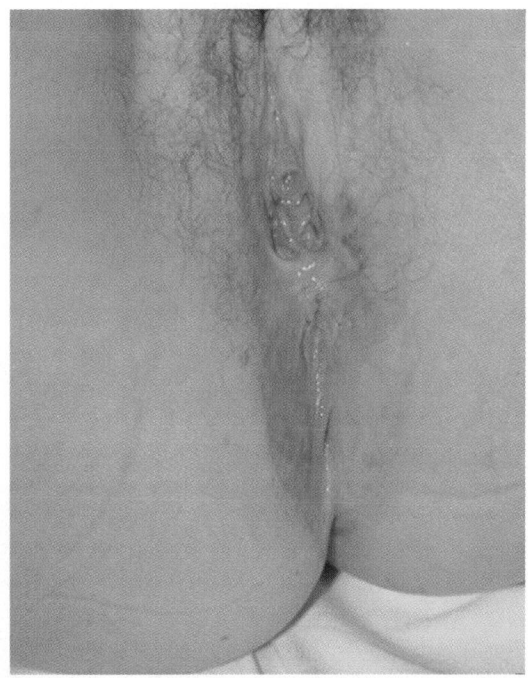

FIGURE 49-26. Bowen's disease. (By permission of Mayo Foundation.)

that women should be evaluated for concomitant genital disorders.

In the absence of an underlying invasive component, the disease can be cured by wide and full-thickness excision of all the affected skin. The extent of the lateral spread of the lesion can be determined by obtaining multiple "mapping" biopsy specimens or by confirming clear surgical margins using intraoperative frozen sections. The resulting defects are often of sufficient size to require wound closure with other than primary approximation; V-Y advancement flaps work well for most defects (Fig. 49-27). Patients who have invasion of the sphincter should be considered for abdominal perineal resection (APR).

Postoperative follow-up is imperative to detect recurrent disease or development of invasive disease.

Paget's Disease

Extramammary Paget's disease of the anus is a rare intraepithelial adenocarcinoma. The presence of intraepithelial adenocarcinoma in an area of squamous epithelium has led to speculation about the origin of Paget's cells. A number of concepts have been proposed, including the possibility that they are derived from pleuripotent epidermal stem cells, arise from apocrine or sweat glands, or are metastatic from underlying adenocarcinomas. Unlike Bowen's disease, Paget's disease is more common in older patients, associated with an underlying carcinoma in 50% to 86% of patients and has a poor prognosis.[75] The typical appearance of Paget's disease is that of well-demarcated eczematoid plaque with whitish-gray ulcerations or papillary lesions (Fig. 49-28).[75] As is true for Bowen's disease, Paget's disease can have a variable and at times subtle appearance and can be confused with other dermatologic conditions, such as hyperkeratosis, eczema, or lichen sclerosus et atrophicus. Histology demonstrates the presence of periodic acid–Schiff–positive Paget's cells, confirming the diagnosis. Treatment is based on the local extent of the disease and on the presence or absence of underlying malignancies. More limited Paget's disease can be widely excised and the defect closed primarily or with V-Y advancement flaps. Biopsies of the proximal anal canal and distal anal skin margins can help map the extent of resection.[75] Patients with underlying rectal adenocarcinoma should undergo APR, whereas those with epider-

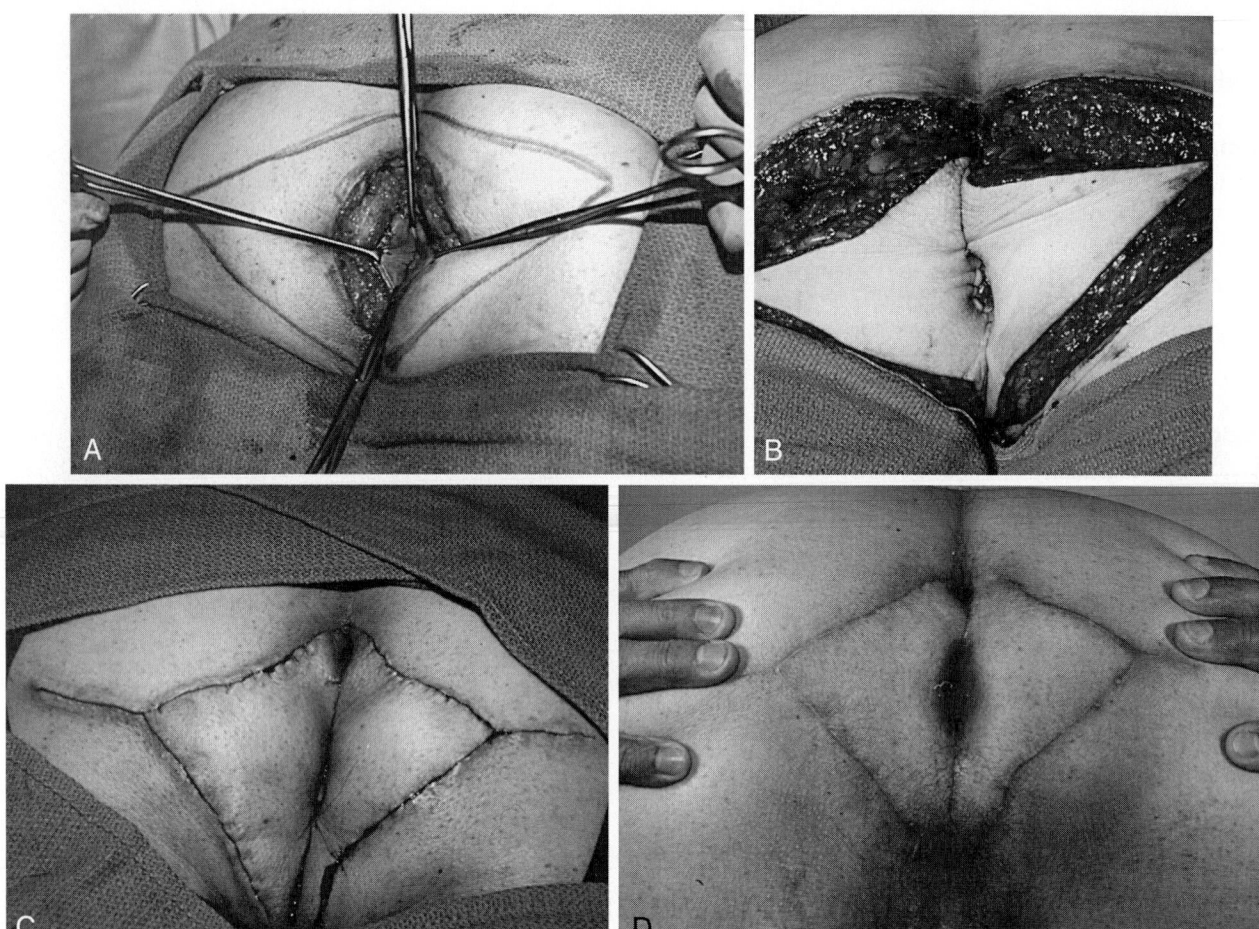

FIGURE 49-27. V-Y advancement flap for perianal Bowen's disease. **A,** Circumferential excision is performed with wide margins, histologically negative for Bowen's disease. The residual defect will be closed by advancing surrounding V-shaped islands of skin and underlying tissue. The Allis clamps expose the anal canal. **B,** The V-shaped flaps are advanced and anastomosed to the residual anal canal at the dentate line. **C,** Closure of the flap wounds converts the V-shaped wounds to Y-shaped suture lines. **D,** Six months after surgery, the perianal scars are soft, compliant, and without stenosis. The patient has normal sphincter tone and a good functional outcome. (**A** to **D,** From Nelson H, Dozois RR: Anal neoplasms. Persp Colon Rectal Surg 7:22, 1994.)

moid anal canal cancer can be treated with combined radiation and chemotherapy.[77] For patients with an invasive component, treated with radical therapy, the 5-year crude survival rate is only 54%.[78] After surgery, patients should be monitored closely for recurrence.

Basal Cell Carcinoma

Basal cell carcinoma is a rare type of anal canal tumor. Macroscopically, these lesions have the same pearly borders with central depression that other basal cell cancers of the skin have (Fig. 49-29). On occasion, it may be difficult to differentiate a cloacogenic (or basaloid) carcinoma arising in the transitional zone from a basal cell cancer arising in the anal skin. The distinction is crucial because of the dramatic behavioral difference and is based on location as well as histologic features.[75] Most often, these tumors can be treated adequately by wide local excision, reserving APR for extensive lesions.[75] Because nearly one third of patients experience recurrence, close follow-up is indicated.

Squamous Cell Carcinoma

Although the oncologic behavior of squamous cell carcinoma resembles that of skin tumors elsewhere, the location of these lesions results in site-specific symptoms, such as a mass, chronic pruritus, bleeding, pain, and associated fistulas and condylomata.[75] Wide local excision is recommended for early anal margin squamous cell carcinoma with excellent results. Recurrences may be managed by re-excision or by APR, especially if locally advanced. Lymphadenectomy is indicated for those rare patients (<10%) presenting with evidence of regional lymph node metastases.

Verrucous Carcinoma

Verrucous carcinoma, also referred to as *giant condyloma acuminatum* or *Buschke-Löwenstein tumors* are poorly defined and best considered as intermediate lesions between condyloma acuminatum and invasive squamous cell carcinomas based on their common HPV etiology.[75]

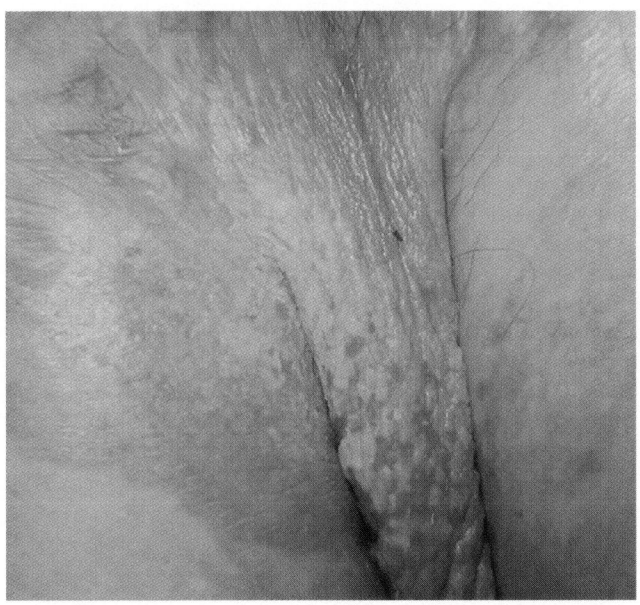

FIGURE 49-28. Paget's disease. (By permission of Mayo Foundation.)

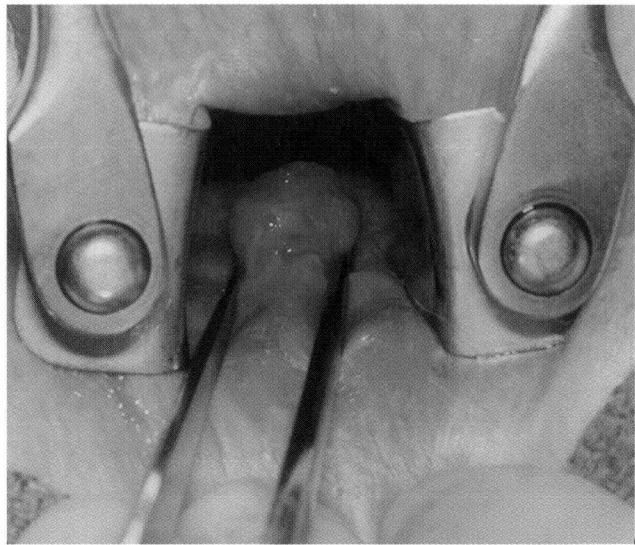

FIGURE 49-30. Squamous cell carcinoma of anal canal. (By permission of Mayo Foundation.)

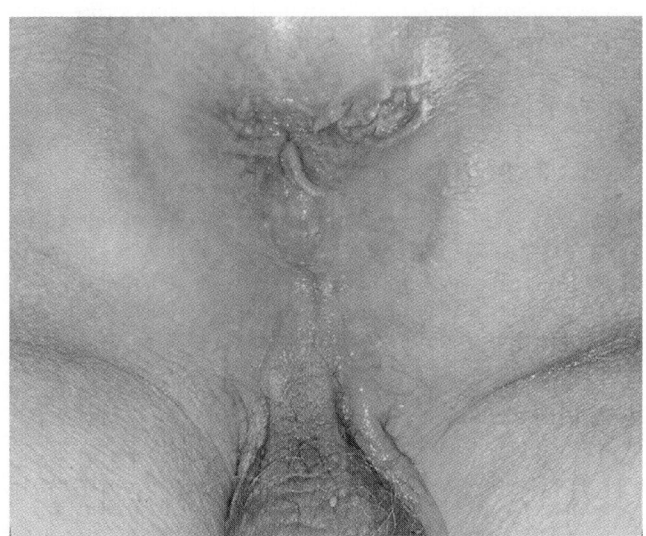

FIGURE 49-29. Basal cell carcinoma of anal margin. (By permission of Mayo Foundation.)

The large, wartlike lesions are soft and slow growing. They may fistulize, become infected, and undergo malignant transformation.[75] Radical wide local excision or APR is recommended. A poor prognosis can be expected for tumors progressing to invasive squamous cell carcinoma, although some may respond favorably to combined irradiation and chemotherapy.

Anal Canal Neoplasms

Epidermoid Carcinoma

Tumors arising in the anal canal or in the transitional zone that have a squamous, basaloid, cloacogenic, or mucoepidermoid epithelium share a similar behavior in clinical presentation, response to treatment, and prognosis[75] and are considered collectively. They typically present as a mass, sometimes with bleeding and pruritus (Fig. 49-30). At the time of diagnosis, nearly one fourth of these are superficial or in situ; half are less than 3 cm in size, and the other half are larger.[75] About 71% have deep tumor penetration; 25% are node positive, and 6% present with distant metastases.

In the past, treatment modalities have included either surgery alone or radiation therapy alone. Patients with tumors confined to epithelial or subepithelial tissue have been treated by local excision and patients with more advanced lesions by APR.[79] The introduction of multimodality therapy combining irradiation and chemotherapy promised to preserve continence, avoid colostomy, and offer similar survival advantage. In keeping with this concept, local excision alone remains an option for superficial, early-stage lesions, which have been associated with variable survivorship (61% to 87%; 100% in at least one study[79]) if the lesion was smaller than 2 cm. Although some small superficial lesions can be treated with local excision, most patients are best treated with combined chemotherapy and irradiation.

Combined-modality therapy has evolved as the preferred alternative to radical surgery because, in theory, surgical mortality and morbidity are largely avoided, intestinal continuity is preserved, and survival compares favorably with that after surgery. Nigro and colleagues[77] were the first to promote radiation therapy plus chemotherapy as definitive treatment for epidermoid anal canal malignancies. The current "Nigro protocol" includes external-beam radiation therapy to the pelvic tumor and pelvic and inguinal nodes, to a total dose of 3000 cGy starting on day 1 using 15 fractions (200 cGy/day).[77] Systemic chemotherapy includes 5-fluorouracil (5-FU), 1000 mg/m^2 for 24 hours as continuous infusion for 4 days, commencing on day 1 and again on day 28 (two cycles total). Mitomycin

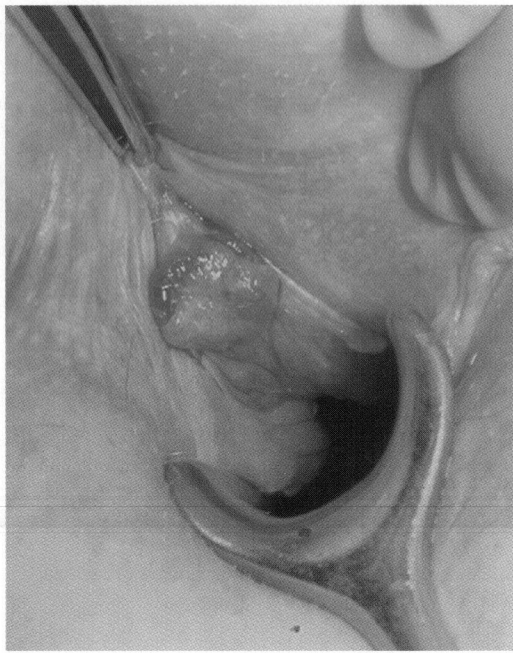

FIGURE 49-31. Anal canal amelanotic melanoma. (By permission of Mayo Foundation.)

C is delivered as an intravenous bolus at 15 mg/m² starting on day 1 only. Many institutions have modified the pelvic radiation doses, approximating the doses typically delivered in rectal cancer. Although some reports have described comparable results using radiation therapy alone, current studies support the continued use of 5-FU and mitomycin C.[80] Although radiation plus chemotherapy has largely replaced the need for APR in anal canal cancers, there remain subsets of patients in whom abdominoperineal resection may be considered appropriate as either single-modality or combined-modality therapy. Such groups would include patients who are already in need of a stoma for fecal incontinence, those for whom chemotherapy or radiation therapy is contraindicated, and those whose disease fails to resolve completely after radiation therapy plus chemotherapy.

Melanoma

Melanoma involving the anal canal can produce a mass, pain, or bleeding and is not infrequently amelanotic (Fig. 49-31). Overall, the outlook of patients with such tumors is poor, with a 5-year survival rate hovering around 10% to, at most, 26%.[81,82] The survivorship, however, depends on the stage of the disease. In general, survival is poor whether the surgery is conservative or radical. APR appears reasonable for advanced lesions if complete resection and palliation are to be achieved. Recent results of local excision and APR seem comparable. Some centers describe better survival for APR and others show no difference; it remains a controversial subject.[81-83] Prophylactic inguinal node dissection offers no benefit.

Adenocarcinoma

True adenocarcinomas of the anal canal are extremely rare. They originate from anal ducts and are often extramucosal in location. Because of their rarity, their diagnosis is frequently delayed. Like melanoma, the tumor is occasionally found incidentally during hemorrhoidectomy. Whether the tumor is locally excised or widely removed by APR, the prognosis is poor.[75] Because it is conceivable that some adenocarcinomas arise in the rectum but appear as in anal adenocarcinomas, it is appealing to give benefit of the doubt and treat these cases as a primary rectal cancer with trimodality therapy, that is, surgery plus irradiation plus chemotherapy. This not only provides appropriate therapy for a misdiagnosed rectal primary but also may improve results for primary anal adenocarcinomas, which are otherwise associated with universally fatal outcomes.

Other Tumors

Connective tissue sarcomas, such as leiomyosarcoma, rhabdomyosarcoma, and myoblastoma, are rare in the anal canal. Lymphoma of the anus is unusual. Carcinoid tumors can occasionally originate from anal canal endocrine cells, and APR may be required, especially for those exceeding 2 cm in size.

Selected References

Hulme-Moir M, Bartolo DC: Hemorrhoids. Gastroenterol Clin North Am 30:183-197, 2001.

> **This article provides a well-referenced, comprehensive review of the classification, etiology, anatomy, diagnosis, and treatment of hemorrhoids.**

McMurrick PJ, Nelson H, Goldberg RM, Haddock MG: Cancer of the anal canal. *In* Torosian MH (ed): Integrated Cancer Management. New York, Marcel Dekker, 1999, pp 195-205.

> **The multidisciplinary authorship of this publication uniquely offers an in-depth description of current practices in the management of anal cancer.**

Nicholls RJ, Dozois RR (eds): Surgery of the Colon and Rectum. New York, Churchill Livingstone, 1997.

> **This well-illustrated compendium of commonly performed colorectal and anal procedures is clearly written and comprehensive.**

Parks AG, Gordon PH, Hardcastle JD: A classification of fistula-in-ano. Br J Surg 63:1-12, 1976.

> **A classic description of anorectal suppurative disease, this article includes the acute phase (abscesses) and chronic phase (fistulas). The anatomic descriptions, data, and classification schema are still relevant today.**

Whitehead WE, Wald A, Norton NJ: Treatment options for fecal incontinence. Dis Colon Rectum 44:131-144, 2001.

> **This article represents a summary review of a Consensus Conference on Treatment Options in Fecal Incontinence.**

References

1. Fozard JBJ, Pemberton JH: Applied surgical anatomy: Pelvic contents. *In* Fielding LP, Goldberg SM (eds): Rob and Smith's Operative Surgery: Surgery of the Colon, Rectum, and Anus, 5th ed. London, Chapman & Hall Medical, 1994, pp 11-23.

2. Nivatvongs S, Gordon PH: Surgical anatomy. *In* Gordon PH, Nivatvongs S (eds): Principles and Practice of Surgery for the Colon, Rectum, and Anus. St. Louis, Quality Medical, 1992, pp 3-37.

3. Ambroze WL, Pemberton JH, Dozois RR, et al: Does retaining the anal transition zone (ATZ) fail to extirpate chronic ulcerative colitis (CUC) after ileal-pouch anal anastomosis (IPAA)? Dis Colon Rectum 34:P20, 1991.

4. Kerremans R: Morphological and Physiological Aspects of Anal Continence and Defecation. Brussels, Arscia, Ultgavon, 1969.

5. Lee SJ, Meagher A, Pemberton JH: Structure and function of the lower gastrointestinal tract. *In* Saclarides T, Brubaker L (eds): The Female Pelvic Floor—Disorders of Function and Support. Philadelphia, FA Davis, 1996, pp 22-32.

6. Ferrara A, Pemberton JH, Levin KE, et al: Relationship between anal canal tone and rectal motor activity. Dis Colon Rectum 36:337-342, 1993.

7. Parks AG: Royal Society of Medicine, Section of Proctology; Meeting 27 November 1974. President's Address. Anorectal incontinence. Proc R Soc Med 68:681-690, 1975.

8. Bartolo DCC, Roe AM, Locke-Edmunds JC, et al: Flap-valve theory of anorectal continence. Br J Surg 73:1012-1014, 1986.

9. Beart RW Jr, Dozois RR, Wolff BG, et al: Mechanisms of rectal continence: Lessons from the ileoanal procedure. Am J Surg 149:31-34, 1985.

10. Sagar PM, Pemberton JH: Anorectal and pelvic floor function: Relevance of continence, incontinence, and constipation. Gastroenterol Clin North Am 25:163-182, 1996.

11. Zetterström J, López A, Anzén B, et al: Anal sphincter tears at vaginal delivery: Risk factors and clinical outcome of primary repair. Obstet Gynecol 94:21-28, 1999.

12. Whitehead WE, Wald A, Norton NJ: Treatment options for fecal incontinence. Dis Colon Rectum 44:131-144, 2001.

13. Rudolph W, Galandiuk S: A practical guide to the diagnosis and management of fecal incontinence. Mayo Clin Proc 77:271-275, 2002.

14. Gilliland R, Altomare DF, Moreira H Jr, et al: Pudendal neuropathy is predictive of failure following anterior overlapping sphincteroplasty. Dis Colon Rectum 41:1516-1522, 1998.

15. Gordon PH: Anal incontinence. *In* Gordon PH, Nivatvongs S (eds): Principles and Practice of Surgery for the Colon, Rectum, and Anus. St. Louis, Quality Medical, 1992, pp 337-359.

16. Matsuoka H, Mavrantonis C, Wexner SD, et al: Postanal repair for fecal incontinence—is it worthwhile? Dis Colon Rectum 43:1561-1567, 2000.

17. Malouf AJ, Vaizey CJ, Nicholls RJ, et al: Permanent sacral nerve stimulation for fecal incontinence. Ann Surg 232:143-148, 2000.

18. Farouk R, Duthie GS: Rectal prolapse and rectal invagination. Eur J Surg 164:323-332, 1998.

19. Theuerkauf FJ Jr, Beahrs OH, Hill JR: Rectal prolapse: Causation and surgical treatment. Ann Surg 171:819-835, 1970.

20. Huber FT, Stein H, Siewert JR: Functional results after treatment of rectal prolapse with rectopexy and sigmoid resection. World J Surg 19:138-143, 1995.

21. Aitola PT, Hiltunen KM, Matikainen MJ: Functional results of operative treatment of rectal prolapse over an 11-year period: Emphasis on transabdominal approach. Dis Colon Rectum 42:655-660, 1999.

22. Birnbaum EH, Stamm L, Rafferty JF, et al: Pudendal nerve terminal motor latency influences surgical outcome in treatment of rectal prolapse. Dis Colon Rectum 39:1215-1221, 1996.

23. Kimmins MH, Evetts BK, Isler J, et al: The Altemeier repair: Outpatient treatment of rectal prolapse. Dis Colon Rectum 44:565-570, 2001.

24. Lechaux JP, Lechaux D, Perez M: Results of Delorme's procedure for rectal prolapse: Advantages of a modified technique. Dis Colon Rectum 38:301-307, 1995.

25. Kim DS, Tsang CBS, Wong WD, et al: Complete rectal prolapse: Evolution of management and results. Dis Colon Rectum 42:460-469, 1999.

26. Bachoo P, Brazzelli M, Grant A: Surgery for complete rectal prolapse in adults. Cochrane Database of Systematic Reviews, Issue 4, 2002.

27. Hämäläinen K-PJ, Raivio P, Antila S, et al: Biofeedback therapy in rectal prolapse patients. Dis Colon Rectum 39:262-265, 1996.

28. Stevenson ARL, Stitz RW, Lumley JW: Laparoscopic-assisted resection-rectopexy for rectal prolapse: Early and medium follow-up. Dis Colon Rectum 41:46-54, 1998.

29. Goh JT, Tjandra JJ, Carey MP: How could management of rectoceles be optimized? ANZ J Surg 72:896-901, 2002.

30. Mimura T, Roy AJ, Storrie JB, et al: Treatment of impaired defecation associated with rectocele by behavorial retraining (biofeedback). Dis Colon Rectum 43:1267-1272, 2000.

31. Van Laarhoven CJ, Kamm MA, Bartram CI, et al: Relationship between anatomic and symptomatic long-term results after rectocele repair for impaired defecation. Dis Colon Rectum 42:204-211, 1999.

32. Karlbom U, Graf W, Nilsson S, et al: Does surgical repair of a rectocele improve rectal emptying? Dis Colon Rectum 39:1296-1302, 1996.

33. Tjandra JJ, Ooi BS, Tang CL, et al: Transanal repair of rectocele corrects obstructed defecation if it is not associated with anismus. Dis Colon Rectum 42:1544-1550, 1999.

34. Hulme-Moir M, Bartolo DC: Hemorrhoids. Gastroenterol Clin North Am 30:183-197, 2001.

35. Perez-Miranda M, Gomez-Cedenilla A, León-Colombo T, et al: Effect of fiber supplements on internal bleeding hemorrhoids. Hepatogastroenterology 43:1504-1507, 1996.

36. MacRae HM, McLeod RS: Comparison of hemorrhoidal treatments: A meta-analysis. Can J Surg 40:14-17, 1997.

37. Shemesh EI, Kodner IJ, Fry RD, et al: Severe complication of rubber band ligation of internal hemorrhoids. Dis Colon Rectum 30:199-200, 1987.

38. Bayer I, Myslovaty B, Picovsky BM: Rubber band ligation of hemorrhoids: Convenient and economic treatment. J Clin Gastroenterol 23:50-52, 1996.

39. Armstrong DN, Ambroze WL, Schertzer ME, et al: Harmonic scalpel versus electrocautery hemorrhoidectomy: A prospective evaluation. Dis Colon Rectum 44:558-564, 2001.

40. Gencosmanoglu R, Sad O, Koc D, et al: Hemorrhoidectomy: Open or closed technique? A prospective, randomized clinical trial. Dis Colon Rectum 45:70-75, 2002.

41. Singer MA, Cintron JR, Fleshman JW, et al: Early experience with stapled hemorrhoidectomy in the United States. Dis Colon Rectum 45:360-369, 2002.

42. Gibbons CP, Read NW: Anal hypertonia in fissures: Cause or effect? Br J Surg 73:443-445, 1986.

43. Lund JN, Binch C, McGrath J, et al: Topographical distribution of blood supply to the anal canal. Br J Surg 86:496-498, 1999.

44. Jensen SL: Treatment of first episodes of acute anal fissure: Prospective randomised study of lignocaine ointment versus hydrocortisone ointment or warm sitz baths plus bran. BMJ 292:1167-1169, 1986.

45. Kocher HM, Steward M, Leather AJ, et al: Randomized clinical trial assessing the side effects of glyceryl trinitrate and diltiazem hydrochloride in the treatment of chronic anal fissure. Br J Surg 89:413-417, 2002.

46. Lund JN, Scholefield JH: A randomised, prospective, double-blind, placebo-controlled trial of glyceryl trinitrate ointment in treatment of anal fissure. Lancet 349:11-14, 1997.

47. Minguez M, Herreros B, Espi A, et al: Long-term follow-up (42 months) of chronic anal fissure after healing with botulinum toxin. Gastroenterology 123:112-117, 2002.

48. Lewis TH, Corman ML, Prager ED, et al: Long-term results of open and closed sphincterotomy for anal fissure. Dis Colon Rectum 31:368-371, 1988.

49. Madoff RD, Fleshman JW: AGA technical review on the diagnosis and care of patients with anal fissure. Gastroenterology 124:235-245, 2003.

50. Henrichsen S, Christiansen J: Incidence of fistula-in-ano complicating anorectal sepsis: A prospective study. Br J Surg 73:371-372, 1986.

51. Parks AG, Gordon PH, Hardcastle JD: A classification of fistula-in-ano. Br J Surg 63:1-12, 1976.

52. Lindsey I, Smilgin-Humphreys MM, Cunningham C, et al: A randomized, controlled trial of fibrin glue versus conventional treatment for anal fistula. Dis Colon Rectum 45:1608-1615, 2002.

53. Gordon PH: Anorectal abscesses and fistula-in-ano. In Gordon PH, Nivatvongs S (eds): Principles and Practice of Surgery for the Colon, Rectum, and Anus. St. Louis, Quality Medical, 1992, pp 221-265.

54. da Silva JH: Pilonidal cyst: Cause and treatment. Dis Colon Rectum 43:1146-1156, 2000.

55. Odili J, Gault D: Laser depilation of the natal cleft—an aid to healing the pilonidal sinus. Ann R Coll Surg Engl 84:29-32, 2002.

56. Senapati A, Cripps NP, Thompson MR: Bascom's operation in the day-surgical management of symptomatic pilonidal sinus. Br J Surg 87:1067-1070, 2000.

57. Urhan MK, Kucukel F, Topgul K, et al: Rhomboid excision and Limberg flap for managing pilonidal sinus: Results of 102 cases. Dis Colon Rectum 45:656-659, 2002.

58. Tsang CB, Madoff RD, Wong WD, et al: Anal sphincter integrity and function influences outcome in rectovaginal fistula repair. Dis Colon Rectum 41:1141-1146, 1998.

59. Saclarides TJ: Rectovaginal fistula. Surg Clin North Am 82:1261-1272, 2002.

60. Hull TL, Fazio VW: Surgical approaches to low anovaginal fistula in Crohn's disease. Am J Surg 173:95-98, 1997.

61. Breese PL, Judson FN, Penley KA, et al: Anal human papillomavirus infection among homosexual and bisexual men: Prevalence of type-specific infection and association with human immunodeficiency virus. Sex Transm Dis 22:7-14, 1995.

62. Olmos L, Vilata J, Rodriguez Pichardo A, et al: Double-blind, randomized clinical trial on the effect of interferon-beta in the treatment of condylomata acuminata. Int J STD AIDS 5:182-185, 1994.

63. El-Attar SM, Evans DV: Anal warts, sexually transmitted diseases, and anorectal conditions associated with human immunodeficiency virus. Prim Care 26:81-100, 1999.

64. Smith LE: Sexually transmitted diseases. In Gordon PH, Nivatvongs S (eds): Principles and Practice of Surgery for the Colon, Rectum, and Anus, 2nd ed. St. Louis, Quality Medical, 1999, pp 341-363.

65. Barrett WL, Callahan TD, Orkin BA: Perianal manifestations of human immunodeficiency virus infection: Experience with 260 patients. Dis Colon Rectum 41:606-612, 1998.

66. Nadal SR, Manzione CR, Galvao VM, et al: Perianal diseases in HIV-positive patients compared with a seronegative population. Dis Colon Rectum 42:649-654, 1999.

67. Viamonte M, Dailey TH, Gottesman L: Ulcerative disease of the anorectum in the HIV-positive patient. Dis Colon Rectum 36:801-805, 1993.

68. Place RJ, Gregorcyk SG, Huber PJ, et al: Outcome analysis of HIV-positive patients with anal squamous cell carcinoma. Dis Colon Rectum 44:506-512, 2001.

69. Boer J, Weltevreden EF: Hidradenitis suppurativa or acne inversa: A clinicopathological study of early lesions. Br J Dermatol 135:721-725, 1996.

70. Mitchell KM, Beck DE: Hidradenitis suppurativa. Surg Clin North Am 82:1187-1197, 2002.

71. Culp CE: Chronic hidradenitis suppurativa of the anal canal: A surgical skin disease. Dis Colon Rectum 26:669-676, 1983.

72. Wiltz O, Schoetz DJ Jr, Murray JJ, et al: Perianal hidradenitis suppurativa: The Lahey Clinic experience. Dis Colon Rectum 33:731-734, 1990.

73. Abcarian H: Perianal Crohn's disease. Semin Colon Rectal Surg 5:210, 1994.

74. Schwartz DA, Pemberton JH, Sandborn WJ: Diagnosis and treatment of perianal fistulas in Crohn disease. Ann Intern Med 135:906-918, 2001.

75. Nelson H, Dozois RR: Anal neoplasms. Perspect Colon Rectal Surg 7:16, 1994.

76. McMurrick PJ, Nelson H, Goldberg RM, et al: Cancer of the anal canal. In Torosian MH (ed): Integrated Cancer Management. New York, Marcel Dekker, 1999, pp 195-205.

77. Nigro ND, Vaitkevicius VK, Considine B Jr: Dynamic management of squamous cell cancer of the anal canal. Invest New Drugs 7:83-89, 1989.

78. Jensen SL, Sjolin KE, Shokouh-Amiri MH, et al: Paget's disease of the anal margin. Br J Surg 75:1089-1092, 1988.

79. Boman BM, Moertel CG, O'Connell MJ, et al: Carcinoma of the anal canal: A clinical and pathologic study of 188 cases. Cancer 54:114-125, 1984.

80. UKCCCR Anal Cancer Trial Working Party: UK Coordinating Committee on Cancer Research: Epidermoid anal cancer: Results from the UKCCCR randomised trial of radiotherapy alone versus radiotherapy, 5-fluorouracil, and mitomycin. Lancet 348:1049-1054, 1996.

81. Brady MS, Kavolius JP, Quan SH: Anorectal melanoma: A 64-year experience at Memorial Sloan-Kettering Cancer Center. Dis Colon Rectum 38:146-151, 1995.

82. Thibault C, Sagar P, Nivatvongs S, et al: Anorectal melanoma—an incurable disease? Dis Colon Rectum 40:661-668, 1997.

83. Bullard KM, Tuttle TM, Rothenberger DA, et al: Surgical therapy for anorectal melanoma. J Am Coll Surg 196:206-211, 2003.

CHAPTER 50

THE LIVER

Michael D'Angelica, M.D., and Yuman Fong, M.D.

Historical Perspective	**Neoplasms**
Anatomy and Physiology	**Hemobilia**
Infectious Diseases	**Viral Hepatitis and the Surgeon**

HISTORICAL PERSPECTIVE

The surface anatomy of the liver was described as early as 2000 years before Christ by the ancient Babylonians.[1,2] Even Hippocrates understood and described the seriousness of liver injury.[3] Francis Glisson, in 1654, was the first physician to accurately describe the essential anatomy of the blood vessels of the liver.[4] The beginnings of liver surgery are accurately described as rudimentary excisions of eviscerated liver from penetrating trauma. The first documented case of a partial hepatectomy is usually credited to Berta in 1716, who amputated a portion of protruding liver in a patient with a self-inflicted stab wound.[5]

In the late 1800s, while the first gastrectomies and cholecystectomies were being performed in Europe, surgery on the liver was regarded as dangerous, if not impossible. J. W. Elliot, in his report on liver surgery for trauma in 1897, wrote that the liver was so "friable, so full of gaping vessels and so evidently incapable of being sutured that it had always seemed impossible to successfully manage large wounds of its substance."[6] European surgeons began to experiment with techniques of elective liver surgery on animals in the late 1800s. The credit for the first elective liver resection is a matter of debate, and many surgeons have been given credit, but it certainly occurred during this time period.[1]

The early 1900s saw some small, but significant advances in liver surgery. Techniques for suturing major hepatic vessels and the use of cautery for small vessels were applied and reported on.[1,2] The most significant advance of that time was probably that of J. Hogarth Pringle, who in 1908 described digital compression of the hilar vessels to control hepatic bleeding from traumatic injuries.[7] The modern era of hepatic surgery was ushered in by the development of a better understanding of

liver anatomy and formal anatomic liver resection. Credit for the first anatomic liver resection is usually given to Lortat-Jacob, who performed a right hepatectomy in 1952 in France.[8] Pack, from New York,[9] and Quattlebaum, from Georgia,[10] performed a similar operation within the next year and were unlikely to have any knowledge of Lortat-Jacob's report. Descriptions of the segmental nature of liver anatomy by Couinaud and by Goldsmith and Woodburne in 1957 opened the door even farther to the modern era of liver surgery.[11,12]

Despite these improvements, hepatic surgery was plagued by tremendous operative morbidity and mortality from the 1950s into the 1980s. Operative mortality rates in excess of 20% were common and usually related to massive hemorrhage.[1] Many surgeons were reluctant to perform hepatic surgery because of these results, and understandably many physicians were reluctant to refer patients for hepatectomy. Nonetheless, with the courage of patients, their families, and persistent surgeons, safe hepatic surgery has been realized. A complete list is not possible here, but courageous hepatic surgeons such as Blumgart,[13,14] Bismuth,[15] Longmire,[16] Fortner,[17] Schwartz, Starzl,[18,19] and Ton deserve mention. Advances in anesthesia, intensive care, and antibiotics have also contributed tremendously to the safety of major hepatic surgery. Total hepatectomy with liver transplantation is now performed routinely. Partial hepatectomy for a large number of indications is now performed throughout the world in specialized centers with mortality rates of 5% or less.[20]

Safe hepatic surgery and its liberal use in the management of a wide variety of diseases is now reality. The future, however, demands improvement and further innovation. Minimally invasive approaches to liver surgery are in their infancy and beckon refinement. The indications and use of regional chemotherapy pump devices also remain to be determined. Lastly, the development of thermal ablative techniques is ongoing, and defining indications and success rates should be a major focus of hepatic surgeons.

ANATOMY AND PHYSIOLOGY

Gross Anatomy

A precise knowledge of the anatomy of the liver is an absolute prerequisite to performing surgery on the liver or biliary tree. With the development of hepatic surgery over the past few decades a greater appreciation for the complex anatomy beyond the misleading minimal external markings has been realized. The days of utilizing the falciform ligament as the only marker of a left and right side of the liver are over, and the anatomic contributions of Couinaud (see later) and the description of the segmental nature of the liver should be embraced and studied by students of hepatic surgery.

General Description and Topography

The liver is a solid gastrointestinal organ whose mass (1200 to 1600 g) largely occupies the right upper quadrant of the abdomen. The costal margin coincides with the lower margin, and the superior surface is draped over by the diaphragm. The large majority of the right liver and most of the left liver is covered by the thoracic cage. The liver extends superiorly to the height of the fifth rib on the right and the sixth rib on the left. The posterior surface straddles the inferior vena cava (IVC). A wedge of liver extends to the left half of the abdomen across the epigastrium to lie above the anterior surface of the stomach and under the central and left diaphragm. The superior surface of the liver is convex and is molded to the diaphragm, whereas the inferior surface is mildly concave and extends to a sharp anterior border.

The liver is invested in peritoneum except for the gallbladder bed, the porta hepatis, and posteriorly on either side of the IVC in two wedge-shaped areas (called the bare area of the liver to the right of the IVC). The peritoneal duplications on the liver surface are referred to as ligaments. The diaphragmatic peritoneal duplications are referred to as the coronary ligament whose lateral margins on either side are the right and left triangular ligaments. From the center of the coronary ligament emerges the falciform ligament, which extends anteriorly as a thin membrane connecting the liver surface to the diaphragm, abdominal wall, and umbilicus. The ligamentum teres (the obliterated umbilical vein) runs along the inferior edge of the falciform ligament from the umbilicus to the umbilical fissure. The umbilical fissure is on the inferior surface of the left liver and contains the left portal triad. The falciform ligament, the most obvious surface marking of the liver, historically was used to mark the division of the right and left lobes of the liver in early descriptions of hepatic anatomy. However, this description is inaccurate and of minimal utility to the hepatobiliary surgeon (see later for detailed segmental anatomy). On the posterior surface of the left liver running from the left portal vein in the porta hepatis toward the left hepatic vein and the IVC is the ligamentum venosum (obliterated sinus venosus), which also runs in a fissure (Fig. 50-1). Hepatic arterial and portal venous blood flow enter the liver at the hilum and branch throughout the liver as a single unit that also includes bile ducts (portal triad). This unit is enclosed in a peritoneal sheath that originates at the hepatic hilum. Venous drainage is through hepatic veins that empty directly into the IVC.[21,22]

Normal Development/Embryology

The liver primordium is formed in the third week of gestation as an outgrowth of endodermal epithelium (known as the hepatic diverticulum or liver bud). The connection between the hepatic diverticulum and the future duodenum narrows to form the bile duct and an outpouching of the bile duct forms into the gallbladder and cystic duct. Hepatic cells develop cords and intermingle with the vitelline and umbilical veins to form hepatic sinusoids. Simultaneously, hematopoietic cells, Kupffer cells, and connective tissue form from the mesoderm of the septum transversum. The mesoderm of the septum transversum connects the liver to the ventral abdominal wall and to the foregut. As the liver protrudes into the abdominal cavity these structures are stretched into thin membranes, ultimately forming the falciform ligament and the lesser omentum, respectively. The mesoderm on the surface of the developing liver differentiates into visceral peritoneum, except superiorly where contact between the liver and mesoderm (future diaphragm) is maintained, forming a bare area devoid of visceral peritoneum (Fig. 50-2).

The primitive liver plays a central role in the fetal circulation. The vitelline veins carry blood from the yolk sac to the sinus venosus and ultimately form a network of veins around the foregut (future duodenum) that drain into the developing hepatic sinusoids. These vitelline veins eventually fuse to form the portal, superior mesenteric, and splenic veins. The sinus venosus that empties into the fetal heart ultimately becomes the hepatocardiac channel and then the hepatic veins and post-hepatic IVC. The umbilical veins that are paired early on carry oxygenated blood to the fetus. Initially, the umbilical veins drain into the sinus venosus, but at 5 weeks they begin to drain into the hepatic sinusoids. The right umbilical vein ultimately disappears, and the left umbilical vein later drains directly into the hepatocardiac channel, bypassing the hepatic sinusoids through the ductus venosus. In the adult liver, the remnant of the left umbilical vein becomes the ligamentum teres, which runs in the falciform ligament into the umbilical fissure, and the remnant of the ductus venosus becomes the ligamentum venosum at the termination of the lesser omentum under the left liver (Fig. 50-3).

The fetal liver plays a very important role in hematopoiesis. In the 10th week of gestation, the liver is

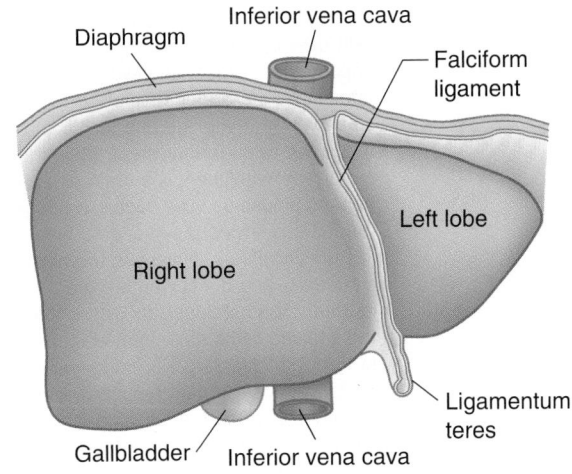

A

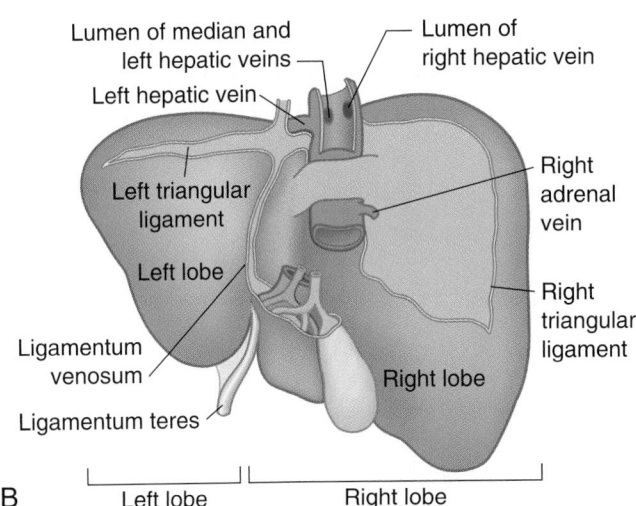

B

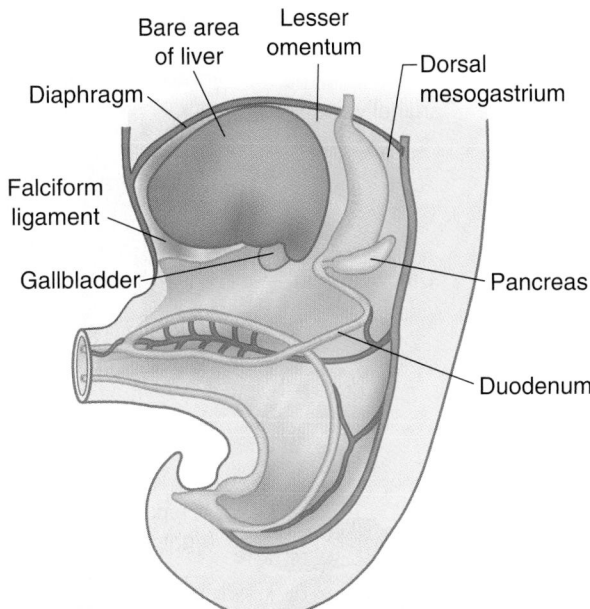

FIGURE 50-2.   An approximately 36-day-old embryo is shown. The extensions of the septum transversum can be seen developing as the liver protrudes into the abdominal cavity stretching out and forming the lesser omentum and the falciform ligament. The liver is completely invested in visceral peritoneum except for a portion next to the diaphragm known as the bare area. (From Sadler TW: Langman's Medical Embryology, 5th ed. Baltimore, Williams & Wilkins, 1985.)

FIGURE 50-1.   A, Historically, the liver was divided into right and left lobes by the external marking of the falciform ligament. On the inferior surface of the falciform ligament, the ligamentum teres can be seen entering the umbilical fissure. B, The posterior and inferior surface of the liver is shown. The liver embraces the inferior vena cava (IVC) posteriorly in a groove. The lumina of the three major hepatic veins (LHV, MHV, RHV) and the right adrenal vein can be seen directly entering the IVC. The bare area, bounded by the right and left triangular ligaments, is illustrated. To the left of the IVC is the caudate lobe, which is bounded on its left side by a fissure containing the ligamentum venosum. The lesser omentum terminates along the edge of the ligamentum venosum, and thus the caudate lobe lies within the lesser sac and the rest of the liver lies in the supracolic compartment. A layer of fibrous tissue can be seen bridging the right lobe to the caudate lobe posterior to the IVC, thus encircling the IVC. This ligament of tissue must be divided on the right side when mobilizing the right liver off of the IVC. (From Blumgart LH, Hann LE: Surgical and radiologic anatomy of the liver and biliary tract. In Blumgart LH, Fong Y [eds]: Surgery of the Liver and Biliary Tract. London, WB Saunders, 2000, pp 3-34.)

10% of the body weight, which is due to developing hepatic sinusoids and active hematopoiesis. During the last 2 months of intrauterine life, hepatic hematopoiesis decreases and the weight of the liver is decreased to 5% of body weight. By the 12th week of gestation, bile forms in hepatic cells along with the simultaneous development of the gallbladder and bile duct, allowing drainage of bile into the foregut.[23]

Lobar Anatomy

Historically, the liver was divided into right and left lobes, determined by portal and hepatic vein branches. Briefly, a plane without any surface markings running from the gallbladder to the left side of the IVC (known as the portal fissure or Cantlie's line) divided the liver into right and left lobes. The right lobe was further divided into anterior and posterior segments. The left lobe was divided into a medial segment (also known as the quadrate lobe) that lies to the right of the falciform ligament and umbilical fissure and a lateral segment lying to the left. This system is sufficient for mobilization of the liver and simple hepatic procedures but does not describe the much more intricate and functional anatomy now embraced by most liver surgeons.[21]

The functional anatomy (Figs. 50-4 and 50-5) of the liver is composed of eight segments that are each supplied by

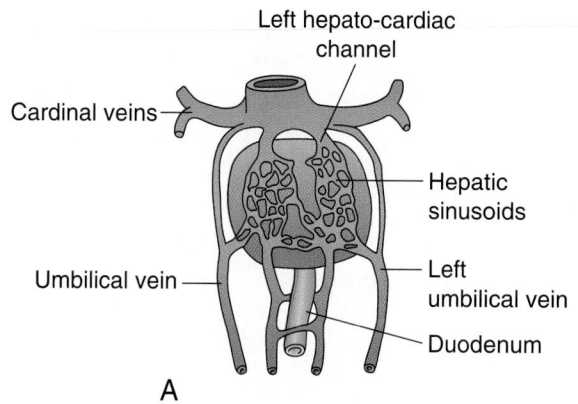

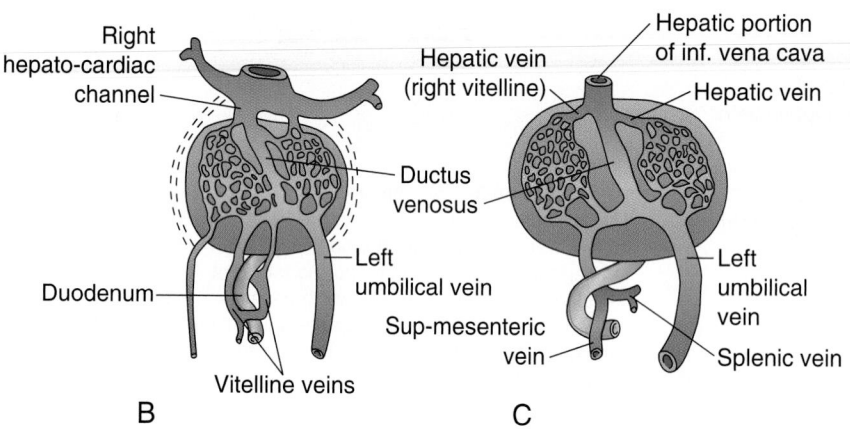

FIGURE 50-3.   A, Umbilical and vitelline vein development of a 5-week-old embryo. The hepatic sinusoids have developed; and although there are channels that bypass these sinusoids, the vitelline and umbilical veins are beginning to drain into them. **B,** In the second month, the vitelline veins drain directly into the hepatic sinusoids. The ductus venosus has formed and accepts oxygenated blood from the left umbilical vein, bypasses the hepatic sinusoids, and directly enters the hepatocardiac channel. **C,** By the third month, the vitelline veins have formed into the portal system (splenic, superior mesenteric, and portal veins). The right umbilical vein has disappeared, and the left umbilical vein (future ligamentum teres) drains into the sinus venosus bypassing the hepatic sinusoids. Note the development of the inferior vena cava and the hepatic veins. (From Sadler TW: Langman's Medical Embryology, 5th ed. Baltimore, Williams & Wilkins, 1985.)

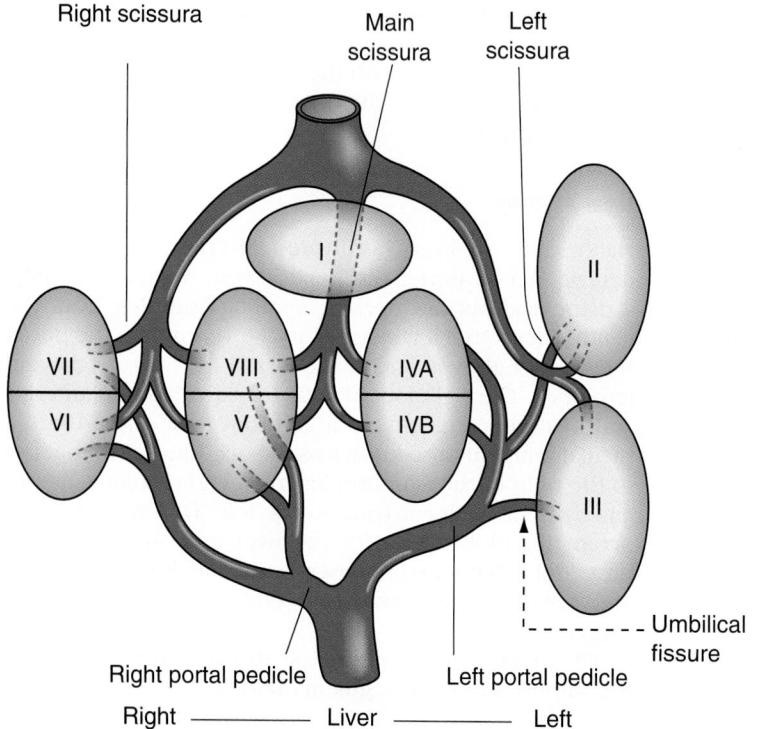

FIGURE 50-4.   Schematic diagram of the segmental anatomy of the liver. Each segment receives its own portal pedicle (triad of portal vein, hepatic artery, and bile duct). The eight segments are illustrated and the four sectors, divided by the three main hepatic veins running in scissurae, are shown. The umbilical fissure (not a scissura) is shown to contain the left portal pedicle. (From Blumgart LH, Hann LE: Surgical and radiologic anatomy of the liver and biliary tract. *In* Blumgart LH, Fong Y [eds]: Surgery of the Liver and Biliary Tract. London, WB Saunders, 2000, pp 3-34.)

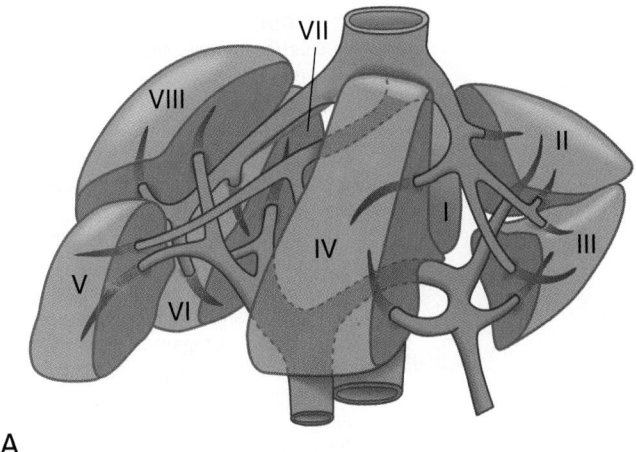

A

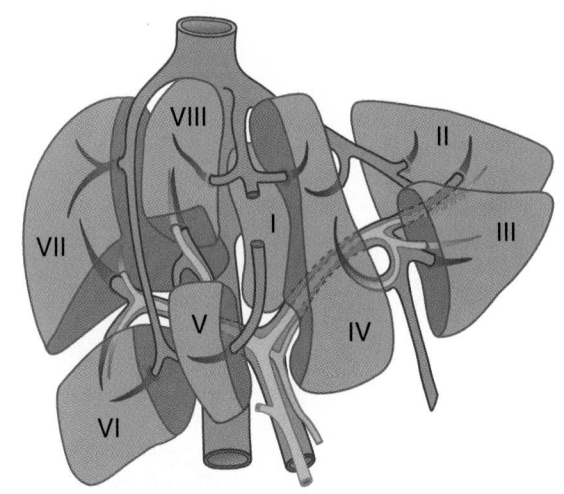

B

FIGURE 50-5. Segmental anatomy of the liver, as seen at laparotomy in the anatomic position **(A)** and in the ex-vivo position **(B)**. (From Blumgart LH, Hann LE: Surgical and radiologic anatomy of the liver and biliary tract. *In* Blumgart LH, Fong Y [eds]: Surgery of the Liver and Biliary Tract. London, WB Saunders, 2000, pp 3-34.)

a single portal triad (pedicle) composed of a portal vein, hepatic artery, and a bile duct. These segments are further organized into four sectors that are separated by scissurae containing the three main hepatic veins. The four sectors are even further organized into the right and left liver (the term *right and left liver* is preferable to *right and left lobe* because there is no external mark that allows the identification of the right and left liver). This system was originally described in 1957 by Goldsmith and Woodburne as well as by Couinaud and defines hepatic anatomy as it is most relevant to surgery of the liver.[11,12]

The main scissura contains the middle hepatic vein that runs in an anteroposterior direction from the gallbladder fossa to the left side of the vena cava and divides the liver into right and left hemilivers. The line of the main scissura is also known as Cantlie's line. The right liver is divided into an anterior (segments V and VIII) and a posterior (segments VI and VII) sector by the right scissura that contains the right hepatic vein. The right portal pedicle composed of the right hepatic artery, portal vein, and bile duct split into right anterior and posterior pedicles that supply the segments of the anterior and posterior sector.

The left liver has a visible fissure along its inferior surface called the umbilical fissure. The ligamentum teres (containing the remnant of the umbilical vein) runs into this fissure. The falciform ligament is contiguous with the umbilical fissure and ligamentum teres. The umbilical fissure is *not* a scissura, does not contain a hepatic vein, and, in fact, contains the left portal pedicle (triad containing the left portal vein, hepatic artery, and bile duct), which runs in this fissure, branching to feed the left liver. The left scissura runs posterior to the ligamentum teres and contains the left hepatic vein. The left liver is split into an anterior (segments III and IV) and posterior (segment II—the only sector composed of a single segment) sector by the left scissura.

At the hilum of the liver, the right portal triad has a short extrahepatic course of approximately 1 to 1.5 cm before entering the substance of the liver and branching into anterior and posterior sectoral branches. The left portal triad, however, has a long extrahepatic course of up to 3 or 4 cm and runs transversely along the base of segment IV in a peritoneal sheath that is the upper end of the lesser omentum. The left portal triad, as it runs along the base of segment IV is separated from the liver substance by connective tissue known as the hilar plate (Fig. 50-6). The continuation of the left portal triad runs anteriorly and caudad in the umbilical fissure and gives branches to segments II and III and recurrent branches to segment IV.

The caudate lobe (segment I) is the dorsal portion of the liver and embraces the IVC on its posterior surface and lies posterior to the left portal triad inferiorly and the left and middle hepatic veins superiorly. The main bulk of the caudate lobe is to the left of the IVC, but inferiorly it traverses between the IVC and left portal triad, where it fuses to the right liver (segments VI and VII). This part of the caudate lobe is known as the right portion and the caudate process. The left portion of the caudate lobe lies in the lesser omental bursa and is covered anteriorly by the gastrohepatic ligament (lesser omentum) that separates it from segments II and III anteriorly. The gastrohepatic ligament attaches to the ligamentum venosum (sinus venosus remnant) along the left side of the left portal triad (Fig. 50-7).

The vascular inflow and biliary drainage to the caudate lobe comes from both the right and left systems. The right side of the caudate and the caudate process largely derive their portal venous supply from the right portal vein or the bifurcation of the main portal vein, whereas the left portion of the caudate derives its portal venous inflow from the left main portal vein. The arterial supply and the biliary drainage of the right portion is generally through the right posterior sectoral system and that of the left portion is through the left main vessels. The hepatic venous drainage of the caudate is unique in that multiple small veins drain directly into the IVC.

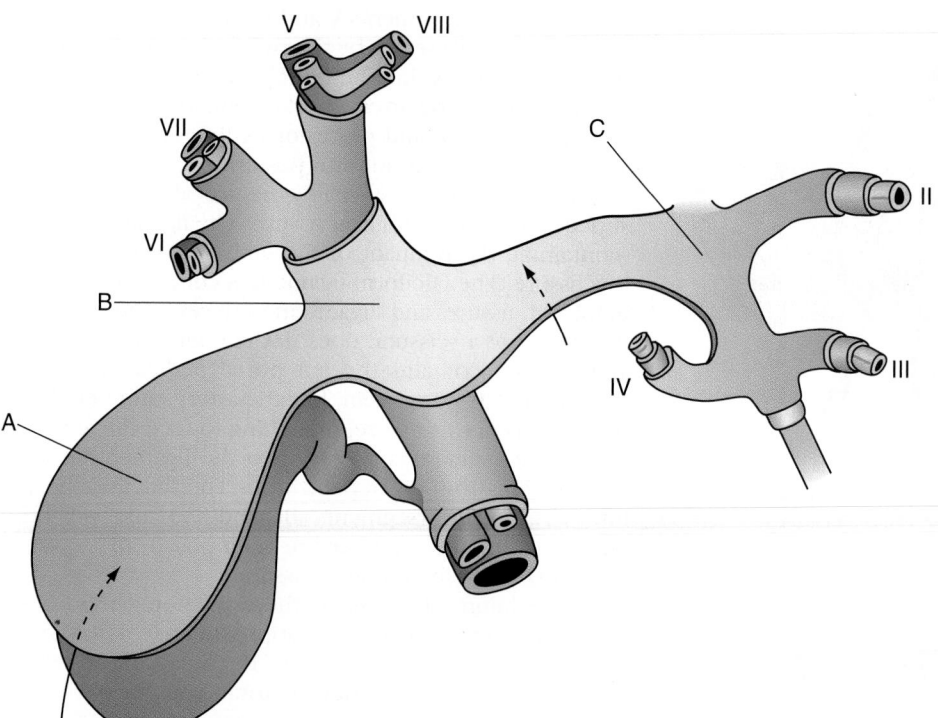

FIGURE 50-6. The plate system is illustrated, including the cystic plate between the gallbladder and the liver (**A**), the hilar plate at the biliary confluence at the base of segment IV (**B**), and the umbilical plate above the umbilical portion of the portal vein (**C**). The *arrows* show the plane of dissection of the cystic plate for cholecystectomy and the hilar plate for exposure of the hepatic duct confluence and the main left hepatic duct. (From Blumgart LH, Hann LE: Surgical and radiologic anatomy of the liver and biliary tract. *In* Blumgart LH, Fong Y [eds]: Surgery of the Liver and Biliary Tract. London, WB Saunders, 2000, pp 3-34.)

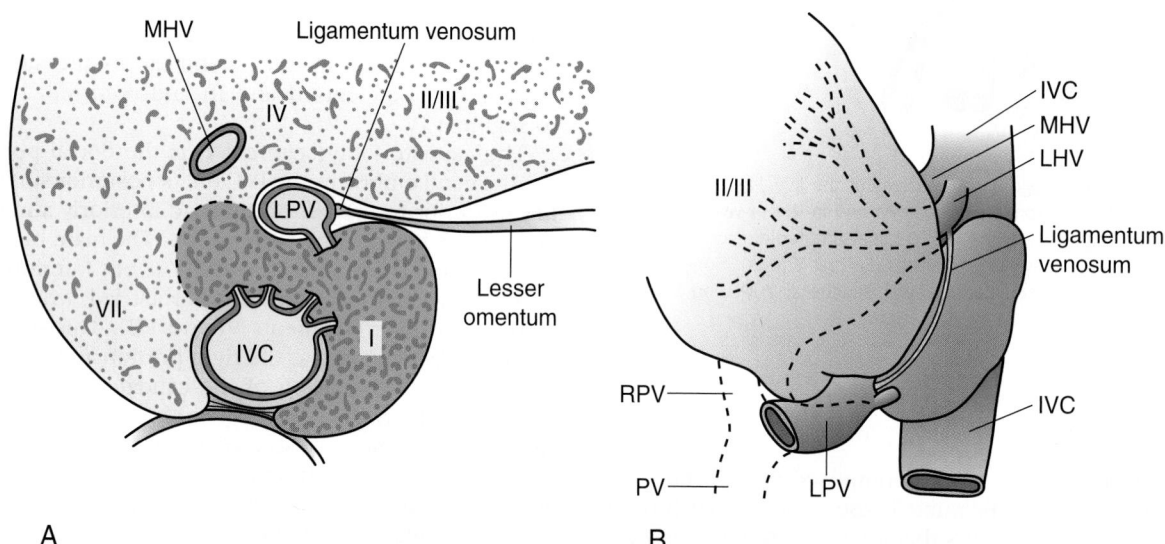

A   B

FIGURE 50-7. The anatomy of the caudate lobe (segment I) is shown. **A,** Seen in cross section, the majority of the caudate is to the left of the inferior vena cava (IVC) and lies posterior to the lesser omentum, which separates the caudate lobe from segments II and III. The termination of the lesser omentum at the ligamentum venosum is demonstrated. The caudate traverses to the right insinuating itself between the IVC and the left portal vein (LPV), where it attaches to the right liver. Note the proximity of the middle hepatic vein to these structures. **B,** Segments II and III have been rotated to the patient's right exposing the left side of the caudate lobe. RPV, Right portal vein; PV, portal vein; LPV, left portal vein; MHV, middle hepatic vein; LHV, left hepatic vein. (From Blumgart LH, Hann LE: Surgical and radiologic anatomy of the liver and biliary tract. *In* Blumgart LH, Fong Y [eds]: Surgery of the Liver and Biliary Tract. London, WB Saunders, 2000, pp 3-34.)

The posterior edge of the left side of the caudate terminates into a fibrous component that attaches to the crura of the diaphragm and also runs posteriorly behind the IVC and attaches to segment VII of the right liver. Up to 50% of the time, this fibrous component is composed either partially or completely of liver parenchyma, and, thus, liver tissue may completely encircle the IVC.

Anomalous development of the liver is uncommonly encountered. Complete absence of the left liver has been reported. A tongue of tissue extending inferiorly off of the right liver has been described (Riedel's lobe). Rare cases of supradiaphragmatic liver in the absence of a hernia sac have been noted.[21,22]

Portal Vein

The portal vein provides about 75% of hepatic blood flow; and although it is postcapillary and largely deoxygenated, its large volume flow rate provides 50% to 70% of the liver's oxygenation. The lack of valves in the portal venous system provides a system that can accommodate high flow at low pressure because of the low resistance and allows measurement of portal venous pressure anywhere along the system.

The portal vein forms behind the neck of the pancreas at the confluence of the superior mesenteric vein and the splenic vein at the height of the second lumbar vertebra. The length of the main portal vein ranges from 5.5 to 8 cm, and its diameter is usually about 1 cm. Cephalad to its formation behind the neck of the pancreas, the portal vein runs behind the first portion of the duodenum and into the hepatoduodenal ligament, where it runs along the right border of the lesser omentum usually posterior to the bile duct and hepatic artery.

The portal vein divides into main right and left branches at the hilum of the liver. The left branch of the portal vein runs transversely along the base of segment IV and into the umbilical fissure, where it gives off branches to segments II and III and feeds back branches to segment IV. The left portal vein also gives off posterior branches to the left side of the caudate lobe. The right portal vein has a short extrahepatic course and usually enters the substance of the liver, where it splits into anterior and posterior sectoral branches. These sectoral branches can occasionally be seen extrahepatically and can come off the main portal vein before its bifurcation. There is usually a small branch off the right portal vein or at the bifurcation that comes off posteriorly to supply the caudate process (Fig. 50-8).[24]

There are a number of connections between the portal venous system and the systemic venous system. Under conditions of high portal venous pressure, these portosystemic connections may enlarge secondary to collateral flow. The most significant portosystemic collateral locations are (1) the submucosal veins of the proximal stomach and distal esophagus, which receive portal flow from the short gastric veins and the left gastric vein and can result in varices with the potential for intestinal hemorrhage; (2) umbilical and abdominal wall veins, which recanalize from flow through the umbilical vein in the

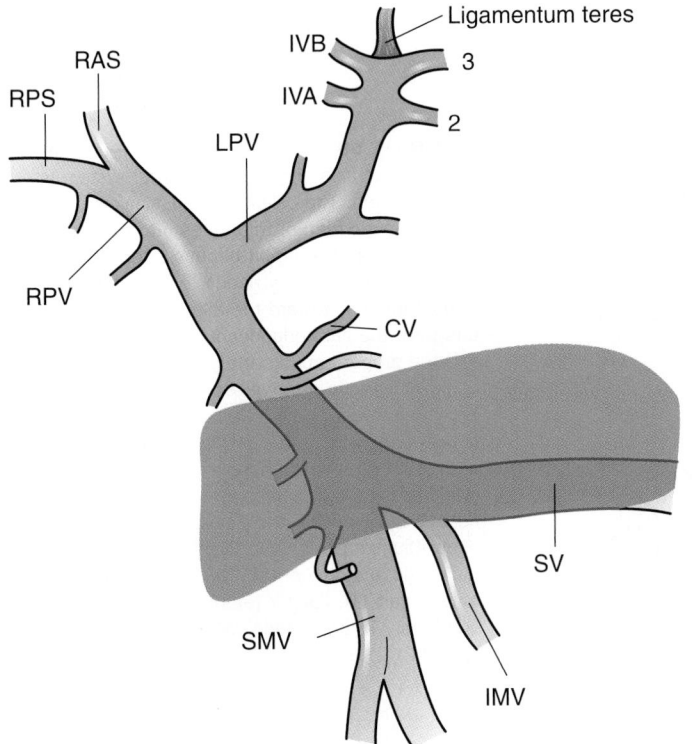

FIGURE 50-8.   The anatomy of the portal vein is demonstrated. The superior mesenteric vein (SMV) joins the splenic vein (SV) posterior to the neck of the pancreas *(shaded)* to form the portal vein. Note the entrance of the inferior mesenteric vein (IMV) into the splenic vein—the most common anatomic arrangement. In its course superiorly in the edge of the lesser omentum posterior to the common bile duct and hepatic artery, the portal vein receives venous effluent from the coronary vein (CV). At the hepatic hilum, the portal vein bifurcates into a larger right portal vein (RPV) and a smaller left portal vein (LPV). The left portal vein runs transversely at the base of segment IV and enters the umbilical fissure to supply the segments of the left liver. Just before the umbilical fissure, the left portal vein usually gives off a sizable branch to the caudate lobe. The right portal vein enters the substance of the liver and splits into anterior and posterior sectoral branches (RAS, RPS). It also gives off a posterior branch to the right side of the caudate lobe/caudate process. (From Blumgart LH, Hann LE: Surgical and radiologic anatomy of the liver and biliary tract. *In* Blumgart LH, Fong Y [eds]: Surgery of the Liver and Biliary Tract. London, WB Saunders, 2000, pp 3-34.)

ligamentum teres resulting in caput medusae; (3) the superior hemorrhoidal plexus, which receives portal flow from inferior mesenteric vein tributaries and yields large hemorrhoids; and (4) other retroperitoneal communications yielding collaterals that can make abdominal surgery hazardous.

The anatomy of the portal vein and its branches is relatively constant and has much less variation than the ductal and hepatic arterial system. The portal vein is rarely found anterior to the neck of the pancreas and the duodenum. Entrance of the portal vein directly into the vena cava has also been described. Very rarely, a pulmonary vein may enter the portal vein. Lastly, there may be a congenital absence of the left branch of the portal vein. In this situation, the right branch courses through the right liver and curves around peripherally to supply the left liver.[21,22]

Hepatic Artery

The hepatic artery, representing high flow oxygenated systemic arterial flow, provides approximately 25% of the hepatic blood flow and 30% to 50% of its oxygenation. A number of smaller perihepatic arteries derived from the inferior phrenic and the gastroduodenal arteries also supply the liver. These vessels are important sources of collateral blood flow in the event of occlusion of the main hepatic arterial inflow. In the case of ligation of the right or left hepatic artery, intrahepatic collaterals almost immediately provide for nutrient blood flow.

The common description of the arterial supply to the liver and biliary tree is only present approximately 60% of the time (Fig. 50-9). The celiac trunk originates directly off the aorta just below the aortic diaphragmatic hiatus

and gives off three branches: the splenic artery, the left gastric artery, and the common hepatic artery. The common hepatic artery passes forward and to the right along the superior border of the pancreas and runs along the right side of the lesser omentum, where it ascends toward the hepatic hilum lying anterior to the portal vein and to the left of the bile duct. At the point that the common hepatic artery begins to head superiorly toward the hepatic hilum, it gives off the gastroduodenal artery, followed by the supraduodenal artery and then the right gastric artery. The common hepatic artery beyond the take-off of the gastroduodenal is called the proper hepatic artery and divides into right and left branches at the hilum. The left hepatic artery heads vertically toward the umbilical fissure to supply segments I, II, and III. The left hepatic artery usually gives off a middle hepatic artery branch that heads toward the right side of the umbilical fissure and supplies segment IV. The right hepatic artery usually runs posterior to the common hepatic bile duct and enters Calot's triangle (bordered by the cystic duct, common hepatic duct, and the liver edge), where it gives off the cystic artery to supply the gallbladder and then continues into the substance of the right lobe.

Unlike portal vein anatomy, hepatic arterial anatomy is extraordinarily variable (Fig. 50-10). An accessory vessel is described as an aberrant origin of a branch that is in addition to the normal branching pattern. A replaced vessel is described as an aberrant origin of a branch that substitutes for the lack of the normal branch. Most often, the hepatic artery originates off of the celiac trunk, but different branches or the entire hepatic arterial system can originate off of the superior mesenteric artery. In this case, the replaced or accessory vessel runs behind the head of the pancreas, to the right of the portal vein and posteri-

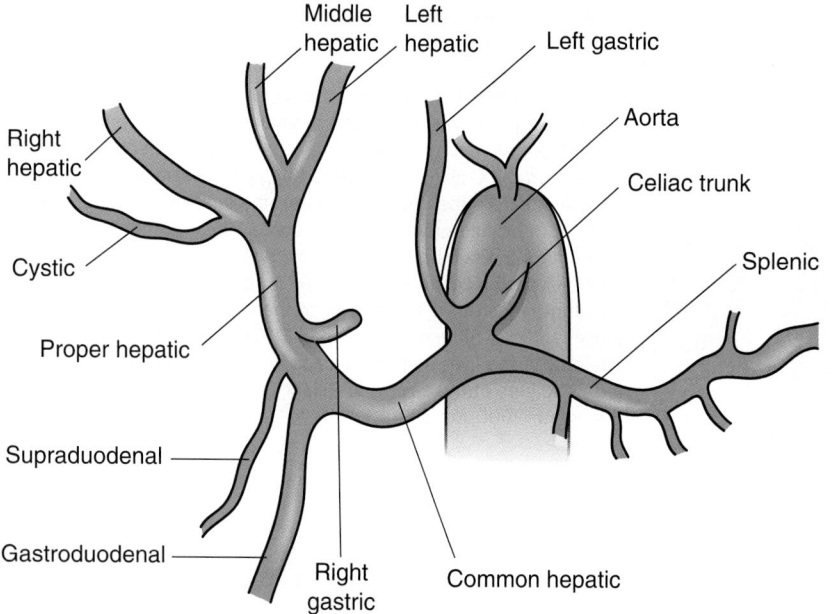

FIGURE 50-9. The most common anatomy of the celiac axis and hepatic arterial system is demonstrated. The celiac axis, just below the diaphragmatic hiatus, trifurcates into the splenic, left gastric, and common hepatic arteries. The common hepatic artery heads to the right and turns superiorly toward the hilum. At the point of this turn, the gastroduodenal artery is given off and the proper hepatic artery is formed. The common hepatic artery gives off right and left hepatic arteries in the hilum. Note the middle hepatic artery off of the proximal left hepatic artery that goes on to supply segment IV. The cystic artery most commonly comes off the right hepatic artery within the triangle of Calot. (From Blumgart LH, Hann LE: Surgical and radiologic anatomy of the liver and biliary tract. *In* Blumgart LH, Fong Y [eds]: Surgery of the Liver and Biliary Tract. London, WB Saunders, 2000, pp 3-34.)

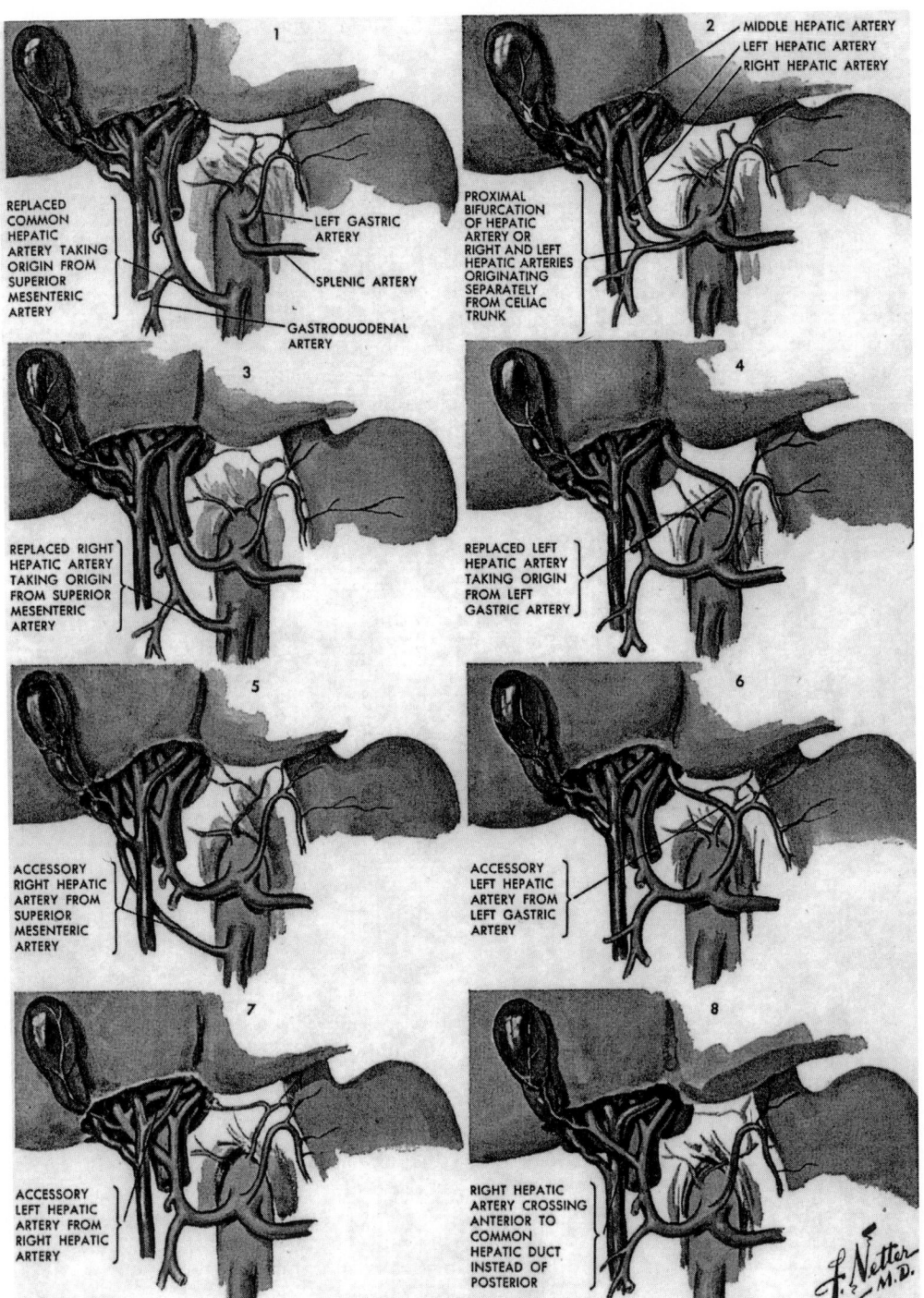

FIGURE 50-10.   The variable anatomy of the hepatic artery is demonstrated. The common hepatic artery can originate off of the superior mesenteric artery instead of the celiac axis. A replaced or accessory right hepatic artery comes off the superior mesenteric artery and runs posterior to the head of the pancreas, to the right of the portal vein and behind the common bile duct into the hilum. A replaced or accessory left hepatic artery originates off of the left gastric artery and runs through the lesser omentum into the umbilical fissure. (From Netter FH: Liver, biliary tract and pancreas. *In* Netter FH: The Netter Collection of Medical Illustrations. Teterboro, NJ, ICON Learning Systems, 2001.)

orly to the right of the common bile duct. The right hepatic artery, in its usual branching pattern, can also course anterior to the common hepatic duct. A replaced or accessory left hepatic artery usually originates from the left gastric artery and is found in the lesser omentum heading toward the umbilical fissure. Other important variations include the origin of the gastroduodenal artery, which has been found to originate from the right hepatic artery and is occasionally duplicated. The anatomy of the cystic artery is also quite variable, and knowledge of these variations is of particular importance in the performance of cholecystectomy (Fig. 50-11). An accessory cystic artery can originate from the proper hepatic artery or the gastroduodenal artery, where it runs anterior to the bile duct. A single cystic artery can originate anywhere off of the proper hepatic artery or the gastroduodenal artery or directly from the celiac axis. These variant cystic arteries can run anterior to the bile duct and are not necessarily present in the triangle of Calot. All of these variations in hepatic arterial anatomy are of obvious importance during

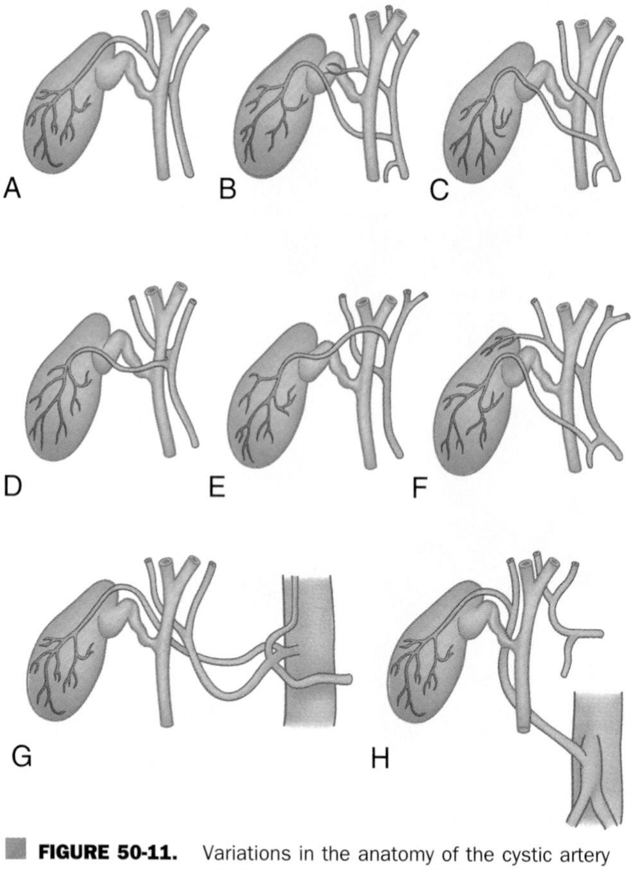

FIGURE 50-11. Variations in the anatomy of the cystic artery are demonstrated. **A,** Most common anatomy. **B,** Double cystic artery—one off the proper hepatic artery. **C,** Origin off the proper hepatic artery and coursing anterior to the bile duct. **D,** Origin off the right hepatic artery and coursing anterior to the bile duct. **E,** Origin from the left hepatic artery and coursing anterior to the bile duct. **F,** Origin off the gastroduodenal artery. **G,** Origin off the celiac axis. **H,** Origin from a replaced right hepatic artery. (From Blumgart LH, Hann LE: Surgical and radiologic anatomy of the liver and biliary tract. In Blumgart LH, Fong Y [eds]: Surgery of the Liver and Biliary Tract. London, WB Saunders, 2000, pp 3-34.)

hepatic resection or for hepatic interventional radiologic procedures.[22,25]

Hepatic Veins

The three major hepatic veins drain from the superior and posterior surface of the liver directly into the IVC (see Figs. 50-4 and 50-5). The right hepatic vein runs in the right scissura (between the anterior and posterior sectors of the right liver) and drains the majority of the right liver after a short (1 cm) extrahepatic course into the right side of the IVC. The left and middle hepatic veins usually join intrahepatically and enter the left side of the IVC as a single vessel, although they may drain separately. The left hepatic vein runs in the left scissura (between segments II and III) and drains segments II and III while the middle hepatic vein runs in the portal scissura (between segment IV and the anterior sector of the right liver) draining segment IV and some of the anterior sector of the right liver. There are, of course, additional hepatic veins. The umbilical vein runs under the falciform ligament, between the left and middle veins, and usually empties into the left hepatic vein. Multiple small venous branches drain posteriorly directly into the IVC, and an inferior accessory right hepatic vein is commonly encountered and can be of substantial size. Venous drainage of the caudate lobe is through multiple small hepatic veins that drain directly into the IVC and a large tributary that drains superiorly into the left hepatic vein.[26]

Biliary System

The intrahepatic bile ducts are terminal branches of the main right and left hepatic ductal branches that invaginate Glisson's capsule at the hilum along with the corresponding portal vein and hepatic artery branches forming the peritoneal covered portal triads (see Fig. 50-5). Along these intrahepatic portal triads, the bile duct branches are usually superior to the portal vein while the hepatic artery branches run inferiorly. The left hepatic duct drains segments II, III, and IV, which constitute the left liver. The ductal branches of the left liver join to form the main left duct along the umbilical fissure where, at its base, the left hepatic duct courses transversely across the base of segment IV to join the right hepatic duct at the hilum. In its transverse portion, the left hepatic duct drains one to three small branches from segment IV. The right hepatic duct drains the right liver (segments V through VIII) and is formed by the joining of the anterior sectoral duct (draining segments V and VIII) and the posterior sectoral duct (draining segments VI and VII). The posterior sectoral duct runs in a horizontal and posterior direction while the anterior sectoral duct runs vertically. The main right hepatic duct bifurcates just above the right portal vein. The short right hepatic duct meets the longer left hepatic duct forming the confluence anterior to the right portal vein, constituting the common hepatic duct. The caudate lobe (segment I) has its own biliary drainage, which is usually through both right and left systems, although in up to 15% of cases drainage is through the left system only and in 5% it is through the right system only.[27]

The confluence of the right and left hepatic duct anterior to the origin of the right portal vein and the portal vein bifurcation forms the common hepatic duct. The common hepatic duct drains inferiorly and below the takeoff of the cystic duct is referred to as the common bile duct. The common bile/hepatic duct runs along the right side of the hepatoduodenal ligament (free edge of the lesser omentum) to the right of the hepatic artery and anterior to the portal vein. The common bile duct continues inferiorly (usually 10 to 15 cm in length and 6 mm in diameter) behind the first portion of the duodenum and into the head of the pancreas in an inferior and slightly rightward direction. The intrapancreatic distal common bile duct then joins with the main pancreatic duct (of Wirsung), with or without a common channel, and enters the second portion of the duodenum through the major papilla of Vater. At the choledochoduodenal junction a complicated muscular complex known as the sphincter of Oddi regulates bile flow and prevents reflux of duodenal contents into the biliary tree. There are three major parts to this sphincter: the sphincter choledochus is a circular muscle that serves to regulate bile flow and the filling of the gallbladder; the pancreatic sphincter, present to variable degrees, surrounds the intraduodenal pancreatic duct; and the sphincter ampullae, made up of longitudinal muscle, serves to prevent duodenal reflux.[21,28]

The gallbladder is a biliary reservoir that lies against the inferior surface of segments IV and V of the liver, usually making an impression against it. A peritoneal layer covers the majority of the gallbladder except for the portion adherent to the liver. Where the gallbladder is adherent to the liver there is a layer of fibrous connective tissue known as the cystic plate that is an extension of the hilar plate (see Fig. 50-6). Variable in size, but usually about 10 cm long and 3 to 5 cm wide, the gallbladder is composed of a fundus, body, infundibulum, and neck that ultimately empties into the cystic duct. The fundus usually projects just slightly beyond the liver edge anteriorly and when folded on itself is described as a "phrygian cap." Continuing toward the bile duct, the body of the gallbladder is usually in close proximity to the second portion of the duodenum and the transverse colon. The infundibulum (or Hartmann's pouch) hangs forward along the free edge of the lesser omentum and can fold in front of the cystic duct. The portion of gallbladder between the infundibulum and the cystic duct is referred to as the neck. The cystic duct is variable in its length, its course, and its insertion into the main biliary tree. The first portion of the cystic duct is usually tortuous and contains mucosal duplications referred to as the fold of Heister that regulate the filling and emptying of the gallbladder. Most commonly, the cystic duct joins the hepatic duct to form the common bile duct.[21,29]

Knowledge of the multiple and frequent variations in the anatomy of the biliary tree is absolutely essential to perform hepatobiliary procedures. Anomalies of the hepatic ductal confluence are common, with the normal anatomy described above present about two thirds of the time. The most common anomalies of the biliary confluence involve variations in the insertion of the right sectoral ducts (more commonly the posterior sectoral duct).

The confluence can be a trifurcation of the right anterior sectoral, right posterior sectoral, and left hepatic ducts. Either of the right sectoral ducts can drain into the left hepatic duct, the common hepatic duct, the cystic duct, or, rarely, the gallbladder (Fig. 50-12). Anomalies of the gallbladder itself are rare. Agenesis of the gallbladder,

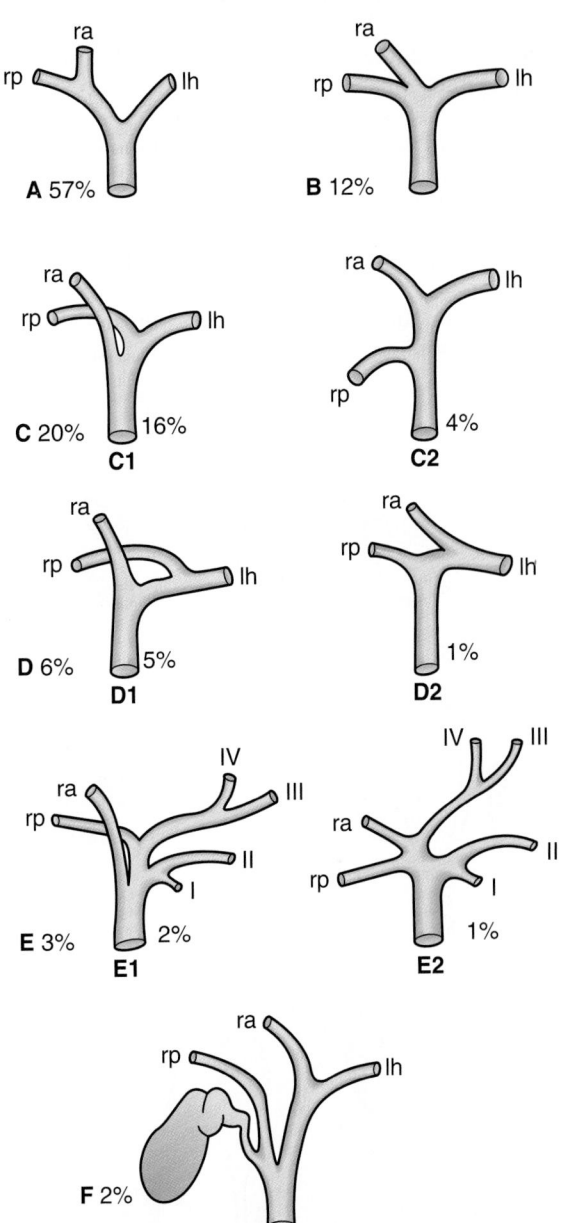

FIGURE 50-12. Variations of the hepatic duct confluence. **A,** Most common anatomy. **B,** Trifurcation at the confluence. Either of the right sectoral ducts drains into the common hepatic duct **(C),** and either of the right sectoral ducts drains into the left hepatic duct **(D). E,** Absence of a hepatic duct confluence. **F,** Absence of right hepatic duct and drainage of right posterior sectoral duct into the cystic duct. ra, right anterior sectoral duct; rp, right posterior sectoral duct; lh, left hepatic duct; *Roman numerals* indicate the segment drained. (From Blumgart LH, Hann LE: Surgical and radiologic anatomy of the liver and biliary tract. *In* Blumgart LH, Fong Y [eds]: Surgery of the Liver and Biliary Tract. London, WB Saunders, 2000, pp 3-34.)

bilobar gallbladder with two ducts or a single duct, septations, and congenital diverticulum of the gallbladder have all been described. Anomalies of the position of the gallbladder are more common and include an intrahepatic position or, rarely, presence on the left side of the liver. The gallbladder can also have a long mesentery, which can predispose to torsion. The position and entry of the cystic duct into the main ductal system is variable. Double cystic ducts draining a unilocular gallbladder and drainage into hepatic duct branches have been reported. Usually, the cystic duct joins the common hepatic duct at an angle, but it can run parallel and enter it more distally. In the latter situation, the cystic duct can be fused to the hepatic duct along its parallel course by connective tissue. The cystic duct can also run a spiral course anteriorly or posteriorly and enter the left side of the hepatic duct. Lastly, the cystic duct can be very short or even absent (Fig. 50-13).[21,22,27]

The supraduodenal and infrahilar bile duct are predominantly supplied by two axial vessels that run in a 3 and a 9 o'clock position. These vessels are derived from the superior pancreaticoduodenal, right hepatic, cystic, gastroduodenal, and retroduodenal arteries. It has been estimated that only 2% of the arterial supply to this portion of the bile duct is segmental and arises directly off of the proper hepatic artery. The bile duct and its bifurcation in the hilum derive their arterial supply from a rich network of multiple small branches from surrounding vessels. Similarly, the retropancreatic bile duct derives its arterial supply from the retroduodenal artery, which provides a rich network of multiple small branches (Fig. 50-14).[30] Venous drainage of the bile duct parallels the arterial supply and drains into the portal venous system. The venous drainage of the gallbladder empties into the veins that drain the bile duct and does not flow directly to the portal vein.

Nerves

The innervation of the liver and biliary tract is via sympathetic fibers originating from T7 through T10 and

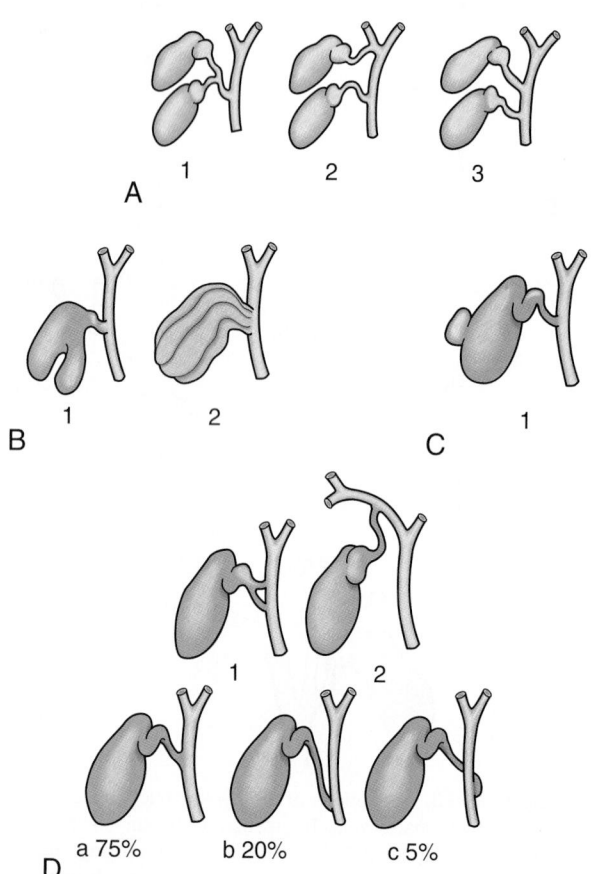

FIGURE 50-13. Variations in the anatomy of the gallbladder and cystic duct. **A,** Bilobar gallbladder. **B,** Septations of the gallbladder. **C,** Diverticulum of the gallbladder. **D,** Variations in cystic duct anatomy. The three types (a, b, c) of union of the cystic duct and common hepatic duct are illustrated. (From Blumgart LH, Hann LE: Surgical and radiologic anatomy of the liver and biliary tract. *In* Blumgart LH, Fong Y [eds]: Surgery of the Liver and Biliary Tract. London, WB Saunders, 2000, pp 3-34.)

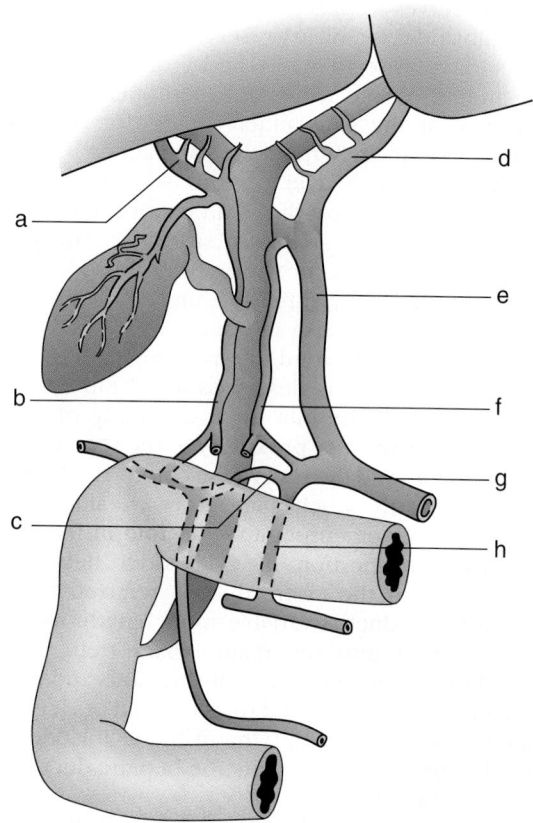

FIGURE 50-14. The blood supply to the common bile duct and common hepatic duct is illustrated: a, right hepatic artery; b, 9:00 artery; c, retroduodenal artery; d, left hepatic artery; e, proper hepatic artery; f, 3:00 artery; g, common hepatic artery; h, gastroduodenal artery. (From Blumgart LH, Hann LE: Surgical and radiologic anatomy of the liver and biliary tract. *In* Blumgart LH, Fong Y [eds]: Surgery of the Liver and Biliary Tract. London, WB Saunders, 2000, pp 3-34.)

parasympathetic fibers from both vagal nerves. The sympathetic fibers pass through celiac ganglia before giving off postganglionic fibers to the liver and bile ducts. The right-sided celiac ganglia and right vagal nerve form an anterior hepatic plexus of nerves that runs along the hepatic artery. The left-sided celiac ganglia and left vagal nerve form a posterior hepatic plexus that runs posterior to the bile duct and portal vein. The hepatic arteries are supplied by sympathetic fibers, whereas the gallbladder and extrahepatic bile ducts receive innervation from both sympathetic and parasympathetic fibers. The clinical significance of these nerves is still not well understood. Pain elicited from acute distention of the liver (and thus the liver capsule) is referred to the right shoulder because of innervation of the capsule from the phrenic nerve.[22]

Lymphatics

The majority of lymph node drainage from the liver is to the hepatoduodenal ligament. From here lymphatic drainage usually continues along the hepatic artery to the celiac lymph nodes and from here to the cisterna chyli. Lymphatic drainage can also follow the hepatic veins to lymph nodes in the area of the suprahepatic IVC and through the diaphragmatic hiatus. The lymphatic drainage of the gallbladder and most of the extrahepatic biliary tract is generally into the lymph nodes of the hepatoduodenal ligament. This drainage can also follow along the hepatic artery to the celiac lymph nodes, but it can also run to lymph nodes behind the head of the pancreas or in the interaortocaval groove.[31]

Microscopic Anatomy

The Functional Unit of the Liver

The organization of hepatic parenchyma into microscopic functional units has been described in a number of ways and referred to as an acinus or a lobule (Fig. 50-15). This was originally described by Rappaport and more recently modified by Matsumoto and Kawakami.[32,33] A lobule is made up of a central terminal hepatic venule surrounded by four to six terminal portal triads forming a polygonal unit. This unit is lined on its periphery (between each terminal portal triad) by terminal portal triad branches. In between the terminal portal triads and the central hepatic

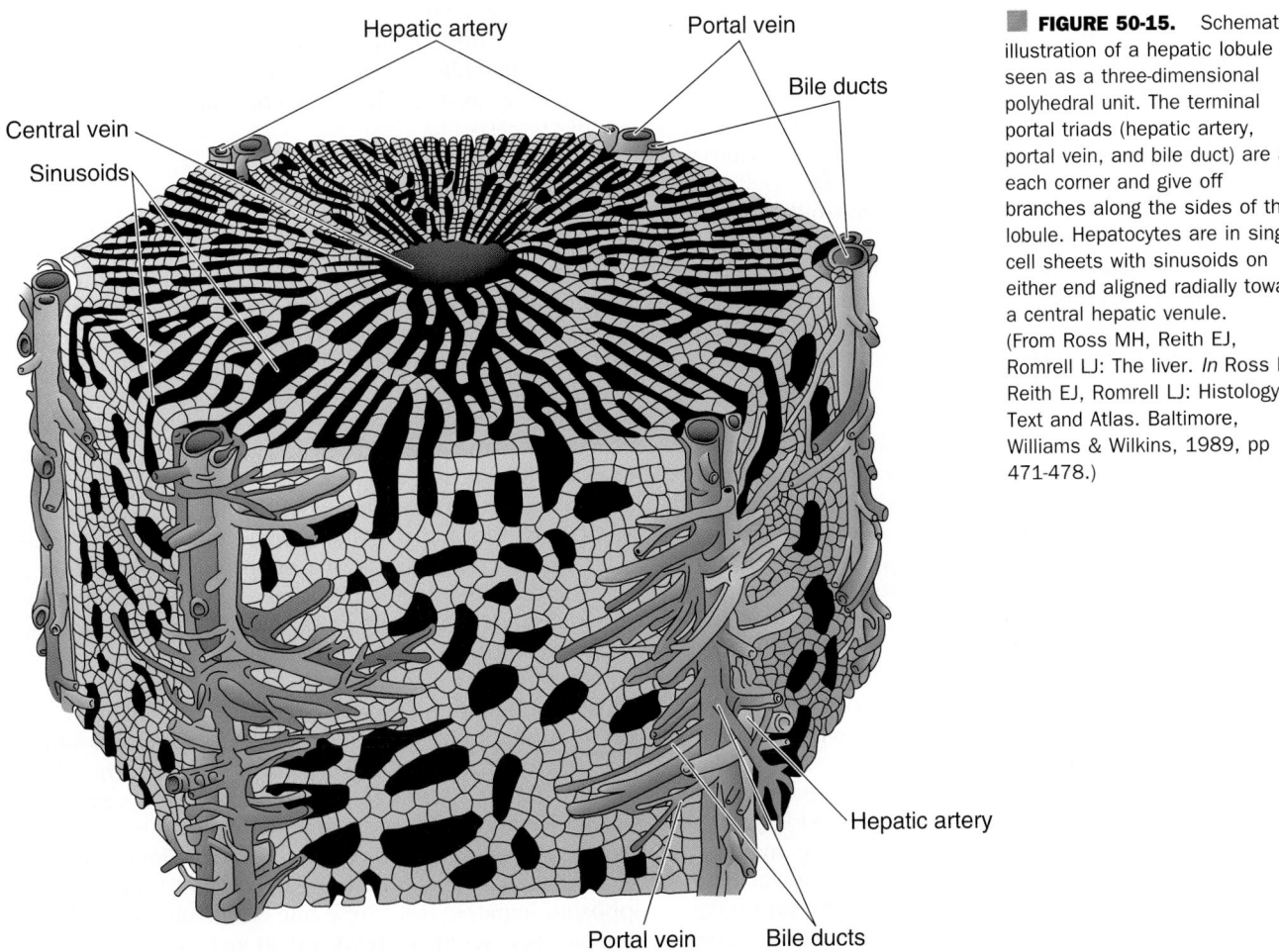

FIGURE 50-15. Schematic illustration of a hepatic lobule seen as a three-dimensional polyhedral unit. The terminal portal triads (hepatic artery, portal vein, and bile duct) are at each corner and give off branches along the sides of the lobule. Hepatocytes are in single cell sheets with sinusoids on either end aligned radially toward a central hepatic venule. (From Ross MH, Reith EJ, Romrell LJ: The liver. *In* Ross RH, Reith EJ, Romrell LJ: Histology: A Text and Atlas. Baltimore, Williams & Wilkins, 1989, pp 471-478.)

Hepatic artery

Portal vein

Bile ducts

Central vein

Sinusoids

Hepatic artery

Portal vein   Bile ducts

venule, hepatocytes are arranged in plates, one cell thick, surrounded on each side by endothelial-lined and blood-filled sinusoids. Blood flows from the terminal portal triad through the sinusoids into the terminal hepatic venule. Bile is formed in the hepatocytes and emptied into terminal canaliculi that form on the lateral walls of the intercellular hepatocyte, ultimately coalescing into bile ducts and flowing toward the portal triads. This functional hepatic unit provides a structural basis for the many metabolic and secretory functions of the liver. Between the terminal portal triad and the central hepatic venule there are three zones that differ in their enzymatic makeup and exposure to nutrients and oxygenated blood. Although there is debate as to the shape of these zones and their relationship to the basic lobular unit, in general, zones 1 through 3 fan out from the terminal portal triad toward the central hepatic venule. Zone 1, known as the periportal zone, is exposed to an environment rich in nutrients and oxygen. Zones 2 (intermediate zone) and 3 (perivenular zone) are exposed to environments less rich in oxygen and nutrients. The cells of the different zones differ enzymatically and respond differently to toxin exposure as well as hypoxia. This anatomic arrangement also explains the phenomenon of centrilobular necrosis from hypotension, with zone 3 being the most susceptible to decreases in oxygen delivery.[34-37]

Hepatic Microcirculation

Terminal portal vessels directly supply sinusoids, providing a constant, but minimal flow into this low volume system. The terminal hepatic arterial branches both empty into the sinusoids and create a plexus of vessels around the terminal small bile ducts, providing nutrients. Arterial branches provide the sinusoids a pulsatile, but low volume flow that enhances flow in the sinusoids. Arterial and portal vein flow vary inversely in the sinusoids and can be compensatory. Local control of blood flow in the sinusoids likely depends on arteriolar sphincters as well as contraction of the sinusoidal lining by endothelial and stellate cells. Blood flow through sinusoids empties directly into terminal hepatic venules at the center of a functional lobule.[38,39]

The endothelial-lined sinusoids of the hepatic lobule provide the functional unit of the liver, where afferent blood flow is exposed to functional hepatic parenchyma before being drained into hepatic venules (Fig. 50-16). The hepatic sinusoids are 7 to 15 μm wide but can increase in size 10-fold, yielding a low-resistance and low-pressure (generally 2 to 3 mm Hg) system. The sinusoidal endothelial cells account for 15% to 20% of the total number of hepatic cells. Sinusoidal endothelial cells are separated from hepatocytes by the space of Disse, which is an extravascular fluid compartment into which hepatocytes project microvilli. Key aspects of these endothelial cells are that they lack intercellular junctions, have no basement membrane, and contain multiple and large fenestrations. This arrangement provides for the maximal contact of hepatocyte membranes, an extravascular fluid compartment (space of Disse), and blood in the sinusoidal space. Thus, this system permits free bidirectional

movement of solutes (high- and low-molecular-weight substances) into and out of hepatocytes, providing tremendous filtration potential. The fenestrations of the endothelial cells restrict movement of molecules between the sinusoids and hepatocytes and vary in response to exogenous as well as endogenous mediators.[34,35,38-42]

Other cell types are found along the sinusoidal lining. Kupffer cells, derived from the macrophage-monocyte system, are irregular stellate-shaped cells that also line the sinusoids, insinuating between endothelial cells. Kupffer cells are phagocytic, can migrate along sinusoids to areas of injury, and play a major role in the trapping of foreign substances and initiating an inflammatory response. Major histocompatibility complex class II antigens are expressed on Kupffer cells but do not confer efficient antigen presentation compared with macrophages elsewhere in the body.[43] Other lymphoid cells also exist in hepatic parenchyma such as natural killer cells and CD4 and CD8 T cells that provide the liver with innate immunity. Hepatic stellate cells (also known as Ito cells or lipocytes) are cells high in lipid content (accounting for their phenotypic identification) found in the space of Disse. They have dendritic processes that contact hepatocyte microvilli and also wrap around endothelial cells. The major function of these stellate cells appears to be vitamin A storage and synthesis of extracellular collagen. In acute and chronic hepatic inflammatory states, these cells are activated to a myofibroblast-like state that is associated with morphologic changes, cellular contractility, decreases in intracellular vitamin A, and production of extracellular collagen. Stellate cells appear to play a central role in the development and progression of hepatic fibrosis.[44]

The Hepatocyte

The hepatocyte is a complex and multifunctional cell that makes up 60% of the cellular mass and 80% of the cytoplasmic mass of the liver (see Fig. 50-16). Morphologically, the hepatocyte is polyhedral with a central spherical nucleus. As mentioned earlier, hepatocytes are arranged in single cell layer plates that are lined on either side by blood-filled sinusoids. Every hepatocyte has contact with adjacent hepatocytes, with the biliary space (bile canaliculus) and the sinusoidal space allowing its broad range of functions. Among the many essential functions performed by the hepatocyte are uptake, storage, and release of nutrients; synthesis of multiple plasma proteins, glucose fatty acids, and lipids; production and secretion of bile (and thus digestion of dietary fats); and degradation and detoxification of toxins. The plasma membrane of the hepatocyte is organized into three specific domains. The sinusoidal membrane is exposed to the space of Disse and has multiple microvilli that provide a surface specialized in the active transport of substances between the blood and hepatocyte. The lateral domain exists between neighboring hepatocytes and contains gap junctions that provide for intercellular communication. The canalicular membrane is a tube containing microvilli formed by two apposing hepatocytes. These bile canaliculi are sealed by zonulae occludentes (tight junctions), which prevent

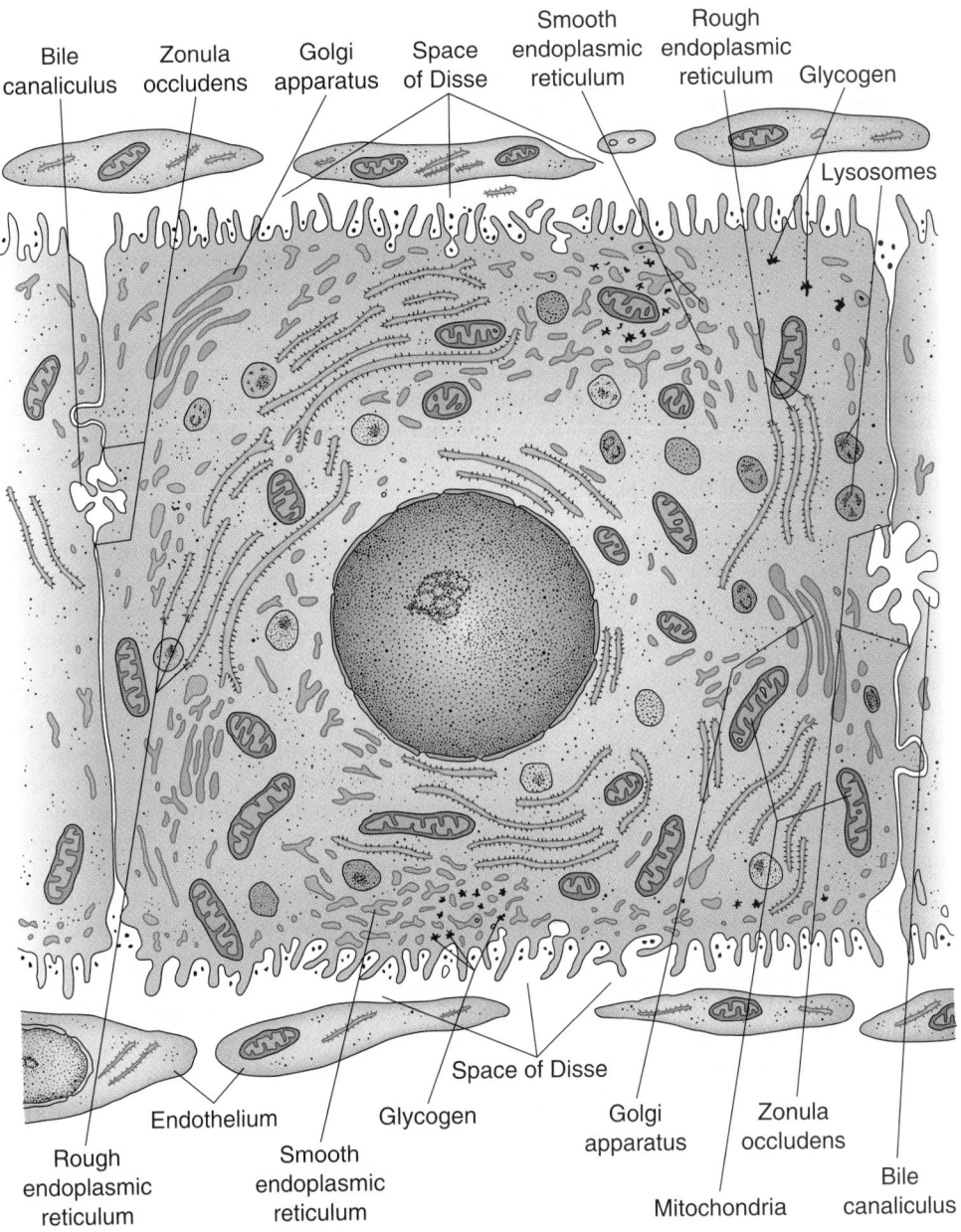

Bile canaliculus — Zonula occludens — Golgi apparatus — Space of Disse — Smooth endoplasmic reticulum — Rough endoplasmic reticulum — Glycogen — Lysosomes

Space of Disse — Glycogen — Golgi apparatus — Zonula occludens — Bile canaliculus — Endothelium — Rough endoplasmic reticulum — Smooth endoplasmic reticulum — Mitochondria

Lumen of Sinusoid

FIGURE 50-16. Illustration of a hepatocyte. Intracellular organelles are depicted. The endothelial-lined sinusoids on two sides of the cell are seen. In between the microvilli of the plasma membrane of the hepatocyte and the sinusoids the extracellular fluid space of Disse is demonstrated. Along the lateral intercellular plasma membrane, bile canaliculi are formed by the apposing cells where microvilli extend into the canaliculus. Envisioning the cell in three dimensions, the bile canaliculi form a ring around each hepatocyte. (From Ross MH, Reith EJ, Romrell LJ: The liver. In Ross RH, Reith EJ, Romrell LJ: Histology: A Text and Atlas. Baltimore, Williams & Wilkins, 1989, pp 471-478.)

escape of bile. The bile canaliculi form a ring around the hepatocyte and drain into small bile ducts known as canals of Hering that ultimately empty into a bile duct at a portal triad. The canalicular membrane contains adenosine triphosphate (ATP)-dependent active transport systems that enable solutes to be secreted into the canalicular membrane against large concentration gradients.[34-36,45]

The hepatocyte is one of the most diverse and metabolically active cells in the body, which is reflected in its abundance of organelles. There are 1000 mitochondria per hepatocyte, occupying 20% of the cell volume. Mitochondria generate energy (ATP) through oxidative phosphorylation and provide the energy for the metabolic demands of the hepatocyte. The hepatocyte mitochondria are also essential for fatty acid oxidation. An extensive system of interconnected membrane complexes composed of smooth and rough endoplasmic reticulum and the Golgi complex make up what is known as the hepatocyte microsomal fraction. These complexes have a diverse range of functions, including synthesis of secretory and structural proteins, metabolism of lipids and glucose, production and metabolism of cholesterol, glycosylation of secretory proteins, bile formation and secretion, and drug metabolism. Lysosomes are intracellular single membrane vesicles that contain a number of enzymes and both store and degrade exogenous and endogenous substances.[32,34,35]

Function

The unique anatomic arrangement of the liver just described provides a remarkable landscape on which the multiple central and critical functions of this organ can be carried out. The liver is the center of metabolic homeostasis. It serves as the regulatory site for energy metabolism by coordinating the uptake, processing, and distribution of nutrients and their subsequent energy products. The liver also synthesizes a large number of proteins, enzymes, and vitamins that participate in a tremendously broad range of bodily functions. Lastly, the liver detoxifies and eliminates many exogenous and endogenous substances, serving as the major filter of the human body.

Energy

The liver is the critical intermediary between dietary sources of energy and the extrahepatic tissues that require this energy. The critical and central nature of the liver in regulating the body's energy metabolism is evidenced by the fact that despite accounting for only 4% of body weight, the liver consumes about 28% of the total body blood flow and 20% of the total oxygen intake. The liver also expends about 20% of the total kilocalories used by the whole body.

The liver receives dietary byproducts through the portal circulation, sorts them, metabolizes them, and distributes them to the systemic circulation. The liver also plays a major role in regulating systemic sources of energy such as fatty acids and glycerol from adipose tissues and lactate, pyruvate, and certain amino acids from skeletal muscle. The two major sources of energy that the liver releases into the extrahepatic circulation are glucose and acetoacetate. Glucose is derived from glycogenolysis of stored glycogen and from gluconeogenesis from lactate, pyruvate, glycerol, propionate, and alanine. Acetoacetate is derived from the oxidation of fatty acids. Storage lipids such as triacylglycerols and phospholipids are synthesized and stored as lipoproteins by the liver as well. These can be carried in the systemic circulation to the peripheral tissues. These complex and essential functions are regulated by hormones, by the overall nutritional state of the organism, and by the needs of obligate glucose-requiring tissues.[46,47]

Functional Heterogeneity

To add to the metabolic complexity of the liver, hepatocytes vary in their function depending on their location within the functional lobule. Additionally, hepatocytes can change their metabolic functionality and be recruited to perform specific functions under varying physiologic conditions. This functional heterogeneity of hepatocytes is anatomically related to their location within the three zones of the lobule and is specifically related to the distance from the incoming portal triad. Cells located in the periportal zone (zone 1) are exposed to a high concentration of substrate and uptake of oxygen and solutes are greater. The sinusoids are also variable in form and function. Sinusoids in the periportal zone are narrower and more tortuous, facilitating increased uptake of substrate by the hepatocyte in this area. In contrast, sinusoids in zone 3 (perivenous) have larger fenestrations, allowing uptake of larger molecules.

Enzymatic makeup, plasma membrane proteins, and ultrastructure are also heterogeneous among the hepatocyte population. This cellular protein variability can also be distinguished based on the hepatocyte location within the lobule. Glucose uptake and release, bile formation, and synthesis of albumin and fibrinogen take place in the periportal zone while glucose catabolism, xenobiotic metabolism, and synthesis of α_1-antitrypsin and α-fetoprotein (AFP) occur in the perivenous zone. Another example of enzymatic heterogeneity according to lobular zones is the location of the urea cycle enzymes in zone 3 adjacent to the terminal hepatic vein. The functional hepatocyte heterogeneity and its anatomic relationship to the lobular unit account for patterns of damage from metabolic or physiologic insults to the liver.[37-39]

Blood Flow

The blood supply to the liver is dual and comes from the portal vein and the hepatic artery. The portal vein provides about 75% of the blood flow to the liver, which is oxygen poor but rich in nutrients. The hepatic artery provides the other 25% of the blood flow and is oxygen rich, representing systemic arterial flow. The large flow rate of the portal vein is still able to provide 50% to 70% of the afferent oxygenation to the liver. Overall, hepatic blood flow represents about one fourth of the cardiac output, demonstrating its central role in whole-body metabolism. Hepatic blood flow is decreased during exercise and increased after ingestion of food (carbohydrates have the most profound effect on hepatic blood flow). Hepatic arterial pressure is representative of systemic arterial pressure. Portal pressures are generally 6 to 10 mm Hg, and sinusoidal pressure is usually 2 to 4 mm Hg.

Hepatic blood flow is regulated by a variety of factors. Differences in afferent and efferent vessel pressures as well as muscular sphincters located at the inlet and outlet of the sinusoids play a major role. Muscular sphincter tone is regulated by the autonomic nervous system, circulating hormones, bile salts, and metabolites. Specific endogenous factors known to affect hepatic blood flow include glucagon, histamine, bradykinin, prostaglandins, nitric oxide, and many gut hormones, including gastrin, secretin, and cholecystokinin. The sinusoids themselves, primarily through contraction and expansion of their endothelial cells, Kupffer cells, and stellate cells, are also primary regulators of hepatic blood flow.[42]

A one-way reciprocal relationship between hepatic artery and portal vein flow has been demonstrated. Increases in hepatic arterial flow accompany decreases in portal vein flow, but the opposite does not occur. Hepatic arterial compensation, however, cannot provide complete compensation to support hepatic parenchyma in the case of total portal vein occlusion. Experimental evidence suggests that the buildup of adenosine in the liver plays an important role in this hepatic arterial compensatory response.

Bile Formation

Bile production and secretion is one of the major functions of the liver. The physiologic role of bile is twofold:

TABLE 50-1. Solute Concentrations of Hepatic Bile in Humans

Solute	Concentration
Na^+	132-165 mEq/L
K^+	4.2-5.6 mEq/L
Ca^{2+}	1.2-4.8 mEq/L
Mg^{2+}	1.4-3.0 mEq/L
Cl^-	96-126 mEq/L
HCO_3^-	17-55 mEq/L
Bile acids	3-45 mM
Phospholipid	25-810 mg/dL
Cholesterol	60-320 mg/dL
Protein	300-3000 mg/L

(1) to dispose of certain substances secreted into bile and (2) to provide enteric bile salts to aid in the digestion of fats. Bile is a substance containing organic and inorganic solutes that is produced by an active process of secretion and subsequent concentration of these solutes. The concentration of inorganic solutes in bile in the main biliary tree resembles plasma (Table 50-1). The osmolality of bile is approximately 300 mOsm/kg and is accounted for by the inorganic solutes. The major organic solutes in bile are bile acids, bile pigments, cholesterol, and phospholipids.

The contents of bile are generally absorbed from the bloodstream through sinusoids into the hepatocyte through the sinusoidal membrane. Bile is initially secreted by hepatocytes into the canaliculi through the specialized microvilli containing lateral membranes of the hepatocytes that form the canaliculi. Tight junctions along the canalicular membranes prevent leakage of bile in the normal state but also provide a route for paracellular secretion of solutes and water into bile. The canaliculi ultimately coalesce into larger bile ductules containing biliary epithelium, which then form the intrahepatic and extrahepatic biliary tree. Thus, the liver, in part, serves as an epithelial structure that moves solutes from blood to bile and provides a route of secretion of bile into the intestines.

Approximately 1500 mL of bile is secreted daily, 80% of which is secreted by hepatocytes into canaliculi. Canalicular bile flow is largely due to water flow in response to active solute transport. Bile acids are transported from the sinusoidal blood into the hepatocyte by ATP-requiring active transport. Intracellular transport to the canalicular membrane is through bile acid–binding proteins that are transported by a vesicular system derived from the Golgi apparatus. The bile acids are then actively pumped into the canaliculus through an ATP-requiring active transport system. It is well recognized that bile flow has a linear association with bile acid secretion, known as *bile acid–dependent flow*. Because bile acids are micellar in bile and do not provide osmotic potential, it is likely

that flow related to bile acid secretion is secondary to ions that accompany the bile acids (counter-ions). Bile flow can also occur in the near absence of bile acid secretion and is known as *bile acid–independent flow*. Experimental evidence suggests that bile acid–independent flow is at least partially the result of biliary glutathione secretion.

Once bile has passed from the canaliculi to the biliary ductules and main bile ducts, bile undergoes further reabsorption and secretion. The epithelial cells of the biliary lining actively reabsorb and secrete water and electrolytes. Secretion is generally through a chloride channel that is activated by secretin (its most powerful activator) and its subsequent activation of cyclic adenosine monophosphate (AMP) production. There is generally a net secretion of water and electrolytes (accounting for the other 20% of biliary secretion), and, in particular, bile becomes highly enriched in bicarbonate ions. Many organic substances such as glutathione are degraded in the biliary tree. Many drugs can be secreted into the biliary tree in a highly concentrated form (e.g., ceftriaxone). The gallbladder acts as the reservoir of the biliary tree whose function is to store bile in the fasting state. The gallbladder reabsorbs water, concentrates stored bile, and secretes mucin. Contraction of the gallbladder is mediated hormonally (largely through cholecystokinin) in response to a meal, with the simultaneous relaxation of the sphincter of Oddi and release of bile into the duodenum.[45,48]

Enterohepatic Circulation

Bile salts are primarily produced in the liver and secreted to be used in the biliary tree and the intestine. The primary bile salts cholic acid and chenodeoxycholic acid are produced in the liver from cholesterol and subsequently conjugated with glycine or taurine within the hepatocyte. Once secreted in the gut, the primary bile acids are modified by intestinal bacteria, forming secondary bile acids deoxycholic acid and lithocholic acid. Bile acids are reabsorbed passively in the jejunum and actively in the ileum into the portal venous system, where up to 90% of the bile acids are extracted by hepatocytes. Only a small fraction spills over into the systemic circulation because of efficient hepatic extraction accounting for low levels of plasma bile acids. After hepatic extraction, bile acids are recirculated into canaliculi and back into the biliary tree, completing the circuit. A small amount of intestinal bile acids are not absorbed by the portal system and are excreted in the stool. Thus, the active secretion of bile salts from hepatocyte to bile and from ileal enterocytes to the portal vein is the engine behind the enterohepatic circulation.

The enterohepatic circulation is more than a unique physiologic mechanism of reusing physiologically valuable bile acids. This circulation of bile constitutes the major mechanism of eliminating excess cholesterol by consuming cholesterol in the production of bile salts as well as accumulating cholesterol in mixed micelles formed by organic biliary solutes with eventual fecal loss. Bile salts also play a critical role in the absorption of dietary fats, fat-soluble vitamins, and lipophilic drugs. Water movement from hepatocytes into bile and water absorption through the small bowel is also regulated by bile salts. Thus, the enterohepatic circulation is central to a number of solubilization, transport, and regulatory functions.[49]

Bilirubin Metabolism

Bilirubin is the result of heme breakdown. An early phase of heme breakdown, accounting for 20% of bilirubin, is from hemoproteins (heme-containing enzymes) and occurs within 3 days of labeling with radioactive heme. A late phase of heme breakdown, accounting for 80% of bilirubin, is from senescent red blood cells and occurs in about 110 days (life span of a red blood cell) after administering labeled radioactive heme. Heme is initially broken down into green-colored biliverdin by heme oxygenase, which is then broken down into the orange-colored bilirubin by biliverdin reductase.

Circulating bilirubin is bound to albumin, which protects many organs from the potentially toxic effects of this compound. The bilirubin-albumin complex enters hepatic sinusoidal blood from which it enters the space of Disse through the large sinusoidal fenestrations and is disassociated in this space. Free bilirubin is then internalized into the hepatocyte, where it is conjugated to glucuronic acid. Conjugated bilirubin is then secreted in an energy-dependent fashion into canalicular bile against a large concentration gradient. Bilirubin is then secreted with bile into the gastrointestinal tract. Within the gastrointestinal tract, bilirubin is deconjugated by intestinal bacteria to a group of compounds known as urobilinogens. These urobilinogens are further oxidized and reabsorbed into the enterohepatic circulation and secreted into bile. A small percentage of the reabsorbed urobilinogens are excreted into urine. It is these oxidized urobilinogens that account for the colored compounds that contribute to the yellow color of urine and the brown color of stool.

Bilirubin has long been known to be a toxic compound and is the agent responsible for neonatal encephalopathy and cochlear damage secondary to severe unconjugated hyperbilirubinemia (kernicterus). The binding of serum bilirubin to albumin protects the tissues from exposure to bilirubin, but binding sites can be overwhelmed by increasing amounts of bilirubin or displaced by other binding agents such as many drugs. The mechanism of bilirubin toxicity appears to be related to a number of its effects. Free bilirubin can uncouple oxidative phosphorylation, inhibit ATPase, reduce glucose metabolism, and inhibit a broad spectrum of protein kinase activity.

Portosystemic shunts, such as those seen with cirrhosis and portal hypertension, decrease the first-pass hepatic clearance of bilirubin, resulting in a mildly increased serum unconjugated hyperbilirubinemia. A number of disorders can result in a serum unconjugated hyperbilirubinemia, such as the aforementioned neonatal hyperbilirubinemia, increased bilirubin load (hemolytic syndromes), and inherited enzymatic deficiencies such as Crigler-Najjar syndrome and Gilbert's syndrome. Disorders presenting with serum conjugated hyperbilirubinemia include cholestasis syndromes, Dubin-Johnson syndrome, and Rotor's syndrome.[50]

Carbohydrate Metabolism

The liver is the center of carbohydrate metabolism because it is the major regulator of storage and distribution of glucose to the peripheral tissues and, in particular, to the glucose-dependent tissues such as the brain and erythrocytes. Both liver and muscle are capable of storing glucose in the form of glycogen, but only the liver is able to break down glycogen to provide glucose for systemic circulation. Broken-down muscular glycogen can only be used within muscle and is therefore not a source of systemically circulated glucose.[51,52]

In the fed state, carbohydrate absorbed through the intestines (mostly glucose) is circulated systemically. Carbohydrate reaching the liver is rapidly converted to its storage form of glycogen (up to 65 g of glycogen per kilogram of liver tissue). Excess carbohydrate is mostly converted to fatty acids and stored in adipose tissue. In the postabsorptive state (between meals/nonfasting), there is no further systemic glucose coming directly from the gut and the liver becomes the primary source of circulating glucose by the breakdown of glycogen. This is crucial for the brain and erythrocytes that rely on glucose for their own metabolism. Most other tissues, in the postabsorptive state, begin to rely on fatty acids derived from adipose tissue as their primary fuel. Highly active muscle may deplete its own glycogen and depend on liver-derived glucose for substrate in the postabsorptive state. After 48 hours of fasting, hepatic glycogen is depleted and the liver shifts from glycogen breakdown to gluconeogenesis. The substrate for hepatic gluconeogenesis is mostly from amino acids (mainly alanine) derived from muscle breakdown, but it also comes from glycerol derived from adipose breakdown. During a prolonged fast, fatty acids from adipose breakdown are beta-oxidized in the liver, releasing ketone bodies that then become the primary fuel of the brain.[53,54]

Transition in and out of these various metabolic states and regulation of carbohydrate metabolism is mostly from glucose concentration in sinusoidal blood and from hormonal (insulin, catecholamines, and glucagon) influence. In the fasting state, during anaerobic metabolism, lactate, largely from muscle, is produced. The liver uses this lactate and by conversion to pyruvate and entrance into gluconeogenic pathways produces glucose. This cycle is known as the Cori cycle.[51]

Derangements of carbohydrate metabolism are common in liver disease. Cirrhotics often demonstrate abnormal glucose tolerance. The mechanism of this is not completely clear but is probably related to an associated insulin resistance. This phenomenon is not due to shunting of glucose containing blood away from the liver. Hypoglycemia is a distinctly uncommon entity in chronic liver disease, owing to the remarkable resilience of the liver and its metabolic function. Only with massive hepatocyte loss in fulminant hepatic failure does gluconeogenesis fail and hypoglycemia ensue.[51,52]

Lipid Metabolism

Fatty acids are synthesized in the liver during states of glucose excess when the liver's ability to store glycogen has been exceeded. Adipocytes have a limited ability to synthesize fatty acids, and, therefore, the liver is the predominant source of synthesized fatty acids, although they are largely stored in adipose tissue. During lipolysis, free fatty acids are transported to the liver, where their metabolism takes place. Fatty acids in the liver either undergo esterification with glycerol to form triglycerides for storage or transportation or they undergo oxidation yielding energy in the form of ATP and ketone bodies. In general, this process is regulated by the nutritional state, with starvation favoring oxidation and the fed state favoring esterification.[51,52,55]

There is a constant cycling of fatty acids between the liver and adipose tissue that is under a delicate balance. This balance can easily be offset, resulting in fatty infiltration of the liver. A few factors influence this balance. Hepatic uptake of fatty acids is a function of plasma concentrations. While there is no limit in the liver's ability to esterify fatty acids, its ability to dispose of or break down fatty acids is limited. The liver is also limited in its ability to secrete triglycerides in the form of lipoproteins. Therefore, conditions of increased circulating fatty acids can easily override the liver's ability to handle them, resulting in fatty accumulation in the liver. Examples of such conditions are diabetes, steroids, and starvation, all of which act through increased lipolysis. Fatty liver associated with alcohol intake is multifactorial and related to increased lipolysis, reduced oxygenation, and augmented esterification of hepatic fatty acids and may also be related to relative starvation in the chronic alcoholic.[56]

Protein Metabolism

The liver is also a central site for the metabolism of proteins and is involved in protein synthesis, catabolism of proteins into energy or storage forms, and managing excess amino acids and nitrogen waste. Ingested protein is broken down into amino acids and circulated throughout the body, where they are used as the building blocks for proteins, enzymes, hormones, and nucleotides. Excess amino acids not used in peripheral tissues are generally handled by the liver, where they are oxidized for energy (providing 50% of the liver's energy needs) or converted into glucose, ketone bodies, or fats. When amino acids are catabolized for energy production throughout the body, ammonia, glutamine, glutamate, and aspartate are produced. These products are largely dealt with in the liver, where the waste nitrogen is converted to urea via the urea cycle. The urea is generally excreted in the urine. The liver, therefore, is central and critical to whole-body nitrogen balance as well as the amino acid metabolism.[57]

While the liver can catabolize most amino acids yielding energy or other storable energy forms such as glucose or fats, a notable exception are the branched-chain amino acids. Branched-chain amino acids cannot be catabolized in the liver and are mostly dealt with by muscle. It has been postulated that this is somewhat of a "safety net" that helps to spare the liver some of the demands of protein and amino acid metabolism.[57,58]

The liver also is the main site of synthesis for many proteins that are involved in such wide-ranging and critical functions as coagulation, transport, iron binding, and protease inhibition. Examples of these proteins are α_1-antitrypsin, ceruloplasmin, and iron storage/binding proteins. Albumin is made exclusively in the liver and is the predominant serum binding protein. Hepatic insufficiency or specific genetic abnormalities can result in altered amounts and function of these proteins with wide-ranging pathologic effects.

The liver is also responsible for the so-called acute phase response, a protein synthetic response by the liver to trauma or infection. The purpose of the response is to restrict organ damage, to maintain vital hepatic function, and to control defense mechanisms. The response is incited by proinflammatory cytokines such as interleukin (IL)-1, IL-6, and tumor necrosis factor (TNF), which induce acute-phase protein gene expression in the liver. Some of the well-known hepatic acute-phase proteins are α_1, α_2, and β globulin, C-reactive protein, and serum amyloid A. An equally important part of this response is its termination. Anti-inflammatory cytokines such as IL-1 receptor antagonist, IL-4, and IL-10 appear to play an important role. The acute phase response is usually over in 24 to 48 hours, but in the context of ongoing injury it can be prolonged.

Vitamin Metabolism

Along with the intestine, the liver is responsible for the metabolism of the fat-soluble vitamins A, D, E, and K. These vitamins are obtained exogenously and absorbed in the intestine. Their adequate intestinal absorption is critically dependent on adequate fatty acid micellization, which requires bile acids. Vitamin A is from the retinoid family and is involved in normal vision, embryonic development, and adult gene regulation. Storage of vitamin A is solely in the liver and believed to be in the stellate cells (Ito cells). Overingestion of vitamin A can result in hepatic toxicity. Vitamin D is involved in calcium/phosphorus homeostasis, and one of its activation steps (25 hydroxylation) occurs in the liver. Vitamin E is a potent antioxidant and protects membranes from lipid peroxidation and free radical formation. Vitamin K is a critical cofactor in the post-translational γ-carboxylation of the hepatically synthesized coagulation factors II, VII, IX, X, protein C, and protein S (so-called vitamin K–dependent factors), which is essential to their activity. Cholestasis syndromes result in inadequate absorption of these vitamins secondary to poor micellization in the intestine. The associated vitamin deficiency syndromes such as metabolic bone disease (D), neurologic disorders (E), and coagulopathy (K) can subsequently occur.[52,59]

The liver is also involved in the uptake, storage, and metabolism of a variety of water-soluble vitamins. These vitamins include thiamine, riboflavin, vitamin B_6, vitamin B_{12}, folate, biotin, and pantothenic acid. The liver is responsible for converting some of these water-soluble vitamins to active coenzymes. It transforms some to storage metabolites, and some are involved in the enterohepatic circulation (vitamin B_{12}).

Coagulation

The liver is responsible for synthesizing almost all of the identified coagulation factors as well as many of the fibrinolytic system components and several plasma regulatory proteins of coagulation and fibrinolysis. As mentioned earlier, the liver is critical in the absorption of vitamin K, synthesizes the vitamin K–dependent coagulation factors, and contains the enzyme that activates these factors. Additionally, the reticuloendothelial system of the liver clears activated clotting factors, activated complexes of the coagulation and fibrinolytic systems, and the end products of fibrin degradation. Diseases of the liver are also often associated with thrombocytopenia, qualitative abnormalities of platelets, vitamin K deficiency, impaired modulation of vitamin K–dependent coagulation factors, and disseminated intravascular coagulation. It is no surprise, therefore, that liver disease is firmly associated with coagulation disorders that are often challenging to deal with.

Warfarin, one of the most commonly dispensed anticoagulants, acts in the liver by blocking vitamin K–dependent activation of factors II, VII, IX, and X. Factor VII has the shortest half-life of the coagulation factors, and its deficiency is manifested clinically as abnormalities of the measured prothrombin time. Patients with hepatic synthetic dysfunction similarly have abnormal prothrombin times.[52,59]

Metabolism of Drugs and Toxins (Xenobiotics)

The human body is exposed to an inordinate amount of foreign chemicals in a lifetime, posing a challenge to our bodies to be able to detoxify and eliminate these potentially harmful chemicals. Many of these chemicals are not incorporated into cellular metabolism and are referred to as xenobiotics. The liver plays a central role in handling these chemicals through an enormously complex and numerous set of enzymes and reaction pathways that are increasingly recognized as newer chemicals are discovered.

Hepatic-based reactions to xenobiotics are broadly classified into phase I and II reactions. Phase I reactions, through oxidation, reduction, and hydrolysis, increase the polarity and thus water solubility of compounds. This, in turn, allows for easier excretion. It is important to realize that phase I reactions do not necessarily detoxify chemicals and may, in fact, create toxic metabolites. An example of phase I reactions is the cytochrome p450 system. Phase II reactions generally act to create a less toxic or less active byproduct. This is generally accomplished through transferase reactions in which a compound is usually coupled to a conjugate, rendering the xenobiotic less dangerous.[60]

Regeneration

The liver possesses the unique quality of adjusting its volume to the needs of the body. This is observed clinically in its regeneration after partial hepatectomy or after toxic injury. It is additionally seen in liver transplant patients in that liver size mismatches adjust to the new host. This quality is highly conserved evolutionarily because of the critical functions of the liver and the fact that the liver is the first line of exposure to ingested toxic agents.

Liver regeneration is a hyperplastic response of all cell types of the liver in which ultimately the microscopic anatomy of the functional liver is maintained. Much of the information we have about the regenerative response of the liver is based on experimental evidence in rodents. Normally quiescent hepatocytes rapidly reenter the cell cycle after partial hepatectomy. Maximal hepatocyte DNA synthesis occurs 24 to 36 hours after partial hepatectomy, and maximal DNA synthesis of the other cell types occurs 48 to 72 hours later. Most of the increase in hepatic mass in rodents is seen by 3 days after partial hepatectomy and is usually nearly complete in 7 days.[61,62]

In the late 1960s it was recognized that circulating factors were responsible, in part, for the regenerative response and over the past 40 years a large amount of research has gone into the humoral and genetic control of hepatic regeneration. The major circulating factors that have been identified (largely from rodent studies) are hepatocyte growth factor, epidermal growth factor, transforming growth factors, insulin, and glucagon, as well as the cytokines TNF, IL-1, and IL-6. These factors when infused into a normal host do not result in hepatic growth, indicating that hepatocytes must be primed in some way before responding to these growth factors. The mediators of this process are not completely known. Ongoing genetic and molecular studies continue to define this remarkable and complex process.[63,64]

Future Developments

The study of the liver and its physiology continues to be a remarkable and exciting field. As the fields of molecular biology and genetic manipulation have exploded, so has the field of hepatology. Given the lack of alternative options to transplantation for patients with end-stage liver failure, tissue engineering and attempts to provide exogenous hepatic functional support continue to be researched. The complexity and wide-ranging functions of the liver make this a very challenging field. Liver repopulation with transplanted cells (hepatocytes or liver stem cells) may provide future options for patients with liver failure as well. Ongoing genetic comparisons of normal and diseased liver will provide clues into the genetic regulation of liver diseases. Great strides have been made in the effectiveness of gene therapy, and many groups continue to study liver-directed gene therapy strategies to treat acquired and inherited disorders. Ongoing molecular biology studies are researching hepatic cell cycle regulation with implications for regeneration and hepatocarcinogenesis.

Assessment of Liver Function

A wide variety of tests are available to evaluate hepatic diseases. Screening for hepatic disease, assessing hepatic function, diagnosing specific disorders, and prognosticating are critical in the management of hepatic pathology. For the surgeon, assessment of hepatic function and estimating the ability of a hepatic remnant to be sufficient after liver resection is also of obvious importance. Unfortunately, most measures of hepatic disease are gross and lack sensitivity, specificity, and accuracy. We have divided these tests into the following categories: routine screening tests, specific diagnostic tests, and quantitative tests of hepatic function.

Screening blood tests are often used to simply ask the question, is there a pathologic process in the hepatobiliary system? Standard liver function tests (LFTs) are generally not tests of function and are not always specific to hepatic pathology. Nonetheless they are valuable as a general screening method that can provide the basic tools to recognize the presence of hepatic disease and give clues about the etiology of that disease. Total bilirubin, direct bilirubin (conjugated), and indirect bilirubin (unconjugated) levels can be affected by a number of processes that are related to the metabolism of bilirubin. Unconjugated hyperbilirubinemia can be a reflection of increased bilirubin production (e.g., hemolysis), drug effects, inherited enzymatic disorders, and the physiologic jaundice of the newborn. Conjugated hyperbilirubinemia is generally a result of cholestasis or mechanical biliary obstruction, but it can also be seen in some inherited disorders or hepatocellular disease. The transaminases alanine aminotransferase (ALT) and aspartate aminotransferase (AST) are the most common serum markers of hepatocellular necrosis, with subsequent leak of these intracellular enzymes into the circulation. AST is found in a variety of other organs (heart, muscle, and kidney), but ALT is liver specific. The level of elevation of these enzymes has never been shown to be of prognostic value. Alkaline phosphatase (ALP) is expressed in liver, bile ducts, bone, intestine, placenta, kidney, and leukocytes. Isoenzyme determinations can sometimes be helpful in distinguishing the source of an elevated ALP. Elevations of ALP in hepatobiliary diseases are generally secondary to cholestasis or biliary obstruction and are caused by increased production of the enzyme. ALP can also be elevated in malignant disease of the liver. γ-Glutamyltranspeptidase (GGT) is an enzyme in many organs aside from the liver (kidney, seminal vesicle, spleen, pancreas, heart, and brain) and can be elevated in diseases affecting any of these. It is induced by alcohol intake and is elevated in biliary obstruction. It is also a nonspecific marker of liver disease, but it can be helpful in determining if an elevated ALP level is from hepatic pathology. 5'-Nucleotidase is also found in a wide variety of organs besides the liver, but increased levels are fairly specific to hepatic pathology. Like GGT, it can be helpful in determining whether an elevated ALP level is secondary to hepatic pathology. Albumin is synthesized exclusively in the liver and can be used as a general measure of hepatic synthetic function. Because chronic malnutrition and acute injury/inflammation can decrease albumin synthesis these factors must be taken into account when evaluating a low serum albumin level. Because of the remarkable protein synthetic capacity of the liver, hypoalbuminemia as a marker of liver

disease lacks sensitivity, and tremendous decreases in hepatic function are required to be reflected in albumin levels. In general, it is most helpful in chronic liver disease. Clotting factors are largely synthesized in the liver, and abnormalities of clotting can be a marker of diminished hepatic synthetic function. Measures of specific clotting factors such as factors V and VII have been used to evaluate hepatic function in the transplant population. The prothrombin time is the best test to measure the effects of hepatic disease on clotting and is usually a marker of advanced chronic liver disease. Hepatic pathology can also affect clotting through intravascular coagulation and vitamin K malabsorption.[49,65,66]

Once screening tests, along with clinical findings, have suggested liver disease, specific tests can be used to help elucidate the etiology and guide treatment if necessary. Serologic studies for hepatitis are important to determine the presence of viral hepatitis. Autoimmune antibodies are used to diagnose primary biliary cirrhosis (antimitochondrial), primary sclerosing cholangitis (antineutrophil), and autoimmune hepatitis. α_1-Antitrypsin and ceruloplasmin levels assist in the diagnosis of α_1-antitrypsin deficiency and Wilson's disease, respectively. Tumor markers such as AFP and carcinoembryonic antigen (CEA) can be helpful in the diagnosis and management of primary and metastatic tumors of the liver.

The LFTs discussed earlier, in general, are gross, nonspecific, and contain little, if any, prognostic value. Many attempts have been made to formulate dynamic and quantitative tests of hepatic function based on the liver's ability to clear various exogenously administered substances. Despite many years of research, it still remains unclear whether these tests of hepatic function are any better than scoring systems derived from simple blood tests and clinical observations.

The aminopyrine breath test is based on the clearance, by the hepatic p450 system, of radiolabeled aminopyrine. A breath test measuring radiolabeled CO_2 as a breakdown product of aminopyrine is performed after administration at a specified time. The results largely depend on the functional hepatic mass, which is generally not depleted until end-stage liver disease. There are varying results of studies comparing the aminopyrine breath test to standard LFTs and scoring systems. Its main value appears to be prognosis in chronic liver disease, but it is clearly not an effective test to detect subclinical hepatic dysfunction. Substances such as antipyrine and caffeine can evaluate liver function in a similar way with similar results. The lidocaine clearance test yields similar information to the aminopyrine test because it is based on its clearance by the hepatic p450 test. Lidocaine clearance is dependent on blood flow and a complex distribution process, but measurement of one of its metabolites, monoethylglycinexylidide (MEGX), has greatly simplified the test. This test has been shown to have some prognostic value in the transplant population. The galactose elimination test is based on the liver's role in phosphorylating galactose and converting it to glucose. The rate at which galactose is eliminated from the bloodstream can be a measure of hepatic function. Problems related to this test are that the enzymes involved are genetically heterogeneous and considerable extrahepatic metabolism occurs. Additionally, multiple blood samples are necessary, making the test cumbersome. The value of this test has also largely been in assessing prognosis in chronic liver disease rather than screening. Indocyanine green is a dye removed by the liver by a carrier-mediated process and excreted into bile. This dye is rapidly cleared from the bloodstream and is not metabolized. This is the only test that has been shown to have some prognostic ability in cirrhotic patients undergoing liver resection, although this is not universally demonstrated in studies, nor is it universally accepted.[49,67]

Lastly, a large number of scoring systems based on clinical observation and standard blood tests have been proposed. The most commonly used system is Pugh's modification of the Child score (Table 50-2). Although all of these systems are less than perfect and not universally accepted, the Child-Pugh score is commonly used in cirrhotic patients who require liver surgery. Mortality and survival rates after hepatectomy have been shown to correlate with this score but are not always related to liver failure. Child's B and C patients generally do not fare well after partial hepatectomy as compared with Child's A patients.[49]

INFECTIOUS DISEASES

Pyogenic Abscess

Epidemiology

Ochsner and DeBakey, in their classic paper on pyogenic liver abscess in 1938, described 47 cases and reviewed the world literature.[68] This was the largest experience of the time and the first serious attempt to study this disease. At that time, pyogenic liver abscess was largely a disease of people in their 20s and 30s and mostly the result of acute appendicitis. With the marked change in medical care over the past 60 years, notably, effective antibiotics, prompt effective treatments for acute inflammatory disorders, and an aging population, the spectrum of this disease has changed. Pyogenic liver abscess is now mostly seen in patients 50 to 60 years old and is more often related to biliary tract disease or is cryptogenic.

The incidence of pyogenic liver abscess has remained similar over 60 years. Ochsner and DeBakey reported an incidence of 8 per 100,000 hospital admissions in 1938,[68] whereas, in 1975, Pitt and Zuidema reported 13 per 100,000 hospital admissions.[69] Two large autopsy studies, one from 1901 and one from 1960, report similar incidences of pyogenic liver abscess: 0.45% and 0.59%, respectively.[70] More recent studies from the 1980s and 1990s have suggested small but significant increases in the incidence of pyogenic liver abscess (as high as 22 per 100,000 hospital admissions).[71,72] This may reflect better, more available, and more frequently used high-quality imaging techniques. Hospital admission practices surely affect these statistics as well. One population-based study calculated the incidence of pyogenic liver abscess to be 11 cases per million persons per year.[70] There are no significant gender, ethnic, or geographic differences in disease frequency, and the male-to-female ratio is approximately 1.5 to 1.

Pathogenesis

The liver is probably exposed to portal venous bacterial loads on a regular basis and clears this bacterial load without problems in the usual circumstance. The development of a hepatic abscess occurs when the inoculum of bacteria, regardless of the route of exposure, exceeds the liver's ability to clear it. This results in tissue invasion, neutrophil infiltration, and the formation of an organized abscess. The potential routes of hepatic exposure to bacteria are (1) biliary tree, (2) portal vein, (3) hepatic artery, (4) direct extension of a nearby focus of infection, and (5) trauma. The relative contribution of these routes to the formation of hepatic abscess is summarized in Table 50-3.[73]

Hepatic infections from the biliary tree are presently the most common identifiable cause of hepatic abscess. Biliary obstruction results in bile stasis, with the potential for subsequent bacterial colonization, infection, and ascension into the liver. This process is known as ascending suppurative cholangitis. The nature of biliary obstruction is mostly related to stone disease or malignancy. In Asia, intrahepatic stones and cholangitis (recurrent pyogenic cholangitis—see later) are a common cause,[74]

TABLE 50-2. Child-Pugh Classification			
	No. of Points*		
Factor	1	2	3
Bilirubin (mg/dL)	<2	2-3	>3
Albumin (g/dL)	>3.5	2.8-3.5	<2.8
Prothrombin time (increased seconds)	1-3	4-6	>6
Ascites	None	Slight	Moderate
Encephalopathy	None	Minimal	Advanced

*Grade A, 5-6 points; grade B, 7-9 points; grade C, 10-15 points.

TABLE 50-3. Percentage of Pyogenic Abscesses Attributable to Specific Cause

	Years/No. Studies		
	1927-1938/1*	1945-1982/8	1970-1995/7
No. Patients	622	521	1131
Portal Vein	42	17	6
Hepatic Artery		9	4
Biliary Tree		38	40
Direct Extension	17	10	1
Trauma	4	4	2
Cryptogenic	20	16	40

*1927-1938 is the Ochsner/DeBakey classic study that reviewed 575 previously reported cases and 47 new cases.

whereas in the Western world, malignant obstruction is becoming a more predominant factor.[75] Other factors associated with increased risk include Caroli's disease, biliary *Ascaris* infection, and biliary tract surgery. The common link between all causes of hepatic abscess from the biliary tree is obstruction and bacteria in the biliary tree. Previous biliary-enteric anastomosis has also been associated with hepatic abscess formation, likely owing to unimpeded exposure of the biliary tree to enteric organisms.

The portal venous system drains the gastrointestinal tract, and therefore any infectious disorder of the gastrointestinal tract can result in an ascending portal vein infection (pyelophlebitis) with exposure of the liver to large amounts of bacteria. Historically, untreated appendicitis was considered the most common cause of hepatic abscess, but with the advent of antibiotics and the development of prompt and effective treatment of acute abdominal infections, portal venous infections of the liver have become less common. The most common causes of pyelophlebitis are diverticulitis, appendicitis, pancreatitis, inflammatory bowel disease, pelvic inflammatory disease, perforated viscus, or omphalitis in the newborn. Hepatic abscess has also been associated with colorectal malignancy.[70,73]

Any systemic infection (e.g., endocarditis, pneumonia, osteomyelitis) can result in bacteremia and infection of the liver via the hepatic artery. Multiple microabscess formation is a relatively common finding at autopsy in patients dying of sepsis, but these patients are generally not included in analyses of pyogenic liver abscess. Hepatic abscess from systemic infections may also reflect an altered immune response, such as in patients with malignancy, acquired immune deficiency syndrome, or disorders of granulocyte function.[71] Children with chronic granulomatous disease are particularly susceptible.

Hepatic abscess can be the result of direct extension of an infective process. Common examples of this include suppurative cholecystitis, subphrenic abscess,

perinephric abscess, or even perforation of the intestine directly into the liver.

Penetrating and blunt trauma can result in an intrahepatic hematoma or an area of necrotic liver that can subsequently develop into an abscess. Bacteria may have been introduced from the trauma, or the affected area may be seeded from systemic bacteremia. Hepatic abscesses associated with trauma can present in a delayed fashion, up to weeks after the injury. Other mechanisms of iatrogenic hepatic necrosis such as hepatic artery embolization or, more recently, thermal ablative procedures can be complicated by abscess. This is an uncommon complication of these procedures but is seen more often when there has been a previous biliary-enteric anastomosis.

Commonly, no cause for a hepatic abscess is found. Cryptogenic abscesses predominate in many series and are more common in recent case series.[68,71-73,75] Possible explanations for cryptogenic hepatic abscess are undiagnosed abdominal pathology, resolved infective process at the time of presentation, or host factors such as diabetes or malignancy rendering the liver more susceptible to transient hepatic artery or portal vein bacteremias. In patients with cryptogenic hepatic abscess, who, in general, have had computed tomography (CT) and ultrasonography, it has been argued that a diligent search for a cause should ensue. In series evaluating colonoscopy and endoscopic retrograde cholangiopancreatography (ERCP) in patients with cryptogenic abscess, the yield has been low and often is only fruitful in patients with some objective finding that might have suggested a subclinical abnormality (e.g., mildly elevated bilirubin).[71,72] In general, these patients should undergo a thorough history, physical examination, and laboratory work-up in search of abnormalities in the intestinal tract or biliary tree. Further invasive procedures should be based on clinical suspicions raised by this work-up.

Pathology and Microbiology

The majority of hepatic abscesses involve the right lobe of the liver, accounting for three fourths of cases. The explanation for this is not known, but preferential laminar blood flow to the right side has been postulated. The left lobe is involved about 20% of the time, and the caudate lobe is uncommonly involved (5%). Bilobar involvement with multiple abscesses is uncommon. About half of hepatic abscesses are solitary. The size of hepatic abscesses can vary from less than a millimeter to several centimeters in diameter and can be multiloculated or a single cavity. At abdominal exploration, hepatic abscesses appear tan and are fluctuant to palpation, although deeper abscesses may not be visible and can be difficult to feel. Surrounding inflammation can cause adhesion to local structures.

Studies on the microbiology of hepatic abscesses have been variable for a number of reasons. In early series, sterile abscesses were commonly reported but probably reflected inadequate culture techniques, whereas in modern series very few abscesses are sampled before the administration of antibiotics. Additionally, the heterogeneity of the routes of infection makes the microbiology variable. Abscesses from pyelophlebitis or cholangitis tend to be polymicrobial, with a high preponderance of gram-negative rods. Systemic infections, on the other hand, usually cause infection with a single organism.[73]

Although the rate of sterility reported by Ochsner's review in 1938 was approximately 50%, series in the 1990s report sterile abscesses in 10% to 20% of cases. Many hepatic abscesses are polymicrobial and account for about 40% of cases. Some authors suggest that solitary abscesses are more likely to be polymicrobial.[71,76] Anaerobic organisms are involved 40% to 60% of the time. The most common organisms cultured are *Escherichia coli* and *Klebsiella pneumoniae*. Other common organisms encountered are *Staphylococcus aureus*, *Enterococcus* species, *Streptococcus viridans*, and *Bacteroides* species. *Klebsiella* is frequently associated with gas-forming abscesses. Enterococci and viridans streptococci are generally found in polymicrobial abscesses whereas staphylococcal infections are typically caused by a single organism. Uncommonly encountered organisms (<10% of cultures) include *Pseudomonas*, *Proteus*, *Enterobacter*, *Citrobacter*, *Serratia*, β-hemolytic streptococci, microaerophilic streptococci, *Fusobacterium*, *Clostridium*, and other rare anaerobes. Blood cultures are positive in 50% to 60% of cases.[73] Of note, highly resistant organisms in patients with indwelling biliary catheters, multiple episodes of cholangitis, and repeated use of antibiotics are being encountered as the use of these catheters becomes more common. Fungal and mycobacterial hepatic abscesses are rare and are almost always associated with immunosuppression, usually from chemotherapy.

Clinical Features

The classic description of the presenting symptoms of hepatic abscess are fever, jaundice, and right upper quadrant pain and tenderness. Unfortunately, this presentation is present only 10% of the time. Fever, chills, and abdominal pain are the most common presenting symptoms, but there is a broad array of nonspecific symptoms that can be found (Table 50-4).[68,70,72,73] Many of these symptoms, such as malaise or vomiting, are constitutional. Involvement of the diaphragm may result in symptoms of cough or dyspnea. Rarely, patients can present with peritonitis secondary to rupture. Cases of rupture into the pleural space or pericardium have been reported but are distinctly uncommon. The duration of presenting symptoms is variable, ranging from an acute illness to a chronic presentation lasting months. It has been suggested that acute presentation is associated with identifiable abdominal pathology whereas a chronic presentation is often associated with a cryptogenic abscess.

On physical examination, fever and right upper quadrant tenderness are the most common findings, with tenderness being present 40% to 70% of the time. Jaundice is found about 25% of the time and is often secondary to underlying biliary disease. Chest findings are often found and are present in about one fourth of cases. Hepatomegaly is also commonly noted and present about half of the time. Ascites, splenomegaly, and severe sepsis are uncommon signs.

TABLE 50-4. Percentage of Pyogenic Abscesses With Noted Symptoms

	Years/No. Studies		
	1927-1938/1*	1945-1982/8	1970-1995/10
No. Patients	333	494	1314
Fever/Chills	94	88	72
Night Sweats		8	9
Malaise		58	25
Anorexia/ Weight Loss		62	33
Nausea/Vomiting	33	40	30
Diarrhea		17	14
Abdominal Pain	92	66	59
Chest Pain		14	16
Cough		13	16

*1927-1938 is the Ochsner/DeBakey classic study that reviewed 286 previously reported cases and 47 new cases.

Nonspecific abnormalities of blood tests are common in pyogenic abscesses. Leukocytosis is present in 70% to 90% of patients, and anemia is commonly encountered. Abnormalities of LFTs are generally present. ALP is mildly elevated in 80% of cases, whereas total bilirubin is elevated 20% to 50% of the time. Transaminases are mildly elevated about 60% of the time. Severe abnormalities of LFTs are almost always associated with underlying biliary disease. Hypoalbuminemia or mild elevations of the prothrombin time can be present and reflect a degree of chronicity. None of these blood tests specifically help to diagnose a hepatic abscess but suggest a liver abnormality that often leads to imaging studies.

The most essential element to making the diagnosis of hepatic abscess is radiographic imaging studies. Chest radiographs are abnormal about 50% of the time, and findings generally reflect subdiaphragmatic pathology such as an elevated right hemidiaphragm, right pleural effusion, or atelectasis. Occasionally, these can be left-sided findings in the case of an abscess involving the left liver. Plain abdominal radiographs, in rare cases, can be helpful. They can show air-fluid levels or portal venous gas (Fig. 50-17).

Ultrasound and CT are the mainstays in diagnostic modalities for hepatic abscess. Ultrasound usually demonstrates a round or oval area that is less echogenic than the liver and can reliably distinguish solid from cystic lesions. The limitations of ultrasound are in its ability to visualize lesions high up in the dome of the liver and the fact that it is a user-dependent modality. The sensitivity of ultrasound in diagnosing hepatic abscess is 80% to 95%. CT demonstrates similar findings to ultrasound, and lesions are of lower attenuation than surrounding hepatic parenchyma. High-quality CT can demonstrate very small abscesses and can more easily pick up multiple small abscesses. The abscess wall usually shows an intense

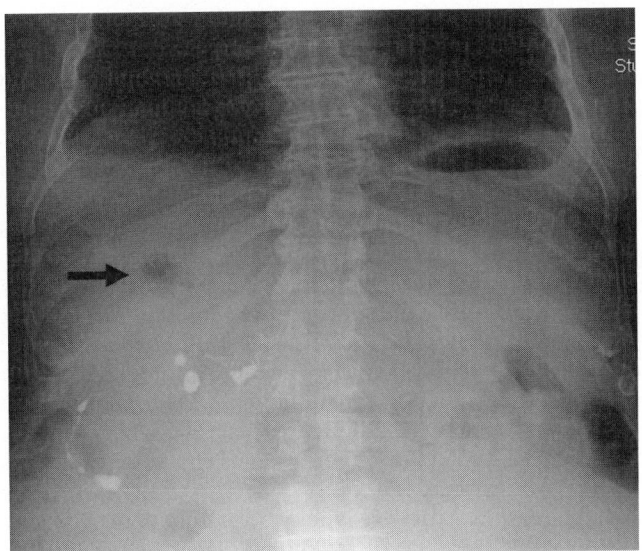

FIGURE 50-17. Plain abdominal radiograph demonstrates an abnormal collection of air in the right upper quadrant consistent with a pyogenic hepatic abscess *(arrow)*.

enhancement on contrast medium–enhanced CT. The sensitivity of CT in diagnosing hepatic abscess is 95% to 100%. Both CT and ultrasound are useful in diagnosing other intra-abdominal pathology, such as biliary disease (ultrasound) or inflammatory disorders such as appendicitis or diverticulitis (CT).[70,72,73] Magnetic resonance imaging (MRI) can be very helpful in distinguishing the etiology of many hepatic masses but does not appear to have any distinct advantage over CT in diagnosing hepatic abscess.

Differential Diagnosis

Differentiating pyogenic abscess from other cystic infective diseases of the liver such as amebic abscess or echinococcal cyst is important because of differences in treatment. Pyogenic abscess (as discussed later) is largely treated by antibiotics and drainage. Amebic abscess is largely treated by antibiotics, and echinococcal cysts often require surgical management. Fortunately, echinococcal cysts can usually be diagnosed by history and characteristic radiologic findings (see later). The presentations of amebic and pyogenic abscess, however, are nearly identical, with some notable exceptions that are critical in distinguishing the two (Table 50-5). Amebic abscesses generally occur in young Hispanic males in North America, whereas pyogenic abscess tends to occur in patients 50 to 60 years of age with no predominant gender or race. Fever is common in both, but chills and symptoms of a severe acute bacteremia are more common in pyogenic abscess. Serologic tests reveal that *Entamoeba histolytica* antibodies are nearly always present in amebic abscesses but are uncommon in patients with pyogenic abscess. Occasionally, differentiating the two is not possible and diagnostic aspiration or a trial of antiamebic antibiotics may be necessary. Unfortunately, aspiration is only diagnostic in amebic abscess 10% to 20% of the time.[77,78]

Treatment

Before the availability of antibiotics and the routine use of drainage procedures, untreated hepatic pyogenic abscess was uniformly fatal. It was not until the classic review by Ochsner and DeBakey in 1938 that routine surgical drainage was employed and dramatic reductions in

TABLE 50-5. Features of Amebic Versus Pyogenic Liver Abscess

Clinical Features	Amebic Abscess	Pyogenic Abscess
Age (yr)	20-40	> 50
Male:female ratio	≥10 : 1	1.5 : 1
Solitary vs. multiple	Solitary ≥80%*	Solitary 50%
Location	Usually right liver	Usually right liver
Travel in endemic area	Yes	No
Diabetes	Uncommon (approx. 2%)	More common (approx. 27%)
Alcohol use	Yes	Yes
Jaundice	Rare	Common
Elevated bilirubin	Uncommon	Common
Elevated alkaline phosphatase	Common	Common
Positive blood culture	No	Common
Positive amebic serology	Yes	No

*In acute amebic abscess 50% are solitary.

mortality were noted. Open surgical drainage of pyogenic abscesses was the sole treatment (with the addition of antibiotics eventually) for hepatic abscess until the 1980s. Since the 1980s less invasive percutaneous drainage techniques along with the use of intravenous antibiotics have been employed. Laparotomy is generally reserved for failures of percutaneous drainage.

Once the diagnosis of pyogenic hepatic abscess is suspected, broad-spectrum intravenous antibiotics should be started immediately to control ongoing bacteremia and its associated complications. Blood cultures and cultures of the abscess from aspiration should be sent for aerobic and anaerobic cultures. In immunosuppressed patients, mycobacterial and fungal cultures of the aspirate should be considered. Patients who are at risk for amebic infections should have blood drawn for amebic serologic studies. Until cultures have specifically identified the offending organism(s), broad-spectrum antibiotics covering gram-negative and gram-positive organisms and anaerobes should be used. Combinations such as ampicillin, an

aminoglycoside, and metronidazole or a third-generation cephalosporin with metronidazole is appropriate. The duration of antibiotic treatment is not well defined and must be individualized depending on the success of the drainage procedure. Antibiotics should certainly be continued while there is evidence of ongoing infection such as fever, chills, or leukocytosis. Beyond this, it is unclear how long to continue antibiotics, but recommendations usually are for 2 or more weeks.

Percutaneous drainage procedures for pyogenic hepatic abscesses were first reported in 1953 but did not gain widespread acceptance until the 1980s with the development of high-quality imaging and expertise in interventional radiologic techniques.[79] Over the past 20 years, percutaneous catheter drainage has become the treatment of choice for most patients (Fig. 50-18). Success rates range from 69% to 90%.[70,72,73,75,76,80] The obvious advantages are the simplicity of treatment (usually employed at the time of radiologic diagnosis) and avoidance of general anesthesia and a laparotomy. Relative

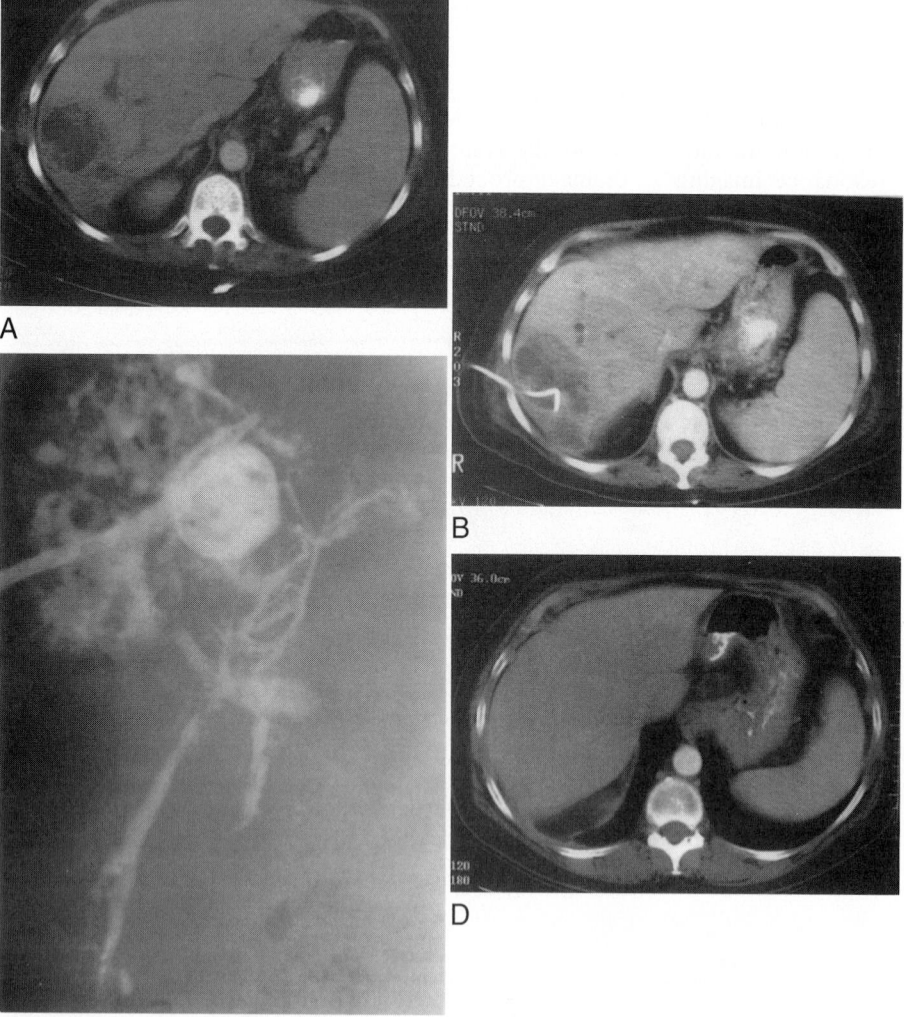

FIGURE 50-18. **A,** CT scan demonstrates multiloculated hepatic abscess in the right liver. **B,** CT scan at the time of percutaneous drainage. **C,** Contrast study through the drainage catheter demonstrating typical irregular loculated type appearance, as well as communication with biliary tree. **D,** Follow-up CT scan 3 months after treatment demonstrating complete resolution of abscess. (From Brown KT, Getrajdman GI: Interventional radiologic techniques in the liver and biliary tract. *In* Blumgart LH, Fong Y [eds]: Surgery of the Liver and Biliary Tract. London, WB Saunders, 2000, pp 575-594.)

contraindications to percutaneous catheter drainage include the presence of ascites, coagulopathy, or proximity to vital structures. Percutaneous drainage of multiple abscesses is usually met with a higher failure rate, but reports demonstrate a high enough success rate that percutaneous approaches should be made first, reserving surgery for percutaneous failures. There has never been a randomized prospective comparison between percutaneous and surgical therapy for hepatic abscess, but case series suggest similar success rates and mortality. Modern series attempting to compare these two techniques retrospectively must be read with caution because the majority of patients treated surgically have failed other less invasive techniques. Surgery should be reserved for patients who require surgical treatment of the primary pathologic process (e.g., appendicitis) or for those who have failed percutaneous techniques. Laparoscopic drainage procedures have been reported with some success, and this can be considered a reasonable option to pursue in selected cases.[81]

Percutaneous aspiration without the placement of a drain has been investigated by a number of groups. Success rates are generally 60% to 90% and are somewhat similar to percutaneous catheter drainage.[70,82] The majority of aspirations, however, require more than one aspiration and one fourth of patients require three or more aspirations. A single randomized trial has evaluated percutaneous aspiration versus percutaneous catheter drainage. Success rates were 60% in the aspiration group and 100% in the catheter group, but all but one patient in the aspiration group had a single aspiration.

Some investigators have reported success with antibiotics alone. The majority of these patients, however, have had a diagnostic aspiration and thus at least a partial drainage. Additionally, other series have reported that antibiotic treatment without drainage carries a prohibitively high mortality (59% to 100%).[70] In patients who are not surgical candidates or who absolutely refuse any invasive procedure, an attempt at antibiotic treatment is reasonable; however, this is not recommended in all other situations.

Liver resection is occasionally required for hepatic abscess. This may be required for an infected hepatic malignancy, hepatolithiasis, or intrahepatic biliary stricture. If hepatic destruction from infection is severe, some patients may benefit from resection.

Outcome

Mortality from pyogenic hepatic abscess has dramatically improved over the past 60 years. Before the routine use of surgical drainage, pyogenic abscess was uniformly fatal. With the routine use of surgical drainage and the use of intravenous antibiotics, mortality was reduced to about 50%, a figure that stayed relatively constant from 1945 until the early 1980s. Since the 1980s, mortality has been reported from 10% to 20%. A number of studies have analyzed factors predictive of a poor outcome in patients with hepatic pyogenic abscess. The presence of malignancy or of factors associated with malignancy (jaundice, markedly elevated LFTs) appears to be a consistent marker of poor

prognosis. Signs of chronic disease such as hypoalbuminemia also are often associated with a poor outcome. Lastly, signs of severe infection such as marked leukocytosis, Acute Physiology and Chronic Health Evaluation (APACHE) II scores, abscess rupture, bacteremia, and shock are also associated with mortality.[70,73]

Amebic Abscess

Epidemiology

Amebiasis is largely a disease of tropical and developing countries but is also a significant problem in developed countries because of immigration and travel between countries. *E. histolytica* is endemic in Mexico, India, Africa, and parts of Central and South America. In 1995, the World Health Organization estimated that 40 to 50 million people suffer from amebic colitis or amebic liver abscess worldwide, resulting in 40,000 to 100,000 deaths each year.[77,83] Prior to this, estimates of amebiasis were unreliable because *E. histolytica* (the pathogenic form) was not differentiated from *E. dispar* (the nonpathogenic form). Male homosexuals with diarrhea previously thought to harbor *E. histolytica* have been found to in fact be infected with *E. dispar*, which requires no treatment.

In contrast to pyogenic hepatic abscesses, patients with amebic liver abscesses tend to be Hispanic males, aged 20 to 40, with a history of travel to (or origination from) an endemic area. A male preponderance of greater than 10:1 has been reported in almost all studies. For unclear reasons, menstruating women have a low incidence of invasive amebiasis and pregnancy appears to abrogate this resistance. Heavy alcohol consumption is commonly reported and may render the liver more susceptible to amebic infection. Impaired host immunity also appears to play a role. Patients with amebic liver abscess without a history of travel to an endemic area often have an associated immunosuppression such as human immunodeficiency virus infection, malnutrition, chronic infection, or chronic corticosteroid use.[77,78,84]

Pathogenesis

E. histolytica is a protozoan and exists as a trophozoite or as a cyst. All other species in the genus *Entamoeba* are considered nonpathogenic, and not all strains of *E. histolytica* are considered virulent. Ingestion of *E. histolytica* cysts through a fecal-oral route is the cause of amebiasis. Humans are the principal host, and the main source of infection is human contact with a cyst-passing carrier. Contaminated water and vegetables are also a route of human infection. Once ingested, the cysts are not degraded in the stomach and pass to the intestines, where the trophozoite is released and passed on to the colon. In the colon, the trophozoite can invade mucosa and result in disease.

It is believed that the trophozoites reach the liver through the portal venous system. There is no evidence for trophozoites passing through lymphatics. As implied by its name, *E. histolytica* trophozoites have the capacity to lyse tissues through a complex set of events, including cell adherence, cell activation, and subsequent release of multiple enzymes resulting in necrosis. The major mechanism is probably enzymatic cellular hydrolysis. Amebic liver abscesses are thus formed by progressing, localized hepatic necrosis, resulting in a cavity containing acellular proteinaceous debris surrounded by a rim of invasive amebic trophozoites. Early development of an amebic liver abscess is associated with an accumulation of polymorphonuclear leukocytes, which are then lysed by the trophozoites.[77,85,86]

Pathology

Hepatic amebic abscess is essentially the result of liquefaction necrosis of the liver, producing a cavity full of blood and liquefied liver tissue. The appearance of this fluid is typically described as "anchovy sauce," and the fluid is odorless unless secondary bacterial infection has taken place. The progressive hepatic necrosis continues until Glisson's capsule is reached because the capsule is resistant to hydrolysis by the amebae, and thus amebic abscesses tend to abut the liver capsule. Because of the resistance of Glisson's capsule, the cavity is typically crisscrossed by portal triads protected by this peritoneal sheath. Early on, the formed cavity is ill-defined with no real fibrous response around the edges but a chronic abscess can ultimately develop a fibrous capsule and may even calcify. Like pyogenic abscesses, amebic abscesses tend to occur mainly in the right liver.[85]

Clinical Features

Approximately 80% of patients with amebic liver abscess present with symptoms lasting from a few days to 4 weeks. The presenting clinical signs and symptoms are summarized in Table 50-6.[77,78,87-89] The typical clinical picture is a patient 20 to 40 years of age who has traveled to an endemic area with fever, chills, anorexia, right upper quadrant pain, and tenderness and hepatomegaly. The abdominal pain is typically constant, dull, and localized to the right upper quadrant. Although some studies report higher numbers, only one third of patients have diarrhea despite an obligatory colonic infection. Synchronous hepatic abscess is found in one third of patients with active amebic colitis. Jaundice, as a result of a large abscess compressing the biliary tree, is a rare presentation. Weight loss and myalgias may occur when symptoms have been present for weeks. Pleuritic or shoulder pain can occur if there is irritation of the diaphragm. Symptoms and tenderness may be epigastric or left sided if the abscess is located in the left liver.

Laboratory abnormalities are common in amebic abscess. Patients typically have a mild to moderate leukocytosis without eosinophilia. Anemia is common. Mild abnormalities of LFTs including albumin, prothrombin time, ALP, AST, and bilirubin levels are typical. The most common LFT abnormality is an elevated prothrombin time.[77,78,87,89] Because greater than 70% of patients with amebic liver abscess do not have detectable amebae in their stool, the most useful laboratory evaluation is the measurement of circulating antiamebic antibodies that are present in 90% to 95% of patients. A number of serologic tests have been devised over the years. An indirect hemagglutinin test was used extensively in the past and has a sensitivity of 90%. This test has largely been replaced by enzyme immunoassays (EIA), which are simple, rapidly performed, and inexpensive. The EIA has a reported sensitivity of 99% and specificity greater than 90% in patients with hepatic abscess. Unfortunately, the presence of antibodies may reflect old infection and interpretation can be difficult in endemic areas. Ongoing studies are focusing on identifying specific *E. histolytia* antigens in an attempt to identify acute infection.[77]

Patients presenting acutely (symptoms less than 10 days) versus those with a chronic presentation (greater than 2 weeks) differ clinically. Acute presentations are typically more dramatic, with high fevers, chills, and significant abdominal tenderness. In the acute presentation, half of patients present with multiple lesions, whereas with the chronic presentation, greater than 80% of patients have a single right-sided lesion. A more complicated course tends to ensue in the acute presentation, but response to therapy is similar in both groups.[90]

Radiologic studies are a critical element in the diagnosis of amebic liver abscess. Plain chest radiographs are abnormal in about half of cases, usually demonstrating elevated right diaphragm, pleural effusion, or atelectasis.[91] Abdominal ultrasound has a reported accuracy of approximately 90% when combined with a typical history and clinical presentation. Typical findings on abdominal ultrasound are a rounded lesion abutting the liver capsule (see earlier) without significant rim echoes interpreted as an abscess wall. The contents of the cavity are usually hypoechoic and nonhomogeneous (Fig. 50-19). These findings on ultrasound appear in 40% to 70% of cases. Abdominal CT is probably more sensitive than ultrasound and is helpful in differentiating amebic from pyogenic abscess,

TABLE 50-6.   Signs and Symptoms in Amebic Liver Abscess in Four Studies Published Between 1986 and 1999 on 241 Patients

Sign/Symptom	Percentage of Patients
Abdominal pain	84-93
Fever	80-93
Chills	41-73
Nausea	45-85
Weight loss	29-45
Diarrhea	17-60
Cough	2-41
Right upper quadrant tenderness	67-80
Hepatomegaly	18-53
Peritoneal signs	18-20
Jaundice	4-12

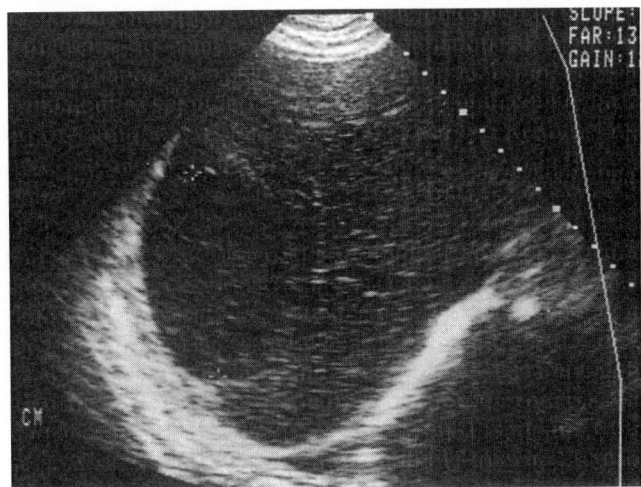

FIGURE 50-19. Typical ultrasound of an amebic hepatic abscess. Note the peripheral location, rounded shape with poor rim, and internal echoes. (From Thomas PG, Ravindra KV: Amebiasis and biliary infection. *In* Blumgart LH, Fong Y [eds]: Surgery of the Liver and Biliary Tract. London, WB Saunders, 2000, pp 1147-1166.)

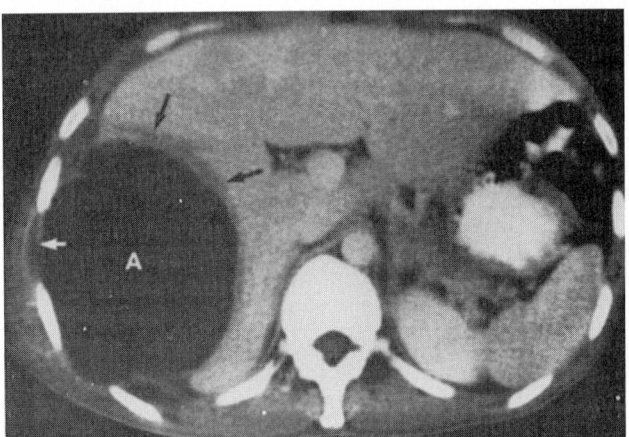

FIGURE 50-20. CT scan of amebic abscess (A). The lesion is peripherally located and round. Rim is nonenhancing but shows peripheral edema *(black arrows)*. Note the extension into the intercostal space *(white arrows)*.

with rim enhancement noted in the latter (Fig. 50-20). CT can also be helpful in identifying simple cysts and necrotic tumors. MRI of the liver has no distinct advantages over CT or ultrasound in typical cases, but it may be helpful in differentiating atypical lesions. Nuclear medicine studies such as gallium scanning or technetium-99m liver scans can be helpful in differentiating pyogenic from amebic abscesses because the latter typically do not contain leukocytes and therefore do not light up on these scans.[77,83,85]

When this work-up is still not definitive and diagnostic uncertainty persists, two options should be considered.

A therapeutic trial of antiamebic drugs in which rapid improvement occurs in most cases of amebic abscess can be helpful. In situations in which amebic serology is inconclusive and a therapeutic trial of antibiotics is either deemed inappropriate or has failed to improve symptoms, consideration should be given to diagnostic aspiration. A pyogenic abscess would have bacteria and leukocytes, whereas an amebic abscess would contain the "anchovy sauce." Cultures of amebic abscess are usually negative and do not contain leukocytes. In cases in which neoplasm or hydatid disease is given serious consideration, aspiration should not be performed.

Differential Diagnosis

The differential diagnosis of an amebic liver abscess can be broad and include such diseases as viral hepatitis, echinococcal disease, cholangitis, cholecystitis, or even other inflammatory abdominal disorders such as appendicitis. Malignant lesions of the liver can also have similar presentations in atypical situations. Occasionally, primary pulmonary disorders must be considered. In the main, the most important distinction to be made is between pyogenic and amebic abscess. The essential elements of this distinction are summarized in Table 50-5 and in the section on pyogenic abscess.[77,78]

Management

The mainstay of treatment for amebic abscesses is metronidazole (750 mg orally three times per day for 10 days), which is curative in over 90% of patients. Clinical improvement is usually seen within 3 days. Other nitroimidazoles (secnidazole, tinidazole) are also as effective and are commonly used outside the United States. If response to metronidazole is poor or the drug is not tolerated, other agents can be used. Emetine is effective against invasive amebiasis (particularly in the liver) but requires intramuscular injections and has serious cardiac side effects. A more attractive option is chloroquine, but this is a less effective agent. After treatment of the liver abscess, it is recommended that luminal agents are administered to treat the carrier state. Luminal agents effective for amebiasis include iodoquinol, paromomycin, and diloxanide furoate.[77,92]

Therapeutic needle aspiration of amebic abscesses has been proposed. In a small randomized trial, therapeutic aspiration combined with metronidazole therapy resulted in more rapid improvement in fever, abdominal pain, and hospital stay.[93] Nonetheless, reasonably rapid improvement is the rule with simple oral metronidazole, and most practitioners do not routinely use aspiration therapeutically. In general, aspiration is recommended for diagnostic uncertainty (see earlier), for failure to respond to metronidazole therapy in 3 to 5 days, or in abscesses believed to be at high risk for rupture. Abscesses larger than 5 cm in diameter are believed to be at high risk of rupture, and, in particular, when they are located in the left lobe with risk of pericardial rupture therapeutic aspiration is recommended.[77,85]

Outcome

Although amebic liver abscess usually has a benign course, there are uncommon complications of which the practitioner must be aware. The most frequent complication of amebic abscess is rupture into the peritoneum, pleural cavity, or pericardium.[77,85] Size of the abscess appears to be the most important risk factor for rupture, and the overall incidence of rupture ranges from 3% to 17%. Most peritoneal ruptures tend to be contained by the diaphragm, abdominal wall, and/or omentum, but rupture can fistulize into a hollow viscus. A peritoneal rupture usually presents as abdominal pain, peritonitis, and either a mass or generalized distention. Laparotomy was advocated in the past for this complication, but now many cases are managed successfully with percutaneous drainage. Laparotomy is indicated in cases of doubtful diagnosis, hollow viscus perforation, fistulization resulting in hemorrhage or sepsis, and failure of conservative therapy. Rupture into the pleural space usually results in a large and rapidly accumulated effusion that collapses the involved lung. Treatment consists of thoracentesis, but if secondary bacterial infection ensues, more aggressive surgical approaches may be necessary. Rupture can occur into the bronchi and is usually self-limited with postural drainage and bronchodilators. Rarely, a left-sided abscess may rupture into the pericardium and can present as an asymptomatic pericardial effusion or even tamponade.[94] This must be treated with aspiration. Other rare complications include compression of the biliary tree or IVC from a very large abscess and the development of a brain abscess.

The mortality for all patients with amebic liver abscess is 2% to 4% and does not appear to be affected by the addition of aspiration to metronidazole therapy or chronicity of symptoms. When an abscess ruptures the mortality is reported to be from 6% to as high as 50%.[85] Factors independently associated with poor outcome are elevated serum bilirubin (>3.5 mg/dL), encephalopathy, hypoalbuminemia (<2.0 g/dL), multiple abscess cavities, abscess volume greater than 500 mL, anemia, and diabetes.[77,85] Although clinical improvement after adequate treatment with antiamebic agents is the rule, radiologic resolution of the abscess cavity is usually delayed. The average time to radiologic resolution is 3 to 9 months and can take as long as years in some patients.[95]

Hydatid Cyst

Hydatid disease or echinococcosis is a zoonosis that occurs primarily in sheep-grazing areas of the world but is common worldwide because the dog is a definitive host. Echinococcosis is endemic in Mediterranean countries, the Middle East, the Far East, South America, Australia, New Zealand, and East Africa. Humans contract the disease from dogs, and there is no human-to-human transmission.[96-98]

There are three species of *Echinococcus* that cause hydatid disease. *E. granulosus* is the most common whereas *E. multilocularis* and *E. oligartus* account for a small number of cases. Dogs are the definitive host of *E. granulosus,* in which the adult tapeworm is attached to the villi of the ileum. Eggs are passed (up to thousands of ova daily) and deposited with the dog's feces. Sheep are the usual intermediate host, but humans are an accidental intermediate host. Humans are an end stage to the parasite. In the human duodenum, the parasitic embryo releases an oncosphere containing hooklets that penetrate the mucosa, allowing access to the bloodstream. In the blood, the oncosphere reaches the liver (most commonly) or lungs, where the parasite develops its larval stage known as the hydatid cyst.[96,98,99]

Three weeks after infection, a visible hydatid cyst develops that then slowly grows in a spherical manner. A pericyst, a fibrous capsule derived from host tissues, develops around the hydatid cyst. The cyst wall itself has two layers, an outer gelatinous membrane (ectocyst) and an inner germinal membrane (endocyst). Brood capsules are small intracystic cellular masses in which future worm heads develop into scoleces. In a definitive host the scoleces would develop into an adult tapeworm, but in the intermediate host they can only differentiate into a new hydatid cyst. Freed brood capsules and scoleces are found in the hydatid fluid and form the so-called hydatid sand. Daughter cysts are true replicas of the mother cyst. Hydatid cysts can die with degeneration of the membranes, development of cystic vacuoles, and calcification of the wall. Calcification of a hydatid cyst, however, does not always imply that the cyst is dead.[96,99]

Hydatid cysts are diagnosed in equal numbers of men and women at an average age of about 45. About three fourths of hydatid cysts are located in the right liver and are singular. The clinical presentation of a hydatid cyst is largely asymptomatic until complications occur. The most common presenting symptoms are abdominal pain, dyspepsia, and vomiting. The most frequent sign is hepatomegaly. Jaundice and fever are each present in about 8% of patients.[100] Infection of a hydatid cyst can occur and present like a pyogenic abscess. Rupture of the cyst into the biliary tree or bronchial tree or free rupture into the peritoneal, pleural, or pericardial cavities can occur. Free ruptures can result in disseminated echinococcosis and/or a potentially fatal anaphylactic reaction. In cases of diagnostic uncertainty a battery of serologic tests are available to evaluate antibody response, but all are plagued by low sensitivity and specificity.[96,101]

Ultrasound is most commonly used worldwide for the diagnosis of echinococcosis because of its availability, affordability, and accuracy. A number of ultrasonographic findings can be diagnostic and depend on the stage of the cyst at the time of the examination. A simple hydatid cyst is well circumscribed with budding signs on the cyst membrane and may contain free floating hyperechogenic hydatid sand. A rosette appearance is seen when daughter cysts are present. The cyst can be filled with an amorphous mass that can be diagnostically misleading. Calcifications in the wall of the cyst are highly suggestive of hydatid disease and can be helpful in the diagnosis (Fig. 50-21).[102] Similar findings are seen on CT or MRI. These studies can also evaluate extrahepatic disease and demonstrate detailed hepatic anatomic relationships to the cyst. In patients with suspected biliary involvement, ERCP or

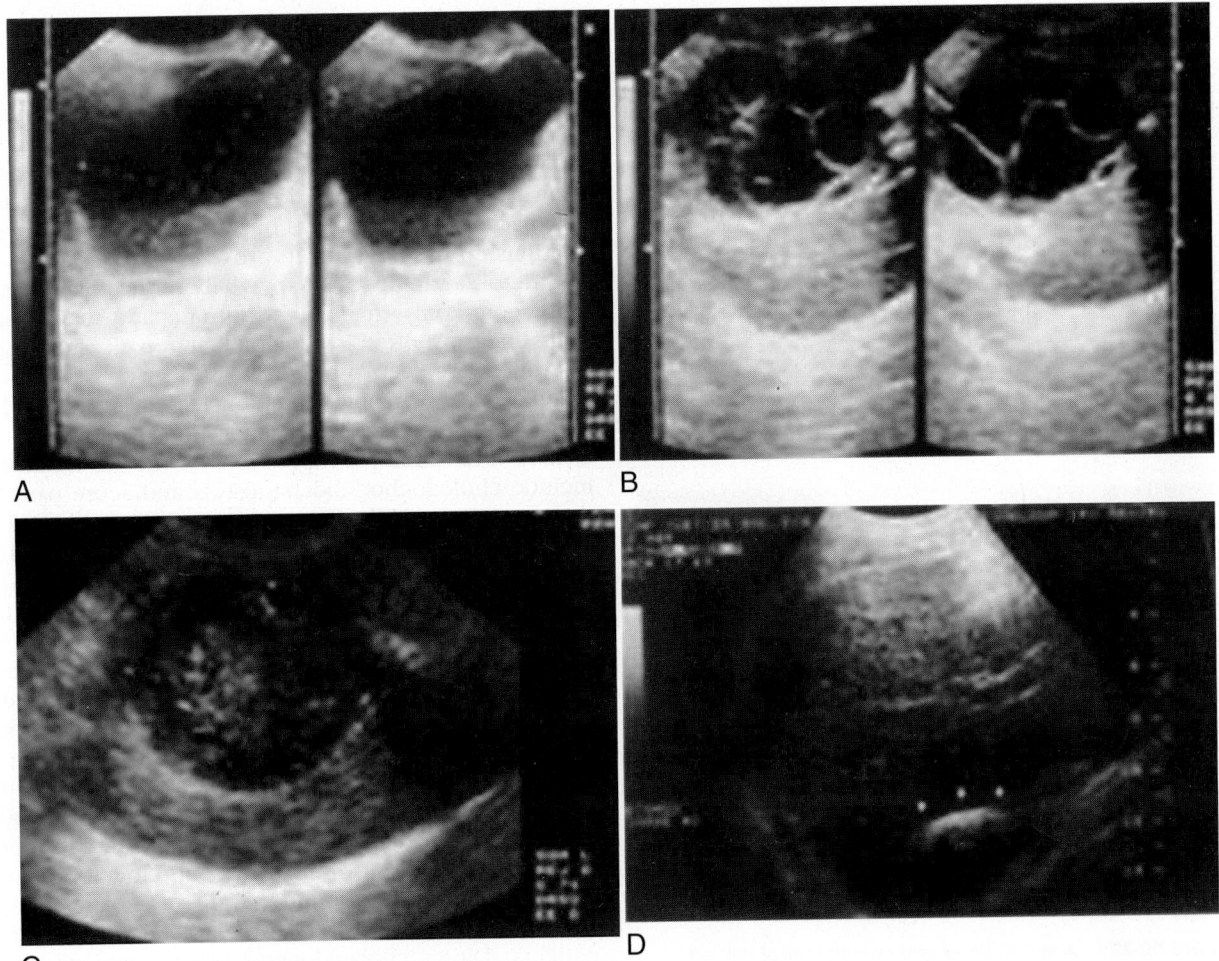

FIGURE 50-21. Ultrasound demonstrating typical characteristics of hydatid cyst at varying stages. **A,** Simple hydatid cyst with "hydatid sand." **B,** Daughter and granddaughter cysts and typical rosette appearance. **C,** Hydatid cyst filled with amorphous mass giving a solid or semi-solid appearance. **D,** Calcified cyst with "eggshell" appearance. (From Thomas PG, Ravindra KV: Amebiasis and biliary infection. *In* Blumgart LH, Fong Y [ed]: Surgery of the Liver and Biliary Tract. London: W.B. Saunders, 2000, pp 1147-1166.)

percutaneous transhepatic cholangiography (PTC) may be necessary.[99,103]

The treatment of hepatic hydatid cysts is primarily surgical. In general, most cysts should be treated, but in elderly patients with small, asymptomatic, calcified cysts, conservative management is appropriate. In preparation for an operation, preoperative corticosteroids have been recommended but are not universally used. The anesthesiologist should have epinephrine and corticosteroids available for the potential of an anaphylactic reaction. A number of operations have been utilized, but, in general, the abdomen is completely explored, the liver mobilized, and the cyst exposed. Packing off of the abdomen is important because rupture can result in anaphylaxis and diffuse seeding. Usually the cyst is then aspirated through a closed suction system and flushed with a scolicidal agent such as hypertonic saline. The cyst is then unroofed, which can then be followed by a number of possibilities, including excision (or pericystectomy), marsupialization

procedures, leaving the cyst open, drainage of the cyst, omentoplasty, or even liver resection. Total pericystectomy can also be performed without entering the cyst (Fig. 50-22).[96,100] When bile duct communication is diagnosed at operation or preoperatively, it must be meticulously searched for. Simple suture repair is often sufficient, but major biliary repairs or approaches through the common bile duct may be necessary.[96,103] Laparoscopic techniques for drainage and unroofing of cysts have been reported in a number of series with encouraging results. Recurrence rates after surgical treatment range from 1% to 20% but are generally 5% or less in experienced centers.[104]

In the past, aspiration of hydatid cysts was contraindicated because of the risk of rupture and uncontrolled spillage. In recent years, however, a number of authors have reported percutaneous aspiration and injection of scolicidal agents with early success rates on the order of 70%.[105,106] This technique has significant limitations and

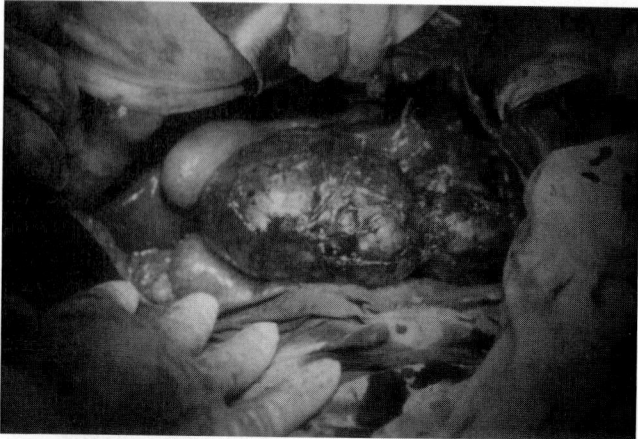

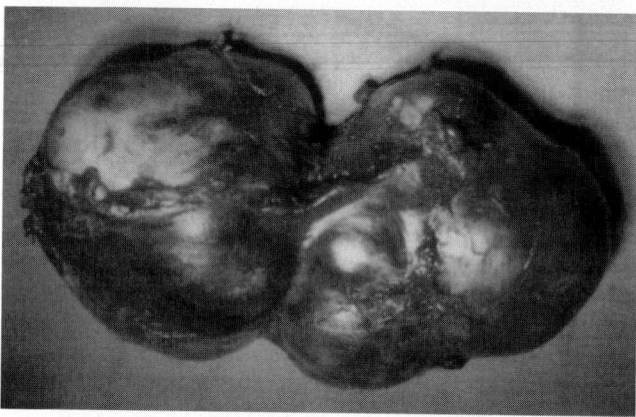

FIGURE 50-22.   **A** and **B,** Peripheral hydatid cyst of the left liver and intact specimen after pericystectomy. Note, the entire pericyst has been removed. (From Milicevic MN: Hydatid disease. *In* Blumgart LH, Fong Y [eds]: Surgery of the Liver and Biliary Tract. London, WB Saunders, 2000, pp 1167-1204.)

should only be used in very well selected cases. Chemotherapy for echinococcosis with albendazole or mebendazole is effective in 20% to 30% of patients infected with *E. granulosus* but requires long-term treatment.[107] Chemotherapy should generally be considered for widely disseminated disease or patients with poor surgical risk.

Recurrent Pyogenic Cholangitis

Recurrent pyogenic cholangitis (RPC) is a syndrome of repeated attacks of cholangitis secondary to biliary stones and strictures that involve the extrahepatic and intrahepatic ducts. The condition has many names but is often referred to as oriental cholangiohepatitis or hepatolithiasis. The disease is almost exclusively found in Asians and therefore is mainly seen in Asian medical centers, but it is also seen in Asian immigrants throughout the world. Males and females are equally affected, and, historically, the disease strikes at an early age (20 to 40) in patients from lower socioeconomic classes.[108,109]

The etiology of RPC is unknown but is related to recurrent infection of biliary radicals with gut bacteria. Ultimately, stones and strictures develop in the biliary tree, but it is not known which occurs first. The stones are bilirubinate stones, and in some patients no stones are found and only biliary sludge is demonstrated. An association between RPC and *Clonorchis sinensis* and *Ascaris lumbricoides* infection has been noted, but a true causal relationship has never been proved.[108]

Strictures can be found anywhere in the biliary tree but more commonly involve the intrahepatic main hepatic ducts and most often involve the left hepatic duct. Dilated bile ducts are seen proximal to the strictures. The gallbladder is only involved in about 20% of cases. Cirrhosis and liver failure are only seen in long-standing disease, usually after multiple operations. Other complications include choledochoduodenal fistula and acute pancreatitis from common bile duct stones. An increased incidence of cholangiocarcinoma has been noted, but a causal relationship is difficult to prove.

The typical patient with RPC is young, Asian, and of a lower socioeconomic background, and presents with repeated bouts of cholangitis. The symptoms and presentation are those of cholangitis: fever, right upper quadrant abdominal pain, and jaundice. Biliary obstruction is usually incomplete, and, therefore, marked jaundice and pruritus are not common. There is usually leukocytosis, and abnormal results of LFTs are consistent with biliary obstruction. Evaluation of the anatomic distribution of disease is critical to formulating a sound therapeutic plan. A combination of ultrasound, CT, direct cholangiography, and MRI is often necessary to completely evaluate these patients. Direct cholangiography performed endoscopically or transhepatically is often a critical study and is complementary to cross-sectional imaging studies. Magnetic resonance cholangiopancreatography (MRCP) can combine cross-sectional imaging and cholangiography in one noninvasive test and may ultimately replace direct cholangiography.[109]

In an acute presentation most patients improve with conservative management, allowing time for radiologic studies and planning of a definitive operation that is necessary in almost all cases. If intervention is necessary during the acute phase it must focus on adequate decompression of the biliary tree through open common bile duct exploration or endoscopic papillotomy.[109] At the definitive operation the goal is to clear the biliary tree of stones and to bypass or enlarge strictures. Many cases only require exploration of the common bile duct with or without hepaticojejunostomy. In complicated cases, providing permanent access to the biliary tree by extending the end of Roux loop hepaticojejunostomy to the skin or subcutaneous space may be necessary. Postoperatively, interventional radiologic procedures can be performed via this hepaticocutaneous jejunostomy (Fig. 50-23).[110] Other potentially necessary procedures include stricturoplasty or partial hepatectomy.[108]

In large series from Hong Kong, mortality rates are 1%, and with aggressive treatment there is almost 100% stone clearance rate and a less than 5% stone recurrence rate. In the long term, most simple cases can be

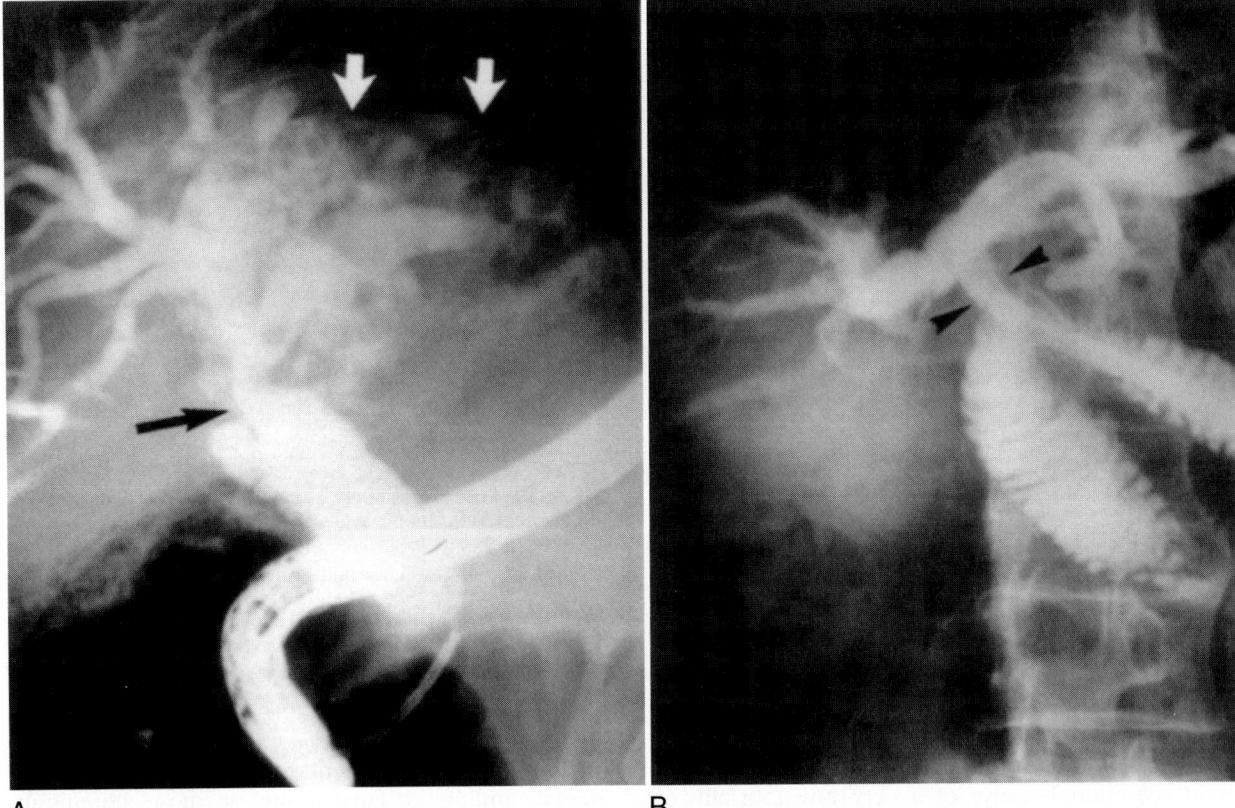

A   B

FIGURE 50-23. **A,** Cholangiogram of a patient with recurrent pyogenic cholangitis and a common hepatic duct stricture *(black arrow).* There are numerous stones inside dilated left ducts *(white arrows).* **B,** A hepaticojejunostomy to the segment III duct *(arrowheads)* has been performed and a flexible choledochoscope is shown passing through the anastomosis into the peripheral left ducts. All stones have been cleared. (From Fan ST, Wong J: Recurrent pyogenic cholangitis. *In* Blumgart LH, Fong Y [eds]: Surgery of the Liver and Biliary Tract. London, WB Saunders, 2000, pp 1205-1225.)

expected to have very low recurrence rates whereas complicated cases have about a 30% rate of recurrent symptoms.[111,112]

NEOPLASMS

Solid Benign Neoplasms

It is estimated that benign focal liver masses are present in about 9% of the population in developed countries. With the increasing use of rapidly improving radiologic examinations these entities are being encountered more frequently. Familiarity with the clinical characteristics, natural history, imaging characteristics, and indications for surgery in these tumors is essential. Many benign lesions can be adequately characterized by modern imaging studies such as CT, ultrasound, and MRI, but in unclear cases, serum tumor markers (AFP, CEA) and a search for a primary tumor (in the case of suspected metastases) should be carried out. Ultimately, a resection might be necessary to make a definitive diagnosis.

Liver Cell Adenoma

Liver cell adenoma (LCA) is a relatively rare benign proliferation of hepatocytes in the context of a normal liver. It is predominantly found in young women (aged 20 to 40), and chronic oral contraceptive use dramatically increases the incidence of this tumor.[113] The female-to-male ratio is approximately 11:1. LCA is usually singular, but multiple lesions have been reported in 12% to 30% of cases. The presence of 10 or more adenomas is termed *adenomatosis.* Interestingly, cases with multiple adenomas are not associated with oral contraceptive use and do not have as dramatic a female preponderance.[114-116] Histologically, LCA are composed of cords of benign hepatocytes containing increased glycogen and fat. The normal architecture of the liver is not present in these lesions.[117]

Patients with LCA present with symptoms about three fourths of the time. Upper abdominal pain is common and may be related to hemorrhage into the tumor or local compressive symptoms. Physical examination is usually unrevealing, and tumor markers are normal. Dramatic presentations with free intraperitoneal rupture and bleeding can occur.[114-116] CT usually demonstrates a well-circumscribed heterogeneous mass. MRI of LCA have specific imaging characteristics, including a well-demarcated mass containing fat or hemorrhage.[118] Although in the past, imaging studies lacked the accuracy to diagnose LCA, modern-day imaging techniques can identify the majority of these tumors. Ultimately, however, resection may be necessary to secure a diagnosis in difficult cases.[115]

The two major risks of LCA are rupture (with potentially life-threatening intraperitoneal hemorrhage) and malignant transformation. Quantifying the risk of rupture is difficult but it has been estimated to be as high as 30% to 50% and may be related to size.[114] Although there are numerous reports of transformation of LCA into hepatocellular carcinoma (HCC) the true risk of transformation is not known.[119]

Patients who present with acute hemorrhage need emergent operation, although hepatic artery embolization can sometimes be a helpful temporizing maneuver. Symptomatic masses, likewise, should be resected. Patients with asymptomatic LCA on oral contraceptives can be watched after stopping the pills, although progression and rupture have been observed in this setting. Behavior of LCA during pregnancy has been unpredictable, and resection before a planned pregnancy is usually recommended. Overall, the surgeon must compare the risks of expectant management with serial imaging studies and AFP measurements against those of resection. Most authorities recommend resection because of a very low mortality in experienced hands and the just-mentioned risks of observation. Margin status is not important in these resections, and limited resections can be performed. The management of adenomatosis is controversial, but large lesions should probably be resected because of the risk of rupture. Occasionally, liver transplant is necessary for aggressive forms of adenomatosis.[114-116]

Focal Nodular Hyperplasia

Focal nodular hyperplasia (FNH) is the second most common benign tumor of the liver and is predominantly discovered in young women. FNH is usually a small (<5 cm) nodular mass arising in a normal liver that involves the right and left liver equally. The mass is characterized by a central fibrous scar with radiating septa, although no central scar is seen in about 15% of cases (Fig. 50-24). Microscopically, FNH contains cords of benign hepatocytes divided by multiple fibrous septa originating from a central scar. Typical hepatic vascularity is not seen, but atypical biliary epithelium is found scattered throughout the lesion. The central scar often contains a large artery that branches out into multiple smaller arteries in a "spoke-wheel" pattern.[114,117]

The etiology of FNH is not known, but the most common theory is that FNH is related to a developmental vascular malformation. Female hormones and oral contraceptive agents have been implicated in the development and growth of FNH, but the association is weak and difficult to prove. Occasional cases of resolution of symptoms after stopping oral contraceptive agents have been reported.

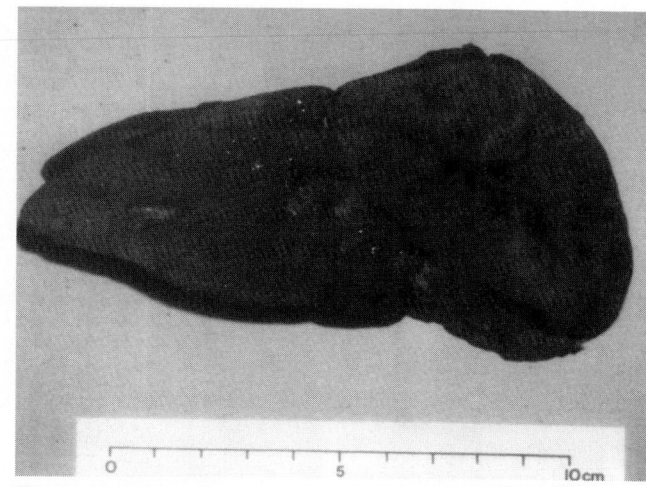

FIGURE 50-24. Cross section of resected focal nodular hyperplasia. Note the well-defined central scar. (From Hugh TJ, Poston GJ: Benign liver tumors and masses. *In* Blumgart LH, Fong Y [eds]: Surgery of the Liver and Biliary Tract. London, WB Saunders, 2000, pp 1397-1422.)

The majority of patients with FNH present as an incidental finding at laparotomy or more commonly on imaging studies. If symptoms are noted, they are most often vague abdominal pain, but a variety of nonspecific symptoms have been described. It is often difficult to ascribe these reported symptoms to the presence of FNH, and therefore other possible causes must be searched for.[115] Physical examination is usually unrevealing, and mild abnormalities of LFT may be found. Serum AFP levels are normal.

With advances in hepatobiliary imaging, the majority of cases of FNH can be diagnosed radiologically with reasonable certainty. Contrast medium–enhanced CT and MRI have become an accurate method of diagnosing FNH. When no central scar is seen, however, radiologic diagnosis is difficult; and differentiating between a benign and malignant mass (especially fibrolamellar HCC) can sometimes be impossible.[118] Occasionally, histologic confirmation is necessary and resection is recommended for definitive diagnosis. Fine-needle aspiration for the diagnosis of FNH is often unrevealing.

The natural history of FNH is not fully understood, but, in the main, FNH is a benign and indolent tumor. Asymptomatic patients mostly remain so over long periods of time. Rupture, bleeding, and infarction are exceedingly rare, and malignant degeneration of FNH has never been reported. The treatment of FNH, therefore, depends on diagnostic certainty and symptoms. Asymptomatic patients with typical radiologic features do not require treatment. If diagnostic uncertainty exists, resection may be necessary for histologic confirmation. Symptomatic patients should be thoroughly investigated to look for other pathology to explain the symptoms. Careful observation of symptomatic FNH with serial imaging is reasonable because symptoms may resolve in a significant number of cases. Patients with persistent symptomatic FNH or an enlarging mass should be considered for resection. Because FNH is a benign diagnosis, resection must be performed with minimal morbidity and mortality.[114-116]

Hemangioma

Hemangioma is the most common benign tumor of the liver. It occurs in women more commonly than men (3:1 ratio) and at a mean age of about 45. Small capillary hemangiomas are of no clinical significance, whereas the larger cavernous hemangiomas more often come to the attention of the liver surgeon (Fig. 50-25). Cavernous hemangiomas have been associated with FNH and are considered congenital vascular malformations. Enlargement of hemangiomas is by ectasia rather than neoplasia. The tumors are usually singular, are less than 5 cm in diameter, and occur equally in the right and left liver. Lesions greater than 5 cm are arbitrarily called giant hemangiomas. Involution or thrombosis of hemangiomas can result in dense fibrotic masses that may be difficult to differentiate from malignancy. Microscopically, they are endothelial lined, blood-filled spaces that are separated by thin fibrous septa.[114,117]

Most commonly, hemangiomas are asymptomatic and incidentally found. Large compressive masses may cause vague upper abdominal symptoms. Symptoms ascribed to a liver hemangioma, however, mandate a search for other pathology because in about half of cases, an alternative cause of symptoms will be found. Rapid expansion or acute thrombosis can, on occasion, cause symptoms. Spontaneous rupture of liver hemangiomas is exceedingly rare. An associated syndrome of thrombocytopenia and consumptive coagulopathy known as Kasabach-Merritt syndrome is rare but well described.[114-116]

LFTs and tumor markers are usually normal in liver hemangiomas. Radiologic investigation can reliably make the diagnosis in the majority of cases. CT and MRI are usually sufficient if a typical peripheral nodular enhancement pattern is seen. Labeled red blood cell scans are an accurate test but are rarely necessary if high-quality CT and MRI are available.[118] Percutaneous biopsy of a suspected hemangioma is potentially dangerous and inaccurate and is therefore not recommended.

Although the natural history of liver hemangioma has not been well documented, it appears that most remain stable over time with a very low risk of rupture or hemorrhage. Growth and development of symptoms do occur, however, occasionally requiring resection. There has never been a report of malignant degeneration of a liver hemangioma. An asymptomatic patient with a secure diagnosis can therefore be simply observed. Symptomatic patients should undergo a thorough evaluation looking for alternative explanations for the symptoms but are candidates for resection if no other cause is found. Rupture, change in size, and development of the Kasabach-Merritt syndrome are indications for resection. In rare cases of diagnostic uncertainty, resection may be necessary to make a definitive diagnosis. Resection of liver hemangiomas should be performed with minimal morbidity and mortality. Resection is mostly performed by enucleation with inflow control, but anatomic resections have been advocated by some. Surgery on large central hemangiomas can be associated with significant morbidity.[114-116]

Liver hemangiomas in children are very common, accounting for about 12% of all childhood hepatic tumors. They are usually multifocal and can involve other organs. Large hemangiomas in children can result in congestive heart failure secondary to arteriovenous shunting. Untreated symptomatic childhood hemangiomas are associated with a 70% mortality, but small capillary hemangiomas almost all resolve. Symptomatic childhood hemangiomas may be treated medically for congestive heart failure with therapeutic embolization. Radiation and chemotherapeutic agents have been used, but experience is limited. Resection may be necessary for symptomatic lesions or for rupture.[120]

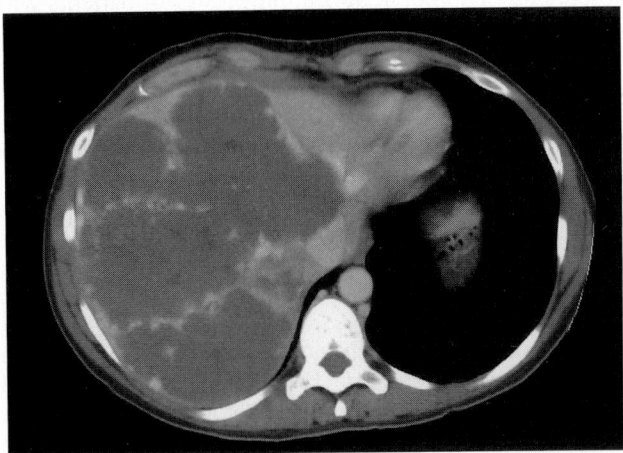

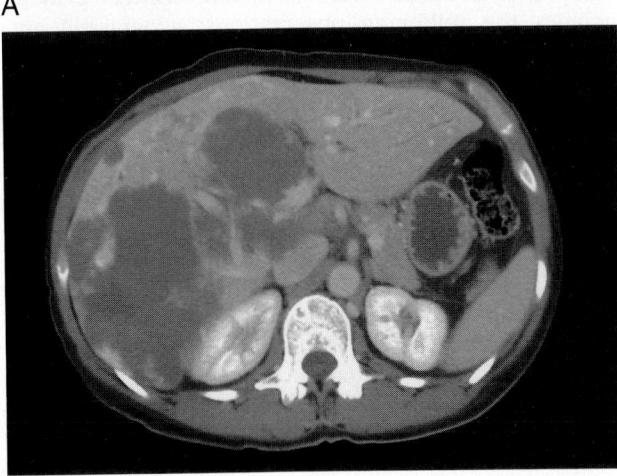

FIGURE 50-25. CT scan of a large cavernous hemangioma showing displacement of left and middle hepatic veins and abutment of the left portal vein. The mass was symptomatic and required an extended right hepatectomy to remove.

Other Benign Tumors

The vast majority of benign solid liver tumors are LCA, FNH, or hemangiomas. An array of other benign hepatic tumors exists but they are rare and can be difficult to differentiate from malignancy. Macroregenerative nodules or adenomatous hyperplasia are single or multiple, well-circumscribed, bile-stained, bulging surface nodules that occur primarily in patients with chronic liver disease. These lesions have varying malignant potential and can be very difficult to distinguish from HCC. Nodular regenerative hyperplasia (NRH) is a diffuse micronodular (usually less than 1.5 cm) process that is associated with portal hypertension and chronic systemic diseases. NRH has no malignant potential and is not associated with cirrhosis. Biopsy may be necessary to distinguish focal nodules from malignancy.[114,117]

Mesenchymal hamartomas (MHs) are rare solitary tumors of childhood that account for 5% of pediatric liver tumors. These are usually large cystic masses found in the right liver that present as progressive painless abdominal distention. Resection of MH may be necessary in the case of large lesions causing a mass effect. Fatty tumors of the liver are rarely encountered but can usually be distinguished by typical characteristics on CT or MRI. Fatty tumors of the liver include primary lipomas, myelolipoma (also containing hematopoietic tissue), angiolipoma (also containing blood vessels), and angiomyolipoma (also containing smooth muscle). Similarly, focal fatty change in the liver can be confused with a neoplastic process. Benign fibrous tumors of the liver exist and can become large and symptomatic, requiring resection. Inflammatory pseudotumors of the liver are a localized mass of inflammatory cells that can mimic a neoplasm. The etiology of these inflammatory lesions is not known but may be related to thrombosed vessels or old abscesses. Other extremely rare benign hepatic tumors include leiomyomas, myxomas, schwannomas, lymphangiomas, and teratomas.[120]

Intrahepatic biliary cystadenomas or bile duct adenomas are extremely rare but can cause biliary symptoms. Biliary hamartomas or biliary hyperplasia are very common and are often seen as small white surface lesions that can mimic small metastatic tumors at abdominal exploration. Adrenal and pancreatic rests have also been found in the liver.[114,117]

Primary Solid Malignant Neoplasms

Hepatocellular Carcinoma

Epidemiology

HCC is the most common primary malignancy of the liver, and one of the most common malignancies worldwide, accounting for over 1 million deaths annually. The geographic distribution of HCC is clearly related to the incidence of hepatitis B virus (HBV) infection. The highest incidence of disease (greater than 10 to 20 per 100,000) is found in Southeast Asia and tropical Africa, and the lowest incidence (1-3 per 100,000) is found in Australia, North America, and Europe. In high incidence areas, rates are variable. For example, Taiwan has an incidence of 150 per 100,000 while Singapore has an incidence of 28 per 100,000. Epidemiologic evidence strongly suggests that HCC is largely related to environmental factors, with

incidence in immigrants eventually taking on that of the local population after several generations. An exception to this observation is that whites living in high-prevalence areas tend to have a low incidence of HCC. This is likely related to the continuation of the lifestyle and environment of their home country. It is probable that the variation in incidence rates among immigrants is related to HBV carrier rates. Recent publications have noted an 80% rise in the incidence of HCC in the United States over the past 30 years, estimating 15,000 new cases annually. The reason for this rising incidence in the United States is not understood, but emergence of hepatitis C virus (HCV) infection and immigration patterns have been suggested.[121,122]

HCC is two to eight times more common in males compared with females in low- and high-incidence areas. Although sex hormones may play a minor role in the development of HCC, the higher incidence in males is probably related to higher rates of associated risk factors, such as HBV infection, cirrhosis, smoking, alcohol abuse, and higher hepatic DNA synthesis in cirrhosis. In general, the incidence of HCC increases with age, but a tendency to develop HCC earlier in high-incidence areas has been noted. For example, in Mozambique 50% of patients with HCC are younger than 30 years of age.[121-123]

Etiology

A large number of associations between hepatic viral infections, environmental exposures, alcohol use, smoking, genetic metabolic diseases, cirrhosis, and the development of HCC have been recognized. What is clear from research is that the development of HCC is a complex and multistep process that involves any number of these risk factors.

Many years of research have documented a clear association between persistent HBV infection and the development of HCC. In one study, a 200-fold greater incidence of HCC in HBV-infected individuals compared with noninfected individuals was observed. Other evidence includes the following observations: geographic areas high in HBV infection have high rates of HCC; HBV infection precedes the development of HCC; the sequence of HBV infection to cirrhosis to HCC is well documented; and the HBV genome is found in the HCC genome. HBV has no known oncogenes, but insertional mutagenesis into hepatocytes may be a contributing factor to the development of HCC. Another proposed mechanism is related to cirrhosis and chronic hepatic inflammation that is present in 60% to 90% of patients with HBV infection and HCC. Cirrhosis, however, is not a prerequisite for the development of HBV-related HCC. The risk of HCC is not simply related to HBV infection but requires chronic infection (i.e., chronically positive hepatitis B surface antigen). There is a higher risk of persistent infection (carrier state) when the infection is acquired at birth or during early childhood. Familial clustering of HCC is probably related to early vertical transmission of the virus and establishment of the chronic carrier state.

Hepatitis C has been discovered to be a major cause of chronic liver disease in Japan, Europe, and the United

States, where there is a relatively low rate of HBV infection. Antibodies to HCV are found in 76% of patients with HCC in Japan and Europe and in 36% of patients in the United States. HBV and HCV infection are both independent risk factors for the development of HCC but may act synergistically when an individual is infected with both viruses. Although the natural history of HCV infection is not completely understood, it appears to be one of chronic infection with a very benign early course but the ultimate development of cirrhosis and HCC. HCV is an RNA virus that does not integrate into the host genome, and therefore the pathogenesis of HCV-related HCC may be more related to chronic inflammation and cirrhosis rather than direct carcinogenesis.

The true relationship of cirrhosis and HCC is very difficult to ascertain, and suggestions of causation remain speculative. Cirrhosis is not required for the development of HCC, and HCC is not an inevitable result of cirrhosis. The relationship of cirrhosis and HCC is further complicated by the fact that they share common associations. Furthermore, some associations (e.g., HBV infection, hemochromatosis) are associated with higher risk of HCC whereas others (e.g., alcohol, primary biliary cirrhosis) are associated with a lower risk of HCC. Research has demonstrated that cirrhotic livers with higher DNA replication rates are associated with the development of HCC.

Chronic alcohol abuse and smoking are both associated with an increased risk of HCC, and there may be a synergistic effect between the two as well as with HBV and HCV infection. Alcohol causes cirrhosis but has never been shown to be directly carcinogenic to hepatocytes and likely acts as a co-carcinogen. Aflatoxin, produced by *Aspergillus* species, is a powerful hepatotoxin. With chronic exposure, aflatoxin acts as a carcinogen and increases the risk of HCC. The offending fungi grow on grains, peanuts, and food products in tropical and subtropical regions, and intake of contaminated foods results in aflatoxin exposure. Levels of aflatoxin in implicated foods are regulated in the United States. A variety of chemicals have been implicated as carcinogens related to HCC and include nitrites, hydrocarbons, solvents, pesticides, and vinyl chloride. Thorotrast (colloidal thorium dioxide) is an angiographic medium that was used in the 1930s that emits high levels of long-lasting radiation and has been associated with hepatic fibrosis, angiosarcoma, cholangiosarcoma, and HCC. Associations with inherited metabolic liver diseases such as hereditary hemochromatosis, α_1-antitrypsin deficiency, and Wilson's disease have also been implicated as risk factors for HCC. Associations with hormonal manipulations such as the use of oral contraceptive agents and anabolic steroids have been suggested but are weak.

CLINICAL PRESENTATION

Most commonly, patients presenting with HCC are men 50 to 60 years of age who complain of right upper quadrant abdominal pain, weight loss, and a palpable mass. Unfortunately, in unscreened populations, HCC tends to present at a late stage because of the lack of symptoms in early stages. Presentation at this advanced stage is often with a vague right upper quadrant abdominal pain that sometimes radiates to the right shoulder. Nonspecific symptoms of advanced malignancy such as anorexia, nausea, lethargy, and weight loss are common. Another common presentation of HCC is hepatic decompensation in a patient with known mild cirrhosis or even in patients without previously recognized cirrhosis.

HCC can rarely present as a rupture with the sudden onset of abdominal pain followed by hypovolemic shock secondary to intraperitoneal bleeding. Other rare presentations include hepatic vein occlusion (Budd-Chiari syndrome), obstructive jaundice, hemobilia, or fever of unknown origin. Less than 1% of cases of HCC present as a paraneoplastic syndrome, most commonly hypercalcemia, hypoglycemia, and erythrocytosis. Small, incidentally noted tumors are becoming a more common presentation because of the knowledge of specific risk factors, screening programs, and the increasing use of high-quality abdominal imaging.[1,121,123]

DIAGNOSIS

Radiologic investigation is a critical part of the diagnosis of HCC. In the past, liver radioisotope scans and angiography were common methods of diagnosis, but ultrasound, CT, and MRI have largely replaced these studies. Ultrasound plays a significant role in screening and early detection of HCC, but definitive diagnosis and treatment planning usually rely on CT and/or MRI. Contrast medium–enhanced CT and MRI protocols aimed at diagnosing HCC take advantage of the hypervascularity of these tumors, and both imaging and enhancement patterns are critical. CT and MRI also evaluate the extent of disease in terms of peritoneal metastases, nodal metastases, and extent of vascular and biliary involvement. Detection of bland or tumor thrombus in the portal venous system is also very important and can be diagnosed with any of the just-described modalities (Fig. 50-26).[118,121]

AFP measurements can be very helpful in the diagnosis of HCC. An AFP level greater than 20 ng/mL is noted in about three fourths of documented cases of HCC. False-positive elevations of serum AFP can be seen in inflammatory disorders of the liver such as chronic active viral hepatitis. Specificity and positive predictive values of AFP improve with higher cutoff levels (such as 400 ng/mL), but at the cost of sensitivity. With the improvements in imaging technology, and the ability to detect smaller tumors, AFP is largely used as an adjunctive test in patients with liver masses. AFP levels are particularly useful in monitoring treated patients for recurrence. Because of accuracy problems, measuring various isoforms of AFP is being researched.[121,123]

Percutaneous needle biopsies of liver lesions suspected of being HCC are only necessary in patients who are being considered for nonoperative therapies. Patients with appropriate risk factors and suggestive radiology (with or without an elevated AFP) who are candidates for potentially curative surgical therapy do not require preoperative biopsy. Percutaneous fine-needle aspiration of HCC does run a small risk of tumor cell spillage (estimated to be about 1%) and rupture/bleeding (especially in cirrhotic

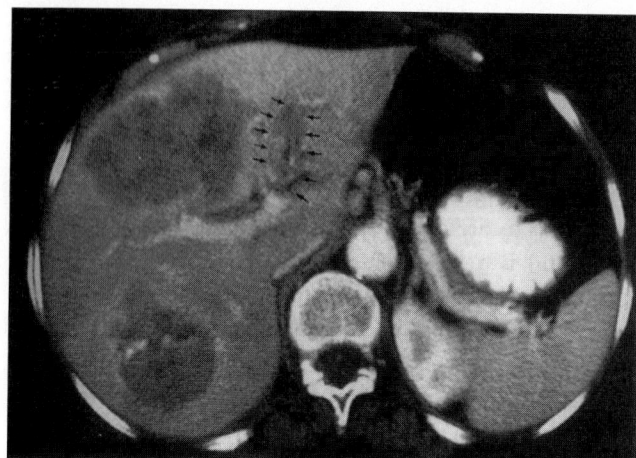

FIGURE 50-26. Contrast medium–enhanced CT scan demonstrating multifocal hepatocellular carcinoma. The left portal vein is invaded and expanded by tumor (arrows). (From Roddie ME, Adam A: Computed tomography of the liver and biliary tree. *In* Blumgart LH, Fong Y [eds]: Surgery of the Liver and Biliary Tract. London, WB Saunders, 2000, pp 309-340.)

livers). In a patient with a suggestive mass on quality imaging and a markedly elevated AFP, biopsy is not required because the diagnosis is obvious.

Once the diagnosis of HCC has been made, an effort to stage the tumor must be made to develop an appropriate treatment plan. Most patients with HCC have two diseases, and survival is as much related to the tumor as it is to cirrhosis. Staging, therefore, includes an extent of disease work-up as well as an "extent of cirrhosis" work-up.

In assessing the extent of disease, the common sites of metastases must be considered. HCC largely metastasizes to the lung, bone, and peritoneum, and preoperative history should focus on symptoms referable to these areas. Extent of disease in the liver including macrovascular invasion and the presence of multiple liver masses must also be considered. Cross-sectional abdominal imaging (see earlier) yields information on extent of disease in the liver as well as peritoneal disease. A preoperative chest radiograph is mandatory and should be followed with CT if any abnormalities are present. Routine bone scans are not performed unless there are suggestive symptoms or signs.

Assessment of liver function is absolutely critical in considering treatment options for a patient with HCC. Liver resection is considered the treatment of choice for HCC, and the risk of postoperative liver failure and/or death must be considered. This risk is related to the degree of cirrhosis, the amount of liver resected (functional liver reserve), and the regenerative response. Other successful treatments are available for HCC, such as ablative techniques, embolization techniques, and liver transplant; therefore, a complete assessment of tumor and liver function must ensue. A number of assessments of liver function are available and are described in an earlier section. Generally, they are divided into a clinical assessment and functional tests. Many clinical assessment schemes are

described (see previous section), but most commonly Child's status (as modified by Pugh) is used. Child's C patients are not candidates for resectional therapy whereas Child's A patients can usually tolerate some extent of liver resection. Many consider Child's B patients candidates for operation, but they are generally borderline and therapy must be individualized. Outside of scoring systems, factors such as an elevated bilirubin, coagulopathy, and thrombocytopenia should be considered. Functional LFTs are well described (see previous section) but are not routinely used in most centers because the results of studies evaluating predictive value have been mixed.

Staging laparoscopy has been employed as a staging tool in HCC and spares about one in five patients a nontherapeutic laparotomy. Laparoscopy yields additional information about extent of disease in the liver, extrahepatic disease, and cirrhosis. Yields of laparoscopy are clearly dictated by the extent of disease on preoperative clinical and radiologic studies but should be considered in all high-risk patients.[124]

A number of staging systems for HCC exist, but none has ever been shown to be particularly superior. The TNM staging system is not routinely used for HCC, and it does not accurately predict survival because it does not take liver function into account. The Okuda staging system is a good example of a system that takes into account liver function and tumor-related factors. It is simple and reliably distinguishes patients with a prohibitively poor prognosis and those with potential for long-term survival (Table 50-7).[121,123]

PATHOLOGY

Histologically, HCC is graded as well, moderately, or poorly differentiated. The grade of HCC, however, has never been shown to accurately predict outcome. Grossly, the growth patterns of HCC have been classified in a number of ways. The most useful scheme divides HCC into three distinct growth patterns that have a distinct relationship to outcome. The hanging type of HCC is connected to the liver by a small vascular stalk and is easily resected without sacrifice of a significant amount of nonneoplastic liver tissue. The hanging type of HCC can grow to substantial size without involving much normal liver

TABLE 50-7.   Okuda Staging System for Hepatocellular Carcinoma*

Clinical Parameters	Cut-off Values	Points
Tumor size	>50%	1
	<50%	0
Ascites	Present	1
	Absent	0
Serum albumin (mg/dL)	>3	0
	<3	1
Serum total bilirubin (mg/dL)	<3	0
	>3	1

*Stage 1 = 0 points; stage 2 = 1-2 points; stage 3 = 3-4 points.

tissue. The pushing type of HCC is well demarcated and often contains a fibrous capsule. It is characterized by growth that displaces vascular structures rather than invading them. The pushing type of HCC is usually resectable. The last type is called the infiltrative type of HCC, which tends to invade vascular structures even at a small size. Resecting the infiltrative type is often possible, but positive histologic margins are common. Small tumors less than 5 cm usually do not fall into any of these groups and are often discussed as separate entities. Lastly, HCC can present in a multifocal manner. Most HCC probably starts as a single tumor, but ultimately multiple satellite lesions can develop secondary to portal vein invasion and metastases. Multifocal tumors throughout the liver probably represent the end stage of HCC with multiple metastases and multiple primary tumors.[117,125]

TREATMENT

There are a large number of treatment options for patients with HCC, reflecting the heterogeneity of this disease as well as the lack of a proven superior treatment excepting complete resection (Box 50-1). Deciding on a treatment regimen for any one patient must take into consideration the stage of malignancy, the condition of the patient, the condition of the liver, and the experience of the treating physicians.

Complete excision of HCC either by partial hepatectomy or by total hepatectomy and transplant is the only treatment modality with curative potential. In general, however, only 10% to 20% of patients are considered to have resectable disease. Mortality rates for partial hepatectomy range from 1% to 20%, but if performed in healthy patients without advanced cirrhosis, most modern series have a mortality rate less than 5%. Advances in surgical

---

Box 50-1. Treatment options for hepatocellular carcinoma

Surgical
    Resection
    Orthotopic liver transplant
Ablative
    Ethanol injection
    Acetic acid injection
    Thermal ablation (cryotherapy, radiofrequency ablation, microwave)
Transarterial
    Embolization
    Chemoembolization
    Radiotherapy
Combination transarterial/ablative
External beam radiation
Systemic
    Chemotherapy
    Hormonal therapy
    Immunotherapy

---

technique have allowed the development of limited segmental resections when appropriate, which preserve functional liver and improve early postoperative recovery. The overall post-resection survival rates for HCC are 58% to 100% at 1 year, 28% to 88% at 3 years, 11% to 75% at 5 years, and 19% to 26% at 10 years. These results obviously depend on the stage of the tumor as well as the degree of cirrhosis in particular series but give a sense of the possibilities. A variety of prognostic factors predictive of survival after resection have been identified, but none is universally agreed on. The most commonly cited negative prognostic factors are tumor size, cirrhosis, infiltrative growth pattern, vascular invasion, intrahepatic metastases, multifocal tumors, lymph node metastases, margin less than 1 cm, and lack of a capsule.[121,123,126]

Theoretically, liver transplantation is the ideal treatment for HCC because it addresses both the liver dysfunction and the HCC. The limitations of transplantation are the need for chronic immunosuppression as well as the lack of organ donors. There is a growing interest in the use of partial hepatectomy from live donors, which addresses the latter point but remains a somewhat controversial approach. Early series of transplantation for HCC had high recurrence rates and relatively poor long-term survival. This has largely been attributed to the fact that most of these patients were being transplanted for advanced disease. Refinements in patient selection, namely, patients with single tumors less than 5 cm or multiple tumors no more than three in number and 3 cm have resulted in improved outcome.[127] Long-term survival rates in recent years have ranged from 25% to 75%. Comparing results of resection to transplantation is difficult, and the two should be viewed as complementary rather than competitive. Patients with advanced cirrhosis (Child's B and C) and early-stage HCC should be considered for transplant, whereas those with Child's A cirrhosis have similar results with transplant and resection and should probably undergo resection.

A number of other nonsurgical local ablative therapies are available for the treatment of HCC. Percutaneous ethanol injection (PEI) is a useful technique for ablating small tumors. The tumor is killed by a combination of cellular dehydration, coagulative necrosis, and vascular thrombosis. Most tumors less than 2 cm can be ablated with a single application of PEI, but larger tumors may require multiple injections. Long-term survival after PEI for tumors less than 5 cm has been reported to range from 24% to 40%, but no randomized trials have compared PEI with resection. Percutaneous injection of acetic acid is a similar technique to PEI but has stronger necrotizing abilities, making it more useful in septated tumors.[128]

Thermal ablative techniques that freeze or heat tumors to destroy them have become very popular in recent years. Cryotherapy uses a specialized cryoprobe to freeze and thaw tumor and surrounding liver tissue with resulting necrosis. Cryotherapy is usually performed at laparotomy or laparoscopically but has recently been performed with percutaneous techniques. One advantage is that the ice ball formed is easily monitored with ultrasound. Disadvantages include a "heat-sink" effect, limiting the utility of freezing near major blood vessels and a relatively high complication rate of 8% to 41%. Reported 2-year survival rates for cryoablation of HCC range from 30% to 60%, but no comparative studies to resection exist. Radiofrequency ablation (RFA) utilizes high-frequency alternating current to create heat around an inserted probe, resulting in temperatures greater than 60°C and immediate cell death. Although initially limited to smaller tumors, improvements in technology have created RFA probes reportedly able to ablate tumors as large as 7 cm. RFA is also limited by the protective effect of blood vessels and does not ablate well in these areas. RFA can easily be performed percutaneously with very low complication rates, and optimal guidance systems are being developed. No long-term data for RFA of HCC exist.[128,129]

Transarterial therapy for HCC is based on the fact that the majority of the tumor's blood supply is from the hepatic artery. Hepatic arterial infusion chemotherapy utilizing 5-fluorouracil–based compounds, cisplatin, and doxorubicin has been studied in limited numbers. Response rates of 25% to 60% have been reported, but the requirement of a laparotomy to place the pump and associated hepatic toxicity limits the applicability of this approach.[128] Percutaneous transarterial embolization can induce ischemic necrosis in HCC, resulting in response rates as high as 50% (Fig. 50-27). Attempts to improve the efficacy of arterial embolization have included adding chemotherapeutic agents (chemoembolization) to the embolization particles and oils such as Lipiodol that are selectively taken up by HCC. Randomized trials have not shown chemoembolization to be superior to embolization alone and additionally have not shown either embolization strategy to be more effective than supportive care alone.[130] Nonetheless, embolization strategies are commonly used in nonoperative candidates.

External beam radiation therapy (EBRT) has a limited role in the treatment of HCC, although occasional dramatic responses are seen. EBRT is limited by damage to normal liver parenchyma and to surrounding organs, but newer methods of conformal radiotherapy and breath-gated techniques are improving the utility of this treatment modality. Intra-arterial injections of iodine-131 with Lipiodol or yttrium-90 in glass microspheres have been utilized to deliver localized radiation to HCC, with reports of dramatic response rates.[131,132] Transarterial radiotherapy is potentially promising therapy for HCC as primary therapy or as adjuvant therapy.

Systemic chemotherapy with a variety of agents has been ineffective for the treatment of HCC and has a minimal role in the treatment of HCC. Response rates are generally under 20% and of short duration. Systemic immunotherapy and hormonal therapy have been used in small numbers of patients with HCC with some early promising results, but further study is necessary to define the role of these therapies.

With the bewildering number of available treatment strategies for HCC it is no surprise that combinations of therapies and adjuvant or neoadjuvant strategies in conjunction with resection have been attempted. Two randomized trials have demonstrated a survival benefit to specific adjuvant strategies after resection of HCC. The first is the use of the retinoid polyprenoic acid,[133] and the second is transarterial iodine-131 Lipiodol treatment.[132] Further studies and larger trials are awaited to confirm these promising strategies.

DISTINCT VARIANTS OF HCC

Fibrolamellar HCC (FHCC) is a variant of HCC with remarkably different clinical features that are summarized in Table 50-8. This tumor generally occurs in younger patients without a history of cirrhosis. The tumor is usually well demarcated, is encapsulated, and may have a central fibrotic area. The central scar can make distinguishing this tumor from FNH difficult. Histologically, FHCC is composed of large polygonal tumor cells embedded in a fibrous stroma forming lamellar structures (Fig. 50-28). FHCC does not produce AFP, but it is associated with elevated neurotensin levels. In general, FHCC has a better prognosis than HCC. This is likely related to high resectability rates and lack of chronic liver disease. Long-term survival can be expected in about 50% of patients with complete resection.[134]

Rarely, HCC can present as a mixed hepatocellular-cholangiocellular tumor with cellular differentiation of both types present. Whether this is two separate tumors growing into each other or mixed differentiation of the same tumor is not known. These mixed tumors tend to take on a worse prognosis than standard HCC. A clear cell variant of HCC exists where the cells contain a clear cyto-

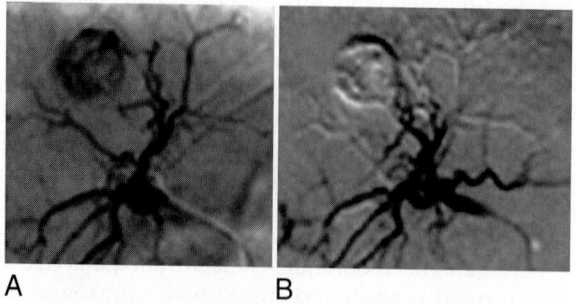

FIGURE 50-27. Angiogram demonstrating hypervascular hepatocellular carcinoma before **(A)** and after **(B)** embolization.

TABLE 50-8.   Comparison of Standard Hepatocellular Carcinoma (HCC) and Fibrolamellar Hepatocellular Carcinoma (FHCC)

Characteristic	HCC	FHCC
Male:female ratio	2:1–8:1	1:1
Median age	55	25
Tumor	Invasive	Well circumscribed
Resectability	<25%	50–75%
Cirrhosis	90%	5%
α-Fetoprotein positive	80%	5%
Hepatitis B positive	65%	5%

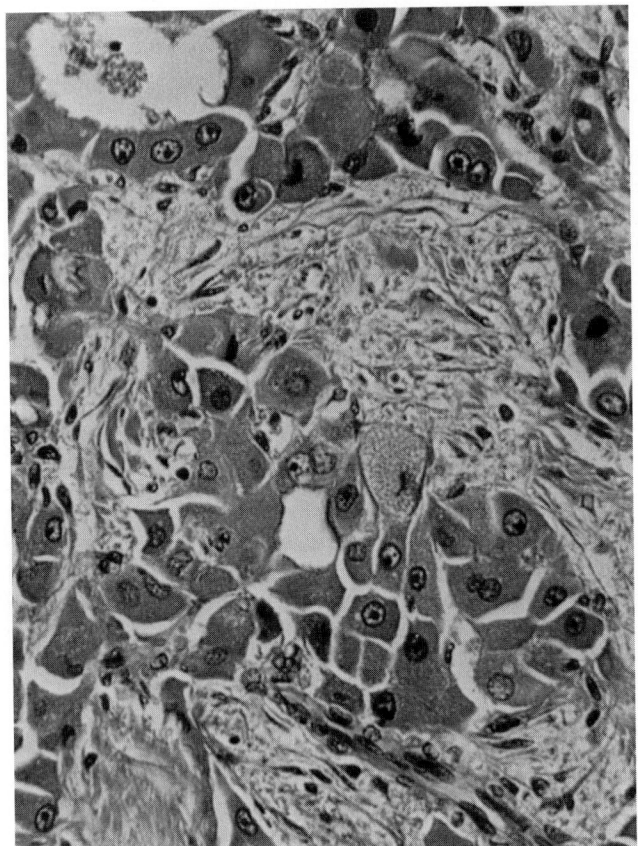

FIGURE 50-28. Fibrolamellar hepatocellular carcinoma. Abundant collagen is evident interconnecting clusters of cells. The cells are often in single-layer sheets. An acinus is present in the left upper field. (From Edmonson HA; Differential diagnosis of tumors and tumor-like lesions in infancy and childhood. Am J Dis Child 91:168, 1956. Copyright 1965, American Medical Association. Courtesy of Dr. Alexander Brunschwig.)

plasm. These tumors can resemble renal cell neoplasms. The clear cell variant may have a better prognosis than standard HCC, but this is a subject of debate. A pleomorphic or giant cell variant of HCC has been reported. Cells in this type are multinucleated, pleomorphic, and large and likely originate from primary hepatic cells. Some HCCs show evidence of sarcomatoid differentiation and are referred to as a sarcomatoid variant or carcinosarcoma. These tumors tend not to produce AFP and have a higher incidence of metastases at presentation.[117,121]

Childhood HCC is a distinct entity that makes up almost one fourth of pediatric liver tumors but rarely occurs in infancy. Viral hepatitis is associated with childhood HCC in Asia, but less so in the United States. Other inherited metabolic liver diseases (see earlier) are often associated with childhood HCC. As in adult HCC, complete resection is the only potentially curative treatment. There is a high incidence of multifocality, vascular invasion, and extrahepatic metastases, resulting in relatively poor long-term survival rates of 10% to 20%.[120]

Intrahepatic Cholangiocarcinoma

Cholangiocarcinoma is an uncommon neoplasm with an incidence of 1 to 2 per 100,000 in the United States and can develop anywhere along the biliary tree from the ampulla of Vater to the peripheral intrahepatic bile ducts. The majority (40% to 60%) of these tumors involve the biliary confluence (Klatskin's tumor), but approximately 10% emanate from intrahepatic ducts, presenting as a liver mass. Intrahepatic cholangiocarcinoma (IHC) is the second most common primary hepatic neoplasm and has also been referred to as peripheral cholangiocarcinoma or cholangiolar carcinoma. Studies on the incidence and natural history of IHC have been confused by the fact that many series include mixed hepatocellular-cholangiocarcinoma (see earlier). Additionally, it is likely that in the past many of these tumors were mistaken for metastatic adenocarcinoma because biopsy is unable to differentiate the two. The most common risk factors for the development of cholangiocarcinoma (all types) include primary sclerosing cholangitis, choledochal cyst disease, and recurrent pyogenic cholangitis.

The clinical presentation of IHC is similar to that of HCC. The most common symptoms are right upper abdominal pain and weight loss. Jaundice occurs in about one fourth of patients. In recent years, patients are more often presenting with incidentally found liver masses on cross-sectional imaging. Unlike in HCC, the AFP level will be normal, although CEA levels can be elevated in some cases. Most often a search for a primary tumor will ensue and will not yield any information. If a biopsy has been performed it is often read as "adenocarcinoma." On CT and MRI, IHC is seen as a focal hepatic mass that may be associated with peripheral biliary dilation. The mass typically has peripheral or central enhancement on contrast medium–enhanced scans. Intrahepatic metastases, lymph node metastases, and growth along the biliary tree are commonly encountered.

Complete resection is the treatment of choice for IHC. Resectability rates generally range from 60% to 90%, and long-term survival in unresected patients is rare. If completely resected, 3-year survival rates range from 16% to 61% and 5-year survival rates range from 24% to 44%. Factors associated with a poor outcome include intrahepatic metastases, lymph node metastases, vascular invasion, and positive margins. There is little known about the utility of radiation and chemotherapy for IHC, and their use is not routine. Chemotherapy is largely considered ineffective for IHC.[123,135]

Other Primary Malignant Neoplasms

Hepatoblastoma is the most common primary hepatic tumor of childhood. There are about 50 to 70 new cases per year in the United States. Rare cases of adult hepatoblastoma have been reported, but, overall, the median age of presentation is 18 months and almost all cases occur before the age of 3. Recently, hepatoblastoma has been associated with the familial polyposis syndrome. There are a number of histologic subtypes, but, in general, the tumor is derived from fetal or embryonic hepatocytes and there are often mesenchymal elements present. Most often this tumor presents as an asymptomatic mass. Mild anemia and thrombocytosis is commonly found at presentation. Serum AFP levels are elevated in 85% to 90% of patients and can serve as useful marker for therapeutic response. Most studies support the use of chemotherapy followed by resection, and survival appears to be dependent on complete resection. Chemotherapy can serve to down-stage tumors, facilitating resection. In patients without metastatic disease or the anaplastic variant, long-term survival rates of 60% to 70% can be expected with complete resection. Interestingly, 50% of patients with pulmonary metastases can be cured with resection of the hepatic tumor and chemotherapy and/or resection of the pulmonary metastases.[117,120]

A variety of sarcomas can rarely present as primary liver tumors but must always be considered metastatic lesions until proved otherwise. Angiosarcoma is probably the best described primary hepatic sarcoma because of its well-known association with vinyl chloride or Thorotrast exposure. Angiosarcoma typically presents as multiple hepatic masses and can present in childhood. Long-term survival is uncommon with primary hepatic angiosarcoma. A variety of other sarcomas, including leiomyosarcoma, malignant fibrous histiocytoma, embryonic sarcoma, and primary hepatic rhabdoid tumor, have been described but are rare. The latter two lesions are typically seen in the pediatric population.

Non-Hodgkin's lymphoma can present primarily in the liver with or without extrahepatic disease. Primary hepatic lymphoma should be treated like lymphoma elsewhere in the body if the diagnosis can be made before a liver resection. Primary hepatic neuroendocrine tumors or carcinoid tumors have been described. Distinguishing the rare primary hepatic neuroendocrine tumor from a metastatic lesion can be difficult because the extrahepatic primary tumor can be radiologically occult and the liver is the most common site of metastases. Malignant germ cell tumors of the liver including teratomas, choriocarcinomas, and yolk sac tumors are very rare and are principally described in the pediatric population. Epithelioid hemangioendothelioma of the liver is a rare malignant vascular tumor that presents as multiple bilateral hepatic masses. Extrahepatic metastases occur in about one fourth of patients, and clinical behavior is unpredictable. Most patients ultimately die of liver failure, but cases of successful transplantation have been reported.

Metastatic Tumors

The most common malignant tumors of the liver are metastatic lesions. The liver is a common site of metastases from gastrointestinal tumors, presumably because of dissemination via the portal venous system. The most relevant metastatic tumor of the liver to the surgeon is colorectal cancer because of the potential for curative resection. However, a large number of other tumors commonly metastasize to the liver. Included among these are tumors of the lung, prostate, breast, pancreas, stomach, kidney, cervix, and ovary. It is important to realize that only a very small percentage of these other metastatic liver tumors occur without evidence of extrahepatic disease, limiting the role of the surgeon to highly selected cases.

Traditionally, when a cancer has spread to a distant site it is considered a systemic disease in which locoregional therapies (i.e., surgery) are not effective. Metastatic tumors to the liver and metastatic colorectal cancer to the liver in particular have been shown to be an exception to this rule. Almost 30 years of clinical research has documented that metastatic colorectal cancer isolated in the liver can be resected with the potential for long-term survival and cure.[136] Advances in systemic and regional hepatic chemotherapy have also broadened the number of patients eligible for surgical therapy and probably improve long-term survival.[137] Patient selection is by far the most important aspect of surgical therapy for metastatic disease in the liver, and clinical follow-up of resected patients has identified those most likely to benefit. Other tumors that present as isolated hepatic metastases can also be resected for potential cure, but data on these other tumors are sparse and less compelling than data for colorectal cancer.

Colorectal

There are over 50,000 cases of colorectal liver metastases a year in the United States. The majority of these cases are associated with widespread disease and/or unresectable hepatic disease, and it is estimated that 5% to 10% of these patients are candidates for a potentially curative liver resection. In the distant past, patients with hepatic colorectal metastases generally presented with symptoms and signs of advanced malignancy, such as pain, ascites, jaundice, weight loss, and a palpable mass. In fact, presentation with such symptoms is a poor prognostic sign and very few of these patients are candidates for therapy outside of chemotherapy or supportive care. This has led most practitioners to carefully follow patients with resected primary colorectal cancer who are potential candidates for aggressive therapy with serial physical examinations, imaging studies, LFTs, and CEA levels. Although not supported by randomized trials, clinical observation has been that patients carefully followed with these tests are the ones often found to have resectable disease. Of course, some patients are found to have synchronous metastatic disease at the time of diagnosis of the primary colorectal cancer on preoperative imaging or at laparotomy.[136,138]

CEA is normally only secreted in utero, but it is secreted by a majority of colorectal cancers. Although an elevated CEA is not specific for recurrent colorectal cancer, a rising CEA on serial examinations and a new solid mass on imaging studies are diagnostic of metastatic disease. Elevated LFTs are common in metastatic colorectal cancer to the liver but are not effective as a screening tool. The most common elevated tests are ALP, GGT, and lactate dehydrogenase (LDH).[136] The best imaging studies for hepatic colorectal metastases are a subject of debate. Most practitioners use contrast medium–enhanced CT, and a triphasic technique is probably best. The most sensitive study is

CT portography, which is a CT performed after cannulation and injection of contrast agent into the hepatic artery during the portal venous phase. Because hepatic metastases obtain their blood supply from the hepatic artery, they show up as dark perfusion defects (Fig. 50-29). Unfortunately, CT portography lacks specificity, is expensive, and is invasive.[139] MRI can be useful to characterize hepatic lesions of uncertain significance (see earlier).

Once a patient who presents with a hepatic colorectal metastasis is considered a candidate for surgical therapy, a complete extent-of-disease work-up must be performed. Colonoscopy should be performed if it has been over a year since the last examination to rule out local recurrence or metachronous lesions. Complete abdominal and pelvic cross-sectional imaging must also be performed. A chest CT is often performed but is of low yield, and a chest radiograph is sufficient. Studies are underway to evaluate the added benefit of PET scans to detect occult extrahepatic disease, and the role of this modality is not completely defined (Fig. 50-30). We have evaluated the role of staging laparoscopy before definitive laparotomy, and about 10% of patients are spared a nontherapeutic laparotomy. The yield of laparoscopy clearly correlates with the number of poor prognostic factors present and can be used selectively.[124]

Because no prospective trial of surgery versus no treatment or chemotherapy has ever been done (or is likely to ever be done) one must understand the natural history of colorectal liver metastases left untreated or treated with systemic chemotherapy alone. Before the 1980s most hepatic metastases were left untreated. A number of investigators have retrospectively studied groups of these patients and documented that these patients had median survivals of 5 to 10 months and long-term survival was rarely seen. The majority of these patients had extensive disease, and most had their primary tumor in place as well.[140,141] Nonetheless, some investigators have been able to identify untreated patients with limited and potentially resectable hepatic disease, and survival in these patients was more favorable.[142] It was clear from these studies that survival is closely related to the amount of disease in the liver. Systemic chemotherapy is largely ineffective as a sole therapy for hepatic colorectal metastases, with median survivals around 12 months and partial response rates of 20% to 30%.[143] Recent developments in chemotherapeutic agents such as irinotecan (CPT-11) and oxaliplatin, with improved response rates, are now approved for use in metastatic colorectal cancer but are unlikely to improve survival by a large amount.

Although performed sporadically before the 1980s, liver resection for isolated hepatic colorectal metastases was viewed with great skepticism. The high morbidity and mortality for liver surgery at that time contributed to this skepticism.[1] Over the past 20 years large series have demonstrated that liver surgery can now be practiced with acceptable safety and that patients with isolated and resectable hepatic metastases have the potential for long-term survival. Five-year survival rates range from 25% to 37%, and mortality in experienced centers is consistently less than 5% (Table 50-9). Almost all series demonstrate that nearly half of patients undergoing a liver resection for metastatic colorectal cancer will survive 3 years and 1 in 5 patients will survive 10 years. Despite the low operative mortality, it must be stated that liver surgery is still associated with significant morbidity rates of 30% to 50%. Complications are most commonly bleeding, bile leak, abscess, and other generalized cardiorespiratory complications.[136,138,144-147]

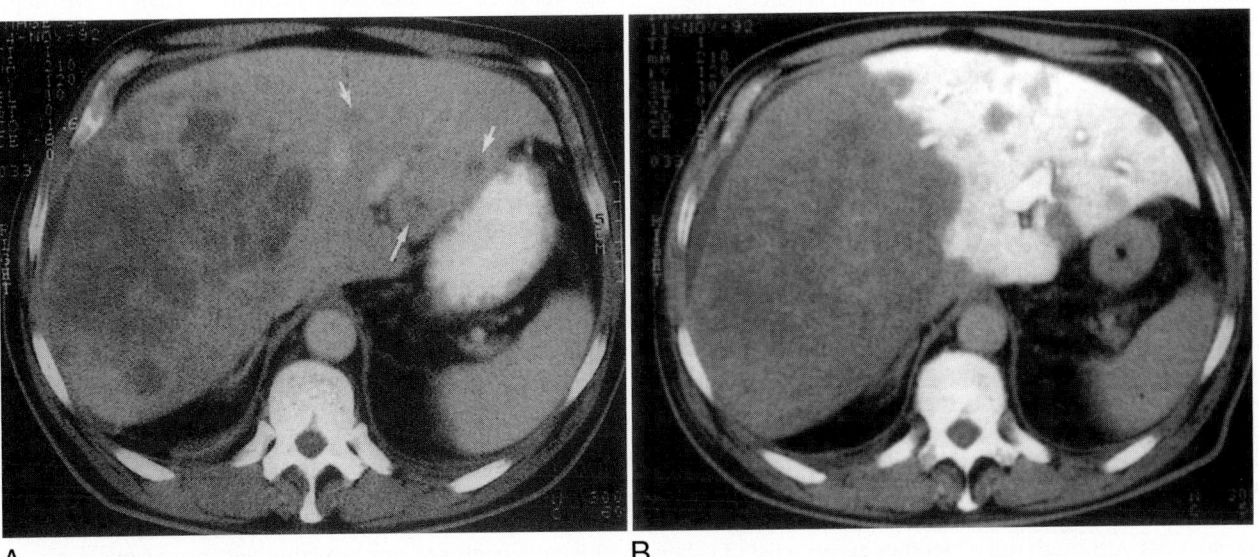

FIGURE 50-29.   Comparison of standard CT and CT portography. **A,** Intravenous contrast medium–enhanced CT demonstrates numerous right-sided metastases and three lesions in the left liver *(arrows)*. **B,** CT portography at the same level demonstrates a straight line sign due to occlusion of the right portal vein and at least 10 lesions in the left liver. (From Roddie ME, Adam A: Computed tomography of the liver and biliary tree. *In* Blumgart LH, Fong Y [eds]: Surgery of the Liver and Biliary Tract. London, WB Saunders, 2000, pp 309-340.)

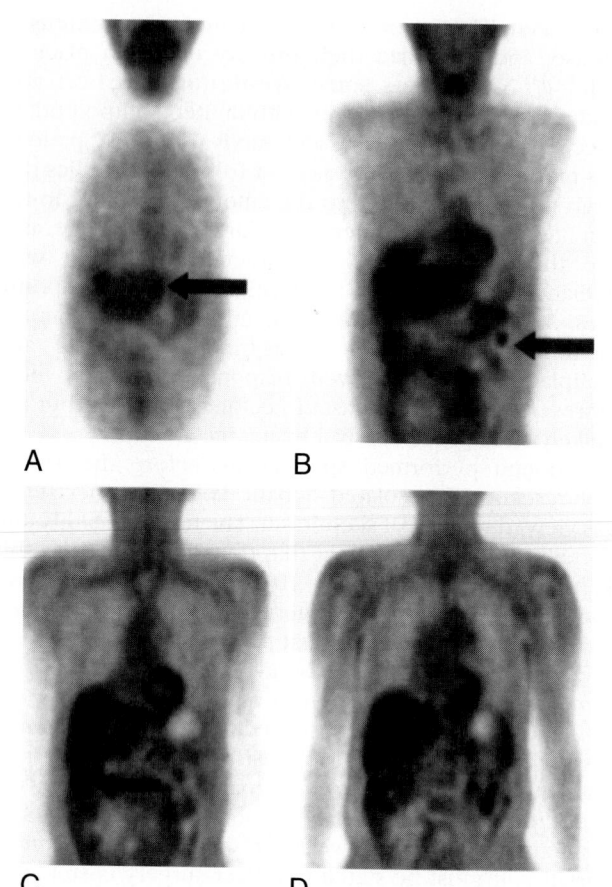

FIGURE 50-30. PET scan in a patient diagnosed with colorectal cancer synchronously metastatic to the liver after resection of the colonic tumor. The scan demonstrates hypermetabolic activity throughout the liver but also shows two areas in the left upper quadrant *(arrows)* consistent with an omental lesion as well as an anastomotic recurrence. A recent CT scan demonstrated liver disease only. (From Akhurst T, Larson SM: The role of nuclear medicine in the diagnosis and management of hepatobiliary diseases. *In* Blumgart LH, Fong Y [eds]: Surgery of the Liver and Biliary Tract. London, WB Saunders, 2000, pp 271-308.)

From these large series, we have learned a lot about prognostic factors and which patients are most likely to benefit from a liver resection for hepatic colorectal metastases. The most commonly cited and most frequently identified negative factors are the presence of extrahepatic disease and the inability to resect all disease in the liver. Most consider these absolute contraindications for liver resection. The exception to this rule is the patient with limited pulmonary metastases or colonic anastomotic recurrence who may undergo combined resections with some success. Although not all studies agree, a list of other poor prognostic factors exist and include involved lymph nodes with the primary colorectal tumor, synchronous presentation (or shorter disease-free interval), larger number of tumors, bilobar involvement, CEA elevation greater than 200 ng/mL, and involved histologic margins.[136,138] In our recent series of 1001 liver resections from the Memorial Sloan-Kettering Cancer Center (MSKCC), a multivariate analysis identified five factors as the most influential on outcome. These included size greater than 5 cm, disease-free interval less than 1 year, more than one tumor, lymph node–positive primary lesion, and a CEA greater than 200 ng/mL. By utilizing these five factors, we have developed a risk score predictive of recurrence after liver resection (Table 50-10).[144]

Although long-term survival after liver resection for hepatic colorectal metastases is clearly possible, recurrence of disease is quite common. In fact, the majority of patients ultimately succumb to recurrent disease. About half of the recurrences are isolated to the liver, and a small number of these patients (about 5% of all patients undergoing liver resection) are candidates for a second liver resection. These highly selected patients who undergo a second liver resection with complete removal of all disease can expect further 5-year survival rates of 30% to 40%. Because of the potential for further effective therapeutic interventions after liver resection, patients eligible for such treatment should be followed with serial CEA and imaging studies to detect recurrences at an early and potentially treatable phase.[138,148]

Adjuvant systemic chemotherapy after liver resection for metastatic colorectal cancer is often given but is not supported by prospective trials. A number of retrospective comparisons have been performed, but no definitive data support the routine use of adjuvant postoperative systemic chemotherapy. The most convincing argument for adjuvant therapy is with the use of hepatic arterial infusion (HAI) chemotherapy. The rationale for hepatic artery chemotherapy is based on the fact that liver tumors derive the majority of their blood supply from the hepatic artery,[149] and regional infusion of chemotherapeutic agents such as fluorodeoxyuridine (FUDR) have hepatic extraction rates of 90%, providing high local concentrations with minimal systemic toxicity. There is clearly a higher response rate with HAI therapy compared with systemic therapy.[150] A trial from the MSKCC comparing HAI therapy with systemic chemotherapy to systemic chemotherapy (5-fluorouracil with or without leucovorin) alone demonstrated significantly lower recurrence rates (9% and 36%) and a survival advantage at 2 years (86% vs. 72%).[151]

Some authors are utilizing a preoperative chemotherapy approach and have shown that some patients initially believed to be unresectable have been rendered resectable by preoperative chemotherapy.[137] Strategies to extend the limits of liver resection have utilized thermal ablative techniques such as cryoablation or RFA. Thus, multiple bilobar tumors can be extirpated by a combination of resection and ablation with preservation of sufficient hepatic parenchyma. Adequate long-term data for this approach are not available yet, however.[138]

In summary, patients with hepatic colorectal metastases have a uniformly poor prognosis with systemic chemotherapy or no treatment. Liver resection, encompassing all gross tumor, in the absence of extrahepatic

TABLE 50-9. Results of Hepatic Resection for Hepatic Colorectal Metastases in Selected Series With More Than 100 Patients

Author/Year	No. Patients	Operative Mortality	1-Yr Survival (%)	5-Yr Survival (%)	10-Yr Survival (%)	Median Survival (mo)
Adson/1984	141	2	82	25		24
Hughes/1986	607			33		
Schlag/1990	122	4	85	30		32
Doci/1991	100	5		30		28
Gayowski/1994	204	0	91	32		33
Scheele/1995	469	4	83	33	20	40
Fong/1995	577	4	85	35		40
Jenkins/1997	131	4	81	25		33
Rees/1997	150	1	94	37		
Jamison/1997	280	4	84	27	20	33
Fong/1999	1001	3	89	37	22	42
Minagawa/2000	235	0		35	26	37
Scheele/2000	597			36		35

TABLE 50-10. Clinical Risk Score and Survival in 1001 Patients Undergoing Liver Resection for Metastatic Colorectal Cancer*

Score	1-Yr Survival (%)	3-Yr Survival (%)	5-Yr Survival (%)	Median Survival (mo)
0	93	72	60	74
1	91	66	44	51
2	89	60	40	47
3	86	42	20	33
4	70	38	25	20
5	71	27	14	22

*Each of the following five risk factors equals one point: node-positive primary, disease-free interval less than 12 months, more than 1 tumor, size greater than 5 cm, carcinoembryonic antigen level greater than 200 ng/mL. Score is total number of points in an individual patient.

disease can result in long-term survival in up to a third of patients. Adjuvant therapies remain unproven, and liver resection in well-selected patients remains the cornerstone of the treatment of these patients.

Neuroendocrine

Liver metastases from neuroendocrine tumors are common but vary according to the primary tumor type. Examples of primary tumors that commonly metastasize to the liver are gastrinomas, glucagonomas, somatostatinomas, and nonfunctional neuroendocrine tumors. Insulinomas and carcinoid tumors metastasize to the liver less commonly. There are two issues to consider when planning therapy for metastatic neuroendocrine tumors. First, these are slow-growing, indolent tumors in which long-term survival is common even in the absence of treatment. Thus, assessing the effects of any treatment is very difficult. Second, these tumors often secrete functional neuropeptides that can create debilitating syndromes of hormonal excess. Thus the goal of treatment is often more focused on quality of life than on prolongation of life.

A number of effective nonsurgical therapies exist for neuroendocrine liver metastases. Long-acting somatostatin analogues are very useful for alleviating hormonal symptoms and may have a therapeutic role as well. Liver tumors can also be treated by hepatic arterial embolization or thermoablative approaches. Combinations of these therapies can be very effective in cytoreducing tumor loads and alleviating symptoms of hormonal excess.

Liver resection can play a role in patients whose tumor can be completely encompassed. Because these tumors are indolent, any therapy must be delivered with minimal mortality; and this has been the case in experienced hepatobiliary units. Five-year survival rates in excess of 50% can be expected if a complete resection is accomplished. Retrospective comparisons have suggested that this survival is better than that in untreated patients, but no prospective data exist. The other role surgery plays is in those patients who have failed medical therapy and have recalcitrant symptoms of hormonal excess. If preoperative staging suggests that at least 90% of tumor can be removed without prohibitive operative risk, surgical cytoreduction is reasonable. Symptom improvement can be expected in the majority of patients if adequate cytoreduction is achieved. Formal resections with wide margins are not necessary for neuroendocrine tumors, and techniques such as enucleations or wedge resections are good options.[148,152] Thermoablative approaches such as cryoablation or radiofrequency ablation are also attractive alternatives in this type of cytoreductive surgery. Recently, laparoscopic RFA has been utilized, although long-term follow-up is not available.[153]

Noncolorectal, Non-neuroendocrine

A number of other tumors can present as isolated liver metastases, but these are uncommon situations and therefore data are sparse. A long list of primary tumors that can present like this exists and includes breast, lung, melanoma, soft tissue sarcoma, Wilms' tumor, ocular melanoma, upper gastrointestinal (gastric, pancreas, esophagus, gallbladder), adrenocortical, urologic tumors (bladder, renal cell, prostate, testicular), and gynecologic tumors (uterine, cervix, ovarian). General principles that should be considered when dealing with these tumors as isolated liver metastases are similar to those of metastatic colorectal cancer. Prognosis tends to be dismal if there is extrahepatic disease, multiple tumors, large tumors, or a short disease-free interval.

Although rare reports of long-term survival after resection of isolated liver metastases from upper gastrointestinal tumor exist, in general, these patients have a dismal prognosis and liver resection is not recommended. In most series, liver resection for genitourinary tumors has the best prognosis and in well-selected patients liver resection should be considered. Breast cancer, melanoma, and sarcoma rarely present as isolated liver metastases; and in the situation of a long disease-free interval and/or long-term stability on chemotherapy, liver resection should be considered. In the main, liver resection for metastatic noncolorectal, non-neuroendocrine tumors has to be considered cytoreductive and should only be used in the most favorable situation, as described earlier. Liver resection can also be an effective therapy for symptomatic tumors in patients who have a reasonable life expectancy and no other effective therapy.[148,154,155]

Cystic Neoplasms

Simple Cyst

Simple cysts of the liver contain serous fluid, do not communicate with the biliary tree, and do not have septations. They are generally spherical or ovoid and can be as large as 20 cm. Large cysts can compress normal liver, inducing regional atrophy and sometimes compensatory hypertrophy. In 50% of cases, the cysts are singular. Histologically, a single layer of cuboidal or columnar cells that have no atypia line these cysts. Simple cysts are generally regarded to be congenital malformations.

Simple cysts are a relatively common finding in adults and in the main are asymptomatic incidental radiologic findings. Occasionally, a large cyst will cause symptoms. Although CT demonstrates anatomic relationships, ultrasound is the test of choice to confirm a single thin-walled simple cyst. Hydatid disease, cystadenoma, and metastatic neuroendocrine tumor are the most important differential diagnoses to consider. The most common complication is intracystic bleeding, but overall, complications are rare. Treatment of simple hepatic cysts is only indicated if they are symptomatic or if there is diagnostic uncertainty. Because most cysts are asymptomatic, a thorough evaluation of the etiology of the symptoms must be carried out before attributing them to the cyst. Nonsurgical treatment consists of aspiration and injection of a sclerosing agent. Few studies have documented long-term follow-up of sclerotherapy for hepatic cysts. Surgical therapy is achieved by fenestration or unroofing the portion of the cyst that is extrahepatic. This can be performed at laparotomy with good long-term results or through laparoscopic approaches. The latter approach is favored, but long-term efficacy is not well documented.[156]

Cystadenoma and Cystadenocarcinoma

Cystadenoma of the liver is a rare neoplasm that usually presents as a large cystic mass (usually 10 to 20 cm). The cyst has a globular external surface with multiple protruding cysts and locules of various sizes. The fluid contained in these cysts is usually mucinous. Microscopically, atypical cuboidal or columnar cells resting on a basement membrane line the cysts. The epithelium often forms polypoid or papillary projections.

Cystadenoma of the liver mainly affects women older than the age of 40. Although many cystadenomas are asymptomatic, symptoms can include abdominal pain, anorexia, nausea, and abdominal distention. The diagnosis is usually suspected by a combination of cross-sectional imaging (CT or MRI) and ultrasound. Ultrasound usually demonstrates a cystic structure with varying wall thickness, nodularity, septations, and fluid-filled locules. Importantly, contrast medium–enhanced CT demonstrates enhancement of the cyst wall and septa. Hydatid disease must always be considered in the differential diagnosis. Cystadenomas tend to grow very slowly but can eventually progress to their malignant counterpart, cystadenocarcinoma. Malignant degeneration is often suggested on imaging with large projections and a markedly thickened wall. The treatment of cystadenoma or cystadenocarcinoma is complete excision. Leaving any disease behind risks recurrence and/or the development of cystadeno-carcinoma.[156]

Polycystic Liver Disease

Liver cysts are commonly seen in patients with the auto-somal dominant inherited adult polycystic kidney disease. Histologically, the cysts are similar to a simple cyst (see earlier), the main difference between the two entities being the number of cysts. When liver cysts are present in patients with adult polycystic kidney disease, they are always multiple. Additionally, there are usually numerous microscopic hepatic cysts as well as the grossly visible macrocysts. Despite the large number of liver cysts, hepatic parenchyma and function are usually preserved. Liver cysts are always preceded by kidney cysts, and the prevalence of liver cysts in adult polycystic kidney disease increases with age. Below the age of 20 the prevalence of liver cysts is 0, whereas it is 80% in those older than the age of 60.

Liver cysts in patients with adult polycystic kidney disease are generally asymptomatic, but in a few patients large numerous cysts may cause abdominal pain and dis-tention. Results of LFTs are almost always normal. Rare complications can occur and include infection or intra-cystic bleeding. Ultrasound and CT show multiple simple cysts throughout the liver and kidneys. Treatment of poly-cystic liver disease is reserved for severe symptoms related to large cysts and complications. Treatment is by percu-taneous aspiration with or without sclerotherapy, fenes-tration (via laparotomy or laparoscopy), hepatic resection, or orthotopic liver transplant. Liver transplant is only uti-lized with progressive disease after fenestration or resec-tion with liver or renal dysfunction. In the context of renal failure a combined kidney and liver transplant may be appropriate.[156]

Bile Duct Cysts

Bile duct cysts or choledochal cysts are congenital dila-tions of the biliary tree that are usually diagnosed in child-hood but can present in adulthood. Because of the risk of malignancy and recurrent cholangitis, treatment is exci-sion with re-establishment of bilioenteric continuity. The majority of bile duct cysts involve the extrahepatic biliary tree, but in type IV cysts there is involvement of the extra-hepatic bile duct and intrahepatic ducts whereas Caroli's disease (type V) is characterized by multiple intrahepatic cysts. Thus, bile duct cysts must be considered in the dif-ferential diagnosis of a patient with multiple hepatic cystic lesions. The intrahepatic lesion of type IV bile duct cysts and Caroli's disease is multifocal dilation of the segmental bile ducts that are separated by portions of normal-caliber bile ducts. About half the cases of Caroli's disease are asso-ciated with congenital hepatic fibrosis, and the cysts are diffusely located throughout the liver. In the other half of cases the dilations may be confined to a part of the liver, usually the left liver. Recurrent bacterial cholangitis usually dominates the clinical course of these diseases, and death usually ensues within 5 to 10 years without

adequate treatment. When intrahepatic bile duct cysts are localized, hepatic resection with or without biliary recon-struction is the treatment of choice. Treatment of diffuse hepatic involvement is poor, and probably the only effec-tive treatment is transplantation in complicated cases.[156]

Principles of Hepatic Resection

Although liver resections were performed in the late 1800s, it was not until 1952 that Lortat-Jacob reported the first true anatomic right hepatectomy.[8] This event ushered in the modern era of hepatic surgery, but early series were plagued by high morbidity and mortality. Series from the 1970s and 1980s often reported mortality rates in excess of 10% and were often as high as 20%, especially for major resections.[1] This high mortality limited the use of liver resection, and there was reluctance to refer patients for such operations. Over the past 2 decades a number of advances have improved perioperative outcome dramati-cally for major hepatic surgery. In experienced centers, perioperative mortality is routinely 5% or less. In a recent review of over 1800 liver resections over a 10-year period from the MSKCC, operative mortality was 3.1%. The median blood loss was 600 mL, and 51% of patients did not require a blood transfusion. Overall postoperative morbidity was 45%, but the median hospital stay was 8 days.[20] As a result of the increasing safety of hepatic surgery, liver resection has become the treatment of choice for a long list of malignant and benign hepatic conditions.

The two most common hazards of liver resection are bleeding and biliary injury. Bile leaks are particularly a problem in cases requiring complex biliary reconstruc-tion. Bleeding has historically been a major problem with liver surgery and usually results from injury to the vena cava and hepatic veins. Because of the regenerative capac-ity of the liver, resections of up to 80% of normal noncir-rhotic livers can be performed with functional compensation within a few weeks. Because many resec-tions encompass tumors as well as normal liver, the concept of "functional liver parenchyma" is important because there is often compensatory hypertrophy of normal liver when tumors occupy a significant amount of the liver volume. The risk of hepatic dysfunction is minimal if the reduction of functional liver parenchyma is less than 50%. Patients with cirrhosis have much higher rates of postoperative liver dysfunction because of impaired regenerative capacity as well as impaired primary liver function. Liver failure, extrahepatic multior-gan failure, and death are serious hazards to performing major liver resections in cirrhotics. Ascites and infectious complications are also common problems after liver resection.[20,157]

Techniques of liver resection differ according to the disease being treated. In benign hepatic diseases requir-ing resection, the indications for operation are usually symptoms or infection. Removal of normal liver should be kept to a minimum in these cases, and techniques such as enucleation are appropriate, although major resections are occasionally necessary. For malignant disease, a margin of normal tissue is critical and formal anatomic resections yield the best results. Techniques such as wedge resections often result in high rates of margin involvement and disease recurrence and should be used carefully and sparingly.

Detailed knowledge of liver anatomy is essential to the practice of safe hepatic surgery and is reviewed in an earlier section. Unfortunately, descriptions of liver anatomy and of common liver resections have yielded a huge number of names that can be confusing to the student (Table 50-11) (Fig. 50-31). In general, one should always revert back to the segmental anatomy of the liver if there is any confusion about the description of a liver resection. Recall that the right liver is composed of segments V through VIII and that *right hepatectomy* and *right hepatic lobectomy* are appropriate terms for resection of these segments. Segments II through IV compose the left liver and *left hepatectomy* or *left hepatic lobectomy* are appropriate terms for resection of these segments. A right hepatectomy can be extended farther to the left to include segment IV, and a left hepatectomy can

be extended farther to the right to include segments V and VIII. Terms such as *extended* or *trisegmentectomy* are often used to describe these resections (see Table 50-11). Resection of segments II and III is a commonly performed sublobar resection and often referred to as a *left lateral segmentectomy,* although this terminology is not based on descriptions of segmental anatomy.[157]

A detailed discussion of the techniques of liver resection is beyond the scope of this chapter, but some general principles should be mentioned. When considering resection of a mass lesion in the liver, two major issues must be addressed. The portion of liver to be resected must be removed safely with consideration of the inflow (portal vein, hepatic artery, and bile duct), outflow (hepatic veins), and parenchymal transection. Proximity of mass lesions to inflow or outflow vessels and plans to safely dissect these areas must be carefully considered. Additionally, a routine technique of transecting liver tissue with minimal blood loss must be employed. The second critical issue is preserving a hepatic remnant with ade-

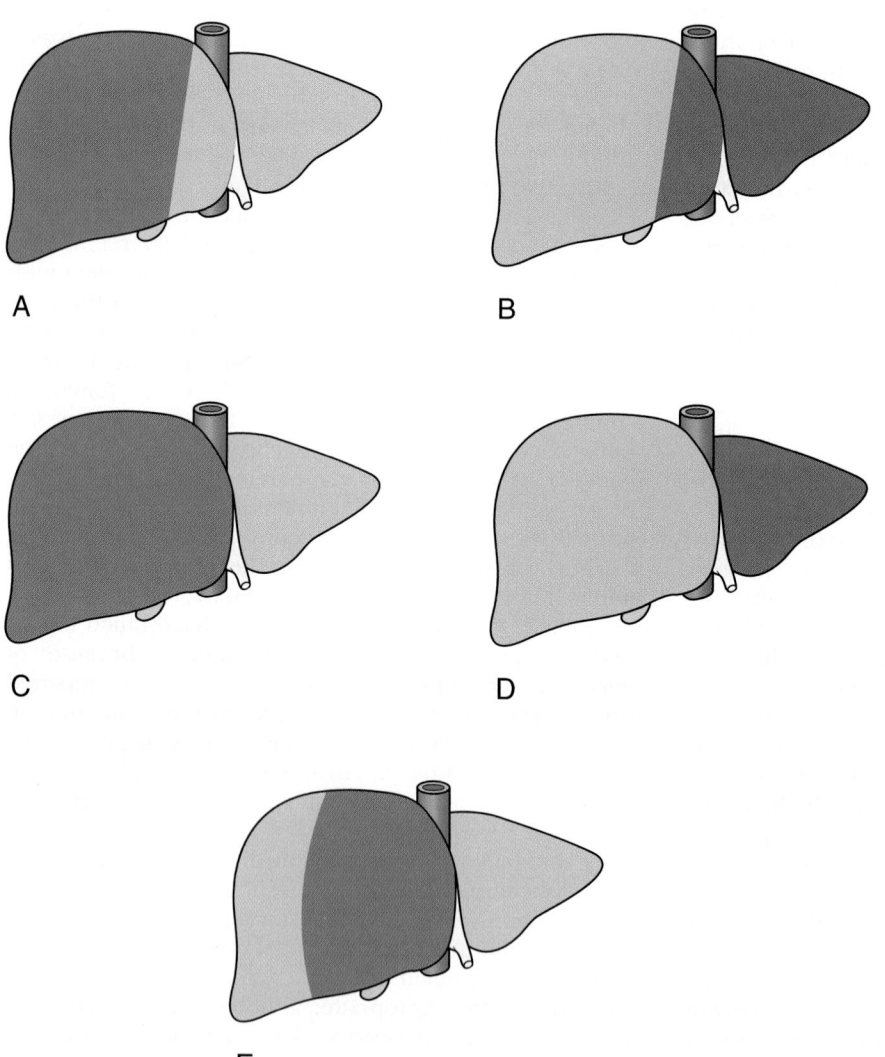

FIGURE 50-31. The commonly performed major hepatic resections are indicated by the shaded areas. **A,** Right hepatectomy or right hepatic lobectomy (segments V-VIII). **B,** Left hepatectomy or left hepatic lobectomy (segments II-IV). **C,** Extended right hepatectomy, extended right hepatic lobectomy, or right trisegmentectomy (segments IV-VIII). **D,** Left lateral segmentectomy or left lobectomy (segments II-III). **E,** Extended left hepatectomy, extended left lobectomy, or left trisegmentectomy (segments II, III, IV, V, VIII). See Table 50-6. (From Blumgart LH, Jarnagin W, Fong Y: Liver resection for benign disease and for liver and biliary tumors. *In* Blumgart LH, Fong Y [eds]: Surgery of the Liver and Biliary Tract. London, WB Saunders, 2000, pp 1639-1714.)

TABLE 50-11. Nomenclature for Major Anatomic Hepatic Resection

Segments	Common Nomenclature
V, VI, VII, VIII	Right hepatectomy, right hepatic lobectomy
IV, V, VI, VII, VIII	Extended right hepatectomy, extended right hepatic lobectomy, right trisegmentectomy
II, III, IV	Left hepatectomy, left hepatic lobectomy
II, III	Left lateral segmentectomy, left lobectomy
II, III, IV, V, VIII	Extended left hepatectomy, extended left lobectomy, left trisegmentectomy

quate blood supply (portal vein, hepatic artery), venous outflow, and biliary drainage. As an example, injury to the only remaining hepatic vein after an extended resection can be fatal and preservation of this vein is as important as performing the resection.[157]

HEMOBILIA

A case of lethal hemobilia secondary to penetrating abdominal trauma was first described by Glisson in 1654.[158,159] It was not until 1948 that Sandblom coined the term *hemobilia* in his seminal paper on the subject.[160] Hemobilia is defined as bleeding into the biliary tree from an abnormal communication between a blood vessel and bile duct. It is a rare condition that is often difficult to distinguish from common causes of gastrointestinal bleeding. The most common causes of hemobilia are iatrogenic trauma, accidental trauma, gallstones, tumors, inflammatory disorders, and vascular disorders. In recent years, iatrogenic trauma dominates as the most common cause of hemobilia and is usually related to interventional radiologic procedures. Major hemobilia is rare, whereas minor inconsequential hemobilia is a common consequence of gallstone disease or interventional hepatic procedures.

Etiology

In recent years, the most common cause of hemobilia has become iatrogenic trauma to the liver and biliary tree. Prior to the 1980s, the ratio of hemobilia attributed to accidental trauma compared with iatrogenic trauma was 2:1. Recent reviews put iatrogenic trauma as the cause of hemobilia in 40% to 60% of cases.[159,161,162] Percutaneous liver biopsy results in hemobilia in less than 1% of cases,[163,164] but percutaneous transhepatic biliary drainage (PTBD) procedures yield an incidence of 2% to 10%.[159] Likewise, surgical exploration of the biliary tree can result in hemobilia from direct injury or arterial pseudoaneurysm. A number of cases of hemobilia after cholecystectomy have been reported in recent years.[158] Hemobilia secondary to accidental trauma is more common with blunt than penetrating abdominal trauma. The incidence

of documented hemobilia after major hepatic trauma ranges from 0.2% to 3%. Risk factors for the development of hemobilia after accidental trauma are central hepatic rupture with a cavity, the use of packs, and inadequate drainage.[165,166]

Extrahepatic causes of hemobilia are rare but must be considered. The gallbladder can be a source of bleeding from trauma, gallstones, or acalculous cholecystitis. Primary vascular pathology such as aneurysm, angiodysplasia, and hemangiomas are rare causes of hemobilia. Malignant tumors of the liver, biliary tree, gallbladder, and pancreas, parasitic infection, hepatic abscess, and cholangitis are uncommon causes of hemobilia.[158,159]

Presentation

Portal venous bleeding into the biliary tree is rare, minor, and self-limited unless the portal pressure is elevated. Arterial hemobilia, the most common source, can be dramatic, however. Clinical sequelae of hemobilia are related to blood loss and the formation of potentially occlusive blood clots in the biliary tree. The classic triad of symptoms and signs of hemobilia are upper abdominal pain, upper gastrointestinal hemorrhage, and jaundice. In a recent review, all three were present in 22% of patients.[159] Minor hemobilia generally runs an uneventful asymptomatic clinical course. The symptoms and signs of major hemobilia are melena (90% of cases), hematemesis (60% of cases), biliary colic (70% of cases), and jaundice (60% of cases).[158,167] Upper gastrointestinal bleeding seen in conjunction with biliary symptoms must always raise the suspicion of hemobilia. One interesting aspect of hemobilia is the tendency for delayed presentations (up to weeks) and recurrent bleeding over months and even years. Blood clots in the biliary tree can masquerade as stones if hemobilia goes unrecognized. These clots can cause cholangitis, pancreatitis, and cholecystitis.

Diagnostic Work-up

Once hemobilia is suspected, the first evaluation should be upper gastrointestinal endoscopy, which rules out other sources of hemorrhage and may visualize bleeding from the ampulla of Vater. Upper endoscopy is only diagnostic of hemobilia in about 10% of cases, however.[164] If upper endoscopy is diagnostic and conservative management is planned, no further studies are necessary. Ultrasound or CT may be helpful in demonstrating intrahepatic tumor or hematoma. Evidence of active bleeding into the biliary tree may be seen on contrast medium–enhanced CT in the form of pooling contrast, intraluminal clots, and biliary dilation. CT may also show risk factors associated with hemobilia, such as cavitating central lesions and aneurysms. Arterial angiography is now recognized as the test of choice when hemobilia is suspected and will reveal the source of bleeding in about 90% of cases.[158,159,168] Cholangiography demonstrates blood clots in the biliary tree, which may appear as stringy defects or smaller spherical defects. The latter may be difficult to distinguish from stones.

Treatment and Outcome

The treatment of hemobilia must be focused on stopping bleeding and relieving biliary obstruction. Many cases of minor hemobilia can be managed conservatively with correction of coagulopathy, adequate biliary drainage, and close observation. In a recent review of 171 reported cases from 1996 to 1999, 43% of cases were successfully managed conservatively.[159] The first line of therapy for major hemobilia is transarterial embolization (TAE), and success rates of 80% to 100% are reported. Angiography with TAE is indicated for major hemobilia requiring blood transfusion (Fig. 50-32).[167,169-171]

Surgery is indicated when conservative therapy and TAE have failed. Even in cases in which a laparotomy may be mandated for other reasons, TAE is still the therapy of choice for hemobilia because of lower morbidity. Surgical approaches generally involve ligation of bleeding vessels, excision of aneurysm, or nonselective ligation of a main hepatic artery. Hepatic resection may be necessary for failed arterial ligation or for cases of severe trauma or tumor.[162,172] Hemorrhage from the gallbladder or hemorrhagic cholecystitis mandates cholecystectomy. There are isolated reports of successful management of hemobilia with endoscopic coagulation, somatostatin, and vasopressin.[159] The management of hemobilia after PTBD usually consists of removal of the catheter or replacement with larger catheters.[172]

At the time of Sandblom's report from 1972, the mortality for hemobilia was at least 25%.[161] A report from 1987 noted a mortality of 12%.[164] In a review of cases from 1996 through 1999, only four deaths were reported.[159] There has clearly been a reduction in mortality from hemobilia that is probably related to two factors. First, the incidence of minor hemobilia has increased secondary to the rising number of percutaneous hepatic procedures. Second, improvements in selective angiography and TAE have greatly improved the treatment.

Bilhemia

Bilhemia is an extremely rare condition in which bile flows into the bloodstream either through the hepatic veins or portal vein branches. This flow occurs in the context of a high intrabiliary pressure exceeding that of the venous system. The cause can be gallstones eroding into the portal vein or accidental/iatrogenic trauma. The condition can be fatal secondary to embolization of large amounts of bile into the lungs. Most often, however, bile flow is low and the fistula spontaneously closes. The clinical presentation is that of rapidly increasing jaundice,

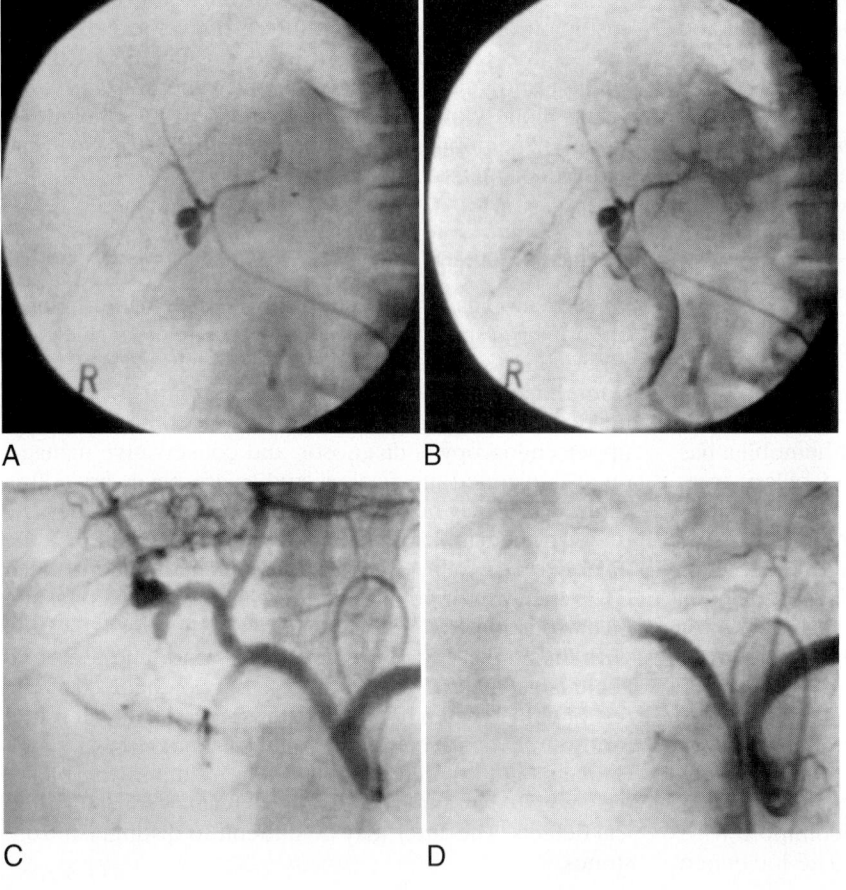

FIGURE 50-32.   Classic findings of hemobilia are demonstrated. After a complicated cholecystectomy an iatrogenic pseudoaneurysm developed and has ruptured into the biliary tree. Exsanguinating hemobilia ensued, and the diagnosis was made by endoscopy and then treated by arterial embolization. **A,** Arteriogram demonstrating a pseudoaneurysm of the hepatic artery at the hilum. **B,** A few seconds later the contrast agent is seen flowing down the hepatic duct with evidence of clot in the biliary tree. **C** and **D,** The same aneurysm before and after successful embolization. (From Sandblom JP: Hemobilia and bilhemia. *In* Blumgart LH, Fong Y [eds]: Surgery of the Liver and Biliary Tract. London, WB Saunders, 2000, pp 1319-1342.)

marked direct hyperbilirubinemia without elevation of hepatocellular enzymes, and septicemia. The best test to make this diagnosis is ERCP. Treatment is directed at lowering intrabiliary pressures either through stents or sphincterotomy.[158]

VIRAL HEPATITIS AND THE SURGEON

Epidemics of jaundice were noted in ancient civilizations and recorded by Hippocrates. During World War II these epidemics were called "catarrhal jaundice," and over 28,000 cases were documented at that time. Epidemiologic studies in the 1940s documented the difference between bloodborne hepatitis (hepatitis B) and enteric hepatitis (hepatitis A).[173,174] The most important discovery was that of the Australia antigen by Blumberg and associates in 1965.[175] This antigen proved to be the hepatitis B surface antigen (HBsAg) and provided a means of differentiating the two types of hepatitis and characterizing the epidemiology of this disease. This discovery also ultimately led to the development of hepatitis B vaccines based on this antigen with obvious and profound effects worldwide. Further research ultimately led to the discovery of the delta virus (hepatitis D)[176] and hepatitis C (explaining cases of non-A, non-B hepatitis).[177] Hepatitis E has been found to be a unique enteral form of infectious hepatitis,[178,179] and recently hepatitis G virus has been discovered and is currently being defined.[180-182]

Viral hepatitis is a major health problem and is the most common cause of liver disease worldwide. Although fulminant acute hepatitis is uncommon, there are over 5 million people who suffer with chronic hepatitis. It is estimated that over 15,000 patients die each year of viral hepatitis in the United States. Viral hepatitis is not a surgical disease but has important consequences for surgeons and surgical patients. For any surgeon performing hepatic surgery, the functional state of the liver is extremely important; and patients with chronic viral hepatitis require special attention before any surgical intervention. Additionally, chronic viral hepatitis is a common cause of HCC. Lastly, the risk of transmission from patient to surgeon and vice versa is an issue all surgeons should be familiar with.[183]

Definition

Viral hepatitis is an infection of the liver by one of six known viruses that have diverse genetic compositions and

structures. Hepatitis viruses A, C, D, E, and G have RNA genomes, whereas hepatitis B has a DNA genome that replicates through RNA intermediates. Hepatitis A (HAV) and E (HEV) virus are both responsible for forms of epidemic hepatitis and are transmitted via a fecal-oral route. The hepatitis B virus (HBV) is the only one with the potential to integrate into host genomes, although this is not required for replication. The hepatitis C (HCV) virus replicates in the cytoplasm of hepatocytes and has complex mechanisms of evading host immunity through hypervariable areas in its genome. The hepatitis D virus (HDV) requires the presence of HBV infection for replication and infectivity and can alter the clinical course of HBV infection. The hepatitis G virus (HGV) has been discovered and has similarities to HCV, but has no definitive association with clinical hepatitis.[183-186]

Diagnosis

Table 50-12 summarizes the serologic tests and their implications for HAV, HBV, and HCV. The diagnosis of HAV infection relies on the determination of antibodies to HAV. Both IgM and IgG antibodies are present early in the infection, but only IgG persists for the long term. HAV antigens and tests for HAV RNA have been developed but are generally restricted to research laboratories.[187,188]

HBV infection has been characterized by a number of antigens and antibodies (Fig. 50-33).[189] Hepatitis B surface antigen (HBsAg) is the hallmark of the diagnosis of HBV infection and appears in the serum from 1 to 10 weeks after infection. HBsAg usually disappears in 4 to 6 months, but persistence in the serum implies chronic infection. Anti-HBs antibodies usually appear during a window period after the disappearance of HBsAg and mark recovery after HBV infection. Anti-HBs antibodies are also induced by the HBV vaccine. The hepatitis core antigen (HBcAg) is an intracellular antigen that is not detectable in serum. Anti-HBc antibodies, however, are detectable early on after infection and persist after recovery and in chronic infections. Hepatitis B e antigen (HBeAg) is a secretory protein that is a marker of HBV replication and infectivity. It is usually present early on and may persist for years in chronic infection but usually disappears within months in the absence of chronic infection. Seroconversion to anti-HBe antibodies is usually associated with the resolution of infection. A small number of cases of chronic HBV infection will have detectable anti-HBe

TABLE 50-12. Serologic Evaluation of the Most Common Viral Hepatitides

Virus	Antigen Name	Interpretation	Antibody Name	Interpretation
Hepatitis A (HAV)	HAV antigen	Acute infection	Anti-HAV IgM	Acute infection
			Anti-HAV IgG	Immunity
Hepatitis B (HBV)	HBsAg	Acute or chronic infection	Anti-HBs	Immunity
	HBeAg	HBV replication/infectivity	Anti-HBc	All phases of infection
			Anti-HBe	Late convalescence
Hepatitis C (HCV)	None		Anti-HCV	Late convalescence or chronic infection

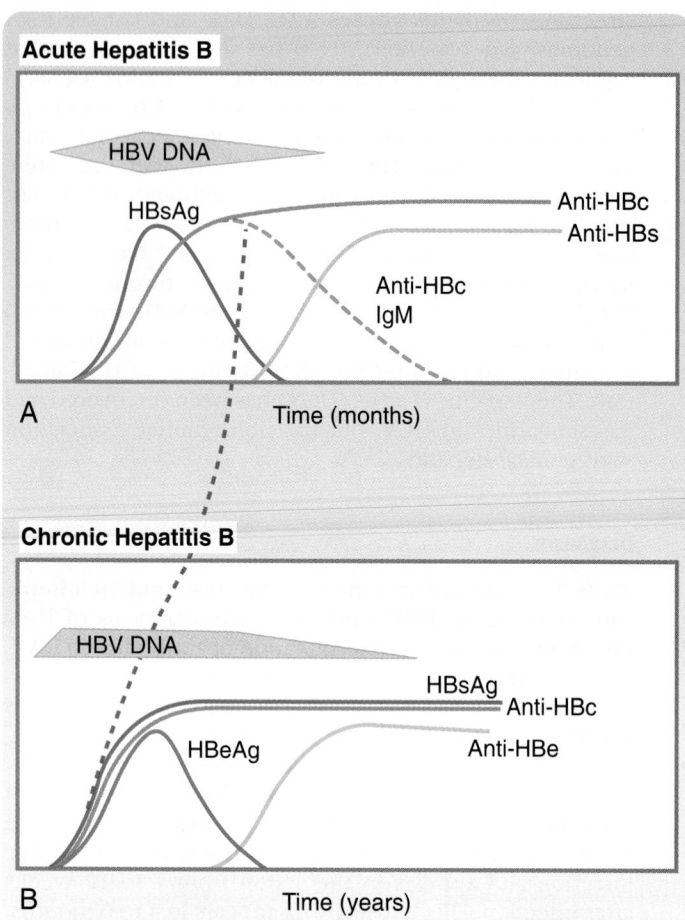

Acute Hepatitis B

HBV DNA

HBsAg

Anti-HBc

Anti-HBs

Anti-HBc
IgM

A   Time (months)

Chronic Hepatitis B

HBV DNA

HBsAg
Anti-HBc

HBeAg

Anti-HBe

B   Time (years)

FIGURE 50-33. Serologic markers in (**A**) acute HBV infection and (**B**) chronic HBV infection. (From Doo EC, Lian TJ: The hepatitis viruses. *In* Schiff ER, Sorrell MF, Maddrey WC [eds]: Schiff's Diseases of the Liver. Philadelphia, Lippincott-Raven, 1999, pp 725-744.)

antibodies. Detection of HBV DNA in the serum is possible by a number of techniques, but its clinical utility is not well defined.

The diagnosis of HCV infection relies on detection of antibodies to multiple HCV antigens.[190] A number of tests have been developed, but the most recent and sensitive tests detect multiple antigens. No specific HCV antigen tests exist, but a variety of quantitative and qualitative tests for HCV RNA exist.[191] These tests of HCV RNA have become very important in confirming the diagnosis as well as assessing responses to therapy.

HDV co-infection of HBV-infected patients is best diagnosed by detection of HDV RNA, which can be measured in serum.[192] The HDV antigen can be detected in liver specimens. HEV infection can be diagnosed by measurement of antibodies in serum or by detection of the virus or its components in feces, serum, or liver.[193]

Epidemiology and Transmission

The epidemiology and modes of transmission for the viral hepatitides are very important to understand for purposes of prevention and identification of patients at the highest risk of carrying such infections. Table 50-13 summarizes the modes of transmission.

Hepatitis A is very common in third world countries, with seropositivity rates approaching 100% in some populations. Infection occurs in childhood and is facilitated by poor hygiene and sanitation. Infection rates are much lower in developed countries. In the United States, approximately 10% of children and 35% of adults have been infected with HAV.[183,194] The primary route of HAV infection is the fecal-oral route. Ingestion of contaminated water or food as well as person-to-person contact accounts for most cases. Parenteral transmission is possible but uncommon. Sexual transmission has been documented in homosexual men.

Hepatitis B is a major worldwide health problem. There are over 300 million carriers and 250,000 associated deaths annually. The prevalence of HBV infection has considerable geographic variation. Low prevalence areas such as the United States and Western Europe have carrier rates of 0.1% to 2%, and transmission is generally sexual or through intravenous drug abuse (IVDA). Carrier rates in intermediate-prevalence areas such as Japan and Singapore range from 3% to 5%. In high-prevalence areas such as Southeast Asia and sub-Saharan Africa, carrier rates range from 10% to 20%. Transmission in high-prevalence areas is largely perinatal and horizontal in childhood.[195]

Transfusion-associated HBV infection was very common in the 1960s, and the risk has been estimated to be as high

TABLE 50-13. Relative Frequency of Modes of Transmission of Viral Hepatitis*

Virus	Major Infectious Body Fluid	Transfusions or Intravenous Drug Use	Fecal-Oral	Sexual	Vertical	Occupational
HAV	Feces	−/−	4+	1+	−	+/−
HBV	Blood	−/4+	+/−	3+	3+	3+
HCV	Blood	2+/4+	+/−	1+	+/−	2+
HDV	Blood	−/4+	1+	3+	3+	+/−
HEV	Feces	−/−	4+	+/−	+/−	Unknown

*Relative frequency rated from − to 4+.

as 50% at that time. Currently, screening programs and limitation of blood donation to voluntary donors has decreased the risk of acquiring HBV from a blood transfusion to 1 in 63,000.[196] Percutaneous transmission through the use of any contaminated needle is a major route of HBV infection and is very common in intravenous drug abusers. Sexual transmission is very common in low-prevalence countries and is estimated to account for approximately 30% of cases in the United States. There is a particularly high incidence in male homosexuals and heterosexuals with multiple sexual partners. Perinatal HBV infection accounts for less than 10% of cases in the United States but is very common in endemic areas, with rates of transmission of 90% in some places. Horizontal transmission among children is common and is probably related to minor breaks in skin and mucous membranes. HBV is the most commonly transmitted virus among health care personnel, and transmission is usually patient to patient or patient to worker. Rare cases of physician to patient transmission have been reported. Needlestick risk has been related to HBeAg positivity.[183]

Hepatitis C is the most common cause of chronic liver disease in the United States, with an estimated prevalence of 1.8%, accounting for 3.9 million infected people. New infection typically occurs at young age (20 to 39), and the most common risk factor is IVDA. Health care workers have higher carrier rates than the general public. Transmission among health care workers is usually related to needlestick incidents, and the risk of transmission is higher than that of HIV and HBV. In the past, blood transfusion was the major cause of HCV infection, accounting for at least 85% of cases. Currently, less than 2% of acute infections are due to transfusions and the risk of transfusion is estimated to be between 0.001% and 0.0001%. Although HCV has never been documented in semen, it is estimated that about 20% of HCV infections are due to sexual transmission. Risk of sexual transmission appears to be related to the number of partners and the presence of other sexually transmitted diseases. Monogamous sexual partners of HCV-infected people occasionally test positive for HCV in the absence of other risk factors, but this appears to be distinctly uncommon. Perinatal transmission has been documented but is rare.

Thirty to 40% of HCV cases have no identifiable risk factors.[197]

HDV infection occurs worldwide, with a variable distribution that parallels HBV infection. About 5% of HBsAg-positive patients also harbor HDV infection. Transmission of HDV is parenteral and can only occur in patients previously infected with HBV.

HEV is endemic in Southeast/Central Asia and occurs with low frequency in other areas of the world. HEV outbreaks are usually large, affecting hundreds to thousands of people at once, and often follow large rains and flooding. There is a particularly high attack rate and mortality in pregnant women. Transmission is fecal-oral and usually related to contaminated drinking water or food. Person to person as well as vertical transmission is rare.[198]

Pathogenesis and Clinical Characteristics

The pathogenesis of hepatic injury from these viral infections is not completely understood. For all the viruses discussed in this section, the hepatic inflammation appears to be due either to direct cytotoxicity or to immune-related phenomena. Combinations of these two mechanisms probably underlie the etiology of hepatitic damage.

Humans are the only host for HAV, and no reservoir of infection has been identified. After oral intake, HAV can survive the acidic gastric pH but the mechanism of hepatic uptake is not known. HAV infection results in acute inflammation of the liver and has no associated chronic sequelae. The majority of children younger than age 2 with HAV infection are asymptomatic, whereas of those patients older than the age of 5, 80% develop symptoms. A fulminant hepatitis develops in 1% to 5% of cases, and mortality is generally under 1%.[199]

Approximately 70% of patients with acute HBV infection have subclinical or anicteric hepatitis, the other 30% having icteric hepatitis. The incubation period for HBV ranges from 1 to 4 months. A prodromal serum-sickness-like syndrome may develop, and this is followed by a multitude of constitutional symptoms, such as malaise, anorexia, and nausea. The constitutional symptoms last about 10 days and are then followed by jaundice in 30%

of patients. Clinical symptoms usually disappear within 3 months. Fulminant hepatic failure develops in 0.1% to 0.5% of cases. Nearly 80% of patients with fulminant HBV-related hepatitis will die unless liver transplantation is performed.[183]

Risk of chronic HBV infection is related to immunocompetence and age. Immunocompetent adults have a risk of less than 5%, whereas 30% of children and 90% of infants will develop chronic disease. Most patients with chronic HBV infection are asymptomatic, but some may experience exacerbations of symptoms. Laboratory tests may be entirely normal in HBV carriers, or mild elevations of ALT and AST may be the only findings. Progression to cirrhosis is marked by hepatic synthetic dysfunction and often cytopenias related to hypersplenism.[200] Extrahepatic manifestations of HBV infection due to circulating immune complexes occur in 10% to 20% of patients and include polyarteritis nodosa, glomerulonephritis, essential mixed cryoglobulinemia, and papular acrodermatitis.[201] The sequelae of chronic HBV infection range from nothing to cirrhosis, to HCC, to hepatic failure, or to death. Although in nonendemic areas the long-term risk appears to be low, in endemic areas chronic HBV infection is a significant cause of morbidity and mortality.[200,202]

Acute HCV infection generally presents as mild elevation of hepatocellular enzymes and 80% of cases occur between 5 and 12 weeks after infection. Symptoms occur in less than 30% of patients and are usually so mild and nonspecific that they do not affect daily life. Jaundice occurs in less than 20% of patients, and fulminant hepatic failure due to HCV is extremely uncommon.[203]

Chronic HCV infection develops in over two thirds of patients. Most patients with chronic HCV infection are asymptomatic without evidence of overt liver disease and only present with mildly elevated hepatocellular enzymes. Despite this quiet clinical course, patients with chronic HCV infection are at risk for developing cirrhosis and HCC. The rate of progression to cirrhosis is a matter of debate, but for the most part it is a slow progression and will generally take decades. The mean duration of HCV infection in patients with associated HCC is 28 years. Several factors appear to speed up progression of HCV infection to cirrhosis, the most important of which is alcohol. Age at acute infection, host genetic factors, and viral genotypes may also play a role.[204,205] A variety of extrahepatic manifestations such as autoimmune disorders and lymphoma can occur with HCV infection and are likely related to circulating immune complexes.

The clinical presentation of HDV infection is related to a complex relationship between the degree of both HBV and HDV infection. Co-infection with high expression of HBV and HDV can result in a fulminant and icteric hepatitis. Conversely, milder forms of acute HDV infection are usually associated with decreased expression of HDV and repression of HBV infection. Occasionally, HDV infection terminates HBV infection. Superinfection of a previous HBV carrier usually results in overt hepatitis.[206,207]

Hepatitis E has a different histologic picture than the other viral hepatitides in that a cholestatic type of hepatitis is seen in over half of patients. HEV is introduced orally, and it is not known how the virus travels to the liver. The incubation period of HEV ranges from 2 to 9 weeks. The most common form of illness is acute icteric hepatis, and most series report jaundice in over 90% of cases. Asymptomatic forms of the disease occur and are probably more common than the icteric form, but the actual frequency is unknown. The disease is usually self-limited, but fulminant hepatic failure can occur in a small percentage of patients. Overall, the mortality rate is probably significantly less than 1%. Pregnant women tend to have a more severe clinical course, and mortality rates range from 5% to 25%.[183]

Prevention

HAV prophylaxis has largely relied on sanitary measures and administration of serum immunoglobulin. Recent development of safe and effective HAV vaccines, however, has made the use of pre-exposure immunoglobulin unnecessary. Serum immunoglobulin is still the therapy of choice for postexposure prophylaxis and may be safely given along with active immunization. Ongoing public health policies are working on vaccination schemes to eradicate HAV in the United States and in high-risk populations throughout the world. Likewise, HEV prophylaxis has focused on sanitary measures, particularly strategies aimed at drinking water. Immunoglobulin has not been successful in pre-exposure or postexposure prevention of HEV infection, but anti-HEV antibodies appear to be effective at attenuating the clinical syndrome. Vaccines for HEV infection have been developed and are being evaluated.

Remarkable advances have been made in the prevention of HBV infection. In the past, prevention of HBV infection was limited to passive immunization with immunoglobulin containing high titers of antibody to HBsAg. Currently, immunoglobulin immunization is only used in postexposure prophylaxis. HBsAg-containing vaccines have been developed with good safety and efficacy profiles.[208] These vaccines are used primarily for pre-exposure prophylaxis but can also be used in a postexposure setting along with immunoglobulin. HBV vaccination is recommended for high-risk groups such as health care workers. There are also schemes for HBV vaccination to prevent perinatal transmission, and currently all children 11 or 12 years old should be vaccinated if not done previously. HBV DNA-based vaccines have been developed, and a combined HBV and HAV vaccine has been approved. Although no vaccine is available for HDV, effective HBV prevention prevents HDV infection.

The only effective preventive strategy for HCV infection relies on public health principles aimed at the major risk factors for transmission. Conventionally prepared anti-HCV immunoglobulin has been evaluated in a number of trials and was never demonstrated to prevent transfusion-related non-A, non-B hepatitis. Screening of blood donors has rendered this issue irrelevant today. Unfortunately, owing to a variety of obstacles, a successful HCV vaccine has not been produced.

Treatment

Treatment of HAV or HEV infection is supportive and is generally aimed at correcting dehydration and providing adequate caloric intake. Although fatigue may mandate significant periods of rest, hospitalization is not usually necessary except in cases of fulminant liver failure.

The treatment of HBV infection is largely aimed at patients with chronic active disease. The two licensed therapies are interferon-α (IFN) and the nucleoside analogue lamivudine. IFN is an immunomodulatory agent with some antiviral properties that can induce a virologic response in 35% to 40% of patients. Long-term benefit with IFN therapy has not definitively been proved. Adverse reactions to IFN are very common, and therapy is difficult, often requiring decreases in dosing or termination of treatment. Corticosteroids given as additional therapy to IFN may be of some clinical benefit. Many nucleoside analogues for the treatment of HBV have been developed and probably work through inhibition of DNA synthesis. They have similar viral response rates to IFN, are inexpensive, and have few side effects. On the other hand, nucleoside analogues often require long-term therapy (>1 year), and the development of resistant HBV mutants has been documented. Ongoing studies are focusing on combination treatments with IFN and nucleoside analogues as well as looking into immunotherapy strategies.[185]

Over the past 15 years tremendous advances in the treatment of HCV infection have occurred. A benefit for IFN in the treatment of non-A, non-B hepatitis was originally demonstrated in 1986 before the discovery of HCV. With current IFN treatment regimens, complete viral response (defined as sustained loss of serum viral RNA) occurs in 12% to 20% of patients. The addition of ribavirin to IFN has resulted in response rates of 35% to 45%. In the most recent trials, treatment with PEG-IFN and ribavirin resulted in viral clearance in 55% of patients. Relapse can occur but usually occurs with monotherapy and shortened courses of therapy. Because therapy with IFN has significant side effects, controversies such as indications for treatment and optimal doses/duration of treatment are still being evaluated.[186]

Selected References

Blumgart LH, Fong Y: Surgical options in the treatment of hepatic metastasis from colorectal cancer. Curr Probl Surg 32:333-421, 1995.

A complete review of the subject clearly outlines the rationale for liver resection of hepatic colorectal metastases.

Blumgart LH, Hann LE: Surgical and radiologic anatomy of the liver and biliary tract. *In* Blumgart LH, Fong Y (eds): Surgery of the Liver and Biliary Tract. London, WB Saunders, 2000, pp 3-34.

A comprehensive and clinically oriented review of hepatobiliary anatomy is provided. The text is specifically oriented toward surgery of the liver and biliary tree.

Fan ST, Wong J: Recurrent pyogenic cholangitis. *In* Blumgart LH, Fong Y (eds): Surgery of the Liver and Biliary Tract. London, WB Saunders, 2000, pp 1205-1225.

A review of the subject from one of the most experienced centers in the world that has led the way in developing treatment strategies for this disease.

Fong Y, Fortner J, Sun RL, et al: Clinical score for predicting recurrence after hepatic resection for metastatic colorectal cancer: Analysis of 1001 consecutive cases. Ann Surg 230:309-321, 1999.

One of the largest single-institution series of liver resection for metastatic colorectal cancer. A very useful prognostic scoring system is presented.

Fortner JG, Blumgart LH: A historic perspective of liver surgery for tumors at the end of the millennium. J Am Coll Surg 193:210-222, 2001.

A recent review of the highlights of the history of liver surgery written by two of the giants in the field.

Foster JH, Berman MM: Solid Liver Tumors. Philadelphia, WB Saunders, 1977.

A classic and comprehensive monograph that contains a complete history of liver surgery.

Friedman LS, Martin P, Munoz SJ: Laboratory evaluation of the patient with liver disease. *In* Zakim D, Boyer TD (eds): Hepatology: A Textbook of Liver Disease. Philadelphia, WB Saunders, 2003, pp 661-708.

A comprehensive review of basic laboratory and quantitative tests of hepatic function.

Green MHA, Duell RM, Johnson CD, et al: Haemobilia. Br J Surg 88:773-786, 2001.

A recent comprehensive and concise review of the subject.

Hoofnagle JH, Heller T: Hepatitis C. *In* Zakim D, Boyer TD (eds): Hepatology: A Textbook of Liver Disease. Philadelphia, WB Saunders, 2003, pp 1017-1062.

An up-to-date and complete review of the subject.

Hughes MA, Petri WA Jr: Amebic liver abscess. Infect Dis Clin North Am 14:565-582, viii, 2000.

A modern review of amebic liver abscess with a complete assessment of current treatment modalities.

Johannsen EC, Sifri CD, Madoff LC: Pyogenic liver abscesses. Infect Dis Clin North Am 14:547-563, vii, 2000.

An excellent and modern review of all aspects of pyogenic liver abscess.

Koff RS: Hepatitis A and E. *In* Zakim D, Boyer TD (eds): Hepatology: A Textbook of Liver Disease. Philadelphia, WB Saunders, 2003, pp 939-959.

A modern complete review of the subject from a comprehensive hepatology textbook.

Lau WY: Primary hepatocellular carcinoma. *In* Blumgart LH, Fong Y (eds): Surgery of the Liver and Biliary Tract. London, WB Saunders, 2000, pp 1423-1450.

Comprehensive review of the subject from an innovative researcher in the field.

Lautt WW, Greenway CV: Conceptual review of the hepatic vascular bed. Hepatology 7:952-963, 1987.

A classic review of the microvascular circulation of the liver.

Milicevic MN: Hydatid disease. *In* Blumgart LH, Fong Y (eds): Surgery of the Liver and Biliary Tract. London, WB Saunders, 2000, pp 1167-1204.

Comprehensive review of hydatid disease by an experienced author in the field.

Nair S, Perrillo RP: Hepatitis B and D. *In* Zakim D, Boyer TD (eds): Hepatology: A Textbook of Liver Disease. Philadelphia, WB Saunders, 2003, pp 959-1016.

A comprehensive and concise review.

Ochsner A, DeBakey M, Murray S: Pyogenic abscess of the liver. Am J Surg 40:292-319, 1938.

A classic landmark study on pyogenic abscesses of the liver. This was the first serious attempt to study hepatic abscesses and ushered in the modern era of treatment.

Poon RT, Fan ST, Tsang FH, et al: Locoregional therapies for hepatocellular carcinoma: A critical review from the surgeon's perspective. Ann Surg 235:466-486, 2002.

An excellent review of locoregional therapies for hepatocellular carcinoma from a very experienced group.

Sandblom P: Hemorrhage into the biliary tract following trauma: "Traumatic hemobilia." Surgery 24:571-586, 1948.

The landmark paper that coined the term hemobilia and described the syndrome.

Sandblom P: Hemobilia (Biliary Tract Hemorrhage): History, Pathology, Diagnosis, Treatment. Springfield, IL, Charles C Thomas, 1972.

A classic paper that reviewed the presentation and treatment of all reported cases of hemobilia at the time.

Saxena R, Zucker SD, Crawford JM: Anatomy and physiology of the liver. *In* Zakim D, Boyer TD (eds): Hepatology: A Textbook of Liver Disease. Philadelphia, WB Saunders, 2003, pp 3-30.

An excellent overview of the microscopic anatomy of the liver and basic hepatic physiology from a comprehensive hepatology textbook.

Stolz A: Liver physiology and metabolic function. *In* Feldman M, Scharschmidt BF, Sleisenger MH (eds): Sleisenger & Fordtran's Gastrointestinal and Liver Disease. Philadelphia, WB Saunders, 1998, pp 1061-1082.

A current basic review of hepatic physiology and the metabolic functions of the liver.

References

1. Foster JH, Berman MM: Solid Liver Tumors. Philadelphia, WB Saunders, 1977.
2. Fortner JG, Blumgart LH: A historic perspective of liver surgery for tumors at the end of the millennium. J Am Coll Surg 193:210-222, 2001.
3. Chen TS, Chen PS: Understanding the Liver—A History. Westport, CT, Greenwood Press, 1984.
4. Glisson F: Anatomia Hepatis. London, Londini: Typis Du-Gardianis, impensis Octaviani Pullein, 1654.
5. Dagradi A, Brearley R: The surgery of hepatic tumours. Postgrad Med J 38:670-687, 1962.
6. Elliot JW: Surgical treatment of tumor of the liver with the report of a case. Ann Surg 26:83, 1897.
7. Pringle JH: Notes on the arrest of hepatic hemorrhage due to trauma. Ann Surg 48:541, 1908.
8. Lortat-Jacob J, Robert H: Hepatectomy droite reglée. Presse Med 60:549-551, 1952.
9. Pack GT, Miller RT, Brasfield R: Total right hepatic lobectomy for cancer of the gallbladder. Am J Surg 91:829-832, 1955.
10. Quattlebaum J: Massive resection of the liver. Ann Surg 137:787-796, 1953.
11. Couinaud C: Le Foi. Études Anatomiques et Chirurgicales. Paris, Masson, 1957.
12. Goldsmith NA, Woodburne RT: Surgical anatomy pertaining to liver resection. Surg Gynecol Obstet 195:310-318, 1957.
13. Blumgart LH, Hadjis NS, Benjamin IS, et al: Surgical approaches to cholangiocarcinoma at confluence of hepatic ducts. Lancet 1:66-70, 1984.
14. Blumgart LH, Drury JK, Wood CB: Hepatic resection for trauma, tumour and biliary obstruction. Br J Surg 66:762-769, 1979.
15. Bismuth H, Houssin D, Castaing D: Major and minor segmentectomies "reglées" in liver surgery. World J Surg 6:10-24, 1982.
16. Longmire WP Jr, Marable SA: Clinical experiences with major hepatic resections. Ann Surg 154:460-474, 1961.
17. Fortner JG, Kim DK, Maclean BJ, et al: Major hepatic resection for neoplasia: Personal experience in 108 patients. Ann Surg 188:363-371, 1978.
18. Starzl TE, Bell RH, Beart RW, et al: Hepatic trisegmentectomy and other liver resections. Surg Gynecol Obstet 141:429-437, 1975.
19. Starzl TE, Groth CG, Brettschneider L, et al: Extended survival in 3 cases of orthotopic liver homografts in man. Am Surg 172:23-32, 1970.
20. Jarnagin WR, Gonen M, Fong Y, et al: Improvement in perioperative outcome after hepatic resection: Analysis of 1,803 consecutive cases over the past decade. Ann Surg 236:397-407, 2002.
21. Blumgart LH, Hann LE: Surgical and radiologic anatomy of the liver and biliary tract. *In* Blumgart LH, Fong Y (eds): Surgery of the Liver and Biliary Tract. London, WB Saunders, 2000, pp 3-34.
22. Netter FH: Liver, biliary tract and pancreas. *In* Netter FH (ed): The Netter Collection of Medical Illustrations, Teteroboro, ICON Learning Systems, 2001.
23. Sadler TW: Langman's Medical Embryology, 5th ed. Baltimore, Williams & Wilkins, 1985.
24. Gillfillan RS: Anatomic study of the portal vein and its branches. Arch Surg 61:449, 1950.
25. Michels NA: Newer anatomy of the liver and its variant blood supply and collateral circulation. Am J Surg 112:337-347, 1966.
26. Nakamura S, Tsuzuki T: Surgical anatomy of the hepatic veins and the inferior vena cava. Surg Gynecol Obstet 152:43-50, 1981.
27. Healey JE Jr, Schroy PC: Anatomy of the biliary ducts within the human liver: Analysis of the prevailing pattern of branchings and the major variations of the biliary ducts. Arch Surg 66:599-616, 1953.

28. Boyden EA: The anatomy of the choledochoduodenal junction in man. Surg Gynecol Obstet 104:641-652, 1957.

29. Gross RE: Congenital abnormalities of the gallbladder: A review of 148 cases with report of a double gallbladder. Arch Surg 32:131-162, 1936.

30. Northover JM, Terblanche J: A new look at the arterial supply of the bile duct in man and its surgical implications. Br J Surg 66:379-384, 1979.

31. Trutmann M, Sasse D: The lymphatics of the liver. Anat Embryol (Berl) 190:201-209, 1994.

32. Rappaport AM, Wanless IR: Physioanatomic considerations. In Schiff L, Schiff ER (eds): Diseases of the Liver. Philadelphia, JB Lippincott, 1993.

33. Matsumoto T, Kawakami M: The unit-concept of hepatic parenchyma—a re-examination based on angioarchitectural studies. Acta Pathol Jpn 32(Suppl 2):285-314, 1982.

34. Ross MH, Reith EJ, Romrell LJ: The liver. In Ross MH, Reith EJ, Romrell LJ (eds): Histology: A Text and Atlas. Baltimore, Williams & Wilkins, 1989, pp 471-478.

35. Saxena R, Zucker SD, Crawford JM: Anatomy and physiology of the liver. In Zakim D, Boyer TD (eds): Hepatology: A Textbook of Liver Disease. Philadelphia, WB Saunders, 2003, pp 3-30.

36. Wanless IR: Anatomy and developmental anomalies of the liver. In Feldman M, Scharschmidt BF, Sleisenger MH (eds): Sleisenger & Fordtran's Gastrointestinal and Liver Disease. Philadelphia, WB Saunders, 1998, pp 1058-1060.

37. Lamers WH, Hilberts A, Furt E, et al: Hepatic enzymic zonation: A reevaluation of the concept of the liver acinus. Hepatology 10:72-76, 1989.

38. Sasse D, Spornitz UM, Maly IP: Liver architecture. Enzyme 46:8-32, 1992.

39. McCuskey RS, Reilly FD: Hepatic microvasculature: Dynamic structure and its regulation. Semin Liver Dis 13:1-12, 1993.

40. Arias IM: The biology of hepatic endothelial fenestrae. In Schaffner F, Popper H (eds): Progress in Liver Diseases. Philadelphia, WB Saunders, 1990, pp 11-26.

41. Smedsrod B, Pertoft H, Gustafson S, et al: Scavenger functions of the liver endothelial cell. Biochem J 266:313-327, 1990.

42. Lautt WW, Greenway CV: Conceptual review of the hepatic vascular bed. Hepatology 7:952-963, 1987.

43. Arii S, Imamura M: Physiological role of sinusoidal endothelial cells and Kupffer cells and their implication in the pathogenesis of liver injury. J Hepatobiliary Pancreat Surg 7:40-48, 2000.

44. Geerts A: History, heterogeneity, developmental biology, and functions of quiescent hepatic stellate cells. Semin Liver Dis 21:311-335, 2001.

45. Arias IM, Che M, Gatmaitan Z, et al: The biology of the bile canaliculus, 1993. Hepatology 17:318-329, 1993.

46. Seifert S, Englard S: Energy metabolism. In Arias IM (ed): The Liver: Biology and Pathobiology. New York, Raven Press, 1994.

47. Felber JP, Golay A: Regulation of nutrient metabolism and energy expenditure. Metabolism 44:4-9, 1995.

48. Muller M, Jansen PLM: Mechanisms of bile secretion. In Zakim D, Boyer TD (eds): Hepatology: A Textbook of Liver Disease. Philadelphia, WB Saunders, 2003, pp 271-290.

49. Zimmermann H, Reichen J: Assessment of liver function in the surgical patient. In Blumgart LH, Fong Y (eds): Surgery of the Liver and Biliary Tract. London, WB Saunders, 2000, pp 35-64.

50. Chowdhury JR, Chowdhury NR, Jansen PLM: Bilirubin metabolism and its disorders. In Zakim D, Boyer TD (eds): Hepatology: A Textbook of Liver Disease. Philadelphia, WB Saunders, 2003, pp 233-270.

51. Zakim D: Metabolism of glucose and fatty acids by the liver. In Zakim D, Boyer TD (eds): Hepatology: A Textbook of Liver Disease. Philadelphia, WB Saunders, 2003, pp 49-80.

52. Stolz A: Liver physiology and metabolic function. In Feldman M, Scharschmidt BF, Sleisenger MH (eds): Sleisenger & Fordtran's Gastrointestinal and Liver Disease. Philadelphia, WB Saunders, 1998, pp 1061-1082.

53. Pilkis SJ, Granner DK: Molecular physiology of the regulation of hepatic gluconeogenesis and glycolysis. Annu Rev Physiol 54:885-909, 1992.

54. Foster DW: Banting lecture 1984. From glycogen to ketones—and back. Diabetes 33:1188-1199, 1984.

55. Bremmer J, Osmundsen H: Fatty acid oxidation and its regulation. In Numa S (ed): Fatty Acid Metabolism and Its Regulation. Amsterdam, Elsevier Science, 1984.

56. Mayes PA, Felts JM: Regulation of fat metabolism of the liver. Nature 215:716-718, 1967.

57. Cooper AJL: Amino acid metabolism and synthesis of urea. In Zakim D, Boyer TD (eds): Hepatology: A Textbook of Liver Disease. Philadelphia, WB Saunders, 2003, pp 81-126.

58. Matthews DE, Fong Y: Amino acid and protein metabolism. In Rombeau JL, Caldwell MD (eds): Clinical Nutrition, Parenteral Nutrition. Philadelphia, WB Saunders, 1993, pp 75-112.

59. Suttie JW: Recent advances in hepatic vitamin K metabolism and function. Hepatology 7:367-376, 1987.

60. Vessey DA: Hepatic metabolism of xenobiotics in humans. In Zakim D, Boyer TD (eds): Hepatology: A Textbook of Liver Disease. Philadelphia, WB Saunders, 2003, pp 185-232.

61. Fausto N, Hadjis NS, Fong Y: Liver hyperplasia, hypertrophy and atrophy and the molecular basis of liver regeneration. In Blumgart LH, Fong Y (eds): Surgery of the Liver and Biliary Tract. London, WB Saunders, 2000, pp 65-84.

62. Michalopoulos GK, DeFrances MC: Liver regeneration. Science 276:60-66, 1997.

63. Haber BA, Mohn KL, Diamond RH, et al: Induction patterns of 70 genes during nine days after hepatectomy define the temporal course of liver regeneration. J Clin Invest 91:1319-1326, 1993.

64. Fausto N: Lessons from genetically engineered animal models: V. Knocking out genes to study liver regeneration: Present and future. Am J Physiol 277:G917-G921, 1999.

65. Friedman LS, Martin P, Munoz SJ: Laboratory evaluation of the patient with liver disease. In Zakim D, Boyer TD (eds): Hepatology: A Textbook of Liver Disease. Philadelphia, WB Saunders, 2003, pp 661-708.

66. Pratt DS, Kaplan MM: Evaluation of abnormal liver-enzyme results in asymptomatic patients. N Engl J Med 342:1266-1271, 2000.

67. Lotterer E, Hogel J, Gaus W, et al: Quantitative liver function tests as surrogate markers for end-points in controlled clinical trials: A retrospective feasibility study. Hepatology 26:1426-1433, 1997.

68. Ochsner A, DeBakey M, Murray S: Pyogenic abscess of the liver. Am J Surg 40:292-319, 1938.

69. Pitt HA, Zuidema GD: Factors influencing mortality in the treatment of pyogenic hepatic abscess. Surg Gynecol Obstet 140:228-234, 1975.

70. Pope IM, Poston GJ: Pyogenic liver abscess. In Blumgart LH, Fong Y (eds): Surgery of the Liver and Biliary Tract. London, WB Saunders, 2000, pp 1135-1145.

71. Branum GD, Tyson GS, Branum MA, et al: Hepatic abscess: Changes in etiology, diagnosis, and management. Ann Surg 212:655-662, 1990.

72. Seeto RK, Rockey DC: Pyogenic liver abscess: Changes in etiology, management, and outcome. Medicine (Baltimore) 75:99-113, 1996.

73. Johannsen EC, Sifri CD, Madoff LC: Pyogenic liver abscesses. Infect Dis Clin North Am 14:547-563, vii, 2000.

74. Chou FF, Sheen-Chen SM, Chen YS, et al: Prognostic factors for pyogenic abscess of the liver. J Am Coll Surg 179:727-732, 1994.

75. Huang CJ, Pitt HA, Lipsett PA, et al: Pyogenic hepatic abscess: Changing trends over 42 years. Ann Surg 223:600-609, 1996.

76. McDonald MI, Corey GR, Gallis HA, et al: Single and multiple pyogenic liver abscesses: Natural history, diagnosis and treatment, with emphasis on percutaneous drainage. Medicine (Baltimore) 63:291-302, 1984.

77. Hughes MA, Petri WA Jr: Amebic liver abscess. Infect Dis Clin North Am 14:565-582, viii, 2000.

78. Barnes PF, De Cock KM, Reynolds TN, et al: A comparison of amebic and pyogenic abscess of the liver. Medicine (Baltimore) 66:472-483, 1987.

79. Gerzof SG, Robbins AH, Johnson WC, et al: Percutaneous catheter drainage of abdominal abscesses: A five-year experience. N Engl J Med 305:653-657, 1981.

80. Petri A, Hohn J, Hodi Z, et al: Pyogenic liver abscess—20 years' experience: Comparison of results of treatment in two periods. Langenbecks Arch Surg 387:27-31, 2002.

81. Tay KH, Ravintharan T, Hoe MN, et al: Laparoscopic drainage of liver abscesses. Br J Surg 85:330-332, 1998.

82. Giorgio A, Tarantino L, Mariniello N, et al: Pyogenic liver abscesses: 13 years of experience in percutaneous needle aspiration with ultrasound guidance. Radiology 195:122-124, 1995.

83. Kimura K, Stoopen M, Reeder MM, et al: Amebiasis: Modern diagnostic imaging with pathological and clinical correlation. Semin Roentgenol 32:250-275, 1997.

84. Mehta RB, Parija SC, Chetty DV, et al: Management of 240 cases of liver abscess. Int Surg 71:91-94, 1986.

85. Thomas PG, Ravindra KV: Amebiasis and biliary infection. In Blumgart LH, Fong Y (eds): Surgery of the Liver and Biliary Tract. London, WB Saunders, 2000, pp 1147-1166.

86. Ravdin JI, Guerrant RL: A review of the parasite cellular mechanisms involved in the pathogenesis of amebiasis. Rev Infect Dis 4:1185-1207, 1982.

87. Conter RL, Pitt HA, Tompkins RK, et al: Differentiation of pyogenic from amebic hepatic abscesses. Surg Gynecol Obstet 162:114-120, 1986.

88. Seeto RK, Rockey DC: Amebic liver abscess: Epidemiology, clinical features, and outcome. West J Med 170:104-109, 1999.

89. Shandera WX, Bollam P, Hashmey RH, et al: Hepatic amebiasis among patients in a public teaching hospital. South Med J 91:829-837, 1998.

90. Katzenstein D, Rickerson V, Braude A: New concepts of amebic liver abscess derived from hepatic imaging, sero-diagnosis, and hepatic enzymes in 67 consecutive cases in San Diego. Medicine (Baltimore) 61:237-246, 1982.

91. DeBakey ME, Ochsner A: Hepatic amebiasis: A 20-year experience and analysis of 263 cases. Surg Gynecol Obstet 92:209-231, 1951.

92. Griffin FM Jr: Failure of metronidazole to cure hepatic amebic abscess. N Engl J Med 288:1397, 1973.

93. Tandon A, Jain AK, Dixit VK, et al: Needle aspiration in large amoebic liver abscess. Trop Gastroenterol 18:19-21, 1997.

94. Ibarra-Perez C: Thoracic complications of amebic abscess of the liver: Report of 501 cases. Chest 79:672-677, 1981.

95. Sharma MP, Dasarathy S, Sushma S, et al: Long term follow-up of amebic liver abscess: Clinical and ultrasound patterns of resolution. Trop Gastroenterol 16:24-28, 1995.

96. Milicevic MN: Hydatid disease. In Blumgart LH, Fong Y (eds): Surgery of the Liver and Biliary Tract. London, WB Saunders, 2000, pp 1167-1204.

97. Dziri C: Hydatid disease—continuing serious public health problem: Introduction. World J Surg 25:1-3, 2001.

98. Bouree P: Hydatidosis: Dynamics of transmission. World J Surg 25:4-9, 2001.

99. Pedrosa I, Saiz A, Arrazola J, et al: Hydatid disease: Radiologic and pathologic features and complications. Radiographics 20:795-817, 2000.

100. Sayek I, Onat D: Diagnosis and treatment of uncomplicated hydatid cyst of the liver. World J Surg 25:21-27, 2001.

101. Biava MF, Dao A, Fortier B: Laboratory diagnosis of cystic hydatic disease. World J Surg 25:10-14, 2001.

102. Gharbi HA, Hassine W, Brauner MW, et al: Ultrasound examination of the hydatic liver. Radiology 139:459-463, 1981.

103. Zaouche A, Haouet K, Jouini M, et al: Management of liver hydatid cysts with a large biliocystic fistula: Multicenter retrospective study. Tunisian Surgical Association. World J Surg 25:28-39, 2001.

104. Ertem M, Uras C, Karahasanoglu T, et al: Laparoscopic approach to hepatic hydatid disease. Dig Surg 15:333-336, 1998.

105. Akhan O, Ozmen MN: Percutaneous treatment of liver hydatid cysts. Eur J Radiol 32:76-85, 1999.

106. Khuroo MS, Wani NA, Javid G, et al: Percutaneous drainage compared with surgery for hepatic hydatid cysts. N Engl J Med 337:881-887, 1997.

107. Saimot AG: Medical treatment of liver hydatidosis. World J Surg 25:15-20, 2001.

108. Fan ST, Wong J: Recurrent pyogenic cholangitis. In Blumgart LH, Fong Y (eds): Surgery of the Liver and Biliary Tract. London, WB Saunders, 2000, pp 1205-1225.

109. Liu CL, Fan ST, Wong J: Primary biliary stones: Diagnosis and management. World J Surg 22:1162-1166, 1998.

110. Fan ST, Choi TK, Lo CM, et al: Treatment of hepatolithiasis: Improvement of result by a systematic approach. Surgery 109:474-480, 1991.

111. Chijiiwa K, Yamashita H, Yoshida J, et al: Current management and long-term prognosis of hepatolithiasis. Arch Surg 130:194-197, 1995.

112. Jan YY, Chen MF, Wang CS, et al: Surgical treatment of hepatolithiasis: Long-term results. Surgery 120:509-514, 1996.

113. Edmondson HA, Henderson B, Benton B: Liver-cell adenomas associated with use of oral contraceptives. N Engl J Med 294:470-472, 1976.

114. Hugh TJ, Poston GJ: Benign liver tumors and masses. In Blumgart LH, Fong Y (eds): Surgery of the Liver and Biliary Tract. London, WB Saunders, 2000, pp 1397-1422.

115. Charny CK, Jarnagin WR, Schwartz LH, et al: Management of 155 patients with benign liver tumours. Br J Surg 88:808-813, 2001.

116. Nagorney DM: Benign hepatic tumors: Focal nodular hyperplasia and hepatocellular adenoma. World J Surg 19:13-18, 1995.

117. Zimmerman A: Tumors of the liver—pathologic aspects. In Blumgart LH, Fong Y (eds): Surgery of the Liver and Biliary Tract. London, WB Saunders, 2000, pp 1343-1396.

118. Fulcher AS, Sterling RK: Hepatic neoplasms: Computed tomography and magnetic resonance features. J Clin Gastroenterol 34:463-471, 2002.

119. Foster JH, Berman MM: The malignant transformation of liver cell adenomas. Arch Surg 129:712-717, 1994.

120. LaQuaglia MP: Liver tumors in children. *In* Blumgart LH, Fong Y (eds): Surgery of the Liver and Biliary Tract. London, WB Saunders, 2000, pp 1397-1422.

121. Lau WY: Primary hepatocellular carcinoma. *In* Blumgart LH, Fong Y (eds): Surgery of the Liver and Biliary Tract. London, WB Saunders, 2000, pp 1423-1450.

122. Beasley RP, Hwang LY: Epidemiology of hepatocellular carcinoma. *In* Vyas GH, Dienstag JL, Hoofnagle JH (eds): Viral Hepatitis and Liver Disease. New York, Grune & Stratton, 1984, pp 209-224.

123. Fong Y, Kemeny N, Lawrence TS: Cancer of the liver and biliary tree. *In* DeVita VT, Hellman S, Rosenberg SA (eds): Cancer Principles and Practice of Oncology. Philadelphia, Lippincott Williams & Wilkins, 2001, pp 1162-1203.

124. D'Angelica M, Fong Y, Weber S, et al: The role of staging laparoscopy in hepatobiliary malignancy: Prospective analysis of 401 cases. Ann Surg Oncol 10:183-189, 2003.

125. Baer HU, Gertsch P, Matthews JB, et al: Resectability of large focal liver lesions. Br J Surg 76:1042-1044, 1989.

126. Fong Y, Sun RL, Jarnagin W, et al: An analysis of 412 cases of hepatocellular carcinoma at a Western center. Ann Surg 229:790-800, 1999.

127. Mazzaferro V, Regalia E, Doci R, et al: Liver transplantation for the treatment of small hepatocellular carcinomas in patients with cirrhosis. N Engl J Med 334:693-699, 1996.

128. Poon RT, Fan ST, Tsang FH, et al: Locoregional therapies for hepatocellular carcinoma: A critical review from the surgeon's perspective. Ann Surg 235:466-486, 2002.

129. Seidenfeld J, Korn A, Aronson N: Radiofrequency ablation of unresectable liver metastases. J Am Coll Surg 195:378-386, 2002.

130. Bruix J, Llovet JM, Castells A, et al: Transarterial embolization versus symptomatic treatment in patients with advanced hepatocellular carcinoma: Results of a randomized, controlled trial in a single institution. Hepatology 27:1578-1583, 1998.

131. Lau WY, Ho S, Leung TW, et al: Selective internal radiation therapy for nonresectable hepatocellular carcinoma with intraarterial infusion of 90-yttrium microspheres. Int J Radiat Oncol Biol Phys 40:583-592, 1998.

132. Lau WY, Leung TW, Ho SK, et al: Adjuvant intra-arterial iodine-131-labelled lipiodol for resectable hepatocellular carcinoma: A prospective randomised trial. Lancet 353:797-801, 1999.

133. Muto Y, Moriwaki H, Ninomiya M, et al: Prevention of second primary tumors by an acyclic retinoid, polyprenoic acid, in patients with hepatocellular carcinoma. Hepatoma Prevention Study Group. N Engl J Med 334:1561-1567, 1996.

134. Craig JR: Fibrolamellar carcinoma: Clinical and pathological features. *In* Okuda K, Tabor E (eds): Liver Cancer. New York, Churchill Livingstone, 1997, pp 255-262.

135. Weber SM, Jarnagin WR, Klimstra D, et al: Intrahepatic cholangiocarcinoma: Resectability, recurrence pattern, and outcomes. J Am Coll Surg 193:384-391, 2001.

136. Blumgart LH, Fong Y: Surgical options in the treatment of hepatic metastasis from colorectal cancer. Curr Probl Surg 32:333-421, 1995.

137. Bismuth H, Adam R, Levi F, et al: Resection of non-resectable liver metastases from colorectal cancer after neoadjuvant chemotherapy. Ann Surg 224:509-522, 1996.

138. McCarter MD, Fong Y: Metastatic liver tumors. Semin Surg Oncol 19:177-188, 2000.

139. Roddie ME, Adam A: Computed tomography of the liver and biliary tree. *In* Blumgart LH, Fong Y (eds): Surgery of the Liver and Biliary Tract. London, WB Saunders, 2000, pp 309-340.

140. Jaffe BM, Donegan WL, Watson F, et al: Factors influencing survival in patients with untreated hepatic metastases. Surg Gynecol Obstet 127:1-11, 1968.

141. Wood CB, Gillis CR, Blumgart LH: A retrospective study of the natural history of patients with liver metastases from colorectal cancer. Clin Oncol 2:285-288, 1976.

142. Wagner JS, Adson MA, Van Heerden JA, et al: The natural history of hepatic metastases from colorectal cancer: A comparison with resective treatment. Ann Surg 199:502-508, 1984.

143. D'Angelica MI, Shoup MC, Nissan A: Randomized clinical trials in advanced and metastatic colorectal carcinoma. Surg Oncol Clin North Am 11:173-191, ix, 2002.

144. Fong Y, Fortner J, Sun RL, et al: Clinical score for predicting recurrence after hepatic resection for metastatic colorectal cancer: Analysis of 1001 consecutive cases. Ann Surg 230:309-321, 1999.

145. Scheele J, Stang R, Altendorf-Hofmann A, et al: Resection of colorectal liver metastases. World J Surg 19:59-71, 1995.

146. Hughes KS, Simon R, Songhorabodi S, et al: Resection of the liver for colorectal carcinoma metastases: A multi-institutional study of patterns of recurrence. Surgery 100:278-284, 1986.

147. Jamison RL, Donohue JH, Nagorney DM, et al: Hepatic resection for metastatic colorectal cancer results in cure for some patients. Arch Surg 132:505-511, 1997.

148. Kavolius J, Fong Y, Blumgart LH: Surgical resection of metastatic liver tumors. Surg Oncol Clin North Am 5:337-352, 1996.

149. Breedis C, Young G: The blood supply of neoplasms in the liver. Am J Pathol 30:969-977, 1954.

150. Koea JB, Kemeny N: Hepatic artery infusion chemotherapy for metastatic colorectal carcinoma. Semin Surg Oncol 19:125-134, 2000.

151. Kemeny N, Huang Y, Cohen AM, et al: Hepatic arterial infusion of chemotherapy after resection of hepatic metastases from colorectal cancer. N Engl J Med 341:2039-2048, 1999.

152. Chamberlain RS, Canes D, Brown KT, et al: Hepatic neuroendocrine metastases: Does intervention alter outcomes? J Am Coll Surg 190:432-445, 2000.

153. Berber E, Flesher N, Siperstein AE: Laparoscopic radiofrequency ablation of neuroendocrine liver metastases. World J Surg 26:985-990, 2002.

154. Harrison LE, Brennan MF, Newman E, et al: Hepatic resection for noncolorectal, nonneuroendocrine metastases: A fifteen-year experience with ninety-six patients. Surgery 121:625-632, 1997.

155. DeMatteo RP, Shah A, Fong Y, et al: Results of hepatic resection for sarcoma metastatic to liver. Ann Surg 234:540-548, 2001.

156. Farges O, Menu Y, Benhamou JP: Non-parasitic cystic diseases of the liver and intrahepatic biliary tree. *In* Blumgart LH, Fong Y (eds): Surgery of the Liver and Biliary Tract. London, WB Saunders, 2000, pp 1245-1260.

157. Blumgart LH, Jarnagin W, Fong Y: Liver resection for benign disease and for liver and biliary tumors. *In* Blumgart LH, Fong Y (eds): Surgery of the Liver and Biliary Tract. London, WB Saunders, 2000, pp 1639-1714.

158. Sandblom JP: Hemobilia and bilhemia. *In* Blumgart LH, Fong Y (eds): Surgery of the Liver and Biliary Tract. London, WB Saunders, 2000, pp 1319-1342.

159. Green MHA, Duell RM, Johnson CD, et al: Haemobilia. Br J Surg 88:773-786, 2001.

160. Sandblom P: Hemorrhage into the biliary tract following trauma: "Traumatic hemobilia." Surgery 24:571-586, 1948.

161. Sandblom P: Hemobilia (Biliary Tract Hemorrhage): History, Pathology, Diagnosis, Treatment. Springfield, IL, Charles C Thomas, 1972.

162. Goodnight JE Jr, Blaisdell FW: Hemobilia. Surg Clin North Am 61:973-979, 1981.

163. Piccinino F, Sagnelli E, Pasquale G, et al: Complications following percutaneous liver biopsy: A multicentre retrospective study on 68,276 biopsies. J Hepatol 2:165-173, 1986.

164. Yoshida J, Donahue PE, Nyhus LM: Hemobilia: Review of recent experience with a worldwide problem. Am J Gastroenterol 82:448-453, 1987.

165. Croce MA, Fabian TC, Spiers JP, et al: Traumatic hepatic artery pseudoaneurysm with hemobilia. Am J Surg 168:235-238, 1994.

166. Olsen WR: Late complications of central liver injuries. Surgery 92:733-743, 1982.

167. Czerniak A, Thompson JN, Hemingway AP, et al: Hemobilia: A disease in evolution. Arch Surg 123:718-721, 1988.

168. Shapiro MJ: The role of the radiologist in the management of gastrointestinal bleeding. Gastroenterol Clin North Am 23:123-181, 1994.

169. Okazaki M, Ono H, Higashihara H, et al: Angiographic management of massive hemobilia due to iatrogenic trauma. Gastrointest Radiol 16:205, 1991.

170. Curet P, Baumer R, Roche A, et al: Hepatic hemobilia of traumatic or iatrogenic origin: Recent advances in diagnosis and therapy, review of the literature from 1976 to 1981. World J Surg 8:2-8, 1984.

171. Richardson A, Simmons K, Gutmann J, et al: Hepatic haemobilia: Non-operative management in eight cases. Aust N Z J Surg 55:447-451, 1985.

172. Dousset B, Sauvanet A, Bardou M, et al: Selective surgical indications for iatrogenic hemobilia. Surgery 121:37-41, 1997.

173. Zuckerman AJ: Viral hepatitis: Laboratory and clinical science. In Deinhardt F (ed): The History of Viral Hepatitis from Antiquity to the Present. New York, Marcel Dekker, 1983, pp 3-32.

174. MacCallum FO: Homologous serum jaundice. Lancet 2:691-692, 1947.

175. Blumberg BS, Gerstley BJ, Hungerford DA, et al: A serum antigen (Australia antigen) in Down's syndrome, leukemia, and hepatitis. Ann Intern Med 66:924-931, 1967.

176. Rizzetto M, Canese MG, Arico S, et al: Immunofluorescence detection of new antigen-antibody system (delta/anti-delta) associated to hepatitis B virus in liver and in serum of HBsAg carriers. Gut 18:997-1003, 1977.

177. Choo QL, Kuo G, Weiner AJ, et al: Isolation of a cDNA clone derived from a blood-borne non-A, non-B viral hepatitis genome. Science 244:359-362, 1989.

178. Balayan MS, Andjaparidze AG, Savinskaya SS, et al: Evidence for a virus in non-A, non-B hepatitis transmitted via the fecal-oral route. Intervirology 20:23-31, 1983.

179. Reyes GR, Purdy MA, Kim JP, et al: Isolation of a cDNA from the virus responsible for enterically transmitted non-A, non-B hepatitis. Science 247:1335-1339, 1990.

180. Laskus T, Wang LF, Radkowski M, et al: Hepatitis G virus infection in American patients with cryptogenic cirrhosis: No evidence for liver replication. J Infect Dis 176:1491-1495, 1997.

181. Linnen J, Wages J Jr, Zhang-Keck ZY, et al: Molecular cloning and disease association of hepatitis G virus: A transfusion-transmissible agent. Science 271:505-508, 1996.

182. Alter HJ, Nakatsuji Y, Melpolder J, et al: The incidence of transfusion-associated hepatitis G virus infection and its relation to liver disease. N Engl J Med 336:747-754, 1997.

183. Doo EC, Lian TJ: The hepatitis viruses. In Schiff ER, Sorrell MF, Maddrey WC (eds): Schiff's Diseases of the Liver. Philadelphia, Lippincott-Raven, 1999, pp 725-744.

184. Koff RS: Hepatitis A and E. In Zakim D, Boyer TD (eds): Hepatology: A Textbook of Liver Disease. Philadelphia, WB Saunders, 2003, pp 939-959.

185. Nair S, Perrillo RP: Hepatitis B and D. In Zakim D, Boyer TD (eds): Hepatology: A Textbook of Liver Disease. Philadelphia, WB Saunders, 2003, pp 959-1016.

186. Hoffnagle JH, Heller T: Hepatitis C. In Zakim D, Boyer TD (eds): Hepatology: A Textbook of Liver Disease. Philadelphia, WB Saunders, 2003, pp 1017-1062.

187. Liaw YF, Yang CY, Chu CM, et al: Appearance and persistence of hepatitis A IgM antibody in acute clinical hepatitis A observed in an outbreak. Infection 14:156-158, 1986.

188. Kao HW, Ashcavai M, Redeker AG: The persistence of hepatitis A IgM antibody after acute clinical hepatitis A. Hepatology 4:933-936, 1984.

189. Hoofnagle JH, Schafer DF: Serologic markers of hepatitis B virus infection. Semin Liver Dis 6:1-10, 1986.

190. Chien DY, Choo QL, Tabrizi A, et al: Diagnosis of hepatitis C virus (HCV) infection using an immunodominant chimeric polyprotein to capture circulating antibodies: Reevaluation of the role of HCV in liver disease. Proc Natl Acad Sci U S A 89:10011-10015, 1992.

191. Pawlotsky JM, Bouvier-Alias M, Hezode C, et al: Standardization of hepatitis C virus RNA quantification. Hepatology 32:654-659, 2000.

192. Jardi R, Buti M, Cotrina M, et al: Determination of hepatitis delta virus RNA by polymerase chain reaction in acute and chronic delta infection. Hepatology 21:25-29, 1995.

193. Lin CC, Wu JC, Chang TT, et al: Diagnostic value of immunoglobulin G (IgG) and IgM anti-hepatitis E virus (HEV) tests based on HEV RNA in an area where hepatitis E is not endemic. J Clin Microbiol 38:3915-3918, 2000.

194. Gust ID: Epidemiological patterns of hepatitis A in different parts of the world. Vaccine 10(Suppl 1):S56-S58, 1992.

195. Gust ID: Epidemiology of hepatitis B infection in the Western Pacific and South East Asia. Gut 38(Suppl 2):S18-23, 1996.

196. Hollinger FB: Comprehensive control (or elimination) of hepatitis B virus transmission in the United States. Gut 38(Suppl 2):S24-30, 1996.

197. Alter MJ: The epidemiology of acute and chronic hepatitis C. Clin Liver Dis 1:559-568, 1997.

198. Krawczynski K: Hepatitis E. Hepatology 17:932-941, 1993.

199. Hadler SC: Global impact of hepatitis A virus infection: Changing patterns. In Hollinger FB, Lemon SM, Margolis HS (eds): Viral Hepatitis and Liver Disease. Baltimore, Williams & Wilkins, 1991, pp 14-20.

200. Fattovich G, Brollo L, Giustina G, et al: Natural history and prognostic factors for chronic hepatitis type B. Gut 32:294-298, 1991.

201. Gocke DJ: Extrahepatic manifestations of viral hepatitis. Am J Med Sci 270:49-52, 1975.

202. Fattovich G, Giustina G, Schalm SW, et al: Occurrence of hepatocellular carcinoma and decompensation in western European patients with cirrhosis type B. The EUROHEP Study Group on Hepatitis B Virus and Cirrhosis. Hepatology 21:77-82, 1995.

203. Hoofnagle JH: Hepatitis C: The clinical spectrum of disease. Hepatology 26:15S-20S, 1997.

204. Seeff LB: The natural history of chronic hepatitis C virus infection. Clin Liver Dis 1:587-602, 1997.

205. Martinot-Peignoux M, Boyer N, Cazals-Hatem D, et al: Prospective study on anti-hepatitis C virus-positive patients with persistently normal serum alanine transaminase with or without detectable serum hepatitis C virus RNA. Hepatology 34:1000-1005, 2001.

206. Wu JC, Chen TZ, Huang YS, et al: Natural history of hepatitis D viral superinfection: Significance of viremia detected by polymerase chain reaction. Gastroenterology 108:796-802, 1995.

207. Ichimura H, Tamura I, Tsubakio T, et al: Influence of hepatitis delta virus superinfection on the clearance of hepatitis B virus (HBV) markers in HBV carriers in Japan. J Med Virol 26:49-55, 1988.

208. Szmuness W, Stevens CE, Harley EJ, et al: Hepatitis B vaccine: Demonstration of efficacy in a controlled clinical trial in a high-risk population in the United States. N Engl J Med 303:833-841, 1980.

SURGICAL COMPLICATIONS OF CIRRHOSIS AND PORTAL HYPERTENSION

Layton F. Rikkers, M.D.

Historical Review
Anatomy, Physiology, and Pathophysiology of
  Portal Hypertension
Evaluation of the Patient With Cirrhosis

Variceal Hemorrhage
Ascites and the Hepatorenal Syndrome
Encephalopathy

HISTORICAL REVIEW

Cirrhosis was first described in a 4th century B.C. hippo-cratic aphorism: In cases of jaundice it is a bad sign when the liver becomes hard.[1] Although the deleterious effect of alcohol on the liver was appreciated by Galen and his contemporaries in the 2nd century A.D., alcoholic liver disease as an entity was first recognized by Baillie and other English writers after the "gin plague" in the 18th century. Shortly thereafter, Laënnec introduced the term *cirrhosis,* which was derived from the Greek word *kirrhos,* meaning "orange-yellow." Nineteenth century European and English pathologists, including Carswell and Rokitansky, described the gross and histopathologic char-acteristics of the disease. Although alcoholic cirrhosis was thought to be due to toxins other than alcohol or to mal-nutrition during much of the 20th century, recent inves-tigations have established alcohol as a hepatotoxin.

Cirrhosis is the end result of a variety of mechanisms causing hepatocellular injury, including toxins (alcohol), viruses (hepatitis B and hepatitis C), prolonged cholesta-sis (extrahepatic and intrahepatic), autoimmunity (lupoid hepatitis), and metabolic disorders (hemochromatosis, Wilson's disease, α_1-antitrypsin deficiency). Although the mechanisms are diverse, the pathologic response is uniform: hepatocellular necrosis followed by fibrosis and nodular regeneration. Each of these elements may exist

alone (necrosis, uncomplicated hepatitis; fibrosis, con-genital hepatic fibrosis; nodular regeneration, partial nodular transformation), but all three are required for the development of cirrhosis. Cirrhosis, always a diffuse process, may be classified either morphologically or by eti-ology. Alcoholic cirrhosis, which is usually micronodular, and posthepatitic cirrhosis, which is generally macro-nodular, are the two most common varieties in the United States. Because the pathologic responses to various mech-anisms of hepatocellular injury are so similar, occasionally the cause cannot be ascertained (cryptogenic cirrhosis).

Cirrhosis causes two major phenomena: hepatocellular failure and portal hypertension. Even after the noxious agent is removed (e.g., abstinence from alcohol), the disease may progress. Although the mechanism is not clear, both ischemia, secondary to extensive fibrosis and intrahepatic and extrahepatic shunts, and autoimmune factors may play roles. The altered hepatic architecture and perisinusoidal fibrosis cause increased hepatic vascu-lar resistance, resulting in portal hypertension and its associated complications of variceal hemorrhage, en-cephalopathy, ascites, and hypersplenism.

Autopsy studies suggest an incidence of cirrhosis of between 3.5% and 5%. Only 10% to 15% of heavy drinkers develop alcoholic cirrhosis. Because of the large number of alcoholic people in the United States, as well as a sig-nificant percentage of patients with nonalcoholic causes of chronic liver disease, cirrhosis presently ranks as the sixth leading cause of death between the ages of 35 and 54 years. Hepatic failure and variceal hemorrhage are the first and second most common causes of death, respectively, in patients with cirrhosis.

Historically, the treatment of cirrhosis has been the treatment of the complications of portal hypertension. Medical treatment of cirrhosis with antifibrogenesis drugs, such as colchicine, has been ineffective. In contrast, since 1980, the surgical management of chronic liver disease with hepatic transplantation has been highly successful, with long-term survival rates generally above 70%. A major challenge to the physician or surgeon managing patients with cirrhosis is to determine when definitive treatment (transplantation) rather than palliative treatment (e.g., interventions to prevent recurrent variceal hemorrhage) should be applied.

ANATOMY, PHYSIOLOGY, AND PATHOPHYSIOLOGY OF PORTAL HYPERTENSION

The liver is a unique organ in that it has a dual blood supply: portal venous and hepatic arterial. The portal vein is formed from the confluence of the superior mesenteric and splenic veins behind the neck of the pancreas and is 6 to 8 cm in length (Fig. 51-1). The left gastric or coronary vein drains the distal esophagus and lesser curvature of the stomach, generally entering the portal vein near its origin. The splenic vein lies beneath the pancreas and is usually joined by the inferior mesenteric vein just before its confluence with the superior mesenteric vein.

The hepatic artery, one of three major branches of the celiac axis, lies medial to the common bile duct and portal vein in the hepatoduodenal ligament. Common variations include origins of the right and left hepatic arteries from the superior mesenteric artery and the left gastric artery, respectively, both of which occur in nearly 20% of the population.

Hepatic blood flow averages 1500 mL/minute, which represents about 25% of the cardiac output. The portal vein contributes two thirds of the total hepatic blood flow, whereas hepatic arterial perfusion accounts for more than half of the liver's oxygen supply. The volume of portal venous flow is indirectly regulated by vasoconstriction and vasodilation of the splanchnic arterial bed. In contrast, hepatic arterioles respond to circulating catecholamines and sympathetic nervous stimulation; thus, hepatic arterial flow is directly regulated. Even intense vasoconstrictive influences, however, can be overcome by a hepatic arterial autoregulatory or *buffer* response, which maintains total hepatic blood flow as near to normal as possible when portal perfusion is decreased in patients with shock or either disease-induced or surgically created portosystemic shunts.[2]

Many splanchnic hormones are important regulators of hepatic metabolism. Insulin is particularly important because it is a hepatotrophic hormone and is essential for maintenance of liver structure and function. Thus, even if the quantity of hepatic blood flow is maintained in the normal range by hepatic arterial compensation for decreased portal flow, hepatic physiology may be impaired.

Because increased portal venous resistance is usually the initiator of portal hypertension, classifications of this disorder are generally based on the site of elevated resistance. However, increased portal venous inflow secondary to a hyperdynamic systemic circulation and splanchnic hyperemia is often a major contributor to the maintenance of portal hypertension. The cause of the elevated cardiac output and splanchnic hyperemia is not known, but splanchnic hormones, such as glucagon, and decreased sensitivity of the splanchnic vasculature to catecholamines probably play a role.[3] Increased production of nitrous oxide and prostacyclin by vascular endothelium is also an important factor.[4] An improved understanding of the pathophysiology of portal hypertension has therapeutic implications because drugs are available that can alter these responses.

The most common cause of prehepatic portal hypertension is portal vein thrombosis, which accounts for about half of cases of portal hypertension in children.

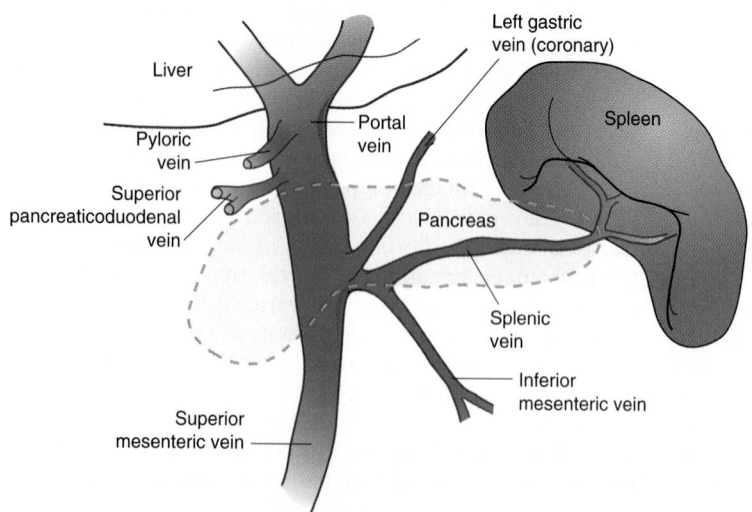

FIGURE 51-1. The extrahepatic portal venous circulation. (From Rikkers LF: Portal hypertension. *In* Goldsmith H [ed]: Practice of Surgery. Philadelphia, Harper & Row, 1981, pp 1-37.)

When the portal vein is thrombosed in the absence of liver disease, hepatopetal (to the liver) portal collateral vessels develop to restore portal perfusion. This combination is termed *cavernomatous transformation of the portal vein.* Isolated splenic vein thrombosis (left-sided portal hypertension) is usually secondary to pancreatic inflammation or neoplasm. The result is gastrosplenic venous hypertension, with superior mesenteric and portal venous pressures remaining normal. The left gastroepiploic vein becomes a major collateral vessel, and gastric, rather than esophageal, varices develop. This variant of portal hypertension is important to recognize because it is easily reversed by splenectomy alone.

The site of increased resistance in intrahepatic portal hypertension may be at the presinusoidal, sinusoidal, or postsinusoidal level. Frequently, more than one level is involved. The most common cause of intrahepatic, presinusoidal hypertension is schistosomiasis. In addition, many causes of nonalcoholic cirrhosis also result in presinusoidal portal hypertension, especially early in their course. Alcoholic cirrhosis, the most common cause of portal hypertension in the United States, usually causes increased resistance to portal flow at the sinusoidal (secondary to deposition of collagen in Disse's space) and postsinusoidal (secondary to regenerating nodules distorting small hepatic veins) levels. Postsinusoidal causes of portal hypertension are rare and include Budd-Chiari syndrome (hepatic vein thrombosis), constrictive pericarditis, and heart failure. Rarely, increased portal venous flow alone, secondary either to massive splenomegaly (idiopathic portal hypertension) or a splanchnic arteriovenous fistula, causes portal hypertension.

Portal hypertension is defined by a portal pressure higher than 5 mm Hg. Somewhat higher pressures (8 to 10 mm Hg) are required to stimulate portosystemic collateralization. Collateral vessels usually develop where the portal and systemic venous circulations are in close proximity (Fig. 51-2). The collateral network through the coronary and short gastric veins to the azygos vein is the most important one clinically because it results in formation of esophagogastric varices; however, other sites include a recanalized umbilical vein from the left portal vein to the epigastric venous system (caput medusae), retroperitoneal collateral vessels, and the hemorrhoidal venous plexus. In addition to extrahepatic collateral vessels, a significant fraction of portal venous flow passes through both anatomic and physiologic (capillarization of hepatic sinusoids) intrahepatic shunts. As hepatic portal perfusion decreases, hepatic arterial flow generally increases (buffer response).[2]

EVALUATION OF THE PATIENT WITH CIRRHOSIS

Key aspects of the assessment of a patient with suspected chronic liver disease or one of the complications of portal hypertension are the following: (1) diagnosis of the underlying liver disease; (2) estimation of functional hepatic reserve; (3) definition of portal venous anatomy and hepatic hemodynamic evaluation; and (4) identification of the site of upper gastrointestinal hemorrhage, if present.

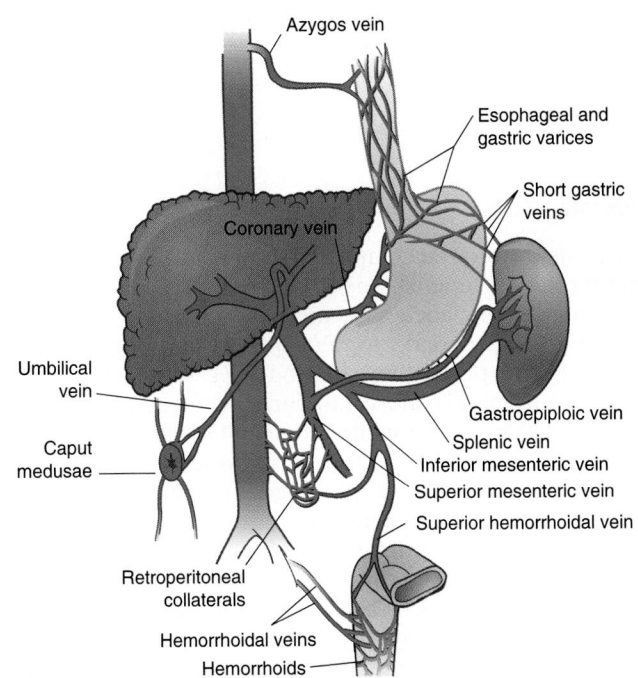

FIGURE 51-2. Portosystemic collateral pathways develop where the portal venous and systemic venous systems are in close apposition. (From Rikkers LF: Portal hypertension. *In* Miller TA [ed]: Physiologic Basis of Modern Surgical Care. St. Louis, CV Mosby, 1988, pp 417-428.)

These diagnostic categories take on varying levels of importance depending on the clinical situation. For example, estimation of functional hepatic reserve is useful in determining the risk associated with therapeutic intervention and whether definitive (hepatic transplantation) or palliative (e.g., endoscopic sclerotherapy or shunt procedure) treatment is indicated. Knowledge of portal anatomy and physiology guides the surgeon in selecting an appropriate operation for control of variceal bleeding. Precise identification of the site of bleeding is essential because hemorrhage secondary to portal hypertension may be from esophageal varices, gastric varices, ectopic varices, portal hypertensive gastropathy (PHG), or portal colopathy and because a significant fraction of patients with portal hypertension bleed from other lesions.

History and Physical Examination

In a patient with nonspecific constitutional complaints such as weight loss, malaise, and weakness, a past history of chronic alcoholism, hepatitis, complicated biliary disease, or exposure to hepatotoxins should lead one to include cirrhosis in the differential diagnosis. Subtle clues to the presence of underlying chronic liver disease on physical examination are spider angiomas, palmar erythema, testicular atrophy, and gynecomastia. A palpable spleen in association with these signs suggests portal hypertension. Confirmatory evidence of cirrhosis is provided by signs of hepatic functional decompensation or advanced portal hypertension, such as jaundice, ascites, palpation of a firm irregular liver edge, dilated abdominal wall veins, impairment of mental status or the presence of asterixis (liver flap).

Laboratory Tests

Cirrhosis is often accompanied by anemia, leukopenia, and thrombocytopenia. Anemia may result from bleeding, nutritional deficiencies, hemolysis, or bone marrow depression secondary to alcoholism. Although many patients with portal hypertension have some degree of hypersplenism, it is unusual to find a platelet count of less than 50,000/mm^3 or a white blood cell count of less than 2000/mm^3. In addition to thrombocytopenia, coagulation may be impaired by a prolonged prothrombin time, because many of the coagulation factors are synthesized by the liver, and by primary fibrinolysis, which is present in many patients with chronic liver disease.

A chemistry profile is helpful in both the diagnosis and assessment of severity of cirrhosis. Hypoalbuminemia and/or a prolonged International Normalized Ratio (INR) are usually reliable indices of chronic rather than acute liver disease. Elevation of the hepatocellular enzymes aspartate aminotransferase and alanine aminotransferase to more than three times their normal level is indicative of significant, ongoing hepatocellular necrosis, which is often present in patients with alcoholic hepatitis and chronic active hepatitis resulting from a variety of causes. Increased disease activity may be an important risk factor in patients who undergo surgery. A ratio of alanine aminotransferase to aspartate aminotransferase of greater than 2 is highly suggestive of alcohol as the cause of liver disease. Although mild elevations of the enzymes alkaline phosphatase and γ-glutamyl transpeptidase are nonspecific, marked increases in these enzymes are indicative of either intrahepatic or extrahepatic cholestasis (primary or secondary biliary cirrhosis). In the absence of prior blood transfusions, a total bilirubin level of greater than 3 mg/100 mL is indicative of severe hepatic decompensation and a high operative risk status.

Hepatitis serology should be obtained in most patients with cirrhosis. A significant fraction of patients with hepatitis B and hepatitis C develop cirrhosis, whereas hepatitis A generally causes only acute liver disease. One of the most common internal malignancies worldwide is hepatocellular carcinoma, which is frequently secondary to hepatitis B or hepatitis C infection. This malignancy, however, frequently develops in patients with other causes of cirrhosis and occasionally in patients without chronic liver disease. Unexpected hepatic functional deterioration in a patient with cirrhosis is often a result of the development of hepatocellular carcinoma, which can be diagnosed in about 60% of patients by an elevated α-fetoprotein level. All newly diagnosed cirrhotic patients should be screened for hepatocellular carcinoma by determination of α-fetoprotein level and by obtaining a computed tomography (CT) scan of the liver.

Common serum electrolyte abnormalities in cirrhosis are hyponatremia, hypokalemia, and metabolic alkalosis.

These metabolic disorders are secondary to hyperaldosteronism, diarrhea, and recurrent emesis, which frequently accompany cirrhosis. Deleterious consequences of metabolic alkalosis are shift of the oxyhemoglobin dissociation curve to the left, which impairs tissue oxygen delivery, and conversion of ammonium chloride to ammonia, which facilitates transport of this purported cerebral toxin across the blood-brain barrier.

Liver Biopsy

Percutaneous liver biopsy is a useful technique for establishing the cause of cirrhosis and for assessing activity of the liver disease. Percutaneous liver biopsy should not be done when either coagulopathy or moderate ascites is present. In these situations, liver tissue can be obtained by means of a transjugular venous approach or laparoscopy. Laparoscopic biopsy reduces the false-negative rate for diagnosing cirrhosis as compared with blind biopsy techniques.

Measurement of Hepatic Functional Reserve

The time-honored method of assessing hepatic functional reserve is Child's classification or one of its modifications. The most commonly used scheme is the Child-Pugh classification (Table 51-1), which includes two clinical variables in addition to three biochemical indices.[5] Although not a direct measure of hepatic functional reserve, no other test has surpassed it with respect to predicting operative outcome or assessing long-term prognosis in the unoperated patient. The serum bilirubin level should be interpreted in the context of recent blood transfusions, which may transiently elevate it but are not indicative of further impairment of hepatic functional reserve. In most clinical series, operative mortality rates for Child-Pugh classes A, B, and C patients are in the range of 0 to 5%, 10% to 15%, and greater than 25%, respectively. Because many patients with acute variceal hemorrhage present with decompensated hepatic function as reflected by their Child-Pugh class, an interval of medical management to improve the patient from class C to class A or B is worth-

TABLE 51-1. Child-Pugh Criteria for Hepatic Functional Reserve

Clinical and Laboratory Measurement	Patient Score for Increasing Abnormality		
	1	2	3
Encephalopathy (grade)	None	1 or 2	3 or 4
Ascites	None	Mild	Moderate
Bilirubin (mg/dL)	1–2	2.1–3	≥3.1
Albumin (g/dL)	≥3.5	2.8–3.4	≤2.7
Prothrombin time (increase, sec)	1–4	4.1–6	≥6.1

Grade A, 5 and 6; grade B, 7–9; grade C, 10–15.

while before surgical intervention if indicated. The Model for End-Stage Liver Disease (MELD) scale that consists of serum bilirubin and creatinine levels, INR, and etiology of liver disease has recently been found to be as predictive of mortality as the Child-Pugh score.[6]

True quantitative measures of hepatocellular function, such as galactose elimination capacity, aminopyrine breath test, indocyanine green clearance, and hepatic clearance of amino acids, are not available in most institutions. These tests, however, may be valuable indicators of limited hepatic reserve in some patients with nearly normal conventional liver function tests. Now that hepatic transplantation has become a realistic option for many patients with cirrhosis, accurate quantitation of hepatocellular function to determine which patients are transplantation candidates has become even more important.

Hepatic Hemodynamic Assessment

In patients with alcoholic cirrhosis and many varieties of nonalcoholic cirrhosis, portal pressure can be indirectly estimated by measurement of hepatic venous wedge pressure (HVWP). Because HVWP is normal in patients with presinusoidal portal hypertension, portal pressure in these patients can be measured only directly by transhepatic or umbilical venous cannulation of the portal venous system or by percutaneous puncture of the spleen.

The portal pressure should be expressed as the portal pressure gradient, which is the difference between the portal pressure and the inferior vena cava pressure. It is an important measurement because a gradient in excess of 10 mm Hg is necessary for varices to form and a pressure higher than 12 mm Hg is required for varices to bleed.

Because splanchnic venous thrombosis may be the cause of portal hypertension or develop as a result of cirrhosis, portal venous anatomy should be defined before performing a portosystemic shunt operation. Although selective visceral angiography has been the most frequently used method for visualization of the portal venous system and for qualitative estimation of hepatic portal perfusion, this relatively invasive approach is presently being replaced in many institutions by less invasive methods such as CT angiography, Doppler ultrasonography, and magnetic resonance imaging. CT angiograms can delineate the location, size, and patency status of all veins (e.g., splenic vein and left renal vein) to be used in creation of a portosystemic shunt (Fig. 51-3).[7] Magnetic resonance imaging has also been successfully used to visualize the portal venous circulation. This technique is particularly appropriate for patients with an allergy to radiopaque contrast agent.

Doppler ultrasonography is a noninvasive technique for assessment of portal venous patency, direction of portal flow, and shunt patency status.[8] Because of its noninvasiveness, Doppler ultrasonography has become a standard for the evaluation of most patients with chronic liver disease because direction of portal flow and its velocity can be diagnostic of associated portal hypertension. Ultrasound is also useful for assessing liver size, spleen size,

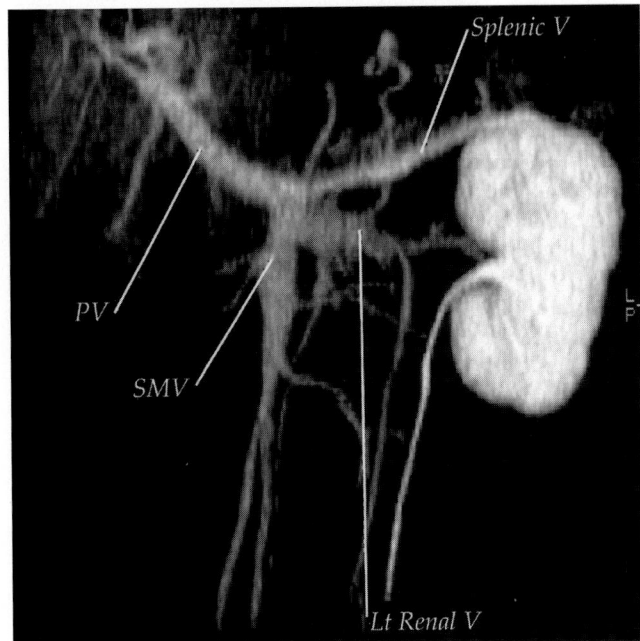

FIGURE 51-3. A three-dimensional reconstruction of a CT angiogram. The portal vein (PV), superior mesenteric vein (SMV), splenic vein, and left renal vein are clearly demonstrated. The ready availability of these scans has decreased the need for more invasive techniques such as visceral angiography.

and the presence of liver masses. It can also detect ascites in its earliest stages (≥100 mL). Doppler ultrasound is less accurate in assessing superior mesenteric and splenic vein anatomy and flow characteristics. Likewise, Doppler ultrasonography usually accurately assesses patency status of surgically constructed shunts unless there is overlying bowel gas. Doppler ultrasound has also been used to evaluate patency and narrowing of transjugular intrahepatic portosystemic shunts (TIPS), but it is less accurate than direct cannulation via a systemic venous approach.

Diagnosis of Bleeding

In the absence of hematemesis, a nasogastric tube should be inserted to determine whether bleeding is from the upper gastrointestinal tract. The key procedure for diagnosing the site of upper gastrointestinal hemorrhage in a patient with portal hypertension is endoscopy. Before endoscopy, the patient should be hemodynamically stabilized and the stomach evacuated of blood clots with a large-bore lavage tube.

Upper gastrointestinal tract bleeding in patients with portal hypertension is caused by the portal hypertension in about 90% of instances. The remaining 10% of patients bleed from Mallory-Weiss tears, gastric ulcers, and duodenal ulcers, all of which are more common in patients with alcoholic cirrhosis than in the general population. Portal hypertensive bleeding is most commonly from esophagogastric varices (esophageal varices, 80%; gastric varices,

20%). Gastric varices most commonly occur in association with esophageal varices, but they occasionally occur alone. Isolated gastric varices should raise the suspicion of splenic vein thrombosis. Hemorrhage from gastric fundal varices can be especially severe and is associated with a higher likelihood of recurrent bleeding and mortality than bleeding from esophageal varices. The endoscopic diagnosis of variceal hemorrhage can be established by either observing a bleeding varix (~25% of patients) or by observation of moderate- to large-sized varices and no other lesions in a patient who has recently experienced a major upper gastrointestinal tract hemorrhage (loss of > 2 units of blood).

The only nonvariceal causes of portal hypertensive bleeding are PHG and, much less commonly, portal colopathy. The frequency of PHG is unknown, but it is probably more common after eradication of varices by endoscopic sclerotherapy or banding. PHG mainly involves the fundus and body of the stomach and, when mild, has an endoscopic appearance of a white reticular network with enclosed erythematous areas. The more severe form of PHG includes granular mucosa and cherry-red spots, both of which indicate a higher risk for bleeding.[9] PHG is associated with increased gastric mucosal perfusion and reflects a hyperemic rather than a congestive pathophysiologic change. Because varices and PHG often coexist, it may be difficult to determine which lesion is responsible for any given episode of bleeding. Occasionally, massive bleeding in a patient with cirrhosis makes an endoscopic diagnosis initially impossible, in which case endoscopy should be repeated after bleeding is controlled. Gastric varices may be difficult to recognize endoscopically even in nonbleeding patients. Endoscopic ultrasound is a more sensitive diagnostic test than endoscopy alone for detection of gastric varices.

VARICEAL HEMORRHAGE

Bleeding from esophagogastric varices is the single most life-threatening complication of portal hypertension, responsible for about one third of all deaths in patients with cirrhosis. Overall, acute variceal bleeding is associated with a mortality rate of about 25% to 30%. Approximately one half of the deaths are due to uncontrolled bleeding. The risk for death from bleeding is mainly related to the underlying hepatic functional reserve. Patients with extrahepatic portal venous obstruction and normal hepatic function rarely die of bleeding varices, whereas those with decompensated cirrhosis (Child-Pugh class C) may face a mortality rate in excess of 50%. The greatest risk for rebleeding from varices is within the first few days after the onset of hemorrhage; the risk declines rapidly between then and 6 weeks after hemorrhage onset, when it returns to the prehemorrhage risk level.[10]

Pathogenesis

Varices in the distal esophagus and proximal stomach are a component of the collateral network that diverts high-pressure portal venous flow through the left and right gastric veins and the short gastric veins to the azygous system. Less commonly, varices develop at other sites in the gastrointestinal tract but are less prone to rupture in those locations. Esophagogastric varices do not bleed until portal pressure exceeds 12 mm Hg, and then they bleed in only one third to one half of patients.[3] The pathogenesis of variceal rupture is incompletely understood but is most likely multifactorial.

Polio and Groszmann[11] have put forth a unifying hypothesis of variceal rupture based on Laplace's law. Although it has been observed that variceal size, magnitude of portal pressure, and thickness of the epithelium overlying the varix all significantly separate bleeders from nonbleeders, the overlap between groups is large when any one of these variables is considered independently. Laplace's law states that variceal wall tension is directly related to transmural pressure and varix radius and inversely related to variceal wall thickness, thus combining all three of these variables. Because all of these parameters cannot be measured clinically, there are inherent inaccuracies in predicting which patients with varices may bleed. The three key variables that are predictive of variceal bleeding are Child-Pugh class, variceal size, and the presence and severity of red wale markings (indicative of epithelial thickness). These factors can be combined into an index that accurately predicts which varices will bleed.[12] The capacity to predict variceal bleeding is especially important when considering prophylactic therapy (treatment of varices that have not previously bled).

Treatment

Therapy for portal hypertension and variceal bleeding has evolved during the past 100 years. The many treatment modalities available suggest that no single therapy is entirely satisfactory for all patients or for all clinical situations. Sequential therapies are often necessary. Nonoperative treatments are generally preferred for acutely bleeding patients because they are often high operative risks because of decompensated hepatic function. Therapies that are effective (a low rebleeding rate) and minimally alter hepatic physiology are optimal for long-term prevention of recurrent bleeding. Only treatments associated with minimal morbidity and mortality can be considered for prophylaxis because many patients will be treated unnecessarily (only one third to one half of patients with varices eventually bleed).

History of Treatment for Portal Hypertension

Table 51-2 presents a chronology of the treatment of portal hypertension, which began with the description of Eck's fistula (end-to-side portacaval shunt) in 1877.[1] Eck's main concerns were to determine whether survival was possible after complete portal flow diversion and to develop a treatment for ascites. Probably the most important contribution to this field was made by Pavlov's group in 1893.[13] These investigators perfected the technique of portacaval shunting and, after carefully observing 20 surviving dogs, described in detail the syndrome of "meat intoxication" or portosystemic encephalopathy, which

TABLE 51-2. History of Treatment of Portal Hypertension	
Investigators, Year of Publication	**Contribution**
Eck, 1877	Portacaval shunt (dog)
Pavlov, 1893	Encephalopathy (dog)
Vidal, 1903	Clinical portacaval shunt (ascites)
Westphal, 1930	Balloon tamponade
Crafoord & Frenckner, 1939	Endoscopic sclerotherapy
Blakemore et al, 1945	Clinical portacaval and splenorenal shunts (bleeding)
Sengstaken & Blakemore, 1950	Balloon tamponade
Kehne, 1956	Vasopressin
Warren et al, 1967	Distal splenorenal shunt
Starzl, 1967	First successful liver transplantation
Inokuchi, 1968	Left gastric–vena caval shunt
Rosch, 1969	TIPS in animals
Johnston & Rodgers, 1973	Reintroduction of endoscopic sclerotherapy
Sugiura & Futagawa, 1973	Extensive esophagogastric devascularization
Calne, 1980	Cyclosporine for transplantation
Lebrec, 1981	Propranolol for bleeding
Colapinto, 1983	TIPS in humans

TIPS, transjugular intrahepatic portosystemic shunt.
Data from Chen TS, Chen PS: Understanding the Liver. Westport, CT, Greenwood Press, 1984, pp 154-155.

they believed was due to intestinally absorbed cerebral toxins bypassing their site of metabolism in the liver. They also found from autopsy studies that dogs with encephalopathy had patent portacaval shunts and atrophic livers, whereas animals with normal cerebral function and preserved hepatic structure had thrombosed shunts and maintenance of hepatic portal perfusion through collateral vessels.

The modern era of treatment of variceal hemorrhage can be dated from the mid-1940s when the portacaval and conventional splenorenal shunts were introduced into clinical practice. Although balloon tamponade and endoscopic sclerosis of varices were initially described in the 1930s, these were found to be only temporizing measures. During the ensuing 20 years, several varieties of nonselective shunts (complete portal decompression and portal flow diversion) were described, and the portacaval shunt was evaluated in randomized, controlled trials. Motivated by the discouraging results of these trials, the concept of selective variceal decompression (distal splenorenal shunt) was introduced in 1967. An initial wave of enthusiasm for the distal splenorenal shunt (partial portal flow diversion) was followed by several randomized trials that produced inconsistent results. A resurgence of interest in endoscopic sclerotherapy occurred in the 1970s, initially in Europe and South Africa and then in the United States.

Although pharmacotherapy with vasopressin was first used for acute hemorrhage in 1956, drug treatment for long-term prevention of initial or recurrent hemorrhage is a phenomenon of the 1980s. Improved immunosuppression (cyclosporine) and surgical techniques have led to the widespread application of hepatic transplantation for patients with end-stage liver disease. Finally, a nonoperative means of portal decompression (TIPS), first described in animals in 1969, has more recently been applied to the problem of variceal bleeding and, along with endoscopic therapy, is presently the most widely used intervention for this complication of portal hypertension.

Treatment of the Acute Bleeding Episode

Because many patients with acute variceal bleeding have decompensated hepatic function secondary to either recent alcoholism or hypotension, they are at high risk for emergency surgical intervention. In addition, these patients often have other complications of chronic liver disease, such as encephalopathy, ascites, coagulopathy, and malnutrition. Therefore, emergency treatment should be nonoperative whenever possible. Endoscopic treatment (sclerosis or ligation), which has become the mainstay of nonoperative treatment of acute hemorrhage in most centers, controls bleeding in more than 85% of patients, allowing an interval of medical management for improvement of hepatic function, resolution of ascites and encephalopathy, and enhancement of nutrition before definitive treatment for prevention of recurrent bleeding. Pharmacotherapy can be initiated in any hospital, and some trials suggest that it is just as effective as endoscopic treatment. Balloon tamponade, which is infrequently used, can be life-saving in patients with exsanguinating hemorrhage and when the other nonoperative methods are not successful. TIPS has replaced operative shunts for managing acute variceal bleeding when pharmacotherapy and endoscopic treatment fail to control bleeding. Emergency surgical intervention in most centers is reserved for selected patients who are not TIPS candidates.

Resuscitation and Diagnosis

The highest priority in emergency management is restoration of circulating blood volume, which should be accomplished before upper gastrointestinal endoscopy. Although initial resuscitation is usually with isotonic crystalloid solutions, a minimum of 6 units of blood should be typed and crossmatched for most patients with variceal bleeding. Volume status is assessed by central venous pressure measurements, urinary output, and a Swan-Ganz pulmonary artery catheter if necessary. If the prothrombin time is prolonged more than 3 seconds, fresh frozen plasma should be a component of the resuscitation volume. Although moderate hypersplenism is a common accompaniment of portal hypertension, platelet transfusions are necessary only when the platelet count is less than 50,000/mm^3.

Endoscopy to determine the cause of bleeding should be performed as soon as the patient is stabilized. If a bleeding esophageal varix is observed or suspected because of an overlying clot, sclerotherapy or variceal ligation should be performed during the initial endoscopy if the expertise is available. Bleeding from gastric varices or from PHG should be treated initially with pharmacotherapy. Because these lesions are often incompletely controlled by nonoperative means, such patients frequently require either insertion of a TIPS or early surgical intervention.

Because infections are common in patients with bleeding varices, prophylactic antibiotics should be initiated. They have been shown to decrease the infection rate by more than 50%.

Pharmacotherapy

Vasopressin, which is a potent splanchnic vasoconstrictor, has been the most commonly used drug in the acute setting and controls hemorrhage in about half of patients. A meta-analysis of multiple trials has shown vasopressin to be more effective than placebo.[14] Vasopressin is usually administered intravenously as a bolus dose of 20 units over 20 minutes and then as a continuous infusion of 0.2 to 0.4 unit/minute. Because vasopressin also constricts systemic arterioles, it frequently causes hypertension, bradycardia, decreased cardiac output, and coronary vasoconstriction. Therefore, the use of this drug should be confined to the intensive care unit, where the patient can be appropriately monitored. Because of the adverse systemic effects of vasopressin, nitroglycerin should be simultaneously infused at an initial rate of 40 µg/minute, which should then be titrated to achieve blood pressure control. The combination of vasopressin and nitroglycerin may also be more effective than vasopressin alone in controlling variceal hemorrhage.[14]

Randomized trials have shown that somatostatin and its longer-acting analogue octreotide are as efficacious as endoscopic treatment for control of acute variceal bleeding.[14] These agents are also associated with fewer adverse side effects than vasopressin. Because of their ease of administration and effectiveness, these newer drugs may return pharmacotherapy to a more central role in the treatment of acute portal hypertensive bleeding, especially when endoscopic treatment is unlikely to be effective (failed chronic endoscopic therapy, gastric varices, and PHG). Somatostatin is administered as a 250-µg intravenous bolus, followed by a continuous infusion of 250 µg/hour for 2 to 4 days. Octreotide is given as an intravenous bolus of 50 µg followed by an infusion of 25 to 50 µg/hour for a similar length of time. Because of the minimal adverse effects and ease of administration, octreotide is now commonly used as an adjunct to endoscopic therapy.

Balloon Tamponade

The major advantages of variceal tamponade with the Sengstaken-Blakemore tube are immediate cessation of bleeding in more than 85% of patients and widespread availability of this device, including small community hospitals (Fig. 51-4). Significant disadvantages of balloon tamponade are frequent recurrent hemorrhage in up to 50% of patients after balloon deflation, considerable discomfort for the patient, and a high incidence of serious complications when the device is used by inexperienced personnel. The potentially lethal complications of esophageal perforation secondary to intraesophageal inflation of the gastric balloon, ischemic necrosis of the esophagus secondary to overinflation of the esophageal balloon, and aspiration can be avoided by using balloon tamponade only in an intensive care unit and adhering to a strict protocol. Controlled trials have demonstrated that balloon tamponade is as effective as pharmacotherapy and endoscopic therapy in controlling acute variceal bleeding.

Because of the effectiveness of endoscopic treatment and pharmacotherapy for acute variceal bleeding, balloon tamponade is infrequently required. It may be life-saving, however, when exsanguinating hemorrhage prevents acute endoscopic treatment and in patients in whom sclerotherapy has failed and who do not respond to pharmacotherapy. Because balloon deflation is followed by a high rebleeding rate, definitive treatment, such as endoscopic therapy, TIPS, or operation, should be planned for most patients in whom the Sengstaken-Blakemore tube is used.

Endoscopic Treatment

Endoscopic treatment (variceal sclerosis or ligation) is the most commonly used therapy for both management of the acute bleeding episode and prevention of recurrent hemorrhage. In the acute setting, sclerotherapy and band ligation have been shown to be equally efficacious. Both techniques require a skilled endoscopist and stop bleeding in 80% to 90% of patients.[14,15]

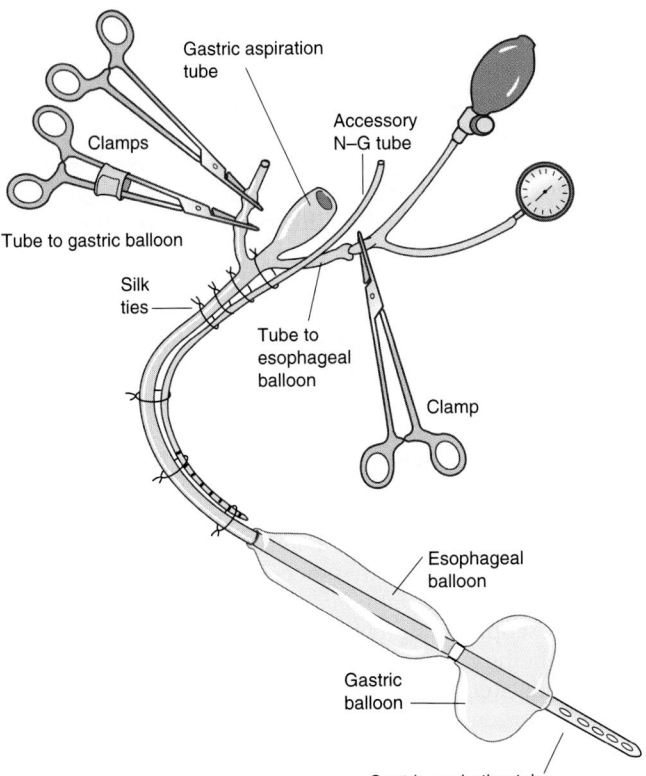

FIGURE 51-4. The modified Sengstaken-Blakemore tube. Note the accessory nasogastric (N-G) tube for suctioning of secretions above the esophageal balloon and the two clamps, one secured with tape, to prevent inadvertent decompression of the gastric balloon. (From Rikkers LF: Portal hypertension. *In* Goldsmith H [ed]: Practice of Surgery. Philadelphia, Harper & Row, 1981, pp 1-37.)

Both intravariceal and paravariceal techniques of sclerosant injection are used, and often these two techniques are purposefully or inadvertently combined (Fig. 51-5). The most commonly used sclerosants in the United States are sodium morrhuate and sodium tetradecyl sulfate.

When experienced personnel are available, the initial sclerotherapy injections can often be done during the endoscopy at which diagnosis of variceal bleeding is made. Each varix is usually injected with 1 to 2 mL of sclerosant just above the esophagogastric junction and 5 cm proximal to it. Alternatively, each varix can be ligated with a rubber band, as shown in Figure 51-6. A subsequent treatment session is planned for 4 to 6 days later. Additional endoscopic treatments depend on the effectiveness of the initial treatments in controlling bleeding and on whether endoscopic therapy has been selected as definitive treatment for that patient.

Minor complications of sclerotherapy, including retrosternal chest pain, esophageal ulceration, and fever, occur commonly. More serious complications, which account for the 1% to 3% mortality rate of this procedure, are esophageal perforation, worsening of variceal hemorrhage, and aspiration pneumonitis. Failure of endoscopic treatment should be declared when two sessions fail to control hemorrhage. Unless urgent surgery is performed in such patients, the mortality rate exceeds 60%.

Transjugular Intrahepatic Portosystemic Shunt

TIPS is a technique that accomplishes portal decompression without an operation. Because of the complexity of the procedure, an experienced interventional radiologist is required. Access is gained to a major intrahepatic portal

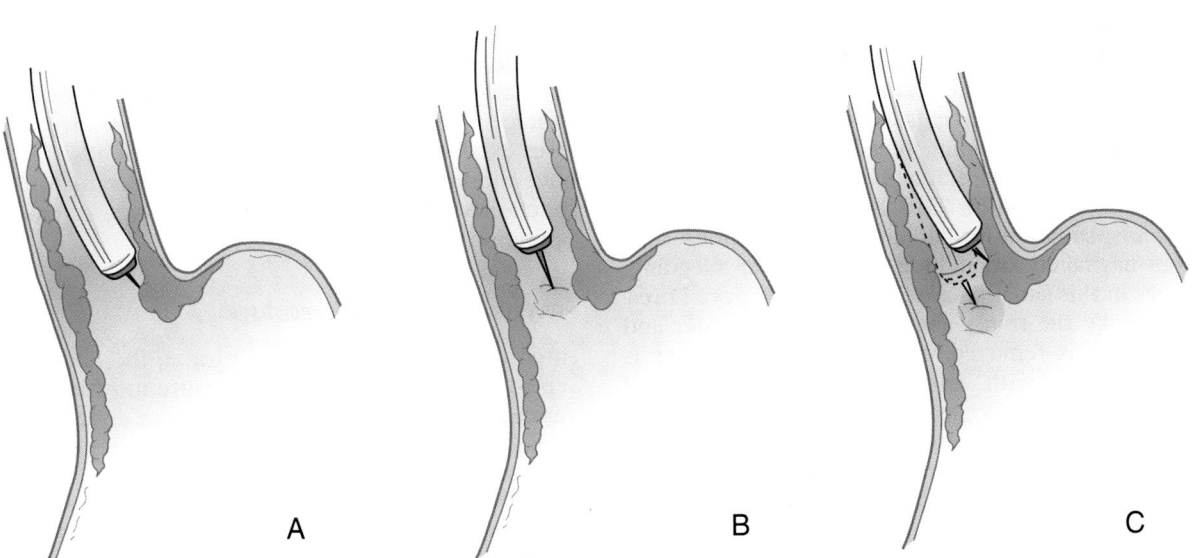

FIGURE 51-5. Techniques of endoscopic sclerotherapy. A flexible endoscope is used for intravariceal injection *(A)*, paravariceal (submucosal) injection *(B)*, and combined paravariceal and intravariceal injection *(C)*. (*A* to *C*, Modified from Terblanche J, Burroughs AK, Hobbs EF: Controversies in the management of bleeding esophageal varices. N Engl J Med 320:1393-1398, 1989.)

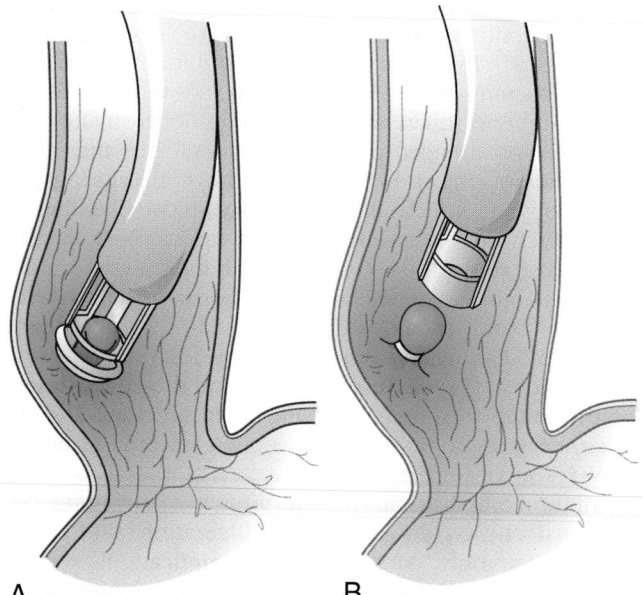

FIGURE 51-6. Endoscopic ligation of esophageal varices. *A,* The varix is drawn into the ligator by suction. *B,* An O ring is applied. (*A* and *B,* From Turcotte JG, Roger SE, Eckhauser FE: Portal hypertension. *In* Greenfield LJ, Mulholland MW, Oldham KT [eds]: Surgery: Scientific Principles and Practice. Philadelphia, JB Lippincott, 1993, p 899.)

venous branch through puncture through a hepatic vein. A parenchymal tract between hepatic and portal veins is then created with a balloon catheter, and a 10-mm expandable metal stent is inserted, thereby creating the shunt (Fig. 51-7).

In large series, the success rate of TIPS has been more than 95%, but experience with this technique is limited in acutely bleeding patients, who generally make up only a small fraction of patients receiving TIPS.[16] At the present time, TIPS should not be recommended as initial therapy for acute variceal hemorrhage but should be used only after less invasive treatments, such as endoscopic therapy and pharmacotherapy, have failed to control bleeding. TIPS is effective in stopping bleeding in this setting.[17] Mortality is related to the status of hepatic function.

One clear indication for TIPS is as a short-term bridge to liver transplantation for patients in whom endoscopic treatment has failed. In addition to controlling bleeding, advantages in this situation are that the lower portal pressure may make the transplantation operation easier and that the shunt is removed when the recipient liver is excised. Patients with advanced hepatic functional decompensation (Child's class C), even those who are not transplantation candidates, may be better served by TIPS than by an emergency operation when less invasive approaches fail to control bleeding.

Hemodynamic studies suggest that TIPS is a nonselective shunt, and several investigations have demonstrated a similar frequency of encephalopathy after TIPS as has been previously reported after nonselective shunts. Another disadvantage of the procedure is that shunt stenosis or occlusion develops in as many as half of patients within 1 year of TIPS insertion. This situation can often be remedied by repeated angiographic intervention, however.

Absolute contraindications to TIPS include right-sided heart failure and polycystic liver disease. Relative contraindications to the procedure are portal vein thrombosis, hypervascular liver tumors, and encephalopathy, which can be worsened by diversion of portal flow.

Emergency Surgery

Although nonoperative therapies are effective in most patients with acute variceal bleeding, emergency operation should be promptly done when less invasive measures fail to control hemorrhage or are not indicated. The most common situations requiring either urgent or emergency surgery are failure of acute endoscopic treatment, failure of long-term endoscopic therapy, hemorrhage from gastric varices or PHG, and failure of TIPS placement. In most institutions, TIPS has become the preferred treatment for acute variceal bleeding when pharmacotherapy and endoscopic treatment have failed, with operative procedures being reserved for those situations in which TIPS is not indicated or not available. Selection of the appropriate emergency operation should mainly be guided by the experience of the surgeon. Esophageal transection with a stapling device is rapid and relatively simple, but rebleeding rates after this procedure are high, and there is little evidence that operative mortality rates are less than after surgical portal decompression.

A commonly performed shunt operation in the emergency setting is the portacaval shunt because it rapidly and effectively decompresses the portal venous circulation. Impressive results have been achieved by Orloff and associates,[18] but not by others, when the emergency portacaval shunt is used as routine therapy for acute variceal bleeding. In patients who are not actively bleeding at the time of surgery and in those in whom bleeding is temporarily controlled by pharmacotherapy or balloon tamponade, a more complex operation, such as the distal splenorenal shunt, may be appropriate. The major disadvantage of emergency surgery is that operative mortality rates exceed 25% in most reported series. Early postoperative mortality is usually related to the status of hepatic functional reserve rather than to the type of emergency operation selected.

Prevention of Recurrent Hemorrhage

After a patient has bled from varices, the likelihood of a repeat episode exceeds 70%. Because most patients with variceal hemorrhage have chronic liver disease, the challenge of long-term management is both prevention of recurrent bleeding and maintenance of satisfactory hepatic function. Options available for definitive treatment include pharmacotherapy, chronic endoscopic treatment, TIPS, three hemodynamic types of shunt operations (nonselective, selective, and partial), a variety of nonshunt procedures, and hepatic transplantation. The most effective treatment regimen usually uses two or more of these therapies in sequence. In most institutions, initial treat-

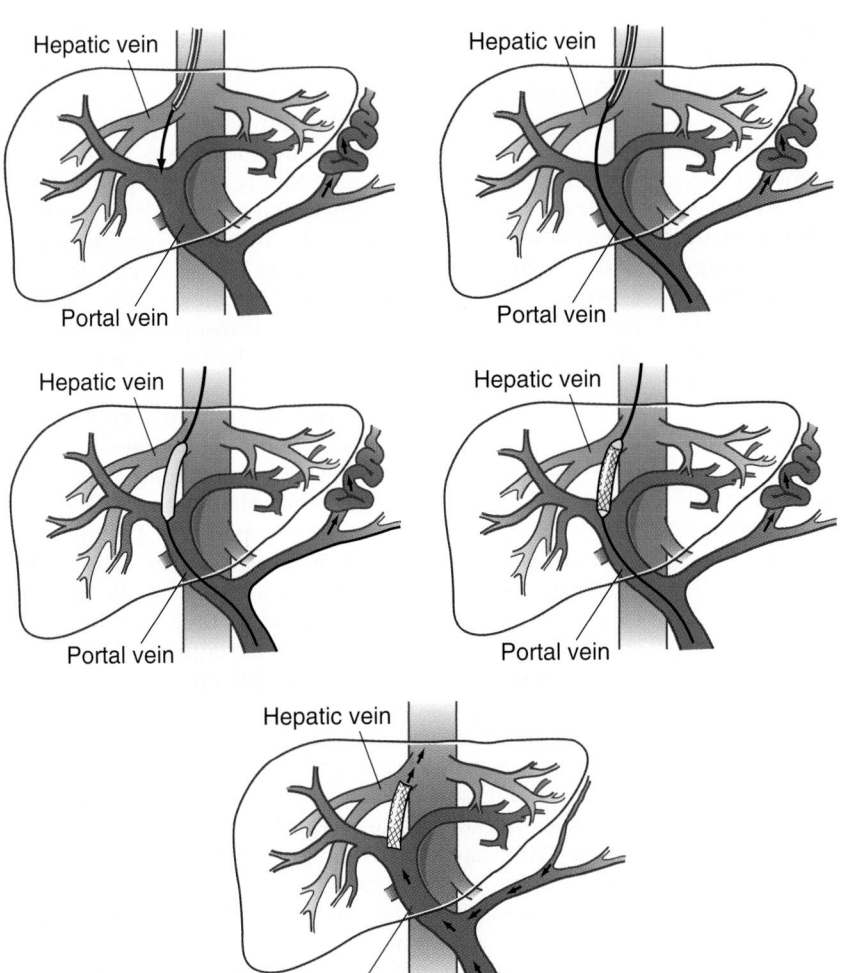

FIGURE 51-7. Transjugular intrahepatic portosystemic shunt. A needle is advanced from a hepatic vein to a major portal vein branch *(top left)* and a guide wire is placed *(top right)*. A hepatic parenchymal tract is created by balloon dilation *(middle left)*, and an expandable metal stent is placed *(middle right)*, thereby creating the shunt *(bottom)*. (From Zemel G, Katzen BT, Becker GJ, et al: Percutaneous transjugular portosystemic shunt. JAMA 266:390, 1991.)

ment consists of pharmacotherapy or endoscopic therapy with portal decompression by means of TIPS or an operative shunt reserved for failures of first-line treatment. Hepatic transplantation is used for patients with end-stage liver disease.

Pharmacotherapy

Pharmacotherapy for the prevention of recurrent variceal bleeding was introduced in 1984 by Lebrec and colleagues,[19] who reported that a dose of propranolol sufficient to decrease the heart rate by 25% resulted in a decreased frequency of recurrent hemorrhage and prolongation of survival in good-risk patients with alcoholic cirrhosis. The objective of pharmacotherapy is to reduce the HVWP below 12 mm Hg, a level at which variceal bleeding does not occur. Invasive hemodynamic monitoring of patients taking propranolol has demonstrated minimal or no reduction of HVWP in many patients and no correlation between decrease in portal pressure and reduction in pulse rate, which has been the parameter used in most studies to assess therapeutic effect. Thus, two obstacles to effective treatment with drugs are variability of response to the drug and lack of an easily measured hemodynamic index to monitor therapy.

A meta-analysis of 11 controlled trials of nonselective β-adrenergic blockade has shown that this treatment significantly decreases the likelihood of recurrent hemorrhage and demonstrates a trend toward decreased mortality.[14] The combination of a β blocker and a long-acting nitrate (isosorbide 5-mononitrate) has been shown to be more effective than sclerotherapy and variceal ligation.[20,21] Combination therapy is probably more effective than β blockade alone. Long-term pharmacotherapy should be used only in compliant patients who are observed closely by their physicians. Although an attractive approach because of its noninvasiveness, pharmacotherapy, like endoscopic therapy, is associated with a high incidence of rebleeding.

Endoscopic Therapy

Since the late 1970s, chronic endoscopic therapy has become the most common treatment for prevention of recurrent variceal hemorrhage. The increasing popularity of endoscopic treatment can be attributed to several factors: (1) several gastroenterologists and surgeons have expressed disenchantment with shunt surgery, (2) endoscopic therapy is less invasive than surgery, (3) there are no adverse hemodynamic effects of endoscopic therapy,

(4) endoscopic treatment can be administered by gastroenterologists to whom most patients are initially referred, and (5) several controlled trials have confirmed its therapeutic efficacy.[14]

The objective of chronic endoscopic therapy is to eradicate esophageal varices (see Figs. 51-5 and 51-6). Although the timing of repeat sessions varies from series to series, variceal eradication is usually successful in about two thirds of patients. After eradication is achieved, diagnostic endoscopy should be performed at 6-month to 1-year intervals because varices do recur and can bleed. Some investigators have noted an increased frequency of bleeding from gastric varices and PHG after eradication of esophageal varices.

Several controlled trials and a meta-analysis comparing endoscopic sclerotherapy to variceal ligation have shown a significant advantage to the latter technique.[22] Complications are less frequent after variceal ligation, and fewer treatment sessions are required to eradicate varices (see Fig. 51-6). Additionally, rebleeding and mortality rates appear to be lower following variceal ligation.

Several controlled trials comparing chronic endoscopic therapy to conventional medical management have been completed.[14] Although fewer patients receiving endoscopic treatment than medical treatment experienced rebleeding in all of the investigations, recurrent bleeding still occurred in about half of endoscopic therapy patients. Rebleeding is most frequent during the initial year, and the rebleeding rate decreases by about 15% per year thereafter. Although a single episode of recurrent hemorrhage does not signify failure of therapy, uncontrolled hemorrhage, multiple major episodes of rebleeding, and hemorrhage from gastric varices and PHG all require that endoscopic therapy be abandoned and another treatment modality substituted. Endoscopic treatment failure secondary to rebleeding occurs in as many as one third of patients.[23,24] Thus, chronic endoscopic therapy is a rational initial treatment for many patients who bleed from esophageal varices, but subsequent treatment with TIPS, a shunt procedure, a nonshunt operation, or hepatic transplantation should be anticipated for a significant percentage of patients. Because of its relatively high failure rate, a course of chronic endoscopic therapy should not be undertaken for noncompliant patients and those living a long distance from advanced medical care.[24]

Transjugular Intrahepatic Portosystemic Shunt

TIPS is being increasingly used as a definitive treatment for patients who bleed from portal hypertension (see Fig. 51-7). A major limitation of TIPS, however, is a high incidence (up to 50%) of shunt stenosis or shunt thrombosis within the first year. Shunt stenosis, which is usually secondary to neointimal hyperplasia, is more common than thrombosis and can often be resolved by balloon dilation of the TIPS or, in some cases, by placement of a second shunt. Total shunt occlusion occurs in 10% to 15% of patients. Both shunt stenosis and shunt thrombosis are often followed by recurrent portal hypertensive bleeding. Except for prosthetic interposition shunts, a surgically created shunt rarely fails in the late postoperative interval.

Until TIPS technology improves, an operative shunt is probably preferable in patients who require long-term portal decompression.

Angiographic and Doppler ultrasound studies suggest that TIPS, when it effectively decompresses varices, is a nonselective shunt and completely diverts portal flow. Clinical evidence of the nonselectivity of TIPS is its effectiveness in resolving medically intractable ascites and a fairly high frequency of post-TIPS encephalopathy (~30%).[25,26] Thus far, all clinical studies regarding TIPS have a relatively brief period of follow-up. It is likely that the frequency of encephalopathy will increase as the interval of follow-up lengthens.

TIPS has been compared to chronic endoscopic therapy in 11 randomized controlled trials.[27] Fewer patients rebled after TIPS (19%) than following endoscopic treatment (47%), but encephalopathy was significantly more common in TIPS patients (34%). TIPS dysfunction developed in 50% of patients. The major advantage of TIPS is that it is nonoperative. Because of this, it would appear to be the ideal therapy when only short-term portal decompression is required. Thus, liver transplantation candidates who fail endoscopic and/or pharmacotherapy are well suited for TIPS followed by transplantation when a donor organ becomes available. The patient is protected from bleeding in the interim, and the transplantation procedure may also be facilitated by the lower portal pressure. Another group of patients in whom TIPS may be advantageous includes those with advanced hepatic functional decompensation who are unlikely to survive long enough for the TIPS to malfunction. Because it functions as a side-to-side portosystemic shunt, TIPS is also effective in the treatment of medically intractable ascites.

Portosystemic Shunts

Portosystemic shunts are clearly the most effective means of preventing recurrent hemorrhage in patients with portal hypertension. These procedures are effective because they all, to some degree, decompress the portal venous system by shunting portal flow into the low-pressure systemic venous system. Diversion of portal blood, however, that contains hepatotropic hormones, nutrients, and cerebral toxins is also responsible for the adverse consequences of shunt operations, namely portosystemic encephalopathy and accelerated hepatic failure. Depending on whether they completely decompress, compartmentalize, or partially decompress the portal venous circulation, portosystemic shunts can be classified as nonselective, selective, or partial. In addition to variceal decompression, the goal of selective and partial portosystemic shunts is preservation of hepatic portal perfusion, thereby preventing or minimizing the adverse consequences of these procedures.

Nonselective Shunts. Commonly used varieties of nonselective shunts, all of which completely divert portal flow, include the end-to-side portacaval shunt (Eck's fistula), the side-to-side portacaval shunt, large-diameter interposition shunts, and the conventional splenorenal shunt (Fig. 51-8). The end-to-side portacaval shunt is the prototype of

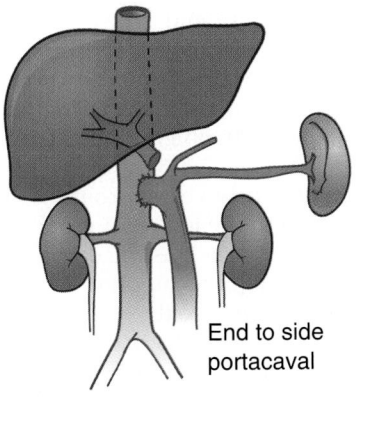

End to side
portacaval

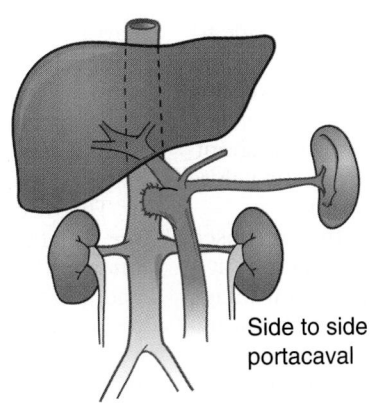

Side to side
portacaval

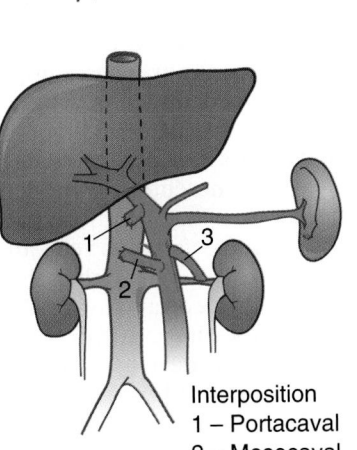

Interposition
1 – Portacaval
2 – Mesocaval
3 – Mesorenal

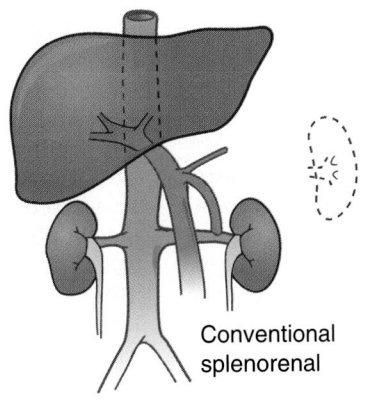

Conventional
splenorenal

FIGURE 51-8.   Nonselective shunts completely divert portal blood flow away from the liver. (From Rikkers LF: Portal hypertension. *In* Moody FG, et al [eds]: Surgical Treatment of Digestive Disease. Chicago, Year Book Medical, 1986, pp 409-424.)

nonselective shunts and is the only shunt procedure that has been compared to conventional medical management in randomized, controlled trials.[14,28] Figure 51-9 combines survival data from the four controlled investigations of the therapeutic portacaval shunt (performed in patients with prior variceal hemorrhage). The most common causes of death in medically treated and shunted patients were rebleeding and accelerated hepatic failure, respectively. Although no survival advantage could be demonstrated for shunt patients, all of these studies had a crossover bias in favor of medically treated patients, several of whom received a shunt when they developed intractable recurrent variceal hemorrhage. In addition, nearly all of the trial patients had alcoholic cirrhosis; therefore, these results do not necessarily apply to other causes of portal hypertension. Other important findings of these randomized trials include reliable control of bleeding in shunted patients, variceal rebleeding in more than 70% of medically treated patients, and spontaneous, often severe, encephalopathy in 20% to 40% of shunted patients.

All of the other nonselective shunts in Figure 51-8 maintain continuity of the portal vein, thereby connecting the portal and systemic venous systems in a side-to-side fashion. Therefore, these procedures decompress both the splanchnic venous circulation and the intrahepatic sinusoidal network. Because the liver and intestines are

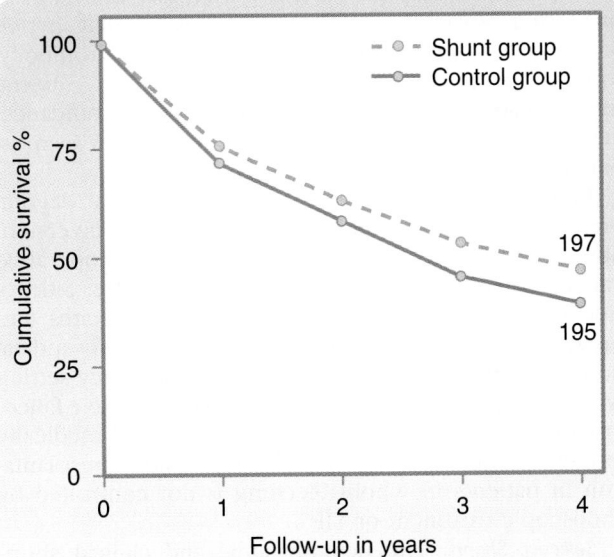

FIGURE 51-9.   Cumulative survival data from four controlled trials of the portacaval shunt versus conventional medical management. (From Boyer TD: Portal hypertension and its complications: Bleeding esophageal varices, ascites, and spontaneous bacterial peritonitis. *In* Zakim D, Boyer TD [eds]: Hepatology: A Textbook of Liver Disease. Philadelphia, WB Saunders, 1982, pp 464-499.)

both important contributors to ascites formation, side-to-side portosystemic shunts are the most effective shunt procedures for relieving ascites as well as preventing recurrent variceal bleeding. Because they completely divert portal flow like the end-to-side portacaval shunt, however, side-to-side shunts also accelerate hepatic failure and lead to frequent postshunt encephalopathy.

Synthetic grafts or autogenous vein may be interposed between the portal and systemic venous circulations at a variety of locations (see Fig. 51-8). A major disadvantage of prosthetic interposition shunts is a high graft thrombosis rate that approaches 35% during the late postoperative interval. This problem can be avoided by using autogenous vein (internal jugular vein) rather than a prosthetic graft. On the other hand, advantages of these shunts are that they are relatively easy to construct; the hepatic hilum is avoided, thereby making subsequent liver transplantation less complicated; and they can be easily occluded if intractable postshunt encephalopathy develops.

The conventional splenorenal shunt consists of anastomosis of the proximal splenic vein to the renal vein. Splenectomy is also done. Because the smaller proximal rather than the larger distal end of the splenic vein is used, shunt thrombosis is more common after this procedure than after the distal splenorenal shunt. Although early series noted that postshunt encephalopathy was less common after the conventional splenorenal shunt than after the portacaval shunt, subsequent analyses have suggested that this low frequency of encephalopathy was probably a result of restoration of hepatic portal perfusion after shunt thrombosis developed in many patients. A conventional splenorenal shunt that is of sufficient caliber to remain patent gradually dilates and eventually causes complete portal decompression and portal flow diversion. A purported advantage of the procedure is that hypersplenism is eliminated by splenectomy. The thrombocytopenia and leukopenia that accompany portal hypertension, however, are rarely of clinical significance, making splenectomy an unnecessary procedure in most patients.

In summary, nonselective shunts effectively decompress varices. Because of complete portal flow diversion, however, they are complicated by frequent postoperative encephalopathy and accelerated hepatic failure. Side-to-side nonselective shunts effectively relieve ascites and prevent variceal hemorrhage. Presently, the only indications for nonselective shunts are in the emergency setting when nonoperative means to control bleeding have failed, in patients with both variceal hemorrhage and medically intractable ascites, and as a bridge to hepatic transplantation in patients in whom bleeding is not controlled by endoscopic treatment or TIPS.

Selective Shunts. The hemodynamic and clinical shortcomings of nonselective shunts stimulated development of the concept of selective variceal decompression. In 1967, Warren and colleagues introduced the distal splenorenal shunt; and in the following year, Inokuchi and associates[29] reported their initial results with the left gastric vena caval shunt. The latter procedure consists of interposition of a vein graft between the left gastric (coronary) vein and the inferior vena cava and, thus, directly and selectively decompresses esophagogastric varices. Only a few patients with portal hypertension, however, have appropriate anatomy for this operation; experience with it has been limited to Japan, and no controlled trials have been conducted.

The distal splenorenal shunt consists of anastomosis of the distal end of the splenic vein to the left renal vein and interruption of all collateral vessels, such as the coronary and gastroepiploic veins, connecting the superior mesenteric and gastrosplenic components of the splanchnic venous circulation (Fig. 51-10). This results in separation of the portal venous circulation into a decompressed gastrosplenic venous circuit and a high-pressure superior mesenteric venous system that continues to perfuse the liver. Although the procedure is technically demanding, it can be mastered by most well-trained surgeons who are knowledgeable in the principles of vascular surgery.

Not all patients are candidates for the distal splenorenal shunt. Because sinusoidal and mesenteric hypertension is maintained and important lymphatic pathways are transected during dissection of the left renal vein, the distal splenorenal shunt tends to aggravate rather than relieve ascites. Thus, patients with medically intractable ascites should not undergo this procedure. However, the larger population of patients who develop transient ascites after resuscitation from a variceal hemorrhage are candidates for a selective shunt. Another contraindication to a distal splenorenal shunt is prior splenectomy. A splenic vein diameter of less than 7 mm is a relative contraindication to the procedure because the incidence of shunt thrombosis is high when using a small-diameter vein.

Although selective variceal decompression is a sound physiologic concept, the distal splenorenal shunt remains

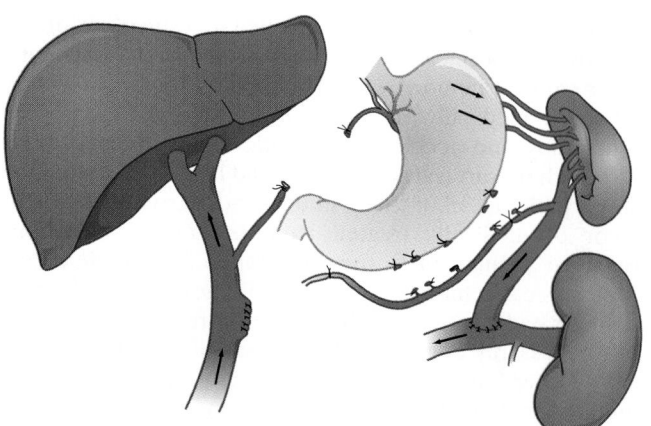

FIGURE 51-10. The distal splenorenal shunt provides selective variceal decompression through the short gastric veins, spleen, and splenic vein to the left renal vein. Hepatic portal perfusion is maintained by interrupting the umbilical vein, coronary vein, gastroepiploic vein, and any other prominent collaterals. (From Salam AA: Distal splenorenal shunts: Hemodynamics of total versus selective shunting. *In* Baker RJ, Fischer JE [eds]: Mastery of Surgery, 4th ed. Philadelphia, Lippincott Williams & Wilkins, 2001, pp 1357-1366.)

controversial after an extensive clinical experience spanning more than 35 years.[30,31] The key questions regarding this procedure are, How effective is it in preserving hepatic portal perfusion? Is it superior to nonselective shunts with respect to duration or quality of survival?

Although the distal splenorenal shunt results in portal flow preservation in more than 85% of patients during the early postoperative interval, the high-pressure mesenteric venous system gradually collateralizes to the low-pressure shunt, resulting in loss of portal flow in about half of patients by 1 year. The degree and duration of portal flow preservation depend on both the cause of portal hypertension and the technical details of the operation (extent to which mesenteric and gastrosplenic venous circulations are separated). Henderson and coworkers[32] have shown that portal flow is maintained in most patients with nonalcoholic cirrhosis and noncirrhotic portal hypertension (e.g., portal vein thrombosis). In contrast, portal flow rapidly collateralizes to the shunt in patients with alcoholic cirrhosis.

Modification of the distal splenorenal shunt by purposeful or inadvertent omission of coronary vein ligation results in early loss of portal flow. Even when all major collateral vessels are interrupted, portal flow may be gradually diverted through a pancreatic collateral network (pancreatic siphon). This pathway can be discouraged by dissecting the full length of the splenic vein from the pancreas (splenopancreatic disconnection), which results in better preservation of hepatic portal perfusion, especially in patients with alcoholic cirrhosis. However, this extension of the procedure makes it technically more challenging, which may be a significant disadvantage in an era when fewer shunts are being done because of increased use of endoscopic therapy, TIPS, and hepatic transplantation.

Six of the seven controlled comparisons of the distal splenorenal shunt with nonselective shunts have included predominantly alcoholic cirrhotic patients.[14,31] None of these trials has demonstrated an advantage to either procedure with respect to long-term survival. Three of the studies have found a lower frequency of encephalopathy after the distal splenorenal shunt, whereas the other trials have shown no difference in the incidence of this postoperative complication. In contrast to survival, encephalopathy is a subjective endpoint that was assessed with a variety of methods in the different trials. Another important endpoint in comparing treatments for variceal hemorrhage is the effectiveness with which recurrent bleeding is prevented. In nearly all uncontrolled and controlled series of the distal splenorenal shunt, this procedure has been equivalent to nonselective shunts in preventing recurrent hemorrhage.[31] Mainly because of these inconsistent results of the controlled trials, there is no consensus as to which shunting procedure is superior in patients with alcoholic cirrhosis. Because the quality of life (encephalopathy rate) was significantly better in the distal splenorenal shunt group in three of the trials, however, there appears to be an advantage to selective variceal decompression even in this population.[33]

Considerably fewer data are available regarding selective shunting in nonalcoholic cirrhosis and in noncirrhotic portal hypertension. Because hepatic portal perfusion after the distal splenorenal shunt is better preserved in these disease categories, one might expect improved results. A single controlled trial in patients with schistosomiasis (presinusoidal portal hypertension) demonstrated a lower frequency of encephalopathy after the distal splenorenal shunt than after a conventional splenorenal shunt (nonselective).[34] The large Emory University series of the distal splenorenal shunt has demonstrated better survival in patients with nonalcoholic cirrhosis than in those with alcoholic cirrhosis.[30] However, this has not been a consistent finding in all centers in which the distal splenorenal shunt is performed.

Several controlled trials have also compared the distal splenorenal shunt with chronic endoscopic therapy.[35] In these investigations, recurrent hemorrhage was more effectively prevented by selective shunting than by sclerotherapy, but hepatic portal perfusion was maintained in a significantly higher fraction of patients undergoing sclerotherapy. Despite this hemodynamic advantage, encephalopathy rates have been similar after both therapies. The two North American trials were dissimilar with respect to the effect of these treatments on long-term survival. Sclerotherapy with surgical rescue for the one third of sclerotherapy failures resulted in significantly better survival than selective shunt alone in one study.[23] In this investigation, 85% of sclerotherapy failures could be salvaged by surgery.

In contrast, a similar investigation conducted in a sparsely populated area (Intermountain West and Plains) showed superior survival after the distal splenorenal shunt.[24] Only 31% of sclerotherapy failures could be salvaged by surgery in this trial. The survival results of these two studies suggest that endoscopic therapy is a rational, initial treatment for patients who bleed from varices if sclerotherapy failure is recognized and such patients promptly undergo surgery or TIPS. However, patients living in remote areas are less likely to be salvaged by shunt surgery when endoscopic treatment fails, and a selective shunt may be preferable initial treatment for such patients.

In a nonrandomized comparison to TIPS, the distal splenorenal shunt had lower rates of recurrent bleeding, encephalopathy, and shunt thrombosis.[36] Ascites was less prevalent after TIPS. A multicenter randomized trial comparing TIPS and the distal splenorenal shunt for the elective treatment of variceal bleeding in good-risk cirrhotic patients is ongoing, but results are not yet available.

Partial Shunts. The objectives of partial and selective shunts are the same: (1) effective decompression of varices, (2) preservation of hepatic portal perfusion, and (3) maintenance of some residual portal hypertension. Initial attempts at partial shunting consisted of small-diameter vein-to-vein anastomoses, but these generally either thrombosed or dilated with time, thereby becoming nonselective shunts.

More recently, a small-diameter interposition portacaval shunt using a polytetrafluoroethylene graft, combined with ligation of the coronary vein and other collateral vessels, has been described (Fig. 51-11). When

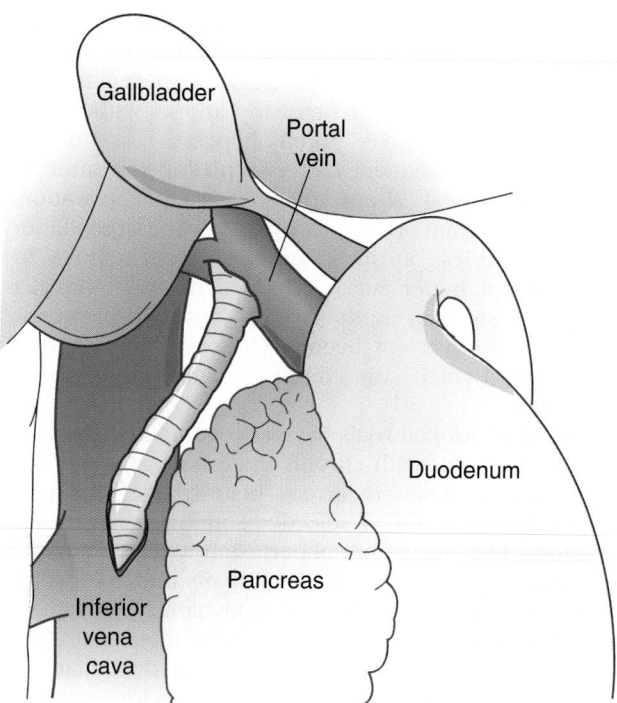

FIGURE 51-11. A small-diameter (8- to 10-mm) interposition portacaval shunt partially decompresses the portal venous system and may preserve hepatic portal perfusion. (From Sarfeh IJ, Rypins EB, Mason GR: A systematic appraisal of portacaval H-graft diameters: Clinical and hemodynamic perspectives. Ann Surg 204:356-363, 1986.)

the prosthetic graft is 10 mm or less in diameter, hepatic portal perfusion is preserved in most patients, at least during the early postoperative interval.[37] Early experience with this small-diameter prosthetic shunt is that fewer than 15% of shunts have thrombosed, and most of these have been successfully opened by interventional radiologic techniques. A prospective, randomized trial of partial (8 mm in diameter) and nonselective (16 mm in diameter) interposition portacaval shunts has shown a lower frequency of encephalopathy after the partial shunt but similar survival after both types of shunts.[38] The number of patients included in this investigation was small, however, and further trials need to be done to confirm this finding. In another controlled trial, the small-diameter interposition shunt was discovered to have a lower overall failure rate than TIPS.[39]

Nonshunt Operations

The objectives of nonshunt procedures are either ablation of varices or, more commonly, extensive interruption of collateral vessels connecting the high-pressure portal venous system with the varices. One exception is splenectomy, which is effective in left-sided portal hypertension caused by splenic vein thrombosis.

The simplest nonshunt operation is transection and reanastomosis of the distal esophagus with a stapling device. This operation, which has generally been used in the emergency setting, is frequently followed by recurrent hemorrhage. The most effective nonshunt operation is extensive esophagogastric devascularization combined with esophageal transection and splenectomy (Fig. 51-12). The Sugiura procedure preserves the coronary and paraesophageal veins to maintain a portosystemic collateral pathway and thus discourage re-formation of varices. In Japan, the results with this operation have been excellent, with rebleeding rates of less than 10%.[40] Extensive devascularization procedures, however, have generally been less successful in North American patients with alcoholic cirrhosis. Long-term follow-up in American series has revealed rebleeding rates of 35% to 55%, which are similar to the endoscopic therapy experience.[41] In many centers, esophagogastric devascularization procedures are mainly used for unshuntable patients with diffuse splanchnic venous thrombosis and for patients with distal splenorenal shunt thrombosis.

Hepatic Transplantation

Liver transplantation is not a treatment for variceal bleeding, per se, but rather needs to be considered for all patients who present with end-stage hepatic failure whether or not it is accompanied by bleeding. Transplantation in patients who have bled secondary to portal hypertension is the only therapy that addresses the underlying liver disease in addition to providing reliable portal decompression. Because of economic factors and a limited supply of donor organs, liver transplantation is not available to all patients. Additionally, transplantation is not indicated for some of the more common causes of variceal bleeding, such as schistosomiasis (normal liver function) and active alcoholism (noncompliance).

There is accumulating evidence that variceal bleeders with well-compensated hepatic functional reserve (Child's classes A and B+) are better served by nontransplantation strategies initially.[42,43] The first-line treatment for such patients should be pharmacologic and endoscopic therapy, with portal decompression by means of an operative shunt or TIPS reserved for those who fail first-line therapy and for circumstances in which pharmacologic or endoscopic treatment would be risky (e.g., patients with gastric varices and those geographically separated from tertiary medical care).

Patients with variceal bleeding who are transplantation candidates include nonalcoholic cirrhotic patients and abstinent alcoholic cirrhotic patients with either limited hepatic functional reserve (Child's classes B and C) or a poor quality of life secondary to their disease (e.g., encephalopathy, fatigue, or bone pain). In these patients, the acute hemorrhage should be treated with endoscopic therapy and the patient's transplantation candidacy should be immediately activated. If sclerotherapy is ineffective, a TIPS should be inserted as a short-term bridge to transplantation.

If a nontransplantation operation (e.g., shunt) is performed initially, these patients should be carefully assessed at 6-month to 1-year intervals and hepatic transplantation considered when other complications of cir-

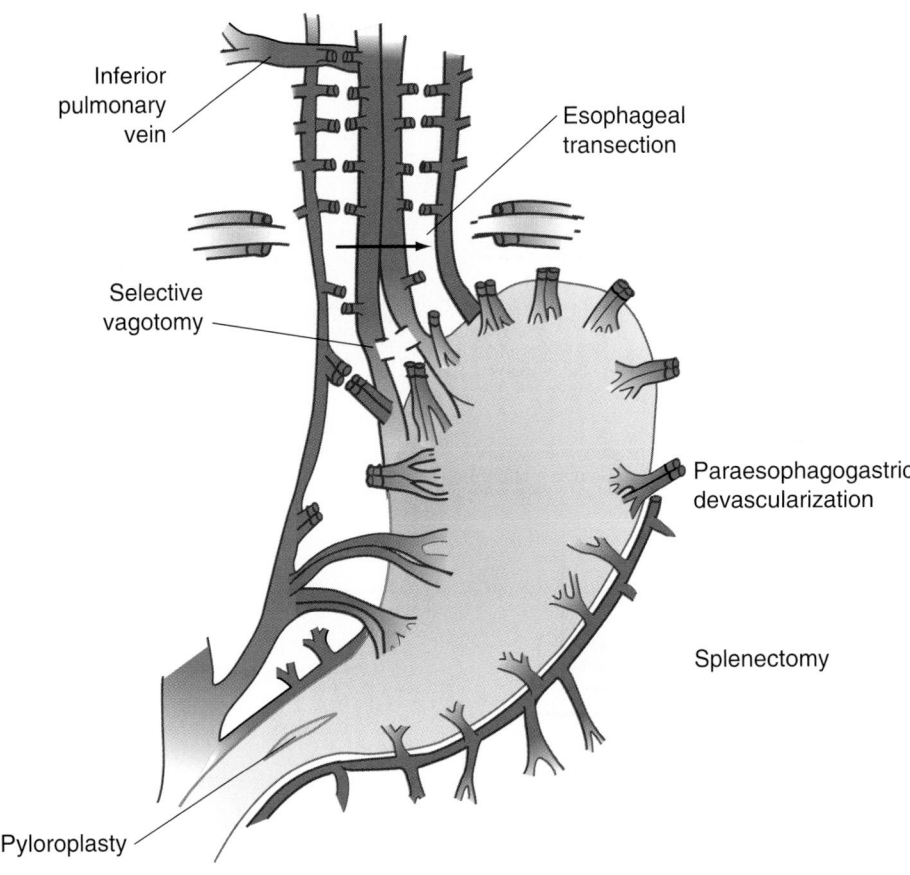

Inferior pulmonary vein

Selective vagotomy

Pyloroplasty

Esophageal transection

Paraesophagogastric devascularization

Splenectomy

FIGURE 51-12. The Sugiura procedure combines esophageal transection, extensive esophagogastric devascularization, and splenectomy. The paraesophageal collateral vessels are preserved to discourage re-formation of varices. (Modified from Sugiura M, Futagawa S: Further evaluation of the Sugiura procedure in the treatment of esophageal varices. Arch Surg 112:1317, 1977.)

rhosis develop or hepatic functional decompensation is evident either clinically or by careful assessment with quantitative tests of liver function.

Overall Treatment Plan

An algorithm for definitive management of variceal hemorrhage is shown in Figure 51-13. Patients are first grouped according to their transplantation candidacy. This decision is based on multiple factors: etiology of portal hypertension, abstinence for alcoholic cirrhotic patients, the presence or absence of other diseases, and physiologic rather than chronologic age. Transplantation candidates with either decompensated hepatic function or a poor quality of life secondary to their liver disease should undergo transplantation as soon as possible. Most future transplantation and nontransplantation candidates should undergo initial endoscopic treatment and/or pharmacotherapy unless they bleed from gastric varices or PHG or live in remote geographic locations and have limited access to emergency tertiary care. Patients who live in remote locations and those who fail endoscopic and drug therapy should receive a selective shunt if they meet the criteria for this operation. Whether TIPS may be just as effective in this setting is presently undergoing investigation. Patients with medically intractable ascites in addition to variceal bleeding are best treated with either

a TIPS or a side-to-side portosystemic shunt. If the TIPS eventually fails, an open side-to-side type shunt can then be constructed if the patient has reasonable hepatic function and is not a transplantation candidate. TIPS is clearly indicated for patients with endoscopic treatment failure who may require transplantation in the near future and for nontransplantation candidates with advanced hepatic functional deterioration. Future transplantation candidates should be carefully monitored so that they undergo transplantation at the appropriate time before they become poor operative risks.

The treatment algorithm for variceal bleeding has changed considerably since the 1970s, during which time endoscopic therapy, liver transplantation, and TIPS have become available to these patients. Nontransplantation operations are now necessary less frequently, the survival results are better because high operative risk patients are managed by other means, and emergency surgery has nearly been eliminated.[44]

Prevention of Initial Variceal Hemorrhage (Prophylactic Therapy)

The rationale for treating patients with varices before they bleed is the high mortality rate associated with the initial hemorrhage. Because only one third of patients with varices eventually bleed, unless potential bleeders

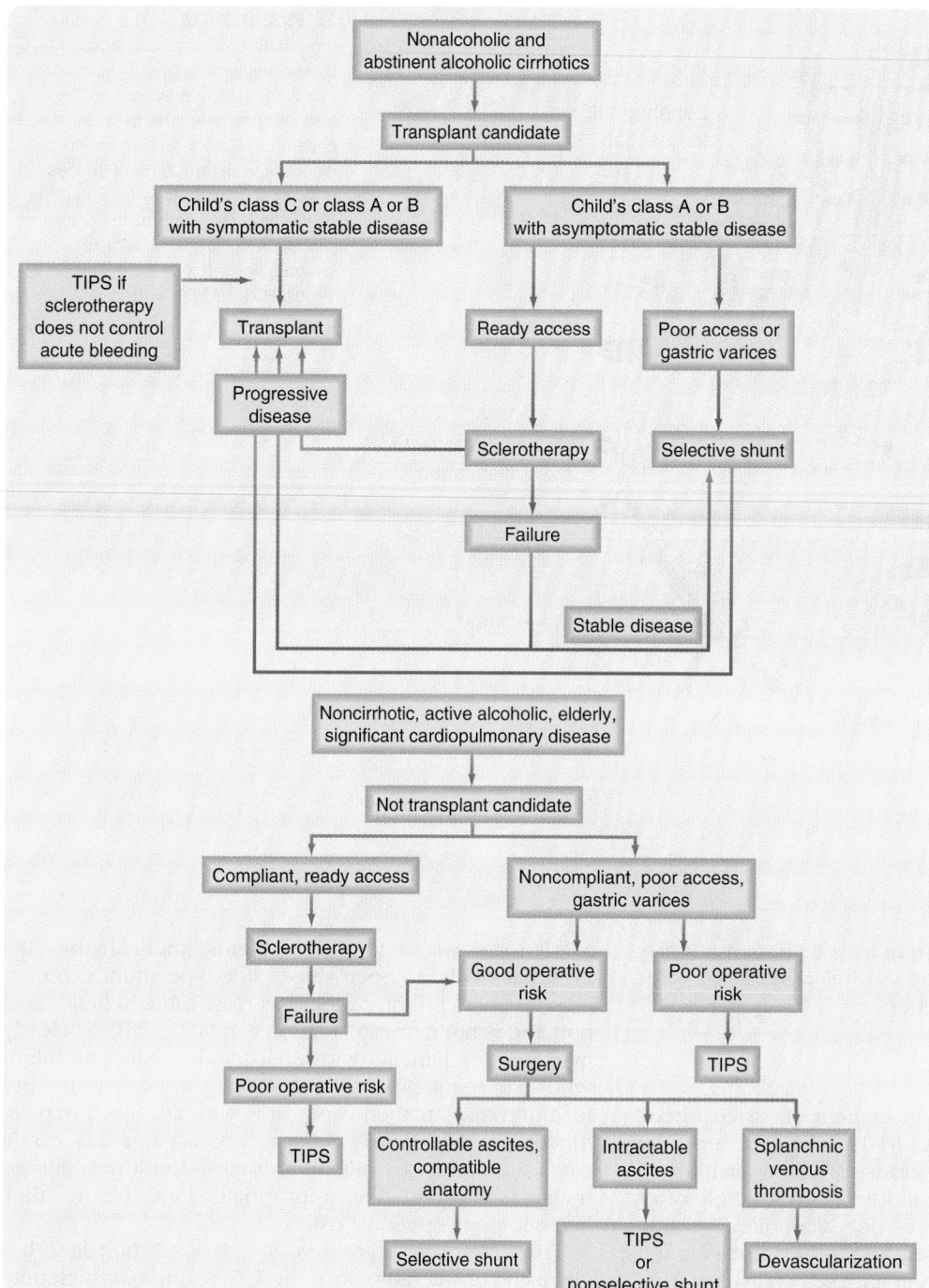

FIGURE 51-13.
Algorithm for definitive therapy of variceal hemorrhage (see text). TIPS, transjugular intrahepatic portosystemic shunt. (Modified from Rikkers LF: Portal hypertension. *In* Levine BA, Copeland E, Howard R, et al [eds]: Current Practice of Surgery, Vol. 3. New York, Churchill Livingstone, 1995.)

are more reliably identified, about two thirds of patients undergoing prophylactic therapy would be treated unnecessarily.

The first trials of prophylaxis for variceal hemorrhage compared the portacaval shunt to conventional medical therapy. In these investigations, survival of shunted patients was actually less than that of medically treated patients because of accelerated hepatic failure secondary to complete portal diversion.[14] In addition, a significant fraction of shunted patients developed postshunt encephalopathy.

The major impetus for reconsideration of prophylactic therapy was the development of relatively noninvasive treatments (endoscopic therapy and pharmacotherapy), which should be associated with less morbidity than major operative procedures, and the development of better methods to identify varices that are likely to bleed.[12] Endoscopic treatment, however, cannot be advocated for prophylaxis because controlled trials have shown no consistent benefit, and some have demonstrated a higher rebleeding rate and a lower survival rate in the sclerotherapy group than in medically treated controls.[14] In contrast, most trials of β blockade as prophylactic therapy have found a reduced incidence of initial variceal hemorrhage in treated patients.[14] In several of these studies, the decreased bleeding rate in the treatment group was statistically significant, and in one study, survival was prolonged in patients receiving β blockade. Because β blockade has been associated with few adverse side effects, it can be recommended for reliable patients with varices that have never bled. Experience with TIPS as a prophylactic procedure is limited.

ASCITES AND THE HEPATORENAL SYNDROME

Ascites is usually an indicator of advanced cirrhosis and is associated with a 1-year survival rate of approximately 50% compared to a 1-year survival rate of greater than 90% for patients with cirrhosis but without ascites.[45] Patients with ascites refractory to medical management, those who develop spontaneous bacterial peritonitis, and those who evolve to the hepatorenal syndrome have a particularly poor prognosis.

Portal hypertensive ascites is initiated by altered hepatic and splanchnic hemodynamics, which cause transudation of fluid into the interstitial space. When the rate of interstitial fluid formation exceeds the lymph drainage capacity, ascites accumulates. This pathophysiologic process results in an intravascular volume deficit, which initiates compensatory mechanisms such as aldosterone secretion, to restore plasma volume. Both the liver and intestine are important sites of ascites formation, and clinically significant ascites is rare in patients with extrahepatic portal hypertension. The hypoalbuminemia that often accompanies advanced chronic liver disease may also contribute to ascites formation.

Since avid sodium retention by the kidneys is one of the key mechanisms in the development of ascites, a central goal of treatment is to achieve a negative sodium balance. A small percentage of patients with ascites can be effectively treated by dietary salt restriction and bed rest alone. More commonly, diuretic therapy is required and will resolve this complication of portal hypertension in greater than 90% of patients. Since secondary hyperaldosteronism is a key pathogenetic mechanism in the formation of ascites, a rational first-line diuretic is spironolactone. A combination of salt restriction (2 g/day) and spironolactone in a dose of 100 to 400 mg/day results in effective diuresis in about two thirds of patients. Clinical trials have shown that spironolactone alone is just as effective as the combination of spironolactone and furosemide.[46] However, diuretic combination therapy should be used in those patients who fail to diurese with spironolactone alone. Diuretic therapy can be associated with significant complications since it can lead to a reduction in intravascular volume and, potentially, renal dysfunction. Serum electrolytes, blood urea nitrogen, and creatinine values should be followed closely in patients on diuretics, which should be discontinued if azotemia develops.

As a general guideline, patients with new-onset ascites that is barely detectable on physical examination should be placed on salt restriction alone. However, patients with more advanced or tense ascites usually require the combination of sodium restriction and diuretic therapy. The preferred initial spironolactone dose is 100 mg/day, and this can be advanced to a maximum dose of 400 mg/day until effective diuresis is achieved. If treatment with spironolactone alone is ineffective or results in hyperkalemia, furosemide in an initial dose of 40 mg/day should be added to the regimen. During diuresis, body weight should be carefully monitored and not allowed to decrease at a rate of more than 1 lb/day in patients with ascites alone and no peripheral edema. More aggressive diuresis usually results in contraction of the intravascular volume and azotemia.

From 5% to 10% of patients with ascites are refractory to medical treatment and require more invasive measures. The two mainstays of therapy in this group of patients are large-volume paracentesis combined with intravenous albumin administration and TIPS. Because it can be done in the outpatient setting and is less invasive, the generally preferred initial treatment for patients with ascites refractory to medical treatment is large-volume paracentesis combined with intravenous albumin infusion in a dose of 6 to 8 g/L of ascites removed.[47] TIPS, which is more effective for the long-term control of ascites than large-volume paracentesis, should be used in patients who require frequent paracentesis for management of their ascites. After large-volume paracentesis, ascites is less likely to recur in patients treated with spironolactone than in those not on a diuretic. Controlled trials have shown either complete or partial resolution of ascites after placement of TIPS in more than 80% of patients with medically intractable ascites.[48] As in patients treated with TIPS for variceal bleeding, major disadvantages of this therapy are a fairly high rate of encephalopathy and eventual TIPS dysfunction in the majority of patients.

Although initially effective in the majority of patients, a surgically placed peritoneovenous shunt is seldom used in the management of medically refractory ascites because of its associated complications such as occlusion, infection, and disseminated intravascular coagulation. Additionally, controlled trials have shown that this relatively simple operation, which can be done under local anesthesia, is no more effective than medical management in prolonging patient survival. A surgically constructed side-to-side portal systemic shunt is also effective in relieving ascites. However, because of the associated morbidity and mortality, these operations are infrequently done and should be used only in ascitic patients who have bled from esophagogastric varices and in whom TIPS is either not indicated or has failed.

Cirrhotic patients with ascites who develop fever, abdominal tenderness, or worsening hepatic and/or renal function should undergo a diagnostic paracentesis to rule out spontaneous bacterial peritonitis. This complication of ascites is associated with a mortality rate of approximately 25% per episode. The diagnosis is made with an ascitic fluid polymorphonuclear leukocyte count of greater than 250/mm^3 or a positive ascites culture. The most common organisms causing spontaneous bacterial peritonitis are aerobic gram-negative ones, which likely come from the bowel via bacterial translocation. Before culture results are available, antibiotic therapy should be initiated when spontaneous bacterial peritonitis is suspected. A 5- to 10-day course of either cefotaxime or a combination of amoxicillin and clavulanic acid have been shown to be effective treatment.[49] Since spontaneous bacterial peritonitis recurs in more than 70% of patients, prophylactic therapy with oral norfloxacin should be initiated as soon as intravenous therapy is completed and continued until ascites is resolved.[50]

Another life-threatening complication of portal hypertension is the hepatorenal syndrome that develops almost exclusively in patients with tense ascites and declining hepatic function. When renal failure is rapidly progressive, the prognosis is poor, with a median survival of approximately 2 weeks. In other patients, renal failure develops more gradually and the prognosis is somewhat better. The only reliable treatment for the hepatorenal syndrome is liver transplantation. Because the renal failure is functional rather than structural, once hepatic function is improved and portal hypertension is relieved, the kidneys recover. A few small series have suggested that renal function may improve in patients with the hepatorenal syndrome after insertion of a TIPS. However, in this setting, TIPS should be regarded as a bridge to liver transplantation in the near future.

ENCEPHALOPATHY

Portal systemic encephalopathy is a psychoneurologic syndrome that may have a variety of manifestations, including alterations in the level of consciousness, intellectual deterioration, personality changes, and neurologic findings such as the flapping tremor, asterixis. Although the pathogenesis of these alterations is unclear, they occur in patients with either significant hepatocellular dysfunction or portal systemic shunting. The shunts may be congenital, spontaneously form secondary to portal hypertension, or surgically or radiologically (TIPS) constructed. The most common setting for the development of encephalopathy is in patients with cirrhosis who undergo a procedural shunt. Nonselective shunts such as the operative portacaval shunt and TIPS are frequently followed by encephalopathy (20% to 40% of patients), whereas this complication is less common in patients who receive a selective shunt, such as the distal splenorenal shunt.

Most theories of the pathogenesis of encephalopathy are based on circulating cerebral toxins that are intestinally absorbed and bypass the liver by means of shunts or fail to be inactivated by the liver's decreased metabolic capacity. Purported cerebral toxins include ammonia, mercaptans, and γ-aminobutyric acid. The false neurotransmitter hypothesis, based on the high ratio of aromatic to branched chain amino acids present in the blood of patients with chronic liver disease, has also been proposed to explain the psychoneurologic disturbances observed. Almost certainly the syndrome is multifactorial, with the bulk of evidence supporting ammonia as the main cerebral toxin. However, the severity of encephalopathy does not correlate well with blood ammonia levels.

Encephalopathy develops spontaneously in less than 10% of patients, and this form of the syndrome is almost entirely confined to those patients who undergo a procedural shunt. More commonly, one or more of the following precipitating factors induce the syndrome: gastrointestinal hemorrhage, excessive diuresis, azotemia, constipation, sedatives, infection, and excess dietary protein. In fact, when encephalopathy develops in a patient with cirrhosis who is otherwise stable, gastrointestinal bleeding or a subtle infection should be suspected. Most of the precipitating factors cause an increase in blood ammonia.

Key to the management of encephalopathy is identifying and then eliminating whatever precipitating factors are responsible. Dietary protein should be restricted, infections should be treated, all sedatives should be discontinued, and intestinal catharsis should be accomplished.

Most episodes of encephalopathy are acute and develop over a period of hours to days. Such episodes may first present with subtle personality changes and sleep disturbances. As encephalopathy progresses, disorientation, slurred speech, confusion, and eventually coma may develop. The characteristic flapping tremor asterixis is commonly present and represents an inability to actively maintain posture or position. Neither asterixis nor the psychoneurologic manifestations of this syndrome are specific to portal systemic encephalopathy and may also be present in other types of metabolic dysfunction such as renal failure. Nearly all cases of acute encephalopathy are induced by one or more precipitating factors that should be identified and eliminated. Chronic encephalopathy is considerably less common than acute encephalopathy and generally occurs in patients with either a surgical nonselective portal systemic shunt or TIPS.

Pharmacologic treatment of encephalopathy is indicated for patients with chronic, intermittent symptoms and for those with persistent, acute psychoneurologic disturbances despite elimination of precipitating factors. The only drugs with proven effectiveness are neomycin, a poorly absorbed antibiotic that suppresses urease-containing bacteria, and lactulose, a nonabsorbable disaccharide that acidifies colonic contents and also has a cathartic effect. A likely mechanism of action of both of these drugs is a decrease in the amount of intestinal ammonia and inhibition of its absorption. Acute episodes of encephalopathy can be treated equally effectively with neomycin and lactulose. Neomycin should be orally administered in a dose of 1.5 g every 6 hours. In the acute setting, lactulose should be given in a dose of 30 g every 1 or 2 hours until a cathartic effect is noted. The patient should then be maintained with 20 to 30 g of lactulose two to four times a day or as needed to result in two soft bowel movements daily. Comatose patients can be treated with lactulose enemas. Lactulose is the mainstay of therapy for chronic encephalopathy because long-term use of neomycin may cause nephrotoxicity or ototoxicity in some patients. Protein restriction is also a component of the therapeutic regimen. The comatose patient should be initially treated exclusively with glucose supplements as intravenous fluids. As encephalopathy lessens, 0.5 to 1.2 g/kg per day of amino acids or proteins should be provided. When an oral diet is resumed, it should initially consist of 40 to 60 g/day of protein, which can then be gradually increased to a maintenance level of 60 to 80 g/day.

Unproven therapies for encephalopathy include the enteral or parenteral administration of branched-chain amino acids and the drug flumazenil, a selective antagonist of benzodiazepine receptors. Neither of these treatments have been clearly established in randomized, controlled trials.

Interventional procedures and surgery have improved cerebral function in some patients with encephalopathy by interrupting a surgically constructed portal systemic shunt or TIPS. Likewise, in isolated cases, occlusion of a major portal systemic collateral, such as the coronary vein, has reversed encephalopathy after the selective distal splenorenal shunt. Although both total colectomy and colonic exclusion have resolved encephalopathy in some patients, the high morbidity and mortality rates after these operations in patients with decompensated hepatic disease have prevented their widespread use.

Selected References

D'Amico G, Pagliaro L, Bosch J: The treatment of portal hypertension: A meta-analytic review. Hepatology 22:332-354, 1995.

> Since the 1960s, countless controlled trials comparing the various treatments for variceal bleeding have been conducted throughout the world. These authors have painstakingly tabulated the results of all these trials and applied meta-analysis when appropriate.

Garcia-Tsao G: Current management of the complications of cirrhosis and portal hypertension: Variceal hemorrhage, ascites, and spontaneous bacterial peritonitis. Gastroenterology. 120:726-748, 2001.

> This is a superb review of the pathophysiology, diagnosis, and treatment of the major life-threatening complications of portal hypertension.

Henderson JM, Barnes DS, Geisinger MA: Portal hypertension. Curr Probl Surg 35:379-452, 1998.

> This is a superb and complete monograph on the pathophysiology, diagnosis, and treatment of complications of portal hypertension. The expertise of the authors represents the disciplines of surgery, gastroenterology, and interventional radiology.

Langer B (ed): World progress in surgery—treatment of portal hypertension, 1994: State of the art. World J Surg 18:169-258, 1994.

> Included in this issue is a compendium of 14 articles on state-of-the-art treatment of the complications of portal hypertension. Eight articles are devoted to surgical treatment (shunts, nonshunt operations, and liver transplantation) of variceal bleeding. Other entries deal with endoscopic treatment, pharmacotherapy, portal hypertension in children, surgical treatment of ascites, and prophylactic therapy for varices that have not bled.

Rikkers LF: The changing spectrum of treatment for variceal bleeding. Ann Surg 228:536-546, 1998.

> A series of 263 consecutive patients undergoing a variety of operations for variceal bleeding from 1978 to 1996 is presented. Four eras, separated by the times when endoscopic treatment, liver transplantation, and TIPS were introduced, are analyzed. The author concludes that these innovations have decreased the need for and improved the results of portal hypertension surgery, which is still indicated for selected patients.

Sharara AI, Rockey DC. Gastroesophageal variceal hemorrhage. N Engl J Med 345:669-681, 2001.

> This is a concise review article devoted to the emergency, elective, and prophylactic treatment of variceal bleeding. Excellent algorithms for treatment are provided.

References

1. Chen TS, Chen PS: Understanding the Liver: A History. Westport, CT, Greenwood, 1984.
2. Lautt WW: The 1995 Ciba-Geigy Award Lecture: Intrinsic Regulation of Hepatic Blood Flow. Can J Physiol Pharmacol 74:223-233, 1996.
3. Bosch J, Garcia-Pagan JC: Complications of cirrhosis: I. Portal hypertension. J Hepatol 32(1 Suppl):141-156, 2000.
4. Pizcueta P, Piqué JM, Fernández M, et al: Modulation of the hyperdynamic circulation of cirrhotic rats by nitric oxide inhibition. Gastroenterology 103:1909-1915, 1992.
5. Pugh RN, Murray-Lyon IM, Dawson JL, et al: Transection of the oesophagus for bleeding oesophageal varices. Br J Surg 60:646-649, 1973.
6. Kamath PS, Wiesner RH, Malinchoc M, et al: A model to predict survival in patients with end-stage liver disease. Hepatology 33:464-470, 2001.
7. Henseler KP, Pozniak MA, Lee FT Jr, et al: Three-dimensional CT angiography of spontaneous portosystemic shunts. Radiographics 21:691-704, 2001.
8. Bolondi L, Gatta A, Groszmann RJ, et al: Baveno II consensus statements: Imaging techniques and hemodynamic measurements in portal hypertension. In De Franchis R (ed): Portal Hypertension II: Proceedings of the Second Baveno International Consensus Workshop on Definitions, Methodology, and Therapeutic Strategies. Oxford, Blackwell Science, 1996, p 67.
9. De Franchis R: Updating consensus in portal hypertension. In Report of the Third Baveno Consensus Workshop on Definitions, Methodology, and Therapeutic Strategies in Portal Hypertension. J Hepatol 18:1082, 1993.
10. Smith JL, Graham DY: Variceal hemorrhage: A critical evaluation of survival analysis. Gastroenterology 82:968-973, 1982.
11. Polio J, Groszmann RJ: Hemodynamic factors involved in the development and rupture of esophageal varices: A pathophysiologic approach to treatment. Semin Liver Dis 6:318-331, 1986.
12. Anonymous: Prediction of the first variceal hemorrhage in patients with cirrhosis of the liver and esophageal varices: A prospective multicenter study. The North Italian Endoscopic Club for the Study and Treatment of Esophageal Varices. N Engl J Med 319:983, 1988.
13. Hahn M, Massen O, Nenki M, et al: De ecksche fistel zwischen der unteren hohlvene und der pfortaden und folgen fur den organismus. Arch Exp Pathol Pharmakol 32:162, 1893.

14. D'Amico G, Pagliaro L, Bosch J: The treatment of portal hypertension: A meta-analytic review. Hepatology 22:332-354, 1995.

15. De Franchis R, Primignani M: Endoscopic treatments for portal hypertension. Semin Liver Dis 19:439-455, 1999.

16. Barton RE, Rosch J, Saxon RR, et al: TIPS: Short- and long-term results—a survey of 1750 patients. Semin Intervent Radiol 12:364, 1995.

17. Sanyal AJ, Freedman AM, Luketic VA, et al: Transjugular intrahepatic portosystemic shunts for patients with active variceal hemorrhage unresponsive to sclerotherapy. Gastroenterology 111:138-148, 1996.

18. Orloff MJ, Orloff MS, Orloff SL, et al: Three decades of experience with emergency portacaval shunt for acutely bleeding esophageal varices in 400 unselected patients with cirrhosis of the liver. J Am Coll Surg 180:257-272, 1995.

19. Lebrec D, Poynard T, Bernuau J, et al: A randomized controlled study of propranolol for prevention of recurrent gastrointestinal bleeding in patients with cirrhosis: A final report. Hepatology 4:355-358, 1984.

20. Villanueva C, Balanzo J, Novella MT, et al: Nadolol plus isosorbide mononitrate compared with sclerotherapy for the prevention of variceal rebleeding. N Engl J Med 334:1624-1629, 1996.

21. Villanueva C, Miñana J, Ortiz J, et al: Endoscopic ligation compared with combined treatment with nadolol and isosorbide mononitrate to prevent recurrent variceal bleeding. N Engl J Med 345:647-655, 2001.

22. Laine L, Cook D: Endoscopic ligation compared with sclerotherapy for treatment of esophageal variceal bleeding: A meta-analysis. Ann Intern Med 123:280-287, 1995.

23. Henderson JM, Kutner MH, Millikan WJJ, et al: Endoscopic variceal sclerosis compared with distal splenorenal shunt to prevent recurrent variceal bleeding in cirrhosis: A prospective, randomized trial. Ann Intern Med 112:262-269, 1990.

24. Rikkers LF, Jin G, Burnett DA, et al: Shunt surgery versus endoscopic sclerotherapy for variceal hemorrhage: Late results of a randomized trial. Am J Surg 165:27-32, 1993.

25. Riggio O, Merlli M, Pedretti G, et al: Hepatic encephalopathy after transjugular intrahepatic portosystemic shunt: Incidence and risk factors. Dig Dis Sci 41:578-584, 1996.

26. Sanyal AJ, Freedman AM, Luketic VA, et al: Transjugular intrahepatic portosystemic shunts compared with endoscopic sclerotherapy for the prevention of recurrent variceal hemorrhage: A randomized, controlled trial. Ann Intern Med 126:849-857, 1997.

27. Papatheodoridis GV, Goulis J, Leandro G, et al: Transjugular intrahepatic portosystemic shunt compared with endoscopic treatment for prevention of variceal rebleeding: A meta-analysis. Hepatology 30:612-622, 1999.

28. Rikkers LF, Sorrell WT, Jin G: Which portosystemic shunt is best? Gastroenterol Clin North Am 21:179-196, 1992.

29. Inokuchi K, Beppu K, Koyanagi N, et al: Fifteen years' experience with left gastric venous caval shunt for esophageal varices. World J Surg 8:716-721, 1984.

30. Henderson JM: Role of distal splenorenal shunt for long-term management of variceal bleeding. World J Surg 18:205-210, 1994.

31. Jin GL, Rikkers LF: Selective variceal decompression: Current status. HPB Surg 5:1-15, 1991.

32. Henderson JM, Millikan WJJ, Wright-Bacon L, et al: Hemodynamic differences between alcoholic and nonalcoholic cirrhotics following distal splenorenal shunt: Effect on survival? Ann Surg 198:325-334, 1983.

33. Rikkers LF: Is the distal splenorenal shunt better? Hepatology 8:1705-1707, 1988.

34. da Silva LC, Strauss E, Gayotto LC, et al: A randomized trial for the study of the elective surgical treatment of portal hypertension in mansonic schistosomiasis. Ann Surg 204:148-153, 1986.

35. Spina GP, Henderson JM, Rikkers LF, et al: Distal splenorenal shunt versus endoscopic sclerotherapy in the prevention of variceal rebleeding: A meta-analysis of four randomized clinical trials. J Hepatol 16:338-345, 1992.

36. Khaitiyar JS, Luthra SK, Prasad N, et al: Transjugular intrahepatic portosystemic shunt versus distal splenorenal shunt—a comparative study. Hepatogastroenterology 47:492-497, 2000.

37. Collins JC, Rypins EB, Sarfeh IJ: Narrow-diameter portacaval shunts for management of variceal bleeding. World J Surg 18:211-215, 1994.

38. Sarfeh IJ, Rypins EB: Partial versus total portacaval shunt in alcoholic cirrhosis: Results of a prospective, randomized clinical trial. Ann Surg 219:353-361, 1994.

39. Rosemurgy AS, Serafini FM, Zweibel BR, et al: Transjugular intrahepatic portosystemic shunt versus small-diameter prosthetic H-graft portacaval shunt: Extended follow-up of an expanded randomized prospective trial. J Gastrointest Surg 4:589-597, 2000.

40. Idezuki Y, Kokudo N, Sanjo K, et al: Sugiura procedure for management of variceal bleeding in Japan. World J Surg 18:216-221, 1994.

41. Jin G, Rikkers LF: Transabdominal esophagogastric devascularization as treatment for variceal hemorrhage. Surgery 120:641-647, 1996.

42. Henderson JM: The role of portosystemic shunts for variceal bleeding in the liver transplantation era. Arch Surg 129:886, 1994.

43. Rikkers LF, Jin G, Langnas AN, et al: Shunt surgery during the era of liver transplantation. Ann Surg 226:51-57, 1997.

44. Rikkers LF: The changing spectrum of treatment for variceal bleeding. Ann Surg 228:536-546, 1998.

45. Gines P, Quintero E, Arroyo V: Compensated cirrhosis: Natural history and prognosis. Hepatology 7:122-128, 1987.

46. Fogel MR, Sawhney VK, Neal A, et al: Diuresis in the ascitic patient: A randomized controlled trial of three regimens. J Clin Gastroenterol 3(Suppl 1):73-80, 1981.

47. Gines P, Arroyo V, Quintero E, et al: Comparison of paracentesis and diuretics in the treatment of cirrhotics with tense ascites: Results of a randomized study. Gastroenterology 93:234-241, 1987.

48. Ochs A, Rossie M, Haag K, et al: The transjugular intrahepatic portosystemic stent-shunt procedure for refractory ascites. N Engl J Med 332:1192-1197, 1995.

49. Ricart E, Soriano G, Novella M, et al: Amoxicillin–clavulanic acid versus cefotaxime in the therapy of bacterial infections in cirrhotic patients. J Hepatol 32:596-602, 2000.

50. Gines P, Rimola A, Planas R, et al: Norfloxacin prevents spontaneous bacterial peritonitis recurrence in cirrhosis: Results of a double-blind, placebo-controlled trial. Hepatology 12:716-724, 1990.

CHAPTER 52

BILIARY TRACT

Steven A. Ahrendt, M.D.   and   Henry A. Pitt, M.D.

Anatomy	**Benign Noncalculous Biliary Disease**
Physiology and Pathophysiology	**Malignant Biliary Disease**
Calculous Biliary Disease	

Although signs and symptoms of gallstones and extrahepatic biliary obstruction have been recognized for centuries, the surgical management of biliary tract disorders has evolved recently. The introduction of general anesthesia and antisepsis in 1848 and 1868, respectively, laid the foundation for the remarkable series of advances that occurred in abdominal surgery during the latter part of the 19th century. Surgery of the biliary tract was no exception.

John Stough Bobb of Indianapolis is credited with performing the first operation on the biliary tract. In 1867, Bobb explored a 32-year-old woman with a large abdominal mass and discovered a massive gallbladder hydrops. Bobb made a cholecystotomy, removed the gallstones, and sutured the gallbladder closed. Carl Langenbuch of Berlin is credited with the first cholecystectomy in 1882. Langenbuch performed the cholecystectomy in a 43-year-old man with a 16-year history of biliary colic. His patient survived the operation and was discharged from the hospital 8 weeks following the operation.

The operative management of extrahepatic biliary obstruction also evolved rapidly in the late 19th century. The first bilioenteric anastomosis was performed by Alexander von Winiwarter (a pupil of Theodore Billroth) in Liège in 1880.[1] Von Winiwarter performed a cholecystocolostomy in a 34-year-old man with choledocholithiasis and common bile duct obstruction. A palliative biliary tract bypass (cholecystojejunostomy) was first performed for malignant biliary obstruction in a patient with periampullary cancer in 1887 by Monastryski. Choledochotomy with stone extraction from the common bile duct was first performed in 1889. However, the high mortality initially associated with this procedure led to the common use of cholecystojejunostomy for biliary obstruction. Ludwig Courvoisier reported his first 10 cases of cholecystojejunostomy in 1890 with an operative mortal-

ity rate of 20% and advocated its use over cholecystostomy for cases of common bile duct obstruction. Choledochoduodenostomy was initially attempted for an impacted common duct stone by Oskar Sprengel in Germany in 1891 and following resection of a periampullary cancer in 1898 by William Stewart Halsted. The use of a Roux-en-Y jejunal limb to create a hepaticojejunostomy as commonly used today was first reported by Robert Dahl of Stockholm in 1909.[1]

A variety of diagnostic and nonoperative modalities have been developed this century that have further refined the management of patients with biliary tract disease. The diagnosis of gallstones was improved considerably by oral cholecystography in 1924. In the 1950s, cholescintigraphy and endoscopic and transhepatic cholangiography were developed permitting nonoperative imaging of the biliary tract. More recently, ultrasonography, computed tomography (CT), and magnetic resonance (MR) imaging have vastly improved the ability to image the biliary tract.

ANATOMY

Extrahepatic Biliary Tract

Normal Anatomy

The extrahepatic biliary tract consists of the bifurcation of the left and right hepatic ducts, the common hepatic duct and common bile duct, and the cystic duct and gallbladder (Fig. 52-1). The left hepatic duct is formed by the ducts draining segments II, III, and IV of the liver, courses horizontally along the base of segment IV, and has an extrahepatic length of 2 cm or more. The right hepatic

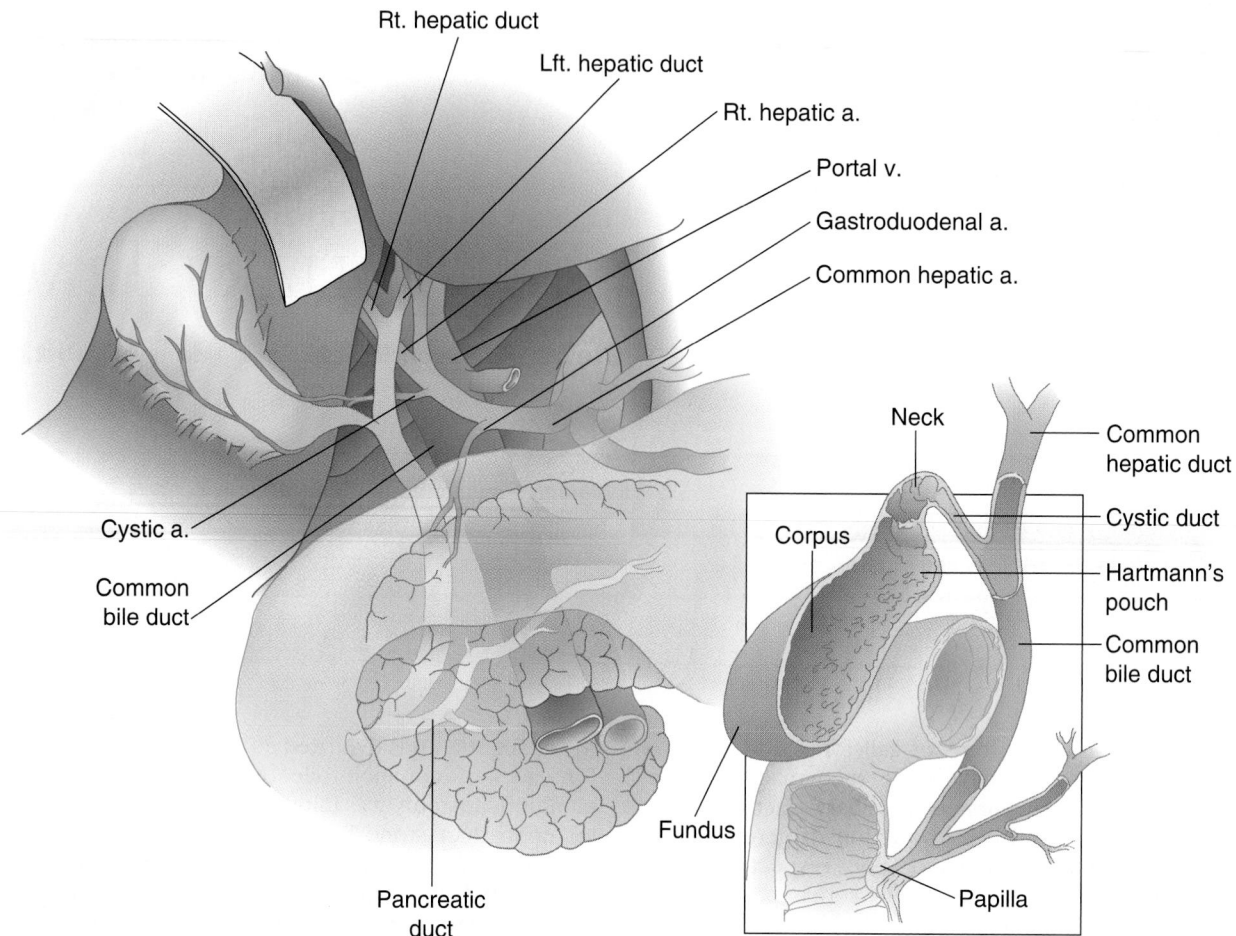

FIGURE 52-1.   Anatomy of the biliary system and its relationship to surrounding structures.

duct is formed by the right posterior (segments VI and VII) and right anterior (segments V and VIII) hepatic ducts and has a short extrahepatic length. The hepatic duct bifurcation is usually extrahepatic and anterior to the portal vein bifurcation. The common hepatic duct lies anteriorly in the hepatoduodenal ligament and joins the cystic duct to from the common bile duct. The common bile duct extends from the cystic duct common hepatic duct junction inferiorly to the papilla of Vater, where it empties into the duodenum. The common bile duct varies in length from 5 to 9 cm depending on its junction with the cystic duct and is divided into three segments: supraduodenal, retroduodenal, and intrapancreatic. The distal common bile duct and pancreatic duct may join outside the duodenal wall to form a long common channel, within the duodenal wall to form a short common channel, or they may enter the duodenum through two distinct ostia.

The gallbladder is a pear-shaped reservoir in continuity with the common hepatic and common bile ducts via the cystic duct. The gallbladder lies on the inferior surface of the liver partially enveloped in a layer of peritoneum. The gallbladder is anatomically divided into the fundus, body, infundibulum, and neck, which empties into the cystic duct. Both the gallbladder neck and the cystic duct contain spirally oriented mucosal folds known as the *valves of Heister*. The cystic duct varies in length from 1 to 4 cm usually joining the common hepatic duct at an acute angle.

Common Anomalies and Variations

Anatomic variations in the cystic duct and hepatic ducts are common. Relatively frequent variations in hepatic ductal anatomy include the right posterior hepatic duct joining the *common hepatic duct* distal to the union of the right anterior and left hepatic ducts (12%) and the *right anterior hepatic duct* joining the common hepatic duct distal to the union of the right posterior and left hepatic ducts (16%) (Fig. 52-2).[2] The cystic duct usually enters the common bile duct at an acute angle. However, the cystic duct may run parallel to the common hepatic duct for a variable distance before joining it on its right side or pass anterior or posterior to the common hepatic duct before joining it on its left side. In addition, the cystic duct may join either the right hepatic duct or a segmental right hepatic duct. An accessory hepatic duct or cholecystohepatic duct may also enter the gallbladder through the gallbladder fossa and, if encountered during a cholecystectomy, should be ligated to prevent a biliary fistula.

Anomalies of the gallbladder are much less frequent than variations in ductal anatomy. Agenesis of the gallbladder is rare (200 reported cases), and duplication of

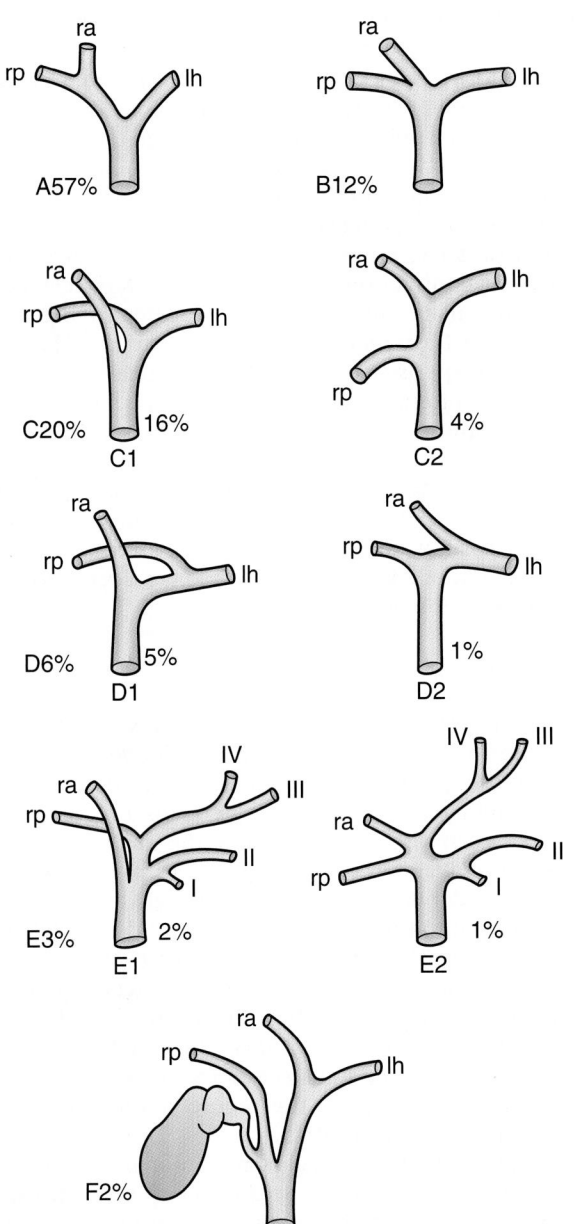

FIGURE 52-2. Main variations in the confluence of the left and right hepatic ducts. **A,** Typical anatomy of the confluence. **B,** Trifurcation of left, right anterior, and right posterior hepatic ducts. **C,** Aberrant drainage of a right anterior (C1) or posterior (C2) sectoral hepatic duct into the common hepatic duct. **D–F,** Less common variations in hepatic ductal anatomy. (**A–F,** From Smadja C, Blumgart L: The biliary tract and the anatomy of biliary exposure. *In* Blumgart L [ed]: Surgery of the Liver and Biliary Tract. New York, Churchill Livingstone, 1994, pp 11-24.)

the gallbladder (two separate gallbladders each with its own cystic duct) occurs in 1 of 4000 births.

Vascular Anatomy

Normal Anatomy and Variations

The gallbladder is supplied by the cystic artery, which most commonly is a single branch of the right hepatic artery. The cystic artery may also originate from the left

hepatic, common hepatic, gastroduodenal, or superior mesenteric arteries. The cystic artery is usually located parallel and medial to the cystic duct, but its course varies with its origin. The cystic artery divides into superficial and deep branches before entering the gallbladder.

The blood supply to the extrahepatic biliary tree originates distally from the gastroduodenal, retroduodenal, and posterior superior pancreatoduodenal arteries and proximally from the right hepatic and cystic arteries. These arteries supply the common bile and common hepatic ducts through branches running parallel to the duct in the 3 and 9 o'clock positions.

PHYSIOLOGY AND PATHOPHYSIOLOGY

Biliary Physiology

Bile Ducts

The bile ducts, gallbladder, and sphincter of Oddi act in concert to modify, store, and regulate the flow of bile. During its passage through the bile ductules and hepatic duct, canalicular bile is modified by the absorption and secretion of electrolytes and water. The gastrointestinal hormone, secretin, increases bile flow primarily by increasing the active secretion of chloride-rich fluid by the bile ducts and ductules. Bile ductular secretion is also stimulated by other hormones such as cholecystokinin (CCK) and gastrin. The bile duct epithelium is also capable of water and electrolyte absorption, which may be of primary importance in the storage of bile during fasting in patients who have previously undergone cholecystectomy.

Gallbladder

The main functions of the gallbladder are to concentrate and store hepatic bile during the fasting state and deliver bile into the duodenum in response to a meal. The usual capacity of the human gallbladder is only about 40 to 50 mL. Only a small fraction of the 600 mL of bile produced each day would be stored were it not for its remarkable absorptive capacity. The gallbladder mucosa has the greatest absorptive capacity per unit area of any structure in the body. Bile is usually concentrated 5-fold to 10-fold by the absorption of water and electrolytes leading to a marked change in bile composition (Table 52-1).[3]

Active NaCl transport by the gallbladder epithelium is the driving force for the concentration of bile. Water is passively absorbed in response to the osmotic force generated by solute absorption. The concentration of bile may affect the solubilities of two important components of gallstones: calcium and cholesterol. Although the gallbladder mucosa does absorb calcium, this process is not nearly as efficient as for sodium or water, leading to greater relative increase in calcium concentration. As the gallbladder bile becomes concentrated, several changes occur in the capacity of bile to solubilize cholesterol. The solubility in the micellar fraction is increased, but the

TABLE 52-1.   Composition of Hepatic and Gallbladder Bile

Characteristic	Hepatic*	Gallbladder*
Na	160.0	270.0
K	5	10
Cl	90	15
HCO$_3$	45	10
Ca	4	25
Mg	2	—
Bilirubin	1.5	15
Protein	150	—
Bile acids	50	150
Phospholipids	8	40
Cholesterol	4	18
Total solids	—	125
pH	7.8	7.2

*All amounts, except pH, are expressed in milliequivalents per liter.

stability of phospholipid-cholesterol vesicles is greatly decreased. Because cholesterol crystal precipitation occurs preferentially by vesicular rather than micellar mechanisms, the net effect of concentrating bile is an increased tendency to nucleate cholesterol (see Gallstone Pathogenesis).[3]

The gallbladder epithelial cell secretes at least two important products into the gallbladder lumen: glycoproteins and hydrogen ions. Secretion of mucus glycoproteins occurs primarily from the glands of the gallbladder neck and cystic duct. The resultant mucin gel is believed to constitute an important part of the unstirred layer (diffusion-resistant barrier) that separates the gallbladder cell membrane from the luminal bile. This mucus barrier may be very important in protecting the gallbladder epithelium from the strong detergent effect of the highly concentrated bile salts found in the gallbladder. However, considerable evidence also suggests that mucin glycoproteins play a role as a pronucleating agent for cholesterol crystallization. The transport of hydrogen ions by the gallbladder epithelium leads to a decrease in gallbladder bile pH through a sodium-exchange mechanism. Acidification of bile promotes calcium solubility, thereby preventing its precipitation as calcium salts. The gallbladder's normal acidification process lowers the pH of entering hepatic bile from 7.5 to 7.8 down to 7.1 to 7.3.[3]

Biliary Motility

Gallbladder

Gallbladder filling is facilitated by tonic contraction of the ampullary sphincter, which maintains a constant pressure in the common bile duct (10 to 15 mm Hg). The gall-

bladder does not, however, simply fill passively and continuously during fasting. Rather, periods of filling are punctuated by brief periods of partial emptying (10% to 15% of its volume) of concentrated gallbladder bile that are coordinated with each passage through the duodenum of phase III of the migrating myoelectric complex (MMC). This process is mediated, at least in part, by the hormone motilin. Following a meal, the release of stored bile from the gallbladder requires a coordinated motor response of gallbladder contraction and sphincter of Oddi relaxation. One of the main stimuli to gallbladder emptying is the hormone CCK, which is released from the duodenal mucosa in response to a meal. When stimulated by eating, the gallbladder empties 50% to 70% of its contents within 30 to 40 minutes. Gallbladder refilling then occurs gradually over the next 60 to 90 minutes. Many other hormonal and neural pathways are also necessary for the coordinated action of the gallbladder and sphincter of Oddi. Defects in gallbladder motility, which increase the residence time of bile in the gallbladder, play a central role in the pathogenesis of gallstones.[3]

Sphincter of Oddi

The human sphincter of Oddi is a complex structure that is functionally independent from the duodenal musculature. Endoscopic manometric studies have demonstrated that the human sphincter of Oddi creates a high-pressure zone between the bile duct and the duodenum. The sphincter regulates the flow of bile and pancreatic juice into the duodenum, prevents the regurgitation of duodenal contents into the biliary tract, and also diverts bile into the gallbladder. This latter function is achieved by keeping pressure within the bile and pancreatic ducts higher than duodenal pressure. The sphincter of Oddi also has very high-pressure phasic contractions. The exact functions of these phasic waves in humans is not known, but they may play a role in preventing the regurgitation of duodenal contents into the biliary tract.

Both neural and hormonal factors influence the sphincter of Oddi. In humans, sphincter of Oddi pressure and phasic wave activity diminish in response to CCK. Thus, sphincter pressure relaxes after a meal, allowing the passive flow of bile into the duodenum. During fasting, high-pressure phasic contractions of the sphincter of Oddi persist through all phases of the MMC. Recent animal studies suggest, however, that sphincter of Oddi phasic waves do vary to some degree in concert with the MMC. Thus, sphincter of Oddi activity is undoubtedly coordinated with the partial gallbladder emptying and increases in bile flow that occur during phase III of the MMC. This activity may be a preventative mechanism against the accumulation of biliary crystals during fasting.[3]

Neurally mediated reflexes link the sphincter of Oddi with the gallbladder and stomach to coordinate the flow of bile and pancreatic juice into the duodenum. The cholecystosphincter of Oddi reflex allows the human sphincter to relax as the gallbladder contracts. Similarly, antral distention causes both gallbladder contraction and sphincter relaxation.

Bacteriology

Bile in the gallbladder or bile ducts in the absence of gall-stones or any other biliary tract disease is normally sterile. In the presence of gallstones or biliary obstruction the prevalence of bactibilia increases. The presence of positive bile cultures is influenced by several factors including the severity or type of biliary disease and the patient's age. The percentage of positive gallbladder bile cultures among patients with symptomatic gallstones and chronic cholecystitis ranges from 11% to 30%. The prevalence of positive gallbladder bile cultures is higher in patients with acute cholecystitis than chronic cholecystitis (46% vs. 22%) and increases further in the presence of common bile duct stones. In a recent study, 46% of patients with acute cholecystitis had positive gallbladder bile cultures.[4] In addition, 58% of patients with gallstones and common bile duct stones but without cholangitis had positive gall-bladder and common duct bile cultures, whereas 94% of patients with gallstones, common bile duct stones, and cholangitis had positive bile cultures.[4] All patients with common bile duct stones after cholecystectomy had bactibilia. Positive bile cultures were significantly more common in elderly (>60 years) patients with symptomatic gallstones than in younger patients (45% vs. 16%). Patients with cholangitis due to malignant biliary obstruction are also more likely to have a positive bile culture than patients with a benign cause of biliary obstruction (stones, stricture, sclerosing cholangitis).[5]

Gram-negative aerobes are the organisms most frequently isolated from bile in patients with symptomatic gallstones, acute cholecystitis, or cholangitis. *Escherichia coli* and *Klebsiella* species are the most common gram-negative bacteria isolated. However, the more resistant organisms *Pseudomonas* and *Enterobacter* are being seen with increased frequency, particularly in patients with malignant biliary obstruction, who may have been treated with antibiotics previously for a biliary tract infection (Table 52-2).[5] Other common isolates include the gram-positive aerobes, *Enterococcus*, and *Streptococcus viridans*. Anaerobes, such as *Bacteroides* species and *Clostridium*, continue to play a small but significant role in biliary infections. The prevalence of anaerobic bacteria is 10% to 13% in patients with acute cholecystitis or cholangitis. *Candida* species are also being increasingly recognized as a significant biliary pathogen particularly in critically ill patients. The majority of patients with symptomatic cholelithiasis, acute cholecystitis, or common bile duct stones in the absence of cholangitis have a single organism isolated in bile cultures. Polymicrobial infections are more common in patients with cholangitis. In analyzing response to therapy, the isolation of *Candida*, panresistant bacteria, and more than two bacteria are associated with treatment failures.

The source of bacteria in patients with biliary tract infections is controversial. The majority of evidence favors an ascending route via the duodenum as the main source of biliary bacteria. The bacterial flora in the small intestine is similar to that detected in the biliary tract. In addition, in the majority of patients gallbladder and common bile duct cultures yield a similar result. Furthermore, the

prevalence of bactibilia is highest in the elderly in whom biliary motility and clearance have decreased.[4]

Antibiotic Selection

Antibiotics should be used prophylactically in most patients undergoing elective biliary tract surgery or other biliary tract manipulations such as endoscopic or percutaneous cholangiography (Box 52-1).[6] The risk of postoperative infectious complications corresponds to the presence of bactibilia, which occurs in 11% to 30% of patients with gallstones, but is difficult to determine preoperatively. In low-risk patients undergoing laparoscopic cholecystectomy for chronic cholecystitis, the incidence of wound infections is low (1%), and several prospective randomized trials have not demonstrated any benefit to prophylactic antibiotics. In high-risk patients (elderly, recent acute cholecystitis, high risk of conversion to open cholecystectomy) a single dose of the first-generation cephalosporin, cefazolin, provides good coverage against the gram-negative aerobes commonly isolated from bile and skin flora.

Therapeutic antibiotics are used in patients with acute cholecystitis and acute cholangitis. In both diseases gram-negative aerobes play a major role and are well covered by the second- or third-generation cephalosporins, aminoglycosides, ureidopenicillins, carbapenems, and the fluoroquinolones. Ureidopenicillins, such as piperacillin, offer the advantage of gram-positive coverage, including the

TABLE 52-2.   Organisms Isolated from Bile of Patients with Either a Benign or Malignant Etiology of Cholangitis

Organisms	Benign Cause (%) (n = 42)	Malignant Cause (%) (n = 54)
GRAM NEGATIVE		
Klebsiella species	31	72*
Escherichia coli	43	35
Enterobacter species	17	48*
Pseudomonas species	12	33†
Citrobacter species	17	24
Proteus species	12	13
GRAM POSITIVE		
Enterococcus	36	33
Streptococcus species	24	48†
Anaerobes		
Bacteroides species	17	13
Clostridium species	2	7
FUNGI		
Candida species	5	28*
OTHERS	19	9
At least one organism isolated	64	96†

*$P < 0.005$ vs. benign.
†$P < 0.025$ vs. benign.
Adapted from Thompson JE Jr, Pitt HA, Doty JE, et al: Broad-spectrum penicillin as an adequate therapy for acute cholangitis. Surg Gynecol Obstet 171:275-282, 1990.

ANTIBIOTIC PROPHYLAXIS

Open Cholecystectomy

Cefazolin (1–2 g single dose)

Laparoscopic Cholecystectomy

Low risk
  None
High-risk*
Cefazolin (1–2 g single dose)

Other Open Biliary Tract Operations

Piperacillin/tazobactam, ampicillin/sulbactam, ticarcillin/
  clavulanate
Ciprofloxacin + metronidazole
Cefoperazone, cefotetan, cefotaxime, ceftriaxone

ERCP—Low Risk

None

ERCP—High Risk†/Percutaneous Biliary Drainage

Piperacillin/tazobactam, ampicillin/sulbactam, ticarcillin/
  clavulanate
Ciprofloxacin + metronidazole
Cefoperazone, cefotetan, cefotaxime, ceftriaxone

THERAPEUTIC ANTIBIOTICS

Acute Cholecystitis

Cefotetan, cefoxitin, ceftizoxime
Ciprofloxacin + metronidazole

Acute Cholangitis

Piperacillin/tazobactam, ampicillin/sulbactam, ticarcillin/
  clavulanate
Ciprofloxacin + metronidazole
Imipenem/cilastatin, meropenem
Cefepime

*Elderly patients, recent acute cholecystitis, jaundiced, increased risk of conversion to open procedure.
†Presence of biliary obstruction or high-risk for developing infective endocarditis.
ERCP, endoscopic retrograde cholangiopancreatography.
Adapted from Cox J, Ahrendt S: Antibiotic selection in biliary tract surgery. In Cameron J (ed): Current Surgical Therapy. St. Louis, Mosby, 2001, p 494.

enterococci and of anaerobic coverage. When combined with a β-lactamase inhibitor such as tazobactam, piperacillin offers extended and improved coverage against organisms with acquired resistance. Most fluoroquinolones such as ciprofloxacin do not cover the anaerobes and should be used in combination with an agent with anaerobic coverage (i.e., metronidazole). *Pseudomonas* has been recovered with increased frequency in patients with cholangitis, particularly with chronic indwelling stents, and should be covered in severely ill patients.

Both mezlocillin and piperacillin have performed as well as combination therapy including an aminoglycoside in prospective, randomized trials in patients with cholangitis.

Obstructive Jaundice

Jaundice is a frequent manifestation of biliary tract disorders, and the evaluation and management of the jaundiced patient are common problems facing the general surgeon. Normal serum bilirubin ranges from 0.5 to 1.3 mg/dL; when levels exceed 2.0 mg/dL, the bilirubin staining of the tissues becomes clinically apparent as jaundice. In addition, the presence of conjugated bilirubin in the urine is one of the first changes noted by patients.

Bilirubin is the normal breakdown product of hemoglobin produced from senescent red blood cells by the reticuloendothelial system. Insoluble unconjugated bilirubin is transported to the liver bound to albumin. Bilirubin is transported across the sinusoidal membrane of the hepatocyte into the cytoplasm. The enzyme uridine diphosphate–glucuronyl transferase then conjugates the insoluble unconjugated bilirubin with glucuronic acid to form the water-soluble conjugated forms, bilirubin monoglucuronide and bilirubin diglucuronide. Conjugated bilirubin is then actively secreted into the bile canaliculus. In the terminal ileum and colon, bilirubin is converted to urobilinogen, 10% to 20% of which is reabsorbed into the portal circulation. This urobilinogen is either re-excreted into the bile or excreted by the kidneys into the urine.

Diagnostic Evaluation

The differential diagnosis of jaundice parallels the metabolism of bilirubin (Table 52-3). Disorders resulting in jaundice can be divided into those causing "medical" jaundice such as increased production, decreased hepatocyte transport or conjugation, or impaired excretion of bilirubin or into those causing "surgical" jaundice through impaired delivery of bilirubin into the intestine. Common causes of increased bilirubin production include the hemolytic anemias and acquired causes of hemolysis including sepsis, burns, and transfusion reactions. Bilirubin uptake and conjugation can be affected by drugs, sepsis, and the aftermath of viral hepatitis. Impaired excretion of bilirubin leads to intrahepatic cholestasis and conjugated hyperbilirubinemia. Common causes of impaired excretion include viral or alcoholic hepatitis, cirrhosis, and drug-induced cholestasis. Extrahepatic biliary obstruction can be caused by a variety of disorders including choledocholithiasis, benign biliary strictures, periampullary cancer, cholangiocarcinoma, or primary sclerosing cholangitis.

While diagnosing jaundice, the physician must be able to distinguish among defects in bilirubin uptake, conjugation, or excretion that are usually managed medically from extrahepatic biliary obstruction, which is usually handled by a surgeon, interventional radiologist, or endoscopist (Fig. 52-3). In most cases, a careful history,

TABLE 52-3. Differential Diagnosis of Jaundice

Abnormality in Bilirubin Metabolism	Predominant Hyperbilirubinemia	Examples
Increased production	Unconjugated	Multiple transfusions, transfusion reaction, sepsis, burns, congenital hemoglobinopathies, hemolysis
Impaired hepatocyte uptake or conjugation	Unconjugated	Gilbert's disease, Crigler-Najjar syndrome, neonatal jaundice, viral hepatitis, drug inhibition, sepsis
Impaired transport and excretion	Conjugated	Dubin-Johnson syndrome, Rotor's syndrome, cirrhosis, amyloidosis, cancer, hepatitis (viral, drug induced, or alcoholic), pregnancy
Biliary obstruction	Conjugated	Choledocholithiasis, benign stricture, periampullary cancer, cholangiocarcinoma, chronic pancreatitis, primary sclerosing cholangitis

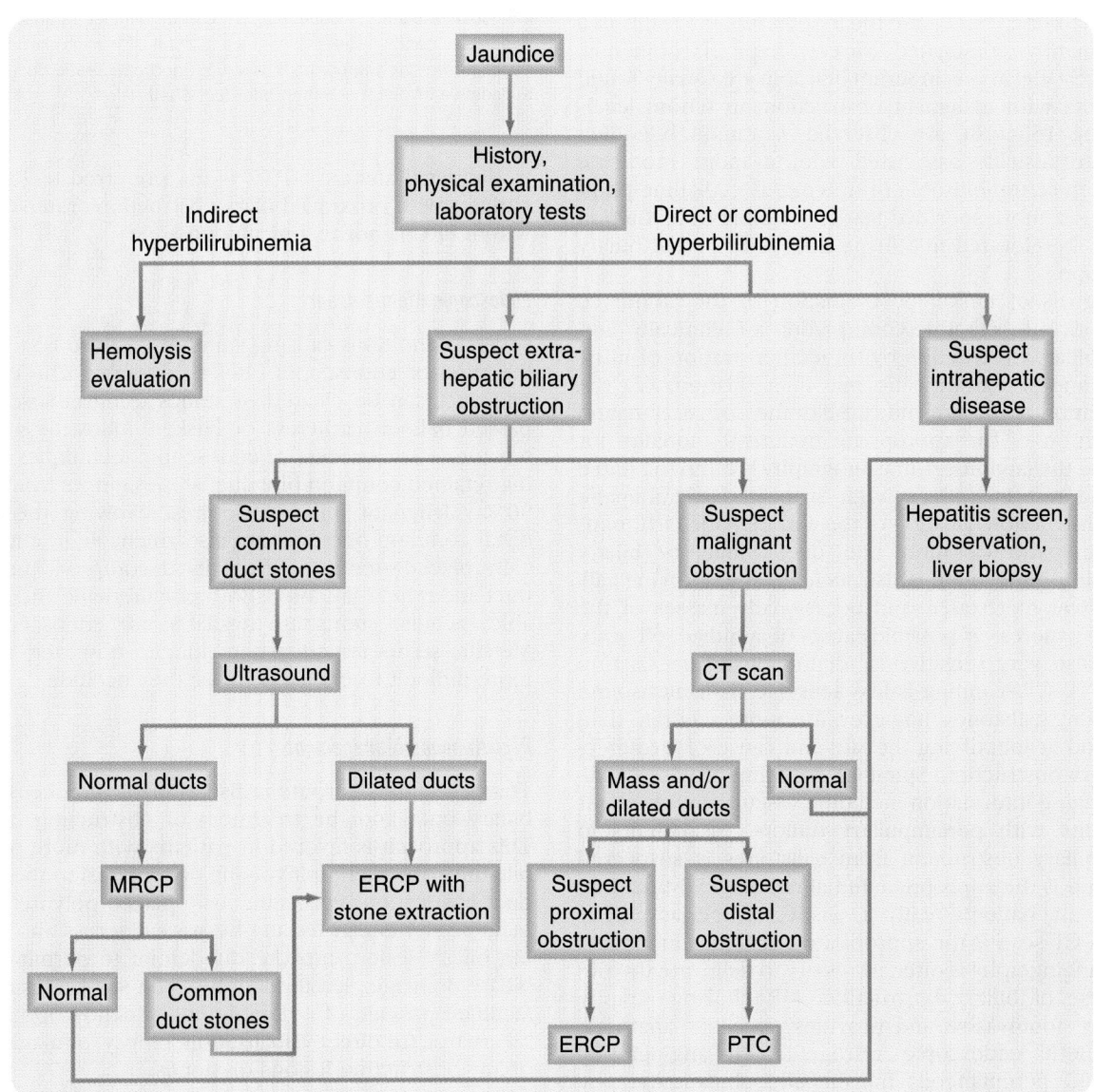

FIGURE 52-3. Diagnostic algorithm for the jaundiced patient. ERCP, endoscopic retrograde cholangiopancreatography; MRCP, magnetic resonance cholangiopancreatography; PTC, percutaneous transhepatic cholangiography.

physical examination, routine laboratory tests, and noninvasive radiologic imaging differentiate extrahepatic biliary obstruction from other causes of jaundice. Cholelithiasis is often associated with right upper quadrant pain and indigestion. Jaundice from common bile duct stones is usually transient and associated with pain and often fever (cholangitis). The gradual onset of painless jaundice with associated weight loss is suggestive of a malignancy. If jaundice occurs after cholecystectomy, retained bile duct stones or an injury to the bile duct should be suspected.

Laboratory tests that should be performed in all jaundiced patients include serum direct and indirect bilirubin, alkaline phosphatase, transaminases, amylase, and a complete blood cell count. Unconjugated (indirect) hyperbilirubinemia occurs when there is an increase in bilirubin production or a decrease in hepatocyte uptake and conjugation. Defects in bilirubin excretion (intrahepatic cholestasis) or extrahepatic biliary obstruction result in a predominantly conjugated (direct) hyperbilirubinemia. The highest elevations in serum bilirubin are usually found in patients with malignant obstruction, in whom levels exceeding 15 mg/dL are observed. Common bile duct stones are usually associated with a more moderate increase in serum bilirubin (4 to 8 mg/dL). Alkaline phosphatase is a more sensitive marker of biliary obstruction and may be elevated first in patients with partial biliary obstruction.

The goals of radiologic evaluation of the jaundiced patient include (1) the confirmation of clinically suspected biliary obstruction by the demonstration of intrahepatic and/or extrahepatic bile duct dilation; (2) the identification of the site and cause of the obstruction; and (3) selection of the appropriate treatment modality for managing the jaundice. Ultrasonography is often the initial screening test in patients with suspected extrahepatic biliary obstruction. Dilation of the extrahepatic (>10 mm) or intrahepatic (>4 mm) bile ducts suggests biliary obstruction. Ultrasound is also accurate at identifying gallstones, liver metastases, and occasionally masses of the liver and pancreas as possible causes of jaundice. CT scanning is also very sensitive at identifying biliary dilation (Fig. 52-4). CT scanning is less sensitive than ultrasound at detecting gallstones; however, it is more accurate than ultrasound at identifying the site and cause of extrahepatic biliary obstruction. Spiral CT scanning provides additional staging information including vascular involvement in patients with periampullary tumors. In patients in whom biliary obstruction from gallstones is suspected ultrasound is the appropriate initial radiologic evaluation, whereas in patients with a suspected periampullary tumor, a CT scan is the appropriate initial imaging study.

Cholangiography is often necessary to delineate the site and cause of biliary obstruction. MR cholangiography (MRC) is noninvasive and provides excellent anatomic detail. Both endoscopic retrograde cholangiography (ERC) and percutaneous transhepatic cholangiography (PTC) are invasive procedures with a 2% to 5% risk of complications but offer the opportunity for a therapeutic intervention (see later). ERC is most useful in imaging patients with periampullary tumors and choledocholithiasis. Occasionally, ERC is not feasible in patients with altered gas-

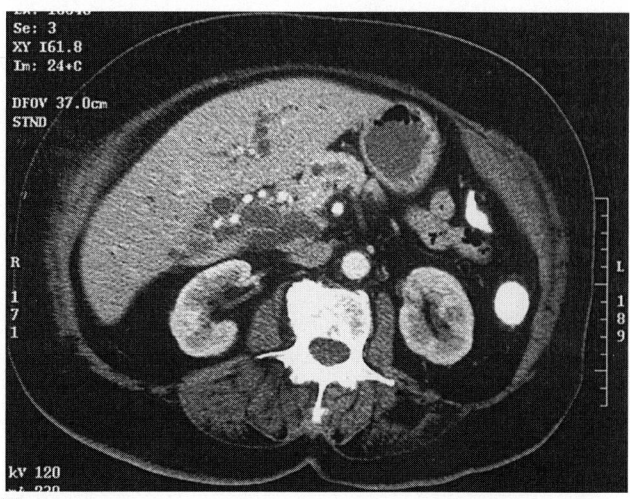

FIGURE 52-4.   Abdominal CT scan in jaundiced patient with pancreatic cancer. The scan shows dilation of the intrahepatic biliary ducts as well as the common bile duct and pancreatic duct, suggestive of distal common bile duct obstruction.

troduodenal anatomy. PTC is the preferred technique in patients with proximal biliary obstruction or in patients in whom ERC is not technically possible.

Endoscopic Management

Several conditions causing jaundice can also be treated at the time of endoscopic cholangiography. The common bile duct can be cleared of stones using endoscopically passed balloon catheters or baskets following a sphincterotomy. The success of endoscopic techniques at clearing retained common bile duct stones ranges from 85% to 90%.[7] Malignant biliary strictures involving the mid or distal common bile duct are also amenable to endoscopically placed stents to internally decompress the biliary tract and relieve jaundice. Both polyurethane and expandable metallic stents are available for endoscopic use. Metallic stents remain patent longer; however, they are more difficult to exchange once they occlude.

Percutaneous Management

The percutaneous route is also available for access to the biliary tract and the treatment of obstructing jaundice. This approach is favored in patients with more proximal bile duct obstruction involving or proximal to the hepatic duct bifurcation. Percutaneously placed polyurethane or metallic stents can usually be passed across an obstructing biliary lesion into the duodenum to permit internal biliary drainage. Serial dilation of the stent tract can also facilitate passage of a flexible choledochoscope into the biliary tree for direct visualization, biopsy, or management of any obstructing lesions or stones.

Operative Risk Factors

A careful evaluation of the overall general medical condition of the patient as well as an accurate staging evaluation are necessary prior to selecting the appropriate management for the patient with obstructive jaundice. The preoperative assessment should include the usual evaluation of cardiac risk factors, respiratory status, and renal function, as well as overall performance status measured by one of several performance scales. In addition, patients with obstructive jaundice have several further physiologic abnormalities, which require careful evaluation. These abnormalities include alterations in hepatic and pancreatic function, the gastrointestinal barrier, immune function, hemostatic mechanisms, and wound healing. Hepatic protein synthesis, hepatic reticuloendothelial function, and other aspects of hepatic metabolism may be significantly altered in patients with obstructive jaundice. In addition, endotoxemia, which occurs frequently with obstructive jaundice, may contribute to renal, cardiac, and pulmonary insufficiency observed in patients with obstructive jaundice.

Altered cell-mediated immunity increases the risk of infection, whereas coagulation disorders make these patients prone to bleeding problems. Several studies have defined preoperative risk factors associated with an increase in morbidity and mortality in patients undergoing treatment for malignant biliary obstruction. Malnutrition (hypoalbuminemia), the presence of sepsis (cholangitis), and renal insufficiency all are associated with an increase in operative morbidity and mortality in biliary tract surgery. Control of sepsis and intensive nutritional support should be undertaken preoperatively in the malnourished patient with cholangiocarcinoma.

Preoperative Biliary Drainage

The preoperative relief of jaundice and the reversal of its systemic effects by either endoscopic or transhepatic biliary decompression have been proposed as a method to decrease the risk of surgery in jaundiced patients. However, several prospective, randomized studies have shown that the routine use of preoperative biliary drainage does not reduce operative morbidity or mortality in patients with obstructive jaundice. In addition, a recent meta-analysis also concluded that preoperative biliary drainage increased rather than decreased overall complications (from surgery and the drainage procedure) and provided no benefit in terms of reduced mortality or decreased hospital stay.[8] In fact, several studies have documented a higher incidence of infectious complications (wound infection, pancreatic fistula) and even mortality in patients undergoing pancreatic or biliary tract resection after preoperative biliary decompression.[8,9] Although preoperative biliary drainage should not be used routinely in the jaundiced patient, it may be useful in carefully selected patients with advanced malnutrition or biliary sepsis.[8,9] Preoperatively placed transhepatic catheters can also be of significant technical help to the surgeon in identifying the intrahepatic ducts in cases of difficult hilar dissections for bile duct strictures or cholangiocarcinoma.

CALCULOUS BILIARY DISEASE

Gallstone Pathogenesis

Bile facilitates the intestinal absorption of lipids and fat-soluble vitamins and represents the route of excretion for certain organic solids, such as bilirubin and cholesterol. The major organic solutes in bile are bilirubin, bile salts, phospholipids, and cholesterol. Bilirubin is the breakdown product of spent red blood cells and is conjugated with glucuronic acid prior to being excreted. Bile salts solubilize lipids and facilitate their absorption. Phospholipids are synthesized in the liver in conjunction with bile salt synthesis. The final major solute of bile is cholesterol, which is also produced primarily by the liver with little contribution from dietary sources. Cholesterol is highly nonpolar and insoluble in water and, thus, in bile. The normal volume of bile secreted daily by the liver is 500 to 1000 mL.

Gallstones represent a failure to maintain certain biliary solutes, primarily cholesterol and calcium salts, in a solubilized state. Gallstones are classified by their cholesterol content as either cholesterol or pigment stones. Pigment stones are further classified as either black or brown. Pure cholesterol gallstones are uncommon (10%), with most cholesterol stones containing calcium salts in their center, or nidus. In most American populations, 70% to 80% of gallstones are cholesterol, and black pigment stones account for most of the remaining 20% to 30%.

An important biliary precipitate in gallstone pathogenesis is biliary "sludge," which refers to a mixture of cholesterol crystals, calcium bilirubinate granules, and a mucin gel matrix. Biliary sludge has been observed clinically in prolonged fasting states or with the use of long-term total parenteral nutrition. Both of these conditions are also associated with gallstone formation. The finding of macromolecular complexes of mucin and bilirubin, similar to biliary sludge in the central core of most cholesterol gallstones, suggests that sludge may serve as the nidus for gallstone growth.

Cholesterol Gallstones

The pathogenesis of cholesterol gallstones is clearly multifactorial but essentially involves three stages: (1) cholesterol supersaturation in bile, (2) crystal nucleation, and (3) stone growth. For many years, gallstones were thought to result primarily from a defect in the hepatic secretion of biliary lipids. More recently, it has become increasingly clear that gallbladder mucosal and motor function also play key roles in gallstone formation. The key to maintaining cholesterol in solution is the formation of both micelles, a bile salt-phospholipid-cholesterol complex, and cholesterol-phospholipid vesicles. Present theory suggests that in states of excess cholesterol production, these large vesicles may also exceed their capability to transport cholesterol, and crystal precipitation may occur. Cholesterol solubility depends on the relative concentration of cholesterol, bile salts, and phospholipid. By plotting the percentages of each component on triangular coordi-

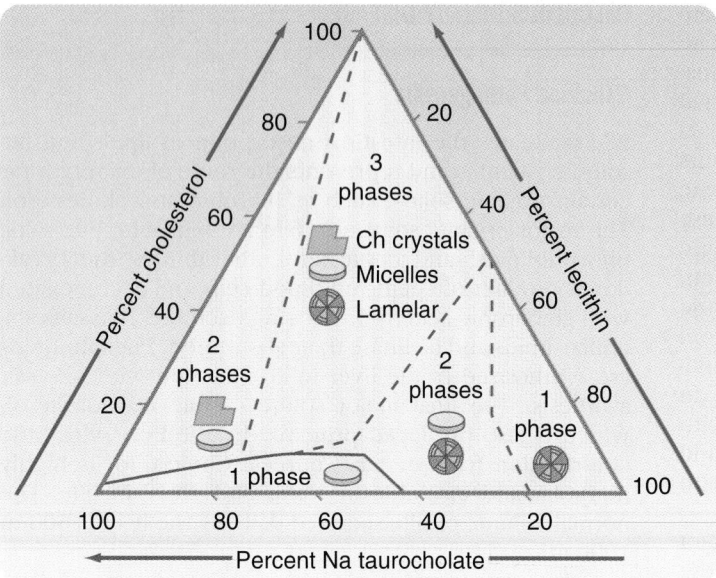

FIGURE 52-5. Triangular-phase diagram with axes plotted in percent cholesterol, lecithin (phospholipid), and the bile salt sodium taurocholate. Below the solid line, cholesterol is maintained in solution in micelles. Above the solid line, bile is supersaturated with cholesterol and precipitation of cholesterol crystals can occur. Ch, cholesterol. (From Donovan JM, Carey MC: Separation and quantitation of cholesterol "carriers" in bile. Hepatology 12:94S, 1990.)

nates, the micellar zone in which cholesterol is completely soluble can be demonstrated (Fig. 52-5). In the area above the curve, bile is supersaturated with cholesterol, and precipitation of cholesterol crystals can occur.

Cholesterol supersaturation is present in many normal humans without gallstones, and a significant overlap exists in cholesterol saturation in patients with and without gallstones. Thus, cholesterol supersaturation results in a metastable state in which cholesterol precipitation may or may not take place and additional factors in bile must be present, therefore, to either enhance or inhibit the nucleation of cholesterol leading to the next stage in gallstone formation.[3]

Nucleation refers to the process in which solid cholesterol monohydrate crystals form and conglomerate. Nucleation occurs more rapidly in gallbladder bile of patients with cholesterol stones than in individuals with cholesterol-saturated bile without stones. As bile is concentrated in the gallbladder, a net transfer of phospholipids and cholesterol from vesicles to micelles occurs. The phospholipids are transferred more efficiently than cholesterol, leading to cholesterol enrichment of the remaining vesicles. These cholesterol-rich vesicles aggregate to form large multilamellar liquid vesicles that then precipitate cholesterol monohydrate crystals. Several pronucleating factors including mucin glycoproteins, immunoglobulins, and transferrin accelerate the precipitation of cholesterol in bile.

For gallstones to cause clinical symptoms, they must obtain a size sufficient to produce mechanical injury to the gallbladder or obstruction of the biliary tree. Growth of stones may occur in two ways: (1) progressive enlargement of individual crystals or stones by deposition of additional insoluble precipitate at the bile-stone interface or (2) fusion of individual crystals or stones to form a larger conglomerate. In addition, defects in gallbladder motility increase the residence time of bile in the gallbladder, thereby playing a role in stone formation. Gallstone formation occurs in clinical states with gallbladder stasis, as

seen with prolonged fasting, the use of long-term parenteral nutrition, after vagotomy, and in patients with somatostatin-producing tumors or in those receiving long-term somatostatin therapy.[3]

Pigment Gallstones

With the recognition that calcium salts are present in most, if not all, cholesterol gallstones, renewed interest has developed in the events leading to the precipitation of calcium with the anions, bilirubin, carbonate, phosphate, or palmitate. Precipitation of these anions as insoluble calcium salts serves as a nidus for cholesterol stone formation. Furthermore, calcium bilirubinate and calcium palmitate also form major components of pigment gallstones.

Pigment gallstones are classified as either black or brown pigment stones. Black pigment stones are typically tarry and are associated frequently with hemolytic conditions or cirrhosis. In hemolytic states, the bilirubin load and concentration of unconjugated bilirubin increases. These stones are usually not associated with infected bile and are located almost exclusively in the gallbladder. In contrast, brown pigment stones are earthy in texture and are typically found in the bile ducts, especially in Asian populations. Brown stones often contain more cholesterol and calcium palmitate and occur as primary common duct stones in Western patients with disorders of biliary motility and associated bacterial infection. In these settings, bacteria-producing slime and those containing the enzyme-glucuronidase cause enzymatic hydrolysis of soluble conjugated bilirubin glucuronide to form free bilirubin, which then precipitates with calcium.[3]

Natural History of Gallstone Disease

Once gallstones develop, they remain silent (asymptomatic) or they can produce biliary pain by obstructing the cystic duct. Additional complications related to gallstones

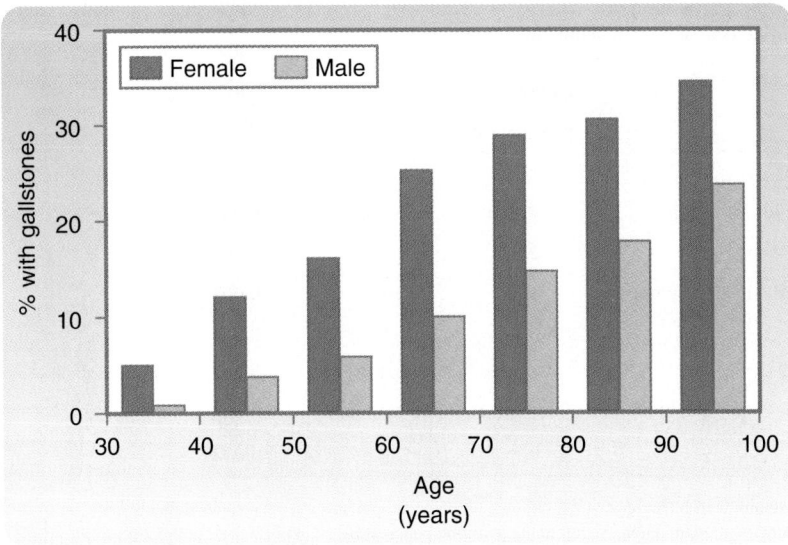

FIGURE 52-6. Influence of age and gender on the incidence of cholelithiasis. Gallstones are more common in females and increase in incidence with aging. (Adapted from Bateson MC: Gallbladder disease and cholecystectomy rate are independently variable. Lancet 2:621-624, 1984.)

include acute cholecystitis, choledocholithiasis with or without cholangitis, gallstone pancreatitis, gallstone ileus, and even gallbladder carcinoma. The prevalence of gallstones is related to a number of factors including age, gender, weight, family history, and ethnic background. The age-related incidence of gallstones among men and women is shown in Figure 52-6.[10] In addition, common dietary factors and medications can also influence the risk of developing symptomatic gallstones. For example, coffee consumption lowers and hormone therapy increases the risk of developing symptomatic gallstones.

Gallstones are common and are frequently identified at laparotomy or on sonography or with other radiologic studies in patients without typical symptoms of biliary tract disease. Several studies have examined the likelihood of developing biliary colic, more significant complications of gallstone disease, or of undergoing cholecystectomy. Approximately 1% to 2% of asymptomatic individuals with gallstones develop serious symptoms or complications related to their gallstones per year, and a similar percentage require cholecystectomy. Over a 20-year period, two thirds of asymptomatic patients with gallstones remain symptom free. The longer stones remain quiescent, the less likely symptoms are to develop.

Patients with mild symptoms (intermittent right upper quadrant pain) have a higher risk of developing gallstone-related complications or requiring cholecystectomy than asymptomatic patients with gallstones. Approximately 1% to 3% of mildly symptomatic patients develop gallstone-related complications per year, and at least 6% to 8% require a cholecystectomy per year to manage their gallbladder symptoms. However, as the magnitude of symptoms attributable to the gallbladder increases, so does the likelihood that those symptoms will persist or recur or that complications of gallstones will develop. For patients with ongoing episodes of biliary colic, 70% will have further episodes of gallbladder pain within the following 1 year.[11] Delay in managing symptomatic gallstones with laparoscopic cholecystectomy may contribute to the high

prevalence of gallstone-related complications. Forty-four percent of cholecystectomies done in California in 1996 were performed for complications of gallstones (acute cholecystitis 36%, gallstone pancreatitis 4%, choledocholithiasis 3%, other 1%), and half of these patients had biliary symptoms and ultrasound confirmation of gallstones prior to developing these complications (Table 52-4).[3]

Diagnosis of Gallbladder Disease

Abdominal Radiograph

The abdominal plain film is often the initial radiologic study performed in patients presenting with acute abdominal pain. In general, abdominal plain films have a low yield in diagnosing biliary tract problems. Gallstones are predominantly cholesterol, which is radiolucent. Only 10% to 15% of gallstones contain sufficient calcium to be radiopaque on abdominal radiographs. Rarely, additional useful information may be obtained (i.e., pneumobilia, calcified gallbladder, and so forth). Abdominal films are most useful in diagnosing or excluding the diagnosis of other causes of acute abdominal pain.

Ultrasound

Ultrasound has become the procedure of choice for documenting gallstones and is also extremely useful at identifying biliary dilation. Ultrasound images are based on reflected high frequency sound waves, which are formed at the interface of two tissues or structures with different acoustic properties. Gallstones have several distinguishing characteristics that are employed in their ultrasonographic diagnosis. The most useful include high-amplitude echodensity, which leaves an acoustic shadow or absence of reflected sound waves behind the gallstone (Fig. 52-7). In addition, gravity-dependent movement of the gallstones with patient repositioning is also a highly specific finding

TABLE 52-4.   Effect of Gallstone Presentation on Treatment Outcome

Variables	Gallstone Presentation		P
	Uncomplicated*	Complicated†	
Percentage of cases	56	44	
Delay: onset symptoms until surgery (days)	728	142	<0.001
Delay: first ultrasound until surgery (days)	210	177	0.56
Percentage of patients with biliary colic as first symptom	100	52	<0.001
Length of hospital stay (days)	3.1	5.1	<0.001
LC/OC ratio	4:1	1.9:1	<0.001
Hospital cost ($)	16,200	22,800	<0.001
Hospital mortality (%)	0.5	0.8	<0.002

*Uncomplicated gallstone disease includes patients with biliary colic.
†Complicated gallstone disease includes patients with acute cholecystitis, acute gallstone pancreatitis, choledocholithiasis, gallbladder cancer, and cholangitis.
LC, laparoscopic cholecystectomy; OC, open cholecystectomy.
Adapted from Glasgow RE, Cho M, Hutter MM, et al: The spectrum and cost of complicated gallstone disease in California. Arch Surg 135:1021-1027, 2000.

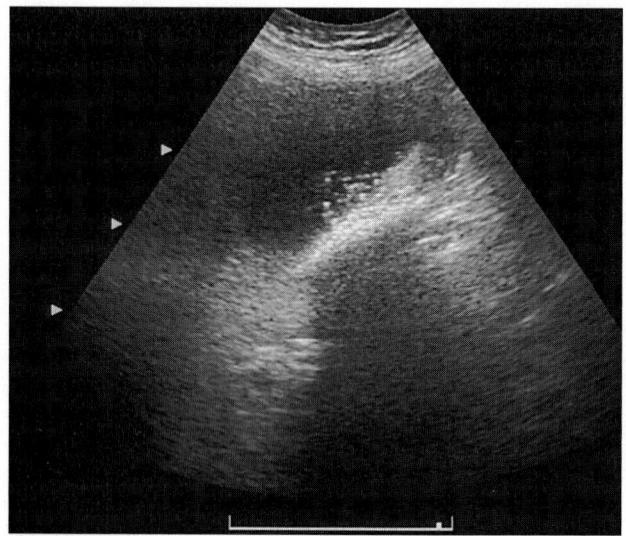

FIGURE 52-7.   Gallbladder ultrasound in patient with biliary colic demonstrating multiple dependent echogenic foci with posterior acoustic shadowing consistent with gallstones.

for gallstones. When these two features are present, the accuracy of ultrasound at diagnosing gallstones approaches 100%.

Several features lower the diagnostic accuracy of ultrasound in detecting gallstones. Small gallstones may not demonstrate an acoustic shadow. Furthermore, a lack of fluid (bile) around the gallstones (stone impacted in cystic duct, gallbladder filled with gallstones) also impairs their detection. In addition, an ileus with increased abdominal gas as occurs with acute cholecystitis may hamper gallbladder visualization. Overall, the false-negative rate for ultrasound in detecting gallstones is approximately 5%.

Cholescintigraphy

Cholescintigraphy provides a noninvasive evaluation of the liver, gallbladder, bile duct, and duodenum with both anatomic and functional information. Technetium-labeled analogues of iminodiacetic acid are currently used for imaging and are excreted into the biliary tract shortly after injection. Uptake by the liver, gallbladder, common bile duct, and duodenum all should be present after 1 hour. Slow uptake of the tracer by the liver suggests hepatic parenchymal disease. Nonvisualization of the gallbladder with prompt filling of the common bile duct and small intestine is consistent with cystic duct obstruction. Filling of the gallbladder and common bile duct with delayed or absent filling of the intestine suggests an obstruction at the ampulla.

The primary use of cholescintigraphy is in the diagnosis of acute cholecystitis. Although used less frequently for this indication than in the past because of the availability and accuracy of ultrasound, cholescintigraphy demonstrates the presence of cystic duct obstruction, which is invariably present in acute cholecystitis. Nonvisualization of the gallbladder 1 hour after the injection of the radioisotope with filling of the common bile duct and duodenum is consistent with total or partial cystic duct obstruction. Increasing sphincter of Oddi and, thus, biliary pressures with morphine may enhance gallbladder filling and lower the incidence of false-positive examinations. The sensitivity and specificity of cholescintigraphy for diagnosing acute cholecystitis are each about 95%. False-positive results are increased in the setting of gallbladder stasis as in critically ill patients or in patients on parenteral nutrition.

Miscellaneous

Abdominal CT scans are more useful in the evaluation of gallbladder cancer than calculous disease. However, like plain abdominal films, calcified gallstones are also identified on CT scans in approximately one half of patients. CT is also a sensitive test for diagnosing acute cholecystitis.

Chronic Calculous Cholecystitis

Pathogenesis

The term *chronic cholecystitis* implies an ongoing or recurrent inflammatory process involving the gallbladder. In the majority of patients (>90%), gallstones are the causative factor and lead to recurrent episodes of cystic duct obstruction manifest as biliary pain or colic. Over time, these recurrent attacks can lead to scarring and a nonfunctioning gallbladder. Histopathologically, chronic cholecystitis is characterized by an increase in subepithelial and subserosal fibrosis and a mononuclear cell infiltrate.

Clinical Presentation

The primary symptom associated with chronic cholecystitis or symptomatic cholelithiasis is pain often labeled biliary colic. The term *biliary colic* is inaccurate and suggests that the pain related to gallstones is intermittent and spasmodic like other colicky pain. However, this pattern is rarely the case. Obstruction of the cystic duct results in a progressive increase in tension in the gallbladder wall, leading to constant pain in most patients. The pain is usually located in the right upper quadrant and/or epigastrium and frequently radiates to the right upper back, right scapula, or between the scapulae. The intensity of the pain is often severe enough to seek immediate medical attention with the first episode. Classically, the pain of biliary colic occurs following a greasy meal, although this situation does not occur in most cases. An association with meals is present in only 50% of patients, and in these patients, the pain often develops more than an hour after eating. In the remaining patients, the pain is not temporally related to meals and often begins at night-time, waking the patient from sleep.

The duration of pain is typically 1 to 5 hours. The attacks rarely persist for more than 24 hours and are rarely shorter than 1 hour. Pain lasting beyond 24 hours suggests that acute inflammation or cholecystitis is present. The attacks are often discrete and severe enough that the patient can accurately recall and number them. The episodes of biliary colic are usually less frequent than one episode per week. Other symptoms such as nausea and vomiting often accompany each episode (60% to 70% of cases). Bloating and belching are also present in 50% of patients. Fever and jaundice occur much less frequently with simple biliary colic.

The physical examination is usually completely normal in patients with chronic cholecystitis, particularly if they are pain free. During an episode of biliary colic, mild right upper quadrant tenderness may be present. Laboratory values such as serum bilirubin, transaminases, and alkaline phosphatase are also usually normal in patients with uncomplicated gallstones.

Diagnosis

The diagnosis of symptomatic cholelithiasis or chronic calculous cholecystitis requires two findings: (1) abdominal pain consistent with biliary colic and (2) the presence of gallstones. The presence of symptoms (usually pain) attributable to the gallbladder is necessary to consider any treatment for gallstones. Patients without symptoms (~ two thirds of patients with gallstones) develop symptoms at a low rate and complications of gallstones at an even lower rate (see Natural History of Gallstone Disease). In most cases treatment is not necessary in these asymptomatic patients. In patients without the episodic pain characteristic of biliary colic, alternate diagnoses should be sought. Other conditions with acute upper abdominal pain that should be included in the differential diagnosis include gastroesophageal reflux disease, acute pancreatitis, peptic ulcer disease, or irritable bowel syndrome. Further studies to exclude these conditions should be performed in patients with gallstones and atypical symptoms.

The presence of gallstones should also be documented. Ultrasound is quite sensitive (95% to 98%) for documenting the presence of gallstones and also provides additional anatomic information—presence of polyps, common bile duct diameter, or any hepatic parenchymal abnormalities. Gallstones are occasionally identified on abdominal radiographs (15%) or CT scans (50%) as gallstones contain enough calcium to be visualized.

Management

The treatment of choice for patients with symptomatic gallstones is elective laparoscopic cholecystectomy. The morbidity and mortality of laparoscopic cholecystectomy are similar to recent large series of patients undergoing elective open cholecystectomy for chronic cholecystitis. The mortality rate for both procedures is approximately 0.1% with cardiovascular complications being the most frequent cause of death. The most significant complication following laparoscopic cholecystectomy is injury to the biliary tract. Overall, complications occur in fewer than 10% of patients. Conversion to an open cholecystectomy is necessary in less than 5% of patients undergoing laparoscopic cholecystectomy for chronic cholecystitis. Conversion rates are increased in elderly, obese, and male patients.

The long-term results of laparoscopic cholecystectomy in appropriately selected patients with chronic cholecystitis are excellent. More than 90% of patients with typical biliary pain and gallstones are rendered symptom free following cholecystectomy. For patients with atypical symptoms or painless dyspepsia (fatty food intolerance, flatulence, belching, or bloating), the percentage of patients experiencing relief of symptoms falls.

Acute Calculous Cholecystitis

Pathophysiology

In 90% to 95% of cases, acute cholecystitis is related to gallstones. Obstruction of the cystic duct by a gallstone leads to biliary colic and is also the first event in acute cholecystitis. If the cystic duct remains obstructed, the gallbladder distends, and the gallbladder wall becomes inflamed and edematous. In the most severe cases (5% to 18%), this process can lead to ischemia and necrosis of the gallbladder wall. More frequently, the gallstone is dislodged and the inflammation gradually resolves. Initially, acute cholecystitis is an inflammatory process. Approximately 50% of patients with uncomplicated acute cholecystitis have positive bile cultures at the time of cholecystectomy. In the most severe cases, generalized sepsis may be present.

Clinical Presentation

Right upper quadrant abdominal pain is the most common complaint in patients with acute cholecystitis. The pain may be similar to previous episodes of biliary colic, but the pain of acute cholecystitis persists for longer than an uncomplicated episode of biliary colic (days vs. several hours). Other common symptoms include nausea, vomiting, and fever. On physical examination, focal tenderness and guarding are usually present inferior to the right costal margin, distinguishing the episode from simple biliary colic. A mass may be present in the right upper quadrant (gallbladder with adherent omentum), and a Murphy's sign (inspiratory arrest with deep palpation in the right upper quadrant) may also be elicited. A mild leukocytosis is usually present (12,000 to 14,000 cells/mm^3). In addition, mild elevations in serum bilirubin (>4 mg/dL), alkaline phosphatase, the transaminases, and amylase may be present.

Diagnosis

Ultrasound is the most useful radiologic examination in the patient with suspected cholecystitis (Fig. 52-8). First, in the patient without known gallstones, ultrasound is a sensitive test for establishing the presence or absence of gallstones. Additional findings suggestive of acute cholecystitis include thickening of the gallbladder wall (>4 mm) and pericholecystic fluid. Focal tenderness directly over the gallbladder (sonographic Murphy's sign) is also suggestive of acute cholecystitis. Ultrasound has a sensitivity and specificity of 85% and 95%, respectively, for diagnosing acute cholecystitis.

Radionuclide scanning is used less frequently for the diagnosis of acute cholecystitis but may provide additional information in the atypical case. Nonfilling of the gallbladder with the radiotracer (^{99}Tc-HIDA) indicates an obstructed cystic duct and, in the right clinical setting, is highly sensitive (95%) and specific (95%) for acute cholecystitis.

Management

Once the diagnosis of acute cholecystitis is made, the patient should have oral intake limited and be started on intravenous antibiotics. An antibiotic appropriate for the common biliary tract pathogens isolated from the bile in patients with acute cholecystitis should be selected (see

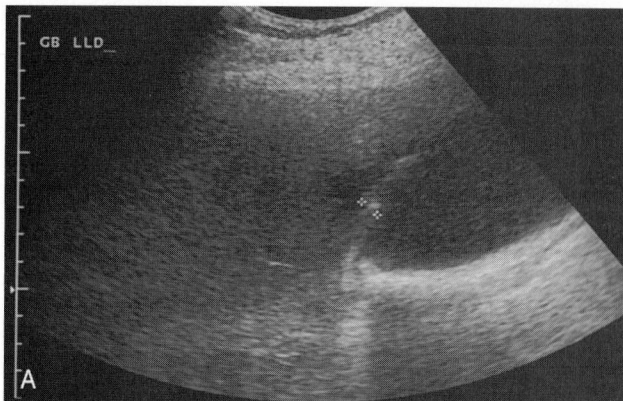

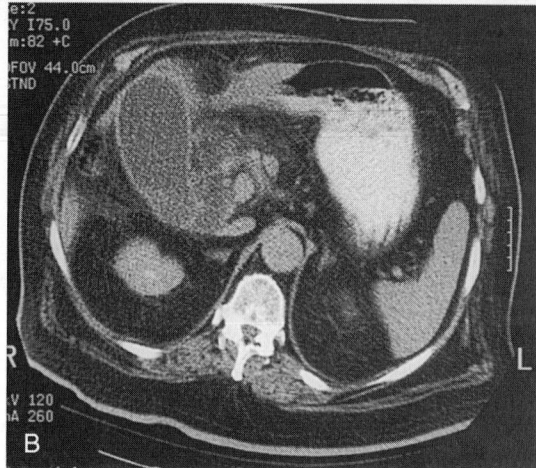

FIGURE 52-8.   **A**, Gallbladder ultrasound in patient with acute cholecystitis demonstrating gallbladder wall thickening (4.2 mm as indicated), and pericholecystic fluid. **B**, Abdominal CT scan in same patient showing distended, thick-walled gallbladder with pericholecystic fluid.

Antibiotic Selection in Biliary Tract Surgery). Parenteral analgesia should also be administered. Unfortunately, narcotics increase biliary pressure, whereas nonsteroidal analgesics, which inhibit prostaglandin synthesis, reduce gallbladder mucin production and therefore relieve pressure and pain.

Open cholecystectomy has been the standard treatment for acute cholecystitis for many years. At the time laparoscopic cholecystectomy was introduced, acute cholecystitis was a relative contraindication. However, with increased experience laparoscopic cholecystectomy has become the preferred approach for most patients with acute cholecystitis. The morbidity rate, hospital stay, and time to return to work all have been lower in patients undergoing laparoscopic cholecystectomy than open cholecystectomy in prospective, randomized trials.[12] However, the conversion rate in the setting of acute cholecystitis (4% to 35%) is higher than with chronic cholecystitis.

The timing of cholecystectomy for acute cholecystitis has been studied for several decades and has been further evaluated recently using laparoscopic cholecystectomy as the primary therapy. Two prospective, randomized trials have compared immediate laparoscopic cholecystectomy versus laparoscopic cholecystectomy after a period of initial medical treatment (6 weeks) to "cool off" the gallbladder.[13,14] Approximately 20% of patients in the delayed surgery arm failed initial medical therapy and had to be operated on during the initial admission or before the end of the planned cooling off period. No significant differences were observed in the conversion rate to open cholecystectomy among patients undergoing early cholecystectomy versus those managed with delayed surgery. No significant differences in the complication rate were observed among early and delayed surgery. However, hospital stay, and therefore cost, was significantly reduced in both trials in the early laparoscopic cholecystectomy group.

Several retrospective series have demonstrated advantages to proceeding with laparoscopic cholecystectomy soon after the diagnosis of acute cholecystitis is made. In one series, patients operated on early in the course of their illness (within 48 hours of presentation) were more likely to have the procedure completed laparoscopically (4% vs. 23%) than patients with a longer duration of symptoms and also had a shorter hospital stay.[15] Additional factors predicting the need to convert to an open cholecystectomy include increased patient age, male gender, elevated American Society of Anesthesiologists class, obesity, and thickened gallbladder wall (>4 mm). Thus, in most patients with acute cholecystitis, laparoscopic cholecystectomy should be attempted soon (24 to 48 hours) after the diagnosis is made. Conversion to an open procedure should be made if the inflammation prevents adequate visualization of important structures.

Complications

Acute cholecystitis may progress to empyema of the gallbladder, emphysematous cholecystitis, or perforation of the gallbladder despite antibiotic therapy. In each case, emergency cholecystectomy is warranted, if the patient can withstand an anesthetic. Empyema occurs with bacterial proliferation in an obstructed gallbladder and results in a pus-filled organ. Patients with empyema of the gallbladder may be toxic with more marked fever and leukocytosis. Laparoscopic cholecystectomy may be attempted, but the conversion rate is high.

Emphysematous cholecystitis develops more commonly in men and patients with diabetes mellitus. Severe right upper quadrant pain and generalized sepsis are frequently present. Abdominal films or CT scans may demonstrate air within the gallbladder wall or lumen. Prompt antibiotic therapy to cover the common biliary pathogens (*E. coli*, *Enterococcus*, *Klebsiella*, and so forth) as well as *Clostridium* species and emergency cholecystectomy are appropriate treatments.

Perforation of the gallbladder occurs in up to 10% of cases of acute cholecystitis. Perforation is a sequelae of ischemia and gangrene of the gallbladder wall and occurs most commonly in the gallbladder fundus. The perforation is most frequently (50% of cases) contained within the subhepatic space by the omentum, duodenum, liver, and hepatic flexure of the colon, and a localized abscess forms. Less commonly, the gallbladder perforates into and adja-

cent viscus (duodenum or colon) resulting in a cholecystoenteric fistula (see Gallstone Ileus). Rarely, the gallbladder perforates freely into the peritoneal cavity leading to generalized peritonitis. With gallbladder perforation, the abdominal tenderness, fever, and white blood cell count are more pronounced or higher than in uncomplicated acute cholecystitis. Localized right upper quadrant pain and tenderness, which becomes diffuse and generalized, should raise the suspicion of free gallbladder perforation. Intravenous fluids, antibiotics, and emergency cholecystectomy are the treatment of choice in patients with gallbladder perforation.

In most patients, cholecystectomy can be performed and is the best treatment of complicated acute cholecystitis. Occasionally, the inflammatory process obscures the structures in the triangle of Calot precluding safe dissection or ligation of the cystic duct. In these patients partial cholecystectomy, cauterization of the remaining gallbladder mucosa, and drainage avoids injury to the common bile duct. In patients considered too unstable to undergo laparotomy because of concurrent medical comorbidities, percutaneous transhepatic cholecystostomy can drain the gallbladder. Success rates approaching 90% have been reported with percutaneous cholecystostomy in managing critically ill patients thought to have acute cholecystitis. However, this procedure leaves in the gallbladder, which may be partially gangrenous and a source of ongoing sepsis. Interval laparoscopic cholecystectomy should then be performed after a delay of 3 to 4 months to allow the patient to recover and the acute inflammation to resolve.

Acute Acalculous Cholecystitis

Acute acalculous cholecystitis accounts for 5% to 10% of all patients with acute cholecystitis and is the diagnosis in approximately 1% to 2% of patients undergoing cholecystectomy. The disease often has a more fulminant course than acute calculous cholecystitis and frequently progresses to gangrene, empyema, or perforation. Acute acalculous cholecystitis usually occurs in the critically ill patient following trauma, burns, long-term parenteral nutrition, and major nonbiliary operations such as abdominal aneurysm repair and cardiopulmonary bypass. The etiology of acute acalculous cholecystitis remains unclear, although gallbladder stasis and ischemia have been most often implicated as causative factors. Stasis is common in critically ill patients not being fed enterally and may lead to colonization of the gallbladder with bacteria. Visceral ischemia is also a common denominator in patients with acute acalculous cholecystitis and may explain the high incidence of gallbladder gangrene. Decreased arteriolar and capillary filling is present in acute acalculous cholecystitis in contrast with the dilation of these vessels observed in acute calculous cholecystitis.

The symptoms and signs of acute acalculous cholecystitis are similar to acute calculous cholecystitis with right upper quadrant pain and tenderness, fever, and leukocytosis most frequently present. However, these findings are often masked by other conditions in the critically ill patient. CT scan and ultrasound findings are similar to calculous cholecystitis and include gallbladder wall thickening and pericholecystic fluid in the absence of gallstones. Cholescintigraphy demonstrates absent gallbladder filling in acute acalculous cholecystitis. However, the false-positive rate (absent gallbladder filling without acute acalculous cholecystitis) may be as high as 40%. Morphine cholescintigraphy has improved the accuracy of this study in the critically ill patient.

Emergency cholecystectomy is the appropriate treatment once the diagnosis is established or the suspicion is high. The incidence of gangrene, perforation, and empyema exceeds 50%; therefore, open cholecystectomy usually is required in this setting. The mortality rate for acute acalculous cholecystitis in recent series remains high (40%) in large part due to the concomitant illnesses in patients who develop this disease.

Biliary Dyskinesia

A subgroup of patients presenting with typical symptoms of biliary colic (postprandial right upper quadrant pain, fatty food intolerance, and nausea) do not have any evidence of gallstones on ultrasound examination. Further investigations have usually been performed in these patients to exclude any other pathology. This work-up often includes an abdominal CT scan, esophagogastroduodenoscopy, or even an ERC. In these patients, the diagnosis of biliary dyskinesia or chronic acalculous cholecystitis should be considered. The CCK-Tc-HIDA scan has been useful in identifying patients with this disorder. CCK is infused intravenously after the gallbladder has filled with the ^{99}Tc-labeled radionuclide. Twenty minutes after the administration of CCK, a gallbladder ejection fraction is calculated. An ejection fraction less than 35% at 20 minutes is considered abnormal.

Patients with symptoms of biliary colic and an abnormal gallbladder ejection fraction should be managed with a laparoscopic cholecystectomy. Between 85% and 94% of patients with a low gallbladder ejection fraction and symptoms of biliary colic will be asymptomatic or improved by cholecystectomy. Most of these patients will have histopathologic evidence of chronic cholecystitis.

Cholecystectomy: Indications and Technique

Cholecystectomy is the most common gastrointestinal operation performed in the United States. Since the introduction of laparoscopic cholecystectomy, the number of cholecystectomies performed in the United States has increased from approximately 500,000 per year to 700,000 per year. Most of these procedures can be safely completed using the laparoscopic technique. Most conditions initially considered to be relative contraindications early in the laparoscopic experience are no longer thought to mandate an open cholecystectomy. Uncontrolled coagulopathy is one of the few current contraindications to laparoscopic cholecystectomy. In addition, patients with severe chronic obstructive pulmonary disease or congestive heart failure may not tolerate the pneumoperitoneum required for performing laparoscopic surgery. Currently, the major contraindication to completing a laparoscopic cholecystectomy is an inability to clearly identify all of the anatomic structures. A liberal policy of converting to an open operation when important anatomic structures cannot be clearly defined represents good surgical judgment rather than a complication. The conversion rate for elective laparoscopic cholecystectomy ranges up to 5%, whereas the conversion rate in the emergency setting for acute cholecystitis may be as high as 30%.[12-14]

The technical difficulty of laparoscopic cholecystectomy is increased in several clinical settings. Laparoscopic cholecystectomy can be performed safely in acute cholecystitis, albeit with a higher conversion rate and operative time than in the elective setting. Morbid obesity, once thought to be a relative contraindication to the laparoscopic approach, is not associated with a higher conversion rate. Longer trocars and instruments and an increase in intra-abdominal pressure may be helpful in these patients. Prior upper abdominal surgery may increase the difficulty of or preclude laparoscopic cholecystectomy. However, placement of a Hasson cannula often reveals few adhesions or adhesions that can be dissected laparoscopically, permitting completion of a laparoscopic cholecystectomy. Elective laparoscopic cholecystectomy has also been completed safely in patients with well-compensated cirrhosis (Childs classes A and B), although difficulty retracting the firm liver and increased bleeding from collaterals have been noted.

Laparoscopic Cholecystectomy

Patients undergoing laparoscopic cholecystectomy are prepared and draped in a similar fashion to open cholecystectomy. Conversion to an open operation should be discussed with the patient, included in the operative consent, and is necessary in up to 5% of patients undergoing elective cholecystectomy and up to 30% of patients undergoing laparoscopic cholecystectomy for acute cholecystitis. A Foley catheter and orogastric tube are inserted to avoid inadvertent injury and improve exposure. Laparoscopic surgery requires a space for visualization and instrument manipulation, and this space is usually created by establishing a pneumoperitoneum with carbon dioxide. Both open and closed methods have been used to establish a pneumoperitoneum. With the open technique, a small incision is made above the umbilicus into the peritoneal cavity. A special blunt-tipped cannula (Hasson) with a gas-tight sleeve is inserted into the peritoneal cavity and anchored to the fascia. This technique is often used following previous abdominal surgery and should avoid infrequent, but potentially life-threatening trocar injuries. In the closed technique a special hollow insufflation needle (Veress) with a retractable cutting sheath is inserted into the peritoneal cavity through a supraumbilical incision and used for insufflation.[16,17]

Once an adequate pneumoperitoneum has been established, an 11-mm trocar is inserted through the supraumbilical incision. The laparoscope with attached video camera is then inserted through the umbilical port, and an examination of the peritoneal cavity is performed. Both forward viewing (0-degree) and angled (30-degree) laparoscopes are available. With either the open or closed techniques, additional trocars are inserted under direct vision. Most surgeons use a second 11-mm trocar–placed subxiphoid and two additional 5-mm trocars positioned subcostally in the right upper quadrant in the midclavicular and anterior axillary lines (Fig. 52-9). Also available are 5-mm cameras and 3-mm instruments.[16,17]

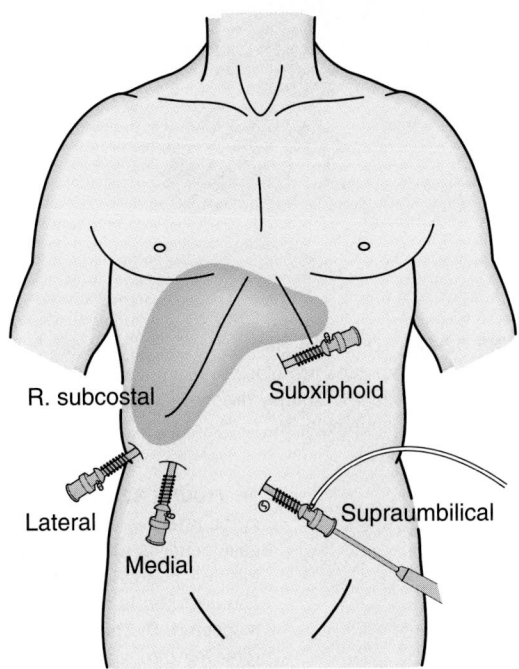

FIGURE 52-9. Trocar placement for laparoscopic cholecystectomy. The laparoscope is placed through a 10-mm port just above the umbilicus. Additional ports are placed in the epigastrium and subcostally in the mid-clavicular and near the anterior axillary lines. (From Cameron J: Atlas of Surgery, Vol 2. Philadelphia, BC Decker, 1994.)

The two smaller ports are used for grasping the gallbladder and placing it in the ideal position for an antegrade cholecystectomy. The lateral port is used to retract the gallbladder cephalad elevating the inferior edge of the liver and exposing the gallbladder and cystic duct (Fig. 52-10). The medial 5-mm cannula is used to grasp the gallbladder infundibulum and retract it laterally to further expose the triangle of Calot. This maneuver may require bluntly taking down any adhesions between the omentum or duodenum and the gallbladder. The junction of the gallbladder and cystic duct is identified by stripping the peritoneum off the gallbladder neck and removing any tissue surrounding the gallbladder neck and proximal cystic duct. This dissection is continued until the triangle of Calot is cleared of all fatty and lymphatic tissue and the gallbladder infundibulum is elevated off the liver bed (Fig. 52-11).[18] At this point two structures (cystic artery and cystic duct) should be seen entering the gallbladder.

Once the cystic duct is identified, an intraoperative cholangiogram may be performed by placing a hemoclip proximally on the cystic duct, incising the anterior surface of the duct, and passing a cholangiogram catheter into the cystic duct. Once the cholangiogram is completed, two clips are placed distally on the cystic duct, which is then divided (Fig. 52-12). Alternatively, the common bile duct may be evaluated for stones using laparoscopic ultrasound. The sensitivity of laparoscopic ultrasound for detecting common bile duct stones is comparable to intraoperative cholangiography (80% to 96% vs. 75% to 99%). A large cystic duct may require placement of a pretied loop ligature to provide a secure closure.[16,17]

The next step is the division of the cystic artery. The artery is usually encountered running parallel to and behind the cystic duct. Once identified and isolated, clips are placed proximally and distally on the artery, which is then divided. Once the artery and any branches are controlled, the gallbladder is dissected out of the gallbladder fossa using either a hook or spatula cautery (Fig. 52-13).

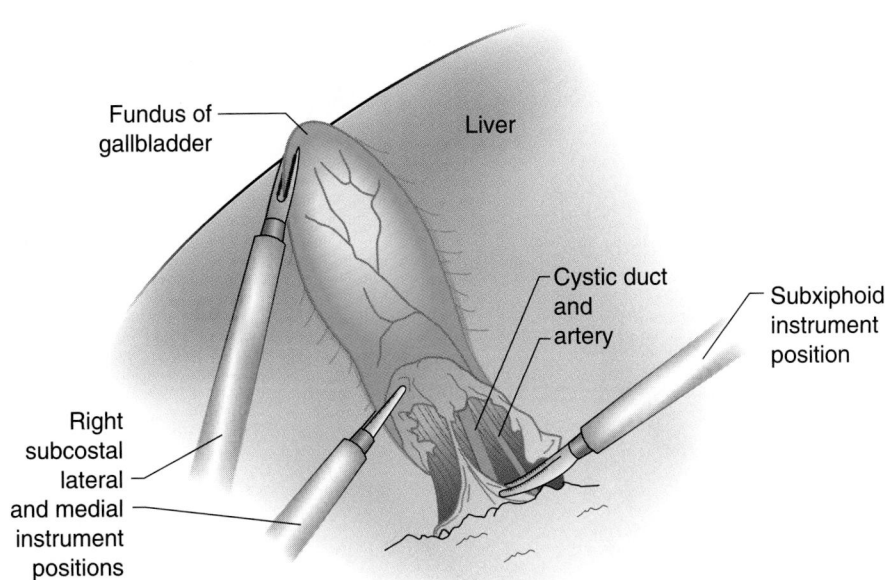

FIGURE 52-10. The gallbladder is retracted cephalad using the grasper on the gallbladder fundus and laterally at the infundibulum. The peritoneum overlying the gallbladder infundibulum and neck and the cystic duct is divided bluntly, exposing the cystic duct. (From Cameron J: Atlas of Surgery, Vol 2. Philadelphia, BC Decker, 1994.)

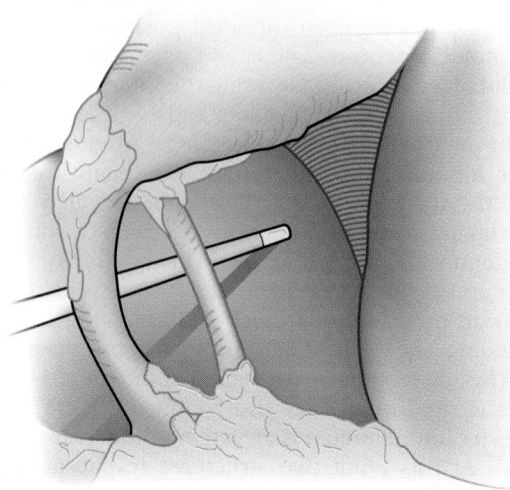

FIGURE 52-11.   View obtained after dissection within the triangle of Calot demonstrating the cystic duct and cystic artery clearly entering the gallbladder. At this point it is safe to ligate and divide the cystic duct. (From Strasberg SM, Hertl M, Soper NJ: An analysis of the problem of biliary injury during laparoscopic cholecystectomy. J Am Coll Surg 180:101-125, 1995.)

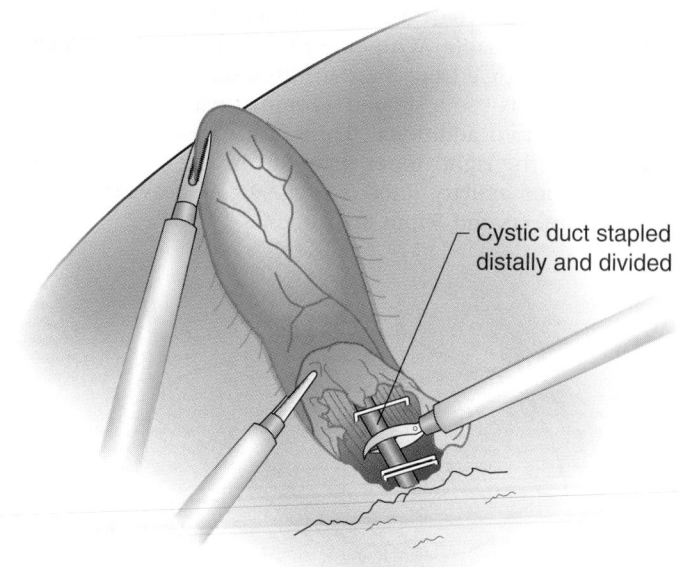

Cystic duct stapled distally and divided

FIGURE 52-12.   Once the gallbladder cystic duct junction has been clearly identified, clips are placed proximally and distally on the cystic duct, and the duct is sharply divided. (From Cameron J: Atlas of Surgery, Vol 2. Philadelphia, BC Decker, 1994.)

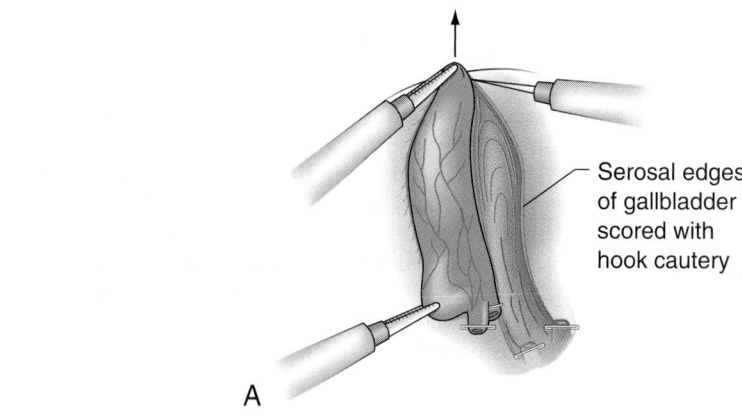

Serosal edges of gallbladder scored with hook cautery

A

FIGURE 52-13.   **A,** After the cystic artery is divided, the gallbladder is dissected out of the liver bed using cautery. **B,** The liver bed is then irrigated and inspected. **C,** The gallbladder is removed through the supraumbilical incision. (**A–C,** From Cameron J: Atlas of Surgery, Vol 2. Philadelphia, BC Decker, 1994.)

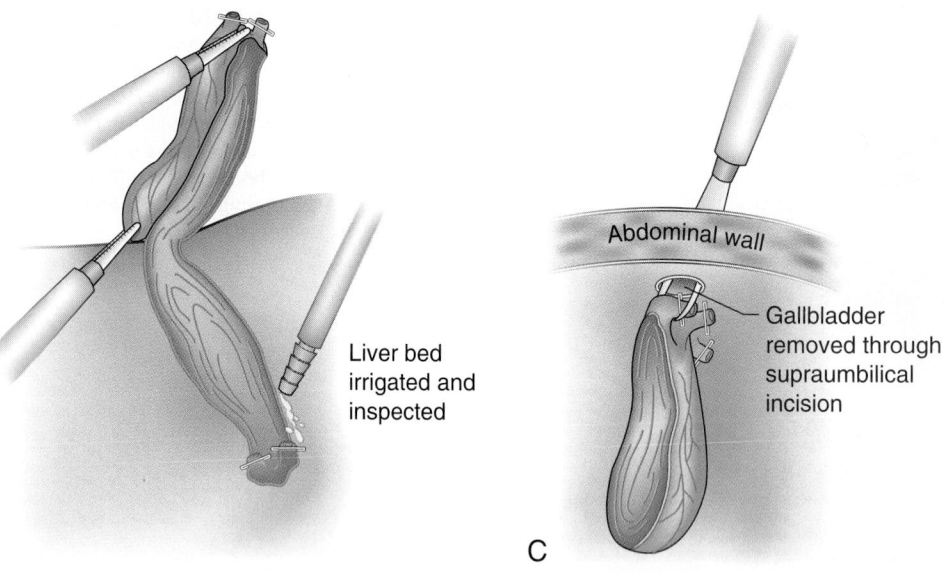

Liver bed irrigated and inspected

Abdominal wall

Gallbladder removed through supraumbilical incision

B   C

The peritoneum overlying the gallbladder is placed on tension using the two grasping forceps, and the peritoneum and adventitia between the gallbladder and liver are divided with the cautery. Just prior to removing the gallbladder from the liver, the operative field is carefully searched for hemostasis, and adequate placement of the cystic duct and artery clips is confirmed. The gallbladder is then dissected off the liver and is usually removed through the umbilical port. The fascial defect and skin incision may need to be enlarged to remove the gallbladder and contained gallstones. If the gallbladder has been entered during the dissection or if it is acutely inflamed or gangrenous, the gallbladder may be placed in a plastic specimen retrieval bag prior to removing it from the peritoneal cavity.[16,17]

Many centers have demonstrated that elective laparoscopic cholecystectomy can be safely performed as an outpatient procedure.[19] Among patients selected for outpatient management, 77% to 97% of patients can be successfully discharged the same day. Factors contributing to overnight admission include uncontrolled pain, nausea and vomiting, operative duration greater than 60 minutes, and cases completed late in the day.

Open Cholecystectomy

Open cholecystectomy can be performed through either an upper midline or right subcostal (Kocher) incision. Identification and division of the cystic duct and artery initially limit bleeding from the gallbladder for the remainder of the dissection. With lateral traction on the gallbladder neck, the peritoneum overlying the triangle of Calot is incised, and the cystic duct is identified and ligated distally (Fig. 52-14A). A cholangiogram is performed at this time if indicated. The cystic duct is then ligated proximally and divided. Similarly, the cystic artery is ligated and divided after carefully tracing it onto the gallbladder (Fig. 52-14B). If the anatomy cannot be clearly identified, the gallbladder should be dissected from the fundus downward toward the gallbladder neck, making the ductal and vascular anatomy easier to identify. The gallbladder is dissected out of the gallbladder bed by incising the overlying peritoneum with cautery (Fig. 52-15A). At this point a cystic duct cholangiogram is performed (Fig. 52-15B). Rarely, a small duct entering the gallbladder from the liver is encountered and then should be ligated. A closed-suction drain is placed if there is concern about the security of the cystic duct closure (i.e., gangrenous cholecystitis).

Choledocholithiasis

Common bile duct stones are classified both by their point of origin as well as the time at which they are discovered relative to cholecystectomy. Most common bile duct calculi in the United States form initially in the gallbladder (see Gallstone Pathogenesis) and migrate through the cystic duct into the common bile duct. These stones are identified as secondary calculi to distinguish them from primary common bile duct calculi, which form within the biliary tract. Common duct stones are also defined as retained, if they are discovered within 2 years of cholecystectomy, or recurrent, if they are detected more than 2 years following cholecystectomy. Retained stones were most likely present at the time of the cholecystectomy.

Primary common duct stones are associated with biliary stasis and infection. Primary stones are usually of the brown pigment type, which are soft and crumble easily when manipulated. The cause of the biliary stasis, which leads to the development of primary duct stones,

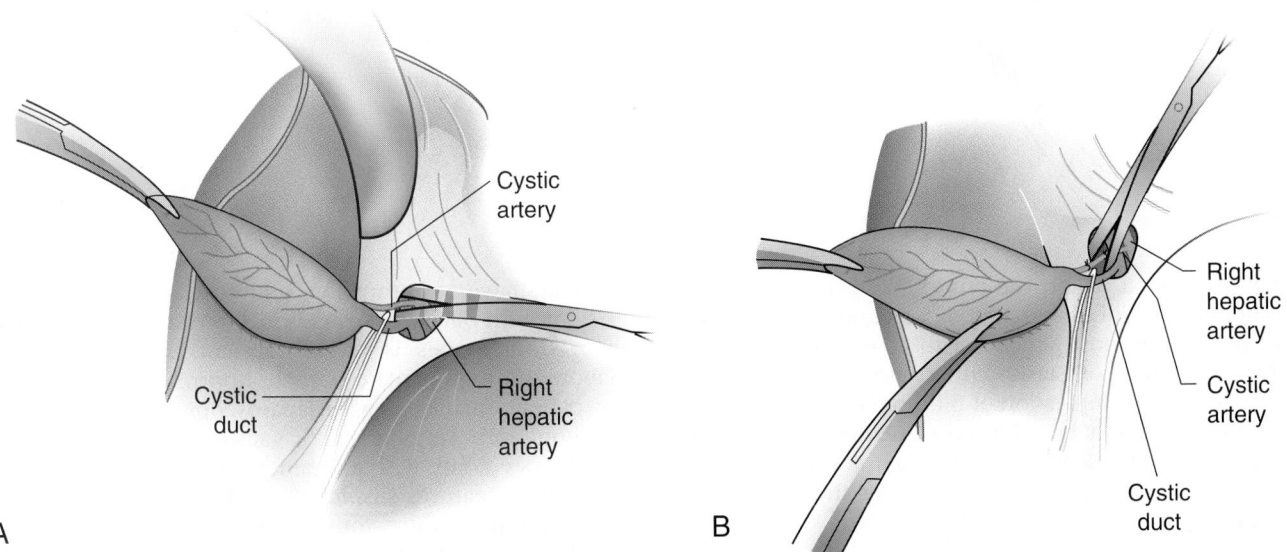

FIGURE 52-14. **A,** Technique of open cholecystectomy. The serosa overlying the triangle of Calot is opened, and the cystic duct and cystic artery are identified. A suture or vessel loop is placed at the gallbladder cystic duct junction to prevent gallbladder stones from passing into the common bile duct during operative manipulation. **B,** The cystic artery is ligated and divided once it is clearly identified. (**A** and **B,** From Cameron J: Atlas of Surgery, Vol 1. Philadelphia, BC Decker, 1994.)

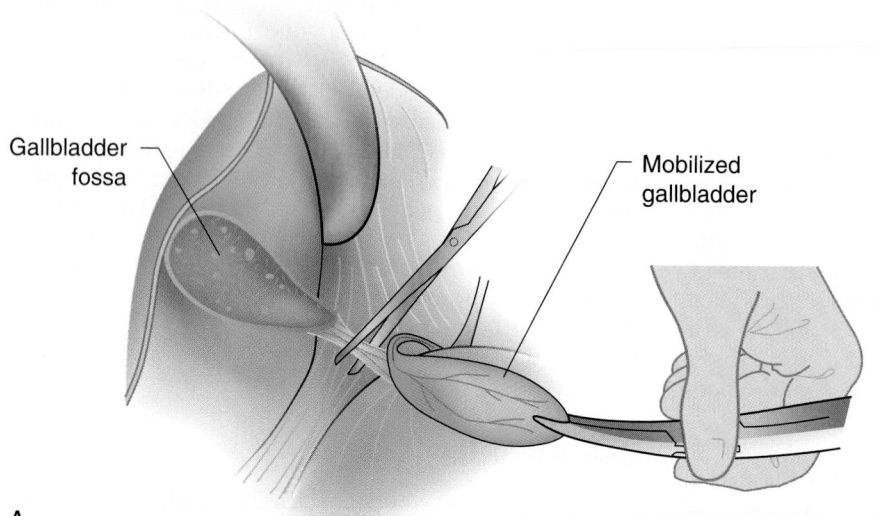

Gallbladder fossa

Mobilized gallbladder

A

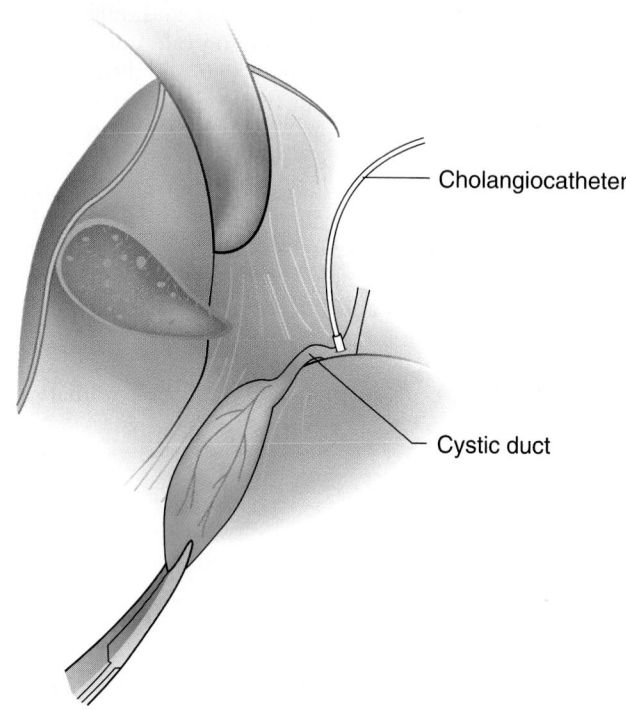

Cholangiocatheter

Cystic duct

B

FIGURE 52-15.   A, Technique of open cholecystectomy (continued from Fig. 52-14). The gallbladder is dissected out of the liver bed after dividing the overlying peritoneum. **B,** Once the gallbladder is mobilized out of the liver bed, a cholangiogram is obtained by inserting a cholangiocatheter through an anterior cystic ductotomy into the common bile duct. Once the cholangiogram is completed, the catheter is removed and the cystic duct is ligated. (**A** and **B,** From Cameron J: Atlas of Surgery, Vol 2. Philadelphia, BC Decker, 1994.)

may include a biliary stricture, papillary stenosis, or sphincter of Oddi dysfunction. In addition, biliary cultures are positive in most patients with common duct stones.[4] The association of stasis with bacterial glucuronidases leads to the deconjugation of bilirubin diglucuronide and the precipitation of bilirubin as its calcium salt. The underlying abnormality leading to biliary stasis usually needs to be identified and corrected to prevent the formation of recurrent stones after removal.

Presentation

Approximately 7% to 15% of patients undergoing chole-cystectomy have common bile duct stones. Many of these

patients have symptoms or laboratory abnormalities consistent with biliary obstruction. However, biliary obstruction from stones is often transient, and preoperative laboratory tests may be normal. Approximately 1% to 2% of patients managed with laparoscopic cholecystectomy without a cholangiogram for gallstones present after the cholecystectomy with a retained stone.

Clinical features suspicious for biliary obstruction due to common bile duct stones include biliary colic, jaundice, lightening of the stools, and darkening of the urine. In addition, fever and chills may be present in patients with choledocholithiasis and cholangitis. Elevated serum bilirubin (>3.0 mg/dL), serum aminotransferases, and alkaline phosphatase all are commonly elevated in patients with biliary obstruction but are neither sensitive nor specific for the presence of common duct stones. Of these, serum bilirubin has the highest positive predictive value (28% to 50%) for the presence of choledocholithiasis. However, laboratory values may be normal in as many as one third of patients with choledocholithiasis.

Standard ultrasound examination can provide additional information supporting the diagnosis of common duct stones. Among patients with gallstones, the prevalence of choledocholithiasis is significantly higher in the setting of a dilated common bile duct (diameter > 5 mm) than in patients with a nondilated duct (58% vs. 1%).[20] However, echogenic shadows consistent with calculi are visible only in 60% to 70% of patients with common duct stones.

Within the past several years several additional noninvasive and invasive modalities have become available to image the biliary tract. MRC provides excellent anatomic detail and has a sensitivity and specificity of 95% and 89% at detecting choledocholithiasis, respectively.[21] MRC has been used to screen patients at low and moderate risk of having common duct stones prior to endoscopic cholangiography. An MRC can avoid the need for an invasive endoscopic cholangiogram in more than 50% of patients. Intravenous cholangiography and spiral CT cholangiography have also been used to detect choledocholithiasis.

Endoscopic cholangiography has been the gold standard for diagnosing common bile duct calculi preoperatively (Fig. 52-16). Endoscopic cholangiography has the advantage of providing a therapeutic option at the time common duct stones are identified. Cannulation of the common bile duct and successful cholangiography is achieved in more than 90% of patients by experienced endoscopists. Complications of diagnostic cholangiography include pancreatitis and cholangitis and occur in up to 5% of patients. Endoscopic ultrasound (EUS) has also been used to identify bile duct stones. Although less sensitive than endoscopic cholangiography, this technique does not require cannulation of the ampulla. Therefore, EUS can be performed in nearly all patients and avoids the risks of pancreatitis and cholangitis.

The choice of radiologic studies to evaluate a patient with suspected choledocholithiasis should be based on the probability of this diagnosis.[22] Patients at highest risk for choledocholithiasis should undergo endoscopic cholangiography (Fig. 52-17). Patients at intermediate risk may be screened with MRC and proceed to laparoscopic cholecystectomy if this study is negative. Those patients at low risk of harboring common duct stones may be evaluated with intraoperative cholangiography at the time of laparoscopic cholecystectomy with laparoscopic common bile duct exploration or postoperative endoscopic stone extraction reserved for the few patients (1.3%) with a positive study.[20]

Endoscopic Management

Endoscopic sphincterotomy and stone extraction was introduced more than 20 years ago and permits common bile duct stones to be removed without the need for conventional surgery. The endoscopic approach is particularly useful for patients prior to cholecystectomy in whom a high suspicion exists for common bile duct calculi, par-

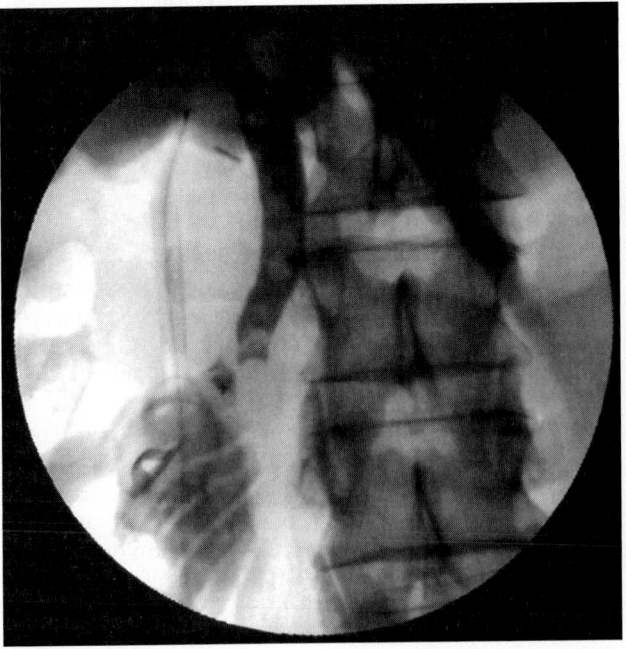

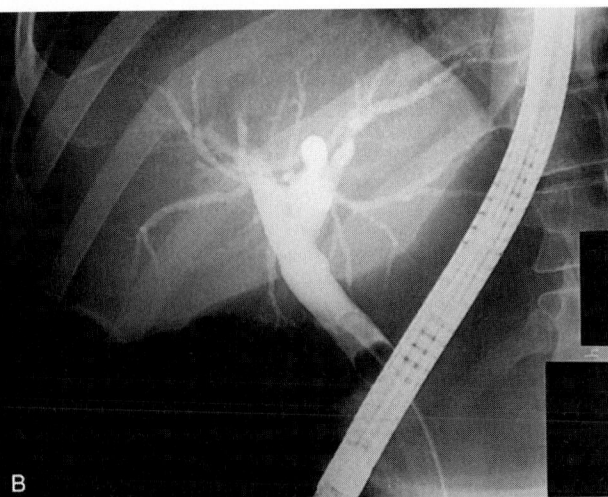

FIGURE 52-16.   **A,** Intraoperative cholangiogram demonstrating several calculi within the distal common bile duct. **B,** Stone removal with a Fogarty catheter.

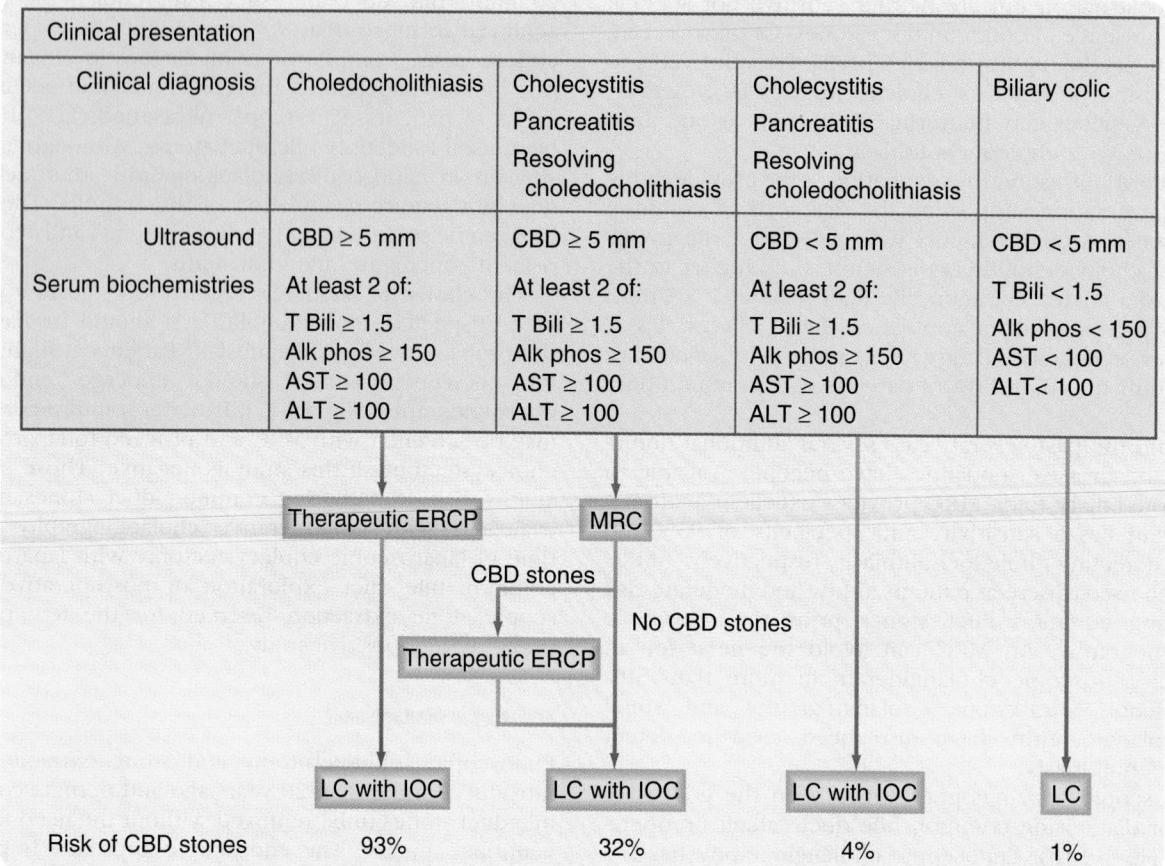

Clinical presentation				

Clinical diagnosis	Choledocholithiasis	Cholecystitis
		Pancreatitis
		Resolving
		  choledocholithiasis
			Cholecystitis
			Pancreatitis
			Resolving
			  choledocholithiasis
				Biliary colic

Ultrasound Serum biochemistries	CBD ≥ 5 mm At least 2 of: T Bili ≥ 1.5 Alk phos ≥ 150 AST ≥ 100 ALT ≥ 100	CBD ≥ 5 mm At least 2 of: T Bili ≥ 1.5 Alk phos ≥ 150 AST ≥ 100 ALT ≥ 100	CBD < 5 mm At least 2 of: T Bili ≥ 1.5 Alk phos ≥ 150 AST ≥ 100 ALT ≥ 100	CBD < 5 mm T Bili < 1.5 Alk phos < 150 AST < 100 ALT < 100

Therapeutic ERCP   MRC

CBD stones   No CBD stones

Therapeutic ERCP

LC with IOC	LC with IOC	LC with IOC	LC

| Risk of CBD stones | 93% | 32% | 4% | 1% |

FIGURE 52-17. A diagnostic and therapeutic algorithm for the management of patients undergoing laparoscopic cholecystectomy (LC). Patients at highest risk of harboring common duct stones should undergo preoperative endoscopic retrograde cholangiography (ERCP). Patients at intermediate risk of choledocholithiasis may be screened using magnetic resonance cholangiography (MRC). Patients at low risk of having common duct stones are managed with laparoscopic cholecystectomy. CBD, common bile duct; T Bili, T-tube bilirubin; Alk phos, alkaline phosphatase; AST, aspartate aminotransferase; ALT, alanine aminotransferase; IOC, intraoperative cholangiography. (Adapted from Liu TH, Consorti ET, Kawashima A, et al: Patient evaluation and management with selective use of magnetic resonance cholangiography and endoscopic retrograde cholangiopancreatography before laparoscopic cholecystectomy. Ann Surg 234:33-40, 2001.)

ticularly if laparoscopic common bile duct exploration is not available. Endoscopic clearance of stones from the common bile duct precholecystectomy can avoid the need for an open operation. Furthermore, if endoscopic stone extraction is not possible (e.g., multiple gallstones, intrahepatic stones, large gallstones, impacted stones, duodenal diverticula, prior gastrectomy, bile duct stricture), this information is known before cholecystectomy, and an open common bile duct exploration or drainage procedure can be performed.

Common bile duct calculi not suspected preoperatively but detected on intraoperative cholangiography may also be suitable for endoscopic management if expertise using endoscopic techniques is available and the equipment and/or ability to perform laparoscopic common bile duct exploration is not. The cholecystectomy is completed laparoscopically, and the endoscopic procedure is sched-

uled soon thereafter. Endoscopic sphincterotomy with stone extraction is also the procedure of choice for patients with retained common bile duct stones after cholecystectomy. The presence of jaundice, biliary-type pain, and biliary dilation on imaging studies should raise the suspicion of either a ductal injury or retained stones.

Endoscopic sphincterotomy with stone extraction is well tolerated in most patients. Complications occur in 5% to 8% of patients and include cholangitis, pancreatitis, perforation, and bleeding. The overall mortality rate is 0.2% to 0.5%. Complete clearance of all common duct stones is achieved endoscopically in 71% to 75% of patients at the first procedure and in 84% to 95% of patients after multiple endoscopic procedures.[7]

Following endoscopic sphincterotomy and stone extraction, patients with a stone-filled gallbladder remain at high risk of developing future biliary symptoms. A recent prospective, randomized trial demonstrated a significantly greater incidence of recurrent biliary symptoms among patients managed with a wait-and-see approach versus laparoscopic cholecystectomy (47% vs. 2%, $P > 0.0001$) following endoscopic stone extraction.[23] A large percentage (37%) of patients managed expectantly later required cholecystectomy.[23]

Laparoscopic Common Bile Duct Exploration

Laparoscopic exploration of the common bile duct for choledocholithiasis enables appropriate patients to undergo complete management of their calculous biliary tract disease with one invasive procedure.[7] The laparoscopic approach is ideal for patients with common bile duct stones identified during intraoperative cholangiography or ultrasound or in patients with suspected choledocholithiasis managed at centers where laparoscopic common bile duct exploration is routinely performed. Intraoperative cholangiography is accomplished via the cystic duct prior to duct exploration.

Once the presence of stones is confirmed, balloon-tipped Fogarty catheters are inserted through the cystic ductotomy into the duodenum and gently withdrawn with the balloon inflated.[19] If this maneuver fails to remove the stone, a wire basket can be inserted under fluoroscopic guidance into the common bile duct to retrieve the stones. A small, flexible choledochoscope is next introduced through one of the 5-mm cannulas and directed into the distal common bile duct (Fig. 52-18). The scope can be used to push stones into the duodenum or to remove stones using the basket under direct vision. Occasionally, the cystic duct needs to be dilated to accept the choledochoscope or to remove larger stones. If the duct can be cleared via the cystic duct, a postoperative T tube is not necessary. If the cystic duct cannot be dilated, an anterior choledochotomy can be used. Postoperative biliary drainage using a T tube is then necessary. Clearance of all common bile duct stones is achieved in 75% to 95% of patients with laparoscopic common bile duct exploration.[7]

The morbidity and mortality of laparoscopic common bile duct exploration are similar to laparoscopic cholecystectomy alone. In a recent prospective, randomized trial comparing laparoscopic common bile duct exploration at the time of laparoscopic cholecystectomy with postoperative endoscopic stone extraction following laparoscopic cholecystectomy, the complication rate and retained stone rate were similar among the two groups. The median hospital stay was significantly shorter for patients managed with the single invasive procedure (1 vs. 3.5 days).[7]

Open Common Bile Duct Exploration

Open common bile duct exploration is performed much less frequently now than 15 years ago with the increased use of endoscopic, percutaneous, and laparoscopic techniques to remove common bile duct stones. Occasionally, when these methods fail, are not available, are not possible due to prior surgery, or when open operation is otherwise necessary, open common bile duct exploration becomes necessary. After mobilizing the duodenum, a longitudinal choledochotomy is made. A combination of techniques including irrigation via soft rubber catheters, passing and retracting balloon-tipped catheters, and the use of Dormia stone baskets all are used to remove stones from the bile duct. Flexible and rigid choledochoscopes are both useful for identifying additional stones. At the completion of the exploration a T tube is placed in the common bile duct via the choledochotomy, and the choledochotomy is closed around the T tube. A completion cholangiogram is performed to be certain all the stones have been removed.

The standard technique for open common bile duct exploration may not be appropriate for all patients. The common bile duct may be explored through a large cystic duct avoiding the need for a postoperative T tube. In patients with a nondilated common bile duct (>4 mm), a transduodenal sphincteroplasty should be performed and the duct explored through the sphincteroplasty. This procedure also avoids the need for a postoperative T tube and the potential for a late bile duct stricture. In patients with definite sphincter stenosis, multiple common bile duct stones, primary common bile duct stones, or intrahepatic stones a drainage procedure (Roux-en-Y choledochojejunostomy, transduodenal sphincteroplasty, or choledochoduodenostomy) should be performed. Open common bile duct exploration is associated with low operative mortality (0 to 2%) and operative morbidity (8% to 16%). With the use of intraoperative choledochoscopy, the rate of retained common bile duct stones is less than 5%.

Postcholecystectomy Pain

Abdominal pain or other symptoms originally attributed to the gallbladder may persist or recur months or years following cholecystectomy. Recurrence of pain or other symptoms following cholecystectomy has been reported in as many as 20% of patients. However, with improvements in biliary imaging over the last decade, the incidence of "postcholecystectomy syndrome" has certainly decreased. Episodic right upper quadrant pain associated with jaundice and chills occurring shortly after cholecystectomy is most commonly associated with a retained common bile duct stone or bile duct injury or leak. Acute epigastric pain not associated with jaundice may be due to unrecognized pancreatitis, peptic ulcer disease, gastroesophageal reflux, wound neuroma, or even irritable bowel syndrome. Formerly, a long cystic duct stump was thought to be a potential source of symptoms following cholecystectomy. However, with the laparoscopic technique, the cystic duct is left long by design to minimize the risk of bile duct injuries, and no increased risk of biliary symptoms has been observed. Finally, a small group of patients have persistent biliary-type pain following

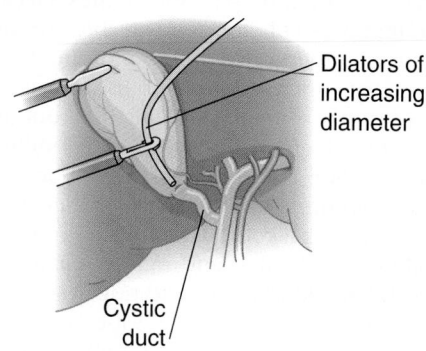

Dilators of
increasing
diameter

Cystic
duct

FIGURE 52-18.   **A,** Laparoscopic common bile duct exploration. After dilation of the cystic duct, the flexible choledochoscope is inserted into the abdomen through the small trocar and maneuvered into the distal common bile duct. **B,** A stone basket is passed through the working channel of the choledochoscope and is used to snare a common duct stone. The stone basket and the choledochoscope are withdrawn together. (**A** and **B** From Curet M, Zucker K: Laparoscopic surgery of the biliary tract and liver. *In* Zuidema G [ed]: Shackelford's Surgery of the Alimentary Tract, 3rd ed. Philadelphia, WB Saunders, 1996, pp 257-278.)

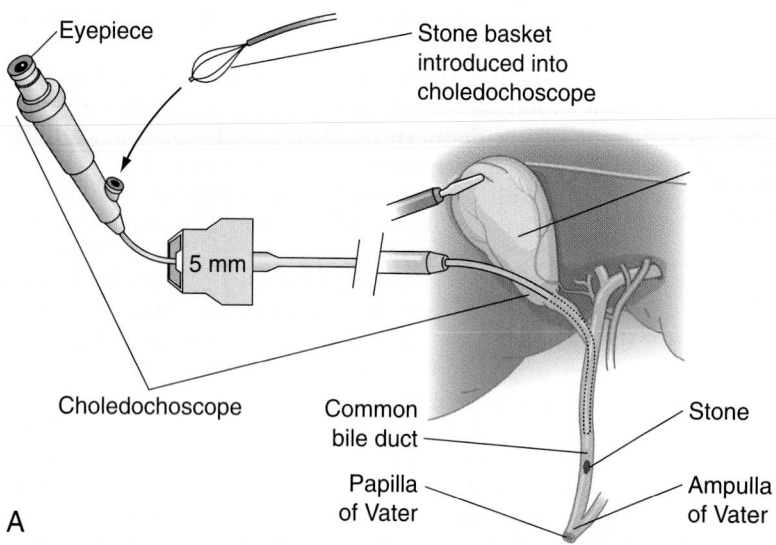

Eyepiece

Stone basket
introduced into
choledochoscope

5 mm

Choledochoscope

Common
bile duct

Stone

Papilla
of Vater

Ampulla
of Vater

A

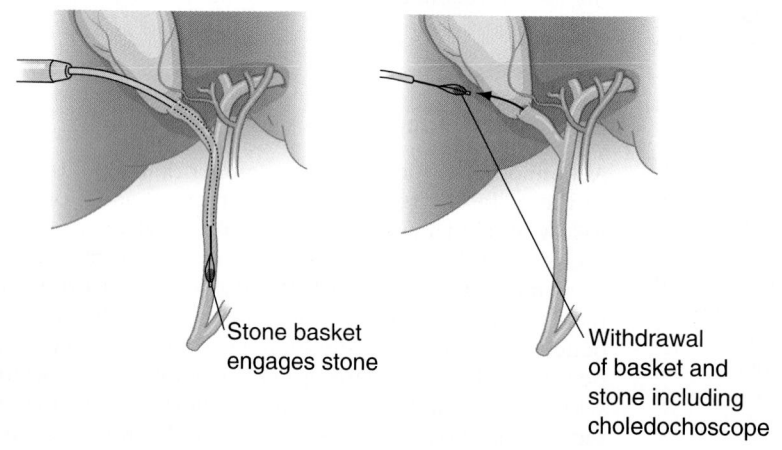

Stone basket
engages stone

Withdrawal
of basket and
stone including
choledochoscope

B

cholecystectomy due to abnormalities in the sphincter of Oddi (stenosing papillitis, sphincter of Oddi dysfunction).[24]

Sphincter of Oddi Dysfunction

The sphincter of Oddi is a complex muscular structure surrounding the distal common bile duct, pancreatic duct, and ampulla of Vater. Pain characteristic of biliary colic and episodes of recurrent acute pancreatitis have been attributed to a poorly defined clinical syndrome described as dysfunction of the sphincter of Oddi. Sphincter of Oddi dysfunction may be caused by either a structural or functional abnormality involving the sphincter. Fibrosis of the sphincter from gallstone migration, operative or endoscopic trauma, pancreatitis, or other nonspecific inflammatory processes can lead to elevated sphincter pressures. Elevated sphincter pressures may also present in the absence of a structural abnormality, and these cases of sphincter of Oddi dyskinesia or spasm are often associated with more diffuse abnormalities of gastrointestinal motility.[24]

Sphincter of Oddi dysfunction should be suspected in patients with typical episodic biliary-type pain without an obvious organic cause. Approximately 1% of patients undergoing cholecystectomy are estimated to have sphincter of Oddi dysfunction. Numerous diagnostic tests have been used to diagnose sphincter of Oddi dysfunction, but none are sensitive or specific. Elevated serum amylase or transaminases may be present in patients with sphincter of Oddi dysfunction. Ultrasound evidence of sphincter of Oddi dysfunction includes a dilated (>12-mm) common bile duct, an increase in common bile duct diameter in response to CCK, or an increase in pancreatic duct diameter in response to secretin. Delayed emptying of contrast medium from the common bile duct after endoscopic retrograde cholangiopancreatography (ERCP) is also indicative of abnormal sphincter function. Endoscopic manometry has also been used to evaluate the sphincter of Oddi, and an elevated basal sphincter pressure (>40 mm Hg) has been correlated with successful response to sphincter ablation.

Both endoscopic sphincterotomy and transduodenal sphincteroplasty with transampullary septectomy have been used to manage patients with sphincter of Oddi dysfunction. Results of both treatments appear to be similar and are more dependent on the presence of objective signs of sphincter dysfunction than on the procedure performed. The surgical approach (transduodenal sphincteroplasty with transampullary septectomy) has the advantage of including division of the transampullary septum, which can impede pancreatic duct drainage when chronically inflamed and fibrotic. A further advantage is that mucosa-to-mucosa apposition can be achieved minimizing the risk of scarring and restenosis. When objective evidence of sphincter dysfunction is present (elevated transaminases, delayed biliary emptying, dilated common bile duct, elevated basal sphincter pressure), 60% to 80% of patients will be pain free or improved following sphincterotomy or sphincteroplasty.[24]

Gallstone Ileus

Gallstone ileus is mechanical obstruction of the gastrointestinal tract from a large gallstone, most commonly following passage of the stone through a spontaneous biliary-enteric fistula. Seventy-five percent of these fistulas develop between the gallbladder and duodenum. Less commonly, fistulas develop between the gallbladder and colon or stomach or between the common bile duct and duodenum. Biliary enteric fistulas usually follow an episode of acute cholecystitis with gangrene and perforation of the gallbladder wall into the adjacent viscus or from pressure necrosis from an impacted gallstone. Gallstone ileus occurs most commonly in the elderly (mean age >70 years). Although gallstone ileus accounts for only 1% of all cases of small bowel obstruction and occurs in fewer than 1% of patients with gallstones, it may account for as many as 25% of cases of intestinal obstruction in elderly patients who have not undergone previous abdominal surgery and do not have a hernia.

Patients with gallstone ileus present with signs and symptoms of intestinal obstruction—nausea, vomiting, and abdominal pain. The pain may be episodic and recurrent as the impacted stone temporarily impacts in the gut lumen and then dislodges and moves distally (tumbling obstruction). A history of gallstone-related symptoms (right upper quadrant pain) may be present in only 50% of these patients. Abdominal films will demonstrate small bowel distension and air-fluid levels and may give additional clues to the source of the obstruction (pneumobilia or a calcified gallstone distant from the gallbladder). The site of obstruction is most frequently in the narrowest part of the small intestine (ileum) or large intestine (sigmoid colon).

The initial management of gallstone ileus includes relieving the obstruction. Most frequently, this goal can be achieved by removing the gallstone through an enterotomy. Additional gallstones should be sought as recurrent obstruction has been reported in up to 10% of patients with gallstone ileus. Takedown of the biliary-enteric fistula and cholecystectomy is warranted because recurrent cholecystitis and cholangitis are common in patients with a biliary-enteric fistula, and gallbladder cancer has been reported in 15% of these patients. However, in patients with a significant inflammatory process in the right upper quadrant or who are too unstable to withstand a prolonged operative procedure, the fistula can be addressed at a second laparotomy.

Intrahepatic Stones

Intrahepatic stones or hepatolithiasis is endemic in East Asia. In the United States the disease is uncommon outside of the East Asian immigrant population. In most cases, hepatolithiasis is associated with more common biliary tract conditions such as benign biliary strictures, primary sclerosing cholangitis, choledochal cyst, and biliary tract tumors. Hepatolithiasis occurs alone in the absence of any other biliary tract pathology in fewer than 10% of cases. Factors important in the pathogenesis of intrahepatic stones include bile stasis, bacterial infection, and biliary mucin. The majority of intrahepatic stones are large, soft, contain bacterial casts and calcium bilirubinate, and are referred to as *brown pigment stones*.[25]

Clinical Presentation

Most patients with hepatolithiasis experience cholangitis (67%) and right upper quadrant pain (63%). Jaundice (39%) and pruritus (6%) are less common symptoms. Intrahepatic stones are diagnosed using ERC, PTC, or MRC. Intrahepatic stones are usually present in both hepatic ducts.[25]

Management

The goal of therapy is correction of the underlying biliary disorder and clearance of all stones from the intrahepatic biliary tree. Often, achieving the latter goal takes several procedures, so long-term biliary access is critical. The surgical approach includes cholecystectomy, resection of the extrahepatic biliary tree to include any strictures, tumors, or choledochal cyst followed by choledochoscopy and extraction of any intrahepatic stones. Biliary-enteric continuity is reestablished with a Roux-en-Y hepaticojejunostomy either over transhepatic stents or as a hepaticocutaneous jejunostomy. In patients with prolonged biliary obstruction and segmental atrophy or cirrhosis, a partial hepatic resection may be required. Approximately 50% of patients require further procedures (percutaneous choledochoscopy or balloon dilation) to clear the intrahepatic ducts of stones or to manage persistent strictures. With this approach, stone clearance rates of 94% have been reported.[25]

BENIGN NONCALCULOUS BILIARY DISEASE

Polypoid Lesions of the Gallbladder

Polypoid lesions of the gallbladder (PLGs) are being identified more frequently as the resolution of ultrasound improves. PLGs are present in 3% to 7% of normal subjects undergoing gallbladder ultrasound and in 2% to 12% of cholecystectomy specimens. Lesions classified as PLGs include benign pseudotumors (cholesterol polyps, adenomyomatosis) and benign (adenoma) and malignant (adenocarcinoma) neoplasms. Cholesterol polyps are the most common PLG, are usually less than 10 mm in size, have a characteristic echogenic pedunculated appearance on ultrasound, and are often multiple (30% of cases).[26] Adenomyomatosis appears as a sessile polyp with characteristic microcysts on ultrasound and is often larger than 10 mm.[26] Adenoma and adenocarcinoma may be sessile or pedunculated, are usually larger than 10 mm, and in the absence of transmural invasion can be difficult to differentiate sonographically. Factors associated with malignancy include age older than 60 years, coexistence of gallstones, a documented increase in size, and size greater than 10 mm. EUS may be more sensitive and specific than transabdominal ultrasound in differentiating among

PLGs.[26] All patients with symptomatic PLGs should undergo laparoscopic cholecystectomy. Patients with asymptomatic PLGs and one or more of the earlier listed risk factors should also undergo cholecystectomy. Asymptomatic PLGs less than 10 mm without ultrasound features of neoplasia may be safely observed provided interval ultrasound documents no change in size.

Benign Stricture/Bile Duct Injury

Benign biliary strictures occur in association with a wide variety of conditions including chronic pancreatitis, primary sclerosing cholangitis, acute cholangitis, several autoimmune diseases, or following either blunt or penetrating abdominal trauma. However, most benign strictures follow iatrogenic bile duct injury, most commonly during laparoscopic cholecystectomy. Most injuries are recognized intraoperatively or during the early postoperative period, and with appropriate management the long-term results are acceptable. However, with unrecognized or inappropriately managed biliary strictures, recurrent cholangitis, secondary biliary cirrhosis, and portal hypertension may eventually develop.

Pathogenesis

The majority of bile duct injuries occur during cholecystectomy. Prior to the widespread use of laparoscopic cholecystectomy, bile duct injuries were relatively infrequent occurring in about 1 in 800 open cholecystectomies. The rate of bile duct injury with laparoscopic cholecystectomy is greater than that observed with open cholecystectomy.[27] Several large studies derived from either state or national databases have estimated the overall rate of bile duct problems at 0.85% or 1 in 120 laparoscopic cholecystectomies. The incidence of major bile duct injuries is about 0.55%, and the incidence of bile leaks or minor injuries is 0.3%.

Several factors have been implicated in the occurrence of bile duct injuries during laparoscopic cholecystectomy. Surgeon training and experience were recognized as factors in early reports of laparoscopic bile duct injuries. As surgeon experience increases beyond 20 cases, the bile duct injury rate decreases. However, recent population-based series do not demonstrate a decrease in bile duct injury rates between the early 1990s and the mid 1990s, suggesting that a steady-state incidence of these injuries has been reached.

Local operative factors can also increase the difficulty of the procedure and, therefore, the risk of injury. The bile duct injury rate is increased in patients with complications of gallstones, including acute cholecystitis, pancreatitis, cholangitis, and obstructive jaundice.[27] Additional factors associated with injury include chronic inflammation, obesity, fat in the periportal area, poor exposure, and bleeding obscuring the operative field. In general, increased patient age, male gender, a long period of symptoms prior to cholecystectomy, and number of attacks all are associated with increased difficulty of the procedure.

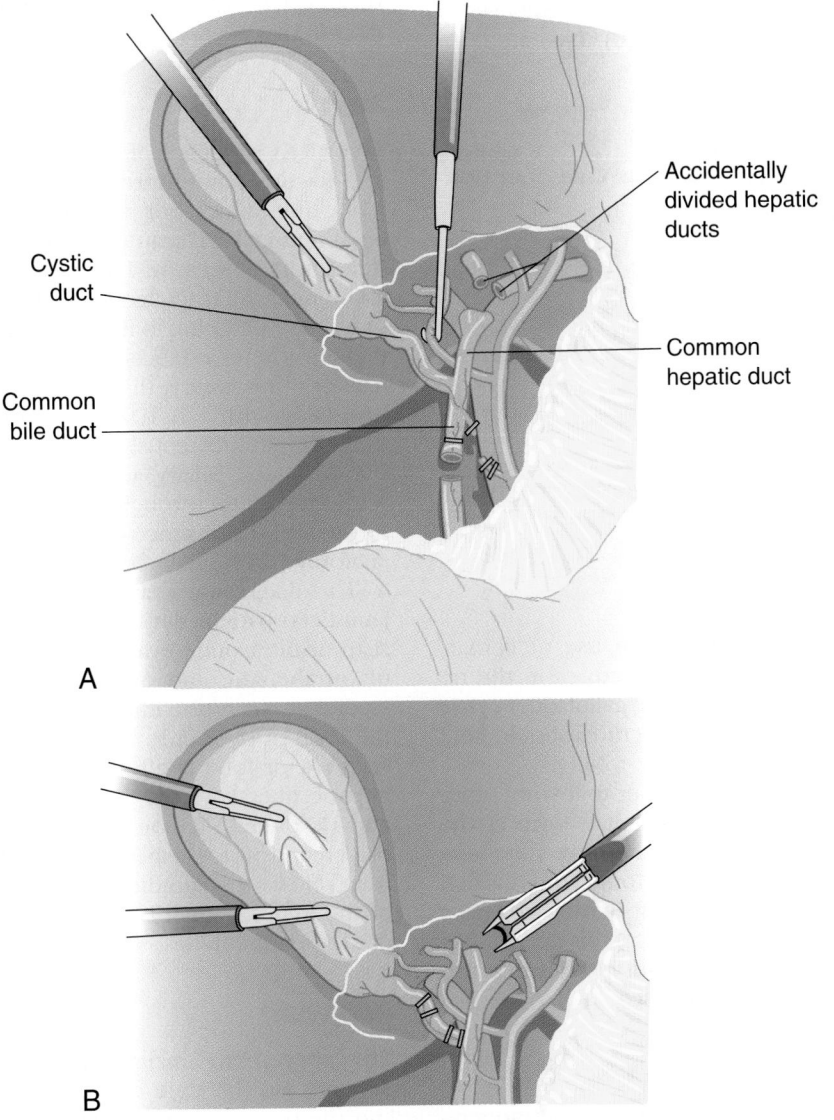

Cystic
duct

Common
bile duct

Accidentally
divided hepatic
ducts

Common
hepatic duct

A

B

FIGURE 52-19. **A,** The classic laparoscopic cholecystectomy bile duct injury. The cystic duct and common bile duct are aligned by traction on the gallbladder. A segment of the common bile and hepatic ducts is resected. **B,** Cephalad traction on the gallbladder may "tent" the common bile duct out of its normal location, leading to clip placement at the cystic duct common bile duct junction. (**A,** From Branum G, Schmitt C, Baillie J, et al: Management of major biliary complications after laparoscopic cholecystectomy. Ann Surg 217:532-541, 1993; **B,** From Curet M, Zucker K: Laparoscopic surgery of the biliary tract and liver. *In* Zuidema G [ed]: Shackelford's Surgery of the Alimentary Tract, 3rd ed. Philadelphia, WB Saunders, 1996, pp 257-278.)

Aberrant biliary anatomy is often cited as a factor in biliary injuries. A common anomaly involved in bile duct injuries is an aberrant right hepatic duct coursing through the triangle of Calot and entering the common hepatic duct. Occasionally, the cystic duct enters a small aberrant right hepatic duct, which is mistaken for the cystic duct and ligated and/or divided.

Intraoperatively, several factors have been implicated in biliary injuries. The classic laparoscopic injury occurs when the cystic duct and common bile duct are brought into alignment, and the common bile duct is mistaken for the cystic duct, is isolated, clipped, and divided (Fig. 52-19A).[28] As the dissection continues cephalad, the common hepatic duct is divided a variable distance from the hilus,

and often the right hepatic artery is injured as well. Other intraoperative factors implicated in bile duct injury include excessive traction on the cystic duct, which can lead to clip placement on the common bile duct (Fig. 52-19B); dissecting too deep in the liver parenchyma, which can injure intrahepatic ducts; poor clip placement on the cystic duct; or injudicious use of cautery.[18]

Routine operative cholangiography has been recommended to decrease or prevent biliary injuries. A recent population-based study demonstrated a 50% reduction in the risk of bile duct injury or bile leak following cholecystectomy in patients evaluated with intraoperative cholangiography (Table 52-5).[27] Cholangiography may define the anatomy and limit the extent of biliary injury,

TABLE 52-5. Proportion of Bile Duct Injuries by Intraoperative Cholangiography (IOC), Type of Surgery, and Case Complexity

	IOC No		IOC Yes	
	Total Cases	Injuries per 1000	Total Cases	Injuries per 1000
Laparoscopic	4140	4.3	3397	2.1
Open	4017	2.7	7632	1.0
Complex*	295	16.9	446	2.2
Not complex*	7862	3.1	10583	1.3

*Complex cases include pancreatitis, cholangitis, obstructive jaundice, and acute cholecystitis.

IOC, intraoperative cholangiography.

Adapted from Fletcher DR, Hobbs MS, Tan P, et al: Complications of cholecystectomy: Risks of the laparoscopic approach and protective effects of operative cholangiography—a population-based study. Ann Surg 229:449-457, 1999.

but injuries certainly occur despite the use of cholangiography. Careful exposure of the structures in the triangle of Calot and clear definition of the gallbladder-cystic duct junction prior to dividing any structures should limit the incidence of these injuries (see Fig. 52-11).[18]

Biliary injuries and stricture also occur following other abdominal operations. Biliary strictures can form at the site of impacted stones or choledochotomy following common bile duct exploration. Gastrectomy with division of the proximal duodenum especially in the presence of acute inflammation from peptic ulcer disease is also associated with a low incidence of injury. Strictures also develop after biliary enteric anastomoses.

Presentation

Patients with bile duct injuries can present intraoperatively, in the early postoperative period or may present months or years after the initial injury. Approximately, 25% of major (common bile or common hepatic) ductal injuries are recognized intraoperatively because of bile leakage, an abnormal cholangiogram, or late recognition of the anatomy. The remaining patients present after a variable time postoperatively. Patients with a bile leak from the cystic duct stump, a transected aberrant right hepatic duct, or a lateral injury to the main bile duct usually present within 1 week of cholecystectomy with pain, fever, and/or mild hyperbilirubinemia (2.5 mg/dL) from a biloma or bile peritonitis. The degree of pain and physical findings may be quite subtle initially.[29] Occasionally, bile begins leaking externally through a drain or surgical incision. The diagnosis of bile leak or bile peritonitis should be considered in any patient with persistent bloating or anorexia more than a few days after laparoscopic cholecystectomy.[29] With injuries involving occlusion of the common hepatic or bile duct without an intraperitoneal bile leak, jaundice with or without abdominal pain is the common mode of presentation. Less commonly, patients present months or years after biliary

surgery with cholangitis or cirrhosis from a remote bile duct injury.[18]

Diagnosis

An orderly sequence of diagnostic tests usually establishes the diagnosis and initiates the treatment of patients with a bile duct injury. For patients with a suspected bile leak, an abdominal CT scan or ultrasound identifies peritoneal fluid or an abscess or biloma. Perihepatic or other intra-abdominal fluid collections should be percutaneously drained.[29] Ongoing biliary drainage through a percutaneous catheter establishes the presence of an active bile leak or, if necessary, this diagnosis can be confirmed noninvasively with a Tc-IDA scan. In patients with a surgical drain or percutaneously placed catheter and an external bile leak, the biliary anatomy can often be determined with a sinogram through the drain after a fibrous tract has formed. In the absence of an external bile leak, the biliary anatomy can be defined with an ERC.[18]

The diagnostic evaluation is slightly different in the jaundiced patient with a suspected bile duct injury. A CT scan or ultrasound evaluation demonstrates the presence of intrahepatic and extrahepatic ductal dilation. These studies also can provide some anatomic information about the level of the injury, whether the ductal system to one segment or lobe is affected or whether the entire intrahepatic ductal system is involved. In patients with intrahepatic ductal dilation from a biliary stricture, PTC and placement of a transhepatic stent decompress the biliary tree, relieve the jaundice, and define the proximal extent of the injury, which is critical in determining the appropriate treatment.

Management

The appropriate management of biliary tract injuries depends on the time of diagnosis after the initial injury and the type, extent, and level of the injury. Cystic duct bile leaks can usually be managed with percutaneous drainage of any intra-abdominal fluid collections, followed by placement of a biliary endoprosthesis. Lateral bile duct (partial transection) injuries recognized at the time of cholecystectomy should be managed with placement of a T tube. The T tube can be placed at the site of the injury if this is similar in size to a choledochotomy. If the biliary rent is more extensive, the injury is repaired primarily and stented with a T tube placed through a proximal or distal choledochotomy. Isolated hepatic ducts smaller than 3 mm or those draining a single hepatic segment can be safely ligated. Ducts larger than 3 mm are more likely to drain several segments or an entire lobe and need to be reimplanted.

Major bile duct injuries including transections of the common bile or common hepatic duct should be repaired if recognized at the time of cholecystectomy. Injuries diagnosed after the early postoperative period should be managed initially with transhepatic catheters for biliary decompression, followed by operative exploration and repair in 6 to 8 weeks when the acute inflammation has resolved. The goal of surgical repair is a tension-free mucosa-to-mucosa duct enteric anastomosis. Duct-to-duct repairs are warranted only in the rare event that no ductal length has been lost with the injury as these repairs have a very high rate of postoperative stricture formation. In most cases either an end-to-side Roux-en-Y choledochojejunostomy or, more commonly, a Roux-en-Y hepaticojejunostomy should be performed (Fig. 52-20).[30] For strictures involving the bifurcation or left or right hepatic ducts, bilateral hepaticojejunostomies may be necessary. Transhepatic stents placed preoperatively are useful technical aids to identify the hepatic ducts particularly with more proximal strictures and are left in postoperatively for several months to stent the anastomosis and provide access to the biliary tract for imaging.[31] Biliary strictures in which the duct remains intact or postoperative anastomotic strictures are also amenable to either percutaneous or endoscopic dilation and/or stenting.

Results

Acceptable results are achieved in most patients undergoing operative repair of bile duct stricture or injury. The operative mortality associated with repair of a bile duct injury has been less than 1% in several large series, and common complications have included cholangitis, subhepatic or subphrenic abscess, bile leak, and hemobilia. Long-term follow-up is necessary to fully evaluate the results of either operative or nonoperative bile duct injury management. Restenosis of a biliary enteric anastomosis can manifest itself many years following operative repair. Two thirds of recurrences, however, will become symptomatic within 2 years after repair.

In one large series, 91% of patients were free of jaundice and cholangitis after undergoing operative repair of a laparoscopic bile duct injury.[31] Several factors may influence the eventual success of biliary reconstruction for bile duct injuries. More proximal strictures (at or proximal to the hepatic duct bifurcation) have a lower success rate, when compared with distal strictures (distal to the hepatic duct bifurcation). Percutaneous balloon dilation with stenting also has a significantly lower success rate (64%) than operative repair.

Although most patients are rendered free of jaundice and the functional consequences of an injured bile duct following biliary reconstruction, the impact of the injury on quality of life may persist. Patients sustaining bile duct injuries continue to score lower on quality of life surveys particularly in the psychological domain than patients undergoing uncomplicated laparoscopic cholecystectomy even years after successful repair.[22]

Acute Cholangitis

Acute cholangitis is a bacterial infection of the biliary ductal system, which varies in severity from mild and self-limited to severe and life threatening. The clinical triad of fever, jaundice, and pain associated with cholangitis was first described in 1877 by Charcot. He postulated that stagnant bile associated with obstructive biliary pathology was a significant factor in the pathogenesis of this disease.

Pathophysiology

Clinical cholangitis results from a combination of two factors: significant bacterial concentrations in the bile and biliary obstruction. Although cultures of the gallbladder and bile ducts are usually sterile, in the presence of common bile duct stones or other obstructing pathology the incidence of positive bile duct cultures increases (see Bacteriology). The most common organisms recovered from the bile in patients with cholangitis include *E. coli*, *Klebsiella pneumoniae*, the enterococci, and *Bacteroides fragilis*.[5] Nevertheless, even in the presence of high biliary bacterial concentrations, clinical cholangitis and bacteremia do not develop unless obstruction causes elevated intraductal pressures.

Normal biliary pressures range from 7 to 14 cm H_2O. In the presence of bactibilia and normal biliary pressures, hepatic vein blood and perihepatic lymph are sterile. However, with partial or complete biliary obstruction, intrabiliary pressures rise to 18 to 29 cm H_2O, and organisms rapidly appear in both the blood and lymph. The fever and chills associated with cholangitis are the result of systemic bacteremia caused by cholangiovenous and cholangiolymphatic reflux.

Etiology

The most common causes of biliary obstruction are choledocholithiasis, benign strictures, biliary enteric anastomotic strictures, and cholangiocarcinoma or periampullary cancer. Prior to 1980, choledocholithiasis was the cause of approximately 80% of the reported cases of cholangitis. In recent years, malignant strictures have become a frequent cause of cholangitis particularly at tertiary referral centers. ERC, PTC, and stent placement via either the endoscopic or percutaneous route all are known to cause bacteremia. These procedures are frequently performed in patients with unresectable malignant obstruction.

Clinical Presentation

Cholangitis may present with a wide spectrum of disease. Patients may have a self-limited illness and never seek attention. At the other end of the spectrum, patients with toxic cholangitis present with a severe illness, including jaundice, fever, abdominal pain, mental obtundation, and hypotension (Reynold's pentad). Fever is the most common presenting symptom and is often accompanied by chills. Jaundice is a frequent physical finding but may be absent, especially in patients with an indwelling endoprosthesis or biliary stent. Pain is also commonly present but is often mild. Severe pain or marked tenderness should prompt consideration of an alternate diagnosis such as acute cholecystitis. Up to 33% of East Asian patients with choledocholithiasis present with toxic cholangitis characterized by septic shock.[32]

Diagnosis

Although cholangitis is a clinical diagnosis, laboratory tests can support evidence of biliary obstruction.

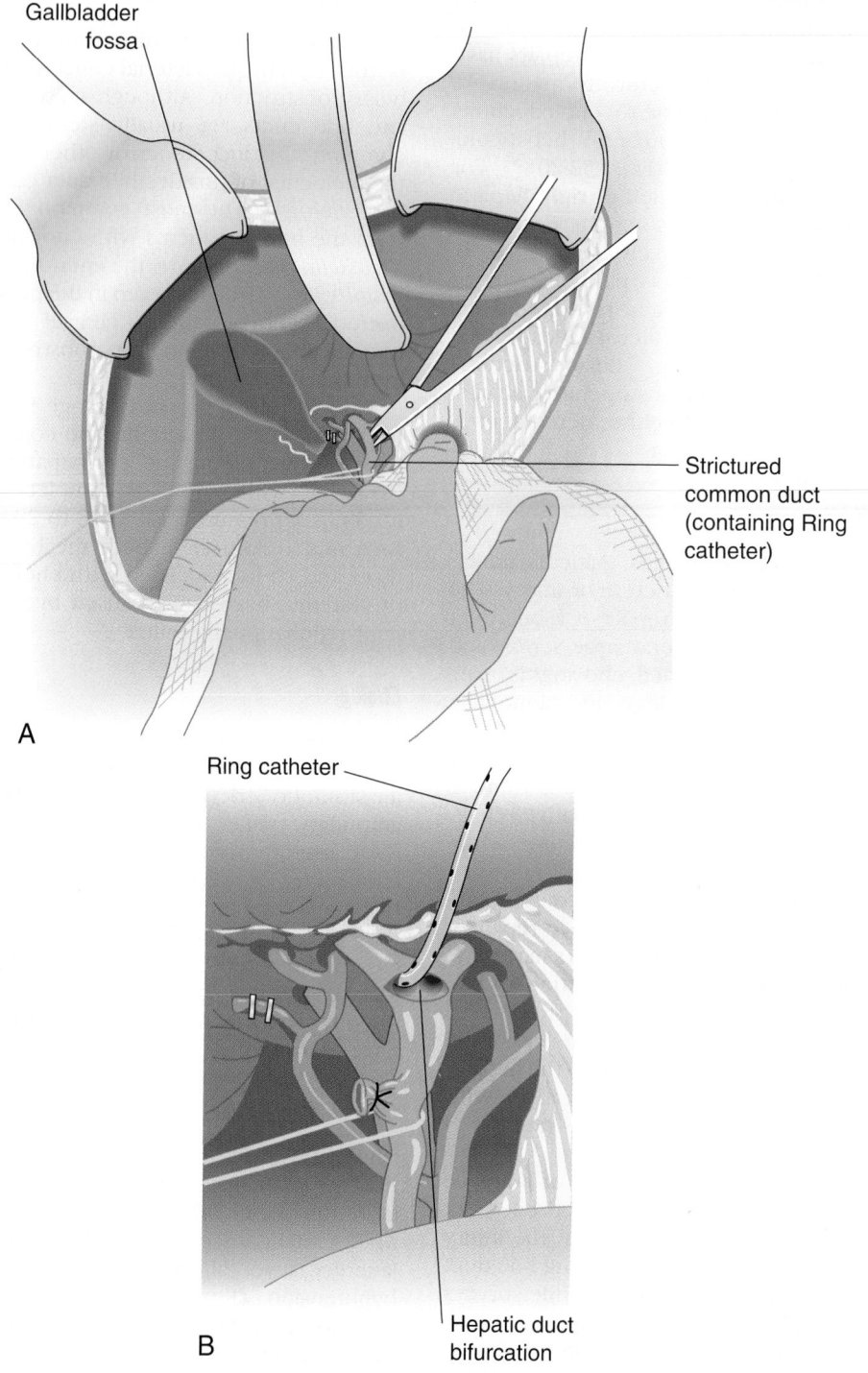

Gallbladder
fossa

Strictured
common duct
(containing Ring
catheter)

A

Ring catheter

Hepatic duct
bifurcation

B

FIGURE 52-20.   **A**, Diagram illustrates operative repair of an operative bile duct injury resulting in a common hepatic duct stricture. The common hepatic duct is identified and encircled. **B**, The common hepatic duct is opened anteriorly where it appears reasonably normal, and the transhepatic catheter is removed from the distal bile duct.

Anterior row of
hepaticojejunostomy

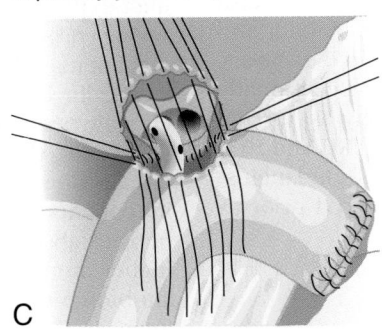

C

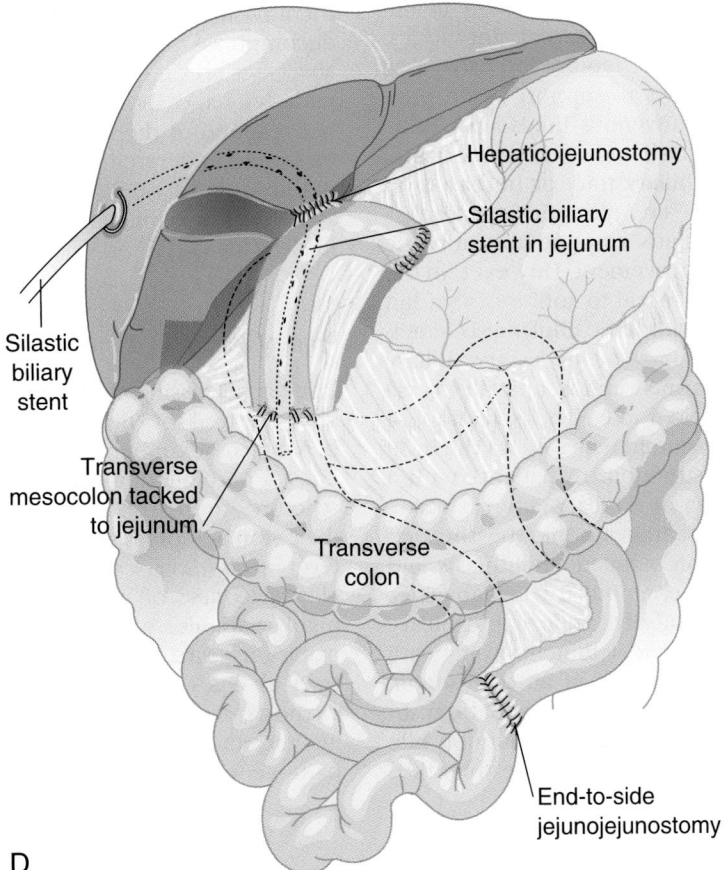

Hepaticojejunostomy

Silastic biliary
stent in jejunum

Silastic
biliary
stent

Transverse
mesocolon tacked
to jejunum

Transverse
colon

End-to-side
jejunojejunostomy

D

FIGURE 52-20. Cont'd C, After resecting the strictured bile duct, a
Roux-en-Y hepaticojejunostomy is performed to the proximal common
hepatic duct over a transhepatic Silastic catheter. **D,** Completed retrocolic
Roux-en-Y hepaticojejunostomy. (**A–D,** From Cameron J: Atlas of Surgery,
Vol 1. Philadelphia, BC Decker, 1994.)

Leukocytosis, hyperbilirubinemia, and elevations of alkaline phosphatase and transaminases all are common in patients with cholangitis. Radiologic studies are also helpful in confirming the diagnosis. CT, ultrasound, and MR scanning can provide noninvasive evidence of biliary ductal dilation, pancreatic masses, and occasionally common bile duct stones. Cholangiography is usually required prior to or as part of therapy. Both ERC and PTC are associated with a 4% to 7% incidence of cholangitis, and systemic antibiotics should be administered prior to these procedures.

Management

The initial treatment of the patient with cholangitis includes antibiotics. Some patients are only mildly ill and can be managed as outpatients with oral antibiotics. Patients with toxic cholangitis may require intensive care unit monitoring and vasopressors to support blood pressure. Most patients require intravenous fluids and antibiotics. The antibacterial regimen should cover the common pathogens isolated from the biliary tract or be based on current or prior bile cultures (see Antibiotic Selection).

Most patients with cholangitis respond to antibiotic therapy alone with clinical improvement. However, in the 15% of patients who do not respond to antibiotics within 12 to 24 hours or in patients with toxic cholangitis, emergency biliary decompression may be necessary. Biliary decompression may be performed endoscopically or via the percutaneous transhepatic route. The selection of which procedure to perform should be based on the level and nature of the biliary obstruction. In patients with a proximal perihilar obstruction or a biliary-enteric anastomotic stricture, percutaneous drainage may be the preferred route of decompression. Choledocholithiasis and cholangitis associated with periampullary malignancies are best approached endoscopically. Endoscopic biliary drainage may include endoscopic sphincterotomy and stone extraction or simply placement of an endoscopic biliary stent in the hemodynamically unstable patient. In experienced hands, successful endoscopic common bile duct stone clearance can be achieved in more than 90% of patients.[33] In settings where either endoscopic or percutaneous biliary drainage is not possible, common bile duct exploration and placement of a T tube remains a lifesaving procedure for seriously ill patients with toxic cholangitis. However, the mortality for patients treated surgically is considerably higher than for patients successfully managed endoscopically.

Overall, the mortality rate associated with an episode of gallstone cholangitis is approximately 2% but is higher in patients with toxic cholangitis (5%). Renal failure, hepatic abscess, and malignancy all are associated with higher morbidity and mortality. The success of the initial antibiotic therapy and biliary drainage is significantly lower in patients with malignant biliary obstruction, and these patients frequently require changes in antibiotic therapy and repeat biliary manipulations to adequately decompress the biliary tract (Fig. 52-21).[5] Hepatic abscesses are frequently observed in patients with biliary pathology and should be considered in patients who do not respond to therapy. Patients with gallstone cholangitis should undergo interval laparoscopic cholecystectomy within 6 to 12 weeks. The incidence of recurrent biliary symptoms is significantly higher if the gallbladder is left in situ (6% vs. 25%).[32]

Primary Sclerosing Cholangitis

Primary sclerosing cholangitis is a cholestatic liver disease characterized by fibrotic strictures involving the intrahepatic and extrahepatic biliary tree in the absence of any known precipitating cause. In cases where diffuse biliary strictures are caused by acute cholangitis, common bile duct stones, operative trauma, or other toxic agents, the term *secondary sclerosing cholangitis* is used. The clinical course of patients with sclerosing cholangitis is highly variable, with some patients remaining asymptomatic for years, whereas in others the obliterative biliary tract changes may progress rapidly to secondary biliary cirrhosis and liver failure. Recent studies suggest that genetic and immunologic factors are important in the pathogenesis of this disorder. Primary sclerosing cholan-

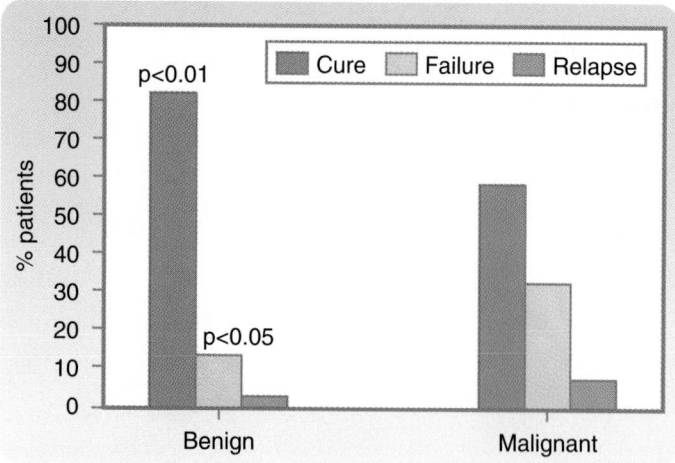

FIGURE 52-21. Cure, failure, and relapse rates among patients with cholangitis caused by either benign or malignant biliary obstruction. The results were significantly worse in patients with malignant obstruction. (From Thompson JE Jr, Pitt HA, Doty JE, et al: Broad-spectrum penicillin as an adequate therapy for acute cholangitis. Surg Gynecol Obstet 171:275-282, 1990.)

gitis is more common in certain HLA haplotypes such as B8/DR3 which is also common in patients with other autoimmune diseases such as insulin-dependent diabetes mellitus, Graves' disease, Sjögren's syndrome, and myasthenia gravis.

Associated Diseases

Several diseases have been associated with primary sclerosing cholangitis. The strongest association exists between inflammatory bowel disease, primarily ulcerative colitis, and sclerosing cholangitis. The incidence of ulcerative colitis in patients with sclerosing cholangitis ranges from 60% to 72%. Patients with sclerosing cholangitis are also at increased risk of developing cholangiocarcinoma.[33] Cholangiocarcinoma can present early in the clinical course of primary sclerosing cholangitis and is often diagnosed simultaneously with this disease. The risk of developing cholangiocarcinoma is approximately 1% per year in patients with sclerosing cholangitis. Most patients with primary sclerosing cholangitis developing cholangiocarcinoma do not have cirrhosis.[33] Between 10% and 15% of patients undergoing liver transplant have an unsuspected cholangiocarcinoma in the hepatectomy specimen.

Clinical Presentation

The natural history of patients with primary sclerosing cholangitis is highly variable with some patients progressing rapidly to hepatic failure and others remaining asymptomatic for years. The mean age at presentation for patients with primary sclerosing cholangitis ranges from 40 to 45 years, and two thirds of patients with primary sclerosing cholangitis are male.[34] Patients present either with signs and symptoms of cholestatic liver disease (jaundice, pruritus, fatigue) or with abnormal serum liver function tests. Approximately 75% of patients are symptomatic at presentation. Symptoms of bacterial cholangitis (pain, fever, and jaundice) are uncommon, especially without preceding biliary tract manipulations. A small percentage of patients present with signs and symptoms of advanced liver disease including ascites, variceal bleeding, and/or splenomegaly. The median survival for patients with primary sclerosing cholangitis from the time of diagnosis ranges from 10 to 12 years.

Diagnosis

The diagnosis of primary sclerosing cholangitis is usually made by ERCP. Diffuse multifocal strictures are most commonly found in both the intrahepatic and extrahepatic bile ducts in patients with primary sclerosing cholangitis (Fig. 52-22). Involvement of the extrahepatic ducts alone without intrahepatic duct involvement occurs in 5% to 10% of patients with primary sclerosing cholangitis. Despite the presence of diffuse disease in most patients with sclerosing cholangitis, the hepatic duct bifurcation is often the most severely strictured segment of the biliary tree. A liver biopsy to determine the degree of hepatic fibrosis or the presence of cirrhosis is also critical in selecting therapy.

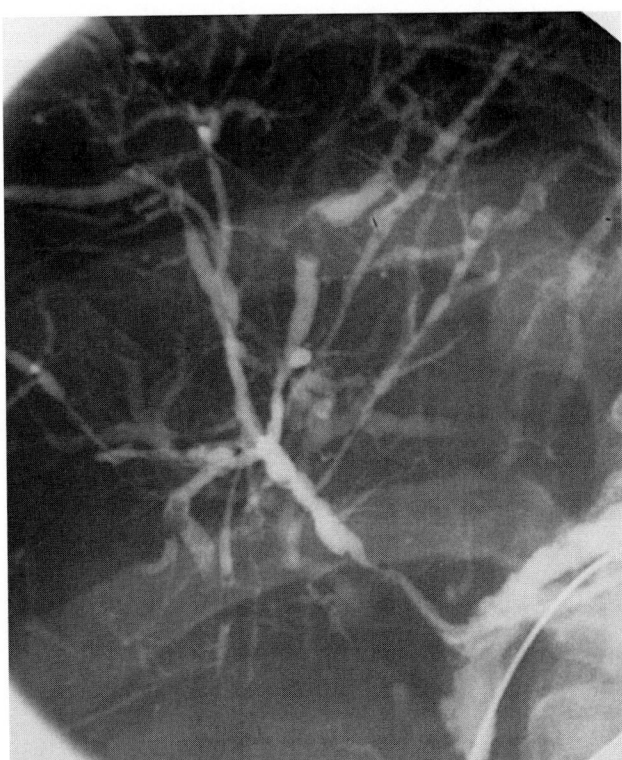

FIGURE 52-22. Percutaneous cholangiogram demonstrating hepatic bifurcation (lower right) and right hepatic ducts in patient with primary sclerosing cholangitis. Cholangiogram demonstrates diffuse strictures of the intrahepatic bile ducts.

Management

Medical therapy for primary sclerosing cholangitis has been disappointing to date. Ursodeoxycholate lowers serum bilirubin and transaminases but has not improved symptoms or delayed disease progression. Biliary strictures in patients with primary sclerosing cholangitis have been dilated or stented using either the percutaneous or endoscopic route. These nonoperative procedures have produced short-term improvements in symptoms and serum bilirubin levels. Symptomatic patients with persistent jaundice are also candidates for surgical therapy. Resection of the extrahepatic biliary tree with bilateral hepaticojejunostomies has yielded reasonable short-term results in patients with significant extrahepatic or bifurcation strictures. Surgical resection should be performed only in patients without cirrhosis or significant hepatic fibrosis on liver biopsy. In addition, patients in whom a cholangiocarcinoma cannot be excluded should also be explored.

Ahrendt and associates recently reported 146 patients with primary sclerosing cholangitis managed with either operative resection or nonoperative biliary dilation.[34] Overall survival was significantly longer in the noncirrhotic patients with primary sclerosing cholangitis managed with surgical resection than in the group of patients managed nonoperatively. Similarly, patients without cirrhosis managed with resection survived significantly longer before needing a liver transplant than patients managed nonoperatively (Table 52-6).[34]

TABLE 52-6. Transplant-Free Survival by Treatment Method: Actuarial Survival in Years (%)

		No. of Years		
		1	3	5
ALL PATIENTS				
Resection	50	86	81	71
ES/BD	35	76	55[†]	36[*]
Percutaneous stenting	19	84	61	49
Combined nonoperative[‡]	54	78	57[†]	40[*]
NONCIRRHOTIC PATIENTS				
Resection	40	95	92	82
ES/BD	26	83	56[*]	42[*]
Percutaneous stenting	17	87	64[†]	51[†]
Combined nonoperative	43	85	59[*]	46[*]

[*]$P < 0.01$ vs. resection.
[†]$P < 0.05$ vs. resection.
[‡]Combined nonoperative includes patients managed with endoscopic balloon dilation or percutaneous stenting.
n, number of patients; ES/BD endoscopic sphincterotomy plus balloon dilation.
Adapted from Ahrendt SA, Pitt HA, Kalloo AN, et al: Primary sclerosing cholangitis: Resect, dilate, or transplant? Ann Surg 227:412-423, 1998.

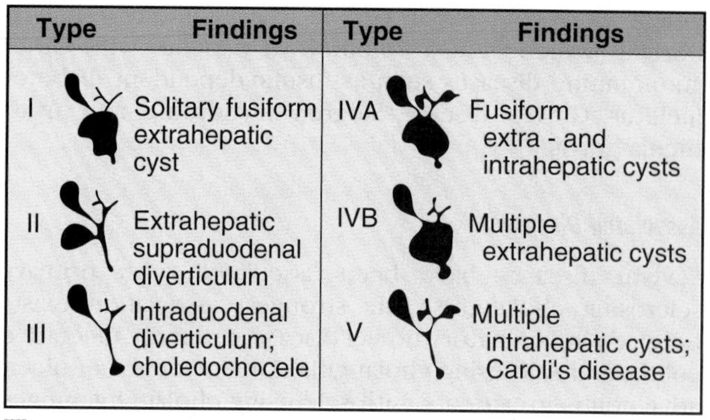

Type	Findings	Type	Findings
I	Solitary fusiform extrahepatic cyst	IVA	Fusiform extra- and intrahepatic cysts
II	Extrahepatic supraduodenal diverticulum	IVB	Multiple extrahepatic cysts
III	Intraduodenal diverticulum; choledochocele	V	Multiple intrahepatic cysts; Caroli's disease

FIGURE 52-23. Todani modification of Alonso-Lej classification of choledochal cysts. (From Chijiiwa K, Koga A: Surgical management and long-term follow-up of patients with choledochal cysts. Am J Surg 165:238-242, 1993.)

Primary sclerosing cholangitis is a progressive disease that eventually results in biliary cirrhosis. Liver transplantation has produced excellent results in patients with primary sclerosing cholangitis and end-stage liver disease. Overall 5-year actuarial patient survival is as high as 85%, and 5-year graft survival of 72% has been reported. Recurrent primary sclerosing cholangitis has been reported in up to 10% of patients and may require retransplantation. Biliary tract surgery prior to liver transplantation does not affect survival following transplantation. Long-term survival in patients with a small incidental cholangiocarcinoma (>1 cm) is similar to patients without cholangiocarcinoma.

Biliary Cysts

Choledochal cyst is a rare congenital dilation of the extrahepatic and/or intrahepatic biliary tract. Although choledochal cysts frequently present in infancy and childhood, the disease is more commonly diagnosed in adults. The incidence of choledochal cyst is only between 1 in 100,000 and 1 in 150,000 people in Western countries but is much more common in Japan. Choledochal cysts are three to eight times more common in women than men.

Etiology and Classification

The frequent presentation of choledochal cysts in infancy supports a congenital origin. An anomalous pancreatobiliary duct junction (APBDJ) has also been documented in between 90% and 100% of patients with choledochal cysts. In APBDJ, the pancreatic duct joins the common bile duct more than 1 cm proximal to the ampulla, resulting in a long common channel and free reflux of pancreatic secretions into the biliary tract. This reflux of pancreatic juice into the biliary tract results in increased biliary pressures and inflammatory changes in the biliary epithelium and may be related to the formation of choledochal cysts.

The current classification of choledochal cysts was initially proposed by Alonso-Lej and was subsequently modified by Todani (Fig. 52-23).[35] Type I cysts (fusiform or cystic dilations of the extrahepatic biliary tract) are the most common and comprise 50% of choledochal cysts. Type IV cysts (cystic dilation of both the intrahepatic and extrahepatic biliary tract) also occur frequently (35% of patients). Type II (saccular diverticulum of extrahepatic bile duct), type III (bile duct dilation within the duodenal wall [choledochocele]), and type V cysts (intrahepatic cysts [Caroli's disease]) are much less common, with each type being diagnosed in fewer than 10% of patients with choledochal cysts.

Clinical Presentation

The classic clinical triad associated with choledochal cysts includes right upper quadrant pain, jaundice, and an abdominal mass; however, this presentation occurs in fewer than 10% of patients. The clinical presentation differs among children and adults. In adults, abdominal pain (87%) and jaundice (42%) are present frequently. Less common clinical findings include nausea (29%), cholangitis (26%), pancreatitis (23%), and an abdominal mass (13%).[36]

Laboratory evaluation may demonstrate mild liver function abnormalities in 60% of adult patients with choledochal cysts, and these findings are not specific. The diagnosis can be established with ultrasound or CT scanning but may be overlooked if the diagnosis is not considered. Cholangiography (endoscopic, transhepatic, or MR) is required to determine the type of choledochal cyst and plan the extent of operative treatment.

Management

Appropriate management of types I and II choledochal cysts should include cholecystectomy, resection of the extrahepatic biliary tract including the choledochal cyst, and Roux-en-Y hepaticojejunostomy. Internal drainage of the cyst into a Roux-en-Y jejunal limb was commonly performed in the past but is associated with a prohibitive risk of cholangitis and hepatolithiasis. In addition, cystenterostomy may increase the risk of cholangiocarcinoma developing in the cyst. Cholangiocarcinoma is uncommon in children with choledochal cysts, but the risk of cholangiocarcinoma may be as high as 30% in adults and supports the role of resection in the management.[36] Resection of the extrahepatic biliary tract is also recommended for type IV cysts. If the intrahepatic cysts are confined to one lobe, hepatic lobectomy may also be considered. Bilobar intrahepatic cysts are associated with a high risk of intrahepatic stones and are managed with long-term transhepatic stenting to provide continuous access to the intrahepatic biliary tree for stone retrieval.

MALIGNANT BILIARY DISEASE

Gallbladder Cancer

Cancer of the gallbladder is an aggressive malignancy that occurs predominantly in the elderly. With the exception of early-stage cases detected incidentally at the time of cholecystectomy for gallstone disease, the prognosis for most patients is poor. Many of these tumors are unresectable at presentation, and most can be managed nonoperatively. Recently, an aggressive surgical approach for patients with localized gallbladder cancer has produced encouraging results with an acceptable morbidity.

Incidence

Gallbladder cancer is the fifth most common gastrointestinal malignancy.[37] Cancer of the gallbladder is two to three times more common in women than men, in part due to the higher incidence of gallstones in women.[38] More than 75% of patients with this malignancy are older than 65 years of age.[38] Approximately 5000 new cases are diagnosed annually in the United States, and the overall incidence of gallbladder cancer is 2.5 cases per 100,000 residents. The incidence of gallbladder cancer varies considerably with both ethnic background and geographic location. In the United States, gallbladder cancer is more common in Native Americans. Similarly, in Chile, the incidence of gallbladder cancer is particularly high.

Etiology

Several factors have been associated with an increased risk of developing gallbladder cancer. Among these factors, gallstones are the most common because of the high prevalence in the general population. The association between an APBDJ, a porcelain gallbladder, and other biliary disorders such as choledochal cysts and primary sclerosing cholangitis and gallbladder cancer has been recognized more recently.

A strong association has long been noted between gallbladder cancer and cholelithiasis, which is present in 75% to 90% of cases. The incidence of gallstones increases with age, and by age 75, about 35% of women and 20% of men in the United States have developed gallstones.[10] The incidence of gallbladder cancer is approximately seven times more common in the presence of cholelithiasis and chronic cholecystitis than in people without gallstones. In addition, the risk of developing gallbladder cancer is higher in patients with symptomatic gallstones than in patients with asymptomatic gallstones. Approximately 1% of all elective cholecystectomies performed for cholelithiasis harbor an occult gallbladder cancer.

Pathology and Staging

Ninety percent of cancers of the gallbladder are classified as adenocarcinoma. Squamous cell, oat cell, undifferentiated, and adenosquamous cancers and carcinoid tumors are much less frequent. Six percent of gallbladder adenocarcinomas demonstrate papillary features histopathologically; these tumors are commonly diagnosed while localized to the gallbladder and are also associated with an improved overall survival. At diagnosis, 25% of cancers are localized to the gallbladder wall, 35% have associated metastases to regional lymph nodes or extension into adjacent organs, and 40% have already metastasized to distant sites.[38]

Lymphatic drainage from the gallbladder occurs in a predictable fashion and correlates with the pattern of lymph node metastases seen in gallbladder cancer. Lymph flow from the gallbladder initially drains to the cystic duct node and then descends along the common bile duct to pericholedochal lymph nodes. Flow then proceeds to nodes posterior to the head of the pancreas and then to interaortocaval lymph nodes. Secondary routes of lymphatic drainage include the retroportal and right celiac lymph nodes. Hepatic involvement with gallbladder cancer can occur by direct invasion through the gallbladder bed, angiolymphatic portal tract invasion, or distant hematogenous spread. The current TNM classification of the American Joint Committee on Cancer (AJCC) is shown in Table 52-7.[39] The appropriate management and overall prognosis are strongly dependent on tumor stage.

Clinical Presentation

Gallbladder cancer most often presents with right upper quadrant abdominal pain often mimicking other more common biliary and nonbiliary disorders. Weight loss, jaundice, and an abdominal mass are less common presenting symptoms. Five different clinical syndromes have been used to describe the presentation of patients with gallbladder cancer (Table 52-8). The largest group of patients present with symptoms of chronic cholecystitis, often with a recent change in the quality or frequency of the painful episodes. Another common presentation is similar to acute cholecystitis with a short duration of pain associated with vomiting, fever, and tenderness. Signs and symptoms of malignant biliary obstruction with jaundice, weight loss, and right upper quadrant pain are also common. Patients can also present with symptoms of a nonbiliary malignancy with anorexia and weight loss in the absence of jaundice or, least commonly, with signs of gastrointestinal bleeding or obstruction. Gallbladder cancer is often misdiagnosed as chronic cholecystitis, pancreatic cancer, acute cholecystitis, choledocholithiasis, or gallbladder hydrops.

Diagnosis

Ultrasonography is often the first diagnostic modality used in the evaluation of patients with right upper quadrant abdominal pain. A heterogeneous mass replacing the gallbladder lumen and an irregular gallbladder wall are common sonographic features of gallbladder cancer. The sensitivity of ultrasound in the detection of gallbladder cancer ranges from 70% to 100%. CT scan usually demonstrates a mass replacing the gallbladder or extending into adjacent organs (Fig. 52-24). Spiral CT also demonstrates the adjacent vascular anatomy. With newer MR techniques, gallbladder cancers may be differentiated from the adjacent liver and biliary obstruction and/or encasement of the portal vein may also be easily visualized.

Cholangiography also may be helpful in diagnosing jaundiced patients with gallbladder cancer. The typical cholangiographic finding in gallbladder cancer is a long stricture of the common hepatic duct. Angiography, spiral CT, or MR imaging may identify encasement of the portal vein or hepatic artery. If radiologic studies suggest that the tumor is unresectable (liver or peritoneal metastases, portal vein encasement, or extensive hepatic invasion), a biopsy of the tumor is warranted and can be performed under ultrasound or CT guidance.

Management

The appropriate operative procedure for the patient with localized gallbladder cancer is determined by the pathologic stage. Patients with tumors confined to the gallblad-

TABLE 52-7.   TNM Staging for Gallbladder Cancer

T1	Tumor invades lamina propria (T1a) or muscular (T1b) layer
T2	Tumor invades perimuscular connective tissue, no extension beyond the serosa or into the liver
T3	Tumor perforates the serosa (visceral peritoneum) and/or directly invades into liver and/or one other adjacent organ or structure such as the stomach, duodenum, colon, pancreas, omentum, or extrahepatic bile ducts
T4	Tumor invades main portal vein or hepatic artery or invades multiple extrahepatic organs and/or structures
N0	No lymph node metastases
N1	Regional lymph node metastases
M0	No distant metastases
M1	Distant metastases

Stage	Stage Grouping
IA	T1 N0 M0
IB	T2 N0 M0
IIA	T3 N0 M0
IIB	T1 N1 M0 T2 N1 M0 T3 N1 M0
III	T4 Any N M0
IV	Any T Any N M1

Adapted from Greene F, Page D, Fleming I, et al (eds): AJCC Cancer Staging Manual, 6th ed. New York, Springer-Verlag, 2002.

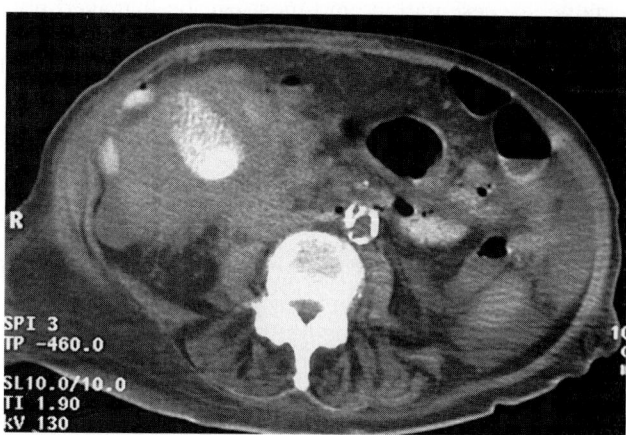

FIGURE 52-24. CT scan demonstrating large gallbladder cancer with extension into duodenum. Gallstones (calcifications) are present within the mass.

TABLE 52-8.   Clinical Presentation of Gallbladder Cancer

Presenting Syndrome	Signs and Symptoms	Percentage of Patients with Gallbladder Cancer*
Chronic cholecystitis (biliary colic)	Postprandial RUQ pain, often with recent change in character	40–45
Acute cholecystitis	Short-duration RUQ pain, nausea, vomiting, fever, tenderness	15–20
Malignant biliary obstruction	Jaundice, weakness, weight loss, anorexia, pain	30–35
Malignant, nonbiliary tract tumor	Anorexia, weight loss, weakness	25–30
Other gastrointestinal problem	Gastrointestinal bleeding or obstruction	<5

*Some overlap among different clinical syndromes present.
RUQ, right upper quadrant.

der mucosa or submucosa (T1a) or confined to the gallbladder muscularis (T1b) are usually identified following cholecystectomy for gallstone disease and have an overall 5-year survival approaching 100% and 85%, respectively. Therefore, cholecystectomy is adequate therapy for patients with T1 tumors. Recurrent cancer at port sites and peritoneal carcinomatosis have been reported following laparoscopic cholecystectomy even for patients with in situ disease. Bile spillage occurs in 26% to 36% of laparoscopic cholecystectomies and appears to be even more common (50%) in cases of gallbladder cancer.[40] Bile spillage is associated with poor survival even in early stage (T1 and T2) gallbladder cancer. Thus, patients with preoperatively suspected gallbladder cancer should undergo open cholecystectomy to minimize the chance of bile spillage and tumor dissemination.[40]

Cancer of the gallbladder with invasion beyond (stages II and III) the gallbladder muscularis is associated with an increasing incidence of regional lymph node metastases and should be managed with an "extended cholecystectomy," including lymphadenectomy of the cystic duct, pericholedochal, portal, right celiac, and posterior pancreatoduodenal lymph nodes. Adequate clearance of the pericholedochal lymph nodes is facilitated by resection of the common bile duct. Extension into the hepatic parenchyma is common, and extended cholecystectomy should incorporate at least a 2-cm margin beyond the palpable or sonographic extent of the tumor. For smaller tumors, this goal can be achieved with a wedge resection of the liver. For larger tumors an anatomic liver resection may be required to achieve a histologically negative margin. Staging laparoscopy should be performed prior to attempted resection in patients with gallbladder cancer because of the high (48% to 55%) incidence of hepatic and peritoneal metastases not detected by noninvasive staging modalities.[41]

In most cases, therapy for gallbladder cancer is palliative. If a tissue diagnosis can be established in patients with an unresectable tumor, nonoperative palliation should be considered. Many of these patients have obstructive jaundice that can be managed with either an endoscopic or percutaneously placed biliary stent. Pain is another problem that should be treated aggressively to improve quality of life. Percutaneous celiac ganglion nerve block may reduce the need for narcotics.

The results of chemotherapy in the treatment of patients with gallbladder cancer have been quite poor. Recently, gemcitabine has demonstrated activity in patients with gallbladder cancer.[42] External beam and intraoperative radiation therapy have both been used in the management of patients with gallbladder cancer.[42] However, no randomized data have demonstrated improved survival with either technique. Trials of chemoradiation in patients with stages II and III disease need to be performed.

Survival

Survival in patients with gallbladder cancer is strongly influenced by the pathologic stage at presentation.[43] Patients with cancer limited to the gallbladder mucosa and submucosa (T1a) have a uniformly excellent prognosis.[43] Invasion into the muscular wall (T1b) of the gallbladder increases the risk of recurrent cancer after curative resection. However, no difference in 10-year survival has been demonstrated following simple cholecystectomy (100%) and extended cholecystectomy (75%) among patients with T1b gallbladder cancer.[44] Invasion into the subserosa (T2) increases the risk of regional lymph node metastases to 33% to 50%.[37,43] Five-year survival in patients with T2 tumors is improved following extended cholecystectomy with lymphadenectomy/liver resection (59% to 61%) versus simple cholecystectomy (17% to 19%) (Fig. 52-25).[37,43] Several groups have recently reported 5-year overall survival for resected patients with stages IIA and IIB gallbladder cancer of 28% to 63% and 19% to 25%, respectively.[43] However, most patients with gallbladder cancer have advanced, unresectable disease at the time of presentation. As a result, fewer than 15% of all patients with gallbladder cancer are alive after 5 years.[38] The median survival for stage IV patients at the time of presentation is only 1 to 3 months.

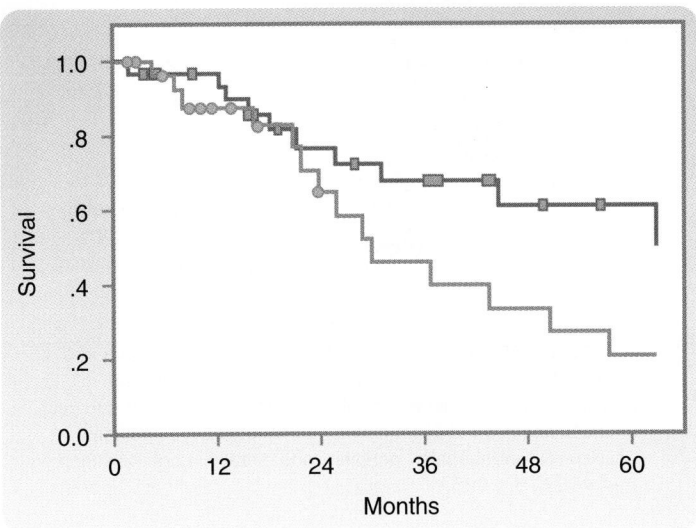

FIGURE 52-25. Survival following surgical resection for T2 gallbladder cancer. Patients undergoing radical resection (boxes) are compared with patients undergoing simple cholecystectomy (circles) ($P > 0.05$). (From Fong Y, Jarnagin W, Blumgart LH: Gallbladder cancer: Comparison of patients presenting initially for definitive operation with those presenting after prior noncurative intervention. Ann Surg 232:557-569, 2000.)

Cholangiocarcinoma

Cholangiocarcinoma is an uncommon tumor, which may occur anywhere along the intrahepatic or extrahepatic biliary tree. These tumors are located most commonly at the hepatic duct bifurcation (60% to 80% of cases). Less commonly, cholangiocarcinomas originate in the distal common bile duct or in the intrahepatic bile ducts. Most cholangiocarcinomas present with jaundice, and the diagnosis of cholangiocarcinoma should be considered in every patient with obstructive jaundice. When possible, surgical resection does offer a chance for long-term disease-free survival. Many patients, however, will be candidates only for palliative bypass or operative or nonoperative intubation aimed to provide biliary drainage and prevent cholangitis and hepatic failure.

Incidence

Between 2500 and 3000 new cases of cholangiocarcinoma are diagnosed annually in the United States. The incidence of cholangiocarcinoma increases with age, and these tumors occur with similar frequency in men and women. Overall, the incidence of cholangiocarcinoma in the United States is approximately 1.0 per 100,000 people per year.[38]

Risk Factors

A number of diseases have been linked to cholangiocarcinoma, including primary sclerosing cholangitis, choledochal cysts, and hepatolithiasis.[25,33,36] Characteristics common to these diseases include bile duct stones, biliary stasis, and infection. Bile duct cancers in patients with primary sclerosing cholangitis are most often extrahepatic, commonly occur near the hepatic duct bifurcation and are difficult to differentiate from the multiple, benign strictures associated with this disease.[33] The mean age at presentation in patients with cholangiocarcinoma and primary sclerosing cholangitis is in the 5th decade of life, and the risk of cholangiocarcinoma does not appear related to the duration of the primary sclerosing cholangitis. Similarly, choledochal cysts are usually diagnosed in childhood or early adult life, and the risk of cholangiocarcinoma increases steadily with patient age.[36] Hepatolithiasis is also a definite risk factor for cholangiocarcinoma, which will develop in 5% to 10% of the patients with intrahepatic stones.[25]

Prior biliary-enteric anastomosis may also increase the future risk of cholangiocarcinoma. Five percent of patients in a large Italian series developed cholangiocarcinoma between 11 and 18 years following a biliary-enteric anastomosis.[45] The risk of bile duct cancer was higher following transduodenal sphincteroplasty and choledochoduodenostomy than hepaticojejunostomy and was most strongly associated with recurrent episodes of cholangitis.[45] Multiple other risk factors for cholangiocarcinoma have been identified including liver flukes, Thorotrast, dietary nitrosamines, and exposure to dioxin.

Staging and Classification

Cholangiocarcinoma is best classified anatomically into three broad groups: (1) intrahepatic, (2) perihilar, and (3) distal (Fig. 52-26).[46] Intrahepatic tumors are treated like hepatocellular carcinoma with hepatectomy, when possible. The perihilar tumors make up the largest group and are managed with resection of the bile duct preferably with hepatic resection. Distal tumors are managed in a fashion similar to other periampullary malignancies with pancreatoduodenectomy.

Cancers of the hepatic duct bifurcation have also been classified according to their anatomic location (Fig. 52-27). In this system, type I tumors are confined to the common hepatic duct, and type II tumors involve the bifurcation without involvement of secondary intrahepatic ducts. Types IIIa and IIIb tumors extend into either the right or left secondary intrahepatic ducts, respectively, and type IV tumors involve the secondary intrahepatic ducts on both sides.

Cholangiocarcinoma is also staged according to the tumor, node, metastasis (TNM) classification of the AJCC (Table 52-9).[39] Using this system, stage IA tumors are limited to the bile duct, whereas stage IB tumors invade periductal tissues. Stage IIA tumors are locally advanced without lymph node metastases, and stage IIB tumors have regional lymph node metastases. Stage III tumors are locally advanced and unresectable, and stage IV tumors have distant metastases.[39]

Clinical Presentation

More than 90% of patients with perihilar or distal tumors present with jaundice.[46] Patients with intrahepatic cholan-

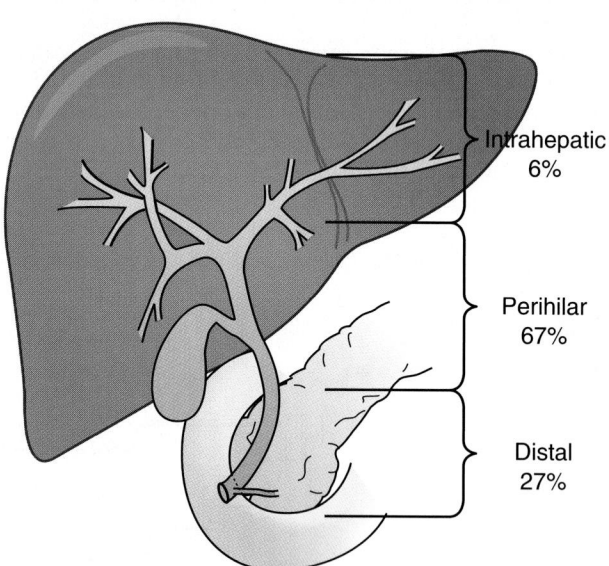

FIGURE 52-26. Classification of cholangiocarcinoma into intrahepatic, perihilar, and distal subgroups, including the percentage of patients with cholangiocarcinoma in each subgroup. (From Nakeeb A, Pitt HA, Sohn TA, et al: Cholangiocarcinoma: A spectrum of intrahepatic, perihilar, and distal tumors. Ann Surg 224:463-475, 1996.)

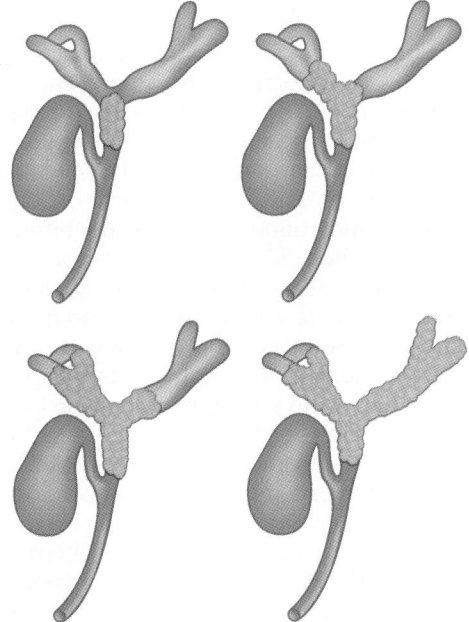

FIGURE 52-27. Bismuth classification of perihilar cholangiocarcinoma by anatomical extent. Type I tumors *(upper, left)* are confined to the common hepatic duct, and type II tumors *(upper, right)* involve the bifurcation without involvement of secondary intrahepatic ducts. Type IIIa and IIIb tumors *(lower, left)* extend into either the right or left secondary intrahepatic ducts, respectively. Type IV tumors *(lower, right)* involve the secondary intrahepatic ducts on both sides.

TABLE 52-9.	TNM Staging for Extrahepatic Cholangiocarcinoma
T1	Tumor confined to bile duct
T2	Tumor invades beyond the wall of the bile duct
T3	Tumor invades the liver, gallbladder, pancreas, and/or unilateral branches of the portal vein (right or left) or hepatic artery (right or left)
T4	Tumor invades any of the following: main portal vein or its branches bilaterally, common hepatic artery, or other adjacent structures, such as the colon, stomach, duodenum, or abdominal wall
N0	No regional lymph node metastasis
N1	Regional lymph node metastasis
M0	No distant metastasis
M1	Distant metastasis

Stage	Stage Grouping
IA	T1 N0 M0
IB	T2 N0 M0
IIA	T3 N0 M0
IIB	T1 N1 M0 T2 N1 M0 T3 N1 M0
III	T4 Any N M0
IV	Any T Any N M1

Adapted from Greene F, Page D, Fleming I, et al (eds): AJCC Cancer Staging Manual, 6th ed. New York, Springer-Verlag, 2002.

giocarcinoma are rarely jaundiced until late in the course of the disease. Less common presenting clinical features include pruritus, fever, mild abdominal pain, fatigue, anorexia, and weight loss. Cholangitis is not a frequent presenting finding but most commonly develops after biliary manipulation. Except for jaundice, the physical examination is usually normal in patients with cholangiocarcinoma.

Diagnosis

At the time of presentation, most patients with perihilar and distal cholangiocarcinoma have a total serum bilirubin level greater than 10 mg/dL. Marked elevations are also routinely observed in alkaline phosphatase. Serum CA 19–9 may also be elevated in patients with cholangiocarcinoma, although levels may fall once biliary obstruction is relieved.

The radiologic evaluation of patients with cholangiocarcinoma should delineate the overall extent of the tumor, including involvement of the bile ducts, liver, portal vessels, and distant metastases. The initial radiographic studies consist of either abdominal ultrasound or CT scanning. Intrahepatic cholangiocarcinomas are easily visualized on CT scans; however, perihilar and distal tumors are often difficult to visualize on ultrasound and standard CT scan. A hilar cholangiocarcinoma gives a picture of a dilated intrahepatic biliary tree and a normal or collapsed gallbladder and extrahepatic biliary tree.

Distal tumors lead to dilation of the gallbladder and both the intrahepatic and extrahepatic biliary tree.

After documentation of bile duct dilation, biliary anatomy has been traditionally defined cholangiographically through either the percutaneous transhepatic or the endoscopic retrograde routes. The most proximal extent of the tumor is the most important feature in determining resectability in patients with perihilar tumors, and the percutaneous route is favored in these patients because it defines the proximal extent of tumor involvement most reliably (Fig. 52-28). Recently, MRC has documented diagnostic accuracy comparable to percutaneous and endoscopic cholangiography.

Prolonged efforts to establish a tissue diagnosis are not indicated unless the patient is not an operative candidate. Percutaneous fine-needle aspiration biopsy, brush and scrape biopsy, and cytologic examination of bile all have been used; however, the sensitivity in detecting a malignancy is low, and a benign result should be considered unreliable. Seven percent to 15% of patients with preoperative symptoms and imaging studies and intraoperative findings consistent with malignant biliary obstruction will ultimately have benign lesions on histologic analysis of resection specimens. However, these patients cannot be reliably identified preoperatively using current imaging or pathologic evaluation.

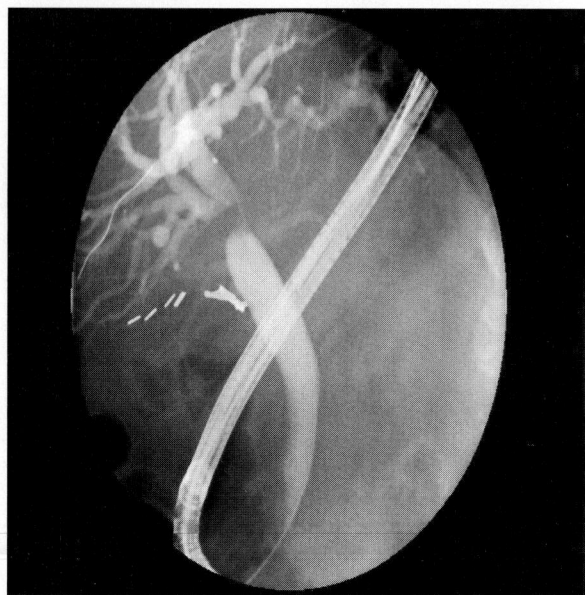

FIGURE 52-28. Endoscopic retrograde cholangiogram demonstrating a perihilar cholangiocarcinoma involving secondary intrahepatic branches on the right as well as the common hepatic duct. The left hepatic duct is not visualized.

Management

Curative treatment of patients with cholangiocarcinoma is possible only with complete resection. The operative approach depends on the site and extent of the tumor. For patients with anatomically resectable intrahepatic cholangiocarcinoma and without advanced cirrhosis, partial hepatectomy is the procedure of choice.[42,46] Patients with perihilar tumors involving the bifurcation or proximal common hepatic duct (Bismuth type I or II) that have no vascular invasion are candidates for local tumor excision. Biliary enteric continuity is restored with bilateral hepaticojejunostomies.[46,47] If preoperative evaluation suggests involvement of the right or left hepatic duct (Bismuth type IIIa or IIIb), right or left hepatic lobectomy, respectively, should be planned (Fig. 52-29).[46,47] To achieve negative margins, resection of the adjacent caudate lobe may be required.[47] A greater percentage of margin negative resections has been achieved with an increased use of combined bile duct and hepatic resection.[47] However, these more extensive procedures have been associated with an increase in operative morbidity and mortality. For patients with resectable distal cholangiocarcinoma, pancreatoduodenectomy is the optimal procedure.

FIGURE 52-29. **A,** Diagram illustrates left hepatic and hilar resection of Bismuth type IIIb cholangiocarcinoma with preoperatively placed transhepatic stents.

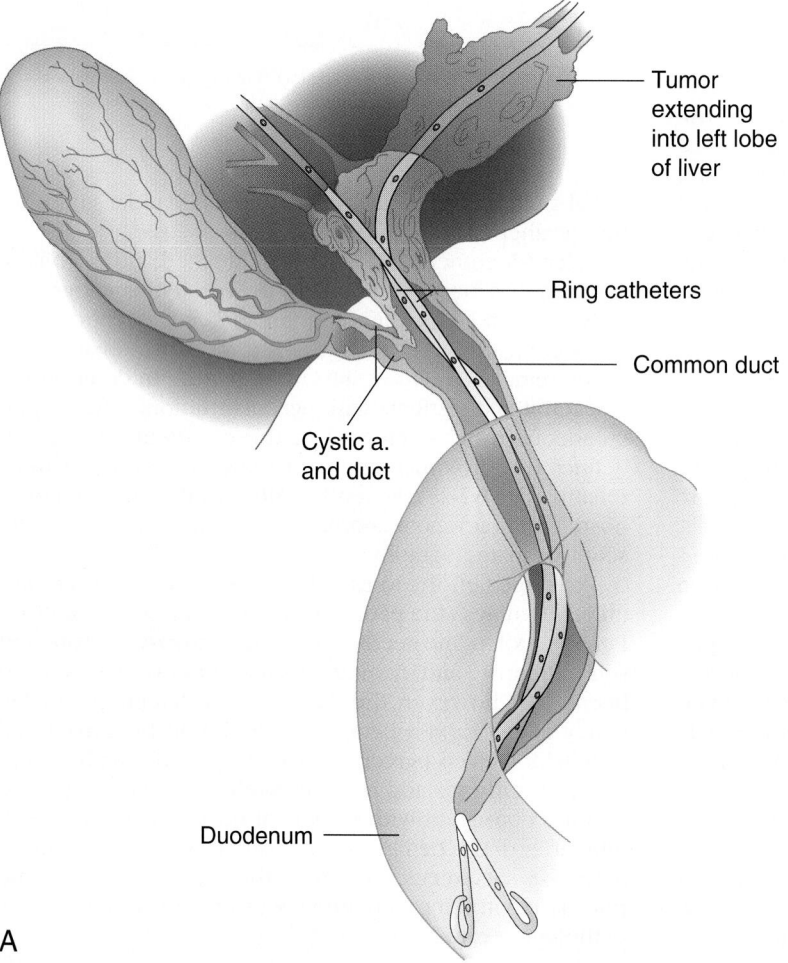

Tumor extending into left lobe of liver

Ring catheters

Common duct

Cystic a. and duct

Duodenum

A

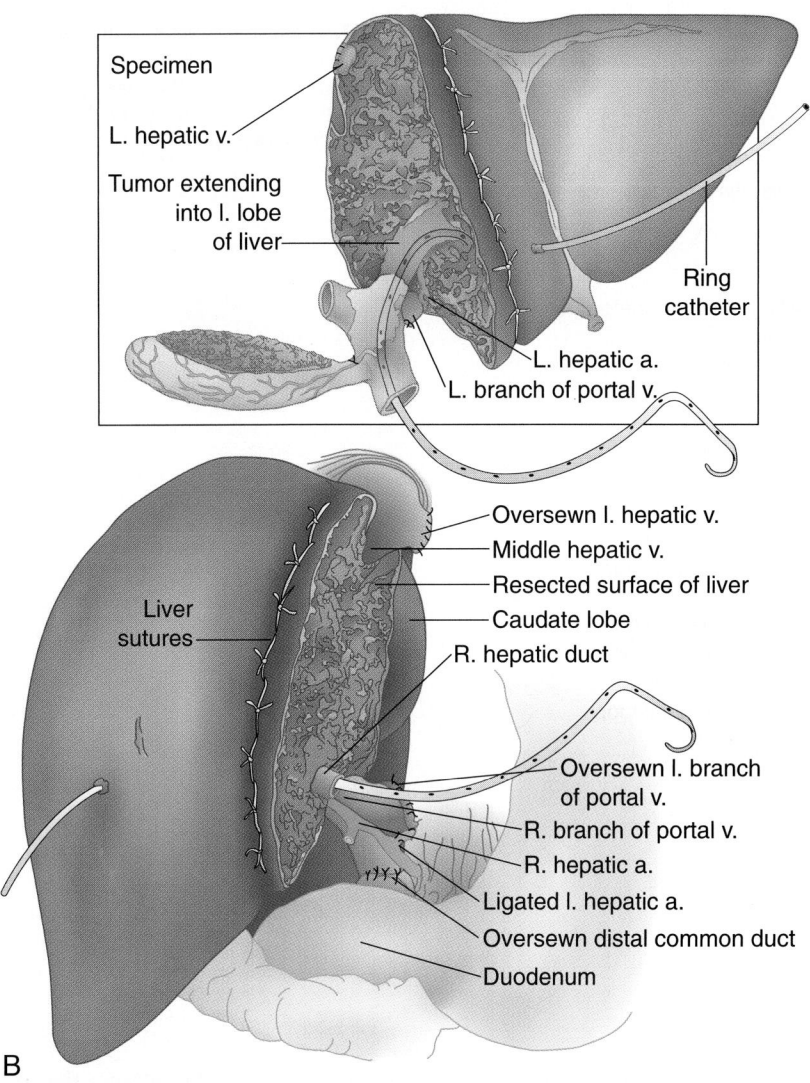

Specimen

L. hepatic v.

Tumor extending
into l. lobe
of liver

Ring
catheter

L. hepatic a.

L. branch of portal v.

Oversewn l. hepatic v.

Middle hepatic v.

Resected surface of liver

Caudate lobe

R. hepatic duct

Liver
sutures

Oversewn l. branch
of portal v.

R. branch of portal v.

R. hepatic a.

Ligated l. hepatic a.

Oversewn distal common duct

Duodenum

B

FIGURE 52-29.   Cont'd B, Diagram demonstrates resected left hepatic lobe and hilum with perihilar cholangiocarcinoma (*top*) and right hepatic lobe with divided right hepatic duct prior to reconstruction (*bottom*).

Surgical exploration should be undertaken in "good-risk" patients without evidence of metastatic or locally unresectable disease; however, intraoperatively more than half of these patients are found to have either peritoneal or hepatic metastases or, more likely, locally unresectable disease.[42,46] Selective use of laparoscopy in patients with locally advanced but potentially resectable perihilar cholangiocarcinoma may avoid laparotomy in some patients with metastatic disease.[41] In patients with extensive metastatic disease preoperative biliary stents may be left in place. However, a cholecystectomy should be performed to avoid the risk of acute cholecystitis, which occurs in patients with long-term indwelling biliary stents. In patients with locally advanced unresectable perihilar tumors, several operative approaches are available for palliation including a Roux-en-Y choledochojejunostomy with intraoperative placement of Silastic biliary catheters or a segment III or V cholangiojejunostomy. Most distal bile duct tumors are resectable; but if resection is not possible due to vascular encasement, cholecystectomy, Roux-en-Y hepaticojejunostomy proximal to

the tumor, and a gastrojejunostomy to prevent gastric outlet obstruction should be performed.

Patients with unequivocal evidence of unresectable cholangiocarcinoma at initial evaluation are palliated nonoperatively. Nonoperative palliation can be achieved both endoscopically and percutaneously. Percutaneous biliary drainage has several advantages over endoscopic management in patients with perihilar cholangiocarcinoma, whereas endoscopic palliation is the preferred approach in patients with distal cholangiocarcinoma. More recently, metallic stents have been used to palliate patients with malignant biliary obstruction. These stents remain patent longer than plastic stents and require fewer subsequent manipulations.

Numerous reports have suggested that radiation therapy improves survival for patients with cholangiocarcinoma, especially when resection is impossible. External-beam radiotherapy has been delivered using a variety of innovative techniques, including intraoperative radiotherapy and brachytherapy with iridium 192 via percutaneous or endoscopic stents. However, no prospective, randomized trials

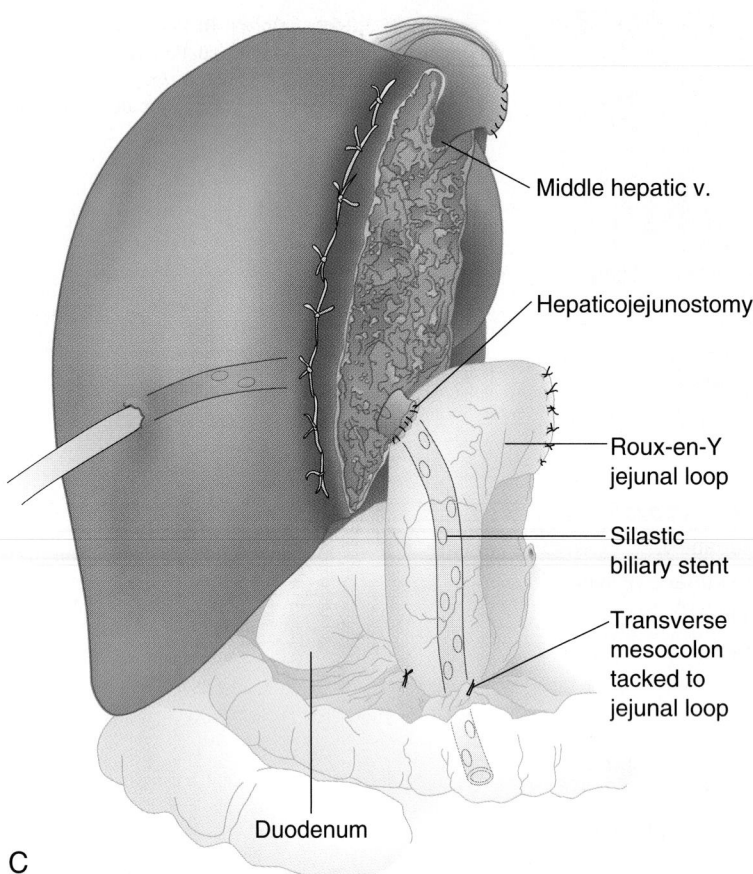

FIGURE 52-29.   Cont'd C, Silastic transhepatic stent is placed through a right Roux-en-Y cholangiojejunostomy after left hepatic lobectomy. (**A–C,** From Cameron J: Atlas of Surgery, Vol 1. Philadelphia, BC Decker, 1990.)

Middle hepatic v.

Hepaticojejunostomy

Roux-en-Y
jejunal loop

Silastic
biliary stent

Transverse
mesocolon
tacked to
jejunal loop

Duodenum

C

have been reported, and a well-controlled, but not randomized, trial reported no benefit for postoperative adjuvant radiation.[48] A survival benefit for postoperative radiation therapy may be limited to patients with local extension into the liver parenchyma and microscopic residual disease following resection.[49] Chemotherapy has also not been shown to improve survival in patients with either resected or unresected cholangiocarcinoma. Given the potential radiosensitization effect of 5-fluorouracil or gemcitabine, the combination of radiation and chemotherapy may be more effective than either agent alone.[42] As with gallbladder cancer, the role of adjuvant chemoradiation needs to be tested in patients with cholangiocarcinoma.

Long-term survival in patients with cholangiocarcinoma is highly dependent on the stage of disease at presentation and on whether the patient is treated by a palliative procedure or complete tumor resection. For resectable intrahepatic cholangiocarcinoma, overall 5-year survival ranges from 30% to 40%. In comparison, overall 5-year survival for patients with resectable perihilar tumors has been only 10% to 20% but may be as high as 24% to 46% in patients with negative microscopic margins (Fig. 52-30).[47,50] Patients with resectable distal bile duct cancer have the highest rate of resection. Those with resectable distal bile duct cancer have a median survival of 32 to 38 months and a 5-year survival rate of 28% to 45%.[46] Even with multimodality adjuvant therapy, median survival for unresectable intrahepatic tumors has been only 6 to 7 months. Similarly, median survival for patients with unresectable perihilar tumors varies between 5 and 8 months.

Metastatic and Other Tumors

Hepatocellular carcinoma and liver metastases can cause obstructive jaundice by direct extension into the perihilar bile ducts. Hepatocellular and metastatic colorectal carcinoma have also both been reported to "embolize" into the biliary tree. This rare phenomenon occurs when tumor cells are shed into the biliary tract and implant distally, leading to biliary obstruction when the tumor embolus increases in size. Hepatic cystadenomas and cystadenocarcinomas arise from the biliary epithelium, and these tumors or the mucin they produce, may also cause bile duct obstruction.

Primary and secondary hepatic tumors can also produce biliary obstruction by metastasizing to hilar or pericholedochal lymph nodes. Hepatocellular carcinoma,

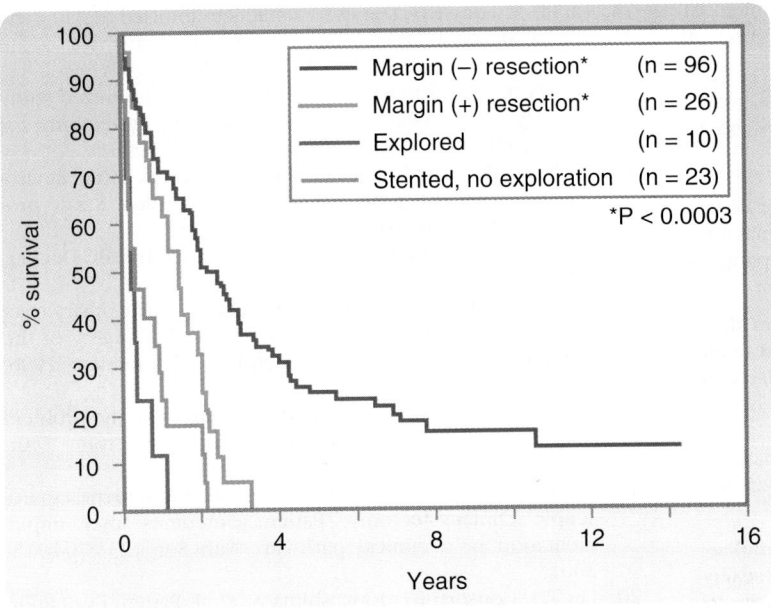

FIGURE 52-30. Actuarial survival following surgical resection for perihilar cholangiocarcinoma. Five-year survival following margin negative resection is significantly longer than following margin positive resection, no resection, or palliative stenting. (From Tsao JI, Nimura Y, Kamiya J, et al: Management of hilar cholangiocarcinoma: Comparison of an American and a Japanese experience. Ann Surg 232:166-174, 2000.)

colorectal carcinoma, and pancreatic carcinoma are the most common primary sites associated with biliary tract obstruction from lymph node metastases, although nodal metastases from a number of tumors including breast and ovarian cancer have been reported to cause bile duct obstruction. Lymphoma can also result in biliary obstruction and mimic either pancreatic cancer or perihilar cholangiocarcinoma. Although commonly extensive, lymphomas usually respond to chemotherapy, leading to resolution of the biliary obstruction.

Selected References

Boerma D, Rauws W, Keulemans Y, et al: Wait-and-see policy or laparoscopic cholecystectomy after endoscopic cholecystectomy for bile-duct stones: A randomized trial. Lancet 360:761-765, 2002.

> Prospective, randomized trial comparing observation versus laparoscopic cholecystectomy following the endoscopic removal of common bile duct stones. Recurrent biliary symptoms developed in 47% of patients in the observation arm, and one third of these patients required cholecystectomy.

Fletcher D, Hobbs M, Tan P, et al: Complications of cholecystectomy: Risks of the laparoscopic approach and protective effects of operative cholangiography—a population-based study. Ann Surg 229:449-457, 1999.

> Large population-based study demonstrating an increased risk of bile duct injury associated with acute cholecystitis, male gender, and procedures done by surgical trainees. Intraoperative cholangiography was associated with a 50% reduction in the risk of bile duct injury.

Fong Y, Jarnagin W, Blumgart L: Gallbladder cancer: Comparison of patients presenting initially for definitive operation with those presenting after prior noncurative operation. Ann Surg 232:557-569, 2000.

> Single-institution series demonstrating long-term survival following extensive resections for patients with advanced gallbladder cancer. Prior noncurative surgery did not preclude long-term survival.

Glasgow R, Cho M, Hutter M, et al: The spectrum and cost of complicated gallstone disease in California. Arch Surg 135:1021-1027, 2000.

> Retrospective series illustrating the continued high rate (44% of all cholecystectomies) of complicated gallstone cases in California in 1996. Half of all patients developing complications of gallstones had symptomatic, radiologically proven gallstones.

Lillemoe K, Melton G, Cameron J, et al: Postoperative bile duct strictures: Management and outcome in the 1990s. Ann Surg 232:430-441, 2000.

> Large series reviewing surgical and radiological methods for managing laparoscopic bile duct injuries. Excellent long term results were achieved with both techniques.

Liu T, Consorti E, Kawashima A, et al: Patient evaluation and management with selective use of magnetic resonance cholangiography and endoscopic retrograde cholangiopancreatography before laparoscopic cholecystectomy. Ann Surg 234:33-40, 2001.

> Single-institution study evaluating a diagnostic and therapeutic algorithm for managing choledocholithiasis.

Rhodes M, Sussman L, Cohen L, et al: Randomized trial of laparoscopic exploration of common bile duct versus postoperative endoscopic retrograde cholangiography for common bile duct stones. Lancet 351:159, 1998.

> Prospective, randomized trial of laparoscopic common bile duct exploration and endoscopic retrograde cholangiography and stone extraction performed postoperatively. Laparoscopic common bile duct exploration was successful in 75% of patients and significantly shortened overall hospitalization.

Strasberg S, Hertl M, Soper N: An analysis of the problem of biliary injury during laparoscopic cholecystectomy. J Am Coll Surg 180:101, 1995.

> **Review article outlining classification, diagnosis, and management of bile duct injuries during laparoscopic cholecystectomy.**

Tocchi A, Mazzoni G, Liotta G, et al: Late development of bile duct cancer in patients who had biliary-enteric drainage for benign disease: A follow-up study of more than 1000 patients. Ann Surg 234:210-214, 2001.

> **Large series of Italian patients followed over 10 years after biliary enteric drainage. Biliary enteric drainage led to an alarming rate of cholangiocarcinoma (5%), particularly in patients with ongoing cholangitis.**

Tsao J, Nimura Y, Kamiya J, et al: Management of hilar cholangiocarcinoma: Comparison of an American and a Japanese experience. Ann Surg 232:166-174, 2000.

> **Large retrospective review of patients with hilar cholangiocarcinoma managed in an American and a Japanese tertiary care center. A more aggressive operative strategy in the Japanese center led to more extensive resections with a higher rate of negative surgical margins and higher long-term survival rate.**

References

1. Ahrendt SA, Pitt HA: A history of the bilioenteric anastomosis. Arch Surg 125:1493-1500, 1990.
2. Smadja C, Blumgart L: The biliary tract and the anatomy of biliary exposure. In Blumgart L (ed): Surgery of the Liver and Biliary Tract. New York, Churchill Livingstone, 1994, pp 11-24.
3. Klein A, Lillemoe K, Yeo C, et al: Liver, biliary tract, and pancreas. In O'Leary J (ed): Physiologic Basis of Surgery. Baltimore, Williams & Wilkins, 1996, pp 441-478.
4. Csendes A, Burdiles P, Maluenda F, et al: Simultaneous bacteriologic assessment of bile from gallbladder and common bile duct in control subjects and patients with gallstones and common duct stones. Arch Surg 131:389-394, 1996.
5. Thompson JE Jr, Pitt HA, Doty JE, et al: Broad-spectrum penicillin as an adequate therapy for acute cholangitis. Surg Gynecol Obstet 171:275-282, 1990.
6. Cox J, Ahrendt S: Antibiotic selection in biliary tract surgery. In Cameron J (ed): Current Surgical Therapy. St. Louis, Mosby, 2001, p 494.
7. Rhodes M, Sussman L, Cohen L, et al: Randomised trial of laparoscopic exploration of common bile duct versus postoperative endoscopic retrograde cholangiography for common bile duct stones. Lancet 351:159-161, 1998.
8. Sewnath ME, Karsten TM, Prins MH, et al: A meta-analysis on the efficacy of preoperative biliary drainage for tumors causing obstructive jaundice. Ann Surg 236:17-27, 2002.
9. Sohn TA, Yeo CJ, Cameron JL, et al: Do preoperative biliary stents increase postpancreaticoduodenectomy complications? J Gastrointest Surg 4:258-268, 2000.
10. Bateson MC: Gallbladder disease and cholecystectomy rate are independently variable. Lancet 2:621-624, 1984.
11. Glasgow RE, Cho M, Hutter MM, et al: The spectrum and cost of complicated gallstone disease in California. Arch Surg 135:1021-1027, 2000.
12. Kiviluoto T, Siren J, Luukkonen P, et al: Randomised trial of laparoscopic versus open cholecystectomy for acute and gangrenous cholecystitis. Lancet 351:321-325, 1998.
13. Lai PB, Kwong KH, Leung KL, et al: Randomised trial of early versus delayed laparoscopic cholecystectomy for acute cholecystitis. Br J Surg 85:764-767, 1998.
14. Lo CM, Liu CL, Fan ST, et al: Prospective randomized study of early versus delayed laparoscopic cholecystectomy for acute cholecystitis. Ann Surg 227:461-467, 1998.
15. Willsher PC, Sanabria JR, Gallinger S, et al: Early laparoscopic cholecystectomy for acute cholecystitis: A safe procedure. J Gastrointest Surg 3:50-53, 1999.
16. Cameron J: Atlas of Surgery, Vol 2. Philadelphia, BC Decker, 1994.
17. Curet M, Zucker K: Laparoscopic surgery of the biliary tract and liver. In Zuidema G (ed): Shackelford's Surgery of the Alimentary Tract, 3rd ed. Philadelphia, WB Saunders, 1996, pp 257-278.
18. Strasberg SM, Hertl M, Soper NJ: An analysis of the problem of biliary injury during laparoscopic cholecystectomy. J Am Coll Surg 180:101-125, 1995.
19. Calland JF, Tanaka K, Foley E, et al: Outpatient laparoscopic cholecystectomy: Patient outcomes after implementation of a clinical pathway. Ann Surg 233:704-715, 2001.
20. Liu TH, Consorti ET, Kawashima A, et al: Patient evaluation and management with selective use of magnetic resonance cholangiography and endoscopic retrograde cholangiopancreatography before laparoscopic cholecystectomy. Ann Surg 234:33-40, 2001.
21. Magnuson TH, Bender JS, Duncan MD, et al: Utility of magnetic resonance cholangiography in the evaluation of biliary obstruction. J Am Coll Surg 189:63-72, 1999.
22. Melton GB, Lillemoe KD, Cameron JL, et al: Major bile duct injuries associated with laparoscopic cholecystectomy: Effect of surgical repair on quality of life. Ann Surg 235:888-895, 2002.
23. Boerma D, Rauws EA, Keulemans YC, et al: Wait-and-see policy or laparoscopic cholecystectomy after endoscopic sphincterotomy for bile-duct stones: A randomised trial. Lancet 360:761-765, 2002.
24. Tzovaras G, Rowlands BJ: Diagnosis and treatment of sphincter of Oddi dysfunction. Br J Surg 85:588-595, 1998.
25. Pitt HA, Venbrux AC, Coleman J, et al: Intrahepatic stones: The transhepatic team approach. Ann Surg 219:527-537, 1994.
26. Sugiyama M, Xie XY, Atomi Y, et al: Differential diagnosis of small polypoid lesions of the gallbladder: The value of endoscopic ultrasonography. Ann Surg 229:498-504, 1999.
27. Fletcher DR, Hobbs MS, Tan P, et al: Complications of cholecystectomy: Risks of the laparoscopic approach and protective effects of operative cholangiography—a population-based study. Ann Surg 229:449-457, 1999.
28. Branum G, Schmitt C, Baillie J, et al: Management of major biliary complications after laparoscopic cholecystectomy. Ann Surg 217:532-541, 1993.
29. Lee CM, Stewart L, Way LW: Postcholecystectomy abdominal bile collections. Arch Surg 135:538-544, 2000.
30. Cameron J: Atlas of Surgery, Vol 1. Philadelphia, BC Decker, 1990.
31. Lillemoe KD, Melton GB, Cameron JL, et al: Postoperative bile duct strictures: Management and outcome in the 1990s. Ann Surg 232:430-441, 2000.
32. Poon RT, Liu CL, Lo CM, et al: Management of gallstone cholangitis in the era of laparoscopic cholecystectomy. Arch Surg 136:11-16, 2001.
33. Ahrendt SA, Pitt HA, Nakeeb A, et al: Diagnosis and management of cholangiocarcinoma in primary sclerosing cholangitis. J Gastrointest Surg 3:357-368, 1999.

34. Ahrendt SA, Pitt HA, Kalloo AN, et al: Primary sclerosing cholangitis: Resect, dilate, or transplant? Ann Surg 227:412-423, 1998.

35. Chijiiwa K, Koga A: Surgical management and long-term follow-up of patients with choledochal cysts. Am J Surg 165:238-242, 1993.

36. Lipsett PA, Pitt HA, Colombani PM, et al: Choledochal cyst disease: A changing pattern of presentation. Ann Surg 220:644-652, 1994.

37. Chijiiwa K, Nakano K, Ueda J, et al: Surgical treatment of patients with T2 gallbladder carcinoma invading the subserosal layer. J Am Coll Surg 192:600-607, 2001.

38. Carriaga MT, Henson DE: Liver, gallbladder, extrahepatic bile ducts, and pancreas. Cancer 75:171-190, 1995.

39. Gallbladder and extrahepatic bile ducts. *In* Greene F, Page D, Fleming I, et al (eds): American Joint Committee on Cancer Staging Manual, 6th ed. New York, Springer-Verlag, 2002, pp 139-150.

40. Weiland ST, Mahvi DM, Niederhuber JE, et al: Should suspected early gallbladder cancer be treated laparoscopically? J Gastrointest Surg 6:50-57, 2002.

41. Weber SM, DeMatteo RP, Fong Y, et al: Staging laparoscopy in patients with extrahepatic biliary carcinoma: Analysis of 100 patients. Ann Surg 235:392-399, 2002.

42. Nakeeb A, Tran KQ, Black MJ, et al: Improved survival in resected biliary malignancies. Surgery 132:555-564, 2002.

43. Fong Y, Jarnagin W, Blumgart LH: Gallbladder cancer: Comparison of patients presenting initially for definitive operation with those presenting after prior noncurative intervention. Ann Surg 232:557-569, 2000.

44. Wakai T, Shirai Y, Yokoyama N, et al: Early gallbladder carcinoma does not warrant radical resection. Br J Surg 88:675-678, 2001.

45. Tocchi A, Mazzoni G, Liotta G, et al: Late development of bile duct cancer in patients who had biliary-enteric drainage for benign disease: A follow-up study of more than 1,000 patients. Ann Surg 234:210-214, 2001.

46. Nakeeb A, Pitt HA, Sohn TA, et al: Cholangiocarcinoma: A spectrum of intrahepatic, perihilar, and distal tumors. Ann Surg 224:463-475, 1996.

47. Tsao JI, Nimura Y, Kamiya J, et al: Management of hilar cholangiocarcinoma: Comparison of an American and a Japanese experience. Ann Surg 232:166-174, 2000.

48. Pitt HA, Nakeeb A, Abrams RA, et al: Perihilar cholangiocarcinoma: Postoperative radiotherapy does not improve survival. Ann Surg 221:788-798, 1995.

49. Todoroki T, Kawamoto T, Koike N, et al: Radical resection of hilar bile duct carcinoma and predictors of survival. Br J Surg 87:306-313, 2000.

50. Klempnauer J, Ridder GJ, von Wasielewski R, et al: Resectional surgery of hilar cholangiocarcinoma: A multivariate analysis of prognostic factors. J Clin Oncol 15:947-954, 1997.

EXOCRINE PANCREAS

Michael L. Steer, M.D.

The pancreas was first mentioned in the writings of Eristratos (310–250 BC) and given its name by Rufus of Ephesus (c.100 AD). The name pancreas (Greek *pan*: all, *kreas*: flesh or meat) was used because the organ contains neither cartilage nor bone. Its main duct was described by Wirsung in 1642, whereas the enlargement of that duct at its junction with the common bile duct and its projection into the duodenum as a papilla were first described by Vater in 1720. Santorini, in 1734, described the accessory duct that bears his name.

ANATOMY

Location

The pancreas lies posterior to the stomach and lesser omentum in the retroperitoneum of the upper abdomen. It extends obliquely, rising slightly as it passes from the medial edge of the duodenal C loop to the hilum of the spleen. It lies anterior to the inferior vena cava, aorta, splenic vein, and left adrenal gland.

Regions

The pancreas is divided into four regions: the head/uncinate process, neck, body, and tail. The head lies within the duodenal C loop, and its uncinate process extends posteriorly and medially to lie behind the portal/superior mesenteric vein and superior mesenteric artery. The neck of the gland extends medially from the head to lie anterior to those vessels. The body extends laterally from the neck toward the spleen, whereas the tail extends into the splenic hilum.

Blood Supply and Lymph Nodes

Both the celiac trunk and the superior mesenteric artery provide the arterial supply to the pancreas. Variations are common but, for the most part, the body and tail are supplied by branches of the splenic artery while the head and uncinate process receive their supply via arcades originating from the hepatic/gastroduodenal branch of the celiac artery and from the first branch of the superior mesenteric artery (Fig.53-1A). Venous drainage is to the splenic, superior mesenteric, and portal veins (Fig. 53-1B). The pancreas is drained by multiple lymph node groups. The major drainage of the pancreatic head and uncinate process is to the subpyloric, portal, mesenteric, mesocolic, and aortocaval nodes. The pancreatic body and tail, for the most part, are drained via nodes in the celiac, aortocaval, mesenteric, and mesocolic groups and via nodes in the splenic hilum.

Innervation

The pancreas is innervated by both sympathetic and parasympathetic components of the autonomic nervous system. The principal, and possibly only, pathway for pancreatic pain involves nociceptive fibers arising in the pancreas. They pass through the celiac ganglia to form the greater, lesser, and least splanchnic nerves that pass to cell bodies in the thoracic sympathetic chain. Efferent visceral motor supply to the pancreas is provided by both the sympathetic and parasympathetic systems. The latter involves preganglionic fibers arising from cell bodies in the vagal nuclei that travel through the posterior vagal trunk to the celiac plexus. Postganglionic fibers then innervate pancreatic islets, acini, ducts, and blood vessels. In general,

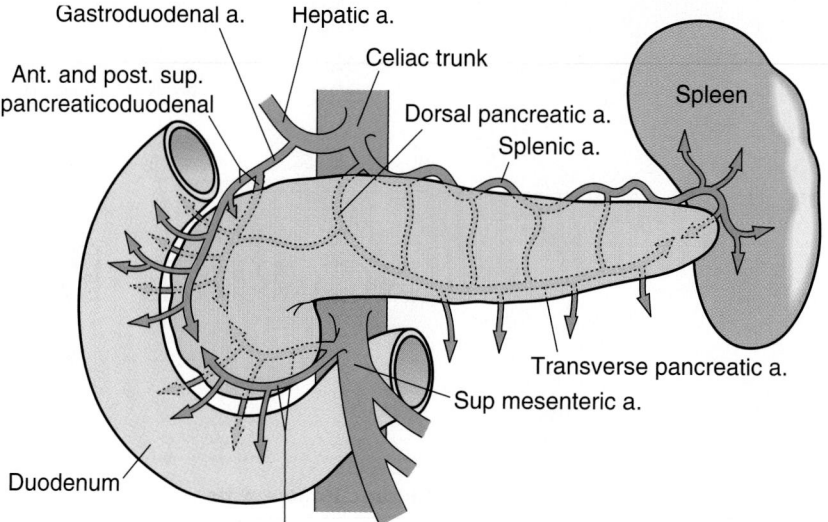

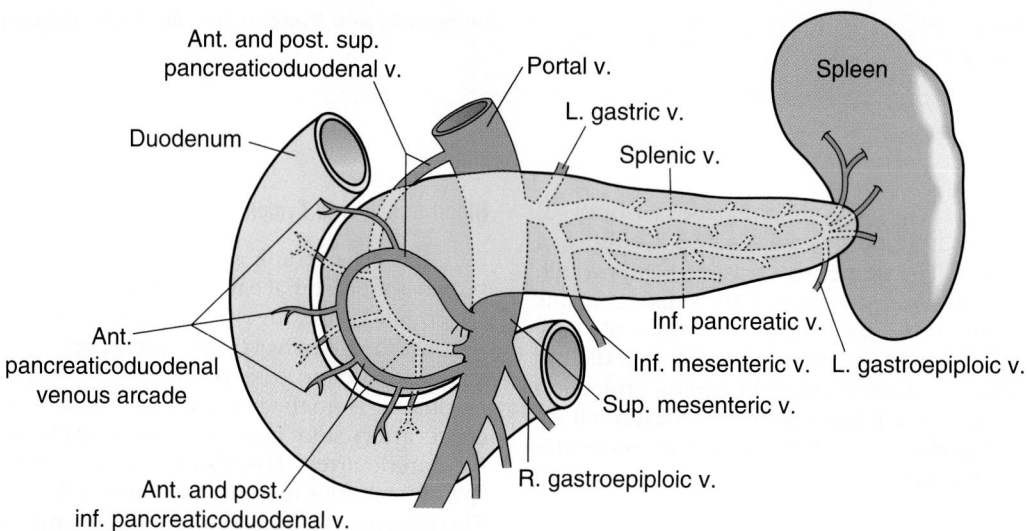

FIGURE 53-1.   Arterial supply to the pancreas (A) and venous drainage of the pancreas (B). The pancreatic head is supplied by branches of the gastroduodenal and superior mesenteric arteries while the body and tail are supplied by branches of the splenic artery. Venous drainage is to the splenic and superior mesenteric/portal veins. (From Skandalakis JE, Gray SW, Rowe JS Jr, et al: Anatomical complications of pancreatic surgery. Contemp Surg 15:17-50, 1979.)

the nerves of the pancreas travel with the blood vessels supplying the organ.

Ducts

The main pancreatic duct, or duct of Wirsung, arises in the tail of the pancreas and terminates at the papilla of Vater in the duodenum. It crosses the vertebral column between T-12 and L-2. Within the body and tail of the pancreas, the duct lies slightly cephalad to a line drawn midway between the superior and inferior edges. The duct is also more posterior than anterior. In adults, the duct within the head measures 3.1 to 4.8 mm in diameter and it gradually tapers, to measure 0.9 to 2.4 mm in the tail. With age, the duct diameter can increase. The duct

of Santorini (i.e., the minor, or accessory, pancreatic duct) is smaller than the main duct. It extends from the main duct to enter the duodenum at the lesser papilla. That papilla lies approximately 2 cm proximal and slightly anterior to the major papilla.

EMBRYOLOGY AND HISTOLOGY

Organogenesis

During the 4th week of gestation, two endodermal buds arise from the duodenum—the hepatic diverticulum, which is destined to form the liver, gallbladder, and bile ducts, and the dorsal pancreatic bud that forms the body

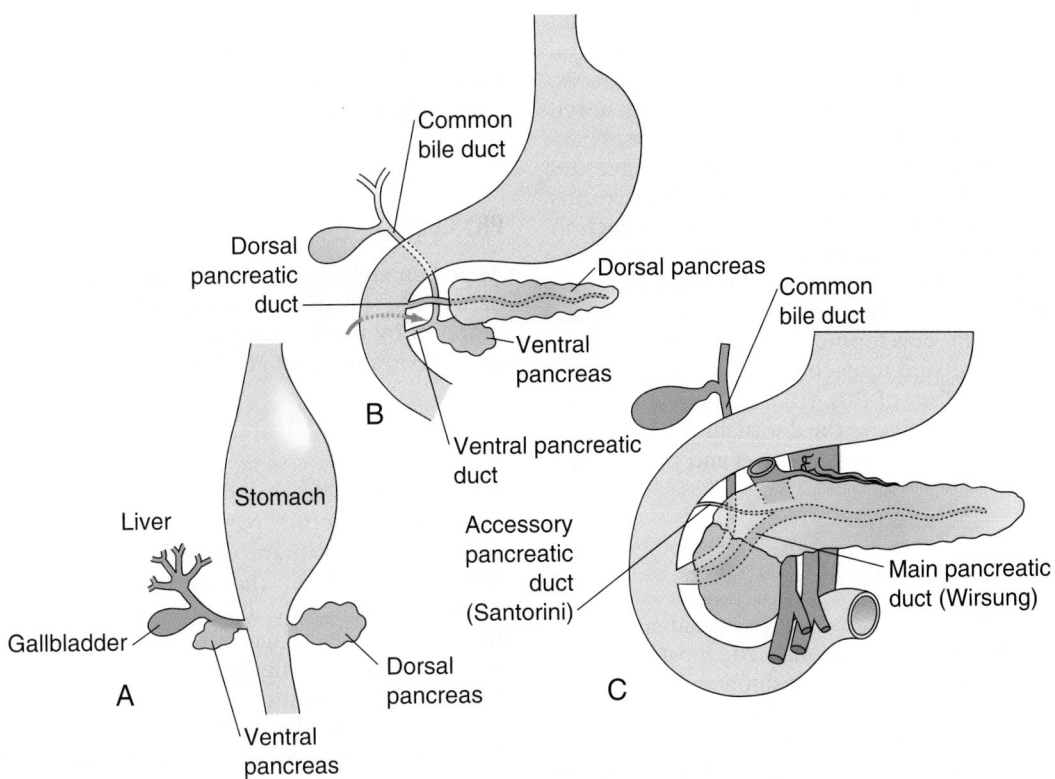

FIGURE 53-2. Organogenesis of the pancreas. *A,* Formation of dorsal and ventral pancreatic buds. *B,* Rotation of the ventral pancreas, distal bile duct, and major papilla. *C,* Fusion of the dorsal and ventral pancreata to form the adult pancreas. (From Skandalakis JE, Gray SW, Rowe JS Jr et al: Anatomical complications of pancreatic surgery. Contemp Surg 15:17-50, 1979.)

and tail of the pancreas (Fig. 53-2). On the 32nd day of gestation, this hepatic diverticulum gives rise to a ventral pancreatic bud that eventually develops into the uncinate process and inferior part of the head of the pancreas. The dorsal pancreatic bud extends transversely across the abdomen, to lie anterior to the portal and mesenteric vessels. With time, as the duodenum rotates to form a C-loop configuration, the ventral pancreas and distal bile duct undergo clockwise rotation around the back of the duodenum to, finally, lie on the medial side of the duodenum, inferior and slightly posterior to the dorsal pancreas and posterior to the portal and mesenteric vessels. On the 37th day of gestation, the two pancreatic buds fuse and, in 90% of individuals, their duct systems also join.

Histology

The mature pancreas is an endocrine organ made up of the islets of Langerhans and an exocrine organ consisting of acinar and ductal cells. The acinar cells, so named because they are clustered like grapes on the stem of a vine, discharge their secretions into a centrally located acinar space that communicates with the main pancreatic duct. Most of the cells in the pancreas are acinar cells, and duct cells make up only 5% of pancreatic mass. Histologically, acinar cells have a high content of endoplasmic reticulum and an abundance of apically located eosinophilic zymogen granules. The cells lining the main

pancreatic duct are tall columnar cells, and many contain mucin granules. With progression from the large ducts to the smaller intralobular and interlobular ducts, the lining cells become flatter, assuming a cuboidal configuration, and mucin granules are no longer seen. Centroacinar cells, located at the junction between ducts and acini, resemble acinar cells in size and shape but lack zymogen granules.

Cell Differentiation

The cells comprising the pancreatic buds are homogeneous and indistinguishable from other endodermal cells of the primitive gut. These endodermal cells undergo stepwise differentiation, from an undifferentiated precursor into committed islet and exocrine cell precursors and then into either acinar cells or ductal cells. Some recently presented evidence has also suggested that transdifferentiation can occur—that differentiated duct cells may give rise to islet and/or acinar cells.

CONGENITAL ANOMALIES

Pancreas Divisum

Failure of the dorsal and ventral pancreatic duct systems to join during embryogenesis (see Fig. 53-2) is referred to as *pancreas divisum.* It results in a pancreas with divided drainage because the dorsal pancreas drains, via the duct of Santorini, to empty at the lesser papilla while the ventral pancreas, composed of the head and uncinate process, drains via Vater's papilla. Pancreas divisum has been noted in as many as 11% of autopsy cases. The significance of pancreas divisum remains controversial. Some have suggested that it may contribute to the development of pancreatitis by establishing a condition of relative outflow obstruction because the major fraction of pancreatic exocrine secretion is obliged to exit through the relatively small orifice of the lesser papilla. On the other hand, the presence of pancreas divisum and the development of pancreatitis are, in most patients, not related to each other in a cause-effect manner and the corollary of this may also be true; that is, attempts to widen the orifice of the dorsal duct at the lesser papilla in patients with pancreas divisum and pancreatitis are unlikely to be of benefit.

Ectopic and Accessory Pancreas

Pancreatic tissue at ectopic sites is not unusual, and most ectopic pancreatic tissue is functional. The most common sites are in the walls of the stomach, duodenum or ileum, in a Meckel's diverticulum, or at the umbilicus. Less common sites include the colon, appendix, gallbladder, omentum, and mesentery. Islet tissue is frequently present when ectopic pancreas is located in the stomach and duodenum but not when it is present elsewhere. For the most part, ectopic pancreatic tissue is a submucosal, irregular nodule of firm, yellow tissue that may have a central umbilication. Pancreatic secretions often exit through this umbilication into the lumen of the stomach or intestine. Ulceration and, on occasion, bleeding can be associated with these lesions. They may also be associated with obstruction or be the lead point for intussusception. Resection or bypass is indicated in such cases.

Annular Pancreas

Annular pancreas refers to the presence of a band of normal pancreatic tissue that partially or completely encircles the second portion of the duodenum and extends into the head of the pancreas. It usually contains a duct that joins the main pancreatic duct. The basis for annular pancreas is uncertain. It may result from failure of normal clockwise rotation of the ventral pancreas, or it may result from expansion of ectopic pancreatic tissue in the duodenal wall. It presents with varying degrees of duodenal obstruction that, in children, is often associated with other congenital anomalies. It may be totally asymptomatic or present later in life with obstructive symptoms if pancreatitis develops in the annular segment. Treatment usually involves bypass, via duodenojejunostomy, rather than resection.

Developmental Pancreatic Cysts

Solitary (congenital, duplication, or dermoid) cysts of the pancreas are rare. In contrast, multiple pancreatic cysts, lined with cuboidal epithelium, are more common. They are frequently associated with polycystic disease of the liver and/or kidney, and they can be seen in up to half of patients with von Hippel-Lindau syndrome. Pancreatic cysts only rarely become symptomatic and, in general, no treatment is indicated.

PHYSIOLOGY

Approximately 2.5 L of clear, colorless, bicarbonate-rich pancreatic juice, containing 6 to 20 g of protein, is secreted by the human pancreas each day. It plays a critical role in duodenal alkalinization and in food digestion.

Protein Secretion

With the possible exception of the lactating mammary gland, the exocrine pancreas synthesizes protein at a greater rate, per gram of tissue, than any other organ. More than 90% of that protein consists of digestive enzymes. Most of the digestive enzymes are synthesized and secreted by acinar cells as inactive proenzymes or zymogens that, in health, are activated only after they reach the duodenum where enterokinase activates trypsinogen and the trypsin catalyses the activation of the other zymogens. Some of the pancreatic digestive enzymes are synthesized and secreted in their active forms without the need for an activation step (e.g., amylase, lipase, ribonuclease). Acinar cells also synthesize proteins, including enzymes, that are not destined for secretion but, rather, are intended for use within the acinar cell itself. Examples of this latter group of proteins include the various structural proteins and lysosomal hydrolases.

Newly synthesized proteins are assembled within the cisternae of the rough endoplasmic reticulum and transported to the Golgi where they are modified by glycosylation. Those destined for secretion pass through the Golgi stacks and are packaged within condensing vacuoles that evolve into zymogen granules as they migrate toward the luminal surface of the acinar cell. By a process involving membrane fusion and fission, the contents of the zymogen granules are then released into the acinar lumen.[1] Other proteins that are not destined for secretion are segregated away from the secretory pathway as they pass through the Golgi, and they are then targeted to their appropriate intracellular site.[2]

Secretion of protein from acinar cells is a regulated process. At rest, secretion occurs at a low or basal rate, but this rate can be markedly increased by secretory stimulation that, in the pancreas, is both hormonal and neural. Pancreatic acinar cells can express receptors for acetylcholine, cholecystokinin, secretin, and vasoactive intestinal peptide. Stimulation of secretion by either acetylcholine or cholecystokinin has been shown to involve activation of phospholipase C, generation of inositol triphosphate and diacyl glycerol, and a rise in intracellular ionized calcium levels that, by yet unidentified mechanisms, upregulates the rate of secretory protein discharge at the apical cell membrane. In contrast, secretin and vasoactive intestinal peptide activate adenylate cyclase, increase cellular levels of cyclic adenosine

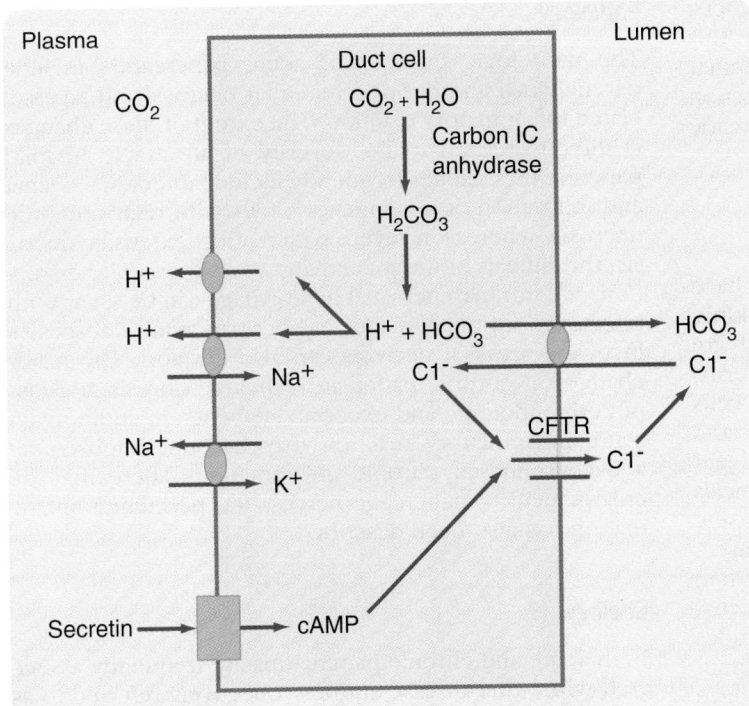

FIGURE 53-3. Secretion of bicarbonate-rich juice by duct cells. CO_2 diffuses into duct cells and is converted to H_2CO_3 by carbonic anhydrase. H_2CO_3 dissociates into HCO_3^- and H^+, which exits at the basal side of the cell. Secretin stimulation increases cyclic adenosine monophosphate (cAMP), which accelerates apical chloride secretion through the cystic fibrosis transmembrane regulator (CFTR) chloride channel. The exchange of luminal Cl^- for cellular HCO_3 results in net HCO_3^- secretion.

monophosphate (AMP), and activate protein kinase A. This also leads to protein secretion at the apical pole. Recent studies indicate that human acinar cells may not possess receptors for cholecystokinin and that, in humans, cholecystokinin stimulation of secretion is mediated by intrapancreatic nerves that express cholecystokinin receptors.

Electrolyte Secretion

Although stimulation of acinar cells results in the secretion of a small amount of serum-like fluid, most of the fluid and electrolytes secreted from the pancreas arise from duct cells (Fig. 53-3).[3] The earliest step in duct cell electrolyte secretion involves diffusion of circulating carbon dioxide into the duct cell and that carbon dioxide is hydrated by carbonic anhydrase to yield carbonic acid. Subsequently, the carbonic acid dissociates into protons and bicarbonate ions. The protons diffuse out of the cell and are carried away in the circulation while the bicarbonate remains inside the cell. The fluid and electrolyte secretagogue secretin acts, via a cyclic AMP–mediated process, to stimulate chloride secretion, at the apical cell surface, via cystic fibrosis transmembrane regulator (chloride) channels. Then, via an apical chloride-bicarbonate exchanger, that actively secreted chloride is re-taken up by the duct cell in exchange for bicarbonate. Taken together, the result of these events is the secretion of a bicarbonate-rich fluid into the duct and the discharge, into the circulation, of protons (see Fig. 53-3). In the absence of secretin stimulation, pancreatic juice has a more plasma-like composition since it is comprised primarily of acinar cell secretions and there is little duct cell secretion of chloride to permit exchange with bicarbonate. With secretin stimulation, chloride secretion is increased, flow rates rise, and chloride-bicarbonate ex-

change results in juice that is rich in bicarbonate and poor in chloride.

Integrated Physiology

During the resting (interdigestive) phase of gastrointestinal function, pancreatic secretion is minimal and may be as low as 2% of that noted with maximal stimulation. The pancreatic response to a meal is a three-phase process that includes a cephalic phase, a gastric phase, and an intestinal phase. The cephalic phase, accounting for 10% to 15% of meal-stimulated pancreatic secretion, reflects the response to the sight, smell, or taste of food. It is believed to be almost exclusively mediated by peripherally released acetylcholine, which directly stimulates pancreatic secretion of enzymes and gastric secretion of acid. The acid indirectly stimulates pancreatic secretion of fluid and electrolytes by causing duodenal acidification and secretin release. The gastric phase of pancreatic secretion, accounting for 10% to 15% of meal-stimulated pancreatic secretion, reflects the response to gastric distention and the entry of food into the stomach. These events can cause release of gastrin and stimulate vagal afferents. By binding to cholecystokinin receptors, gastrin is itself a weak stimulant of pancreatic enzyme secretion. Vagal stimulation also increases enzyme secretion. More important, however, gastrin and vagal stimulation cause gastric acid secretion, and this leads to duodenal acidification, release of secretin from the duodenum, and pancreatic secretion of fluid and electrolytes. The intestinal phase of pancreatic secretion reflects the response to food and gastric secretions entering the proximal intestine. Acidification of the duodenum and the presence of bile in the duodenum promote secretin release. In addition, in the duodenum and proximal small intestine, the presence of fat and protein, as well as their partial breakdown products, stimulates the release of cholecystokinin, and this cholecystokinin stimulates enzyme secretion from acinar cells. The intestinal phase of pancreatic secretion accounts for 70% to 75% of meal-stimulated pancreatic secretion.

Feedback Loop

Luminal proteins, referred to as *releasing factors*, have been described that can also stimulate cholecystokinin and secretin release. The most well characterized are the releasing factors for cholecystokinin.[4] Two forms are known, one apparently synthesized by duodenal cells *(cholecystokinin-releasing factor)* and the other secreted by the pancreas *(monitor peptide)*. Both forms are subject to degradation by trypsin. Thus, with high-protein meals that quench intraduodenal tryptic activity, the releasing factor remains intact, cholecystokinin release is increased, and pancreatic secretion is stimulated. In contrast, when food is absent from the duodenum, the proteolytic activity that remains unquenched within the lumen degrades the releasing factor and, as a result, cholecystokinin release and pancreatic secretion are reduced. Some have argued that this feedback loop may, at least in part, explain the pain of chronic pancreatitis since, with pancreatic insufficiency, intraluminal proteolytic activity would be low and cholecystokinin release would increase. Based on this concept, some have advocated administration of exogenous pancreatic enzymes as a treatment for the chronic pain of pancreatitis. Presumably, administration of exogenous enzymes to such patients would result in degradation of the releasing factor and reduce pancreatic stimulation. However, evidence supporting a physiologic role for these releasing factors comes almost exclusively from experiments using rodents, and the actual existence of a physiologic feedback loop in humans has not been established.

PANCREATITIS

Definition and Classification

Pancreatitis can be classified as either *acute* or *chronic* based on its clinical characteristics, pathologic changes, and natural history. Clinically, acute pancreatitis is usually characterized by the acute onset of symptoms in a previously healthy individual and the disappearance of those symptoms as the attack resolves. In contrast, patients with chronic pancreatitis may have had prior attacks or symptoms of either exocrine or endocrine insufficiency prior to the current attack, and their symptoms may persist even after resolution of the current attack. From a clinical standpoint, however, attacks of *either* acute or chronic pancreatitis can be characterized by the abrupt onset of symptoms that are often similar. Thus, without the test of time or a tissue sample, it may be difficult or impossible to determine if a first attack is one of acute or chronic pancreatitis.

Pathology

The pathologic changes of acute pancreatitis include parenchymal and peripancreatic fat necrosis and an associated inflammatory reaction. The extent of these changes is directly related to the severity of an attack. In mild pancreatitis, changes frequently include interstitial edema and infiltration of inflammatory cells with relatively little necrosis, whereas in severe pancreatitis, extensive necrosis, thrombosis of intrapancreatic vessels, vascular disruption, and intraparenchymal hemorrhage can be seen. With infection, intrapancreatic or peripancreatic abscesses involving areas of necrosis can also develop. The major changes of chronic pancreatitis include fibrosis and loss of both endocrine and exocrine elements. In addition, an acute inflammatory reaction may be superimposed on a background of chronic inflammation. There may be enlargement of pancreatic nerves, and perineural inflammation has also been described.

Etiology

Both acute and chronic pancreatitis are frequently associated with other disease entities collectively referred to as the *etiologies of pancreatitis* (Box 53-1). In developed countries, roughly 70% to 80% of patients with pancreatitis have their pancreatitis in association with either biliary tract stone disease or ethanol abuse. For the most part, biliary tract stone disease is associated with acute pancreatitis, whereas chronic pancreatitis is associated with the intake of large amounts of ethanol over protracted

---

Box 53-1.   Etiologies of Pancreatitis

Acute Pancreatitis

Biliary tract stones
Drugs
ERCP
Ethanol abuse
Hypercalcemia
Hyperlipidemia
Idiopathic
Infections
Ischemia
Parasites
Postoperative
Scorpion sting
Trauma

Chronic Pancreatitis

Autoimmune
Duct obstruction
Ethanol abuse
Hereditary
Hypercalcemia
Hyperlipidemia
Idiopathic

ERCP, endoscopic retrograde cholangiopancreatography.

periods. In 10% to 15% of pancreatitis cases, no etiology can be identified, and those individuals are said to have idiopathic pancreatitis. In the remaining 10% to 15% of patients, pancreatitis is associated with one of many possible miscellaneous etiologies. In underdeveloped countries, particularly in Africa and Southeast Asia, pancreatitis is frequently termed either *tropical* or *nutritional*. Recent reports indicate that many patients with tropical pancreatitis have a form of hereditary pancreatitis caused by mutations of the genes that code for pancreatic secretory trypsin inhibitors.[5] Affected individuals often complain of painful attacks, and they frequently develop pancreatic calcifications as well as diabetes. Ketoacidosis is uncommon.

Biliary Tract Stones

The onset of acute pancreatitis is frequently associated with the passage of biliary tract stones through the terminal biliopancreatic duct into the duodenum. Stones can be retrieved from the stools of roughly 90% of patients with stone-induced pancreatitis. There has been much speculation regarding the mechanisms by which such stones might cause pancreatitis. In 1901, Opie, a pathologist at Johns Hopkins University, noted a stone lodged in the terminal biliopancreatic duct of a patient who had died of severe pancreatitis. He suggested that the stone might have caused outflow obstruction from a *common biliopancreatic channel*, allowing bile to reflux into the pancreatic duct.[6] In a second publication based on observations made at another autopsy, Opie suggested that biliary pancreatitis could also occur when a stone, or the edema and inflammation caused by its passage, caused outflow obstruction of the pancreatic duct even in the absence of bile reflux. Although the bile reflux theory, often referred to as the "common channel theory," was originally favored, subsequent studies have cast doubt on its validity, and most observers now believe that it is stone-induced pancreatic duct obstruction and ductal hypertension, rather than bile reflux, that triggers acute pancreatitis. Recent data derived from experiments using a model of pancreatitis induced in opossums also support the duct obstruction theory. Those experiments indicate that pancreatic duct obstruction, without bile duct obstruction or bile reflux, can cause pancreatitis and that the severity of pancreatitis is not worsened by bile reflux into the pancreatic duct.[7]

Abuse of Ethanol

The most frequent cause of morphologically defined chronic pancreatitis is ethanol abuse, but occasionally ethanol can also induce acute pancreatitis. There is no threshold rate of consumption below which ethanol consumption is not associated with an increased incidence of pancreatitis. The mean ethanol consumption among patients with ethanol-induced pancreatitis is 150 to 175 g/day. The mean duration of ethanol abuse for men is 18 ± 11 years and, for women, it is 11 ± 8 years. Ethanol-induced pancreatitis, like ethanol abuse itself, is more common in men than in women. Dietary factors, such as consumption of a high-protein diet with either high- or low-fat content, may contribute to the development of pancreatitis. Most observers currently believe that the chronic pancreatitis that follows prolonged ethanol abuse reflects repeated, but subclinical, episodes of acute pancreatic injury. These repeated episodes of pancreatic injury with necrosis eventually lead to the fibrosis that characterizes chronic pancreatitis.[8] A number of theories have been advanced to explain the mechanism by which ethanol might cause pancreatic injury. According to one theory, ethanol consumption causes hypertriglyceridemia and the generation of fatty acids as well as their ethyl ester metabolites that can injure the pancreas. Another theory suggests that ethanol ingestion causes intrapancreatic generation of oxygen-derived free radicals that can injure the pancreas. Others believe that ethanol acts directly on pancreatic acinar cells to cause injury or that it promotes secretion of pancreatic juice that is high in proteolytic enzyme content but low in enzyme inhibitor content. Theoretically, enzyme activation could occur under these conditions and that activation could cause pancreatic injury. Secretion of an enzyme-rich fluid deficient in enzyme inhibitors could also lead to protein precipitation and the formation of intraductal plugs. Those plugs, by causing duct obstruction and ductal hypertension, could subsequently trigger pancreatic injury. Ethanol ingestion has also been reported to cause sphincter of Oddi spasm, and this could also contribute to ethanol-induced pancreatitis if it resulted in ductal hypertension. Each of these various theories has attractive features and its own proponents, but, at present, the actual mechanisms by which ethanol causes pancreatitis remain unclear.

Drugs

Exposure to certain drugs is, perhaps, the third most frequent cause of pancreatitis (Box 53-2), but the mechanisms by which those drugs cause pancreatitis is not known. Although many different drugs have been implicated, the strength of the data supporting a cause-effect relationship in pancreatitis varies considerably. Drugs associated with pancreatitis can be divided into the following three groups: (1) those considered to be definite causes of pancreatitis because their use has been associated with the onset of pancreatitis and the disease has recurred when patients have been rechallenged with the drug; (2) those considered to be probable causes of pancreatitis because the incidence of disease is increased in individuals exposed to the drug; and (3) those whose relationship to pancreatitis is just "suspected" because only anecdotal evidence has been presented to support such a relationship. In the past, there have been claims that steroids as well as H_2-histamine antagonists can cause pancreatitis, but there is little evidence to support those claims.

Obstruction

Even in the absence of biliary tract stones, pancreatic duct obstruction can cause pancreatitis. Thus, pancreatitis has been associated with duodenal lesions such as duodenal

Box 53-2.   Drugs Associated with Pancreatitis

Definite Cause

5-Aminosalicylate
6-Mercaptopurine
Azathioprine
Cytosine arabinoside
Dideoxyinosine
Diuretics
Estrogens
Furosemide
Metronidazole
Pentamidine
Tetracycline
Thiazide
Trimethoprim-sulfamethoxide
Valproic acid

Probable Cause

Acetaminophen
α-Methyl-DOPA
Isoniazid
L-Asparaginase
Phenformin
Procainamide
Sulindac

DOPA, dihydroxyphenylalanine.

ulcers, duodenal Crohn's disease, and periampullary tumors. It can also be triggered by a periampullary diverticulum, particularly if that diverticulum is filled with debris or food particles. Pancreatitis can also be the result of a pancreatic duct stricture or disruption following blunt pancreatic trauma or duct obstruction caused by a pancreatic tumor. Most patients with obstruction-induced pancreatitis have chronic, rather than acute, pancreatitis. That chronic pancreatitis affects only the obstructed portion of the pancreas, and it can be cured by removing that part of the pancreas. Post-traumatic strictures, the result of blunt abdominal trauma, can cause pancreatitis. They usually occur where the pancreas passes over the vertebral column. Parasites such as *Ascaris* and *Clonorchis* can also cause pancreatitis by obstructing the pancreatic duct. Pancreas divisum has also been described as a cause of "obstructive" pancreatitis. Presumably, that pancreatitis results from the relative obstruction that might occur at the lesser papilla when the major fraction of pancreatic secretion is forced to exit via that orifice. Most observers believe that pancreas divisum, which occurs in roughly 10% of individuals, is rarely the cause of pancreatitis.

Hereditary and Autoimmune Pancreatitis

There has been considerable recent interest in the few patients who develop pancreatitis on a hereditary basis.[9]

It is generally believed that spontaneous trypsinogen activation normally occurs to a slight degree within the pancreas but that, in health, the pancreas is protected from injury by the presence of trypsin inhibitors. In hereditary pancreatitis, genetic mutations are believed to cause this protective process to fail either because a trypsin that is resistant to inhibition is synthesized or because the trypsin inhibitors themselves are defective. In either case, the end result could be expected to be further intrapancreatic activation of trypsin and, possibly, other digestive enzymes, eventually leading to repeated episodes of pancreatitis. In hereditary pancreatitis, those attacks begin at a young age and lead to chronic changes including fibrosis, calcifications, and loss of both exocrine and endocrine function. The incidence of pancreatic cancer is also markedly increased in patients with hereditary pancreatitis. Hereditary pancreatitis is an autosomal dominant disease with incomplete penetrance. Pancreatic cancer most frequently develops in those with a paternal pattern of inheritance.

Pancreatitis can be the result of an autoimmune process, and, in those patients, it is frequently associated with other autoimmune diseases such as primary sclerosing cholangitis, Sjögren's syndrome, and primary biliary cirrhosis. Recently, a distinct form of autoimmune pancreatitis has been described in which there is a severe, sclerosing process characterized by intense lymphocyte and plasmacyte infiltration. It is frequently associated with bile as well as pancreatic duct strictures, pancreatic inflammation, and a pancreatic mass. Some refer to the disease as *lymphoplasmacytic autoimmune pancreatitis*. Most patients with this form of pancreatitis have elevated circulating IgG levels, and that elevation is mostly due to an elevation in the levels of IgG_4.[10] Perhaps the most important feature of this form of autoimmune pancreatitis is the fact that it frequently presents as an otherwise unexplained mass in the head of the pancreas and the sclerotic process can result in bile as well as pancreatic duct strictures (i.e., a "double-duct" sign). Thus, it can easily be confused with pancreatic cancer. If correctly diagnosed, the mass as well as the strictures can completely resolve with steroid treatment.

Other Miscellaneous Causes of Pancreatitis

Pancreatitis can result from pancreatic trauma even without major duct disruption or stricture. In those cases, the inflammatory process is usually related to contusion or laceration of the gland and possibly disruption of small ducts. Pancreatitis can occur during the postoperative period in patients undergoing procedures on or near the pancreas or procedures associated with either hypoperfusion or atheroembolism (cardiopulmonary bypass, cardiac transplantation, renal transplantation). The injection of the pancreatic duct that occurs during endoscopic retrograde pancreatography or during sphincter of Oddi manometry can also cause pancreatitis. Both acute and chronic pancreatitis can be caused by metabolic abnormalities, especially those leading to hypercalcemia (i.e., hyperparathyroidism) and those leading to hyperlipidemia (type I, IV, or V hyperlipoproteinemias). Hypercalcemia may result in pancreatitis by facilitating intrapancreatic digestive enzyme activation. Hyperlipidemia may lead to pancreatitis if the accompanying hyperchylomicronemia interferes with the pancreatic microcirculation or results in release of free fatty acids in the pancreatic microcirculation. Both hypercalcemia-induced pancreatitis and hyperlipidemia-induced pancreatitis can be prevented if the underlying metabolic abnormality is corrected by either parathyroidectomy or by drug and dietary management of the hyperlipidemia. In places such as Trinidad, scorpion stings are a frequent cause of pancreatitis. Scorpion toxin contains a potent pancreatic secretagogue and, presumably, the excessive pancreatic stimulation that follows exposure to this toxin leads to pancreatic injury.

Idiopathic Pancreatitis

In most series, roughly 20% of patients have pancreatitis without an identifiable etiology. Some of those individuals have gallbladder sludge or microcrystals, and further attacks can be prevented by either cholecystectomy or biliary sphincterotomy. Other patients have been found to have sphincter of Oddi malfunction, sometimes associated with increased pressures in the pancreatic duct system, and they can be effectively treated by sphincterotomy with pancreatic septotomy. Therefore, these patients have forms of biliary pancreatitis rather than truly idiopathic pancreatitis. There remains, however, a significant group of patients with no identifiable cause for their pancreatitis. Recent studies by several independent groups have suggested that some of these patients may have subclinical mutations of the cystic fibrosis gene.[11] In its most severe form, cystic fibrosis can cause pancreatic fibrosis and the loss of both exocrine and endocrine function as a result of the blockade of ducts with inspissated secretions. However, the patients with idiopathic pancreatitis related to cystic fibrosis have subclinical mutations of the cystic fibrosis transmembrane regulator gene. They do not have inspissated secretion and their pancreatitis probably develops on another basis.

Pathophysiology of Acute and Chronic Pancreatitis

It is generally believed that acute pancreatitis is triggered by obstruction of the pancreatic duct and that the injury begins within pancreatic acinar cells. That injury is believed to include, and possibly be the result of, intra-acinar cell activation of digestive enzyme zymogens including trypsinogen. Chronic pancreatitis is believed to reflect repeated episodes of subclinical acute pancreatitis with unrecognized pancreatic necrosis evolving into pancreatic fibrosis.

One of the central issues in our understanding of the cellular events leading to acute pancreatitis is how duct obstruction could result in intra-acinar cell enzyme activation. Perhaps one of the most widely accepted theories to explain this coupling is the so-called colocalization hypothesis.[12] This hypothesis is based on a number of studies that have used experimental models of pancreatitis induced in laboratory animals. In those studies, one of the earliest changes noted has been the colocalization of digestive enzyme zymogens such as trypsinogen with lysosomal hydrolases such as cathepsin B inside cytoplasmic vacuoles. Under these conditions, cathepsin B can activate trypsinogen and trypsin can activate the other zymogens. According to the colocalization hypothesis, cathepsin B–mediated intra-acinar cell activation of the digestive enzymes leads to acinar cell injury and triggers an intrapancreatic inflammatory response. The intensity of that inflammatory response appears to regulate the severity of the pancreatitis and to couple pancreatitis to extrapancreatic events such as lung and renal injury.

Presentation of an Acute Attack

The clinical presentation, diagnosis, and management of an acute attack of pancreatitis are similar regardless of whether that attack is *acute* or *chronic* pancreatitis. In fact, many describe patients with chronic pancreatitis who present with acute symptoms as having *acute on chronic* pancreatitis. On the other hand, the long-term management of patients with acute and chronic pancreatitis may differ considerably. The former primarily involves elimination of the inciting cause whereas, for chronic pancreatitis, irreversible changes have usually occurred prior to diagnosis and long-term management primarily involves treatment of pain and pancreatic exocrine/endocrine insufficiency. For these reasons, this discussion of clinical presentation focuses on issues relevant to an acute attack and does not make distinctions based on whether that is an attack of acute or chronic pancreatitis.

Symptoms

Abdominal pain, nausea, and vomiting are the dominant symptoms of pancreatitis. Typically, the pain is located in the epigastrium, but it may also involve both upper quadrants, the lower abdomen, or the lower chest. It may have a pleuritic component and be felt in one or both shoulders. Most patients describe the pain as being knifelike and radiating straight through to the mid-central back. It is usually abrupt in onset and slowly increases in magnitude to reach a maximal level. The pain is usually constant, although it may be somewhat relieved by leaning forward or lying on the side with the knees drawn upward. Patients with chronic pancreatitis frequently describe similar prior attacks that are often noted to occur within 12 to 24 hours of ethanol consumption. The nausea and vomiting of pancreatitis usually persists even after the stomach has been emptied. The vomiting may lead to gastroesophageal tears (i.e., Mallory-Weiss syndrome) and upper gastrointestinal bleeding. Although vomiting and retching may be relieved by passage of a nasogastric tube, the pain usually persists even after gastric decompression. Some patients, especially those with postoperative pancreatitis who are already receiving analgesic medications, may not experience abdominal pain and, therefore, the diagnosis of pancreatitis may be particularly difficult.

Physical Findings

Pancreatitis patients are frequently noted to be rolling or moving around in search of a more comfortable position and, in this sense, they are unlike patients with a perforated viscus who often remain motionless because movement worsens their pain. Patients with severe pancreatitis usually appear ill and anxious. Hyperthermia is common and may be explained by the release of proinflammatory factors, including cytokines and chemokines, from the injured pancreas. Tachycardia, tachypnea, and hypotension caused by hypovolemia are common. Hypovolemia can also result in collapsed neck veins, dry skin, dry mucous membranes, and diminished subcutaneous elasticity. Because pleuritic and abdominal pain may make breathing difficult, breath sounds in the lower lung fields are usually diminished and atelectasis may be present. A pleural effusion can often be detected on either side, although it is more commonly found on the left. Patients with severe pancreatitis frequently develop an acute lung injury that can clinically present as the adult respiratory distress syndrome (ARDS). Occasionally, patients with pancreatitis have alterations in their mental status as a result of drug or ethanol exposure, hypotension, hypoxemia, or release of circulating toxic agents from the inflamed pancreas. Some degree of jaundice is common. In gallstone-induced acute pancreatitis, the jaundice may reflect distal bile duct obstruction, but jaundice can also occur in nonbiliary pancreatitis either as a result of duct obstruction caused by the inflamed pancreas or as a result of cholestasis induced by the severe illness itself. As a result of ileus, bowel sounds are usually diminished during an attack of pancreatitis and the abdomen may become distended and tympanitic. Direct, percussion, and rebound abdominal tenderness as well as both voluntary and involuntary guarding are common. These findings may be localized to the epigastrium or they may be diffusely present throughout the abdomen. An epigastric mass, reflecting the inflamed pancreas and surrounding tissues, may be felt in the upper abdomen or left upper quadrant. On rare occasions, flank ecchymoses (Grey Turner's sign) or periumbilical ecchymoses (Cullen's sign), which result from retroperitoneal hemorrhage, can be seen during severe pancreatitis. Occasionally, patients develop areas of tender subcutaneous induration and erythema that resemble erythema nodosum but that, in the case of pancreatitis, are caused by subcutaneous fat necrosis.

Diagnosis

Routine Blood Tests

Pancreatitis can induce a diffuse capillary leak syndrome that, when combined with vomiting, can result in significant fluid losses. The resulting hypovolemia can be marked. It usually leads to an increased hematocrit, hemoglobin, blood urea nitrogen, and creatinine. Serum albumin levels may be markedly depressed, particularly if fluid losses are corrected by administration of albumin-free crystalloid solutions. The serum electrolytes may be normal but, with significant vomiting, a hypochloremic metabolic alkalosis can develop. The white blood cell count is usually elevated with an associated left shift in the differential count. Blood glucose may be elevated either due to associated diabetes mellitus or as a result of increased glucagon and catecholamine release combined with diminished insulin release. Hyperbilirubinemia is relatively common during the early stages of pancreatitis. It can be caused by either a biliary tract stone or by the inflamed (and possibly fibrotic) pancreas causing bile duct obstruction and, in this setting, cholangitis with positive blood cultures can be superimposed on the pancreatitis. On the other hand, the hyperbilirubinemia of pancreatitis can also reflect the nonobstructive cholestasis that often accompanies any severe illness. Hypertriglyceridemia is routinely noted in patients who have hyperlipidemia-induced pancreatitis. Hypertriglyceridemia can also be induced by exposure to ethanol and therefore, the diagnosis of pancreatitis should always be suspected when lactescent serum is found when evaluating an alcoholic patient with abdominal pain. Many patients with pancreatitis appear to have hypocalcemia but, for the most part, that hypocalcemia can be explained by the hypoalbuminemia that accompanies pancreatitis. Occasionally however, patients with severe pancreatitis have a reduction in their free, ionized calcium that is not a reflection of hypoalbuminemia. This type of hypocalcemia is associated with a poor prognosis. Some of these patients manifest tetany and carpopedal spasm, making treatment with calcium mandatory. The mechanisms responsible for this type of pancreatitis-associated hypocalcemia are not clear. Most likely, it occurs because bone calcium stores do not respond to circulating parathormone. Patients with severe pancreatitis can also develop disseminated intravascular coagulation. In those cases, thrombocytopenia, elevated levels of fibrin degradation products, a decreased fibrinogen level, prolonged partial thromboplastin time, and a prolonged prothrombin time can be observed.

Amylase Measurement

Serum amylase activity is usually, but not always, elevated during pancreatitis, but the magnitude of that elevation does not parallel the severity of the attack. In fact, as many as 10% of patients with lethal pancreatitis may have near-normal or normal amylase levels. This could reflect the fact that pancreatitis-associated hyperamylasemia can be transient. Typically, amylase levels rise 2 to 12 hours after the onset of symptoms and then decline so that, 3 to 6 days after the onset of an attack, the serum amylase levels are usually normal. Elevations that persist beyond a week suggest either ongoing inflammation or the development of a complication such as pseudocyst, abscess, or pancreatic ascites. Urinary amylase levels remain elevated longer than serum amylase levels and, thus, measurement of urinary amylase levels may be of diagnostic help in patients who present long after the onset of symptoms. Although amylase can enter the circulation from nonpancreatic sites, including the salivary glands, lung, prostate, and ovary, it is pancreatic amylase that accounts for the rise in circulating amylase activity during pancreatitis.

The mechanisms responsible for the hyperamylasemia of pancreatitis are not clear. Some have suggested that, during pancreatitis, amylase and other digestive enzymes may be secreted from the basolateral, as opposed to the apical, surface of acinar cells and, in this manner, they could gain access to the lymphatic and vascular system. On the other hand, some recent studies have indicated that cell-cell contacts are loosened during pancreatitis.[13] This could allow enzymes in the duct to reach periacinar, lymphatic, and intravascular spaces.

The overall sensitivity and specificity of serum amylase determination in the diagnosis of pancreatitis depend on both the clinical presentation and the cut-off value chosen for the upper limit of normal. In some series, sensitivity and specificity values in the low-to-mid 90% range have been reported. Hyperamylasemia can be associated with acute cholecystitis, perforated viscus, bowel obstruction, and bowel infarction. These states can also be clinically confused with pancreatitis since they are also characterized by abdominal pain, nausea, vomiting, and abdominal tenderness. In most cases, patients with hyperamylasemia that is not due to pancreatitis have only mild elevations in the circulating amylase level (i.e., twofold to threefold elevations from the normal value), whereas those with pancreatitis usually have greater elevations. At one time, measurement of the clearance ratio between amylase and creatinine was advocated as a method by which pancreatitis-associated hyperamylasemia could be distinguished from non–pancreatitis-associated elevations of amylase activity. It was claimed that an elevated clearance rate was diagnostic of pancreatitis. Unfortunately, the so-called amylase-to-creatinine clearance ratio has not proven to be clinically useful since changes in this ratio are not specific to pancreatitis and elevated clearance ratios can be seen in other diseases. Occasionally, serum amylase activity may be normal, even during the early stages of an attack. The basis for this phenomenon is not certain. In some cases, it may reflect overwhelming necrosis of the gland. Some patients with acute pancreatitis superimposed on advanced chronic pancreatitis do not develop hyperamylasemia because there is little residual and functional pancreatic exocrine tissue and, therefore, little pancreatic amylase to be released into the circulation. In some patients with hyperlipidemia-induced pancreatitis, hyperamylasemia may be masked by circulating amylase inhibitors. This is particularly true of patients with lactescent serum in whom the circulating amylase activity may appear to be normal.

Macroamylasemia is a form of pancreatitis-independent hyperamylasemia that affects 0.5% of individuals. It occurs when amylase binds to an abnormal circulating albumin-like protein. Because of its large size, this protein prevents the normal clearance of amylase and, as a result, circulating levels of amylase rise. In some patients, episodes of abdominal pain can also occur raising the suspicion that they have pancreatitis. In this situation, macroamylasemia can be distinguished from the hyperamylasemia of pancreatitis by simple measurement of urinary amylase activity. In the former, urinary amylase levels are very low.

Other Blood Tests

In addition to amylase, other enzymes and inflammatory mediators are released into the circulation during pancreatitis, and many have been the target of diagnostic or prognostic tests. Circulating lipase levels usually increase during pancreatitis. That increase usually parallels the rise in amylase activity, but the elevations of lipase activity may persist even after amylase activity has returned to normal. Thus, serum lipase measurement may be particularly helpful when patients are first seen several days after the onset of symptoms. Circulating levels of other pancreatic enzymes including trypsinogen, phospholipase, elastase, and chymotrypsinogen increase during pancreatitis, but measurement of these circulating enzymes is usually not performed since they add little to the information gained by the easier and more straightforward measurement of amylase activity. The activation peptides released during either trypsinogen, procarboxypeptidase, or prophospholipase activation are increased in the urine of patients with acute pancreatitis, and several studies have indicated that measurement of those activation peptides may aid in predicting the severity of an attack.[14] Although methemalbumin levels sometimes rise during attacks of severe pancreatitis, and methemalbuminemia is indicative of a poor prognosis, methemalbumin levels are usually not measured. Circulating levels of several inflammatory mediators and acute-phase reactants (e.g., interleukin [IL]-1, IL-6, tumor necrosis factor-alpha, and C-reactive protein) also increase during pancreatitis, and the magnitude of those increases can be used to predict the severity of an attack.

Imaging Studies

In general, the plain chest and abdominal radiographs are not particularly helpful in the diagnosis of pancreatitis, although they may be useful in patient management by revealing other causes for the patient's symptoms (e.g., pneumonia, perforated hollow viscus, mechanical bowel obstruction). In patients with pancreatitis, radiographs of the chest frequently reveal basal atelectasis and elevation of the diaphragm caused by splinting of respiration. Pleural effusions, most common on the left, can also be seen. Plain abdominal films usually show the gas pattern of a paralytic ileus but, occasionally, retroperitoneal gas bubbles indicating infection with gas-forming organisms can be seen. Pancreatic calcifications that are pathognomonic of chronic pancreatitis and are caused by the formation of calcified intraductal protein plugs may be seen on the routine abdominal films. Transcutaneous ultrasound may be useful in demonstrating the presence of gallbladder stones and/or dilated bile ducts, but ultrasound examination has limited value because of the presence of intestinal gas in the upper abdomen.

Computed tomography (CT) has been shown to be particularly helpful in the diagnosis and management of patients with pancreatitis. During the early stages of an attack, CT can image the upper abdomen and pancreas without being obscured by overlying or surrounding intestinal gas. When combined with bolus administration of intravenous contrast material, helical CT can detect the subtle changes of mild pancreatitis (i.e., pancreatic swelling and edema) as well as the changes of more severe pancreatitis (i.e., varying degrees of pancreatic necrosis and the presence of peripancreatic or intrapancreatic fluid collections). Both clinical and experimental studies have demonstrated the close parallel that exists between non-perfused pancreas seen on CT examination and necrosis seen on morphologic examination of the pancreas. At later times during the evolution of an attack, CT can be used to detect and follow pseudocysts and to permit fine-needle aspiration of areas suspected of harboring pancreatic infection. The timing of CT during an attack of pancreatitis is a matter of considerable controversy. One study, using an experimental model of pancreatitis in rodents, suggested that early CT with administration of intravenous contrast material could adversely affect the course of pancreatitis and worsen outcome,[15] but this conclusion has not been borne out by other studies,[16] and, at present, it is generally believed that early performance of contrast-enhanced CT does not worsen pancreatitis. On the other hand, there may be little or no value in obtaining a CT in patients with obvious pancreatitis since early CT is unlikely to alter treatment. Early CT may be particularly helpful when the diagnosis of pancreatitis is in doubt. A normal pancreas imaged in a patient thought to have severe pancreatitis would prompt further diagnostic studies. Magnetic resonance imaging (MRI), which has the same sensitivity and specificity as CT in pancreatitis, has also been used in these patients. It provides information that is similar to that obtained by CT but, because of its ease of interpretation and ready availability, most clinicians prefer to use CT, rather than MRI, for the diagnosis and management of patients with pancreatitis.

Differential Diagnosis

The differential diagnosis of acute pancreatitis includes any process that can cause upper abdominal pain and tenderness, nausea, and vomiting (Box 53-3). Usually, but not always, the serum amylase and/or lipase levels are elevated in pancreatitis, but those enzymes can also be elevated in other conditions including cholecystitis/cholangitis, perforated hollow viscus, bowel obstruction, and bowel infarction. In those patients, the CT does not

suggest pancreatitis and, for the most part, enzyme elevations in those conditions are usually only twofold or three-fold above normal. Occasionally, however, it may be difficult or even impossible to be certain that the patient actually has pancreatitis and, in those cases, a diagnostic exploratory laparotomy may be indicated.

Prognosis of an Acute Attack

The ultimate severity of an attack appears to be determined by events that occur within the first 24 to 48 hours. Most patients experience only a mild self-limited illness that can be expected to resolve with only supportive care, but approximately 10% of patients experience a severe attack. Severe attacks are more common in acute pancreatitis, but they can also occur when an acute attack is superimposed on chronic pancreatitis, that is, the so-called acute on chronic pancreatitis. Severe attacks are also more common in patients older than 60 years of age; those experiencing a first attack; those with postoperative pancreatitis; and those with methemalbuminemia, hypocalcemia, Grey Turner's sign, or Cullen's sign. The observation that the ultimate severity is determined by events that occur during the early stages of pancreatitis has prompted several groups of investigators to undertake studies designed to determine which clinical, chemical, or radiologic parameters might be used to identify those patients destined to experience a severe illness. As a result, a number of prognostic schemes have been developed. Among the clinical scoring systems, the most widely used are those developed in New York by Ranson's group[17] (Table 53-1), and, in Glasgow, by Imrie's group.[18] Patients with fewer than three of the prognostic criteria can be expected to have a mild attack with little morbidity and a mortality rate of less than 1%. On the other hand,

---

Box 53-3.   Differential Diagnosis of Acute Pancreatitis

Bowel obstruction
Cholecystitis/cholangitis
Mesenteric ischemia/infarction
Perforated hollow viscus

TABLE 53-1.   Ranson's Prognostic Signs

Admission	Initial 48 Hours
Gallstone Pancreatitis	
Age > 70 yr	Hct fall > 10
WBC > 18,000/mm³	BUN elevation > 2 mg/100 mL
Glucose > 220 mg/100 mL	Ca²⁺ > 8 mg/100 mL
LDH > 40 IU/L	Base deficit > 5 mEq/L
AST > 250 U/100 mL	Fluid sequestration > 4 L
Non-Gallstone Pancreatitis	
Age > 55 yr	Hct fall > 10
WBC > 16,000/mm³	BUN elevation > 5 mg/100 mL
Glucose > 200 mg/100 mL	Ca²⁺ > 8 mg/100 mL
LDH > 350 IU/L	Pao₂ > 55 mm Hg
AST > 250 U/100 mL	Base deficit > 4 mEq/L
	Fluid sequestration > 6 L

WBC, white blood count; LDH, lactic dehydrogenase; AST, aspartate transaminase; HCT, hematocrit; BUN, blood urea nitrogen; Ca²⁺, calcium; Pao₂, arterial oxygen.
Adapted from Ranson JHC, Rifkind KM, Roses DF, et al: Prognostic signs and the role of operative management in acute pancreatitis. Surg Gynecol Obstet 139:69-81, 1974' and Ranson JHC. Etiological and prognostic factors in human acute pancreatitis: A review. Am J Gastroenterol 77:633-, 1982.

with the presence of more prognostic factors, increased morbidity and mortality can be expected so that, with three or four of Ranson's criteria, the mortality rate may reach 15%, and 50% of patients may need to be treated in an intensive care unit. Most patients with five or six signs will require intensive care and, with seven or eight of Ranson's signs, the mortality rate may reach 90%. As an alternative to using clinical criteria, Balthazar and coworkers developed radiologic criteria for predicting a severe attack. In a prospective study employing contrast-enhanced CT examination,[19] they noted that the severity of an attack was related to the number of pancreatic fluid collections and the extent of pancreatic nonperfusion (i.e., necrosis) seen on CT examination. In addition to clinical and radiologic criteria, high levels of certain circulating factors can also be used to predict the evolution of a severe attack. Those factors include the following: C-reactive protein, phospholipase A_2, polymorphonuclear elastase, immunoreactive trypsin, IL-6, and pancreatitis-associated protein. High urinary levels of the activation peptides for trypsinogen, procarboxypeptidase, and prophospholipase also indicate a severe attack. The second version of the Acute Physiology and Chronic Health Evaluation (APACHE-II) scoring system has also been used to predict the severity of a pancreatitis attack. An APACHE-II score of 8 or more is generally indicative of a severe attack. The APACHE-II scoring system has the advantage of continually quantifying disease severity. Although the APACHE-II system can be used at the time of admission, recent studies have suggested that an admission score that worsens over the initial 48 hours of hospitalization in spite of aggressive treatment, or the score itself 48 hours after admission, may be particularly accurate in predicting the severity of the attack and a poor outcome.[20]

Although each of these scoring systems may predict the severity of an attack, there is also evidence that a good examination by an experienced clinician can accurately discriminate between mild and severe pancreatitis. Furthermore, none of the prognostic schemes are intended for use as a diagnostic tool in pancreatitis. Their ultimate value is in triaging patients to their appropriate care settings. In addition, they may be useful in clinical studies by permitting comparison of therapeutic outcomes for comparable patients stratified to different treatments.

Treatment of an Acute Attack

An acute attack of pancreatitis evolves in two, somewhat overlapping, phases. The initial phase, which lasts for 1 to 2 weeks, involves an acute inflammatory and auto-digestive process that takes place within and around the pancreas. It may have systemic effects as well. In patients with severe pancreatitis, this initial phase of pancreatitis seamlessly evolves into a later phase that may last for weeks or months. This later phase of pancreatitis is primarily characterized by the development of local complications that are, themselves, the result of necrosis, infection, and pancreatic duct rupture.

Initial Treatment

The initial management of patients with pancreatitis should focus on establishing the diagnosis, estimating its severity, addressing the major symptoms (i.e., pain, nausea, vomiting, and hypovolemia), and limiting its progression. Ideally, the diagnosis should be established without exploratory surgery since exploration may increase the incidence of later pancreatic infection. On occasion, however, exploration may be required to establish the diagnosis with certainty, especially when the diagnosis is uncertain and the patient has not responded favorably to aggressive nonoperative treatment. For the most part, patients with predicted severe pancreatitis should be treated in an intensive care setting since it is in this group that fluid and respiratory management may be particularly challenging and both morbidity and mortality are, essentially, confined to this group.

Management of Pain

The pain of pancreatitis may be severe and difficult to control. Most patients require narcotic medications. Meperidine or its analogues are probably preferable to morphine in this setting since morphine can induce spasm of the sphincter of Oddi and that could, at least theoretically, worsen biliary pancreatitis.

Fluid and Electrolyte Management

Aggressive fluid and electrolyte repletion is the most important element in the initial management of pancreatitis. Fluid losses can be enormous and can lead to marked hemoconcentration as well as hypovolemia. Inadequate fluid resuscitation during the early stages of pancreatitis can worsen the severity of an attack and lead to subsequent complications. The fluid depletion that occurs in pancreatitis results from the additive effects of losing fluid both externally and internally. The external fluid losses are caused by repeated episodes of vomiting and worsen by nausea that limits fluid intake. Repeated vomiting can result in a hypochloremic alkalosis. Internal fluid losses, which are usually even greater than the external losses, are caused by fluid sequestration into areas of inflammation (i.e., the peripancreatic retroperitoneum) and into the pulmonary parenchyma and soft tissues elsewhere in the body. These latter losses result from the diffuse capillary leak phenomenon that is triggered by proinflammatory factors released during pancreatitis. Total fluid losses may be so great that they lead to hypovolemia and hypoperfusion and, as a result, a metabolic acidosis can develop. Many of the patients with chronic pancreatitis are alcoholics who, even before the onset of pancreatitis, had hypoalbuminemia and hypomagnesemia. Those problems are exacerbated by the losses of pancreatitis. The measured values for serum albumin may be even further depressed as fluid losses are treated with albumin-free crystalloid solutions. Although hypocalcemia is common particularly during a severe attack, the low total serum calcium is usually attributable to the low levels of circulating albumin and no treatment is needed when ionized calcium is normal. Occasionally, however, ionized calcium levels may also be depressed and tetany as well as carpopedal spasm can occur. Under those circumstances, aggressive calcium repletion is indicated.

During the first several days of a severe attack, circulating levels of many proinflammatory factors, including cytokines and chemokines, are elevated. This "cytokine storm," in many cases, triggers the systemic immune response syndrome and, as a result, the hemodynamic parameters of these patients may resemble those of sepsis associated with other disease states. Heart rate, cardiac output, and cardiac index usually rise and total peripheral resistance falls. Hypoxemia can also occur as a result of the combined effects of increased intrapulmonary shunting and a pancreatitis-associated lung injury that closely resembles that seen in other forms of the ARDS. Fluid management, although critical, may be particularly difficult when hypovolemia is combined with the respiratory failure of ARDS.

Treatment requires meticulous replacement of fluid and electrolyte losses. A fluid balance flow sheet is helpful, but parameters such as pulse rate, blood pressure, oxygen saturation, and urine output are notoriously unreliable for determining fluid needs in this setting. The hematocrit, however, can be quite useful as increased levels usually are accurate indicators of the magnitude of extracellular fluid loss. However, in a setting of blood loss or hemolysis, hematocrit measurements may lose their value in fluid management. Measurement of central filling pressures, using a Swan-Ganz or central venous pressure catheter, can be helpful in guiding fluid management, particularly when hypovolemia is combined with lung injury.

Role of Nasogastric Decompression

The nausea and vomiting of pancreatitis can result in significant fluid as well as electrolyte losses. Furthermore, retching can lead to gastroesophageal mucosal tears and result in upper gastrointestinal bleeding (i.e., the Mallory-Weiss syndrome). To increase patient comfort, nasogastric decompression may be needed, although the institution of nasogastric drainage has not been shown to alter the eventual outcome of an attack.

Role of Prophylactic Antibiotics

Over the past decade, three separate studies have indicated that prophylactic antibiotics are useful in the management of patients with severe pancreatitis[21-23] but no benefit was observed when prophylactic antibiotics were given to patients with mild pancreatitis. They postulated that patients with mild pancreatitis almost invariably recover quickly and without infectious complications. In patients with severe pancreatitis, benefit was observed with regimens that included imipenem alone, imipenem with cilastatin, and cefuroxime. Selective gut decontamination with a combination of norfloxacin, colistin, and amphotericin has also been found to be beneficial,[24] although that approach is labor intensive and not readily available. Although these recent studies argue strongly for administration of prophylactic antibiotics to patients with severe pancreatitis, there is an opposing view that is becoming increasingly widespread. According to that

school of thought, administration of prophylactic antibiotics favors emergence of resistant organisms in the area of pancreatic injury. That may be particularly true for fungal strains such as *Candida*. Some have advocated adding antifungal agents such as fluconazole to the prophylactic antibiotic regimen, whereas others have argued that, because of the risk of infection with resistant organisms or fungi, antibiotics should not be prophylactically used in the management of a severe attack.

Nutritional Support

Patients with severe pancreatitis may be unable to eat for prolonged periods and an alternative route for providing nutrition is required. Traditionally, these patients have been given parenteral nutrition administered via a central venous catheter. Widely differing opinions exist regarding the time that total parenteral nutrition should be started. Some advocate starting within the first day or two, whereas others delay starting total parenteral nutrition until the early phase of pancreatitis, characterized by extensive fluid shifts and high fluid requirements, has been completed. I favor the latter approach.

Several investigative groups have recently demonstrated that most patients with pancreatitis, including those with severe pancreatitis, can actually tolerate small amounts of enterally administered nutrients. They have shown that those nutrients can be tolerated if given either into the stomach (via a nasogastric tube) or into the small intestine (via a nasojejunal tube). Pancreatic infections are believed to occur because gut bacteria are translocated across the injured bowel wall adjacent to areas of pancreatic injury. Theoretically, enteral nutrition exerts a trophic effect on the injured bowel wall that could reduce this translocation and, thus, reduce the incidence of pancreatic infections. Studies evaluating this concept are currently underway, but, even in the absence of definitive results, I favor administration of trophic amounts of nutrients to patients with severe pancreatitis and begin that treatment within 72 hours of hospitalization.

Treatments of Limited or Unproved Value

Peritoneal dialysis, designed to eliminate the proinflammatory factors released into the abdomen during pancreatitis, might theoretically be expected to reduce the severity of pancreatitis. Indeed, early anecdotal studies did support the use of peritoneal dialysis in patients with severe pancreatitis, but a more recent, prospective, randomized multi-institutional study showed that peritoneal dialysis was of no benefit. Nasogastric decompression does not appear to alter the course or outcome of a pancreatitis attack, although it may provide for greater patient comfort during the early stages when nausea and vomiting are common. Other attempts to reduce gastrointestinal and/or pancreatic secretion (i.e., H_2 blockers, proton-pump inhibitors, antacids, atropine, somatostatin, glucagon, calcitonin) have not been shown to be beneficial in the treatment of pancreatitis. Similarly, the use of anti-inflammatory agents (i.e., steroids, prostaglandins, and indomethacin) has not been helpful although recent experimental studies have suggested that specific inhibition of cyclooxygenase-2 might be beneficial. Many attempts to treat pancreatitis with agents designed to inhibit activated proteolytic enzymes (e.g., aprotinin, gabexate mesylate) have failed to alter the course of pancreatitis unless their use is begun prior to the onset of the attack. Hypothermia, thoracic duct drainage, and plasmapheresis have been evaluated in experimental models of pancreatitis but, to date, there is little evidence that these modes of therapy are clinically useful. Many other approaches have also been tried (e.g., procainamide, isoproterenol, heparin, dextran, vasopressin). Although these forms of treatment have been supported by experimental animal studies, particularly when the treatment is begun prior to the onset of pancreatitis, human clinical trials have failed to show a beneficial effect on the course of patients with established pancreatitis and, at present, none of these treatments are commonly employed. Platelet-activating factor (PAF) is a proinflammatory factor that has been shown to promote worsening of experimental pancreatitis in animal models. Recently, several clinical trials have evaluated the effects of interfering with PAF action during severe clinical pancreatitis, but they have failed to show these anti-PAF agents beneficially alter the outcome of patients with severe pancreatitis. Therefore, anti-PAF agents are not currently used.

Treatment of Early Systemic Complications of Pancreatitis

The pathogenesis and management of the cardiovascular collapse, respiratory failure, renal failure, metabolic encephalopathy, gastrointestinal bleeding, and disseminated intravascular coagulation that complicate severe pancreatitis appear to be identical to those involved when these processes are superimposed on other disease states that are characterized by peritonitis and hypovolemia. Cardiovascular collapse is largely caused by hypovolemia, and its management requires aggressive fluid and electrolyte repletion. This may necessitate placement of a central venous or Swan-Ganz monitoring catheter. Changes in hematocrit, filling pressures, and cardiac output can be used to monitor the adequacy of treatment, but changes in blood pressure, pulse, and urine output do not accurately and reliably reflect the adequacy of fluid replacement.

The pulmonary manifestations of pancreatitis include atelectasis and acute lung injury. The latter appears to be similar to the acute lung injury caused by other systemic processes including septic shock, ischemia/reperfusion, and massive blood transfusion. Management includes good pulmonary toilet combined with close monitoring of pulmonary function. For many patients, intubation and respiratory support may be required. Renal failure in pancreatitis is usually prerenal and is associated with a poor prognosis. In severe cases, dialysis, usually hemodialysis, may be required. Stress-induced gastroduodenal erosions account for most of the gastrointestinal bleeding in pancreatitis and prophylaxis with antacids, H_2 receptor antagonists, or proton-pump inhibitors may be appropriate. Rarely, massive bleeding can result from injury to peripancreatic vascular structures leading to hemorrhage into the retroperitoneum. The peripancreatic inflammatory process can also cause thrombosis of major gastrointestinal vessels and result in ischemic lesions involving the stomach, small intestine, or colon that can cause bleeding. Management of these complications of pancreatitis is similar to that involved when they occur in the absence of pancreatitis. Some patients with severe pancreatitis develop disseminated intravascular coagulation, but it rarely causes bleeding and prophylactic heparinization is usually not indicated.

Role of Early Endoscopy and Stone Extraction

Patients with mild pancreatitis may ultimately require endoscopic duct clearance to prevent recurrent attacks, but they rarely benefit from early endoscopy because their pancreatitis generally resolves spontaneously within several days. On the other hand, the role of early endoscopic duct clearance in the initial management of patients with severe biliary pancreatitis is more controversial. Three randomized, controlled, prospective studies have differing results.[25-27] One study indicated that early stone clearance reduced the severity and mortality of biliary pancreatitis, whereas a second study indicated that early duct clearance reduced the incidence of infectious complications. The third study concluded that early endoscopy and duct clearance actually adversely affected the course of pancreatitis because it was associated with a high incidence of complications. At the present time, most experts would favor early (i.e., < 48 hours after the onset of symptoms) endoscopic intervention in severe biliary pancreatitis, but further studies are needed.

Role and Timing of Cholecystectomy in Patients with Gallstone Pancreatitis

In general, patients with gallstone pancreatitis should undergo some form of definitive treatment prior to discharge from the hospital, and that intervention should take place as soon as possible after resolution of their attack. Further delaying the intervention would increase the chances that additional stones might be passed and another attack of pancreatitis might be triggered. Intervening sooner, on the other hand, could introduce infection into the inflamed peripancreatic area and/or worsen the pancreatitis.

For purposes of therapeutic decision making, patients with gallstone pancreatitis can be divided into two groups: those who have or have had gallbladder-derived problems (cholecystitis or biliary colic) and those whose only problems are purely related to stones in the biliary ductal system (i.e., cholangitis and pancreatitis). Patients in the first group should undergo cholecystectomy since that operation will prevent additional gallbladder attacks as well as eliminating the source of stones that might trigger another attack of pancreatitis. Patients in the second group, however, do not necessarily require cholecystectomy since their problem relates only to ductal stones. Theoretically they could be treated simply by endoscopic stone clearance combined with endoscopic sphincterotomy so that future stones are passed without becoming impacted in the ampulla and triggering either pancreatitis or cholangitis. Indeed, for poor surgical risk patients, the endoscopic approach is generally recommended. On the other hand, roughly 25% of patients treated in this manner will go on to develop gallbladder symptoms over the next 3 to 5 years. Thus, good surgical risk patients are better managed by cholecystectomy.

Treatment of Later Complications

Definitions

In 1992, an international symposium was held to resolve the confusion that had arisen concerning the terminology used to describe the local complications of pancreatitis and the value of specific treatments for those complications.[28] The following definitions were agreed on at that conference:

1. *Acute fluid collections.* These occur during the early stages of severe pancreatitis in 30% to 50% of patients, lack a wall of granulation or fibrous tissue, and more than half regress spontaneously. Most are peripancreatic, but some are intrapancreatic. Those that do not regress may evolve into pseudocysts or involve areas of necrosis.
2. *Pancreatic and peripancreatic necrosis.* These are areas of nonviable pancreatic or peripancreatic tissue that may be either sterile or infected. They typically include areas of fat necrosis, and the necrotic tissue has a putty-like or paste-like consistency. Some necrotic regions may evolve into pseudocysts, whereas others may be replaced by fibrous tissue.
3. *Pancreatic pseudocyst.* These are collections of pancreatic juice, usually rich in digestive enzymes, that are enclosed by a nonepithelialized wall composed of fibrous and granulation tissue (Fig. 53-4). Pseudocysts can be intrapancreatic but are more commonly extrapancreatic and occupy the lesser peritoneal sac. Pseudocysts are usually round or oval in shape and are not present before 4 to 6 weeks after the onset of an attack. Prior to that time, the fluid collection lacks a defined wall and is usually either an acute fluid collec-

tion or a localized area of necrosis (see earlier). Pseudocysts may be colonized by microorganisms, but infection, as evidenced by the presence of pus, is less common. When pus is present, the infected pseudocyst is referred to as a *pancreatic abscess.* Leakage or rupture of a pseudocyst into the peritoneal cavity results in *pancreatic ascites.* A *pancreaticopleural fistula* results from erosion of a pseudocyst into the pleural space.

4. *Pancreatic abscess.* These are circumscribed intra-abdominal collections of pus, usually in proximity to the pancreas, which contain little or no necrotic tissue but arise as a consequence of pancreatitis. An infected pseudocyst should be considered a pancreatic abscess. Pancreatic abscess and infected pancreatic necrosis represent the extremes of a spectrum that include lesions with varying amounts of necrosis. Thus, in a pancreatic abscess, there is little necrosis and the material has a liquid consistency, whereas in infected pancreatic necrosis, necrosis predominates and the material is paste or putty-like.

Diagnosis

Contrast-enhanced CT is particularly valuable as a means of quantifying the extent of pancreatic necrosis (i.e., nonenhancement). The maturation of a pseudocyst can be followed by both contrast-enhanced CT and endoscopic ultrasound. Management of local pancreatitis complications is dependent on whether the lesion is sterile or infected (see later). Occasionally, infection can be diagnosed when plain abdominal films or CT scans reveal extraintestinal gas bubbles or air either within the area of inflammation or elsewhere in the retroperitoneum. When the clinical suspicion of infection is high, fine-needle aspiration of peripancreatic or intrapancreatic fluid for culture and Gram stain analysis may be particularly helpful.[29] The procedure is most frequently done with CT guidance, and it is safe when performed by experienced radiologists.

Management of Sterile and Infected Acute Fluid Collections

Sterile acute fluid collections usually resolve spontaneously and no specific treatment is indicated. Attempts to drain acute fluid collections, either by using percutaneously placed drains or by intervening surgically, should be discouraged as they are usually unnecessary, and, furthermore, they are likely to lead to infection. Even without instrumentation, these fluid collections can become infected but, since they contain liquid pus with little or no necrotic tissue, they are amenable to transcutaneous catheter drainage along with antibiotic therapy. It is generally believed that aspirating fluid from any site near the pancreas yields information that is relevant to all of the fluid collections and that sampling multiple sites is unnecessary.

Management of Sterile and Infected Necrosis

The role of surgical intervention in the management of patients with *sterile* pancreatic or peripancreatic necrosis

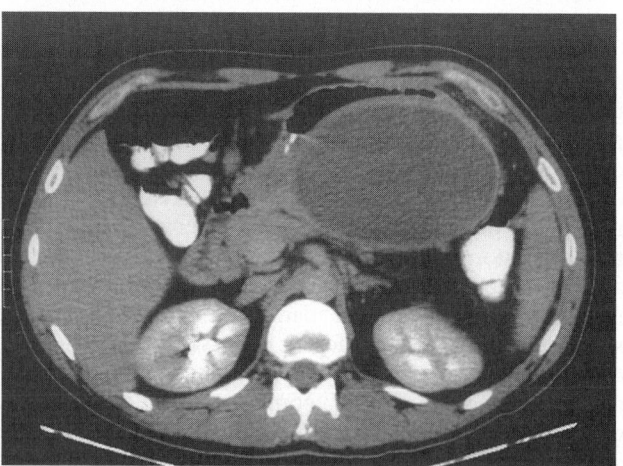

FIGURE 53-4.   CT scan of pancreatic pseudocyst.

has been the subject of considerable controversy. Opinions range from those advocating aggressive débridement for patients with sterile necrosis who fail to rapidly improve on nonoperative treatment to those who claim that surgical intervention is virtually never indicated when the necrosis is sterile. Those taking the former position claim that removing the necrotic tissue (i.e., necrosectomy) reduces morbidity and speeds recovery, whereas those taking the latter position, including me, base their position on the fact that most people treated nonoperatively will eventually recover and some who undergo operation may actually be made worse by the operation.

There is, however, a general consensus that patients with *infected* necrosis require some form of intervention. Prospective studies have indicated that infection of areas of necrosis can occur at any time but that it usually occurs during the initial 3 to 4 weeks of an attack. Although some recent reports have indicated that highly selected patients might be adequately treated with antibiotics alone,[30] simple antibiotic therapy is generally considered to be inadequate because the necrotic tissue acts as a foreign body, making it impossible to sterilize the area with antibiotics alone. Combining antibiotic therapy with percutaneous catheter drainage may also not be adequate treatment because the pastelike necrotic tissue does not pass through the small-bore drainage catheters and, therefore, drainage is usually incomplete. Other methods of removing the necrotic tissue, either via a transpapillary endoscopic route or using minimally invasive surgical approaches with an operating nephroscope, have been tried, but experience with these techniques has been limited and essentially anecdotal. The conventional approach to managing infected necrosis involves laparotomy and surgical débridement of the infected, devitalized tissue. Repeated operations and débridement may be needed. The timing of the initial débridement appears to be closely related to the outcome; that is, those undergoing later operations do better and require fewer repeat operations than those undergoing early operation.

The goal of operation in patients with infected necrosis is to remove as much as possible of the infected, necrotic tissue and to provide drainage for the remaining viable exocrine tissue. Many different ways of achieving these goals have been described (Box 53-4) and, although each has its advocates, none has been proven to be superior to the others. My practice is to perform repeated operations, each of which involves débridement and abdominal wall closure. At the time of the final débridement, drains and a feeding jejunostomy are placed. For the most part, the repeated laparotomies are performed every 2 to 3 days until no further débridement is possible or necessary.

Management of Pancreatic Pseudocysts

Most pseudocysts communicate with the pancreatic ductal system and contain a watery fluid that is rich in pancreatic digestive enzymes. Typically, patients with pseudocysts have persistent elevations of circulating pancreatic enzymes. Recent reports have shown that many pseudocysts eventually resolve without complications and

---

BOX 53-4. Management Options for Infected Pancreatic Necrosis

Conventional Approach

Débridement with reoperation when clinically indicated or at planned intervals
Débridement with open or closed packing and reoperation when clinically indicated or at planned intervals
Débridement with continuous lavage

Unconventional Approach

Antibiotics alone
Antibiotics with percutaneous drainage
Antibiotics with endoscopic drainage
Antibiotics with surgical drainage but not débridement
Antibiotics with débridement via minimally invasive surgery

---

that intervention is not mandatory in all cases unless the pseudocysts are symptomatic, enlarging, or associated with complications. The likelihood that a pseudocyst will resolve spontaneously, however, is dependent on its size. Large pseudocysts (i.e., > 6 cm in diameter) are more likely to become symptomatic either because they are tender or because of their mass effect on adjacent organs. Those that compress the stomach or duodenum may cause gastric outlet obstruction with nausea and vomiting. Those that reduce the capacity of the stomach frequently cause early satiety, whereas those impinging on the bile duct can cause obstructive jaundice. Pancreatic pseudocysts that erode into a neighboring vessel can result in formation of a pseudoaneurysm with *hemosuccus pancreaticus* and upper gastrointestinal bleeding.

Symptomatic or enlarging pseudocysts can be treated by several methods. Those in the tail can be treated by excision (i.e., distal pancreatectomy) but excision in the setting of recent acute inflammation may be hazardous. Most patients who develop symptomatic pseudocysts are best managed by pseudocyst drainage. In poor surgical risk patients, percutaneous catheter drainage can be considered, but in my experience, that approach leads to considerable morbidity because of catheter-induced infection and the development of a prolonged external pancreatic fistula. Internal drainage can avoid these problems and seems preferable. Internal drainage can be accomplished either endoscopically (via transpapillary drainage, cyst-gastrostomy or cyst-duodenostomy) or surgically (via cyst-gastrostomy, cyst-duodenostomy, or Roux-en-Y cyst-jejunostomy). The approach chosen depends primarily on the locally available expertise as well as the location of the pseudocyst, but endoscopic drainage may be preferable in poor surgical risk patients.

Pseudocysts that are directly adjacent to either the stomach or duodenum can be safely drained endoscopically if there are no intervening vessels. After endoscopic ultrasound and preliminary aspiration of the cyst fluid to confirm the diagnosis and exclude intervening vessels, endoscopic drainage is achieved by making an incision into the pseudocyst through the wall of the stomach or duodenum. To facilitate decompression, the opening should be relatively large and a pigtail catheter may be placed. Transpapillary drainage might be more appropriate for patients with pancreatic head pseudocysts whose CT and endoscopic ultrasound suggest that incising into the pseudocyst could be hazardous. At the time of endoscopic retrograde cholangiopancreatography (ERCP), a stent is passed into the pseudocyst through the papilla of Vater. Unfortunately, transpapillary drainage, particularly when incomplete, can allow bacteria to enter the pseudocyst and lead to development of an infected pseudocyst. Another transpapillary approach involves placing a stent across the duct defect rather than into the cyst through the defect. By excluding pancreatic juice from the pseudocyst, this bridging intraductal stent may permit the duct disruption to heal and the pseudocyst to resolve without drainage. Further experience with this technique will be needed before its ultimate use can be determined.

Surgical internal drainage of pseudocysts is usually accomplished by creating either a Roux-en-Y cyst-jejunostomy, a side-to-side cyst-gastrostomy, or a side-to-side cyst duodenostomy. The former is usually accomplished by directly anastomosing a defunctionalized Roux-en-Y limb of jejunum to the opened pseudocyst. Surgical cyst-gastrostomy (or cyst-duodenostomy) has traditionally been accomplished by laparotomy and anterior gastrotomy (or lateral duodenotomy). A generous incision is then made through the posterior wall of the stomach (or medial wall of the duodenum) into the pseudocyst. Some surgeons now perform cyst-gastrostomy using a laparoscopic approach.

Management of Pancreatic Ascites and Pancreaticopleural Fistulas

Pancreatic ascites occurs when pancreatic juice gains entry into the peritoneal cavity either from a pancreatic duct disruption or from a leaking pseudocyst. The diagnosis can usually be made when high amylase levels are found in the ascitic fluid. The initial treatment usually is nonoperative and involves attempts to decrease pancreatic secretion by elimination of enteral feeding, institution of nasogastric drainage, and administration of the antisecretory hormone somatostatin. Repeated paracentesis may also be helpful. Roughly 50% to 60% of patients can be expected to respond to this treatment with resolution of pancreatic ascites within 2 to 3 weeks. Persistent or recurrent ascites can be treated either endoscopically or surgically. Endoscopic treatment involves endoscopic pancreatic sphincterotomy with or without placement of a transpapillary pancreatic duct stent. By reducing the resistance to drainage into the duodenum, and by bridging the site of duct disruption, this approach is designed to allow the site of leakage to seal. Surgical treatment of pancreatic ascites, usually preceded by performance of an ERCP to identify the site of duct disruption, involves either resection (for leaks in the pancreatic tail) or internal Roux-en-Y drainage (for leaks in the head/neck region). It seems most appropriate to attempt endoscopic treatment initially and to reserve surgical treatment for those patients who do not respond to endoscopic therapy.

The genesis of pancreaticopleural fistula is similar to that of pancreatic ascites, but in this case the duct disruption is usually posterior and the extravasated juice travels in a cephalad direction through the retroperitoneum to reach the thoracic cavity. Although the incidence of pancreaticopleural fistula is lower than that of pancreatic ascites, the management of both is similar.

Management of Pancreatitis-Induced False Aneurysms

Rarely, pancreatic pseudocysts or areas of pancreatic necrosis can erode into pancreatic or peripancreatic vascular structures. This results in the formation of a false aneurysm since the vessel communicates with the pseudocyst. That false aneurysm may either communicate with the ductal system or rupture into the free peritoneal cavity. The former leads to bleeding into the pancreatic duct (*hemosuccus pancreaticus*) and presents as transpapillary upper gastrointestinal bleeding. Rupture into the peritoneal cavity can lead to hemoperitoneum. Therapeutic angiographic embolization is most appropriate for the unstable patient, and this approach may also provide definitive treatment, particularly for those patients whose false aneurysm is in the pancreatic head. For those whose false aneurysm is in the tail of the pancreas, subsequent distal pancreatectomy, once the patient is stabilized, may provide more secure hemostasis.

Management of Pancreaticoenteric Fistulas

Pancreatic pseudocysts or areas of pancreatic necrosis can erode into the small intestine, duodenum, stomach, bile duct, or splenic flexure of the colon. Occasionally, this results in resolution of the pseudocyst and no further treatment is needed. More often, however, such an event is accompanied by significant bleeding and/or signs of sepsis, and surgical intervention is usually required. Management of these fistulas is determined by the gastrointestinal organ involved.

Management of Pancreatitis-Induced Splenic Vein Thrombosis

Because of the close proximity of the splenic vein to the pancreas, splenic vein thrombosis is not unusual in cases of severe pancreatitis. For the most part, it does not result in early symptoms, but it may eventually result in the formation of gastroesophageal varices. Splenectomy provides effective and definitive treatment when these sinistral varices bleed, but because bleeding occurs in fewer than 10% of these patients, prophylactic splenectomy is not generally performed.

CHRONIC PANCREATITIS

Pathology and Etiology of Chronic Pancreatitis

Chronic pancreatitis is characterized by irreversible changes including pancreatic fibrosis and the loss of functional pancreatic exocrine and/or endocrine tissue. Most patients develop chronic pancreatitis as a result of prolonged ethanol abuse. It is generally believed that, in its earliest stages, chronic pancreatitis is an acute inflammatory process and that repeated episodes of subclinical acute pancreatic injury and necrosis lead to the fibrosis of chronic pancreatitis.

Diagnosis of Chronic Pancreatitis

There has been considerable confusion concerning the clinical distinction between chronic and acute pancreatitis. To a great extent, this confusion results from the fact that, from a clinical standpoint, attacks of chronic pancreatitis may be indistinguishable from those of acute pancreatitis. Fortunately, the initial management of acute or chronic pancreatitis attacks is identical, as is the management of complications such as infection, necrosis, and pseudocyst (see Treatment section, earlier). On the other hand, the two forms of pancreatitis have natural histories that differ considerably, and the long-term management of chronic pancreatitis presents challenges that are not inherent to the management of acute pancreatitis.

History

Patients with chronic pancreatitis may describe prior episodes of pancreatic-type abdominal pain, and 60% to 80% of patients have a long history of ethanol abuse. There may be a family history of pancreatitis suggestive of the presence of hereditary pancreatitis or a history of autoimmune diseases including primary sclerosing cholangitis and Sjögren's syndrome that should raise suspicion of pancreatitis on an autoimmune basis. Diabetes mellitus and/or a history suggestive of malabsorption (i.e., steatorrhea) indicate that significant pancreatic endocrine and/or exocrine function has been lost and this is most compatible with the diagnosis of chronic pancreatitis. Typically, patients with chronic pancreatitis have upper abdominal pain radiating to the back. It can be constant or episodic and triggered by drinking alcohol or eating. Repeated use of heating pads or hot water bottles to treat the chronic pain may result in skin lesions (erythema *ab igne*) that define the distribution of the pain (Fig. 53-5). Some patients experience no pain.

Imaging Studies

Radiographs or CT scans showing pancreatic calcifications are diagnostic of chronic pancreatitis (Fig. 53-6). Those calcifications reflect the deposition of calcium carbonate in the intraductal protein plugs that frequently, but not invariably, occur in chronic pancreatitis. Thus, the absence of pancreatic calcifications does not rule out a diagnosis of chronic pancreatitis. Perhaps the most sensitive methods for diagnosing chronic pancreatitis are those that provide images of the pancreatic ductal system. ERCP, CT cholangiopancreatography, or MR cholangiopancreatography may be particularly valuable in the diagnosis of chronic pancreatitis. Chronic pancreatitis is characterized by irregularities of the pancreatic ducts, ductal strictures, and areas of duct dilation (Fig. 53-7). The

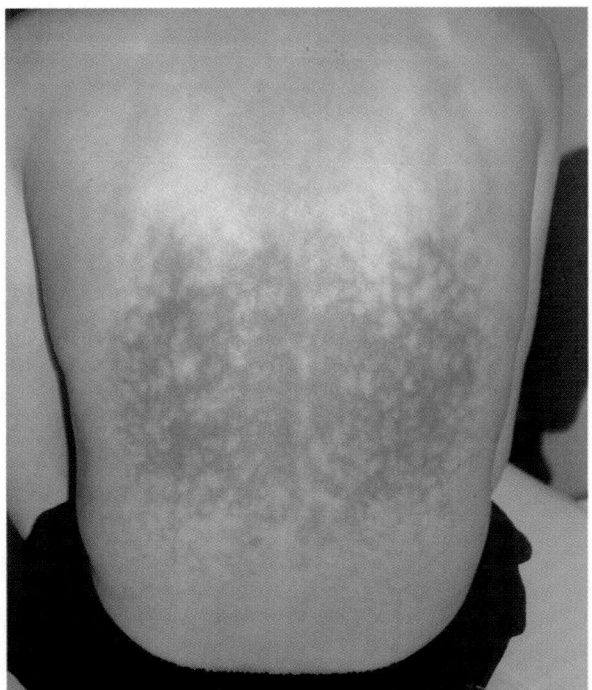

FIGURE 53-5. *Erythema ab igne.* Skin injury, characterized by keratinocyte injury and melanocyte activation, is induced by mild and repeated exposure to infrared sources. This patient with chronic pancreatitis repeatedly applied a heating pad to the painful area on his back.

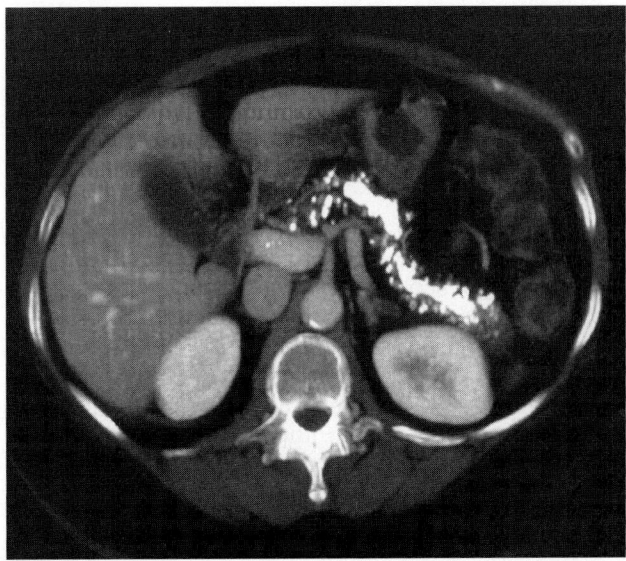

FIGURE 53-6. Pancreatic calcifications. CT scan showing multiple, calcified, intraductal stones in a patient with hereditary chronic pancreatitis.

major as well as the side-branch ducts may be involved. For unexplained reasons, some patients with chronic pancreatitis develop dilated main pancreatic ducts ("large duct disease"), whereas others retain ducts of normal or even smaller than normal caliber ("small duct disease"). Some patients with chronic pancreatitis can be shown to

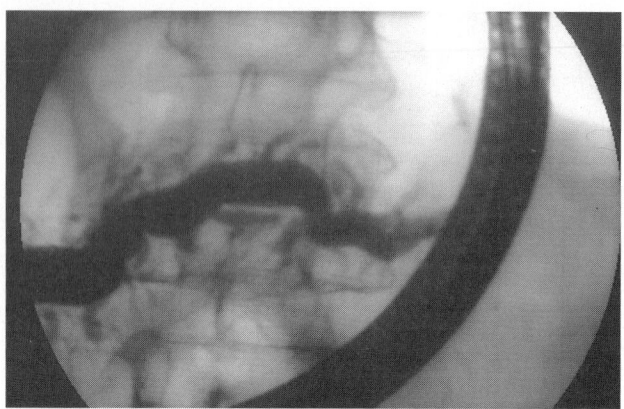

FIGURE 53-7. Endoscopic retrograde cholangiopancreatography (ERCP) in chronic pancreatitis. The pancreatic duct and its side branches are irregularly dilated.

Box 53-5.   Pancreatic Function Tests

Tubeless Tests

Fecal tests
  Fat stain
  72-hour fat content
  Chymotrypsin, trypsin, elastase content
Indirect tests
  Bentiromide test
  Pancreolauryl test
  Breath tests

Tube Tests

Lundh test meal
Secretin/cholecystokinin test

---

have major ducts that have the appearance of a "chain of lakes" or a "string of pearls" that is the result of segments of dilated duct separated by areas of ductal stricture. Transcutaneous and endoscopic ultrasound can also be used to diagnose chronic pancreatitis if duct dilation, calcifications, pseudocysts, or parenchymal fibrosis are seen. Ultrasound examination is more operator dependent and perhaps less sensitive than either CT or MRI.

Pancreatic Function Tests

The pancreas has considerable functional reserve, and more than 90% of exocrine function must be lost before steatorrhea develops. More subtle losses may be identified by performance of pancreatic function tests that can be either noninvasive ("tubeless tests") or invasive ("tube tests") (Box 53-5). Tubeless tests involve measuring the stool content of fat, measuring stool content of digestive enzymes, or orally administering a pancreatic digestive enzyme substrate and quantitating enzyme activity in the gut by measuring metabolic product in either the urine or exhaled gases. These tests, although nonintrusive, are notoriously insensitive and, therefore, normal results are

not too helpful. The more invasive tube tests involve placement of a collecting tube in the duodenum and measuring pancreatic bicarbonate or enzyme output after meal or hormone stimulation of the pancreas. These tests are more specific and sensitive than the tubeless tests, but they are still relatively insensitive and they have a relatively high rate of false-negative results

Natural History

Some patients with chronic pancreatitis have a painless disease that remains unrecognized until complications or loss of pancreatic function lead to the diagnosis. Most patients, however, have intermittent or constant pain that may limit lifestyle and/or mandate repeated hospitalizations. Ammann and coworkers[31] have suggested that the painful pancreatitis experienced by many of these patients evolves into a painless disease as pancreatic function is lost, but the existence of this "burn-out" phenomenon is highly controversial. More often, the disease remains painful, addicting doses of narcotics are required, and loss of function results in diabetes, steatorrhea, and profound weight loss.

Treatment of Pancreatic Malabsorption

The loss of pancreatic exocrine function in chronic pancreatitis affects the output of all pancreatic digestive enzymes, but it is mostly fat absorption that is abnormal, and it is the delivery of lipolytic enzyme activity to the small intestine that determines the success of treatment. In health, roughly 300,000 IU of lipase is secreted by the pancreas within 4 hours of ingesting a typical meal, but only 10% (30,000 IU) of secreted lipase is needed to allow for normal fat digestion/absorption. Theoretically, pancreatic malabsorption of fat should be corrected by oral administration of exogenous lipase. Unfortunately, most orally administered lipase is inactivated as it traverses the acidic environment of the stomach, allowing only 8% to 15% of ingested lipase activity to reach the duodenum. Some of that lipase may be ineffective, either because of low duodenal pH (caused by inadequate pancreatic secretion of bicarbonate) or because the exogenously administered lipase arrives in the duodenum before or after the ingested fat. The use of acid-inhibiting agents (e.g., proton-pump inhibitors) and enterically coated microsphere delivery systems can partially compensate for these problems. Thus, treatment involves acid suppression, a low-fat diet, and lipase doses of 90 to 150,000 IU per meal, although control of steatorrhea is often incomplete even with this treatment.

Treatment of Pain in Chronic Pancreatitis

Medical Management

Complete abstinence from ethanol is advised for patients with alcohol-induced pancreatitis, but symptoms may persist even after complete abstinence. Attacks of hyperlipidemia-induced pancreatitis can be prevented by normalizing lipid levels with medication and/or dietary changes. Some patients with autoimmune pancreatitis are cured by administration of steroids. For most patients with painful chronic pancreatitis, intermittent or persistent pain remains a major issue and analgesics of increasing potency are needed. Toskes and coworkers[32] have noted that some of their patients with painful chronic pancreatitis have diminished pain if pancreatic secretion is reduced either by oral administration of pancreatic enzymes or by administration of the inhibitory hormone somatostatin. However, the clinical results achieved using exogenous pancreatic enzymes to reduce the pain of chronic pancreatitis have been variable and, at this time, the role of enzyme administration for pain relief in these patients is highly controversial.

Endoscopic Management

The endoscopic treatment of chronic pancreatitis has not been tested by well-designed prospective, randomized trials; therefore, the ultimate value of these treatments remains to be established. Several endoscopic approaches have been described. Endoscopic pancreatic sphincterotomy has been reported to benefit some patients with elevated sphincter of Oddi pressures. Endoscopic minor pancreatic sphincterotomy has been used to treat patients with pancreatitis and pancreas divisum. Pancreatic duct stones have also been removed or fragmented using an endoscopic approach with reported benefits. Finally, some patients with pancreatic duct strictures have been treated with endoscopically placed stents that pass across the stricture, but the value of this treatment is unclear since the stents themselves can cause strictures.

Neuroablative Procedures

Pain from the pancreas is carried in sympathetic fibers that traverse the celiac ganglia, reach the sympathetic chain through the splanchnic nerves, and then ascend to the cortex. Celiac plexus nerve blocks performed either percutaneously or endoscopically have been employed to abolish this pain with inconsistent results. Recently, splanchnicectomy performed in the chest via a thoracoscopic approach has been used with reports of transient improvement in 70% of patients and long-lasting pain control in 50%.[33] Experience with thoracoscopic splanchnicectomy has been only anecdotal, and randomized, prospective trials will be needed to determine its ultimate value.

Surgical Treatment of Chronic Pancreatitis

The two indications for surgical intervention are pain and concern over the possible presence of cancer. After the diagnosis of chronic pancreatitis has been established, surgical intervention should be considered when (1) the pain is severe enough to limit the patient's lifestyle and/or reduce productivity and (2) the pain persists in spite of complete abstinence from alcohol and administration of non-narcotic analgesics. Imaging studies should be performed to define pancreatic and ductal anatomy since that will determine the surgical options. Finally, the risks and benefits of planned procedures should be clearly explained to the patient because, even with a technically successful operation, the pain may persist and further deterioration in exocrine and endocrine function can still occur.

Drainage Procedures for Patients With Small Ducts

Patients with small (>4- to 5-mm) pancreatic ducts, particularly those whose pancreatitis is caused by obstruction at the ampullary level, may benefit from transduodenal sphincteroplasty of the common bile duct with division of the septum that lies between the pancreatic duct and bile duct (pancreatic septotomy). Sphincteroplasty of the lesser papilla might be appropriate for patients with pancreas divisum. On the other hand, most patients with chronic pancreatitis have multiple areas of duct stricture throughout the pancreas and are unlikely to benefit from these transduodenal procedures.

Drainage Procedures for Patients With Dilated Ducts

The ideal treatment for these patients involves creating an anastomotic connection between the dilated duct and the intestinal lumen. There is little agreement concerning the minimum duct size needed to perform these anastomoses. Ducts larger than 1 cm in diameter are, clearly, large enough, but many surgeons perform duct-to-intestine drainage procedures with ducts as small as 5 mm. Duct drainage operations were pioneered by Duval, who described a procedure that involved splenectomy, resection of the pancreatic tail, and then creation of an end-to-end anastomosis between the transected end of the pancreas and a Roux-en-Y limb of jejunum. This procedure often failed because the presence of multiple pancreatic duct strictures interfered with complete ductal decompression. Puestow and Gillesby, in 1958, described an operation that involved longitudinally opening the entire duct and then invaginating the opened pancreas into a Roux-en-Y loop of jejunum. This allowed for more complete decompression but still required splenectomy. Later, Partington and Rochelle[34] modified the Puestow procedure by creating a side-to-side anastomosis between the opened duct and jejunum, thus eliminating the need for splenectomy (Fig. 53-8). In appropriately selected patients (i.e., those with large ducts and those with intraductal stones), longitudinal pancreaticojejunostomy, performed according to the Partington and Rochelle modification of the Puestow procedure, has been reported to result in immediate pain relief in more than 80% of patients and long-term pain relief in roughly 60% of patients. More recently, Ho and Frey[35] further modified the procedure by including removal of part of the pancreatic head, thereby marsupializing the duct as it dives deeply in the pancreas to reach the ampulla of Vater. This allows for an even more complete duct decompression and a longer longitudinal pancreaticojejunostomy. Both short- and long-term pain relief appear to be improved, and the procedure can be performed when the duct is only moderately dilated.

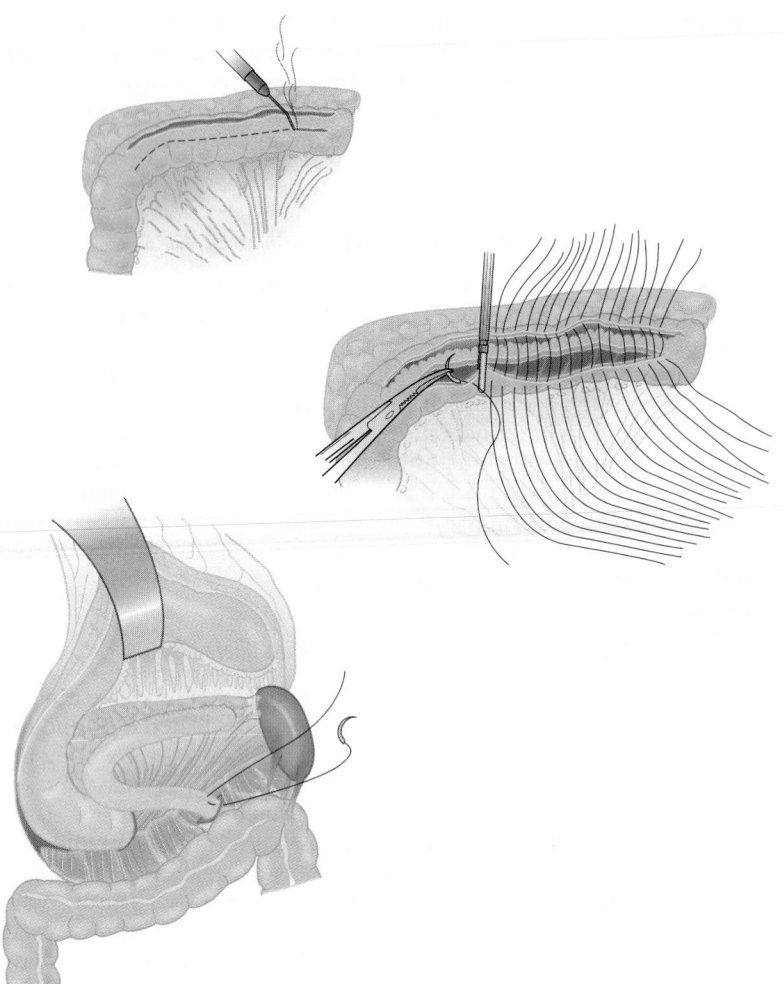

FIGURE 53-8.   Partington and Rochelle modification of the Puestow procedure. The pancreatic duct is opened from the tail of the pancreas to the edge of the duodenum and a side-to-side anastomosis is created joining a Roux-en-Y limb of jejunum to the opened pancreatic duct. (From Carey LC: Pancreatico-jejunostomy with cystoduodenostomy. *In* Malt RA [ed]: Surgical Techniques Illustrated. New York, WB Saunders, 1985, 396-405.)

Resective Procedures

Painful chronic pancreatitis can be treated with resection of the body and tail of the pancreas (distal pancreatectomy), resection of the head and uncinate process of the pancreas (Whipple procedure), with subtotal pancreatectomy that spares a rim of pancreas along the inner curve of the duodenum, and with total pancreatectomy. Each of these procedures can either cause or worsen pancreatic exocrine and endocrine insufficiency and, in the case of total pancreatectomy, a brittle form of diabetes can occur. Most experts believe that it is the inflammatory process in the pancreatic head that controls both the severity of symptoms and the further progression of the disease in the remainder of the gland. Perhaps because of this, resection of the pancreatic head has been shown to completely relieve the pain of chronic pancreatitis in 70% to 80% of patients. Resection of the pancreatic head can be accomplished by a standard pancreaticoduodenectomy (Whipple procedure) or by its pylorus-preserving modification (pylorus-preserving Whipple procedure) (Fig. 53-9).[36] Relief of symptoms by either procedure is com-

parable, but some claim that the quality of life and gastrointestinal function are better after the pylorus-preserving operation. Beger and colleagues have modified the Whipple procedure even further by coring out the head of the pancreas and preserving the duodenum and distal bile duct.[37] They claim that this "duodenum-preserving pancreatic head resection" yields results that are as good as or better than those achieved with the standard Whipple procedure.

Distal pancreatectomy is the ideal surgical procedure for patients whose chronic pancreatitis is confined to the pancreatic tail. This occurs in patients who develop a mid-duct stricture either as a result of necrotizing acute pancreatitis or as a result of trauma that injures the gland and duct as they cross the spine. Usually, distal pancreatectomy is combined with splenectomy for technical reasons but, in fact, the spleen can be preserved if its vascular supply is secure. Distal pancreatectomy should not be performed for patients with diffuse, chronic pancreatitis that involves the entire gland, even if the pancreatic tail is the area most severely involved, since recurrence of pancreatitis in the head can be anticipated and further resection

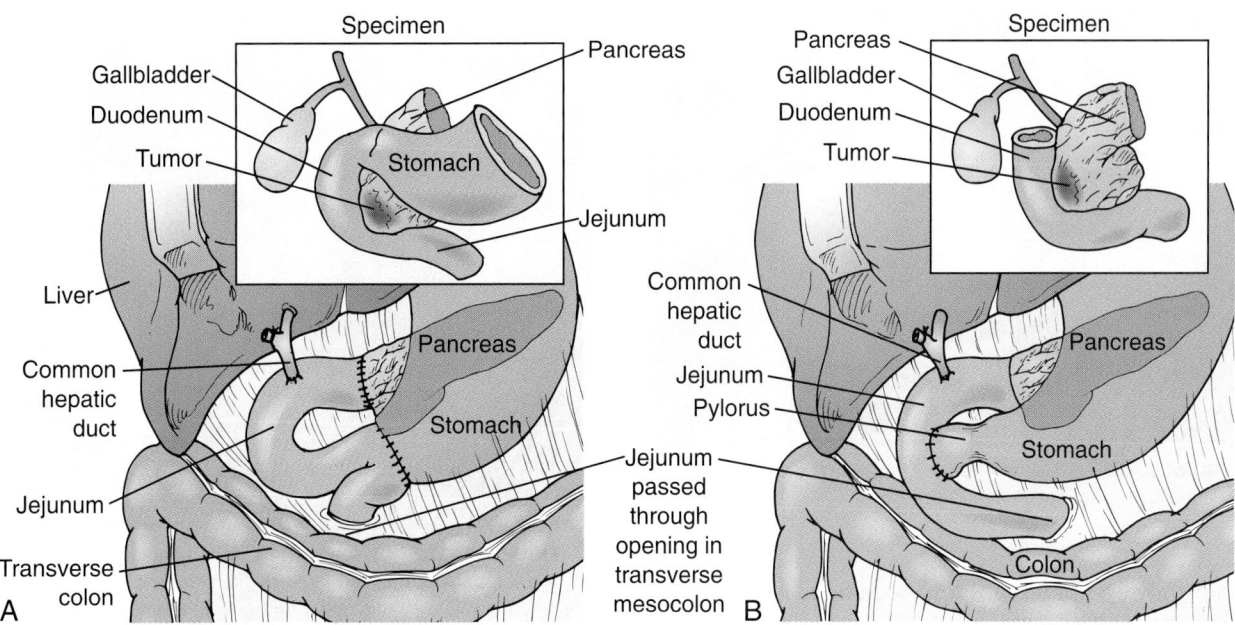

FIGURE 53-9.   Standard and pylorus-preserving Whipple procedure. The "standard Whipple" (A) involves resection of the gastric antrum, head of pancreas, distal bile duct, and entire duodenum with reconstruction as shown. The "pylorus-preserving Whipple" (B) does not include resection of the distal stomach, pylorus, or proximal duodenum. Gl. bl., gallbladder; duod., duodenum; stom., stomach; trans., transverse. (From Cameron, JL: Current status of the Whipple operation for periampullary carcinoma. Surg Rounds 77-87, 1988.)

of the pancreas, in that case, would leave the patient without functioning pancreatic endocrine tissue.

The role of total or near-total pancreatectomy in the treatment of patients with chronic pancreatitis is not clear. These procedures may represent the only surgical option for patients who have failed drainage procedures or those with small ducts who have already undergone distal pancreatectomy. Some patients continue to experience severe "pancreatic" pain even after total pancreatectomy, and, for this reason, the effects of total pancreatectomy on pain in chronic pancreatitis cannot be accurately predicted. On the other hand, it can be expected that patients undergoing total or near-total pancreatectomy will have brittle diabetes and severe steatorrhea. In combination with ongoing ethanol or drug abuse, the brittle diabetes and malnutrition may be unmanageable problems, and a high late mortality rate in these patients has been reported. In an attempt to avoid brittle diabetes in these patients, some surgeons have advocated harvesting and autotransplanting islets of Langerhans from the resected specimen. Modest success at insulin independence has been achieved using this approach, but the ultimate role of islet reimplantation remains to be established. In the past, some surgeons have reimplanted the entire resected pancreas with mixed results, and the procedure is performed only rarely now.

BENIGN EXOCRINE TUMORS

Most benign pancreatic exocrine tumors are cystic, but not all cystic tumors are benign. Benign cystic tumors, which account for 10% to 15% of pancreatic tumors, are usually asymptomatic but, when symptoms develop, they are usually related to pressure or obstruction of an adjacent organ.

Serous Cystadenoma

These tumors account for 20% to 40% of cystic pancreatic neoplasms. They are lined by a flattened epithelium with glycogen-rich cytoplasm that does not stain for mucins, and the finding of glycogen-rich cells on cytologic examination is diagnostic of a serous cystadenoma. Rare cases of malignant serous cystic lesions have been reported, but most are benign and have no malignant potential. Typically, they are large, spherical masses that contain a watery fluid and have a central, calcified stellate scar (Fig. 53-10). Oligocystic varieties, with large cystic spaces, can occur, but most are microcystic. They usually occur in the body or tail and are asymptomatic but, when located in the head, even benign serous cystadenomas can become symptomatic if they enlarge and compress adjacent structures. Resection is indicated when the diagnosis is in doubt or when they become symptomatic.

Mucinous Tumors

These tumors account for 20% to 40% of cystic tumors. Even if benign at the time of diagnosis, they are usually considered to have malignant potential. Two types have been described, but neither type usually communicates with the pancreatic duct. One form contains areas of ovarian-like stroma, is almost always found in women, and

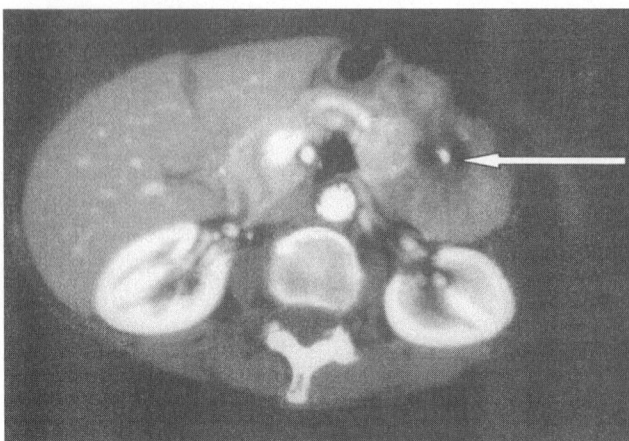

FIGURE 53-10.   CT scan of serous (microcystic) cystadenoma. Note scar with central calcification *(arrow)*.

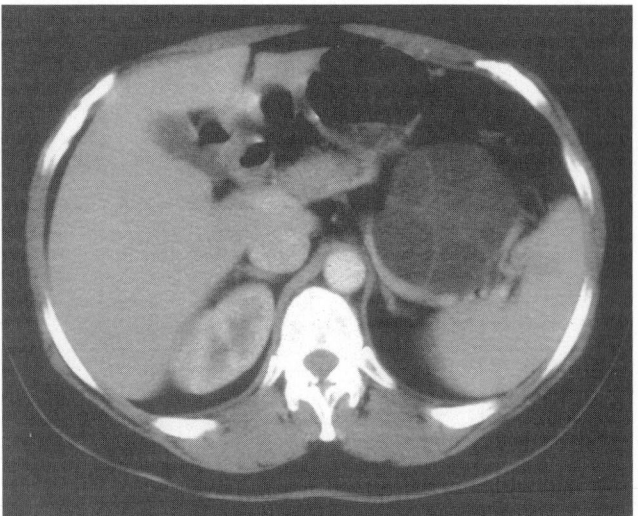

FIGURE 53-11.   CT scan of mucinous (macrocystic) cystadenoma. Note multiple large cystic spaces. Microscopic examination revealed multiple areas of ovarian-like stroma.

is almost always found in the pancreatic tail (Fig. 53-11). The more common type, however, lacks ovarian stroma and it can be found anywhere in the pancreas. It occurs equally in both sexes. For both types, imaging studies usually indicate that the lesion is composed of one or more very large cysts (i.e., macrocystic), although microcystic mucinous tumors can also occur. The cysts are lined by a columnar, mucin-producing, and sometimes papillary epithelium. Prolonged survival (i.e., >5 years) can be anticipated in more than 50% of patients if these tumors are resected prior to the development of invasive malignancy, but even after the development of malignant changes and invasion, long-term survival is still better than for ductal adenocarcinoma.

Intraductal Papillary Mucinous Tumor

Intraductal papillary mucinous tumor (IPMT), also known as *intraductal papillary mucinous neoplasm*, is another type of cystic pancreatic neoplasm. Although first described in Japan in the 1980s, it is now being recognized worldwide and its incidence appears to be rapidly increasing. Both men and women are equally affected. IPMT can involve the major ducts ("main duct variety"), the smaller ducts ("branch duct variety") or both types of ducts. It can be located in any or all parts of the pancreas, although involvement of the head appears to be its most common form. IPMT patients can experience pancreatitis when mucus, secreted by the tumor, transiently obstructs the orifice of the pancreatic duct. The diagnosis of IPMT can be made with near certainty if mucus is seen extruding through a large, fish-mouth–like papillary orifice at the time of endoscopy. The main or side-branch ducts involved with IPMT are usually lined by columnar mucin-producing cells that develop papillary projections. Other areas of the duct, although lined by normal epithelium, may be dilated as a result of prior obstructive episodes. IPMT is believed to follow an adenoma-carcinoma sequence, and it can be classified according to the Pan-IN classification scheme (Fig. 53-12) that categorizes tumors as having minimal or no dysplasia (PanIN-1), moderate

dysplasia (PanIN-2), or severe dysplasia/carcinoma in situ (PanIN-3).[38] The natural history of tumors with only mild or no dysplasia is not known, but those with severe dysplasia and/or carcinoma in situ are likely to become locally invasive and metastasize if left unresected. Resection with, at worst, PanIN-1 changes at the margin, prior to development of invasive malignancy, is usually curative. This may mandate total pancreatectomy. When resection is performed after development of invasive malignancy, cure rates are relatively low.

Management of Cystic Pancreatic Neoplasms

A recent history of pancreatitis, enzyme-rich fluid in the cyst, and communication between the cyst and the pancreatic duct suggests that the cystic lesion is a postpancreatitic (i.e., inflammatory) pseudocyst. Patients with asymptomatic pseudocysts can be left untreated. However, occasionally these features can also be associated with neoplastic cystic lesions; therefore, these patients should be closely followed. Serous cystadenomas, diagnosed by finding glycogen-rich cells on fine-needle aspiration biopsy, can also be followed without resection if they are not symptomatic. The major challenge is distinguishing pseudocysts and serous cystadenomas from the other, malignant or potentially malignant, types of cystic pancreatic tumors. The finding of mucin in the cyst, mucin-secreting cells on biopsy, a high cyst fluid viscosity, or a high cyst fluid carcinoembryonic antigen (CEA) is suggestive, but not diagnostic, of a potentially malignant tumor.[39] Failure to observe these changes, however, does not exclude a malignant or potentially malignant mass. Because of these uncertainties, all neoplastic cysts should be resected unless the diagnosis of a serous cystadenoma can be made with certainty. For those located in the pancreatic tail, a distal pancreatectomy is ideal, whereas cystic lesions in the pancreatic head present a greater

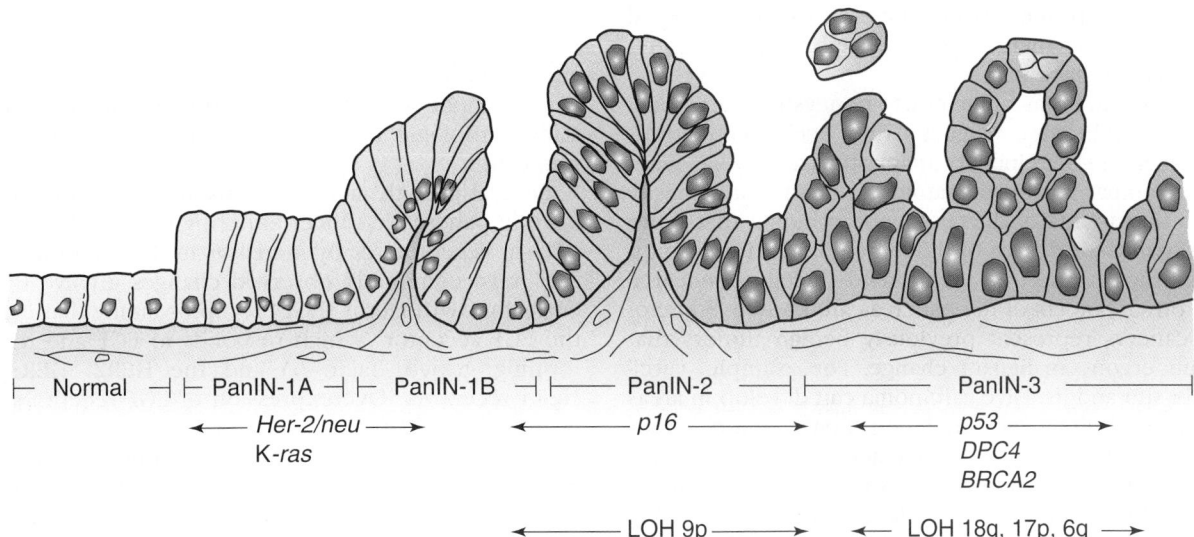

| ⊢ Normal ⊣ ⊢ PanIN-1A ⊣ ⊢ PanIN-1B ⊣ ⊢ PanIN-2 ⊣ ⊢ PanIN-3 ⊣ |

← Her-2/neu →
K-ras

← p16 →

← p53 →
DPC4
BRCA2

← LOH 9p → ← LOH 18q, 17p, 6q →

FIGURE 53-12. Progression model for pancreatic cancer. The progression from histologically normal ductal epithelium to low-grade pancreatic intraepithelial neoplasia (PanIN) to high-grade PanIN (left to right) is associated with the accumulation of specific genetic changes. Early changes include *Her-2*/neu and K-*ras* mutations; intermediate changes include *p16* mutations; and changes associated with either in situ or early invasive cancer include *p53, BRCA2,* and *DPC4* mutations. (From Wilentz RE, Iacobuzio-Donahoe CA, Argani P, et al: Loss of expression of *DPC4* in pancreatic intraepithelial neoplasia: Evidence that *DPC4* inactivation occurs late in neoplastic progression. Cancer Res 60:2002-2006, 2000.)

decision-making challenge because resection would require pancreaticoduodenectomy. Cytologic examination of aspirated tissue, removed either transcutaneously or with endoscopic ultrasonographic guidance, may aid in the difficult management decision, but not infrequently, doubt persists, and in good surgical risk patients, pancreaticoduodenectomy is probably indicated.

Solid-Pseudopapillary Tumor of the Pancreas

Solid-pseudopapillary tumor, a relatively uncommon tumor, often occurs in young women and follows a benign course. Local resection is usually curative, although incomplete removal can result in local recurrence, and malignant varieties have been described. The tumors are usually large, round, and well-demarcated masses that can occur in any part of the pancreas. Histologically, the tumor is mostly solid and consists of monomorphous eosinophilic or clear cells that demonstrate a pseudopapillary architecture. In suitable operative candidates, solid-pseudopapillary tumors of the pancreas should be resected.

MALIGNANT PANCREATIC TUMORS

Incidence and Epidemiology

Pancreatic cancer affects 25,000 to 30,000 people in the United States each year and is the fourth or fifth leading cause of cancer-related death in this country. It occurs more frequently in men than in women and it is more common among blacks than whites. Roughly 80% of cases occur between 60 and 80 years of age, whereas less than 2% occur in people younger than 40. Other risk factors include a history of hereditary or chronic pancreatitis, cigarette smoking, and occupational exposure to carcinogens. The incidence of diabetes mellitus is increased in patients with pancreatic cancer, but the relationship of diabetes to pancreas cancer is controversial. Some studies have indicated that diabetes is a risk factor for the development of pancreas cancer, whereas others have argued that diabetes may be a manifestation of the cancer. Coffee drinking, which was once considered a risk factor, is no longer thought to play a role in the development of pancreatic cancer.

Pathology

Ductal adenocarcinoma and its variants account for 80% to 90% of all pancreatic neoplasms and for an even greater fraction of the malignant tumors. Roughly 70% of ductal cancers arise in the pancreatic head or uncinate process. Grossly, they appear as hard, irregular, gritty masses that are yellow-gray and are usually poorly demarcated. At the time of diagnosis, they are usually larger than 3 cm in diameter and both nodal and distant metastases are also frequently present. Those originating in the body or tail of the pancreas are often larger and more likely to have spread before their presence is known. Microscopically, the degree of differentiation, mitotic index, and amount of mucous may vary considerably. They are frequently associated with an intense desmoplastic stromal reaction and fibrosis. A halo of chronic pancreatitis frequently surrounds the tumor, presumably caused by tumor-induced obstruction of neighboring ducts. Areas of vascular and lymphatic invasion within and around the tumor are commonly seen. In addition, perineural growth of the tumor is highly characteristic of this cancer and may account for the propensity of pancreatic cancer to extend into neighboring neural plexus causing both upper abdominal and back pain.

Cancers such as mucinous noncystic carcinoma (colloid carcinoma), signet ring cell carcinoma, adenosquamous carcinoma, anaplastic carcinoma, giant cell carcinoma, and sarcomatoid carcinoma are considered to be variants of ductal adenocarcinoma that differ primarily in their degree of differentiation and their morphologic appearance. In addition to ductal adenocarcinoma, other cancers of the pancreas are known. Some of those cancers represent previously benign tumors that have undergone malignant change. For example, carcinoma in situ and invasive carcinoma can develop in areas of IPMT or within areas of mucinous cystic tumors. Other forms of pancreas cancer include acinar cell carcinomas, which are most common in the 5th to 7th decade of life and most frequently present as large masses in the body or tail of the pancreas. Pancreatoblastoma is a rare form of pancreas cancer that usually presents in young children. Nonepithelial cancers of all types, including leiomyosarcomas, liposarcomas, plasmacytomas, and lymphomas, can also develop within the pancreas, but these tumors are quite rare. Lymphomas of the pancreas, if diagnosed prior to resection, are usually best treated with chemoradiation.

Development and Molecular Biology

The following three types of genetic abnormalities have been observed in pancreatic cancers: activation of growth-promoting oncogenes, mutations that result in the inactivation of tumor suppressor genes, and excessive expression of growth factors and/or their receptors.[40] Almost all pancreatic cancers and most of the precursor lesions demonstrate codon 12 mutations of the K-*ras* oncogene. These and other mutations of K-*ras* are believed to be early events in pancreatic tumorigenesis. K-*ras* normally plays a key role in regulating many cellular events, including growth. Its activation is a guanosine triphosphate (GTP)-dependent event, terminated by GTP hydrolysis and dissociation of GDP. Oncogenic point mutations of K-*ras* interfere with that termination event, and, as a result, K-*ras* becomes permanently activated and a continuous growth signal is transmitted to the nucleus.

Mutation of the *p53* tumor suppressor gene is the most common genetic event in all human cancers, and it is observed in 75% of pancreatic cancers. The gene encodes a 53-kD nuclear phosphoprotein that plays an important role in regulating the cell cycle, DNA synthesis and repair, apoptosis, and cell differentiation. Although mutation of *p53* results in the loss of its function, *p53* mutations alone are not believed to be sufficient to cause malignant transformation. Mutations resulting in the functional loss of other tumor suppressor genes, including *p16*, *SMAD-4*, *DPC*, and *DCC* are also commonly observed in pancreatic cancer. Other much less frequent tumor suppressor gene deletions that have been observed in pancreatic cancers result in the loss of the retinoblastoma gene and the adenomatous polyposis coli (*APC*) gene. DNA mismatch repair genes have also been reported to be mutated and functionally deleted in pancreatic cancers. These genes encode for enzymes that function to repair potentially pathologic DNA changes that occur during DNA replication.

Several growth factor systems are commonly upregulated in pancreatic cancer either by increased expression of their receptors or by increases in the relevant ligands. The most commonly observed changes involve the epidermal growth factor (EGF) receptor family that includes the EGF receptor (which responds to EGF and to transforming growth factor-α) and the HER2, HER3, and HER4 receptors. Overexpression of EGF receptors or its ligands is correlated with tumor invasiveness, enhanced potential for metastasis, and a poorer prognosis. Increased expression of HER2 is associated with a better differentiated phenotype. Other growth factor systems implicated in pancreatic cancer development include those for hepatocyte growth factor and for transforming growth factor-β.

It is now generally believed that pancreas cancer evolves in a progressive, step-wise fashion, much like that observed for colon cancer. Precursor ductal lesions (see Fig. 53-12) have been identified, and the step-wise progression toward invasive cancer and metastasis has been related to the accumulated presence of multiple genetic abnormalities. K-*ras* mutations and *HER2*/neu overexpression are the earliest changes to occur. Alterations in *p16* are found primarily in *PanIN-2* and *PanIN-3*. *DPC4*, *BRCA2*, and *p53* are inactivated during the later stages of cancer progression and are found almost exclusively in invasive lesions.

Hereditary Pancreatic Cancer Syndromes

Pancreatic cancer has been observed to be increased in families with hereditary nonpolyposis colon cancer (HNPCC), those with familial breast cancer (associated with the *BRCA2* mutation), those with Peutz-Jeghers syndrome, those with ataxia-telangiectasia, and those with the familial atypical multiple mole melanoma (FAMMM) syndrome. Patients with hereditary pancreatitis are also at increased risk of developing pancreatic cancer. This is particularly true in those with a paternal pattern of inheritance who may have a 75% risk of developing pancreatic cancer.[41] Even in the absence of one of these familial cancer syndromes or hereditary pancreatitis, individuals with a family history of pancreatic cancer, especially those with two or more pancreatic cancer–affected first-degree relatives, have an increased risk of developing pancreatic cancer.

Symptoms and Signs

Pancreatic cancers are insidious tumors that can be present for long periods and grow extensively before they produce symptoms. The symptoms, once they develop, are determined by the location of the tumor in the

TABLE 53-2. Signs and Symptoms of Pancreatic Cancer	
Frequent	**Infrequent**
Pancreatic Head Cancers	
Weight loss (92%)	Nausea (37%)
Pain (72%)	Weakness (35%)
Jaundice (82%)	Pruritus (24%)
Dark Urine (63%)	Vomiting (37%)
Light stools (62%)	
Anorexia (64%)	
Pancreatic Body/Tail Cancers	
Weight loss (100%)	Jaundice (7%)
Pain (87%)	Dark urine (5%)
Weakness (43%)	Light stool (6%)
Nausea (45%)	Pruritus (4%)
Anorexia (33%)	
Vomiting (37%)	

pancreas (Table 53-2). Those in the head or uncinate process of the pancreas make their presence known by causing bile duct, duodenal, or pancreatic duct obstruction. Symptoms include unexplained episodes of pancreatitis, painless jaundice, nausea, vomiting, steatorrhea, and unexplained weight loss. With further spread beyond the pancreas, these patients may note upper abdominal and/or back pain when peripancreatic nerve plexus are involved and ascites when peritoneal carcinomatosis or portal vein occlusion develops. Patients with tumors arising in the neck, body, or tail of the pancreas usually do not develop jaundice or gastric outlet obstruction. Their symptoms may be limited to unexplained weight loss and vague upper abdominal pain until the tumor has grown extensively and spread beyond the pancreas. New-onset diabetes mellitus is occasionally the first symptom of an otherwise occult pancreatic cancer. Recent studies have suggested that this form of diabetes may be mediated by a factor released from the tumor that either inhibits insulin release from islets or induces peripheral insulin resistance. Unexplained migratory thrombophlebitis (Trousseau's syndrome) may be associated with pancreatic and other types of malignancy. It is probably a paraneoplastic phenomenon that results from a tumor-induced hypercoagulable state.

The physical findings in patients with pancreas cancer are also dependent on the location, size, and extent of the tumor. Liver nodules indicative of metastases can sometimes be felt. Metastatic subumbilical ("Sister Mary Joseph node") and pelvic peritoneal ("Blummer's shelf") deposits as well as left supraclavicular lymphadenopathy ("Virchow's node") indicate the presence of distant metastases. Malignant ascites, caused by peritoneal carcinomatosis, may also be present. With portal, splenic, or superior mesenteric vein occlusion, mesenteric venous pressures may be increased and collateral channels, including gastroesophageal varices and a caput medusae, may develop. Distal common bile duct obstruction caused by the tumor often leads to bile duct and gallbladder distention. Thus, a palpable gallbladder in a patient with painless jaundice (i.e., Courvoisier's sign) should suggest the presence of a periampullary neoplasm.

Blood Tests

Patients with pancreatic head lesions frequently have elevated bilirubin and alkaline phosphatase levels suggestive of obstructive jaundice. Other routine laboratory studies are usually normal. The two most widely used pancreatic cancer serum markers are the CEA and the Lewis blood group carbohydrate antigen CA 19-9. Both are frequently elevated in patients with advanced disease, but, unfortunately, the circulating levels of these tumor markers are often normal in patients with early, potentially curable, tumors. Thus, using these tumor markers to screen patients with vague symptoms or those in high-risk groups has not been shown to be useful in detecting early disease. With a cutoff value of 37 U/mL, CA 19-9 has been reported to have a sensitivity of 86% and a specificity of 87%.[42] CA 19-9 can also be elevated in patients with cholangitis and jaundice not caused by pancreatic cancer. Extremely high levels of either the CA 19-9 or CEA usually indicate unresectable and/or metastatic disease.

Imaging Studies

For most patients, the initial imaging study is a transcutaneous ultrasound examination. It may reveal a pancreatic mass and indicate whether that mass is solid or cystic. It can also aid in the diagnosis of jaundiced patients by revealing the presence of extrahepatic ductal dilation in the absence of demonstrable biliary tract stones. Transcutaneous ultrasound, regardless of its findings, is usually followed by helical contrast-enhanced CT, performed in conjunction with intravenous infusion of contrast material. Timed images are taken to permit visualization of the pancreas during the arterial phase, the parenchymal phase, and finally the venous phase of contrast perfusion. Pancreatic cancer usually appears as a hypodense mass with poorly demarcated edges. It may have a more hypodense center, indicating either central necrosis or cystic change, and the pancreatic duct to the left of the lesion may be dilated. When performed and interpreted by experienced radiologists, CT has a specificity for diagnosing pancreatic tumors of 95% or better. Its sensitivity depends on the size of the tumor exceeding 95% for tumors larger than 2 cm in diameter. Much, if not all, of the information provided by CT can also be obtained with high-quality MRI. Although the sensitivity and specificity of MRI appear to equal those of CT, CT is currently more widely employed perhaps because it is cheaper, more user friendly, and more easily interpreted by clinicians. Positron emission tomography (PET) may be of value in diagnosing small pancreatic tumors that escape CT or MRI detection, but the sensitivity and specificity of PET scanning remain to be established.

ERCP may be particularly helpful in evaluating patients with obstructive jaundice without a detectable mass on CT or MRI. It can identify stones or other nonmalignant causes of obstructive jaundice, define the location of the bile duct obstruction, identify ampullary and periampullary lesions, and establish the diagnosis of IPMT if mucous is seen extruding through a fish-mouth papillary opening. The finding of superimposable bile duct and pancreatic duct strictures (i.e., the double-duct sign) on ERCP is highly suggestive of a pancreatic head cancer (Fig. 53-13) but benign processes, such as chronic pancreatitis or autoimmune pancreatitis, can also produce a double-duct sign. The role of ERCP in the management of patients with a mass on CT is more controversial. Many surgeons (including me) would argue that ERCP is not helpful since a malignant lesion cannot be entirely excluded by ERCP. Thus, resection is indicated, regardless of the ERCP findings.

The Role of Biopsy

Biopsy to confirm the presence and identify the type of cancer is usually required before chemoradiation therapy of unresectable pancreatic tumors or neoadjuvant treatment of resectable tumors. Percutaneous biopsy, performed with either CT or ultrasound guidance, or transduodenal biopsy, performed with endoscopic ultrasound guidance, is routinely employed in these situations. Considerable controversy, however, surrounds the question of whether all patients with potentially resectable tumors should undergo preoperative biopsy. That biopsy might yield false-negative results, and, at least theoretically, transcutaneous biopsy could promote intraperitoneal dissemination of the tumor. Performing the biopsy via a transduodenal approach would eliminate the concern of tumor dissemination, but even with this approach a positive biopsy merely confirms the decision

for resection and a negative biopsy is inconclusive. For these reasons, most surgeons would not recommend routine preoperative biopsy for confirmation of the diagnosis in the management of patients with potentially resectable lesions. However, if this policy of not performing preoperative biopsy is followed, 5% to 10% of patients undergoing resection for suspected cancer will be found to have benign lesions.

Staging of Pancreatic Cancer

The American Joint Committee on Cancer (AJCC) staging system is widely used to stage pancreatic cancer (Table 53-3). This system uses the TNM classification to define the *t*umor extent, *n*odal metastases, and distant *m*etastases.[43] Tis, which denotes in situ cancer, corresponds to PanIN-3, that is, the most advanced of the ductal cancer precursor lesions (see Fig. 53-12). T1 and T2 cancers are confined to the pancreas and either less than 2 cm or greater than 2 cm in diameter. T3 and T4 lesions extend beyond the pancreas. T3 lesions are considered to be potentially resectable because they do not involve the celiac axis or superior mesenteric artery. They may involve the portal/superior mesenteric vein and resection of the tumor may mandate venous resection and reconstruction. Long-term survival of patients undergoing major venous resection is poor, and it is not clear that those patients actually benefit from resection. T4 lesions are considered to be unresectable because they involve the critical peripancreatic arteries. N1 lesions have positive regional nodes and M1 lesions have distant metastases, whereas N0 and M0 lesions lack both of these features. Distant metastases are common, and they are most frequently located in the liver or lung or on the peritoneal surfaces of the abdomen.

Stages 1 and 2 cancers are amenable to resection. Poor prognostic signs include aneuploidy, large tumor size (T2), the presence of positive regional nodes (N1), and an incomplete resection at the pancreatic or retroperitoneal margin. The latter is most closely associated with poor

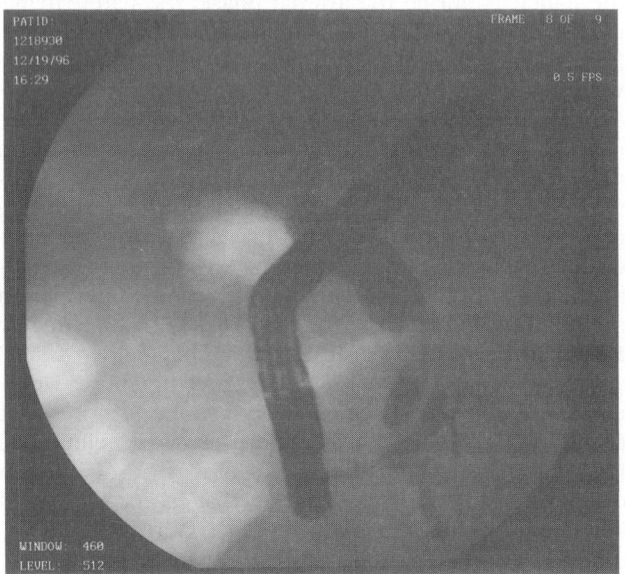

FIGURE 53-13. Endoscopic retrograde cholangiopancreatography (ERCP) showing double-duct sign. A stent traverses the bile duct stricture. Note closely adjacent bile and pancreatic duct strictures in patient with adenocarcinoma of the pancreatic head.

TABLE 53-3. American Joint Committee on Cancer: TNM System for Staging of Pancreatic Cancer

Stage	T Status	N Status	M Status
Stage 0	Tis	N0	M0
Stage IA	T1	N0	M0
Stage IB	T2	N0	M0
Stage IIA	T3	N0	M0
Stage IIB	T1	N1	M0
	T2	N1	M0
	T3	N1	M0
Stage III	T4	Any N	M0
Stage IV	Any T	Any N	M1

Adapted from AJCC Cancer Staging Handbook, 6th ed. New York, Springer, 2002, pp 179-188.

survival. Stages 3 and 4 cancers are considered to be unresectable, either because of distant metastases (stage 4) or because of major arterial involvement (stage 3). Mean survival for patients with stage 3 tumors ranges from 8 to 12 months, whereas that for patients with stage 4 tumors is only 3 to 6 months.

Preoperative staging of pancreatic cancers is usually accomplished using one or more of the standard imaging techniques, such as CT, MRI, or ultrasonography. High-resolution helical CT, with phased imaging for visualization of the pancreas and major peripancreatic vessels, is the most widely used method of evaluating tumor resectability. Circumferential encasement, invasion, or occlusion of the portal vein/superior mesenteric vein and/or the superior mesenteric artery is generally considered to be a sign of unresectability although, strictly speaking, resection is still technically possible if only the venous structures are involved. Partial encasement (i.e., involvement of 30% to 60% of the circumference of the vein) may result in distortion of the vein and the appearance of a teardrop-shaped rather than a round structure. In our experience, this is associated with a low resectability rate. Other CT changes suggestive of unresectability include extension beyond the pancreatic capsule and into the retroperitoneum, involvement of neural or nodal structures surrounding the origin of either the celiac axis or superior mesenteric artery, and extension of the tumor along the hepatoduodenal ligament. MRI provides information that is similar to that obtained by CT, but combining MRI with CT does not seem to provide additional information. There have been recent claims that endoscopic ultrasound may provide staging information that is superior to that obtained by either CT or MRI[44] since it permits better visualization of nodal structures and allows for determination of the depth of invasion for tumors involving the duodenal wall. Unfortunately, endoscopic ultrasound is operator dependent, and its applicability to preoperative staging is dependent on the locally available expertise. Theoretically, PET scanning might be useful in staging pancreatic cancers by permitting detection of small metastatic lesions that escape detection by standard cross-sectional imaging techniques, but the sensitivity and specificity of PET scans in this setting are not currently known.

The Role of Laparoscopy in Staging

The role of staging laparoscopy in the management of pancreatic cancer is controversial. Proponents claim that 20% to 40% of patients believed to have stage 1 or 2 disease have unrecognized small metastases to peritoneal surfaces (such as diaphragm, liver) and that those metastases can be laparoscopically detected, thus preventing a needless laparotomy. Our own experience indicates that, with high-quality modern imaging techniques, few patients with pancreatic head tumors are deemed unresectable at operation merely because they are found to have metastases that might have been found by laparoscopy. More commonly, unappreciated vascular involvement is the operative finding that prevents resection and, in those

patients, benefit can still be provided by performance of bilioenteric, and possibly a gastroenteric, bypass. The argument for preliminary laparoscopy would be more compelling in the case of patients with body or tail lesions since, with left-sided lesions, neither obstructive jaundice nor gastric outlet obstruction are likely to develop and, therefore, there is no role for surgical bypass in those patients. For these reasons, it is my practice to perform staging laparoscopy for potentially resectable body or tail lesions. For pancreatic head lesions that are deemed resectable by preoperative routine staging, laparoscopy is not advocated.

Resectional Surgery for Pancreatic Head and Uncinate Process Tumors

Tumors of the head, neck, and uncinate process of the pancreas account for approximately 70% of pancreatic tumors. They are generally resected by pancreaticoduodenectomy, with or without preservation of the pylorus and proximal duodenum (see Fig. 53-10). The two procedures yield similar survival rates and have similar morbidity. The pylorus-preserving operation is technically easier and faster, but it may be associated with a higher incidence of and more prolonged delayed gastric emptying. Both operations can be performed through a midline, bilateral subcostal, or right subcostal incision. After a preliminary search for metastases or other reasons to abort resection, the retroperitoneal area behind the pancreatic head, the hepatoduodenal ligament, and the base of the transverse mesocolon should be carefully examined. The finding of involved peripancreatic nodes, even along the cephalad border of the pancreas near the portal vein, does not preclude resection although it worsens prognosis. A tunnel (the "tunnel of love") should be developed behind the neck of the pancreas and anterior to the underlying visceral vessels before concluding that the lesion can be resected. Once it is deemed resectable, irreversible steps can be taken. The gallbladder is usually removed and the common bile duct is divided above the duodenum. The proximal gastrointestinal tract is divided at the level of the gastric antrum (standard Whipple) or first part of the duodenum (pylorus-preserving Whipple). The proximal jejunum is divided and the neck of the pancreas is transected. Finally, the uncinate process of the pancreas is resected from the retroperitoneum along the lateral surface of the superior mesenteric artery and the specimen is removed. Reconstruction can be accomplished in a variety of ways but the most common involves a pancreaticojejunostomy (as an end-to-end or as an end-to-side), an end-to-side hepaticojejunostomy, and then an antecolic end-to-side gastrojejunostomy (standard Whipple) or duodenojejunostomy (pylorus-preserving Whipple) (see Fig. 53-10). Frequently, drains and a feeding jejunal tube are placed, the latter in anticipation of the delayed gastric emptying that frequently occurs, and the abdomen is closed.

Several reports, mostly from Japan, have suggested extending the Whipple procedure to include an extensive retroperitoneal lymphadenectomy and, in some cases, total pancreatectomy along with possible major venous resection, can result in increased long-term patient survival. This so-called extended radical pancreaticoduodenectomy is frequently followed by a prolonged delay in the return of gastrointestinal function and, on occasion, with incapacitating and persistent diarrhea. A recent prospective, randomized study in the United States has failed to show a survival benefit for this extended radical operation and it is rarely performed in the United States.[45]

Complications of Pancreaticoduodenectomy

When performed by experienced surgeons in high-volume centers, the operative mortality of pancreaticoduodenectomy is 2% to 4%. Anastomotic leaks, intra-abdominal abscesses, and delayed gastric emptying account for most of the perioperative complications after pancreaticoduodenectomy. Leakage from the pancreatic anastomosis, resulting in a pancreatic fistula, occurs in 15% to 20% of patients. With adequate drainage, these fistulas usually heal within several weeks. Some pancreatic surgeons have claimed that administration of a somatostatin analogue to patients undergoing pancreaticoduodenectomy for cancer could reduce the incidence and/or duration of pancreatic fistula, but a recent randomized trial addressing this subject concluded that prophylactic administration of a somatostatin analogue in this setting is not beneficial. Biliary fistulas are much less common than pancreatic fistulas after pancreaticoduodenectomy, but they also usually heal if adequate drainage is achieved. Delayed gastric emptying occurs in 15% to 40% of patients and almost always resolves with time. Its occurrence is unpredictable and it may persist for several weeks or even months. The basis for delayed gastric emptying after pancreaticoduodenectomy is not clear. Some have suggested that it is the result of removing the cells in the duodenum that secrete the promotility hormone motilin. Erythromycin, which has a structure that resembles motilin, acts as an agonist at motilin receptors and has been used to treat these patients. Success has been reported using this approach, but my experience with this use of erythromycin has been disappointing.

The endocrine pancreas has considerable functional reserve and, for that reason, most patients do not develop diabetes after resection of the pancreatic head. In fact, some patients with tumor-induced diabetes may have resolution of their diabetes after resection. In contrast pancreatic malabsorption and steatorrhea are relatively common long-term problems. It may reflect exocrine secretory insufficiency, an obstruction at the pancreatic-jejunal anastomosis, or poor postoperative mixing of secreted enzymes with food. Although distressing, postoperative malabsorption and steatorrhea are rarely incapacitating but require exogenously administered pancreatic enzymes.

Results of Pancreaticoduodenectomy for Pancreatic Cancer

Long-term survival, when the operation is performed for ductal adenocarcinoma, is unusual. Five-year survival rates of 15% to 20% have been reported from some centers, but rates of 10% to 15% are more common, and most of those patients who survive for 5 years succumb over the subsequent 5 years. A number of factors affect the survival rate. Perhaps the most influential is the presence or absence of tumor at the resection margin. Negative margins, in one study, were associated with a 26% 5-year survival, whereas positive margins were associated with an 8% 5-year survival. Extending the resection to a total pancreatectomy or to include more radical retroperitoneal lymph node resection does not appear to increase long-term survival. Other factors that affect long-term survival include tumor diameter, diploid/aneuploid DNA content, and lymph node status. The 5-year survival of node-positive patients, in one series, was reported to be 14%, whereas 5-year survival of node-negative patients was 36%.

Resectional Surgery for Pancreatic Body and Tail Tumors

Most body and tail cancers have already metastasized to distant sites or extended locally to involve nodes, nerves, or major vessels by the time of diagnosis. Splenic vein involvement and/or occlusion is not uncommon and, by itself, is not a sign of nonresectability. On the other hand, involvement of the splenic/superior mesenteric vein confluence generally precludes resection. Resection involves a distal pancreatectomy either with or without concomitant splenectomy. Splenectomy should be performed for malignant tumors, but splenic preservation is not contraindicated when benign tumors are being removed. After a thorough search for metastatic disease, the operation starts by dividing the gastrocolic omentum, short gastric vessels, and peritoneal reflections around the body and tail of the pancreas to elevate the spleen and pancreatic tail out of the retroperitoneum. The splenic artery and vein, in that order, are ligated and the pancreas is transected, to the right of the tumor leaving an uninvolved margin. The resection margin can be either closed with a stapler or imbricated with sutures. Ideally, the transected duct should be suture ligated separately.

Complications of distal pancreatectomy include subphrenic abscess, which may occur in 5% to 10% of patients, and pancreatic duct leak, which has been reported to occur in up to 20% of patients. Both complications can usually be managed nonoperatively by percutaneous drainage and reoperation is rarely required. Pancreatic duct leak usually results in the formation of a fluid collection that resembles a pseudocyst and that, following drainage, becomes a pancreaticocutaneous fistula. Some surgeons have advocated prophylactic administration of a somatostatin analogue to reduce the incidence or duration of pancreatic fistula after distal pancreatectomy, but there are no convincing data to support this practice. Somatostatin administration frequently reduces the output of these pancreatic fistulas, but it does not appear to alter the time of fistula closure.

Only 10% of cancers involving the tail or body of the pancreas are resectable at the time of diagnosis. The 5-year survival of patients who are deemed resectable is somewhat lower than that of patients with resectable cancer of the pancreatic head (8% to 14%). Factors affecting long-term survival are similar to those for pancreatic head cancers.

Palliative Nonsurgical Treatment for Pancreatic Cancers

Establishing the diagnosis and relieving symptoms of jaundice, gastric outlet obstruction, and pain are the goals of palliative nonsurgical treatment. Tissue diagnosis can usually be made by CT- or ultrasound-guided percutaneous fine-needle aspiration of either the tumor or its metastases. Transduodenal fine-needle aspiration of the tumor with endoscopic ultrasound guidance and duct cytology obtained by brushings are alternative, but less frequently successful, methods of establishing the diagnosis. Decompression of the obstructed biliary tract can be achieved using either an endoscopic or a percutaneous-transhepatic approach. The former has been shown, in randomized trials, to yield better results with fewer associated complications. At the time of ERCP, a transpapillary stent is placed across the obstructed segment of bile duct. Either plastic or expandable metal stents can be used, but metal stents give more complete and more long-lasting relief of jaundice. Plastic stents can become obstructed by tumor or debris and, as a result, they must be changed every 2 to 3 months. The percutaneous-transhepatic approach to duct decompression is usually reserved for patients in whom, for technical reasons, a stent cannot be placed endoscopically. Pancreatic tumors can extend into and obstruct the duodenum leading to gastric outlet obstruction. This commonly occurs in the second portion of the duodenum in patients with pancreatic head cancers. Pancreatic body tumors can invade the third or fourth portion of the duodenum and also cause obstruction. Recent reports indicate that many of these patients can be palliated by endoscopic placement of expandable endoluminal metal stents into the duodenum.[46] For lesions that are not amenable to stents, surgical gastrojejunostomy may be required. Pain, which is a common symptom of pancreatic cancer, is usually caused by tumor invasion of the peripancreatic neural plexus. Most patients can be adequately treated with orally or transcutaneously administered analgesics. Narcotic medications may be required. When or if this fails, percutaneous CT-guided or endoscopic ultrasound–guided celiac plexus block may be helpful.

Palliative Surgical Management of Pancreatic Cancer

Most of the symptoms experienced by patients with unresectable pancreatic cancer can be relieved by nonsurgical means. Surgical palliation is, for the most part, employed for patients who are undergoing laparotomy for anticipated resectable disease and found to be unresectable at the time of surgery. In that situation, biliary tract decompression can be achieved by creating either a cholecystojejunostomy or a choledochojejunostomy. The former is most appropriate for patients with nondilated ducts in whom the cystic duct–common bile duct junction is far

from the pancreatic tumor. Choledochojejunostomy, on the other hand, should be performed when the tumor is close to or at the cystic duct–common bile duct junction and the bile duct is dilated. Either a loop or a Roux-en-Y segment of jejunum can be used with similar results. Duodenal obstruction can be managed by creation of a side-to-side gastrojejunostomy in which an antecolic jejunal loop is anastomosed to the posterior wall of the gastric antrum. Duodenal obstruction, even in advanced pancreatic cancer, occurs in less than 25% of patients and, therefore, considerable controversy surrounds whether a prophylactic gastrojejunostomy should be performed prior to the development of gastric outlet obstruction. The issue is further complicated by the fact that a gastrojejunostomy can cause delayed gastric emptying and result in symptoms identical to those experienced by patients with duodenal obstruction. It is my practice to perform gastrojejunostomy selectively (i.e., for patients whose tumor is locally advanced but without distant metastases [stage 3 lesions]) since they have an expected survival of 8 to 12 months. I would not perform prophylactic gastrojejunostomy for patients with distant metastasis (stage 4 lesions) since their expected survival is only 3 to 6 months and they are less likely to develop duodenal obstruction prior to death. Palliation of pain can be achieved, intraoperatively, by injecting alcohol into the celiac plexus and some surgeons routinely perform operative celiac plexus block at the time of surgical palliation. This is usually accomplished by injecting 15 to 20 mL of 50% ethanol into the celiac plexus on either side of the aorta and, in one randomized, prospective trial, this treatment has been reported to reduce postoperative pain and the need for postoperative analgesics in patients with unresectable pancreatic cancers. However, many patients with unresectable pancreatic cancer can be successfully managed with minimal or no narcotic analgesics and, when more severe pain occurs, results similar to those achieved by intraoperative chemical splanchnicectomy can be achieved using a percutaneous approach. For these reasons, many surgeons do not routinely perform intraoperative celiac plexus blocks.

Chemoradiation Therapy

Many different protocols for chemoradiation treatment of recurrent or unresectable pancreatic cancer have been described. The body of literature on this subject is quite large and beyond the scope of this review. For the most part, the best results have been achieved using radiation therapy combined with either 5-fluorouracil or gemcitabine. Patients undergoing resection may also benefit from adjuvant chemoradiation therapy. The frequently quoted Gastrointestinal Tumor Study Group (GITSG) report suggested that the combination of 5-fluorouracil with radiation therapy could increase the 2-year survival rate for patients with tumor-free resection margins from 18% to 43%.[47] This approach, although based on the experience with a very small group of patients, has been generally accepted and is widely employed. Recently, the European Study Group for Pancreatic Cancer (ESPAC) has reported a different experience.[48] They conducted a large study evaluating adjuvant chemotherapy (5-fluorouracil), radiation therapy, both, or neither. A survival benefit was observed for those undergoing chemotherapy but not for those receiving either radiation therapy alone or combined chemoradiotherapy. Intraoperative radiation therapy, as adjuvant treatment, has been evaluated but no benefit has been found. Neoadjuvant chemoradiation has also been used for patients believed to have resectable lesions, but good prospective, randomized studies have not been reported. Some have claimed up to 15% of selected patients with locally advanced lesions deemed to be unresectable can be made resectable by aggressive administration of chemoradiation therapy. Although the specimens ultimately resected in these cases have frequently contained relatively little viable tumor, the long-term benefits achieved by resecting these advanced tumors are not known.

PANCREATIC AND PANCREATICODUODENAL TRAUMA

Three percent to 12% of patients with severe abdominal trauma have pancreatic injury. On average, these patients have 3.5 other organs injured and isolated pancreatic injury is uncommon. Roughly two thirds of pancreatic injuries are the result of penetrating trauma, and the remaining one third are due to blunt trauma. Blunt abdominal trauma can cause damage that ranges from a mild contusion to a severe crushing injury. Classically, blunt injury is the result of midline upper abdominal trauma inflicted by objects as diverse as automobile seatbelts and bicycle handlebars. In these cases, the neck and body of the pancreas can be injured as they pass over the vertebral column. The mortality rate for pancreatic trauma is closely related to the nature of the injury. Thus, the mortality rate associated with blunt trauma is 17% to 19%, whereas, with stab wounds, it is 3% to 5%, with gunshot wounds it is 15% to 22%, and with shotgun wounds it is 46% to 56%.

Diagnosis

Serum amylase levels are elevated in most patients with significant pancreatic trauma, but they are also increased in up to 90% of severe abdominal trauma patients who do not have pancreatic injury. Thus, measurement of amylase at the time of hospital admission is not helpful in identifying those with pancreatic injury. On the other hand, a progressive rise in serum amylase activity is a more specific indicator of pancreatic injury. Contrast-enhanced CT, which is increasingly being used as a screening test of patients with major abdominal trauma, is the most useful noninvasive method of evaluating patients with suspected pancreatic injury, but even high-quality CT examinations may be either falsely negative or falsely positive. Changes suggestive of pancreatic injury include the presence of peripancreatic fluid collections, focal or diffuse enlargement of the gland, parenchymal disruption, and areas of diminished contrast perfusion. Frequently, serial CT exam-

inations are needed because the changes indicative of pancreatic injury may not be present on examinations performed very soon after injury.

Ultimately, the management of pancreatic injuries depends on the presence of pancreatic duct disruption, major associated vascular injury, and/or significant injury to peripancreatic organs, especially the duodenum. Vascular and duodenal injury can be evaluated at the time of exploratory laparotomy, but the integrity of the pancreatic duct may be difficult to determine at the time of operation unless the pancreas is transected or pancreatic juice is seen to be extravasating from the region of the duct. In the absence of these findings, pancreatography is required to localize or exclude a duct injury. Intraoperative ductography can be performed either transduodenally after duodenotomy or, in a prograde fashion, from the cut end of the duct after resection of the pancreatic tail. Both of these approaches are difficult and dangerous since, if the suture line fails, they can result in either a pancreatic or a duodenal fistula. Thus, if the patient is stable and duct injury is suspected, the surgeon should consider preoperative ERCP to determine whether or not the duct is intact. ERCP may have an even more important role in the evaluation of patients managed by delayed exploratory laparotomy after abdominal trauma since, in this setting, delineation of the site and extent of duct injury helps plan a definitive procedure.

Management

The Pancreas Organ Injury Scale,[49] developed by the American Association for the Surgery of Trauma, can be used to grade pancreatic injuries (Box 53-6). Management of pancreatic injuries is determined by the site and grade of that injury. Grade I injuries, which involve minor contusions or lacerations of the gland without duct injury,

---

BOX 53-6.   Grading and Treatment of Pancreatic Injuries

Grade 1: Minor contusion or laceration without duct injury
   Treatment: Observation alone
Grade II: Major contusion or laceration without duct injury
   Treatment: Débridement, drainage, possible repair
Grade III: Distal transection or injury with duct injury
   Treatment: Distal resection, possible Roux-en-Y drainage
Grade IV: Proximal transection or injury involving ampulla

or

Grade V: Massive disruption of the pancreatic head
   Treatment: Damage control, hemostasis/drainage; resection and possible Roux-en-Y drainage; triple-tube decompression; duodenal diverticularization; pancreaticoduodenectomy

Adapted from Moore EE, Cogbill TH, Malangoni MA, et al: Organ injury scaling: II. Pancreas, duodenum, small bowel, colon, and rectum. J Trauma 30:1427-1429, 1990.

should be treated expectantly. Drainage is usually not needed. On the other hand, grade II injuries, which involve major contusions or lacerations of the gland without duct injury, are traditionally treated by débridement, adequate hemostasis, and placement of sump drains. Some surgeons advocate repairing the disrupted capsule and placing an omental patch into areas of devitalized parenchyma. Transection of the neck/body/tail of the pancreas or parenchymal injury to those areas accompanied by duct injury is considered a grade III injury. The critical feature of these injuries is violation of the major pancreatic duct. Preoperative ERCP in stable patients may identify the presence and location of the duct injury in some patients but, because most patients are not stable enough to undergo preoperative ERCP, the status of the duct is uncertain at the time of operation. Occasionally, in such patients, the intraoperative finding of a transected gland, fat necrosis, and/or extravasation of clear fluid from the region of the duct establishes the presence of a duct injury. The classic treatment of grade III injuries involves resection of the pancreas to the left of the injury along with splenectomy. Because of the fear of overwhelming postsplenectomy sepsis, splenic conservation might be considered for children with grade III injuries. When the location of a grade III injury is to the right of the pancreatic neck, the surgeon should consider débriding the site of injury and conserving, rather than resecting, the uninjured body and tail by anastomosing it to a Roux-en-Y jejunal limb.

Grades IV and V injuries present the greatest surgical challenge because they involve the head of the pancreas and, in addition, they also usually involve the adjacent duodenum and/or papilla of Vater. Because of their location, grades IV and V injuries are also the ones that are most likely to involve major adjacent vascular structures. The initial goal in managing these multiply injured patients is that of obtaining hemostasis, minimizing contamination by repairing torn bowel, and repairing associated injuries. In unstable patients or in those with major associated injuries, this "damage control" approach may be all that is done at the initial operation, and definitive

repair may be postponed until the patient's condition has improved. On the other hand, some patients may require emergent pancreaticoduodenectomy as the initial procedure if they have uncontrollable hemorrhage from the head of the pancreas, injury to adjacent major vessels that can only be controlled by removing the pancreatic head, or devitalization of the duodenal C loop and pancreatic head. Short of radical resection, however, other options designed to divert gastric, pancreatic, and biliary secretions away from the duodenum should be considered for the management of patients with grades IV and V injuries. These include duodenal diverticularization, pyloric exclusion/gastrojejunostomy, and triple-tube decompression. Duodenal diverticularization is accomplished by performing antrectomy and gastrojejunostomy to achieve gastric diversion, choledochostomy to divert bile if the ampulla is injured, tube duodenostomy for decompression of the duodenum, suture repair of any duodenal injuries, and extensive periduodenal and peripancreatic drainage. Pyloric exclusion with gastrojejunostomy (Fig. 53-14) is a simpler method of protecting the injured duodenum, and it does not permanently alter function.[50] Through a gastrotomy, the pylorus is closed with a purse-string suture and an antecolic gastrojejunostomy is performed at the site of the gastrotomy. As with duodenal diverticularization, duodenal injuries should be closed and the area should be extensively débrided. Use of a slowly absorbable suture for pyloric closure results in diversion of gastric secretions from the duodenum for approximately 2 to 3 weeks but, after 21 days (i.e. dissolution of the suture), more than 90% of patients are found to have a patent and functioning pylorus. Triple-tube decompression involves placement of a gastrostomy tube for drainage of the stomach, drainage of the duodenum via a tube passed retrogradely through a jejunostomy, and antegrade passage of a jejunostomy tube for provision of enteral nutrition. The rapidity and ease of this procedure make it an attractive choice, but subsequent dislodgment of the duodenal tube and/or inadequate diversion provided by the gastrostomy tube may limit its effectiveness.

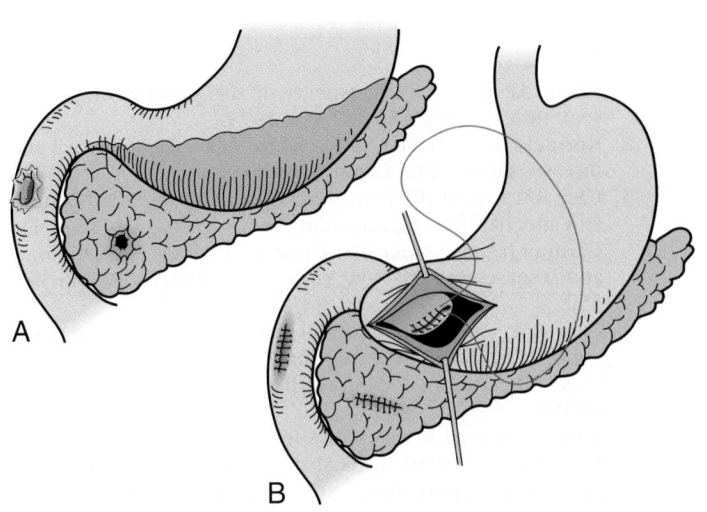

FIGURE 53-14. Pyloric exclusion with gastrojejunostomy. *A,* After repairing the duodenal injury, débriding the area of pancreatic injury, and achieving adequate hemostasis, a gastrotomy is performed and the pylorus is closed with a slowly reabsorbable suture. *B,* A gastrojejunostomy is performed and the area of injury is widely drained. (©1978 Baylor College of Medicine.)

Delayed Complications

The major delayed complications of severe pancreatic injuries involve the development of sterile or infected pseudocysts or other fluid collections and the ultimate development of a pancreatic duct stricture at a site of duct injury or transection. Classically, the duct stricture usually develops in the portion of the pancreas that overlies the spinal column. In many patients, the initial injury may go undetected, and even the trauma itself may be forgotten until the patient returns months or years later with recurrent episodes of obstructive chronic pancreatitis involving the pancreatic tail but sparing the pancreatic head. Management involves distal pancreatectomy.

Selected References

Bradley EL III: A clinically based classification system for acute pancreatitis: Summary of the International Symposium on Acute Pancreatitis. Atlanta, GA, September 11–13, 1992. Arch Surg 128:586-590, 1993.

> A conference summary article that outlines the definitions of terms currently used to describe the complications of pancreatitis.

Burch JM, Moore EE: Duodenal and pancreatic trauma. In Taylor MB, Gollan JL, Steer ML, Wolfe MM (eds): Gastrointestinal Emergencies. Baltimore, Williams & Wilkins, 1997, pp 995-1001.

> A recent review of current surgical treatment for pancreatic and duodenal injuries.

Case RM: Pancreatic exocrine secretion mechanisms and control. In Beger HG, Warshaw AW, Buchler MW, et al (eds): The Pancreas. Oxford, Blackwell Science, 1998, pp 63-100.

> An up-to-date summary of current concepts regarding the physiology of pancreatic exocrine secretion.

Chey WY, Chang TM: Neural hormonal regulation of exocrine pancreatic secretion. Pancreatology 1:320-335, 2001.

> An up-to-date review of pancreatic exocrine physiology.

Hamano H, Kawa S, Akira H, et al: High serum IgG4 concentrations in patients with sclerosing pancreatitis. N Engl J Med 344:732-738, 2001.

> Report describing elevated IgG4 levels in patients with autoimmune pancreatitis and their favorable response to treatment with steroids.

Hruban RH, Adsay NV, Albores-Saavedra J, et al: Pancreatic intraepithelial neoplasia: A new nomenclature and classification system for pancreatic duct lesions. Am J Surg Pathol 25:579-586, 2001.

> A detailed description of criteria used to define ductal cancer precursor lesions in the pancreas.

Kloppel G, Kosmahl M: Cystic lesions and neoplasms of the pancreas: The features are becoming clearer. Pancreatology 1:648-655, 2001.

> A review of cystic exocrine pancreatic lesions that focuses on their pathology and growth characteristics.

Opie EL: The etiology of acute hemorrhagic pancreatitis. Bull Johns Hopkins Hosp 12:182-192, 1901.

> The classic paper by Opie that led to the common channel theory as an explanation for gallstone pancreatitis.

Skandalakis LJ, Rowe JS Jr, Gray SW, et al: Surgical embryology and anatomy of the pancreas. Surg Clin North Am 73:661-697, 1993.

> A comprehensive overview of embryology and anatomy focused on issues relevant to pancreatic disease and pancreatic surgery.

Steer ML: The early intra-acinar cell events which occur during acute pancreatitis: The Frank Brooks Memorial Lecture. Pancreas 17:31-37, 1998.

> A summary of recent experimental data defining the early events that occur within pancreatic acinar cells and that ultimately lead to pancreatitis.

Steer ML, Waxman I, Freedman S: Chronic pancreatitis. N Engl J Med 332:1482-1490, 1995.

> A review of current concepts regarding the pathophysiology, diagnosis, and treatment of chronic pancreatitis.

Whipple AO, Parsons WB, Mullens CR: Treatment of carcinoma of the ampulla of Vater. Ann Surg 102:763-769, 1935.

> The first successful two-stage radical pancreaticoduodenectomy for periampullary carcinoma.

Whitcomb DC, Gorry MC, Preston RA, et al: Hereditary pancreatitis is caused by a mutation in the cationic trypsinogen gene. Nat Genet 14:141-145, 1996.

> Initial report defining the genetic abnormality underlying the most common form of hereditary pancreatitis.

Yeo CJ, Cameron JL, Lillemoe KD, et al: Pancreaticoduodenectomy with or without distal gastrectomy and extended retroperitoneal lymphadenectomy for periampullary adenocarcinoma: II. Randomized controlled trial evaluating survival, morbidity, and mortality. Ann Surg 236:355-368, 2002.

> Randomized, prospective trial of conventional Whipple resection versus extended Whipple resection for pancreatic cancer showing no benefit for the more radical procedure.

References

1. Palade G: Intracellular aspects of the process of protein secretion. Science 189:347-358, 1975.
2. Kornfeld S: Trafficking of lysosomal enzymes in normal and disease states. J Clin Invest 77:1-6, 1986.
3. Case RM Argent BE: Pancreatic duct cell secretion: Control and mechanisms of transport. In Go VLW, DiMagno EP, Gardner JD, et al (eds): The Pancreas: Biology, Pathobiology, and Disease, 2nd ed. New York, Raven Press, 1993, pp 301-350.
4. Case RM: Pancreatic exocrine secretion: Mechanisms and control. In Beger HG, Warshaw AW, Buchler MW, et al (eds): The Pancreas. Oxford, Blackwell Science, 1998, pp 63-100.
5. Rossi L, Pfutzer RH, Parvin S, et al: SPINK/PSTI mutations are associated with tropical pancreatitis in Bangladesh: A preliminary report. Pancreatology 1:242-245, 2001.

6. Opie EL: The etiology of acute hemorrhagic pancreatitis. Bull Johns Hopkins Hosp 12:182-192, 1901.

7. Lerch MM, Saluja AK, Runzi M, et al: Pancreatic duct obstruction triggers acute necrotizing pancreatitis in the opossum. Gastroenterology 104:853-861, 1993.

8. Kloppel G: Progression from acute to chronic pancreatitis: A pathologist's view. Surg Clin North Am 79:801-814, 1999.

9. Gates LD, Ulrich CD, Whitcomb DC, et al: Hereditary pancreatitis gene defects and their implications. Surg Clin North Am 79:711-722, 1999.

10. Hamano H, Kawa S, Horiuchi A, et al: High serum IgG4 concentrations in patients with sclerosing pancreatitis. N Engl J Med 344:732-738, 2001.

11. Cohn JA, Friedman KJ, Noone PG, et al: Relation between mutations of the cystic fibrosis gene and idiopathic pancreatitis. N Engl J Med 339:653-658, 1998.

12. Steer ML: The early intra-acinar cell events which occur during acute pancreatitis: The Frank Brooks Memorial Lecture. Pancreas 17:31-37, 1998.

13. Fallon M, Gorelick F, Anderson JM, et al: Effect of caerulein hyperstimulation on the paracellular barrier of rat exocrine pancreas. Gastroenterology 108:1863-1873, 1995.

14. Gudgeon AM, Heath DI, Hurley P, et al: Trypsinogen activation peptide assays in the early prediction of severity of acute pancreatitis. Lancet 335:4-8, 1990.

15. Foitzik T, Bassi DG, Schmidt J, et al: Intravenous contrast medium accentuates the severity of acute necrotizing pancreatitis in the rat. Gastroenterology 106:207-214, 1994.

16. Kaiser AM, Grady T, Gerdes D, et al: Intravenous contrast medium does not increase the severity of acute necrotizing pancreatitis in the opossum. Dig Dis Sci 40:1547-1553, 1995.

17. Ranson JHC, Rifkind KM, Roses DF, et al: Prognostic signs and the role of operative management in acute pancreatitis. Surg Gynecol Obstet 139:69-81, 1974.

18. Imrie CW, Benjamin IS, Ferguson JC, et al: A single-centre double-blind trial of Trasylol therapy in primary acute pancreatitis. Br J Surg 65:337-341, 1978.

19. Balthazar EJ, Ranson JHC, Naidich DP, et al: Acute pancreatitis: Prognostic value of CT. Radiology 156:767-772, 1985.

20. Khan AA, Parekh D, Young C, et al: Improved prediction of outcome in patients with severe acute pancreatitis by the APACHE II score at 48 hours after hospital admission compared with the APACHE II score at admission. Arch Surg 137:1136-1140, 2002.

21. Pederzoli P, Bassi C, Vesentini S, et al: A randomized multicenter clinical trial of antibiotic prophylaxis of septic complications in acute necrotizing pancreatitis with imipenem. Surg Gynecol Obstet 176:480-483, 1993.

22. Sainio V, Kemppainen E, Puolakkainen P, et al: Early antibiotic treatment in acute necroitizing pancreatitis. Lancet 346:663-667, 1995.

23. Golub R, Siddiqi F, Pohl D: Role of antibiotics in acute pancreatitis: A meta-analysis. J Gastrointest Surg 115:1513-1517, 1998.

24. Luiten EJ, Hop WC, Lange JF, et al: Controlled clinical trial of selective decontamination for the treatment of severe acute pancreatitis. Ann Surg 222:57-65, 1995.

25. Neoptolemos JP, Carr-Locke DL, London NJ, et al: Controlled trial of urgent endoscopic retrograde cholangiopancreatography and endoscopic sphincterotomy versus conservative treatment for acute pancreatitis due to gallstones. Lancet 2:979-983, 1988.

26. Folsch OR, Nitsche R, Ludtke R, et al: Early ERCP and papillotomy compared with conservative treatment for acute biliary pancreatitis. The German Study Group on Acute Biliary Pancreatitis. N Engl J Med 336:237-242, 1997.

27. Fan ST, Lai CS, Mok FPT, et al: Early treatment of acute biliary pancreatitis by endoscopic papillotomy. N Engl J Med 328:228-232, 1993.

28. Bradley EL: A clinically based classification system for acute pancreatitis: Summary of the International Symposium on Acute Pancreatitis. Atlanta, GA, September 11-13, 1992. Arch Surg 128:586-590, 1993.

29. Gerzof SG, Banks PA, Robbins AH, et al: Early diagnosis of pancreatic infection by computed tomography–guided aspiration. Gastroenterology 93:1315-1320, 1987.

30. Runzi M, Layer P: Nonsurgical management of acute pancreatitis: Use of antibiotics. Surg Clin North Am 79:759-765, 1999.

31. Ammann RW, Muellhaupt B: The natural history of pain in alcoholic chronic pancreatitis. Gastroenterology 116:1252-1257, 1999.

32. Toskes PP: Medical management of chronic pancreatitis. Scand J Gastroenterol Suppl 208:74-80, 1995.

33. Buscher HC, Jansen JB, van Dongen R: Long-term results of bilateral thoracoscopic splanchnicectomy in patients with chronic pancreatitis. Br J Surg 89:158-162, 2002.

34. Partington PF, Rochelle EL: Modified Puestow procedure for retrograde drainage of pancreatic duct. Ann Surg 152:1037-1043, 1960.

35. Ho HS, Frey CF: The Frey procedure: Local resection of pancreatic head combined with lateral pancreaticojejunostomy. Arch Surg 136:1353-1358, 2001.

36. Traverso LW, Longmire WP: Preservation of the pylorus during pancreaticoduodenectomy. Surg Gynecol Obstet 146:959-962, 1978.

37. Beger HG, Schlosser W, Friess H, et al: Duodenum-preserving head resection in chronic pancreatitis changes the normal course of the disease: Single-center 26-year experience. Ann Surg 230:512-519, 1999.

38. Hruban RH, Adsay V, Albores-Saavedra J, et al: Pancreatic intraepithelial neoplasia: A new nomenclature and classification system for pancreatic duct lesions. Am J Surg Pathol 25:579-586, 2001.

39. Lewandrowski K, Lee J, Southern J: Cyst fluid analysis of the differential diagnosis of pancreatic cysts: A new approach to the preoperative assessment of pancreatic cystic lesions. AJR Am J Roentgenol 164:815-819, 1995.

40. McCormick CSF, Lemoine NR: Molecular biological events in the development of pancreatic cancer. In Beger HG, Warshaw AL, Buchler MW, et al (eds) : The Pancreas. Oxford, Blackwell Science, 1998, pp 907-921.

41. Lowenfels AB, Maisonneuve P, Whitcomb DC: Risk factors for cancer in hereditary pancreatitis. International Hereditary Pancreatitis Study Group. Med Clin North Am 84:565-573, 2000.

42. Safi F, Schlosser W, Falkenreck S, et al: Ca 19-9 serum course and prognosis of pancreatic cancer. Int J Pancreatol 20:155-162, 1996.

43. AJCC Cancer Staging Handbook, 6th ed. New York, Springer, 2002, pp 179-188.

44. Wiersema MJ: Accuracy of endoscopic ultrasound in diagnosing and staging pancreatic carcinoma. Pancreatology 1:625-632, 2001.

45. Yeo CJ, Cameron JL, Lillemoe KD, et al: Pancreaticoduodenectomy with or without distal gastrectomy and extended retroperitoneal lymphadenectomy for periampullary adenocarcinoma: II. Randomized controlled trial evaluating survival, morbidity, and mortality. Ann Surg 236:355-368, 2002.

46. Adler DG, Baron TH: Endoscopic palliation of malignant gastric outlet obstruction using self-expanding metal stents: Experience in 36 patients. Am J Gastroenterol 97:72-80, 2002.

47. Kalser NH, Ellenberg SS: Pancreatic cancer: Adjuvant combined radiation and chemotherapy following curative resection. Arch Surg 120:899-903, 1985.

48. Neoptolemos JP, Dunn JA, Stocken DD, et al: Adjuvant chemoradiotherapy and chemotherapy in resectable pancreatic cancer: A randomized controlled trial. Lancet 358:1576-1585, 2001.

49. Moore EE, Cogbill TH, Malangoni MA, et al: Organ injury scaling: II. Pancreas, duodenum, small bowel, colon, and rectum. J Trauma 30:1427-1429, 1990.

50. Burch JM, Moore EE: Duodenal and pancreatic trauma. *In* Taylor MB, Gollan JL, Steer ML, Wolfe MM (eds): Gastrointestinal Emergencies. Baltimore, Williams & Wilkins, 1997, pp 995-1001.

CHAPTER 54

SPLEEN

R. Daniel Beauchamp, M.D., Michael D. Holzman, M.D., M.P.H., and Timothy C. Fabian, M.D.

Splenic Anatomy	Splenectomy for Miscellaneous Benign Conditions
Splenic Function	Splenic Trauma
Splenectomy for Benign Hematologic Conditions	Elective Laparoscopic Splenectomy
Splenectomy for Malignancy	Late Morbidity after Splenectomy

SPLENIC ANATOMY

The spleen develops from mesenchymal cells in the dorsal mesogastrium during the 5th week of gestation. The spleen is located in the posterior left upper quadrant of the abdomen. The convex smooth surface of the spleen faces superiorly, posteriorly, and to the left in relation to the abdominal surface of the diaphragm. The diaphragm separates the spleen from the pleura; the left lower lobe of the lung; and the adjacent 9th, 10th, and 11th ribs. The costodiaphragmatic recess of the pleura extends down as far as the inferior border of the normal-sized spleen. The normal size and weight vary somewhat; in adults, the approximate size of the spleen is 12 cm in length, 7 cm in width, and 3 to 4 cm in thickness. The average spleen weight in an adult is 150 g, with a range of 80 to 300 g.

The visceral relationships of the spleen are with the proximal greater curvature of the stomach, the tail of the pancreas, the left kidney, and the splenic flexure of the colon (Fig. 54-1). The parietal peritoneum adheres firmly to the splenic capsule, except at the splenic hilum. The peritoneum extends superiorly, laterally, and inferiorly, creating folds that form the suspensory ligaments of the spleen. The splenophrenic and splenocolic ligaments are usually relatively avascular. The splenorenal ligament extends from the anterior left kidney to the hilum of the spleen as a two-layered fold in which the splenic vessels and the tail of the pancreas are invested. These two layers continue anteriorly and superiorly to the greater curvature of the stomach to form the two leaves of the gastrosplenic ligament through which the short gastric arteries and veins course.

A fibroelastic capsule commonly known as the *splenic capsule* invests the organ, and from it trabeculae pass into the parenchyma, branching to form a trabecular network that subdivides the organ into small compartments.

The splenic artery is a tortuous vessel that arises from the celiac trunk; it courses along the superior border of the pancreas (Fig. 54-2). The branches of the splenic artery include the numerous pancreatic branches, the short gastric arteries, the left gastroepiploic artery, and the terminal splenic branches. The splenic artery divides into several branches within the splenorenal ligament before entering the splenic hilum, where they branch again into these trabeculae as they enter the splenic pulp. Small arteriolar branches leave the trabeculae, and their adventitial coat becomes replaced by a sheath of lymphatic tissue that accompanies the vessels and their branches until they divide into capillaries. It is these lymphatic sheaths that make up the white pulp of the spleen and that are interspersed along the arteriolar vessels as lymphatic follicles. The interface between the white pulp and the red pulp is known as the *marginal zone*. As the arterioles lose their sheaths of lymphatic tissue, they traverse the marginal zone and enter the red pulp, which is composed of large branching, thin-walled blood vessels called *splenic sinuses* and *sinusoids,* and thin plates of cellular tissue comprising the splenic chords.

The venous sinusoids empty into the veins of the red pulp, and these veins drain back along the trabecular veins that empty into at least five major tributaries, ultimately joining to form the splenic vein in the splenorenal ligament. The splenic vein runs inferior to the artery and posterior to the pancreatic tail and body. It receives several

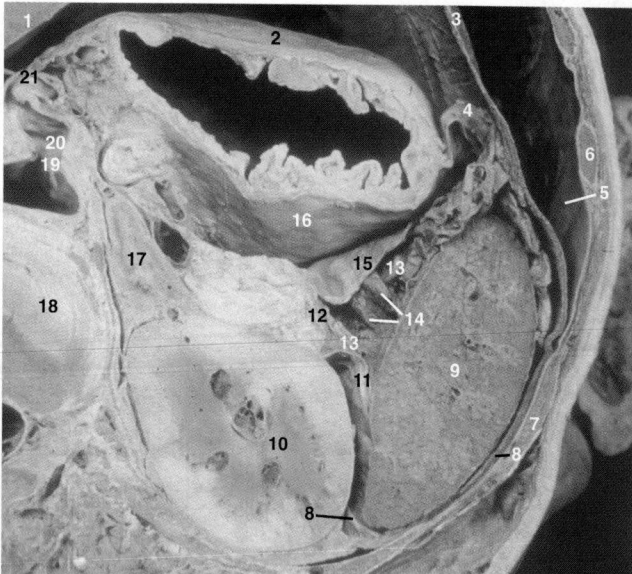

■ FIGURE 54-1.   A, Spleen, from the front: (1) diaphragm, (2) stomach, (3) gastrosplenic ligament, (4) gastric impression, (5) superior border, (6) notch, (7) diaphragmatic surface, (8) inferior border, (9) left colic flexure, (10) costodiaphragmatic recess, (11) thoracic wall. The left upper abdominal and lower anterior thoracic walls have been removed and part of the diaphragm (1) turned upward to show the spleen in its normal position, lying adjacent to the stomach (2) and colon (9), with the lower part against the kidney (*B*9 and 10, opposite). **B,** Spleen, in a transverse section of the left upper abdomen: (1) left lobe of liver, (2) stomach, (3) diaphragm, (4) gastrosplenic ligament, (5) costodiaphragmatic recess of pleura, (6) 9th rib, (7) 10th rib, (8) peritoneum of greater sac, (9) spleen, (10) left kidney, (11) posterior layer of lienorenal ligament, (12) tail of pancreas, (13) splenic artery, (14) splenic vein, (15) anterior layer of lienorenal ligament, (16) lesser sac, (17) left suprarenal gland, (18) intervertebral disc, (19) abdominal aorta, (20) coeliac trunk, (21) left gastric artery. The section is at the level of the disc (18) between the 12th thoracic and 1st lumbar vertebrae and is viewed from below looking toward the thorax. The spleen (9) lies against the diaphragm (3) and left kidney (10) but separated from them by peritoneum of the greater sac (8). The peritoneum behind the stomach (2) forming part of the gastrosplenic (4) and ileorenal (15) ligaments belongs to the lesser sac (16).   (*A* and *B,* From McMinn RMH, Hutchings RT, Pegington J, Abrahams PH: Color Atlas of Human Anatomy, 3rd ed. St. Louis, Mosby–Year Book, 1993, pp 230-231.)

short tributaries from the pancreas. The splenic vein joins the superior mesenteric vein at a right angle behind the neck of the pancreas to form the portal vein. The inferior mesenteric vein often empties into the splenic vein; it may also empty into the superior mesenteric vein at or near the confluence of the splenic vein and superior mesenteric vein.

SPLENIC FUNCTION

The spleen has important hematopoietic functions during early fetal development, with both red and white blood cell production. By the 5th month of gestation, the bone marrow assumes the predominant role in hematopoiesis, and normally there is no significant hematopoietic function left in the spleen. Under certain pathologic conditions, however, such as myelodysplasia, the spleen can reacquire its hematopoietic function. Removal of the spleen does not usually result in anemia or leukopenia in

an otherwise healthy person. Although the hematopoietic function is usually lost during fetal development, the spleen continues to function as a sophisticated filter because of the unique circulatory system and lymphoid organization, and it has both blood cell monitoring and management functions as well as important immune functions throughout life.

The functions of the spleen are closely linked to splenic structure and its unique circulatory system. The arteries flow through the white pulp (lymphoid tissues), after which part of the blood flow goes directly through endothelial cell–lined capillaries into the venous system ("closed" theory). Most of the blood flow, however, enters the macrophage-lined reticular meshwork, and the blood flows slowly back to the venous circulation through the venous sinuses ("open" theory). The formed blood elements must pass through slits in the lining of the venous sinuses; if they cannot pass, they are trapped in the spleen and ingested by splenic phagocytes[1] (Fig. 54-3). Experimental animal studies have demonstrated that an intact

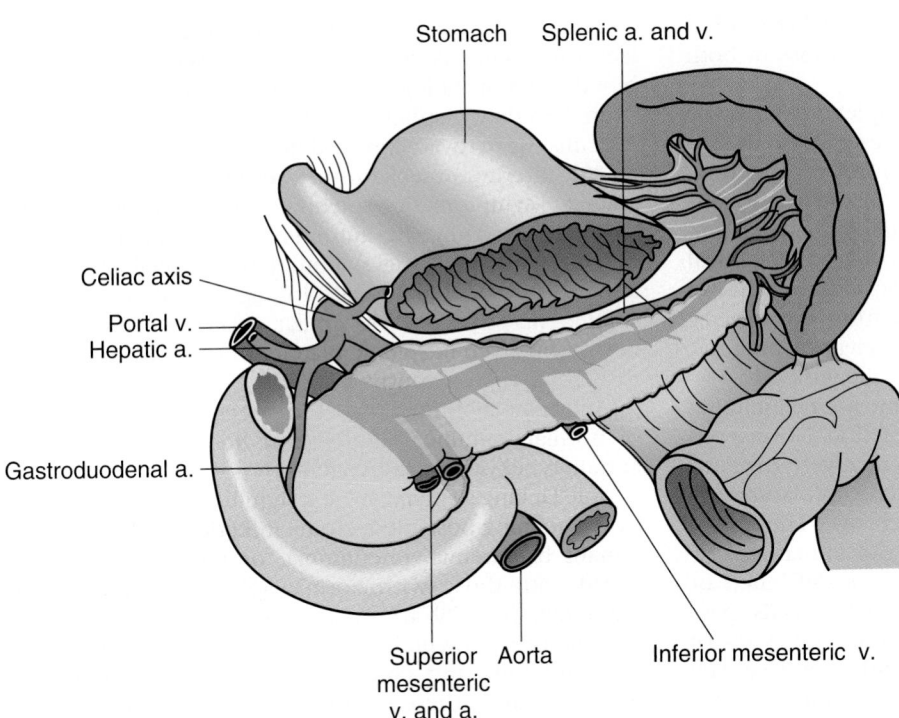

FIGURE 54-2. The anatomic relationships of the splenic vasculature. (From Economou SG, Economou TS: Atlas of Surgical Techniques. Philadelphia, WB Saunders, 1966, p 562.)

Stomach

Splenic a. and v.

Celiac axis

Portal v.

Hepatic a.

Gastroduodenal a.

Superior mesenteric v. and a.

Aorta

Inferior mesenteric v.

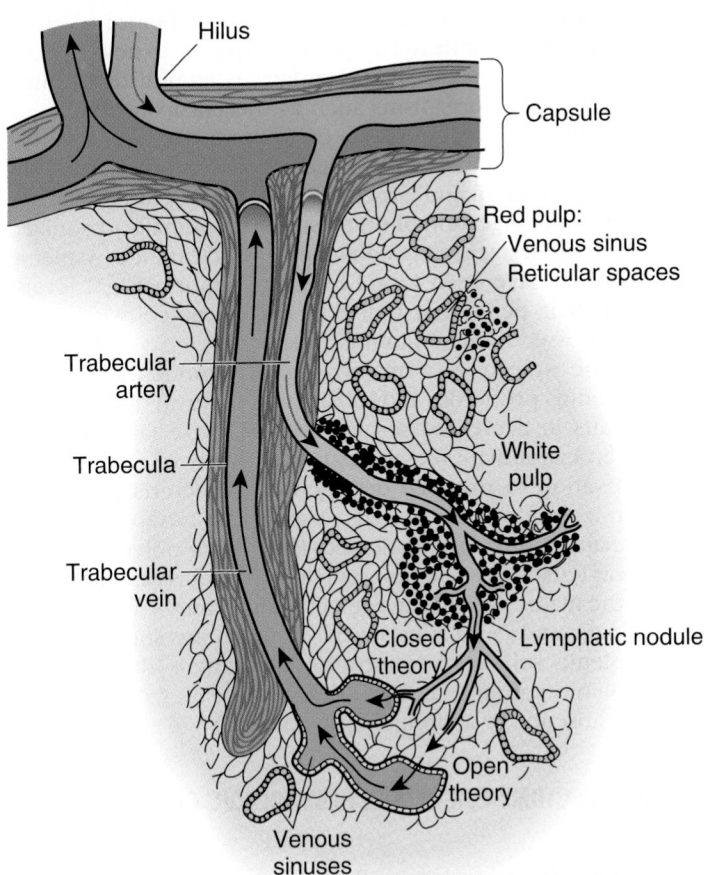

FIGURE 54-3. Structure of the sinusoidal spleen shows the open and closed blood flow routes. (From Bellanti JA: Immunology: Basic Processes. Philadelphia, WB Saunders, 1979.)

Hilus

Capsule

Red pulp:
Venous sinus
Reticular spaces

Trabecular artery

White pulp

Trabecula

Trabecular vein

Closed theory

Lymphatic nodule

Open theory

Venous sinuses

splenic arterial system is necessary for optimal control of infection.[2] Removal of the spleen results in loss of both the immunologic and filtering functions.

The most important function of the spleen is probably its mechanical filtration, which removes senescent erythrocytes and likely contributes to control of infection. The spleen is important in clearing circulating pathogens that reside within erythrocytes, for example, malarial parasites or bacteria such as *Bartonella* species. Mechanical filtration by the spleen may also be important for removal of unopsonized, noningested bacteria from the circulation. It may be particularly important for clearing microorganisms for which the host has no specific antibody.

Splenic-filtering function is important for maintaining normal erythrocyte morphology and function. Normal red blood cells are biconcave and deform relatively easily to facilitate both passages through the microvasculature and optimal oxygen and carbon dioxide exchange. The spleen is an important site for the processing of immature erythrocytes and for repair or destruction of deformed or aged erythrocytes. As immature red blood cells pass through the spleen, they may undergo several types of repair, including removal of nuclei and excessive cell membrane from immature cells to convert them from a spherical nucleated to a biconcave anucleated mature morphology. Erythrocytes may also undergo repair by having surface abnormalities such as pits or spurs removed. In the asplenic condition, there are several characteristic alterations in the morphologic appearance of the peripheral red blood cells, with the presence of target cells (immature cells), Howell-Jolly bodies (nuclear remnant), Heinz bodies (denatured hemoglobin), Pappenheimer bodies (iron granules), stippling, and spur cells. Aged red blood cells (120 days) that have lost enzymatic activity and membrane plasticity are trapped and destroyed in the spleen (Box 54-1).

Box 54-1. Biologic Substances Removed by the Spleen

In Normal Subjects

Red blood cell membrane
Red blood cell surface pits and craters
Howell-Jolly bodies
Heinz bodies
Pappenheimer bodies
Acanthocytes
Senescent red blood cells
Particulate antigen

In Patients with Disease

Spherocytes (hereditary spherocytosis)
Sickle cells, hemoglobin C cells
Antibody-coated red blood cells
Antibody-coated platelets
Antibody-coated white blood cells

Modified from Eichner ER: Splenic function: Normal, too much and too little. Am J Med 66:311, 1979.

The filtering function of the spleen is also an important factor in anemic conditions associated with abnormal red blood cell morphology. Abnormal erythrocytes that result from hereditary spherocytosis, sickle cell anemia, thalassemia, or pyruvate kinase deficiency are trapped by the splenic-filtering mechanism, resulting in worsening anemia, symptomatic splenomegaly, and occasionally splenic infarction. In autoimmune hemolytic anemia, immunoglobulin G (IgG) bound to the cell membrane targets the red blood cells for splenic destruction by splenic macrophages. A similar IgG-dependent mechanism is involved in splenic platelet destruction in immune thrombocytopenic purpura (ITP).

Another major function of the spleen is the maintenance of normal immune function and host defenses against certain types of infectious agents. It is well established that people lacking a spleen are at a significantly higher risk for overwhelming postsplenectomy infection (OPSI) with fulminant bacteremia, pneumonia, or meningitis, as compared with those with normal splenic function. Major pathogens in OPSI are organisms such as *Streptococcus pneumoniae,* in which polysaccharide capsules requiring both antibody and complement are important in host defense against these organisms. Asplenic subjects have defective activation of complement by the alternative pathway, leaving them more susceptible to infection.

Asplenic patients have a normal response to reimmunization to an antigen first encountered before splenectomy but do not have an optimal response to new antigen exposure, especially if the antigen is administered intravenously. For organisms such as the encapsulated bacteria, much higher quantities of antibody are necessary for effective clearance. The spleen, with its specialized circulatory system and large supply of macrophages that are capable of ingestion of organisms not optimally opsonized with antibody, greatly enhances their clearance. Asplenic subjects have been found to have subnormal IgM levels, and their peripheral blood mononuclear cells exhibit a suppressed immunoglobulin response.[3]

The spleen is a major site of production for the opsonins properdin and tuftsin, and removal of the spleen results in decreased serum levels of these factors. Properdin can initiate the alternative pathway of complement activation to produce destruction of bacteria as well as foreign and abnormal cells. Tuftsin is a tetrapeptide that enhances the phagocytic activity of both polymorphonuclear leukocytes and mononuclear phagocytes. The spleen is the major site of cleavage of tuftsin from the heavy chain of IgG, and circulating levels of tuftsin are suppressed in asplenic subjects.[4] Neutrophil function is decreased in asplenic patients, and the defect appears to result from the absence of a circulating mediator.[5]

SPLENECTOMY FOR BENIGN HEMATOLOGIC CONDITIONS

Immune Thrombocytopenic Purpura

Immune thrombocytopenic purpura is also referred to as *idiopathic* thrombocytopenic purpura. A low platelet count, a normal bone marrow, and the absence of other causes of thrombocytopenia characterize this disease. ITP is principally a disorder of increased platelet destruction mediated by autoantibodies to platelet membrane antigens that results in platelet phagocytosis by the reticuloendothelial system.[6] Bone marrow megakaryocytes are present in normal or sometimes increased numbers; however, there is relative marrow failure in that the marrow does not increase production sufficiently to compensate for platelet destruction in the spleen. In adults, ITP is more common in young women than men. Seventy-two percent of patients older than 10 years of age are women, and 70% of affected women are younger than 40 years of age. In children, ITP is manifested somewhat differently. It affects both sexes equally, and its onset is typically abrupt, with severe thrombocytopenia; however, spontaneous permanent remissions are the rule, occurring in about 80% of affected children. Children who develop chronic thrombocytopenia are usually girls older than 10 years of age and present with a longer history of purpura.

Patients with ITP often present with a history of purpura, epistaxis, and gingival bleeding. Hematuria and gastrointestinal bleeding occur less commonly, and intracerebral hemorrhage is a rare but sometimes fatal event. The diagnosis of ITP requires exclusion of other causes of thrombocytopenia (Box 54-2).[6] Apparent thrombocytopenia may be an artifactual report on a complete blood count because of in vitro platelet clumping or the presence of giant platelets. Mild thrombocytopenia may occur in 6% to 8% of otherwise normal pregnant women and in up to one fourth of women with preeclampsia. Several drugs are known to induce thrombocytopenia, including heparin, quinidine, quinine, and sulfonamides. Human immunodeficiency virus (HIV) infection and other viral infections may cause thrombocytopenia that may be mistaken for ITP. Other conditions that may be associated with thrombocytopenia include myelodysplasia, congenital thrombocytopenia, thrombotic thrombocytopenic purpura, chronic disseminated intravascular coagulation, autoimmune diseases such as systemic lupus erythematosus, and lymphoproliferative disorders such as chronic lymphocytic leukemia (CLL) and non-Hodgkin's lymphoma (NHL).

Management of patients with ITP varies according to the severity of the thrombocytopenia.[7] Patients with asymptomatic disease and platelet counts higher than 50,000/mm³ may simply be followed with no specific treatment. Platelet counts higher than 50,000/mm³ are seldom associated with spontaneous clinically important bleeding, even with invasive procedures. Patients with platelet counts between 30,000 and 50,000/mm³ who do not have symptoms may also be observed without treatment; however, careful follow-up is essential in these patients because they are at risk for more severe thrombocytopenia. The initial medical treatment is with glucocorticoids, usually prednisone (1 mg/kg body weight per day). About two thirds of patients treated in this manner experience an increase in their platelet count to more than 50,000/mm³, usually within 1 week of treatment, although it sometimes requires as long as 3 weeks. As many as 26% of patients may have a complete response with glucocorticoid therapy. Patients with platelet counts

---

Box 54-2. Differential Diagnosis of Immune Thrombocytopenic Purpura

Falsely Low Platelet Count

In vitro platelet clumping caused by ethylenediamine tetra-acetic acid (EDTA)-dependent or cold-dependent agglutinins
Giant platelets

Common Causes of Thrombocytopenia

Pregnancy (gestational thrombocytopenia, preeclampsia)
Drug-induced thrombocytopenia (common drugs include heparin, quinidine, quinine, and sulfonamides)
Viral infections, such as human immunodeficiency virus, rubella, infectious mononucleosis
Hypersplenism due to chronic liver disease

Other Causes of Thrombocytopenia That Have Been Mistaken for Immune Thrombocytopenic Purpura

Myelodysplasia
Congenital thrombocytopenias
Thrombotic thrombocytopenic purpura and hemolytic-uremic syndrome
Chronic disseminated intravascular coagulation

Thrombocytopenia Associated With Other Disorders

Autoimmune diseases, such as systemic lupus erythematosus
Lymphoproliferative disorders (chronic lymphocytic leukemia, non-Hodgkin's lymphoma)

From George JN, El-Harake MA, Raskob GE: Chronic idiopathic thrombocytopenic purpura. N Engl J Med 331:1207-1211, 1994.

---

greater than 20,000/mm³ who are symptom free or who have only minor purpura do not require hospitalization. Treatment of ITP is indicated in patients with platelet counts of less than 20,000 to 30,000/mm³ or for those with platelet counts of less than 50,000/mm³ and significant mucus membrane bleeding or risk factors for bleeding, such as hypertension, peptic ulcer disease, or a vigorous lifestyle.

Hospitalization is often required for patients with platelet counts of less than 20,000/mm³ who have significant mucus membrane bleeding and is necessary for all patients who experience severe life-threatening hemorrhage. Although platelet transfusions are necessary for controlling severe hemorrhage, they are seldom indicated in patients with ITP in the absence of severe hemorrhage. Intravenous immunoglobulin is important in the management of acute bleeding and for the preparation of patients for operation or delivery in the case of pregnancy. The usual dose is 1 g/kg per day for 2 days. This dose increases the platelet count in most patients within 3 days. It also increases the efficacy of transfused platelets. Administration of intravenous immunoglobulin is also appropriate in patients with platelet counts of less than 20,000/mm³ who are being prepared for splenectomy.

Splenectomy was the first effective treatment described for ITP and was an established therapeutic modality long before glucocorticoid therapy was introduced in 1950.[7] About two thirds of patients achieve a complete response with normalization of platelet counts after splenectomy and require no further therapy. Splenectomy is indicated in patients with refractory severe symptomatic thrombocytopenia, in patients requiring toxic doses of steroids to achieve remission, and in patients with a relapse of thrombocytopenia after initial glucocorticoid treatment. Splenectomy is an appropriate consideration for patients who have had the diagnosis of ITP for 6 weeks and continue to have a platelet count of less than 10,000/mm³ whether or not bleeding symptoms are present. Splenectomy is also indicated for patients who have had the diagnosis of ITP for as long as 3 months and have experienced a transient or incomplete response to primary therapy and have a platelet count of less than 30,000/mm³. Splenectomy should be considered for women in the second trimester of pregnancy who have failed glucocorticoid and intravenous immunoglobulin therapy and have platelet counts of less than 10,000/mm³ or who have platelet counts of less than 30,000/mm³ and bleeding problems. Splenectomy is probably not indicated in nonbleeding patients who have had a diagnosis of ITP for 6 months, have platelet counts of greater than 50,000/mm³, and are not engaged in high-risk activities.

The success rate of splenectomy in achieving complete and permanent response was reported to be 65% in a cumulative study of 1761 patients.[7] The site of platelet destruction on preoperative indium 111 (¹¹¹In)-labeled platelet scintigraphy was also reported to be predictive of the efficacy of splenectomy. The best long-term cure rates have been when predominantly splenic sequestration is present. In a cumulative study of 564 patients with ITP, a predominant splenic sequestration site was associated with an 87% to 93% rate of good response after splenectomy. In comparison, in patients with hepatic sequestration, the response rate was significantly lower (7% to 30%).[8]

Most patients who respond to splenectomy with increased platelet counts do so within the first 10 days after their operation. Durable platelet responses have been correlated with platelet counts greater than 150,000/mm³ by the 3rd postoperative day or greater than 500,000/mm³ on the 10th postoperative day. The immediate response rates among series collected between 1980 and 1998 range from 71% to 95%, with relapse rates of 4% to 12% (Tables 54-1 and 54-2).[9]

For patients with chronic ITP who fail to achieve complete response after splenectomy, the options range from simple observation in patients with no bleeding symptoms and platelet counts of more than 30,000/mm³ to continued long-term prednisone therapy (Table 54-3).[6] Single-agent treatment with azathioprine or cyclophosphamide may be considered, but response to these agents may require up to 4 months of treatment. Patients who fail to respond to splenectomy or have relapsing disease after an initial response should be investigated for the presence of accessory spleen. Accessory spleen may be found in as many as 10% of these patients. The presence of an accessory spleen may be suggested by the absence of asplenic red blood cell morphologic features and may also be identified by radionuclide imaging. Identification of an accessory spleen in a patient who remains severely thrombocytopenic and is otherwise fit for operation warrants surgical excision of the accessory spleen.

TABLE 54-1.   Hematologic Response after Laparoscopic Treatment of Immune Thrombocytopenia Purpura

Study	Patients (n)	ITP (n)	AS (n [%])	IR (n [%])	RR (n [%])
Cadiere et al, 1994[118]	17	8	2 (11.8)	NA	NA
Emmermann et al, 1995[119]	27	20	2 (7.4)	19 (95.0)	0 at 14 mo
Poulin et al, 1995[120]	22	22	6 (27.2)	NA	NA
Yee and Akpata, 1995[96]	25	14	2 (8.0)	11 (76.0)	NA
Brunt et al, 1996[121]	26	17	3 (11.5)	13 (76.0)	NA
Flowers et al, 1996[97]	43	22	4 (9.3)	18 (82.0)	0 at 21 mo
Gigot et al, 1996[122]	18	16	7 (39.0)	NA	2 (12.5) at 14 mo
Smith et al, 1996[123]	10	8	2 (20.0)	NA	0
Friedman et al, 1997[82]	63	28	11 (17.5)	NA	NA
Park et al, 1997[108]	22	8	2 (9.0)	NA	NA
Tsiotos and Schlinkert, 1997[124]	18	18	1 (5.6)	17 (94.0)	0
Katkhouda et al, 1998[9]	103	67	17 (16.5)	56 (83.6)	4 (6.0) at 38 mo
Total	394	237	59/394 (15.0)	134/158 (85.0)	6/151 (4.0)

AS, total number of patients with accessory spleens; IR, immediate response in immune thrombocytopenic purpura (ITP); RR, relapse rate in ITP; NA, data not available.

From Katkhouda N, Hurwitz MB, Rivera RT, et al: Laparoscopic splenectomy: Outcome and efficacy in 103 consecutive patients. Ann Surg 228:568-578, 1998.

TABLE 54-2. Results in 749 Collected Cases of Open Splenectomy

Study	Patients (n)	Morbidity (n [%])	Mortality (n [%])	ITP (n)	AS (n [%])	IR (n [%])	RR (n [%])
DiFino et al, 1980[125]	37	9 (24.3)	0	37	2 (5.4)	27 (73.0)	9 (24.3)
Mintz et al, 1981[126]	66	13 (14.1)	1 (1.4)	66	20 (28.2)	56 (84.8)	6 (9.0)
Musser et al, 1984[89]	306	118 (24.0)	18 (6.0)	65	58 (19.0)	50 (77.0)	NA
Jacobs et al, 1986[127]	102	15 (14.7)	0	102	NA	95 (93.1)	11 (10.7)
Akwari et al, 1987[128]	100	8 (8.0)	0	100	18 (18.0)	71 (71.0)	4 (4.0)
Julia et al, 1990[129]	138	NA	NA	138	NA	114 (83.0)	23 (17.0)
Total	749	163/611 (26.7)	19/611 (3.1)	508	98/611 (16.0)	413/508 (81.3)	53/443 (12.0)

ITP, immune thrombocytopenic purpura; AS, total number of patients with accessory spleens; IR, immediate response in ITP; RR relapse rate in ITP; NA, data not available.
From Katkhouda N, Hurwitz MB, Rivera RT, et al: Laparoscopic splenectomy: Outcome and efficacy in 103 consecutive patients. Ann Surg 228:568-578, 1998.

TABLE 54-3. Treatment Options for Patients with Chronic Immune Thrombocytopenic Purpura Unresponsive to Initial Glucocorticoid Therapy and Splenectomy

Intervention	Indication	Outcome
Observation	No bleeding symptoms; platelet count of ≥ 30,000-50,000/mm³	Platelet count may remain stable, but the risk for more severe thrombocytopenia with serious bleeding is unknown
Prednisone	Symptomatic thrombocytopenia, with bleeding symptoms; platelet count of ≤ 30,000-50,000/mm³	Goal is a safe platelet count with a minimal dose, such as 10 mg every other day; steroid toxicity is the limiting factor
Azathioprine or cyclophosphamide	Symptomatic thrombocytopenia, with bleeding symptoms; platelet count of ≤ 30,000-50,000 mm³	Response may require 4 months of treatment; complete recovery may occur in 10-40% of patients
Other regimens	Symptomatic thrombocytopenia, with bleeding symptoms; platelet count of ≤ 30,000-50,000 mm³	Some regimens promising in small, preliminary studies; in others, few patients recover completely
Resection of accessory spleen or spleens	Symptomatic thrombocytopenia in a patient who is a good candidate for surgery	Complete recoveries reported in a few patients; symptomatic improvement in some others
Observation (with glucocorticoid or intravenous immune globulin as needed to treat or prevent bleeding)	Unresponsive to treatment	Some patients require frequent supportive therapy; others have minimal symptoms despite severe thrombocytopenia; spontaneous remissions may occur

From George JN, El-Harake MA, Raskob GE: Chronic idiopathic thrombocytopenic purpura. N Engl J Med 331:1207-1211, 1994.

In a summary of splenectomy series for hematologic disease using either a laparoscopic or open approach, Katkhouda and colleagues[9] found that among 394 patients treated with laparoscopic splenectomy, 237 (60%) had ITP and 59 (15%) had an accessory spleen (see Tables 54-1 and 54-2). From the combined series of patients treated for ITP, there was an immediate response rate to splenectomy of 85% and a relapse rate of 4%. These series spanned from 1994 through 1998. The same authors also summarized another six series of open splenectomy for hematologic disease spanning from 1980 to 1990 and totaling 749 patients, of which 508 patients underwent splenectomy for ITP. The incidence of accessory spleen in these combined series was 16%. For treatment of ITP, the immediate response rate was 81.3%, and the relapse rate was 12%.

About 10% to 20% of otherwise symptom-free patients infected with HIV develop ITP.[10] Splenectomy may be performed safely in this cohort of patients and produces sustained increases in platelet levels in more than 80%. Splenectomy does not increase the risk of progression to acquired immunodeficiency syndrome (AIDS), and a recent cohort study suggested that the absence of a spleen during the asymptomatic phase of HIV infection may delay disease progression.[10]

Hereditary Spherocytosis

Hereditary spherocytosis is an autosomal dominant disease that results from a deficiency of spectrin, a red blood cell cytoskeletal protein.[11,12] This protein defect causes a membrane abnormality in the red blood cells resulting in small, spherical, and rigid erythrocytes. These cells have increased osmotic fragility. These spherocytes are more susceptible to becoming trapped in the spleen and destroyed. The clinical features of this disease include anemia, occasionally with jaundice, and splenomegaly. The diagnosis is made by identification of spherocytes on the peripheral blood smear, an increased reticulocyte count, increased osmotic fragility, and a negative Coombs' test.

Splenectomy decreases the rate of hemolysis and usually leads to resolution of the anemia. Splenectomy is usually performed in childhood shortly after diagnosis. Although splenectomy does not normalize the morphology of the red blood cells, it does reduce the trapping and premature destruction of them. It is generally recommended that the operation be delayed until after the 4th year of life to preserve immunologic function of the spleen in young children who are most at risk for OPSI. There is a high incidence of pigmented gallstones among patients with spherocytosis, similar to other hemolytic anemias, and ultrasound should be performed before splenectomy. If gallstones are present, it is appropriate to perform cholecystectomy at the time of the splenectomy.

Other anemias associated with erythrocyte structural abnormalities include hereditary elliptocytosis, hereditary pyropoikilocytosis, hereditary xerocytosis, and hereditary hydrocytosis. All of these conditions result in abnormalities of the erythrocyte cellular membrane and increased red blood cell destruction. Splenectomy is indicated for the severe hemolytic anemia that commonly occurs in these conditions. An exception to this is the mild anemia that is usually of limited clinical significance in the condition of hereditary xerocytosis, in which splenectomy is not usually indicated.

Hemolytic Anemia due to Erythrocyte Enzyme Deficiency

Glucose-6-phosphate dehydrogenase deficiency and pyruvate kinase deficiency are the two predominant hereditary conditions associated with hemolytic anemia. These deficiencies result in abnormal glucose use and metabolism, leading to increased hemolysis. Pyruvate kinase deficiency is an autosomal recessive condition in which there is decreased red blood cell deformability resulting in increased hemolysis. The spleen is the site of erythrocyte entrapment and destruction in patients with deficiency of pyruvate kinase. These patients often have splenomegaly, and splenectomy has been shown to decrease their transfusion requirements. For the previously mentioned reasons of preserving immunologic function, splenectomy is usually delayed until after 4 years of age in patients with this condition.

Glucose-6-phosphate dehydrogenase deficiency is an X-linked hereditary condition that is most frequently seen in people of African, Middle Eastern, or Mediterranean ancestry. Hemolytic anemia occurs in most patients after exposure to certain drugs or chemicals. Splenectomy is rarely indicated in patients with glucose-6-phosphate dehydrogenase deficiency.[13]

Hemoglobinopathies

Thalassemia and sickle cell disease are hereditary hemolytic anemias that result from abnormal hemoglobin molecules. This results in abnormal shape of the erythrocyte, which may be subject to splenic sequestration and destruction. Sickle cell anemia is the result of the homozygous inheritance of hemoglobin S. Hemoglobin S has a single amino acid substitution of a valine for a glutamic acid in the sixth position of the beta chain of hemoglobin A.

Sickling of erythrocytes may also occur in patients who coinherit hemoglobin S and other hemoglobin variants, such as hemoglobin C or sickle cell β thalassemia.[14] Sickle cell disease results in patients who are homozygous for hemoglobin S. About 0.5% of African Americans are homozygous for hemoglobin S, whereas about 8% are heterozygous for hemoglobin S. The heterozygotes have the sickle cell trait. Under conditions of reduced oxygen tension, hemoglobin S molecules crystallize within the cell, which results in an elongated, distorted cell with a crescent shape. These altered erythrocytes are rigid and incapable of deforming in microvasculature. This lack of deformation results in capillary occlusion and thrombosis, ultimately leading to microinfarction. This occurs with particular frequency in the spleen. The spleen is enlarged during the 1st decade of life in most patients with sickle cell disease and then with progressive infarction caused by repeated attacks of vaso-occlusion and infarction, resulting in autosplenectomy. The spleen in patients with sickle cell disease usually atrophies by adulthood, although splenomegaly may occasionally persist into adult life.

Thalassemias constitute a group of hemoglobin disorders that also result in hemolytic anemia. Thalassemias are inherited as autosomal dominant traits and occur as a result of a defect in hemoglobin synthesis. This results in variable degrees of hemolytic anemia. Splenic infarction, splenomegaly, and hypersplenism may be predominant features of either sickle cell disease or thalassemia.

Hypersplenism and acute splenic sequestration are life-threatening disorders in children with sickle cell anemia and thalassemia. In these conditions, there may be rapid splenic enlargement, resulting in severe pain and requiring multiple blood transfusions.[14,15] In addition to acute splenic sequestration crisis, these patients may suffer from symptomatic massive splenomegaly causing discomfort and interfering with daily activities. Indications for splenectomy in patients with sickle cell disease include acute splenic sequestration crisis, hypersplenism, and splenic abscess.[14] Children with sickle cell anemia often exhibit weight loss and poor growth; these conditions may be improved after splenectomy as the result of decreased whole-body total protein turnover and decreased resting metabolic rate.[16] Sickle cell disease–associated hypersplenism is characterized by anemia-requiring transfusions as well as leukopenia and thrombocytopenia. Splenectomy reduces the need for transfusions in these patients.

Splenic abscesses are not uncommon in patients with sickle cell anemia and are characterized by fever, abdominal pain, and a tender, enlarged spleen. Many patients with splenic abscess have leukocytosis. Thrombocytosis and Howell-Jolly bodies also occur in these patients, indicating functional asplenia. Common organisms involved in splenic abscess in patients with sickle cell anemia are *Salmonella* species, *Enterobacter* species, and other enteric organisms. In acute splenic sequestration crisis, the patients have severe anemia, splenomegaly, and an acute bone marrow response with erythrocytosis. They may exhibit a dramatic decrease in their hemoglobin levels along with abdominal pain and may undergo circulatory collapse. These patients should be stabilized with hydration and transfusion and may require urgent splenectomy after stabilization.

SPLENECTOMY FOR MALIGNANCY

Lymphomas

Hodgkin's Disease

Hodgkin's disease is a malignant lymphoma that typically affects young adults in their 20s and 30s. Most patients have asymptomatic lymphadenopathy at the time of diagnosis, and most present with cervical node enlargement. A few patients, usually with more advanced disease, may present with constitutional symptoms such as night sweats, weight loss, and pruritus. Hodgkin's disease is histologically classified as either lymphocyte-predominant, nodular-sclerosing, mixed-cellularity, or lymphocyte-depleted Hodgkin's disease.

The disease is pathologically staged according to the Ann Arbor classification. Stage I represents disease in a single lymphatic site, whereas stage II indicates the presence of disease in two or more lymphatic sites on the same side of the diaphragm. Stage III indicates the presence of lymphatic disease (includes splenic involvement) on both sides of the diaphragm. Stage IV disease is disseminated into extralymphatic sites such as liver, lung, or bone marrow. Subscript E indicates single or contiguous extralymphatic involvement in stages I to III, and subscript S represents splenic involvement. Patients with constitutional symptoms are classified as B (presence) or A (absence), for example, stage IIA or IIB.

Historically, staging laparotomy including splenectomy provided essential pathologic staging information that was necessary to select appropriate therapy for Hodgkin's disease. The purpose of staging laparotomy is to pathologically stage the presence and extent of disease below the diaphragm. In one of the larger reported series from 1985, 38.9% of 825 splenectomy specimens tested positive for involvement with Hodgkin's disease.[17] In half of the patients with splenic involvement, the spleen was the only site of intra-abdominal disease. The spleen was also involved in all of the 6.2% of patients with liver involvement. In this important series by Taylor and colleagues,[17] the clinical stage was changed in 43% of cases by laparotomy.

Advances in imaging techniques, with widespread availability of dynamic helical computed tomography (CT) scan and lymphangiography and increasing availability of fluorodeoxyglucose positron-emission tomography imaging, have improved nonoperative staging of Hodgkin's disease. The improved nonoperative staging, along with the use of less toxic systemic chemotherapeutics for earlier stages of Hodgkin's disease, has led to a dramatic decrease in the numbers of patients requiring staging laparotomy. Patients at high risk for relapse, especially those with B symptoms and those with evidence of intra-abdominal involvement on one or more of the diagnostic imaging studies, require systemic chemotherapy and should not undergo a staging laparotomy. Staging laparotomy and splenectomy are appropriate for selected patients with an early clinical stage of disease (stage IA or IIA) in whom pathologic staging of the abdomen will significantly influence the therapeutic management. Early-stage Hodgkin's disease is often cured with radiation therapy alone.

When indicated, the staging laparotomy for Hodgkin's disease should include a thorough abdominal exploration, splenectomy with splenic hilar lymphadenectomy, bilateral wedge and core-needle liver biopsies, retroperitoneal lymphadenectomy, iliac crest bone marrow biopsy, and in premenopausal women, oophoropexy. The perioperative mortality rate for staging laparotomy should be less than 1%, and the risk for major complications has been less than 10%.[17]

Non-Hodgkin's Lymphomas

Splenomegaly or hypersplenism is a common occurrence during the course of NHL. Splenectomy is indicated for patients with NHL for treatment of massive splenomegaly when the bulk of the spleen contributes to abdominal pain, fullness, and early satiety. Splenectomy may also be effective in the treatment of patients who develop hypersplenism with associated anemia, thrombocytopenia, and neutropenia.[18]

Splenectomy occasionally plays an important role in the diagnosis and staging of patients who present with isolated splenic disease. The most common primary splenic neoplasm is NHL. The spleen is involved in 50% to 80% of NHL patients, but fewer than 1% of patients present with splenomegaly without peripheral lymphadenopathy.[19] Disease that appears clinically confined to the spleen has been called *malignant lymphoma with prominent splenic involvement.* Most affected patients have low-grade NHL. There is frequent involvement of the splenic hilar lymph nodes, extrahilar nodes, bone marrow, and liver in these patients. About 75% exhibit clinical evidence of hypersplenism. In a series of 59 such patients reported by Morel and associates,[19] 40 underwent splenectomy, and 19 did not. Eighty-two percent of the cytopenic patients who underwent splenectomy had correction of their hematologic abnormalities postoperatively. For those patients with low-grade NHL who had spleen-predominant features, survival was significantly improved after splenectomy (median, 108 months) as compared with patients receiving similar treatment without splenectomy (median, 24 months).

Leukemia

Hairy Cell Leukemia

Hairy cell leukemia is a rare disease that represents about 2% of adult leukemias. Splenomegaly, pancytopenia, and neoplastic mononuclear cells in the peripheral blood and bone marrow characterize the disease.[20,21] The "hairy" cells are usually B lymphocytes that have cell membrane ruffling, which appears as cytoplasmic projections under the light microscope. The patients are usually elderly men with palpable splenomegaly. About 10% of cases have an indolent course requiring no specific therapy, but most require therapy for cytopenias such as symptomatic anemia, infectious complications from neutropenia, or hemorrhage from thrombocytopenia. The pancytopenia results from the combined effects of hypersplenism and bone marrow replacement by leukemic cells. Therapy may also be required for massive splenomegaly. Patients with hairy cell leukemia have a twofold to threefold increased risk for diagnosis of a second primary malignancy at a median interval of 40 months after the diagnosis of hairy cell leukemia.[20] Most of the second malignancies are solid tumors, and the types of tumors include prostate cancer, skin cancers, lung cancer, and gastrointestinal adenocarcinomas.

Splenectomy and interferon-α_2 have been the standard treatment of hairy cell leukemia until recently; this approach is being replaced with systemic administration of purine analogues, such as 2-chlorodeoxyadenosine and deoxycoformycin, as initial treatment.[22,23] Splenectomy is still indicated for some patients with massive enlargement of the spleen or with evidence of hypersplenism that is refractory to medical therapy. Splenectomy provides a highly effective and sustained palliation of these problems, and most patients show definite hematologic improvement after the procedure. About 40% of patients experience normalization of their blood counts after splenectomy. The responses to splenectomy usually last for 10 years or longer, and about half of patients require no further therapy. Patients with diffusely involved bone marrow who do not have significant splenomegaly are far less likely to achieve a significant benefit from splenectomy. The current 4-year survival rate after diagnosis of hairy cell leukemia is about 80%, as compared with 60% for patients diagnosed in the 1970s.[24]

Chronic Lymphocytic Leukemia

CLL is a B-cell leukemia that is characterized by the progressive accumulation of relatively mature, but functionally incompetent, lymphocytes. CLL occurs more frequently in men and usually occurs after 50 years of age. Staging of CLL is according to the Rai staging system, which correlates well with prognosis.[25] Stage 0 includes bone marrow and blood lymphocytosis only; stage I includes lymphocytosis and enlarged lymph nodes; stage II includes lymphocytosis and enlarged spleen, liver, or both; stage III includes lymphocytosis and anemia; and stage IV includes lymphocytosis with thrombocytopenia. Chlorambucil has long been the mainstay of medical

therapy and was useful for the palliation of symptoms; however, there is increasing interest in using purine analogues, such as fludarabine, as first-line therapy, with some studies showing improved rates of remission.[24] Bone marrow transplantation has also become increasingly used in the treatment of CLL, and both allotransplantation and autotransplantation approaches are being investigated.

The role of splenectomy in the treatment of CLL continues to be for palliation of symptomatic splenomegaly and for treatment of cytopenia related to hypersplenism. Relief of bulk symptoms from splenomegaly is virtually always successful, whereas the hematologic response rates for correction of anemia and thrombocytopenia are between 60% and 70%.[26,27] Cusack and colleagues[26] reported a review of 77 consecutive patients with CLL (76% Rai stage III or IV) who underwent splenectomy at the University of Texas M. D. Anderson Cancer Center and who were compared with an age- and gender-matched cohort of CLL patients treated with fludarabine and no splenectomy. In this retrospective review, the patients with profound anemia and thrombocytopenia who underwent splenectomy had significantly better survival rates than the nonsplenectomy group.

Chronic Myelogenous Leukemia

Chronic myelogenous leukemia (CML) is a myeloproliferative disorder that results from neoplastic transformation of myeloid elements. CML was the first leukemic subset for which a chromosomal marker (the Philadelphia chromosome) was discovered.[28] The Philadelphia chromosome is caused by a fusion of fragments of chromosomes 22 and 9 and results in the expression of an abnormal chimeric oncogenic protein called $p210^{bcr-abl}$. The disease is characterized by a progressive replacement of the normal diploid elements of the bone marrow with mature-appearing neoplastic myeloid cells.

CML may occur from childhood to old age. CML usually presents with an indolent or chronic phase that is asymptomatic. Progression to the accelerated phase is marked by the onset of symptoms such as fever, night sweats, and progressive splenomegaly; however, this phase may also be asymptomatic and detectable only from changes in the peripheral blood or bone marrow. The accelerated phase may give rise to the blastic phase, which is characterized by the previously listed symptoms as well as anemia, infectious complications, and bleeding. Splenomegaly with splenic sequestration of blood elements often contributes to these symptoms.

Treatment of CML is primarily medical and may include hydroxyurea, interferon-alfa, and high-dose chemotherapy with bone marrow transplantation. Symptomatic splenomegaly and hypersplenism in patients with CML may be effectively palliated by splenectomy.[29] Otherwise, the role of splenectomy in the treatment of CML has been controversial. Randomized studies of patients with CML have demonstrated no survival benefit when splenectomy is performed during the early chronic phase.[30,31] Splenectomy has also not resulted in a survival benefit when performed before allogeneic bone marrow transplantation.[32] Thus, splenectomy before allogeneic bone marrow transplantation is recommended only for patients with significant splenomegaly.

Nonhematologic Tumors of the Spleen

The spleen is a site of metastatic tumor in up to 7% of autopsies of cancer patients. The primary solid tumors that most frequently metastasize to the spleen are carcinomas of the breast, lung, and melanoma; however, virtually any primary malignancy may metastasize to the spleen.[33] Metastases to the spleen are often asymptomatic but may be associated with symptomatic splenomegaly or even spontaneous splenic rupture. Splenectomy may provide effective palliation in carefully selected symptomatic patients with splenic metastasis.

Vascular neoplasms are the most common primary splenic tumors that include both benign and malignant variants. Hemangiomas are usually incidental findings identified in spleens removed for other reasons. Angiosarcomas (or hemangiosarcomas) of the spleen have been associated with environmental exposure to thorium dioxide or monomeric vinyl chloride, but they most often occur spontaneously. Patients with these tumors may present with splenomegaly, hemolytic anemia, ascites, and pleural effusions or with spontaneous splenic rupture. These are highly aggressive tumors that have a poor prognosis. Lymphangiomas are usually benign endothelium-lined cysts that may become symptomatic by causing splenomegaly. Lymphangiosarcoma within a cystic lymphangioma has been reported.[34] Splenectomy is appropriate for diagnosis, treatment, or palliation of the conditions cited earlier.

SPLENECTOMY FOR MISCELLANEOUS BENIGN CONDITIONS

Splenic Cysts

Cystic lesions of the spleen have been recognized with increasing frequency since the advent of CT scanning and ultrasound imaging. Splenic cysts are classified as true cysts, which may be either nonparasitic or parasitic, and pseudocysts. Cystic-appearing tumors of the spleen include cystic lymphangiomas and cavernous hemangiomas, as discussed earlier.[35,36] Primary true cysts of the spleen account for about 10% of all nonparasitic cysts of the spleen. Most nonparasitic cysts are pseudocysts and are secondary to trauma. The diagnosis of true splenic cysts is commonly made in the 2nd and 3rd decades of life. True cysts are characterized by a squamous epithelial lining, and many are considered congenital. These epithelial cells are often positive for CA 19–9 and carcinoembryonic antigen by immunohistochemistry, and patients with epidermoid cysts of the spleen may have elevated serum levels of one or both of these tumor-associated antigens.[35] Despite the presence of these tumor markers, these cysts are benign and apparently do not have malignant potential greater than any other native tissue.

Often, true splenic cysts are asymptomatic and found incidentally. When symptomatic, patients may complain of vague upper abdominal fullness and discomfort, early satiety, pleuritic chest pain, shortness of breath, left back or shoulder pain, or renal symptoms from compression of the left kidney. A palpable abdominal mass may be present. The presence of symptoms is often related to the size of the cysts, and cysts smaller than 8 cm are rarely symptomatic.[36] Rarely, these cysts may present with acute symptoms related to rupture, hemorrhage, or infection. The diagnosis of splenic cysts is best made with CT imaging. Operative intervention is indicated for symptomatic cysts and for large cysts. Either total or partial splenectomy may provide successful treatment. The clear advantage of partial splenectomy is the preservation of splenic function. Preservation of at least 25% of the spleen appears sufficient to protect against pneumococcal pneumonia.[37] Most recent reports describe successful experience with partial splenectomy, cyst wall resection, or partial decapsulation, which may be accomplished with either an open or laparoscopic approach.[35,36,38]

Most true splenic cysts are parasitic cysts in areas of endemic hydatid disease (*Echinococcus* species). Radiographic imaging may reveal cyst wall calcifications or daughter cysts. Although hydatid cysts are uncommon in North America, this diagnosis should always be excluded before the performance of invasive diagnostic or therapeutic procedures that may risk spillage of cyst contents. Serologic tests for *Echinococcus* species are often helpful in verifying the presence of parasites. As with hydatid cysts of the liver, spillage of cyst contents may precipitate an anaphylactic shock and risks intraperitoneal dissemination of infective scolices. Splenectomy is the treatment of choice, and great care should be taken to avoid rupture of the cysts intraoperatively. The cysts may be sterilized by injection of a 3% sodium chloride solution, alcohol, or 0.5% silver nitrate, as has been recommended for hydatid cysts of the liver.[39]

Pseudocysts account for 70% to 80% of all nonparasitic cysts of the spleen. A history of prior trauma can usually be elicited. Splenic pseudocysts are not epithelial lined. Radiographic imaging may demonstrate focal calcifications in up to half of cases. Most splenic pseudocysts are unilocular, and the cysts are smooth and thick walled. Small asymptomatic splenic pseudocysts (<4 cm) do not require treatment and may undergo involution over time. When the pseudocysts are symptomatic, patients often present with left upper quadrant and referred left shoulder pain. Symptomatic pseudocysts should be treated surgically. If the spleen can be safely and completely mobilized and partial splenectomy accomplished to include the cystic portion of the spleen, this technique offers effective therapy that preserves splenic function.[40] Presented with less favorable conditions, the surgeon should not hesitate to perform total splenectomy. Successful percutaneous drainage has also been reported for splenic pseudocysts, although the success rate with this approach as compared with surgical intervention has not been determined. The 90% success rate of image-guided percutaneous drainage of unilocular splenic abscesses suggests that this may be a reasonable initial approach for the management of symptomatic splenic pseudocysts.[40]

Splenic Abscess

Splenic abscess is an uncommon and potentially fatal illness. The incidence in autopsy series approximates 0.7%.[41] The mortality for splenic abscess ranges from about 80% for multiple abscesses in immunocompromised patients to about 15% to 20% in previously healthy patients with solitary unilocular lesions. Predisposing illnesses include malignancies, polycythemia vera, endocarditis, previous trauma, hemoglobinopathy (such as sickle cell disease), urinary tract infection, intravenous drug abuse, and AIDS.[42,43] About 70% of splenic abscesses result from hematogenous spread of the infecting organism from another location, as occurs with endocarditis, osteomyelitis, and intravenous drug abuse. Splenic abscess may also occur as the result of infection of a contiguous structure, such as the colon, kidney, or pancreas. Gram-positive cocci, such as *Staphylococcus, Streptococcus,* or *Enterococcus* species, and gram-negative enteric organisms are often the infectious agents. Splenic abscesses may also be caused by other fastidious organisms, including *Mycobacterium tuberculosis, Mycobacterium avium,* and *Actinomyces* species. Immunosuppressed patients may develop multiple fungal abscesses, typically from *Candida* species infection.

The clinical presentation of splenic abscess is often nonspecific and insidious, including abdominal pain, fever, peritonitis, and pleuritic chest pain. The abdominal pain is localized in the left upper quadrant less than half the time and is more often vague abdominal pain. Splenomegaly is present in a minority of patients. The diagnosis is made most accurately by CT; however, it may also be made with ultrasonography. Two thirds of splenic abscesses in adults are solitary, and the remaining one third are multiple. These ratios are reversed in children.[42,44,45]

The initial approach to treatment of splenic abscess depends on whether it is unilocular or multilocular. Unilocular abscesses are amenable to CT-guided drainage, and this approach, along with systemic antibiotic administration, has a success rate that is in excess of 75%[46] and that may be as high as 90% when only patients with unilocular collections are considered.[47] Failure of a prompt clinical response to percutaneous drainage should lead to splenectomy without delay. Multilocular abscesses should usually be treated by splenectomy, with drainage of the left upper quadrant and antibiotic administration.

Wandering Spleen

Wandering spleen is a rare finding, accounting for only a fraction of a percentage of all splenectomies. The spleen normally has peritoneal attachments (called *suspensory ligaments*) that fix the spleen in its usual anatomic position. Failure to form these attachments has been postulated to result from failure of the dorsal mesogastrium to fuse to the posterior abdominal wall during embryonic development. The result is an unusually long splenic pedicle. It has also been postulated that an acquired defect in splenic attachment may occur in multiparous women secondary to hormonal changes during pregnancy and associated abdominal laxity. Wandering spleen is most often diagnosed in children or women between the ages of 20 and 40 years.

Most patients with wandering spleen are asymptomatic. Symptomatic patients often present with recurrent episodes of abdominal pain. This is likely related to tension on the vascular pedicle or intermittent torsion. Torsion of the splenic vessels may lead to venous congestion and splenomegaly. Severe and persistent pain is suggestive of splenic torsion and ischemia. On examination, a mobile abdominal mass may be present along with abdominal tenderness. The diagnosis may be most readily confirmed with a CT scan of the abdomen. The typical finding is the absence of a spleen in its normal position and the presence of a spleen in an ectopic location. Intravenous contrast injection during the CT scan provides valuable information. Lack of contrast enhancement of the spleen suggests splenic torsion, as does a whorled appearance to the splenic pedicle. Lack of splenic perfusion on the CT scan may be helpful in guiding the operative decision for splenectomy versus splenopexy.[48,49]

SPLENIC TRAUMA

The most significant contemporary issue in managing splenic trauma is the role of nonoperative management. Advances in diagnostic techniques that have occurred since the early 1980s have led to alternative approaches to managing these injuries. In recent years, abdominal ultrasound and CT have permitted observation of the location and relative quantification of the amount of intra-abdominal hemorrhage (ultrasound and CT), and CT has provided relatively good definition of the degree of anatomic splenic disruption. The main thrust of this section of the chapter is to trace those diagnostic developments in conjunction with the issues of clinical presentation and splenic anatomy to develop a logical platform for decision making.

General Considerations

Injury to the spleen is the most common indication for laparotomy after blunt mechanisms of injury. Motor vehicular crashes continue to be the major source of injury in industrialized nations. Other common mechanisms include motorcycle crashes, falls, pedestrian and vehicular incidents, bicycle accidents, and sports. Significant abdominal pain produced in the setting of nonvehicular blunt trauma is associated with a high incidence of significant intra-abdominal injury, with the spleen being the most commonly injured organ.

Directly surrounding the spleen are the left hemidiaphragm, splenic flexure of the colon, kidney, distal pancreas, and stomach (see Fig. 54-1). The relatively avascular ligaments described earlier in this chapter (splenophrenic, splenorenal, splenocolic, and gastrosplenic) secure the spleen in this left upper quadrant niche somewhat protected by the lower costal margins (see Fig. 54-1). Splenic injuries are produced by rapid deceleration, compression, energy transmission through the posterolateral chest wall over the spleen, or puncture from an adjacent rib fracture. Rapid deceleration results in the spleen continuing in a forward motion while being tethered at the point of attachment. Injuries produced by deceleration forces result in capsular avulsion along the various ligamentous attachments and linear or stellate fractures of varying depths. Because of its solid structural characteristics and density, energy transfer to the spleen is relatively efficient. Injuries caused by assaults or falls are usually a result of direct blows over the lower chest wall, with transmission of energy resulting in splenic lacerations and fractures.

The blood supply to the spleen is considerable. The spleen receives about 5% of the cardiac output. The blood supply is through the splenic artery and the short gastric vessels (see Fig. 54-2). The splenic arteries divide into several segmental vessels supplying the poles and midportion, and these arteries divide into second- and third-order vessels that course transversely within the spleen. Because of this extensive arterial supply, even superficial lacerations and capsular avulsions often yield substantial hemorrhage.

Diagnosis

The history and physical examination continue to be the basis from which splenic injury should be diagnosed. Details concerning the mechanism of injury delineated in the previous section should be sought. On physical examination, evidence of peritoneal irritation (tenderness, guarding, rebound) is sometimes apparent. Recently extravasated blood, however, is a fairly benign peritoneal irritant, and large amounts of blood may be contained in the free peritoneal cavity with minimal physical findings. In the era before diagnostic peritoneal lavage (DPL), physical examination was found to be accurate only 42% to 87% of the time.[50-53] Perhaps more helpful than examination directed at the abdominal cavity is that focused in the left upper quadrant. Percussion tenderness or evidence of bruising and soft tissue contusion in the posterior left lower costal margin is usually present when direct blows have produced splenic injury. Complaints of left upper quadrant pain or of pain referred to the left shoulder (Kehr's sign) are highly correlated with injury. At least one fourth of patients with left lower rib fractures have associated injury to the spleen.

Significant injury producing hemorrhage is indicated by the hemodynamic status of the patient. Hypotension or tachycardia should alert the clinician to the potential for splenic injury. At the initial trauma assessment, apparent injuries that may yield enough blood loss individually or in aggregate to produce physiologic changes in hemodynamics should be noted. If blood loss from long bone or pelvic fractures or from external losses from lacerations cannot be attributed, an intra-abdominal source must be assumed, and the spleen is the most common source. Indeed, since the classic study by West and associates[54] of preventable deaths that directly contributed to the development of trauma systems in the United States, mortality from missed or delayed recognition of splenic hemorrhage has remained near the top of the list of causes of preventable death.

The diagnosis becomes more difficult in the presence of multiple injuries, which are both distracting to examination and confounding to interpretation of potential sources and volumes of blood loss. Furthermore, associated neurologic injury and substance abuse often add to the diagnostic difficulty. Closed-head injury is associated in 30% to 40% of cases and compromises or eliminates the reliability of the physical examination. Spinal cord injury also eliminates reliance on abdominal examination. Substance abuse has been documented in about 40% of patients involved in motor vehicle crashes. Because of the unreliability of physical examination accounted for by these several concerns, more objective means of diagnosis have evolved.

Diagnostic Peritoneal Lavage

DPL was introduced by Root and colleagues in 1965.[55] That modality remained the standard diagnostic procedure for blunt abdominal trauma evaluations for the subsequent 20 years. Initially, results were interpreted from a grossly positive examination or from quantification of red and white blood cells in the large effluent. A positive DPL consisted of either 10 mL of gross blood aspirated with catheter insertion or a microscopically positive examination. For microscopic examination in adults, 1 L of crystalloid solution is instilled through a periumbilical catheter inserted by either open or closed technique. Assuming complete instillation of the liter, positive examinations consisted of a red blood cell count higher than 100,000/mm^3 or a white blood cell count higher than 500/mm^3 in the completely mixed effluent. The dilution factor that produces a red blood cell count of more than 100,000/mm^3 accounts for about 30 to 40 mL of blood in the peritoneal cavity. A microscopically positive examination by white blood cell count criteria is indicative of peritoneal inflammation generally produced by hollow viscus injury.

After the introduction of DPL, multiple investigators demonstrated sensitivities approaching 99% and specificities in the range of 95% to 98%. Subsequent refinements included enzyme analysis of the effluent to enhance diagnostic accuracy of hollow viscus and pancreatic injury. An extraordinary amount of clinical research has been done on DPL-related issues. For several years, one could expect at least one presentation on DPL at any surgical meeting dealing with clinical trauma topics, and often multiple papers were presented.

Reliance on DPL as a standard screening procedure, however, came into scrutiny from two fronts. As CT began to be applied for trauma diagnostics, it was observed that small splenic injuries had occurred and that the patient remained hemodynamically stable. It was further noted that enough blood was present to have caused a positive lavage. Coincident with that development was the observation by surgeons that many of the positive DPL procedures led to laparotomies in which there was indeed a splenic injury, but often of a relatively trivial nature without active bleeding. Based on these parallel observations, the term *nontherapeutic laparotomy* began surfacing in the splenic injury literature, and it began to be appreciated that DPL was perhaps too sensitive.

Computed Tomography

Application of this technology for diagnosing abdominal injuries began in the early 1980s. The group at San Francisco General Hospital provided the early leadership in this area.[56] Initial observation consisted of examinations done for other injuries at some interval after initial trauma evaluation (e.g., chest or pelvic CT). Injuries to the spleen and liver were noted incidentally and, although initially unrecognized, produced no sequelae. This led to questioning of both the routine reliance on DPL for screening and the necessity of operating on all splenic injuries. As opposed to DPL, CT permitted not only identification of intraperitoneal blood but also definition of individual organ injuries. This actually revolutionized the management of splenic injury. Heretofore, it was assumed that once injured, the spleen invariably continued bleeding. It was generally taught in surgical training programs that if the spleen was incidentally injured from retraction during elective celiotomy, splenectomy was required because of the high risk for continued or recurrent hemorrhage. The early incidental CT observations of damaged spleens in stable patients ushered in the era of nonoperative management.

The anatomic definition of injury provided objective criteria for classification of degrees of splenic injury. The American Association for the Surgery of Trauma developed a splenic injury grading scale through a consensus methodology (Table 54-4).[57] This scale has been useful for comparison of data among institutions. It has also provided a structure for a logical approach to management decisions. Advances in CT technology have continued to increase the value of evaluating intra-abdominal and retroperitoneal injury. The current generation of helical and spiral scanning technology is both rapid and high resolution. Previous technology required 15 to 20 minutes for complete examination, but current technology requires 1 to 2 minutes. The resolution permits more precise delineation of organ fracture and intraparenchymal vascular disruption. The newest generation of CT technology is multislice scanning. That approach allows for scanning of the torso in less than 10 seconds and, owing to a much higher number of accumulated images compared to standard helical technology, an even higher resolution is obtained. This technology is highly promising to replace diagnostic angiography and may have profound importance in better defining solid-organ injury and further minimizing failures of nonoperative management.

Ultrasonography

During the 1990s, ultrasonography was introduced and firmly established as an important diagnostic tool for evaluating blunt abdominal trauma. It was first used in Europe in the early 1980s.[58-60] A few years later, it was adopted by physicians in the United States. Its advantages include noninvasiveness, rapidity, and low cost. Ultrasound provides similar but somewhat more information than DPL. The presence of free intraperitoneal fluid can be identified and semiquantitated. Acoustic windows are noted around solid interfaces. Those solid interfaces for trauma evaluation include the spleen, kidneys, liver, heart, and distended urinary bladder. The acronym FAST (*f*ocused *a*bdominal *s*onography for *t*rauma) has been applied to this quick survey, which takes about 3 minutes to complete in experienced hands. Significant bowel distention, obesity, and subcutaneous emphysema compromise the examination. Initial concerns were with the sensitivity and reproducibility of FAST. There was also a question of whether this technology could be grasped easily enough to permit widespread application by surgeons or whether the difficulty was such that only radiologists who had more extensive training could be relied on for accuracy.

Tso and colleagues[61] reported in 1992 on 163 stable patients evaluated by ultrasound before either DPL or CT and found a 91% sensitivity, with all cases of clinically significant hemoperitoneum being identified. A subsequent study by Bode and associates[62] involved 353 blunt abdominal trauma patients evaluated with ultrasound by a radiologist. These investigators reported a 93% specificity rate, 99% accuracy rate, and no nontherapeutic laparotomies. Rothlin and coworkers[63] reported a study of 290 patients in which ultrasound was performed by a surgeon. They found a 90% sensitivity rate and a 99% specificity rate

Grade	Type	Injury Description
TABLE 54-4.	**American Association for the Surgery of Trauma Splenic Injury Scale (1994 Revision)**	
I	Hematoma	Subcapsular, < 10% surface area
	Laceration	Capsular tear, < 1-cm parenchymal depth
II	Hematoma	Subcapsular, 10–50% surface area; intraparenchymal, < 5 cm in diameter
	Laceration	1–3 cm parenchymal depth, which does not involve a trabecular vessel
III	Hematoma	Subcapsular, > 50% surface area or expanding; ruptured subcapsular or parenchymal hematoma Intraparenchymal hematoma > 5 cm or expanding
	Laceration	>3 cm parenchymal depth or involving trabecular vessels
IV	Laceration	Laceration involving segmental or hilar vessels producing major devascularization (>25% of spleen)
	Vascular	Hilar vascular injury that devascularizes spleen

Adapted from Moore EE, Cogbill TH, Jurkovich GJ, et al: Organ injury scaling: Spleen and liver (1994 revision). J Trauma 38:323, 1995.

for intra-abdominal injury. They also noted the ease of repeatability for follow-up of these patients. The reported data would suggest that with a structured training format, FAST can be expeditiously taught to practicing surgeons. The American College of Surgeons is vigorously involved in evaluating new technologies and is developing structured courses for teaching surgeons the applications of ultrasound for evaluation of breast disease, intra-abdominal pathology, and trauma.

Ultrasound has emerged as a replacement for DPL. It appears to be as sensitive in detecting free intraperitoneal blood and is less invasive and quicker. The most important application is in evaluating the hemodynamically unstable patient with multiple injuries. A positive ultrasound would generally mandate expeditious exploratory laparotomy. The place for ultrasound use in the stable patient has been less clear. As nonoperative management has become so prominent, CT has become indispensable in defining the location and degree of organ injury. Ultrasound is not capable of accurately defining those anatomic characteristics. Technology is advancing rapidly, however, and it is likely that future generations of ultrasonography equipment will significantly improve resolution and anatomic definition. Furthermore, ultrasound may have a more positive impact on cost than is immediately apparent. As ultrasound has become more widely adopted and confidence in the modality has developed, it has become apparent that ultrasound can be applied for screening as an alternative to the more costly CT evaluation.

In a prospective study, Branney and associates[64] used ultrasound in the emergency department for screening stable patients. Their findings included a reduction in the number of CT examinations in patients with significant injury because those with negative examinations required no further studies. Sixty-five percent of the patients had no further studies, the number of admissions for observation decreased significantly, and no significant injuries were missed.

Issues Concerning Operation

Indications for Exploration

The clearest indication for urgent operation is hemodynamic instability. Unfortunately, this is not a binomial or discrete factor. The definition of stability is clearly associated with some degree of arbitrary assignment. This problem is underscored in the face of multiorgan system injury in which blood loss accumulates from external losses from lacerations, internal losses in fractures and soft tissues, and thoracic and abdominal cavities. Optimal decisions become apparent in retrospect. Nonetheless, when in doubt, abdominal exploration should be performed. The risks associated with nontherapeutic laparotomy are outweighed by the risks associated with shock secondary to prolonged intraperitoneal hemorrhage and the associated consequences of immunocompromise, multiorgan system dysfunction, and death.

Because there can be no *standard* criteria for hemodynamic instability, a general guideline is to operate for a systolic blood pressure below 90 mm Hg or a pulse of more than 120 beats/min if there is not immediate response to 1 to 2 L of crystalloid resuscitation and when physical examination, ultrasound, or DPL indicates intra-abdominal blood loss. Indications for operation based on CT findings are delineated in a subsequent section of this chapter on nonoperative management.

Technical Issues

A midline incision is usually preferred for trauma exploration. This approach is expeditious and provides access to all areas of the abdominal cavity, including the retroperitoneum. A left subcostal approach may be preferred when laparotomy is directed by CT findings. The small bowel and lesser sac are easily evaluated from this incision. Extension to the right side provides outstanding exposure of the liver and access to all of the abdomen with the exception of the deepest portion of the pelvis. Both incisions are adequate, but the performance of a midline incision is quicker.

After rapid evacuation of free blood and clots to assess other sources of injury, including the liver and mesentery, the spleen should be mobilized into the wound. Splenic mobilization should be accomplished by the fundamental operative principle of traction and countertraction. In the case of splenic mobilization, traction and countertraction are based on the spleen and its suspensory ligaments. The operating surgeon should apply dorsal and medial traction on the spleen with the hand splayed widely over the splenic surface to stretch and define clearly the splenorenal and splenophrenic ligaments. It appears that there is a natural tendency to place ventral traction on the spleen to "lift" it from the left upper quadrant, a maneuver that results in decapsulation over the posterior splenic surface and along the splenocolic ligament, producing iatrogenic trauma and increasing hemorrhage. After exposure of the splenorenal and splenophrenic ligaments, which is facilitated by the first assistant providing countertraction with tissue forceps, the ligaments can be divided under direct vision.

The incision begins at the phrenocolic ligament, continuing through the ligaments to the stomach in the vicinity of the highest short gastric vessels. Division should occur 1 to 2 cm from the spleen to avoid injury to both spleen and diaphragmatic muscle. Continued tension on the tissues allows gradual mobilization anterior to the spleen as deeper layers of filmy connective tissue planes are placed under tension and easily visualized and divided. The dissection should progress such that the left adrenal gland is visualized and left undisturbed in its posterior location. As this dissection progresses through these thin connective tissue planes, the posterior surface of the pancreas and the splenic vein densely adherent to the pancreas are visualized. The spleen-pancreas complex can be mobilized over the top of the aorta, taking care to avoid injury of the superior mesenteric artery. After this mobilization, the spleen and distal pancreas are delivered to the level of the subcutaneous tissue. Laparotomy pads are placed in the left upper quadrant to maintain the spleen in the wound. At this point, the degree of injury can be clearly evaluated and the decision for extirpation or repair made.

Splenectomy is usually indicated under the following circumstances: (1) the patient is unstable; (2) other injuries require prompt attention; (3) the spleen is extensively injured with continuous bleeding; and (4) bleeding is associated with hilar injury. There are both anterior (short gastric arteries) and posterior (splenic artery) blood supplies. After complete splenic mobilization, traction can be placed on the gastrosplenic ligament that places tension on and exposes the short gastric arteries. These are rapidly divided; with appropriate traction, the gastric wall is easily visualized, avoiding clamp injury. The spleen can then be grasped and elevated by the surgeon or assistant and the splenic artery identified at the superior border of the pancreas. The artery and vein are separately divided and ligated. Not infrequently, the tail of the pancreas extends right into the hilum, in which case it is generally more practical and safer to ligate the splenic vessels after they have divided to avoid the morbid complication of injury to the pancreatic tail. In the absence of pancreatic injury, drainage of the splenic fossa is not necessary.

As noted earlier in this chapter, thrombocytosis occurs in about half of postoperative patients in the initial weeks after splenectomy. The thrombocytosis may increase the risk for deep venous thrombosis. When the platelet count rises higher than 750,000/mm^3, many surgeons treat the patient with antiplatelet therapy, low-dose heparin, or low-molecular-weight heparin. Pimpl and colleagues[65] reviewed 37,000 autopsies over 20 years of adults who died after splenectomy and compared them with a deceased population of 403 who did not have splenectomy. These investigators found higher incidence rates of lethal pneumonia, sepsis with multiorgan failure, purulent pyelonephritis, and pulmonary embolism in the splenectomy group. They concluded that splenectomy carries a considerable lifelong risk for severe infection and thromboembolism.

Splenorrhaphy

Attempts at splenic repair were initiated with appreciation of the entity of OPSI (see previous section). Additionally, splenic absence provides a relative dead space in the left upper quadrant, which often becomes occupied with blood clot or serum, creating a potential for subphrenic abscess. This occurrence is especially pronounced in the face of hollow viscus or pancreatic injuries. Those scenarios provide for bacterial colonization and culture media.

Splenorrhaphy techniques became widely applied in the late 1970s, reaching a peak in the mid-1980s. Their application has gradually decreased since that time in association with the rise of nonoperative management. Splenorrhaphy was applied to nearly half of splenic injuries at the height of its use. A general rule is that if more than 1 unit of blood is required for salvage, splenectomy should be performed. Beyond that, the risks associated with transfusion generally outweigh the risks of OPSI. Four types of splenorrhaphy have been used: (1) superficial hemostatic agents (cautery, oxidized cellulose,

absorbable gelatin sponge, topical thrombin); (2) suture repair; (3) absorbable mesh wrap; and (4) resectional débridement.

Superficial hemostatic approaches are useful for American Association for the Surgery of Trauma grades I and II injuries (see Table 54-4). They may also be adjunctive in higher grades of injury. The argon-beam coagulator has received some support, but there is no clinical evidence that it is superior to other approaches.

Suture repair of lacerations in grades II and III injuries has become common. When feasible, temporary occlusion of the splenic artery may reduce blood loss and facilitate repair. A problem with suture repair is the tendency for the sutures to tear the spleen further when tied. Pledgeted repairs reduce that occurrence. Many surgeons have used Teflon pledgets. The use of pledgets constructed of 2- to 3-cm absorbable gelatin sponge wrapped in oxidized cellulose and secured with suture ties to resemble a cigarette has been commonly applied (Fig. 54-4). These are placed along each edge of the laceration and secured with a running polypropylene suture. That approach has proved effective for both splenic and hepatic lacerations.

Mesh wrapping has been effectively used for grade III and some grade IV injuries. Investigators from Cook County Hospital provided some of the earliest data and description of this technique.[66] Disposable mesh, composed of either polyglycolic acid or polyglactin, has been used. If knitted mesh is used, a keyhole about 1 to 2 cm in diameter is cut in the middle of the mesh and is stretched, so that the spleen can be delivered through it, resulting in the keyhole around the splenic hilum. The edges of the mesh are then approximated with a running suture over the top, so that the spleen is effectively enclosed in a mesh sac. If woven mesh is used, it will not stretch; thus, the keyhole for surrounding the hilum is designed by dividing one side of a square piece of mesh to the center and constructing an appropriately sized circular hole. The mesh is tightened around the hilum by reapproximating the severed mesh. The mesh is secured

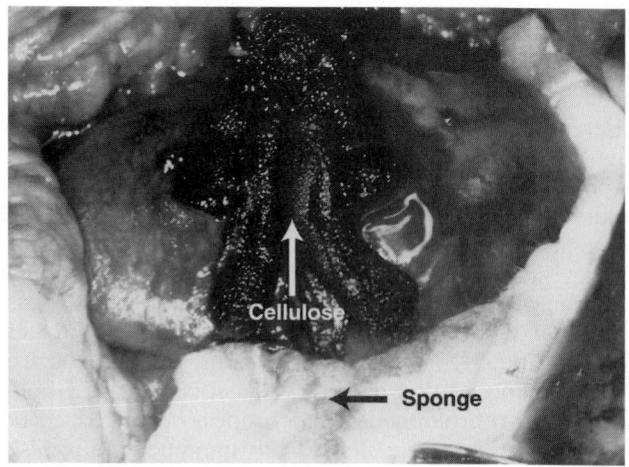

■ FIGURE 54-4.   Pledgets constructed of gelatin sponge wrapped in oxidized cellulose are used to suture-repair a grade III splenic laceration.

over the top of the spleen as described previously (Fig. 54-5). This technique works surprisingly well, apparently through a tamponade effect.

Resectional débridement has been applied for major fractures, usually involving the upper or lower pole (grade II or IV). The raw surfaces are approximated. Pledgeted materials are of considerable benefit for reapproximating those edges. At least one third of the splenic mass is necessary to maintain immunocompetence.

As noted previously, in the past, splenic conservation through splenorrhaphy was applied to nearly half of all splenic injuries. That percentage decreased substantially in the 1990s and probably now accounts for no more than 10%. A high percentage of splenorrhaphy was accounted for by simple techniques for repair of grades I and II injuries. Most of those types of injury are now being managed nonoperatively. Most patients who currently undergo operation for splenic injury have active bleeding or destructive injuries requiring splenectomy. Heightened awareness of risk for transmission of viral disease, especially hepatitis, with blood transfusion has also dampened enthusiasm for splenic repair.

Nonoperative Management

The basis for nonoperative management can be traced to OPSI and incidental notation of splenic injury in the early years of CT scanning for trauma. Nonoperative management originated in pediatric surgery. For several years, general surgeons questioned the judgment of their pediatric surgical colleagues. With the passage of time, it has become clear that nonoperative management is logical. Nonoperative management in adults is somewhat more controversial but is gaining continuously wider acceptance as data accumulate.

Currently, 70% to 90% of children with splenic injury are successfully treated without operation, and 40% to 50% of adult patients with splenic injury are managed nonoperatively in large-volume trauma centers. The lower

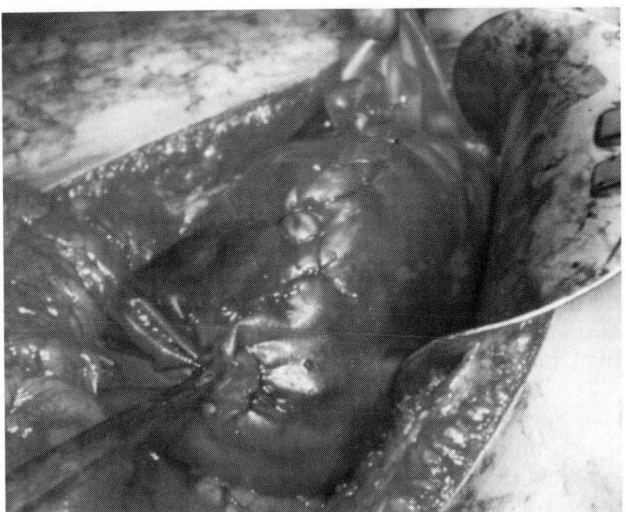

FIGURE 54-5. Splenorrhaphy of grade IV splenic laceration is accomplished by wrapping with woven polyglactin.

percentage of nonoperatively managed splenic injury in adults than in children has been a source of speculation. It has been suggested that anatomic differences between adults and children are responsible, including a more elastic, cartilaginous rib cage providing protection and more elastin in the spleen producing contraction and some degree of hemostasis in children. Powell and colleagues,[67] however, have produced data demonstrating that the differences in management of splenic injury between adults and children are most likely related to mechanisms of injury. Their analysis of 411 patients (293 adults and 118 children) found major differences in mechanism of injury in adults and children ($P < .05$), including the following: motor vehicle crash (67% in adults vs. 24% in children), motorcycle crash (9% vs. 1%), sports-related injury (2% vs. 17%), falls (9% vs. 25%), pedestrian and auto collision (4% vs. 11%), and bicycle crash (1% vs. 9%). Higher injury severity scores, lower Glasgow Coma Scale scores, and higher mortality rates indicated that adults were more severely injured.

A fundamental rule for consideration of nonoperative management is the requirement that the patient be hemodynamically stable. Additionally, institutional resources should be such that the patient can be monitored in a critical care environment and that operating room facilities and personnel are available in the event of sudden bleeding that requires splenectomy. Most grades I and II injuries can be managed nonoperatively; these account for about 60% to 70% of cases of nonoperative management.[68] Although CT scanning is the fundamental measure for selecting nonoperative management, it has shortcomings that must be taken into consideration. A report by Sutyak and coworkers[69] involving CT in 49 patients with splenic injury correlated surgical with CT findings. These investigators found that CT matched surgical grading in 10 patients, underestimated it in 18, and overestimated it in 6. They also reported that 5 injuries were missed by CT and that radiologists disagreed in their interpretations of 20% of scans. Note, however, that the CT scan used in this study was not the current state-of-the-art helical CT scan.

In early reports, most investigators expressed extreme caution regarding nonoperative management of grades III and IV, even with hemodynamic stability. As experience has accumulated, most feel comfortable with observing stable grade III injuries, and many have begun observing grades IV and V injuries.[68,70,71] Most of the early reports of nonoperative management in the 1980s were anecdotal, noting occasional successful management in highly selected cases. Since the 1990s, nonoperative management has become a more standardized approach. In a review in 1990, Shackford and Molin[72] reported on 1866 splenic injuries in which 13% were managed nonoperatively. Subsequently, Smith and colleagues[73] reported a 47% nonoperative management rate among 166 splenic injuries. These and most other reports have reserved nonoperative management for injury grades I through III.

Analysis of failure rates is important in evaluating criteria for selecting appropriate patients for nonoperative management. Although age older than 55 years has been reported to be associated with high failure rates,[74] others have refuted that observation.[68,70,71] Nonoperative man-

TABLE 54-5.   Comparison of Results of Nonoperative Management of Blunt Splenic Injuries from Published Series

Study	Splenic Injuries (*n*)	Cases Planned Nonoperatively Managed (%)	Nonoperative Success (%)	Failure (%)
Shackford and Molin, 1990[72]	1866	13	69	31
Schurr et al, 1995[75,*]	309	25	87	13
Smith et al, 1996[73,*]	166	47	97	3
Morrell et al, 1996[74]	135	18	52	48
Davis et al, 1998[68]	524	61	94	6
Myers et al, 1999[76]	204	68	93	7
Cocanour et al, 1999[70]	368	57	86	14
Bee et al, 2001[77]	558	77	92	8

*Excluded grade IV and V injuries.

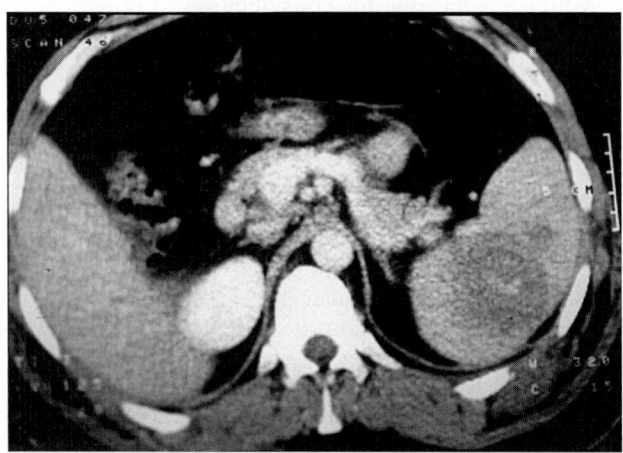

FIGURE 54-6.   CT scan demonstrates "vascular blush" in an injured spleen.

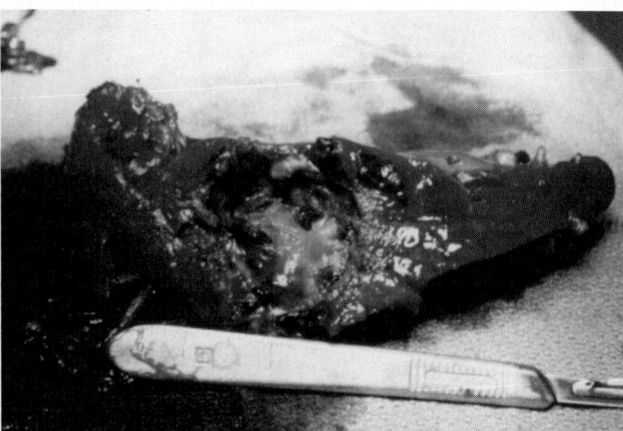

FIGURE 54-7.   After splenectomy, the sectioned spleen demonstrated a false aneurysm, which corresponds to the vascular blush in Figure 54-6.

agement failure rates from recent series are shown in Table 54-5.

An important finding that has been correlated with failed nonoperative management is the presence of a vascular blush on CT examination. Schurr and associates[75] reported on 309 blunt splenic injuries, of which 29% were managed nonoperatively. They noted a 13% failure rate; two thirds of the failures were associated with a vascular blush (Fig. 54-6). Those vascular blushes were proved to represent false aneurysms of intraparenchymal branches of the splenic artery (Fig. 54-7). The cause of failure from false aneurysms is gradual enlargement of the aneurysm, with rupture of the aneurysm and spleen. This pathophysiology most likely accounts for many of the instances of "delayed splenic rupture" noted from the past. Not all of these pseudoaneurysms rupture, however. It appears likely that 30% to 40% spontaneously thrombose.[75] A subsequent study from the same institution by Davis and colleagues[68] dealt with 524 blunt splenic injuries during a 4.5-year period. In that report, a protocol was followed in which vascular blushes identified by CT were followed by

angiography with embolization of the false aneurysm (Fig. 54-8). That approach yielded a failure rate of 5% for nonoperative management, a rate significantly lower (*P* < .03) than their prior experience.

Controversy exists concerning the need for follow-up CT evaluations. Some institutions have suggested that follow-up scans are unnecessary.[70,76] Davis and colleagues,[68] however, noted that 74% of vascular blushes were seen only in follow-up studies. Because a high rate of failure was noted with the finding, these investigators recommend follow-up scans within 2 to 3 days for all but the most trivial lesions. The reasons for absence of vascular blush on initial scans include missed 1-cm-cut protocol and lysis of initial clot.

The cause of other failures is less clear. Investigators have become more aggressive by including patients with higher injury grades (IV and V). Fifty-six of 106 grades IV and V injuries were nonoperatively managed with a failure rate of 18%.[68] This and subsequent reports have also correlated a higher failure rate with large amounts of free intraperitoneal blood on the admission CT scan

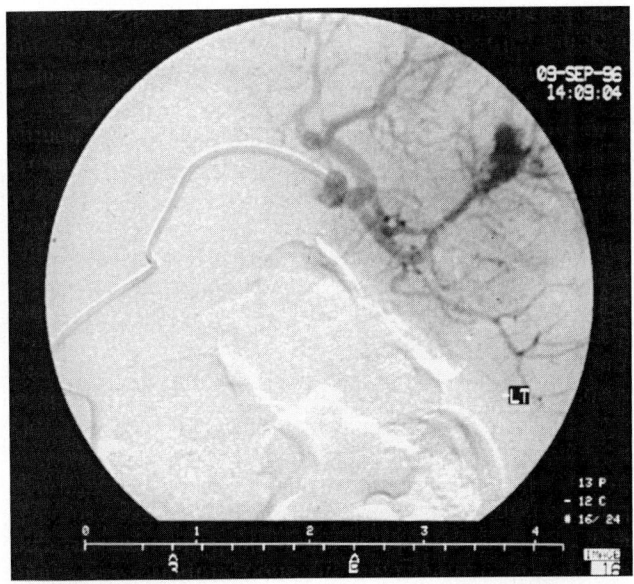

A

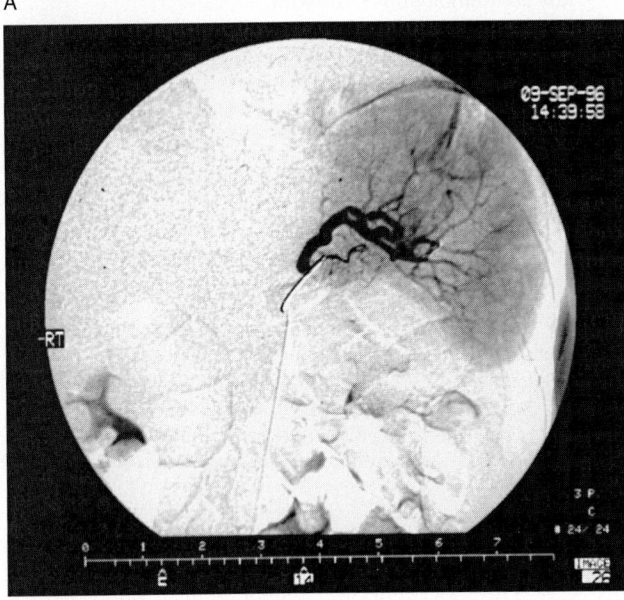

B

FIGURE 54-8. A and **B**, Angiographic embolization of a false aneurysm, which was demonstrated by helical CT.

(perisplenic and perihepatic and gutter and pelvis).[68,70,76] It seems intuitive that larger degrees of splenic injury as indicated by CT scan and by volume of intraperitoneal blood would be associated with higher failure rates. In a recent report published by Bee and coworkers, the published contraindications to nonoperative management (NOM) of blunt splenic injury were reviewed and compared with their experience with nonoperative failures.[77] The published indications that were reviewed included age of 55 years, Glasgow Coma Scale score of 13, admission blood pressure lower than 100 mm Hg, major (grades III through V) injuries, and large amounts of hemoperitoneum in their evaluation of 430 consecutive patients who were observed. The nonoperative management failure rate was 8%. Multivariate analysis identified age of

55 in grades III to V as independent predictors of failure. They noted the highest failure rate (30% to 40%) occurred in patients older than 55 years with major injury or moderate to large amounts of hemoperitoneum. They noted a mortality rate for successful nonoperative management of 12% compared to 9% for failed nonoperative management and concluded that failed nonoperative management was not significantly associated with adverse outcome. An ideal situation would be for 70% to 80% of cases to be manageable nonoperatively, with a 1% to 2% failure rate. This may not be possible. Future clinical studies should be designed to address these important issues of selection, causes of failure, and use of adjunctive techniques, including embolization. We believe that advancing CT technology, which will better define the injuries combined with clinical trials, will ultimately approach those numbers—high nonoperative management rates coupled with very low failure rates.

No objective data are available related to recommendations for return to activity after splenic injury. For grades I and II injuries, 2 to 3 weeks is probably adequate healing time. For higher-grade injuries, 6 to 8 weeks is probably more appropriate, and many surgeons would obtain a CT scan at that time to evaluate degree of healing before return to excessive physical activity.

Evidence-Based Medicine Evaluation

The use of evidence-based medicine (EBM) to address optimal management of clinical problems is gaining increased acceptance. One of the most important applications of EBM is to develop practice management guidelines. There are two basic methodologies. The first is through statistical methodology centered on meta-analysis. Rigorous meta-analytic techniques require randomized, controlled trials for analysis; however, there are relatively few randomized, controlled trials for addressing most questions in surgery. Therefore, a second methodology for EBM addresses questions through data classification and assessment of confidence levels for recommendations. Extensive work on data classification has been done by the Canadian and U.S. Preventive Task Forces and by the Agency for Health Care Policy and Research of the U.S. Department of Health and Human Services.[78] A classification system based on that work is outlined in Box 54-3.

The Agency for Health Care Policy and Research has also developed a system of assessing confidence levels for recommendations based on that data classification system, which is presented in Box 54-4. Using those methodologies for data evaluation and assessment, the Eastern Association for the Surgery of Trauma (EAST) has published 11 patient management guidelines on their Internet website (*www.east.org*). One of those evidence-based guidelines addresses nonoperative management of splenic injury. To develop the guidelines for splenic injury, a study group consisting of seven surgeons identified 50 English-language clinical articles published between 1976 and 1996 addressing pertinent questions about blunt splenic injury management. The recommendations based on the classification and assessment of those published data are listed in

Box 54-3. Evidence-Based Classification of Medical Literature Adapted from Recommendations by the Agency for Health Care Policy and Research

Class I Evidence

Prospective, randomized controlled trials—the gold standard of clinical trials. Some may be poorly designed, have inadequate numbers, or suffer from other methodologic inadequacies and thus may not be clinically significant.

Class II Evidence

Clinical studies in which the data were collected prospectively and retrospective analyses that were based on clearly reliable data. These types of studies include observational studies, cohort studies, prevalence studies, and case-control studies.

Class III Evidence

Studies based on retrospectively collected data. Evidence used in this class includes clinical series, databases or registries, case reviews, case reports, and expert opinion.

Box 54-4. Categorization of Strengths of Recommendations Based on a Medical Literature Review of a Specified Topic* According to Methodologies Derived from the Agency for Health Care Policy and Research

Level 1

This recommendation is convincingly justifiable based on the available scientific information alone. It is usually based on class I data; however, strong class II evidence may form the basis for a level 1 recommendation, especially if the issue does not lend itself to testing in a randomized format. Conversely, weak or contradictory class I data may not be able to support a level 1 recommendation.

Level 2

This recommendation is reasonably justifiable by available scientific evidence and strongly supported by expert critical care opinion. It is usually supported by class II data or a preponderance of class III evidence.

Level 3

This recommendation is supported by available data, but adequate scientific evidence is lacking. It is generally supported by class III data. This type of recommendation is useful for educational purposes and in guiding future studies.

*See Table 54-1.

Box 54-5. Eastern Association for the Surgery of Trauma* Recommended Patient Management Guidelines for the Nonoperative Management (NOM) of Blunt Injuries to the Liver and the Spleen

Level I

There are insufficient data to suggest NOM as a level I recommendation for the initial management of blunt injuries to the liver and/or spleen in the hemodynamically stable patient.

Level II

1. There are class II and mostly class III data to suggest that NOM of blunt hepatic and/or splenic injuries in a hemodynamically stable patient is reasonable.
2. Severity of hepatic or splenic injury (as suggested by CT grade or degree of hemoperitoneum), neurologic status, and/or the presence of associated injuries are not contraindications to NOM.
3. Abdominal CT is the most reliable method to identify and assess the severity of the injury to the spleen or liver.

Level III

1. The clinical status of the patient should dictate the frequency of follow-up scans.
2. Initial CT of the abdomen should be performed with oral and intravenous contrast agents to facilitate the diagnosis of hollow-viscus injuries.
3. Medical clearance to resume normal activity status should be based on evidence of healing.
4. Angiographic embolization is an adjunct in the NOM of the hemodynamically stable patient with hepatic and splenic injuries and evidence of ongoing bleeding.

*See their website at www.east.org.

Box 54-5. The EAST evidence-based analysis demonstrates that there are neither class I data nor level I recommendations. Those findings make it clear that splenic injury management must be addressed by prospective, multi-institutional trials. A strong case for such trials can be made because splenic injury occurs at a high incidence and is associated with substantial cost and morbidity.

The intent of EBM-derived guidelines is that they be adopted at the local level into management schemes through clinical pathways and algorithms that consider resource availability and practice patterns. An algorithm developed from the EAST recommendations and their accompanying literature review is represented in Figure 54-9.

ELECTIVE LAPAROSCOPIC SPLENECTOMY

The technique of open splenectomy was described in detail in the previous section on splenic trauma. Many surgeons now prefer to use the laparoscopic approach for

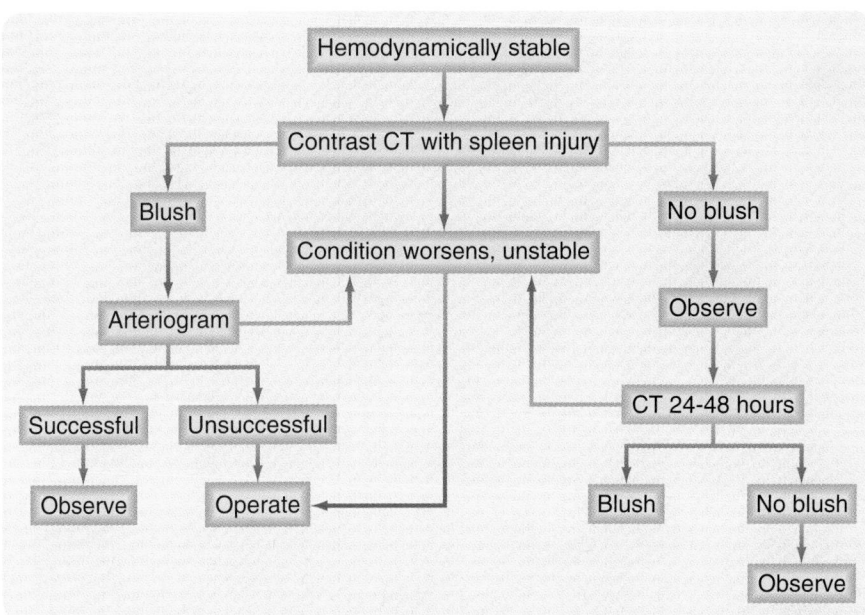

FIGURE 54-9. Algorithm for nonoperative management of splenic injuries in the hemodynamically stable patient. (From Bee TK, Croce MA, Miller PR, et al: Failures of splenic nonoperative management: Is the glass half empty or half full? J Trauma 50:231, 2001.)

most elective splenectomies. The technique of laparoscopic splenectomy was first described in 1992.[79-81] In experienced hands, laparoscopic splenectomy can be performed as safely and effectively as open splenectomy, particularly for hematologic diseases in which the spleen size is normal or only slightly enlarged.[9,82,83] Early experiences with laparoscopic splenectomy have demonstrated many similarities to the early days of laparoscopic cholecystectomy. Operative time is longer for laparoscopic splenectomy, but the procedure offers the advantages of more rapid postoperative recovery and shorter duration of hospital stay, leading some to consider laparoscopic splenectomy the standard of care for some hematologic disorders requiring splenectomy.[83]

Results of laparoscopic splenectomy for benign hematologic diseases, such as ITP, should be compared with the standard of open splenectomy, which is technically feasible in 100% of patients and is associated with a hospital mortality rate of less than 1% and a morbidity rate of 10% to 20%. In a retrospective literature review of 1358 patients who underwent open splenectomy, the rate of wound-related complications was estimated to be 3%. The mean postoperative hospital stay ranged from 7.5 to 11 days.[84-90] In patients with splenomegaly secondary to malignant hematologic disorders, however, the operative mortality rates are increased in the range of 0 to 18% and morbidity rates are increased in the range of 19% to 56%, respectively.[91-93]

In comparison, laparoscopic splenectomy can be completed in about 90% of properly selected patients. The incidence of conversion to open splenectomy is between 0 and 20%. Most of the conversions are caused by intraoperative bleeding, but lack of surgical experience,[82,94-96] extensive adhesions,[95,97] large splenomegaly,[82,94,95,98-101] and obesity[80,82,94,102] are also involved. A significant learning curve is observed with laparoscopic splenectomy, and with increasing experience, the conversion rate has been reported to decrease dramatically.[96,103] Yee[96] and

Glasgow[103] and their associates reported a conversion rate of 36% during the initial 11 laparoscopic splenectomies; during the subsequent operations, the conversion rate dropped to 0% to 5%.

In two reviews[8,9] of laparoscopic series that included 418 and 948 patients, respectively, the mean operative time for laparoscopic splenectomy ranged from 88 to 261 minutes, with an open conversion rate ranging from 0 to 30% (Table 54-6). In a multivariate analysis by Friedman and coworkers,[82] operative time was significantly related to patient age, hematologic diagnosis, operative technique, and splenic weight. The perioperative morbidity rates averaged 8% and 12%, respectively (range, 0 to 30%), and the mortality rate was 0.7% (0 to 6%). Most deaths were attributable to the patient's underlying diseases or hematologic disorder. In the review by Gigot and associates[8] of 984 patients, 119 had reported complications. Bleeding was the most frequent perioperative complication and has been significantly linked to the surgeon's learning curve.[97] The mean number of patients requiring intraoperative or postoperative transfusions was 13%, ranging from 0 to 40%. Local complications, including wound-related complication (seroma, hematoma, infection, evisceration, or incisional hernia) occurred in 1.5%. Postoperative bleeding occurred in 1% of patients, and 73% of these cases required re-exploration. Pancreatic complications (pancreatitis or pancreatic fistula) occurred in 0.6% and subphrenic abscess in 0.5%. General postoperative complications occurred in 7.4%; most (3.2%) were pleuropulmonary.

Postoperative recovery after laparoscopic splenectomy is surprisingly fast, as has previously been observed with laparoscopic cholecystectomy. The length of stay ranged from 1.8 to 6 days after laparoscopic splenectomy.[8,9] Most patients are able to return to full activities within 1 week if their underlying hematologic disorder allows. In the study by Flowers and coworkers,[97] 9% of patients returned to work in 7 days, and all patients with uncomplicated

TABLE 54-6. Retrospective Case-Control Series Comparing Open and Laparoscopic Splenectomies in Adults

	Yee et al, 1995[130]		Rhodes et al, 1995[131]		Brunt et al, 1996[121]		Watson et al, 1997[132]		Diaz et al, 1997[133]		Friedman et al, 1997[82]		Delaitre & Pitre, 1997[102]		Smith et al, 1996[123]		Glasgow et al, 1997[103]		Hashizume et al, 1996[134]	
	OS	LS	OS	LS	OS	LS	OS	LS	OS	LS	OS	LS	OS	LS	OS	LS	OS	LS	OS	LS
Patients	25	25	11	24	20	26	47	13	15	15	74	63	28	28	10	10	28	52	41	10
Operative time (min)	156	198[†]	75	120	134	202[†]	84	88	116	196[†]	121	153	127	183[*]	131	261[*]	156	196[†]	249	100[†]
Delay before regular diet (days)	4.3	2.1[†]	—	—	4.1	1.4[‡]	—	—	—	—	3.2	1.5[*]	—	—	4.4	1.9[*]	4.3	2	—	—
Blood loss (mL)	273	319	—	—	222	376	—	—	359	385	437	259	—	—	—	—	274	320	512	176[*]
Transfusion rate	12	16	—	—	15	10	13	0	—	—	27	3.5	36	29	20	40	18	27	—	—
Complications (%)	12	8	8	27	23	23	19	0	13	6.7	22	12	32	11	20	0	14	10	46	0
POHS	6.7	5.1[*]	7	3[‡]	5.8	2.5[‡]	10	2[‡]	8.8	2.3[†]	6.7	3.5[*]	8.6	5.1[*]	5.8	3[*]	6.7	4.8[*]	20	8.2
Total hospital costs USD × 10³	13,433	9207	—	—	—	—	4224	2238	16,362	18,015	10,900	9700[*]	—	—	13,196	17,071	17,876	20,295	9264	6438[†]
Cure rate at FU in ITP (%)	76	81	—	—	75	75	83	92	75	80	—	—	86	93	—	81	81	74	63	80
Mean FU (mo)	—	—	—	—	6.5	6.5	60	14	—	—	—	—	—	—	—	—	—	—	—	—
AS detected (%)	24	8	—	—	5	5	6	15	20	29	13.5	19	18	11	30	21	21	16	—	—
Return to full activity (days)	—	—	—	—	—	—	—	—	23	12[*]	—	—	—	—	6 wk	—	—	1-2 wk	—	—

FU, follow-up; ITP, immune thrombocytopenic purpura; LS, laparoscopic splenectomy; OS, open splenectomy; POHS, postoperative hospital stay; USD, U.S. dollars.

*P < .05.

†P < .001.

‡P = .0005.

From Gigot JF, Lengele B, Gianello P, et al: Present status of laparoscopic splenectomy for hematologic diseases: Certitudes and unresolved issues. Semin Laparosc Surg 5:159, 1998.

laparoscopic splenectomy were fully recovered by 21 days, regardless of profession. Although a prospective, randomized comparison has not been conducted, several retrospective case-control series have compared the laparoscopic approach to an open splenectomy (see Table 54-6). Even though it is difficult to extrapolate definitive data from these series because of potential selection bias (patient age, diagnosis and indication, splenic weight, and major comorbid conditions), the results are consistently in favor of the laparoscopic approach. Each series has demonstrated an earlier resumption of diet, reduced postoperative analgesics, and decreased postoperative hospital stay.

Despite the promising technical results of laparoscopic splenectomy, the hematologic response and long-term cure rates are the most important. Open splenectomy for the treatment of ITP achieves a long-term cure rate of 65% to 90%. In clinical series of laparoscopic splenectomy, the mean follow-up is usually limited to 1 to 2 years. During this short follow-up, reports of 76% to 100% success rates have been published. Similarly, Katkhouda and associates[9] reported that the treatment of ITP appears to be at least as good after laparoscopic surgery as after the open technique in comparisons of separate series (see Tables 54-1 and 54-2). Gigot and colleagues[8] reported on 279 patients with ITP where an absence of initial response and/or recurrent thrombocytopenia occurred in approximately 15% (Table 54-7).

The causes of recurrence in patients with ITP are multifactorial, but residual accessory spleens are well known to be one of the factors of recurrence. There have been several reported cases of recurrent thrombocytopenia secondary to retained accessory spleens (see Table 54-7). This issue of accessory spleens has been prominent in the discussion of the role of laparoscopic splenectomy. Autopsy studies have demonstrated that the incidence of accessory spleens in the normal population is about 10%. In clinical series, however, accessory spleens have been reported in 15% to 30% of patients. The incidence of accessory spleen in recently reviewed splenectomy series since 1980 is 15% to 16%.[9] The incidence probably correlates with the diligence of the search and is higher than commonly estimated because small accessory spleens are easily missed or mistaken for lymph nodes. Because accessory spleens are often easier felt than seen, it is likely that the incidence of missed splenunculi is higher at laparoscopic than open splenectomy. The reliability of laparoscopic exploration in dealing with the problem of accessory spleens is a key factor in establishing the long-term credibility of the laparoscopic approach.[8]

Though the indications for a laparoscopic splenectomy remain the same as open splenectomy, some cases require caution in performing laparoscopically. Absolute contraindications to the laparoscopic approach include severe cardiopulmonary disease, cirrhosis, and pregnancy.[104] Variceal short gastric vessels compounded by

TABLE 54-7.   Long-Term Hematologic Cure Rate after Laparoscopic Treatment of Immune Thrombocytopenic Purpura Patients

Study	Patients (n)	Mean Follow-Up (mo [range])	Absence of Initial Response and/or Recurrent Thrombocytopenia	Residual Accessory Spleen Detected
Emmermann et al, 1995[119]	20	14 (1–28)	1	?
Yee et al, 1995[130]	14	At discharge	4	1
Liew and Storey, 1995[135]	6	?	1	1
Legrand et al, 1996[95]	9	12 (1–26)	1	?
Parent et al, 1995[136]	11	— (6–9)	1	?
Flowers et al, 1996[97]	22	21 (3–36)	4	?
Dexter et al, 1996[137]	6	24 (17–33)	0	—
Zamir et al, 1996[138]	15	— (2–36)	0	—
Katkhouda et al, 1996[139]	20	20 (1–46)	0	—
Watson et al, 1997[132]	13	14 (5–21)	1	1
Tsiotos and Schinkert, 1997[124]	18	15 (1–30)	1	?
Lee and Kim, 1997[140]	15	?	3	?
Glasgow et al, 1997[103]	16	?	4	1
Delaitre and Pitre, 1997[102]	26	— (3–48)	2	?
Decker et al, 1998[99]	17	12.5 (1–28)	4	?
Trias et al, 1998[101]	32	12 (1–50)	9	3
Gigot, 1998*	19	45 (22–63)	6	3

*Unpublished data.

?, data not given despite treatment failures—not assessed; —, no treatment failures, therefore not assessed.

the coagulopathy of liver disease present an unacceptable risk of operative hemorrhage and temper enthusiasm for the laparoscopic approach in patients with portal hypertension. Thrombocytopenia in pregnancy is frequently gestational. Surgery is reserved for the failure of medical management and associated with a fetal mortality of 31%.[105] Though laparoscopic cholecystectomy has been shown to be safe in the second trimester of pregnancy, results of laparoscopic splenectomy in this rare patient population have not been reported.

Initially, splenomegaly was thought to be an absolute contraindication to the laparoscopic approach. Increasing experience and improvement of surgical devices have made this a relative contraindication. Splenic size and surgeon experience are the determining factors. Though technically feasible, laparoscopic splenectomy in the patient with splenomegaly can be a challenge. The introduction of hand-assisted laparoscopic surgery has led some surgeons to approach these larger spleens with outcomes similar to the totally laparoscopic approach.[106]

The laparoscopic technique may be performed with the patient in the supine (or modified lithotomy) position[107] or in the right lateral decubitus position.[108] After induction of general anesthesia and endotracheal intubation, a nasogastric tube and a urinary catheter are inserted, and pneumatic compression stockings are applied. Appropriate patient positioning is of paramount importance to the successful completion of a laparoscopic splenectomy. With either the lateral or the supine approach, the patient is placed so that the kidney rest can be raised to maximize the space between the iliac crest and the costal margin. The patient is positioned so that the table may be flexed to create a wider working space. The patient is then placed in a reverse Trendelenburg position to facilitate gravity retraction of the viscera away from the left upper quadrant.

In the supine approach, the surgeon stands to the left of the patient, and the first assistant and camera assistants stand to the right.[97] It is often easier for a right-handed surgeon to work from a position between the patient's legs, with the patient in a modified lithotomy position. The scrub nurse stands to the patient's left side near the foot of the table. Alternatively, the patient may be placed on a beanbag in a 60-degree right lateral decubitus position, with a right axillary roll. The left arm should be supported by a splint. In this approach, the surgeon and the scrub nurse stand to the patient's right, and the assistants stand to the left. The spleen is suspended from its diaphragmatic attachments, and gravity retracts the stomach, transverse colon, and greater omentum, while placing the splenic hilum under tension. For both approaches, the video monitors are placed on each side of the table, at or above the level of the patient's shoulders.

Pneumoperitoneum is established to a pressure of 12 to 15 mm Hg, and three to five 2- to 12-mm diameter operating ports are used, with the camera port at the umbilicus or offset between the umbilicus and the left costal margin. The other port sites are arrayed in the positions depicted in Figure 54-10. The operation is begun with a thorough search of the abdominal cavity for the presence

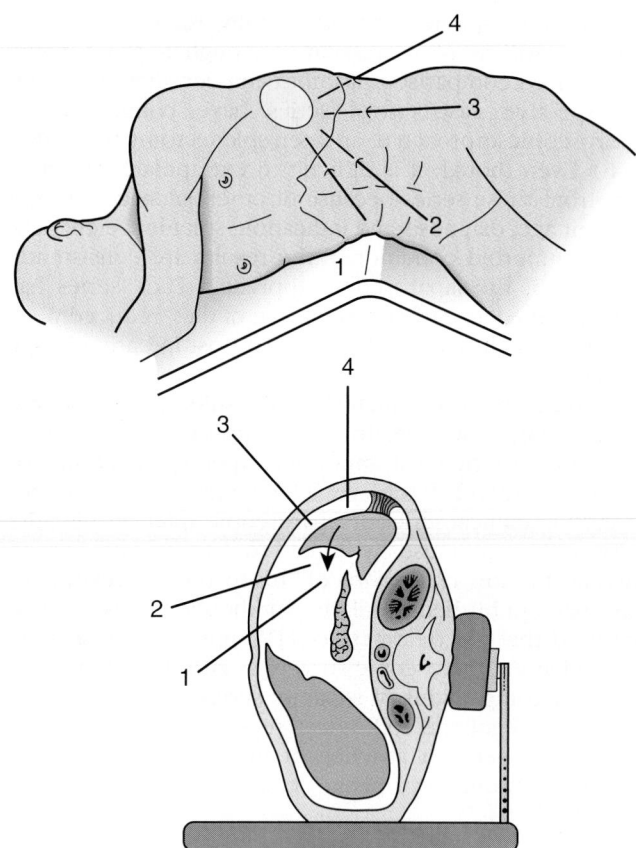

FIGURE 54-10. Strict lateral position of the patient for laparoscopic splenectomy. The table is angulated, giving forced lateral flexion of the patient to open the costophrenic space. Trocars are inserted along the left costal margin more posteriorly. The spleen is hanged by its peritoneal attachments. The numbered lines show the position of laparoscopic ports. (From Gigot JF, Lengele B, Gianello P, et al: Present status of laparoscopic splenectomy for hematologic diseases: Certitudes and unresolved issues. Semin Laparosc Surg 5:149, 1998.)

of accessory splenic tissue (Fig. 54-11). The stomach is retracted to the right to facilitate inspection of the gastrosplenic ligament. The splenocolic ligament, the greater omentum, and the phrenosplenic ligament are then carefully inspected. The small and large bowel mesenteries, the pelvis, and the adnexal tissues all should be inspected. The gastrosplenic ligament should be opened and the area of the pancreatic tail inspected.

Our preference has been to use the lateral decubitus approach.[108] The initial dissection is begun by mobilization of the splenic flexure of the colon. The splenocolic ligament is divided using sharp dissection. This mobilizes the inferior pole of the spleen and allows the spleen to be retracted cephalad. Great care is taken to avoid rupture of the splenic capsule during retraction.

The lateral peritoneal attachments of the spleen are then incised using either sharp dissection or ultrasonic shears. A 1-cm cuff of peritoneum is left along the lateral aspect of the spleen to be grasped if the spleen needs to be drawn medially. The lesser sac is entered along the medial border of the spleen. With the spleen elevated, the

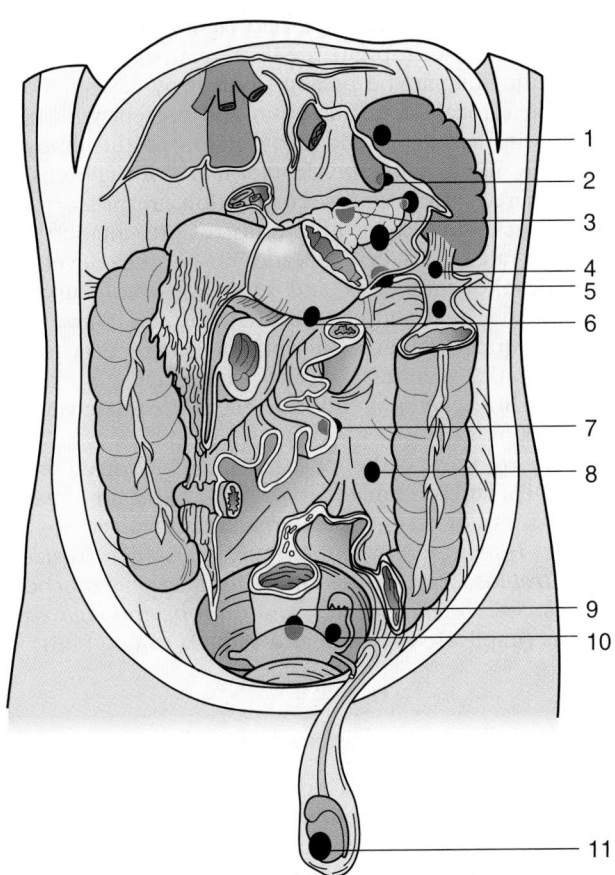

FIGURE 54-11. Usual location of accessory spleens: (1) gastrosplenic ligament, (2) splenic hilum, (3) tail of the pancreas, (4) splenocolic ligament, (5) left transverse mesocolon, (6) greater omentum along the greater curvature of the stomach, (7) mesentery, (8) left mesocolon, (9) left ovary, (10) Douglas pouch, (11) left testis. (From Gigot JF, Lengele B, Gianello P, et al: Present status of laparoscopic splenectomy for hematologic diseases: Certitudes and unresolved issues. Semin Laparosc Surg 5:156, 1998.)

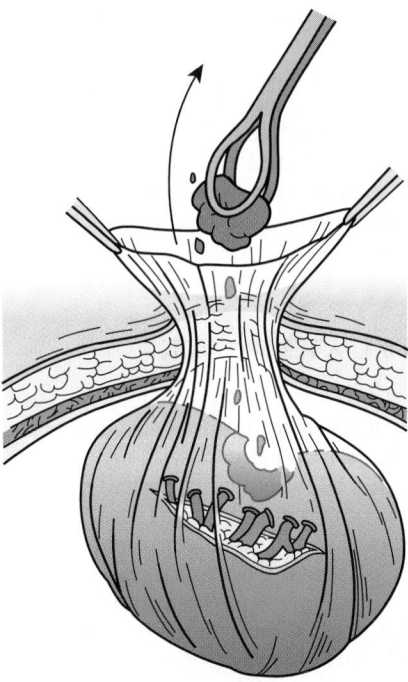

FIGURE 54-12. Extraction of the spleen within a heavy plastic bag. Instrumental morcellation of the organ with forceps. (From Gigot JF, Lengele B, Gianello P, et al: Present status of laparoscopic splenectomy for hematologic diseases: Certitudes and unresolved issues. Semin Laparosc Surg 5:154, 1998.)

short gastric vessels and main vascular pedicle are visualized. The tail of the pancreas is also visualized and avoided at this point as it approaches the splenic hilum. The short gastric vessels are divided. This can be accomplished with several different modalities as long as the surgeon has familiarity with the device and its application. Currently available instrumentation for the control of splenic vessels include ultrasonic dissector, hemoclips, bipolar devices, Ligasure, or an endovascular stapling device. The use of hemoclips should be minimized throughout the procedure and especially around the hilum because the clips may interfere with future applications of a stapling device. The stapler will not function if a clip is caught within its jaws, and this can result in significant bleeding from hilar vessels.

After the short gastric vessels have been divided, the splenic pedicle may be carefully dissected from both the medial and lateral aspects (an advantage over the anterior approach). After the artery and vein are dissected, the vessels are divided by application of endoscopic vascular staplers or suture ligatures. In the more common distributed mode, there are multiple vascular branches that enter

the spleen; these arise from the main vascular trunks about 2 to 3 cm from the hilum.[9] For this reason, we generally try to keep our dissection 2 cm from the splenic capsule. Several branches may still be encountered, however, and should be controlled individually if necessary. A pedicle formed by the artery and vein that enters the hilum as a compact bundle is known as the *magistral mode*. In this circumstance, the pedicle should be transected en bloc using a linear vascular stapler. The tail of the pancreas is well visualized as the staplers are applied to avoid injury to this structure. The surgeon should be acutely aware of the position of the tail of the pancreas during the hilar division. The pancreatic tail lies within 1 cm of the splenic hilum in 75% of patients and touches the splenic hilum in 30%.[109]

After the hilar vessels have been controlled, the completely devascularized spleen is suspended by a small cuff of avascular superior pole splenophrenic attachments. This is left in place to facilitate entrapment of the spleen into the retrieval bag. To remove the detached spleen, a puncture-resistant nylon extraction bag is introduced through one of the trocar sites, typically the left lateral site. The bag is opened within the abdominal cavity, and the spleen is placed into the bag. The drawstring is grasped and the bag is closed, leaving only the superior pole attachments to be divided at this stage. The open end of the closed bag is brought outside the abdomen through the supraumbilical or epigastric trocar site. The spleen is then morcellated with ring forceps and with finger fracture and is removed in fragments (Fig. 54-12).

In conditions requiring pathologic evaluation of an intact spleen, an incision adequate to enable removal of the bag containing the intact spleen is made. Care must be taken to avoid spillage of any fragments of spleen into either the abdominal cavity or the wound. The laparoscope is reinserted, and the splenic bed is assessed for hemostasis. At this point, drains may be placed if deemed necessary. The fascia of all trocar ports larger than 5 mm should be closed.

LATE MORBIDITY AFTER SPLENECTOMY

Postsplenectomy thrombocytosis may be associated with both hemorrhagic and thromboembolic phenomena. This occurs particularly in patients with myeloproliferative disorders such as CML, agnogenic myeloid dysplasia, essential thrombocytosis, and polycythemia vera. Thrombosis of the mesenteric, portal, and renal veins may be a life-threatening sequela of postsplenectomy thrombocytosis.[110] The lifelong risk of deep venous thrombosis and pulmonary embolism has not been well defined but may be significant. In review of 37,012 autopsies over a 20-year period, Pimpl and colleagues[65] identified 202 deceased adults who had a history of splenectomy and matched them with a cohort of 403 deceased patients who had not undergone splenectomy. Pulmonary embolism was the major or contributory cause of death more often in the splenectomy group (35.6%) than in the control group (9.7%).[65]

OPSI is among the more devastating sequelae of asplenia and is the most common fatal late complication of splenectomy.[111] Hyposplenism in the neonatal period has been suggested to contribute to the poor outcomes from neonatal sepsis. The exact incidence of OPSI has been difficult to determine. The incidence of infection in postsplenectomy patients is likely to be under-reported. In the same autopsy series by Pimpl and colleagues mentioned in the previous paragraph, lethal pneumonia was identified twice as often in autopsies of splenectomized patients than in controls (57.9% vs. 24.1%) and lethal sepsis with multiorgan failure occurred in 6.9% of splenectomized versus 1.5% of autopsies on controls.[65] One consistent observation is that the risk for OPSI is greater after splenectomy for malignancy or hematologic disease than for trauma. The risk also appears to be greater in young children (<4 years of age). The risk for fatal OPSI is estimated to be 1 per 300 to 350 patient-years follow-up for children and 1 per 800 to 1000 patient-years follow-up for adults.[112] The incidence of nonfatal infection and sepsis is likely to be significantly greater. A recent review of selected reported splenectomy series of 7872 total cases inclusive of both children and adults revealed 270 episodes of sepsis (3.5%), with 169 septic fatalities (2.1%).[113] Infection may occur at any time after splenectomy; in one recent series, most infections occurred more than 2 years after splenectomy, and 42% occurred more than 5 years after splenectomy.[114]

OPSI typically begins with a prodromal phase characterized by fever and chills and nonspecific symptoms, including sore throat, malaise, myalgias, diarrhea, and vomiting. Patients may have had rigors for 1 to 2 days before seeking appropriate medical treatment. Pneumonia and meningitis may be present, but many cases have no identifiable focal site of infection and present with high-grade primary bacteremia. Progression of the illness is classically rapid, with the development of hypotension, disseminated intravascular coagulation, respiratory distress, coma, and death within hours of presentation. The mortality rate is between 50% and 70% for fully developed OPSI despite antibiotics and intensive care. Survivors often have a long and complicated hospital course with severe sequelae, such as peripheral gangrene requiring amputation, deafness from meningitis, mastoid osteomyelitis, bacterial endocarditis, and cardiac valvular destruction.

S. pneumoniae is the most frequently involved organism in OPSI and is estimated to be responsible for between 50% and 90% of cases. Other organisms involved in OPSI include *Haemophilus influenzae*, *Neisseria meningitidis*, *Streptococcus* species and other than pneumococcal species, *Salmonella* species, and *Capnocytophaga canimorsus* (implicated in OPSI as a sequela of dog bites).

Prophylactic Treatment of Splenectomized Patients

The spleen is important for generating responses to thymus-independent antigens. In elective procedures, immunization should be administered before splenectomy whenever possible; the Advisory Committee on Immunization Practices has recommended that the immunization precede splenectomy by at least 2 weeks.[115] Presplenectomy immunization is not possible in cases of splenic trauma. The immunizations should be administered to these patients during the hospitalization in which their splenectomy occurred rather than waiting until they return for a follow-up visit. Many of these patients become lost to follow-up, and clinical studies have demonstrated adequate antibody response to immediate immunization.[116,117] High-risk patients without spleens should be considered for revaccination if they received the earlier 14-valent vaccine rather than the more current 23-valent preparation or if more than 3 to 6 years have elapsed since primary immunization.[117] Simultaneous immunization with *H. influenzae* type b, meningococcal serogroup C, and polyvalent pneumococcal vaccine is both immunogenic and well tolerated. Unfortunately, rare cases of OPSI have been reported in vaccinated patients.

Penicillin prophylaxis is commonly practiced in children during the first few years after splenectomy, and some authorities have advocated this form of prophylaxis in adults, although data showing the efficacy of this treatment are lacking. OPSI has been reported in both adults and children taking prophylactic penicillin, despite penicillin-sensitive pneumococci infection.[112] Available data do not support the practice of long-term penicillin prophylaxis in asplenic adults. Another approach that appears rational is to provide the asplenic patient with a supply of oral antibiotics, such as amoxicillin, with instructions to begin taking the medication at the onset of rigor or a febrile illness if appropriate medical evaluation is not immediately available. Fever and rigor in an asplenic patient should prompt immediate aggressive, empirical treatment with antibiotic coverage, even in the absence of culture data.

Selected References

Advisory Committee on Immunization Practices: Prevention of pneumococcal disease: Recommendations of the Advisory Committee on Immunization Practices (ACIP). MMWR Morb Mortal Wkly Rep 46:1-24, 1997.

> This report of the Advisory Committee on Immunization Practices provides a summary of the epidemiology of pneumococcal infections as well as treatment and prophylaxis recommendations. Groups at high risk are discussed in detail, including patients who have undergone splenectomy.

Bohnsack JF, Brown EJ: The role of the spleen in resistance to infection. Annu Rev Med 37:49-59, 1986.

> This is a comprehensive review of the roles played by the spleen in protection from infection. The roles of opsonins and splenic bacterial clearance are well covered.

George JN, Woolf SH, Raskob GE, et al: Idiopathic thrombocytopenic purpura: A practice guideline developed by explicit methods for the American Society of Hematology. Blood 88:3-40, 1996.

> This report comprehensively summarizes the practice guideline recommendations for the treatment of idiopathic thrombocytopenic purpura (ITP) as established by the American Society of Hematology in 1994. This comprehensive review provides the evidence for the current treatment recommendations and the data for treatment outcomes for children and adults with ITP.

Gigot JF, Lengele B, Gianello P, et al: Present status of laparoscopic splenectomy for hematologic diseases: Certitudes and unresolved issues. Semin Laparosc Surg 5:147-167, 1998.

> Gigot and colleagues nicely summarized the published experience on the role of laparoscopic splenectomy in the management of hematologic disorders. The authors provide useful technical tips for the practicing surgeon.

Katkhouda N, Hurwitz MB, Rivera RT, et al: Laparoscopic splenectomy: Outcome and efficacy in 103 consecutive patients. Ann Surg 228:568-578, 1998.

> Katkhouda and colleagues show the safety and efficacy of laparoscopic splenectomy in a large series of patients. The discussion section of this article provides an extensive review of previously published series and provides helpful tables comparing the outcomes of open versus laparoscopic splenectomy.

Schwartz SI: Role of splenectomy in hematologic disorders. World J Surg 20:1156-1159, 1996.

> This review is by one of the recognized surgical authorities on splenic diseases and their management. This is a comprehensive review of the role of splenectomy in hematologic disorders.

Styrt B: Infection associated with asplenia: Risks, mechanisms, and prevention. Am J Med 88:5-33N, 1990.

> This is an excellent review of the risks, mechanisms, and prevention of infections that are associated with the condition of asplenia. The mechanisms by which the spleen protects from certain infectious organisms are well covered. Data regarding the level of risk to asplenic patients are provided. Specific recommendations regarding antibiotic and vaccine prophylaxis are also provided.

References

1. Groom AC: The Microcirculatory Society Eugene M. Landis Award Lecture: Microcirculation of the spleen—new concepts, new challenges. Microvasc Res 34:269-289, 1987.
2. Horton J, Ogden ME, Williams S, et al: The importance of splenic blood flow in clearing pneumococcal organisms. Ann Surg 195:172-176, 1982.
3. Drew PA, Kiroff GK, Ferrante A, et al: Alterations in immunoglobulin synthesis by peripheral blood mononuclear cells from splenectomized patients with and without splenic regrowth. J Immunol 132:191-196, 1984.
4. Bohnsack JF, Brown EJ: The role of the spleen in resistance to infection. Annu Rev Med 37:49-59, 1986.
5. Foster PN, Bolton RP, Cotter KL, et al: Defective activation of neutrophils after splenectomy. J Clin Pathol 38:1175-1178, 1985.
6. George JN, el-Harake MA, Raskob GE: Chronic idiopathic thrombocytopenic purpura. N Engl J Med 331:1207-1211, 1994.
7. George JN, Woolf SH, Raskob GE, et al: Idiopathic thrombocytopenic purpura: A practice guideline developed by explicit methods for the American Society of Hematology. Blood 88:3-40, 1996.
8. Gigot JF, Jamar F, Ferrant A, et al: Inadequate detection of accessory spleens and splenosis with laparoscopic splenectomy: A shortcoming of the laparoscopic approach in hematologic diseases. Surg Endosc 12:101-106, 1998.
9. Katkhouda N, Hurwitz MB, Rivera RT, et al: Laparoscopic splenectomy: Outcome and efficacy in 103 consecutive patients. Ann Surg 228:568-578, 1998.
10. Tsoukas CM, Bernard NF, Abrahamowicz M, et al: Effect of splenectomy on slowing human immunodeficiency virus disease progression. Arch Surg 133:25-31, 1998.
11. Croom RD III, McMillan CW, Orringer EP, et al: Hereditary spherocytosis: Recent experience and current concepts of pathophysiology. Ann Surg 203:34-39, 1986.
12. Schwartz SI: Role of splenectomy in hematologic disorders. World J Surg 20:1156-1159, 1996.
13. Schwartz LH, Ginsberg MS, Burt ME, et al: MRI as an alternative to CT-guided biopsy of adrenal masses in patients with lung cancer. Ann Thorac Surg 65:193-197, 1998.
14. al-Salem AH, Qaisaruddin S, Nasserallah Z, et al: Splenectomy in patients with sickle cell disease. Am J Surg 172:254-258, 1996.
15. al-Salem AH: The role of splenectomy in patients with sickle cell disease. Ann Saudi Med 17:1997.
16. Badaloo AV, Singhal A, Forrester TE, et al: The effect of splenectomy for hypersplenism on whole-body protein turnover, resting metabolic rate, and growth in sickle cell disease. Eur J Clin Nutr 50:672-675, 1996.
17. Taylor MA, Kaplan HS, Nelsen TS: Staging laparotomy with splenectomy for Hodgkin's disease: The Stanford experience. World J Surg 9:449-460, 1985.

18. Brodsky J, Abcar A, Styler M: Splenectomy for non-Hodgkin's lymphoma. Am J Clin Oncol 19:558-561, 1996.

19. Morel P, Dupriez B, Gosselin B, et al: Role of early splenectomy in malignant lymphomas with prominent splenic involvement (primary lymphomas of the spleen): A study of 59 cases. Cancer 71:207-215, 1993.

20. Au WY, Klasa RJ, Gallagher R, et al: Second malignancies in patients with hairy cell leukemia in British Columbia: A 20-year experience. Blood 92:1160-1164, 1998.

21. Golomb HM, Ratain MJ: Recent advances in the treatment of hairy cell leukemia. N Engl J Med 316:870-872, 1987.

22. Gollard R, Lee TC, Piro LD, et al: The optimal management of hairy cell leukaemia. Drugs 49:921-931, 1995.

23. Saven A, Burian C, Koziol JA, et al: Long-term follow-up of patients with hairy cell leukemia after cladribine treatment. Blood 92:1918-1926, 1998.

24. Montserrat E: Chronic lymphoproliferative disorders. Curr Opin Oncol 9:34-41, 1997.

25. Rai KR, Sawitsky A, Cronkite EP, et al: Clinical staging of chronic lymphocytic leukemia. Blood 46:219-234, 1975.

26. Cusack JC Jr, Seymour JF, Lerner S, et al: Role of splenectomy in chronic lymphocytic leukemia. J Am Coll Surg 185:237-243, 1997.

27. Seymour JF, Cusack JD, Lerner SA, et al: Case/control study of the role of splenectomy in chronic lymphocytic leukemia. J Clin Oncol 15:52-60, 1997.

28. Khouri I, Sanchez FG, Deisseroth A: Leukemias. In DeVita VT Jr, Hellman S, Rosenberg SA (eds): Cancer: Principles and Practice of Oncology, 5th ed. Philadelphia, Lippincott-Raven, 1997, pp 2285-2321.

29. Bouvet M, Babiera GV, Termuhlen PM, et al: Splenectomy in the accelerated or blastic phase of chronic myelogenous leukemia: A single-institution, 25-year experience. Surgery 122:20-25, 1997.

30. Medical Research Council's Working Part for Therapeutic Trials in Leukaemia: Randomized trial of splenectomy in P$_H$1-positive chronic granulocytic leukaemia, including an analysis of prognostic features. Br J Haematol 54:415-430, 1983.

31. The Italian Cooperative Study Group on Chronic Myeloid Leukemia: Results of a prospective randomized trial of early splenectomy in chronic myeloid leukemia. Cancer 54:333-338, 1984.

32. Gratwohl A, Goldman J, Gluckman E, et al: Effect of splenectomy before bone marrow transplantation on survival in chronic granulocytic leukaemia. Lancet 2:1290-1291, 1985.

33. Morgenstern L, Rosenberg J, Geller SA: Tumors of the spleen. World J Surg 9:468-476, 1985.

34. Feigenberg Z, Wysenbeek A, Avidor E, et al: Malignant lymphangioma of the spleen. Isr J Med Sci 19:202-204, 1983.

35. Sardi A, Ojeda HF, King D Jr: Laparoscopic resection of a benign true cyst of the spleen with the harmonic scalpel producing high levels of CA 19–9 and carcinoembryonic antigen. Am Surg 64:1149-1154, 1998.

36. Tsakayannis DE, Mitchell K, Kozakewich HP, et al: Splenic preservation in the management of splenic epidermoid cysts in children. J Pediatr Surg 30:1468-1470, 1995.

37. Goldthorn JF, Schwartz AD, Swift AJ, et al: Protective effect of residual splenic tissue after subtotal splenectomy. J Pediatr Surg 13:587-590, 1978.

38. Touloukian RJ, Maharaj A, Ghoussoub R, et al: Partial decapsulation of splenic epithelial cysts: Studies on etiology and outcome. J Pediatr Surg 32:272-274, 1997.

39. Little JM, Deane SA: Hydatid disease. In Blumgart LH (ed): Surgery of the Liver and Biliary Tract. Edinburgh, Churchill Livingstone, 1988, pp 955-966.

40. Pachter HL, Hofstetter SR, Elkowitz A, et al: Traumatic cysts of the spleen—the role of cystectomy and splenic preservation: Experience with seven consecutive patients. J Trauma 35:430-436, 1993.

41. Gadacz TR: Splenic abscess. World J Surg 9:410-415, 1985.

42. Alonso Cohen MA, Galera MJ, Ruiz M, et al: Splenic abscess. World J Surg 14:513-517, 1990.

43. Wolff MJ, Bitran J, Northland RG, et al: Splenic abscesses due to Mycobacterium tuberculosis in patients with AIDS. Rev Infect Dis 13:373-375, 1991.

44. Faught WE, Gilbertson JJ, Nelson EW: Splenic abscess: Presentation, treatment options, and results. Am J Surg 158:612-614, 1989.

45. Keidl CM, Chusid MJ: Splenic abscesses in childhood. Pediatr Infect Dis J 8:368-373, 1989.

46. van der Laan RT, Verbeeten B Jr, Smits NJ, et al: Computed tomography in the diagnosis and treatment of solitary splenic abscesses. J Comput Assist Tomogr 13:71-74, 1989.

47. Gleich S, Wolin DA, Herbsman H: A review of percutaneous drainage in splenic abscess. Surg Gynecol Obstet 167:211-216, 1988.

48. Gayer G, Zissin R, Apter S, et al: CT findings in congenital anomalies of the spleen. Br J Radiol 74:767-772, 2001.

49. Sayeed S, Koniaris LG, Kovach SJ, et al: Torsion of a wandering spleen. Surgery 132:535-536, 2002.

50. Ahmad W, Polk HC Jr: Blunt abdominal trauma: A study of relationship between diagnosis and outcome. South Med J 66:1127-1130, 1973.

51. Engrav LH, Benjamin CI, Strate RG, et al: Diagnostic peritoneal lavage in blunt abdominal trauma. J Trauma 15:854-859, 1975.

52. Olsen WR, Redman HC, Hildreth DH: Quantitative peritoneal lavage in blunt abdominal trauma. Arch Surg 104:536-543, 1972.

53. Perry JF Jr, Strate RG: Diagnostic peritoneal lavage in blunt abdominal trauma: Indications and results. Surgery 71:898-901, 1972.

54. West JG, Trunkey DD, Lim RC: Systems of trauma care: A study of two counties. Arch Surg 114:455-460, 1979.

55. Root HD, Hauser CW, McKinely CR: Diagnostic peritoneal lavage. Surgery 57:633-637, 1965.

56. Federle MP, Crass RA, Jeffrey RB, et al: Computed tomography in blunt abdominal trauma. Arch Surg 117:645-650, 1982.

57. Moore EE, Cogbill TH, Jurkovich GJ, et al: Organ injury scaling: Spleen and liver (1994 revision). J Trauma 38:323-324, 1995.

58. Aufschnaiter M, Kofler H: Sonographic acute diagnosis in polytrauma. Aktuelle Traumatol 13:55-57, 1983.

59. Halbfass HJ, Wimmer B, Hauenstein K, et al: Ultrasonic diagnosis of blunt abdominal injuries. Fortschr Med 99:1681-1685, 1981.

60. Hauenstein KH, Wimmer B, Billmann P, et al: Sonography of blunt abdominal trauma (author's transl). Radiologe 22:106-111, 1982.

61. Tso P, Rodriguez A, Cooper C, et al: Sonography in blunt abdominal trauma: A preliminary progress report. J Trauma 33:39-44, 1992.

62. Bode PJ, Niezen RA, van Vugt AB, et al: Abdominal ultrasound as a reliable indicator for conclusive laparotomy in blunt abdominal trauma. J Trauma 34:27-31, 1993.

63. Rothlin MA, Naf R, Amgwerd M, et al: Ultrasound in blunt abdominal and thoracic trauma. J Trauma 34:488-495, 1993.

64. Branney SW, Moore EE, Cantrill SV, et al: Ultrasound-based key clinical pathway reduces the use of hospital resources

for the evaluation of blunt abdominal trauma. J Trauma 42:1086-1090, 1997.

65. Pimpl W, Dapunt O, Kaindl H, et al: Incidence of septic and thromboembolic-related deaths after splenectomy in adults. Br J Surg 76:517-521, 1989.

66. Rogers FB, Baumgartner NE, Robin AP, et al: Absorbable-mesh splenorrhaphy for severe splenic injuries: Functional studies in an animal model and an additional patient series. J Trauma 31:200-204, 1991.

67. Powell M, Courcoulas A, Gardner M, et al: Management of blunt splenic trauma: Significant differences between adults and children. Surgery 122:654-660, 1997.

68. Davis KA, Fabian TC, Croce MA, et al: Improved success in nonoperative management of blunt splenic injuries: Embolization of splenic artery pseudoaneurysms. J Trauma 44:1008-1015, 1998.

69. Sutyak JP, Chiu WC, D'Amelio LF, et al: Computed tomography is inaccurate in estimating the severity of adult splenic injury. J Trauma 39:514-518, 1995.

70. Cocanour CS, Moore FA, Arteaga BS: Age should not be a consideration for nonoperative management of blunt splenic injury. J Trauma 47:220, 1999.

71. Myers JG, Dent DL, Stewart RM: Nonoperative management of blunt splenic injuries: Dedicated trauma surgeons can achieve a high rate of success in patients of all ages [Abstract]. J Trauma 47:220, 1999.

72. Shackford SR, Molin M: Management of splenic injuries. Surg Clin North Am 70:595-620, 1990.

73. Smith JS Jr, Cooney RN, Mucha P Jr: Nonoperative management of the ruptured spleen: A revalidation of criteria. Surgery 120:745-750; discussion 750-741, 1996.

74. Morrell DG, Chang FC, Helmer SD: Changing trends in the management of splenic injury. Am J Surg 170:686-690, 1995.

75. Schurr MJ, Fabian TC, Gavant M, et al: Management of blunt splenic trauma: Computed tomographic contrast blush predicts failure of nonoperative management. J Trauma 39:507-513, 1995.

76. Myers LK, Tang B, Rosloniec EF, et al: Characterization of a peptide analog of a determinant of type II collagen that suppresses collagen-induced arthritis. J Immunol 161:3589-3595, 1998.

77. Bee TK, Croce MA, Miller PR, et al: Failures of splenic nonoperative management: Is the glass half empty or half full? J Trauma 50:230-236, 2001.

78. Agency for Health Care Policy and Research: Interim Manual for Clinical Practice Guideline Development. Rockville, MD, U.S. Department of Health and Human Services, Public Health Service, 1991.

79. Carroll BJ, Phillips EH, Semel CJ, et al: Laparoscopic splenectomy. Surg Endosc 6:183-185, 1992.

80. Delaitre B, Maignien B: Laparoscopic splenectomy—technical aspects. Surg Endosc 6:305-308, 1992.

81. Thibault C, Mamazza J, Letourneau R, et al: Laparoscopic splenectomy: Operative technique and preliminary report. Surg Laparosc Endosc 2:248-253, 1992.

82. Friedman RL, Hiatt JR, Korman JL, et al: Laparoscopic or open splenectomy for hematologic disease: Which approach is superior? J Am Coll Surg 185:49-54, 1997.

83. Gigot JF, Lengele B, Gianello P, et al: Present status of laparoscopic splenectomy for hematologic diseases: Certitudes and unresolved issues. Semin Laparosc Surg 5:147-167, 1998.

84. Berchtold P, McMillan R: Therapy of chronic idiopathic thrombocytopenic purpura in adults. Blood 74:2309-2317, 1989.

85. Chirletti P, Cardi M, Barillari P, et al: Surgical treatment of immune thrombocytopenic purpura. World J Surg 16:1001-1005, 1992.

86. Coon WW: Splenectomy for idiopathic thrombocytopenic purpura. Surg Gynecol Obstet 164:225-229, 1987.

87. Dawson AA, Jones PF, King DJ: Splenectomy in the management of haematological disease. Br J Surg 74:353-357, 1987.

88. Eraklis AJ, Filler RM: Splenectomy in childhood: A review of 1413 cases. J Pediatr Surg 7:382-388, 1972.

89. Musser G, Lazar G, Hocking W, et al: Splenectomy for hematologic disease: The UCLA experience with 306 patients. Ann Surg 200:40-45, 1984.

90. Naouri A, Feghali B, Chabal J, et al: Results of splenectomy for idiopathic thrombocytopenic purpura: Review of 72 cases. Acta Haematol 89:200-203, 1993.

91. Danforth DN Jr, Fraker DL: Splenectomy for the massively enlarged spleen. Am Surg 57:108-113, 1991.

92. Goldstone J: Splenectomy for massive splenomegaly. Am J Surg 135:385-388, 1978.

93. Schwartz SI, Bernard RP, Adams JT, et al: Splenectomy for hematologic disorders. Arch Surg 101:338-347, 1970.

94. Friedman RL, Fallas MJ, Carroll BJ, et al: Laparoscopic splenectomy for ITP: The gold standard. Surg Endosc 10:991-995, 1996.

95. Legrand MJ, Honore P, Joris J, et al: Techniques of laparoscopic morcellation of the spleen. Minim Invasive Ther Allied Tech 5:143-146, 1996.

96. Yee JC, Akpata MO: Laparoscopic splenectomy for congenital spherocytosis with splenomegaly: A case report. Can J Surg 38:73-76, 1995.

97. Flowers JL, Lefor AT, Steers J, et al: Laparoscopic splenectomy in patients with hematologic diseases. Ann Surg 224:19-28, 1996.

98. Bove T, Delvaux G, Van Eijkelenburg P, et al: Laparoscopic-assisted surgery of the spleen: Clinical experience in expanding indications. J Laparoendosc Surg 6:213-217, 1996.

99. Decker G, Millat B, Guillon F, et al: Laparoscopic splenectomy for benign and malignant hematologic diseases—35 consecutive cases. World J Surg 22:62-68, 1998.

100. Trias M, Targarona EM, Balague C: Laparoscopic splenectomy—an evolving technique: A comparison between anterior and lateral approaches. Surg Endosc 10:389-392, 1996.

101. Trias M, Targarona EM, Espert JJ, et al: Laparoscopic surgery for splenic disorders: Lessons learned from a series of 64 cases. Surg Endosc 12:66-72, 1998.

102. Delaitre B, Pitre J: Laparoscopic splenectomy versus open splenectomy: A comparative study. Hepatogastroenterology 44:45-49, 1997.

103. Glasgow RE, Yee LF, Mulvihill SJ: Laparoscopic splenectomy: The emerging standard. Surg Endosc 11:108-112, 1997.

104. Katkhouda N, Mavor E: Laparoscopic splenectomy. Surg Clin North Am 80:1285-1297, 2000.

105. Moise KJ Jr: Autoimmune thrombocytopenic purpura in pregnancy. Clin Obstet Gynecol 34:51-63, 1991.

106. Romanelli JR, Kelly JJ, Litwin DE: Hand-assisted laparoscopic surgery in the United States: An overview. Semin Laparosc Surg 8:96-103, 2001.

107. Phillips EH, Carroll BJ, Rosenthal RJ: Laparoscopic splenectomy. In Cameron J (ed): Current Surgical Therapy. St. Louis, CV Mosby, 1995.

108. Park A, Gagner M, Pomp A: The lateral approach to laparoscopic splenectomy. Am J Surg 173:126-130, 1997.

109. Michels NA: The variational anatomy of the spleen and the splenic artery. Am J Anat 70:21-72, 1942.

110. Gordon DH, Schaffner D, Bennett JM, et al: Postsplenectomy thrombocytosis: Its association with mesenteric, portal, and/or renal vein thrombosis in patients with myeloproliferative disorders. Arch Surg 113:713-715, 1978.

111. Horowitz J, Smith JL, Weber TK, et al: Postoperative complications after splenectomy for hematologic malignancies. Ann Surg 223:290-296, 1996.

112. Styrt B: Infection associated with asplenia: Risks, mechanisms, and prevention. Am J Med 88:33N-42N, 1990.

113. Hansen K, Singer DB: Asplenic-hyposplenic overwhelming sepsis: Postsplenectomy sepsis revisited. Pediatr Dev Pathol 4:105-121, 2001.

114. Cullingford GL, Watkins DN, Watts AD, et al: Severe late postsplenectomy infection. Br J Surg 78:716-721, 1991.

115. Advisory Committee on Immunization Practices: Prevention of pneumococcal disease: Recommendations of the Advisory Committee on Immunization Practices (ACIP). MMWR Morb Mortal Wkly Rep 46:1-24, 1997.

116. Caplan ES, Boltansky H, Snyder MJ, et al: Response of traumatized splenectomized patients to immediate vaccination with polyvalent pneumococcal vaccine. J Trauma 23:801-805, 1983.

117. Rutherford EJ, Livengood J, Higginbotham M, et al: Efficacy and safety of pneumococcal revaccination after splenectomy for trauma. J Trauma 39:448-452, 1995.

118. Cadiere GB, Verroken R, Himpens J, et al: Operative strategy in laparoscopic splenectomy. J Am Coll Surg 179:668-672, 1994.

119. Emmermann A, Zornig C, Peiper M, et al: Laparoscopic splenectomy: Technique and results in a series of 27 cases. Surg Endosc 9:924-927, 1995.

120. Poulin EC, Thibault C, Mamazza J: Laparoscopic splenectomy (see Discussion). Surg Endosc 9:172-177, 1995.

121. Brunt LM, Langer JC, Quasebarth MA, et al: Comparative analysis of laparoscopic versus open splenectomy. Am J Surg 172:596-601, 1996.

122. Gigot JF, de Ville de Goyet J, Van Beers BE, et al: Laparoscopic splenectomy in adults and children: Experience with 31 patients. Surgery 119:384-389, 1996.

123. Smith CD, Meyer TA, Goretsky MJ, et al: Laparoscopic splenectomy by the lateral approach: A safe and effective alternative to open splenectomy for hematologic diseases. Surgery 120:789-794, 1996.

124. Tsiotos G, Schlinkert RT: Laparoscopic splenectomy for immune thrombocytopenic purpura. Arch Surg 132:642-646, 1997.

125. DiFino SM, Lachant NA, Kirshner JJ, et al: Adult idiopathic thrombocytopenic purpura: Clinical findings and response to therapy. Am J Med 69:430-442, 1980.

126. Mintz SJ, Petersen SR, Cheson B, et al: Splenectomy for immune thrombocytopenic purpura. Arch Surg 116:645-650, 1981.

127. Jacobs P, Wood L, Dent DM: Results of treatment in immune thrombocytopenia. Q J Med 58:153-165, 1986.

128. Akwari OE, Itani KM, Coleman RE, et al: Splenectomy for primary and recurrent immune thrombocytopenic purpura (ITP): Current criteria for patient selection and results. Ann Surg 206:529-541, 1987.

129. Julia A, Araguas C, Rossello J, et al: Lack of useful clinical predictors of response to splenectomy in patients with chronic idiopathic thrombocytopenic purpura. Br J Haematol 76:250-255, 1990.

130. Yee LF, Carvajal SH, de Lorimier AA, et al: Laparoscopic splenectomy: The initial experience at University of California, San Francisco (see Discussion). Arch Surg 130:874-879, 1995.

131. Rhodes M, Rudd M, O'Rourke N, et al: Laparoscopic splenectomy and lymph node biopsy for hematologic disorders. Ann Surg 222:43-46, 1995.

132. Watson DI, Coventry BJ, Chin T, et al: Laparoscopic versus open splenectomy for immune thrombocytopenic purpura. Surgery 121:18-22, 1997.

133. Diaz J, Eisenstat M, Chung R: A case-controlled study of laparoscopic splenectomy. Am J Surg 173:348-350, 1997.

134. Hashizume M, Ohta M, Kishihara F, et al: Laparoscopic splenectomy for idiopathic thrombocytopenic purpura: Comparison of laparoscopic surgery and conventional open surgery. Surg Laparosc Endosc 6:129-135, 1996.

135. Liew SC, Storey DW: Laparoscopic splenectomy. Aust N Z J Surg 65:743-745, 1995.

136. Parent S, Bresler L, Tortuyaux JM, et al: Splenectomy under celioscopy. Ann Chir 49:477-481, 1995.

137. Dexter SP, Martin IG, Alao D, et al: Laparoscopic splenectomy: The suspended pedicle technique. Surg Endosc 10:393-396, 1996.

138. Zamir O, Szold A, Matzner Y, et al: Laparoscopic splenectomy for immune thrombocytopenic purpura. J Laparoendosc Surg 6:301-304, 1996.

139. Katkhouda N, Waldrop DJ, Feinstein D, et al: Unresolved issues in laparoscopic splenectomy. Am J Surg 172:585-590, 1996.

140. Lee WJ, Kim BR: Laparoscopic splenectomy for chronic idiopathic thrombocytopenic purpura. Surg Laparosc Endosc 7:209-212, 1997.

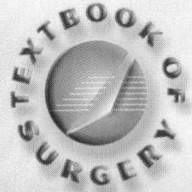

CHAPTER 55

CHEST WALL AND PLEURA

Jeanne M. Lukanich, M.D. and **David J. Sugarbaker, M.D.**

Historical Perspectives	Pleura
Chest Wall	

HISTORICAL PERSPECTIVES

Chest wall abscesses, tumors, and trauma were described as long ago as 2900 BC in the *Edwin Smith Surgical Papyrus.* Later, drainage of empyema and penetrating chest wall trauma and their sequelae were recorded.[1,2] However, the modern treatment of diseases of the chest wall and pleura would await several important medical developments and discoveries. The understanding of ventilatory physiology was of foremost importance. Forced respiration through the trachea was practiced for respiratory arrest such as drowning or morphine poisoning in the 19th century. The first working iron lung was developed in 1876 by Wille for negative-pressure ventilation. Techniques for positive-pressure ventilation by tracheal intubation were described in the early 1900s but were not used clinically until much later in the century. Roentgen's discovery of the x-ray in 1895 was crucial for diagnosis because of limitations in clinical examination. During World War I, experience with open incision for empyema secondary to influenza led to physiologic studies by the Empyema Commission, which defined the problem of open pneumothorax and its consequences.[3] On the basis of these studies, closed aspiration or drainage of the pleural space, which prevented the introduction of air, was developed. Over the next 50 years, surgery of the thorax became commonplace. The discovery and development of antibiotics during World War II, as well as advances in anesthesiology, greatly lessened the morbidity and mortality of transpleural procedures and operations. Basic thoracic surgical techniques primarily focused on the treatment of pulmonary and pleural tuberculosis and suppurative diseases of the chest wall, pleura, and lung. Variations of these techniques are still widely employed today. Most recently, in the 1990s, the introduction of thoracoscopy into the specialty has altered the standard of practice in the treatment of diseases of the chest wall and pleura.

CHEST WALL

Anatomy

The thorax is a rigid, noncollapsible structural frame that houses and protects the thoracic organs and supports the upper extremities. Owing to specialized mechanics that allow for limited expansion, it provides for ventilation and phonation. The bony thorax consists of 12 paired ribs, multiple cartilages, and the sternum and clavicles arranged about the thoracic vertebrae. The ribs and sternum determine the size and shape of the thoracic cavity. The upper seven ribs (numbered 1 to 7) are true ribs because they articulate directly with the sternum by means of cartilages. The lower five ribs (numbered 8 to 12) are false ribs; they do not directly connect to the sternum anteriorly but, in most cases, connect with the costocartilage above them. Ribs 11 and 12 are floating ribs. They can be diminutive or large; they articulate only with the thoracic spine. Each rib is composed of a head, neck, and shaft. Each head has an upper facet, which articulates with the vertebral body above it, and a lower facet, which articulates with the corresponding thoracic vertebra to that rib, establishing the costovertebral joint. The neck of the rib has a tubercle with an articular facet; this articulates with the transverse process, creating the costotransverse joint and imparting strength to the posterior rib cage.

The sternum is a flat bone, 15 to 20 cm in length, divided superiorly to inferiorly into the manubrium, body, and xiphoid. The manubrium articulates with the clavicles and first costal cartilage at its rostral aspect. The manubrium joins the body of the sternum at the angle of Louis, which corresponds to the anterior aspect of the junction of the second rib. The anterior cartilaginous attachments of the true ribs to the sternum, along with intercostal muscles and the hemidiaphragms, allow for movement of the ribs with respiration.

Beneath skin and subcutaneous tissue, the bony thorax is covered by three groups of muscles: the primary and secondary muscles for respiration and those attaching the upper extremity to the body. The primary muscles include the diaphragm and intercostal muscles. The intercostal muscles of the intercostal spaces include the external, internal, and transverse or innermost muscles. Eleven intercostal spaces, each associated numerically with the rib superior to it, contain the intercostal bundles (vein, artery, and nerve) that travel along the lower edge of each rib. All intercostal spaces are wider anteriorly, and each intercostal bundle falls away from the rib posteriorly to become more centrally located within each space.

The secondary muscles consist of the sternocleidomastoid, the serratus posterior, and the levatores costarum. The third muscle group attaches the upper extremity to the body. The pectoralis major and minor muscles lie anteriorly and superficially. Posterior superfi-cial musculature includes the trapezius and latissimus dorsi. Deep muscles include the serratus anterior and posterior, the levatores, and the major and minor rhomboids. These superficial and deep muscles help to hold the scapulae to the chest wall (Fig. 55-1).[4] In respiratory distress, the deltoid, pectoralis, and latissimus dorsi muscles form a tertiary system for ventilatory assistance through fixation of the upper extremities.[4]

Chest Wall Deformities

Infants and children present with a wide range of congenital chest wall deformities (Box 55-1). Although most of these young patients are asymptomatic, some defects can be life threatening and may be associated with other congenital malformations.

Depression Deformities (Pectus Excavatum)

Pectus excavatum (also called funnel chest) is the most common chest wall deformity, occurring in 1 of 400 children. Males are affected more frequently than females (4:1). Although a familial predisposition is not confirmed,

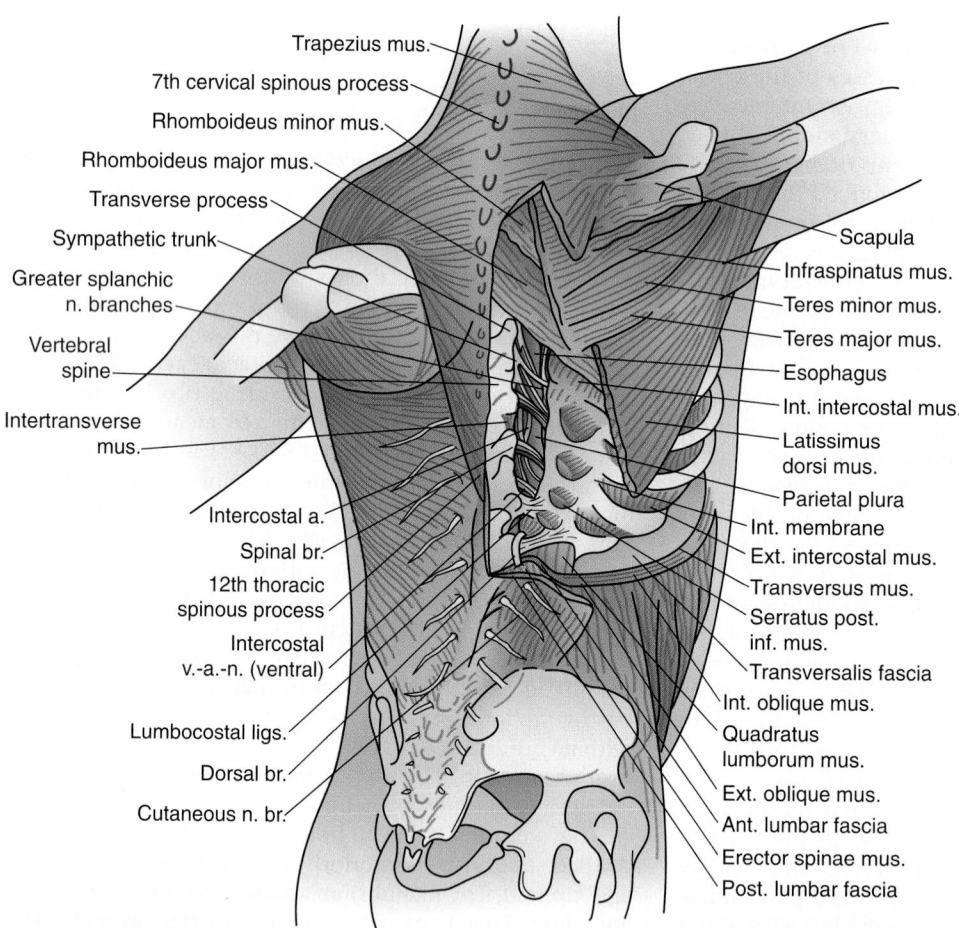

FIGURE 55-1. Musculature of the chest wall. (From Ravitch MM, Steichen FM: Atlas of General Thoracic Surgery. Philadelphia, WB Saunders, 1988.)

Trapezius mus.
7th cervical spinous process
Rhomboideus minor mus.
Rhomboideus major mus.
Transverse process
Sympathetic trunk
Greater splanchic n. branches
Vertebral spine
Intertransverse mus.
Intercostal a.
Spinal br.
12th thoracic spinous process
Intercostal v.-a.-n. (ventral)
Lumbocostal ligs.
Dorsal br.
Cutaneous n. br.

Scapula
Infraspinatus mus.
Teres minor mus.
Teres major mus.
Esophagus
Int. intercostal mus.
Latissimus dorsi mus.
Parietal plura
Int. membrane
Ext. intercostal mus.
Transversus mus.
Serratus post. inf. mus.
Transversalis fascia
Int. oblique mus.
Quadratus lumborum mus.
Ext. oblique mus.
Ant. lumbar fascia
Erector spinae mus.
Post. lumbar fascia

Box 55-1. Chest Wall Abnormalities

Depression deformities/pectus excavatum
Protrusion deformities/pectus carinatum
Poland's syndrome
Sternal defects
Cervical ectopia cordis
Thoracic ectopia cordis
Thoracoabdominal ectopia cordis
Bifid sternum

over 30% of cases have a family history of chest wall anomalies.[5] Pectus excavatum arises from imbalanced or excessive growth of the lower costal cartilages, causing posterior sternal depression. The depression can often be deeper on the right side than the left, causing a rotation of the sternum. Typically, the defect is diagnosed within the first year of life and worsens over time. A wide range of depression abnormalities is reported, varying from a mildly depressed sternum to sternal depression abutting the vertebral column with displacement of mediastinal organs. Approximately 20% of cases are associated with other musculoskeletal abnormalities such as scoliosis (15%) and Marfan's syndrome, whereas congenital heart disease is seen in 1.5% of patients.[6]

The majority of patients with pectus excavatum are asymptomatic at the time of presentation; however, some subjects report a decrease in respiratory reserve or pain along the costal cartilages with exercise. Occasionally, palpitations or murmurs are noted, particularly in the presence of mitral valve prolapse. Evaluation of baseline pulmonary function can be obtained with pulmonary function testing, exercise radiologic or physiologic studies, and ventilation-perfusion scans.[7] Cardiovascular assessment can be performed using echocardiography or angiography. In severe cases, decreased stroke volume and cardiac output have been documented, along with a restrictive pattern (decreased maximal breathing capacity) on pulmonary function testing.

To assess the severity of this defect, a variety of methods have been used based on measurements obtained from chest radiography or chest computed tomography (CT).[8] Most methods use the distance between the sternum and spine to create a ratio to compare the depth of the depression. Examples of these methods include a ratio of the sternovertebral distance divided by the anteroposterior diameter of the chest at the sternomanubrial joint or, alternatively, the depth of the chest wall defect and the maximal anteroposterior distance of the thorax.

The indications for operative intervention include cosmesis, psychosocial factors, and the presence of respiratory or cardiovascular insufficiency. Poor self-image is an important concern for many patients, particularly children and adolescents or young adults who are taunted by peers. Frequently, these individuals attempt to cover the defect with clothing and abstain from participating in activities that require their chests to be bare, such as swimming. Because of these concerns, early repair is supported, with best results reported between 2 and 5 years of age.[9]

Surgical repair of pectus excavatum has evolved from techniques developed by surgeons over the past 50 years. Four procedures are mentioned here. The first involves repositioning the sternum anteriorly by sternal osteotomy. The second is a modification of this procedure that involves supporting the repositioned sternum with a posterior strut (sternal strut). The third technique involves removing the sternum and repositioning it in a front-to-back rotated position before stabilization. The fourth technique for correction employs a Silastic mold that is implanted into the subcutaneous space to fill the defect without altering the thoracic cage.[10]

The most frequently used operative technique employs a small transverse inframammary or midline incision. Electrocautery is used to mobilize the soft tissue and to reflect the pectoralis muscles laterally and the rectus muscle inferiorly. Once the involved costal cartilages are exposed, the deformed segments of cartilage are isolated subperichondrially for the length of the deformity and resected. The perichondrium is preserved to allow for growth of new cartilage over several months, creating a firm anterior chest wall. Once the cartilages are removed, the pleura is mobilized away from the posterior surface of the sternum by blunt dissection. This maneuver allows the sternum to be completely freed from its attachments once the intercostal muscles laterally are divided.[11] A transverse osteotomy is made through the sternomanubrial joint, permitting the sternum to be straightened.[5] Fixation of the sternum in a slightly overcorrected position is essential to ensure good repair. A number of techniques for stabilizing the sternum have been used, including bioabsorbable struts, Marlex mesh, Dacron vascular grafts, and metallic wires and struts.[12] At present, little evidence exists to support one technique over another. Drainage of the mediastinum is routinely performed postoperatively. Complications of surgical repair are rare and include wound infection and pneumothorax. Improvement of respiratory function and exercise capacity after repair has been reported. Early (1-year) cosmetic results are excellent (80% to 90%) (Fig. 55-2),[13] with recurrence varying from 5% to 15% with long-term follow-up.[7,14] A lengthy follow-up period is indicated in these patients, especially with regard to recurrence, because the rapid growth phase of puberty can alter dramatically the appearance of the chest wall.

Protrusion Deformities (Pectus Carinatum)

Pectus carinatum (also called pigeon breast) is a defect characterized by an anterior protrusion deformity of the sternum and costal cartilages. This condition affects males more than females (4:1) and presents less frequently than pectus excavatum by a ratio of approximately 1:5.[15] The defect, which worsens as the child grows, typically is not appreciated until after the first decade of life. Similar to

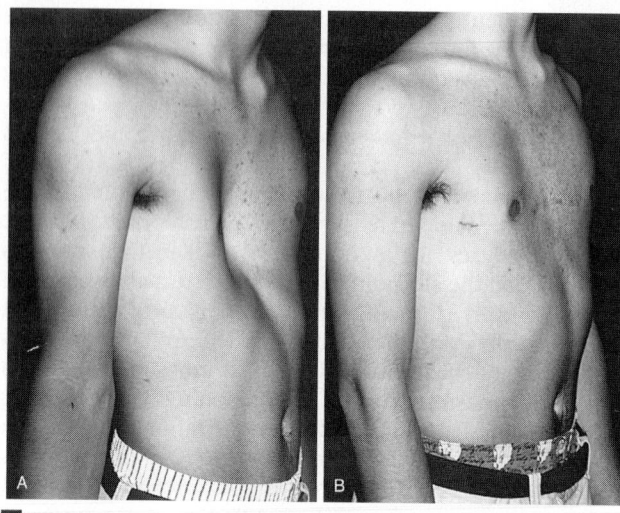

FIGURE 55-2. Patient with pectus excavatum. **A,** Preoperative. **B,** After repair. (**A** and **B,** From Shamberger RC, Hendren WH III. Congenital deformities of the chest wall and sternum. In Pearson FG, Cooper JD et al. [eds]: Thoracic Surgery, 2nd ed. Philadelphia, Churchill Livingstone, 2002, p 1352).

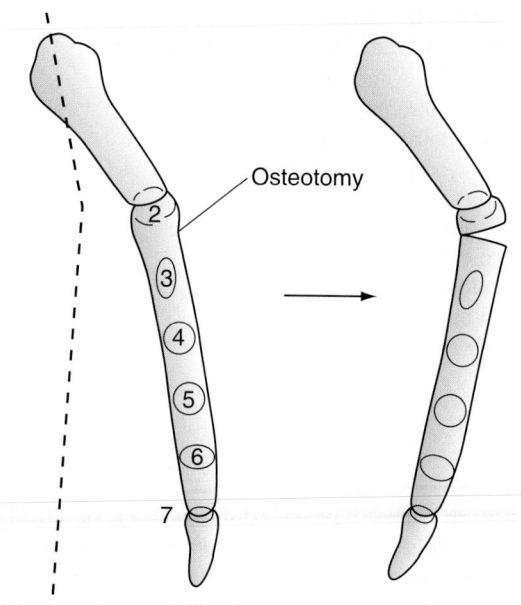

FIGURE 55-3. A single or double osteotomy after resection of the costal cartilage allows posterior displacement of the sternum to an orthotopic position in pectus carinatum. (From Shamberger RC: Congenital chest wall deformities. Curr Probl Surg 33:471, 1996.)

pectus excavatum, a familial predisposition (30%) and an association with scoliosis (15%) and congenital heart disease (20%) are reported.[15]

Three types of defects have been described in pectus carinatum. The most frequent variant, an anterior displacement of the body of the sternum and symmetrical concavity of the costal cartilages, is termed *chondrogladiolar protrusion.* The second variety involves a lateral depression of the ribs on one or both sides of the sternum; Poland's syndrome frequently is associated with this type. The third and least common type, the pouter pigeon breast, consists of an upper or chondromanubrial prominence with protrusion of the manubrium and depression of the sternal body.

Symptoms are uncommon but may include exertional dyspnea or cardiac arrhythmias. Pulmonary function tests and echocardiography are useful for determining the extent of cardiopulmonary compromise. Frequently, distinguishing this defect from a neoplasm is a concern of the patient and family.

The initial repair of pectus carinatum involves mobilization of the skin and pectoralis muscle flaps through a transverse incision. The subsequent surgical correction is modified depending on the extent of the deformity. In patients with the chondrogladiolar or chondromanubrial deformity, the sternum can be straightened using an osteotomy (sometimes two) of the sternal table (Fig. 55-3).[8] In the mixed deformity, the protrusion of the costal cartilages is corrected by using a subperichondrial resection of the involved costal cartilages. The oblique position of the sternum subsequently is fixed using a wedge-shaped osteotomy in the anterior sternal plate. Complications arising from surgical intervention such as pneumothorax, wound infection, or dehiscence are rare.

Excellent results commonly are obtained with few recurrences reported.

Poland's Syndrome

Poland's syndrome is a rare, nonfamilial disease of unknown cause that occurs in 1 per 30,000 births. The components of the syndrome include absence of the pectoralis major muscle, absence or hypoplasia of the pectoralis minor muscle, absence of costal cartilages, hypoplasia of breast and subcutaneous tissue (including the nipple complex), and a variety of hand anomalies. Occasionally, Poland's syndrome has been associated with Möbius' syndrome (facial palsy and abducens oculi palsy) or childhood leukemia.[16]

Patients who present with absent ribs are considered candidates for surgical repair. Although a variety of surgical techniques have been described to correct this anomaly, an approach using a latissimus dorsi muscle flap with autologous rib grafts to reconstruct the chest wall commonly is used.[17]

Sternal Defects

During embryologic development, the body of the sternum arises from migrating cells (sixth week) originating in the lateral plate mesoderm, which form two bands that fuse by the tenth week of gestation. The manubrium arises from primordia between the ventral ends of the clavicles. Abnormalities in the development of the sternum lead to four types of sternal clefts.

The upper sternal defects (cervical ectopia cordis) are associated with a broad defect that extends to the fourth costal cartilage in a U- or V-shaped appearance. Repair entails joining the sternal bands in the midline after performing oblique chondrotomies to provide protective coverage for the heart and great vessels. In severe cases, reconstruction of the defect with prosthetic material (e.g., Marlex mesh) is necessary to avoid excessive compression of the heart that would lead to bradycardia or hypotension. Complete clefts (thoracic ectopia cordis) are more extensive and frequently are associated with a crescentic anterior diaphragmatic defect and diastasis recti, which results in free communication between the peritoneum and pericardial cavities. Distal sternal clefts (thoracoabdominal ectopia cordis) are the most extensive defects and are associated with Cantrell's pentalogy. This group of anomalies is characterized by a distal cleft in the sternum, omphalocele, diaphragmatic cleft, pericardial defect, and congenital heart defect (ventricular septal defect, tetralogy of Fallot).[18] Bifid sternum is the least severe anomaly of the sternum and may be associated with facial hemangiomas.

Chest Wall Tumors

Chest wall tumors are rare neoplasms. They include tumors originating in the bone, cartilage, or soft tissue of the chest wall. Most bony chest wall tumors arise in the ribs (85%), with the remainder arising from the scapula, sternum, and clavicle.[19] These chest wall neoplasms commonly are classified as benign or malignant tumors of bone and soft tissue (Table 55-1). Malignant lesions are further divided into primary or secondary (metastatic) tumors. Although metastatic disease to the ribs is the most common malignant chest wall tumor, primary bone tumors account for 7% to 8% of all chest wall tumors.

The clinical presentation of chest wall tumors ranges from an asymptomatic lump to a painful and sometimes ulcerated mass.[20] Pain usually indicates periosteal invasion and more commonly is associated with malignancy. The correct diagnosis of chest wall lesions relies on a thorough clinical evaluation (history and physical examination) and radiologic tests. In particular, chest radiography with rib tomograms and chest CT are helpful in delineating soft tissue or bony involvement. Magnetic resonance imaging (MRI) is useful in determining neural and vascular invasion. Bone scanning also may aid in the differential diagnosis to rule out the presence of satellite or metastatic disease.

The correct treatment of chest wall tumors requires pathologic confirmation to be obtained. Excisional rather than incisional biopsy, with a minimum of a 1- to 2-cm margin, is preferred. Incisional biopsy occasionally may be appropriate for a large tumor. Frequently, surgical resection is the treatment of choice and often requires a multidisciplinary team approach (e.g., plastic surgery, neurosurgery, orthopedic surgery, and thoracic surgery).

Bone

Benign

Fibrous dysplasia of bone accounts for over 30% of benign chest wall tumors. Typically, these lesions present in the third or fourth decade of life, with equal frequency in men and women. They are slow growing and most com-

---

TABLE 55-1.   Classification of Tumors of the Chest Wall

	Benign	Malignant
Bone Tumors		
Bone	Osteoid osteoma	Osteosarcoma
	Aneurysmal bone cyst	Ewing's sarcoma
Cartilage	Enchondroma	Chondrosarcoma
	Osteochondroma	
Fibrous	Fibrous dysplasia	Malignant fibrous histiocytoma
Marrow	Eosinophilic granuloma	Plasmacytoma
Vascular	Hemangioma	Hemangiosarcoma
Soft Tissue		
Adipose	Lipoma and its variations	Liposarcoma
Muscle	Leiomyoma	Leiomyosarcoma
	Rhabdomyoma	Rhabdomyosarcoma
Neural	Neurofibroma	Neurofibrosarcoma
	Neurilemoma	Malignant schwannoma
		Askin's tumor (primitive neuroectodermal tumor)
Fibrous	Desmoid	Fibrosarcoma

Adapted from Faber LP, Somers J, Templeton AC: Chest wall tumors. Curr Probl Surg 32:663, 1995.

monly present as an asymptomatic mass in the lateral or posterior aspect of the rib. Pain may develop as the tumor enlarges and causes pressure symptoms or develops pathologic fractures. Albright's syndrome should be suspected if these lesions are multiple and associated with precocious puberty and skin pigmentation. The diagnosis is assisted by the appearance of a lytic lesion in the posterior aspect of the rib with a characteristic "soap bubble" or "ground glass" appearance on chest radiography. Excision is indicated for symptom relief (pain) and to confirm the diagnosis.

Chondromas account for 15% to 20% of benign chest wall lesions. These lesions present in the second or third decade of life as asymptomatic, slowly growing tumors at the anterior costochondral junction. Males and females are affected equally. The tumors can arise in the medulla (enchondroma) or the periosteum (periosteal chondroma). On chest radiography, the neoplastic growth appears as a lytic lesion with sclerotic margins that may be difficult to distinguish from chondrosarcomas. As a result, wide excision of the lesion is necessary to rule out a malignant component.

Osteochondroma presents as a mass originating from the cortex of the rib. Symptoms depend on the direction of tumor growth. Inward-growing tumors are usually asymptomatic, whereas outward-growing tumors present as a painless mass. Young males are most commonly affected. A characteristic finding on chest radiography is a pedunculated bony mass capped with viable cartilage. Familial osteochondromatosis should be suspected if multiple lesions are noted. Complete excision is the treatment of choice; recurrences are rare.

Eosinophilic granuloma is a benign component of malignant fibrous histiocytosis, which primarily affects men. Patients present with skull and rib involvement that appears as expansile bone lesions on radiographic evaluation. Excisional biopsy is indicated for solitary lesions; radiotherapy is reserved for patients who present with multiple lesions.

Osteoid osteomas are rare tumors that arise in the bony cortex of the rib or vertebral arches. Young males most commonly are affected and present with sharp pain that is worse at night and is relieved by aspirin. A small radiolucent nidus encircled by a sclerotic margin is frequently seen on a chest radiograph. Indications for resection include cosmesis and relief of pain; resection of the entire rib is recommended.

Aneurysmal bone cysts commonly occur in the ribs and may arise as the result of chest wall trauma. The characteristic pattern of a blow-out lytic lesion frequently is seen on chest radiography. Complete excision is warranted for relief of pain.

Malignant

Chondrosarcoma is the most common malignant tumor of the chest wall, accounting for 20% of all bone tumors. These lesions arise in the third and fourth decades of life and may be associated with trauma to the chest or represent malignant degeneration of benign chondromas or osteochondromas. On chest radiography, a poorly defined tumor mass that is destroying cortical bone is observed. The anterior costochondral junctions of the sternum most frequently are involved. Resection with wide margins is the treatment of choice, with a 70% 5-year survival rate reported for complete excision.[21] Radiotherapy may be effective for control of local recurrences.

Osteosarcoma (osteogenic sarcoma) is a tumor that arises most frequently in the long bones of adolescents and young adults. In the chest, osteosarcomas account for 10% to 15% of malignant tumors. Typically, the tumor presents as a rapidly enlarging mass with a characteristic sunburst pattern on chest radiography. Because metastases are common at presentation, a complete radiographic evaluation of the lungs, liver, and bones is indicated. Five-year survival with complete excision and adjuvant chemotherapy approaches 60%.

Ewing's sarcoma is a bone tumor that arises most commonly in the pelvis, humerus, or femur of young males. It is the third most common malignant chest wall tumor (5% to 10%). A mass that is intermittently painful is a common presentation in this disease. A characteristic onion peel appearance caused by periosteal elevation and bony remodeling is seen on the chest radiograph. Survival is approximately 50% at 5 years with multimodality therapy (chemotherapy, radiotherapy, and surgery).[22]

Solitary plasmacytoma is a rare tumor arising from plasma cells. Multiple myeloma is the same tumor arising in more than one location. The tumor commonly presents as pain without a mass in older men. A diffuse, punched-out appearance of the bone caused by myelogenous deposits is seen on chest radiography. Systemic disease can be confirmed using serum electrophoresis, urinalysis (Bence Jones protein), and bone marrow aspiration. Incisional biopsy frequently is used to confirm the diagnosis, although a solitary plasmacytoma should be resected completely. Radiotherapy is the primary mode of therapy, with a 5-year survival of 30% reported.[23]

Soft Tissue

Many benign tumors arise from the chest wall. These rare tumors are listed in Table 55-1 and are discussed in detail elsewhere in the text. Malignant degeneration rarely has been observed in some of these tumors, such as neurofibromas. Surgical excision is the preferred mode of therapy.

Soft tissue sarcomas are the most common malignant primary chest wall tumors. These lesions can arise anywhere in the thorax and usually are graded as low or high grade based on mitotic rate, cellular pleomorphism, and nuclear-cytoplasmic ratio. Incisional biopsy is performed to establish the diagnosis, and surgical excision with wide margins is used for definitive therapy. Of note, the pseudocapsule that surrounds the tumor and frequently contains microscopic disease should be avoided during the resection to decrease the chance of local recurrence. Chemotherapy and radiotherapy are used frequently as adjuvant therapeutic modalities.

Metastatic

Metastatic neoplasms may involve the chest wall by direct extension, by progression of lymphatic disease or by metastases from blood-borne deposits, with the latter being most common. Tumors that involve the chest wall by direct extension include breast and lung cancer. In breast cancer, locoregional recurrence involving the chest wall can occur in over 10% of stage II lesions after mastectomy.[24,25] Recurrences are treated with resection and adjuvant radiotherapy and chemotherapy.

Chest wall invasion is reported in 5% of primary non–small cell lung cancer patients. Historically, these tumors have the best prognosis of all T3 lesions because they are readily amenable to resection. In 1985, a report by McCaughan and colleagues[26] noted that the actuarial 5-year survival rate for patients with chest wall invasion without lymph node involvement (T3N0-stage IIB) was 56%, whereas patients with tumors with N1 or N2 nodal invasion had a survival of 35% and 16%, respectively. In 1987, similar findings were reported by the Mayo Clinic. A 59% 5-year survival rate for patients with resected T3N0 chest wall lesions was noted, compared with a 7% rate for patients with T3N1-N2 disease.[27] Therefore, nodal involvement is a strong prognostic determinant of survival. An evaluation of other prognostic factors from this series indicated that long-term survival was additionally affected by the extent of chest wall involvement and the ability to completely resect the tumor. For these reasons, the use of adjuvant radiotherapy for these patients has been investigated[28,29]; however, a large trial has yet to confirm a survival advantage in this subset of patients with T3 tumors.

In 1924, Pancoast described posteroapical chest tumors characterized by arm pain, atrophy of hand muscles, bone destruction, and Horner's syndrome.[30] These tumors, which account for less than 5% of all non–small cell lung cancer, have been associated with a favorable survival, with cumulative 5-year survival over 30%.[31] Controversy regarding the importance of nodal status in the survival of these patients exists; however, most series rarely report long-term survival with N2 disease.[32,33] For this reason, careful preoperative mediastinal lymph node staging is important to exclude inoperable N2 or N3 disease. Recently, efforts have focused on improving local control by using preoperative radiotherapy in conjunction with surgery. Most series report local control rates of 70% to 85% using this bimodality approach.[34,35] Currently, neoadjuvant chemotherapy also is being used clinically.

Secondary chest wall metastases arise from sarcomas and breast, lung, kidney, and thyroid cancers. Surgical resection is uncommon, except for diagnosis. These lesions usually are treated palliatively with radiotherapy.

Reconstruction

Reconstruction of the chest wall requires an intricate knowledge of the anatomy of the chest defect and the availability of soft tissues and prosthetic materials to repair the defect. Defects in the anterior, superior, and lateral chest wall commonly are reconstructed if the defect is greater than 5 cm. Skeletal stabilization is obtained using a prosthetic mesh or patch or with methyl methacrylate. Posterior defects generally do not require reconstruction, particularly if they are adequately covered by the scapula in superior defects. Soft tissue reconstruction can be accomplished using a variety of techniques, such as myocutaneous flaps (latissimus dorsi, pectoralis major, rectus abdominis, trapezius, serratus anterior), omental transposition, tissue expansion, and microvascular composite tissue transfer. Frequently, the assistance of other surgical specialties is beneficial in the reconstruction of complex defects.[36]

Chest Wall Infections

Chest wall infections encompass those infections arising from skin, soft tissue, cartilage, and bony structures of the chest wall. Frequently, these infections occur after surgical intervention. Infections caused by tuberculosis or fungi are less common than those caused by bacteria but may be more difficult to eradicate. Management of chest wall infections ranges from antibiotic therapy to radical resection and débridement for more advanced or complicated infections.

Soft tissue infections commonly include superficial abrasions, carbuncles, or furuncles. Herpes zoster (shingles) also may present as painful lesions distributed along cutaneous nerve dermatomes and usually is self-limited, although antiherpes medications generally improve the time course and diminish the severity of symptoms. Life-threatening necrotizing (clostridial, streptococcal or *Escherichia coli*) infections also may appear in diabetic or immunocompromised patients and require aggressive débridement with systemic antibiotic therapy.[37] Inflammatory breast carcinoma may mimic chest wall infection or breast abscess and requires a high index of suspicion to make the appropriate diagnosis. Although Mondor's disease frequently is misdiagnosed as a chest wall infection, it is actually a thrombophlebitis of the superficial veins of the breast and anterior chest wall. Ultrasound may be helpful in confirming this diagnosis.

Cartilage and bony structures occasionally may be the source of a chest wall infection. Costochondritis usually is self-limited, as in Tietze's syndrome. However, because the poor vascular supply of cartilage limits the exposure to systemic antibiotics, a small indolent infection may fester or progress and subsequently require radical débridement and reconstruction. Consideration should be given for early débridement in these situations. Bone infections arise primarily from surgical interventions such as median sternotomy. Although relatively uncommon today in the postantibiotic era, sternal wound infection or thoracotomy infection occurs in 1% to 2% of operative cases.[38] Thoracotomy infection is rare. Risk factors include trauma, chronic obstructive pulmonary disease, diabetes, prolonged mechanical ventilation, age, general debilitation, and division or use for revascularization of the internal thoracic arteries. Diagnosis can be confirmed with chest CT or gallium scan. Treatment of sternal osteomyelitis includes radical débridement, irrigation systems, systemic antibiotics, and muscle flap reconstruction. Occasionally, chest wall infections can arise from fungal infections, such as actinomycosis or nocardiosis, and frequently lead to chest wall fistulae. Tuberculous chest wall infections are uncommon; however, the entity of lytic chest wall lesions arising from tuberculosis is becoming more common with the increased incidence of multidrug-resistant tuberculosis or mycobacterial organisms, more widespread use of immunosuppression, and the rising prevalence of HIV infection.

Radiotherapy is an effective modality in the treatment of malignancies arising in the thorax such as Hodgkin's lymphoma, lung cancer, breast cancer, and other chest wall malignancies. It may be used to treat a tumor as first-line therapy, as adjuvant therapy, or for treatment of metastasis or local recurrences. Radiotherapy works by releasing free radicals and peroxidases into cells. These intermediaries cause destruction of rapidly dividing cells, such as neoplastic cells, by fracturing DNA molecules. These ionizing rays also cause a nonspecific injury and hence can damage surrounding normal tissue. Endothelial cells in blood vessels are particularly susceptible to injury, leading to arteritis and ischemic fibrosis. Therefore, poorly vascularized tissues such as bone and cartilage are very susceptible to radiation injury. A wide spectrum of injuries has been reported, ranging from erythema of the skin (radiodermatitis) to soft tissue ulceration with osteoradionecrosis and chondroradionecrosis.[38] Although the severity of the injuries is dose dependent, standard doses of 45 to 50 Gy given over 4 to 6 weeks appear to limit complications. Prevention is the best treatment of radionecrosis. Currently, new techniques in administrating radiotherapy that increase the therapeutic effect while limiting toxicities are being explored. If radionecrosis develops in the chest wall, partial or full-thickness resection with vascularized soft tissue flap reconstruction may be necessary if more conservative therapy fails.[39]

Thoracic Outlet Syndrome

Thoracic outlet syndrome (TOS) refers to compression of the subclavian vessels and nerves of the brachial plexus in the region of the thoracic inlet. These neurovascular structures of the upper extremity may be compressed by a variety of anatomic structures, such as bone (cervical rib, long transverse process of C7, abnormal first rib, osteoarthritis), muscles (scalenes), trauma (neck hematoma, bone dislocation), fibrous bands (congenital and acquired), or neoplasm. Symptoms most commonly develop secondary to neural compromise; however, vascular or neurovascular symptoms are reported.[40] The patient population most commonly affected by TOS is middle-aged women. To understand the pathophysiology of TOS, knowledge of the relevant anatomy is essential.

At the apex of the thorax, the subclavian vessels and nerves of the brachial plexus traverse the cervicoaxillary canal en route to the upper extremity. The cervical

portion of the canal is divided into two portions by the first rib. The first portion, the scalene triangle, is bound by the scalenus anticus anteriorly, scalenus medius posteriorly, and the first rib inferiorly. The clavicle and the first rib bind the second portion, the costoclavicular space (Fig. 55-4).[41] The route of neurovascular structures through these anatomic regions helps to explain the variable symptomatology that may be noted in patients with TOS.

The subclavian artery exits the chest behind the sternoclavicular joints and passes between the scalenus anticus and medius muscles. The trunks of the five spinal nerves (C5-C8, T1) accompany the artery after they exit their intervertebral foramina. The trunks become cords as the nerves run posterior to the pectoralis minor tendon. Distal to the pectoralis tendon, the cords subsequently divide into the major motor and sensory nerves of the upper extremity (Fig. 55-5).[42] The axillary vein passes posteriorly to the costocoracoid ligament and pectoralis minor tendons. The axillary vein becomes the subclavian vein as it passes anteriorly over the first rib. The subclavian vein joins the jugular venous system after passing between the scalenus anterior muscle and clavicle.

These subclavian vessels and the brachial plexus can be compressed at a variety of locations as they pass between the thoracic inlet and the upper extremity. From medial to lateral, these anatomic regions are (1) the interscalene triangle (artery and nerves), (2) the costoclavicular space (vein), and (3) the subcoracoid area (artery, vein, nerves).[43]

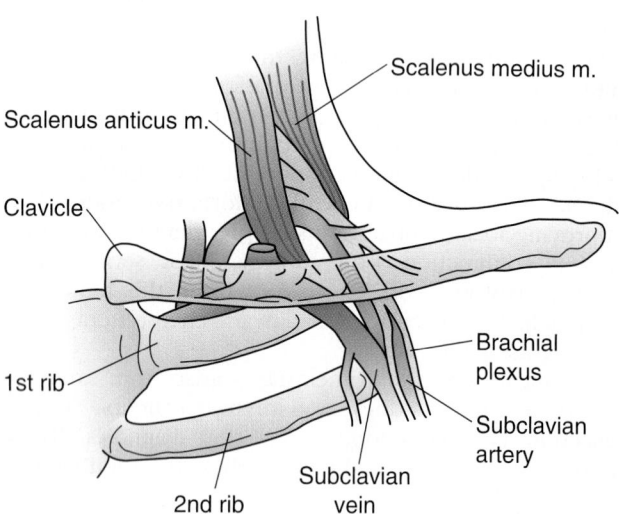

FIGURE 55-4.   Relationship of the neurovascular bundle to the scalenus muscles, clavicle, and first rib. (From Urschel HC: Thoracic outlet syndromes. *In* Baue AE, Geha AS, Hammond GL, et al [eds]: Glenn's Thoracic and Cardiovascular Surgery, 6th ed. Stamford, CT, Appleton & Lange, 1996, p 567. With permission of The McGraw-Hill Companies.)

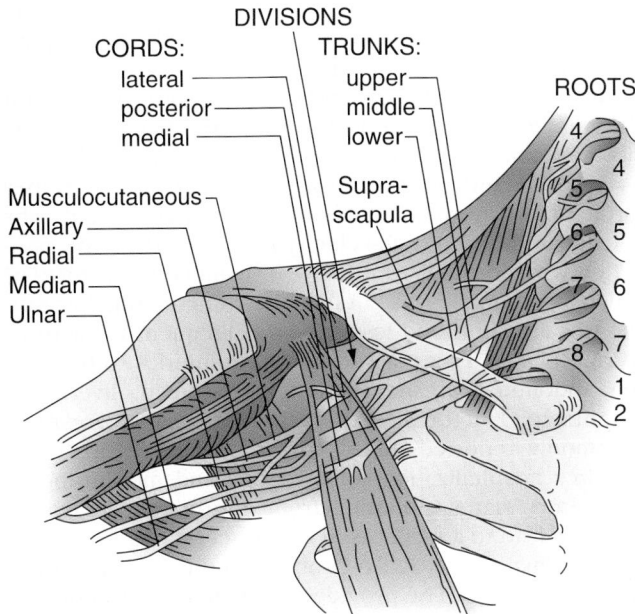

DIVISIONS

CORDS:
lateral
posterior
medial

TRUNKS:
upper
middle
lower

Supra-
scapula

ROOTS

Musculocutaneous
Axillary
Radial
Median
Ulnar

FIGURE 55-5. Detailed view of brachial plexus. (From Urschel HC, Razzuk M: Upper plexus thoracic outlet syndrome: Optimal therapy. Ann Thorac Surg 63:935-939, 1997. Reprinted with permission from the Society of Thoracic Surgeons.)

Diagnosis

The symptoms associated with TOS vary depending on the anatomic structure that is compressed. In over 90% of cases, neurogenic manifestations are reported. Ulnar nerve (C8-T1) involvement is associated with motor weakness and atrophy of the hypothenar and interosseous muscles, as well as pain and paresthesia along the medial aspect of the arm and hand, the fifth finger, and the medial aspect of the fourth finger. Median nerve (C5-8, T1) involvement produces symptoms in the index and middle fingers, as well as in the flexor compartment of the forearm. Symptoms of subclavian artery compression include fatigue, weakness, coldness, ischemic pain, and paresthesia. Exercise or cold weather may precipitate or potentiate these symptoms. Thrombosis with distal embolization rarely can occur, producing vasomotor symptoms (Raynaud's phenomenon) in the hand or ischemic changes. Atypical chest pain (pseudoangina) also has been reported. Edema, venous distention, collateral formation, and cyanosis of the affected limb are manifestations of venous compression or occlusion. Patients with Paget-Schroetter syndrome present with effort-induced thrombosis of the axillary or subclavian vein secondary to unusual, repetitive, or excessive arm exertion or exercise.

Four provocative clinical maneuvers to evaluate a patient suspected of having TOS have been described.[44] The loss or decrease of radial pulse or the reproduction of neurologic symptoms suggests a positive test. (1) The Adson (scalene) test causes narrowing of the space between the scalenus anticus and medius, resulting in compression of the subclavian artery and the brachial plexus. The patient is instructed to inspire maximally and hold his or her breath while the neck is fully extended and the head is turned toward the affected side. A decrease or loss of the ipsilateral radial pulse suggests compression. (2) The Halsted (costoclavicular) test is used to narrow the costoclavicular space between the first rib and the clavicle, thereby causing neurovascular compression. The patient is instructed to place his or her shoulders in a military position (drawn backward and downward). This maneuver causes changes in the radial pulse if compression of one or both subclavian arteries is present. (3) The Wright (hyperabduction) test causes the neurovascular structures to be compressed in the subcoracoid region by the pectoralis tendon, the head of the humerus, or the coracoid process. To perform the test, the patient's arm is hyperabducted 180 degrees. Compression is suspected with decrease or loss of the radial pulse. (4) The Roos test is performed by having the patient abduct his or her arm 90 degrees with external rotation of the shoulder. Maintaining this body position, the modified Roos test is performed by opening and closing the hand rapidly for 3 minutes in an attempt to reproduce symptoms. Additionally, neurogenic compromise also may be detected using provocative tests such as percussion of the nerve (Tinel's sign) or flexion of the elbow or wrist (Phalen's sign).

The radiologic evaluation of a patient suspected of having TOS includes chest and cervical spine radiography. Occasionally, these tests reveal bony abnormalities such as a cervical rib or bony degenerative changes. CT, MRI, or cervical myelograms are sometimes helpful to rule out narrowing of the intervertebral foramina or cervical disc pathology. Doppler studies or vascular imaging (angiogram/venogram) may be indicated if the extent of vascular impairment cannot be determined clinically or if an aneurysm or venous thrombosis is suspected.

Nerve conduction velocities can be very useful in differentiating the causes of neurologic symptoms reported by patients. Using electrodiagnostic testing, the velocity of action potential progression can be measured over proximal and distal segments of specific nerves, such as the median, ulnar, radial, and musculocutaneous nerves. By varying the points of stimulation along these nerves from the supraclavicular fossa to the wrist, the site of compression can be identified.[45]

Management

Once the diagnosis of TOS has been confirmed, the initial method of management is nonsurgical.[46] Improvements in postural sitting, standing, and sleeping positions are recommended first, along with behavior modification at work. Many patients also benefit from muscle stretching and strengthening exercises, as instructed by physiotherapists. With these measures and patient education, 50% to 90% of patients can be successfully treated.[47]

Indications for surgical intervention include failure of conservative management, progression of sensory or motor symptoms, the presence of excessively prolonged ulnar or median nerve conduction velocities, narrowing or occlusion of the subclavian artery, and thrombosis of the axillary/subclavian vein. The initial operation for TOS should include complete removal of the first rib. A first rib resection can be accomplished through a variety of approaches, including transaxillary, supraclavicular, infraclavicular, transthoracic, and posterior.[48] A review by Urschel and Razzuk[42] of more than 2200 procedures suggested that the transaxillary approach alone is required to obtain satisfactory symptom relief from upper (median nerve) and lower plexus (ulnar nerve) compression. Brachial plexus injuries, vascular injuries, pleural effusion, winged scapula, and infection are complications that may arise secondary to first rib removal. Recurrence of symptoms is documented in approximately 1% of patients.[42] Reoperation with removal of a persistent bony remnant or neurolysis of the brachial plexus then may be required.

Aneurysmal dilatation of the subclavian artery requires close follow-up. Treatment using graft reconstruction occasionally is required for large aneurysms or thrombosis. Treatment of subclavian vein thrombosis is accomplished with thrombolytic and anticoagulant therapy and simultaneous surgical decompression.

Chest Wall Trauma

Trauma to the chest wall is common and can range from an isolated single rib fracture to flail chest. Approximately 30% of patients presenting with significant trauma have a chest wall injury.[49] Guidelines of the Advanced Trauma Life Support program (Airway, Breathing, Circulation, Disability, Exposure) always should be followed in the preliminary assessment of these patients.[50] This organized approach helps to rule out injuries to the underlying viscera such as the lungs, heart, liver, and spleen, all of which frequently are associated with chest wall injury.

Soft Tissue

Blunt chest wall trauma commonly results in contusion with localized tissue swelling and hematoma formation. In severe cases, these injuries can progress to soft tissue infections or necrosis that require antibiotic therapy and débridement. Initially, it often is difficult to distinguish between deep muscle injury and bony fractures, given the pain that is caused by these injuries. Chest radiography and chest CT can be helpful in making this distinction. When subcutaneous emphysema is palpable on the chest wall, injury to the airway or lung parenchyma leading to a pneumothorax or esophageal perforation should be suspected. Circumferential burns to the chest wall require escharotomy to allow adequate chest wall expansion.

Ribs

Rib fractures are a common injury sustained after blunt chest wall trauma. A higher incidence of fractures is observed in the elderly owing to the loss of chest wall compliance from ossification of costal cartilage and osteoporosis. Symptoms include pain on inspiration and localized tenderness. Chest and rib radiographs can help to confirm the diagnosis in an acute setting but cannot completely rule out this injury. Three to 6 weeks after injury, callus formation around the fracture site is evident on repeat films. The management of rib fractures depends on the number and location of the injuries. Upper thoracic rib fractures (T1-T5) are uncommon because of the relatively protected position of these ribs below the upper girdle musculature. Fractures of the first two thoracic ribs usually are seen in high-velocity injuries and can be associated with aortic disruption (6%).[51] Similarly, fractures of the lower thoracic ribs (T11-T12) are uncommon because the ribs are short and less exposed. Frequently, fractures to ribs 11 and 12 are associated with injuries to underlying abdominal organs such as the spleen, liver, and diaphragm. Fractures to thoracic ribs 5 to 10 are most commonly reported. Injury to three or more ribs often requires hospitalization for analgesia and monitoring of respiratory status. Splinting from improperly controlled pain can lead to atelectasis, retained secretions, and pneumonia. This is a particular problem in the elderly population. Analgesia can be provided using oral, intravenous, or intramuscular opioid analgesics for mild-to-moderate injuries, or epidural analgesia or intercostal nerve blocks for more severe injuries. Delayed healing or chronic pain may be an issue for patients who present with fractures or dislocation of the costochondral junction.

Flail chest is a unique injury in which rib fractures lead to an unstable chest wall that results in a paradoxical motion during respiration. The injuries must occur along the same rib to produce the free-floating segment. This injury arises from blunt chest wall trauma such as direct impact from a steering wheel column.[52] The diagnosis of flail chest is made on clinical examination. Pulmonary contusion is the most commonly associated injury. Maintenance of adequate ventilation is the goal of therapy. Stabilization of the chest wall has been attempted using weights and rib binders, as well as fixation devices such as pins and plates. Mechanical ventilation with positive-pressure ventilation also occasionally is used to treat injuries in the elderly or in those patients with underlying pulmonary disease. Some centers report a more rapid wean from mechanical ventilation with the use of internal fixation.[53]

Sternum

Although relatively uncommon, sternal injuries can occur secondary to blunt trauma of the anterior chest. Commonly, fracture of the sternomanubrial joint occurs and leads to severe localized pain. A step deformity may be palpable if fracture dislocation of the sternum has occurred. The diagnosis is made by clinical evaluation with the assistance of a lateral chest radiograph. Operative stabilization using internal fixation is indicated in isolated injuries to achieve analgesia or long-term cosmetic improvement. The main concern of sternal injuries is the potential for associated underlying injuries that can be life threatening, such as aortic disruption, cardiac contusion, and pericardial effusion.[54] Serial electrocardiograms with cardiac enzymes and echocardiography are used to rule out these injuries.

Clavicles and Scapulae

Clavicular fractures may be associated with injury to the brachial plexus or subclavian vessels that can lead to TOS with improper healing. The usual mechanism of injury is either a direct blow or shoulder-restraint injury. Scapular fracture is a high-velocity injury associated with injuries to the lung (contusion and pneumothorax) and ribs (fractures). Clavicular and scapular fractures generally are treated expectantly, except if joint function is impaired or pain is excessive.

Chest Wall Defects

A defect in the chest wall may create a direct communication between the pleural space and the exterior of the patient. If the wound is of sufficient size, an open pneumothorax develops. Clinical examination and chest radiography can confirm the diagnosis. Treatment involves closure of the defect with a dressing and chest tube drainage of the affected hemithorax. Occasionally, a flap-valve mechanism (sucking chest wound) is created by the soft tissue that surrounds the chest wall defect, resulting in lung collapse and paradoxical shifting of the mediastinum. The resulting tension pneumothorax is life threatening because of the diminished cardiac output that accompanies the mediastinal shift. Prompt needle decompression via the second intercostal space (midclavicular line) is required, followed by chest tube insertion to restore the mediastinum to midline. Very rarely, a problem of lung herniation through a chest wall defect that leads to strangulation has been observed. Lung herniation, which occasionally occurs after thoracic surgical procedures, is rarely clinically symptomatic.

PLEURA

Anatomy

The pleural cavity appears between the fourth and seventh gestational weeks and is lined by the splanchnopleurae and somatopleurae, which later form the visceral and parietal pleurae and account for anatomic differences in vascular, nervous, and lymphatic structure.[55] The pleural space is a potential cavity lining the chest wall and into which each lung protrudes. The visceral and parietal pleurae are smooth, serous membranes, continuous with each other at the lung hila and pulmonary ligaments.[56] Humans have a divided pleural space or two individual pleural spaces, unlike some other mammals, because of the development of a complete mediastinum. Under normal circumstances, the pleural space contains only a small amount of pleural fluid.

The parietal pleura is divided into four areas.[55] The cervical pleura, or cupula, covers the apex of the hemithorax and extends above the level of the first rib to join stronger connective tissue known as the Sibson fascia. The costal pleura lines the inner surface of the sternum, ribs, and vertebrae and is attached to the chest wall by the endothoracic fascia, a layer of loose connective tissue. The mediastinal pleura covers the pericardium and other mediastinal structures. The diaphragmatic pleura lines the diaphragm, where it is tightly bound to the central tendon of the diaphragm. It forms the floor of the pleural cavity.

The visceral pleura covers both lungs and follows all fissures. The pleural spaces oppose one another anteriorly at the sternal angle but diverge to accommodate the heart. Under normal conditions, the parietal and visceral pleural membranes are separated by a thin layer of fluid, which functions as a lubricant and transmits the forces of breathing between lung and chest wall.[56] This fluid is formed as an ultrafiltrate of plasma but contains molecules secreted by mesothelial cells of the pleura that have surfactant-like properties. The parietal pleura derives its arterial blood supply from systemic arteries, including the posterior intercostal, internal mammary, anterior mediastinal, and superior phrenic arteries. Its drainage is through venules and corresponding systemic veins. The dual blood supply of the visceral pleura is both systemic and pulmonary. Typically, pulmonary capillaries form a subpleural network for the visceral pleura. However, fibrosis and inflammation increase the contribution of radicular branches of the bronchial arteries to the visceral pleural arterial supply. Venous drainage is only by the low-pressure pulmonary veins. The lymphatic drainage of the parietal pleura is into regional lymph nodes, including intercostal, mediastinal, and phrenic nodes. Visceral pleural lymphatics form a subpleural plexus when they mesh with superficial lung lymphatics. This subpleural plexus subsequently drains into mediastinal lymph nodes.[57,58] Parietal pleura is richly innervated by the intercostal nerves, except the mediastinal and central diaphragmatic parietal pleurae, which are innervated by the phrenic nerves. The visceral pleura is insensitive and is innervated by vagal branches and the sympathetic system.

Pleural Effusions

The movement of fluid across the pleural membranes is complicated but in general is governed by Starling's law of capillary exchange. This suggests that the flux of fluid is controlled by the balance of both oncotic and hydrostatic pressures within the pleural capillaries and pleural space. The net pressure difference moves fluid primarily from the parietal pleura into the pleural space.[59] Five to 10 L of fluid transgresses the pleural space over a 24-hour period. However, the amount of fluid within the normal pleural space is quite small.[60] The balance of forces favors fluid reabsorption from the pleural cavity across the visceral pleura. Nevertheless, under physiologic conditions, most pleural fluid reabsorption is via lymphatics of the parietal pleura because protein that enters the pleural space cannot enter the relatively impermeable visceral pleural capillaries. The parietal pleura, with its lymphatics, has an enormous capacity for both protein and fluid removal.[56] In addition, this pleural homeostasis is affected by other factors, including gravity, pleural fluid viscosity, pleural membrane thickness, and the distribution of lymphatic drainage sites throughout the parietal pleura.[55] Even a small imbalance of accumulation and absorption of

Box 55-2. Etiology of Transudative Effusions

Congestive heart failure	Fluid retention/overload
Cirrhosis	Pulmonary embolism
Nephrotic syndrome	Lobar collapse
Hypoalbuminemic conditions	Meigs' syndrome

Box 55-3. Etiology of Exudative Effusions

Malignant

Bronchogenic carcinoma
Metastatic carcinoma
Lymphoma
Mesothelioma
Pleural adenocarcinoma

Infectious

Bacterial/parapneumonic
Empyema
Tuberculosis
Fungal
Viral
Parasitic

Collagen-Vascular Disease Related

Rheumatoid arthritis
Wegener's granulomatosis
Systemic lupus erythematosus
Churg-Strauss syndrome

Abdominal/Gastrointestinal Disease Related

Esophageal perforation
Subphrenic abscess
Pancreatitis/pancreatic pseudocyst
Meigs' syndrome

Others

Chylothorax
Uremia
Sarcoidosis
Post coronary artery bypass grafting
Post irradiation
Trauma
Dressler's syndrome
Pulmonary embolism with infarction
Asbestosis related

pleural fluid will lead to the development of a pleural effusion. The mechanisms of this imbalance include (1) increased hydrostatic pressure, (2) increased negative intrapleural pressure, (3) increased capillary permeability, (4) decreased plasma oncotic pressure, and (5) decreased or interrupted lymphatic drainage.[61,62]

Approximately 300 mL of fluid is required for the development of costophrenic angle blunting seen on an upright chest radiograph. At least 500 mL of effusion is necessary for detection on clinical examination.[63] Pleural effusions are classified as either transudates or exudates based on fluid protein and lactate dehydrogenase (LDH) concentrations. Transudative effusions occur as the result of a change in fluid balance in the pleural space. Exudative effusions suggest the disruption or integrity loss of pleura or lymphatics. An effusion is considered exudative if it meets any one of the following criteria[64]:

- Pleural fluid protein/serum protein greater than 0.5
- Pleural fluid LDH/serum LDH greater than 0.6
- Pleural fluid LDH 1.67 times normal serum

The etiology of pleural effusions is quite varied.[65-67] Some of the many causes are listed in Boxes 55-2 and 55-3.

Benign

Many, but not all, benign pleural effusions are transudates. With chronicity, however, even initially transudative effusions may be exudative. Benign transudative effusions tend to be free flowing and layer dependently. Benign, noninfectious, pleural effusions should be drained completely by thoracentesis for diagnosis. Treatment of benign pleural effusions is directed toward treatment of the underlying disease, such as congestive heart failure or ascites.[66,68]

Recurrent benign pleural effusions are not uncommon and should be treated aggressively. Repeat thoracenteses can be carried out. Medical management of the underlying cause should be maximized. Despite these efforts, some pleural effusions tend to recur and cause symptoms of dyspnea or chest pain or heaviness. Tube thoracostomy or thoracoscopic drainage with or without chemical pleurodesis then is warranted. Chest tube insertion is carried out in such a way (angled chest tube, low insertion site) that drainage is as complete as possible. Pleurodesis can be carried out through the chest tube once chest tube outputs have decreased to less than 150 to 200 mL/day. Because tetracycline is no longer being manufactured for this purpose, alternatives are being used that are equally effective.[69,70] Doxycycline and minocycline can be

instilled through the chest tube, as can sterile talc in slurry form. Typically, 300 mg of doxycycline or 2 to 5 g of talc in 100 to 200 mL of saline solution is instilled, and the chest tube is clamped at its exit site. The patient is turned at intervals for 1 hour to assist with distribution, and then the chest tube is replaced to suction drainage.

Thoracoscopic drainage of effusions with intraoperative chemical pleurodesis is currently widely used with excellent results.[71,72] Talc or doxycycline can be insufflated in its powdered form to cover all pleural surfaces. This procedure has the added advantage of being diagnostic in a pleural effusion whose cause is undiagnosed. The procedure does require general anesthesia with lung separation, and all patients may not be candidates (Fig. 55-6).

Thoracoscopy or thoracotomy with mechanical pleurodesis or pleurectomy is reserved for only the most recalcitrant effusions. A chronic pleural effusion

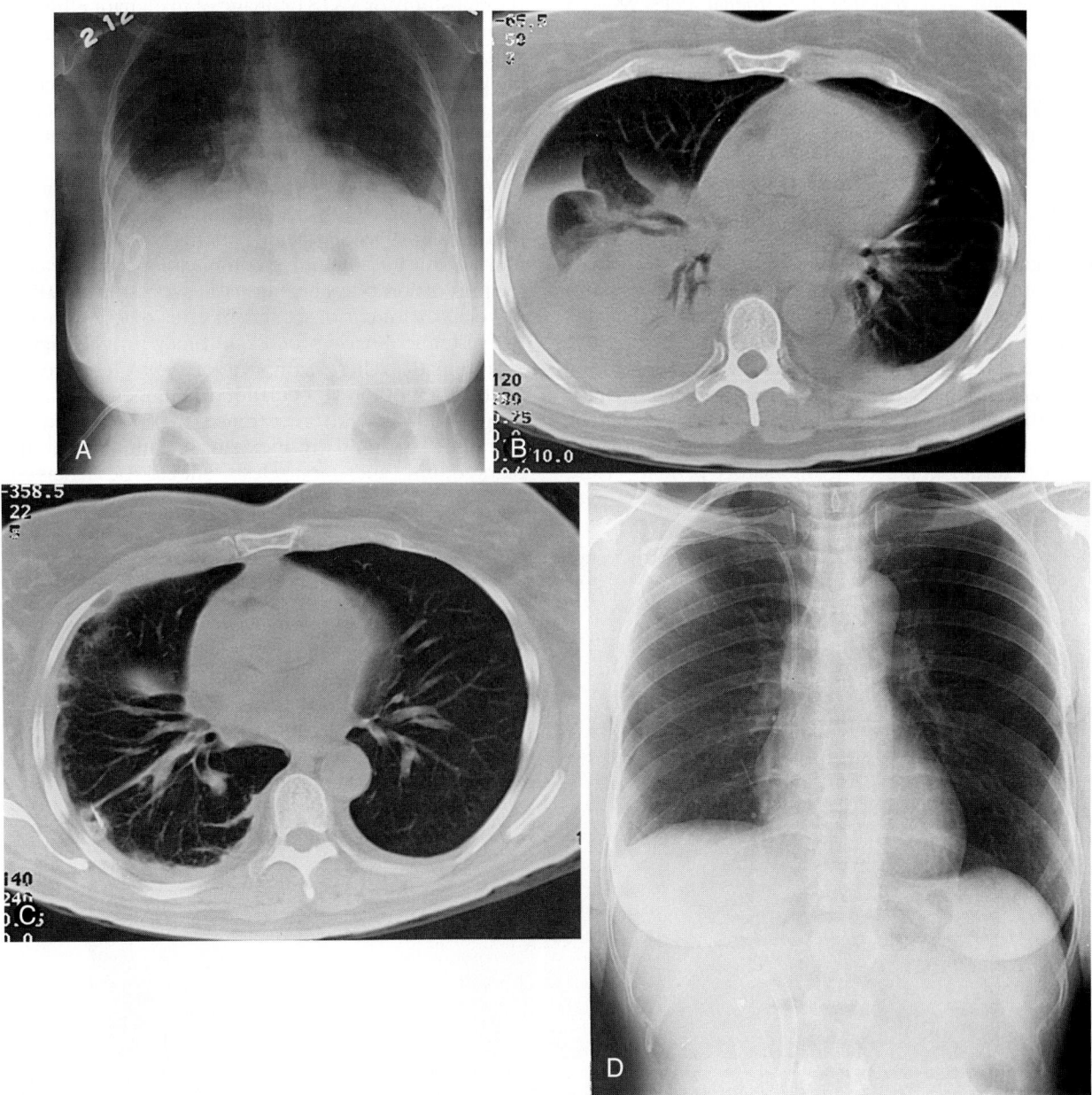

FIGURE 55-6. A, Chest radiograph demonstrates right pleural effusion after laparoscopic cholecystectomy. **B,** CT scan shows complicated (loculated) inflammatory effusion. **C,** CT scan from the postoperative period, after thoracoscopic débridement and decortication; note location of basilar chest tube. **D,** Follow-up chest radiograph after complete resolution.

may cause lung entrapment and not be amenable to procedures other than thoracotomy with decortication. Therefore, prompt attention to all benign pleural effusions is recommended.

Malignant

Malignancy is a common cause of pleural effusion. Most malignant pleural effusions are exudative. They are the second most common exudative effusive process. Metastatic breast and lung cancers are the most common malignancies that cause malignant effusions.[73] Metastatic ovarian carcinoma is not uncommon. Lymphomas are an

important cause of malignant effusion and account for 10% to 14% of all malignant pleural effusions.

Malignant pleural effusion is an effusion with positive cytopathology. Not all pleural effusions associated with malignancy are caused by direct or metastatic pleural involvement. Other mechanisms for their development (bronchial or lymphatic obstruction, hypoproteinemia, and sympathetic accumulation from infradiaphragmatic involvement) exist.[69,74,75] Although repeated cytologic evaluation of a pleural effusion achieves high positive and negative predictive values, limitations are important. It is unreliable in establishing a diagnosis of lymphoma. Inflammation makes cytologic examination difficult and inaccurate. Malignant and reactive mesothelial cells have a similar appearance.

A malignant pleural effusion is best approached with a combination of treatment of the underlying disease (if available) and specific intervention on the effusion itself. Initial complete thoracentesis of a suspected malignant effusion should be carried out for diagnostic (type of effusion, expansibility of the lung) and therapeutic purposes.[76] If the effusion reaccumulates, either repeat thoracentesis, chest tube insertion, or video-assisted thoracic surgery (VATS) drainage is indicated. Thoracentesis may be appropriate if the patient is minimally symptomatic, is symptomatic but expected to have a prompt response to other therapy, is receiving chemotherapy and chest tube insertion is contraindicated (neutropenia), or is not a candidate for a more aggressive approach because of comorbid disease or stage of malignancy. A permanent pleural drainage catheter (Hickman, Groshong) can facilitate repeated thoracenteses in ambulatory patients. Tube

thoracostomy or VATS drainage of malignant effusions not only allows for continued emptying of the pleural space with visceral and parietal pleural apposition and possible adherence but also allows for chemical or mechanical pleurodesis. VATS drainage has the added benefit of obtaining a definitive diagnostic biopsy if the pleural effusion is of an indeterminate cause (Fig. 55-7).[74]

Yim and coworkers[77] reported their experience with thoracoscopic (VATS) management of malignant pleural effusions in 1996. Sixty-nine patients were treated without mortality or intraoperative complications; talc insufflation for prevention of recurrence was successful in 94%.

Local treatment of malignant effusions does not affect the systemic disease process, but may provide significant symptomatic relief. Complications of these treatments include hemothorax, loculation of fluid, empyema, failure of pleurodesis with recurrence of effusion, and lung entrapment caused by inexpansile lung. Open surgical pleurectomy and pleurodesis should be reserved for

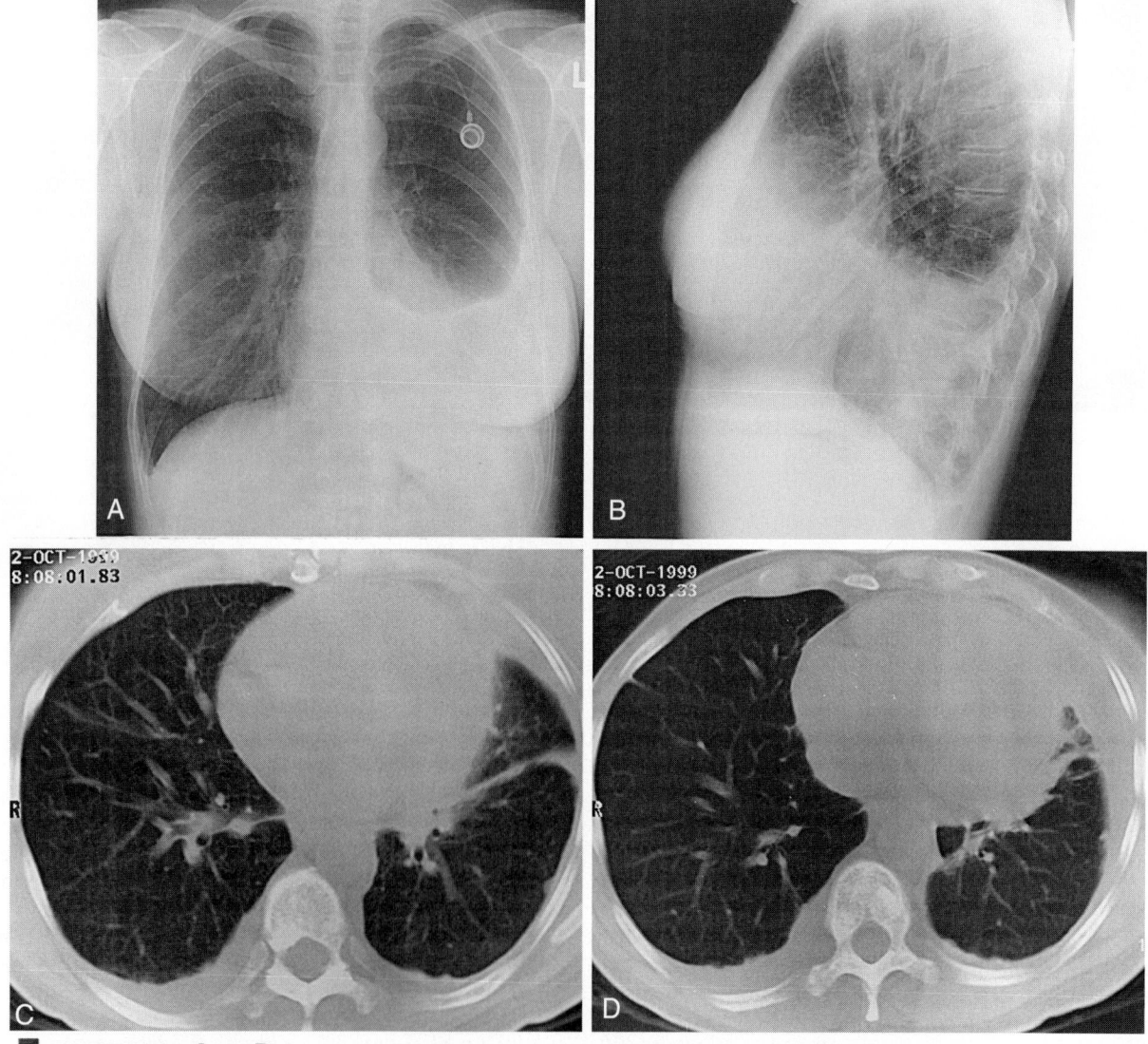

■ **FIGURE 55-7.**   **A** and **B,** Posteroanterior lateral chest radiograph demonstrates left malignant pleural effusion. **C** and **D,** CT scan cuts after video-assisted thoracic surgery (VATS) drainage and talc pleurodesis.

patients who fail other therapies and who have a reasonably long life expectancy.

Empyema

Empyema is a pyogenic or suppurative infection of the pleural space. Empyemas are the most common exudative type of pleural effusion. They may be classified into three categories based on the chronicity of the disease process.[78] The acute phase is characterized by pleural effusion of low viscosity and cell count. The transitional or fibrinopurulent phase, which can begin after 48 hours, is characterized by an increase in white blood cells in the pleural effusion. The effusion is turbid, begins to loculate, and is associated with fibrin deposition on visceral and parietal pleurae and progressive lung entrapment. The organizing or chronic phase occurs after as little as 1 to 2 weeks and is associated with an ingrowth of capillaries and fibroblasts into the pleural rind and inexpansile lung.

An empyema may occur by direct contamination of the pleural space through wounds of the chest (trauma or surgery), by hematologic spread (bacteremia or sepsis), by direct extension from lung parenchymal infection (parapneumonic or postpneumonic), by rupture of an intrapulmonary abscess or infected cavity, or by extension from the mediastinum (esophageal perforation). Most often, empyemas are the result of a primary infectious process in the lung. Historically, these infections were commonly due to *Streptococcus* or *Pneumococcus pneumoniae*; today gram-negative and anaerobic organisms are common causes of empyema. Tuberculous empyema has had a recent resurgence.[66]

Most patients with acute or transitional phase empyema present with symptoms of their primary lung infection (cough, fever, sputum production), followed by symptoms of pleural effusion (chest pain and dyspnea) and systemic illness (anorexia, malaise, and sweats). Fever from empyema can be very high. Without intervention, a septic course will ensue. Chest radiography demonstrates a pleural effusion; chest CT may demonstrate a complicated effusion with loculations and a heterogeneous appearance to the effusion.

Treatment of empyema is dependent on its phase but involves the identification and systemic treatment (antibiotics) of the causative organism and complete drainage of the pleural space. In the acute and early fibrinopurulent phases, complete thoracentesis can be both diagnostic and therapeutic if the effusion is drained entirely. The prior administration of antibiotics may lead to a sterile tap, but Gram stain (organisms), cell count (polymorphonuclear leukocytic predominance in bacterial empyema and lymphocytic predominance in tuberculous empyema), chemistries (protein, LDH, amylase, and glucose), and pH (<7.3) all can be useful in making the diagnosis.

Tube thoracostomy may be indicated for pleural drainage if thoracentesis fails or the empyema has progressed beyond its earliest stages. Chest tube insertion, however, can be ineffective if the empyema has become loculated or organized (Fig. 55-8). VATS empyema drainage with early pleural débridement has the added advantage of more complete pleural drainage by visualizing and breaking down loculations. Full lung expansion and the prevention of complications is the goal of the procedural intervention. Occasionally, radiologically guided catheter drainage can be a useful adjunct to these surgical procedures. Thoracotomy with débridement or formal decortication in later-stage empyema is reserved for treatment failures with persistent sepsis.

Complications of empyema include empyema necessitans (spontaneous decompression of pus through the chest wall), chronic empyema (with entrapped lung and pulmonary restrictive disease), osteomyelitis or chondritis of the ribs or vertebrae, pericarditis, mediastinitis, the development of a bronchopleural fistula, or disseminated infection of the central nervous system. Complications are best treated with prompt complete pleural drainage and débridement of infected tissues. Long-term (6 weeks or more) antibiotic therapy is required. Nutritional optimization plays an important role in treatment.

Chronic empyema is the result of failure to recognize or properly treat acute pneumonia or acute empyema, or failure (or incompleteness) of earlier intervention, and usually is associated with lung entrapment by a thick pleural peel or fibrothorax. This process can begin as early as 1 to 2 weeks and as late as 6 weeks after the onset of the acute illness. Chronic empyema can mimic other systemic illnesses with symptoms of anorexia, weight loss, and lethargy. Debilitation is both a contributing factor to and an end result of this disease. Anemia is a common sign.

With chronic empyema, chest radiography demonstrates opacification of the affected hemithorax, particularly laterally and inferiorly, where thickened pleura abuts compressed lung. The interspaces are narrowed, and the hemithorax becomes contracted. CT of the chest is useful for defining the extent of pleural thickening and the exact location of the empyema cavity and to rule out other associated parenchymal disease.

The open surgical approaches for chronic empyema include variations of an open thoracostomy with rib resection or full thoracotomy with empyema evacuation and lung decortication.[78] The appropriate procedure depends on the patient's overall status and comorbidities. Open drainage involves removal of a portion of a rib or ribs at the most dependent portion of the empyema cavity. The pus is evacuated. This space can then be drained with a tube, packed with dressings (thoracic window), irrigated, or lined with a mobilized skin flap to prevent closure (Eloesser flap). Open drainage usually allows the cavity to constrict and eventually obliterate itself, although this can take many months. Delayed muscle flap closure of the space may be an option in selected patients.

Empyema evacuation and decortication is indicated for relatively young patients who are in otherwise good health and without significant underlying lung parenchymal disease. Resection of the thickened peel or cortex over the chest wall and lung permits expansion of chronically collapsed lung. Resolution of sepsis (early) and improvement in pulmonary function (late) are the expected results of this surgery. Often, extrapleural resection of the parietal pleura is necessary. Occasionally, pleuropneumonectomy is indicated in

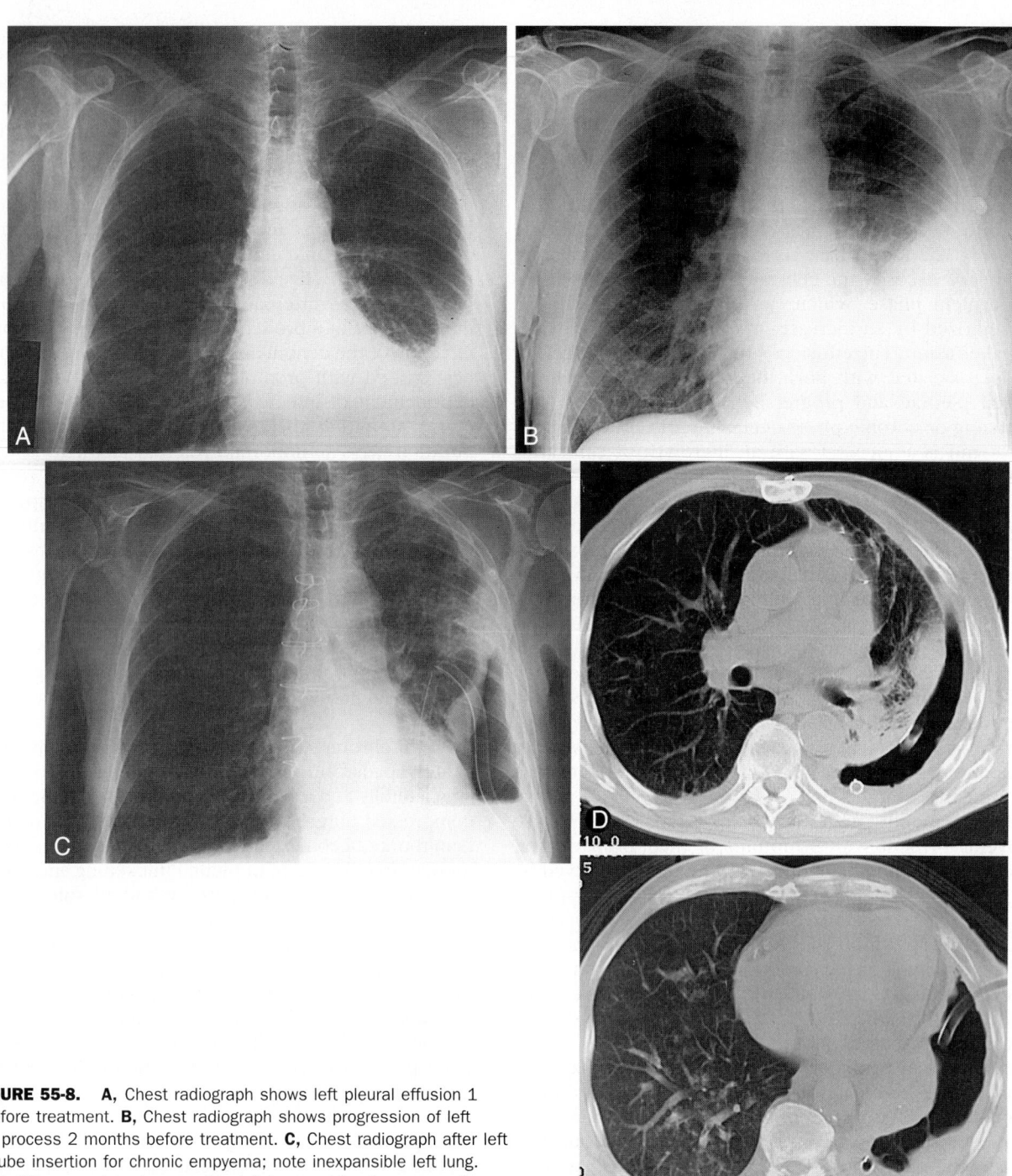

FIGURE 55-8. **A,** Chest radiograph shows left pleural effusion 1 year before treatment. **B,** Chest radiograph shows progression of left pleural process 2 months before treatment. **C,** Chest radiograph after left chest tube insertion for chronic empyema; note inexpansible left lung. **D** and **E,** CT scans show inexpansible left lung and basilar space with residual fluid.

empyema with underlying destroyed lung (tuberculosis or bronchiectasis).

Chylothorax

Chylothorax is the accumulation of lymph within the pleural space. The incidence of chylothorax may be increasing, because the number of thoracic surgical procedures and chest traumas continues to rise. Chylothorax

characteristically is milky white fluid that contains a high concentration of emulsified fats (triglycerides, chylomicrons) and a lymphocytic predominance on cell count.[66] However, depending on the nutritional and dietary status of the patient, the effusion can be only slightly cloudy or even clear. Chylothorax occurs when the contents of the thoracic duct empty into the pleural space. It is more common on the left side because of the anatomy of the thoracic duct. The underlying causes of chylothorax are numerous (Box 55-4).

Box 55-4. Etiology of Chylothorax

Traumatic (Chest and Neck)

Blunt
Penetrating

Iatrogenic

Catheterization, particularly subclavian venous
    Postsurgical
    Excision of cervical/supraclavicular lymph nodes
    Radical lymph node dissections of the neck
    Radical lymph node dissections of the chest
    Esophagectomy
    Lobectomy or pneumonectomy
    Mediastinal tumor resection
    Thoracic aneurysm repair
    Sympathectomy
    Congenital cardiovascular surgery

Neoplasms

Lymphoma
Lung cancers
Esophageal cancers
Mediastinal malignancies
Metastatic carcinomas

Infectious

Tuberculous lymphadenosis
Mediastinitis
Ascending lymphangitis

Other

Lymphangioleiomyomatosis
Venous thrombosis

Congenital

Symptoms of chylothorax may mimic the effects of a pleural effusion (dyspnea, chest pain, fatigue), be attributable to underlying disease (infectious or neoplastic causes), or may be the result of chronic metabolic effects of a thoracic duct leak (loss of fat, protein, antibodies, and fat-soluble vitamins). Losses in fluid volume may be large (>3 L/day) and produce hemodynamic instability if not adequately replaced.

After diagnosis, management of a chylothorax consists initially of tube thoracostomy drainage (chest tube insertion) with complete lung re-expansion and supportive measures such as a low-fat or fat-free diet supplemented by medium-chain triglycerides and aggressive fluid, electrolyte, and nutritional replacement or correction. Often, these measures are enough to promote closure of the thoracic duct pleural fistula. If the chylothorax is caused by malignancy, primary treatment of the neoplasm may be necessary. Radiation therapy to the mediastinum has been useful in managing chylothorax secondary to lymphoma.

Conservative measures for the treatment of chylothorax generally are maintained for 1 to 2 weeks. If the chylous effusion has not responded to this management,

surgical intervention is indicated.[78] The most common procedures are ligation of the thoracic duct or mass ligation of tissue at the diaphragmatic hiatus (generally through a right thoracotomy) or direct closure of the duct injury. Instillation of olive oil or cream via nasogastric tube at the time of surgery can help to identify the duct and area of leakage. Rarely, pleurectomy and pleurodesis are useful adjuncts to these other surgical procedures or recalcitrant chylothorax. Most recently, minimally invasive techniques for thoracic duct obliteration via cisterna chyli cannulation have been championed by interventional radiologists.

Pneumothorax

Pneumothorax is the accumulation of air within the pleural space. Pneumothoraces may be spontaneous or occur secondary to a traumatic, surgical, therapeutic, or disease-related event. A pneumothorax compresses lung tissue and reduces pulmonary compliance, ventilatory volumes, and diffusing capacity. These pathophysiologic consequences depend primarily on the size of the pneumothorax and condition of the underlying lung. If air enters the pleural space repeatedly (as with inspiration) and is unable to escape, positive pressure develops in the pleural space, causing compression of the entire lung, shifting of the mediastinum and heart away from the pneumothorax, and severe respiratory compromise with hemodynamic collapse. This situation is called a tension pneumothorax and requires immediate decompressive treatment. It may be the sequela of a pneumothorax from many causes.

Pneumothoraces may be classified as shown in Box 55-5. A primary spontaneous pneumothorax occurs without known cause or evidence of diffuse pulmonary disease or from subpleural blebs.[49,79] A secondary spontaneous pneumothorax occurs as the result of an underlying pulmonary process that predisposes to pneumothorax. Iatrogenic pneumothoraces are common and may be caused by thoracentesis, central venous catheterization, surgery, mechanical ventilation, or diagnostic lung biopsy.

Patients with pneumothorax most commonly present with chest pain. It is often sharp and pleuritic and may lead to severe respiratory embarrassment or become dull and persistent. Dyspnea is the second most common symptom in patients with pneumothorax. Less common symptoms include nonproductive cough and orthopnea.

The diagnosis of primary spontaneous pneumothorax usually is established by history and physical examination and confirmed with chest radiography. Patients are often tall, thin men from 25 to 40 years of age. Physical findings may be normal if the pneumothorax is less than 25%. Characteristic physical findings include diminished chest excursion and hyperresonance on percussion of the affected side. Breath sounds are diminished to absent. Rarely, subcutaneous emphysema may be palpated or pneumomediastinum auscultated on cardiac examination.[80]

A pneumothorax usually is seen on the standard posteroanterior chest radiograph with displacement of the

---

Box 55-5. Classifications of Pneumothorax

Spontaneous

Primary
Secondary
   Chronic obstructive pulmonary disease (COPD)
   Bullous disease
   Cystic fibrosis
   Pneumocystis-related congenital cysts
   Idiopathic pulmonary fibrosis (IPF)
   Pulmonary embolism
Catamenial
Neonatal

Traumatic

Penetrating
Blunt

Iatrogenic

Mechanical ventilation
Thoracentesis
Lung biopsy
Venous catheterization
Postsurgical

Other

Esophageal perforation

---

visceral pleura from the parietal pleura by air in the pleural space. The area appears hyperlucent with absent pulmonary markings. An end-expiratory chest radiograph may appear to increase the size of the pneumothorax because of reduction in lung volume during forced expiration. Recognition of a pneumothorax may be difficult on portable supine or semirecumbent chest radiographs obtained in trauma or critically ill patients because of both the location of the least dependent pleural spaces (anterior, subdiaphragmatic) and associated radiographic findings. Patients with bullous disease also may have chest radiographs that are difficult to interpret; chest CT may be useful in these situations. The routine use of CT in patients with spontaneous primary pneumothorax is not warranted because the confirmation of apical blebs does not change treatment recommendations. The occurrence of apical blebs and bullae in these patients has been found to be greater than 85% in most recent surgical series.[81]

The treatment of a first-time spontaneous pneumothorax depends on the size of pneumothorax, associated symptoms, and pulmonary history. Small pneumothoraces (<20%) that are stable may be monitored if the patient has few symptoms. Follow-up of a pneumothorax should include a chest radiograph to assess stability within 24 to 48 hours. An uncomplicated pneumothorax should reabsorb at a rate of approximately 1% per day. Indications for intervention include progressive pneumothorax, delayed pulmonary expansion, or development of symptoms.

Moderate (20% to 40%) and large (>40%) pneumothoraces nearly always are associated with persistent symptoms that cause physical limitations and require intervention. Simple needle aspiration of a pneumothorax may relieve symptoms and can promote quicker lung re-expansion.[79] It also may help to determine whether the initial fistula that caused the pneumothorax has sealed or if there is an ongoing air leak that requires chest tube insertion. This method is carried out using a standard thoracentesis kit and either an evacuated bottle or hand aspiration via a three-way stopcock and syringe. The needle generally is placed either anteriorly or laterally. The needle aspiration may be repeated, or a chest tube or needle catheter/thoracic vent drainage system may be inserted. It provides excellent management of iatrogenic pneumothoraces after central venous access or lung needle biopsy. This approach conservatively treats a sealed pneumothorax and identifies those with an active air leak for chest tube insertion.

Emergent needle decompression for tension pneumothorax is carried out on the affected side by placing an 18-gauge needle or angiocatheter into the hemithorax at the midclavicular line in the second anterior intercostal space. This emergency maneuver relieves the tension created within the thorax. It does not treat the pneumothorax; subsequent chest tube insertion is required.

Tube thoracostomy (chest tube insertion) and underwater seal drainage are the mainstays of treatment for spontaneous pneumothorax. Full re-expansion of the lung, even in the presence of a continuous leak, usually can be achieved with the application of suction to the thoracostomy drainage system. The classic location for chest tube insertion is the same as for emergency needle decompression because the tube can be inserted quickly and easily without the need for patient positioning. The preferred approach is through the fourth, fifth, or sixth intercostal space in the mid-to-anterior axillary line. This can be done under local anesthetic employing rib blocks or under intravenous procedural sedation. The chest tube should be directed upward to the apex of the hemithorax. Care should be taken to avoid the subcutaneous placement of a chest tube. Digital pleural dilatation is recommended to confirm entrance into the chest cavity, appreciate any adhesions, and allow passage of the chest tube without need for a stylet, which can cause damage to the lung or other intrathoracic structures.

Needle catheter/thoracic vent drainage systems may be employed for the treatment of a pneumothorax.[82] This system is comparable to a chest tube and drainage system, although the tube is of much smaller diameter and is inserted by means of the Seldinger technique or stylet. The end of the needle catheter drain is modified to be completely compatible with the many underwater seal drainage systems available. Many kits also include a Heimlich valve (also available separately), which can be used in conjunction with either a catheter drain or conventional chest tube. The Heimlich valve and thoracic vent function as a one-way valve that lets air escape from the hemithorax, similar to an underwater seal. Patients may be discharged with these in place, to be removed at a later time after the leak has stopped.

Complications of chest tube insertion for pneumothorax are infrequent but include laceration of an intercostal vessel, laceration of the lung, intrapulmonary or extrathoracic placement of the chest tube, and infection. Re-expansion pulmonary edema is a rare complication that can be seen after treatment of a pneumothorax. It was first reported by Carlson and colleagues[83] in 1958 in this setting. Risk factors for this complication have not been consistently identified. Although re-expansion pulmonary edema is thought to be secondary to a sudden increase in capillary permeability, the exact mechanism of this increased permeability is unknown. Most cases have been reported after rapid lung re-expansion.

An air leak may be present for a variable amount of time after tube thoracostomy. Should the air leak persist for more than 72 hours or the lung not completely re-expand, surgical intervention is warranted. Primary spontaneous pneumothorax tends to recur with increasing frequency after each episode. The risk of first-time recurrence is on the order of 25% to 30%. Surgery is recommended for a recurrence or the development of a contralateral pneumothorax. Surgical intervention for a first-time pneumothorax is recommended in situations that include bilateral simultaneous pneumothoraces, complete (100%) pneumothorax, pneumothorax associated with tension, and borderline cardiopulmonary reserve and in patients in high-risk professions or activities involving significant variations in atmospheric pressure, such as pilots or scuba divers. Surgery for complications of pneumothorax (empyema, hemothorax, or chronic pneumothorax) also is recommended in patients with first-time spontaneous pneumothorax.

Surgery for primary spontaneous pneumothorax has evolved over recent years from open thoracotomy (axillary or posterolateral) to a minimally invasive video-assisted technique (Fig. 55-9).[84-86] The surgery carried out is identical, despite the differences in approach. Apical blebs are resected. The parietal pleura over the apex of the hemithorax can be removed (pleurectomy), abraded (mechanical pleurodesis), or treated with talc or tetracycline-like agents (chemical pleurodesis or poudrage). The recurrence rate for these procedures, performed open or closed, is less than 5%. Naunheim and colleagues[87] reported their results on 113 consecutive patients treated with VATS blebectomy and pleurodesis in 1995. Their recurrence rate was 4%. More importantly, they found a reduced drainage time and complication rate and a shorter hospital stay with this approach. Patients also had a high acceptance rate of this procedure.

Treatment options for primary and secondary spontaneous pneumothorax are similar. However, patients with secondary pneumothorax generally are debilitated from a respiratory standpoint and may have other significant comorbid diseases.[88] Treatment with tube thoracostomy alone has a high recurrence rate. Effective treatment must be individualized but should include chemical or surgical pleurodesis in combination with complete lung re-expansion and effective sealing of air leaks.

Mesothelioma

Mesothelioma is a rare neoplasm that arises from mesothelial cells lining the parietal and visceral pleura and can present in a localized or diffuse manner. The localized variant (solitary fibrous tumor) is very uncommon and usually presents as a well-defined, encapsulated tumor that is not associated with exposure to asbestos. Typically, the lesions are diagnosed as an asymptomatic mass on a chest radiograph. Complete surgical resection is the treatment of choice.

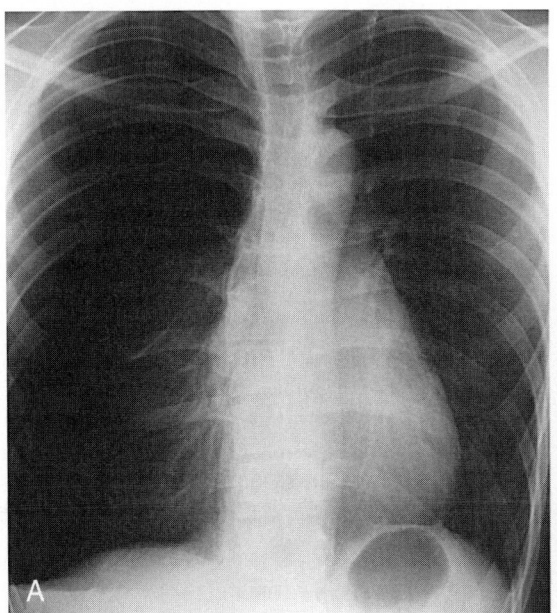
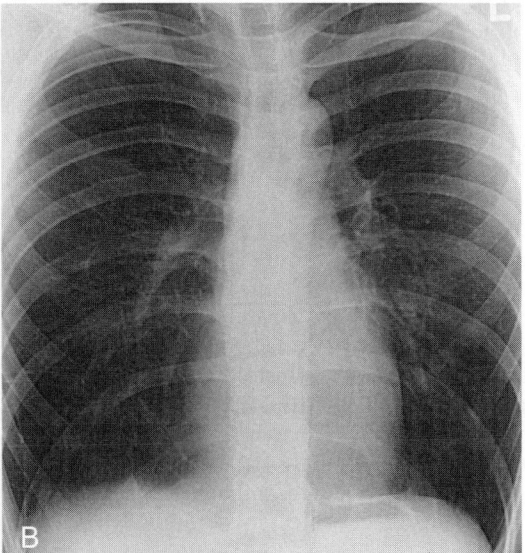

■ FIGURE 55-9.   A, Chest radiograph demonstrates spontaneous right pneumothorax. Note left apical scarring from previous surgery for spontaneous left pneumothorax. **B,** Chest x-ray after thoracoscopic blebectomy and apical pleurectomy.

The diffuse variant presents as a locally aggressive tumor commonly associated with asbestos exposure (75%).[89] A long latency period between asbestos exposure and the development of the disease has been reported.[90] Although smoking alone is not a reported risk factor, other factors such as radiation therapy and various occupational exposures have been implicated.[89] In the late 1990s an association between simian virus 40 (SV 40) and mesothelioma was investigated.[91,92]

The clinical presentation of a patient with diffuse malignant pleural mesothelioma (MPM) is variable; therefore, a thorough clinical evaluation is essential. Dyspnea secondary to pleural effusion or encasement of the lung and chest pain from tumor infiltration into the chest wall and adjacent organs are the most commonly reported symptoms. Nonspecific symptoms such as weight loss, anorexia, night sweats, and weakness also frequently are noted. Physical signs vary depending on the stage of the neoplasm. Early in the disease, decreased breath sounds secondary to pleural effusion may be noted. In advanced stages of the disease, palpable tumor invading the chest wall and abdomen or nodal involvement may be identified.

Radiographic tests such as chest radiography, chest CT, and MRI play a major role in the evaluation of the patient with mesothelioma. Depending on the extent of disease, the chest radiographic findings may be quite variable. Typically, chest radiography demonstrates pleural thickening with or without pleural effusion. Chest CT and MRI are particularly effective in determining the presence of advanced disease, such as transdiaphragmatic involvement or mediastinal organ invasion.[93] Echocardiography also is helpful in ruling out pericardial invasion. In the future, positron emission tomography (PET) also may prove to be a useful tool in determining the extent of tumor invasion.

A number of techniques are used to confirm the diagnosis of MPM, including thoracocentesis of pleural effusion and pleural biopsy (open, VATS, and closed).[94,95] Open or VATS biopsy provides the best method to obtain a tumor sample sufficient to distinguish mesothelioma from other tumors such as adenocarcinoma and to determine the specific subtype of MPM. Frequently, immunohistochemistry techniques and electron microscopy performed by an experienced pathologist are required to confirm the diagnosis of MPM.[96]

Microscopically, malignant mesothelioma originates from mesothelial cells that line the pleural cavity. Three histologic subtypes of mesothelioma have been identified; these are epithelial, sarcomatous, and mixed histologies.[97] The histologic subtype has been shown to affect survival dramatically, with epithelial histology having a more favorable prognosis than the other two subtypes.[98,99]

Several staging systems for mesothelioma are used throughout the world. Although the Butchart tumor node metastasis (TNM) and Brigham staging systems are the most commonly used classifications, neither has been widely accepted.[98,100,101]

With supportive care, survival for mesothelioma ranges between 4 to 12 months.[102] Attempts to improve survival have been made using a wide variety of therapeutic modalities. Treatment of this tumor using single-modality therapy such as radiotherapy, chemotherapy, or surgery has not demonstrated any improvement in survival.[103]

Two surgical cytoreductive procedures, extrapleural pneumonectomy (EPP) or pleural pneumonectomy and pleurectomy/decortication, have been used in the treatment of MPM.[104] In our experience, EPP is the more effective cytoreductive procedure because decorticating the tumor from the fissures and other recesses during pleurectomy can be difficult. The published results of pleurectomy/decortication in a multimodality setting indicate a median survival between 9 and 21 months and a mortality rate ranging from 1.5% to 5%.[105] Controversy surrounding the use of EPP is based on published trials that report high operative morbidity and mortality with no impact on patient survival when used as a single-modality therapy.[106-109] With advances in perioperative management and the development of multimodality approaches, long-term survival can, however, be obtained with EPP with perioperative mortality rates of less than 3%.[98,105,110]

At the Brigham and Women's Hospital, a series of 183 patients who underwent trimodality therapy for MPM from 1980 to 1997 was reviewed in 1999.[98] The patients had undergone EPP followed by sequential chemotherapy (carboplatin/paclitaxel) and radiotherapy (55 Gy). Results from this series identified a favorable subgroup of patients who had epithelial histology, tumor-free resection margins, and negative extrapleural lymph nodes. This group of patients had a 46% 5-year survival and a median survival of 51 months. More recently, novel chemotherapeutic approaches have been advocated. Promising new agents are undergoing clinical trial for single modality and adjuvant therapy. Intraoperative intracavitary heated chemotherapy (cisplatin) administered at the time of either EPP or pleurectomy/decortication is being clinically utilized under protocol.[111]

Despite the overall improvement in survival with multimodality therapy, only 15% to 25% of patients are candidates for EPP.[112] Thus, novel treatment strategies are being developed for this locally aggressive tumor using an intracavitary approach. These strategies include intracavitary chemotherapy, photodynamic therapy, immunotherapy, gene therapy, and vaccination therapy.

Selected References

Martin T, Fontana G, Olak J, et al: Use of pleural catheter for the management of simple pneumothorax. Chest 110:1169-1172, 1996.

> Retrospective review of 84 patients treated with a pleural catheter for iatrogenic or spontaneous pneumothorax demonstrates an 85% resolution rate with this therapy alone.

Naunheim KS, Mack MJ, Hazelrigg SR, et al: Safety and efficacy of video-assisted thoracic surgical techniques for the treatment of spontaneous pneumothorax. J Thorac Cardiovasc Surg 109:1198-1204, 1995.

Review of 113 consecutive patients undergoing VATS treatment of spontaneous pneumothorax demonstrates low morbidity and recurrence rates. Univariate and multivariate analyses identify failure of bleb identification at surgery as the only significant independent predictor of recurrence.

Shamberger RC, Welch KJ: Surgical repair of pectus excavatum. J Pediatr Surg 23:615-622, 1988.

Three-decade review of 704 patients with corrected pectus excavatum. Long-term follow-up documented major recurrence in 2% to 7% and identified total preservation of the perichondrial sheaths (resulting in full cartilage regeneration) as the key to a successful repair.

Sugarbaker DJ, Flores RM, Jaklitsch MT, et al: Resection margins, extrapleural nodal status, and cell type determine postoperative long-term survival in trimodality therapy of malignant pleural mesothelioma: Results in 183 patients. J Thorac Cardiovasc Surg 117:54-65, 1999.

Review of 183 patients undergoing trimodality therapy for MPM demonstrated a 3.8% mortality rate and extended survival in patients with epithelial type, margin-negative, and extrapleural node-negative resection.

Webb WR, Ozmen V, Moulder PV, et al: Iodized talc pleurodesis for the treatment of pleural effusions. J Thorac Cardiovasc Surg 103:881-886, 1992.

Prospective study of talc slurry pleurodesis in 34 patients demonstrating safety and efficacy for pleurodesis of benign or malignant pleural effusions.

Yim AP, Chung SS, Lee TW, et al: Thoracoscopic management of malignant pleural effusions. Chest 109:1234-1238, 1996.

Single-institution experience of VATS management of malignant pleural effusions in 69 patients showing feasibility and safety.

References

1. Celsus: De Medicina. Spencer GW (trans). Cambridge, Harvard University Press, 1938.
2. Hippocrates: The Genuine Works of Hippocrates. Adams F (trans). New York, William Wood, 1929.
3. Graham EA, Bell RD: Open pneumothorax: Its relation to the treatment of acute empyema. Am J Med Sci 156:839, 1918.
4. Ravitch MM, Steichen FM: Atlas of General Thoracic Surgery. Philadelphia, WB Saunders, 1988.
5. Shamberger RC, Welch KJ: Surgical repair of pectus excavatum. J Pediatr Surg 23:615-622, 1988.
6. Shamberger RC, Welch KJ, Castaneda AR, et al: Anterior chest wall deformities and congenital heart disease. J Thorac Cardiovasc Surg 96:427-432, 1988.
7. Ellis DG: Chest wall deformities. Pediatr Rev 11:147-151, 1989.
8. Shamberger RC: Congenital chest wall deformities. Curr Probl Surg 33:469-542, 1996.
9. Shamberger RC, Welch KJ: Chest wall deformities. *In* Ashcraft KW, Holder TM (eds): Pediatric Surgery, 2nd ed. Philadelphia, WB Saunders, 1993, p 146.
10. Crump HW: Pectus excavatum. Am Fam Physician 46:173-179, 1992.
11. Ravitch MM: Pectus excavatum. *In* Rob C, Smith R (eds): Operative Surgery: Cardiothoracic Surgery, 3rd ed. London, Butterworth & Co, 1978.
12. Shamberger RC: Chest wall deformities. *In* Shields TW (ed): General Thoracic Surgery, 4th ed. Baltimore, Williams & Wilkins, 1994, p 529.
13. Baue AE: Chest wall, pleura, lungs, and diaphragm. *In* Davis JH, Drucker WR, Gann DS, et al (eds): Clinical Surgery. St. Louis, CV Mosby, 1987, p 1190.
14. Kowalewski J, Brocki M, Zolynski K: Long-term observation in 68 patients operated on for pectus excavatum: Surgical repair of funnel chest. Ann Thorac Surg 67:821-824, 1999.
15. Shamberger RC, Welch KJ: Surgical correction of pectus carinatum. J Pediatr Surg 22:48-53, 1987.
16. Beiser GD, Epstein SE, Stampfer M, et al: Impairment of cardiac function in patients with pectus excavatum, with improvement after operative correction. N Engl J Med 287:267-272, 1972.
17. Shamberger RC, Welch KJ, Upton J III: Surgical treatment of thoracic deformity in Poland's syndrome. J Pediatr Surg 24:760-766, 1989.
18. Cantrell JR, Haller JA, Ravitch MM: A syndrome of congenital defects involving the abdominal wall, sternum, diaphragm, pericardium, and heart. Surg Gynecol Obstet 107:1958.
19. Anderson BO, Burt ME: Chest wall neoplasms and their management. Ann Thorac Surg 58:1774-1781, 1994.
20. Graeber GM, Jones DR, Pairolero PC: Primary neoplasms. *In* Pearson FG, Deslauriers J, Ginsberg RJ, et al (eds): Thoracic Surgery. New York, Churchill Livingstone, 1995, p 1237.
21. Burt M, Fulton M, Wessner-Dunlap S, et al: Primary bony and cartilaginous sarcomas of chest wall: Results of therapy. Ann Thorac Surg 54:226-232, 1992.
22. Miser JS, Kinsella TJ, Triche TJ, et al: Preliminary results of treatment of Ewing's sarcoma of bone in children and young adults: Six months of intensive combined modality therapy without maintenance. J Clin Oncol 6:484-490, 1988.
23. Faber LP, Somers J, Templeton AC: Chest wall tumors. Curr Probl Surg 32:661-747, 1995.
24. McCormack PM, Bains MS, Burt ME, et al: Local recurrent mammary carcinoma failing multimodality therapy: A solution. Arch Surg 124:158-161, 1989.
25. Pairolero PC, Arnold PG: Chest wall reconstruction. Ann Thorac Surg 32:325-326, 1981.
26. McCaughan BC, Martini N, Bains MS, et al: Chest wall invasion in carcinoma of the lung: Therapeutic and prognostic implications. J Thorac Cardiovasc Surg 89:836-841, 1985.
27. Pairolero PC, Trastek VF, Payne WS: Treatment of bronchogenic carcinoma with chest wall invasion. Surg Clin North Am 67:959-964, 1987.
28. Patterson GA, Ilves R, Ginsberg RJ, et al: The value of adjuvant radiotherapy in pulmonary and chest wall resection for bronchogenic carcinoma. Ann Thorac Surg 34:692-697, 1982.
29. Piehler JM, Pairolero PC, Weiland LH, et al: Bronchogenic carcinoma with chest wall invasion: Factors affecting survival following en bloc resection. Ann Thorac Surg 34:684-691, 1982.
30. Pancoast H: Superior pulmonary sulcus tumor: Tumor characterized by pain, Horner's syndrome, destruction of bone and atrophy of hand muscles. JAMA 99:1391, 1932.
31. Paulson DL: Carcinomas in the superior pulmonary sulcus. J Thorac Cardiovasc Surg 70:1095-1104, 1975.

32. Hilaris BS, Martini N, Wong GY, et al: Treatment of superior sulcus tumor (Pancoast tumor). Surg Clin North Am 67:965-977, 1987.

33. Taylor LQ, Williams AJ, Santiago SM: Survival in patients with superior pulmonary sulcus tumors. Respiration 59:27-29, 1992.

34. Neal CR, Amdur RJ, Mendenhall WM, et al: Pancoast tumor: Radiation therapy alone versus preoperative radiation therapy and surgery. Int J Radiat Oncol Biol Phys 21:651-660, 1991.

35. Wright CD, Moncure AC, Shepard JA, et al: Superior sulcus lung tumors. Results of combined treatment (irradiation and radical resection). J Thorac Cardiovasc Surg 94:69-74, 1987.

36. Mathes SJ: Chest wall reconstruction. Clin Plast Surg 22:187-198, 1995.

37. Urschel JD, Takita H, Antkowiak JG: Necrotizing soft tissue infections of the chest wall. Ann Thorac Surg 64:276-279, 1997.

38. Lee RB, Miller JI Jr.: Radionecrosis and infection. *In* Pearson FG, Deslauriers J, Ginsberg RJ, et al (eds): Thoracic Surgery. New York, Churchill Livingstone, 1995, p 1253.

39. Granick MS, Larson DL, Solomon MP: Radiation-related wounds of the chest wall. Clin Plast Surg 20:559-571, 1993.

40. Abe M, Ichinohe K, Nishida J: Diagnosis, treatment, and complications of thoracic outlet syndrome. J Orthop Sci 4:66-69, 1999.

41. Urschel HC: Thoracic outlet syndromes. *In* Baue AE, Geha AS, Hammond GL, et al (eds): Glenn's Thoracic and Cardiovascular Surgery, 6th ed. Stamford, CT, Appleton & Lange, 1996, p 567.

42. Urschel HC Jr, Razzuk MA: Upper plexus thoracic outlet syndrome: Optimal therapy. Ann Thorac Surg 63:935-939, 1997.

43. Harding A, Silver D: Thoracic outlet syndrome. *In* Sabiston DC Jr (ed): Textbook of Surgery: The Biological Basis of Modern Surgical Practice, 14th ed. Philadelphia, WB Saunders, 1991, p 1757.

44. Mackinnon SE, Patterson GA, Novak CB: Thoracic outlet syndrome: A current overview. Semin Thorac Cardiovasc Surg 8:176-182, 1996.

45. Rayan GM: Thoracic outlet syndrome. J Shoulder Elbow Surg 7:440-451, 1998.

46. Novak CB: Conservative management of thoracic outlet syndrome. Semin Thorac Cardiovasc Surg 8:201-207, 1996.

47. Pang D, Wessel HB: Thoracic outlet syndrome. Neurosurgery 22:105-121, 1988.

48. Mackinnon SE, Patterson GA: Supraclavicular first rib resection. Semin Thorac Cardiovasc Surg 8:208-213, 1996.

49. Pate JW: Chest wall injuries. Surg Clin North Am 69:59-70, 1989.

50. Feliciano DV: The diagnostic and therapeutic approach to chest trauma. Semin Thorac Cardiovasc Surg 4:156-162, 1992.

51. Poole GV: Fracture of the upper ribs and injury to the great vessels. Surg Gynecol Obstet 169:275-282, 1989.

52. Miller HAB, Taylor GA: Flail chest and pulmonary contusion. *In* McMurtry RY, McLellan BA (eds): Management of Blunt Trauma. Baltimore, Williams & Wilkins, 1990, p 186.

53. Ahmed Z, Mohyuddin Z: Management of flail chest injury: Internal fixation versus endotracheal intubation and ventilation. J Thorac Cardiovasc Surg 110:1676-1680, 1995.

54. Krasna MJ, Flancbaum L: Blunt cardiac trauma: Clinical manifestations and management. Semin Thorac Cardiovasc Surg 4:195-202, 1992.

55. Lee KF, Olak J: Anatomy and physiology of the pleural space. Chest Surg Clin North Am 4:391-403, 1994.

56. Boggs DS, Kinasewitz GT: Review: Pathophysiology of the pleural space. Am J Med Sci 309:53-59, 1995.

57. Henschke CI, Davis SD, Romano PM, et al: The pathogenesis, radiologic evaluation, and therapy of pleural effusions. Radiol Clin North Am 27:1241-1255, 1989.

58. Kinasewitz GT: Transudative effusions. Eur Respir J 10:714-718, 1997.

59. Owens MW, Milligan SA: Pleuritis and pleural effusions. Curr Opin Pulm Med 1:318-323, 1995.

60. Miserocchi G: Physiology and pathophysiology of pleural fluid turnover. Eur Respir J 10:219-225, 1997.

61. Gitt SM: Acute dyspnea in a woman with a chronic pleural mass. Hosp Pract (Off Ed) 27:181-182, 1992.

62. Sahn SA: The pathophysiology of pleural effusions. Annu Rev Med 41:7-13, 1990.

63. Muller NL: Imaging of the pleura. Radiology 186:297-309, 1993.

64. Light RW, Macgregor MI, Luchsinger PC, et al: Pleural effusions: The diagnostic separation of transudates and exudates. Ann Intern Med 77:507-513, 1972.

65. Ansari T, Idell S: Management of undiagnosed persistent pleural effusions. Clin Chest Med 19:407-417, 1998.

66. Hammar SP: The pathology of benign and malignant pleural disease. Chest Surg Clin North Am 4:405-430, 1994.

67. Joseph J, Sahn SA: Connective tissue diseases and the pleura. Chest 104:262-270, 1993.

68. Leuallen EC, Carr DT: Pleural effusion: A statistical study of 436 patients. N Engl J Med 252:79, 1955.

69. Grossi F, Pennucci MC, Tixi L, et al: Management of malignant pleural effusions. Drugs 55:47-58, 1998.

70. Robinson LA, Fleming WH, Galbraith TA: Intrapleural doxycycline control of malignant pleural effusions. Ann Thorac Surg 55:1115-1122, 1993.

71. Fentiman IS, Rubens RD, Hayward JL: A comparison of intracavitary talc and tetracycline for the control of pleural effusions secondary to breast cancer. Eur J Cancer Clin Oncol 22:1079-1081, 1986.

72. Webb WR, Ozmen V, Moulder PV, et al: Iodized talc pleurodesis for the treatment of pleural effusions. J Thorac Cardiovasc Surg 103:881-886, 1992.

73. Berkman N, Kramer MR: Diagnostic tests in pleural effusion—an update. Postgrad Med J 69:12-18, 1993.

74. DeCamp MM Jr, Mentzer SJ, Swanson SJ, et al: Malignant effusive disease of the pleura and pericardium. Chest 112:291S-295S, 1997.

75. Hausheer FH, Yarbro JW: Diagnosis and treatment of malignant pleural effusion. Semin Oncol 12:54-75, 1985.

76. Ruckdeschel JC: Management of malignant pleural effusion: An overview. Semin Oncol 15:24-28, 1988.

77. Yim AP, Chung SS, Lee TW, et al: Thoracoscopic management of malignant pleural effusions. Chest 109:1234-1238, 1996.

78. DeMeester TR, LaFontaine E: The pleura. *In* Sabiston DC Jr, Spencer FC (eds): Surgery of the Chest, 5th ed. Philadelphia, WB Saunders, 1990, p 444.

79. Sassoon CS: The etiology and treatment of spontaneous pneumothorax. Curr Opin Pulm Med 1:331-338, 1995.

80. Paape K, Fry WA: Spontaneous pneumothorax. Chest Surg Clin North Am 4:517-538, 1994.

81. Schramel FM, Postmus PE, Vanderschueren RG: Current aspects of spontaneous pneumothorax. Eur Respir J 10:1372-1379, 1997.

82. Martin T, Fontana G, Olak J, et al: Use of pleural catheter for the management of simple pneumothorax. Chest 110:1169-1172, 1996.

83. Carlson RI, Classen KL, Gollan F, et al: Pulmonary edema following the rapid re-expansion of a totally collapsed lung

due to a pneumothorax: A clinical and experimental study. Surg Forum 9:367, 1958.

84. Berrisford RG, Page RD: Video assisted thoracic surgery for spontaneous pneumothorax. Thorax 51(Suppl 2):S23-S28, 1996.

85. Janssen JP: Thoracoscopy in the management of spontaneous pneumothorax. Int Surg 81:339-342, 1996.

86. Massard G, Thomas P, Wihlm JM: Minimally invasive management for first and recurrent pneumothorax. Ann Thorac Surg 66:592-599, 1998.

87. Naunheim KS, Mack MJ, Hazelrigg SR, et al: Safety and efficacy of video-assisted thoracic surgical techniques for the treatment of spontaneous pneumothorax. J Thorac Cardiovasc Surg 109:1198-1204, 1995.

88. Boutin C, Astoul P, Rey F, et al: Thoracoscopy in the diagnosis and treatment of spontaneous pneumothorax. Clin Chest Med 16:497-503, 1995.

89. McDonald JC, McDonald AD: The epidemiology of mesothelioma in historical context. Eur Respir J 9:1932-1942, 1996.

90. Price B: Analysis of current trends in United States mesothelioma incidence. Am J Epidemiol 145:211-218, 1997.

91. Pass HI, Donington JS, Wu P, et al: Human mesotheliomas contain the simian virus-40 regulatory region and large tumor antigen DNA sequences. J Thorac Cardiovasc Surg 116:854-859, 1998.

92. Pass HI, Kennedy RC, Carbone M: Evidence for and implications of SV 40-like sequences in human mesotheliomas. *In* DeVita VT, Hellman S, Rosenberg SA (eds): Important Advances in Oncology. Philadelphia, Lippincott-Raven, 1996, p 89.

93. Patz EF Jr, Shaffer K, Piwnica-Worms DR, et al: Malignant pleural mesothelioma: Value of CT and MR imaging in predicting resectability. AJR Am J Roentgenol 159:961-966, 1992.

94. Gottehrer A, Taryle DA, Reed CE, et al: Pleural fluid analysis in malignant mesothelioma. Prognostic implications. Chest 100:1003-1006, 1991.

95. Sugarbaker DJ, Norberto JJ, Swanson SJ: Surgical staging and work-up of patients with diffuse malignant pleural mesothelioma. Semin Thorac Cardiovasc Surg 9:356-360, 1997.

96. Soosay GN, Griffiths M, Papadaki L, et al: The differential diagnosis of epithelial-type mesothelioma from adenocarcinoma and reactive mesothelial proliferation. J Pathol 163:299-305, 1991.

97. Sugarbaker DJ, Mentzer SJ, DeCamp M, et al: Extrapleural pneumonectomy in the setting of a multimodality approach to malignant mesothelioma. Chest 103:377S-381S, 1993.

98. Sugarbaker DJ, Flores RM, Jaklitsch MT, et al: Resection margins, extrapleural nodal status, and cell type determine postoperative long-term survival in trimodality therapy of malignant pleural mesothelioma: Results in 183 patients. J Thorac Cardiovasc Surg 117:54-65, 1999.

99. Sugarbaker DJ, Garcia JP, Richards WG, et al: Extrapleural pneumonectomy in the multimodality therapy of malignant pleural mesothelioma: Results in 120 consecutive patients. Ann Surg 224:288-296, 1996.

100. George SL, Desu MM: Planning the size and duration of a clinical trial studying the time to some critical event. J Chronic Dis 27:15-24, 1974.

101. Rusch VW: A proposed new international TNM staging system for malignant pleural mesothelioma. From the International Mesothelioma Interest Group. Chest 108:1122-1128, 1995.

102. Pass HI, Pogrebniak HW: Malignant pleural mesothelioma. Curr Probl Surg 30:921-1012, 1993.

103. Boutin C, Schlesser M, Frenay C, et al: Malignant pleural mesothelioma. Eur Respir J 12:972-981, 1998.

104. Sugarbaker DJ, Norberto JJ, Bueno R: Current therapy for mesothelioma. Cancer Control 4:326-334, 1997.

105. Sugarbaker DJ, Norberto JJ, Swanson SJ: Extrapleural pneumonectomy in the setting of multimodality therapy for diffuse malignant pleural mesothelioma. Semin Thorac Cardiovasc Surg 9:373-382, 1997.

106. Butchart EG, Ashcroft T, Barnsley WC, et al: Pleuropneumonectomy in the management of diffuse malignant mesothelioma of the pleura: Experience with 29 patients. Thorax 31:15-24, 1976.

107. Faber LP: Malignant pleural mesothelioma: Operative treatment by extrapleural pneumonectomy. *In* Kittle CF (ed): Current Controversies in Thoracic Surgery. Philadelphia, WB Saunders, 1986, p 80.

108. Rusch VW, Piantadosi S, Holmes EC: The role of extrapleural pneumonectomy in malignant pleural mesothelioma: A Lung Cancer Study Group trial. J Thorac Cardiovasc Surg 102:1-9, 1991.

109. Worn H: [Chances and results of surgery of malignant mesothelioma of the pleura (author's transl)]. Thoraxchir Vask Chir 22:391-393, 1974.

110. Sugarbaker DJ, Strauss GM, Lynch TJ, et al: Node status has prognostic significance in the multimodality therapy of diffuse, malignant mesothelioma. J Clin Oncol 11:1172-1178, 1993.

111. Sugarbaker DJ, Richards W, Jaklitsch M, et al: Prevention, early detection and management of complications following 328 consecutive extrapleural pneumonectomies. Presented before the American Association for Thoracic Surgery, 83rd Annual Meeting. Boston, 2003.

112. Kaiser LR: New therapies in the treatment of malignant pleural mesothelioma. Semin Thorac Cardiovasc Surg 9:383-390, 1997.

CHAPTER 56

THE MEDIASTINUM

Christine L. Lau, M.D. and R. Duane Davis, Jr., M.D.

Anatomic Landmarks

Mediastinal Emphysema

Mediastinitis

Mediastinal Hemorrhage

Superior Vena Cava Obstruction

Primary Neoplasms and Cysts

The mediastinum is an anatomic division of the thorax extending from the diaphragm to the thoracic inlet. It is the site of many localized disorders and is involved in a number of systemic diseases. Localized disorders that occur in this region include primary tumors and cysts as well as infection, hemorrhage, emphysema, and aneurysms. Systemic diseases include metastatic neoplasms and granulomatous and other inflammatory disorders. Lesions that originate in the esophagus, great vessels, trachea, and heart may present as a mediastinal mass and are relevant in the differential diagnosis of the various primary mediastinal disease processes. Mediastinal disorders present as a number of clinical features. Many cases are asymptomatic, and the disorder is identified on routine chest radiographs. Most patients, however, have clinical features related to local involvement of adjacent structures, tumor secretory factors, or immunologic factors.

ANATOMY

The mediastinum is defined by the following borders: the thoracic inlet superiorly, the diaphragm inferiorly, the sternum anteriorly, the vertebral column posteriorly, and the parietal pleura laterally. Many mediastinal tumors and cysts occur in characteristic locations; therefore, the mediastinum has been subdivided artificially for the convenience of localizing specific types of lesions. Some subdivide the mediastinum into four compartments: superior, anterior, middle, and posterior; however, the frequency with which tumors occurring in the anterior or posterior compartments extend into the superior mediastinum has prompted a division of the mediastinum into three subdivisions: the anterosuperior, middle, and posterior (Fig. 56-1).

MEDIASTINAL EMPHYSEMA

Air may enter the mediastinum from the esophagus, trachea, bronchi, lung, neck, or abdomen, producing mediastinal emphysema or pneumomediastinum. Injury to these structures can occur from blunt or penetrating trauma, intraluminal injury (e.g., during endoscopy), and barotrauma. Mediastinal emphysema may also be caused by intra-abdominal air dissecting through the diaphragmatic hiatus. Spontaneous pneumomediastinum is usually seen in patients with exacerbation of bronchospastic disease.

The clinical manifestations of pneumomediastinum include substernal chest pain, which may radiate into the back, and crepitation in the region of the suprasternal notch, chest wall, and neck. With increasing pressure, the air can dissect into the neck, face, chest, arms, abdomen, and retroperitoneum. Frequently, pneumomediastinum and pneumothorax occur simultaneously. Auscultation over the pericardium demonstrates a characteristic crunching sound that is accentuated during systole and is termed Hamman's sign. The diagnosis of pneumomediastinum is confirmed by the presence of air in the mediastinum as visualized on the chest radiographs or computed tomographic (CT) scans. Air is usually also present in the pectoral muscles, neck, and upper extremities. To evaluate the esophagus and large airways as potential sources, contrast studies of the esophagus, initially using a water-soluble contrast material, and bronchoscopy are best. Perforations of these structures usually require urgent surgical treatment. Spontaneous mediastinal emphysema and pneumomediastinum secondary to barotrauma usually respond to conservative measures that treat bronchospasm and minimize further barotrauma without sequelae. Surgical decompression is rarely necessary. In patients with pneumomediastinum and pneumothorax, tube thoracostomy is indicated in the affected

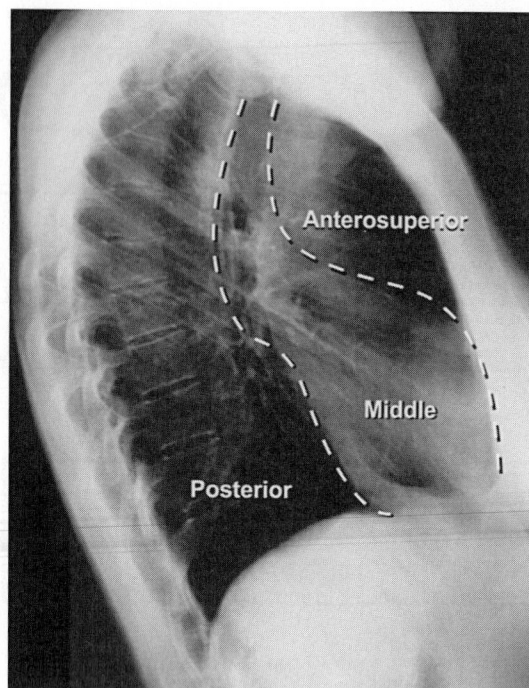

FIGURE 56-1. Lateral chest radiograph divided into three anatomic subdivisions, with the tumors and cysts that occur most frequently in each region.

pleural space. Patients with pneumomediastinum secondary to barotrauma continuing to require high levels of ventilator support may require bilateral tube thoracostomies to prevent the development of tension pneumothorax. In patients who are distressed by the inability to open their eyes, 5-mm incisions in the skinfolds of the eyelids and neck can be made using local anesthesia. With gentle pressure on the surrounding soft tissue, sufficient air can be removed to provide symptomatic relief.

MEDIASTINITIS

Infection of the mediastinal space is a serious and potentially fatal process. Etiologic factors responsible for the development of acute mediastinitis include perforation of the esophagus resulting from instrumentation, foreign bodies, penetrating or, more rarely, blunt trauma, spontaneous esophageal disruption (Boerhaave's syndrome), leakage from an esophageal anastomosis, tracheobronchial perforation, and mediastinal extension from an infectious process originating in the pulmonary parenchyma, pleura, chest wall, vertebrae, great vessels, or neck. Mediastinitis occurs most often after median sternotomy for cardiac operations.

Mediastinitis is manifested clinically by fever, tachycardia, leukocytosis, and pain that may be localized to the chest, back, or neck, although in some patients the clinical course remains indolent for long periods. In postoperative patients, wound cellulitis and instability of the sternal closure are often present.

Treatment of mediastinitis requires correction of the inciting cause and aggressive supportive therapy. After obtaining cultures, appropriate antimicrobial coverage should be initiated, with modification after results of culture and sensitivity testing are available. In patients with mediastinal infections in continuity or communication with empyema, subphrenic abscess, or neck abscess, drainage of the empyema with tube thoracostomy or percutaneous drainage of the abscess in conjunction with appropriate antimicrobial therapy is frequently successful. Similarly, mediastinitis associated with catheter sepsis can often be treated with removal of the catheter and antimicrobial therapy. In patients who do not respond to these initial measures or in whom mediastinitis occurs from most other causes, thorough débridement of necrotic and infected tissue is necessary in conjunction with surgical drainage. When costal cartilage is infected, it is necessary to excise the cartilage back to bleeding bone.

Postoperative mediastinitis after median sternotomy has been successfully treated with a number of different techniques. The best results have been obtained using a variety of tissue flaps to obliterate dead space and to provide immediate coverage of the heart, bypass grafts, and great vessels after effective surgical control of the wound. Débridement of infected and necrotic sternum, cartilage, and soft tissue in conjunction with wound care is necessary to provide a clean wound to optimize results. The omentum has also been used successfully.

MEDIASTINAL HEMORRHAGE

Mediastinal hemorrhage is most frequently caused by blunt or penetrating trauma, thoracic aortic dissection, rupture of aortic aneurysm, or surgical procedures within the thorax. The clinical presentation varies with the underlying etiology. Retrosternal pain radiating to the back or neck is common. With increased accumulation of blood in the mediastinum, signs and symptoms related to compression of mediastinal structures (primarily the great veins) develop, including dyspnea, venous distention, cyanosis, and cervical ecchymosis resulting from blood dissecting into soft tissue planes. Diagnostic measures include chest radiographs, which may indicate superior mediastinal widening, loss of the normal aortic contour, and soft tissue density in the anterosuperior mediastinum; echocardiography; and magnetic resonance imaging (MRI) or CT, which may better characterize a mass and its relationship to vascular structures, particularly if a false lumen is present. Arteriography may be useful in localizing the site of bleeding or intimal disruption. Therapy is directed toward evacuation of existing clot and repair of the underlying process. In patients who have suffered penetrating trauma with associated profound hypotension, emergency thoracotomy or sternotomy is indicated without initial arteriography.

SUPERIOR VENA CAVA OBSTRUCTION

A number of benign and malignant processes may cause obstruction of the superior vena cava, leading to superior vena caval syndrome. The pathophysiology of the syndrome involves the increased pressure in the venous system draining into the superior vena cava, producing the characteristic features of the syndrome, which include edema of the head, neck, and upper extremities; distended neck veins with dilated collateral veins over the upper extremities and torso; cyanosis; headache; and confusion. Superior vena caval obstruction may arise from compression, invasion, or thrombosis. The cause may be the primary tumor or mass but is often paratracheal lymph node metastases. In adults the most frequent cause is a malignant neoplasm, usually a bronchogenic carcinoma; in children, however, the syndrome is most common after cardiac surgical procedures. Contrast medium–enhanced CT or MRI is usually adequate to establish the diagnosis of superior vena cava obstruction and to assist in the differential diagnosis of probable cause. Rarely are the malignant processes responsible for the superior vena caval syndrome surgically resectable. Percutaneous needle biopsy is usually the initial diagnostic modality used to establish a histologic diagnosis, which is attempted before the initiation of empirical therapy because of the alteration of the morphologic appearance after therapy. Open biopsy in patients able to tolerate anesthesia may be necessary to establish a diagnosis. These patients, however, are at an increased risk for cardiorespiratory compromise during general anesthesia.

The most useful types of therapy include percutaneous stenting, irradiation, corticosteroid therapy, multiagent chemotherapy, and anticoagulant or fibrinolytic therapy. The optimal therapeutic regimen is dependent on the histologic diagnosis. In patients in whom the syndrome develops rapidly or neurologic symptoms are present, therapy may be necessary on an emergency basis.

The use of percutaneous stents has shown great promise in the treatment of superior vena cava syndrome, especially in cases associated with malignant tumors.[1,2] Excellent results have been reported, with responses seen in 68% to 100% of patients treated. One major advantage of these self-expandable stents is that they can be placed under local anesthesia with radiologic manipulation. Complications are rare. Recurrence of symptoms is uncommon and can usually be treated with anticoagulation, angioplasty of the stented area, or new stent placement.[1]

Superior vena caval syndromes that are caused by benign disease usually respond to medical therapy consisting of diuretics, upright positioning, and fluid restriction until collateral channels develop and allow clinical regression.

PRIMARY NEOPLASMS AND CYSTS

A large number of neoplasms and cysts may arise from multiple anatomic sites in the mediastinum and present as myriad clinical signs and symptoms. The natural history varies from those that are asymptomatic, to those with benign slow growth causing minimal symptoms, to aggressive, invasive neoplasms that are often widely metastatic, rapidly resulting in death. With improvements in treatment modalities, the observation of a mediastinal mass, except in rare circumstances, cannot be justified. A classification of primary mediastinal tumors and cysts is

shown in Box 56-1. The relative incidence with which they occurred in a combined series of 2504 patients is shown in Table 56-1.[3-16] Although differences in the relative incidence of neoplasms and cysts exist in some series, the most common mediastinal masses are neurogenic tumors (20%), thymomas (19%), primary cysts (18%), lymphomas (13%), and germ cell tumors (10%).

Mediastinal masses are most frequently located in the anterosuperior mediastinum (56%), with the posterior (25%) and middle mediastinum (19%) being less frequently involved. Many of the mediastinal lesions occur in characteristic sites within the mediastinum. The masses that occur most commonly in each of the three anatomic subdivisions and the relative incidence with which they occurred in a series of 514 patients from the Duke University Medical Center are shown in Table 56-2. In addition, the location of the mass explains some of the typical symptoms related to a mediastinal mass because of compression or invasion of adjacent mediastinal structures. The common symptoms related to mechanical involvement with mediastinal structures are listed in Box 56-2.

Malignant neoplasms represent 25% to 42% of mediastinal masses. Lymphomas, thymomas, germ cell tumors, primary carcinomas, and neurogenic tumors are the most common. The relative frequency of mediastinal mass malignancy varies with the anatomic site in the mediastinum. Anterosuperior masses are most likely malignant (59%), relative to middle mediastinal masses (29%) and posterior mediastinal masses (16%). The relative percentage of lesions that are malignant also varies with age. Patients in the second through fourth decades of life have a greater proportion of malignant mediastinal masses. This period corresponds to the peak incidence of lymphomas and germ cell tumors. In contrast, in the first decade of life, a mediastinal mass is most likely benign (73%).

The incidence of mediastinal masses varies in infants, children, and adults. In a combined series of 723 children with mediastinal masses, neurogenic tumors (35%), lymphomas (25%), germ cell tumors (10%), and primary cysts (16%) were diagnosed most frequently. The neurogenic tumors in children most commonly originate from sympathetic ganglion cells: gangliomas, ganglioneuroblastomas, and neuroblastomas. In contrast, neurilemomas and neurofibromas are the most common neurogenic tumors in adults. The childhood lymphomas are usually of a non-Hodgkin's lymphoma variety. The germ cell tumors are most frequently benign teratomas. Pericardial cysts and thymomas are uncommon in children.

Clinical Features

The clinical presentation varies from asymptomatic disease (the diagnosis is made by routine chest radiographs) to symptoms related to mechanical effects of invasion or compression to systemic symptoms. Of patients with a mediastinal mass, 56% to 65% have symptoms at presentation. Patients with a benign lesion are more often symptom free (54%) than are patients with a malignant neoplasm (15%). The most common features in a series of 514 patients were chest pain, fever, cough, and

Box 56-1. Classification of Primary Mediastinal Tumors and Cysts

Neurogenic Tumors

Neurofibroma
Neurilemoma
Neurosarcoma
Ganglioneuroma
Neuroblastoma
Chemodectoma
Paraganglioma

Thymoma

Benign
Malignant

Lymphoma

Hodgkin's disease
Lymphoblastic lymphoma
Large cell lymphoma

Germ Cell Tumors

Teratodermoid
  Benign
  Malignant
Seminoma
Nonseminoma
  Embryonal
  Choriocarcinoma
  Endodermal

Primary Carcinomas

Mesenchymal Tumors

Fibroma/fibrosarcoma
Lipoma/liposarcoma

Leiomyoma/leiomyosarcoma
Rhabdosarcoma
Xanthogranuloma
Myxoma
Mesothelioma
Hemangioma
Hemangioendothelioma
Hemangiopericytoma
Lymphangioma
Lymphangiomyoma
Lymphangiopericytoma

Endocrine Tumors

Intrathoracic thyroid
Parathyroid adenoma/carcinoma
Carcinoid

Cysts

Bronchogenic
Pericardial
Enteric
Thymic
Thoracic duct
Nonspecific

Giant Lymph Node Hyperplasia

Castleman's disease

Chondroma

Extramedullary Hematopoiesis

TABLE 56-1.   Primary Mediastinal Tumors and Cysts in 2504 Patients

Type of Tumor	Sabiston and Scott,[3] 1952	Heimburger et al,[4] 1965	Burkell et al,[5] 1969	Fontanelle et al,[6] 1971	Benjamin et al,[7] 1972	Conkle and Adkins,[8] 1972	Rubush et al,[9] 1973
Neurogenic tumor	20	21	13	17	49	8	36
Thymoma	17	10	12	17	34	11	42
Lymphoma	11	9	12	16	32	10	14
Germ cell neoplasm	9	10	3	7	27	2	14
Primary carcinoma	10	11	0	2	0	10	3
Mesenchymal tumor	1	4	4	0	24	2	10
Endocrine tumor	2	8	4	0	24	0	13
Other	14	0	0	0	0	0	0
Cysts	17	24	13	23	19	0	21
Pericardial	2	4	4	2	3	0	10
Bronchogenic	5	12	9	13	11	0	6
Enteric	2	5	0	4	1	0	2
Other	8	3	0	4	4	0	3
Total	101	97	61	82	209	43	153

Continued

TABLE 56-1. Primary Mediastinal Tumors and Cysts in 2504 Patients—*Cont'd*

Vidne and Levy,[10] 1973	Ovrum and Birkeland,[11] 1979	Nandi et al,[12] 1980	Adkins et al,[13] 1984	Parish et al,[14] 1984	Duke Medical Center,[15] 1998	Total	Incidence (%)
9	19	27	8	212	71	510	20
9	10	18	4	206	94	484	19
6	11	4	7	107	77	316	13
3	5	7	11	99	53	250	10
2	9	0	5	25	37	114	5
4	4	2	0	60	29	144	6
2	21	6	2	56	19	157	6
1	2	1	1	36	10	65	3
8	10	9	0	196	124	464	18
2	7	2	0	72	45	153	6
2	0	0	0	54	48	160	6
1	0	0	0	29	12	56	2
3	3	7	0	41	19	95	4
44	91	74	38	997	514	2504	

TABLE 56-2. Anatomic Location of Primary Tumors and Cysts of the Mediastinum

Type of Tumor or Cyst	Percentage
ANTEROSUPERIOR MEDIASTINUM (n = 287)	
Thymic neoplasms	33
Lymphomas	19
Germ cell tumors	17
Benign	9
Malignant	8
Carcinoma	11
Cysts	8
Mesenchymal	4
Endocrine	6
Other	2
MIDDLE MEDIASTINUM (n = 98)	
Cysts	61
Lymphomas	21
Mesenchymal	8
Carcinoma	6
Other	4
POSTERIOR MEDIASTINUM (n = 129)	
Neurogenic	53
Benign	41
Malignant	12
Cysts	32
Mesenchymal	9
Endocrine	2
Other	4

Box 56-2. Clinical Manifestations of Anatomic Compression or Invasion by Neoplasms of the Mediastinum

Spinal cord compressive syndrome
Vena caval obstruction
Pericardial tamponade
Congestive heart failure
Dysrhythmias
Pulmonary stenosis
Tracheal compression
Esophageal compression
Vocal cord paralysis
Horner's syndrome
Phrenic nerve paralysis
Chylothorax
Chylopericardium
Spinal cord compressive syndrome
Pancoast's syndrome
Postobstructive pneumonitis

are more indicative of a malignant histologic diagnosis, although patients with a benign lesion, on occasion, present in this manner.

A number of primary mediastinal lesions produce hormones or antibodies that cause systemic symptoms, which may characterize a specific syndrome (Table 56-4). Examples of these syndromes include Cushing's syndrome, caused by ectopic production of adrenocorticotropic hormone, most frequently by neuroendocrine tumors; thyrotoxicosis, which is caused by a mediastinal goiter; hypertension and a hyperdynamic state, caused by

dyspnea (Table 56-3). Infants and children are more likely to present with symptoms or findings (78%) because of the relatively small space within the mediastinum.

Symptoms related to compression or invasion of mediastinal structures, such as the superior vena caval syndrome, Horner's syndrome, hoarseness, and severe pain,

TABLE 56-3.   Presenting Symptoms in Patients With a Mediastinal Mass

Symptoms	Percentage of Patients (n = 514)
Chest pain	33
Dyspnea	20
Cough	18
Fever, chills	19
Weight loss	9
Superior vena caval syndrome	8
Myasthenia gravis	7
Fatigue	6
Dysphagia	4
Night sweats	3

TABLE 56-4.   Systemic Syndromes Caused by Mediastinal Neoplasm Hormone Production

Syndrome	Tumor
Hypertension	Pheochromocytoma, chemodectoma, ganglioneuroma, neuroblastoma
Hypoglycemia	Mesothelioma, teratoma, fibrosarcoma, neurosarcoma
Diarrhea	Ganglioneuroma, neuroblastoma, neurofibroma
Hypercalcemia	Parathyroid adenoma/carcinoma, Hodgkin's disease
Thyrotoxicosis	Thyroid adenoma/carcinoma
Gynecomastia	Nonseminomatous germ cell tumors

TABLE 56-5.   Systemic Syndromes Associated With Mediastinal Neoplasms

Tumor	Syndrome
Thymoma	Myasthenia gravis Red blood cell aplasia White blood cell aplasia Aplastic anemia Hypogammaglobulinemia Progressive systemic sclerosis Hemolytic anemia Megaesophagus Dermatomyositis Systemic lupus erythematosus Myocarditis Collagen vascular disease
Lymphoma	Anemia, myasthenia gravis
Neurofibroma	Von Recklinghausen's disease
Carcinoid	Cushing's syndrome
Carcinoid, thymoma	Multiple endocrine adenomatosis
Thymoma, neurofibroma, neurilemoma, mesothelioma	Osteoarthropathy
Enteric cysts	Vertebral anomalies
Hodgkin's disease	Alcohol-induced pain Pel-Ebstein fever
Neuroblastoma	Opsomyoclonus Erythrocyte abnormalities
Enteric cysts	Peptic ulcer

pheochromocytoma; and hypercalcemia secondary to increased parathyroid hormone release from a mediastinal parathyroid adenoma.

In other syndromes, the pathophysiology is not as well understood (Table 56-5). Autoimmune mechanisms have been implicated in the association of myasthenia gravis and red blood cell aplasia with thymoma. In other cases the pathophysiology is less defined: osteoarthropathy and neurogenic tumors; pain after ingestion of alcohol and the cyclic Pel-Ebstein fevers associated with Hodgkin's disease; and the opsomyoclonus syndrome and neuroblastoma.

Diagnosis

The goal of the diagnostic evaluation in a patient with a mediastinal mass is a precise histologic diagnosis so that optimal therapy can be performed. The preoperative evaluation of a patient with a mediastinal mass should achieve the following: (1) differentiate a primary mediastinal mass from masses of other causes that have a similar radiographic appearance; (2) recognize associated systemic manifestations that may affect the patient's perioperative course; (3) evaluate for possible compression by the mass of the tracheobronchial tree, pulmonary artery, or superior vena cava; (4) ascertain whether the mass extends into the spinal column; (5) determine whether the mass is a nonseminomatous germ cell tumor; (6) assess the likelihood of resectability; and (7) identify significant factors of medical comorbidity and optimize overall medical condition.

The initial diagnostic intervention should be a careful history and physical examination. The recognition of associated systemic syndromes with many neoplasms is necessary to avoid potentially serious intraoperative and postoperative complications. Although most systemic syndromes listed in Table 56-5 may be of little consequence regarding the planned surgical management, the association of myasthenia gravis, malignant hypertension, hypogammaglobulinemia, hypercalcemia, and thyrotoxicosis with mediastinal neoplasms markedly affects appropriate management.

The posteroanterior and lateral chest radiographs provide important information concerning anatomic location and size of the tumor. CT with contrast medium enhancement should be done routinely in patients with a mediastinal mass. In patients with a contraindication to the use of contrast dye and in those with surgical clips in the anatomic region of interest, MRI is useful. Considerable information can be obtained regarding the relative invasiveness and malignant nature of the mediastinal mass with either CT or MRI. Tumor disruption of fat planes;

irregularity of pleural, vascular, or pericardial margins by tumor; and infiltration into muscle or periosteum are useful for differentiating tumor compression from invasion. Resectability is better assessed than nonresectability using CT or MRI. MRI may be more useful than CT with certain posterior mediastinal masses in terms of evaluating their involvement with the spinal canal, and it has been shown to be superior to CT in diagnosing various cysts.[17] Additionally, MRI may provide information regarding the involvement of the tumor with major vascular structures and may help detect whether the tumor is actually a vascular abnormality. Angiographic studies may be required when there is a question of a vascular abnormality and the MRI is unable to determine vessel involvement.

Echocardiography may be useful in the evaluation of mediastinal masses, especially tumors, that occur in the middle mediastinum or in patients with tamponade or pulmonary stenosis. Echocardiography delineates the cystic nature of lesions, and it has been used to guide needle biopsy, especially with lesions adjacent to the chest wall. Although echocardiography is not as sensitive as MRI or CT, it is useful in determining the physiologic effect of tumor involvement of the pericardium, heart, or great vessels.

FDG (2-deoxy-2-[^{18}F]fluoro-D-glucose) positron-emission tomography (PET) has played an adjunctive role in evaluation of mediastinal neoplasms, especially in determining the malignant potential of a mediastinal mass. One series reported the sensitivity and specificity of CT and PET in diagnosing tumor invasion and found PET to be superior (sensitivity, 90%; specificity, 92%; accuracy, 91%) to CT (sensitivity, 70%; specificity, 83%; accuracy, 77%). With thymic neoplasms, high FDG uptake was reflective of invasiveness and was seen in thymic carcinomas and invasive thymomas.[18] FDG-PET has a significantly higher sensitivity compared with gallium-67 (^{67}Ga) scintigraphy in pretherapy imaging of aggressive non-Hodgkin's lymphomas and Hodgkin's disease.[19]

Serologic evaluation is indicated in certain patients. Male patients in their second through fifth decades who have an anterosuperior mediastinal mass should have α-fetoprotein and β-human chorionic gonadotropin (β-HCG) serologic studies obtained. A positive serology is indicative of a nonseminomatous germ cell tumor.

Patients with a mediastinal mass and a history of significant hypertension or hypermetabolism should have measurement of urinary excretion of vanillylmandelic acid and catecholamines. This enables the initiation of appropriate perioperative adrenergic blockers in patients with hormonally active intrathoracic pheochromocytoma, paraganglioma, and neuroblastoma, limiting perioperative complications secondary to episodic catecholamine release. In these patients, nuclear scans using metaiodobenzylguanidine (MIBG) are useful in tumor location and in identifying sites of metastatic disease, particularly when located in the middle mediastinum.

Patients with contrast medium–enhancing lesions in the superior mediastinum who do not have symptoms should be evaluated with an iodine-131 (^{131}I) scan. In a patient who does not have symptoms but has a positive scan indicative of a thyroid lesion and no identifiable active thyroid tissue elsewhere, careful observation without excision using serial CT scans to evaluate for growth is indicated.

Increased success has been reported in making a cytologic diagnosis preoperatively by using fine-needle biopsy techniques (18- to 22-gauge needle) with low morbidity and almost no mortality. CT, echocardiography, and, recently, endoscopic ultrasound,[20] because of better localization of the mass and improved placement of the needle, have increased the sensitivity of the technique. Although a cytologic diagnosis of benign or malignant differentiation between masses can be made in about 90% of patients, a precise histologic diagnosis is not always possible. Obtaining core biopsy specimens using cutting needles increases the accuracy of the precise histologic diagnosis and differentiation between benign and malignant lesions. Core biopsy techniques particularly are useful in the diagnosis of lymphomas, thymomas, and neural tumors. Recent advances in immunohistochemical and core biopsy techniques have allowed it to become more accurate for establishing the initial diagnosis of lymphoma, but it is probably better utilized for confirming recurrent disease.[21] Complications related to the procedure include pneumothorax in 20% to 25% of patients, with about 5% requiring tube thoracostomy; hemoptysis in 5% to 10%, with rare occurrences of significant hemorrhagic complications; and tumor seeding along the needle tract, which is a theoretical but extremely rare complication. Needle biopsy techniques are particularly useful for evaluating patients in whom excisional therapy is not indicated but have limited yield in tumors with marked associated desmoplastic reaction, such as nodular sclerosing Hodgkin's lymphoma.

Poorly differentiated malignant tumors of the anterosuperior mediastinum, particularly thymomas, lymphomas, germ cell tumors, and primary carcinomas, can have remarkably similar cytologic and morphologic appearances. In addition to light microscopy using special staining techniques, immunostaining techniques and electron microscopy of multiple sections of the tumor may be necessary to establish an accurate diagnosis. The characteristic ultrastructural features as evaluated by electron microscopy are shown in Table 56-6. Monoclonal anti-

TABLE 56-6. Ultrastructural Characteristics of Mediastinal Tumors

Tumors	Ultrastructure
Carcinoid	Dense core granules, fewer tonofilaments and desmosomes
Lymphoma	Absence of junctional attachments and epithelial features
Thymoma	Well-formed desmosomes, bundles of tonofilaments
Germ cell	Prominent nucleoli, even chromatin, scant desmosomes, rare tonofilaments
Neuroblastoma	Neurosecretory granules, synaptic endings

bodies for surface antigens specific to a cell line of origin and for tumor secretory products can be useful in establishing a precise diagnosis. Chromosomal analysis of tumor tissue is often useful at differentiating histology.[22]

When needle biopsy techniques are contraindicated or do not produce sufficient tissue for the histologic diagnosis, more invasive procedures are often required, such as mediastinoscopy, mediastinotomy, thoracoscopy, thoracotomy, or median sternotomy. Mediastinoscopy is a useful technique to evaluate and biopsy lesions of the middle mediastinum. This technique is often used to evaluate associated lymphadenopathy in this region. Biopsy of lesions in the anterosuperior mediastinum that are unresectable is best done using a limited anterior second or third interspace parasternal mediastinotomy or using thoracoscopy. Similarly, unresectable lesions in the superior mediastinum, hilar, or paratracheal regions can be sampled through a small lateral thoracotomy in the third or fourth interspace after retracting the apex of the lung inferiorly. Unresectable posterior mediastinal masses may be approached thoracoscopically or through a limited posterolateral thoracotomy. A representative section of the tissue obtained should be submitted for immediate frozen-section analysis to establish adequacy of the biopsy before closing. Importantly, the incision should not be made in the portals for potential radiation therapy. Lesions that appear resectable should be excised. Median sternotomy provides optimal exposure for lesions in the anterosuperior mediastinum. A transcervical approach using sternal elevators has been successfully used to resect tumors in the superior aspect of the anterosuperior mediastinum. Occasionally for extensive tumors of the anterosuperior mediastinum, a trans-sternal bilateral thoracotomy (clam shell) incision is indicated. Middle and posterior mediastinal masses are usually best excised through a posterolateral thoracotomy. Thoracoscopic and thoracoscopically assisted procedures are increasingly attaining a leading role in diagnosing and treating a variety of mediastinal lesions in carefully selected patients.[23,24] Thoracoscopy is also useful in evaluating, sampling, and resecting mediastinal lesions in infants and children.[25]

Although most patients undergo surgical procedures safely, patients with large anterosuperior or middle mediastinal masses, particularly children, have an increased risk for severe cardiorespiratory complications during general anesthesia. Patients with posture-related dyspnea and superior vena caval syndrome are at increased risk. Patients with a reduction in tracheal cross-sectional area of more than 35% assessed by CT or a reduction in peak expiratory flow assessed by pulmonary flow mechanics are at risk for airway compression.[26] In patients with airway compression or superior vena caval obstruction, the risk associated with general anesthesia is markedly increased, and attempts to obtain a histologic diagnosis should be limited to needle biopsies or open procedures done with local anesthesia. If it is not possible to obtain a diagnosis without general anesthesia, some suggest that before induction of anesthesia all patients with a 50% or more reduction of the cross-sectional area of the airway should be readied for possible cardiopulmonary bypass by having their femoral vessels cannulated under local anesthesia.[27] An awake fiberoptic intubation should be performed, rigid bronchoscopy available, and, if at all possible, anesthesia provided with inhalational agents only; muscle paralysis should be avoided.[27]

Neurogenic Tumors

Neurogenic tumors are the most common neoplasm, constituting 20% of all primary tumors and cysts. These tumors are usually located in the posterior mediastinum and originate from the sympathetic ganglia (ganglioma, ganglioneuroblastoma, and neuroblastoma), the intercostal nerves (neurofibroma, neurilemoma, and neurosarcoma), and the paraganglia cells (paraganglioma). Tumors arising from the sympathetic ganglia, known as neuroblastic tumors, have recently been assigned to one of four basic morphologic categories: neuroblastoma, ganglioneuroblastoma intermixed, ganglioneuroma, and ganglioneuroblastoma, nodular.[28,29] Only rarely are neurogenic tumors located in the anterosuperior mediastinum. Although the peak incidence occurs in adults, neurogenic tumors make up a proportionally greater percentage of mediastinal masses in children (34%). Although most neurogenic tumors in adults are benign, a greater percentage of neurogenic tumors are malignant in children.

Many of these tumors are found on routine chest radiographs in patients who do not have symptoms. When present, symptoms are usually caused by mechanical factors, such as chest and back pain resulting from compression or invasion of intercostal nerve, bone, and chest wall; cough and dyspnea resulting from compression of the tracheobronchial tree; Pancoast's syndrome; and Horner's syndrome resulting from involvement of the brachial and the cervical sympathetic chain. Symptoms may be systemic and related to production of neurohormonal agents.

Thoracoscopy has played an increasing role in both diagnosis and treatment of neurogenic tumors (Fig. 56-2). Benign neurogenic tumors are particularly amenable to thoracoscopic removal, and more rapid postoperative recovery is seen with thoracoscopic removal than with open excision.[30,31] Robot-assisted thoracoscopic techniques for resection of benign neurogenic tumors are being utilized.[32] For malignant tumors, the standard of care remains thoracotomy.

About 10% of neurogenic tumors have extensions into the spinal column. These tumors are termed *dumbbell tumors* because of their characteristic shape resulting from the relatively large paraspinal and intraspinal portions connected by a narrow isthmus of tissue traversing the intervertebral foramen. Although 60% of patients with a dumbbell tumor have neurologic symptoms related to spinal cord compression, the significant proportion of patients without symptoms underscores the importance of evaluating all patients with a posterior mediastinal mass for possible intraspinal extension. MRI is preferred to evaluate the presence and extent of the intraspinal component. The recommended surgical approach to dumbbell tumors is a one-stage excision of the intraspinal component before resecting the thoracic component to minimize any spinal column hematoma. The incision used for

Access around lung assisted with gravity
and 45-degree forward rotation
of patient from lateral position

Posterior mediastinal tumor

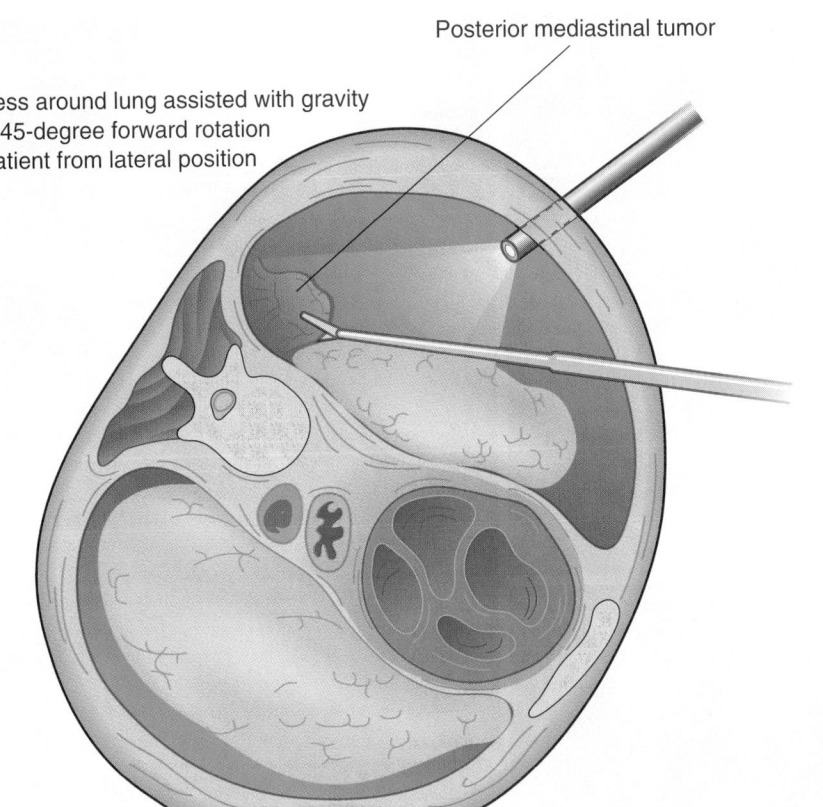

FIGURE 56-2. The endoscopic dissector, scissors, and grasper can be introduced into the pleural cavity through the accessory intercostal space access sites to complete the tumor resection. The resected tumor can be put into a plastic bag and withdrawn through one of the access sites. The access site may have to be extended to allow tumor removal. Adequate hemostasis is essential. A chest tube (28 French) is inserted into the pleural cavity through the lowest access site for underwater sealed drainage. The other incisions are closed with sutures. (From Sabiston DC Jr: Atlas of Cardiothoracic Surgery. Philadelphia, WB Saunders, 1995, p 560.)

the posterior laminectomy is extended into the appropriate interspace to allow resection of the mediastinal component. Anterior video-assisted thoracoscopy for removal of the intrathoracic component of the tumor has been combined with a posterior laminectomy for microneurosurgical removal of the spinal component.[33]

Neuroblastoma

Neuroblastomas originate from the sympathetic nervous system. The most common location for a neuroblastoma is in the retroperitoneum; however, 10% to 20% occur primarily in the mediastinum. These are highly invasive neoplasms that have frequently metastasized before diagnosis. Biologically they can behave quite uniquely and have been known to spontaneously regress, mature, or proliferate aggressively. Unfortunately the majority present at advanced stages and do not regress spontaneously or mature. Common sites of metastases are the regional lymph nodes, bone, brain, liver, and lung. Most of these tumors occur in children, and 75% occur in children younger than 4 years of age. The tumor is composed of small, round, immature cells organized in a rosette pattern. These tumors can be undifferentiated, poorly differentiated, or differentiating.[28] On ultrastructural examination the presence of neurosecretory granules is characteristic. Patients usually have symptoms. Paraplegia and other neurologic symptoms related to spinal cord compression were present in one third of children with mediastinal neuroblastoma in one series.[34] A variety of paraneoplastic syndromes have been reported, including profuse watery diarrhea and abdominal pain related

to vasoactive intestinal polypeptide production, the opsoclonus-polymyoclonus syndrome (an unexplained symptom complex characterized by cerebellar and truncal ataxia with rapid, darting eye movements [dancing eyes] that is possibly related to an autoimmune mechanism), and pheochromocytoma syndrome caused by catecholamine secretion. A 24-hour urine collection to measure catecholamines should be obtained in children with a posterior mediastinal mass.

Neuroblastoma[35-37] and ganglioneuroblastoma are staged as follows:

Stage I—well-circumscribed, noninvasive tumor; complete gross excision ± residual microscopic disease; microscopically negative nodes

Stage IIA—tumor invasion locally without extension across the midline; incomplete gross excision; microscopically negative nodes

Stage IIB—tumor invasion locally without extension across the midline; complete or incomplete gross resection; positive nodes ipsilaterally but negative microscopically contralateral lymph nodes

Stage III—unresectable tumor spread across the midline ± node involvement (regional); or no extension across the midline with contralateral lymph nodes positive; or midline tumor with bilateral nodes positive

Stage IV—tumor with metastasis (except as in stage IVS).

Stage IVS—primary tumor localized, metastatic disease limited to liver, skin, and/or bone marrow in infants younger than 1 year of age

Therapy is determined by the stage of the disease: stage I, surgical excision; stage II, excision and radiation

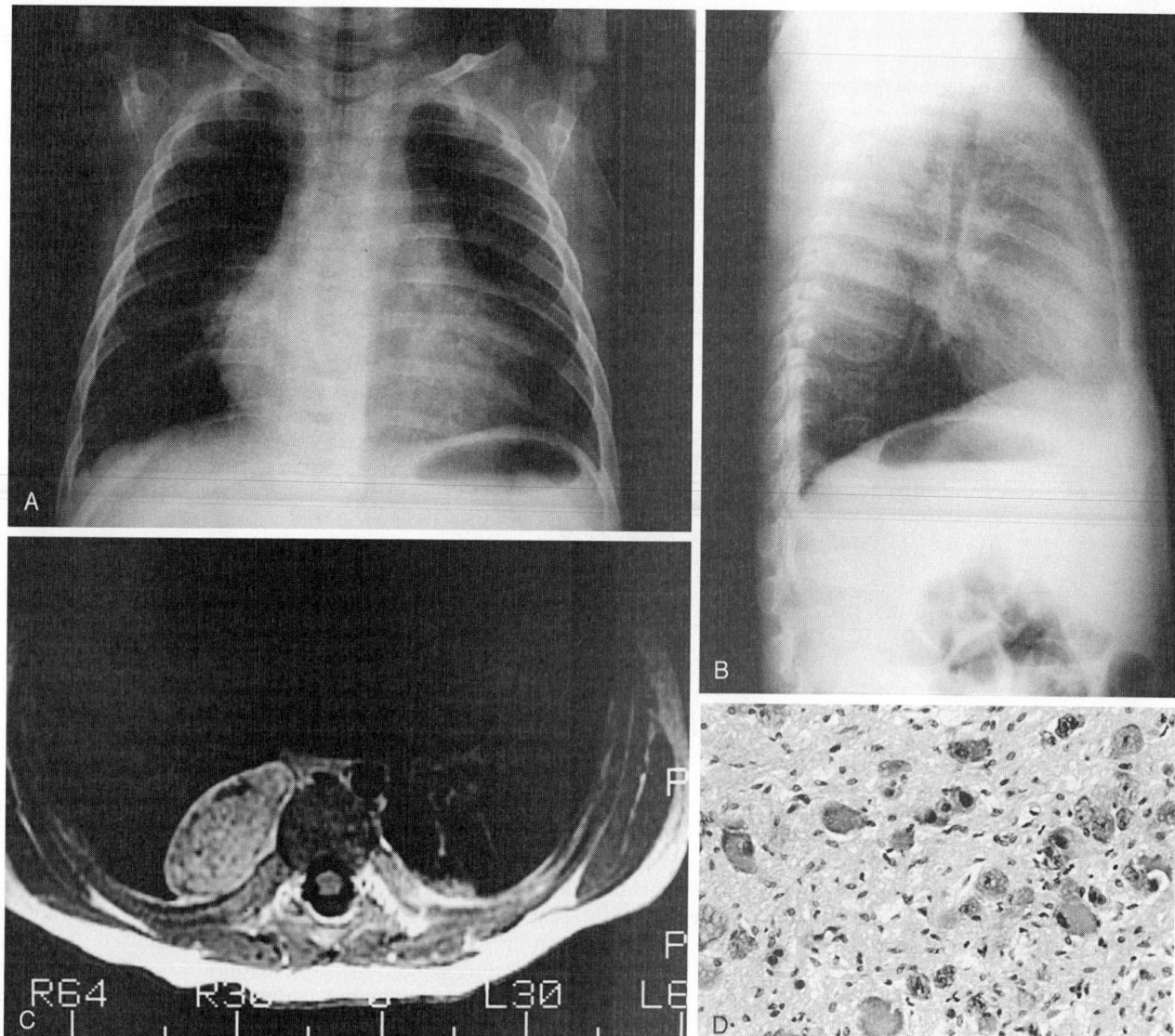

■ FIGURE 56-3. **A** and **B,** Chest radiographs of patient with ganglioneuroblastoma. **C,** Magnetic resonance image (cross-sectional) of tumor. **D,** Histopathologic examination of ganglioneuroblastoma shows mature component of tumor (H&E, ×250).

therapy; stages III and IV, multimodality therapy using surgical debulking, radiation therapy, and multiagent chemotherapy as well as a second-look exploration to resect residual disease when necessary. The usual chemotherapeutic agents used include cisplatin, vincristine, doxorubicin, cyclophosphamide, and etoposide. Children younger than 1 year of age have an excellent prognosis even when widespread disease is present. With increasing age and extent of involvement, however, the prognosis worsens. Genetic abnormalities have been identified in neuroblastomas, with allelic loss of chromosome 1p, and N-*myc* gene amplification associated with an unfavorable prognosis.[38,39] Certain morphologic criteria (grade of neuroblastic differentiation and mitosis-karyorrhexis index) have age-linked prognostic effects.[40] In the subset of patients with high-risk neuroblastomas, dose-intensive chemotherapy and autologous bone marrow transplantation resulted in improved event-free survival but not

overall survival compared with conventional chemotherapy.[41] Treatment of patients with 13-*cis*-retinoic acid, a differentiating agent, after initial therapy also appeared to confer a benefit.[41] Patients with neuroblastomas resistant to therapy and in those whose disease relapses also have seen some success with ablative chemotherapy and autologous bone marrow transplantation or stem cell rescue. Developing treatments in this group include ^{131}I-MIBG therapy,[42] immunotherapy,[43] and allogenic tumor vaccines.[44] Interestingly, mediastinal neuroblastomas appear to have a better prognosis than neuroblastomas occurring elsewhere.

Ganglioneuroblastoma

Ganglioneuroblastomas exhibit an intermediate degree of differentiation between ganglioneuromas and neuroblastomas (Fig. 56-3). They are composed of mature and

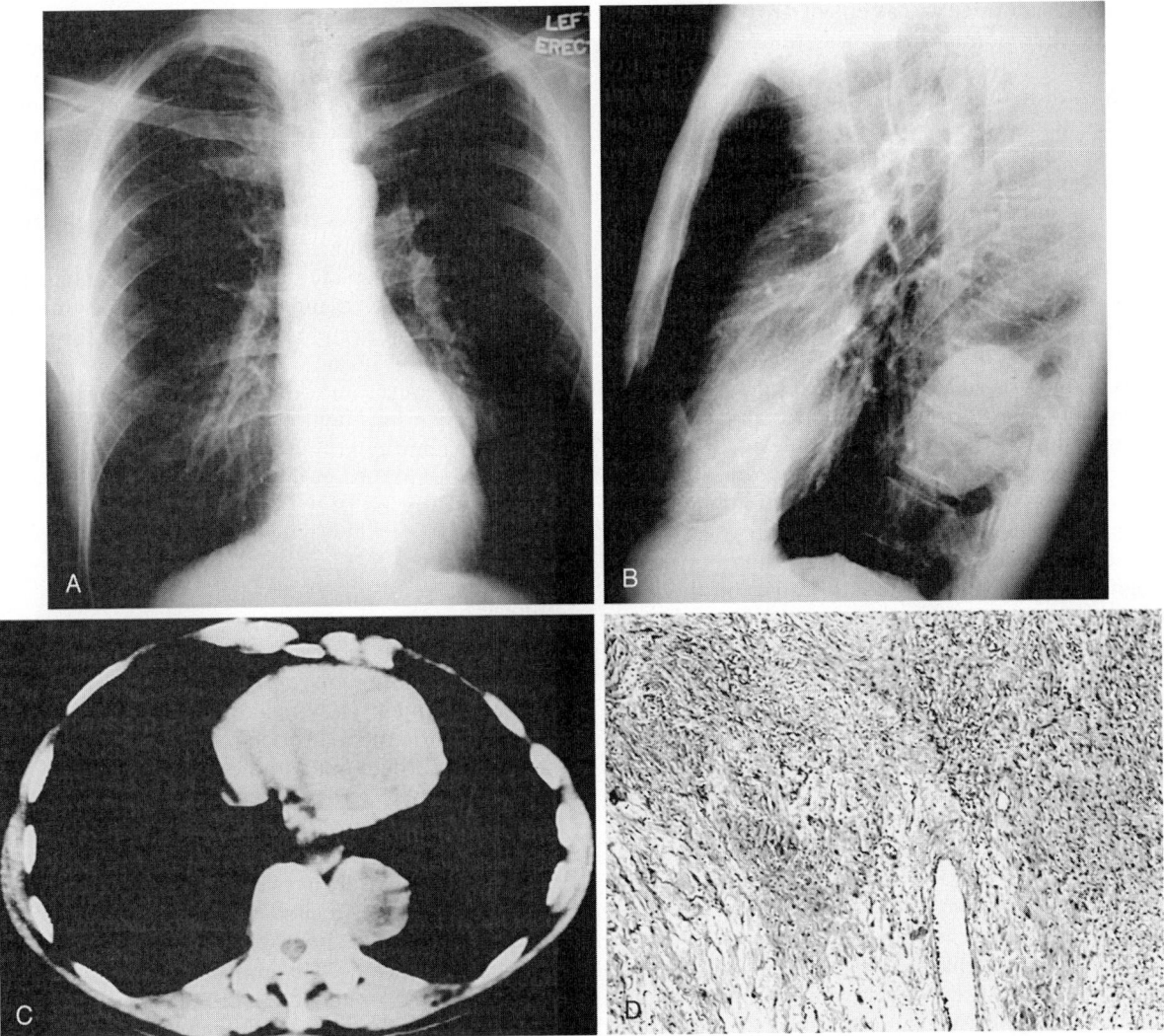

FIGURE 56-4.   A and **B,** Chest radiograph of patient with a neurilemoma. **C,** CT scan of the tumor in the posterior mediastinum. **D,** Histopathologic examination of neurilemoma shows the highly cellular Antoni A areas and the less cellular Antoni B areas (H&E, ×68).

immature ganglion cells. Two different histologic patterns occur: intermixed subtype–ganglioneuroblastoma (neuroblastic component seen as multiple microscopic foci) and nodular subtype ganglioneuroblastoma (neuroblastic component seen in distinct macroscopic and commonly hemorrhagic nodules).[28] Patients diagnosed with the intermixed subtype ganglioneuroblastoma (100% overall 5-year survival) have a significantly better prognosis than those with the nodular category (59.1% overall 5-year survival).[40] Recently it has been shown that there is a subset of patients in nodular subtype group that have a more favorable prognosis (based on age, grade of neuroblastic differentiation, and mitosis-karyorrhexis index). The less favorable subgroup in the nodular subtype of ganglioneuroblastomas presented with distant metastatic disease 63% of the time.[45] Treatment of ganglioneuroblastomas ranges from surgical excision alone to various chemotherapeutic strategies depending on histologic characteristics, age at diagnosis, and stage of disease.

Ganglioneuroma

Ganglioneuromas are benign tumors originating from the sympathetic chain that are composed of ganglion cells and nerve fibers. These tumors typically present at an early age and are the most common neurogenic tumors occurring during childhood. The usual location is the paravertebral region. These tumors are well encapsulated and, when cross-sectioned, frequently exhibit areas of cystic degeneration. Two subtypes exist: maturing and mature.[28] Surgical excision provides cure.

Neurilemoma, Neurofibroma, and Neurosarcoma

The most common neurogenic tumor is the neurilemoma (Fig. 56-4), which originates from perineural Schwann cells. These tumors are well circumscribed and have a defined capsule. There are two morphologic patterns: Antoni type A, which has organized architecture with a cellular palisading pattern of growth; and Antoni type B, which has a loose reticular pattern of growth. The peak incidence of these tumors is in the third through fifth decades of life.

In contrast to neurilemomas, neurofibromas are poorly encapsulated and consist of randomly arranged spindle-shaped cells. These tumors originate as a proliferation of all the elements of the peripheral nerve. Although both neurilemomas and neurofibromas occur as a manifestation of neurofibromatosis (von Recklinghausen's disease), they must be differentiated from the two other common entities in the posterior mediastinum: meningioma and meningocele. With both neurilemoma and neurofibroma, surgical excision results in cure.

Neurosarcomas originate by malignant degeneration of either neurilemomas or neurofibromas, in addition to developing de novo. These tumors usually occur in adults; however, patients with neurofibromatosis may develop neurosarcomas as children. These are rapidly growing tumors that frequently invade vital structures, preventing attempts at resection. Unless tumor excision is possible, the prognosis is extremely poor because of the unresponsiveness to adjuvant therapies.

Paraganglioma (Pheochromocytoma)

Mediastinal paragangliomas are rare tumors, representing less than 1% of all mediastinal tumors and less than 2% of all pheochromocytomas. Although most are found in the paravertebral sulcus, an increasing number of middle mediastinal paragangliomas occur in the branchial arch structures, coronary and aortopulmonary paraganglia, atria, and islands of tissue in the pericardium. The likelihood of functional activity of a paraganglioma is related to the site of origin: adrenal medulla, high likelihood; branchiomeric and intravagal, very low likelihood; and aortosympathetic and visceral autonomic, intermediate likelihood. Catecholamine production causes the classic constellation of symptoms associated with pheochromocytomas, including periodic or sustained hypertension, often accompanied by orthostatic hypotension, hypermetabolism manifested by weight loss, hyperhidrosis, palpitations, and headaches. Measurement of elevated levels of urinary catecholamines or their metabolites, the metanephrines and vanillylmandelic acid, usually establishes the diagnosis. Although adrenal pheochromocytomas often produce both epinephrine and norepinephrine, extra-adrenal paragangliomas rarely secrete epinephrine.

Tumor localization has improved remarkably through the use of CT and ^{131}I-MIBG scintigraphy, particularly when the tumors are hormonally active. Hormonally active tumors may be located with an 85% sensitivity using the ^{131}I-MIBG scan. Because of the high vascularity of these lesions, enhancement with contrast medium administration occurs during CT. Because of the accuracy of CT and MIBG scanning, rarely is selective venous angiography with serial sampling for catecholamine levels necessary for preoperative localization. Tumor localization using MRI has been reported.

When appropriate, surgical resection is the optimal therapy. In patients with tumors involving the middle mediastinum, cardiopulmonary bypass may be necessary to enable resection. Recently, preoperative embolization to reduce perioperative bleeding followed by surgical resection has been described.[46] Although half of tumors appear malignant morphologically, metastatic disease develops in only 3% of patients. In those with metastatic disease, α-methyltyramine, a tyrosine hydroxylase inhibitor that blocks the synthesis of catecholamines, is helpful in controlling symptoms.

About 10% of patients have multiple paragangliomas. They are more common in patients with multiple endocrine neoplasia syndrome, a family history of disease, and Carney's syndrome (pulmonary chondroma, gastric leiomyosarcoma, and extra-adrenal paraganglioma). In patients who have had excision of an adrenal pheochromocytoma and continue to have symptoms, a search for an extra-adrenal lesion should be undertaken, with careful attention directed to the evaluation of the mediastinum.

Thymoma

Thymoma is the most common neoplasm of the anterosuperior mediastinum and the second most common mediastinal mass (19%; see Table 56-1). The peak incidence is in the third through fifth decades, but this tumor may occur throughout adulthood. Thymoma is rare in the first two decades of life. On a radiograph it may appear as a small, well-circumscribed mass or as a bulky lobulated mass confluent with adjacent mediastinal structures (Fig. 56-5). Patients usually have symptoms at presentation, and symptoms may be related to local mass effects causing chest pain, dyspnea, hemoptysis, cough, and the superior vena caval syndrome. Thymomas, however, are frequently associated with systemic syndromes caused by immunologic mechanisms. Although the most common syndrome is myasthenia gravis, many other syndromes have been associated with thymomas, including red blood cell aplasia, pure white blood cell aplasia, aplastic anemia, Cushing's syndrome, hypogammaglobulinemia and hypergammaglobulinemia, dermatomyositis, systemic lupus erythematosus, progressive systemic sclerosis, hypercoagulopathy with thrombosis, rheumatoid arthritis, megaesophagus, and granulomatous myocarditis. These systemic syndromes often do not improve after successful control of the thymoma.

Most patients with myasthenia gravis do not have thymoma. The incidence is 10% to 42%, depending on the reporting medical center. Although red blood cell aplasia occurs in only 5% of patients with thymoma, 33% to 50% of adults with red blood cell aplasia have a thymoma. Because of the significant association between thymoma and these syndromes, an evaluation of the mediastinum with CT or MRI is recommended in all patients with myasthenia gravis and red blood cell aplasia.

Thymomas are histologically classified either by the predominance of epithelial or lymphocytic cells (lymphocytic, epithelial, mixed, and spindle) or by the morphologic resemblance to cortical or medullary epithelium.[47] Unfortunately, a wide variance in the cellular composition is often present within the tumor and a consistent

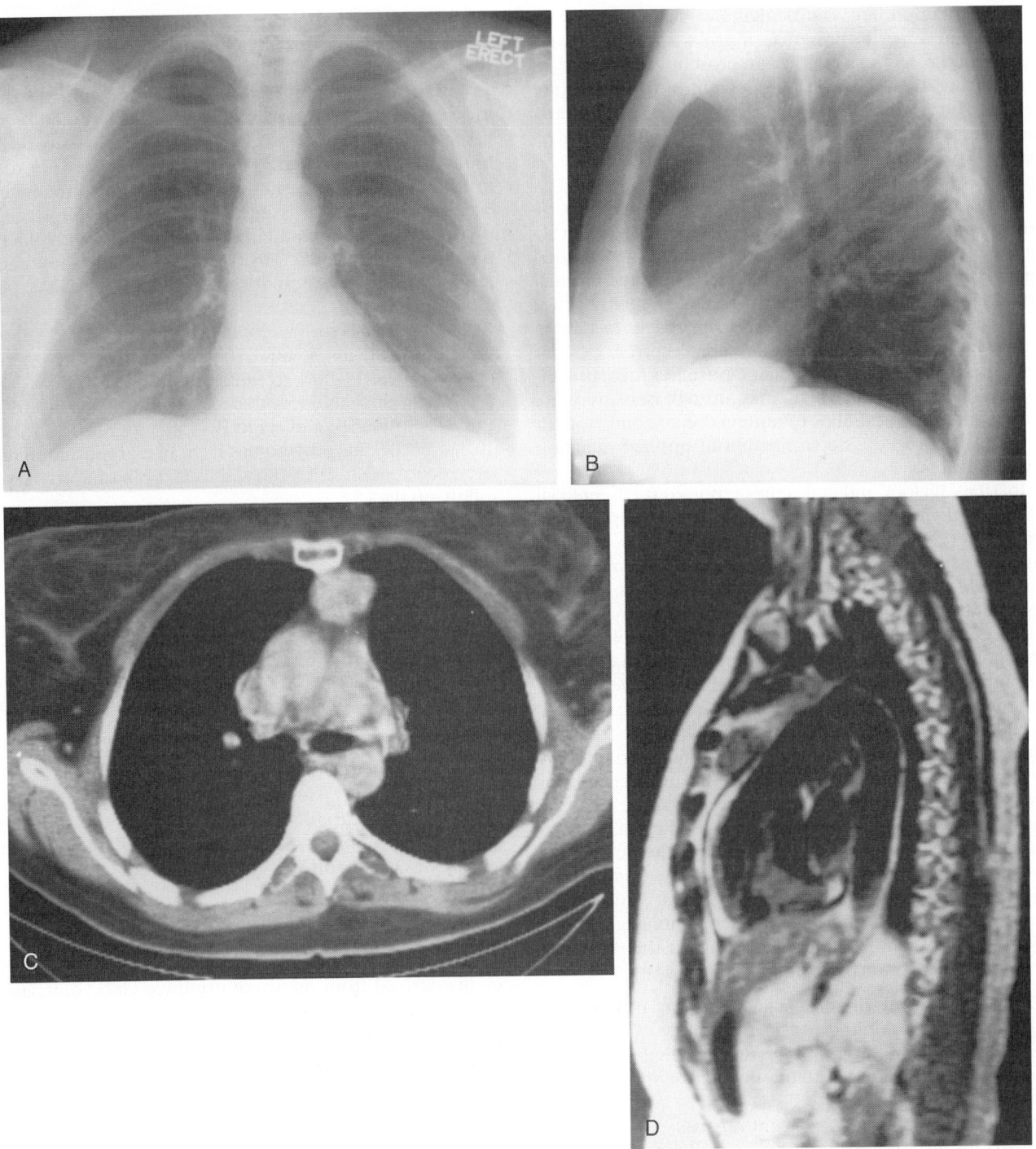

FIGURE 56-5. **A** and **B,** Chest radiographs of a patient with myasthenia gravis who had a benign thymoma. The tumor is poorly visualized, manifested only by an irregularity of the anterior cardiac border. **C,** CT scan clearly illustrates the tumor in the anterior mediastinum. **D,** Sagittal MR image of the mediastinum demonstrates a separation between the tumor and the pericardium. (**A** to **D,** From Davis RD Jr, Oldham HN Jr, Sabiston DC Jr: The mediastinum. *In* Sabiston DC Jr, Spencer FC [eds]: Surgery of the Chest, 5th ed. Philadelphia, WB Saunders, 1990.)

relationship is not present between the microscopic appearance and biologic behavior, with regard to either tumor invasiveness or association with systemic syndromes. In one series, however, an improved 10-year survival rate was reported in patients with spindle cell or lymphocyte-rich thymomas (75%), as compared with dif-ferentiated epithelial type (50%) and undifferentiated type (0%).[48] Similarly, the differentiation into medullary and cortical types has been shown to offer no prognostic information in one series,[49] whereas in another series, the presence of cortical morphology was associated with a malignant clinical course.[50]

Differentiation between benign and malignant disease is determined by the presence of gross invasion of adjacent structures, metastasis, or microscopic evidence of capsular invasion. Fifteen to 65 percent of thymomas are benign. The relative percentage is partially related to early surgical treatment of myasthenia gravis; when thymectomy is performed early in the course of myasthenia gravis, a greater percentage of thymomas are benign.

Whenever possible, the therapy for thymoma is surgical excision without removing or injuring vital structures. Even with well-encapsulated thymomas, extended thymectomy with eradication of all accessible mediastinal fatty areolar tissue should be performed to ensure removal of all ectopic thymic tissue. This approach has been shown to lower the number of tumor recurrences. The best operative exposure is obtained using a median sternotomy. Because many thymomas are radiosensitive, the placement of surgical clips to outline the anatomic extent of disease aids in the determination of optimal radiation portals.

In 1939, Blalock and colleagues reported the beneficial effect of thymectomy in the treatment of myasthenia gravis.[51] For patients with myasthenia gravis without thymomas, extended transcervical thymectomy offers comparable results to trans-sternal procedures.[52,53] The perioperative management in patients with myasthenia gravis is extremely important to prevent complications. Anticholinesterase inhibitors are discontinued to decrease the amount of pulmonary secretions and prevent inadvertent cholinergic weakness. Plasmapheresis is used routinely within 72 hours of thymectomy. In most patients, plasmapheresis is effective in controlling generalized weakness. Also, careful attention to the maintenance of pulmonary function with chest physiotherapy, endotracheal suctioning, and bronchodilators is the mainstay of postoperative management. Although myasthenic patients with thymoma had a worse prognosis in past series, improvements in therapy for myasthenia gravis have allowed prognosis to be dependent on the stage of the disease rather than on the presence of myasthenia gravis.

Staging of thymoma is as follows.[54]

Stage I—tumor is well encapsulated without evidence of gross or microscopic capsular invasion.

Stage II—tumor exhibits pericapsular growth into adjacent fat or mediastinal pleura or microscopic invasion of the thymic capsule.

Stage III—tumor invades adjacent organs.

Stage IVa—intrathoracic metastatic spread occurs.

Stage IVb—extrathoracic metastatic spread occurs (uncommon).

Complete surgical resection for stage I is sufficient treatment. The adjunctive use of radiation therapy with a dose of 50 Gy had previously been recommended for stage II and III disease.[55] Recently, however, it has been reported based on retrospective data that most patients with stage II thymomas do not need adjuvant radiation therapy.[56] Tumors greater than 5 cm, locally invasive tumors, unresectable tumors, and metastatic tumors should be treated by protocols that include chemotherapy[57,58] followed by surgical exploration with the goal of complete resection and postoperative radiation therapy. The best results are seen with cisplatin-based regimens, with overall response rates of 70% to 100%.[58]

An aggressive surgical approach is recommended for invasive thymomas that includes radical resection and vascular reconstruction of the superior vena cava or its branches when invaded.[59] Using this aggressive approach to obtain complete resection, a significant difference in 5-year survival rates is seen in patients with stage III thymomas (94%) compared with those with incomplete resections (35%). Thymomas frequently show recurrence, and reoperation for recurrent disease has been recommended.[59]

The prognosis for patients with thymoma is dependent on clinical stage; 5- and 10-year survival rates are as follows: stage I—90% to 96.2% and 66.7% to 86%; stage II—70% to 96% and 55% to 75%; stage III—50% to 69.6% and 21% to 58.3%; and stage IV—50% to 100% and 0% to 40%.[54,55,57] Because thymomas have been reported to have late recurrences, cure rates should be based on 10-year follow-up data.

Germ Cell Tumors

Germ cell tumors are benign and malignant neoplasms thought to originate from primordial germ cells that fail to complete the migration from the urogenital ridge and come to rest in the mediastinum. These tumors are classified as shown in Box 56-3. Although these lesions are identical histologically to germ cell tumors originating in the gonads, they are not considered to be metastatic from primary gonadal tumors. The current recommendations for evaluating the testes of a patient with mediastinal germ cell tumor is careful physical examination and ultrasonography. Biopsy is reserved for positive findings. Blind biopsy or orchiectomy is contraindicated.

Teratomatous Lesions

Teratomas are neoplasms composed of multiple tissue elements derived from the three primitive embryonic layers

---

BOX 56-3. Classification of Germ Cell Tumors

Benign

Mature teratomas
Dermoid cysts

Malignant

Seminomas
Nonseminomatous germ cell tumors
  Immature teratoma
  Teratoma with malignant components
  Choriocarcinomas
  Embryonal cell carcinomas
  Endodermal cell (yolk sac) tumors
  Mixed germ cell tumors

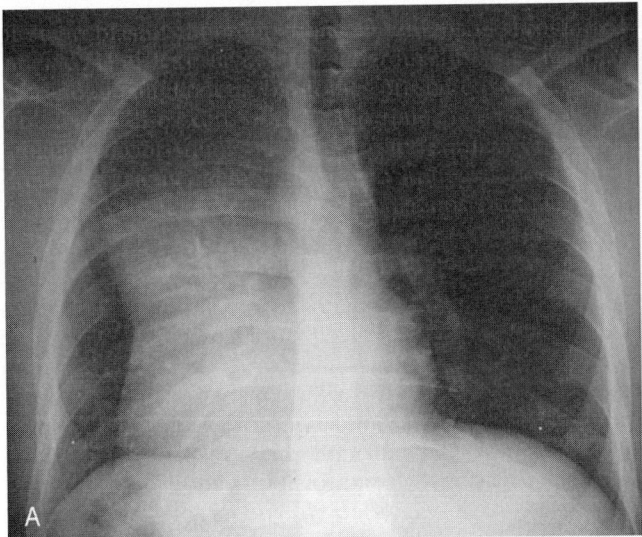

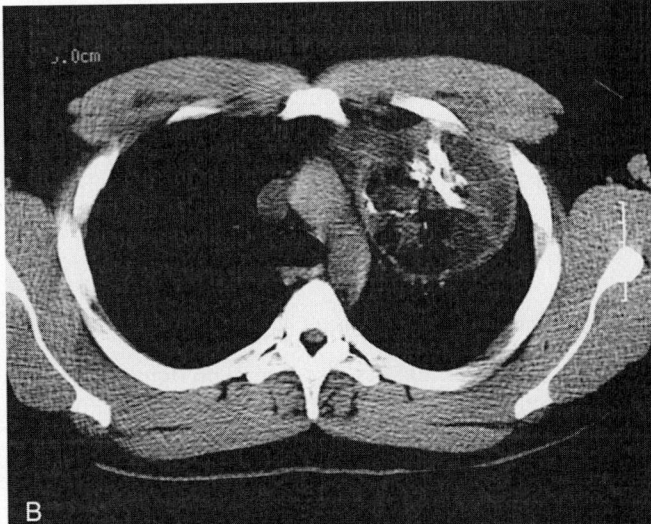

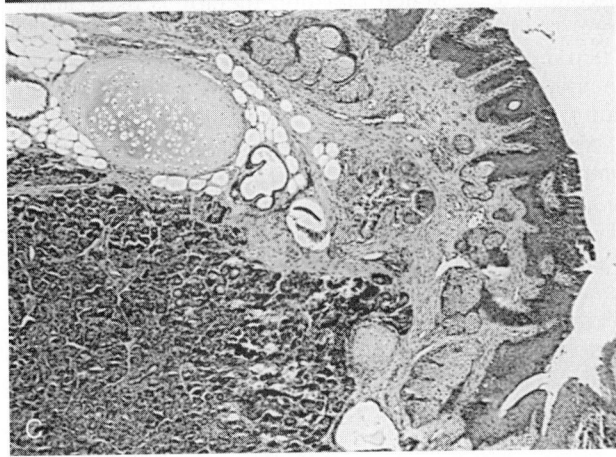

FIGURE 56-6. **A,** Chest radiograph of patient with teratoma. **B,** CT scan of tumor. **C,** Histopathologic examination of benign teratoma (H&E, ×52).

foreign to the area in which they occur. The peak incidence is in the second and third decades of life. There is no gender predisposition. These tumors are located most commonly in the anterosuperior mediastinum, although 3% to 8% are found in the posterior mediastinum. Symptoms, when present, are related to mechanical effects and include chest pain, cough, dyspnea, or symptoms related to recurrent pneumonitis. If a communication between the tumor and the tracheobronchial tree develops, the pathognomonic finding of a cough productive of hair or sebaceous material may result. Unusual presentations include recurrent pericarditis or pericardial tamponade after invasion or rupture into the pericardium. Rupture into the pleural space may cause respiratory distress as a result of the markedly irritative nature of the cyst fluid.

Although germ cell tumors are rare, the diagnosis can be made on routine chest radiography by the identification of well-formed teeth. CT findings of a predominantly fatty mass with a denser dependent portion containing globular calcifications, bone, or teeth and a solid protuberance into a cystic cavity are considered specific. Despite occasional characteristic appearances using various imaging techniques, the diagnosis usually depends on microscopic examination.

The teratodermoid (dermoid) cyst is the simplest form. It is composed predominantly of derivatives of the epidermal layer, including dermal and epidermal glands, hair, and sebaceous material. Teratomas are histologically more complex (Fig. 56-6). The solid component of the tumor often contains well-differentiated elements of bone, cartilage, teeth, muscle, connective tissue, fibrous and lymphoid tissue, nerve, thymus, mucous and salivary glands, lung, liver, or pancreas. Malignant tumors are differentiated from benign tumors by the presence of primitive (embryonic) tissue or by the presence of malignant components. Immature teratomas contain combinations of mature epithelial and connective tissues with immature areas of mesenchymal and neuroectodermal tissues. Teratomas with malignant components are divided into categories based on the elements present. Subclassification of these tumors into those with malignant components containing sarcomatous elements, another germ cell tumor, an epithelial neoplasm, or a combination of any of these has been recommended.[60] The most common presentation is teratoma with another germ cell tumor, most often a yolk sac tumor.

Diagnosis and therapy rely on surgical excision. For those benign tumors of such large size or with involvement of adjacent mediastinal structures such that complete resection is impossible, partial resection has led to resolution of symptoms, frequently without relapse. Late sequelae after excision of a childhood teratoma may include impaired spermatic function and decreased serum levels of testosterone and luteinizing hormone.[61] For malignant teratomas, chemotherapy and radiation therapy, combined with surgical excision, are individualized for the type of malignant components contained in the tumors. The overall prognosis is poor for malignant tumors.

Malignant Nonteratomatous Germ Cell Tumors

Malignant germ cell tumors also occur predominantly in the anterosuperior mediastinum. Unlike benign teratomas there is a marked male predominance. The peak incidence is in the third and fourth decades of life. Most cases are symptomatic, with chest pain, cough, dyspnea, and hemoptysis; the superior vena caval syndrome occurs commonly. The chest radiograph usually demonstrates a large anterior mediastinal mass that is often multilobular; frequently, there is evidence of intrathoracic spread of disease. CT and MRI are most helpful in defining the extent of involvement for the purpose of providing a means of following response to therapy and diagnosing relapses. These imaging modalities are also useful in determining impingement on vital structures that may contraindicate the use of general anesthesia. Serologic measurements of α-fetoprotein and β-HCG are useful for the following tasks: differentiating seminomas from nonseminomas, quantitatively assessing response to therapy in hormonally active tumors (the plasma half-life of α-fetoprotein and β-HCG is 5 days and 12 to 24 hours, respectively), and diagnosing relapse or failure of therapy before changes that can be observed in gross disease. Seminomas rarely produce β-HCG (less than 7%) and never produce α-fetoprotein; in contrast, more than 90% of nonseminomas secrete one or both of these hormones. This differentiation is important because of the marked radiosensitivity of seminomas and the relative radiosensitivity of nonseminomas. Chromosomal analysis of tumor tissue is useful for differentiating germ cell tumors from other tumors with a similar histologic appearance. A characteristic isochromosome of chromosome 12 has been identified as a karyotypic abnormality of all germ cells.[22]

Seminomas

Seminomas constitute 50% of malignant germ cell tumors and 2% to 4% of all mediastinal masses. Unlike other malignant germ cell tumors, seminomas usually remain intrathoracic with local extension to adjacent mediastinal and pulmonary structures. Although metastatic spread occurs first through lymphatics, hematogenous spread with extrathoracic involvement may develop late in the course of disease. Bone and lung are the most common sites of metastatic spread. Patients usually develop symptoms related to the mechanical effects of the tumor on adjacent structures. The superior vena caval syndrome occurs in 10% to 20% of patients. The histologic appearance of this tumor is characterized by large cells with round nuclei, scant cytoplasm, and abundant glycogen.

Therapy is determined by the stage of the disease. Occasionally, excision is possible without injury to vital structures (22%) and is recommended when possible. When complete resection is possible, the use of adjuvant therapy is unnecessary. Careful follow-up with serial CT examinations is required to diagnose recurrences. When excision is not possible, a biopsy sample of sufficient size to establish the diagnosis should be obtained. Because these tumors are sensitive to irradiation and chemotherapy, cytoreductive resection before chemotherapy or radiation therapy is unnecessary and is contraindicated when vital structures are involved or when the procedure is technically difficult. Treatment varies somewhat based on extent of disease and usually consists of chemotherapy with or without secondary surgery or combination chemotherapy and radiation therapy. Radiation therapy alone is occasionally used for localized disease, but inferior results have been reported and its sole use should be discouraged.[62,63] When radiation therapy is used alone a dose of 40 to 45 Gy is usually given versus 25 to 35 Gy when combined with chemotherapy.[63] Cisplatin-based chemotherapy is the treatment of choice; alternatively, carboplatin-based regimens can be used.

As discussed in the subsequent section on nonseminomatous mediastinal germ cell tumors, residual disease should be surgically resected after chemotherapy. FDG-PET is of no apparent benefit in evaluation of postchemotherapy residual masses in patients with seminomas.[64] Recurrent disease is treated with salvage chemotherapy and selective consolidation. Excellent long-term survival rates have been seen with mediastinal seminoma, with a recent large multi-institutional series reporting an 88% 5-year survival.[63]

Nonseminomatous Tumors

Malignant nonseminoma tumors include choriocarcinomas, embryonal cell carcinomas, immature teratomas, teratomas with malignant components, and endodermal cell (yolk sac) tumors, of which 40% are a mixture of tissue types. Malignant teratomas have already been discussed with other teratomatous lesions. The nonseminomas differ from seminomas in several aspects: they are more aggressive tumors that are frequently disseminated at the time of diagnosis; they are rarely radiosensitive; and more than 90% produce either β-HCG or α-fetoprotein. All patients with choriocarcinoma and some patients with embryonal cell tumors have elevated levels of β-HCG. α-Fetoprotein is most commonly elevated in patients with embryonal cell carcinomas and yolk sac tumors.

Like seminomas, most nonseminomatous neoplasms are symptomatic with chest pain, dyspnea, weight loss, cough, hemoptysis, fever, chills, and the superior vena caval syndrome (20%). Children with these tumors may present with precocious puberty. Patients are predominantly men in their third or fourth decades. Chest radiographs usually reveal a large anterior mediastinal mass with frequent extension into lung parenchyma and adjacent mediastinal structures. In addition to superior vena caval obstruction, they may cause pulmonary stenosis and coarctation of the aorta. Characteristically, these tumors have extensive intrathoracic involvement and frequently have metastasized outside the thorax. Frequent sites of metastatic disease include brain, lung, liver, bone, and the lymphatic system, particularly the supraclavicular nodes. Chest wall involvement is common.

A number of chromosomal abnormalities are associated with an increased incidence of nonseminomatous germ cell tumors, including Klinefelter's syndrome, trisomy 8, and 5q deletion. In one series of patients with germ cell tumors, the incidence of Klinefelter's syndrome was 22%.[65] Additionally, mediastinal nonseminomas but not testicular germ cell tumors are associated with the development of rare hematologic malignancies, such as acute megakaryocytic leukemia, systemic mast cell disease, and malignant histiocytosis, as well as other hematologic abnormalities, including myelodysplastic syndrome and idiopathic thrombocytopenia refractory to treatment. One explanation, and probably the most plausible, for this association is that the hematologic malignancy results from the multipotential differentiation ability of germ cell tumors.[66] The diagnosis of a hematologic disorder in a patient with a primary mediastinal nonseminomatous germ cell tumor has been shown to have a statistically significant negative impact on survival.[67]

The local invasiveness of these tumors and their frequent metastasis usually preclude surgical resection of all disease at the time of diagnosis. Initially, operative intervention is necessary only to establish the histologic diagnosis in patients without elevations in serum α-fetoprotein or β-HCG.

Treatment of these nonseminomatous tumors currently is with cisplatin and etoposide-based regimens.[68] Evaluation of these regimens followed by high-dose chemotherapy (cyclophosphamide, carboplatin, etoposide) and peripheral blood stem cell support is ongoing.[68]

Serum markers, α-fetoprotein, and β-HCG are followed to assess response to treatment. If a complete serologic and radiologic response is achieved, patients are closely observed. If the disease progresses during therapy, salvage chemotherapy is initiated. If there is a serologic response but a radiographic abnormality remains, the patient is taken to the operating room and surgical removal of as much of the remaining tumor as possible is performed. The pathology of the resected post-chemotherapy specimen appears to be the most significant predictor of survival.[68,69] The presence of residual disease after chemotherapy portends a poor prognosis and the need for additional chemotherapy. When tumor necrosis or a benign teratoma is found during surgical exploration after chemotherapy, an excellent and intermediate prognosis is conferred.[70] Overall 45% of patients with mediastinal nonseminomas are alive at 5 years.[71] Attempts to reduce the relapse rate have encouraged investigation into the use of first-line high-dose chemotherapy at the time of initial diagnosis.[72]

Although salvage therapies have achieved cures in 20% to 50% of patients with relapsing or refractory testicular nonseminomatous tumors, salvage treatment protocols have been disappointing in those with mediastinal nonseminomatous tumors.[73,74] Currently used salvage therapies are adapted based on initial chemotherapeutic regimens and include regimens containing cisplatin, ifosfamide, etoposide, gemcitabine, vinblastine, paclitaxel, or high-dose chemotherapy based on carboplatin and etoposide followed by autologous bone marrow transplantation.[75] Residual tumor masses after salvage therapy are treated with secondary resection. In a recent series only 11% of patients with primary mediastinal nonseminomatous germ cell tumors treated with salvage therapies were long-term disease free. There was no survival difference between patients treated with conventional salvage regimens and dose-intensive chemotherapy with autologous bone marrow transplantation.[75]

Lymphomas

Although the mediastinum is frequently involved in patients with lymphoma at some time during the course of their disease (40% to 70%), it is infrequently the sole site of disease at the time of presentation. Only 5% to 10% of patients with Hodgkin's and non-Hodgkin's lymphoma present solely with symptoms related to local mass effects, such as mediastinal involvement. Patients usually have symptoms; chest pain, cough, dyspnea, hoarseness, and superior vena caval syndrome are the most common clinical manifestations. Nonspecific systemic symptoms of fever and chills, weight loss, and anorexia are frequently noted and are important in the staging of patients with Hodgkin's lymphoma. Symptoms characteristic of Hodgkin's lymphoma include chest pain after consumption of alcohol and the cyclic fevers that were first described by Pel and Ebstein.

Characteristically, these tumors occur in the anterosuperior mediastinum or in the hilar region of the middle mediastinum. CT and MRI are useful in delineating the extent of disease, determining invasiveness into contiguous structures, differentiating the lesions from cardiovascular abnormalities, aiding the selection of radiation portals, following the response to therapy, and diagnosing relapse. Also, differentiation from thymomas and germ cell tumors, which usually are solitary masses, may be possible because lymphomas are usually composed of multiple nodules that appear as separate masses on CT.

Hodgkin's Lymphoma

The classification of Hodgkin's lymphoma was updated from the previous Rye classification in 1994 by the International Lymphoma Study Group.[76] This updated classification, the Revised European-American Lymphoma (REAL) classification, incorporated new immunologic and molecular data and divides Hodgkin's disease into two main groups: nodular lymphocyte predominant and classic Hodgkin's disease.[76] More recently, the new World Health Organization (WHO) classification of hematologic malignancies has incorporated the REAL concepts.[77]

Classic Hodgkin's disease is composed of nodular sclerosing, mixed cellularity, lymphocyte-rich classic disease, and lymphocyte-depleted types. The nodular sclerosing type is the most common type of Hodgkin's lymphoma (Fig. 56-7) seen in the mediastinum, occurring 55% to 75%

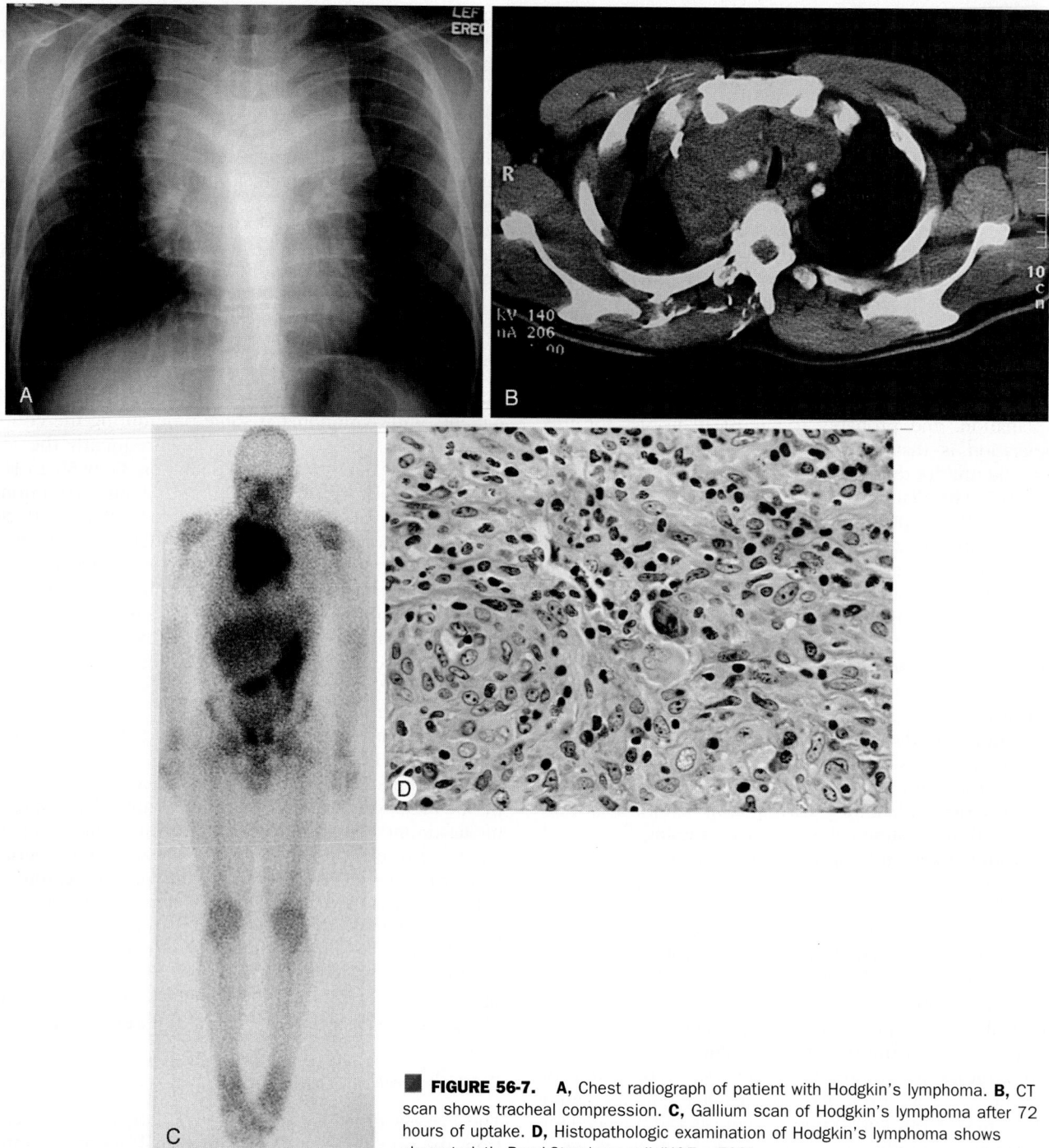

FIGURE 56-7. **A,** Chest radiograph of patient with Hodgkin's lymphoma. **B,** CT scan shows tracheal compression. **C,** Gallium scan of Hodgkin's lymphoma after 72 hours of uptake. **D,** Histopathologic examination of Hodgkin's lymphoma shows characteristic Reed-Sternberg cell (H&E, ×520).

of the time, followed by the lymphocyte-predominant type (40%). Nodular sclerosing lymphoma has a predilection for the thymus, whereas other variants tend to affect mediastinal lymph nodes and are not seen as commonly as an isolated mediastinal mass. The neoplastic cells in Hodgkin's disease are Reed-Sternberg cells or Reed-Sternberg variants that have been shown recently to be derived in most cases from germinal center B cells.[78]

Treatment of Hodgkin's lymphoma is determined by the stage of disease and the prognostic factors related to the patient and the tumor. The Cotswold classification,[79] a modification of the Ann Arbor classification, is used for staging. Treatment is based on radiation therapy and chemotherapy. Surgical excision of all disease is rarely possible, and the surgeon's primary role is to provide sufficient tissue for diagnosis and to assist in pathologic staging. A needle biopsy is often unsuccessful because larger tissue samples are needed to make a histologic diagnosis, particularly with nodular sclerosing lesions. Thoracoscopy, mediastinoscopy, or mediastinotomy and, rarely, thoracotomy or median sternotomy may be necessary to obtain sufficient tissue. The role of staging laparotomy has been minimized, and its only current indication now is for patients with clinically limited disease who opt for limited treatment.[80]

Early- and intermediate-stage Hodgkin's disease is generally treated with combined chemotherapy and involved-field irradiation. Care should be taken that the heart does not receive more than 30 Gy of radiation. Early-stage disease with favorable prognostic factors was traditionally treated with radiation alone, but this treatment is currently not recommended because of high relapse rates.[81] Patients with more advanced disease at presentation or with adverse prognostic factors are treated with extensive chemotherapy alone or with multimodality therapy. When bulky mediastinal disease is present, involved field or regional field irradiation is added.

Chemotherapeutic regimens used in Hodgkin's disease consist of various combinations, including MOPP (nitrogen mustard, vincristine [Oncovin], procarbazine, prednisone), ABVD (doxorubicin [Adriamycin], bleomycin, vinblastine, dacarbazine), MOPP plus ABVD, and other various combination regimens selected on an individual basis with attention to the toxicity of each regimen. Furthermore, dose-intensified chemotherapy has been introduced to treat advanced Hodgkin's disease and BEACOPP (bleomycin, etoposide, doxorubicin [Adriamycin], cyclophosphamide, vincristine [Oncovin], procarbazine, prednisone) has shown improved survival and thus may be used in advanced disease over MOPP/ABVD regimens.[82] If cure is not achieved with conventional-dose chemotherapy, patients with Hodgkin's disease should be considered candidates for high-dose chemotherapy with hematopoietic support.[37,83] Patients with disease that does not respond to salvage therapy can be tried in clinical protocols on experimental treatments.

Today most patients with Hodgkin's disease, whether localized or advanced, can be cured. Looking at all stages of Hodgkin's lymphoma with appropriate treatment, 5-year survival rates around 90% can be achieved.[81] Unfortunately, as the cure rate has improved over the past several decades the long-term complications of treatment (secondary malignancies, coronary artery disease, and late pulmonary toxicity) have become more apparent. It has become increasingly possible to tailor specific treatments to individual risks of the patient, with patients with more favorable disease receiving less intensive and toxic therapy and more aggressive treatment protocols reserved for those with unfavorable disease.[82]

Non-Hodgkin's Lymphoma

Non-Hodgkin's lymphoma, like Hodgkin's disease, is classified now by the WHO classification of lymphoid malignancies adopting the REAL concepts to define clinically relevant entities.[77] Mediastinal non-Hodgkin's lymphoma is usually of either lymphoblastic (60%) or large cell morphology (40%). Patients with non-Hodgkin's lymphoma usually have symptoms because of involvement of adjacent mediastinal structures. Superior vena caval syndrome is relatively common. Lymphoblastic lymphoma occurs predominantly in children, adolescents, and young adults and represents 60% of cases of mediastinal non-Hodgkin's lymphoma. These tumors usually arise from the thymus, and patients often present with respiratory difficulties from a rapidly enlarging anterior mediastinal mass. This disease is two to four times more common in men and has an aggressive course with rapid dissemination to the central nervous system and bone marrow involvement that often progresses to a leukemic phase, gonads, and other visceral sites. Consensus now exists that lymphoblastic lymphoma and acute lymphoblastic leukemia represent different clinical presentations of the same biologic disease.[77] Differentiation of lymphoblastic lymphoma from acute lymphoblastic leukemia is arbitrary, determined by more than 25% bone marrow infiltration; higher degrees of bone marrow involvement are classified as acute lymphoblastic leukemia.[84] Because lymphoblastic lymphoma infiltrates the thymus and is diffuse in appearance, it can be confused with a lymphocyte-predominant thymoma if not carefully studied.[85]

Twenty percent of lymphoblastic lymphomas are from B-cell precursors; the remainder are from T-cell precursors and phenotypically express various stages of T-cell differentiation. High levels of terminal deoxynucleotidyl transferase activity are often present in lymphoblastic lymphoma. Histologically, these tumors are divided into convoluted, nonconvoluted, and large cell subtypes according to the appearance of the neoplastic cell nucleus. The convoluted type is present in 80% of cases, and the convoluted and nonconvoluted types preferentially involve the mediastinum.

Large cell non-Hodgkin's lymphomas of the mediastinum are a diverse group of lymphomas arising from both B-cell and T-cell lineage. These tumors are subdivided into primary mediastinal (thymic) large B-cell lymphoma and anaplastic large cell lymphoma of T-cell and null cell types. Additional variants of mediastinal large cell lymphomas have been identified: large cell lymphoma with marked tropism for germ centers and low-grade mucosa-associated lymphoma of the thymus.[86]

Primary mediastinal B-cell lymphoma is by far the most common of the large cell lymphomas seen in the mediastinum. Studies have reported a slight female predominance and a young adult age at onset.[87] Primary mediastinal B-cell lymphomas present with a rapidly growing mass located in the anterior mediastinum. These lymphomas likely originate from a native population of B cells located in the thymus.[87,88] At diagnosis these tumors are often limited to intrathoracic organs, but recurrence at extrathoracic sites including the liver, kidneys, and central nervous system is common.[87] Histologically, mediastinal large B-cell lymphoma tumors are often composed of large clear cells, which may appear compartmentalized by associated connective tissue (sclerosis). Because of this compartmentalization pattern, large cell lymphomas can be mistaken for seminomas, thymic undifferentiated carcinomas, or Hodgkin's lymphoma based on light microscopic appearance. The degree of B-cell differentiation found in these tumors varies, ranging from early B cells negative for surface immunoglobulin to well-differentiated surface cells positive for immunoglobulin (usually IgG or

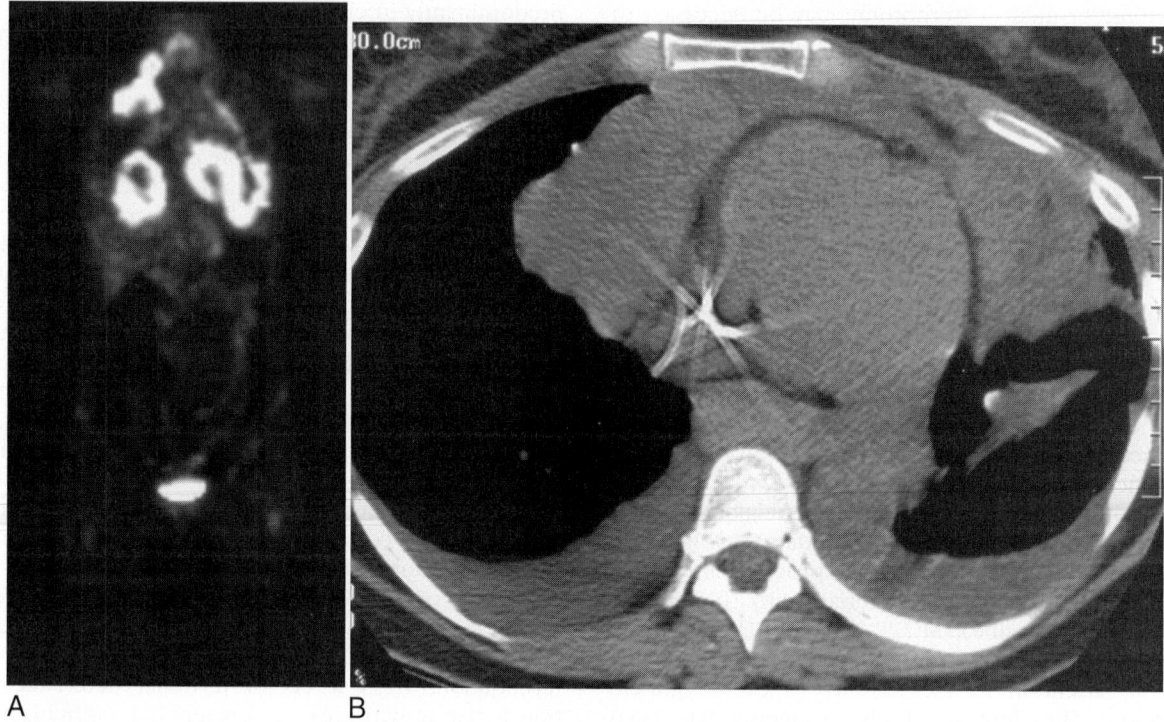

FIGURE 56-8. **A,** FDG-PET scan showing relapse of Hodgkin's disease evidenced by increased uptake in the mediastinum, along left chest wall, and in right neck. **B,** Chest CT scan of same patient as in **A.**

IgA).[85] Primary mediastinal B-cell lymphoma stains positive for CD20 and negative for CD3.[87]

The anaplastic large cell lymphoma of T-cell and null cell types was initially recognized by its expression of antigen for the Ki-1 (CD30) antibody.[76] These tumors have only rarely been located primarily in the mediastinum; however, up to 75% of patients with these tumors have bulky mediastinal involvement in addition to their extrathoracic disease.[86] Histologically, these tumors are composed of large cells and show marked nuclear pleomorphism.

Treatment of non-Hodgkin's lymphoma consists of aggressive anthracycline-containing chemotherapeutic regimens. After intensive chemotherapy, consolidation-involved field radiotherapy may be given.[87,89-92] In lymphoblastic lymphoma, central nervous system prophylaxis is given in conjunction with the standard chemotherapeutic regimen and consists of intrathecal chemotherapy, with or without cranial irradiation. Prophylactic treatment of the central nervous system is not needed in large cell lymphoma because of its infrequent involvement. Recently, the chimeric anti-CD20 monoclonal antibody rituximab combined with standard chemotherapy has shown promise in the initial treatment of diffuse large B-cell lymphoma.[93] Poor response to initial doxorubicin-containing chemotherapy was a predictor of nonresponsiveness to subsequent chemotherapies. Bulky mediastinal disease at presentation or residual abnormality after initial chemotherapy were risk factors for relapse.[92] Patients in first response with poor prognostic factors, with refractory disease, or with recurrent lymphoma can be treated with high-dose chemotherapy and with either autologous bone marrow or peripheral stem cell transplantation.[94,95] Anti-CD20 antibody may have

a role in salvage therapy of patients with primary mediastinal B-cell lymphoma.[96] With an aggressive approach, cure rates of 50% and greater have been achieved in patients with non-Hodgkin's lymphomas.

Residual Masses After Lymphoma Treatment

After treatment of lymphomas, residual abnormalities within the mediastinum are commonly noted radiographically (64% to 88%). Residual radiographic abnormalities are seen more commonly in patients with initial bulky mediastinal disease. Residual mediastinal abnormalities were not significantly associated with eventual disease relapse, except when treatment was with chemotherapy alone. CT cannot differentiate fibrosis or necrosis from residual tumor. MRI can differentiate residual malignant tissue from fibrosis based on different signal characteristics; however, it has a low sensitivity and is not proven very useful for lymphoma.[97]

[67]Ga scintigraphy is a metabolic imaging technique and has proved valuable in the determination of neoplastic disease in residual mediastinal abnormalities post therapy. A negative ^{67}Ga scintigraphic scan has been predictive of absence of residual disease.[89,98] In order to be useful post therapy, avidity of the lymphoma for ^{67}Ga should be confirmed before treatment.

Recently the use of metabolic imaging with FDG-PET has shown promise as a noninvasive way to detect active mediastinal disease and predict relapse in patients with lymphoma (Fig. 56-8). One study evaluated 28 patients with Hodgkin's disease and a residual mediastinal mass 2 cm or larger after treatment with 29 FDG-PET scans.

After FDG-PET patients were observed for signs of relapse over a minimum time period of 1-year. In the 19 patients with a negative PET scan, 16 remained in remission and 3 relapsed (negative predictive value of PET was 95% at 1 year). Of the 10 patients with positive scans, 6 experienced progression or relapse whereas 4 remained in remission (positive predictive value of PET 60% at 1 year). Clearly from this study a positive PET indicates a significant relapse risk and closer follow-up and diagnostic tests should be undertaken.[99] A study by Spaepen and colleagues concluded in non-Hodgkin's lymphoma patients that a positive FDG-PET after chemotherapy was highly predictive of residual disease.[100]

Jerusalem and colleagues have shown the use of FDG-PET can detect preclinical relapse of Hodgkin's disease, which may allow earlier treatment of patients with salvage chemotherapy when minimal disease is present.[101] More studies are required to determine whether earlier detection of relapse by FDG-PET will alter treatment management, be cost effective, and improve survival. As in ^{67}Ga scintigraphy, rebound thymus hyperplasia can result in false-positive FDG-PET results.[102]

Interestingly, FDG-PET appears to be able to differentiate responders from nonresponders early after treatment in patients with lymphoma. This may be useful in determining who can proceed with standard chemotherapeutic agents and which patients should undergo more intense treatments. In one study 95% of patients with an increased uptake by FDG-PET after 1 cycle of chemotherapy relapsed compared with 15% of patients with a negative FDG-PET after 1 cycle.[103] Progression-free survival was significantly different in the patients with positive versus negative FDG-PET scans after 1 cycle of chemotherapy. Further studies are needed to determine whether therapy modifications should be made based on FDG-PET results.[104]

Primary Carcinoma

Primary carcinomas of the mediastinum constitute between 3% and 11% of primary mediastinal masses in most series and represent 4% of the mediastinal masses in the collected series. The origin of these tumors is unknown. It is important to differentiate them from malignant thymomas, germ cell tumors, carcinoid tumors, lymphomas, mediastinal extension of bronchogenic carcinomas, and metastatic tumors, which may have a similar light microscopic appearance. Metastatic disease in mediastinal lymph nodes is usually from bronchogenic or esophageal malignancies and rarely occurs with extrathoracic malignancies. The tumors most likely to metastasize to the mediastinum include those originating in the breast, head, neck, and genitourinary tract as well as melanomas. Primary carcinomas are usually of the large cell, undifferentiated morphology, although small cell and squamous cell tumors have been described. The use of electron microscopic examination of the tumor ultrastructure and immunostaining for surface antigens and cellular proteins better define the origin of some of these primary carcinomas and decrease the reported incidence.

These tumors occur with equal frequency in either sex. Most patients have symptoms from the local mass effects of the tumor. Extensive involvement within the thorax and often metastatic disease outside the thorax characterize this disease. Surgical excision is rarely possible. Unfortunately, the routine use of radiation therapy and chemotherapy has been unsuccessful in prolonging survival. Overall, the mean survival is less than 1 year.

Endocrine Tumors

Thyroid Tumors

Although substernal extension of a cervical goiter is common, totally intrathoracic thyroid tumors are rare and make up only 1% of all mediastinal masses in the collected series. These tumors arise from heterotopic thyroid tissue, which occurs most commonly in the anterosuperior mediastinum but may also occur in the middle mediastinum between the trachea and esophagus as well as in the posterior mediastinum. Although there may be a demonstrable connection with the cervical gland (usually a fibrous connective tissue band), a true intrathoracic thyroid gland derives its blood supply from thoracic vessels.

The peak incidence is in the sixth and seventh decades. Women are more commonly affected. When these lesions occur in the anterosuperior or middle mediastinum, symptoms related to tracheal compression are often present, such as dyspnea, cough, wheezing, and stridor. When these tumors occur in the posterior mediastinum, esophageal compression manifested by dysphagia is common. Rarely, symptoms related to thyrotoxicosis may be the initiating factor for a patient to seek medical attention. On chest radiography, these lesions appear as sharply circumscribed, dense masses, occurring more frequently on the right. The administration of iodinated contrast material causes prolonged enhancement of thyroid tissue, and intrathoracic goiters are contrast medium–enhancing lesions when visualized by CT. When functioning thyroid tissue is present, the ^{131}I scan is usually diagnostic. Some of these neoplasms, however, are functionally inactive and are not identified by ^{131}I scanning.

Most of these tumors are adenomas, but carcinomas have been reported. If the lesion is identified as the sole functioning thyroid tissue and the patient does not have symptoms, surgical exploration and excision is not indicated. In these patients, frequent follow-up radiographic examinations are indicated to evaluate changes in the size and nature of the lesion. Otherwise, these lesions should be resected because of their propensity to enlarge and compress adjacent structures. Because of the thoracic derivation of the blood supply, intrathoracic thyroid tumors should be approached through the thorax, using either an anterolateral thoracotomy or a median sternotomy for anterior lesions or a posterolateral thoracotomy for posterior lesions. Substernal extensions of a cervical goiter can usually be excised using a cervical approach.

Parathyroid Tumors

Although parathyroid glands may occur in the mediastinum in 10% of patients, they are usually accessible through the cervical incision. A sternotomy is necessary to excise a hyperfunctioning parathyroid gland in about 2.5% of all patients and in 15% to 30% of those with a mediastinal gland.[105,106] Most often, these adenomas are found in the anterosuperior mediastinum (80%) embedded in or near the superior pole of the thymus. This anatomic relationship is the result of the common embryogenesis of the inferior parathyroid glands from the third branchial cleft. The superior parathyroid glands and the lateral lobes of the thyroid gland are derived from the fourth branchial pouch. Because they migrate with the lateral lobes of the thyroid gland to a paraesophageal position, parathyroid adenomas can also be found in the posterior mediastinum (20%).[105]

The clinical manifestations of a mediastinal parathyroid tumor are similar to those that occur with tumors of the cervical region; symptoms are related to the excess secretion of parathyroid hormone causing the hyperparathyroid syndrome. Preoperative attempts at anatomic localization are indicated. In patients whose preoperative studies have failed to locate the site of the responsible parathyroid gland, exploration of the mediastinum is often unsuccessful. Because of their small size, these neoplasms rarely cause symptoms related to mechanical effects and are not often visualized using conventional radiography. Using CT, MRI, thallium and technetium scanning, technetium-sestamibi scintigraphy, selective arteriography, and more recently FDG-PET, preoperative localization of these tumors can be made in greater than 80% of patients.[107] Venous angiography with selective sampling is useful for determining the size of the adenoma but is usually inadequate for defining the anatomic location.

Most frequently, the mediastinal adenoma may be excised after a negative exploration of the cervical region through the existing cervical incision. Usually, the vascular supply to the adenoma extends from cervical blood vessels. In patients with persistent hyperparathyroidism, after cervical exploration if localization studies show residual parathyroid in the mediastinum, mediastinal exploration using a median sternotomy is indicated. Alternatively, successful removal has been performed thoracoscopically.[108] Additionally, ethanol ablation of mediastinal parathyroids can be performed with long-term success in a select number of patients.[107]

Parathyroid carcinomas have been reported and are usually hormonally active. Patients differ in clinical presentation in that they often have higher serum calcium levels and manifest more severe symptoms of hyperparathyroidism. When possible, surgical resection is the optimal therapy.

Unlike parathyroid adenomas and carcinomas, parathyroid cysts are usually not hormonally active. These cysts are defined by the presence of parathyroid cells identifiable within the cyst wall. Because these lesions are frequently larger than adenomas, symptoms related to local mass effects are more common, as is visualization on chest film. Surgical excision yields a cure.

Neuroendocrine Tumors

Mediastinal neuroendocrine tumors, previously known as carcinoid tumors, arise from cells of Kulchitsky located in the thymus. These tumors show a predilection for males in their 40s and 50s, are usually located in the anterosuperior mediastinum, and behave aggressively.[109] Metastatic spread to mediastinal and cervical lymph nodes, liver, bone, skin, and lungs is present in at least 20% at presentation.[109] Fifty percent of thymic neuroendocrine tumors are hormonally active, often associated with Cushing's syndrome[110] because of production of adrenocorticotropic hormone, less frequently associated with multiple endocrine neoplasia syndromes, and only rarely associated with carcinoid syndrome (0.6%).[109]

In patients with hormonally inactive tumors, symptoms are related to local mass effects, leading to chest pain, dyspnea, cough, and the superior vena caval syndrome. Hormonally inactive neuroendocrine tumors tend to be larger and are frequently invasive locally.

Often neuroendocrine tumors are difficult to differentiate from other common anterior mediastinal masses, particularly thymomas and germ cell tumors. Positive immunohistochemical staining of thymic neuroendocrine tumors for cytokeratins and often other markers including chromogranin, leu-7, neurospecific enolase, bombesin, synaptophysin, and adrenocorticotropic hormone may help confirm the diagnosis.[109] Neuroendocrine tumors are characterized by the ultrastructural findings of dense-core neurosecretory granules. These tumors appear to be part of a continuous spectrum ranging from well-differentiated lesions to small cell carcinomas.[111]

The best chance for cure is surgical excision, but local invasion or metastatic spread often precludes complete excision. Adjuvant therapy is controversial, but irradiation should probably be added particularly in patients with capsular invasion. Therapies that exploit the somatostatin receptors present on these tumors, such as radiolabeled octreotide, may hold promise.[109] A recent large series of neuroendocrine tumors reported a 29% 5-year and a 10% 10-year survival.[112] Patients with tumors associated with an endocrinopathy have a particularly poor prognosis. Late recurrences are possible.

Mesenchymal Tumors

Mediastinal mesenchymal tumors originate from the connective tissue, striatal and smooth muscle, fat, lymphatic tissue, and blood vessels present within the mediastinum, giving rise to a diverse group of neoplasms. Relative to other sites in the body, these tumors occur less commonly within the mediastinum. Mesenchymal tumors constituted 7% of the primary masses in the collected series. There is no apparent difference in incidence between genders. The soft tissue neoplasms include lipomas, liposarcomas, fibrosarcomas, fibromas, xanthogranulomas, leiomyomas, leiomyosarcomas, benign and malignant mesenchymomas, rhabdomyosarcomas, and mesotheliomas. These tumors have a similar histologic appearance and generally follow the same clinical course as the soft tissue tumors found elsewhere in the body. Fifty-five percent of these tumors are malignant. Surgical resection remains the primary therapy because poor results have been obtained using radiation therapy and chemotherapy.

Similarly, the mesenchymal tumors derived from blood and lymph vessels are common elsewhere in the body but rare in the mediastinum. Although these tumors occur anywhere in the mediastinum, the most frequent location is in the anterosuperior mediastinum. They include capillary, cavernous, and venous hemangiomas; hemangioendotheliomas; hemangiopericytomas; lymphangiomas; and the derivatives of lymphangiomas. Symptoms are related to the size and invasiveness of the lesion. Occasionally, hemorrhage into the lesion may lead to a rapid increase in the size. Rupture of hemangiomas into the pleural space may cause exsanguination; rupture into the mediastinum may cause tamponade.

Between 10% and 30% of vascular tumors are malignant, although the differentiation may be difficult because of the histologic appearance, number of mitotic figures, and even the gross appearance are often similar. Vascular tumors are not well encapsulated, and even benign tumors may exhibit local invasion. The incidence of metastatic spread is low, however, about 3%. Hemangiopericytomas have the highest incidence of malignancy, and these tumors usually occur in older patients. Because these neoplasms are not supplied by large vessels, tumor opacification usually does not occur during angiographic studies. Excision remains the only effective means of therapy, although radiation therapy has been used with mixed results. Successful treatment of an extensive mediastinal hemangioma with interferon alfa-2a followed by resection has been reported.[113]

Tumors originating from lymph vessels are differentiated from tumors of blood vessel origin by using indirect evidence, such as the absence of red blood cells within the lumen of the tumor vasculature, extrusion of chylous fluid from the cut edges, and the tumor's relationship to documented lymphatic tissue. Also, these tumors usually occur in the anterior mediastinum, appearing as round or lobulated cystic densities on chest radiograph. The most common lymphatic tumor is the lymphangioma (also called *cystic hygroma, lymphatic cyst,* and *lymphatogenous cyst*), which in most patients occurs in the superior mediastinum as an extension of a cervical lesion. Only 17% of mediastinal lymphangiomas are completely within the mediastinum, whereas 10% of cervical lymphangiomas have a mediastinal extension. Lymphangiomas are usually diagnosed in children, and they frequently cause symptoms related to obstruction of the trachea, including stridor, dyspnea, recurrent pulmonary infection, and tachypnea. Lymphangiomas have characteristic appearances on ultrasound and CT. Growth of these tumors is by proliferation of endothelium-lined buds that spread along tissue planes. The local ingrowth of vessels and fibrous reaction to the endothelial buds prevent easy surgical removal resulting from the lack of well-defined tissue planes. Because radiation therapy and sclerotherapy have not been successful, however, operative resection is the optimal treatment. Total excision is not indicated when nerves and vital structures are involved. Multiple procedures may be necessary.

Extramedullary Hematopoiesis

Extramedullary hematopoiesis occurs in all age groups, usually as a result of altered hematopoiesis. In the adult, this is typically a result of massive hemolysis, myelofibrosis, spherocytic anemia, or thalassemia. These lesions appear as bilateral, asymmetrical paravertebral masses and enhance with contrast medium. Radionuclide imaging using ^{99m}Tc sulfur colloid is a noninvasive method of diagnosing intrathoracic extramedullary hematopoiesis.[114] Surgical resection is unnecessary unless there is invasion or compression of mediastinal structures. Radiation therapy can produce rapid shrinkage of these masses.

Giant Lymph Node Hyperplasia (Castleman's Disease)

Giant lymph node hyperplasia was initially described by Castleman.[115] Although the mediastinum was the site of disease in the initial report and in most patients, these tumors may develop wherever lymph nodes are present; the retroperitoneum and cervical, axillary, and pelvic regions are the most common nonmediastinal sites. Although these tumors are usually located in the anterosuperior mediastinum, they are also found in the posterior mediastinum and at the pericardiophrenic angle, where they may be confused with neurogenic tumors and pericardial cysts, respectively. Two distinct histologic entities exist: (1) hyaline vascular, characterized by small hyaline follicles and interfollicular capillary proliferation, and (2) plasma cell, characterized by large follicles with intervening sheets of plasma cells. Increasingly, it appears that there are different causes for the distinct histologic variants.[116] The tumors most frequently appear as single, well-demarcated lesions. The hyaline vascular type represents 90% of Castleman's tumors, and these are most often discovered in patients without symptoms on a routine chest radiograph. Patients with the plasma cell type often exhibit systemic features, including fever, night sweats, anemia, and hypergammaglobulinemia. Surgical excision effects cure, although resection of the hyaline vascular type may be associated with significant hemorrhage because of extreme vascularity.

Castleman's disease may also be multicentric, characterized by generalized lymphadenopathy with morphologic features of giant lymph node hyperplasia. Patients most often have symptoms, including fever, chills, weight loss, and hepatosplenomegaly, and exhibit disordered immunity and autoimmune phenomena. Multicentric Castleman's disease has been associated with HIV infection and human herpesvirus 8.[117] Unlike the benign clinical course of classic Castleman's disease, multicentric disease is a much more malignant disease, with death often occurring after infectious complications. Patients with multicentric disease of the plasma cell variant and the presence of systemic features have recently shown promising responses to treatment with anti–IL-6 receptor antibody.[118]

Chordoma

Chordomas are rare malignant tumors that may occur in the posterior mediastinum and originate from the primitive notochord. Men are affected twice as often as women, with the peak age of incidence in the fifth through seventh decades. Chest pain, cough, and dyspnea are the most common features. Spinal cord compression may follow extension into the spinal canal. Radical surgical excision is the only effective therapy. Despite resection, chordomas tend to recur at the surgical site, and 70% of patients die of their disease.[119]

Primary Cysts

Primary cysts of the mediastinum make up 18% of the mediastinal masses in the collected series. These cysts can be bronchogenic, pericardial, enteric, or thymic or may be of an unspecified nature. More than 75% of cases are asymptomatic, and these tumors rarely cause morbidity. Because of the proximity of vital structures within the mediastinum, however, with increasing size, even benign cysts may cause significant morbidity. In addition, these masses need to be differentiated from malignant tumors. Benign mediastinal cysts can be removed thoracoscopically and techniques have been developed to help prevent cystic rupture.[120]

Bronchogenic cysts are the most common primary cysts of the mediastinum. They originate as sequestrations from the ventral foregut, the antecedent of the tracheobronchial tree. The bronchogenic cyst may lie within the lung parenchyma or the mediastinum. The cyst wall is composed of cartilage, mucous glands, smooth muscle, and fibrous tissue with a pathognomonic inner layer of ciliated respiratory epithelium. When bronchogenic cysts occur in the mediastinum, they are usually located proximal to the trachea or bronchi and may be just posterior to the carina. Rarely, a true communication between the cyst and the tracheobronchial tree exists, and an air-fluid level may be observed on chest radiograph.

Two thirds of bronchogenic cysts are asymptomatic. In infants, these cysts may cause severe respiratory compromise by compressing the trachea or the bronchus; compression of the bronchus may cause bronchial stenosis and recurrent pneumonitis. In children with recurrent pulmonary infections, CT may be useful in assessing the subcarinal space for possible bronchogenic cyst, an area that is poorly visualized using standard radiography. More often, bronchogenic cysts occur in older children and adults, in whom these cysts may cause symptoms of chest pain, dyspnea, cough, and stridor. Bronchogenic cysts appear as a smooth density at the level of the carina that may compress the esophagus on barium swallow. Differentiation from hilar structures may be difficult.

Surgical excision is recommended in all patients to provide definitive histologic diagnosis, alleviate symptoms, and prevent the development of associated complications. Malignant degeneration has been reported, as has the presence of a bronchial adenoma within the cysts.

Pericardial cysts are the second most frequently encountered cysts within the mediastinum. These cysts classically occur in the pericardiophrenic angles (Fig. 56-9), with 70% in the right pericardiophrenic angle, 22% in the left, and the remainder in other sites in the peri-

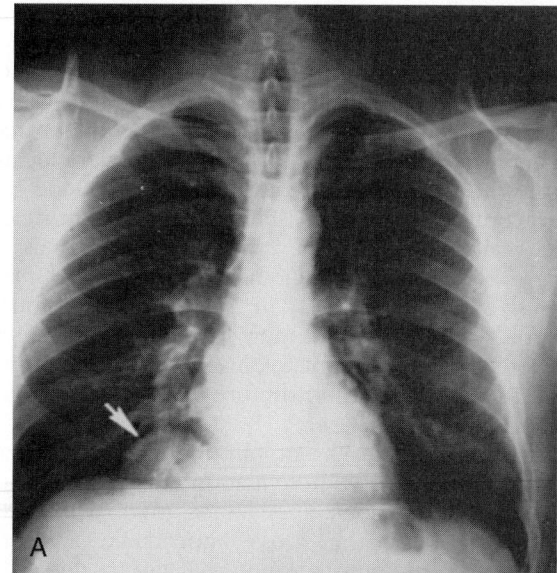

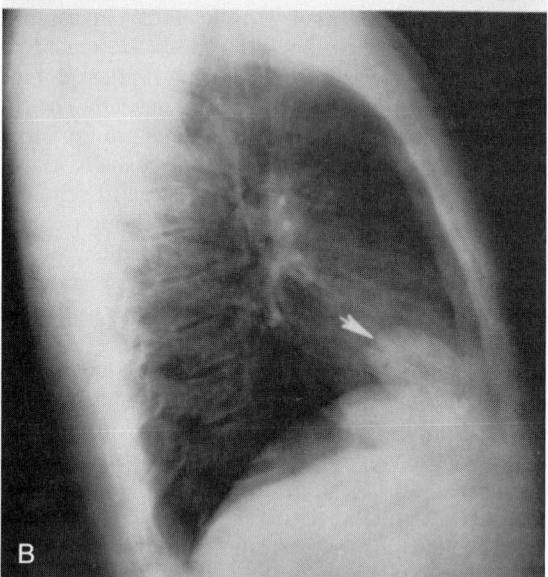

FIGURE 56-9. **A** and **B,** Chest radiographs show the typical location of a pericardial cyst in the right cardiophrenic angle. (**A** and **B,** From Sabiston DC Jr, Oldham HN Jr: The mediastinum. *In* Sabiston DC Jr, Spencer FC [eds]: Gibbon's Surgery of the Chest, 4th ed. Philadelphia, WB Saunders, 1983.)

cardium. Pericardial cysts may or may not have a communication with the pericardium. Numerous reports have described the characteristic CT appearance of pericardial cysts: pericardiophrenic location, near-water attenuation value, and smooth borders. Lesions demonstrating classic CT characteristics of pericardial cysts have been managed with needle aspiration and follow-up with serial CT rather than surgical excision. Surgical excision of pericardial cysts is indicated primarily for diagnosis and to differentiate these cysts from malignant lesions.

Enteric cysts (duplication cysts) arise from the posterior division of the primitive foregut, which develops into the upper division of the gastrointestinal tract. These cysts are found less frequently than bronchogenic or pericardial cysts and are most frequently located in the posterior mediastinum, usually adjacent to the esophagus. These lesions are composed of smooth muscle with an inner epithelial lining of esophageal, gastric, or intestinal mucosa. When gastric mucosa is present, peptic ulceration with perforation into the esophageal or bronchial lumina may occur, producing hemoptysis or hematemesis. Usually, enteric cysts have an attachment to the esophagus and may be embedded within the muscularis layer. Symptoms are usually related to compression of the esophagus, leading to obstruction that commonly presents as dysphagia. Compromise of the tracheobronchial tree with symptoms of cough, dyspnea, recurrent pulmonary infections, and chest pain also may result. Most enteric cysts are diagnosed in children, who are also more likely to have symptoms.

When enteric cysts are associated with anomalies of the vertebral column, they are referred to as *neuroenteric cysts.* Such cysts may be connected to the meninges, or, less frequently, a direct communication with the dural space may exist. In patients with neuroenteric cysts, preoperative evaluation for potential spinal cord involvement is mandatory. The vertebral anomalies associated with this syndrome include spina bifida, hemivertebrae, and a widened neural canal. Treatment is surgical excision, providing a definite histologic diagnosis as well as alleviating symptoms and preventing potential complications.

Nonspecific cysts include those lesions in which a specific epithelial or mesothelial lining cannot be identified. These lesions may originate in any of the aforementioned cysts by the destruction of the inner epithelial lining by an inflammatory or digestive process. Other causes include postinflammatory cysts and hemorrhagic cysts.

Selected References

Blalock A, Mason MF, Morgan HJ, Riven SS: Myasthenia gravis and tumors of the thymic region. Ann Surg 110:544-561, 1939.

> This landmark paper substantiates the use of thymectomy in the treatment of myasthenia gravis. In this paper, Blalock reports the successful removal of a 6 × 5 × 3-cm thymic tumor from a 19-year-old woman. Follow-up of this patient over a 3-year period demonstrated significant improvement in her symptoms of myasthenia.

Bokemeyer C, Nichols CR, Droz J-P, et al: Extragonadal germ cell tumors of the mediastinum and retroperitoneum: Results from an international analysis. J Clin Oncol 20:1864-1873, 2002.

> This article characterizes the clinical and biologic features of extragonadal germ cell tumors. Based on currently available treatment strategies it shows that, independent of primary tumor site, patients with pure seminomatous histology have an almost 90% long-term chance of cure. Unfortunately only 45% of patients with mediastinal nonseminomas are alive at 5 years. Patients with nonseminomatous mediastinal primary tumors have a significantly inferior outcome compared with patients with nonseminomatous retroperitoneal primary tumors.

Davis RD, Oldham HN, Sabiston DC: Primary cysts and neoplasms of the mediastinum: Recent changes in clinical presentation, methods of diagnosis, management, and results. Ann Thorac Surg 44:229-237, 1987.

> This study of 400 patients with mediastinal tumors is one of the largest in the literature. It emphasizes the major changes that have occurred in clinical presentation, diagnosis, and management of primary lesions of the mediastinum.

Masaoka A, Monden Y, Nakahara K, Tanioka T: Follow-up study of thymomas with special reference to their clinical stages. Cancer 48:2485-2492, 1981.

> This article proposes the clinical staging system for thymomas that is most widely used today. This staging system allows for comparison between studies.

Shimosato Y, Mukai K: Atlas of Tumor Pathology, 3rd series, fascicle 21. Washington, DC, Armed Forces Institute of Pathology, 1997.

> This comprehensive fascicle provides one of the best overall reviews available on tumors of the mediastinum, with special emphasis on thymic tumors.

Weihrauch MR, Re D, Scheidhauer K, et al: Thoracic positron emission tomography using ^{18}F-fluorodeoxyglucose for the evaluation of residual mediastinal Hodgkin disease. Blood 98:2930-2934, 2001.

> This article shows the value of using FDG-PET to evaluate residual mediastinal masses after treatment of Hodgkin's disease. Hodgkin's disease patients with residual mediastinal masses with negative post-treatment FDG-PET are unlikely to relapse before 1 year. Positive post-treatment FDG-PET scans in patients with residual masses indicate a significantly higher risk of relapse and warrant further diagnostic procedures and closer follow-up.

References

1. Hochrein J, Bashore TM, O'Laughlin MP, Harrison JK: Percutaneous stenting of superior vena cava syndrome: A case report and review of the literature. Am J Med 104:78-84, 1998.
2. Tanigawa N, Sawada S, Mishima K, et al: Clinical outcome of stenting in superior vena syndrome associated with malignant tumors: Comparison with conventional treatment. Acta Radiol 39:669-674, 1998.
3. Sabiston DC, Scott HW: Primary neoplasms and cysts of the mediastinum. Ann Surg 136:777-797, 1952.
4. Heimburger IL, Battersby JS: Primary mediastinal tumors of childhood. J Thorac Cardiovasc Surg 50:92-103, 1965.
5. Burkell CC, Cross JM, Kent HP, Nanson EM: Mass lesions of the mediastinum. Curr Prob Surg 2:57, 1969.
6. Fontenelle LJ, Armstrong RG, Stanford W, et al: The asymptomatic mediastinal mass. Arch Surg 102:98-102, 1971.
7. Benjamin SP, McCormack LJ, Effler DB, et al: Primary lymphatic tumors of the mediastinum. Cancer 30:708-712, 1972.
8. Conkle DM, Adkins RB: Primary malignant tumors of the mediastinum. Ann Thorac Surg 14:553-567, 1972.
9. Rubush JL, Gardner IR, Boyd WC, Ehrenhaft JL: Mediastinal tumors: Review of 186 cases. J Thorac Cardiovasc Surg 65:216-222, 1973.

10. Vidne B, Levy MJ: Mediastinal tumors: Surgical treatment in forty-five consecutive cases. Scand J Thorac Cardiovasc Surg 7:59-65, 1973.

11. Ovrum E, Birkeland S: Mediastinal tumors and cysts: A review of 91 cases. Scand J Thorac Cardiovasc Surg 13:161-168, 1979.

12. Nandi P, Wong KC, Mok CK, Ong GB: Primary mediastinal tumors: Review of 74 cases. J R Coll Surg Edinb 25:460-466, 1980.

13. Adkins RB, Maples MD, Hainsworth JD: Primary malignant mediastinal tumors. Ann Thorac Surg 38:648-659, 1984.

14. Parish JM, Rosenow EC III, Muhm JR: Mediastinal masses: Clues to interpretation of radiologic studies. Postgrad Med 76:173-182, 1984.

15. Duke Medical Center: Updated data from unpublished 1998 data.

16. Davis RD, Oldham HN, Sabiston DC: Primary cysts and neoplasms of the mediastinum: Recent changes in clinical presentation, methods of diagnosis, management, and results. Ann Thorac Surg 44:229-237, 1987.

17. Nakata H, Egashira K, Watanabe H, et al: MRI of bronchogenic cysts. J Comput Assist Tomogr 17:267-270, 1993.

18. Kubota K, Yamada S, Kondo T, et al: PET imaging of primary mediastinal tumours. Br J Cancer 73:882-886, 1996.

19. Kostakoglu L, Leonard JP, Kuji I, et al: Comparison of fluorine-18 fluorodeoxyglucose positron emission tomography and Ga-67 scintigraphy in evaluation of lymphoma. Cancer 94:879-888, 2002.

20. Panelli F, Erickson RA, Prasad VM: Evaluation of mediastinal masses by endoscopic ultrasound and endoscopic ultrasound-guided fine needle aspiration. Am J Gastroenterol 96:401-408, 2001.

21. Protopapas Z, Westcott JL: Transthoracic hilar and mediastinal biopsy. Radiol Clin North Am 38:281-91, 2000.

22. Motzer RJ, Bosl GJ, Geller NL, et al: Advanced seminoma: The role of chemotherapy and adjunctive surgery. Ann Intern Med 108:513, 1988.

23. Cirino LM, Milanez de Campos JR, Fernandez A, et al: Diagnosis and treatment of mediastinal tumors by thoracoscopy. Chest 117:1787-1792, 2000.

24. Roviaro G, Varoli F, Nucca O, et al: Videothoracoscopic approach to primary mediastinal pathology. Chest 117:1179-1183, 2000.

25. Partrick DA, Rothenberg SS: Thoracoscopic resection of mediastinal masses in infants and children: An evaluation of technique and results. J Pediatr Surg 36:1165-1167, 2001.

26. Azizkhan RG, Dudgeon DL, Buck JR, et al: Life-threatening airway obstruction as a complication to the management of mediastinal masses in children. J Pediatr Surg 20:816, 1985.

27. Goh MH, Liu XY, Goh YS: Anterior mediastinal masses: An anaesthetic challenge. Anaesthesia 54:670-674, 1999.

28. Shimada H, Ambros IM, Dehner LP, et al: Terminology and morphologic criteria of neuroblastic tumors: Recommendations by the international neuroblastoma pathology committee. Cancer 86:349-363, 1999.

29. Shimada H, Ambros IM, Dehner LP, et al: The International Neuroblastoma Pathology Classification (the Shimada system). Cancer 86:364-372, 1999.

30. Bousamra M, Haasler GB, Patterson GA, Roper CL: A comparative study of thoracoscopic vs open removal of benign neurogenic mediastinal tumors. Chest 109:1461-1465, 1996.

31. Zierold D, Halow KD: Thoracoscopic resection as the preferred approach to posterior mediastinal neurogenic tumors. Surg Laparosc Endosc Percutan Tech 10:222-225, 2000.

32. Ruurda JP, Hanlo PW, Hennipman A, Broeders IA: Robot-assisted thoracoscopic resection of a benign mediastinal neurogenic tumor: Technical note. Neurosurgery 52:462-464; discussion 464, 2003.

33. Vallieres E, Findlay JM, Frazer RE: Combined microneurosurgical and thoracoscopic removal of neurogenic dumbbell tumors. Ann Thorac Surg 59:469-472, 1995.

34. Simpson I, Campbell PE: Mediastinal masses in childhood: A review from a pediatric pathologist's point of view. Prog Pediatr Surg 27:93, 1991.

35. Evans AE, D'Angio GJ, Sather HN, et al: A comparison of four staging systems for localized and regional neuroblastoma: A report from the Children's Cancer Study Group. J Clin Oncol 8:678-688, 1990.

36. Brodeur GM, Pritchard J, Berthold F, et al: Revisions of the international criteria for neuroblastoma diagnosis, staging, and response to treatment [comment]. J Clin Oncol 11:1466-1477, 1993.

37. Kaufman D, Longo DL: Hodgkin's disease. In Abeloff MD, Armitage JO, Lichter AS, Niederhuber JE (eds): Clinical Oncology, 2nd ed. New York, Churchill Livingstone, 2000, pp 2620-2657.

38. Seeger RC, Brodeur GM, Sather H, et al: Association of multiple copies of the N-myc oncogene with rapid progression of neuroblastomas. N Engl J Med 313:1111-1116, 1985.

39. Caron H, van Sluis P, de Kraker J, et al: Allelic loss of chromosome 1p as a predictor of unfavorable outcome in patients with neuroblastoma. [comment]. N Engl J Med 334:225-230, 1996.

40. Shimada H, Umehara S, Monobe Y, et al: International neuroblastoma pathology classification for prognostic evaluation of patients with peripheral neuroblastic tumors: A report from the Children's Cancer Group. Cancer 92:2451-2461, 2001.

41. Matthay KK: Intensification of therapy using hematopoietic stem-cell support for high-risk neuroblastoma. Pediatr Transplant 3:72-77, 1999.

42. Yanik GA, Levine JE, Matthay KK, et al: Pilot study of iodine-131-metaiodobenzylguanidine in combination with myeloablative chemotherapy and autologous stem-cell support for the treatment of neuroblastoma. J Clin Oncol 20:2142-2149, 2002.

43. Valteau-Couanet D, Leboulaire C, Maincent K, et al: Dendritic cells for NK/LAK activation: Rationale for multicellular immunotherapy in neuroblastoma patients. Blood 100:2554-2561, 2002.

44. Rousseau RF, Haight AE, Hirschmann-Jax C, et al: Local and systemic effects of an allogeneic tumor cell vaccine combining transgenic human lymphotactin with interleukin-2 in patients with advanced or refractory neuroblastoma. Blood 101:1718-1726, 2003.

45. Umehara S, Nakagawa A, Matthay KK, et al: Histopathology defines prognostic subsets of ganglioneuroblastoma, nodular. Cancer 89:1150-1161, 2000.

46. Rakovich G, Ferraro P, Therasse E, Duranceau A: Preoperative embolization in the management of a mediastinal paraganglioma. Ann Thorac Surg 72:601-603, 2001.

47. Marino M, Müller-Hermelink HK: Thymoma and thymic carcinoma: Relation of thymoma epithelial cells to the cortical and medullary differentiation of thymus. Virchows Arch 407:119-149, 1985.

48. Verley JM, Hollmann KH: Thymoma: A comparative study of clinical stages, histologic features, and survival in 200 cases. Cancer 55:1074-1086, 1985.

49. Kornstein MJ, Curran WJ, Turrisi AT, Brooks JJ: Cortical versus medullary thymomas: A useful morphologic distinction? Hum Pathol 19:1335, 1988.

50. Elert O, Buchwald J, Wolf K: Epithelial thymus tumors—therapy and prognosis. Thorac Cardiovasc Surg 36:109, 1988.

51. Blalock A, Mason MF, Morgan HJ, Riven SS: Myasthenia gravis and tumors of the thymic region. Ann Surg 110:544-561, 1939.

52. Calhoun RF, Ritter JH, Guthrie TJ, et al: Results of transcervical thymectomy for myasthenia gravis in 100 consecutive patients. Ann Surg 230:555-559; discussion 559-561, 1999.

53. Shrager JB, Deeb ME, Mick R, et al: Transcervical thymectomy for myasthenia gravis achieves results comparable to thymectomy by sternotomy. Ann Thorac Surg 74:320-327, 2002.

54. Masaoka A, Monden Y, Nakahara K, Tanioka T: Follow-up study of thymomas with special reference to their clinical stages. Cancer 48:2485-2492, 1981.

55. Wilkins EW, Grillo HC, Scannell G, et al: Role of staging in prognosis and management of thymoma. Ann Thorac Surg 51:888-892, 1991.

56. Mangi AA, Wright CD, Allan JS, et al: Adjuvant radiation therapy for stage II thymoma. Ann Thorac Surg 74:1033-1037, 2002.

57. Blumberg D, Port JL, Weksler B, et al: Thymoma: A multivariate analysis of factors predicting survival. Ann Thorac Surg 60:908-914, 1995.

58. Loehrer PJ, Kim K, Chen M, et al: Phase II trial of cisplatin (P), adriamycin (A), cyclophosphamide (C) plus radiotherapy in limited stage unresectable thymoma. Proc Am Soc Clin Oncol 14:433, 1995.

59. Yagi K, Hirata T, Fukuse T, et al: Surgical treatment for invasive thymoma, especially when the superior vena cava is invaded. Ann Thorac Surg 61:521-524, 1996.

60. Moran CA, Suster S: Primary germ cell tumors: I. Analysis of 322 cases with special emphasis on teratomatous lesions and a proposal for histopathologic classification and clinical staging. Cancer 80:681-690, 1997.

61. Lahdenne P: Late sequelae of gonadal, mediastinal and oral teratomas in childhood. Acta Paediatr 81:235, 1992.

62. Fizazi K, Culine S, Droz JP, et al: Initial management of primary mediastinal seminoma: Radiotherapy or cisplatin-based chemotherapy? Eur J Cancer 34:347-352, 1998.

63. Bokemeyer C, Droz JP, Horwich A, et al: Extragonadal seminoma: An international multicenter analysis of prognostic factors and long term treatment outcome. Cancer 91:1394-1401, 2001.

64. Ganjoo KN, Chan RJ, Sharma M, Einhorn LH: Positron emission tomography scans in the evaluation of postchemotherapy residual masses in patients with seminoma. J Clin Oncol 17:3457-3460, 1999.

65. Nichols CR, Heerema NA, Palmer C, et al: Klinefelter's syndrome associated with mediastinal germ cell neoplasms. J Clin Oncol 5:1290-1294, 1987.

66. Nichols CR: Mediastinal germ cell tumors: Clinical features and biologic correlates. Chest 99:472-479, 1991.

67. Hartmann JT, Nichols CR, Droz JP, et al: Hematologic disorders associated with primary mediastinal nonseminomatous germ cell tumors. J Natl Cancer Inst 92:54-61, 2000.

68. Ganjoo KN, Rieger KM, Kesler KA, et al: Results of modern therapy for patients with mediastinal nonseminomatous germ cell tumors. Cancer 88:1051-1056, 2000.

69. Vuky J, Bains M, Bacik J, et al: Role of postchemotherapy adjunctive surgery in the management of patients with nonseminoma arising from the mediastinum. J Clin Oncol 19:682-688, 2001.

70. Kesler KA, Rieger KM, Ganjoo KN, et al: Primary mediastinal nonseminomatous germ cell tumors: The influence of postchemotherapy pathology on long-term survival after surgery. J Thorac Cardiovasc Surg 118:692-701, 1999.

71. Bokemeyer C, Nichols CR, Droz JP, et al: Extragonadal germ cell tumors of the mediastinum and retroperitoneum: Results from an international analysis. J Clin Oncol 20:1864-1873, 2002.

72. Bokemeyer C, Kollmannsberger C, Meisner C, et al: First-line high-dose chemotherapy compared with standard-dose PEB/VIP chemotherapy in patients with advanced germ cell tumors: A multivariate and matched-pair analysis. J Clin Oncol 17:3450-3456, 1999.

73. Hartmann JT, Kanz L, Bokemeyer C: Diagnosis and treatment of patients with testicular germ cell cancer. Drugs 58:257-281, 1999.

74. Saxman SB, Nichols CR, Einhorn LH: Salvage chemotherapy in patients with extragonadal nonseminomatous germ cell tumors: The Indiana University experience. J Clin Oncol 12:1390-1393, 1994.

75. Hartmann JT, Einhorn L, Nichols CR, et al: Second-line chemotherapy in patients with relapsed extragonadal nonseminomatous germ cell tumors: Results of an international multicenter analysis. J Clin Oncol 19:1641-1648, 2001.

76. Harris NL, Jaffe ES, Stein H, et al: A revised European-American classification of lymphoid neoplasms: A proposal from The International Lymphoma Study Group. Blood 84:1361-1392, 1994.

77. Harris NL, Jaffe ES, Diebold J, et al: The World Health Organization classification of hematological malignancies report of the Clinical Advisory Committee Meeting, Airlie House, Virginia, November 1997. Mod Pathol 13:193-207, 2000.

78. Marafioti T, Hummel M, Foss HD, et al: Hodgkin and Reed-Sternberg cells represent an expansion of a single clone originating from a germinal center B cell with functional immunoglobulin gene rearrangements but defective immunoglobulin transcription. Blood 95:1443, 2000.

79. Lister TA, Crowther D, Sutcliffe SB, et al: Report of a committee convened to discuss the evaluation and staging of patients with Hodgkin's disease: Cotswold Meeting. J Clin Oncol 7:1630, 1989.

80. Diehl V, Mauch PM, Harris NL: Hodgkin's disease. In DeVita VT, Hellman S, Rosenberg SA (eds): Cancer: Principles & Practice of Oncology, vol 2. Philadelphia, Lippincott Williams & Wilkins, 2001, pp 2339-2387.

81. Yung L, Linch D: Hodgkin's lymphoma. Lancet 361:943-951, 2003.

82. Sieber M, Engert A, Diehl V: Treatment of Hodgkin's disease: Results and current concepts of the German Hodgkin's Lymphoma Study Group. Ann Oncol 11:81-85, 2000.

83. Josting A, Katay I, Rueffer U, et al: Favorable outcome of patients with relapsed or refractory Hodgkin's disease treated with high-dose chemotherapy and stem cell rescue at the time of maximal response to conventional salvage therapy (Dex-BEAM). Ann Oncol 9:289-295, 1998.

84. Hoelzer D, Gokbuget N, Digel W, et al: Outcome of adult patients with T-lymphoblastic lymphoma treated according to protocols for acute lymphoblastic leukemia. Blood 99:4379-4385, 2002.

85. Shimosato Y, Mukai K: Atlas of Tumor Pathology, 3rd series, fascicle 21. Washington, DC, Armed Forces Institute of Pathology, 1997.

86. Suster S, Moran CA: Pleomorphic large cell lymphomas of the mediastinum. Am J Surg Pathol 20:224-232, 1996.

87. van Besien K, Kelta M, Bahaguna P: Primary mediastinal B-cell lymphoma: A review of pathology and management. J Clin Oncol 19:1855-1864, 2001.

88. Suster S: Primary large-cell lymphomas of the mediastinum. Semin Diagn Pathol 16:51-64, 1999.

89. Zinzani PL, Martelli M, Magagnoli M, et al: Treatment and clinical management of primary mediastinal large B-cell lymphoma with sclerosis: MACOP-B regimen and medi-

astinal radiotherapy monitored by (67)Gallium scan in 50 patients. Blood 94:3289-3293, 1999.

90. Zinzani PL, Martelli M, Bendandi M, et al: Primary mediastinal large B-cell lymphoma with sclerosis: A clinical study of 89 patients treated with MACOP-B chemotherapy and radiation therapy. Haematologica 86:187-191, 2001.

91. Dabaja BS, Ha CS, Thomas DA, et al: The role of local radiation therapy for mediastinal disease in adults with T-cell lymphoblastic lymphoma. Cancer 94:2738-2744, 2002.

92. Lazzarino M, Orlandi E, Paulli M: Treatment outcome and prognostic factors for primary mediastinal (thymic) B-cell lymphoma: A multicenter study of 106 patients. J Clin Oncol 15:1646-1653, 1997.

93. Coiffier B: Immunochemotherapy: The new standard in aggressive non-Hodgkin's lymphoma in the elderly. Semin Oncol 30:21-27, 2003.

94. Sehn LH, Antin JH, Shulman LN, et al: Primary diffuse large B-cell lymphoma of the mediastinum: Outcome following high-dose chemotherapy and autologous hematopoietic cell transplantation. Blood 91:717-723, 1998.

95. Cairoli R, Grillo G, Tedeschi A, et al: Efficacy of an early intensification treatment integrating chemotherapy, autologous stem cell transplantation and radiotherapy for poor risk primary mediastinal large B cell lymphoma with sclerosis. Bone Marrow Transplant 29:473-477, 2002.

96. Ratei R, Matylis A, Krahl D, et al: Salvage therapy for relapsed mediastinal B-cell lymphoma with allogeneic HLA-identical related donor bone marrow transplantation, donor lymphocyte infusion and IDEC-C2B8. Leuk Lymphoma 40:133-140, 2000.

97. Hill M, Cunningham D, Mac-Vicar D, et al: Role of magnetic resonance imaging in predicting relapse in residual masses after treatment of lymphoma. J Clin Oncol 11:2273, 1993.

98. Weiner M, Leventhal B, Cantor A, et al: Gallium-67 scans as an adjunct to computed tomography scans for the assessment of a residual mediastinal mass in pediatric patients with Hodgkin's disease. Cancer 68:2478-2480, 1991.

99. Weihrauch MR, Re D, Scheidhauer K, et al: Thoracic positron emission tomography using ^{18}F-fluorodeoxyglucose for the evaluation of residual mediastinal Hodgkin disease. Blood 98:2930-2934, 2001.

100. Spaepen K, Stroobants S, Dupont P, et al: Prognostic value of positron emission tomography (PET) with fluorine-18 fluorodeoxyglucose ([^{18}F]FDG) after first-line chemotherapy in non-Hodgkin's lymphoma: Is [18F]FDG-PET a valid alternative to conventional diagnostic methods? J Clin Oncol 19:414-419, 2001.

101. Jerusalem G, Beguin Y, Fassotte MF, et al: Early detection of relapse by whole-body positron emission tomography in the follow-up of patients with Hodgkin's disease. Ann Oncol 14:123-130, 2003.

102. Weinblatt ME, Zanzi I, Belakhlef A, et al: False-positive FDG-PET imaging of the thymus of a child with Hodgkin's disease. J Nucl Med 38:888-890, 1997.

103. Kostakoglu L, Coleman M, Leonard JP, et al: PET predicts prognosis after 1 cycle of chemotherapy in aggressive lymphoma and Hodgkin's disease. J Nucl Med 43:1018-1027, 2002.

104. Kostakoglu L, Goldsmith SJ: ^{18}F-FDG PET evaluation of the response to therapy for lymphoma and for breast, lung, and colorectal carcinoma. J Nucl Med 44:224-239, 2003.

105. Clark OH: Mediastinal parathyroid tumors. Arch Surg 123:1096, 1988.

106. Wang C, Gaz RD, Moncure AC: Mediastinal parathyroid exploration: A clinical and pathologic study of 47 cases. World J Surg 10:687-695, 1986.

107. Hopkins CR, Reading CC: Thyroid and parathyroid imaging. Semin Ultrasound CT MR 16:279-295, 1995.

108. O'Herrin JK, Weigel T, Wilson M, Chen H: Radioguided parathyroidectomy via VATS combined with intraoperative parathyroid hormone testing: The surgical approach of choice for patients with mediastinal parathyroid adenomas? J Bone Miner Res 17:1368-1371, 2002.

109. Chaer R, Massad MG, Evans A, et al: Primary neuroendocrine tumors of the thymus. Ann Thorac Surg 74:1733-1740, 2002.

110. de Perrot M, Spiliopoulos A, Fischer S, et al: Neuroendocrine carcinoma (carcinoid) of the thymus associated with Cushing's syndrome. Ann Thorac Surg 73:675-681, 2002.

111. Klemm KM, Moran CA: Primary neuroendocrine carcinomas of the thymus. Semin Diagn Pathol 16:32-41, 1999.

112. Moran CA, Suster S: Neuroendocrine carcinomas (carcinoid tumor) of the thymus: A clinicopathologic analysis of 80 cases. Am J Clin Pathol 114:100-110, 2000.

113. Kumar P, Judson I, Nicholson AG, Ladas G: Mediastinal hemangioma: Successful treatment by alpha-2a interferon and postchemotherapy resection. J Thorac Cardiovasc Surg 124:404-406, 2002.

114. Bolaman Z, Polatli M, Cildag O, et al: Intrathoracic extramedullary hematopoiesis resembling posterior mediastinal tumor. Am J Med 112:739-741, 2002.

115. Castleman B, Iverson L, Menendez VP: Localized mediastinal lymphoid hyperplasia resembling thymoma. Cancer 9:822, 1956.

116. Day JRS, Bew D, Ali M, et al: Castleman's disease associated with myasthenia gravis. Ann Thorac Surg 75:1648-1650, 2003.

117. Cesarman E: The role of Kaposi's sarcoma–associated herpesvirus (KSHV/HHV-8) in lymphoproliferative diseases. Recent Results Cancer Res 159:27-37, 2002.

118. Nishimoto N, Sasai M, Shima Y, et al: Improvement in Castleman's disease by humanized anti-interleukin-6 receptor antibody therapy. Blood 95:56-61, 2000.

119. Rahman AM, Farahat IG, Ali WA, Mansour KA: Giant mediastinal chordoma. Ann Thorac Surg 73:1952-1954, 2002.

120. Iwasaki A, Hiratsuka M, Kawahara K, Shirakusa T: New technique for the cystic mediastinal tumor by video-assisted thoracoscopy. Ann Thorac Surg 72:632-633, 2001.

CHAPTER 57

LUNG (INCLUDING PULMONARY EMBOLISM AND THORACIC OUTLET SYNDROME)

Joe B. Putnam, Jr., M.D.

ANATOMY

The development of the respiratory system begins at 21 to 28 days' gestation as a ventral groove in the foregut. The bronchial tree is complete at approximately 16 weeks of gestation, and the lungs have subdivided into 15 to 26 divisions. The alveoli are lined by cuboidal cells to about the fourth month. These cells become flattened and capillary buds develop at 4 to 6 months. The true alveolar stage, with air sacs surrounded on all sides by capillaries, develops from approximately 7 months' (26 to 28 weeks') gestation to term. Alveolar proliferation continues to occur after birth. There are approximately 20 million alveoli at birth, which increase to approximately 300 million by age 10 years with no more increase after that time. Eighty percent of the lung volume is air, 10% of the lung volume is blood, and approximately 10% of the lung volume is solid tissue.

The alveolar-capillary membrane consists of approximately five layers: the alveolar epithelium, the basement membrane, ground substance, basal membrane, and capillary endothelium. The pores of Kohn perforate and connect the alveoli, although it is unknown whether they can actually serve for collateral ventilation. Twenty-three generations of bronchi occur between the trachea and terminal alveoli. Alveoli make up approximately 50% of the entire lung volume. The ciliated tall columnar epithelium, as a single layer, lines the larger airways. These cells maintain a cuboidal shape in bronchioles and are flattened, thinned epithelial cells in alveoli.

The interstitium is a narrow space between basement membrane of capillary endothelium and alveolar epithelium where gas exchange takes place in alveoli. The space is wider in submucosa, muscle, and cartilage in larger airways.

The alveoli are composed of type I and type II cells in approximately equal number. However, type I cells constitute approximately 40% of the number of cells lining the alveoli but cover more than 90% percent of the alveolar lining and are for gas exchange. Type II alveolar cells are the granular pneumocyte with lipid inclusion bodies and manufacture surfactant, a lipoprotein (idpalmitoyl-lecithin), which decreases surface tension. This substance maintains alveolar stability and fluid balance, preventing atelectasis and edema. Capillary endothelial cells have a nonspecific response to lung injury with edema, hyaline membrane formation, cellular infiltrates, and granuloma formation. Chronically, this process of lung injury is marked by diffuse fibrosis and honeycombing.

The bony thorax consists of 12 ribs. The 11th and 12th ribs are "floating" ribs and are not attached directly to the sternum. Ribs 1 to 5 are directly attached to the sternum by costal cartilages. The lower ribs (6 to 10) coalesce by way of the costal cartilages into the costal arch. The first rib is flat and travels from the first thoracic vertebra to the manubrium at the manubrium-clavicular junction. Through this relatively small area pass the great vessels, trachea, esophagus, and nerves. The remaining ribs gradually slope downward. The intercostal muscle layers assist with respiration and protect the thoracic structures. The extrinsic muscles of the chest, the latissimus dorsi muscle, the serratus anterior muscle, the pectoralis major and minor muscles, and the cervical muscles (sternocleidomastoid, scalene muscles) attach to the bony thorax and protect the chest wall itself.

The right lung is composed of three lobes: the upper, middle, and lower. Two fissures separate these lobes. The major, or oblique, fissure separates the lower lobe from the upper and middle lobes. The minor or horizontal fissure separates the upper lobe from the middle lobe. The left lung has two lobes—the upper lobe and the lower lobe; the lingula is a portion of the left upper lobe and corresponds embryologically to the right middle lobe. A single oblique fissure separates the lobes (Fig. 57-1).

The bronchopulmonary segments are divisions of each lobe that contain anatomically separate arterial, venous, and bronchial supply. There are 10 bronchopulmonary segments on the right and 8 bronchopulmonary segments on the left (Fig. 57-2).

The blood supply of the lung is twofold. Unoxygenated blood is pumped to the lung from the right ventricle by way of the pulmonary artery. After oxygenation in the lung, the blood is returned to the left atrium by way of the pulmonary veins. Blood supply to the bronchi is from the systemic circulation by bronchial arteries arising from the aorta.

Lymphatic vessels are present throughout the parenchyma and gradually coalesce toward the hilar areas of the lungs. Generally, lymphatic drainage from the lung affects the ipsilateral lymph nodes; however, flow of lymph from the left lower lobe may drain to the right mediastinal lymph nodes. Lymphatic drainage within the mediastinum moves cephalad. The pulmonary parenchyma does not contain a nerve supply; however, the parietal pleura has rich nerve endings. Generous local anesthesia is therefore necessary for chest tube insertion.

Anatomic variations within the lung usually cause no clinical difficulty. The azygous lobe can be identified on approximately 0.5% of routine chest radiographs. In this normal variant the azygous vein lies within the substance of the right lung. Because of the position of the azygous vein, the development of the right upper lobe continues around the azygous vein in an inferior to superior direction. The lung develops a double fold of visceral pleura associated with the azygous lobe that can be identified on a chest radiograph. A "reverse comma sign" is evident on chest radiography. The azygous lobe is not a true anatomic lobe, in that it does not have a separate segmental bronchus, although it may be involved by tuberculosis, cancer, or pulmonary metastasis, without involving the other portions of the lung.

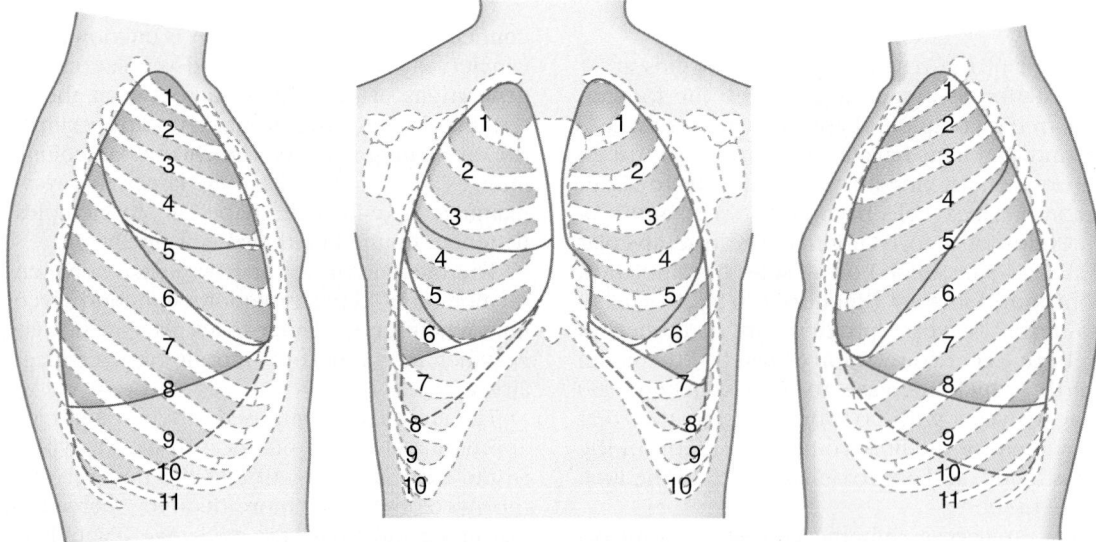

■ **FIGURE 57-1.** The relationships of the pleural reflections and the lobes of the lung to the ribs. The topographic anatomy and the relationship of the fissures of the lobes to ribs in inspiration and expiration are important in evaluation of the routine posteroanterior and lateral chest film.

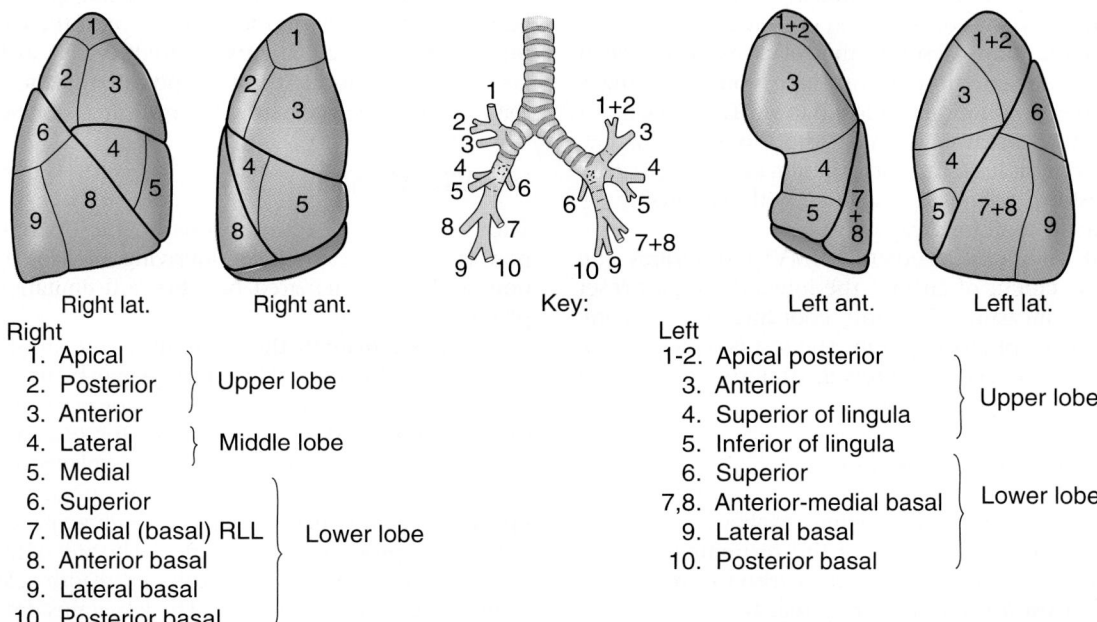

Right lat.   **Right ant.**   **Key:**   **Left ant.**   **Left lat.**

Right
1. Apical ⎫
2. Posterior ⎬ Upper lobe
3. Anterior ⎭
4. Lateral ⎫ Middle lobe
5. Medial ⎭
6. Superior ⎫
7. Medial (basal) RLL ⎬ Lower lobe
8. Anterior basal ⎪
9. Lateral basal ⎪
10. Posterior basal ⎭

Left
1-2. Apical posterior ⎫
3. Anterior ⎬ Upper lobe
4. Superior of lingula ⎪
5. Inferior of lingula ⎭
6. Superior ⎫
7,8. Anterior-medial basal ⎬ Lower lobe
9. Lateral basal ⎪
10. Posterior basal ⎭

■ FIGURE 57-2.   Segments of the pulmonary lobes. (Modified from Jackson CL, Huber JF: Correlated applied anatomy of the bronchial tree and lungs with a system of nomenclature. Dis Chest 9:319, 1943.)

PULMONARY FUNCTION TESTS AND CARDIOPULMONARY EXERCISE TESTING

Before pulmonary resection, patients are evaluated by a combination of spirometry and pulmonary function tests (Fig. 57-3).[1,2] Each of these tests measures a specific component of the patient's pulmonary function and, in some cases, measures the combined function of both the heart and the lungs. Pulmonary function testing measures the lung volumes and mechanical properties of lung elasticity, recoil, and compliance. It also evaluates gas exchange functions. Occasionally, this combined measurement of the cardiorespiratory axis serves as a more appropriate study to assess the patient's physiologic reserve.[3,4] Elevated PCO_2 is also associated with increased risk. A PCO_2 greater than 43 to 45 mm Hg suggests severe disease with nearly a 50% functional loss of the lung.

The predicted postoperative forced expiratory volume in 1 second (FEV_1) is the most common and important predictor of postoperative pulmonary reserve. Typically, this should be greater than 0.8 L. FEV_1 may be expressed as an actual value, such as 0.9 L/sec, or as a percentage, such as 68% of that predicted. The predicted value is based on height and weight in normal patients. In addition, FEV_1 of less than 0.8 L/min suggests an increased risk of postoperative pulmonary morbidity. Patients with an FEV_1 of less than 0.5 liter have the greatest risk of postoperative pulmonary complications.

The forced expiratory volume in one second to vital capacity ratio (FEV_1/FVC) describes the relationship between the FEV_1 and the total lung volume. In obstructive disease, the ratio is low (FEV_1 is low and the FVC is high); in restrictive disease, the ratio is about normal because both FEV_1 and FVC are reduced. For patients with marginal pulmonary function, a quantitative xenon ventilation-perfusion lung scan should be performed to evaluate the impact of the planned extent of resection on the specific lobe or lung to be resected and to estimate the remaining pulmonary reserve. Other techniques of evaluating the patients for pulmonary reserve include obtaining maximal ventilatory volume, stair-climbing two flights

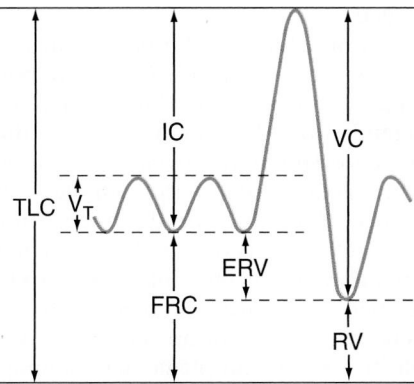

■ FIGURE 57-3.   Spirometry. Subdivisions of lung volumes. ERV, expiratory reserve volume; FRC, functional residual capacity, that is, lung volume at end-expiration; IC, inspiratory capacity; RV, residual volume, that is, lung volume after forced expiration from FRC; TLC, total lung capacity; VC, vital capacity, that is, the maximal volume of gas inspired from RV; VT, tidal volume.

or greater, carbon monoxide diffusing capacity (DLCO), and maximal oxygen consumption (V_{O_2} max).

Flow-volume loops describe the relationship between lung volume and air flow as the lung volume changes during a forced expiration and inspiration. The typical test consists of tidal breathing at rest, then maximal inspiratory effort to total lung capacity, then maximal expiratory effort to residual volume, concluding with maximal inspiratory effort to total lung capacity.

Maximal voluntary ventilation (MVV) describes the maximal movement of air into the lungs during a preset interval. MVV measures the effort, coordination, and compliance of the respiratory system. The test is typically conducted over a 12-second interval, and the results are expressed in liters per minute.

CARDIOPULMONARY EXERCISE TESTING

Cardiopulmonary exercise testing evaluates the cardiopulmonary axis, the ability of the respiratory system to take up oxygen in exchange for carbon dioxide, and the ability of the cardiovascular system to transport this oxygen to the tissues. The body's ability to accomplish this task at rest and when stressed with exercise can be measured by DLCO, and V_{O_2} max.

DLCO can be measured by several methods, although the single breath test is most commonly performed. Variability in the DLCO may be as much as 12% or greater. The DLCO measures the rate at which test molecules such as carbon monoxide move from the alveolar space to combine with hemoglobin in the red blood cells. The DLCO is determined by calculating the difference between inspired and expired samples of gas. DLCO levels less than 50% are associated with increased perioperative risk.[5]

V_{O_2} max can also be measured. Physiologic limits to the elevation in cardiac output depend on cardiac reserve and oxygen extraction. Typically, additional work is accompanied by an elevation in oxygen extraction. At some point, a plateau in the oxygen extraction is identified. Low values of V_{O_2} max (<15 mL/min/kg) are associated with increased risk of surgical morbidity and mortality.[6,7]

The quantitative xenon-133 ventilation-perfusion lung scan is used to evaluate lung function and to predict postoperative pulmonary function after pulmonary resection. Tumors that compress the pulmonary artery may cause decreased perfusion to that lung. Tumors that impair ventilation by partial or complete obstruction of the bronchus have a corresponding reduction in ventilation values. The surgeon can calculate or predict the postoperative FEV_1 by multiplying the preoperative value of the noninvolved lung by the percentage of activity within the noninvolved lung (Fig. 57-4).

Some thoracic surgeons have advocated stair-climbing as a suitable measure of preoperative cardiopulmonary assessment.[8] If the patient can walk up one flight of stairs, a wedge resection should be appropriate. If the patient can walk up two flights of stairs, a lobectomy is appropriate; and if three flights of stairs can be achieved, a pneumonectomy is done. The surgeon subjectively assesses breathlessness. This subjective evaluation is difficult to quantitate. In patients undergoing evaluation for lung volume reduction surgery or for lung transplantation, a 6-minute walk test is used for a measure of the cardiac and pulmonary reserve. Patients are told to walk as far and as fast as they can during this time period. Distances of more than 1000 feet suggest an uncomplicated course.

THORACIC INCISIONS

The choice of incision depends on the operation to be performed, the patient's underlying physiologic condition, and the anticipated benefits and limitations of the planned approach.[9-11]

The posterolateral thoracotomy is the most frequent thoracic incision used. This incision may be used for operations on a single thorax, for pulmonary resection, for esophageal surgery or resection, or for resection of portions of the chest wall. The patient is placed in a lateral decubitus position with the side to be operated on placed up. An incision is made obliquely from a space between the spinous processes and the medial border of the scapula inferiorly to approximately one fingerbreadth below and in front of the tip of the scapula. The latissimus dorsi muscle may be divided; however, many surgeons prefer to spare this muscle and mobilize its lateral and inferior edge to facilitate additional exposure. The serratus anterior muscle is typically not divided but is simply mobilized along its lateral border. The chest is entered through the fifth intercostal space (the interspace just above the sixth rib) by dividing the intercostal muscles. The posterior portion of the sixth rib is often divided to facilitate exposure and to minimize the risk of breaking the rib. A thoracic epidural catheter is used to minimize postoperative pain.

The axillary thoracotomy may be created in two ways. A small transverse incision 3 to 4 cm underneath the axillary hairline (bordered posteriorly by the latissimus dorsi muscle and anteriorly by the pectoralis major muscle) is made. The chest is entered through the fourth intercostal space. Another technique creates a vertical incision extending from just below the axillary hair to just above the costal arch. The latissimus dorsi muscle is mobilized posteriorly, and the chest is entered through the fifth intercostal space. The serratus anterior muscle is mobilized as needed.

The anterior or anterolateral thoracotomy is created by a curvilinear incision underneath the inferior border of the pectoralis major muscle at the inframammary fold. The incision extends from 2 to 3 cm medial to the sternum and then extends superiorly toward the anterior axillary line. The chest is then entered through the fourth or fifth intercostal space depending on the operation to be performed. The pectoralis major muscle may be mobilized to assist in obtaining the selected interspace. This approach is good for open lung biopsies in that all lobes of the lung can be reached; however, the apex of the upper lobe may be difficult to reach. Supplemental techniques using video-assisted devices may be considered in addition to, or as an alternative to, open techniques.

A median sternotomy is performed using a vertical incision from the sternal notch to the xiphoid. A sternal saw is then used to divide the sternum in the midline. With gentle retraction, the sternum can be spread 4 or 5 inches

Section of Pulmonary Medicine
Pulmonary Function Report

Last Name: First Name:
Identification:
Age: 56 years   Room: Out-patient
Sex: male   Race: Caucasian
Height: 65 inches   Physician:
Weight: 177 lbs   Operator:
Date
Time

Spirometry		Pred	Pre BD	%Pred	Post BD	%Pred	%Chg
FVC	[l]	3.48	3.07	88	3.07	88	0
FEV$_1$	[l]	2.83	2.23	79	2.26	80	1
FEV$_1$/VC	[%]	80.81	72.26	89	69.78	86	−3
FEF 25–75	[l/s]	3.01	1.37	45	1.46	49	7
PEF	[l/s]	7.57	6.43	85	7.10	94	10
FIVC	[l]	3.48	3.09	89	3.24	93	5
FIV$_1$	[l]		3.09		3.24		5
FIV$_1$/FVC	[%]		100.00		100.00		0

Lung Volumes		Pred	Measured	%Pred
SVC	[l]	3.48	3.04	87
TLC	[l]	5.51	5.54	101
RV	[l]	1.96	2.49	127
RV/TLC	[%]	35.9	45.0	125
FRC-Box	[l]	2.24	3.01	134

Diffusion SB		Pred	Measured	%Pred
D$_{LCO}$ SB	[ml/min/mm Hg]	22.59	23.81	105
D$_{LCO}$ Hb Corr	[ml/min/mm Hg]	22.6	24.2	107
VA	[l]		5.27	
D$_{LCO}$/VA	[ml/min/mm Hg/l]	3.93	4.52	115
Hb	[g/100ml]		14.1	

Interpretation

Spirometry reveals an isolated reduction in mid-expiratory flows consistent with an obstructive small airways defect. Increased residual volume (RV) is consistent with air trapping. Following the inhalation of a bronchodilator, there is no improvement of the obstructive airway defect. The diffusing capacity is normal.

A

FIGURE 57-4. Pulmonary function report. **A,** The pulmonary function report provides complete spirometry data based on predicted values for height and weight. In this patient, the forced expiratory volume in 1 second (FEV$_1$) is 2.26 L after bronchodilators, which is 80% of predicted. The carbon monoxide diffusing capacity (DL$_{CO}$) is measured as 23.81 mL/min/mm Hg, which is 105% of predicted. FEF, forced expiratory flow; FIV$_1$, forced inspiratory volume in 1 second; FIVC, forced inspiratory vital capacity; FRC, functional reserve capacity; FVC, forced vital capacity; Hb, hemoglobin; PEF, peak expiratory flow; SB, single breath; SVC, slow vital capacity; TLC, total lung capacity; VA, alveolar volume; VC, vital capacity.

Figure continued on next page

to allow access to both the right and left thorax. The pleura is opened in its anteromedial aspect. This approach is used for operations on the anterior mediastinum, for bilateral pulmonary metastasis, or when both lungs need to be explored or inspected. The sternum is closed with stainless steel wire.

The thoracoabdominal incision is infrequently used for pulmonary operations although it provides access to both the thorax and abdomen and lower chest. This incision is most frequently used for operations on the thoracic and upper abdominal aorta. Because of the division of the costal arch, the incision may be more painful than others that do not divide the costal arch.

The transverse sternotomy or "clamshell" incision is performed as an alternative to median sternotomy. This incision is larger and combines two anterior thoracotomy incisions with transverse division of the sternum at the fourth intercostal space. Both internal

Patient Name:

Patient Number:

Date of Test:

REGIONAL PULMONARY FUNCTION STUDY (XENON-133)

Referring Physician: Patient's Age: 56 yrs Sex: Male   Height: 65 inches Weight: 177 lb

(Distribution of Volume, Ventilation and Perfusion expressed in %)

VOLUME, %

Right			Left
4	1	1	5
23	2	2	6
26	3	3	8
24	4	4	4
77			23

VENTILATION, %

Right			Left
3	1	1	4
23	2	2	4
29	3	3	6
29	4	4	2
84			16

PERFUSION, %

Right			Left
4	1	1	5
20	2	2	4
29	3	3	6
31	4	4	1
84			16

V̇/Q̇ INDICES

Right			Left
0.8	1	1	0.8
1.1	2	2	1.0
1.0	3	3	1.0
0.9	4	4	2.0

VENTILATORY CLEARANCE (T1/2 in seconds)

VENT GAS

Right			Left
17	1	1	99
11	2	2	99
11	3	3	99
9	4	4	26

PERFUSED GAS

Right			Left
19	1	1	218
16	2	2	21
20	3	3	16
12	4	4	20

INTERPRETATION:

There is severe, generalized hypoventilation and hypoperfusion throughout the left lung. Apical reduction in ventilation and perfusion is also noted on the right lung. The left lung contributes to approximately 16% of overall ventilation and 16% of overall perfusion. Estimated post left pneumonectomy FEV$_1$ = 52 (1.5 L) If indicated, resection of up to a left pneumonectomy should be functionally tolerated.

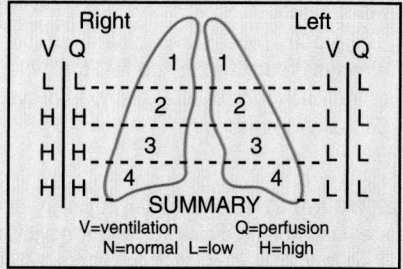

Right				Left	
V	Q			V	Q
L	L	1	1	L	L
H	H	2	2	L	L
H	H	3	3	L	L
H	H	4	4	L	L

SUMMARY

V=ventilation   Q=perfusion
N=normal L=low   H=high

Post BD FEV$_1$: 62% Pred   1.76 Liters

Involved lung: Left

B

■ **FIGURE 57-4.**—*Cont'd.*   **B,** The quantitative xenon ventilation-perfusion lung scan report provides the lung volume, the ventilation, and the perfusion to each lung. In this patient with a large hilar tumor, both ventilation and perfusion are reduced in the involved left lung compared with the uninvolved right lung. The predicted post–left pneumonectomy right lung function can be obtained by multiplying the right lung percent perfusion (84%) by the observed best FEV$_1$ (2.26 L). The resulting value, 1.9 L as a post–left pneumonectomy FEV$_1$, suggests that a left pneumonectomy would be functionally well tolerated.

mammary arteries require ligation. The pectoralis major muscles of both sides generally need to be mobilized to access the appropriate (fourth) interspace. This approach is ideal for accessing both the right and the left hilum, as well as providing additional exposure for large mediastinal tumors, bilateral hilar dissections, lung transplant surgery, or posterior-based metastases in both lungs.

Video-assisted thoracoscopic surgery (VATS) or other minimally invasive techniques have been developed to treat some benign pulmonary conditions such as pneumothorax, to perform open lung biopsy, and to facilitate diagnosis and staging of thoracic malignancies.[12-14] The use of VATS for treatment of thoracic malignancies is being investigated. Although the use of minimally invasive techniques does minimize surgical trauma from the incisions, the individual surgeon must ensure that fundamentals of the operation are not compromised by such a limited approach, particularly for patients with known or suspected thoracic neoplasms. VATS is performed with the patient under general anesthesia with a double-lumen endotracheal tube, typically with the patient in a lateral decubitus position. A 1-cm incision is made over the central thorax, the muscles are gently spread, a trochar is inserted, and the thorax is entered. The thoracoscope is then introduced. One or more additional incisions are made to facilitate manipulation of the lung or other thoracic structures. The advantage of this approach is the limited surgical trauma that occurs compared with lateral thoracotomy. However, the surgeon is limited by visualization in two dimensions. Tactile feedback is limited, although studies are ongoing to improve tactile sensory feedback.

PERIOPERATIVE RISK

Certain comorbidities are associated with increased pulmonary risk, including smoking, poor overall health, increasing age, poorer pulmonary function or chronic obstructive pulmonary disease (COPD), asthma, and obesity. Optimization of medical care for these problems should be coordinated with planned pulmonary resection.[3,4,15,16]

Preoperative preparation begins with the first visit. If the patient is a smoker, he or she should stop smoking immediately! If possible, patients should be smoke free for a minimum of 2 weeks and preferably for 4 to 8 weeks before surgery. Smoking cessation programs and nicotine patches may be helpful in these patients. Smoking is an addiction and should be treated as such. Patients with COPD or asthma should be medically optimized with bronchodilators for their pulmonary function before surgery. Obstructive pneumonia typically clears with antibiotic treatment of 7 to 10 days. Occasionally, patients require intravenous antibiotics to clear infection before pulmonary resection. Corticosteroids may be required in some patients. Patients are taught to use incentive spirometry before surgery. The device is given to the patient for practice at home before surgery and is brought to the hospital for postoperative lung expansion. Patients are also educated as to the rationale for their surgery and what to expect during their convalescence. Before surgery and during the perioperative period, deep venous thrombosis prophylaxis is provided by subcutaneous heparin or by sequential compression stocks. As well, perioperative antibiotics are used to minimize complications from infections.

Postoperative morbidity may also be minimized by adequate pain control with intravenous analgesics, usually patient-controlled analgesia (PCA), or by use of the thoracic epidural catheter. Some surgeons have successfully used intercostal nerve blocks after thoracotomy for postoperative pain relief. Pulmonary exercises to expand the lungs are performed by all patients after pulmonary resection. Incentive spirometry assists in expanding the lung and reducing the incidence of pulmonary morbidities. Postoperative positive airway pressure may be used effectively in some patients. Nasal bilevel positive airway pressure may delay or eliminate the need for intubation or reintubation after pulmonary resection.

CONGENITAL LESIONS OF THE LUNG, TRACHEA, AND BRONCHI

Various congenital lung abnormalities can occur.[17,18] Bilateral agenesis of the lungs is fatal. Unilateral agenesis may occur more frequently on the left than on the right (approximately 70/30), with more than a 2:1 male-to-female ratio. Fifty percent of cases are isolated and compatible with life; however, 50% are associated with other abnormalities. The chest radiograph may demonstrate a small lucency on the involved side with a mediastinal shift. Isolated lobar agenesis is rare.

Hypoplasia of the lungs may occur as a result of interference with the development of the alveolar system during the last 2 months of gestation. This problem is seen in conjunction with lesions that compete with the lung for space in the pleural cavity. When this occurs, the number of branches in the airway decrease as does the lining of the airways with cuboidal cells. Bochdalek hernia is the most frequent cause of hypoplasia. Reversal of this condition in utero is being investigated.

Conditions associated with hypoplasia of the lungs include oligohydramnios, prune-belly syndrome (deficiency in the abdominal musculature, genitourinary abnormalities), scimitar syndrome (abnormal pulmonary vein draining into the inferior vena cava, demonstrated as a crescent along the right heart border on cardiac angiography), and dextrocardia. Isolated pulmonary hypoplasia is rare.

Hyaline membrane disease (or infant respiratory distress syndrome) is frequent in premature infants (24 to 28 weeks' gestation) and infants of diabetic mothers. At that gestation, the infants have an immature surfactant system. Hyaline membrane disease develops in the alveoli, causing congestion and a grossly deep purple–appearing lung. Respiratory distress frequently ensues, requiring high concentrations of oxygen. The chest radiographs demonstrate a ground-glass appearance from the interstitial edema. As needs for oxygen and ventilator pressure increase to counteract this interstitial edema, pneumothorax frequently occurs. Ten to 30 percent of these infants do not survive.

Congenital cystic lesions generally occur secondary to separation of the pulmonary remnants from airway branchings. Diffuse cystic disease is a rare male-predominant (2:1) abnormality. This disease may usually involve one lobe or a portion of a lobe. Occasionally, the condition may be more generalized and consist of innumerable small cystic cavities lined with ciliated epithelium and containing clear mucus. The distribution within each of the lobes is approximately equal. Clinically, approximately one third of patients are without symptoms; one third have cough; and one third have infection or, rarely, hemoptysis. Treatment may be with antibiotics or, for more severe localized cases, with resection.

The differential diagnosis of cystic disease in the lung may be challenging. Various categories should be considered. Cystic fibrosis is an autosomal recessive disorder that is found in white Americans. Approximately 20% of patients with cystic fibrosis survive to the age of 30 years. Lung failure is the most frequent cause of death in most patients. Excessively thick mucus leads to inspissation, recurrent infections, bronchitis, and bronchiectasis. Pneumothorax secondary to air trapping is also found. Fibrosis and cystic changes on pathologic examinations are identified.

Tension cyst may be a complication of cystic disease. A rapid increase in the size of the cyst may yield to mechanical ventilation problems as well as mediastinal shift. Resection, usually lobectomy, corrects this problem.

Pneumatoceles may develop as a result of childhood *Staphylococcus aureus* infection. They can be very large and may cause mechanical complications. These problems may resolve completely as the pneumonia resolves.

Congenital cystic adenomatoid malformations are closely related to a hamartoma without cartilage. Terminal bronchioles proliferate, yielding the "adenomatoid" malformation. The lung has the appearance of Swiss cheese and feels like a large rubbery mass. With air trapping and overdistention, respiratory distress may occur, which is optimally relieved by lobectomy.

Lobar emphysema frequently occurs as a congenital or infantile process. It rarely occurs after 6 months of age. Fifty percent of patients do not have an obvious cause. Twenty-five percent of patients have bronchial cartilage dysplasia, and 25% are thought to be secondary to a variety of causes, such as bronchial atresia, mucosal valves, bronchostenosis, enlarged lymph nodes, and abnormal vessels. Bronchiolitis is probably the most common cause overall. The onset of rapidly progressive respiratory distress usually occurs from 4 to 5 days to several weeks after birth. Treatment is lobectomy.

Pulmonary sequestration occurs most commonly in the lower lobes (L > R) and within an area of embryonic lung tissue that has its blood supply from an anomalous systemic artery. This condition occurs secondary to an accessory lung bud caudad to the normal lung, but with a lack of absorption of primitive surrounding splanchnic vessels. During lung development, interlobar sequestration (75%) occurs early. Later, after the pleura forms, extralobar sequestration occurs (25%). The blood supply is from the systemic artery to the pulmonary vein (intralobar) or to the systemic veins (extralobar). Ninety-five percent of the systemic blood supply to the pulmonary sequestration comes from the thoracic aorta.

Kartagener's syndrome, an autosomal recessive condition, consists of sinusitis, bronchiectasis, and situs inversus. Dyskinetic cilia are a hallmark sign of this syndrome and affect both sperm and respiratory epithelium. Because of these dyskinetic cilia, bronchiectasis occurs in 20% to 25% of patients; however, with good medical supervision, these patients may live a full life span.

CONGENITAL ABNORMALITIES OF THE TRACHEA AND BRONCHI

Esophageal atresia with tracheal-esophageal fistula is the most frequent abnormality of the trachea in infants. This topic is discussed under pediatric surgery.

Bronchial atresia is the second most frequent congenital pulmonary lesion after tracheal-esophageal fistula. The lung tissue distal to the atresia expands and becomes emphysematous as a result of air entry through the pores of Kohn. With no exit for air or mucus because of this blind bronchial stump, emphysema from air trapping or development of a mucocele may occur. The chest radiographs may demonstrate hyperinflation of a lobe or a segment. The oval density may be identified between the hyperinflated lung and the hilum. The left upper lobe is the most frequently involved of all lobes within the lung. Diagnosis may be confirmed with bronchography or computed tomography (CT). The surgeon must rule out a mucous plug, adenoma, vascular compression, or sequestration.

Tracheal agenesis is a rare phenomenon and is fatal. The trachea is absent from the larynx to the carina, and bronchi communicate with the esophagus.

Tracheal stenosis is also rare and consists of generalized hypoplasia, a funnel-like trachea, and bronchial and segmental malformations. The right upper lobe bronchus may come from the trachea directly and may be associated with an aberrant left pulmonary artery ("pulmonary artery sling"). Completely circular vascular rings are common. Repair is by incision of the trachea vertically and widening of the tracheal lumen.

Tracheomalacia can be identified by bronchoscopy. The surgeon will notice marked variation of the tracheal lumen with inspiration and expiration. The tracheal rings are ineffective in maintaining the lumen of the trachea; and with negative intrathoracic pressure, the trachea collapses. With the positive pressure exerted by exhalation, the trachea expands. Respiratory difficulty ensues from the intermittently collapsing trachea. Stent placement in adults or primary repair is required.

CONGENITAL BRONCHOPULMONARY MALFORMATIONS

Various congenital bronchopulmonary malformations include pulmonary sequestration, bronchogenic cysts, congenital lobar emphysema, and congenital cystic adenomatoid malformation. Lobectomy is commonly required. Any thoracic cystic lesion that is enlarging on serial radiographs should be considered for resection. Asymptomatic cystic lesions may eventually produce compression of lung parenchyma, infection, or malignant degeneration.[19,20]

A bronchogenic cyst arises from a tracheal or bronchial diverticulum.[21,22] This diverticulum becomes completely separated from the trachea and is frequently found as an asymptomatic mass on routine chest radiographs. CT of the chest demonstrates this abnormality as a homogeneous-type mass, well circumscribed, and adjacent to the trachea (Fig. 57-5).

The bronchogenic cyst accounts for 10% of mediastinal masses in children and is located in the mid-medi-

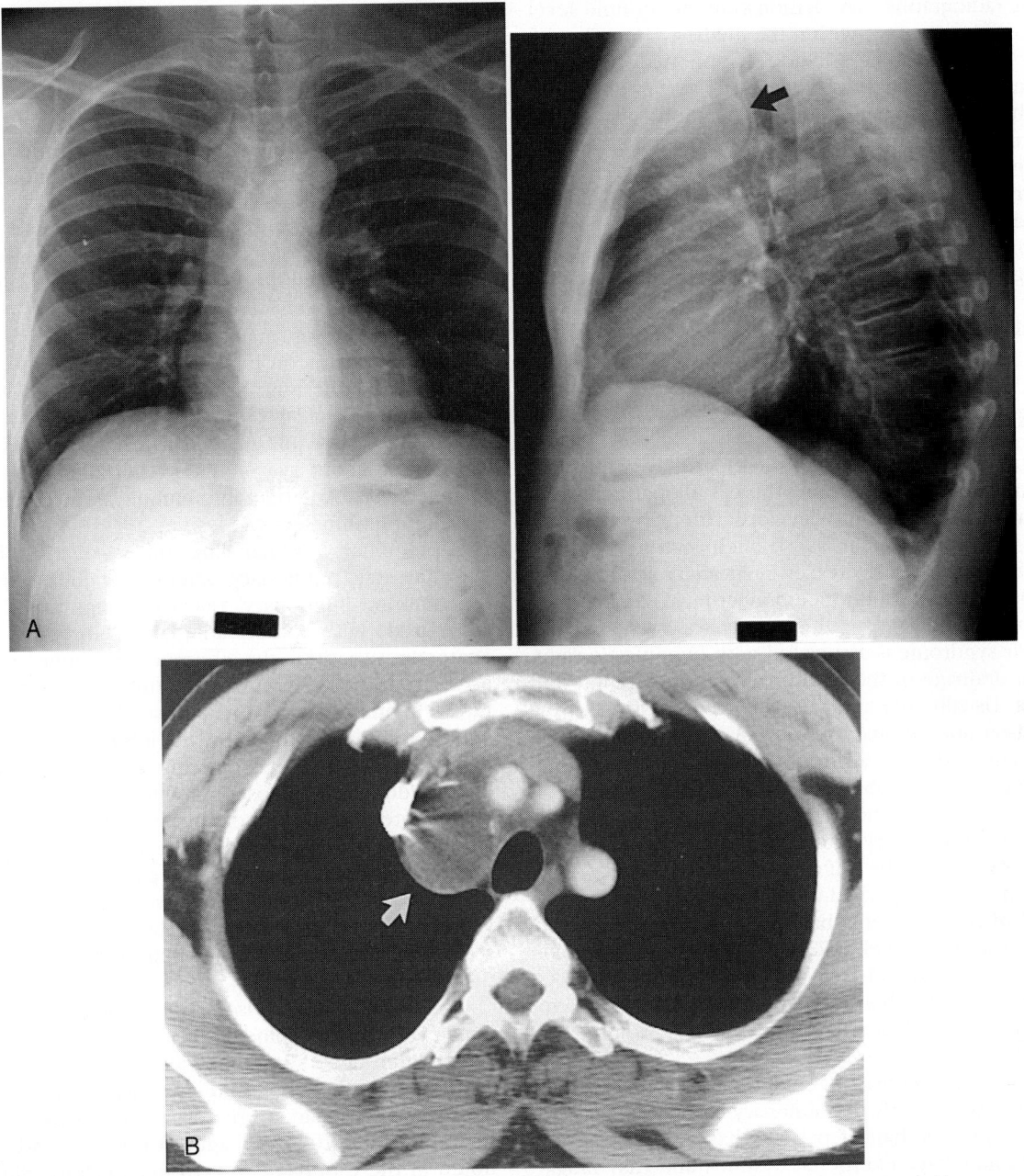

FIGURE 57-5. Two chest roentgenograms (**A**) and a computed tomogram of the chest (**B**) of a patient with a bronchogenic cyst (*arrow*).

astinum. The bronchogenic cyst arises from nests of cells that become isolated from the primitive lung bud. They are usually found in close association with the major bronchi or trachea but are not usually connected. The cyst may be adjacent to or involving the esophagus, or it may be located within the pulmonary substance. It is typically 2 to 10 cm in size, and the fluid is usually clear, although it may be cloudy. The wall of the system is of variable thickness and composed of fibrous tissue. This cyst wall may also have muscle-elastin cartilage in its composition. The inner lining usually consists of pseudostratified ciliated columnar epithelium. It may also have squamous or gastric mucosa, and it may or may not have a bronchial

communication. Usually a bronchial or tracheal communication cannot be identified.

Clinically, the bronchogenic cyst occurs more frequently within the right mediastinum and is more frequent in men. Where there is no bronchial communication, the bronchogenic cyst typically is without symptoms, although tracheal compression, pain, and secondary infection may exist. The chest radiograph may identify a circle or ovoid density in proximity to a major air passage, or it may be noted simply as a mediastinal mass. With bronchial communication, the bronchogenic cyst is almost always asymptomatic. Cough, fever, sputum production, or hemoptysis may occur. If a connection occurs, the chest radiographs may demonstrate an air-fluid level within a cystic structure within the mediastinum. The differential diagnosis may include lymphoma, teratoma, hamartoma, granuloma, and saccular aortic aneurysm (although these frequently have calcification).

Treatment consists of excision, even if the patient is asymptomatic, to confirm the diagnosis. Care is needed to protect the phrenic nerve, the superior vena cava, and the esophagus during the dissection because some fibrosis may be present from chronic inflammation. Typically, the bronchogenic cyst is simply enucleated from the mediastinum. If attached to a bronchus by a stalk, this stalk must be ligated.

CONGENITAL VASCULAR DISORDERS

Congenital vascular disorders of the lungs may occur.[23] In Swyer-James-Macleod syndrome, there is idiopathic hyperlucent lung. This problem develops from chronic pulmonary infections such as bronchiectasis. As the consolidation persists, decreased pulmonary artery blood supply may cause an "autopneumonectomy" and a hyperlucent lung.

Scimitar syndrome is associated with hypoplastic right lung with drainage of the pulmonary vein to the inferior vena cava. Usually, the anomaly is corrected using extracorporeal cardiopulmonary support. A patch from the pulmonary vein to the left atrium by way of an atrial septal defect corrects this problem.

Pulmonary arteriovenous malformations may exist as one or more pulmonary artery to pulmonary vein connections, bypassing the pulmonary capillary bed. This connection results in a right-to-left shunt. Approximately one third of these patients have hereditary hemorrhagic telangiectasia (Osler-Weber-Rendu syndrome). Approximately 50% are small (<1 cm) and tend to be multiple. As well, 50% are greater than 1 cm and usually less than 5 cm and tend to be subpleural. Local resection is required for these.

Clinical features consist of small arteriovenous malformations (shunting < 25% of pulmonary blood flow). There is no true cyanosis; half of patients have no symptoms, and others may have exertional dyspnea and easy fatigability. Larger arteriovenous malformations (which may shunt > 25% of pulmonary blood flow) may present as cyanosis, dyspnea, and fatigability. The onset is frequently in adolescence or adulthood. With severe shunting, cyanosis, and clubbing, polycythemia (found in 20% overall) may occur. The differential diagnosis includes primary pulmonary hypertension, right-to-left cardiac shunts, or methemoglobinemia. Complications include pneumothorax, hemoptysis, cerebral thrombosis, or brain abscess. Cardiac output is not increased because resistance of the arteriovenous malformation is equivalent to the pulmonary vascular resistance; therefore, no congestive heart failure or cardiac enlargement occurs. There is a continuous bruit present in approximately half of the patients with cyanosis. The chest radiograph may demonstrate a lobulated density frequently with larger lesions. On fluoroscopy, pulsations may be identified; as well, the size of the arteriovenous malformation may decrease with the Valsalva maneuver. For diagnosis, CT with contrast medium enhancement may be sufficient, although angiography is best. The entire lungs are reviewed. A perfusion scan of the lung may demonstrate a cold spot in the area of the arteriovenous malformation. Angiography is required to find multiple arteriovenous malformations or to plan for resection. The surgeon should consider resection of the arteriovenous malformation if symptoms are present, the lesions are enlarging, or the lesion is large and is sufficiently localized. If the patient has hereditary hemorrhagic telangiectasia, resection may be considered even if the lesions are of small size because solitary lesions will enlarge. The surgeon may consider lobectomy or wedge excision if adhesions are noted at the chest wall or diaphragm. Vascular control before excision is critical. Observation is recommended if lesions are small (<1 to 1.5 cm), without symptoms, or hereditary hemorrhagic telangiectasia. Angiographic embolization can be helpful for multiple unresectable lesions.

A pulmonary vascular sling consists of an anomalous or aberrant left pulmonary artery, which causes airway obstruction. Pulmonary vascular slings are commonly associated with other anomalies. In this particular anatomic variation, the aberrant left pulmonary artery arises from the right ("main") pulmonary artery. The aberrant left pulmonary artery courses between the trachea and the esophagus to supply the left lung. More than 90% of patients have serious difficulty consisting of wheezing and stridor. Esophagoscopy will show the anomalous vessel anterior to the esophagus; bronchoscopy or bronchography will demonstrate the vessel posterior to the trachea. Surgical correction requires exploration of the left chest, division of the artery, and oversewing of the vessel as far as possible distal within the mediastinum. The reanastomosis to the main pulmonary artery is then performed.

Vascular rings comprise 7% of all congenital heart problems. The most common vascular ring is double aortic arch, which occurs in 60% of all cases. The right, or posterior arch, is the larger and gives rise to the right carotid and right subclavian arteries. The ring wraps around both the trachea and the esophagus. A posterior indentation is noted in the esophagus on barium swallow. Simple division corrects the anomaly.

A right aortic arch with retroesophageal left subclavian artery and left ligamentum arteriosum occurs in 25% to 30% of patients with vascular rings. Intracardiac defects occur with double aortic arch. Most of these infants require operation within the first weeks or months of life.

Most patients with vascular rings require only a careful history and a barium swallow for diagnosis. Typically, one does not need bronchoscopy or esophagoscopy, because it may be harmful; aortography adds little additional information. Repair is performed through the left chest. Division of the smaller arch, usually the left, is undertaken. The ligamentum is divided and the trachea and the esophagus are freed from the surrounding tissues. When a retroesophageal right subclavian artery with left ligament occurs, the patient may complain of dysphagia. This clinical anomaly is often referred to as dysphagia lusoria. The differential diagnosis includes neuromotor diseases of the esophagus or stricture.

LUNG CANCER

Lung cancer is a significant public health problem in the United States and the world. In 2004, an estimated 173,770 new cases of cancer of the lung and bronchus was estimated to occur. Lung cancer is the most frequent cause of cancer death and accounts for 14% of all cancer diagnoses and 28% of all cancer deaths. Lung cancer is the most common cause of cancer death in women and the second most common cause of cancer death in men. The deaths attributed to lung cancer in 2004 were approximately 160,440, exceeding the combined total deaths of breast, prostate, and colorectal cancer patients (Fig. 57-6).

For men, the mortality rate for lung cancer declined significantly (decreasing 1.6% per year) in the period 1991 to 1995. However, since 1987, more women have died of lung cancer than breast cancer, which for almost 50 years was the major cause of death in women. The decrease in lung cancer incidence and the mortality rate probably reflects decreasing cigarette smoking over the previous 30 years. However, smoking cessation in women has lagged behind smoking cessation in men, and the incidence of lung cancer in women continues to climb (Figs. 57-7 and 57-8).

One-year survival rates for lung cancer have improved from 32% in 1973 to 41% in 1994; however, the 5-year survival rate for all stages combined is only 14%. For localized disease, 5-year survival can approach 50% (stages I and II); for regional disease, 20%; and for distant disease, 2%. Only a small percentage (15%) are discovered when localized.

Although local and systemic interventions may improve survival rates in these patients, accurate treatment depends on accurate and histologic staging before treatment and following resection. Anatomic resection of the involved lobe of the lung and mediastinal lymph node dissection provide optimal material for pathologic staging and optimal treatment (local control) for patients with stages I and II lung cancer. In advanced-stage (IIIA) patients, a multidisciplinary approach to the patient's treatment plan (with evaluation and recommendations by the surgeon, the medical oncologist, and radiation oncologist before treatment) ensures an optimal treatment recommendation in a planned and structured manner. Earlier-staged patients (IB, IIA, and IIB) may eventually achieve similar benefit. In the future, knowledge of molecular changes that predispose to the development of lung cancer may provide strategies for chemoprevention or

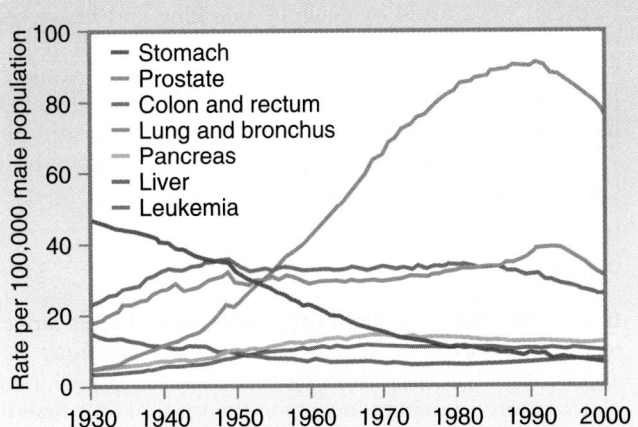

FIGURE 57-7. Age-adjusted cancer death rates for men, by site, in the United States (1930-2000) per 100,000, age-adjusted to the 2000 US standard population. (From http://www.cancer.org/downloads/STT/CAFF2003PWSecured.pdf. Reprinted by permission of the American Cancer Society, Inc.)

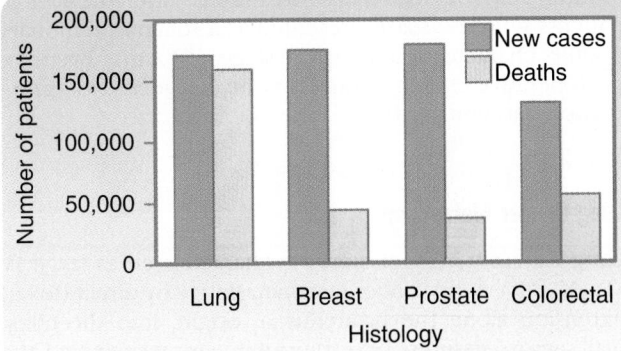

FIGURE 57-6. Cancer statistics, United States, 2004. New cases of cancer and cancer deaths for the four leading cancers in the United States. (Data from http://www.cancer.org/statistics/.)

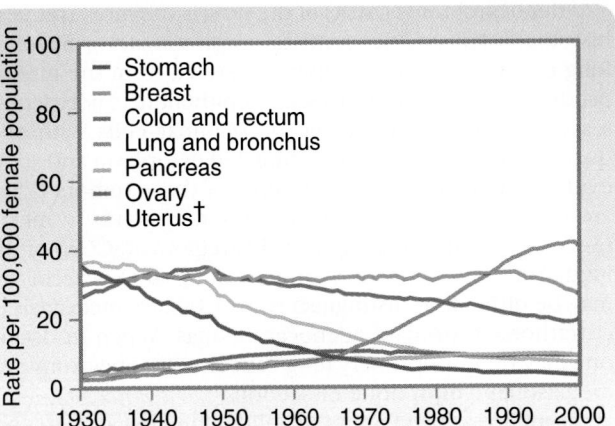

FIGURE 57-8. Age-adjusted cancer death rates for women, by site, in the United States (1930-2000) per 100,000, age-adjusted to the 2000 US standard population. †Uterus cancer death rates are for uterine cervix and uterine corpus combined. (From http://www.cancer.org/downloads/STT/CAFF2003PWSecured.pdf. Reprinted by the permission of the American Cancer Society, Inc.)

other treatments directed at genetic alterations in the cancer itself. Many prospective protocols have been initiated through the efforts of oncologists throughout the world in an attempt to better understand and evaluate various combinations of multidisciplinary treatments.

Etiology

Cigarette smoking is unequivocally the most important risk factor in the development of lung cancer. Other environmental factors that may predispose to lung cancer include industrial substances such as asbestos, arsenic, chromium, or nickel; organic chemicals; radon or iatrogenic radiation exposure; air pollution; and other environmental (secondary) smoke in nonsmokers.

If cancers caused by cigarette smoking and heavy use of alcohol could be prevented a significant number of lives would be saved. The American Cancer Society estimates that approximately 175,000 cancer deaths are attributed to tobacco use and an additional 19,000 cancer deaths per year are related to excessive alcohol use (frequently in combination with tobacco use).

Pathology

In general, there is a slight preponderance of lung cancer to develop in the right lung because the right lung has approximately 55% of the lung parenchyma. As well, lung cancer more frequently occurs in the upper lobes than in lower lobes. The blood supply to these tumors, which arise from the bronchial epithelium, is from the bronchial arteries. A small percentage of patients may have a second focus or metastasis of lung cancer that increases the stage of the patient (see Staging of Lung Cancer). A progression of histologic changes in the lung occurs from smoking from (1) proliferation of basal cells, (2) to development of atypical nuclei with prominent nucleoli, (3) to stratification, (4) to development of squamous metaplasia and (5) carcinoma in situ, to (6) invasive carcinoma.

Adenocarcinoma (ACA) of the lung is the most frequent histologic type and accounts for approximately 45% of all lung cancers. ACA of the lung is derived from the mucus-producing cells of the bronchial epithelium. Microscopic features consist of cuboidal to columnar cells with adequate to abundant pink or vacuolated cytoplasm and some evidence of gland formation. Most of these tumors (75%) are peripherally located. ACA of the lung tends to metastasize earlier than squamous cell carcinoma (SCCA) of the lung. Differentiation of a primary lung adenocarcinoma may be difficult to distinguish from a solitary metastasis of extrathoracic primary adenocarcinomas. When in doubt, one may treat for primary lung cancer with lobectomy and mediastinal lymph node dissection.

Bronchoalveolar carcinoma of the lung is a subcategory of ACA but is a more indolent disease. It has the best prognosis of any kind of lung cancer because it is highly differentiated and spreads along alveolar walls. Bronchoalveolar carcinoma may present as a solitary nodule, multiple nodules, or diffuse parenchymal infiltrates. It may require resection to confirm the diagnosis. A solitary focus of bronchoalveolar carcinoma should be treated in a similar manner to ACA.

SCCA of the lung occurs in approximately 30% of patients with lung cancer. Approximately two thirds of these tumors are centrally located and tend to expand against the bronchus, causing extrinsic compression. These tumors are prone to undergo central necrosis and cavitation. SCCA tends to metastasize later than does ACA. Microscopically in SCCA, keratinization, stratification, and intercellular bridge formation are exhibited. SCCA may be more readily detected on sputum cytology than ACA.

A diagnosis of large cell undifferentiated carcinoma may be made in approximately 10% of all lung tumors. Specific cytologic features of SCCA or ACA are lacking. These tumors tend to occur peripherally and may metastasize relatively early. Microscopically, these tumors show anaplastic, pleomorphic cells with vesicular or hyperchromatic nuclei and abundant cytoplasm.

Small cell lung cancer represents approximately 20% of all lung cancers; about 80% are centrally located. The disease is characterized by a very aggressive tendency to metastasize. It spreads very early to mediastinal lymph nodes and distant sites, especially bone marrow and brain. Small cell lung cancer appears to arise in cells derived from the embryologic neural crest. Microscopically they appear as sheets or clusters of cells with dark nuclei and very little cytoplasm. This "oat-like" appearance under the microscope provides the term *oat cell carcinoma* to this disease. Neurosecretory granules are evident on electron microscopy.

Most of these tumors are typically not treated by surgery because of extensive disease at presentation and their aggressive tendency to metastasize; chemotherapy is preferred. Complete responses may occur in approximately 30% of patients; however, 5-year survival rate is only 5%. Radiation may be used for palliation of symptoms or metastasis. Patients with limited disease may have a better survival rate.

Surgery is not the primary treatment for small cell carcinoma. Surgical techniques may be helpful for staging or diagnosis (such as bronchoscopy) in rare cases in which questions persist after fine-needle aspiration and radiographic staging.[24] Pulmonary resection (e.g., wedge resection or lobectomy and mediastinal lymph node dissection) may be viewed as "treatment" after the fact in patients whose disease presented as a solitary pulmonary nodule characterized as early stage (≤3 cm). Even so, postoperative chemotherapy may be considered as appropriate treatment for this diagnosis.

Lung Cancer Metastases

Lung cancer with metastases is characterized as stage IV ($T_{any}N_{any}M_1$). Lung cancer may metastasize by direct (local) extension along the bronchus of origin, into the chest wall, across fissures, into the pulmonary vessels and the pericardium, and into the diaphragm. Lung cancer can involve other thoracic structures such as the superior vena cava, recurrent or phrenic nerves, or the esophagus by direct extension.

Lung cancers most commonly metastasize to the pulmonary and mediastinal lymph nodes (lymphatic spread). Small cell carcinoma is the most aggressive tumor to metastasize to the lymph nodes. Typically, the pattern of spread is first to the hilar lymph nodes and then into the mediastinal (usually ipsilateral) lymph nodes. Tumors of the left lower lobe that metastasize to the mediastinal nodes often involve the contralateral mediastinum in approximately 25% of patients.

Hematogenous spread of lung cancer to the liver, adrenals, lung, bone, kidneys, and brain may occur. Bone metastases are usually osteolytic. Lung cancer is the second most common cause of bone metastasis after breast cancer. Metastases rarely occur distal to the elbow or distal to the knee.

Aerogenous spread (spread through the "air") of lung cancer to another discontinuous area is extremely rare and frequently difficult to prove. Second endobronchial primary lung cancers are more frequent.

Detection Of Lung Cancer

Patients with lung cancer typically are first seen with symptoms and in advanced stage (stages III and IV). Because the pulmonary parenchyma does not contain nerve endings, many lung cancers grow to a large size before they cause local symptoms of hemoptysis, a change in sputum production, dyspnea, obstruction, or pain. Obstruction of a mainstem bronchus or lobar bronchus may impair mucus passage. With this partial obstruction and bacterial overgrowth, pneumonia may develop. Frequently, patients are seen by their local physician with clinical evidence of pneumonia of several days' onset. The pneumonia may be treated intermittently with antibiotics for a period of several weeks. If the clinical pneumonia does not clear, a chest radiograph is obtained, which frequently identifies the lung cancer. Earlier stages of lung cancer are occasionally found on a screening chest radiography that is obtained when the patient goes to the physician for a routine physical examination or other non–thoracic-related problem.

Cytologic examination of sputum, chest radiography, fiberoptic bronchoscopy, or fine-needle aspiration of the mass may further assist the clinician in making the diagnosis and establishing a more precise stage of the patient's lung cancer.

Screening of patients at high risk of lung cancer by sputum cytology or by chest radiography does not provide a sensitive examination in the presence of small, resectable lung cancer. More recently, however, low-resolution CT of the chest has revealed small nodules undetectable on routine chest radiography in some patients. Some of these nodules have the potential to be lung cancer. Such early detection may improve subsequent survival rates. Patients with benign nodules and patients identified with high likelihood of early stage lung cancer were excluded. It is hoped that long-term survival rates will result from complete resection.

Staging of Lung Cancer

Patients with lung cancer may have specific treatment based on their physical characteristics and their anticipated survival outlook. These groupings have been described within the International System for Staging Lung Cancer. The system was adopted in 1986 and supported by the American Joint Committee on Cancer (AJCC) and the Union Internationale Contre Le Cancer (UICC). In 1997, the International System for Staging Lung Cancer was revised. This international staging system classified patients with lung cancer based on TNM characteristics (T corresponds to characteristics of the primary tumor, N to the regional and extrathoracic lymph nodes, and M to metastasis). Patients with similar survival outlooks were grouped together and their clinical characteristics examined.[25,26]

Stage I disease is divided into stage IA and IB. Prior stage IIIA (T3N0) patients had survival characteristics more like those with stage IIB. In 1997, these patients (T_3N_0) were moved from stage IIIA to stage IIB to reflect this survival advantage.

The TNM definitions and stage groupings of the TNM subsets are listed in Boxes 57-1 and 57-2 and Table 57-1. Descriptions of T (tumor) and N (nodal) characteristics are given in Table 57-1. Stage grouping definitions are listed in Box 57-2 and Table 57-1. Representative descriptions of stages IA, IB, IIA, IIB, IIIA, and IIIB are shown in

TABLE 57-1. TNM Subsets by Stage

A

Stage 0	Carcinoma in situ
Stage 1A	T1 N0 M0
Stage 1B	T2 N0 M0
Stage IIA	T1 N1 M0
Stage IIB	T2 N1 M0
	T3 N0 M0
Stage IIIA	T3 N1 M0
	T1 N2 M0
	T2 N2 M0
	T3 N2 M0
Stage IIIB	T4 N0 M0
	T4 N1 M0
	T4 N2 M0
	T1 N3 M0
	T2 N3 M0
	T3 N3 M0
	T4 N3 M0
Stage IV	Any T, any N, M1

B. Simplified Mnemonic for TNM Subsets by Stage of Lung Cancer

	N0	N1	N2	N3
T1	IA	IIA	IIIA	IIIB
T2	IB	IIB	IIIA	IIIB
T3	IIB	IIIA	IIIA	IIIB
T4	IIIB	IIIB	IIIB	IIIB

Data from Mountain CF: Revisions in the International System for Staging Lung cancer. Chest 111:1710-1717, 1997; and Mountain CF, Dressler CM: Regional lymph node classification for lung cancer staging. Chest 111:1718-1723, 1997.

Box 57-1. TNM Definitions

T—Primary tumor

TX Tumor proven by the presence of malignant cells in bronchopulmonary secretions but not visualized roentgenographically or bronchoscopically, or any tumor that cannot be assessed, as in a re-treatment staging

T0 No evidence of primary tumor

TIS Carcinoma in situ

T1 A tumor that is 3 cm or less in greatest dimension, surrounded by lung or visceral pleura, and without evidence of invasion proximal to a lobar bronchus at bronchoscopy*

T2 A tumor more than 3.0 cm in greatest dimension, or a tumor of any size that either invades the visceral pleura or has associated atelectasis or obstructive pneumonitis extending to the hilar region. At bronchoscopy, the proximal extent of demonstrable tumor must be within a lobar bronchus or at least 2 cm distal to the carina. Any associated atelectasis or obstructive pneumonitis must involve less than an entire lung.

T3 A tumor of any size with direct extension into the chest wall (including superior sulcus tumors), diaphragm, or the mediastinal pleura or pericardium without involving the heart, great vessels, trachea, esophagus, or vertebral body, or a tumor in the main bronchus within 2 cm of the carina without involving the carina, or associated atelectasis or obstructive pneumonitis of entire lung

T4 A tumor of any size with invasion of the mediastinum or involving heart, great vessels, trachea, esophagus, vertebral body, or carina or presence of malignant pleural or pericardial effusion,† or with satellite tumor nodules within the ipsilateral, primary tumor lobe of the lung

N—Nodal involvement

N0 No demonstrable metastasis to regional lymph nodes

N1 Metastasis to lymph nodes in the peribronchial or the ipsilateral hilar region, or both, including direct extension

N2 Metastasis to ipsilateral mediastinal lymph nodes and subcarinal lymph nodes

N3 Metastasis to contralateral mediastinal lymph nodes, contralateral hilar lymph nodes, or ipsilateral or contralateral scalene or supraclavicular lymph nodes

M—Distant metastasis

M0 No (known) distant metastasis

M1 Distant metastasis present.‡ Specify site(s).

*The uncommon superficial tumor of any size with its invasive component limited to the bronchial wall, which may extend proximal to the main bronchus, is classified as T1.

†Most pleural effusions associated with lung cancer are due to tumor. There are, however, some few patients in whom cytopathologic examination of pleural fluid (on more than one specimen) is negative for tumor and the fluid is nonbloody and is not an exudate. In such cases in which these elements and clinical judgment dictate that the effusion is not related to the tumor, the patients should be staged T1, T2, or T3, excluding effusion as a staging element.

‡Separate metastatic tumor nodules in ipsilateral nonprimary tumor lobes of the lung also are classified M1.

Data from Mountain CF: Revisions in the International System for Staging Lung Cancer. Chest 111:1710-1717, 1997; and Mountain CF, Dressler CM: Regional lymph node classification for lung cancer staging. Chest 111:1718-1723, 1997.

Figure 57-9. The lymph node map definitions are shown in Box 57-3. The regional lymph node classification schema is presented in Figure 57-10. This map presents a graphic representation of the mediastinal and pulmonary lymph nodes in relationship to other thoracic structures for optimal dissection and correct anatomic labeling by the surgeon.

Lung cancer can be roughly grouped into three major categories:

1. Stages I and II tumors are completely contained within the lung and may be completely resected with surgery.
2. Stage IV disease includes metastatic disease and is not typically treated by surgery, except in those patients requiring surgical palliation.
3. "Resectable" stage IIIA and IIIB tumors are locally advanced tumors with metastasis to the ipsilateral mediastinal (N2 lymph nodes; stage IIIA) or involving mediastinal structures (T4N0M0). These tumors, by

their advanced nature, may be mechanically removed with surgery; however, surgery does not control the micrometastases that exist within the general area of the operation nor systemically.

A clinical pathway for lung cancer treatment in use at The University of Texas M. D. Anderson Cancer Center is presented in Figure 57-11.

Despite current surgical efforts, 5-year survival rates by stage are approximately 65% for patients with stage I disease, 40% for those with stage II disease, 15% for those with stage III disease, and 5% for those with stage IV disease.[27] Lung cancer staging allows physicians to group patients based on the extent of their disease and prospective survival, so that therapy can be applied in a systematic manner for which the patients will benefit. Staging also assists the physician in counseling the patient and the family as to potential therapy and prognosis. Table 57-2 demonstrates the survival based on the TNM subsets.[25,28]

Box 57-2. Stage Grouping of the TNM Subsets

The TNM subsets are combined in seven stage groups, in addition to stage 0, reflecting fairly precise levels of disease progression and their implications for treatment selection and prognosis. Staging is not relevant for occult carcinoma TXN0M0.

Stage 0 is assigned to patients with carcinoma in situ, which is consistent with the staging of all other sites.

Stage IA includes only patients with tumors 3 cm or less in greatest dimension and no evidence of metastasis, the anatomic subset T1N0M0.

Stage IB includes only patients with a T2 primary tumor classification and no evidence of metastasis, the anatomic subset T2N0M0.

Stage IIA is reserved for patients with a T1 primary tumor classification and metastasis limited to the intrapulmonary, including hilar, lymph nodes, the anatomic subset T1N1M0.

Stage IIB includes two anatomic subsets: patients with a T2 primary tumor classification and metastasis limited to the ipsilateral intrapulmonary, including hilar, lymph nodes, the anatomic subset T2N1M0; and patients with primary tumor classification of T3 and no evidence of metastasis, the anatomic subset T3N0M0.

Stage IIIA includes four anatomic subsets that reflect the implications of ipsilateral, limited, extrapulmonary extension of the lung cancer. Patients included are those with a T3 primary tumor classification and metastasis limited to the ipsilateral intrapulmonary, including hilar, lymph nodes, T3N1M0 disease, and patients with T1, T2, or T3 primary tumor classifications and metastasis limited to the ipsilateral mediastinal and subcarinal lymph nodes—the T1N2M0, T2N2M0, and T3N2M0 subsets.

Stage IIIB designates patients with extensive primary tumor invasion of the mediastinum and metastases to the contralateral mediastinal, contralateral hilar, and ipsilateral and contralateral scalene/supraclavicular lymph nodes. Patients with a T4 primary tumor classification or N3 regional lymph node metastasis, but no distant metastasis, are included.

Stage IV is reserved for patients with evidence of distant metastatic disease, M1, such as metastases to brain, bone, liver, adrenal gland, contralateral lung, pancreas, and other distant organs, and metastases to distant lymph node groups such as axillary, abdominal, and inguinal. Patients with metastasis in ipsilateral nonprimary tumor lobes of the lung are also designated M1.

Data from Mountain CF: Revisions in the International System for Staging Lung Cancer. Chest 111:1710-1717, 1997; and Mountain CF, Dressler CM: Regional lymph node classification for lung cancer staging. Chest 111:1718-1723, 1997.

TABLE 57-2. Postsurgical Survival Based on TNM Subsets from Mountain and Dresler[25,26] and Naruke[28]

TNM Subset	Mountain, 1997		Naruke, 1988	
	n	5-Yr Survival (%)	n	5-Yr Survival (%)
T1 N0 M0	511	67.0	245	75.5
T2 N0 M0	549	57.0	241	57.0
T1 N1 M0	76	55.0	66	52.5
T2 N1 M0	288	39.0	153	40.0
T3 N0 M0	87	38.0	106	33.3
T3 N1 M0	55	25.0	85	39.0
Any N2 M0	344	23.0	368	15.1

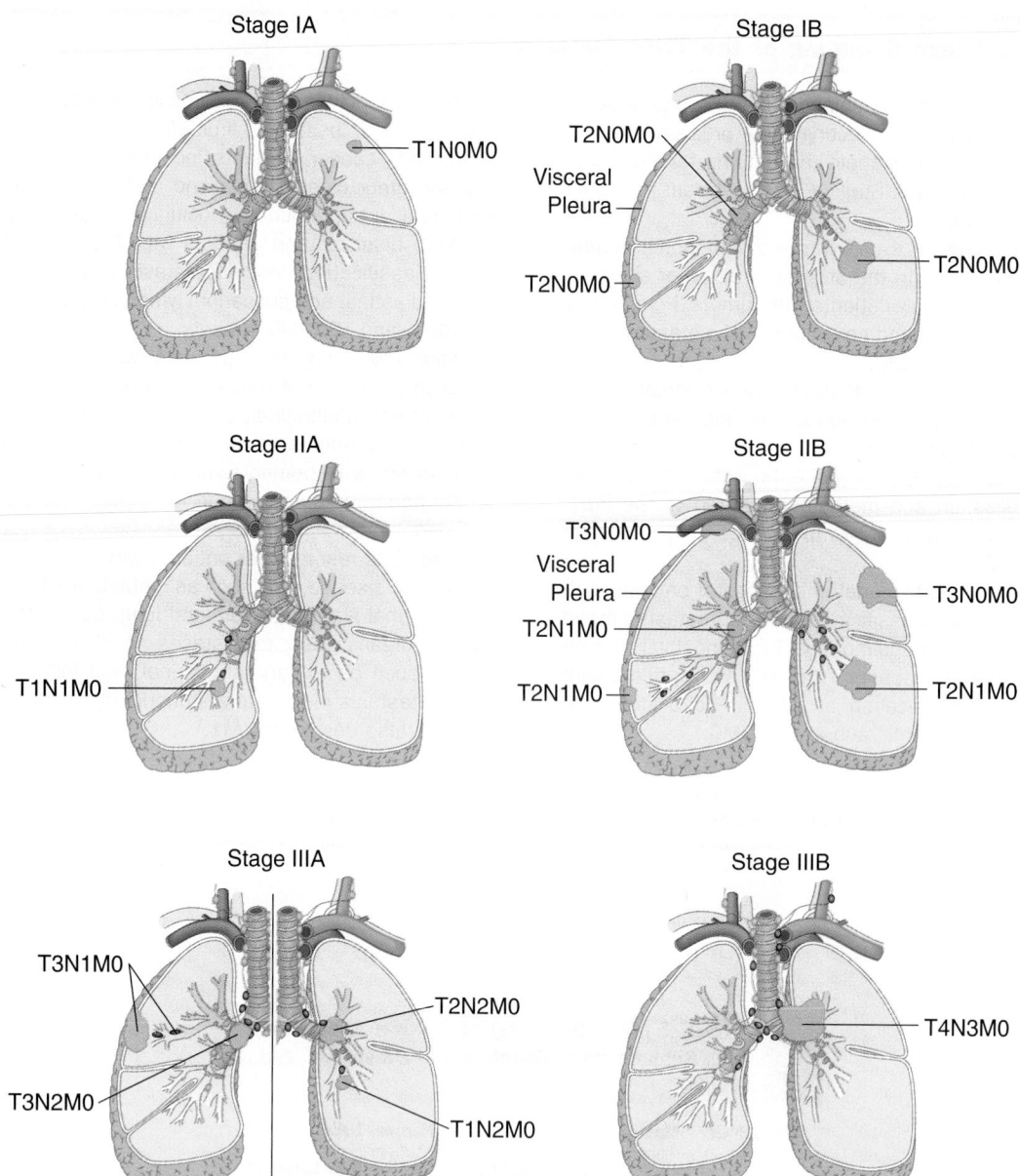

FIGURE 57-9.   Stage groups based on (TNM) subsets. (From Mountain CF, Libshitz HI, Hermes KE: Lung Cancer: A Handbook for Staging, Imaging, and Lymph Node Classification. Houston, TX, Mountain, 1999, pp 1-71.)

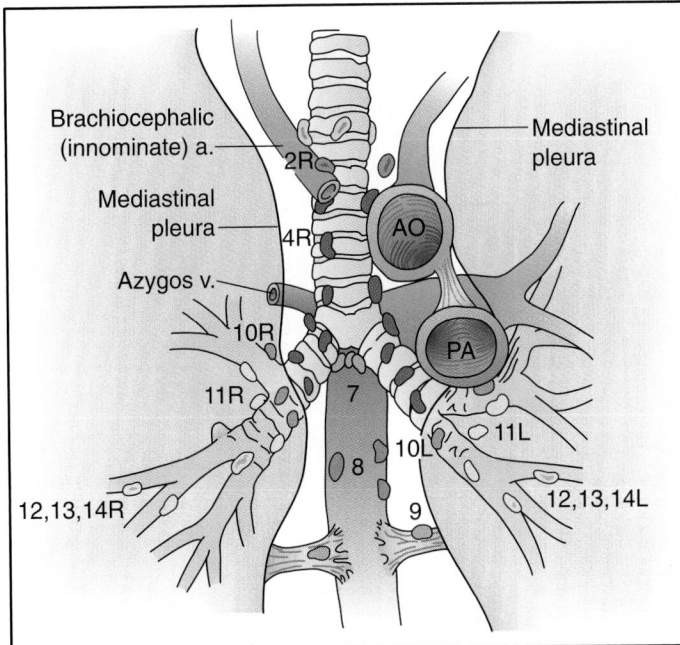

Superior mediastinal nodes
- 1 Highest mediastinal
- 2 Upper paratracheal
- 3 Pre-vascular and retrotracheal
- 4 Lower paratracheal
   (including azygos nodes)

Aortic nodes
- 5 Subaortic (A-P window)
- 6 Para-aortic
   (ascending aorta or phrenic)

Inferior mediastinal nodes
- 7 Subcarinal
- 8 Paraesophageal
   (below carina)
- 9 Pulmonary ligament

N1 nodes
- 10 Hilar
- 11 Interlobar
- 12 Lobar
- 13 Segmental
- 14 Subsegmental

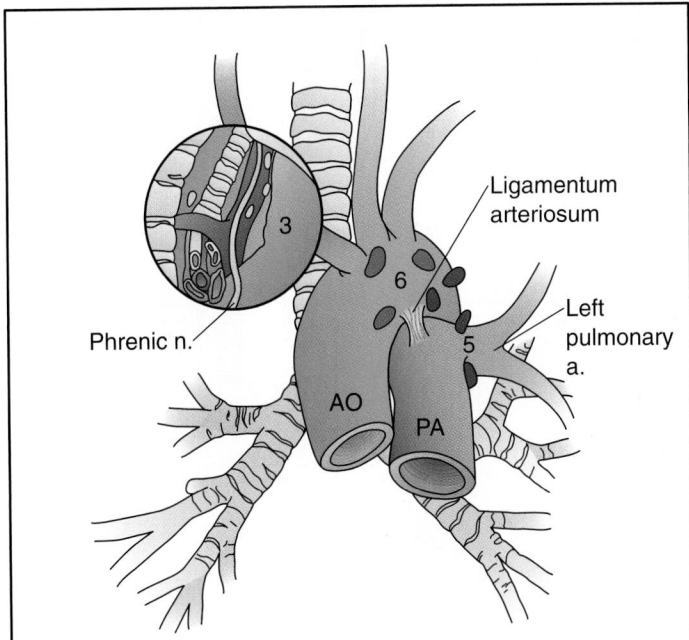

FIGURE 57-10. Regional lymph node station location. AO, aorta; PA, pulmonary artery. (From Mountain CF, Libshitz HI, Hermes KE: Lung Cancer: A Handbook for Staging, Imaging, and Lymph Node Classification. Houston, TX, Mountain, 1999, pp 1-71.)

Surveillance:
For Stages I and II: Should include postoperative visit every 6 months for two visits, then annually; chest x-ray (posteroanterior and lateral) annually.

For Stage III: Chest x-ray, history and physical, and laboratory tests every 3 months for 2 years; then every 6 months for 3 years, then annually.

For Stage IV (not on treatment or in home hospice): History and physical, complete blood count, chest x-ray, and other tests as clinically indicated every 2 to 3 months.

FIGURE 57-11. **A,** Postoperative guidelines for follow-up of patients with non–small-cell lung cancer based on TNM grouping. CBC, complete blood count; CT, computed tomography; CXR, chest x-ray; ECG, electrocardiogram; LDH, lactase dehydrogenase; SGPT, serum glutamic pyruvic transaminase (alanine aminotransferase). (Copyright © The University of Texas M.D. Anderson Cancer Center, 1999.)

A

Figure continues on following pages

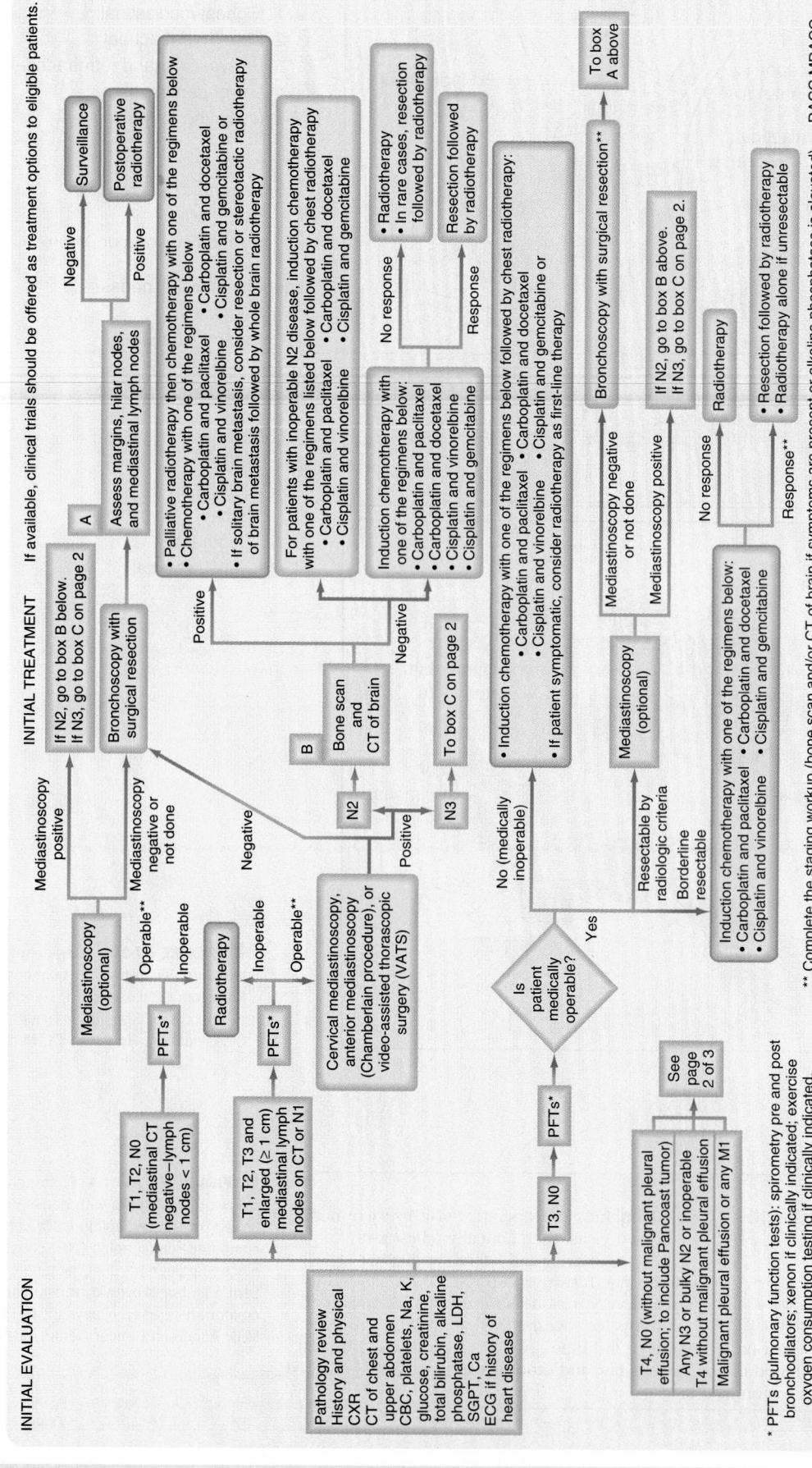

FIGURE 57-11. *Continued* **B,** Postoperative guidelines for follow-up of patients with non–small-cell lung cancer based on TNM grouping.

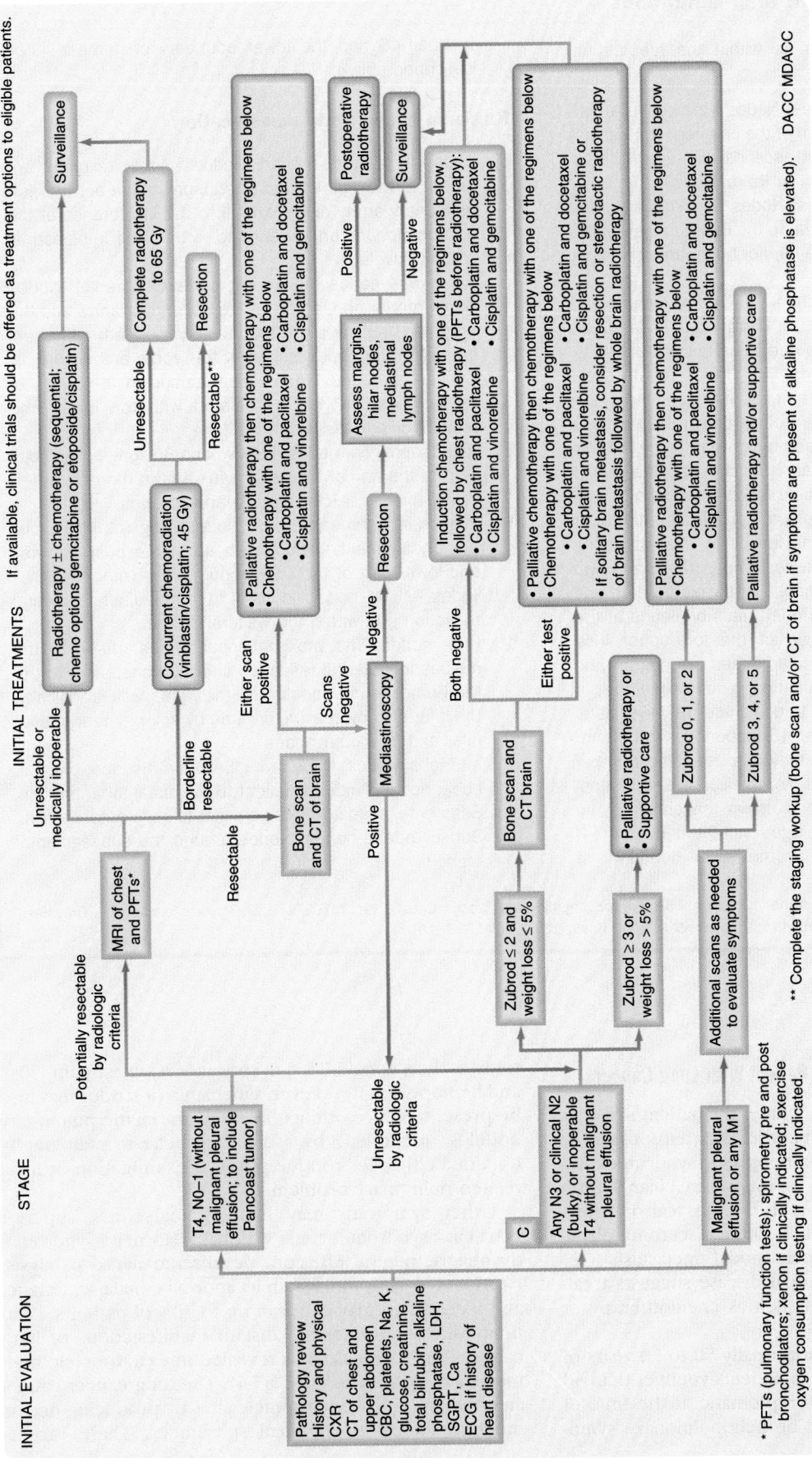

FIGURE 57-11.—Continued

Box 57-3. Lymph Node Map Definitions

N2 Nodes—All N2 nodes lie within the mediastinal pleural envelope.

1. Highest mediastinal nodes: Nodes lying above a horizontal line at the upper rim of the bracheocephalic (left innominate) vein where it ascends to the left, crossing in front of the trachea at its midline.
2. Upper paratracheal nodes: Nodes lying above a horizontal line drawn tangential to the upper margin of the aortic arch and below the inferior boundary of number 1 nodes.
3. Prevascular and retrotracheal nodes: Pretracheal and retrotracheal nodes may be designated 3A and 3P. Midline nodes are considered to be ipsilateral.
4. Lower paratracheal nodes: The lower paratracheal nodes on the right lie to the right of the midline of the trachea between a horizontal line drawn tangential to the upper margin of the aortic arch and a line extending across the right main bronchus at the upper margin of the upper lobe bronchus and contained within the mediastinal pleural envelope; the lower paratracheal nodes on the left lie to the left of the midline of the trachea between a horizontal line drawn tangential to the upper margin of the aortic arch and a line extending across the left main bronchus at the level of the upper margin of the left upper lobe bronchus, medial to the ligamentum arteriosum and contained within the mediastinal pleural envelope.

   Researchers may wish to designate the lower paratracheal nodes as number 4S (superior) and number 4I (inferior) subsets for study purposes; the number 4S nodes may be defined by a horizontal line extending across the trachea and drawn tangential to the cephalic border of the azygos vein; the number 4I nodes may be defined by the lower boundary of number 4S and the lower boundary of number 4, as described above.

Regional lymph node classification

5. Subaortic (aortopulmonary window): Subaortic nodes are lateral to the ligamentum arteriosum or the aorta or left pulmonary artery and proximal to the first branch of the left pulmonary artery and lie within the mediastinal pleural envelope.
6. Para-aortic nodes (ascending aorta or phrenic): Nodes lying anterior and lateral to the ascending aorta and the aortic arch or the innominate artery, beneath a line tangential to the upper margin of the aortic arch.
7. Subcarinal nodes: Nodes lying caudad to the carina of the trachea, but not associated with the lower lobe bronchi or arteries within the lung.
8. Paraesophageal nodes (below carina): Nodes lying adjacent to the wall of the esophagus and to the right or left of the midline, excluding subcarinal nodes.
9. Pulmonary ligament nodes: Nodes lying within the pulmonary ligament, including those in the posterior wall and lower part of the inferior pulmonary vein.

N1 Nodes—All N1 nodes lie distal to the mediastinal pleural reflection and within the visceral pleura.

10. Hilar nodes: The proximal lobar nodes, distal to the mediastinal pleural reflection and the nodes adjacent to the bronchus intermedius on the right; radiographically, the hilar shadow may be created by enlargement of both hilar and interlobar nodes.
11. Interlobar nodes: Nodes lying between the lobar bronchi.
12. Lobar nodes: Nodes adjacent to the distal lobar bronchi.
13. Segmental nodes: Nodes adjacent to segmental bronchi.
14. Subsegmental nodes: Nodes around the subsegmental bronchi.

Data from Mountain CF: Revisions in the International System for Staging Lung Cancer. Chest 111:1710-1717, 1997; and Mountain CF, Dressler CM: Regional lymph node classification for lung cancer staging. Chest 111:1718-1723, 1997.

Preoperative Assessment of the Patient With Lung Cancer

The preoperative assessment includes the patient's history and physical examination with particular attention paid to the presence or absence of paraneoplastic syndromes and to the presence of cervical or supraclavicular lymph nodes. It is these lymph nodes in the cervical or supraclavicular areas that may provide, to the discerning physician, evidence of extrathoracic nodal metastasis (N3 disease). This extrathoracic nodal disease suggests treatment with nonsurgical means such as chemotherapy or radiation therapy.

Patients with lung cancer are usually 50 to 70 years of age; lung cancer is rarely seen in patients younger than 30 years old. Few patients are asymptomatic at the time of diagnosis. Most patients have bronchopulmonary symptoms such as cough, 75%; dyspnea, 60%; chest pain, 50%; and hemoptysis, 30%. Fever, wheezing, or stridor may also be present. Some patients have asymptomatic pulmonary nodules identified by screening chest radiography obtained either for routine physical examination or for a related pulmonary problem.

Other symptoms may include hoarseness, superior vena cava syndrome, chest wall pain, Horner's syndrome, dysphagia, pleural effusion, or phrenic nerve paralysis. Nonspecific symptoms such as anorexia, malaise, fatigue, and weight loss may occur in up to 70% of patients. Paraneoplastic syndromes are distant manifestations of lung cancer (not metastases) as revealed in extrathoracic nonmetastatic symptoms (Box 57-4). The lung cancer causes an effect on these extrathoracic sites by producing one or more biological/biochemical substances. These various

Box 57-4. Extrathoracic Nonmetastatic Symptoms (Paraneoplastic Syndromes)

General

Weight loss/cachexia
Fatigue
General malaise

Endocrine

Cushing's syndrome from adrenocorticotropic hormone secretion
Inappropriate antidiuretic hormone causing hyponatremia
Carcinoid syndrome
Hypercalcemia
Rarely, hypoglycemia or ectopic gonadotropins

Skeletal

Clubbing, 10% to 20%
Hypertrophic pulmonary osteoarthropathy—5% painful periosteal proliferation at the ends of long bones

Neuromuscular (approximately 15% and most common with small cell carcinoma)

Polymyositis
Myasthenia-like syndrome (Eaton-Lambert)
Peripheral neuropathy
Subacute cerebellar degeneration
Encephalopathy

Vascular thrombophlebitis

Box 57-5. Criteria for Nonresectability

Recurrent laryngeal nerve paralysis
Superior vena cava syndrome
Involvement of main pulmonary artery
Contralateral or supraclavicular node involvement
Ipsilateral mediastinal nodes if high (2R)
Malignant (or bloody) pleural effusion, which may cause dyspnea or pleuritic chest pain or may be asymptomatic
Malignant pericardial effusion
Phrenic nerve paralysis (relative contraindication)
Extrathoracic metastatic disease typically involving the brain, bone, adrenals, or liver
Involvement of trachea, heart, great vessel
Insufficient pulmonary reserve
Other signs may suggest a more advanced tumor:
  Chest wall pain that may be described by the patient as dull, deep, and persistent
  Horner's syndrome causing compression of the splanchnic nerve with unilateral ptosis, meiosis, anhidrosis, and enophthalmos
  Phrenic nerve paralysis, with elevation of a hemidiaphragm from nerve paralysis
  Esophageal compression, yielding symptoms of dysphagia from extrinsic compression from enlarged subcarinal left nodes or direct invasion into the left mainstem/carina junction yielding a tracheoesophageal fistula

effects are grouped into paraneoplastic syndromes. Various criteria for nonresectability have been proposed as listed in Box 57-5.

Radiographic Staging of Lung Cancer

The standard chest radiograph and CT scan of the chest and upper abdomen (to include the adrenals) are the most frequent diagnostic imaging studies performed in patients with lung cancer. The chest radiograph provides information on the size, shape, density, and location of the tumor in relationship to the mediastinal structures. The chest radiograph is performed to evaluate the location of the mass, the presence or absence of thoracic lymphadenopathy, pleural effusion, pericardial effusion, pulmonary infiltrates, pneumonia, or consolidation. Changes in the contour of the mediastinum secondary to lymphadenopathy and metastasis to ribs or other bone structure may be visualized. Clues to the histology may also be provided. Squamous carcinomas have a tendency to be large and central in location, adenocarcinoma tends to be more peripheral in its initial presentation, and a small cell carcinoma tends to have bulky mediastinal lymphadenopathy as well as large hilar and central tumors.

Specific attention should be paid to whether the mass has cavitation or not and its relationship to the thoracic structures and mediastinum, and whether it is limited or diffuse in appearance. Also sought is the presence or absence of segmental or lobar collapse or consolidation, hilar and mediastinal enlargement, or evidence of intrathoracic metastasis or extrapulmonary intrathoracic extension.

CT of the chest provides more detail than chest radiography on the surface characteristics of the tumor, relationships of the tumor to the mediastinum and mediastinal structures, and metastasis to lung, bone, liver, and adrenals. Enlargement of the mediastinal lymph nodes can be identified if present. Although CT cannot accurately or consistently predict invasion, it can identify size and the density of mediastinal nodes. CT of the chest has a 65% specificity and a 79% sensitivity for identifying positive mediastinal lymphadenopathy. When lymph nodes are greater than 1.5 cm in diameter, CT is approximately 85% specific in identifying metastasis to mediastinal lymph nodes.

A high-quality CT evaluation of the chest and upper abdomen to include the adrenals is mandatory. This examination evaluates the presence or absence of enlarged (≥1 cm) mediastinal lymph nodes and evaluates the liver, adrenals, and kidneys for metastasis. If mediastinal lymph nodes are enlarged (≥1 cm), invasive staging is required to define the extent of involvement of these lymph nodes with metastases from lung cancer. The evaluation may consist of cervical mediastinoscopy, extended cervical mediastinoscopy, video-assisted thoracoscopy, fine-needle aspiration, or other staging modalities. These enlarged lymph nodes must be sampled and the pathology report reviewed before initiation of treatment. Other causes for enlarged lymph nodes include various infections and inflammatory processes.

Invasive Staging and Other Tests

Invasive staging such as bronchoscopy, mediastinoscopy, or fine-needle aspiration is usually considered after obtaining a chest radiograph or CT scan. These staging procedures may be required for diagnosis to assist in the pretreatment planning for patients with a lung mass. Invasive staging of lung cancer is part of the clinical staging work-up (cTNM) and typically includes bronchoscopy, mediastinoscopy, thoracoscopy, or other intrathoracic staging, as well as the complementary pathologic and histologic examinations that are done before definitive surgical resection. Surgical or pathologic staging (pTNM) provides the most accurate staging of the TNM status of the tumor. Invasive staging identifies those patients with high likelihood of complete resection and those patients with metastases to mediastinal nodes for prospective clinical studies (protocols) or for definitive chemotherapy and radiation therapy.

Bronchoscopy is recommended before any planned pulmonary resection if the sputum is positive with a negative chest radiograph or if atelectasis or an infiltrate fails to clear with medical management. The surgeon always performs a bronchoscopy before resection to independently assess the endobronchial anatomy, exclude secondary endobronchial primary tumors, and ensure that all known cancer will be encompassed by the planned pulmonary resection. Bronchoscopy may be "positive" based on the location of the lesion. For example, more centrally located lung cancers are more likely to be biopsy positive by bronchoscopy, whereas smaller and more peripheral lung cancers are more likely to be "negative" on bronchoscopy. The surgeon always performs a bronchoscopy just before thoracotomy unless the same surgeon has performed the bronchoscopy previously.

The surgeon must take a personal responsibility to ensure that no additional occult endobronchial lesions exist before resection. In addition, the precise location of the endobronchial tumor may modify the planned operation. For example, if the tumor is located in the right upper lobe orifice and involves a portion of the right mainstem bronchus or portion of the right bronchus intermedius, a sleeve lobectomy may be required to conserve the right middle and lower lobe, thereby avoiding a pneumonectomy.

Transbronchial biopsy may be performed with a special 21-gauge needle through the flexible bronchoscope. This technique may be used to biopsy mediastinal nodes or other masses adjacent to the larger bronchi. As well, a transbronchial biopsy may obtain pulmonary parenchyma by forcing the flexible bronchoscope biopsy forceps through the terminal bronchioles into the lung parenchyma. Potential for hemorrhage and a pneumothorax exists. Use of fluorescence bronchoscopy after intravenous injection of hematoporphyrin derivatives localizes in situ and superficial tumors. These tumors fluoresce when illuminated with the light from a special laser.

Positron-emission tomography evaluation is being investigated as an alternative to mediastinoscopy for defining metastatic involvement of mediastinal nodes with lung cancer and other occult sites of metastases.[29]

Various other studies are indicated selectively. Sputum cytology may yield a diagnosis if the patient is a poor operative risk or has suggestive symptoms of cancer or if a transthoracic needle biopsy may cause increased risk. A fine-needle aspiration via a transthoracic route may be approximately 95% accurate in patients with a poor operative risk. Fine-needle aspiration is not always needed in the patient with good physiologic reserve who is otherwise an appropriate candidate for surgery (e.g., stages I and II patients). If the patient does have hard palpable lymph nodes in the cervical or supraclavicular area, fine-needle aspiration or biopsy may provide an accurate diagnosis of metastatic (N3) involvement. Otherwise, a superficial lymph node biopsy or a scalene node biopsy could be performed to obtain tissue for further evaluation. If this N3 lymph node is positive, the patient is stage IIIB and surgery is not recommended.

A mediastinoscopy or anterior mediastinotomy (Chamberlain procedure) or VATS should be performed in all patients with enlarged (≥1 cm) lymph nodes based on the location of the enlarged lymph nodes. This specific staging (pathologic staging) of mediastinal nodes is required before initiating surgical or medical management. Enlarged lymph nodes (≥1 cm) are more likely to be involved with metastases from lung cancer. Other causes of mediastinal lymphadenopathy include mediastinal inflammation, peripheral pulmonary obstruction, atelectasis, consolidation, bronchitis, pneumonitis, or pneumonia, or some patients may have normally enlarged lymph nodes. In one series of patients with N2-positive lymph nodes, the 5-year survival rate with enlarged lymph nodes on CT scan was 6.6%; with a negative scan, it was 13.5%.[30]

Large mediastinal lymph nodes are more likely to be associated with metastasis (>70%); however, normal size lymph nodes (<1 cm) have a 7% to 15% chance of being involved.[30] Some thoracic surgeons use CT to select patients for mediastinoscopy with enlarged lymph nodes (≥1 cm) because 90% of patients with a normal mediastinum have negative N2 lymph nodes after mediastinoscopy and pathologic examination. Some thoracic surgeons perform mediastinoscopy on every patient with lung cancer because small lymph nodes sometimes harbor metastasis (approximately 11%); for example, reliance on radiologic staging may miss occult nodal metastases in 11% of patients with a radiographically "negative" mediastinum.[31]

Mediastinoscopy is recommended before the planned resection if the cancer is proximal, if pneumonectomy may be required, if the patient is at increased risk for the planned surgery or resection, if enlarged lymph nodes are noted on CT scan, or if neoadjuvant therapy is planned. Mediastinoscopy provides a means to assess the mediastinal lymph nodes by palpation and by biopsy for histologic diagnosis.[32] The surgeon may decide to perform mediastinoscopy in all patients undergoing cervical mediastinoscopy or may decide to select patients for mediastinoscopy based on the CT identification of lymph nodes greater than 1.0 cm or greater in diameter. Sensitivity for mediastinoscopy in this situation is 89%, and specificity is 100%. Anterior mediastinotomy or Chamberlain procedure provides adequate assessment of the left-sided para-aortic and aortopulmonary window lymph nodes. VATS or VATS techniques may also be used to biopsy left hilar lymph nodes and to evaluate the intrathoracic manifestations of a cancer.

Mediastinoscopy can evaluate levels 2R and 2L, 4R and 4L, and 7 nodal stations. Aortopulmonary window (level 5) or anterior mediastinum (level 6) can be evaluated using a left parasternal incision, the Chamberlain procedure, or extended mediastinoscopy anterior to the innominate artery. VATS techniques can evaluate enlarged level 5 or 6 lymph nodes and enlarged level 8 or 9 or low level 7 lymphadenopathy.

In the patient with a right upper lobe cancer, pathologically confirmed metastasis to region 5 (aortopulmonary window) or 6 (left anterior mediastinal) mediastinal lymph nodes (clinical stage IIIB) in the absence of extensive subcarinal adenopathy is extremely unlikely. However, region 4R lymphadenopathy may occur in 10% of patients with left lower lobe cancers. Left upper lobe cancers are unlikely to have 4R (right paratracheal) adenopathy in the absence of extensive subcarinal disease.

Transesophageal ultrasound may assist the clinician in evaluating lung cancer that may abut the esophagus, heart, or aorta. Directed transesophageal biopsies of subcarinal lymph nodes may also be obtained.

In resectable lung cancer patients (with stages I and II disease), a bone scan or a CT scan of the brain is not recommended in the absence of related symptoms such as bone pain or neurologic findings. A bone scan should be performed only if the patient complains of bone pain. Plain films of the affected area should supplement this examination. If questions still exist after the studies are completed, magnetic resonance imaging (MRI) of this area may also be performed. Finally, biopsy of the involved bony area may be required. Similarly, a CT scan or MR image of the brain should be performed only if the patient has neurologic symptoms or if the diagnosis of small cell carcinoma is suspected. It is not cost effective to perform CT of the brain in an otherwise asymptomatic patient who is physiologically fit and stage-appropriate for surgery.

MRI is frequently used to complement CT in evaluating the location of tumors within the chest.[33] Specifically, MRI is helpful for evaluating bony invasion of the chest wall or of other mediastinal structures. In patients with superior sulcus tumors or patients with tumors involving the first and second or third ribs, MRI may provide additional information as to the extent of the tumor's involvement with the brachial plexus, thoracic inlet, great vessels, or other mediastinal structures.[34]

Positron-emission tomography (PET) determines the presence or absence of cancer based on the differential metabolism of glucose in cancer cells (increased) compared to normal tissues.[29,35,36] Using 18-fluorodeoxyglucose (FDG) intravenously as a substrate, cancer cells phosphorylate this compound, and FDG-phosphate with tracer is trapped within the cell. It is subsequently imaged with various nuclear scanning devices. Areas of increased uptake are commonly associated with cancer metastasis. The American College of Surgeons Oncology Group evaluated the role of PET after routine staging of lung cancer.[37] PET was better than CT for detection of N1 and N2/N3 disease (42% vs. 13%, p=0.0177; and 58% vs. 32%, p=0.0041). Negative predictive value for mediastinal disease (nodal metastases) was 87%. Unsuspected FDG-avid lesions were confirmed as metastases in 6.3% of patients and benign in 6.6% of patients. PET coupled with CT may yield increased sensitivity and specificity in determining the stage of patients with lung cancer before treatment interventions. Active inflammation may yield false positives, and such areas must be histologically evaluated. FDG PET scanning may assist in distinguishing recurrent or persistent lung cancer and radiation fibrosis in patients having previous radiation therapy for their disease.

Despite the widespread use of CT and MRI, questions may still arise: Does the lung cancer involve structures of the mediastinum, chest wall, and vertebral bodies? Chest CT and MRI can describe the location of the primary tumor with respect to the other mediastinal structures; however, it is difficult to determine whether lung cancer invades specific structures on some scans. Frank invasion may not be determined with accuracy. When there is a question of invasion the patient should undergo exploration. Frequently, these tumors may simply abut the structure without invasion.

Patients with local extension of lung cancer at the apex of the lung into the thoracic inlet may have characteristics of shoulder and arm pain, Horner's syndrome, and, occasionally, paresthesia in the ulnar nerve distribution of the hand (fourth and fifth fingers). Patients with all these characteristics may be classified as having "Pancoast's syndrome."[38-41] Pain comes from the C8 and T1 nerve roots. Sympathetic nerve involvement may result in Horner's syndrome (miosis, ptosis, anhidrosis, and enophthalmos). Typically, the first, second, and third ribs are involved and require resection. Reconstruction of the defect is not required because the scapula and arm protect the defect. CT and MRI are used to assist in selecting treatment options.

Solitary Pulmonary Nodule

A solitary pulmonary nodule (SPN) is frequently a diagnostic and therapeutic dilemma.[42-44] An SPN may be defined as an asymptomatic mass within the lung parenchyma that is less than 3 cm and is circumscribed. Overall, 33% of these masses are malignant; 50% are malignant if the patient's age is older than 50 years. In general, a patient with an SPN should undergo resection for definitive diagnosis and treatment. The exceptions to this general statement are (1) those patients who have a mass unchanged for greater than 2 years (documented on serial radiographic examinations), (2) patients with benign patterns of calcification such as in hamartoma, (3) patients with masses clearly caused by an inflammatory process such as tuberculosis, (4) those patients with prohibitive operative risk, or (5) those patients in whom small cell carcinoma is suspected. If the mass represents active tuberculosis or other infectious process, the lesion may disappear after therapy.

A fine-needle aspiration for diagnosis of a new SPN in a patient who is otherwise physiologically fit is often not needed or superfluous. A fine-needle aspiration should only be done if the surgeon is trying to identify a reason not to operate (especially in high-risk patients) or if small cell carcinoma is expected. If the fine-needle aspiration is positive, resection of the nodule is recommended; if the result is nondiagnostic, the results should not always be trusted and surgery should be recommended. Sputum cytology is frequently nondiagnostic in this situation, whereas the sensitivity of transthoracic fine-needle aspiration approaches 100%.

A wedge resection may not always be possible, particularly if an SPN is located centrally within the lobe. For an SPN in the absence of a cancer diagnosis, a lobectomy is appropriate for a diagnosis (and treatment) in the patient who is physiologically fit to undergo a lobectomy. If a cancer diagnosis is obtained, a mediastinal lymph node resection should be performed. A pneumonectomy should not be performed without a cancer diagnosis. I perform a mediastinal lymph node dissection, not sampling, to optimize pathologic staging of the mediastinal lymph nodes (Box 57-6).

Box 57-6. Mediastinal Nodes to Be Dissected During Pulmonary Resection for Lung Cancer

The following mediastinal nodal stations should be inspected and dissected, and identified lymph nodes resected during a pulmonary resection for lung cancer.

Right side (level)

[2R]	If possible
4R	Paratracheal
7	Subcarinal
8R	Periesophageal
9R	Pulmonary ligament

Left side (level)

[2L]	If possible
[4L]	If possible
5	Aortopulmonary window
6	Anterior mediastinal, anterior to the ligamentum arteriosum
7	Subcarinal
8L	Periesophageal
9L	Pulmonary ligament

Molecular Markers

Various molecular characteristics may be associated with a worse prognosis in patients with lung cancer.[45] DNA aneuploidy is associated with poor survival rate. Oncogenes (*KRAS, MYC, NEU*) serve to regulate, in a positive sense, growth of tumors. *KRAS* mutation is the most frequent mutation, accounting for 90% of genetic mutations in ACA. This oncogene codes for a protein associated with signal transduction. Mutations in *KRAS* are associated with poor survival outlook.[46] Overexpression of *HER2* oncogenes is associated with worse survival rate in patients with lung cancer.

Tumor suppressor genes, such as *p53*, normally provide a negative influence on cell growth. If a tumor suppressor gene, such as *p53*, is mutated, then this negative influence is removed and the tumor growth occurs unchecked. Gene therapy trials to replace or modify this mutation have been shown to be safe when used in a clinical environment.[47,48] Mutations in the retinoblastoma *(RB)* gene are also associated with poor survival. If both *p53* and *RB* mutations are present, survival expectation is only 12 months compared with 46 months in patients with normal expression of these proteins.

Treatment of Lung Cancer

Treatment options include surgery for localized disease, chemotherapy for metastatic disease, and radiation therapy for local control in patients whose condition is not amenable to surgery. Radiation therapy and chemotherapy together are better than chemotherapy or radiation therapy alone for primary treatment of advanced-stage lung cancer. Protocols evaluating chemotherapy, radiation, and surgery for advanced stage lung cancer are ongoing.

Small cell lung cancer is frequently disseminated at diagnosis. Surgery is not the primary treatment for small cell carcinoma. Chemotherapy can provide patients with a survival advantage over no treatment. In patients with an SPN and no evidence of metastatic disease, resection (with wedge resection and frozen section) may reveal cancer. Lobectomy would be appropriate along with mediastinal lymph node dissection. If a wedge resection cannot be performed, lobectomy for diagnosis would be appropriate in a physiologically fit individual.

The clinician treats non–small cell lung cancer based on the clinical stage at presentation. Survival depends on the cumulative mechanical and biological effects of that treatment on the primary tumor and micrometastases. Despite the clinician's best efforts, survival expectations for advanced-stage lung cancer remain dismal for most patients. Even in earlier stage cases (stages IB, 2A, and 2B), 5-year survival may only reach 55%, 50%, and 40%, respectively. In selected patients, combinations of surgery, chemotherapy, and radiation therapy may provide better survival results than a single modality alone. The choice of initial therapy (whether single modality or multimodality therapy) depends on the patient's clinical stage at presentation and the availability of prospective protocols.

TABLE 57-3.   Results of Randomized Trials for Advanced Stage Lung Cancer

Investigators	Treatment	Patients (n)	Resection Rate	Median Survival (mo)	3-Yr Survival
Rosell et al, 1994[52]	Surgery (+ radiation therapy)	30	90	8.0	0
	Chemosurgery (+ radiation therapy)	29	85	26.0	29
Roth et al, 1994[53]	Surgery	32	66	11.0	15
	Chemotherapy	28	61	64.0	56
Pass et al, 1992[51]	Surgery	14	13	86	85
	Chemotherapy + surgery	15.6	28.7	23	50

However, treatment options may vary even among different subsets of patients within the same clinical stage. Pretreatment staging remains the critical step before initiating therapy.

Treatment of Early-Stage Lung Cancer: Stages IA, IB, IIA, IIB, and Early IIIA

Early stage lung cancer (stages I and II) may successfully be treated with surgery alone and, in most patients, yields long-term survival rates. Lobectomy is the procedure of choice for lung cancer confined to one lobe. Certain patients with lung cancer with chest wall involvement (T3N0M0) may be treated well with surgery alone as a local control modality. En bloc resection of the lung and involved chest wall with mediastinal lymphadenectomy results in approximately a 50% 5-year survival rate. In addition, T3N0M0 patients (with tumors < 2 cm from the carina) have a 36% 5-year survival rate with surgical resection alone. Such improved survival rates based on the 1986 staging system have prompted the AJCC and UICC to propose the current (1997) staging system to account for such survival. This stage (T3N0M0) has been designated stage IIB.

Based on the favorable results of trials with advanced-stage disease, application of chemotherapy in earlier stages of lung cancer may improve survival expectations. Depierre and colleagues[49] conducted a randomized trial evaluating whether preoperative chemotherapy would improve survival in patients with resectable non-small-cell lung cancer (clinical stage IB, II, and IIIA) compared to surgery alone. The preoperative chemotherapy was two cycles of mitomycin (6 mg/m^2, day 1), ifosfamide (1.5 g /m^2, days 1 to 3) and cisplatin (30 mg/m^2, days 1 to 3). Responding patients received an additional two cycles of chemotherapy after resection. Postoperative radiation for enhanced local control was used for patients with pT3 or pN2 status. Three hundred and sixty-five patients were randomized. Overall response rate was 64%. Mortality was similar in both arms (6.7% chemotherapy arm; 4.5% resection arm, p=0.38). Median survival was 37 months (chemotherapy) and 26.0 months (surgery alone), p=0.15. Although earlier-stage disease had a decrease in the relative risk in the chemotherapy group compared to the surgery alone group (RR=0.68; p=0.027), overall disease-free survival time was significantly longer in the chemotherapy group (p=0.033). In this study, observable

but not statistically significant differences in survival were noted, except for stage I and II disease. Additional studies are warranted. Recently, a randomized trial identified a 4% survival advantage and decreased hazard ratio for death (0.86, 95% C.I. 0.76-0.98, p<0.003) in patients receiving post-resection chemotherapy (cisplatin-based) to observation alone.[50]

Treatment of Advanced Stage Lung Cancer (Stages IIIA [N2], IIIB, IV)

Treatment decisions require accurate and complete staging as an integral component of pulmonary resection for lung cancer. For postoperative treatment decisions, mediastinal lymphadenectomy determines pathologic stage and provides information to the clinician as to potential survival and the need for postresection therapy. For nodal stations to be identified and dissected during each lung cancer operation, see Box 57-6.

Most patients with histologically confirmed N2 disease have a biologically aggressive tumor with probable occult metastatic disease. While pulmonary resection and mediastinal lymphadenectomy can provide some patients with improved survival rate and enhanced local control, most patients will not benefit from surgery as a sole modality for the treatment of p-stage IIIa non–small cell lung cancer. Neoadjuvant therapy (platinum based) before surgery for p-stage IIIA (N2) disease improves survival expectations over surgery alone (Table 57-3).[51-53] Currently, a prospective trial for stage IIIA (N2) patients (RTOG 93-09) comparing neoadjuvant chemoradiotherapy and surgical resection with definitive chemotherapy and radiation therapy is being analyzed.

Advanced-stage lung cancer, particularly with nodal spread, cannot typically be considered a disease effectively treated with a single modality (i.e., chemotherapy or radiation therapy). Surgery alone for stage IIIA (N2), IIIB, or IV lung cancer is infrequently performed because the risks of surgery usually exceed the benefits of surgery. The surgeon must balance the value of mechanical extirpation of the local disease (local disease control, pain relief, potential for improved survival) with the risks of a surgical procedure and potential improvement in survival length or quality of life. Typically, the risks exceed the benefits and surgery is not considered; however, in some patients, surgery for advanced-stage lung cancer may receive benefit by local tumor control, palliation of symptoms, improved quality of life, and the potential for longer survival. Resection for isolated brain metastasis is warranted for improvement in quality of life and survival rate.[54,55] The primary lung tumor can then be treated according to T and N stage.

Chemotherapy

Combination chemotherapy has been well tolerated and associated with a modest improvement in survival rate. Quality of life analysis in patients undergoing chemotherapy has demonstrated maintenance or improvement in quality of life.

Induction chemotherapy followed by radiation appears to improve survival rate in patients with locally advanced lung cancer, as shown in prospective randomized studies.[56-59] In these studies cisplatin-based combination chemotherapy has been shown to improve survival expectation over and above that achieved with radiation alone.

Dillman and colleagues[56,57] showed that patients given cisplatin at 100 mg/m^2 body surface area and vinblastine, 5 mg/m^2, before radiation therapy (60 Gy over 6 weeks) were better off than patients who received the same radiation therapy but began it immediately and received no chemotherapy. This study was reviewed again in 1996. Dillman and colleagues provided data for 7 years of follow-up of induction chemotherapy before radiation therapy. The radiographic response was 56% for the chemotherapy and radiation therapy group and only 43% for the radiation therapy alone group ($P = .092$). Median survival rate was greater for the chemotherapy-radiation therapy group at 13.7 months compared with the radiation alone group at 9.6 months ($P = .012$). The authors concluded that sequential chemotherapy radiation increased survival rate compared with radiation alone.

Le Chevalier and colleagues[58] reported the results of a large prospective study evaluating radiation therapy (65 Gy) compared with radiation therapy and chemotherapy of cisplatin, vindesine, cyclophosphamide, and lomustine. The 2-year survival rate was 14% for radiation therapy alone and 21% for chemotherapy and radiation therapy ($P = .08$). Distant metastasis was significantly lower in the combined treatment group. Local control at 1 year was poor in both groups (17% in radiation therapy alone and 15% in those receiving combined therapy).

Sause and colleagues[59] examined three treatment groups of locally advanced, surgically unresectable lung cancer patients: (1) standard radiation therapy, (2) induction chemotherapy followed by standard radiation therapy, and (3) twice-daily radiation therapy. They observed that chemotherapy plus radiation was superior to the other treatment arms (log rank $P = .03$). One-year survival and median survival rates were 46% and 11.4 months, respectively, for standard radiation therapy; 51% and 12.3 months for hyperfractionated radiation therapy; and 60% and 13.8 months for chemotherapy plus radiotherapy.

Concurrent chemotherapy and radiation therapy may provide better patient tolerance and improved survival rate compared with sequential chemotherapy and radiation therapy. A prospective multi-institutional trial is ongoing to evaluate chemotherapy, radiation, and surgery versus chemotherapy and radiation only to define the role of surgery in improving local control beyond that obtained with radiation alone.

Radiation Therapy

Like surgery, radiation therapy is a local control treatment modality. Prospective studies of preoperative radiation therapy alone in clinically resectable cases show that postoperative survival rates do not improve over surgery alone.[60,61]

Postoperative radiation therapy may provide a local control advantage but no survival advantage in patients with complete resection of lung cancer. Postoperative radiation therapy has no significant survival benefit for patients without evidence of lymphatic metastasis. In a prospective randomized trial by the Lung Cancer Study Group (LCSG) (LCSG 773), local recurrence rates were reduced; however, survival rate was not improved.[62] Radiation therapy can be effective palliative therapy in patients with symptomatic disease such as metastases to the bones or brain.

Complications of radiation therapy include esophagitis and fatigue. Radiation-induced myelitis of the spinal cord is devastating and can be minimized or eliminated by careful administration of the radiotherapy to avoid the spinal cord. Three-dimensional (conformal) radiotherapy may further concentrate dose to the treated area while minimizing radiation injury to surrounding tissues.

Lung Cancer Summary

The histologic (not radiologic) diagnosis of metastatic involvement of the enlarged (≥ 1 cm) mediastinal lymph nodes for lung cancer is the single most important piece of information to determine before treatment decisions are made. For lung cancer patients with negative mediastinal lymph nodes, anatomic pulmonary resection and intrathoracic mediastinal lymph node dissection should be performed. For lung cancer patients with positive mediastinal lymph nodes, pulmonary resection is not performed alone, nor is it performed as the initial intervention in a combined treatment program. Rather, a combined program of chemotherapy and radiation therapy would provide these patients with the best chance of improved survival. Entry of these patients into prospective protocols is preferred.

PULMONARY METASTASES

Isolated pulmonary metastases represent a unique manifestation of systemic spread of a primary neoplasm. These patients, with metastases isolated only within the lungs, may have biologic make-up more amenable to local or local and systemic treatment options than do other patients with multiorgan metastases. Although primary tumors can be locally controlled with surgery or radiation, extraregional metastases are usually treated with systemic chemotherapy. Radiation therapy may be used to treat or palliate the local manifestations of metastatic disease, particularly when metastases occur within the bony skeleton and cause pain.

One of the first long-term survivors of any pulmonary metastasectomy was reported by Barney and Churchill[63] after resection of a metastasis from a patient with renal cell carcinoma. Local control of the primary tumor was achieved and the patient survived for 23 years after resection of the metastasis; the patient died of unrelated causes. Other authors have noted that certain clinical characteristics (prognostic indicators) may enable clinicians to identify patients with more favorable disease-free and overall survival expectations. Resection of solitary and multiple pulmonary metastases from sarcomas and various other primary neoplasms have been performed with improved long-term survival rates in up to 40% of patients so treated.[64]

Isolated pulmonary metastases, therefore, should not be viewed as untreatable. Patients who have complete resection of all metastases have associated longer survival expectations than those patients whose metastases are unresectable. Long-term survival (greater than 5 years) may be expected in 20% to 30% of all patients with resectable pulmonary metastases (Box 57-7). Optimal (and more consistent) survival statistics await improvements in local control, systemic therapy, or regional drug delivery to the lungs.[65]

Symptoms

Symptoms rarely occur from pulmonary metastases; therefore, diagnosis of metastases is routinely made on chest radiographs after primary tumor resection. Few (<5%) patients with metastases are first seen with symptoms of dyspnea, pain, cough, or hemoptysis. Rarely, pneumothorax from disruption of the peripheral pulmonary parenchyma develops in patients with peripheral sarcomatous metastases.

Box 57-7. Criteria for Resection of Pulmonary Metastases

Pulmonary parenchymal nodules or changes consistent with metastases
Absence of uncontrolled extrathoracic metastases
Control of the patient's primary tumor
Potential for complete resection
Sufficient pulmonary parenchymal reserve following resection

Additional criteria for partial or complete resection

Provide a diagnosis
Evaluate the effects of chemotherapy on residual disease
Obtain tumor for markers, immunohistochemical studies, vaccine, and so on
Palliate symptoms
Decrease tumor burden

Diagnosis and Identification of Pulmonary Metastases

Routinely, clinicians may evaluate patients for pulmonary metastases based on screening chest radiographs. Although the specificity of chest radiographs exceeds 95% when nodules consistent with metastases are identified, their sensitivity (compared with chest CT) has prompted some clinicians to screen patients at high risk of recurrent metastases with chest CT. CT of the chest is quite sensitive and identifies smaller nodules earlier than conventional linear tomography, although these nodules may or may not be a metastasis.

MRI is not routinely helpful for the radiographic diagnosis of pulmonary metastases; rather, CT of the chest is preferred. MRI may assist the surgeon in planning the approach needed for resection of these complex intrathoracic neoplasms.

Benign granulomatous diseases may mimic metastases; however, in patients with a prior diagnosis of malignancy, these nodules are most likely metastases (>95%). Clinical stage I or II primary lung carcinoma may be indistinguishable from a solitary metastasis, particularly if the original tumor was SCCA or ACA. For these two histologies with solitary lesions, thoracotomy and lobectomy may be the procedure of choice. Mediastinal lymph node dissection would complete the staging. Fine-needle aspiration of thoracoscopic wedge excision may be helpful for diagnosis or staging of pulmonary changes in high-risk patients. In patients with lymphangitic spread of cancer, biopsy may be required to differentiate neoplasm from infection.

Selection of Patients for Surgery

Predictors for improved survival rate have been studied retrospectively for various tumor types. These predictors may allow the clinician to identify selected patients who will optimally benefit from pulmonary metastasectomy. These "prognostic indicators" are clinical, biologic, and molecular criteria, which describe the biologic interaction between the metastases and the patient and their association with prolonged survival. Pastorino and colleagues[64] retrospectively reviewed more than 5000 patients with metastases treated with resection. Overall, actuarial 5-year survival rate was 36%, 10-year survival rate was 26%, and 15-year survival rate was 22%. Cancer could generally be staged by the presence of favorable clinical indicators. These indicators included a disease-free interval of greater than 3 years, an SPN, and germ cell histology.

Surgical Incisions

Surgical procedures for resection include single thoracotomy, staged bilateral thoracotomy, and median sternotomy. These procedures have almost no associated mortality rate and minimal morbidity. There are various advantages and disadvantages inherent to each incision. Patients with pulmonary metastases may also undergo multiple procedures for re-resection of metastases with prolonged survival expectations after complete resection.[66]

Thoracoscopy may readily be used for diagnosis of metastatic disease; however, its use in treatment of metastatic disease is more controversial.[67] In an elegant study, McCormack and colleagues[68] conducted a prospective study of VATS resection for treatment of pulmonary metastases. Patients were screened with CT, followed by VATS, followed by open exploration. The authors found more nodules by thoracotomy and noted that VATS failed to identify all nodules. VATS is not the standard approach for resection in patients with pulmonary metastases. At present, VATS can be advocated only for diagnosis or staging of the extent of metastases. Follow-up on all patients is necessary at regular intervals because the likelihood of recurrence remains for a period of years.

Various prognostic indicators have been studied (Box 57-8). Regardless of histology, patients with pulmonary metastases isolated to the lungs that are *completely resected* have improved survival rates when compared with patients with unresectable metastases. Resectability consistently correlates with improved post-thoracotomy survival rates for patients with pulmonary metastases.

Molecular and Genetic Strategies

Restoration of normal W*T-p53* (wild-type) in soft tissue sarcomas may provide for more controlled cell growth or

---

Box 57-8. Prognostic Indicators for Pulmonary Metastases

1. Age and gender do not usually influence post-thoracotomy survival and, generally, should not be considered as prognostic factors.

2. Use of multivariate analysis may allow more accurate prediction of postresection survival expectations and allow better patient selection.

3. Separate prognostic variables may be combined to enhance the predictive value for survival:
   Resectability
   Histology, location, and stage of the primary tumor
   Disease-free interval (from primary to initial evidence of metastasis)
   Number of nodules on preoperative imaging studies: unilateral or bilateral metastases
   Number of metastases resected
   Tumor doubling time (TDT) (see formula). TDT only reflects the growth rate during the interval measured and may be affected by the size of the tumor or ongoing chemotherapy. A formula may be used to precisely calculate TDT:

$$TDT = T \left[1n\ 2/3 \times 1n\ (M_2/M_1) \right]$$
$$= 0.231 \times T/1n\ (M_2/M_1)$$

   where M_1 = first measurement, M_2 = second measurement, and T = number of days between measurements.

---

even programmed cell death (apoptosis). In one in vitro study, transduction of wild-type (wt) *p53* into soft tissue sarcomas bearing mutated *p53* genes altered the malignant potential of the tumor. After transduction, transfected cells expressed wild-type *p53* and decreased cell proliferation occurred.[69]

Novel drug delivery systems may enhance chemotherapy treatment effects by increasing drug concentration in lung tissues and minimizing systemic effects of such treatment. Regional drug delivery to the lungs minimizes systemic drug delivery, preventing systemic toxicity; however, this technique requires a significant concentration of drug delivered to the lung over a short time period.

Preclinical studies in rodents with experimental pulmonary metastases have shown that chemotherapy may be delivered to pulmonary tissue in significantly higher concentrations than with systemic delivery. Minimal to no systemic toxicity was noted. In this model, isolated single lung perfusion with doxorubicin (Adriamycin) was safe and effective.[70] The technique was also effective as follows: 9 of 10 animals given 320 μg/L had complete eradication of metastases from an implanted methylcholanthrene-induced sarcoma.[70]

Previous clinical studies of lung perfusion have shown higher drug concentrations in pulmonary tissue, although clinical tumor response has been mixed. Johnston and colleagues[71] described a continuous perfusion of the lungs with doxorubicin (single lung, continuous perfusion) as a safe technique and subsequently applied their technique clinically. Drug concentrations in normal lung and tumor generally increased with higher drug dosages. No objective responses occurred (0/4 patients with sarcomas). Phase I studies of isolated lung perfusion in patients with unresectable pulmonary metastases from soft tissue sarcomas are underway at various national and international centers.

Surgery alone for treatment of pulmonary metastases will fail in a significant number of patients. Use of neoadjuvant or adjuvant therapy may allow for further prolonged survival or cure. Novel therapies such as identification of molecular events for therapy, gene transfer, or regional delivery of therapeutic agents to the lung by way of an isolated pulmonary system (isolated lung perfusion) may provide better and more directed therapy for patients with metastases. Cure in most patients represents a serendipitous occurrence in which the host biology, spread of tumor, response to chemotherapy, and surgical resection, together render the patient disease free.

MISCELLANEOUS LUNG TUMORS

Slow-growing lung tumors may arise from the epithelium, ducts, and glands of the bronchial tree. Most are of low-grade malignant potential and account for 1% to 2% of all lung neoplasms.

Carcinoid tumors (1% of lung neoplasms) arise from Kulchitsky (APUD) cells in bronchial epithelium. They have positive histologic reactions to silver staining and to chromogranin. Special stains and examination can identify neurosecretory granules by electron microscopy. These "typical carcinoid" tumors (least malignant) are the most indolent of the spectrum of pulmonary neuroendocrine tumors that include atypical carcinoid, large cell undifferentiated carcinoma, and small cell carcinoma (most malignant). Histologic findings include less than 2 to 10 mitoses/10 high-power fields (HPF).

Peripheral tumors are usually without symptoms, although central tumors may produce cough, hemoptysis, recurrent infection or pneumonia, bronchiectasis, lung abscess, pain, or wheezing. Symptoms may persist for many years without diagnosis, particularly if only an endobronchial component partially obstructs the airway. Stridor is often the presenting symptom of adenoid cystic tumors because they are most often found in the trachea and mainstem bronchi. Carcinoid syndrome itself is not frequent and occurs with large tumors or extensive metastatic disease. The chest radiograph may reveal the tumor mass or the results of tracheobronchial traction, but approximately 25% are normal. CT may assist in localizing the tumor. Bronchoscopy is usually positive unless the nodule or mass is peripheral. Ninety-eight percent of adenoid cystic carcinomas can be identified with CT and bronchoscopy with biopsy. Seventy-five percent of carcinoids can be identified in this manner; and although they tend to bleed, they can usually be sampled safely.

Atypical carcinoid may have lymph node or vascular invasion with metastasis. The location is in the mainstem bronchi (20%), lobar bronchi (70% to 75%), or peripheral bronchi (5% to 10%). They rarely occur in the trachea. There is often some local invasion with involvement of peribronchial tissue. At bronchoscopy, most carcinoids are sessile, although a few are polypoid. The histology is that of small uniform cells with oval nuclei and interlacing cords of vascular connective tissue stroma. Mitoses are infrequent but occasionally bizarre cells are noted. Atypical carcinoids are more pleomorphic and have more mitoses (>2 to 10 mitoses/HPF) than typical carcinoid. They have more prominent nucleoli but are more monotonous and have more cytoplasm than oat cell carcinoma. These tumors are more aggressive with a 5-year survival rate of approximately 60%. These tumors tend to metastasize to the liver, bone, or adrenal. Electron microscopy can be used to identify neurosecretory granules.

Carcinoid syndrome is uncommon with lung carcinoids, although it might occur with very large or metastatic tumors. Carcinoid syndrome is related to the body's reaction to various vasoactive amines such as serotonin, substance P, bradykinin, and histamine. Clinical manifestations include flushing, tachycardia, wheezing, or diarrhea. These tumors can produce other substances such as adrenocorticotropic hormone, melanocyte-stimulating hormone, and antidiuretic hormone.

Surgical resection of typical carcinoid and atypical carcinoid is standard, with complete removal of the tumor and as much preservation of lung as possible. Lobectomy is the most common procedure; endoscopic removal is performed only for rare polypoid tumors if thoracotomy is contraindicated. Survival rate is typically 85% at 5 to 10 years. Patients with metastases tend to die of their disease. Large cell neuroendocrine tumors and small cell cancer are not typically treated with surgery and may be best treated with combinations of chemotherapy and radiation; survival of these patients is poor.

Adenoid cystic carcinoma is a slow-growing malignancy involving the trachea and mainstem bronchi that is similar to salivary gland tumors.[72] Adenoid cystic carcinoma is more malignant than carcinoid tumors and has a slight female preponderance. The tumor typically involves the lower trachea, carina, and takeoff of the mainstem bronchi. One third of tumors may occur in the major bronchi; it is rarely peripheral. One third of patients have tumors that have metastasized at the time of treatment. These patients typically have involvement of the perineural lymphatics, regional nodes, or liver, bone, or kidneys. The tumor arises from ducts in the submucosa and spread in that plane. Microscopic examination demonstrates cells with large nuclei and a small cytoplasm and surrounding cystic spaces (pseudoacinar type) and a Swiss cheese appearance for medullary type.

Treatment is wide en bloc resection with conservation of as much lung tissue as possible. Mediastinal lymph node dissection and frozen section control may be required to resect all tumor. Radiation treatment alone may cure approximately one third of patients who are not amenable to surgical resection.

Mucoepidermoid carcinoma is rare in the bronchi, although the location is the same as carcinoid. This tumor may be of either high-or low-grade malignancy. Most are polypoid avascular submucosal masses that are gray to pink. Histologic examination reveals epidermoid cells with keratinization, mucin-producing cells lining cystic spaces, and intermediate cells in the cords. Treatment of these low-grade tumors is like that for carcinoid. The tumor is locally resected. High-grade tumors are treated like lung cancer with equivalent survival rates.

Benign tumors of the lung account for less than 1% of all lung neoplasms and arise from mesodermal origins (Box 57-9). Hamartomas are the most frequent benign lung tumor; hamartomas consist of normal tissue elements found in an abnormal location. Most commonly, hamartomas are manifested by overgrowth of cartilage. Hamartomas are typically identified at 40 to 60 years of age and have a 2:1 male-to-female predominance. They are usually peripheral. They slowly grow in the lung. The chest radiograph usually demonstrates a 2- to 3-cm mass that is sharply demarcated and frequently lobulated. It is usually not calcified, but the "popcorn" appearance on chest radiography may provide the diagnosis of hamartoma. Cystic adenomatoid malformation may represent adenomatous hamartoma. The lesion usually occurs in infants as cysts or immature elements in the lung.

Very low-grade malignancies include hemangiopericytoma or pulmonary blastoma that arises from embryonic lung tissue. Treatment is resection. Tumorlets are epithelial proliferative lesions that may resemble oat cell or carcinoid. These are typically incidental findings noted on examination of resected lung specimens. They rarely metastasize.

Primary sarcomas of the lung occur rarely. They rarely break through the bronchial epithelium, and a cytologic evaluation by sputum is typically negative. The tumors are

Box 57-9. Miscellaneous Lung Tumors

Hamartoma

Epithelial origin tumors

Papilloma: Single or multiple, squamous epithelium, occurs in childhood, probably viral, may require bronchial resection but frequently recur

Polyp: Inflammatory—squamous metaplasia on a stalk; bronchial resection may be needed; these do not usually recur

Mesodermal Origin Tumors

Fibroma: Most frequent mesodermal tumor

Chondroma

Lipoma

Leiomyoma: Intrabronchial or peripheral; conservative resection

Granular cell tumor

Rhabdomyoma

Neuroma

Hemangioma: Subglottic larynx or upper trachea of infants; radiation therapy

Lymphangioma: Similar to cystic hygroma—upper airway obstruction in neonates

Hemangioendothelioma: Newborn lungs, often progressive and lethal

Lymphangiomyomatosis: Rare, slowly progressive—death from pulmonary insufficiency; fine, multinodular lesions, loss of parenchyma and honeycombing; usually women in their reproductive years

Arteriovenous fistula: Congenital, right to left shunt; cyanosis, dyspnea on exertion, clubbing, brain abscess; associated with hereditary hemorrhagic telangiectasia of lower lobes

Inflammatory/Pseudotumors

Plasma cell granuloma

Pseudolymphoma

Xanthoma

Teratoma

usually well circumscribed, asymptomatic, and solitary. Local invasion most frequently occurs, with blood-borne metastasis or lymphatic metastasis occurring less commonly. Resection, similar to lung carcinoma, is feasible in 50% to 60% of patients. The prognosis of patients with leiomyosarcoma is excellent, with approximately 50% survival rate at 5 years; all others have poor survival expectations.

Lymphoma of the lung most commonly occurs as disseminated lymphoma involving the lung. The disseminated lymphoma occurs in 40% of patients with Hodgkin's disease and 7% in non-Hodgkin's disease. Primary lymphoma of the lung is rare. The diagnosis is usually made at surgery. A thorough evaluation for other primary sites of lymphoma should be made if primary pulmonary lymphoma is suspected preoperatively.

TRACHEA

The trachea is about 11.8 cm long and ranges from 10 to 13 cm. There are 18 to 22 cartilaginous rings with each ring being about 0.5 cm wide. The internal diameter in adults is 2.3 cm laterally and 1.8 cm anteroposteriorly. The larynx ends with the inferior edge of cricoid cartilage. The cricoid is the only complete cartilaginous ring in the trachea. The trachea begins about 1.5 cm below the vocal cords and is not rigidly fixed to surrounding tissues. Vertical movement is easily possible. The most rigid point of fixation is where the aortic arch forms a sling over the left mainstem bronchus. The innominate artery crosses over the anterior trachea in a left inferolateral to high right anterolateral direction. The azygous vein arches over the proximal right mainstem bronchus as it travels from posterior to anterior to empty into the superior vena cava. The esophagus is closely applied to the membranous trachea throughout its course. The esophagus is not a midline structure but more frequently lies just to the left from the midline of the trachea. The recurrent laryngeal nerves run in the tracheoesophageal groove on both the right and the left. Most commonly, the left recurrent laryngeal nerve lies close to the tracheoesophageal groove on the left and is a bit more laterally displaced on the right.

The trachea is up to 50% cervical with hyperextension in the young patient. The location of the carina is at the level of the angle of Louis anteriorly and the T4 vertebra posteriorly.

The blood supply to the trachea is lateral and segmental from the inferior thyroid, the internal thoracic, the supreme intercostal, and the bronchial arteries. One should never circumferentially dissect more than 1 to 2 cm of trachea that will remain in the patient before or after reconstruction. The potential for tracheal necrosis is increased with circumferential dissection.

Stenosis of the trachea implies significant functional impairment. A normal, 2-cm trachea has a 100% peak expiratory flow rate. A 10-mm opening provides an 80% peak expiratory flow rate. At 5 to 6 mm, only a 30% expiratory flow rate is obtained.

Congenital lesions of the trachea may be lethal (e.g., tracheal atresia) or may provide significant functional impairment, depending on the extent of the stenosis. Stenosis may be generalized, funnel type, segmental (which is most common), or weblike. Treatment consists of dilation for resection of webs. For localized or segmental stenosis, resection and reanastomosis should be performed. One should limit resection to one third or less of the trachea. A pericardial patch for a generalized or funnel-type stenosis may be required.

Vascular rings such as double aortic arch (right aortic arch with left ligamentum) may cause pulmonary insufficiency or dyspnea. The trachea is normal, and release of the ring provides relief of symptoms. This is in contrast to pulmonary artery sling, consisting of the left pulmonary artery coming from the right pulmonary artery traveling between the trachea and esophagus, which is identified by anterior indentation of the esophagus on barium swallow and by compression of the trachea. Approximately 50% of patients have a separate tracheal stenotic problem (most commonly circumferential rings) and correction of the vascular sling alone would not correct the respiratory distress: the tracheal stenosis must also be treated. Treatment of congenital tracheomalacia, identified as a collapsible wall seen on bronchoscopy, may be related to chronic compression by the innominate artery and treated with aortopexy.

Tracheostomy is one of the most commonly performed operations. The technique is shown in Figure 57-12. For an elective procedure, the incision should be made 1 to 2 cm above the sternal notch. The strap muscles are separated in the midline to expose the trachea. Division of two tracheal cartilages (usually rings 2 and 3) is performed in a longitudinal (vertical) manner to insert the tracheostomy appliance. Occasionally, the thyroid isthmus must be divided. Rarely, a high innominate artery is encountered and should be protected.

Primary neoplasms of trachea include squamous cell carcinoma in approximately two thirds of patients and adenoid cystic carcinoma in other patients. Squamous cell carcinoma may be focal, diffuse, or multiple. The physical appearance may be exophytic or ulcerative. One third of these primary tracheal tumors have extensive local spread or metastases at initial presentation. Adenoid cystic carcinoma (previously called cylindroma) has a propensity for intramural and perineural spread. In adenoid cystic carcinoma, negative margins are important. Margin evaluation with frozen section control should be performed with stricture resection. Clinical features include dyspnea on exertion, wheezing, cough with or without hemoptysis, and recurrent pulmonary infections.

Secondary neoplasms of the trachea may include those related to laryngeal carcinomas with distal or inferior extension, recurrence of these laryngeal carcinomas at the tracheal stomal site, or other skip metastases. In patients with previous laryngectomy, anterior mediastinal tracheostomy may be required. Five centimeters of uninvolved trachea (i.e., negative margins at a minimum of 5 cm above the carina) is the minimal length of trachea that should remain to ensure optimal potential for recovery. To minimize innominate artery fistula, the trachea may be moved under the innominate artery. Cervical exenteration, with resection of tumor recurrence and portion of trachea, requires resection of the breastplate (manubrium, first rib, clavicles to the angle of Louis) before anterior mediastinal tracheostomy.

Involvement of the trachea because of local extension from bronchogenic carcinoma may contraindicate resection. Involvement of the trachea because of local extension of esophageal carcinoma may require palliative external-beam radiation therapy or endoscopic palliation with laser, bronchoscopy, or esophagoscopy, or perhaps intraluminal brachytherapy. For thyroid carcinoma, resection of a short segment of trachea in continuity with thyroid may be performed with primary repair. However, resection is contraindicated for extensive anaplastic thyroid tumors because recurrence is rapid and risks often exceed anticipated benefits.

Infection and inflammation are uncommon causes of tracheal obstruction.

Tracheal Trauma

Penetrating injuries to the trachea are usually cervical; penetrating injuries that involve the mediastinal trachea are often lethal. Penetrating cervical injuries often involve the esophagus, and concurrent esophageal injury should be excluded by barium esophagram or esophagoscopy. Neck exploration may be required.

Blunt trauma to the neck or trachea can produce lacerations, transections, or shattering injuries of both the cervical and mediastinal trachea.

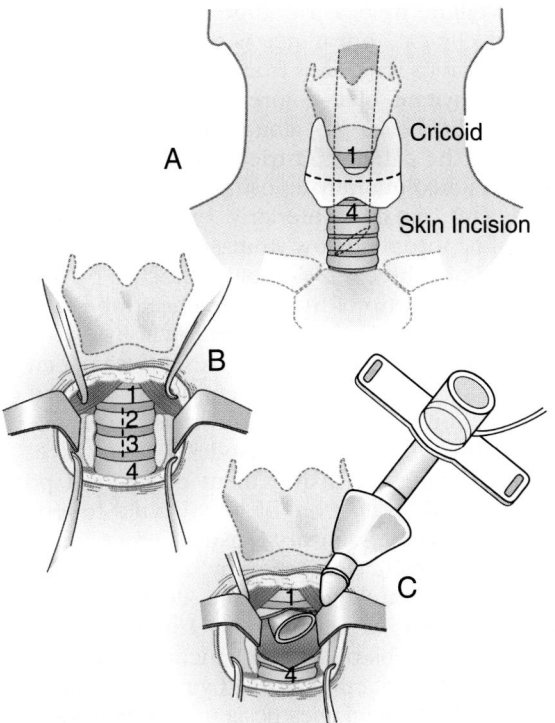

■ FIGURE 57-12. Technique of tracheostomy. **A,** An endotracheal airway is in place. With the patient's neck extended and centered in the midline, a short horizontal incision is made over the second or third tracheal ring after the level of the cricoid cartilage has been carefully palpated. The first and fourth tracheal cartilages are numbered. **B,** After horizontal division of the platysma, the strap muscles are separated in the midline, the cricoid is identified, and the thyroid isthmus usually is divided and sutured to allow easy access to the second and third tracheal rings. The second and third rings are incised vertically. Occasionally, an additional partial incision of the fourth ring is necessary. **C,** Smooth thyroid pole retractors are used to spread the opening in the trachea. The endotracheal tube is withdrawn to a point just above the incision. The tracheostomy tube is introduced with a small amount of water-soluble lubricant and with its large-volume cuff collapsed. The endotracheal airway is not removed until it is demonstrated that the tracheostomy tube is properly seated and permits suitable gas exchange. Closure is made with simple skin sutures. The flange of the tracheostomy tube is both sutured to the skin and tied with the usual tapes around the neck. On a rare occasion when an airway cannot be established from above, an emergency incision may be necessary over the cricothyroid membrane for rapid establishment of a temporary airway.

Clinical features of a cervical injury are suggested by subcutaneous air in neck, respiratory distress, and hemoptysis. Diagnosis is made by bronchoscopy.

Injury to the mediastinal trachea may be suggested by mediastinal or subcutaneous emphysema, pneumothorax of the lung that fails to expand after chest tube insertion, or a large air leak. Other clinical signs include respiratory distress and hemoptysis. Diagnosis is made by bronchoscopy. A chest tube may be inserted as initial management of a pneumothorax on screening trauma chest radiography. If the lung does not completely inflate, a second chest tube may be inserted. If the pneumothorax or a continuous air leak persists, a bronchoscopy is recommended to exclude a mediastinal tracheal or bronchial injury. Anesthetic management with laryngeal mask airway may be helpful for initial examination for full visualization of the airway before endotracheal intubation.

Management of tracheal injuries includes control of airway, endotracheal intubation (using flexible bronchoscopy as a guide), or emergency tracheostomy. If emergency tracheostomy is considered, it should be performed through the area of the tracheal tear (because this area is likely to be resected during the definitive reconstruction procedure). Cervical injuries may be treated conservatively. The endotracheal tube is placed distal to the lesion, and the cuff is kept inflated for approximately 2 days. This approach is indicated only if a small partial laceration is identified, there is little subcutaneous air, there is good apposition of lacerated tissue, and there are no other associated injuries. Cervical injury to trachea may also be treated with primary repair without tracheostomy. This approach is indicated with most knife wounds, many gunshot wounds, and occasional cases of blunt transections.

Primary repair of tracheal injury may be accomplished with tracheostomy, if the tracheostomy is performed distal to the repair. This approach is indicated for some blunt transections and some gunshot wounds. Alternatively, one may consider initial tracheostomy along with delayed repair. The tracheostomy may be best done through the damaged trachea. This approach is indicated for complex shattering injuries of the trachea, especially with significant laryngeal involvement.

For injuries to the mediastinal trachea, the surgical approach is thoracotomy through the right fourth intercostal space. Tracheostomy is rarely needed. Most patients have selective intubation of the left mainstem bronchus, double lumen tube, or jet ventilation. Associated esophageal injuries should be repaired primarily. Some tissue (e.g., the sternocleidomastoid or strap muscle) should be interposed between the two structures.

Postintubation injuries occur because of laryngeal or tracheal irritation from an indwelling endotracheal tube. This condition is usually reversible. Vocal cord fusion must occasionally be treated by division of the fissure. The cricoid is rarely injured but is difficult to repair if injury does occur. For patients with a tracheostomy stoma, postintubation injuries are common. Granulation tissue occurs, as does anterolateral stricture of the trachea. There are various predisposing factors, including too large a stoma, infection in the stoma, and excessive pressure from connecting systems. The cricoid may be damaged either by cricothyroidostomy or by too proximal a tracheostomy.

Low-pressure cuffs on the endotracheal tube have reduced cuff injuries. Pathogenesis is directly proportional to pressure necrosis. A wide spectrum of injury may occur, depending on depth of damage, to include mucosal-tracheal stenosis, tracheomalacia, and full-thickness stricture. Clinical features of tracheal stenosis include dyspnea on exertion, stridor or wheezing, which is easily noted, and perhaps episodes of obstruction with small amounts of mucus.

Acquired tracheoesophageal fistula is the result of prolonged erosion posteriorly. Patients also usually have an indwelling nasogastric tube posteriorly. The most common clinical appearance is that of a sudden appearance of copious secretions from the tracheobronchial tree or of methylene blue–colored tube feedings promptly appearing in the airway along with increasing difficulty ventilating the patient. Gastric distention also may occur.

The tracheoinnominate fistula may result from prolonged cuff erosion inferiorly and anteriorly to the trachea. Inappropriate low stoma may further increase the likelihood of a direct erosion of the trachea by the innominate artery. The tip of the endotracheal tube may predispose to erosions or granulomas within the trachea. Tracheoinnominate fistula may present as sudden exsanguinating hemorrhage. The patient usually has had one or more previous sentinel hemorrhages. Investigation of these sentinel hemorrhage episodes is imperative.

The principles of management of tracheal problems include a full evaluation of the larynx to ensure its integrity before tracheal repair. Direct or indirect endoscopy as well as fluoroscopy may be needed. A tracheal stenosis rarely demands a definitive procedure, either electively or emergently. However, emergency management of obstruction may include sedation, humidified air, or racemic epinephrine by nebulizer. In addition, dilation under general anesthesia may be helpful. The first choice of placement of the tracheostomy is through the stricture, then through the old tracheostomy site, then remote from the lesion. Exceptions include those stenoses immediately above the carina, because they cannot readily be stented. Conservative measures can be supplemented on a chronic basis with a stent, especially if the patient is considered poor risk or if the patient has a partial thickness lesion with potential for regression.

Contraindications to trachea repair include (1) inadequately treated laryngeal problem (which does not include single vocal cord paralysis), (2) need for ventilatory support or permanent tracheostomy for patients with amyotropic lateral sclerosis, myasthenia gravis, or quadriplegia, (3) use of high-dose steroids, or (4) inflamed or recent tracheostomy. Poor pulmonary reserve is not a contraindication for repair in patients who have been weaned from the ventilator.

Various techniques may be considered for diagnosis of tracheal abnormalities. Plain films of the trachea and routine chest roentgenograms (posteroanterior, lateral, and obliques) are critical first steps. CT of the trachea is good for examining luminal compromise; however, it is less suitable than linear tomograms for longitudinal abnormalities. Fluoroscopy may be helpful for the diagnosis of tracheomalacia. A contrast tracheogram is not always necessary. If the patient has symptoms of dysphagia or if an esophageal cancer is suspected, a barium swallow is helpful to evaluate the extent of esophageal involvement.

Bronchoscopy is generally best deferred to the time of the proposed treatment. This approach avoids precipitating an acute episode of tracheal obstruction in an outpatient area. Exceptions to this rule may include highly complicated situations such as attempted previous repair or the need for urgent dilation. Both flexible and rigid bronchoscopes should be available, and the surgeon should be adept at their use.

The surgical management of tracheal problems may be complex. General inhalational anesthesia is used and induction may take a long time if the stenosis is tight. If the stenosis is less than 5 to 6 mm, dilation may be required before passing the endotracheal tube. This may

be performed with rigid bronchoscopy. If the stenosis is greater than 5 to 6 mm, the endotracheal tube may be positioned to a point above the stricture for induction. Stenoses that are subglottic must be dilated for intubation. The endotracheal tube often goes alongside tumors.

Surgical approaches to the trachea include (1) purely cervical for the upper third, (2) cervicothoracic (with upper sternal split) (Fig. 57-13), and (3) cervical approach plus upper sternal split plus right fourth anterior thoracotomy to expose the entire trachea posteriorly and inferiorly. (This approach is rarely used.) The right fourth posterolateral thoracotomy provides the best exposure of the lower trachea and carina (Fig. 57-14).

The cervical approach with or without an upper sternal split is usually used for tumors of the upper half of the trachea plus all benign tracheal stenoses (because these usually occur as a result of endotracheal tube placement). The posterolateral thoracotomy is used for tumors of the lower half of the trachea plus carinal reconstruction. Rigid

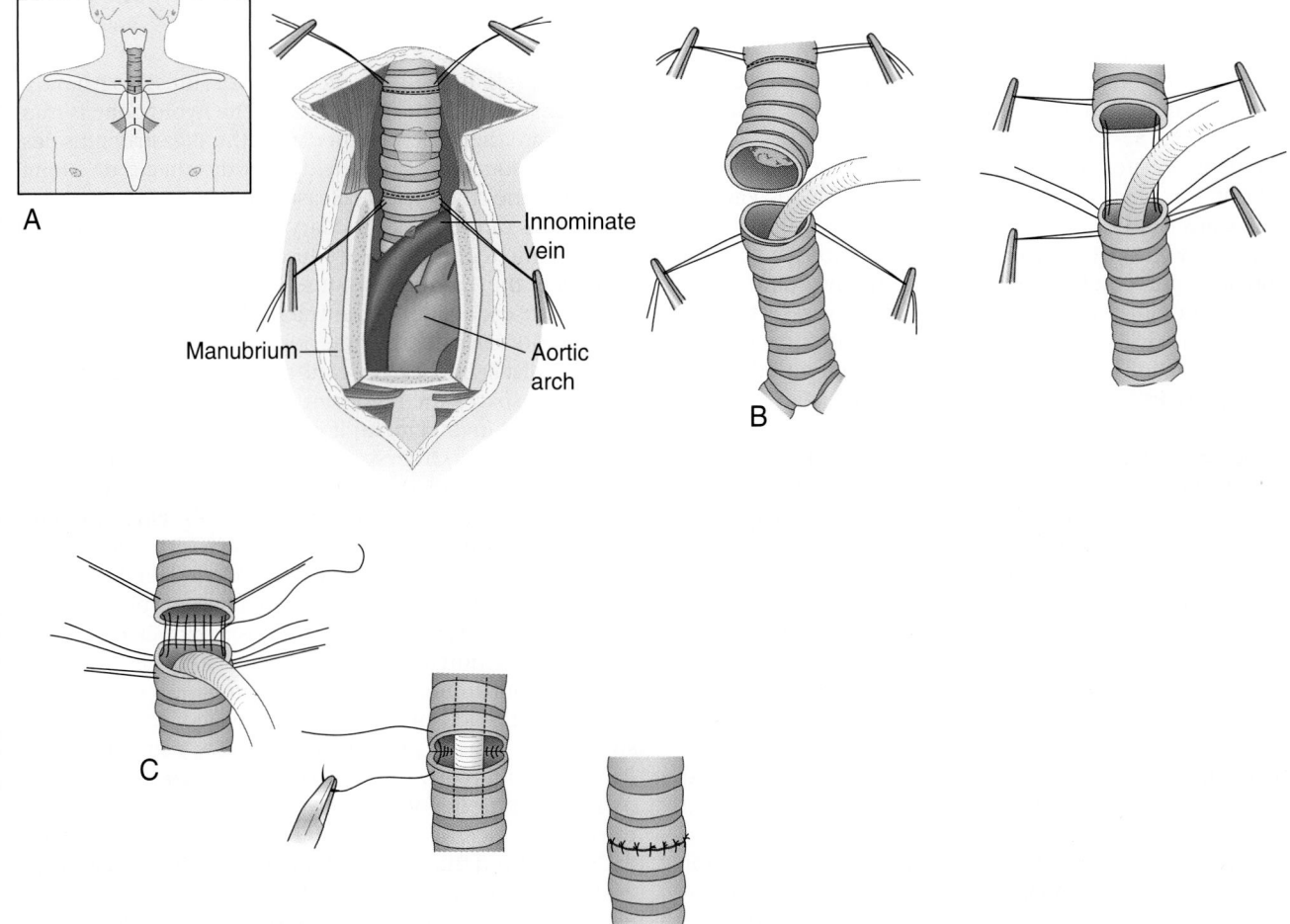

FIGURE 57-13. **A,** Exposure of the midtrachea through a cervical and partial sternal-splitting incision. The extent of the resection has been marked by sutures. After distal division, a sterile, armored endotracheal tube is placed. **B,** After proximal resection, two mattress sutures are placed in the edges of the cartilaginous rings. A simple, running suture completes the membranous anastomosis. **C,** At this point, the original endotracheal tube is positioned in the distal trachea so that the anastomosis can be completed with interrupted, simple sutures between cartilaginous rings.

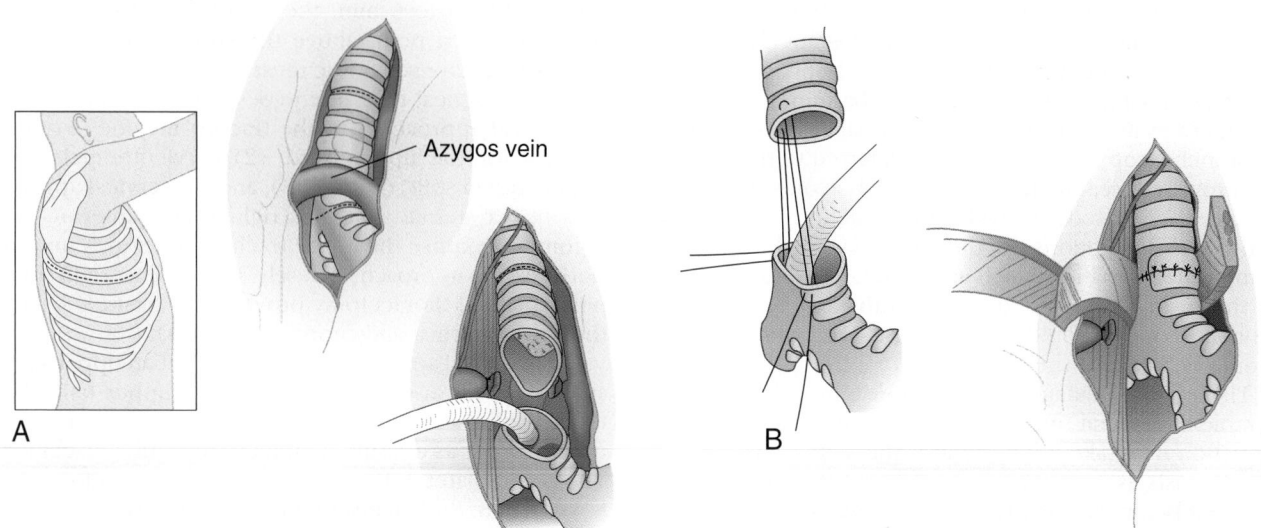

Azygos vein

A

B

■ FIGURE 57-14.   A right serratus-sparing posterolateral thoracotomy is extended behind the scapula. Proximal and distal exposure shows a tracheal tumor near the bifurcation. **A,** After division of the azygos vein and the distal trachea, a sterile, armored endotracheal tube is placed into the left mainstem bronchus. After proximal resection, the interrupted mattress sutures are placed at the edges of the tracheal rings. **B,** After completion of the anastomosis (see Fig. 57-13), a vascularized intercostal muscle flap is placed around the anastomosis.

bronchoscopy for diagnosis, biopsy, dilation, or treatment may be required if the tumor cannot be immediately resected (Fig. 57-15).

In general, the amount of trachea that can be resected is about 5 cm but varies from person to person. Various techniques can be used to achieve this resection without undue tension on the anastomosis. The anterior cervical approach plus mobilization of the trachea and neck flexion can allow for 4 to 5 cm of trachea resection. A suprahyoid release may achieve 1 cm of additional length, and mobilization of the right hilum, together with division of the pericardium around the right hilum, may achieve an additional 1.4 cm.

The reconstruction of the upper trachea may be performed through a collar incision through an old tracheostomy site, which is convenient. Skin flaps are created superiorly to the thyroid prominence and inferiorly to the suprasternal notch. The sternal split is performed whenever indicated. The entire anterior length of the trachea is exposed, close to the tracheal wall. Limited circumferential dissection is performed around the trachea just below the lesion. Silk stay sutures are placed on either side below and later above the lesion. The trachea is transected just below the stricture or tumor. The endotracheal tube is placed across the operative field into the distal trachea. The diseased trachea is dissected superiorly and then transected above the lesion. Posterior mobilization and neck flexion are performed. Posterior sutures are placed with knots on the outside, and then the patient is reintubated through the trachea. Anterior sutures are then placed and tied. No tracheostomy is performed. If ventilation is necessary, an endotracheal tube is used with the cuff away from the anastomosis.

A suprahyoid release as described by Montgomery achieves a little over 1 cm of length by cutting the mylo-

hyoid, the geniohyoid, and genioglossus muscles from the superior surface of the hyoid bone. The hyoid bone is transected on either side just medial to the digastric muscles. This technique probably yields less dysphagia or aspiration than the thyrohyoid release procedure.

Stenosis of the subglottic larynx or cricoid stenosis is a challenging technical procedure. The recurrent nerves innervate the larynx just superior to the posterolateral cricoid on each side. If the tracheal lesions only involve the anterior surface, the anterior cricoid can be removed and the distal trachea beveled to match the defect. This maneuver spares the recurrent laryngeal nerves. With circumferential involvement, it may be necessary to perform a laryngectomy. Otherwise, an attempt to preserve the larynx could be made. The anterior cricoid is removed with a rectangle of posterior cricoid. This leaves the posterolateral portions of the cricoid intact to protect the recurrent laryngeal nerves. The beveled trachea may be brought up to this level along with a flap of membranous trachea posteriorly to match the posterior defect.

Reconstruction of the lower trachea is performed in the right fourth intercostal space. Intubation of the distal trachea or the left mainstem is performed. Carinal reconstruction is usually performed for tumor and is the most feasible of alternative reconstructions chosen.

The technique of tracheostomy is best approached through cervical incision and a vertical incision through the second and third or the third and fourth tracheal rings. The tracheostomy should not be placed too low because erosion of the innominate artery by the tracheostomy prosthesis may occur.

If a tracheoinnominate fistula occurs, this fistula may be controlled initially by inflating the cuff on the endotracheal tube to tamponade and decrease the bleeding. The innominate artery is divided, ligated, and covered

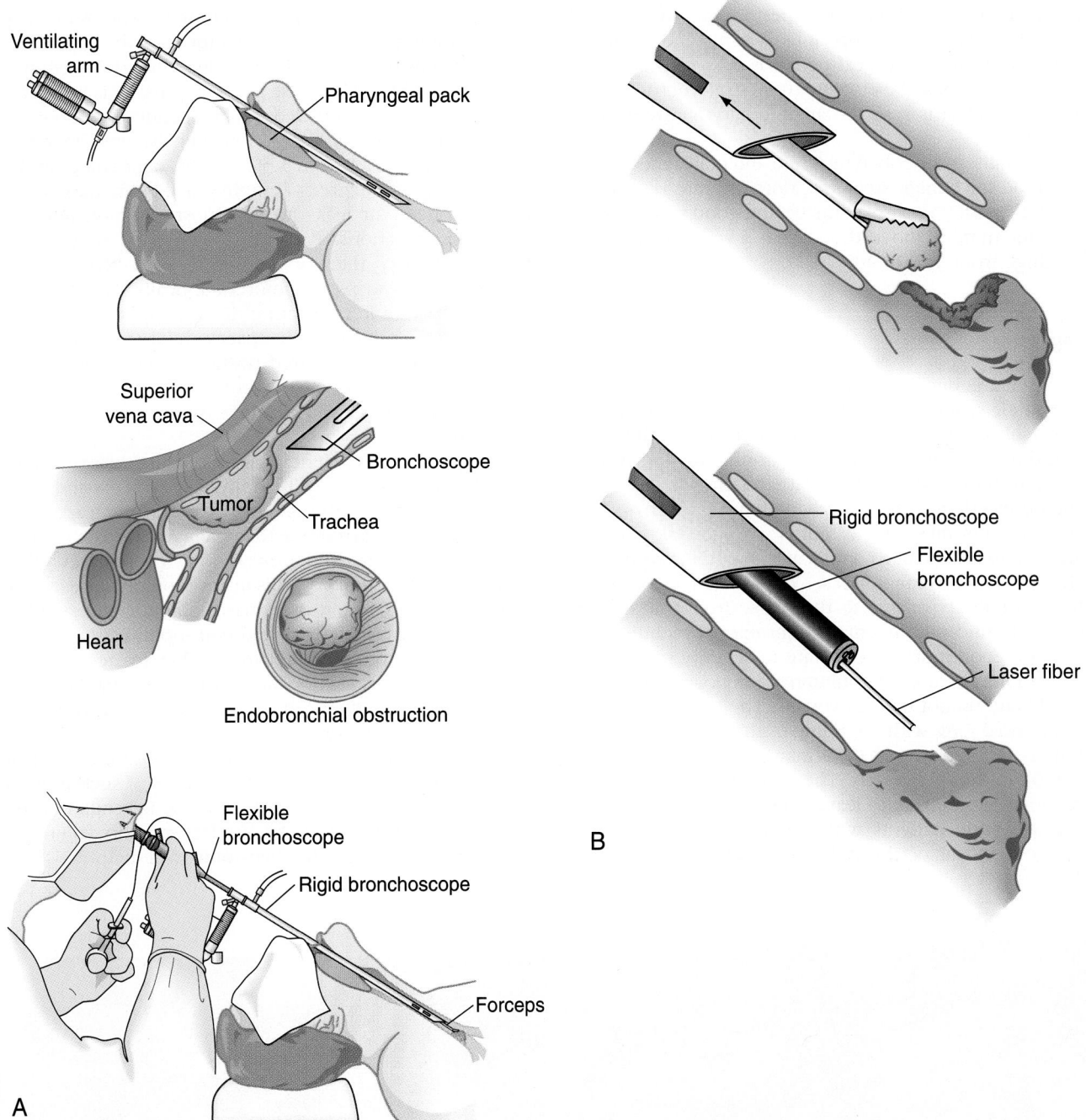

FIGURE 57-15. **A,** Proper technique for rigid bronchoscopy in a patient with a tracheal mass. *Top,* Pharyngeal packing is used to protect the esophagus. *Middle,* A nearly obstructing tumor is shown. *Bottom,* A flexible bronchoscope is placed into the rigid scope for the biopsy. This protects the airway. **B,** A technique for endoscopic resection of a tracheal mass with a rigid bronchoscope without *(top)* and with *(bottom)* use of the laser. (From Sugarbaker DJ, Mentzer SJ, Strauss G, Fried MP: Laser resection of endobronchial lesions: Use of the rigid and flexible bronchoscopes. Oper Tech Otolaryngol Head Neck Surg 3:93, 1992.)

with muscle, thymus, or fat. Resection of the damaged trachea with primary reanastomosis is performed. The endotracheal tube is placed with the cuff away from the anastomosis. If the tracheoinnominate fistula occurs from tube erosion, the surgeon tamponades the bleeding with digital pressure or packing anterior and inferior to the tube or tracheostomy prosthesis. This maneuver is easier with an endotracheal tube placed through the mouth or

stoma. One may simply perform a median sternotomy, divide the innominate artery, and cover as described earlier. Potential for a neurologic event does exist.

A tracheoesophageal fistula from cuff erosion may also occur. If the patient is ventilator dependent, then delayed repair may be necessary. The nasogastric tube should be removed, a gastrostomy and jejunostomy should be placed, and a low-pressure cuff should be used and placed below the lesion. If the patient is off the ventilator, then immediate repair should be performed. A cervical approach is used. The esophagus is separated from the trachea, and the esophageal defect is closed in layers. A muscle is interposed between the two structures. The damaged trachea is resected and primary anastomosis is performed.

The results as described by Grillo and colleagues[73] have been good for benign stenoses. Mortality rate is approximately 2% with 93% of patients having good results. With malignant tumors above the carina, 5-year survival rate may range from 25% to 40%.

EMPHYSEMA

Emphysema is defined as dilation and destruction of the terminal air spaces. These air cavities may be defined as blebs—subpleural air space separated from the lung by a thin pleural covering with only minor alveolar communications—or bullae—"larger than a bleb" with some destruction of the underlying lung parenchyma.

Bullous emphysema is either congenital without general lung disease or a complication of COPD with more or less generalized lung disease. The challenge is to separate the disability related to the bullae from that caused by the chronic emphysema or chronic bronchitis. The DLco is a good index of the state of severity of the generalized lung disease. On pulmonary angiography, bullae are cold and do not contain vessels. The bullae may compress normal lung with crowding of the relatively normal pulmonary vasculature. COPD may show abrupt narrowing and tapering of vessels. The surgical option includes resection of the bullae to leave functioning lung tissue.

Symptomatic patients with progressive dyspnea may undergo removal of the bullae with good results. The disease must be localized with the air space occupying at least 40% to 50% of one hemithorax. The remaining "good" lung parenchyma is compressed by the bulla. Simple removal of the bulla alone is required. Lobectomy is seldom indicated because good lung tissue is removed, which is frequently needed for independent function by these patients with significant lung impairment. Operative mortality rate varies from 1.5% to 10%, depending on the patient's age and degree of emphysema. Pulmonary sepsis and prolonged air leaks are the most common nonfatal major complications. Proper treatment and preparation with pulmonary therapy before surgery, exercise programs, and thin strips to reinforce surgically stapled suture lines are helpful in preventing these complications.

Cysts are congenital air spaces lined by epithelium; pneumatoceles are acquired postinflammatory air spaces with an epithelial lining. The cause is probably the result of biochemical alterations that permit alveolar wall destruction.

α_1-Antitrypsin deficiency is an autosomal recessive trait that affects 1% to 2% of all emphysema patients and commonly begins before the age of 40 years. Women are more likely to have this syndrome than men. Antitrypsin inhibits neutrophil elastase and other serine proteinases. This homeostatic function controls major proteolytic cascades. Absence of this serine proteinase inhibitor allows intrapulmonary elastase activity and neutrophil elastase activity (released from inflammatory cells) to act without control, thereby causing panacinar emphysema. Smoking significantly worsens α_1-antitrypsin deficiency actions and worsens this panacinar emphysema.

Pneumothorax may occur with emphysema. Conservative therapy often requires days to weeks of suction with chest tubes to obtain pleural symphysis. Resection of the bleb may be required (Fig. 57-16). If respiratory failure for pneumonia develops, tracheostomy will help in some

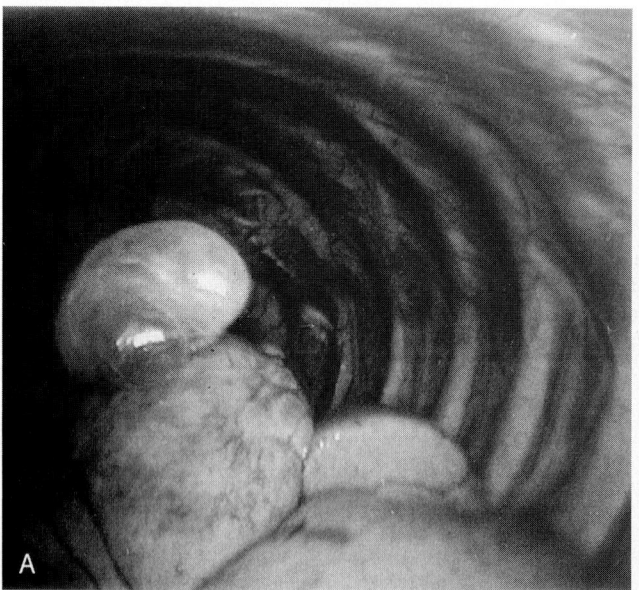
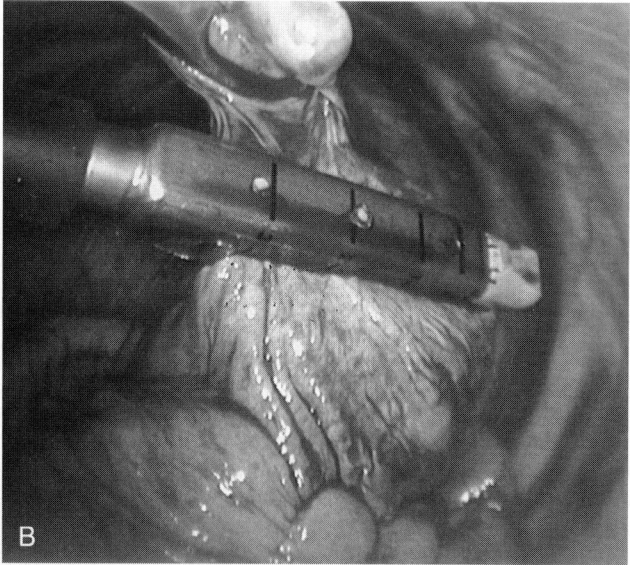

■ **FIGURE 57-16.** **A,** Thoracoscopic view of a typical apical bleb in a young patient who was first seen with spontaneous pneumothorax. **B,** Initial application of a linear stapler in excision of an apical bleb.

patients but makes it impossible for the patient to cough. Respiratory care and pulmonary hygiene are critical components of successful outcome.

Indications for surgical intervention include a significantly large bulla (one third to one half of a hemithorax) with symptoms and only mild diffuse lung disease. The surgical treatment must be individualized, because no criteria exist for predicting with certainty which patients will benefit from resection. Asymptomatic patients are generally observed, and infected bullae are resected. The mortality rate varies and the patients experience variable improvement.

Surgical therapy for emphysema exists. Although emphysema is diffuse within the lung, some areas may be worse than others. These areas may be identified by CT and subsequently resected. Lung volume reduction surgery (LVRS) removes areas of greater emphysematous involvement. The remaining lung tissue expands with improved elastic recoil and improved aeration and perfusion of the remaining lung. A recent prospective trial compared LVRS to medical treatment. Patients with predominantly upper lobe emphysema and low exercise capacity had lower mortality with LVRS than medical therapy (RR=0.47; p=0.005). In patients with non-upper lobe emphysema and high exercise capacity, mortality was higher in the LVRS group (RR=2.06, p=0.02).[74]

Lung transplantation is performed for COPD, including α_1-antitrypsin deficiency. Pulmonary fibrosis, primary pulmonary hypertension, and cystic fibrosis are other indications for lung transplantation. The recipient is required to have a significant functional disability but be ambulatory. The recipient should be free of chronic and debilitating disease (e.g., no hepatic, renal, or cardiac disease), have no other effective therapy available, have a stable nutritional status, have good social and psychological support, and have several years of life potentially remaining. Survival rate after lung transplantation is approximately 75% at 1 year, 60% at 2 years, and 50% at 5 years. The annual lung transplantation rate has begun to level off, and waiting times for lung transplants are currently approximately 18 months. Chronic immunosuppression with cyclosporine, azathioprine, and prednisone is required. Routine follow-up and screening for rejection is required. Transbronchial biopsy may be performed for diagnosis of acute rejection. Acute rejection usually occurs within 3 months of transplantation and is manifested with dyspnea, chest radiography with perihilar infiltrates, leukocytosis, and mild fever. FEV$_1$ is reduced. High-dose corticosteroids may be used for treatment. Chronic lung rejection problems include bronchiolitis obliterans and reduction in FEV$_1$.

Unilateral lung transplantation is more readily tolerated than double lung transplant. Early mortality rate ranges from 8% to 21% as a result of infection or organ failure. The 5-year survival rate approaches 60%.[75]

DIFFUSE LUNG DISEASE AND OPEN LUNG BIOPSY

The surgeon's role in diffuse lung disease is to obtain a diagnosis, typically by open lung biopsy. The patient has usually undergone several diagnostic bronchoscopies and often a transbronchial biopsy. The chest radiograph may demonstrate an alveolar pattern (fluffy with air bronchograms) or an interstitial pattern (ground-glass or granular appearance, indicating a diffuse increase in interstitial tissue) (Box 57-10).

Sarcoidosis affects the lungs in 90% of patients with this diagnosis, causing symptoms of dyspnea and dry cough. Foci of noncaseating epithelioid granulomas may be found in any part of the body. Ten to 20 percent of patients are asymptomatic, 20% to 40% are first seen with an acute form with fever and other significant symptoms, and 40% to 50% have insidious respiratory complaints without constitutional symptoms. Severe progressive pulmonary fibrosis may develop in 10% to 20%. Bilateral hilar mediastinal lymph nodes are involved in 60% to 80% of patients. Biopsy of these mediastinal lymph nodes may be required for diagnosis and often may be the only surgical procedure that is needed. Skin lesions such as erythema nodosum, plaques, squamous nodules, and maculopapular eruption occur in approximately 25% of patients, and eye involvement (uveitis) may occur in 25% of patients.

For diagnosis, clinical criteria and biopsy are needed. Bronchoscopy and transbronchial biopsy are good, and open lung biopsy is rarely needed. Corticosteroids may be used for treatment. An open lung biopsy is generally not necessary when the lung picture is typical of a previously known cause; however, open lung biopsy is generally necessary for those diseases for which the cause is not known.

In an acute setting, an open lung biopsy is often not warranted for diffuse lung disease or patients with chronic ventilatory requirements. The value of open lung biopsy in this clinical setting is low and typically no better than the best medical management in intensive care. An open lung biopsy should not be performed unless the results of open lung biopsy will modify subsequent treatment, such as the initiation of protocol-based treatment for experimental antibiotics.

ACUTE RESPIRATORY DISTRESS SYNDROME

The acute, or adult, respiratory distress syndrome (ARDS) is a complex biologic and clinical process. This acute deterioration of pulmonary function occurs exclusive of pulmonary edema, pneumonia, or exacerbation of COPD. Approximately 50,000 cases occur each year in the United States, with a mortality rate of 30% to 70%. Some causes of ARDS are listed in Box 57-11.

The initial clinical presentation of dyspnea, tachypnea, hypoxemia, and mild hypocapnia is nonspecific. A chest radiograph may show diffuse bilateral infiltrates secondary to increased interstitial fluid. Pathologically, vascular congestion occurs with alveolar collapse, edema, and inflammatory cell infiltration. The underlying mechanism is increased pulmonary capillary permeability with extravasation of intravascular fluid and protein into the interstitium and alveoli. The leukocyte is the most prominent mediator of this injury. Stimuli such as sepsis activate the complement pathway, causing recruitment of leukocytes to the site of the infection. The lung releases potent

Box 57-10. Classification of Diffuse Lung Diseases

Infections (more commonly cause focal disease, granuloma formation)

Viruses—especially influenza, cytomegalovirus
Bacteria—tuberculosis, all kinds of regular bacteria, Rocky Mountain spotted fever
Fungi—all types can cause diffuse disease
Parasites—*Pneumocystis,* toxoplasmosis, paragonimiasis, among others

Occupational causes

Mineral dusts
Chemical fumes—NO_2 (silo filler's disease), Cl, NH_3, SO_2, CCl_4, Br, HF, HCl, HNO_3, kerosene, acetylene

Neoplastic disease

Lymphangitic spread
Hematogenous metastases
Leukemia, lymphoma, broncholoalveolar cell cancer

Congenital—familial

Niemann-Pick, Gaucher's, neurofibromatosis, and tuberous fibrosis

Metabolic/unknown

Liver disease, uremia, inflammatory bowel disease

Physical agents

Radiation, O_2 toxicity, thermal injury, blast injury

Heart failure/multiple pulmonary emboli

Immunologic causes

Hypersensitivity pneumonia

Inhaled antigens
Farmer's lung (actinomycosis)
Bagassosis (sugar cane)
Malt workers (*Aspergillus*)
Byssinosis (cotton)

Drug reactions

Hydralazine, busulfan, nitrofurantoin (Macrodantin), hexamethonium, methysergide, bleomycin

Collagen diseases

Scleroderma, rheumatoid, systemic lupus erythematosus, dermatomyositis, Wegener's granulomatosis, Goodpasture's syndrome

Other

Sarcoidosis
Histiocytosis
Idiopathic hemosiderosis
Pulmonary alveolar proteinosis
Diffuse interstitial fibrosis, idiopathic pulmonary fibrosis
Desquamative interstitial pneumonia
Eosinophilic pneumonia (*Note:* some are caused by drugs, actinomycosis, parasites)
Lymphangioleiomyomatosis

Box 57-11. Causes of Adult Respiratory Distress Syndrome

Extrathoracic sepsis
Blunt chest trauma
Nonthoracic trauma
Shock
Burns
Aspiration pneumonia
Diffuse infectious pneumonia
Nonbacterial pneumonia (viral, mycoplasma, legionnaires' disease, *Pneumocystis carinii*)
Miscellaneous events
    Smoke inhalation
    Oxygen toxicity
    Neurogenic pulmonary edema
    Ingestion of toxic drugs
    Acute hypersensitivity reactions

mediators such as oxygen free radicals, arachidonic acid metabolites, and proteases. If the underlying disease is not controlled, these changes progress to vascular thromboses and interstitial fibrosis and to hyaline membrane deposition in the alveoli. This process causes hypoxemia, pulmonary hypertension, CO_2 retention, secondary infections, and eventually right-sided heart failure, hypoxia, and death. Other criteria include impaired oxygenation with the PaO_2/FIO_2 ratio less than 200 mm Hg. As well, pulmonary edema is present without cardiac failure and a pulmonary capillary wedge pressure is less than 18 mm Hg (noncardiac pulmonary edema).

The outcome of ARDS is related to the initial injury stimulus. Treatment is directed to improve oxygenation with optimal pulmonary hygiene, intubation, and pressure ventilation. Maintaining an inspired oxygen concentration as low as possible and positive end-expiratory pressure as low as possible to maintain adequate oxygenation and CO_2 exchange is helpful. A Swan-Ganz catheter to optimize hemodynamics, to reduce pulmonary artery pressure, and to improve coronary perfusion can be considered. Inotropes, corticosteroids, prostaglandin inhibitors, and oxygen free radical scavengers have been examined, yet, to date, they have failed to consistently improve pulmonary function or mortality rate for patients with ARDS.

HIGH-PRESSURE JET VENTILATION

High-pressure jet ventilation can be used during bronchoscopy and carinal resection and to improve oxygenation in patients with bronchopleural fistula or in the noncompliant lung in patients with respiratory failure. Complications include pneumothorax, hypotension at high driving pressures, blocked endotracheal tube from encrustation at the end of the tube, and a decrease in cardiac output, which may be prevented with inotropes.

Its most frequent use is in managing respiratory failure in neonates.

BACTERIAL INFECTIONS

Bronchiectasis is an infection of the bronchial wall and surrounding lung with sufficient severity to cause destruction and dilation of the air passages. This condition is decreasing in frequency and severity because of the use of antibiotics. There are numerous predisposing factors, including cystic fibrosis, α_1-antitrypsin deficiency, various immunodeficiency states, Kartagener's syndrome (sinusitis, bronchiectasis, situs inversus, and hypomotile cilia), and bronchial obstruction from foreign body, extrinsic lymph nodes that compress the bronchus, neoplasm, or mucous plug. The distribution is primarily in the basal segments of the lower lobes. Destructive changes and dilation of the bronchi accompany the infection.

With use of antibiotics, it has become rare to see an emaciated febrile patient coughing up large amounts of foul sputum accompanied by clubbing, cyanosis, and hemoptysis. Currently, frequent respiratory infections are typical and sputum production is minimal except during exacerbations and acute infections. Mild hemoptysis may occur; massive hemoptysis is rare. Frequently, symptoms can be controlled with medical management. Patients can be evaluated with chest radiography and CT. CT of the chest is good at showing bronchiectasis.

Bronchoscopy cannot differentiate bronchitis from bronchiectasis. Bronchoscopy can be performed to clear secretions and, when the diagnosis is suspected, to rule out cancer, foreign body, or stricture. Cultures may be obtained to facilitate antibiotic treatment. Bronchography is a method of diagnosis and may be required when surgery is being considered, although it (Fig. 57-17) has generally been replaced by CT. Dilation of the bronchi and no feathering of distal airways can be visualized. Medical treatment should be optimized; this includes discontinuation of smoking and institution of postural drainage, bronchodilator medications, and oral antibiotics.

Surgical management may be performed if the disease is irreversible or if there is failure of medical therapy with recurrent pneumonia, hemoptysis affecting a normal lifestyle, or persistent sputum production greater than 1 to 2 ounces daily. The disease should be localized and the patient should be physiologically suitable for resection. One segment of involvement with bronchiectasis is not enough to consider resection. Disease limited to but involving one lobe is best treated surgically. If bilateral bronchiectasis exists, medical management should continue. Results of treatment are good in 80% to 90% of patients.

Lung Abscess

The incidence of lung abscess is decreasing in frequency as a result of use of antibiotics.[76] A lung abscess may occur from an infection behind a blocked bronchus. The infection is usually anaerobic and may be associated with alcohol abuse, a debilitated or elderly individual, or esophageal disease with aspiration. Lung abscess used to occur after tonsillectomy or tooth extraction, but this has become a rare event. Hematogenous spread from bacteremia may occur if congestive heart failure or debilitating disease is present, such as in the very old, the very young, patients who use intravenous drugs, and patients on corticosteroids. These areas of infection are usually multiple and rarely require operative intervention. *Staphylococcus* bacteremia is frequently associated with lung abscess. Necrotizing pneumonia from *Klebsiella* may rapidly destroy the involved lung with minimal surrounding reaction. This cause is decreasing with use of antibiotics. Rupture of a lung abscess may yield empyema and pneumothorax. Lung abscess may also be superimposed on structural abnormalities, for example, as a bronchogenic cyst, sequestration, bleb, or tuberculosis or fungal cavities.

In patients with aspiration progressing to lung abscess, the location is more commonly found on the right than the left. The location may occur in the lateral divisions of the anterior and posterior segments of the upper lobe, the axillary subsegment, or the superior segment of the lower lobe. Clinical features are similar to those of pneumonia, including fever, cough, leukocytosis, pleuritic pain, and sputum production. The chest radiograph and the CT scan of the chest may demonstrate a rounded area of consolidation early and an air-fluid level on upright or decubitus chest radiography later.

The differential diagnosis includes loculated empyema, which may be treated with drainage, epiphrenic diverticulum (in which the patient is not septic), or tuberculosis or fungus cavity. These cavities do not retain fluid, so no air-fluid level is present; however, they may contain debris or a fungus ball. *Aspergillus* may present in this manner (Fig. 57-18). Medical management is with antibiotics and pulmonary care (e.g., re-expansion). Bronchoscopy may be performed for diagnosis to rule out foreign body, stenosis, or cancer. It also may be used for treatment to assist in drainage of the cavity either directly or by way of transbronchial catheterization of the cavity. Most patients (85% to 95%) respond to medical management with rapid decrease in fluid, collapse of the walls, and complete healing in 3 to 4 months. Patients with long-standing symptoms greater than 3 months before treatment or cavities greater than 4 to 6 cm are less likely to respond.

Surgical therapy is indicated for persistent cavity (>2 cm and thick walled) after 8 weeks of medical therapy, failure to clear sepsis, hemoptysis (often small sentinel hemorrhage before a massive hemorrhage), and to exclude cancer. If a lung abscess ruptures into the pleural cavity, simple drainage may suffice, with the patient being managed for empyema or bronchopleural fistula. Lobectomy is typically required; the mortality rate is 1% to 5%. Occasionally, external drainage may be required in critically ill patients if pleural symphysis has occurred.

Other Bronchopulmonary Disorders

Bronchopulmonary disorders caused by inflammatory lymph node disease are usually caused by tuberculosis or

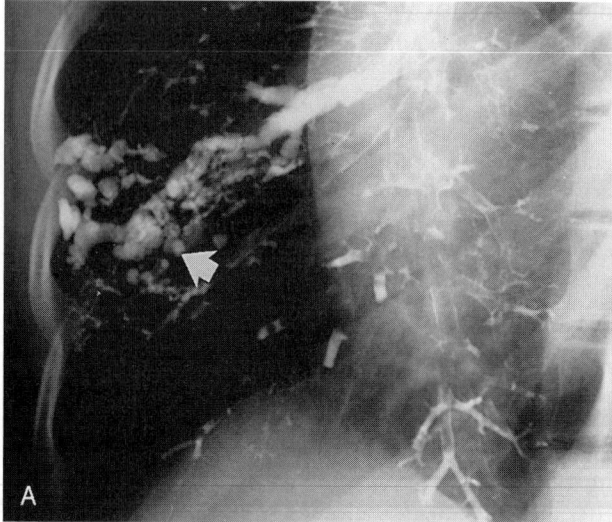

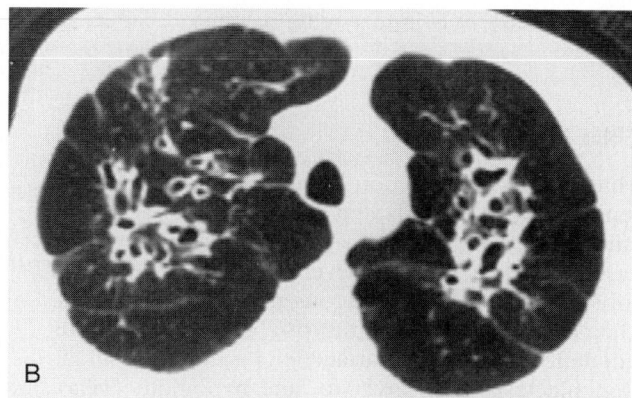

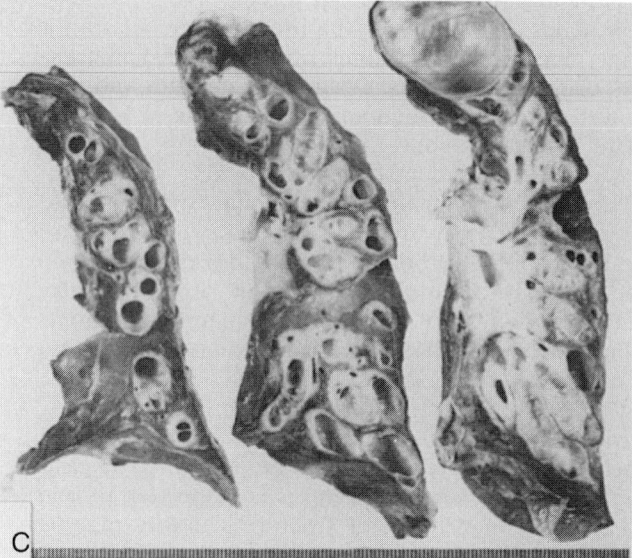

FIGURE 57-17. **A,** Contrast bronchography in a patient with saccular bronchiectasis *(arrow)* in the middle lobe. **B,** Computed tomogram of the chest of a 30-year-old man with multisegmental bronchiectasis involving both lungs. Note the abnormally dilated airways extending into the lung parenchyma bilaterally. **C,** Lung specimen demonstrating grossly dilated subsegmental bronchi caused by bronchiectasis. (**C** From Bolman RM, Wolfe WG: Bronchiectasis and bronchopulmonary sequestration. Surg Clin North Am 60:867, 1980.)

histoplasmosis. Lobar atelectasis, hemoptysis, or broncholithiasis can occur. Bronchial compressive disease typically occurs most commonly in the middle lobe. More than 20% is caused by cancer. This condition results in repeated infection in the same area of the lung, which usually responds to antibiotics. The differential diagnosis includes endobronchial tumors in adults and foreign body aspiration in children. Bronchoscopy is essential to rule out cancer and foreign body and to evaluate for stricture. Medical management is required to treat infection. Surgery is indicated to treat bronchostenosis, irreversible bronchiectasis, or severe recurrent infection.

Broncholithiasis is a calcified node tightly adherent to a bronchus. Innocent hemoptysis may occur even with a negative chest radiograph. Sudden bleeding caused by erosion of a small bronchial artery and mucosa by a spicule in the calcified node causes this hemoptysis. Bright red blood occurs, ranging from 5 to 500 mL and generally always stops with sedation. This hemoptysis is almost never massive (>600 mL in 24 hours). Bronchoscopy is possible during a bleeding episode to locate the lobe or site of the bleeding. Nasal or pharyngeal lesions should be excluded.

Organizing pneumonia may replace lung parenchyma with scar tissue or persistent atelectasis or consolidation. Initially, an acute pneumonia develops and then a persistent shadow. If the shadow or mass does not clear in 6 to 8 weeks, then resection should be performed to exclude carcinoma. The differential diagnosis includes pneumonia, congenital abnormality, and aneurysm of the aorta.

Mycobacterial Infections

Tuberculosis infects approximately 7% of patients exposed, and it develops in 5% to 10% of those patients infected. A primary infection develops. The exudative

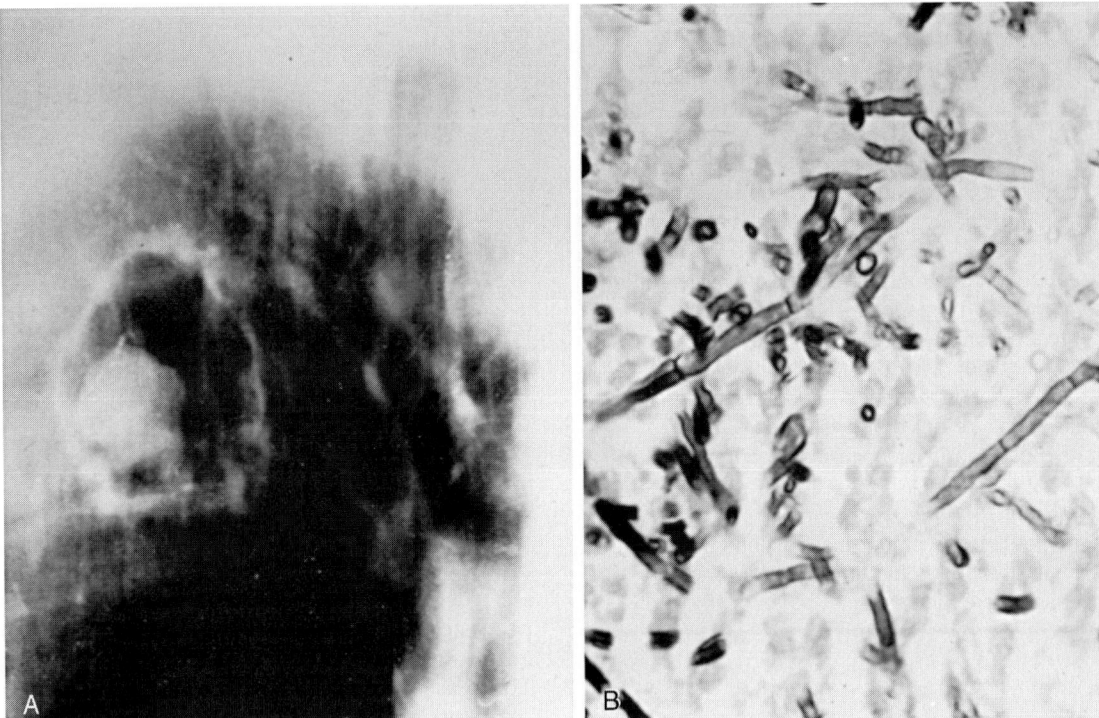

■ FIGURE 57-18. **A,** Linear tomogram of the lung demonstrates an aspergilloma ("fungus ball") within a large cavitary lesion within the lung parenchyma. The fungus ball is often unattached within the cavity and is located in the most gravity-dependent area of the cavity. It can alter its position as the patient changes position. **B,** The coarse, fragmented, septate mycelia of *Aspergillus fumigatus.* (**A** from Aslam PA, Larkin J, Eastridge CA, Hughes FA Jr: Endocavitary infusion through percutaneous endobronchial catheter. Chest 57:94, 1970. **B** from Takaro T: Thoracic mycotic infections. *In* Lewis' Practice of Surgery. New York, Hoeber Medical Division, Harper & Row, 1968.)

response progresses to caseous necrosis. Postprimary tuberculosis tends to occur in apical and posterior segments of the upper lobes and superior segments of the lower lobes. Healing occurs with fibrosis and contracture. Extensive caseation with cavitation may occur early. Coalescing areas of caseous necrosis may form cavities. There are frequently incomplete septations and lobulations. Septations supplied by bronchial arteries can cause hemoptysis if eroded and may be secondarily infected by other organisms.[77]

Bronchoscopy may be required for patients not responding to medical management. Cancer should be excluded with a newly identified mass on chest radiography even with a positive TB skin test and acid-fast bacillus–negative sputum. Medical management is with isoniazid, rifampin, ethambutol, streptomycin, or pyrazinamide. The initial treatment for the disease is combination therapy (e.g., isoniazid plus rifampin or other drugs).

Surgical therapy may be considered when medical therapy fails and persistent tuberculosis-positive sputum remains as well as when surgically correctable residua of tuberculosis may be of potential danger to the patient.[78,79] This is not the same management as for atypical mycobacteria; many of these patients remain clinically well even with positive sputum. Some indications for surgery are listed in Box 57-12.

Surgical options include resection, which is the procedure of choice in most instances. Pleural adhesions and granulomas in peribronchial nodes and chronic inflammation make resection difficult. Preservation of lung tissue should be a goal of the treatment. Surgical complications are doubled if the sputum is positive for mycobacteria tuberculosis and decreased if remaining lung tissue is fully expanded. Infectious complications include empyema, bronchopleural fistula, endobronchial spread of the disease, and higher mortality.

Thoracoplasty or collapse therapy is infrequently required. Thoracoplasty may be used to control the postresection empyema space and, rarely, if ever, to manage parenchymal disease alone. This technique may be used in patients who fail medical management and who were not otherwise candidates for resection. Patients with extensive disease and positive sputum or chronic active endobronchial disease may also be considered. Plombage may be preferred over staged conventional thoracoplasty, because it requires only one operation; there is no paradoxical chest motion and chest wall deformity. Cavernostomy, or external drainage of a tuberculous cavity with a

Box 57-12. Potential Indications for Surgery for Pulmonary Tuberculosis

Open positive cavity after 3 to 6 months of chemotherapy, especially if resistant mycobacteria

Persistent positive sputum with pathology (destroyed lung, atelectasis, bronchiectasis, bronchostenosis) amenable to resection

Negative sputum *but* destroyed lung, blocked cavity, tuberculoma—consider for resection

Localized infection with atypical mycobacteria

Tuberculous bronchiectasis of lower and middle lobes (usually occurs in upper lobes—good drainage; lower and middle lobes do not drain well)

Open negative cavities if thick walled, slow response, or unreliable patient

To exclude cancer

Recurrent or persistent hemoptysis: resection if greater than 600 mL of blood is lost in 24 hours or less

Pleural disease where indicated

TABLE 57-4.   Extrapulmonary Manifestations of Fungal Infections

Actinomycosis	Cervicofacial, chest wall
Nocardiosis	Chest wall, central nervous system (CNS)
Histoplasmosis	Marrow, adrenal
Coccidioidomycosis	Bone (however, usually just lung)
Blastomycosis	Skin > genitourinary system
Cryptococcosis	CNS
Aspergillosis	CNS, blood vessels
Mucormycosis	Rhinocerebral, blood vessels

chest tube or open drainage, may be used to control a large cavity with positive sputum or massive bleeding in a patient who was unable to tolerate resection or collapse therapy.

Fungal and Parasitic Infections

The surgical management of fungal infections includes diagnosis and management of complications of fungal disease. Frequently, cancer has to be excluded or other infectious or benign conditions confirmed. Medical management may be considered an initial treatment for fungal diseases in the lung and as part of the patient's overall management.

Immunocompromised patients suffer from aspergillosis as the most frequent opportunistic infection, followed by candidiasis, nocardiosis, and mucormycosis. Normal, or immunocompetent, patients may be affected by histoplasmosis, coccidioidomycosis, or blastomycosis. Both groups may be affected by actinomycosis and cryptococcosis. Diagnosis is most often made by sputum examination using potassium hydroxide preparations. Cultures are poor and may take some time for results to be obtained; Papanicolaou smear cytology may be best. Silver methenamine stain is key to the evaluation. Extrapulmonary involvement of various fungal diseases is listed in Table 57-4. Most infections are self-limited and do not require treatment. Intravenous or oral antifungal agents may be used for treatment of the diseases.

Histoplasmosis is the most common of all fungal infections in the United States and is most frequently a serious systemic fungal disease.[80] *Histoplasma capsulatum* is endemic to the Mississippi Valley as well as portions of the southwestern United States. A high percentage of patients are affected, usually with a subclinical form of this disease. An inoculum (from the mycelial form found in soil, decaying materials, and bat or bird guano) can produce an acute pneumonic illness in immunocompetent hosts and usually resolves without specific treatment. The yeast form exists in macrophages or within the cytoplasm of the alveoli. Pathologic examination demonstrates granulomas (like tuberculosis) or caseating epithelioid granulomas. Calcified nodes in the lung, mediastinum, spleen, and liver may occur. The chest radiograph may demonstrate central or target calcification or concentric laminar calcification. Any form can have arthralgias or erythema nodosum or erythema multiforme. The localized form is usually an acute pneumonia, self-limited, and rarely severe. A solitary pulmonary nodule may be a residual finding of acute pneumonia and should be resected unless proper calcification is identified. The lymphogenous reaction to *Histoplasma* causes mediastinal lymph node enlargement and may cause middle lobe syndrome, bronchiectasis, esophageal traction diverticulum, tracheoesophageal fistula, constrictive pericarditis, or fibrosing mediastinitis with superior vena cava syndrome, or other problems relating to compression of mediastinal structures.

Coccidioidomycosis is endemic to the Southwest and is localized in the soil. It is second only to histoplasmosis in frequency. Inhaling the organism results in a primary lung disease that is usually self-limited (Fig. 57-19).

Actinomyces is a bacterium that is not found free in nature. It produces a chronic anaerobic endogenous infection, actinomycosis, deep within a wound. "Sulfur granules" draining from infected sinuses are microcolonies (Fig. 57-20). The cervicofacial form is the most common. The thoracic form usually occurs as pulmonary parenchymal disease resembling cancer. The treatment is most commonly penicillin. Surgery may occasionally be required for radical excision of the chest wall disease and empyema.

Nocardia is an aerobic bacterium widely disseminated in soil and domestic animals; it was formerly rare, although it is increasing in immunocompromised patients. Nocardiosis resembles actinomycosis in invading the chest wall and produces subcutaneous abscesses and

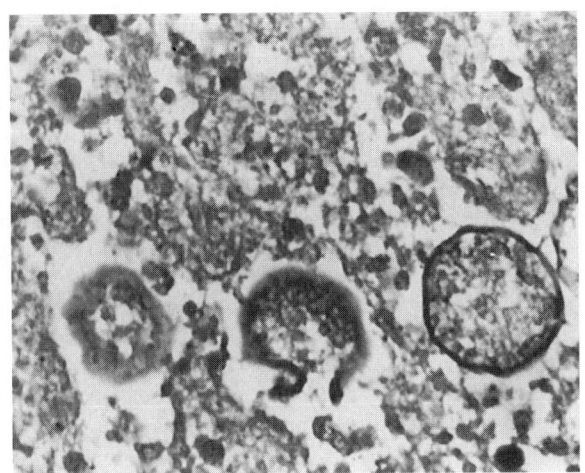

FIGURE 57-19. Microscopic sections of a coccidioidal granuloma (×400) show spherules packed with endospores. (From Scott S, Takaro T: Thoracic mycotic and actinomycotic infections. *In* Shields TW [ed]: General Thoracic Surgery, 4th ed. Baltimore, Williams & Wilkins, 1994.)

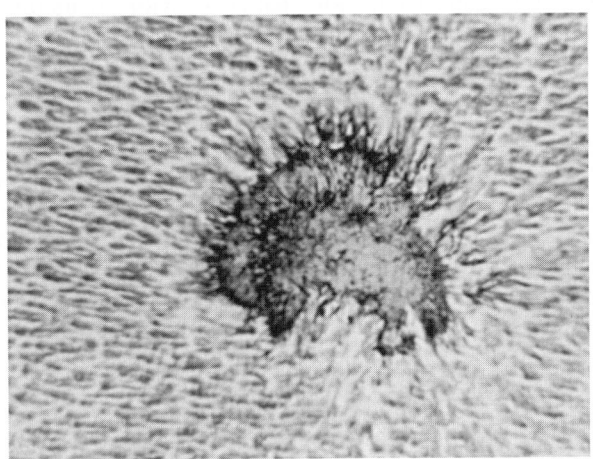

FIGURE 57-20. Actinomycotic granule shows branching filaments of a microscopic colony of *Actinomyces israelii*. Gomori stain, ×250.

Open lung biopsy may be required to make a diagnosis of cryptococcosis, which is widely disseminated in soil, dust, and pigeon guano. Pathologically, the organism appears as round, budding yeasts, with wide capsules and granulomas. It is the second most frequent lethal fungus after histoplasmosis. Lungs are frequently involved. The disease is usually mild. Meningitis is the most frequent cause of death. Surgery may be required for open lung biopsy for diagnosis or to exclude lung cancer.

Aspergillosis is an opportunistic infection, characterized by coarse fragmented septa; hyphae are noted. The chest radiograph may demonstrate a crescent radiolucency next to a rounded mass. Cavities may form because of destruction of the underlying pulmonary parenchyma; and debris and hyphae may coalesce and form a fungus ball, which lies free in the cavity and can roll around. Prophylactic resection is controversial, although some recommend resection if isolated disease is present in good risk patients.

Surgery is infrequently used in the management of mucormycosis other than to establish a diagnosis. Mucormycosis is rare, opportunistic, and rapidly progressive. The appearance is that of a black mold; it has wide nonseptate branching hyphae. The infection causes blood vessels to thrombose and lung tissue to infarct. Clinically, the rhinocerebral form occurs much more frequently than the pulmonary form of consolidation and cavities. Medical management is with cessation of corticosteroids and antineoplastic drugs and initiation of amphotericin, and control of diabetes is undertaken. The disease is often too advanced for effective treatment.

Candida is a small, thin-walled budding yeast that occurs in immunocompromised patients (Fig. 57-21). Lung involvement alone is rare. Surgery may be required to confirm the diagnosis of the infection.

Surgery may also be used to manage the sequelae and complications of parasitic infections. Infections with

sinuses draining sulfur granules. Surgery is performed to exclude cancer, to obtain a diagnosis, or to treat complications of the disease.

Treatment is often with amphotericin for those patients who are severely ill, such as those who are immunocompromised and have positive sputum cultures. Other options include ketoconazole or itraconazole for non–life-threatening disease.

Surgery may be considered for treatment of cavitary disease or complications of cavitary disease. Amphotericin should be used perioperatively. Indications for surgery include thick-walled or greater than 2-cm cavities, enlarging cavities, ruptured cavities, secondary bacterial infections, and severe recurrent hemoptysis.

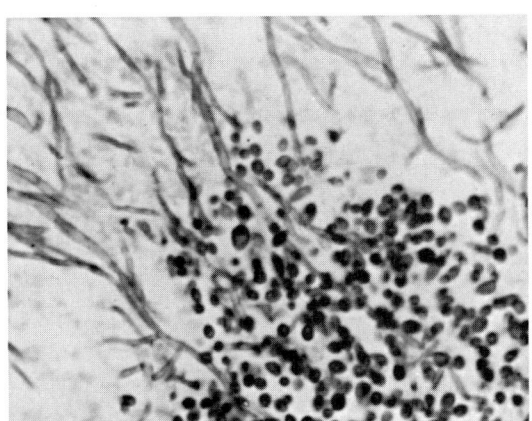

FIGURE 57-21. *Candida albicans* with both the mycelial and the yeast forms. (From Takaro T: Thoracic mycotic infections. *In* Lewis' Practice of Surgery. New York, Hoeber Medical Division, Harper & Row, 1968.)

Entamoeba histolytica are usually confined to the right lower thorax and are related to extension from a liver abscess below the diaphragm by way of direct extension or lymphatics to the right thorax. Metronidazole (Flagyl) is usually effective, although Flagyl and tube drainage may be required for treatment of empyema. Open resection is infrequently required. Similarly, infection with *Echinococcus* may occur. The hydatid cyst may rupture, flooding the lung or producing a severe hypersensitivity reaction. A lung abscess could occur with compression of the airway, great vessels, or esophagus. Surgery, if feasible, may include simple enucleation by way of a cleavage of planes between the cyst and the normal tissue. Aspiration and hypertonic saline 10% may be performed before enucleation. Positive pressure on the lung should be maintained until the cyst is out to prevent contamination, soilage, or hypersensitivity reaction. Nonoperative therapy for small asymptomatic calcified cyst may be considered. Paragonimiasis is another common infection and common cause of hemoptysis in Asia.[81] In endemic areas, prevalence may reach 5%, and hemoptysis from paragonimiasis in one Asian population (16%) exceeded that from tuberculosis (3%).[82,83]

Pneumocystis carinii is an opportunistic infection that is positive on silver methenamine stain. Bronchoalveolar lavage obtains the diagnosis in more than 90% of patients. However, lung biopsy may be required to confirm the diagnosis.

MASSIVE HEMOPTYSIS

Massive hemoptysis may be defined as greater than 500 to 600 mL of blood loss from the lungs in 24 hours.[84] The current mortality rate is approximately 13% and is related to drowning or suffocation rather than exsanguination. Causes of hemoptysis are listed in Box 57-13.

Diagnosis and treatment of massive hemoptysis typically include a chest radiograph and emergency bronchoscopy. Rigid bronchoscopy with an 8.5-mm or larger bronchoscope is needed. A 10-mm scope is preferred.

Flexible bronchoscopy is usually inadequate for treatment of hemoptysis, but it may be considered for observation if active bleeding has stopped. Blood should be drawn for type and crossmatch, and the interventional radiologist should be notified if angiographic embolization is anticipated. Often, patients have been seen previously with slight hemoptysis and have undergone diagnostic evaluation consisting of a chest radiograph and CT of the chest. These studies may provide additional information to guide the surgeon in palliating hemoptysis.

Treatment options must be guided by the clinical situation and findings. Bronchoscopy under general anesthesia is performed, and bleeding is controlled so as to prevent soiling the contralateral (uninvolved) lung. Conservative management may consist simply of bronchoscopy, clearing the airway of blood, cough suppression (with codeine), and rest (Box 57-14).

Patients with hemoptysis from cystic fibrosis may do well with expectant treatment of hemoptysis, which may require tamponade using a balloon catheter. Patients with aspergilloma fungus balls are at high risk for fatal hemorrhage and should be treated aggressively and undergo resection when possible.

Angiographic catheterization for massive hemoptysis may be considered for patients with hemoptysis and inability to localize a bleeding site.[85] A relative contraindication to angiographic catheterization and embolization is the contribution of the bronchial arteries to the blood supply of the spinal cord or a common origin of the blood supply to the bronchi and the spinal cord. The risk of quadriplegia must be considered in light of the overall patient condition. Embolization is carried out with small particles of polyvinyl alcohol or other synthetic embolic material to occlude vessels at a peripheral level. Some reports show that bleeding is controlled in 70% of patients, but 50% rebleed. Re-embolization may be

---

Box 57-13. Causes of Hemoptysis

Lung cancer
Lung abscess
Cavitary aspergillosis
Tuberculosis
Bronchiectasis
Swan-Ganz catheterization
Cystic fibrosis
Broncholithiasis
Foreign body
Transbronchial lung biopsy
Tuberculosis

Box 57-14. Treatment Options for Massive Hemoptysis

Treatment of intrabronchial lesion by laser or topical epinephrine (transient effect only)
Definitive surgical resection (probably most applicable)
Expectant management (observation, cough suppression, rest)
Bronchoscopic lavage with iced saline
Fogarty catheter tamponade
Intracavitary instillation of antimicrobial medications for poor-risk patients with mycetomas
Cavernostomy with packing for patients too sick to undergo resection
Plombage (for active cavitary tuberculosis)
Bronchial arterial embolization by interventional radiology
Mass resection with large stapler (*last resort*)

Box 57-15. Potential Indications for Angiographic Catheterization

Cystic fibrosis
Bilateral chronic pulmonary disease and inability to localize a bleeding site
Nonresectable malignancy, primary or metastatic
Vital capacity of less than 40% of predicted value
Recurrent hemoptysis after surgery

repeated. Angiographic catheterization indications are given in Box 57-15.

PULMONARY EMBOLISM

Pulmonary embolism is a spectrum of disease that ranges from the clinically insignificant pulmonary microembolus to a catastrophic instantaneously fatal massive pulmonary thrombus obstructing both pulmonary arteries.[86] Thrombi most commonly develop in the veins of the lower leg from stasis and a hypercoagulable state, and they propagate proximally to the deep veins of the leg and pelvis. As these clots become larger and as the veins become larger, the propensity for these clots to dislodge and embolize to the lungs increases. When this occurs, a chain reaction of events takes place: the pulmonary artery blood supply to those sections of the lung is occluded, vasoactive agents are released with elevation of pulmonary vascular resistance, a shunt develops as the pulmonary blood flow is redistributed, and pulmonary edema may occur. Alveolar dead space is increased and gas exchange is impaired. Depending on the size of the thrombus or the patient's reaction to the embolic event, right ventricular work is increased. With increased afterload, right ventricular dysfunction or failure may occur. Right ventricular hypokinesis with a normal arterial blood pressure is a poor prognostic indicator. Paradoxical embolus from a patent foramen ovale may occur.

Pulmonary embolism may account for up to 3% of postoperative surgical deaths and has been found in 24% of 5477 patients in an autopsy series.[87] Untreated pulmonary embolism has a 30% hospital mortality rate, whereas treated patients have a mortality rate estimated at approximately 2%.[88] In the general population, the incidence of pulmonary embolus is estimated to be 1 in 1000 per year. Pulmonary embolism may occur in more than 250,000 patients annually in the United States with mortality rate of 15% to 17%.[86]

Risk factors for pulmonary embolus may include high body-mass index, cigarette smoking, hypertension, and surgery. Activated protein C is an extremely potent anticoagulant. Resistance to activated protein C may be transmitted as an autosomal dominant trait in some patients with a propensity for venous thrombosis.[89] Routine laboratory tests in the past for a hypercoagulable state or pulmonary embolus included an assay of antithrombin III, protein C, and protein S; however, deficiencies in these proteins rarely occur.[86] Currently, recommended testing should include (1) factor V Leiden mutation (the most common hypercoagulable state), (2) hyperhomocystinemia (readily treated with B vitamins), and (3) lupus anticoagulant (because intensive anticoagulation may be required).

Activated protein C is a potent endogenous anticoagulant. The genetic changes responsible for resistance to activated protein C are transmitted in an autosomal dominant manner. A point mutation occurs in the gene coding for coagulation factor V (which is responsible for activated protein C resistance). This is the "factor V Leiden mutation," which makes activated factor V more difficult for activated protein C to cleave and inactivate. The risk of venous thrombosis in patients with this trait is increased twofold to fourfold. Plasma hyperhomocystinemia is caused by deficiencies of folate and an inadequate supply of B vitamins (B_6 and B_{12}). Risk of deep vein thrombosis is increased two to three times in patients with hyperhomocystinemia. When both hyperhomocystinemia and factor V Leiden mutation are present, the risk of venous thrombosis is increased 10-fold. As well, patients with antiphospholipid antibodies or the lupus anticoagulant are associated with an increased risk of venous thrombosis. These patients may not have systemic lupus.

The clinical presentation of pulmonary embolus ranges from dyspnea, tachypnea, and chest pain to instant death. Chest pain, hypotension, hemoptysis, or cyanosis may occur. Physical examination may include signs of right ventricular dysfunction such as enlarged neck veins and an accentuated second pulmonary sound on cardiac examination. About 40% of patients with pulmonary embolism have right ventricular dysfunction.[90] The normal right ventricle with acute pulmonary embolism cannot tolerate a sustained mean positive air pressure of more than 40 mm Hg. These patients may be unresponsive to medical therapy with persistent hypotension, hypoxia, and mean positive airway pressure greater than 25 to 30 mm Hg despite anticoagulation and inotropes. Initial studies to be obtained include arterial blood gases, electrocardiogram, and chest roentgenograms.

The electrocardiogram may demonstrate right ventricular hypertrophy with strain, right bundle branch block, tachycardia, and T-wave inversion in the anterior chest leads (V_1 to V_4). Chest radiographic results are frequently normal. A Westermark sign (decreased pulmonary vascular markings peripherally) or a Palla sign (enlarged right descending pulmonary artery) may be present.

If the clinical likelihood is low, then a D-dimer enzyme-linked immunosorbent assay and ultrasound study of the lower extremities may be performed. The D-dimer is elevated in a number of conditions other than pulmonary embolism; however, a negative D-dimer assay suggests that the likelihood of pulmonary embolism is low. As well, hypoxia or hypercapnia is suggestive but not diagnostic of pulmonary embolism.

Other studies include ultrasound examination or impedance plethysmography of the lower extremities, ventilation-perfusion lung scan, echocardiography, high-resolution spiral CT of the chest, and pulmonary angiogram.

Ultrasound study of leg veins, even if negative, does not rule out pulmonary embolism. Ventilation-perfusion lung scans are usually performed for any hemodynamically stable patient with suspicion of pulmonary embolism. If normal, the likelihood of pulmonary embolism is low. If decreased perfusion is matched by normal ventilation, a high probability of pulmonary embolism exists and the patient should receive treatment. Nondiagnostic results are difficult to interpret, and further studies may be required. The pulmonary arteriogram remains the "gold standard" for diagnosis. High-resolution helical CT of the chest with contrast may assist in defining the presence of thrombus in the proximal pulmonary arteries. The use of magnetic resonance pulmonary angiography is being studied.

The definitive study for pulmonary embolism is pulmonary arteriography, particularly for patients with cardiovascular collapse and hypotension, or when other studies are inconclusive. Lower extremity deep venous thrombosis itself may be an indication for treatment with anticoagulants.

Treatment of Pulmonary Embolus

Treatment of pulmonary embolus includes anticoagulation, oxygen, and analgesia. Intravenous fluids, monitoring of central venous pressures, or use of inotropes may be required as dictated by the clinical situation. Heparin is the mainstay of treatment for pulmonary embolus. Heparin enhances antithrombin III activity to prevent propagation of the clot and to facilitate fibrinolysis. A bolus of heparin of 5000 to 10,000 units intravenously is given and followed by a continuous infusion of heparin (18 U/kg/hr; not to exceed 1600 U/hr). After therapeutic partial thromboplastin times have been achieved (ratio of activated partial thromboplastin time to the control ranges from 1.5 to 2.5), oral anticoagulation may be started with warfarin. At least 3 to 5 days of therapy with heparin and warfarin (Coumadin) are needed before adequate oral anticoagulation is achieved with the warfarin to remove the intravenous heparin. Warfarin should be started at 5 mg/day to achieve an international normalized ratio (INR) of 2.0 to 3.0 (unfractionated heparin usually adds 0.5 to the INR). Routine anticoagulation monitoring is required. The duration of warfarin therapy should be 3 months or longer.[91] Treatment greater than 6 months may carry increased risk.[92]

Use of an inferior vena cava filter should be considered in patients with pulmonary embolism where anticoagulation would carry increased risk (e.g., recent surgery, < 24 hours post operation, brain metastasis) or in patients with recurrent pulmonary emboli. The filter is placed below the renal veins at approximately the L3 vertebra level by way of the femoral or right jugular vein. The efficacy is 95%, and the risk of recurrent pulmonary embolism is 2% to 4%.

In patients with a serious hemodynamic and hypoxic response to pulmonary embolism (cardiogenic shock or hemodynamic instability) who do respond to resuscitation, heparin is initiated as standard therapy. In addition, thrombolytics (streptokinase or urokinase) may be given. Thrombolysis of clots occurs more quickly with thrombolytics than with heparin.[93] Multivariate analysis suggests that thrombolysis and anticoagulation have better clinical outcomes than anticoagulation alone; however, the value of such treatment must be weighed against the risk of major hemorrhage.[94] No prospective study has shown that the benefits of thrombolytic therapy in acute pulmonary embolism exceed the risks. Intracranial bleeding may occur in 3% of treated patients.[95] Other authors propose thrombolytic therapy in patients with right ventricular dysfunction.[96]

Further therapy may include catheter suction embolectomy for patients in whom thrombolytic therapy is ineffective. Venous (suction) or open (surgical) embolectomy may be performed to extract or obliterate the clot. Intravenous pressors are frequently required. The open technique is infrequently performed and requires sternotomy (with consideration of femoral vein to femoral artery extracorporeal support before sternotomy) and bicaval cannulation, if possible, after sternotomy. The pulmonary artery is opened with a longitudinal incision, and gallstone forceps are used to extract proximal emboli followed by use of Fogarty balloon catheters to extract emboli that are more distal.

Inferior vena cava interruption may be considered if all alternatives have been exhausted. Complications include chronic venous insufficiency of the lower extremities.

Chronic pulmonary embolism may develop with failure of the usual resolution of acute pulmonary emboli. Whereas most emboli will lyse, some become fibrotic and adhere to the pulmonary arterial wall. Symptoms of cor pulmonale, chronic dyspnea, right ventricular hypertrophy, and high right-sided pressures are all indications of chronic pulmonary embolism. Indications for surgery include (1) proximal pulmonary artery occlusion, (2) adequate collaterals with filling of distal pulmonary artery, (3) high right-sided cardiac pressures and hypoxia, and (4) minimally impaired lung function. The surgical approaches include (1) unilateral thoracotomy without cardiopulmonary bypass, (2) standard cardiopulmonary bypass with proximal and distal control of pulmonary arteries, and (3) cardiopulmonary bypass with total circulatory arrest (intermittent). Incisions are patched with pericardium unless they are on the main pulmonary artery.

Prevention

Prevention of pulmonary embolism should be considered in all patients having a major surgical procedure. All hospitalized patients must be evaluated and stratified for their risk of pulmonary embolism and the appropriate prophylaxis applied. Unfractionated heparin is most commonly used for perioperative prophylaxis and effectively reduces the rate of fatal pulmonary embolism. The dose is typically 5000 units twice daily and is continued until the patient is discharged and ambulatory. Low-molecular-weight heparins are an alternative to unfractionated heparin because of their characteristics of improved bioavailability, improved absorption, once-daily injection, and reduced rates of heparin-induced thrombocytopenia. Mechanical compression devices to stimulate fibrinolysis (from stimulation of the venous endothelium) are effective in patients who are bed-bound; however, ambulatory patients are usually not compliant in their use within a general ward environment.

Pulmonary embolus, even in its treatable form, carries high morbidity and potential mortality risks. Patients with pulmonary embolism are given heparin, oral anticoagulants, or fractionated low-molecular-weight heparin. Subsequent anticoagulation after discharge is required for periods up to 6 months. Patients with specific genetic characteristics are at increased risk for venous thrombolic events. Prevention of pulmonary embolism with some type of prophylaxis should be initiated in all patients having major surgical procedures.

THORACIC OUTLET SYNDROME

Thoracic outlet syndrome may occur in 5% of the population in a mild form. Vascular compression may be documented; neurogenic compression and pain or paresthesias may require electromyelogram for diagnosis. The syndrome occurs more frequently in women than in men. The anatomy of thoracic outlet syndrome includes compression of the subclavian artery, the subclavian vein, or the brachial plexus where it passes between the scalene muscles and over the first rib. Anomalous fibromuscular bands and cervical ribs may also compress the brachial plexus or subclavian vessels.[11]

Clinical features of thoracic outlet syndrome include intermittent symptoms of nerve compression in most patients, which include pain, paresthesias, and weakness. If the upper brachial plexus is involved, symptoms may be increased by turning or tilting the head. If the lower brachial plexus (C8 to T1) is involved, pain may be noted in the supraclavicular fossa extending to the inner arm and involving the ring and small fingers.

Diagnosis is primarily clinical. A history and physical examination as well as a cervical spine radiographic series can be performed to evaluate for cervical spine disease. Electromyelogram or nerve conduction studies are helpful to rule out carpal tunnel syndrome. A venogram may be performed for significant venous symptoms. Noninvasive arterial studies may be helpful. Angiography may be performed if aneurysm, thrombus, or emboli are suspected.

Treatment is physical therapy for 2 to 12 months. Exercises to strengthen the shoulder girdle, neck stretching, hot and cold packs, and muscle relaxants are used. Repetitive mechanical and muscular trauma is avoided. Surgery is used as a last resort for severe pain, impaired motor function or atrophy, treatment failure, or need to improve quality of life.

If surgery is required, transaxillary first rib resection allows complete resection with a good cosmetic result.[97] Cervical ribs are also removed. The assistant must relax the arm and shoulders intermittently (every 5 minutes for at least 30 seconds). An anterior scalenectomy (total) may be performed through an anterior supraclavicular approach and is usually indicated for significant symptoms of upper plexus involvement. The results of surgical treatment are mixed, with 50% to 60% of patients having a good to excellent result, 20% to 30% having a fair or improved result, and 10% having no improvement. Recurrent symptoms may prompt surgical treatment in approximately one third of patients.[98]

Selected References

Arriagada R, Bergman B, Dunant A, et al: Cisplatin-based adjuvant chemotherapy in patients with completely resected non-small-cell lung cancer. N Engl J Med 350:351–360, 2004.

> Recently, a randomized trial identified a 4% survival advantage and decreased hazard ratio for death (0.86, 95% C.I. 0.76-0.98, p < 0.003) in patients receiving postresection chemotherapy (cisplatin-based) to observation alone.

Depierre A, Milleron B, Moro-Sibilot D, et al: Preoperative chemotherapy followed by surgery compared with primary surgery in resectable stage I (except T1N0), II, and IIIA non-small-cell lung cancer. J Clin Oncol 20:247–253, 2002.

> This prospective randomized trial demonstrated an observable survival difference using preoperative chemotherapy followed by resection, compared to resection alone, but the difference was not statistically significant. In a subset analysis of early-stage disease (IB and II) patients with preoperative chemotherapy followed by resection had a statistically significant improvement in survival compared to resection alone.

Fishman A, Martinez F, Naunheim K, et al: A randomized trial comparing lung-volume-reduction surgery with medical therapy for severe emphysema. N Engl J Med 348:2059–2073, 2003.

> This recent prospective trial compared lung-volume-reduction surgery (LVRS) to medical treatment. Patients with predominantly upper lobe emphysema and low exercise capacity had lower mortality with LVRS than medical therapy (RR 0.47; p = 0.005). In patients with non-upper lobe emphysema and high exercise capacity, mortality was higher in the LVRS group (RR 2.06, p = 0.02).

Long-term results of lung metastasectomy: Prognostic analyses based on 5206 cases. The International Registry of Lung Metastases. J Thorac Cardiovasc Surg 113:37–49, 1997.

> The results of this international registry confirmed the survival benefit associated with complete resection of pulmonary metastases. Multiple histologies were examined and complete resection was consistently identified as a critical factor in post-thoracotomy survival. The actuarial 5-year and 10-year survival was 36% and 26%, respectively. Multivariate analysis revealed a better prognosis for patients with germ cell tumor histology, a disease-free interval of 36 months or greater, and single metastasis. Resection of pulmonary metastases is a safe and potentially curative procedure.

Pisters KM, Ginsberg RJ, Giroux DJ, Putnam JB Jr, et al: Induction chemotherapy before surgery for early-stage lung cancer: A novel approach. Bimodality Lung Oncology Team. J Thorac Cardiovasc Surg 119:429–439, 2000.

> The authors examined the feasibility of perioperative chemotherapy (paclitaxel and carboplatin) in patients with early-stage (IB, IIA, IIB, and selected IIIA [T3N1]) non-small-cell lung carcinoma. Ninety-four percent of patients underwent surgical exploration and 86% underwent complete resection. Preoperative chemotherapy was well tolerated in 96% of patients; however, only 46% of patients received the planned postoperative chemotherapy. No unexpected chemotherapy or surgical morbidity occurred. The 1-year survival was estimated at 85%. This study provides the basis for the current intergroup prospective randomized trial comparing induction chemotherapy and surgery with surgery alone in early-stage non-small-cell lung carcinoma.

Reed CE, Harpole DH, Posther KE, et al: Results of the American College of Surgeons Oncology Group Z0050 trial: The utility of positron emission tomography in staging potentially operable non-small cell lung cancer. J Thorac Cardiovasc Surg 126:1943–1951, 2003.

> The American College of Surgeons Oncology Group evaluated the role of positron emission tomography with 18F-fluorodeoxyglucose (PET) in detecting lesions that would preclude pulmonary resection surgically in resectable lung cancer patients. PET was better than CT for nodal disease detection. The negative predictive value for mediastinal nodal disease was 86%. "Distant" FDG-avid lesions required histologic confirmation as some were benign.

Rosell R, Gomez-Codina J, Camps C, et al: A randomized trial comparing preoperative chemotherapy plus surgery with surgery alone in patients with non-small-cell lung cancer. N Engl J Med 330:153–158, 1994.

Roth JA, Fossella F, Komaki R, et al: A randomized trial comparing perioperative chemotherapy and surgery with surgery alone in resectable stage IIIA non-small-cell lung cancer. J Natl Cancer Inst 86:673–680, 1994.

> These two small, single-institution, prospective randomized studies demonstrated the value of perioperative chemotherapy in patients with advanced stage (IIIA and selected IIIB) lung cancer. Although small numbers of patients were entered (60 in each study), a survival advantage was demonstrated in patients having perioperative chemotherapy compared to surgery alone. In the Rosell study, the median period of survival was 26 months in patients treated with chemotherapy plus surgery as compared with 8 months in patients treated with surgery alone (p < 0.001). In the Roth et al. study, patients treated with perioperative chemotherapy and surgery had an estimated median survival of 64 months compared with 11 months for patients who had surgery alone (p < 0.008 by long-rank test; p < 0.018 by Wilcoxon text). Both studies conclude that preoperative chemotherapy increases the median survival in patients with non-small-cell lung cancer.

References

1. Crapo RO: Pulmonary function testing. N Engl J Med 331:25, 1994.

2. Gass GB, Olsen GN: Preoperative pulmonary function testing to predict postoperative morbidity and mortality. Chest 89:127, 1986.

3. Weisman IM: Cardiopulmonary exercise testing in the preoperative assessment for lung resection surgery. Semin Thorac Cardiovasc Surg 13:116-125, 2001.

4. Pate P, Tenholder MF, Griffin JP, et al: Preoperative assessment of the high-risk patient for lung resection. Ann Thorac Surg 61:1494-1500, 1996.

5. Wang J, Olak J, Ferguson MK: Diffusing capacity predicts operative mortality but not long-term survival after resection for lung cancer. J Thorac Cardiovasc Surg 117:581-586, 1999.

6. Morice RC, Peters EJ, Ryan MB, et al: Exercise testing in the evaluation of patients at high risk for complications from lung resection. Chest 101:356-361, 1992.

7. Walsh GL, Morice RC, Putnam JBJ, et al: Resection of lung cancer is justified in high-risk patients selected by exercise oxygen consumption. Ann Thorac Surg 58:704-710, 1994.

8. Brunelli A, Al Refai M, Monteverde M, et al: Stair climbing test predicts cardiopulmonary complications after lung resection. Chest 121:1106-1110, 2002.

9. Bains MS, Ginsberg RJ, Jones WG2, et al: The clamshell incision: An improved approach to bilateral pulmonary and mediastinal tumor. Ann Thorac Surg 58:30-33, 1994.

10. Cina G, Marra R, Di Stasi C, Macis G: Epidemiology, pathophysiology and natural history of venous thromboembolism. Rays 21:315-327, 1996.

11. Roos DB: Transaxillary approach for first rib resection to relieve thoracic outlet syndrome. Ann Surg 163:354, 1966.

12. Brown WT: Atlas of Video-Assisted Thoracic Surgery. Philadelphia, WB Saunders, 1994.

13. Lewis RJ: Video-assisted thoracic surgery. Chest Surg Clin North Am 3:2, 1993.

14. Mack MJ, Scruggs GR, Kelly KM, et al: Video-assisted thoracic surgery: Has technology found its place? Ann Thorac Surg 64:211, 1997.

15. Goldman L, Caldera DL, Nussbaum SR, et al: Multifactorial index of cardiac risk in noncardiac surgical procedures. N Engl J Med 297:845, 1977.

16. Zeldin RA, Math B: Assessing cardiac risk in patients who undergo noncardiac surgical procedures. Can J Surg 27:402, 1984.

17. Azizkhan RG: Congenital pulmonary lesions in childhood. Chest Surg Clin North Am 3:547, 1993.

18. Bogers AJ, Hazebroek FW, Molenaar J, Bos E: Surgical treatment of congenital bronchopulmonary disease in children. Eur J Cardiothorac Surg 7:117-120, 1993.

19. Evrard V, Ceulemans J, Coosemans W, et al: Congenital parenchymatous malformations of the lung. World J Surg 23:1123-1132, 1999.

20. Luck SR, Reynolds M, Raffensperger JG: Congenital bronchopulmonary malformations. Curr Probl Surg 23:245-314, 1986.

21. Bower RJ, Kiesewetter WB: Mediastinal masses in infants and children. Arch Surg 112:1003-1009, 1977.

22. McAdams HP, Kirejczyk WM, Rosado-de-Christenson ML, Matsumoto S: Bronchogenic cyst: imaging features with clinical and histopathologic correlation. Radiology 217:441-446, 2000.

23. Pegolio W, Mattei P, Colombani PM: Congenital intrathoracic vascular abnormalities in childhood. Chest Surg Clin North Am 3:529, 1993.

24. Lassen U, Hansen HH: Surgery in limited-stage small cell lung cancer. Cancer Treat Rev 25:67-72, 1999.

25. Mountain CF: Revisions in the International System for Staging Lung Cancer. Chest 111:1710-1717, 1997.

26. Mountain CF, Dresler CM: Regional lymph node classification for lung cancer staging. Chest 111:1718-1723, 1997.

27. Nesbitt JC, Putnam JBJ, Walsh GL, et al: Survival in early-stage non–small cell lung cancer. Ann Thorac Surg 60:466-472, 1995.

28. Naruke T, Tomoyuki G, Tsuchiya R, Suemasu K: Prognosis and survival in resected lung carcinoma based on the new international staging system. J Thorac Cardiovasc Surg 96:440-447, 1988.

29. Boiselle PM, Patz EF Jr, Vining DJ, et al: Imaging of mediastinal lymph nodes: CT, MR, and FDG PET. Radiographics 18:1061-1069, 1998.

30. Cybulsky IJ, Lanza LA, Ryan MB, et al: Prognostic significance of computed tomography in resected N2 lung cancer. Ann Thorac Surg 54:533-537, 1992.

31. Ginsberg RJ: Evaluation of the mediastinum by invasive techniques. Surg Clin North Am 67:1025-1035, 1987.

32. Pearson FG, Nelems JM, Henderson RD, et al: The role of mediastinoscopy in the selection of treatment for bronchial carcinoma with involvement of superior mediastinal lymph nodes. J Thorac Cardiovasc Surg 54:382-390, 1972.

33. Stiglbauer R, Schurawitzki H, Klepetko W, et al: Contrast-enhanced MRI for the staging of bronchogenic carcinoma: Comparison with CT and histopathologic staging: Preliminary results. Clin Radiol 44:293-298, 1991.

34. Komaki R, Mountain CF, Holbert JM, et al: Superior sulcus tumors: Treatment selection and results for 85 patients without metastasis (M_0) at presentation. Int J Radiat Oncol Biol Phys 19:31-36, 1990.

35. Coleman RE: PET in lung cancer. J Nucl Med 40:814-820, 1999.

36. Al Sugair A, Coleman RE: Applications of PET in lung cancer. Semin Nucl Med 28:303-319, 1998.

37. Reed CE, Harpole DH, Posther KE, et al: Results of the American College of Surgeons Oncology Group Z0050 trial: The utility of positron emission tomography in staging potentially operable non-small cell lung cancer. J Thorac Cardiovasc Surg 126:1943-1951, 2003.

38. Dartevelle PG, Chapelier AR, Macchiarini P: Anterior trans-cervical-thoracic approach for radical resection of lung tumors invading the thoracic inlet. J Thorac Cardiovasc Surg 105:1025, 1993.

39. Deslauriers J, Beaulieu M, Despres JP: Transaxillary thoracotomy for the treatment of spontaneous pneumothorax. Ann Thorac Surg 30:35, 1980.

40. Detterbeck FC: Pancoast (superior sulcus) tumors. Ann Thorac Surg 63:1810, 1997.

41. Ginsberg RJ: Resection of superior sulcus tumors. Chest Surg Clin North Am 5:315, 1995.

42. Gould MK, Lillington GA: Strategy and cost in investigating solitary pulmonary nodules. Thorax 53(Suppl 2):S32-S37, 1998.

43. Libby DM, Henschke CI, Yankelevitz DF: The solitary pulmonary nodule: Update 1995. Am J Med 99:491-496, 1995.

44. Gambhir SS, Shepherd JE, Shah BD, et al: Analytical decision model for the cost-effective management of solitary pulmonary nodules. J Clin Oncol 16:2113-2125, 1998.

45. Fong KM, Sekido Y, Minna JD: Molecular pathogenesis of lung cancer. J Thorac Cardiovasc Surg 118:1136-1152, 1999.

46. Slebos RJ, Habets GG, Evers SG, et al: Allele-specific detection of K-ras oncogene expression in human non–small-cell lung carcinomas. Int J Cancer 48:51-56, 1991.

47. Roth JA, Nguyen D, Lawrence DD, et al: Retrovirus-mediated wild-type p53 gene transfer to tumors of patients with lung cancer. Nat Med 2:985-991, 1996.

48. Swisher SG, Roth JA, Nemunaitis J, et al: Adenovirus-mediated p53 gene transfer in advanced non–small-cell lung cancer. J Natl Cancer Inst 91:763-771, 1999.

49. Depierre A, Milleron B, Moro-Sibilot D, et al: Preoperative chemotherapy followed by surgery compared with primary surgery in resectable stage I (except T1N0), II, and IIIa non-small-cell lung cancer. J Clin Oncol 20:247-253, 2002.

50. Arriagada R, Bergman B, Dunant A, et al: Cisplatin-based adjuvant chemotherapy in patients with completely resected non-small-cell lung cancer. N Engl J Med 350:351-360, 2004.

51. Pass HI, Pogrebniak HW, Steinberg SM, et al: Randomized trial of neoadjuvant therapy for lung cancer: Interim analysis. Ann Thorac Surg 53:992-998, 1992.

52. Rosell R, Gomez-Codina J, Camps C, et al: A randomized trial comparing preoperative chemotherapy plus surgery with surgery alone in patients with non-small-cell lung cancer. N Engl J Med 330:153-158, 1994.

53. Roth JA, Fossella F, Komaki R, et al: A randomized trial comparing perioperative chemotherapy and surgery with surgery alone in resectable stage IIIA non–small-cell lung cancer. J Natl Cancer Inst 86:673-680, 1994.

54. Andrews RJ, Gluck DS, Konchingeri RH: Surgical resection of brain metastases from lung cancer. Acta Neurochir 138:382-389, 1996.

55. Figlin RA, Piantadosi S, Feld R: Intracranial recurrence of carcinoma after complete surgical resection of Stage I, II, and III non–small-cell lung cancer. N Engl J Med 318:1300-1305, 1988.

56. Dillman RO, Herndon J, Seagren SL, et al: Improved survival in Stage III non–small-cell lung cancer: Seven-year follow-up of cancer and leukemia group B (CALGB) 8433 trial. J Natl Cancer Inst 88:1210-1215, 1996.

57. Dillman RO, Seagren SL, Propert KJ, et al: A randomized trial of induction chemotherapy plus high-dose radiation versus radiation alone in Stage III non–small-cell lung cancer. N Engl J Med 323:940-945, 1990.

58. Le Chevalier T, Arriagada R, Quoix E, et al: Radiotherapy alone versus combined chemotherapy and radiotherapy in nonresectable non-small-cell lung cancer: First analysis of a randomized trial in 353 patients. J Natl Cancer Inst 83:417-423, 1991.

59. Sause WT, Scott C, Taylor S, et al: Radiation Therapy Oncology Group (RTOG) 88-08 and Eastern Cooperative Oncology Group (ECOG) 4588: Preliminary results of a phase III trial in regionally advanced, unresectable non-small-cell lung cancer. J Natl Cancer Inst 87:198-205, 1995.

60. Komaki R: Preoperative and postoperative irradiation for cancer of the lung. J Belge Radiol 68:195-198, 1985.

61. Komaki R, Cox JD, Hartz AJ, et al: Characteristics of long-term survivors after treatment for inoperable carcinoma of the lung. Am J Clin Oncol 8:362-370, 1985.

62. The Lung Cancer Study Group: Effects of postoperative mediastinal radiation on completely resected stage II and stage III epidermoid cancer of the lung. The Lung Cancer Study Group. N Engl J Med 315:1377-1381, 1986.

63. Barney JD, Churchill EJ: Adenocarcinoma of the kidney with metastasis to the lung cured by nephrectomy and lobectomy. J Urol 42:269-276, 1939.

64. Long-term results of lung metastasectomy: Prognostic analyses based on 5206 cases. The International Registry of Lung Metastases. J Thorac Cardiovasc Surg 113:37-49, 1997.

65. Putnam JB Jr: New and evolving treatment methods for pulmonary metastases. Semin Thorac Cardiovasc Surg 14:49-56, 2002.

66. Casson AG, Putnam JB, Natarajan G, et al: Efficacy of pulmonary metastasectomy for recurrent soft tissue sarcoma. J Surg Oncol 47:1-4, 1991.

67. McCormack PM, Ginsberg KB, Bains MS, et al: Accuracy of lung imaging in metastases with implications for the role of thoracoscopy. Ann Thorac Surg 56:863-866, 1993.

68. McCormack PM, Bains MS, Begg CB, et al: Role of video-assisted thoracic surgery in the treatment of pulmonary metastases: Results of a prospective trial. Ann Thorac Surg 62:213-216, 1996.

69. Pollock R, Lang A, Ge T, et al: Wild-type p53 and a p53 temperature-sensitive mutant suppress human soft tissue sarcoma by enhancing cell cycle control. Clin Cancer Res 4:1985-1994, 1998.

70. Weksler B, Lenert J, Ng B, Burt M: Isolated single lung perfusion with doxorubicin is effective in eradicating soft tissue sarcoma lung metastases in a rat model. J Thorac Cardiovasc Surg 107:50-54, 1994.

71. Johnston MR, Minchen RF, Dawson CA: Lung perfusion with chemotherapy in patients with unresectable metastatic sarcoma to the lung or diffuse broncholoalveolar carcinoma. J Thorac Cardiovasc Surg 110:368-373, 1995.

72. Regnard JF, Fourquier P, Levasseur P: Results and prognostic factors in resections of primary tracheal tumors: A multicenter retrospective study. The French Society of Cardiovascular Surgery. J Thorac Cardiovasc Surg 111:808-814, 1996.

73. Grillo HC, Donahue DM, Mathisen DJ, et al: Postintubation tracheal stenosis: Treatment and results. J Thorac Cardiovasc Surg 109:486-493, 1995.

74. Fishman A, Martinez F, Naunheim K, et al: A randomized trial comparing lung-volume-reduction surgery with medical therapy for severe emphysema. N Engl J Med 348:2059-2073, 2003.

75. Arcasoy SM, Kotloff RM: Lung transplantation. N Engl J Med 340:1081-1091, 1999.

76. Hirshberg B, Sklair-Levi M, Nir-Paz R, et al: Factors predicting mortality of patients with lung abscess. Chest 115:746-750, 1999.

77. Reed CE, Parker EF, Crawford FA Jr: Surgical resection for complications of pulmonary tuberculosis. Ann Thorac Surg 48:165-167, 1989.

78. Pomerantz M: Surgery for tuberculosis. Chest Surg Clin North Am 3:723, 1993.

79. Treasure RL, Seaworth BJ: Current role of surgery in *Mycobacterium* tuberculosis. Ann Thorac Surg 59:1405, 1995.

80. Garrett HE Jr, Roper CL: Surgical intervention in histoplasmosis. Ann Thorac Surg 42:711-722, 1986.

81. Blair D, Xu ZB, Agatsuma T: Paragonimiasis and the genus *Paragonimus*. Adv Parasitol 42:113-222, 1999.

82. Belizario V, Guan M, Borja L, et al: Pulmonary paragonimiasis and tuberculosis in Sorsogon, Philippines. Southeast Asian J Trop Med Public Health 28(Suppl 1):37-45, 1997.

83. Kum PN, Nchinda TC: Pulmonary paragonimiasis in Cameroon. Trans R Soc Trop Med Hyg 76:768-772, 1982.

84. Knott-Craig CJ, Oostuizen JG, Rossouw G, et al: Management and prognosis of massive hemoptysis: Recent experience with 120 patients. J Thorac Cardiovasc Surg 105:394-397, 1993.

85. Uflacker R, Kaemmerer A, Picon PD, et al: Bronchial artery embolization in the management of hemoptysis: Technical aspects and long-term results. Radiology 157:637-644, 1985.

86. Goldhaber SZ: Pulmonary embolism. N Engl J Med 339:93-104, 1998.

87. Bergqvist D, Lindblad B: A 30-year survey of pulmonary embolism verified at autopsy: An analysis of 1274 surgical patients. Br J Surg 72:105-108, 1985.

88. Carson JL, Kelley MA, Duff A, et al: The clinical course of pulmonary embolism. N Engl J Med 326:1240-1245, 1992.

89. Cattaneo M, Franchi F, Zighetti ML, et al: Plasma levels of activated protein C in healthy subjects and patients with previous venous thromboembolism: Relationships with plasma homocysteine levels. Arterioscler Thromb Vasc Biol 18:1371-1375, 1998.

90. Miller A: Acute pulmonary embolism: Practical guidelines. Br J Hosp Med 58:385-388, 1997.

91. Kearon C, Gent M, Hirsh J, et al: A comparison of three months of anticoagulation with extended anticoagulation for a first episode of idiopathic venous thromboembolism [published erratum appears in N Engl J Med 22:34:298, 1999]. N Engl J Med 340:901-907, 1999.

92. Schulman S, Granqvist S, Holmstrom M, et al: The duration of oral anticoagulant therapy after a second episode of venous thromboembolism. The Duration of Anticoagulation Trial Study Group. N Engl J Med 336:393-398, 1997.

93. Konstantinides S, Geibel A, Olschewski M, et al: Association between thrombolytic treatment and the prognosis of hemodynamically stable patients with major pulmonary embolism: Results of a multicenter registry. Circulation 96:882-888, 1997.

94. Mikkola KM, Patel SR, Parker JA, et al: Increasing age is a major risk factor for hemorrhagic complications after pulmonary embolism thrombolysis. Am Heart J 134:69-72, 1997.

95. Elliott G: Thrombolytic therapy for venous thromboembolism. Curr Opin Hematol 6:304-308, 1999.

96. Goldhaber SZ: Thrombolytic therapy. Adv Intern Med 44:311-325, 1999.

97. Urschel HC Jr, Razzuk MA: Upper plexus thoracic outlet syndrome: Optimal therapy. Ann Thorac Surg 63:935-939, 1997.

98. Urschel HC Jr, Razzuk MA: Neurovascular compression in the thoracic outlet: Changing management over 50 years. Ann Surg 228:609-617, 1998.

CHAPTER 58

CONGENITAL HEART DISEASE

Roger B. B. Mee, M.B., Ch.B.   and
Jonathan J. Drummond-Webb, M.B.B.Ch.

Anatomy and Terminology	**Congenital Lesions**
Cardiopulmonary Bypass and Myocardial Protection	**Other Anomalies**

In this brief review, the impressive historical contributions are not discussed. The knowledge base of congenital cardiac disease has undergone a quantum leap impossible to detail in this chapter. The development of pediatric and congenital cardiac surgery as a separate specialty has resulted in superior outcomes in institutions adopting this policy. Congenital cardiac disease accounts for 0.8% to 1.0% of all live births. The spectrum of anomalies ranges from isolated defects to complex lesions, with or without associated systemic abnormalities. Documentation of chromosomal abnormalities has opened new vistas in this field, especially chromosome 22 microdeletions (velocardiofacial syndrome and DiGeorge's syndrome variants) as well as the association of many syndromes (e.g., Turner's, Marfan's, Williams') with congenital cardiac abnormalities.[1]

Diagnosis relies on noninvasive methods, especially transthoracic echocardiography. This technology has advanced to such a degree that catheterization is required in only certain circumstances, that is, when pressure measurement and specific morphologic details are required or for intervention. Prenatal echocardiographic diagnosis of congenital lesions allows preemptive planning. Developments in echocardiography include three-dimensional and spin-echo capabilities. Magnetic resonance imaging (MRI) and nuclear scanning have enhanced noninvasive diagnosis. Interventional catheterization has become established as a management option, with balloon atrial septostomy, pulmonary and aortic valve dilation, device closure of defects, and major blood vessel dilation and stenting.

ANATOMY AND TERMINOLOGY

The assessment of congenital heart disease involves a systematic approach to the heart and its connections. The segmental approach involves description and analysis of three elements (atria, ventricles, and outlet) and analysis of the nature of the junctions (Fig. 58-1). Connections are described as concordant or discordant (abnormal); chambers as left or right sided (morphologically); and the valve connections between chambers as normal, absent, overriding, or straddling. Abnormal communications and specific morphologic anomalies are then described. The shorthand nomenclature of Van Praagh[2] allows some detail to be communicated effectively and succinctly. The system utilizes a name followed by a sequence of three letters. The first letter denotes the situs of atrial chambers and usually the abdominal and thoracic organs: *S,* solitus or normal; *I,* inversus or inverse; and *A,* ambiguus or unknown. The second letter denotes the ventricular loop: d, right-hand topology and l, left-hand topology. The third letter denotes the aortic valve position relative to the pulmonary valve position: d, right-sided and l, left-sided. The possible combinations are shown in Figure 58-2.

CARDIOPULMONARY BYPASS AND MYOCARDIAL PROTECTION

Cardiopulmonary bypass (CPB) in congenital heart surgery is very different from that used in adult cardiac surgery, which relates to the smaller size and the mini-

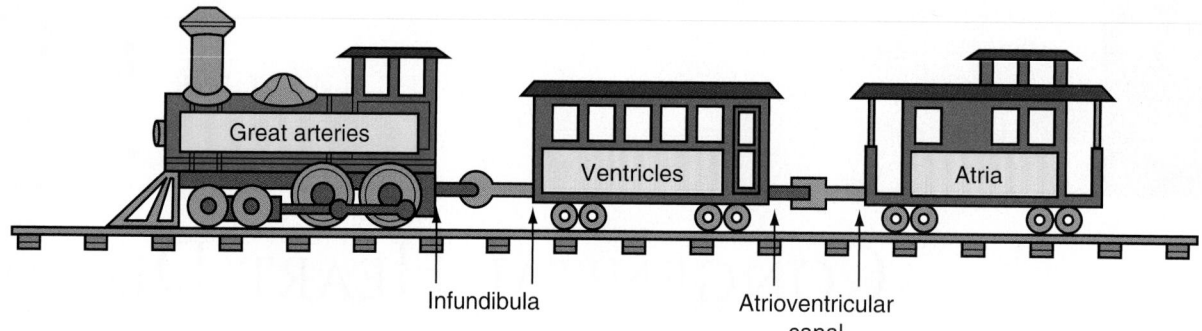

FIGURE 58-1.   Cartoon illustrates how the cardiac segments (atria, ventricles, great arteries) are analogous to a train and how the segmental approach analyzes the connection and alignment of these segments. (From Freedom RM: The application of a segmental nomenclature. *In* Freedom RM, Culham JAG, Moes CAF [eds]: Angiocardiography of Congenital Heart Disease. New York, Macmillan, 1984, p 18. Reproduced with permission of The McGraw-Hill Companies.)

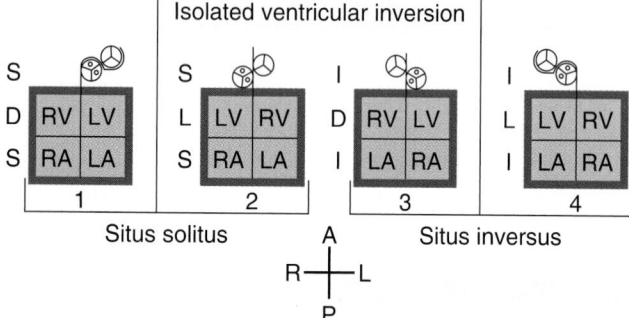

FIGURE 58-2.   Model of four normal hearts (excluding situs ambiguus) in the convention of Van Praagh. See text for details. A, anterior; L, left; LA, left atrium; LV, left ventricle; P, posterior; R, right; RA, right atrium; RV, right ventricle. (From Kirklin JW, Barratt-Boyes BG: General considerations: Anatomy, dimensions, and terminology. *In* Cardiac Surgery, 2nd ed. New York, Churchill Livingstone, 1993.)

mization of technology and circuitry needed to achieve appropriate flows. Vulnerability of immature, neonatal organ systems to the stresses imposed by the heart lesion, the insult of nonphysiologic CPB flow, and the inflammatory response of CPB require highly specialized techniques of perfusion and postoperative management.[3] Differences in neonates, infants, and children do not translate into linear reductions of adult protocols; rather, these are very specific, individualized needs.

Neonates have different myocardial metabolic properties than those of older children and adults.[4] These differences require alternative myocardial protection strategies. Cardioplegia infusion pressures are adjusted to patient size and weight. In neonates, immaturity of myocardial calcium sequestration leads to a dependency on extracellular calcium for calcium-dependent excitation-contraction coupling, as does the exclusive dependency of neonatal myocardium on glucose for metabolic substrate. Complex reconstruction and small patient size

may require deep hypothermic circulatory arrest (DHCA). The consequences of low-flow CPB and DHCA in infants are now becoming apparent, and neurologic outcomes are of concern in congenital heart surgery.[5]

CONGENITAL LESIONS

Lesions Resulting in Increased Pulmonary Blood Flow

Increased pulmonary blood flow, particularly at high pressure, decreases lung compliance. Pulmonary congestion can be added when there is increased resistance to adequate pulmonary venous outflow. The amount of increased pulmonary blood flow will depend on the absolute size of the defect, the resistances of the pulmonary and systemic vascular beds, and the total pumping capacity of the ventricular mass.

Patent Ductus Arteriosus and Aorticopulmonary Window

Patent Ductus Arteriosus

Patent ductus arteriosus (PDA) is a common isolated defect affecting 1 in 2000 births, with an increased incidence in premature neonates. In complex lesions, the PDA may be the only source of pulmonary blood supply. This discussion is limited to isolated PDA.

Anatomy and Pathophysiology The ductus arteriosus is a fetal structure that allows blood to divert away from the lungs and into the descending aorta. The PDA arises from the junction between the left and the main pulmonary artery and joins the underside of the distal aortic arch beyond the origin of the left subclavian artery. The recurrent laryngeal nerve is intimately related to the PDA (Fig. 58-3). Right-sided, bilateral PDAs and connections to the subclavian artery have been described. After birth, closure of the ductus is an important transition. Functional closure occurs first, mediated by the removal of the placental source of prostaglandin and its metabolism in the lungs. Functional closure is due to muscular contraction and is reversible. Anatomic closure is irreversible and develops

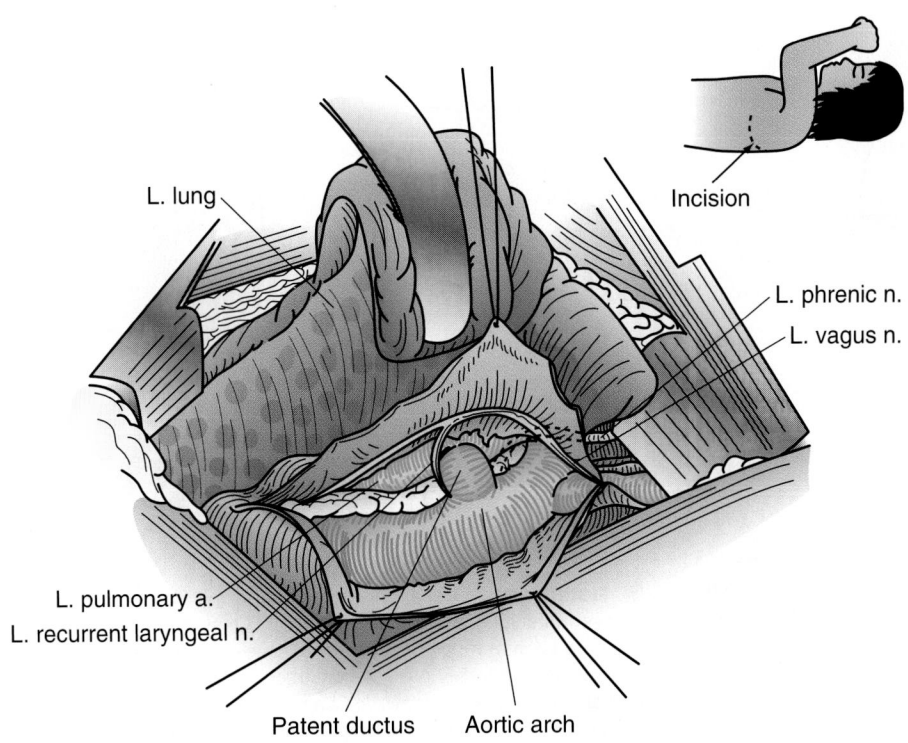

FIGURE 58-3. The anatomic relationships of a patent ductus arteriosus, exposed from a left thoracotomy. The parietal pleura is incised and reflected medially. The course of the recurrent laryngeal nerve is shown. (From Castaneda AR, Jonas RA, Mayer JE Jr, Hanley FL: Patent ductus arteriosus. *In* Cardiac Surgery of the Neonate and Infant. Philadelphia, WB Saunders, 1994.)

over weeks, involving degenerative changes. Spontaneous closure is rare before birth. A ductus that fails to close after 3 months of age is considered pathologic. Any PDA causing congestive cardiac failure or preventing ventilator weaning is also pathologic. The physiology of a PDA is left-to-right shunting and increased pulmonary blood flow with left atrial and ventricular volume overload. Complications of a PDA in older patients include aneurysm formation, infective endocarditis, calcification, and the risk of pulmonary vascular obstructive disease.

Diagnosis and Intervention The typical "machinery" murmur is heard in older children. In neonates and infants, pulmonary congestion and failure to thrive and, in premature infants, difficulty in weaning from ventilatory support should prompt echocardiographic examination. In premature infants, surgical closure is considered after medical failure (three doses of indomethacin). In older infants, closure of the PDA should be considered in the first 6 months of life. Echocardiography is diagnostic. Cardiac catheterization is reserved for patients in whom irreversible pulmonary hypertension is suspected.

Closure of the PDA Inhibition of prostaglandin synthesis in premature infants by indomethacin induces ductal closure. Transcutaneous catheter closure of the PDA is achieved in older children using coils and occluder devices. Patients with large, calcified, and aneurysmal ducts are not suitable for this approach. Small patients pose vascular access difficulties. Surgery is through a left posterolateral thoracotomy. The recurrent laryngeal nerve is preserved. The duct is ligated or, in the case of premature infants, either clipped with a metal clip or ligated. Video-assisted thoracoscopic closure of the PDA has been described.[6] A very large PDA may require division. In cal-

cified, infected, or aneurysmal PDAs, CPB and patch closure from the aortic or pulmonary artery side are safer. The mortality rate for uncomplicated PDA ligation approaches 0%.[7] Complications relate to duct trauma with bleeding, recurrent laryngeal nerve injury, pneumothoraces, and chylothorax.

Aorticopulmonary Window

Aorticopulmonary window, a rare defect, is a conotruncal anomaly, producing a window or communication between the aorta and the pulmonary artery.

Anatomy and Pathophysiology A defect of the conotruncal ridges results in this communication between the great vessels. The window is variable in size and situation. Three types of aorticopulmonary window are recognized (Fig. 58-4). Associated lesions include ventricular septal defect (VSD), coarctation of the aorta, and aortic arch interruption.[8] Physiology of the defect is similar to that of a large PDA with pulmonary overcirculation, pulmonary hypertension, left ventricular volume overload, and possible diastolic steal from the coronary circulation.

Diagnosis and Indications for Intervention Patients present in heart failure when the pulmonary vascular resistance (PVR) falls after birth. Pulmonary vascular disease is an early risk because of the usual nonrestrictive size of the defect. Echocardiography is diagnostic. Cardiac catheterization is not indicated, unless high PVR is suspected. Intervention is indicated at the time of diagnosis, unless irreversible pulmonary vascular obstructive disease is already established.

Intervention Surgical intervention usually requires a median sternotomy and CPB. After aortic cross-clamping

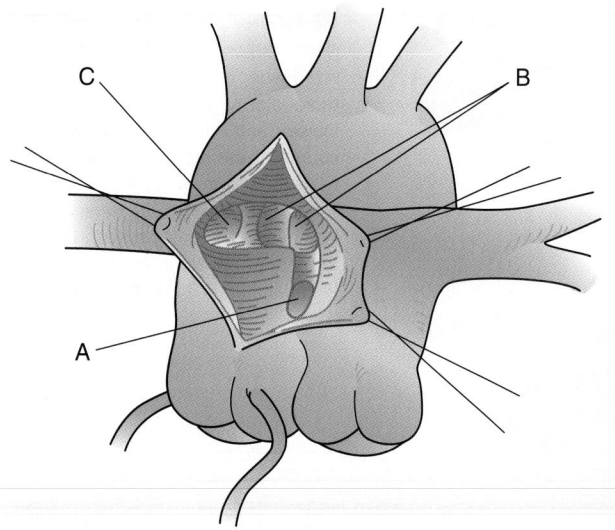

FIGURE 58-4. The types of aorticopulmonary window. Type A is the simplest. In type B, both the main pulmonary artery and the left pulmonary artery are involved. In type C, the right pulmonary artery arises separately from the aorta. (From Chang AC, Wells W: Aorticopulmonary window. *In* Chang AC, Lee FL, Wernovsky G, Wessel DL [eds]: Pediatric Cardiac Intensive Care. Baltimore, Williams & Wilkins, 1998.)

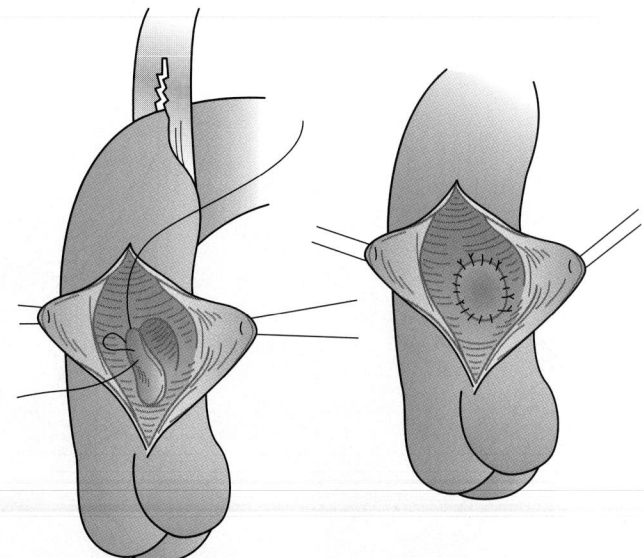

FIGURE 58-5. Repair of a type A aorticopulmonary window, exposed through a longitudinal aortotomy. Closure is by means of a patch. In infants, a patch is usually unnecessary. Types B and C may require pulmonary artery reconstruction. (From Chang AC, Wells W: Aorticopulmonary window. *In* Chang AC, Lee FL, Wernovsky G, Wessel DL [eds]: Pediatric Cardiac Intensive Care. Baltimore, Williams & Wilkins, 1998.)

and cardioplegic arrest, the defect is incised and exposed. Direct suture closure or patch closure with branch pulmonary artery reconstruction is performed (Fig. 58-5). Postoperative management requires monitoring of the pulmonary artery pressures (PAPs) and alertness to possible pulmonary hypertensive episodes. The operative mortality rate should approach 0%. Distortion of the repaired pulmonary artery is possible in the long term.[9]

Atrial Septal Defects

Isolated atrial septal defects (ASDs) are the most commonly encountered congenital cardiac anomalies, occurring in 10% to 15% of patients. These are the most common isolated cardiac defects encountered in the adult population. ASDs are also associated with complex congenital cardiac anomalies.

Anatomy and Pathophysiology The atrial septum consists of the septum primum and the septum secundum. These structures merge superiorly and inferiorly with the caval orifices. Defects are caused by failure of the septum primum to develop or regression of the interatrial folds at the level of the superior or inferior vena cavae. Developmentally, a patent foramen ovale allows the placentofetal circulation to function. A defect of the septum primum is classified as an ostium secundum defect. The ostium primum type of ASD is a form of atrioventricular (AV) canal defect. Other ASDs are either the sinus venosus type—with the defect at the level of the superior vena cava or inferior vena cava—or the coronary sinus type of ASD. Sinus venosus defects occur in association with partial anomalous pulmonary venous drainage. Coronary sinus ASD is rare and is due to a defect in the wall between the coronary sinus and the left atrium. The types of ASDs are shown in Figure 58-6.

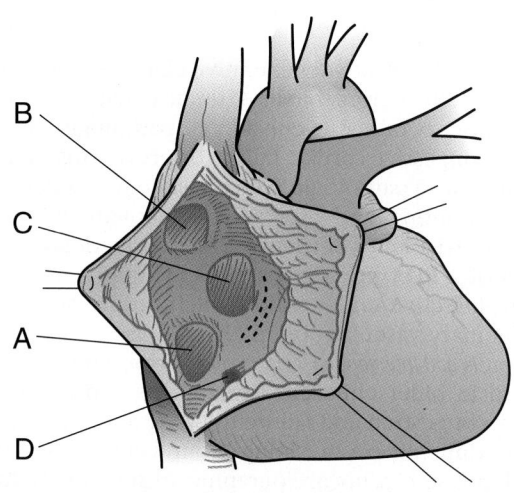

FIGURE 58-6. Types of atrial septal defects (ASDs). The anatomy of various ASDs is shown from the right atrial perspective. A, Ostium secundum defect. B, Superior vena caval, sinus venosus type of ASD. C, Ostium primum with partial atrial ventricular canal defect. D, The site of the coronary sinus in the right atrium. (From Chang AC, Jacobs J: Atrial septal defect. *In* Chang AC, Lee FL, Wernovsky G, Wessel DL [eds]: Pediatric Cardiac Intensive Care. Baltimore, Williams & Wilkins, 1998.)

The direction and amount of shunting depends on the size of the defect as well as the relative diastolic compliance of the ventricles. The shunt is left to right, resulting in increased flow to the right side of the heart and increased pulmonary blood flow. Congestive heart failure usually occurs after the second or third decade of life. Pulmonary hypertension is rare in children, but it can occur. The risks of ASD in older patients include paradoxical embolism and stroke, atrial fibrillation and flutter, sinus node dysfunction, as well as pulmonary vascular obstructive disease. Bacterial endocarditis is very rare.[10]

Diagnosis and Indications for Intervention Younger patients are asymptomatic, and the defect is found on routine physical examination. Older patients tend to be symptomatic with subtle signs of heart failure, exercise intolerance, palpitations, and arrhythmias. Complications such as cryptogenic stroke or pulmonary hypertension may be the presenting feature. Transthoracic echocardiography is usually diagnostic. Cardiac catheterization is needed to assess pulmonary pressure and PVR in patients with suspected significant pulmonary hypertension and to exclude coronary artery disease in older patients.

Surgery Indications for closure of small defects remain controversial. Spontaneous closure of a small patent foramen ovale occurs in up to 80% of infants within the first year. Closure is indicated in all symptomatic patients and all children with a significant ASD. Adults with a left-to-right shunt greater than 1.5:1 are candidates for closure, provided comorbid conditions do not add excessive risk to the procedure. Severe pulmonary vascular obstructive disease (resistance greater than 8.0 Wood units/m²)[11] is a contraindication to closure.

An ASD may be closed surgically or, if appropriate, by percutaneous transcatheter device closure. Surgery requires CPB. A median sternotomy is used, although a bilateral submammary incision or right anterolateral thoracotomy have all been used. Port access and limited (mini) median sternotomies have gained popularity. Most surgeons utilize aortic cross-clamping and cardioplegia to operate on a motionless heart, whereas others prefer to fibrillate the heart. The defect is closed by direct suture or pericardial or other prosthetic patch. For sinus venosus defects, techniques that route the anomalous veins to the left atrium are used. The surgical risk for death approaches 0% in isolated ASDs. Postoperative complications include pericardial effusions, postpericardiotomy syndrome, postoperative dysrhythmias, and residual ASDs.

Ventricular Septal Defects

Congenital defects of the interventricular septum may be single, multiple, or part of more complex cardiac anomalies. Congenital VSDs occur in 1 to 2 per 1000 live births, and of those requiring surgical repair, 50% will have another cardiac anomaly.

Anatomy and Pathophysiology VSDs are classified by the position they occupy in the ventricular septum. This classification is important because, by defining the position of the defect, the path of the conducting system can be reliably predicted and avoided during surgery.[12] In addition, the probability of spontaneous closure or of the predisposition to secondary cardiac pathology can be factored into the management decision making. The ventricular septum is described from the morphologic right side. The septum is divided into four parts: the membranous septum, the inlet, the trabecular, and the outlet parts of the muscular septum (the outlet septum is also called the conal or infundibular septum).

Perimembranous or Paramembranous Defects Perimembranous or paramembranous defects occur around the membra-

nous septum and the fibrous trigone of the heart. The defect is near the aortic valve, and the annulus of the tricuspid valve contributes to the rim of the defect. The defect may extend into any of the other components of the septum. The conduction tissue passes along the posteroinferior rim of the defect.

Muscular Defects Muscular defects have muscular rims. They may be single, but they are commonly multiple. Most commonly, multiple defects occur in the apical trabecular septum. The term *Swiss cheese septum* is used for associated spongiform myocardium and not for multiple muscular defects alone.[13] Prediction of the conducting system depends on whether the defect extends to the membranous septum.

Subarterial, Outlet, or Conal Defects Subarterial, outlet, or conal defects are located in the outlet portions of the left and right ventricles. The superior edge of the VSD is the conjoined annulus of the aortic and pulmonary valves. These are also called juxta-arterial or supracristal defects. This VSD is associated with prolapse of the unsupported aortic valve cusps and progressive aortic regurgitation.

Malalignment Defects Malalignment defects are created by malalignment between the infundibular and the trabecular muscular septum. This malalignment can be anterior, as in tetralogy of Fallot (TOF), or posterior. Associated defects occur frequently and include PDA, pulmonary stenosis, ASD, persistent left superior vena cava, and coarctation of the aorta.

The hemodynamic effect of a VSD is left-to-right shunting leading to increased pulmonary blood flow, left atrial dilation, and left ventricular volume overload. The size of the shunt is determined by the size of the defect (restrictive is smaller than the aortic root diameter) and the PVR. Compared with an ASD, the shunting in a VSD occurs mainly during systole. It is useful to quantify the shunt by the ratio of systemic to pulmonary blood flow (Qp:Qs). At cardiac catheterization, the Qp:Qs can be estimated from the equation:

$$Qp:Qs = \text{aortic } O_2 \text{ \%sat} - \text{central venous } O_2 \text{ \%sat}$$

$$\text{pulmonary vein } O_2 \text{ \%sat} - \text{pulmonary artery } O_2 \text{ \%sat}$$

The severity of pulmonary vascular disease correlates with the size of the shunt. In time, as the PVR increases, histologic changes occur within the pulmonary vascular bed, which may be irreversible. The time of onset and the severity of pulmonary vascular disease correlate with the size of the shunt but are also subject to considerable individual variation. As the PVR increases, the left-to-right shunt decreases, causing unloading of the left ventricle. Congestive heart failure improves, and the patient feels better! If untreated, a reversal of the flow occurs, leading to a right-to-left shunt with the development of increasing cyanosis (Eisenmenger's syndrome).

Diagnosis and Indications for Intervention The clinical presentation depends on the size of the shunt and the PVR. The clinical picture varies from an asymptomatic patient with a murmur, to a patient in fulminant heart failure, to a cyanosed patient with irreversible pulmonary vascular obstructive disease. Associated abnormalities determine the findings, especially if aortic regurgitation is present.

The echocardiogram is diagnostic, and the defect, as well as associated cardiac abnormalities, can be assessed. The echocardiogram can also provide an estimation of RV pressure (and PAP in the absence of pulmonary stenosis) by obtaining the Doppler velocity (V) of the jet through the VSD and/or the regurgitant jet through the tricuspid valve, using the modified Bernoulli equation:

$$\text{Pressure change (mm Hg)} = 4 \times V^2.$$

Cardiac catheterization is indicated when reversibility of the PAP is questionable. The Qp:Qs can be documented, and a dynamic assessment is possible, obtaining the PVR before and after pulmonary vasodilation. A PVR of more than 8.0 Wood units/m^2 with vasodilation is inoperable.

Management The ideal is to intervene when the likelihood of spontaneous VSD closure is lowest and the risk of irreversible pulmonary vascular disease and ventricular dysfunction are minimized. Perimembranous and muscular defects tend to close with time. Eighty percent of VSDs seen at 1 month of age will close spontaneously. Spontaneous closure of malalignment and subarterial defects is unlikely. Bacterial endocarditis is more common with small and moderate-sized VSDs with an incidence of 0.15% to 3% per year. In subarterial VSDs, the risk of irreversible aortic valve damage owing to cusp prolapse leads to earlier intervention.[14] Single-stage closure is recommended early, when the defect is large and symptoms and signs of congestive heart failure and failure to thrive are found.[15] With perimembranous and muscular defects, if the infant is thriving and it is known that the PAP is near normal, surgery may be delayed reasonably up to 1 year or more. Other defects should be closed. The younger patient with a small defect may be followed. The ideal management of a small defect (Qp:Qs < 1.5:1; normal PAP) in a patient older than 10 years of age is controversial. Multiple VSDs present a different problem: if a large shunt is present and persists beyond 6 to 8 weeks, pulmonary artery banding and removal after 2 years of age with an attempt at septation is reasonable. Banding is also reasonable in VSDs complicated by straddling or overriding of the AV valves. In VSDs associated with coarctation, aortic arch hypoplasia, or interruption, single-stage repair of both defects through the midline is recommended, provided this can be achieved with low risk.

Surgery VSDs are closed using CPB with bicaval cannulation. Circulatory arrest may be required for simultaneous arch reconstruction. Most VSDs can be repaired through a right atrial approach, except for subarterial defects, which are approached through the pulmonary valve, and multiple apical trabecular defects, which are sometimes easier to approach through a small apical right ventriculotomy.[13] Prosthetic patch closure using Dacron, Teflon, or Gore-Tex is recommended (Fig. 58-7). Transcatheter device closure and intraoperative device placement have been used in unusual circumstances to achieve VSD closure. Postoperatively, monitoring the left atrial and PAP simplifies management in those with large defects, preexisting heart failure, and known pulmonary hypertension. Precautions are taken to limit the responsiveness of the pulmonary vascular bed, and ventilatory

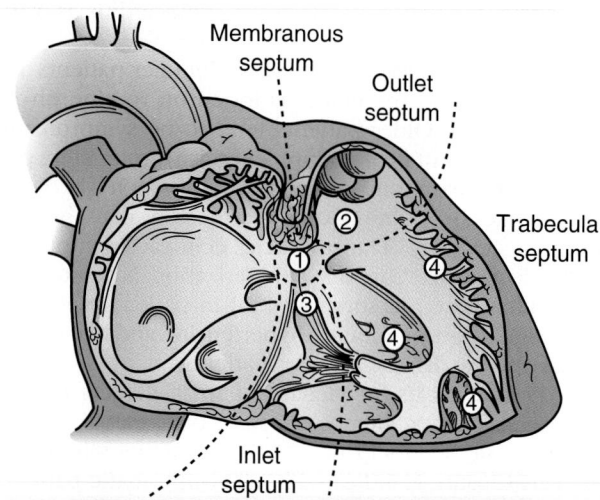

FIGURE 58-7. The location of various ventricular septal defects (VSDs) in the ventricular septum. (This is a view of the ventricular septum from the right side.) 1, Perimembranous VSD. 2, Subarterial VSD. 3, Atrioventricular canal-type VSD. 4, Muscular VSD. (From Tchervenkov CI, Shum-Tim D: Ventricular septal defect. *In* Baue AE, Geha AS, Hammond GL [eds]: Glenn's Thoracic and Cardiovascular Surgery, 6th ed. Stamford, CT, Appleton & Lange, 1996. Reproduced with permission of The McGraw-Hill Companies.)

management becomes an important tool. With persistent, severe pulmonary hypertension, nitric oxide is available.[16]

For uncomplicated VSD repair, the operative mortality rate should approach 0%. The overall risk for VSD repair is less than 5%. Mortality and morbidity increase with multiple VSDs, pulmonary hypertension, and complex associated anomalies. Postoperative problems are residual VSDs that may require reoperation if hemodynamically significant. Heart block is infrequent and approaches zero in many centers.

Atrioventricular Canal Defects

AV canal defects are also known as endocardial cushion defects or AV septal defects. There is a high incidence of Down's syndrome with endocardial cushion defects. A spectrum of anomalies occurs depending on the presence of atrial and ventricular defects. AV canal defects are either partial (PAVC) or complete (CAVC). Intermediate types occur. Additionally, hypoplasia of either the left or the right ventricular chamber can lead to an unbalanced AV canal, which may preclude biventricular repair. Associated anomalies include heterotaxy syndromes, TOF, double-outlet right ventricle (DORV), and total anomalous venous return.

Anatomy and Pathophysiology The actual embryologic origin of this defect remains unclear. Three principal components are found in CAVC: a defect of the AV septum, a defect of the interventricular septum, and an abnormal AV valve.

An ostium primum defect or PAVC consists of an ASD associated with abnormal AV valve anatomy, a cleft leaflet of the left-sided and right-sided AV valves. Left-sided AV valve regurgitation is not uncommon. Two separate AV valve orifices are present (Fig. 58-8). There is in fact also

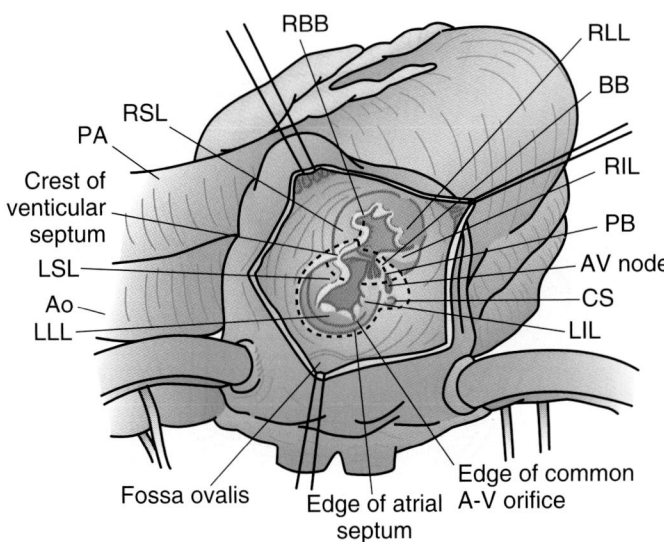

FIGURE 58-8. The position of the conducting system in complete atrioventricular canal defect (CAVC). The anatomic relationships and morphology of the common atrioventricular (AV) valve are shown. The view is through a right atriotomy. Ao, aorta; BB, left bundle branch; CS, coronary sinus; LIL, left inferior leaflet; LLL, left lateral leaflet; LSL, left superior leaflet; PA, pulmonary artery; PB, penetrating bundle; RBB, right bundle branch; RIL, right inferior leaflet; RLL, right lateral leaflet; RSL, right superior leaflet. (From Bharati S, Lev M, Kirklin JW: Cardiac Surgery and the Conduction System. New York, Churchill Livingstone, 1983.)

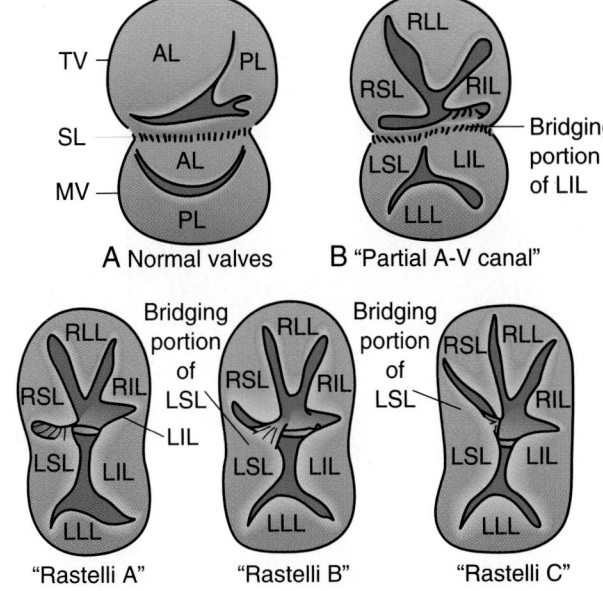

FIGURE 58-9. The Rastelli classification type A, B, or C. **A** to **C**, The difference in valve morphology in a normal, partial canal and complete canal defect is illustrated. AL, anterior leaflet; A-V, atrioventricular; MV, mitral valve; PL, posterior leaflet; RIL, right interior leaflet; RLL, right lateral leaflet; RSL, right superior leaflet; TV, tricuspid valve. (From Kirklin JW, Pacifico AD, Kirklin JK: The surgical treatment of atrioventricular canal defects. *In* Arciniegas E [ed]: Pediatric Cardiac Surgery. Chicago, Year Book Medical, 1985.)

a deficiency of the interventricular septum similar to that of CAVC, but in the PAVC the tissues of both AV valves are continuously adherent to the septal crest. A transitional or intermediate AV canal defect is an ostium primum defect, with the AV valve only partially adherent to the septal crest. Classification of CAVC into Rastelli types A, B, and C relates to the superior AV valve leaflet chordal attachments to the ventricular septum. In type A, the superior leaflet chords are attached to the septum; in type B, the superior leaflet is attached to an abnormal papillary muscle in the right ventricle; and in type C, the superior leaflet is free floating (Fig. 58-9). Pathophysiology depends on whether all three components are present. In PAVC, the pathophysiology is that of an ASD, with or without left-sided AV valve regurgitation. In CAVC, the pathophysiology is that of a VSD with an associated ASD. This results in a large left-to-right shunt at two levels, equalization of right ventricular and left ventricular pressures, and volume overload of all cardiac chambers. With additional AV valve regurgitation, there is further volume overload.

Diagnosis These children usually present in congestive heart failure. In PAVC, this is uncommon before 6 months of age but is quite common in CAVC by the age of 2 months. Of concern is the development of irreversible pulmonary vascular obstructive disease, which may occur before 1 year of age. Down's syndrome children with chronic upper airway obstruction have a predilection for pulmonary vascular obstructive disease. Echocardiography is diagnostic with demonstration of the typical cleft in the anterior leaflet of the AV valve. Cardiac catheteri-

zation is indicated in patients older than 3 to 4 months of age in whom elevated PVR is suspected. On left ventriculography, the "goose-necked deformity" of the elongated left ventricular outflow tract is seen.

Surgery For PAVC, surgery has been recommended at preschool age. This may be performed earlier, usually after the age of 8 to 12 months. For CAVC, the ideal age for surgery relates to the risk for the development of pulmonary vascular obstructive disease. Elective repair in patients by 3 months of age is a reasonable compromise between heart size and risk of irreversible complications. A median sternotomy and CPB are used. The common denominator in all forms of endocardial cushion defect is that the fibrous center of the heart is deficient and the conduction system is thus found in an abnormal position. Careful suture placement for the ASD and VSD patch is essential to avoid heart block (Fig. 58-10). For PAVC, the ASD is closed with an autologous pericardial patch, leaving the coronary sinus ostium in the right atrium. In CAVC, a one- or two-patch technique is used. The two-patch technique may be advantageous in a small heart, by minimizing loss of leaflet tissue in the suture line.[17] The VSD portion of the patch is completed first, with care taken to avoid obstructing the left ventricular outflow tract. The valve leaflets are then attached to the patch, and the ASD is closed with the pericardial patch (see Fig. 58-10).

For PAVC, the mortality approaches zero. CAVC mortality rates in the last 5 to 10 years have been reported between 0 and 10%.[18] Other surgical procedures include

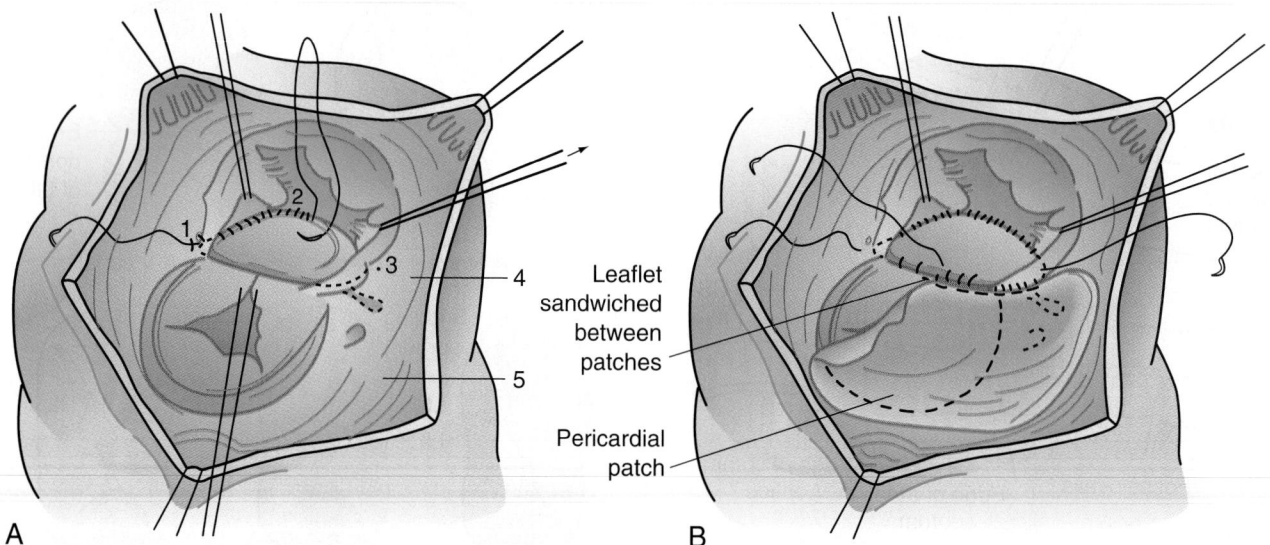

A

B

Leaflet
sandwiched
between
patches

Pericardial
patch

FIGURE 58-10.   The two-patch closure of CAVC. A ventricular septal patch is placed first (**A**), and a separate patch is used to close the ASD component (**B**). Note the position of the coronary sinus and conducting system relative to the ASD patch suture line, to avoid injury to the AV node. (From Kirklin JW, Barratt-Boyes BG: Cardiac Surgery. New York, Churchill Livingstone, 1986.)

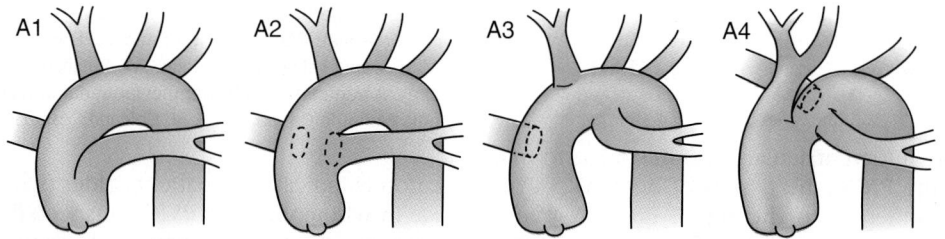

FIGURE 58-11.   Classification of truncus arteriosus according to Van Praagh. Type *A*, with a VSD; Type B, without a VSD. A1, Partially separate main pulmonary artery. A2, Absent aorticopulmonary septum, both branch pulmonary arteries arise from the common trunk. A3, Absence of either branch pulmonary artery. A4, Hypoplasia, coarctation, atresia, or absence of the aortic isthmus in association with a large patent ductus arteriosus. (From Hernanz-Schulman M, Fellows KE: Persistent truncus arteriosus: Pathologic, diagnostic and therapeutic considerations. Semin Roentgenol 20:121-129, 1985.)

pulmonary artery banding, which has a role in patients with respiratory compromise from viral illness, extremely small babies, and patients who have an unbalanced AV canal with excessive pulmonary blood flow in whom a biventricular repair may or may not be possible.

Truncus Arteriosus

A single arterial trunk arises from both ventricles, from which the coronary and pulmonary arteries originate. It is usually associated with a conotruncal VSD. There is an association with microdeletion of chromosome 22q11 and the DiGeorge syndrome.

Anatomy and Pathophysiology   The classification of Van Praagh is useful from a surgical perspective (Fig. 58-11). Failure of the embryologic truncus arteriosus to septate into the aorta and the pulmonary artery gives rise to the characteristic single arterial trunk from both ventricles.

Associated lesions include aortic arch obstruction, right aortic arch, interrupted aortic arch, and ASDs. The single truncal valve is often dysmorphic and can be either stenotic or regurgitant or both. Variability of the leaflets is common, and the number of leaflets can vary from two to six, with truncal valve incompetence more common with four or more leaflets.[19] Associated coronary artery abnormalities may be present. Pathophysiology relates to a pressure and volume overload to both right and left ventricles, with pulmonary overflow dependent on the PVR. The effect of volume and pressure overload is worsened by truncal valve stenosis or regurgitation. The fall in PVR after birth causes significant pulmonary overflow and congestive heart failure. Heart failure is more severe with truncal valve regurgitation. These patients are at risk of early development of pulmonary vascular obstructive disease and of subendocardial ischemia from coronary diastolic steal.

Diagnosis and Presentation Echocardiography is diagnostic. In addition to the obvious conotruncal defect, attention should be focused on the number of VSDs, the anatomy of the truncal valve, and coronary artery anomalies. These patients should be assumed as having a component of DiGeorge's syndrome, and only irradiated blood products are used. Cardiac catheterization is indicated in older infants when pulmonary vascular disease is suspected. Presentation is usually in the neonatal period.

Surgery Complete repair is recommended in the neonatal period for severe heart failure, but this can be safely delayed up to 3 months in patients with easily controlled heart failure. Again, this is a compromise between attaining increased heart size and the development of irreversible complications. The only absolute contraindication for surgery is the presence of Eisenmenger physiology. Palliative pulmonary artery banding is difficult and is high risk.[20] Median sternotomy with CPB and DHCA is limited to the period of arch repair if required. The pulmonary arteries are detached from the truncal root, and the defect is closed. Through a right ventriculotomy, the VSD is closed and a conduit is placed from the right ventricle to the transected pulmonary arteries (Fig. 58-12). Mortality in truncus arteriosus depends on the associated

conditions. The most important factor for nonsurvival is severe incompetence of the truncal valve. Uncomplicated truncus mortality should be less than 5% and perhaps higher in patients with arch obstruction, severe truncal valve stenosis or regurgitation, and coronary artery abnormalities. Low birth weight is an independent predictor of nonsurvival. Conduit obstruction requiring replacement or revision is usual.[21]

Abnormalities of Venous Return: Systemic and Pulmonary

Abnormal Systemic Venous Return

Abnormal systemic venous return is a frequent finding in complex congenital disease and in the normal population. A persistent left superior vena cava draining to the coronary sinus may be associated with hypoplasia or atresia of the mitral valve but is harmless in isolation. Absence of an innominate vein is a clue to this anomaly. More complex variations are found in the heterotaxy (isomeric) syndromes with interrupted inferior vena cava and azygos or hemiazygos continuations. Implications of these abnormalities are that they complicate cannulation for CPB and may preclude septation of the heart.

Anomalous Pulmonary Venous Return

Anomalous pulmonary venous return may be either partial or complete.

Partial The most common anomalies are right upper pulmonary veins draining to the superior vena cava (associated with a superior sinus venosus ASD); the "scimitar" syndrome with partial or complete drainage of the right-sided pulmonary veins to the inferior vena cava; and isolated left upper pulmonary veins draining to the left innominate vein via a vertical vein.

DIAGNOSIS AND PRESENTATION Diagnosis depends on the magnitude of the associated shunt, the degree of systemic desaturation, and the presence or absence of pulmonary vein obstruction. Echocardiography is often diagnostic, but catheter study may be required.

SURGERY Redirection of the pulmonary venous return with closure of the ASD or reconnecting the pulmonary veins to the left atrium and division of the systemic venous connection are performed. Surgery is low risk, and late complications are stenosis of the reconnected pulmonary vein or baffle obstruction.

Cor Triatriatum Cor triatriatum is a rare anomaly that has a diaphragm or membrane separating either the right or left atrium into two chambers. On the left side the superior chamber connects all four pulmonary veins and the inferior chamber contains the orifice of the left atrial appendage and the orifice of the mitral valve. The pathophysiology is similar to mitral stenosis and is affected by the size of the communication between the chambers and the size and position of the ASD if present. Operative correction involves excision of the obstructing membrane through the fossa ovalis or existing ASD, followed by closure of the ASD. On the right side the membrane represents a filling in of the Chiari network presumably derived from the venous valves and mimics tricuspid valve

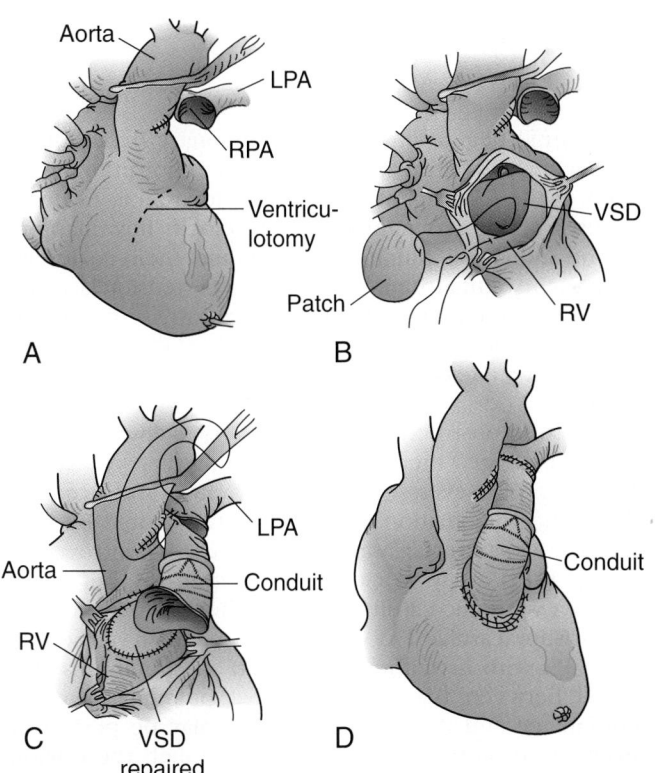

FIGURE 58-12. Surgical repair of truncus arteriosus. **A,** Origin of truncus arteriosus is excised and the truncal defect closed with direct suture. The incision is made high in the right ventricle (RV). LPA, left pulmonary artery; RPA, right pulmonary artery. **B,** Ventricular septal defect (VSD) is closed with a prosthetic patch. **C,** Placement of a valved conduit into the pulmonary arteries. **D,** Proximal end of conduit is anastomosed to the RV. (From Wallace RB: Truncus arteriosus. *In* Sabiston DC Jr, Spencer FC [eds]: Gibbons Surgery of the Chest, 3rd ed. Philadelphia, WB Saunders, 1976.)

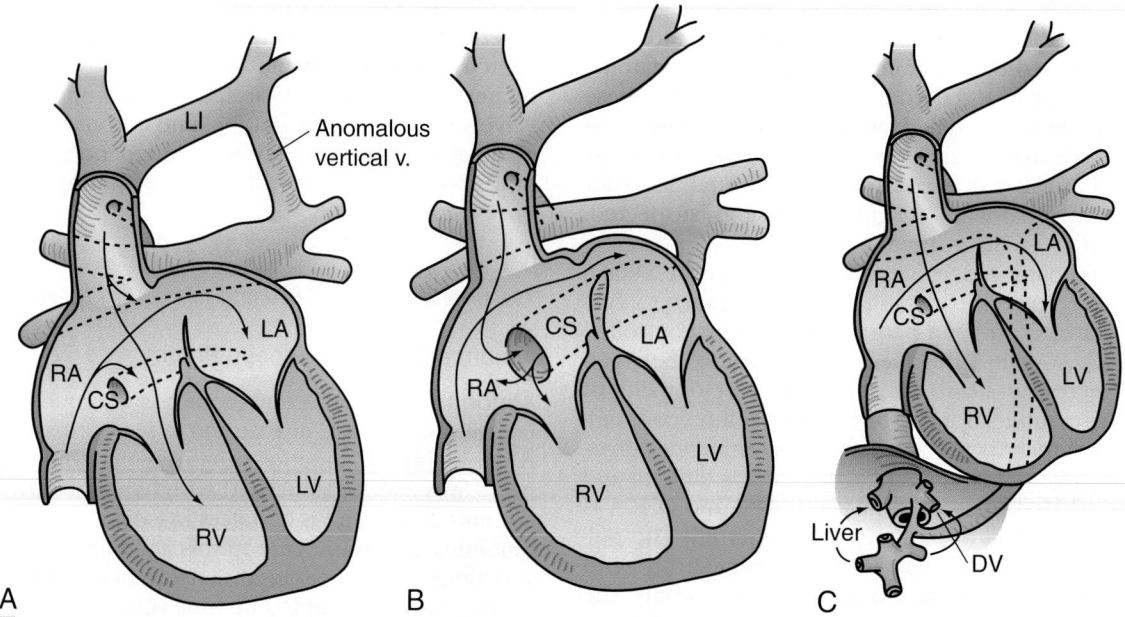

FIGURE 58-13. Types of total anomalous pulmonary venous connection (TAPVC). **A,** Supracardiac type with a vertical vein joining the left innominate vein. CS, coronary sinus; LA, left atrium; LV, left ventricle; RA, right atrium; RV, right ventricle. **B,** Intracardiac type with connection to the coronary sinus. **C,** Infracardiac type with drainage through the diaphragm via an inferior connecting vein. (From Hammon JW Jr, Bender HW Jr: Anomalous venous connections: Pulmonary and systemic. *In* Baue AE [ed]: Glenn's Thoracic and Cardiovascular Surgery, 5th ed. Norwalk, CT, Appleton & Lange, 1991. Reproduced with permission of The McGraw-Hill Companies.)

stenosis. Operative mortality approaches zero with good long-term results.[22]

Total Anomalous Pulmonary Venous Connection Total anomalous pulmonary venous connection (TAPVC) results in abnormal drainage of all the pulmonary veins directly or indirectly to the systemic venous atrium. Thirty percent of patients will have associated cardiac defects. Classification of TAPVC is based on the site of the connection to the systemic venous system and may be supracardiac, cardiac, infracardiac, or mixed (Fig. 58-13). Supracardiac is the most common (approximately 50%) and mixed the rarest.

PATHOPHYSIOLOGY All the pulmonary venous return is to the right atrium, and the physiology depends on whether the veins or the ASD is obstructed. With obstructed TAPVC, the obstructed pulmonary venous return causes pulmonary congestion or edema and pulmonary hypertension. The obstruction is due to a number of mechanisms. With the supracardiac type, the vertical vein may be compressed between the pulmonary artery and the left bronchus (vascular vice), or anatomic narrowing of the pulmonary venous confluence and stenosis of the pulmonary veins themselves may occur. In the absence of a VSD, left ventricular filling depends on the size of the ASD. A restrictive ASD adds the pathophysiology of low systemic arterial output.

DIAGNOSIS AND PRESENTATION Obstructed TAPVC requires immediate surgical intervention. These neonates present with cyanosis, various levels of pulmonary venous congestion, respiratory compromise, and acidosis. If the ASD is obstructive, systemic cardiac output is also low. In unobstructed TAPVC with an unobstructed ASD, the clinical presentation is usually similar to that of a large ASD

with some degree of cyanosis. Pulmonary hypertension can occur as a late consequence. On echocardiography, each of the four pulmonary veins is identified. Evidence for obstruction is obtained through velocity flow mapping of the individual pulmonary veins and their coalescing path to the right atrium. Pulmonary hypertension is always present when pulmonary venous return is obstructed. Cardiac catheterization is not usually indicated, unless uncertainty exists over the site of pulmonary venous drainage.

SURGERY In obstructed TAPVC, surgery is an emergency. Without surgery, mortality is 100% in the first year of life. Because of severe pulmonary venous obstruction, mechanical ventilation is necessary and should be instituted quickly. Prostaglandin E_1 (PGE$_1$) use is controversial. An open PDA may worsen systemic cyanosis, but it may improve systemic cardiac output if the ASD is restrictive.

For supracardiac TAPVC, through a median sternotomy and CPB with or without DHCA, an anastomosis is fashioned between the retropericardial pulmonary venous confluence and the left atrium. This may be performed from the posterior aspect working through the oblique pericardial sinus or utilizing the techniques of Schumacher and Tucker (Fig. 58-14A).[23] The ASD is closed as well.

For the intracardiac type repair requires the huge coronary sinus to be unroofed into the left atrium. The ASD and coronary sinus ostium are closed primarily or patched separately.

For the infracardiac type the pulmonary venous confluence and left atrium are anastomosed in a side-to-side fashion (see Fig. 58-14B). The descending vertical vein is

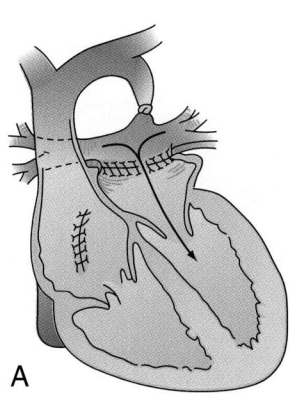
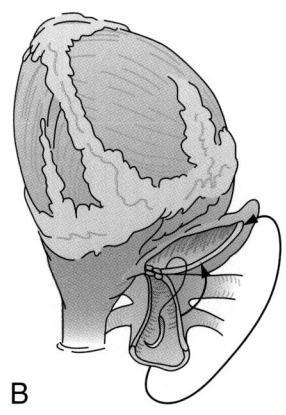

FIGURE 58-14. A, Repair of supracardiac TAPVC through a superior approach. **B,** Repair of infracardiac TAPVC. Elevating the apex of the heart to the right side exposes the left atrium and pulmonary confluence. Anastomosis is created as shown. (From Lupinetti FM, Kulik TJ, Beekman RH, et al: Correction of total anomalous pulmonary venous connection in infancy. J Thorac Cardiovasc Surg 106:880, 1993.)

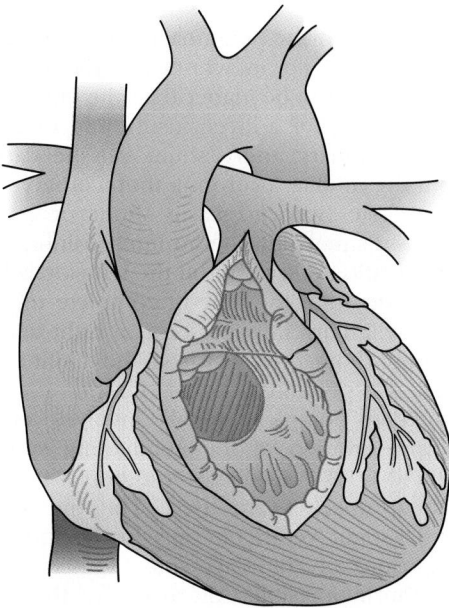

FIGURE 58-15. Anatomy of tetralogy of Fallot. A cutaway of the right ventricular free wall reveals the four components: ventricular septal defect, aortic override, hypertrophied right ventricular muscle, and infundibular stenosis, with small hypoplastic pulmonary annulus. (From Spray TL, Wernovsky G: Right ventricular outflow tract obstruction. *In* Chang AC, Lee FL, Wernovsky G, Wessel DL [eds]: Pediatric Cardiac Intensive Care. Baltimore, Williams & Wilkins, 1998.)

divided. The current overall mortality is quite low for obstructed TAPVC, around 5%. This correlates directly with preoperative morbidity. Postoperative pulmonary venous obstruction occurs in 5% to 10% of patients. This is associated with a poor outcome if it involves the individual veins.[24]

Lesions Resulting in Decreased Pulmonary Blood Flow

These lesions reduce pulmonary blood flow by obstruction at, below, or above the pulmonary valve. The obstruction may be at a single level (e.g., pulmonary valve stenosis) or may be a more complex, multilevel obstruction, such as TOF.

Tetralogy of Fallot

TOF is a conotruncal defect resulting from anterior malalignment of the infundibular septum. This single morphologic defect gives rise to the four components of TOF: the VSD, aortic valve override, and narrowing of the right ventricular outflow tract resulting in secondary right ventricular hypertrophy (Fig. 58-15). Complex forms of TOF include TOF with pulmonary atresia with or without major aortopulmonary collateral arteries, absent pulmonary valve, and CAVC defects.[25]

Anatomy and Pathophysiology The right ventricular outflow tract obstruction (RVOTO) may be at subpulmonary level, pulmonary valve level, main pulmonary artery level, or pulmonary artery bifurcation level or may involve branch pulmonary arteries. In some cases, obstruction is present at all levels. A right-sided aortic arch occurs in 25% (associated with chromosome 22q11 microdeletion); particularly in the presence of anomalous origin of the left subclavian artery. Preoperative physiology depends on the degree of RVOTO. Patients with minimal obstruction present with a left-to-right shunt owing to the VSD. These patients have pulmonary overcirculation; this is called *acyanotic TOF*. These patients present with congestive heart failure. At the other end of the spectrum, severe obstruction to pulmonary blood flow causes profound cyanosis.

Indications for Intervention The nature of the RVOTO dictates management. In cyanotic TOF, hypercyanotic episodes may occur with agitation or irritability. If profound, blood pressure falls with an altered level of consciousness; this is a classic TOF spell. A single spell is an indication for surgery. Ideally, referral should precede the spell. Conservative management is knee-to-chest positioning, administration of supplemental oxygen, sedation, volume expansion, and other measures that increase cardiac preload and systemic resistance. β Blockade is helpful. The chest radiograph may be classic in terms of a "boot-shaped" heart. Echocardiography is diagnostic, and associated anomalies can be excluded. Cardiac catheterization is indicated before repair of TOF with previous palliation and under those circumstances in which the presence of aortic pulmonary collaterals and pulmonary artery branching abnormalities are suspected. Timing is controversial regarding management of asymptomatic TOF. In asymptomatic patients, elective repair has been advocated from the neonatal period up until 1 year of age. In symptomatic or cyanotic patients, depending on institutional preferences, complete repair can be performed as a single-stage procedure or as a two-stage approach, with initial systemic-to-pulmonary artery shunting.[26,27]

Surgical Intervention

PALLIATION A systemic-to-pulmonary artery shunt is indicated in those patients in whom the risk of complete repair is considered to be higher than the cumulative risk of two-stage repair for a given institution. Creation of a systemic-to-pulmonary artery shunt can be carried out either from the midline or from a thoracotomy. Methods include a classic Blalock-Taussig shunt or a modified Blalock-Taussig shunt utilizing an interposition Gore-Tex tube graft. Creation of a shunt on the left side is more difficult to take down at the time of complete repair. Most institutions will currently perform a right-sided shunt through a right thoracotomy or from the midline, creating a central-to-right pulmonary artery shunt.[27]

COMPLETE REPAIR Complete repair involves closure of the VSD, preservation of the conducting system, and relief of the RVOTO. A median sternotomy is utilized with CPB. Two approaches are used. The transventricular repair with a right ventriculotomy in the infundibulum allows exposure of the VSD and a patch closure of the infundibular incision. Alternatively, the VSD and subpulmonary obstruction can be approached from a transatrial direction.[28] Muscle resection is carried out to relieve the RVOTO. Assessment of the pulmonary annulus, utilizing predicted mean-normal diameters of the pulmonary valve annulus corrected for body surface area, provide some guidance for enlarging the pulmonary annulus (transannular patching) (Fig. 58-16).[29] The transventricular repair is less popular today with increasing use of the transatrial-transpulmonary repair. In severe multilevel obstruction and hypoplasia, a conduit connection of the right ventricle to the pulmonary arteries is preferred in some centers. Distal pulmonary arteries and branch pulmonary artery stenosis are dealt with at the time of surgery, utilizing autologous pericardial patch enlargement.

Today, the mortality risk for uncomplicated TOF repair should approach 0%. Specific postoperative problems are a residual or previously undiagnosed VSD. Residual RVOTO may be progressive and may require repeat resection. Acute right ventricular dysfunction is quite frequent after TOF repair utilizing a transventricular approach but usually recovers. Residual VSDs, residual RVOTO, and long-standing pulmonary and tricuspid valve regurgitation all contribute to right ventricular dysfunction. The risk of reoperation for various reasons within 2 to 5 years is 3% to 5%. Other forms of complex TOF (e.g., absent pulmonary valve and CAVC) are managed as follows:

TOF with absent pulmonary valve is usually associated with massive enlargement of the main and branch pulmonary arteries. There is a characteristic "to-and-fro" murmur. The airway is abnormal, with areas of tracheomalacia or malformed cartilage. Three basic symptom groups are identified. The first group is neonates in extremis with immediate postnatal respiratory distress. The second group comprises older infants who develop significant airway compromise more remotely from birth. The third group experiences no significant airway problems. The neonatal group presents early with marked respiratory distress, cyanosis, and air trapping owing to tracheobronchial compression. The hypoxemia is largely

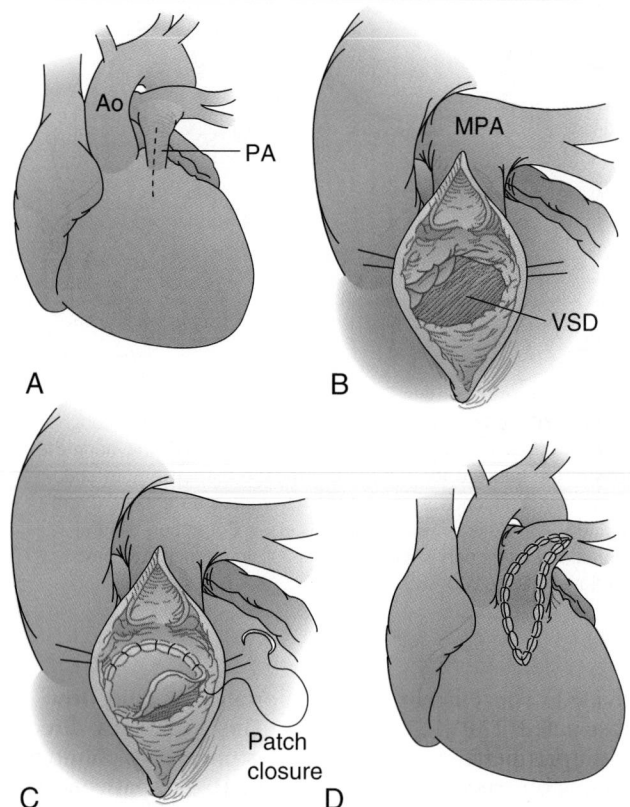

■ FIGURE 58-16.   Complete repair of tetralogy of Fallot. **A,** Enlargement of the right ventricle to main pulmonary artery (PA) connection with a transannular incision if necessary. Ao, aorta. **B,** Resection of muscle from the outflow tract and identification of edges of the ventricular septal defect (VSD). MPA, main pulmonary artery. **C,** Patch closure of the VSD. **D,** Placement of a transannular patch if required.

due to impaired ventilation because it is unusual to have severe RVOTO. Early repair of this subgroup is necessary, with anterior and posterior reduction of the pulmonary arteries and complete TOF repair, but results may be disappointing because of the intrinsic small and large airway disease.[30] Older infants are repaired when airway obstruction becomes evident and usually do well. The third group is electively repaired by 1 year of age.

The combination of TOF with CAVC has resulted in a very widespread incidence of reported surgical and postoperative mortality. The management of the RVOTO is as been described for TOF, but it is important to avoid narrowing of the left ventricular outflow tract at the time of patch placement for the VSD. Right-sided AV valve regurgitation is of more concern when pulmonary valve incompetence is created by a transannular patch.[31]

Another subgroup that should be included briefly is the group of "extreme tetralogy" or TOF with pulmonary atresia and duct-dependent pulmonary blood flow. Neonatal surgical intervention is required, either shunt or complete repair. A further subgroup of TOF with pulmonary atresia has hypoplastic or absent central pulmonary arteries and multiple aortopulmonary collateral arteries

(MAPCAs). In this variant, the intracardiac anatomy is that of TOF. However, the heterogeneity of the pulmonary artery anatomy complicates the condition. Essentially three patterns of pulmonary supply are recognized:

Absent central pulmonary arteries with MAPCAs; small central pulmonary arteries and MAPCAs; and diminutive central pulmonary arteries usually with significant arborization defects and MAPCAs. The approach is to provide a stable source of pulmonary blood flow and attempt to recruit the MAPCAs into the central pulmonary artery system (unifocalization). Complete or biventricular repair is achieved when enough unobstructed segments have been unifocalized to allow VSD closure and placement of a conduit between the right ventricle and the reconstructed pulmonary arteries, with a postrepair right ventricular pressure less than 70 mm Hg. The optimal choice of surgery is controversial, with many groups still preferring a staged approach,[32] whereas others prefer a single-stage, midline complete unifocalization and an attempt at VSD closure.[33]

Pulmonary Atresia and Intact Ventricular Septum

Pulmonary atresia and intact ventricular septum (PAIVS) is a heterogeneous group of lesions. The spectrum ranges from patients with small right ventricles and small tricuspid valves with associated coronary artery abnormalities placing them at high risk for survival. At the other end of the spectrum, patients have nearly normal-sized right ventricles with a well-developed infundibulum and absent coronary anomalies. These patients have a favorable prognosis.

Anatomy and Pathophysiology Associated with atresia of the pulmonary valve is an intact ventricular septum and variable hypoplasia of the right ventricle and tricuspid valve. The main pulmonary artery is present, somewhat smaller than normal, and pulmonary blood flow is supplied by a PDA. The tricuspid valve is variably hypoplastic and usually morphologically abnormal. Right ventricular cavity-to-coronary artery connections are almost always seen in patients with a particularly small right ventricle and tricuspid valve and a tiny or absent infundibulum. The physiology is similar to that of other forms of functional single ventricle with a duct-dependent pulmonary circuit. Depending on the degree of sinusoid and fistula formation, part or all of the coronary circuit may exhibit so-called right ventricular dependency.

Diagnosis can be made on echocardiography. Ductal patency can be confirmed and the degree of right ventricular hypertension estimated by the gradient across the regurgitant tricuspid valve. Abnormal flow patterns into the right ventricle are suggestive of coronary artery fistula. The presence and size of the infundibulum, inflow, and the trabeculated portion of the right ventricle are determined. Cardiac catheterization is indicated for an assessment of coronary artery anatomy when sinusoids and fistula formation are suspected,[34] or this investigation may be deferred until before planned CPB operations. PAIVS associated with Ebstein's anomaly and a large right ventricle constitutes a separate subgroup warranting a separate therapeutic approach.

Management This condition necessitates a staged approach toward either a univentricular or a biventricular repair. Decision making is based initially on the size of the infundibulum.[35] In patients with an absent infundibulum and significant coronary-to-right ventricle fistulas in whom biventricular repair is unlikely, the first stage would be a palliative modified Blalock-Taussig shunt with or without ligation of the PDA in the neonatal period. If the PDA remains open without PGE$_1$, the PDA should be ligated at the time of shunting. With favorable anatomy, relief of the RVOTO by means of a surgical valvotomy, a systemic-to-pulmonary artery shunt (left subclavian to main pulmonary artery), and PDA ligation through a left thoracotomy is an option. Alternatively, if the right ventricle is less hypoplastic, the pulmonary valve may be opened in the catheterization laboratory and the duct kept open with PGE$_1$ for 2 to 4 weeks. If saturations are inadequate with trial duct closure, a shunt is added surgically.

Depending on the response to the initial procedures, either a Fontan-type track is chosen or a biventricular repair is aimed for. If the RVOTO can be adequately relieved and the tricuspid valve and right ventricle grow to adequate size, the shunt can be taken down surgically and the ASD closed. About 80% of patients with a well-formed infundibulum will eventually achieve biventricular repair. The remainder may benefit from 1$^{1/2}$ ventricle repair (ASD closure and a superior vena cava-to-right pulmonary artery shunt [bidirectional Glenn]).[36] The Fontan operation is indicated in those cases with severe right ventricular hypoplasia and a right ventricle-dependent coronary circuit. Surgical mortality depends on the anatomic variant of PAIVS; some of these patients will require subsequent cardiac transplantation.[37]

Pulmonary Valve Stenosis

Isolated pulmonary valve stenosis usually occurs with a nearly normal-sized, hypertrophied right ventricle and a normal tricuspid valve, but some have significant right ventricular hypoplasia. The distal pulmonary artery anatomy is also usually normal. The morphology of the pulmonary valve is variable and can be morphologically abnormal with a unicuspid, bicuspid, or tricuspid valve with commissural fusion. In these patients, a biventricular outcome can be expected. Balloon valvuloplasty has become the initial procedure of choice. In some patients with severely dysplastic pulmonary valves, surgical valvotomy may be required. If properly managed, these patients have a low mortality

Other Abnormalities of the Conotruncus

Transposition of the great arteries (TGA) accounts for 5% to 7% of all congenital cardiac malformations. Congenitally corrected TGA is a condition in which, in addition to ventricular arterial discordance, AV discordance is present.[38]

Transposition of the Great Arteries

TGA is defined as an aorta arising from the morphologic right ventricle and the pulmonary artery arising from the morphologic left ventricle. Associated abnormalities include VSD (40%), coarctation or interrupted aortic arch (10%), left ventricular outflow tract obstruction (5% to 10%), and abnormal coronary artery branching patents in one third of patients.[39] Classification of TGA is into simple and complex TGA.

Simple Transposition

The interventricular septum is intact or almost intact. Profound cyanosis presents soon after birth, worsened by closure of the PDA. Early survival depends on the size of the ASD. Reopening of a closing ductus arteriosus with PGE_1 infusion enhances mixing at the atrial level. The dominant physiologic abnormality in TGA is reduced oxygenation with increased right and left ventricular volume load.

Complex TGA

The physiology is essentially unchanged from that of simple transposition, aside from the fact that a VSD or VSDs allow mixing at an additional level, with a tendency to higher systemic saturations than occurs in simple TGA and adding congestive heart failure to the symptoms.

Diagnosis In the neonatal period, diagnosis is made with echocardiography. Formal catheterization is rarely needed. If balloon atrial septostomy is required, this can be done in the catheter laboratory, or preferably in the intensive care unit under echocardiographic guidance. Cardiac catheterization may be requested in complex TGA in the absence of adequate echocardiographic detail or in delayed diagnosis to measure pulmonary resistance.

Surgical Intervention The current "gold standard" is the arterial switch operation. Previously, atrial level repair with either a Senning or a Mustard procedure was used (Fig. 58-17). The atrial level repair is no longer the procedure of choice owing to associated atrial arrhythmias, baffle obstruction, and late deterioration of the morphologic right ventricular function in the systemic circuit.[40] Fundamental to the arterial switch operation is the fact that the left ventricle must be able to handle the systemic workload. In simple TGA, closure of the PDA in the postnatal period decreases PAPs, which causes the left ventricle to involute or decondition. Currently, experience indicates that the left ventricle remains adequately prepared for at least 1 month after closure of the PDA.[41] Patients with a large VSD will have a higher pressure in the left ventricle.

Surgery can be undertaken when the infant is a little older but, in the absence of a pulmonary artery band, should be achieved by 3 months of age. The arterial switch is performed on CPB through a median sternotomy. In simple TGA, circulatory arrest is avoided or utilized only for ASD closure. The great vessels are transected, and the orifices and course of the coronary arteries are inspected. The coronary arteries are reimplanted into the neoaorta. The posteriorly located pulmonary artery bifurcation is brought anterior to the aorta (Lecompte maneuver) and aortic reconstruction is completed. Pulmonary artery reconstruction of the excised coronary artery buttons is with autologous pericardium. Continuity between the right ventricle and the pulmonary arteries is reestablished (Fig. 58-18). Any associated defects are repaired at the time of arterial switch.

Results In some centers, mortality for simple TGA approaches 0%, whereas for TGA with VSD it is reported at between 3% and 5%. Factors shown to increase the mortality in some series include intramural course of the left coronary artery, a retropulmonary course of the left coronary artery, multiple VSDs, and hypoplasia of a ventricle.[42]

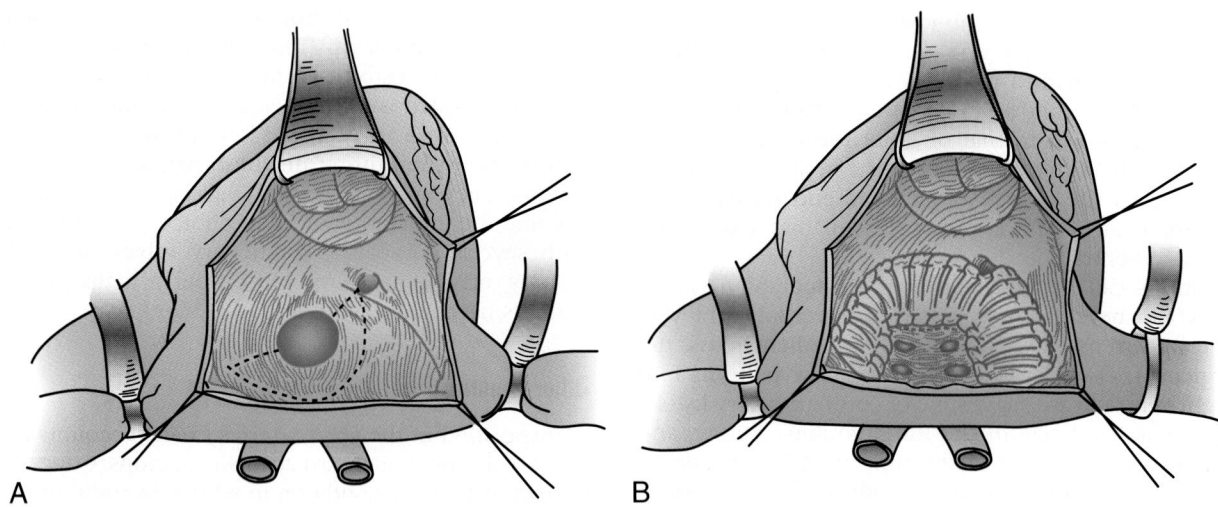

A   **B**

■ **FIGURE 58-17.**   The Mustard operation. **A,** Interior of the right atrium is shown after a longitudinal right atriotomy is performed. The interatrial septum is excised along the *dotted lines.* The coronary sinus is cut back toward the left atrial side. **B,** A baffle is used to divert the venal caval blood to the left atrium and across the mitral valve. Completion of the right atrial suture line will allow systemic venous blood to enter the right atrium, cross the tricuspid valve, and exit into the transposed aorta. (From Trusler GA, Freedom RM: Transposition of the great arteries: The Mustard procedure. *In* Sabiston DC Jr, Spencer FC [eds]: Gibbons Surgery of the Chest. Philadelphia, WB Saunders, 1983, p 1138.)

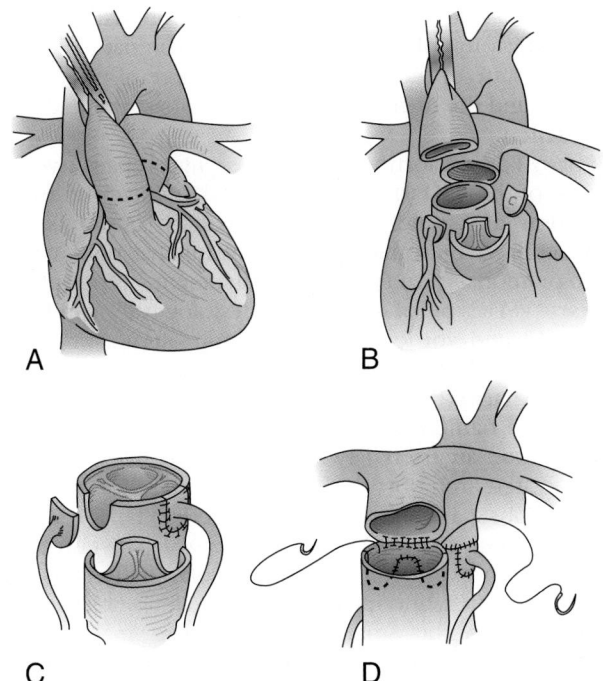

FIGURE 58-18. The arterial switch procedure for transposition of the great arteries. **A,** The external anatomy is shown, with sites of transection of the two great vessels delineated by the *dotted lines.* **B,** The aorta and main pulmonary arteries are transected and the coronary buttons have been removed from the native aortic root. **C,** The coronary buttons are transferred to the neoaorta. **D,** The coronary button reimplantation sites are repaired with a pericardial patch, and the neopulmonary artery is anastomosed to the distal main pulmonary artery. The distal pulmonary artery has been moved anterior to the ascending aorta (Lecompte maneuver). (From Wernovsky G, Jonas RA: Other conotruncal lesions. *In* Chang CA, Hanley FL, Wernovsky G, Wessell DL [eds]: Pediatric Cardiac Intensive Care. Baltimore, Williams & Wilkins, 1998.)

Postoperatively, reevaluation for supravalvular, aortic, and pulmonary stenosis should be followed with echocardiography. Long-term follow-up of patients has so far been notable for the low incidence of complications or need for reoperation in many series.[42] Late coronary artery obstruction has been reported in some series.

Congenitally Corrected Transposition (ccTGA)

In this rare condition there is atrioventricular and ventriculoarterial discordance or DORV at the transposition end of the DORV spectrum. Saturated and desaturated blood streams through this kind of heart to the appropriate destination but the morphologic RV is in the systemic circuit and is prone to a high incidence of Ebsteinoid malformation of the tricuspid valve (systemic AV valve). The systemic RV tends to fail with time in much the same way that the systemic RV tends to fail after atrial repair (Mustard or Senning) for TGA. Similarly in ccTGA the incidence and earliness of systemic RV failure is related to associated lesions, and particularly the presence of a large VSD that has been previously patched. In addition the prevalence of an Ebsteinoid type malformation of the tri-

cuspid valve ensures a high incidence of early or progressive systemic AV valve regurgitation in ccTGA compared with atrially repaired TGA. Spontaneous or surgical heart block occurs, adding to the burden of the morphologic RV.

In theoretical terms, a combined atrial repair (Mustard or Senning) and arterial switch in patients without significant pulmonary stenosis, or a combined atrial repair and Rastelli operation for those with significant pulmonary stenosis, will extract the morphologic RV from the systemic circuit and decrease the back pressure on a defective tricuspid valve. This has been called the "double switch operation." However, this is a long operation with at least significant theoretic hazards in terms of myocardial protection and ability to achieve a nonobstructed atrial repair particularly in the commonly found configuration of a ventricular apex in a position discordant with the atrial situs. In this situation the morphologic RA lies behind the ventricular mass and has a much smaller anteroposterior width of the free wall. Interestingly, this form of cardiac positional discordance appears to present more frequently in the presence of severe pulmonary stenosis or atresia. In addition, the tricuspid valve appears less likely to be deformed compared with when the apex of the heart is pointing in the appropriate direction for the type of atrial situs and is also less likely to be incompetent when significant PS or pulmonary atresia is present.

There are two types of ccTGA. The most common is with atrial situs solitus and an L-loop of the ventricles (ccTGA SLL), and much more rarely (2% to 3% of a ccTGA) there is atrial situs inversus with a D-loop of the ventricles (ccTGA IDD). When the pulmonary valve comes largely off the RV (DORV) there is nearly always severe pulmonary stenosis or atresia and the aorta is further from the VSD, making the Rastelli part of the double switch more difficult, particularly if the VSD is somewhat restrictive. The usual VSD enlargement for a Rastelli by enlarging superiorly is not possible without creating complete heart block in a ccTGA (SLL), because of the superiorly placed AV mode and conducting bundle. In ccTGA (IDD) the conducting system is inferior and superior VSD enlargement is feasible.

If patients with ccTGA present with RV and TV failure with an intact interventricular septum (either congenitally or after previous VSD closure), without LV outflow obstruction, the morphologic LV has involuted and is thin walled. Before achieving a double switch, the LV requires retraining by pulmonary artery banding to a point where it is operating comfortably at near systemic pressure and with good function, before double switching is feasible. It is clearly easier to retrain a morphologic LV in patients younger than 12 to 14 years of age than in late adolescence or adulthood, particularly when full retraining must be achieved from an LV starting pressure that is of a normal pulmonary artery systolic pressure. The double switch after LV retraining appears more hazardous and is more likely to be associated with late LV failure particularly in older patients. LV failure either during retraining or after the double switch is an indication to consider heart transplantation at the appropriate clinical timing.

Despite the magnitude of the double switch (0 to 8%) operations, the 30-day mortality has been acceptable particularly in the three centers with the largest current experience (the author's personal series,[43] Birmingham Children's Hospital, UK,[44] and Tokyo Women's Hospital[45]). Intermediate-term results also appear encouraging, but long-term results are not yet available.

Double-Outlet Right Ventricle

DORV is a conotruncal malformation in which both great arteries arise or mostly arise from the right ventricle. DORV is a spectrum of abnormalities with variable physiology and surgical options.

Anatomy and Pathophysiology By one definition, all of one and more than 50% of the other great artery arise from the right ventricle. Four types of DORV can be described based on the relationship of the VSD to the great vessels (Fig. 58-19): (1) subaortic VSD with or without pulmonary stenosis; (2) subpulmonary VSD with or without subaortic stenosis (SAS) and associated arch obstruction; (3) doubly committed VSD; and (4) remote or noncommitted VSD. Associated abnormalities occur frequently, including right or left ventricular hypoplasia, straddling or common AV valves, mitral or tricuspid valve stenosis or atresia, multiple VSDs, and an association with heterotaxy.[46] The physiology will depend on the nature of the VSD, the state of the AV valves, the degree of pulmonary stenosis, and the degree of subaortic obstruction and arch obstruction.

Surgery For subaortic VSD, biventricular repair involves closure of the VSD to baffle the left ventricular outflow to the aorta and relief of the pulmonary outflow tract obstruction, which may or may not involve right ventricle-to-pulmonary artery conduit placement.[47] The subpulmonary VSD type of DORV is physiologically similar to TGA. SAS and aortic arch obstruction often complicate this subtype. In the absence of significant pulmonary or subpulmonary stenosis, surgical repair involves closure of the VSD to baffle the left ventricular outflow to the pulmonary root, an arterial switch operation, and correction of associated arch obstruction and SAS. Surgical mortality for this subset is higher, around 10%. For DORV with a doubly committed VSD or a remote VSD, biventricular repair is more difficult. Intraventricular baffling is frequently complex, and intracardiac obstruction may result, particularly in the smaller heart. Staged management should be considered. Frequently, pulmonary artery banding or a palliative systemic-to-pulmonary artery shunt allows somatic growth and a reassessment of the feasibility of a biventricular repair. If septation is possible but the right ventricle is small, a one and one-half ventricle repair may be considered. If septation of the heart is impossible or very difficult, it may be safer to perform a Fontan type of repair.

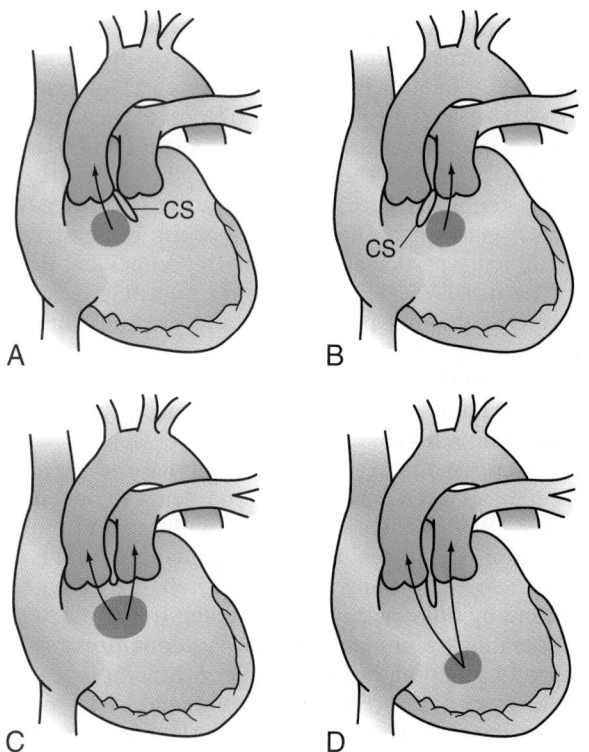

FIGURE 58-19. The four types of VSD in double-outlet right ventricle (DORV). A view of the right-sided ventricular septum. CS, conal septum. **A,** Subaortic VSD. **B,** Subpulmonary VSD. **C,** Doubly committed VSD. **D,** Remote or noncommitted VSD. (From Thompson WR, Nichols DG, Ungerleider RM: Double outlet right ventricle and double outlet left ventricle. *In* Nichols DG, Cameron DE, Greeley WJ, et al [eds]: Critical Heart Disease in Infants and Children. St. Louis, Mosby, 1995.)

Left Ventricular Outflow Tract Obstruction

Left ventricular outflow tract obstruction (LVOTO) can occur at any level from the subaortic area to the descending aorta. These lesions may be isolated or combined; and when combined with mitral and left ventricular hypoplasia, the eponym Shone's syndrome is attached. Significant hypoplasia of the left ventricle, mitral valve, and aortic valve may preclude a biventricular repair. Various degrees of left ventricular hypertrophy accompany LVOTO.

In severe LVOTO, endocardial fibroelastosis may be present at birth, further impairing contractile function and significantly affecting short- and long-term survival. Neonates with critical or severe LVOTO present in a low cardiac output state and with multiple organ dysfunction. Adequate systemic output requires an open duct, and PGE_1 infusion is needed for resuscitation and stabilization. Older patients have time for the left ventricle to hypertrophy. Concentric hypertrophy, if severe enough, can lead to subendocardial ischemia, which will present as an abnormal exercise response. If the condition is untreated, left ventricular failure or sudden death supervenes. Surgery is directed at establishing unobstructed systemic blood flow, and a wide variety of procedures are variously indicated: from the conservative LVOTO resection, through the radical Konno procedure, which includes aortic valve replacement, to the Norwood-type procedure for overall uncorrectable left heart inadequacy.

Aortic Stenosis

Valvular Aortic Stenosis

The degree of stenosis varies, and symptoms are usually seen only when the stenosis is severe. In symptomatic neonates, the valve leaflets are often markedly thickened and nodular. The valve may be tricuspid, bicuspid, or unicuspid, and this has a bearing on the anticipated effectiveness of the different forms of intervention. In older children, gross nodular myxomatous changes are less frequently seen. Multiple additional levels of LVOTO may accompany valvular stenosis.

Diagnosis and Presentation The echocardiogram is usually diagnostic. Neonates and infants present with congestive heart failure or circulatory collapse. Older infants present with signs of congestive heart failure or a murmur. Surgery in the neonate can be briefly delayed for resuscitation with PGE_1, inotropes, and positive-pressure ventilation. Urgent relief of the obstruction should be considered. In older infants, a measured gradient of greater than 50 mm Hg, a positive exercise test, or symptoms (even in the presence of normal left ventricular function) are indications for intervention.

Surgery Balloon dilation is considered by some centers as a valid alternative to surgical valvotomy. Surgical valvotomy is undertaken under CPB. The aortic valve is incised through an aortotomy (Fig. 58-20). Patients with severe multiple left heart obstructions may be better served with a Norwood-type procedure.[48] In older patients, aortic valvuloplasty is undertaken. Aortic valve replacement is the less preferable option. Replacement may be with a bioprosthetic, mechanical valve, or a homograft. Another option is the Ross procedure, which involves translocation of the excised, native pulmonary valve into the aortic position with coronary artery relocation. The right ventricular outflow tract is then reconstructed utilizing a pulmonary homograft (Fig. 58-21). The Ross operation has risks, and those reported include coronary artery insufficiency, aortic insufficiency, ventricular dysfunction, RVOTO, and LVOTO. Additionally, the conduit in the pulmonary position will have to be replaced in time.[49]

For patients with severe complex LVOTO, aortoventriculoplasty or a Konno procedure is an option. An incision is made into the aorta, and a right ventriculotomy is extended into the septum. The aortic annulus is enlarged with a prosthetic patch. A patch is used to close the right ventriculotomy separately. A modification of this procedure includes the Ross-Konno operation.[50]

Results In expert hands, there is little difference in mortality between balloon valvuloplasty and surgical valvotomy.[51] Surgical valvotomy provides the opportunity of a more precise valvotomy and débridement of thickened nodular leaflets. Mortality for the Ross-Konno operation in selected centers can be less than 5% but is higher in neonates and infants.[50]

Subaortic Stenosis

SAS is divided into three groups: discrete membranous, fibromuscular tunnel type, and hypertrophic type. Discrete membranous SAS consists of a fibrous ring located below the level of the aortic valve. The aortic valve is often distorted, owing to abnormal flow patterns, and aortic insufficiency is common. So-called discrete membranous SAS is nearly always associated with a muscular abnormality of the LVOTO, and membrane removal should be combined with muscle wedge excision. The fibromuscular tunnel type is less common. The hypertrophic type is a dynamic outflow tract obstruction with hypertrophy of the underlying interventricular septum (idiopathic hypertrophic SAS). The characteristics of this are asymmetrical septal hypertrophy and the presence of systolic anterior motion of the anterior leaflet of the mitral valve. A posteriorly malaligned VSD may contribute postoperatively to a degree of subaortic obstruction. Associated lesions include malalignment VSD defects, coarctation of the aorta, and CAVC.

Physiology These lesions have in common a pressure overload on the left ventricle associated with progressive left ventricular hypertrophy and eventual dysfunction. Additionally, with SAS, the turbulence created below the valve leaflets causes thickening and distortion of the aortic valve with an increased risk of aortic regurgitation. Echocardiography can identify the anatomic site of obstruction as well as the degree of obstruction. Cardiac catheterization is rarely indicated. Serial exercise testing is useful for borderline cases.

Surgery Indications for surgical intervention include a gradient of more than 25 mm Hg, the presence of underlying aortic insufficiency, and coexisting lesions. Surgery removes the LVOTO and preserves the aortic valve (Fig. 58-22). In Figure 58-22B the authors would recommend that the muscular wedge incision is made more to the left than shown in this illustration to avoid complete heart

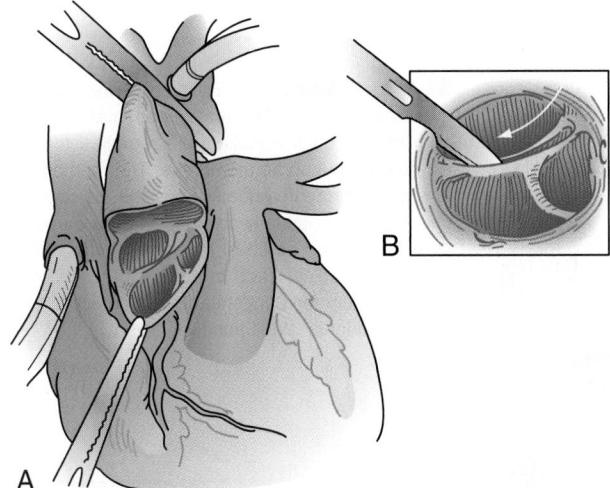

■ FIGURE 58-20. Close-up of the aortic valve demonstrates a surgical valvotomy. **A,** The valve is bicuspid with a prominent raphe in the anterior valve leaflet. **B,** The orifice is enlarged by incising the fused commissure between the two leaflets. (From Chang AC, Burke RP: Left ventricular outflow tract obstruction. *In* Chang AC, Hanley FL, Wernovsky G, Wessell DL [eds]: Pediatric Cardiac Intensive Care. Baltimore, Williams & Wilkins, 1998.)

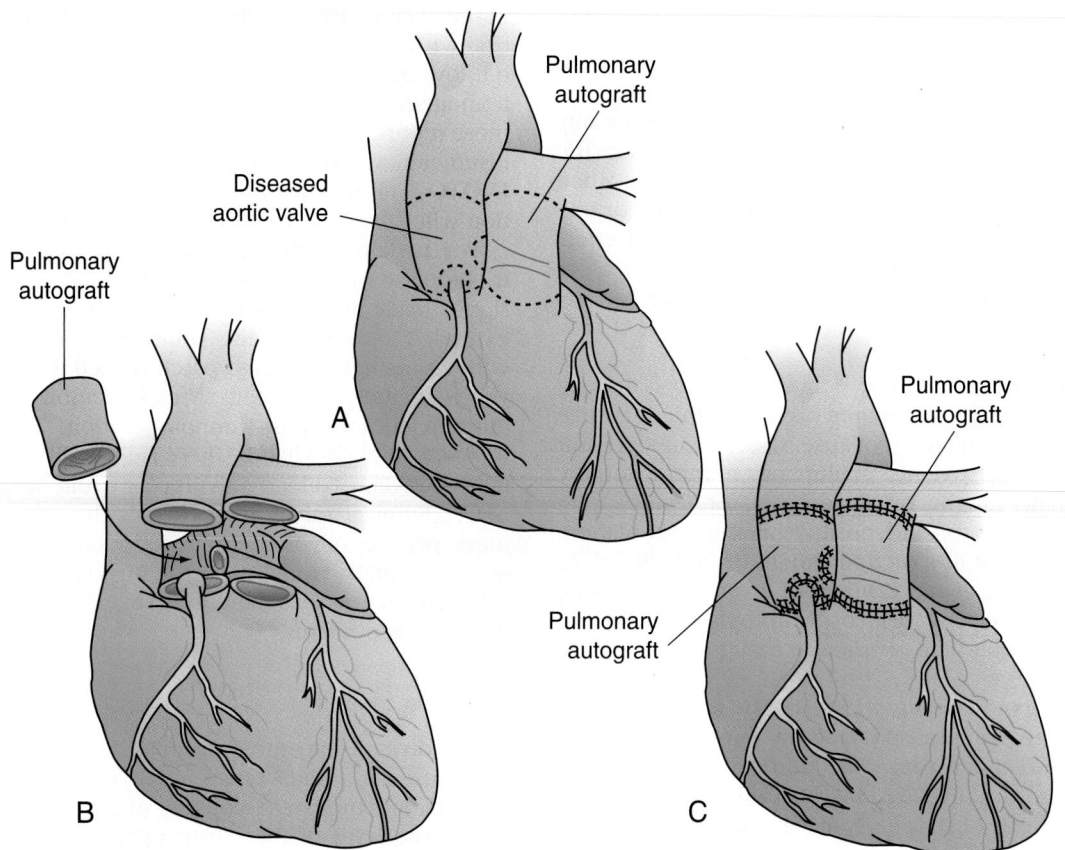

FIGURE 58-21.   The Ross procedure. **A,** The anatomy is shown with the lines of transection of the pulmonary autograft and the diseased aortic valve root. **B,** The pulmonary autograft is removed and is placed into the aortic root with coronary artery transfer. **C,** A pulmonary allograft is placed to reestablish right ventricular-to-pulmonary artery continuity. (From Kouchoukos NT, Davila-Roman VT, Spray TL, et al: Replacement of the aortic root with a pulmonary autograft in children and young adults with aortic valve disease. N Engl J Med 330:1, 1994. Copyright 1994 Massachusetts Medical Society. All rights reserved.)

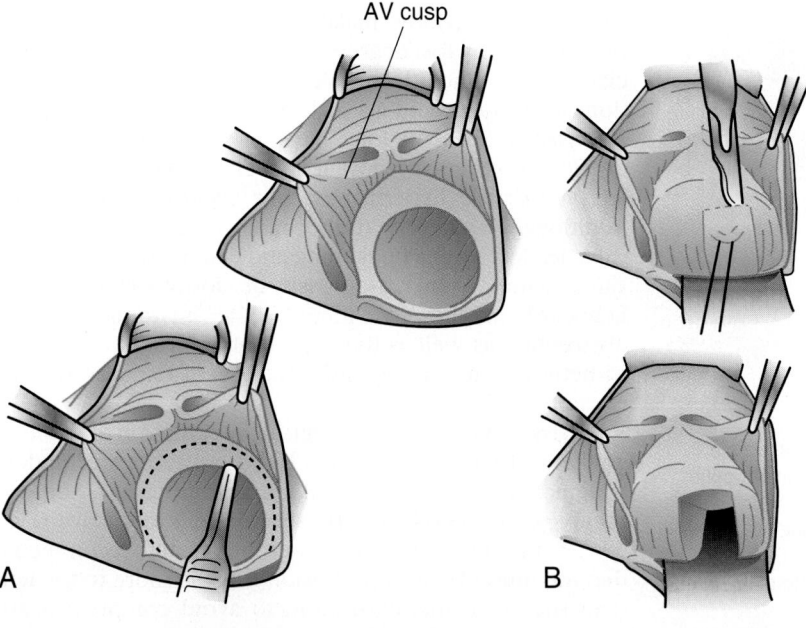

FIGURE 58-22.   **A,** Excision of discrete subaortic stenosis. The aorta is opened obliquely, and the aortic valve leaflets are retracted to expose the subaortic membrane. The membrane is excised circumferentially along the *indicated line.* **B,** This is usually combined with a muscle resection. (From de Leval M: Surgery of the left ventricular outflow tract. *In* Stark J, de Leval M [eds]: Surgery for Congenital Heart Defects, 2nd ed. Philadelphia, WB Saunders, 1994.)

block. Aortic insufficiency may be addressed by repair, but replacement may be necessary. For the tunnel-type SAS, a more radical procedure has to be undertaken; this would be a Konno or a modified Ross-Konno procedure. Current mortality is less than 5% for uncomplicated SAS. With a fibromuscular tunnel and other extensive surgeries, the mortality rate is higher. Recurrence and reoperation for SAS vary between 5% and 10%, with recurrence rates higher in the younger patient with severe stenosis.[52]

Supravalvular Aortic Stenosis

Supravalvular is rare and consists of a localized or diffuse narrowing from the level of the sinotubular junction. It is often associated with Williams' syndrome. A narrowing occurs above the aortic valve and the sinuses of Valsalva associated with a generalized vessel wall thickening. The aortic valve leaflets may or may not be abnormal. The coronary orifices may be obstructed by the thickened ring of tissue at the sinotubular junction.[53] Two types of supravalvular stenosis are described. Branch vessels from the ascending or descending aorta may be stenotic or hypoplastic. Associated lesions are pulmonary stenosis (valvular, supravalvular, or peripheral), aortic valve stenosis, and coarctation of the aorta. The pathophysiology is that of pressure overload and progressive left ventricular hypertrophy and eventual dysfunction.

Diagnosis Echocardiography is usually diagnostic. In association with Williams' syndrome, right-sided obstruction should be excluded. Cardiac catheterization is probably indicated to identify coronary artery origin narrowing, other systemic artery origin stenosis, and peripheral pulmonary artery stenosis.

Surgery Indications for surgery are a gradient of more than 50 mm Hg in an asymptomatic patient or positive exercise testing. Coronary artery stenosis is an indication for surgery. Through a median sternotomy and under CPB, patch angioplasty of the ascending aorta has been satisfactory (Fig. 58-23). Mortality for surgery is lower for the discrete type of supravalvular aortic stenosis (<5%). With the diffuse form, the risk of recurrence and re-intervention is quite high.[53]

Aortic Arch Interruption

Aortic arch interruption is a rare lesion with loss of continuity between the ascending and the descending aorta. Blood flowing to the descending aorta is maintained through a large ductus arteriosus. Interrupted arch is rarely isolated, and in 80% of cases there is an associated large, malalignment VSD. Other associated abnormalities include a bicuspid aortic valve, LVOTO, DiGeorge's syndrome, truncus arteriosus, single ventricle, TGA, DORV, and aorticopulmonary window.

Anatomy and Pathophysiology Aortic arch interruption is classified into the three types of Celoria and Patton, types A, B, and C. Type A (interruption beyond the left subclavian artery) occurs in approximately 25% of patients. Type B (interruption between the left carotid and the subclavian arteries) is the most common form, occurring in approximately 70% of patients. Type C (interruption

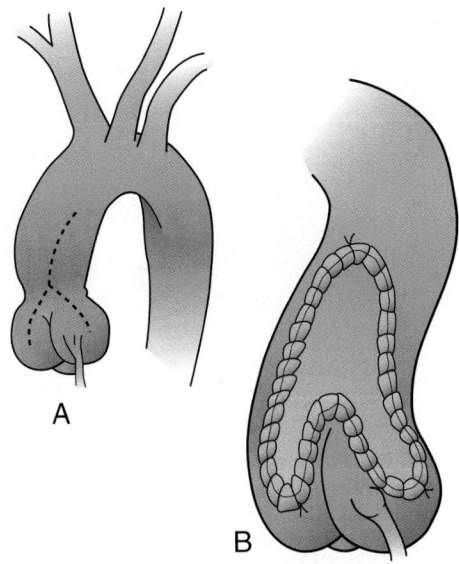

FIGURE 58-23. Surgical repair of discrete supravalvular aortic stenosis. **A,** The autotomy is performed extending into both the noncoronary and the right coronary sinuses. **B,** After the supravalvular ridge and obstructive tissue are excised, a Y-shaped, pantaloon-shaped patch of pericardium is sutured in place. (From Van Son JA, Danielson GK, Puga FJ, et al: Supravalvular aortic stenosis: Long term results of surgical treatment. J Thorac Cardiovasc Surg 107:103, 1994.)

between the innominate and the left carotid arteries) is the rarest, occurring in less than 5% of patients (Fig. 58-24). Interrupted aortic arch is thought to occur as a result of disappearance of a normally persisting connection between the left fourth and the left sixth aortic arches. Most infants with interrupted aortic arch present within the first few days of life. Reduced systemic blood flow to the lower extremities causes acidosis, renal failure, hepatic ischemia, and necrotizing enterocolitis. Additionally, the pulmonary circulation is flooded as the PVR drops. These patients develop rapid congestive heart failure. Pulse oximetry may reveal a differential between left upper body, right upper body, and lower body saturations. PGE_1 allows reopening of the duct, providing a period for recovery before undertaking complete repair. Ventilatory management is used to limit pulmonary blood flow. The DiGeorge syndrome or variant occurs in 15% to 30% of infants with interrupted aortic arch. Hypocalcemia can be problematic, and blood products should be irradiated. Echocardiography is diagnostic.

Surgery In the current era, a single-stage complete repair is preferable to a staged approach. Utilizing CPB and DHCA, resection of all ductal tissue followed by anastomosis between the separated aortic segments is performed. The VSD and other defects are repaired on CPB to limit the period of DHCA. The VSD is closed, and other

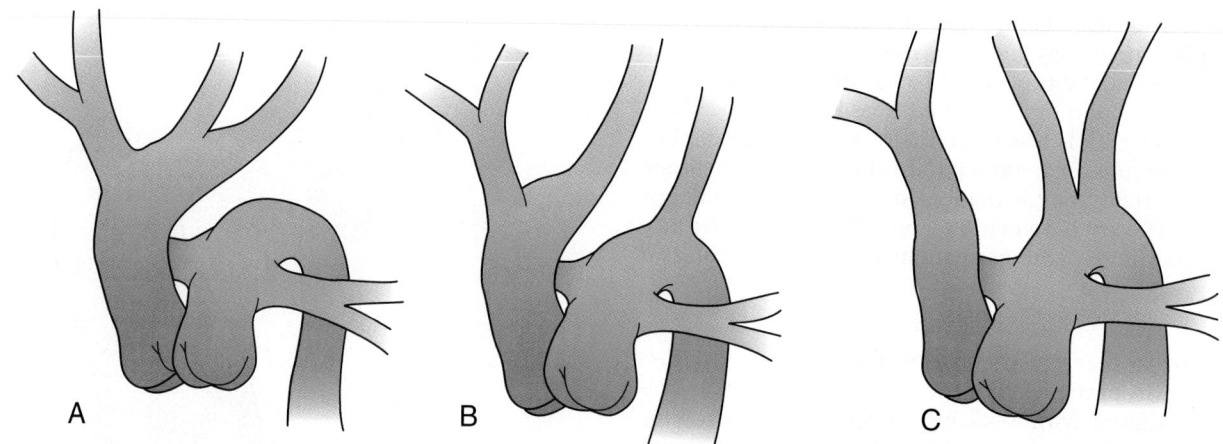

FIGURE 58-24.   The types of interrupted aortic arch. **A,** The interruption is at the aortic isthmus between the left subclavian artery and the ductus arteriosus. **B,** The interruption is at the distal aortic arch between the left carotid and the left subclavian arteries. **C,** The interruption is located at the proximal aortic arch between the innominate and the left carotid arteries. (From Chang AC, Starnes VA: Interrupted aortic arch. *In* Chang AC, Hanley FL, Wernovsky G, Wessell DL [eds]: Pediatric Cardiac Intensive Care. Baltimore, Williams & Wilkins, 1998.)

defects are treated accordingly. Surgical management of interrupted aortic arch continues to have a relatively high mortality rate owing to associated defects. Reported mortality rates vary between 10% and 38%. Risk factors for mortality are low birth weight, interrupted aortic arch type B, and SAS.[54]

Coarctation of the Aorta

Coarctation of the aorta is a congenital narrowing of the thoracic aorta, usually occurring distal to the left subclavian artery, at the point of insertion of the ductus arteriosus. Coarctation represents 5% to 8% of all cases of congenital heart disease. It is associated with other congenital heart defects, specifically PDA, VSD, bicuspid aortic valve, subaortic obstruction, and mitral valve abnormalities.

Anatomy and Pathophysiology The site of coarctation is always juxtaductal, with or without associated arch or isthmic hypoplasia. Two theories for the development of coarctation are the flow theory and the ductal sling theory. Coarctation of the aorta occurs in two groups of patients: infants with associated cardiac anomalies and those with isolated severe coarctation of the aorta, with the blood flow to the lower extremities dependent on the ductus arteriosus. Patients with severe coarctation and duct-dependent descending aortic flow present with cardiovascular collapse at the time of spontaneous ductal closure. PGE_1 opens and maintains the patency of the ductus arteriosus, preserving distal organ perfusion. Surgical intervention can be delayed until stabilization of the child has been achieved. Older patients are often asymptomatic or present with claudication on exercise or with upper body hypertension. Alterations in renal function, baroreceptor function, and the renin-angiotensin axis contribute to the proximal systemic hypertension. Later in life, these patients may develop aortic aneurysms proximal or distal to the coarctation, aortic dissection, cerebral aneurysm rupture, and increased atherosclerotic disease.

Diagnosis and Indications for Intervention Physical findings of absent femoral pulses and poor distal perfusion are highly suggestive of the diagnosis in an infant. Echocardiography is diagnostic in most instances. This study can document the branching pattern of the head and neck vessels and determine the aortic arch and isthmus size. In the older child who is asymptomatic, upper extremity hypertension and a differential between upper and lower body pressures should be diagnostic. The echocardiogram in most instances will confirm the diagnosis. Cardiac catheterization may be required for associated cardiac anomalies. Other modalities that may be useful include computed tomography (CT) and MRI. In the older patient, diagnosis is an indication for elective intervention.

Surgery The surgical approach is through a left posterolateral thoracotomy. The exception is with important associated intracardiac anomalies, when the defect is repaired simultaneously through the midline. Surgical options include resection and end-to-end anastomosis (Fig. 58-25), prosthetic patch aortoplasty, and subclavian flap aortoplasty. In the current era, the re-coarctation rate for end-to-end anastomosis is less than previously reported. The re-coarctation rate in neonates is about 10%. Prosthetic patch aortoplasty was introduced owing to the high rate of re-coarctation with the earlier end-to-end technique. Aneurysm formation has been reported in 5% to 30% of these patients. Subclavian flap aortoplasty utilizes the subclavian artery as an onlay graft. Variations of this technique include a reverse subclavian flap for repair of a coarctation proximal to the left subclavian artery. In older children, left arm ischemia after ligation of the subclavian artery can occur and sacrifice of the left subclavian artery may affect long-term growth and function of the limb. Prosthetic interposition graft placement has been used but has disadvantages in a growing child.

Potential complications during and after coarctation repair include hemorrhage, recurrent laryngeal nerve injury, Horner's syndrome, paraplegia, stroke, aneurysm formation, and recoarctation. Postoperatively, paradoxic

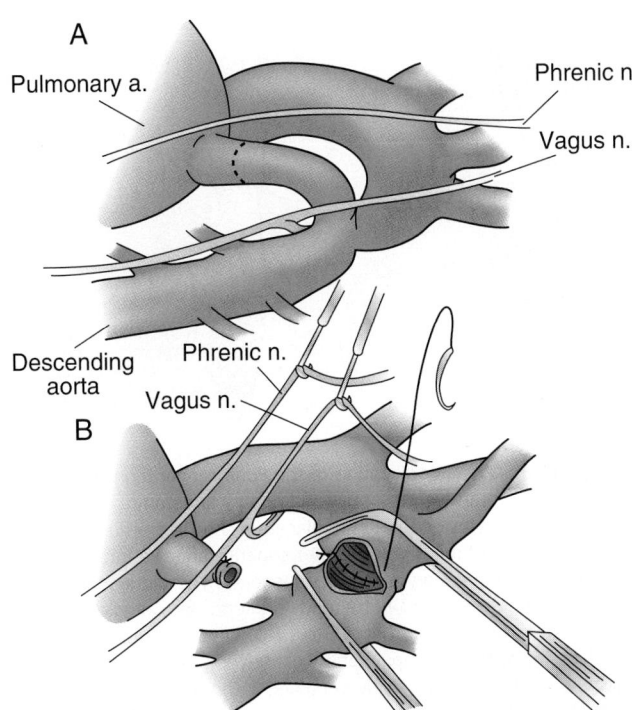

A

Pulmonary a.

Phrenic n.

Vagus n.

Descending aorta

Phrenic n.

Vagus n.

B

■ **FIGURE 58-25.** Repair of discrete coarctation by end-to-end anastomosis. **A,** The lines of resection of the coarctation are shown, as is the relationship of the vagus and recurrent laryngeal nerves. **B,** Completion of the anterior suture line. Note the clamp positioning preserving upper body flow. (From Castaneda AR, Jonas RA, Mayer JE, Hanley FL: Aortic coarctation. *In* Cardiac Surgery of the Neonate and Infant. Philadelphia, WB Saunders, 1994.)

hypertension is a common occurrence. It relates to the release of pressure on the baroceptors in the carotid arteries and aortic arch after removing the obstruction, as well as dissection around the sympathetic plexus of the aorta. This has to be carefully controlled postoperatively because reperfusion of the mesenteric arteries at a high pressure is potentially hazardous. Children are particularly prone to the development of mesenteric ischemia with severe abdominal pain, distention, and the development of an ileus. Hypertension usually resolves within 2 to 4 weeks postoperatively.

Paraplegia is a feared complication of aortic adult coarctation surgery, with an incidence of up to 1.5%. The incidence in neonates and children is closer to 0.2%. Paraplegia correlates with the length of aortic cross-clamping. Prevention of paraplegia requires the shortest possible cross-clamp time, moderate hypothermia intraoperatively (34°C to 35°C), a high-enough proximal blood pressure, and the avoidance of acute blood loss or acidosis. Aneurysms are related to all types of coarctation repair but especially prosthetic patch aortoplasty. Risk of aneurysms is greater over the age of 15 years or in patients undergoing operation for re-coarctation. Reoperation is required for a postoperative peak systolic pressure gradient over 20 mm Hg across the repair.[55] In recurrent coarc-

tation, balloon angioplasty is the procedure of choice; initial success rates are high, with a low incidence of complications.[56]

Unseptatable Hearts and the Fontan Principle

When it is estimated that one of the ventricles is inadequate for supporting total cardiac output, attempts at septation become too risky. A large number of diverse pathologic processes fall into this category. In unseptatable hearts, the aim of palliation is to ensure adequate, but not excessive, pulmonary blood flow, unobstructed systemic outflow from the ventricular mass, and unobstructed pulmonary venous return to the ventricular mass. If the early and subsequent palliative procedures are well conceived and executed, each patient will then fulfill criteria controlling eligibility for a Fontan-type repair. The Fontan principle requires that providing the total resistance to blood flow through the lungs and into the ventricular cavity is nearly normal; the systemic venous return can be connected directly to the pulmonary arteries without an intervening pump. This will separate oxygenated and nonoxygenated blood. Systemic venous blood will then flow continuously through the lungs with a mean pressure of between 8 and 14 mm Hg. The Fontan procedure has many modifications to separate the systemic and pulmonary circuits and achieve full oxygen saturation of systemic arterial blood. An often used preliminary procedure before completing the Fontan connection is the bidirectional cavopulmonary shunt (superior vena cava connected to pulmonary artery) or bidirectional Glenn shunt (Fig. 58-26). This intermediate procedure reduces volume load on the ventricle. The initial selection criteria by Fontan were stringent,[57] and these principles remain largely valid. Improved understanding of Fontan physiology has allowed modifications to the selection of patients and the classification of risk.[58] Complications of the Fontan procedure are frequent in the postoperative period: increased incidence of atrial arrhythmias, pleural effusions, and, with bad Fontan physiology, ascites with protein-losing enteropathy and progressive ventricular dysfunction. Currently, the theoretical hemodynamic advantages of the lateral tunnel Fontan procedure (Fig. 58-27) are being evaluated.[59]

Tricuspid Atresia

Tricuspid atresia is characterized by the absence of a communication between the right atrium and the right ventricle. Associated with this anomaly are an ASD, enlargement of the mitral valve and left ventricle, and a varying degree of right ventricular hypoplasia. Tricuspid atresia is a relatively common cyanotic heart lesion, occurring in 0.3% to 3.7% of patients with congenital heart disease.

Anatomy and Physiology Tricuspid atresia has been classified into three types. In type 1 (70% of patients), the great arteries are in concordance with the ventricles. Type 2 (20% of patients) comprises hearts with TGA. Type 3 (<10%) includes hearts with AV discordance and TGA.

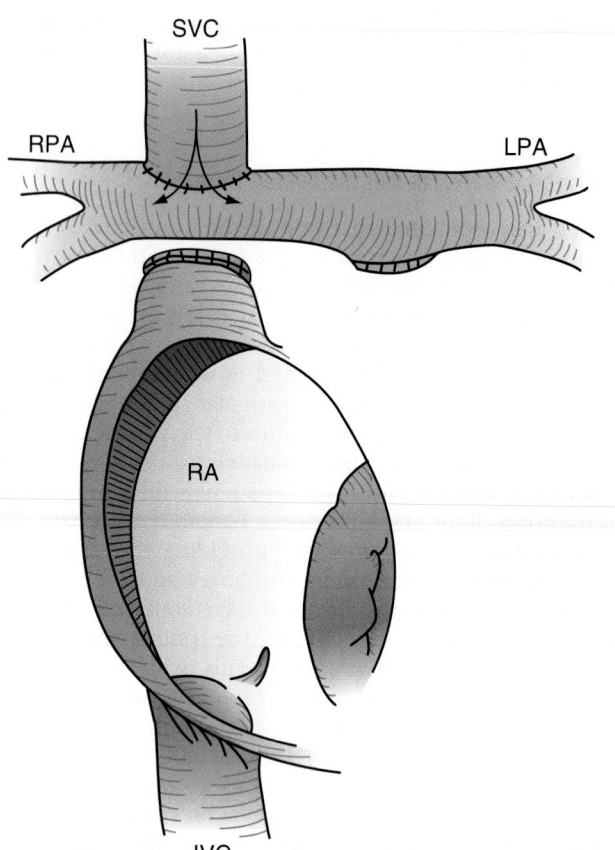

FIGURE 58-26.   The cavopulmonary shunt or bidirectional Glenn shunt. An end-to-side anastomosis of the superior vena cava (SVC) to the right pulmonary artery (RPA) is performed. The proximal end of the SVC is divided at the cavoatrial junction. IVC, inferior vena cava; LPA, left pulmonary artery; RA, right atrium. (From Bridges ND, Jonas RA, Mayer JE, et al: Bidirectional cavopulmonary anastomosis as interim palliation for high-risk Fontan candidates: Early results. Circulation 82[Suppl IV]:IV-170, 1990. Copyright 1990, American Heart Association.)

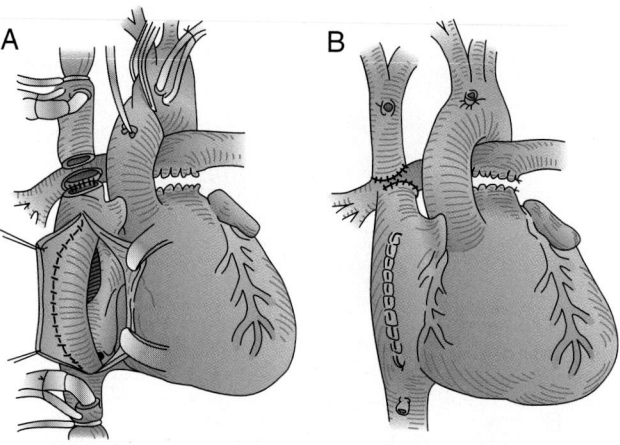

FIGURE 58-27.   Modification of the Fontan operation—the lateral tunnel Fontan with total cavopulmonary anastomosis. **A,** Polytetrafluoroethylene patch is placed in the right atrium, creating a uniform tunnel between the superior and the inferior vena cava. The main pulmonary artery is transected. The bidirectional Glenn is then performed (if not already present). **B,** Completed total cavopulmonary connection. (From Stein DG, Laks H, Drinkwater DC, et al: Results of total cavopulmonary connection in the treatment of patients with a functional single ventricle. J Thorac Cardiovasc Surg 102:280, 1991.)

Physiology depends on the degree of obstruction to pulmonary blood flow. As a rule, patients with obstruction to pulmonary blood flow have unobstructed systemic blood flow. In contrast, patients with unobstructed pulmonary blood flow tend to have some obstruction to systemic flow.

Diagnosis and Management Echocardiography is diagnostic of the cardiac morphology. Cardiac catheterization is required for assessment of PVR and to assess the anatomy of the pulmonary arteries in patients subjected to either pulmonary artery banding or previous shunt placement.

Surgery The ultimate goal for these patients is to achieve anatomy and physiology favorable for an eventual Fontan circuit. Patients with inadequate pulmonary blood flow will require shunting, and care is taken to avoid overshunting. With unobstructed pulmonary blood flow, a pulmonary artery band is applied early in life. Atrial septectomy can be performed at the same time, but in general, neonates will have already been subjected to balloon atrial septostomy. Survival and mortality rates reflect the complexity of the lesion, the effectiveness of initial palliation, and correct decision making at the time

of assessment for completing the Fontan circuit. Most centers report an early mortality of around 5% for tricuspid atresia. The actuarial survival after the Fontan operation deviates significantly from that of normal people. Failing Fontans are managed by residual lesions or by heart transplantation.

Hypoplastic Left Heart Syndrome

Hypoplastic left heart syndrome (HLHS) encompasses a constellation of features: severe aortic valve hypoplasia or atresia, hypoplasia of the ascending aorta, stenosis or atresia of the mitral valve, and hypoplasia or atresia of the left ventricle. Associated noncardiac abnormalities are frequent and affect survival. HLHS accounts for 25% of cardiac mortality in the first week of life, with an incidence of 7% of all cardiac anomalies. Norwood[60] was the first to describe an operative method for successful palliation. These principles have led to an option for managing other forms of single-ventricle, complex lesions with LVOTO. The staged operative strategy for long-term palliation involves creation of an unobstructed outlet to the systemic circuit and adequate pulmonary blood flow, followed a few months later by a bidirectional cavopulmonary shunt and, finally, completion of the Fontan.

Anatomy and Pathophysiology There are variations in the degree of stenosis or atresia of the aortic and mitral valves. The ascending aorta ranges from 1 to 2 mm to near normal in size (Fig. 58-28). In neonates, the duct must be kept open with PGE_1 infusion. As PVR falls, in the setting of parallel circulations, available cardiac output preferentially goes to the lungs. This leads to progressive acidosis from reduced systemic perfusion. The key to managing these patients is to balance the pulmonary and systemic

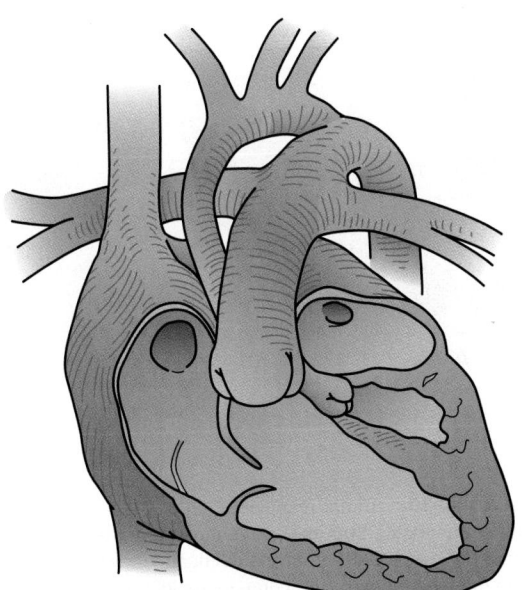

■ FIGURE 58-28. Anatomy of the hypoplastic left heart syndrome. The tiny ascending aorta is seen, arising from a markedly hypoplastic left ventricle. The ductus arteriosus is large, providing forward flow to the systemic circuit. The right ventricle is hypertrophied, and the pulmonary artery is enlarged. (From Wernovsky G, Bove EL: Single ventricle lesions. *In* Chang AC, Hanley FL, Wernovsky G, Wessell DL [eds]: Pediatric Cardiac Intensive Care. Baltimore, Williams & Wilkins, 1998.)

blood flows. This is achieved by controlling ventilation to adjust the PVR by increasing the hematocrit and pharmacologically by manipulating the systemic vascular resistance and PVR.[61]

Diagnosis Echocardiography is diagnostic and cardiac catheterization is not usually indicated, unless associated anomalies require further delineation and clarification.

Surgery First-stage palliation is accomplished with the Norwood procedure or a modification. Important to achieving survival is aggressive preoperative management and optimizing all organ systems before surgery. This is achieved by balancing the systemic and pulmonary blood flow ratios. Surgical attainment of the Norwood operation usually involves a period of circulatory arrest, although, recently, almost complete avoidance of cerebral circulatory arrest has been achieved by regional perfusion through the upper end of a preplaced PTFE shunt. A modification of the Norwood operation has been described,[62] without using homograft material for arch reconstruction but using all native tissue (Fig. 58-29). A stable source of pulmonary blood supply is provided by the creation of a shunt. More recently, Sano[63] has described placement of a small RV to distal MPA PTFE conduit instead of systemic shunt. Theoretically, this poses an advantage in that there is no diastolic steal from the aorta, compared with the use of systemic shunt. This new approach is rapidly gaining acceptance. Postoperative management involves balancing the pulmonary and systemic circulation again. Pro-

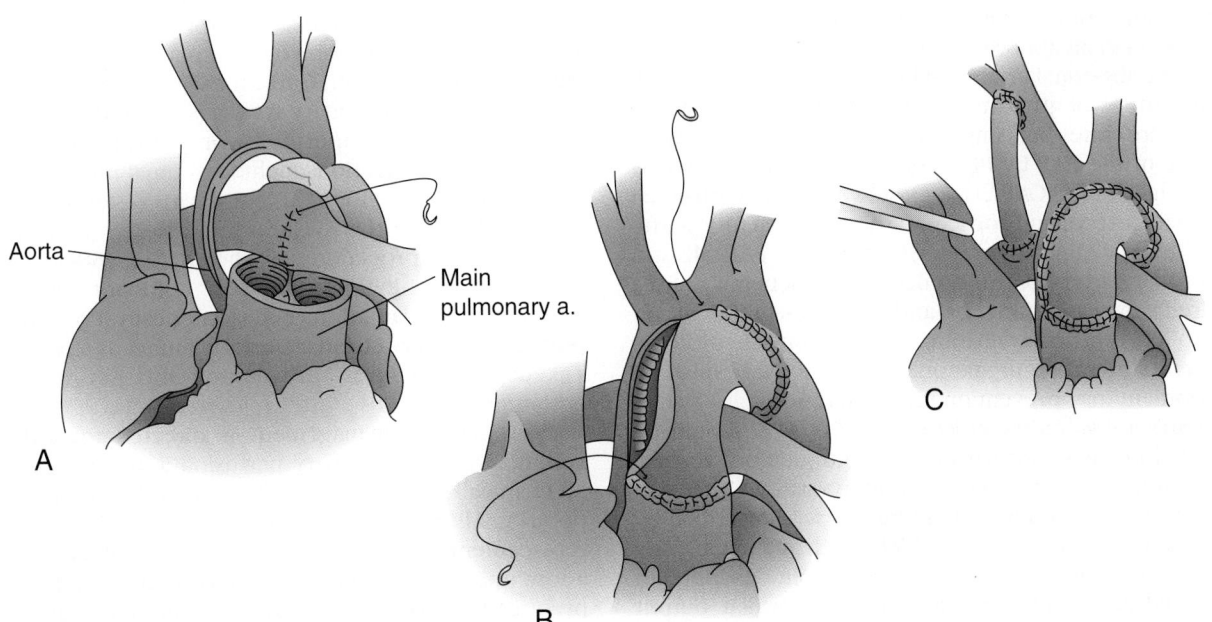

■ FIGURE 58-29. The Norwood procedure for first-stage palliation of the hypoplastic left heart syndrome. **A,** The main pulmonary artery (MPA) is divided proximal to the bifurcation, the ductus arteriosus is ligated and divided, and the aortic arch is opened from the level of the transected MPA to a point distal to the ductal insertion in the descending aorta. **B,** A segment of homograft is cut to an appropriate size and shape. This is sutured into place, creating an unobstructed outflow from the right ventricle to the pulmonary artery and aorta. **C,** Polytetrafluoroethylene tube graft is placed from the innominate artery to the right pulmonary artery. The atrial septectomy is done while the patient is under circulatory arrest as well. (From Castaneda AR, Jonas RA, Mayer JE, Hanley FL: Hypoplastic left heart syndrome. *In* Cardiac Surgery of the Neonate and Infant. Philadelphia, WB Saunders, 1994.)

vided aortic arch and pulmonary artery growth is satisfactory, the second stage is undertaken when the child
outgrows the shunt. The ventricle is unloaded by a bidirectional cavopulmonary shunt, and this is later converted
to a lateral tunnel Fontan or a modification thereof at $1\frac{1}{2}$
to 5 years of age. Some centers prefer to utilize primary
heart transplantation for HLHS.[64] This approach is hindered by the lack of donor availability.

Results Current reviews indicate that survival after surgical intervention for both transplantation and staged palliation is approximately 67% at 1 month and 52% at 12
months.[64] An advantage of staged palliation with use of
the Fontan is that transplantation may be avoided for a
number of years.

OTHER ANOMALIES

Coronary Artery Anomalies

Anomalies occur as a result of anomalous origin, termination, courses, and aneurysm formation. Of these variables,
only anomalous left coronary artery rising from the pulmonary artery (ALCAPA) and coronary artery fistulas are
discussed. An ALCAPA is a rare lesion often lethal in early
infancy. Untreated, the mortality approaches 90%.

Anomalous Left Coronary Artery Rising from the Pulmonary Artery

Anatomy and Pathophysiology Developmentally, failure of the
normal connection of the left coronary artery bud to the
aorta results in an abnormal connection to the pulmonary
artery. The abnormal origin can be situated in the main pulmonary artery or proximal branches. Associated abnormalities are rare but important to recognize because
lowering of the PAP by PDA ligation or closure of a VSD
can be fatal if the ALCAPA is not noted. In utero, with equal
pulmonary arterial and aortic pressures, satisfactory perfusion of the ALCAPA can occur. After birth, the PAP falls and
left coronary artery perfusion decreases. Ischemia causes
impaired ventricular function and myocardial infarcts and
leads to left ventricular dilation. Papillary muscle dysfunction causes mitral regurgitation. Early coronary collateral
development may prevent ongoing infarction.

Diagnosis and Indications for Intervention ALCAPA should be
suspected in any infant with mitral regurgitation, ventricular dysfunction, or dilated cardiomyopathy. The syndrome of angina with feeding in infants was described by
Bland and colleagues,[65] with sudden death and angina precipitated by feeding. Sudden death has been described in
older children. Infants present with a low cardiac output
and systemic heart failure. The electrocardiogram may
reflect ischemic changes. The echocardiogram is usually
diagnostic, but because this diagnosis is often confused
with dilated cardiomyopathy there is an argument in favor
of catheterizing all patients with dilated cardiomyopathy
in whom the coronary artery anatomy cannot be clearly
defined on echocardiography. Secondary findings of
dilated cardiac chambers and segmental wall motion

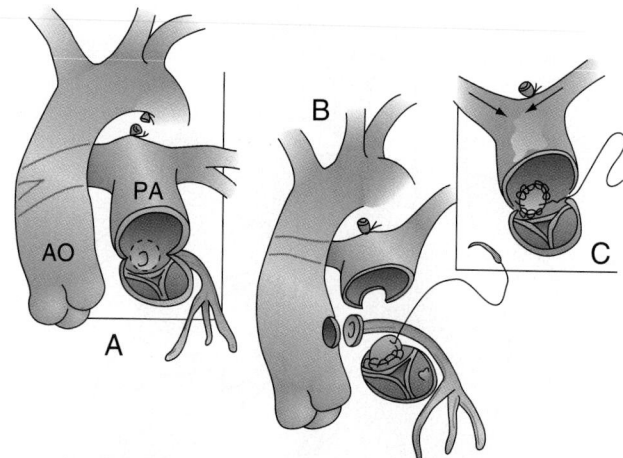

FIGURE 58-30. Direct reimplantation of the anomalous left
coronary artery arising from the pulmonary artery (ALCAPA).
A, Excision of the ALCAPA from the pulmonary artery (PA). AO, aorta.
B, Aortic reimplantation of the coronary ostium into the aorta.
C, Reconstruction of the PA with autologous pericardium. (From
Vouhe PR, Tamisier D, Sidi D, et al: Anomalous left coronary artery
from the pulmonary artery: Results of isolated aortic reimplantation.
Ann Thorac Surg 54:621, 1992. Reprinted with permission from the
Society of Thoracic Surgeons.)

abnormalities together with mitral regurgitation should
prompt a search for an ALCAPA. Diagnosis of an ALCAPA
is an indication for intervention.

Surgery A degree of ventricular dysfunction is usually
present. Preoperative inotropic support and optimization
of hemodynamics may be required before surgical intervention. Severe cardiomyopathy may rarely necessitate
cardiac transplantation. Current experience indicates that
creation of a dual coronary system is safe and reproducible
and offers the best opportunity for recovery of function.[65]
Operative considerations include optimal myocardial protection and prevention of left heart distention. Direct
reimplantation of the ALCAPA into the ascending aorta is
currently the procedure of choice (Fig. 58-30). Sometimes, limited mobility of the coronary artery will
preclude reimplantation, and a surgically created aorta-
pulmonary artery-coronary artery tunnel is created: the
Takeuchi procedure.[66] Ligation of the ALCAPA is not
recommended.

Postoperative management is directed toward maintaining adequate coronary perfusion and cardiac output.
Mechanical support of the heart may be required temporarily. Mitral regurgitation usually improves, and valve
replacement is rarely necessary. Current intervention has
a low operative mortality. Risks for nonsurvival relate to
preoperative ventricular dysfunction and cardiogenic
shock. The Takeuchi repair is associated with tunnel complications such as obstruction, leak, aortic valve damage,
and RVOTO in the long term.

Coronary Arteriovenous Fistula and Aneurysms

Isolated coronary artery fistula is rarer than ALCAPA.
Aneurysms are associated with Kawasaki's disease.

Drainage of coronary artery fistula is reported to terminate more commonly in the right side of the heart or pulmonary artery than in the left side of the heart. A shunt from the high-pressure coronary artery system into a low-pressure cardiac chamber may result in coronary steal and some degree of cardiac volume overload.

Diagnosis and Indications for Intervention Presentation depends on the amount of functional compromise produced by the ischemia and volume overload. Echocardiography may be able to delineate the anomaly, but coronary angiography is diagnostic. Details of coronary anatomy are essential for determining intervention. Interventional catheterization is useful for the obliteration of fistulas and terminal aneurysms.[67]

Surgery If the lesion is not amenable to transcatheter intervention, surgery is indicated. The options include suture ligation without bypass, CPB, and aneurysmectomy with closure of the fistula. Early and late mortality are low. Risk factors for death and ventricular dysfunction relate to coronary artery insufficiency and infarction after fistula ligation or aneurysmectomy.

Vascular Rings and Pulmonary Artery Sling

Vascular rings and pulmonary artery sling are abnormalities of the aortic arch and its branches, compressing the trachea and or esophagus. The ring may be either complete or partial. A pulmonary artery sling occurs when the left pulmonary artery arises from the right pulmonary artery, passing leftward between the trachea and the esophagus. The trachea may be compressed, the cartilage may be soft, or there may be intrinsic stenosis of the trachea in the form of complete cartilage rings.

Anatomy Categorization of the defects is useful for description:

Complete Vascular Rings
  Double arch: equal arches or left or right arch dominant
  Right arch: left ligamentum arteriosus from anomalous left subclavian artery
  Right arch: mirror image branching, with left ligamentum from descending aorta
Partial Vascular Rings
  Left arch: aberrant right subclavian artery
  Left arch: innominate artery compression
Pulmonary Artery Slings

Understanding of aortic arch formation has been enhanced by the hypothetical model of paired segmental structures and a double aortic arch in the embryo.[68] The final configuration of the aortic arch and its branching pattern depends on the regression and preservation of specific segments (Fig. 58-31). The double aortic arch is the most common form of complete ring. Two arches arise from the ascending aorta, forming a true ring. The left arch is usually smaller. The right arch-left ligamentum complex is formed from persistence of the right fourth arch and regression of the left fourth arch. The anomalously arising left subclavian artery is often associated with a diverticulum at its base (Kommerell). In partial rings, the most common form is an aberrant right subcla-

vian artery arising distal to the left subclavian artery with a left arch. The right subclavian artery passes behind the esophagus from left to right. Innominate artery compression arises from a more posterior and leftward origin of the innominate artery from a left arch, leading to anterior compression of the trachea.

Diagnosis and Indications for Intervention Symptoms reflect the degree of tracheal and esophageal compression, as well as the presence of coexistent tracheomalacia or stenosis from complete rings. Upper respiratory symptoms predominate, with a characteristic brassy cough, recurrent respiratory infections, failure to thrive, and, sometimes, esophageal motility problems. In children, documentation of a ring is an indication for surgery. Older patients are often asymptomatic. Initially, diagnosis is made by a high index of suspicion and the barium swallow as the first investigation. Nowadays, echocardiography can document an abnormal head and neck vessel branching pattern, excluding intracardiac abnormalities. MRI provides complete anatomic detail.

Surgery Most vascular rings are accessible through a left posterolateral thoracotomy (the exception is a left arch with right-sided ligamentum). Division of the ring and, in the case of double arch, preservation of the dominant arch is performed. Preservation of the recurrent laryngeal nerve is of importance. Pulmonary artery slings are approached through the midline, and currently the use of CPB facilitates tracheal reconstruction and relocation of the right pulmonary artery (Fig. 58-32).[69] Repair can be achieved with low risk. Symptoms may take months to resolve, with slow resolution of the underlying tracheomalacia.

Ebstein's Anomaly of the Tricuspid Valve

Ebstein's anomaly of the tricuspid valve is a rare defect in which the tricuspid valve attachments are displaced into the right ventricle to varying degrees. Ebstein's anomaly comprises a spectrum of abnormalities involving a degree of displacement of the tricuspid valve, variable right ventricular size, and variable pulmonary outflow obstruction. Associated abnormalities are an ASD, pulmonary atresia, and congenitally corrected transposition. The tricuspid valve's posterior and septal leaflets are variably displaced to the apex of the right ventricle. This results in an atrialized portion of the right ventricle. The anterior leaflet remains large and sail-like. The major hemodynamic issue is tricuspid incompetence with decreased pulmonary blood flow and, if an ASD is present, right-to-left shunting causing cyanosis. Long-standing tricuspid incompetence leads to volume overload of an abnormal right ventricle. Variable pulmonary outflow tract obstruction will limit effective pulmonary blood flow. If adequate pulmonary blood flow requires continued ductal patency, then the need for neonatal intervention is almost certain.

Diagnosis and Intervention The more severe forms of Ebstein's anomaly present with cyanosis in infancy. Ill neonates tend to have a severe form of the disease, with a grossly inefficient right ventricle compounded by the high pulmonary resistance of the neonate or by pul-

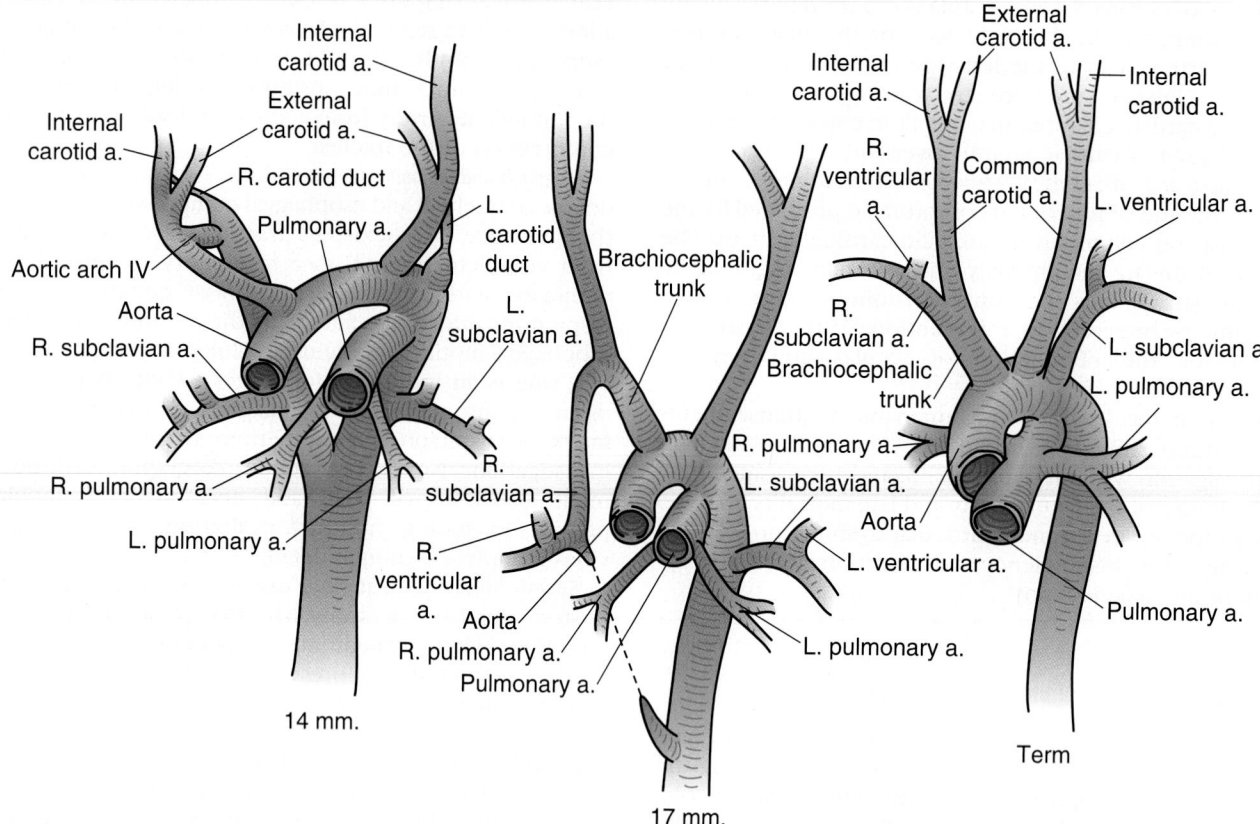

FIGURE 58-31. The process of resorption and fusion of the paired first to the sixth branchial arches with paired dorsal aortas results in the formation of the normal aorta, aortic arch, and pulmonary artery. The appearance of the aorta at various embryo crown-rump lengths is shown. (From Castaneda AR, Jonas RA, Mayer JE, Hanley FL: Vascular rings, slings, and tracheal anomalies. *In* Cardiac Surgery of the Neonate and Infant. Philadelphia, WB Saunders, 1994.)

monary valve atresia. The mortality rate in this group is high. Older patients present in heart failure and may have cyanosis. Supraventricular arrhythmias and the preexcitation syndrome (Wolff-Parkinson-White) are associated with Ebstein's anomaly. Echocardiography is diagnostic. Critically ill neonates have poor survival rates, and surgery is indicated only after stabilization with PGE$_1$ and controlled ventilation. In the older patient, cyanosis and heart failure are indications to intervene, although recently earlier intervention in the asymptomatic patient, before excessive RV dilation, is being more actively pursued.

Surgery In critically ill neonates, after stabilization, palliation with a systemic-to-pulmonary artery shunt may be required. The Starnes operation has allowed salvage in previously hopeless cases. This operation consists of patch closure of the tricuspid orifice, atrial septectomy, and a systemic-to-pulmonary artery shunt.[70] This approach commits the child to a Fontan-type repair in the future. In patients with less severe forms of this disease, options include tricuspid valve repair using several ingenious methods (Fig. 58-33)[71] and tricuspid valve replacement. Surgery should be performed when heart size increase is documented.

Results Neonates have poor survival rates after palliative surgery. Older patients have a reported operative mortality of 0% to 25%.

Mitral Valve Anomalies

Most abnormalities of the mitral valve are associated with other complex lesions, for example, Shone's complex. More commonly, mitral disease in the pediatric population will be inflammatory in nature, that is, rheumatic disease or infective endocarditis. It may also be associated with collagen vascular disease and Marfan's syndrome.

Mitral Stenosis

Mitral stenosis is caused by obstruction at a supravalvular, valvular, or subvalvular level, singly or in combination. Supravalvular stenosis is due to a ring of fibrous tissue above the annulus of the mitral valve or attached to the proximal leaflets. Valvular stenosis involves the leaflets, with commissural fusion occurring with or without hypoplasia of the valve ring. Hypoplasia of the mitral valve is often associated with left ventricular hypoplasia. Frequently, the leaflets and subvalvular apparatus are dysplastic as well. Fusion of the leaflets can lead to an accessory orifice and produce mitral stenosis at a pure valvular level (so-called double-orifice mitral valve). Three types of subvalvular stenosis have been recognized: parachute mitral valve, hammock valve, and absence of one or both papillary muscles.

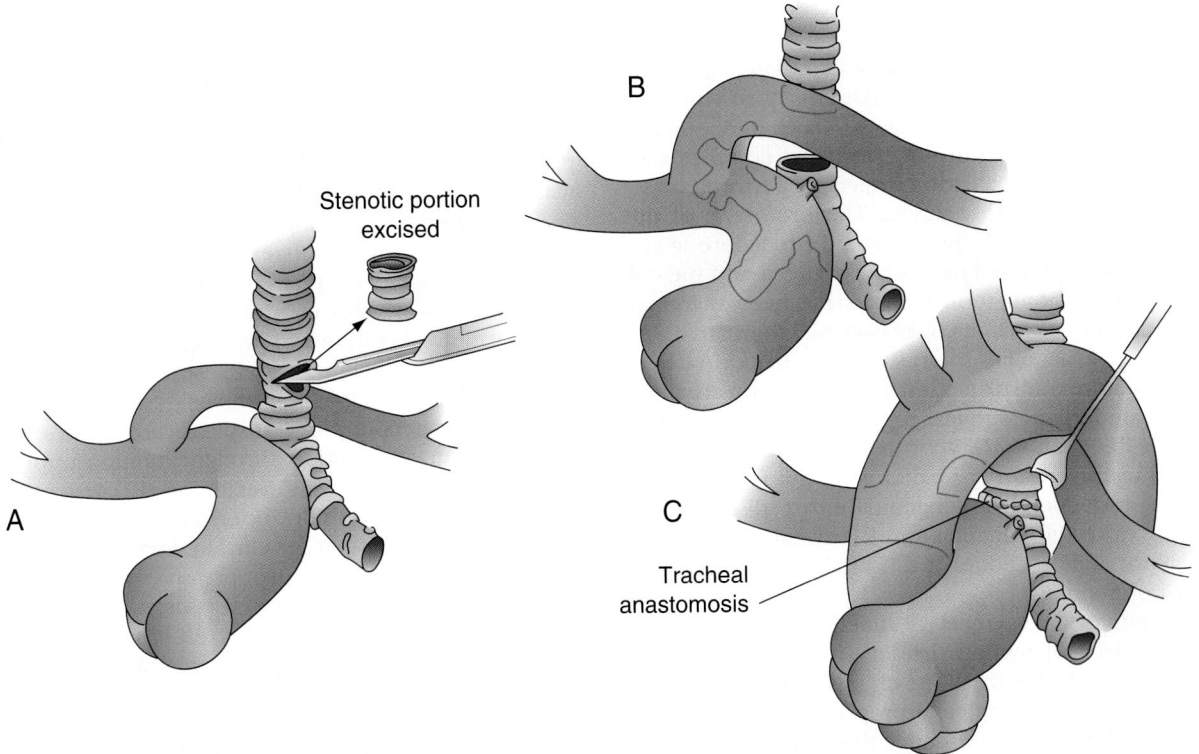

Stenotic portion excised

A

B

C

Tracheal anastomosis

FIGURE 58-32. Method for the management of a pulmonary artery sling with associated tracheal stenosis, using cardiopulmonary bypass. **A,** Tracheal resection of the involved segment. **B,** Anterior translocation of the left pulmonary artery after transection of the trachea. **C,** Direct anastomosis of the trachea. (From Castaneda AR, Jonas RA, Mayer JE, Hanley FL: Vascular rings, slings, and tracheal anomalies. *In* Cardiac Surgery of the Neonate and Infant. Philadelphia, WB Saunders, 1994.)

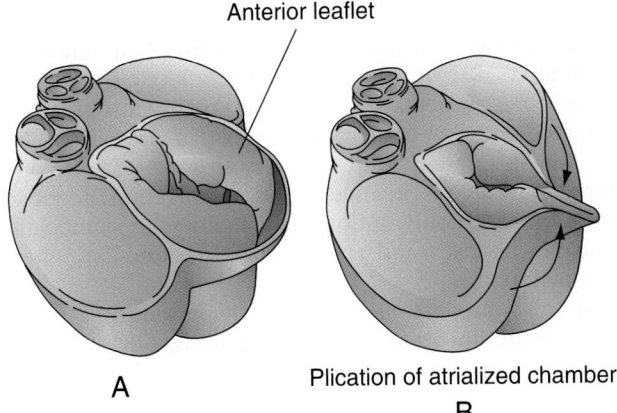

Anterior leaflet

A

Plication of atrialized chamber

B

FIGURE 58-33. Repair of Ebstein's malformation using the Carpentier method. **A,** The anterior and posterior leaflets of the tricuspid valve are detached from the annulus. **B,** The atrium is plicated, reducing the annular diameter. The detached leaflets are reattached to the annulus. (From Ebstein's anomaly. *In* Castaneda AR, Jonas RA, Mayer JE, Hanley FL [eds]: Cardiac Surgery of the Neonate and Infant. Philadelphia, WB Saunders, 1994.)

Mitral regurgitation is a result of secondary annular dilation, congenital isolated clefts of the valve, and prolapse of the leaflets from abnormal chordae or papillary muscle insertion.

Echocardiography is diagnostic. Intervention includes balloon valvuloplasty, particularly for selected forms of rheumatic mitral stenosis, and surgical intervention. Inter-

vention is timed to avoid irreversible sequelae related to either chronic volume overload or pulmonary hypertension. Surgical intervention in children is aimed at preserving the mitral valve. Valvuloplasty techniques have a valuable place in children. Prosthetic valves are the least desirable option. Bioprosthetic or tissue valves should be avoided in children. Supra-annular placement of the prosthesis may be necessary. Repeat replacement is ensured.[72]

Thoracic Transplantation in Congenital Cardiac Disease

The philosophy of transplantation is to maximize survival and improve quality of life. Transplantation is in itself not curative and carries time-related attrition rates from acute and chronic rejection, infection, and other complications associated with long-term immunosuppression. Pretransplant evaluation and contraindications to transplant are identical to those of the adult population. Additionally, the need for providing a stable home environment and reliable medication administration (immunosuppression) becomes crucial.

Heart Transplantation

Pediatric heart transplant candidates fall into two categories: primary or secondary cardiomyopathy and congenital heart disease not amenable to standard surgery. In the pediatric age group, the specific risk factor for heart transplantation is an elevated PVR. There is a significantly increased risk of mortality when indexed PVR exceeds 6 Wood units/m^2, under which circumstances heart-lung transplantation or heterotopic transplantation is a consideration. Approximately 10% of all patients born with congenital heart disease are unable to have a reasonable anatomic surgical repair. In some forms of complex congenital heart disease, palliative surgery is performed as a bridge to cardiac transplantation. The prototype of this group is HLHS, in which the Norwood procedure is currently offered in a limited number of centers, and the collective short- and long-term results have been marginal. Transplantation has become a reasonable alternative, but lack of donor availability has resulted in attrition rates of up to 40% before transplantation. Another group are those who have undergone surgical repair but have developed an irreversible abnormality or myocardial dysfunction. Examples in this group are patients with a failed Fontan operation and complex congenital heart disease with severe AV valve regurgitation and RV dysfunction following the Norwood procedure or the atrial switch procedure (Mustard or Senning).

Preoperative management is aimed at optimizing the patient for transplantation. Under some circumstances and depending on the size of the child, implantable bridge to transplant devices may be appropriate. In smaller children, particularly infants younger than 6 months of age, extracorporeal membrane oxygenation is used as a bridge for transplantation. In this group of patients, the time constraints are imposed by the complications related to longer duration of extracorporeal support. Anatomic considerations with regard to aortic arch hypoplasia, heterotaxy syndromes, and varying degrees of previous palliative procedures on pulmonary artery and interatrial anatomy pose different surgical challenges for this group. In the infant group, donor size greater than 300% of the recipient can be successfully used; in other pediatric recipients, the body weight of the donor can be 50% to 250% greater than that of the recipient.

As a general rule, a donor weighing more than 25% less than the recipient is not acceptable. The transplanted heart grows proportionately, maintaining a cardiac output sufficient to sustain normal growth. It is preferable to use an oversized donor heart or a donor heart with a conditioned right ventricle for preexisting, elevated PVR. Heart transplantation is performed utilizing an orthotopic heart transplant technique or variations as imposed by the congenital anomalies.[73]

Lung and Heart-Lung Transplantation

The cumulative experience with pediatric lung and heart-lung transplantation has increased since the mid-1990s. Potential candidates for lung transplantation are those with end-stage pulmonary vascular disease or bronchopulmonary pathology. Bronchopulmonary pathology includes those patients with cystic fibrosis and severe bronchopulmonary dysplasia. Patients with repairable congenital heart lesions who have Eisenmenger's syndrome with long-standing, irreversible cardiomyopathy are candidates for heart-lung transplantation. Lung transplantation (cadaveric and living-related) is another option

for pediatric patients.[74] Decreased right ventricular function in a setting of pulmonary hypertension is not a contraindication to isolated lung transplantation.

Single-lung transplantation can generally be performed through a thoracotomy without CPB. Double-lung transplantation exposure is provided with a transverse submammary, clamshell incision. A median sternotomy can also be used. Heart-lung transplantation exposure is through either a midline sternotomy or a clamshell incision. Postoperative management in transplantation follows the principles of postcardiac surgery care. Variable organ preservation and prolonged ischemia, together with reperfusion injury, may cause a delay in return of function of the transplanted organs.

Special aspects of post-transplant care involve the prevention of graft rejection through immunosuppression. Standard triple therapy is usually used (corticosteroids, cyclosporine, and azathioprine). Some centers favor a corticosteroid-free regimen for chronic immunosuppression, if feasible. Newer immunosuppressives (mycophenolate and tacrolimus [FK-506]) are also used in the pediatric group. Immunosuppression may result in infectious complications that are often more severe and may sometimes be fatal in the pediatric population.[75]

Results Heart transplantation for children has a 30-day perioperative mortality of 15% to 20% with 1- and 5-year actuarial survival rates of 75% to 80% and 60% to 75%, respectively. Pediatric heart and lung transplantation provides 1- and 5-year survival rates of 60% and 40%, respectively. The 24-month survival rate for double-lung transplantation is approximately 60%.[75] The leading cause of early death in these patients is infection, whereas bronchiolitis obliterans accounts for many late deaths in lung and heart-lung transplantation. Post-transplant lymphoproliferative disease is a malignancy affecting approximately 10% of pediatric transplant recipients. This is associated with infection with the Ebstein-Barr virus.[76] In heart transplantation, graft coronary artery disease is considered to be a consequence of chronic rejection. Retransplantation is the only option for patients with significant coronary disease and myocardial dysfunction after transplantation.

Other complications include hypertension, renal failure, hyperlipidemia, and postoperative cytomegalovirus infection.

Selected References

Castaneda AR, Jonas RA, Mayer JE, Hanley FL (eds): Cardiac Surgery of the Neonate and Infant. Philadelphia, WB Saunders, 1994.

> This book details an experience of the Children's Hospital in Boston over a 20-year period. Congenital cardiac defects with special emphasis on neonatal and infant applications are discussed in detail. The heart defects themselves are very well covered, and the strength of this particular reference is in the general considerations, which cover in detail cardiopulmonary bypass, myocardial preservation, and perioperative management of the infant and neonate with congenital heart disease.

Kirkland JW, Barratt-Boyes BG: Cardiac Surgery, 2nd ed. New York, Churchill Livingstone, 1993.

> This remarkable book is the standard reference for cardiac surgeons. It catalogs the experiences of two well-known experts in the field of congenital heart surgery. The material is well organized, well presented, and exquisitely illustrated. This reference provides an in-depth review of all aspects of congenital cardiac surgery.

Stark J, de Leval M: Surgery for Congenital Heart Defects, 2nd ed. Philadelphia, WB Saunders, 1994.

> This book is a readable, well-illustrated, and in-depth synopsis of congenital cardiac disease. Chapters are written by experts in the various fields. A perspective on the management of all congenital lesions is presented.

References

1. Johnson MC, Hing A, Wood MK, et al: Chromosome abnormalities in congenital heart disease. Am J Med Genet 70:292-298, 1997.
2. Van Praagh R: Terminology of congenital heart disease: Glossary and commentary [Editorial]. Circulation 56:139-143, 1977.
3. Elliott MJ: Perfusion for pediatric open heart surgery. Semin Thorac Cardiovasc Surg 2:332-340, 1990.
4. Julia P, Kofsky ER, Buckberg GD, et al: Studies of myocardial protection in the immature heart: III. Models of ischemic and hypoxic/ischemic injury in the immature puppy heart. J Thorac Cardiovasc Surg 101:14-22, 1991.
5. Bellinger DC, Jonas RA, Rappaport LA, et al: Developmental and neurologic status of children after heart surgery with hypothermic circulatory arrest or low-flow cardiopulmonary bypass. N Engl J Med 332:549-555, 1995.
6. Laborde F, Folliguet TA, Etienne PY, et al: Video-thoracoscopic surgical interruption of patent ductus arteriosus: Routine experience in 332 pediatric cases. Eur J Cardiothorac Surg 11:1052-1055, 1997.
7. Hawkins JA, Minich LL, Tani LY, et al: Cost and efficacy of surgical ligation versus transcatheter coil occlusion of patent ductus arteriosus. J Thorac Cardiovasc Surg 112:1634-1639, 1996.
8. Kutsche LM, Van Mierop LH: Anatomy and pathogenesis of aorticopulmonary septal defect. Am J Cardiol 59:443-447, 1987.
9. Tkebuchava T, von Segesser LK, Vogt PR, et al: Congenital aortopulmonary window: Diagnosis, surgical technique and long-term results. Eur J Cardiothorac Surg 11:293-297, 1997.
10. Lechat P, Mas JL, Lascault G, et al: Prevalence of patent foramen ovale in patients with stroke. N Engl J Med 318:1148-1152, 1988.
11. Steele PM, Fuster V, Cohen M, et al: Isolated atrial septal defect with pulmonary vascular obstructive disease—long-term follow-up and prediction of outcome after surgical correction. Circulation 76:1037-1042, 1987.
12. Anderson RH, Becker AE: The anatomy of ventricular septal defects and their conduction tissues. In Stark J, de Leval MR (eds): Surgery for Congenital Heart Defects, 2nd ed. Philadelphia, WB Saunders, 1994, pp 115-138.
13. Seddio F, Reddy VM, McElhinney DB, et al: Multiple ventricular septal defects: How and when should they be repaired? J Thorac Cardiovasc Surg 117:134-140, 1999.
14. Komai H, Naito Y, Fujiwara K, et al: Surgical strategy for doubly committed subarterial ventricular septal defect with aortic cusp prolapse. Ann Thorac Surg 64:1146-1149, 1997.

15. Hardin JT, Muskett AD, Canter CE, et al: Primary surgical closure of large ventricular septal defects in small infants. Ann Thorac Surg 53:397-401, 1992.
16. Fullerton DA, Jaggers J, Piedalue F, et al: Effective control of refractory pulmonary hypertension after cardiac operations. J Thorac Cardiovasc Surg 113:363-370, 1997.
17. Weintraub RG, Brawn WJ, Venables AW, et al: Two-patch repair of complete atrioventricular septal defect in the first year of life: Results and sequential assessment of atrioventricular valve function. J Thorac Cardiovasc Surg 99:320-326, 1990.
18. Hanley FL, Fenton KN, Jonas RA, et al: Surgical repair of complete atrioventricular canal defects in infancy: Twenty-year trends. J Thorac Cardiovasc Surg 106:387-397, 1993.
19. Elami A, Laks H, Pearl JM: Truncal valve repair: Initial experience with infants and children. Ann Thorac Surg 57:397-402, 1994.
20. Ebert PA, Turley K, Stanger P, et al: Surgical treatment of truncus arteriosus in the first 6 months of life. Ann Surg 200:451-456, 1984.
21. Hanley FL, Heinemann MK, Jonas RA, et al: Repair of truncus arteriosus in the neonate. J Thorac Cardiovasc Surg 105:1047-1056, 1993.
22. Oglietti J, Cooley DA, Izquierdo JP, et al: Cor triatriatum: Operative results in 25 patients. Ann Thorac Surg 35:415-420, 1983.
23. Lupinetti FM, Kulik TJ, Beekman RH III, et al: Correction of total anomalous pulmonary venous connection in infancy. J Thorac Cardiovasc Surg 106:880-885, 1993.
24. Sano S, Brawn WJ, Mee RB: Total anomalous pulmonary venous drainage. J Thorac Cardiovasc Surg 97:886-892, 1989.
25. Anderson RH, Allwork SP, Ho SY, et al: Surgical anatomy of tetralogy of Fallot. J Thorac Cardiovasc Surg 81:887-896, 1981.
26. Hennein HA, Mosca RS, Urcelay G, et al: Intermediate results after complete repair of tetralogy of Fallot in neonates. J Thorac Cardiovasc Surg 109:332-344, 1995.
27. Karl TR, Sano S, Pornviliwan S, et al: Tetralogy of Fallot: Favorable outcome of nonneonatal transatrial, transpulmonary repair. Ann Thorac Surg 54:903-907, 1992.
28. Mee RBB: Trans atrial transpulmonary repair of tetralogy of Fallot. In Yacoub M, Pepper JR (eds): Annual of Cardiac Surgery 1997, 10th ed. London, Rapid Science, 1997, pp 141-147.
29. Blackstone EH, Shimazaki Y, Maehara T, et al: Prediction of severe obstruction to right ventricular outflow after repair of tetralogy of Fallot and pulmonary atresia. J Thorac Cardiovasc Surg 96:288-293, 1988.
30. Snir E, de Leval MR, Elliott MJ, et al: Current surgical technique to repair Fallot's tetralogy with absent pulmonary valve syndrome. Ann Thorac Surg 51:979-982, 1991.
31. Ilbawi M, Cua C, DeLeon S, et al: Repair of complete atrioventricular septal defect with tetralogy of Fallot. Ann Thorac Surg 50:407-412, 1990.
32. Iyer KS, Mee RB: Staged repair of pulmonary atresia with ventricular septal defect and major systemic to pulmonary artery collaterals. Ann Thorac Surg 51:65-72, 1991.
33. Reddy VM, Liddicoat JR, Hanley FL: Midline one-stage complete unifocalization and repair of pulmonary atresia with ventricular septal defect and major aortopulmonary collaterals. J Thorac Cardiovasc Surg 109:832-845, 1995.
34. Freedom RM, Benson LN, Trusler GA: Pulmonary atresia and intact ventricular septum: A consideration of the coronary circulation and ventriculocoronary artery connections. In Yacoub M (ed): Annual of Cardiac Surgery 1989, 2nd ed. London, Current Science, 1989, pp 38-44.

35. Pawade A, Capuani A, Penny DJ, et al: Pulmonary atresia with intact ventricular septum: Surgical management based on right ventricular infundibulum. J Card Surg 8:371-383, 1993.

36. Miyaji K, Shimada M, Sekiguchi A, et al: Pulmonary atresia with intact ventricular septum: Long-term results of "one and a half ventricular repair." Ann Thorac Surg 60:1762-1764, 1995.

37. Hanley FL, Sade RM, Blackstone EH, et al: Outcomes in neonatal pulmonary atresia with intact ventricular septum: A multiinstitutional study. J Thorac Cardiovasc Surg 105:406-427, 1993.

38. Van Praagh R, Papagiannis J, Grunenfelder J, et al: Pathologic anatomy of corrected transposition of the great arteries: Medical and surgical implications. Am Heart J 135:772-785, 1998.

39. Planche C, Lacour-Gayet F, Serraf A: Arterial switch. Pediatr Cardiol 19:297-307, 1998.

40. Puley G, Siu S, Connelly M, et al: Arrhythmia and survival in patients >18 years of age after the Mustard procedure for complete transposition of the great arteries. Am J Cardiol 83:1080-1084, 1999.

41. Mee RBB: The arterial switch operation. In Stark J, de Leval M (eds): Surgery for Congenital Heart Defects, 2nd ed. Philadelphia, WB Saunders, 1994, pp 483-500.

42. Kirklin JW, Blackstone EH, Tchervenkov CI, et al: Clinical outcomes after the arterial switch operation for transposition: Patient, support, procedural, and institutional risk factors. Congenital Heart Surgeons Society. Circulation 86:1501-1515, 1992.

43. Duncan BW, Mee RBB, Mesia CI, et al: Results in double switch operation for congenitally corrected transposition of the great arteries. Eur J Cardiothorac Surg 24:11-20, 2003.

44. Stumper O, Brawn WJ: Anatomic repair of double discordant hearts [Editorial]. Heart 80:424-425, 1998.

45. Imai Y, Seo K, Aoki M, et al: Double-switch operation for congenitally corrected transposition. Semin Thorac Cardiovasc Surg Pediatr Card Surg Annu 4:16-33, 2001.

46. Wilkinson JL, Wilcox BR, Anderson RH: The anatomy of double outlet right ventricle. In Anderson RH, Macartney FJ, Shinebourne EA, et al (eds): Paediatric Cardiology, 5. Edinburgh, Churchill Livingstone, 1983, pp 397-407.

47. Kleinert S, Sano T, Weintraub RG, et al: Anatomic features and surgical strategies in double-outlet right ventricle. Circulation 96:1233-1239, 1997.

48. Gates RN, Laks H, Elami A, et al: Damus-Stansel-Kaye procedure: Current indications and results. Ann Thorac Surg 56:111-119, 1993.

49. Rubay JE, Shango P, Clement S, et al: Ross procedure in congenital patients: Results and left ventricular function. Eur J Cardiothorac Surg 11:92-99, 1997.

50. Reddy VM, Rajasinghe HA, Teitel DF, et al: Aortoventriculoplasty with the pulmonary autograft: The "Ross-Konno" procedure. J Thorac Cardiovasc Surg 111:158-167, 1996.

51. Zeevi B, Keane JF, Castaneda AR, et al: Neonatal critical valvar aortic stenosis: A comparison of surgical and balloon dilation therapy. Circulation 80:831-839, 1989.

52. Serraf A, Zoghby J, Lacour-Gayet F, et al: Surgical treatment of subaortic stenosis: A seventeen-year experience. J Thorac Cardiovasc Surg 117:669-678, 1999.

53. van Son JAM, Edwards WD, Danielson GK: Pathology of coronary arteries, myocardium, and great arteries in supravalvular aortic stenosis: Report of five cases with implications for surgical treatment. J Thorac Cardiovasc Surg 108:21-28, 1994.

54. Serraf A, Lacour-Gayet F, Robotin M, et al: Repair of interrupted aortic arch: A ten-year experience. J Thorac Cardiovasc Surg 112:1150-1160, 1996.

55. Quaegebeur JM, Jonas RA, Weinberg AD, et al: Outcomes in seriously ill neonates with coarctation of the aorta: A multi-institutional study. J Thorac Cardiovasc Surg 108:841-854, 1994.

56. Hijazi ZM, Fahey JT, Kleinman CS, et al: Balloon angioplasty for recurrent coarctation of aorta: Immediate and long-term results. Circulation 84:1150-1156, 1991.

57. Fontan F, Baudet E: Surgical repair of tricuspid atresia. Thorax 26:240-248, 1971.

58. Driscoll DJ, Offord KP, Feldt RH, et al: Five- to fifteen-year follow-up after Fontan operation. Circulation 85:469-496, 1992.

59. de Leval MR, Kilner P, Gewillig M, et al: Total cavopulmonary connection: A logical alternative to atriopulmonary connection for complex Fontan operations: Experimental studies and early clinical experience. J Thorac Cardiovasc Surg 96:682-695, 1988.

60. Norwood WI Jr: Hypoplastic left heart syndrome. Ann Thorac Surg 52:688-695, 1991.

61. Riordan CJ, Randsback F, Storey JH, et al: Balancing pulmonary and systemic arterial flows in parallel circulations: The value of monitoring system venous oxygen saturations. Cardiol Young 7:74-79, 1997.

62. Fraser CD Jr, Mee RB: Modified Norwood procedure for hypoplastic left heart syndrome. Ann Thorac Surg 60:S546-549, 1995.

63. Sano S, Ishino K, Kawada M, et al: Right ventricle-to-pulmonary artery shunt in first-stage palliation of hypoplastic left heart syndrome. Presented before the AATS 82nd annual meeting, 2002.

64. Jacobs ML, Blackstone EH, Bailey LL: Intermediate survival in neonates with aortic atresia: A multi-institutional study. The Congenital Heart Surgeons Society. J Thorac Cardiovasc Surg 116:417-431, 1998.

65. Schwartz ML, Jonas RA, Colan SD: Anomalous origin of left coronary artery from pulmonary artery: Recovery of left ventricular function after dual coronary repair. J Am Coll Cardiol 30:547-553, 1997.

66. Takeuchi S, Imamura H, Katsumoto K, et al: New surgical method for repair of anomalous left coronary artery from pulmonary artery. J Thorac Cardiovasc Surg 78:7-11, 1979.

67. Reidy JF, Anjos RT, Qureshi SA, et al: Transcatheter embolization in the treatment of coronary artery fistulas. J Am Coll Cardiol 18:187-192, 1991.

68. Edwards JE: Anomalies of the derivatives of the aortic arch system. Med Clin North Am 52:925-949, 1948.

69. Backer CL, Idriss FS, Holinger LD, et al: Pulmonary artery sling: Results of surgical repair in infancy. J Thorac Cardiovasc Surg 103:683-691, 1992.

70. Starnes VA, Pitlick PT, Bernstein D, et al: Ebstein's anomaly appearing in the neonate: A new surgical approach. J Thorac Cardiovasc Surg 101:1082-1087, 1991.

71. Quaegebeur JM, Sreeram N, Fraser AG, et al: Surgery for Ebstein's anomaly: The clinical and echocardiographic evaluation of a new technique. J Am Coll Cardiol 17:722-728, 1991.

72. Collins-Nakai RL, Rosenthal A, Castaneda AR, et al: Congenital mitral stenosis: A review of 20 years' experience. Circulation 56:1039-1047, 1977.

73. Chartrand C: Pediatric cardiac transplantation despite atrial and venous return anomalies. Ann Thorac Surg 52:716-721, 1991.

74. Starnes VA, Barr ML, Cohen RG: Lobar transplantation: Indications, technique, and outcome. J Thorac Cardiovasc Surg 108:403-411, 1994.

75. Boucek MM, Novick RJ, Bennett LE, et al: The Registry of the International Society of Heart and Lung Transplantation: Second Official Pediatric Report—1998. J Heart Lung Transplant 17:1141-1160, 1998.

76. Bernstein D, Baum D, Berry G, et al: Neoplastic disorders after pediatric heart transplantation. Circulation 88:II230-II237, 1993.

CHAPTER 59

SURGICAL TREATMENT OF CORONARY ARTERY DISEASE

Phillip C. Camp, Jr., M.D. and **Robert M. Mentzer, Jr., M.D.**

Coronary Artery Anatomy

Coronary Circulation and Regulation of Blood Flow

Mechanics of Pump Function

Coronary Artery Disease

Ischemia and Myocardial Cell Injury

Clinical Manifestations and Diagnosis of Coronary Artery Disease

Coronary Artery Bypass Surgery: Technical Aspects

Indications for CABG Surgery and Outcomes After Revascularization

Prediction of CABG Surgery Outcomes Using Risk Stratification Models

Alternative Methods for Myocardial Revascularization

Future Developments

CORONARY ARTERY ANATOMY

The coronary arteries originate at the root of the aorta, behind the left and right cusps of the aortic valve. They provide the blood supply to the myocardium via the main epicardial conductance vessels and enter the myocardium by penetrating vessels called *resistance arteries*. These vessels then branch into a plexus of capillaries that are essentially contiguous with every myocyte (intercapillary distance at rest is 17 μm). The left main coronary artery (LMCA) rises from the left coronary sinus; it averages 2 cm in length, and varies from 1 to 4 cm. After coursing between the pulmonary artery and the left atrial appendage, it bifurcates into two major branches, the left anterior descending coronary artery (LAD) and the left circumflex coronary artery (LCA). In many instances, the vessel trifurcates; this occurs when the ramus medianus vessel originates between the anterior descending and the circumflex arteries. Occasionally, the LMCA is absent, and the LAD and LCA arise from common or separate ostia. Less commonly, a single coronary vessel arises from a common orifice and provides all cardiac blood flow (Fig. 59-1).

In general, the LAD supplies the anterior and left lateral portions of the left ventricle. The LAD proceeds distally behind the pulmonary trunk into the anterior intraventricular sulcus and provides a number of anterior perfo-

rating branches to the anterior interventricular septum. In most cases, the LAD wraps around the apex of the heart and forms an anastomosis with the posterior descending coronary artery (PDA), a branch of the right coronary artery (RCA). As the LAD follows the interventricular groove, it may give rise to one or more branches that course diagonally over the left anterior ventricular free wall. The first diagonal branch and the first septal perforator are usually the largest vessels arising from the LAD, and both the septals and the diagonals become smaller as the vessel progresses distally.

The LCA originates from the LMCA and follows a course posteriorly under the left atrial appendage and along the left atrioventricular (AV) groove. In most cases, the circumflex terminates as an obtuse marginal branch. It can, however, be the primary source of blood flow to the PDA. One to four obtuse marginal branches of varying size emerge from the main circumflex artery and course along the lateral and posterolateral aspects of the left ventricle. The branches that arise most distally are often referred to as *posterolateral branches of the circumflex artery*. These branches course parallel to the PDA but provide no perforating branches into the intraventricular septum. In 10% of patients, the circumflex artery supplies the posterior descending and the AV nodal arteries as it courses along the posterior intraventricular sulcus. This

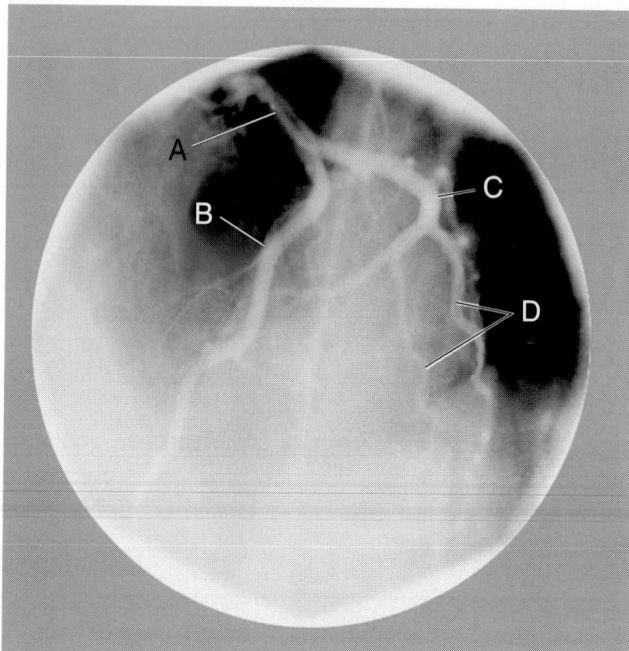

FIGURE 59-1.   Left main coronary artery (A), left anterior descending coronary artery (B), left circumflex coronary artery (C); and obtuse marginal vessels (D). (Courtesy of David Booth, MD, Division of Cardiology, University of Kentucky, 2003.)

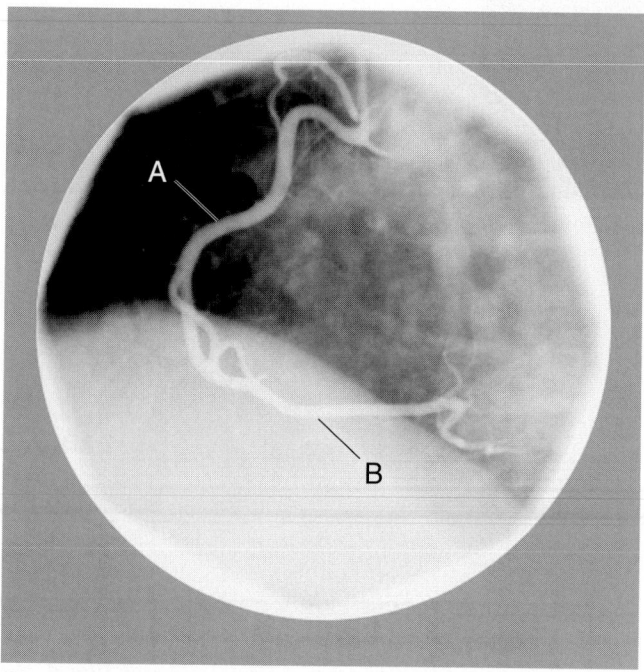

FIGURE 59-2.   Right coronary artery (A) and posterior descending artery (B). (Courtesy of David Booth, MD, Division of Cardiology, University of Kentucky, 2003.)

pattern of circulation is referred to as a *left dominant circulation* (see Fig. 59-1).

The RCA supplies most of the right ventricle, as well as the posterior part of the left ventricle. The RCA emerges from its ostium in the right coronary sinus, passes deep in the right AV groove, and then proceeds to course over the anterior surface of the heart. At the superior end of the acute margin of the heart, the RCA turns posteriorly toward the crux and usually bifurcates into the PDA and the right posterolateral artery. The RCA also supplies multiple right ventricular branches (acute marginals) as wells as branches to the AV node, although the latter may also arise from the left circumflex artery. In approximately 90% of patients, the RCA passes through the AV sulcus to the posterior interventricular sulcus and becomes the PDA. This pattern of circulation is referred to as a *right dominant system*. Occasionally, the PDA arises from both the RCA and the LCA, and the circulation is considered to be *codominant* (Fig. 59-2). The sinoatrial node artery arises from the proximal RCA in 50% of patients, and many other small atrial branches arise from the RCA, but they are rarely of significance. Other prominent branches arising from the RCA include the acute marginal artery and anterior ventricular branches. Although the source of the PDA is often used clinically to define dominance of circulation in the heart, anatomists define it based on where the sinoatrial node artery arises. In 90% of patients, the RCA bifurcates into the posterior descending and the right posterolateral arteries. The AV node artery arises from the RCA in approximately 90% of patients.

The incidence of coronary artery anomalies is approximately 1%, and these congenital anomalies may or may not be clinically significant. Hemodynamically significant anomalies include coronary fistulas or origin of the coronary artery from the pulmonary artery. Both may result in abnormal coronary perfusion. The most common congenital variation encountered during angiography is the origin of the circumflex artery from the RCA or the right coronary sinus, which occurs in approximately 0.5% of patients. Anomalous origin of the anterior descending artery from the right sinus of Valsalva or from the RCA is another common anomaly and is associated with tetralogy of Fallot.

A network of veins drains the coronary circulation, and the venous circulation can be divided into three systems: the coronary sinus and its tributaries, the anterior right ventricular veins, and the thebesian veins. Occlusive disease is uncommon in the venous system.

The coronary sinus predominantly drains the left ventricle and receives 85% of coronary venous blood. It lies within the posterior AV groove and empties into the right atrium. The anterior right ventricular veins travel across the right ventricular surface to the right AV groove, where they enter directly into the right atrium or form the small cardiac vein, which enters into the right atrium directly or joins the coronary sinus just proximal to its orifice. The thebesian veins are small venous tributaries that drain directly into the cardiac chambers and exit primarily into the right atrium and right ventricle.

CORONARY CIRCULATION AND REGULATION OF BLOOD FLOW

Coronary Blood Flow

The coronary arteries deliver oxygen and other metabolic substrates to the myocardium and simultaneously remove carbon dioxide and metabolic degradation products through the process of transcapillary exchange. Relative to most other organ systems, the myocardium has a high rate of energy utilization. Normal coronary blood flow averages 225 mL/min or 0.7 to 0.9 mL/g of myocardium per minute and delivers 0.1 mL of oxygen per gram per minute to the myocardium. Oxygen extraction in the coronary capillary bed averages 75% under normal conditions and has the capacity to increase to 100% during stress. In response to strenuous exercise, the healthy heart can increase myocardial blood flow fourfold to sevenfold.

Factors Influencing Coronary Vascular Resistance

Metabolic

Local myocardial metabolism is the primary regulator of coronary blood flow (Fig. 59-3). There is a strong correlation between myocardial metabolic activity and the magnitude of coronary blood flow changes (Fig. 59-4). The mechanism by which increased myocardial metabolism promotes coronary blood flow has not yet been clearly elucidated. It is hypothesized that the decrease in oxygen supply to oxygen demand triggers release of a vasodilator substance from the myocardium, which in turn, initiates relaxation of the coronary resistance vessels. This results in increased delivery of oxygen-rich blood. An example of this is the phenomenon of reactive hyperemia. When blood flow is transiently stopped by the occlusion of a vessel in the beating heart, blood flow immediately exceeds the normal baseline flow when the occlusion is removed. Blood flow returns to the baseline level over a period of time proportional to the duration of the occlusion. Several metabolic factors that have been implicated as the mediator of reactive hyperemia include CO_2, decreased O_2 tension, hydrogen ions, lactate, potassium ions, and adenosine. Of these, adenosine is one of the strongest candidates. In the setting of ischemia or increased metabolic activity, adenosine, a potent vasodilator and degradation product of adenosine triphosphate, is produced, accumulates in the interstitial space, and releases the vascular smooth muscle. This results in vasomotor relaxation, coronary vasodilation, and increased blood flow. Although adenosine is a leading candidate, it may be only part of the process, since adenosine receptor antagonists do not completely block reactive hyperemia. Another factor that may play an important role is nitric oxide (NO). In the absence of the endothelium, a source of NO production, coronary arteries do not autoregulate.

Physical

Aortic pressure is a key factor responsible for myocardial perfusion. The coronary vasculature can compensate and maintain normal coronary perfusion pressures between systolic pressures of 60 and 180 mm Hg via the process of autoregulation. This is a process whereby baroreceptors promote local vasodilation or vasoconstriction through alterations in coronary diameter, so that coronary blood flow is maintained at a constant level. Extravascular compression of the coronaries during systole is another factor that plays an important role in the regulation of blood flow. During systole, the intracavitary pressures generated within the left ventricular wall exceeds intracoronary pressure and nutrient flow is impeded. This may result in the transient reversal in the direction of blood flow in the epicardial vessels (see Fig. 59-3). The heart rate

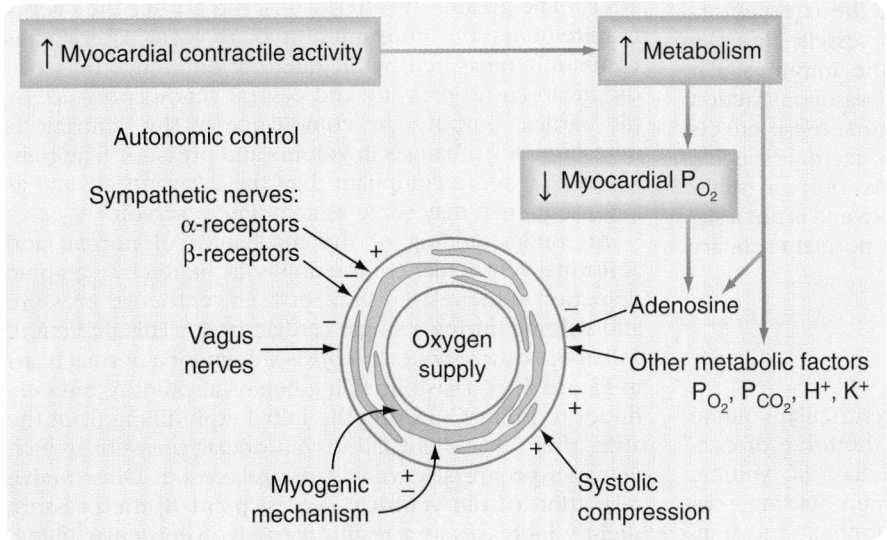

FIGURE 59-3. Schematic representation of factors that increase (+) or decrease (–) coronary vascular resistance. (From Berne RM, Levy MN [eds]: Physiology, 4th ed. St. Louis, Mosby, 1998, p 483.)

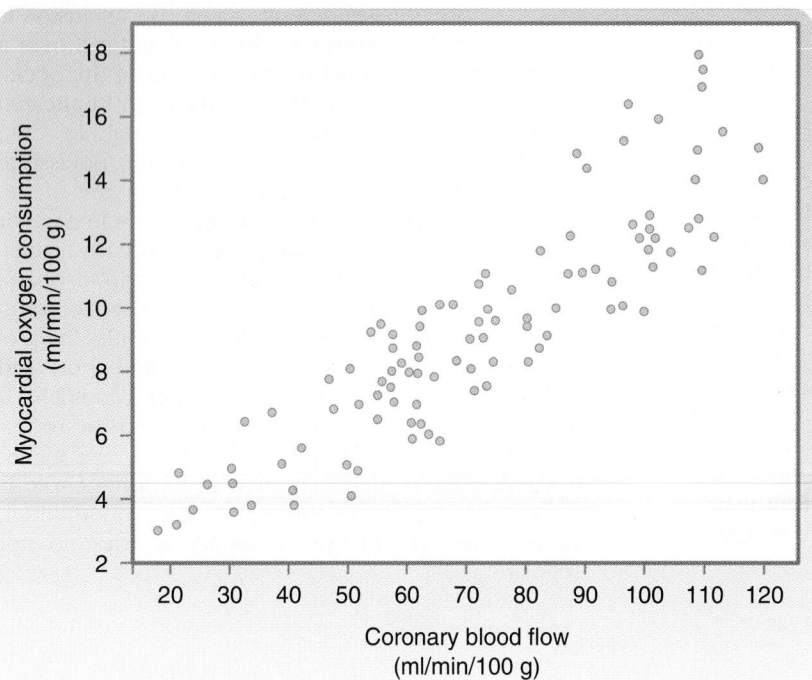

FIGURE 59-4. Relationship between myocardial oxygen consumption and coronary blood flow during a variety of interventions that increased or decreased myocardial metabolic rate. (From Berne RM, Levy MN [eds]: Physiology, 4th ed. St. Louis, Mosby, 1998, p 482.)

also affects coronary artery blood flow. Tachycardia increases the proportion of the cardiac cycle in systole and results in the restriction of blood flow. In general, this is compensated by coronary vasodilation that occurs as a result of an increase in metabolic activity. Bradycardia prolongs diastole, and thus coronary flow and nutrient delivery is increased (see Fig. 59-3).

Neural and Neurohumoral

Stimulation of the cardiac sympathetic nerves indirectly increases coronary blood flow as a result of increased metabolic activity secondary to augmented myocardial contractility and tachycardia. Although α- and β-adrenergic receptors do exist in coronary vessels, the α receptors are more prominent in the epicardial vessels, and the β receptors are more prominent in the intramuscular vessels. Although both vasodilation and vasoconstriction can occur with activation of the receptors, these effects play a less important role than metabolic factors (see Fig. 59-3). Parasympathetic stimulation has only a slight vasodilatory effect on the coronary arteries and is not a significant contributor to the regulation of normal coronary blood flow.

MECHANICS OF PUMP FUNCTION

In the normal heart, an increase in intraventricular volume during diastole leads to an increase in the force of contraction. The association between end-diastolic volume and systolic pressure, known as the Frank-Starling relationship, is under the influences of hormonal and neuronal stimulation. For example, an increase in circulating catecholamines may result in more forceful contractions (inotropy), a rapid heartbeat (chronotropy), and more efficient relaxation (lusitropy). Ventricular performance is also determined, in part, by changes in preload and afterload. Preload varies as a result of changes in intravascular volume caused by alterations in systemic venous capacitance, pulmonary vascular capacitance, and ventricular compliance. *Preload* is a term that describes the intraventricular pressure immediately prior to contraction and is commonly referred to as the *filling pressure*. *Afterload* refers to the amount of pressure developed during ventricular systole that is required to eject blood against the pressure of the receiving vessel, the aorta, or pulmonary artery. The greater the afterload is, the greater the energy requirements and consumption of oxygen. Afterload is commonly measured by dividing the difference between the mean aortic pressure and central venous pressure by the cardiac output. The compliance of the ventricle is determined by changes in volume and pressure. The right ventricle is more compliant than the left ventricle and as a consequence may serve as a volume reservoir.

An understanding of the mechanics of normal and abnormal ventricular contraction is facilitated by a graphic depiction of the relationship between ventricular pressure and volume during a single cardiac cycle. This depiction, called a *pressure-volume loop*, is shown for a normal heart in Figure 59-5. Diastolic filling begins at point A and continues to point C. During the initial rapid filling from the atria, there is a slight fall in ventricular pressure, which demarks progressive ventricular relaxation. Once active relaxation of the ventricle ceases, point B, the pressure slightly increases as a result of passive ventricular filling.

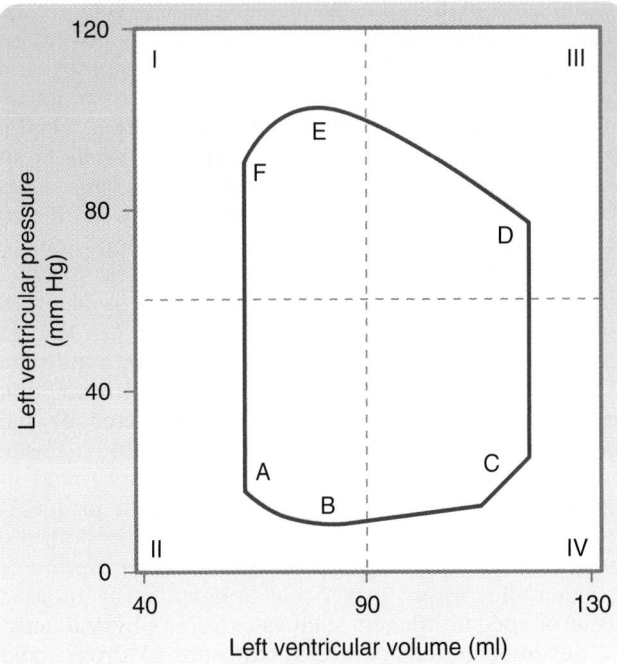

FIGURE 59-5. Pressure-volume loop during a single cardiac cycle. A variety of pathologic conditions bring about a shift in the pressure-volume loop to quadrants, here identified as quadrants I to V. A to C, diastolic filling; C to D, isovolumetric contraction; D to F, ventricular ejection; F to A, isovolumetric relaxation. (Courtesy of the Division of Cardiothoracic Surgery, University of Kentucky, 2003.)

Just prior to completion of filling, point C, an atrial contraction adds additional volume, the atrial kick. During isovolumetric contraction, from point C to D, the ventricular pressure rapidly increases with no change in ventricular volume. When the pressure in the ventricle exceeds the pressure in the aorta, the aortic valve opens, point D, and the rapid phase of ejection begins. Between point D and E, ventricular pressure increases while ventricular volume declines. Between points E and F, both pressure and volume decline until ejection is complete and the aortic valve closes, point F. Once the aortic valve is closed, a phase of isovolumetric relaxation occurs, point F to A, which is characterized by a rapid fall in pressure with no change in ventricular volume. When the ventricular pressure falls below the atrial pressure, the mitral valve opens, point A, and ventricular filling begins completing the cardiac cycle.

Pressure-volume loops are useful in understanding various physiologic and pathophysiologic conditions. The shape of the pressure-volume loop during systole is determined by the contractility of the heart and the afterload against which the ventricle is ejecting. In the setting of adrenergic stimulation, the pressure-volume loop is shifted to the left (see Fig. 59-5, quadrant II). Assuming all other variables remain constant, the positive inotropic and lusitropic effects of adrenergic stimulation promote an improved ejection fraction (EF) that is associated with a lower end-diastolic filling pressure. An increase in after-

load, as might be seen with hypertension or with aortic valve stenosis, is associated with a shift of the loop upward and to the right (see Fig. 59-5, quadrant III). If the stroke volume remains constant, the EF decreases slightly. In the setting of myocardial ischemia, there is a reduction in myocardial contractility and ventricular compliance. If the stroke volume is maintained, the pressure-volume loop shifts to the right (see Fig. 59-5, quadrant IV). This results in an acute decline in the EF and an increase in filling pressure. Myocardial fibrosis secondary to chronic ischemia and infarction can lead to decreased ventricular compliance. If systolic function is preserved, the stroke volume can be maintained if the filling pressures are increased. In this setting the pressure-volume loop is shifted upward. As ventricular function begins to deteriorate and the ventricle dilates, the pressure-volume loop also shifts to the right and higher filling pressures are required to maintain cardiac output (see Fig. 59-5, quadrant IV).

CORONARY ARTERY DISEASE

Pathogenesis

Coronary artery atherosclerosis is a progressive disease that begins early in life. Epicardial vessels are the most susceptible, intramyocardial arteries the least. Initially, the internal elastic membrane undergoes rupture, degeneration, and regeneration. This is accompanied by a deposition of mucopolysaccharides and proliferation of endothelial cells and fibroblasts. Later, growth lesions appear in the form of small deposits of lipoid material visible beneath the intima. This ultimately progresses to plaque formation and obstruction of the arterial lumen. In the final stages of the disease, patients become symptomatic or die from a myocardial infarct as a result of marked narrowing or closure of the vessel lumen, plaque rupture, or coronary artery thrombosis.

Role of Inflammation

Although several mechanisms and many risk factors for disease development have been implicated, it appears that the primary causes of atherosclerotic coronary artery disease (CAD) are endothelial injury induced by an inflammatory wall response and lipid deposition. There is evidence that an inflammatory response is involved in all stages of the disease, from early lipid deposition to plaque formation, plaque rupture, and coronary artery thrombosis. Early after initiation of an atherogenic diet in animals, endothelial cells begin to express selected adhesion molecules, such as the vascular cell adhesion molecule-1, that bind various classes of leukocytes, monocytes, and T lymphocytes. Once the leukocytes adhere to the endothelium, chemoattractant molecules promote transmigration, and they penetrate the intima where they participate in and perpetuate a local inflammatory response. The monocytes express scavenger receptors for modified lipoproteins, which allow them to ingest lipids. These modified lipids induce the expression of numerous adhesion molecules, chemokines, proinflammatory cytokines, and other mediators of inflammation in macrophages and vascular wall cells. The activated macrophages also release mitogens and chemoattractants, such as macrophage colony–stimulating factor, and monocyte chemoattractant protein-1. These molecules promote and perpetuate ongoing mobilization of monocytes into the evolving plaque. Tissue signals likewise stimulate T cells to elaborate inflammatory cytokines, such as interferon-γ and tumor necrosis factor-β, which further stimulate the inflammatory process.[1] Activated leukocytes also release fibrogenic mediators, which promote elaboration by local cells of a dense extracellular matrix. In addition to promoting the initiation of the atheroma, the inflammation precipitates the evolution of acute thrombotic complications. For instance, activated macrophages secrete proteolytic enzymes that degrade the collagen that lends strength to the plaque's protective fibrous cap. This in turn renders the cap thin, weak and prone to rupture.

Plaque Rupture

Several studies have shown that 70% to 80% of coronary thrombi occur where the fibrous cap of an atherosclerotic plaque has fissured or ruptured. Subsequent extension of the thrombus into the plaque with propagation of the thrombus downstream leads to an acute coronary event. According to the current paradigm, rupture of the fibrous cap leads to exposure of thrombogenic components of the plaque with subsequent activation of the platelets and coagulation pathways that result in thrombus formation and acute luminal compromise (Figs. 59-6 and 59-7).[2] Although the exact mechanism responsible for plaque rupture is unknown, the five features of vulnerable or high-risk plaques that are disruption prone are (1) a large, eccentric, soft lipid core; (2) a thin, fibrous cap; (3)

inflammation within the cap and adventitia; (4) increased plaque neovascularity; and (5) evidence of outward or positive vessel remodeling. Thinner fibrous caps are at a higher risk for rupture. This is probably due to an imbalance between the synthesis and degradation of the extracellular matrix in the fibrous cap that results in an overall decrease in the collagen and matrix components (Fig. 59-8). Increased matrix breakdown may be due to matrix degradation as a result of metalloproteinase expressed by inflammatory cells within the plaque. Reduced production of extracellular matrix is likely to contribute as well. Although plaque rupture can lead to thrombosis and manifest as an acute coronary syndrome (ACS), not all ruptures are symptomatic. The thrombotic response to plaque rupture is likely regulated by the thrombogenicity of the plaque's components. Tissue factor, secreted by activate macrophages and found in high concentrations within the lipid core of the plaque, is one of the most potent thrombogenic stimuli in both the intrinsic and extrinsic pathways. Spontaneous rupture of a vulnerable plaque may occur spontaneously or as a result of specific triggers such as extreme physical activity, severe emotional distress, exposure to drugs, cold exposure, and acute infections. There are also circadian components to the onset of ACSs.[3-5]

Lipid Metabolism

Epidemiologic evidence suggests that coronary artery atherosclerosis is closely linked to lipid metabolism, specifically cholesterol. Numerous studies have demonstrated that hydroxymethylglutaryl coenzyme-A reductase inhibitor (statin) therapy, aimed at lowering lipids, has resulted in a significant reduction in mortality.[6] In one observational study of patients who received statin therapy and were known to have CAD, statin treatment was associated with improved survival in all age groups.[7]

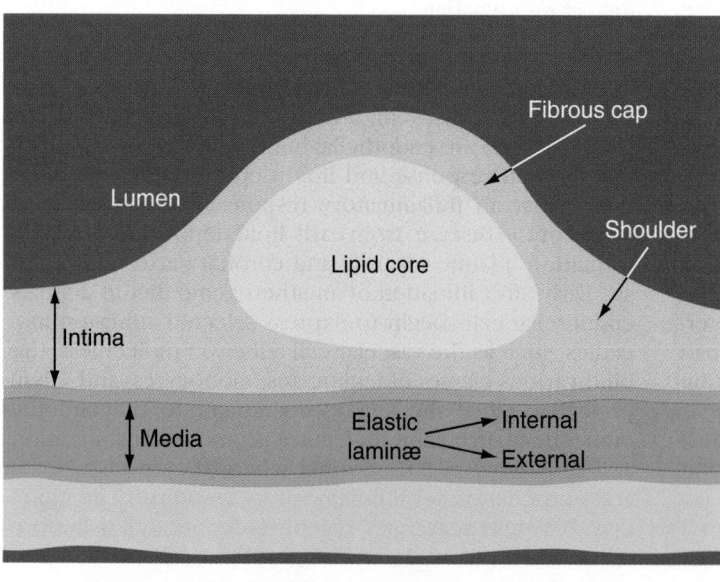

FIGURE 59-6. Anatomy of the atherosclerotic plaque. After the leukocytes have accumulated in the lesion, they often undergo death, sometimes by apoptosis, which can lead to a lipid core covered by a fibrous cap. (From Lipids Online—www.lipidsonline.org.)

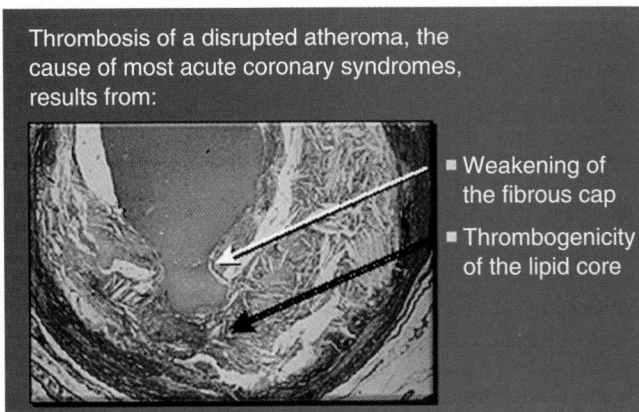

Thrombosis of a disrupted atheroma, the cause of most acute coronary syndromes, results from:

- Weakening of the fibrous cap
- Thrombogenicity of the lipid core

FIGURE 59-7. Thrombosis of a disrupted atheroma: weakening of the fibrous cap. Most coronary syndromes are caused by thrombosis of a disrupted atheroma, which can result from weakening of the fibrous cap and enhanced thrombogenicity of the lipid core. (Courtesy of Michael J. Davies, MD. Source: Lipids Online—www.lipidsonline.org.)

There was a 30% adjusted risk reduction in mortality for those younger than 65 years of age, 44% for patients aged 65 to 79, and a 50% reduction in patients who were older than 79 years old. The greatest survival benefit was derived in those patients with the highest quartile of high-sensitivity C-reactive protein (hs-CRP), a biomarker of inflammation and CAD.[8] Animal and human studies have demonstrated that statin therapy also modifies the lipid composition within plaques by lowering the amount of low-density lipoprotein (LDL) cholesterol and by stabilizing the plaque through a variety of mechanisms, including reduction in macrophage accumulation, collagen degradation, reduction in smooth muscle cell protease expression, and decrease in tissue factor expression.[9] Thus, more aggressive statin use after coronary artery bypass grafting (CABG) surgery may be indicated.

Fixed Coronary Obstructions

More than 90% of patients with symptomatic ischemic heart disease have advanced coronary atherosclerosis due to a fixed obstruction. Atherosclerotic plaques of the coronary arteries are either concentric (25%) or eccentric (75%). Eccentric lesions compromise only a portion of the lumen and, through vascular remodeling, the arterial lumen may remain patent until late in the disease process. The impact of an arterial stenosis on coronary blood flow can be appreciated in the context of Poiseuille's law. The volume of a homogeneous fluid passing per unit time through a tube is directly proportional to the pressure difference between its ends and to the fourth power of its internal radius, and inversely proportional to its length and to the viscosity of the fluid. Clinically, reductions in luminal diameter up to 60% have minimal impact on flow. Once the cross-sectional area of the vessel decreases by 75% or more, however, coronary blood flow is significantly compromised. Clinically, this often coincides with the onset of exertional angina. With a 90% reduction in luminal diameter, resistance is 256 times greater than a 60% stenosis, and coronary flow may be inadequate at rest.

ISCHEMIA AND MYOCARDIAL CELL INJURY

Myocardial ischemia can lead to reversible and/or irreversible injury. Ischemia of 15 to 20 minutes' duration is associated with postischemic myocardial dysfunction that lasts from hours to days despite the restoration of normal coronary blood flow. This reversible injury is referred to as *myocardial stunning*. The mechanisms underlying stunning are complex but in general appear to be related to intracellular calcium overload and oxidative stress induced by reactive oxygen species (ROS) released at the time of reperfusion. Although intracellular calcium may

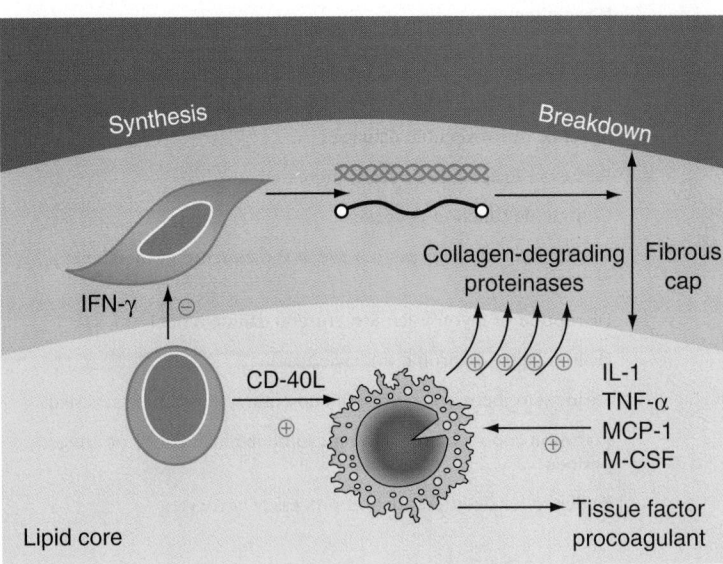

FIGURE 59-8. Matrix metabolism and integrity of the plaque's fibrous cap. This figure depicts the current understanding of the dynamics of the plaque's stability and thrombogenicity. The inflammatory cells can send molecular messages to the smooth muscle cells (interferon-γ) that inhibit the ability of this cell type to synthesize new collagen to strengthen the plaque's fibrous cap. In addition, the inflammatory cells can release proteolytic enzymes capable of degrading collagen and other structurally important constituents of the plaque's fibrous cap. Thus, when there is inflammation in the intima, the collagen responsible for the integrity of the plaque's fibrous cap is under double attack, subject to both decreased synthesis and increased degradation. This sets the stage for plaque disruption. The inflammatory cells also are responsible for signaling and producing increased quantities of tissue factor, a potent procoagulant deemed responsible for thrombosis of ruptured plaques. (From Libby P: Molecular bases of the acute coronary syndromes. Circulation 91:2844-2850, 1995. Source: Lipids Online—www.lipidsonline.org.)

return to normal levels early during reperfusion, transient increases can activate a variety of proteases, including protein kinase C, whose activation and subsequent action on contractile proteins can lead to myofibrillar injury. The incidence of myocardial stunning in patients after CABG surgery ranges from 20% to 80%, depending on its definition and/or clinical manifestation. For example, as many as 75% of patients after CABG surgery may be administered some form of inotropic support in the immediate postoperative period to maintain a satisfactory cardiac index, mixed venous saturation, blood pressure, and/or urinary output. In most patients, this is not associated with specific adverse outcomes. In the patient with severe preoperative myocardial dysfunction and limited cardiac reserve, however, myocardial stunning may result in a more profound reduction in cardiac output. These patients may require intensive inotropic support postoperatively and insertion of an intra-aortic balloon pump (IABP). In these patients the mortality rate secondary to stunning may be as high as 10% to 15%.

Reversible contractile dysfunction that matches a reduction in resting coronary artery blood flow is termed *hibernating myocardium*. It is characterized by a balanced reduction in myocardial contractility and oxygen consumption and is typically found in patients with severe CAD who present with stable or unstable angina (UA), myocardial infarction, or congestive heart failure. By definition, it is reversible on restoration of normal coronary blood flow. Human tissue biopsies obtained from hibernating myocardium have shown a loss of myofibrils, glycogen accumulation, and interstitial fibrosis. Whether the contractile dysfunction in the hibernating myocardium is due to a reduction in coronary blood flow or a reduction

in coronary reserve is unclear. It is also controversial whether chronic contractile dysfunction is caused by repetitive episodes of myocardial stunning or is an adaptive mechanism to chronic myocardial ischemia. Characteristics that differentiate these two phenomena are summarized in Table 59-1.

Myocardial infarction represents cell death and necrosis. It is an irreversible injury that is associated with ischemia lasting more than 20 minutes. Since a gradient of ischemia may exist within the myocardium, not all cells are equally at risk for injury. Cells around the periphery of an ischemic zone and adjacent to the oxygen-rich blood in the ventricular chamber may remain viable. In the absence of adequate collateral flow, sustained ischemia often results in a transmural infarction within 6 to 12 hours. Cell death leads to an inflammatory process that involves the migration of polymorphonuclear leukocytes into the ischemic area and removal of necrotic tissue by macrophages over days. This is followed by a fibroblastic response and neovascularization. Because the myocytes are incapable of regeneration, the infarcted tissue is ultimately replaced with noncontractile fibrous tissue.

Another cause of cardiomyocyte cell loss associated with ischemia is apoptosis, or programmed cell death. This phenomenon is a noninflammatory process that occurs as a result of reperfusion and may be associated with early and delayed cardiac muscle dysfunction. Some of the proposed mechanisms underlying apoptosis are the same mechanisms proposed for myocardial stunning, hibernation, and infarction, namely, generation of intracellular ROS, and/or intracellular calcium overload. Apoptosis has been observed in humans with hibernating myocardium, acute myocardial infarction (AMI), and

TABLE 59-1.   Characteristics of Reversible Postischemic Myocardial Dysfunction

Stunning	Hibernation
Dysfunctional myocardium with normal or near-normal blood flow	Dysfunctional myocardium with reduced blood flow
Contractile abnormality reversible with time	Contractile abnormality reversible on reperfusion
Absence of irreversible damage	Absence of irreversible damage
Perfusion imaging (PET scan) normal or increased	Perfusion imaging (PET scan) increased
Contractile function decreased	Contractile function decreased
No metabolic deterioration during inotropic stimulation	Recruitment of inotropic reserve at the expense of metabolic recovery
Disruption of myofibrillar structure in canine model	Disruption of myofibrillar structure in canine model
Heart does not adapt to chronic underperfusion	Heart adapts to chronic underperfusion
Steady-state between perfusion and contraction not achieved	Steady-state between perfusion and contraction can be reached
Perfusion-contraction mismatching lasts from hours to days to months	Perfusion-contraction matching can be maintained for prolonged periods
Lack of evidence for dedifferentiation process in myocytes	Evidence for dedifferentiation process in myocytes

PET, positron-emission tomography.

chronic heart failure. The characteristics of apoptotic death are morphologically and biochemically different from cell death secondary to cell necrosis. With necrosis, cell death is associated with swelling and rupture of the sarcolemmal, mitochondrial, and nuclear membranes, and nuclear chromatin clumping, and the dead cells are removed via an inflammatory process. In contrast, the apoptotic cell shrinks, the nucleus condenses and breaks into nucleosomes and DNA fragments and the cells are phagocytized. There is some evidence that not all apoptotic cells are committed to cell death in the early stages of the process. Apoptosis represents one aspect of a continuum of ischemia. Its contribution to myocardial dysfunction after ischemia may be more relevant to the process of postischemic ventricular remodeling.

Finally, there is preclinical and circumstantial evidence in humans that an ischemic adaptive phenomenon exists in the human heart. This phenomenon is known as *ischemic preconditioning* (IPC). It is associated with a reduction in infarct size, apoptosis, and reperfusion-associated arrhythmias. IPC occurs when the heart is exposed to brief periods of sublethal ischemia prior to a period of prolonged ischemia. The underlying mechanism(s) is unclear but most likely involves activation of cell surface receptors and intracellular transduction signaling pathways. If the phenomenon can be mimicked pharmacologically, this could lead to the development of pharmacologic agents that are effective in increasing the heart's tolerance to ischemia.

CLINICAL MANIFESTATIONS AND DIAGNOSIS OF CORONARY ARTERY DISEASE

Clinical Presentation

One of the most typical manifestations of CAD is angina pectoris, a discomfort or sensation of heaviness, tightening, squeezing, or constricting in the chest. This discomfort is often retrosternal or left precordial and may radiate from the chest. It is also characterized as discomfort in the jaw, shoulder, back, or arm. Patients often experience a disagreeable feeling similar to that of indigestion and/or experience shortness of breath. It often presents while the patient is exercising, eating, or under emotional duress and usually subsides with rest. Patients with UA typically have pain at rest or with minimal exertion that lasts more than 20 minutes. It is often severe in nature, new in onset (within 1 month), and occurs in a crescendo pattern. Angina is not, however, always present with myocardial ischemia. As many as 15% of patients with significant CAD do not present with angina. This silent ischemia occurs most frequently in patients with diabetes mellitus and is detected during electrocardiographic (ECG) and/or echocardiographic monitoring during stress testing. In patients at risk for the disease, angina pectoris is graded according to a variety of classification systems, such as the New York Heart Association Functional Classification, and Canadian Cardiovascular Society Classification System (CCSCS). The latter is more specific for patients with

angina pectoris. Using the CCSCS schema, class I patients are asymptomatic, class II patients experience slight limitation of ordinary activity, class III patients experience marked limitation of activity with ordinary physical activity, and class IV patients are unable to undertake any activity without discomfort. Classifications allow for the evaluation of the patient's condition followed over time and the assessment of therapeutic interventions.

In contrast to angina pectoris, a myocardial infarction often presents as crushing chest pain that may be associated with nausea, diaphoresis, anxiety, and dyspnea. Symptoms also include dizziness, fatigue, and vomiting. The pain or associated paresthesias often radiate to the neck and/or jaw and down the arm. Heart rate and blood pressure may be initially normal, but both increase in response to the duration and severity of pain.

Physical Examination

It is possible for a patient to have extensive CAD and the physical examination to be unremarkable. Pertinent physical findings are more frequently associated with manifestations of atherosclerosis in general. The patient's mental status can vary from normal, to anxious, to confused. Eye examination may reveal a copper-wire sign, retinal hematoma or thrombosis secondary to vascular occlusive disease, and hypertension. The presence of neck bruits and thrills may reflect significant underlying carotid artery disease. Abnormal neck vein pulsations may be seen in patients with second- or third-degree heart block. The pulse may be weak or thready and suggest ectopic or premature ventricular beats. Often a precordial ectopic impulse may be palpated along the left lower sternal border, demarking enlargement of the left ventricle due to increase chamber compliance and bulging. A third heart sound can be noted with elevated left ventricular filling pressures. A fourth heart sound is commonly heard in patients with acute and chronic CAD, and heart murmurs may reflect ischemic papillary muscles and mitral valve insufficiency, aortic stenosis/insufficiency, and ventricular septal rupture. In patients with more advanced ischemic heart disease, auscultation of the chest may reveal rales, and examination of the abdomen may reveal hepatomegaly, right upper abdominal quadrant tenderness, ascites, and marked peripheral and presacral edema.

Laboratory Studies

Patients suspected of having CAD should undergo appropriate blood testing, including a lipid profile (cholesterol, triglycerides, LDL, high-density lipoprotein [HDL]) and perhaps an hs-CRP level. Elevated serum cholesterol level is associated with an elevated risk of coronary heart disease. A 10% increase in serum cholesterol is associated with a 20% to 30% increase in heart disease. Clear benefits have been shown for dietary and drug regimens that lower serum cholesterol, and statins have been shown to reduce fatal and nonfatal coronary heart disease and slow the progression of bypass graft plaque progression.

There are also several markers of inflammation that are useful at predicting the development of coronary heart disease. These include hs-CRP, the adhesion molecule ICAM-1, and cytokines such as interleukin (IL)-6 and tumor necrosis factor. hs-CRP adds to the predictive value of total and HDL cholesterol in determining risk of future myocardial infarction. Whether these markers can be used to better identify patients at risk and target therapeutic intervention remains to be determined.

Diagnostic Studies

There are numerous methods and technologies that are available to detect the presence of hemodynamically

significant coronary artery stenoses and to assess cardiac function and myocardial viability. The information ultimately determines whether a patient should be treated medically, with percutaneous transluminal coronary angioplasty (PTCA), percutaneous coronary intervention (PCI), or with CABG surgery (Fig. 59-9). Many of these studies can be performed even if the patient is unable to exercise. The strengths and weaknesses of each method are shown in Box 59-1.

Chest Radiograph

The chest radiograph is helpful in identifying causes of chest discomfort or pain other than that due to CAD. With

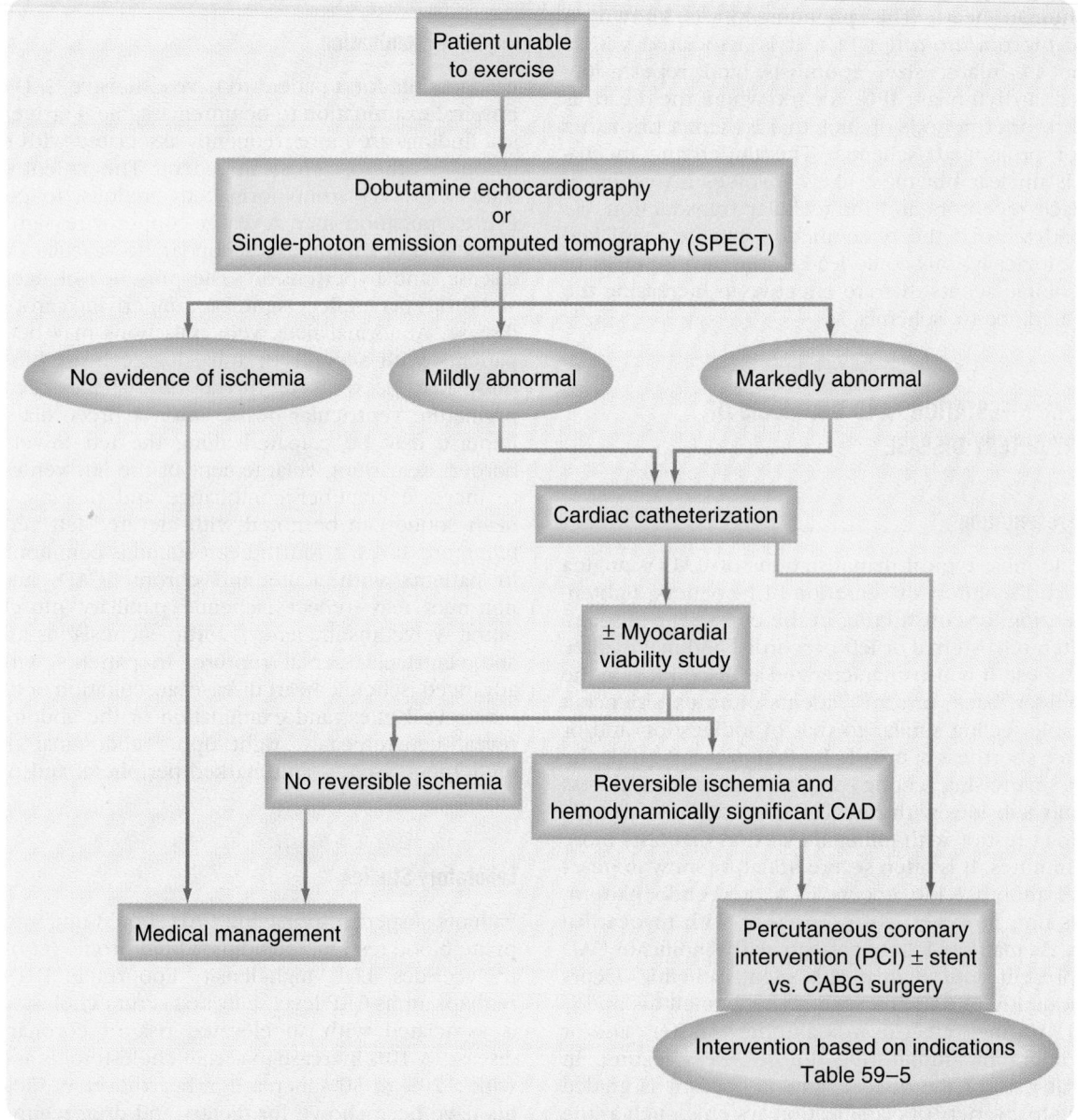

■ FIGURE 59-9.   A strategy for evaluating patients with suspected coronary artery disease (CAD) and unable to exercise. CABG, coronary artery bypass graft. (Courtesy of the Division of Cardiothoracic Surgery, University of Kentucky, 2003.)

Box 59-1. Strengths and Limitations of Diagnostic Techniques

DETECTING CORONARY ARTERY DISEASE AND ASSESSING PROGNOSIS

Exercise ECG

Strengths: Low cost; short duration; functional status evaluated; high sensitivity in three-vessel or left main coronary artery disease; prognostic (e.g., ischemia at low workload)

Limitations: Suboptimal sensitivity; low detection rate of one-vessel disease; nondiagnostic with abnormal baseline ECG; poor specificity in premenopausal women; must achieve $\geq$ 85% of maximum heart rate for accuracy

Exercise/Pharmacologic SPECT Perfusion Imaging

Strengths: Simultaneous evaluation of perfusion and function (gated SPECT); higher sensitivity and specificity than exercise ECG; high specificity with ^{99m}Tc; can be performed in most patients; added prognostic value; comparable accuracy with pharmacologic stress; viability and ischemia simultaneously assessed; quantitative image analysis

Limitations: Suboptimal specificity with ^{201}Tl; long procedure time with 99^{m}Tc; higher cost than exercise ECG; radiation exposure; poor-quality images in obese patients

Exercise/Pharmacologic Stress Echocardiography

Strengths: Higher sensitivity and specificity than exercise ECG; added prognostic value; comparable value with dobutamine stress; short examination time; identification of structural cardiac abnormalities; simultaneous evaluation of perfusion with contrast agents; relatively lower cost; no radiation

Limitations: Decreased sensitivity for detection of one-vessel disease or mild stenosis with postexercise imaging; inability to image all of the left ventricle in some patients; highly operator dependent; no quantitative image analysis; poor acoustic window in some patients (e.g., chronic obstructive lung disease); infarct zone ischemia less well detected

ASSESSMENT OF MYOCARDIAL VIABILITY

SPECT Imaging

Strengths: High sensitivity for predicting improved function after revascularization; quantitative objective criteria (e.g., >60% segmental uptake); LVEF quantitated on ^{99m}Tc-sestamibi or ^{99m}Tc-tetrofosmin imaging; predictive of clinical outcomes

Limitations: Reduced resolution and sensitivity compared to PET; less quantitative than PET; areas of attenuation (e.g., inferior wall on ^{99m}Tc-sestamibi scans) misconstrued as nonviability; cannot differentiate endocardial from epicardial viability; no absolute measurement of blood flow; lower specificity than dobutamine echocardiography for predicting improved function after revascularization

PET Imaging

Strengths: Simultaneous assessment of perfusion and metabolism; more sensitive than other techniques; good specificity; no attenuation problems; absolute blood flow can be measured; predictive of outcomes

Limitations: Lower specificity than dobutamine echocardiography or MRI; cannot separate endocardial from epicardial viability; high cost and highly sophisticated technology; limited availability

Dobutamine Echocardiography

Strengths: Higher specificity than nuclear techniques; viability assessed at low doses and ischemia at higher doses; evaluation of mitral regurgitation on baseline echocardiography; predictive of outcomes; widely available; lower cost than dobutamine MRI

Limitations: Poor windows in 30% of patients; lower sensitivity than nuclear techniques; myocardium with poor flow may not show increased during stimulation; reliance on visual assessment of wall thickening

Contrast Echocardiography

Strengths: Microcirculatory integrity evaluated as well as systolic thickening; better estimation of extent of viability than functional assessment alone; precise delineation of area of necrosis; resolution of endocardial vs. epicardial perfusion; viability assessed in presence of total coronary occlusion

Limitations: Difficult windows in 30% of patients; attenuation problems; scant clinical data available

Dobutamine MRI

Strengths: Evaluate inotropic reserve in endocardium with tagging; measurement of wall thickness more accurate than with TTE; better image quality than echocardiography for contractile reserve; simultaneous assessment of perfusion using contrast enhancement; good sensitivity and specificity for viability

Limitations: Higher cost than echocardiography; limited availability; less sensitive than nuclear techniques but may be more specific; imaging information not available in real time; patients with pacemakers or implantable cardioverter defibrillators cannot be imaged

ECG, electrocardiogram; LVEF, left ventricular ejection fraction; MRI, magnetic resonance imaging; PET, positron-emission tomography; SPECT, single-photon emission computed tomography; TTE, transesophageal echocardiography.

Adapted from Braunwald E, Zipes DP, Libby P (eds): Heart Disease: A Textbook of Cardiovascular Medicine, 6th ed. Philadelphia, WB Saunders, 2001, pp 435, 437.

advanced CAD there may be evidence of cardiomegaly, pulmonary edema, or pleural effusions, which are indicative of heart failure. Evidence of calcification in the coronary arteries, aortic or mitral valves, or aorta is also consistent with presumptive evidence of generalized atherosclerosis.

Electrocardiogram

A 12-lead resting ECG should be obtained in patients suspected of having CAD and in those with episodes of chest discomfort or angina pectoris. The ECG is evaluated for evidence of left ventricular hypertrophy, ST-segment depression or elevation, ectopic beats, or Q waves. In addition, arrhythmias (atrial fibrillation or ventricular tachycardia) and conduction defects (left anterior fascicular block, right bundle branch block, left bundle branch block) are suggestive of CAD and myocardial infarction. Persistent ST-segment elevation or an evolving Q wave is consistent with myocardial injury and ongoing ischemia. Fifty percent of patients have normal ECGs despite the existence of significant CAD, and 50% of ECGs obtained during chest pain are normal at rest. An exercise stress ECG is helpful in determining the extent of CAD and prognosis. Exercise protocols, typically using a treadmill or bicycle, increase myocardial oxygen demand to elicit an ischemic threshold. A positive exercise ECG may show progressive flattening of the ST-segment or ST-segment depression as exercise progresses. During the recovery phase, ST depression may persist, with down-sloping segments and T-wave inversion. Additional findings associated with an adverse prognosis and presence of multivessel occlusive disease include duration of symptom-limited exercise less than 6 metabolic equivalents, failure to increase systolic blood pressure higher than 120 mm Hg, or appearance of ventricular arrhythmias. For detection of CAD, the sensitivity and specificity of an exercise ECG approaches 70% and 80%, respectively. The accuracy of exercise ECG testing is dependent on a patient achieving 85% to 90% of their age-predicted maximum exercise (see Box 59-1).

Echocardiography

Surface and transesophageal echocardiography (TEE) use reflected acoustic waves for cardiac imaging. Common indications for a resting echocardiogram include heart murmurs and suggested diagnoses such as aortic stenosis or insufficiency, hypertrophic cardiomyopathy, mitral valve stenosis or regurgitation, and congestive heart failure. Rest echocardiography can also reveal regional wall motion abnormalities, ventricular dilation, and wall thinning. The sensitivity and specificity of echocardiography can be enhanced with the administration of intravenous dobutamine in incremental doses and is helpful in differentiating stunned, hibernating, and infarcted myocardium. A reduced inotropic response and evidence of new wall motion abnormalities are also indicative of myocardial ischemia (see Box 59-1).

Single-Photon Emission Computed Tomographic Imaging

Exercise or pharmacologic stress ^{201}Tl or ^{99m}Tc-sestamibi single-photon emission computed tomographic (SPECT) imaging has a sensitivity for detecting CAD of 85% to 96% and, when gated with ECG, has a specificity of 90%. Compared to exercise ECG, both techniques are more accurate. They are particularly useful in patients with left ventricular hypertrophy and/or conduction abnormalities and for patients unable to achieve 85% of their maximum predicted exercise response. In conjunction with ECG gating, ^{201}Tl SPECT imaging also provides useful data on regional wall thickening, global left ventricular EF, and myocardial perfusion. For the patient who cannot exercise, administration of vasodilators (adenosine, dipyridamole) or inotropes (dobutamine) allows similar data acquisition with comparable sensitivity and specificity (see Fig. 59-9).

Positron-Emission Tomography

Positron-emission tomography (PET) scanning is a useful technique for assessing myocardial viability and metabolism and evaluating myocardial blood flow. Since myocardial extraction of glucose is elevated in ischemic myocytes, the glucose analog radiotracer ^{18}F-2-fluoro-2-deoxyglucose (FDG) can be used to image the heart; PET is reported to be superior to thallium SPECT, ^{99m}Tc perfusion, and stress-dobutamine echocardiography in the evaluation of myocardial viability.[10] The positive predictive value (PPV) and negative predictive value (NPV) approach 95%. Perfusion of nonmetabolic tracers through the myocardium can identify two basic patterns: normal/uniform perfusion and underperfused myocardium. The combination of abnormal perfusion with a positive PET study indicates viable myocardium in an area of coronary artery stenosis. In addition, FDG PET is a highly accurate predictor of improvement in regional wall motion and global left ventricular EF after myocardial revascularization. For patients with abnormal perfusion and greater than 75% of normal PET uptake, the PPV value of left ventricular recovery is 65% to 90%. Uptake less than 75% generally indicates unlikely recovery of left ventricular function (NPV, 75% to 95%) after revascularization. Limitations to PET include cost, availability of cardiac PET, and inability to interpret the study in diabetic patients who have significant insulin resistance (see Box 59-1).

Magnetic Resonance Imaging (MRI)—Gadolinium MRI

Due to the radiation exposure of SPECT scanning, and the limited availability of cardiac PET imaging, myocardial first-pass magnetic resonance imaging (MRI) perfusion is a good alternative for evaluating the myocardial viability. One prospective study of 31 patients with confirmed CAD and reduced left ventricular function (EF < 0.35) showed that MRI had a sensitivity and specificity of 86% and 94%, respectively, when PET was used as the standard for identifying segments of myocardium with matched flow/metabolism defects.[11] Quantitative assessment of infarct mass also correlated well with PET. In another study, 48 patients with CAD were prospectively evaluated with gadolinium-enhanced multislice hybrid echo-planar pulse-sequence MRI versus PET, and compared to 18 normal patients.[12] Receiver-operator characteristic analysis of CAD (as defined by PET) had a sensitivity and specificity of 91% and 94%, respectively. Compared to quantitative coronary angiography, MRI detected lesions greater than 50% with a specificity and sensitivity of 87% and 85%, respectively. These findings suggest that cardiac MRI is an excellent alternative diagnostic method that can be used to determine the presence and extent of CAD and myocardial viability (see Box 59-1).

ECG-Gated Multidetector Spiral Computed Tomography/Electron-Beam Computed Tomography

ECG-gated multidetector spiral computed tomography (CT) is a potential tool for functional and ischemic cardiac imaging. It can identify regional myocardial wall thinning and the presence of mural thrombus. Contrast-enhanced electron-beam CT (EBCT) is used to detect hemodynamically significant lesions, although 30% to 40% of patients cannot be imaged due to unacceptable cardiac motion artifact. There is variation in efficacy for specific coronary arteries, with an overall sensitivity and specificity of 90% and 80%, respectively. EBCT quantification of coronary artery calcium has been reported to predict abnormal SPECT findings and correlate with existing asymptomatic myocardial ischemia in clinically high-risk patients. This suggests that EBCT may be a good screening test for CAD.

Cardiac Catheterization

Anatomy of the coronary arteries, ascending aorta, aortic and mitral valves, and left ventricle can be readily evaluated at the time of left heart catheterization. High-quality coronary angiography is essential for the identification of CAD and the assessment of its extent and severity. Cardiac catheterization that includes ventriculogram also permits assessment of systolic and diastolic function, diagnosis of intracardiac shunts, differentiation of myocardial restriction from pericardial constriction, and assessment of valve dysfunction. Right heart catheterization is used to measure central venous, right atrial, right ventricular, pulmonary artery, and pulmonary wedge pressures, as well as cardiac output. It can also be used to evaluate the presence of intracardiac shunts, assess arrhythmias, and initiate temporary cardiac pacing.

CORONARY ARTERY BYPASS SURGERY: TECHNICAL ASPECTS

Cardiopulmonary Bypass

The basic components of an extracorporeal heart pump circuit consist of one or more venous cannulae, a venous reservoir that collects blood by gravity, an oxygenator and heat exchanger, a perfusion pump, a blood filter in the arterial line, and an arterial cannula (Fig. 59-10). The cardiopulmonary bypass (CPB) machine is constructed from a variety of biocompatible materials that can include polycarbonate, polyvinyl chloride, Teflon, polyethylene, stainless steel, titanium, silicone rubber, and polyurethane. The blood conduits are designed to minimize turbulence, cavitation, changes in blood flow velocity, and the volume of nonblood solutions necessary to prime the pump and tubing. The circuitry has multiple access ports or sites to obtain blood samples for laboratory studies and the infusion of blood, blood products, crystalloids, and/or drugs.

Supplemental components include a cardiotomy suction system to collect undiluted or "clean" blood from open cardiac chambers and the surgical field. This blood is filtered, de-aired, and returned to the bypass pump. Diluted field blood and blood that has been exposed to potentially harmful elements (e.g., inflammatory cytokines, fat) are collected via a separate system device that concentrates washed red blood cells before returning them directly to the patient. A cardioplegia infusion device consists of a separate pump, reservoir, and heat exchanger. It is used to deliver a cold potassium-enriched blood or crystalloid solutions into the coronary circulation to protect the heart during ischemic arrest. Approximately 2 L of solution are required to prime the heart pump for adults. The priming solution consists of a balanced salt solution and often a starch solution. Homologous blood is not usually added unless the patient is anemic (i.e., the hematocrit is <25 mL/dL). Use of CPB requires suppression of the clotting cascade with heparin since the components of the bypass pump and the surgical wound are powerful stimuli for thrombus formation. Systemic heparinization may, however, result in increased blood loss and the requirements for homologous blood and blood product transfusions. Heparin can also induce transient hypotension as a result of an allergic reaction.

The oxygen consumption of a patient on CPB at normal temperatures averages 80 to 125 mL/min/m² similar to the anesthetized adult not on bypass.[13] Although a pump flow rate of 2.2 L/min/m² meets the metabolic needs of most patients and avoids acidosis, a flow rate of 2.5 L/min/m² ensures perfusion of the microcirculation and adds a margin of safety. If hypothermia is employed, the flow rate can be reduced to less than 2.2 L/min/m². This is because the mean oxygen consumption of the body decreases by 50% for every 10°C decrease in body temperature.[14] Below 28°C, a flow rate of 1.6 L/min/m² may be safe for as long as 2 hours. Significant disadvantages of using systemic hypothermia to accommodate lower flow rates include the extra time required to rewarm the patient and associated alterations that occur in the reactivity of blood elements, particularly platelets. The latter may result in a greater propensity for bleeding once the patient has been rewarmed. During CPB, the systemic blood pressure is maintained by adjusting the speed of the roller pump, manipulating the patient's intravascular volume, and adjusting the peripheral vascular resistance by infusing vasodilators such as nitroprusside or nitroglycerin or vasoconstrictors like ephedrine. In general, the mean normothermic blood pressure should be maintained between 50 and 70 mm Hg. The perfusion pressure may

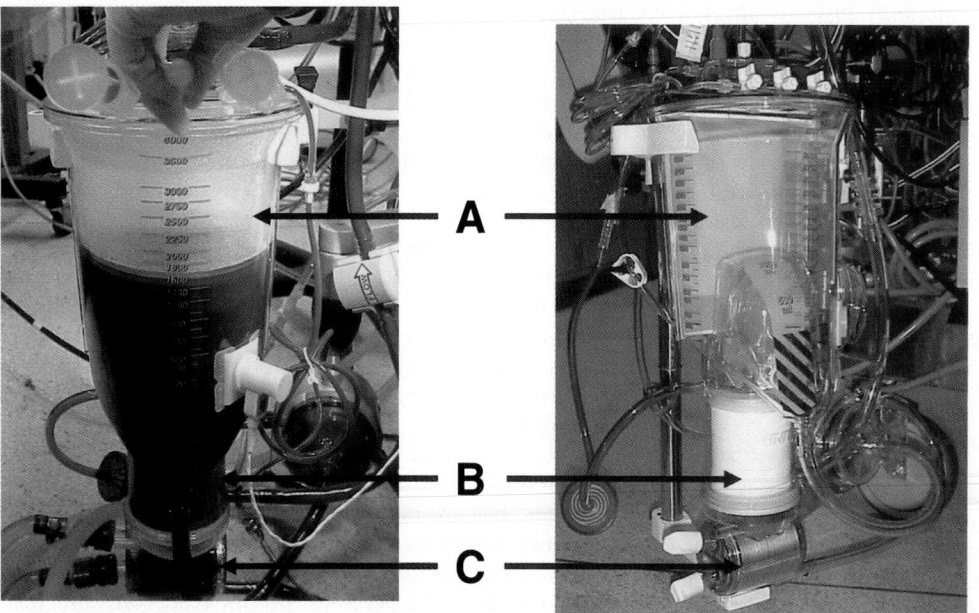

FIGURE 59-10.

Components of cardiopulmonary bypass (CPB) system: A indicates the venous reservoir and blood filter; B indicates the membrane oxygenator; and C indicates the heat exchange coil. D shows the following components: (1) CPB control console, (2) roller pump for infusing oxygenated blood, (3) cardioplegia, and (4) controlling suction catheters. E is the cardioplegia reservoir and heat exchanger. (Courtesy of the Division of Cardiothoracic Surgery, University of Kentucky, 2003.)

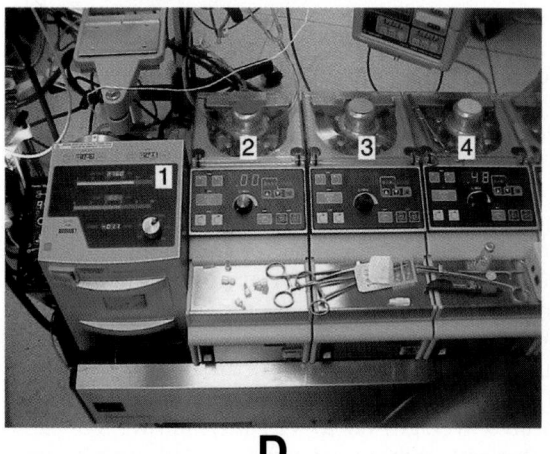

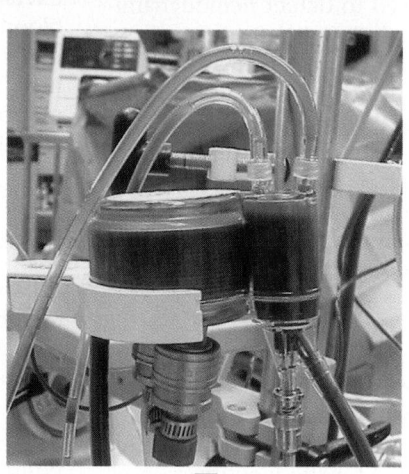

be maintained 10 to 15 mm Hg higher if a patient is known to have significant obstructive intracranial or carotid artery disease.

Myocardial Protection Techniques

With the advent of CABG surgery, it was evident that some patients experienced varying degrees of myocardial injury and necrosis despite adequate myocardial revascularization. Many of these patients died of heart failure or experienced prolonged periods of low cardiac output. Ultimately, it was determined that this necrosis occurred as a result of ischemic damage sustained during the time of aortic cross-clamping and ischemic arrest. As a result, a number of methodologies and techniques have evolved over the past 50 years to prevent this complication (Table 59-2). The cornerstone, however, is the use of systemic hypothermia and the infusion of cold hyperkalemic crystalloid or blood solutions directly into the proximal ascending aorta after placement of the aortic cross-clamp.[15] The latter results in diastolic arrest of the heart, a marked reduction in myocardial oxygen consumption, and a quiescent operative field.

Currently, there are a number of different ways to deliver cardioplegic solutions (Table 59-3). One technique involves a balanced approach; that is, the cardioplegic solution is administered first antegrade via the proximal ascending aorta and then retrograde via a coronary sinus catheter inserted through a pursestring suture placed in the right atrium. The extensive collateralization among the coronary veins and arteries and the paucity of valves within the coronary vein system ensures a relatively homogeneous distribution of cardioplegia when the retrograde approach is used. Patients with high-grade proximal lesions, especially those with suboptimal collateral

TABLE 59-2. Innovations in the Field of Myocardial Protection

Name	Year	Innovation
Bigelow WG	1950	Studied the application of hypothermia to cardiac surgery in canines
Melrose DG & Bentall HH	1955	Introduced the concept of reversible chemical cardiac arrest in canines
Lillehei CW	1956	Detailed a method for delivering hypothermic crystalloid cardioplegia by cannulating coronary arteries
Gerbode F & Melrose DG	1958	Used potassium citrate to induce cardiac arrest in humans
Bretschneider HJ	1964	Developed a sodium-poor, calcium-free, procaine-containing solution to arrest the heart
Sondergaard KT	1964	Adopted Bretschneider's cardioplegic solution and was one of the first to routinely use it for myocardial protection in clinical practice
Gay WA & Ebert PA	1973	Credited with revival of potassium-induced cardioplegia; demonstrated that potassium solution could arrest a canine heart for 60 minutes without cellular damage
Hearse DJ	1975	Emphasized preischemic infusions to negate ischemic injuries in rats; this formula became known as St. Thomas solution No. 1
Braimbridge MV	1975	One of the first to use St. Thomas solution No. 1 clinically
Buckberg GD	1979	Introduced the use of blood as the vehicle for infusing potassium into coronary arteries
Akins CW	1984	Utilized technique of hypothermic fibrillatory arrest for coronary revascularization without cardioplegia
Lichenstein SV & Salemo TA	1991	Introduced warm-blood cardioplegia

TABLE 59-3. Methods and Delivery of Cardioplegic Solutions

Infusion Types	Infusion Temperatures	Infusion Intervals
Antegrade	Tepid	Continuous
Retrograde	Warm	Intermittent
Combined retrograde/antegrade	Cold	

vessels, may benefit from the application of both techniques. Following the initial administration of cardioplegia, additional doses are usually administered every 15 to 20 minutes. The temperature of the myocardium can be continuously monitored with an intracardiac probe. For patients with significant ventricular hypertrophy, and those without obvious adequate collateral vessels, shorter intervals between infusions may be required.

Conduits for Coronary Artery Bypass Grafting

The internal thoracic arteries (ITAs) (left and/or right) are the preferred conduits since their patency rates exceed 90% at 10 years.[16] The left ITA is generally used to graft the LAD, and reversed saphenous vein segments are used to graft the remaining vessels. The right ITA pedicle can be used to graft the RCA; if it is of sufficient length, it can be used to graft the PDA or branches of the LCA. The advantage of using these conduits must be weighed

against the potential risks in specific subsets of patients. For example, the diabetic patient may be at increased risk of infections. In these patients bilateral ITA mobilization has been associated with a 14-fold increase in the risk of sternal wound infections. Since there is some evidence that there may be a survival benefit associated with using only arterial grafts,[17] the radial artery is often used in conjunction with ITA grafts to revascularize the heart. Use of arterial grafts only has the added advantages of eliminating the need for lower extremity incisions and the risk of leg wound infections.[18] Prior to making a forearm incision, an Allen's test is performed, and the palmar arch is evaluated using ultrasound to confirm the presence of adequate collateral circulation in the hand. The radial artery is then procured using a no-touch technique. Prior to its removal, the adequacy of arterial flow to the respective hand can be assessed by direct compression of the proximal end of the vessel. Systemic vasodilators, such as nitroglycerin, are frequently used during the dissection to minimize vasospasm. The free graft is then stored in a solution containing heparin and papaverine. Another pedicled arterial conduit that can be used is the gastroepiploic artery. This conduit is more appropriate for vessels in the inferior and lateral portions of the left ventricle. Limitations associated with the use of this graft include its predilection for vasospasm, twisting, kinking, and vulnerability to technical error at the anastomotic site due to its thin arterial wall. In general, the gastroepiploic artery is reserved for patients with limited conduit options.

The most commonly used conduit is the greater saphenous vein. Whether the right or left leg is chosen depends on a variety of factors such as evidence of previous saphenous vein stripping, venous stasis disease, arterial vascular insufficiency, presence of nonhealing wounds, varicose veins, or history of superficial thrombophlebitis. The adequacy of the vein can be assessed preoperatively using Doppler ultrasound. This technique can also be used to map the anatomic location of the vessel to minimize the extent of the lower extremity incision. Techniques that are used to procure the saphenous vein include a single long incision over the vein, multiple small incisions with bridges of intact skin, and endoscopic dissection. In general, the ideal saphenous vein should have a diameter of 3.5 mm, no varicosities, or areas of stricture. The bridged or endoscopic technique minimizes the length of the skin incision and is associated with lower infection rates and less postoperative pain. Stretching or manipulation of the vessel is minimized to avoid endothelial injury and thrombosis. Side branches are clipped or ligated to avoid bleeding complications in the postoperative period. The leg incisions are closed in layers to eliminate dead space and avoid hematoma formation and decrease the risk of infection. The vein conduit is then stored in heparinized saline or blood until it is needed. Vein graft patency rates have been reported to be 88% early after grafting, 81% at 1 year, 75% at 5 years, and 50% at 15 years. Venous graft occlusion rate is approximately 2% per year.[19] If the saphenous vein is inadequate or unavailable, the lesser saphenous vein can be used.

Anesthesia for Myocardial Revascularization

Major advances in cardiac anesthesia in the past 5 years primarily reflect improvements in techniques and methodologies. For example, high-dose narcotic anesthesia, which was routinely used a decade ago, has evolved into a method of balanced anesthesia. This involves the judicious use of shorter-acting narcotics, such as remifentanil, supplemented by safer volatile agents, such as sevoflurane, and/or short-acting intravenous agents, such as propofol. The use of short-acting agents has resulted in less ventilatory support time, shorter intensive care unit (ICU) stay, and a decrease in hospital length of stay. There is also an increase in the use of supplemental techniques, such as regional, epidural, and paraspinal blocks to reduce the use of systemic agents and improve analgesic control and postoperative pulmonary function. Maintaining control of the mean arterial blood pressure to preserve the cerebral perfusion pressure minimizes postoperative neuropsychometric and neurocognitive dysfunction. Also, real-time cerebral bispectral index monitoring, although somewhat controversial, can be used to predict anesthetic depth and avoid excess narcotic anesthesia. Adequate oxygen delivery is ensured by maintaining a hematocrit 25% or higher during and after CPB. Finally, there is evidence that tight glycemic control in diabetic patients undergoing CABG surgery may improve survival and decrease recurrent ischemic events. Perioperative serum glucose levels should be maintained between 100 and 150 mg/dL.

The use of intraoperative TEE represents another major advance in cardiac anesthesia. It is particularly useful in assessing myocardial function before and after CPB. Perioperative myocardial ischemia manifest by new regional wall motion abnormalities can often be detected prior to ischemic changes in the ECG and elevation in pulmonary artery pressures. TEE can also be used to determine the presence of intracavitary air and the ventricular response to increasing intravascular volume. This information can be helpful in deciding the optimum time to wean the patient from CPB.

With off-pump CABG (OPCAB) surgery, there is, in general, a greater requirement for increased monitoring and circulatory support, particularly during cardiac manipulation and periods of isolated coronary occlusion. This includes a more dynamic administration of inotropic and chronotropic agents, intravascular volume loading, and the administration of antiarrhythmic medications. This has enabled myocardial revascularization to be performed safely without CPB and is responsible, in part, for the wider application of OPCAB surgery.

The Operation

Preparation for CABG surgery includes the administration of preoperative antibiotics (e.g., cefuroxime 1.5 g intravenously or vancomycin 1 g intravenously for a patient with penicillin allergy) at least 30 minutes prior to making the skin incision. After the appropriate hemodynamic monitoring lines have been placed and a Foley catheter inserted, the patient is positioned in a frog-leg position and padded appropriately to minimize pressure points. The patient is prepared and draped, and a median sternotomy incision is performed (Fig. 59-11). Typically, the left half of the sternum is retracted and elevated to expose the ITA. Once identified and pulsatility verified, the endothoracic fascia is opened medial to the artery. Minimal traction and a no-touch technique are employed to protect the vessel. The use of a headlight and magnification provided by surgical loupes allows precise dissection. A radiofrequency device or electrocautery can be used to mobilize the pedicle and identify the arterial and venous branches. The advantage of a radiofrequency device is the lack of transmitted thermal energy with its associated risk of heat-induced vascular injury. Side branches are clipped on the arterial side, and the other side is clipped or cauterized. The pedicle is mobilized from the subclavian artery and vein beneath the manubrium to the bifurcation of the superior epigastric and musculophrenic branches distally at the level of the diaphragm. Following anticoagulation with heparin, the ITA is divided at the distal bifurcation and flow is measured. A free flow rate greater than 60 mL/min is desirable. The vessel is then gently occluded distally with a clamp, and the pedicle is inoculated with a stream of papaverine solution to promote arterial dilation and prevent vascular spasm. The distal end of the vessel is prepared for grafting at this time or deferred to just prior to performing the anastomosis. If the diameter of the ITA appears adequate but the vessel lacks adequate inflow or pulsatility, the pedicle can be used as a free graft. In this case, the pedicle is divided at the level of the subclavian artery and stored in a papaverine solution until needed. Another surgical

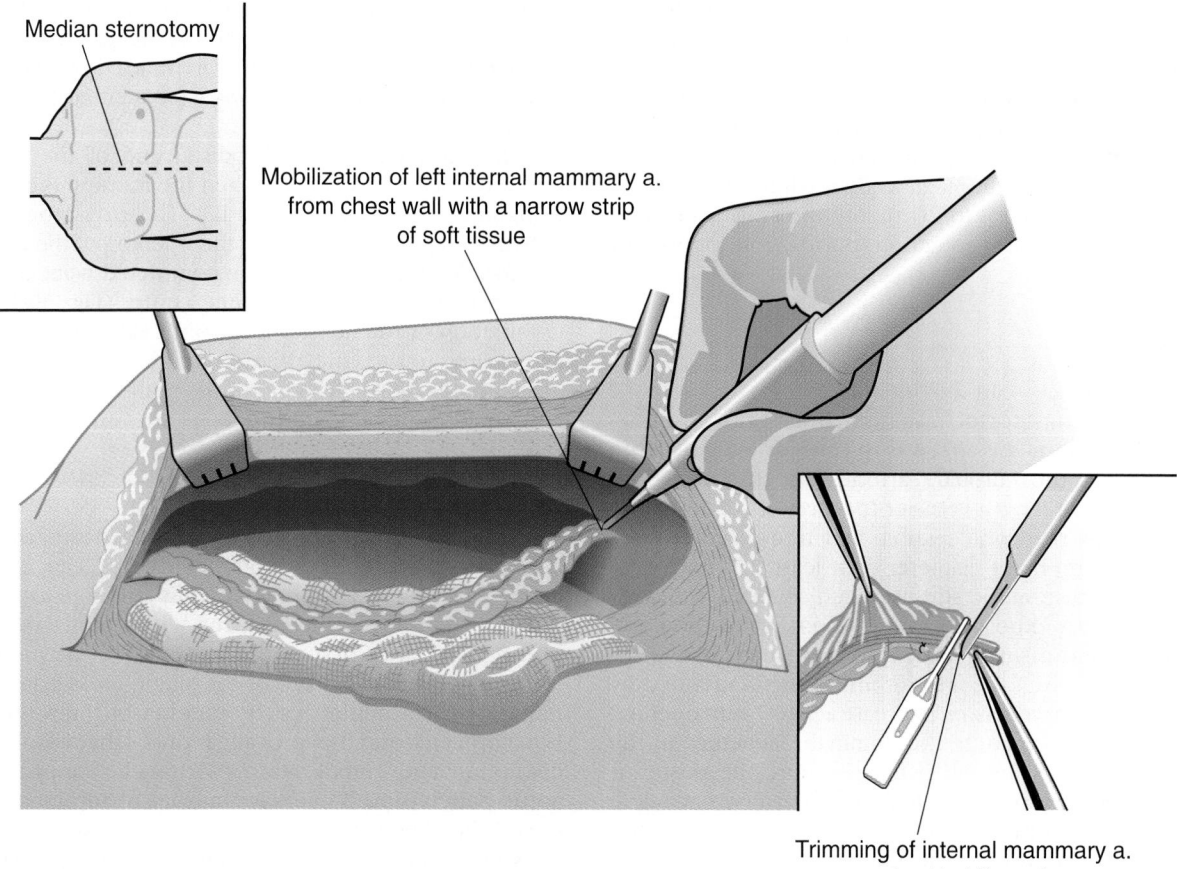

Median sternotomy

Mobilization of left internal mammary a. from chest wall with a narrow strip of soft tissue

Trimming of internal mammary a. proximal to bifurcation

■ FIGURE 59-11. Coronary artery bypass procedures are performed through a median sternotomy *(left inset)*. The divided sternum is lifted by controlled retraction that provides exposure but must not be so excessive as to fracture the sternum or ribs. The section proceeds proximally and distally until adequate length is obtained for the intended graft and usually terminates at the bifurcation of the internal mammary artery *(right inset)*. Heparin is then administered systemically before the internal mammary artery is occluded. The internal mammary artery is prepared for grafting after transection. (From Jones RH: Coronary artery bypass grafts. *In* Sabiston DC Jr [ed]: Atlas of Cardiothoracic Surgery. Philadelphia, WB Saunders, 1995.)

team can procure the greater saphenous vein or radial artery simultaneously.

Next, the patient is systemically heparinized (300 units/ kg) with a target activated clotting time (ACT) greater than 400 seconds. The aorta is examined to detect areas of calcification and determine the site of cannulation and cross-clamping. Epiaortic echocardiography can be used to identify calcific plaques and help plan the site of cannulation to minimize disruption of atherosclerotic plaques and reduce the risk of embolization and stroke. The ascending aorta is then cannulated proximal to the innominate artery using double-pursestring sutures placed anterolaterally. When the cannula is introduced into the aorta, it is important that the tip is directed distally. The aortic cannula is then secured in place by tightening the pursestring sutures with Rumel tourniquets; these are then secured to the side of the cannula. The open end of the cannula is back-flushed to de-air and remove any atherosclerotic debris in the cannula. It is then attached to the arterial perfusion line from the CPB machine. The proximal end of the aortic cannula is then secured to the wound edges. Venous cannulation is performed by introducing a cannula into the right atrium through a single pursestring suture in the right atrial appendage. If a dual-stage venous drainage cannula is used, the tip is directed into the inferior vena cava. The venous pursestring sutures are tightened using a Rumel tourniquet and then secured to the venous cannula. The open end is then interfaced with the venous tubing from the bypass pump. If retrograde cardioplegia is to be administered, a pursestring suture is placed near the AV groove, the atrium is incised, and a retrograde cardioplegia cannula is introduced into the coronary sinus.

After heparinization, the patient is placed on CPB and cooled to a core temperature of 30°C to 32°C. During cooling, a cardioplegic cannula can be inserted into the aorta through a separate pursestring suture. It is sufficiently distanced from the aortic cannula to allow room for the aorta to be cross-clamped. In addition to infusing cardioplegic solutions, the cannula can be used to decompress the left ventricle. Once acceptable pump flows (2.2 L/min/m²) have been achieved, and the mean blood pressure has been stabilized (50 to 70 mm Hg), the aorta is cross-clamped and cold cardioplegic solution is infused.

The heart is also cooled topically using a saline slush solution. The phrenic nerve can be protected by covering it with an insulating pad. If both antegrade and retrograde cardioplegia are to be used, two thirds of the solution is administered antegrade, with the remainder given via the retrograde cannula. Antegrade and/or retrograde cold oxygenated blood cardioplegia is then administered intermittently, usually at 15- to 20-minute intervals, to ensure adequate myocardial protection during the period of ischemic arrest.

Distal Anastomoses

The target vessels can be identified and the sites of the distal anastomoses determined either prior to cross-clamping the aorta or afterward. The advantage of the former is that the coronary arteries are distended and appropriate graft length is easier to assess. The ideal anastomotic site is readily accessible and free of atherosclerotic disease and has a diameter of at least 1.5 mm.

After the anastomotic site has been selected, a Beaver blade is used to expose the anterior aspect of the coronary artery, and a small, sharp, pointed lance is used to puncture the vessel; the arteriotomy is then extended by using fine coronary scissors to create a 3- to 7-mm opening that is scaled to match the luminal diameter of the conduit. Care must be taken not to injure the posterior wall. An endarterectomy of the coronary artery is avoided, if possible, because this is associated with a higher graft/native artery thrombosis rate.

When a reversed saphenous vein segment graft is used, the anastomosis is performed with either interrupted sutures or a continuous running 7-0 or 8-0 polypropylene suture. With the latter, care is taken to avoid pursestringing the suture line and narrowing the anastomotic site. A 1.0- or 1.5-mm vessel probe is often used to evaluate the patency of the anastomosis. The graft is then pressurized with heparinized blood or cardioplegic solution to evaluate the anastomosis for hemostasis or evidence of stricture. If multiple vessels are to be grafted, a single conduit (e.g., saphenous vein) can be used by performing multiple side-to-side anastomoses (sequential grafting) to conserve graft length.

When using the ITA, the distal end of the vessel is beveled at a sharp angle and then the incision is extended using fine iris scissors (Fig. 59-12). The arteriotomy of the native vessel is sized to match the opening of the ITA. The end-to-side anastomosis can be completed using a continuous running 8-0 polypropylene suture (Fig. 59-13). On completion of the anastomosis, both sides of the pedicle are sutured to the epicardium to minimize tension on the anastomosis and/or twisting of the graft when the patient is weaned from CPB and the lungs are ventilated.

Proximal Anastomoses

If the proximal anastomoses are completed after the distal anastomoses have been completed, this can be done either while the aortic cross-clamp is still in place or after it has been removed and replaced with a partial occlusion clamp. The latter allows the heart to be perfused and rewarmed. The advantage of the single cross-clamp technique is that it minimizes the number of times the aorta is manipulated and theoretically reduces the risk of plaque disruption and embolization. With either approach, an aortic punch is used to excise buttons of aortic tissue and create the sites for the proximal graft anastomoses. The proximal opening of the conduits are then spatulated to create a hood, and each anastomosis is completed using a running 6-0 or 7-0 polypropylene suture. The same technique can be used if the proximal aortic anastomoses are performed prior to placing the patient on CPB using a partial aortic occlusion clamp. After completing the anastomoses, small bulldog clamps are placed on each graft and the patient is placed in a head-down position. Pump flow is transiently reduced as the aortic cross-clamp is

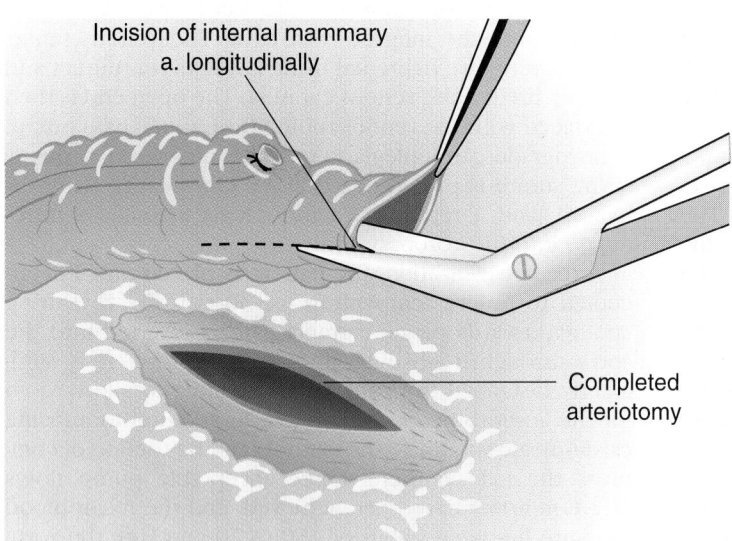

Incision of internal mammary
a. longitudinally

Completed
arteriotomy

FIGURE 59-12. The technique of anastomosis between the left internal mammary artery and the left anterior descending coronary artery illustrates the general principles used to construct all proximal and distal anastomoses. The graft is opened longitudinally to match or exceed the length of the coronary arteriotomy. This opening prevents kinking at the site of the anastomosis of the internal mammary artery and aorta to the saphenous vein. This opening is not necessary at the distal vein anastomotic site, but a slight bevel cut of the distal vein helps prevent kinking of the saphenous vein to the coronary artery anastomosis. (From Jones RH: Coronary artery bypass grafts. *In* Sabiston DC Jr [ed]: Atlas of Cardiothoracic Surgery. Philadelphia, WB Saunders, 1995.)

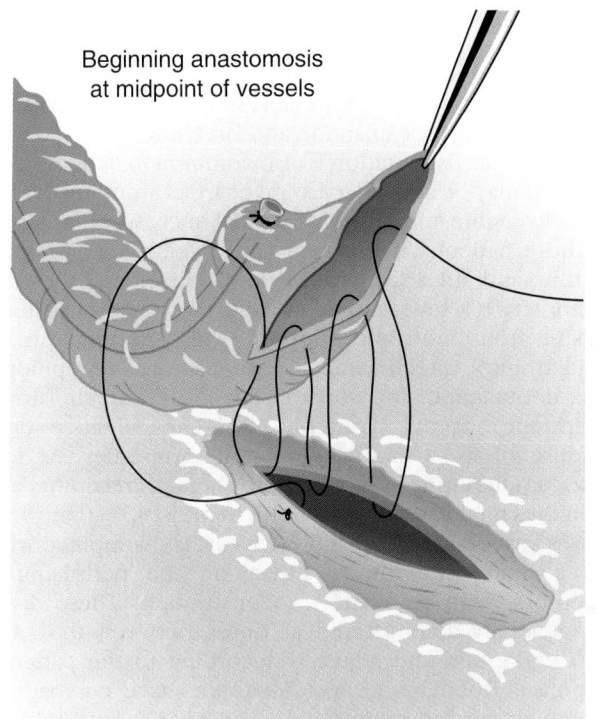

Beginning anastomosis
at midpoint of vessels

■ FIGURE 59-13. The anastomosis begins midway along the side of the graft so that the final knot will not be at the most distal or proximal portion of the anastomosis, thereby decreasing the chances of technical error that would impede graft flow. The polypropylene suture permits a portion of the anastomosis to be completed before the two vessels are joined. (From Jones RH: Coronary artery bypass grafts. *In* Sabiston DC Jr [ed]: Atlas of Cardiothoracic Surgery. Philadelphia, WB Saunders, 1995.)

removed and the heart is reperfused. After the grafts have filled with blood, small punctures are made in the veins using a 25-gauge needle for de-airing. The bulldog clamps are then removed, and the heart is perfused via both the grafts and the native vessels. All anastomotic sites are re-examined and bleeding sites are oversewn.

Termination of Cardiopulmonary Artery Bypass

Systemic rewarming is usually initiated after completion of the last distal anastomosis. Blood that has accumulated in the pleural spaces is evacuated and reprocessed using a Cell Saver for later reinfusion. After removing the aortic cross-clamp, the heart usually starts to beat spontaneously within a short time. Although a normal sinus rhythm may develop, it frequently deteriorates into ventricular fibrillation and requires cardioversion using internal defibrillating paddles. If the heart rate is less than 70 beats/min, temporary atrial and ventricular pacing wires can be attached to the surface of the heart, usually the right atrium or right ventricle, and pacing is commenced at approximately 90 beats/min. Once the patient has been adequately rewarmed (~36.5°C), normal sinus rhythm has been restored, and ventilation has been re-established,

then the patient is weaned from CPB by gradually reducing the pump flow rates to zero while maintaining adequate intravascular volume via transfusion. It is often necessary to manipulate the contractile state of the heart and the peripheral vascular resistance (afterload) by infusing inotropic agents such as dobutamine and vasodilators or vasoconstrictors such as nitroglycerin and ephedrine, respectively. Once the patient has been stabilized off CPB, protamine is administered to reverse the heparin-induced anticoagulation. The aortic and venous cannulae are removed and pursestring sutures tied. Pleural and mediastinal chest tubes are inserted (along with temporary epicardial atrial and ventricular pacing wires if not placed earlier) and after hemostasis has been achieved, the sternum is closed using large-caliber stainless steel wire in simple and/or figure-of-eight patterns. The presternal fascia and area around the xiphoid is then approximated with Vicryl sutures and the remaining tissue closed in layers. The skin can be approximated with a running subcuticular monofilament suture and Steri-Strips or staples. Dry sterile dressings are placed over all incisions, lines, wires, and drains and the patient is transferred to the surgical ICU.

Postoperative Care

Postoperative care begins with the transport of the patient to the cardiac surgery ICU.[20] A directed physical examination should be performed on arrival. This includes the assessment of level of consciousness, respiratory sounds, peripheral pulses, and body temperature. Mediastinal chest tube drainage should be recorded and assessed hourly. Initial ventilator settings should be set to match those in the operating room. Alternatively, the ventilator can be set at a tidal volume of 12 mL/kg, an intermittent mandatory ventilation rate of 8 to 10 breaths/min, a fraction of inspired oxygen of 60% and a 5 cm H_2O positive end-expiratory pressure to provide an adequate margin of safety. A portable chest radiograph is obtained to confirm the position of the endotracheal tube and identify a pneumothorax, atelectasis, pulmonary edema, or pleural effusions. Initial laboratory studies should include hemoglobin, hematocrit, electrolytes, blood urea nitrogen, creatinine, platelet count, prothrombin time, partial thromboplastin time, and arterial blood gases. With respect to continuous monitoring devices, the patient should have an ECG with the ability to assess ST-T wave abnormalities, an arterial line to measure arterial blood pressure, a line to measure central venous pressure, pulse oximetry, capnography, and a core temperature. In select patients, pulmonary artery pressures and cardiac output are monitored continuously using a Swan-Ganz catheter.

The primary considerations during the first 12 hours after the operation should be the maintenance of adequate blood pressure, cardiac output, correction of coagulation defects, correction of ionized hypocalcemia, stabilization of intravascular volume, and normalization of the peripheral vascular resistance. This often involves the administration of crystalloid solutions, blood or blood products, inotropic agents, calcium, and vasodilators and/or vasoconstrictors.

In the immediate postoperative period it is desirable to avoid marked elevations in blood pressure (mean arterial pressure > 100 mm Hg). Significant hypertension results in increased myocardial oxygen consumption and tension on arterial suture lines. In patients with significant preexisting left ventricular dysfunction, this can also lead to a reduction in the cardiac index. The hypertension may be due to hypoxemia, hypercarbia, hypothermia with shivering, and inadequate sedation and analgesia. It can be treated by clearing the endotracheal tube of secretions, adjusting ventilator settings, warming the patient with forced hot-air blankets, administering analgesics, and infusing vasodilators. Since low cardiac output occurs frequently after CPB, a Swan-Ganz catheter can be used to assess the adequacy of systemic perfusion by measuring the cardiac index and monitoring mixed venous oxygenation. In general, the aim is to maintain a cardiac index of 2.2 L/min/m^2 and a mixed venous oxygenation of 60%. The most common causes of low cardiac output are myocardial ischemia, hypovolemia, abnormal heart rate/rhythm, myocardial dysfunction, and cardiac tamponade. Myocardial ischemia can range from asymptomatic ST-segment changes to infarction with profound hypotension. The former may be due to coronary artery spasm, ITA hypoperfusion, or early graft occlusion. Coronary artery spasm occurs in about 1% of patients, and it can be treated with intravenous nitroglycerin or calcium-channel blockade. In the meantime, α-adrenergic agents may be required to support the blood pressure. If the ischemia is severe and the patient does not respond to pharmacologic support, the patient may require emergent coronary angiography or reoperation and/or regrafting. With hypovolemia, there is a variety of opinion as to which resuscitation fluid should be used postoperatively. Generally, lactated Ringer's solution is appropriate but can be supplemented with up to 1.5 L of hydroxy-ethyl starch (Hetastarch) or blood products. The latter depends on whether the patient is anemic or there is evidence of active bleeding.

In the immediate postoperative period, most patients are tachycardic. If they have been treated prior to surgery with β blockers, they may be bradycardic (<60 beats/min). In general, the desirable rhythm and heart rate is sinus and a rate between 70 and 100 beats/min. A normal sinus rhythm ensures AV synchrony and maintenance of the atrial kick, which can contribute up to 25% of the cardiac output. If the patient is bradycardic or has evidence of heart block, atrial or AV pacing via temporary pacing wires should be initiated to increase the rate and/or restore synchrony. Arrhythmias are common and may result from abnormal electrolytes, acidosis, high circulating catecholamine levels, and myocardial ischemia. Supraventricular tachyarrhythmias associated with hemodynamic instability should be treated immediately with cardioversion. Hemodynamically stable patients with re-entrant supraventricular tachyarrhythmias should be treated with adenosine in incremental doses. Atrial flutter can be treated using overdrive pacing if the rapid atrial rate can be captured and controlled. Atrial fibrillation responds to intravenous digoxin, procainamide, diltiazem, β blockers, amiodarone,

and cardioversion. The hemodynamically unstable patient with ventricular arrhythmias needs immediate defibrillation and an intravenous bolus infusion of lidocaine followed by a continuous infusion. Other alternative agents include procainamide and bretylium.

Myocardial dysfunction is also common in patients after CPB and may be secondary to myocardial stunning (a transient reversible injury) or myocardial necrosis (infarction). In these patients, if the heart rate, ventricular preload, rhythm, and afterload have been optimized and they still demonstrate a low cardiac output, they will most likely benefit from inotropic support. This support can be divided into catecholamine (epinephrine, norepinephrine, dobutamine, and dopamine) and noncatecholamine (milrinone) agents. Epinephrine is an effective drug because of its α- and β-adrenergic properties. At low doses, epinephrine stimulates peripheral β$_2$ receptors and promotes mild vasodilation. At higher doses, α stimulation causes vasoconstriction and tachycardia. Norepinephrine has a more pronounced effect on the peripheral α receptors, with resultant vasoconstriction. These drugs are generally administered at doses between 0.01 and 0.10 µg/kg/min and adjusted according to the patient's response. Dobutamine and dopamine have comparable effects on cardiac output and are similar to epinephrine and norepinephrine but, in general, are less arrhythmogenic. Dobutamine is also a vasodilator and is used to reduce both left ventricular preload and afterload. Milrinone is a phosphodiesterase inhibitor and slows the degradation of cyclic adenosine monophosphate (cAMP). Its mechanism of action complements that of catecholamines, which stimulate cAMP. This drug is often used in combination with other inotropic agents to achieve a synergistic outcome.

Intra-aortic Balloon Pump. For patients who demonstrate profound myocardial dysfunction, and are unresponsive to volume resuscitation, intense pharmacologic therapy treatment with an IABP may be indicated. Intra-aortic balloon pumping improves mean blood pressures and coronary artery perfusion and decreases cardiac work/oxygen demand. If the IABP was used to control chest pain preoperatively, it is often removed within 24 hours after the operation. However, if used preoperatively for hemodynamic instability, weaning from the IABP may be more difficult and require more time.

Tamponade. In the postoperative period, pericardial tamponade is due to formation of pericardial clot and compression of the heart. The condition should be suspected if the patient exhibits evidence of low cardiac output and hypotension, fails to respond to intravenous fluid infusions, and requires increasing levels of inotropic support. Often there has been a marked decline in mediastinal chest tube drainage prior to the onset of signs of tamponade. The diagnosis can be made on the basis of widening of the mediastinum on chest radiograph and evidence of a pericardial effusion by echocardiography. Surface echocardiography is helpful but may be compromised due to the presence of wound dressings and chest tubes. TEE is more reliable but may not be immediately available. If a Swan-Ganz catheter is in place and right and left heart pressures are monitored, the central venous pressure and pulmonary capillary wedge pressure are usually elevated and equal. Once the diagnosis is made, the patient should be returned to the operating room for evacuation of the clot and relief of the compression. If the patient's condition is rapidly deteriorating, a simple subxiphoid approach can be performed at the bedside and result in a dramatic improvement in hemodynamics.[21]

Postoperative Bleeding. The combination of heparinization, hypothermia, CPB, and protamine reversal is associated with increased risk of bleeding after CABG surgery. Bleeding after CABG surgery requiring transfusion and/or reoperation to stop the bleeding is associated with a significant increase in morbidity and mortality. Bleeding, more than 500 mL in the first hour or persistent bleeding more than 200 mL an hour for 4 hours, are indications for mediastinal exploration. Exploration is also indicated if a large hemothorax is identified on chest radiograph or pericardial tamponade occurs. In 20% of the cases, a specific site of bleeding can be identified. The typical sources of surgical bleeding include the cannulation sites, the proximal/distal anastomoses, and branches of the ITAs and the vein grafts. Most of the time, however, a specific bleeding site is not identified, and it is related to inadequate heparin neutralization; qualitative or quantitative platelet dysfunction; fibrinolysis; and deficiencies in factors V, VIII, XIII, and fibrinogen and plasminogen. In the setting of suspected nonsurgical postoperative bleeding, one approach is to obtain an ACT and administer protamine to return the ACT to baseline.[22] In general, red blood cells are administered if the patient is actively bleeding and/or anemic (hematocrit $\leq$25%). Platelets are administered if there is evidence of thrombocytopenia (<50,000/mm^3) or platelet dysfunction (abnormal thromboelastography). Cryoprecipitate can be used to treat low fibrinogen levels (<100 mg/dL). Desmopressin,[23] epsilon aminocaproic acid,[24] and aprotonin[25] can also be used, although these are generally restricted to high-risk patients.

Extubation. It is desirable to initiate the process of ventilator weaning as soon as the patient awakens, is hemodynamically stable with minimal chest tube drainage, and can maintain a satisfactory spontaneous tidal volume and respiratory rate. In general, the cardiac index should be 2.2 L/min/m^2 or higher and the mean arterial pressure should exceed 70 mm Hg. The patient should be comfortable on continuous positive airway pressure support with minimal secretions and have a spontaneous respiratory rate of 20 or more breaths/min. The ability to maintain an arterial pH greater than 7.35 while the intermediate mandatory ventilation rate is reduced to zero is a reliable test. After extubation the patient needs to be encouraged to breathe deeply and use incentive spirometry. Suboptimal postoperative pulmonary function may require additional therapy, including the use of bronchodilators, mucolytics, and chest physical therapy. After extubation it is important to provide the patient with sufficient pain relief to minimize emotional distress, poor coughing, and the reluctance to begin ambulation. Unrelieved pain can also be a source of tachycardia, hypertension, and myocardial ischemia. Prior to leaving the ICU, unnecessary lines and catheters should be removed.

Removal of temporary atrial and ventricular pacing wires is often deferred to the third postoperative day.[26-28]

INDICATIONS FOR CABG SURGERY AND OUTCOMES AFTER REVASCULARIZATION

The aim of medical treatment for patients with symptomatic CAD is to reduce the heart's demand for oxygen by slowing the heart rate, decreasing myocardial contractility, and reducing systemic vascular resistance. The objective of interventional therapy is to increase the supply of oxygen and nutrients by dilating or bypassing the coronary artery obstructions. Although medical therapy can be effective, in many cases the optimal treatment is angioplasty with or without stents and/or CABG surgery. Since interventional therapy is not without risk, it is important to understand the relative survival benefits and risks associated with them. The survival benefit of CABG surgery patients was initially studied in patients with chronic stable angina.

Chronic Stable Angina

CABG Surgery Versus Medical Management

In the 1970s and 1980s several prospective, randomized clinical trials evaluated the survival benefit of CABG surgery in patients with chronic stable angina (Table 59-4). These studies showed significant benefit and resulted in the widespread application of CABG surgery for the treatment of patients with CAD. They also helped to identify specific categories of patients with angina who were most likely to benefit from CABG surgery, namely patients with LMCA disease; one-, two-, or three-vessel disease with proximal LAD involvement; and three-vessel disease with impaired left ventricular function.[29,30] These observations were confirmed in a meta-analysis of these studies (see Table 59-4) (Fig. 59-14). These trials were conducted in an era in which fewer than 50% of the patients were treated with β blockers, fewer than 40% were administered aspirin (ASA), and fewer than 10% of the patients received an ITA graft. Also, calcium-channel blockers, angiotensin-converting enzyme inhibitors, and lipid-lowering agents were not available. Women were excluded in all but one of the trials, and only patients younger than 65 years of age were studied. Nevertheless, as a direct result of these clinical studies, CABG surgery is now accepted as an appropriate therapeutic modality for the treatment of specific subsets of patients with chronic stable angina (Table 59-5).

PTCA Versus Medical Management

In the 1980s PTCA was introduced as an alternative to CABG surgery. The first successful PTCA was performed by Gruntzig and colleagues.[31] Initially the procedure was performed in patients with one-vessel disease and isolated lesions. With improvements in catheter technology, increasing experience, and the advent of stent-based

TABLE 59-4. Foundation Studies of Patients with Stable Ischemic Heart Disease Used to Evaluate CABG Surgery Outcomes*

Study	Reference Source	Conclusions
Veterans Administration Coronary Artery Bypass Surgery Cooperative Study Group: Eleven-year survival in the Veterans Administration randomized trial of coronary bypass surgery for stable angina.	N Engl J Med 311:1333-1339, 1984	Survival advantage was associated with CABG surgery when CAD included LM and/or 3VD with impaired LV function.
Varnauskas E, European Coronary Surgery Study Group: Twelve-year follow-up of survival in the randomized European Coronary Surgery Study.	N Engl J Med 319:332-337, 1988	CABG surgery was associated with increased survival in patients with LM disease, 3VD, decreased LV function, and proximal LAD stenosis 12 years from randomization. Peak advantage was observed at 5 years.
Coronary Artery Surgery Study (CASS) principal investigators and associates: CASS: A randomized trial of coronary bypass surgery.	Circulation 68:939-950, 1983	CABG surgery and nonoperative management was associated with similar survival rates. Surgery could be safely deferred until onset of symptoms.
Norris RM, Agnew TM, Brandt PWT, et al: Coronary surgery after recurrent myocardial infarction: Progress of a trial comparing surgical with nonsurgical management for asymptomatic patients with advanced coronary disease.	Circulation 63:785-792, 1981	CABG surgery conferred survival advantage in patients with LM disease and/or 3VD with decreased LV function.
Mathur VS, Guinn GA: Prospective randomized study of the surgical therapy of stable angina.	Cardiovasc Clin 8:131-144, 1977	CABG surgery was associated with superior improvement in symptoms and quality of life.
Kloster FE, Kremkau EL, Ritzman LW, et al: Coronary bypass for stable angina.	N Engl J Med 300:149-157, 1979	CABG surgery resulted in greater functional improvement and less UA compared to medical therapy, no difference in death or myocardial infarction after 3 years.

*Used by Yusuf and associates[30] in meta-analysis.

LM, left main; 3VD, three-vessel disease; CAD, coronary artery disease; LAD, left anterior descending artery; CABG, coronary artery bypass grafting; UA, unstable angina; LV, left ventricular.

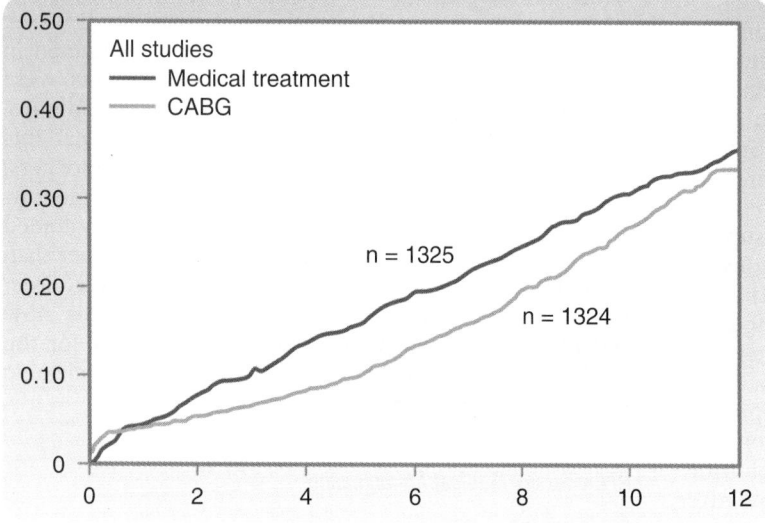

FIGURE 59-14. Cumulative total mortality for 12 years after coronary artery bypass grafting (CABG) surgery versus noninterventional management for patients with chronic stable angina. (Adapted from Yusuf S, Zucker D, Peduzzi P, et al: Effect of coronary artery bypass graft surgery on survival: Overview of 10-year results from randomised trials by the Coronary Artery Bypass Graft Surgery Trialists Collaboration. Lancet 344:563-570, 1994.)

TABLE 59-5. Indications for CABG Surgery Alone in Patients with Stable Angina, Unstable Angina, and Acute Myocardial Infarction

Condition	Class*			
	I	**IIa**	**IIb**	**III**
Asymptomatic or mild angina	1. LMCA stenosis ≥ 60% 2. LMCA equivalent: proximal LAD and LCA stenoses > 70% 3. 3VD (survival benefit > with abnormal LV function: EF < 0.50)	Proximal LAD stenosis with 1VD or 2VD†	1VD or 2VD not involving the proximal LAD‡	None
Chronic stable angina	1. LMCA stenosis ≥ 60% 2. LMCA equivalent: proximal LAD and LCA stenoses > 70% 3. 3VD (survival benefit > with abnormal LV function: EF < 0.50) 4. 2VD with significant proximal LAD stenosis: either EF < 0.50 or ischemia on noninvasive testing 5. 1VD or 2VD without significant proximal LAD stenosis, but with a large area of viable myocardium and high-risk criteria on noninvasive testing 6. Disabling angina despite maximal medical therapy (acceptable-risk patient)	1. Proximal LAD stenosis with 1VD† 2. 1VD or 2VD without significant proximal LAD stenosis, moderate area of viable myocardium, and demonstrable ischemia on noninvasive testing	None	1. 1VD or 2VD without significant proximal LAD stenosis, in patients who have mild symptoms that are unlikely due to myocardial ischemia or have not received an adequate trial of medical therapy and (1) have only a small area of viable myocardium or (2) no demonstrable ischemia on noninvasive testing 2. Borderline stenoses (50–60%) other than in the LCMA, no demonstrable ischemia on noninvasive testing 3. <50% coronary stenosis
UA/NSTEMI	1. LMCA stenosis ≥ 60% 2. LMCA equivalent: proximal LAD and LCA stenoses > 70% 3. Ongoing ischemia unresponsive to maximal nonsurgical therapy	Proximal LAD stenosis with 1VD or 2VD†	1VD or 2VD not involving the proximal LAD‡	None
STEMI/AMI	None	Ongoing ischemia/infarction unresponsive to maximal nonsurgical therapy	1. Progressive LV pump failure with coronary stenosis compromising viable myocardium outside the initial infarct area 2. Primary reperfusion in the early hours (≤6–12 hr) of an evolving STEMI	Primary reperfusion late (>12 hr) in evolving STEMI without ongoing ischemia

*Class I: Conditions for which there is evidence and/or general agreement that a given procedure/treatment is useful and effective.
Class IIa: Weight of evidence/opinion is in favor of usefulness/efficacy.
Class IIb: Usefulness/efficacy is less well established by evidence/opinion.
Class III: Conditions for which there is evidence and/or general agreement that the procedure/treatment is not useful/effective and in some cases may be harmful.
†Becomes class I if extensive ischemia documented by noninvasive study and/or an LVEF < 0.50.
‡If there is a large area of viable myocardium and high-risk criteria on noninvasive testing, becomes class I.
§Becomes class I if arrhythmia is resuscitated sudden cardiac death or sustained ventricular tachycardia.
1VD, one-vessel disease; 2VD, two-vessel disease; 3VD, three-vessel disease; LMCA, left main coronary artery; LAD, left anterior descending coronary artery; LCA, left coronary artery; LV, left ventricular; EF, ejection fraction; STEMI/AMI, ST-elevation myocardial infarction/acute myocardial infarction; UA/NSTEMI, unstable angina/non–ST-elevation myocardial infarction.
Adapted from Eagle KA, Guyton RA, Davidoff R, et al: ACC/AHA guidelines for coronary artery bypass graft surgery: Executive summary and recommendations. Circulation 100:1464-1480, 1999.

interventions, angioplasty is now performed in patients with multivessel disease. Although the short-term symptomatic success rate for PTCA approaches 85% to 90%, the role of PTCA in the management of patients with angina whose symptoms are adequately controlled with medical therapy remains controversial.[32,33] In the Angioplasty Compared to Medicine (ACME) trial,[32] the efficacy of PTCA was compared to best medical management in 212 patients with proven ischemia, one-vessel disease, and stenoses greater than 70%.[34] In this study, patients undergoing PTCA demonstrated better relief from angina, reduced need for antianginal medications, a better quality of life, and improved exercise tolerance; there was no difference in mortality. Some PTCA patients (19%), however, required additional catheter-based interventions, and 7% underwent CABG surgery. In the medically managed group of patients, 11% progressed to PTCA, and none underwent CABG surgery. At 4 years, the patients who were initially randomized to PTCA had a better quality of life and significantly fewer episodes of UA. Thus, in this trial the increased number of reinterventions in the first year and higher costs for the PTCA-treated group appeared to be justified owing to the lower incidence of late procedures and lower costs in the extended follow-up period. In the Coronary Angioplasty Versus Medical Therapy for Angina: The Second Randomised Intervention Treatment of Angina (RITA-2) trial,[33] PTCA provided better early symptomatic relief from angina compared to medical treatment. This, however, was not sustained over time and at 2.9 years the PTCA group had a 3% greater risk of death or myocardial infarction (Table 59-6).

A major limitation of these studies was the absence of preprocedural cardiac stress and myocardial viability testing. Without this information, it is difficult to know whether the PTCA and medical therapy groups were equally matched. It is also difficult to extrapolate the findings to current practice since the studies were performed prior to the use of coronary stents. Nevertheless, it appears that patients with angina may be treated relatively safely with either medical management or PTCA intervention. The risk of early complications associated with PTCA, however, needs to be taken into consideration prior to proceeding with the interventional approach in this group of patients.

CABG Surgery Versus PTCA

One of the first large-scale, prospective, randomized studies comparing PTCA and CABG surgery was the Bypass Angioplasty Revascularization Investigation (BARI) trial reported in 1996.[35] Patients with multivessel disease were randomly assigned to either CABG surgery ($n = 914$) or PTCA ($n = 915$) and followed for a mean of 5.4 years. In the short term, the incidence of Q-wave myocardial infarction was higher in the CABG surgery group (4.6% vs. 2.1%); the stroke rates were similar (0.8% vs. 0.2%). At the end of 5 years, the survival rate was 89.3% for the CABG surgery cohort and 86.3% for the PTCA cohort ($P = 0.19$). Among the PTCA patients, however, 54% required additional revascularization procedures. Thirty-one percent underwent CABG surgery, 34% underwent additional

PTCA, and 11% underwent both interventions. In contrast, only 8% of the CABG surgery patients required repeat revascularization. Thus it appears that although PTCA did not compromise the 5-year survival rate in patients with multivessel disease, subsequent revascularization including CABG surgery was required more often. Among the diabetic patients, the 5-year survival rate for the CABG surgery patients was markedly greater (80.6% vs. 65.5%) (see Table 59-6). In the Emory Angioplasty versus Surgery Trial (EAST), the primary endpoints were death, myocardial infarction, or the presence of a large myocardial ischemic defect at 3 years. Secondary endpoints included all-cause mortality and the requirement for repeat revascularization procedures after extended follow-up. After the 3-year anniversary visit, patients were contacted and medical records examined until death or the 8-year anniversary. The results showed that after 3 years the number of repeat interventions was similar. At 8 years, the survival rate for both groups was also similar: angioplasty, 79.3%, and CABG surgery, 82.7%. There was a tendency for patients with proximal LAD stenosis and those with diabetes to have better late survival with CABG surgery (see Table 59-6). Owing to the relatively small number of patients enrolled, however, the study was underpowered to detect significant survival differences.

A strength of the BARI trial was that the myocardial infarction classification methodology was based on symptoms, ECG results obtained at predetermined time intervals, and a core laboratory was used to measure myocardial enzyme levels. The entry criteria, however, resulted in the selection of patients preferentially suited for PTCA. Thus the, findings may not be fully applicable to patients with complex multivessel disease. Also, in both the BARI and EAST studies, few CABG surgery patients underwent extensive arterial grafting, and they were performed when stents and new pharmacologic agents, such as clopidogrel and other glycoprotein (GP) IIb/IIIa inhibitors, were not available. Despite these limitations, it appears that CABG surgery clearly confers a survival benefit to diabetic patients that is superior to angioplasty. With respect to quality of life and economic issues, although the data collected in 934 of the 1829 patients enrolled in the BARI trial showed that PTCA patients returned to work sooner, CABG surgery patients had better functional status scores (Duke Activity Status Index). Also, although the cost of angioplasty was 95% that of CABG surgery ($P = 0.047$), the actual difference between the two interventions was less than $3000, and this was observed only in patients with two-vessel disease. PTCA appeared to be more expensive in patients with three-vessel disease.

In summary, patients with stable angina can safely undergo PTCA as a first intervention for CAD. CABG surgery confers a superior long-term survival benefit in patients with specific anatomic lesions and is associated with an increased freedom from angina, a significant reduction in antianginal medications, and fewer subsequent PCIs. CABG surgery is the treatment of choice in diabetic patients. Although controversial, the economic impact appears to be comparable when the frequency of repeat PCI is taken into consideration.

TABLE 59-6. Pertinent Studies Comparing PTCA and CABG Surgery

Study, No. of Patients (N), and Follow-Up (F/U)	Reference	Purpose	Findings
Arterial Revascularization Therapies Study (ARTS) N = 205 F/U = 400 days	J Am Coll Cardiol 39:559-564, 2002	Evaluated effectiveness of revascularization on event-free survival	Complete revascularization more frequently accomplished by CABG surgery. Patients randomized to stenting with incomplete revascularization had greater need for subsequent bypass surgery
	N Engl J Med 344:1117-1124, 2001	Compared CABG surgery and stenting for multivessel disease	Coronary stenting was less expensive than bypass surgery ($3000/patient) and conferred same degree of protection against death, stroke, and myocardial infarction. Stenting was associated with greater need for repeat revascularization.
Bypass Angioplasty Revascularization Investigation (BARI) N = 1829 F/U = 5.4 years	N Engl J Med 335:217-225, 1996	Compared CABG surgery with angioplasty in patients with multivessel disease	Initial strategy of PTCA did not compromise 5-year survival of overall population but was associated with more frequent subsequent revascularizations. Five-year survival for treated diabetics was better after CABG surgery (PTCA 65.5%, CABG 80.6%).
	JAMA 277:715-721, 1997	Analyzed clinical and functional outcomes in patients with multivessel disease	Angina-free episodes were greater in CABG patients. Use of anti-ischemic medications was higher in PTCA group. Need for revascularization was greater in PTCA patients (52%) vs. CABG surgery (6%).
	Circulation 96:1761-1769, 1997	Assessed influence of diabetes in CABG and PTCA patients with multivessel disease	Patients with treated diabetes mellitus assigned to initial strategy of CABG had a marked improvement in survival (CABG 94.2%, PTCA 79.4%). Survival benefit of CABG surgery was confined to patients receiving at least one ITA graft.
	N Engl J Med 336:92-99, 1997	Analyzed cost and quality of life	CABG surgery was associated with better quality of life. PTCA had a lower 5-year cost than CABG surgery only in patients with 2VD.
	Circulation 98:1279-1285, 1998	Analyzed outcome for women	The 5-year unadjusted mortality rate for women and men undergoing CABG and PTCA was similar. Due to higher risk profiles, female gender was an independent predictor of improved 5-year survival after adjusting for risk factors.
F/U = 7.8 years	J Am Coll Cardiol 35:1122-1129, 2000	Assessed long-term outcomes in diabetic patients	Survival benefit of CABG surgery over PTCA was more pronounced at 7 years (CABG 76.4%, PTCA 55.7%).
Emory Angioplasty Versus Surgery Trial (EAST) N = 392 F/U = 8 years	J Am Coll Cardiol 35:1116-1121, 2000	Evaluated long-term outcome	Patients with proximal LAD stenosis and those with diabetes tended to have better late survival with CABG surgery (did not reach statistical significance).
Randomized Intervention Treatment of Angina (RITA)-1 N = 1011 F/U = 2.5 years	Lancet 341:573-580, 1993	Examined long-term effects of PTCA vs. CABG in patients with 1VD, 2VD, and 3VD	Prevalence of angina was three times higher in the PTCA group at 6 months and 1.5 times higher at 2 years. Antianginal drugs were more frequent in the PTCA group. CABG surgery was associated with a lower risk of angina and fewer additional diagnostic and therapeutic interventions.
F/U = 2 years	Lancet 344:927-930, 1994	Analyzed cost of intervention	Cost of PTCA was 80% of CABG surgery at 2 years.
F/U 6.5 year	Lancet 352:1419-1425, 1998	Analyzed clinical outcomes and cost	No difference in mortality. In the PTCA group, the prevalence of angina was higher and 26% underwent CABG. PTCA and CABG surgery costs were similar after 5 years.
RITA-2 Coronary Angioplasty Versus Medical Therapy for Angina N = 1018 F/U = 2.7 years	Lancet 350:461-468, 1997	Compared long-term effects of PTCA and conservative care	Early intervention with PTCA was associated with greater symptomatic improvement but also with small but real excess hazard due to procedure-related complications.

CABG, coronary artery bypass grafting; PTCA, percutaneous transluminal coronary angioplasty; LAD, left anterior descending coronary artery; ITA, internal thoracic artery; 1VD, one-vessel disease; 2VD, two-vessel disease; 3VD, three-vessel disease.

Whether this will remain the case with drug-eluting stents is unknown.

Acute Coronary Artery Syndromes

Patients with ACSs represent a cohort of patients who have signs and symptoms that require expedited evaluation and treatment. It characterizes a constellation of clinical conditions that reflect acute myocardial ischemia and includes the categories of UA, non–ST-elevation myocardial infarction (NSTEMI), and ST-elevation myocardial infarction (STEMI). UA with an enzyme leak is termed an NSTEMI. More than 1.5 million patients with UA or NSTEMI are admitted to the hospital annually, and 800,000 are admitted with STEMI. Of those suffering from an AMI, 213,000 will die; and half of these patients do so within an hour after onset of symptoms. Arrhythmias, usually ventricular fibrillation, are the cause of early death. The categories of AMI are NSTEMI, STEMI, non–Q-wave myocardial infarction (NQWMI) and Q-wave myocardial infarction (QWMI). Most patients with ST elevation go on to develop an acute QWMI. Depending on presentation and diagnosis, the interventional management and outcomes may differ greatly among patients with UA/NSTEMI and STEMI/AMI.

UA/NSTEMI

PCI Versus Medical Management

The Thrombolysis In Myocardial Ischemia (TIMI) IIIB trial[36] studied the effectiveness of thrombolytic therapy with tissue plasminogen activator (t-PA) and early PTCA in the treatment of patients with UA. The results showed that thrombolysis conferred no treatment benefit; in fact, there was some evidence that intravenous t-PA administration prior to PTCA increased the risk of periprocedural myocardial infarction. PTCA, however, did achieve a high rate of angiographic success and at 1-year follow-up, the cumulative mortality was only 2.0%. The recurrent ischemia rate, however, was frequent; rehospitalization was required in more than one third of the patients, and repeat revascularization was performed in 28%. Ten percent of the patients underwent CABG surgery within 12 months. Thus, it appears that although PTCA may be an acceptable therapeutic option in patients with UA, it is associated with the need for repeat revascularization procedures. Most patients in this study had one-vessel disease and left ventricular function was only mildly compromised.

Adjunctive Therapy to PCI

To minimize the complications of acute coronary occlusion and restenosis after PTCA (35% to 45% at 6 months), contemporary catheter-based revascularization now includes coronary stenting and the adjuvant use of platelet GP IIb/IIIa receptor inhibitors. The platelet GP IIb/IIIa receptor is a site for fibrinogen binding and promotes platelet aggregation. Binding of more than 80% of these receptors results in potent antithrombosis. The ready availability of these inhibitors (abciximab, tirofiban, eptifibatide) has led to several multicenter clinical trials to address their efficacy. In the Evaluation of Platelet IIb/IIIa Inhibitor for Stenting (EPISTENT) trial, patients who underwent PTCA for UA/NSTEMI were randomized to stent use and abciximab therapy versus placebo.[37] The stent patients also received ASA and the thienopyridine, ticlopidine. Adjunctive use of abciximab was associated with a reduction in death, myocardial infarction, and urgent revascularization at 30 days. It was also associated, however, with a higher incidence of severe bleeding. At 1 year, the mortality for the stented patients with abciximab was also less in the diabetic patients. In contrast, in a meta-analysis of six randomized, placebo-controlled trials of patients with UA/NSTEMI receiving GP IIb/IIIa antagonists, there was only a slight reduction in death or myocardial infarction in patients undergoing stenting. Major bleeding complications, however, remained a problem.

Thienopyridines, adenosine diphosphate (ADP) inhibitors, such as ticlopidine and clopidogrel, are also used to prevent the activation of platelets and thrombosis and have been studied in patients treated conservatively and with PCI. The Clopidogrel in Unstable Angina to Prevent Recurrent Ischemic Events (CURE) trial evaluated the effectiveness of clopidogrel in the noninterventional management of patients with UA.[38] Treatment was associated with a lower rate of death, myocardial infarction, and stroke but a higher rate of major bleeding. In the PCI-CURE trial, patients were randomized to clopidogrel and ASA, or placebo and ASA, preprocedurally and for 1 month after the procedure. PCI with adjuvant clopidogrel and ASA demonstrated a reduction in cardiac death and myocardial infarction.[39] Although promising, it is premature to conclude that all patients with UA/NSTEMI with or without PCI should be treated with IIb/IIIa receptor or ADP inhibitors. This is due, in part, to the differences in clinical trial design that pertain to entry criteria and definable endpoints and the lack of sufficient long-term follow-up. It does appear, though, that coronary stenting and antiplatelet therapy improve the efficacy and durability of PCI in managing patients with UA/NSTEMI. A major advantage to using thienopyridines as adjunct therapy is the lower bleeding complication rates compared to the GP IIb/IIIa inhibitors.

CABG Surgery Versus Medical Management

One of the first studies to evaluate the role of CABG surgery in the treatment of patients with UA/NSTEMI was reported by Parisi and associates.[40] Patients were stratified by clinical presentation and invasive evaluation of left ventricular function. Clinical presentations included progressive or new-onset angina and prolonged episodes of angina unrelieved by medication. Abnormal left ventricular function was defined as an EF of less than 0.50. Five-year follow-up revealed important survival differences in patients with three-vessel disease. The survival rate for the CABG surgery patients was 89%, whereas it was only 75% for medically treated patients. CABG surgery was also associated with fewer subsequent hospitalizations. At 8 years' follow-up, Sharma and colleagues[41] reported that the cumulative survival rates for patients with severe rest angina associated with ST-T changes on the ECG and abnormal left ventricular function were higher in surgical patients compared to medically treated patients (87% vs. 54%). In another analysis of the data, medical therapy was determined to be the preferred therapy with UA patients with only one- or two-vessel disease and normal EF, whereas surgery enhanced survival in patients with three-vessel disease or low EF.[42] These and other studies demonstrate that CABG surgery is an effective treatment for the management of UA and is associated with sustained symptom relief and excellent long-term survival (see Table 59-5).

CABG Surgery Versus PCI

With increasing evidence that PCI can be performed safely with good long-term survival rates in patients with chronic stable angina, PCI has now been expanded to treat patients with UA. This has led to clinical trials designed to compare the survival rates between CABG surgery and PCI for patients with UA/NSTEMI. The Angina with Extremely Serious Operative Mortality Evaluation (AWESOME) trial[43] randomized patients with medically refractory myocardial ischemia and risk factors for adverse outcomes with CABG surgery into two groups: CABG surgery or PCI. The 30-day survival rates for CABG surgery and PCI were 95% and 97%, respectively. At 3 years the survival rates were 79% and 80%, respectively. Thus, PCI appeared to be an acceptable alternative to CABG surgery in patients with medically refractory myocardial ischemia. In a subanalysis of the Arterial Revascularization Therapies Study (ARTS), patients with multivessel disease and UA were compared to patients with stable angina randomized to either PCI with stent implantation or CABG surgery using arterial grafts.[44] Similar to the AWESOME trial, there was no difference in the rate of major adverse events at 1 year. The need, however, for repeat revascularization was higher in the stented PCI patients. Whether long-term survival and symptom relief in UA patients with multivessel disease treated with stented angioplasty will be comparable to CABG surgery is unknown.

STEMI/AMI

PCI Versus Medical Management for AMI

The role of primary angioplasty in the treatment of patients with STEMI/AMI is controversial. In a meta-analysis that included PTCA as an adjunct to primary thrombolysis, there was no improvement in survival with delayed PTCA following thrombolytics.[45] In this analysis, there was a trend toward an increase in the combined endpoints of death and myocardial infarction for patients who underwent deliberate PTCA within a few days of infarction. When PTCA as an initial therapy was compared to the use of thrombolytics, however, there was a significant reduction in both in-hospital and 6-week mortality and

combined myocardial infarction/mortality in the PTCA patients. These findings suggest that PTCA has a survival advantage over thrombolytics as an initial treatment for STEMI/AMI, and that use of delayed PTCA as an adjunct to therapy, including thrombolytics, does not affect survival. In the Global Use of Strategies to Open Occluded Coronary Arteries in Acute Coronary Syndromes (GUSTO) IIb trial,[46] the composite endpoint of death, nonfatal myocardial infarction, and nonfatal disabling stroke at 30 days was 9.6% for PTCA and 13.7% for thrombolytics. At 6 months, however, the outcomes were similar. This study suggests that although PTCA may confer a short-term benefit over medical management and thrombolytics, the benefit does not persist over time. In contrast, a retrospective review of the National Registry of Myocardial Infarction (NRMI)-2,[47] comparing PTCA and thrombolytic therapy for STEMI/AMI, showed no difference in in-house mortality (5.2% vs. 5.4%) or reinfarction rates (2.5% vs. 2.9%). However, in the cohort of patients who presented in cardiogenic shock, there was a survival advantage of 68% for PTCA versus 48% for thrombolytics. In general, however, there appears to be no major advantage to PTCA for patients with STEMI/AMI.

Role of CABG Surgery

In patients with AMI, CABG surgery is usually performed in conjunction with an operation to treat a specific complication. Examples include refractory postinfarction angina, papillary muscle rupture with mitral regurgitation, and infarction ventricular septal defect. The rationale for urgent or emergent surgery is often based on high early mortality due to mechanical complications. Since there are an increasing number of patients who undergo catheterization early after AMI, it is not surprising that there has been an increase in the number of patients who are identified as candidates for surgery. The controversial aspect is the timing, since early operative mortality may be as low as 5% in patients with a subendocardial infarction or as high as 25% in patients with poor ventricular function.[48]

In general, patients who were operated on early after AMI are sicker, refractory to medical therapy, have a higher incidence of renal insufficiency, require IABP insertion, are older, or have sustained a previous myocardial infarction. In one study, the mortality rate for patients undergoing urgent or emergent CABG surgery less than 6 hours, 6 hours to 2 days, 2 to 14 days, 2 to 6 weeks, and more than 6 weeks following myocardial infarction was 9.1%, 8.3%, 5.2%, 6.5%, and 2.9%, respectively.[49] There was also a twofold higher mortality in patients undergoing CABG surgery in less than 48 hours versus more than 48 hours. The use of preoperative IABP was associated with an improvement in operative mortality. Thus, CABG surgery after uncomplicated myocardial infarction can be accomplished with acceptable mortality rates provided appropriate supportive interventions, including IABP, are used early to stabilize the patient prior to surgery. In STEMI/AMI patients who cannot be stabilized with aggressive medical therapy and nonsurgical interventional support, CABG surgery should be entertained if the coronary anatomy is acceptable and a specific mechanical defect can be corrected.

CABG Surgery and Special Patient Populations

Diabetes Mellitus

Patients with diabetes mellitus are at increased risk for developing CAD. This is a significant problem since CAD accounts for 75% of deaths in diabetic patients. Likewise, the mortality rate after CABG surgery is higher in diabetic patients than it is for the general population. In the prospective, randomized BARI trial (see Table 59-6), CABG surgery mortality rates in diabetic patients receiving saphenous vein grafts only or PTCA were high, 18.2% and 20.6%, respectively. The mortality rate was considerably lower, however, in surgery patients who received ITA grafts (2.9%). In the EAST trial (see Table 59-6), the findings were less conclusive, but there was a similar trend that favored surgery. Thus, CABG surgery that includes ITA grafts appears to be the treatment of choice for diabetic patients. Currently the Bypass Angioplasty Revascularization Investigation 2 Diabetes (BARI 2D) trial is underway to determine whether treatment targeted to attenuate insulin resistance can arrest or retard progression of CAD and whether early revascularization reduces the mortality and morbidity in patients with type II diabetes whose symptoms are mild and stable.[50]

Women

While women for every age group have a lower incidence of CAD than men, it is still the leading cause of death in women in the United States. Historically, serious manifestations and associated complications of CAD in women were considered uncommon. This may explain, in part, why women have received less intensive management and invasive treatment. For these reasons, and the fact that the early studies evaluating the efficacy of CABG surgery focused primarily on men, the objective of more recent studies has been to determine whether female gender is an independent risk factor for complications after interventional therapy. In the TIMI IIIB registry, the rates of myocardial infarction and death at 6 weeks after thrombolytics and PCI for UA/NSTEMI were similar for women and men.[51] This was true even though the women were older and had significantly more comorbidities (hypertension, diabetes). Multivessel disease was, however, less common in women: they had fewer critical coronary lesions with 60% or more stenosis, and their mean EF was higher. This may explain why fewer women (19%) underwent CABG surgery than men (27%). Among the CABG surgery patients, the 6-week mortality rate, however, was higher for women (albeit the total number of deaths in the study was only 7). When age was factored into a multivariate analysis of the data, gender was not linked to outcome.

In contrast, examination of the Society of Thoracic Surgeons (STS) database in two separate studies revealed that the operative mortality rate was higher in women, namely

3.15% versus 2.61%.[52,53] The database consisted of 97,153 women and 247,760 men. In this analysis, the mean left ventricular function was better in women; they received fewer ITA grafts, were older, and had more comorbidities (diabetes, hypertension, peripheral vascular disease).

Similar findings were observed in a retrospective age-stratified analysis of 51,187 patients (women = 15,178, 29.7%) in the National Cardiovascular Network database.[54] In this study, women experienced a nearly twofold increase in hospital mortality after CABG surgery (5.3% vs. 2.9%). Gender-based adjusted mortality, however, decreased inversely with age. Specifically, although women younger than 50 years of age had a twofold increase in mortality, this differential decreased with age and disappeared in patients older than 79 years of age. Women also experienced more postoperative complications such as renal failure (5.0% vs. 4.0%), neurologic complications (5.3% vs. 3.8%), and postoperative myocardial infarction (1.7% vs. 1.3%). Although these findings suggest that women do experience more complications and are at a higher risk of death after CABG surgery, it is unclear why the mortality was inversely related to age and the complication occurred most frequently in women younger than 50 years of age. It is also important to recognize that retrospective studies using a voluntary database have inherent limitations.

In a prospective study by Vaccarino and coworkers,[55] women were found to be older, underwent urgent operation more commonly (64.3% vs. 56.9%), had a higher angina score, and presented more frequently with UA and congestive heart failure. Women also received fewer total bypass grafts and ITA grafts. Although the hospital course for women and men were similar, women had a higher rate of hospital readmissions and more persistent problems such as angina, dyspnea, incisional infection, decreased SF-36 physical function scores, and depressive symptoms. Thus, although still controversial, the preponderance of evidence indicates that female gender is an independent risk factor for increased morbidity and mortality after CABG surgery.

Renal Disease

Renal insufficiency is also an independent risk factor for survival after CABG surgery. A serum creatinine level higher than 2.0 mg/dL is associated with a twofold increase in mortality.[56] It has been estimated that approximately 14% of patients undergoing CABG surgery have some degree of renal insufficiency when it is defined as a serum creatinine level higher than 1.5 mg/dL.[57] In one retrospective study[58] of 59,576 patients who underwent either CABG surgery or PCI, a survival benefit with CABG surgery in patients with a serum creatinine level higher than 2.5 mg/dL was demonstrated. The one-, two-, and three-year survival rates were 84.1%, 77.4%, and 65.9% for CABG surgery compared to 70.8%, 51.9%, and 46.1% for PCI. This survival differential was not attributed to differences in left ventricular function, severity of CAD, and incidence of comorbidities. In another retrospective study[59] of 15,784 hemodialysis-dependent patients undergoing CABG surgery, PTCA alone, and PTCA with stent, there was also a survival advantage for CABG surgery. Although early mortality was higher for CABG surgery (8.6%) versus PTCA (6.4%) or stenting (4.1%), mortality equalized at 6 to 9 months. At 2 years, survival was demonstrably better with CABG surgery. Compared to PTCA, CABG surgery provided a 20% reduction in death risk, whereas PTCA with stenting provided only a 6% survival advantage. This effect was more dramatic in diabetic patients, in which CABG surgery was associated with a 27% lower risk of death. Thus, although CABG surgery in patients with renal insufficiency and failure is associated with increased morbidity and mortality, CABG surgery is associated with better survival when compared to PCI.

Obesity

Obesity is a known risk factor for CAD, diabetes, hypertension, and stroke and is associated with a 50% to 100% higher risk of all-cause mortality when compared to age-matched peers. Thus it is not surprising that obesity is generally assumed to be a risk factor for adverse events after CABG surgery. However, contrary to various assumptions, there is a lack of agreement as to whether obesity per se is an independent predictor of mortality. In one retrospective, multicenter study of 11,101 patients undergoing CABG surgery,[60] the mortality was similar in nonobese (body mass index [BMI] < 31), moderately obese (BMI 31 to 36), and severely obese patients (BMI > 36). Although sternal wound infections were more frequent in the moderately and severely obese patients, the incidences of bleeding complications and cerebral vascular accidents were the same. In contrast, an adjusted multivariate analysis of data in the STS National Cardiac Database revealed that operative mortality was elevated in both the moderately and severely obese patient.[61] In addition, the incidences of postoperative renal failure, prolonged ventilation, and sternal wound infection were also significantly higher. In this analysis, obesity was defined as normal/mild (BMI < 35), moderate (BMI 35 to 39.9), and extreme (BMI ≥ 40). Thus, although obesity may affect morbidity, its impact on mortality is unclear. This may be due to the marked variability of the definition of obesity, a reliance on anecdotal experience, and the observational nature of the studies to date.

Reoperation for Coronary Artery Disease

Within 5 years, 15% of CABG surgery patients experience a recurrence of symptoms, typically angina. This increases to about 40% within 10 years. Recurrent symptoms almost always indicate progression of disease in the native coronary circulation or graft disease. In most cases the indications to proceed with coronary angiography, PCI with or without stenting, and/or repeat CABG surgery are the same as for the first operation. Patients who are considered candidates for reoperative CABG surgery are usually older, have more diffuse CAD, and have diminished ventricular function. Factors that increase the risk of reoperation include the absence of an ITA graft, younger age at the time of primary surgery, prior incomplete revascularization, congestive heart failure, and New York Heart

Association class III or IV angina.[62] Reoperative CABG surgery differs from that of the primary procedure in that care is taken to avoid injury to the patent grafts. Manipulation of the old grafts is kept to a minimum to avoid distal coronary bed microembolization. The mortality of reoperative CABG surgery may exceed that of primary CABG surgery; in some series it has been reported to be as high as 10%. Although reoperative CABG surgery can be performed safely, overall patient survival and freedom from angina over time are diminished. Maximal survival and freedom from reoperation are best achieved in patients by aggressive management of risk factors such as diabetes mellitus, hypercholesterolemia, hypertension, and smoking.

Complications of CAD Amenable to Surgery

A region of the ventricular wall that is akinetic or dyskinetic and results in a reduction in left ventricular EF is termed a *ventricular aneurysm*. Surgical treatment is designed to improve ventricular geometry and thus function, and often includes the use of prosthetic materials to restore normal ventricular geometry and chamber volume and normalize ventricular wall tension. The incidence of ventricular aneurysm after AMI has been reported to be as high as 35%. This has been declining due, in part, to the early and aggressive application of interventional therapies. Ninety percent of left ventricular aneurysms are the result of a transmural myocardial infarction secondary to an acute occlusion of the LAD. Patients may develop an aneurysm as early as 48 hours after infarction, but most patients do so within weeks. Approximately two thirds of patients who develop ventricular aneurysms remain asymptomatic. The 10-year survival rate of these patients may exceed 90%. In contrast, the 10-year survival for symptomatic patients is less than 50%. The most common causes of death are arrhythmias (>40%), congestive heart failure (>30%), and recurrent myocardial infarction (>10%). Mortality is influenced by the patient's age, onset of heart failure, extent of CAD, presence of mitral regurgitation, incidence and types of ventricular arrhythmias, and reduced left ventricular function. The risk of thromboembolism is low, and long-term anticoagulation is not recommended, with the exception of those patients who have evidence of a mural thrombus. The diagnosis is usually made by echocardiography. Thallium imaging or PET is useful in detecting the extent of the aneurysm and viability of adjacent regions. In general, patients with symptoms of angina, congestive heart failure, and/or who have refractory arrhythmias should be considered candidates for CABG surgery and resection of the aneurysm. Patients with a contained rupture and/or evidence of a false aneurysm should undergo surgery soon after the diagnosis is made since these have a tendency to rupture spontaneously. Patients experiencing thromboembolic events despite anticoagulation are also candidates for surgery. The most common cause of postoperative death is heart failure. The 5-year survival rate after surgery has been reported to range between 60% and 80%. In general, surgical repair/resection in conjunction with CABG surgery results in angina relief and resolution of heart failure symptoms for most patients.

Another complication of AMI is a postinfarction ventricular septal defect. This occurs in approximately 5% of patients and is associated with an acute vessel occlusion. The defect is more common in men (3:2) and typically presents within 2 to 4 days of the infarction. The VSD is usually located in the anterior or apical aspect of the ventricular septum. About 25% of patients present with a defect in the posterior aspect of the ventricular septum. This is more commonly associated with an inferior wall myocardial infarction and is secondary to an occlusion of the RCA system or a distal branch of the LCA. Approximately one third of the patients have evidence of a transient AV conduction block prior to the onset of septal rupture. A new, loud systolic cardiac murmur after a myocardial infarction suggests the diagnosis and is an indication for echocardiography. The echocardiogram is effective in determining the size and character of the VSD, as well as the degree of left-to-right shunting. Right heart catheterization typically shows a step-up in oxygen saturation levels in the right ventricle and pulmonary artery. Once the diagnosis is established, patients should undergo immediate left heart catheterization to characterize the degree of CAD, the magnitude of left ventricular dysfunction, and presence of mitral valve insufficiency. Approximately 60% of patients with an infarction VSD have significant CAD in an unrelated vessel. The mortality rate in the untreated patient is high, with 25% of the patients dying within 24 hours from refractory heart failure. Patient survival at 1 week, 1 month, and more than 1 year is 50%, 20%, and less than 10%, respectively. Patients who are considered candidates for surgery should be managed early with closure of the defect and concomitant CABG surgery. In the absence of refractory heart failure and hemodynamic instability, the survival rate may be as high as 75%.

Ischemic mitral regurgitation (IMR) may occur early or late and, depending on the severity of left ventricular dysfunction, may be life threatening. Approximately 40% of patients who sustain an AMI develop IMR that is detectable by color-flow Doppler echocardiography. In 3% to 4% of the cases the degree of mitral regurgitation is moderate or severe. Acute IMR may occur as a result of a papillary muscle necrosis and rupture due to occlusion of overlying epicardial arteries that give rise to penetrating vessels that supply the papillary muscles. The posterior papillary muscle is involved three to six times more often than the anterior muscle, and either the entire trunk of the muscle or one of the heads to which chordae attach may partially or totally rupture. Another cause of IMR is ischemic papillary muscle dysfunction. The pathogenesis of acute and chronic IMR in the absence of papillary muscle rupture is not completely understood but appears to be related to deformations of ventricular geometry. Patients usually present with chest pain and shortness of breath and evidence of pulmonary edema, hypotension, and a heart murmur that radiates into the left axilla. The chest radiograph shows signs of pulmonary congestion with interstitial pulmonary edema and cardiomegaly. A

right heart catheterization demonstrates elevated pulmonary artery pressures with prominent V waves, low mixed venous oxygen saturation, and a low cardiac output. Transthoracic echocardiography or TEE is often diagnostic, but left heart catheterization is helpful in defining coronary artery anatomy. In most cases, prompt surgical intervention provides the best chance for survival. Predictors of in-hospital death include congestive heart failure, renal insufficiency, and multivessel CAD. Emergent surgical treatment usually involves mitral valve replacement and concomitant CABG surgery. The hospital mortality may be as high as 50%, although in selected patients the mortality may be as low as 10% to 15%. The operation for chronic IMR is usually performed on an elective basis and more often consists of complete myocardial revascularization and mitral valve repair rather than replacement.

PREDICTION OF CABG SURGERY OUTCOMES USING RISK STRATIFICATION MODELS

Improvements in operative technique and the anesthetic management of cardiac surgery patients have resulted in the application of CABG surgery to sicker and more complex patients. Since there are few absolute contraindications to CABG surgery, it is important to understand hospital mortality and morbidity in the context of preoperative risk. This has resulted in the creation of risk stratification models that are designed to provide a better understanding of variations in institutional outcomes and a more accurate prediction of short-term mortality and morbidity. Examples of risk-adjusted, multi-institutional databases include the Department of Veterans Affairs (VA) Continuous Improvement in Cardiac Surgery Program, the STS National Database, and the Northern New England (NNE) Database. Risk stratification outcomes are provided to both participating institutions and surgeons. This information is then used as a screening tool to evaluate and improve quality of care.

Risk-adjusted databases are particularly helpful in identifying and prioritizing preoperative variables predictive of outcomes. A meta-analysis[63] of seven large databases of patients identified 7 core (unequivocally related to operative mortality) and 13 level 1 (likely relation to short-term CABG surgery mortality) risk factors. The core variables included acuity of operation, prior heart operation, age, EF, gender, severity of CAD, and presence of LMCA disease. These variables were acknowledged as predictive of mortality after CABG surgery in all seven databases. The presence of elevated serum creatinine levels, PTCA during index admission, recent myocardial infarction less than 1 week, history of angina, ventricular arrhythmia, congestive heart failure, mitral regurgitation, diabetes, cerebrovascular disease, peripheral vascular disease, chronic obstructive pulmonary disease, height, and weight were considered less predictive.

To determine differences between voluntary and mandatory databases, a 2001 10-year comparative analysis of CABG surgery risk factors and outcomes was performed using the voluntary STS National Database ($n = 1.1$ million) and the mandatory VA Continuous Improvement in Cardiac Surgery Program (CICSP) ($n = 74,000$).[16] Although there were differences in demographics, both datasets produced similar risk factors, with similar odds ratios for 30-day mortality after CABG surgery. The three strongest predictors of risk for mortality in the STS and VA databases were serum creatinine level higher than 3.0 mg/dL, need for preoperative IABP, and prior heart surgery. In the 1990s, CABG surgery mortality in both databases declined from 3.8% to 2.7% in the STS registry and from 4.3% to 2.7% in the CICSP registry. This occurred despite an increase in preoperative risk factors in both databases. This explains, in part, the significant decline over time in the observed-to-expected mortality ratios in both databases. These risk-adjusted databases provide an opportunity for hospitals and surgeons to identify system problems and address them with the intent to improve outcomes and enhance patient care. There are, however, subtle but important regional, institutional and provider variances that cannot be entirely accounted for in a generalized model of risk stratification.

ALTERNATIVE METHODS FOR MYOCARDIAL REVASCULARIZATION

Off-Pump Coronary Artery Bypass Grafting Surgery

The use of CPB is reportedly associated with a whole-body inflammatory response (WIR), a response mediated, in part, by activation of complement, macrophages, and cytokines. This phenomenon has been related to the contact of blood components with the surface of the bypass circuit. It has been hypothesized that the WIR contributes to postoperative bleeding, neurocognitive dysfunction, thromboembolism, fluid retention, and reversible organ dysfunction. In an attempt to minimize these complications, OPCAB surgery is used with increasing frequency and is currently considered an acceptable alternative method for myocardial revascularization. A number of studies and clinical trials have been performed to evaluate the efficacy and safety of this operation and define the subsets of patient who are most likely to benefit from this approach (Table 59-7). The findings to date have been mixed.

In one retrospective multicenter analysis of 7867 registry patients published in 2001,[64] OPCAB patients had a lower incidence of IABP use (2.3% vs. 3.41%), lower incidence of postoperative atrial fibrillation (21.2% vs. 26.3%), and a shorter length of stay (5 vs. 6 days) compared to CABG surgery with CPB. The incidences of stroke, mediastinitis, and bleeding requiring reoperation were similar, however, and there was no difference in mortality, namely 2.5% for off-pump and 2.6% for on-pump. In another observational study involving 1570 patients, OPCAB surgery was associated with less blood loss, higher postoperative hemoglobin levels, fewer blood transfusions, and the length of stay in the ICU and hospital was

shorter.[65] In this study, there was no difference in perioperative myocardial infarction, use of inotropic agents, incidence of postoperative atrial fibrillation, neurologic complications, prolonged ventilation, renal failure, or death. Thus, it appears that the operation may be a safe alternative to conventional CABG surgery with CPB.

To address CPB-mediated WIR more directly, Ascione and associates conducted a prospective, randomized OPCAB surgery trial to examine the relationship between biomarkers of WIR and postoperative morbidity and mortality in OPCAB surgery and CABG surgery patients (see Table 59-7). Serum neutrophil elastase, IL-8, C3a, and C5a levels were higher in the CABG surgery with CPB group immediately after surgery. These elevated levels were also associated with a higher incidence of infection, longer intubation time, greater blood loss, greater transfusion requirements, and longer ICU and hospital length of stay. There was no difference, however, in the incidence of postoperative myocardial infarction, acute renal failure, stroke, or death. The failure to demonstrate a reduction in the WIR and the incidence of death and myocardial infarction could have been due, in part, to the relatively small number of patients studied. Alternatively, there may be no direct relationship between CPB-induced WIR, as assessed by certain biomarkers, and death and myocardial infarction.

With respect to neurocognitive dysfunction, a prospective, randomized trial was performed to determine the possible relationship between the number of high intensive transient signals (HITSs) using transcranial Doppler ultrasound (as a surrogate marker of cerebrovascular microemboli) in patients undergoing conventional CABG surgery versus OPCAB surgery patients.[66] The results suggested that the occurrence of microemboli and incidence of cognitive impairment were increased in the patients subjected to CPB. The median number of HITSs in the OPCAB patients was 11 versus 394 in the patients undergoing conventional CABG surgery. This correlated with two of three neurologic tests, which indicated the incidence of neuropsychiatric and neurocognitive dysfunction was greater in the on-pump CABG surgery patients. These findings support the hypothesis that OPCAB surgery is associated with a reduction in the occurrence of microemboli and adverse neurocognitive outcomes. Using a different approach, Patel and colleagues[67] studied 2327 consecutive patients and divided them into three groups: on-pump, off-pump with aortic manipulation (aorta used as source of graft inflow), and off-pump without aortic manipulation (pedicle-based inflow). In this study, CPB was a risk factor for focal neurologic deficit, but there were no differences in focal deficits between the OPCAB surgery patients with or without aortic manipulation. Although this study also supports the concept that CPB may be associated with more neurologic events, it does not appear to be related to aortic manipulation as defined by the investigators. Other investigators, however, have not demonstrated superior neurocognitive protection with OPCAB surgery (see Table 59-7). Whether OPCAB surgery results in greater cerebral protection will have to await the results of the VA

TABLE 59-7. Representative Prospective, Randomized Studies Comparing Results of OPCAB Surgery to CABG Surgery with CPB

Study, No. of Patients (N), and Follow-up (F/U)	Reference	Purpose	Findings
LOW-RISK PATIENTS			
Beating Versus Arrested Heart Revascularization: Evaluation of Myocardial Function in a Prospective, Randomized Trial N = 80 F/U = 1 week	Eur J Cardiothorac Surg 15:685-690, 1999	Evaluated efficacy and safety	OPCAB is safe and effective and associated with reduction in troponin I release.
On-Pump Versus Off-Pump Revascularization: Evaluation of Renal Function N = 50 F/U = 1 week	Ann Thorac Surg 68:493-498, 1999	Analyzed postoperative renal function	Glomerular filtration, as assessed by creatinine clearance and microalbumin/creatinine ratio, was significantly reduced below preoperative levels in CABG patients compared with OPCAB subjects at 24 and 48 hours after surgery. There were no instances of acute renal failure, death, or myocardial infarction in either group.
Economic Outcome of Off-Pump Coronary Artery Bypass Surgery: A Prospective, Randomized Study N = 200 F/U = 1 week	Ann Thorac Surg 68:2237-2242, 1999	Safety and cost analysis	OPCAB was safe and effective. On average, the cost was 30% lower with OPCAB. Total mean cost per patient for operating materials, bed occupancy, and transfusion requirements was $3731 for on-pump and $2615 for off-pump.
Inflammatory Response After Coronary Revascularization With or Without Cardiopulmonary Bypass N = 60 F/U = 1 week	Ann Thorac Surg 69:1198-1204, 2000	Effect of surgery on the inflammatory response	OPCAB was associated with reduced inflammatory response and postoperative infection (24 and 60 hours postoperatively).
Serum S-100 Protein Release and Neuropsychologic Outcomes During Coronary Revascularization on the Beating Heart: A Prospective, Randomized Study N = 60 F/U = 12 weeks	J Thorac Cardiovasc Surg 119:148-154, 2000	Evaluated S-100 protein release up to 24 hours after operation and neuropsychologic outcomes	Brain and/or blood-brain barrier may be more adversely affected during CABG surgery with CPB. This was not reflected in detectable neuropsychologic deterioration at 12 weeks.
Cognitive Outcome After Off-Pump and On-Pump Coronary Artery Bypass Surgery N = 281 F/U = 3 and 12 months	JAMA 287:1405-1412, 2002	Analyze effect of procedures on cognitive outcome	OPCAB patients had improved cognitive outcomes at 3 months after surgery, but effects were limited and became negligible at 12 months.
Complete Revascularization in Coronary Artery Bypass Grafting With and Without Cardiopulmonary Bypass N = 80 F/U = 2 weeks	Ann Thorac Surg 71:165-169, 2001	Evaluate the feasibility of CABG surgery without CPB to achieve complete revascularization	OPCAB was safe and effective, but the rate of incomplete revascularization was higher.
Early Outcome After Off-Pump Versus On-Pump Coronary Bypass Surgery N = 281 F/U = 1 month	Circulation 104:1761-1766, 2001	Evaluate cardiac outcome and quality of life	OPCAB is safe and results in a similar short-term cardiac mortality and quality-of-life outcome similar to CABG surgery with CPB. Note that creatine kinase-MB release was 41% less in the OPCAB group.
HIGH-RISK PATIENTS			
Different CABG Methods in Patients With Chronic Obstructive Pulmonary Disease N = 37 F/U = 2 months	Ann Thorac Surg 71:152-157, 2001	Determine effect of different CABG techniques on pulmonary function	OPCAB procedures were more advantageous than on-pump procedures for patients with chronic obstructive pulmonary disease.

CABG, coronary artery bypass grafting; OPCAB, off-pump CABG; CPB, cardiopulmonary bypass.

Prospective Randomized Cooperative Study when it concludes in 2007.

Another rationale for performing OPCAB surgery is the potential for reducing the incidence of postoperative renal failure. In one prospective, randomized trial, patients were studied to determine whether OPCAB surgery patients were at lower risk of elevations in creatinine clearance and the urinary microalbumin/creatinine ratio in the immediate postoperative period.[68] In the OPCAB surgery patients, the values were lower and N-acetyl-β-glucosaminidase levels, a sensitive marker of renal injury, were less (see Table 59-7). This difference was observed despite the use of mannitol and the maintenance of normal mean arterial blood pressure in the patients undergoing conventional CABG surgery. Neither group, however, demonstrated any clinical manifestations of renal failure. Thus, it is unclear whether OPCAB surgery actually reduces the risk of significant clinical renal failure compared to CABG surgery with CPB.

Robotics

Rapid advances in technology have led to the application of robotic CABG surgery. Robotically assisted microsurgical systems have the theoretical advantage of enhancing surgical dexterity and minimizing the invasive nature of conventional coronary artery surgery.[69] One major system currently in use is the da Vinci system by Intuitive Surgical (Mountain View, CA). It consists of three major components: the surgeon-device interface module, the computer controller, and the specific patient interface instrumentation. Both allow real-time surgical manipulation of tissue, advanced dexterity, and optical magnification of the operative field via minimal access ports. Although only a few preliminary studies have been initiated, the results to date suggest that CABG surgery can be safely performed with satisfactory graft patency rates. Current limitations include its lack of applicability to all patients, prolonged operating room time, limited applicability to access all vessels, cost, and limited training opportunities.

Transmyocardial Laser Revascularization

Patients with UA and diffuse multivessel disease are candidates for transmyocardial laser revascularization (TMLR). This controversial surgical therapy is employed for the surgical treatment of end-stage ischemic heart disease not amenable to percutaneous or conventional surgical operations.[70-72] TMLR uses a high-energy laser beam to create myocardial transmural channels that were originally thought to provide direct access to oxygenated blood in the left ventricular cavity. This is no longer considered the mechanism by which TMLR results in a reduction in symptoms of ischemic heart disease. Although some local neovascularization has been documented, the magnitude of changes do not account for any substantive increases in myocardial perfusion. Despite reports of anginal relief, SPECT ^{201}Tl imaging, PET imaging, and other perfusion studies have failed to show any significant improvement in regional blood flow.[73,74] One mechanism that has been proposed relates to a local effect on cardiac neuronal signaling. It has been hypothesized that local tissue injury by TMLR damages ventricular sensory neurons and autonomic efferent axons, and this leads to local cardiac denervation and anginal relief. Regardless, TMLR therapy is associated with a reproducible improvement in symptoms; patients undergoing TMLR have shown a persistent improvement in angina class using the Canadian Cardiovascular System.[72] This improvement is achieved in 60% to 80% of patients within 6 months after the operation. The procedure is usually performed on patients in conjunction with other revascularization procedures.

FUTURE DEVELOPMENTS

CABG surgery has evolved into a mature treatment modality for the management of patients with ischemic heart disease. It is now the safest and most reliable method for completely revascularizing the ischemic heart and is associated with excellent medium- and long-term outcomes. Preclinical and clinical studies are now underway to develop and evaluate new methodologies that will make the operation even safer and more effective. This includes use of less-invasive techniques, testing of smaller extracorporeal circulation devices, developing methods to improve myocardial protection, and techniques to enhance graft patency. With respect to less-invasive operative techniques, new enabling technologies are being developed to facilitate the performance of more precise surgical maneuvers within more confined spaces. There are already a variety of bypass graft coupling devices under investigation that are designed to facilitate proximal and distal coronary artery graft anastomoses. These include interrupted clips, magnetic docking ports, and specialized metallic intracoronary stents. Hopefully, a usable device will be available within the next few years. Also, clinical trials are underway to determine whether normalization of left ventricular geometry in patients with dilated ischemic heart disease will enhance the beneficial effects of complete myocardial revascularization. The development of smaller, more efficient ventricular assist devices, without a propensity for infection and thromboembolic complications, could lead to circulatory support systems that will obviate the need for orthotopic heart transplantation for ischemic left ventricular dysfunction. In regard to myocardial protection, there is increasing evidence that even mild necrosis during the CABG surgery operation (as measured by creatine kinase (CK) and CK-MB) occurs not only more frequently than previously appreciated but is also associated with a decrease in medium- and long-term survival. This has led to renewed interest in developing more effective methods for protecting the heart. One such strategy under intense investigation is to mimic the phenomenon of IPC pharmacologically.[75]

Finally, it is now known that vascular intimal hyperplasia (VIH) is an important component of vein graft occlusive disease. Gene-based therapies may make it possible to transfect human saphenous veins prior to grafting and prevent VIH. It also may be possible to manipulate hs-CRP and slow the progression of the atherosclerotic heart disease process in native coronary arteries. Likewise, since statins have been shown to increase survival in patients with CAD, it may be possible to use these agents to promote endothelial protection and induce reversal of the inflammatory response cascade that leads to atherosclerotic plaque formation. If all of these efforts are successful, it may be that the current survival benefit of CABG surgery to patients with advanced CAD will be extended twofold within the near future.

Selected References

Allen Maycock CA, Muhlestein JB, Horne BD, et al: Intermountain Heart Study: Statin therapy is associated with reduced mortality across all age groups of individuals with significant coronary disease, including very elderly patients. J Am Coll Cardiol 40:1777-1785, 2002.

> Numerous clinical trials have demonstrated that statin therapy reduces the instance of myocardial infarction, stroke, and cardiovascular death among patients with coronary artery disease (CAD). The results of this study revealed that statin therapy is associated with reduced mortality in all age groups of patients with advanced CAD, especially very elderly patients. Since older patients are less likely to receive statin therapy, more aggressive statin use in this patient population may be warranted.

BARI Investigators: Influence of diabetes on 5-year mortality and morbidity in a randomized trial comparing CABG and PTCA in patients with multivessel disease: The Bypass Angioplasty Revascularization Investigation (BARI). Circulation 96:1761-1769, 1997.

> In 1987, the NHLBI initiated the BARI trial to compare the results of coronary artery bypass grafting (CABG) surgery and percutaneous transluminal coronary angioplasty (PTCA) in patients with multivessel disease. One of the initial findings revealed that the mortality rate of patients with diabetes mellitus treated with oral hypoglycemic agents or insulin was lower in patients who underwent CABG surgery than in PTCA patients. The present report examined cause-specific mortality and CABG surgery efficacy by use of internal mammary artery (IMA) grafts versus saphenous vein grafts only. The investigators reported a much better 5-year survival with CABG surgery compared to PTCA, which was due to reduced cardiac mortality (5.8% vs.20.6%, P = 0.0003). This was confined to those patients receiving at least one IMA graft.

Chamberlain MH, Ascione R, Reeves BC, Angelini GD: Evaluation of the effectiveness of off-pump coronary artery bypass grafting in high-risk patients: An observational study. Ann Thorac Surg 73:1866-1873, 2002.

> In this nonrandomized study of 1570 consecutive patients, off-pump coronary artery bypass surgery (332 patients) was associated with less blood loss, fewer blood transfusions, and a shorter length of stay in the intensive care unit and hospital when compared to conventional coronary artery bypass grafting surgery (1238 patients). Despite these observations, there was no difference in neurologic complications or death between the two groups.

Fitzgibbon GM, Kafka HP, Leach AJ, et al: Coronary bypass graft fate and patient outcome: Angiographic follow-up of 5065 grafts related to survival and reoperation in 1388 patients during 25 years. J Am Coll Cardiol 28:616-626, 1996.

> Coronary bypass graft disease and occlusion are common after CABG surgery and increase with time. The purpose of this study was to evaluate the long-term fate of venous coronary bypass grafts angiographically and to correlate graft patency and disease with patient survival and reoperation. In this study the graft occlusion rate was 12% for 4592 saphenous vein grafts and 5% for 456 internal mammary artery (IMA) grafts early after operation. This increased to 51% for vein grafts after 12 years and 20% for IMA grafts. Overall survival from the time of the first bypass procedure was enhanced in patients who underwent reoperation.

Grover FL, Shroyer AL, Hammermeister K, et al: A decade's experience with quality improvement in cardiac surgery using the Veterans Affairs and Society of Thoracic Surgeons national databases. Ann Surg 234:464-472, 2001.

> The objective of this report was to evaluate the similarities and differences between the Department of Veterans Affairs (mandatory) and the Society of Thoracic Surgeons national (voluntary) risk-adjusted databases. Both databases showed a reduction in the risk-adjusted surgical death rate over the course of 10 years despite the fact that patients presented with an increasing risk factor profile. Risk factors that predicted surgical death for coronary artery bypass grafting surgery were similar in the two databases.

Higgins TL, Yared JP, Ryan T: Immediate postoperative care of cardiac surgical patients. J Cardiothorac Vasc Anesth 10:643-658, 1996.

> This review article addresses important aspects of postoperative management of patients undergoing cardiac surgery. It emphasizes that postoperative care begins with the preoperative visit and ends when the patient is ambulatory.

Parisi AF, Khuri S, Deupree RH, et al: Medical compared with surgical management of unstable angina: Five-year mortality and morbidity in the Veterans Administration Study. Circulation 80:1176-1189, 1989.

> Early reports regarding the role of coronary artery bypass grafting (CABG) surgery in the treatment of patients with unstable angina suggested that there was no advantage of surgical therapy over medical therapy other than superior symptom relief. The purpose of this prospective, randomized Veterans Administration study was to examine survival rates for the two groups of patients in the context of intermediate and long-term outcomes. Clinical presentations included (1) progressive or new-onset angina relieved by medication and (2) prolonged bouts of angina poorly or incompletely relieved by medication. Of 468 patients, 237 were assigned to medical therapy and 231 to surgical therapy. Left ventricular function was abnormal in 134 patients and was defined as an ejection fraction less than 0.50. Five-year follow-up indicated a superior survival rate with CABG surgery in patients with unstable angina and reduced ejection fraction or three-vessel coronary artery disease suitable for surgical revascularization.

Passamani E, Davis KB, Gillespie JF, Killip T: A randomized trial of coronary artery bypass surgery: Survival of patients with a low ejection fraction. N Engl J Med 312:1665-1671, 1985.

> This report from the Coronary Artery Surgery Study sponsored by the National Heart, Lung, and Blood Institute was one of the first to demonstrate that coronary artery bypass grafting (CABG) surgery for chronic stable angina was associated with a superior survival rate in a specific subset of patients when compared to medical therapy. Specifically, the survival rate at the end of 7 years in patients with chronic stable coronary artery disease with triple-vessel disease and ejection fractions higher than 0.34 but lower than 0.50 was 84% with CABG surgery compared to 70% for medically treated patients. In patients with one-vessel and two-vessel disease, there was no difference in survival rates between the two treatment groups.

Shah PK: Pathophysiology of coronary thrombosis: Role of plaque rupture and plaque erosion. Prog Cardiovasc Dis 44:357-368, 2002.

> The development of a coronary thrombus is the immediate cause of most acute coronary syndromes of unstable angina, acute myocardial infarction, and sudden death. The major mechanism appears to be plaque rupture. This article addresses triggers for plaque rupture, consequences of plaque rupture, and the concept of plaque stabilization.

Sharma GV, Deupree RH, Luchi RJ, Scott SM: Identification of unstable angina patients who have favorable outcome with medical or surgical therapy (eight-year follow-up of the Veterans Administration Cooperative Study). Am J Cardiol 74: 454-458, 1994.

> In this report of the Veterans Administration Cooperative Study, the 468 patients who had been randomized in the Veterans Administration Cooperative Study of unstable patients noted in the Parisi report[40] were risk stratified and analyzed using angiographic criteria of the number of coronary arteries diseased and left ventricular ejection fraction (LVEF). At 8 years' follow-up, the investigators reported that medical therapy appeared to be the preferred therapy for unstable angina patients with only one-vessel or two-vessel disease and normal LVEF, and surgical therapy was associated with a superior survival advantage in patients with unstable angina, three-vessel disease, or abnormal LVEF.

Yusuf S, Zucker D, Peduzzi P, et al: Effect of coronary artery bypass graft surgery on survival: Overview of 10-year results from randomised trials by the Coronary Artery Bypass Graft Surgery Trialists Collaboration. Lancet 344:563-570, 1994.

> In this meta-analysis of six randomized foundation trials, the authors compared the strategy of initial coronary artery bypass grafting (CABG) surgery with that of initial medical therapy for the treatment of patients with stable coronary heart disease. The findings demonstrated that initial CABG surgery is associated with lower mortality than medical management with delayed surgery, especially in high-risk and medium-risk patients. The improvement in survival was greatest for patients with left main coronary artery disease, intermediate for those with three-vessel disease, and least for those with one-vessel or two-vessel disease. Greater survival prolongation was also found among patients with abnormal exercise test and abnormal left ventricular function.

References

1. Corti R, Fuster V, Badimon JJ: Pathogenetic concepts of acute coronary syndromes. J Am Coll Cardiol 41:7S-14S, 2003.
2. Shah PK: Pathophysiology of coronary thrombosis: Role of plaque rupture and plaque erosion. Prog Cardiovasc Dis 44:357-368, 2002.
3. Muller JE, Abela GS, Nesto RW, et al: Triggers, acute risk factors and vulnerable plaques: The lexicon of a new frontier. J Am Coll Cardiol 23:809-813, 1994.
4. Muller JE, Mangel B: Circadian variation and triggers of cardiovascular disease. Cardiology 85(Suppl 2):3-10, 1994.
5. Virmani R, Burke AP, Farb A, et al: Pathology of the unstable plaque. Prog Cardiovasc Dis 44:349-356, 2002.
6. Horne BD, Muhlestein JB, Carlquist JF, et al: Statin therapy, lipid levels, C-reactive protein, and the survival of patients with angiographically severe coronary artery disease. J Am Coll Cardiol 36:1774-1780, 2000.
7. Allen Maycock CA, Muhlestein JB, Horne BD, et al: Statin therapy is associated with reduced mortality across all age groups of individuals with significant coronary disease, including very elderly patients. J Am Coll Cardiol 40:1777-1785, 2002.
8. de Winter RJ, Heyde GS, Koch KT, et al: The prognostic value of pre-procedural plasma C-reactive protein in patients undergoing elective coronary angioplasty. Eur Heart J 23:960-966, 2002.
9. Asztalos BF, Schaefer EJ: High-density lipoprotein subpopulations in pathologic conditions. Am J Cardiol 91:12E-17E, 2003.
10. Segall G: Assessment of myocardial viability by positron emission tomography. Nucl Med Commun 23:323-330, 2002.
11. Klein C, Nekolla SG, Bengel FM, et al: Assessment of myocardial viability with contrast-enhanced magnetic resonance imaging: Comparison with positron emission tomography. Circulation 105:162-167, 2002.
12. Schwitter J, Nanz D, Kneifel S, et al: Assessment of myocardial perfusion in coronary artery disease by magnetic resonance: A comparison with positron emission tomography and coronary angiography. Circulation 103:2230-2235, 2001.
13. Hickey RF, Hoar PF: Whole-body oxygen consumption during low-flow hypothermic cardiopulmonary bypass. J Thorac Cardiovasc Surg 86:903-906, 1983.
14. Davies LK: Hypothermia: Physiology and clinical use. In Gravlee GP, Davis RF, Utley JR (eds): Cardiopulmonary Bypass. Baltimore, Williams & Wilkins, 1975, p 140.
15. Mentzer RM Jr, Jahania S, Lasley RD: Myocardial protection. In Cohn LH, Edmunds LH Jr (eds): Cardiac Surgery in the Adult, 2nd ed. New York, McGraw-Hill, 2003, pp 413-438.
16. Grover FL, Shroyer AL, Hammermeister K, et al: A decade's experience with quality improvement in cardiac surgery using the Veterans Affairs and Society of Thoracic Surgeons national databases. Ann Surg 234:464-474, 2001.
17. Hata M, Seevanayagam S, Manson N, et al: Radial artery 2000—risk analysis of mortality for coronary bypass surgery with radial artery. Ann Thorac Cardiovasc Surg 8:354-357, 2002.
18. Modine T, Al-Ruzzeh S, Mazrani W, et al: Use of radial artery graft reduces the morbidity of coronary artery bypass graft surgery in patients aged 65 years and older. Ann Thorac Surg 74:1144-1147, 2002.
19. Fitzgibbon GM, Kafka HP, Leach AJ, et al: Coronary bypass graft fate and patient outcome: Angiographic follow-up of 5,065 grafts related to survival and reoperation in 1,388

patients during 25 years. J Am Coll Cardiol 28:616-626, 1996.

20. Higgins TL, Yared JP, Ryan T: Immediate postoperative care of cardiac surgical patients. J Cardiothorac Vasc Anesth 10:643-658, 1996.

21. Hoit BD, Gabel M, Fowler NO: Cardiac tamponade in left ventricular dysfunction. Circulation 82:1370-1376, 1990.

22. Martin P, Horkay F, Gupta NK, et al: Heparin rebound phenomenon—much ado about nothing? Blood Coagul Fibrinolysis 3:187-191, 1992.

23. Porte RJ, Leebeek FW: Pharmacological strategies to decrease transfusion requirements in patients undergoing surgery. Drugs 62:2193-2211, 2002.

24. Daily PO, Lamphere JA, Dembitsky WP, et al: Effect of prophylactic epsilon-aminocaproic acid on blood loss and transfusion requirements in patients undergoing first-time coronary artery bypass grafting: A randomized, prospective, double-blind study. J Thorac Cardiovasc Surg 108:99-108, 1994.

25. Murkin JM, Lux J, Shannon NA, et al: Aprotinin significantly decreases bleeding and transfusion requirements in patients receiving aspirin and undergoing cardiac operations. J Thorac Cardiovasc Surg 107:554-561, 1994.

26. Engelman RM, Rousou JA, Flack JE III, et al: Fast-track recovery of the coronary bypass patient. Ann Thorac Surg 58:1742-1746, 1994.

27. Higgins TL: Early endotracheal extubation is preferable to late extubation in patients following coronary artery surgery. J Cardiothorac Vasc Anesth 6:488-493, 1992.

28. Mangano DT, Siliciano D, Hollenberg M, et al: Postoperative myocardial ischemia: Therapeutic trials using intensive analgesia following surgery. The Study of Perioperative Ischemia (SPI) Research Group. Anesthesiology 76:342-353, 1992.

29. Passamani E, Davis KB, Gillespie MJ, et al: A randomized trial of coronary artery bypass surgery: Survival of patients with a low ejection fraction. N Engl J Med 312:1665-1671, 1985.

30. Yusuf S, Zucker D, Peduzzi P, et al: Effect of coronary artery bypass graft surgery on survival: Overview of 10-year results from randomised trials by the Coronary Artery Bypass Graft Surgery Trialists Collaboration. Lancet 344:563-570, 1994.

31. Gruntzig AR, Senning A, Siegenthaler WE: Nonoperative dilatation of coronary-artery stenosis: Percutaneous transluminal coronary angioplasty. N Engl J Med 301:61-68, 1979.

32. Parisi AF, Folland ED, Hartigan P: A comparison of angioplasty with medical therapy in the treatment of single-vessel coronary artery disease. Veterans Affairs ACME Investigators. N Engl J Med 326:10-16, 1992.

33. RITA-2 Trial Participants: Coronary angioplasty versus medical therapy for angina: The Second Randomised Intervention Treatment of Angina (RITA-2) trial. Lancet 350:461-468, 1997.

34. Hartigan PM, Giacomini JC, Folland ED, et al: Two- to three-year follow-up of patients with single-vessel coronary artery disease randomized to PTCA or medical therapy (results of a VA cooperative study). Veterans Affairs Cooperative Studies Program ACME Investigators: Angioplasty Compared to Medicine. Am J Cardiol 82:1445-1450, 1998.

35. BARI Investigators: Influence of diabetes on 5-year mortality and morbidity in a randomized trial comparing CABG and PTCA in patients with multivessel disease: The Bypass Angioplasty Revascularization Investigation (BARI). Circulation 96:1761-1769, 1997.

36. Williams DO, Braunwald E, Thompson B, et al: Results of percutaneous transluminal coronary angioplasty in unstable angina and non-Q-wave myocardial infarction: Observations from the TIMI IIIB Trial. Circulation 94:2749-2755, 1996.

37. Topol EJ, Mark DB, Lincoff AM, et al: Outcomes at 1 year and economic implications of platelet glycoprotein IIb/IIIa blockade in patients undergoing coronary stenting: Results from a multicentre randomised trial. EPISTENT Investigators—Evaluation of Platelet IIb/IIIa Inhibitor for Stenting. Lancet 354:2019-2024, 1999.

38. Budaj A, Yusuf S, Mehta SR, et al: Benefit of clopidogrel in patients with acute coronary syndromes without ST-segment elevation in various risk groups. Circulation 106:1622-1626, 2002.

39. Mehta SR, Yusuf S, Peters RJ, et al: Effects of pretreatment with clopidogrel and aspirin followed by long-term therapy in patients undergoing percutaneous coronary intervention: The PCI-CURE study. Lancet 358:527-533, 2001.

40. Parisi AF, Khuri S, Deupree RH, et al: Medical compared with surgical management of unstable angina: Five-year mortality and morbidity in the Veterans Administration Study. Circulation 80:1176-1189, 1989.

41. Sharma GV, Deupree RH, Khuri SF, et al: Coronary bypass surgery improves survival in high-risk unstable angina: Results of a Veterans Administration Cooperative study with an 8-year follow-up. Veterans Administration Unstable Angina Cooperative Study Group. Circulation 84:III260-267, 1991.

42. Sharma GV, Deupree RH, Luchi RJ, et al: Identification of unstable angina patients who have favorable outcome with medical or surgical therapy (eight-year follow-up of the Veterans Administration Cooperative Study). Am J Cardiol 74:454-458, 1994.

43. Morrison DA, Sethi G, Sacks J, et al: Percutaneous coronary intervention versus coronary artery bypass graft surgery for patients with medically refractory myocardial ischemia and risk factors for adverse outcomes with bypass: A multicenter, randomized trial. Investigators of the Department of Veterans Affairs Cooperative Study No. 385, the Angina With Extremely Serious Operative Mortality Evaluation (AWESOME). J Am Coll Cardiol 38:143-149, 2001.

44. van den Brand MJ, Rensing BJ, Morel MA, et al: The effect of completeness of revascularization on event-free survival at one year in the ARTS trial. J Am Coll Cardiol 39:559-564, 2002.

45. Michels KB, Yusuf S: Does PTCA in acute myocardial infarction affect mortality and reinfarction rates? A quantitative overview (meta-analysis) of the randomized clinical trials. Circulation 91:476-485, 1995.

46. Berger PB, Ellis SG, Holmes DR Jr, et al: Relationship between delay in performing direct coronary angioplasty and early clinical outcome in patients with acute myocardial infarction: Results from the global use of strategies to open occluded arteries in Acute Coronary Syndromes (GUSTO-IIb) trial. Circulation 100:14-20, 1999.

47. Tiefenbrunn AJ, Chandra NC, French WJ, et al: Clinical experience with primary percutaneous transluminal coronary angioplasty compared with alteplase (recombinant tissue-type plasminogen activator) in patients with acute myocardial infarction: A report from the Second National Registry of Myocardial Infarction (NRMI-2). J Am Coll Cardiol 31:1240-1245, 1998.

48. Kaul TK, Fields BL, Riggins SL, et al: Coronary artery bypass grafting within 30 days of an acute myocardial infarction. Ann Thorac Surg 59:1169-1176, 1995.

49. Creswell LL, Moulton MJ, Cox JL, et al: Revascularization after acute myocardial infarction. Ann Thorac Surg 60:19-26, 1995.

50. Sobel BE, Frye R, Detre KM: Burgeoning dilemmas in the management of diabetes and cardiovascular disease: Rationale for the Bypass Angioplasty Revascularization Investiga-

tion 2 Diabetes (BARI-2D) Trial. Circulation 107:636-642, 2003.

51. Hochman JS, McCabe CH, Stone PH, et al: Outcome and profile of women and men presenting with acute coronary syndromes: A report from TIMI IIIB. TIMI Investigators. Thrombolysis in Myocardial Infarction. J Am Coll Cardiol 30:141-148, 1997.

52. Hartz RS, Rao AV, Plomondon ME, et al: Effects of race, with or without gender, on operative mortality after coronary artery bypass grafting: A study using the Society of Thoracic Surgeons National Database. Ann Thorac Surg 71:512-520, 2001.

53. Edwards FH, Carey JS, Grover FL, et al: Impact of gender on coronary bypass operative mortality. Ann Thorac Surg 66:125-131, 1998.

54. Vaccarino V, Abramson JL, Veledar E, et al: Sex differences in hospital mortality after coronary artery bypass surgery: Evidence for a higher mortality in younger women. Circulation 105:1176-1181, 2002.

55. Vaccarino V, Lin ZQ, Kasl SV, et al: Gender differences in recovery after coronary artery bypass surgery. J Am Coll Cardiol 41:307-314, 2003.

56. Nakayama Y, Sakata R, Ura M, et al: Long-term results of coronary artery bypass grafting in patients with renal insufficiency. Ann Thorac Surg 75:496-500, 2003.

57. Mangano CM, Diamondstone LS, Ramsay JG, et al: Renal dysfunction after myocardial revascularization: Risk factors, adverse outcomes, and hospital resource utilization. The Multicenter Study of Perioperative Ischemia Research Group. Ann Intern Med 128:194-203, 1998.

58. Szczech LA, Reddan DN, Owen WF, et al: Differential survival after coronary revascularization procedures among patients with renal insufficiency. Kidney Int 60:292-299, 2001.

59. Herzog CA, Ma JZ, Collins AJ: Comparative survival of dialysis patients in the United States after coronary angioplasty, coronary artery stenting, and coronary artery bypass surgery and impact of diabetes. Circulation 106:2207-2211, 2002.

60. Birkmeyer NJ, Charlesworth DC, Hernandez F, et al: Obesity and risk of adverse outcomes associated with coronary artery bypass surgery. Northern New England Cardiovascular Disease Study Group. Circulation 97:1689-1694, 1998.

61. Prabhakar G, Haan CK, Peterson ED, et al: The risks of moderate and extreme obesity for coronary artery bypass grafting outcomes: A study from the Society of Thoracic Surgeons database. Ann Thorac Surg 74:1125-1131, 2002.

62. Lytle BW, McElroy D, McCarthy P, et al: Influence of arterial coronary bypass grafts on the mortality in coronary reoperations. J Thorac Cardiovasc Surg 107:675-683, 1994.

63. Jones RH, Hannan EL, Hammermeister KE, et al: Identification of preoperative variables needed for risk adjustment of short-term mortality after coronary artery bypass graft surgery. The Working Group Panel on the Cooperative CABG Database Project. J Am Coll Cardiol 28:1478-1487, 1996.

64. Hernandez F, Cohn WE, Baribeau YR, et al: In-hospital outcomes of off-pump versus on-pump coronary artery bypass procedures: A multicenter experience. Northern New England Cardiovascular Disease Study Group. Ann Thorac Surg 72:1528-1534, 2001.

65. Chamberlain MH, Ascione R, Reeves BC, et al: Evaluation of the effectiveness of off-pump coronary artery bypass grafting in high-risk patients: An observational study. Ann Thorac Surg 73:1866-1873, 2002.

66. Diegeler A, Hirsch R, Schneider F, et al: Neuromonitoring and neurocognitive outcome in off-pump versus conventional coronary bypass operation. Ann Thorac Surg 69:1162-1166, 2000.

67. Patel NC, Deodhar AP, Grayson AD, et al: Neurological outcomes in coronary surgery: Independent effect of avoiding cardiopulmonary bypass. Ann Thorac Surg 74:400-406, 2002.

68. Ascione R, Lloyd CT, Underwood MJ, et al: On-pump versus off-pump coronary revascularization: Evaluation of renal function. Ann Thorac Surg 68:493-498, 1999.

69. Shennib H, Bastawisy A, Mack MJ, et al: Computer-assisted telemanipulation: An enabling technology for endoscopic coronary artery bypass. Ann Thorac Surg 66:1060-1063, 1998.

70. Schofield PM, Sharples LD, Caine N, et al: Transmyocardial laser revascularisation in patients with refractory angina: A randomised controlled trial. Lancet 353:519-524, 1999.

71. Burns SM, Sharples LD, Tait S, et al: The Transmyocardial Laser Revascularization International Registry report. Eur Heart J 20:31-37, 1999.

72. Horvath KA, Aranki SF, Cohn LH, et al: Sustained angina relief 5 years after transmyocardial laser revascularization with a CO2 laser. Circulation 104:I81-84, 2001.

73. Nagele H, Stubbe HM, Nienaber C, et al: Results of transmyocardial laser revascularization in non-revascularizable coronary artery disease after 3 years follow-up [see Comments]. Eur Heart J 19:1525-1530, 1998.

74. Landolfo CK, Landolfo KP, Hughes GC, et al: Intermediate-term clinical outcome following transmyocardial laser revascularization in patients with refractory angina pectoris. Circulation 100:II128-133, 1999.

75. Mentzer RM Jr: Does size matter? What is your infarct rate after coronary artery bypass grafting? J Thorac Cardiovasc Surg 126:326-328, 2003.

CHAPTER 60

ACQUIRED HEART DISEASE: VALVULAR

author block

David A. Fullerton, M.D., and Alden H. Harken, M.D.

Valvular heart diseases may be considered surgical diseases. Stenotic or regurgitant cardiac valves create hemodynamic demands on one or both ventricles of the heart. The compensatory mechanisms of the ventricles permit the heart to tolerate these lesions for varying periods of time, sometimes years, before surgical intervention is required. Significant valvular lesions, however, ultimately produce systolic and/or diastolic ventricular dysfunction, leading to heart failure. As a general rule, surgery for stenotic valve lesions may be deferred until the patient develops symptoms. Regurgitant valve lesions, however, may produce significant ventricular dysfunction before symptoms develop; surgery in patients who do not have symptoms may be indicated. Among the heart's valves, the aortic and mitral valves are by far the most likely to acquire disease and thus are the focus of this chapter.

HISTORICAL PERSPECTIVE

Heart failure from mitral stenosis was well recognized by the late 19th century, and efforts at surgical correction began well before the heart-lung machine was available.[1] As early as 1897, Samways suggested (but never acted on) the possibility of dilating the stenotic mitral valve. Based on his own postmortem studies of rheumatic heart disease in London, Brunton in 1902 proposed surgical intervention for mitral stenosis by passing a dilator through the wall of the left ventricle retrograde into the mitral valve orifice; his proposal was shunned by London physicians, and Brunton never tried this maneuver. The concept, however, was applied 20 years later in Boston when the

first report of successful surgical correction of mitral stenosis appeared in 1923; Cutler and Levine reported successful relief of mitral stenosis by incision of the valve with a knife introduced through an apical left ventriculotomy. In 1925, Soutter performed the first successful closed mitral commissurotomy at the London Hospital by introducing his index finger through the left atrial appendage. Despite Soutter's success, he received no more patient referrals, and another 20 years elapsed before the procedure became widespread. In June 1948, Bailey in Philadelphia and Harken in Boston each performed a successful closed mitral commissurotomy. Thereafter, it became widely used for mitral stenosis.

By the mid 1970s, the closed technique was supplanted by open mitral commissurotomy. Although closed mitral commissurotomy did achieve good palliation of mitral stenosis for its era, open mitral commissurotomy offers several advantages. First, the valvuloplasty may be performed under direct vision. The primary reason for failure of closed mitral commissurotomy is residual stenosis, not restenosis. In up to 75% of patients, the subvalvular apparatus of the mitral valve contributes significantly to the stenosis. The open technique permits precise and maximal division of fused commissures as well as fused chordae. In addition, calcium may be sharply débrided from the valve and any residual mitral insufficiency may be corrected at the time of operation. Finally, the closed technique has the disadvantage of potentially dislodging a left atrial thrombus, resulting in intraoperative embolization and stroke.

Surgical attempts to correct aortic stenosis also began in the early 20th century.[1] In 1912, Tuffier, in Paris, attempted transaortic digital dilatation of a stenotic aortic valve. In 1947, Smithy (who died of aortic stenosis at 43 years of age) and Parker at the University of South Carolina described an experimental model of aortic valvotomy. Three years later in Philadelphia, Bailey reported successful aortic valvulotomy by insertion of a mechanical dilator across the stenotic valve of patients to open fused commissures. In 1952, Hufnagel and Harvey, at Georgetown University, placed the first prosthetic ball valve into the descending aorta of a patient with aortic insufficiency. Surgery on the aortic valve under direct vision required the development of cardiopulmonary bypass by Gibbon in 1954. In 1955, Swann performed the first successful aortic valvotomy using hypothermia and inflow occlusion. Initially, open aortic valve operations were limited to aortic valve commissurotomy and débridement of calcified aortic valve leaflets. Harken, in Boston in 1960, and Starr, in Portland in 1963, however, reported replacement of the aortic valve with a ball-valve prosthesis. In 1962, Ross, in London, successfully performed orthotopic homograft valve replacement. In 1967, Ross performed the first pulmonary autograft procedure (Ross procedure) for correction of aortic stenosis. In the mid 1960s, stent-mounted porcine aortic valves were implanted, but these formaldehyde-fixed valves rapidly degenerated. In 1974, Carpentier, in Paris, reported superior longevity of the glutaraldehyde-preserved porcine valve.

DIAGNOSTIC CONSIDERATIONS

Valvular heart disease may be suggested by a patient's history or by a heart murmur detected on physical examination. Regardless of the valve lesion in question, echocardiography should be employed to assess the severity of the stenosis, regurgitation, or both. Information available from the echocardiogram includes definition of valve anatomy, assessment of ventricular contractile function, determination of the magnitude of valve regurgitation using color flow Doppler imaging, and determination of the severity of valve stenosis.

Transthoracic two-dimensional echocardiography is completely noninvasive and may provide the necessary information. If more information is needed, transesophageal echocardiography may provide better definition of aortic and mitral valve anatomy; it is also a more sensitive imaging modality for detection of mitral regurgitation.

Although most valve lesions may be accurately diagnosed by echocardiography, cardiac catheterization may be necessary to confirm the diagnosis or to provide additional information pertaining to ventricular function. Before surgery, it may be necessary to exclude the presence of coronary artery disease. Mitral or aortic valve areas may be determined at cardiac catheterization using the Gorlin formula,[2] which permits calculation of the valve area as follows:

$$\text{Valve area} = \text{Flow across the valve} \div (C \times \sqrt{\text{Mean transvalvular gradient}})$$

where C is an empirical constant: 44.5 for the aortic valve and 38 for the mitral valve.

MITRAL VALVE

Surgical Anatomy of the Mitral Valve

The normal function of the mitral valve is dependent on coordinated interaction of the mitral valve apparatus, which includes the mitral valve annulus, the valve leaflets, the valve chordae tendineae, and the left ventricular papillary muscles. The normal mitral valve has two leaflets: the anterior (or aortic leaflet) and the posterior (or mural leaflet). Two papillary muscles arise from the left ventricular wall: the posterior (or posteromedial) and the anterior (or anterolateral). Each of the leaflets of the mitral valve is connected to each of the papillary muscles by tendons, the chordae tendineae.

The leaflets are suspended from the mitral annulus, a collagenous structure that encircles the orifice between the left atrium and ventricle. Although the two leaflets have about the same surface area, they have very different shapes (Fig. 60-1). The anterior leaflet is rectangular. Its base is attached to the mitral annulus anteriorly, and the width of the base is about one third the circumference of the mitral annulus. This attachment of the anterior leaflet to the mitral annulus extends to the aortic annulus through fibrous tissue, providing "fibrous continuity" between the aortic and mitral valves; the anterior leaflet of the mitral valve is immediately visible as the surgeon looks down through the aortic valve. The posterior leaflet is rectangular, and its attachment to the mitral annulus extends for about two thirds of the circumference of the mitral annulus. The two leaflets are separated by two distinct commissures.

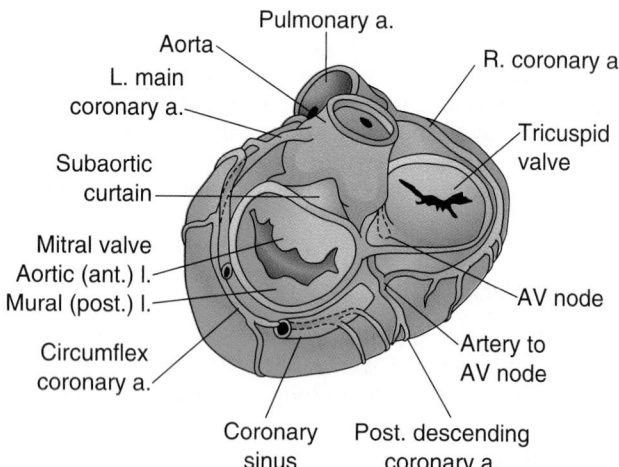

FIGURE 60-1. Anatomy of the mitral valve as it relates to other cardiac structures. Important surgical landmarks include the relationship of the mitral valve to the aortic valve, the circumflex coronary artery, and the atrioventricular (AV) node. (From Buchanan SA, Tribble CG: Reoperative mitral replacement. *In* Kaiser LR, Kron IL, Spray TL [eds]: Mastery of Cardiothoracic Surgery. Philadelphia, Lippincott-Raven, 1998, p 351.)

There are three important surgical landmarks (see Fig. 60-1). First, the circumflex coronary artery runs along the epicardial surface of the heart overlying the posterior mitral annulus. Just millimeters of left atrial muscle separate the artery from the annulus, making it susceptible to injury during mitral valve surgery. Second, the aortic valve is in close approximation to the anterior leaflet of the mitral valve (aortomitral continuity). The noncoronary leaflet of the aortic valve is therefore susceptible to injury during mitral surgery. Third, the atrioventricular node is located deep to the posteromedial commissure of the mitral valve.

Mitral Stenosis

Etiology

Rheumatic fever is the principal cause of mitral stenosis, and about two thirds of patients with rheumatic mitral stenosis are female. Rheumatic fever usually occurs in childhood or adolescence (mean age, 8 to 12 years) and creates an inflammatory infiltration of the myocardium and valves. Perhaps because the disease afflicts young people and many years pass before symptoms are manifest, a prior history of rheumatic fever is often difficult to confirm. As the mitral valve heals after acute rheumatic fever, the mitral apparatus may slowly become deformed, and the disease typically remains asymptomatic for at least 10 years; symptoms most commonly appear during the patient's third or fourth decade of life. Healing of the inflammation from rheumatic fever ultimately causes the cusps and commissures of the mitral valve to thicken and fuse, with concomitant fusion and shortening of the chordae tendineae. The structure of the valve apparatus then calcifies and narrows, becoming funnel shaped. Such thickening and fusion of the valve not only creates stenosis but also often prevents complete closure of the valve. In fact, of all patients with rheumatic mitral valve disease, about half have combined mitral stenosis and mitral regurgitation.[3]

Other causes of mitral stenosis that are far less common than rheumatic fever include malignant carcinoid, systemic lupus erythematosus, and rheumatoid arthritis. Rarely, congenital malformation of the valve may cause mitral stenosis, and congenital mitral stenosis is almost never an isolated congenital cardiac lesion.

Pathophysiology

The cross-sectional area of the normal mitral valve is 4 to 6 cm^2. A mitral valve area of 2 cm^2 is considered "moderate" mitral stenosis, and an area of 1 cm^2 is considered "severe" mitral stenosis.[4] Under normal conditions, there is no pressure gradient across the mitral valve, and the left atrial pressure is normally less than 15 mm Hg. As the mitral valve becomes more narrowed, an increasing pressure gradient is required to move the blood across the mitral valve from the left atrium into the left ventricle during diastole; a transvalvular gradient of 10 mm Hg indicates severe mitral stenosis. The significance of the trans-valvular gradient is that left atrial pressure progressively increases, as the mitral valve becomes more stenotic. In turn, the increased left atrial pressure is transmitted retrograde into the pulmonary veins, pulmonary capillaries, and ultimately pulmonary arteries. A left atrial pressure of about 25 mm Hg increases pulmonary capillary pressure enough to produce pulmonary edema.

The severity of obstruction across the valve is determined by the transvalvular gradient and the flow rate across the valve. The flow rate is a function of both the cardiac output and the heart rate; because flow across the mitral valve occurs during diastole and diastole is shortened as heart rate increases, a faster heart rate at any given cardiac output increases the transvalvular gradient and raises left atrial pressure. The contribution of the atrial contraction ("kick") to cardiac output is particularly important in mitral stenosis; it accomplishes as much as 30% of the transvalvular gradient. For these reasons, the onset of symptoms is generally associated with exertional activities or with the onset of atrial fibrillation.

To maintain adequate left ventricular filling across a 1-cm^2 valve, for example, a pressure gradient of 20 mm Hg is required. A normal left ventricular end-diastolic pressure of 5 mm Hg results in a left atrial pressure of 25 mm Hg. Left atrial pressure rises farther if flow rate across the valve increases (increased cardiac output), transit time across the valve is shortened (decreased diastolic time), or atrial kick is lost (atrial fibrillation).

Pulmonary hypertension is an important component of the pathophysiology of mitral stenosis and, when severe, may dominate the clinical picture. At least three pathophysiologic mechanisms contribute to the pulmonary hypertension seen in long-standing mitral valvular disease: (1) increased left atrial pressure transmitted retrograde into the arterial circulation, (2) vascular remodeling of the pulmonary vasculature in response to chronic obstruction to pulmonary venous drainage ("fixed component"), and (3) pulmonary arterial vasoconstriction ("reactive component").

Diagnosis

SYMPTOMS

Dyspnea is the principal symptom of mitral stenosis. Dyspnea is typically brought on with exertion or associated with the abrupt onset of atrial fibrillation. The increased cardiac output or heart rate with exertion or the loss of atrial kick and tachycardia with atrial fibrillation result in an increased transvalvular gradient. This, in turn, increases left atrial pressure, and the pulmonary veins and capillaries become engorged, producing the sensation of dyspnea and promoting pulmonary edema. If the left atrium enlargement is sufficient to compress surrounding structures, the patient may complain of dysphagia or hoarseness. Marked elevation in left atrial pressure may produce hemoptysis.

PHYSICAL EXAMINATION

The left ventricle is typically normal in size, and the apex is therefore not displaced. The murmur of mitral stenosis is best heard at the apex. It is a low-pitched, rumbling diastolic murmur that is decreased with inspiration and increased during expiration; it may be markedly decreased by Valsalva maneuver. An opening snap precedes the murmur, is heard at the apex, and represents the completed excursion of the mitral valve leaflets. If the mitral leaflets are stiff or calcified, an opening snap may not be heard. In patients with pulmonary hypertension, signs of elevated right ventricular and central venous pressure may predominate the clinical picture. Physical findings, such as distended neck veins, hepatomegaly, ascites, and peripheral edema, combined with a loud pulmonary valve component of the second heart sound (P_2) heard on cardiac auscultation, all suggest significant pulmonary hypertension.

CHEST RADIOGRAPH

Several findings may be noted on the chest radiograph. The cardiac silhouette may be normal in size, but the left atrium is enlarged. The enlarged left atrium may be seen as a double density behind the right atrium on the posteroanterior projection, or it may be seen to displace the left mainstem bronchus superiorly. On the lateral projection, the enlarged left atrium may displace the esophagus posteriorly. Calcification of the mitral leaflets or the mitral annulus may be seen. Pulmonary venous hypertension should be suspected when the pulmonary arteries are enlarged and there is cephalization of pulmonary blood flow.

ECHOCARDIOGRAM

The echocardiogram is the principal tool used to confirm the diagnosis.[5] Using the echocardiogram, the mitral valve area may be determined by two mechanisms. First, the mitral valve area may be determined directly from the echocardiogram by planimetry. Second, measurement of the velocity of blood flow across the valve by Doppler echocardiography permits calculation of the transvalvular gradient. Because the transvalvular gradient persists longer with greater stenosis of the valve, the time required for the transvalvular gradient to decline may be measured and is referred to as the *pressure half-time*. The mitral valve area may then be calculated using the following formula:

$$\text{Mitral valve area} = 220 \div \text{pressure half-time}$$

CARDIAC CATHETERIZATION

Mitral stenosis may also be diagnosed by cardiac catheterization. In fact, before undergoing surgical correction of mitral stenosis, cardiac catheterization should be performed in patients with a history of angina and in those who are older than 40 years of age to exclude coronary artery disease. At the time of cardiac catheterization, left atrial pressure may be determined directly (by transatrial puncture) or inferred from pulmonary capillary wedge pressure. Simultaneous measurement of the left ventricular diastolic pressure permits calculation of the transvalvular gradient; a transvalvular gradient of greater than

10 mm Hg is consistent with significant mitral stenosis. Using the Gorlin formula, the mitral valve area (MVA) may be calculated as follows:

$$\text{MVA} = F \div 38 \ (\sqrt{\Delta P})$$

where ΔP is the mean diastolic transvalvular gradient (mm Hg), F is the mean diastolic mitral flow in milliliters per second (derived from the measured cardiac output and a determination of diastolic duration), and 38 is a constant.

Natural History

The natural history of mitral stenosis has been altered by successful surgical intervention. Data collected from the era before widespread surgery for mitral stenosis, however, indicate that after diagnosis, the mean survival among patients with asymptomatic mitral stenosis was 15 to 20 years; on the other hand, patients with symptoms had a mean survival of only 2 to 7 years.[6] Left atrial distention predisposes to atrial fibrillation and its associated intra-atrial thrombus formation. As many as 20% of patients with mitral stenosis and atrial fibrillation may sustain systemic embolization, especially strokes.

Treatment

The symptom-free patient in sinus rhythm requires only prophylaxis against bacterial endocarditis.[5] When symptoms appear, medical treatment of mitral stenosis includes diuretics to lower left atrial pressure and efforts to maintain sinus rhythm with β-blocking agents or calcium-channel blocking agents. Digoxin is helpful in controlling ventricular rate in patients who do go into atrial fibrillation. Patients in atrial fibrillation should be anticoagulated with chronic warfarin sodium (Coumadin) therapy because the risk for systemic embolization is high.

Mechanical relief of mitral stenosis should be considered when patients develop symptoms, when evidence of pulmonary hypertension appears, or when the mitral valve area is reduced to about 1 cm^2. Other conditions that should prompt surgical consideration include systemic embolization, worsening pulmonary hypertension, and endocarditis. The options for mechanical relief of mitral stenosis include balloon mitral valvuloplasty, open surgical mitral valvuloplasty (commissurotomy), and mitral valve replacement.

BALLOON MITRAL VALVULOPLASTY

First performed in 1984, balloon mitral valvuloplasty has become the treatment of choice for selected patients with mitral stenosis.[7] Echocardiography may be used to determine patients considered to be good candidates, including those with pliable valve leaflets but without valvular calcification or deformation of the chordae tendineae. Contraindications to this procedure include the presence of moderate mitral regurgitation, thickening and calcification of the mitral leaflets, and scarring and calcification of the subvalvular apparatus.[8] Performed in the cardiac catheterization suite under fluoroscopic guidance, the technique entails advancement of one or two balloon catheters across the interatrial septum and inflation of the balloon within the stenotic mitral valve.

Balloon mitral valvuloplasty has provided good short-term and intermediate-term results in appropriately selected patients. Balloon inflation should increase the mitral valve area to about 2 cm². This increase in mitral valve area is usually associated with a significant decline in left atrial pressure and transvalvular gradient and with at least a 20% increase in cardiac output. The mortality rate associated with balloon mitral valvuloplasty is 0.5% to 2%. Other risks associated with this procedure include systemic embolism, cardiac perforation, and creation of mitral regurgitation; the risk of each of these complications is 1% to 2%. Increased pulmonary vascular resistance has been shown to normalize after successful balloon valvuloplasty. About 10% of patients are left with a residual interatrial septal defect. Three years after balloon valvuloplasty, at least 66% of patients are free of subsequent intervention. In appropriately selected patients, the results of balloon valvuloplasty compare favorably with surgical valvuloplasty.[9]

OPEN MITRAL COMMISSUROTOMY

Open surgical valvuloplasty (commissurotomy) permits careful examination of the mitral valve and the chordae tendineae under direct vision as well as removal of left atrial thrombus. Because thrombus typically originates in the left atrial appendage, its orifice may be surgically oversewn from within the left atrium, reducing the risk for subsequent embolization. The surgeon may then sharply divide fused commissures and leaflets, mobilize scarred chordae, and débride calcification. Furthermore, reconstruction of the valve may eliminate preexistent mitral regurgitation. The presence of significant mitral regurgitation, however, should prompt consideration of mitral valve replacement.

The mortality rate associated with open mitral valvuloplasty is less than 2%.[10] When performed in appropriately selected patients, the freedom from subsequent mitral valve intervention is about 75% at 5 years.[9] Nonetheless, because of less procedure-related morbidity, balloon valvuloplasty is the procedure of choice.

MITRAL VALVE REPLACEMENT

The mitral valve should be replaced when valvuloplasty is precluded by dense calcification of the leaflets or subvalvular apparatus or because of concomitant mitral regurgitation. Regardless of whether a tissue or mechanical prosthesis is implanted, efforts should be made to preserve the continuity between the left ventricular apex and the mitral annulus provided by the chordae tendineae. This may be readily accomplished by preservation of the posterior leaflet of the native mitral valve.

The contribution of the mitral apparatus to left ventricular function has become appreciated in recent years.[11,12] A mechanical advantage is afforded the left ventricle by the connection of its apex (by way of the papillary muscles) to the mitral annulus through the chordae tendineae; elimination of this connection by removal of the entire mitral apparatus leads to loss of left ventricular function. Convincing data from laboratory animals and humans demonstrate that preservation of at least some of the chordae tendineae at the time of mitral valve replacement results in much better long-term left ventricular function than mitral valve replacement with chordal separation. Therefore, if mitral valve replacement is required, efforts should be made to preserve the posterior and, in some cases, the anterior leaflets of the native mitral valve.

The operative mortality rate associated with mitral valve replacement for mitral stenosis is 2% to 10%.[10,13] Operative mortality is increased with advanced age and the presence of coronary disease. Pulmonary hypertension typically resolves after valve replacement, but several weeks or months may be required. The 5-year survival rate after replacement is 70% to 90%.[9,10,14]

Mitral Regurgitation

Etiology

Competency of the mitral valve requires an intact mitral valve apparatus. Abnormalities of any component of the mitral valve apparatus may produce mitral regurgitation: the mitral leaflets, the chordae tendineae, the mitral valve annulus, or the papillary muscles. Worldwide, rheumatic fever remains the most common cause of mitral regurgitation; it results in deformity and retraction of the leaflets and shortening of the chordae. The leaflets may be perforated by trauma or infective endocarditis. Calcification of the mitral annulus may result in annular rigidity and may prevent valve closure, and mitral annular dilatation resultant to left ventricular dilatation may likewise preclude leaflet apposition during systole. Chordal rupture may result from trauma, endocarditis, rheumatic fever, or diseases of collagen formation; chordae to the posterior leaflet rupture more frequently than those to the anterior leaflet. Mitral valve prolapse is found in about 2% of the U.S. population, and up to 5% of patients with mitral valve prolapse develop mitral regurgitation secondary to chordal elongation or rupture. Coronary arterial disease may produce infarction of the papillary muscle, resulting in mitral regurgitation. Infarction in the distribution of the anterior descending coronary artery may necrose the anterolateral papillary muscle, whereas the posteromedial muscle may infarct if blood flow through the posterior descending coronary artery is interrupted. Mitral regurgitation resultant to myocardial infarction typically presents as a new murmur several days after infarction.

Pathophysiology

The regurgitant mitral valve offers an alternative route by which blood may exit the left ventricle. During both isovolumetric contraction and systole, blood is preferentially ejected into the low-pressure left atrium. The volume of the regurgitant flow (regurgitant fraction) is dependent on the size of the regurgitant orifice and the pressure gradient between the left ventricle and left atrium.

Increased left ventricular afterload or decreased forward left ventricular stroke volume increases left ventricular pressure and thereby increases the pressure gradient between left ventricle and atrium. The mitral valve annulus is enlarged by dilatation of the left ventricle. Therefore, the size of the regurgitant orifice is increased by diminished left ventricular contractility as well as increased left ventricular preload and increased afterload. Because the valve leaks during systole, the volume of regurgitant flow also increases as heart rate (number of systoles per minute) increases.

The compensatory mechanism by which the left ventricle adapts to maintain an adequate systemic blood flow (forward cardiac output) is volume overload; it must pump the combined volume of systemic and regurgitant flows (Fig. 60-2). Volume overload leads to cardiac dilatation as well as left ventricular hypertrophy. Because the left ventricle ejects into the reduced resistance of the left atrium, parameters of systolic function (ejection fraction)

are *increased* in mitral regurgitation. As with aortic insufficiency, however, the left ventricle ultimately fails with chronic volume overload. In fact, *normal* parameters of systolic function indicate significant contractile dysfunction of the left ventricle. An ejection fraction of less than 40% in the setting of mitral regurgitation indicates significant left ventricular contractile dysfunction.

As in mitral stenosis, left atrial hypertension results from mitral regurgitation. This pressure is transmitted retrograde into the pulmonary circulation and, if high enough, produces pulmonary hypertension. The magnitude of the left atrial pressure is a function of the compliance of the left atrium. Normal or low compliance of the left atrium, such as may occur in acute mitral regurgitation, results in a relatively rapid rise in left atrial pressure. On the other hand, chronic, left atrial volume overload that develops slowly may create significant enlargement of a compliant left atrium with relatively low left atrial pressure.

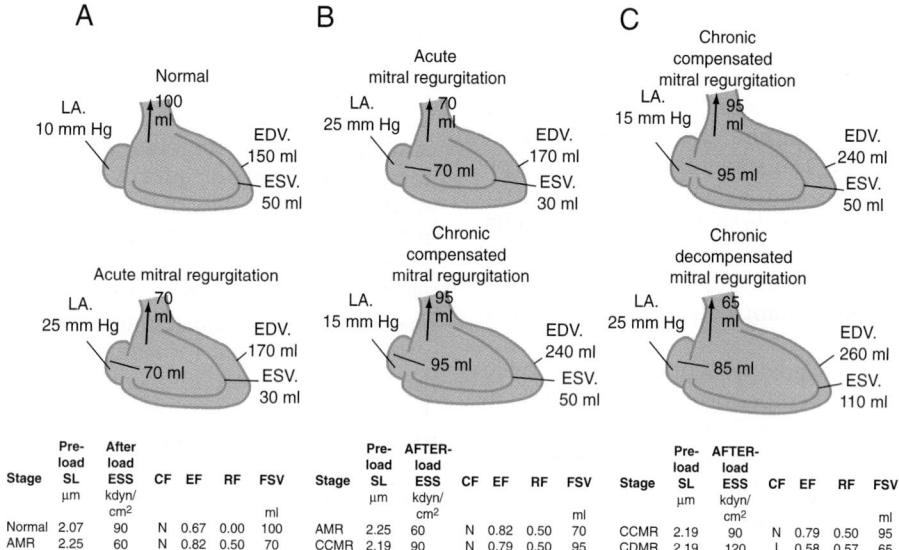

FIGURE 60-2. Pathophysiology and compensation for acute and chronic mitral regurgitation. **A,** With acute mitral regurgitation, end-diastolic volume (EDV) increases from 150 to 170 mL. Because the left ventricle ejects blood into both the aorta and the left atrium (LA), end-systolic volume (ESV) decreases from 50 to 30 mL. The ejection fraction therefore increases acutely; but because a significant percentage is ejected into the LA, the volume of blood flow into the aorta (forward stroke volume [FSV]) decreases from 100 to 70 mL. The regurgitant volume into the LA increases LA pressure. **B,** Myocardial compensation for chronic mitral regurgitation includes eccentric left ventricular hypertrophy. Left ventricular EDV increases from 170 to 240 mL. The larger ventricle results in an increased total stroke volume as well as FSV. Enlargement of the LA increases in capacitance, which accommodates the regurgitant volume at a lower pressure. The left ventricular ejection fraction is supernormal. **C,** Ultimately, the heart decompensates and the contractile force (CF) of the left ventricle declines; the ESV increases from 50 to 110 mL as FSV declines. The left ventricle dilates, which further compromises the ability of the mitral valve apparatus to close; the regurgitant volume increases. The ejection fraction remains above normal until contractile function declines further. SL, sarcomere length; ESS, end-systolic stress; RF, regurgitant fraction; EF, ejection fraction. (From Carabello BA: Mitral regurgitation: Basic pathophysiologic principles. Mod Concepts Cardiovasc Dis 57:53, 1988.)

Diagnosis

SYMPTOMS

The symptoms of mitral regurgitation are those of heart failure: shortness of breath, dyspnea on exertion, orthopnea, pulmonary edema, and diminished exercise tolerance. Symptoms are determined by the degree of mitral regurgitation, the rate of its progression, the degree of pulmonary hypertension, and the magnitude of left ventricular contractile dysfunction. For example, patients with mild mitral regurgitation may remain symptom free for most of their lives. At the other extreme, patients with acute, severe mitral regurgitation, such as may occur with endocarditis or a ruptured chordae tendineae, may have pulmonary edema and require urgent surgery. The onset of atrial fibrillation does impair the patient's functional status, but not to the same degree as with mitral stenosis. With chronic, moderate to severe mitral regurgitation, patients may be symptom free for long periods of time. Lack of symptoms, however, may be very deceiving because the contractile function of the left ventricle may be slowly deteriorating from volume overload. When symptoms occur, left ventricular contractile dysfunction may be irreversible.

PHYSICAL EXAMINATION

On cardiac auscultation, a holosystolic murmur is heard best at the apex and radiates to the axilla and left scapular region. The pulmonary examination may be significant for rales and bronchospasm caused by increased pulmonary interstitial fluid. In fact, mitral valve pathology should be considered in the differential diagnosis of patients with adult-onset asthma.

ELECTROCARDIOGRAM

The electrocardiogram is notable for left atrial enlargement and, frequently, atrial fibrillation.

CHEST RADIOGRAPH

The chest radiograph is significant for cardiomegaly and left atrial enlargement. Pulmonary venous hypertension may manifest as cephalization of pulmonary blood flow and pulmonary edema.

ECHOCARDIOGRAM

The diagnosis is confirmed by echocardiography. Transesophageal echocardiography is particularly effective in providing an anatomic explanation for the regurgitation, such as perforated leaflets, poor leaflet coaptation, or ruptured chordae. Doppler echocardiography reveals a high-velocity jet of regurgitant blood flow into the left atrium during systole.

Unfortunately, the determination of the severity of mitral regurgitation is only semiquantitative. The severity of the regurgitation is gauged as a function of the distance from the mitral annulus that the jet can be visualized (e.g., into the pulmonary veins) and by the width of the regurgitant jet. The regurgitation is scored subjectively on a scale from 1 (mild) to 4 (severe). The chronicity of the regurgitation may be inferred from the size of the left atrium; an enlarged left atrium suggests chronic mitral regurgitation. Contrast ventriculography, performed at cardiac catheterization, likewise demonstrates mitral regurgitation during systole.

Natural History

The natural history of the disease is variable, determined by the cause of mitral regurgitation, the regurgitant volume, and the magnitude of left ventricular systolic dysfunction. Patients with mild mitral regurgitation typically remain symptom free for years and rarely go on to develop severe mitral regurgitation. As is the situation with most valve diseases, the natural history of mitral regurgitation is obscure because surgical intervention has effectively altered this history. In the presurgical era, however, about 80% of patients with severe mitral regurgitation survived 5 years and 60% survived 10 years.[15,16] Patients with combined mitral stenosis and regurgitation had a worse prognosis, with a 5-year survival rate of only 67%.

Treatment

The cornerstone of medical management is diuresis and afterload reduction with angiotensin-converting enzyme inhibitors. The importance of afterload reduction cannot be overemphasized. Because blood leaving the left ventricle travels the path of least resistance, lowering systemic vascular resistance increases systemic cardiac output. In the setting of heart failure from acute mitral regurgitation, intravenous vasodilators (nitroprusside) may be needed. When a patient's condition is stabilized, conversion to oral angiotensin-converting inhibitors may be achieved. Diuretics function not only to relieve pulmonary edema but also to reduce left ventricular diameter. The size of the mitral annulus is thereby diminished and the regurgitant fraction reduced.

The indications for surgical intervention include symptoms despite medical management; severe mitral regurgitation in the presence of an identified structural abnormality, such as a ruptured chorda tendinea; development of pulmonary hypertension; or evidence of deteriorating left ventricular contractile function as determined by echocardiography or contrast ventriculography.

It is difficult to judge left ventricular function in patients without symptoms, making close follow-up with serial echocardiograms essential. In fact, asymptomatic left ventricular dysfunction may develop insidiously. Two parameters of left ventricular function are useful in making the decision regarding timing of surgery: ejection fraction (EF) and end-systolic diameter (ESD). Because mitral regurgitation lowers the total impedance against left ventricular ejection, the EF should be supernormal in the presence of normal myocardial contractile function. An EF of less than 60% suggests myocardial dysfunction, and operative mortality increases.[17] The other useful parameter of left ventricular function is the left ventricular ESD.[17] ESD is less preload dependent than is EF, and

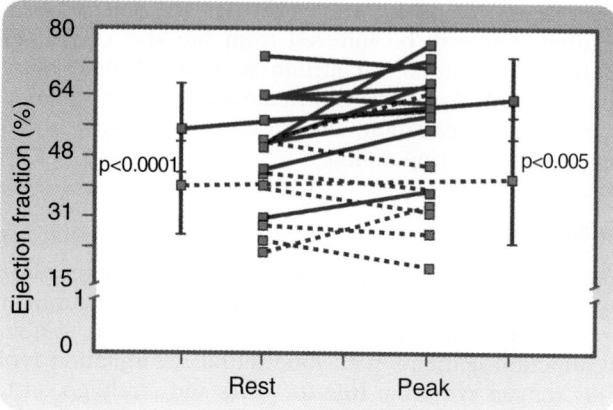

FIGURE 60-3. Left ventricular (LV) ejection fraction after mitral valve repair *(white squares)* versus replacement *(black squares)*. Ejection fraction is greater at rest and with exercise after repair. (From Tishler MD, Cooper KA, Rowen M, LeWinter MM: Mitral valve replacement versus mitral repair: A Doppler and quantitative stress echocardiograph study. Circulation 89:132, 1994. Copyright 1994, the American Heart Association.)

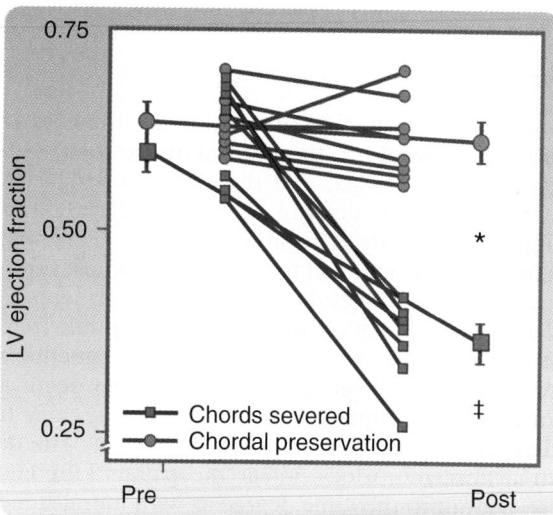

FIGURE 60-4. Postoperative ejection fraction after mitral valve replacement with *(circles)* and without *(squares)* preservation of the chordae tendineae. Ejection fraction decreases significantly without chords severed but is preserved with choral preservation. (From Roseate JD, Carabello BA, Ushere BW, et al: Mitral valve replacement with and without chordal preservation in patients with chronic mitral regurgitation. Circulation 86:1718, 1992. Copyright 1992, the American Heart Association.)

the information it implies is complementary. When left ventricular ESD exceeds 45 mm, the prognosis after surgery is worse.[18,19] Even in the absence of symptoms, therefore, patients should be referred for surgery when the left ventricular EF is less than 60% or when the left ventricular ESD is more than 45 mm.[20]

In those cases, there are two surgical options: mitral valve repair or replacement. When possible, the valve should be repaired. The final decision about which of these options to employ is made intraoperatively after valve inspection. Mitral valve repair has several advantages over replacement. First, left ventricular function is better preserved after repair (Fig. 60-3).[21,22] Valve repair preserves the continuity between the mitral annulus and ventricular papillary muscle provided by the chordae tendineae; this provides the left ventricle a mechanical advantage and optimizes its function. When the chordae tendineae are sacrificed during a mitral valve replacement, the postoperative ejection fraction typically decreases (Fig. 60-4). Therefore, even when mitral valve replacement is necessary for mitral regurgitation, the chordae tendineae should be preserved if possible.[23]

Second, mitral valve replacement subjects the patient to the risks associated with the valve prosthesis, such as thromboembolism and the risk for prosthetic valve endocarditis. Bioprosthetic valves may ultimately experience structural deterioration, and mechanical prosthetic valves obligate the patient to lifelong anticoagulation with warfarin sodium. After mitral valve repair, patients in sinus rhythm do not require long-term warfarin sodium therapy.

Third, the operative mortality rate associated with mitral valve repair (0% to 2%) is significantly less than that for replacement (4% to 8%).[10] Long-term survival appears better with repair as well. These outcomes likely derive from the superior left ventricular function after mitral repair than after replacement.

Significant left ventricular dysfunction has long been recognized as a significant risk factor for operative death after surgical correction for mitral regurgitation. Recently, however, several investigators have achieved excellent results with mitral valve repair even in patients with severe heart failure and left ventricular ejection fractions below 20%.[24] Functional status of the patients has been significantly improved, and the need for hospital admission for treatment of heart failure has been markedly decreased. Preservation of the mitral apparatus at the time of repair is essential to achieve those results.

AORTIC VALVE

Surgical Anatomy of the Aortic Valve

The normal aortic valve is composed of three thin, pliable leaflets, or cusps, attached to the heart at the junction of the aorta and the left ventricle. The leaflets are attached within the three sinuses of Valsalva of the proximal aorta and join together in three commissures, which create the shape of a coronet. Because the coronary arteries arise from two of the three sinuses of Valsalva, the aortic leaflets are named after their respective sinuses as the *left coronary leaflet,* the *right coronary leaflet,* and the *noncoronary leaflet.* There are two important surgical landmarks. First, the commissure between the left and noncoronary leaflets is positioned over the anterior leaflet of the mitral valve. Second, the commissure between the noncoronary and the right coronary leaflets is positioned over the left bundle of His. Injury to this conduction bundle during aortic valve surgery may create heart block (Fig. 60-5).

Aortic Stenosis

Etiology

Acquired aortic stenosis usually results from calcification of the aortic valve associated with advanced age. Although the process is most often idiopathic,[25] rheumatic fever may affect the aortic valve in a process similar to that of the mitral valve. In rheumatoid aortic stenosis, inflammation produces adhesions and fusion of the commissures and leaflets with thickening and calcification. Retraction of the leaflets often makes these valves both regurgitant and stenotic. The inflammatory process of rheumatic fever rarely involves the aortic valve alone, usually involving the mitral valve as well. In idiopathic degenerative or senile aortic stenosis, grossly normal leaflets become calcified as a result of normal leaflet stress at the flexion points, causing leaflet immobility. This calcification may extend down onto the anterior mitral valve leaflet or upward along the aorta, occasionally causing coronary ostial stenosis.

Congenital valvular abnormalities may be clinically significant immediately after birth, as with unicuspid and dome-shaped valves. Patients born with a congenitally bicuspid aortic valve are uncommonly symptomatic in childhood but are prone to develop aortic stenosis early in adulthood. The bicuspid valve produces turbulent flow across the leaflets, leading to fibrosis, calcification, and stiffening. Patients with a bicuspid aortic valve are prone to develop aortic stenosis at an earlier age (fifth and sixth decades of life) than those with a tricuspid valve (seventh, eighth, and ninth decades) (Fig. 60-6).

Pathophysiology

In acquired aortic stenosis, there is a chronic, progressive narrowing of the aortic valve. As the valve narrows, the appropriate compensatory response of the left ventricle is hypertrophy. As the ventricle hypertrophies, it becomes stiffer as its compliance decreases; a higher left ventricular-end-diastolic pressure is needed to maintain the same volume of cardiac output. To achieve a sufficiently high left ventricular end-diastolic pressure (diastolic loading), the heart becomes increasingly dependent on the atrial kick; loss of the atrial kick, as occurs with atrial fibrillation, may result in a significant decline in cardiac output and acute hemodynamic decompensation.

Although left ventricular hypertrophy is an appropriate biologic response to an increasing afterload, it has detrimental effects. The combined effects of any of the following will culminate in increased myocardial oxygen demand: greater left ventricular muscle mass; decreased left ventricular compliance, resulting in greater ventricular wall tension; higher systolic ventricular pressure; and longer systolic ejection time. At the same time, coronary artery blood flow is compromised by increased wall tension compressing the vessels and by higher left ventricular diastolic pressure, which lowers the coronary artery perfusion pressure. These factors contribute to inadequate coronary arterial perfusion of the subendocardium, leading to chronic ischemia. In turn, chronic ischemia leads to cell death and fibrosis.

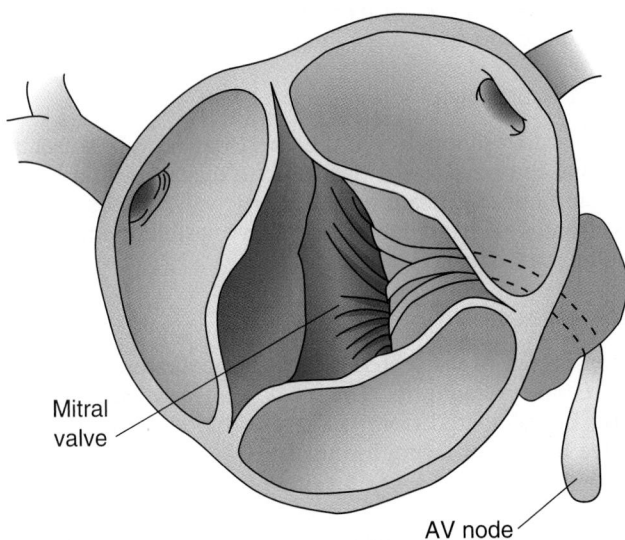

FIGURE 60-5. Surgical anatomy of the aortic valve. The commissure between the noncoronary and the left coronary leaflets lies anterior to the left bundle of His. Injury to this conduction tissue during aortic valve surgery may result in heart block. AV, atrioventricular.

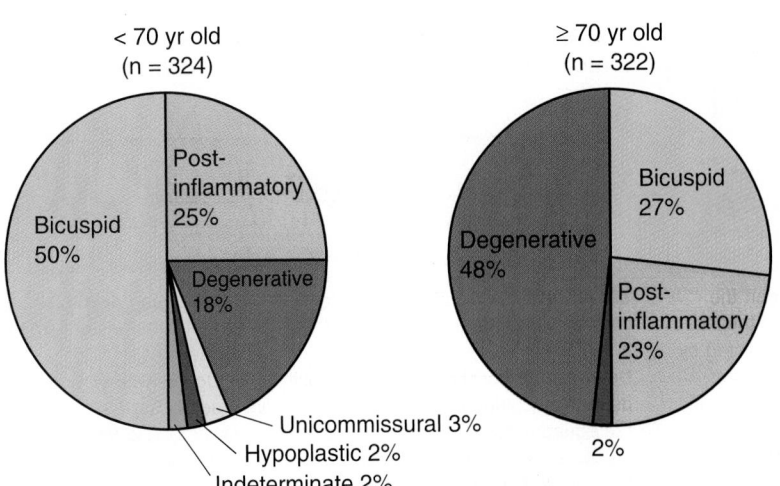

< 70 yr old
(n = 324)

Bicuspid 50%
Post-inflammatory 25%
Degenerative 18%
Unicommissural 3%
Hypoplastic 2%
Indeterminate 2%

≥ 70 yr old
(n = 322)

Bicuspid 27%
Degenerative 48%
Post-inflammatory 23%
2%

FIGURE 60-6. Causes of aortic stenosis as a function of age. (From Passik CS, Ackermann DM, Pluth JR, Edwards WD: Temporal changes in the causes of aortic stenosis: A surgical pathologic study of 646 cases. Mayo Clin Proc 62;119, 1987.)

Left ventricular hypertrophy may allow the heart to achieve a normal cardiac output under resting conditions.[26] To do so, however, a pressure gradient across the valve is required, and, as the aortic valve area becomes smaller, the gradient across the valve from left ventricle to aorta increases. This relationship of flow across the valve, valve area, and transvalvular pressure gradient is expressed in the Gorlin formula,[2] as follows:

$$AVA = F \div 44.5 \ (\sqrt{\Delta P})$$

where ΔP is the mean pressure gradient across the valve. Aortic valve flow (F) equals cardiac output in milliliters per minute divided by systolic ejection period in seconds per minute. AVA is the aortic valve area in square centimeters, and C is an empirical orifice constant, 44.5.

For quick calculations, this simplifies to the following:

$$AVA = Cardiac \ output \div \sqrt{Mean \ pressure \ gradient}$$

The relationship of flow across the aortic valve and the transvalvular pressure gradient is shown in Figure 60-7. As the valve area decreases to 1 cm², there is little change in the transvalvular gradient needed to generate the same flow, and patients frequently experience no symptoms. With a valve area of 0.8 cm², patients invariably develop symptoms.[5]

Diagnosis

SYMPTOMS

The classic symptoms of aortic stenosis are angina, syncope, and heart failure. Patients may not develop symptoms until the aortic valve area is about 1 cm²; this usually requires years. When this degree of stenosis has

been reached, however, it may quickly narrow farther, with rapid onset of symptoms and occasionally sudden death.

PHYSICAL EXAMINATION

Auscultation of the chest in patients with aortic stenosis reveals a systolic murmur best heard at the base of the heart that radiates into the carotid arteries; it may be difficult to distinguish the murmur of aortic stenosis from a bruit in the carotid artery. This murmur is associated with a slow, prolonged rise in the arterial pulse, called *pulsus parvus et tardus*. The murmur of severe aortic stenosis is soft and high pitched and is often described as a "sea gull" murmur.

ELECTROCARDIOGRAM

The electrocardiogram is notable for left ventricular hypertrophy in 85% of patients and evidence of left atrial enlargement in 80% of patients. T-wave inversion and ST-segment depression are common.

CHEST RADIOGRAPH

The cardiac silhouette on the chest radiograph is usually normal but may reveal poststenotic dilatation of ascending aorta or calcification of the aortic valve. Patients with symptoms of heart failure may have visible evidence of pulmonary edema.

ECHOCARDIOGRAM

The severity of aortic stenosis may be accurately estimated by echocardiography. The peak transvalvular gradient may be calculated from velocity of blood traversing the valve by the following formula:

$$Gradient = 4V^2$$

where V is the maximal measured blood velocity (in meters per second) across the valve. Echocardiographic determination of the velocity across the valve may also be used to calculate the aortic valve area using the continuity equation (Fig. 60-8).[27]

CARDIAC CATHETERIZATION

The most accurate measure of aortic stenosis is determined by cardiac catheterization. A catheter may be

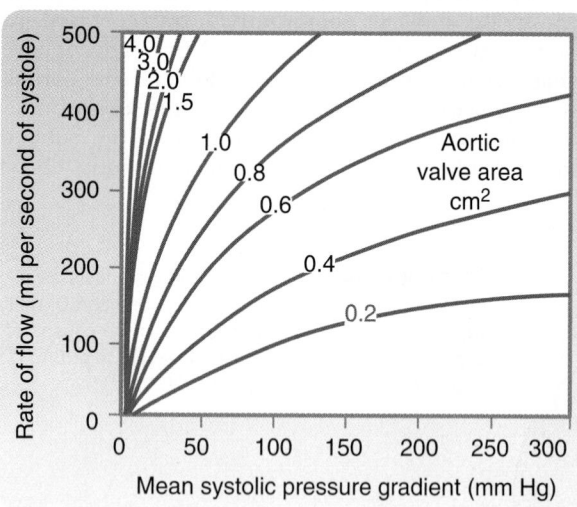

FIGURE 60-7. Chart illustrates the relationship between the mean systolic pressure gradient across the aortic valve and the rate of flow across the aortic valve per second of systole, as predicted by the Gorlin formula. As the valve area is reduced to about 0.7 cm², little increase in flow is achieved despite marked increases in mean gradient, thus defining "critical" aortic stenosis. (From Hurst JW, Logue RB, Schlant RC, Wenger NK (eds): Hurst's The Heart: Arteries and Veins, 3rd ed. New York, McGraw-Hill, 1974, p 811.)

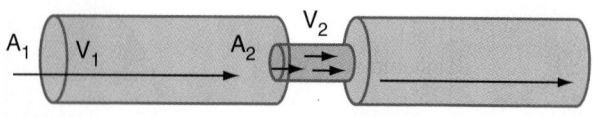

$$A_1 \times V_1 = A_2 \times V_2$$

FIGURE 60-8. Determination of aortic valve area using the continuity equation. For blood flow ($A_1 \times V_1$) to remain constant when it reaches a stenosis (A_2), velocity must increase to V_2. Determination of the increased velocity V_2 by Doppler ultrasound permits calculation of both the aortic valve gradient and solution of the equation for A_2. A, area; V, velocity. (From Carabello BA: Aortic stenosis. In Crawford MH [ed]: Current Diagnosis and Treatment in Cardiology. Norwalk, CT, Appleton & Lange, 1995, p 87.)

pulled back from the left ventricle to the aorta to determine the transvalvular pressure gradient. Simultaneous aortic and ventricular pressure measurements are more precise, however, and they are, in fact, mandatory when the patient is in atrial fibrillation. Patients older than 40 years of age should have coronary angiography before aortic valve surgery to exclude coronary artery disease.

Natural History

The natural history of aortic stenosis was reported by Ross and Braunwald.[28] Patient survival is not diminished until patients develop symptoms, which is associated with reduction in the aortic valve area from the normal 3 to 4 cm^2 to less than 1 cm^2. After symptoms develop, patient survival is limited. The three principal symptoms of aortic stenosis are angina, syncope, and congestive heart failure (Fig. 60-9).[28] Angina is usually the earliest symptom, and the mean survival of a patient with aortic stenosis and angina is 4.7 years. When a patient experiences syncope, survival is typically less than 3 years. Patients with dyspnea and congestive heart failure, in keeping with their associated left ventricular dysfunction, have a mean survival of 1 to 2 years. Congestive heart failure is the presenting symptom in nearly one third of patients.

Treatment

Aortic stenosis is a mechanical obstruction to flow from the left ventricle. The only effective therapy is aortic valve replacement. The existence of symptoms is an indication for valve replacement. Angina and syncope warrant elective surgical therapy, whereas congestive heart failure mandates urgent intervention. The issue of aortic valve replacement in patients with aortic stenosis who do not have symptoms is less clear. A small number of symptom-free patients do precipitously develop symptoms and then experience sudden death. Investigators agree, however, that in patients with aortic stenosis without symptoms, survival is excellent.[29-31] The risk for sudden death in symptom-free patients with a transvalvular gradient greater than or equal to 50 mm Hg or a valve area of less than 0.5 cm^2 is about 4% per year.[32] In one study of 113 symptom-free patients with critical aortic stenosis, 38 developed symptoms within 2 years. There were no sudden cardiac deaths in 118 patient-years of follow up.[31] To identify better those symptom-free patients likely to develop symptoms, a group of 123 adults (mean age, 63 years) with asymptomatic aortic stenosis with an initial mean transvalvular gradient of 30 mm Hg were prospectively followed. During 2.5 years of follow-up, there were no sudden deaths. Among patients with an initial transvalvular velocity of more than 4 m/sec, however, only 21% were alive and free of valve replacement at 2 years of follow-up.[33] Therefore, aortic valve surgery should be recommended to patients with symptomatic and asymptomatic disease who have evidence of left ventricular decompensation or a transvalvular gradient of more than 4 m/sec.

In patients with good ventricular function, aortic valve replacement is associated with an operative mortality rate of 2% to 8%.[10] Independent perioperative risk factors include age, left ventricular function, New York Heart Association class, and pulmonary function. After aortic valve replacement, the projected 10-year age-matched survival rate is 80% to 85%.[34] Symptoms are relieved in nearly all patients; however, improvement in ejection fraction and resolution of ventricular hypertrophy may require months to occur. Surgical mortality increases exponentially with decreasing left ventricular ejection fraction. Aortic valve replacement in patients with congestive heart failure carries a mortality rate of up to 24%.[10] In patients with aortic stenosis and coronary artery disease, valve replacement and myocardial revascularization should be performed concurrently. Perioperative mortality is higher in patients who do not undergo simultaneous coronary artery bypass grafting.

For patients with severe aortic stenosis who are not candidates for aortic valve replacement, percutaneous aortic balloon valvuloplasty may provide some palliation of aortic stenosis. In this procedure, either one or two balloon catheters may be passed through the aortic orifice and then inflated in an effort to "crack" the calcium that is retarding leaflet motion. The immediate results show an increase in the aortic valve area of only 50%, with a 3% to 10% mortality rate. The long-term results are even more

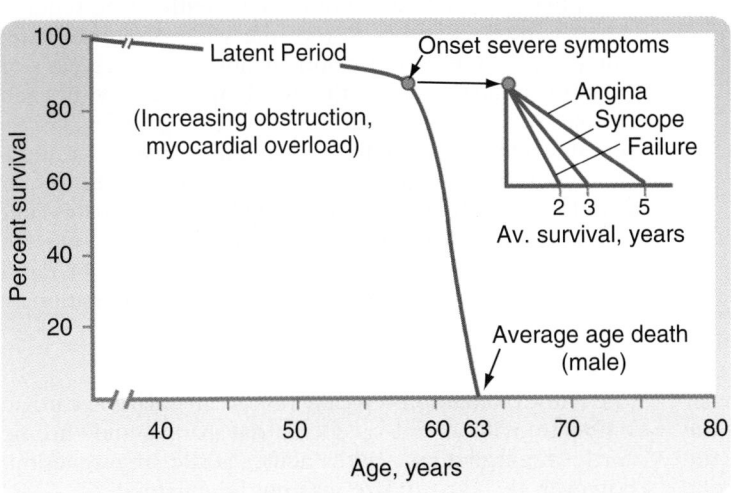

FIGURE 60-9. The natural history of medically treated aortic stenosis. (From Ross J, Braunwald E: Aortic stenosis. Circulation 37:V61, 1968. Copyright 1968, the American Heart Association.)

disappointing: 30% to 35% of patients have recurrent symptoms within 6 months, and the mortality rate is 60% within 18 months after the procedure.[35] There is a recurrence of symptoms, death, aortic valve restenosis, or a combination of these in more than half of patients within 6 months. The only potential role of aortic balloon valvuloplasty may be in aged, frail, and possibly senile patients whose long-term survival is poor.

Aortic Insufficiency

Etiology

Aortic insufficiency may result from disease of the valve leaflets or of the aortic root. Rheumatic fever may affect the leaflets by shortening the distance from the leaflet-free edge to the aortic annulus rather than by leading to commissural fusion. This prevents coaptation of the leaflets during diastole and results in a central leak. Congenital bicuspid aortic valves typically lead to aortic stenosis but may become regurgitant if a leaflet prolapses. Endocarditis may destroy leaflets.

Dilatation of the aortic root produces aortic regurgitation despite normal leaflet morphology by precluding leaflet coaptation. The most common of these conditions is annuloaortic ectasia, an idiopathic dilatation of the aortic root and annulus; as the sinuses of Valsalva and the proximal aorta dilate, diastolic coaptation of the leaflets is precluded, resulting in valvular insufficiency. Similarly, myxoid degeneration of the aortic root may lead to dilatation of the root, as seen in Marfan's syndrome, Ehlers-Danlos syndrome, and cystic medial necrosis. Those conditions may lead to leaflet redundancy, progressive prolapse, and regurgitation. Trauma or dissection of the aortic wall may produce aortic regurgitation if it leads to loss of commissural suspension and leaflet prolapse.

Pathophysiology

The aortic valve leaks during diastole, which lowers diastolic pressure and widens the pulse pressure. Because coronary blood flow occurs primarily in diastole, the lower diastolic blood pressure lowers coronary perfusion pressure. Unlike aortic stenosis, in which the pathologic process is left ventricular pressure overload, the pathophysiology of aortic insufficiency derives from left ventricular volume overload. The increased left ventricular end-diastolic volume (preload) results from filling through the mitral valve as well as the incompetent aortic valve. Patients with chronic aortic insufficiency may have the greatest left ventricular end-diastolic volume of any form of heart disease. Because left ventricular compliance is often increased, however, left ventricular end-diastolic pressure may or may not be elevated. With left ventricular dilatation, normal forward stroke volume and ejection fraction may be maintained by increased left ventricular end-diastolic and end-systolic volumes. According to the law of Laplace, this left ventricular dilatation increases the left ventricular wall tension required to develop systolic pressure. Such increased wall stress not only increases myocardial oxygen demand but also initiates left ventricular hypertrophy and increases left ventricular wall mass. Ultimately, myocardial fibrosis occurs.

With well-compensated aortic insufficiency, exercise may be tolerated because peripheral vascular resistance declines, lowering left ventricular afterload and increasing effective forward flow. At the same time, heart rate increases, which shortens diastolic time, thereby decreasing the regurgitant flow. Because the ventricle ultimately decompensates, however, the left ventricular end-diastolic volume increases even without an increase in aortic regurgitant volume. The end-systolic volume increases as the forward stroke volume declines because ventricular emptying is impaired; the ventricle fails (Fig. 60-10).

In severe aortic regurgitation, increased myocardial oxygen demand exceeds myocardial oxygen supply, causing ischemia despite normal coronary arteries. Increased left ventricular mass and wall tension occur concurrently with low diastolic pressures (low coronary perfusion pressure). Consequently, and particularly with exercise when the diastolic period shortens, coronary blood flow may not meet demand.

Diagnosis

SYMPTOMS

The compensatory mechanisms of aortic regurgitation may permit patients to remain symptom free for long periods. When these compensatory mechanisms begin to fail, however, left ventricular dysfunction becomes manifest, and patients experience symptoms of heart failure. Symptoms, generally the result of an elevation in left atrial pressure, include dyspnea on exertion, orthopnea, and paroxysmal nocturnal dyspnea. Nocturnal angina occurs occasionally as a result of a slow heart rate and an exceedingly low diastolic pressure with resultant poor coronary flow.

PHYSICAL EXAMINATION

The physical examination of patients with aortic regurgitation is distinctive because of the wide pulse pressure. The peripheral pulses rise and fall abruptly (Corrigan's or "water-hammer" pulse), the head may bob with each systole (de Musset's sign), and the capillaries visibly pulsate (Quincke's sign). Auscultation reveals a high-frequency decrescendo diastolic regurgitant murmur. A middle to late diastolic rumble may be heard (Austin-Flint murmur) and represents rapid antegrade flow across the mitral valve that closes prematurely as a result of rapid ventricular filling secondary to the aortic regurgitation.

CHEST RADIOGRAPH

The chest radiograph typically reveals an enlarged cardiac silhouette with an enlarged left atrial shadow and chronic aortic regurgitation. With acute aortic regurgitation, however, the cardiac size may not be enlarged.

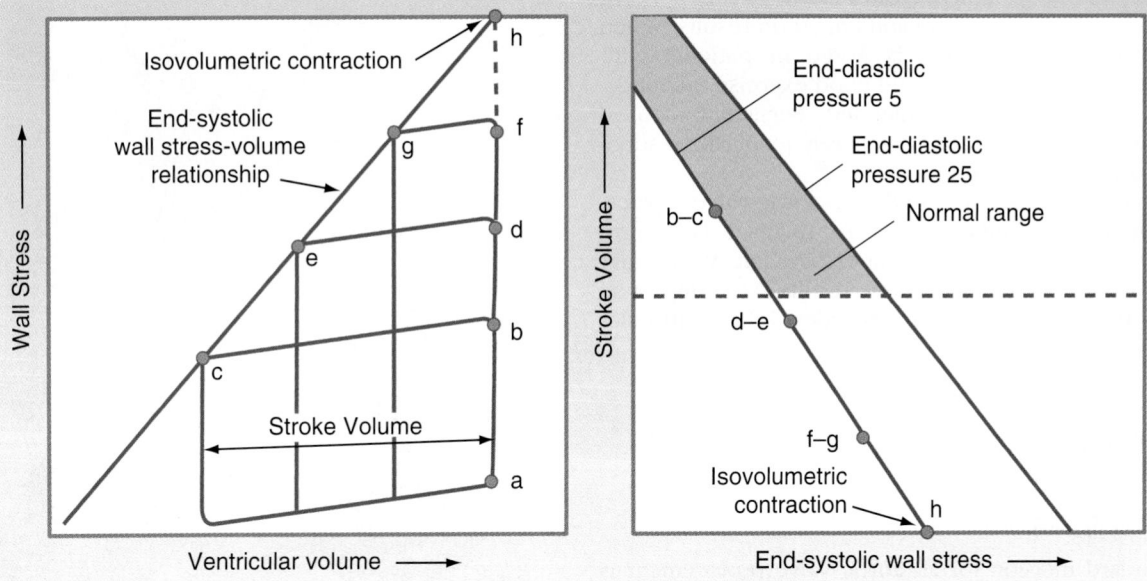

FIGURE 60-10. A series of stress-volume loops is shown. As afterload is progressively increased, wall stress is increased such that ejection, which initially occurred at b, now occurs at d, and then f. Stroke volume diminishes from b to c to d to e and then to f to g. At maximal wall stress h, there is no stroke volume but rather simply isovolumic contraction. On the right, the inverse relationship between stroke volume and end-systolic wall stress is portrayed. The two negative slopes represent families of stroke volumes generated with a left ventricular end-diastolic pressure of 5 mm Hg. (From Weber KT, Janicki JS, Shroff SG, Laskey W: The mechanics of ventricular function. Hosp Pract 18:113, 1983.)

ELECTROCARDIOGRAM

The electrocardiogram is usually nonspecific but may reveal left ventricular hypertrophy and left atrial enlargement.

ECHOCARDIOGRAPHY

Doppler echocardiography is the most accurate noninvasive technique to confirm the diagnosis of aortic regurgitation and to determine the severity of aortic insufficiency. As with mitral regurgitation, the severity is graded semiquantitatively as mild, moderate, or severe.

CARDIAC CATHETERIZATION

The severity of the aortic regurgitation may be visualized angiographically at cardiac catheterization. As with echocardiography, the severity is graded subjectively from mild to severe.

Natural History

Because of the compensatory mechanisms discussed previously, patients with chronic aortic regurgitation may be symptom free for long periods of time. In fact, patients with mild to moderate aortic regurgitation have an excellent long-term prognosis; the 10-year survival rate after diagnosis is 85% to 95%. Studies in which patients with severe aortic regurgitation have been included revealed a 70% 10-year survival rate and a 50% 20-year survival rate. Once symptoms of congestive heart failure occur, survival is markedly decreased; almost 50% of patients with left ventricular failure die within 2 years.

Treatment

Medical therapy for aortic regurgitation is based on a combination of afterload reduction and diuretics. Afterload reduction with nifedipine has been demonstrated to delay the need for aortic valve replacement.[20,36] Chronic use of angiotensin-converting enzyme inhibitors is more common for afterload reduction.

Patients with symptomatic aortic insufficiency require surgical therapy because their prognosis when treated medically is only a few years. Optimal timing of surgical intervention in patients with or without symptoms, however, may be a very difficult clinical decision.[32,37] Such patients may be successfully managed with diuretics and afterload reduction for long periods of time. Significant irreversible left ventricular systolic dysfunction may develop insidiously and before clinical evidence of congestive heart failure.

Therefore, symptom-free patients should be carefully followed noninvasively with serial echocardiography or radionuclide ventriculography for evidence of systolic dysfunction or decreasing ejection fraction. Aortic valve replacement should be performed before the left ventricle has irreversibly dilated. An end-systolic dimension greater than 55 mm Hg estimated by echocardiography has been associated with irreversible left ventricular dysfunction even after aortic valve replacement,[32,37] and aortic valve replacement should be performed before the ventricular dimension exceeds this. At cardiac catheterization, the end-systolic volume may help in determining management for these symptom-free patients. When end-systolic volume is less that 30 mL/m^2, prognosis after surgical therapy is excellent. Progressive systolic dysfunction with end-systolic volumes greater than 90 mL/m^2 have poor intermediate short-term and long-term results. When left ventricular dysfunction is noted in patients with diminished ejection fraction and good exercise tolerance, elective operation is recommended. Persistent medical management of these patients severely jeopardizes surgical outcome and ultimate prognosis.[20]

The mortality rate associated with aortic valve replacement for aortic insufficiency is 4% to 6%.[10] Long-term survival is dependent on preoperative left ventricular function. Both early and late results are improved when surgical intervention precedes left ventricular decompensation.

OPERATIVE TECHNIQUE

Aortic Valve Replacement

The standard incision for an aortic valve replacement is a median sternotomy. Once the incision has been made, the patient is connected to the cardiopulmonary bypass circuit by cannulation of the distal ascending aorta and the right atrium. Myocardial protection is achieved by topical myocardial cooling and retrograde cardioplegia. Most surgeons employ moderate systemic hypothermia (28°C to 32°C) during the operation.

After the heart fibrillates and the aortic cross-clamp has been applied, a transverse aortotomy is performed about 4 cm distal to the origin of the right coronary artery. The aortotomy is extended to the left and right, thus exposing the aortic valve (Fig. 60-11). The native aortic valve leaflets are excised, with great care to remove any particles of calcium. Once the leaflets have been removed, an appropriately sized prosthetic valve is sewn in place (see Fig. 60-11). The aortotomy is closed, cardiac function is resumed, and the patient is weaned from cardiopulmonary bypass.

Mitral Valve Replacement and Repair

The standard incision for mitral valve replacement is a median sternotomy, although a right thoracotomy may sometimes be appropriate for reoperations. The patient is connected to the arterial limb of the cardiopulmonary bypass circuit by cannulation of the distal ascending aorta. Venous drainage for the cardiopulmonary bypass is established by cannulation of the superior and inferior vena cavae (bicaval cannulation). Myocardial protection is achieved by topical myocardial cooling and retrograde cardioplegia. Most surgeons employ moderate systemic hypothermia (28°C to 32°C) during the operation.

Surgical exposure of the mitral may be particularly difficult and may be achieved by using several different incisions on the heart. The most common incision used to expose the valve is a transverse left atriotomy made in the right lateral wall of the left atrium, just anterior to the left pulmonary veins. An alternative surgical approach to the mitral valve is through an incision in the right

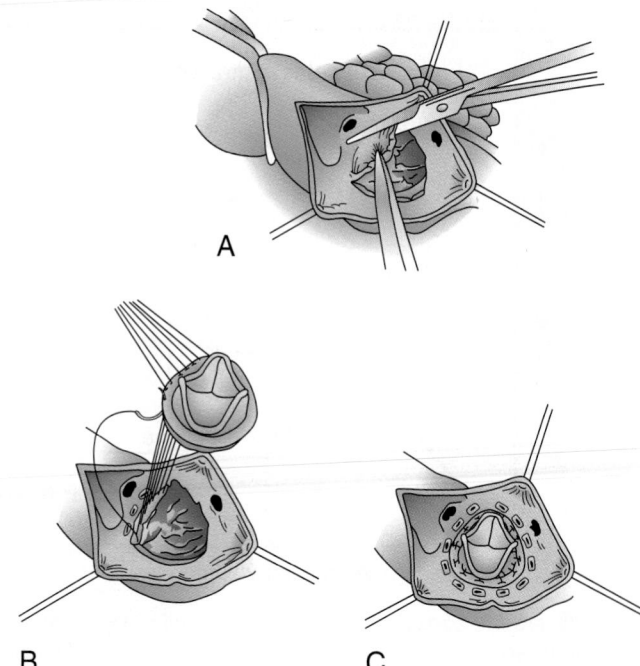

FIGURE 60-11.   Aortic valve replacement. The diseased leaflets are excised (**A**), and the prosthetic valve is sewn in place with interrupted pledgeted mattress stitches (**B** and **C**). (From Albertucci M, Karp RB: Prosthetic valve replacement. *In* Al Zaibag M, Duran CMG [eds]: Valvular Heart Disease. New York, Marcel Dekker, 1994, p 615.)

atrium, then through the interatrial septum, which provides excellent exposure to the left atrium and the mitral valve.

Once the mitral valve has been exposed, it must be carefully examined to determine whether it may be repaired or must be replaced. If the valve must be replaced, efforts should be made to preserve the native mitral valve apparatus if possible to preserve the mechanical continuity between the mitral valve annulus and the left ventricular apex. This may usually be accomplished by imbricating the leaflets of the mitral valve with sutures and placing an appropriately sized prosthetic valve within the annulus of the native valve (Fig. 60-12).

If the valve can be repaired, a variety of surgical techniques may be applied to restore valve competency. In most cases, an incompetent portion of one or both of the mitral valve leaflets must be resected and the leaflet then reapproximated (Fig. 60-13). At the time of mitral valve repair, the specific pathology responsible for the regurgitation is addressed. For example, a common cause of mitral regurgitation is a ruptured chorda tendinea. At the time of surgery, the prolapsed or flail leaflet subtended by the ruptured chorda tendinea is resected, the leaflet is primarily reapproximated, and the circumference of the mitral annulus is reduced by use of an annuloplasty ring. The adequacy of the repair is judged under direct vision by filling the left ventricle with saline under modest pressure. After the patient has been weaned from cardiopulmonary bypass, a final determination about the

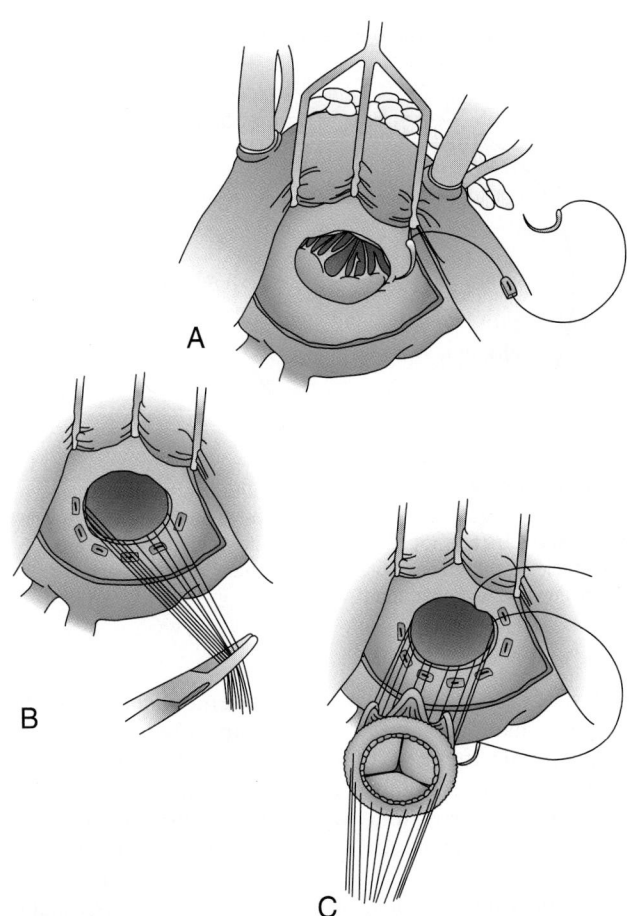

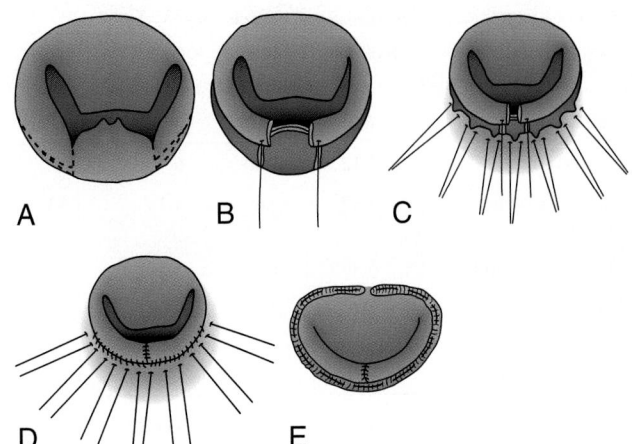

FIGURE 60-13. **A** to **E,** Example of mitral valve repair. In this example, the specific pathology is a flail posterior leaflet. It is repaired by resection of the flail segment, reapproximations of the leaflet, and reduction of the mitral annulus circumference using an annuloplasty ring. (From Perier P, Clausnizer B, Mistarz K: Carpentier "sliding leaflet" technique for repair of mitral valve: Early results. Ann Thorac Surg 57:383, 1994.)

FIGURE 60-12. **A** to **C,** Mitral valve replacement with preservation of the posterior leaflet. This preserves the annular-apical connection by means of the chordae tendineae. (From Albertucci M, Karp RB: Prosthetic valve replacement. *In* Al Zaibag M, Duran CMG [eds]: Valvular Heart Disease. New York, Marcel Dekker, 1994, p 613.)

TABLE 60-1.	Operative Mortality Rates			
	AVR	**MVR**	**AVR/CAB**	**MVR/CAB**
Society of Thoracic Surgeons	4.0	6.0	6.8	13.3
New York Cardiac Surgery Reporting System	3.3	6.2	7.1	12.8
Department of Veterans Affairs	3.9	5.9	7.3	11.8

AVR, Aortic valve replacement; MVR, mitral valve replacement; CAB, coronary artery bypass grafting.
From Grover FL, Edwards FH: Similarity between STS and New York State databases for valvular heart disease. Ann Thorac Surg 70:1143, 2000.

competency of the repair is made with use of intraoperative transesophageal echocardiography. The durability of a given mitral valve repair is largely dependent on the pathology responsible for the regurgitation. In most series, however, the failure rate of mitral valvuloplasty for mitral regurgitation is less than 1% per year. The mitral annulus is invariably dilated in surgical cases of mitral regurgitation, contributing to poor coaptation of the anterior and posterior mitral valve leaflets during systole. To return the enlarged mitral annular diameter to normal and to reinforce the leaflet repair, an annuloplasty ring is sewn to the perimeter of the mitral annulus.

SURGICAL OUTCOMES

According to the Society of Thoracic Surgeons (STS) National Cardiac Surgery Database, approximately 70,000 valve operations are performed in the United States annually.[38] The operative mortality rate for valve replacement

surgery is influenced by several variables, including which valve is replaced, whether coronary bypass surgery is performed at the same operation, and other patient-specific variables.

As shown in Table 60-1, the operative mortality rate in the STS Database for isolated aortic valve replacement is approximately 4%. On the other hand, the operative mortality rate for combined mitral valve replacement and coronary bypass grafting is much higher at 13%.[39,40] Other databases, including the New York State Department of Health Cardiac Surgery Reporting System and the Department of Veteran Affairs Cardiac Surgery Database, have found very similar mortality rates for cardiac valve operations.

The inherent risks all surgical procedures is influenced by patient-specific risk factors, and large databases such as those just mentioned provide the statistical power to identify patient-specific factors contributing to the risks of valve surgery. Table 60-2 lists some the major patient-specific risk factors for the most common valve operations from the STS Database.[38]

TABLE 60-2. Independent Risk Factors for Operative Mortality (Odds Ratios) for Valve Replacements				
Risk Factor	AVR	AVR+CAB	MVR	MVR+CAB
Salvage status	7.12	7.00	6.39	3.40
Dialysis-dependent renal failure	4.32	4.60	4.74	1.83
Emergency status	3.46	1.89	3.57	2.38
Non–dialysis-dependent renal failure	2.20	2.11	2.31	
First reoperation	1.70	2.40	1.45	1.31

AVR, Aortic valve replacement; MVR, mitral valve replacement; CAB, coronary artery bypass grafting.

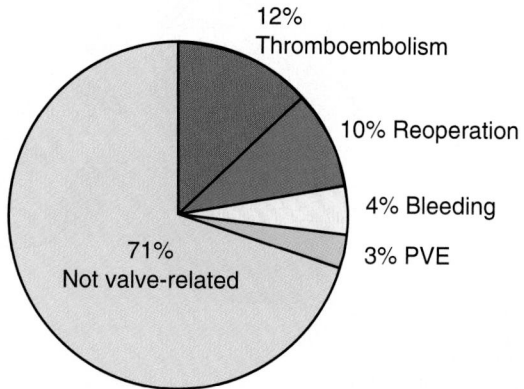

Cause of Valve-Related Death

12% Thromboembolism

10% Reoperation

4% Bleeding

3% PVE

71% Not valve-related

■ **FIGURE 60-14.** Causes of valve-related deaths after valve replacement surgery. Of all deaths after valve surgery 29% are valve related and 71% are not valve related. Valve-related deaths are attributable to thromboembolism, reoperation, bleeding, and prosthetic valve endocarditis (PVE).

CHOICE OF PROSTHETIC VALVES

For replacement of either the aortic or the mitral valve, there are two principal choices of cardiac valve prostheses: mechanical and bioprosthetic. Bioprosthetic valves are either porcine valves or bovine pericardial valves. The hemodynamic performances of the valves are similar. The operative risks associated with cardiac valve replacement are unassociated with the choice of prosthesis.

The choice of prosthetic valve must be patient specific. Mechanical valves have excellent durability and will perform indefinitely without structural deterioration, but because they are thrombogenic, mechanical valves obligate the patient to lifelong anticoagulation (warfarin sodium). Hence, the patient with a mechanical valve incurs the risks of chronic anticoagulation. Bioprosthetic valves do not require anticoagulation but will undergo structural deterioration. The durability of a bioprosthetic valve is inversely related to the patient's age at the time the valve is implanted. Should a bioprosthetic valve structurally deteriorate, the patient will require reoperation and valve re-replacement. It is important to recognize that approximately 80% of all aortic and mitral valve replacements in the United States are performed in patients above the age of 60 years. The patient's age should be considered because it may be dangerous to commit a geriatric patient to chronic anticoagulation.

The 10-year survival for patients after aortic valve replacement ranges from 40% to 70%, with an average in the literature of 50%.[42] The type of prosthesis does not impact survival, but other patient-specific factors such as age at operation and presence or absence of coronary artery disease do impact survival after valve replacement. Regardless of the type of prosthetic valve implanted, approximately one third of patients die of valve-related causes. An important consideration for the choice of valve for any patient is therefore how the individual patient may be affected by valve-related morbidity or mortality.

As shown in Figure 60-14, the principal causes of valve-related death after valve implantation include thromboembolism, reoperation, bleeding, and prosthetic valve endocarditis. The leading cause of valve-related death is thromboembolism. Largely because mechanical valves are thrombogenic, the risk of thromboembolism is greater with mechanical valves. At 10 years after aortic valve replacement, the risk of thromboembolism is 20% for mechanical valves[43] and 9% for bioprosthetic valves.[44]

The risk of prosthetic valve endocarditis is not different between mechanical or tissue valves. It is approximately 4% spread over the patient's lifetime. However, if prosthetic valve endocarditis does occur, it is associated with a 50% mortality rate.[45]

The choice of prosthetic valve must consider the risks of anticoagulation (mechanical valve) and the likelihood and risks of reoperation for structural valve deterioration (bioprosthetic valve). The risk of bleeding complications from chronic anticoagulation is between 1% and 2% per year. In fact, 4% of valve-related deaths result from bleeding (see Fig. 60-14). Bioprosthetic valves are indicated in patients with contraindications to anticoagulation because of occupation or because of coexistent medical conditions. Likewise, patients who are medically noncompliant or whose level of anticoagulation may not be closely monitored should not receive mechanical valves. Ten percent of valve-related deaths result from reoperation, and this fact steers some patients and physicians away from bioprosthetic valves. However, data demonstrate that if actual rather that actuarial statistical methodology is used to evaluate the likelihood of reoperation for structural valve deterioration of a bioprosthetic valve, the incidence of reoperation is less than 15% for patients older than 60 years (Fig. 60-15).[46] A joint task force from the American Heart Association and the American College of Cardiology has provided some recommendations to help balance these risks. The task force recommended that tissue valves be placed in the aortic position in patients older than 65 years and in the mitral position in patients older than 70 years.[20]

An advance in the treatment of aortic valve disease in young patients is the pulmonary autograft procedure (Ross procedure).[46] Initially performed by Ross in 1967,

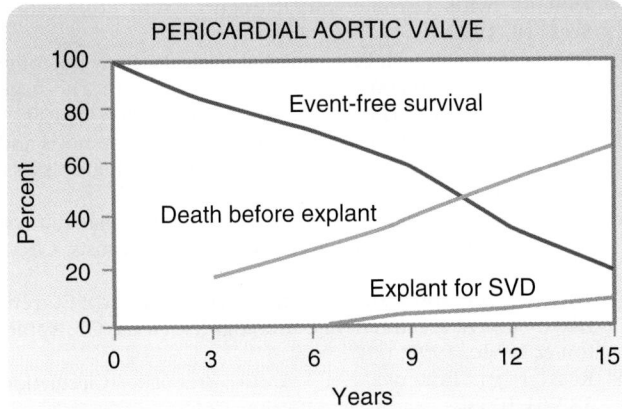

FIGURE 60-15. After aortic valve replacement with a bovine pericardial bioprosthesis, the risk of undergoing reoperation for structural valve deterioration (SVD) is less than 15% at 15 years. (From Banbury MK, Cosgrove DM III, White JA, et al: Age and valve size effect on the long-term durability of the Carpentier-Edwards aortic pericardial bioprosthesis. Ann Thorac Surg 72:753, 2001.)

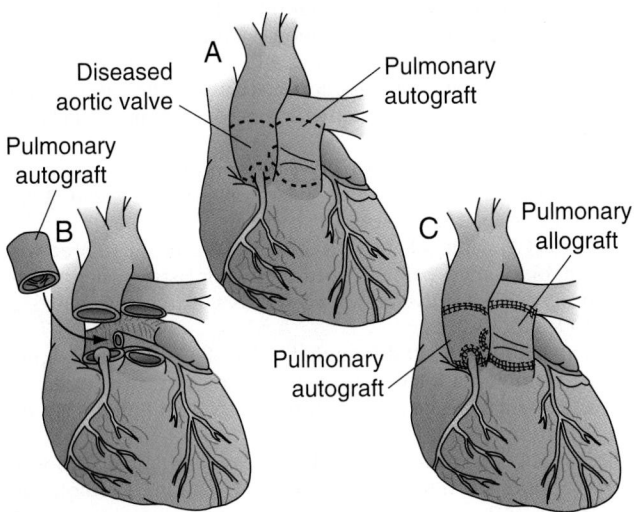

FIGURE 60-16. **A** to **C,** Pulmonary autograft (Ross) procedure. The diseased aortic valve and proximal aortic root are excised. The pulmonary valve and the main pulmonary artery (autograft) are excised, and the autograft is used to replace the aortic root. The coronary artery buttons are reimplanted into the pulmonary root. A pulmonary homograft is then used to reconstruct the right ventricular outflow tract. (From Kouchoukos NT, Davila-Roman VG, Spray TL, et al: Replacement of the aortic root with a pulmonary autograft in children and young adults with aortic-valve disease. N Engl J Med 330:1, 1994.)

the procedure has gained wider acceptance during the past two decades. The procedure entails use of the patient's own pulmonary root as an autograft to replace the diseased aortic valve and root. A cryopreserved pulmonary homograft is then used to replace the patient's pulmonary root (Fig. 60-16). Although it is a technically demanding procedure, the operative mortality rate associated with the Ross procedure is 5% or less and is not dif-

ferent from that associated with isolated aortic valve replacement when performed by experienced surgeons.[48] Intermediate-term data suggest excellent function of the pulmonary autograft; need for autograft reoperation is rare within the first postoperative decade.[49] The durability of the pulmonary homograft is excellent; 80% of patients are free of homograft dysfunction at 16 years.[49] Chronic anticoagulation is not required, and the risk of valve-related complications is extremely low.[50]

Selected References

Banbury MK, Cosgrove DM III, White JA, et al: Age and valve size effect on the long-term durability of the Carpentier-Edwards aortic pericardial bioprosthesis. Ann Thorac Surg 72:753, 2001.

> **This study highlights the importance of using actual rather than actuarial statistical methodology in the assessment valve-related events after prosthetic valve implantation. The paper highlights the fact that even though bioprosthetic valves may structurally deteriorate, the likelihood of reoperation is low because a majority of patients may die before that.**

Bonow RO, Carabello B, De Leon AC, et al: ACC/AHA guidelines for the management of patients with valvular heart disease. J Am Coll Cardiol 32:1486, 1998.

> **This is a very comprehensive reference that addresses virtually all aspects of valvular heart disease, including indications for surgery.**

Jamieson WRE, Edwards FH, Bero J, et al: Cardiac valve replacement surgery: The Society of Thoracic Surgeons national database experience. Ann Thorac Surg 67:43, 1999.

> **Using the power of the STS database, this report provides the foundation for risk-stratification for valve replacement surgery.**

Ross J Jr, Braunwald E: Aortic stenosis. Circulation 38:V61, 1968.

> **This classic study provides the natural history of aortic stenosis.**

Zellner JL, Kratz JM, Crumbly AJ III, et al: Long-term experience with the St. Jude Medical valve prosthesis. Ann Thorac Surg 68:1210, 1999.

> **The majority of valves implanted are mechanical valves. This report provides a comprehensive picture of valve-related morbidity and mortality after mechanical valve implantation.**

References

1. Westaby S, Bosher C: Development of surgery for valvular heart disease. *In* Westaby S, Bosher C: Landmarks in Cardiac Surgery. Oxford, England, Isis Medical Media, 1997, p 139.
2. Gorlin R, Gorlin SG: Hydraulic formula for calculation of area of stenotic mitral valve, other cardiac valves, and central circulatory shunts. Am Heart J 41:1, 1951.
3. Delahaye F, Delahaye J, Ecochard R, et al: Influence of associated valvular lesions on long-term prognosis of mitral stenosis: A 20-year follow-up of 202 patients. Eur Heart J 12(Suppl B):77, 1991.

4. Kawanishi DT, Rahimtoola SH: Mitral stenosis. *In* Rahimtoola SH (ed): Valvular Heart Disease and Endocarditis. Atlas of Heart Diseases. St. Louis, CV Mosby, 1996.

5. Carabello BA, Crawford FA: Valvular heart disease. N Engl J Med 337:32, 1997.

6. Olesen KH: The natural history of 271 patients with mitral stenosis under medical treatment. Br Heart J 24:349, 1962.

7. Reyes VP, Raju BS, Wynne J, et al: Percutaneous balloon valvuloplasty compared with open surgical commissurotomy for mitral stenosis. N Engl J Med 331:229, 1994.

8. Palacios IF, Sanchez PL, Harrell LC, et al: Which patients benefit from percutaneous mitral balloon valvuloplasty? Prevalvuloplasty and post valvuloplasty variables that predict long-term outcome. Circulation 105:1465-1471, 2002.

9. Cohen JM, Glower DD, Harrison JK, et al: Comparison of balloon valvuloplasty with operative treatment for mitral stenosis. Ann Thorac Surg 56:1254,1993.

10. Kirklin JW, Barratt-Boyes BG: Mitral valve disease with or without tricuspid valve disease. *In* Kirklin JW, Barratt-Boyes BG (ed): Cardiac Surgery, 2nd ed. New York, Churchill Livingstone, 1993, p 425.

11. David TE, Omran A, Armstrong S, et al: Long-term results of mitral valve repair for myxomatous disease with and without chordal replacement with expanded polytetrafluoroethylene sutures. J Thorac Cardiovasc Surg 115:1279, 1998.

12. Hetzer R, Drews T, Siniawski H, et al: Preservation of papillary muscles and chordae during mitral valve replacement: Possibilities and limitation. J Heart Valve Disease 4(Suppl II):115, 1995.

13. Straub U, Feindt P, Huwer H, et al: Mitral valve replacement with preservation of the subvalvular structures where possible: An echocardiographic and clinical comparison with cases where preservation not possible. J Thorac Cardiovasc Surg 42:2, 1994.

14. Lee SJK, Bay KS: Mortality risk factors associated with mitral valve replacement: A survival analysis of 10 year follow-up data. Can J Cardiol 7:11,1991.

15. Rapaport E: Natural history of aortic and mitral valve disease. Am J Cardiol 35:221, 1975.

16. Rosen SF, Borer JS, Hochreiter C, et al: Natural history of the asymptomatic patient with severe mitral regurgitation secondary to mitral valve prolapse and normal right and left ventricular performance. Am J Cardiol 74:374, 1994.

17. Carabello BA: Clinical assessment of systolic dysfunction. ACC Curr J Rev 3:25, 1994.

18. Crawford MH, Souchek J, Oprian CA, et al: Determinants of survival and left ventricular performance after mitral valve replacement: Department of Veterans Affairs Cooperative Study on valvular heart disease. Circulation 81:1173, 1990.

19. Wisenbaugh T, Skudicky D, Sareli P: Prediction of outcome after valve replacement for rheumatic mitral regurgitation in the era of chordal preservation. Circulation 89:191, 1994.

20. Bonow RO, Carabello B, De Leon AC, et al: ACC/AHA guidelines for the management of patients with valvular heart disease. J Am Coll Cardiol 32:1486, 1998.

21. Horskotte D, Schulte HD, Bircks W, Strauer BE: The effect of chordal preservation on late outcome after mitral valve replacement: A randomized study. J Heart Valve Dis 2:148, 1993.

22. Tishler MD, Cooper KA, Rowen M, LeWinter MM: Mitral valve replacement versus mitral valve repair: A Doppler and quantitative stress echocardiographic study. Circulation 89:132, 1994.

23. Rozich JD, Carabello BA, Usher BW, et al: Mitral valve replacement with and without chordal preservation in patients with chronic mitral regurgitation. Circulation 86:1718, 1992.

24. Bolling SE, Deeb GM, Brunsting LA, Bach DS: Early outcome of mitral valve reconstruction in patients with end-stage cardiomyopathy. J Thorac Cardiovasc Surg 109:676, 1995.

25. Waller B, Howard J, Fess S: Pathology of aortic stenosis and pure aortic regurgitation: A clinical morphologic assessment. Clin Cardiol 17:85, 1994.

26. Laskey WK, Kussmaul WG, Noordergraaf A: Valvular and systemic arterial hemodynamics in aortic valve stenosis. Circulation 91:473, 1995.

27. Carabello BA: Aortic stenosis. *In* Crawford MH (ed): Current Diagnosis and Treatment in Cardiology. Norwalk, CT, Appleton & Lange, 1995, p 87.

28. Ross J Jr, Braunwald E: Aortic stenosis. Circulation 38:V61,1968.

29. Carabello BA: Evaluation and management of patients with aortic stenosis. Circulation 105:1746, 2002.

30. Carabello BA: Indications for valve surgery in asymptomatic patients with aortic and mitral stenosis. Chest 108:1678, 1995.

31. Pellikka PA, Nishimura RA, Bailey KR, Tajik AJ: The natural history of adults with asymptomatic hemodynamically significant aortic stenosis. J Am Coll Cardiol 15:1012, 1990.

32. Bonow RO, Lakatos E, Maron BJ, Epstein SE: Serial long-term assessment of the natural history of asymptomatic patients with chronic aortic regurgitation and normal left ventricular systolic function. Circulation 84:1625, 1991.

33. Otto CM, Burwash IG, Legget ME, et al: Prospective study of asymptomatic valvular aortic stenosis: Clinical, echocardiographic, and exercise predictors of outcome. Circulation 95:2262, 1997.

34. Lindblom D, Lindblom U, Qvist J, Lundstrom H: Long-term relative survival rates after heart valve replacement. J Am Coll Cardiol 15:566, 1990.

35. Otto CM, Mickel MC, Kennedy JW, et al: Three-year outcome after balloon aortic valvuloplasty: Insights into prognosis of valvular aortic stenosis. Circulation 89:642, 1994.

36. Scognamiglio R, Rashimtoola SH, Fasoli G, et al: Nifedipine in asymptomatic patients with severe aortic regurgitation and normal left ventricular function. N Engl J Med 331:689, 1994.

37. Zile MR: Chronic aortic and mitral regurgitation: Choosing the optimal time for surgical correction. Cardiol Clin 9:239,1991.

38. Jamieson WRE, Edwards FH, Bero J, et al: Cardiac valve replacement surgery: The Society of Thoracic Surgeons national database experience. Ann Thorac Surg 67:43, 1999.

39. Grover FL, Edwards FH: Similarity between the STS and New York state databases for valvular heart disease. Ann Thorac Surg 70:1143, 2000.

40. Edwards FH, DeLong ER, Shroyer AL, et al: Prediction of operative mortality following valve replacement surgery. J Am Coll Cardiol 35(Suppl A):529, 2000.

41. Hannan EL, Racz MJ, Jones RH, et al: Predictors of mortality for patients undergoing cardiac valve replacements in New York State. Ann Thorac Surg 70:1212, 2000.

42. Peterseim DS, Cen YY, Cheruvu S, et al: Long-term outcome after biologic versus mechanical aortic valve replacement in 841 patients. J Thorac Cardiovasc Surg 117:890, 1999.

43. Zellner JL, Kratz JM, Crumbley AJ III, et al: Long-term experience with the St. Jude Medical valve prosthesis. Ann Thorac Surg 68:1210, 1999.

44. Cosgrove DM, Lytle BW, Taylor PC, et al: The Carpentier-Edwards pericardial aortic valve: Ten-year results. J Thorac Cardiovasc Surg 110:651, 1995.

45. Grover FL, Cohen DJ, Oprian C, et al: Determinants of the occurrence of and survival from prosthetic valve endocarditis: Experience of the Veterans Affairs Cooperative Study on Valvular Heart Disease. J Thorac Cardiovasc Surg 108:207, 1994.

46. Banbury MK, Cosgrove DM III, White JA, et al: Age and valve size effect on the long-term durability of the Carpentier-Edwards aortic pericardial bioprosthesis. Ann Thorac Surg 72:753, 2001.

47. Kouchoukos NT, Davila-Roman VG, Spray TL, et al: Replacement of the aortic root with a pulmonary autograft in children and young adults with aortic-valve disease. N Engl J Med 330:1, 1994.

48. Elkins RC: Pulmonary autograft. *In* Franco KL, Verier ED (eds): Advanced Therapy in Cardiac Surgery. St. Louis, BC Decker, 1999, p 1283.

49. Elkins RC, Lane MM, McCue C: Pulmonary autograft reoperations: Incidence and management. Ann Thorac Surg 62:450,1996.

50. Fullerton DA, Fredericksen JW, Sundaresan RS, Horvath KA: The Ross procedure in adults: Intermediate-term results. Ann Thorac Surg 76:471-476, 2003; discussion 476-477.

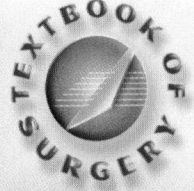

CHAPTER 61

THORACIC VASCULATURE (WITH EMPHASIS ON THE THORACIC AORTA)

Tam T. T. Huynh, M.D., Anthony L. Estrera, M.D., Charles C. Miller III, Ph.D., and Hazim J. Safi, M.D.

EMBRYONIC DEVELOPMENT

During embryonic development, the thoracic vasculature undergoes many stages of formation. Vascular connections may form and then vanish, capillaries fuse and produce veins or arteries, and blood flow may reverse direction several times. None of the major vessels of the adult, other than the aorta, manifest as single trunks in the embryo. During this period aortic anomalies may arise as a result of structures that fail to regress or to develop.[1]

The systemic arterial system originates from the heart and aortic sac as six pairs of ventrally situated arteries, or aortic arches, that pass laterally around the gut to form paired dorsal vessels, or dorsal aortae (Fig. 61-1). The two dorsal aortae are initially separated by the neural tube and notochord, which is in contact with the gut. With separation from the gut, cross connections develop between the two dorsal aortae until a plexus of vessels is formed. Progression of this plexus leads to coalescence and then fusion of the aorta dorsally.

The six paired embryonic aortic arches develop and regress during maturation to eventually become distinct structures of the thoracic aorta. The first and second arches are nearly gone by the time the third arch appears.

The dorsal end of the second arch becomes the stem of the stapedial artery, while the remainder of this arch also disappears. The third pair of arches becomes the common carotid and proximal portion of the internal carotid arteries. The right fourth arch becomes the proximal portion of the right subclavian artery, while the left fourth arch constitutes a portion of the aortic arch between the left common carotid and left subclavian arteries. The fifth embryonic arch ultimately disappears on both sides. The right sixth arch becomes the proximal part of the right pulmonary artery, and the left sixth arch becomes the proximal part of the left pulmonary artery while the distal portion persists as the ductus arteriosus.

Toward the end of the fourth week the connection between the bulbus cordis, the foremost of the three parts of the primitive heart of the embryo, and the first pair of arches extends and becomes the truncus arteriosus. The truncus arteriosus becomes the aortic and pulmonary roots. The aortic sac becomes the ascending aorta, brachiocephalic artery, and aortic arch up to the origin of the left common carotid. The cranial portion of the right dorsal aorta becomes the right subclavian artery, and the left dorsal aorta becomes the distal arch. The remaining

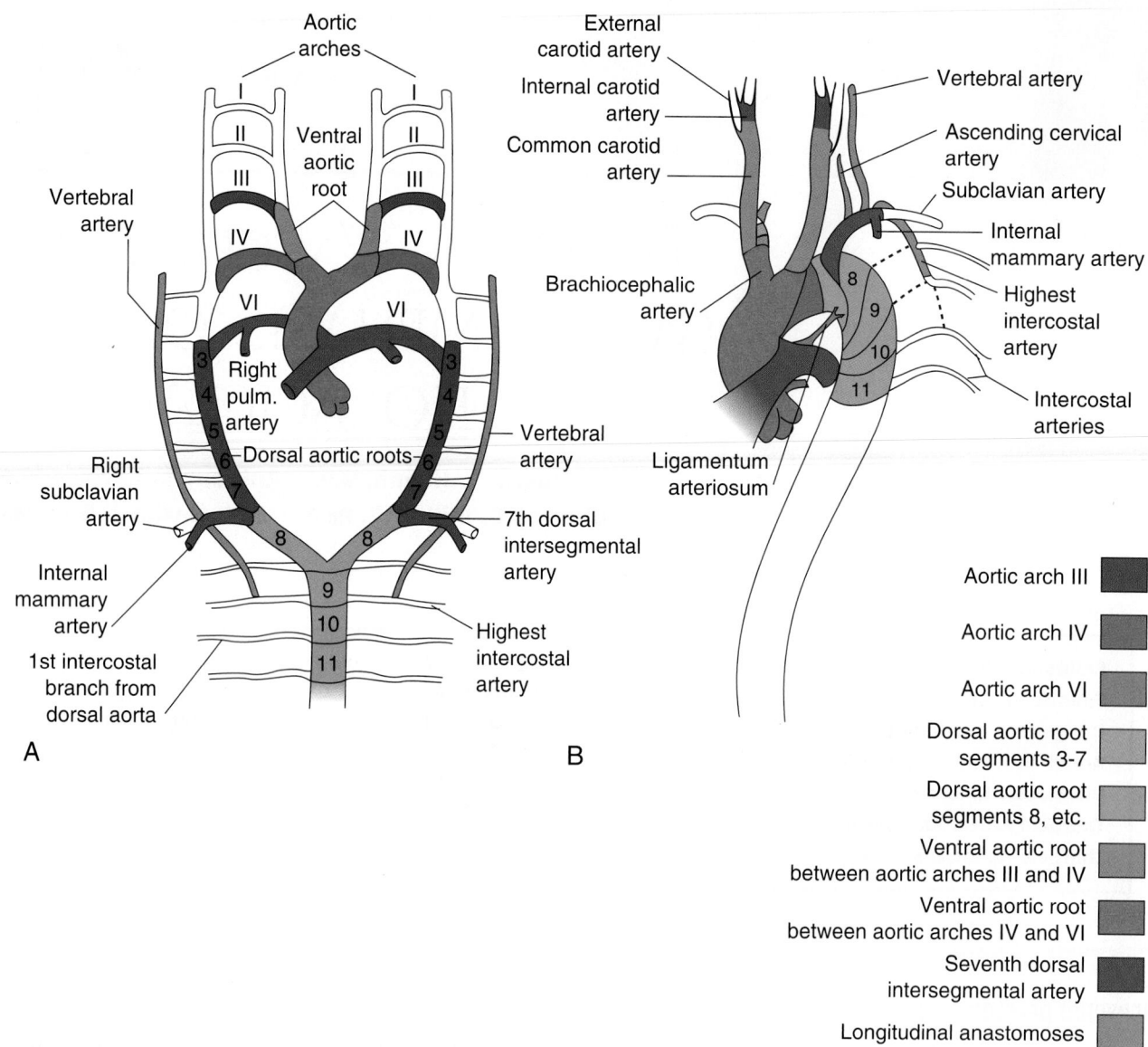

Aortic arches

Ventral aortic root

Vertebral artery

Right pulm. artery

Dorsal aortic roots

Right subclavian artery

Internal mammary artery

1st intercostal branch from dorsal aorta

A

Vertebral artery

7th dorsal intersegmental artery

Highest intercostal artery

External carotid artery

Internal carotid artery

Common carotid artery

Brachiocephalic artery

Ligamentum arteriosum

B

Vertebral artery

Ascending cervical artery

Subclavian artery

Internal mammary artery

Highest intercostal artery

Intercostal arteries

Aortic arch III

Aortic arch IV

Aortic arch VI

Dorsal aortic root segments 3-7

Dorsal aortic root segments 8, etc.

Ventral aortic root between aortic arches III and IV

Ventral aortic root between aortic arches IV and VI

Seventh dorsal intersegmental artery

Longitudinal anastomoses

FIGURE 61-1. A diagram of the various components of the aortic arch in the human embryo (**A**). Portions that regress are shown in outline; portions that develop into adult human aorta and branches (**B**) correspond by cross-hatching and gray tones. (Redrawn from illustration by Carl Clingman after Barry A: Aortic arch derivatives in the human adult. Anat Rec 111:221-228, 1951.)

right and left dorsal aortae fuse to create the descending thoracic and abdominal aorta. The right and left seventh intersegmental arteries develop into the respective subclavian arteries.

Early embryonic veins can be segregated into three main groups: the vitelline, umbilical, and cardinal vein complexes. At about the same time as the arterial system develops, the venous system arises from a capillary network that eventually coalesces to form channels, then distinct vessels. The primitive cardinal system, from which the veins of the thorax arise, is formed by anastomoses with umbilical veins and vitelline veins at the posterior end of the developing heart. The early symmetrical disposition of the common cardinal vein, right and left precardinal, postcardinal, subcardinal, and supracardinal

veins eventually enlarge, combine, or retrogress to become the asymmetrical arrangement of the inferior and superior vena cavae, brachiocephalic, azygos, and hemiazygos veins.

FUNCTIONAL ANATOMY

The base or root of the aorta begins in the ventricular outflow tract of the heart and ends in the abdomen at the aortic bifurcation, which divides into the right and left common iliac arteries. The aortic root houses the aortic valve, sinuses of Valsalva, and the right and left coronary arteries. The anterior tubular segment or ascending aorta emerges from the root. The ascending aorta curves posteriorly and to the left as the aortic arch, from which emerge the brachiocephalic, left common carotid, and left subclavian arteries. The descending thoracic aorta begins distal to the left subclavian artery and ends at the 12th intercostal space. Branches of the descending thoracic aorta are the intercostal, bronchial, and esophageal arteries. The artery of Adamkiewicz is the main source of blood to the lower part of the anterior spinal artery, which in turn supplies much of the blood to the spinal cord. There is significant variability in the origin of this critical artery, but it usually branches from an intercostal artery that connects to the aorta between the 9th and 12th intercostal space. As the aorta exits the thorax, it enters the abdomen through the aortic hiatus. The *thoracoabdominal aorta* refers to the entire descending thoracic and abdominal aorta.

CONGENITAL ANOMALIES

Aortic anomalies are often multiple and frequently occur in siblings. The most common right-to-left branching pattern of the aortic arch is brachiocephalic artery, left common carotid artery, and left subclavian artery (75%). Less frequently, (20%), the brachiocephalic and left common carotid artery share a common origin from the arch proximal to the left subclavian artery (bovine arch). Least common (3%) are separate starting points for the brachiocephalic, left common carotid, left vertebral, and left subclavian arteries. Fourteen other configurations have been described in cadavers, with as many as four primary branches or as few as two primary branches.[2]

A vascular ring is a condition in which the anomalous configuration of the arch and/or associated vessels forms a partial or complete ring around the trachea or esophagus, causing compression. Anomalies of the aortic arch may be characterized as left, right, or double aortic arch. These arch configurations may be associated with a left or right ligamentum arteriosum and a left or right retroesophageal subclavian artery. Patients with a right aortic arch and left ligamentum frequently develop a diverticulum known as *Kommerell's diverticulum* associated with the left retroesophageal subclavian artery. A retroesophageal or aberrant right subclavian artery forms as the result of a persistent right eighth segmental artery and regression of the right fourth aortic arch, which is the opposite of normal development. The aberrant right subclavian artery arises from the descending thoracic aorta, distal to the left subclavian artery, traversing posterior to the trachea and esophagus in front of the vertebral column. As originally described by the English surgeon, David Bayford, in 1787, this anomaly may lead to compression of the esophagus by the right subclavian artery, promoting obstructed deglutition, or dysphagia lusoria.

Patent ductus arteriosus is the most common vascular anomaly. The ductus arteriosus, which carries fetal blood from the left ventricle to the aorta, constricts at birth due to raised oxygen tension. At 1 month the ductus arteriosus is usually obliterated, ultimately forming the fibrous ligamentum arteriosum. A patent ductus arteriosus can prompt shunting from the systemic to the pulmonary circulation, leading to pulmonary hypertension.

Coarctation refers to a narrowing of the aortic wall and lumen. The most common of these anomalies is the postductal type, which occurs distal to the ligamentum, compared to the preductal type that occurs just proximal to a patent ductus arteriosus. The etiologic mechanism of coarctation is unknown, but constriction is thought to occur as the result of the incorporation of oxygen-sensitive ductal tissue into the wall of the thoracic aorta. Chronic coarctation generates extensive formation of intercostal artery collaterals, proximal hypertension, and rib notching.

Venous Anomalies

Venous anomalies can occur in connections of either the systemic or pulmonary veins. The most common is persistent left superior vena cava, which drains into the right atrium through an enlarged orifice of the coronary sinus. The persistent left superior vena cava forms when the left anterior cardinal vein fails to regress, but it communicates with the right atrium via the left horn of the sinus venosus, which becomes the coronary sinus. The absence of a left brachiocephalic vein (innominate vein) and a small right superior vena cava can signal the presence of persistent left superior vena cava. The most common anomaly of the inferior vena cava is an interruption of its abdominal course with drainage to the heart via the azygos or hemiazygos venous system. Anomalies of the pulmonary veins connect to sites individually or in combination. A totally anomalous connection is usually a confluence of veins behind the left atrium that joins either to the superior vena cava, the coronary sinus, or the portal venous system crossing the diaphragm.

AORTIC DISEASES AND ETIOLOGY

Aortic Aneurysm and Dissection

The most common diseases of the aorta are aneurysm and dissection, which are classified by anatomic location (Figs. 61-2 to 61-4). An *aortic aneurysm* is defined as a localized or diffuse aortic dilation that exceeds 50% of the normal aortic diameter. Factors associated with aneurysm formation include advanced age, hypertension, smoking, arteriosclerosis, and aortic dissection. Acute aortic dissection is the most common catastrophic event involving the aorta. A tear in the intima allows blood to escape from the true lumen of the aorta, dissects the aortic layers, and reroutes some of the blood through a newly formed false channel. The weakened aortic wall is highly susceptible to acute rupture and chronically prone to progressive dilation. Arterial hypertension and connective tissue disorders (particularly Marfan syndrome) may predispose patients to dissection. The cause of the initial tear remains unknown, but the histology of the aortic wall typically exhibits medial degeneration.

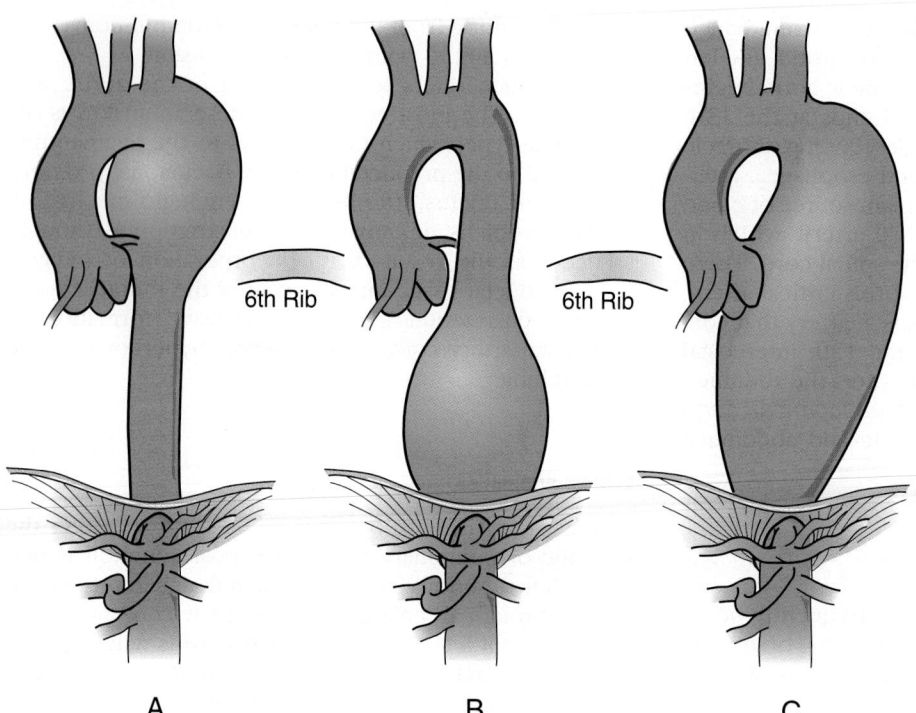

FIGURE 61-2. Classification of descending thoracic aortic aneurysm: Type **A,** distal to the left subclavian artery to the 6th intercostal space. Type **B,** 6th intercostal space to above the diaphragm (12th intercostal space). Type **C,** entire descending thoracic aorta, distal to the left subclavian artery to above the diaphragm (12th intercostal space). (©2002 Carl Clingman.)

6th Rib   6th Rib

A   B   C

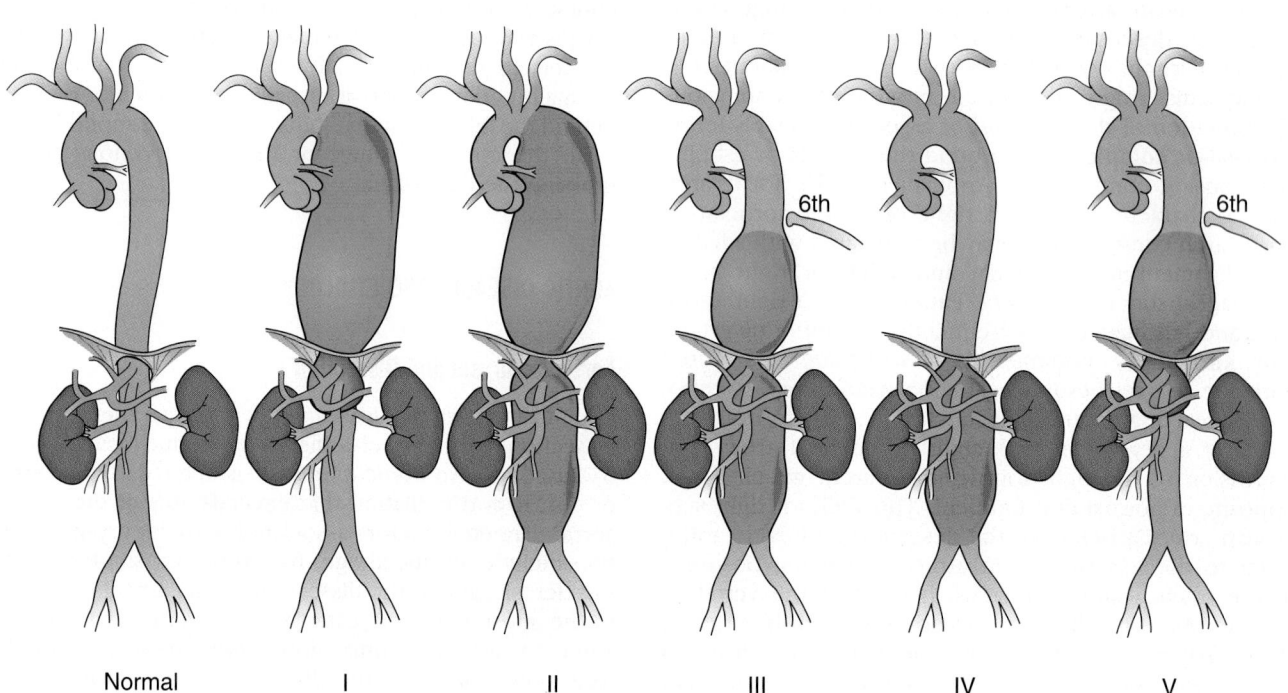

Normal   I   II   III   IV   V

FIGURE 61-3. Normal thoracoabdominal aorta *(far left)* and aneurysm classification: Extent I, distal to the left subclavian artery to above the renal arteries; extent II, distal to the left subclavian artery to below the renal arteries; extent III, from the 6th intercostal space to below the renal arteries; extent IV, the 12th intercostal space to below the renal arteries (total abdominal aortic aneurysm); and extent V, below the 6th intercostal space to just above the renal arteries. (Redrawn from illustration by Carl Clingman.)

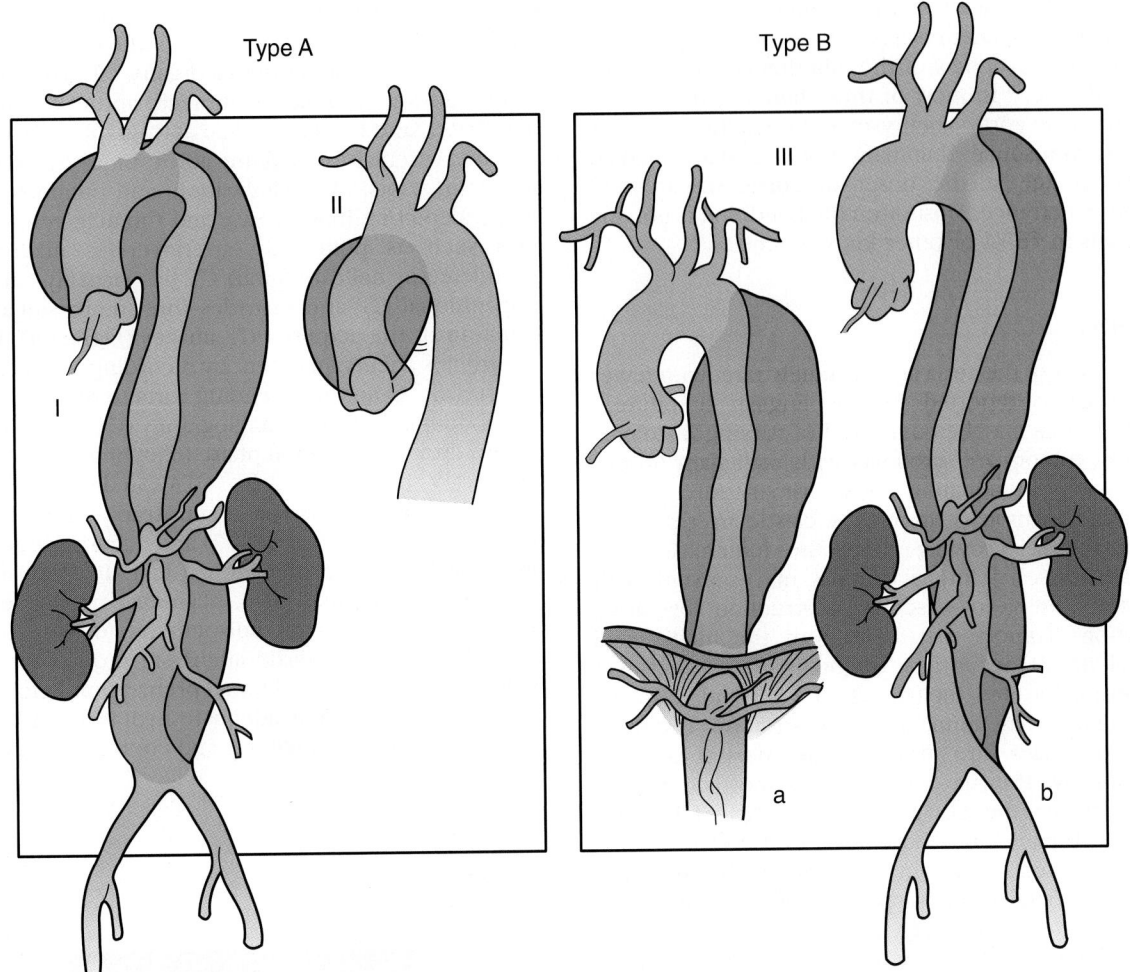

FIGURE 61-4.   Aortic dissection classification based on the site of the intimal tear. *Left,* Stanford type A, DeBakey types I and II. *Right,* Stanford type B, DeBakey type III. (Redrawn from illustration by Carl Clingman.)

Conventionally, aortic dissection is termed *acute* when a clinical diagnosis is made within 14 days following the onset of symptoms and *chronic* after 14 days. When a dissection involves the ascending aorta, it is commonly referred to as a *Stanford type A*. Dissection without involvement of the ascending aorta—most often with the intimal tear in the descending thoracic aorta—is referred to as a *Stanford type B* or *DeBakey type III*. DeBakey classification further distinguishes ascending aortic dissection *with* involvement of the descending thoracic aorta (DeBakey type I) from ascending aortic dissection *without* involvement of the descending thoracic aorta (DeBakey type II).

Approximately 20% of aortic aneurysms and dissections are related to hereditary connective tissue disorders.[3] Marfan syndrome is the most common of these disorders, occurring in the worldwide population at a frequency of 1 in 5000.[4] Skeletal, ocular, and cardiovascular complications characterize Marfan syndrome, with aortic aneurysm and dissection as the major cause of morbidity and mortality.

Aortic dilation observed in Marfan patients is the result of defects in a specific component of elastic fibers known as *fibrillin-1* (*FBN1*). Although inherited in an autosomal dominant manner, one fourth of patients do not have a family history and have the syndrome as the result of a new mutation.[5] One hundred thirty-seven mutations have been entered in the international Marfan database (*http://www.umd.necker.fr*). Some patients who do not fulfill the usual diagnostic criteria may still have *FBN1* mutations and thoracic aortic aneurysm and dissection.[6]

A number of other known genetic syndromes predispose individuals to thoracic aortic aneurysm and dissection, such as Turner's syndrome, Ehlers-Danlos syndrome, and polycystic kidney disease. Mutations in fibrillin-2, or *FBN2*, cause congenital contractural arachnodactyly, a syndrome closely related to Marfan syndrome. Familial aggregation studies have indicated that up to 19% of thoracic aortic aneurysm and dissection patients without one of the genetic syndromes described earlier have other affected family members.[7,8] These studies support the hypothesis that genetic factors predispose individuals who do not have a known genetic syndrome to thoracic aortic aneurysm and dissection.[9]

Families in which multiple members have thoracic aortic aneurysm and dissection have been reported in the literature. Aortic imaging of family members of patients with thoracic aortic aneurysm and dissection has provided us with the best overview of the inheritance and features of this syndrome.[10] In most of these families, the phenotype for thoracic aortic aneurysm and dissection is inherited in an autosomal dominant manner with marked variability in age at the onset of aortic disease and decreased penetrance. Most often the condition is not due to mutations in FBN1 or other known genes.

Aortic Tumors

Primary tumors of the aorta are extremely rare, with fewer than 100 cases reported in the English literature.[11] Although tumors may be composed of varying histologic types, most tumors are sarcomas with malignant fibrous histiocytoma predominating. Most primary sarcomas of the aorta and pulmonary artery (the elastic arteries) arise from the intima, growing along the lumen, forming polypoidal masses.[12] Intimal tumors may present with symptoms related to vascular obstruction or distal embolization. Tumors that arise from the medial and adventitial layers occur less frequently. Symptoms are often nonspecific and include chest pain and dyspnea. Because tumors may mimic aneurysm or aortic occlusive disease, diagnoses are often made postmortem or intraoperatively. Primary aortic tumors most commonly present between the 6th and 7th decades of life and involve the thoracic and abdominal aorta equally. Malignant tumors, such as sarcomas, are generally associated with a poor prognosis and respond poorly to chemotherapy or radiation. However, surgical resection of any sarcoma of the vasculature, when feasible, may result in cure or palliation of symptoms.[13]

DIAGNOSTIC IMAGING

Before computed tomography (CT) scanning and, later, magnetic resonance (MR) imaging became widely available, aortography was performed routinely in aortic aneurysm and aortic dissection patients. In acute traumatic aortic injury, aortography typically can identify irregularity of the aorta, focal outpouching, and accumulation of contrast medium at the region of irregularity. The aortogram can detect aortic root dilation and define the condition of the coronary arteries. Aortography used to be the gold standard imaging modality for confirming the diagnosis of aortic dissection, because it can identify the aorta's true and false lumen and determine tear sites and the extent of dissection. However, false-negative aortograms may occur when the false lumen is not opacified, when there is simultaneous opacification of the true and false lumen, or when the intimal flap is not seen. CT scan has replaced aortography for the evaluation of the thoracic aorta and its branches. Aortography is currently reserved for patients with suspected aortic branch occlusive disease and is often performed in conjunction with cardiac catheterization.

Over the past decade technical advances in CT and MR have vastly improved thoracic vasculature imaging.

CT, a digitally based radiographic technique, can quickly produce images of multiple slices of the body's soft tissue, neurovasculature, and internal organs. CT is our preferred technique for imaging the thoracic aorta. It is less invasive, faster, and less costly than aortography. CT evaluates systemic vasculature, defining aortic anomalies, dissection aneurysm, clots, and calcification; and pulmonary vasculature, depicting lung disease and thoracic venous anomalies such as pulmonary arteriovenous malformation. Multidetector helical (spiral) CT has virtually supplanted conventional CT and provides three-dimensional reconstruction of the acquired CT images (Fig. 61-5). CT scan determines aneurysm extent by recording the aortic diameter serially, from the ascending aorta to the arch and thoracoabdominal aorta. CT angiography (CTA) acquires axial images during the arterial phase following a bolus of intravenous (IV) contrast medium. CTA can distinguish the difference between the false and true lumen in aortic dissection (Figs. 61-6 and 61-7) and accurately detect the proximal location of the intimal tear. It can also reveal associated thrombus and/or inflammatory changes in the aortic wall. CT scans are indispensable for patient followup and tracking of aortic aneurysm growth rate. Some patients may require additional preparation before undergoing CT scan, such as adequate hydration and premedication for renal insufficiency and contrast allergy.

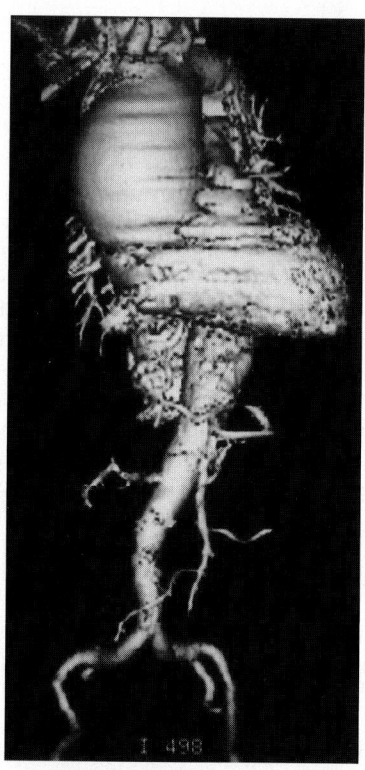

FIGURE 61-5. Reformatted three-dimensional CT image of the aorta and its major branches in a patient with large ascending aortic aneurysm.

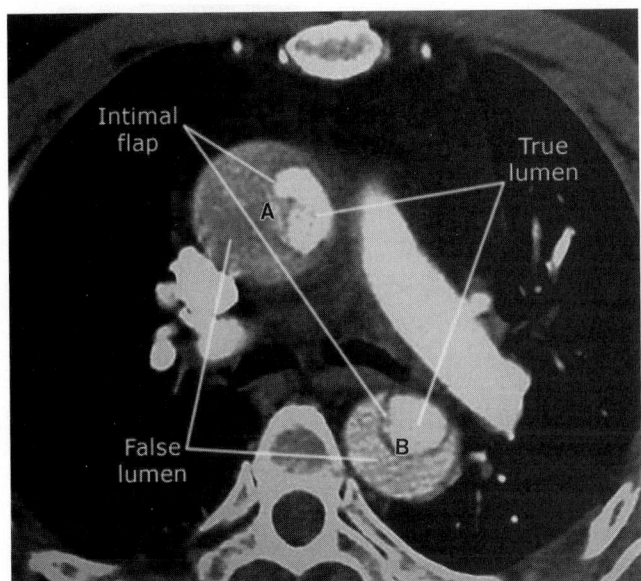

FIGURE 61-6. CT scan of type A aortic dissection with intimal flap in the ascending (A) and descending (B) segments of the aorta.

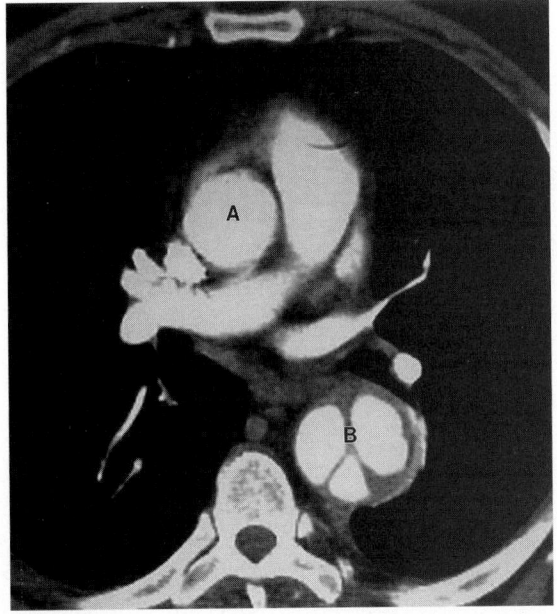

FIGURE 61-7. CT scan of type B aortic dissection with normal ascending aorta (A) and multiple partitions of the lumen in the descending thoracic aorta (B).

MR does not require iodinated contrast medium and can be performed safely in patients with impaired renal function. An image is detected by radiofrequency signals when the body's hydrogen atoms react to the MR's strong magnetic field. MR, particularly three-dimensional gadolinium-enhanced MR angiography, can clearly identify the morphology of the aortic and pulmonary vascula-

ture. MR can reliably assess the site and extent of nonvalvular obstructive lesions of the aorta (i.e., coarctation, interruption of the aortic arch, and supravalvular stenosis). MR is the imaging modality of choice for aortic tumors because of its diverse capabilities, which include multiplanar imaging for excellent anatomic definition of the heart, pericardium, mediastinum, and lungs and improved morphologic differentiation between tumor tissue and surrounding cardiovascular, mediastinal, or pulmonary tissues. Patients with internal metallic hardware (such as pacemakers and orthopedic rods) cannot undergo MR. Higher cost and longer examination times are other limitations of MR.

Other imaging modalities for thoracic vasculature include transesophageal echocardiography (TEE), intravascular ultrasound (IVUS), and intraoperative epiaortic ultrasound (IEUS). IVUS can provide an image of the anatomy within the aortic walls. A miniature catheter tip inserted percutaneously, incorporated with an ultrasound device, can identify intimal defects, atheromatous plaques, calcification, and laminated thrombi. TEE uses a miniature high-frequency ultrasound transducer placed on a probe and inserted into the lower esophagus. Because the lower esophagus is located close to the posterior of the heart, there is no image interruption by lung tissue. TEE has the advantage of portability and quick execution. TEE is highly sensitive in aortic pathology diagnosis (Fig. 61-8) and is an excellent intraoperative tool, able to report cardiac structure and function. It can assess ventricular function and reliably survey aortic valve disease, aortic dilation, ascending aortic aneurysm, dissection, thrombi, atherosclerotic disease, and mitral valve disease. Of particular value during cardiac operations that employ cardiopulmonary bypass, TEE and IEUS can detect atheromas of the thoracic aorta. Aortic aneurysms of the transverse aortic arch cannot be identified by TEE because of the interposition of the air-filled trachea and bronchi. Although TEE can be done at the bedside or intraoperatively, the technique requires a skilled anesthesiologist or cardiologist to interpret study data. Contraindications are esophageal obstruction, diverticulum, or varices, active upper gastrointestinal bleed, or cervical spine disease.

THORACIC AORTIC ANEURYSMS

Natural History and Incidence

Population screening for thoracic aneurysm is not a practical endeavor; consequently, we have no prospective or randomized analyses of the natural history of aortic aneurysms or dissection. However, population rates can be estimated by monitoring a defined population for health system utilization, which was the approach taken by Bickerstaff and associates[14] in the well-described population of Rochester, Minnesota.[15] The study was conducted on a population-based historical cohort from records collected between 1951 and 1980. Only 11% underwent surgical treatment. The time of diagnosis was abstracted from medical records, and patients were

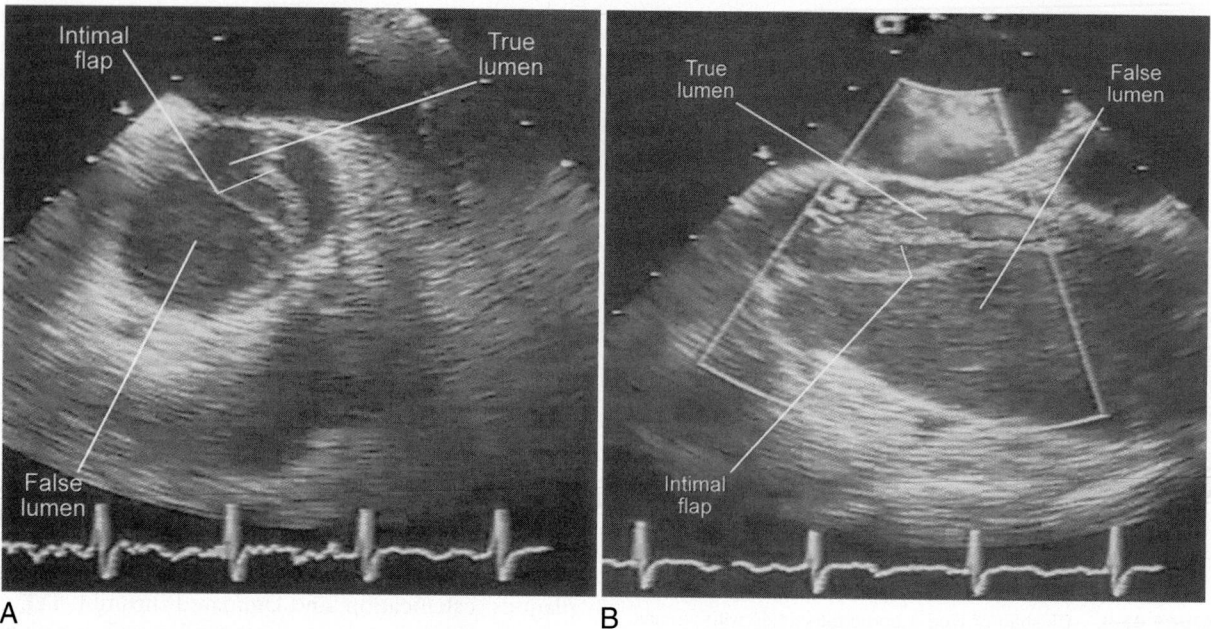

FIGURE 61-8. Transesophageal echocardiography of dissection of the ascending aortic aorta in cross-section (**A**) and saggital color-Doppler mode view demonstrate no flow in the large false lumen (**B**). (**A** and **B**, Courtesy of Mihai Croitaru, MD, University of Texas–Houston.)

"followed" historically until death. This study reported a population incidence of detected thoracic aortic aneurysms estimated to be 5.9 new aneurysms per 100,000 person-years in 1982. In a follow-up to Bickerstaff, Clouse and colleagues studied the same Rochester, Minnesota, cohort starting in 1980, where the previous study had left off, through 1994.[16] These authors estimated the incidence to be 10.4 per 100,000 person-years, or twice higher than the 1951 to 1980 rate after age adjustment. The significant difference from the 1982 study was almost certainly due to improved case ascertainment brought about by the increased use of thoracic CT scanning after 1980.

Untreated, 75% to 80% of thoracic aortic aneurysms will eventually rupture (Fig. 61-9). Five-year untreated survival ranges between 10% and 20%, with a median time to rupture in nondissecting aneurysms between 2 and 3 years. Although women develop thoracic aortic aneurysms 10 to 15 years later than men, rupture occurs more frequently in women. Age has also been associated with increased risk of rupture. Aneurysm size significantly influences the rate of rupture. When an ascending aortic aneurysm reaches a diameter of 6 cm, the risk of rupture is 31%. For the descending thoracic aorta the critical size is around 7 cm with a 43% risk of rupture.[17]

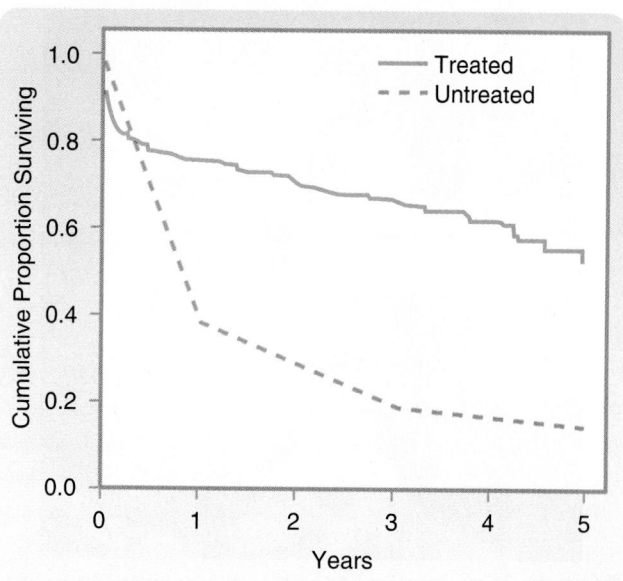

FIGURE 61-9. Thoracoabdominal aortic aneurysm: comparison of survival rates in untreated (Bickerstaff and associates[15]) versus surgically treated patients (Safi and colleagues[40]).

Clinical Presentation

The clinical manifestations of thoracic aortic aneurysms vary widely. In most patients an aortic aneurysm is discovered incidentally without specific symptoms, because the slow growth of aneurysms is typically silent. Chronic

back pain is a frequent complaint in patients, but pain related to musculoskeletal causes is usually difficult to differentiate from pain related to aneurysm. Large aortic aneurysms can put pressure on adjacent structures and can create symptoms such as hoarseness due to vocal cord paralysis related to compression of the left recurrent laryngeal or vagus nerves, dyspnea from mild to severe upper airway compromise from compression of the tracheo-bronchial tree, pulmonary hypertension due to pressure on the pulmonary artery, and dysphagia caused by compression of the esophagus. Direct erosion of the aneurysm into the adjacent tracheobronchial tree and/or esophagus results in fistulization and bleeding (hemoptysis or hematemesis). A thoracoabdominal aortic aneurysm may press against the stomach and cause weight loss related to early satiety. Associated atherosclerotic occlusive disease of the visceral or renal arteries may cause intestinal angina or arterial hypertension, respectively. A widened pulse pressure with a diastolic murmur may alert the physician to an ascending aortic aneurysm with aortic valve insufficiency.

When to Operate

Patients who are diagnosed with aneurysms greater than 5 cm or larger or with rapid aneurysm enlargement are considered for surgical repair. A sudden change in the characteristics or the severity of the pain is significant and should alert clinicians to the possibility of rapid aneurysm expansion, leakage, or rupture. When considering aneurysm growth rate and the risk of rupture, the Marfan patient or other patients with inherited collagen vascular disorders or familial patterns of aortic dissection must be given special attention. More than 90% of deaths in Marfan patients are related to complications of aneurysms or dissections of the thoracic aorta. Marfan patients are often considered for surgery at an earlier stage of aneurysm development due to faster rates of aneurysm growth and rupture at smaller diameters.[18]

THORACIC AORTIC DISSECTION

Clinical Presentation

Abrupt excruciating pain epitomizes the onset of acute aortic dissection.[19] Chest pain is present in about two thirds of patients and back pain invariably accompanies dissections that begin distal to the aortic arch. Pain may migrate as the dissection progresses distally. Patients with ascending aortic dissections may have associated aortic valve insufficiency with dyspnea and a diagnostic loud pansystolic murmur. Other acute symptoms and signs related to aortic branch occlusion can cause cerebral infarction, myocardial infarction, abdominal malperfusion, limb ischemia, and paraplegia. The distinctions between acute and chronic aortic dissections, types A and B, have important clinical implications (Fig. 61-10). The 14-day period after onset of dissection has been empirically designated the acute phase because mortality and morbidity rates are highest, and surviving patients usually stabilize at the end of this period. Serious life-threatening complications typically occur during the acute phase, and

surgery on the acutely dissected aorta is high risk, associated with considerable bleeding due to the friability of the aortic wall.

Acute Phase

Acute type A dissection most often requires emergency surgical repair because of the associated high risk of death due to rupture, tamponade, and/or aortic valve insufficiency (see later section, Surgical Treatment and Results: Proximal Thoracic Aorta).[20] The patient who is unstable with suspected type A acute aortic dissection is immediately transferred to the operating room and evaluated by TEE. If dissection is confirmed then repair is undertaken at once (Fig. 61-11). Surgery in the case of the hemodynamically stable patient is less urgent, and the patient is first transferred to an acute care setting until confirmation of the diagnosis is made.

For acute type B aortic dissection the treatment of choice is generally medical therapy aimed at pain control and the correction of hypertension (see later section, Medical Treatment). Patients are admitted to an intensive care unit and observed closely. Surgical repair is most often reserved for dissection complicated by aortic rupture, abdominal malperfusion, limb ischemia, intractable pain, or uncontrollable hypertension. Approximately 20% of patients with acute type B aortic dissection require surgical therapy (see later section, Surgical Treatment and Results: Distal Thoracic Aorta).

MEDICAL TREATMENT

We initiate antihypertensive or so-called anti-impulse therapy for all patients with acute dissection, whether type A or type B. An arterial line is placed for close monitoring of the systemic arterial blood pressure. We use esmolol for IV β blockade (range 50 to 300 μg/kg/min) titrated to heart rate (60 to 80 beats/min), systolic blood pressure (<120 mm Hg), and mean arterial blood (80 mm Hg). We prefer esmolol, a β₁ selective agent, because of its ease of titration due to its short-acting nature. β Blockade can also be achieved with propranolol, nonselective β₁ and β₂ blocker, (2 to 5 mg IV every 4 to 6 hours) or labetolol, a nonselective β₁ and β₁ as well as α₁ blocker (20 mg IV slow injection followed by 40 mg IV every 10 minutes).

Patients whose hypertension is refractory to β blockade may require combination therapy with other agents. Our choice with combination therapy includes a calcium-channel blocker, nicardipine (5 to 15 mg/hour IV infusion), nitroglycerin (5 μg/min IV infusion), and sodium nitroprusside (0.5 to 5 μg/kg/min IV infusion). Since potent unloading agents such as sodium nitroprusside may actually cause an increase in the dp/dt (rate of rise of aortic pressure) when used alone, it is important to use it in combination with a β-blocking agent. In addition, sodium nitroprusside must be used with caution since it may be associated with cyanide toxicity and paraplegia.

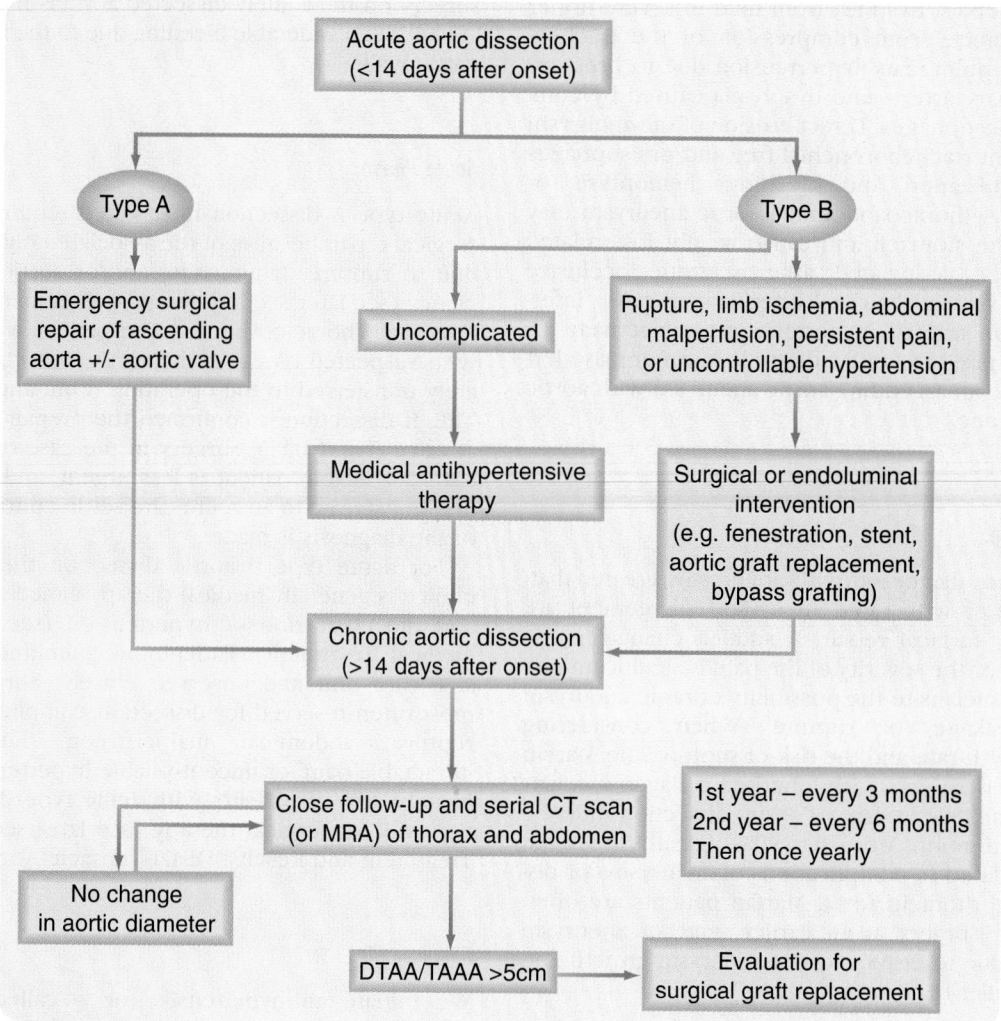

FIGURE 61-10. Algorithm for treatment of aortic dissection. MRA, magnetic resonance angiography; DTAA, descending thoracic aortic aneurysm; TAAA, thoracoabdominal aortic aneurysm.

Chronic Phase

All patients who survive the acute phase of aortic dissection, whether type A or type B, must be followed closely. Serial imaging of the dissected aorta should be obtained prior to discharge from the acute-care hospital, and then at 1 month, 3 months, 6 months, 12 months, and yearly thereafter. Compliance with chronic antihypertensive therapy decreases the incidence of subsequent hospitalization and may reduce the progression of aortic dilation. In most patients, acute pain resolves and symptoms subside. Recurrent chest and back pain may indicate sudden aortic expansion and/or impending rupture. All symptomatic patients should be evaluated for surgical repair. Approximately 20% to 40% of patients who survive the acute phase of aortic dissection will develop significant aneurysmal dilation of the aorta within 2 to 5 years, requiring surgical graft replacement when the maximal aortic diameter reaches 5 to 6 cm to prevent rupture. The extent of surgical graft replacement depends on the extent of the aortic aneurysm. In general, we replace all

aneurysmal aortic segments, leaving the nonaneurysmal part (with or without dissection) in situ.

SURGICAL TREATMENT AND RESULTS: PROXIMAL THORACIC AORTA

Aortic Root

The technical innovations of the early 1950s permitted the first successful operations of the aortic root. Cardiopulmonary bypass, which replaces the pumping action of the heart and the gas exchange function of the lungs, was essential. The patient is placed on cardiopulmonary bypass after the chest is opened with a median sternotomy (Fig. 61-12) and either the femoral artery or ascending aorta is cannulated. Retrograde cardioplegic perfusion via the coronary sinus provides myocardial protection throughout the procedure, keeping the myocardial temperature below 15°C. Venting through the left superior

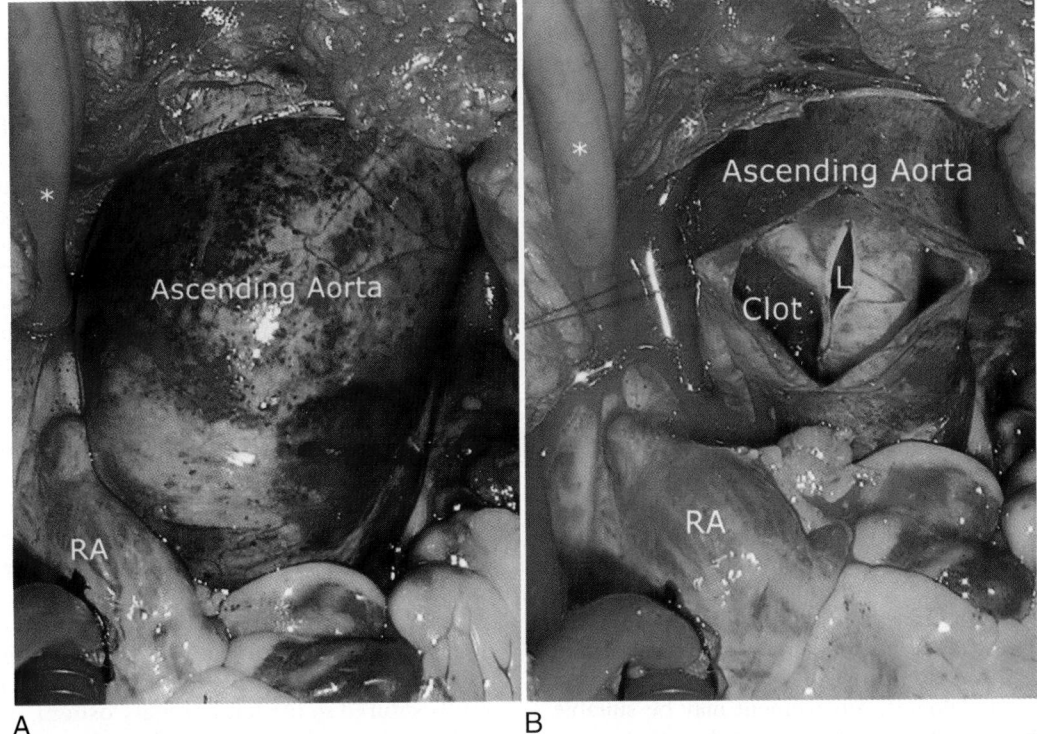

A   B

FIGURE 61-11. **A,** Operative photograph of acute type A aortic dissection with hematoma in the aortic wall. **B,** After opening the aorta, a large clot was cleared from the false lumen; true lumen (L) is seen after division of the intimal flap. RA, right atrium; the asterisks indicate Rumel tourniquet around superior vena cava.

FIGURE 61-12. Median sternotomy. (©1996 Hazim J. Safi, MD.)

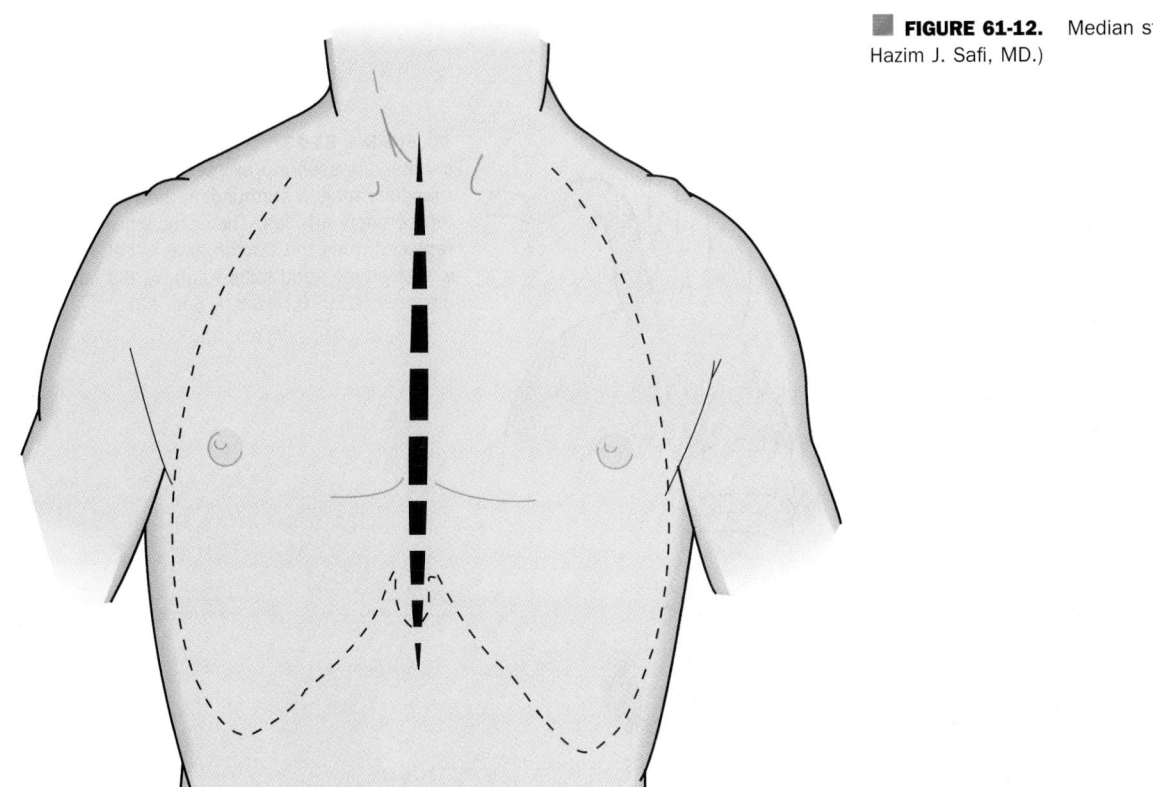

pulmonary vein prevents ventricular distention and allows optimal decompression of the left ventricle. Profound hypothermia and circulatory arrest are required in cases of acute aortic dissection or aneurysms that extend into the aortic arch; otherwise, the ascending aorta can be safely clamped without profound hypothermia.

The extent of prosthetic valve and/or graft replacement depends on patient presentation and is determined at the time of surgery. Patients who have intrinsic abnormalities in the valve leaflets, bicuspid aortic valve, or Marfan syndrome often require aortic valve replacement. Separate valve and graft replacement, or the Wheat technique (Fig. 61-13), rather than a composite valve/graft may be applicable for older patients with minor to moderate sinus dilation. Unlike the Bentall, Cabrol, or button techniques described later, the Wheat technique does not require reattachment of the coronary arteries. The sinuses are excised, the tissue surrounding the coronary arteries is left intact, and the aortic graft is cut in a scalloped fashion to accommodate reattachment of the coronary arteries and replacement of the sinuses. Although two suture lines in the proximal aorta increase the potential for bleeding, the Wheat technique avoids the problem of sinus of Valsalva dilation that can lead to rupture into the right or left ventricle of the heart. Allograft replacement may be suitable for physically active patients who do not wish to take anticoagulants or patients with native or prosthetic valve endocarditis. Valve resuspension, rather than replacement, may be adequate in cases of acute aortic dissection and a normal aortic valve. Patients who have Marfan syndrome and/or aortic root dilation most often require a composite valve graft.

Bentall and de Bono in 1968 and Edwards and Kerr in 1970 created the composite valve graft. In the Bentall technique (Fig. 61-14) a composite valve graft is placed in the aortic annulus after the walls of the aorta have been opened longitudinally and the aortic valve leaflets excised. The distal end of the graft is cut and sewn end-to-end to the distal ascending aorta. Openings are cut in the graft opposite the right and left coronary arteries. The coronary ostia are tightly sutured to their corresponding openings in the composite graft and wrapped with aortic aneurysmal wall to prevent immediate postoperative bleeding (the inclusion technique). However, the side-to-side attachment of the coronary arteries to the valve prosthesis can bring the anastomosis under tension, which can lead to pseudoaneurysm. Although a few groups continue to use the Bentall technique, the report of pseudoaneurysm in 7% to 25% of patients prompted many surgeons to adopt new techniques for coronary artery reattachment.[21]

Christian Cabrol in 1981 devised an ingenious method for replacing the aortic root without having to mobilize the coronary arteries (Fig. 61-15). A small Dacron tube graft is sutured to the left coronary ostium, passed behind the larger ascending aortic graft, and anastomosed to the right coronary ostium. The small Dacron graft is then anastomosed side-to-side to the composite graft. Bleeding is minimized because suture line tension is significantly reduced, but kinking can occur at the side-to-side anasto-

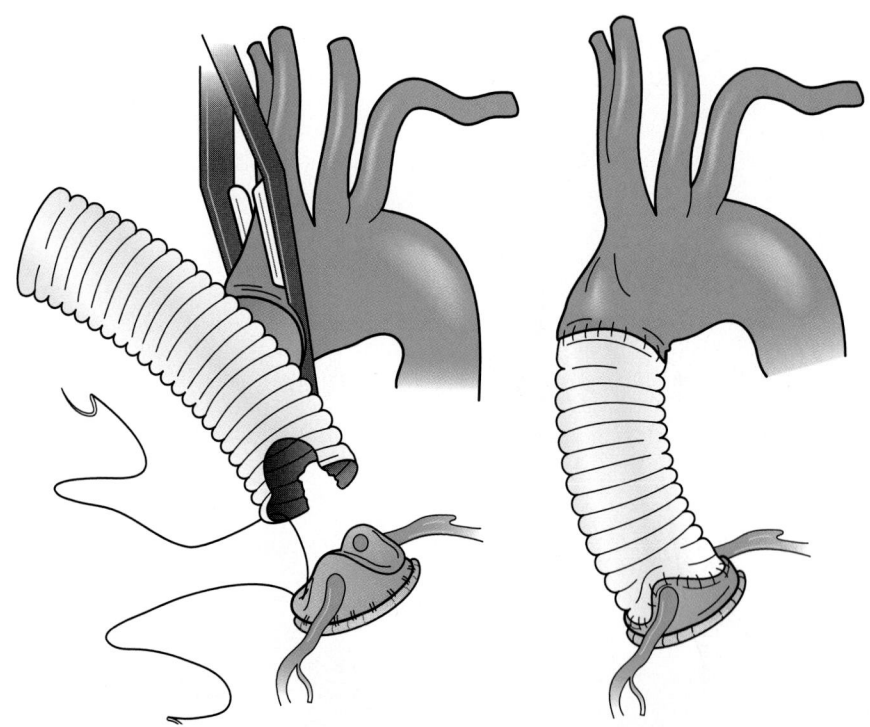

FIGURE 61-13. Wheat technique: The coronary sinuses are excised, leaving a triangular tongue surrounding the right and the left coronary arteries. The aortic valve is replaced, then the Dacron graft is cut in two wedge shapes and sutured above the coronary arteries. (©1996 Hazim J. Safi, MD.)

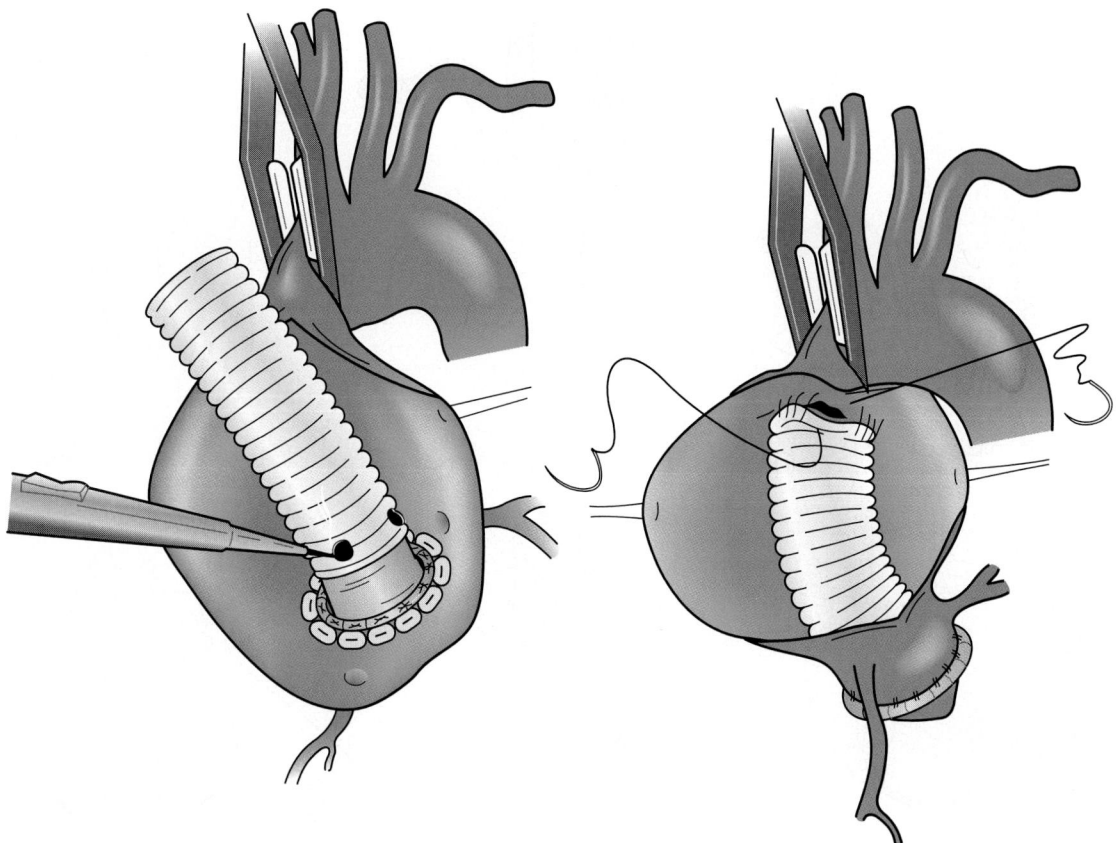

FIGURE 61-14. Bentall technique: The coronary ostia are tightly sutured to openings in the graft. (©1996 Hazim J. Safi, MD.)

mosis or right ostium. Modification of the Cabrol technique consists of an end-to-side anastomosis of the left main coronary Dacron graft, with a button attachment of the right coronary artery directly to the composite graft or replaced by separate vein or Dacron graft (Fig. 61-16). Graft kinks or graft occlusion at the angle of the right coronary artery ostium are avoided because the smaller graft is not restrained by a side-to-side anastomosis. We most often use the button technique (Fig. 61-17) or Carrel patch for right and left coronary artery reattachment. It is more time consuming than the Cabrol technique but complications are fewer. The right and left coronary artery ostia are dissected from the aorta, preserving a circle of tissue or button, and anastomosed directly to the composite graft.

Results: Aortic Root

A lack of reporting standards in the literature makes interpretation of aortic root surgical results difficult to summarize. In general, both etiology (dilation, Marfan syndrome, aortic dissection) and reconstructive technique (Cabrol, Wheat, Bentall, button) appear to influence outcome. Repair of a diseased aortic root can be accomplished safely, depending on risk factors, with an overall operative mortality rate in the range of 2% to 15%. Major operative complications of the surgery are bleeding at the anastomotic site—requiring reoperation—and throm-

boembolism. Long-term complications include endocarditis, thromboembolic events, and pseudoaneurysm.

Ascending Aorta and Arch

If aneurysmal disease is limited to the tubular portion of the ascending aorta profound hypothermia is not required and we use the closed technique (i.e., with aorta clamped). If, however, the aneurysm extends beyond the ascending aorta into the arch or there is acute dissection, we use the open distal anastomosis technique—with profound hypothermic circulatory arrest. The dry surgical field of the open technique permits the surgeon to clearly view all diseased portions of the ascending aorta to within a few millimeters of the great vessels. Cardiopulmonary bypass, circulatory arrest, and retrograde cerebral perfusion are also used. Retrograde cerebral perfusion is begun after the patient has been cooled to between 15°C and 20°C (nasopharyngeal temperature) and the electroencephalogram monitor shows an isoelectric flat line. Oxygenated blood is perfused in a retrograde direction through the superior vena cava to the brain. Another technique that has been used for cerebral protection during the circulatory arrest period is antegrade cerebral perfusion. This technique employs cannulae inserted directly into the ostia of the innominate and left common carotid arteries during the period of arrest.

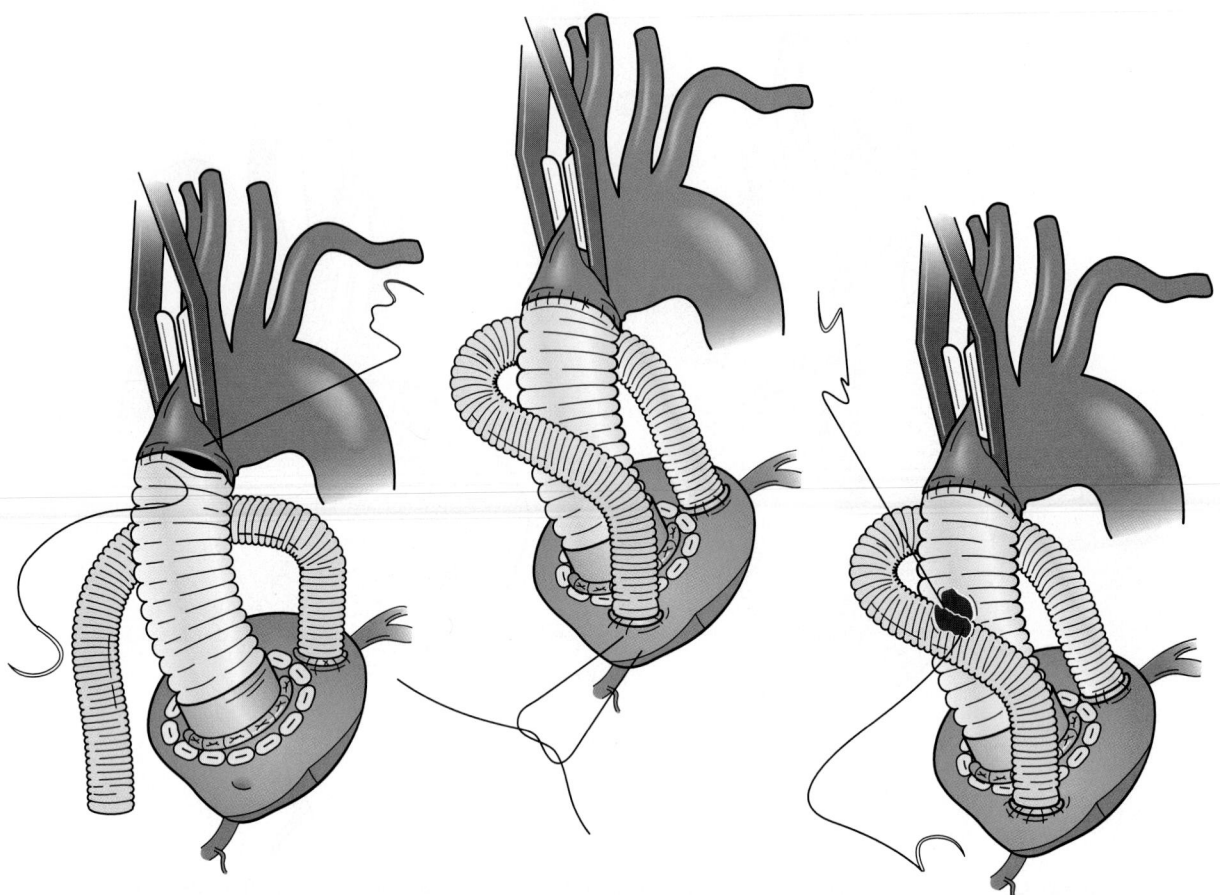

FIGURE 61-15.   Cabrol technique: A graft is sutured to the left coronary ostium, passed behind the ascending aortic graft, and anastomosed to the right coronary ostium. The coronary graft is then sewn side-to-side to the composite aortic graft. (©1996 Hazim J. Safi, MD.)

The brachiocephalic, left common carotid, and left sub-clavian arteries are preserved as a patch while the ascend-ing aorta and transverse arch are excised. After a graft is sutured to the descending thoracic aorta just distal to the left subclavian artery, the brachiocephalic arteries are anastomosed to a side hole cut in the superior arch portion of the graft. The aortic valve and aortic sinuses are inspected and repaired if necessary (see earlier section, Aortic Root). The graft is then sutured to the supracoro-nary ascending aorta.

Surgery for type A dissection and for aneurysms of the root, ascending aorta, and arch is similar except for the additional suturing necessitated by false lumen in aortic dissection (Fig. 61-18). The partition between the true and false lumen is cut. The false lumen is obliterated by sewing together the dissected walls using running 4-0 polypropy-lene suture. The graft is sutured to the proximal aortic arch. The aortic arch is replaced if a hematoma, fragmen-tation of the aortic wall, or free rupture is identified. Intimal tears are either excised or repaired. The aortic root is reconstructed by placing 4-0 Prolene pledgeted sutures along the sinotubular junction to prevent retrograde dissection.

Results: Ascending and Arch

Before profound hypothermic circulatory arrest became a regular part of aortic surgery, arch replacement carried an extremely high mortality rate of up to 75%. The intro-duction of profound hypothermia and circulatory arrest reduced operative mortality to between 10% and 15%. The development of additional circulatory adjuncts has reduced operative mortality to around 5%. Retrograde cerebral perfusion has been shown to decrease the inci-dence of stroke (Fig. 61-19) and is currently the most widely adopted perfusion adjunct. There exists a renewed interest in antegrade perfusion at some centers.[23] The major risk factors associated with stroke and encephalopa-thy following ascending/arch repair are circulatory arrest time and involvement of the transverse arch.

SURGICAL TREATMENT AND RESULTS: DISTAL THORACIC AORTA

Despite remarkable improvements in morbidity and mor-tality rates, surgical repair of the descending thoracic and thoracoabdominal aorta remains one of the most

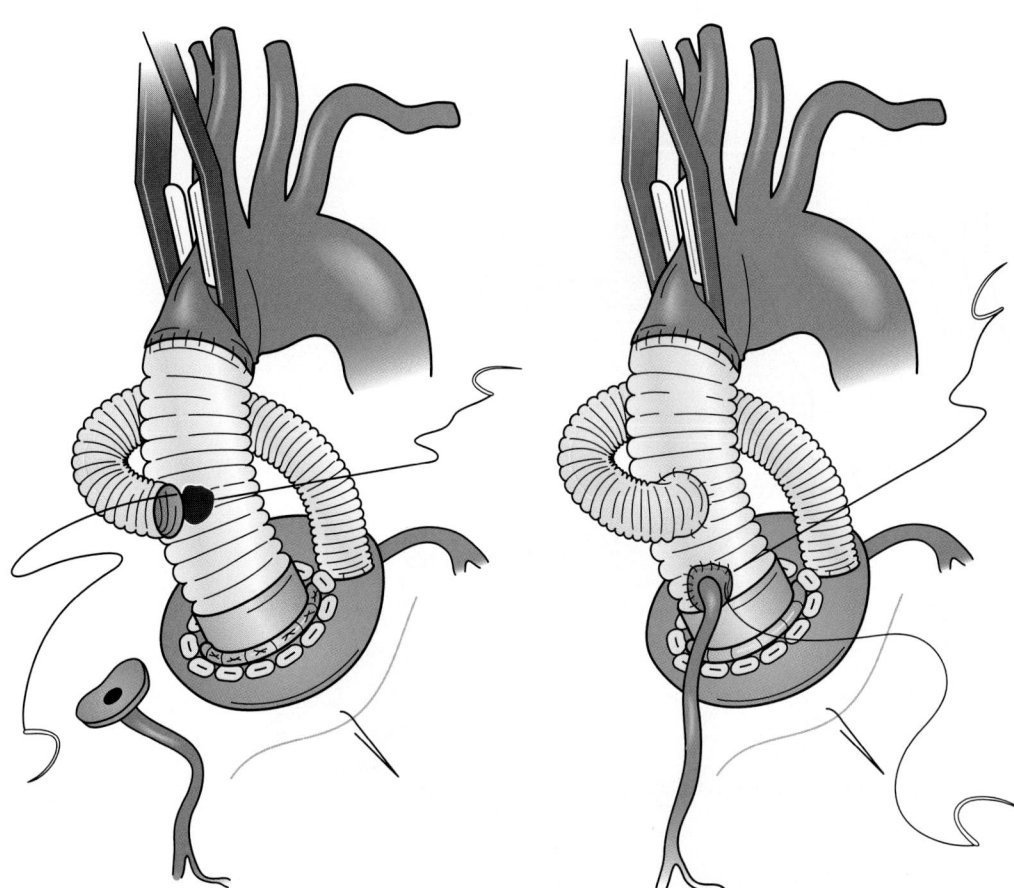

■ **FIGURE 61-16.**
Modified Cabrol technique: The left coronary graft is anastomosed end-to-side to the composite aortic graft, and the right coronary artery attached as a button. (©1996 Hazim J. Safi, MD.)

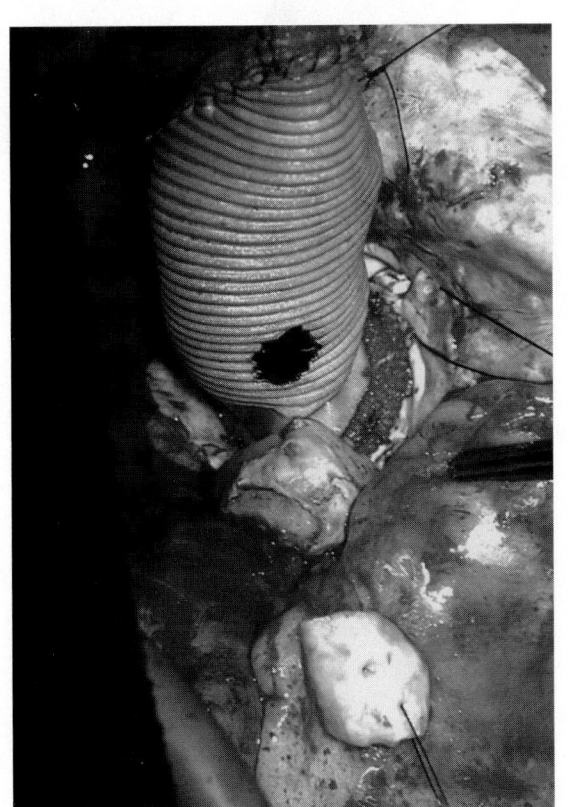

■ **FIGURE 61-17.**   Button reattachment of the right coronary artery (left coronary artery reattachment done in a similar fashion not shown).

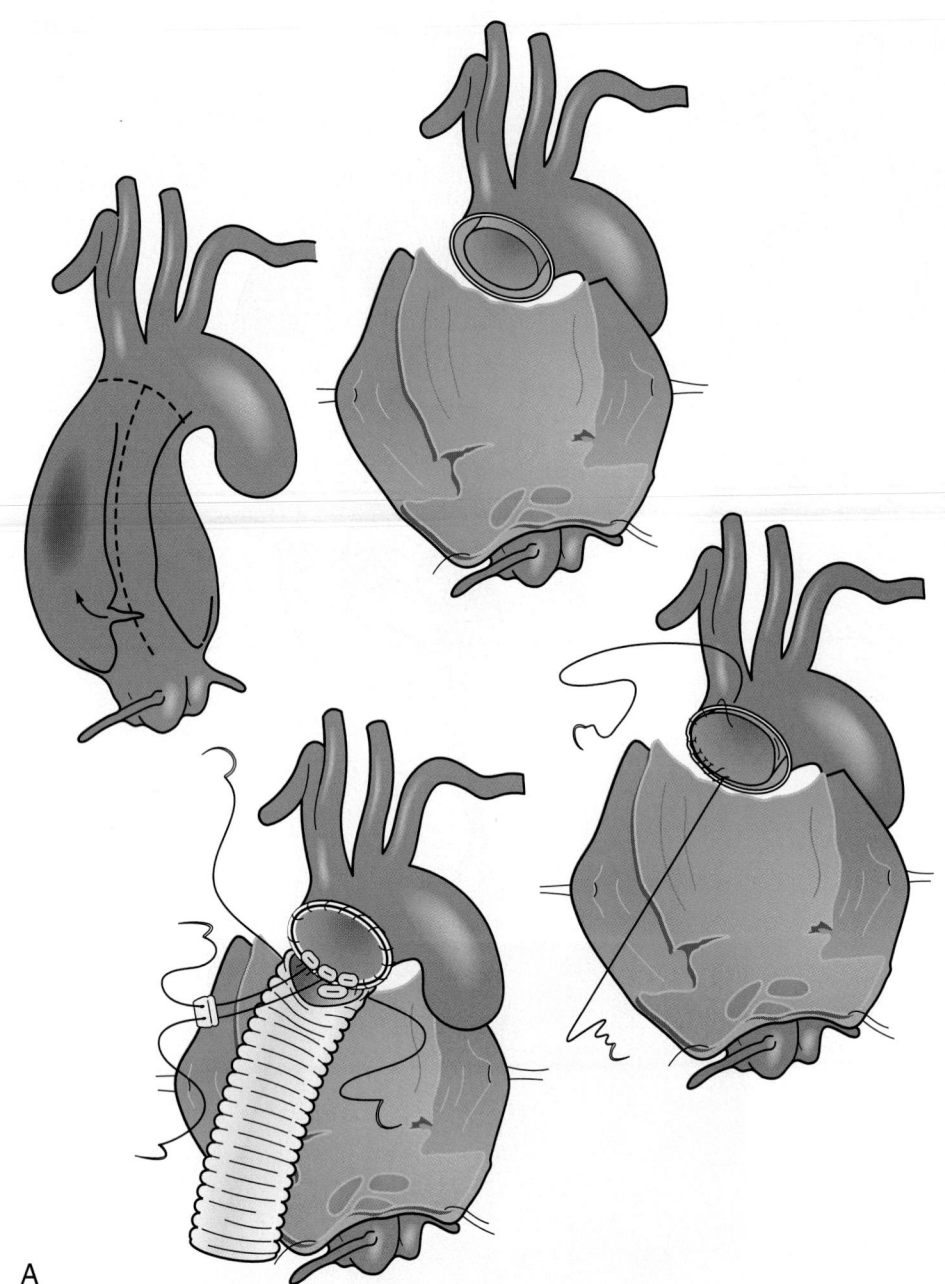

A

FIGURE 61-18.   Ascending aortic dissection repair. **A,** Proximal tear site, aortic valve inspection, intima and adventitial suture, inner distal anastomosis with pledgeted polypropylene suture reinforcement.

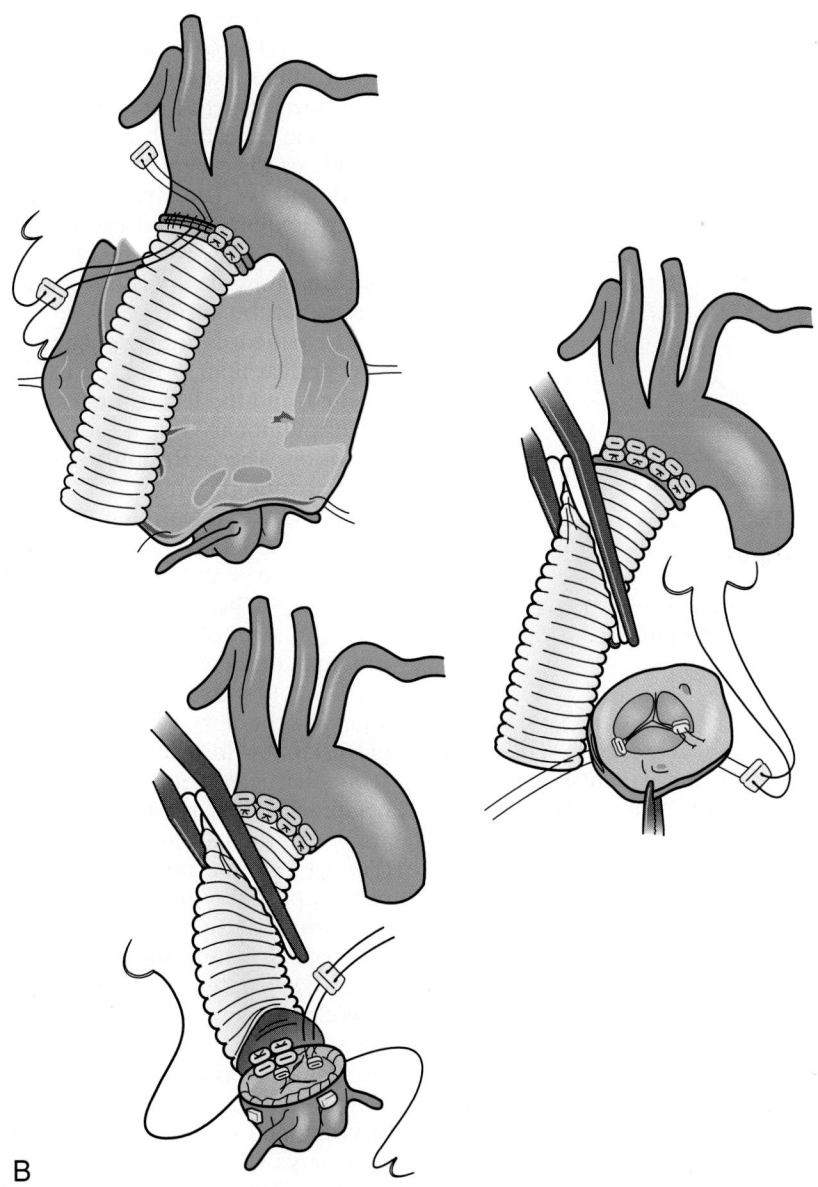

B

FIGURE 61-18.—Cont'd   B, Outer distal anastomosis with pledgeted polypropylene suture reinforcement, aortic valve resuspension, and proximal reinforced anastomosis. (**A** and **B**, ©1996 Hazim J. Safi, MD.)

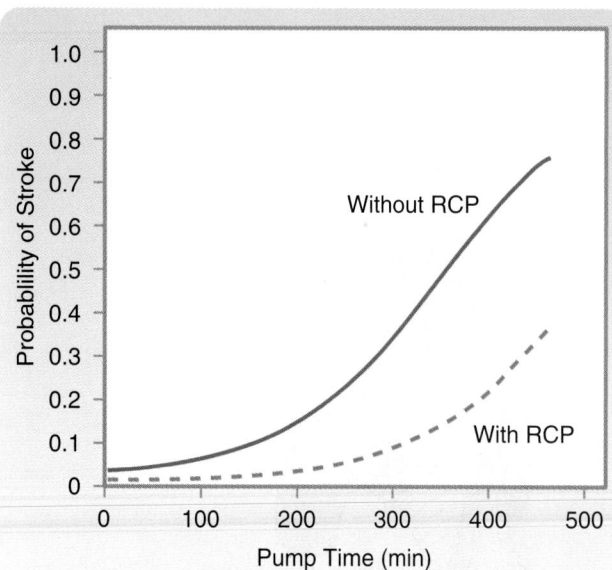

FIGURE 61-19. Probability of stroke according to pump time, with and without retrograde cerebral perfusion (RCP).

formidable tasks in cardiovascular surgery. Following induction of general anesthesia, the patient is intubated with a double-lumen endotracheal tube to permit right lung ventilation during surgery. Monitoring cardiac function, oxygenation, blood pressure, urine output, and coagulation is critical to the prevention of intraoperative and postoperative complications related to cardiac dysfunction, renal failure, paraplegia, pulmonary failure, and hemorrhage. Electrodes attached to the scalp for electroencephalogram and along the spinal cord for somatosensory-evoked potential assess cerebral and spinal cord function. A radial artery catheter checks arterial pressures. A Swan-Ganz catheter floated through a catheter placed in the internal jugular or subclavian vein monitors the central venous and pulmonary artery pressures. Large-bore central and peripheral venous lines are inserted for fluid and blood replacement therapy. Probes placed in the patient's nasopharynx, bladder, and rectum record temperatures.

During the period of aortic cross-clamp, the spinal perfusion pressure is markedly decreased due to interruption of aortic flow and increased cerebrospinal fluid (CSF) pressure. We use distal aortic perfusion and CSF drainage to provide spinal cord protection.[24] Distal aortic perfusion, or left atrial to femoral bypass, partially combats the effect of the clamp by raising the distal aortic pressure, thereby increasing the spinal perfusion pressure (Fig. 61-20). CSF drainage complements distal aortic perfusion by lowering CSF pressure and further improving spinal cord perfusion. A CSF catheter is placed in the 3rd or 4th lumbar space (Fig. 61-21). CSF pressure is monitored and kept below 10 mm Hg throughout the procedure.

The patient is positioned in the right lateral decubitus position with the hip flexed 45 degrees for accessibility of the left and right groins. The common femoral artery is dissected out and isolated with umbilical tape. We tailor the chest incision to complement the extent of the aneurysm (Fig. 61-22)—a modified thoracoabdominal incision to below the costal margin for the descending thoracic aorta, extent I, and extent V thoracoabdominal aortic aneurysm, and full thoracoabdominal exploration to the umbilicus for extent I and V, and to the pubis for extent II, III, and IV. The sixth rib is removed for all aneurysms except extent IV, and the left lung is collapsed. Taking care to avoid injury to the phrenic nerve, the aortic hiatus and the muscular portion of the diaphragm are cut for passage of the aortic graft.

The patient is anticoagulated with 1 mg/kg of heparin. The pericardium posterior to the left phrenic nerve is opened, and the left atrium is cannulated through the left lower pulmonary vein or atrial appendage for distal aortic perfusion. The perfusionist attaches the cannula to a Bio-Medicus pump, which has an in-line heat exchanger for postoperative rewarming. Arterial inflow is established through the left common femoral artery, or the descending thoracic or abdominal aorta if the femoral artery is not accessible. The descending thoracic aorta is dissected from the level of the hilum of the lung, cephalad to the proximal descending thoracic aorta. We identify the *ligamentum arteriosum* and transect it, taking care to avoid injury to the left recurrent laryngeal nerve. Distal aortic perfusion is initiated. The aorta is cross-clamped in sequential segments to minimize organ ischemic time, beginning either proximal or distal to the left subclavian artery and then again at the mid-descending thoracic aorta (Fig. 61-23). We no longer use the inclusion technique of wrapping the graft with the aneurysmal aortic wall in the proximal anastomosis because of the danger of esophageal fistula. Instead, we completely transect the aorta to separate it from the underlying esophagus.

We prefer a woven Dacron graft for aortic replacement. We suture the graft in end-to-end fashion to the descending thoracic aorta, using a running 3-0 or 2-0 monofilament polypropylene suture. We check the anastomosis for bleeding and use pledgeted sutures for reinforcement, if necessary. The lower clamp is then moved down to the distal thoracic aorta at the diaphragm level, and the remainder of the aneurysm is opened. For descending thoracic aortic aneurysms, the graft is cut in a beveled fashion and sewn to the distal thoracic aorta, using 3-0 or 2-0 monofilament polypropylene suture, incorporating the patent lower intercostal arteries that are in close proximity to the graft.

Before the use of the adjuncts distal aortic perfusion and CSF drainage, during the period sometimes referred to as "cross-clamp and go," the speed of the operation was intricately linked to probability of good neurologic outcome. Reimplantation of intercostal arteries was controversial because it prolonged clamp time. After analyzing data collected over several years of thoracoabdominal surgery, we found that ligation of patent lower intercostal arteries (T9 to T12) increased the risk of paraplegia.[25] Therefore we reattach all patent lower intercostal arteries from T9 to T12, either together as a patch to a side hole made in the Dacron graft or individually. Substantial back-bleeding from patent intercostal arteries can be minimized with temporary placement and inflation of balloon

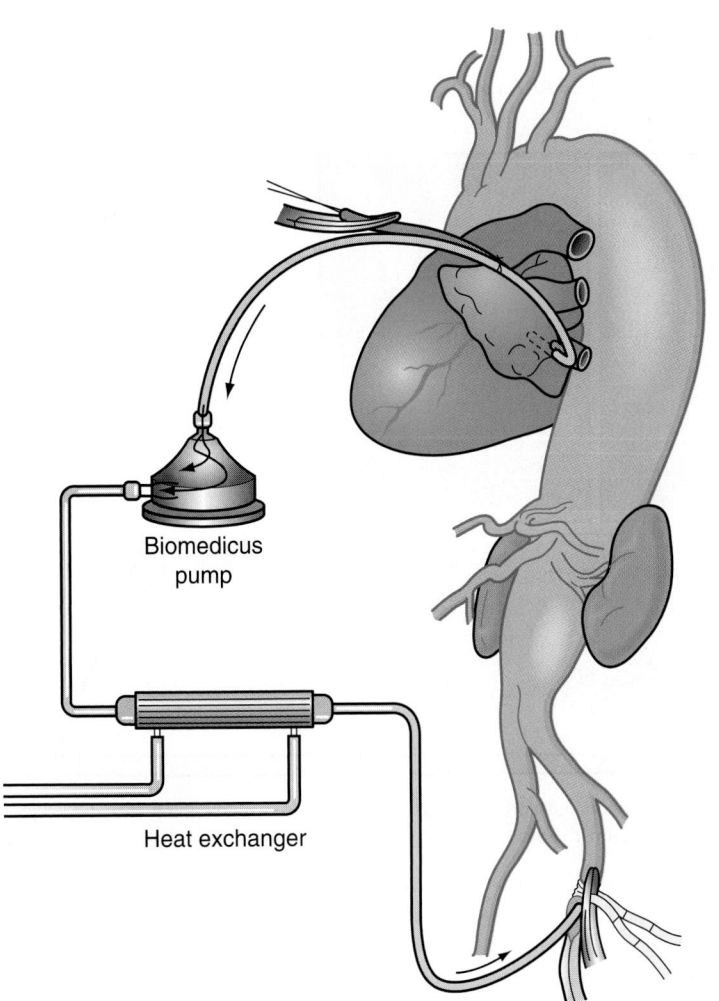

FIGURE 61-20.   Distal aortic perfusion. Outflow is from the left atrium, and inflow is to the left femoral artery. (Redrawn from illustration by Carl Clingman.)

Biomedicus pump

Heat exchanger

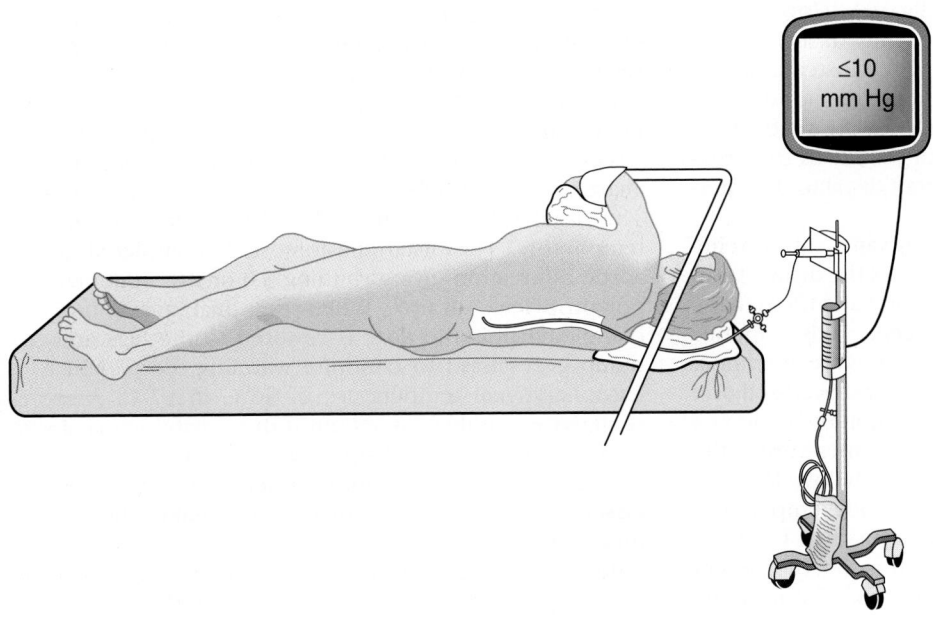

FIGURE 61-21.   Cerebrospinal fluid (CSF) drainage is initiated intraoperatively and maintained for 3 days postoperatively to keep CSF pressure below 10 mm Hg. (Redrawn from illustration by Carl Clingman.)

≤10 mm Hg

DTAA
TAAA Ext. I and V
(Celiac)

TAAA Ext. I and V
(Celiac and SMA)

TAAA Ext. II, III and IV

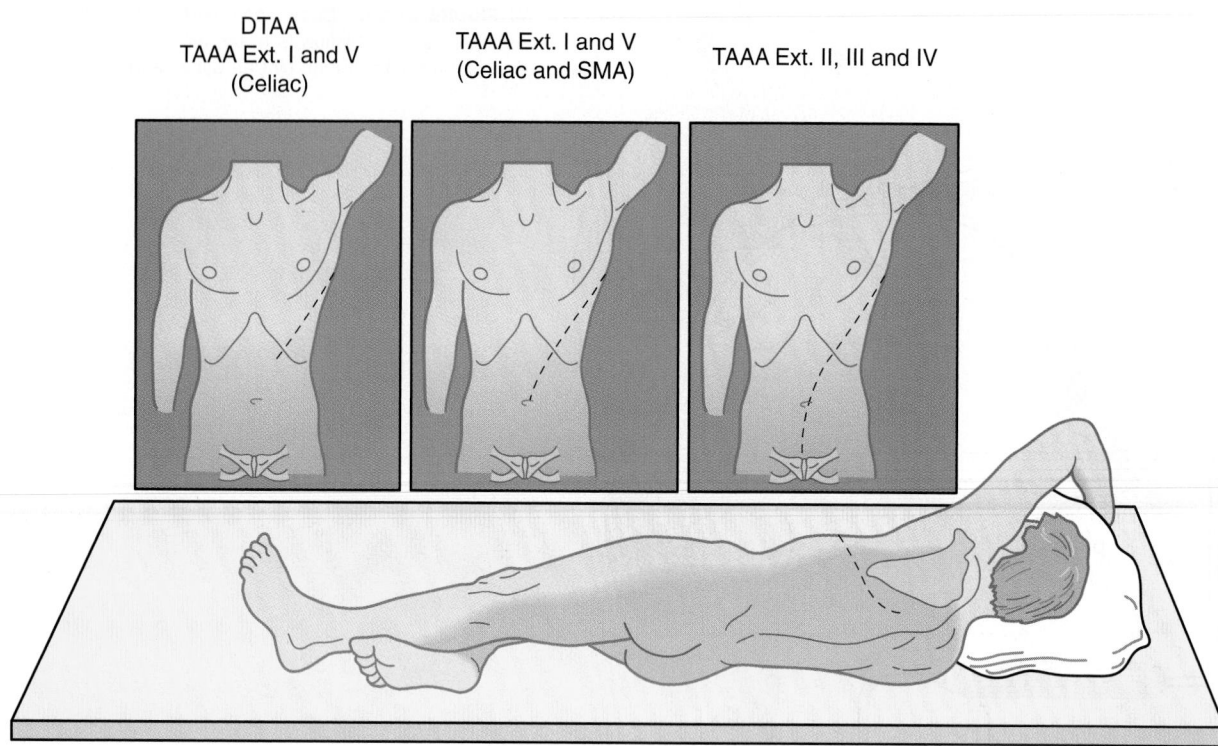

FIGURE 61-22. Incision is tailored to the extent of the thoracoabdominal aortic aneurysm (TAAA). DTAA, descending thoracic aortic aneurysm; SMA, superior mesenteric artery. (©2002 Hazim J. Safi, MD.)

catheters (3 French) prior to reimplantation. The upper intercostal arteries are generally ligated. However, if the lower intercostal arteries are occluded, any patent upper intercostal arteries are reimplanted instead, having assumed a more important role in supplying blood to the spinal cord. Once the intercostal arteries are reattached, pulsatile flow is restored to the spinal cord with the proximal clamp repositioned across the graft distal to the intercostal anastomosis.

For thoracoabdominal aortic aneurysms, after reimplantation of the lower intercostal arteries the distal clamp is moved to the infrarenal abdominal aorta and the remainder of the aneurysm is opened. The celiac axis, superior mesenteric, right renal, and left renal arteries are identified, cannulated with 9 French Pruitt catheters, perfused and cooled using either Ringer's lactate solution or blood at a flow rate of 300 to 600 mL/minute. The temperature of the left kidney is directly monitored and kept below 15°C. At the same time, we maintain the patient's body temperature at about 33°C by warming the lower circulation. If we are unable to warm the lower body, we do not cool the viscera due to the risk of severe hypothermia (<32°C core body temperature) and ventricular fibrillation.

The visceral anastomosis has to be evaluated intraoperatively. If the celiac axis, superior mesenteric, and both renal arteries are in close proximity, they can be reim-

planted as a single patch to a side hole made in the aortic graft, using running 3-0 or 2-0 monofilament polypropylene suture. Not infrequently, however, the left or right renal artery is more caudad and is reattached as a Carrel patch or use of a short interposition bypass graft. Patent lumbar arteries are usually ligated. After completion of the visceral anastomosis, the graft is clamped distal to the anastomosis and pulsatile flow is restored to the viscera. The distal clamp is removed and the pump is stopped temporarily. The distal anastomosis is completed at the aortic bifurcation, using running 3-0 or 2-0 monofilament polypropylene suture. When the final anastomosis is completed pulsatile flow is restored to the legs and the pump is restarted to continue warming the patient to a nasopharyngeal temperature of 36°C to 37°C. A representative example of an extent II thoracoabdominal aortic aneurysm repair is shown in Figure 61-24.

The operative techniques for acute or chronic type B dissection and aneurysm of the descending thoracic or thoracoabdominal aorta are similar.[26] However, dissection requires identification of the true lumen versus the false lumen. The partition or septum between the two lumina must be excised to redirect the flow of blood into the true lumen of the distal aorta. In acute aortic dissection, both the proximal and distal ends of the dissected aorta are first reinforced with running 4-0 polypropylene suture before

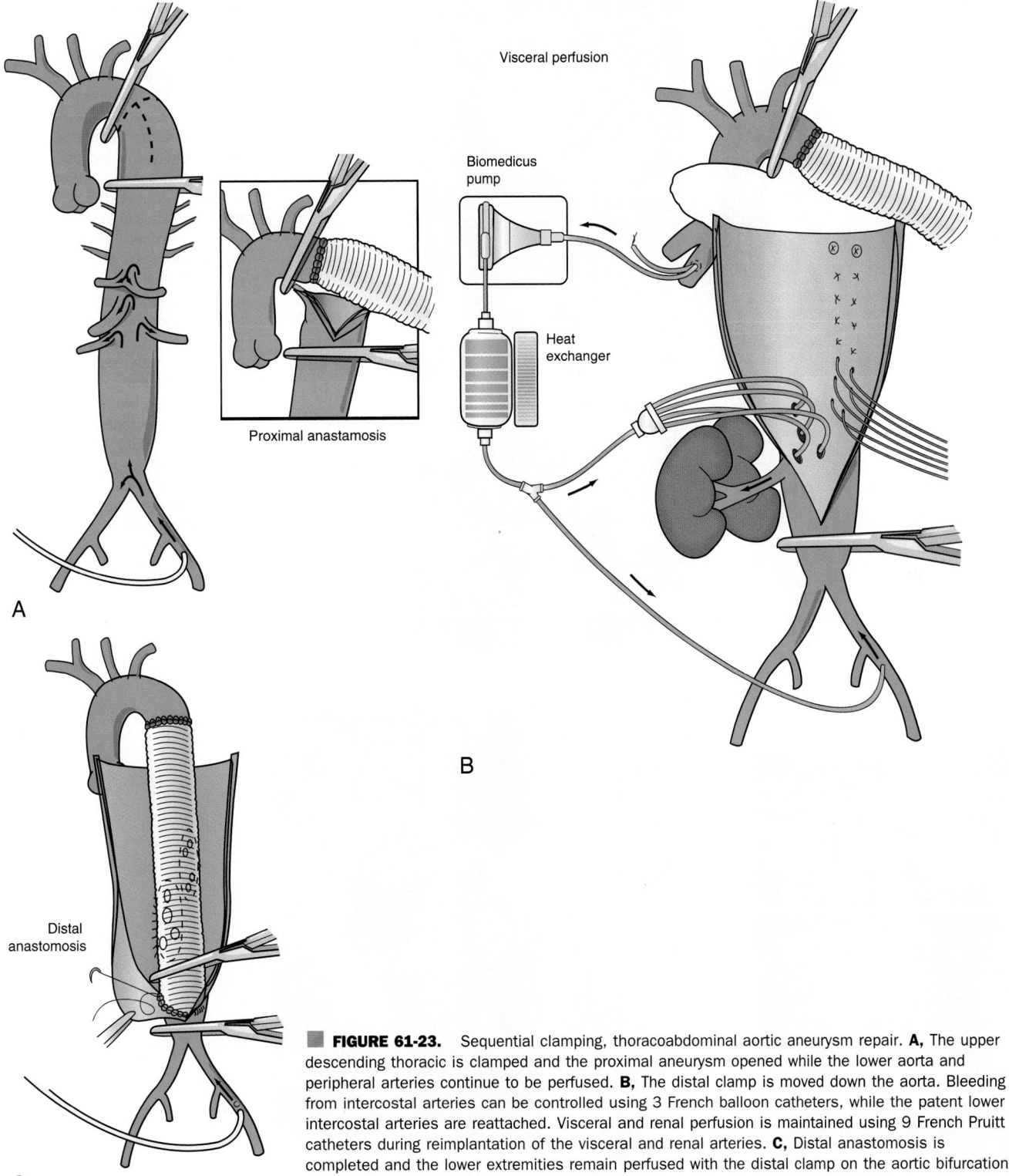

Visceral perfusion

Biomedicus
pump

Proximal anastamosis

Heat
exchanger

Distal
anastomosis

A

B

C

FIGURE 61-23. Sequential clamping, thoracoabdominal aortic aneurysm repair. **A,** The upper descending thoracic is clamped and the proximal aneurysm opened while the lower aorta and peripheral arteries continue to be perfused. **B,** The distal clamp is moved down the aorta. Bleeding from intercostal arteries can be controlled using 3 French balloon catheters, while the patent lower intercostal arteries are reattached. Visceral and renal perfusion is maintained using 9 French Pruitt catheters during reimplantation of the visceral and renal arteries. **C,** Distal anastomosis is completed and the lower extremities remain perfused with the distal clamp on the aortic bifurcation. (**A-C,** ©1995 Hazim J. Safi, MD.)

attaching the graft. Additional interrupted pledgeted polypropylene sutures are then sewn into the posterior and anterior walls for reinforcement. In chronic dissection, patent lower intercostal arteries are reattached. For acute dissection, however, because of the friability of the aortic tissue we advocate ligatures of all intercostal and lumbar arteries to avoid catastrophic bleeding.

Results: Descending and Thoracoabdominal Aorta

Mortality rates for repair of descending thoracic and thoracoabdominal aortic aneurysms currently range between 5% and 21%. Multivariable analyses by different groups, including ours, have found age, renal failure, symptomatic, and extent II aneurysms to be significant

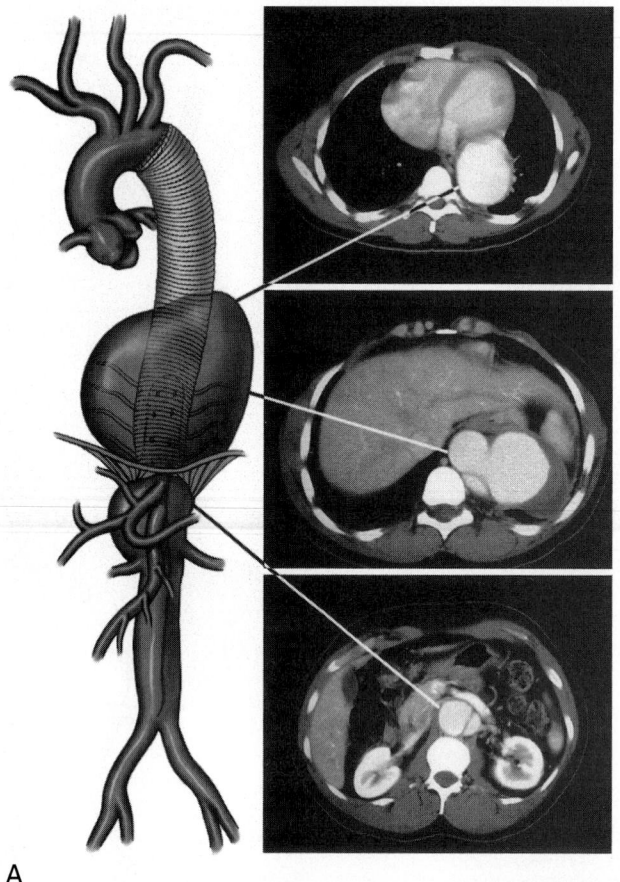

A

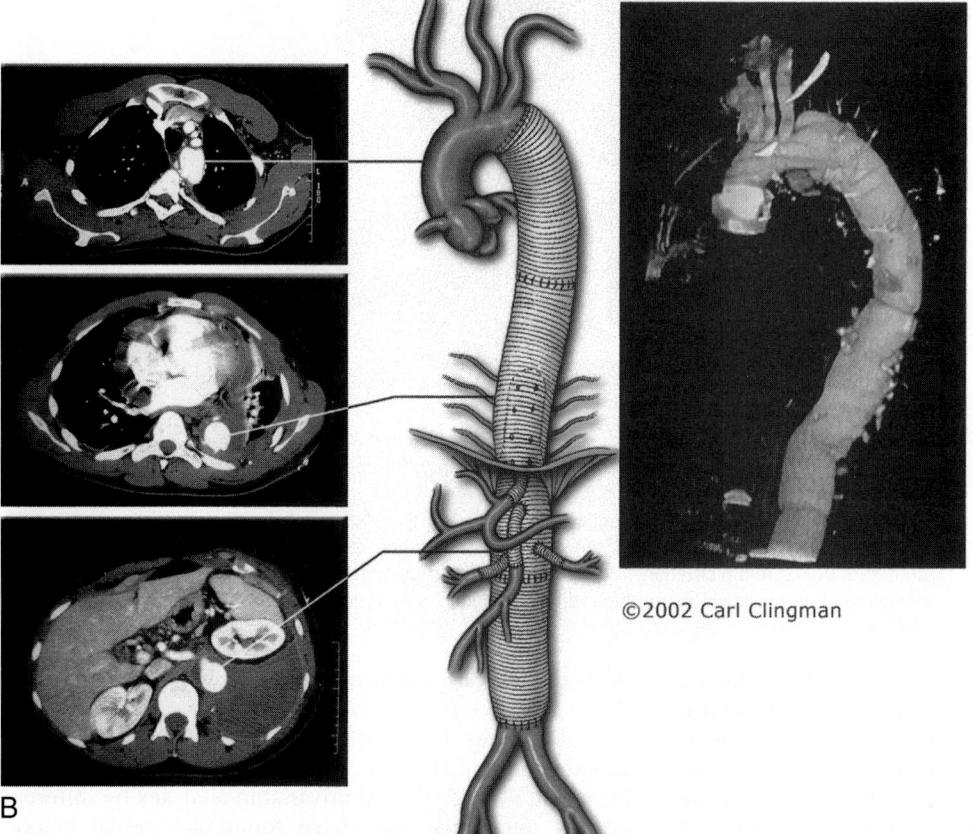

B

FIGURE 61-24. Repair of extent II thoracoabdominal aortic aneurysm with chronic dissection. **A,** Status post–descending thoracic aortic aneurysm repair (type C); the patient presented with aneurysmal enlargement of the remaining thoracoabdominal aorta to below the renal arteries; artist's diagram of the thoracoabdominal aortic aneurysm extent II (*left*) and corresponding CT axial images (*right*). **B,** Postoperative complete graft replacement of the thoracoabdominal aorta from the left subclavian artery to the aortic bifurcation, with reattachment of the lower intercostal arteries, and reimplantation of the celiac axis, superior mesenteric, right and left renal arteries, using separate interposition bypass grafts (*center*, artist's diagram); corresponding CT axial images (*left*) and reformatted three-dimensional sagittal view (*right*). (A and B, © 2002 Carl Clingman.)

©2002 Carl Clingman

risk factors for mortality.[27-31] Patients who undergo elective graft replacement at high-volume centers of excellence fare best, with mortality rates between 5% and 15%.[32] Our current mortality rate for elective repair is between 5% and 12%, as opposed to rates of 20% to 25% in the early 1990s.

Spinal Cord Complications

Adjuncts (distal aortic perfusion and CSF drainage) have reduced our overall incidence of spinal cord complications to 0.9% for descending thoracic aortic aneurysm repair and to 3.3% for thoracoabdominal aortic aneurysm repair. With adjuncts our rate of neurologic deficit for the most troublesome extent II thoracoabdominal aortic aneurysms has also declined and is now between 7% and 12% compared with rates between 30% and 40% in the era of cross-clamp and go (Fig. 61-25).

Immediate neurologic deficit is defined as paraplegia or paraparesis that occurs as the patient awakens from anesthesia. *Delayed-onset neurologic deficit* refers to paraplegia or paraparesis that develops after a period of normal neurologic function. We have observed delayed neurologic deficit as early as 2 hours and as late as 2 weeks following surgery (median, 3 days), in 2.4% of patients.[33] No single risk factor explains the onset of either deficit, but researchers have become more and more interested in how a patient can emerge from surgery neurologically intact but later develop paraplegia. Using multivariable analysis, we found that acute dissection, extent II thoracoabdominal aortic aneurysm, and renal insufficiency were independent preoperative predictors.[34] In another study examining postoperative factors independent of preoperative risk factors, we found lowest postoperative mean arterial pressure (<60 mm Hg) and CSF drain complications to be significant predictors.[35] We speculate that delayed neurologic deficit after thoracoabdominal aortic repair may result from a "second-hit" phenomenon. Although adjuncts may protect the spinal cord intraoperatively and reduce the incidence of immediate neurologic deficit, the spinal cord remains vulnerable during the early postoperative period. Additional ischemic insult caused by hemodynamic instability and CSF drainage catheter malfunction may constitute a second hit, causing delayed neurologic deficit. Because postoperative factors associated with delayed neurologic deficit are likely related to arterial blood pressure and oxygen delivery, we keep the mean arterial pressure above 90 to100 mm Hg, hemoglobin above 10 mg/dL, and cardiac index greater than 2.0 L/min. If delayed neurologic deficit occurs while the CSF drain is in place, the patient is placed supine, and CSF is drained freely until the CSF pressure drops below 10 mm Hg. If the drain has been removed and delayed neurologic deficit occurs, the CSF drainage catheter is reinserted and drained for 72 hours. With this protocol, we have observed partial recovery from neurologic deficit in more than 50% of patients and complete recovery in 40%.

Renal Failure

The incidence of renal failure after thoracoabdominal aortic repair ranges between 4% and 29%. Renal failure increases morbidity, length of stay, and mortality. We have shown that the presence of preoperative renal insufficiency and the development of postoperative renal failure are associated with increased 30-day mortality and neurologic deficit.[36] Our current incidence of renal failure varies between 7% and 15%, depending on the extent of the aneurysm and the patient's preoperative renal function. About 15% of patients with postoperative renal failure require hemodialysis. Risk factors associated with renal failure are increased preoperative creatinine level (>2.0 mg/dL), direct left renal artery reattachment, and the use of simple cross-clamp technique. Good strategies to protect renal function during thoracoabdominal aortic repair remain elusive. The goals of perioperative renal protection are to maintain adequate renal oxygen delivery, reduce renal oxygen utilization, and reduce direct renal tubular injury. Thus far these goals have been addressed most effectively by active renal cooling, directly maintaining renal perfusion, suppressing renal vasoconstriction, preventing micro-occlusion by particulate emboli, and preventing postischemic reperfusion injury.

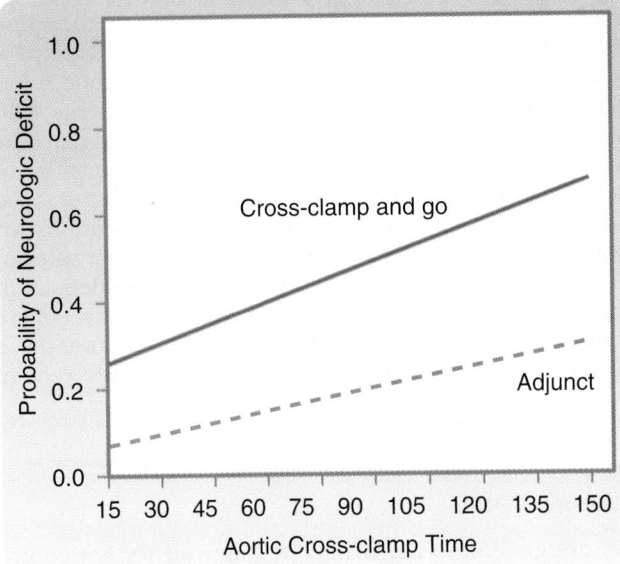

FIGURE 61-25. The probability of neurologic deficit increases as clamp time increases in extent II thoracoabdominal repair: "cross-clamp and go" repair *(solid line)* versus repair with adjuncts, distal aortic perfusion and CSF drainage *(dashed line).*

Impact of Dissection

Acute aortic dissection substantially raises the risk of paraplegia following graft replacement of the descending thoracic or thoracoabdominal aorta. Because dissection patients are critically ill and undergo surgery emergently with little time for preparation, the method of spinal cord protection during surgery for acute dissection is often less than optimal. Reported in-hospital death rates vary from 30% to 50% compared to 10% to 20% of patients treated medically. Survival outcome for "uncomplicated" patients treated with early surgical repair resembles the outcome of patients treated medically. However, surgery during the acute phase is associated with more significant bleeding from the dissected aorta and a higher rate of paraplegia (14% to 32%).

Chronic dissection was previously considered a risk factor for paraplegia or paraparesis in patients undergoing repair of the descending thoracic and thoracoabdominal aorta, particularly during the era of cross-clamp and go. However, when we analyzed recent data we found no appreciable difference in the rate of neurologic deficit for patients with or without chronic dissection who underwent descending thoracic or thoracoabdominal aortic repair (3.6% vs. 4.7%, respectively).[37] Chronic dissection undoubtedly makes surgical repair of descending thoracic and thoracoabdominal aortic aneurysms more difficult, but survival and neurologic outcome do not differ from that of aneurysm surgery without dissection. Several factors are likely responsible for the good neurologic outcome of our patients with chronic dissection, including better surgical techniques and anesthetic care, the use of moderate hypothermia, and reimplantation of intercostal arteries. However, the key element in improved spinal cord protection is the use of the adjuncts distal aortic perfusion and CSF drainage.

EXTENSIVE AORTIC ANEURYSM AND THE ELEPHANT TRUNK TECHNIQUE

Aneurysmal disease occurs in more than one part of the aorta in approximately 20% of cases. Extensive aortic aneurysm (also known as *mega-aorta*) refers to aneurysmal involvement of the entire ascending, transverse aortic arch and thoracoabdominal aorta. Although associated factors include Marfan syndrome and chronic aortic dissection, the cause of extensive aortic aneurysm remains unknown. Single-stage repair of extensive aneurysms can greatly increase risks. The patient is submitted to a lengthy procedure that requires multiple incisions, a daunting array of protective surgical adjuncts, protracted clamp times, and considerable blood loss. Staged repair would seem to be a logical solution. But prior to the introduction of the elephant trunk technique by Borst in 1983, staged repair was fraught with complications, particularly excessive bleeding in the second stage. Because the elephant trunk technique permits the surgeon to avoid cross-clamping the proximal native descending thoracic aorta in the second stage, this problem was resolved.

Since 1991 we have routinely used the elephant trunk technique for extensive aortic aneurysm repair (Fig. 61-26).[38] The ascending aorta and transverse arch are usually operated first and, following a recovery period of 4 to 6

weeks, repair of the descending thoracic or thoracoabdominal aortic aneurysm is performed. The first stage is performed in a similar fashion to standard surgery of the ascending aorta and transverse arch (see earlier section, Surgical Treatment and Results: Proximal Thoracic Aorta) except for graft replacement of the aortic arch. The replacement graft is partially inverted on itself and the doubled graft is positioned 7 to 10 cm into the descending aorta. The folded edge of the graft is sutured to the descending thoracic aorta just distal to the left subclavian artery. When this anastomosis is completed, the inner portion of the tube graft is pulled out toward the ascending aorta and the outer portion is left to dangle in the descending aorta, (resembling an elephant's trunk). The brachiocephalic, left common carotid, and left subclavian arteries are then reimplanted to a side hole made in the superior arch portion of the graft.

Following a recovery period of 4 to 6 weeks, the patient undergoes second-stage repair. The second stage of the elephant trunk technique is much like standard repair of descending thoracic or thoracoabdominal aortic aneurysms (see earlier section, Surgical Treatment and Results: Distal Thoracic Aorta). CSF drainage is utilized. Distal aortic perfusion is established from the left atrial appendage or pulmonary vein to the left common femoral artery. The proximal descending thoracic aorta is opened, and the elephant trunk portion of the graft (inserted in the descending thoracic aorta during stage 1), is promptly grasped and clamped. A new graft is sutured to the "elephant trunk." The elephant trunk technique obviates the need to clamp the proximal descending thoracic aorta and reduces the risk of excessive bleeding.

Results: Elephant Trunk Technique

We have performed the elephant trunk procedure in nearly 200 patients. Mortality rates range from 5% to 9% after stage 1, and 6% to 7% for stage 2. During the interval between surgeries, or approximately 31 days to 6 weeks after stage 1, mortality has averaged around 6.5%. When we performed a 5-year follow-up of patients who failed to return for second-stage repair, we found that 32% had died. Although we were able to obtain the cause of death in only a small percentage of patients, most of these were due to aneurysm rupture. Major complications for both stages have been relatively low, with stroke rates of about 2% in the first stage and no neurologic deficits in the second. Determining the optimum length of recovery time between stages has been difficult. Because these patients are vulnerable to rupture, we currently recommend no more than a 6-week period of recovery.

Acknowledgments

We are grateful to Dr. Dianna M. Milewicz for her contribution to the genetic section of this chapter, and we thank our editor, Amy Wirtz Newland, and our illustrator, Carl Clingman.

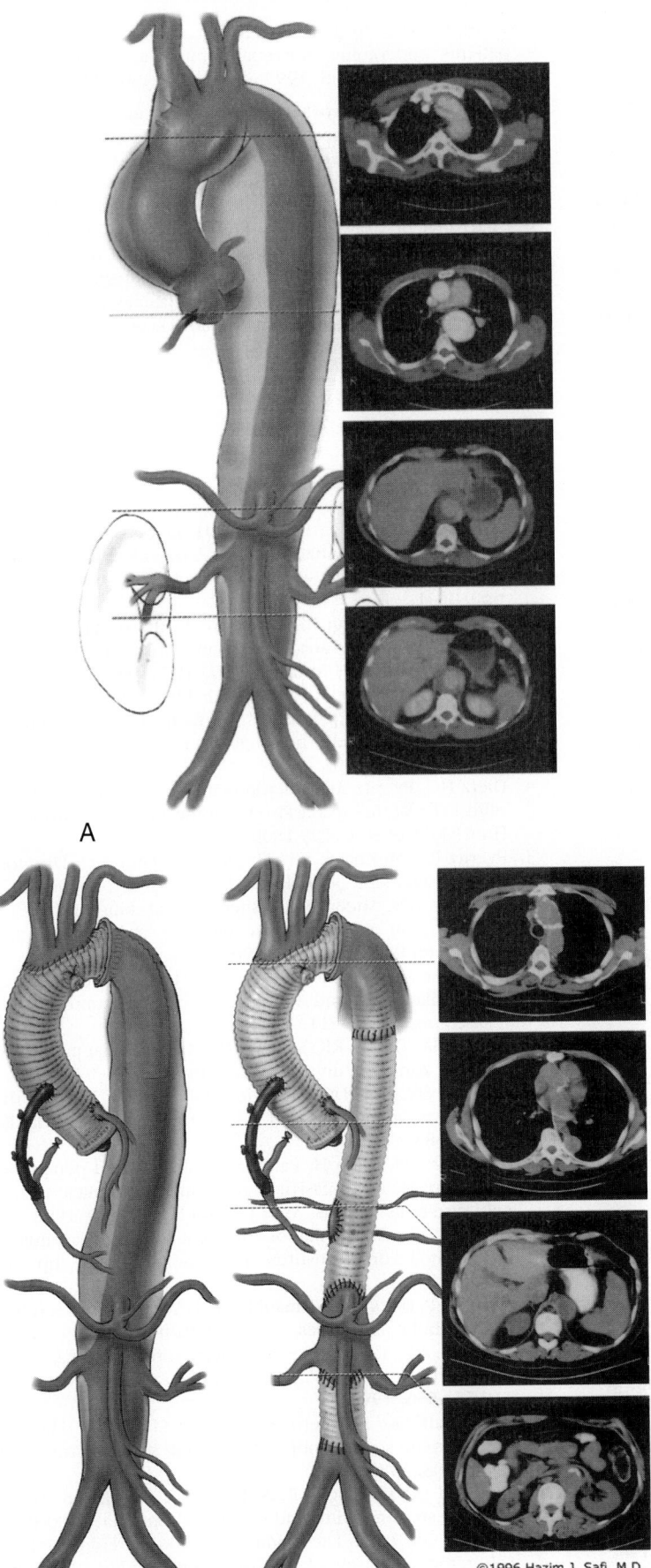

FIGURE 61-26. Repair of extensive aortic aneurysm and chronic dissection. **A,** Artist's diagram *(left)*, and corresponding CT axial images *(right)* of preoperative aneurysm. **B,** Stage 1 elephant trunk repair with graft replacement of ascending/arch, reimplantation of great vessels, bypass of the right coronary artery, and Carrel patch of the left coronary artery; the "trunk" is inside the descending thoracic aorta *(left)*; stage 2 completion of elephant trunk repair with extent II thoracoabdominal aortic graft replacement, reattachment of lower intercostal arteries, reimplantation of visceral and renal arteries *(center)*, and corresponding CT axial images *(right)*. (*A* and *B*, ©1996 Hazim J. Safi, MD.)

A

©1996 Hazim J. Safi, M.D.

B

Selected References

Clouse WD, Hallett JW Jr, Schaff HV, et al: Improved prognosis of thoracic aortic aneurysms: A population-based study. JAMA 280:1926-1929, 1998.

In this update of Bickerstaff's classic study on the natural history of thoracic aortic aneurysms, Clouse and associates examine the possible causes of the poor prognosis of this disease when untreated. From their population-based cohort study of 133 patients, they found an increased incidence of thoracic aortic aneurysm compared to Bickerstaff's study, but they also observed improved survival. They discuss the causes for these phenomena and provide a good look at a difficult and underexplored subject.

Hagan PG, Nienaber CA, Isselbacher EM, et al: The International Registry of Acute Aortic Dissection (IRAD): New insights into an old disease. JAMA 283:897-903, 2000.

Acute aortic dissection is a life-threatening medical emergency associated with high rates of morbidity and mortality. The International Registry of Acute Aortic Dissection culled the data of 464 patients from 12 international referral centers to increase our knowledge of the effect of recent technical advances on patient care and outcome. Physical findings previously regarded as typical are noted in only a third of patients, and clinicians are alerted to the wide range of manifestations in acute aortic dissection. A detailed analysis of data for type A and type B acute and chronic aortic dissection treated surgically or medically affords an excellent overview of the outcome of modern dissection patients.

Hasham SN, Guo DC, Milewicz DM: Genetic basis of thoracic aortic aneurysms and dissections. Curr Opin Cardiol 17:677-683, 2002.

Hasham and colleagues have extensively studied the molecular genetics of cardiovascular disease, particularly in the Marfan syndrome. This article explores the identity of genes that predispose patients without known syndromes to aortic aneurysms and dissections. The article provides a look at the future and how characterization of these genes will enhance our ability to determine persons at risk for aortic aneurysms and dissections.

Safi HJ, Miller CC III, Estrera AL, et al: Staged repair of extensive aortic aneurysms: Morbidity and mortality in the elephant trunk technique. Circulation 104:2938-2942, 2001.

Borst introduced the elephant trunk technique—the two-stage repair of extensive aortic aneurysms that involve the ascending aorta, aortic arch, and descending or thoracoabdominal aorta—in the 1980s. This article describes one of the largest series of elephant trunk patients from the group that continues to study the peculiar characteristics and surgical requirements of the patients with extensive aortic aneurysm or mega-aorta. The article investigates patient outcome and provides a sound argument in favor of two-stage versus single-stage repair of the entire aorta.

Svensson LG, Crawford ES, Hess KR, et al: Experience with 1509 patients undergoing thoracoabdominal aortic operations. J Vasc Surg 17:357-368, 1993; discussion 368-370.

Svensson and coworkers' study of E. Stanley Crawford's extensive patient series closely examines a wide range of risk factors associated with early death and postoperative complications in patients undergoing thoracoabdominal aortic operations. The size of the series permits solid comparisons of Crawford's four types of thoracoabdominal aortic aneurysm and analysis of the effect of aneurysm extent on complications such as paraplegia and renal failure. The study is a classic and continues to be cited by thoracoabdominal aortic aneurysm researchers.

References

1. Gray H, Williams PL, Bannister LH: Embryology and development. In Gray's Anatomy: The Anatomical Basis of Medicine and Surgery. New York, Churchill Livingstone, 1995, pp 91-341.
2. McDonald JJ, Anson BJ: Variations in the origin of arteries derived from the aortic arch in American whites and negroes. Am J Phys Anthrop 27:97-107, 1940.
3. Vaughan CJ, Casey M, He J, et al: Identification of a chromosome 11q23.2-q24 locus for familial aortic aneurysm disease, a genetically heterogeneous disorder. Circulation 103:2469-2475, 2001.
4. Dietz HC, Pyeritz RE: Mutations in the human gene for fibrillin-1 (FBN1) in the Marfan syndrome and related disorders. Hum Mol Genet 4:1799-1809, 1995.
5. Pyeritz RE, McKusick VA: The Marfan syndrome: Diagnosis and management. N Engl J Med 300:772-777, 1979.
6. Milewicz DM, Michael K, Fisher N, et al: Fibrillin-1 (FBN1) mutations in patients with thoracic aortic aneurysms. Circulation 94:2708-2711, 1996.
7. Biddinger A, Rocklin M, Coselli J, et al: Familial thoracic aortic dilatations and dissections: A case control study. J Vasc Surg 25:506-511, 1997.
8. Coady MA, Davies RR, Roberts M, et al: Familial patterns of thoracic aortic aneurysms. Arch Surg 134:361-367, 1999.
9. Hasham SN, Guo DC, Milewicz DM: Genetic basis of thoracic aortic aneurysms and dissections. Curr Opin Cardiol 17:677-683, 2002.
10. Milewicz DM, Chen H, Park ES, et al: Reduced penetrance and variable expressivity of familial thoracic aortic aneurysms/dissections. Am J Cardiol 82:474-479, 1998.
11. Burke A, Virmani R: Tumors of Great Vessels. Washington, DC, Armed Forces Institute of Pathology, 1996, pp 211-226.
12. Wright EP, Glick AD, Virmani R, et al: Aortic intimal sarcoma with embolic metastases. Am J Surg Pathol 9:890-897, 1985.
13. Sekine S, Abe T, Seki K, et al: Primary aortic sarcoma: Resection by total arch replacement. J Thorac Cardiovasc Surg 110:554-556, 1995.
14. Bickerstaff LK, Pairolero PC, Hollier LH, et al: Thoracic aortic aneurysms: A population-based study. Surgery 92:1103-1108, 1982.
15. Kurtland LT, Elveback LR, Nobrega FT: Population studies in Rochester and Olmstead County, Minnesota, 1900-1968. In Levin ML (ed): The Community and an Epidemiologic Laboratory: A Casebook of Community Studies. Baltimore, Johns Hopkins Press, 1970, pp 47-52.

16. Clouse WD, Hallett JW Jr, Schaff HV, et al: Improved prognosis of thoracic aortic aneurysms: A population-based study. JAMA 280:1926-1929, 1998.

17. Elefteriades JA: Natural history of thoracic aortic aneurysms: Indications for surgery, and surgical versus nonsurgical risks. Ann Thorac Surg 74:S1877-S1880, 2002; discussion S1892-S1898.

18. Davies RR, Goldstein LJ, Coady MA, et al: Yearly rupture or dissection rates for thoracic aortic aneurysms: Simple prediction based on size. Ann Thorac Surg 73:17-27, 2002; discussion 27-28.

19. Hagan PG, Nienaber CA, Isselbacher EM, et al: The International Registry of Acute Aortic Dissection (IRAD): New insights into an old disease. JAMA 283:897-903, 2000.

20. Estrera AL, Huynh TT, Porat EE, et al: Is acute type A aortic dissection a true surgical emergency? Semin Vasc Surg 15:75-82, 2002.

21. Kouchoukos NT, Marshall WG Jr, Wedige-Stecher TA: Eleven-year experience with composite graft replacement of the ascending aorta and aortic valve. J Thorac Cardiovasc Surg 92:691-705, 1986.

22. Estrera AL, Miller CC III, Huynh TT, et al: Replacement of the ascending and transverse aortic arch: Determinants of long-term survival. Ann Thorac Surg 74:1058-1064, 2002; discussion 1064-1065.

23. Di Eusanio M, Schepens MA, Morshuis WJ, et al: Antegrade selective cerebral perfusion during operations on the thoracic aorta: Factors influencing survival and neurologic outcome in 413 patients. J Thorac Cardiovasc Surg 124:1080-1086, 2002.

24. Safi HJ, Miller CC III: Spinal cord protection in descending thoracic and thoracoabdominal aortic repair. Ann Thorac Surg 67:1937-1939, 1999; discussion 1953-1958.

25. Safi H, Miller CC III, Carr C, et al: The importance of intercostal artery reattachment during thoracoabdominal aortic aneurysm repair. J Vasc Surg 27:58-68, 1998.

26. Safi HJ: How I do it: Thoracoabdominal aortic aneurysm graft replacement. Cardiovasc Surg 7:607-613, 1999.

27. Svensson LG, Crawford ES, Hess KR, et al: Experience with 1509 patients undergoing thoracoabdominal aortic operations. J Vasc Surg 17:357-368, 1993; discussion 368-370.

28. Safi HJ, Campbell MP, Ferreira ML, et al: Spinal cord protection in descending thoracic and thoracoabdominal aortic aneurysm repair. Semin Thorac Cardiovasc Surg 10:41-44, 1998.

29. Estrera AL, Miller CC III, Huynh TT, et al: Neurologic outcome after thoracic and thoracoabdominal aortic aneurysm repair. Ann Thorac Surg 72:1225-1230, 2001; discussion 1230-1231.

30. Coselli JS, LeMaire SA, Miller CC III, et al: Mortality and paraplegia after thoracoabdominal aortic aneurysm repair: A risk factor analysis. Ann Thorac Surg 69:409-414, 2000.

31. Cambria RP, Davison JK, Carter C, et al: Epidural cooling for spinal cord protection during thoracoabdominal aneurysm repair: A five-year experience. J Vasc Surg 31:1093-1102, 2000.

32. Derrow AE, Seeger JM, Dame DA, et al: The outcome in the United States after thoracoabdominal aortic aneurysm repair, renal artery bypass, and mesenteric revascularization. J Vasc Surg 34:54-61, 2001.

33. Huynh TT, Miller CC III, Safi HJ: Delayed onset of neurologic deficit: Significance and management. Semin Vasc Surg 13:340-344, 2000.

34. Estrera AL, Miller CC III, Huynh TT, et al: Preoperative and operative predictors of delayed neurologic dificit following repair of thoracoabdominal aortic aneurysm repair. J Thorac Cardiovasc 126:1288-1295, 2003.

35. Azizzadeh A, Huynh TT, Miller CC III, et al: Postoperative risk factors for delayed neurologic deficit after thoracic and thoracoabdominal aortic aneurysm repair: A case-control study. J Vasc Surg 37:750-754, 2003.

36. Safi HJ, Harlin SA, Miller CC, et al: Predictive factors for acute renal failure in thoracic and thoracoabdominal aortic aneurysm surgery [published erratum, J Vasc Surg 25:93, 1997]. J Vasc Surg 24:338-344, 1996; discussion 344-345.

37. Safi HJ, Miller CC III, Estrera AL, et al: Chronic aortic dissection not a risk factor for neurologic deficit in thoracoabdominal aortic aneurysm repair. Eur J Vasc Endovasc Surg 23:244-250, 2002.

38. Safi HJ, Miller CC III, Estrera AL, et al: Staged repair of extensive aortic aneurysms: Morbidity and mortality in the elephant trunk technique. Circulation 104:2938-2942, 2001.

39. Safi HJ, Miller CC III, Huynh TT, et al: Distal aortic perfusion and cerebrospinal fluid drainage for thoracoabdominal and descending thoracic aortic repair: Ten years of organ protection. Ann Surg 238:372-381, 2003.

CHAPTER 62

ENDOVASCULAR SURGERY

Ross Milner, M.D., and **Elliot L. Chaikof**, M.D.

Vascular Access | Intravascular Stents and Endoprostheses
Guide Wires and Catheters | Image-Guided Therapy
Balloon Catheters |

Endovascular surgery occupies an increasingly central role in the management of patients with peripheral vascular disease as the preeminent form of minimally invasive vascular therapy, with associated reductions in periprocedural morbidity and mortality as well as in hospital stays. Although the efficacy and durability of catheter-based image-guided therapy varies with approach, application of adjunctive techniques, and disease entity, there is little doubt that the continued development of innovative technologies will extend the accepted indications for these techniques, through improvements in early technical success and long-term outcome.[1] In this chapter a framework is provided for the technical aspects of endovascular therapy with an emphasis on the fundamentals of percutaneous techniques pertinent to a range of arterial and venous disorders. Appropriate indications for catheter-based therapy and current outcomes are discussed in detail elsewhere in this textbook.

VASCULAR ACCESS

Percutaneous access can be achieved by a single- or double-wall puncture technique. In the former approach a beveled needle is introduced and a guide wire is passed after confirmation of arterial or venous access by visual inspection of backbleeding with or without use of direct pressure measurement and inspection of arterial or venous waveforms.[2] As a routine, we initially gain vascular access using a 21-gauge micropuncture needle and an 0.018-inch wire (Fig. 62-1). The double-wall technique requires the use of a blunt needle with an inner cannula. The needle is inserted through the vessel, after which the inner cannula is removed, the introducer needle then withdrawn until backbleeding is obtained, and a wire

introduced. Although percutaneous access can be routinely achieved in nearly all patients, those with scarred access sites from prior interventions or patients with decreased pulses due to occlusive disease represent an especially challenging subset that may benefit from ultrasound guidance with Doppler insonation or B-mode visualization of the target vessel.[3] Indeed, access site needles have been developed with integrated Doppler probes.

The initial goal of vascular access is to facilitate wire placement for subsequent insertion of an introducer sheath. At this stage of an endovascular procedure, the most commonly used wire is a 0.035-inch Benston guide wire that has an atraumatic floppy tip, which decreases the risk of an arterial dissection, and a stiff main body that allows passage of a sheath. Fluoroscopic visualization of free wire passage confirms appropriate placement and likewise minimizes the risk of inadvertent vessel wall dissection.[4] Characteristically, a 5-French sheath is adequate for most diagnostic procedures, whereas larger sheaths are often required for catheter-based interventions (Fig. 62-2). Although closure devices[5,6] have been used to facilitate the percutaneous introduction of large sheaths, we advocate direct arterial or venous cutdown for insertion of sheaths that exceed 12 French in outer diameter.

The femoral artery is the most commonly used site of arterial entry and allows access to almost any arterial bed with an associated low complication rate. In addition to palpation of an arterial pulse, bony landmarks, as opposed to skin creases, are most helpful in achieving femoral access. Specifically, when imaged fluoroscopically, the common femoral artery typically overlies the middle third of the femoral head. Skin puncture over the lower portion of the femoral head is recommended. In the absence of femoral pulses or for those patients in need of visceral

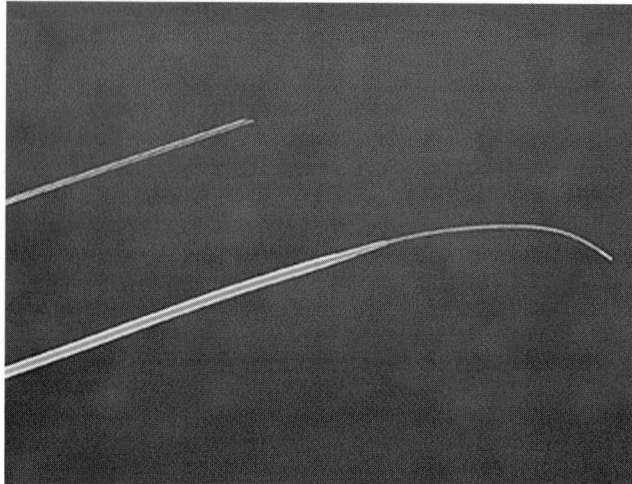

FIGURE 62-1. Micropuncture needle with dilator and wire system shown below the introducer needle. The needle is 21 gauge and the dilator is 5 French.

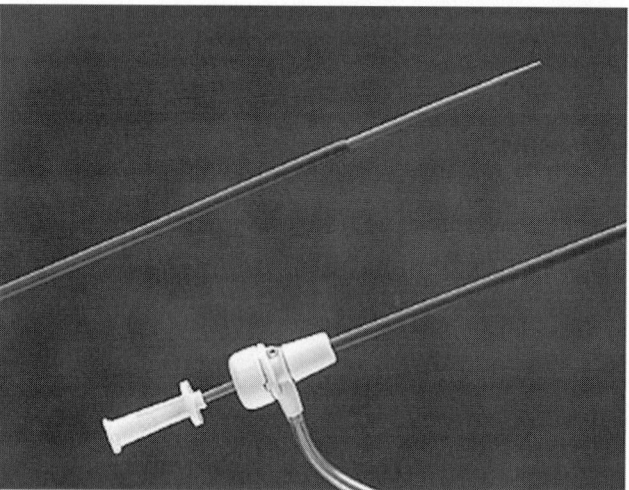

FIGURE 62-2. A hemostatic arterial sheath showing the inner dilator and hemostatic valve.

or arch vessel intervention, the brachial artery may provide a preferable point of entry.[7] This approach is especially advantageous for the patient with acute downward angulation of renal or visceral arteries. However, care is required when accessing the brachial artery to minimize the risk of median nerve injury, owing to brachial sheath hematoma or, rarely, needle-induced nerve trauma.

Retrograde femoral artery puncture with passage of sheaths, wires, and catheters in a cephalad direction is the standard approach for access to the suprainguinal arterial circulation, whereas antegrade puncture with caudal orientation of the puncture needle is often used when the intended site of treatment is at a distal infrainguinal location.[8] Fluoroscopic visualization of guide wire passage into the superficial femoral artery is mandatory for planned antegrade cannulation to avoid unintended catheterization of the profunda femoris artery.

GUIDE WIRES AND CATHETERS

Once arterial access is obtained, the success of an endoluminal intervention is based, in part, on proper selection of guide wires and catheters. After arterial cannulation, guide wires are used to navigate the diseased arterial bed. Multipurpose angled (MPA) or Berenstein catheters are often used to assist passage of a wire across a stenosis or occlusion or into a branch vessel. If unable to cross a stenosis with a standard wire, use of guide wires or catheters with hydrophilic coatings is indicated, although the use of these systems carries a greater risk of arterial dissection. Guide wires range from 0.014 to 0.035 inch in diameter, with a recent trend toward increased use of systems that utilize 0.014 inch or 0.018-inch wires.

Significantly, although hydrophilic wires may be critical in achieving access to a target location, they are not suitable for performing interventions because they are easily dislodged during placement or withdrawal of angioplasty balloons or vascular stents. Thus, exchange is usually made for a Bentson or other stiff wire, such as an Amplatz, Meier, or Lunderquist wire.[9] It is important to fluoroscopically visualize placement of these wires because their stiffness increases the risk of arterial perforation. Stiff wires are especially useful when inserting large sheaths or devices required for the endovascular management of aortoiliac aneurysms. Other stiff wires exist for specific interventions. For example, the Rosen wire has a stiff body and floppy J-tip, which is used for renal artery angioplasty and stenting.[10] The J-tip design prevents the wire from perforating the renal parenchyma as the wire is advanced into the terminal arterial branches. More recently, 0.014- and 0.018-inch wires are being used with increasing frequency for renal artery interventions. The smaller-diameter design allows balloons and stents to be placed using lower-profile delivery systems that more easily traverse tortuous anatomy or a high-grade stenosis. As a final rule of thumb, when using a coaxial balloon catheter or stent delivery system in which the wire passes through a central lumen, the lengths of the guide wires should be twice that of the intended catheter. In contrast, use of a monorail system in which the wire passes through a distal side lumen of the balloon catheter or stent deployment device allows employment of shorter wires.

A plethora of catheters have been designed for specific arterial beds and designated by configuration, length, and French size (Fig. 62-3). Most catheters range from 4 to 8 French with smaller catheters used for smaller vessels. As previously mentioned, MPA or Berenstein catheters have a slightly angled tip and are used for straightforward vessel cannulation or guide wire exchange. A Kumpe (KMP) catheter can serve a similar purpose but has a slightly greater degree of angulation at the tip. Additional selective catheters include the Contra, SOS Omni, and Motarjeme catheters, which may be used for cannulating the contralateral iliac artery, ipsilateral hypogastric artery, or other visceral vessel. We prefer to use the SOS Omni or Motarjeme catheters for an "over the horn" maneuver into the contralateral iliac artery. By cannulating the contralateral iliac artery a variety interventions can be per-

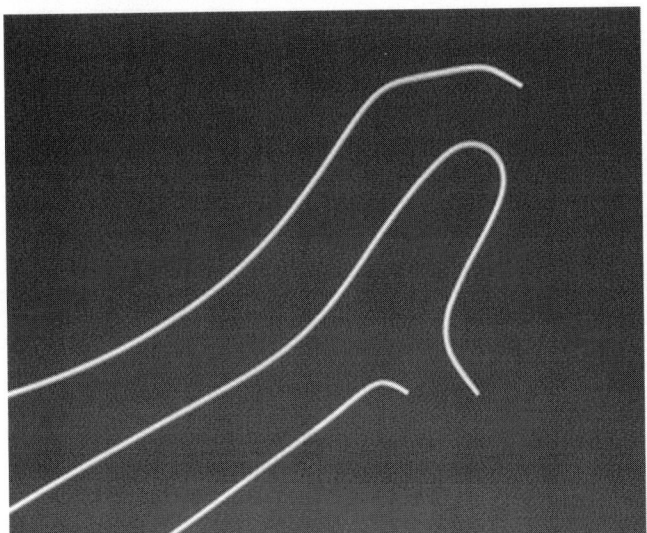

FIGURE 62-3.   A variety of selective catheters that are used for peripheral interventions.

formed, including hypogastric artery embolization in preparation for endovascular aneurysm repair with an aneurysmal common iliac artery, pull-back pressure measurements to determine if an intervention is needed, and treatment of proximal disease in a common or superficial femoral artery.

As endoluminal techniques have improved and more durable results are being demonstrated, angioplasty and stenting are now more commonly used for the management of visceral vessel lesions, as well as renovascular disease.[11,12] In addition to the SOS Omni and Motarjeme catheters, Cobra or renal double curve catheters may also be used for selective catheterization of the celiac axis, superior mesenteric artery, and renal arteries.

Aortic arch branch vessels can be accessed via femoral or brachial artery puncture sites with catheterization of subclavian or innominate arteries using a Kumpe or MPA catheter. Placement of a stent within the subclavian artery mandates careful identification of branch vessels so as to avoid compromising antegrade flow through the internal mammary or vertebral artery. The carotid artery, when approached by the femoral artery, is selected using a Headhunter (H1) or Vitek catheter. Angioplasty and stenting of carotid lesions and use of adjunctive embolization protection devices are areas of active investigation.

BALLOON CATHETERS

Once the diseased arterial bed has been selected with the appropriate catheter and wire, the presence of the anticipated lesion needs to be confirmed and, where appropriate, its hemodynamic significance determined. An arteriogram is obtained by hand injection of contrast agent through the selective catheter and a "road map" acquired that creates a virtual image of the effected arterial segment through which repeated passes of catheters, wires, or stents can be visualized.

The contrast load is always minimized and tailored to the specific patient according to the intervention being performed. For patients with an elevated serum creatinine level (≥1.4 mg/dL), pre-intervention hydration, minimization of contrast load, and/or use of fenoldopam have been advocated to limit the nephrotoxic effects of the contrast agent. Fenoldopam is administered as a continuous infusion at a rate of 0.01 to 1.6 µg/kg/min. A steady-state concentration is usually reached within 20 minutes. Other options for lesion localization when the baseline serum creatinine exceeds 2 mg/dL include use of gadolinium, CO_2 contrast, or intravascular ultrasound. Of note, the total administered volume of gadolinium should not exceed 0.2 to 0.4 mmol/kg, which is equivalent to 30 to 60 mL in a 75-kg person.

There is no consensus as to whether an intervention should be based on a pressure gradient difference measured by an intra-arterial catheter. We suggest that a mean pressure gradient greater than 10 mm Hg is sufficiently significant to require treatment. If no difference is detected in the resting state, then 100 µg of nitroglycerin can be infused intra-arterially to mimic the increased demand that occurs with walking. A gradient can be checked after the infusion is complete. It has been suggested that accuracy may be improved by simultaneous measurement of aortic pressure through a guide catheter and pressure distal to the stenosis with a pressure wire (Radi Medical Systems, 0.014 inch, 175 cm).

Whereas systemic anticoagulation or use of antiplatelet agents is not required for diagnostic procedures, appropriate pre-interventional therapy is a prerequisite for optimizing the likelihood of a successful treatment outcome. Patients are routinely hydrated overnight and no oral intake is permitted 8 hours before the procedure. Aspirin (81 mg) is initiated 24 hours before intervention and, in the case of renal artery interventions, all antihypertensive medications are held the morning of the procedure to avoid a precipitous decrease in blood pressure that may occur after angioplasty. Before angioplasty or stenting, we administer 5000 units of heparin intravenously and a single dose of cefazolin or vancomycin is given if a vascular stent or prosthesis is to be inserted. Once the intervention is completed and the activated clotting time falls below 150 to 160 seconds, the arterial sheath can safely be removed. Our current practice is to place all patients on aspirin and clopidogrel (Plavix) with an initial 300-mg loading dose followed by 75 mg/day for 3 to 6 months. Most studies involving the use of thienopyridines, such as clopidogrel or ticlopidine, and arterial stents have focused on their application in coronary artery disease. In the STARS trial, 1965 patients undergoing coronary stenting were randomized to aspirin alone, aspirin and warfarin, and aspirin and ticlopidine.[13] Patients who received aspirin and ticlopidine had a significantly lower rate of stent thrombosis compared with the other two groups. The clinical benefit was noticed for up to 12 months, although no reduction in restenosis was observed.

For a given lesion, a balloon catheter is selected on the basis of balloon diameter (millimeters) and length (centimeters), as well as the length of the catheter shaft, which

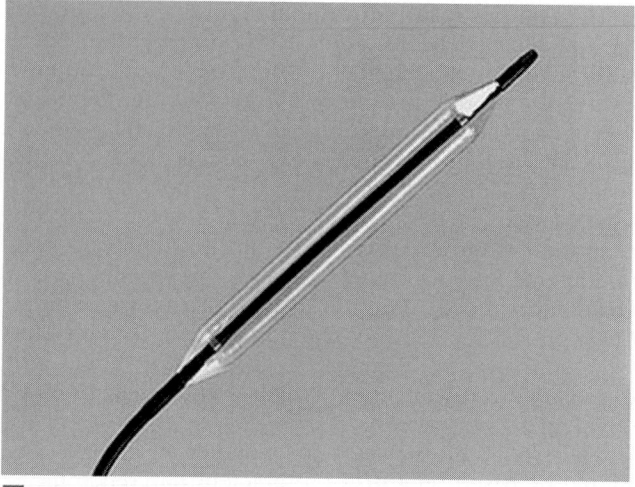

FIGURE 62-4.   An inflated angioplasty balloon catheter.

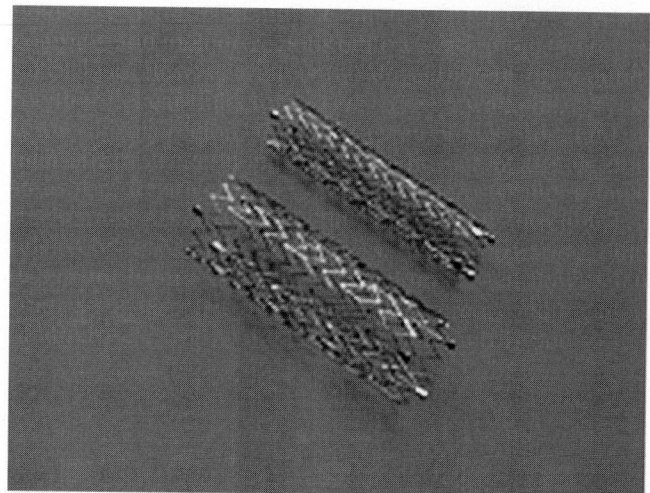

FIGURE 62-5.   Two sizes of intravascular stents.

is dictated by lesion location and chosen access site (Fig. 62-4). Characteristically, angioplasty balloons are produced from a noncompliant plastic, such as polyethylene, which facilitates high-pressure inflation to a predetermined maximum shape and size. Pressure required for inflation may vary widely from 4 to 16 atmospheres and is dependent on the compliance of the vascular lesion to be dilated. Higher pressures are typically required for relatively stiff venous stenoses. The ability to respond to an inflation pressure without balloon disruption is dictated by the material properties of a given balloon and, as a consequence, is also a factor in selection of an appropriate balloon catheter. Balloons that are composed of a compliant plastic, such as Silastic, have a much greater range of potential final diameters, with continued balloon expansion dictated as a function of the inflated volume. Embolectomy balloons fall in this category, as well as occlusion balloons that may be used to seat an aortic stent graft or temporarily facilitate proximal aortic occlusion in the presence of a ruptured aneurysm. Both balloon types are capable of inadvertently perforating a vessel wall. Cutting balloon technology has been primarily utilized in the coronary circulation. A recent report from England demonstrated the short-term efficacy of a 6-mm cutting balloon in the periphery.[14] Further studies of cutting balloons for applications in peripheral arterial disease are underway.

Selection of the appropriate balloon size is primarily dictated by the diameter of the normal vessel in which a given lesion is located. Iliac and subclavian arteries, for example, may range in diameter from 6 to 10 mm and are typically smaller in women than in men. The infrarenal aorta varies from 14 to 20 mm, and renal and superficial femoral arteries are usually 4 to 5 mm in diameter. The diameters of infrageniculate vessels are often 3 mm. Stenotic lesions in the iliac and subclavian veins and inferior vena cava may also require angioplasty; and whereas these vessels are generally larger than their accompanying arteries, similar rules apply. With experience, balloon selection can be made on the basis of the appearance of

the arteriogram, but more accurate measurement techniques exist, including use of integrated image-based software programs referenced to a fluoroscopically visualized catheter of known French size. Alternatively, intravascular ultrasound[15] also provides a very accurate means for defining vessel size, and marker catheters that contain radiopaque marks at known intervals can also be used for a more accurate assessment of vessel diameter. Balloon shaft lengths are commonly 75 cm or 120 cm, and, depending on the system, can be coaxial or monorail and designed to be inserted over 0.014-inch, 0.018-inch, or 0.035-inch wires.

The balloon inflating solution is usually a mixture of saline and contrast solution. Whereas most balloons are best imaged using a 50-50 mix, larger aortic balloons can be easily visualized using 20% to 30% (v/v) of contrast agent, which decreases viscosity of the solution and allows the balloon to be more rapidly inflated or deflated. To accurately pre-position an angioplasty catheter before inflation, balloons are designed with a radiopaque marker at each end at the cylindrical portion of the balloon. However, balloons may be designed with differing degrees of taper, and a significant "shoulder" may protrude past these marks. In this regard, when treating a lesion that lies near a branch point, it is important to account for balloon taper and limit inadvertent extension of the terminal portion of the balloon into a smaller branch vessel with attendant risk or vessel rupture or dissection.

INTRAVASCULAR STENTS AND ENDOPROSTHESES

Vascular stents are commonly used after an inadequate angioplasty with dissection or elastic recoil of an arterial stenosis (Fig. 62-5). Appropriate indications for primary stenting of a lesion without an initial trial of angioplasty alone are evolving in a manner that are dependent on the extent and site of the lesion. Vascular stents are classified into two basic categories: balloon-expandable and self-expanding. Balloon-expandable stents are usually composed of stainless steel, mounted on an angioplasty balloon, and deployed by balloon inflation. They can be manually placed on a chosen balloon catheter or obtained premounted on a balloon catheter. The capacity of a balloon expandable stent to shorten in length during deployment depends on both stent geometry and the final diameter to which the balloon is expanded. Self-expanding stents are deployed by retracting a restraining sheath and usually consist of Elgiloy, a cobalt, chromium, nickel alloy, or Nitinol, a shape memory alloy composed of nickel and titanium, which will contract and assume a heat-treated shape above a transition temperature that depends on the composition of the alloy. Self-expanding stents will expand to a final diameter that is determined by stent geometry, hoop strength, and vessel size. In particular, if the vessel diameter is significantly less than that of the stent, final stent length may be longer than the anticipated unconstrained length.

Several recent innovations in stent technology are worthy of comment. Covered stents have been designed with either a surrounding polytetrafluoroethylene or polyester fabric[16] and have been used predominantly for treatment of traumatic vascular lesions, including arterial disruption and arteriovenous fistulas. However, these devices may well find a growing role in treatment of iliac or femoral arterial occlusive disease as well as of popliteal aneurysms.[17] A second important development has been the development of drug-eluting stents, which transiently release antiproliferative agents into the vessel wall so as to reduce intimal hyperplasia and restenosis.[18-22] Efficacy has been demonstrated for local delivery of selected agents, such as rapamycin and paclitaxel, in the coronary circulation. Data remain limited for the benefit of these agents in the peripheral circulation.[23] Brachytherapy has played a significant role in the management of restenosis in the coronary circulation. One trial thus far has demonstrated a benefit of brachytherapy in the periphery,[24] and two additional brachytherapy trials, the PARIS trial and the Vienna 3 trial, are ongoing. The impact of any of these evolving technologies will require further evaluation in the peripheral circulation.

Endovascular aneurysm repair was initiated by Parodi in 1991.[25] Since that time, a large number of endografts have been inserted under the auspice of clinical trials at first and now as Food and Drug Administration–approved devices. The AneuRx (Medtronic AVE, Santa Rosa, CA), Ancure (Guidant Corp., Menlo Park, CA), Excluder (W.L.Gore & Associates, Flagstaff, AZ), and Zenith (Cook Inc., Bloomington, IN) devices have all been approved for clinical use. All of these devices require that patients have an infrarenal aneurysm with at least a 1-cm neck and not greater than 60 degrees of angulation. For those patients with associated common iliac artery aneurysmal disease, endovascular treatment can be achieved by initial coil embolization of the ipsilateral hypogastric artery with extension of the endovascular device into the external iliac artery. Clinical trials are underway with devices that will expand indications to aneurysms involving the visceral segment of the abdominal aorta.

Commercially available endografts for treatment of thoracic aortic disease are not yet available. However, experience with experimental devices is rapidly accumulating.[26] Thoracic aortic devices have been used to treat descending thoracic aneurysms, traumatic aortic transections, and aortic dissections. A larger experience with these devices exists in both Europe and Asia, and trials are underway in the United States with several devices.

IMAGE-GUIDED THERAPY

Excellent imaging is the key to endoluminal therapies regardless of whether the intervention is performed in an imaging suite or an operating room. Fluoroscopy is the modality used for digital subtraction angiography. Fluoroscopy functions via an image intensifier that receives, concentrates, and brightens an x-ray image to produce an electronic image that can be displayed on a screen. The larger size of an image intensifier usually allows for better quality imaging. A standard imaging suite image intensifier is 15 inches in diameter, whereas a standard image intensifier on a portable C arm is 12 inches in diameter. Both portable and stationary equipment have specialized functions that are commonly used during interventions. Magnified views are obtained when focusing on a limited area such as the aortic bifurcation for kissing stent deployment. Another feature is the road map technique. This allows for a representation of the arterial tree by contrast angiography on one digital screen with real-time fluoroscopy on another screen. Road mapping facilitates crossing high-grade stenosis or occlusions. It is also useful when deploying vascular stents.

Fluoroscopic images can be obtained in many different angles. Anteroposterior (AP), right anterior oblique (RAO), and left anterior oblique (LAO) are the most common views. The oblique views allow better visualization of portions of the vascular tree, such as the internal iliac arteries. For example, the oblique angles allows the origin of this vessel to be visualized so that it does not overlap with the common iliac artery. This is especially important with iliac arterial interventions to prevent stenting across the origin of the internal iliac artery. Additional views such as craniocaudal correction can also be obtained. This is particularly useful for correcting angulation in difficult aortic necks during endovascular aneurysm repair.

It is important for all vascular surgeons working with fluoroscopy to be aware of its potential deleterious effects. Radiation exposure can lead to short-term effects on the hematopoietic, gastrointestinal, and central nervous systems, which can be lethal if the exposure is high. Long-term radiation effects include sterility and the development of malignancies. It is important that everyone exposed to the radiation field be protected by appropriate lead gowns. Some surgeons routinely wear lead glasses as well as lead gloves to minimize their exposures and risks from the radiation.

Selected References

Mackrell PJ, Langan EM III, Sullivan TM, et al: Management of renal artery stenosis: Effects of a shift from surgical to percutaneous therapy on indications and outcomes. Ann Vasc Surg 17:54-59, 2003.

> This article demonstrates the change in thought in treating renal artery occlusive disease. Percutaneous therapy has broadened the patient population that can be safely treated.

Parodi JC, Palmaz JC, Barone HD: Transfemoral intraluminal graft implantation for abdominal aortic aneurysms. Ann Vasc Surg 5:491-499, 1991.

> This pioneering work revolutionized the field of vascular surgery.

Sousa JE, Serruys PW, Costa MA: New frontiers in cardiology: Drug-eluting stents: I. Circulation 107:2274-2279, 2003.

Sousa JE, Serruys PW, Costa MA: New frontiers in cardiology: Drug-eluting stents: II. Circulation 107:2383-2389, 2003.

> The two articles by Sousa and coworkers demonstrate the tremendous impact that drug-eluting stents have had on the coronary circulation. Trials are underway to investigate their potential efficacy in the peripheral circulation.

Steinmetz E, Tatou E, Favier-Blavoux C, et al: Endovascular treatment as first choice in chronic intestinal ischemia. Ann Vasc Surg 16:693-699, 2002.

> This report highlights the paradigm shift that is occurring in the management of chronic intestinal ischemia. Patients who were previously too high risk for a surgical intervention are considered candidates for an endoluminal approach.

Tielliu IF, Verhoeven EL, Prins TR, et al: Treatment of popliteal artery aneurysms with the Hemobahn stent-graft. J Endovasc Ther 10:111-116, 2003.

> This technology requires further investigation but is a promising approach to the management of peripheral arterial aneurysmal disease.

References

1. Faries P, Morrissey NJ, Teodorescu V, et al: Recent advances in peripheral angioplasty and stenting. Angiology 53:617-626, 2002.
2. Robinson JD, Eikens PH, Smith TP, et al: A stepless needle-dilator for expedient percutaneous catheterization: Technical note. Cardiovasc Intervent Radiol 13:329-332, 1990.
3. Yeow KM, Toh CH, Wu CH, et al: Sonographically guided antegrade common femoral artery access. J Ultrasound Med 21:1413-1416, 2002.
4. Gorog DA, Watkinson A, Lipkin DP: Treatment of iatrogenic aortic dissection by percutaneous stent placement. J Invasive Cardiol 15:84-85, 2003.
5. Rickli H, Unterweger M, Sutsch G, et al: Comparison of costs and safety of a suture-mediated closure device with conventional manual compression after coronary artery interventions. Catheter Cardiovasc Interv 57:297-302, 2002.
6. Chevalier B, Lancelin B, Koning R, et al: Effect of a closure device on complication rates in high-local-risk patients: Results of a randomized multicenter trial. Catheter Cardiovasc Interv 58:285-291, 2003.
7. Kaukanen ET, Manninen HI, Matsi PJ, et al: Brachial artery access for percutaneous renal artery interventions. Cardiovasc Intervent Radiol 20:353-358, 1997.
8. Nice C, Timmons G, Bartholemew P, et al: Retrograde vs. Antegrade puncture for infra-inguinal angioplasty. Cardiovasc Intervent Radiol, Jun 25, 2003 [Epub ahead of print].
9. Cardella JF, Kotula F, Hunter DW, et al: Very stiff guidewire with a floppy tip. Radiology 156:837, 1985.
10. Rosen RJ, McLean GK, Oleaga JA, et al: A new exchange guidewire for transluminal angioplasty. Radiology 140:242-243, 1981.
11. Mackrell PJ, Langan EM III, Sullivan TM, et al: Management of renal artery stenosis: Effects of a shift from surgical to percutaneous therapy on indications and outcomes. Ann Vasc Surg 17:54-59, 2003.
12. Steinmetz E, Tatou E, Favier-Blavoux C, et al: Endovascular treatment as first choice in chronic intestinal ischemia. Ann Vasc Surg 16:693-699, 2002.
13. Leon M, Baim DS, Popma JJ, et al: A clinical trial comparing three antithrombotic-drug regimens after coronary-artery stenting. N Engl J Med 339:1665-1671, 1998.
14. Engelke C, Sandhu C, Morgan RA, et al: Using 6-mm cutting balloon angioplasty in patients with resistant peripheral artery stenosis: Preliminary results. AJR Am J Roentgenol 179:619-623, 2002.
15. Arko F, McCollough R, Manning L, et al: Use of intravascular ultrasound in the endovascular management of atherosclerotic aortoiliac occlusive disease. Am J Surg 172:546-549; discussion 549-550, 1996.
16. Rzucidlo EM, Powell RJ, Zwolak RM, et al: Early results of stent-grafting to treat diffuse aortoiliac occlusive disease. J Vasc Surg 37:1175-1180, 2003.
17. Tielliu IF, Verhoeven EL, Prins TR, et al: Treatment of popliteal artery aneurysms with the Hemobahn stent-graft. J Endovasc Ther 10:111-116, 2003.
18. Sonoda S, Honda Y, Kataoka T, et al: Taxol-based eluting stents from theory to human validation: Clinical and intravascular ultrasound observations. J Invasive Cardiol 15:109-114, 2003.
19. Finkelstein A, McClean D, Kar S, et al: Local drug delivery via a coronary stent with programmable release pharmacokinetics. Circulation 107:777-784, 2003.
20. Virmani R, Kolodgie FD, Farb A, et al: Drug eluting stents: Are human and animal studies comparable? Heart 89:133-138, 2003.
21. Sousa JE, Serruys PW, Costa MA: New frontiers in cardiology: Drug-eluting stents: II. Circulation 107:2383-2389, 2003.
22. Sousa JE, Serruys PW, Costa MA: New frontiers in cardiology: Drug-eluting stents: I. Circulation 107:2274-2279, 2003.
23. Duda SH, Poerner TC, Wiesinger B, et al: Drug-eluting stents: Potential applications for peripheral arterial occlusive disease. J Vasc Interv Radiol 14:291-301, 2003.
24. Minar E, Pokrajac B, Budinsky A, et al: Endovascular brachytherapy in peripheral arteries. Vasa 32:3-9, 2003.
25. Parodi JC, Palmaz JC, Barone HD: Transfemoral intraluminal graft implantation for abdominal aortic aneurysms. Ann Vasc Surg 5:491-499, 1991.
26. Milner R, Bavaria JE, Baum RA, et al: Thoracic aortic stent grafts. Semin Roentgenol 36:340-350, 2001.

CHAPTER 63

CEREBROVASCULAR DISEASE

G. Patrick Clagett, M.D.

Stroke Epidemiology	**Current Indications for Carotid Endarterectomy**
Pathology and Pathophysiology	**Operative Management**
Clinical Presentation and Work-up	**Postoperative Complications**
Carotid Endarterectomy: Historical Perspective	**Ongoing Issues**
Carotid Endarterectomy in Modern Times	

STROKE EPIDEMIOLOGY

Stroke mortality is the third leading cause of death in the United States, accounting for one in every 15 deaths in 1992.[1] There has been a dramatic and striking 60% decline in United States' stroke mortality between 1960 and 1990. Despite this decline, nearly 150,000 Americans died of stroke during 1995, which corresponds to one death every 3.5 minutes. The distribution of stroke morbidity and mortality is heterogeneous in the United States population, and the burden of stroke is greater among elderly men and African Americans. In the southeastern United States, stroke risk is approximately 1.4 times that of other regions. The mortality after stroke remains substantial in that about 25% of those who have strokes die in the year following the stroke.

Besides mortality, morbidity in the more than 3 million surviving stroke victims is substantial. Stroke is the leading cause of serious disability in the United States and accounts for approximately half of the patients hospitalized for acute neurologic disease. Among long-term stroke survivors, 48% have hemiparesis, 22% cannot walk, 24% to 53% are completely or partially dependent for normal daily activities, 12% to 18% are aphasic, and 32% are clinically depressed.[1] The average health care cost in the United States exceeds $10 billion annually. Inpatient and outpatient costs for each of the following conditions are as follows: cerebral infarction, $8,000 to $16,500; subarachnoid hemorrhage, $27,000 to $33,000; and intracerebral hemorrhage, $11,000 to $13,000.

Strong risk factors for stroke that are modifiable include hypertension, cigarette smoking, sickle cell disease, transient ischemic attack (TIA), asymptomatic carotid stenosis, and cardiac diseases, including atrial fibrillation, infective endocarditis, mitral stenosis, and recent large myocardial infarction. Hypertension is the single most important modifiable risk factor for ischemic stroke. Most estimates for hypertension indicate a relative risk of stroke of approximately four times normal when hypertension is defined as systolic pressure of 160 mm Hg and/or diastolic blood pressure of 95 mm Hg.[1] Meta-analysis of trials of hypertension throughout the world have demonstrated a 38% reduction in all strokes and a 40% reduction in fatal strokes with systematic treatment of hypertension.

Atrial fibrillation is the most powerful and treatable cardiac precursor of stroke. It is estimated that almost half of the cardioembolic strokes occur in the setting of atrial fibrillation. Warfarin anticoagulation reduces the risk of stroke by 68% in pooled analyses of atrial fibrillation trials.[2] Cigarette smoking increases the relative risk of ischemic stroke nearly two times, with a clear dose-response relation. Major trials of smoking cessation have documented a prompt reduction in stroke risk. Moderate consumption of alcohol may reduce cardiovascular disease, including stroke; however, heavy alcohol consumption increases the risk of stroke, particularly from brain hemorrhage.

PATHOLOGY AND PATHOPHYSIOLOGY

Atherosclerosis of arteries supplying the brain is a leading cause of ischemic stroke in North America and Europe (Figs. 63-1 and 63-2). Large-artery atherosclerosis, most often involving the carotid bifurcations, causes stroke by three principal mechanisms: embolization of atherosclerotic and thrombotic material (artery-to-artery emboli); thrombotic occlusion; and hypoperfusion from advanced, hemodynamically significant stenoses (see Fig. 63-2).

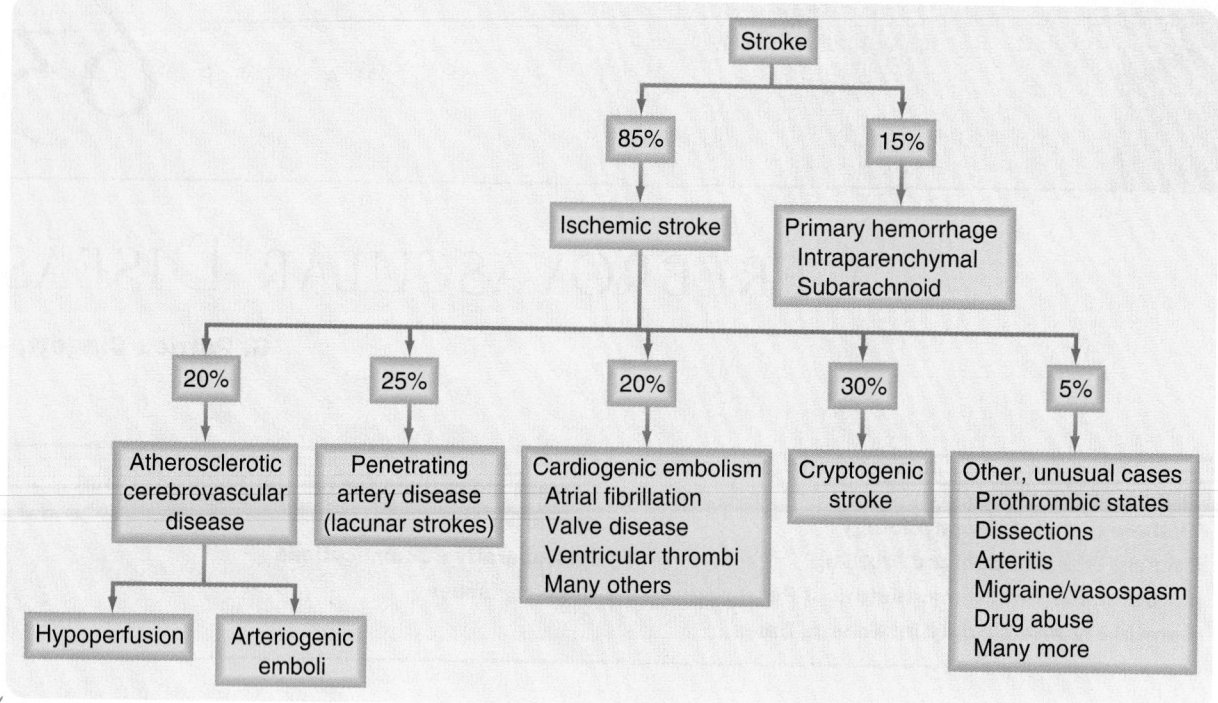

FIGURE 63-1.   Proportion of strokes caused by different etiologies.

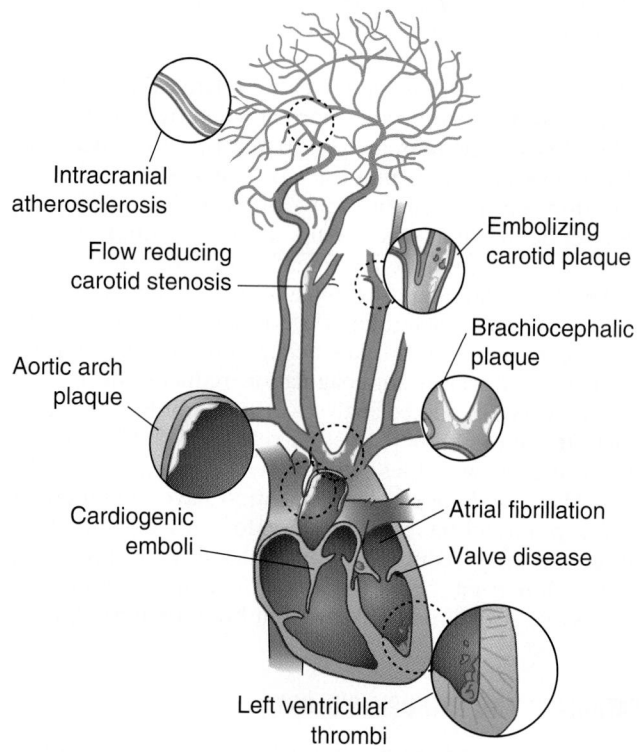

FIGURE 63-2.   Cardiogenic and arterial atherosclerotic sources for stroke.

Aortic arch atherosclerosis may also be a source of cerebral emboli and is increasingly being implicated with wider application of transesophageal echography in the evaluation of stroke patients. Small-vessel atherosclerosis, also called *lipohyalinosis*, leading to occlusion of small penetrating brain arteries is the leading cause of subcortical or lacunar infarcts. About 20% of ischemic strokes are due to cardiogenic embolism, most commonly from atrial fibrillation (see Figs. 63-1 and 63-2). Despite thorough evaluation, the exact cause of about 30% of ischemic strokes is unknown, and these are termed *cryptogenic strokes*. Serial cerebral angiography in patients with cryptogenic stroke often reveals occlusions of intracranial arteries that resolve within days. This implicates embolic occlusion, although the source of embolism is unknown.

Localization of advanced atherosclerosis along the outer wall of the carotid sinus has been noted in postmortem specimens, on angiograms of patients with carotid stenosis, and in carotid bifurcation plaques removed during carotid endarterectomy. In rheologic studies involving glass models of the carotid bifurcation, fluid-flow patterns along the outer wall of the sinus are complex and include regions of flow separation and reversal of axial flow as well as the development of counter-rotating helical trajectories (Fig. 63-3).[3] Wall shear stress is low in this region. In contrast, regions of moderate-to-high shear stress, along the inner border of the carotid sinus, are relatively free of atherosclerosis and intimal thickening. Atherosclerosis develops largely in regions of relatively low wall shear stress, flow separation, and departure from axially aligned, unidirectional flow. Such studies suggest that the unique and stereotyped location of atherosclerosis at the carotid bifurcation is due to the

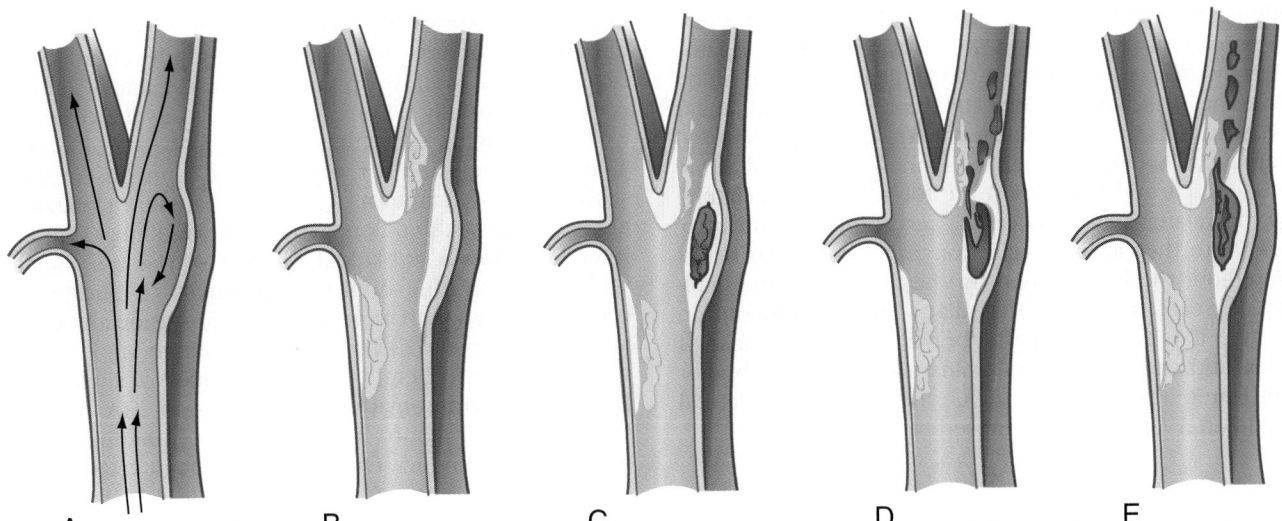

FIGURE 63-3.   A, Simplified flow patterns at the carotid bifurcation demonstrate complex reversal of flow along the posterior wall of the carotid sinus. This region is most vulnerable to plaque development. B, Established plaque at the carotid bifurcation. C, Soft, central necrotic core with an overlying thin fibrous cap. This area is prone to plaque rupture. D, Disruption of the fibrous cap allows necrotic cellular debris and lipid material from the central core to enter the lumen of the internal carotid artery, thus becoming atherogenic emboli. The patient may experience symptoms (transient ischemia, stroke, or amaurosis fugax) or remain asymptomatic depending on the site of lodgment and the extent of tissue compromise. E, The empty necrotic core becomes a deep ulcer in the plaque. The walls of the ulcer are highly thrombogenic and reactive with platelets. This leads to thromboembolism in the internal carotid artery circulation.

unusual geometry of this area that gives rise to hemodynamic and rheologic disturbances.[3] The relatively sluggish flow in such areas may lead to vessel wall metabolic disturbances that are cumulative over time. In contrast to high-shear areas, these areas might be more likely to have prolonged exposure to plasma lipids, circulating white blood cells and platelets, activated coagulation factors, and other mitogenic stimuli.

Established carotid bifurcation plaques have features in common with other complex atherosclerotic lesions. There is a soft central core of necrotic cellular elements and lipid material sometimes associated with fibrin thrombus, red blood cells, hemosiderin, and other evidence of previous hemorrhage into the plaque (see Fig. 63-3). A fibrous cap of varying thickness that is composed of collagen, glycosaminoglycans, vascular smooth muscle cells, and fibroblasts covers the central core and is a vulnerable region of the plaque. The remainder of the plaque consists of vascular smooth muscle cells, fibroblasts, collagen, and scattered regions of calcification. Lipid-laden macrophages may be found in several areas of the plaque but are usually concentrated in the central core.

Plaque destabilization with rupture of the plaque results in embolization of debris from the central core, producing symptoms of TIA, amaurosis fugax, and stroke (see Fig. 63-3). Atherosclerotic plaque rupture occurs as a result of interactions between external mechanical triggers and vulnerable regions of the plaque when force is acting on the plaque and its fibrous cap exceeds the tensile strength of these structures. Along with causing symptoms, plaque rupture with dissection of blood into its interior can lead to dramatic growth of the plaque.

In addition to external mechanical forces, the integrity of the fibrous cap is a balance between synthesis and degradation of the extracellular matrix. Inflammatory cells consisting mainly of macrophages and T lymphocytes appear at the borders of the necrotic core and of the fibrous cap; these cells secrete metalloproteinases, cysteine proteases, growth factors, and cytokines that degrade matrix and make the fibrous cap vulnerable to rupture.[4,5] Cytokines released by inflammatory cells may also contribute to this process by inducing adjacent smooth muscle cells to secrete proteases. A substantial percentage of cells within the plaque have been found to have positive markers of apoptosis, and most apoptotic cells are found near or within the necrotic core and in the fibrous cap.[6] Inflammatory cytokines from macrophages may also contribute to induction of apoptosis. Loss of cells in the fibrous cap along with matrix degradation may accelerate fibrous cap disruption.

Once the fibrous cap has ruptured and the debris from the central core has escaped, a deep ulcer remains in the plaque (see Fig. 63-3). The surface lining the ulcer is highly thrombogenic and stimulates platelet aggregation and blood coagulation. This process is promoted by stasis of blood within the depths of the ulcer. Platelet thrombogenesis at this site is a dynamic process, with platelets accumulating and embolizing into the internal carotid artery. These events may be microembolic, causing TIA and amaurosis fugax, or they may lead to large emboli or thrombosis of the entire internal carotid artery, causing major stroke.

Tracer studies in animal models employing radioactive microemboli have documented that emboli introduced at the carotid bifurcation lodge preferentially in the ophthalmic and middle cerebral arteries.[7] Furthermore, there is a predictable regularity in the distribution of the paths taken by these emboli due to the laminar nature of blood flow. These findings account for the repetition of similar TIA symptoms in an individual patient. If the contralateral internal carotid artery is ligated, emboli introduced at the ipsilateral carotid bifurcation are found in the ipsilateral and contralateral anterior cerebral territories. Emboli introduced into the cardiac circulation are equally distributed throughout the brain. Based on these experimental findings, one can conclude that cardiac sources of emboli can produce TIAs anywhere in the brain. In contrast, those of the carotid artery cause predominantly middle cerebral or ophthalmic artery territory TIAs unless the contralateral carotid artery is severely stenosed or occluded.

CLINICAL PRESENTATION AND WORK-UP

Symptomatic patients present with TIAs, amaurosis fugax, or stroke. TIAs are defined as brief episodes of focal loss of brain function due to ischemia that can usually be localized to that portion of the brain supplied by one vascular system (left or right carotid or vertebrobasilar).[8] By convention, episodes lasting less than 24 hours are classified as TIAs, although the longer the episode, the greater the likelihood of finding a cerebral infarct on computed tomography (CT) or magnetic resonance imaging (MRI). TIAs commonly last 2 to 15 minutes and are rapid in onset (no symptoms to maximal symptoms in < 5 minutes and usually in < 2 minutes). Fleeting episodes lasting only a few seconds are not likely to be TIAs. Each TIA leaves no persistent deficit, and there are often multiple attacks.

Left carotid system TIAs manifest as (1) motor dysfunction (dysarthria, weakness, paralysis, or clumsiness of the right extremities and/or face); (2) loss of vision in the left eye (amaurosis fugax), or, rarely, the right field of vision (homonymous hemianopsia); (3) sensory symptoms (numbness, including loss of sensation or paresthesia involving the right upper and/or lower extremity and/or face); and (4) aphasia (language disturbance).

Right carotid system TIAs produce similar symptoms on the opposite side, except that aphasia occurs only when the right hemisphere is dominant for speech (left-handed individual).

Vertebrobasilar system TIAs are characterized by the rapid onset of (1) motor dysfunction (weakness, paralysis, or clumsiness) of any combination of upper and lower extremities and face (left and/or right); (2) sensory symptoms (loss of sensation, numbness, or paresthesia involving the left, right, or both sides); (3) loss of vision in one or both homonymous visual fields; and (4) loss of balance, vertigo, unsteadiness or disequilibrium, diplopia, or dysarthria.[8] These last symptoms are characteristic but are not considered as a TIA when any of these symptoms are alone. Dysarthria can accompany either carotid or vertebrobasilar TIAs.

Most patients have TIAs that include motor symptoms. Sensory symptoms involving only part of one extremity or only one side of the face during a single attack not accompanied by other symptoms are difficult to interpret with

certainty. Occasionally, patients have only episodes of aphasia. An attack that does not include either motor defect, visual loss, or aphasia is unusual and should be reviewed carefully before accepting TIA as the diagnosis.

The following symptoms are not to be considered as TIAs: (1) march of a sensory deficit; (2) unconsciousness without other symptoms; (3) vertigo alone; (4) dizziness alone; (5) dysarthria alone; (6) diplopia alone; (7) incontinence of bowel or bladder; (8) loss of vision associated with alteration of level of consciousness; (9) focal symptoms associated with migraines; (10) confusion alone; (11) amnesia alone; and (12) drop-attacks alone.

A reversible ischemic neurologic deficit or small stroke has similar symptomatic components to TIA but lasts longer than 24 hours. Full neurologic function returns within 48 to 72 hours. On careful neurologic examination, there may be some lingering deficits, in which case the patient is said to have suffered a small stroke.

Amaurosis fugax is best defined as a transient monocular visual disturbance. Symptoms are sudden in onset and last for minutes. They are usually shorter in duration than cortical TIAs. Patients often describe the visual disturbance as being like a curtain shade descending to the horizontal mid-visual field and then ascending. The opposite can occur with the curtain shade ascending to the mid-horizontal visual field and then descending. Whether the curtain shade involves the top or bottom half of the visual field depends on whether the inferior or superior retinal artery is embolized with the corresponding portion of retina rendered ischemic. If the entire central retinal artery is transiently occluded, patients will complain of almost complete loss of vision in the eye. Because the macula lutea and fovea centralis have a separate blood supply, they often retain this small portion of the visual field and patients describe their vision as telescoped or as looking out of a tunnel. The visual impairment itself may be complete absence of vision in the involved portion or blurriness or "graying" of vision.

The diagnosis of TIA and amaurosis fugax is based on history. It is rare for a physician to actually witness one of these episodes. It is therefore incumbent on the physician to carefully probe and document the characteristics of the event. Often it is helpful to question the patient's spouse or friend who may have been present during the episode.

Once the diagnosis of TIA, amaurosis fugax, or small stroke is established, urgent work-up is required because these are warning symptoms of major stroke. The first priority is to rule out carotid artery occlusive disease, and this can be effectively done with duplex ultrasonography (Fig. 63-4). Duplex ultrasonography allows determination of whether or not significant carotid occlusive disease is present and the severity of the stenosis at the origin of the internal carotid artery. If advanced carotid stenosis is present ipsilateral to the symptoms, carotid endarterectomy is generally indicated and no further testing is required except for a brain imaging study (CT scan or MRI) to rule out intracranial pathology. Contrast arteriography is helpful for lesser degrees of stenosis because duplex ultrasonography frequently underestimates or overestimates levels of stenosis in the moderate (40% to 59%) range.[9] Contrast arteriography is also indicated when

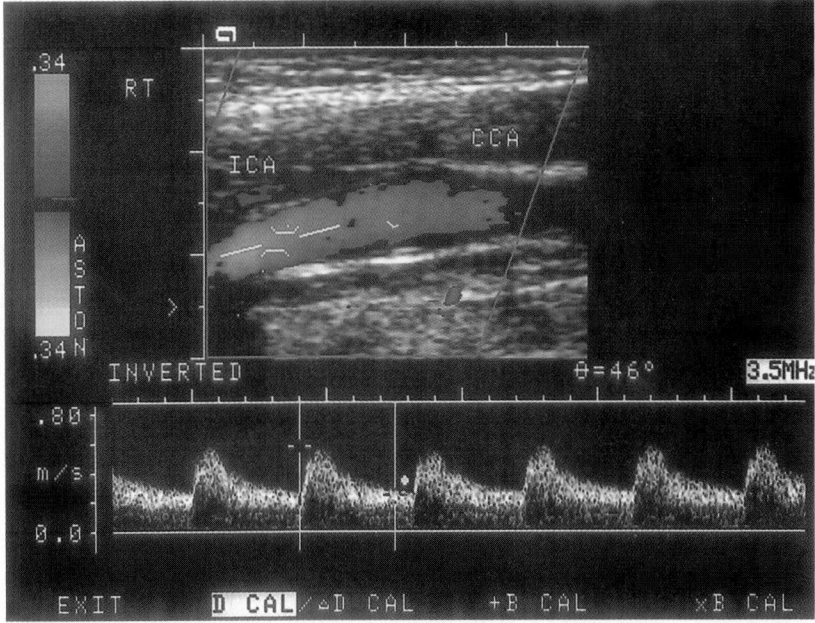

A

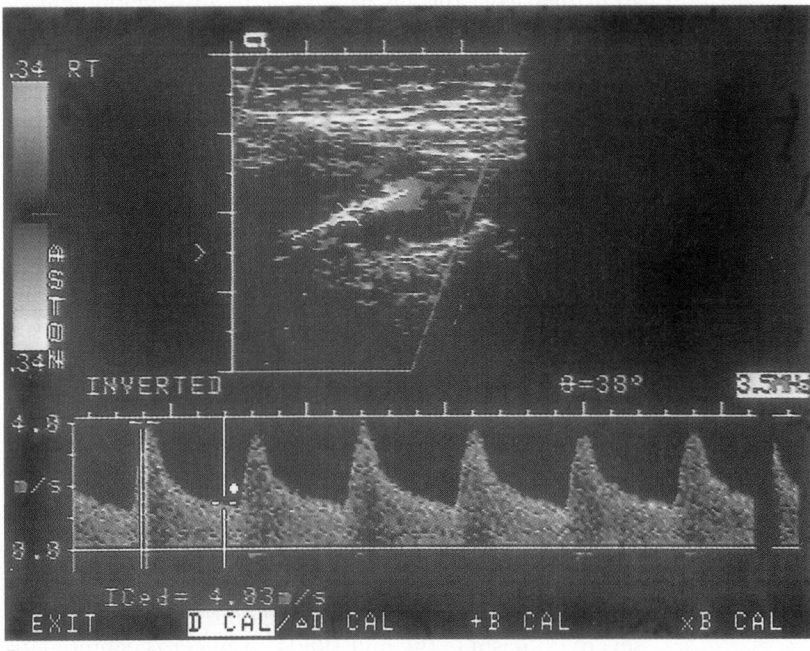

B

FIGURE 63-4. A duplex scan combines two diagnostic modalities. Anatomic information from the B-mode scan and the physiologic information of flow velocities from the Doppler scan define morphologic and hemodynamic abnormalities at the carotid bifurcation. Pulsed Doppler technology allows sampling of flow velocities within a particular area of the vessel lumen. Color-flow imaging allows determination of blood flow direction and velocity within the vessel lumen and is projected as colors displayed within the vessel image formed from the B-mode scan. Thus, vessels with blood flowing in the arterial direction are displaced as one color, generally red, and blood flow in the opposite direction (venous flow) is displayed as blue. Variations of color shading indicate changes in velocity, with lighter shades of color indicating higher velocities. This technology is useful in allowing the examiner to choose the areas of greatest disease and flow disturbance in the real-time B-mode image to measure velocities and perform spectral analysis at the point of maximal stenosis. Further information is derived from spectral waveform analysis. The returning Doppler signal consists of multiple frequencies that are representative of the velocities of the cellular elements of the blood within the sample volume. If the cells are moving at similar velocities and in similar directions, the resulting frequencies when displayed graphically as velocities on the Y axis produce a narrow waveform. This type of waveform is seen with unidirectional, laminar flow. Luminal irregularities, such as plaque, not only increase the peak velocities within the sample volume but also increase the range of frequencies within it, as the resulting flow disturbances cause variations in the velocity and direction of the cellular components of the blood. This results in broadening of the spectral waveform and is characteristic of significant stenosis of the lumen.

A, Arterial flow (red) is displayed in the internal (ICA) and common (CCA) carotid arteries. Sampling for flow velocities and spectral waveform analysis is carried out in the center stream of the internal carotid artery, as displayed on the diagram, and the waveform is shown below. Peak systolic and end-diastolic velocities are measured on a representative wave, and in the example, these are 0.58 m/sec (58 cm/sec) and 0.25 m/sec (25 cm/sec), respectively. These are well within normal limits. B, The same general area is being interrogated in a diseased internal carotid artery. The lumen appears to narrow and the red color becomes variegated and lighter. Arterial flow is sampled in the area of maximal disturbance and narrowing, and the resultant waveform is displayed below. The peak systolic velocities approach 4 m/sec (400 cm/sec) and the end-diastolic velocity is 1.41 m/sec (141 cm/sec). These values are elevated, indicating abnormally increased flow velocities in the area of stenosis. In addition, spectral analysis shows broadening from nonlaminar flow. These findings are characteristic of significant stenosis. By applying validated criteria, the severity of the stenosis can be estimated accurately.

more proximal atherosclerotic disease is suspected involving the branches coming off the aortic arch. In patients with negative findings on duplex ultrasonography, arteriography is useful to eliminate intracranial vascular disease and unusual arteriopathies such as fibromuscular dysplasia. If the source for TIA has not been identified after duplex ultrasonography, brain imaging tests, and complete arteriography, cardiac sources must be ruled out with echography and arrhythmia monitoring. Work-up for hypercoagulable disorder may also be indicated. A full algorithm for a diagnostic work-up of patients presenting with TIA is shown in Figure 63-5.

CAROTID ENDARTERECTOMY: HISTORICAL PERSPECTIVE

The goal of surgical therapy for cerebrovascular disease in general and carotid endarterectomy in particular is to prevent stroke. The first individual to realize the potential of surgical therapy was a neurologist. In seminal papers in the early 1950s, Fisher focused attention on the relationship between extracranial carotid disease and cerebral

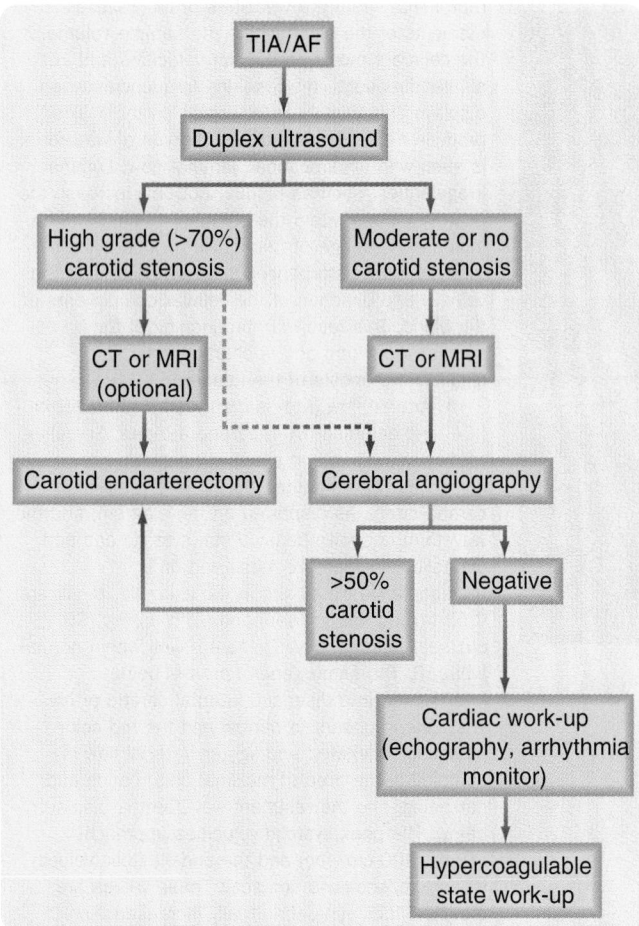

FIGURE 63-5. Diagnostic algorithm for patients presenting with transient ischemic attack (TIA) and/or amaurosis fugax (AF). The dashed line indicates that cerebral angiography is unnecessary in most patients presenting with clear-cut symptoms and high-grade stenosis on duplex ultrasonography. However, under certain circumstances (see text), angiography may be necessary.

infarction and made several important observations about the nature of carotid occlusive disease that led directly to the development of the concept of surgical reconstruction of the extracranial vessels.[10,11] He defined the basic nature of the lesion as atherosclerosis of the extracranial vessels, pointing out the predilection for atheroma to occur at the carotid bifurcation in the neck, and he also observed that the internal carotid artery distal to the bifurcation and the intracranial vessels were usually free of disease. To Fisher, these observations not only indicated that extracranial carotid disease was, indeed, an important cause of strokes but also suggested the possible form of therapy to prevent stroke. He speculated that "it is even conceivable that someday vascular surgery will find a way to bypass the occluded portion of the artery during the period of ominous, fleeting symptoms. Anastomosis of the external carotid artery . . . with the internal carotid artery above the area of narrowing should be feasible."

As a result of Fisher's publications, Carrea, Mollins, and Murphy performed the first successful surgical reconstruction of the carotid artery in Buenos Aires on October 20, 1951.[12] The first successful carotid endarterectomy was performed by DeBakey on August 7, 1953. The operation that gave the greatest impetus to development of surgery for carotid occlusive disease was that of Eastcott, Pickering, and Robb, which was performed in London on May 19, 1954.[12] The case was a woman who had recurrent TIAs associated with stenosis of the left carotid bifurcation. She underwent resection of the bifurcation with restoration of blood flow by anastomosis of the internal carotid artery to the common carotid artery. The patient was completely relieved of symptoms, and the operation dramatically demonstrated that removal of carotid bifurcation atherosclerosis could halt TIAs and, presumably, prevent strokes.

CAROTID ENDARTERECTOMY IN MODERN TIMES

In the decades following the seminal developments in the 1950s, carotid endarterectomy became one of the most common cardiovascular operations performed. The number of patients undergoing endarterectomy in hospitals in the United States rose from 15,000 in 1971 to 107,000 in 1985 (Fig. 63-6).[13] However, the efficacy and appropriateness of carotid endarterectomy sustained severe criticism in the mid 1980s.[14] Concerns centered on the effectiveness of the operation and marked geographic variation in rates of endarterectomy. Adding to this uncertainty was the decline in the number of nonfatal and fatal strokes, the influence of risk factor management in reducing strokes, and the emerging recognition of aspirin and other antiplatelet drugs in preventing stroke.[15] Early randomized trials in the 1970s evaluating carotid endarterectomy yielded negative results, most likely because of a combination of poor selection criteria and high perioperative morbidity and mortality.[16] When a contemporary randomized trial demonstrated that extracranial-intracranial bypass was ineffective in preventing stroke,[17] this presented an opportunity to re-examine the efficacy of carotid endarterectomy, and several randomized trials were begun in both symptomatic and asymptomatic patients.

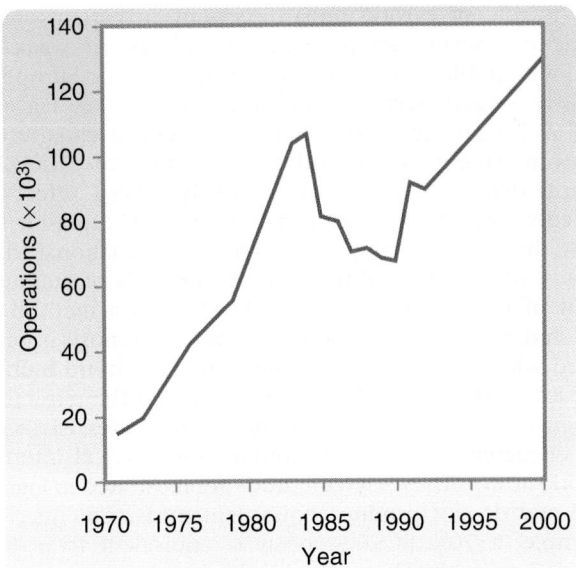

FIGURE 63-6. Number of carotid endarterectomies performed annually in the United States.

A summary of the most important randomized trials is presented in Figure 63-7.[18-25] In all trials, carotid endarterectomy was compared with best medical therapy. Trials involving symptomatic patients are displayed in the top and middle panels, and trials dealing with asymptomatic patients are displayed in the bottom panel. Several important points are apparent by examining the results in Figure 63-7. First, the risk of stroke and death with medical therapy was much greater in symptomatic patients than in asymptomatic patients, thereby yielding a more striking relative risk reduction with endarterectomy. Second, because of the more benign prognosis with medical therapy in asymptomatic patients, it was much more difficult to demonstrate a clear-cut, positive benefit of operation. In fact, only one trial, the Asymptomatic Carotid Atherosclerosis Study (ACAS), was able to show conclusive benefit of carotid endarterectomy in asymptomatic patients.[21] In contrast, almost all trials in symptomatic patients demonstrated an important benefit of carotid endarterectomy that was most apparent in patients with advanced, high-grade stenoses. Although the stroke and death rate with medical therapy in asymptomatic patients was similar in all three trials, the significant benefit of endarterectomy in the ACAS study was the result of a low, perioperative stroke and death rate. These data underscore the need for careful selection for operation of relatively fit patients with asymptomatic disease as well as the critical importance of skill and experience in performing this operation.

The most influential trial was the North American Symptomatic Carotid Endarterectomy Trial (NASCET).[18,24] Patients randomized either to medical or surgical therapy for TIA or mild, disabling stroke ipsilateral to a 70% to 99% narrowing of the internal carotid artery were unequivocally shown to be best treated by surgical therapy. Among the symptomatic patients with high-grade stenosis, carotid endarterectomy reduced the overall risk of fatal and non-

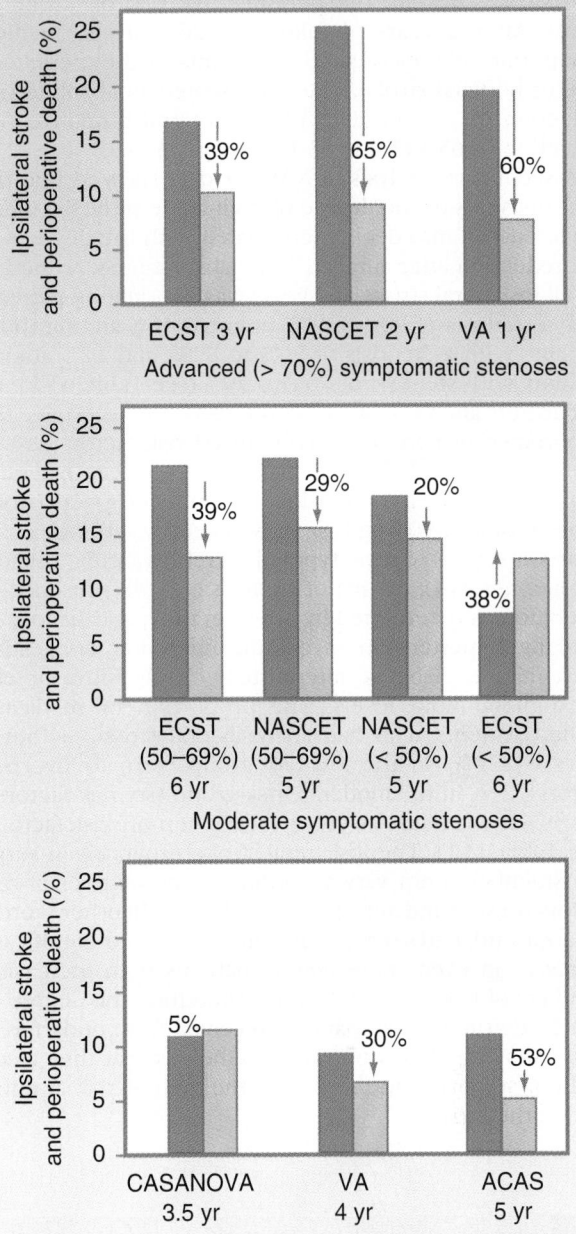

FIGURE 63-7. Randomized trials comparing carotid endarterectomy (cross-hatched bars) to medical therapy (open bars) in symptomatic (top and middle graphs) and asymptomatic (bottom graph) patients. Principal endpoints include ipsilateral stroke and death with operation or initiation of medical treatment. The percentage relative risk reduction from carotid endarterectomy is indicated by the downward-pointing arrows. The length of follow-up for each trial is indicated below the bars. ACAS, Asymptomatic Carotid Atherosclerosis Study; CASANOVA, Carotid Artery Stenosis with Asymptomatic Narrowing: Operation Versus Aspirin; ECST, European Carotid Surgery Trial; NASCET, North American Symptomatic Carotid Endarterectomy Trial; VA, Veterans Administration Trial.

fatal stroke, despite the perioperative risk of stroke or death. After 2 years of follow-up, 26% of the medical group, but only 9% of surgical patients, had experienced fatal or nonfatal stroke. This represented an absolute risk reduction of 17% in favor of surgery and a relative risk reduction of 65% (Table 63-1; see Fig. 63-7).

A secondary analysis of NASCET data showed that the finer divisions of the degree of high-grade stenosis, when broken down into deciles, correlated with the degrees of risk reduction after surgery.[24] The absolute risk reduction for all ipsilateral stroke at 2 years was 26% among patients with a stenosis of 90% to 99% at entry, 18% among those patients with a stenosis of 80% to 89%, and 12% among patients with stenosis of 70% to 79% (see Table 63-1).

Further analyses were conducted to ascertain the importance of commonly recognized risk factors associated with stroke.[24] These included age (>70 years); gender (male); systolic hypertension (>160 mm Hg); diastolic hypertension (>90 mm Hg); how recent was the onset of symptoms (<30 days); type of cerebrovascular events (stroke, not TIA); degree of stenosis (>80%); presence of ulceration as determined by arteriography; and history of smoking, hypertension, myocardial infarction, congestive heart failure, diabetes, intermittent claudication, or elevated blood lipid levels. The proportion of medically treated patients who had an ipsilateral stroke within 2 years was 17% in the low-risk group (zero to five risk factors), 23% in the moderate-risk group (six risk factors), and 39% in the high-risk group (seven or more risk factors) (see Table 63-1). The ipsilateral stroke prognosis in surgical patients did not vary according to the number of risk factors present and averaged 9% at 2 years. In other words, after carotid endarterectomy, there were no significant increases in event rates among patients with increasing numbers of baseline risk factors. Therefore, the degree of benefit that individual patients received from endarterectomy was directly proportional to the risk that they faced without surgery, and those with the highest risk at entry gained the most.

The role of carotid endarterectomy in patients with moderately severe, symptomatic carotid stenoses was clarified with publication of further results from the European Carotid Surgery Trial (ECST)[19] and NASCET (see Fig. 63-7).[18] Although the ECST found no benefit of endarterectomy in patients with moderate stenoses, the NASCET clearly demonstrated a significant beneficial effect in patients with stenoses greater than 50%. The reason for these discordant findings in two major international trials is most likely due to differences in methods of measurement of carotid stenoses. The ECST used a method in which the angiographic point of maximal stenosis is compared with the *estimated* diameter of the carotid bulb at that level. The NASCET method compared the minimum lumen diameter at the point of maximal stenosis with the diameter of the distal, nontapering cervical internal carotid artery. These two methods are illustrated in Figure 63-8 and do not produce equivalent measurements. For example, a 70% ECST stenosis is equivalent to a 40% NASCET stenosis. Therefore, it is likely that more patients with lesser degrees of stenosis were present in the ECST, thus making it more difficult to show a benefit of carotid endarterectomy. When corrections are made for differences in measurement of stenosis, the results of the two trials are in broad agreement.

Discrepancies among the major carotid endarterectomy trials have been clarified pooling the data from the NASCET and the ECST in the form of meta-analysis.[26] Reanalysis of the trials with the same measurements and definitions yielded highly consistent results. Carotid endarterectomy is of modest but significant benefit for patients with 50% to 69% symptomatic stenosis and highly beneficial for those with 70% symptomatic stenosis or greater. Patients with near occlusion (≥95% stenosis) receive less benefit from carotid endarterectomy, possibly due to collateral development.

In the NASCET, symptomatic patients with moderate stenoses were divided into two categories: those with 50% to 69% stenoses (high to moderate) and those with less

TABLE 63-1.   Benefit of Carotid Endarterectomy in Different Patient Categories

Stenosis (%)	Ipsilateral Stroke*		Follow-up (yr)	Relative Risk Reduction (%)	Absolute Risk Reduction (%)	P Value	No. Needed to Treat†
	Medical Treatment (%)	Carotid Endarterectomy (%)					
Symptomatic Disease							
70-99	26	9	2	65	17	.001	6
70-99 + multiple risk factors	39	9	2	77	30	.001	3
70-99 + contralateral occlusion	55	20	2	64	35	.001	3
90-99	35	9	2	88	26	.001	4
80-89	27	9	2	80	18	.001	6
70-79	21	9	2	65	12	.001	8
50-69	22	16	5	29	6.5	.05	15
<50	19	15	5	20	4	.16	25
Asymptomatic Disease							
60-99	11	5	5	53	6	.004	17

*Includes perioperative stroke and strokes occurring during follow-up period.
†This value represents the theoretical number of patients in this category who would have to undergo carotid endarterectomy to prevent one stroke.

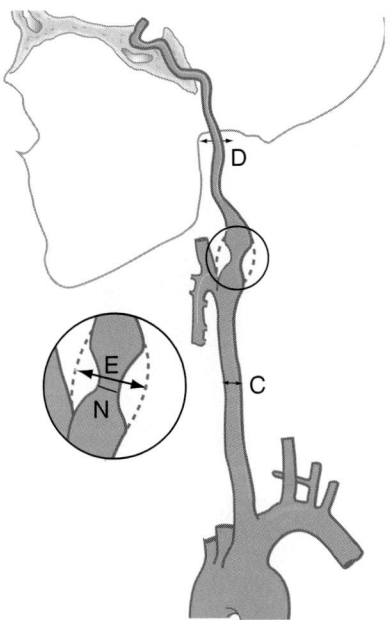

FIGURE 63-8. Measurement of diameters used in calculating percentage of stenosis for three methods. C, common carotid artery; D, distal normal internal carotid artery; E, estimate of unseen carotid artery bulb wall; N, narrowest portion. Percentage of stenosis was calculated as follows: North American Symptomatic Carotid Endarterectomy Trial method = [1 − (N/D)] × 100%; European Carotid Surgery Trial method = [1 − (N/E)] × 100%; common carotid artery method = [1 − (N/C)] × 100%. (From Eliasziw M, Smith RF, Singh N, et al: Further comments on the measurement of carotid artery stenosis from angiograms. Stroke 25:2445-2449, 1994.)

than 50% stenoses (low to moderate).[18] Endarterectomy was of significant benefit in preventing ipsilateral stroke in the high-to-moderate patients; in patients with less than 50% stenoses, medical treatment produced equivalent results (see Fig. 63-7).

In addition to clearly delineating the biologic significance of severity of stenosis in symptomatic patients, the NASCET also has determined that other factors are important in determining stroke prognosis with medical therapy and the potential benefit of endarterectomy. Contralateral carotid occlusion, angiographic findings of ulceration, intracranial stenoses, and hemispheric as opposed to retinal ischemic events all increase the risk of stroke with medical therapy for a given level of stenosis (see Table 63-1).[27-32] Elderly patients (>75 years) with 50% to 99% symptomatic stenoses also benefit more from carotid endarterectomy than younger patients.[33] Furthermore, the long-term benefit of surgery is greater and the risk of stroke with medical treatment is higher for men than for women and for patients who have had stroke rather than for those with TIAs.[18] NASCET data have also delineated perioperative risk factors that increase the risk of stroke or death with operation. These include diabetes mellitus, elevated blood pressure, contralateral occlusion, left-sided disease, or a lesion that is evident on CT or MRI.[34] All of these factors must be taken into account before recommending carotid endarterectomy in a given patient. Although the severity of stenosis may be the most important determi-

nant in selecting patients for surgery, the ultimate threshold may be adjusted upward or downward, depending on the absence or presence of other risk factors.

CURRENT INDICATIONS FOR CAROTID ENDARTERECTOMY

In clinical settings where the risk of carotid endarterectomy is acceptably low according to published guidelines, the operation can be recommended in patients with carotid stenosis of 50% or greater with ipsilateral TIAs, amaurosis fugax, a reversible neurologic deficit, or small stroke and in selected cases of recurrent, symptomatic carotid stenosis.[35,36] Patients with lesser degrees of symptomatic stenosis may be considered for operation if they have failed medical therapy (have ongoing symptoms), particularly if there is evidence of ulceration of the lesion or if contralateral occlusion is present.

Individualized patients may require surgery for progressive stroke, progressive retinal ischemia, acute carotid occlusion, symptomatic carotid stump syndrome (treated with external carotid reconstruction), global cerebral ischemia caused by multiple large-vessel occlusive disease, and in certain cases of symptomatic carotid dissection and true or false aneurysm. The procedure is generally not indicated in patients presenting with vertebrobasilar distribution TIAs, or multi-infarct dementia, patients with severe neurologic deficits, and those with evidence of intracranial hemorrhage or large infarcts. Medical contraindications include the presence of uncontrolled congestive heart failure, recent myocardial infarction, unstable angina, dementia, advanced malignancy, and uncertain diagnosis.

The indications for endarterectomy in asymptomatic patients remain less clear cut. Although ACAS demonstrated significant benefit for all patients randomized to operation with 60% to 99% carotid stenoses, it is likely that those with advanced stenoses benefited most. This assumption is based on the strong, positive correlation between the degree of stenosis and subsequent risk of stroke and death in symptomatic and asymptomatic populations. Because the benefit-to-risk ratio in asymptomatic patients is much less than that of symptomatic patients, it is appropriate to reserve carotid endarterectomy only for *good risk*, asymptomatic patients with advanced stenoses. Once again, the presence of ulceration or contralateral occlusion may lower the threshold for recommending operation.

In reviewing all the data from randomized trials (see Fig. 63-7 and Table 63-1), several important points are apparent in weighing the risks versus benefit of carotid endarterectomy. First, symptomatic patients benefit most from carotid endarterectomy because they are much more likely to experience stroke or death with medical therapy. Second, symptomatic patients with severe stenoses (70% to 99%) are more at risk than those with moderate stenoses (50% to 69%); patients with mild stenoses (<50%) are best treated medically. Third, asymptomatic patients with advanced stenoses (>60% to 70%) have a comparatively benign prognosis, and a significant benefit from carotid endarterectomy can be realized only if the morbidity and mortality rates with intervention are low.

Finally, the complication rate from carotid endarterectomy in symptomatic patients is higher than in asymptomatic patients.

OPERATIVE MANAGEMENT

Preoperative Evaluation

Although myocardial infarction is a leading cause of death after carotid endarterectomy, the overall incidence is low (0.3% from NASCET data[34]), and extensive preoperative cardiac testing is unnecessary and cost ineffective. A detailed cardiac history and electrocardiogram suffice in most patients. Patients with frequent, severe, or unstable angina pectoris or other advanced cardiac conditions may require cardiac catheterization independent of the need for carotid endarterectomy. In these unusual patients, staged or combined operations may be necessary depending on the severity of the coronary and carotid disease. Patients who have sustained a transmural myocardial infarction within the past 3 months or who have uncontrolled congestive heart failure should have operation delayed and intensive medical therapy to control failure. If such individuals have preocclusive carotid lesions and frequent TIAs, operation may be necessary despite the medical risk. In these circumstances, monitoring with a pulmonary artery catheter and special anesthetic techniques to optimize cardiac performance are indicated.

Aspirin therapy should be started at the time of diagnosis of TIA, amaurosis fugax, or stroke.[37] Data from the prospective Aspirin and Carotid Endarterectomy (ACE) trial has documented that low-dose aspirin (80 to 325 mg/daily) is optimal in preventing thromboembolic events after carotid endarterectomy.[38] Patients who cannot take aspirin because of allergy or active peptic ulcer disease should be given clopidogrel (Plavix) 75 mg daily. If patients continue to have frequent TIAs despite antiplatelet therapy and also have severe, preocclusive stenosis, intravenous continuous heparin therapy keeping the partial thromboplastin time at 1.5 times control is recommended.

Poorly controlled hypertension and diabetes mellitus are risk factors for complications following carotid endarterectomy. Intensive medical treatment of these conditions is important prior to carotid endarterectomy.

Positioning

The operating table should be horizontal without head elevation and the head turned partially to the opposite side. In some patients it is helpful to place a rolled towel under the shoulders to exaggerate neck extension. Gentle preparation of the operative site and minimal manipulation of the carotid bifurcation area decrease the likelihood of dislodging fragments from a fragile carotid plaque.

Initial Dissection

An oblique incision along the anterior border of the sternocleidomastoid provides optimal exposure (Fig. 63-9).

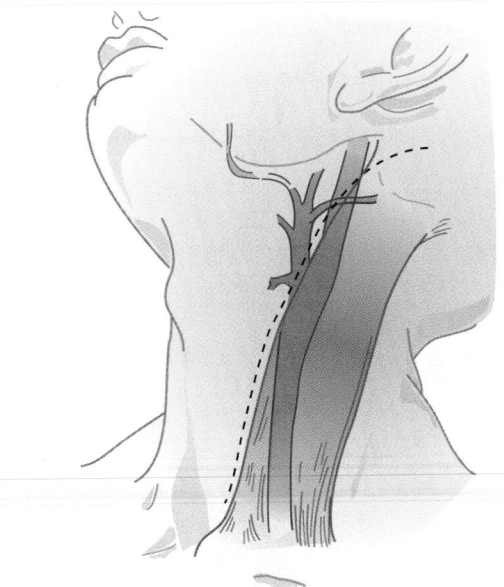

FIGURE 63-9. Position of incision for optimal exposure of the extracranial carotid artery.

The line of incision begins at the level of the mastoid process, extends anteriorly along the anteriomedial border of the sternocleidomastoid muscle and ends about 1 to 2 fingerbreaths above the sternal notch. The incision is about 10 cm in length and can be shifted cephalad or caudad along this line depending on the location of the carotid bifurcation. The location of the carotid bifurcation can be determined preoperatively by duplex ultrasonography or arteriography. After sectioning the platysma muscle in the line of the incision, the plane of dissection is anteromedial to the sternocleidomastoid beginning inferiorly and proceeding superiorly. In the upper mid portion of the incision, the transverse cervical nerve, which is responsible for the skin innervation medial to the incision and along the lower jaw, is divided. The approach to the carotid sheath begins inferiorly along the anterior border of the sternocleidomastoid muscle and proceeds superiorly.

The carotid sheath is a fascial sheath formed by extensions of the deep cervical fascia and prevertebral fascia. The sheath contains the carotid artery, the internal jugular vein, the vagus nerve, and the deep cervical lymphatic chain. To expose the carotid sheath, the medial and inner borders of the sternocleidomastoid muscle are dissected and retracted posteriorly (Fig. 63-10). Dissection and medial mobilization of the sternocleidomastoid should continue cephalad until the aponeurotic portion of this muscle is clearly visible. The internal jugular vein is next identified, and the carotid sheath is opened along the anterior and medial border of this vein. Branches of the internal jugular vein coursing anteriorly are ligated and divided throughout the extent of the incision. It is important to keep the dissection along the anterior border of this vein during this portion of the operation to avoid injury to the spinal accessory nerve in the superior portion of the

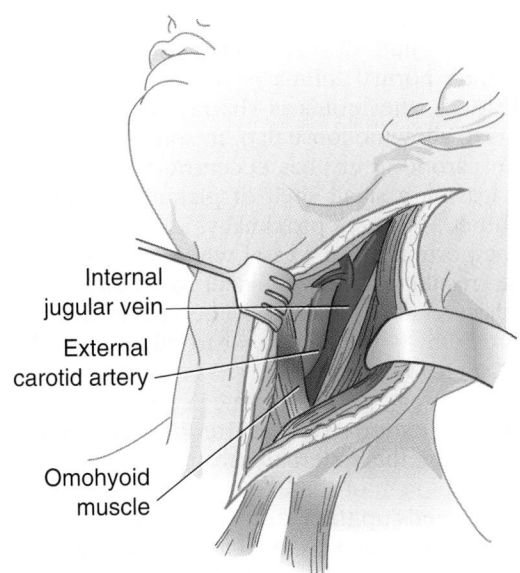

Internal jugular vein

External carotid artery

Omohyoid muscle

FIGURE 63-10.   The sternocleidomastoid muscle is retracted posteriorly to expose the carotid sheath.

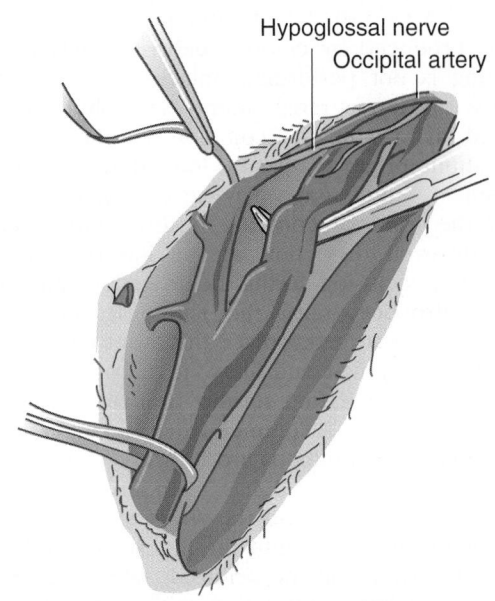

Hypoglossal nerve
Occipital artery

FIGURE 63-12.   The common carotid, internal carotid, and external carotid arteries are exposed and mobilized with minimal dissection and manipulation of the disease-bearing segment of the distal, common, and proximal internal carotid arteries (carotid bulb).

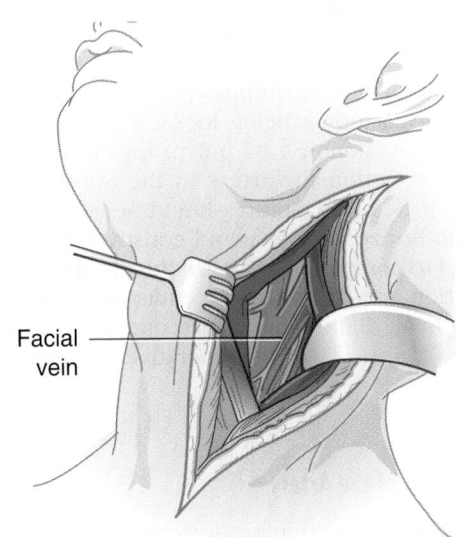

Facial vein

FIGURE 63-11.   The common facial vein branch of the internal jugular vein marks the site of the carotid bifurcation. After dividing the facial vein, the internal jugular vein is retracted posteriorly to expose the carotid bifurcation.

wound. The internal jugular vein is retracted posteriorly with the sternocleidomastoid muscle (Fig. 63-11).

Prevention of Intraoperative Embolization

The major danger in this portion of the operation is embolization produced by excessive manipulation of the carotid bifurcation. One must be intensely aware of the fragile nature of an atherosclerotic plaque, particularly with ulceration or intraluminal thrombus. A "no touch" technique is employed whereby the common carotid, internal carotid, and external carotid arteries all are exposed in that sequence and dissected free with minimal manipulation of the disease-bearing carotid bifurcation area (Fig. 63-12). The common facial vein enters the internal jugular vein usually at the level of the bifurcation of the common carotid artery and provides a landmark to identify the general location of most of the atherosclerotic disease. The common carotid artery is dissected first with sharp technique in the periadventitial plane to prevent injury to the vagus nerve, which usually is found lateral and posterior to the common carotid artery. On occasion, the vagus nerve can be found anteriorly on the common carotid artery and, for this reason, the dissection should proceed along the medial border of the common carotid artery to prevent injury to this nerve.

A major difficulty is encountered in achieving exposure for lesions extending high into the internal carotid artery of patients with high carotid bifurcations. When exposure is required above the second cervical vertebra or a line drawn between the tip of the mastoid and the angle of the mandible, special techniques are required. Anterior subluxation of the mandible can extend the exposure to above the body of the first cervical vertebra. This is almost always accompanied by sectioning of the posterior belly of the digastric muscles and sometimes by styloidectomy. Multiple techniques for mandibular subluxation have been described, but the most commonly favored is that of circummandibular/transnasal wiring manipulations that fix the mandible in a subluxated anterior location for the duration of the operation.[39]

Many surgeons routinely use monitoring with electroencephalography (EEG) to determine the need for shunting and to also detect intraoperative episodes of ischemia produced by embolic debris. If EEG or other monitoring is not performed, most surgeons routinely introduce an intra-arterial shunt. The shunt may be employed as a straight, common carotid–to–internal carotid shunt or an externally looped shunt. Embolus as a result of shunt usage may be produced by intimal injury to the proximal, common, or distal internal carotid arteries or even dissection of the intima. The shunt may undergo occlusion during the procedure, and emboli may be introduced into the shunt at the time of placement. Most surgeons place the shunt into the internal carotid artery first and allow it to backbleed freely before carefully inserting it into the common carotid artery. Some have recommended placement of the shunt first into the common carotid artery, making certain that any embolic material has been flushed from the common carotid artery and the shunt allowed to bleed slightly before placing it into the internal carotid artery. Soaking the shunt in heparinized saline before use may retard thrombus formation within the shunt and prevent air bubbles from being in the shunt at the time of placement.

Prior to arteriotomy and shunt insertion, Rummel tourniquets are used for vascular control. A large Rummel tourniquet is placed around the common carotid artery, and small Rummel tourniquets are placed around the external and internal carotid arteries. Again, manipulation of the disease-bearing segment of the carotid bifurcation is avoided during these maneuvers. Some surgeons temporarily occlude the internal carotid artery with a Silastic vascular loop or a small aneurysm clip. Instead of Rummel tourniquets, fine vascular clamps are preferred by some surgeons to obtain proximal and distal control. Whether or not a proximal clamp or Rummel tourniquet is used, every effort should be made to avoid carotid plaque at the bifurcation and to apply these constricting devices on normal artery. All of these maneuvers are designed to prevent not only damage to normal intima but also fracture of atherosclerotic plaque with subsequent stenosis or subintimal dissection or a site for thrombus formation with distal embolization intraoperatively or postoperatively. Prior to application of tourniquets or clamps, the patient is heparinized with 100 to 150 units/kg of intravenous heparin.

Endarterectomy

The arteriotomy begins in the proximal common carotid artery and extends into the internal carotid artery. A No. 11 scalpel blade is used to open the common carotid artery at the site below the plaque, and angled Potts scissors are used to incise the artery through the plaque into normal internal carotid artery. It is important to extend the arteriotomy above and below gross intimal disease. If an internal shunt is used, careful backbleeding of the shunt to completely flush air and other debris, along with placement of the shunt proximally and distally in areas free of gross atherosclerotic debris, minimizes the potential for embolization during these manipulations.

The plaque is carefully dissected from the arterial wall using a blunt dissector such as a Penfield instrument. When normal intima is reached in the common carotid artery, the intima is sharply dissected and transected as to allow no loose flap. In some cases, the entire common carotid artery has eccentric thickening, necessitating leaving a small shelf of plaque. The endarterectomy should proceed proximally as far as possible to reach the portion of the vessel where plaque is minimal, and the resulting shelf is small at the point where the endarterectomy ends. On occasion, this requires endarterectomy in the common carotid artery to the level of the clavicle.

At the bifurcation, the plaque is peeled from below upward to the external carotid artery, where it is carefully dissected from the external carotid artery by everting proximal 2 to 3 cm of the external carotid artery. As this process proceeds up the external carotid artery, it is wise to release the occluded Rummel tourniquet temporarily to allow the plaque to be carefully removed. It is important to make certain that the external carotid artery is left patent and free of gross disease. If there is any uncertainty, it may be necessary to fashion a separate arteriotomy on the external carotid artery, remove external carotid artery plaque, and patch the arteriotomy with vein or prosthetic material. Subsequently, the plaque is peeled out of the internal carotid artery, and it will usually peel out quite smoothly distally. If the distal intima remains thickened and infiltrated with plaque, it is necessary to remove this to the point of normal intima. If there is any question about the distal intima being loose, it should be tacked down with 6-0 double-arm polypropylene sutures proceeding from within the artery to the outer wall where the suture is tied. The suture should be placed vertically rather than horizontally to avoid constricting the lumen. It is critical to completely visualize the distal endpoint and the transition area between the endarterectomy site and normal intima. "Blind" endarterectomy may invite distal flaps that can lead to postoperative thromboembolic phenomena.

Reconstruction of the Artery

Once the vessel is meticulously cleaned, primary closure or closure with a vein or prosthetic patch ensues. The experience reported in the literature supports the use of patch over primary closure.[40,41] In addition to protecting against postoperative occlusion and ischemic events, the incidence of restenosis may be minimized. In occasional cases in which plaque is focally confined to the carotid bulb with minimal extension into the internal carotid artery, primary closure can be recommended if the arteriotomy does not extend above the bulb. Just prior to completing closure, the shunt is removed and all vessels are allowed to flush; the closure is then completed. Flushing is important to remove air and debris. After closure, the external and common carotid arteries are first opened and then the internal carotid artery is opened to minimize air or particulate embolization into the internal carotid artery system.

The arterial wall is then palpated to determine the presence of a thrill, which would indicate a loose intimal flap or some obstructive intraluminal mass. If a thrill is present, an arteriogram should be performed to determine the characteristics of the endarterectomy site. If clot or debris is found inside the lumen, the vessel must be reoccluded and opened and all debris removed. Many surgeons routinely insonate the carotid bifurcation area with a continuous-wave Doppler probe. One should hear unimpeded diastolic flow in the internal carotid artery. Irregular and high-pitched flow may indicate stenosis or other problems and would lead to intraoperative arteriography. Duplex ultrasonography is increasingly being used to assess the flow and luminal characteristics after endarterectomy, and it has high sensitivity for detecting residual stenoses and flaps.[42] If these are present, the artery should be reopened and the problem corrected.

Reversal of heparin with protamine sulfate is subject to wide practice variations. Some surgeons stress nonreversal of heparin, or waiting a period of at least 20 minutes to reverse the heparin with protamine sulfate. Studies in animals suggest that this practice reduces thrombus formation at the endarterectomy site. Regardless of reversal or nonreversal, meticulous hemostasis is important. Because most of these patients have been medicated with aspirin, residual heparin effects are accentuated and wound hematomas may result.[43] Although these hematomas are usually minor, airway compromise can occur with large hematomas. If heparin reversal is used, a 0.5- to 1-mg equivalent reversal of dose is appropriate (0.5 to 1 mg of protamine sulfate for every 100 units of heparin).

POSTOPERATIVE COMPLICATIONS

Stroke or Transient Neurologic Deficit

Neurologic deficits within the first 12 hours of operation are almost always the result of thromboembolic phenomena stemming from the endarterectomy site or damaged internal, common, or external carotid arteries.[34] Immediate heparinization and exploration are indicated without the need for confirmatory arteriography or noninvasive tests.[44] Neurologic deficits that begin beyond 12 to 24 hours of operation are usually due to thromboembolic phenomena stemming from the endarterectomy site, but these deficits may also be caused by postoperative hyperperfusion syndrome or intracerebral hematoma. These latter conditions may be worsened by immediate heparinization and re-exploration. Therefore, deficits occurring 12 to 24 hours after operation should be promptly investigated with a CT scan and arteriography.

If on reopening the wound, an excellent pulse is present in the internal carotid artery and flow is present on Doppler ultrasound examination, an on-the-table arteriogram is performed. If the arteriogram reveals an intimal flap or irregular mural thrombus at the endarterectomy site, then appropriate vessel isolation and reopening of the vessel are indicated. Thrombus is removed and back-bleeding is allowed. At this point, the mechanical cause

of thrombosis is usually defined as an intimal flap and this is repaired. If there is no pulse on initial inspection of the artery, the vessel is obviously thrombosed and a preliminary arteriogram is not necessary prior to opening the vessel and extracting thrombus.

Prior to restoration of flow, an internal carotid arteriogram is done by placing a small catheter into the distal internal carotid artery and injecting a small amount of contrast agent to ensure that the distal internal carotid artery is patent and to determine whether there is an embolus in the middle cerebral artery. If the vessel is patent with or without middle cerebral artery embolus, flow can be restored after reconstruction of the vessel. If an embolus exists in the intracranial carotid or middle cerebral artery, local infusion of a lytic agent should be considered.[45]

Hyperperfusion Syndrome and Intracerebral Hematoma

The incidence of hyperperfusion syndrome following carotid endarterectomy is reported to be between 0.3% and 1.0%.[46] The pathophysiology appears to be secondary to paralysis of autoregulation from chronic ischemia.[47] Restoration of internal carotid flow leads to hyperperfusion in the ipsilateral cerebrovascular bed. Isotopic regional cerebral blood flow studies and transcranial Doppler examinations have documented marked increases in ipsilateral cerebral blood flow.[47] Pathologic changes include a spectrum of findings ranging from mild cerebral edema to petechial hemorrhages to frank intracerebral hemorrhage. This syndrome is often heralded by ipsilateral frontal headache within the first week after endarterectomy. However, ipsilateral headache is not specific for hyperperfusion syndrome and, in fact, is not uncommon following endarterectomy. In patients with the hyperperfusion syndrome, headache may be followed by focal motor seizures that are often difficult to control. Even more alarming is the postictal Todd's paralysis that can mimic post-endarterectomy stroke from internal carotid artery thrombosis. Angiography, along with CT or MRI, may be necessary to distinguish between these disorders. Risk factors for the hyperperfusion syndrome include a high-grade (>70%) stenosis; poor collateral hemispheric flow; contralateral carotid occlusion; evidence of chronic ipsilateral hypoperfusion; preoperataive and postoperative hypertension; preexisting ipsilateral cerebral infarction; and preoperative anticoagulation or antiplatelet therapy.[48]

Seizures from the hyperperfusion syndrome are usually successfully treated with phenytoin (Dilantin). Aspirin and anticoagulants should be avoided, and hypertension should be carefully controlled. The most catastrophic complication stemming from hyperperfusion is intracerebral hemorrhage that can be massive and fatal.[49] Intracranial hemorrhage has been reported to occur in 0.5% to 0.7% of patients undergoing carotid endarterectomy and may account for up to 20% of perioperative strokes.[50]

Hypertension/Hypotension

Fluctuations in blood pressure with postoperative hypertension or hypotension are common after endarterectomy, occurring in up to one third to one half of patients. Fortunately, the postoperative instability in blood pressure usually disappears within 12 to 24 hours. It is important that the blood pressure be maintained below a maximum systolic level of approximately 140 mm Hg. This may require the intravenous use of nitroprusside or nitroglycerin. Hypertension has been implicated in the development of the hyperperfusion syndrome, intracerebral hemorrhage, and cardiac complications. Postoperative hypotension may be as disastrous as postoperative hypertension. The instability of blood pressure is caused by carotid sinus malfunction. Patients with atherosclerosis of the carotid body often lose effective baroreceptor activity. Following endarterectomy, the carotid bulb can again distend, and the carotid sinus reflex can over-respond, producing postoperative hypotension. Significant postoperative hypotension may produce cerebral ischemic complications and can be best treated by ensuring that volume replacement is adequate and by the use of vasopressors. Phenylephrine increases left ventricular work and myocardial oxygen demands and may be associated with myocardial ischemia. Dopamine is preferred when a pressor is needed.

Wound Complications

Most patients undergoing carotid endarterectomy have been treated with preoperative aspirin and are continued on antithrombotic therapy in the postoperative period. Bleeding complications, particularly wound hematomas, occur in 1.4% to 3% of patients undergoing endarterectomy and are associated with incomplete heparin reversal with protamine, hypertension, and perioperative antiplatelet therapy.[43] If intraoperative heparin is not fully reversed or continuous heparin anticoagulation is administered postoperatively, perioperative aspirin therapy would potentially increase the incidence of hematomas and other bleeding complications.[51] The combination of aspirin plus clopidogrel markedly prolongs the bleeding time beyond that of either antiplatelet agent alone and causes wound hematomas and other bleeding complications. Aspirin plus clopidogrel should be avoided in patients undergoing carotid endarterectomy, and clopidogrel should be discontinued at least 5 days before operation.

Although most postoperative hematomas are minor and of no clinical consequence, large hematomas cause pain, tracheal deviation, and airway compromise and require emergency drainage.[34] An important symptom suggesting the presence of a significant hematoma that may lead to airway embarrassment is the inability to swallow. When the airway is acutely and severely compromised, the wound must be opened in bed but, if possible, the patient should be returned to the operating room. If the airway is stable, the neck should be prepared and draped and the wound opened under local anesthesia prior to intubation. Often the hematoma can be evacuated without the necessity of general anesthesia. Rapid induction of anesthesia with attempt at intubation

should be avoided because of major difficulty in placing an endotracheal tube without prior evacuation of the hematoma.

The overall incidence of saphenous vein patch rupture is 0.5% and occurs 1 to 7 days after operation.[50] There appears to be a higher incidence in women, and it is more common when ankle saphenous vein is used. There is a linear correlation between the diameter of intact veins and rupture pressure, and biomechanical studies would suggest that saphenous veins smaller than 4 to 5 mm in diameter should not be used for vein patch reconstruction.[52] This finding may explain the apparent difference in vein patch strength between proximal and distal saphenous veins. The major stroke and death rate associated with vein patch rupture is 48%.[53]

Operative Damage to Nerves

The sensory branches of the cervical plexus, namely the transverse cervical nerve and the greater auricular nerve, are frequently severed or injured during the course of carotid endarterectomy. The resulting ipsilateral numbness of the upper face, lower neck, and lower ear is vexing to some patients but is generally well tolerated. Permanent hypesthesia in this area is common after carotid endarterectomy. Of much greater consequence is injury to cranial nerves in the field of dissection because the resulting neurologic deficits can produce serious complications (Fig. 63-13). Fortunately, cranial nerve injury is infrequent and is usually reversible, with neurologic deficits lasting weeks to months.[54] The approximate frequencies of clinically significant injury to cranial nerves are as follows: recurrent laryngeal nerve, 5% to 7%; hypoglossal nerve, 4% to 6%; marginal mandibular nerve,

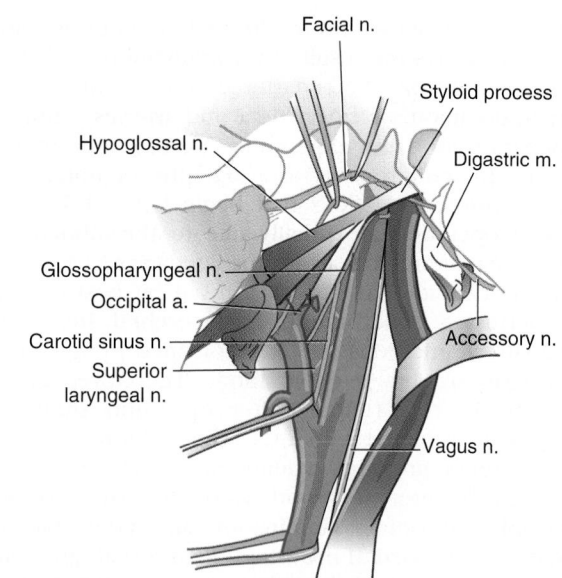

FIGURE 63-13. Cranial nerves vulnerable to injury during carotid endarterectomy.

1% to 3%; superior laryngeal nerve, 1% to 3%; and spinal accessory nerve, 0.5% to 1%.[34,55]

Vagal Nerve Injury

Injury to the main trunk of the vagus trunk is rare. It may be injured in high exposure and by careless use of the cautery. In rare circumstances, the right recurrent laryngeal branch of the vagus nerve arises at the level of the bifurcation and crosses anteriorly. This anatomic variation is termed a "nonrecurrent" recurrent laryngeal nerve and is almost always associated with an aberrant origin of the right subclavian artery from the distal aortic arch. Identification of this vascular anomaly on preoperative arteriography should alert one to the presence of an anomalous recurrent laryngeal nerve. On occasion, an anterior vagus nerve is present, and the nerve and its recurrent branch are at jeopardy when mobilizing the common carotid artery. The policy of beginning dissection medially and maintaining circumferential dissection within the periadventitial plane facilitates displacement and mobilization of the nerve away from the artery. The fibers of the recurrent laryngeal nerve run in the medial aspect of the main trunk of the vagus nerve, and injury to the medial portions of the vagus nerve can result in recurrent laryngeal nerve injury.

The right recurrent laryngeal nerve arises from the vagus trunk at the root of the neck and loops around the right subclavian artery. The left recurrent laryngeal nerve arises from the vagal trunk in the mediastinum and loops around the aortic arch at the level of the ligamentum arteriosum. Both the right and left nerves ascend in the neck behind the common carotid artery in the groove between the trachea and the esophagus. The recurrent laryngeal nerve supplies intrinsic muscles of the larynx that control the ipsilateral vocal cord. Damage results in unilateral vocal cord paralysis. This nerve is rarely, if ever, exposed during carotid endarterectomy and is usually damaged by traction or cautery. Bilateral recurrent laryngeal nerve injury results in midline vocal cord apposition that can severely compromise the airway. Because of this possibility, many recommend indirect laryngoscope prior to the second stage of bilateral staged carotid endarterectomies.

The superior laryngeal nerve is a branch of the vagus nerve at the lower margin of the first cervical vertebra and runs posteriorly and medially to the internal and external carotid arteries. The nerve divides into internal and external branches. The internal branch is responsible for the sensory supply of the epiglottis and the larynx above the vocal cords. The external branch is responsible for the motor supply to the cricothyroid muscle and the inferior pharyngeal constrictor. The nerve is covered by loose fascia posterior and medial to the carotid arteries and can best be seen just medial and deep to the carotid bifurcation. It is usually damaged in unusual circumstances when complete mobilization of the carotid bifurcation is required. It also may be damaged by high exposure of the internal carotid artery at and above C1, where the medial aspect of the vagus nerve may be in jeopardy. Damage to

the superior laryngeal nerve leads to voice fatigue and difficulty in swallowing.

Hypoglossal Nerve Injury

The hypoglossal nerve is responsible for total innervation of the tongue. Paralysis of the nerve produces slight impairment of speech and deviation of the tongue to the side of the paralysis with subsequent ipsilateral tongue atrophy. The descending hypoglossal branch leaves the nerve at its inferior curve and runs anterior and medial to the jugular vein and anterior to the internal carotid artery. Section of the descendens hypoglossi above the cervical branch, which forms the ansa cervicalis, produces no clinical syndrome. This branch, along with the cervical branch, is responsible for the motor supply of the deep strap muscles of the neck. As an external landmark, the hypoglossal nerve is usually found at the level of the occipital artery. It is invariably crossed superiorly by the branch of the occipital artery to the sternocleidomastoid muscle. Occasionally, the nerve is crossed by an aberrant vein, and this vein may be closely adherent to the nerve.

Facial Nerve Injury

Total facial nerve paralysis is rare and occurs only when high exposure of the internal carotid artery is required. To expose the internal carotid artery at C2 and above, some surgeons recommend extending the incision anterior to the tragus of the ear and reflecting the superficial lobe of the parotid superiorly and anteriorly. In the process of this extensive dissection, traction on the main facial nerve may produce a complete facial nerve paralysis. This potential complication can be avoided by using alternative methods to gain high exposure of the internal carotid artery such as mandibular subluxation.[39]

The more common injury involves that of the marginal mandibular branch of the facial nerve, and this usually occurs with anterior and superior retraction along the angle of the mandible where the marginal mandibular nerve is vulnerable. Injury to this branch produces asymmetry of the mouth secondary to paralysis of the depressor muscle of the lip. This is annoying to the patient in speech, and when eating the patient may bite the lower lip. The deficit is usually transient and often clears within 3 months.

Glossopharyngeal Nerve Injury

The glossopharyngeal nerve is usually more remote from the field of dissection during carotid endarterectomy but may be injured during high exposure of the internal carotid at the base of the skull. It exits the skull via the jugular foramen and passes between the internal and external carotid arteries just below the stylopharyngeus muscle near its insertion into the styloid process. This nerve provides sensory fibers to the mucosa of the pharynx and motor fibers to elevate the larynx and pharynx during swallowing. Injury results in defective swallowing with dysphagia and recurrent aspiration.

Spinal Accessory Nerve Injury

The spinal accessory nerve is a motor nerve that is rarely injured during carotid endarterectomy. After exiting the jugular foramen, the nerve lies superficial to the internal jugular vein and courses into the sternocleidomastoid muscle. The nerve is usually injured by misdirected exposure of the carotid artery into the posterior triangle of the neck, by traction, or by cautery injury in superior exposures of the internal carotid artery. Damage results in complete paralysis of the sternocleidomastoid and trapezius muscles, which causes a dropped shoulder. This can result in discomfort in the neck and shoulder and can be debilitating for active individuals.

ONGOING ISSUES

Surgical Expertise and Training

With the publication of results from randomized trials demonstrating benefit of carotid endarterectomy in patients with symptomatic and asymptomatic disease, the overall rate of this operation performed in the United States has increased dramatically (see Fig. 63-6).[13] Much of the increase is in patients with asymptomatic disease.[56,57] However, the benefits of carotid endarterectomy will not be realized if perioperative morbidity and mortality are excessive. The reported risk of endarterectomy shows wide variation, and concerns have been raised about whether the results from NASCET and other randomized trials can be extrapolated for the nation as a whole.[58]

In a report published in 1998, the national mortality for Medicare beneficiaries undergoing carotid endarterectomy was found to be 1.6%.[59] Using ratios derived from NASCET data, one can estimate that the national incidence of combined *major, disabling* stroke and death is approximately 5% (3 times the mortality rate) and the incidence of all strokes (major and minor) and death may be as high as 16% (10 times the mortality rate).[60] If the perioperative morbidity and mortality were this high in NASCET and other trials, these studies would have shown no benefit of endarterectomy. These considerations are sobering and point to the importance of ongoing quality improvement audits in institutions where patients are subjected to carotid endarterectomy.[61,62]

A consensus of a selected committee of neurologists, neurosurgeons, and vascular surgeons made recommendations that carotid endarterectomy should be performed with low morbidity and mortality in selected patients with appropriate symptoms and that the limits of perioperative morbidity and mortality should be categorized by clinical presentation.[63] The combined morbidity and mortality of the procedure should not exceed 3% for asymptomatic patients, 5% for TIAs, and 7% for ischemic stroke. In addi-

tion, the 30-day mortality rate from all causes related to endarterectomy should not exceed 2%. Concomitantly, ongoing audits should be completed in an institution where endarterectomy is being performed to ensure adherence to these guidelines. Unfortunately, there is no evidence that widespread quality assurance/improvement audits are being conducted in U.S. hospitals. Because of the failure of the current voluntary system, a group of prominent stroke neurologists and surgeons have editorialized that auditing the complication rates of carotid endarterectomy should be mandated as a condition of hospital certification by the Joint Commission of Accreditation of Health Care Organizations.[64]

Many recent studies have documented an inverse relationship between morbidity and mortality with carotid endarterectomy and hospital and surgeon volumes.[65-68] In general, the morbidity and mortality rates are higher in small hospitals where the procedures are infrequently performed. More important, individual surgeon volume has a more direct impact on results. In one study, surgeons performing fewer than 5 carotid endarterectomies per year had twice the mortality in comparison to surgeons performing more than this number.[67] Other studies have documented that 10 to 12 carotid endarterectomies per year are necessary to maintain surgical expertise and reduce complications to a minimum.

Surgeons participating in NASCET and ACAS were all board-certified vascular surgeons or neurosurgeons. Does this mean that the performance of this operation should be restricted to individuals with these credentials to realize the benefits of carotid endarterectomy? There are many surgeons from other backgrounds, including general surgery and cardiothoracic surgery, who are well trained to perform this operation and have commendable results. The main point is that regardless of training environment, one must obtain in-depth experience in the management of patients with cerebrovascular disease and the performance of carotid endarterectomy. Most important, all surgeons must participate in quality assurance programs, submit their results on an ongoing basis, and be willing to have them reviewed by an independent audit group.[63,69]

Increasing the Benefit/Cost Ratio of Carotid Endarterectomy

In response to increasing costs of health care, physicians have been challenged to conserve hospital resources, minimize cost, and continue to provide quality care. The length of stay following carotid endarterectomy has decreased dramatically, with many groups reporting 24-hour admissions for most of their patients.[70,71] Traditionally, patients have been observed in an intensive care unit for 12 to 24 hours after the operation. In retrospective analyses, many have pointed out that only 10% to 20% of patients required this expensive monitoring. Predictors of the need for intensive care unit observation include preoperative history of hypertension, myocardial infarction, arrhythmia, recent stroke, and chronic renal failure.[72] Patients not having these risk factors have been successfully observed for short periods (2 to 4 hours) in a postanesthetic recovery room setting.[73] Following this, patients can be monitored on a standard hospital unit and discharged the next day. Some have pointed out that local anesthesia for the performance of carotid endarterectomy is important in the success of this approach; however, others have used this care algorithm successfully in patients having general anesthesia.

A more controversial cost-saving approach has relied on duplex ultrasonography alone or in combination with magnetic resonance angiography (MRA) and the elimination of contrast angiography in the preoperative work-up of patients undergoing endarterectomy.[74-76] In addition to being expensive, contrast angiography has a 0.5% to 1% incidence of major neurologic complications. Angiography also results in complications at the arterial puncture site in approximately 5% of patients as well as contrast-induced renal dysfunction in 1% to 5%. Several centers have reported the results of carotid endarterectomy performed with duplex examination alone or in combination with MRA.

All groups advocating the noninvasive approach stress that optimal results can be realized only with a fully equipped vascular laboratory with well-trained personnel and an established quality control record. Laboratories should maintain ongoing protocols to correlate angiographic and duplex findings to ensure continued diagnostic accuracy. Although committed vascular laboratories may report excellent results, few prospective studies have been performed with angiographic validation. Furthermore, excellent results reported from single centers cannot be extrapolated to national practice. The duplex ultrasound findings from NASCET and ACAS demonstrated that there was significant variability between centers and machinery in the determination of stenosis severity.[9,77] Mismanagement of even a small number of patients incorrectly categorized by duplex ultrasonography could have major economic and medical consequences that would quickly abolish the cost-effectiveness of eliminating angiography.[78] As an example, a symptomatic patient with a 70% stenosis identified by duplex ultrasonography as having a less than 50% stenosis might be denied carotid endarterectomy and be at risk of stroke with inappropriate medical therapy.

In addition to validation of individual vascular laboratory results with a high degree of accuracy, all experts recommend limiting carotid endarterectomy based on duplex ultrasonography alone or coupled with MRA to patients with clear-cut history and physical findings that correlate with duplex findings.[74] Furthermore, a CT scan or MRI should be obtained to rule out other intracranial explanations for a patient's symptoms. Indications for adjunctive arteriography include the following:

1. Discrepancy among the history, physical examination, duplex scan, and CT scan
2. Patients presenting with vertebrobasilar symptoms, since they often have proximal brachiocephalic disease
3. Patients suspected of proximal disease involving branches of the aortic arch (patients with unequal arm blood pressures or duplex ultrasonographic evidence

of abnormal flow characteristics in the proximal common carotid arteries)
4. Patients presenting with focal cerebrovascular symptoms and a stenosis in the 40% to 59% (moderate) range according to duplex criteria (this is the range where even slight overestimation or underestimation may inaccurately categorize the patient)
5. Patients with duplex findings suggestive of distal internal carotid artery or carotid siphon disease
6. Patients with duplex evidence of total carotid occlusion in the presence of ongoing ipsilateral hemispheric symptoms (patients may have near-total occlusion or a "string sign")
7. Patients with contralateral carotid occlusion or severe carotid stenosis since ipsilateral duplex results are often overestimated because of increased ipsilateral flow velocities
8. Patients with nonatherosclerotic disease such as fibromuscular dysplasia and patients with recurrent carotid stenosis because plaque morphology and extent of disease are sometimes unusual in these patients
9. Patients with duplex scans that are equivocal or of poor quality

Recurrent Carotid Stenosis

Recurrent stenosis is infrequent but not rare.[79] The overall risk appears to be about 10% in the first year after primary endarterectomy, 3% in the second year, and 2% in the third year.[80] Long-term risk has been estimated to be approximately 1% per year. Symptomatic recurrent carotid disease occurs in about 0.6% to 3% of patients after endarterectomy. Asymptomatic lesions occur with a much greater frequency (7% to 49%), depending on the method used in detection. In reported series, the need for reoperative carotid endarterectomy is 0.5% for asymptomatic lesions and 1.4% for symptomatic lesions.[79] Medical treatment with antiplatelet therapy has no influence on the development of clinical manifestations of recurrent carotid stenosis.[81]

The etiology of recurrent disease can be broadly categorized into local or systemic factors. One of the most important local determinants is residual defects at the endarterectomy site.[42,82] The most important risk factor seems to be the degree of residual plaque left at the time of the original endarterectomy. Flaps or other technical defects may also be important. Systemic factors that have been associated with the development of recurrent disease include female sex, continued smoking after endarterectomy, hypercholesterolemia, diabetes mellitus, hypertension, young age at original endarterectomy, and associated severe atherosclerotic disease.[83,84] Female sex is the most consistently reported risk factor for the recurrence of disease.[85] The high incidence of recurrence in women may be related to the smaller vessel size in these patients.

The histopathology of recurrent lesions is interesting, because late recurrent lesions have atherosclerotic features and are more likely to be symptomatic than earlier lesions, which are often bland and asymptomatic. Serial observations in a large number of patients have shown that early and late recurrent lesions are a continuum of atherosclerotic changes.[86] Early lesions (recurrence < 2 to 3 years) are predominantly neointimal fibromuscular hyperplasia consisting of proliferating smooth muscle cells surrounded by proteoglycans. Late recurrent lesions (recurrence interval > 2 to 3 years) tend to have elements of atherosclerosis with foam cells, cholesterol crystals, abundant collagen, and calcium.[86] Late recurrent lesions tend to be easier to endarterectomize in comparison with earlier recurrent lesions.[87]

Reoperation for recurrent disease can be technically challenging; however, the overall incidence of major morbidity and mortality approximates those of primary endarterectomy except for the incidence of cranial nerve injury. In general, the mean risk of stroke with reoperation is approximately 4%, with a death rate of approximately 1.2% and cranial nerve injury of approximately 12%.[79,87]

Closure Technique of Carotid Arteriotomy

The rationale for vein patch closure following carotid endarterectomy is to improve the safety and durability of the procedure.[88] By increasing lumen size, reconstructing a portion of the endarterectomy site with endothelialized tissue, and altering the hemodynamic configuration of the carotid bifurcation, vein patch closure theoretically would reduce thrombus accumulation and could prevent perioperative stroke and asymptomatic occlusion of the internal carotid artery. Recurrent carotid stenosis also might be prevented or delayed in causing hemodynamically significant compromise because of the increase in lumen size. Despite the attractiveness of these theoretical considerations, vein patch closure has some drawbacks. In addition to increasing operative time, vein patch closure is associated with its own unique set of complications, including patch rupture, false aneurysm formation, and thromboembolism stemming from the dilated aneurysmal reconstructed bifurcation. The use of Dacron or other prosthetic material for the patch avoids some of these complications; however, the potential for infection is present, albeit small, and infection of a prosthetic patch in this location can lead to catastrophic complications.

The results from randomized, prospective studies would suggest that the routine use of vein or prosthetic patch closure decreases perioperative stroke morbidity and asymptomatic occlusion only when stroke morbidity and mortality exceed 5% to 7%.[89] In settings where perioperative morbidity and mortality rates are less than 2% to 3%, there is no significant difference between primary closure and vein or prosthetic patch angioplasty in perioperative morbidity and mortality.[90] In men, the use of vein patch closure does not significantly reduce the long-term follow-up incidence of recurrent carotid disease.[91] However, in women, who have a higher incidence of recurrent carotid stenosis, vein patch closure significantly reduces the incidence of this long-term complication.[92] Whether or not vein is superior to prosthetic material for

patch closure has not been answered definitively. A recent large randomized trial demonstrated equivalence between these two materials[93]; however, a systematic overview of all randomized trials demonstrated that carotid endarterectomy patch reconstruction with saphenous vein had better perioperative stroke and restenosis outcomes than those obtained with Dacron and polytetrafluoroethylene.[40]

Considerations bearing on the decision of whether or not to use patch closure are broadly categorized into three major groups.[89] First, in clinical settings in which the incidence of perioperative ischemic stroke and carotid thrombosis is unacceptably high, consideration should be given to employing routine patch closure. Once again, ongoing quality improvement audits are necessary to define unacceptably high results that trigger reassessment of multiple technical and patient selection factors that may influence these rates. One factor that may reduce these rates is the more liberal use of vein or prosthetic patch closure.

Next, local or anatomic risk factors need to be considered. These factors require careful intraoperative assessment. Among these, the size of the internal carotid artery is critical. Some studies have defined 5 mm in external diameter as measured with calipers as being the lower limit acceptable for primary closure.[90] Redundant carotid arteries with loops or kinks that are at or near the site of endarterectomy are also problematic. Resection or imbrication of redundant portions of the vessel is necessary under these circumstances, and the long arteriotomy should be closed with a patch. Vein patch closure is also recommended when extensive disease is present and when a longer arteriotomy in the internal carotid artery is necessary. The need for distal tacking sutures also implies that diseased intima is left behind. In such cases, the arteriotomy is extended well above the diseased intima, and a vein patch closure is used. Likewise, if extensive disease is present in the common carotid artery, extending the arteriotomy proximally and closing with a vein patch may be important to prevent recurrent stenosis at this site. The inability to obtain a smooth transition between an endarterectomized and an unendarterectomized vessel wall, either proximally or distally, may give rise to unstable, nonlaminar flow phenomena that favor thrombogenesis. The transition area with a pronounced shelf of intima should be covered with a vein patch if the shelf cannot be removed. Other local problems that would be helped with a patch closure include a crooked or spiral-shaped arteriotomy and failure to obtain precise and even arteriotomy closure.

Finally, systemic risk factors for recurrent carotid disease have already been mentioned. In all major studies, women have been found to have a much higher than expected rate of recurrent carotid stenosis. Vein patch closure is recommended in all women unless the internal carotid artery is larger than 5 mm in diameter and the arteriotomy is short and confined to the bulb. In addition, if multiple systemic atherosclerotic risk factors are present in a patient, one should consider using patch closure to prevent or delay recurrent carotid disease.

Local Versus General Anesthesia for Carotid Endarterectomy

Performance of carotid endarterectomy in awake patients under local or regional anesthesia has the advantage of accurate neurologic assessment of the patient during surgery and in the early postoperative period.[94] Neurologic deterioration can be detected early and allow appropriate use of selective shunting. In addition, the cardiac and pulmonary morbidity of general anesthesia is avoided, and there is also a suggestion that operation under local anesthesia is associated with shorter hospital stays.[73] Blood pressure appears to be more stable under local anesthesia, and wide swings that can occur during operation and in the early postoperative period may be less than with general anesthesia. However, carotid endarterectomy under local anesthesia has some disadvantages. The operation may be more hurried and technically more difficult. Patients may also suffer pain and stress during the operation, and this may increase the risk of myocardial ischemia. Also, some surgeons find performing the operation under local anesthesia stressful. There are many advantages associated with general anesthesia, including a more stable operative field and salutary effects of some general anesthetics on cerebral circulation and protection against ischemic damage.

There are many retrospective, nonrandomized series in the literature that support routine general or local anesthesia for carotid endarterectomy.[73,94] Critical review of these data document no superiority of either approach over the other.[95,96] Routine use of general or local anesthesia for carotid endarterectomy is usually based on training and experience, and either approach is acceptable.

Carotid Shunt and Monitoring

The main benefit of using an internal shunt during carotid endarterectomy is the re-establishment of some blood flow in the few patients who might need it. A second benefit associated with the use of shunt comes with closure of the arteriotomy. The shunt may serve as a stent over which the arteriotomy closure, either primary or with a patch, can be facilitated. The principal risk of using a shunt involves technical complications associated with its placement. With increasing familiarity in the use of a shunt, these risks may be reduced. The major risk is the introduction of emboli into the internal carotid artery resulting in cerebral embolization. Careful backbleeding of the shunt to completely flush air and other debris, along with placement of the shunt proximally and distally in areas free of gross atherosclerotic debris, minimizes the potential for this complication. The second complication that occurs with the shunt is intimal injury. With soft, plastic material specifically designed for use in the internal carotid artery and with the availability of different sizes of shunts, these complications have also been minimized. Another potential complication associated with shunt use is that it may interfere with carotid endarterectomy and prevent the surgeon from visualizing the distal endpoint.

When a shunt is in place, a longer arteriotomy is required to ensure adequate visualization of the distal endpoint.

Advocates of routine shunting point to excellent results in large series and argue persuasively that expensive monitoring techniques are unnecessary because facility and familiarity are enhanced by routine shunting.[97] Those who prefer selective shunting point out that only 10% to 15% of patients who are intolerant of temporary carotid clamping benefit from an internal shunt.[98-101] The problem comes in identifying these 10% to 15% of patients who might require a shunt. Methods used include monitoring neurologic status during temporary carotid occlusion in an awake patient under local anesthesia, measurement of internal carotid artery back pressure ("stump pressure" of <50 mm Hg is the generally accepted criterion for need for shunt placement), isotopic regional blood flow measurements, transcranial Doppler monitoring, somatosensory evoked potential monitoring, and EEG monitoring. All of these techniques have their limitations, and some are expensive and cumbersome. From data in the literature, patients most vulnerable to intraoperative cerebral infarct related to hypoperfusion are those who have had prior strokes, those who had a contralateral carotid occlusion, and those who show changes during intraoperative EEG monitoring. A shunt would be necessary in most patients with prior infarcts and/or contralateral carotid occlusion and mandatory in all who show EEG changes or who develop a neurologic deficit during regional anesthesia.

The controversy surrounding selective shunt use based on monitoring versus routine shunt use will continue as long as surgeons perform carotid endarterectomy, and it is unlikely that it will be laid to rest by a randomized trial because of the low incidence of perioperative stroke with either approach. Both approaches are valid and depend primarily on training, local availability, and the expense of monitoring techniques. The only approach that is not valid is *routine nonshunt* use.

Timing of Operation After Stroke

The early experience with carotid endarterectomy resulted in a generally accepted policy to delay the operation for 4 to 6 weeks in patients diagnosed with acute stroke, regardless of its severity, for fear of clinical deterioration associated with conversion of a bland infarct into a hemorrhagic one. Recent reports have suggested that an early operation without waiting 4 to 6 weeks is safe in patients with minor, nondisabling stroke.[102,103] On the other hand, a higher incidence of perioperative stroke has been reported in patients undergoing operation within 5 to 6 weeks after presenting with stroke.[104] A compelling reason for not delaying the operation is that patients may be placed at risk for recurrent stroke during the waiting period, particularly in circumstances where the stenosis is advanced or preocclusive. This reasoning is supported by the fact that, in the NASCET, 4.9% of the medically treated patients diagnosed with symptoms of stroke on entry had recurrent ipsilateral stroke within 30 days after randomization.[24]

The NASCET database provides further information.[102] Subgroup analysis was carried out on 100 surgical patients with 70% to 99% stenosis who were diagnosed with nondisabling hemispheric stroke at entry into the trial. Of these patients, 40% had carotid endarterectomy performed within 30 days, and the remainder had their endarterectomy performed at delayed times. There was no significant difference in the perioperative stroke and death rate and delayed stroke and death rate, and no association was found between an abnormal preoperative CT scan result and the subsequent risk of stroke when an early operation was performed. Based on these results, early carotid endarterectomy for severe carotid stenosis after nondisabling stroke can be done with rates of morbidity and mortality comparable with those who receive a delayed operation. Delaying the procedure for 4 to 6 weeks for patients with symptomatic high-grade stenosis exposes them to risk of recurrent stroke, which may be avoidable by earlier surgery.

From available data, one can draw the following conclusions about timing of carotid endarterectomy after stroke.[105] Patients with severe neurologic deficits, including altered consciousness, are not candidates for early carotid endarterectomy or carotid endarterectomy at any time unless they have considerable clinical recovery and, therefore, have brain tissue that can be preserved. Patients with a stable, nondisabling acute stroke, a normal CT scan, and a normal level of consciousness can probably undergo carotid endarterectomy shortly after the diagnosis is made and evaluation is complete. Patients with a small stroke on CT without significant midline shift, a stable neurologic deficit, and a normal level of consciousness have low risk with early surgery. If these individuals have an advanced (>70%) stenosis, they should undergo early operation. If the stenosis is moderate (50% to 69%) delaying operation for 4 to 6 weeks may be prudent. Patients with large strokes on CT with a midline shift may be at higher risk, particularly if they have a depressed level of consciousness. Operation should be delayed until these patients improve and plateau in their clinical recovery.

Simultaneous Carotid Endarterectomy and Coronary Artery Bypass

It is generally accepted that coronary artery disease is highly prevalent in patients presenting with carotid atherosclerotic stenosis. Many studies have documented that one fourth to one third of patients undergoing carotid endarterectomy have severe underlying coronary artery disease. The converse, however, is not true. The incidence of hemodynamically significant carotid stenosis in screening studies of patients undergoing coronary artery bypass is 5% to 11%.[106] Special problems arise in patients who have advanced disease in both territories. Although many centers have reported favorable experiences in combined carotid endarterectomy and coronary artery bypass procedures performed simultaneously, others point out that the overall stroke and death rate with this approach is higher than with either procedure alone. It is not clear whether this is due to the increased magnitude of the operation or the poor overall risk in such patients with advanced disease in both territories.

Simultaneous operation is generally restricted to patients whose carotid lesions appear to present a real threat in the postoperative period after coronary artery bypass. It should be considered in patients with precarious coronary artery disease such as unstable angina or high-grade left main lesions who have symptomatic high-grade carotid stenoses, bilateral high-grade asymptomatic stenoses, or ipsilateral advanced, asymptomatic stenosis and contralateral occlusion.[107] Staged approaches are appropriate in most patients. Initial carotid endarterectomy followed by coronary artery bypass is frequently applied to patients who present with symptomatic, high-grade carotid lesions who have stable coronary artery disease. In patients undergoing urgent or emergent coronary artery bypass grafting who have advanced carotid disease, a reversed staged approach may be employed, whereby carotid endarterectomy is carried out later. There appears to be an increased morbidity from performing carotid endarterectomy immediately after coronary artery bypass grafting, and available data would suggest that the operation should be delayed for at least 2 weeks.[107] Little data exist from prospective studies or randomized trials to guide the decision making for these complex patients, and most require individualized attention.

Eversion Carotid Endarterectomy

Eversion carotid endarterectomy was introduced in the late 1950s. The technique involves division of the common carotid artery below the bifurcation and eversion endarterectomy of both the external and internal carotid arteries.[108,109] Most recent modifications of the technique involve transection of the internal carotid artery at the level of the bifurcation and reimplantation of the internal carotid artery after endarterectomy into the common carotid artery.[110] Purported advantages of the eversion technique include simplicity, faster operating times, ease of correction of elongated and tortuous internal carotid arteries and, possibly, a lower rate of carotid restenosis. Disadvantages of the technique include difficulty in shunting, the possibility of incomplete removal of distal intimal flaps, difficulties in obtaining complete endarterectomy of the external and common carotid arteries when these are extensively involved with the disease, and frequent need for extensive distal mobilization of the internal carotid artery with a higher rate of cranial nerve injury in some series. Randomized studies to date demonstrate no differences in the major outcomes of stroke, death, and recurrent stenosis.[111,112]

Carotid Angioplasty/Stent Placement

During the years that carotid endarterectomy trials were being conducted, the techniques of balloon angioplasty and subsequently of stenting were being perfected for the coronary and peripheral arteries. Most recently, the technique has been extended to arteries supplying the brain.

This procedure in cerebral arteries is now performed by cardiologists, radiologists, and surgeons with increasing frequency and a reported decline in periprocedural complications.[113]

Angioplasty/stenting has been reported in many case series with extracranial and intracranial atherosclerotic and nonatherosclerotic disease affecting the carotid and the vertebrobasilar arteries. The quality of these studies is variable because of their retrospective nature, the heterogeneity of patients (asymptomatic and symptomatic patients) and disease processes (atherosclerosis, restenoses, fibromuscular disease, and others), the lack of controls and independent neurologic assessment, inaccuracy in reporting neurologic outcomes, the absence of long-term follow-up, and the lack of objective assessment of restenosis.

With these limitations noted, contemporary series of carotid angioplasty and stenting report a technical success rate of 97% to 98% and a stroke and death rate of 0% to 7.1%.[113-117] Cerebral protection devices that capture atherothrombotic debris at the time of angioplasty and stent deployment reduce the overall rate of periprocedural neurologic deficits by 40% to 50%.[114,118-121] Four randomized trials have compared carotid endarterectomy to carotid angioplasty and stenting.[122-125] Two demonstrated equivalent results with both interventions,[123,124] and the others were halted because of the high rate of adverse events from angioplasty and stenting.[122,125] Cerebral protection devices were not utilized routinely in any of these trials.

Large-scale, properly designed randomized trials of carotid endarterectomy versus angioplasty/stenting that feature cerebral protection devices are needed. Just as randomized trials have provided clear guidelines for the selection of patients to be treated with carotid endarterectomy, the same methodology will be required to define the role of angioplasty/stenting in stroke prevention. Major trials are currently underway. Until data from such trials are available, the procedure of carotid angioplasty/stenting should be reserved for patients requiring carotid revascularization who are not candidates for carotid endarterectomy because of anatomic, technical, or medical reasons.[113,118,126]

Selected References

Barnett HJM, Taylor DW, Eliasziw M, et al: Benefit of carotid endarterectomy in patients with symptomatic moderate or severe stenosis. North American Symptomatic Carotid Endarterectomy Trial Collaborators. N Engl J Med 339:1415-1425, 1998.

This paper presents the NASCET results in symptomatic patients with moderate stenoses (<70%) randomized to carotid endarterectomy plus medical therapy versus medical therapy alone. In patients with 50% to 69% stenoses, carotid endarterectomy was superior to medical therapy; however, in patients with less than 50% stenoses, medical and surgical therapy were equivalent. The paper also presents long-term follow-up in patients with severe stenoses (>70%) randomized to carotid endarterectomy. These patients had sustained benefit over the entire 7-year period of follow-up.

Beneficial effect of carotid endarterectomy in symptomatic patients with high-grade carotid stenosis. North American Symptomatic Carotid Endarterectomy Trial Collaborators. N Engl J Med 325:445-453, 1991.

This landmark article was the first major randomized, prospective trial to demonstrate the superiority of carotid endarterectomy over medical therapy for symptomatic patients with severe carotid stenosis. In addition to confirming the benefit of surgical intervention, the study documented the extraordinary high risk of stroke with medical treatment.

Clagett GP: When should I reoperate for recurrent carotid stenosis? In Naylor R, MacKay WC (eds): Carotid Artery Surgery: A Problem-Based Approach. London, Bailliere Tindall, 2000.

This chapter reviews the incidence, pathogenesis, indications for intervention, and operative techniques for recurrent carotid stenosis.

Counsell CE, Salinas R, Naylor R, et al: A systematic review of the randomised trials of carotid patch angioplasty in carotid endarterectomy. Eur J Vasc Endovasc Surg 13:345-354, 1997.

A meta-analysis confirms the superiority of patch angioplasty over primary closure in carotid endarterectomy. Perioperative stroke and recurrent carotid stenosis are reduced by the use of patch angioplasty to close the arteriotomy. However, there are not sufficient data to judge which patch material (vein, Dacron, and expanded polytetrafluoroethylene vascular sutures) is superior.

Endarterectomy for asymptomatic carotid artery stenosis. Executive Committee for the Asymptomatic Carotid Atherosclerosis Study. JAMA 273:1421-1428, 1995.

Patients with greater than 60% asymptomatic carotid stenosis were shown to benefit from carotid endarterectomy in this study. However, the results remain somewhat controversial because, although statistically significant, the absolute risk reduction in stroke and death was only 6%.

Ferguson GG, Eliasziw M, Barr HW, et al: The North American Symptomatic Carotid Endarterectomy Trial: Surgical results in 1415 patients. Stroke 30:1751-1758, 1999.

A detailed analysis of perioperative morbidity and mortality of surgical patients in the NASCET study is presented. A major conclusion was that thromboembolism stemming from the endarterectomy site is a major cause of postoperative stroke.

Hsia DC, Moscoe LM, Krushat WM: Epidemiology of carotid endarterectomy among Medicare beneficiaries: 1985–1996 update. Stroke 29:346-350, 1998.

In this sobering analysis, the authors document that the national stroke and death rate among patients undergoing carotid endarterectomy who are also Medicare beneficiaries remains unacceptably high. The authors question whether the beneficial results of carotid endarterectomy can be extrapolated nationally.

Jackson MR, Clagett GP: Antithrombotic therapy in peripheral arterial occlusive disease. Chest 114:6665, 1998.

This review critically assesses the benefit of antithrombotic therapy for peripheral arterial occlusive disease, including carotid artery disease.

Moore WS, Barnett HJ, Beebe HG, et al: Guidelines for carotid endarterectomy: A multidisciplinary consensus statement from the Ad Hoc Committee, American Heart Association. Circulation 91:566-579, 1995.

> **A group of prominent vascular surgeons, neurosurgeons, and neurologists details indications for carotid endarterectomy as well as relative contraindications in patients who may be better treated medically.**

Pritz MB: Timing of carotid endarterectomy after stroke. Stroke 28:2563-2567, 1997.

> **This thoughtful review addresses the risks/benefits of early versus late carotid endarterectomy for patients presenting with stroke. Early intervention is advocated for patients who are neurologically stable with relatively minor deficits.**

Tangkanakul C, Counsell CE, Warlow CP: Local versus general anaesthesia in carotid endarterectomy: A systematic review of the evidence. Eur J Vasc Endovasc Surg 13:491-499, 1997.

> **In this meta-analysis, the authors critically review available data on outcomes following general or local anesthesia for carotid endarterectomy. They conclude that there is no superiority of either approach over the other.**

Thompson JE: Carotid surgery: The past is prologue. The John Homans Lecture. J Vasc Surg 25:131-140, 1997.

> **This is an outstanding account of the history of carotid endarterectomy, as well as the operation's current status. The author is one of the pioneers of carotid surgery.**

References

1. Sacco RL, Benjamin EJ, Broderick JP, et al: American Heart Association Prevention Conference: IV. Prevention and rehabilitation of stroke: Risk factors. Stroke 28:1507-1517, 1997.
2. Laupacis A, Albers G, Dalen J, et al: Antithrombotic therapy in atrial fibrillation. Chest 114:579S-589S, 1998.
3. Zarins CK, Giddens DP, Bharadvaj BK, et al: Carotid bifurcation atherosclerosis: Quantitative correlation of plaque localization with flow velocity profiles and wall shear stress. Circ Res 53:502-514, 1983.
4. Carr SC, Farb A, Pearce WH, et al: Activated inflammatory cells are associated with plaque rupture in carotid artery stenosis. Surgery 122:757-764, 1997.
5. Jander S, Sitzer M, Schumann R, et al: Inflammation in high-grade carotid stenosis: A possible role for macrophages and T cells in plaque destabilization. Stroke 29:1625-1630, 1998.
6. Konstadoulakis MM, Kymionis GD, Karagiani M, et al: Evidence of apoptosis in human carotid atheroma. J Vasc Surg 27:733-739, 1998.
7. Svensson LG, Robinson MF, Esser J, et al: Influence of anatomic origin on intracranial distribution of microemboli in the baboon. Stroke 17:1198-1202, 1986.
8. Whisnant JP, Basford JR, Bernstein EF, et al: Classification of cerebrovascular diseases: III. Stroke 21:638, 1990.
9. Eliasziw M, Rankin RN, Fox AJ, et al: Accuracy and prognostic consequences of ultrasonography in identifying severe carotid artery stenosis. North American Symptomatic Carotid Endarterectomy Trial (NASCET) Group. Stroke 26:1747-1752, 1995.
10. Fisher M: Occlusion of the carotid arteries. Arch Neurol Psychiatry 72:187, 1954.
11. Fisher M: Occlusion of the internal carotid artery. Arch Neurol Psychiatry 65:346, 1951.
12. Thompson JE: Carotid surgery: The past is prologue. The John Homans Lecture. J Vasc Surg 25:131-140, 1997.
13. Tu JV, Hannan EL, Anderson GM, et al: The fall and rise of carotid endarterectomy in the United States and Canada. N Engl J Med 339:1441-1447, 1998.
14. Barnett HJM, Plum F, Walton JN: Carotid endarterectomy—an expression of concern. Stroke 15:941-943, 1984.
15. Barnett HJM, Eliasziw M, Meldrum HE: Drugs and surgery in the prevention of ischemic stroke. N Engl J Med 332:238-248, 1995.
16. Fields WS, Maslenikov V, Meyer JS, et al: Joint study of extracranial arterial occlusion: V. Progress report of prognosis following surgery or nonsurgical treatment for transient cerebral ischemic attacks and cervical carotid artery lesions. JAMA 211:1993-2003, 1970.
17. Failure of extracranial-intracranial arterial bypass to reduce the risk of ischemic stroke: Results of an international randomized trial. The EC/IC Bypass Study Group. N Engl J Med 313:1191-1200, 1985.
18. Barnett HJM, Taylor DW, Eliasziw M, et al: Benefit of carotid endarterectomy in patients with symptomatic moderate or severe stenosis. North American Symptomatic Carotid Endarterectomy Trial Collaborators. N Engl J Med 339:1415-1425, 1998.
19. Endarterectomy for moderate symptomatic carotid stenosis: Interim results from the MRC European Carotid Surgery Trial. Lancet 347:1591-1593, 1996.
20. MRC European Carotid Surgery Trial: Interim results for symptomatic patients with severe (70–99%) or with mild (0–29%) carotid stenosis. European Carotid Surgery Trialists' Collaborative Group. Lancet 337:1235-1243, 1991.
21. Endarterectomy for asymptomatic carotid artery stenosis. Executive Committee for the Asymptomatic Carotid Atherosclerosis Study. JAMA 273:1421-1428, 1995.
22. Hobson RW II, Weiss DG, Fields WS, et al: Efficacy of carotid endarterectomy for asymptomatic carotid stenosis. The Veterans Affairs Cooperative Study Group. N Engl J Med 328:221-227, 1993.
23. Mayberg MR, Wilson SE, Yatsu F, et al: Carotid endarterectomy and prevention of cerebral ischemia in symptomatic carotid stenosis. Veterans Affairs Cooperative Studies Program 309 Trialist Group. JAMA 266:3289-3294, 1991.
24. Beneficial effect of carotid endarterectomy in symptomatic patients with high-grade carotid stenosis. North American Symptomatic Carotid Endarterectomy Trial Collaborators. N Engl J Med 325:445-453, 1991.
25. Carotid surgery versus medical therapy in asymptomatic carotid stenosis. The CASANOVA Study Group. Stroke 22:1229-1235, 1991.
26. Rothwell PM, Eliasziw M, Gutnikov SA, et al: Analysis of pooled data from the randomised controlled trials of endarterectomy for symptomatic carotid stenosis. Lancet 361:107-116, 2003.
27. Benavente O, Eliasziw M, Streifler JY, et al: Prognosis after transient monocular blindness associated with carotid artery stenosis. N Engl J Med 345:1084-1090, 2001.
28. Eliasziw M, Streifler JY, Fox AJ, et al: Significance of plaque ulceration in symptomatic patients with high-grade carotid stenosis. North American Symptomatic Carotid Endarterectomy Trial. Stroke 25:304-308, 1994.
29. Gasecki AP, Eliasziw M, Ferguson GG, et al: Long-term prognosis and effect of endarterectomy in patients with symptomatic severe carotid stenosis and contralateral

carotid stenosis or occlusion: Results from North American Symptomatic Carotid Endarterectomy Trial (NASCET) Group. J Neurosurg 83:778-782, 1995.

30. Kappelle LJ, Eliasziw M, Fox AJ, et al: Importance of intracranial atherosclerotic disease in patients with symptomatic stenosis of the internal carotid artery. The North American Symptomatic Carotid Endarterectomy Trial. Stroke 30:282-286, 1999.

31. Streifler JY, Eliasziw M, Benavente OR, et al: The risk of stroke in patients with first-ever retinal versus hemispheric transient ischemic attacks and high-grade carotid stenosis. North American Symptomatic Carotid Endarterectomy Trial. Arch Neurol 52:246-249, 1995.

32. Streifler JY, Eliasziw M, Fox AJ, et al: Angiographic detection of carotid plaque ulceration: Comparison with surgical observations in a multicenter study. North American Symptomatic Carotid Endarterectomy Trial. Stroke 25:1130-1132, 1994.

33. Alamowitch S, Eliasziw M, Algra A, et al: Risk, causes, and prevention of ischaemic stroke in elderly patients with symptomatic internal carotid artery stenosis. Lancet 357:1154-1160, 2001.

34. Ferguson GG, Eliasziw M, Barr HW, et al: The North American Symptomatic Carotid Endarterectomy Trial: Surgical results in 1415 patients. Stroke 30:1751-1758, 1999.

35. Barnett HJM, Meldrum HE, Eliasziw M: The appropriate use of carotid endarterectomy. Can Med Assoc J 166:1169-1179, 2002.

36. Moore WS, Barnett HJ, Beebe HG, et al: Guidelines for carotid endarterectomy: A multidisciplinary consensus statement from the Ad Hoc Committee, American Heart Association. Circulation 91:566-579, 1995.

37. Jackson MR, Clagett GP: Antithrombotic therapy in peripheral arterial occlusive disease. Chest 119:283S-299S, 2001.

38. Taylor DW, Barnett HJ, Haynes RB, et al: Low-dose and high-dose acetylsalicylic acid for patients undergoing carotid endarterectomy: A randomised controlled trial. ASA and Carotid Endarterectomy (ACE) Trial Collaborators. Lancet 353:2179-2184, 1999.

39. Fisher DF Jr, Clagett GP, Parker JI, et al: Mandibular subluxation for high carotid exposure. J Vasc Surg 1:727-733, 1984.

40. Archie JP Jr: Patching with carotid endarterectomy: When to do it and what to use. Semin Vasc Surg 11:24-29, 1998.

41. Counsell CE, Salinas R, Naylor R, et al: A systematic review of the randomised trials of carotid patch angioplasty in carotid endarterectomy. Eur J Vasc Endovasc Surg 13:345-354, 1997.

42. Papanicolaou G, Toms C, Yellin AE, et al: Relationship between intraoperative color-flow duplex findings and early restenosis after carotid endarterectomy: A preliminary report. J Vasc Surg 24:588-596, 1996.

43. Clagett GP, Krupski WC: Antithrombotic therapy in peripheral arterial occlusive disease. Chest 108:431S-443S, 1995.

44. Koslow AR, Ricotta JJ, Ouriel K, et al: Re-exploration for thrombosis in carotid endarterectomy. Circulation 80:III73-III78, 1989.

45. Comerota AJ, Eze AR: Intraoperative high-dose regional urokinase infusion for cerebrovascular occlusion after carotid endarterectomy. J Vasc Surg 24:1008-1016, 1996.

46. Youkey JR, Clagett GP, Jaffin JH, et al: Focal motor seizures complicating carotid endarterectomy. Arch Surg 119:1080-1084, 1984.

47. Jorgensen LG, Schroeder TV: Defective cerebrovascular autoregulation after carotid endarterectomy. Eur J Vasc Surg 7:370-379, 1993.

48. Naylor AR, Ruckley CV: The post-carotid endarterectomy hyperperfusion syndrome. Eur J Vasc Endovasc Surg 9:365-367, 1995.

49. Pomposelli FB, Lamparello PJ, Riles TS, et al: Intracranial hemorrhage after carotid endarterectomy. J Vasc Surg 7:248-255, 1988.

50. Riles TS, Imparato AM, Jacobowitz GR, et al: The cause of perioperative stroke after carotid endarterectomy. J Vasc Surg 19:206-216, 1994.

51. Treiman RL, Cossman DV, Foran RF, et al: The influence of neutralizing heparin after carotid endarterectomy on postoperative stroke and wound hematoma. J Vasc Surg 12:440-446, 1990.

52. Archie JP Jr, Green JJ Jr: Saphenous vein rupture pressure, rupture stress, and carotid endarterectomy vein patch reconstruction. Surgery 107:389-396, 1990.

53. Riles TS, Lamparello PJ, Giangola G, et al: Rupture of the vein patch: A rare complication of carotid endarterectomy. Surgery 107:10-12, 1990.

54. Ballotta E, Da Giau G, Renon L, et al: Cranial and cervical nerve injuries after carotid endarterectomy: A prospective study. Surgery 125:85-91, 1999.

55. Bergqvist D: Peripheral nerve injuries associated with carotid endarterectomy. Semin Vasc Surg 4:47, 1991.

56. Cebul RD, Snow RJ, Pine R, et al: Indications, outcomes, and provider volumes for carotid endarterectomy. JAMA 279:1282-1287, 1998.

57. Huber TS, Durance PW, Kazmers A, et al: Effect of the Asymptomatic Carotid Atherosclerosis Study on carotid endarterectomy in Veterans Affairs medical centers. Arch Surg 132:1134-1139, 1997.

58. Kresowik TF, Bratzler D, Karp HR, et al: Multistate utilization, processes, and outcomes of carotid endarterectomy. J Vasc Surg 33:227-235, 2001.

59. Hsia DC, Moscoe LM, Krushat WM: Epidemiology of carotid endarterectomy among Medicare beneficiaries: 1985–1996 update. Stroke 29:346-350, 1998.

60. Rothwell PM, Slattery J, Warlow CP: A systematic review of the risks of stroke and death due to endarterectomy for symptomatic carotid stenosis. Stroke 27:260-265, 1996.

61. Kresowik TF, Hemann RA, Grund SL, et al: Improving the outcomes of carotid endarterectomy: Results of a statewide quality improvement project. J Vasc Surg 31:918-926, 2000.

62. Wong JH, Lubkey TB, Suarez-Almazor ME, et al: Improving the appropriateness of carotid endarterectomy: Results of a prospective city-wide study. Stroke 30:12-15, 1999.

63. Beebe HG, Clagett GP, DeWeese JA, et al: Assessing risk associated with carotid endarterectomy: A statement for health professionals by an Ad Hoc Committee on Carotid Surgery Standards of the Stroke Council, American Heart Association. Stroke 20:314, 1989.

64. Goldstein LB, Moore WS, Robertson JT, et al: Complication rates for carotid endarterectomy: A call to action. Stroke 28:889-890, 1997.

65. Feasby TE, Quan H, Ghali WA: Hospital and surgeon determinants of carotid endarterectomy outcomes. Arch Neurol 59:1877-1881, 2002.

66. Hannan EL, Popp AJ, Tranmer B, et al: Relationship between provider volume and mortality for carotid endarterectomies in New York state. Stroke 29:2292-2297, 1998.

67. Kantonen I, Lepantalo M, Salenius JP, et al: Influence of surgical experience on the results of carotid surgery. The Finnvasc Study Group. Eur J Vasc Endovasc Surg 15:155-160, 1998.

68. Wennberg DE, Lucas FL, Birkmeyer JD, et al: Variation in carotid endarterectomy mortality in the Medicare population: Trial hospitals, volume, and patient characteristics. JAMA 279:1278-1281, 1998.

69. Barnett HJM: Efficacy of carotid endarterectomy translates to being efficacious with appropriate surgical skill. Arch Neurol 59:1866-1868, 2002.

70. Collier PE: Fast-tracking carotid endarterectomy: Practical considerations. Semin Vasc Surg 11:41-45, 1998.

71. Hirko MK, Morasch MD, Burke K, et al: The changing face of carotid endarterectomy. J Vasc Surg 23:622-627, 1996.

72. Lipsett PA, Tierney S, Gordon TA, et al: Carotid endarterectomy: Is intensive care unit care necessary? J Vasc Surg 20:403-410, 1994.

73. Back MR, Harward TR, Huber TS, et al: Improving the cost-effectiveness of carotid endarterectomy. J Vasc Surg 26:456-464, 1997.

74. Erdoes LS, Marek JM, Mills JL, et al: The relative contributions of carotid duplex scanning, magnetic resonance angiography, and cerebral arteriography to clinical decision making: A prospective study in patients with carotid occlusive disease. J Vasc Surg 23:950-956, 1996.

75. Patel MR, Kuntz KM, Klufas RA, et al: Preoperative assessment of the carotid bifurcation: Can magnetic resonance angiography and duplex ultrasonography replace contrast arteriography? Stroke 26:1753-1758, 1995.

76. Purcell PN, Brewster DC: When should carotid endarterectomy be performed on the basis of carotid noninvasive examination alone? Perspect Vasc Surg 9:1, 1998.

77. Howard G, Chambless LE, Baker WH, et al: A multicenter validation study of Doppler ultrasound versus angiography. J Stroke Cerebrovasc Dis 1:166, 1991.

78. Kent KC, Kuntz KM, Patel MR, et al: Perioperative imaging strategies for carotid endarterectomy: An analysis of morbidity and cost-effectiveness in symptomatic patients. JAMA 274:888-893, 1995.

79. Clagett GP: When should I reoperate for recurrent carotid stenosis? In Mackey WC, Naylor R (eds): Carotid Artery Surgery: A Problem-Based Approach. Philadelphia, WB Saunders, 2000, pp 375-382.

80. Frericks H, Kievit J, van Baalen JM, et al: Carotid recurrent stenosis and risk of ipsilateral stroke: A systematic review of the literature. Stroke 29:244-250, 1998.

81. Harker LA, Bernstein EF, Dilley RB, et al: Failure of aspirin plus dipyridamole to prevent restenosis after carotid endarterectomy. Ann Intern Med 116:731-736, 1992.

82. Reilly LM, Okuhn SP, Rapp JH, et al: Recurrent carotid stenosis: A consequence of local or systemic factors? The influence of unrepaired technical defects. J Vasc Surg 11:448-460, 1990.

83. Clagett GP, Rich NM, McDonald PT, et al: Etiologic factors for recurrent carotid artery stenosis. Surgery 93:313-318, 1983.

84. Valentine RJ, Myers SI, Hagino RT, et al: Late outcome of patients with premature carotid atherosclerosis after carotid endarterectomy. Stroke 27:1502-1506, 1996.

85. Healy DA, Zierler RE, Nicholls SC, et al: Long-term follow-up and clinical outcome of carotid restenosis. J Vasc Surg 10:662-669, 1989.

86. Clagett GP, Robinowitz M, Youkey JR, et al: Morphogenesis and clinicopathologic characteristics of recurrent carotid disease. J Vasc Surg 3:10-23, 1986.

87. Rossi PJ, Myers SI, Clagett GP: Reoperative approaches for carotid restenosis. Semin Vasc Surg 7:195-200, 1994.

88. Archie JP Jr: Early and late geometric changes after carotid endarterectomy patch reconstruction. J Vasc Surg 14:258-266, 1991.

89. Clagett GP: Vein patch graft closure for carotid endarterectomy. In Ernst CB, Stanley JC (eds): Current Therapy in Vascular Surgery, 2nd ed. Philadelphia, BC Decker, 1991, p 85.

90. Clagett GP, Patterson CB, Fisher DF Jr, et al: Vein patch versus primary closure for carotid endarterectomy: A randomized prospective study in a selected group of patients. J Vasc Surg 9:213-223, 1989.

91. Myers SI, Valentine RJ, Chervu A, et al: Saphenous vein patch versus primary closure for carotid endarterectomy: Long-term assessment of a randomized prospective study. J Vasc Surg 19:15-22, 1994.

92. Eikelboom BC, Ackerstaff RG, Hoeneveld H, et al: Benefits of carotid patching: A randomized study. J Vasc Surg 7:240-247, 1988.

93. Abu Rahma AF, Robinson PA, Saiedy S, et al: Prospective randomized trial of carotid endarterectomy with primary closure and patch angioplasty with saphenous vein, jugular vein, and polytetrafluoroethylene: Long-term follow-up. J Vasc Surg 27:222-234, 1998.

94. Lawrence PF, Alves JC, Jicha D, et al: Incidence, timing, and causes of cerebral ischemia during carotid endarterectomy with regional anesthesia. J Vasc Surg 27:329-337, 1998.

95. McCleary AJ, Maritati G, Gough MJ: Carotid endarterectomy: Local or general anaesthesia? Eur J Vasc Endovasc Surg 22:1-12, 2001.

96. Tangkanakul C, Counsell CE, Warlow CP: Local versus general anaesthesia in carotid endarterectomy: A systematic review of the evidence. Eur J Vasc Endovasc Surg 13:491-499, 1997.

97. Thompson JE: Role of shunting during carotid endarterectomy. In Ernst CB, Stanley JC (eds): Current Therapy in Vascular Surgery, 3rd ed. St. Louis, Mosby, 1995, p 57.

98. Halsey JH Jr: Risks and benefits of shunting in carotid endarterectomy. The International Transcranial Doppler Collaborators. Stroke 23:1583-1587, 1992.

99. Harada RN, Comerota AJ, Good GM, et al: Stump pressure, electroencephalographic changes, and the contralateral carotid artery: Another look at selective shunting. Am J Surg 170:148-153, 1995.

100. Imparato AM, Ramirez A, Riles T, et al: Cerebral protection in carotid surgery. Arch Surg 117:1073-1078, 1982.

101. Sundt TM Jr, Sharbrough FW, Piepgras DG, et al: Correlation of cerebral blood flow and electroencephalographic changes during carotid endarterectomy: With results of surgery and hemodynamics of cerebral ischemia. Mayo Clin Proc 56:533-543, 1981.

102. Gasecki AP, Ferguson GG, Eliasziw M, et al: Early endarterectomy for severe carotid artery stenosis after a nondisabling stroke: Results from the North American Symptomatic Carotid Endarterectomy Trial. J Vasc Surg 20:288-295, 1994.

103. Piotrowski JJ, Bernhard VM, Rubin JR, et al: Timing of carotid endarterectomy after acute stroke. J Vasc Surg 11:45-52, 1990.

104. Giordano JM: The timing of carotid endarterectomy after acute stroke. Semin Vasc Surg 11:19-23, 1998.

105. Pritz MB: Timing of carotid endarterectomy after stroke. Stroke 28:2563-2567, 1997.

106. Berens ES, Kouchoukos NT, Murphy SF, et al: Preoperative carotid artery screening in elderly patients undergoing cardiac surgery. J Vasc Surg 15:313-323, 1992.

107. Hertzer NR, Loop FD, Beven EG, et al: Surgical staging for simultaneous coronary and carotid disease: A study including prospective randomization. J Vasc Surg 9:455-463, 1989.

108. Ballotta E, Da Giau G, Saladini M, et al: Carotid endarterectomy with patch closure versus carotid eversion endarterectomy and reimplantation: A prospective randomized study. Surgery 125:271-279, 1999.

109. Cao P, Giordano G, De Rango P, et al: A randomized study on eversion versus standard carotid endarterectomy: Study design and preliminary results—the Everest Trial. J Vasc Surg 27:595-605, 1998.

110. Shah DM, Leather RP, Darling RC, et al: Technique of eversion carotid endarterectomy and contemporary results. Perspect Vasc Surg 9:49, 1998.

111. Cao P, De Rango P, Zannetti S: Eversion versus conventional carotid endarterectomy: A systematic review. Eur J Vasc Endovasc Surg 23:195-201, 2002.

112. Cao P, Giordano G, De Rango P, et al: Eversion versus conventional carotid endarterectomy: Late results of a prospective multicenter randomized trial. J Vasc Surg 31:19-30, 2000.

113. New G, Roubin GS, Iyer SS, et al: Safety, efficacy, and durability of carotid artery stenting for restenosis following carotid endarterectomy: A multicenter study. J Endovasc Ther 7:345-352, 2000.

114. Al-Mubarak N, Colombo A, Gaines PA, et al: Multicenter evaluation of carotid artery stenting with a filter protection system. J Am Coll Cardiol 39:841-846, 2002.

115. Baudier JF, Licht PB, Roder O, et al: Endovascular treatment of severe symptomatic stenosis of the internal carotid artery: Early and late outcome. Eur J Vasc Endovasc Surg 22:205-210, 2001.

116. Bergeron P, Becquemin JP, Jausseran JM, et al: Percutaneous stenting of the internal carotid artery: The European CAST I Study. Carotid Artery Stent Trial. J Endovasc Surg 6:155-159, 1999.

117. Gray WA, White HJ Jr, Barrett DM, et al: Carotid stenting and endarterectomy: A clinical and cost comparison of revascularization strategies. Stroke 33:1063-1070, 2002.

118. Kastrup A, Groschel K, Krapf H, et al: Early outcome of carotid angioplasty and stenting with and without cerebral protection devices: A systematic review of the literature. Stroke 34:813-819, 2003.

119. Parodi JC, La Mura R, Ferreira LM, et al: Initial evaluation of carotid angioplasty and stenting with three different cerebral protection devices. J Vasc Surg 32:1127-1136, 2000.

120. Tubler T, Schluter M, Dirsch O, et al: Balloon-protected carotid artery stenting: Relationship of periprocedural neurological complications with the size of particulate debris. Circulation 104:2791-2796, 2001.

121. Whitlow PL, Lylyk P, Londero H, et al: Carotid artery stenting protected with an emboli containment system. Stroke 33:1308-1314, 2002.

122. Alberts M: Results of a multicenter prospective randomized trial of carotid artery stenting versus carotid endarterectomy: For the publications committee of the WALLSTENT [Abstract]. Stroke 32:325, 2001.

123. Brooks WH, McClure RR, Jones MR, et al: Carotid angioplasty and stenting versus carotid endarterectomy: Randomized trial in a community hospital. J Am Coll Cardiol 38:1589-1595, 2001.

124. Brown MM, Rogers J, Bland JM: Endovascular versus surgical treatment in patients with carotid stenosis in the Carotid and Vertebral Artery Transluminal Angioplasty Study (CAVATAS): A randomised trial. Lancet 357:1729-1737, 2001.

125. Naylor AR, Bolia A, Abbott RJ, et al: Randomized study of carotid angioplasty and stenting versus carotid endarterectomy: A stopped trial. J Vasc Surg 28:326-334, 1998.

126. Fox DJ Jr, Moran CJ, Cross DT III, et al: Long-term outcome after angioplasty for symptomatic extracranial carotid stenosis in poor surgical candidates. Stroke 33:2877-2880, 2002.

CHAPTER 64

ANEURYSMAL VASCULAR DISEASE

**Christopher K. Zarins, M.D.,   Maarit A. Heikkinen, M.D., Ph.D.,
and   Bradley B. Hill, M.D.**

An *arterial aneurysm* is defined as a permanent localized enlargement of an artery to more than 1.5 times its expected diameter.[1] Aneurysms can develop at any location in the arterial tree but are most commonly found in the human aorta, iliac, popliteal, and femoral arteries, in decreasing order of frequency. The carotid, renal, visceral, and upper extremity arteries can also develop aneurysms. Intracranial cerebrovascular aneurysms are distinct from extracranial arterial aneurysms with regard to age, risk factors, manifestations, and treatment, and they are not considered here.

Arterial ectasia refers to localized arterial enlargement less than 50% of normal diameter. *Arteriomegaly* refers to generalized arterial enlargement including the aorta, iliac, and femoral arteries and usually includes arteries that are normally not prone to develop aneurysms, such as the external iliac artery and the profunda femoris artery. Although arteriomegalic arteries can become quite large, they are usually not prone to rupture.

The primary clinical significance of centrally located aneurysms (intrathoracic and intra-abdominal) is related to the risk of aneurysm rupture, whereas the primary clinical significance of peripheral aneurysms is related to the risk of thrombosis or embolism.

Aneurysms are classified according to anatomic site, morphology, and etiology. The most common aneurysm morphology is a fusiform, symmetrical circumferential enlargement involving all layers of the artery wall.

Aneurysms may also be saccular with aneurysmal degeneration affecting only part of the arterial circumference.

The most common etiology of aneurysms is atherosclerotic degeneration of the arterial wall. The pathogenesis is a multifactorial process involving genetic predisposition, aging, atherosclerosis, inflammation, and localized proteolytic enzyme activation. Most aneurysms occur in elderly people, and the prevalence of aneurysms increases with increasing age. Aneurysms can also occur in younger, genetically susceptible individuals with Ehlers-Danlos and Marfan syndromes. Other etiologies include localized infection that results in mycotic aneurysms and the rare tertiary stage of syphilis.

Aortic aneurysms may also occur with aortic dissection. Aortic dissections usually occur in the thoracic aorta with an intimal tear and separation of the layers of the aortic wall. This results in the creation of a false lumen within the aortic wall with compression of the true lumen. The term *dissecting aneurysm* is applied to aortic dissections with aneurysmal dilation of the false lumen. This can result in rupture of the aorta.

Aneurysmal enlargement can also result from hemodynamic causes such as poststenotic arterial dilation or arteriovenous fistulas. Long-standing poststenotic dilation at sites such as in the subclavian artery distal to a cervical rib or thoracic outlet compression, or in the aorta distal to coarctation or aortic valvular stenosis, may result in aneurysmal degeneration. Once the artery becomes aneurysmal, reversal of the hemodynamic aberration does not result in regression of the aneurysm. Similarly, arteries supplying a long-standing high-flow arteriovenous fistula, either congenital or acquired, can become aneurysmal. Additional types of aneurysms include those associated with pregnancy and childhood or congenital aneurysms.

Pseudoaneurysms (false aneurysms) are localized arterial disruptions caused by blunt or penetrating trauma, vascular intervention, or anastomotic disruption. Blood is contained by adjoining tissues and fibrous reaction. Pseudoaneurysms are distinguished from true aneurysms involving a pathologic process of the arterial wall.

HISTORICAL PERSPECTIVE

Early attempts at repairing aneurysms included (1) ligation (Cooper, 1817); (2) induction of thrombosis by inserting steel wire (Moore, 1864); (3) passing an electrical current within the vessel wall; (4) cellophane wrapping (Rea, 1948); and (5) endoaneurysmorrhaphy, which consisted of imbrication of the opened aneurysm edges (Matas, 1906).

The first modern repair of an abdominal aortic aneurysm was performed in 1951 in Paris by Charles Dubost, who used the retroperitoneal approach and replaced the aneurysm with a freeze-dried thoracic aortic homograft. Repair of a ruptured abdominal aortic aneurysm was first reported by Bahnson at Johns Hopkins in 1953. Initially, aneurysm repair involved excision of the aneurysm and replacement of the aorta with a graft. The term *aneurysmectomy* persists in the surgical lexicon to denote aortic aneurysm repair, although aneurysms are rarely excised. In the late 1950s, it was realized that removal of the aneurysm was unnecessary, and aortic aneurysm repair is currently performed "intrasaccularly" by opening the aneurysm sac and suturing a prosthetic graft to the nonaneurysmal proximal aorta and distal vessels. Numerous technical advances have been made since the 1960s and have resulted in improvement in grafts, sutures, instruments, clamps, and techniques. Furthermore, significant advances have been made in areas of anesthesia, blood transfusion, and preoperative and postoperative care. Surgical repair of aneurysms can be performed safely and is effective in preventing death from rupture of abdominal aortic aneurysms.[2]

The unreliable early aortic homografts were replaced through pioneering efforts of Vorhees, DeBakey, and others using a variety of prosthetic cloth grafts, of which the crimped Dacron polyester graft has proven to be the most durable and is still used.

Repair of a thoracoabdominal aneurysm was first reported in 1954 by Etheredge, followed by four cases in 1956 by DeBakey and colleagues. Throughout the 1960s, 1970s, and 1980s, Crawford laid the foundation for the treatment of thoracoabdominal aneurysm, Marfan syndrome, and the surgical treatment of aortic dissection.[3,4] Ongoing evolutionary changes in patient management included improvement in perioperative cardiopulmonary management, modification of the approach to coronary artery comorbidity, and improvement in the ways to reduce spinal cord ischemia and paraplegia after thoracoabdominal aneurysm repair.

In 1991, Parodi introduced a revolutionary minimally invasive endovascular approach to the treatment of abdominal aortic aneurysms. This involved transfemoral endoluminal placement of a stented prosthesis within the aneurysm sac to exclude the aneurysm from the circulation. Endovascular stent graft repair offers the advantage of reduced patient morbidity by avoiding direct transabdominal or transthoracic aneurysm surgical exposure. A number of commercial bifurcated stent graft devices have been developed for the abdominal aorta, and these have largely replaced the early "homemade" devices. Three commercially available devices have received U.S. Food and Drug Administration (FDA) approval for clinical use for abdominal aortic aneurysms. Several thoracic stent graft devices are in clinical trials for thoracic aneurysms.

PATHOGENESIS

The pathogenesis of aortic aneurysms is complex and not well defined. A number of theories have been proposed, but no single theory has been universally accepted. It is likely that aneurysm formation is the consequence of the interaction of multiple factors rather than a single process. Histologically, the aneurysm wall is thinned with a marked decrease in the amount of medial and adventitial elastin. An inflammatory infiltrate has been observed in some abdominal aneurysms, with a relative preponderance of plasma cells in the media of some and a chronic infiltrate with a preponderance of T cells in the adventitia in others. Because of the frequent coexistence with generalized atherosclerosis, degenerative aneurysms are often referred to as *atherosclerotic aneurysms*. Although aneurysmal and occlusive disease demonstrate common pathologic features and share common risk factors, a common pathogenesis has not been proved. The etiologic role of atherosclerosis in the development of these aneurysms has been questioned, and alternative or additional mechanisms have been proposed. However, the similarity of the pathologic processes involving artery degeneration suggests that common disease mechanisms between atherosclerotic occlusive disease and aneurysmal disease will be found (Fig. 64-1).

The following mechanisms are not mutually exclusive, and, most likely, all of them play a part in the formation of aneurysms.

Genetic

Abdominal as well as thoracic aneurysms exhibit familial clustering and occur in 10% to 20% of first-degree relatives. Specific genetic abnormalities have been linked to aneurysm formation in patients with Marfan syndrome (fibrillin) and in patients with Ehlers-Danlos type 4 (procollagen type III). However, the aneurysms in these patients appear at an earlier age and are often different from the usual variety of degenerative aneurysms, and the relevance of these abnormalities to the latter is doubtful.

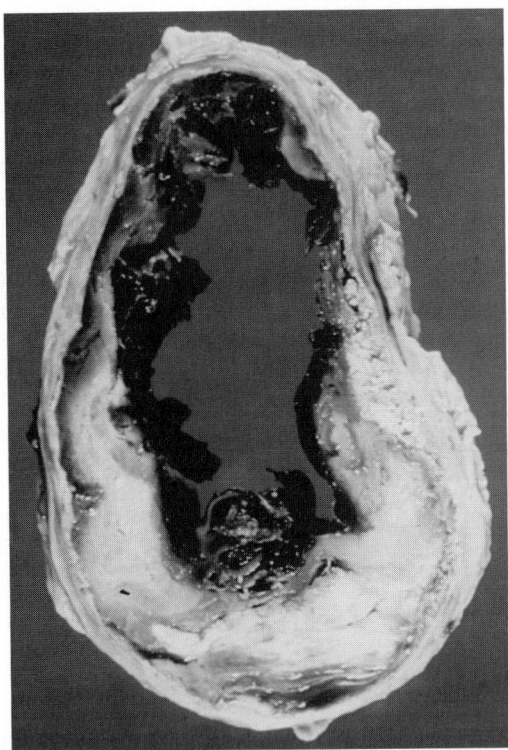

FIGURE 64-1. Cross section of abdominal aortic aneurysm reveals dilated arterial wall with posterior atherosclerotic plaque and laminated mural thrombus.

Less specific genetic abnormalities include decreased type III collagen in the aortic media of familial aneurysms and more common polymorphisms on the gene for pro-alpha$_1$(III) chain of type III collagen and the haptoglobin alpha' allele in patients with aneurysms. In addition, abnormalities on the long arm of chromosome 16 have been found. Because most patients with aneurysms do not have a known family history, a genetic predisposition as the sole or principal cause of degenerative aneurysms is unlikely.

Proteolytic

The primary determinants of aortic structural integrity and stability are the musculoelastic fascicles in the media and the collagen scaffold structure of the adventitia. Degradation of these structures is expected to result in aneurysmal degeneration and, indeed, experimental enzymatic destruction of the aortic wall results in the formation of aneurysms. Many changes in aneurysm wall have been described, including a marked decrease in the quantity of elastin in the aneurysm wall while the quantity of collagen remains unchanged. There is increased activity of elastase in the aneurysm wall, which may be related to matrix metalloproteinase (MMP)-9 or other proteases. Increased collagenase activity (MMP-1) has also been found in abdominal aortic aneurysm wall as well as MMP-3 (an activator of MMP-9 and MMP-1) and plasmin. A decrease in the concentration of protease inhibitors tissue inhibitor of metalloproteinase (TIMP)-1 and TIMP-2 has also been reported. Interleukin-1β and tumor necrosis factor-α, which are secreted by inflammatory cells, were also found to be elevated in aneurysm wall. The causative role of these and other derangements has not been proved, and they may represent secondary changes related to degeneration of the arterial wall.

Atherosclerosis

Atherosclerosis is epidemiologically linked to aneurysmal disease. Both occur in older individuals, predominantly in men and in smokers. Pathologically, atherosclerosis is characterized by focal intimal thickening encroaching on the lumen and consequent compensatory arterial dilation. This remodeling occurs by thinning of the media underneath the plaque and loss of normal arterial architecture, a change identical to the process underlying aneurysmal degeneration.[5,6] Experimentally, aneurysms can be induced in nonsusceptible primates by exogenous cholesterol feeding and induction of atherosclerosis, and their formation can be further enhanced by plaque regression.

EPIDEMIOLOGY

Distribution of Aortic Aneurysms

Aortic aneurysms are most commonly located in the infrarenal aorta (Fig. 64-2). The segment immediately below the renal arteries is usually spared. Aneurysms involving the immediate infrarenal segment are known as juxtarenal aneurysms. Suprarenal aneurysms are those that extend above the renal arteries. Thoracoabdominal aneurysms occur in a minority of cases (2%) and involve the thoracic aorta in addition to the abdominal aorta, including the segment involving the celiac, superior mesenteric, and renal arteries.

The iliac arteries are involved in 40% of patients with abdominal aortic aneurysms. In 90% of these, the common iliac arteries are involved, whereas 10% involve the hypogastric arteries. The external iliac arteries are almost never involved. Occasionally, iliac aneurysms occur in an isolated fashion.

Prevalence of Abdominal Aortic Aneurysms

The prevalence of abdominal aortic aneurysms at autopsy is 1.8% to 6.6%. In one large autopsy study, the prevalence of abdominal aortic aneurysms in men was 4.3%, increasing rapidly after the age of 55 years and peaking at the age of 80 years, whereas the prevalence in women was 2.1%, increasing after age 70 years and continuing to do so beyond age 90 years.[7] The most common location of aortic aneurysms is in the abdominal aorta, and up to 40% of patients with infrarenal aneurysms have an aneurysm elsewhere in the aorta. The incidence of newly diagnosed aortic aneurysms is 21 in 100,000 patient-years. Since 1970, there has been a more than threefold increase in overall as well as age-specific prevalence of abdominal

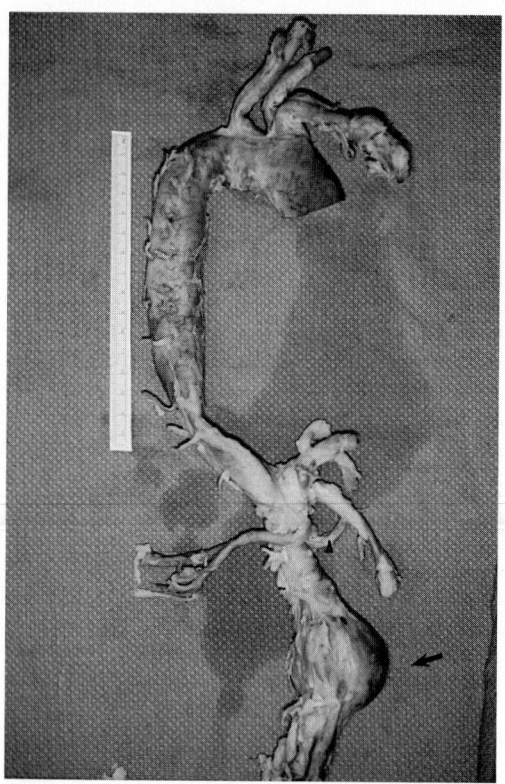

FIGURE 64-2. Human anatomic specimen containing thoracic and abdominal aorta. Note the 5.5-cm abdominal aortic aneurysm (arrow) at a typical location below the renal arteries (arrowhead).

aneurysms, whereas death rates from strokes and heart disease have been declining.

The average age of patients with abdominal aortic aneurysms is 75 years, about 10 years older than the average age of patients with clinically significant arterial occlusive disease. Abdominal aortic aneurysms are more common in men than in women, with a male-to-female ratio of approximately 8:1. White men have a higher prevalence than black men or women. In 50- to 75-year-old men, aneurysms larger than 4 cm occur at a rate of 1.4%; in patients older than 60 years of age, the prevalence of aneurysms larger than 3 cm is 3%. Smoking is the most important risk factor and is associated with 78% of aneurysms discovered on screening.[8,9] Prevalence of aneurysms is approximately 10% in men with hypertension or with clinical evidence of peripheral, carotid, or coronary arterial disease. There is a definite familial incidence, with a rate of 10% to 20% and an 11.6-fold increase in relative risk in first-degree relatives of patients with abdominal aortic aneurysm. Familial aneurysms affect patients at a younger age, and more women are affected.

Aneurysm rupture is the cause of death in 1.2% of men and 0.6% of women in the United States. It is the 13th most common cause of death in the United States and is the cause of deaths in 15,000 people annually. In 12% of the ruptured aneurysms, the aneurysm has not been previously diagnosed. About 46,000 abdominal aneurysms were repaired in 1992 in the United States and, of these, approximately 10% were ruptured.

Thoracic aortic aneurysms are diagnosed at a rate of 5.9 in 100,000 per year. In 12% to 25%, they are multisegmental, and the most common combination (44% of cases) is a descending thoracic and an infrarenal aortic aneurysm. Thoracic aneurysms are more equally distributed between the genders than are abdominal aortic aneurysms, with a male-to-female ratio of 2:1. There is familial clustering, and patients with a family history tend to be younger.

Aortic dissection has an incidence of approximately 10 in 100,000 per year; as a cause of death, 2 in 100,000 are listed annually for men and 0.8 in 100,000 for women. The incidence is declining, possibly because of better control of hypertension. It is estimated that only one third to two thirds of aortic dissections are diagnosed before death and that this may be the most common aortic catastrophe. The median age for dissection is 60 years (range 13 to 87 years), and 77% of the patients are men. It may occur in younger women during the third trimester of pregnancy.

NATURAL HISTORY

Abdominal Aortic Aneurysms

The natural history of abdominal aortic aneurysms is to enlarge and rupture. Treatment strategies are designed to prevent this complication. The survival statistics after rupture of an aortic aneurysm have not changed significantly since the 1980s. Following rupture of an abdominal aortic aneurysm, only 50% of patients arrive at the hospital alive. Of these, 24% or more die before surgery and 42% die after the operation, for an overall mortality rate of 78% to 94%.

Aneurysms enlarge at an average rate of 0.4 cm per year, with a high individual variability.[10] Enlargement may be discontinuous, and 25% of aneurysms remain stationary over prolonged periods. Higher enlargement rates have been associated with arterial hypertension, chronic obstructive lung disease, family history, and increased aneurysmal thrombus.

In less than 5% of abdominal aneurysms, the first clinical manifestation is embolization to the lower extremity. This complication is not related to the size of the aneurysm and constitutes an independent indication for repair.

Risk of Rupture

The single most important factor associated with rupture is maximal cross-sectional aneurysm diameter. Maximal aneurysm diameter correlates best to the probability of rupture. Equal in significance is maximal cross-sectional area.[11] The fate of large aneurysms was initially investigated in the 1950s and 1960s. Overall survival rate and the risk of rupture were related to maximal transverse diameter, and 50% of those with large aneurysms (>6 cm) died of rupture whereas the other half died from underlying diseases, most commonly ischemic heart disease. The risk of rupture is estimated at 1% to 3% per year for aneurysms 4 to 5 cm, 6% to 11% per year for 5- to 7-cm aneurysms, and 20% per year for aneurysms larger than 7 cm. Aneurysms smaller than 4 cm appear to be at a very low risk of rupture. The most powerful factors that increase the risk of rupture are chronic obstructive pulmonary disease and pain. Even vague and uncharacteristic pain has been found to be significantly associated with subsequent rupture. Advanced age, female gender, and renal failure have been linked to an increased risk of rupture.[1-4,8-25,27]

Thoracic Aneurysms

The natural history of thoracic aortic aneurysms is less well defined. Dissecting aneurysms carry a worse prognosis and expand more rapidly than degenerative aneurysms. Ascending and arch aneurysms fare worse than descending aortic aneurysms of either the dissecting or degenerative variety. The expansion rate is 0.42 cm per year for descending thoracic aneurysms and 0.56 cm per year for arch aneurysms. In a population-based study, 95% of patients with dissecting aneurysms and 51% of patients with degenerative aneurysms eventually ruptured.[28] Following rupture, only 11% underwent surgery (with a mortality rate of 43%) for an overall mortality rate of 94%.

Natural history data on thoracoabdominal aneurysms are sparse. The natural history seems to parallel that of thoracic and abdominal aneurysms. In the largest series, 24% of unoperated patients with large thoracoabdominal aneurysms were alive at 2 years and more than 50% died of aneurysm rupture, whereas of those who underwent surgical repair, 59% survived 5 years.[29]

ABDOMINAL AORTIC ANEURYSMS

Clinical Presentation

Most abdominal aortic aneurysms are asymptomatic before rupture. Because no large-scale screening programs for abdominal aortic aneurysm are in place, most aneurysms are discovered on routine physical examination with the palpation of a pulsatile abdominal mass or on imaging while investigating an unrelated problem. Approximately 80% of aneurysms are identified incidentally on abdominal ultrasound, computed tomography (CT), magnetic resonance imaging (MRI), or plain abdominal radiograph.

Aneurysms can be associated with vague abdominal and back discomfort. Occasionally, spinal erosion is the cause of back pain, and large aneurysms may be associated with early satiety and occasionally vomiting. Acutely expanding aneurysms produce severe, deep back pain or abdominal pain radiating to the back. This may be accompanied by tenderness to palpation of the aneurysm. This presentation often precedes rupture and urgent treatment is required. Less than 5% of patients with abdominal aortic aneurysm have evidence of embolization, usually small, to the distal arteries of the lower extremities. As many as 12% of aneurysms present for the first time with acute aneurysm rupture.

About 5% of aneurysms present with nonspecific, idiopathic retroperitoneal inflammation and fibrosis. These aneurysms are referred to as *inflammatory aneurysms*. They are often associated with pain, fever, and fibrosis, which may involve the ureters and cause ureteral obstruction.

Diagnosis

Physical examination is useful for the diagnosis of abdominal aortic aneurysms, especially in thin patients and patients with large aneurysms. An important feature on physical examination is detection of expansile pulsation, where the gap between both hands placed on either side of the aneurysm widens with each systole. This finding separates the aneurysm from normal aortic pulsations, which can be normally palpated in thin subjects, particularly those with lordotic spines, and young women, and whenever a mass overlies the aorta and transmits them.

However, most patients with aneurysms are not thin, and most aneurysms are less than 6 cm. Under these circumstances, physical examination may be unreliable, resulting in 50% false-positive and 50% false-negative results. Extension of an aortic aneurysm into the iliac arteries or the presence of isolated iliac aneurysms cannot be appreciated on physical examination. Large hypogastric aneurysms can sometimes be palpated on rectal examination.

Abdominal aortic aneurysms are occasionally discovered on plain abdominal or on a lumbar spine radiograph by the characteristic "eggshell" pattern of calcification. However, most aneurysms are not sufficiently calcified to be identified on these films, and this is not a reliable method for diagnosis or exclusion.

Abdominal ultrasound is the most widely used noninvasive test for diagnosing and following up abdominal aortic aneurysms. Ultrasound is accurate in demonstrating the presence of an aortic aneurysm and in measuring transverse aneurysmal diameter (Fig. 64-3). Diameter measurements correlate well with dimensions measured on CT scan and at operation. The quality of the examination may be influenced by patient factors such as obesity and bowel gas and by the expertise of the examiner. Because of its low cost, wide availability, and lack of risk, ultrasound is particularly useful for screening and for surveillance of small aneurysms and may prove useful for follow-up after endovascular repair. Duplex ultrasound is inconsistent in visualization of the renal and iliac arteries and is not reliable in demonstrating accessory renal arteries or other anomalies; it is, therefore, less useful as a preoperative planning tool.

CT is the most precise test for imaging aortic aneurysms (Fig. 64-4). CT scanning with a timed intravenous contrast infusion provides good images of the aorta, aortic lumen, branch vessels, and adjacent retroperitoneal structures. Modern spiral CT scanners acquire complete volumetric data and may be reproduced as serial cross sections at specified intervals, as well as a full data set, which can be used for special image processing. The data set can be used for three-dimensional image rendering, which may

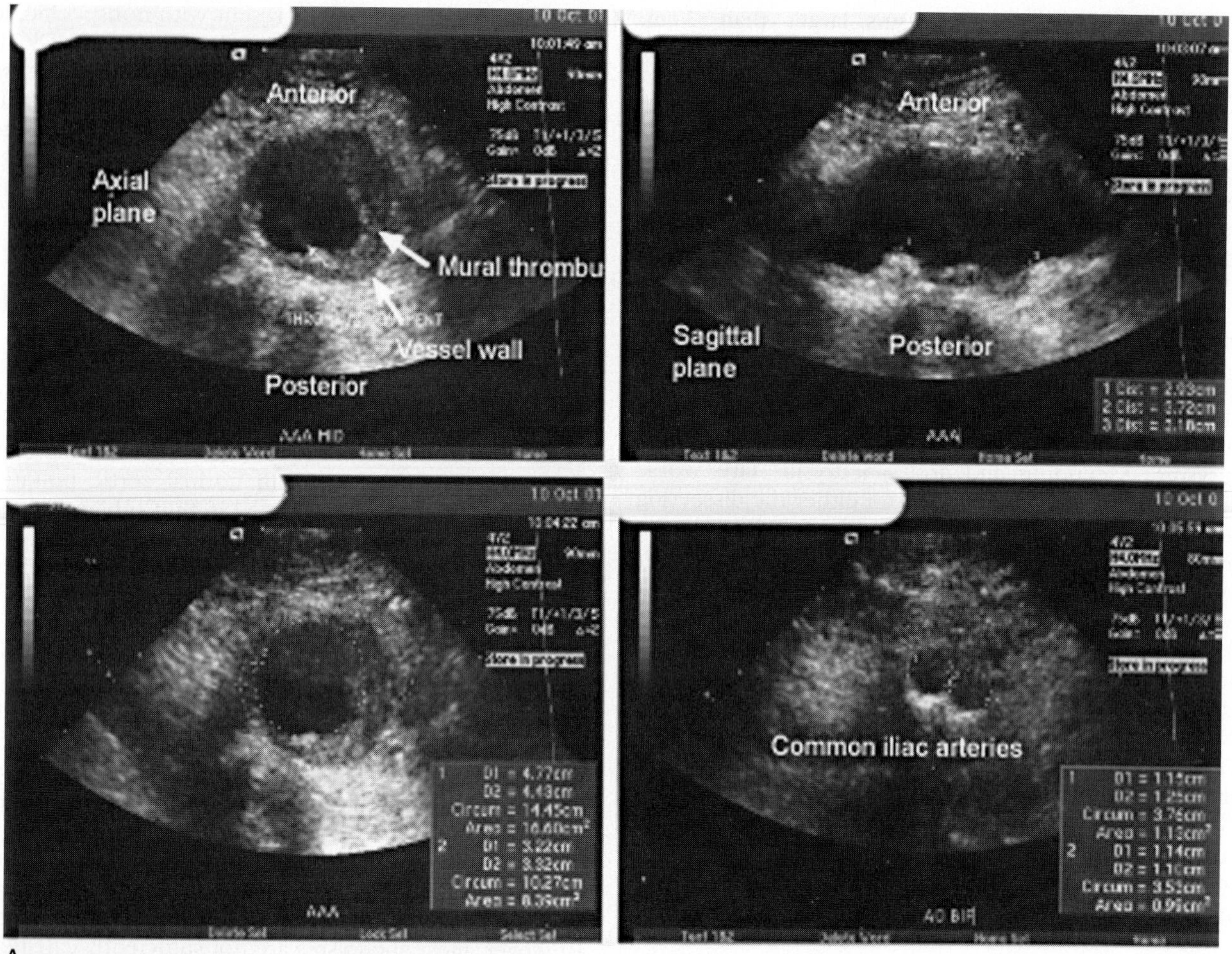

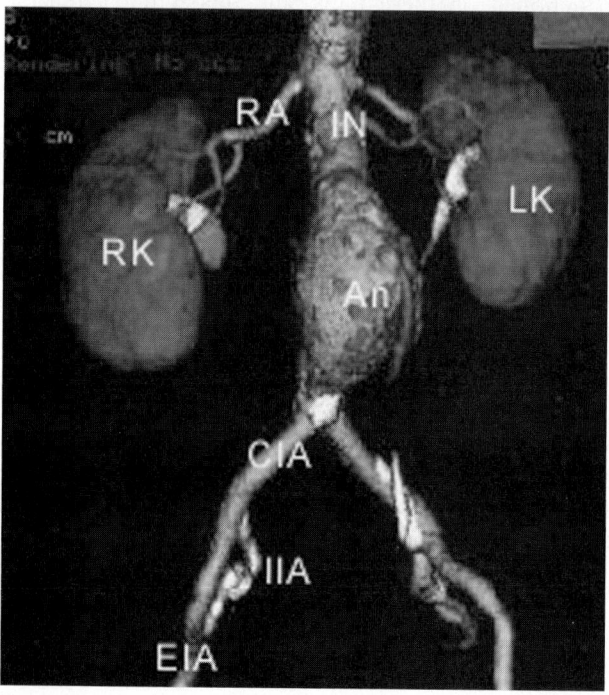

FIGURE 64-3.   A, Ultrasonography demonstrates an abdominal aortic aneurysm. Note the posterior mural thrombus within the aneurysm sac. B, Three-dimensional CT image illustrates the presence of an infrarenal abdominal aortic aneurysm. RK, right kidney; LK, left kidney; RA, renal artery; IN, infrarenal neck; An, aneurysm; CIA, common iliac artery; IIA, internal iliac artery; EIA, external iliac artery.

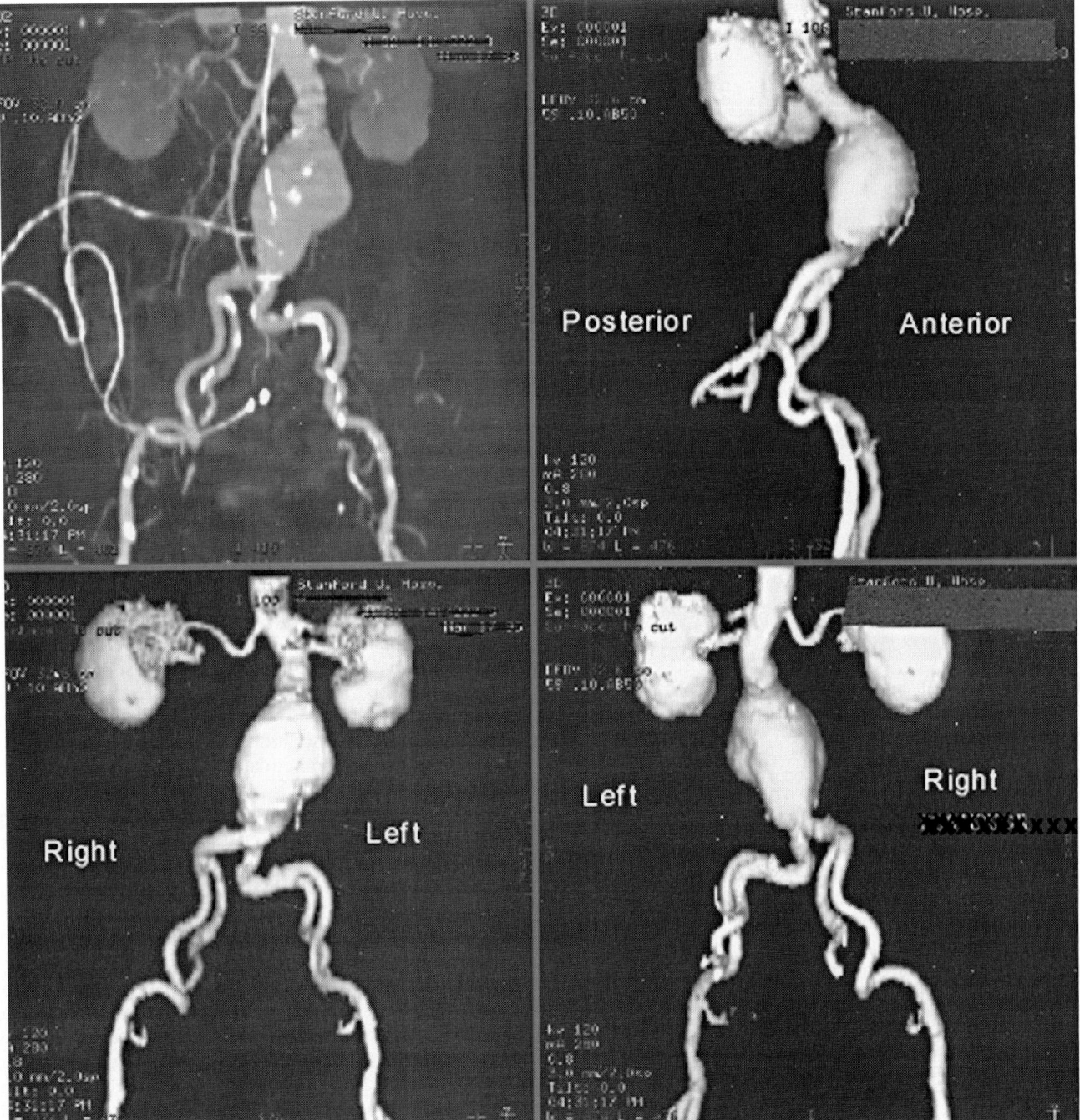

FIGURE 64-4. CT image illustrates an infrarenal abdominal aortic aneurysm from lateral (*top, right*), anterior (*bottom, left*), and posterior (*bottom, right*) views.

be important for understanding the particular arterial anatomy and for planning treatment (Fig. 64-5). CT scanning clearly demonstrates the size and extent of aortic aneurysms and their relation to renal and iliac arteries. Renal artery stenoses, accessory renal arteries, and renal and renal vein anomalies are clearly evident. CT scanning demonstrates the thickened wall typical of inflammatory aneurysms and demonstrates a contained rupture. At this time, CT is the most versatile of the noninvasive tests and has largely replaced arteriography for evaluation of aortic aneurysmal disease.

MRI is the newest of the noninvasive imaging techniques used for evaluation of aortic aneurysmal disease. Technologic advances such as fast acquisition times short enough for suspended respiration and use of intravenous contrast agents (gadolinium chelates) have made it possible to produce high-quality images of the aorta that rival the quality CT scan. MR angiography accurately demonstrates aortoiliac aneurysmal disease and is useful for planning and for follow-up of endovascular repair. It is less sensitive than CT scanning in identifying accessory renal arteries and grading renal artery stenoses.

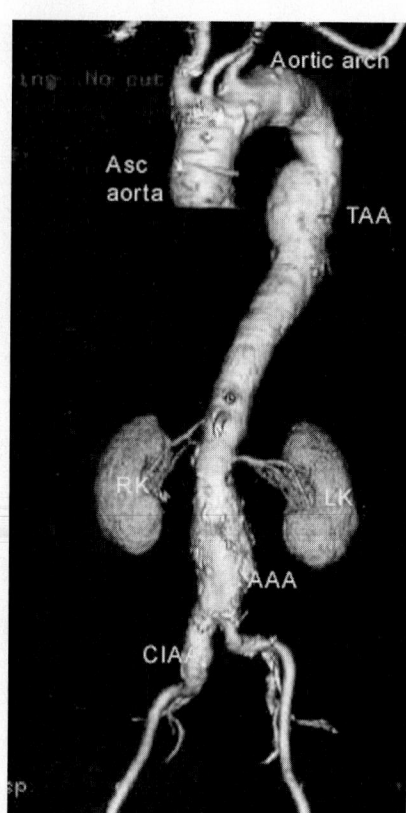

FIGURE 64-5. Three-dimensional CT image showing an aneurysmal aortic wall in the descending thoracic aorta, abdominal aorta, and right common iliac artery. Asc aorta, ascending aorta; TAA, thoracic aortic aneurysm; RK, right kidney; LK, left kidney; CIAA, common iliac artery aneurysm; AAA, abdominal aortic aneurysm.

Arteriography provides reliable information on artery lumen caliber and branch vessel disease. However, because most aneurysms contain a variable amount of thrombus lining the aneurysm wall, assessment of the size of the aneurysm by arteriography is unreliable. Even so, arteriography is widely used in planning treatment strategies, particularly in evaluating the renal arteries, visceral branch vessels, and iliac and femoral arteries. With the availability of high-quality contrast CT scanning that can demonstrate branch vessels, arteriography is beginning to be replaced for preoperative planning. Arteriography is important in the investigation of aortic dissection and, in conjunction with CT, can demonstrate the area of the intimal tear, delineate the true and false lumen, and assist in planning interventional or operative treatment.

Preoperative Evaluation

Patients with aneurysms are most often elderly and frequently have coexisting cardiac, pulmonary, or renal disease, which increases the risk of aneurysm repair. Complete preoperative evaluation and careful patient selection can reduce perioperative risk. With current perioperative management strategies, even individuals with significant comorbidities can undergo endovascular or surgical repair of abdominal aortic aneurysms with very low morbidity

and mortality rates. Especially endovascular repair can be safely performed in very old patients, and repair is not denied on the basis of chronologic age alone.

The most important step in preparing for invasive treatment of aortic disease is the cardiac evaluation. Severe coronary artery disease is present in 50% of patients in whom it is suspected and in 20% of patients without clinical indications of the disease. The presence of uncorrected coronary artery disease raises the risk of death from less than 3% to 5% to 10%, the risk of fatal myocardial infarction to 4.7%, and the risk of nonfatal myocardial infarction to 16%. In comparison, the perioperative mortality rate in patients without coronary artery disease is 1.1% and in those after coronary revascularization is 0.4%.[18]

Because history, physical examination, and electrocardiography (ECG) do not identify all patients at risk, noninvasive tests have been used to identify patients who may benefit from a change in strategy or from coronary revascularization. Exercise ECG testing has been largely superseded by stress or dipyridamole thallium cardiac scintillation scan and the dobutamine echocardiogram. Other tests include measurement of the ejection fraction by echocardiogram or multigated acquisition scan and continuous portable ECG monitoring. These tests are applied to patients at risk, including older patients and those with a history of myocardial infarction, angina pectoris, congestive heart failure, abnormal baseline ECG, and diabetes mellitus. Selection of patients for preoperative cardiac screening may be based on a variety of indices, including the Detsky modified Goldman risk index, Eagle's criteria, and the recommendations of the American Heart Association.

Patients who are found to have significant coronary artery disease may be referred for catheter-based or surgical coronary revascularization before surgical repair of the aneurysm. In addition to decreasing perioperative cardiac morbidity, this approach may decrease the 39% 5-year mortality rate associated with underlying coronary disease in these patients.

Other important risk factors for surgical repair of abdominal aortic aneurysms include chronic obstructive pulmonary disease and impaired renal function. Pulmonary function studies can serve as a rough prognostic guide and should be optimized before surgical intervention. Preoperative renal function is an important determinant of perioperative morbidity and influences the use of contrast agents in diagnostic tests or at the time of endovascular repair.

Selection of Patients for Aneurysm Repair

The selection of patients for aneurysm repair of aortic aneurysms is based on assessments of the risks of rupture and of the procedure. When the maximal diameter reaches 5.5 cm, risk of rupture increases rapidly and aneurysm repair is indicated. Anatomy of the aneurysm, infrarenal aorta, and iliac arteries usually determines the type of reconstruction: open surgical repair or endovascular repair. Patients with significant comorbidities should be treated with endovascular graft. However, if anatomy is unsuitable for endovascular repair in high-risk patients, an open surgical procedure may be considered if the aneurysm is large (>6 to 7 cm). Patients with aneurysms between 4 and 5 cm are candidates for repair if there is evidence of more than a 0.5-cm enlargement over a 6-month period. Patients with evidence of rapid expansion, tenderness in the region of the aneurysm, and back or abdominal pain, which may originate in the aneurysm, should undergo urgent aneurysm repair. Peripheral embolization originating from the aneurysm is an indication for repair, regardless of aneurysm size.

Endovascular repair does introduce morphologic criteria for patient selection in that only aneurysms with a suitable infrarenal neck and iliac arteries can be treated with endovascular stent grafts. Patients requiring additional abdominal or pelvic revascularization procedures, patients with narrow femoral and external iliac access vessels, and patients with a short or tortuous neck and common iliac aneurysms are not candidates for endovascular repair and should undergo open surgical repair.

Operative Technique of Open Surgical Repair

Open surgical repair of abdominal aortic aneurysms is performed through a transperitoneal or retroperitoneal exposure of the aorta under general endotracheal anesthesia. Preoperative preparation to optimize cardiopulmonary function, administration of operative antibiotics, and careful intraoperative hemodynamic monitoring with fluid management and appropriate blood transfusion can significantly reduce the risks of surgery. Patients with cardiac disease should be monitored throughout surgery with a pulmonary artery catheter, cardiac output monitoring, and transesophageal echocardiography. Epidural anesthesia may be combined with general anesthesia to decrease drug dosage intraoperatively, and it may be used for postoperative pain management. Before aortic cross-clamping, volume loading is combined with vasodilation and lost blood may be returned to the patient with an autotransfusion system to prevent declamping hypotension.

The aortic aneurysm may be exposed through a long midline incision for transperitoneal approach, an oblique flank incision for retroperitoneal exposure, or an upper abdominal transverse incision for either transperitoneal or retroperitoneal exposure. Equivalent results can be obtained using each of these approaches. The transabdominal approach is preferred when exposure of the right renal artery is required, when access to intra-abdominal organs is necessary, or when extensive access to the distal right iliac system is required. The retroperitoneal exposure offers advantages when there are extensive peritoneal adhesions, intestinal stomas, underlying pulmonary disease, or the need for suprarenal exposure. The retroperitoneal approach may be associated with a shorter duration of ileus, reduced pulmonary complications, and a shorter stay in the intensive care unit.

When using the transperitoneal approach, the small bowel is mobilized to the right and the posterior peritoneum overlying the aortic aneurysm is divided to the left of the midline (Fig. 64-6). The duodenum is mobilized and the left renal vein is identified and exposed. The nonaneurysmal infrarenal neck, immediately below the left renal vein, is exposed and encircled to obtain proximal control. The common iliac arteries are then mobilized and controlled, taking care to avoid the underlying iliac veins and ureters that cross over the iliac bifurcation. If the common iliac arteries are aneurysmal, control of the internal and external iliac arteries is obtained. The inferior mesenteric artery arising from the anterior aspect of the aneurysm is exposed and controlled for possible reimplantation into the graft after aneurysm repair (Fig. 64-7). The retroperitoneal approach involves a transverse left abdominal or flank incision and reflection of the peritoneal sac anteriorly. The left kidney may be left in place or mobilized anteriorly to expose the posterolateral aspect of the aorta. Exposure of the right iliac system is facilitated by division of the inferior mesenteric artery. Control of the infrarenal aorta and iliac arteries and aneurysm repair are the same regardless of abdominal incision or approach.

After systemic anticoagulation with intravenous heparin, the infrarenal aorta and iliac arteries are cross-clamped. The aneurysm is opened longitudinally; mural thrombus is removed and backbleeding lumbar arteries are oversewn. Depending on its backflow and on patency of hypogastric arteries, the inferior mesenteric artery may be ligated or clamped and left with a rim of aortic wall for subsequent reimplantation. The aneurysm neck is partially or completely transected, and an appropriately sized tubular or bifurcated prosthetic graft is sutured to the normal infrarenal aorta with monofilament, permanent nonabsorbable suture. In the case of juxtarenal aneurysms in which there is a very short or absent neck, suprarenal aortic clamping may be necessary to perform the proximal anastomosis. The distal graft anastomosis is performed to the aortic bifurcation when the aneurysm is confined to the aorta. This is known as *tube graft reconstruction*. Tube grafts are used in 30% to 50% of patients. Patients with iliac aneurysms are reconstructed with bifurcated grafts anastomosed to the distal common iliac arteries or to the common femoral arteries in the case of significant associated external iliac disease. The open aneurysm sac is sutured closed over the aortic graft to separate the graft from the duodenum and viscera, preventing the possibility of late aortoenteric fistula formation.[30]

Endovascular Aortic Aneurysm Repair

Endovascular aneurysm repair differs from open surgical repair in that the prosthetic graft is introduced into the aneurysm through the femoral arteries and fixed in place to the nonaneurysmal infrarenal neck and iliac arteries with self-expanding or balloon-expandable stents rather than sutures (Fig. 64-8). A major abdominal incision is thus avoided, and patient morbidity related to the procedure is much reduced. The first endovascular abdominal aortic aneurysm repair was carried out by Parodi and associates in 1991 using a Dacron graft sutured onto balloon-expandable Palmaz stents.[24] The effectiveness of endovascular repair was demonstrated in the 1990s using a variety of

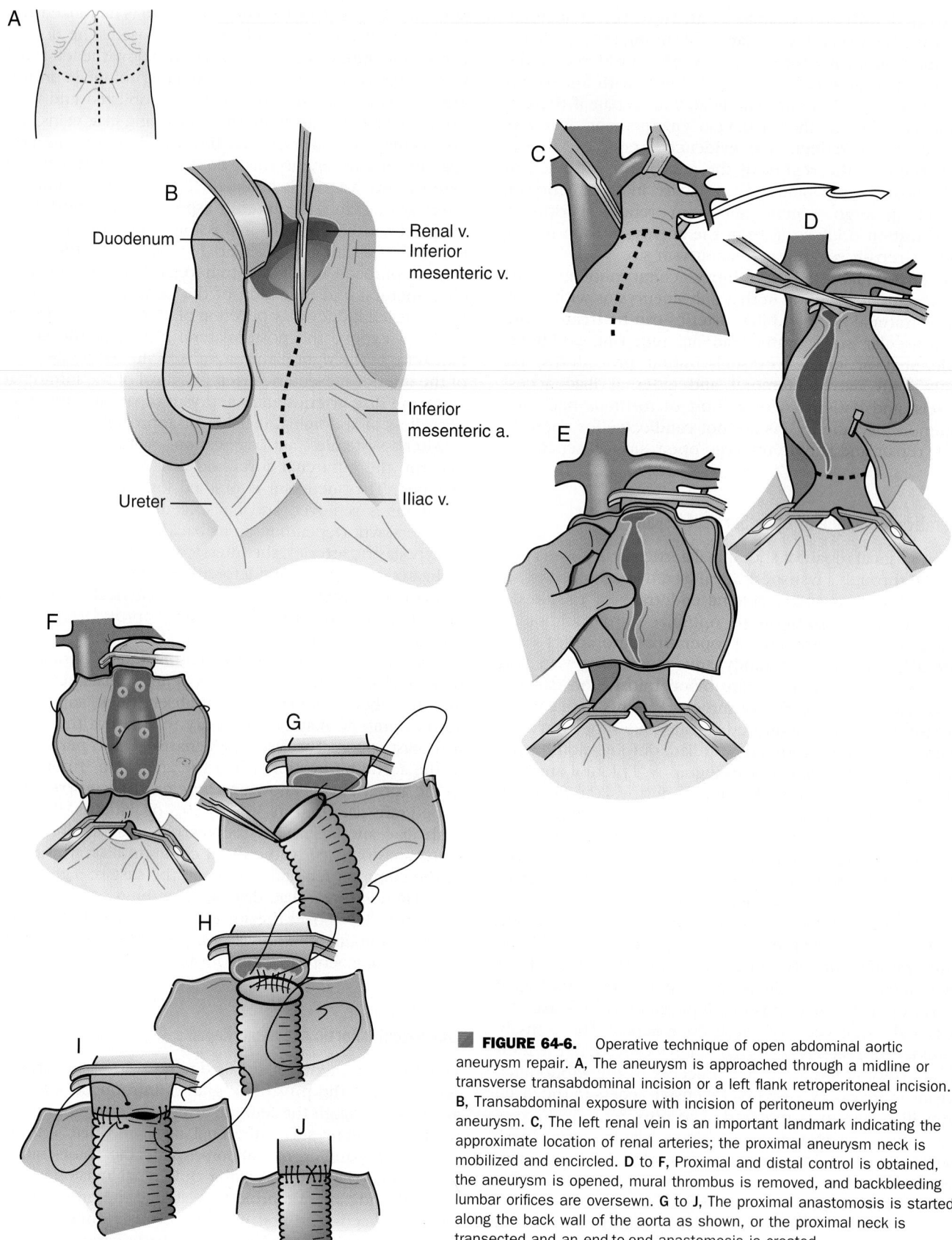

FIGURE 64-6.   Operative technique of open abdominal aortic aneurysm repair. **A,** The aneurysm is approached through a midline or transverse transabdominal incision or a left flank retroperitoneal incision. **B,** Transabdominal exposure with incision of peritoneum overlying aneurysm. **C,** The left renal vein is an important landmark indicating the approximate location of renal arteries; the proximal aneurysm neck is mobilized and encircled. **D to F,** Proximal and distal control is obtained, the aneurysm is opened, mural thrombus is removed, and backbleeding lumbar orifices are oversewn. **G to J,** The proximal anastomosis is started along the back wall of the aorta as shown, or the proximal neck is transected and an end-to-end anastomosis is created.

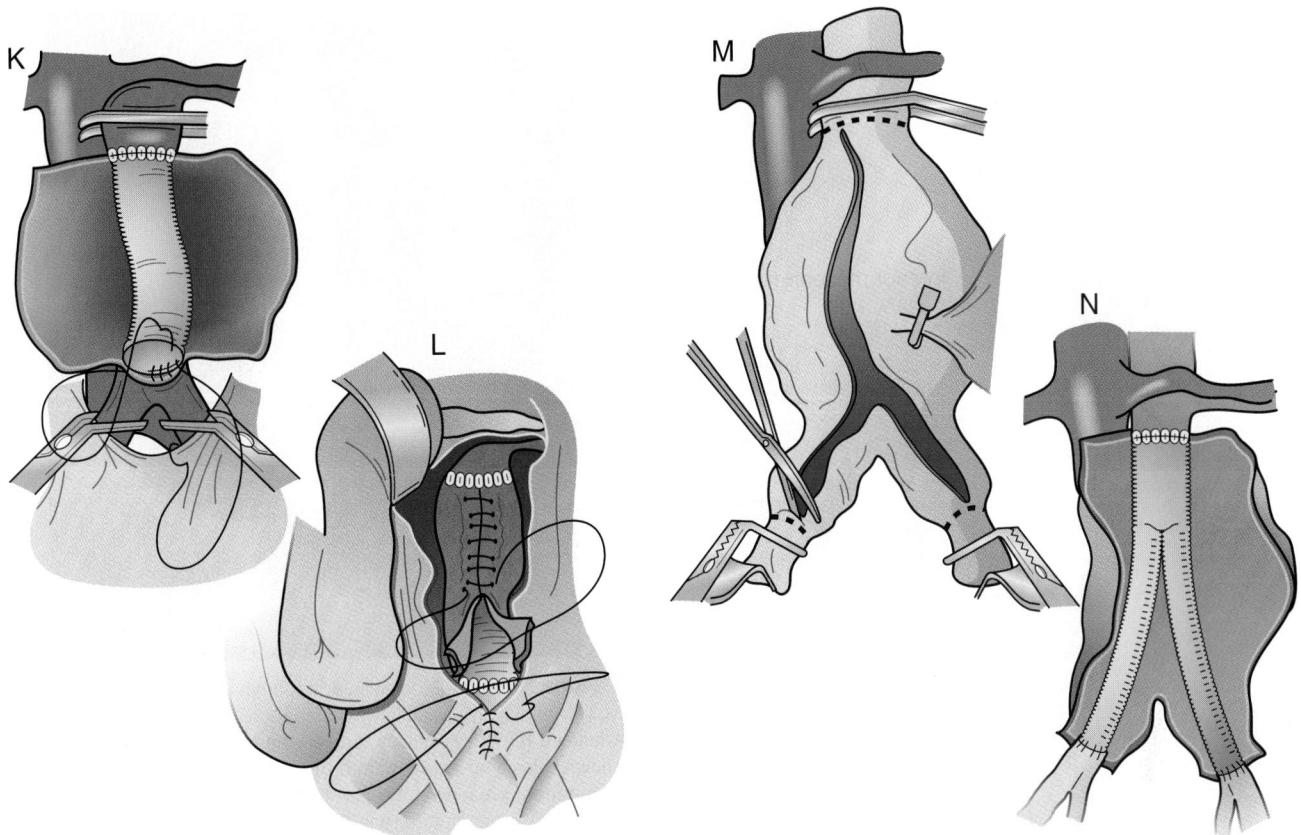

FIGURE 64-6.—Cont'd. **K,** The distal anastomosis is constructed in a similar fashion; if backbleeding from the inferior mesenteric artery (IMA) is pulsatile and the hypogastric arteries are patent, the IMA may be oversewn. **L,** The aneurysm sac is sewn over the tube graft, thereby completing the repair. **M** and **N,** If the iliac arteries are aneurysmal, a bifurcated prosthetic graft is used.

homemade devices. A number of commercially manufactured stent grafts have since been developed. Early tubular grafts have been replaced by modular bifurcated grafts that have expanded the applicability of this therapy. Clinical trials comparing endovascular repair to open surgical repair are underway with favorable short-term results. Presently, there are three FDA-approved endovascular devices for infrarenal abdominal aortic aneurysm (Medtronic, AneuRx; Gore, Excluder; Cook, Zenith) in the United States, and approval of additional devices is anticipated soon.

The technical details of endovascular repair vary with each specific device, but the general principles are similar. In most cases, a self-expanding stent graft is inserted into the aorta by way of the femoral arteries. Presently, the insertion requires surgical exposure of another or both common femoral arteries. The arteries are cannulated and guide wires are inserted into the aorta. Most stent grafts are made of two pieces: (1) a main module, including the body, and (2) one of the limbs with a gate for the separate contralateral limb. The appropriately sized primary module is inserted under fluoroscopic guidance and deployed just below the renal arteries. The opening in the bifurcated module for the contralateral limb is cannulated by way of the other femoral artery, and the contralateral limb is deployed to create a bifurcated stent graft that

excludes the aneurysm from the circulation. Technical success rate is 99% to 100%.[31-37]

Candidates for this procedure include patients with a proximal infrarenal neck at least 1.5 to 2 cm in length and common iliac arteries for proximal and distal fixation of an endograft, without excessive tortuosity and with appropriate iliofemoral access. The benefits of this procedure are decreased blood loss, quicker recovery, and lesser morbidity with shorter stay in the hospital, and it may be applicable to high-risk patients,[31,34-36] so mid-term recovery (3 months after surgery) has been found to be significantly better after endovascular repair compared to open surgical repair.[31] There are few studies with long-term follow-up, up to 5-years, comparing endovascular and surgical procedures. Long-term survival after endovascular aneurysm repair has been comparable to that with open repair.[32,33,38,39]

RUPTURED ABDOMINAL AORTIC ANEURYSM

The most dreaded complication of abdominal aortic aneurysms is aneurysm rupture. Aneurysms can rupture freely into the peritoneal cavity or into the retroperitoneum. Free intraperitoneal rupture is usually an anterior rupture and is usually accompanied by immediate hemo-

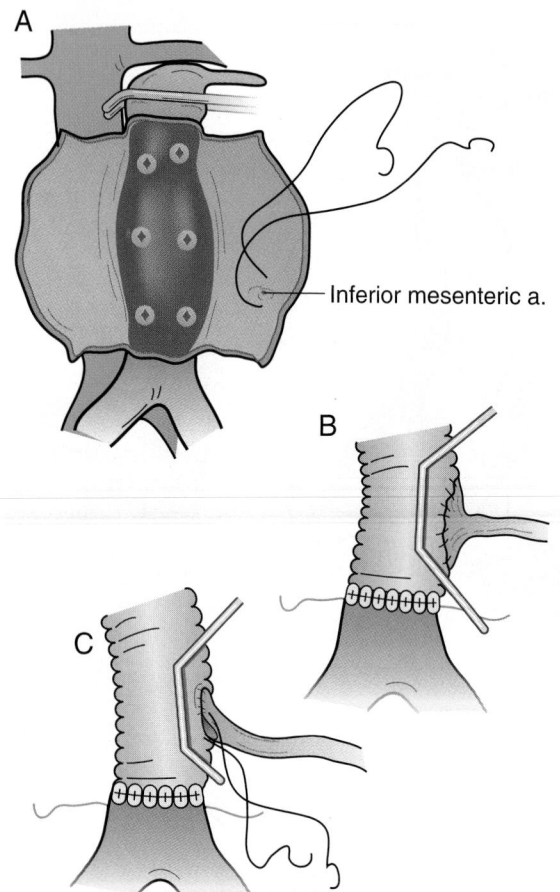

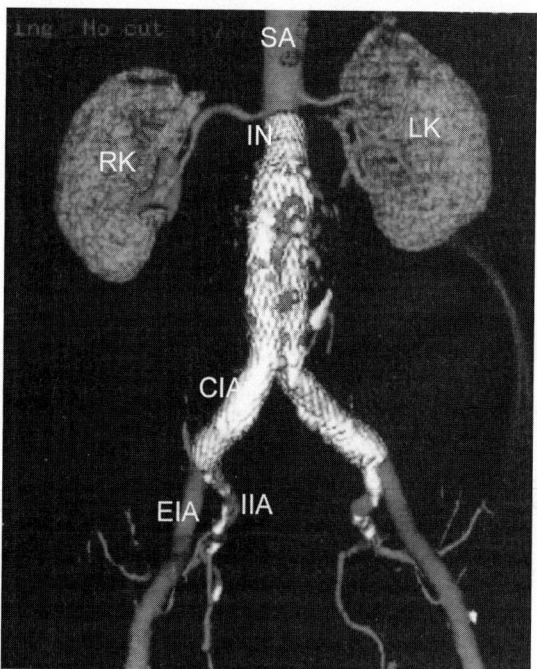

FIGURE 64-8. Endovascular abdominal aortic aneurysm repair involves aneurysm exclusion with an endoluminal aortic stent-graft introduced remotely, usually through the femoral artery. An endovascular graft extends from the infrarenal aorta to both common iliac arteries, preserving the flow to the internal iliac arteries. SA, suprarenal aorta; IN, infrarenal aortic neck; CIA, common iliac artery; IIA, internal iliac artery; RK, right kidney; LK, left kidney.

FIGURE 64-7. A to C, The inferior mesenteric artery (IMA) is reimplanted into the side of the aortic graft with a button of surrounding aorta or reconstructed with an interposition autologous vein, artery, or prosthetic graft. Reimplantation is particularly important if the IMA is large (>3 mm in diameter), if collateral blood flow is compromised (hypogastric artery occluded or oversewn), or if backbleeding from the artery is poor.

dynamic collapse and a very high mortality rate. Retroperitoneal ruptures are usually posterior and may be contained by the psoas muscle and adjacent periaortic and perivertebral tissue. This type of rupture may occur without significant blood loss initially, and the patient may be hemodynamically stable. Both types of rupture present with acute excruciating back and abdominal pain, accompanied by pallor, diaphoresis, syncope, and other symptoms and signs related to blood loss and hypovolemic shock. Occasionally, patients may have chest pain induced by retroperitoneal blood loss or hypovolemia, misleading the physician to suspect primary myocardial ischemia. Rarely, an aortic aneurysm may rupture into the inferior vena cava to produce an acute massive arteriovenous fistula or into the duodenum with upper gastrointestinal bleeding. In all its variations, rupture of the aorta, unless corrected, is fatal.

Patients with ruptured aortic aneurysms require immediate surgical repair. If the patient is unstable and an abdominal aortic aneurysm has been previously diagnosed or a pulsatile abdominal mass is present, no further eval-

uation is performed and the patient is transferred to the operating room without additional tests. Stable patients with a questionable diagnosis may undergo CT scanning, which can confirm the presence of an aneurysm as well as demonstrate its extent, the site of rupture, and the degree of iliac involvement. In patients not stable enough to undergo CT scanning, the presence of an aneurysm can be confirmed by bedside ultrasound. This does not demonstrate aortic rupture but does confirm the presence of an aortic aneurysm. Acutely expanding aneurysms may present with abdominal pain and tenderness on palpation. These are prone to rupture and should be repaired on an emergent basis.

Surgical repair of ruptured aneurysms is most commonly undertaken transperitoneally. In cases of contained rupture, supraceliac control should be achieved before infrarenal dissection and, once the aneurysm neck is dissected, the aortic clamp can be moved to the infrarenal level. In cases of free rupture, an attempt at obtaining control may include compression of the aorta at the hiatus and infrarenal control with a clamp or an intraluminal balloon. Heparin is not usually given in these cases. Once proximal and distal control is achieved, the operation is conducted in a manner similar to elective aneurysm repair.

Results after open repair of ruptured aneurysm vary. For patients in stable condition with a contained rupture, the mortality rate is less than 50%. For patients with free intraperitoneal rupture who arrive in shock with possible cardiac arrest, the outlook is grim and mortality rates exceed 90%.[17] Most patients do not die on the operating table; rather, they succumb to the sequelae of shock and resuscitation with progressive multiorgan dysfunction that occurs in the intensive care unit.

Ruptured abdominal aortic aneurysm is thought to be less suitable for endovascular repair, because it needs preoperative measurements of the aneurysm and adjacent arterial anatomy to determine the appropriate size and type of graft and also because of the inherent delay to obtain proximal occlusion. Veith and Ohki reported the results of 25 endovascular repairs of ruptured abdominal aortic aneurysms.[40] Patients were treated with restricted fluid resuscitation (hypotensive hemostasis), rapid transportation to operating room, placement of transbrachial or transfemoral guide wire under local anesthesia, and urgent arteriography. In this small series, total operative mortality was 9.7%. Also, high-risk patients were treated successfully. Operative mortality rates after endovascular repair of ruptured abdominal aortic aneurysm vary from 10% to 45%.[40-42] The number of studies and patients is low so far, and the final role of endovascular treatment in ruptured abdominal aortic aneurysms will be seen in the future.

RESULTS AND COMPLICATIONS OF AORTIC ANEURYSM REPAIR

The perioperative mortality rate for elective surgery for abdominal aortic aneurysms was 14% to 19% in the 1960s. The mortality rate for open aneurysm repair has been greatly reduced by improvements in preoperative evaluation and perioperative care, and published series report a mortality rate of 0 to 5% in leading centers.[43] The overall population-wide mortality rate for open aneurysm repair is estimated to be higher, in the range of 5% to 10%. Mortality rates following repair of inflammatory aneurysms and emergent repair for symptomatic, nonruptured aneurysms remain higher at 5% to 10%, primarily as a result of less thorough preoperative evaluation. The current perioperative mortality rate for thoracoabdominal aortic aneurysm repair is 8.5% to 15%. Mortality rate after endovascular repair of abdominal aortic aneurysms is 1% to 3%, not different from open surgical repair of selected patients.

The overall morbidity rate after elective aneurysm repair is 10% to 30%. The most frequent complication is myocardial ischemia, which occurs in 3% to 16% (mean 7%) of cases, usually within the first 2 days after surgery. Myocardial infarction is also the most common cause of postoperative death.[15] Mild renal failure is the second most frequent complication and occurs following 6% of elective open aneurysm repairs. It is more frequent with preexisting renal disease and may occur as a result of hypoperfusion, contrast administration, and, occasionally, atheroembolism. Severe renal failure requiring dialysis is rare. The third most common group of complications is pulmonary, and the postoperative pneumonia rate is approximately 5%. However, with proper patient selection and care, pulmonary failure as the principal cause of death is rare.

Postoperative bleeding may occur occasionally and may be related to the anastomotic suture lines, to inadequately recognized venous injuries, and to coagulopathy that may result from intraoperative hypothermia or excessive blood loss. Evidence of ongoing postoperative bleeding should lead to early re-exploration. Lower limb ischemia may occur secondary to emboli or thrombosis of the graft and may require reoperation and thrombectomy. Occasionally, microemboli propagated to the distal circulation result in a "trash foot," which manifests with pain, muscle tenderness, and patchy skin changes without loss of the peripheral pulse.

Postoperative paralytic ileus may last for 3 to 4 days, but occasionally duodenal or small bowel obstruction persists longer. Colon ischemia occurs after 1% of aneurysm repairs and presents with bloody diarrhea, abdominal pain, and distention and leukocytosis with findings of mucosal sloughing on sigmoidoscopy. In case of transmural colonic necrosis, colon resection and exteriorization of stomas are warranted. Mortality rate in patients with colon ischemia is 50% and increases to 90% when full-thickness gangrene and peritonitis have developed.

Paraplegia is rare after infrarenal aortic aneurysm repair, with an incidence of 0.2%. Most of the cases occur after repair of ruptured aneurysms or when the pelvis has been devascularized. Approximately 50% of patients recover some neurologic function.

Postoperative sexual dysfunction is frequent and may manifest with impotence, which may be psychogenic, neurologic, or related to hypogastric artery perfusion, or with retrograde ejaculation, which is related to nerve injury in the vicinity of the left common iliac artery.

Late complications are rare but may include pseudoaneurysms at the proximal or distal suture lines, graft or graft limb thrombosis, and graft infection, which may become manifest months to years after aneurysm repair. It may be associated with graft enteric fistula and is notoriously difficult to diagnose and treat.

Long-term survival rate following successful aortic aneurysm repair is less than that in the general population, primarily because of associated coronary artery disease. Late deaths are generally due to cardiac causes. Five-year survival rate after repair of abdominal aortic aneurysms is 67% with a range of 49% to 84% compared with a rate of 80% to 85% in age-matched control subjects. The mean duration of survival has been reported to be 7.4 years after aortic aneurysm repair.

Endovascular aneurysm repair is associated with a unique set of complications. Incomplete exclusion of the aneurysm sac with continued perfusion is referred to as *endoleak* and occurs in 9% to 44% of cases. There are several types of endoleaks. Endoleaks related to the endovascular stent graft or its attachment sites (type I) may be associated with continued aneurysm expansion and risk of rupture. Such endoleaks can often be fixed by endovascular methods. Other complications include graft migration and stent-graft occlusion. Migration can cause graft kinking and occlusion and endoleaks and lead to conversion to open aneurysm repair. In early devices migration was more common, but in development of new devices, attention has been paid to stability. In current devices, 1-year migration rates have varied between 0 and 4% during the first 2 years after endografting.[33,34,44] Endograft limb occlusion usually presents with acute, severe ischemic symptoms. Cumulative risk for limb occlusion is about 4% at 2 years after the procedure.[44] Postoperative persistent renal impairment has occurred in 9% after endovascular repair, and preoperative renal dysfunction has been found to be the only predictive factor for that.[45] Conversion to open repair has to be done sometimes during or immediately after endovascular repair (primary conversion) owing to access problems or improper graft position, and the rate has varied between 0 and 3.8%.[33,46] Late conversion rates vary from 1.5% to 4% during 2-year follow-up and the most common reasons have been endoleaks.[47-49] Late aneurysm ruptures are rare and are associated with types I and III endoleaks.[46] Kaplan-Meier estimates for the freedom from all-cause rupture has been 99.5% at 1 year, 98.5% at 2 years, and 98.4% at 3 and 4 years.[37]

Iliac Aneurysms

Iliac aneurysms occur in conjunction with aortic aneurysms in 40% of patients. Isolated iliac aneurysms are uncommon (<2% of aortoiliac aneurysms) and affect the common iliac or the hypogastric arteries (Figs. 64-9 and 64-10). Most of these aneurysms are atherosclerotic in origin. Because of their location, they are not easily palpable and are not readily identified on ultrasound. Consequently, most go undetected and as many as 50% present with rupture. Iliac aneurysm rupture is associated with a 50% to 60% mortality rate. Elective repair of iliac artery aneurysm prevents aneurysm rupture.

COMPLICATING FEATURES OF ANEURYSM REPAIR

Occasionally, repair of abdominal aneurysms is complicated by a concurrent disease process. Successful treatment requires careful evaluation and a correct decision whether to treat the two entities sequentially or concurrently. The most common disease entities that coexist with aortic aneurysms include hepatobiliary, pancreatic, gastrointestinal, gynecologic, and genitourinary disorders and structural abnormalities of the abdominal wall. As a

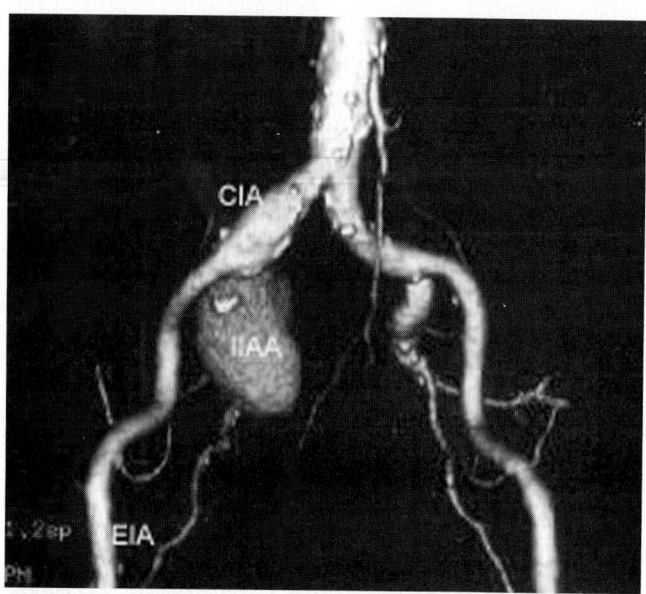

FIGURE 64-9. Three-dimensional CT image from a right internal iliac artery aneurysm of 6.4 cm in diameter. CIA, common iliac artery; IIAA, internal iliac artery aneurysm; EIA, external iliac artery aneurysm.

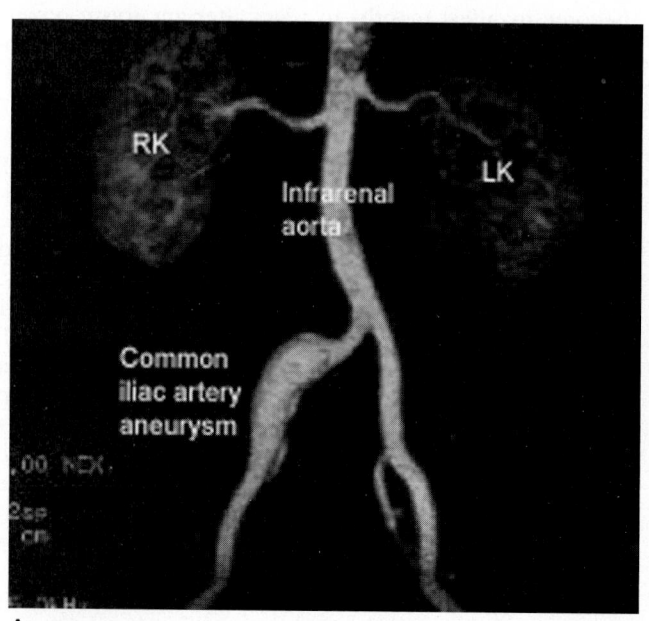

A

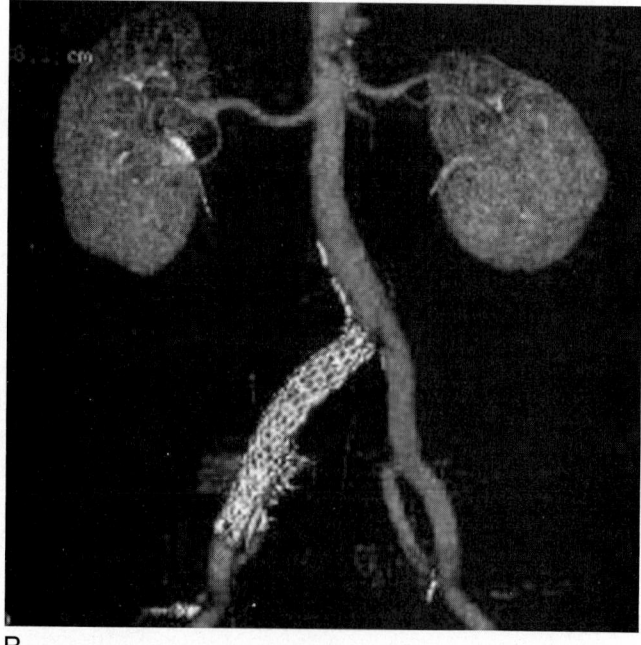

B

FIGURE 64-10. A, Three-dimensional CT image illustrates a fusiformal aneurysm in the right common iliac artery. B, Aneurysm is treated with an endovascular graft, which excludes the aneurysm from circulation. RK, right kidney; LK, kidney.

rule, the most life-threatening process is treated first, and if both processes are symptomatic, they both should be treated concomitantly.

The following principles are applicable when managing patients with aortic aneurysms and concurrent diseases:

1. Preoperative diagnostic work-up usually delineates unusual anatomic variants and concomitant diseases
2. In emergency situations such as a ruptured or symptomatic aneurysm when preoperative images (CT scan) are unavailable, the aneurysm always takes priority unless the other condition is life threatening and the aneurysm is clearly not the cause of the patient's symptoms
3. A retroperitoneal approach to the abdominal aorta can avoid concomitant intraperitoneal conditions, including adhesions and scarring from previous operations
4. Endovascular aneurysm repair can avoid concomitant intra-abdominal problems, but it will not resolve intestinal obstruction or other life-threatening conditions

Anatomic variants that may be encountered during repair of abdominal aneurysms include horseshoe kidney, accessory renal arteries, and venous anomalies.

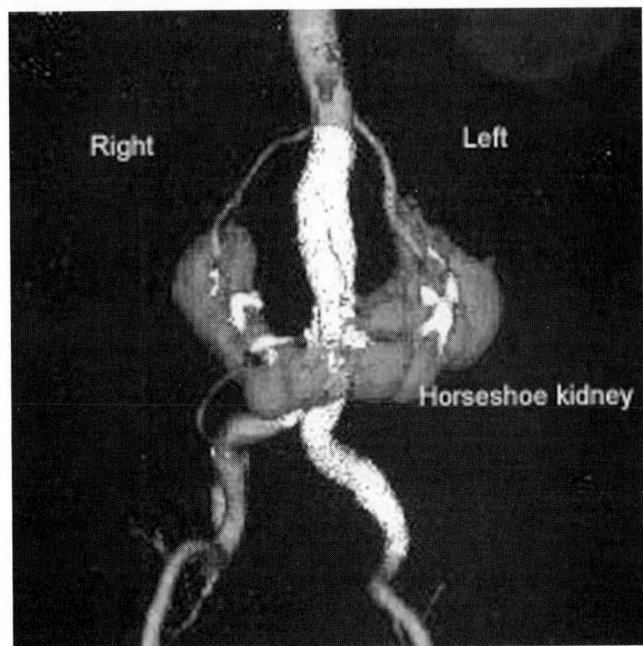

FIGURE 64-11. Three-dimensional CT image showing a horseshoe kidney and an abdominal aortic aneurysm treated with an endovascular graft.

Horseshoe Kidney

Less than 0.3% of the general population have horseshoe kidneys. Papin's autopsy study of 139 horseshoe kidneys served as the basis for a classification system consisting of three groups[23]: Group 1 kidneys have normal renal arteries and account for 20% of all horseshoe kidneys; group 2 kidneys have three to five renal arteries and account for 66% of cases; and group 3 kidneys have more than five renal arteries and account for 14%. To preserve renal function, renal arteries arising from the aneurysm should be reimplanted. Horseshoe kidneys with more than five renal arteries often have multiple small accessory arteries, some of which originate from the aneurysm or the iliac arteries, or both. In this situation, repair of the aneurysm with preservation of renal function may be difficult or even impossible. Creatinine clearance should be determined preoperatively for evaluation of renal function. To help prevent significant renal tubular damage, furosemide and mannitol may be administered before renal ischemia, and renal arteries should be reimplanted quickly after aortic reconstruction.

Endovascular repair can be performed in the normal way to these patients (Fig. 64-11). However, if the patient is unsuitable for endovascular repair, the presence of a horseshoe kidney may complicate but does not preclude an anterior approach for repairing an infrarenal aortic aneurysm.[49] The left retroperitoneal approach, however, is preferable and can provide excellent exposure of the infrarenal aorta in these patients. This approach requires that the surgeon dissect the space between the aneurysm and the left portion and isthmus of the kidney. The entire kidney can then be reflected to the right and the aneurysm thereby fully exposed. The left ureter crosses the iliac arteries from the right with the kidney in this position,

and duplication of ureters may be present. The surgeon must carefully mobilize the ureters and renal arteries. Damage to the ureters, renal pelvis, or calices can cause urinary leak in the region of the vascular reconstruction, a complication that must be avoided. If a urinary leak is detected during the course of operation, the source must be identified and repaired with absorbable suture.

Accessory Renal Arteries

Accessory renal arteries are present in 20% to 40% of patients. They are important considerations when planning aortic reconstructions. If a portion of one kidney is devascularized, glomerular filtration rate decreases and renal insufficiency or hyper-reninemia with associated hypertension may occur. Accessory renal arteries can be detected by duplex ultrasound, CT scanning, MR angiography, and conventional invasive angiography. The decision to use one imaging modality over another may depend on the imaging resources that are available and on which modality is best for evaluating additional features. For instance, a patient with a known abdominal aortic aneurysm and aortoiliac artery occlusive disease who is noted to have an accessory renal artery on duplex ultrasonography might best be evaluated by conventional angiography in one institution, whereas at another institution, CT scanning or MR angiography might be sufficient.

Accessory renal arteries should be preserved when possible during aortic reconstruction. This can usually be achieved by either incorporating the artery into a beveled proximal graft anastomosis, by reimplanting the artery onto the aortic graft distal to the proximal anastomosis, or by placing an interposition graft between the aortic graft and the accessory renal artery.

Venous Anomalies

The surgeon must be aware of anatomic variations and abnormalities. Left-sided vena cava and retroaortic left renal vein are the most common anomalies. Trigaux and colleagues[50] reviewed more than 1000 abdominal spiral CT scans and detected left renal vein variants in 10% of patients (4% were retroaortic left renal veins and 6% were circumaortic venous rings). Azygous continuation of the inferior vena cava was seen in one patient (0.1%) and bilateral inferior vena cava was detected in three patients (0.3%). Preoperative CT scanning and angiographic imaging may reveal these variants; however, the surgeon can avoid unnecessary bleeding without prior knowledge by adhering to the principles of careful dissection and meticulous technique.

Inflammatory Aneurysms

Inflammatory aneurysms represent approximately 5% of all infrarenal abdominal aortic aneurysms.[11] They typically have a dense fibroinflammatory rind that is usually adherent to the fourth portion of the duodenum and often involves the inferior vena cava and left renal vein. One or more ureters may also be involved.

The etiology of the inflammatory tissue is not clearly understood. One theory is that lymphatic obstruction occurs during aneurysm expansion, producing stasis, edema, and secondary fibrosis.[24] Other possible etiologies include inflammation as a result of remodeling within the aortic wall during aneurysm expansion, autoimmune disorder, infection, and reaction from chronic, contained aortic rupture.

Patients with inflammatory aneurysms frequently are seen with abdominal or flank pain; they often have associated weight loss, and erythrocyte sedimentation rate is elevated in 75% of cases. Rupture of inflammatory aneurysms is unusual. This is likely because most inflammatory aneurysms are symptomatic and are treated before rupture. Whether the inflammatory process provides a protective effect is not known.

Diagnosis is best made by CT scanning. Timed contrast injection for CT angiography provides the highest resolution images. Typically, four separate layers are identified, including the aortic lumen, mural thrombus, thickened aortic wall, and periaortic inflammatory tissue.

Repair of these aneurysms can be challenging from a technical standpoint because of the involvement of adjacent structures. A retroperitoneal approach to repairing inflammatory aneurysms has been advocated.

Associated Abdominal Malignancy

As previously stated, when an abdominal malignancy or other intra-abdominal process coexists with a symptomatic or ruptured aortic aneurysm, treatment of the aneurysm must take priority if the immediate survival of the patient is to be ensured.

Liver tumors that coexist with aortic aneurysms should be treated on an independent basis, and judgment regarding treatment must be guided by the relative risk of the two diseases. Incidental discovery of a liver mass at the time of elective abdominal aneurysm repair should be documented and the planned aneurysm repair should be carried out. After retroperitonealizing the graft, the liver mass may be biopsied, at the discretion of the surgeon, and small liver tumors may be resected as long as blood loss does not complicate the aneurysm repair.

When a colonic neoplasm coexists with abdominal aortic aneurysm, the most life-threatening problem should be treated first. An obstructing, bleeding, or perforated colon cancer should be resected before electively repairing a stable, asymptomatic 4.5-cm aneurysm, and a symptomatic or ruptured aneurysm should be treated before an elective colon resection is undertaken. When both entities are asymptomatic, treatment generally should be based on the size of the aneurysm. If large (≥5 cm in diameter), the aneurysm should be repaired initially, and, if small, the colonic lesion should be resected first. If a symptomatic or ruptured aneurysm and an obstructing colon cancer are encountered concurrently, one acceptable treatment strategy would be aneurysm repair and externalization of a colonic loop proximal to the tumor at the same operation, gastrointestinal nasogastric tube decompression, and colostomy maturation the next day to avoid vascular graft contamination.

Concurrent renal or bladder neoplasm and abdominal aortic aneurysm deserve independent assessment and treatment by their respective specialists. The most life-threatening entity should be treated first. Partial, total, or radical nephrectomy may be indicated in cases of renal malignancy, and the vascular surgeon should involve urologic and oncologic colleagues preoperatively to facilitate a multidisciplinary approach to treatment. When an incidental renal mass is encountered during repair of a symptomatic or ruptured abdominal aortic aneurysm, the aneurysm should be repaired and the renal mass addressed on its own merits as soon as the patient has recovered.

Incidental ovarian cysts and tumors are occasionally encountered during abdominal aortic aneurysm surgery. Simple ovarian cysts can be safely excised; however, women with abdominal aortic aneurysm are almost always postmenopausal or have had hysterectomy, and the lifetime risk of development of ovarian cancer is approximately 1.8%. Bilateral oophorectomy is justified if a solid ovarian abnormality is encountered, and staging of the tumor should include peritoneal washings for cytologic testing and biopsy of periaortic lymph nodes, omentum, and undersurface of the diaphragm. Positive findings may be an indication for postoperative chemotherapy. Hysterectomy is indicated in cases of solid ovarian tumors, but this should not be performed in conjunction with aneurysm repair because of the increased risk of graft contamination and additional blood loss. Uterine tumors found incidentally at the time of abdominal aortic aneurysm repair should be documented and treated later. Tubulo-ovarian abscess and pelvic inflammatory disease are rare in the aortic aneurysm population; however, these disorders may cause symptoms and should be treated before elective repair of abdominal aortic aneurysm.

Other neoplasms that may be encountered during evaluation or treatment of abdominal aortic aneurysm include lymphoma, adrenal neurogenic lesions, soft tissue tumors, metastatic lesions, and small bowel neoplasms. Small tumors can be excised and diagnosis of larger tumors can be made by true-cut or incisional biopsy with later definitive treatment as indicated.

THORACIC AORTIC ANEURYSMS

Aortic aneurysms isolated to the thoracic aorta are becoming increasingly prevalent as the population ages. Slightly less common than abdominal aortic aneurysms, thoracic aortic aneurysms may involve the ascending, arch, or descending thoracic aorta, or a combination of these segments (Fig. 64-12). Thoracic aortic aneurysms are classified as being atherosclerotic or degenerative. Atherosclerotic aneurysms result from aortic wall remodeling and dilation, whereas degenerative aneurysms result from abnormal collagen metabolism. The two main degenerative types seen are associated with Marfan syndrome and Ehlers-Danlos syndrome. Marfan syndrome is an autosomal dominant disorder with variable penetrance. It has been found to be associated with an abnormal synthesis of fibrillin, a major constituent of microfibrils, and a defective gene on the long arm of chromosome 15.

The rupture rate in unoperated patients with thoracic aortic aneurysm has been 40% to 70%. Most of the other deaths are related to cardiovascular disease. Mortality of

the ruptured thoracic aortic aneurysm is almost 100%. Most patients die before reaching the operating room. Results of elective open thoracic aortic aneurysm repair are influenced by surgeons or team case load volume and patient selection. Published series are often selected single institutional reports, which have lower mortality than unselected multicenter series. Mortality rates of open elective aneurysm repair vary between 10% and 20%, and the mortality rate of emergency operation for ruptured aneurysm is about 50%.[22,25]

Most thoracic aneurysms are discovered incidentally during evaluation for other medical problems. Most frequently, calcium in the aneurysm wall is detected on a plain chest radiograph. CT angiography can be used to measure aneurysm dimensions and to determine the aneurysm location relative to the arch vessels and celiac axis. The presence and extent of aortic dissection and mural thrombus can be evaluated. MR angiography is also available at many hospitals, and three-dimensional reconstruction of both CT and MR data can provide additional information about tortuosity and angulation of the aorta, which is especially important when planning endovascular repair. Conventional angiography is sometimes needed to define arch vessel disease and can best delineate intercostal arteries and the relationship between the true and false lumen of aortic dissection if CT findings are unclear.

The goal of thoracic aortic aneurysm repair is to prevent death from rupture. Open repair of these aneurysms carries a higher risk of significant complications than does open repair of abdominal aortic aneurysm. Because most patients have associated comorbidities, including chronic obstructive pulmonary disease and coronary artery disease, elective repair of thoracic aortic aneurysm should involve

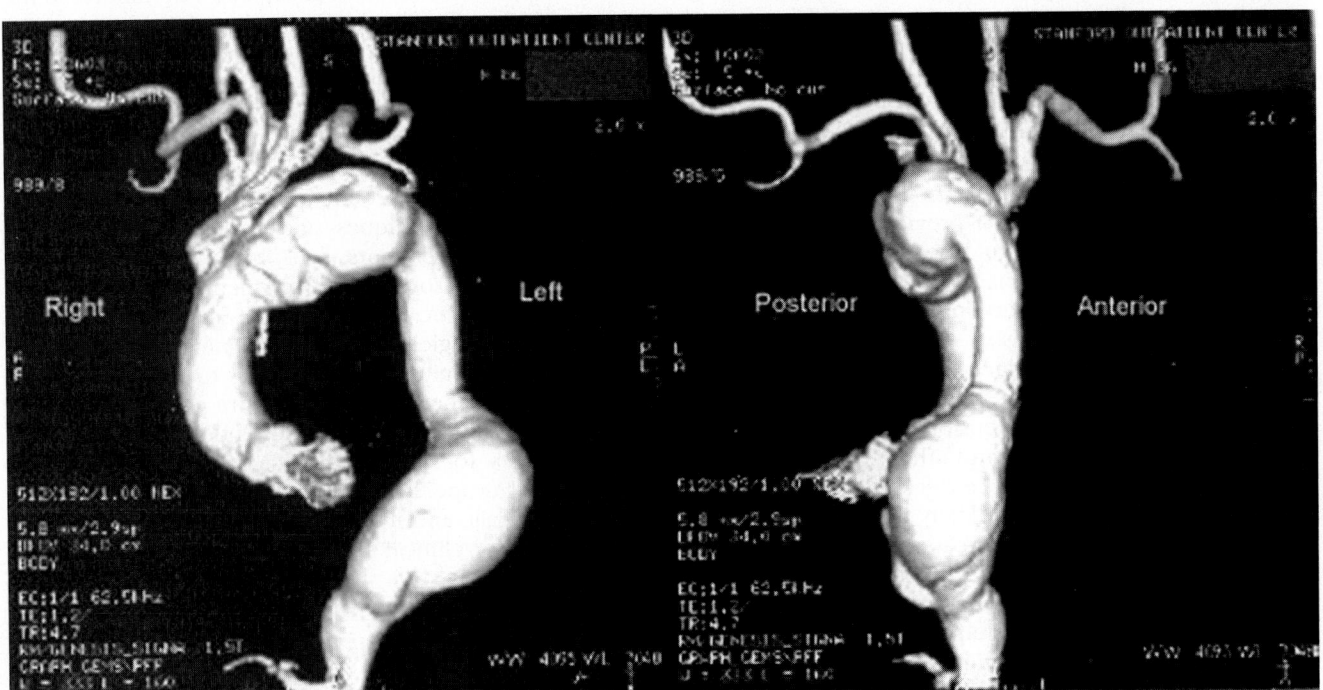

FIGURE 64-12.   Three-dimensional MR images showing anterior (left) and lateral (right) views of tandem thoracic aortic aneurysms. Aneurysmatic changes in the aortic arch and descending thoracic aorta are seen.

a thorough preoperative evaluation, and steps should be taken to optimize cardiac and pulmonary function. Signs and symptoms of aneurysm expansion or rupture including syncope, hypotension, unexplained chest pain, hoarseness, stridor, dysphagia, hemoptysis, or hematemesis should prompt immediate evaluation and aneurysm repair. Elective aneurysm repair may be warranted when an aneurysm reaches a diameter equal to or greater than 2.5 times the diameter of adjacent normal aorta or when the aneurysm becomes more than 6 to 7 cm in diameter.

The technique of open surgical repair of thoracic aortic aneurysms varies depending on the location and histologic type of the aneurysm—degenerative versus atherosclerotic. Woven polyester tube grafts are most commonly used for replacing the aneurysmal aortic segment, and monofilament polypropylene suture is used for suturing the anastomoses. Degenerative aneurysms of the thoracic aorta as seen in patients with Marfan syndrome typically involve the entire aorta, including the aortic root beginning at the aortic annulus. Repair of these aneurysms requires replacement of the entire aortic root with a valved conduit and reimplantation of the coronary ostia or a bypass to them with a separate graft. Atherosclerotic aneurysms involving the ascending aorta are repaired through a median sternotomy incision, and the aorta is replaced from the sinotubular ridge to the innominate artery or to the undersurface of the aortic arch under conditions of cardiopulmonary bypass, full heparin anticoagulation, and moderate systemic hypothermia. Aortic arch aneurysms are typically repaired during a period of circulatory arrest and profound hypothermia (18°C). Atherosclerotic aneurysms of the descending thoracic aorta are repaired through a posterolateral thoracotomy with double-lumen endotracheal intubation. The proximal cross-clamp is usually applied distal to the left common carotid artery. A properly sized graft is interposed between full-thickness aortic cuffs created proximal and distal to the aneurysm. Descending aortic aneurysms can be performed under conditions of full cardiopulmonary bypass or partial bypass, with a "clamp-and-go" technique, or with heparin bonded shunts. Left atrial to femoral artery bypass with a centrifugal pump and minimal heparin is another method to provide distal perfusion. Further steps designed to avoid paraplegia include cerebrospinal fluid (CSF) drainage, localized spinal cord cooling, administration of corticosteroids and free radical scavengers, and somatosensory evoked potential monitoring. None of these measures provides complete protection, however. Ensuring adequate resuscitation and avoiding perioperative hypotension are critical for minimizing the risk of paraplegia and other complications.

Remarkable progress has been made in the treatment of thoracic aortic aneurysms. Many advances in cardiovascular anesthesia and critical care have contributed to the improved success with lower operative mortality rates and reduced perioperative morbidity, including paraplegia. A 5-year study that concluded in 1996 included 45 patients who underwent aortic root replacement with composite valve grafts for Marfan syndrome. There were no intraoperative deaths, two early deaths (4.4%), and no postoperative strokes.[20] LeMaire and Coselli studied 198 consecutive descending thoracic aortic aneurysm repairs over an 8-year period: 62% of patients had aneurysmal disease involving at least two thirds of the descending aorta. Repair was achieved by the simple-clamp technique in 77% with a mean clamping time of 25 minutes. High-risk patients underwent atrium-to-femoral bypass (13%), and profound hypothermia with circulatory arrest occurred in 10%. Operative mortality rate was 5.1% ($n = 10$). Postoperative paraplegia occurred in three patients (1.5%) and renal failure, pulmonary complications, and paraplegia were determined to be important predictors of death by regression analysis.

In 1997, Mitchell and colleagues[21] reported the results of 108 patients receiving thoracic aortic stent grafts at Stanford University Medical Center. Mean aneurysm diameter was 6.3 cm. Twenty percent of patients had stent-grafts placed in conjunction with abdominal aortic aneurysm repair. Ten patients (9%) died within 30 days from the time of surgery, and four deaths were directly attributable to the procedure. Four patients had postoperative paraplegia and four had strokes. Patients in whom paraplegia developed either had stent-graft repair of thoracic aneurysms in conjunction with suprarenal abdominal aortic aneurysm repair or had deployment of the thoracic stent-graft across the orifices of intercostal arteries at the T10 level. An Austrian comparative study of endovascular versus open repair of thoracic aortic aneurysms was reported by Ehrlich and colleagues[16] in 1997. Sixty-eight patients were deemed good candidates for stent-graft repair. Because of limited device availability, 10 patients (15%) underwent stent-graft repair and 58 (85%) had open repair. The 30-day mortality rate was 30% for patients who underwent open surgery and 10% for endovascular repair. Mean procedural time was 320 minutes in the conventional group and 150 minutes in the stent-graft group. Paraplegia developed in five patients (12%) in the open surgical group compared with no paraplegia or neurologic sequelae in the stent-graft group. Hospital stay was 26 days in the open surgical group versus 10 days in the stent-graft group.

Endovascular repair appears to have a promising role in the treatment of descending thoracic aortic aneurysms. Refinement of techniques and devices will continue; however, many patients will have morphology not amenable to endovascular treatment, and aneurysms involving the aortic root, ascending aorta, and arch will require open surgical repair. Maintaining the highly specialized open surgical skills necessary to correct complex thoracic aortic aneurysms is therefore critical for continued progress in the current era of endovascular intervention. Devices for use in thoracic aortic aneurysm are available in Europe. In the United States they are currently in clinical trials, and it is anticipated that they will soon be available for clinical use.

THORACOABDOMINAL ANEURYSMS

Etheredge and colleagues[17] reported the first thoracoabdominal aneurysm repair in 1955. The tremendous advances in surgical technique, anesthetic management, and intensive care technology since that time have greatly improved the surgeon's ability to extend the success of these challenging operations beyond the operating room. A program capable of thoracoabdominal aneurysm repair with good results on a consistent basis depends on the integrity of an organized and dedicated team that includes highly skilled surgeons, cardiovascular anesthesiologists, and a state-of-the-art intensive care unit. Outside academic centers, these procedures are rarely undertaken because of the extraordinary effort required by the surgeons and critical care physicians during the perioperative period both to avoid complications and to successfully manage them when they arise.

Crawford and associates[12] proposed a classification scheme for thoracoabdominal aneurysms that has become widely recognized. All varieties of aneurysms are described, including atherosclerotic, degenerative, and dissecting, as follows:

- Type I aneurysms involve most of the descending thoracic aorta and abdominal aorta proximal to the renal arteries.
- Type II aneurysms involve most of the descending thoracic aorta and abdominal aorta distal to the renal arteries.
- Type III aneurysms involve the distal half or less of the descending aorta and the abdominal aorta distal to the renal arteries.
- Type IV aneurysms involve all or most of the abdominal aorta, including the paravisceral segment.

The Crawford classification has facilitated stratification for risk assessment and type-specific comparison of results including paraplegia and mortality rates.

Most thoracoabdominal aortic aneurysms are discovered incidentally during evaluation for other medical problems or they are palpated on routine physical examination if the aneurysm extends below the renal arteries. As with isolated abdominal and thoracic aortic aneurysms, CT scanning and MR angiography are useful for measuring aneurysm dimensions and determining the extent of aortic involvement relative to important branch vessels. Conventional angiography is helpful for defining arch vessel disease and delineating intercostal arteries.

As with other aortic aneurysms, selection of patients for repair of thoracoabdominal aortic aneurysms is dependent on a thorough risk assessment, with emphasis given to preexisting cardiac and pulmonary comorbidities. The risk of rupture must be weighed against the risk of serious operative morbidity and death, and patients who undergo repair must have optimization of their cardiac and pulmonary function preoperatively. Patients with signs and symptoms of aneurysm expansion or rupture should prompt immediate evaluation and aneurysm repair. Elective repair may be warranted when an aneurysm reaches a diameter two times or more than the diameter of adjacent normal aorta.

The technique of open surgical repair of thoracoabdominal aortic aneurysms varies depending on the extent of the aneurysm. Double-lumen endotracheal intubation is performed. The patient is positioned on a bean bag with shoulders at 60 degrees and hips at 30 degrees, and operative exposure is obtained through a thoracoabdominal incision with the level of the incision determined by the proximal extent of the aneurysm in the thoracic aorta. Aneurysms that extend from the proximal and mid descending thoracic aorta to the infrarenal aorta (types II and III) are approached through the 6th intercostal space, with the incision carried through the costal margin into the abdomen, whereas type I aneurysms can be approached through a thoracic incision and type IV aneurysms can be approached retroperitoneally through a left flank incision made from the 9th or 10th interspace toward the umbilicus. After exposure of the thoracic and abdominal aorta as well as the visceral and renal arteries, the proximal cross-clamp is applied with careful control of blood pressure to avoid hypertension proximal to the clamp. A properly sized graft is selected and sewn end-to-end to a full-thickness cuff of normal aorta above the aneurysm. After completing the proximal anastomosis, reimplantation of intercostal, visceral, and renal arteries is carried out in a sequential fashion. The distal end of the graft is typically sewn to the distal aorta in an end-to-end fashion, although a bifurcated extension is sometimes required to the bilateral iliac or femoral arteries. Dissecting aneurysms of the thoracic and abdominal aorta that are considered chronic or "mature" are treated similarly to nondissecting aneurysms. However, during surgical repair, the septum between true and false lumina is excised, and care is taken to ensure the patency of branch vessels.

As with descending thoracic aortic aneurysms, repair of thoracoabdominal aortic aneurysms can be performed under conditions of full cardiopulmonary bypass or partial bypass, with a clamp-and-go technique, with heparin-bonded shunts, or with left atrial to femoral artery centrifugal pump bypass. CSF drainage, localized spinal cord cooling, administration of corticosteroids and free radical scavengers, and somatosensory-evoked potential monitoring have also been advocated to minimize paraplegia risk. Adequate resuscitation must be ensured and perioperative hypotension must be avoided to minimize the risk of paraplegia and other serious complications.

The results of E. Stanley Crawford's series of more than 1500 thoracoabdominal aortic aneurysm repairs greatly improved modern understanding of surgical outcome following these operations. Survival rate for all patients was 90% or higher, regardless of the extent of aneurysm involvement. The risk of paraplegia was highest in patients with types I and II (15% and 31%) and lowest in patients with types III and IV (7% and 4%). Overall, renal failure occurred in 9% of patients with less dramatic differences between aneurysm types.[51]

FEMORAL AND POPLITEAL ARTERY ANEURYSMS

Popliteal aneurysms are the most frequent peripheral aneurysms, accounting for 70% of all such aneurysms. They are followed in frequency by femoral aneurysms, and together they constitute 90% of the peripheral aneurysms not involving the aortoiliac arteries. The majority of these aneurysms are of the degenerative type. Men outnumber women 20 to 30:1, and the mean age at presentation is 65 years. More than 50% are bilateral, and 75% of those with femoral aneurysm and 33% of those with popliteal aneurysm also have an aortic aneurysm. The susceptibility of popliteal arteries to aneurysm formation is unclear, and factors such as turbulence beyond a relative stenosis at the tendinous hiatus of the adductor magnus and repeated flexion at the knee have been considered. However, these do not account for the association with other aneurysms elsewhere or the striking male preponderance.

Popliteal and femoral aneurysms are commonly asymptomatic when discovered. The most important manifestation of femoral and popliteal aneurysms is distal embolization. In 10% of femoral aneurysms, evidence of distal embolization is found. Evidence of embolization is found in 25% of popliteal aneurysms, and the most common symptom is distal ischemia, which is limb threatening in 44% of cases. Thrombosis of the aneurysm is more common in popliteal aneurysms (40%) than in femoral aneurysms (1% to 16%). Approximately 25% of patients with distal thromboembolism arising in femoral popliteal aneurysms come to amputation primarily because of progressive chronic occlusion of the runoff vessels before thrombosis. Rupture of these aneurysms is rare and occurs at a rate of 1% to 14% in femoral aneurysms and at a rate less than 5% in popliteal aneurysms. Other symptoms include local pain related to nerve compression and compression of adjacent veins with resultant venous thrombosis or edema.

Femoropopliteal aneurysms can usually be diagnosed on physical examination. In the groin, appreciation of aneurysm size is easier, whereas over the popliteal fossa, because of the deep location of the artery, only an abnormally pronounced pulse is palpated and may be confused with a Baker's cyst or a tumor. Duplex ultrasonography is the best initial study for evaluation of femoropopliteal aneurysm. It offers the ability to accurately measure diameter and determine the extent of mural thrombus. This is also the examination of choice for acute femoropopliteal occlusion when previously undiagnosed popliteal aneurysmal disease is suspected. Both CT and MR scanning can demonstrate femoropopliteal aneurysms but are usually unnecessary. Angiography is important to demonstrate the extent of the involved segment, to evaluate the patency and quality of the runoff vessels, and to detect distal embolic occlusions. Further evaluation should include a search for aneurysmal disease elsewhere because 40% of patients have abdominal aortic aneurysm and 70% have contralateral femoral popliteal aneurysms.

Indications for treatment include acute lower limb ischemia resulting from acute occlusion, distal emboli, and a transverse diameter larger than 2 cm for popliteal aneurysms and larger than 2.5 cm for common femoral aneurysms. Treatment of femoral and popliteal aneurysms consists of exclusion of the aneurysm and restoration of blood supply. In case of multiple aneurysms, the one posing the biggest threat is repaired first. Femoral aneurysms are often replaced with a prosthetic graft in conjunction with other procedures. Popliteal aneurysms can be approached medially or posteriorly. They are pref-

erentially replaced with an autogenous conduit such as the greater saphenous vein when available. Resection of the aneurysm is unnecessary and may be hazardous. When the aneurysm is thrombosed or when part of the distal runoff bed has been obliterated by emboli, thromboembolectomy or thrombolysis may be necessary for establishing distal and arterial runoff. Endovascular treatment of femoral and popliteal aneurysms is being evaluated and may become an available treatment modality.

Following repair of femoral and popliteal aneurysms, death is rare and, for asymptomatic patients, limb salvage rate is 90% to 98%. For symptomatic patients, the early graft patency rate is 59% to 85% and the limb salvage rate 70% to 80%.

UPPER EXTREMITY ANEURYSMS

Aneurysms of the upper extremities are rare compared with aneurysms in other peripheral locations. However, they are important, and their presence should be evaluated and treated promptly because of the potential for serious complications, including digit and limb loss, stroke from embolization into more proximal vertebral and right carotid arteries, and exsanguinating hemorrhage depending on the location and nature of the aneurysm.

Subclavian artery aneurysms are the most common of the upper extremity aneurysms. They are caused by atherosclerosis, compression at the thoracic outlet, and trauma. Aneurysms involving the proximal subclavian artery most commonly are associated with atherosclerosis, and as many as 50% of patients have aortoiliac or other peripheral aneurysms. Aneurysms involving the distal subclavian artery are typically associated with a cervical rib or other causes of thoracic outlet syndrome.

Patients with subclavian aneurysms may have neck, chest, and shoulder pain from aneurysm expansion or rupture; acute and chronic ischemic symptoms, transient ischemic attacks, or stroke from thromboembolism; or hoarseness, impaired motor or sensory function, or respiratory insufficiency from recurrent laryngeal nerve, brachial plexus, or tracheal compression, respectively. Patients may also have Horner's syndrome from compression of the stellate ganglion or hemoptysis from erosion into the lung. Patients may also complain of a pulsating sensation in the neck or shoulder region without pain or other compelling symptoms. The diagnosis can be established by duplex ultrasound or CT. Aortic arch and upper extremity angiography is necessary to define the extent of the aneurysm and its position relative to the vertebral artery, common carotid artery (right side), and thoracic outlet structures and to evaluate the nature and extent of thromboembolitic arterial occlusion if present. Surgical repair of subclavian artery aneurysms involves resection of the aneurysm and re-establishment of arterial continuity, usually with an arterial interposition graft. A median sternotomy with extension of the incision into the supraclavicular fossa provides excellent exposure for repair of proximal right subclavian aneurysms, and a left anterior thoracotomy may be required for repair of proximal left subclavian aneurysms. Aneurysms involving the mid and distal subclavian artery can usually be repaired through combined supraclavicular and infraclavicular incisions, although some surgeons advocate resecting the middle one third of the clavicle for exposure. Decompression of the thoracic outlet may also be necessary depending on the etiology, and reimplantation of a vertebral artery may be prudent if the origin arises from the aneurysm. If recent extremity thromboembolism has occurred, balloon thromboembolectomy should be performed to restore distal perfusion.

An aberrant right subclavian artery originating from the proximal descending thoracic aorta is sometimes associated with aneurysmal change at the origin of the artery (Kommerell's diverticulum). Complications associated with this abnormality include dysphagia from esophageal compression, dyspnea from tracheal compression, pain from expansion and rupture, and ischemic symptoms in the extremity from thromboembolism. Elective repair of aberrant right subclavian arteries with Kommerell's diverticulum is recommended regardless of aneurysm size because of the risk of rupture and other serious complications.

Aneurysms and pseudoaneurysms of the axillary arteries are typically associated with a history of previous blunt or penetrating trauma, although rare congenital cases do occur. Symptoms are related to nerve compression and ischemia from thrombosis or thromboembolism. Repair involves resection of the aneurysmal artery and primary repair, if a short segment is involved, or reconstruction with an interposition vein graft using, preferably, greater saphenous vein.

The ulnar artery also occasionally gives rise to upper extremity aneurysms. Such aneurysms are typically associated with repetitive trauma to the dominant hand, a disease entity termed the *hypothenar hammer syndrome*. Complications include ulnar artery thrombosis and distal thromboembolism with associated rest pain, numbness, cyanosis, and gangrene of the hand or digits (usually third and fourth) and ulnar nerve compression symptoms. Treatment consists of resection of the aneurysm and microvascular reconstruction with a vein interposition graft.

VISCERAL ARTERY ANEURYSMS

Visceral or splanchnic artery aneurysms are relatively uncommon, but they are important to recognize and treat because roughly 25% present as emergencies and 8.5% result in death. Involved arteries and their relative frequencies include the splenic (60%), hepatic (20%), superior mesenteric (5.5%), and other arterial (each < 5%).

Splenic artery aneurysms occur most frequently in women, with a female-to-male ratio of 4:1 (Fig. 64-13). This unusual sex predilection is likely related to acquired derangements of the arterial wall influenced by a number of processes, including medial fibrodysplasia, portal hypertension, repeated pregnancy, penetrating or blunt abdominal trauma, pancreatitis, and infection. Women of childbearing age who have splenic artery aneurysms are at particularly high risk of death as a result of aneurysm

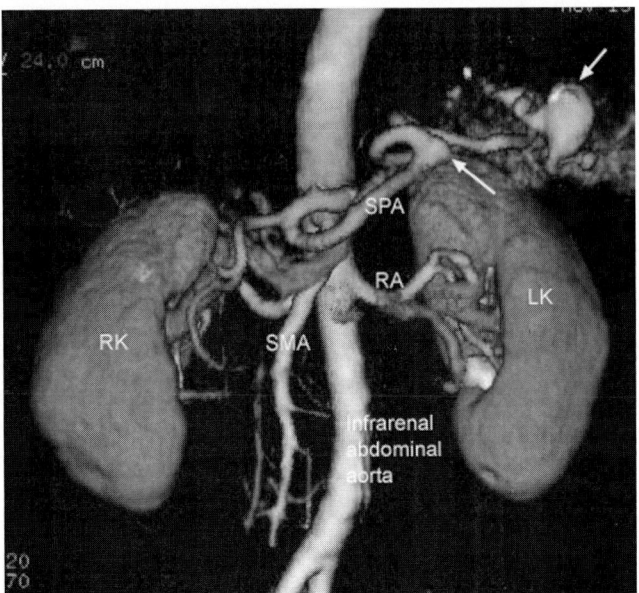

FIGURE 64-13. Multiple aneurysms of the splenic artery (arrowheads). SPA, splenic artery; SMA, superior mesenteric artery; RA, renal artery; RK, right kidney; LK, left kidney.

rupture and should have elective repair. Symptomatic or ruptured aneurysms also warrant immediate repair. Surgical techniques for treating splenic artery aneurysms include simple proximal and distal ligation without arterial reconstruction for proximal aneurysms and splenectomy versus aneurysm exclusion and vascular reconstruction for salvage of the spleen.

Hepatic artery aneurysms are more common in men, with a male-to-female ratio of 2:1. There are multiple causes of hepatic artery aneurysm, including previous abdominal trauma, history of intravenous drug abuse, medial degeneration of the arterial wall, and periarterial inflammatory process. An aggressive approach to treating these aneurysms regardless of size appears justified because of a high risk of eventual rupture and a mortality rate of more than 35% when rupture occurs. Aneurysm repair can be carried out by simple excision and interposition vein graft repair or by aortohepatic bypass to restore normal hepatic arterial perfusion.

Other splanchnic artery aneurysms generally warrant surgical repair because of the high mortality rate associated with rupture as long as the patient is not a prohibitive risk. Patients who are deemed to be at prohibitive risk for operation may undergo transluminal embolization to ablate the aneurysm. However, this approach is not definitive and may not prevent aneurysm rupture.

MYCOTIC ANEURYSMS

Mycotic aneurysms result from localized infection, which may be blood-borne or associated with a localized infectious process. They can occur anywhere, but the most common location is the femoral artery, followed by the aorta. The most common pathogens for blood-borne infection are *Salmonella* and *Staphylococcus*. Syphilitic aneurysms, which were common at the turn of the 20th century, are currently extremely rare. Localized infection is often the result of direct injury with superimposed infection and may follow intravascular drug abuse.

The classic presentation is pain in the region of the aneurysm and a pulsatile mass accompanied by fever and chills. Often, particularly in aortic infection, presentation is nonspecific with fever of unknown origin. Peripheral evidence of septic emboli such as petechial skin lesions and splinter hemorrhages in the fingers or toenails may be seen. CT and MR studies may demonstrate a saccular aneurysm often of lobulated and irregular configuration. In the groin, duplex ultrasonography is the preferred diagnostic modality.

Management goals are eradication of the infection and preservation of adequate blood supply. Infected tissue should be débrided and, if arterial, reconstruction should be performed when the integrity of the artery or distal arterial perfusion is compromised. Depending on the location and extent of infection, arterial reconstruction may precede excision. Reconstruction and excision can be carried out simultaneously, taking care to avoid contamination of the reconstruction, or arterial reconstruction can be performed after excision. Previously, avoidance of the region of infection was a basic principle of management and conduits were routed through extra-anatomic planes (e.g., lateral thigh or transobturator for femoral infections). More recently, several groups have shown that in situ reconstruction following aggressive débridement and wound care can have good results. The conduits of choice are autologous veins including superficial femoral veins. When no autologous conduit can be used, homografts may be considered. Patients are placed on long-term, or in case of aortic *Salmonella* infection, lifelong antibiotic therapy.

PSEUDOANEURYSMS

Pseudoaneurysms are contained arterial disruptions that can be categorized to two main types: those that result from a perforation of an artery by traumatic or iatrogenic injury and those that result from dehiscence of a surgical vascular anastomosis. Both types are most prevalent in the femoral artery.

Traumatic pseudoaneurysms may occur acutely or, more commonly, they may be discovered following unrecognized arterial injury. In all such cases, infection has to be ruled out. Management includes direct surgical repair or, in selected instances involving less accessible large arteries, exclusion of the pseudoaneurysm with a stent-graft. Pseudoaneurysms arising in small, nonvital arteries may be treated with ligation, compression, or coil embolization.

Iatrogenic pseudoaneurysms occur most commonly after arterial puncture for angiography or for vascular intervention, and the most frequently affected site is the common femoral artery. With the increasing number of interventional procedures that involve large-bore devices and full anticoagulation, the incidence is not decreasing and occurs after 0.05% to 0.4% of punctures, depending on the complexity of the procedure. The common site for the development of pseudoaneurysms is at the bifurcation of the superficial and the deep femoral artery, where compression is less effective. Pseudoaneurysms manifest with pain, a pulsatile mass, and compression of adjacent structures. The natural history of these is variable. Large, expanding, and painful pseudoaneurysms are at significant risk of rupture and should be repaired, whereas smaller, stable ones can be observed. The imaging modality of choice is duplex ultrasonography, which can define the size, morphology, and location of the pseudoaneurysm compression while preserving flow in the common femoral artery. Pseudoaneurysms less than 2 cm in diameter have a 70% likelihood of spontaneous thrombosis with compression therapy, whereas larger ones and those in anticoagulated patients are likely to persist. During the last decade, ultrasound-guided thrombin injection has become a treatment option. During injection of thrombin into a pseudoaneurysm, immediate thrombosis can be demonstrated. Surgery is required in some patients with infected and rapidly expanding pseudoaneurysms. Surgical repair involves exposing the arterial defect or puncture and repairing it, usually with one or two stitches.

Anastomotic pseudoaneurysms occur as a result of partial or complete disruption of a vascular anastomotic suture line. They occur most commonly in the femoral anastomosis of aortofemoral bypass grafts and are most common with prosthetic conduits. Pseudoaneurysms develop in 3% of all femoral anastomoses after a mean interval of 6 years. Anastomotic pseudoaneurysms may result from material fatigue of the suture (formerly silk) or graft or from pull-through of the suture from the arterial wall. Infection is an important cause of anastomotic disruption and needs to be ruled out. Common femoral pseudoaneurysms manifest as pulsatile groin masses. In deeper locations, pseudoaneurysms may be associated with pain or free rupture or they may be discovered incidentally. All graft anastomoses should be evaluated by CT, duplex ultrasound, or MR scanning, and the presence of multiple pseudoaneurysms increases the likelihood of an infectious etiology. Preoperative work-up should include arteriography to define inflow and outflow anatomy. Surgical repair of anastomotic pseudoaneurysms is indicated and consists of patching or, preferentially, graft replacement of the disrupted region. Bacterial cultures should be obtained at the time of reconstruction, and, if gross evidence of infection exists, proper débridement and an appropriately planned reconstruction must be performed. Mortality after repair of pseudoaneurysm is rare, and the recurrence rate is lower after graft interposition than after primary repair. Graft patency at 2 years is 98%, and the amputation rate is 2%.

HIV-RELATED ARTERIAL ANEURYSMS

Patients with human immunodeficiency virus (HIV)-related aneurysms are typically young and lack the usual risk factors associated with vascular diseases. HIV-related aneurysms are often multiple and occur at unusual sites, particularly in the common carotid and superficial femoral arteries. Abdominal aorta has been the third most frequent site.[52] On angiography, they may appear saccular or have the appearance of large pseudoaneurysms.[52] In ultrasound, features are typical of pseudoaneurysms with a blow-out defect, thickening, and hyperechoic spotting of the vessel wall.[53] Microscopically, the features of HIV vasculopathy are typical of a leukocytoclastic vasculitis that affects vasa vasorum.[54] The inflammatory infiltrate is restricted to the adventitia, with sparing of the inner layers of the artery.

If the disease is limited to seropositivity only, patient should be offered the same treatment as a seronegative patient. In patients with advanced HIV infection and short life expectancy, the use of minimal or no surgical intervention may be justifiable. Severely symptomatic aneurysms or life-threatening complications should be treated. Reconstructions should be made with autogenous graft if available.

Selected References

Beckman JA, O'Gara PT: Diseases of the aorta. Adv Intern Med 44:267-291, 1999.

> This article reviews the current knowledge of aortic diseases, including etiology, pathogenesis, and diagnosis. Special emphasis is given to aortic aneurysms.

Gewertz BL, Schwartz LB (eds): Surgery of the Aorta and Its Branches. Philadelphia, WB Saunders, 2000.

> This text addresses the full range of aortic pathology with special sections dedicated to branch vessel disease and endoluminal grafting. It is particularly useful for physicians interested in the intricacies of various treatment strategies.

Rehm JP, Grange JJ, Baxter BT: The formation of aneurysms. Semin Vasc Surg 11:193-202, 1998.

> The authors summarize the dynamic interactions within a diseased vessel in the fields of immunology, biochemistry, cell biology, and genetics. The roles of local inflammatory infiltrates and their destructive proteolytic enzymes are reviewed. New therapeutic measures are presented that may control the critical matrix changes that contribute to the formation of aortic aneurysms.

Svensson LD, Crawford ES: Aortic dissection and aortic aneurysm surgery: Clinical observations, experimental observations, and statistical analyses. Part I, Curr Probl Surg 29:817-911, 1992; Part II, Curr Probl Surg 29:913-1057, 1992; Part III, Curr Probl Surg 30:1-163, 1993.

> This three-part review provides a broad perspective on aneurysmal disease of the thoracic and abdominal aorta, from etiology and demographics to treatment and long-term outcome.

White RA, Fogarty TJ (eds): Peripheral Endovascular Interventions, 2nd ed. New York, Springer-Verlag, 1999.

> This text is a comprehensive review of the numerous technologies now available for treating vascular diseases in a minimally invasive fashion. It is a valuable reference for the endovascular specialist.

Zarins CK, Glagov S. Artery wall pathology in atherosclerosis. *In* Rutherford RB (ed): Vascular Surgery, 5th ed, Vol. 1. Philadelphia, WB Saunders, 2000, pp 313-333.

> This book chapter reviews the problem of atherosclerosis and its effects on the functional biomechanical properties of the artery wall. The evolution of atherosclerotic lesions and the associated arterial wall responses, normal and pathologic, are outlined. Local differences that may account for the propensity of certain areas to form extensive and complex plaques or aneurysms are also explored.

References

1. Johnston KW, Rutherford RB, Tilson MD, et al: Suggested standards for reporting on arterial aneurysms. Subcommittee on Reporting Standards for Arterial Aneurysms, Ad Hoc Committee on Reporting Standards, Society for Vascular Surgery and North American Chapter, International Society for Cardiovascular Surgery [see comments]. J Vasc Surg 13:452-458, 1991.
2. Killen DA, Reed WA, Gorton ME, et al: Twenty-five–year trends in resection of abdominal aortic aneurysms. Ann Vasc Surg 12:436-444, 1998.
3. Svensson LD, Crawford ES: Aortic dissection and aortic aneurysm surgery: Clinical observations, experimental observations, and statistical analyses: III. Curr Prob Surg 30:5-163, 1993.
4. Baumgartner WA, Cameron DE, Redmond JM, et al: Operative management of Marfan syndrome: The Johns Hopkins experience. Ann Thorac Surg. 676:1859-1860, 1999.
5. Xu C, Zarins CK, Glagov S: Aneurysmal and occlusive atherosclerosis of the human abdominal aorta. J Vasc Surg. 33:91-96, 2001.
6. Zarins CK, Xu C, Glagov S: Atherosclerotic enlargement of the human abdominal aorta. Atherosclerosis 155:157-164, 2001.
7. Coady MA, Rizzo JA, Goldstein LJ, Elefteriades JA: Natural history, pathogenesis, and etiology of thoracic aortic aneurysms and dissections. Cardiol Clin 17:615-635, 1999.
8. Lederle FA, Johnson GR, Wilson SE, et al: Prevalence and associations of abdominal aortic aneurysm detected through screening. Aneurysm Detection and Management (ADAM) Veterans Affairs Cooperative Study Group. Ann Intern Med 126:441-449, 1997.
9. Lederle FA, Johnson GR, Wilson SE, et al: The Aneurysm Detection and Management Study screening program: Validation cohort and final results. Aneurysm Detection and Management Veterans Affairs Cooperative Study Investigators. Arch Intern Med 160:1425-1430, 2000.
10. The U.K. Small Aneurysm Trial Participants, Brown LC, Powell JT: Risk factors for aneurysm rupture in patients kept under ultrasound surveillance. Ann Surg 230:289-297, 1999.
11. Englund R, Hudson P, Hanel K, Stanton A: Expansion rates of small abdominal aortic aneurysms. Aust N Z J Surg 68:21-24, 1998.
12. Crawford ES, Snyder DM, Cho GC, Roehm JO Jr: Progress in treatment of thoracoabdominal and abdominal aortic aneurysms involving celiac, superior mesenteric, and renal arteries. Ann Surg 188:404-422, 1978.
13. Crawford Rasmussen TE, Hallett JW Jr: Inflammatory aortic aneurysms: A clinical review with new perspectives in pathogenesis. Ann Surg 225:155-164, 1997.
14. Powell JT, Brown LC: The natural history of abdominal aortic aneurysms and their risk of rupture. Acta Chir Belg 101:11-16, 2001.

15. Diehl JT, Cali RF, Hertzer NR, Beven EG: Complications of abdominal aortic reconstruction: An analysis of perioperative risk factors in 557 patients. Ann Surg 197:49-56, 1983.

16. Ehrlich M, Grabenwoeger M, Cartes-Zumelzu F, et al: Endovascular stent graft repair for aneurysms on the descending thoracic aorta. Ann Thorac Surg 25:332-340, 1997.

17. Etheredge SN, Yee J, Smith JV, et al: Successful resection of a large aneurysm of the upper abdominal aorta and replacement with homograft. Surgery 38:1171-1181, 1955.

18. Hertzer NR, Beven EG, Young JR, et al: Coronary artery disease in peripheral vascular patients: A classification of 1000 coronary angiograms and results of surgical management. Ann Surg 199:223-233, 1984.

19. Alric P, Ryckwaert F, Picot MC, et al: Ruptured aneurysm of the infrarenal abdominal aorta: Impact of age and postoperative complications on mortality. Ann Vasc Surg 17:277-283, 2003.

20. LeMaire SA, Coselli JS: Aortic root surgery in Marfan syndrome: Current practice and evolving techniques. J Card Surg 12(Suppl 2):137-141, 1997.

21. Mitchell RS, Miller DC, Dake MD: Stent-graft repair of thoracic aortic aneurysms. Semin Vasc Surg10:257-271, 1997.

22. Moreno-Cabral CE, Miller DC, Mitchell RS, et al: Degenerative and atherosclerotic aneurysms of the thoracic aorta: Determinants of early and late surgical outcome. J Thorac Cardiovasc Surg 88:1020-1032, 1984.

23. Papin E: Chirurgie du Rein: Anomalies du Rein. Paris, G. Doin, 1928, pp 205-220.

24. Parodi JC, Palmaz JC, Barone HD: Transfemoral intraluminal graft implantation for abdominal aortic aneurysms. Ann Vasc Surg 5:491-499, 1991.

25. Heijmen RH, Deblier IG, Moll FL, et al: Endovascular stent grafting for descending thoracic aortic aneurysms. Eur J Cardiothorac Surg 21:5-9, 2002.

26. Rasmussen TE, Hallett JW Jr: Inflammatory aortic aneurysms: A clinical review with new perspectives in pathogenesis. Ann Surg 225:155-164, 1997.

27. Juvonen T, Ergin MA, Galla JD, et al: Prospective study of the natural history of thoracic aortic aneurysms. Ann Thorac Surg 63:1533-1545, 1997.

28. Svensjo S, Bengtsson H, Bergqvist D: Thoracic and thoracoabdominal aortic aneurysm and dissection: An investigation based on autopsy. Br J Surg 83:68-71, 1996.

29. Coselli JS, Conklin LD, LeMaire SA: Thoracoabdominal aortic aneurysm repair: Review and update of current strategies. Ann Thorac Surg 74:S1881-S1884; discussion, S1892-S1898, 2002.

30. Zarins CK, Harris EJ Jr: Operative repair for aortic aneurysms: The gold standard. J Endovasc Surg 4:232-241, 1997.

31. Arko FR, Hill BB, Olcott C, et al: Endovascular repair reduces early and late morbidity compared to open surgery for abdominal aortic aneurysm. J Endovasc Ther 9:711-718, 2002.

32. Moore WS, Matsumura JS, Makaroun MS, et al, EVT/Guidant Investigators: Five-year interim comparison of the Guidant bifurcated endograft with open repair of abdominal aortic aneurysm. J Vasc Surg 38:46-55, 2003.

33. Matsumura JS, Brewster DC, Makaroun MS, Naftel DC: A multicenter controlled clinical trial of open versus endovascular treatment of abdominal aortic aneurysm. J Vasc Surg 37:262-271, 2003.

34. Hill BB, Wolf YG, Lee WA, et al: Open versus endovascular AAA repair in patients who are morphological candidates for endovascular treatment. J Endovasc Ther 9:255-261, 2002.

35. Lee WA, Wolf YG, Hill BB, et al: The first 150 endovascular AAA repairs at a single institution: How steep is the learning curve? J Endovasc Ther 9:269-276, 2002.

36. Zarins CK, Shaver DM, Arko FR, et al: Introduction of endovascular aneurysm repair into community practice: Initial results with a new Food and Drug Administration–approved device. J Vasc Surg 36:226-233, 2002.

37. Zarins CK, White RA, Schwarten D, et al: AneuRx stent graft versus open surgical repair of abdominal aortic aneurysms: Multicenter prospective clinical trial. J Vasc Surg 29:292-305, 1999.

38. Arko FR, Lee WA, Hill BB, et al: Aneurysm-related death: Primary endpoint analysis for comparison of open and endovascular repair. J Vasc Surg 36:297-304, 2002.

39. Zarins CK, for the AneuRx Clinical Investigators: The US AneuRx Clinical Trial: Six-year clinical update 2002. J Vasc Surg 37:904-908, 2003.

40. Veith FJ, Ohki T: Endovascular approaches to ruptured infrarenal aorto-iliac aneurysms. J Cardiovasc Surg (Torino) 43:369-378, 2002.

41. Yilmaz N, Peppelenbosch N, Cuypers PW, et al: Emergency treatment of symptomatic or ruptured abdominal aortic aneurysms: The role of endovascular repair. J Endovasc Ther 9:449-457, 2002.

42. Hinchliffe RJ, Yusuf SW, Machierewicz JA, et al: Endovascular repair of ruptured abdominal aortic aneurysm—a challenge to open repair? Results of a single-centre experience in 20 patients. Eur J Vasc Endovasc Surg 22:528-534, 2001.

43. Crawford ES, Saleh SA, Babb JW III, et al: Infrarenal abdominal aortic aneurysm: Factors influencing survival after operation performed over a 25-year period. Ann Surg 193:699-709, 1981.

44. Sampram ES, Karafa MT, Mascha EJ, et al: Nature, frequency, and predictive factors of secondary procedures after endovascular repair of abdominal aortic aneurysm. J Vasc Surg 31:134-146, 2003.

45. Alric P, Hinchliffe RJ, Picot MC, et al: Long-term renal function following endovascular aneurysm repair with infrarenal and suprarenal aortic stent-grafts. J Endovasc Ther 10:397-405, 2003.

46. Vallabhaneni SR, Harris PL: Lessons learnt from the EUROSTAR registry on endovascular repair of abdominal aortic aneurysm repair. Eur J Radiol 29:34-41, 2001.

47. Terramani TT, Chaikof EL, Rayan SS, et al: Secondary conversion due to failed endovascular abdominal aortic aneurysm repair. J Vasc Surg 38:473-477, 2003.

48. Zarins CK, White RA, Hodgson KJ, et al: Endoleak as a predictor of outcome after endovascular aneurysm repair: AneuRx multicenter clinical trial. J Vasc Surg 32:90-107, 2000.

49. Zarins CK, Gewertz BL: Atlas of Vascular Surgery. New York, Churchill Livingstone, 1988.

50. Trigaux JP, Vandroogenbroek S, De Wispelaere JF, et al: Congenital anomalies of the inferior vena cava and left renal vein: Evaluation with spiral CT. J Vasc Intervent Radiol 9:339-345, 1998.

51. Coselli JS: Thoracoabdominal aortic aneurysm. In Rutherford RB (ed): Vascular Surgery, 4th ed. Philadelphia, WB Saunders 1995, pp 1069-1087.

52. Nair R, Robbs JV, Naidoo NG, Wooglar J: Clinical profile of HIV-related aneurysms. Eur J Vasc Endovasc Surg 20:235-240, 2000.

53. Woolgar JD, Ray R, Maharaj K, Robbs JV: Colour Doppler and grey scale ultrasound features of HIV-related vascular aneurysms. Br J Radiol 75:884-888, 2002.

54. Chetty R, Batitang S, Nair R: Large-vessel vasculopathy in HIV-positive patients: Another vasculitic enigma? Hum Pathol 31:374-379, 2000.

CHAPTER 65

PERIPHERAL ARTERIAL OCCLUSIVE DISEASE

Michael Belkin, M.D.,   Anthony D. Whittemore, M.D.,

Magruder C. Donaldson, M.D.,   Michael S. Conte, M.D.,

and   Edwin Gravereaux, M.D.

Basic Considerations

Acute Thromboembolic Disease

Chronic Occlusive Disease of the Lower Extremities

Chronic Visceral Ischemia

BASIC CONSIDERATIONS

Arterial occlusive diseases are highly prevalent in Western societies, where they constitute the leading overall cause of death. Adverse events are due to the effects of impaired circulation on critical end organs (e.g., brain, heart, abdominal viscera) or extremities. In addition to death, which is most commonly caused by myocardial infarction or stroke, significant disability and loss of function is incurred at a substantial cost to society. Atherosclerosis accounts for the overwhelming majority of causative lesions and, with the increasing longevity and changing demographics of the U.S. population, assumes top priority as a national health issue.

Atherosclerosis

General Observations and Risk Factors

Atherosclerosis is a complex, chronic inflammatory process that affects the elastic and muscular arteries. The disease is both systemic and segmental, with clear predilections for certain locations within the arterial tree and relative sparing of others. The earliest lesions (i.e., fatty streaks) may be detected in childhood in susceptible individuals. Lesions progress through a series of well-characterized pathologic stages before clinical manifestations develop. Population-based studies have demonstrated a number of important risk factors that have become targets for preventive therapy as well as potential clues into the pathogenesis of the disease (Box 65-1). The most important independent risk factors for atherosclerosis are hypercholesterolemia, hypertension, cigarette smoking, and diabetes mellitus.

Hypercholesterolemia (e.g., total serum cholesterol greater than 200 mg/dL) is clearly associated with increased risk. Of great prognostic significance is the relative apportioning between the subclasses of cholesterol-carrying lipoproteins: the low density fraction (LDL), which is atherogenic, and the high-density lipoprotein fraction (HDL), which exerts an atheroprotective effect by "reverse transport" of cholesterol. Studies have demonstrated a strong positive correlation between atherosclerotic cardiovascular disease and elevated total and LDL cholesterol and an equally strong negative correlation with HDL levels. Despite these known relationships between serum lipid profiles and cardiovascular risk, the association with dietary intake remains complex in that individual metabolism is highly variable. Genetic variability in cholesterol metabolism provides one important mechanism for the well-known familial clustering of premature atherosclerotic disease. An important role for diet is strongly suggested by the variation in prevalence noted among different nations and ethnic groups, with a clear increase associated with consumption of the so-called Western diet (i.e., high fat, low fiber). The potential effects of numerous dietary components, both protective and atherogenic, have been intensely investigated with only limited consensus. Of these, a causative role of dietary lipid, particularly cholesterol and saturated fats, has been most well defined.

Box 65-1. Risk Factors for Atherosclerosis

Firmly Established

Hypercholesterolemia
Cigarette smoking
Hypertension
Diabetes mellitus

Relative Factors

Advanced age
Male gender
Hypertriglyceridemia
Hyperhomocysteinemia
Sedentary lifestyle
Family history

Box 65-2. Guidelines for Risk Factor Modification

Lipid Management

Goal: Primary—serum LDL <100 mg/dL; secondary—HDL >35 mg/dL, TG <200 mg/dL
Approach: Diet <30% fat, <7% saturated fat, <200 mg/day cholesterol; specific drug therapy targeted to lipid profile

Weight Reduction

Goal: <120% of ideal body weight
Approach: Physical activity, diet as outlined

Smoking

Goal: Complete cessation
Approach: Behavior modification, counseling, nicotine analogues

Blood Pressure

Goal: <140/90
Approach: Weight control, physical activity, sodium restriction, antihypertensive drugs

Physical Activity

Goal: At least 30 min of moderate exercise 3 to 4 times/wk
Approach: Walking, cycling, jogging, lifestyle and work activities

---

HDL, high-density lipoprotein; LDL, low-density lipoprotein; TG, triglycerides.
Data from the American Heart Association Council Newsletter, Fall 1995.

Cigarette smoking is strongly associated with the incidence of atherosclerosis, as well as with increased morbidity and mortality rates from its coronary, cerebral, and peripheral manifestations. The mechanism for the effects of smoking is likely to involve direct toxicity of tobacco metabolites on the vascular endothelium, probably by creating oxidant stress. Diabetic patients are also at markedly increased risk for atherosclerosis, often manifesting a particularly virulent form of the disease, leading to higher rates of myocardial events, stroke, and amputation. Hypertension is another important independent risk factor for coronary atherosclerosis, with a continuous increase in relative risk associated with each increment of pressure.

Age and gender also demonstrate an important influence. The implications of age as a risk factor are clear: prevalence will continue to increase with the advancing age of the U.S. population. In addition, initial end organ manifestations tend to cluster at different ages, with coronary events often presaging peripheral disease by a decade or more. The increased risk associated with male gender and postmenopausal states in women has led to tremendous interest in the potential "atheroprotective" effects of estrogen. Hypertriglyceridemia, elevated serum fibrinogen, and hyperhomocysteinemia have also been associated with cardiovascular risk. Moderate amounts of daily physical activity appear to induce a protective effect, whereas a sedentary lifestyle has been associated with higher incidence of clinical disease. Guidelines for risk factor modification have been published and regularly updated by the American Heart Association (Box 65-2).

Pathology and Theories of Atherogenesis

The pathologic hallmark of atherosclerosis is the atherosclerotic plaque. There are several major components of plaque: smooth muscle cells, connective tissue (matrix), lipid, and inflammatory cells (predominantly macrophages). The presence of lipid within these lesions is a prominent distinguishing feature in comparison to other arteriopathies. Atherosclerotic lesions have been categorized by the varying extent of each of these components in addition to complicating features such as calcification and ulceration, which can occur in advanced plaques. An important concept linking plaque morphology with clinical events is the relationship between the fibrous cap—a layer of smooth muscle cells and connective tissue of variable thickness—and the underlying necrotic lipid core, composed of amorphous extracellular lipid, plasma proteins, and hemostatic factors.[17] The contents of this central region are markedly thrombogenic when exposed to circulating blood, such as occurs when a thin fibrous cap ruptures or ulcerates. This phenomenon is thought to be an important mechanism whereby lesions of relatively mild hemodynamic significance may be responsible for acute thrombosis and downstream tissue infarction. In fact, this sequence may be more typical for some clinical endpoints (e.g., myocardial infarction) than slow progression of lesion size, producing hemodynamic failure downstream. Longitudinal study of plaque morphology has not been possible until recently, and with further refinements in ultrasound and magnetic resonance imaging these types of data will assume an important role in clinical decision making. For the present, it is sufficiently clear that both the mechanical characteristics of the plaque as well as the degree of luminal encroachment (stenosis) it produces are of clinical importance.

The anatomic distribution of atherosclerosis is remarkably constant and is thought to reflect an important role

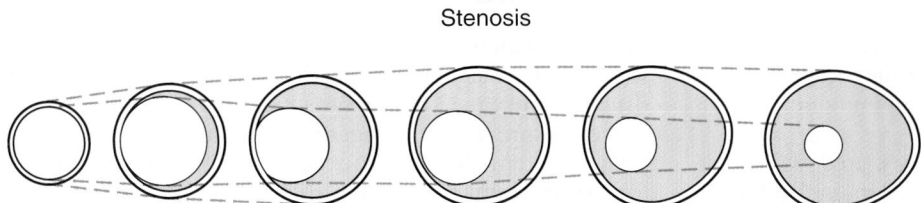

~40%
Stenosis

FIGURE 65-1. Adaptive arterial enlargement in atherosclerosis preserves luminal caliber until a critical plaque mass is reached. (Adapted from Glagov S, Weisenberg E, Zarins CK, et al: Compensatory enlargement of human atherosclerotic coronary arteries. N Engl J Med 316:1371-1375, 1987.)

for hemodynamic stresses.[19] An underlying influence of embryologic development (e.g., topographically distinct lineages of arterial smooth muscle cells in the developing circulatory system) may also be involved in this regional vulnerability. Plaques tend to be concentrated at bifurcations or bends, where local alterations in shear stress, flow separation, turbulence, and stasis are known to occur. The infrarenal abdominal aorta, proximal coronary arteries, iliofemoral arteries (especially the superficial femoral artery), carotid bifurcation, and popliteal arteries are commonly involved. Upper extremity vessels, as well as the common carotid, renal, and mesenteric arteries (beyond their origins), are usually spared.

Atherosclerotic plaques are dynamic lesions that may undergo progression or regression over time. Similarly, the underlying arterial wall also undergoes adaptive remodeling. Arterial enlargement is a well-established feature of atherosclerosis and often results in relative preservation of luminal area until plaque volume reaches a threshold size (approximately 40% stenosis) beyond which compensation fails and lumen narrowing becomes progressive (Fig. 65-1).[18] Medial atrophy may also occur, in which case mechanical stability of the wall may be impaired. This has been suggested as one possible mechanism for the known association with aneurysmal disease.

The "response to injury" hypothesis and its more recent modifications, which include the concept of endothelial cell dysfunction, is the leading theory of pathogenesis.[31] This hypothesis incorporates important roles for lipid, inflammation, and thrombosis in addition to proliferation and dysfunction of the residing cells in the arterial wall. In the earlier versions of this theory, the triggering event was thought to be a focal denuding injury to the endothelium. More recently, a widened definition of endothelial injury has been espoused to include a mechanically intact but phenotypically altered endothelial monolayer as a substrate. The source of the initial mechanical or toxic injury may be variable, with a partial list including hemodynamic stress, toxic metabolites (e.g., cigarette smoke, homocysteine), hypoxia, or infectious agents (cytomegalovirus, *Chlamydia,* herpesvirus). The final common pathway is a loss of the numerous atheroprotective effects of normal endothelium, which include its barrier function, potent antiadhesive properties, and antiproliferative influence on the underlying smooth muscle cells.

The vascular smooth muscle cell (SMC) plays a central role in the developing lesion. Migration and proliferation of medial SMCs result in a cellular neointima. The intimal SMC undergoes a phenotypic change from a contractile to a

secretory state, producing the extracellular matrix constituents of the plaque. Lipid entry and accumulation in the vessel wall is an important early event. Oxidation of lipid, particularly LDL particles, produces metabolites that potentiate the "activated" endothelial phenotype characterized by the expression of proinflammatory (e.g., leukocyte adhesion molecules) and procoagulant (e.g., tissue factor) molecules as well as producing a decrease in protective substances (e.g., nitric oxide). Circulating monocytes are recruited by adhesion to activated endothelium or to exposed matrix, enter the wall to become macrophages, and scavenge lipid. T lymphocytes are also recruited, and together these inflammatory cells elaborate an array of cytokines (especially interleukin-1, tumor necrosis factor-α, and transforming growth factor-β), which potentiate the inflammation. In addition, macrophages are important sources of matrix degrading enzymes, which may be involved in wall remodeling and plaque stability.

Platelets may adhere to dysfunctional endothelium, exposed matrix, and monocytes/macrophages. An important role for platelets and their growth-promoting and vasoactive products has long been espoused. The prototypic growth factor known as platelet-derived growth factor (PDGF) is a potent stimulator of both migration and proliferation of SMCs, and it has been identified in abundance in atherosclerotic plaques. Platelets are not the only source of PDGF: different isoforms of PDGF may also be produced by endothelial cells and by SMCs themselves. Other locally produced growth factors, in particular basic fibroblast growth factor (bFGF), are likely to play a role in the SMC hyperplasia that occurs. Amplification occurs by means of numerous potential positive feedback loops between cytokines and growth factors (both autocrine and paracrine) in which persistent inflammatory activation is the central feature.

An alternative explanation is offered by the "monoclonal hypothesis," which hinges on the intriguing observation that many atherosclerotic plaques appear to contain a clonally expanded population of SMCs.[6] The developing plaque is viewed as a benign SMC neoplasm with an associated alteration in SMC phenotype to the secretory state. Even though the observation of plaque monoclonality remains intriguing, this theory falls short in explaining all of the epidemiologic and pathologic features of atherosclerosis and is currently less favored.

Other Arteriopathies

Other causes of arterial occlusive disease, although far less common than atherosclerosis in Western societies, must also be considered, especially in patients who do not fit the risk factor profile outlined. These include thromboangiitis obliterans (Buerger's disease), Takayasu's arteritis, giant cell/temporal arteritis, and other less common vasculitides. Each of these disorders has unique clinical, radiographic, and anatomic features.[30]

Buerger's disease is exclusively associated with cigarette smoking. The disease is more prevalent in the Middle East and Asia. Occlusive lesions are predominantly seen in the muscular arteries, with a predilection for the tibial vessels. Rest pain, gangrene, and ulceration are the typical presentations. Recurrent superficial thrombophlebitis ("phlebitis migrans") is a characteristic feature. The diagnosis is suspected in younger patients who are heavy smokers and do not have other atherosclerotic risk factors. Angiography often reveals diffuse occlusion of the distal extremity vessels. The arterial involvement appears to progress in a distal to proximal fashion. Revascularization options are therefore usually limited. The disease virtually always shows clinical remission if smoking cessation can be achieved. Sympathectomy has a limited role in patients with ulcerations.

Takayasu's arteritis ("pulseless disease") commonly afflicts younger female patients and has a higher prevalence in those of Eastern European or Asian descent. There is often a prodrome marked by systemic inflammatory signs and symptoms. The arterial pathology is focused on the aorta and its major branches; several patterns of involvement are described. The brachiocephalic vessels of the arch are often diffusely involved, leading to symptoms of global cerebral hypoperfusion or upper extremity claudication. Initial management focuses on the active inflammation and is predominantly medical. Surgical treatment is often indicated for ischemic manifestations and should only be undertaken when active inflammation is under control (i.e., normalized erythrocyte sedimentation rate).

Temporal arteritis (sometimes referred to as giant cell arteritis) predominantly afflicts patients older than 50 years of age, with a slight (2:1) female preponderance. The incidence increases for each decade over age 50 years. The superficial temporal, vertebral, and major aortic arch branches may be involved. As in Takayasu's disease, there are often signs of systemic inflammation. Ischemic symptoms are common, including claudication of facial or extremity muscles and retinal ischemia. Headache is a common symptom. Blindness, usually irreversible, is a dreaded complication. Once the clinical diagnosis is suspected, treatment must be prompt and consists of high-dose corticosteroid therapy. Surgery is rarely indicated except in cases of major aortic branch involvement with ischemic symptoms.

Raynaud's phenomenon is characterized by recurrent, episodic vasospasm of the digits brought on by cold exposure or emotional stress.[10] Exposure to cold initially produces pallor of the digits, followed by cyanosis, and is accompanied by pain and paresthesias. Rewarming leads to marked rubor caused by a hyperemic response. The clinical spectrum of severity is broad and may include ulceration or loss of digits in patients with protracted periods of ischemia. Progression to tissue loss implies persistent vascular occlusions beyond the vasospastic component. Primary (Raynaud's disease) and secondary causes are recognized. Secondary Raynaud's phenomenon has been associated with a variety of rheumatologic, hematologic, and traumatic disorders, as well as a number of drugs and toxins. Treatment is centered around minimizing exposure to the triggering stimulus and pharmacologic (calcium channel blockers, sympatholytics) therapy. Sympathectomy may play a role in patients with severe digital ischemia and ulceration.

Diagnostic Modalities in Peripheral Arterial Occlusive Disease

Noninvasive Hemodynamic Assessment

Atherosclerotic plaques produce local and downstream alterations in pressure and flow that may be quantitated by a variety of noninvasive methods. A key principle in the treatment of peripheral atherosclerosis is the hemodynamic assessment of circulatory impairment, which assumes paramount importance in comparison to the anatomic presence or distribution of lesions. In current practice, the noninvasive vascular laboratory is able to provide a combination of physiologic measurements and lesion mapping, which is critical for longitudinal surveillance, patient selection for interventions, and postprocedural follow-up.

In the lower extremities, measurement of pressure plays a central role in the assessment of disease severity. Segmental pressure measurements in the limb can be used to localize and grade hemodynamically significant lesions, as well as the overall degree of circulatory impairment. The single most useful index is the ankle pressure, which can be obtained simply at the bedside with a handheld Doppler probe and pressure cuff. The cuff is placed around the lower calf just above the malleolus and the Doppler probe is positioned over the dorsalis pedis or posterior tibial arteries to obtain a flow signal. The cuff is inflated and then slowly deflated, and the examiner records the pressure at which the audible signal returns. Because the ankle pressure varies with central aortic pressure, it is commonly indexed to the brachial artery pressure as a ratio (ankle-brachial index [ABI]). The ABI is quite reproducible in a given patient and is therefore extremely useful for longitudinal surveillance of obstructive disease. In normal resting subjects, the ABI is slightly greater than unity (1.0 to 1.2). There is a correlation between the severity of signs and symptoms of arterial insufficiency and the ABI (Fig. 65-2), such that claudicants usually fall in the 0.5 to 0.7 range, whereas critical ischemia (rest pain or tissue necrosis) most commonly is associated with an ABI less than 0.4.[40] In addition to preoperative assessment, the ABI can be used to follow up patients after arterial reconstruction as a measure of technical success or subsequent graft failure. The most common source of error in the ABI is false elevation resulting from extensive vascular calcification, as is common in diabetic patients or those with chronic renal failure. In these instances, other measures of distal perfusion (e.g., toe pressures, transmetatarsal pulse volume recording,

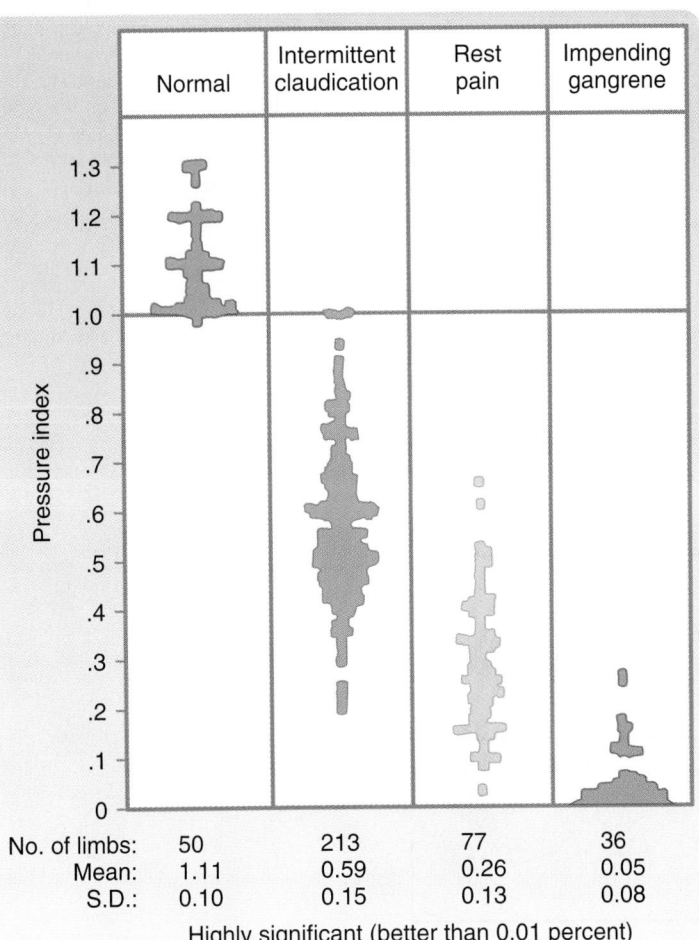

FIGURE 65-2. Correlation between signs and symptoms of lower extremity arterial insufficiency and the ankle-brachial index (ABI). (Adapted from Yao JST: Hemodynamic studies in peripheral arterial disease. Br J Surg 57:761, 1970.)

	Normal	Intermittent claudication	Rest pain	Impending gangrene
No. of limbs:	50	213	77	36
Mean:	1.11	0.59	0.26	0.05
S.D.:	0.10	0.15	0.13	0.08

Highly significant (better than 0.01 percent)

transcutaneous oximetry) may be more reliable indicators of physiologic impairment.

A more complete assessment of infrainguinal arterial disease may be obtained by the segmental pressure technique. Pneumatic cuffs are placed at several levels in the lower extremity, typically the upper thigh, lower thigh, calf, and ankle. The technique is facilitated by automated systems, which sequentially inflate and deflate the cuffs, while a Doppler probe is used to record distal flow as in the ABI technique (Fig. 65-3). Upper thigh pressures in normal patients exceed brachial pressure, and a high thigh index of less than 1.0 is highly suggestive of aortoiliac disease. Pressure gradients between adjacent levels of 30 mm Hg or greater are usually indicative of occlusion of the intervening segment. Again, false-positive results may be obtained in patients with extensive calcification. Digital (finger or toe) pressures may be obtained with appropriately sized cuffs and the use of a photoplethysmography probe on the pulp of the distal digit. Digital pressures are useful in patients with disease confined to the distal vessels (e.g., advanced Raynaud's disease with fixed obstructive lesions) or, more commonly, to help predict the likelihood of healing of forefoot procedures, ulcerations, or toe amputations. A toe pressure of greater than 30 mm Hg is predictive of successful healing in approximately 90% of cases, whereas values less than

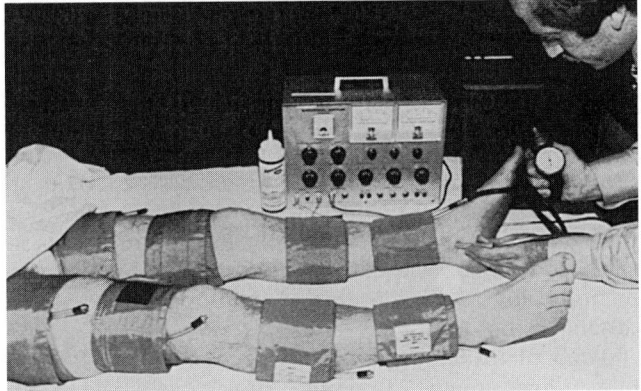

FIGURE 65-3. Technique of recording segmental limb pressures in the lower extremity. (From Summer DS, Thiele BL: The vascular laboratory. *In* Rutherford RB [ed]: Vascular Surgery, 4th ed. Philadelphia, WB Saunders, 1995, p 54.)

10 mm Hg are highly predictive of poor outcome. Values in the midrange of 10 to 30 mm Hg are not highly predictive and must be interpreted in the context of careful physical examination and clinical assessment.

Exercise (treadmill) testing may be used in patients with claudication. It is particularly useful in the evaluation of patients with atypical symptoms, normal resting pulse

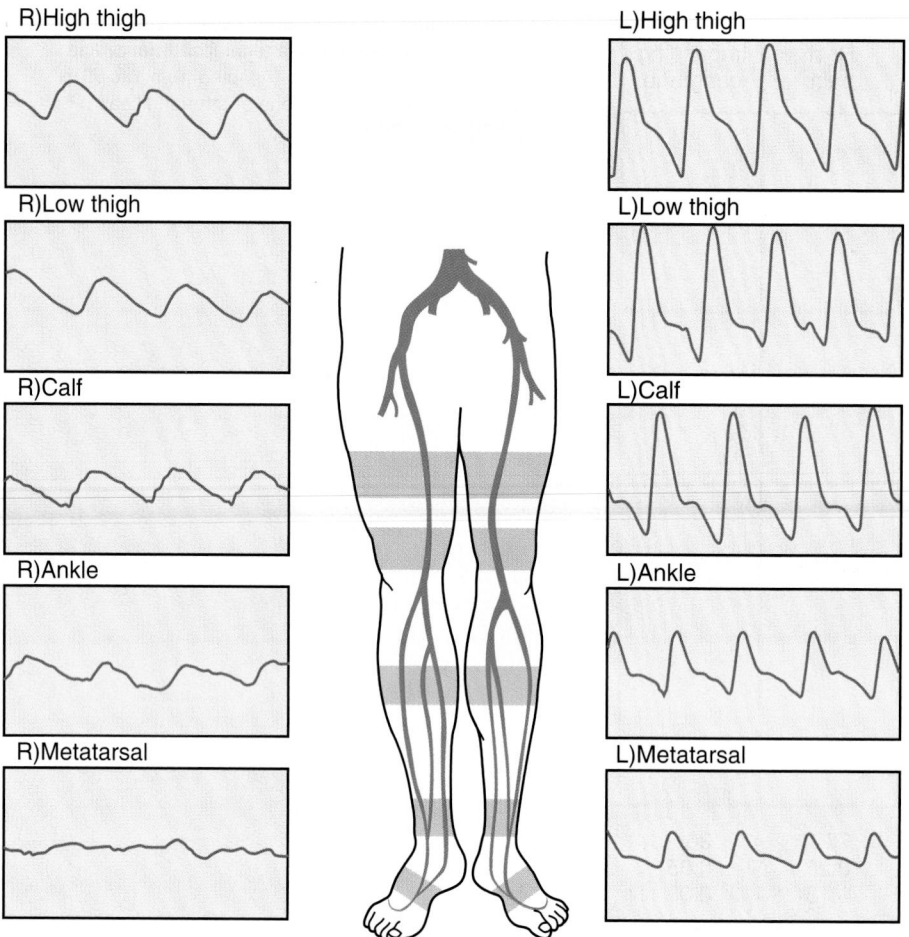

R)High thigh

R)Low thigh

R)Calf

R)Ankle

R)Metatarsal

L)High thigh

L)Low thigh

L)Calf

L)Ankle

L)Metatarsal

FIGURE 65-4. Example of PVR recordings from a normal lower extremity (left) and a patient with rest pain (right). The tracings on the right are consistent with combined aorto-iliac and femoropopliteal disease with minimal distal collateralization.

examinations, or clinical suspicion of lumbar spine disease, in which case both neurogenic and arterial causes may be present to varying extents. Patients with calf claudication resulting from superficial femoral arterial disease uniformly demonstrate a marked decrease in ankle pressure at the time of symptom occurrence as a result of the increased gradient produced by a fixed resistance in the setting of increased blood flow. A normal exercise test rules out arterial insufficiency explicitly. In addition, exercise testing has been used to quantify the degree of impairment in arterial claudication; self-reporting of walking distance is notoriously unreliable.

Limb plethysmography, which measures the fluctuation in limb volume during the cardiac cycle, is a useful adjunct to segmental pressure measurements. The most common technique involves segmental air plethysmograph cuffs, commonly referred to as a pulse volume recording (PVR). Waveform analysis (contour and amplitude) is highly predictive of upstream arterial stenosis or occlusion (Fig. 65-4). Transmetatarsal PVRs, obtained with a cuff across the forefoot, are particularly useful in diabetic patients with falsely elevated segmental limb pressures. In clinical practice, segmental pressures and PVRs are often obtained simultaneously and the information integrated by comparing adjacent segments as well as corresponding levels in the contralateral

limb. Combined with a careful history and physical examination, these basic noninvasive studies usually provide adequate data for most clinical decision making regarding the selection of patients for lower extremity revascularization.

Doppler and Duplex Ultrasonography

Ultrasound technology has revolutionized vascular imaging. The availability of high-resolution portable scanners, with scan heads accommodating a range of tissue depths, allows for noninvasive longitudinal assessment of virtually the entire circulatory tree outside of the thoracic aorta. Duplex ultrasound combines the traditional B-mode two-dimensional image with Doppler measurement of blood flow parameters. Doppler relies on a measured frequency shift, which correlates with the velocity of flow. The B-mode image is used to guide placement of the Doppler sampling volume at different locations, and the resulting frequency or velocity profile can be used to grade the severity of obstructive lesions. A color scale can also be used to visually assess locations of low velocity, high velocity, or turbulence (Fig. 65-5).

Duplex ultrasound plays a central role in several areas of vascular practice. The most common application is for carotid bifurcation disease, which is discussed in Chapter

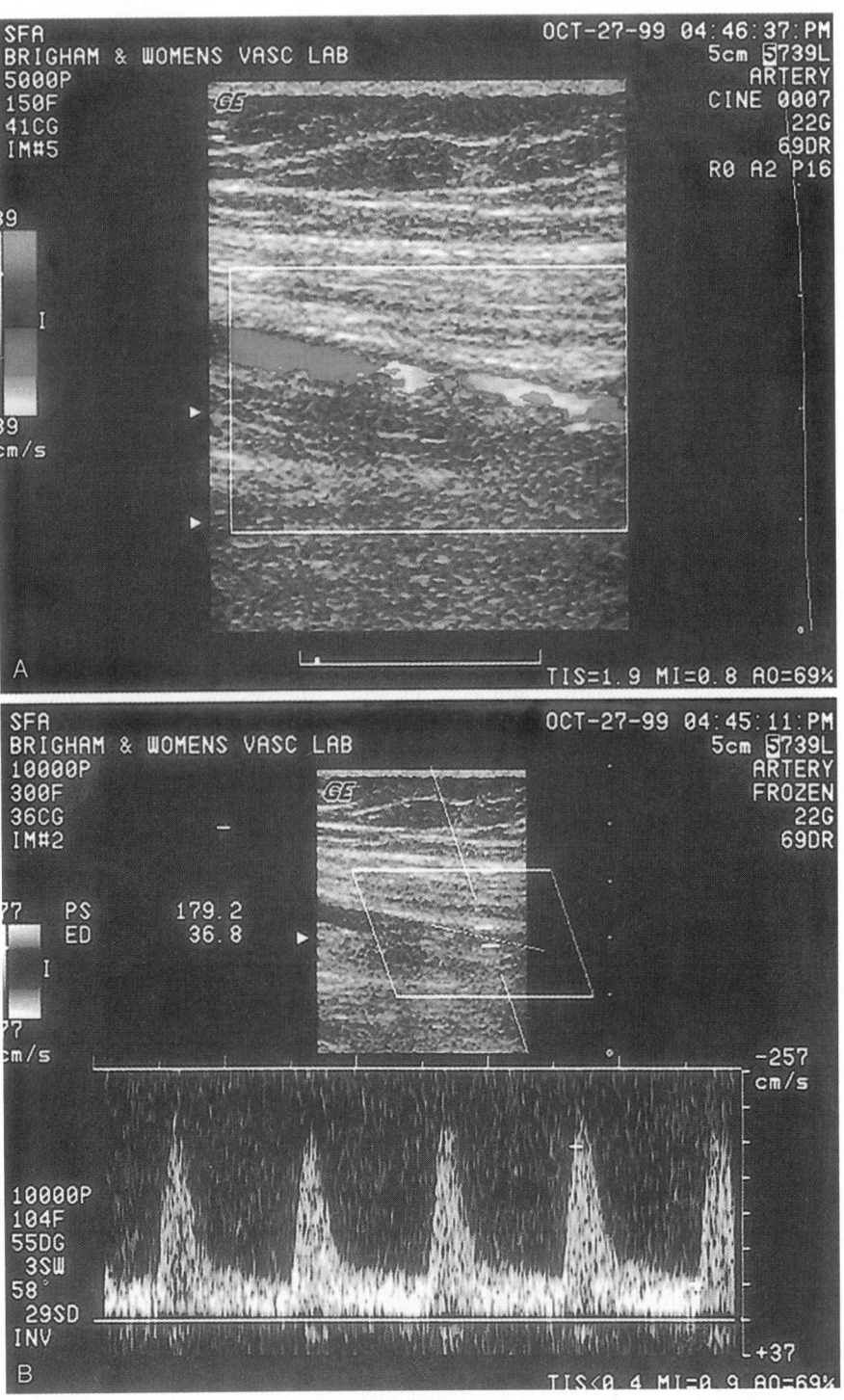

FIGURE 65-5.   Color Duplex ultrasound images with Doppler velocity profiles. **A,** High-grade lesion in the superficial femoral artery as demonstrated by turbulent flow and high peak systolic velocities (PSV). **B,** A focal vein graft stenosis is identified by elevated PSV compared with adjacent segment.

63. In abdominal and extremity vascular disease, its use is continually expanding. Compared with the other noninvasive techniques discussed earlier, duplex scanning allows for precise anatomic localization of lesions, quantitates their severity, and, with the development of higher-resolution systems, can assess plaque morphology. Color-flow imaging facilitates the examination by allowing the technician to rapidly identify deeper vessels and by demonstrating areas of turbulence where high-grade lesions are likely to reside. Although the instrumentation has undergone tremendous technologic refinement, operator skill and training remains an important variable in accuracy. The abdominal aorta, renal and mesenteric vessels, iliac arteries, and infrainguinal vessels can all be visualized. Overlying bowel gas is a common technical limitation for the abdominal vessels. Lower extremity duplex arterial mapping has been touted as an imaging strategy to determine patient suitability for angioplasty or

bypass; however, the examination of an entire extremity is time consuming and has significant operator-dependent variables. It does not provide the same global measure of limb perfusion as segmental pressures or PVRs, and it remains inferior to angiographic techniques for pre-operative planning. In summary, duplex imaging is most useful to assess the anatomy and severity of native arterial lesions in defined locations within the vascular tree, particularly the carotid bifurcation and the renal and femoral arteries.

A critical application of duplex scanning is in the postoperative assessment of lower extremity vein bypass grafts. Numerous studies have demonstrated improved long-term graft patency and limb salvage when failing (i.e., stenotic) grafts are detected and revised before occlusion. Identification of patent but failing vein grafts by clinical examination alone, including serial ABI measurement, is relatively insensitive. Color-flow imaging of the entire graft, including proximal and distal arteries and anastomotic regions, provides a complete map of any flow disturbances or developing stenoses. Velocity criteria have been developed for high-grade lesions that may warrant either more intensive surveillance, arteriography, or intervention to prevent failure. Focal areas of high velocity (peak systolic velocity >300 cm/sec or velocity ratio [lesion/upstream] >3.5) or overall low velocity (<40 cm/sec) throughout the graft are usually indicative of a critical hemodynamic lesion.[3] By generating detailed velocity maps of a given graft, individual lesions can be followed up over time for progression. In most high-volume vascular surgery practices, this technique has proved valuable in identifying and treating focal hyperplastic lesions with a variety of surgical (patch angioplasty, jump or interposition grafting) or radiologic (angioplasty) techniques, thereby improving long-term patency and reducing the need for difficult "re-do" bypass surgery.

Transcutaneous Oximetry

Transcutaneous measurement of oxygen tension (tcPo$_2$) is another technique for assessing tissue perfusion. Small polarographic electrodes are applied to the skin in a number of locations, usually including the torso (control), thigh, calf, and dorsum of the foot. The electrodes measure oxygen diffused to the skin, which is a reflection of underlying tissue perfusion but is also affected by numerous other variables, including skin temperature, sympathetic tone, skin conditions such as cellulitis or hyperkeratosis, and edema. These variables limit the reproducibility of the examination. Nonetheless, tcPo$_2$ measurement has a role in the assessment of critical ischemia, particularly in diabetic patients with extensive vascular calcification. Normal tcPo$_2$ levels in the foot are in the 50 to 60 mm Hg range. Values greater than 40 mm Hg are predictive for healing of foot lesions or primary forefoot amputations; values less than 10 mm Hg are almost universally associated with failure to heal. As in the case of toe pressures, values in the middle range are not particularly useful as isolated measurements and must be placed in clinical context.

Arteriography

The modern era of arterial reconstruction was made possible by the development of contrast arteriography (Moniz, 1927; dos Santos, 1929), which allowed for anatomic localization of aneurysmal and occlusive lesions and their relationship to symptoms. Technologic advances in catheters, contrast agents, radiographic equipment, and image processing have led to greatly improved safety and high-resolution imaging of virtually the entire circulatory tree.

Aortic and lower extremity arteriograms are generally performed by needle puncture of the femoral or brachial arteries, followed by guide wire placement and catheter insertion using the Seldinger technique. Most diagnostic studies are performed using catheters passed through 5-French (1.7 mm outer diameter) sheaths. After fluoroscopic catheter positioning, radiopaque contrast medium is injected by a timed mechanical injector, and images are obtained rapidly by digital acquisition. Full examination of the abdominal aorta and lower extremities usually requires multiple injections because there is a need for different catheter positions, projections, and patient stations to obtain optimal images. A large variety of highly specialized guide wires and catheters have been developed to assist surgeons in selective cannulation of remote vessels (e.g., renal, mesenteric, cerebral, and pulmonary vasculature). Postprocessing of digital images allows for subtraction of overlying bone and other enhancements to facilitate visualization of the vessels and lesions in question.

Complications of arteriography can be divided into those related to the catheterization and those related to the injected contrast agent (Box 65-3). The major complications of catheter placement are atheroembolization and puncture site problems (bleeding, pseudoaneurysm, or arteriovenous fistula). Distal embolization may occur by dislodgment of plaque by the catheter as it is passed or manipulated within the arterial system. Atheroemboli from the proximal (thoracic or upper abdominal) aorta can produce devastating effects if they shower into the

---

Box 65-3. Complications of Contrast Arteriography

Puncture Site or Catheter Related

Hemorrhage/hematoma
Pseudoaneurysm
Arteriovenous fistula
Atheroembolization
Local thrombosis

Contrast Agent Related

Major (anaphylactoid) sensitivity reaction
Minor sensitivity reactions
Vasodilation/hypotension
Nephrotoxicity
Hypervolemia (osmotic load)

renal or mesenteric circulations where bowel infarction or renal failure may ensue. Debris traveling into the lower extremities usually lodges in the most distal vessels of the toes, resulting in the classic appearance of "blue toe syndrome." The skin lesions produced are usually exquisitely painful and the extent of tissue loss, which is often overestimated by the initial appearance, may ultimately require toe or even forefoot amputation. This complication occurs in only a small fraction of cases.

Puncture site complications are relatively infrequent after diagnostic studies, being more commonly associated with the larger-caliber sheaths required for catheter-based interventions (i.e., angioplasty, stents). The key is prevention, which begins with appropriate selection of the arterial site for cannulation, a minimally traumatic needle/guide wire/catheter insertion, and adequate management of hemostasis after catheter removal. Significant bleeding or pseudoaneurysm formation can almost always be attributed to either a technical difficulty or to the need for persistent systemic anticoagulant or antiplatelet drugs. An arteriovenous fistula can result from inadvertent passage of the needle and guide wire through an adjacent vein en route to the artery. Diagnosis is suggested by the physical findings of a pulsatile mass or continuous bruit and is easily confirmed by duplex imaging. The management of these various puncture site complications is individualized and depends on the stability of the patient, the requirement for continuous anticoagulation, and other factors. Patients with hemodynamically significant bleeding, expanding hematomas, large pseudoaneurysms, or local complications caused by pressure on adjacent nerves or skin or patients requiring intensive continuous anticoagulation are best managed with early surgery. The vessel is exposed and the puncture site repaired by direct suture. Rarely, a prosthetic patch repair may be required, usually in the setting of severe injury to a badly calcified atherosclerotic vessel where primary repair is either impossible or would produce narrowing. For stable pseudoaneurysms in patients without coagulopathy, ultrasound-guided compression has been highly successful as sole therapy. Most recently, ultrasound-directed thrombin injection into the sac has been reported as a rapid and highly successful technique for pseudoaneurysms.

Contrast agents may produce both minor and major adverse reactions.[1] Conventional iodinated agents have direct toxic effects on endothelium because of their high osmolarity (five to eight times normal plasma osmolarity). Newer low-osmolarity (nonionic) agents have approximately one third the osmolarity of the older media. Intravascular injection of contrast agent causes vasodilation (sensation of heat) with a concomitant decrease in blood pressure. Many patients experience discomfort during injection, which is thought to be attributable to the osmolarity. Idiosyncratic reactions to the contrast medium occur in approximately 4% of patients. They are not dose related and may be either serious (anaphylaxis) or minor (nausea, urticaria, pruritus). Major reactions are rare; they must be recognized and treated promptly with airway control, corticosteroids, and cardiopulmonary support. The incidence of minor reactions appears to be reduced with low-osmolarity agents. Patients with a prior history of allergy to contrast agents or iodine (e.g., shellfish) or those with asthma are at higher risk.

Renal toxicity is an important adverse consequence of contrast arteriography. The mechanism is unknown and may involve renal ischemia resulting from the osmotic diuresis produced or direct toxic effects on tubular epithelium. Assessment of risk and preangiography preparation are critical. Factors associated with elevated risk include chronic renal insufficiency (baseline creatinine >1.5), diabetes, dehydration, age older than 60 years, recent surgery, and larger doses of contrast medium. The risk factors appear additive. Maintenance of adequate hydration before, during, and after contrast injection is absolutely critical and is best accomplished by continuous intravenous administration of isotonic crystalloid. Nonionic agents appear to have less renal toxicity and should be selected in high-risk patients. The major limitation of these agents is their markedly increased cost compared with conventional media.

Computed tomography (CT) with intravenous contrast medium administration can also delineate vascular anatomy. Specific protocols for timed injection and rapid image acquisition (i.e., spiral CT angiography) have improved the resolution. Three-dimensional reconstructions are possible that may be particularly helpful in highly tortuous vessels and aneurysms. The technique has been most useful for the thoracoabdominal aorta and carotid bifurcations (Fig. 65-6). Dissection and aneurysmal

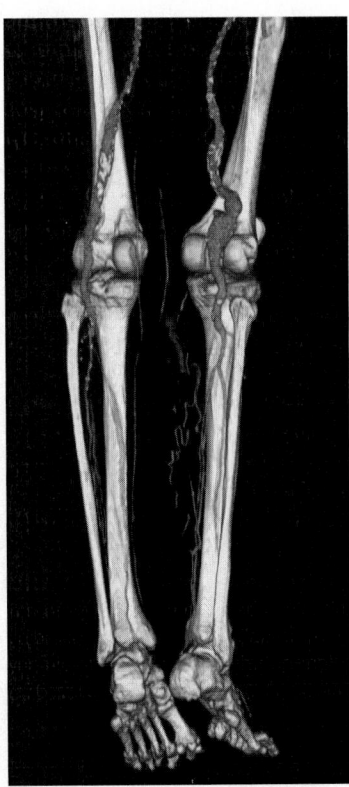

FIGURE 65-6. CT angiogram of lower extremity arteries with three-dimensional reconstruction reveals bilateral popliteal artery aneurysms. (Courtesy of Joseph Schoepf, M.D., and Edgar K. Yucel, M.D., Brigham and Women's Hospital.)

diseases of the aorta are particularly well suited, in that the pathologic process spans a longer segment and is less likely to be missed between adjacent slices. It has had limited use in aortoiliac or infrainguinal occlusive disease.

Magnetic resonance angiography (MRA) is an important technique that is gaining application by virtue of rapidly improving technology. It offers the distinct advantages of being noninvasive and avoiding contrast exposure. The most common technique used for obtaining vascular enhancement is time-of-flight (TOF), in which brightness is directly related to the velocity of blood entering the slice. As a result, lesion severity is often overestimated, which is an important limitation. The technique has had its greatest application thus far in evaluating the carotid and intracranial circulation, thoracoabdominal aorta, renal arteries, and lower extremity vessels (Fig. 65-7). It is the test of choice for studying arteriovenous malformations or the major abdominal veins (e.g., for planning portal decompression procedures). Lower extremity studies are primarily limited by the prolonged acquisition times required if the equivalent of an aortogram with leg runoff is needed. When the examination can be more limited, as in the preoperative assessment of distal runoff in a patient with a normal femoral pulse, its utility is increased. MRA is particularly useful in patients who are at high risk for contrast-induced nephropathy, particularly elderly diabetics.

Therapeutic Interventions in Arterial Occlusive Disease

The modern therapeutic armamentarium for treating arterial occlusive diseases is barely half a century old. Its devel-

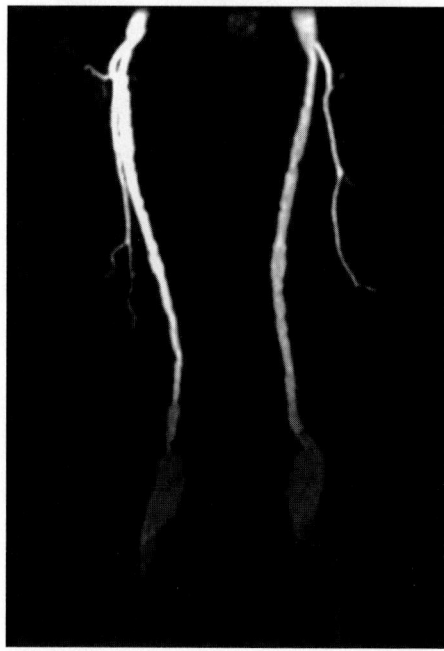

FIGURE 65-7.   MR angiogram with gadolinium enhancement of femoropopliteal vessels in a patient with bilateral popliteal artery aneurysm. (Courtesy of Servet Tatli, M.D., and Edgar K. Yucel, M.D., Brigham and Women's Hospital.)

opment is marked by several key advances: the discovery of heparin, arteriography (Moniz, 1927), arterial homografts (DeBakey, 1950s), prosthetic grafts (Voorhees, 1952), balloon angioplasty (Gruntzig, 1974), and stents (Dotter, 1969), combined with a continuous improvement in instruments and suture materials to facilitate vascular anastomoses.

Medical Management

The medical management of atherosclerosis is targeted to reduce progression, induce regression, and prevent morbid endpoints of lesion formation. Risk factor management is the primary approach. Lipid-lowering therapy uses both dietary treatment and an increasing pharmacopeia with specific effects on different lipid subclasses. These drugs include niacin, bile acid–binding resins, HMG-CoA reductase inhibitors (the statins), clofibrate, and gemfibrozil. The specific dietary and drug regimen is tailored to the lipid profile abnormality of the individual patient. Smoking cessation is clearly of paramount importance. Newer nicotine analogues, available in a variety of sustained-release delivery forms, may be helpful, but long-term success hinges on behavior modification.

Antiplatelet therapy constitutes the other major medical treatment option. The goal is to prevent thrombosis, embolization, and perhaps even the progression of atherosclerotic disease given the possible role of platelets as an etiologic factor. Aspirin remains the cornerstone of platelet therapy, with a well-established track record of compliance, low risk, and minimal cost. Large meta-analyses have demonstrated beneficial effects of aspirin in patients with prior myocardial infarctions, carotid atheroembolism, and peripheral arterial surgery.[2] Newer antiplatelet agents have been developed with ever-increasing potency and more specific antiaggregative effects. These include ticlopidine and clopidogrel, both of which have shown efficacy in reducing some cardiovascular endpoints. Oral antagonists of the platelet glycoprotein IIb/IIIa receptor for fibrinogen, the critical interaction required for aggregation, are being extensively studied primarily in patients with coronary interventions. The long-term roles for these newer agents remains to be defined, especially given their increased cost and lower safety profile as compared with aspirin. For the present, low-dose aspirin (325 mg/day) is the most widely accepted antiplatelet prophylaxis for patients with cardiovascular disease.

Basic Techniques of Arterial Surgery

Technical success in arterial reconstructive surgery hinges on the meticulous application of basic techniques of handling and suturing blood vessels. Arterial incisions are preferentially placed in soft areas of the vessel wall spared of disease. The choice of orientation (i.e., longitudinal or transverse) of the arteriotomy depends on the vessel size, the local extent of disease, and the reconstructive technique being used. Primary closure of longitudinal incisions may result in narrowing; hence these are often closed with a vein or prosthetic patch. In the case of thromboembolectomy of otherwise normal arteries, transverse incisions are often used in the larger (e.g., iliofemoral) vessels; longitudinal incisions with patch angioplasty are more forgiving in smaller vessels. In general, the longitudinal incision offers more flexibility for extension to deal with local disease or to accommodate a bypass graft anastomosis.

Suture materials for vascular surgery are nonabsorbable (e.g., polypropylene). A practice of minimal handling of the arterial wall, using specially designed vascular forceps (e.g., DeBakey), minimizes separation or fragmentation of plaque that can complicate the exercise. Suture bites must incorporate all layers of the vessel wall, with care taken to ensure the intima is included. The needle should pass through the wall at a right angle and then be gently rotated along its curvature to draw the suture through. Shallow angled bites, levering of the needle, or rough handling of the suture can produce a localized linear tear in an atherosclerotic vessel. In performing a primary closure of an arteriotomy, the bites are closely spaced and of appropriate depth to produce hemostasis without narrowing. Slight, gentle eversion of the edges is important and is facilitated by the assistant who maintains traction on the suture. In the case of a vein or prosthetic patch, the edges must be carefully everted onto the arterial wall to avoid leaks between sutures. The choice of suturing technique (i.e., continuous or interrupted) is dependent on vessel size and surgical preference. Interrupted sutures may be preferred in small-caliber vessels because they avoid the "pursestring" effect of a continuous stitch, which may produce a degree of narrowing. For larger arteries and in most cases of patch angioplasty or bypass grafting, a carefully done continuous suture works well and is more efficient. In either case, sutures are usually first placed at either corner of the arteriotomy, then progressively continued to the middle. Flushing and backbleeding by release of clamps is an important maneuver to be done before completing the anastomosis, to remove any small amounts of thrombus, air, or debris.

Surgical Bypass Grafting

Surgical bypass grafting has evolved as the most widely applicable technique for the treatment of arterial occlusive lesions. It has found broad application in the coronary, abdominal, and peripheral vascular beds. In comparison to other techniques such as angioplasty, stent-

ing, or endarterectomy, bypass is far less restrictive in terms of the anatomic nature of lesions amenable to treatment (Table 65-1). Although each of these other modalities is limited in treating longer occlusions and smaller caliber vessels, these areas are precisely those where surgical bypass excels. The specific choice of percutaneous or surgical approach must be tailored to the individual patient, lesion, and the skill and experience of the operator. In current practice, a combination of these methods is frequently required to achieve the best therapeutic result; thus, familiarity with all of the techniques is fundamental to the discipline of vascular surgery. A brief discussion of general techniques and graft materials follows; for more detailed technical descriptions the reader is referred to one of the standard vascular surgical texts or atlases.[32]

Anatomic exposure of the selected inflow and outflow arteries is obtained through standard incisions in the abdomen or extremities. Complete circumferential dissection is not always required and, in some situations (e.g., aorta, iliac arteries, reoperative exposures), carries unnecessary additional risk because of the presence of immediately adjacent major venous structures. Despite arteriographic appearances, the presence of significant plaque or calcification may require modifying the original operative strategy. Whenever possible, segments bearing minimal disease are selected for anastomotic sites because this greatly facilitates both vascular occlusion as well as suturing. The outflow site is selected to be downstream from all hemodynamically significant disease, in the most readily accessible vessel that can provide downstream perfusion. Shorter grafts are preferable, particularly when autogenous vein conduit is in limited supply. Numerous techniques are available for occlusion and depend to great extent on the size of the vessel, the arterial pressure, and the presence or severity of plaque (especially calcification). These methods include the application of atraumatic vascular clamps, elastic vessel loops, intraluminal occluders, or an extremity tourniquet.

Systemic anticoagulation, by intravenous administration of heparin sodium, is achieved before vascular occlusion. Standard heparin doses are in the range of 70 to 100 units/kg as a bolus. Repeated doses may be necessary depending on the length of the operation and the requirement for additional periods of flow occlusion. The half-life of heparin ranges from 60 to 90 minutes in most patients, which is a suitable interval for redosing with smaller

TABLE 65-1. Comparison of Arterial Reconstructive Techniques by Most Favorable Anatomic Features of Treated Lesions

	Bypass	Endarterectomy	PTA/Stenting
Stenosis vs. occlusion	Either	Stenosis > occlusion	Stenosis > occlusion
Length of segment	Not a factor	Preferably short	Preferably short
Vessel caliber	>2 mm	Preferably >5-6 mm	Preferably >4 mm
Anatomic sites most suitable	Aortic arch through distal extremity	Carotid bifurcation, common femoral, aortic branch lesions	Distal abdominal aorta and iliacs, aortic branch lesions (?? femoral/popliteal, carotid)

PTA, percutaneous transluminal angioplasty; ??, controversial application of PTA.

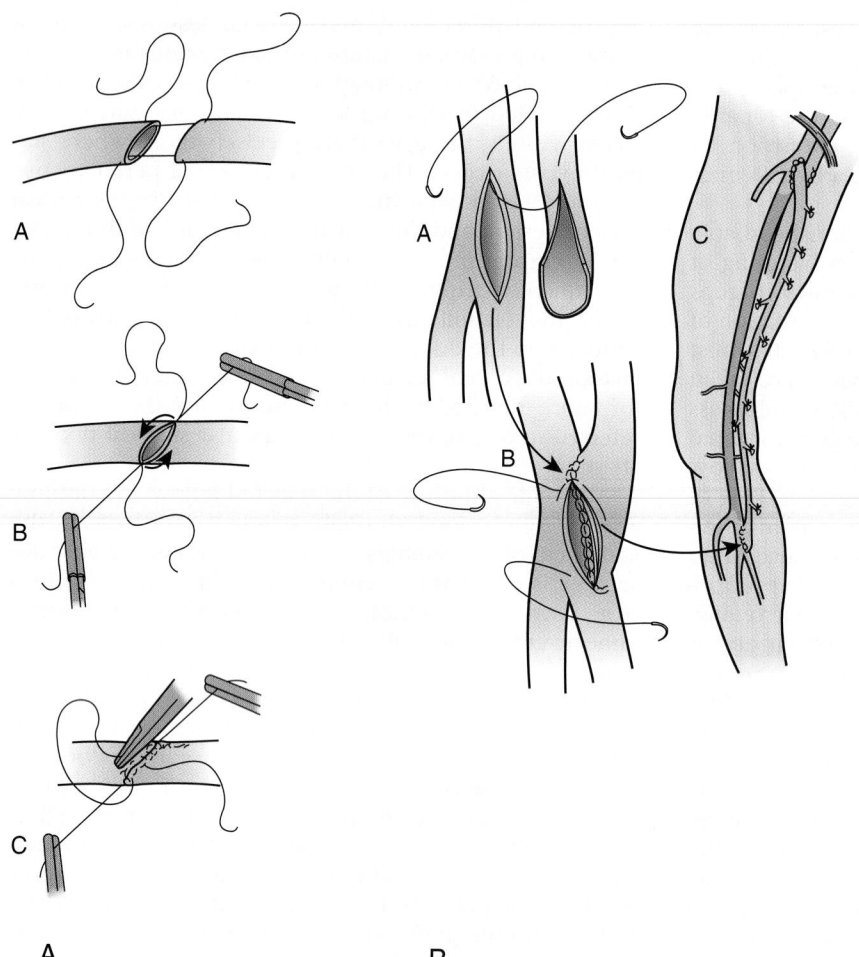

FIGURE 65-8. Techniques of constructing artery-to-graft anastomoses. **A,** End-to-end technique employing spatulation and corner sutures. **B,** End-to-side anastomosis employing a two-suture, continuous technique.

boluses (one third to one half the initial dose is typical). Measurement of the activated clotting time (ACT) is readily accomplished using standard equipment available in most cardiovascular operating suites and facilitates appropriate heparin dosing during longer procedures. For peripheral vascular operations, an ACT in the 250- to 350-second range is adequate. At the conclusion of the procedure, when hemostasis is desired, it may be necessary to reverse the effects of heparin by administration of protamine sulfate (dose: 1 mg/100 units of circulating heparin).

The arteriotomy is preferably made in a disease-free area; poorly chosen sites or ill-advised extension into areas of heavy plaque may greatly complicate the operation. Anastomoses are most commonly performed either in an end-to-side or end-to-end configuration (Fig. 65-8). The end-to-side approach has broader application and is somewhat more forgiving technically. End-to-end anastomoses are facilitated by slightly beveling the two ends (45 degrees) to enlarge the opening and by the use of interrupted sutures to avoid a pursestring effect of continuous suture. End-to-side configurations are usually made at an entry angle of less than 45 degrees to minimize turbulence. The graft is appropriately beveled, and the heel sutures are placed first. One or two sutures may

be used to complete the anastomosis; in the two-suture technique, a separate stitch is placed at the toe, which is the most critical point at which one must avoid narrowing.

Intraoperative assessment of the bypass is critical to both short- and long-term outcome. For lower extremity bypass, completion arteriography is the "gold standard." Duplex scanning is finding an ever-increasing role in the operating suite and provides greater resolution of intraluminal defects as well as flow velocity mapping. In either case, the anastomotic sites, conduit, and distal runoff are examined for intraluminal defects (thrombus, valves, plaque, emboli), extrinsic compression or kinks (tunneling errors), and technical adequacy.

The optimal choice of graft material depends on the anatomic location, size, and hemodynamic environment of the bypass. The "ideal" vascular graft would be characterized by both its mechanical attributes and postimplantation healing responses. Mechanical strength is a paramount issue in that grafts placed in the arterial circulation must be capable of withstanding long-term hemodynamic stress without material failure, which might be catastrophic. Availability, suturability, and simplicity of handling are desirable for minimizing operating time, risk, and expense. The graft should be resistant to both thrombosis and infection and, optimally, would be completely incorporated by the body to yield a neovessel resembling a native artery in structure and function. Given the economic considerations, low cost and long-term durability are issues of great importance as well.

For large-caliber arterial reconstructions, currently available synthetic grafts made of either Dacron or expanded polytetrafluoroethylene (PTFE) offer a reasonable approximation of these ideals and proven clinical efficacy. Long-term results of synthetic grafts for replacement of the thoracic and abdominal aorta, arch vessels, and iliac and common femoral arteries for either aneurysmal or occlusive disease are generally excellent using any of a number of materials and manufacturing processes. Whereas graft infection, occlusion, and dilatation are important clinical problems, the majority of patients can expect durable patency and a low frequency of repeat procedures. However, prosthetic grafts have generally proven unfavorable as small-caliber (<6 mm) arterial substitutes. In these demanding, low-flow environments, the primary factor influencing long-term patency is the conduit itself, and the thromboresistance of endothelialized autogenous materials becomes paramount.

Autogenous vein, particularly the greater saphenous, has proven to be a durable and versatile arterial substitute. In the lower extremity, long-term results with saphenous vein bypass (used in either the in situ or reversed configurations) to below-knee popliteal, tibial, and even pedal arteries have been excellent and serve as the standard of reference for other conduits. Ectopic (i.e., lesser saphenous, arm veins) or composite vein grafts for infrapopliteal bypass are generally inferior to a single segment saphenous vein, although they are still superior to the performance of synthetic grafts in the hands of most surgeons. Randomized trials of prosthetic grafts in the femoropopliteal position have demonstrated reasonable patency rates, particularly in the above-knee position, where they provide a viable alternative. Tibial bypass with prosthetics has generally achieved markedly inferior results and should only be considered in extreme circumstances.

The most important complications of surgical bypass are graft occlusion and infection. Graft occlusion is covered in detail later in this chapter. Infection of vascular grafts may be catastrophic and poses immediate threat to both life and limb. Death may occur by sudden and massive hemorrhage internally or externally. Limb loss may result from secondary thrombosis or failure of attempted redo procedures after graft removal. Prosthetic grafts may become infected by break in sterile technique at implantation, hematogenous seeding from other sources, or wound complications resulting secondarily in exposure of the graft. By and large, these often require complete excision of the infected prosthetic and alternative revascularization approaches that avoid the contaminated field. Vein grafts are far less commonly afflicted by infection, which occurs almost exclusively in the context of a local wound complication resulting in exposed graft. These are best treated aggressively by operative wound débridement, segmental graft replacement if necessary, and adequate soft tissue coverage.

Surgical Endarterectomy

Endarterectomy is a direct disobliterative technique that takes advantage of the pathologic localization of atherosclerosis to the intima and inner media. This allows a cleavage plane to be easily developed between the plaque and the underlying deeper media (Fig. 65-9). Surprisingly, the residual deep media and adventitia normally retain sufficient mechanical strength to resist disruption or progressive enlargement under arterial pressure. The various techniques used all involve blunt separation of the plaque, termination by spontaneous tapering or sharp division, and careful attention to the distal endpoint, which must be firmly adherent to resist dissection or flap elevation leading to thrombosis. The most common and technically simplest technique is the open method, performed by way of a longitudinal arteriotomy with direct vision of both endpoints as well as the entire endarterectomized surface. Extraction, eversion, and semiclosed methods are applicable in specific situations as well.

Endarterectomy is most feasible and durable when applied to focal stenotic lesions in large-caliber, high-flow vessels. The carotid bifurcation, visceral artery origins, and common femoral artery are particularly well suited to this approach. The use of endarterectomy for longer-segment disease in the aortoiliac and femoropopliteal systems has fallen into disfavor because of the technical difficulty, higher failure rates, and clear advantages demonstrated for bypass grafting in these locations. It offers the advantage of an autogenous reconstruction, avoiding the risk of infection associated with prosthetics.

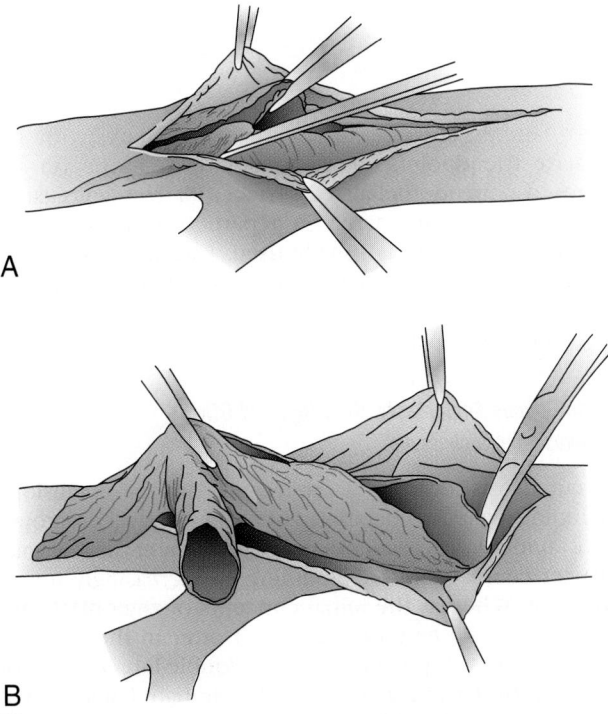

FIGURE 65-9. Technique of endarterectomy. **A,** Initial separation of plaque in the appropriate cleavage plane with mobilization facilitated by a fine spatula. **B,** Termination of endarterectomy by feathering to a tapered endpoint.

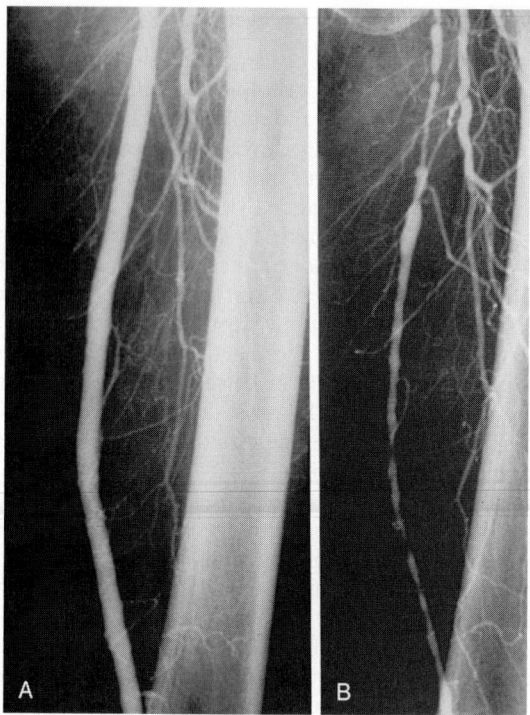

FIGURE 65-10.   Restenosis after long-segment endarterectomy of the superficial femoral artery (SFA). **A,** Completion operative angiogram after semi-closed endarterectomy of SFA using a loop stripper. **B,** Follow-up arteriogram 8 months later, when symptoms of claudication had recurred. A vigorous intimal hyperplastic response is evident.

Early failures are due to technical problems with the imperfect endpoints or to in situ thrombosis on the exposed nonendothelialized surface. Platelet aggregation to the collagenous matrix is a particular problem, and antiplatelet therapy is usually used. Late failures are due to exuberant intimal hyperplasia, which is a more frequent occurrence in longer segments of muscular arteries (e.g., superficial femoral) (Fig. 65-10).

Percutaneous Angioplasty, Stenting, and Other Endovascular Techniques

Percutaneous techniques for treating arterial occlusions, including balloon dilatation, stenting, and atherectomy, have undergone tremendous development in the past quarter century and are assuming an increasingly important role. Whereas the initial concepts of angioplasty and stenting can be first attributed to Dotter in the 1960s, it was the development of the double-lumen balloon catheter by Gruntzig in 1974 that initiated widespread clinical application. The use of balloon angioplasty in the treatment of coronary, renal, iliac, and lower extremity disease has come to be accepted as a standard alternative to open surgical therapy.

The mechanism of dilation in balloon angioplasty is thought to involve fracture and displacement of plaque and overstretch of the media and perhaps the adventitia as well. Specific guide wires, catheters, and balloons have been designed for different anatomic sites. The initial technical feat is to accomplish crossing of the lesion with a guide wire, followed by appropriate positioning of the balloon catheter. The balloon must be of adequate length to encompass the lesion and its diameter matched to that of the normal vessel to avoid overdistention (leading to rupture) or inadequate dilation. Low-profile balloon systems have allowed for smaller introducer sheaths, reducing puncture site complications.

Similar to endarterectomy, percutaneous transluminal angioplasty (PTA) has found its greatest success in the treatment of focal stenoses in large-caliber, high-flow arteries. The 5-year patency rate for PTA (without stenting) of common iliac lesions, for example, is in the 70% to 80% range. Excellent results have also been reported for suitable aortic, arch vessel, renal, and mesenteric lesions. Results in the femoropopliteal system are inferior to bypass overall, but carefully selected lesions, primarily in claudicants, may be durably treated. In all anatomic locations, both early and late success is increased for shorter lesions and stenoses as compared with occlusions.

Restenosis after angioplasty may be due to both elastic recoil and intimal hyperplasia. In the coronary circulation, clinically significant restenosis may develop in as many as 40% of patients within the first year, necessitating repeat revascularization. Promising methods for limiting restenosis include the more liberal use of stents to minimize elastic recoil and constrictive remodeling and approaches targeting the cellular response by local delivery of antiproliferative agents (e.g., drug-eluting stents) or ionizing radiation (brachytherapy).

Intravascular stents have secured an important niche in the vascular armamentarium. The mechanical concept is to maintain luminal patency by exerting persistent radial force on the vessel. Metallic stents come in a variety of design configurations and sizes. For purposes of placement, they may be grouped into those that require balloon inflation (e.g., the Palmaz stent) and those that do not (e.g., the Wallstent). Stents are most commonly used as an adjunct to PTA, although their application as a primary modality is increasing. Localized dissections, elastic recoil, or residual stenoses after PTA are situations in which stent placement can often improve the technical result. The superiority of stents over PTA alone remains to be proven but appears likely for longer-segment iliac lesions as well as ostial lesions of the aortic branch vessels. Recent interest has developed in the use of stents to treat carotid bifurcation disease, although long-term data and results from randomized trials are pending. The anatomic sites most suitable for stenting are similar to those mentioned for endarterectomy. Because stent application is increasing and recurrences are no longer amenable to endarterectomy, the benefits of either approach must be carefully evaluated to avoid harming patients. Longer-term data are clearly needed to determine the appropriate indications.[49]

Another technique is catheter-directed atherectomy. This involves the use of specially designed catheter devices to remove atherosclerotic plaque from the arterial wall by shaving, cutting, or high-speed rotational ablation. Laser energy has also been advocated to vaporize and debulk plaque in heavily stenosed or occluded vessels before PTA. In general, long-term results in the lower extremity vessels have been poor and there does not appear to be an advantage over PTA alone, which is less expensive and has fewer complications. Atherectomy is sometimes used for debulking of restenotic lesions, particularly in the coronary circulation, but repeated treatments are not infrequently required as a result of recurrence of the hyperplastic response. Further applications will require substantial progress in the prevention and treatment of intimal hyperplasia.

Thrombolytic Therapy

Fibrinolytic drugs enhance conversion of plasminogen to plasmin, which is then capable of degrading fibrin clot. These agents have been used in both systemic and local fashion to achieve lysis of both arterial and venous thrombi. Except for acute embolic events, thrombolytic therapy for arterial occlusive disease is not a sole modality. Rather, it is used as an important adjunct to PTA or surgical interventions that directly address the underlying atherosclerotic lesions, restoring perfusion to the downstream bed. The two major drugs in current use are urokinase and tissue plasminogen activator (tPA).

For arterial occlusions, regional therapy by means of an angiographically guided catheter is most effective. Compared with systemic administration, directed intra-clot infusion has been shown to reduce the dose and duration of therapy required to achieve complete lysis. The catheter may be positioned just proximal to or directly into the thrombus. Different dosing regimens and catheters have been espoused for the available agents. Generally, an initial high-dose infusion (lacing-dose) is followed by a lower-dose regimen, with frequent follow-up angiograms to document progressive lysis to a satisfactory endpoint. Systemic anticoagulation with continuous heparin administration must be maintained throughout, so that new thrombus is not formed on, around, or distal to the catheter as lysis is taking place. Because of the significant risks of bleeding as well as the need for careful monitoring of the infusion catheters, patients requiring extended therapy (in some cases up to 48 hours) are best managed in an intensive care setting.

Appropriate selection of patients is critical for reducing the incidence of serious complications and improving the likelihood of successful lysis. Even with regional delivery, a state of systemic fibrinolysis is induced; therefore, patients at high risk for serious bleeding are not candidates (Box 65-4). These include patients with recent surgery, trauma, gastrointestinal or other internal bleeding, intracranial tumors, pregnancy, or recent stroke. Relative contraindications include remote gastrointestinal bleeding, hemostatic disorders, severe hypertension, or intracardiac thrombus. The risk of serious bleeding (5% to 15%) is increased with longer durations of therapy and a

---

Box 65-4. Contraindications to Thrombolytic Therapy

Absolute

Recent major bleeding
Recent stroke
Recent major surgery or trauma
Irreversible ischemia of end organ
Intracranial pathology
Recent ophthalmologic procedure

Relative

History of gastrointestinal bleeding or active peptic ulcer disease
Underlying coagulation abnormalities
Uncontrolled hypertension
Pregnancy
Hemorrhagic retinopathy

---

decrease in fibrinogen levels to less than 100 mg/dL or to less than 50% of baseline, which is associated with the development of a systemic lytic state. Fresh thrombi are the most easily lysed. Although no clear upper limit of chronicity has been established, most clinicians believe that thrombotic occlusions more than 2 weeks old are unlikely to respond well to lytic therapy.

An important consideration in evaluating patients for thrombolytic therapy is the severity of ischemia and the time interval for restoring perfusion before irreversible tissue injury has occurred. Patients with signs of irreversibility such as major neurologic impairment should not undergo attempted thrombolysis. In addition, patients with acute, rapid deterioration to advanced ischemia are often poorly collateralized and may not tolerate the time required to achieve reperfusion with this approach.

Recent large-scale trials have supported a potential useful role for thrombolytic therapy in the treatment of arterial occlusions, although many controversies remain concerning specific indications.[37] In appropriately selected patients and with a lesion-specific strategy of percutaneous or surgical intervention, thrombolytic therapy has an important role in the management of arterial occlusive disease.

ACUTE THROMBOEMBOLIC DISEASE

The management of acute extremity ischemia remains a major surgical challenge. Even with optimal surgical management, acute lower extremity ischemia resulting from thromboembolic disease continues to cause significant morbidity and mortality. Limb loss rates of 8% to 22% and perioperative mortality rates of 10% to 17% continue to be reported.[4,15,24,28] Maximization of limb salvage, while simultaneously minimizing associated morbidity and mortality, requires expeditious diagnosis and restoration of perfusion.

Pathophysiology

Compared with other organs and tissues, the extremities are relatively resistant to the effects of ischemia. Unlike the brain, which suffers infarction after only 4 to 8 minutes of ischemia, or the myocardium, which infarcts after 17 to 20 minutes, the lower extremity may be salvaged after up to 5 to 6 hours of profound ischemia.

Evaluation of the effect of ischemia on the extremity is complicated by the fact that the various tissues that comprise the extremity have different susceptibilities to ischemic injury and they manifest this injury in different fashions. Skin and bone are relatively resistant to the effects of ischemia and may survive injuries that, by their effect on other tissues, have rendered the limb painful and useless. Nervous tissue is generally the most sensitive component of the extremity to the effects of ischemia. Significant morbidity may therefore result from isolated ischemic nerve injury in an otherwise intact limb.

Skeletal muscle is the major structural component of the extremity and, for a variety of reasons, plays a key role in the pathophysiology of extremity ischemia. Skeletal muscle constitutes more than 40% of the body mass and approximately 75% of the lower extremity weight. Although skeletal muscle has a relatively slow resting metabolic rate compared with other tissues, it accounts for 90% of the metabolic activity of the lower extremity. Skeletal muscle receives 71% of the resting lower extremity blood flow and a larger proportion during reperfusion hyperemia. Skeletal muscle plays a pivotal role in the numerous local and systemic manifestations of extremity ischemia-reperfusion injury.

Reperfusion Syndrome

The profound effects of revascularization of the ischemic lower extremity were described as early as the 1950s by Haimovici.[20] As ischemic skeletal muscles reperfuse, a variety of intracellular ions, structural proteins, enzymes, and other components are released through the damaged sarcolemma into the circulation. The resulting "myonephropathic syndrome," with its associated hemodynamic instability, lactic acidosis, and hyperkalemia, is well recognized by surgeons. Myoglobin released from injured muscle cells into the circulation is cleared through the kidneys, resulting in dark urine (without red blood cells). Myoglobinuria may persist for 2 to 4 days after reperfusion. Acute renal failure may ensue from myoglobin casts developing in the renal tubules as well as direct toxic effects of the myoglobin on the tubules. Serum creatinine phosphokinase levels may increase dramatically (to greater than 10,000 units) after reperfusion of ischemic muscle. Myocardial contractility may become depressed; increased cardiac irritability in the setting of electrolyte disturbances (typically hyperkalemia) may lead to life-threatening dysrhythmias.

When a lower extremity is subjected to severe ischemia, cellular membrane dysfunction results. In this setting, the reperfusion phase is marked by the development of both intracellular and interstitial edema. Intracellular edema results from membrane damage and failure of the membrane-bound adenosine triphosphatase (ATPase). Interstitial edema results from increased microvascular membrane permeability to ions, water, and proteins. This edema may appear within minutes, progressing significantly over the next 24 hours. The amount of edema is dependent on the period of ischemia, the underlying occlusive disease, and the adequacy of revascularization. When muscle edema occurs within the confines of an osseofascial compartment, interstitial pressure continues to increase. Acute compartment syndrome results as pressure increases beyond capillary perfusion pressure (30 mm Hg) and tissue perfusion is impaired. Unless recognized and decompressed by fasciotomy, compartment syndromes will lead to prolonged tissue ischemia despite apparent successful revascularization.

Occasionally, prolongation of the ischemic injury may also occur as a result of microvascular obstruction to blood flow. Endothelial cell edema may predispose to white blood cell and platelet sludging, leading to the so-called no-reflow phenomenon. Similarly, prolonged vascular occlusion can lead to small-vessel thrombosis in the muscle and skin, which prevents tissue reperfusion when blood flow is restored to the larger vessels.

Although current understanding of the systemic effects of limb revascularization and compartment syndrome is well developed, understanding of ischemia-reperfusion injury at the tissue level is only beginning to evolve. The pathophysiology of the ischemic injury is complex and involves a variety of factors, including decreased cellular energy charge, inadequate oxygen and substrate delivery, altered ion compartmentalization, and membrane permeability changes. More recently, attention has focused on "reperfusion injury" (i.e., cellular injury that occurs or is manifested at the time perfusion is restored to ischemic tissue). Most of this injury is believed to be induced by oxygen-derived free radicals, which are formed as oxygen is reintroduced into ischemic tissue. These oxygen-derived free radicals are generated by neutrophils through an NADPH oxidase enzyme on the plasma membrane. These radicals are highly reactive compounds that result from the univalent reduction of molecular oxygen. The most important free radical species include the superoxide radical, hydrogen peroxide, and the extremely reactive hydroxyl radical. These unstable compounds attack the unsaturated bonds of fatty acids within the phospholipid membranes, causing both mechanical and functional derangements within the reperfused tissue.

Etiology

Embolism

Embolic occlusion of a previously unobstructed vessel generally results in the most severe forms of acute ischemia. The most common sources of arterial emboli are reviewed in Table 65-2. Approximately 80% of arterial emboli are cardiac in origin. In the past, the majority of these emboli were due to complications of rheumatic heart disease, including emboli from diseased valves as well as atrial fibrillation. More recently, atherosclerotic

TABLE 65-2. Sources of Peripheral Emboli

Source	Percentage
Cardiogenic	80%
Atrial fibrillation	50%
Myocardial infarction	25%
Other	5%
Noncardiac	10%
Aneurysmal disease	6%
Proximal artery	3%
Paradoxical emboli	1%
Other or Idiopathic	10%

TABLE 65-3. Site of Peripheral Embolization

Site	Percentage
Aortic bifurcation	10-15
Iliac bifurcation	15
Femoral bifurcation	40
Popliteal	10
Upper extremities	10
Cerebral	10-15
Mesenteric/visceral	5

cardiovascular disease has become the major contributor. Approximately 70% of patients with cardiogenic emboli have atrial fibrillation, with the emboli arising in atrial mural thrombus. Atrial fibrillation is currently the most common source of cardiogenic emboli. Acute myocardial infarction is the second most common cause of cardiogenic emboli, preceding approximately one third of peripheral embolic events. Ventricular mural thrombus, which occurs after acute myocardial injury, is often the source of emboli. Mural thrombus can form within hours of a myocardial infarction but may develop weeks after myocardial infarction and ultimately occurs in more than a third of cases. Peripheral embolization may often be the first sign of a previously "silent" myocardial infarction. Although readily available, standard echocardiographic techniques are often insensitive to the detection of thrombus within the atrium. Transesophageal echocardiography is more sensitive in the detection of both atrial and ventricular mural thrombus.

Although rheumatic valvular heart disease has declined in importance as a source of emboli, emboli from prosthetic heart valves have become an increasingly important source of embolization. Patients with prosthetic heart valves who have sudden onset of lower extremity ischemia should be suspected of having valvular embolization, particularly in the setting of inadequate anticoagulation.

Bacterial or fungal endocarditis can result in peripheral embolization. Such emboli tend to be more peripheral and result in septic complications rather than large vessel occlusion and ischemia. Intravenous drug abuse remains a major risk factor for endocarditis and subsequent embolic complications. These smaller emboli often result in digital lesions and peripheral infected pseudoaneurysms. More rare forms of cardiogenic emboli include embolization from intracardiac tumors, most commonly, atrial myxomas. Pathologic examination of unusual appearing emboli is essential for making the diagnosis in this situation. An unusual form of peripheral embolization, termed *paradoxical embolization,* may occur in the setting of patients with intracardiac defects (e.g., patent foramen ovale) and elevated right-sided cardiac pressures. In such patients, venous emboli to the heart may gain access to the arterial circulation through the patent foramen ovale and thereby embolize to the distal arterial circulation. Although rare, such emboli should be considered in patients with concurrent deep venous thrombosis, pulmonary emboli, or appropriate cardiac defects.

Arterial to arterial embolization is another cause of extremity ischemia. The majority of such cases arise from atherosclerotic plaque of the aorta. In most situations, such atheroembolization results in diffuse microembolization, resulting in the picture of painful, bluish discoloration of the toes with cutaneous gangrene, livedo reticularis, and often transient muscular pain. This so-called blue toe syndrome generally appears in the setting of palpable peripheral pulses right down to the pedal level. Although this syndrome most frequently occurs after intraluminal catheterization, it may occur spontaneously. Such microembolization may also affect the renal and mesenteric circulations, resulting in progressive renal failure and intestinal infarction. More rarely, artery to artery emboli may be sufficiently large to result in macroembolization with distal ischemia. This may occur both from mural thrombus or plaque from an atherosclerotic aorta or from the mural thrombus lining an aneurysmal artery.

In 10% to 15% of cases, the source of embolization ultimately cannot be determined. Such emboli should not be designated as idiopathic until a detailed history and physical examination, as well as complete cardiac and peripheral imaging, fail to identify an embolic source.

The most common sites of embolization are reviewed in Table 65-3. Cardiogenic emboli most commonly travel to the distal aorta and lower extremities (70% to 90% of all emboli). Within vessels, the emboli tend to lodge at branch points where vessel diameter decreases. Ten to 15 percent of large cardiogenic emboli lodge at the aortic bifurcation (Fig. 65-11). Such "saddle emboli" may result in profound bilateral lower extremity ischemia as well as neurologic ischemic injury. Another 15% embolize to the iliac bifurcation. The most common site of lower extremity embolization is the femoral bifurcation (Fig. 65-12), constituting more than 40% of cases. Smaller emboli lodge at the distal popliteal artery level at the level of the tibioperoneal artery trunk (Fig. 65-13) in 10% to 15% of cases. The upper extremities are affected in approximately 10% of cases in which the embolus most typically settles in the brachial artery.

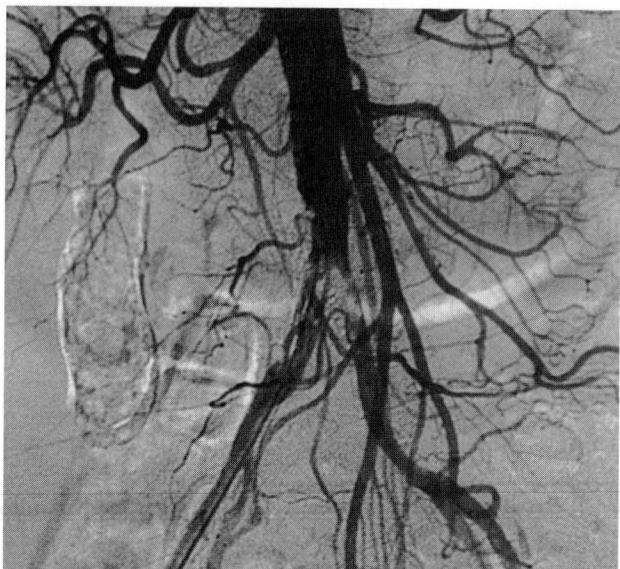

FIGURE 65-11. Large cardiogenic embolus lodged at the aortic bifurcation known as a "saddle embolus."

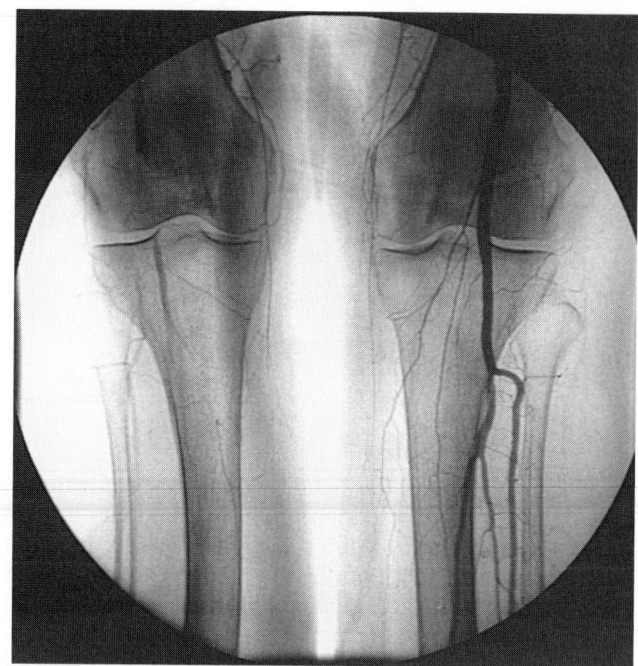

FIGURE 65-13. Distal embolus occluding the right popliteal artery.

Thrombosis

Acute thrombosis generally occurs in vessels affected by preexistent atherosclerosis. As such, there is generally some degree of collateral vessel development and the resultant ischemia is often less severe than with acute embolic disease. The most common extremity vessel affected is the superficial femoral artery, which is often affected by long segments of atherosclerosis. Popliteal artery aneurysms are also prone to thrombosis and may result in severe ischemia, particularly when associated with embolization to the tibial vessels.

A particularly severe form of ischemia results from distal vascular thrombosis of the extremities, which may occur in the setting of sepsis or with hypercoagulable states.[14] The most common hypercoagulable states associated with acute arterial thrombosis are antithrombin III deficiency, lupus anticoagulant (antiphospholipid antibody), and protein C deficiency. Although usually associated with venous thrombosis, activated protein C resistance caused by the spontaneous mutations of factor V Leiden may also cause arterial thrombosis. Exposure to heparin may lead to heparin-induced thrombosis in patients with heparin-induced antibodies. These antibodies cross-react with the platelet surface, leading to granular, white, platelet-laden thrombi and thrombocytopenia.

Acute thrombosis of a previous arterial bypass graft may also lead to recurrent ischemia. The degree of ischemia depends on the location of the graft and the original indication for surgery. Early graft occlusions (within 2 months of surgery) are usually caused by technical or judgmental errors. Intermediate graft occlusions (within 2 years) are generally attributable to the formation of intimal hyperplasia at the anastomoses or within the graft (for vein grafts).

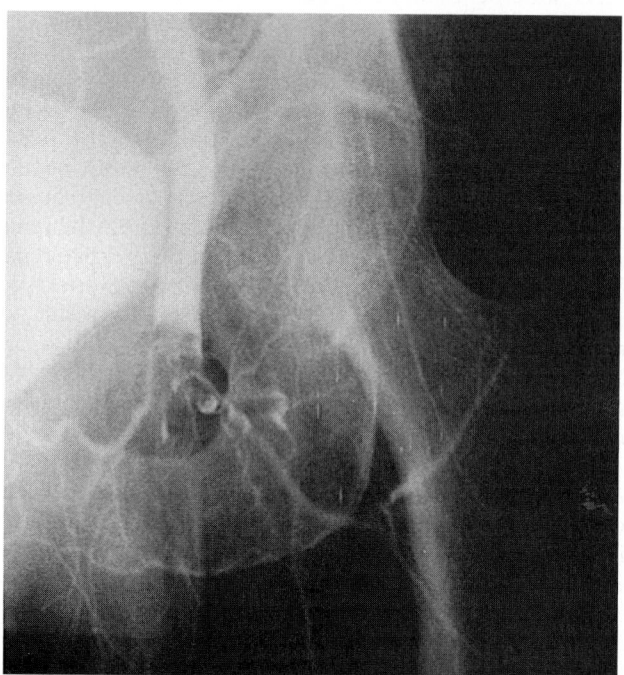

FIGURE 65-12. This arteriogram demonstrates an occlusive left femoral embolus with a typical rounded "meniscus" along its upper border.

Cardiogenic emboli are less likely to occur to the cerebral or visceral circulation. Embolization to the cerebral circulation occurs in approximately 13% of cases with potentially devastating results. Mesenteric and renal embolization to the vessels occurs in approximately 5% of peripheral emboli. Although often clinically silent, such emboli can result in acute catastrophes, such as mesenteric ischemia secondary to a superior mesenteric artery embolus.

Presentation and Evaluation

The classic presentation of patients with acute ischemia of the extremities may be recalled by the "five Ps": *pain, pallor, pulselessness, paresthesias,* and *paralysis.*

Pain is the most common complaint in alert patients. The degree of pain depends on the severity of ischemia, which is generally determined by the location of the occlusion and the degree of collateral flow. Ischemic pain can be severe and difficult to relieve with even large doses of narcotics. The sudden onset of severe ischemic pain in a previously asymptomatic patient is most suggestive of an embolic occlusion. Patients with spontaneous thrombosis often have had chronic symptoms of claudication or various degrees of pain before the acute event. Obtunded patients may have severe ischemia without complaints of pain. This is most commonly encountered in intubated, postoperative patients with spontaneous or iatrogenic arterial thrombosis.

Pallor is a common but relative finding that depends on the degree of ischemia and the underlying skin color. A sudden and complete embolic occlusion may result in a cool, waxy-appearing white extremity with no signs of cutaneous blood flow. Conversely, a partial occlusion may result in only delayed capillary refill with pallor on elevation of the extremity and rubor on dependency.

The absence of arterial pulses on examination will alert the surgeon to both the location of the arterial occlusion and the degree of ischemia. Patients with acute arterial embolism generally have normal palpable pulses above the occlusion with a complete absence below. The pulse immediately above the occlusion (e.g., the common femoral pulse in a patient with a femoral bifurcation embolus) may be particularly prominent with a "water-hammer" quality that results from limited arterial outflow. The presence of normal arterial pulses in the contralateral extremity is most suggestive of an acute embolus because patients with acute thrombosis generally have some degree of symmetrical pulse deficit, owing to long-standing atherosclerosis. A handheld continuous-wave Doppler examination plays an important role in the initial evaluation of patients with acute vessel occlusion. The presence of even monophasic Doppler signals over the pedal vessels affirms distal vascular patency and at least short-term viability of the distal tissues. Conversely, a complete absence of arterial flow is most suggestive of profound ischemia and calls for immediate revascularization.

As mentioned previously, within the extremities, the peripheral nerve is the tissue that is most sensitive to ischemia. As such, the degree of neurologic dysfunction is a sensitive barometer of the degree of ischemia. With mild ischemia, the findings may be subjective and subtle. Early paresthesias may be characterized as a numbness of the toes or a slight decrease of sensation of the foot compared with the contralateral extremity to light touch or pinprick. With severe ischemia, however, profound sensory loss may lead to complete anesthesia of the foot, indicative of impending tissue loss without early revascularization. Paradoxically, these patients with the most severe ischemia and complete anesthesia complain of less pain than those with more mild ischemia and intact sensation.

Weakness of the extremity is another important sign of neurologic ischemia of the extremity. Mild ischemia results in a weakness or subjective "stiffness" of the toes and foot, which may be easily appreciated on physical examination. As ischemia becomes more progressively severe, the weakness may progress to frank paralysis of the effected extremity. It is not unusual for the patient with a sudden complete embolic occlusion to suffer the immediate onset of paralysis of the affected extremity. Patients with an aortic saddle embolus may have bilateral paralysis and anesthesia from the waist down. In patients with severe ischemia characterized by anesthesia and paralysis, it is important to distinguish reversible from irreversible ischemic changes. Patients with prolonged ischemia have palpable firmness to the extremity muscle and stiffness to the extremity indicative of muscle rigor. Reperfusion of such an extremity does not restore function and can result in severe systemic injury. Primary amputation is the safest form of management in such cases.

The acute embolic occlusion of an extremity artery can be accurately diagnosed by a careful history and physical examination in most cases; emboli to the cerebral and visceral bed may be more difficult to identify and treat. The diagnosis in these cases is based on a high index of suspicion based on the patient's complaints and history. For example, a patient with the sudden onset of severe aching abdominal pain coupled with risk factors for cardiogenic emboli and a relative lack of physical findings should be presumed to have suffered a superior mesenteric artery embolus until proven otherwise.

Because evaluation of patients with acute arterial occlusion generally differs for patients who have suffered embolic versus thrombotic occlusion, it is important to make the appropriate clinical distinction. As outlined previously, patients with emboli tend to have risk factors (e.g., atrial fibrillation, recent myocardial infarction, prosthetic heart valve), a more sudden onset of symptoms (no prior claudication), and unilateral findings (normal contralateral extremity). Despite these guidelines, the distinction can be difficult to make at times. Certainly, patients with recent myocardial infarctions or atrial fibrillation may have concurrent peripheral vascular occlusive disease and patients with peripheral vascular occlusive disease may suffer cardiogenic emboli. Thus, the evaluation of each patient must be individualized to supply enough information to effectively treat the patient without jeopardizing limb salvage or function by delaying revascularization.

When the history and physical examination implicates an embolus as the source of occlusion, the subsequent evaluation should be simple and direct. Routine preoperative blood work and a chest radiograph are obtained, and a 12-lead electrocardiogram is performed to document atrial fibrillation, cardiac ischemia, or a previous (and perhaps unsuspected) myocardial infarction. Because arterial emboli are removed by direct arterial cutdown and removal of the embolus (as described later), there is generally no need for preoperative arteriography. When the diagnosis of embolus is questionable or the site for simple arterial cutdown and arteriotomy unclear, a preoperative arteriogram may be useful to define the anatomy and guide the revascularization procedure. The management of distal extremity emboli (below the brachial or popliteal artery) may be assisted by detailed preoperative angiograms in selected cases. For example, very distal emboli within the distal tibial or pedal vessels may be best treated by catheter-based thrombolytic therapy (described later) rather than surgical extraction. Arteriograms of intra-arterial emboli often demonstrate an abrupt cutoff of the artery with a rounded meniscus at the site of the embolus (see Fig. 65-12). Conversely, the embolus may appear as an intraluminal defect with partial flow around it (see Fig. 65-11). Postoperatively, when the embolus has been removed and the limb revascularized, and the patient is stable, the evaluation should be completed by documentation of the source of the embolus. In most cases, this involves transesophageal echocardiography.

The surgical management of patients with acute arterial thrombosis is generally more complex than the simple arteriotomy and clot extraction used for embolic occlusion. Patients suffering thrombotic occlusion often have diffuse atherosclerotic disease at multiple arterial levels, various degrees of collateral blood vessel development, and unpredictable levels of distal arterial reconstitution. These patients are best evaluated with complete arteriography to define the optimal approach to revascularization. Rarely, arterial thrombosis results in such profound ischemia that the patient is taken immediately to the operating room and intraoperative arteriography is performed after arterial exposure.

Management

Embolic Occlusion

Patients with acute arterial occlusion should be anticoagulated with an intravenous heparin bolus (5000 to 10,000 units) and begun on a continuous infusion at 1000 units/hr. The primary goal of anticoagulation is to prevent thrombosis resulting from stagnant flow beyond the primary embolic or thrombotic occlusion. Furthermore, short- and long-term anticoagulation is indicated in patients with cardiogenic emboli to prevent additional embolic events. Recurrent embolization occurs in approximately 7% of patients who are chronically anticoagulated versus 21% of those who are not.[28]

The most important initial decision focuses on the viability and potential salvage in the ischemic limb. Rarely, patients have such long-standing and severe ischemia that irreversible ischemic injury to the extremity (manifesting as rigor of the muscles or frank gangrenous changes to the foot) has occurred. Such cases are best treated with primary extremity amputation.

In most cases, however, early revascularization for restoration of limb function is indicated. As mentioned earlier, immediate progression to the operating room after minimal and expeditious evaluation is indicated for patients who have suffered occlusive emboli to the extremities. For patients with emboli to the lower extremity, the entire extremity is prepped and draped into the field. This allows immediate evaluation of success of the revascularization as well as ready access for more distal arterial exposure if necessary to complete the procedure. Emboli to the iliac and femoral vessels are approached through a femoral cutdown. Femoral artery cutdowns can be performed under local anesthesia with intravenous sedation. Often, however, regional or general anesthesia is preferable, particularly when popliteal artery exposure is necessary.

A standard longitudinal or oblique skin incision is made with the common femoral artery as well as profunda femoris and superficial femoral arteries all independently controlled. Normal arteries, free of significant atherosclerosis, are best incised transversely just above the femoral bifurcation. In patients with significant atherosclerosis, however, longitudinal arteriotomies afford the best exposure and most reliable closure (often with an arterial patch). Patients with iliac level emboli often have an absence of a femoral pulse. Inflow is restored by retrograde passage of a No. 4 or 5 balloon thrombectomy catheter. The catheter is passed in 10-cm increments. Gentle inflation of the catheter as it is withdrawn engages and extracts the thrombus without causing arterial wall injury. Each passage should extend an additional 10 cm until pulsatile arterial inflow is restored. Passages are continued until no additional thrombus is recovered. Attention is then turned to the outflow vessels. Antegrade passage of a No. 3 Fogarty catheter, 3 to 5 cm down the profunda, generally extracts any impacted thrombus and restores good backflow. The catheter is then passed down the superficial femoral artery in increments until no further thrombus is extracted. This may necessitate passage to the popliteal level or beyond. Blind passage of the Fogarty catheter from the groin to below the popliteal artery almost always results in cannulation of the peroneal artery. Specific cannulation of the anterior tibial and posterior tibial arteries requires more distal, below-knee popliteal artery exposure. Alternatively, selective passage of balloon catheters over guide wires using fluoroscopic control has facilitated selective cannulation of distal vessels. When good inflow and backbleeding has been restored, the transverse arteriotomy is closed with 5-0 polypropylene sutures and flow is restored.

For patients with a palpable popliteal pulse and a distal emboli, exposure is best obtained at the level of the below-knee popliteal artery through a standard medial incision. The soleus muscle is carefully taken down off the tibia, exposing the tibioperoneal trunk. The anterior tibial veins may be divided to facilitate individual control of the anterior tibial, posterior tibial, and peroneal arteries. A distal popliteal arteriotomy may then be performed and retrograde passage of a No. 3 catheter used to restore normal inflow to the popliteal level. Selective cannulation of the anterior and posterior tibial vessels, as well as the peroneal artery, may be performed with a No. 2 or 3 thrombectomy catheter, restoring good backflow. At the conclusion of the embolectomy and closure of the arteriotomy, reperfusion of the extremity is assessed. In most cases, restoration of palpable pedal pulses and pink, well-perfused toes reassures the surgeon of a successful and complete embolectomy. In some cases, however, spasm of the distal vessels secondary to passage of the Fogarty catheter may delay the return of normal perfusion. Even in these cases, however, restoration of strong Doppler signals should be present at the pedal level. After several minutes, palpable pulses and well-perfused skin are re-established. In any case in which there is a doubt as to the success of the embolectomy, completion arteriography should be performed to assess the distal vasculature for spasm and retained thrombus. For those rare patients who have restoration of patent vessels down to the mid-tibial level, with occlusions of the distal tibial and pedal vessels, direct intraoperative arterial infusion of urokinase (50,000 to 250,000 units) may help lyse distal thrombus and restore perfusion to the foot. Occasionally, direct cutdown and thrombectomy of the distal tibial and pedal levels is necessary to remove distally impacted thrombus.

Patients with a saddle embolus to the aortic bifurcation with bilateral lower extremity ischemia are approached through simultaneous bilateral femoral artery cutdowns. The femoral arteries are simultaneously clamped and opened, and retrograde thrombectomies are performed to both limbs simultaneously to prevent fragmentation of the thrombus and distal embolization to the extremity contralateral to the thrombectomy. Once normal inflow is obtained, the remainder of the procedure is similar to that for an iliac level embolectomy.

Patients with upper extremity emboli are approached in a similar fashion. The entire extremity is prepped and draped into the field. Usually the entire embolectomy can be performed under local anesthesia through a longitudinal incision performed just above the elbow. The brachial artery is carefully dissected from its companion structures, and a transverse arteriotomy is performed. Most emboli impact just above the elbow and are easily extracted by passage of a No. 3 Fogarty catheter both proximally and distally. Emboli that have lodged at the subclavian level are generally easy to remove by retrograde passage of the No. 3 Fogarty catheter from the elbow proximally to the subclavian level. Arterial closure and assessment are similar to that performed for the lower extremity.

Recently, several authors have reported on the adjunctive use of fluoroscopy for accurate passage of the thrombectomy catheter. Similarly, others have found angioscopy to be useful in the evaluation of completeness of the thrombectomy (particularly during thrombectomies of occluded prosthetic grafts).

Thrombotic Occlusion

As mentioned previously, patients with thrombotic arterial occlusion undergo an initial arteriogram to delineate the arterial anatomy and define the best mode of revascularization. In most cases, the site of thrombotic occlusion is well delineated. In patients with a satisfactory inflow and outflow vessel with a long segment of occluded vessel, the best option is generally to proceed to surgery and perform a surgical bypass procedure. Inflow to the femoral artery can be restored with either a direct aortofemoral revascularization or various forms of extra-anatomic bypass (femorofemoral bypass, axillo-femoral bypass, or iliofemoral bypass) depending on the patient's anatomy. Infrainguinal arterial occlusions are best treated with femoral-distal bypass operations with autogenous vein. When short-segment thrombotic occlusions are identified, a catheter-directed infusion of thrombolytic therapy may recanalize the vessel, revealing an appropriate underlying lesion for balloon angioplasty. Recent studies have suggested that aggressive thrombolytic therapy is most beneficial when the ischemic interval is short and that initial thrombolysis may reduce the magnitude of subsequent surgical procedures.[29,37] When the arteriogram reveals no distal arterial reconstitution appropriate for bypass, catheter-based thrombolysis may restore sufficient perfusion to establish or reveal a distal vessel suitable for bypass.

Compartment Syndrome

As described previously, extremities subjected to prolonged periods of ischemia followed by reperfusion suffer reperfusion injury manifesting as both intracellular and interstitial edema. This reperfusion injury occurs regardless of the cause of arterial occlusion (embolus or thrombosis) or mode of revascularization (balloon embolectomy, surgical bypass, or catheter-based thrombolytic recanalization). When muscular swelling occurs within the confines of an unyielding osseofascial bound space, increased compartmental pressures occur. These increased pressures can occur in either the arm or leg. In the lower extremity, the calf is the most frequently affected area. The anterior compartment of the calf, followed by the lateral, deep posterior, and superficial posterior compartments are involved with decreasing frequency. Within the thigh, the anterior quadriceps compartment is the most frequently involved area. In the upper extremity, the anterior or volar forearm compartment is most frequently involved but the dorsal forearm as well as hand and upper arm may also be involved by reperfusion edema.

When the intracompartmental pressures increase to more than the level of capillary perfusion pressure, both venous outflow and capillary perfusion may become impaired. This may result in recurrent and prolonged ischemia unless the affected compartment is decompressed. As with the initial ischemic injury, the nerve tissue is most susceptible to the effects of compartment syndrome. The diagnosis of compartment syndrome is based on a high degree of suspicion and careful evaluation for signs and symptoms. Extremities that are revascularized after 4 to 6 hours of severe ischemia are most at risk for development of compartment syndrome. The early signs and symptoms must be carefully watched for, particularly in patients with decreased sensorium. The typical clinical findings of early compartment syndrome are severe pain that is disproportionate to the relative paucity of physical findings. Patients usually have marked tenderness on compression of the edematous calf and severe discomfort on passive extension of the calf with dorsiflexion or plantarflexion of the foot. Because the anterior compartment is the most commonly affected space within the calf, the first neurologic findings are

TABLE 65-4.   Natural History of Intermittent Claudication

Study	Patients (n)	Follow-up (yr)	Stable/Improved (%)	Amputation (%)	Survival (%)
Boyd	1476	5	80	7.2	73
		10	60	12	38
Imparato	104	2.5	79	5.8	—
McAllister	100	6	78	7.0	89

Adapted from Braunwald E: Atlas of heart diseases. *In* Craeger MA (ed): Vascular Disease, vol VII. Philadelphia, Current Medicine, 1996, p 3.5.

often numbness in the area of the great toe web space, attributable to pressure on the deep peroneal nerve. Palpable pulses and strong Doppler signals may be well preserved despite progressive compartment syndrome and should not lead to a false sense of security. When the diagnosis of compartment syndrome is in question, direct measures of the pressure within the compartment may be performed. A needle cannula placed directly into the compartment and attached to a pressure transducer gives an accurate measure of the intracompartmental pressure. There are also portable, handheld devices designed for measurement of intracompartmental pressures. Although somewhat controversial, it is generally agreed that, as compartmental pressure reaches 30 mm Hg, capillary perfusion is impaired and neurologic and muscular injury occurs.

Although significant calf swelling and increased compartment pressures can often be managed with extreme elevation of the extremity, marked elevation of compartment pressures with neurologic changes necessitates early and effective decompression to prevent a permanent and disabling injury. Most vascular surgeons prefer a two-incision, four-compartment fasciotomy. The medial-based longitudinal incision is made just posterior to the tibia and is carried down through the fascia into the superficial posterior space. The soleus muscle is then incised longitudinally, near its tibial insertion, and the deep fascia is incised longitudinally to decompress the deep posterior compartment. A second anterolateral calf incision is made longitudinally and carried down through the fascia into the anterior compartment. A second longitudinal fascial incision is made over the lateral compartment, decompressing the peroneus muscles. Severe compartment syndrome is manifest by an immediate pouting of the muscles as they swell beyond the fascial incision. The skin incision should be long enough to prevent any restriction on the underlying muscle.

When patients undergo revascularization after a prolonged interval (6 hours or more) of severe ischemia, consideration for a prophylactic fasciotomy in anticipation of impending compartment syndrome should be entertained. Such prophylactic fasciotomies may be performed through more limited skin incisions with blind extension of the fascial incisions by sliding a slightly opened Metzenbaum scissors along the cut edge of the fascia. The skin incisions can be extended later if full-blown compartment syndrome develops.

An alternative surgical approach to four-compartment fasciotomy, favored by many orthopedic surgeons, involves resection of a portion of the fibula or parafibular dissection of all soft tissues away from a section of the fibula. Because the fascia of all four compartments inserts on the fibula, disruption of these fibular attachments may adequately decompress the various calf compartments.

CHRONIC OCCLUSIVE DISEASE OF THE LOWER EXTREMITIES

Presentation and Natural History

Patients with arterial claudication suffer from reproducible ischemic muscle pain resulting from inadequate oxygen delivery during exercise. Studies suggest that patients with claudication, while having an increased risk of cardiovascular mortality, have a low risk of limb loss (Table 65-4).[8,23,27] Recent reports using noninvasive studies and multivariate analysis have more accurately defined the natural history of arterial claudication. The annual risk of mortality and limb loss in patients with claudication is approximately 5% and 1%, respectively. More than half of these patients either remain stable or have improvement in their symptoms with conservative management, consisting of increased exercise, weight loss, and risk factor modification. Twenty to 30 percent of patients with claudication come to operation within 5 years because of disease progression.

As opposed to the patient with claudication, who has cramping in the thigh, buttock, or calf with exercise, the patient with more advanced critical ischemia complains of pain at rest. Rest pain occurs when blood flow is inadequate to meet metabolic requirements. In the lower extremity, ischemic rest pain is localized to the forefoot and should be easily distinguished from benign nocturnal muscle cramps in the calf, which are also common in older patients. The patient with rest pain is often awakened by severe discomfort in the forefoot and hangs the affected extremity off the bed for temporary relief of symptoms. Patients often have trophic changes, such as muscle wasting, thinning of skin, thickening of nails, and hair loss in the distal affected limb. Rest pain is an ominous symptom and usually requires revascularization because this form of advanced ischemia generally progresses to tissue loss.

The patient with critical ischemia is at risk for tissue infection or gangrene resulting from arterial insufficiency. Patients with diabetes or renal failure are more susceptible to the development of ischemic pedal ulcers. Minor trauma to the forefoot leads to ulcer formation and skin breakdown that, with diminished tissue perfusion, are unable to heal. The simple friction between adjacent ischemic toes may result in breakdown termed *kissing ulcers*. Bacterial superinfection of pedal and leg ulcers, as well as osteomyelitis of the underlying bone, frequently complicates the management of these patients. The depth and pattern of ulcer penetration, the degree of bone involvement, the location of the ulcer, the presence of infection, the presence of neuropathy, and the degree of arterial insufficiency all may impact on the management of the complex patient with lower extremity arterial insufficiency.

Evaluation

Vascular Laboratory

Noninvasive testing may aid in predicting the location and severity of atherosclerotic occlusive disease. Noninvasive evaluation is also helpful to establish a preoperative baseline assessment for subsequent comparison postoperatively. Routine segmental Doppler pressure ABI determinations are the standard studies, but results may be spuriously elevated in diabetics and patients with renal failure. In this select group of patients with heavily calcified vessels, metatarsal and digital PVRs may be more helpful in evaluating peripheral vascular disease.

Patients with known risk factors and symptoms consistent with occlusive disease pose little diagnostic challenge. However, many patients with occlusive disease may have normal perfusion at rest and may require provocative testing to reproduce their symptoms and demonstrate abnormal laboratory findings. Treadmill testing may be used to enhance symptoms of claudication, at which point re-examination of the patient with measurement of PVRs and Doppler signals should help delineate vascular insufficiency.

Angiography

The standard angiographic approach for patients with lower extremity occlusive disease should be by transfemoral catheterization. The aorta, iliacs, femorals, and distal runoff arteries from both lower extremities should be evaluated. The aorta should be imaged in two planes, and views of the celiac and superior mesenteric arteries are also obtained. If the hemodynamic significance of a lesion is called into question, pressure gradients across the lesion before and after infusion with a vasodilator (e.g., tolazoline [Priscoline] or nitroglycerin) should be obtained. If the patient is an appropriate candidate for balloon angioplasty, interventional therapy may be performed at that time.

As discussed earlier, both MRA and duplex ultrasonography are assuming an increased role in the delineation of central and peripheral vascular anatomy. These noninvasive modalities may be of particular value in minimizing the use or dosage of contrast media in patients at risk for dye-induced nephropathy. An important limitation as compared with contrast arteriography is the inability to simultaneously treat lesions by catheter-based techniques (e.g., PTA). The use of duplex scanning or MRA as a screening test to predict the likelihood of a lesion amenable to PTA or stenting is another potential algorithm aimed at reducing the morbidity of conventional arteriography.

Cardiac Risk Assessment

Risk factors for occlusive disease are similar to those for atherosclerosis in general and include cigarette smoking, hypertension, hypercholesterolemia, diabetes, and male sex. Many of these patients have overt cardiac disease, and work-up of these patients has been well described in the literature. Because myocardial ischemia remains the leading cause of death after vascular surgery, patients should undergo preoperative risk factor assessment and selective stress testing before undergoing major vascular surgery. The initiation and optimization of medical therapy (particularly β-adrenergic blockade) before elective vascular surgery has been of paramount importance in minimizing perioperative morbidity and death in this group of patients.

Management

Aortoiliac Occlusive Disease

Many patients with aortoiliac occlusive disease (AOD) can be managed conservatively with risk factor modification and an aggressive walking regimen. Only patients who suffer disabling claudication or limb-threatening ischemia should be considered for arteriography and intervention.

PERCUTANEOUS TRANSLUMINAL ANGIOPLASTY

During the 1990s, the indications for PTA have become more liberal as the effectiveness of PTA of the iliac arteries has been increasingly well documented. PTA is performed under local anesthesia with minimal sedation, as a day surgery admission, with significantly less morbidity and productivity reduction. Although initially performed only in the common iliac artery for stenosis, PTA is routinely used to treat short-segment occlusions as well as external iliac lesions. Iliac artery PTA may be particularly useful to help improve inflow before a more distal surgical reconstruction.

The use of iliac artery stents has also begun to play an increasing role in the management of patients with AOD. Iliac artery stents are most useful after initial suboptimal results from PTA. Occasionally, however, they are used primarily in the treatment of complex lesions. For example, bilateral proximal common iliac lesions are problematic for standard PTA and are best managed with simultaneous bilateral common iliac stenting ("kissing"

PTA and stenting technique). Overall, reports from numerous series suggest that the results of percutaneous therapies for aortoiliac disease are more favorable for common (versus external) iliac lesions and less favorable for long occlusions as opposed to short stenoses; stents appear to improve the results of isolated PTA in some situations, but the data are less clear. Application of advances in stent design and materials as well as reduction in delivery profile improved early patency results. Five-year patency rates for common iliac PTA alone are typically in the range of 80% and are notably inferior (50% to 60%) for external iliac disease. Importantly, complication rates are low and failure rarely changes the available surgical options.

When PTA is not an option, a number of surgical alternatives are available. The technique of combined open surgical common femoral artery exposure with endovascular recanalization and balloon angioplasty of severely diseased iliac artery segments has been described, primarily in patients with comorbidities prohibiting major surgery or general anesthesia. This treatment strategy includes femoral endarterectomy and subsequent endoluminal deployment of a stent-graft to re-line the balloon-dilated artery, with the ability to post-dilate the vessel to a larger caliber and to surgically fashion the distal anastomosis to the femoral outflow vessels.[50] Depending on the condition of the patient and the patient's pathologic anatomy, the options include aortobifemoral bypass, aortoiliac thromboendarterectomy, axillofemoral bypass, iliofemoral bypass, and femorofemoral bypass.

AORTOFEMORAL BYPASS

Aortofemoral bypass is performed under general endotracheal anesthesia. An epidural catheter is placed preoperatively to improve pain control and facilitate early postoperative extubation. The patient is prepped and draped from the chest to the mid thighs with the groins exposed. The femoral vessels are exposed first through bilateral longitudinal, oblique incisions. Preliminary exposure of the femoral vessels minimizes the time that the abdomen is open and improves the efficiency of the operation. In patients with significant occlusive disease of the femoral arteries, a broad exposure of the profunda femoris for potential profundaplasty should be performed before entry into the abdomen. Once the femoral vessels have been dissected, retroperitoneal tunnels are gently developed underneath the inguinal ligament on the anterior surface of the external iliac artery. The groins are packed with antibiotic-soaked sponges and attention is turned to the abdomen. Either a direct transperitoneal or lateral (flank) retroperitoneal aortic exposure may be used; generally, the anterior approach is preferred because graft tunneling to the right groin is far easier. The abdomen is entered through a longitudinal midline incision, and the patient is explored for any intra-abdominal abnormalities. The transverse colon is pulled cephalad, and the entire small bowel is retracted to the right of the patient. The ligament of Treitz is incised, and the duodenum is mobilized to the right for standard infrarenal aortic exposure. The dissection is carried up to the level of renal vein to allow for optimal cross-clamping and improved conditions

for a proximal anastomosis. The dissection is completed down to the level of the inferior mesenteric artery. Anticoagulation with heparin (5000 to 7000 units) is performed after creating retroperitoneal tunnels anterior to both iliac arteries and posterior to the ureters. Great care is taken to avoid trauma to the autonomic nervous plexus (particularly over the proximal left common iliac artery). Atraumatic vascular clamps are placed above the inferior mesenteric artery and below the renal arteries.

The proximal anastomosis may be completed with either an end-to-end or end-to-side configuration. The end-to-end technique is preferred in most cases and has the advantage of not requiring flow to be re-established in the more distal aorta, thereby avoiding potential intraoperative emboli to the lower extremities. The end-to-end technique may also decrease the incidence of aortoenteric fistula postoperatively because retroperitonealization of the graft is facilitated. To perform an end-to-end proximal anastomosis, the aorta is divided in a beveled fashion just above the distal clamp. The distal aorta is closed with either a running nonabsorbable monofilament suture or a surgical stapler. If there is associated aneurysmal disease of the aorta, the aorta may be incised longitudinally and the bifurcation oversewn to achieve complete exclusion of the dilated segment. The end-to-side technique for the proximal anastomosis of the aortofemoral bypass graft is generally reserved for patients with occlusion of the external iliac arteries who would lack retrograde perfusion of important collaterals in the pelvis. The proximal anastomosis is completed using a running 3-0 polypropylene suture.

On completion, the proximal clamps are released and a vascular clamp is placed proximally across the graft limbs. The limbs of the graft are then passed through the previously created retroperitoneal tunnels to the femoral arteries. The femoral vessels are controlled in the groins with atraumatic vascular clamps. For those patients with normal femoral vessels and a widely patent profunda, the anastomosis is performed to the common femoral artery. Many patients with AOD have associated occlusive disease of the femoral arteries, and it is essential that blood flow to the profunda femoris artery be optimized. In this instance, the toe of anastomosis is placed onto the profunda femoris artery. If necessary, a complete profunda endarterectomy and profundaplasty may be performed. Before tying down the anastomosis, the inflow and outflow vessels are flushed in an attempt to remove any atherosclerotic debris or clot that may have collected in the graft or native vessels. On completion of both anastomoses in the groin, the abdomen and proximal anastomosis are reinspected for evidence of bleeding. Once hemostasis is attained, the proximal anastomosis and graft are covered with autogenous material. If an end-to-end anastomosis has been performed, the retroperitoneum is closed over the graft. If an end-to-side anastomosis was performed, the omentum may be used to wrap around the anastomosis and to partially cover the graft. The abdomen and groins are closed in a standard fashion.

Aortobifemoral bypass grafting has generally resulted in patency rates among the highest reported for any major arterial reconstruction. Primary patency rates of ABF grafts at 5 years are reported to be 70% to 88% with 10-year rates of 66% to 78%.[9] Patients operated on for claudication with good infrainguinal outflow have superior patency rates compared with those operated on for limb-threatening ischemia with associated infrainguinal occlusive disease. Studies have demonstrated that younger patients (<50 years) and those with smaller aortas have inferior patency rates to older patients and those with larger aortas.[43] In patients with significant profunda femoris disease, simultaneous profundaplasty improves graft patency. In addition to excellent patency rates after aortobifemoral bypass grafting, most patients have significant relief of their symptoms. Perioperative mortality rates average about 4% with a 5-year cumulative survival rate for patients undergoing aortobifemoral bypass grafting of 70% to 75%, which is significantly poorer than an age-matched control population but typical of claudicant patients in general.

Rarely, patients have isolated terminal aorta and proximal common iliac artery occlusive disease. These patients are primarily female smokers in their fourth or fifth decade of life. In these patients, when the AOD is localized at the aortic bifurcation, an aortoiliac endarterectomy may be performed. This procedure offers the advantage of not requiring prosthetic material; however, it is fraught with more numerous potential technical pitfalls and has largely been replaced by percutaneous options for such localized lesions. Aortoiliac endarterectomy is contraindicated in AOD patients with arterial ectasia or aneurysmal disease.

EXTRA-ANATOMIC BYPASS

Blaisdell[7] and others, using polyester (Dacron) grafts, pioneered the performance of extra-anatomic axillary to ipsilateral femoral artery bypass for occlusive disease. Originally, the use of extra-anatomic bypasses was used for patients with complications after aortoiliac reconstruction. Currently, extra-anatomic bypasses are important alternatives in the selective management of AOD. Extra-anatomic bypass is most useful when femoral inflow is required and a direct transabdominal reconstructive approach is contraindicated because of patient comorbidities or intra-abdominal pathology, or because the aorta is thought to be an unsatisfactory inflow source. Extra-anatomic bypass grafting may also be preferable in patients with uncontrolled malignancy or in patients in whom other diseases might limit their life expectancy.

Axillofemoral (or bifemoral) bypass is performed with the patient under general anesthesia. The patient is placed in the supine position with the arm tucked or abducted no more than 90 degrees. The axillary artery on the side with the least evidence of upper extremity atherosclerosis (higher blood pressure, strongest pulse) is selected as the donor site. If the disease burden is equal in both upper extremities, the right axillary artery should be used as the preferred donor vessel because it has a lower risk of developing subclavian occlusive disease than the left. Axillary exposure is gained through a transverse incision over the deltopectoral groove. The axillary artery, which is deep to the axillary vein and inferior to the brachial plexus, is identified and dissected free. Occasionally, division of the pectoralis minor tendon aids in axillary artery exposure. The

femoral arteries are dissected in the standard fashion. A subcutaneous tunnel is made between the axillary and femoral artery with a tunneling device. The tunnel should course laterally from the axillary artery deep to the pectoralis major, inferiorly along the midaxillary line (superficial to the external oblique fascia), and then medial to the anterior-superior iliac spine because this prevents kinking of the graft when the patient sits up. An extrafascial, suprapubic tunnel is then made between the two femoral incisions. After completion of the tunnels, the patient is anticoagulated with heparin. A 6- or 8-mm externally supported PTFE graft is the preferred conduit. The anastomoses are performed in a sequential fashion with the axillary anastomosis first, followed by the ipsilateral femoral artery and subsequently those of the femorofemoral bypass. If an axillobifemoral graft is to be performed, the inflow for the femorofemoral bypass originates off the hood of the femoral anastomosis of the axillofemoral graft. Flow is re-established, hemostasis is attained, and the wounds are irrigated with antibiotic solution and closed with an absorbable suture. Because patients undergoing axillofemoral grafting often have increased comorbidities, the mortality rate after axillofemoral bypass grafting ranges up to 13%. Five-year primary patency rates vary widely in the literature and range from 19% to 79%, with secondary patency rates as high as 85%.[16]

FEMOROFEMORAL BYPASS

In the patient with unilateral iliac occlusive disease, the contralateral femoral artery may serve as a source of inflow. Even though a femorofemoral bypass is best performed under general or regional anesthesia, it may be completed under local anesthesia in selected circumstances. Bilateral groin incisions are made parallel to the femoral arteries, and the vessels are isolated. Before heparin is administered, a subcutaneous tunnel superficial to the external oblique fascia between the two incisions is created. Polyester (Dacron) or PTFE graft material may be used with similar results. If significant femoral occlusive disease is present, it is important to establish unrestricted flow to the profunda femoris. The graft is anastomosed to the femoral arteries in the standard fashion with a running monofilament suture. Cumulative patency rates range from 60% to 80% at 5 years after femorofemoral bypass.[16]

ILIOFEMORAL BYPASS

In addition to femorofemoral bypass, iliofemoral bypass may be used to treat unilateral iliac artery disease. An iliofemoral bypass is best suited for patients with occluded or stenosed external iliac arteries and a relatively disease-free proximal common iliac artery. This procedure may be performed under general or regional anesthesia with the patient in the supine position. The common iliac artery is exposed through an oblique lower abdominal incision. The retroperitoneal plane is entered, the abdominal contents are retracted medially, and the proximal common iliac artery is isolated. A femoral incision is made as described previously. A tunnel under the inguinal ligament is created before heparin administration. The iliac artery anastomosis is performed first in an end-to-side fashion. PTFE or polyester (Dacron) grafts are equally suitable for use. The graft is passed under the inguinal ligament and anastomosed to the femoral artery as described earlier. The abdominal and femoral artery incisions are closed in a standard fashion after hemostasis is attained. Three-year patency rates for iliofemoral bypass are 90% or greater in several reports.

Infrainguinal Occlusive Disease

Infrainguinal arterial occlusive disease represents the most common manifestation of chronic arterial occlusive disease confronted by the vascular surgeon. Isolated superficial femoral artery occlusive disease generally presents as claudication of the calf muscles. Patients with multilevel occlusions of the superficial femoral, popliteal, and tibial arteries generally have rest pain or ischemic tissue loss. These ischemic ulcerations initially present as small, dry ulcers of the toes or heel area but may progress to frank gangrenous changes of the forefoot or heel. Most smokers initially have isolated superficial femoral artery occlusive disease and claudication. On the other hand, diabetics more often harbor distal occlusions of the popliteal and tibial arteries; these patients may initially have frank tissue necrosis with no prior history of claudication if the superficial femoral artery is spared.

Patients with symptoms of claudication are generally managed conservatively with risk factor modification and an aggressive walking regimen. Medical treatment has had a limited role, although newer agents (e.g., the phosphodiesterase inhibitor cilostazol) currently being marketed may find a potential niche. Patients with truly disabling claudication, such as those who are unable to perform their occupation because of claudication symptoms, should be considered for arteriography and interventional therapy. Once the ischemic symptoms have progressed to the point of rest pain or tissue ulceration, surgical therapy is generally indicated for the purposes of pain relief and limb salvage. In the patient considered a candidate for interventional therapy, an arteriogram is performed to delineate the anatomy. Occasionally, patients have isolated lesions of the superficial femoral artery that may be appropriate for PTA (described later). In most cases, however, long-segment occlusions require femoral to distal artery bypass surgery to improve the distal circulation. Any such infrainguinal bypass operation requires normal inflow to the level of the groin. Patients with associated iliac occlusive disease should have these lesions corrected with either PTA or surgical bypass before the infrainguinal reconstructive operation. In many cases, correction of the occlusions within the inflow vessels will relieve the patient's symptoms and obviate the need for infrainguinal reconstruction.

In general, infrainguinal bypass surgery is best performed with autogenous vein conduit, preferably the ipsilateral greater saphenous. The superiority of autogenous vein reconstructions is most evident for bypass grafts performed to the below-knee popliteal, tibial, or pedal vessels. When bypass grafts are performed to the above-

knee popliteal artery for claudication, prosthetic grafts (i.e., Dacron or PTFE) may be used with the expectation of results approaching those achieved with greater saphenous vein.

Reversed Vein Graft

The original technique for infrainguinal bypass surgery, an approach still preferred by many surgeons, uses the greater saphenous vein in a reversed configuration. The operation may be performed under general or regional anesthesia. The patient's entire extremity from the umbilicus to the foot is prepped and draped into the wound. A longitudinal incision is made in the groin and deepened down through the fascia. The femoral vessels are carefully dissected from their companion veins and individually controlled.

Lymphatic tissue overlying the femoral vessels is best ligated and divided to prevent lymph fistulas or lymphoceles postoperatively. The greater saphenous vein is then dissected from the saphenofemoral junction and exposed through either a single, continuous, longitudinal incision along the thigh or through separate, shorter incisions leaving skin bridges between each incision. More recently, endoscopic saphenous vein harvest has allowed vein preparation through minimal incisions. Sufficient greater saphenous vein is exposed to reach the distal outflow vessel. The above-knee popliteal artery is exposed through a medial thigh incision and carried anterior to the sartorius muscle and posterior to the vastus medialis muscle entering the above-knee popliteal space. The popliteal artery is carefully dissected from its companion vein and nerves. Similarly, the below-knee popliteal artery is dissected through a medial upper calf incision just posterior to the tibia and is carried down through the fascia into the below-knee popliteal space. There, the below-knee popliteal artery is easily dissected from the companion structures. The tibioperoneal trunk may be exposed by dissecting distally and dividing the soleus insertion from the tibia. The posterior tibial and peroneal arteries are dissected through a similar, more distal medial incision, which is deepened down through the investing fascia of the calf. The soleus is then taken off the tibia, exposing the posterior tibial artery within the deep space of the calf. The peroneal artery is located more laterally and is exposed by reflecting the flexor hallucis longus muscle posteriorly. The anterior tibial artery is exposed through a separate, anterolateral calf incision, which is carried down through the fascia and just lateral to the anterior tibialis muscle, thereby exposing the anterior tibial vessels lying directly over the intraosseous membrane. Once the proximal and distal vessels are exposed, the greater saphenous vein is gently removed from its bed by ligating its side branches with silk ties and gently dilating the vein with crystalloid solution containing heparin and papaverine. The patient is anticoagulated with 5,000 to 10,000 units of heparin, and the femoral vessels are clamped and opened longitudinally. Because of the orientation of the greater saphenous vein valves, the vein is reversed such that the distal end of the vein is sewn to the proximal inflow artery and the proximal end of the

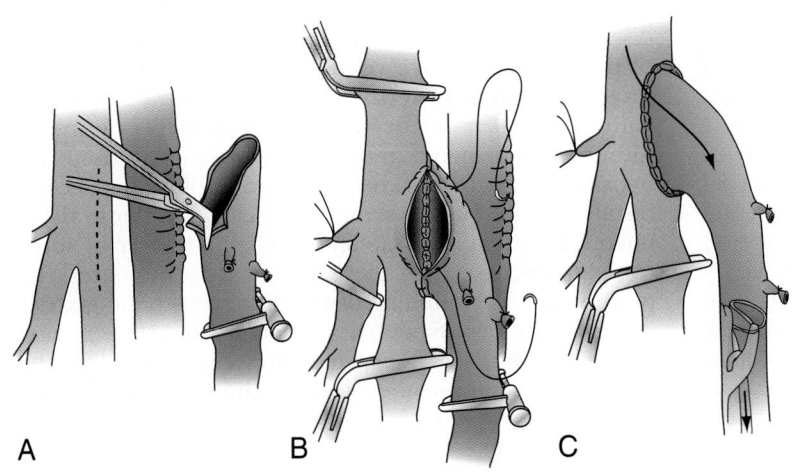

FIGURE 65-14. **A**, In the in situ method of infrainguinal reconstruction, the saphenofemoral junction is transected in the groin, the venotomy in the femoral vein is oversewn, and the proximal end of the saphenous vein is prepared for anastomosis. **B**, After the first venous valve is excised under direct vision, the graft is anastomosed end-to-side to the femoral artery. **C**, Flow is then restored through the vein graft, and the valvotome is inserted through side branches at appropriate intervals to lyse residual valve cusps.

vein is sewn to the outflow distal artery. The vein graft is spatulated appropriately, and the anastomosis is completed with 5-0 polypropylene suture, using standard anastomotic techniques. Before completion of the anastomosis, all vessels are flushed and the anastomosis is tied down; flow is restored to the native vessels, and flow through the graft is assessed. The reversed vein graft may be placed directly in the subcutaneous plane as it travels from the proximal to distal anastomosis. Conversely, a more anatomic, subsartorial plane may be preferable, particularly in patients in whom wound healing may be a problem. When bypass grafts are performed at the below-knee popliteal artery, it is often preferable to tunnel the graft directly through the popliteal fossa to facilitate a favorable distal anastomotic configuration. Bypass grafts to the anterior tibial artery may be tunneled through the intraosseous membrane or, if preferred, subcutaneously over the anterolateral thigh, lateral to the knee, and directly to the anterior tibial artery exposure site on the anterolateral calf. The distal vessels are clamped with atraumatic bulldog clamps and opened longitudinally. The vein graft is trimmed to an appropriate length and bevel, and the anastomosis is completed with 6-0 or 7-0 polypropylene suture. It is often preferable to "parachute" the heel of the distal anastomosis, particularly when the artery is deep within the calf. Before completion of the anastomosis, all vessels are flushed and patency at each end of the anastomosis is verified with a fine coronary artery dilator. The anastomosis is tied down, and flow is restored. Recent reported results with reversed saphenous vein grafting using modern surgical techniques have been excellent, with 5-year primary and secondary patency rates of 75% and 80%, respectively, and limb salvage rates of 90%.[36]

IN SITU GREATER SAPHENOUS VEIN BYPASS

The in situ greater saphenous vein bypass technique differs in that the saphenous vein is left in its own bed (i.e., in situ) rather than removing it and reversing its orientation. This approach requires disruption of the competent saphenous vein valves to allow flow down the vein. Although the in situ greater saphenous vein bypass was originally introduced in the 1960s, the tedious nature of the procedure and mixed results prevented its widespread adoption. In the early 1970s, however, Leather and Karmody developed a new technique for lysing the valves, leading to new interest and eventual widespread adoption of this technique.[25] Although there are a number of theoretical advantages to the in situ technique, including maintenance of the vasa vasorum and the endothelial layer of the vein graft, these have never been proven to offer a clear advantage in terms of patency or vein graft function. There are several practical advantages to the in situ technique, however, that offer technical benefits to the surgeon. Maintaining the vein graft in the in situ configuration allows the surgeon to sew the large end of the greater saphenous vein to the larger femoral vessels and to sew the smaller distal saphenous vein to the smaller tibial vessels. This size match at the proximal and distal ends facilitates the completion of precise technical anastomoses. Preservation of the saphenous vein hood offers particular advantages when sewing to a thick-walled, diseased femoral artery. Given these technical advantages, it is possible to successfully use smaller greater saphenous veins, which may not be serviceable for the reversed vein technique.

The preparation and arterial exposure for in situ bypass is similar to that for reversed vein bypass grafting. Most surgeons prefer to expose the entire greater saphenous vein through a continuous thigh and calf incision. After anticoagulation with heparin and performance of the arteriotomy, the saphenous vein hood is divided flush with the common femoral vein, using a Satinsky clamp. The common femoral vein is then oversewn with a 5-0 Prolene suture (Fig. 65-14). The proximal valve of the greater saphenous vein can be excised under direct vision with a fine forceps and Potts scissors. The proximal anastomosis of the saphenous vein hood to the femoral artery (see Fig. 65-14B) is performed with standard surgical techniques. Again, all vessels are flushed and flow is restored to the femoral vessels after tying down the anastomosis.

Pulsatile flow is restored to the vein graft, and the first site of a competent valve is obvious as the vein graft distends to that point and remains decompressed below. A valvulotome is then used to lyse the valves and therefore allow antegrade flow through the graft (see Fig. 65-14C). A number of valvulotomes are currently available. Most surgeons prefer the modified Mills valvulotome, which is a short, hockey-stick–shaped cutter that is serially introduced through side branches of the greater saphenous vein and pulled inferiorly, thereby lysing each pair of valves as they are encountered. The consistent orientation of the vein valves parallel to the skin facilitates precise, atraumatic valve lysis. The most distal valves are lysed by introducing the valvulotome through the open distal end of the vein graft and pulling inferiorly. A number of modifications of the in situ technique have been introduced to improve the simplicity and precision of the operation while decreasing morbidity. For example, long, self-centering valvulotomes, which may be introduced through the distal open end of the vein, may be used to lyse the valves in a single pass. Once all of the valves have been lysed and excellent pulsatile flow through the graft is ensured, the various side branches of the greater saphenous vein must be occluded with surgical clips or ties to prevent the formation of arteriovenous fistulas. Most recently, intra-arterial angioscopy has been combined with specially designed valvulotomes and coil embolization of the side branches to allow the in situ technique to be performed through limited proximal and distal incisions without exposing the entire length of vein. Recent series using the in situ greater saphenous vein have reported 5-year cumulative graft patency rates in the 80% range with limb salvage rates of 84% to 90%.[13]

On completion of the bypass with either a reversed or in situ saphenous vein, flow through the graft as well as outflow arteries is assessed with a continuous-wave Doppler study. A completion arteriogram is performed by direct cannulation of the proximal graft to demonstrate the bypass conduit, distal anastomosis, and outflow bed. Unsuspected technical defects, such as intraluminal thrombus, kinking or twisting of the graft, or unlysed valves, should be immediately repaired. More recently, intraoperative duplex ultrasonography has proved to be a sensitive completion study for detecting hemodynamically significant abnormalities at either anastomosis or within the graft conduit.

PROSTHETIC BYPASS

As mentioned previously, both polyester (Dacron) and PTFE graft material may be selectively used for infrainguinal arterial reconstructive surgery, particularly when the distal anastomosis is to the above-knee popliteal artery. Better results can be anticipated when the operations are performed to large-caliber vessels with good outflow (two to three open tibial vessels). The conduct of the operation is similar to that of reversed vein greater saphenous vein bypass grafting except that the longitudinal incision for saphenous vein harvest is unnecessary. The ability to perform a prosthetic bypass graft through two small proximal and distal arterial exposure incisions is a distinct advantage of the technique. The arteriotomy and proximal anastomosis is performed using standard techniques, and the graft is tunneled through a subsartorial plane down to the above-knee popliteal artery. The

distal anastomosis is then performed. Aggressive flushing of the graft and native vessels is imperative when using prosthetic bypass materials. Depending on the size of the native vessels, a 6- or 8-mm graft may be desirable. Although prosthetic grafts are occasionally used for bypasses to the below-knee popliteal or tibial vessels, the results achieved in this setting are clearly inferior to those obtained with greater saphenous vein. A variety of surgical adjuncts, including the creation of a distal arteriovenous fistula, the patching of the distal prosthetic graft to native artery bypass with a vein patch, and the creation of a cuff of autogenous vein interposed between the native artery and prosthetic graft at the distal anastomotic site, have all been proposed as useful techniques for improving the results of prosthetic bypass grafts performed to the below-knee level.

REOPERATIVE BYPASS SURGERY

Increasingly, patients are having failure of previous arterial reconstructions and recurrence of their limb-threatening ischemia symptoms. Reoperative infrainguinal arterial reconstruction offers a number of challenges. In most cases, the ipsilateral greater saphenous vein has previously been used and is no longer available for the secondary bypass procedure. Extensive scarring around the inflow and outflow vessels resulting from the previous surgical dissection complicates the surgical exposure. A number of strategies are useful in dealing with these complex cases. Whenever possible, alternative arterial inflow sites above or below the previous scarred arteries should be used to avoid dissection in areas of previous scarring.

The contralateral greater saphenous vein, if available, constitutes the optimal conduit for secondary bypass surgery. Recent studies have also demonstrated minimal short- or long-term impact on the contralateral leg in these situations.[44] Depending on the length of the bypass and the size of the greater saphenous vein, the graft may be used in either the reversed or nonreversed configuration with lysed valves. Frequently, however, because of contralateral bypass surgery or previous coronary artery bypass surgery, no greater saphenous vein is available for this secondary procedure. In these situations, a preliminary survey of the arm veins and lesser saphenous veins, using duplex ultrasound, reveals the best autogenous vein available for reconstruction. Although arm veins may be scarred or small below the elbows, the deeper upper arm veins, including cephalic and basilic veins, are often of excellent caliber and quality. Although these veins are thin walled and tedious to work with, they are strong and are generally of excellent caliber and quality. Because these various ectopic veins are usually relatively short, it is often necessary to perform a venovenostomy to create composite vein grafts of sufficient length to complete the arterial reconstruction.[45] Ample spatulation of each vein and the use of fine monofilament and sutures facilitate the completion of widely patent anastomoses within these composite vein grafts. Depending on the size and taper of these ectopic veins, they may be placed in either the reversed configuration or nonreversed configuration with lysed valves. When autogenous vein is in short supply it is often advantageous to originate the bypass graft from a more distal vessel such as the distal superficial femoral or popliteal artery. Such distal origin grafts work particularly well in diabetic patients who often have relative preservation of flow to the knee level.[46]

Despite improvements in operative techniques, the results of redo infrainguinal bypass surgery remain inferior to those obtained with primary operation. When autogenous vein is available for secondary bypass, 5-year patency rates of 60% and limb salvage rates of 72% have been achieved.[5]

After completion of any autogenous vein bypass graft, potential graft failure remains a major problem. Early failure vein grafts (within 30 days) generally represents a judgmental or technical error within the conduct of surgery. These include simple technical errors, such as a kink or twist within the graft, or failure to completely lyse the valves. Judgmental errors include the use of a small or poor-quality vein conduit or the construction of an anastomosis to an inadequate outflow artery. Intermediate failures (30 days to 2 years) are generally caused by intimal hyperplastic lesions that form at anastomotic sites or valve sites within the graft. Late graft failures (beyond 2 years) are most often caused by progression of atherosclerotic occlusive disease within the inflow or outflow vessels. Because of the importance of vein graft patency in maintaining both limb function and salvage, and because of the inability to restore durable patency to vein grafts once they have thrombosed, it is important to maintain a surveillance program to ensure that vein grafts are functioning well and not harboring stenotic lesions that threaten graft patency. Serial postoperative examinations with a duplex scan have proven extremely accurate in identifying significant vein graft lesions that threaten the graft patency. Recognition and repair of such lesions before graft thrombosis ensures continued durable graft patency in most cases.

PERCUTANEOUS TRANSLUMINAL ANGIOPLASTY

The role of PTA in the management of infrainguinal occlusive disease is considerably more limited than in the management of AOD. The smaller vessel size, more diffuse nature of the disease, and more limited outflow significantly impair the long-term results of infrainguinal angioplasty compared with those achieved in the larger iliac vessels. Whereas short, isolated, stenotic lesions, or even short-segment occlusions within the superficial femoral artery, may be successfully treated with PTA, most patients with such isolated lesions are well managed with conservative treatment. Unlike the management of iliac lesions in which stents have proven to be useful after technically complicated angioplasties, stents have not significantly improved the patency of femoral or popliteal angioplasties. Newer and more flexible self-expanding stent design, smaller-caliber delivery systems, and medicated or drug-eluting stent technology may improve patency.[51] In patients with limited autogenous vein, a short-segment angioplasty of a superficial femoral artery lesion may allow the bypass graft to originate more distally from the superficial femoral artery or popliteal artery.

CHRONIC VISCERAL ISCHEMIA

Renovascular Occlusive Disease

Chronic occlusive disease of the main renal artery results in reduced blood flow to the kidney. When the level of occlusion exceeds 60% of the diameter of the main renal artery, changes in pressure and flow distally result in increased secretion of renin and subsequent shifts in peripheral vasoconstriction and extracellular fluid volume, which result in hypertension. It has been estimated that less than 5% of hypertensive people have renovascular hypertension. Patients with clinically apparent atherosclerosis have a somewhat higher prevalence of renal artery disease. For example, among patients with coronary disease who underwent abdominal arteriography, 11% have significant unilateral renal artery disease with stenosis greater than 50% and 4% have significant bilateral disease.[21] Among patients with diastolic blood pressure greater than 115 mm Hg, the prevalence of renovascular hypertension is 15% to 20%; and among children younger than 5 years of age, the prevalence approximates 75%.

When there is significant bilateral renal artery involvement, total glomerular filtration rate is reduced sufficiently to decrease creatinine clearance. Renal insufficiency from reduced renal perfusion is a late manifestation of advanced arterial occlusive disease involving both kidneys. It has been estimated that up to 30% of patients on dialysis for end-stage renal disease have significant renovascular occlusive disease as a contributing factor. Nephrosclerosis, diabetic nephropathy, atheroembolism, glomerulonephritis, and other conditions may coexist with renovascular disease in many patients with chronic renal insufficiency.

Recognition and correction of large artery renal occlusive disease can result in impressive improvement in blood pressure control and preservation of renal function.

Pathology

Atherosclerosis accounts for nearly 90% of cases of renovascular hypertension (Box 65-5). This cause is twice as

---

Box 65-5. Causes of Renovascular Occlusive Disease

Atherosclerosis
Fibromuscular dysplasia
Takayasu's arteritis
Radiation vasculitis
Neurofibromatosis
Thromboembolism

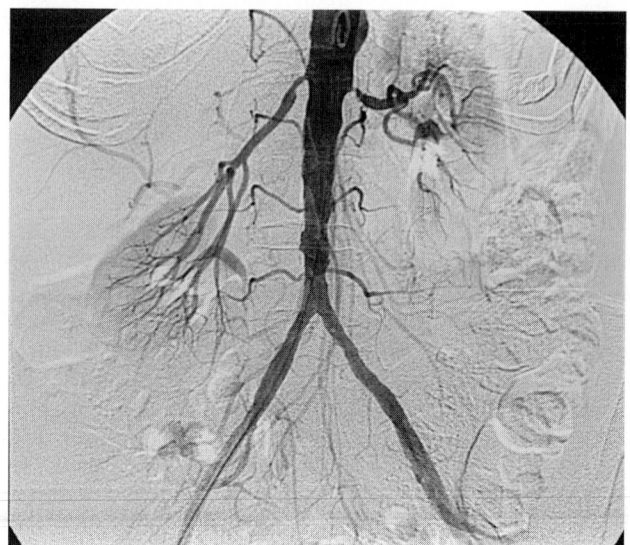

FIGURE 65-15. Arteriogram demonstrating proximal atherosclerotic involvement of both renal arteries. Most typically aortic plaque encroaches on the renal ostium as is seen in this example of bilateral orificial renal artery occlusive disease.

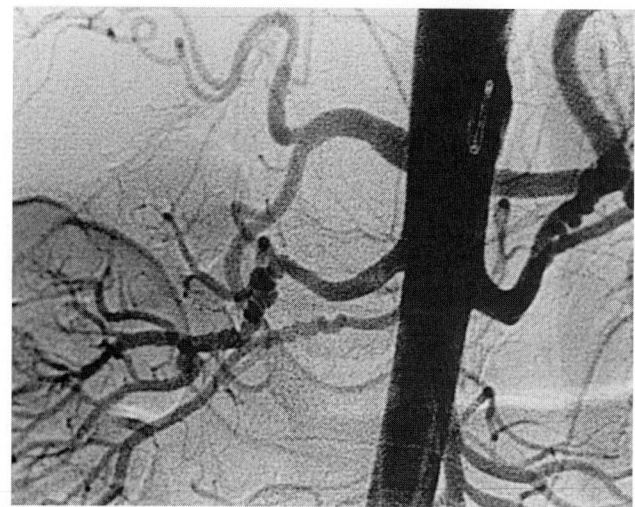

FIGURE 65-16. Arteriogram demonstrating bilateral fibromuscular dysplasia with involvement of the left renal artery and anomalous upper and lower pole arteries on the right. Note typical "string of beads" appearance in all three vessels.

common in men as in women, although as age increases, the sex distribution becomes more equal. Most commonly, the atherosclerotic process begins in the adjacent aorta with "spillover" plaque that encroaches into the proximal renal artery, resulting in "orificial" renal artery stenosis (Fig. 65-15). Plaque extends into the proximal third of the artery, but the more distal vessel remains relatively free of disease. Atherosclerosis involves the renal artery origins bilaterally in more than half of patients. Plaque is subject to fracture and subintimal hemorrhage with associated increase in stenosis or abrupt occlusion as well as atheroembolism, which produces small branch occlusion in the renal parenchyma. Studies using serial angiography and renal ultrasound have elucidated the natural history of atherosclerotic renal occlusive disease. Arteries detected to have more than 60% stenosis progress over the next several years to increased stenosis and ultimate occlusion.[42]

Fibromuscular dysplasia is the second most common type of renal artery disease. Three subtypes are distinguished on the basis of the layer of the arterial wall most involved. Medial fibroplasia is by far the most common, accounting for 85% of dysplastic lesions. It nearly always affects women, most commonly appearing between the ages of 25 and 45 years. The etiology is unknown. The condition involves the main renal artery with either a solitary stenosis or multiple stenoses with intervening dilatations that may appear like a "string-of-beads" (Fig. 65-16). True aneurysms may occur in approximately 10% of patients with this condition, most often at branch points of the peripheral arterial arcade. Lesions are bilateral in 70%, and medial fibroplasia can also affect other arteries, most commonly the internal carotid and external iliac arteries. Perimedial dysplasia accounts for about 10% of dysplastic lesions, also nearly exclusively in women

between 30 and 50 years of age. Intimal fibroplasia accounts for the remaining 5% of dysplastic lesions. This subtype is more common in children and young adults of either sex. Fibromuscular dysplasia is generally self-limited and does not progress after it reaches a clinically recognizable threshold.

A small number of patients in the pediatric age group have developmental anomalies that result in impaired renal artery flow. These lesions usually involve the origin of the renal artery with fibrous stricture, sometimes in association with abdominal aortic coarctation.

Pathophysiology

An association between hypertension and renal disease was noted in 1836. A pressor substance was discovered in the rabbit in 1897 and called renin. In 1934, Goldblatt showed that unilateral renal artery constriction produced hypertension in the dog. Cure of hypertension by nephrectomy was reported in 1937 and by restoration of flow to the kidney using thromboendarterectomy in 1954.

Hypertension occurs after reduction in mean renal artery perfusion pressure by greater than 60% diameter or 75% cross-sectional area of the proximal renal artery. Renal baroreceptors in the afferent arterioles sense the reduction in mean arterial pressure, leading to release of renin by the juxtaglomerular apparatus. Renin appears in the renal vein and hydrolyzes angiotensinogen, produced in the liver, to form angiotensin I. This decapeptide is inactive but is converted to the octapeptide angiotensin II in the lungs by angiotensin-converting enzyme (ACE). Angiotensin II is a strong vasoconstrictor with a half-life of 4 minutes and acts directly on vascular smooth muscle. ACE inhibitors such as captopril are particularly effective in treating hypertension related to high renin and subsequent high angiotensin II levels (Fig. 65-17).

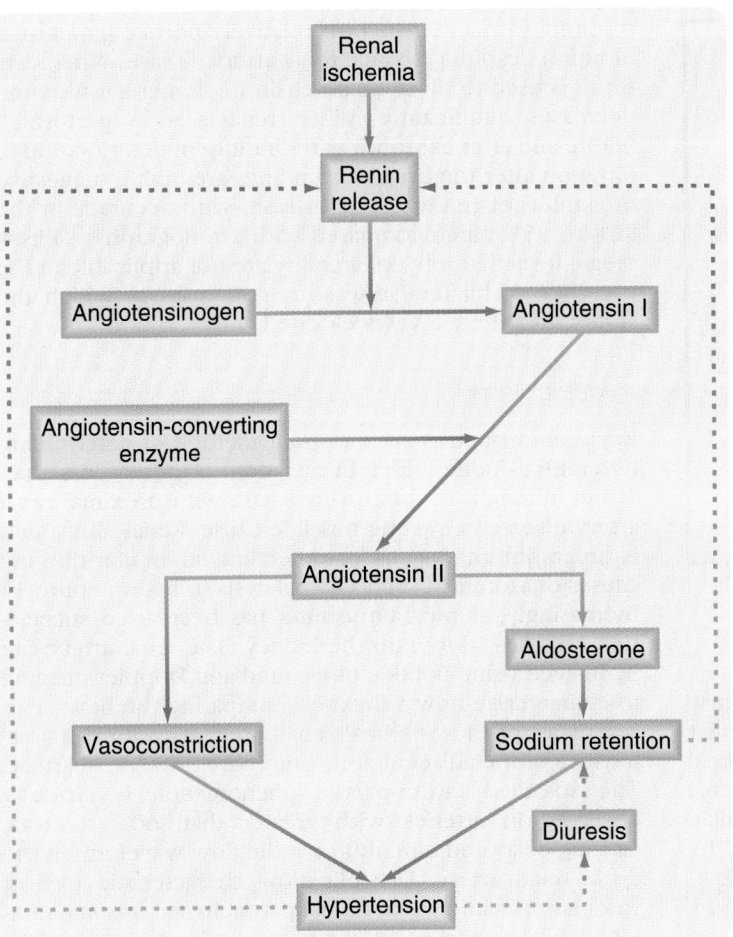

FIGURE 65-17. Consequences of renin hypersecretion as result of renal ischemia. *Dotted arrows* represent inhibitory influence. (Adapted from Pickering TG: Renal vascular disease. *In* Braunwald S, Creager MA [eds]: Atlas of Heart Diseases, vol 7. St. Louis, CV Mosby, 1996, p 4.3)

Angiotensin II also facilitates formation of aldosterone by the adrenal cortex. Aldosterone causes conservation of salt and water by the kidney, resulting in increased extracellular fluid volume contributing to hypertension. Diuretics are beneficial in controlling hypertension because they help correct hypervolemia.

When one renal artery is involved with occlusive disease, increased renin secretion from the affected kidney results in hypertension, which suppresses renin secretion from the contralateral kidney. Increased glomerular filtration occurs in the normal kidney, resulting in relatively normal or low extracellular volume. When both kidneys are involved, or in circumstances of a solitary affected kidney, overall renal hypoperfusion results in hypervolemic hypertension. With increasing severity, decreased creatinine clearance occurs and azotemia supervenes.

Renovascular hypertension has a significant impact on the heart and vascular tree. Nephrosclerosis affects renal tissue "unprotected" by proximal renal artery disease and thus exposed to hypertension, as in a relatively normal kidney opposite a kidney with significant occlusive disease. Hypertension also contributes significantly to progression of atherosclerosis in the peripheral, coronary, and carotid arteries as well as to hypertensive retinopathy. The heart itself is affected with left ventricular hypertrophy and reduced ventricular compliance. In the presence of bilateral renal artery occlusive disease and resulting hypervolemia superimposed upon hypertension, a sudden hypertensive crisis may occur with acute left ventricular failure precipitating so-called flash pulmonary edema.

Diagnosis

CLINICAL PRESENTATION

The clinical presentation is an important clue to the presence of renovascular occlusive disease (Box 65-6). Hypertensive patients in the pediatric age group, among whom renovascular causes are more prevalent, should be investigated for correctable causes. Females between the ages of 25 and 50 years should similarly be considered. Patients in the older age group with recent significant change in blood pressure control or renal function and in whom there are coexistent risk factors for atherosclerosis should also undergo screening. Patients who respond dramatically to ACE inhibitors are more likely to have high renin hypertension related to renovascular disease. If azotemia becomes worse on antihypertensive therapy, bilateral renal artery disease should be suspected. Patients with a hypertensive crisis and flash pulmonary edema and left ventricular failure are highly suspect, particularly if blood pressure control results in increased renal insufficiency.

Box 65-6. Clinical Correlates of Increased Prevalence of Renovascular Disease

Severe hypertension—diastolic >115 mm Hg

Refractory hypertension

New onset of sustained hypertension at age younger than 20 yr, female age younger than 50, either sex age older than 50

Hypertension and epigastric or flank bruit

Moderate progressive or severe hypertension in patients with manifestations of systemic atherosclerosis and unexplained stable or progressive renal insufficiency

Malignant hypertension or hypertensive crisis

Dramatic normalization of blood pressure by angiotensin-converting enzyme inhibitor

Increase in serum creatinine with blood pressure improvement

PHYSIOLOGIC TESTS

Much work has been done in an effort to perfect the use of the renin assay to make the diagnosis of renovascular hypertension. Selective sampling of blood from each renal vein and comparing each to samples from the infrarenal and suprarenal vena cava can indeed demonstrate unilateral hypersecretion of renin from the kidney affected by the diseased renal artery. The best accuracy requires cessation of β blockers and stimulation of renin secretion by limiting sodium intake and administering a diuretic for a few days before the assay, as well as tilting the patient into an upright position during sampling. These logistical problems have made selective renin assay impractical in most centers. Peripheral venous renin assay has also been used, but values are most helpful only when similarly stimulated and indexed against serum sodium balance. Because many antihypertensive drugs have an impact on renin and sodium and because such drugs must be stopped for as long as 3 weeks to obtain a precise measurement, this approach has also been generally impractical.

Demonstration of asymmetrical renal function is another physiologic approach to diagnosis. Split renal function studies use selective ureteral catheterization to sample urine from each kidney. If decreased amounts of urine with higher concentrations of sodium, creatinine, or administered *p*-aminohippuric acid are detected on one side, the involved kidney is likely ischemic. This method is somewhat cumbersome and rarely used. Hypertensive intravenous pyelography can demonstrate delayed appearance of intravenous contrast dye in the involved kidney, a difference in renal size, and delayed hyperconcentration of contrast agent in the collecting system as well as occasional "nicking" of the ureter caused by large periureteral arterial collaterals.

More currently, radionuclide tracer is used to assess renal blood flow and excretory function. The ACE inhibitor captopril has enhanced the accuracy of radionuclide scanning. Angiotensin II in the involved kidney leads to selective vasoconstriction of the efferent arterioles, resulting in maintenance of relatively normal glomerular filtration despite proximal renal artery disease. When captopril is used to block angiotensin II, glomerular filtration decreases significantly. When renal scan is performed before and after captopril with findings of deterioration in filtration after the drug, the findings are highly suggestive of significant renovascular disease, with accuracy in the 90% to 95% range compared with arteriography.[11] Physiologic tests that rely on laterality are not applicable in the presence of bilateral disease nor in cases in which the serum creatinine level is elevated above 3 mg/dL.

ANATOMIC TESTS

Renal ultrasound is an important method of determining differential kidney size. In an adult, a kidney less than 10 cm in length is abnormally small, with proximal renal artery disease being one possible cause. Renal ultrasound is an important means of detecting other contributing causes of azotemia, such as renal cysts or hydronephrosis. Increasingly, duplex ultrasound has been used successfully to assess flow into the kidney. The renal artery can be imaged using B-mode ultrasound and Doppler imaging to characterize flow velocities, comparing the flow characteristics of the proximal renal artery with flow characteristics of the adjacent aorta and more distal renal artery. The so-called tardus-parvus phenomenon is typically observed in arteries with greater than 60% stenosis, causing delay and diminution in the flow waveform in the distal renal artery. Diastolic flow characteristics reflect vascular resistance in the renal parenchyma. In some noninvasive laboratories, duplex ultrasound is more than 90% accurate in detecting significant large vessel renal artery disease.[11]

MRI is becoming the anatomic imaging modality of choice in many centers where gadolinium-enhanced scanning has provided an expeditious, objective, and safe means of identifying renal artery disease.[47] Although tortuosity and obliquity of the renal artery origins may result in artifacts that may make images difficult to interpret, scans are generally sufficiently accurate to allow MRI an important role in the initial phases of patient evaluation. CT is also available, using spiral technique for high-resolution imaging of the renal arteries. This method is very accurate but requires use of intravenous contrast material with a small risk of renal toxicity.

Arteriography is the most precise diagnostic tool. Intravenous digital subtraction arteriography, although less invasive, requires a relatively large dose of iodinated contrast and often yields comparatively poor images. Selective intra-arterial study using computer enhancement allows precise anatomic definition, usually with minimal dye exposure. An even safer variant involves use of carbon dioxide as a radiographic contrast medium in patients with advanced renal insufficiency.

Routine screening using a single laboratory study such as peripheral renin or a single anatomic study such as MRI on the broad population of hypertensive patients is inappropriate. Evaluation requires consideration of the clinical presentation and setting, followed by a logical sequence of confirmatory studies designed to uncover the diagnosis

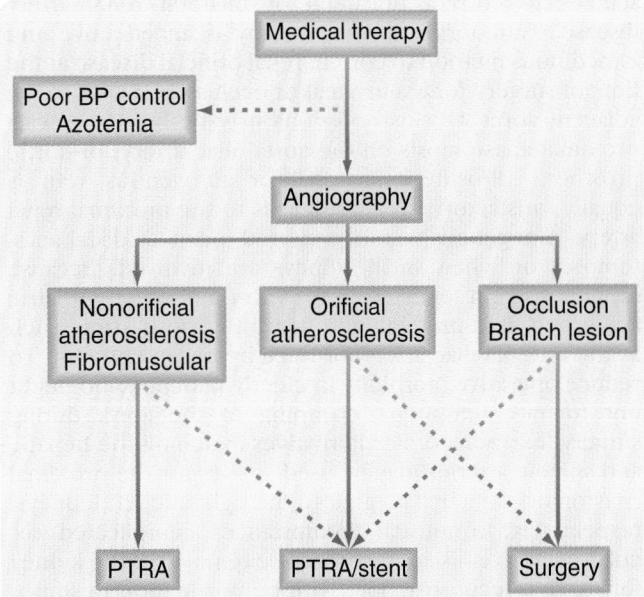

FIGURE 65-18. Therapeutic scheme for patients with proven renal artery occlusive disease. *Dotted arrows* represent secondary therapeutic options.

with minimal cost and risk. Because they are logistically cumbersome, physiologic studies have increasingly yielded to anatomic diagnosis, relying on ultrasound and MRI for initial detection of disease and then arteriography for confirmation and possible catheter-based intervention if appropriate (Box 65-7). In the proper clinical setting, the presence of a small kidney with arterial stenosis greater than 60%, poststenotic dilatation, and evidence of delayed parenchymal function is highly predictive of therapeutic success after revascularization. Increasingly, percutaneous methods of revascularization are available with minimal risk to the patient, making absolute precision in diagnosis less compelling than it would be if the only therapeutic solution involved more risky and arduous surgery.

Treatment

Initial therapy of renovascular hypertension is medical. β-Adrenergic blockers, diuretics, vasodilators, and ACE inhibitors are commonly used with success. A more aggressive therapeutic approach is justifiable if blood pressure control requires increasing doses of two or three medications or if renal function deteriorates while on antihypertensive medications, particularly ACE inhibitors (Fig. 65-18). Under these circumstances, noninvasive imaging with ultrasound or MRI should be performed, followed by arteriography as appropriate with plans to proceed at the same sitting with percutaneous endovascular renal artery therapy if favorable lesions are confirmed.

Percutaneous transluminal renal angioplasty is an important therapeutic tool. Balloon dilatation is the procedure of choice for patients with fibromuscular dysplasia involving the main renal artery, reserving surgical revascularization for more complicated lesions involving branches of the renal artery. Percutaneous transluminal renal angioplasty is also successfully applicable to patients with focal nonorificial atherosclerotic renal artery disease. Nonorificial atherosclerosis or dysplasia can be treated with greater than 90% technical success rate and long-term benefit in 70% to 90% of cases.[33] Orificial atherosclerotic lesions are much less likely to respond to balloon dilatation alone because they are essentially composed of aortic plaque, which cannot be effectively cracked and remodeled in a durable manner by a balloon alone. Technical success for orificial atherosclerosis is no greater than 50%, and long-term success rate is 40% among those initially successfully treated by angioplasty.[33] The immediate and long-term success of balloon angioplasty can be

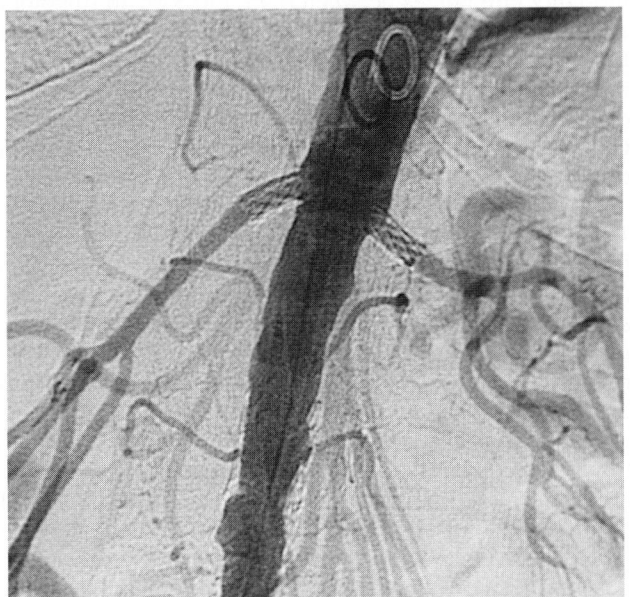

FIGURE 65-19. Completion arteriogram after percutaneous transluminal angioplasty and stenting for orificial left renal artery disease in patient illustrated in Figure 62-15.

improved by using arterial stenting (Fig. 65-19).[39] Although not necessary for most nonorificial lesions, stents have extended the usefulness of percutaneous therapy to orificial atherosclerosis. The morbidity rate after percutaneous therapy is below 10%, with severe morbidity including arterial rupture or occlusion occurring in 1% to 2%.

A direct approach to the renal artery is possible using a variety of surgical techniques.[34] Isolated renal endarterectomy may be performed in unusual circumstances to correct unilateral or bilateral renal artery disease. Transaortic endarterectomy is an effective and expeditious method to correct renal orificial disease at the time of surgery for aneurysmal or occlusive disease of the adjacent aorta. Occlusive lesions may be bypassed with proximal anastomosis on the aorta, iliac artery, or aortic prosthesis. Prosthetic material or autogenous vein is equally satisfactory for anastomosis to the proximal renal artery. Autogenous vein is preferred for more distal anastomoses or when small kidneys are involved. Because saphenous vein tends to dilate with time in the pediatric age group, it is preferable to use autogenous artery such as the internal iliac artery for renal bypass in children. To reduce operative morbidity in elderly patients who might not tolerate temporary clamping of the aorta during surgery, extra-anatomic alternatives including the hepatic and splenic arteries may be used as sites for the proximal anastomosis of a bypass graft to the right and left kidneys, respectively. In unusual circumstances, complicated vascular occlusive disease may require removal of the kidney for ex vivo reconstruction, with reimplantation in situ or in the pelvis using the iliac artery and vein as in a renal transplant procedure. Major morbidity occurs in 5% to 10% of patients after contemporary surgery. Perioperative death is unusual in pediatric and dysplastic patients, and mortality rate ranges between 0.9% and 5.8% in the older atherosclerotic group. Although it was initially thought that combining renal artery surgery with aortic surgery increased morbidity and mortality rates, recent experience indicates that renal artery endarterectomy can be performed in conjunction with aortic aneurysm resection or aortic bypass without increasing the mortality risk.[12]

The presence of an occluded artery is not necessarily a contraindication to revascularization. Percutaneous therapy may be attempted, and, if a wire can be passed through the occlusion, balloon angioplasty and stent may succeed. More typically, surgery is necessary, at which time a short segmental occlusion is usually found with reconstitution of a virtually normal artery within 1 to 2 cm. If the kidney is more than 7 to 8 cm in length, there is a significant chance of recovery of function and reduction in renin secretion after revascularization. Kidneys that are smaller than 6 cm are generally not salvageable, and nephrectomy may be considered. Nephrectomy is much less frequent than in past years because of the success of revascularization and the efficacy of ACE inhibitors for high renin hypertension.

Results of Revascularization

Long-term results after percutaneous transluminal renal angioplasty are excellent for patients with fibromuscular dysplasia. Recurrent stenosis occurs in approximately 10% of patients but is most often amenable to repeat angioplasty. Lesions involving branch arteries or bifurcation areas are less likely to be successfully treated and more likely to be associated with complications after attempted angioplasty. Among patients with atherosclerotic renal artery disease, appropriate selective use of balloon angioplasty and stents results in generally excellent success after several years with cure of hypertension in 20% to 25% of cases, improvement or stabilization in 50% to 60%, and failure in 15% to 20%.[38,39,52]

Surgical revascularization for fibromuscular dysplasia results in cure or improvement of hypertension at rates similar to percutaneous therapy. Among children, surgical therapy is highly successful, resulting in cure of hypertension in 70% to 85% of cases and improvement in another 10% to 25%, with failure in less than 10%. Among patients with atherosclerosis, hypertension is cured in roughly one third and improved in 50%, with failure in 10% to 20%.[12] Endarterectomy of the renal artery orifice is a very durable procedure. Serial study of bypass patency indicates as many as 88% of grafts remain patent for as long as 20 years after surgery. Vein graft dilatation occurs in 3% to 5%, particularly among the pediatric age group.

Renal function has been reported to improve in 40% of patients who had revascularization for azotemia. Such patients almost always underwent revascularization bilaterally or had a solitary kidney, with the therapeutic goal of increasing blood flow to as much renal parenchyma as possible. Follow-up evaluation of natural history indicates that, even among patients with no significant immediate improvement in renal insufficiency, the rate at which renal function deteriorates appears to be reduced by revascularization. On rare occasions, patients who have been placed on dialysis have been taken off support after intervention.

Renal artery occlusive disease is responsible for hypertension and renal failure in a significant number of patients. Clinical suspicion and appropriate diagnostic study may direct patients toward therapy designed to improve flow to the kidneys, increasingly using relatively safe percutaneous methods. Results of such therapy offer substantial benefit to carefully selected and managed patients.

Mesenteric Ischemia

Vascular occlusive disease of the mesenteric vessels is a relatively rare but often catastrophic problem. When acute occlusion of a major artery occurs, profound illness usually results and survival is fortunate. Nonocclusive mesenteric insufficiency and mesenteric venous occlusion occur in the presence of severe concurrent illness of variable causes. Chronic intestinal ischemia often presents a diagnostic challenge, but results are gratifying with timely therapy.

Pathophysiology

Mesenteric arterial anatomy is notable for rich collateral flow (Fig. 65-20). As a result, gradual occlusion of one or even two of the main mesenteric trunks is usually tolerated, as long as there is time for a collateral vessel from uninvolved branches to enlarge. On the other hand, sudden occlusion of a main branch or more peripherally beyond the largest collateral vessels may be poorly tolerated, with profound consequences. Acute vascular occlusion results in tissue injury with release of intracellular contents and byproducts of anaerobic metabolism to the

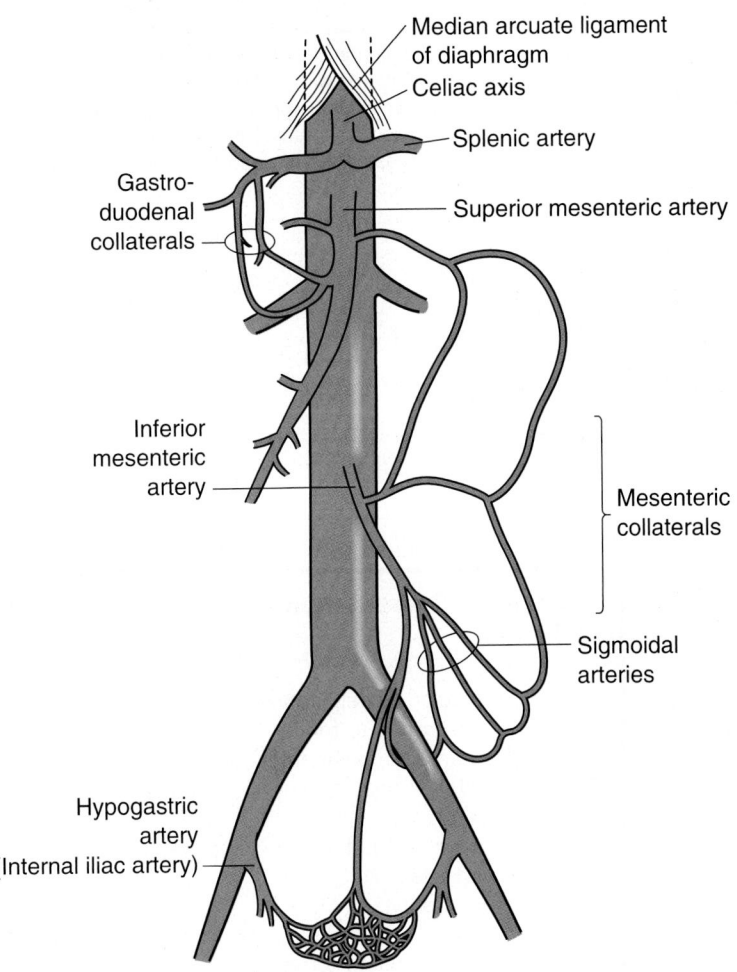

FIGURE 65-20. Mesenteric arterial anatomy demonstrating extensive collateral channels between major branches. (Adapted from Stoney RJ, Wylie EJ: Surgery of celiac and mesenteric arteries. *In* Haimovici HH [ed]: Vascular Surgery: Principles and Techniques. New York, McGraw-Hill, 1976, pp 668-679.)

general circulation. Compromised bowel mucosa allows unrestricted influx of toxic materials from the bowel lumen with systemic consequences. If serosal surfaces are affected by full-thickness necrosis, bowel perforation and peritonitis ensue. Associated heart disease or systemic atherosclerosis often compounds the complexity of acute arterial occlusion. Nonocclusive ischemia and mesenteric venous occlusion are usually complicated by significant or life-threatening concurrent abdominal or systemic illness.

Acute mesenteric artery occlusion most frequently results from a cardiogenic embolus and usually involves the superior mesenteric artery. Embolic occlusion most often occurs distal to the origin of the superior mesenteric artery because the embolus is pushed into the artery to a point where arborization reduces the lumen to a diameter less than that of the embolus (Fig. 65-21). Less commonly, thrombotic occlusion at the site of chronic atherosclerotic plaque occurs at the origin of the vessel adjacent to ostial disease. In both instances, secondary stasis thrombosis may occur in adjacent proximal and distal vessels to the point where flow from collaterals is maintained. Acute embolic occlusion is generally a more profound and damaging insult than thrombosis at the site of chronic disease because of (1) lack of protection by chronically enlarged collaterals from the other mesenteric arteries, (2) occlusion at levels beyond the point of inflow

of larger collaterals, and (3) occlusion of multiple branches to adjacent segments at the point of arterial arborization.

Acute nonocclusive mesenteric insufficiency accompanies profound illness with sepsis and cardiovascular collapse with consequent vasoconstriction of the mesenteric vascular bed. Use of vasopressors for hemodynamic support exacerbates the problem. If prolonged, such illness may result in hemodynamic compromise of nutrient flow to the bowel and mesenteric viscera. Mesenteric venous occlusion results in vascular compromise on the basis of reduced venous drainage of the bowel.

Chronic mesenteric insufficiency is almost exclusively a problem in the older age group with diffuse atherosclerosis that involves the aorta and the proximal mesenteric arteries. Because collaterals are usually abundant between the three main mesenteric vessels, at least two, most often the celiac and superior mesenteric artery, are severely compromised before symptoms arise (Table 65-5). Relative ischemia occurs after meals when there is increased demand for flow into the mesenteric bed. Vasodilation after eating reduces peripheral resistance, but flow cannot increase in the presence of proximal fixed occlusive lesions, creating transient ischemic pain that has been appropriately termed *intestinal angina*. Chronic abdominal pain occurs among an unusual group of generally

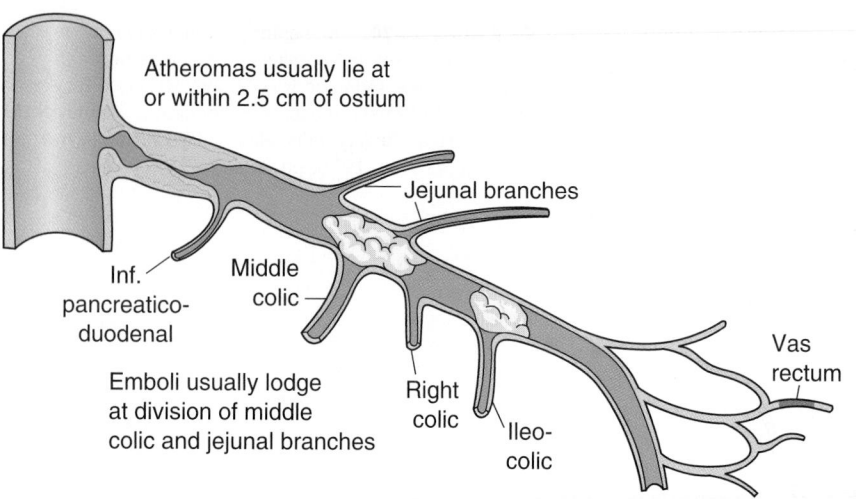

Atheromas usually lie at or within 2.5 cm of ostium

Jejunal branches

Inf. pancreatico-duodenal

Middle colic

Emboli usually lodge at division of middle colic and jejunal branches

Right colic

Ileo-colic

Vas rectum

FIGURE 65-21. Typical location of superior mesenteric artery obstruction in patients with embolic and thrombotic occlusion. (From Donaldson MC: Mesenteric vascular disease. *In* Braunwald S, Creager MA [eds]: Atlas of Heart Diseases. St. Louis, Mosby, 1996, p 5.6.)

TABLE 65-5. Extent of Obstruction in Chronic Mesenteric Arterial Insufficiency

Site	Percentage
Celiac/SMA/IMA	41-75
Celiac/SMA	29-82
Celiac/IMA	2
SMA/IMA	5
Celiac	0-14
SMA	1.4-9

IMA, inferior mesenteric artery; SMA, superior mesenteric artery.

Box 65-8. Presentation of Acute Mesenteric Ischemia

Concurrent cardiac or debilitating disease
Pain out of proportion to tenderness
Abdominal distention, gastrointestinal dysfunction
Evidence of "third" spacing—oliguria, hemoconcentration
Blood in stool
Elevated white cell count—often >20,000
Metabolic acidosis
Elevated serum enzymes
Bowel distention, wall thickening on kidney-ureter-bladder imaging and computed tomography
Endoscopic findings in colon
Specific findings on arteriogram

younger and otherwise healthy patients who have compression of the celiac artery by the median arcuate ligament of the diaphragm.

Presentation and Management

ACUTE MESENTERIC ARTERIAL OCCLUSION

The most common cause of acute mesenteric arterial occlusion is embolus to the superior mesenteric artery and rarely the celiac artery. Severe pain is always present and prominent, centered in the periumbilical region (Box 65-8). Abdominal examination typically reveals relatively little tenderness during the early stages, only to become more impressive as ischemic bowel produces visceral peritonitis and finally parietal peritonitis. The white blood cell count is generally elevated, and metabolic acidosis may be present. A plain radiograph of the abdomen may demonstrate fluid-filled bowel loops with evidence of edema in the bowel wall. Underlying cardiac disease is responsible for the embolus in 90% of cases, and manifestations of arrhythmia, recent myocardial infarction, or valvular disease may be present.

Early management relies critically on prompt diagnosis, which requires a high index of suspicion. Alternative diagnoses such as acute pancreatitis, perforated viscus, ruptured aneurysm, or kidney stone should be rapidly excluded while fluid resuscitation and antibiotics are instituted. Arteriography can identify the site of occlusion but is not crucial if the patient has compelling clinical evidence and if surgical therapy will be inordinately delayed as a result.

Surgery offers the best chance of successful treatment.[26] Exploratory laparotomy allows rapid confirmation of the diagnosis and exclusion of other conditions. If the entire bowel is frankly necrotic, the likelihood of survival is virtually nil and no further therapy should be pursued in most cases. If there is patchy or segmental necrosis or generalized ischemia that appears reversible, the proximal superior mesenteric artery is exposed at the base of the transverse mesocolon. Pulsation and flow are assessed in the main artery and its arcades using intraoperative Doppler ultrasound. In general, an embolus creates an accessible occlusion distal to the origin of the superior mesenteric artery, lodging in the first bifurcation point of the artery. Most often, the proximal superior mesenteric artery should be opened longitudinally and thromboembolectomy performed using a patch angioplasty to close the artery (Fig. 65-22).[41] If the artery is soft and free of ath-

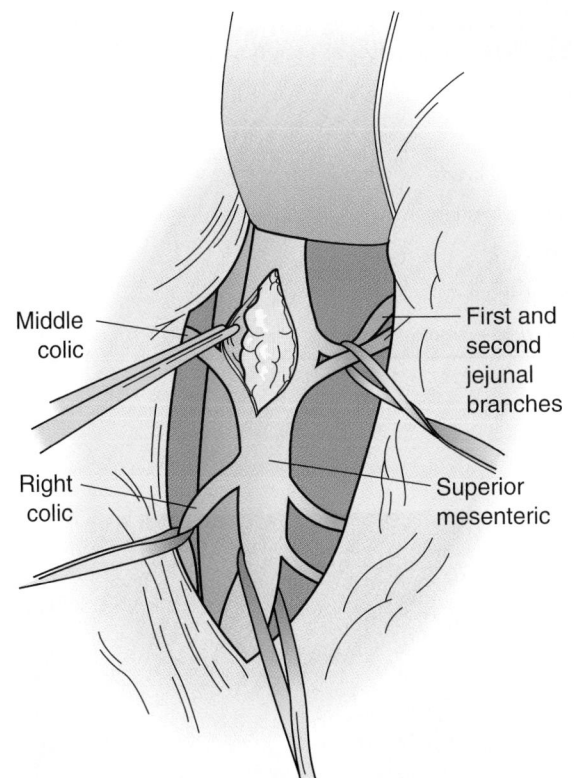

Middle colic

First and second jejunal branches

Right colic

Superior mesenteric

■ FIGURE 65-22. Longitudinal arteriotomy of the superior mesenteric artery for thromboembolectomy. Arteriotomy is closed either by patch angioplasty or by anastomosis to a bypass graft from a suitable source of inflow. (Adapted from Yao JST, Bergan JJ, Pearce WH, Flinn WR: Operative procedures in visceral ischemia. *In* Bergan JJ, Yao JST [eds]: Techniques in Arterial Surgery. Philadelphia, WB Saunders, 1990, pp 284-293.)

erosclerotic changes, a transverse arterotomy may be used and closed primarily without a patch. In patients with significant associated chronic arterial disease in whom thrombosis has occurred, a simple thromboembolectomy may fail to restore normal inflow. In such cases, the superior mesenteric artery arterotomy is used as the site for distal anastomosis of a bypass. Most often, autogenous vein is preferred to avoid the risk of infection of a prosthetic graft. The bypass may originate from the aorta or an iliac artery, depending on which is least involved with disease. After flow is established, frankly necrotic regions of bowel should be resected. Regions where there is potential for recovery may be observed for 24 to 36 hours and reassessed at a "second look" operation. The mortality rate reported for patients undergoing surgery for acute intestinal ischemia is as high as 85%, although with aggressive diagnosis and intervention, mortality rates may be reduced to the range of 25%.[26]

NONOCCLUSIVE MESENTERIC INSUFFICIENCY

Patients suffering from nonocclusive mesenteric insufficiency are frequently seriously ill and often have been in an intensive support setting before development of mesenteric insufficiency. If the patient is obtunded, intubated, or heavily narcotized, the presentation may be subtle and the diagnosis thus delayed. Diffuse abdominal pain is prominent and out of proportion to tenderness. Acidosis may be profound. Abdominal flat plate, ultrasound, and CT help to exclude other diagnoses such as perforated ulcer or acute cholecystitis. Arteriography is a valuable confirmatory diagnostic step. Classic arteriographic findings include absence of large vessel occlusion and a pattern of sequential focal vasospasm with "beading" of the major mesenteric branches and a "pruned tree" appearance to the distal vasculature.

In addition to making the diagnosis, arteriography facilitates valuable early therapy with continuous selective infusion of vasodilators such as papaverine into the superior mesenteric artery. Fluid resuscitation, withdrawal of vasoconstrictors, antibiotics to combat portal transmigration of bacteria, and angiographic monitoring of vasospasm are important components of patient management. Surgery should be reserved for patients who experience clinical deterioration or evidence of peritonitis suggesting bowel infarction. Success is possible only with control of the underlying illness that precipitated the mesenteric insufficiency. Because of the complexity of the illness, patients with nonocclusive mesenteric insufficiency have a grim prognosis.

MESENTERIC VENOUS OCCLUSION

Mesenteric venous occlusion occurs in patients with a number of concurrent illnesses, including liver disease and portal hypertension, pancreatitis, intraperitoneal inflammatory conditions, hypercoagulable states, and systemic low-flow states (Box 65-9). Venous thrombosis is less dramatic than arterial occlusion, and early diagnosis is typically difficult because the presentation is subtle (Table 65-6).[22] Abdominal pain is usually vague, and tenderness is mild or equivocal. CT may demonstrate thickened bowel wall with delayed passage of intravenous contrast agent into the portal system and lack of opacification of the portal vein. Arteriography may demonstrate venous congestion and lack of prompt filling of the portal system.

Therapy should consist of hemodynamic support, anticoagulation, and serial examination. If peritonitis develops, exploratory laparotomy is appropriate to assess bowel viability with segmental bowel resection as necessary. Surgical thrombectomy is not likely to be successful. Fibrinolytic therapy is hazardous because the congested bowel wall is susceptible to hemorrhage. In general, prognosis is good because collateral venous outflow develops and partial or even complete recanalization of the mesenteric veins may occur in many instances.

CHRONIC MESENTERIC INSUFFICIENCY

Patients with advanced chronic mesenteric artery disease most commonly have a stereotypical pattern of postprandial pain in a periumbilical location that occurs within 30 minutes of a meal (Table 65-7). It gradually resolves thereafter, only to recur with subsequent meals. Because eating causes pain, patients reduce the size of meals and develop a pattern of "food fear" abstinence that results in weight

Box 65-9. Conditions Associated With Mesenteric Venous Thrombosis

Portal Hypertension

Cirrhosis
Congestive splenomegaly

Inflammation

Peritonitis
Inflammatory bowel disease
Pelvic or intra-abdominal abscess
Diverticular disease

Postoperative State and Trauma

Splenectomy and other postoperative states
Blunt abdominal trauma

Hypercoagulable States

Neoplasms (colon, pancreas)
Oral contraceptives
Pregnancy
Migratory thrombophlebitis
Antithrombin III, protein C/S deficiency
Peripheral deep vein thrombosis
Polycythemia vera
Thrombocytosis

Other Conditions

Renal disease (nephrotic syndrome)
Cardiac disease (congestive failure)

TABLE 65-6. Presentation of Mesenteric Venous Thrombosis Pancreatic Cancer

Pain (insidious)	81%
Gastrointestinal bleed	19%
Guaiac + stool	63%
Anorexia	44%
Previous deep vein thrombosis	44%
Pancreatic cancer	13%
Hepatitis	25%
Thrombocytosis	25%
Increased fibrinogen	13%
Decreased proteins C, S	50%

TABLE 65-7. Signs and Symptoms of Chronic Mesenteric Arterial Insufficiency

Pain	100%
Weight loss	80-98%
Abdominal bruit	68-75%
Nausea, vomiting	54-84%
Diarrhea	35%
Constipation	13%-26%
Hemoccult + stool	8%

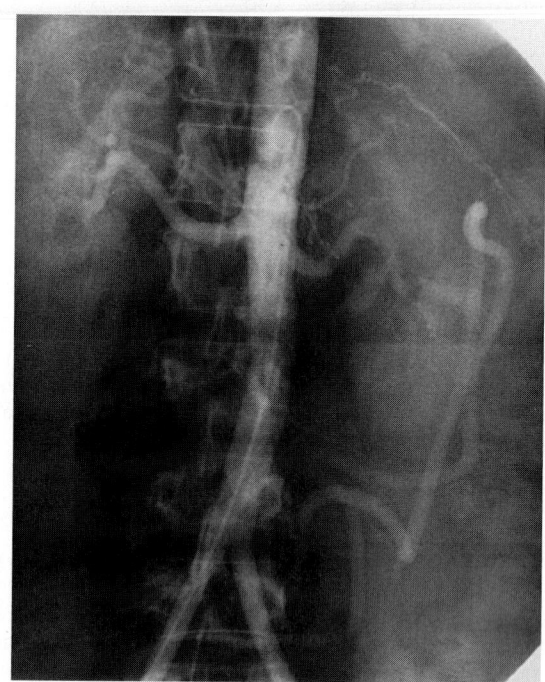

FIGURE 65-23. Arteriogram of patient with chronic intestinal ischemia demonstrating large meandering artery forming collateral within the mesentery of the colon.

loss. Malabsorption is rarely, if ever, a component of this disease.

Diagnosis requires a careful history and exclusion of other illnesses such as malignancy, chronic pancreatitis, and gastric ulcer. Often, a series of diagnostic studies is performed to exclude these entities and the diagnosis of chronic mesenteric ischemia is made late by exclusion. Duplex ultrasound has been used with increasing success to document occlusive disease in the proximal superior mesenteric artery and celiac arteries. The definitive diagnostic study is arteriography, which invariably reveals occlusion of at least two of the three major mesenteric arteries. Patterns of collateral vessels are often prominent, including a large meandering artery in the mesentery of the colon (Fig. 65-23).

In selected circumstances, revascularization by balloon angioplasty or stent placement may be successful, a strategy particularly applicable among elderly patients who may be poor candidates for surgery. More commonly,[48] definitive therapy requires surgery using either a direct approach to proximal arterial occlusions through transaortic endarterectomy or bypass grafting. Bypass may be performed using a prosthetic graft originating in the supraceliac aorta and connecting to both the celiac and superior mesenteric arteries. Alternatively, retrograde bypass from the infrarenal aorta or iliac artery may be used. Surgical exploration and therapy is usually facilitated because the patient has lost a significant amount of weight preoperatively. Results of surgery are generally highly gratifying in properly selected patients, with rapid resolution of symptoms and return of weight. Long-term patency of the grafts is excellent, exceeding 90%.

A small subset of patients without atherosclerosis and generally of younger age experience postprandial pain on the basis of celiac artery compression from the median arcuate ligament of the diaphragm. In general, such patients have a long history of chronic complaints. They often have been evaluated by numerous physicians and may have developed dependency on pain medications. Evaluation using MRI or arteriography reveals extrinsic compression of the proximal celiac artery with post-stenotic dilatation. Images during inspiration and expiration demonstrate a dynamic constriction of the artery. Therapy should be directed at highly selected patients. Percutaneous methods are not successful in relieving extrinsic compression. Surgery involves release of the median arcuate ligament. A minority of patients may have secondary fibrous thickening of the proximal celiac artery, which should be treated with a short bypass or patch angioplasty. A hemodynamic cause for pain is not always clear, and some therapeutic benefit may result from ablation of the celiac nerve plexus during surgery. Results of surgery are generally favorable in carefully selected patients.

Selected References

Antiplatelet Trialists' Collaboration: Collaborative overview of randomised trials of antiplatelet therapy: II. Maintenance of vascular graft or arterial patency by antiplatelet therapy. BMJ 308:159-168, 1994.

> Second of a series of meta-analyses of published trials of antiplatelet therapy, focused on the issues of peripheral vascular disease and bypass grafts.

Boley SJ, Brandt LJ, Veith FJ: Ischemic disorders of the intestines. Curr Prob Surg 14, 1978.

> This excellent overview emphasizes the important role of angiographic diagnosis and therapy, particularly for nonocclusive mesenteric disease.

Glagov S, Zarins C, Giddens DP, Ku DN: Hemodynamics and atherosclerosis: Insights and perspectives gained from studies of human arteries. Arch Pathol Lab Med 112:1018-1031, 1988.

> Authored by a pioneer in this field, this is an excellent introduction to the conceptual and experimental framework linking hemodynamic forces and atherosclerosis.

Goldblatt H: Studies on experimental hypertension. J Exp Med 59:347, 1934.

> This classic paper first describes the mechanism behind renovascular hypertension.

Haimovici H: Muscular, renal and metabolic complications of acute arterial occlusions: Myonephropathic-metabolic syndrome. Surgery 85:461-473, 1979.

> A classic description of the systemic effects of revascularization of the severely ischemic extremity.

Pohl MA: The ischemic kidney and hypertension. Am J Kidney Dis 21(Suppl 2):22-28, 1993.

> This paper is an excellent review of renovascular disease from the kidney's point of view.

Ross R: Atherosclerosis: An inflammatory disease. N Engl J Med 340:115-126, 1999.

> A concise, updated overview of current hypotheses of atherogenesis with an excellent reference list.

Sos T, Pickering T, Sniderman K, et al: Percutaneous transluminal renal angioplasty in renovascular hypertension due to atheroma or fibromuscular dysplasia. N Engl J Med 309:274, 1983.

> This paper was the first to carefully describe techniques and results of percutaneous therapy for renovascular disease, differentiating between ostial and nonostial disease.

STILE Investigators: Results of a prospective randomized trial evaluating surgery versus thrombolysis for ischemia of the lower extremity. The STILE Trial. Ann Surg 220:251-268, 1994.

> A large randomized evaluation of the role of thrombolysis in the management of acute lower extremity ischemia.

Stoney RJ, Cunningham CG: Acute mesenteric ischemia. Surgery 114:489-490, 1993.

> An authoritative review of a challenging subgroup of patients with mesenteric disease.

References

1. Altman SD, Kumpe DA, Redmond PL, et al: Principles of angiography. In Rutherford RB (ed): Vascular Surgery, 4th ed. Philadelphia, WB Saunders, 1995.
2. Antiplatelet Trialists' Collaboration: Collaborative overview of randomised trials of antiplatelet therapy: II. Maintenance of vascular graft or arterial patency by antiplatelet therapy. BMJ 308:159-168, 1994.
3. Bandyk DF, Schmitt DD, Seabrook GR, et al: Monitoring patency of in situ vein grafts: The impact of a surveillance program and elective revision. J Vasc Surg 9:286-296, 1989.
4. Baxter-Smith D, Ashton F, Slaney G: Peripheral arterial embolism: A 20-year review. J Cardiovasc Surg 29:453-457, 1988.
5. Belkin M, Conte MS, Donaldson MC, et al: Preferred strategies for secondary infrainguinal bypass: Lessons learned from 300 consecutive reoperations. J Vasc Surg 21:282-295, 1995.
6. Benditt EP: Implications of the monoclonal character of human atherosclerotic plaques. Am J Pathol 86:693, 1977.
7. Blaisdell FW: Extra-anatomic bypass procedures. World J Surg 12:798-804, 1988.
8. Boyd AM: The natural history of atherosclerosis of the lower extremities. Proc R Soc Med 55:591, 1962.

9. Crawford ES, Bomberger RA, Glaeser DH, et al: Aortoiliac occlusive disease: Factors influencing survival and function following reconstructive operation over a 25-year period. Surgery 90:1555, 1981.

10. Creager MA, Halpern JL, Coffman JD: Raynaud's phenomenon and other vascular disorders related to temperature. In Loscalzo J, Creager MA, Dzau VJ (eds): Vascular Medicine. Boston, Little, Brown, 1996.

11. Davidson DS, Wilcox C: Newer tests for the diagnosis of renovascular disease. JAMA 268:3353-3358, 1992.

12. Dean RH, Benjamin ME, et al: Surgical management of renovascular hypertension. Curr Prob Surg 34:209-308, 1997.

13. Donaldson MC, Mannick JA, Whittemore AD: Femoral-distal bypass with in situ greater saphenous vein: Long term results using the Mills valvulotome. Ann Surg 213:457-465, 1991.

14. Donaldson MC, Weinberg DS, Belkin M, et al: Screening for hypercoagulable states in vascular surgical practice: A preliminary study. J Vasc Surg 11:825-831, 1990.

15. Elliot JP, Hageman JM, Szialagyi DE, et al: Arterial embolization: Problems of source, multiplicity, recurrence, and delayed treatment. Surgery 93:377-380, 1983.

16. Fann JI, Harris J, Dalman RL: Extra-anatomic bypass. In Porter JM, Taylor LM (eds): Basic Data Underlying Clinical Decision Making in Vascular Surgery. St. Louis, Quality Medical, 1994.

17. Fuster V (ed): Syndromes of Atherosclerosis: Correlations of Clinical Imaging and Pathology. New York, Futura, 1996.

18. Glagov S, Weisenberg E, Zarins CK, et al: Compensatory enlargement of human atherosclerotic coronary arteries. N Engl J Med 316:1371-1375, 1987.

19. Glagov S, Zarins C, Giddens DP, Ku DN: Hemodynamics and atherosclerosis: Insights and perspectives gained from studies of human arteries. Arch Pathol Lab Med 112:1018-1031, 1988.

20. Haimovici H: Muscular, renal and metabolic complications of acute arterial occlusions: Myonephropathic-metabolic syndrome. Surgery 85:461-473, 1979.

21. Harding M, Smith L, et al: Renal artery stenosis: Prevalence and associated risk factors in patients undergoing routine cardiac catheterization. J Am Soc Nephrol 2:1608-1616, 1992.

22. Harward T, Green D, et al: Mesenteric venous thrombosis. J Vasc Surg 9:328-333, 1989.

23. Imparato AM, Kim GE, Davidson T, et al: Intermittent claudication: Its natural course. Surgery 78:795-799, 1975.

24. Jivegar LE, Arfvidsson B, Holm J, et al: Selective conservative and routine early operative treatment in acute limb ischemia. Br J Surg 74:798-801, 1987.

25. Leather RP, Shah DM, Chang BB, et al: Resurrection of the in situ saphenous vein bypass. Ann Surg 208:435-442, 1988.

26. Park WM, Gloviczki P, Cherry KJ, et al: Contemporary management of acute mesenteric ischemia: Factors associated with survival. J Vasc Surg 35:445-452, 2002.

27. McAllister FF: The fate of patients with intermittent claudication managed conservatively. Am J Surg 132:593, 1976.

28. Mills JL, Porter JM: Acute limb ischemia. In Porter JM, Taylor LM (eds): Basic Data Underlying Clinical Decision Making in Vascular Surgery. St. Louis, Quality Medical, 1994.

29. Ouriel KO, Veith FJ, Sasahara AS: A comparison of recombinant urokinase with vascular surgery as initial treatment for acute arterial occlusion of the legs. N Engl J Med 338:1105-1111, 1998.

30. Porter JM, Taylor LM, Harris EJ: Nonatherosclerotic vascular disease. In Moore WS (ed): Vascular Surgery: A Comprehensive Review. Philadelphia, WB Saunders, 1991.

31. Ross R: Atherosclerosis: An inflammatory disease. N Engl J Med 340:115-126, 1999.

32. Rutherford RB: Atlas of Vascular Surgery: Basic Techniques and Exposures. Philadelphia, WB Saunders, 1993.

33. Sos TA: Angioplasty for the treatment of azotemia and renovascular hypertension in atherosclerotic renal artery disease. Circulation 83(Suppl 2):I162-I166, 1991.

34. Stanley JC, Ernst CB: Renal artery occlusive disease and renovascular hypertension. In Callow AD, Ernst CB (eds): Vascular Surgery: Theory and Practice. Stamford, CT, Appleton & Lange, 1995, pp 653-676.

35. Stoney RJ, Wylie EJ: Surgery of celiac and mesenteric arteries. In Haimovici HH (ed): Vascular Surgery: Principles and Techniques. New York, McGraw-Hill, 1976, pp 668-679.

36. Taylor LM, Edwards JM, Porter JM: Present status of reversed vein bypass grafting: Five-year results of a modern series. J Vasc Surg 11:193-206, 1990.

37. The STILE Investigators: Results of a prospective randomized trial evaluating surgery versus thrombolysis for ischemia of the lower extremity. The STILE Trial. Ann Surg 220:251-268, 1994.

38. Tullis M, Zierler E, et al: Results of percutaneous transluminal angioplasty for atherosclerotic renal artery stenosis: A follow-up study with duplex ultrasonography. J Vasc Surg 25:46-54, 1997.

39. Rodriguez-Lopez JA, Werner A, Ray LI, et al: Renal artery stenosis treated with stent deployment: Indications, technique, and outcome for 108 patients. J Vasc Surg 29:617-624, 1999.

40. Yao JST: Hemodynamic studies in peripheral arterial disease. Br J Surg 57:761, 1970.

41. Yao JST, Bergan JJ, Pearce WH, Flinn WR: Operative procedures in visceral ischemia. In Bergan JJ, Yao JST (eds): Techniques in Arterial Surgery. Philadelphia, WB Saunders, 1990, pp 284-293.

42. Zierler R, Bergelin R, et al: Natural history of atherosclerotic renal artery stenosis: Prospective study with duplex ultrasonography. J Vasc Surg 19:250-258, 1994.

43. Reed AB, Conte MS, Donaldson MC, et al: The impact of patient age and aortic size on the results of aortobifemoral bypass grafting. J Vasc Surg 37:1219-1225, 2003.

44. Chew DKW, Owens CD, Belkin M, et al: Bypass in the absence of ipsilateral greater saphenous vein—safety and superiority of the contralateral greater saphenous vein. J Vasc Surg 35:1085-1092, 2002.

45. Chew KW, Conte MS, Donaldson MC, et al: Autogenous composite vein bypass graft for infrainguinal arterial reconstruction. J Vasc Surg 33:259-265, 2001.

46. Reed AB, Conte MS, Belkin M, et al: Utility of autogenous bypass grafts originating distal to the groin. J Vasc Surg 35:48-55, 2002.

47. Cambria RP, Kaufman JL, Brewster DC, et al: Surgical renal artery reconstruction without contrast angiography: The role of clinical profiling and magnetic resonance angiography. J Vasc Surg 29:1012-1021, 1999.

48. Kasirijan K, O'Hara PJ, Gray BH, et al: Chronic mesenteric ischemia: Open surgery versus percutaneous angioplasty and stenting. J Vasc Surg 33:63-71, 2001.

49. Faries PF, Morrissey NJ, Teodorescu V, et al: Recent advances in peripheral angioplasty and stenting. Angiology 53:617-626, 2002.

50. Gravereaux EC, Marin ML: Endovascular repair of diffuse atherosclerotic occlusive disease using stented grafts. *In* Kupfer S (ed): Minimally Invasive Surgery Monograph. New York, The Mount Sinai Journal of Medicine, 2003.

51. Duda SH, Poerner TC, Wiesinger B, et al: Drug-eluting stents: Potential applications for peripheral arterial occlusive disease. J Vasc Interv Radiol 14:291-301, 2003.

52. Lim ST, Rosenfield K: Renal artery stent placement: Indications and results. Curr Interv Cardiol Rep 2(2):130-139, 2000.

CHAPTER 66

VASCULAR TRAUMA

Asher Hirshberg, M.D. and **Kenneth L. Mattox, M.D.**

Key Concepts	Abdominal Vascular Injuries
Operative Principles	Peripheral Vascular Trauma
Truncal Vascular Trauma	Conclusion

KEY CONCEPTS

Despite dramatic advances in trauma care during the two last decades of the 20th century, injuries to blood vessels present some of the most challenging problems to the trauma surgeon. The effective management of vascular injuries hinges on successfully merging the principles of modern trauma care with the current approach to vascular therapy as outlined in the previous chapters of this section.

The fundamental difference between elective vascular surgery and vascular trauma is the physiology of the wounded patient. A lacerated major vessel is typically only one component of multiorgan trauma. These patients are often critically ill and rapidly approaching a point of physiologic irreversibility.[1] In these situations, the key to a favorable outcome is maintaining correct priorities.

The surgeon must keep in mind that while major hemorrhage (typical of truncal vascular injuries) is an immediate threat to the patient's life, ischemia (commonly from peripheral arterial injury) is a threat to limb viability, a much lower priority. Furthermore, although control of hemorrhage is usually mandatory, rapid, and life saving, the detailed reconstruction of an injured vessel may be neither. As the injured patient is approaching the boundaries of his or her physiologic envelope, a simpler, sometimes temporary technical solution will often be a much safer option than a complex and time-consuming reconstruction.[2] In the severely traumatized patient, all that is technically feasible is not always in the patient's best interest.

The first part of this chapter focuses on key concepts and fundamental principles in the diagnosis and management of vascular trauma. The second part deals with injuries to specific vessels based on their anatomic location. A special emphasis is placed on the convergence of innovative surgical strategies with cutting-edge technology, offering the surgeon an expanded array of management options in the management of injuries to major vessels.

Patterns of Injury

Vascular trauma occurs in a limited number of patterns, which are determined primarily by the mechanism of injury.[3] Penetrating trauma typically results in varying degrees of laceration or transection of the vessel. The severed ends of a completely transected artery often retract and undergo spasm with subsequent thrombosis. Therefore, a lacerated or incompletely transected vessel typically bleeds more profusely than a completely transected one.

Blunt trauma results in disruption of the arterial wall, ranging in severity from small intimal flaps to extensive transmural damage with either extravasation or thrombosis. Deceleration injury causes deformation of the arterial wall. In a small vessel (e.g., the renal artery) this leads to intimal disruption and subsequent thrombosis, while in a large vessel the result will be full-thickness injury with only a thin layer of adventitia temporarily bridging the gap, as typically occurs in the descending thoracic aorta.

Bleeding from a lacerated vessel can be free or contained, the latter leading to pseudoaneurysm formation. An arteriovenous fistula is the result of a traumatic communication between an injured artery and vein.

Limb loss is more likely to result from blunt trauma and high-velocity gunshot injuries, mainly because of the significantly greater damage to bone and soft tissue of the injured extremity. Low-velocity gunshot injuries and stab wounds rarely lead to limb loss.

The rapidly increasing use of invasive diagnostic, monitoring, and therapeutic modalities in many fields of medicine brought with it a corresponding dramatic increase in iatrogenic vascular trauma. Every cardiac catheterization or arterial line insertion is, in fact, a form of vascular injury, where the physician relies on the patient's hemostatic mechanism to plug the hole and repair the damage. Iatrogenic injury may occur either at the target site of the intervention (e.g., a coronary artery) or at the access site (e.g., the common femoral artery). The latter is more common and sometimes requires surgical repair.

Minimal Injury and Nonoperative Management

Not all arterial injuries require operative management. During the past decade, a series of studies have convincingly demonstrated that nonocclusive intimal flaps, segmental narrowing, small false aneurysms, and small arteriovenous fistulas generally have a benign natural history and are very likely to either heal or improve without intervention. These asymptomatic angiographic findings have been named minimal arterial injuries. Contrary to previous belief, only about 10% of minimal injuries progress with time and eventually require a surgical intervention.[4] Nonoperative management and careful follow-up is therefore a safe and cost-effective course of action for these patients. However, currently there are no objective criteria to precisely define what constitutes a "minimal" lesion. The size of the angiographic defect and the patient's overall trauma burden and, most importantly, the patient's availability for follow-up are factors to consider in making the decision to treat a minimal lesion nonoperatively. In rare instances when a nonocclusive minimal injury progresses and eventually requires surgical intervention, morbidity is not increased by the delay.

Endovascular Therapy

With recent amazingly rapid progress in the field of endovascular therapy of arterial disease, it is not surprising that endovascular stent-grafts are gaining in popularity as an alternative to open repair in selected patients with arterial injuries. In the hemodynamically stable patient with a nonbleeding traumatic arterial lesion, percutaneous placement of an endovascular stent-graft across a defect in the arterial wall is a low-morbidity solution to a problem that may otherwise require a technically challenging surgical procedure in a patient with a severely compromised physiology. In fact, endovascular therapy has revolutionized the management of delayed complications of trauma such as arteriovenous fistulas and pseudoaneurysms, especially in inaccessible sites.[5]

For some arterial injuries, the endovascular option is proving to be the preferred approach. The technical difficulties of gaining access to the vertebral artery in the bony canal or obtaining distal control of a distal injury to the internal carotid artery make the endovascular one an extremely attractive alternative. In nonocclusive blunt injuries to the renal artery, endovascular stenting offers great expediency as compared with an open repair, albeit at the risk of yet unknown long-term patency. Similarly, blunt subclavian artery injury is often part of multiorgan trauma and an endovascular stent-graft may well be the quickest and least hazardous solution for the patient.

The endovascular approach to blunt injuries to the descending thoracic aorta is currently the focus of much interest.[6] The clinical experience with endovascular stent-grafting of the aorta is showing promise and is rapidly accumulating. The procedure provides an effective solution for a potentially lethal type of trauma and is especially applicable in patients with multiple associated injuries who are poor candidates for a major aortic reconstruction. It may well become the procedure of choice for the repair of blunt aortic injuries in the near future.

OPERATIVE PRINCIPLES

Access, Exposure, and Control

Initial control of hemorrhage is achieved by direct pressure over the bleeding site typically using digital or manual compression. Blind clamping of a bleeding vessel is usually ineffective and may damage adjacent structures in the neurovascular bundle. The surgeon can then choose which definitive hemostatic technique to deploy from the wide array of hemostatic options. These include, among others, the insertion of a hemostatic suture, ligation, reconstruction of the vessel, and temporary shunt insertion.[7-9] Balloon catheter tamponade using a Foley catheter inserted into the missile tract is a very useful adjunct to obtaining rapid temporary control of torrential bleeding from relatively inaccessible sites, such as high in the neck, deep in the pelvis, and in the groin (Fig. 66-1).

A cardinal operative principle in managing major vascular trauma is to first obtain proximal (and if possible also distal) control of the injured vessel before entering the surrounding hematoma. In the extremities and in the neck, control is achieved using standard extensible vascular exposure techniques.[9,10] In the chest, control of a vascular injury hinges on correct selection of a thoracotomy incision, because each incision provides access to a different thoracic visceral compartment. In the abdomen, the major vessels are located in the retroperitoneum, and therefore exposure is based on operative maneuvers that mobilize the intraperitoneal viscera off the underlying retroperitoneal structures.[11,12]

Assessing the Injury and the Patient

The anatomic extent of injury is revealed only when the traumatized vessel is carefully dissected, isolated, and opened. External inspection often does not reflect the full

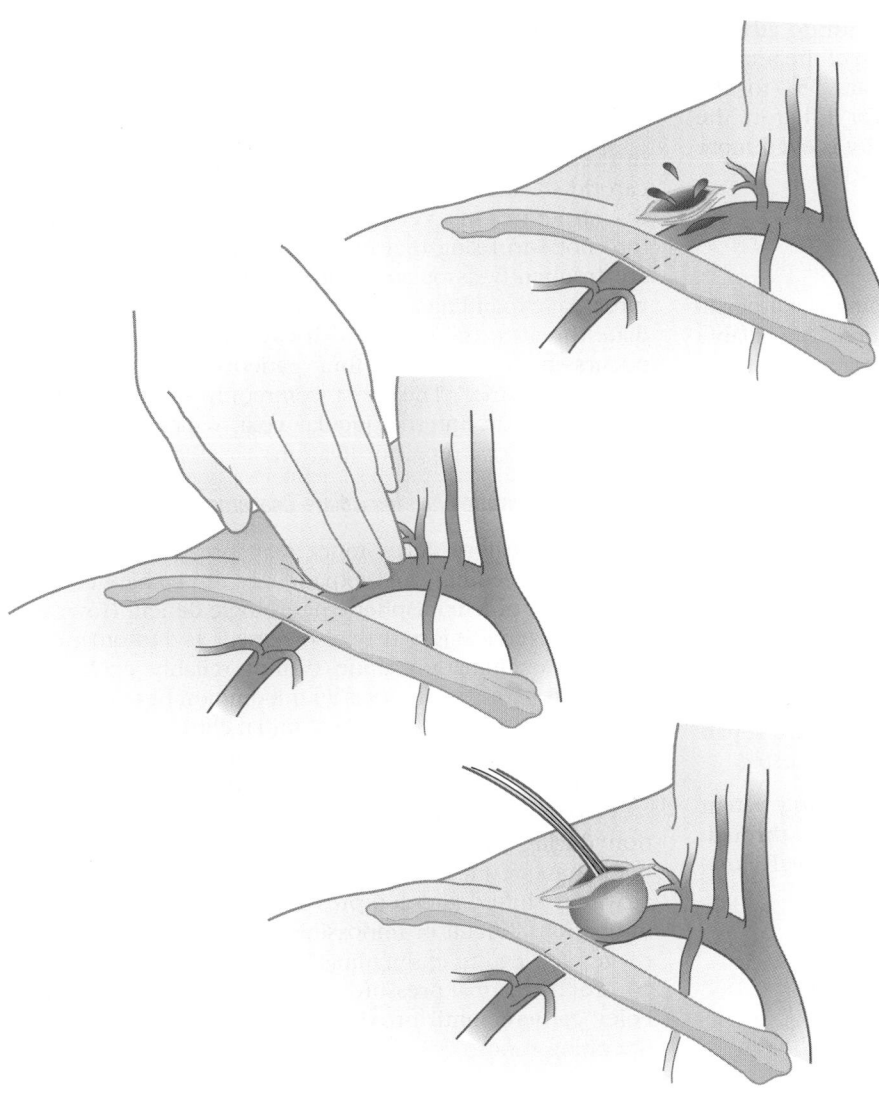

FIGURE 66-1. Use of a balloon tamponade for temporary hemostasis of subclavian artery injury. (Illustration by Jan Redden. © Kenneth L. Mattox, M.D.)

extent of intimal damage, especially in blunt trauma. An important principle in the operative management of vascular trauma is that selection of the vascular repair technique is heavily influenced not only by the anatomic situation but also by the patient's physiologic condition, associated injuries, and overall clinical trajectory.

The massively bleeding patient rapidly develops a self-propagating triad of hypothermia, coagulopathy, and acidosis that leads to an irreversible physiologic insult and death. From the vascular perspective, coagulopathy means a suture line that will continue to bleed after completion as well as diffuse oozing all over the operative field. The hypothermia-coagulopathy-acidosis syndrome effectively marks the boundaries of the patient's physiologic envelope beyond which there is diffuse coagulopathic bleeding, persistent ventricular arrhythmias, and death from irreversible shock. The operative management of a vascular injury must focus not only on restoration of anatomy but also on the patient's physiologic envelope: The complexity and duration of the planned repair should

be inversely proportional to the physiologic insult that the patient has already sustained.

Simple and Complex Repairs

Based on these considerations, it is important to distinguish between two categories of vascular repairs. Simple repairs are very rapid and include ligation, lateral repair, and shunt insertion. Complex repairs are patch angioplasty, end-to-end anastomosis, and graft interposition, all of which are time consuming and typically entail the creation of a long suture line. Simple repairs are feasible even under adverse physiologic circumstances, whereas complex repairs are usually not.

Ligation of an injured vessel in a critically injured patient is a marker of good surgical judgment rather than an admission of defeat. All peripheral veins and the majority of truncal veins can be ligated with impunity. The external carotid, celiac axis, and internal iliac arteries are examples of arteries that can be ligated with no adverse effects. The risk of amputation after ligation of the femoral vessels was 81% for the common femoral and 55% for the superficial femoral artery during World War II (before the advent of fasciotomy). The upper extremity is even more tolerant to ligation of the subclavian artery.

Temporary Intraluminal Shunts

A shunt is a temporary means of maintaining distal perfusion through an injured artery.[13] A commercially available carotid shunt, endotracheal suction catheter, or sterile intravenous tubing trimmed to the appropriate length is inserted into both ends of a disrupted vessel and held in place with vessel loops or ligatures (Fig. 66-2). An intraluminal shunt can be used in three clinical situations:

1. Transfer of a patient with peripheral arterial injury from the field (or from a remote facility) for vascular reconstruction at a trauma center
2. Repair of combined vascular and orthopedic extremity injuries, when skeletal alignment is accomplished before vascular repair in an ischemic limb
3. As a "damage control" technique in a critically injured patient who is unlikely to survive a complex repair because physiologic reserves have been exhausted

There are reports of temporary shunts remaining patent for more than 24 hours after insertion. Blood flow through the shunt is approximately half of the normal flow, enough to maintain limb viability.

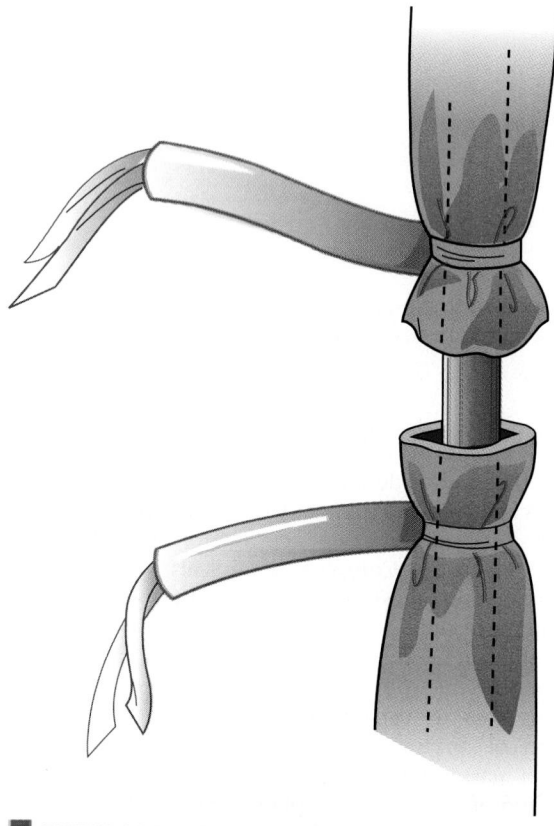

■ FIGURE 66-2. Temporary intravascular shunt.
(Illustration by Jan Redden. © Kenneth L. Mattox, M.D.)

TRUNCAL VASCULAR TRAUMA

The Neck

In the neck, two large neurovascular bundles within the carotid sheaths are closely adherent to midline aerodigestive structures in a very compact arrangement. It is therefore not surprising that injuries to major cervical vessels are frequently associated with trauma to adjacent structures. An expanding cervical hematoma presents an immediate threat to the patient's airway. Major vascular injury occurs in one of every four patients with penetrating cervical trauma.[9] The most commonly injured vascular structure is the internal jugular vein, which is amenable to simple lateral repair or ligation.

Clinical Presentation and Immediate Concerns

Major cervical vascular injury may present as vigorous external bleeding, an expanding or stable cervical hematoma, or a hemispheric neurologic deficit. However, a major arterial injury may also remain asymptomatic, so physical examination alone cannot reliably exclude it. Blunt carotid artery injury is an uncommon but potentially devastating injury.[14-20] The only initial clinical clue may be a gross hemispheric neurologic deficit without computed tomographic (CT) evidence of cerebral trauma.

Two immediate concerns are the focus of clinical attention during the initial evaluation. A rapidly expanding hematoma requires rapid intubation before the upper airway is shifted and compressed, making an orotracheal intubation difficult or impossible. Severe ongoing hemorrhage may lead to exsanguination and requires temporary control by manual pressure or balloon tamponade using a Foley catheter until proximal control is obtained in the operating room.

Diagnostic Studies

The actively bleeding unstable patient with a penetrating neck injury is immediately taken to the operating room for neck exploration. Management of the hemodynamically stable patient with a suspected vascular injury depends on the zone of cervical penetration. Asymptomatic patients with penetrating injuries to the base of the neck (zone I) require a four-vessel arch angiography either to exclude major arterial injury or to plan the operative approach if an injury is present. The same applies to penetrating injuries above the angle of the mandible (zone III), where both exploration and distal control are technically difficult; therefore, an endovascular solution, if feasible, may be the safest option.

Patients with asymptomatic midcervical injuries (zone II) may undergo either formal neck exploration (a straightforward procedure associated with very low morbidity) or a combination of four-vessel angiography, esophagoscopy, and barium swallow to rule out significant arterial and esophageal injury. Both alternatives are acceptable, and thus choice reflects individual preferences and/or institutional policies.

Duplex ultrasonography is an excellent imaging modality for major cervical arterial trauma. However, lack of immediate availability around the clock in the trauma resuscitation area prevents it from being widely used as a substitute for angiography in most emergency centers.

Operative Management

Safe exploration of an anatomically hostile neck distorted by an expanding hematoma hinges on a systematic progression from one key structure to the next. The standard cervical incision is along the anterior border of the sternocleidomastoid muscle. After division of the platysma, dissection proceeds along the anterior border of the sternocleidomastoid to identify the internal jugular vein. Dissection along the anterior border of this large vein identifies the facial vein, which is divided between ligatures to gain access to the carotid bifurcation.

The *carotid arteries* are reconstructed using standard vascular techniques. There are no good data to support preference for vein or synthetic interposition grafts in the neck, nor is there evidence to support routine shunting. A synthetic graft has the advantage of immediate availability, and a shunt can be threaded through the graft and then inserted into the internal and common carotids to facilitate construction of the anastomoses with the shunt in place. Control of the distal internal carotid artery at the base of the neck may be impossible even with adjunctive measures such as dividing the posterior belly of the digastric muscle. Balloon catheter tamponade through the missile tract followed by ligation and division of the internal carotid artery at the carotid bifurcation, with removal of the balloon 3 days later, affords a simple solution to a very difficult technical problem (Fig. 66-3).

The need to reconstruct the carotid artery of a patient with a clear preoperative hemispheric neurologic deficit has been the subject of debate. Current evidence supports revascularization regardless of the patient's neurologic status, accepting that prognosis is poor in the presence of

a profound neurologic deficit (i.e., coma) with or without revascularization.

Vertebral artery injuries present in the operative field as vigorous bleeding emanating from a hole between the transverse processes of the cervical vertebrae, posterolateral to the carotid sheath.[21-24] Although several elaborate techniques have been described for operative exposure of the extracranial vertebral artery, none is a practical option in the presence of severe and life-threatening hemorrhage. The artery is best controlled by simple means, such as tightly filling the bleeding hole in the transverse process with bone wax. If extravasation from the vertebral artery is encountered during arteriography, angiographic control of this inaccessible vessel is clearly the preferred course of action.

Blunt Carotid and Vertebral Artery Injury

The estimated incidence of clinically important blunt injury to the carotid and vertebral arteries is 1 to 3 patients per 1000 admitted to major trauma centers.[14-19,25] However, with increased awareness and screening of asymptomatic patients it is possible to identify these injuries in up to 1% of blunt trauma admissions. The typical mechanism is either hyperextension and contralateral rotation of the neck or a direct blow to the neck, but in some patients no such mechanism can be elicited. The key pathophysiologic event is an intimal tear that can remain asymptomatic or progress to local thrombosis, embolization, or distal dissection.

The clinical hallmark of blunt carotid artery injury is a hemispheric neurologic deficit that is incompatible with CT findings. A salient clinical feature of this injury is that in approximately one half of the patients there is a latent period of hours or days before neurologic deficit appears. Maintaining a high index of suspicion in patients with severe maxillofacial trauma, a mechanism of cervical hyperextension, and evidence of direct trauma to the neck or fractures of the skull base or cervical spine in proximity to the relevant vessels should enable early diagnosis of these lesions. The standard diagnostic modality is angiography, because duplex scanning is not sensitive enough. The treatment of blunt carotid and vertebral artery injury remains controversial and primarily nonoperative. Most patients are treated with systemic anticoagulation (if not prohibited by associated injuries), although the benefits of intravenous heparin are less clear in low-grade nonobstructing luminal irregularities. Hemodynamically significant dissection or inaccessible pseudoaneurysms are amenable to endovascular therapy.

Penetrating Thoracic Vascular Trauma

The patient with a major penetrating thoracic vascular injury typically presents in shock, with either a massive hemothorax or an expanding hematoma at the thoracic inlet. The need for urgent operation is usually obvious. Less commonly, the patient may be hemodynamically stable and a nonbleeding injury (e.g., a pseudoaneurysm, an arteriovenous fistula, or an occluded artery) is

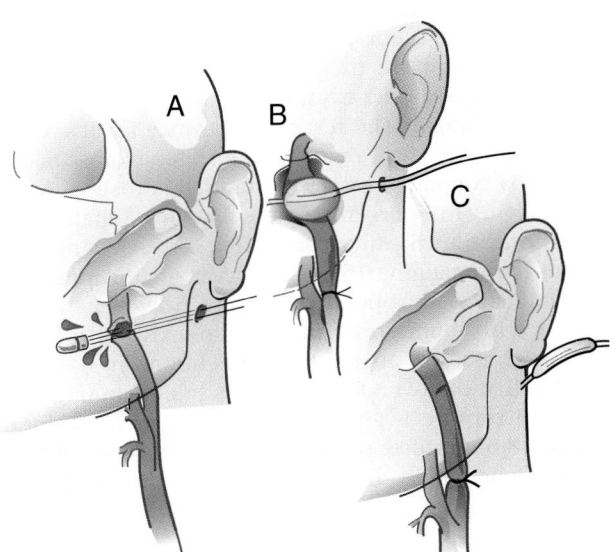

FIGURE 66-3. **A** to **C**, Balloon tamponade of inaccessible internal carotid artery injury.
(**A** to **C**, © Baylor College of Medicine, 1980.)

suspected on clinical grounds and then delineated angiographically.

Choice of Incision

Patient positioning and the choice of thoracotomy incision are central considerations in the management of thoracic vascular injuries because an incorrectly placed incision will often convert a straightforward procedure into a difficult one. In stable patients, the choice of thoracotomy incision is dictated by angiographic findings. In the actively bleeding, hemodynamically unstable patient, the incision is based on the presumed location of the vascular injury. As a general rule, an anterolateral thoracotomy on the injured side is the incision of choice for patients with ongoing bleeding into the pleural cavity. This incision, performed immediately below the nipple in men or below the manually retracted breast in women, does not require special patient positioning, nor does it limit access to the contralateral hemithorax or to the abdomen. The only exception is a penetrating injury to the right lower chest (below the nipple) where bleeding will most commonly emanate from an injured liver, so the initial operative approach should be through a midline laparotomy. An anterolateral thoracotomy can be rapidly extended across the sternum to provide access to the mediastinal great vessels and the contralateral hemithorax, albeit at the cost of additional morbidity associated with this "clam shell" incision.

Penetrating injuries to the base of the neck (thoracic outlet) present special access problems. Right-sided injuries to the base of the neck are approached through a median sternotomy, which provides access to the innominate artery and the proximal right carotid and subclavian arteries. The proximal part of the left subclavian artery is intrapleural and posterior, so the most expeditious way to obtain proximal control is through a separate left anterolateral thoracotomy incision through the third intercostal space (above the nipple).

A supraclavicular incision is used to gain access to the more distal parts of both subclavian arteries. The incision entails careful division of two muscle layers, the sternocleidomastoid and the anterior scalene muscle posterior to it. The phrenic nerve, which crosses the latter muscle, is the key to the dissection and must be identified and preserved. Exposure of the subclavian vessels can be facilitated by subperiosteal resection of the medial half of the clavicle.

Management of Specific Injuries

Penetrating injuries to the innominate vessels and proximal carotid arteries present intraoperatively as a mediastinal hematoma. Much like any other hematoma resulting from a major vascular injury, plunging into it without proximal control is a recipe for disaster. Proximal control can be obtained from within the pericardium where the anatomy is not obscured by the hematoma. Exposure is enhanced by division of the innominate vein. The bypass exclusion technique for innominate artery injuries is described in the next section.

In patients who are massively bleeding from pulmonary hilar injuries, the mortality rate is in excess of 70%. In practice, these injuries usually involve more than one element of the pulmonary hilum. Instead of attempting vascular repair of the pulmonary artery or vein in these exsanguinating patients, a rapid pneumonectomy using a linear stapler may prove lifesaving.

For injuries of the subclavian arteries the exposure required is almost always more extensive than initially anticipated, and the incision can be extended laterally to expose the proximal axillary artery. Special care must be taken to avoid injury to the phrenic nerve and brachial plexus. Most subclavian artery injuries are repaired using a synthetic interposition graft. Subclavian vein injuries are repaired with lateral venorrhaphy or are ligated. Penetrating injuries to the intrapericardial great vessels and to the vena cava are very rare, and repair requires cardiopulmonary bypass. In practice, these injuries are almost invariably fatal.

Blunt Thoracic Vascular Trauma

The Aorta

Blunt aortic injury is the great nemesis of blunt trauma, having caused or contributed to 10% to 15% of motor vehicle–related deaths for nearly 30 years.[26] It is a lethal injury that provides the surgeon with a window of opportunity for effective surgical intervention. This window may be missed because the injury remains asymptomatic until catastrophic bleeding suddenly occurs. In most cases (54% to 65%), the involved aortic segment is the proximal descending aorta just distal to the origin of the left subclavian artery. Less common is involvement of the aortic arch (10% to 14%), the distal thoracic aorta at the diaphragm (12%), or multiple sites (13% to 18%).

The dominant pathophysiologic event in blunt aortic injury is sudden deceleration with creation of a shear force between a relatively mobile part of the thoracic aorta and an adjacent fixed segment. The three major points of fixation are the atrial attachments of the pulmonary veins and vena cava, the ligamentum arteriosum, and the diaphragm. The resulting tear may involve either part of the aortic wall or may be a full-thickness disruption that is contained by periadventitial and surrounding tissues. Eighty-five percent of patients with a full-thickness blunt thoracic aortic injury die before arrival at a hospital. Most of the remaining 15% have a contained rupture and are candidates for operative repair. However, 15% of patients with blunt aortic injury who arrive at a trauma center die before operative intervention. It has been reported that the overall free rupture rate of an untreated contained rupture is approximately 1% per hour during the first 48 hours after presentation. The majority of these deaths occur within the first few hours, thus underscoring the urgency of a timely diagnosis and a prompt operative repair.[18,27,28]

The classic mechanism of blunt aortic injury is sudden deceleration during a frontal impact motor vehicle collision or a fall from height. However, recent data show a considerable number of cases secondary to other mechanisms, such as side-impact collisions, vehicular-pedestrian accidents, and crush and blast injuries. Certainly, the possibility of blunt aortic injury should be considered in all victims of motor vehicle collision, regardless of the point of impact.

As a general rule, a contained blunt aortic injury is not an explanation for hemodynamic instability. If the patient with a suspected or proven blunt aortic injury is hemodynamically unstable, the explanation almost always lies in other associated injuries, typically in the abdomen. This source of active bleeding is an immediate threat to the patient's life and should be addressed before the aortic injury. Very rarely, the aortic disruption itself may present as an ongoing nonexsanguinating hemorrhage causing hemodynamic instability. The window of opportunity to salvage these patients is extremely narrow, and the surgeon is often forced to operate without an angiographic definition of the injury. The mortality rate in these patients is 90%.

Physical examination of the patient with blunt aortic injury is rarely helpful because the classically described signs such as upper extremity hypertension, diminished femoral pulses ("pseudo-coarctation"), and an intrascapular murmur are distinctly uncommon. The most important aspect of the physical examination is not to miss associated injuries that may either have priority over the aortic injury or may have a major impact on the operative risk.

Several radiographic findings on a supine chest radiograph should suggest the diagnosis of blunt aortic injury. The most significant ones are a widened mediastinum (>8 cm), an obscured or indistinct aortic knob, deviation of the left main stem bronchus, an off-midline position of a nasogastric tube, and obliteration of the aortopulmonary window. The diagnosis of blunt aortic injury remains notoriously elusive. In 5% of patients, the mechanism of injury is, in fact, the only clue to the diagnosis; and, in others, radiographic signs may be so subtle that even an experienced interpreter will not discern them.

The role of CT in the diagnosis of blunt aortic injury has been the focus of debate. Spiral or helical scans of the chest have a high negative predictive value and can be used to rule out an aortic injury.[25,29-32] However, demonstration of a mediastinal hematoma does not obviate the need for subsequent aortography to clearly define the site and extent of injury. At least 10 aortic arch anomalies exist that are *not* demonstrated by CT, and the surgeon is best advised to know of these anomalies before thoracotomy.

Helical CT angiography is rapidly becoming an imaging modality that rivals aortography as being more expedient and noninvasive. Three-dimensional reconstructions of the aorta provide accurate anatomic detail that obviates the need for a subsequent aortography. However, these reconstructions are time consuming and use massive computing resources. As this technology matures, it may replace aortography as the imaging modality of choice.

Transesophageal echocardiography (TEE) is a bedside procedure that can rapidly diagnose blunt aortic injury in the emergency center, operating room (during surgery in another visceral cavity), and intensive care unit. TEE is contraindicated in patients with suspected cervical spine injury, and diagnostic accuracy is compromised in the presence of atherosclerotic disease and pneumomediastinum. Injuries to the ascending aorta and arch are not well visualized. All these considerations limit the usefulness of TEE in the diagnosis of blunt aortic injury.

The correct and timely identification of blunt aortic injury hinges on a low threshold for aortography when the mechanism of injury, relevant physical findings, or an abnormal chest radiograph suggests the diagnosis. Aortography remains the "gold standard" imaging modality to which all other modalities are compared. It provides valuable information, not only about precise location and extent of the injury but also about other details that may affect the operative plan. Two classic pitfalls in interpretation of aortograms are ductus diverticulum and vascular ring remnant.

The management of blunt aortic injury is prompt operative repair of the injured aortic segment. However, in some patients, a purposeful delay or even nonoperative management may be indicated.[26,27,33] Patients with severe head injury or complex multisystem injury and those about to breach their physiologic envelope are bad candidates for an aortic reconstruction. The estimated risk of free rupture of 1% per hour pales into insignificance when compared with the risk of aortic surgery under these circumstances. Patients with severe comorbid factors are also poor candidates for aortic reconstruction. Evidence is now accumulating that in stable patients purposeful delay of surgery combined with pharmacologic control of the blood pressure (similar to a nontraumatic type B aortic dissection) and careful monitoring of the mediastinal hematoma may be an acceptable course of action. This purposeful delay allows the surgeon to assess the total injury burden of the patient and select the optimal timing for operative intervention. "Minimal" blunt aortic injuries, such as a small intimal flap or a small pseudoaneurysm, may be amenable to nonoperative management. However, the long-term behavior of these lesions is still not well defined, so careful follow-up by serial imaging is mandatory whenever nonoperative management is selected for a "nonthreatening" lesion.

The use of endovascular stent-grafts to treat blunt aortic injury is under intense scrutiny.[6] One major concern has been the close proximity of the classic aortic tear to the takeoff of the left subclavian artery. As a result, the orifice of the left subclavian artery is covered during deployment of the device. However, only approximately 1 in 10 patients develops left upper extremity ischemia that requires revascularization. The current worldwide experience is less than 100 cases, but the concept is certainly valid. With further experience and refinement of the technique, it is rapidly becoming a standard alternative to operative repair.

The descending thoracic aorta is approached through a left posterolateral thoracotomy in the fourth intercostal space. A midline sternotomy with full cardiopulmonary bypass is used for repair of the ascending aorta. The standard operative repair of aortic injuries uses clamp and direct reconstruction and can be achieved by using one of three adjuncts: pharmacologic control of central hypertension, a temporary passive shunt, or pump-assisted atriofemoral bypass. The latter can be achieved either by a traditional pump bypass (which requires full heparinization) or by using a centrifugal pump without heparin.

The use of temporary shunts or pump bypass is more complex than direct reconstruction with pharmacologic control. While some reports suggest that preservation of distal perfusion by using a shunt or partial bypass may improve morbidity and mortality, no clear-cut advantage over the clamp-repair technique has been demonstrated in a prospective study.[26,28]

Proximal control of the injury is obtained by encircling the subclavian artery and the aortic arch (between the carotid and left subclavian arteries). The latter is the most difficult part of the dissection. The pleura between the vagus and phrenic nerves is incised, and using a combination of blunt and sharp dissection a plane is developed between the pulmonary artery and the inferior aspect of the aortic arch. A large curved vascular clamp can then be carefully brought around the aorta, making just enough space for an aortic clamp. The distal descending aorta is encircled after opening the mediastinal pleura, taking care not to injure an intercostal vessel. Clamps are placed on the isolated vessels, and extreme blood pressure fluctuations are avoided by careful pharmacologic control. After clamping, the hematoma is entered and the extent and configuration of the tear is assessed through a careful longitudinal aortotomy. Direct primary repair is possible in only 15% of patients, while the rest require an interposition graft.

The reported operative mortality of blunt aortic injury repair is 5% to 25% and is related not only to the procedure itself but also to the presence of associated injuries and their late sequelae. The most dreaded complication is paraplegia or paraparesis, which occurs in approximately 8% of patients. The incidence of spinal cord damage is affected neither by choice of operative technique nor by the method chosen to deal with central hypertension and distal ischemia. There is also no direct proven correlation between aortic cross clamp time and the incidence of spinal cord damage.

The Innominate Artery

The second most common blunt thoracic vascular injury is a tear at the origin of the innominate artery. The artery is either sheared off the aortic arch, as with blunt aortic injury, or "pinched" between the sternum and the spine during frontal impact. Blunt innominate artery injury is akin to a side hole in the thoracic aorta because operative repair requires obtaining control at the aortic arch.

The clinical presentation is similar to that of blunt aortic injury in that most patients are hemodynamically stable and asymptomatic. Radiologic evidence of mediastinal widening at the aortic outlet and leftward deviation of the trachea suggest the diagnosis, but angiography is the definitive diagnostic modality.

The operative repair of blunt innominate artery injury is based on the "bypass and exclusion" principle, thus eliminating the need for cardiopulmonary bypass, shunts, or the use of heparin.[20,26] After median sternotomy the ascending aorta is exposed inside the pericardium while deliberately avoiding the traumatized segment. Using a partially occluding clamp on a segment of normal aorta, a graft is sewn to it in an end-to-side configuration, away from the injury. The distal innominate artery is exposed and clamped proximal to the bifurcation, and the distal anastomosis is constructed (Fig. 66-4). Only then is the injured segment of the aortic arch addressed and repaired.

ABDOMINAL VASCULAR INJURIES

Most abdominal vascular injuries result from penetrating trauma and are associated with other abdominal injuries.[3] Vascular injuries are much more common after abdominal gunshot wounds (25% of patients) as compared with stab wounds (10%). Major abdominal vascular trauma presents clinically either as free intraperitoneal hemorrhage or as a contained retroperitoneal hematoma.[34,35] The patient with free hemorrhage usually presents in shock, whereas the patient with a contained retroperitoneal hematoma may be hemodynamically stable or unstable but responsive to fluids. The latter presentation is typical of patients with a single venous injury and usually carries a better prognosis.

Occasionally there are clinical hints to the presence of an abdominal vascular injury. Examples are a bullet trajectory across the abdominal midline in a hypotensive patient or rarely an absent femoral pulse. In most patients, the indication for urgent celiotomy is obvious and the diagnosis is made at operation. Time should not be wasted on unnecessary diagnostic tests or on futile attempts to "stabilize" the patient because volume loading before achieving surgical control of the bleeding vessel may augment bleeding and adversely affect the outcome.

Immediate Concerns

The typical situation encountered at celiotomy is vigorous bleeding or an expanding hematoma at a relatively inaccessible site, combined with other abdominal visceral injuries. Temporary control of hemorrhage is the obvious first priority. Direct manual or digital pressure achieves initial control of ongoing hemorrhage, whereas formal proximal and distal control is obtained later. Once bleeding has been temporarily controlled, the surgeon should stop and organize the operative attack on the injury. The natural urge to immediately proceed with definitive repair is the worst possible mistake at this point. Instead, the time interval should be used to transfuse and resuscitate the patient, to obtain additional instruments and an autotransfusion device, to optimize exposure, and to organize the operating room team. Only then should the definitive repair begin.

Once the total injury burden of the patient is determined, the surgeon must choose between the traditional operative profile of definitive repair and a "damage control" profile. The latter consists of a rapid initial operation wherein only temporary "bail out" measures to control hemorrhage and spillage are employed. The patient is then transferred to the surgical intensive care unit for rewarming and stabilization, with definitive repair performed at a planned reoperation after 24 to 48 hours.

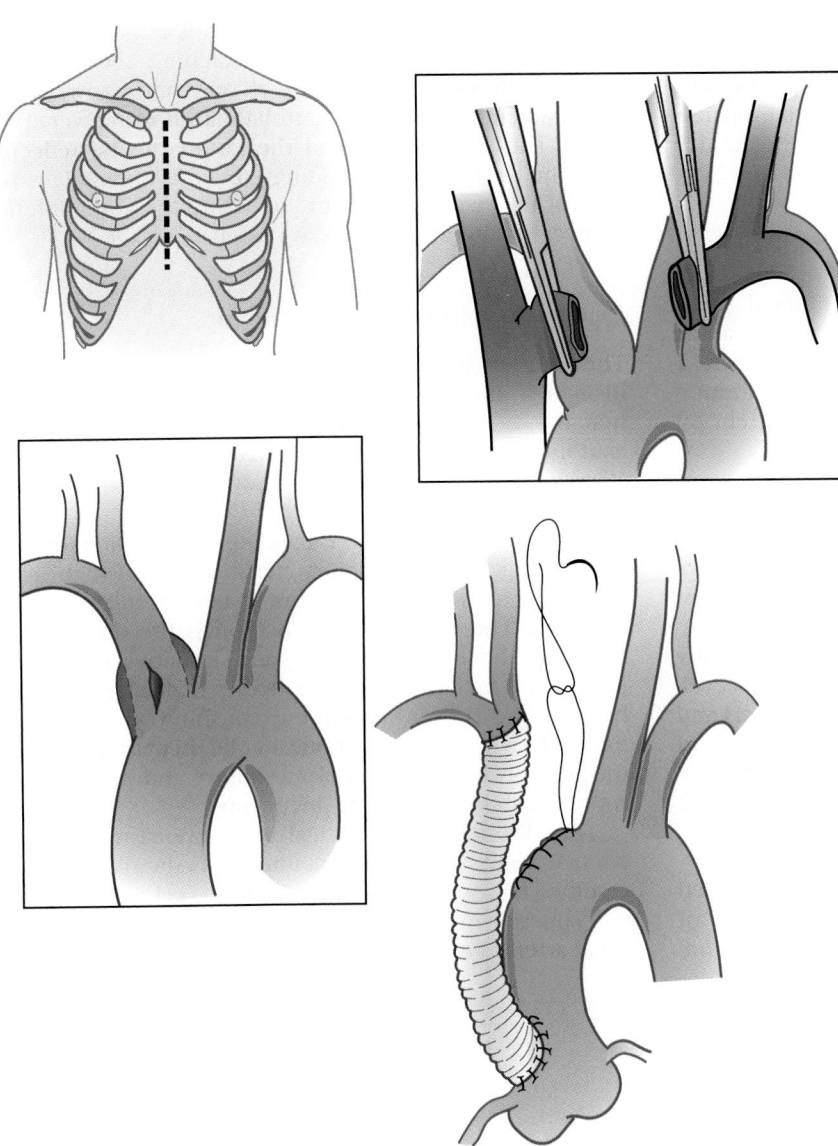

FIGURE 66-4. The "bypass and exclusion" technique for repair of innominate artery injuries.
(Illustration by Jan Redden. © Kenneth L. Mattox, M.D.)

The "damage control" approach temporarily sacrifices anatomic integrity so as to avoid the irreversible physiologic insult that presents as the hypothermia-coagulopathy-acidosis syndrome. This operative strategy is particularly suitable for the patient with major abdominal vascular injury in conjunction with hollow or solid abdominal visceral trauma, in whom formal repair of all injuries will not be tolerated by the patient's fragile physiology. In these circumstances, the surgeon may decide to address the vascular injury using only simple repair techniques such as ligation or temporary shunt placement. Another option is to perform a definitive repair of the vascular injury and use "bail out" techniques for the hollow visceral damage.

Aortic Clamping

Aortic cross-clamping is both an adjunct to resuscitation and a means of obtaining "global" proximal control to reduce torrential hemorrhage in the abdomen. The supraceliac aorta is most expediently clamped at the diaphragmatic hiatus. Rapid blunt creation of an opening in the lesser omentum allows the surgeon to approach the left diaphragmatic crus and open it longitudinally in the direction of its fibers. This is done by finger dissection, and the purpose is to create just enough space on both sides of the aorta to accommodate an aortic clamp. This transcrural route avoids the dense periaortic tissue of the suprarenal abdominal aorta. Alternatively, the aorta can be clamped in the lower chest (through a left anterolateral thoracotomy). Clamping the aorta through the lesser sac is typically performed blindly in a pool of blood. It is therefore often much safer to compress the aorta manually at the hiatus than to risk iatrogenic damage to the celiac axis, esophagus, or even the aorta itself by a blindly and incorrectly placed clamp.

Aortic clamping has profound physiologic consequences. Although the maneuver elevates the patient's blood pressure, it also causes sudden afterload augmentation and visceral and peripheral ischemia, all of which may be detrimental to the patient's borderline physiology. Thus, aortic clamping, while at times a life-saving maneuver in a rapidly deteriorating patient, should be used judiciously and performed carefully.

Maneuvers for Retroperitoneal Exposure

The major abdominal vessels are retroperitoneal structures that lie posterior to the content of the peritoneal sac and close to the midline. Rapid exposure of these relatively inaccessible structures hinges on two mobilization maneuvers that rotate the abdominal visceral content off the midline retroperitoneal structures.

Left-sided medial visceral rotation (Mattox maneuver) exposes the entire length of the abdominal aorta and its branches (except the right renal artery).[12] The correct plane is entered by incising the lateral peritoneal attachment of the sigmoid and left colon, and the hand is swept upward lateral to the left colon, kidney, and spleen (Fig. 66-5). The presence of a retroperitoneal hematoma greatly facilitates the dissection. The plane of dissection is developed bluntly in front of the left common iliac vessels and behind the kidney, with the back of the dissecting hand sliding on the posterior abdominal wall muscles. The left-sided viscera (left colon, kidney, spleen, and pancreas) are brought to the midline, and the entire length of the abdominal aorta is thus exposed.

Right-sided medial visceral rotation ("extended Kocher" maneuver) consists of medial reflection of the right colon and duodenum by incising their lateral

peritoneal attachments (Fig. 66-6). This exposure can be extended farther medially by detaching the posterior attachments of the small bowel mesentery toward the duodenojejunal ligament (Cattell-Braasch maneuver) (Fig. 66-7). The small bowel and the colon can be reflected onto the lower chest, providing the widest possible exposure of the retroperitoneum, including the aorta, inferior vena cava, and iliac and renal vessels.

Approach to Retroperitoneal Hematoma

The location of a retroperitoneal hematoma and mechanism of injury guide the decision to explore the hematoma. The retroperitoneum is divided into three anatomic zones: the midline retroperitoneum (zone 1), (Fig. 66-8), the perinephric space (zone 2), and the pelvic retroperitoneum (zone 3).

Any hematoma in zone 1 mandates exploration for both penetrating and blunt injury because of the high likelihood and unforgiving nature of major vascular injury in this area. The transverse mesocolon is the dividing line between the supramesocolic and inframesocolic compartments. A central supramesocolic hematoma presents behind the lesser omentum, pushing the stomach forward, whereas an inframesocolic hematoma pushes the root of the small bowel mesentery and presents as a ruptured abdominal aortic aneurysm.[2,36]

This distinction has critical implications on proximal control and exposure. A supramesocolic hematoma is the result of injury to the suprarenal aorta, celiac axis, proximal superior mesenteric artery, or the proximal part of a renal artery. Proximal control is obtained by clamping or

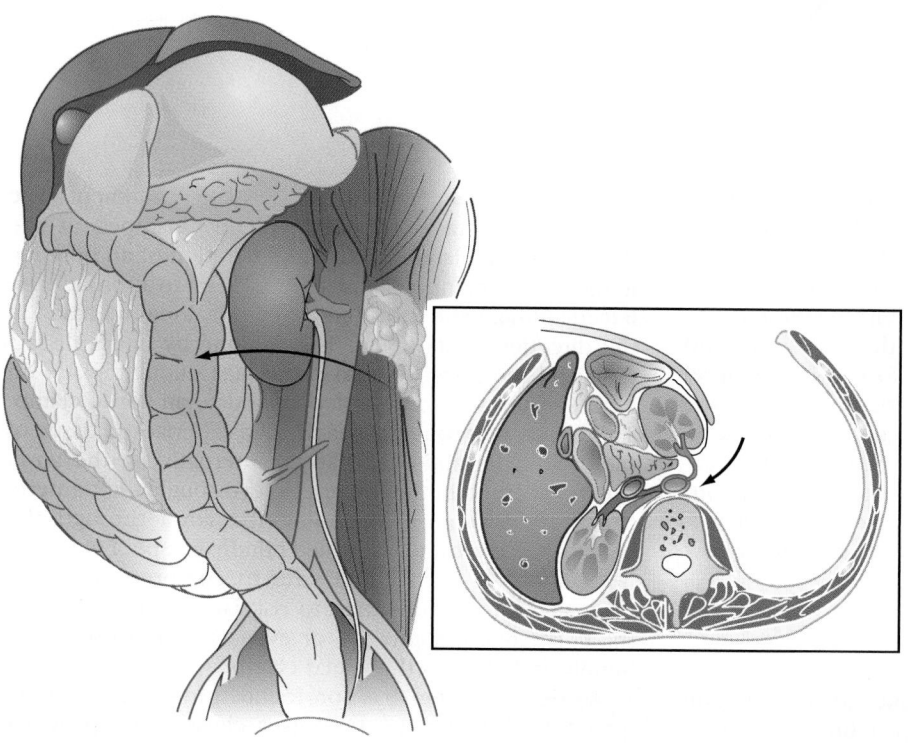

FIGURE 66-5. Left-sided medial visceral rotation (Mattox maneuver). (Illustration by Jan Redden after Jim Schmidt. © Kenneth L. Mattox, M.D.)

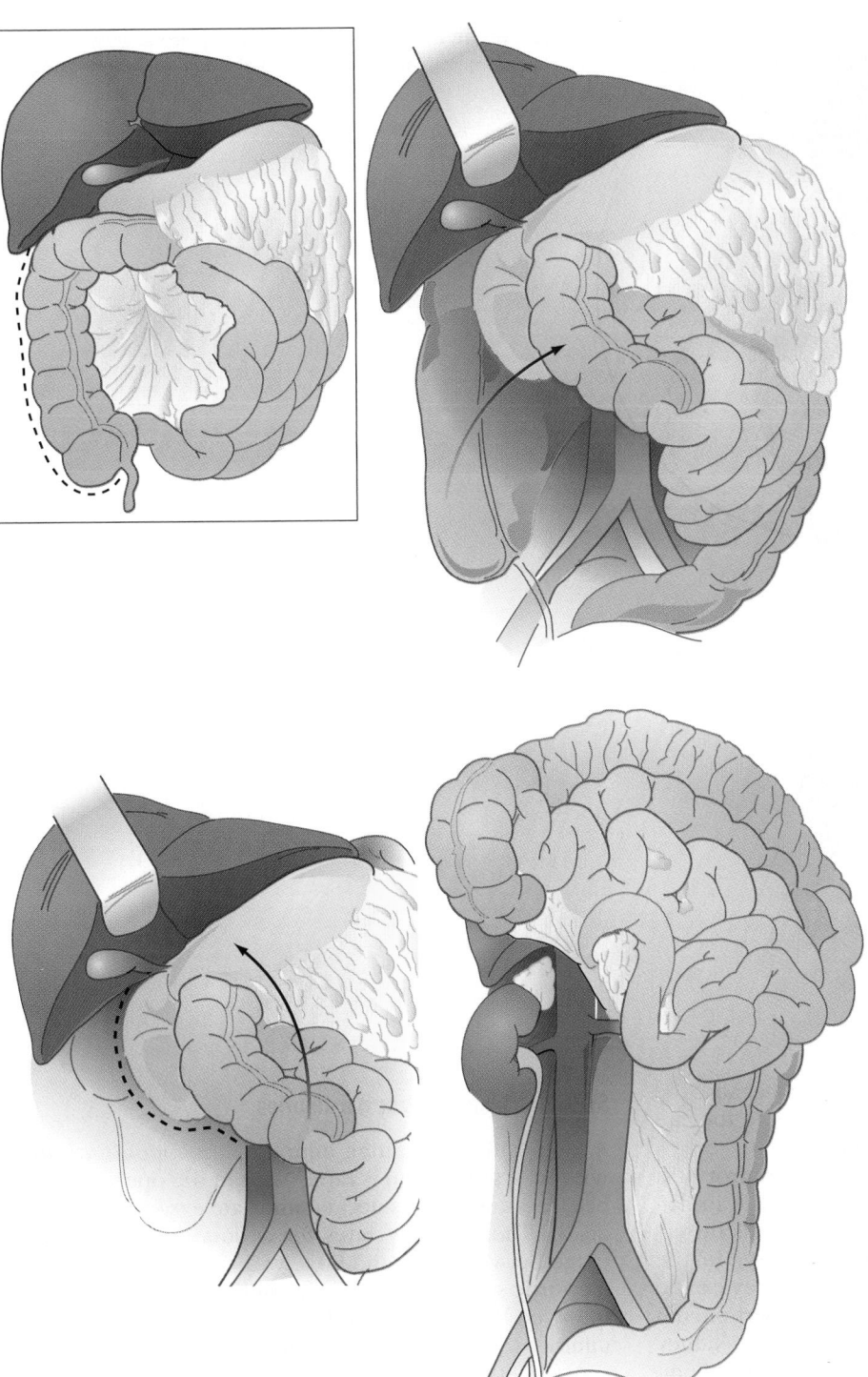

FIGURE 66-6. Right-sided medial visceral rotation (extended Kocher maneuver).
(Illustration by Jan Redden. © Kenneth L. Mattox, M.D.)

FIGURE 66-7. Extensive retroperitoneal exposure by the Cattell-Braasch maneuver.
(Illustration by Jan Redden. © Kenneth L. Mattox, M.D.)

compressing the aorta at the diaphragmatic hiatus, and exposure of the injured vessels is provided by left-sided medial visceral rotation. A central inframesocolic hematoma is the result of injury to the infrarenal aorta or inferior vena cava. Proximal control is achieved at the supraceliac aorta, and exposure is provided by opening the midline posterior peritoneum, in much the same way as for an infrarenal aortic aneurysm.

A hematoma in zone 2 is the result of injury to the renal vessels and/or parenchyma and mandates exploration for penetrating trauma. A nonexpanding stable hematoma resulting from a blunt trauma is better left unexplored because opening Gerota's fascia may result in further damage to the traumatized renal parenchyma and subsequent loss of the kidney. In the critically injured patient with a stable hematoma from a penetrating injury, it may

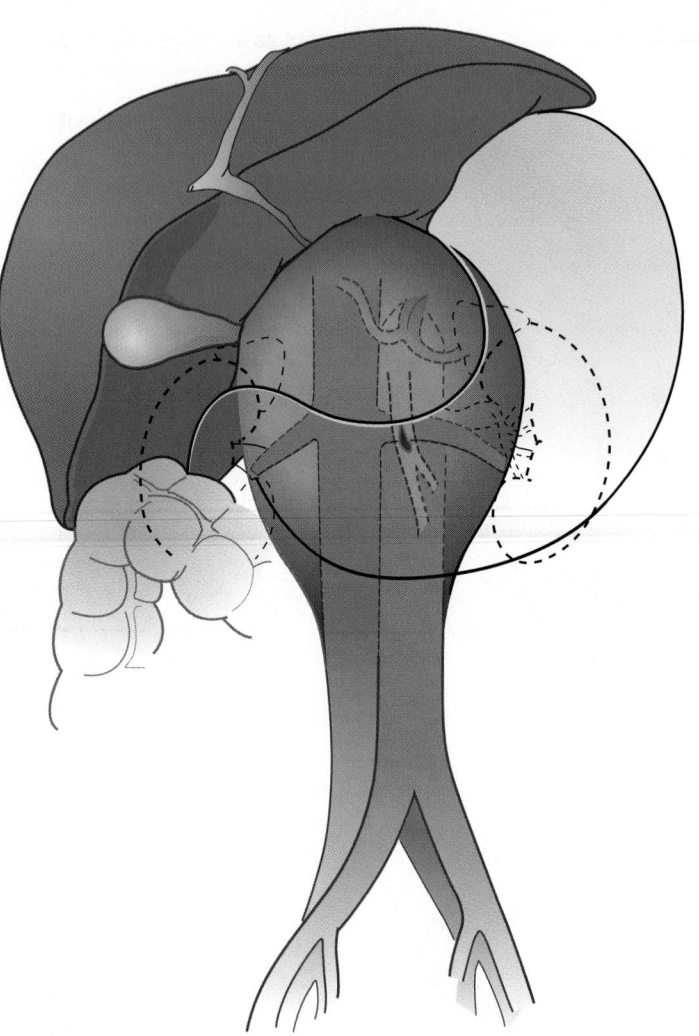

FIGURE 66-8. Retroperitoneal hematoma, zone 1. (Illustration by Jan Redden after Jim Schmidt. © Kenneth L. Mattox, M.D.)

be advisable not to explore the injured kidney because the patient may not have the physiologic reserves to tolerate an elaborate and time-consuming repair.

Traditional teaching advocates proximal control of a perinephric hematoma by midline looping of the ipsilateral artery and vein at the midline. However, this dissection is time consuming and often unnecessary. In the presence of active hemorrhage, the injured kidney can be rapidly mobilized by incising the posterior peritoneum and Gerota's fascia lateral to it, rotating the injured kidney medially and up and then clamping the entire renal hilum.

A pelvic retroperitoneal hematoma (zone 3) secondary to penetrating trauma mandates exploration because of the likelihood of iliac vessel injury. However, zone 3 hematomas resulting from blunt trauma are usually associated with a pelvic fracture and should not be explored because the effective management of this type of bleeding is based not on operative control (which rarely proves effective) but on external fixation and/or angiographic embolization of the bleeding vessels. The only exception is a rapidly expanding hematoma where the surgeon suspects a major iliac vascular injury that requires operative repair.

Specific Abdominal Vascular Injuries

A high-grade penetrating injury to the *abdominal aorta* with near-transection is rarely seen in the operating room because it usually results in immediate exsanguination and death. The mortality rates for abdominal aortic injuries range between 50% and 90%, with injuries to the perirenal aortic segment being the most lethal (>80% mortality), followed by suprarenal (50% to 70%) and infrarenal injuries (50% to 60%).[26] Clean lacerations of the aorta can sometimes be primarily repaired by transverse approximation of the lumen, but more often extensive destruction of the aortic wall mandates prosthetic graft interposition. Despite theoretical concerns that spillage of intestinal content may cause synthetic graft infection, a synthetic graft is the only practical option, and graft infections after placement for penetrating trauma to the aorta have not been reported.

Blunt trauma to the abdominal aorta is very rare, usually the result of motor vehicle collision with impingement of the steering wheel or a seatbelt. The most common location is the origin of the inferior mesenteric artery, and clinical presentation is that of acute aortic thrombosis secondary to intimal disruption. The diagnosis is made at angiography, and operative repair usually requires a synthetic interposition graft.

Penetrating injuries to the *iliac vessels* carry high mortality rates (25% to 40%), because exposure and control can be difficult and associated injuries to adjacent abdominal organs are the rule rather than the exception.[37-40] Initial proximal control is obtained on the inframesocolic aorta and vena cava, and distal control is achieved on the external iliac vessels at the inguinal ligament by "towing in" with a large retractor over the inferior edge of the abdominal incision, thus compressing the iliac vessels against the edge of the bony pelvis. Reflection of the colon from its lateral peritoneal attachment on the relevant side unroofs the pelvic hematoma, and control can then be optimized by sequentially advancing the clamps closer to the injury as dissection proceeds. The "damage control" approach reduces mortality from iliac vessel injuries because the vessels are amenable to "bail out" solutions such as temporary shunt insertion, balloon tamponade of a venous injury, or arterial ligation with a delayed extra-anatomical reconstruction. Occasionally, the only way to gain access to an injured iliac vein is to divide the overlying common iliac artery and then reconstruct it after the venous repair has been completed.

The use of a polytetrafluoroethylene (PTFE) graft for iliac artery reconstruction in the presence of peritoneal contamination is a cause for concern.[41] In the presence of limited spillage of small bowel content, use of a PTFE graft (after the bowel injury has been repaired and the field irrigated) is an acceptable option. However, with gross fecal contamination, ligation of the injured iliac artery and a subsequent femorofemoral bypass is a safe course of action.

A low threshold for fasciotomy should be maintained after iliac vessel injuries because leg edema is common (particularly with iliac vein ligation) and ischemia from iliac artery trauma can be prolonged. The hypotensive critically injured patient is particularly susceptible to the devastating effects of elevated compartment pressures.

Injuries to the *superior mesenteric vessels* present as either exsanguinating hemorrhage from the root of the mesentery, a supra-mesocolic central retroperitoneal hematoma, or ischemic bowel. The origin of the superior mesenteric artery is exposed by left-sided medial visceral rotation, whereas the infrapancreatic part of the vessel is accessed by pulling the small bowel down and to the left and incising the peritoneum of the root of the mesentery. Another option for exposure of the infrapancreatic part is the Cattell-Braasch maneuver. The anatomic location of the mesenteric vessels in close proximity to the pancreatoduodenal complex, inferior vena cava, and the right renal pedicle means that severe associated injuries are the rule with mesenteric vascular trauma, opportunities for complex reconstructions are rare, and mortality is very high. The successful use of a temporary shunt in the superior mesenteric artery as a "damage control" technique has been reported. If graft interposition is required to reconstruct the superior mesenteric artery, a takeoff from the distal aorta above the bifurcation keeps the suture line away from an injured pancreas. A second-look exploratory

laparotomy is mandatory to assess the viability of the bowel. The injured superior mesenteric vein should be repaired by lateral venorrhaphy when possible. Often the only technical option is ligation, which requires aggressive postoperative fluid resuscitation to compensate for ensuing massive splanchnic sequestration and may lead to venous gangrene of the bowel. A second-look laparotomy is mandatory.

Penetrating injuries to the *renal arteries* usually result in nephrectomy, because associated injuries make complex vascular reconstruction of the renal artery an unattractive option. Blunt renovascular deceleration trauma is usually asymptomatic and is discovered when a kidney does not opacify on excretory urography or CT. Arteriography is required for diagnosis and may document a spectrum of injuries ranging from intimal tear to complete renal artery thrombosis. Because blunt renovascular trauma is characteristically associated with more life-threatening injuries, a significant diagnostic delay is common, and attempted renal salvage by major vascular reconstruction is usually not an option. For possible suitable operative candidates, the time limit that precludes a successful revascularization remains controversial. If 4 to 6 hours have elapsed since the injury and the renal artery is occluded, repair should not be undertaken.

Injuries to the inferior vena cava (IVC) remain highly lethal, with mortality rates consistently in excess of 50%, particularly for the least accessible segments of the vein (iliac bifurcation, suprarenal and retrohepatic IVC).[2,42-47] The IVC is exposed by a right-sided medial visceral rotation (Fig. 66-9), and initial control is achieved by direct pressure above and below the injury (Fig. 66-10). The technical options for the infrarenal IVC are lateral repair or ligation. A posterior laceration can be repaired from inside the vein through an anterior venotomy.

Retrohepatic IVC injuries are especially unforgiving, presenting the surgeon with some of the most challenging abdominal vascular injuries.[48] Typical operative find-

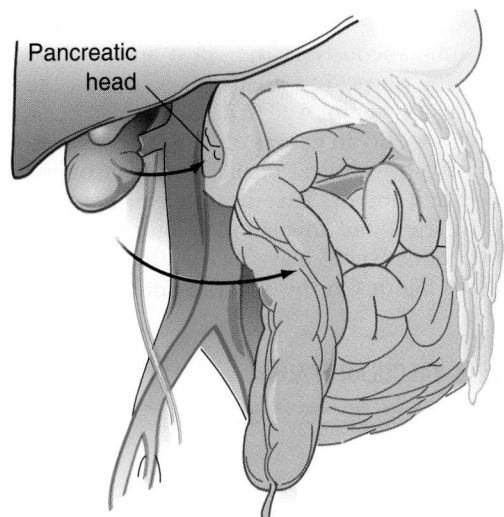

FIGURE 66-9. Right-sided medial rotation of the viscera to expose the inferior vena cava.
(© Baylor College of Medicine, 1981.)

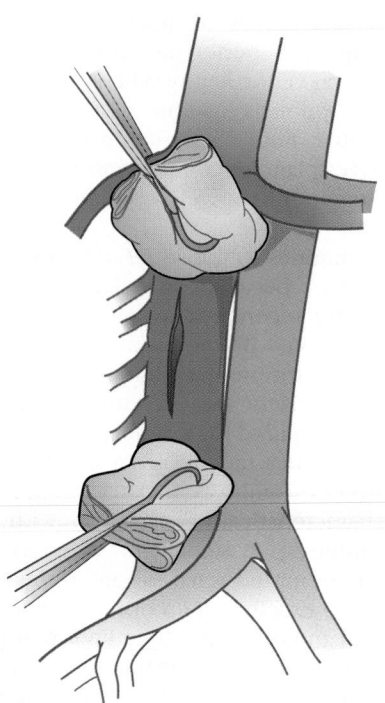

FIGURE 66-10. Compressing the inferior vena cave above and below the injury.

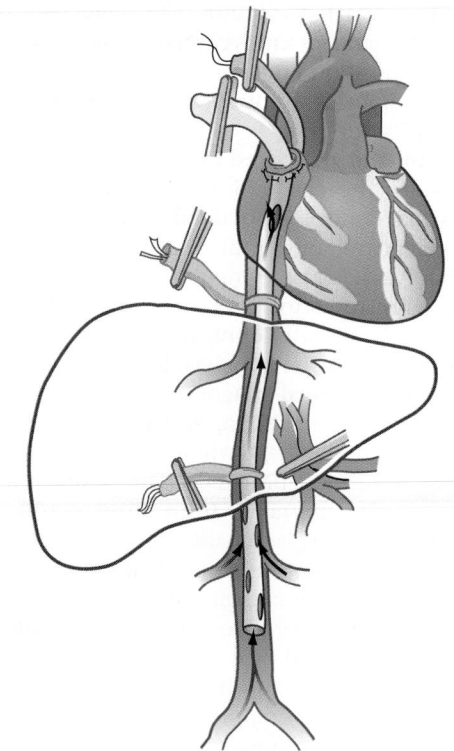

FIGURE 66-11. The atriocaval shunt.
(© Baylor College of Medicine, 1984.)

ings are massive venous bleeding either through a deep hepatic wound or from the posterior aspect of a severely injured liver. The bleeding is unaffected by a Pringle maneuver. Usually by the time the injury is identified, the patient has already sustained massive blood loss and is in profound shock. Direct repair options for the retrohepatic IVC are complex and have dismal results. The most widely known technique is the atriocaval shunt first described by Schrock in 1968.[42,47] The atriocaval shunt uses either a chest tube or an endotracheal tube inserted through the right atrium to exclude the injured segment without compromising cardiac preload (Fig. 66-11). This technically demanding procedure requires familiarity with cardiac cannulation and is usually performed by two teams working simultaneously in the chest and abdomen. It is therefore not surprising that this elaborate technical maneuver, usually employed in dire circumstances, carries a reported mortality in excess of 80%. There is no optimal solution for the technical challenge of retrohepatic IVC trauma. Several authors have reported successful packing of these injuries, and this simple solution, if performed early and effectively, may prove the most practical approach to injuries in this low-pressure system.

PERIPHERAL VASCULAR TRAUMA

General Principles

Initial Assessment

Initial assessment and care of the patient with peripheral vascular trauma focuses on control of external hemorrhage and the diagnosis of limb ischemia. In an ischemic extremity, the severity of ischemia and the arterial segment involved are the key considerations. It is extremely important to document the neurologic status of the injured extremity and to assess it for compartment syndrome. In the hemodynamically unstable trauma patient, a diminished arterial pulse or cold and pale extremity is difficult to assess, and diagnosis of ischemia depends on a comparison to the contralateral extremity.[25]

Although it is stated that restoration of arterial perfusion in less than 6 hours improves limb salvage rates, the window of opportunity for salvage is not a rigid interval. Instead, it is a flexible time frame that is heavily influenced by the site and nature of injury, the presence of efficient collaterals, and the patient's age and hemodynamic status. Of all the symptoms and signs of acute limb ischemia, a sensorimotor deficit conveys the greatest urgency because it signifies an imminent threat of irreversible ischemic insult.

Noninvasive Vascular Diagnosis

The hand-held Doppler flow detector provides limited but useful qualitative information, especially in the hemodynamically unstable, cold, and vasoconstricted patient in whom diagnosis of limb ischemia is often difficult. The hand-held Doppler is a reliable screening tool for significant arterial obstruction after both blunt and penetrating trauma, and arteriography is indicated for any significant difference (>10 mm Hg) in ankle pressures between extremities. The hand-held Doppler is also useful in assessing severity of ischemia by determining the presence of an arterial and venous Doppler signal. Absence of the latter signifies grave ischemia.

Duplex scanning has an overall accuracy rate of around 98% in detecting clinically significant injuries. It can also detect "minimal" arterial injuries such as intimal flaps and small pseudoaneurysms. However, the routine use of Duplex ultrasonography in the acute admission area of many trauma centers is limited by logistical constraints such as cost and the availability of trained personnel. It remains a very valuable tool for follow-up in patients with suspected or "minimal" vascular injuries, postoperative patients, and those with late complications of vascular trauma such as pseudoaneurysm and arteriovenous fistula.

Role of Arteriography

Arteriography is the definitive modality for diagnosing extremity arterial injuries in hemodynamically stable patients. It is indicated when the information gained can alter or facilitate the operative approach. In patients with multiple penetrations in an ischemic extremity and in those with blunt trauma (especially if several fractures are present) preoperative arteriography eliminates the need for extensive exposure and tedious dissection by precisely pinpointing the site of injury. In the actively bleeding patient, immediate surgical exploration without angiography is the correct course of action.

The use of arteriography to "rule out" arterial trauma in asymptomatic patients with penetrating wounds in proximity to the neurovascular bundle has changed in the past decade. While previously considered a standard practice, current evidence shows that physical examination is very accurate in detecting arterial injuries that require operative repair, and arteriography for proximity is therefore no longer indicated. If exclusion arteriography is routinely performed for proximity injuries, approximately 10% of patients will have an angiographic abnormality, but these lesions are "minimal" injuries that do not require operative repair and have a benign natural history. Based on these considerations, there is now enough evidence to avoid routine arteriography in asymptomatic patients with "proximity" injuries.

The Mangled Extremity

The decision to immediately amputate a severely wounded extremity rather than attempt to salvage it is difficult and emotionally charged, especially because vascular reconstruction is usually technically feasible, being one of the less problematic aspects of the injury. The mangled extremity is defined as injury to an extremity that involves at least three of the four major tissue systems of a limb, consisting of bone, soft tissue, vessels, and nerves. Several scoring systems have been proposed that attempt to predict the ultimate fate of the limb based on the severity of injury and the patient's associated injuries and premorbid factors. However, in practice the decision to proceed with amputation hinges on surgical judgment and the patient's individual circumstances. It is a team decision and should be made only after careful examination and consideration.

The decision is usually made in the operating room, where the mangled extremity can be meticulously examined under optimal conditions. This is the only reliable way to assess the full extent of the damage, especially to nerve continuity, a critical factor in the decision process. While the vascular injury is usually a less critical component than the neural or soft tissue damage, the total ischemia time is a major consideration in the decision to amputate. As a general rule, a totally interrupted distal innervation, extensive soft tissue destruction, and bone loss exceeding 6 cm in length all portend a grave prognosis for the limb.

Operative Technique

While control of active hemorrhage is always a top priority, reconstruction of injured vessels must be carefully orchestrated in the management of bone and soft tissue injuries. As a general rule, it is preferable to achieve bone alignment before vascular reconstruction because orthopedic manipulation and reconstruction takes time and may disrupt the vascular repair. Thus, if the limb is not grossly ischemic, reduction and fixation of fractures is performed first. If the limb is ischemic, a temporary intraluminal shunt can be inserted to maintain perfusion while the orthopedic procedure is performed.

As in any type of vascular trauma, the first priority with peripheral vascular injuries is to obtain proximal and distal control. This is achieved outside the hematoma or area of active bleeding. The underlying technical principle in access to the extremity vessels is to use *extensile exposures* that can be carried proximally and distally as necessary.

The next step is dissection to define the full extent of the injury and plan necessary reconstruction. In a contused vessel that remains in continuity, the key factor is integrity of the intima. An overlooked segment of injured intima can easily frustrate an otherwise meticulous arterial repair. The injury should be carefully débrided and a reconstruction technique chosen.

Because of the relatively small diameter of the peripheral arteries, lateral repair is feasible only in a minority of patients: those with iatrogenic lacerations or a simple stab wound. Most injuries require end-to-end anastomosis or an interposition graft. The completely transected artery of a young patient typically retracts a surprising distance, making interposition graft the only practical option.

Before the actual repair is performed, a Fogarty catheter thrombectomy should be performed on both ends of the injured vessel to remove intraluminal thrombus and ascertain the presence of good inflow and backflow. The vessel ends are then irrigated with heparinized saline. Full systemic anticoagulation is not used in the repair of vascular trauma because it is unnecessary and often contraindicated in the patient with multiple injuries. If there is any uncertainty about the integrity or adequacy of the outflow tract, an intraoperative angiogram is performed before the reconstruction.

The small diameter of arteries in the arm and below the knee prohibits the use of synthetic material, making a segment of greater saphenous vein the ideal conduit in these locations. PTFE is the preferred conduit in the thoracic outlet and above the groin. There is some controversy surrounding graft interposition of the femoral artery.[41] The traditional view that autogenous vein grafts have a better outcome in contaminated traumatic wounds is not supported by clinical or experimental data. Considerable evidence has accumulated to support the use of PTFE grafts in a contaminated operative field because the material is resistant to dissolution by bacterial collagenase and fares better than a vein graft if soft tissue cover is lost. Use of a synthetic graft also expedites the operative procedure, an important additional consideration in severely injured patients.

Graft protection by adequate soft tissue cover is a fundamental principle in vascular surgery that is especially relevant in trauma. The graft must be routed through a noncontaminated field and must also be adequately covered with viable soft tissue. An exposed graft, even if patent, represents a serious threat, not only to the viability of the limb but also to the patient's life. Therefore, considerations of graft protection may dictate the use of a longer extra-anatomical route rather than a shorter but contaminated route and may also affect the operative sequence.

Vein Injuries

The need to repair an injured peripheral vein and the long-term results of vein ligation in trauma patients remain the focus of active debate. The available evidence supports the repair of venous injuries encountered during exploration for an associated arterial trauma, but only if the patient is hemodynamically stable and the repair will not jeopardize or delay management of other significant injuries. Long-term patency rates of complex venous repairs (including interposition grafts using either saphenous vein or synthetic material) are poor, whereas best results are achieved by simple lateral repair that does not narrow the lumen or by end-to-end anastomosis. Contrary to previously held views, peripheral veins (including the popliteal vein) can be ligated without compromising adjacent arterial repairs or affecting limb salvage rates. The risk of long-term leg edema or chronic venous insufficiency is also very low.

Fasciotomy

Multiple factors contribute to the rapid development of elevated compartment pressures in the patient with peripheral vascular injury: direct muscular trauma, hypotension, reperfusion of the ischemic extremity, and ligation of injured veins.[49,50] Compartment syndrome is common in these patients but is also notoriously difficult to diagnose early. Generalized edema, swelling of the injured extremity, and lack of communication with the patient all combine to deprive the surgeon of vital early clues. Arbitrary definitions of ischemic times are poor guidelines to the need for fasciotomy. Pressure measurement using a hand-held transducer is problematic in the hemodynamically labile patient, where the critical compartment pressure that compromises capillary perfusion may be significantly lower than in the stable patient.

Therefore, the safest course of action is to maintain a low threshold for fasciotomy and decide based on individual clinical circumstances and operative findings.

A combined arterial and venous trauma, a long delay between injury and revascularization, and extensive bone and soft tissue destruction are examples of clinical circumstances where early fasciotomy is in the patient's best interest. In lower extremity fasciotomy, the four compartments of the leg should all be decompressed and is most commonly achieved through two longitudinal incisions (Fig. 66-12). The anterior and lateral compartments are approached through a longitudinal incision lateral to the tibial crest, whereas the superficial and deep posterior compartments are decompressed through a medial incision slightly posterior to the edge of the tibia.

Iatrogenic Trauma

The various types of iatrogenic trauma to the femoral vessels in the groin can serve as a model of similar iatrogenic injuries in other anatomic locations. Bleeding from a groin puncture wound is often the result of inadequate groin compression after catheter removal. Ongoing hemorrhage into the subcutaneous tissue presents as an expanding hematoma, where the major concern is not so much massive blood loss as pressure necrosis of the skin overlying the expanding hematoma and compression of the branches of the cutaneous branches of the femoral nerve with a resulting painful neuralgia. The management is by operative exploration and repair of the injured femoral artery through a longitudinal groin incision. Proximal control can usually be obtained at or immediately above the inguinal ligament, and a simple hemostatic suture is all that is required.

An inadvertently high cannulation of the external iliac artery is difficult to compress effectively and may result in a retroperitoneal hematoma. The patient typically presents with flank or groin pain and clinical signs of ongoing blood loss without a groin hematoma. Abdominal CT reveals the hematoma, and bleeding is usually self-limited. Rarely, hemodynamic deterioration leads to urgent operative repair of the injured external iliac artery.

Despite effective compression, a pseudoaneurysm may still develop at the puncture site. The presentation is usually with groin pain and hematoma that may appear hours and even days after the arterial cannulation. With a large pseudoaneurysm, a pulsatile hematoma may be noted. Diagnosis of a pseudoaneurysm is made by color-flow Doppler ultrasound, and the initial treatment is by ultrasound-guided manual compression. Groin compression is applied directly over the ultrasound-defined arterial laceration with the aim of inducing thrombosis of the pseudoaneurysm. The reported success rate of ultrasound-guided compression is 80% to 90% for small acute pseudoaneurysms but significantly lower for large pseudoaneurysms and in anticoagulated patients. Thus, 20% to 30% of patients with iatrogenic femoral pseudoaneurysms still require operative repair.

Iatrogenic arteriovenous fistula is typically the result of a low groin puncture that perforates the superficial or deep femoral artery and an adjacent vein. The resulting

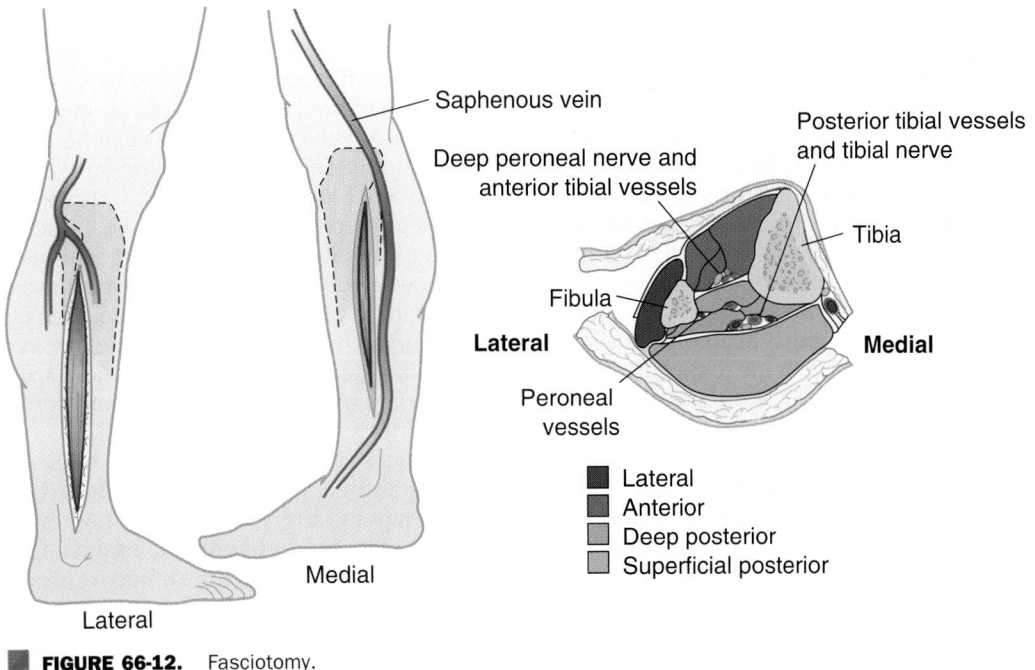

FIGURE 66-12. Fasciotomy.

arteriovenous fistula is often asymptomatic and is incidentally discovered during color Doppler evaluation of a groin hematoma. A larger fistula may be associated with a continuous murmur and a palpable thrill. Small incidentally discovered fistulas usually have a benign natural history. They either close spontaneously or remain asymptomatic and do not require treatment. A large or symptomatic fistula may require surgical repair.

Arterial thrombosis is another frequently encountered type of iatrogenic injury. It is more common with large-bore cannulations in patients with atherosclerosis of the femoral artery. The underlying mechanism is an intimal flap or fracture of a small segment of the arterial wall that leads to thrombosis. Understanding this pathophysiologic mechanism is the key to an effective repair because simple thrombectomy will not suffice. The underlying intimal injury must be identified and repaired, sometimes by means of a patch angioplasty of the common femoral artery.

Management of Specific Injuries

Most injuries to the *common or superficial femoral arteries* are penetrating. Proximal control for a high thigh or groin wound is usually obtained through a longitudinal groin incision using the inguinal ligament as a guide to dissection. The inguinal ligament limits the upward spread of a groin hematoma and, by carrying the dissection through the inguinal ligament and into the preperitoneal fat behind and above it, the surgeon can rapidly identify and control the distal external iliac artery before addressing the hematoma itself. Alternatively, the external iliac

artery can be exposed through a separate oblique incision above and parallel to the inguinal ligament, using a retroperitoneal approach. Dissection can then proceed inside the femoral triangle to expose the injured vessels. The deep femoral artery should be identified and preserved during reconstruction of an injured common femoral artery.

The superficial femoral artery in Hunter's canal is exposed through a medial thigh incision. The sartorius muscle is mobilized and retracted, exposing the roof of Hunter's canal. Special care must be taken to preserve the saphenous nerve lying on the anterior aspect of the artery.

Popliteal artery injuries result in limb loss more often than any other peripheral vascular injury. Amputation rates as high as 20% have been reported, especially from blunt trauma. The collateral arterial system around the knee is not well developed and is very susceptible to interruption by significant trauma, making delays in diagnosis and treatment of popliteal injuries particularly unforgiving. Posterior dislocation of the knee is associated with popliteal artery injury in one of every three patients, but other types of blunt trauma around the knee, such as a "bumper" injury to the proximal tibia or any injury that causes an unstable knee joint, are also likely to damage the artery. The majority of patients present with a clearly ischemic extremity, for which the indication for an urgent surgical exploration is obvious. In the absence of associated injuries, some surgeons administer intravenous heparin preoperatively to prevent thrombosis of the distal capillary bed, a major concern with popliteal injuries. A full fasciotomy is performed before the vascular exploration in a grossly ischemic leg. In approximately 30% of

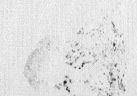

patients, the clinical presentation is less clear because the limb is not grossly ischemic. The key to avoiding undue delays is a high index of suspicion and a low threshold for angiography whenever significant blunt trauma has affected the area around the knee.

The proximal popliteal artery is exposed through an incision along the anterior border of the sartorius muscle above the knee. The deep fascia is incised and the sartorius is retracted, providing access to the popliteal space between the semimembranosus muscle and the adductor magnus tendon. The distal artery is approached through a medial incision immediately behind the posterior border of the tibia. The crural fascia is incised, and the popliteal space is entered between the medial head of the gastrocnemius and the soleus muscles. Wide exposure of the entire length of the popliteal artery is often required and is achieved by joining the incisions and dividing the tendons of the semitendinosus, semimembranosus, gracilis, and sartorius and then dividing the medial head of the gastrocnemius. In the majority of patients, the artery is repaired using a saphenous vein interposition graft from the contralateral extremity. On completion of reconstruction, an intraoperative angiogram is obtained. An associated vein injury is repaired if the clinical circumstances allow, but venous reconstruction does not affect the eventual outcome of the arterial repair. A fasciotomy is frequently performed after the reconstruction, especially when concomitant arterial and venous injury is present.

Penetrating injuries to the *lower leg arteries* below the popliteal trifurcation usually present with bleeding and progressive swelling of the calf. If one of the three shank arteries is involved, hemostasis can be achieved either by angiographic embolization or operative ligation. Patients with severe blunt trauma to the lower leg usually present with a combination of extensive bone and soft tissue damage as well as diminished or absent pedal pulses. Physical examination is unreliable under these circumstances, and angiography is used to diagnose or exclude an arterial injury. The traditional teaching that it is advisable to maintain patency of at least two shank arteries after blunt trauma is unproven. Exploration and repair of the lower leg arteries can be technically difficult in the hostile circumstances created by adjacent bone and soft tissue injuries and can safely be avoided in the presence of a single patent artery. There is, however, evidence to suggest that if the only remaining intact vessel is the peroneal artery, this may not suffice to prevent ischemia of the foot.

Exposure of the lower leg arteries is best begun proximally, away from the area of injury (Fig. 66-13). The distal popliteal artery is exposed below the knee through a

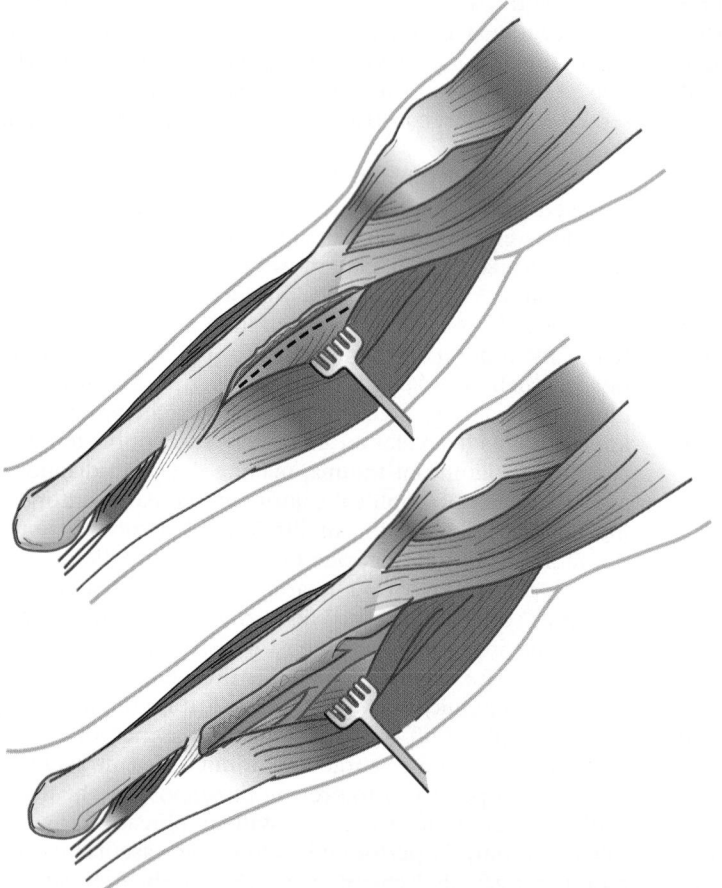

FIGURE 66-13.   Exposure of tibial vessels. (Illustration by Jan Redden. © Kenneth L. Mattox, M.D.)

medial approach, and dissection is continued distally by detaching the soleus muscle from the posterior border of the tibia, thus providing access to the posterior tibial and peroneal arteries. The anterior tibial artery is approached through a separate anterolateral incision between the tibialis anterior and the extensor hallucis longus muscles.

The great majority of *axillary artery injuries* are penetrating, resulting in hemorrhage or distal ischemia. In most published series, injuries to the subclavian and axillary vessels are treated as a single clinical entity. Extending a subclavian incision into the medial aspect of the abducted upper arm exposes the axillary artery. The incision is carried through the pectoral fascia, and the pectoralis major muscle can be either split or divided (near its insertion into the humerus) depending on the exposure required. The pectoralis minor muscle is either retracted or divided, and the clavipectoral fascia is opened, exposing the neurovascular bundle in the axillary sheath.

Injuries to the *brachial artery* account for 20% to 30% of peripheral arterial injuries, making this vessel the most frequently injured artery in the body. The artery is exposed through a medial arm incision in the groove between the biceps and triceps muscles. The first structure encountered in the neurovascular bundle is the median nerve, which must be isolated and preserved. If the brachial artery is exposed in the proximal arm, the deep brachial artery should be identified and controlled at the lateral border of the teres major muscle.

Most isolated *ulnar or radial artery injuries* can be ligated with impunity. An ischemic hand (due to an incomplete palmar arch or injury to both arteries) requires an arterial reconstruction. In the presence of associated bone and soft tissue injury, it is often safest to begin the exposure of a radial artery proximally at the brachial bifurcation and then proceed distally to the injured segment. A lower medial arm incision is carried into the antecubital fossa in an S-shaped configuration so as to avoid a longitudinal incision across the antecubital skin crease. The bicipital aponeurosis is divided to expose the brachial bifurcation, and the radial artery is identified and isolated. Exposure of the ulnar artery in the proximal forearm is more difficult because of the deeper location of the artery at this level. It is found deep to the antebrachial fascia, between the flexor carpi ulnaris and flexor digitorum superficialis muscles.

CONCLUSION

This chapter highlights several important differences between vascular trauma and other types of vascular disease. One salient feature of vascular trauma is the constant need to consider the injury and the various therapeutic options within the context of the patient's overall trauma burden. Purposeful delay in the operative repair of blunt aortic injury and the decision to employ "damage control" tactics during laparotomy for combined vascular and hollow visceral injury are but two examples of this key principle.

In the severely injured patient, management priorities change constantly and the surgeon must not only tailor the technical solution to the specific clinical circumstances but also be prepared to modify it or improvise a new solution as the circumstances change. The sequencing of the orthopedic and vascular repairs in the severely wounded extremity illustrates this need for flexibility.

The successful management of major vascular trauma hinges on the adaptation of standard vascular surgical techniques to nonstandard situations. The use of temporary intraluminal shunts and balloon catheter tamponade demonstrates how standard technical adjuncts have been adapted to new situations.

Endovascular therapy offers a new array of solutions for vascular trauma, and its minimally invasive nature is particularly suited to the critically injured patient with strained physiologic reserves. Endovascular solutions will play an increasing part in the management of truncal vascular injuries in nonbleeding patients.

Current advances in understanding the pathophysiology of trauma and innovative technology for vascular diagnosis and therapy are rapidly converging to provide the trauma surgeon of the future with an exciting selection of new tools. These tools will be used to further push the therapeutic envelope and continuously improve outcome in the management of the patient with major vascular injury.

Selected References

Aucar JA, Hirshberg A: Damage control for vascular injuries. Surg Clin North Am 77:853-862, 1997.

> **A summary of the "damage control" strategy in trauma and its application to the operative management of vascular injuries.**

Bickell WH, Wall MJ Jr, Pepe PE, et al: Immediate versus delayed fluid resuscitation for hypotensive patients with penetrating torso injuries. N Engl J Med 331:1105-1109, 1994.

> **The only prospective randomized study in the literature that examined delayed fluid resuscitation in penetrating torso trauma and showed that delayed fluid resuscitation favorably affects outcome.**

Biffl WL, Moore EE, Elliott JP, et al: Blunt cerebrovascular injuries. Curr Probl Surg 36:505-599, 1999.

> **A detailed summary of the current state of knowledge on blunt cerebrovascular trauma.**

Burch JM, Richardson RJ, Martin RR, et al: Penetrating iliac vascular injuries: Recent experience with 233 consecutive patients. J Trauma 30:1450-1459, 1990.

> **The largest series in the literature, with a detailed discussion of the various technical options for control and repair of these devastating injuries.**

Fabian TC, Richardson JD, Croce MA, et al: Prospective study of blunt aortic injury: Multicenter Trial of the American Association for the Surgery of Trauma. J Trauma 42:374-383, 1997.

> **This study showed that aortic clamp times under 30 minutes and that bypass techniques that provide for distal aortic perfusion are associated with a lower risk of paraplegia.**

Mattox KL, Feliciano DV, Burch J, et al: Five thousand seven hundred sixty cardiovascular injuries in 4459 patients: Epidemiologic evolution 1958 to 1987. Ann Surg 209:698-707, 1989.

The largest epidemiologic study in the literature on civilian vascular injuries.

Parker MS, Matheson TL, Rao AV, et al: Making the transition: The role of helical CT in the evaluation of potentially acute thoracic aortic injuries. AJR Am J Roentgenol 176:1267-1272, 2001.

Helical CT has a sensitivity and negative predictive value comparable to aortography.

Valentine RJ, Wind GG: Anatomic Exposures in Vascular Surgery. Philadelphia, Lippincott Williams & Wilkins, 2003.

A modern text on exposure and access techniques in vascular surgery.

References

1. Bickell WH, Wall MJ Jr, Pepe PE, et al: Immediate versus delayed fluid resuscitation for hypotensive patients with penetrating torso injuries. N Engl J Med 331:1105-1109, 1994.
2. Asensio JA, Chahwan S, Hanpeter D, et al: Operative management and outcome of 302 abdominal vascular injuries. Am J Surg 180:528-534, 2000.
3. Mattox KL, Feliciano DV, Burch J, et al: Five thousand seven hundred sixty cardiovascular injuries in 4459 patients: Epidemiologic evolution 1958 to 1987. Ann Surg 209:698-707, 1989.
4. Hirshberg A, Wall MJ Jr, Allen MK, et al: Causes and patterns of missed injuries in trauma. Am J Surg 168:299-303, 1994.
5. Villas PA, Cohen G, Putnam SG III, et al: Wallstent placement in a renal artery after blunt abdominal trauma. J Trauma 46:1137-1139, 1999.
6. Orford VP, Atkinson NR, Thomson K, et al: Blunt traumatic aortic transection: The endovascular experience. Ann Thorac Surg 75:106-112, 2003.
7. Aucar JA, Hirshberg A: Damage control for vascular injuries. Surg Clin North Am 77:853-862, 1997.
8. Feliciano DV, Burch JM, Mattox KL, et al: Balloon catheter tamponade in cardiovascular wounds. Am J Surg 160:583-587, 1990.
9. Hirshberg A, Wall MJ, Johnston RH Jr, et al: Transcervical gunshot injuries. Am J Surg 167:309-312, 1994.
10. Valentine RJ, Wind GG: Anatomic Exposures in Vascular Surgery. Philadelphia, Lippincott Williams & Wilkins, 2003.
11. Fry WR, Fry RE, Fry WJ: Operative exposure of the abdominal arteries for trauma. Arch Surg 126:289-291, 1991.
12. Mattox KL, McCollum WB, Jordan GL Jr, et al: Management of upper abdominal vascular trauma. Am J Surg 128:823-828, 1974.
13. Dawson DL, Putnam AT, Light JT, et al: Temporary arterial shunts to maintain limb perfusion after arterial injury: an animal study. J Trauma 47:64-71, 1999.
14. Biffl WL, Moore EE, Offner PJ, et al: Optimizing screening for blunt cerebrovascular injuries. Am J Surg 178:517-522, 1999.
15. Biffl WL, Moore EE, Elliott JP, et al: The devastating potential of blunt vertebral arterial injuries. Ann Surg 231:672-681, 2000.
16. Biffl WL, Moore EE, Elliott JP, et al: Blunt cerebrovascular injuries. Curr Probl Surg 36:505-599, 1999.
17. Biffl WL, Moore EE, Mestek M: Patients with blunt carotid and vertebral artery injuries. J Trauma 47:438-439, 1999.
18. Biffl WL, Moore EE, Offner PJ, et al: Blunt carotid arterial injuries: Implications of a new grading scale. J Trauma 47:845-853, 1999.
19. Biffl WL, Moore EE, Ryu RK, et al: The unrecognized epidemic of blunt carotid arterial injuries: Early diagnosis improves neurologic outcome. Ann Surg 228:462-470, 1998.
20. Miller PR, Fabian TC, Bee TK, et al: Blunt cerebrovascular injuries: Diagnosis and treatment. J Trauma 51:279-286, 2001.
21. Giacobetti FB, Vaccaro AR, Bos-Giacobetti MA, et al: Vertebral artery occlusion associated with cervical spine trauma: A prospective analysis. Spine 22:188-192, 1997.
22. Sturzenegger M: Headache and neck pain: The warning symptoms of vertebral artery dissection. Headache 34:187-193, 1994.
23. Weller SJ, Rossitch E Jr, Malek AM: Detection of vertebral artery injury after cervical spine trauma using magnetic resonance angiography. J Trauma 46:660-666, 1999.
24. Willis BK, Greiner F, Orrison WW, et al: The incidence of vertebral artery injury after midcervical spine fracture or subluxation. Neurosurgery 34:435-442, 1994.
25. Britt LD, Weireter LJ, Cole FJ: Newer diagnostic modalities for vascular injuries: The way we were, the way we are. Surg Clin North Am 81:1263-1279, xii, 2001.
26. Mattox KL: Red River anthology. J Trauma 42:353-368, 1997.
27. Fabian TC, Richardson JD, Croce MA, et al: Prospective study of blunt aortic injury: Multicenter Trial of the American Association for the Surgery of Trauma. J Trauma 42:374-383, 1997.
28. von Oppell UO, Dunne TT, De Groot MK, et al: Traumatic aortic rupture: Twenty-year meta-analysis of mortality and risk of paraplegia. Ann Thorac Surg 58:585-593, 1994.
29. Berland LL, Smith JK: Multidetector-array CT: Once again, technology creates new opportunities. Radiology 209:327-329, 1998.
30. Crawford CR, King KF: Computed tomography scanning with simultaneous patient translation. Med Phys 17:967-982, 1990.
31. Horrocks JA, Speller RD: Short communication: Helical computed tomography: Where is the cut? Br J Radiol 67:107-111, 1994.
32. Parker MS, Matheson TL, Rao AV, et al: Making the transition: The role of helical CT in the evaluation of potentially acute thoracic aortic injuries. AJR Am J Roentgenol 176:1267-1272, 2001.
33. Pate JW, Fabian TC, Walker WA: Acute traumatic rupture of the aortic isthmus: Repair with cardiopulmonary bypass. Ann Thorac Surg 59:90-99, 1995.
34. Carrillo EH, Bergamini TM, Miller FB, et al: Abdominal vascular injuries. J Trauma 43:164-171, 1997.
35. Coimbra R, Hoyt D, Winchell R, et al: The ongoing challenge of retroperitoneal vascular injuries. Am J Surg 172:541-545, 1996.
36. Jurkovich GJ, Hoyt DB, Moore FA, et al: Portal triad injuries. J Trauma 39:426-434, 1995.
37. Burch JM, Richardson RJ, Martin RR, et al: Penetrating iliac vascular injuries: Recent experience with 233 consecutive patients. J Trauma 30:1450-1459, 1990.
38. Carrillo EH, Spain DA, Wilson MA, et al: Alternatives in the management of penetrating injuries to the iliac vessels. J Trauma 44:1024-1030, 1998.

39. Cushman JG, Feliciano DV, Renz BM, et al: Iliac vessel injury: Operative physiology related to outcome. J Trauma 42:1033-1040, 1997.

40. Degiannis E, Velmahos GC, Levy RD, et al: Penetrating injuries of the iliac arteries: A South African experience. Surgery 119:146-150, 1996.

41. Feliciano DV, Mattox KL, Graham JM, et al: Five-year experience with PTFE grafts in vascular wounds. J Trauma 25:71-82, 1985.

42. Burch JM, Feliciano DV, Mattox KL: The atriocaval shunt: Facts and fiction. Ann Surg 207:555-568, 1988.

43. Burch JM, Feliciano DV, Mattox KL, et al: Injuries of the inferior vena cava. Am J Surg 156:548-552, 1988.

44. Ciresi KF, Lim RC Jr: Hepatic vein and retrohepatic vena caval injury. World J Surg 14:472-477, 1990.

45. Kuehne J, Frankhouse J, Modrall G, et al: Determinants of survival after inferior vena cava trauma. Am Surg 65:976-981, 1999.

46. Porter JM, Ivatury RR, Islam SZ, et al: Inferior vena cava injuries: Noninvasive follow-up of venorrhaphy. J Trauma 42:913-918, 1997.

47. Schrock T, Blaisdell FW, Mathewson C Jr: Management of blunt trauma to the liver and hepatic veins. Arch Surg 96:698-704, 1968.

48. Cue JI, Cryer HG, Miller FB, et al: Packing and planned re-exploration for hepatic and retroperitoneal hemorrhage: Critical refinements of a useful technique. J Trauma 30:1007-1113, 1990.

49. Feliciano DV, Cruse PA, Spjut-Patrinely V, et al: Fasciotomy after trauma to the extremities. Am J Surg 156:533-536, 1988.

50. Fainzilber G, Roy-Shapira A, Wall MJ Jr, et al: Predictors of amputation for popliteal artery injuries. Am J Surg 170:568-571, 1995.

CHAPTER 67

VENOUS DISEASE

Niren Angle, M.D., and Julie A. Freischlag, M.D.

Anatomy	**Deep Venous Thrombosis**
Venous Insufficiency	**Treatment**
Diagnostic Evaluation of Venous Dysfunction	**Conclusion**

Disorders of the vascular system can broadly be classified, in anatomic terms, into arterial, venous, or lymphatic diseases. Although there is undoubtedly overlap of these etiologies in some patients, for the most part, a clear understanding of the symptoms, signs, clinical presentation, as well as the history, can usually classify the problem discretely into one of those categories.

The focus of this chapter is on disorders of the venous system, which affect, according to some estimates, 40% of the U.S. population. The significance of venous disease, in terms of scope, cost, and implications, is not appreciated by most physicians since it is scarcely life or limb threatening, except for the notable exception of pulmonary embolism. Disorders of the venous system can be divided into thrombotic or thromboembolic disease and venous insufficiency. Thrombotic disease of the veins can and does frequently lead to venous insufficiency, the consequences of which are quite disabling. Another factor in truly assessing the prevalence of venous disease, in particular venous insufficiency, is that the range of venous insufficiency can span a vast array of manifestations, from mildly symptomatic varicose veins to severe chronic venous insufficiency (CVI) with ulceration. For accurate prevalence data, the essential requirement is that a uniform classification scheme be used, and, more important, the success of various therapeutic options can be properly gauged only if the clinician is knowledgeable about accurately classifying the disease, almost analogous to staging systems in oncology.

ANATOMY

A clear understanding of the anatomy of the venous system in the legs is essential to understanding pathophysiology as well as treatment. Venous drainage of the legs is the function of two parallel and connected systems: the deep and the superficial systems. The nomenclature of the venous system of the lower limb has undergone a revision, and the most relevant changes are addressed here.[1] The revised nomenclature is shown in Boxes 67-1 and 67-2 and is used in this chapter.

Superficial Venous System

The superficial veins of the sole form a network that connects to the superficial dorsal veins of the foot and the deep plantar veins. The dorsal venous arch, into which empty the dorsal metatarsal veins, is continuous with the greater saphenous vein medially and the lesser saphenous vein laterally (Fig. 67-1).

The greater saphenous vein, in close proximity to the saphenous nerve, ascends anterior to the medial malleolus, crosses, and then ascends medial to the knee (Fig. 67-2). It ascends in the superficial compartment and empties into the common femoral vein after entering the fossa ovalis. Before its entry into the common femoral vein, it receives medial and lateral accessory saphenous veins, as well as small tributaries from the inguinal region, pudendal region, and anterior abdominal wall. The posterior arch vein drains the area around the medial malleolus, and as it ascends up the posterior medial aspect of the calf, it receives medial perforating veins, termed *Cockett's perforators*, before joining the greater saphenous vein at or below the knee.

The lesser saphenous vein arises from the dorsal venous arch at the lateral aspect of the foot and ascends posterior to the lateral malleolus, and it empties into the popliteal vein after penetrating the fascia. The exact entry of the lesser saphenous vein into the popliteal vein is vari-

Box 67-1. Superficial Veins

Terminologica Anatomica	Proposed Terminology
Greater or long saphenous vein	Great saphenous vein
	Superficial inguinal veins
External pudendal vein	External pudendal vein
Superficial circumflex vein	Superficial circumflex iliac vein
Superficial epigastric vein	Superficial epigastric vein
Superficial dorsal vein of clitoris or penis	Superficial dorsal vein of clitoris or penis
Anterior labial veins	Anterior labial veins
Anterior scrotal veins	Anterior scrotal veins
Accessory saphenous vein	Anterior accessory great saphenous vein
	Posterior accessory great saphenous vein
	Superficial accessory great saphenous vein
Smaller or short saphenous vein	Small saphenous vein
	Cranial extension of small saphenous vein
	Superficial accessory small saphenous vein
	Anterior thigh circumflex vein
	Posterior thigh circumflex vein
	Intersaphenous veins
	Lateral venous system
Dorsal venous network of the foot	Dorsal venous network of the foot
Dorsal venous arch of the foot	Dorsal venous arch of the foot
Dorsal metatarsal veins	Superficial metatarsal veins (dorsal and plantar)
Plantar venous network	Plantar venous subcutaneous network
Plantar venous arch	
Plantar metatarsal veins	Superficial digital veins (dorsal and plantar)
Lateral marginal vein	Lateral marginal vein
Medial marginal vein	Medial marginal vein

able. The sural nerve closely accompanies the lesser saphenous vein.

Deep Venous System

The plantar digital veins in the foot empty into a network of metatarsal veins that comprise the deep plantar venous arch. This continues into the medial and lateral plantar veins that then drain into the posterior tibial veins. The dorsalis pedis veins on the dorsum of the foot form the paired anterior tibial veins at the ankle.

The paired posterior tibial veins, adjacent to and flanking the posterior tibial artery, run under the fascia of the deep posterior compartment. These veins enter the soleus and join the popliteal vein, after joining with the paired peroneal and anterior tibial veins. There are large venous sinuses within the soleus muscle—the soleal sinuses—that empty into the posterior tibial and peroneal veins. There are bilateral gastrocnemius veins that empty into the popliteal vein distal to the point of entry of the lesser saphenous vein into the popliteal vein.

The popliteal vein enters a window in the adductor magnus, at which point it is termed the *femoral vein*, previously known as the superficial femoral vein in the old nomenclature. The femoral vein ascends and receives venous drainage from the profunda femoris vein, or the deep femoral vein, and after this confluence, it is called the *common femoral vein*. As the common femoral vein crosses the inguinal ligament, it is called the *external iliac vein*.

Perforating veins connect the superficial venous system to the deep venous system at various points in the leg—the foot, the medial and lateral calf, the mid- and distal thigh (Fig. 67-3). The perforating veins in the foot are either valveless or with valves directing blood from the deep to the superficial venous system.

Varicose Veins

The term *varicose veins* is, in the common parlance, a term that encompasses a spectrum of venous dilation that ranges from minor telangiectasia to severe dilated, tortu-

Box 67-2. Deep Veins

Terminologica Anatomica	Proposed Terminology
Femoral vein	Common femoral vein
	Femoral vein
Profunda femoris vein or deep vein of thigh	Profunda femoris vein or deep femoral vein
Medial circumflex femoral vein	Medial circumflex femoral vein
Lateral circumflex femoral vein	Lateral circumflex femoral vein
Perforating veins	Deep femoral communicating veins (accompanying veins of perforating arteries)
	Sciatic vein
Popliteal vein	Popliteal vein
	Sural veins
	Soleal veins
	Gastrocnemius veins
	Medial gastrocnemius veins
	Lateral gastrocnemius veins
	Intergemellar vein
Genicular veins	Genicular venous plexus
Anterior tibial veins	Anterior tibial veins
Posterior tibial veins	Posterior tibial veins
Fibular or peroneal veins	Fibular or peroneal veins
	Medial plantar veins
	Lateral plantar veins
	Deep plantar venous arch
	Deep metatarsal veins (plantar and dorsal)
	Deep digital veins (plantar and dorsal)
	Pedal vein

ous varicose veins. As stated earlier, for a proper categorization, as well as for appropriate treatment options to be considered, certain definitions must be agreed on.

Varicose veins refer to any dilated, tortuous, elongated vein of any caliber. Telangiectasias are intradermal varicosities that are small and tend to be cosmetically unappealing but not symptomatic in and of themselves. Reticular veins are subcutaneous dilated veins that enter the tributaries of the main axial or trunk veins. Trunk veins are the named veins, such as the greater or lesser saphenous veins or their tributaries.

Risk Factors

A combination of risk factors, rather than any one specific risk factor, is a better predictor of the likelihood of a given patient developing symptomatic varicose veins. Heredity undoubtedly plays a significant role in the development of varicose veins. Once again, factors such as lack of clear classification, variability in reporting including patient self-reporting, and variability in definitions limit the accuracy

of any accurate assessment of incidence, prevalence, and thus, predisposing etiologic factors.

Venous Function

The venous wall is composed of the intima, the media, and the adventitia. The vein is thinner and has less smooth muscle and elastin than does an artery. The venous intima has an endothelial cell layer resting on a basement membrane, whereas the media is composed of smooth muscle cells and elastin/connective tissue. It is not generally appreciated that the adventitia of the venous wall contains adrenergic fibers, particularly in the cutaneous veins. Central sympathetic discharge and brain stem thermoregulatory centers can alter venous tone, as can other stimuli such as temperature changes, pain, emotional stimuli, and volume changes.

The histologic features of veins vary depending on the caliber of the veins. The venules, the smallest veins ranging from 0.1 to 1 mm, contain mostly smooth muscle cells, whereas the larger extremity veins contain relatively

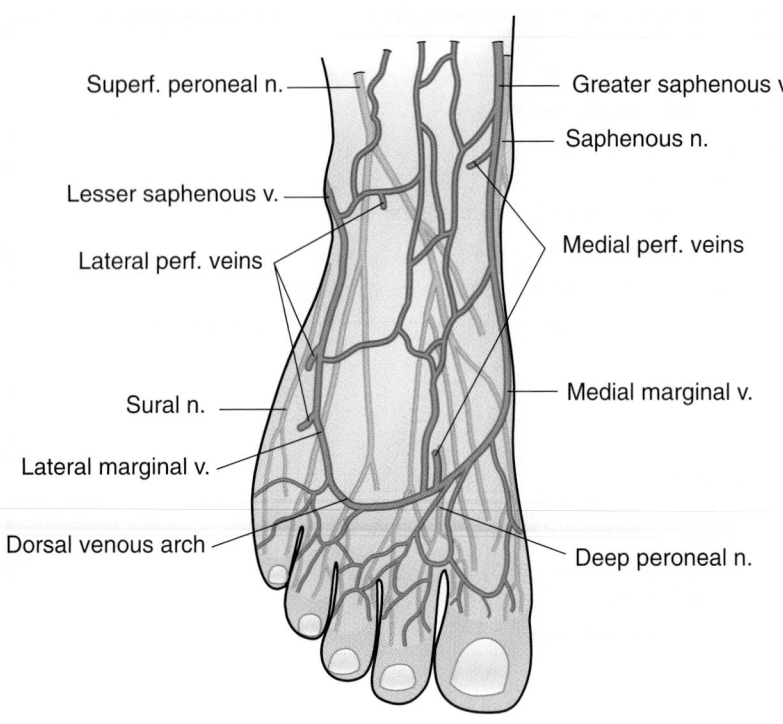

FIGURE 67-1.   Venous drainage of the foot.

Superf. peroneal n.

Greater saphenous v.

Saphenous n.

Lesser saphenous v.

Medial perf. veins

Lateral perf. veins

Sural n.

Medial marginal v.

Lateral marginal v.

Dorsal venous arch

Deep peroneal n.

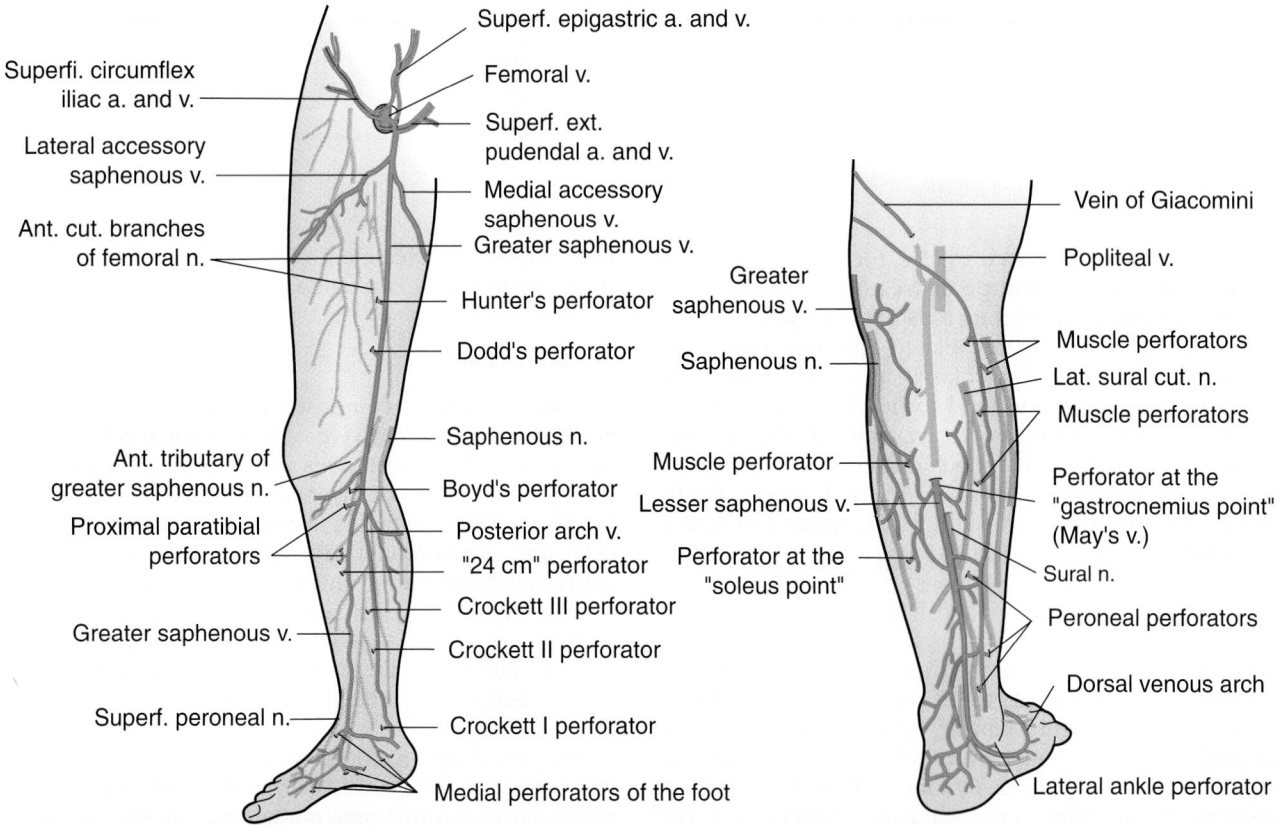

Superf. epigastric a. and v.

Superfi. circumflex
iliac a. and v.

Femoral v.

Lateral accessory
saphenous v.

Superf. ext.
pudendal a. and v.

Ant. cut. branches
of femoral n.

Medial accessory
saphenous v.
Greater saphenous v.

Vein of Giacomini

Popliteal v.

Hunter's perforator

Greater
saphenous v.

Muscle perforators

Dodd's perforator

Saphenous n.

Lat. sural cut. n.

Muscle perforators

Saphenous n.

Ant. tributary of
greater saphenous n.

Muscle perforator

Perforator at the
"gastrocnemius point"
(May's v.)

Boyd's perforator

Lesser saphenous v.

Proximal paratibial
perforators

Posterior arch v.

"24 cm" perforator

Perforator at the
"soleus point"

Sural n.

Crockett III perforator

Peroneal perforators

Greater saphenous v.

Crockett II perforator

Dorsal venous arch

Superf. peroneal n.

Crockett I perforator

Lateral ankle perforator

Medial perforators of the foot

FIGURE 67-2.   Venous drainage of the lower limb.

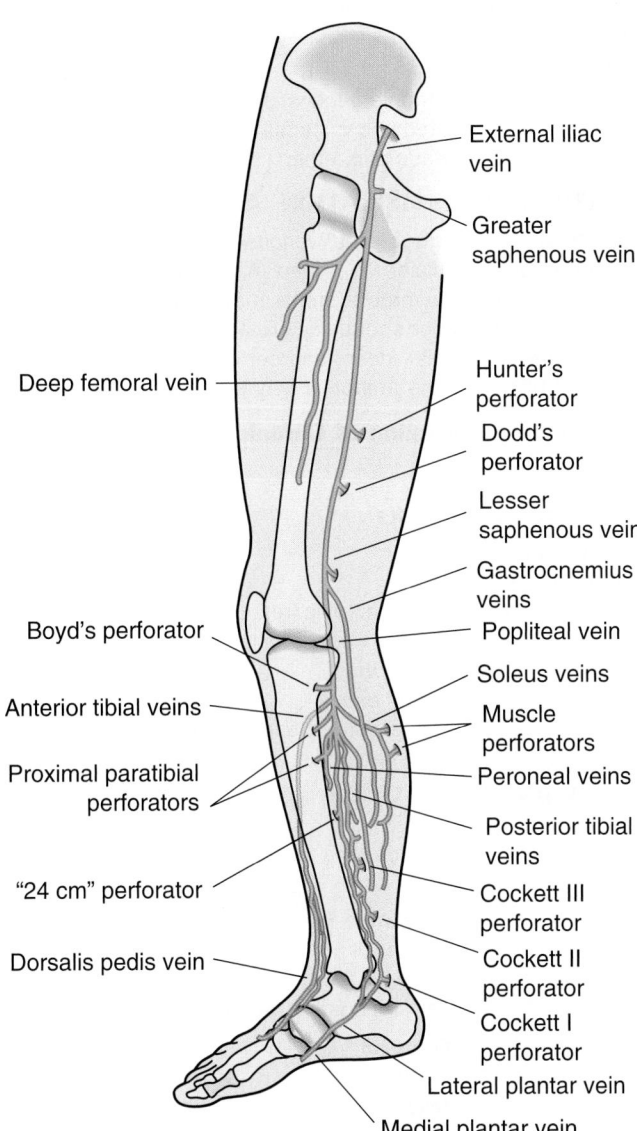

External iliac vein

Greater saphenous vein

Deep femoral vein

Hunter's perforator

Dodd's perforator

Lesser saphenous vein

Gastrocnemius veins

Boyd's perforator

Popliteal vein

Soleus veins

Anterior tibial veins

Muscle perforators

Proximal paratibial perforators

Peroneal veins

Posterior tibial veins

"24 cm" perforator

Cockett III perforator

Dorsalis pedis vein

Cockett II perforator

Cockett I perforator

Lateral plantar vein

Medial plantar vein

FIGURE 67-3. Perforating veins of the lower limb.

few smooth muscle cells. These larger caliber veins have limited contractile capacity in comparison to the thicker-walled greater saphenous veins. The venous valves prevent retrograde flow, and it is the failure of the valves that leads to reflux and associated symptoms. Venous valves are most prevalent in the distal lower extremity, whereas as one proceeds proximally, the number of valves decreases to the point that in the superior and inferior vena cava, no valves are present.

Most of the capacitance of the vascular tree is in the venous system. Because of the thin walls relatively devoid of elastin, the venous system is able to accommodate large changes in volume with virtually no increase in pressure up to a point. A vein has a normal elliptical configuration until the limit of its capacitance is reached, at which point the vein assumes a round configuration.

The calf muscles augment venous return by functioning as a pump. In the supine state, the resting venous pressure in the foot is the sum of the residual kinetic energy minus the resistance in the arterioles and precapillary sphincters.

There is thus generated a pressure gradient to the right atrium of approximately 10 to 12 mm Hg. In the upright position, the resting venous pressure of the foot is a reflection of the hydrostatic pressure from the upright column of blood extending from the right atrium to the foot.

The return of the blood to the heart from the lower extremity is facilitated by the muscle pump function of the calf—a mechanism whereby the calf muscle, functioning as a bellows during exercise, compresses the gastrocnemius and soleal sinuses and propels the blood toward the heart. The normally functioning valves in the venous system prevent retrograde flow; it is when one or more of these valves become incompetent that symptoms of venous insufficiency can develop. During calf muscle contraction, the venous pressure of the foot and ankle drops dramatically. The pressures developing in the muscle compartments during exercise range from 150 to 200 mm Hg, and when there is failure of perforating veins, these high pressures are transmitted to the superficial system.

VENOUS INSUFFICIENCY

The important fact about venous varicosities is that symptoms can be experienced by the patient in all the various forms of venous insufficiency. As noted earlier, the anatomy of venous drainage of the lower extremity is such that the superficial and the deep venous system independently or in concert may exhibit valvular dysfunction and insufficiency of a degree severe enough to cause symptoms.

Before examining the cause of the symptoms, it is useful to try to identify factors that may predispose one to developing varicose veins and associated symptoms. It is clear that despite the limitations in epidemiologic studies, the main influences that affect the development of varicose veins are the female sex, heredity, gravitation hydrostatic force, and hydrodynamic forces due to muscular contraction.

Telangiectasia, reticular varicosities, and varicose veins all are physiologically similar despite the variations in caliber. The unifying end result is dilated, tortuous, elongated veins with dysfunctional or nonfunctional valves.

The end result of CVI can range from aching, heaviness, pain, and swelling with prolonged standing or sitting in the case of symptomatic varicose veins, to severe lipo-dermatosclerosis with edema and ulceration in the patient with severe CVI.

The C-E-A-P classification is a recent scoring system that stratifies venous disease based on *c*linical presentation, *e*tiology, *a*natomy, and *p*athophysiology. This classification scheme, listed in Box 67-3, is useful in helping the physician coherently and thoughtfully assess a limb afflicted with venous insufficiency and then arrive at an appropriate treatment plan.

Symptoms

The patient with symptomatic varicose veins relates, most often, symptoms of aching, heaviness, discomfort, and sometimes outright pain in the calf of the affected limb.

Box 67-3. Classification of Chronic Lower Extremity Venous Disease

C   Clinical signs (grade$_{0-6}$), supplemented by "A" for asymptomatic and "S" for symptomatic presentation

E   Etiologic classification (*congenital*, *primary*, *secondary*)

A   Anatomic distribution (*superficial*, *deep*, or *perforator*, alone or in combination)

P   Pathophysiologic dysfunction (*reflux* or *obstruction*, alone or in combination)

CLINICAL CLASSIFICATION (C$_{0-6}$)

Any limb with possible chronic venous disease is first placed into one of seven clinical classes (C$_{0-6}$) according to the objective signs of disease.

Clinical Classification of Chronic Lower Extremity Venous Disease

Class 0   No visible or palpable signs of venous disease
Class 1   Telangiectasia, reticular veins, malleolar flare
Class 2   Varicose veins
Class 3   Edema without skin changes
Class 4   Skin changes ascribed to venous disease (e.g., pigmentation, venous eczema, lipodermatosclerosis)
Class 5   Skin changes as defined above with healed ulceration
Class 6   Skin changes as defined above with active ulceration

Limbs in higher categories have more severe signs of chronic venous disease and may have some or all of the findings defining a less severe clinical category. Each limb is further characterized as asymptomatic (A), for example, C$_{0-6,A}$, or symptomatic (S), for example, C$_{0-6,S}$. Symptoms that may be associated with telangiectatic, reticular, or varicose veins include lower extremity aching, pain, and skin irritation. Therapy may alter the clinical category of chronic venous disease. Limbs should therefore be reclassified after any form of medical or surgical treatment.

ETIOLOGIC CLASSIFICATION (E$_C$, E$_P$, or E$_S$)

Venous dysfunction may be congenital, primary, or secondary. These categories are mutually exclusive. Congenital venous disorders are present at birth but may not be recognized until later. The method of diagnosis of congenital abnormalities must be described. Primary venous dysfunction is defined as venous dysfunction of unknown cause but not of congenital origin. Secondary venous dysfunction denotes an acquired condition resulting in chronic venous disease, for example, deep venous thrombosis.

Etiologic Classification of Chronic Lower Extremity Venous Disease

Congenital (E$_C$)   Cause of the chronic venous disease present since birth
Primary (E$_P$)   Chronic venous disease of undetermined cause

Secondary (E$_S$)   Chronic venous disease with an associated known cause (post-thrombotic, post-traumatic, other)

ANATOMIC CLASSIFICATION (A$_S$, A$_D$, or A$_P$)

The anatomic site(s) of the venous disease should be described as superficial (A$_S$), deep (A$_D$), or perforating (A$_P$) vein(s). One, two, or three systems may be involved in any combination. For reports requiring greater detail, the involvement of the superficial, deep, and perforating veins may be localized by use of the anatomic segments.

Segmental Localization of Chronic Lower Extremity Venous Disease

Segment No.	Vein(s)
Superficial Veins (A$_{S1-5}$)	
1	Telangiectasia/reticular veins
	Greater (long) saphenous vein
2	*Above knee*
3	*Below knee*
4	Lesser (short) saphenous vein
5	Nonsaphenous
Deep Veins (A$_{D6-16}$)	
6	Inferior vena cava
	Iliac
7	*Common*
8	*Internal*
9	*External*
10	Pelvic: gonadal, broad ligament
	Femoral
11	*Common*
12	*Deep*
13	*Superficial*
14	Popliteal
15	Tibial (anterior, posterior, or peroneal)
16	Muscular (gastrointestinal, soleal, other)
Perforating Veins (A$_{P17,18}$)	
17	Thigh
18	Calf

PATHOPHYSIOLOGIC CLASSIFICATION (P$_{R,O}$)

Clinical signs or symptoms of chronic venous disease result from reflux (P$_R$), obstruction (P$_O$), or both (P$_{R,O}$).

Pathophysiologic Classification of Chronic Lower Extremity Venous Disease

Reflux (P$_R$)
Obstruction (P$_O$)
Reflux and obstruction (P$_{R,O}$)

This is particularly worse at the end of the day, most likely due to prolonged sitting or standing that results in venous distention and associated pain. The symptoms are typically reduced or absent in the morning owing to the fact that the limb has not been in a dependent position through the night.

In the case of women, the symptoms are often most troubling and exacerbated during the menstrual period, particularly during the first day or two. It is not unusual for a patient to have significant reflux at the saphenofemoral junction and yet not have impressive varicose veins on physical examination. Additionally, the patient may have combined superficial and deep venous insufficiency, and thus a clear diagnosis, with the aid of the CEAP system, is useful in determining treatment.

Primary varicose veins consist of elongated, tortuous, superficial veins that are protuberant and contain incompetent valves. These produce the symptoms of mild swelling, heaviness, and easy fatigability. Primary varicose veins merge imperceptibly into more severe CVI. Swelling is moderate to severe, an increased sensation of heaviness occurs with larger varicosities, and early skin changes of mild pigmentation and subcutaneous induration appear.

When CVI becomes severe, marked swelling and calf pain occur after standing, sitting, or walking. Multiple dilated veins are seen associated with various clusters and heavy medial and lateral supramalleolar pigmentation.

Pathogenesis

Cutaneous venectasia develops under the same influences and may become symptomatic similarly. Textbooks of venous disease in the past and recent present have referred to venectasias as cosmetic and not symptomatic, yet ample documentation exists to the contrary. Effective treatment of venectasia can relieve symptoms of venostasis.

Fundamental defects in the strength and characteristics of the venous wall enter into the pathogenesis of varicose veins. These defects may be generalized or localized and consist of deficiencies in elastin and collagen. Gandhi and colleagues[2] compared the collagen and elastin content of varicose veins with those of normal greater saphenous veins and discovered a significant increase in the collagen content and a significant reduction in the elastin content of varicose veins. No difference in proteolytic activity was demonstrated, thereby diminishing the likelihood that enzymatic degradation is an essential component of varicose vein formation.

Anatomic differences in the location of the superficial veins of the lower extremities may contribute to the pathogenesis. For example, the main saphenous trunk is not always involved in varicose disease. Perhaps this is because it contains a well-developed medial fibromuscular layer and is supported by fibrous connective tissue that binds it to the deep fascia. In contrast, tributaries to the long saphenous vein are less supported in the subcutaneous fat and are superficial to the membranous layer of superficial fascia (Fig. 67-4). These tributaries also contain less muscle mass in their walls. Thus, these, and not the main trunk, may become selectively varicose.[3]

When these fundamental anatomic peculiarities are recognized, the intrinsic competence or incompetence of the valve system becomes important. For example, failure of a valve protecting a tributary vein from the pressures of the long saphenous vein allows a cluster of varicosities to develop. This is not an uncommon history for pregnant women who describe a sudden development of a cluster of varicosities of unknown cause. Failure of the protective valve is the mechanism for such development.

The Middlesex Hospital (London, England) group has carried those observations into the clinical situation, where the micronized purified flavonoids were given as treatment for 60 days to patients with chronic venous disease.[4] Monitoring soluble endothelial adhesion molecules revealed that there was a reduction in the level of intercellular adhesion molecule-1, vascular cell adhesion molecules, and plasma lactoferrin.

Furthermore, communicating veins connecting the deep with the superficial compartment may have valve failure. Pressure studies show that two sources of venous hypertension exist. The first is gravitational and is a result of venous blood coursing in a distal direction down linear axial venous segments. This is referred to as *hydrostatic*

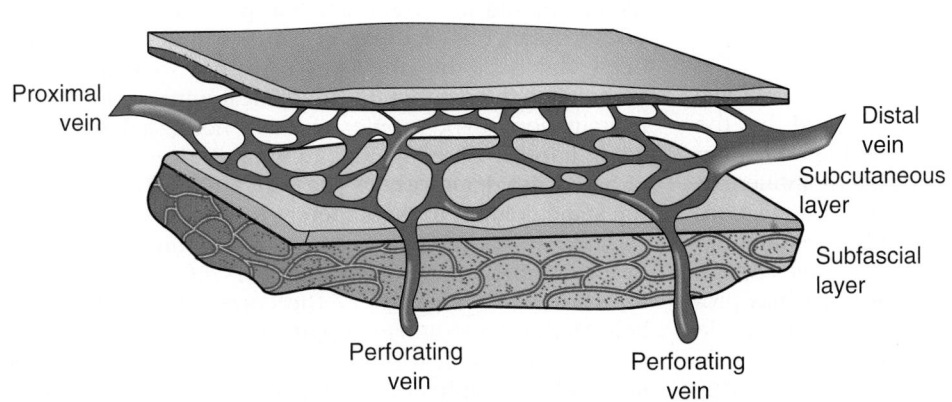

FIGURE 67-4. Dilation of superficial venous tributaries due to increased transmission of pressure via the perforating veins.

Proximal vein

Distal vein

Subcutaneous layer

Subfascial layer

Perforating vein

Perforating vein

pressure and is the weight of the blood column from the right atrium. The highest pressure generated by this mechanism is evident at the ankle and foot, where measurements are expressed in centimeters of water or millimeters of mercury. The second source of venous hypertension is dynamic. It is the force of muscular contraction, usually contained within the compartments of the leg. If a perforating vein fails, high pressures (ranging from 150 to 200 mm Hg) developed within the muscular compartments during exercise are transmitted directly to the superficial venous system. Here, the sudden pressure transmitted causes dilation and lengthening of the superficial veins. Progressive distal valvular incompetence may occur. If proximal valves such as the saphenofemoral valve become incompetent, systolic muscular contraction pressure is supplemented by the weight of the static column of blood from the heart. Furthermore, this static column becomes a barrier. Blood flowing proximally through the femoral vein spills into the saphenous vein and flows distally. As it refluxes distally through progressively incompetent valves, it is returned through perforating veins to the deep veins. Here, it is conveyed once again to the femoral veins, only to be recycled distally. Changes also occur at the cellular level. In the distal liposclerotic area, capillary proliferation is seen and extensive capillary permeability occurs as a result of the widening of interendothelial cell pores. Transcapillary leakage of osmotically active particles, the principal one being fibrinogen, occurs. In CVI, venous fibrinolytic capacity is diminished and the extravascular fibrin remains to prevent the normal exchange of oxygen and nutrients in the surrounding cells.[5,6] However, little proof exists for an actual abnormality in the delivery of oxygen to the tissues.[7] Instead, research suggests that many pathologic processes are involved, and at present difficulty exists in identifying which are active and which are bystanders. Fundamental investigations into this problem in the future should improve the care of patients with severe venous stasis disease. An understanding of the source of venous hypertension and its differentiation into hydrostatic and hydrodynamic reflux is important. The presence of hydrostatic reflux implies the need for surgical correction of this abnormality, and the presence of hydrodynamic reflux implies the need for ablation of the perforating venous mechanism allowing exposure of the subcutaneous circulation to compartment pressures.

Hormonal Influence

Venous function is undoubtedly influenced by hormonal changes. In particular, progesterone liberated by the corpus luteum stabilizes the uterus by causing relaxation of smooth muscle fibers.[8,9] This effect directly influences venous function. The result is passive venous dilation, which, in many instances, causes valvular dysfunction. Although progesterone is implicated in the first appearance of varicosities in pregnancy, estrogen also has profound effects. It produces the relaxation of smooth muscle and a softening of collagen fibers. Further, the estrogen-progesterone ratio influences venous distensibility. This

ratio may explain the predominance of venous insufficiency symptoms on the first day of a menstrual period when a profound shift occurs from the progesterone phase of the menstrual cycle to the estrogen phase.

Symptoms

Many causes of leg pain are possible, and most may coexist. Therefore, defining the precise symptoms of venostasis is necessary. These symptoms may be of gradual onset or may be initiated by a lancinating pain, and they may precede the clinical appearance of the varicosity. Discomfort usually occurs during warm temperatures and after prolonged standing. Varicose vein symptoms are often disproportionate to the degree of pathologic change. Patients with small, early varices may complain more than those with large, chronic varicosities. The initial symptoms may vary from a pulsating pressure or burning sensation to a feeling of heaviness. The pain is characteristically dull, does not occur during recumbency or early in the morning, and is exacerbated in the afternoon, especially after long standing. The discomforts of aching, heaviness, fatigue, or burning pain are relieved by recumbency, leg elevation, or elastic support.

Cutaneous itching is also a sign of venostasis and is often the hallmark of inadequate external support. It is a manifestation of local congestion and may precede the onset of dermatitis. This, and nearly all the symptoms of stasis disease, can be explained by the irritation of superficial nerve fibers by local pressure or accumulation of metabolic end products with a consequent pH shift. External hemorrhage may occur as superficial veins press on overlying skin within this protective envelope.

DIAGNOSTIC EVALUATION OF VENOUS DYSFUNCTION

The most important of all noninvasive tests available to study the venous system are the physical examination and a careful history that elucidates the symptoms mentioned earlier. Clinical examination of the patient in good light provides nearly all the information necessary. It determines the nature of the venostasis disease and ascertains the presence of intercutaneous venous blemishes and subcutaneous protuberant varicosities, the location of principal points of control or perforating veins that feed clusters of varicosities, the presence and location of ankle pigmentation and its extent, and the presence and severity of subcutaneous induration. After these facts have been obtained, the physician may turn to noninvasive techniques to corroborate the clinical impression. Visual examination can be supplemented by noting a downward-going impulse on coughing. Tapping the venous column of blood also demonstrates pressure transmission through the static column to incompetent distal veins.

The Perthes test for deep venous occlusion and the Brodie-Trendelenburg test of axial reflux have been replaced by in-office use of the continuous-wave, handheld Doppler instrument supplemented by duplex evaluation.[10] The handheld Doppler instrument can confirm an impression of saphenous reflux, and this, in turn, dictates the operative procedure to be performed in a given patient. A common misconception is belief that the Doppler instrument is used to locate perforating veins. Instead, it is used in specific locations to determine incompetent valves (e.g., the handheld, continuous-wave, 8-MHz flow detector placed over the greater and lesser saphenous veins near their terminations). With distal augmentation of flow and release, with normal deep breathing, and with performance of a Valsalva maneuver, accurate identification of valve reflux is ascertained. Formerly, the Doppler examination was supplemented by other objective studies. These included the photoplethysmograph, the mercury stain-gauge plethysmograph, and the photorheograph. These are no longer in common use.

Another instrument reintroduced to assess physiologic function of the muscle pump and the venous valves is the air-displacement plethysmograph.[11] This instrument was discarded after its use in the 1960s because of its cumbersome nature. Computer technology has allowed its reintroduction as championed by Christopoulos and coworkers.[12] It consists of an air chamber that surrounds the leg from knee to ankle. During calibration, leg veins are emptied by leg elevation, and the patient is then asked to stand so that leg venous volume can be quantitated and the time for filling recorded. The filling rate is then expressed in milliliters per second, thus giving readings similar to those obtained with the mercury strain-gauge technique.

Duplex technology more precisely defines which veins are refluxing by imaging the superficial and deep veins. The duplex examination is commonly done with the patient supine, but this gives an erroneous evaluation of reflux. In the supine position, even when no flow is present, the valves remain open. Valve closure requires a reversal of flow with a pressure gradient that is higher proximally than distally.[13] Thus, the duplex examination should be done with the patient standing or in the markedly trunk-elevated position.[14,15]

Imaging is obtained with a 10- or 7.5-MHz probe, and the pulsed Doppler consists of a 3.0-MHZ probe. The patient stands with the probe placed longitudinally on the groin. After imaging, sample volumes can be obtained from the femoral or saphenous vein. This flow can be observed during quiet respiration or by distal augmentation. Sudden release of augmentation allows assessment of valvular competence. The short saphenous vein and popliteal veins are similarly examined. Imaging improves the accuracy of the Doppler examination. For example, short saphenous venous incompetence can be differentiated from gastrocnemius venous valvular incompetence by the imaging and flow detection of the duplex or triplex scans.

Widespread use of duplex scanning has allowed a comparison of findings between standard clinical examinations with duplex Doppler studies.[16] In a study in which each patient was examined by three surgeons using different techniques (one using clinical examination, a second using the handheld Doppler instrument, and a third using a color duplex scanner), it was found that clinical examination failed in assessing main axial reflux at the saphenofemoral junction and saphenopopliteal junction.

Whenever a Doppler instrument was added to the examination, the evaluation became more accurate. Based on preoperative assessments using clinical examination alone, inappropriate surgery would have been performed in 20% of the limbs. Clinical examination plus Doppler study would have produced a 13% incidence of inappropriate surgery.

Phlebography

In general, phlebography is unnecessary in diagnosis and treatment of primary venostasis disease and varicose veins. In the complex problems of severe CVI, phlebography has specific utility. Ascending phlebography defines obstruction. Descending phlebography identifies specific valvular incompetence suspected on B-mode scanning and clinical examination.

Treatment

Indications for treatment are pain, easy fatigability, heaviness, recurrent superficial thrombophlebitis, external bleeding, and appearance. Treatment of venous insufficiency is similar to surgical treatment elsewhere; that is, it may be ablative or restorative. Most of the restorative venous surgical techniques remain experimental, and only a few can be considered standard therapy. On the other hand, ablative treatment has not been employed sufficiently for such a long time that the operations have undergone marked improvement and modernization.

Nonoperative Management

The cornerstone of therapy for patients with CVI is external compression, and most patients are treated nonoperatively. Patients with CVI have lower extremity edema as part of their clinical complex. Compression that relieves the leg edema generally controls the CVI. Although the exact mechanism by which compression is of benefit is not entirely known, a number of physiologic alterations have been observed with compression. These include reduction in ambulatory venous pressure, improvement in skin microcirculation, and increase in subcutaneous pressure, which counters transcapillary fluid leakage. Most patients with severe CVI and those with venous ulceration are treated with local wound care and elastic compression.

A triple-layer compression dressing, with a zinc oxide paste gauze wrap in contact with the skin, is utilized most commonly from the base of the toes to the anterior tibial tubercle with snug, graded compression. This is an iteration of what is known most commonly as an *Unna's boot*. A recent 15-year review of 998 patients with one or more venous ulcers treated with a similar compression bandage demonstrated that 73% of the ulcers healed in patients who returned for care. The median time to healing for individual ulcers was 9 weeks. In general, snug, graded-pressure triple-layer compression dressings effect more rapid healing than compression stockings alone.

For most patients, well-applied, sustained compression therapy offers the most cost-effective and efficacious therapy in the healing of venous ulcers. After healing, most cases of CVI are controlled with elastic compression stockings to be worn during waking hours. Occasionally, patients who are elderly and those with arthritic conditions cannot apply the compression stocking required, and control must be maintained by triple-layer zinc oxide compression dressings, which can usually be left in place and changed once a week.

Venous Ablation: Sclerotherapy

Cutaneous venectasia with vessels smaller than 1 mm in diameter do not lend themselves to surgical treatment. If their cause is saphenous or tributary venous incompetence, these conditions can be treated surgically. The venectasia themselves can be ablated successfully using modern sclerotherapy technique. Dilute solutions of sclerosant (e.g., 0.2% sodium tetradecyl) can be injected directly into the vessels of the blemish. Care should be taken to ensure that no single injection dose exceeds 0.1 mL but that multiple injections completely fill all vessels contributing to the blemish. When all of the ramifications of the blemish have been filled with sclerosant, and before the subsequent inflammatory reaction has progressed, a pressure dressing can be applied to keep vessels free of return blood for 24 to 72 hours. At 14 to 21 days' postinjection, incision and drainage of entrapped blood are performed, and a second pressure dressing is applied for 12 to 18 hours. This liberation of entrapped blood is as important to success as the primary injection. Such therapy is remarkably successful in achieving an excellent cosmetic result and relief of stasis symptoms.

In allergic patients, a solution of hypertonic saline can be used for sclerotherapy. On the other hand, the use of newer technologies such as the laser in treatment of telangiectasia has proved disappointing. Venules larger than 1 mm and smaller than 3 mm in size can also be injected with sclerosant of slightly greater concentration (e.g., 0.5% sodium tetradecyl), but limiting the amount injected to less than 0.5 mL. Pressure dressings for these venules must be in place for 72 hours or longer. Evacuation of entrapped blood is of paramount importance to prevent recanalization of these vessels after treatment.

Surgical Management

Surgical treatment may be used to remove clusters with varicosities greater than 4 mm in diameter. Ambulatory phlebectomy may be performed using the stab avulsion technique with preservation of the greater and lesser saphenous veins, if they are unaffected by valvular incompetence (Fig. 67-5).[17] When greater or lesser saphenous incompetence is present, the removal of clusters is preceded by limited removal of the saphenous vein (stripping). Stripping techniques are best done from above downward to avoid lymphatic and cutaneous nerve damage (Fig. 67-6). A number of techniques have been described that adapt new instruments to minimally invasive removal of the saphenous vein.[18,19]

At the present time, when the greater saphenous vein is used for coronary artery bypass and peripheral arterial reconstruction, there has been an interest in preserving the saphenous vein while relieving the symptoms of venous insufficiency, with little evidence to justify such an approach. However, a number of studies have shown

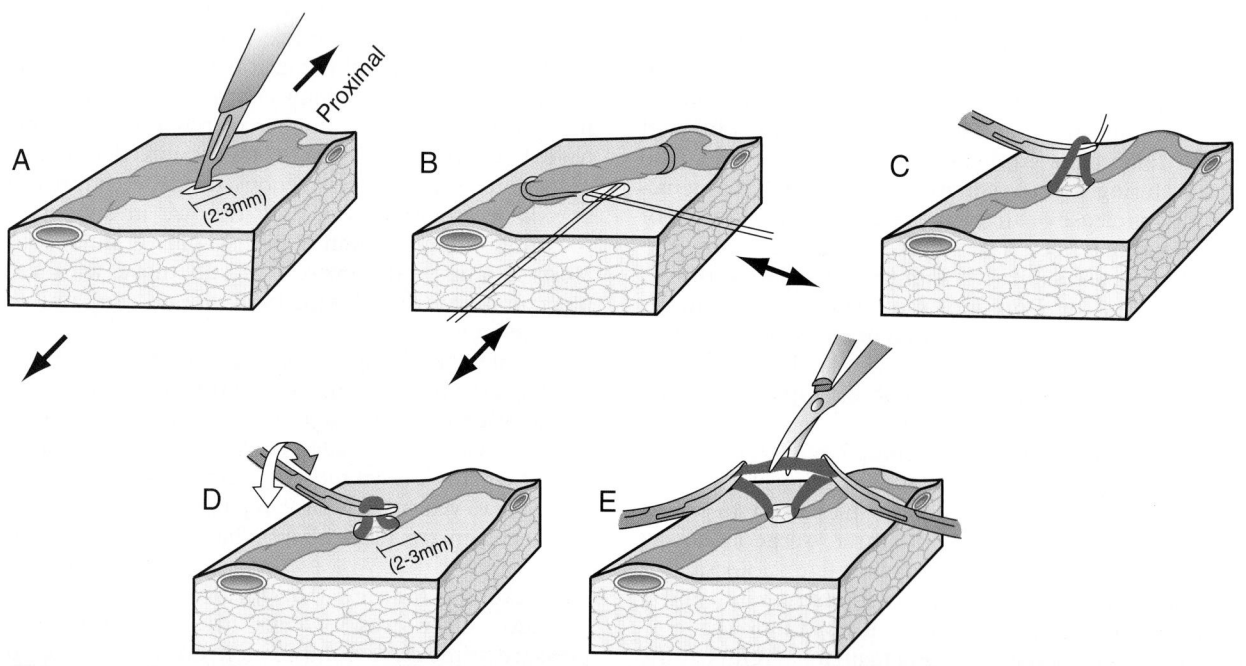

FIGURE 67-5.   **A to E,** Technique of ambulatory phlebectomy, otherwise known as *stab avulsions of varicosities.*

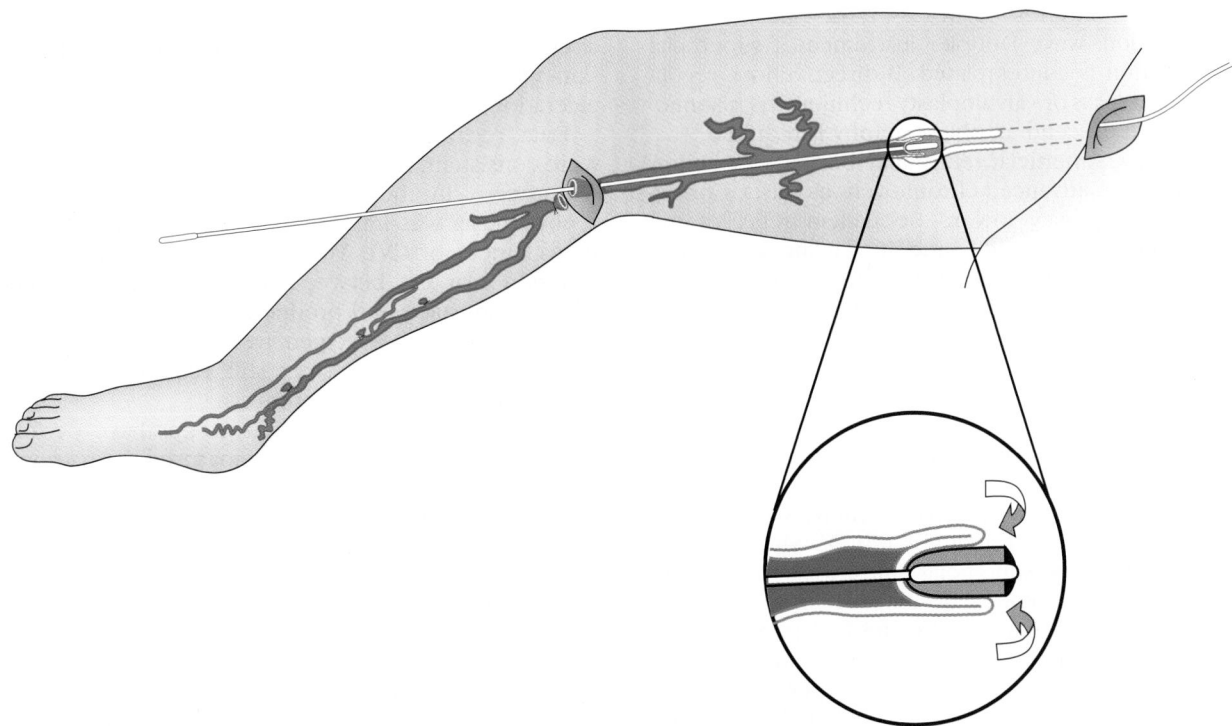

■ FIGURE 67-6.   Inversion stripping of the saphenous vein for superficial venous reflux due to an incompetent saphenofemoral junction.

the advantage of stripping in prevention of varicose vein recurrence.

The question of preservation or stripping of the saphenous vein is an important one; therefore, a 5-year clinical and duplex scan follow-up examination of a group of patients has been performed.[20] Patients were randomized to stripping of the long saphenous vein during varicose vein surgery versus saphenofemoral ligation with stab avulsion of varices. It was found that reoperation, either done or awaited, was necessary for only 3 of 52 legs that underwent stripping as compared with 12 of 58 limbs in which proximal ligation had been done. Neovascularization at the saphenofemoral junction was responsible for 10 of 12 recurrent varicose veins that underwent reoperation, and it was the cause of recurrence of saphenofemoral incompetence in 12 of the 52 limbs that were stripped versus 30 of the 58 limbs in which ligation was done. Clearly, the problem of neovascularization and recurrent varicose veins was not solved by the stripping operation, but stripping reduced the risk of reoperation by two thirds after 5 years of observation. It was the conclusion of the authors of the study that stripping "should be routine for primary long saphenous varicose veins."[20]

Modern treatment of varicose veins is fundamentally centered on the principle of ablation of the reflux source, sometimes termed the *escape point*. In most cases, this escape point is the incompetent valve at the saphenofemoral junction. It is clear to those who study this disease that unless the anatomic problem of reflux and the source of the reflux are dealt with, secondary procedures

such as injection sclerotherapy are plagued with a high rate of recurrence. For this reason, the fundamental precept in the treatment of superficial venous insufficiency is to treat the escape point and then treat the secondary varicosities. A recent addition to the armamentarium of the treatment of varicose veins is that of radiofrequency ablation of the saphenous vein. This method of treatment uses a radiofrequency ultrasound probe to obliterate the saphenous vein endoluminally throughout its length as well as at the junction. The preliminary data suggest that it may be as effective as ligation and stripping in the short to medium term. However, this modality has by no means been universally embraced as equivalent in outcomes or advantageous in cost.

Surgery for Severe Chronic Venous Insufficiency

What is new in the treatment of venous stasis is a rearranging of, and modifications to, older methods.[21] What has not changed is that conservative treatment of CVI always precedes consideration of intervention. Such conservative treatment relies on limb compression to counteract the effects of venous hypertension.

While conservative therapy is being pursued or ulcer healing achieved, appropriate diagnostic studies should reveal patterns of venous reflux or segments of venous occlusion so that specific therapy can be prescribed for the individual limb being examined. Imaging by duplex suffices for detection of reflux if the examination is carried out in the standing individual. Such noninvasive imaging may prove the only testing necessary beyond the hand-held, continuous-wave Doppler instrument if superficial venous ablation is contemplated. If direct venous reconstruction by bypass or valvuloplasty techniques is planned, ascending and descending phlebography is required.

Surprisingly, superficial reflux may be the only abnormality present in advanced chronic venous stasis. Correction goes a long way toward permanent relief of the chronic venous dysfunction and its cutaneous effects. Using duplex technology, Hanrahan and colleagues found that in 95 extremities with current venous ulceration, 16.8% had only superficial incompetence, and another 19% showed superficial incompetence combined with perforator incompetence.[22] Similarly, the Middlesex group, in a study of 118 limbs, found that "in just over half of the patients with venous ulceration, the disease was confined to the superficial venous system."[23]

Walsh and associates studied 58 limbs with class 3 venous insufficiency.[24] Ten limbs (17%) exhibited only superficial reflux, and superficial reflux was a major contributor to chronic venous dysfunction in another 17 limbs. Of some importance is the fact that primary, non-thrombotic deep (superficial femoral vein and popliteal vein) incompetence may accompany superficial reflux. This is explained by reflux proceeding distally down the greater saphenous vein and overloading the deep venous system. One would presume this causes dilation and elongation of the deep vessels so that their valves become incompetent. A study of limbs following greater saphenous vein stripping in which superficial femoral and popliteal venous incompetence was present has revealed correction of the deep reflux by superficial venous stripping in most limbs. Clearly, a significant proportion of patients with venous ulceration have normal function in the deep veins, and surgical treatment is a useful option that can definitively address the hemodynamic derangements. Maintaining that all venous ulcers are surgically incurable is not reasonable when these data suggest that superficial vein surgery holds the potential for ameliorating the venous hypertension.

In the early 1940s, Linton[25] emphasized the importance of perforating veins, and direct surgical interruption of these was advocated. This has fallen into disfavor because of a high incidence of postoperative wound healing complications. However, video techniques that allow direct visualization through small-diameter scopes have made endoscopic subfascial exploration and perforator vein interruption the desirable alternative to the Linton technique, minimizing morbidity and wound complications. The connective tissue between the fascia cruris and the underlying flexor muscles is so loose that this potential space can be opened up easily and dissected with the endoscope. This operation, done with a vertical proximal incision, accomplishes the objective of perforator vein interruption on an outpatient basis.

The availability of subfascial endoscopic perforator vein surgery had an impact on the care of venous ulcers in Western countries, albeit not as dramatic as its proponents had hoped. As patient limbs with severe CVI were studied accurately, the term *post-thrombotic syndrome* had to give way to the term *chronic venous insufficiency,*

and a link to platelet and monocyte aggregates in the circulation reflected the leukocytic infiltrate of the ankle skin with its lipodermatosclerosis and healed and open ulcerations.[26]

Data regarding leukocytes in CVI accumulated and were consistent, showing that the activation of leukocytes sequestered in the cutaneous microcirculation during venous stasis was important to the development of the skin changes of CVI. This is reflected in the finding of adhesion markers between leukocytes and endothelial cells and an increased production of leukocyte degranulation enzymes and oxygen free radicals. Nevertheless, experimental evidence was still required for decisive proof of the leukocyte hypothesis.

In the United States, several groups have performed perforating vein division using laparoscopic instrumentation. Initial data suggested that perforator interruption produced rapid ulcer healing and a low rate of recurrence. The North American Registry, which voluntarily recorded the results of perforating venous surgery, confirmed a low 2-year recurrence rate of ulcers and a more rapid ulcer healing.[27]

A comparison of the three methods of perforator vein interruption, including the classic Linton procedure, the laparoscopic instrumentation procedure, and the single open-scope procedure, revealed that the endoscopic techniques produced results comparable with those of the open Linton operation, with much less scarring and much greater tendency toward a fast recovery. More perforating veins were identified with the open technique. However, the mean hospital stay and the period of convalescence were more favorable with the scope procedures.[28]

In general, the registry reports and individual institution clinical experience showed that patients with true post-thrombotic limbs were disadvantaged by the procedure, enough so that at Leicester (England), the students of the procedure said, "We conclude that perforating vein surgery is not indicated for the treatment of venous ulceration in limbs with primary deep venous incompetence."[29] Nevertheless, studies were reported in which previous superficial reflux was corrected with failures of such treatment. Rescue of such limbs with perforating vein division produced satisfactory results and verified that perforating veins are important in the genesis of venous ulceration and that their division accelerates healing and may reduce recurrence of ulceration.

Part of the difficulty in understanding the need for perforating vein division is the disparity between venous hemodynamics and the severity of cutaneous changes. This should not be surprising because the cutaneous changes of CVI are dependent on leukocyte-endothelial interactions, and these may not be directly related to venous hemodynamics. Yet, endoscopic perforator vein division has improved venous hemodynamics in some limbs, as would be expected, by removing superficial reflux and perforating vein outflow.[30]

Direct Venous Reconstruction

Historically, the first successful procedures done to reconstruct major veins were the femorofemoral crossover graft of Eduardo Palma and the saphenopopliteal bypass described by him and used also by Richard Warren of Boston.[31] These operations were elegant in their simplicity, use of autogenous tissue, and reconstruction by a single venovenous anastomosis.

With regard to femorofemoral crossover grafts, the only group to provide long-term physiologic study of a large number of patients is Halliday and colleagues from Sydney, Australia.[32] Although phlebography was used in selecting patients for surgery, no other details of preoperative indications are given. They were able to document that 34 of 50 grafts remained patent in the long term as assessed by postoperative phlebography. They believed the best clinical results were achieved in relief of postexercise calf pain, but they had the impression that a patent graft also slowed the progression of distal liposclerosis and controlled recurrent ulceration. No proof of this was given in their report. The history of application of bypass procedures for venous obstruction is a fascinating one. Nevertheless, the advent of endovascular techniques has made those operations nearly obsolete.[33]

Perforator interruption combined with superficial venous ablation has been effective in controlling venous ulceration in 75% to 85% of patients. However, emphasis on failures of this technique led to Kistner's significant breakthrough in direct venous reconstruction with valvuloplasty in 1968 and the general recognition of this procedure after 1975.[34] Late evaluation of direct valve reconstruction indicates good to excellent long-term results in more than 80% of the patients.[35]

One cannot overestimate the contributions of Kistner. The technique of directing the incompetent venous stream through a competent proximal valve via venous segment transfer was his next achievement. After Kistner's contributions, surgeons were provided with an armamentarium that included Palma's venous bypass, direct valvuloplasty (of Kistner), and venous segment transfer (of Kistner). Moreover, external valvular reconstruction as performed by various techniques, including monitoring by endoscopy, holds the promise of a renewed interest in this form of treatment of venous insufficiency.

Axillary-to-popliteal autotransplantation of valve-containing venous segments has been considered since the early observations of Taheri and colleagues.[36] Verification in the long term of some preliminary excellent results has not been accomplished.

The advent of perforator vein surgery and the fine results achieved with it have displaced direct valvuloplasty into a position of less importance and even less interest than the procedure had called for during the 1980s.

DEEP VENOUS THROMBOSIS

Acute deep venous thrombosis (DVT) is a major cause of morbidity and mortality in the hospitalized patient, particularly in the surgical patient. The triad of venous stasis, endothelial injury, and hypercoagulable state first posited by Virchow in 1856 has held true a century and a half later.

Acute DVT poses several risks and has significant morbid consequences. The thrombotic process initiating in a venous segment can, in the absence of anticoagulation or in the presence of inadequate anticoagulation, propagate to involve more proximal segments of the deep venous system, thus resulting in edema, pain, and immobility. The most dreaded sequel to an acute DVT is that of pulmonary embolism, a condition of potentially lethal consequence. The late consequence of DVT, particularly of the iliofemoral veins, can be CVI due to valvular dysfunction in the presence of luminal obstruction.

For these reasons, understanding the pathophysiology, standardizing protocols to prevent or reduce DVT, and instituting optimal treatment promptly all are critical to reducing the incidence and morbidity of this unfortunately common condition.

Etiology

The triad of stasis, hypercoagulable state, and vessel injury all exist in most surgical patients. It is also clear that increasing age places a patient at a greater risk, with those older than 65 years of age representing a higher risk population.

Stasis

Labeled fibrinogen studies in patients as well as autopsy studies have demonstrated quite convincingly that the soleal sinuses are the most common sites for initiation of venous thrombosis. The stasis may contribute to the endothelial cellular layer contacting activated platelets and procoagulant factors, thereby leading to DVT. Stasis, in and of itself, has never been shown to be a causative factor for DVT.

The Hypercoagulable State

Our knowledge of hypercoagulable conditions continues to improve, but it is still undoubtedly embryonic. The standard array of conditions screened for when searching for a "hypercoagulable state" is listed in Box 67-4. Should any of these conditions be identified, a treatment regimen of anticoagulation is instituted for life, unless specific contraindications exist. It is generally appreciated that the postoperative patient, following major operative procedures, is predisposed to formation of DVT. Following

---

Box 67-4. Hypercoagulable States

- Factor V Leiden mutation
- Prothrombin gene mutation
- Protein C deficiency
- Protein S deficiency
- Antithrombin III deficiency
- Homocysteine
- Antiphospholipid syndrome

major operations, large amounts of tissue factor may be released into the bloodstream from damaged tissues. Tissue factor is a potent procoagulant expressed on leukocyte cell surface as well as in a soluble form in the bloodstream. Increases in platelet count, adhesiveness, changes in coagulation cascade, and endogenous fibrinolytic activity all result from physiologic stress such as major operation or trauma and have been associated with an increased risk of thrombosis.

Venous Injury

It has been clearly established that venous thrombosis occurs in veins that are distant from the site of operation; for instance, it is well known that patients undergoing total hip replacement frequently develop contralateral lower extremity DVT.

In a set of elegant experiments,[36a,36b] animal models of abdominal and total hip operations were used to study the possibility of venous endothelial damage distant from the operative site. In these experiments, jugular veins were excised after the animals were perfusion fixed. These experiments demonstrated that endothelial damage occurred after abdominal operations and were much more severe after hip operations. There were multiple microtears noted within the valve cusps that resulted in the exposure of the subendothelial matrix. The exact mechanism by which this injury at a distant site occurs, and what mediators, whether cellular or humeral, are responsible is not clearly understood but that the injury occurs and occurs reliably is evident from these and other studies.

Diagnosis

Incidence

Venous thromboembolism occurs for the first time in approximately 100 persons per 100,000 each year in the United States. This incidence increases with increasing age with an incidence of 0.5% per 100,000 at 80 years of age. More than two thirds of these patients have DVT alone, and the rest have evidence of pulmonary embolism. The recurrence rate with anticoagulation has been noted to be 6% to 7% in the ensuing 6 months.

In the United States, pulmonary embolism causes 50,000 to 200,000 deaths per year. A 28-day case fatality rate of 9.4% after first-time DVT and 15.1% after first-time pulmonary thromboembolism has been observed. Aside from pulmonary embolism, secondary CVI (that resulting from DVT) is significant in terms of cost, morbidity, and lifestyle limitation.

If the consequence of DVT, in terms of pulmonary embolism and CVI, is to be prevented, the prevention, diagnosis, and treatment of DVT must be optimized.

Clinical Diagnosis

The diagnosis of DVT requires, to use an overused phrase, a high index of suspicion. Most are familiar with Homans' sign, which refers to pain in the calf on dorsiflexion of the foot. It is certainly true that although the absence of this sign is not a reliable indicator of the absence of venous thrombus, the finding of a positive Homans' sign should prompt one to attempt to confirm the diagnosis. Certainly, the extent of venous thrombosis in the lower extremity is an important factor in the manifestation of symptoms. For instance, most calf thrombi may be asymptomatic unless there is proximal propagation. This is one of the reasons that radiolabeled fibrinogen testing demonstrates a higher incidence of DVT than incidence studies using imaging modalities. Only 40% of patients with venous thrombosis have any clinical manifestations of the condition.

Major venous thrombosis involving the iliofemoral venous system results in a massively swollen leg with pitting edema, pain, and blanching, a condition known as *phlegmasia alba dolens*. With further progression of disease, there may be such massive edema that arterial inflow can be compromised. This condition results in a painful blue leg, the condition called *phlegmasia cerulea dolens*. With this evolution of the condition, unless flow is restored, venous gangrene can develop.

Venography. Injection of contrast material into the venous system is obviously and understandably the most accurate method of confirming DVT and the location. The superficial venous system has to be occluded with tourniquet, and the veins in the foot are injected for visualization of the deep venous system. Although this is a good test for finding occlusive and nonocclusive thrombus, it is also invasive, subject to risks of contrast, and requires interpretation with 5% to 10% error rate.

Impedance Plethysmography. Impedance plethysmography measures the change in venous capacitance and rate of emptying of the venous volume on temporary occlusion and release of the occlusion of the venous system. A cuff is inflated around the upper thigh until the electrical signal has plateaued. Once the cuff is deflated, there should be rapid outflow and reduction of volume. With a venous thrombosis, one notes a prolongation of the outflow wave. It is not very useful clinically for the detection of calf venous thrombosis and in patients with prior venous thrombosis.

Fibrin Fibrinogen Assays. The basis of fibrin and/or fibrinogen can be assayed by measuring the degradation of intravascular fibrin. The D-dimer test measures cross-linked degradation products, which is a surrogate of plasmin's activity on fibrin. It is shown that in combination with clinical evaluation and assessment, the sensitivity exceeds 90% to 95%. The negative predictive value is 99.3% for proximal evaluation and 98.6% for distal evaluation. In the postoperative patient, D-dimer is causally elevated due to surgery, and, as such, a positive D-dimer assay for evaluating for DVT is of no use. However, a negative D-dimer test in patients with suspected DVT has a high negative predictive value, ranging from 97% to 99%.[37]

Duplex Ultrasound. The modern diagnostic test of choice for the diagnosis of DVT is the duplex ultrasound, a modality that combines Doppler ultrasound and color-flow imaging. The advantage of this test is that it is noninvasive, comprehensive, and without any risk of contrast angiography. This test is also highly operator dependent, and this is one of the potential drawbacks.

The Doppler ultrasound is based on the principle of the impairment of an accelerated flow signal due to an intraluminal thrombus. A detailed interrogation begins at the calf with imaging of the tibial veins and then proximally over the popliteal and femoral veins. A properly done examination evaluates flow with distal compression that should result in augmentation of flow and with proximal compression that should interrupt flow. If any segment of the venous system being examined should fail to demonstrate augmentation on compression, venous thrombosis should be suspected.

Real time B-mode ultrasonography with color-flow imaging has improved the sensitivity and specificity of ultrasound scanning. With color-flow duplex imaging, blood flow can be imaged in the presence of a partially occluding thrombus. The probe is also used to compress the vein: A normal vein should be easily compressed, whereas in the presence of a thrombus, there is resistance to compression. In addition, the chronicity of the thrombus can be evaluated based on its imaging characteristics, namely, increased echogenicity and heterogeneity. Duplex imaging is significantly more sensitive than indirect physiologic testing.

Magnetic Resonance Venography. With major advances in technology of imaging, magnetic resonance venography has come to the forefront of imaging for proximal venous disease. The cost and the issue of patient tolerance due to claustrophobia limit the widespread application, but this is changing. It is a useful test for imaging the iliac veins and the inferior vena cava, an area where duplex ultrasound is limited in its usefulness.

Prophylaxis

The patient who has undergone either major abdominal surgery, major orthopedic surgery, has sustained major trauma, or has prolonged immobility (>3 days) represents a patient who has an elevated risk for the development of venous thromboembolism. The specific risk factor analysis and epidemiologic studies dissecting the etiology of venous thromboembolism are beyond the scope of this chapter. The reader is referred to more extensive analysis of this problem.[38]

The methods of prophylaxis can be mechanical or pharmacologic. The simplest method is for the patient to be able to walk. Activation of the calf pump mechanism is an effective means of prophylaxis as evidenced by the fact that few active people without underlying risk factors develop venous thrombosis. A patient who is expected to be up and walking within 24 to 48 hours is at low risk of developing venous thrombosis. The practice of having a patient "out of bed into a chair" is one of the most thrombogenic positions that one could order a patient into. Sitting in a chair with the legs in a dependent position causes venous pooling, which in the postoperative milieu could be easily a predisposing factor in the development of thromboembolism.

The most common method of prophylaxis in the surgical universe has traditionally revolved around sequential compression devices, which periodically compress the calves and essentially replicate the calf bellows mechanism. This has clearly reduced the incidence of venous thromboembolism in the surgical patient. The most likely mechanism for the efficacy of this device is most likely from prevention of venous stasis. There is some literature that suggests that fibrinolytic activity systemically is enhanced by sequential compression device. However, this is by no means established, because there are a considerable number of studies demonstrating no enhancement of fibrinolytic activity.[39]

Another traditional method of thromboprophylaxis is the use of fixed "minidose" heparin. The dose traditionally used is 5000 units of unfractionated heparin every 12 hours. However, analysis of trials comparing placebo versus fixed-dose heparin shows that the stated dose of 5000 units subcutaneously every 12 hours is no more effective than placebo. When subcutaneous heparin is used on an every-8-hour dosing, rather than every 12 hours, there is a reduction in the development of venous thromboembolism.

More recently, a wealth of literature has revealed the efficacy of fractionated low-molecular-weight heparin (LMWH) for prophylaxis and treatment of venous thromboembolism. LMWH inhibits factors Xa and IIA activity, with the ratio of antifactor Xa to antifactor IIA activity ranging from 1:1 to 4:1. LMWH has a longer plasma half-life and has significantly higher bioavailability. There is much more predictable anticoagulant response than in fractionated heparin. No laboratory monitoring is necessary because the partial thromboplastin time (PTT) is unaffected. A variety of analyses, including a major meta-analysis, have clearly shown that LMWH results in equivalent, if not better, efficacy with significantly less bleeding complications.

Comparison of LMWH with mechanical prophylaxis demonstrates superiority of LMWH in reduction of the development of venous thromboembolic disease.[40-42] Prospective trials evaluating LMWH in head-injured and trauma patients have also proven the safety of LMWH, with no increase in intracranial bleeding or major bleeding at other sites.[43] In addition, LMWH shows significant reduction in the development of venous thromboembolism compared to other methods.

In short, LMWH should be considered the optimal method of prophylaxis in moderate and high-risk patients. Even the traditional reluctance to use heparin in high-risk groups such as the multiply injured trauma patient and the head-injured patient must be re-examined, given the efficacy and safety profile of LMWH in multiple prospective trials.

TREATMENT

Once a diagnosis of venous thrombosis is made, a decision must be made about whether to treat it or not. The treatment of calf venous thrombosis is controversial in most circles. It is true that the risk of pulmonary embolism from calf venous thrombosis is extremely low. However, propagation of calf venous thrombi occurs in up to 30% of hospitalized patients. The long-term sequelae of venous thrombosis involving more proximal venous segments certainly is reason enough to consider anticoagulation. If untreated, recurrent venous thromboembolism occurs in up to 30% of patients. For this reason, we would strongly advocate anticoagulant therapy of the patient with calf venous thrombosis, especially if the cause of the DVT has not been eliminated. If a decision not to anticoagulate is made, repeat duplex in 3 days is recommended, and if proximal propagation is noted, anticoagulation should be instituted.

Any venous thrombosis involving the femoropopliteal system should be treated with full anticoagulation. Traditionally, the treatment of DVT centers around heparin treatment to maintain the PTT at 60 to 80 seconds, followed by warfarin therapy to obtain an International Normalized Ratio (INR) of 2.5 to 3.0. If unfractionated heparin is used, it is important to use a nomogram-based dosing therapy. The incidence of recurrent venous thromboembolism increases if the time to therapeutic anticoagulation is prolonged. For this reason, it is important to reach therapeutic levels within 24 hours. A widely used regimen is 80 U/kg bolus of heparin, followed by a 15 U/kg infusion. The PTT should be checked 6 hours after any change in heparin dosing. Warfarin is started the same day. If warfarin is initiated without heparin, the risk of a transient hypercoagulable state exists, because proteins C and S levels fall before the other vitamin K–dependent factors are depleted. With the advent of LMWH, it is no longer necessary to admit the patient for intravenous heparin therapy. It is now accepted practice to administer LMWH to the patient as an outpatient, as a bridge to warfarin therapy, which also is monitored on an outpatient basis.

The recommended duration of anticoagulant therapy continues to undergo evolution. A minimum treatment time of 3 months is advocated in most cases. The recurrence rate is the same with 3 versus 6 months of warfarin therapy. If, however, the patient has a known hypercoagulable state or has experienced episodes of venous thrombosis, then lifetime anticoagulation is required, in the absence of contraindications. The accepted INR range is 2.0 to 3.0; a recent randomized, double-blind study confirmed that a goal INR of 2.0 to 3.0 was more effective in preventing recurrent venous thromboembolism than a low-intensity regimen with a goal INR of 1.0 to 1.9.[44] Additionally, the low-intensity regimen did not reduce the risk of clinically important bleeding.

Oral anticoagulants are teratogenic and thus cannot be used during pregnancy. In the case of the pregnant woman with venous thrombosis, LMWH is the treatment of choice, and this is continued through delivery and can be continued postpartum if needed.

Thrombolysis

The advent of thrombolysis has resulted in increased interest in thrombolysis for DVT. The purported benefit is preservation of valve function with subsequently lesser chance of developing CVI. However, to date, little definitive, convincing data exist to support the use of thrombolytic therapy for DVT.

One exception is the patient with phlegmasia in whom thrombolysis is advocated for relief of significant venous obstruction. In this condition, thrombolytic therapy probably results in better relief of symptoms and less long-term sequelae than heparin anticoagulation alone. The alternative for this condition is surgical venous thrombectomy. No matter which treatment is chosen, long-term anticoagulation is indicated. The incidence of major bleeding is higher with lytic therapy.

Vena Caval Filter

The most worrisome and potentially lethal complication of DVT is pulmonary embolism. The symptoms of pulmonary embolism, ranging from dyspnea, chest pain, and hypoxia to acute cor pulmonale are nonspecific and require a vigilant eye for the diagnosis to be made. The gold standard remains the pulmonary angiogram, but increasingly this is being displaced by the computed tomographic angiogram.

Adequate anticoagulation is usually effective in stabilizing venous thrombosis, but if a patient should develop a pulmonary embolism in the presence of adequate anticoagulation, a vena cava filter is indicated. The general indications for a caval filter are listed in Box 67-5. The modern filters are placed percutaneously over a guide wire. The Greenfield filter, with the most extensive use and data, has a 95% patency rate and a 4% recurrent embolism rate. This high patency rate allows for safe suprarenal placement if there is involvement of the inferior vena cava up to the renal veins or if it is placed in a woman of childbearing potential.

The device-related complications are wound hematoma, migration of the device into the pulmonary artery, and caval occlusion due to trapping of a large embolus. In the latter situation, the dramatic hypotension that accompanies acute caval occlusion can be mistaken for a massive pulmonary embolism. The distinction between the hypovolemia of caval occlusion versus the right heart failure from pulmonary embolism can be arrived at by measuring filling pressures of the right side of the heart. The treatment of caval occlusion is volume resuscitation.

CONCLUSION

Venous disease, in a surgical perspective, is unglamorous and frustrating. However, the consequence of both

---

Box 67-5. Indications for a Vena Cava Filter

- Recurrent thromboembolism despite "adequate" anticoagulation
- Deep venous thrombosis in a patient with contraindications to anticoagulation
- Chronic pulmonary embolism and resultant pulmonary hypertension
- Complications of anticoagulation
- Propagating iliofemoral venous thrombus in anticoagulation

venous insufficiency as well as venous thrombosis is debilitating, expensive, and associated with significant morbidity in terms of the initial condition as well as its sequelae. A thorough knowledge of the disease, the risk factors, and treatment will hopefully result in more effective prevention and treatment of this pervasive disease in the near future. The last 20 years have seen major advances in our diagnostic abilities, in terms of imaging, as well as our understanding of hypercoagulable states. Surgical advances, such as subfascial endoscopic perforator surgery, have had mixed results, but the general trajectory is forward, albeit with small steps.

Selected References

American Venous Forum: Classification and grading of chronic venous disease in the lower limb: A consensus statement. Vasc Surg 30:5, 1996.

> Interpretation based on external evidence alone, with regard to chronic venous disease, can be highly error prone, and this consensus statement by an international group of experts in chronic venous disease is an attempt to clearly identify the etiologic, anatomic, pathophysiologic, and clinical features of the limb with chronic venous disease.

Caggiati A, Bergan JJ, Gloviczki P, et al: Nomenclature of the veins of the lower limbs: An international interdisciplinary consensus statement. J Vasc Surg 36:416-422, 2002.

> A revision in the nomenclature of the venous system that seeks to eliminate some confusion about the superficial and the deep venous system, as commonly understood. It is unclear whether this advances the cause, but it is an attempt to standardize the nomenclature.

Christopolous D, Nicolaides AN, Cook A, et al: Pathogenesis of venous ulceration in relation to the calf muscle pump function. Surgery 106:829, 1989.

> Ulceration due to venous insufficiency is accompanied by increasing reflux and decreasing calf ejection fraction. The authors elegantly demonstrate that the combination of venous reflux and ejection fraction with exercise, expressed as the residual volume fraction, correlated well with the incidence of ulceration and the measurement of ambulatory venous pressure.

Lippman HI, Fishman LM, Farrar RH, et al: Edema control in the management of disabling chronic venous insufficiency. Arch Phys Med Rehabil 75:436, 1994.

> A 15-year experience demonstrating the efficacy of compression therapy, in particular Unna's boot, in healing ulceration of the limb, with 90% success in healing in compliant patients.

Rutgers PH, Kitslaar PJ: Randomized trial of stripping versus high ligation combined with sclerotherapy in the treatment of the incompetent saphenous vein. Am J Surg 168:311, 1994.

> This study demonstrated convincingly that the saphenous vein ligation and stripping in combination with stab avulsions were superior to high ligation without stripping and sclerotherapy with regard to cosmetic, functional, and duplex outcome criteria.

References

1. Caggiati A, Bergan JJ, Gloviczki P, et al: Nomenclature of the veins of the lower limbs: An international interdisciplinary consensus statement. J Vasc Surg 36:416-422, 2002.
2. Gandhi RH, Irizarry E, Nackman GB, et al: Analysis of the connective tissue matrix and proteolytic activity of primary varicose veins. J Vasc Surg 18:814-820, 1993.
3. Mashiah A, Rose SS, Hod I: The scanning electron microscope in the pathology of varicose veins. Isr J Med Sci 27:202-206, 1991.
4. Shoab SS, Porter J, Scurr JH, et al: Endothelial activation response to oral micronised flavonoid therapy in patients with chronic venous disease—a prospective study. Eur J Vasc Endovasc Surg 17:313-318, 1999.
5. Burnand KG, O'Donnell TF Jr, Thomas ML, et al: The relative importance of incompetent communicating veins in the production of varicose veins and venous ulcers. Surgery 82:9-14, 1977.
6. Burnand KG, Whimster I, Clemenson G, et al: The relationship between the number of capillaries in the skin of the venous ulcer–bearing area of the lower leg and the fall in foot vein pressure during exercise. Br J Surg 68:297-300, 1981.
7. Scurr JH, Coleridge-Smith PD: Pathogenesis of venous ulceration. Phlebologie I 1(Suppl):3-16, 1992.
8. Wahl LM: Hormonal regulation of macrophage collagenase activity. Biochem Biophys Res Commun 74:838-845, 1977.
9. Woolley DE: On the sequential changes in levels of oestradiol and progesterone during pregnancy and parturition and collagenolytic activity. *In* Pez KA, Eddi AH (eds): Extracellular Matrix Biochemistry. New York, Elsevier, 1984.
10. Hoare MC, Royle JP: Doppler ultrasound detection of saphenofemoral and saphenopopliteal incompetence and operative venography to ensure precise saphenopopliteal ligation. Aust N Z J Surg 54:49-52, 1984.
11. Christopoulos D, Nicolaides AN: Noninvasive diagnosis and quantitation of popliteal reflux in the swollen and ulcerated leg. J Cardiovasc Surg (Torino) 29:535-539, 1988.
12. Christopoulos D, Nicolaides AN, Szendro G: Venous reflux: Quantification and correlation with the clinical severity of chronic venous disease. Br J Surg 75:352-356, 1988.
13. van Bemmelen PS, Beach K, Bedford G, et al: The mechanism of venous valve closure: Its relationship to the velocity of reverse flow. Arch Surg 125:617-619, 1990.
14. van Bemmelen PS, Bedford G, Beach K, et al: Quantitative segmental evaluation of venous valvular reflux with duplex ultrasound scanning. J Vasc Surg 10:425-431, 1989.
15. Vasdekis SN, Clarke GH, Nicolaides AN: Quantification of venous reflux by means of duplex scanning. J Vasc Surg 10:670-677, 1989.
16. Singh S, Lees TA, Donlon M, et al: Improving the preoperative assessment of varicose veins. Br J Surg 84:801-802, 1997.
17. Bishop CCR, Jarrett PEM: Outpatient varicose vein surgery under local anaesthesia. Br J Surg 73:821-822, 1986.
18. Conrad P: Groin-to-knee downward stripping of the long saphenous vein. Phlebology 7:20-22, 1992.
19. Neglen P, Einarsson E, Eklof B: The functional long-term value of different types of treatment for saphenous vein incompetence. J Cardiovasc Surg (Torino) 34:295-301, 1993.
20. Dwerryhouse S, Davies B, Harradine K, et al: Stripping the long saphenous vein reduces the rate of reoperation for recurrent varicose veins: Five-year results of a randomized trial. J Vasc Surg 29:589-592, 1999.
21. Bergan JJ: New developments in the surgical treatment of venous disease. Cardiovasc Surg 1:624-631, 1993.

22. Hanrahan LM, Araki CT, Rodriguez AA, et al: Distribution of valvular incompetence in patients with venous stasis ulceration. J Vasc Surg 13:805-812, 1991.

23. Shami SK, Sarin S, Cheatle TR, et al: Venous ulcers and the superficial venous system. J Vasc Surg 17:487-490, 1993.

24. Walsh JC, Bergan JJ, Beeman S, et al: Femoral venous reflux abolished by greater saphenous vein stripping. Ann Vasc Surg 8:566-570, 1994.

25. Linton RR: The communicating veins of the lower legs and the operative technique for their ligation. Ann Surg 107:582, 1938.

26. Powell CC, Rohrer MJ, Barnard MR, et al: Chronic venous insufficiency is associated with increased platelet and monocyte activation and aggregation. J Vasc Surg 30:844-851, 1999.

27. Gloviczki P, Bergan JJ, Rhodes JM, et al: Mid-term results of endoscopic perforator vein interruption for chronic venous insufficiency: Lessons learned from the North American Subfascial Endoscopic Perforator Surgery Registry. The North American Study Group. J Vasc Surg 29:489-502, 1999.

28. Murray JD, Bergan JJ, Riffenburgh RH: Development of open-scope subfascial perforating vein surgery: Lessons learned from the first 67 cases. Ann Vasc Surg 13:372-377, 1999.

29. Scriven JM, Bianchi V, Hartshorne T, et al: A clinical and haemodynamic investigation into the role of calf perforating vein surgery in patients with venous ulceration and deep venous incompetence. Eur J Vasc Endovasc Surg 16:148-152, 1998.

30. Rhodes JM, Gloviczki P, Canton L, et al: Endoscopic perforator vein division with ablation of superficial reflux improves venous hemodynamics. J Vasc Surg 28:839-847, 1998.

31. Palma EC, Esperon R: Vein transplants and grafts in the surgical treatment of the postphlebitic syndrome. J Cardiovasc Surg (Torino) 1:94-107, 1960.

32. Halliday P, Harris J, May J: Femorofemoral crossover grafts (Palma operation): A long-term follow-up study. In Bergan JJ, Yao JST (eds): Surgery of the Veins. Orlando, Grune & Stratton, 1985, pp 225-265.

33. Molina JE, Hunter DW, Yedlicka JW: Thrombolytic therapy for iliofemoral thrombosis. Vasc Surg 39, 1992.

34. Kistner RL: Surgical repair of the incompetent femoral vein valve. Arch Surg 110:1336-1342, 1975.

35. Kistner RL: Late results of venous valve repair. In Yao JST, Pearce WL (eds): Long-Term Results of Vascular Surgery. Philadelphia, WB Saunders, 1993, p 451.

36. Taheri SA, Lazar L, Elias S, et al: Surgical treatment of postphlebitic syndrome with vein valve transplant. Am J Surg 144:221-224, 1982.

36a. Schaub RG, Lynch PR, Stewart GJ: The response of canine veins to three types of abdominal surgery: A scanning and transmission electron microscopic study. Surgery 83:411, 1978.

36b. Stewart GJ, Alburger PD, Stone EA, Soszka TW: Total hip replacement induces injury to remote veins in a canine model. J Bone Joint Surg Am 65-A:97, 1983.

37. Kovacs MJ, MacKinnon KM, Anderson D, et al: A comparison of three rapid D-dimer methods for the diagnosis of venous thromboembolism. Br J Haematol 115:140-144, 2001.

38. Anderson FA Jr, Spencer FA: Risk factors for venous thromboembolism. Circulation 107:I9-I16, 2003.

39. Killewich LA, Cahan MA, Hanna DJ, et al: The effect of external pneumatic compression on regional fibrinolysis in a prospective randomized trial. J Vasc Surg 36:953-958, 2002.

40. Bernardi E, Prandoni P: Safety of low-molecular-weight heparins in the treatment of venous thromboembolism. Expert Opin Drug Saf 2:87-94, 2003.

41. Couturaud F, Julian JA, Kearon C: Low-molecular-weight heparin administered once versus twice daily in patients with venous thromboembolism: A meta-analysis. Thromb Haemost 86:980-984, 2001.

42. Mismetti P, Laporte S, Darmon JY, et al: Meta-analysis of low-molecular-weight heparin in the prevention of venous thromboembolism in general surgery. Br J Surg 88:913-930, 2001.

43. Norwood SH, McAuley CE, Berne JD, et al: Prospective evaluation of the safety of enoxaparin prophylaxis for venous thromboembolism in patients with intracranial hemorrhagic injuries. Arch Surg 137:696-702, 2002.

44. Kearon C, Ginsberg JS, Kovacs MJ, et al: Comparison of low-intensity warfarin therapy with conventional-intensity warfarin therapy for long-term prevention of recurrent venous thromboembolism. N Engl J Med 349:631-639, 2003.

CHAPTER 68

THE LYMPHATICS

Iraklis I. Pipinos, M.D., and B. Timothy Baxter, M.D.

Embryology and Anatomy	**Diagnostic Tests**
Function and Structure	**Therapy**
Pathophysiology and Staging	**Chylothorax**
Differential Diagnosis	**Chyloperitoneum**
Classification	**Tumors of the Lymphatics**

EMBRYOLOGY AND ANATOMY

The primordial lymphatic system is first seen during the sixth week of development in the form of lymph sacs located next to the jugular veins. During the eighth week, the cisterna chyli forms just dorsal to the aorta, and, at the same time, two additional lymphatic sacs corresponding to the iliofemoral vascular pedicles begin forming. Communicating channels connecting the lymph sacs, which will become the thoracic duct, develop during the ninth week.

From this primordial lymphatic system sprout endothelial buds that grow with the venous system to form the peripheral lymphatic plexus (Fig. 68-1). Failure of one of the initial jugular lymphatic sacs to develop proper connections and drainage with the lymphatic and, subsequently, venous system may produce focal lymph cysts (cavernous lymphangiomas) also known as cystic hygromas.[1] Similarly, failure of embryologic remnants of lymphatic tissues to connect to efferent channels leads to the development of cystic lymphatic formations (simple capillary lymphangiomas) that, depending on their location, are classified as truncal, mesenteric, intestinal, and retroperitoneal lymphangiomas. Hypoplasia or failure of development of drainage channels connecting the lymphatic systems of extremities to the main primordial lymphatic system of the torso may result in primary lymphedema of the extremities.

FUNCTION AND STRUCTURE

The lymphatic system is composed of three elements: (1) the initial or terminal lymphatic capillaries, which absorb lymph; (2) the collecting vessels, which serve primarily as conduits for lymph transport; and (3) the lymph nodes, which are interposed in the pathway of the conducting vessels, filtering the lymph and serving a primary immunologic role.

The terminal lymphatics have special structural characteristics that allow entry not only of large macromolecules but even cells and microbes. Their most important structural feature is a high porosity resulting from a very small number of tight junctions between endothelial cells, a limited and incomplete basement membrane, and anchoring filaments tethering the interstitial matrix to the endothelial cells. These filaments, once the turgor of the tissue increases, are able to pull on the endothelial cells and essentially introduce large gaps between them, which then allow for very low resistance influx of interstitial fluid and macromolecules in the lymphatic channels. The collecting vessels ascend alongside the primary blood vessels of the organ or limb, pass through the regional lymph nodes, and drain into the main lymph channels of the torso. These channels eventually empty into the venous system through the thoracic duct. There are additional communications between the lymphatic and the venous system. These smaller lymphovenous shunts mostly occur at the level of lymph nodes and around major venous structures, such as the jugular, subclavian, and iliac veins. Several structures in the body contain no lymphatics. Specifically, lymphatics have not been found in the epidermis, cornea, central nervous system, cartilage, tendon, and muscle.

The lymphatic system has three main functions. First, tissue fluid and macromolecules ultrafiltrated at the level of the arterial capillaries are reabsorbed and returned to the circulation through the lymphatic system. Every day,

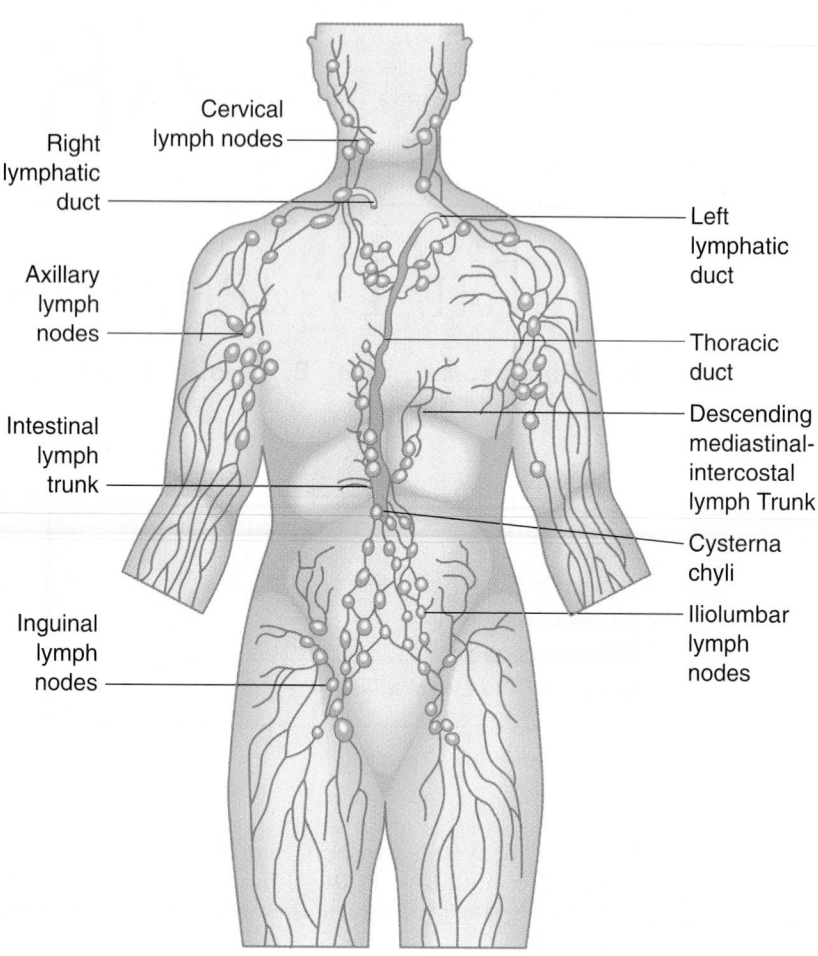

Right
lymphatic
duct

Cervical
lymph nodes

Axillary
lymph
nodes

Intestinal
lymph
trunk

Inguinal
lymph
nodes

Left
lymphatic
duct

Thoracic
duct

Descending
mediastinal-
intercostal
lymph Trunk

Cysterna
chyli

Iliolumbar
lymph
nodes

FIGURE 68-1. Major anatomic pathways and lymph node groups of the lymphatic system.

50% to 100% of the intravascular proteins are filtered this way in the interstitial space. Normally they then enter the terminal lymphatics and are transported through the collecting lymphatics back into the venous circulation. Second, microbes arriving in the interstitial space enter the lymphatic system and are presented to the lymph nodes, which represent the first line of the immune system. Last, at the level of the gastrointestinal tract, lymph vessels are responsible for the uptake and transport of most of the fat absorbed from the bowel.

In contrast to what happens with venous forward flow, lymph's centripetal transport occurs mainly through intrinsic contractility of the individual lymphatic vessels, which in concert with competent valvular mechanisms is effective in establishing constant forward flow of lymph. In addition to the intrinsic contractility, other factors, such as surrounding muscular activity, negative pressure secondary to breathing, and transmitted arterial pulsations, have a lesser role in the forward lymph flow. These secondary factors appear to become more important under conditions of lymph stasis and congestion of the lymphatic vessels.

PATHOPHYSIOLOGY AND STAGING

Lymphedema is the result of an inability of the existing lymphatic system to accommodate the protein and fluid entering the interstitial compartment at the tissue level.[2] In the first stage of lymphedema, impaired lymphatic drainage results in protein-rich fluid accumulation in the interstitial compartment. Clinically, this manifests as soft pitting edema. In the second stage of lymphedema, the clinical condition is further exacerbated by accumulation of fibroblasts, adipocytes, and, perhaps most importantly, macrophages in the affected tissues, which culminate in a local inflammatory response. This results in important structural changes from the deposition of connective tissue and adipose elements at the skin and subcutaneous level. In the second stage of lymphedema, tissue edema is more pronounced, is nonpitting, and has a spongy consistency. In the third and most advanced stage of lymphedema, the affected tissues sustain further injury as a result of both the local inflammatory response as well as recurrent infectious episodes that typically result from minimal subclinical skin breaks in the skin. Such repeated episodes injure the incompetent, remaining lymphatic channels, progressively worsening the underlying insufficiency of the lymphatic system. This eventually results in excessive subcutaneous fibrosis and scarring with associated severe skin changes characteristic of lymphostatic elephantiasis (Fig. 68-2).

DIFFERENTIAL DIAGNOSIS

In most patients with second- or third-stage lymphedema, the characteristic findings on physical examination can usually establish the diagnosis. The edematous limb has a firm and hardened consistency. There is loss of the normal perimalleolar shape, resulting in a "tree trunk" pattern. The dorsum of the foot is characteristically swollen, resulting in the appearance of the "buffalo hump," and the toes become thick and squared (Fig. 68-2). In advanced lymphedema, the skin undergoes characteristic changes, such as lichenification, development of peau d'orange, and hyperkeratosis.[3] Additionally, the patients give a history of recurrent episodes of cellulitis and lymphangitis after trivial trauma and frequently present with fungal infections affecting the forefoot and toes. Patients with isolated lymphedema usually do not have the hyperpigmentation or ulceration one typically sees in patients with chronic venous insufficiency. Lymphedema does not respond significantly to overnight elevation, whereas edema secondary to central organ failure or venous insufficiency does.

The evaluation of a swollen extremity should start with a detailed history and physical examination. The most common causes of bilateral extremity edema are of systemic origin. The most common etiology is cardiac failure,

followed by renal failure.[4] Hypoproteinemia secondary to cirrhosis, nephrotic syndrome, and malnutrition can also produce bilateral lower extremity edema. Another important cause to consider with bilateral leg enlargement is lipedema. Lipedema is not true edema but rather excessive subcutaneous fat found in obese women. It is bilateral, nonpitting, and greatest at the ankle and legs, with characteristic sparing of the feet. There are no skin changes, and the enlargement is not affected by elevation. The history usually indicates that this has been a lifelong problem that "runs in the family."

Once the systemic causes of edema are excluded, in the patient with unilateral extremity involvement, edema secondary to venous and lymphatic pathology should be entertained. Venous pathology is overwhelmingly the most common cause of unilateral leg edema. Leg edema secondary to venous disease is usually pitting and is greatest at the legs and ankles with a sparing of the feet. The edema responds promptly to overnight leg elevation. In the later stages, the skin is atrophic with brawny pigmentation. Ulceration associated with venous insufficiency occurs above or posterior and beneath the malleoli.

CLASSIFICATION

Lymphedema is generally classified as primary when there is no known etiology and secondary when its cause is a known disease or disorder.[5] Primary lymphedema has generally been classified on the basis of the age at onset and presence of familial clustering. Primary lymphedema with onset before the first year of life is called congenital. The familial version of congenital lymphedema is known as Milroy's disease and is inherited as a dominant trait. Primary lymphedema with onset between the ages of 1 and 35 years is called lymphedema praecox. The familial version of lymphedema praecox is known as Meige's disease. Finally, primary lymphedema with onset after the age of 35 is called lymphedema tarda. The primary lymphedemas are relatively uncommon, occurring in one of every 10,000 individuals. The most common form of primary lymphedema is praecox, which accounts for approximately 80% of the patients. Congenital and tarda lymphedemas each account for 10%. Worldwide the most common cause of secondary lymphedema is infestation of the lymph nodes by the parasite *Wuchereria bancrofti* in the disease state called filariasis. In the developed countries the most common causes of secondary lymphedema involve resection or ablation of regional lymph nodes by surgery, radiation therapy, tumor invasion, direct trauma, or, less commonly, an infectious process.

DIAGNOSTIC TESTS

The diagnosis of lymphedema is relatively easy in the patient who presents in the second and third stages of the disease. It can however, be a difficult diagnosis to make in the first stage, particularly when the edema is mild, pitting, and relieved with simple maneuvers such as elevation.[6,7] For patients with suspected secondary forms of lym-

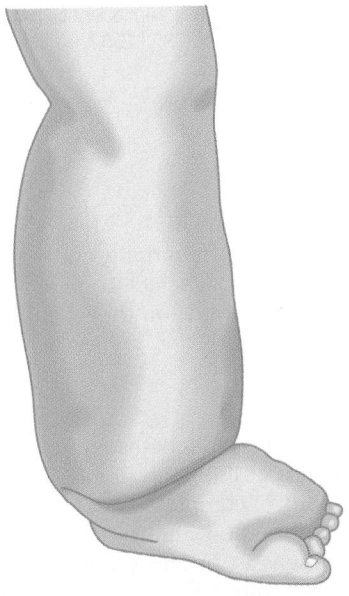

FIGURE 68-2. Lymphedema with characteristic loss of the normal perimalleolar shape resulting in a "tree trunk" pattern. Dorsum of the foot is characteristically swollen, resulting in the appearance of the "buffalo hump."

phedema, computed tomography (CT) and magnetic resonance imaging (MRI) are valuable and indeed essential for exclusion of underlying oncologic disease states.[8,9] In patients with known lymph node excision and radiation treatment as the underlying problem of their lymphedema, additional diagnostic studies are rarely needed except as these studies relate to follow-up of an underlying malignancy. For patients with edema of unknown etiology and a suspicion for lymphedema, lymphoscintigraphy is the diagnostic test of choice. When lymphoscintigraphy confirms that lymphatic drainage is delayed, the diagnosis of primary lymphedema should never be made until neoplasia involving the regional and central lymphatic drainage of the limb has been excluded through CT or MRI. If a more detailed diagnostic interpretation of lymphatic channels is needed for operative planning, then contrast lymphangiography may be considered.

Lymphoscintigraphy has emerged as the test of choice in patients with suspected lymphedema.[10-12] It cannot differentiate between primary and secondary lymphedemas; however, it has a sensitivity of 70% to 90% and a specificity of nearly 100% in differentiating lymphedema from other causes of limb swelling. The test assesses lymphatic function by quantitating the rate of clearance of a radiolabeled macromolecular tracer (Fig. 68-3). The advantages of the technique are that it is simple, safe, and reproducible with small exposure to radioactivity (approximately 5 mCI). It involves the injection of a small amount of radioiodinated human albumin or ^{99}Tc-labeled sulfide colloid into the first interdigital space of the foot or hand. Migration of the radiotracer within the skin and subcutaneous lymphatics is easily monitored with a whole-body gamma camera, thus producing clear images of the major lymphatic channels in the leg as well as measuring the amount of radioactivity at the inguinal nodes 30 and 60 minutes after injection of the radiolabeled substance in the feet. An uptake value that is less than 0.3% of the total injected dose at 30 minutes is diagnostic of lymphedema. The normal range of uptake is between 0.6% and 1.6%. In patients with edema secondary to venous disease, isotope clearance is usually abnormally rapid, resulting in more than 2% ilioinguinal uptake. Importantly, variation in the degree of edema involving the lower extremity does not appear to significantly change the rate of the isotope clearance.

Direct contrast lymphangiography provides the finest details of the lymphatic anatomy.[13] However, it is an invasive study that involves exposure and cannulation of lymphatics at the dorsum of the forefoot, followed by slow injection of contrast medium (ethiodized oil). The procedure is tedious, the cannulation often necessitates aid of magnification optics (frequently an operating microscope is needed), and the dissection requires some form of anesthetic. After cannulation of a superficial lymph vessel, contrast material is slowly injected into the lymphatic system. A total of 7 to 10 mL of contrast medium is ideal for lower extremity evaluation and 4 to 5 mL for upper extremity evaluation. Potential complications include damage of the visualized lymphatics, allergic reactions, and pulmonary embolism if the oil-based contrast medium enters the venous system through lymphovenous anasto-

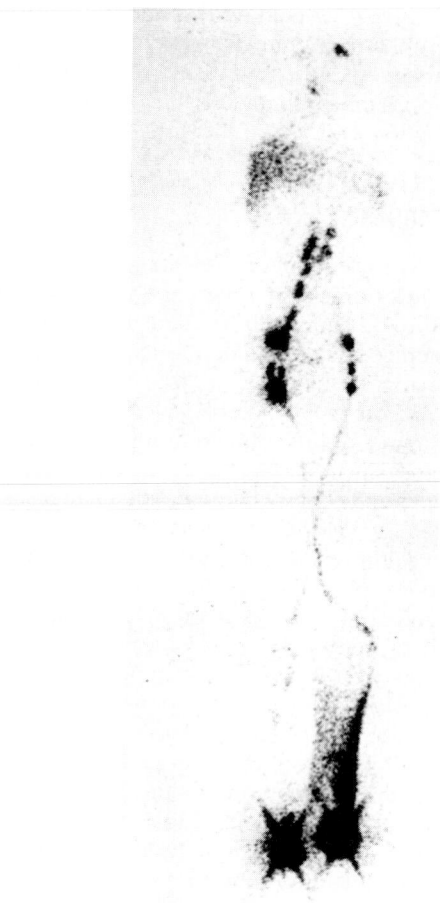

FIGURE 68-3. Lymphoscintigraphic pattern in primary lymphedema. Note area of dermal backflow on the left and diminished number of lymph nodes in the groin.
(From Cambria RA, Gloviczki P, Naessens JM, Wahner HW: Noninvasive evaluation of the lymphatic system with lymphoscintigraphy: A prospective, semiquantitative analysis in 386 extremities. J Vasc Surg 18:773-782, 1993.)

moses. Lymphangiography in the present practice of vascular surgery is used infrequently and reserved for the preoperative evaluation of selected patients that are candidates for direct operations on their lymphatic vessels.

THERAPY

The large majority of lymphedema patients can be treated with a combination of limb elevation, a high-quality compression garment, complex decongestive physical therapy, and compression pump therapy. A new class of medications known as benzopyrones is still under investigation in the United States but may find a place in the care of lymphedema in the near future. Operative treatment may be considered for patients with advanced complicated lymphedema that fail management with nonoperative means.

General Therapeutic Measures

All patients with lymphedema should be educated in meticulous skin care and avoidance of injuries.[14] The patients should always be instructed to see their physicians early for signs of infections because these may progress rapidly in a serious systemic manner.[15] Infections should be aggressively and promptly treated with appropriate antibiotics directed at gram-positive cocci.[16] Eczema at the level of the forefoot and toes requires treatment, and hydrocortisone-based creams may be considered. Additionally, basic range-of-motion exercises for the extremities have been shown to be of value in the management of lymphedema in the long term. Finally, the patients should make every effort to maintain ideal body weight.

Elevation and Compression Garments

For lymphedema patients in all stages of disease, management with high-quality elastic garments is necessary at all times except when the legs are elevated above the heart.[17,18] The ideal compression garment is custom fitted and delivers pressures in the range of 30 to 60 mm Hg. Such garments may have the additional benefit of protecting the extremity from injuries such as burns, lacerations, and insect bites. The patients should avoid standing for prolonged periods and should elevate their legs at night by supporting the foot of the bed on 15-cm blocks.

Complex Decongestive Physical Therapy

This specialized massage technique for patients with lymphedema is designed to stimulate the still functioning lymph vessels, evacuate stagnant protein-rich fluid by breaking up subcutaneous deposits of fibrous tissue, and redirect lymph fluid to areas of the body where lymph flow is normal.[19] The technique is initiated on the normal contralateral side of the body evacuating excessive fluid and preparing first the lymphatic zones of the nonaffected extremity, followed by the zones in the trunk quadrant adjacent to the affected limb before attention is turned to the swollen extremity. The affected extremity is massaged in a segmental fashion, with the proximal zones being massaged first, proceeding to the distal limb. The technique is time consuming but effective in reducing the volume of the lymphedematous limbs.[20] After the massage session is complete the extremity is wrapped with a low stretch wrap and then the limb is placed in the custom-fitted garment to maintain the decreased girth obtained with the massage therapy. This kind of therapy is appropriate for patients with all stages of lymphedema.[21]

When the patient is first referred for complex decongestive physical therapy, the patient undergoes daily to weekly massage sessions for up to 8 to 12 weeks. Limb elevation and elastic stockings are a necessary adjunct in this phase. After maximal volume reduction is achieved, then the patient returns for maintenance massage treatments every 2 to 3 months.

Compression Pump Therapy

Pneumatic compression pump therapy is another effective method of reducing the volume of the lymphedematous limb using a similar principle to massage therapy. The device consists of a sleeve containing several compartments. The lymphedematous limb is positioned inside the sleeve, and the compartments are serially inflated so as to milk the stagnant fluid out of the extremity.[22]

When a patient with advanced lymphedema is first referred for therapy, an initial approach with hospitalization for 3 to 4 days involving strict limb elevation, daily complex decongestive physical therapy, and compression pump treatments may be necessary to achieve optimal control of the lymphedema. Patients with cardiac or renal dysfunction should be monitored for fluid overload. After this initial period of intensive therapy the patients are fitted with high-quality compression garments to maintain the limb volume. Maintenance sessions are then prescribed for the patients on an as-needed basis.

Drug Therapy

Benzopyrones have attracted interest as potentially effective agents in the treatment of lymphedema. This class of medications, with the main representative being coumarin (1,2-benzopyrone), is thought to reduce lymphedema through stimulation of proteolysis by tissue macrophages and stimulation of the peristalsis and pumping action of the collecting lymphatics. Benzopyrones have no anticoagulant activity. The first randomized, crossover trial of coumarin in patients with lymphedema of the arms and legs was reported in 1993.[23] The study concluded that coumarin was more effective than placebo in reducing not only volume but also other important parameters, including skin temperature, attacks of secondary acute inflammation and discomfort of the lymphedematous extremities, skin turgor, and suppleness. A second randomized, crossover trial was reported in 1999.[24] This study focused on effects of coumarin in women with secondary lymphedema after treatment of breast cancer. The trial investigators found that coumarin was not effective therapy for the specific group of women. Because of the disagreement between these two major trials, the enthusiasm for use of benzopyrones in the United States has been tempered. Additional trials should be undertaken to clarify the potential effects of the medications on primary and secondary lymphedemas in different extremities and stages.

Diuretics may temporarily improve the appearance of the lymphedematous extremity with stage I disease, leading patients to request continuous therapy. However, other than producing temporary intravascular volume depletion, there is no long-term benefit. Thus, diuretics have no role in the treatment of lymphedema at any stage.

Operative Treatment

Ninety-five percent of patients with lymphedema can be managed nonoperatively. Surgical intervention may be considered for patients with stage II and III lymphedema who have severe functional impairment, recurrent episodes of lymphangitis, and severe pain despite optimal medical therapy. Two main categories of operations are available for the care of patients with lymphedema: reconstructive and excisional.

Reconstructive operations should be considered for those patients with proximal (either primary or secondary) obstruction of the extremity lymphatic circulation with preserved, dilated lymphatics distal to the obstruction.[25-27] In these patients the residual dilated lymphatics can be anastomosed either to nearby veins or to transposed healthy lymphatic channels (usually mobilized or harvested from the contralateral extremity) in an attempt to restore effective drainage of the lymphedematous extremity. Treatment of selected lymphedema patients with lymphovenous anastomoses has resulted in objective improvement in 30% to 40% of the patients with an average initial reduction in the excess limb volume of 40% to 50%.[28,29]

For those patients with primary lymphedema who have hypoplastic and fibrotic distal lymphatic vessels, such reconstruction is not an option. For such patients, surgical strategy involving transfer of lymphatic-bearing tissue (portion of the greater omentum) into the affected limb has been attempted. This is intended to connect the residual hypoplastic lymphatic channels of the leg to competent lymphatics in the transferred tissue. Omental flap operations have been found to have poor results.[30] Alternatively, a segment of the ileum can be disconnected from the rest of the bowel, stripped of its mucosa, and mobilized to be sewn onto the cut surface of residual ilioinguinal nodes in an attempt to bridge the lower extremity with mesenteric lymphatics. When this enteromesenteric bridge procedure was applied to a group of eight carefully selected patients, the outcomes were promising, with six patients showing sustained clinical improvement in long follow-up.[31]

Excisional operations are essentially the only viable option for patients without residual lymphatics of adequate size for reconstructive procedures. For patients with recalcitrant stage II and early stage III lymphedema in whom the edema is moderate and the skin is relatively healthy, an excisional procedure that removes a large segment of the lymphedematous subcutaneous tissues and overlying skin is the procedure of choice. This palliative procedure was introduced by Kontoleon in 1918 and was later popularized by Homans as "staged subcutaneous excision underneath flaps" (Fig. 68-4). The operative approach starts with a medial incision extending from the level of the medial malleolus through the calf into the mid thigh.[32-34] Flaps 1 to 2 cm thick are elevated anteriorly and posteriorly, and all subcutaneous tissue beneath the flaps along with the underlying medial calf deep fascia is removed with the redundant skin. The sural nerve is preserved. After the first-stage procedure is completed and if additional lymphedematous tissue removal is necessary, then a second operation is performed usually 3 to 6 months later. The second-stage operation is performed using similar techniques through an incision on the lateral aspect of the limb.

In a recent long-term, follow-up study, 80% of patients undergoing staged subcutaneous excision underneath flaps had significant and long-lasting reduction in extremity size associated with improved function and extremity contour. Wound complications were encountered in 10% of the patients.[32]

When the lymphedema is extremely pronounced and the skin is unhealthy and infected, the simple reducing operation of Kontoleon is not adequate. In this case, the classic excisional operation originally described by Charles in 1912 is performed (Fig. 68-5). The procedure involves complete and circumferential excision of the skin, subcutaneous tissue, and deep fascia of the involved leg and dorsum of the foot.[35] The excision is usually performed in one stage, and coverage is provided preferably by full-thickness grafting from the excised skin. In a recent follow-up report, patients subjected to Charles' operation had immediate volume and circumference reduction. Skin graft take was 88% and complications of operation consisted primarily of wound infections, hematomas, and necrosis of skin flaps. The hospital stay was 21 to 36 days.[36] Although this is a very successful and radically reducing operation, the behavior in the healing skin graft is unpredictable. Between 10% and 15% of the grafted segments do not take and can be difficult to manage because of frequent localized sloughing, excessive scarring, focal recurrent infections, and hyperkeratosis or dermatitis. These complications seem to be worse in patients when leg resurfacing is performed using split-thickness grafts from the opposite extremity. In advanced cases the exophytic changes within the grafted skin, chronic cellulitis, and skin breakdown may eventually lead to leg amputation.[37]

CHYLOTHORAX

Chylous pleural effusion is usually secondary to thoracic duct trauma (usually iatrogenic after chest surgery) and rarely a manifestation of advanced malignant disease with lymphatic metastasis.[38] Chylomicrons on lipoprotein analysis and a triglyceride level of more than 110 mg/dL in the pleural fluid are diagnostic. Initially, patients can be treated nonoperatively with tube thoracostomy and a medium-chain triglyceride diet or total parenteral nutrition. For patients with thoracic duct injury and an effusion that persists after 1 week of drainage, video-assisted thoracoscopy or thoracotomy should be employed to identify and ligate the thoracic duct above and below the leak. The site of the leak can be identified if cream is given to the patient a few hours before operation. For patients with cancer-related chylothorax and persistent drainage despite optimal chemotherapy and radiation therapy, pleurodesis is highly successful in preventing recurrences.[39]

CHYLOPERITONEUM

In contrast to chylothorax, the most common causes of chylous ascites are congenital lymphatic abnormalities in children and malignancy involving the abdominal lymph nodes in adults. Postoperative injury to abdominal lymphatics resulting in chylous ascites is rare.[40] Presence of

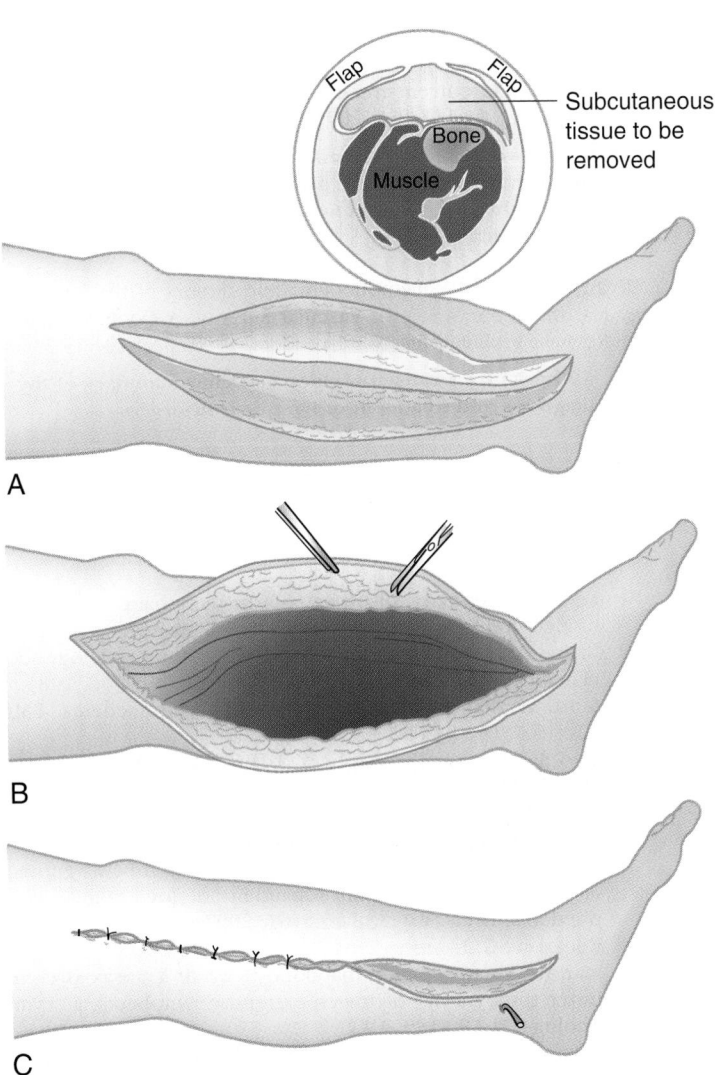

FIGURE 68-4. A to C, Schematic representation of Kontoleon's or Homans' procedure. Relatively thick skin flaps are raised anteriorly and posteriorly, and all subcutaneous tissue beneath the flaps and the underlying medial calf deep fascia are removed along with the necessary redundant skin.

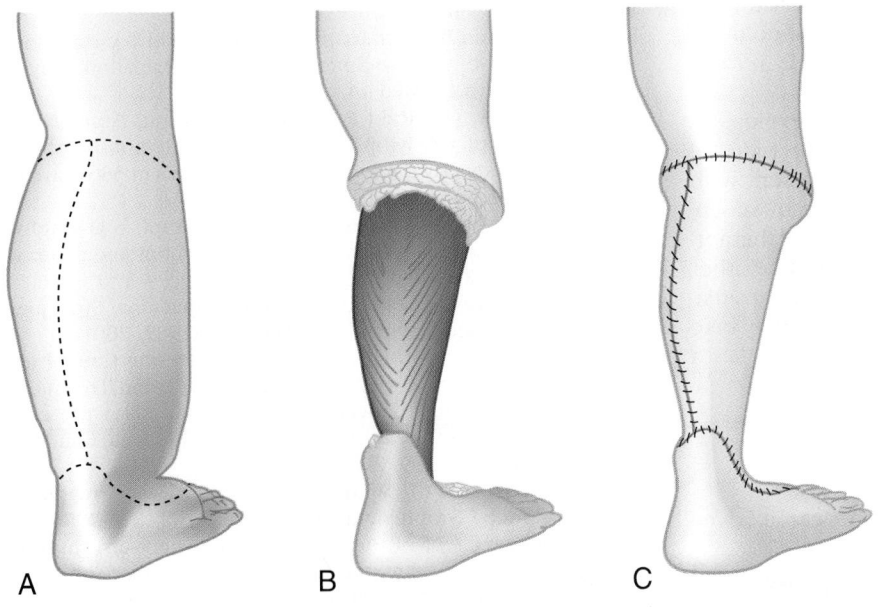

FIGURE 68-5. A to C, Schematic representation of Charles' procedure. It involves complete and circumferential excision of the skin, subcutaneous tissue, and deep fascia of the involved leg and dorsum of the foot. Coverage is provided preferably by full-thickness grafting from the excised skin.

chylomicrons on lipoprotein analysis and a triglyceride level of more than 110 mg/dL are again diagnostic. Initial treatment includes paracentesis followed by a medium-chain triglyceride diet or total parenteral nutrition. In patients with postoperative chyloperitoneum, if ascites does not respond after 1 to 2 weeks of nonoperative management, exploration should be employed to identify and ligate the leaking lymphatic duct. Congenital and malignant causes should be given longer periods (up to 4 to 6 weeks) of nonoperative management. If ascites persists in patients with congenital ascites, lymphoscintigraphy or lymphangiography is performed before making an attempt to control the leak with celiotomy. At the time of exploration, control of the leak can be achieved by ligation of leaking lymphatic vessels or resection of the bowel associated with the leak. Patients with malignancies should receive aggressive management for their underlying disease, which generally is effective at controlling the chyloperitoneum.

TUMORS OF THE LYMPHATICS

Lymphangiomas are the lymphatic analogue of the hemangiomas of blood vessels. They are generally divided into two types: simple or capillary lymphangioma and cavernous lymphangioma or cystic hygroma.[41] They are thought to represent isolated and sequestered segments of the lymphatic system that retain the ability to produce lymph. As the volume of lymph inside the cystic tumor increases, they grow larger within the surrounding tissues. The majority of these benign tumors are present at birth, and 90% of them can be identified by the end of the first year of life. The cavernous lymphangiomas almost invariably occur in the neck or the axilla and very rarely in the retroperitoneum. The simple capillary lymphangiomas also tend to occur subcutaneously in the head and neck region as well as the axilla. Rarely, however, they can be found in the trunk within the internal organs or the connective tissue in and about the abdominal or thoracic cavities. The treatment of lymphangiomas should be surgical excision, taking care to preserve all normal surrounding infiltrated structures.

Lymphangiosarcoma is a rare tumor that develops as a complication of long-standing (usually more than 10 years) lymphedema.[42] Clinically, the patients present with acute worsening of the edema and appearance of subcutaneous nodules that have a propensity toward hemorrhage and ulceration. The tumor can be treated, like other sarcomas, with preoperative chemotherapy and irradiation followed by surgical excision, which usually may take the form of radical amputation. Overall, the tumor has a very poor prognosis.[43]

Selected References

Gloviczki P: Principles of surgical treatment of chronic lymphoedema. Int Angiol 18:42-46, 1999.

> Comprehensive review summarizes the important elements in the management of patients with lymphedema.

Rockson SG: Lymphedema. Am J Med 110:288-295, 2001.

Tiwari A, Cheng KS, Button M, et al: Differential diagnosis, investigation, and current treatment of lower limb lymphedema. Arch Surg 138:152-161, 2003.

> These two current reviews illustrate the current knowledge and controversies in the pathophysiology, classification, natural history, differential diagnosis, and treatment of lymphedema

Wyatt LE, Miller TA: Lymphedema and tumors of the lymphatics. *In* Moore WS (ed): Vascular Surgery, A Comprehensive Review. Philadelphia, WB Saunders, 1998, pp 829-843.

> Authoritative treatise provides a succinct summary of the diagnosis and treatment of lymphatic disorders.

References

1. Levine C: Primary disorders of the lymphatic vessels—a unified concept. J Pediatr Surg 24:233-240, 1989.
2. Browse NL, Stewart G: Lymphoedema: Pathophysiology and classification. J Cardiovasc Surg (Torino) 26:91-106, 1985.
3. Mortimer PS: Swollen lower limb: II. Lymphoedema. BMJ 320:1527-1529, 2000.
4. Cho S, Atwood JE: Peripheral edema. Am J Med 113:580-586, 2002.
5. Szuba A, Rockson SG: Lymphedema: Classification, diagnosis and therapy. Vasc Med 3:145-156, 1998.
6. Tiwari A, Cheng KS, Button M, et al: Differential diagnosis, investigation, and current treatment of lower limb lymphedema. Arch Surg 138:152-161, 2003.
7. Rockson SG: Lymphedema. Am J Med 110:288-295, 2001.
8. Marotel M, Cluzan R, Ghabboun S, et al: Transaxial computer tomography of lower extremity lymphedema. Lymphology 31:180-185, 1998.
9. Werner GT, Scheck R, Kaiserling E: Magnetic resonance imaging of peripheral lymphedema. Lymphology 31:34-36, 1998.
10. Burnand KG, McGuinness CL, Lagattolla NR, et al: Value of isotope lymphography in the diagnosis of lymphoedema of the leg. Br J Surg 89:74-78, 2002.
11. Szuba A, Shin WS, Strauss HW, et al: The third circulation: Radionuclide lymphoscintigraphy in the evaluation of lymphedema. J Nucl Med 44:43-57, 2003.
12. Cambria RA, Gloviczki P, Naessens JM, et al: Noninvasive evaluation of the lymphatic system with lymphoscintigraphy: A prospective, semiquantitative analysis in 386 extremities. J Vasc Surg 18:773-782, 1993.
13. Weissleder H, Weissleder R: Interstitial lymphangiography: Initial clinical experience with a dimeric nonionic contrast agent. Radiology 170:371-374, 1989.
14. Cohen SR, Payne DK, Tunkel RS: Lymphedema: Strategies for management. Cancer 92(4 Suppl):980-987, 2001.
15. Harris SR, Hugi MR, Olivotto IA, et al: Steering Committee for Clinical Practice Guidelines for the Care and Treatment of Breast Cancer. Clinical practice guidelines for the care and treatment of breast cancer: 11. Lymphedema. Can Med Assoc J 164:191-199, 2001.
16. Bernas MJ, Witte CL, Witte MH: The diagnosis and treatment of peripheral lymphedema: Draft revision of the 1995 Consensus Document of the International Society of Lymphology Executive Committee for discussion at the September 3-7, 2001, XVIII International Congress of Lymphology in Genoa, Italy. Lymphology 34:84-91, 2001.

17. Yasuhara H, Shigematsu H, Muto T: A study of the advantages of elastic stockings for leg lymphedema. Int Angiol 15:272-277, 1996.

18. Badger CM, Peacock JL, Mortimer PS: A randomized, controlled, parallel-group clinical trial comparing multilayer bandaging followed by hosiery versus hosiery alone in the treatment of patients with lymphedema of the limb. Cancer 88:2832-2837, 2000.

19. Lerner R: What's new in lymphedema therapy in America? Int J Angiol 7:191-196, 1998.

20. Franzeck UK, Spiegel I, Fischer M, et al: Combined physical therapy for lymphedema evaluated by fluorescence micro lymphography and lymph capillary pressure measurements. J Vasc Res 34:306-311, 1997.

21. Ko DS, Lerner R, Klose G, et al: Effective treatment of lymphedema of the extremities. Arch Surg 133:452-458, 1998.

22. Richmand DM, O'Donnell TF Jr, Zelikovski A: Sequential pneumatic compression for lymphedema: A controlled trial. Arch Surg 120:1116-1119, 1985.

23. Casley-Smith JR, Morgan RG, Piller NB: Treatment of lymphedema of the arms and legs with 5,6-benzo-[alpha] pyrone. N Engl J Med 329:1158-1163, 1993.

24. Loprinzi CL, Kugler JW, Sloan JA, et al: Lack of effect of coumarin in women with lymphedema after treatment for breast cancer. N Engl J Med 340:346-350, 1999.

25. Campisi C, Boccardo F: Lymphedema and microsurgery. Microsurgery 22:74-80, 2002.

26. Gloviczki P: Principles of surgical treatment of chronic lymphoedema. Int Angiol 18:42-46, 1999.

27. Tanaka Y, Tajima S, Imai K, et al: Experience of a new surgical procedure for the treatment of unilateral obstructive lymphedema of the lower extremity: Adipolymphaticovenous transfer. Microsurgery 17:209-216, 1996.

28. O'Brien BM, Mellow CG, Khazanchi RK, et al: Long-term results after microlymphaticovenous anastomoses for the treatment of obstructive lymphedema. Plast Reconstr Surg 85:562-572, 1990.

29. Gloviczki P, Fisher J, Hollier LH, et al: Microsurgical lymphovenous anastomosis for treatment of lymphedema: A critical review. J Vasc Surg 7:647-652, 1988.

30. Goldsmith HS: Long-term evaluation of omental transposition for chronic lymphedema. Ann Surg 180:847-849, 1974.

31. Hurst PA, Stewart G, Kinmonth JB, Browse NL: Long-term results of the enteromesenteric bridge operation in the treatment of primary lymphoedema. Br J Surg 72:272-274, 1985.

32. Miller TA, Wyatt LE, Rudkin GH: Staged skin and subcutaneous excision for lymphedema: A favorable report of long-term results. Plast Reconstr Surg 102:1486-1498, 1998.

33. Wyatt LE, Miller TA: Lymphedema and tumors of the lymphatics. In Moore WS (ed): Vascular Surgery, A Comprehensive Review. Philadelphia, WB Saunders, 1998, pp 829-843.

34. Miller TA: Surgical management of lymphedema of the extremity. Plast Reconstr Surg 56:633-641, 1975.

35. Dellon AL, Hoopes JE: The Charles procedure for primary lymphedema: Long-term clinical results. Plast Reconstr Surg 60:589-595, 1977.

36. Dandapat MC, Mohapatro SK, Mohanty SS: Filarial lymphoedema and elephantiasis of lower limb: A review of 44 cases. Br J Surg 73:451-453, 1986.

37. Miller TA: Charles procedure for lymphedema: A warning. Am J Surg 139:290-292, 1980.

38. Johnstone DW: Postoperative chylothorax. Chest Surg Clin North Am 12:597-603, 2002.

39. Romero S: Nontraumatic chylothorax. Curr Opin Pulm Med 6:287-291, 2000.

40. Aalami OO, Allen DB, Organ CH Jr: Chylous ascites: A collective review. Surgery 128:761-778, 2000.

41. Fonkalsrud EW: Congenital malformations of the lymphatic system. Semin Pediatr Surg 3:62-69, 1994.

42. Nakazono T, Kudo S, Matsuo Y, et al: Angiosarcoma associated with chronic lymphedema (Stewart-Treves syndrome) of the leg: MR imaging. Skel Radiol 29:413-416, 2000.

43. Sordillo PP, Chapman R, Hajdu SI, et al: Lymphangiosarcoma. Cancer 48:1674-1679, 1981.

CHAPTER 69

ACCESS AND PORTS

Carl E. Haisch, M.D., Frank M. Parker, D.O., and Philip M. Brown, Jr., M.D.

| Vascular Access | Peritoneal Dialysis |

VASCULAR ACCESS

History

Access to the vascular system is necessitated by the therapy required for the complex medical conditions that occur in many patients. Frequent access to the bloodstream is required for patients undergoing parenteral nutrition, chemotherapy for malignant disease, plasmapheresis, and short-term and long-term dialysis.

Without adequate vascular access, hemodialysis would not have developed as we know it today. The first significant research to investigate dialysis was begun in the 19th century by Thomas Graham. George Haas, in 1924, continued Graham's work when he attempted dialysis in the first human patient. The patient tolerated the procedure well, but the amount of dialysis was inadequate for the patient to gain a therapeutic effect, and the patient died. In the early 1940s, Willem Johan Kolff designed a dialysis machine using cellulose tubing, and when heparin became available, he dialyzed his first patient. The patient eventually died after 26 days of treatment when vascular access became unavailable after repeated surgical cutdowns.

The breakthrough in long-term access for dialysis occurred when Quinton and colleagues used a Teflon conduit to construct arteriovenous connections in 1960. This advance allowed the first long-term dialysis of patients and was not improved on until 1966, when Brescia and associates[1] constructed a natural arteriovenous fistula between the radial artery and the cephalic vein. The Brescia-Cimino fistula is still considered the "gold standard" for dialysis. For patients without an adequate cephalic vein, saphenous vein was used but found to be unsatisfactory. Artificial materials were eventually developed, and the current standard material is polytetrafluoroethylene (PTFE).

The need to infuse irritating solutions into a patient required a high-flow system. Aubaniac used the subclavian vein for vascular access in 1952, and Dudrick and Wilmore used it later for nutritional support. This vein was selected for its high flow and easy accessibility. The Broviac catheter and, later, the Hickman catheter were used for nutritional support and for chemotherapy and blood drawing, respectively. Currently, double-lumen and triple-lumen catheters are available for access in monitoring, dialysis, and numerous other applications. Catheters such as the Port-A-Cath and Infus-A-Port are designed so the entire catheter and access port are totally covered by skin. To use these catheters, access is gained through a septum in an access port with a special needle.

Indications

Hemoaccess through a fistula, jump graft, or external angioaccess is appropriate when frequent access to the vascular system is required, when a high-flow system is needed, when the ability to withstand multiple needle punctures is required, or when highly sclerotic solutions are administered intravenously. The most common uses are for acute and chronic renal failure, administration of chemotherapeutic agents and other drugs, hyperalimentation, and administration of blood and blood products. Angioaccess is also frequently required in patients with AIDS who need medications for treatment of cytomegalovirus infection or who need access for blood drawing.

Vascular access is an extremely important part of medicine. In the end-stage renal disease budget, maintaining and placing vascular access devices and fistulas cost over $1 billion per year in the United States. This amount comprises up to 17% of the budget for patients with end-stage renal failure. An estimated 240,000 patients require dialysis and the number continues to increase, as does the age of these patients. Currently, 40% of all patients who undergo dialysis are 65 years old or older and the percentage of patients older than age 65 continues to increase.

External Angioaccess

Dialysis

The first successful shunt for repeated hemodialysis was the Scribner shunt, which used a Teflon tip inserted into both the artery and the vein. Silastic tubing, attached to the Teflon tip, was placed through the skin by means of a skin incision, both ends were connected, and continuous blood flow was established. These shunts are used infrequently now, primarily for plasmapheresis or for acute, continuous renal replacement therapy.

Dialysis Through Major Vessels

Short-term angioaccess for hemodialysis may be obtained by insertion of a non-tunneled catheter into the subclavian, external jugular, internal jugular, or femoral vein. These percutaneously placed catheters may make construction of an autogenous or internal arteriovenous fistula more difficult or impossible. After placement of a subclavian catheter for even as short a period as 2 weeks, up to 50% of subclavian veins have a significant stenosis that causes either clotting of the fistula or a swollen arm after fistula placement. The incidence of stenosis is much lower, less than 10%, with use of the internal jugular vein, but this complication must be considered nonetheless. Stenoses may not be clinically evident because of collateral circulation, but a fistula will make the stenosis evident. While the patient is undergoing dialysis, the fistula or graft may have a high venous pressure. For this reason, if the patient has had a subclavian or internal jugular catheter in place, a Doppler study of the central veins should be done before an internal access is placed. The gold standard is still a venogram, which allows the subclavian vein to be seen behind the clavicular head. Femoral catheters may be placed at the patient's bedside; ideally, they are removed after dialysis, to prevent infection or venous thrombosis. Repeated use of these catheters may cause iliofemoral thrombosis, local bleeding, or arterial puncture and injury.

The most commonly used catheters today are dual-lumen, silicone rubber, or polyurethane catheters. These catheters are soft and therefore are usually placed percutaneously in the external jugular or internal jugular vein, with the help of a peel-away sheath. A cutdown will be necessary infrequently. These catheters can be placed in the veins listed earlier, but they also have been placed in the inferior vena cava via a translumbar or transhepatic approach. The dual-lumen design imparts a low incidence of recirculation (2% to 5%), except when short catheters are placed in the femoral vein, where recirculation is unacceptably high (18% to almost 40% at higher blood flows of 400 mL/min) (Fig. 69-1).[2] Because these catheters are soft and pliable, endothelial damage is less than with stiff catheters and the incidence of thrombosis is lower.

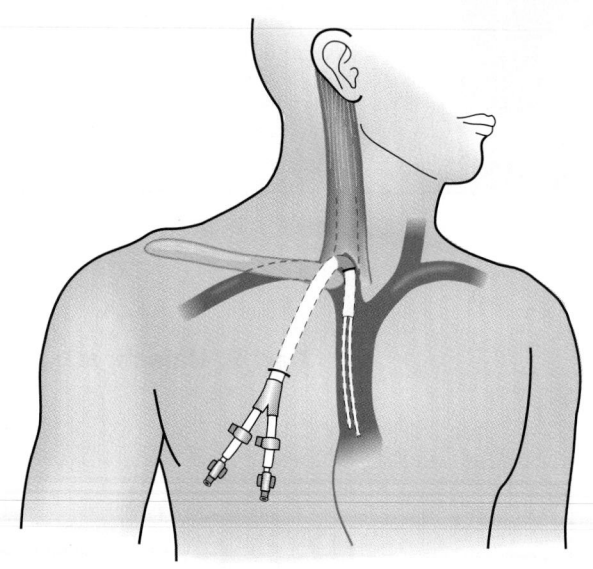

FIGURE 69-1.   Position of a soft Silastic internal jugular catheter for dialysis. (From Uldall R, DeBruyne M, Besley M, et al: A new vascular access catheter for hemodialysis. Am J Kidney Dis 21:270, 1993.)

Patients who will require long-term access should have a tunneled catheter placed. The Dacron cuff allows tissue ingrowth that helps reduce the risk of infection when compared with noncuffed catheters. Many different types of catheters can be used in patients who are undergoing dialysis. Most catheters have both lumens in a single unit; however, the Tesio catheter is really two separate catheters that are placed through two separate needle sticks.[3] These catheters allow blood flows of up to 400 mL/min and thus allow high-flux dialysis. The catheter tip should be in the right atrium to prevent recirculation and decrease the incidence of clot forming on the catheter tip. Stiff catheters should be placed at the junction of the right atrium and the superior vena cava to prevent arrhythmias or venous puncture. The incidence of central stenosis is approximately the same with these soft catheters as it is with the stiffer catheters described earlier. There are also recently approved implantable ports that in initial reports have less thrombotic and infectious complications than tunneled catheters and have comparable performance to Tesio catheters.[4] However, these catheters are still not proven and probably only have a place in selected patients.

Some patients are not candidates for placement of a fistula or a PTFE graft. In these patients, a silicone rubber catheter may be adequate. McLaughlin and colleagues[5] showed that approximately 50% of catheters placed in the right subclavian position survive for 1 year. This finding is consistent with the data of Mosquera and associates,[6] who showed that the cumulative PermCath survival rate was 74% at 1 year and 43% at 2 years. One of the major problems with these catheters is that they become dysfunctional due to clot or fibrin sheath formation. The use of tissue plasminogen activator for opening the catheters has been discussed. This agent is safe and nonallergenic and, although expensive, may prolong catheter life. Urokinase can again be used; a volume sufficient to fill the catheter with 5000 IU of urokinase and left to dwell for 1 hour is usually adequate to open a catheter. Should this low-dose therapy fail, a 4-hour infusion with 60,000 IU urokinase can reopen many catheters, and this is as effective as percutaneous fibrin sheath stripping.[7]

Nutrition, Blood Access, and Chemotherapy

Access to the venous system for chemotherapy, parenteral nutrition, antibiotics, and blood products is most frequently obtained through the central vessels such as the subclavian, internal jugular, external jugular, or basilic vein. When no other site can be found, a catheter can be placed in the inferior vena cava by using a translumbar or transhepatic approach. If a patient has had multiple previous catheters, ultrasound-guided access to collateral veins with fluoroscopically monitored central advancement can assist in catheter placement. Venography done before attempted catheter placement is unnecessary because this can be done concomitantly. The catheters used are either totally implantable, such as Port-A-Cath or Infus-A-Port, or external, such as Broviac, Hickman, and Groshung catheters. Groshung catheters have a valve on the end to prevent blood flow into the catheter. These catheters can be placed in the operating room or can be safely placed in the angiography suite with no increased infectious risk.

The peripherally inserted central catheter line is placed through an arm vein at the bedside. This catheter may have an open tip and may require heparin, or it may have a Groshung tip. These catheters are constructed with a port, similar to that of a Port-A-Cath, which is placed under the skin.

Complications

Complications can be divided into those that occur secondary to catheter placement and those that occur later. The early complications of subclavian or internal jugular placement include pneumothorax, arterial injury, thoracic duct injury, air embolus, inability to pass the catheter, bleeding, nerve injury, and great vessel injury. These complications all decrease in incidence as the physician gains more experience in placing these catheters. A chest radiograph must be taken after catheter placement to rule out pneumothorax and injury to the great vessels and to check for position of the catheter. The incidence of pneumothorax is 1% to 4%, and the incidence of injury to the great vessels is less than 1%.[8] A widened mediastinum is an indication of injury to the great vessels. Injury most commonly occurs when the catheter is placed from the right side. In patients who have had catheters placed previously or in whom finding the vein is difficult, ultrasonography is recommended. This allows determination of the anatomic location of the vein and pathologic processes that may be present from previous invasive procedures, such as occlusion, thrombosis, or stenosis. The use of ultrasound in one study resulted in successful venous cannulation in 100% of patients.[9]

Other complications are mechanical, thrombotic, and infectious. Mechanical complications include catheter malposition, inability to pass fluid or withdraw blood, and catheter shearing between the clavicle and the first rib. If one has a question regarding the catheter lumen or the inability to flush the catheter secondary to potential shearing between the clavicle and first rib, the catheter must be removed, to prevent division of the catheter and the need to retrieve it from the heart.

Thrombotic complications occur in 4% to 10% of patients. Thrombosis may occur secondary to venous wall irritation caused by the catheter, as a result of a hypercoagulable state in the patient, or from irritation to the venous wall by the chemotherapeutic agents. The initial sign of thrombosis is the inability to draw blood from the catheter. However, the catheter may draw up against the vessel wall and thereby may also cause an inability to withdraw blood. Initial therapy for catheter thrombosis is intraluminal instillation of 5000 IU of urokinase, which usually resolves the problem. If this is unsuccessful, a contrast radiograph is indicated to determine catheter position and integrity. Thrombosis of the vein itself is not adequately treated with low doses of urokinase. When fresh thrombus surrounds the catheter but patient care requirements preclude its removal, mechanical or pharmacologic thrombectomy should be considered. If the catheter can be removed and placed elsewhere the patient will still need to be treated for the deep venous thrombosis.

The second most common catheter problem is infection. It may occur soon after placement (3 to 5 days) or late in the life of the catheter and may be at the exit site or the cause of catheter-related sepsis. In spite of the use of antibiotics, infection can be a catastrophic complication and result in epidural abscess, osteomyelitis, bacterial endocarditis, or septic arthritis. The diagnosis of infection is difficult. The best techniques to determine whether a catheter is infected require that the catheter be removed. Maki and associates (as reported by Whitman[8]) described a semiquantitative culture that is considered positive with 15 colony-forming units.[8] Another technique calls for a Gram stain of the catheter tip.[8] A third technique quantifies colony counts of bacteria in blood cultures taken from the central venous catheter and from a peripheral intravenous catheter. If the ratio is 10:1 catheter to blood colonies, the catheter is considered infected.

The exact incidence of catheter-related infection is difficult to ascertain, but reports indicate a rate of between 0.5 and 3.9 episodes per 1000 catheter-days.[10] Many patients who have catheters in place are immunocompromised secondary to chemotherapy, nutritional status, or underlying disease. Multilumen catheters and catheter thrombosis both increase the incidence of catheter sepsis.[8]

When the catheter is placed, strict sterile technique must be used. A report by Darouiche and colleagues[11] indicated that catheters with minocycline and rifampin on the external and luminal surfaces had a lower infection rate than those with chlorhexidine and silver sulfadiazine on the external surface only. This finding indicates that the antibiotic combination may be important but also that the intraluminal route remains important in central catheter-related bloodstream infections.

Infections are most often caused by skin flora. Early infection (3 to 5 days) most often results from infection of the subcutaneous tract. Later infections may have the same cause or may occur by hematogenous spread. The most common bacteria are *Staphylococcus epidermidis* and *S. aureus. Candida* species can also be involved but less frequently. The exit site should be covered with dry gauze impregnated with iodophor ointment. This method is effective against both bacteria and fungi, and the dressing can be changed three times a week.

The most common therapy for suspected catheter infection is removal of the catheter. However, because catheter sites may be few, consideration has been given to catheter exchange over a guide wire. Beathard and colleagues outlined an approach to catheter exchange. The exit site was examined; if clean, the catheter was simply changed over a guide wire. If the exit site was thought to have an infection, a guide wire was used for the catheter but a new exit site was chosen. When the infection was severe the catheter was removed, the patient allowed to improve, and a new catheter was placed.[12]

Internal Angioaccess

Natural Fistulas

Prosthetic material, regardless of type, has a greater tendency toward thrombosis than autogenous tissue. Thus, the development of arteriovenous fistulas by direct anastomosis without the use of intervening prosthetic material represented one of the major advances in the management of patients undergoing hemodialysis. The fistula most frequently used, the standard by which all other fistulas are measured, is the Brescia-Cimino fistula. An Allen test should be performed before operation to ensure adequate collateral flow from the ulnar artery to minimize hand ischemia. The artery and vein are isolated through a longitudinal incision, with care taken to avoid the superficial branch of the radial nerve. The artery and vein can be anastomosed in a number of ways, including from side to side, from end artery to side vein, from side artery to end vein, or from end artery to end vein (Fig. 69-2). A side-to-side anastomosis can cause venous hypertension in the hand, which can be corrected by ligation of the vein distal to the anastomosis. The end-to-end anastomosis appears to be accompanied by a higher initial thrombosis rate because fewer collateral channels are present. Dilatation of the artery and vein at the time of creation of the fistula by insertion of a coronary dilator seems to diminish the initial thrombosis rate of these anastomoses.

Types of Natural Fistulas

Arteriovenous fistulas have several different anastomotic possibilities, the names of which have been standardized.[13] In addition to the autogenous radial-cephalic direct wrist access (Brescia-Cimino fistula) other possibilities include the autogenous posterior radial branch-cephalic

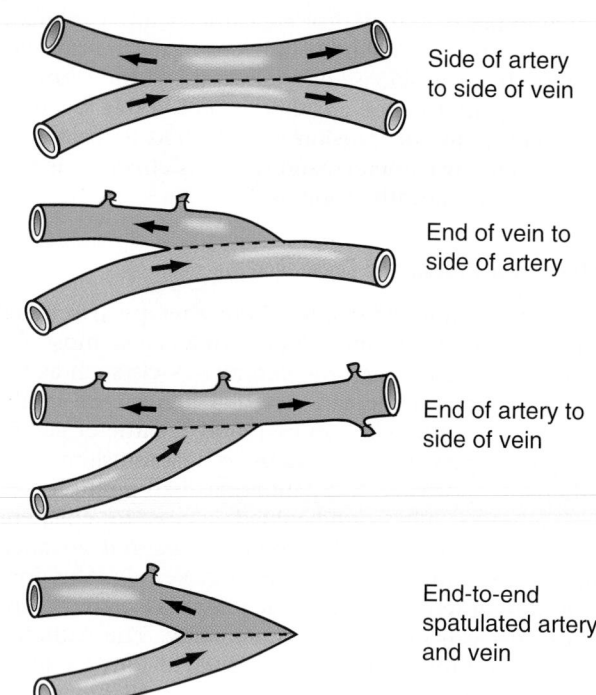

FIGURE 69-2. Four different anastomoses commonly constructed between the radial artery and cephalic vein. (From Ozeran RS: Construction and care of external arteriovenous shunts. *In* Wilson SE, Owens ML [eds]: Vascular Access Surgery. Chicago, Year Book Medical, 1980.)

direct access (snuffbox fistula), autogenous ulnar-cephalic forearm transposition, autogenous brachial-cephalic upper arm direct access (antecubital vein to the brachial artery), and autogenous brachial-basilic upper arm transposition (basilic vein transposition). The last fistula calls for dissection of the basilic vein and transfer to a superficial position on the medial portion of the upper extremity (Fig. 69-3).[14] If at all possible, these options should be exhausted before nonautogenous material is used for dialysis access.

Because of the high propensity for infection among patients with the acquired immunodeficiency syndrome (AIDS), natural vein is the preferred conduit for construction of vascular access for hemodialysis. Frequently, these patients have no usable veins in their arms. Gorksi and colleagues[15] described their experience using the saphenous vein in the lower leg in these patients. The vein was dissected free of its bed and was anastomosed to the superficial femoral artery just below the profunda femoris to form a loop of saphenous vein to be used for dialysis.[15]

At present, the number of natural fistulas is thought to be too low. Therefore, the National Kidney Foundation's Dialysis Outcome Quality Initiative Guidelines have called for a much higher use of natural fistulas.[16] The call is for approximately 50% of new accesses to be natural fistulas. Doppler mapping of vessels has been done to determine what vessels can be used for the construction of a natural

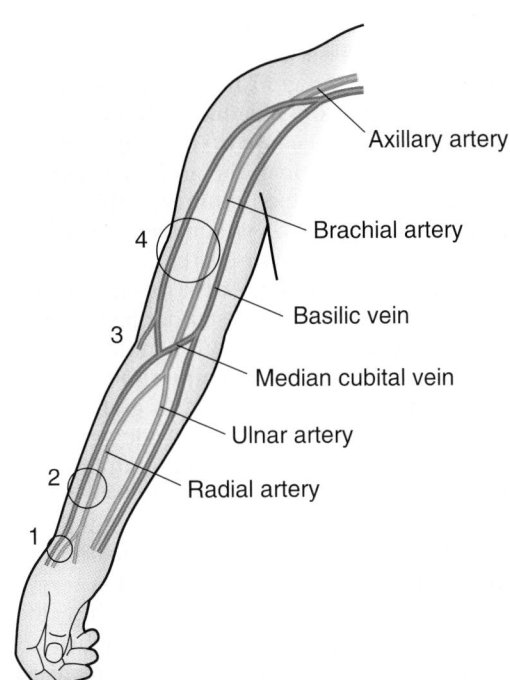

Axillary artery

Brachial artery

Basilic vein

Median cubital vein

Ulnar artery

Radial artery

■ FIGURE 69-3. Four possible anastomotic sites for arteriovenous fistulas in the upper extremity. (Redrawn from Tilney NL, Lazarus JM [eds]: Surgical Care of the Patient with Renal Failure. Philadelphia, WB Saunders, 1982; as shown in Haisch CE: Chronic vascular and peritoneal access. In Davis JH, Sheldon GF [eds]: Clinical Surgery. St. Louis, CV Mosby, 1995.)

fistula. Silva and colleagues[17] showed that an artery had to be 2 mm or more in diameter and a vein had to be 2.5 mm or more in diameter to be useful for a fistula. Using these size criteria based on Doppler studies, the authors were able to improve patency rates of natural fistulas. Parmley and associates showed that a large percentage of patients could have natural fistulas placed despite half having had previous access attempts (less than 5% required prosthetic).[18] Allon and Robbin have described an approach to venous mapping and planning access.[19] These authors have also shown that venous mapping has improved maturation rates in diabetics and women but have also shown that certain patients have inadequate veins for fistula construction.[20] Investigators also believe that this type of information will make possible a greater number of natural fistulas.

The patency of these fistulas depends on the anatomic type. The autogenous radial-cephalic direct wrist access (Brescia-Cimino arteriovenous wrist fistula) has a patency at 2 years of 55% to 89%. One analysis combined a collective series of more than 1400 autogenous radial-cephalic direct wrist accesses and found an overall patency rate of 65% at 1 year.[14] Studies 20 to 25 years ago showed a failure rate of 10% after construction of a fistula compared with more recent studies, which have shown failure rates up to 50%.[19] This failure rate is attributed to poor vessels in an aging population, poor venous outflow,

excessive dehydration, or hypotension. The patency rate for autogenous brachial-cephalic upper arm direct accesses (brachiocephalic fistulas) is approximately 80%. The use of the autogenous brachial-basilic upper arm transposition (basilic vein transposition) is also impressive, with a 24-month patency rate of 73%. All patients who are potential candidates for dialysis should have an arm vein preserved for future placement of dialysis access.

COMPLICATIONS

Several complications occur with arteriovenous fistulas. The most common is failure to mature (i.e., enlarge to a size that can be used for dialysis). After the fistula has been in place, the most common complication is stenosis at the proximal venous limb (48%). Aneurysms (7%) and thrombosis (9%) are the next most common complications.[14] Aneurysms from repeated needle punctures are more likely to occur when venous access is obtained repeatedly in the same location, a maneuver that weakens the vessel wall. Heart failure can occur in those patients with a marginal cardiac reserve and a fistula flow rate of more than 500 mL/min. The cardiac failure may be reversed by placing a Teflon band around the outflow tract of the fistula until the blood flow is decreased to less than 500 mL/min. Occasionally the fistula requires ligation. The arterial steal syndrome and its ensuing ischemia occur in about 1.6% of patients with arteriovenous fistulas. This problem is unusual in patients with wrist fistulas (0.25%), but it is relatively common in patients with the more proximal fistulas (approximately 30%).[21] The steal syndrome is caused by blood flow from the anastomosed artery to the low-resistance vein, with additional blood flowing in retrograde fashion from the hand and forearm to create ischemia.

The complication of venous hypertension distal to the fistula results from high-pressure arterial blood flow into the low-pressure venous system; this situation causes venous hypertension with distal tissue swelling, hyperpigmentation, skin induration, and eventual skin ulceration similar to that seen in the legs of patients with venous stasis.[21] With normal unobstructed venous outflow this is a rare condition. When there is a proximal venous stenosis in a side-to-side anastomosis, this condition can occur. Both the steal syndrome and distal venous hypertension occur more frequently in patients with side-to-side anastomosis. Ligation of the distal limb of a side-to-side shunt corrects the problem, but this maneuver often causes shunt occlusion because the proximal vein is usually at least partially occluded. This proximal partial occlusion can be detected clinically by balloting the vein to feel a transmitted pulse wave in the proximal vein or by using duplex scanning to map the veins of the arm.[22] These complications can be avoided by performing an endvenous to side-arterial anastomosis in all cases. Infection of an autogenous radial-cephalic direct wrist access (Brescia-Cimino arteriovenous fistula) is rare (less than 3%). Rarely, a patient develops clinical steal syndrome characterized by pain, weakness, paresthesia, muscle atrophy, and, if left untreated, gangrene. These conditions can be reversed by closure of the fistula.

Prosthetic Grafts

The construction of vascular access using subcutaneously placed prosthetic material to join an artery to a vein is becoming increasingly necessary in patients with poor peripheral veins or previously failed arteriovenous fistulas. The material ideally should be easy to handle and to suture, it should allow graft-host biocompatibility, and it should be minimally thrombogenic and resist infection. It should be inexpensive, it should seal after repeated needle punctures, and it should allow tissue ingrowth.

Several different prosthetic materials were used for jump grafts in the past, including Dacron, bovine graft, and polytetrafloroethylene (PTFE). PTFE is the most popular material. It permits ingrowth of tissue through the interstices of the graft and thus incorporates the graft into viable tissue. A neointima formed in the graft presumably lessens the likelihood of thrombosis and infection. PTFE grafts have a lower incidence of aneurysm formation than do bovine grafts, and PTFE grafts do not always have to be removed when they become infected. Recently, a polyurethane graft has become available (Vectra) that has similar characteristics to PTFE but can be accessed within 24 hours of implantation.[23]

Technique of Prosthetic Jump Grafts

Successful creation of vascular access using prosthetic material requires good arterial inflow and venous outflow. Duplex scanning can help outline the arterial and venous vasculature. In patients who have had multiple venous punctures and subsequent venous stenosis, the site of the venous anastomosis must be chosen carefully so it is proximal to these areas of obstruction. Rotation or pinching of the graft in the tunnel must be avoided. The graft must be large enough to permit needle puncture readily. The usual sizes used are a 6-mm graft or a rapid-taper 4- to 7-mm graft. The latter gives approximately 20% of the maximum flow of the straight 6-mm graft at the same pressure and length. Dialysis can usually be performed relatively promptly after the graft has been placed; however, hematoma formation from bleeding at the puncture site is a serious complication because of the propensity for infection and pressure occlusion of the graft. Allowing the graft to mature for 1 to 2 weeks minimizes this problem by permitting tissue ingrowth, which facilitates sealing of the graft at the needle puncture site.

Several graft configurations have been developed for dialysis and names have been standardized.[13] Just as in natural arteriovenous fistulas, the nondominant arm should be used first and an attempt should be made to start as distal in the arm as possible. A graft between the radial artery at the wrist and the cephalic vein just below the elbow accomplishes this end. This graft has the lowest primary patency rate of any configuration because of the low flow through the radial artery. A prosthetic brachial-antecubital forearm loop access (forearm loop graft) is easily constructed to join the brachial artery to the cephalic vein or the brachial vein at the elbow. In the upper arm, an approach from the brachial artery to the axillary vein may be used (prosthetic brachial-axillary access—new nomenclature). A loop between the axillary artery and the ipsilateral axillary vein is also possible (Fig. 69-4). These upper arm grafts have a high flow rate and a low incidence of thrombosis. However, they do have a higher incidence of ischemia in the hand compared with other grafts because of preferential flow of arterial blood through the graft rather than to the peripheral circulation (Fig. 69-5). After graft placement, swelling is frequently seen secondary to surgical trauma and changes in venous outflow. Both these problems usually resolve with arm elevation and time.

Interposition grafts in the lower extremity are used for patients who have no usable vessels available in the upper arms. A loop graft in the thigh (superficial femoral artery

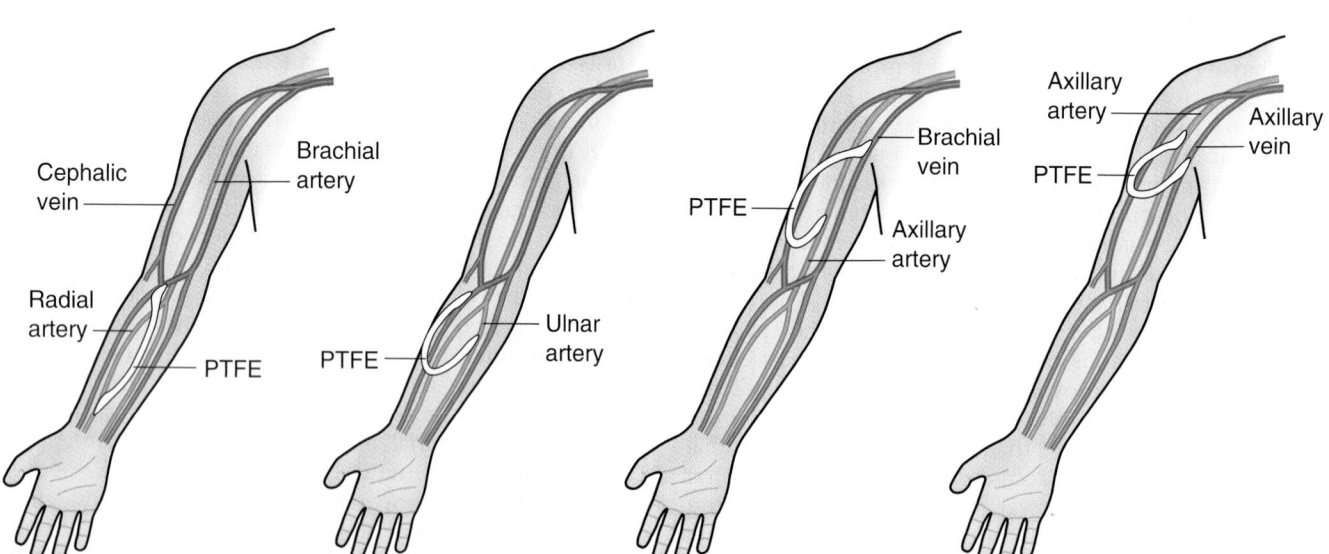

FIGURE 69-4. Four most common sites for placement of a jump graft in the upper extremity. PTFE, polytetrafluoroethylene. (From Haisch CE: Chronic vascular and peritoneal access. *In* Davis JH, Sheldon GF [eds]: Clinical Surgery. St. Louis, CV Mosby, 1995.)

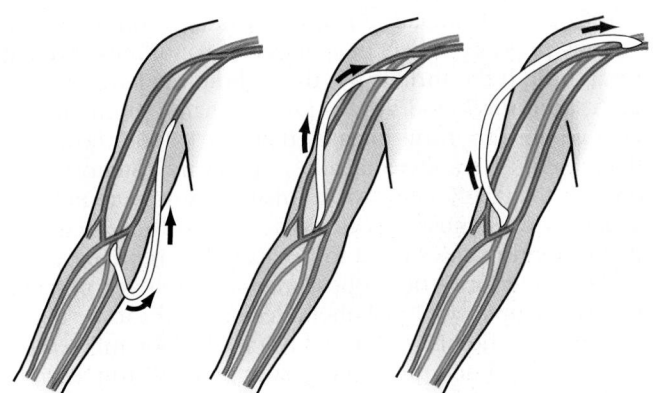

FIGURE 69-5. Three possible graft configurations for jump grafts in which standard sites have been used. (Redrawn from Tilney NL, Lazarus JM [eds]: Surgical Care of the Patient with Renal Failure. Philadelphia, WB Saunders, 1982; as shown in Haisch CE: Chronic vascular and peritoneal access. *In* Davis JH, Sheldon GF [eds]: Clinical Surgery. St. Louis, CV Mosby, 1995.)

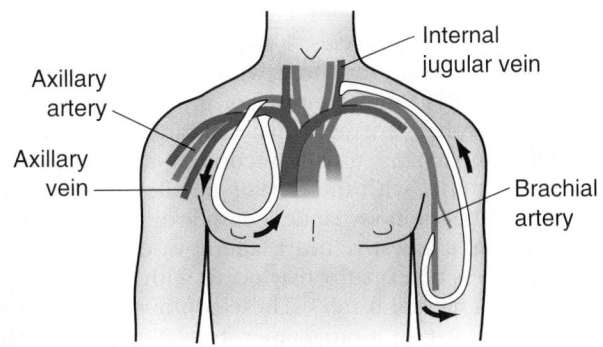

FIGURE 69-6. A graft from axillary artery to axillary vein with a loop on the chest. (Redrawn from Haimov M: Vascular access for hemodialysis: New modifications for the difficult patient. Surgery 92:109, 1982; as shown in Haisch CE: Chronic vascular and peritoneal access. *In* Davis JH, Sheldon GF [eds]: Clinical Surgery. St. Louis, CV Mosby, 1995.)

to saphenous vein—prosthetic femoral-saphenous looped inguinal access—new nomenclature) and a jump graft between the popliteal artery and the femoral vein are the two most common configurations. They are especially poor choices in patients with diabetes and in elderly patients, who frequently have peripheral arterial insufficiency. When a leg graft is considered in a patient with no other sites for construction of a jump graft, one must realize that 18 months after graft placement, one third of these patients will have died of the systemic complications of renal failure.[24]

In patients who have exhausted all previously described sites, other sites can be used for the creation of an arteriovenous jump graft. These possibilities include grafting from the axillary artery to the axillary vein across the chest, creating a loop on the anterior chest, grafting from the axillary artery to the iliac vein, or grafting from artery to artery (Fig. 69-6). The last type of graft requires narrowing the artery between the graft anastomoses with the prosthesis to allow adequate flow through the graft itself and thus to prevent graft thrombosis, which would potentially result in acute limb-threatening ischemia.

Complications

Early hemorrhage can occur at the anastomotic site, whereas late hemorrhage is usually secondary to needle puncture of the graft and bleeding into the perigraft space. Early thrombosis usually occurs for technical reasons, such as narrowing of inflow or outflow. Later thrombosis is secondary to venous intimal hyperplasia at or distal to the anastomosis. Outflow stenosis or occlusion may be repaired by a patch graft, balloon dilatation of the strictured area, or graft bypass of the obstruction.

Low blood pressure or excessive external pressure applied to graft puncture sites can contribute to the incidence of thrombosis. Thrombosis unaccompanied by narrowing of either inflow or outflow is often corrected by

simple thrombectomy of the graft or by simple urokinase injection into the graft. Occasionally, no anatomic or blood pressure-related reason exists for a patient to have recurrent episodes of thrombosis. The cause is frequently thought to be hypercoagulability. Pharmacologic intervention for prevention of thrombosis has been largely unsuccessful. Some early studies indicated that dipyridamole was of use in new grafts but was of no use in preventing subsequent clotting. One approach to a patient whose graft seems to clot for no anatomic reason has been to perform a coagulation evaluation and then to treat with an appropriate medication. These studies include evaluations of protein S, protein C, antithrombin III, plasminogen, factor V Leiden, and antiphospholipid antibodies. No pharmacologic interventions have satisfactorily prevented intimal hyperplasia; however both cilostazol (Pletal) and clopidogrel (Plavix) have been shown to reduce the incidence of intimal hyperplasia in animal models. Local application of numerous agents bound to stents as well as brachytherapy is being investigated and results are promising.

Infection is a major problem in patients with prosthetic jump grafts. Local drainage and wound care may resolve the problem in a number of grafts, if the suture line is not involved. In some cases, the infected area may be bypassed with a short graft or may be covered with a skin flap. The major reasons for removal of the entire graft for infection are involvement of the suture line, tunnel infection, clotting of the graft, or lack of success with local wound therapy. The salvage rate of infected grafts is low (25% to 50%). Old clotted prosthetic grafts can be a source of future infection especially in those patients who have a low serum albumin concentration. Nassar and Ayus speculate that leaving old clotted PTFE grafts in place may predispose a number of hemodialysis patients to the risk of developing a serious infection that originates from the PTFE graft.[25] In patients infected with the human immunodeficiency virus, the leading complication is infection; 32% of grafts in these patients become infected within

30 days. The organisms are *S. aureus* or coagulase-negative staphylococcal species.[26] Patients with a history of intravenous drug use or those with AIDS have an infection rate with PTFE grafts in place of approximately 40%.[27]

PTFE and other prosthetic materials are also associated with false aneurysms, usually secondary to laceration of the graft material with the dialysis needle; these can be bypassed. The hemodynamic complications of venous hypertension, congestive heart failure, vascular steal, and vascular access neuropathy may occur with jump grafts as they do with natural fistulas. These complications can be decreased by use of a rapid-taper 4- to 7-mm graft. This method decreases the flow rate in the graft and has been used in elderly patients and in those with diabetes. The steal syndrome is more likely to occur in upper arm fistulas than in forearm fistulas. Katz and Kohl[28] described their experience in a small group of patients with a technique to increase flow to the distal arm in the presence of steal syndrome. A saphenous vein graft was placed proximal to the arterial anastomosis of the graft. The distal end of the saphenous vein was placed distal to the arterial takeoff of the graft. The artery was then ligated between the arterial takeoff of the graft and the distal end of the saphenous vein graft.[28] This technique resolved the steal completely in five of six patients. The remaining patient kept the PTFE in place and had minimal numbness.

Patency

The patency rate of jump grafts is less than that of autogenous arteriovenous fistulas. Marx and colleagues,[14] in an evaluation of numerous articles, showed that the 1-year secondary patency rate for PTFE grafts is 80% and the 2-year rate is 69%. This is approximately the same rate as for natural fistulas; however, most of the losses, as with natural fistulas, are early, and the rate of loss decreases after the first 3 to 6 months. Therefore, a natural fistula should always be attempted if vessels are available. Raju[22] reported a 93% patency of PTFE at 1 year and a 77% patency at 2 years. Munda and associates[29] analyzed their experience with PTFE and showed that the location of the graft affects patency rates. In an upper arm location, the patency rate was 60% at 12 months; a straight forearm graft produced a 35% patency rate at 12 months, compared with a 78% patency for a forearm loop.[29] Thigh grafts have been shown to have a 12-month patency rate of 80%. Overall, the patency rate appears to be related to the magnitude of arterial inflow and the size and distensibility of the venous outflow.

Radiographic Intervention and Screening for Stenosis

Schwab and associates[30] showed that early intervention for graft stenosis with percutaneous luminal angioplasty reduced the incidence of graft thrombosis. These investigators measured venous pressure with an inline three-way stopcock attached to a 16-gauge venous return needle. The measurements were performed with a flow rate in the dialysis machine of 200 to 250 mL/min. A pressure greater than 150 mm on three separate occasions correlated with a venous stenosis of 50% or greater. Monitoring of grafts

and fistulas has included Doppler examination, checking venous pressure, checking for recirculation, and feeling for a thrill. If the thrill is felt throughout the length of the graft, then the blood flow is greater than 450 mL/min. A change in the thrill means that the blood flow has decreased. Hemodynamically significant stenoses of greater than 50% need to be dilated; however, no data suggest that stenoses greater than 50% without hemodynamic abnormalities need to be dilated or repaired.

The superiority of surgical intervention over percutaneous angioplasty of peripheral lesions is yet to be determined. Dilatation is performed using a balloon inflated for up to 10 to 15 minutes at a pressure up to 20 atm. Peripheral dilatation by angioplasty has a good success rate with both long and short stenotic lesions.[12] The diameter of the balloon used may also be important for long-term results (a 6-mm graft distal stenosis may need dilation to 7 or 8 mm). Cutting balloons may also have some role in very resistant lesions. The length of time the lesions stay open varies, but at 90 days, patency was 90%, and at 1 year, it was 40%. Most series have published a 6-month patency of 40% to 50% without additional intervention. In contrast to the findings of other investigators, Beathard[31] was able to show that subsequent dilatations gave the same patency rate as did initial dilatations (Fig. 69-7).

When a graft is clotted, the clot can be dissolved with a thrombolytic therapy, broken up mechanically, removed with a rheolytic catheter, or removed with a Fogarty catheter through an open method. Some of these treatments may result in pulmonary emboli, which can be significant in patients with compromised pulmonary reserve. Some studies have shown no significant difference in success or long-term patency between those grafts opened surgically and those treated percutaneously. A recent meta-analysis examining surgical versus endovascular treatment of clotted access grafts found seven acceptable studies with a total of 479 patients and showed a clear superiority of surgical therapy at 30, 60, and 90 days and 1 year.[32]

Few studies have compared surgery and radiology in a randomized prospective manner. Marston and colleagues[33] showed that in patients with both venous stenosis and long-segment venous outflow stenosis, surgical therapy resulted in a longer functional life of the graft when compared with the endovascular group (36% vs. 11% at 6 months). The arguments against surgical therapy are that additional vein is used and that surgery requires central catheters before the access is reused. This article indicates a possible place for both types of therapy, and selection of the best type of therapy for both long stenotic lesions and short lesions at the anastomosis is yet to be determined.[33] Despite shorter patency of endovascular therapy in the present studies, surgical jump graft revision may still be employed after failure of endovascular therapy. Hence, using the two techniques as complementary may potentially extend the life span of an access site.

Angioplasty plays an important role in central stenosis that occurs after placement of a subclavian catheter. Given the number of comorbidities these patients frequently have, only high-risk surgical intervention can be

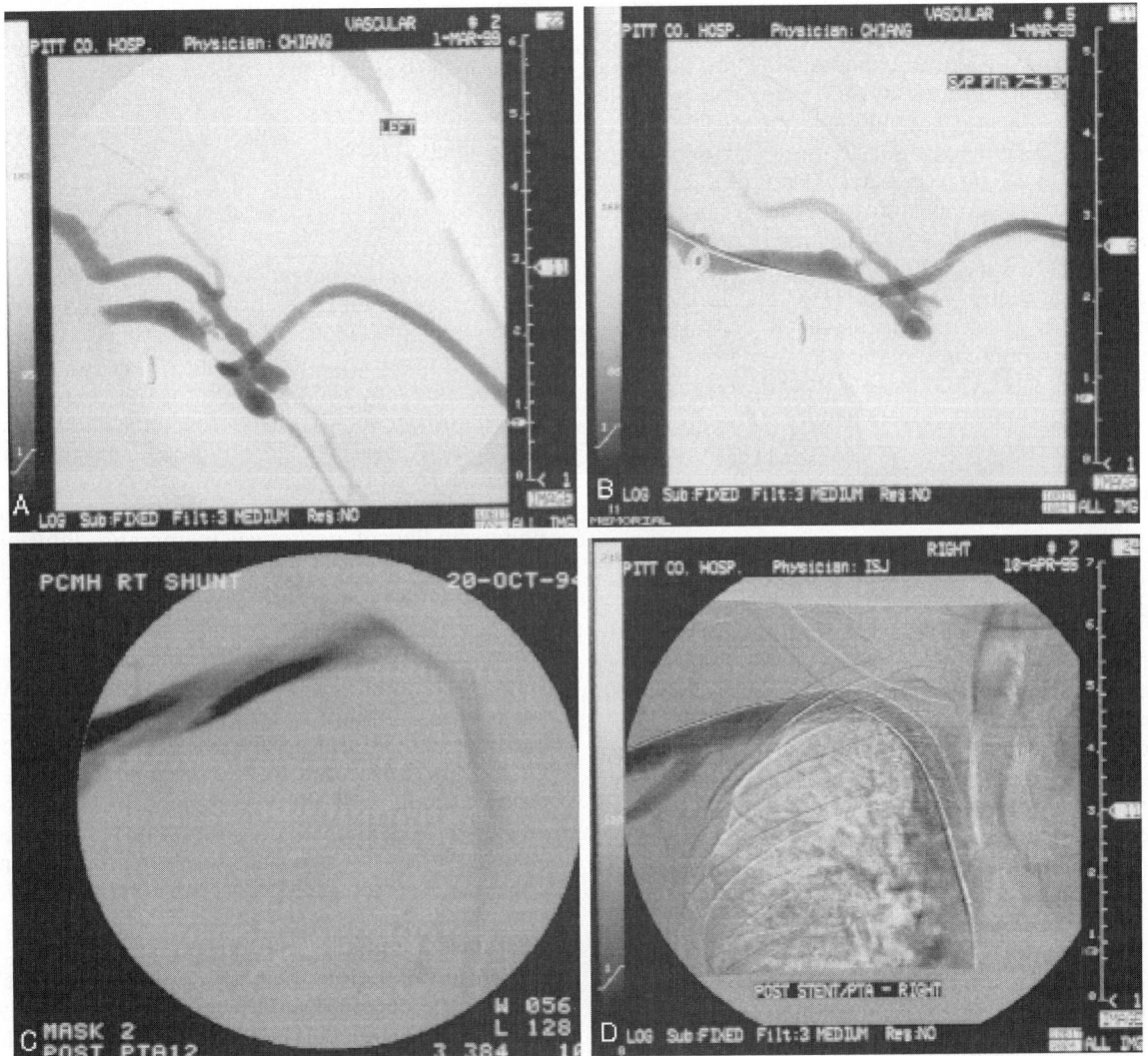

FIGURE 69-7. **A,** A fistulogram showing a short-segment stenosis and the venous anastomosis of a polytetrafluoroethylene graft that has caused thrombosis of the graft. **B,** Successful dilatation of the stenosis using balloon dilatation. **C,** Subclavian vein stenosis caused by a central catheter. This stenosis is so significant that collateral vessels have been formed. **D,** Successful dilatation of the stenosis with placement of a Wallstent.

undertaken. Lumsden and associates[34] showed that balloon dilatation was successful in 17 of 22 patients with central stenosis, with a 42% patency at 6 months. The authors used a stent in 5 patients and had good initial success.[34] Similar results were obtained by Vesely and colleagues.[35] These authors used three different stents and stated that the indications for and the type of stent to be placed are not yet determined.[35] The most common cause of stent failure is intimal hyperplasia in or around the stent. These stents seem to be most effective in patients with a large vein without a venous confluence, such as occurs in the central venous system (see Fig. 69-7).

Physiology

The physiologic consequences of arteriovenous fistulas depend on the size of the proximal and distal arteries and veins, the collateral flow around the fistula, and the diameter of the fistula. The length of the fistula has little influence on the flow when this length is less than 20% or greater than 75% of the arterial diameter. Between these two values, however, small changes in the size of the fistula can change flow dramatically. Most fistulas for clinical use are constructed so the fistula is larger than the arterial diameter to allow some margin for subsequent stenosis.[36] Blood flow through a side-to-side or an end vein-to-side artery wrist fistula is contributed by both the proximal arteries and the distal arteries, with as much as one third of the flow coming from the distal artery.[37]

A large, functioning arteriovenous fistula may cause a fall in both systolic and diastolic blood pressure, an increase in cardiac output, an increase in venous blood pressure both proximal and distal to the fistula, an increase in pulse rate, and a slight increase in the size of the heart. Increases also occur in blood volume in patients with chronic arteriovenous fistulas. These changes are all reversible with fistula closure.[36]

Platelets and fibrin may accumulate in a chronic fistula, with eventual closure of the lumen. Patients with a larger fistula usually have progressive lengthening and dilatation of both the proximal artery and the vein. The proximal artery elongates and dilates, and smooth muscle hypertrophy occurs. Eventually, smooth muscle atrophy develops and additional elongation and dilatation occur. This situation produces an aneurysmal dilatation and a tortuous vessel. The outflow vein has increases in smooth muscle, fibrous tissue, and collagen and also enlarges significantly. Blood flow around the fistula is increased to maintain flow distal to the fistula. A corresponding increase in temperature also occurs. However, blood flow distal to the fistula may be decreased, with resulting cool temperatures, particularly in the hand.[36]

Pathophysiology of Venous Hyperplasia

The turbulent flow at the anastomosis of an arteriovenous fistula or PTFE graft has an influence on venous hyperplasia. The Reynolds number changes when the flow of fluid is not straight. When a fistula or an H-graft between an artery and vein is in place the Reynolds number will increase. An increased Reynolds number correlates with increased turbulence and consequent hyperplasia.

The changes that occur at the molecular level at the anastomosis of the arteriovenous fistula and the venous end of a PTFE graft have been examined. Stracke and colleagues[38] have compared levels of transforming growth factor-β (TGF-β) and insulin growth factor-1 (IGF-1) in stenotic veins of arteriovenous fistulas and nonstenosed control veins from patients who were uremic but not on dialysis. Another control was from normal saphenous veins of patients who had undergone coronary artery bypass grafting. The stenosed veins showed markedly increased levels of TGF-β and IGF-1 in the neointimal and medial layers compared with control veins. Both of these growth factors have been shown to correlate with neointimal formation and are known to be involved with local inflammation.

Changes in the venous intima have also been examined in the PTFE-vein anastomosis from patients with intimal hyperplasia with a PTFE graft in place. One descriptive study found an increase in the amount of platelet-derived growth factor (PDGF), basic fibroblast growth factor (bFGF), and vascular endothelial growth factor (VEGF) compared with unaffected vein. These factors were expressed in the smooth muscle cells in the neointima of the vein and in the macrophages lining the PTFE graft.[39]

Summary

The development of convenient vascular access made long-term hemodialysis possible. Clearly, the three major improvements in the development of adequate vascular access were the development of the external shunt with prosthetic material penetrating the skin, the development of the arteriovenous wrist fistula, and the use of a subcutaneous prosthetic material to connect the artery and the vein. These techniques have been associated with an increasing success rate and decreasing morbidity.

However, for some patients, hemodialysis is not clinically appropriate. For patients with these and other indications, peritoneal dialysis is now widely used.

PERITONEAL DIALYSIS

Physiology

The exact surface and mechanism responsible for hemofiltration in peritoneal dialysis remain unknown. Investigators widely believe that the capillary vessels in the peritoneum are critical, with diffusion across the capillary membrane being the primary transport barrier. The peritoneal surface approximates the total body surface area. The effective surface area depends on the number of transcellular pores available for transport corresponding to the number of perfused capillaries.[40] Much of our understanding of peritoneal membrane diffusion comes from comparison with hemodialysis, in which the exact membrane pore size and surface area are known. Clearance of various molecules is different between the two techniques. For example, clearance of urea exceeds 100 L/wk in hemodialysis, whereas continuous ambulatory peritoneal dialysis (CAPD) yields 70 L/wk of urea clearance (604 L/wk for normal kidneys).[41] The current targets for weekly dialysis is a Kt/V of greater than 2 and a creatinine clearance of more than 60 L/1.73m². The differences are well documented and can be summarized by stating that CAPD appears more effective at removal of large solutes (more than 500 daltons) and less effective at removal of small solutes than does hemodialysis.[41] The peritoneal lymphatics and mesothelial cells play a lesser role in ultrafiltration. Measurement of lymphatic absorption can be accomplished using intraperitoneally administered macromolecular tracer. Regardless of the exact contributions, overall ultrafiltration in CAPD depends on Starling forces and lymphatic drainage.

Indications

The only absolute indication for peritoneal dialysis as renal replacement therapy is the inability to undergo hemodialysis. Poor vascular access, an unstable cardiovascular system, and bleeding diatheses are the most frequent reasons to avoid hemodialysis. CAPD therapy has many relative advantages, including increased patient mobility and independence, fewer dietary restrictions, increased patient satisfaction, and no requirement for systemic anticoagulation.

The absolute contraindications for CAPD are few and include obliteration of the peritoneal space from previous surgery, inadequate peritoneal clearance, and lack of diaphragmatic integrity. Relative contraindications include respiratory insufficiency secondary to dialysate infusion, large abdominal hernias, or malignant peritoneal disease.

Technical Procedures

Several types of catheters are available for use in peritoneal dialysis. Three frequently used types are the

Tenckhoff catheter, the Toronto Western catheter, and the curl-tip catheter. Variations on catheter design include straight versus coiled intra-abdominal configurations, single and double cuffs, and preformed intercuff bends (Swan neck). Prospective studies have not demonstrated significant differences in catheter survival or catheter complications between coiled and straight catheters.

Peritoneal dialysis catheters can be placed using open surgical technique, percutaneously, or laparoscopically. In experienced hands, percutaneous placement is safe and can be accomplished at the bedside. The catheter is inserted aseptically below the umbilicus and using local anesthesia and is directed toward the pelvis. The catheter is brought out through a subcutaneous tunnel on the side of the insertion site, with the Dacron cuff placed in the tunnel at least 1 inch from the skin surface. The percutaneous approach is being used more frequently by interventionallists in the interventional suite but still requires a 2-cm long incision for the deep cuff placement.[42] Surgeons typically can perform an open placement through an incision of the same size.

In the surgical approach, the Tenckhoff or curl-tip catheter is placed by making a paramedian incision below the umbilicus longitudinally through the anterior rectus sheath and muscle. The posterior fascia and the peritoneum are exposed, and a pursestring suture is placed. The catheter is directed toward the pelvis with a metal guide. Care is taken to avoid bowel or bladder injury. The deep Dacron cuff is left in the muscle just above the posterior fascia and is sutured into place with the pursestring suture. The anterior fascia is closed, and the second cuff is placed in the subcutaneous tunnel with the catheter exiting distally. If necessary, placement and fixation of the catheter in the pelvis under direct vision may decrease the incidence of nonfunctioning straight catheters. Omentectomy may also be necessary in some instances (Fig. 69-8).

The role of laparoscopy in peritoneal dialysis catheter placement is being developed. Single-port and double-port laparoscopic techniques have been successfully described for catheter placement.[43] Patency and complication rates are comparable to those seen with the open approach. However, the cost effectiveness of the laparoscopic approach has not been evaluated. Peritoneoscopy has a definite role in evaluation and salvage of malfunctioning catheters.[44] The incidence of catheter malfunction ranges from 12% to 73% of patients, and obstruction is a common cause of catheter loss.[45] Multiple studies have demonstrated successful laparoscopic manipulation of obstructed catheters, with salvage rates between 50% and 80%.[44]

Dialysis Fluids

Dialysis fluids are glucose based and vary in concentration. As stated earlier, peritoneal dialysis depends on Starling forces. The largest contribution in peritoneal dialysis comes from osmotic forces. Therefore, dialysis fluid with low osmolarity (1.5%) causes little fluid removal (200 mL per 2-L exchange), whereas the greatest concentration (4.5%) treats or prevents fluid overload (800 mL per 2-L exchange). High-concentration dialysis fluid is more

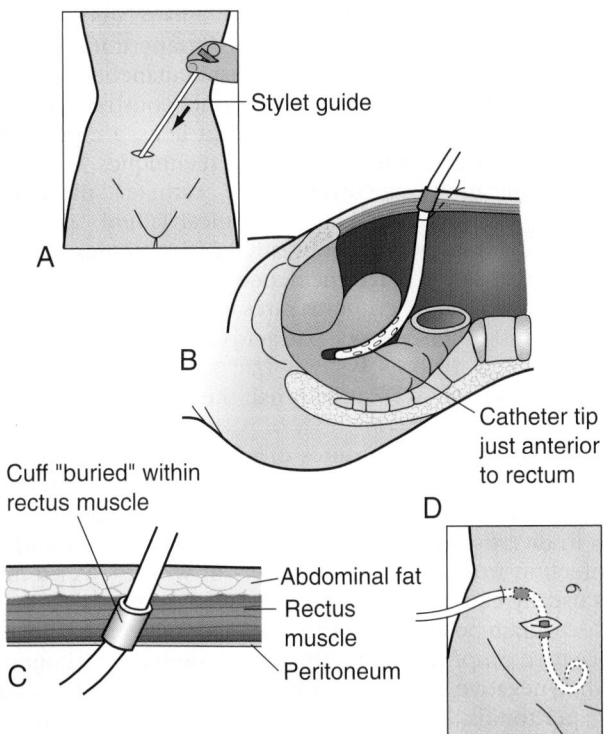

FIGURE 69-8.   Location of the chronic ambulatory peritoneal dialysis catheter. **A,** Location of the surgical incision. **B,** Location of the catheter in the pelvis. **C,** Dacron cuff at the level of the posterior rectus sheath. **D,** Exit site shown with final placement. (Redrawn from Simmons RL, Finch ME, Ascher NL, Najarian JS [eds]: Manual of Vascular Access, Organ Donation and Transplantation. New York, Springer-Verlag, 1984; as shown in Haisch CE: Chronic vascular and peritoneal access. *In* Davis JH [ed]: Clinical Surgery. St. Louis, CV Mosby, 1987.)

irritating to the peritoneal surface. Glycosylation of the peritoneal vascular walls occurs over time and reduces the intrinsic filtering ability of the peritoneum.[40] These changes are likely similar to the microangiopathy that occurs in patients with diabetes.[40] Lower concentration dialysis fluid should be used routinely when possible. Glucose polymers have been in clinical trials since the early 1990s, with emphasis on reducing the glucose concentration.[46] Electrolyte components are adjusted based on the patient's needs. A typical exchange is 2 L four times per day.

Research is ongoing to produce more biocompatible dialysis fluids. Insulin is often added to the dialysis fluid of patients with diabetes to allow for steady absorption. Intraperitoneal amino acids are being studied in an attempt to reduce malnutrition in patients undergoing peritoneal dialysis.[46] Administration of glycosaminoglycans has improved ultrafiltration in animal models, but results in humans are inconclusive.[46]

Complications

Complications can be divided into those related to surgical placement of the catheter and those occurring after catheter placement. Technical problems related to placement include leakage of dialysate, intraperitoneal bleeding, bowel or bladder perforation, subcutaneous bleeding with hematoma formation from tunnel construction, and ileus. All these complications, except ileus, are preventable with close attention to surgical technique.

Complications occurring after catheter placement include exit-site infection, mechanical failure, and peritonitis. Peritonitis is a potentially life-threatening complication with an average incidence of 1.3 to 1.4 episodes per patient-year.[47] Peritonitis rates have decreased in some series to 0.9 episode per patient-year with the introduction of Y-set dialysis systems that allow flushing of the catheter before use.[48] At least half the peritonitis episodes are experienced by only 25% of patients undergoing peritoneal dialysis.[47] Five routes of infection are recognized: through the dialysis tubing and peritoneal catheter; from tissue around the catheter; from fecal contamination, such as in diverticulitis; blood-borne infections; and ascending infection from the fallopian tubes in women. Peritonitis is usually caused by a single pathogen. In 60% to 70% of cases, gram-positive cocci are the culprits, with coagulase-negative *Staphylococcus* the most common pathogen.[47] Gram-negative bacilli account for 20% to 30% of the cases of peritonitis. *Pseudomonas aeruginosa* is not uncommon, occurring in 5% to 10% of the cases.[47] Uncommon causes are tuberculosis and fungal infection. However, fungal peritonitis is increasing in relative frequency. Risk factors for fungal peritonitis include recent hospitalization, immunologic compromise, and bacterial peritonitis. Combination therapy using both peritoneal and parenteral antibiotics treats peritonitis. Therapy should be directed by Gram stain and culture of peritoneal fluid. Synergistic double coverage is indicated for *P. aeruginosa* peritonitis. A biofilm containing microorganisms is thought to be the reason that some catheter infections are refractory to therapy. In these cases catheter removal is required.[49] Catheter removal is also required for fungal infections.[47]

Exit-site infections occur at a rate of 0.80 per patient-year.[48,50] Most are caused by gram-positive organisms (80%), with *S. aureus* accounting for 90% of these cases.[50] Catheter infection precedes peritonitis in about 20% of cases.[48]

Catheter malfunction may be caused by a number of factors and is manifested by poor inflow or total obstruction. Poor inflow is caused by displacement, omental wrapping, or partial blockage of the catheter holes. Total obstruction is caused by kinking of the catheter, blockage of all catheter holes, or omental wrapping of the entire intra-abdominal portion of the catheter. If the catheter flips out of the pelvis, it can be repositioned under fluoroscopic guidance or with peritoneoscopy. Other complications such as hernia formation, fluid loculation, or dialysate leaks can be detected using computed tomography.[51]

Catheter Longevity

CAPD catheters function for 1 year in 85% of patients with an expectation of a 3-year catheter survival of 80%. However, catheter survival is significantly shorter in patients with diabetes than in other patients. Infection is the leading reason for discontinuation of CAPD. Abdominal surgical events and social reasons have surpassed infection as a cause of treatment failure in some centers.[52]

Summary

Peritoneal dialysis allows the patient to be at home and to work with minimal disruption of activities. This approach to the management of chronic renal failure is gaining popularity because of the decreasing incidence of catheter infections, the decrease in cardiac complications, the lower incidence of anemia, and the greater convenience than hemodialysis. Some studies indicate a slight decrease in mortality relative to hemodialysis.[53] Infection and mechanical failure are the major factors that cause patients to switch to hemodialysis. Because these techniques may produce uncertain results, renal transplantation is still the therapy of choice for suitable patients with end-stage renal failure. Superb patient compliance is a basic requirement of paramount importance.

Selected References

Brescia MJ, Cimino JE, Appel D, Harwich BJ: Chronic hemodialysis using venipuncture and a surgically created arteriovenous fistula. N Engl J Med 275:1089, 1966.

> **This article is the original description of the wrist fistula, which revolutionized dialysis and allowed patients long-term vascular access with fewer complications than occurred with external shunts. The article describes the fistula against which all other methods of vascular access for dialysis are measured.**

Davidson IJA: Access for Dialysis: Surgical and Radiologic Procedures, 2nd ed. Georgetown, TX, Landes Biosciences, 2002.

> **This book has information on management of hemodialysis access procedures and radiologic approaches to access for dialysis. There are a large number of case reports as learning exercises. There is also a section on coding for access procedures.**

Eerola R, Kaukinen L, Kaukinen S: Analysis of 13,800 subclavian vein catheterizations. Acta Anaesthesiol Scand 29:193, 1985.

> **The results of a large study are presented on the practice of subclavian catheterization. Complications are discussed.**

Gray RJ, Sands JJ (eds): Dialysis Access: A Multidisciplinary Approach. Philadelphia, Lippincott, Williams & Wilkins, 2002.

> **A comprehensive volume covering surgery, radiology, and peritoneal dialysis.**

Haimov M, Baex A, Neff M, Slifkin R: Complications of arteriovenous fistulas for hemodialysis. Arch Surg 110:708, 1975.

> **This article reports on a group of more than 400 patients with more than 500 arteriovenous fistulas. The vascular complications are examined. Complications including ischemia, steals, gangrene, aneurysms, and venous hypertension are outlined, and their incidence is noted. The therapy and outcome are discussed for these complications.**

Henry ML: Vascular Access for Hemodialysis V. WL Gore and Associates, Precept, 2001.

> The publication is from a meeting on dialysis access held in 2000. The symposium reviewed physiology, pathology, and results of clinical care of dialysis patients. This good review covers a wide variety of topics.

National Kidney Foundation: Dialysis outcomes quality initiatives (DOQI) guidelines. Am J Kidney Dis 37(Suppl):137-179, 2001.

> These are group guidelines that recommend care to be given to patients in renal failure. These include peritoneal dialysis guidelines and care to be given to patients who need vascular access through a fistula or a graft.

Nolph KD: Peritoneal anatomy and transport physiology; and Mion CM: Practical use of peritoneal dialysis. *In* Drukker W, Parson FM, Maher JF (eds): Replacement of Renal Function by Dialysis. Boston, Martinus Nijhoff, 1983.

> These two chapters give an excellent overview of peritoneal physiology and anatomy and the practical uses and limitations of peritoneal dialysis. The chapter on physiology compares peritoneal dialysis with hemodialysis and gives its limitations. The chapter on the use of peritoneal dialysis includes sections on solutions and catheter insertion, complications, and catheter longevity.

Whitman ED: Complications associated with the use of central venous access devices. Curr Probl Surg 33:311, 1996.

> This good review of the best current venous access devices includes a description of current devices and their development. The article has sections on complications that occur with insertion and also discusses long-term complications.

References

1. Brescia MJ, Cimino JE, Appel K, et al: Chronic hemodialysis using venipuncture and a surgically created arteriovenous fistula. N Engl J Med 275:1089-1092, 1966.
2. Leblanc M, Fedak S, Mokris G, et al: Blood recirculation in temporary central catheters for acute hemodialysis. Clin Nephrol 45:315-319, 1996.
3. Tesio F, De Baz H, Panarello G, et al: Double catheterization of the internal jugular vein for hemodialysis: Indications, techniques, and clinical results. Artif Organs 18:301-304, 1994.
4. Sandhu J: Dialysis ports: A new totally implantable option for hemodialysis access. Tech Vasc Interv Radiol 5:108-113, 2002.
5. McLaughlin K, Jones B, Mactier R, et al: Long-term vascular access for hemodialysis using silicon dual-lumen catheters with guidewire replacement of catheters for technique salvage. Am J Kidney Dis 29:553-559, 1997.
6. Mosquera DA, Gibson SP, Goldman MD: Vascular access surgery: A 2-year study and comparison with the Permcath. Nephrol Dial Transplant 7:1111-1115, 1992.
7. Gray RJ, Levitin A, Buck D, et al: Percutaneous fibrin sheath stripping versus transcatheter urokinase infusion for malfunctioning well-positioned tunneled central venous dialysis catheters: A prospective, randomized trial. J Vasc Interv Radiol 11:1121-1129, 2000.
8. Whitman ED: Complications associated with the use of central venous access devices. Curr Probl Surg 33:309-378, 1996.
9. Denys BG, Uretsky BF, Reddy PS: Ultrasound-assisted cannulation of the internal jugular vein: A prospective comparison to the external landmark-guided technique. Circulation 87:1557-1562, 1993.
10. Marr KA, Sexton DJ, Conlon PJ, et al: Catheter-related bacteremia and outcome of attempted catheter salvage in patients undergoing hemodialysis. Ann Intern Med 127:275-280, 1997.
11. Darouiche RO, Raad II, Heard SO, et al: A comparison of two antimicrobial-impregnated central venous catheters. Catheter Study Group. N Engl J Med 340:1-8, 1999.
12. Beathard GA: Management of bacteremia associated with tunneled-cuffed hemodialysis catheters. J Am Soc Nephrol 10:1045-1049, 1999.
13. Sidawy AN, Gray R, Besarab A, et al: Recommended standards for reports dealing with arteriovenous hemodialysis accesses. J Vasc Surg 35:603-610, 2002.
14. Marx AB, Landmann J, Harder FH: Surgery for vascular access. Curr Probl Surg 27:1-48, 1990.
15. Gorski TF, Nguyen HQ, Gorski YC, et al: Lower-extremity saphenous vein transposition arteriovenous fistula: An alternative for hemodialysis access in AIDS patients. Am Surg 64:338-340, 1998.
16. National Kidney Foundation: Dialysis outcomes quality initiative (DOQI) guidelines. Am J Kidney Dis 37:S139-S179, 2001.
17. Silva MB Jr, Hobson RW II, Pappas PJ, et al: A strategy for increasing use of autogenous hemodialysis access procedures: Impact of preoperative noninvasive evaluation. J Vasc Surg 27:302-308, 1998.
18. Parmley MC, Broughan TA, Jennings WC: Vascular ultrasonography prior to dialysis access surgery. Am J Surg 184:568-572, 2002.
19. Allon M, Robbin ML: Increasing arteriovenous fistulas in hemodialysis patients: Problems and solutions. Kidney Int 62:1109-1124, 2002.
20. Allon M, Lockhart ME, Lilly RZ, et al: Effect of preoperative sonographic mapping on vascular access outcomes in hemodialysis patients. Kidney Int 60:2013-2020, 2001.
21. Haimov M, Baez A, Neff M, et al: Complications of arteriovenous fistulas for hemodialysis. Arch Surg 110:708-712, 1975.
22. Raju S: PTFE grafts for hemodialysis access: Techniques for insertion and management of complications. Ann Surg 206:666-673, 1987.
23. Glickman M, Gheissari A, Money S, et al: A polymeric sealant inhibits anastomotic suture hole bleeding more rapidly than Gelfoam/thrombin: Results of a randomized controlled trial. Arch Surg 137:326-332, 2002.
24. Taylor SM, Eaves GL, Weatherford DA, et al: Results and complications of arteriovenous access dialysis grafts in the lower extremity: A five-year review. Am Surg 62:188-191, 1996.
25. Nassar GM, Ayus JC: Infectious complications of the hemodialysis access. Kidney Int 60:1-13, 2001.
26. Nannery WM, Stoldt HS, Fares LG II: Hemodialysis access operations performed upon patients with human immunodeficiency virus. Surg Gynecol Obstet 173:387-390, 1991.
27. Brock JS, Sussman M, Wamsley M, et al: The influence of human immunodeficiency virus infection and intravenous drug abuse on complications of hemodialysis access surgery. J Vasc Surg 16:904-912, 1992.
28. Katz S, Kohl RD: The treatment of hand ischemia by arterial ligation and upper extremity bypass after angioaccess surgery. J Am Coll Surg 183:239-242, 1996.
29. Munda R, First MR, Alexander JW, et al: Polytetrafluoroethylene graft survival in hemodialysis. JAMA 249:219-222, 1983.

30. Schwab SJ, Raymond JR, Saeed M, et al: Prevention of hemodialysis fistula thrombosis. Early detection of venous stenoses. Kidney Int 36:707-711, 1989.

31. Beathard GA: Percutaneous transvenous angioplasty in the treatment of vascular access stenosis. Kidney Int 42:1390-1397, 1992.

32. Green LD, Lee DS, Kucey DS: A meta-analysis comparing surgical thrombectomy, mechanical thrombectomy, and pharmacomechanical thrombolysis for thrombosed dialysis grafts. J Vasc Surg 36:939-945, 2002.

33. Marston WA, Criado E, Jaques PF, et al: Prospective randomized comparison of surgical versus endovascular management of thrombosed dialysis access grafts. J Vasc Surg 26:373-381, 1997.

34. Lumsden AB, MacDonald MJ, Isiklar H, et al: Central venous stenosis in the hemodialysis patient: Incidence and efficacy of endovascular treatment. Cardiovasc Surg 5:504-509, 1997.

35. Vesely TM, Hovsepian DM, Pilgram TK, et al: Upper extremity central venous obstruction in hemodialysis patients: Treatment with Wallstents. Radiology 204:343-348, 1997.

36. Dow P, Hamilton WF: Handbook of Physiology, section 2, vol 3. Circulation. Washington, DC, American Physiological Society, 1965.

37. Anderson CB, Etheredge EE, Harter HR, et al: Local blood flow characteristics of arteriovenous fistulas in the forearm for dialysis. Surg Gynecol Obstet 144:531-533, 1977.

38. Stracke S, Konner K, Kostlin I, et al: Increased expression of TGF-beta1 and IGF-I in inflammatory stenotic lesions of hemodialysis fistulas. Kidney Int 61:1011-1019, 2002.

39. Roy-Chaudhury P, Kelly BS, Miller MA, et al: Venous neointimal hyperplasia in polytetrafluoroethylene dialysis grafts. Kidney Int 59:2325-2334, 2001.

40. Krediet RT, Ho-Dac-Pannekeet MM, Struijk DG: Preservation of peritoneal membrane function. Kidney Int Suppl 56:S62-68, 1996.

41. Nolph KD: Comparison of continuous ambulatory peritoneal dialysis and hemodialysis. Kidney Int Suppl 24:S123-131, 1988.

42. Georgiades CS, Geschwind JF: Percutaneous peritoneal dialysis catheter placement for the management of end-stage renal disease: Technique and comparison with the surgical approach. Tech Vasc Interv Radiol 5:103-107, 2002.

43. Nijhuis PH, Smulders JF, Jakimowicz JJ: Laparoscopic introduction of a continuous ambulatory peritoneal dialysis (CAPD) catheter by a two-puncture technique. Surg Endosc 10:676-679, 1996.

44. Kimmelstiel FM, Miller RE, Molinelli BM, et al: Laparoscopic management of peritoneal dialysis catheters. Surg Gynecol Obstet 176:565-570, 1993.

45. Bernardini J: Peritoneal dialysis catheter complications. Perit Dial Int 16(Suppl 1):S468-S471, 1996.

46. Medcalf JF, Walls J: New frontiers in continuous ambulatory peritoneal dialysis. Kidney Int Suppl 62:S108-110, 1997.

47. Johnson CC, Baldessarre J, Levison ME: Peritonitis: Update on pathophysiology, clinical manifestations, and management. Clin Infect Dis 24:1035-1045; quiz 1046-1037, 1997.

48. Paquay YC, Jansen JA, Goris RJ, et al: Long-term clinical experience with continuous ambulatory peritoneal dialysis: Access-related problems. J Invest Surg 9:81-93, 1996.

49. Giangrande A, Allaria P, Torpia R, et al: Ultrastructure analysis of Tenckhoff chronic peritoneal catheters used in continuous ambulatory peritoneal dialysis patients. Perit Dial Int 13(Suppl 2):S133-135, 1993.

50. Piraino B: Management of catheter-related infections. Am J Kidney Dis 27:754-758, 1996.

51. Hollett MD, Marn CS, Ellis JH, et al: Complications of continuous ambulatory peritoneal dialysis: Evaluation with CT peritoneography. AJR Am J Roentgenol 159:983-989, 1992.

52. Rodriguez-Carmona A, Garcia Falcon T, Perez Fontan M, et al: Survival on chronic peritoneal dialysis: Have results improved in the 1990s? Perit Dial Int 16(Suppl 1):S410-S413, 1996.

53. Fenton SS, Schaubel DE, Desmeules M, et al: Hemodialysis versus peritoneal dialysis: A comparison of adjusted mortality rates. Am J Kidney Dis 30:334-342, 1997.

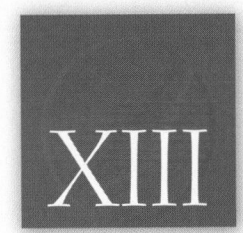
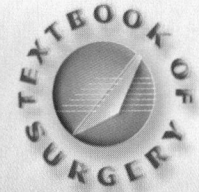

CHAPTER 70

PEDIATRIC SURGERY

Brad W. Warner, M.D.

Newborn Physiology	**Abdominal Wall**
Fluids/Electrolytes/Nutrition	**Congenital Diaphragmatic Hernia**
Extracorporeal Life Support	**Congenital Chest Wall Deformities**
Trauma	**Bronchopulmonary Malformations**
Lesions of the Neck	**Hepatobiliary Conditions**
Alimentary Tract	**Childhood Solid Tumors**

Pediatric surgery is a subspecialty that is both exciting and rewarding for multiple reasons. First, the range of problems encountered may be quite dramatic and are not limited to specific anatomic boundaries. Further, the pathogenesis of many significant pediatric surgical conditions remains unknown. As such, the challenge for intense, active investigation is ever-present. Finally, the approach to the child, interactions with concerned parents, and lifelong consequences of operative interventions demand a unique sensitivity and attention to detail, the impact of which is often profound.

In contrast with prior editions, this chapter has been significantly truncated, both in references and text to emphasize the most important components of the more common pediatric surgical conditions. In addition, a discussion of several common pediatric conditions (e.g., appendicitis, inflammatory bowel disease) is intentionally omitted to avoid redundancy with other chapters.

NEWBORN PHYSIOLOGY

The newborn infant is both physically and physiologically distinct from the adult patient in several respects. The smaller size, immature organ systems, and differing volume capacities present unique challenges toward perioperative management. In utero, the cardiovascular system essentially pumps blood from the placenta and bypasses the lungs via the patent foramen ovale and the ductus arteriosus. With clamping of the umbilical cord at the time of delivery, the foramen ovale closes and there is an abrupt fall in pulmonary arterial pressure. The ductus

arteriosus begins to close soon thereafter. These factors serve to promote pulmonary blood flow. Persistent pulmonary hypertension, which is associated with hypoxemia, acidosis, or sepsis, may contribute toward ductal patency, and right-to-left shunting may occur. In addition, prematurity is a risk factor for failure of the ductus arteriosus to close. As such, attempts to close the ductus pharmacologically using indomethacin or by direct surgical ligation may be necessary. Before the ductus is closed, there may be a higher partial pressure and saturation of oxygen in the blood when sampled from the right arm (preductal) when compared with the other extremities (postductal) due to the flow of unoxygenated blood from the pulmonary artery through the ductus into the aorta.

Cardiac perfusion is best monitored clinically by capillary refill, which should to be less than 1 second. A capillary refill longer than 1 to 2 seconds is associated with significant shunting of blood from the skin to the central organs as may occur with cardiogenic shock or significantly reduced intravascular volume from dehydration or bleeding. In neonates, the size of the liver is a reasonable gauge of intravascular volume. Finally, it should be noted that cardiac output in the newborn period is rate dependent, and the heart has a limited capacity to increase stroke volume to compensate for bradycardia.

The lungs are not completely developed at birth and continue to form new terminal bronchioles and alveoli until about 8 years of age. In premature infants, lung immaturity is one of the greatest contributors toward morbidity and mortality. In addition to reduced alveoli, immature lungs have reduced production of surfactant, which is critical for maintaining surface tension within the alveoli and gas exchange. A major contribution in the management of premature infants has therefore been the ability to provide exogenous surfactant. This has resulted in improved survival and less bronchopulmonary dysplasia (defined as the need for supplemental oxygen beyond the first 28 days of life). In addition to pulmonary parenchymal issues, the airway of the newborn is quite small (tracheal diameter, 2.5 to 4 mm) and easily plugged with secretions. The respiratory rate for a normal newborn may range from 40 to 60 breaths/min. Respiratory distress is heralded by nasal flaring, grunting, intercostal and substernal retractions, and cyanosis. Finally, infants preferentially breathe through their nose and not their mouth.

Newborn infants must be maintained in a neutral thermal environment since they are at great risk for cold stress. The major risk factors for the development of hypothermia in infants include their relatively large body surface area, lack of hair and subcutaneous tissue, and increased insensible losses. Neonates that are cold stressed respond by nonshivering thermogenesis. Metabolic rate and oxygen consumption are augmented by brown fat mobilization. Continued cold exposure leads to decreased perfusion and acidosis. Radiant heat warmers are usually necessary in very small premature infants, and this may contribute to further insensible water losses.

The neonate is relatively immunodeficient, with reduced levels of immunoglobulins and the C3b component of complement. As such, premature infants are at significantly increased risk for severe infection. Sepsis may result from multiple interventions that are necessary to care for these premature infants, including prolonged endotracheal intubation and central vein or bladder catheterization. Empiric antibiotic therapy to prevent overwhelming sepsis may be lifesaving and may be based on simple clinical judgment of subtle alterations in factors such as reduced tolerance of enteral feeding, temperature instability, reduced capillary refill, tachypnea, or irritability.

FLUIDS/ELECTROLYTES/NUTRITION

Several basic principles must be understood prior to assuming the responsibility for the metabolic needs for an infant or child. First, the margin for error is narrower when compared with adults. The consequences of too much or too little intravenous glucose in a neonate may be devastating and even life threatening. As such, the fluid, electrolyte, and parenteral nutrition orders should be considered as important as writing for any medication that has the potential for serious side effects. Second, on a body weight basis, protein and energy requirements are much greater in younger children and decrease with age. Not only are calories utilized for higher baseline metabolic rates but also a significant proportion of energy in the diet must be allocated for growth. Third, in contrast with adults, daily weight gain in neonates is an important indicator of providing sufficient calories. Infants who are losing weight, or even failing to gain weight, should mandate a careful reassessment of metabolic needs and amount of nutrition provided.

Fluid Requirements

Because of increased insensible water losses through thinner, less mature skin, the fluid requirements for premature infants are substantial. Insensible water losses are directly related to gestational age and range from 45 to 60 mL/kg/day for premature infants weighing less than 1500 g to 30 to 35 mL/kg/day for term infants. In contrast, insensible water losses in an adult are roughly 15 mL/kg/day. Other factors such as radiant heat warmers, phototherapy for hyperbilirubinemia, and respiratory distress further increase losses.

At 12 weeks' gestation, 94% of the fetal body weight is composed of water. This amount declines to about 78% by term (40 weeks/ gestation) and reaches adult levels (60%) by 1 ½ years of age. In the first 3 to 5 days of life, there is a physiologic water loss of up to 10% of the body weight of the infant. This is the singular exception to the general principle that infants are expected to gain weight each day. As such, fluid replacement volumes are less over the first several days of life. Recommended fluid volume replacements are shown in Table 70-1. These fluid volumes should be regarded as estimates and may change given differing environmental or patient factors.

The best two indicators of sufficient fluid intake are urine output and osmolarity. The minimum urine output in a newborn and young child is 1 to 2 mL/kg/day. Although adults can concentrate urine in the 1200-mOsm/kg range, an infant responding to water deprivation is able to concentrate urine only to a maximum of 700 mOsm/kg. Clinically, this means that a greater fluid intake and urine output are necessary to excrete the solute load presented to the kidney during normal metabolism.

Electrolyte Requirements

In general, the daily requirements for sodium are 2 to 4 mEq/kg and for potassium are 1 to 2 mEq/kg. These requirements are usually met with a solution of 5% dextrose in 0.2% normal saline with 20 mEq KCl added per liter at the calculated maintenance rate as noted earlier.

Caloric Requirements

Energy requirements from birth through childhood are partitioned into maintenance of existing body tissues,

TABLE 70-1. Daily Fluid Requirements for Neonates and Infants	
Weight	**Volume**
Premature < 2.0 kg	140–150 mL/kg/day
Neonates and infants 2–10 kg	100 mL/kg/day for first 10 kg
Children 10–20 kg	1000 mL + 50 mL/kg/day for weight 10–20 kg
Children > 20 kg	1500 mL + 20 mL/kg/day for weight > 20 kg

Adapted from Coran AG: The pediatric surgical patient. In Wilmore DW, Cheung LY, Harken AH, et al (eds): Scientific American Surgery, Sect. VII, Subsect. 12. New York, Healtheon/WebMD, 2000.

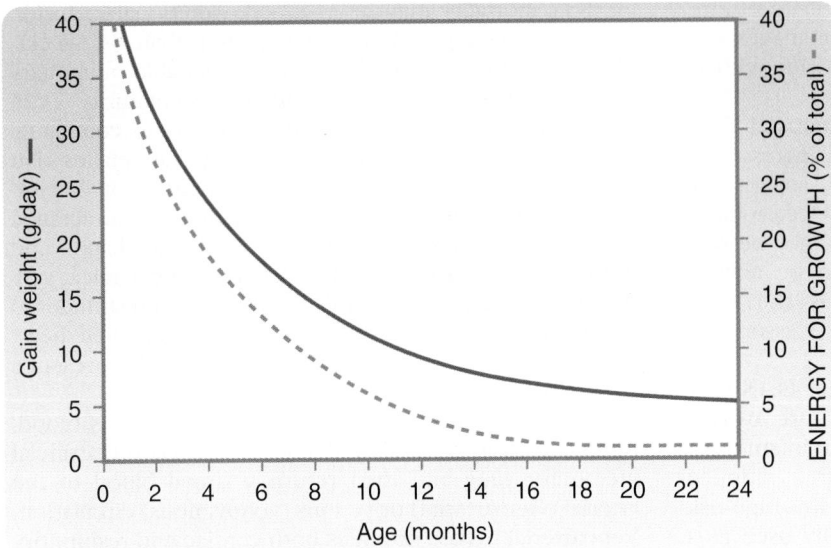

FIGURE 70-1.   Daily gain in body weight and percentage of energy intake used for growth at 2 weeks to 2 years of age. *Solid line*, weight gain (g/day); *dashed line*, percentage of energy used for growth. (From Anderson TA: Birth through 24 month. *In* Rudolph AM [ed]: Pediatrics, 18th ed. Norwalk, CT, Appleton & Lange, 1987, p 158.)

growth, and physical activity. As depicted in Figure 70-1, the amount of energy from the diet required for growth alone may be as high as 40% in neonates. The parameter that is most indicative of sufficient provision of calories in neonates is daily weight gain. As such, infants should gain roughly 30 g/day. The expected daily weight gain decreases with age. Total daily caloric requirements, which range from 100 to 120 kcal/kg/day during infancy, steadily decrease with age.

Protein

The average intake of protein should comprise approximately 15% of the total daily calories and range from 2 to 3.5 g/kg/day in infants. This protein requirement is reduced in half by 12 years of age and approaches adult requirement levels (1 g/kg/day) by 18 years of age. The provision of greater amounts of protein, relative to nonprotein calories, results in rising blood urea nitrogen levels. The nonprotein calorie (carbohydrate plus fat calories) to protein calorie ratio (when expressed in grams of nitrogen) should therefore not be less than 150:1. For infants on parenteral nutrition, the amount of protein provided is usually begun at 0.5 g/kg/day and advanced in daily increments of 0.5 g/kg/day to the target goal.

Carbohydrate

When oral nutrition cannot be provided to infants, it is critical that intravenous fluids are provided to supply water, electrolytes, and glucose. Failure to provide glucose for prolonged periods will result in the rapid (within hours) development of hypoglycemia. In turn, this may lead to seizures, neurologic impairment, or even death. The absolute minimum intravenous glucose infusion rate for neonates is 4 to 6 mg/kg/minute. This rate should be calculated daily for every neonate receiving parenteral nutrition. During total parenteral nutrition, the amount of glucose provided is increased daily to a maximum of 10 to 12 mg/kg/min. These are general guide-

lines and should be tailored to each individual patient. The amount of weight gain dictates the need to continue advancing glucose calories. Further, hyperglycemia from either too rapid advancement or underlying sepsis should be avoided as this will lead to rapid hyperosmolarity and dehydration. In contrast with adults, the addition of insulin to the parenteral nutrition solution in children is very high risk and is generally not indicated in routine practice.

Fat

In adults, parenteral fat is provided either as a daily infusion as a source of calories or given intermittently to prevent the development of essential fatty acid deficiency. In the pediatric population, fat is always provided as a daily infusion for both purposes. The lipid requirements for growth are significant, and fat is a robust caloric source. Similar to protein, fat infusions are done starting at 0.5 g/kg/day and advanced up to 2.5 to 3 g/kg/day. In infants with unconjugated hyperbilirubinemia, fat administration should be done with caution, because fatty acids may displace bilirubin from albumin. The free unconjugated bilirubin may then cross the blood-brain barrier and lead to kernicterus and resultant mental retardation.

EXTRACORPOREAL LIFE SUPPORT

Extracorporeal life support (ECLS), formerly referred to as *extracorporeal membrane oxygenation* (ECMO), is a type of heart-lung bypass that provides short-term (days to weeks) support for the critically ill patient with acute life-threatening respiratory and/or cardiac failure. ECLS is a purely supportive, nontherapeutic intervention that maintains adequate gas exchange and circulatory support while "resting" the injured lungs or heart. Although the use of ECLS has been described in both pediatric and adult populations, the greatest experience has been reported in neonatal respiratory failure.[1] Since the mid-1970s when the first neonatal survival was reported, ECLS has become the standard of care for neonatal respiratory failure unresponsive to maximum conventional medical management. It is practiced in more than 90 centers worldwide with an overall survival rate of 80%.

The major indications for initiation of neonatal ECLS include meconium aspiration, respiratory distress syndrome, persistent pulmonary hypertension, sepsis, and congenital diaphragmatic hernia (CDH). Occasionally, neonates with congenital cardiac anomalies may be supported with ECLS until surgical repair can be accomplished. Meconium aspiration syndrome is the most common indication for neonatal ECLS and is associated with the highest survival rate (>90%).

Selection criteria for initiation of neonatal ECLS vary slightly from institution to institution and are usually derived from historical controls. Generally, an infant must have at least 80% predicted mortality with continued conventional medical management to justify this high-risk therapy. Two formulas have been historically used as a means to predict survival without ECLS. One formula is the alveolar-arterial oxygen gradient ($AaDO_2$) and is calculated as (atmospheric pressure − 47) − (PaO_2 + $PaCO_2$). An $AaDO_2$ that is greater than 620 for 12 hours or an $AaDO_2$ greater than 620 for 6 hours associated with extensive barotrauma and/or severe hypotension requiring inotropic support is considered to be criteria for ECLS.

The oxygen index (OI) likewise may be used to predict mortality, where the OI is calculated as the fraction of inspired oxygen (usually always 1.0) multiplied by the mean airway pressure × 100) + PaO_2. If the OI is more than

40, 80% mortality may be assumed. Additional inclusion criteria include gestational age greater than 34 weeks, birth weight more than 2 kg, and a reversible pulmonary process. Exclusion criteria include prematurity (<24 weeks' gestation), the presence of cyanotic congenital heart disease or other major congenital anomalies that preclude survival, intractable coagulopathy or hemorrhage, sonographic evidence of a significant intracranial hemorrhage (>grade I intraventricular hemorrhage), and more than 10 to 14 days of high-pressure mechanical ventilation. Before initiation of ECLS, all infants must undergo a cardiac echocardiogram to rule out congenital heart disease and a cranial ultrasound to exclude the presence of significant intracranial hemorrhage.

The basic concept of ECLS is to drain venous blood, remove carbon dioxide, and add oxygen via the artificial membrane lung and then return warmed blood to the arterial (venoarterial) or venous (venovenous) circulation. Venoarterial bypass provides both cardiac and respiratory support, whereas venovenous bypass provides only respiratory support. Venoarterial bypass is used most commonly, and the right internal jugular vein and common carotid artery are typically chosen for cannulation because of their large size, accessibility, and adequate collateral circulation. The ECLS circuit (Fig. 70-2) is composed of a silicone rubber collapsible bladder (which collapses if there is low venous return), a roller pump, a membrane oxygenator, a heat exchanger, tubing, and connectors. Venous blood from the right atrium drains through the venous cannula to the bladder and is pumped to the

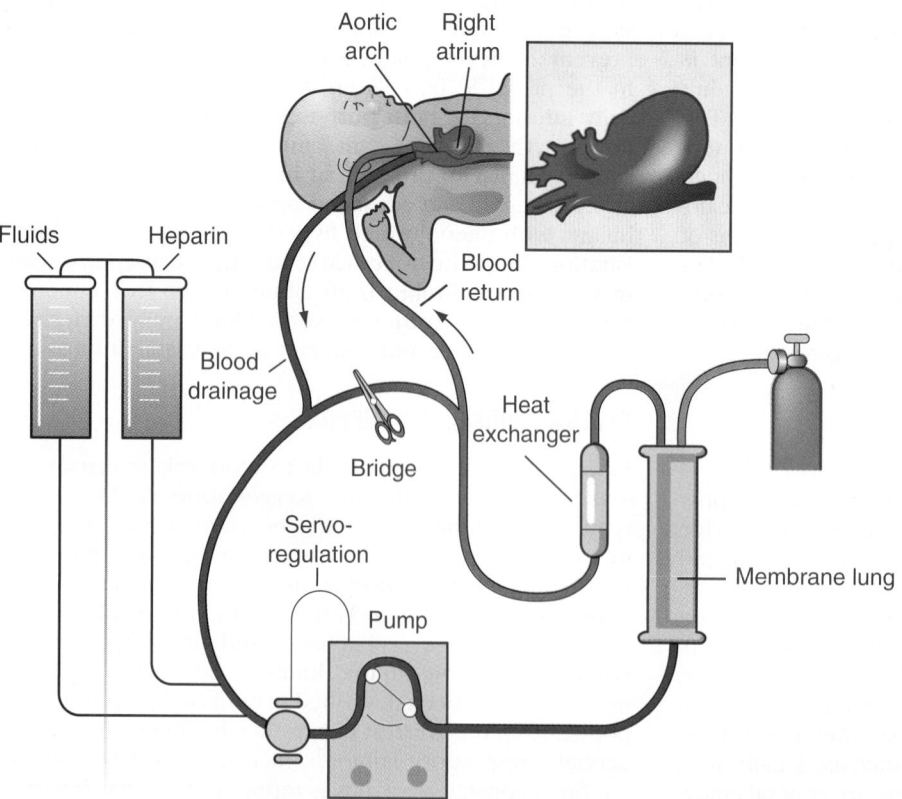

FIGURE 70-2. Diagrammatic representation of venoarterial extracorporeal life support circuit. (From Shanley CJ, Bartlett RH: Extracorporeal life support: Techniques, indications, and results. *In* Cameron JL (ed): Current Surgical Therapy, 4th ed. St. Louis, Mosby–Year Book, 1992, pp 1062-1066).

membrane oxygenator where carbon dioxide is removed and oxygen is added. The oxygenated blood then passes through the heat exchanger and is returned to the patient through the arterial cannula.

To prevent clotting of the ECLS circuit, systemic anticoagulation is maintained. The fully heparinized patient is at risk for serious bleeding complications. As such, hematocrit levels are followed closely. Similarly, platelet counts and fibrinogen level must be monitored and normal levels maintained. Daily cranial ultrasound evaluations are obtained to monitor for hemorrhage.

Extracorporeal flow is gradually weaned as native cardiac or pulmonary function improves. Indicators of lung recovery include an increasing PaO_2, improved lung compliance, and clearing of the chest radiograph. Once the extracorporeal flow rates are at minimal levels, the venous and arterial cannulas may be clamped to give the patient a trial off bypass. If the patient remains hemodynamically stable with adequate oxygenation and ventilation while the cannulas are clamped, the cannulas are surgically removed and conventional ventilatory support is continued. The mean duration of ECLS in neonates is roughly 5 to 6 days. Patients with CDH and sepsis tend to have the longest required duration of bypass.

In addition to bleeding, ECLS is associated with significant morbidity and mortality. Multiple factors contribute to the risk of this technology and include ligation and cannulation of the right common carotid artery and right internal jugular vein, systemic heparinization, exposure to multiple blood products, and potential for mechanical failure of the circuit. Bleeding is the most common complication and may be either medical (too few platelets, too much heparin, intracranial) or surgical (neck cannulation site, intrathoracic, gastrointestinal, and so forth). Birth weight and gestational age are the most significant correlates of intracranial hemorrhage on ECLS, with infants weighing less than 2.2 kg and younger than 35 weeks' gestational age at the highest risk. Other significant complications associated with ECLS include seizures, neurologic impairment, renal failure requiring hemofiltration or hemodialysis, hypertension, infection, and mechanical malfunction (such as failure of the membrane oxygenator, pump, or heat exchanger).

TRAUMA

In children between 1 and 15 years of age, trauma is the leading cause of death. Although motor vehicle accidents account for the majority of traumatic deaths, falls, bicycle accidents, and child abuse comprise a substantial component as well. Violence-related penetrating injury from firearms is becoming increasingly common. Much emphasis on trauma research is directed toward prevention. Since a large percentage of motor vehicle accident–related injury occurs because of absent or improper use of child restraint devices, community outreach education programs are vital. Along these lines, programs for distribution and education on the use of safety helmets for bike riding and skateboarding are extremely important in reducing injury severity. Finally, active participation by

pediatric surgeons in legislative efforts toward factors such as firearm safety locks or use of all-terrain vehicles by young children are critical.[2]

The management of trauma in children is similar to that of adults and beyond the scope of the present chapter. However, several caveats are important to consider. Just as in adults, the priorities during the resuscitation phase are airway, breathing, and circulation. In general, a child who is crying on arrival to the emergency department is reassuring, since the airway and breathing are more than likely to be intact. If endotracheal intubation is required, an uncuffed endotracheal tube should be used in children younger than 8 to 10 years of age because of the small size of the trachea. The appropriate endotracheal tube size can be estimated visually as being equivalent to the diameter of the child's little finger. Alternatively the appropriate endotracheal tube inner diameter can be calculated by the following formula

$$4 + (patient's\ age\ in\ years) \div 4$$

Because of the soft and easily injured trachea of young children, surgical cricothyroidotomy should never be attempted in a child who is younger than 12 years of age.

With regard to fluid resuscitation, crystalloid is given as a rapid intravenous bolus in increments of 20 mL/kg. The ability to secure reliable intravenous access in young children may be quite challenging. In children younger than 6 years of age in whom an intravenous line cannot be secured within a reasonable period, intraosseous access should be considered. This is accomplished with a specially designed needle placed under sterile conditions through the flat, anteromedial surface of the tibia, 1 to 2 cm below the anterior tibial tuberosity. Virtually any intravenous drug or fluid that may be required during a trauma resuscitation can be safely administered by the intraosseous route. Blood transfusion is warranted in pediatric trauma patients who demonstrate persistent evidence of hypovolemic shock after two boluses (total of 40 mL/kg) of crystalloid fluid. An estimate of a child's entire blood volume is roughly 80 mL/kg. As a general rule, if the need for blood transfusion within the first 24 hours following blunt abdominal trauma exceeds half the estimated blood volume, active hemorrhage is presumed and is usually an indication for laparotomy.

Imaging of the pediatric blunt trauma patient is predominately by computed tomography (CT) of the abdomen and pelvis. The indications for CT include the presence of a distracting injury such as an associated arm or leg fracture, significant closed head injury, if the examination is unclear or cannot be obtained because of an uncooperative or very young child, or if the serum glutamic-oxaloacetic transaminase or serum glutamic-pyruvic transaminase levels are higher than 200 or 100 IU/L, respectively. A significant amount of peritoneal fluid in the absence of solid organ injury should raise the suspicion for a small bowel injury and should prompt further investigation. Although significant spleen and/or liver injuries are frequently identified, the need for operative intervention is rare. The major indications for laparotomy in these circumstances include obvious hemodynamic instability, the need for blood transfusion in amounts greater than half the child's calculated blood volume (40 mL/kg) within the first 24 hours following injury, or obvious extravascular blush of intravenously administered contrast material. Recently, specific treatment guidelines based on CT grade of liver or spleen injury have been prospectively validated by the Liver/Spleen Trauma Study Group of the American Pediatric Surgical Association.[3] According to these guidelines, a patient with an isolated grade I liver or spleen injury may be managed without the need for admission to an intensive care unit (ICU), require no more than 2 days of hospitalization, and resume full activities and contact sports after 3 weeks. At the other end of the spectrum, patients with isolated grade IV injuries should be carefully monitored in an ICU for at least the first 24 hours and remain hospitalized for no less than 5 days. Return to full activities should not take place until 6 weeks following injury. Regardless of the injury grade and in the absence of specific indications, follow-up imaging either at the time of discharge or prior to resumption of normal activities is not indicated.

LESIONS OF THE NECK

Cystic Hygroma

A cystic hygroma is a lymphatic malformation that occurs as a result of a maldeveloped localized lymphatic network, which fails to connect or drain into the venous system. The vast majority (75%) involve the lymphatic jugular sacs and present in the posterior neck region (Fig. 70-3). Another 20% occur in the axilla, and the remainder is found throughout the body, including the retroperitoneum, mediastinum, pelvis, and inguinal area. Roughly 50% to 65% of hygromas present at birth, with most becoming apparent by the second year of life.

Since hygromas are multiloculated cystic spaces lined by endothelial cells, they usually present as soft, cystic masses that distort the surrounding anatomy. The indications for therapy are obviously cosmetic. In addition, the

hygroma may expand to compress the airway, resulting in acute airway obstruction. Prenatal recognition of a large cystic mass of the neck is associated with significant risk to the airway, greater association with chromosomal abnormalities, and higher mortality.[4] Improved fetal imaging modalities may allow for intervention at the time of delivery based on the principle of maintaining placental circulation until endotracheal intubation is achieved.[5] In addition to accumulating lymph fluid, hygromas are prone to infection and hemorrhage within the mass. Thus, rapid changes in the size of the hygroma may necessitate more urgent intervention.

Complete surgical excision is the preferred treatment; however, this may be impossible due to the hygroma infiltrating within and around important neurovascular structures. Careful preoperative magnetic resonance imaging (MRI) to define the extent of the hygroma is crucial. Operations are routinely performed with the aid of loupe magnification and a nerve stimulator. Since hygromas are not neoplastic tumors, radical resection with removal of major blood vessels and nerves is not indicated. Postoperative morbidity includes recurrence, lymphatic leak, infection, and neurovascular injury.

Injection of sclerosing agents such as bleomycin or the derivative of *Streptococcus pyogenes* OK-432[6] have also been reported to be effective in the management of cystic hygromas. Intracystic injection of sclerosants seems to be most effective for macrocystic hygromas, as opposed to the microcystic variety.

Branchial Cleft Remnants

The mature structures of the head and neck are embryologically derived from six pairs of branchial arches, their intervening clefts externally, and pouches internally. Congenital cysts, sinuses, or fistulas result from failure of these structures to regress or persist in an aberrant location. The location of these remnants generally dictates their embryologic origin and guides the subsequent operative approach. Failure to understand the embryology may result in incomplete resection or injury to adjacent structures.

By definition, all branchial remnants are present at the time of birth although they may not become clinically evident until later in life. In children, fistulas are more common than external sinuses, which are more frequent than cysts. In adults, cysts predominate. The clinical presentation may range from a continuous mucoid drainage from a fistula or sinus to the development of a cystic mass that may become infected. Branchial remnants may also be palpable as cartilaginous lumps or cords corresponding with a fistulous tract. Dermal pits or skin tags may also be evident.

First branchial remnants are typically located in the front or back of the ear or in the upper neck in the region of the mandible. Fistulas typically course through the parotid gland, deep, or through branches of the facial nerve, and end in the external auditory canal.

Remnants from the second branchial cleft are the most common. The external ostium of these remnants is located along the anterior border of the sternocleidomas-

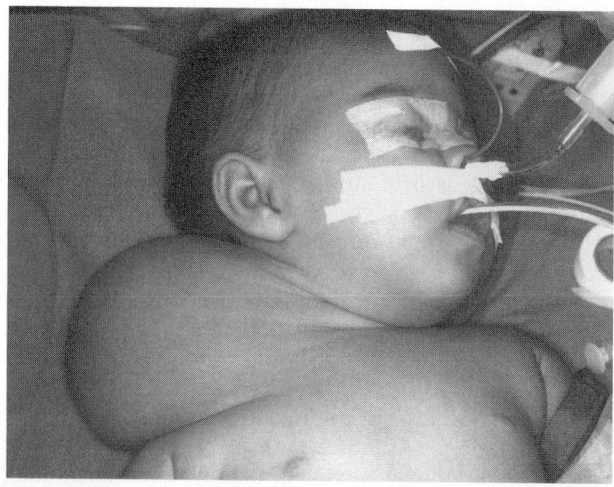

FIGURE 70-3.   Cystic hygroma.

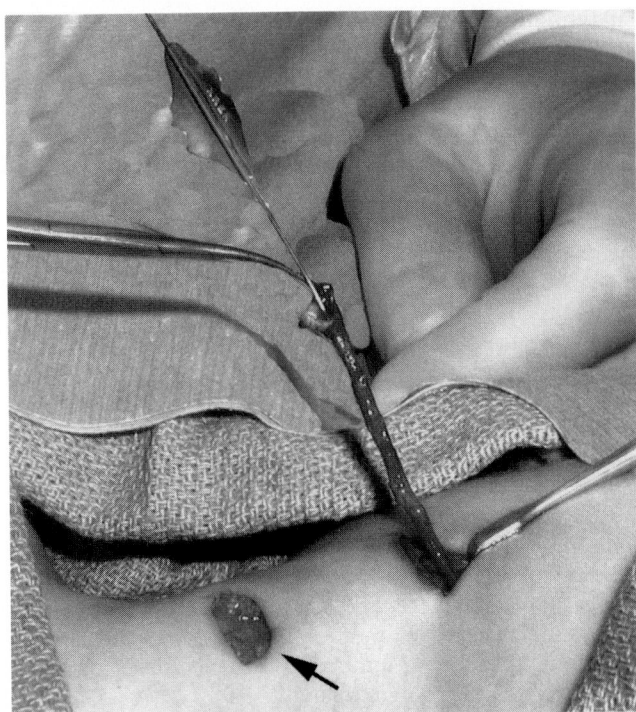

FIGURE 70-4. Branchial cleft fistula. The original site of the fistula in the lower neck *(arrow)* has been elliptically excised and a step-ladder counterincision has been made higher in the neck to remove the entire tract. A lacrimal probe has been inserted into the tract to define its course.

toid muscle, usually in the vicinity of the upper half to the lower third of the muscle. The course of the fistula must be anticipated preoperatively, as step-ladder counterincisions are often necessary to completely excise the fistula (Fig. 70-4). Typically, the fistula penetrates the platysma, ascends along the carotid sheath to the level of the hyoid bone and then turns medially to extend between the carotid artery bifurcations. The fistula then courses behind the posterior belly of the digastric and stylohyoid muscles to end in the tonsillar fossa.

Third branchial cleft remnants usually do not have associated sinuses or fistulas and are located in the suprasternal notch or clavicular region. These most often contain cartilage and present clinically as a firm mass or as a subcutaneous abscess.

Thyroglossal Duct Cyst

One of the most common lesions in the midline of the neck is the thyroglossal duct cyst, which most commonly presents in preschool-age children. Thyroglossal remnants are involved with the embryogenesis of the thyroid gland, tongue, and hyoid bone and produce midline masses extending from the base of the tongue (foramen cecum) to the pyramidal lobe of the thyroid gland. Complete failure of thyroid migration results in a lingual thyroid. Ultrasound or radionuclide imaging may therefore be useful to identify the presence of a normal thyroid gland within the neck. This information would be useful to prevent performing an inad-

vertent complete thyroidectomy during treatment of a presumed thyroglossal remnant.

Thyroglossal duct cysts may be located in the midline of the neck anywhere from the base of the tongue to the thyroid gland. Most, however, are found at or just below the hyoid bone. The indications for surgery include increasing size, the risk for cyst infection, or the presence (1% to 2%) of carcinoma. The classic treatment has remained unchanged since it was described by Sistrunk in 1928 and involves complete excision of the cyst in continuity with its tract, the central portion of the hyoid bone, and the tissue above the hyoid bone extending to the base of the tongue.[7] Failure to remove these tissues results in a high risk of recurrence, since multiple sinuses have been histologically identified in these locations (Fig. 70-5).

Torticollis

Torticollis simply refers to a "twisted neck," which may be either congenital or acquired. In infants with congenital torticollis, the head is typically tilted toward the side of the affected muscle and rotated in the opposite direction. In many cases, a mass can be palpated within the affected muscle. Although the true etiology is unknown, birth trauma is most frequently considered. The typical onset of congenital torticollis is 4 to 6 weeks of age in an otherwise healthy infant. The diagnosis is purely clinical.

The treatment for congenital torticollis is initially conservative. Range-of-motion exercises consist of passive stretching of the affected muscle and are curative in most infants. The average duration of required treatment is

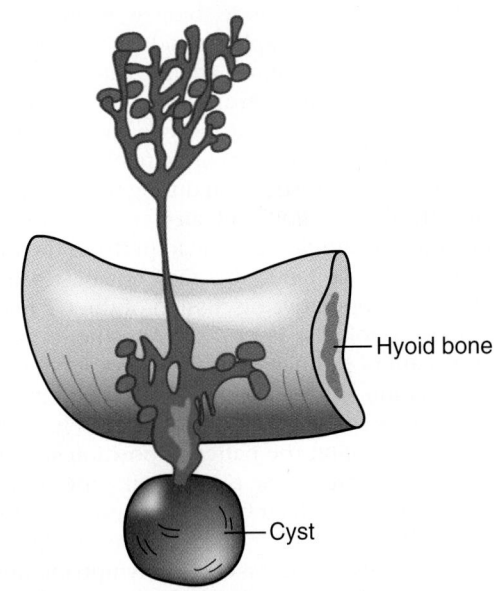

FIGURE 70-5. Thyroglossal duct cyst. There are usually branches from the cyst that are intimate with the hyoid bone and extend cephalad for variable distances. The Sistrunk procedure, which involves en bloc removal of the cyst, central portion of the hyoid bone, and tissue above to the base of the tongue, is required to minimize recurrence. (From Horisawa M, Niinomi N, Ito T: What is the optimal depth for core-out toward the foramen cecum in a thyroglossal duct cyst operation? J Pediatr Surg 27:710-713, 1992.)

roughly 4 to 5 months. Surgical resection or division of the involved muscle is rarely necessary but indicated if symptoms persist beyond 1 year.

Congenital torticollis should be distinguished from acquired torticollis. In the former, the onset is fairly soon (within weeks) after birth and associated problems are rare. Acquired torticollis occurs later and is associated with a range of conditions including acute myositis, brain stem tumors, atlantoaxial subluxation, or infectious causes such as retropharyngeal abscess, cervical adenitis, or tonsillitis.

Cervical Lymphadenopathy

Enlarged cervical lymph nodes occur frequently in the pediatric population, and referral to a surgeon for biopsy is common. The etiology is overwhelmingly infectious; however, it is important to be aware of several other causative factors. Decisions regarding diagnostic testing and therapy are based largely on clinical judgment and should be derived from a thoughtful history and physical examination.[8]

The distribution of enlarged lymph nodes is important, since most healthy children have small, mobile, rubbery palpable lymph nodes in the anterior cervical triangle. On the other hand, nontender, fixed nodes in the supraclavicular region are worrisome for malignancy. Further, concern should be raised regarding nodes that are larger than 2 cm, hard, nontender, and fixed to surrounding structures. Additional concerns for an underlying neoplasm should be raised by a history of weight loss, night sweats, and progressive nodal enlargement.

If a diagnostic lymph node biopsy is indicated, a preoperative chest radiograph should be performed to exclude associated mediastinal adenopathy. If enlarged anterior mediastinal nodes are seen, CT of the chest should be done to determine if there is airway compression. Failure to recognize this preoperatively may result in life-threatening airway obstruction during the induction of general anesthesia. If significant airway compression is seen, every attempt should be made to perform the biopsy under local anesthesia. Since this may not be feasible in some children, preoperative discussion of the CT findings with the anesthesiologist is critical. Anesthetic admonitions for this patient population includes preserving spontaneous ventilation during intubation, induction in the sitting position, securing intravenous access in a lower extremity, and changing the patient's position whenever cardiorespiratory compromise is apparent. Fiberoptic and rigid bronchoscopy, a skilled bronchoscopist, and longer endotracheal tubes must be immediately available.

Patients with acute, bilateral cervical lymphadenitis are usually managed conservatively, since infection with respiratory viruses is so common. These include adenovirus, influenza virus, and respiratory syncytial virus and are often associated with symptoms of cough, rhinorrhea, and sinus congestion. Acute unilateral pyogenic lymphadenitis is caused by *Staphylococcus aureus* and group A *Streptococcus* species in more than 80% of cases. In early cases, an oral antibiotic directed primarily toward gram-positive organ-

isms is indicated. Once the nodes become fluctuant, needle aspiration or incision and drainage will be necessary.

Cat-scratch disease is thought to account for as much as 3% of acute cervical lymphadenopathy and is caused by the organism *Bartonella henselae*. A history of exposure to cats is helpful but not always present. The diagnosis may be made by polymerase chain reaction from nodal tissue. Antibiotic therapy is not recommended because the disease is self-limiting in most cases.

A less common infectious cause for cervical lymphadenitis is nontuberculous *Mycobacteria*. Typically, the nodes are fluctuant, and the overlying skin has a violaceous appearance but is not particularly tender. Occasionally, the nodes drain spontaneously with the formation of mature sinus tracts. The diagnosis is made by positive cultures for nontuberculous acid-fast bacilli together with a positive tuberculin skin test. Since most of the nontuberculous *Mycobacteria* are resistant to conventional chemotherapy, surgical excision is the treatment of choice.[9] Incision and drainage alone is associated with a high rate of recurrence and poor healing of the wound. In contrast with patients with active tuberculous infections, there is no indication for isolation of patients with nontuberculous lymphadenitis.

ALIMENTARY TRACT

Esophageal Atresia and Tracheoesophageal Fistula

Esophageal atresia (EA) is a congenital interruption or discontinuity of the esophagus resulting in esophageal obstruction. Tracheoesophageal fistula (TEF) is an abnormal communication (fistula) between the esophagus and trachea. EA may be present with or without a TEF. Alternatively, a TEF can occur without EA. The incidence and range of anatomic variants are depicted in Figure 70-6.

The prevalence of EA/TEF is 2.6 to 3 per 10,000 births and with a slight male predominance. The etiology of the disturbed embryogenesis is presently unknown. Roughly one third of infants with EA/TEF have low birth weight, and two thirds of infants have associated anomalies. There is a nonrandom, nonhereditary association of anomalies in patients with EA/TEF that must be considered under the acronym VATER (*v*ertebral, *a*norectal, *t*racheal, *e*sophageal, *r*enal or *r*adial limb). Another acronym that is commonly used is VACTERL (*v*ertebral, *a*norectal, *c*ardiac, *t*racheal, *e*sophageal, *r*enal, *l*imb).

The diagnosis of EA should be entertained in an infant with excessive salivation along with coughing or choking during the first oral feeding. A maternal history of polyhydramnios is often present. In a baby with EA and TEF, acute gastric distention may occur due to air entering the distal esophagus and stomach with each inspired breath. Reflux of gastric contents into the distal esophagus traverses the TEF and spills into the trachea, resulting in cough, tachypnea, apnea, or cyanosis. The presentation of isolated TEF without EA may be more subtle and often beyond the newborn period. In general, these infants have choking and coughing associated with oral feeding.

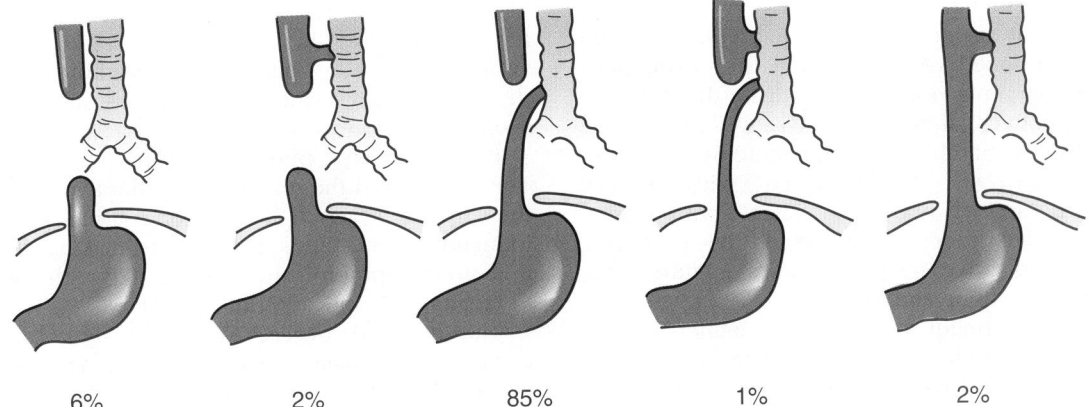

6%   2%   85%   1%   2%

■ FIGURE 70-6. The main anatomic variants and incidence of esophageal atresia and tracheoesophageal fistula.

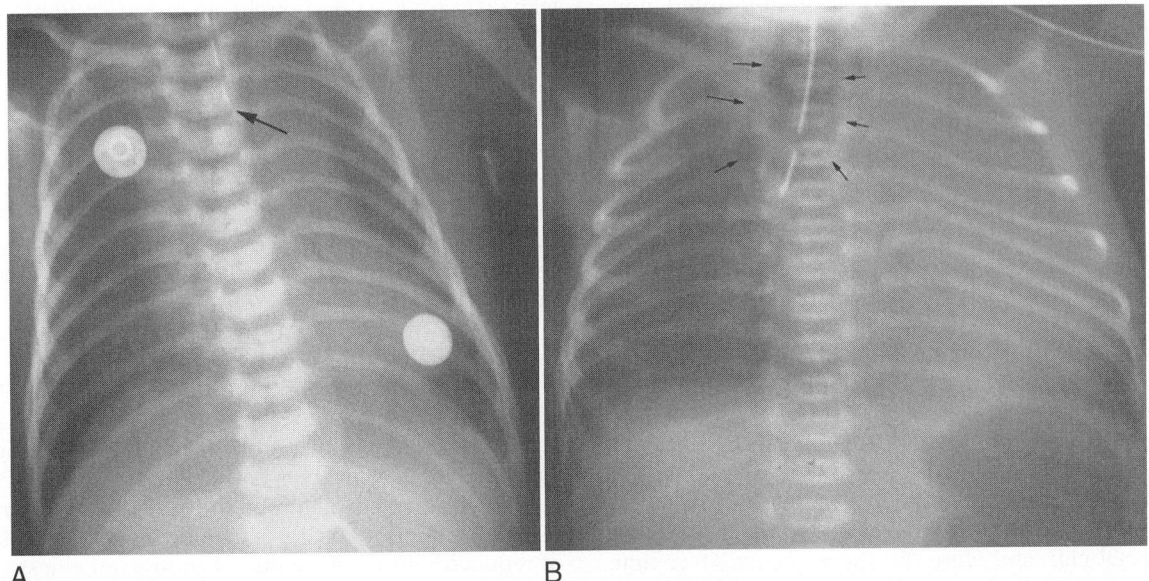

A   B

■ FIGURE 70-7. **A,** Plain chest radiograph of infant with pure esophageal atresia. Note the inability to pass the nasogastric tube *(arrow)* into the stomach and absence of gas within the abdomen. **B,** Plain chest radiograph of infant with esophageal atresia and tracheoesophageal fistula (TEF). The esophageal atresia is suggested by the inability to pass the nasogastric tube into the stomach and the surrounding gas-filled proximal esophagus *(arrows).* The TEF is verified by the presence of gas within the abdomen.

The inability to pass a nasogastric tube into the stomach of the neonate is a cardinal feature for the diagnosis of EA. Inability to pass a nasogastric tube in an infant with absent radiographic evidence for gastrointestinal gas is virtually diagnostic of an isolated EA without TEF (Fig. 70-7A). On the other hand, if gas is present in the gastrointestinal tract below the diaphragm, an associated TEF is confirmed (Fig. 70-7B). These simple rules provide the correct diagnosis in most cases. Occasionally, a small amount of isotonic contrast may be given by mouth to demonstrate the level of the proximal EA pouch and/or the presence of a TEF, but this is rarely necessary. In fact, the risk of aspiration with studies of this type is generally high.

The immediate care of an infant with EA/TEF includes decompression of the proximal EA pouch with a sump-type of tube placed to continuous suction. This prevents spillover of oral secretions into the trachea. The presence of the TEF may be life threatening because positive-pressure ventilation may be inadequate to inflate the lungs, since air is directed into the TEF via the path of least resistance. Ventilation may further be compounded by the resultant gastric distention. In theses circumstances, manipulation of the endotracheal tube distal to the TEF may minimize the leak and permit adequate ventilation. Further, placement of an occlusive balloon (Fogarty) catheter into the fistula via a bronchoscope may be useful. In these cases, performance of a gastrostomy to decompress the distended stomach should be avoided, since it may result in the abrupt inability to ventilate the patient. Finally, urgent thoracotomy with direct ligation of the fistula but without repair of the EA may be required.

In the preoperative period, it is necessary to perform a thorough physical examination, with particular attention to the aforementioned VACTERL anomalies. A preoperative echocardiogram is essential to evaluate the presence or absence of congenital heart disease as well as to define the side of the aortic arch. A right thoracotomy is typically done for the repair of EA/TEF in patients with a normal left-sided aortic arch. However, for infants with a right-sided arch, a left thoracotomy would be preferred. Additional preoperative imaging studies include ultrasonography of the spine and kidneys.

The surgical treatment for the most common EA/TEF involves an extrapleural thoracotomy through the 4th intercostal space. A bronchoscopy should be done prior to the thoracotomy to identify the relative site of the fistula, exclude the presence of a second fistula, and delineate the bronchial anatomy. On the right side, the azygous vein is divided to reveal the underlying TEF. The TEF is dissected circumferentially and then ligated using interrupted, nonabsorbable sutures. The proximal esophageal pouch is then mobilized as high as possible to afford a tension-free esophageal anastomosis. The blood supply to the upper esophageal pouch is generally robust and based on arteries derived from the thyrocervical trunk. On the other hand, the blood supply to the lower esophagus is more tenuous and segmental, originating from intercostal vessels. As such, significant mobilization of the lower esophagus should not be done, so as to avoid ischemia at the site of the esophageal anastomosis. The anastomosis is performed using either a single- or double-layer technique. The rates of anastomotic leak are slightly higher with the single-layer anastomosis, whereas the rates of esophageal stricture are higher with the double-layer technique.

If the two ends of the esophagus cannot be joined without significant tension, there are several options. The first would be to suture the divided end of the distal esophagus to the prevertebral fascia, mark its location with a metal clip, and close the thoracotomy. Over time (2 to 3 months), the proximal esophageal pouch may grow such that a subsequent thoracotomy may permit a primary esophageal anastomosis. A circular or spiral esophagomyotomy[10] of the upper pouch may also be done to gain esophageal length and facilitate a primary anastomosis. Another technique involves placement of traction sutures through the proximal and distal ends of the esophagus and brought out through the chest. These sutures are progressively tightened, and a primary esophageal anastomosis is performed after several days.[11] Alternatively, a cervical esophagostomy may be constructed, and a formal esophageal replacement is performed later.

In patients with pure EA, the gap between the two esophageal ends is frequently wide, thus preventing a primary anastomosis in the newborn period. In these patients, the traditional approach is to perform a cervical esophagostomy for drainage of oral secretions and insertion of a gastrostomy for enteral feeding. An esophageal replacement using the stomach, small intestine, or colon is then performed at about 1 year of age. More recently, it has become apparent that the two ends of the esophagus may spontaneously grow such that a primary anastomosis may be accomplished by 3 months of age.[12] Thus, insertion of a gastrostomy in the neonatal period for feeding may be the only necessary intervention. The swallowing of saliva may actually promote elongation of the upper pouch and an esophagostomy is therefore avoided.

In patients with pure TEF without EA, the site of the TEF is usually in the region of the thoracic inlet. As such, the surgical approach is via a cervical incision. After the induction of anesthesia, but prior to making the incision, it is often helpful to cannulate the TEF with a guide wire to facilitate identification of the TEF.

The mortality of EA/TEF is directly related to the associated anomalies, particularly cardiac defects and chromosomal abnormalities. In the absence of these factors, survival of 90% to 95% is expected.[13] Postoperative complications unique to EA/TEF include esophageal motility disorders, gastroesophageal reflux (GER) (25% to 50%), anastomotic stricture (15% to 30%), anastomotic leak (10% to 20%), and tracheomalacia (8% to 15%).

Gastroesophageal Reflux

Vomiting during infancy is a common occurrence and can be difficult to distinguish from chronic GER that ultimately requires surgical correction. Although the diagnosis and surgical management of GER are similar between adults and children, there are several major differences that must be understood.

Although the symptoms of GER can often be obtained easily in adults, the recognition of symptoms in young children may be more subtle. Rather than complain of heartburn, children with significant GER tend to associate pain with eating. As such, they may be irritable during or after feeding or limit their formula intake altogether. This may be identified by failure to thrive (FTT). Another cause of FTT in infants with GER is the nutritional consequences of reduced caloric intake due to protracted emesis. Other unique symptoms include life-threatening episodes of apnea termed *near-miss sudden infant death syndrome* (SIDS). In a child with documented GER, an episode of near-miss SIDS is an absolute indication for antireflux surgery. Respiratory symptoms of GER in children may manifest as chronic cough, hoarseness, recurrent pneumonias, or asthma. Persistent asthma may be due to GER in up to 75% of children, a significant proportion who have no other apparent symptoms of GER.[14]

Many children referred for antireflux surgery are neurologically impaired, usually secondary to factors such as metabolic conditions, head trauma, and birth asphyxia. As such, most of these patients require permanent feeding access in the form of a gastrostomy tube. Thus, antireflux surgery is often entertained at the time of the gastrostomy tube insertion, especially in patients who are unable to reliably protect their airway or who already have significant vomiting associated with intragastric tube feeding.

The evaluation of the child with GER involves several studies, each designed to provide different information. The initial study includes an upper gastrointestinal (UGI) radiographic series. The UGI does not correlate well with the presence or absence of GER but is important to exclude other causes of vomiting in children. These would include malrotation, antral web, foregut duplication cysts, and pyloric or duodenal stenosis. The gold standard test for delineating pathologic from physiologic GER is continuous (18- to 24-hour) esophageal pH monitoring.[15] Risk assessment for the development of esophagitis can be derived from a reflux index, which takes into account the percentage of time the lower esophageal pH is less than 4. A reflux index of greater than 11% in infants up to 1 year or greater than 6% in older children is considered pathologic. The limitation of this study is that it nicely delineates risk for acid injury to the esophagus but may fail to detect pathologic GER in patients who have symptoms related to pulmonary aspiration. In these circumstances, the episode of reflux may be of sufficient magnitude to cause pneumonia or bronchospasm, but cleared efficiently from the esophagus so as to be interpreted as normal. Nuclear scintigraphy involves labeling food or formula with a radioisotope and then measuring the number of postprandial episodes of GER and aspiration events. The advantages of this technique include the ability to identify nonacid GER events and to quantitate gastric emptying. A drawback is that it is extremely sensitive and therefore is unable to distinguish between pathologic and nonpathologic GER. Further, the normative data for the pediatric population are lacking. Finally, endoscopic visualization of the esophagus, larynx, and trachea all are complementary studies to confirm the presence of acid injury.

Nonoperative measures to reduce GER include thickening of formula with cereal, reducing the volume of feeding, and postural maneuvers. In addition, pharmacologic acid suppression may be useful. Indications for surgical intervention include severe GER that is unresponsive to aggressive medical management. In addition, surgery is generally warranted in patients with life-threatening near-miss SIDS episodes, FTT, or esophageal stricture. Other relative indications include those requiring complex surgical airway reconstruction,[16] patients with neurologic impairment requiring permanent feeding access, or a history of recurrent pneumonias or persistent asthma.

As in adults, multiple operations have been designed for children with GER. The gold standard procedure remains the Nissen fundoplication. In the pediatric population, this can be done open or laparoscopically[17] with similar results. In severely neurologically impaired patients, a complete esophagogastric disconnection with Roux-en-Y esophagojejunostomy has been proposed.[18] This procedure is certainly definitive but may be associated with significant perioperative morbidity.

The overall results for anti-reflux surgery in children are excellent. The risk for recurrent GER and other morbidity are highest in the neurologically impaired population[19] and the presence of chronic cough associated with severe underlying lung disease.

Hypertrophic Pyloric Stenosis

Hypertrophic pyloric stenosis (HPS) is one of the most common gastrointestinal disorders during early infancy, with an incidence of 1:3000 to 4000 live births. This condition is most common between the ages of 2 and 8 weeks. In HPS, hypertrophy of the circular muscle of the pylorus results in constriction and obstruction of the gastric outlet. Gastric outlet obstruction leads to nonbilious, projectile emesis, loss of hydrochloric acid with the development of hypochloremic, metabolic alkalosis, and ultimate dehydration. The treatment of this condition is by surgical mechanical distraction of the pyloric ring. There is currently no place for medical management of HPS.

The cause for pyloric stenosis is unknown because multiple factors have been implicated. Ethnic origin is important as the highest incidence is found among whites of Scandinavian decent and lowest risk in African Americans and Chinese. Males outnumber females in every series by a ratio of 4 to 5:1. There is a higher risk for developing HPS in offspring of parents with this condition, and in many series, firstborn males are frequently encountered.

The clinical presentation of infants with HPS present is projectile and/or frequent episodes of *nonbilious* emesis. Occasionally, the vomitus may be brown or blood-streaked but it is always nonbilious. Visible gastric peristalsis may be seen as a wave of contraction from the left upper quadrant to the epigastrium. The infants usually feed vigorously between episodes of vomiting.

Palpation of the pyloric tumor (also called the *olive*) in the epigastrium or right upper quadrant by a skilled examiner is pathognomonic for the diagnosis of HPS. If the olive is palpated, no additional diagnostic testing is necessary. The sensitivity of the clinical examination alone appears to range from 72% to 74%, the positive predictive value ranges from 98% and 99.3%, and the specificity is 97%.[20]

When the olive cannot be palpated, the diagnosis of HPS can be made with an ultrasound examination or fluoroscopic UGI series. These imaging tests are similar in terms of sensitivity and specificity for the diagnosis of HPS. The UGI series is useful for the evaluation of other causes of vomiting, whereas the absence of radiation exposure and cost make the ultrasound the usual preferred study. A persistent pyloric muscle thickness more than 3 to 4 mm or pyloric length longer than 15 to 18 mm in the presence of functional gastric outlet obstruction is generally considered to be diagnostic.[21]

The treatment of HPS is by a pyloromyotomy. This consists of cutting across the abnormal pyloric musculature while preserving the underlying mucosa (Fig. 70-8). This can be done through a traditional right upper quadrant incision, through a periumbilical incision, or laparoscopically. Prior to surgery, it is important that the infant is hydrated with intravenous fluids to establish a normal urine output. It is important that the underlying metabolic alkalosis is slowly corrected with normal saline. Potassium should not be given until the intravascular volume has been restored and normal urine output has resumed. Since the infant with underlying metabolic alkalosis compensates with respiratory acidosis, postoperative apnea may occur. Thus, the serum bicarbonate level should be normalized prior to surgery.

Postoperatively, infants are usually allowed to resume enteral feedings. Vomiting after surgery occurs frequently

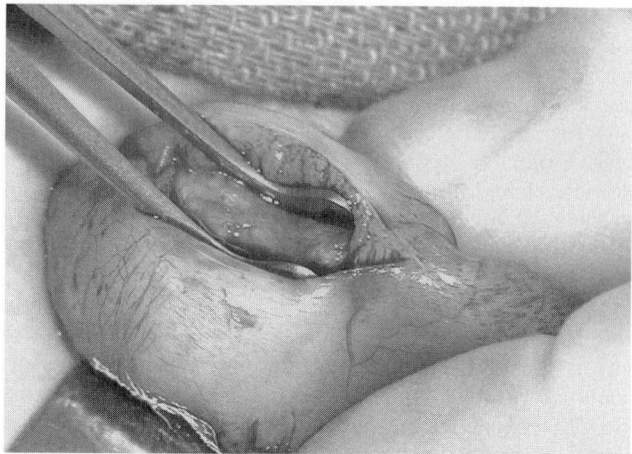

FIGURE 70-8. Pyloromyotomy for hypertrophic pyloric stenosis. The thickened pyloric musculature has been cut and then spread apart to reveal the underlying mucosa.

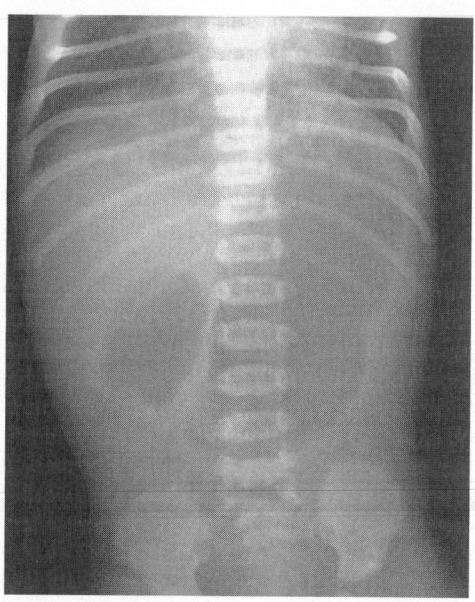

FIGURE 70-9. Plain abdominal radiograph demonstrating the typical double-bubble appearance of duodenal atresia. The large gas-filled stomach is visualized along with the dilated proximal duodenum. There is no gas beyond the duodenum.

but is usually self-limited. Complications specific to the pyloromyotomy include incomplete myotomy; mucosal perforation, usually at the duodenal end; or wound infection. These complications may be slightly higher when the incision is made in the umbilicus.[22]

Intestinal Atresia

Duodenal Atresia

In contrast with more distal intestinal atresias, duodenal atresia (DA) is believed to occur as a result of failure of vacuolization of the duodenum from its solid cord stage. The range of anatomic variants includes duodenal stenosis, mucosal web with intact muscular wall ("windsock" deformity), two ends separated by a fibrous cord, or complete separation with a gap within the duodenum.

DA is associated with several conditions, including prematurity, Down syndrome, maternal polyhydramnios, malrotation, annular pancreas, and biliary atresia (BA). Other anomalies such as cardiac, renal, esophageal, and anorectal are also frequent. In most, the duodenal obstruction is distal to the ampulla of Vater and infants present with bilious emesis in the neonatal period. In patients with a mucosal web, the symptoms of postprandial emesis may occur later in life.

The classic plain abdominal radiograph of DA is termed the *double-bubble sign* (air-filled stomach and duodenal bulb) (Fig. 70-9). In cases whereby there is no distal air, the diagnosis is secured and no further studies are necessary. On the other hand, if distal air is present, a UGI contrast study should be performed fairly rapidly. This study is important not only to confirm the diagnosis of duodenal stenosis or atresia but also to exclude midgut volvulus, which would constitute a surgical emergency.

The treatment of DA is by surgical bypass of the duodenal obstruction as either a side-to-side or proximal transverse to distal longitudinal (diamond-shaped) duo-

denoduodenostomy. When the proximal duodenum is markedly dilated, a tapering duodenoplasty may be performed to reduce the duodenal caliber and may improve postoperative gastric emptying. In patients with a duodenal mucosal web, the web is excised transduodenally. The ampulla is often associated with the web itself and must therefore be identified and preserved during the web excision.

Jejunoileal Atresia

Although several mechanisms have been proposed to explain the findings of jejunoileal atresia (JIA), the prevailing theory is that of an intrauterine focal mesenteric vascular accident. The spectrum of gross pathologic findings includes simple stenosis, complete interruption of the intestinal lumen with or without a fibrous cord attached to the distal bowel, a missing segment of bowel and mesentery, or multiple atresias. One final type is referred to as the "apple peel" or "Christmas tree" deformity (Fig. 70-10). This atresia is unique from the standpoint that the obstruction is usually in the proximal jejunum, which is supplied by the entire superior mesenteric artery (SMA). There is then a gap in the mesentery and the remainder of the small intestine is coiled around the ileocolic branch of the SMA, which is perfused retrograde from the middle colic artery. This tenuous blood supply has obvious implications for reanastomosis and the potential for ischemic necrosis due to an antenatal volvulus. As such, many of these infants with this type of atresia are born with reduced intestinal length.

The clinical presentation is typically dependent on the level of obstruction. In proximal atresia, abdominal

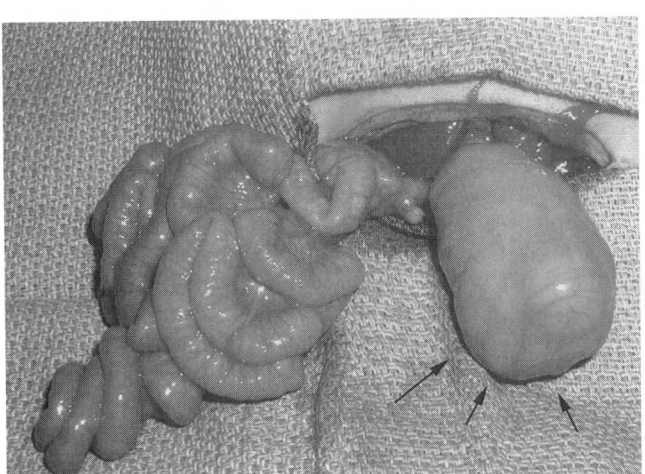

FIGURE 70-10. Proximal jejunal atresia of the "apple peel" or "Christmas tree" variant. The dilated proximal jejunum *(arrows)* is supplied by the superior mesenteric artery (SMA). There is a gap in the mesentery, and the remainder of the small intestine is coiled around the ileocolic branch of the SMA, which is perfused retrograde from the middle colic artery.

distention is less frequent and bilious emesis is usually present. Plain abdominal radiographs typically reveal air-fluid levels with absent distal gas. If the atresia is distal, abdominal distention may be present. A preoperative barium enema may be useful to exclude multiple atresias, which may be present in 10% to 15% of cases. In contrast with DA, JIA is usually not associated with other anomalies. One exception is cystic fibrosis (CF), which may be present in roughly 10% of cases.

The treatment of JIA is to re-establish intestinal continuity. In the presence of multiple atresias, it is imperative to preserve as much intestinal length as possible. This may require multiple anastomoses over an endoluminal stent. If the proximal intestine is significantly dilated, peristalsis will be perturbed. As such, a tapering enteroplasty of the dilated bowel should be performed if the remnant intestinal length is short. On the other hand, the dilated bowel should be resected if the remnant small bowel length is normal. The overall survival for infants with JIA atresia should be higher than 90%[23] and unrelated to the type of atresia encountered. The most significant associated morbidity is the short gut syndrome.

Anomalies of Intestinal Rotation/Fixation

Most intestinal rotation and fixation abnormalities become clinically evident during infancy and childhood. The true incidence of rotational anomalies of the midgut is difficult to determine and has been reported to occur with a frequency of 1 in 6000 live births. An understanding of the embryology of the intestine is essential in the recognition and appropriate surgical management of these conditions.

The midgut normally herniates out of the abdominal cavity through the umbilical ring at approximately the 4th week of development in all human fetuses. By the 10th week of gestation, the intestine returns to the abdominal cavity and rotates around the axis of the SMA for 270 degrees in a counterclockwise direction. The final position of the ligament of Treitz is in the left upper quadrant and the cecum in the right lower quadrant of the abdomen. Interruption or reversal of any of these coordinated movements permits an embryologic explanation for the range of anomalies that are seen.

Complete nonrotation of the midgut is the most frequently encountered anomaly and occurs when neither the duodenojejunal limb nor the cecocolic limb undergo rotation. As a result, there is no duodenal C loop and the ligament of Treitz is located on the right side of the abdomen. Likewise, the cecum has failed to rotate and is present in the left side of the abdomen. In nonrotation, the proximal jejunum and ascending colon are fused together as one pedicle, through which the blood supply to the entire midgut (SMA) is located. It is this pedicle on which a midgut volvulus occurs, leading to ischemic necrosis of the entire midgut.

Nonrotation of the duodenojejunal limb followed by normal rotation and fixation of the cecocolic limb results in duodenal obstruction due to mesenteric (Ladd's) bands originating from the colon and extending over the duodenum to end in the retroperitoneum. In this situation, a midgut volvulus is less likely, since the base of the mesentery is relatively wide and fixed to the posterior abdomen. Duodenal obstruction from Ladd's bands is usually heralded by bilious emesis. Several other abnormalities are possible with any combination of incomplete, absent, or reverse rotation of the duodenojejunal limb followed by varied rotation patterns of the cecocolic limb.

Rotational anomalies may manifest clinically in several different ways: however, the main symptom complexes may be grouped together as those related to volvulus, duodenal obstruction, or intermittent or chronic abdominal pain or as an incidental finding in an otherwise asymptomatic patient. Most patients develop symptoms during the first month of life.

Midgut volvulus is a true surgical emergency since delay in operative correction is associated with a high risk of intestinal necrosis and subsequent death. The sudden appearance of bilious emesis in a newborn is the classic presentation. Although bilious emesis is most often due to other causes, it is critical to exclude midgut volvulus. Once clinical signs of intestinal compromise begin to appear, the ability to salvage the patient or any significant length of small bowel may be gone.

Midgut volvulus may also be incomplete or intermittent. Patients may complain of chronic abdominal pain or have intermittent episodes of emesis (which may be nonbilious), early satiety, weight loss, FTT, or malabsorption/diarrhea. With partial volvulus, the resultant mesenteric venous and lymphatic obstruction may impair nutrient absorption and produce protein loss into the gut lumen as well as mucosal ischemia and melena as a result of arterial insufficiency.

The preoperative evaluation of a child with a suspected rotational anomaly of the intestine should include plain abdominal radiographs and a UGI contrast series. Occasionally, plain abdominal radiographs may reveal evidence for intestinal obstruction; however, the most common findings are nonspecific. The UGI contrast series remains the gold standard for the diagnosis. A key element for the diagnosis of rotational abnormalities of the intestine is the position of the ligament of Treitz. This should normally be located to the left of midline and at the level of the gastric antrum. In the presence of a volvulus, the site of obstruction is usually the third portion of the duodenum and has the appearance of a "bird's beak."

In the acutely ill child with midgut volvulus/obstruction, urgent operative correction is indicated and little time should be needed for intravenous fluid resuscitation, placement of a nasogastric tube and Foley catheter, type and crossmatch for blood, and administration of broad-spectrum antibiotics. Time is critical in terms of intestinal salvage.

The operative management for most rotational anomalies of the intestine is Ladd's procedure. On entering the peritoneal cavity, the entire bowel should be immediately exposed. If a volvulus is encountered, in most cases the volvulus twists in a clockwise direction; thus, it should be untwisted in a counterclockwise manner ("turning back the hand's of time"). After detorsion, the intestine may be congested and edematous, and some areas may appear necrotic. Placement of warm sponges and observation for awhile may improve the appearance of the intestine when the vascular integrity has been compromised. If areas of the bowel are obviously necrotic, resection with creation of a stoma(s) is performed. Since it is imperative to preserve as much intestine as possible, marginal or questionable segments of bowel should be left in place and a second-look procedure performed within 24 to 36 hours. Next, Ladd's bands are divided as they extend from the ascending colon across the duodenum and attach to the posterior aspect of the right upper quadrant. To prevent extramural compression of the duodenum and recurrent obstruction, the bands must be lysed completely on both lateral and medial aspects of the duodenum. In dividing the medial bands, the distance between the duodenum and ascending colon is increased. Broadening this mesenteric base reduces the tendency of the bowel to volvulize. There has been no demonstrated benefit to pexing the cecum or duodenum to the abdominal wall. In neonates, a balloon catheter may be passed through the mouth and advanced beyond the pylorus into the distal duodenum to exclude an intraluminal obstruction. An incidental appendectomy is then performed since the cecum will ultimately lie on the left side of the abdomen after this procedure. The intestine should be replaced into the abdominal cavity with the small bowel lying entirely on the right side while the colon is positioned on the left.

Recurrent volvulus is relatively infrequent but should be of prime concern in patients presenting with obstructive symptoms at any time postoperatively. More commonly, the cause for postoperative obstruction is adhesive bands. Gastrointestinal motility disturbances are also frequent. Midgut volvulus accounts for roughly 18% of cases of short gut syndrome in the pediatric population. Urgent recognition and management are the most important factors in preventing this complication.

Necrotizing Enterocolitis

Necrotizing enterocolitis (NEC) is the most common gastrointestinal emergency in the neonatal period. Prematurity is the single most important risk factor, although other factors such as ischemia, bacteria, cytokines, and enteral feeding all are likely significant. The advent of exogenous surfactant and improved methods of mechanical ventilation are contributing to greater numbers of premature infants at risk for developing NEC. Despite the tremendous impact of NEC on neonatal morbidity and mortality, progress in understanding this condition is hampered by the fact that a reliable animal model for NEC does not exist.

The development of NEC is unusual in the first few days of life. Approximately 80% of cases occur, however, within the first month of life. The clinical presentation of NEC is often nonspecific and unpredictable. Clinical signs include irritability, temperature instability, poor feeding, or episodes of apnea or bradycardia. More specific signs include abdominal distention, vomiting, feeding intolerance, or passage of a bloody stool. As NEC progresses, systemic sepsis develops, with cardiorespiratory deterioration, coagulopathy, and death. The radiographic hallmark of NEC is pneumatosis intestinalis (Fig. 70-11). Pneumatosis is comprised of hydrogen gas generated by bacterial fermentation of luminal substrates. Other radiographic findings may include portal venous gas, ascites, fixed loops of small bowel, or free air. The distal ileum and ascending colon are the usual sites affected, although the entire gastrointestinal tract (NEC totalis) may also be involved.

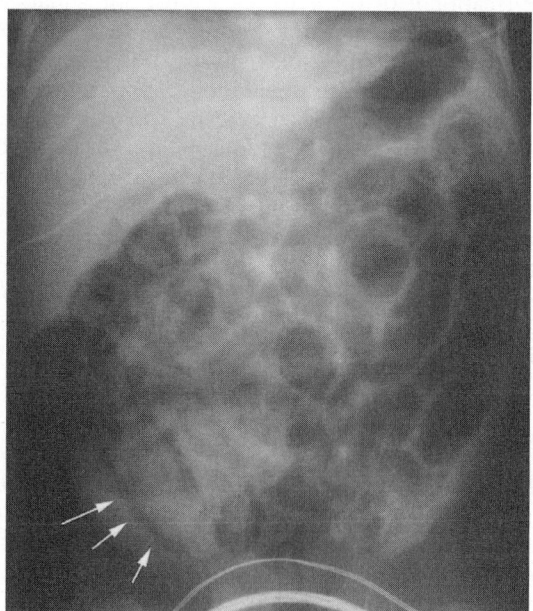

■ FIGURE 70-11. Plain abdominal radiograph of an infant with necrotizing enterocolitis demonstrating diffuse pneumatosis intestinalis. In addition to the typical "ground glass" appearance, linear gas corresponding with the submucosal plane of the bowel wall is easily visualized *(arrows)*.

Once the diagnosis of NEC has been established, initial management consists of bowel rest with nasogastric tube decompression, fluid resuscitation, blood and/or platelet transfusion, and administration of broad-spectrum antibiotics. Medical management continues for 7 to 10 days and is successful in about 50% of cases. The absolute indication for operative management of NEC is the presence of intestinal perforation as revealed by the identification of free air on plain abdominal radiographs. Other relative indications for surgery include overall clinical deterioration, abdominal wall cellulitis, worsening acidosis, falling white blood cell or platelet count, palpable abdominal mass, or a persistent fixed loop on repeated abdominal radiographs. The decision to proceed with surgery can be difficult and must be weighed against the risks of laparotomy in an already compromised premature infant.

The general principles of surgical management of NEC include resection of all nonviable segments of intestine with creation of a stoma. All efforts should be made to preserve as much intestinal length as possible. As such, it may be necessary to resect multiple sites of necrotic bowel, preserve intervening segments of viable intestine, and create multiple stomas. In cases where the bowel is ischemic, but not frankly necrotic, a second-look operation may be performed after 24 hours. Bowel resection with primary reanastomosis may be considered in the rare infant with focal involvement of NEC, with minimal peritoneal contamination, and who is stable in the operating room. The risks for anastomotic leak and stricture formation have tempered widespread enthusiasm for this approach.

Another, more recent operative approach to the management of the infant with NEC whose intestine has perforated is bedside placement of peritoneal drains under local anesthesia. Drainage of the contaminated peritoneal fluid may improve ventilation and halt the progression of sepsis in select very ill, preterm infants. Surprisingly, drainage of the peritoneum may be the only necessary intervention in a few patients. The data to support peritoneal drainage as an accepted mode of treatment for NEC are currently sparse and are the subject of an ongoing multicenter trial.

The overall mortality from surgically managed NEC ranges from 10% to 50%. NEC is currently the single most common cause of the short gut syndrome in children.[24] Intestinal strictures may develop after either medical or surgical management of NEC in about 10% of infants. The most common site for involvement is the splenic flexure of the colon. Because of the risk for stricture, a radiographic contrast study of the distal intestine should be done prior to elective stoma closure. Neurodevelopmental delay is also a frequent long-term problem in these infants.

Meconium Syndromes

The meconium syndromes of infancy represent a complex group of gastrointestinal conditions associated with CF, with considerable overlap in clinical presentation and management. CF results from a mutation within the cystic fibrosis transmembrane regulator *(CFTR)* gene and is autosomal recessive. Therefore, both parents must be carriers. It is estimated that 3.3% of whites in the United States are asymptomatic carriers of the mutated CF gene. The abnormal chloride transport in patients with CF results in tenacious, viscous secretions affecting a wide variety of organs, including the intestine, pancreas, lungs, salivary glands, reproductive organs, and biliary tract. The clinical presentation of the meconium syndromes ranges from a meconium plug to simple and complicated meconium ileus.

Meconium Plug

Meconium plug syndrome is a frequent cause of neonatal intestinal obstruction and associated with multiple conditions including Hirschsprung's disease, maternal diabetes, hypothyroidism, and CF. Although most children with meconium plug syndrome are normal, further studies to exclude Hirschsprung's disease and CF are warranted. Typically, affected infants are often preterm and present with signs and symptoms of distal intestinal obstruction. Abdominal distention is a prominent feature. Plain abdominal radiographs reveal multiple dilated loops of intestine. The diagnostic and therapeutic procedure of choice is a water-soluble contrast enema. This often results in the passage of a plug of meconium and relief of the obstruction (Fig. 70-12).

Simple Meconium Ileus

Meconium ileus in the newborn represents the earliest clinical manifestation of CF and affects about 15% of patients with this inherited disease. In North America, virtually all white neonates with meconium ileus have CF. In simple meconium ileus; the terminal ileum is dilated and filled with thick, tarlike, inspissated meconium. Smaller

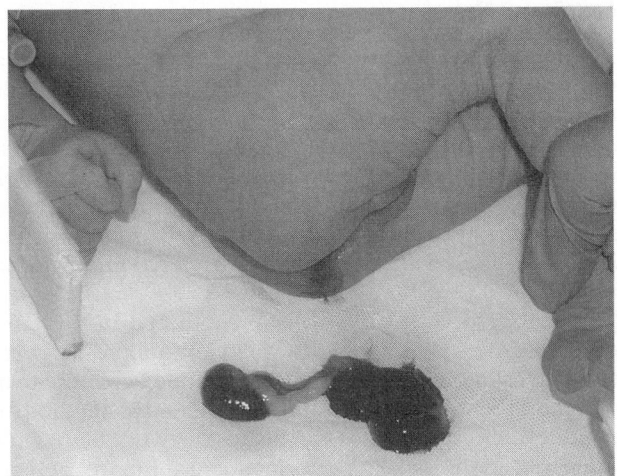

■ FIGURE 70-12. Meconium plug. This plug of meconium was passed following a contrast enema performed in an infant with abdominal distention and obstipation for 48 hours. After passage of the plug, the infant began to stool normally.

pellets of meconium are found in the more distal ileum leading into a relatively small colon. In patients with simple meconium ileus, important plain abdominal radiographic findings include dilated, gas-filled loops of small bowel, absence of air-fluid levels, and a mass of meconium within the right side of the abdomen mixed with gas to give a "ground glass" or "soap bubble" appearance.

The initial diagnostic study of choice is a contrast enema using water-soluble, ionic contrast solution. Gastrografin is probably the most frequently used.[25] Since the contrast agents are typically hypertonic relative to serum, it is important that the infants are well hydrated and electrolytes and vital signs are carefully monitored following the procedure. It is important that the contrast medium reach the ileum into the area of inspissated meconium. This is successful in relieving the obstruction in up to 75% of cases, with a bowel perforation rate of less than 3%.

The operative management of simple meconium ileus is required when the obstruction cannot be relieved with contrast enema. Historically, the dilated terminal ileum was resected and various types of stomas were created. This allowed for a very sick neonate to recover who would have otherwise died. More recently, simple evacuation of the luminal meconium without the need to create a stoma is all that is necessary in most cases. This is accomplished via open laparotomy, and a small enterotomy is made in the dilated terminal ileum. A red rubber catheter is used to irrigate the proximal and distal bowel with either warmed saline solution or 4% N-acetylcysteine. The latter solution serves to break the disulfide bonds within the meconium and facilitate separation from the bowel mucosa. The meconium is either manipulated into the distal colon or removed through the enterotomy, with care taken to avoid peritoneal contamination. Once the obstruction is relieved, the procedure is concluded by closure of the enterotomy in two layers. In cases where the meconium evacuation is incomplete, a T tube may be left in place within the ileum to facilitate continued postoperative irrigation.

Complicated Meconium Ileus

Meconium ileus is considered complicated when perforation of the intestine has taken place. This may occur in utero or the early neonatal period. Meconium within the peritoneal cavity results in severe peritonitis with a dense inflammatory response and calcification. The presentation of complicated meconium ileus is variable and includes formation of a meconium pseudocyst, adhesive peritonitis with or without secondary bacterial infection, or ascites.

The diagnosis of CF is usually confirmed in the postoperative period. The pilocarpine iontophoresis sweat test revealing a chloride concentration greater than 60 mEq/L is the most reliable and definitive method to confirm the diagnosis of CF. This test may not be reliable in infants and is usually performed later. A more immediate test includes detection of the mutated CFTR gene. This test, coupled with a careful family history and clinical presentation, permits confirmation of the diagnosis in most infants.

The long-term outcome of patients with CF with or without meconium ileus is probably not different, although gastrointestinal complications continue throughout life. A meconium ileus equivalent (distal ileal obstructive syndrome) may develop as a consequence of noncompliance with oral enzyme replacement therapy or bouts of dehydration. This is managed nonoperatively in most patients with enemas and/or oral polyethylene glycol purging solutions. Other diagnoses must also be considered, including simple adhesive intestinal obstruction. Further, with the introduction of enteric-coated, high-strength pancreatic enzyme replacement therapy, a fibrosing cholangiopathy has been described. Resection of the inflammatory colon stricture may be necessary.

Intussusception

Intussusception is the telescoping of one portion of the intestine into the other and is the most common cause of intestinal obstruction in early childhood. In most pediatric intussusceptions, the cause is unknown, the location is at the ileocecal junction, and there is no identifiable pathologic lead point. Invariably, there is marked swelling of the lymphoid tissue within the region of the ileocecal valve. It is unknown as to whether this represents the cause or the effect of the intussusception. Evidence to implicate a role for lymphoid swelling in the pathogenesis of intussusception is suggested by the association of this condition with a history of recent episodes of viral gastroenteritis, upper respiratory infections, and recently, administration of rotavirus vaccine.

The incidence of a pathologic lead point is up to 12% in most pediatric series and increases directly with age. The most common lead point for intussusception is a Meckel's diverticulum; however, other causes must be considered including polyps, the appendix, intestinal neoplasm, submucosal hemorrhage associated with Henoch-Schönlein purpura, foreign body, ectopic pancreatic or gastric tissue, and intestinal duplication. Intussusception may also occur within the small bowel in the absence of a lead point in children who undergo abdominal surgery for a variety of reasons. This diagnosis should be entertained in a child with crampy abdominal pain and emesis in the early postoperative period.

Intussusception classically produces severe, cramping abdominal pain in an otherwise healthy child. The child often draws his or her legs up during the pain episodes and is usually quiet during the intervening periods. After some time, the child becomes lethargic. Vomiting is almost universal. Although frequent bowel movements may occur with the onset of pain, the progression of the obstruction results in bowel ischemia with passage of dark blood clots mixed with mucus, commonly referred to as "currant jelly" stool. An abdominal mass may be palpated.

In about half of cases, the diagnosis of intussusception can be suspected on plain abdominal radiographs. Suggestive radiographic abnormalities include the presence of a mass, sparse gas within the colon, or complete distal small bowel obstruction. In cases where there is a low index of suspicion for intussusception based on clinical findings, an abdominal ultrasound may be the initial diagnostic test. The characteristic sonographic findings of intussusception include the "target" of the intussuscepted layers of bowel on transverse view or the "pseudokidney" sign when seen longitudinally.

When the clinical index of suspicion for intussusception is high, hydrostatic reduction by contrast agent or air enema is the diagnostic and therapeutic procedure of choice. Contraindications to this study include the presence of peritonitis or hemodynamic instability. Further, an intussusception that is located entirely within the small intestine is unlikely to be reached by enema and more likely to have an associated lead point. Hydrostatic reduction using barium has been the mainstay of therapy; however, more recently, the use of air enema has become more widespread. Successful reduction is accomplished in more than 80% of cases and is confirmed by resolution of the mass, along with reflux of air into the proximal ileum. To avoid radiation exposure altogether, intussusception reduction by saline enema under ultrasound surveillance may be employed. Recurrence rates after hydrostatic reduction are about 11% and usually occur within the first 24 hours. Recurrence is usually managed by another attempt at hydrostatic reduction. A third recurrence is usually an indication for operative management.

The indications for operation in patients with intussusception include the presence of peritonitis and/or a clinical examination consistent with necrotic bowel. The presence of complete small bowel obstruction, small bowel location, failure of hydrostatic complete reduction, or history of several recurrences should also direct surgical intervention. Laparoscopy may be useful as a first step to confirm the presence of an incompletely reduced intussusception and to facilitate reduction, thus avoiding a larger incision.[26] The intussusceptum is delivered through a transverse incision in the right side of the abdomen and reduced by squeezing the mass retrograde from distal to proximal until completely reduced. Warm laparotomy pads may be placed over the bowel, and a period of observation may be warranted in cases of questionable bowel viability. Adhesive bands around the ileocecal junction are divided, and an appendectomy is then performed. Invariably, the lymphoid tissue within the ileocecal valve region is thickened and edematous and may be mistaken for a tumor within the small bowel. Experience with this condition may prevent an unnecessary bowel resection. The recurrence rates are quite low following surgical reduction. Bowel resection is required in cases when the intussusception cannot be reduced, the viability of the bowel is uncertain, or if a lead point is identified. An ileocolectomy with primary reanastomosis is the usual procedure performed.

Hirschsprung's Disease

Hirschsprung's disease occurs in 1:5000 live births and is characterized pathologically by absent ganglion cells in the myenteric (Auerbach's) and submucosal (Meissner's) plexus. This neurogenic abnormality is associated with muscular spasm of the distal colon and internal anal sphincter resulting in a functional obstruction. Hence, the abnormal bowel is the contracted, distal segment, whereas the normal bowel is the proximal, dilated portion. The area between the dilated and contracted segments is referred to as the *transition zone*. In this area, ganglion cells begin to appear, but in reduced numbers. The aganglionosis always involves the distal rectum and extends proximally for variable distances. The rectosigmoid is affected in about 75% of cases, splenic flexure or transverse colon in 17%, and the entire colon with variable extension into the small bowel in 8%. The risk for Hirschsprung's disease is greater if there is a positive family history and in patients with Down syndrome.

In most, infants are symptomatic within the first 24 hours of life with progressive abdominal distention and bilious emesis. Failure to pass meconium in the first 24 hours is highly significant and a cardinal feature of this condition. In some infants, diarrhea may develop due to the presence of enterocolitis. The diagnosis of Hirschsprung's disease may also be overlooked for prolonged periods. In these cases, older children may present with a history of poor feeding, chronic abdominal distention, and a history of significant constipation. Since constipation is a frequent problem among normal children, referral for surgical biopsy to exclude Hirschsprung's disease is relatively frequent. Enterocolitis is the most common cause of death in patients with uncorrected Hirschsprung's disease and may present with diarrhea alternating with periods of obstipation, abdominal distention, fevers, hematochezia, and peritonitis.

The initial diagnostic step in a newborn with radiographic evidence for a distal bowel obstruction is a barium enema. Prior to this study, rectal examination and enemas should be avoided so as not to interfere with the identification of a transition zone. In a normal barium enema study, the rectum is wider than the sigmoid colon. In patients with Hirschsprung's disease, spasm of the distal rectum usually results in a smaller caliber when compared with the more proximal sigmoid colon. Identification of a transition zone may be quite helpful (Fig. 70-13); however, determination of the location of the transition zone is considered to be relatively inaccurate. Failure to completely evacuate the instilled contrast material after 24 hours would also be consistent with Hirschsprung's disease and may provide additional diagnostic yield. An important goal of this study is to exclude other causes of constipation in the newborn such as meconium plug, small left colon syndrome, and atresia.

Anorectal manometry may also suggest the diagnosis of Hirschsprung's disease. The classic finding is failure of the internal sphincter to relax when the rectum is distended with a balloon. The advantage of this method is that it can be done in an outpatient setting, without the need for general anesthesia. This is more often useful in an older patient and is seldom used in neonates.

A rectal biopsy is the gold standard for the diagnosis of Hirschsprung's disease. In the newborn period, this is done at the bedside with minimal morbidity using a special suction rectal biopsy instrument. It is important to obtain the sample at least 2 cm above the dentate line so as to avoid sampling the normal transition from ganglion-

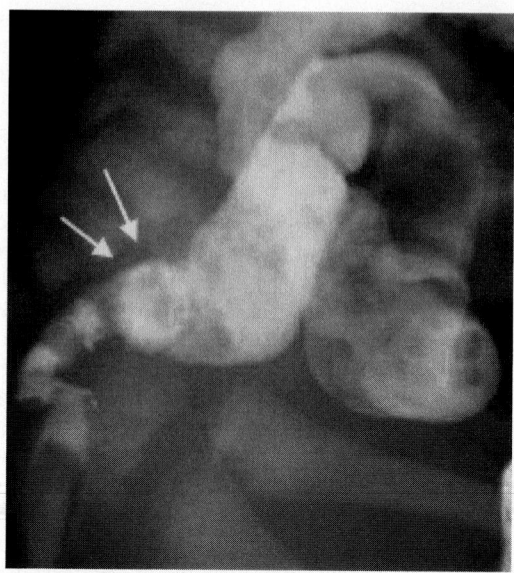

FIGURE 70-13. Hirschsprung's disease. A barium enema demonstrating the zone of transition *(arrows)* from the dilated proximal normal colon to the reduced caliber of the distal aganglionic colon.

ated bowel to the paucity or absence of ganglia in the region of the internal sphincter. In older children, because the rectal mucosa is thicker, a full-thickness biopsy should be obtained under general anesthesia. Absent ganglia, hypertrophied nerve trunks, and robust immunostaining for acetylcholinesterase are the pathologic criteria to make the diagnosis.

Multiple surgical options exist for the management of Hirschsprung's disease. Traditionally, a leveling procedure is done, followed by proximal diversion. This consists of a formal laparotomy, which is usually performed through a small incision in the left lower quadrant of the abdomen. The location of the transition zone is then identified and confirmed by multiple seromuscular biopsies. A diverting colostomy is then performed in the region of normal ganglionated bowel. A definitive procedure is performed later.

The definitive management of Hirschsprung's disease involves variations among three main procedures. In the Swenson procedure, the aganglionic bowel is removed down to the level of the internal sphincters and a coloanal anastomosis is performed on the perineum. In the Duhamel procedure, the aganglionic rectal stump is left in place and the ganglionated, normal colon is pulled behind this stump. A GIA stapler is then inserted through the anus with one arm within the normal, ganglionated bowel posteriorly and the other in the aganglionic rectum anteriorly. Firing of the stapler therefore results in formation of a neorectum that empties normally, due to the posterior patch of ganglionated bowel. Finally, the Soave technique involves an endorectal mucosal dissection within the aganglionic distal rectum. The normally ganglionated colon is then pulled through the remnant mus-

cular cuff and a coloanal anastomosis is performed. More recently, the Soave procedure has been performed in the newborn period as a primary procedure and without an initial ostomy.[27] Further, the same procedure has been described in infants completely via a transanal approach with or without laparoscopic guidance.[28] The overall survival of patients with Hirschsprung's disease is excellent; however, long-term stooling problems are not infrequent. Constipation is the most frequent postoperative problem, followed by soiling and incontinence.

Imperforate Anus

The spectrum of anorectal malformations ranges from simple anal stenosis to the persistence of a cloaca; incidence ranges from 1 in 4000 to 5000 live births and is slightly more common in boys. The most common defect is an imperforate anus with a fistula between the distal colon and the urethra in boys or to the vestibule of the vagina in girls.

By 6 weeks' gestation, the urorectal septum moves caudally to divide the cloaca into the anterior urogenital sinus and posterior anorectal canal. Failure of this septum to form results in a fistula between the bowel and urinary tract (in boys) or the vagina (in girls). Complete or partial failure of the anal membrane to resorb results in an anal membrane or stenosis. The perineum also contributes to development of the external anal opening and genitalia by formation of cloacal folds, which extend from the anterior genital tubercle to the anus. The perineal body is formed by fusion of the cloacal folds between the anal and urogenital membranes. Breakdown of the cloacal membrane anywhere along its course results in the external anal opening being anterior to the external sphincter (i.e., anteriorly displaced anus).

An anatomic classification of anorectal anomalies is based on the level at which the blind-ending rectal pouch ends in relationship to the levator ani musculature (Box 70-1). Historically, the level of the end of the rectal pouch was determined by obtaining a lateral pelvic radiograph (i.e., invertogram) after the infant is held upside down for several minutes to allow air to pass into the rectal pouch. This examination is highly subjective and no longer used. Inspection of the perineum alone determines the pouch level in 80% of boys and 90% of girls. Clinically, if an anocutaneous fistula is seen anywhere on the perineal skin of a boy or external to the hymen of a girl, a low lesion can be assumed, which allows a primary perineal repair procedure to be performed, without the need for a stoma. Most all other lesions are high or intermediate, and they require proximal diversion by a sigmoid colostomy. This is followed by a definitive repair procedure at a later date. If required, the level of the rectal pouch can be detailed more definitively by ultrasonography or MRI.

Rectal atresia refers to an unusual lesion in which the lumen of the rectum is either completely or partially interrupted, with the upper rectum being dilated and the lower rectum consisting of a small anal canal. A *persistent cloaca* is defined as a defect in which the rectum, vagina, and urethra all meet and fuse to form a single, common

Box 70-1. Classification of Congenital Anomalies of the Anorectum

Female

High: anorectal agenesis with or without rectovaginal fistula, rectal atresia
Intermediate: anorectal agenesis with or without rectovaginal fistula, anal agenesis
Low: anovestibular or anocutaneous fistula (anteriorly displaced anus), anal stenosis
Cloaca

Male

High: anorectal agenesis with or without rectoprostatic urethral fistula, rectal atresia
Intermediate: anorectal agenesis with or without rectobulbar urethral fistula, anal agenesis
Low: anocutaneous fistula (anteriorly displaced anus), anal stenosis

---

channel. In girls, the type of defect may be determined by the number of orifices at the perineum. A single orifice would be consistent with a cloaca. If two orifices are seen (i.e., urethra and vagina), the defect represents either a high imperforate anus or, less commonly, a persistent urogenital sinus comprising one orifice and a normal anus as the other orifice.

Congenital anorectal anomalies often coexist with other lesions, and the VATER or VACTERL association must be considered. Bony abnormalities of the sacrum and spine occur in about one third of patients and consist of absent, accessory, or hemivertebrae and/or an asymmetrical or short sacrum. Two or more absent vertebrae are associated with a poor prognosis for bowel and/or bladder continence. Occult dysraphism of the spinal cord also may be present, and it consists of tethered cord, lipomeningocele, or fat within the filum terminale. Clinical evaluation should therefore include plain radiographs of the spine, as well as an ultrasound of the spinal cord. Genitourinary abnormalities other than the rectourinary fistula occur in 26% to 59% of patients. Vesicoureteral reflux and hydronephrosis are the most common, but other findings such as horseshoe, dysplastic, or absent kidney as well as hypospadias or cryptorchidism also must be considered. In general, the higher the anorectal malformation, the greater the frequency of associated urologic abnormalities. In patients with a persistent cloaca or rectovesical fistula, the likelihood of a genitourinary abnormality is approximately 90%. In contrast, the frequency is only 10% in children with low defects (i.e., perineal fistula). Radiographic evaluation of the urinary tract should include renal ultrasonography and voiding cystourethrography; a rectourinary fistula (if present) likely will be demonstrated by the latter procedure.

In addition to these tests just discussed, a plain chest radiograph and careful clinical evaluation of the heart should be conducted. If a cardiac defect is suspected, echocardiography should be performed before any surgical procedure. Before feeding, a nasogastric tube should be placed, and its presence within the stomach confirmed, to exclude EA.

The newborn infant with a low lesion can have a primary, single-stage repair procedure without need for a colostomy. Three basic approaches may be used. For anal stenosis in which the anal opening is in a normal location, serial dilation alone is usually curative. Dilations are performed daily by the caretaker and the size of the dilator should be increased progressively (beginning with 8 or 9 French and increased slowly to 14 to 16 French). If the anal opening is anterior to the external sphincter (i.e., anteriorly displaced anus) with a small distance between the opening and the center of the external sphincter, and the perineal body is intact, a *cutback* anoplasty is performed. This consists of an incision extending from the ectopic anal orifice to the central part of the anal sphincter, thus enlarging the anal opening. Alternatively, if there is a large distance between the anal opening and the central portion of the external anal sphincter, a *transposition* anoplasty is performed in which the aberrant anal opening is transposed to the normal position within the center of the sphincter muscles, and the perineal body is reconstructed.

Infants with intermediate or high lesions traditionally require a colostomy as the first part of a three-stage reconstruction. The colon is completely divided in the sigmoid region, with the proximal bowel as the colostomy and the distal bowel as a mucous fistula. Complete division of the bowel minimizes fecal contamination into the area of a rectourinary fistula, and it may lessen the risk of urosepsis. Furthermore, the distal bowel can be evaluated radiographically to determine the location of the rectourinary fistula. The second-stage procedure usually is performed 3 to 6 months later and consists of surgically dividing the rectourinary or rectovaginal fistula with a "pull-through" of the terminal rectal pouch into the normal anal position. A posterior sagittal approach as championed by Peña is the procedure most frequently performed.[29] This consists of determination of the location of the central position of the anal sphincter by electrical stimulation of the perineum. An incision is then made in the midline extending from the coccyx to the anterior perineum and through the sphincter and levator musculature until the rectum is identified. The fistula from the rectum to the vagina or urinary tract is divided. The rectum is then mobilized, and the perineal musculature is reconstructed. The third and final stage is closure of the colostomy, which is performed a few months later. Anal dilations are begun 2 weeks after the pull-through procedure and continue for several months after the colostomy closure.

More recently, a single-stage procedure using a transabdominal laparoscopic approach has been described for treatment of intermediate and high imperforate anus anomalies.[30] This technique offers the theoretical advantages of placement of the neorectum within the central position of the sphincter and levator muscle complex under direct vision and avoids the need to cut across these structures. The long-term outcome of this new approach when compared with the standard posterior sagittal method is presently unknown.

Most of the morbidity in patients with anorectal malformations is related to the presence of associated anomalies. Fecal continence is the major goal regarding correction of the defect. Prognostic factors for continence include the level of the pouch and whether the sacrum is normal. Globally, 75% of all patients have voluntary bowel movements. Half of this group still soil their underwear occasionally, whereas the other half are considered totally continent.[29] Constipation is the most common sequela. A bowel management program consisting of daily enemas is an important postoperative plan to reduce the frequency of soilage and improve the quality of life for these patients.

ABDOMINAL WALL

Abdominal Wall Defects

Defects of the anterior abdominal wall are a relatively frequent anomaly managed by pediatric surgeons. During normal development of the human embryo, the midgut herniates outward through the umbilical ring and continues to grow. By the 11th week of gestation, the midgut returns back into the abdominal cavity and undergoes normal rotation and fixation, along with closure of the umbilical ring. If the intestine fails to return, the infant is born with abdominal contents protruding directly through the umbilical ring and is termed an *omphalocele* (Fig. 70-14A). Most commonly, a sac is still covering the bowel, thus protecting it from the surrounding amniotic fluid. Occasionally, the sac may be torn at some point in utero, thus creating confusion with the other major type of abdominal wall defect termed *gastroschisis* (Fig. 70-14B). In contrast with omphalocele, the defect seen with gastroschisis is always on the right side of the umbilical ring with an intact umbilical cord, and there is never a sac covering the abdominal contents. The major morbidity and mortality with either anomaly are not as much with surgical repair of the abdominal defect as they are with the associated abnormalities. In the absence of other major anomalies, the long-term survival is excellent.[31]

Omphalocele

The abdominal contents with an omphalocele are covered with a membrane comprising the peritoneum on the inside and amnion on the outside. The size of the defect is variable, ranging from a small opening through which a small portion of the intestine is herniated to a large one in which the entire bowel and liver are included. In contrast with gastroschisis, karyotype abnormalities are present in roughly 30% of infants, including trisomies 13, 18, and 21. More than half of infants with omphalocele have other major or minor malformations, with cardiac being the most common, followed by musculoskeletal, gastrointestinal, and genitourinary. There is also a close

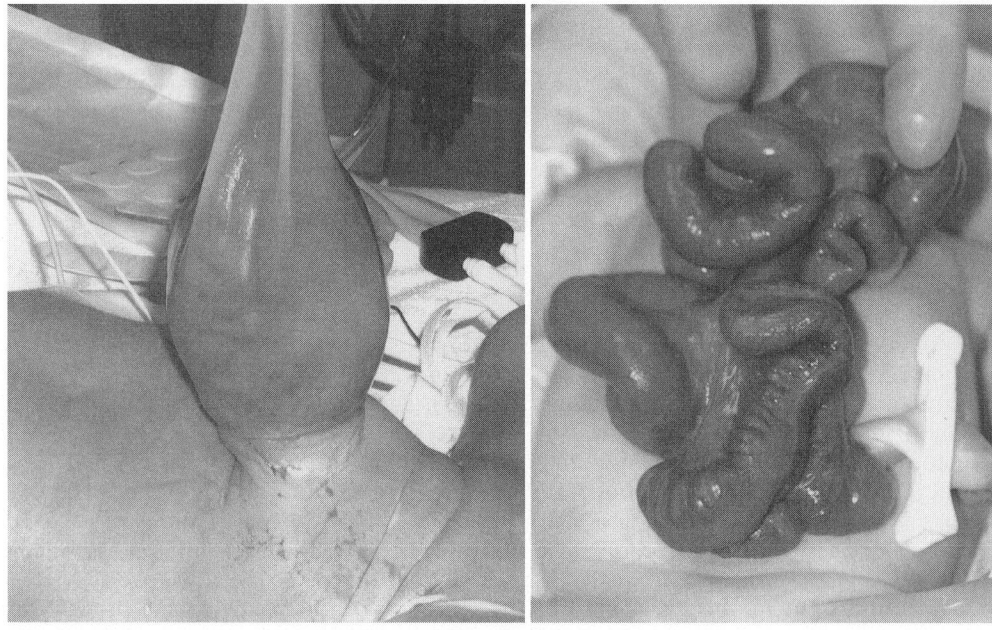

A   B

■ FIGURE 70-14.   The two major abdominal wall defects. An omphalocele *(A)* originates in the center of the umbilical ring and contains a sac covering the bowel, and there is a high incidence of other associated anomalies in the infant. In contrast, a gastroschisis *(B)* defect originates on the right side of the umbilical ring, there is no sac covering the viscera, and associated anomalies are relatively infrequent.

association with Beckwith-Wiedemann syndrome (omphalocele, hyperinsulinemia, macroglossia).

The treatment of an omphalocele consists of a nasogastric or orogastric tube decompression for prevention of visceral distention due to swallowed air. An intravenous line should be secured for administration of fluids and broad-spectrum antibiotics. The sac should be covered with a sterile, moist dressing and the infant transported to a tertiary care pediatric surgery facility. Prior to operative repair, the infant should be evaluated for potential chromosomal and developmental anomalies by a careful physical examination, plain chest radiograph, echocardiography if the physical examination suggests underlying congenital heart disease, and renal ultrasonography. Since the viscera are covered by a sac, operative repair of the defect may be delayed so as to allow thorough evaluation of the infant.

Several options exist for the surgical management of an omphalocele and are largely dictated by the size of the defect. In most cases, the contents within the sac are reduced back into the abdomen, the sac is excised with care to individually ligate the umbilical vessels, and the fascia and skin are closed. Fascial closure may be facilitated by stretching the anterior abdominal wall as well as milking out the contents of the bowel proximally and distally.

In giant omphaloceles, the degree of visceroabdominal disproportion prevents primary closure and the operative management becomes more challenging. Construction of a Silastic silo allows for gradual reduction of the viscera into the abdominal cavity over several days. Monitoring of intra-abdominal pressure during reduction may prevent the development of an abdominal compartment syndrome. Once the abdominal contents are returned to the abdomen, the infant is taken back to the operating room for formal fascia and/or skin closure. Occasionally, closure of the fascia may be impossible. In these cases, the skin is closed and a large hernia is accepted. This is repaired after 1 or 2 years. When the skin cannot be closed over the defect, several options exist, including the topical application of an antimicrobial solution to the outside of the sac such as silver nitrate or silver sulfadiazine. Over time, this results in granulation tissue and subsequent epithelialization of the sac. A repair of the large hernia is then performed a few years after this.

Gastroschisis

In contrast with patients with an omphalocele, the risk for associated anomalies with gastroschisis is infrequent. One major exception to this general rule is the association of gastroschisis with intestinal atresia, which may be present in up to 15%. Atresias may involve the small and/or large intestine. The cause of gastroschisis is presently unknown, but a prevailing theory is that it results from an abdominal wall defect associated with normal involution of the second umbilical vein. In addition, babies with gastroschisis are more often small for gestational age and born to mothers with a history of cigarette, alcohol, and recreational drug use, intake of aspirin, ibuprofen, and pseudoephedrine during the first trimester, and an 11-fold increase in risk in mothers younger than 20 years of age.

The surgical management of gastroschisis is similar to omphalocele. Considerations for third-space fluid losses from the exposed intestine and risk of infection dictate more expedient coverage. The presence of an atresia in a patient with gastroschisis may be managed in a number of ways. The bowel can simply be placed into the abdomen with a planned reoperation after several weeks. Another approach would be to perform a proximal diverting stoma. Finally, a primary anastomosis may be attempted. This is rarely advised, because of the possibility of other atresias as well as the overall condition of the bowel.

In patients with gastroschisis, the intestine is often thickened, edematous, matted together, and foreshortened. It is unclear as to whether this represents damage from the amniotic fluid or ischemia from the small, constricting abdominal wall defect. The short gut syndrome may be a consequence of the attenuated intestinal length. Even with adequate length, the remnant bowel may be damaged to the point that motility, digestion, and/or absorption are markedly impaired. This prenatal intestinal injury accounts for most of the postoperative morbidity and mortality. Virtually all infants have a prolonged postoperative ileus. Parenteral nutrition is life saving but also associated with the development of cholestasis, cirrhosis, portal hypertension, and ultimate liver failure.

Inguinal Hernia

Repair of an inguinal hernia (IH) represents one of the most frequent surgical procedures performed in the pediatric age group. Virtually all IH in children are indirect and congenital in origin. The variable persistence of the embryonic processus vaginalis offers a spectrum of abnormalities including a scrotal hernia, communicating hydrocele, a hydrocele of the cord, or a simple hydrocele (Fig. 70-15).

The incidence of IH has been reported to range between 0.8% and 4.4%, which roughly translates into 10 to 20 per 1000 live births. In preterm infants, the incidence may be as high as 30%. Approximately one third of children with IH are younger than 6 months of age, and males are affected approximately six times more often than females. The right side is involved in 60%, the left in 30%, and bilateral hernias are seen in 10%. The higher incidence on the right side compared with the left is probably related to the later descent and obliteration of the processus vaginalis of the right testis.

Most IH present as a bulge in the region of the external ring extending downward for varying distances to the scrotum or labia. Often, the hernia is detected by a pediatrician during a routine physical examination or observed by the parents. Inguinal pain may also be a presenting complaint. Incarceration and possible strangulation are the most feared consequences of IH and occur more frequently in premature infants. Because of the risk for these complications, all IH in children should be repaired.

Hydroceles represent fluid around the testicle and/or cord. A hydrocele that fills with fluid from the peritoneum

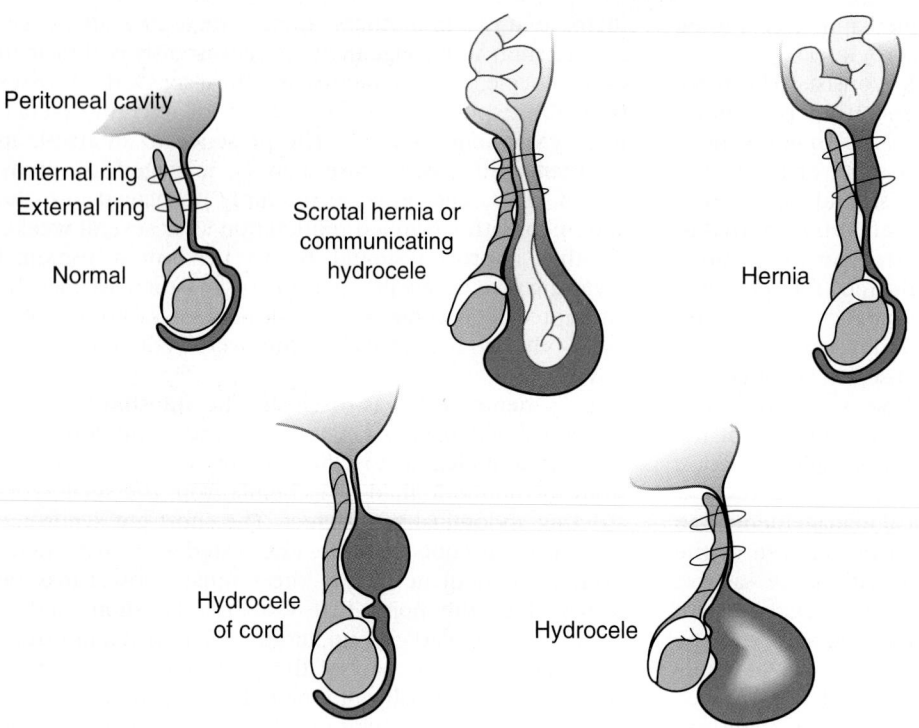

FIGURE 70-15. Anatomic variants of inguinal hernia and hydrocele. (From Cox JA: Inguinal hernia of childhood. Surg Clin North Am 65:1331-1342, 1985.)

is termed *communicating*. This is distinguished from a *noncommunicating* hydrocele by the history of variation in size throughout the day and palpation of a thickened cord above the testicle on the affected side. A communicating hydrocele is basically a small IH in which fluid but not peritoneal structures traverses the processus vaginalis. As such, all communicating hydroceles should be repaired in the same manner as an indirect IH. In contrast, non-communicating hydroceles are common among infants and can be observed for several months. The indications for repair of a noncommunicating hydrocele include failure to resolve and increase in size to one that is large and tense. The acute development of a hydrocele might be associated with the onset of epididymitis, testicular tumor, trauma, and torsion of a testicular appendage. An ultrasound of the scrotum may provide important diagnostic information in cases of an acute hydrocele in which examination of the testicle is difficult.

The timing for IH repair in premature infants is controversial. Early repair may be associated with a higher risk for injury to the cord structures, greater recurrence rate, and anesthetic-related apnea. These factors must be weighed against the higher risk for incarceration and strangulation, the potential for losing the patient during follow-up, and the development of a larger IH with loss of domain in the abdominal cavity. Taking these factors into account, most pediatric surgeons perform herniorrhaphy before the neonate is discharged to home from the nursery.[32] If the infant has already been discharged home, most pediatric surgeons wait until the infant is older than 60 weeks postconception (gestational age + postnatal age). After this age, the risk for postoperative apnea is diminished.

The timing for repair of incarcerated IH is another important point and dependent on the sex of the patient and contents within the hernia sac. In girls, the most common structure present in an IH that cannot be reduced is an ovary. The ovary within the sac is at significant risk for torsion and strangulation. Although this is not a true surgical emergency, IH repair should be done relatively soon (within a few days).

In patients with incarcerated IH containing bowel, attempts should be made to reduce the hernia, unless there is clinical evidence of peritonitis. This may require intravenous sedation and careful monitoring. If the reduction is successful, the child is admitted and observed for 24 to 48 hours. The IH repair should be done after the period of observation to allow for tissue edema to subside. On the other hand, if the IH cannot be reduced, the child should be promptly taken to the operating room for inguinal exploration. If an intestinal resection is required, it can usually be done through the opened hernia sac prior to IH repair.

There is much controversy over the management of the opposite groin of the child with a unilateral IH. The major advantage of contralateral exploration is that it determines the presence of a patent processus vaginalis. Although a patent processus is not the same as an IH, an indirect IH cannot occur without it. Since there is a higher incidence of a contralateral patent processus within the first year of life, many surgeons restrict exploration of the other side to children younger than 1 year of age. In addition, many surgeons believe that contralateral exploration should be performed in all girls presenting with a clinically obvious unilateral IH, since the likelihood of injury to reproductive structures is rare. Laparoscopic evaluation of the contralateral groin through the opened sac at the time of repair may be a safe and accurate method of identifying the presence of a patent processus vaginalis.[33]

The technical details of IH repair in infants have been well described[34] and consist of high ligation of the hernia sac at the level of the internal ring. A repair of the floor of the inguinal canal is usually not necessary. In most cases, this is an outpatient procedure with minimal morbidity. Recurrence, injury to the vas deferens, wound infection, and postoperative hydrocele are recognized complications associated with IH repair but should occur with a frequency of less than 1%.

Undescended Testes

The incidence of undescended testes (UDT) among males in the first year of life is roughly 1% to 2%. In the newborn period, this incidence is higher, but a few have spontaneous descent by 3 months of age. If descent of the testicle has not occurred after this time interval, further descent is unlikely. It is important to differentiate a true UDT from a retractile testis. In the former, the testicle cannot be manipulated into a scrotal position, whereas in the latter the testicle is able to be pulled down into the scrotum. The retractile testis does not typically require any further therapy beyond parental reassurance.

Most (~90%) UDT are palpable within the inguinal canal, and the treatment is by surgical orchidopexy. It is not completely clear as to whether the abnormal UDT is the cause or the result of maldescent. However, since the severity of histologic abnormalities of the testes is directly related to patient age, most pediatric surgeons perform orchidopexy at around the first year of life. The effect of higher temperatures and other factors on the developing UDT results in several abnormalities, including attenuated spermatogenesis, infertility, and increased risk for malignancy. The risk for these problems is greater in bilateral when compared with unilateral UDT. Although the risk for malignancy is not completely abrogated by orchidopexy, the resulting scrotal testis is in a more favorable position to clinically monitor for the development of abnormalities. In addition to histologic abnormalities within the testicle, UDT is typically associated with an ipsilateral IH and is at greater risk for trauma.

The customary surgical procedure for treatment of UDT that are palpated within the inguinal canal is by orchidopexy along with repair of the associated IH. This is accomplished through a transverse inguinal incision. After division of the external oblique aponeurosis in the direction of its fibers through the external ring, the testicle is identified. The hernia sac is opened and the cord structures are separated from the sac. The hernia sac is then dissected up to the level of the internal ring and ligated. This is the maneuver in which the cord structures are able to be mobilized to gain sufficient length for the UDT to reach the base of the scrotum. The testicle is passed through a subcutaneous tunnel and sutured into a pocket between the dartos muscle and skin of the scrotum with nonabsorbable suture material.

The nonpalpable testis poses a difficult problem. These are typically not able to be located at the time of simple inguinal exploration, and the relatively short blood vessels to the testicle are the main limiting factor for the testicle to reach the scrotum. Although preoperative localization of the intra-abdominal UDT using CT, MRI, or ultrasound may be helpful, laparoscopy is currently the procedure of choice.[35] Obviously atrophic testes may be removed or division of the superiorly based blood supply will permit moving the testicle into a scrotal position (based on the inferiorly based blood supply to the vas and cremasteric fibers) at a later stage (so-called Fowler-Stephens procedure). As another option, the testicle may be autotransplanted into the scrotal position based on a microvascular anastomosis of the spermatic artery and vein to the epigastric vessels.[36]

Umbilical Hernia

An umbilical hernia (UH) occurs as a result of persistence of the umbilical ring. Complete closure of this ring can be anticipated by 4 to 6 years of age in up to 80% of cases. In contrast with IH, a UH is rarely associated with significant complications. As such, most pediatric surgeons defer UH repair until the child is old enough to begin kindergarten. Exceptions to this general rule are a large UH defect (>2 cm) since the likelihood for spontaneous resolution is lower. Further, a history of incarceration, a large skin proboscis, or in a patient with a ventriculoperitoneal shunt are other relative indications for repair. The technique for UH repair generally involves an infraumbilical semicircular incision, separation of the hernia sac from the overlying umbilical skin, repair of the fascial defect, pexing of the base of the umbilical skin to the fascia, and skin closure.

Epigastric Hernia

Epigastric hernias (EHs) represent the third most common hernia in children. These are found anywhere along the midline of the abdomen between the umbilicus and xiphoid process. Not to be confused with a broad defect of a diastasis rectus, the fascial defect of an EH is quite small but allows herniation of properitoneal fat through the defect. Although this does not pose a significant risk to the patient, strangulation of the fat often results in pain, redness, and swelling. This scenario often directs urgent operative exploration to exclude incarceration of other, more important structures. Because of this and the likelihood for continued enlargement, most pediatric surgeons recommend elective repair. This is accomplished via a small transverse incision overlying the palpable mass. The herniated fat is excised, and the fascia is repaired.

CONGENITAL DIAPHRAGMATIC HERNIA

CDH represents one of the most enigmatic diseases encountered in pediatric surgery. The reported incidence of CDH is in the range of 1 in 2000 to 5000 live births. Most CDH defects are on the left side (80%); however, up to 20% may occur on the right side. A CDH may also be bilateral, but this is distinctly rare. Despite multiple innovative treatment strategies, including in utero diaphragm repair, fetal tracheal occlusion, high-frequency oscillation or partial liquid ventilation, ECLS, exogenous surfactant, and inhaled nitric oxide, survival rates for this condition have not been significantly impacted. The exact survival rate for CDH is difficult to determine but in the range of 60% to 70%.[37] Calculation of true survival is complicated by the fact that many infants with CDH are stillborn, and many reports tend to exclude infants with complex associated anomalies from survival calculations.

The cause for CDH is unknown but is believed to result from failure of normal closure of the pleuroperitoneal canal in the developing embryo. As a result, abdominal contents herniate through the resultant defect in the posterolateral diaphragm and compress the ipsilateral developing lung. The posterolateral location of this hernia is known as *Bochdalek's hernia* and distinguished from the congenital hernia of the anteromedial, retrosternal diaphragm, which is known as *Morgagni's hernia*. Compression of the lung results in pulmonary hypoplasia involving both lungs, with the ipsilateral lung being the most affected. In addition to the abnormal airway development, the pulmonary vasculature is distinctly abnormal in that the medial muscular thickness of the arterioles is excessive and extremely sensitive to the multiple local and systemic factors known to trigger vasospasm. Thus, the two main factors that affect morbidity and mortality are pulmonary hypoplasia and pulmonary hypertension.

The most frequent clinical presentation of CDH is respiratory distress due to severe hypoxemia. The infant appears dyspneic, tachypneic, and cyanotic, with severe retractions. The anteroposterior diameter of the chest may be large, and the abdomen may be scaphoid. There are three general presentations of infants with CDH. In the first scenario, signs of severe respiratory distress are present immediately at the time of birth. As such, if the diagnosis is known prenatally, delivery within an institution capable of providing ECLS, high-frequency ventilation, and sophisticated neonatal care is crucial. In these infants, pulmonary hypoplasia may be severe enough to be incompatible with life. The infant may also have a reversible cause for immediate hypoxia such as hypovolemia and severe pulmonary vasospasm. Unfortunately, there are no known criteria capable of distinguishing infants with severe lung hypoplasia from those with reversible conditions. As such, many infants with irreversible lung hypoplasia are placed on ECLS for prolonged periods before it becomes apparent that their underlying lung condition is incurable.

In the second and most common presentation, the infant does well for several hours after delivery (so-called honeymoon period) and then begins to deteriorate from a respiratory standpoint. Patients in this category may benefit from therapy to reduce pulmonary hypertension and hypoxemia. Theoretically, these patients are ideal candidates for ECLS because their lung development has progressed enough to sustain life. Unfortunately, this is not always the case since many infants in this group do not survive, even with ECLS support.

The third and final clinical presentation of CDH is beyond the first 24 hours of life, which occurs in about 10% to 20% of cases. Many of these children present with feeding difficulties, chronic respiratory disease, pneumonia, or intestinal obstruction. This group of patients enjoys the best prognosis.

The diagnosis of CDH is frequently made at the time of a prenatal ultrasound during an otherwise unremarkable pregnancy. The postnatal diagnosis is relatively straightforward because a plain chest radiograph demonstrates the gastric air bubble or loops of bowel within the chest (Fig. 70-16). There may also be a mediastinal shift away from the side of the hernia or polyhydramnios from the obstructed stomach. Rarely is a UGI contrast study necessary.

The management of CDH that has been detected in utero has directed open fetal surgery as a strategy to remove the compression of the abdominal viscera and allow for improved lung development. Unfortunately, this intervention is high risk to both the mother and fetus and has failed to demonstrate any survival advantage.[38] Subsequent to this was the realization that occlusion of the fetal trachea might result in accumulation of lung fluid with stimulation of lung growth. Although several techniques for occlusion of the trachea have been described, including the use of balloons, sponges, or external clip application, the overall result is larger but persistently abnormal lungs.[39] Currently, there appears to be no rationale for fetal intervention for the diagnosis of CDH.

The postnatal management of CDH is complex, but all efforts should be directed toward stabilization of the car-

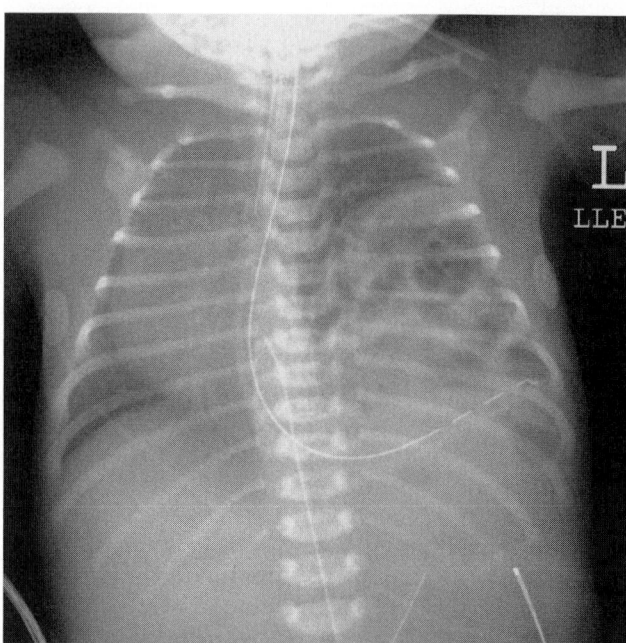

■ **FIGURE 70-16.** Congenital diaphragmatic hernia. The tip of the nasogastric tube and obvious loops of gas-filled bowel are located in the left hemithorax.

diorespiratory system while minimizing iatrogenic injury from therapeutic interventions. Endotracheal intubation is critical to optimize ventilation. Placement of a nasogastric tube is also important to prevent gastric distention, which may worsen the lung compression, mediastinal shift, and ability to ventilate. Acute deterioration of an infant with CDH may be due to a number of factors including inadvertent extubation. However, a pneumothorax may develop during aggressive attempts at ventilation. As such, the pneumothorax in patients with CDH always occurs on the side *contralateral* to the side of the CDH. Needle decompression of the contralateral chest during an acute deterioration event may be life saving and necessary before a chest radiograph can be obtained.

Although used traditionally, pharmacologic pulmonary vasodilators (tolazoline), surfactant, high-frequency ventilation, and inhaled nitric oxide all have demonstrated inconsistent success. One of the more important recent contributions to the management of infants with CDH has been the concept of gentle ventilation with permissive hypercapnea and stable hypoxemia (tolerance of preductal oxygen saturations above 80%). Using this strategy, Boloker and associates have reported a survival of 76%.[40]

Historically, the surgical repair of a CDH was considered to be a surgical emergency because it was believed that the abdominal viscera within the chest prevented the ability to ventilate. More recently, it has become realized that the physiologic stress associated with early repair probably adds more insult and that survival is not improved when compared with delayed repair. Thus, most pediatric surgeons wait for a variable period (24 to 72 hours) to allow for stabilization of the infant before embarking on surgical repair.

Most pediatric surgeons repair a posterolateral CDH via an abdominal subcostal incision, although a thoracotomy also provides adequate exposure. The viscera are reduced into the abdominal cavity and the posterolateral defect in the diaphragm is closed using interrupted, nonabsorbable sutures. In most cases (~80% to 90%), a hernia sac is not present. If identified, however, it should be excised at the time of repair. Occasionally, the defect is too large to permit primary closure, and a number of reconstructive techniques are available, including various abdominal or thoracic muscle flaps. The use of prosthetic material such as Gore-Tex has become more widespread. The advantage of a prosthetic patch is that a tension-free repair can be frequently obtained. The major problems with prosthetic patches are the risk for infection and recurrence of the hernia. Occasionally, the abdominal compartment may be too small to accommodate the viscera that has developed within the thoracic cavity. In these circumstances, an abdominal silo may need to be constructed as in the management of congenital abdominal wall defects.

Beyond the early postoperative period, many infants with CDH have continued morbidity, which demands careful long-term follow-up.[41] Many children who survive aggressive management of severe respiratory failure manifest neurologic problems, such as abnormalities in both motor and cognitive skills, developmental delay, seizures, and hearing loss. Other problems include a high incidence of GER and foregut dysmotility. Other morbidity associated with CDH survivors includes chronic lung disease, scoliosis, and pectus excavatum deformities.

CONGENITAL CHEST WALL DEFORMITIES

Although several categories for congenital chest wall deformities exist, the two major types include *pectus excavatum* and *pectus carinatum* (Fig. 70-17). Pectus excavatum is also referred to as a funnel, or sunken, chest and is the most common deformity encountered (~ five times more common than carinatum deformities). It is three times more frequent in males and is identified in the first year of life in roughly 90% of cases. Although the etiology is unknown, abnormalities of costal cartilage development have been most frequently implicated. Several conditions are known to be associated with pectus excavatum and must be considered in the preoperative evaluation. Roughly 15% of patients have scoliosis. In addition, the possibility of Marfan syndrome must be considered, and ophthalmologic evaluation along with an echocardiogram should be obtained. Mitral valve prolapse may be seen in about half of patients, and structural congenital heart disease occurs in about 2%. Asthma is also frequent, but it is unknown whether it contributes to the development of the defect or occurs as a result of it.

The most common indication for surgery in patients with pectus deformities is cosmetic. This is not a minor issue, particularly for adolescents with significant concerns regarding body image and development of self-esteem. Theoretically, correction of a severe excavatum deformity significantly improves cardiopulmonary function. However, notwithstanding many decades of experience with this condition, no appreciable consensus has been reached regarding the degree of cardiopulmonary impairment, if any, this common chest wall deformity produces. Despite this, it is important to screen for underlying cardiopulmonary conditions before embarking on operative correction. Standard anteroposterior and lateral chest radiographs are essential to serve as a baseline of the degree of deformity as well as to detect the presence of thoracic scoliosis. Pulmonary function studies are important to document either restrictive or obstructive abnormalities. The latter is particularly important if this component is reversible with bronchodilators. If a heart murmur is detected on physical examination, an echocardiogram is indicated. Finally, a CT scan permits the calculation of an index by dividing the measured transverse diameter of the chest by the anteroposterior diameter to more objectively document the severity of the defect.

The surgical correction of a pectus excavatum should not be done prior to the age of 5 years as a severe, postoperative restrictive chest wall deformity may result. Presently, there are two main methods for operative correction. The original technique was originally described in 1949 by Ravitch and remains as the standard by which all other procedures are compared. This procedure is applied to patients with either excavatum or carinatum deformities and consists of a transverse skin incision overlying the deformity, bilateral subchondral resection of abnormal costal cartilages, sternal osteotomy, and anterior

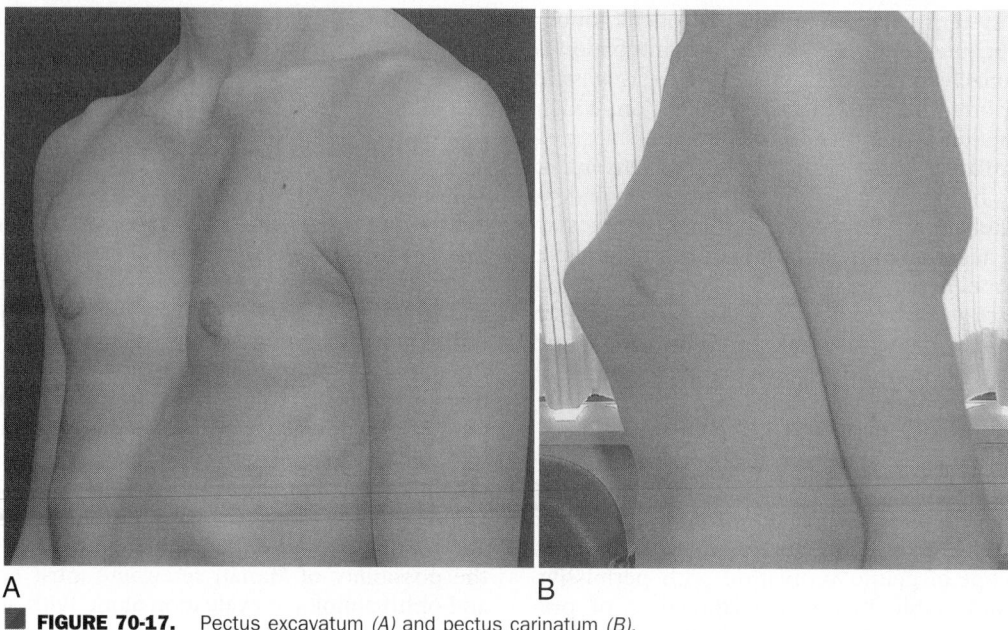

FIGURE 70-17.   Pectus excavatum *(A)* and pectus carinatum *(B)*.

fixation of the sternum with a retrosternal stainless-steel strut. The strut is removed as a secondary procedure in 6 months to a year. The results with this operation are excellent. More recently, a minimally invasive technique has been described for excavatum defects in which a C-shaped bar is passed in a retrosternal plane from one hemithorax into the other via two lateral intercostal incisions. The bar is then "flipped" such that the convexity is outward and the chest wall defect is immediately corrected. As originally described by Nuss and colleagues,[42] this technique avoids the creation of pectoral flaps, cartilage resection, and sternal osteotomy. The bar must be left in place for 2 years, after which it is removed. Although this new technique has gained considerable popularity among the lay public, the advantages of this technique over the standard Ravitch procedure have yet to be conclusively demonstrated. A multicenter, prospective trial to address this issue is currently ongoing.

BRONCHOPULMONARY MALFORMATIONS

Dramatic improvements in prenatal ultrasonography have led to a more frequent recognition of developmental abnormalities of the lungs and major bronchi. Some lesions may be associated with in utero death unless fetal intervention is performed, some infants may have respiratory compromise at birth, and some patients may present later in life with a persistent infection or neoplasm.

Bronchogenic Cyst

Bronchogenic cysts are usually solitary and lined by cuboidal or columnar ciliated epithelium and mucus glands. Roughly two thirds of cysts are within the lung parenchyma, and the remainder are found within the mediastinum. Cysts within the pulmonary parenchyma typically communicate with a bronchus, whereas those in the mediastinum usually do not. Although up to a third of patients are asymptomatic and the diagnosis is made on a routine chest radiograph, many patients present with respiratory complaints including recurrent pneumonia, cough, hemoptysis, or dyspnea. Because of these symptoms as well as the reports of neoplasm occurring within these cysts, the treatment for all bronchogenic cysts is resection. Frequently, mediastinal cysts may be amenable to resection using minimally invasive techniques.

Pulmonary Sequestration

Sequestrations represent malformations of the lung in which there is usually no bronchial communication and there is frequently an aberrant systemic blood supply. Sequestrations are discriminated on the basis of being either intralobar, in which they reside within the lung parenchyma, or extralobar, in which they are surrounded by a separate pleural covering. Intralobar sequestrations are infrequently associated with other anomalies and are found within the medial or posterior segments of the lower lobes, with about two thirds occurring on the left side. In approximately 85% of cases, the intralobar sequestration is supplied by an anomalous systemic vessel arising from the infradiaphragmatic aorta and located within the inferior pulmonary ligament. Anticipation of this structure is therefore critical during attempted resection of this malformation. The venous drainage is usually via the inferior pulmonary vein but may also occur by way of systemic veins. Because of the risk for infection and/or bleeding, intralobar sequestrations are usually removed, either by segmentectomy or lobectomy. Historically, angiography was considered to be an important preoperative study before embarking on resection of a sequestration. More recently, CT or MRI have replaced the need for angiography and provide excellent mapping of the blood supply.

In contrast with those that are intralobar, extralobar sequestrations occur predominantly in males (3:1) and are found three times more frequently on the left side. In about 40% of cases, multiple other anomalies are encountered, including posterolateral diaphragmatic hernia, eventration of the diaphragm, pectus excavatum and carinatum, enteric duplication cysts, and congenital heart disease. Extralobar sequestrations are usually asymptomatic, and since there is usually no bronchial communication, the risk for infection is low. As such, many of these malformations may be observed. Frequently, their discovery during other procedures or inability to make the correct diagnosis by noninvasive imaging dictates their removal.

Congenital Lobar Emphysema

Congenital lobar emphysema (CLE) results from overdistention of one or more lobes within a histologically normal lung due to abnormal cartilaginous support of the feeding bronchus. This focal area of bronchial collapse results in a check-valve with air trapping and a progressive increase in lobar distention. Most often, the cartilage within the bronchus is abnormal; however, extrinsic compression of the bronchus from an aberrant vessel may also cause the same findings. The left upper lobe is involved in roughly half of cases, with the remainder evenly distributed between the right middle and lower lobes.

The symptoms of CLE range from none to severe respiratory distress within the neonatal period. Asymptomatic patients are often identified during a routine chest radiograph as an area of hyperlucency. In these cases, observation without pulmonary resection may be prudent. Occasionally, CLE is identified in a patient with recurrent or persistent pneumonia or with progressive dyspnea. Resection of the involved lung is therapeutic and well tolerated. The presentation of CLE in a neonate may include severe respiratory distress. In these cases, the clinical and radiographic pictures may mimic a tension pneumothorax with severe mediastinal shift. Inadvertent placement of a chest tube into the distended lung would be catastrophic. Immediate thoracotomy with resection of the involved lobe may be lifesaving.

Congenital Cystic Adenomatoid Malformation

A congenital cystic adenomatoid malformation (CCAM) typically involves a single lobe and represents a multicystic mass of pulmonary tissue in which there is proliferation of bronchial structures at the expense of alveoli. Unlike sequestrations, a CCAM does typically have a bronchial communication, and the arterial and venous drainage is classically from the normal pulmonary circulation. There are three general types segregated on the basis of cyst size. A type I CCAM is considered the macrocystic variety and includes single or multiple cysts larger than 2 cm. Type I lesions account for about 50% of all cases and usually have no associated anomalies. A type II CCAM contains respiratory epithelial lined cysts, but they

are smaller than 1 cm. Type II lesions are associated with other anomalies such as renal agenesis, cardiac malformations, CDH, or skeletal abnormalities. The outcome of patients with type II CCAM is dependent on the associated conditions. A type III CCAM is considered microcystic, and on gross inspection may appear to be solid; however, microscopic analysis has multiple cysts. Type III CCAMs are often associated with mediastinal shift, the development of nonimmune hydrops, and a generally poor prognosis. In utero surgery has been applied with some success in the management of large CCAMs. The development of nonimmune hydrops is one of the main predictors of survival, since 100% mortality has been reported once this develops.[43] The postnatal management for the symptomatic patient is relatively straightforward by pulmonary resection in the newborn period. In asymptomatic patients with small lesions detected by fetal ultrasound, the rationale for resection becomes less clear. Since there have been reports of malignancy developing within these lesions as well as the potential for infection and enlargement, they should probably all be resected.

HEPATOBILIARY CONDITIONS

Biliary Atresia

BA is characterized by progressive (not static) obliteration of the extrahepatic and intrahepatic bile ducts. The cause is presently unknown, and the incidence is approximately 1 in 15,000 live births. Presently, there is no medical therapy to reverse the obliterative process, and patients who are not offered surgical treatment uniformly develop biliary cirrhosis, portal hypertension, and death by 2 years of age.

Pathologically, the biliary tracts contain inflammatory and fibrous cells surrounding minuscule ducts that are probably remnants of the original ductal system. Bile duct proliferation, severe cholestasis with plugging, and inflammatory cell infiltrate are the pathologic hallmarks of this disease. Over time, these changes progress to fibrosis with end-stage cirrhosis. This histology is usually distinct from the giant cell transformation and hepatocellular necrosis that are characteristic of neonatal hepatitis, the other major cause of direct hyperbilirubinemia in the newborn. There are variants of BA ranging from fibrosis of the distal bile ducts with proximal patency (5%, considered *correctable* form), fibrosis of the proximal bile ducts with distal patency (15%), or fibrosis of both proximal and distal bile ducts (80%).

A serum direct bilirubin level higher than 2.0 mg/dL or greater than 15% of the total bilirubin level defines cholestasis and is distinctly abnormal, and further evaluation is mandatory. Delay in diagnosis of BA is associated with a worse prognosis. Success with surgical correction is much improved if undertaken prior to 60 days of life when compared with surgical correction undertaken after 90 days of life.[44] Thus, the initial opportunity for success in the management of this disease relies on the *early* recognition of abnormal direct hyperbilirubinemia.

The list of potential causes for cholestasis in infants is relatively long; however, an organized, systematic approach usually permits the establishment of an accurate diagnosis within a few days. In addition to a careful history and physical examination, blood and urine should be obtained for bacterial and viral cultures, reducing substances in the urine to rule out galactosemia, serum IgM titers for syphilis, cytomegalovirus, herpes, and hepatitis B, serum α_1-antitrypsin level and phenotype, serum thyroxine level, and a sweat chloride test done to exclude CF.

Ultrasonography of the liver and gallbladder is important in the evaluation of the infant with cholestasis. In BA, the gallbladder is typically shrunken or absent, and the extrahepatic bile ducts cannot be visualized. The next diagnostic step is to perform a percutaneous liver biopsy if the hepatic synthetic function is normal. This is well tolerated under local anesthesia, and the diagnostic accuracy is in the range of 90%.[45] In cases where the ultrasound and biopsy findings are inconclusive, hepatobiliary scintigraphy, using iminodiacetic acid analogues, may demonstrate normal hepatic uptake but absent excretion into the intestine. Pretreatment of the infant with phenobarbital may improve the sensitivity of this test.

If the needle biopsy and/or the abdominal ultrasound are consistent with BA, exploratory laparotomy is then performed expeditiously. The initial goal at surgery is to confirm the diagnosis. This requires the demonstration of the fibrotic biliary remnant and definition of absent proximal and distal bile duct patency by cholecystocholangiography. The classic technique for correction of BA is the Kasai hepatoportoenterostomy. In this procedure, the distal bile duct is transected and dissected proximally up to the level of the liver capsule, whereby it is excised, along with the gallbladder remnant (Fig. 70-18). A Roux-en-Y hepaticojejunostomy is then constructed by anastomosis of the jejunal Roux-limb to the fibrous plate above the portal vein. Some surgeons prefer to monitor postoperative bile flow by constructing a distal double-barrel stoma. Although it has been considered that this may lessen the risk for cholangitis, this has yet to be definitively established.

Postoperatively, the use of oral choleretic bile salts such as ursodeoxycholic acid may facilitate bile flow.[46] In addition, methylprednisolone is employed as an anti-inflammatory agent, and trimethoprim-sulfamethoxazole is administered for long-term antimicrobial prophylaxis. Cholangitis is a serious but common problem after hepatoportoenterostomy and may be associated with cessation of bile flow. Episodes of cholangitis are managed by hospitalization, rehydration, broad-spectrum intravenous antibiotics, steroids, and occasionally surgical exploration of the portoenterostomy.

Approximately 30% of infants undergoing hepatoportoenterostomy prior to 60 days of age have a long-term successful outcome and do not require liver transplantation. Older children and those with preoperative evidence for bridging fibrosis seen on liver biopsy predictably do less well. As such, some surgeons may forgo performing a portoenterostomy procedure and simply place the patient on a waiting list for liver transplantation. The remaining patients undergoing portoenterostomy develop progressive hepatic fibrosis with resultant portal hypertension and progressive cholestasis. In this group, liver transplantation is lifesaving and associated with an 82% 5-year survival.[47] BA currently represents the most common indication for pediatric liver transplantation.

Choledochal Cyst

A cystic enlargement of the common bile duct is referred to as a *choledochal cyst*. The initial anatomic organization was proposed by Alonso-Lej and coworkers in 1959[48] and has been updated to the current classification as depicted in Figure 70-19. Type I cysts represent 80% to 90% of cases and are simply cystic dilations of the common bile duct. Type II cysts are represented as a diverticulum arising from the common bile duct. Type III cysts are also referred to as *choledochoceles* and are isolated to the intrapancreatic portion of the common bile duct and frequently involve the ampulla. Type IV cysts are second in frequency and represent dilation of both intrahepatic and extrahepatic bile ducts. In type V cysts, only the intrahepatic ducts are dilated.

The pathophysiology of choledochal cysts remains poorly understood. In one theory, reflux of pancreatic digestive enzymes into the bile duct via an anomalous pancreaticobiliary ductal junction results in damage to the duct. In another theory, persistent or transient obstruction of the distal bile duct may be present.

Although choledochal cysts can produce symptoms in any age group, most become clinically evident within the 1st decade of life. The triad of a right upper quadrant mass, abdominal pain, and jaundice is highly suggestive of the diagnosis. In some patients, pancreatitis may be

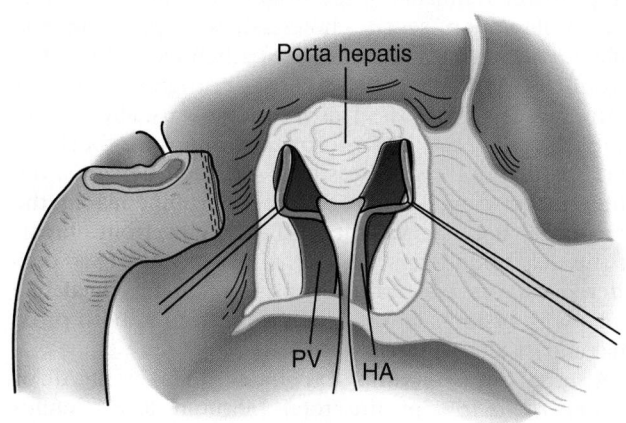

FIGURE 70-18. Kasai's hepatoportoenterostomy procedure for biliary atresia. The extrahepatic bile ducts and gallbladder have been removed. The fibrous plate of the hepatic duct is transected above the bifurcation of the portal vein (PV) and hepatic artery (HA), and a Roux limb of jejunum is sewn to this plate to achieve drainage of bile. (From Grosfeld JL, Fitzgerald JF, Predaina R, et al: The efficacy of hepatoportoenterostomy in biliary atresia. Surgery 106:692-700, 1989.)

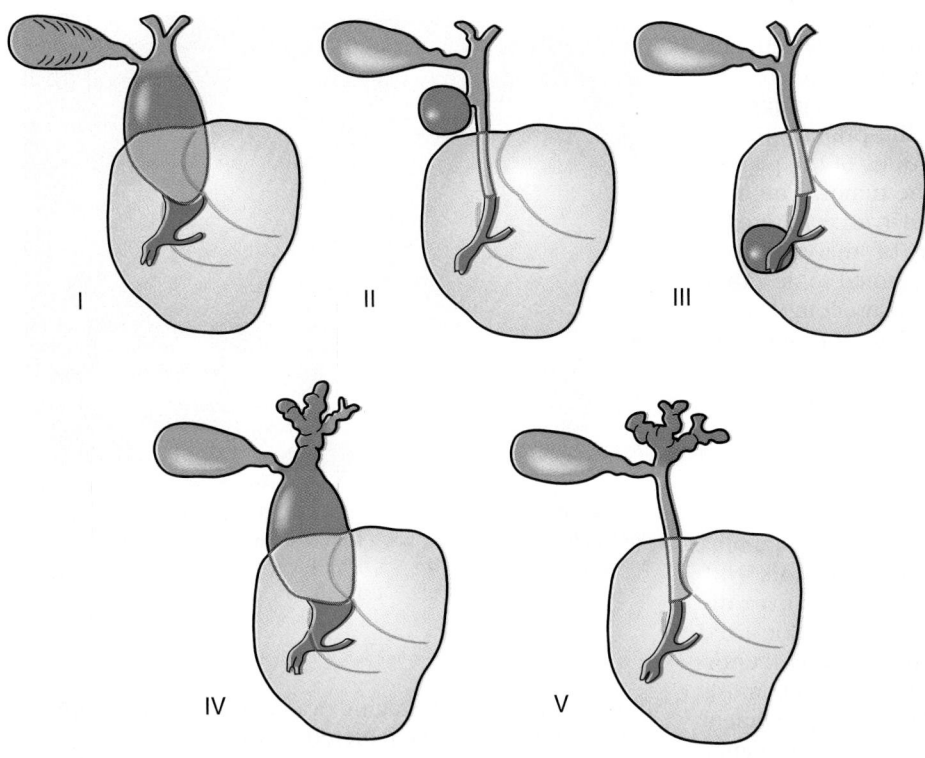

FIGURE 70-19. The anatomic classification of choledochal cyst: Types I to V. (From Sigalet DL: Biliary tract disorders and portal hypertension. *In* Ashcraft KW, Sharp RJ, Sigalet DL, Snyder CL [eds]: Pediatric Surgery, 3rd ed. Philadelphia, WB Saunders, 2000, p 588.)

present. In older children and adults, the presentation may be more insidious and include choledocholithiasis, cholangitis, and cirrhosis with progression to portal hypertension. Malignant degeneration is also found in up to 16% of adults with choledochal cysts.

In addition to routine measurement of serum bilirubin, alkaline phosphatase, and amylase levels, the most useful diagnostic test for choledochal cysts is ultrasonography. Once dilation of the extrahepatic biliary ducts is demonstrated, no further testing is usually necessary in children. Although seldom necessary, preoperative endoscopic retrograde cholecystopancreatography may provide additional information regarding the pancreaticobiliary ductal anatomy to guide intraoperative decision making.

Total cyst excision with Roux-en-Y hepaticojejunostomy is the definitive procedure for management of types I and II choledochal cysts. In cases whereby there is significant inflammation, it may be impossible to safely dissect the entire cyst way from the anterior surface of the portal vein. In these circumstances, the internal lining of the cyst can be excised, leaving the external portion of the cyst wall intact. Type III cysts are typically approached by opening the duodenum, resecting the cyst wall with care to reconstruct and marsupialize the remnant pancreaticobiliary ducts to the duodenal mucosa. In type IV cysts, the bile duct excision is coupled with a lateral hilar dissection to perform a jejunal anastomosis to the lowermost intrahepatic cysts. If the intrahepatic cysts are confined to a single lobe or segment, hepatic resection may be indicated. The treatment of type V cysts involving both lobes is usually palliative with transhepatic or U tubes until liver transplantation can be performed. The postoperative outcomes following excision of choledochal cysts are excellent.[49]

CHILDHOOD SOLID TUMORS

Neuroblastoma

Neuroblastoma (NBL), the most common abdominal malignancy in children, accounts for 6% to 10% of all childhood cancers and 15% of all pediatric cancer deaths in the United States. The overall incidence in an unscreened population is 1 case per 10,000 persons, with about 525 new cases diagnosed in the United States each year.

These tumors are of neural crest origin and, as a result, may arise anywhere along the sympathetic ganglia or within the adrenal medulla. Although these tumors may occur at any site from the brain to the pelvis, 75% originate within the abdomen or pelvis, and half of these occur within the adrenal medulla. Twenty percent of NBLs originate within the posterior mediastinum, and 5% are within the neck. The median age at diagnosis is 2 years. Nearly 35% occur in children younger than 1 year of age, and fewer than 5% of cases present in children older than 10 years of age.

NBL is an enigmatic tumor that is capable of rapid progression in some children and spontaneous regression in others, particularly those younger than 1 year of age. Approximately 25% of patients present with a solitary mass that may be cured by surgical therapy, whereas most present with extensive locoregional or metastatic disease. In this latter group of patients, the prognosis is generally poor, with an overall survival of less than 30%.

The presenting symptoms of NBL are dependent on several factors, including the site of the primary tumor, the presence of metastatic disease, the age of the patient, as well as the metabolic activity of the tumor. The most common presentation is a fixed, lobular mass extending from the flank toward the midline of the abdomen. Although the abdominal mass may be noted in an otherwise asymptomatic child, patients may complain of abdominal pain, distention, weight loss, or anorexia. Bowel or bladder dysfunction may arise from direct compression of these structures by the tumor. Cervical tumors may be discovered as a palpable or visible mass or be associated with stridor or dysphagia. Posterior mediastinal masses are usually detected by plain chest radiographs in a child with Horner's syndrome, dyspnea, or pneumonia. Further, the tumor may extend into the neural foramina and cause symptoms of spinal cord compression. NBL tends to metastasize to cortical bones, bone marrow, and liver. As such, patients may present with localized swelling and tenderness, lump, or refusal to walk. Periorbital metastasis accounts for proptosis and ecchymosis (termed "panda" or "raccoon" eyes). Marrow replacement by tumor may result in anemia and weakness. In infants, liver metastasis may rapidly expand, causing massive hepatomegaly and respiratory distress that require mechanical ventilation and surgical decompression. Metastatic lesions to the skin produce a characteristic "blueberry muffin" appearance.

Numerous paraneoplastic syndromes can occur in conjunction with NBL. Cerebellar ataxia, involuntary movements, and nystagmus are the hallmark of the "dancing eyes and feet" syndrome. Excess secretion of vasoactive intestinal polypeptide may stimulate an intractable watery diarrhea. Hypertension may be significant, owing to excessive catecholamine production by the tumor.

Although histologic evaluation of tissue is necessary for establishing the definitive diagnosis, a high level of suspicion may arise from the history and physical examination. Initial laboratory evaluation should include a complete blood count, serum electrolytes, blood urea nitrogen, creatinine, and liver function studies. A spot urine should be tested for the catecholamine metabolites homovanillic and vanillylmandelic acid. In addition, several other biochemical markers harbor prognostic significance. A serum lactate dehydrogenase level higher than 1500 IU/mL, serum ferritin level higher than 142 ng/mL, and neuron-specific enolase levels higher than 100 ng/mL correlate with advanced disease and reduced survival.

CT and/or MRI are the preferred modalities for characterizing the location and extent of the NBL. This tumor frequently infiltrates through vascular structures (Fig. 70-20). As such, many tumors that cross the midline are generally not resectable. A CT scan of the chest should be done to exclude pulmonary metastasis, and a bone scan should be done to identify potential bone metastasis. In addition, radiolabeled metaiodobenzyl guanidine (MIBG) is one of the single best studies to document the presence of metastatic disease. Finally, a bone marrow aspirate and

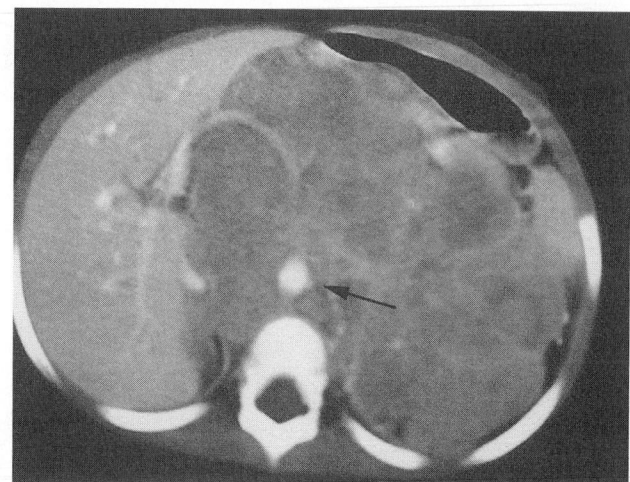

FIGURE 70-20. Neuroblastoma. A CT scan of the abdomen demonstrating a large neuroblastoma surrounding the aorta (arrow) and displacing the liver to the right. Punctate areas of calcium can be seen dispersed throughout the tumor.

biopsy complete the staging evaluation. The international NBL staging system is depicted in Table 70-2.

Although imaging at the time of presentation of most tumors reveals unresectability, the definitive diagnosis requires tissue. This can be obtained via an incisional or needle biopsy of the tumor. NBL identified within bone marrow aspirate or biopsy may also be sufficient. Cytogenetic studies provide significant prognostic information that may affect treatment. Amplification of the N-*myc*

TABLE 70-2.	International Neuroblastoma Staging System	
Stage	**Definition**
1	Localized tumor with complete gross excision, with or without microscopic residual disease; representative ipsilateral lymph nodes negative for tumor microscopically (nodes attached to and removed with the primary tumor may be positive)
2A	Localized tumor with incomplete gross excision; representative ipsilateral nonadherent lymph nodes negative for tumor microscopically
2B	Localized tumor with or without complete gross excision, with ipsilateral nonadherent lymph nodes positive for tumor; enlarged contralateral lymph nodes must be negative microscopically
3	Unresectable unilateral tumor with contralateral regional lymph node involvement; or midline tumor with bilateral extension by infiltration (unresectable) or by lymph node involvement
4	Any primary tumor with dissemination to distant lymph nodes, bone, bone marrow, liver, skin, and/or other organs (except as defined for stage 4S)
4S	Localized primary tumor (as defined for stage 1, 2A, or 2B), with dissemination limited to skin, liver, and/or bone marrow (limited to infant < 1 year of age)

oncogene is one of the classic factors associated with rapid tumor progression and poor prognosis. In addition, gain of genetic material from chromosome arm 17q is associated with deletion of chromosome 1p and N-*myc* amplification and is highly predictive of poor outcome.[50] Diploid tumors have an unfavorable prognosis, whereas hyperdiploid tumors have a better prognosis. Further, expression of the *TRK* protooncogene is inversely associated with N-*myc* amplification and has a more favorable prognosis. Finally, expression of the multidrug resistance–associated protein is associated with a poor outcome. In addition to the cytogenetic studies, prognosis may be derived from the pathologic classification as proposed by Shimada and colleagues, taking into account the degree of differentiation, the mitotic-karyorrhexis index, and presence or absence of stroma.[51]

Current therapy for NBL is multimodal, incorporating surgery, chemotherapy, radiation, and occasionally immunotherapy. Surgical resection of the primary tumor and adjacent lymph nodes should be the goal and may be curative for localized stages 1 and 2 disease. In most situations in which the tumor is unresectable, exploration with incisional biopsy is the initial procedure, with re-evaluation for resection following a course of adjuvant therapy. Following cytoreductive therapy, attempts at resection may be the only option for long-term survival. Meticulous dissection of major blood vessels, which often course through the tumor, is required. These procedures are frequently prolonged and associated with significant blood loss.

Children of any age with localized NBL and infants younger than 1 year of age with advanced disease and favorable disease characteristics have a high likelihood of long-term, disease-free survival. Older children with advanced-stage disease, however, have a significantly decreased chance for cure despite intensive therapy. Prognosis resides in stratification of patients into low-, intermediate-, or high-risk categories (Table 70-3). These are associated with survival rates of greater than 90%, greater than 80%, and 10% to 20%, respectively.[52]

Wilms' Tumor

Wilms' tumor (WT) is an embryonal tumor of renal origin and is the most common primary malignant kidney tumor of childhood. About 500 new cases of WT are diagnosed in the United States each year. This tumor is most frequently seen in children between the ages of 1 and 5 years (~80%) with a peak incidence between 3 and 4 years. Bilateral WT is present in up to 13% of cases and, when present, is synchronous in 60%.

Despite the number of genes implicated in the genesis of this neoplasm, hereditary WT is uncommon.[53] Specific germline mutations in one of these genes (WT gene-1, *WT1*) located on the short arm of chromosome 11, are not only associated with WT but also cause a variety of genitourinary abnormalities such as cryptorchidism and hypospadias. A gene that causes aniridia is located near the *WT1* gene on chromosome 11p13, and deletions encompassing the *WT1* and aniridia genes may explain the

TABLE 70-3. Schema of Clinical Factors Combined for Patient Risk Group Assignment in Future Neuroblastoma Studies*

Risk Group	Stage	Factors
Low	1	
	2	< 1 year
		> 1 year, low N-*myc*
		> 1 year, amplified N-*myc*; favorable histology
	4S	Favorable biology
Intermediate	3	< 1 year, low N-*myc*
		> 1 year, favorable biology
	4	< 1 year, low N-*myc*
	4S	Low N-*myc*
High	2	> 1 year, all unfavorable biology
	3	< 1 year, amplified N-*myc*
		> 1 year, any unfavorable biology
	4	< 1 year, amplified N-*myc*
		> 1 year
	4S	Amplified N-*myc*

*Favorable biology denotes low N-*myc*, favorable histology, and hyperdiploidy (infants).

association between these two conditions. There appears to be a second WT gene at or near the Beckwith-Wiedemann gene locus, also on chromosome 11. Children with Beckwith-Wiedemann syndrome (omphalocele, visceromegaly, macroglossia, hypoglycemia) are at increased risk for developing WT. Approximately one fifth of patients with Beckwith-Wiedemann syndrome who develop WT present with bilateral disease at the time of diagnosis.

Most patients (60%) with WT present clinically with a palpable abdominal mass (Fig. 70-21). Often, the patient has no symptoms and the parents discover the mass during bathing or the pediatrician finds it during a routine physical examination. Hypertension is present in about 25% of patients and hematuria in 15%. Since WT is associated with several syndromes, including Denys-Drash syndrome (WT, intersex disorder, and progressive nephropathy), WAGR syndrome (*W*T, *a*niridia, *g*enitourinary anomalies, mental *r*etardation), and Beckwith-Wiedemann syndrome, patients with these phenotypes should be screened closely into adulthood for the potential development of WT.

The initial evaluation of the child with an abdominal mass and suspected WT is by ultrasonography. This is useful not only in confirming that the mass originates from the kidney but also whether the mass is cystic or solid. In addition, ultrasonography assists in the detection of potential tumor thrombus within the renal vein and inferior vena cava (IVC). Frequently, it is difficult to distinguish WT from NBL. CT or MR imaging is frequently useful in this regard (Fig. 70-22) because WT originates from the kidney and NBL develops in the adrenal or sympathetic ganglia. In cases whereby the origin of the mass is difficult to determine, urinary catecholamine measurements distinguish WT from NBL, since they are elevated in most

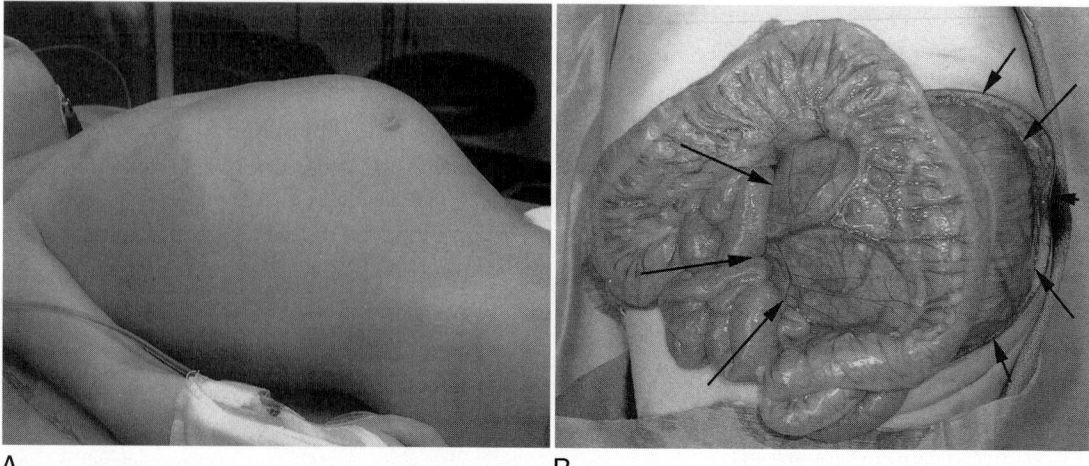

A   B

FIGURE 70-21.   Wilms' tumor. *A,* The large left-sided flank mass is obvious on visual inspection. *B,* On entering the peritoneal cavity, the large Wilms' tumor within the left kidney (outlined by *arrows*) can be seen behind the descending colon, displacing it anterior and medially.

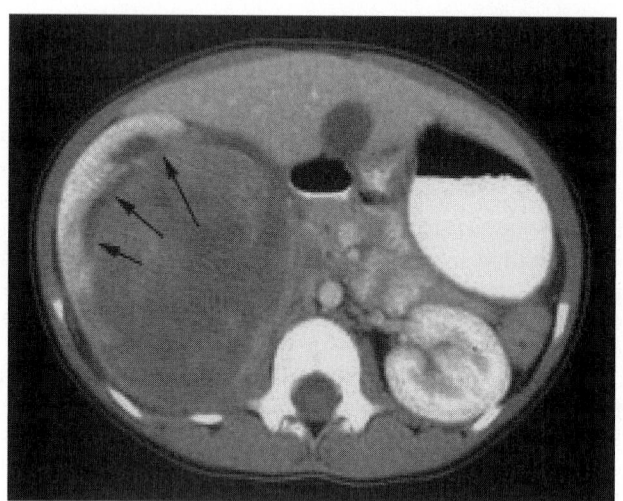

FIGURE 70-22.   CT scan of a Wilms' tumor involving the right kidney. Remnants of the remaining functional kidney (*arrows*) are noted at the periphery of the tumor.

cases of NBL but not in WT. The CT and/or MR studies are also indicated preoperatively to identify bilateral WT, characterize potential invasion into surrounding structures, document liver and/or lung metastasis, and detect tumor thrombus within the IVC. A preoperative plain chest radiograph is also necessary for staging purposes.

After the preoperative evaluation is completed as outlined earlier, exploratory laparotomy is crucial for both staging and treatment of WT. Preoperative chemotherapy may be indicated in cases where WT is present within a solitary or horseshoe kidney, in both kidneys, the presence of respiratory distress from extensive metastatic tumor, or when IVC tumor thrombus has extended above the level of the hepatic veins. In these situations, chemotherapy-induced tumor shrinkage may allow for a more complete resection with less morbidity and with the potential to salvage maximal functional renal parenchyma.

The goals for operative therapy for WT are to confirm the diagnosis, assess the opposite kidney and other abdominal organs for metastatic spread, and completely resect the primary tumor, ureter, and adjacent lymph nodes. This is achieved through a generous transverse or midline transperitoneal incision. At some point during the exploration, Gerota's fascia of the opposite kidney must be opened to more definitively exclude bilateral tumor. The anterior and posterior surfaces of the opposite kidney must be carefully inspected and palpated. Despite the large size of the tumor, complete resection by radical nephroureterectomy can be safely performed. Care should be taken to avoid tumor rupture because this increases the stage of the tumor and mandates additional postoperative adjuvant therapy. Frequently, the ipsilateral adrenal gland is removed en bloc with the kidney. Invasion into surrounding organs such as the pancreas, spleen, or liver may direct their removal as well.

Surgical exploration, coupled with the preoperative imaging studies and histology, permits accurate staging of WT, which correlates with prognosis and guides postoperative adjuvant therapy. The pathologic evaluation of WT involves inspection of the three elements of normal renal development (blastemal, epithelial, and stromal) and identification of the absence or presence of anaplasia, which distinguishes the classification of either favorable histology (FH) or unfavorable histology (UH), respectively. The current staging scheme as proposed by the National Wilms' Tumor Study Group (NWTS) is depicted in Table 70-4.

The treatment of WT represents one of the greatest triumphs in the field of pediatric oncology. In contrast with what used to be a lethal malignancy, the current overall survival exceeds 85%. The successful treatment of this tumor is a direct result of collaboration between multiple

TABLE 70-4. Staging System Used by the National Wilms' Tumor Study Group

Stage	Definition
I	Tumor limited to the kidney and completely excised without rupture or biopsy; surface of the renal capsule is intact
II	Tumor extends through the renal capsule but is completely removed with no microscopic involvement of the margins; vessels outside the kidney contain tumor; also placed in stage II are cases in which the kidney has been biopsied before removal or where there is "local" spillage of tumor (during resection) limited to the tumor bed
III	Residual tumor is confined to the abdomen and of nonhematogenous spread; also included in stage III are cases with tumor involvement of the abdominal lymph nodes, "diffuse" peritoneal contamination by rupture of the tumor extending beyond the tumor bed, peritoneal implants, and microscopic or grossly positive resection margins
IV	Hematogenous metastases at any site
V	Bilateral renal involvement

Box 70-2. NWTS-5 Treatment Recommendations for Wilms' Tumor

Stage I (FH): surgery, no radiotherapy, dactinomycin + vincristine for 18 weeks

Stage I focal anaplasia: surgery, no radiation therapy, dactinomycin + vincristine for 18 weeks

Stage II (FH): surgery, no radiation therapy, dactinomycin + vincristine for 18 weeks

Stage II focal anaplasia: surgery, 1080 cGy to tumor bed, dactinomycin + vincristine + doxorubicin for 24 weeks

Stage III (FH): surgery, 1080 cGy to tumor bed, dactinomycin + vincristine + doxorubicin for 24 weeks

Stage III focal anaplasia: surgery, 1080 cGy to tumor bed, dactinomycin + vincristine + doxorubicin for 24 weeks

Stage IV (FH) *focal anaplasia:* surgery, 1080 cGy to tumor bed according to local tumor stage, 1200 cGy to lung and/or other metastatic sites, dactinomycin + vincristine + doxorubicin for 24 weeks

Stage II-IV diffuse anaplasia: surgery, radiation therapy (whole lung; abdominal 1080 cGy), cyclophosphamide + etoposide + vincristine + doxorubicin + mesna for 24 weeks

Stage I-IV (clear cell sarcoma): surgery, radiation therapy (abdominal 1080 cGy; whole lung, stage IV only), cyclophosphamide + etoposide + vincristine + doxorubicin + mesna for 24 weeks

Stage I-IV (rhabdoid tumor): surgery, radiation therapy, carboplatinum + etoposide + cyclophosphamide + mesna for 24 weeks

Infants < 11 months of age are given half the recommended dose of all drugs. Full doses lead to prohibitive hematologic toxicity in this age group. Full doses of chemotherapeutic agents should be administered to those > 12 months of age
NWTS, National Wilms' Tumor Study; FH, favorable histology.

disciplines to form two major associations (the NWTS group and the International Society of Pediatric Oncology) in which there has been a systematic organization of multicenter trials designed to address focused, highly relevant questions. The recommended treatment for WT based on stage is shown in Box 70-2. The survival of patients with stage I or II FH or stage I UH is the same and is about 95%. For all stages, the overall survival of patients with FH is 90%. For patients with UH, stages II to IV are associated with 70% and 56%, and 17% 4-year survival, respectively.[54]

Rhabdomyosarcoma

Rhabdomyosarcoma (RMS) is a soft tissue malignant tumor of skeletal muscle origin and accounts for approximately 3.5% of the cases of cancer among children younger than 14 years of age. It is a curable disease in most children, with more than 60% surviving 5 years after diagnosis. The most common primary sites for RMS are the head and neck (parameningeal, orbit, pharyngeal), the genitourinary tract, and the extremities. Other less common primary sites include the trunk, gastrointestinal (including liver and biliary) tract, and intrathoracic or perineal region. Most cases of RMS occur sporadically with no recognized predisposing factors, although a small proportion is associated with other genetic conditions. These include Li-Fraumeni cancer susceptibility syndrome (with germline *p53* mutations), neurofibromatosis-1, and Beckwith-Wiedemann syndrome.

The prognosis for a child or adolescent with RMS is related to patient age, site of origin, extent of tumor at time of diagnosis or after surgical resection, and tumor histology.[55] Age younger than 10 years is considered a more favorable prognosis. With regard to tumor site, a more favorable prognosis is afforded when tumors are located in the orbit and nonparameningeal head and neck, genitourinary (excluding bladder and prostate), and the biliary tract.

Patients with smaller tumors (<5 cm) have improved survival when compared to children with larger tumors, whereas children with metastatic disease at diagnosis have the worst prognosis. The prognostic significance of metastatic disease is further modulated by tumor histology, patient age, and primary site. Patients younger than 10 years of age with metastatic disease and with embryonal histology have 5-year survival rates greater than 50%, whereas those older than 10 years of age or with alveolar histology have a much poorer outcome. The presence of regional lymph node involvement is also associated with a worse prognosis. The ability to completely resect the tumor is associated with a better outcome when compared with patients with gross residual disease after initial surgery.

From a histologic standpoint, the botryoid and spindle cell subtypes are associated with a more favorable outcome. Embryonal and pleomorphic subtypes are inter-

---

Box 70-3. Staging for Rhabdomyosarcoma

Group I: localized disease that is completely resected with no regional node involvement (13%)

Group II (~20%)

    IIA: localized, grossly resected tumor with microscopic residual disease but no regional nodal involvement

    IIB: locoregional disease with tumor-involved lymph nodes with complete resection and no residual disease

    IIC: locoregional disease with involved nodes, grossly resected, but with evidence of microscopic residual tumor at the primary site and/or histologic involvement of the most distal regional node (from the primary site)

Group III: localized, gross residual disease including incomplete resection, or biopsy only of the primary site (~48%)

Group IV: distant metastatic disease present at the time of diagnosis (~18%)

---

mediate, and alveolar, or undifferentiated, subtypes are generally associated with a worse prognosis. Favorable prognostic groups have been identified by previous Intergroup Rhabdomyosarcoma Studies, and treatment plans have been designed based on assignment of patients to different groups based on prognosis (Box 70-3).

The diagnostic work-up generally involves CT or MRI. Because there are no useful markers at present, an accurate diagnosis depends on incisional biopsy of the tumor. In the extremity, the direction of the incision should allow it to be incorporated into the wound created by a subsequent wide local excision.

All children with RMS require multimodality therapy. This entails surgical resection, if possible, followed by chemotherapy, followed by second-look surgery for some patients with initially unresectable tumors. Depending on original histologic type, extent of disease, and extent of resection, radiation therapy may be indicated.

The basic surgical principles for the treatment of RMS are complete resection of the primary tumor with a surrounding margin of normal tissue, coupled with sampling of the adjacent lymph nodes. This may not be feasible in patients with obvious metastatic disease but should be done if possible. Because RMS can arise from so many primary muscle sites, surgical care must be tailored to the unique aspects of each site. Surgical management of the more common primary sites is provided in the following sections.

Head and Neck

For those tumors that are superficial and nonorbital, wide excision of the primary tumor with ipsilateral neck lymph node sampling of clinically involved nodes is appropriate.

Because of cosmetic and functional concerns, margins less than 1 mm are acceptable. For patients with tumors that are considered unresectable, chemotherapy and radiation therapy become the primary management. RMS of the orbit requires a biopsy to establish diagnosis and then chemotherapy and radiation therapy. Orbital exenteration is reserved for the small number of patients with local, persistent, or recurrent disease.

Extremity

The definitive surgical procedure involves wide local excision with en bloc of normal tissue. If it is anatomically feasible, a re-excision procedure is associated with better outcome in patients whose initial surgical procedure left microscopic residual disease on pathologic examination. Amputation is reserved for selected patients with lesions involving major neurovascular structures in addition to the muscle of origin. Owing to the significant incidence of nodal spread for extremity primary tumors (often without clinical evidence of involvement), and because of the prognostic and therapeutic implications of nodal involvement, surgical assessment for regional nodal involvement is important.[56] For clinically negative nodes, axillary or femoral node sampling should be done for upper or lower extremity tumors, respectively. If clinically positive nodes are present, biopsy of more proximal nodes is recommended prior to sampling of the involved nodal region.

Trunk

As with RMS in other locations, wide local excision and an attempt to achieve negative microscopic margins should be the goal. Reconstruction may require use of prosthetic materials. Extremely large masses are initially biopsied, followed by a course of chemotherapy and/or radiation. This may shrink the tumor enough to permit a subsequent margin-negative resection with successful reconstruction.

Genitourinary

The initial surgical procedure in most patients consists of a biopsy, which often can be performed via a cystoscope, transanally, or under direct vision. Bladder salvage is an important goal of therapy for patients with tumors arising in the prostate and bladder. Occasionally, when the tumor is confined to the dome of the bladder, it can be completely resected. Otherwise, preresection chemotherapy and radiation therapy allow preservation of a functional bladder in most patients. For patients with biopsy-proven, residual, malignant tumor following chemotherapy and radiation therapy, appropriate surgical management may include partial cystectomy, prostatectomy, or anterior exenteration.

Testis or spermatic cord RMS should be removed by radical orchiectomy and resection of the entire spermatic cord. Resection of hemiscrotal skin may be necessary when there is tumor fixation or invasion, or if a previous transscrotal biopsy has been performed. Since paratesticular tumors are associated with a relatively high incidence of lymphatic spread, all patients with paratesticular primary tumors should have thin-cut abdominal and pelvic CT scans with contrast medium to evaluate nodal involvement. Retroperitoneal lymph node sampling is needed for patients with suggestive or positive CT scans for patients younger than 10 years of age. In contrast, an ipsilateral retroperitoneal lymph node dissection is currently required for all children older than 10 years of age with paratesticular RMS for staging.

Liver Tumors

Liver cancer is rare in childhood and essentially comprises either hepatoblastoma (HBL) or hepatocellular carcinoma (HCC). Several important differences exist between these two subtypes. HBLs usually occur before 3 years of age, whereas HCC may be found in children and adults of all ages. HBL is most often unifocal, whereas HCC is often extensively invasive or multicentric at the time of diagnosis. Complete resection is therefore more often possible in patients with HBL. Childhood HBLs frequently have associated mutations in the β-catenin gene, the function of which is closely related to the development of familial adenomatous polyposis. In addition, HBL is associated with hemihypertrophy, very low birth weight, and Beckwith-Wiedemann syndrome. In contrast, HCC is associated with a history of perinatally acquired hepatitis B and C infection; mutations in the hepatocyte growth factor receptor gene (Met); and tyrosinemia, biliary cirrhosis, and α_1-antitrypsin deficiency. The serum tumor marker α-fetoprotein levels parallel disease activity for both HBL and HCC. The overall survival rate for children with HBL is 70% compared with 25% for HCC. A general staging scheme for hepatic tumors in children is depicted in Table 70-5. Children diagnosed with stages I and II HBL have a cure rate of greater than 90%, whereas stage III is associated with a 60% survival. Children with stage IV disease have a survival of roughly 20%. Children diagnosed with stage I HCC generally have a good outcome. Stage II is too rarely seen to predict outcome, and stages III and IV are usually fatal.

Complete resection of the primary tumor with negative surgical margins is one of the most critical factors in prognosis. Preoperative chemotherapy can convert an unresectable tumor into one that is resectable and may lessen the incidence of postoperative morbidity.[57] Preoperative chemotherapy is more effective in the treatment of HBL when compared with HCC. Surgical resection of distant disease has also contributed to the cure of children with HBL. Resection of pulmonary metastases is recommended when the number of metastases is limited. Liver transplantation may be useful therapy for patients with unresectable hepatic tumors. Five-year survival rates approximating 83% for children with HBL and 63% for children with HCC have been reported.[58] Owing to the worse prognosis in patients with HCC, liver transplant should be considered early in the course for disorders such as tyrosinemia and familial intrahepatic cholestasis prior to the development of liver failure and malignancy. The fibrolamellar variant of HCC may have a better prognosis with liver transplant than other types.

Teratoma

Teratomas are tumors that contain elements derived from more than one of the three embryonic germ layers. In addition, teratomas must contain tissue that is foreign to the anatomic site in which they occur. Teratomas can occur anywhere in the body and present as cystic, solid, or mixed lesions. When they occur during infancy and early childhood, they are most commonly extragonadal. In contrast, in older children teratomas most frequently involve the gonads.

Teratomas occur most frequently in the neonatal period and the sacrococcygeal region is the most common site. Sacrococcygeal teratoma (SCT) is four times more common in females and is most often an obvious external presacral mass (Fig. 70-23). Although most of the tumor is usually external with a minimal intrapelvic presacral component, there is a spectrum of tumor distribution and ranges to the extent of being entirely presacral, with no visible external component. As such, a digital rectal examination of a neonate with care to feel the normal presacral space may be an important screening technique. Occasionally, SCTs are identified during routine prenatal ultrasonography. It is important that these lesions be carefully followed with serial sonography until delivery, since the blood supply to the tumor may grow to the point of stealing a significant proportion of placental blood flow to the fetus. The development of hydrops or placentomegaly is associated with a poor prognosis. In these situations, in utero resection of the tumor may be lifesaving.[59]

Most neonatal SCTs are benign. The incidence of malignancy is related to age at time of diagnosis and represented as endodermal sinus tumors (yolk sac tumors) or embryonal carcinomas. In addition, the likelihood of malignancy is slightly increased in males.

The treatment for SCT is complete surgical excision via a chevron-shaped buttock incision. Most tumors can be completely removed via a sacral approach. If preoperative imaging demonstrates significant intra-abdominal extension of the tumor, a combined abdominosacral approach may be needed. Resection of the coccyx is critical, since

Stage	Definition
TABLE 70-5.	**Liver Tumor Staging**
I	No metastases, tumor completely resected
II	No metastases, tumor grossly resected with microscopic residual disease (i.e., positive margins); or tumor rupture, or tumor spill at the time of surgery
III	No distant metastases, tumor unresectable or resected with gross residual tumor, or positive lymph nodes
IV	Distant metastases regardless of the extent of liver involvement

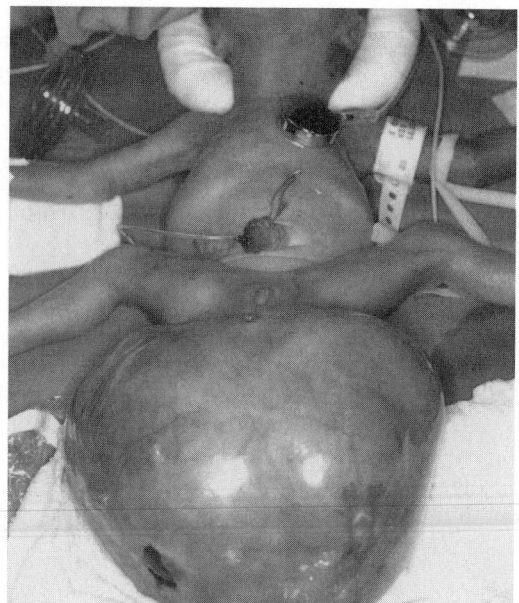

FIGURE 70-23. Sacrococcygeal teratoma. Despite its large size, this tumor is benign in most cases.

failure to remove this structure results in significantly higher local recurrence rates. Care must be taken to individually ligate the vessels supplying the tumor, including the middle sacral artery and branches of the hypogastric arteries. After the tumor is excised, the levator muscle complex is secured to the presacral fascia and the remaining wound is closed in layers. Careful follow-up is necessary because recurrence may be significant, even for benign tumors.

Selected References

Ashcraft KW, Murphy JP, Sharp RJ, et al (eds): Pediatric Surgery, 3rd ed. Philadelphia, WB Saunders, 2000.

> An excellent reference source for most pediatric surgical conditions. Although most topics are not covered as in-depth as the O'Neill text in this list, this book is easy to read and serves as an outstanding practical resource.

Bianchi DW, Crombleholme TM, D'Alton ME: Fetology: Diagnosis and Management of the Fetal Patient. New York, McGraw-Hill, 2000.

> This outstanding reference covers diagnosis and management of prenatally identified conditions. This is a terrific resource to have on hand when counseling parents and provides an excellent overview of the field of fetal therapeutics.

Mattei P (ed): Surgical Directives: Pediatric Surgery. Philadelphia, Lippincott Williams & Wilkins, 2003.

> This is a beautiful reference text for senior surgical residents, fellows, and general surgeons. The chapters are short, to the point, and written to provide a practical approach to most of the common pediatric surgery conditions.

Oldham KT, Colombani PM, Foglia RP (eds): Surgery in Infants and Children: Scientific Principles and Practice. Philadelphia, Lippincott-Raven, 1997.

> This is an excellent reference book that tends to integrate more pathophysiology and basic science discussions of pediatric surgical conditions.

O'Neill JA, Rowe MI, Grosfeld JL, et al (eds): Pediatric Surgery, 5th ed. St. Louis, Mosby, 1998.

> This two-volume monograph provides a comprehensive review of the field of pediatric surgery. This book is considered to be the most authoritative and is the gold standard textbook for pediatric surgeons.

Ziegler MM, Azizkhan RG, Weber TR (eds): Operative Pediatric Surgery. New York, McGraw-Hill, 2003.

> One of the most current, authoritative texts emphasizing operative technique. The illustrations are extremely well done, and this is a beautiful reference for pediatric-specific procedures.

References

1. Conrad SA, Rycus PT: Extracorporeal life support 1997. ASAIO J 44:848-852, 1998.
2. Brown RL, Koepplinger ME, Mehlman CT, et al: All-terrain vehicle and bicycle crashes in children: Epidemiology and comparison of injury severity. J Pediatr Surg 37:375-380, 2002.
3. Stylianos S: Compliance with evidence-based guidelines in children with isolated spleen or liver injury: A prospective study. J Pediatr Surg 37:453-456, 2002.
4. Gallagher PG, Mahoney MJ, Gosche JR: Cystic hygroma in the fetus and newborn. Semin Perinatol 23:341-356, 1999.
5. Liechty KW, Crombleholme TM, Flake AW, et al: Intrapartum airway management for giant fetal neck masses: The EXIT (ex utero intrapartum treatment) procedure. Am J Obstet Gynecol 177:870-874, 1997.
6. Hall N, Ade-Ajayi N, Brewis C, et al: Is intralesional injection of OK-432 effective in the treatment of lymphangioma in children? Surgery 133:238-242, 2003.
7. Sistrunk WE: Technique of removal of cysts and sinuses of the thyroglossal duct. Surg Gynecol Obstet 46:109-112, 1928.
8. Peters TR, Edwards KM: Cervical lymphadenopathy and adenitis. Pediatr Rev 21:399-405, 2000.
9. Flint D, Mahadevan M, Barber C, et al: Cervical lymphadenitis due to non-tuberculous mycobacteria: Surgical treatment and review. Int J Pediatr Otorhinolaryngol 53:187-194, 2000.
10. Livaditis A, Radberg L, Odensjo G: Esophageal end-to-end anastomosis: Reduction of anastomotic tension by circular myotomy. Scand J Thorac Cardiovasc Surg 6:206-214, 1972.
11. Foker JE, Linden BC, Boyle EM Jr, et al: Development of a true primary repair for the full spectrum of esophageal atresia. Ann Surg 226:533-543, 1997.
12. Puri P, Khurana S: Delayed primary esophageal anastomosis for pure esophageal atresia. Semin Pediatr Surg 7:126-129, 1998.
13. Engum SA, Grosfeld JL, West KW, et al: Analysis of morbidity and mortality in 227 cases of esophageal atresia and/or tracheoesophageal fistula over two decades. Arch Surg 130:502-509, 1995.

14. Balson BM, Kravitz EK, McGeady SJ: Diagnosis and treatment of gastroesophageal reflux in children and adolescents with severe asthma. Ann Allergy Asthma Immunol 81:159-164, 1998.

15. Lee P, Rudolph C: Gastroesophageal reflux in infants and children. Adv Pediatr 48:301-329, 2001.

16. Dedivitis RA, Camargo DL, Peixoto GL, et al: Thyroglossal duct: A review of 55 cases. J Am Coll Surg 194:274-277, 2002.

17. Rothenberg SS: Experience with 220 consecutive laparoscopic Nissen fundoplications in infants and children. J Pediatr Surg 33:274-278, 1998.

18. Danielson PD, Emmens RW: Esophagogastric disconnection for gastroesophageal reflux in children with severe neurological impairment. J Pediatr Surg 34:84-87, 1999.

19. Fonkalsrud EW, Ashcraft KW, Coran AG, et al: Surgical treatment of gastroesophageal reflux in children: A combined hospital study of 7467 patients. Pediatrics 101:419-422, 1998.

20. White MC, Langer JC, Don S, et al: Sensitivity and cost minimization analysis of radiology versus olive palpation for the diagnosis of hypertrophic pyloric stenosis. J Pediatr Surg 33:913-917, 1998.

21. Rohrschneider WK, Mittnacht H, Darge K, et al: Pyloric muscle in asymptomatic infants: Sonographic evaluation and discrimination from idiopathic hypertrophic pyloric stenosis. Pediatr Radiol 28:429-434, 1998.

22. Leinwand MJ, Shaul DB, Anderson KD: The umbilical fold approach to pyloromyotomy: Is it a safe alternative to the right upper-quadrant approach? J Am Coll Surg 189:362-367, 1999.

23. Kumaran N, Shankar KR, Lloyd DA, et al: Trends in the management and outcome of jejuno-ileal atresia. Eur J Pediatr Surg 12:163-167, 2002.

24. Warner BW, Ziegler MM: Management of the short bowel syndrome in the pediatric population. Pediatr Clin North Am 40:1335-1350, 1993.

25. Kao SC, Franken EA Jr: Nonoperative treatment of simple meconium ileus: A survey of the Society for Pediatric Radiology. Pediatr Radiol 25:97-100, 1995.

26. Hay SA, Kabesh AA, Soliman HA, et al: Idiopathic intussusception: The role of laparoscopy. J Pediatr Surg 34:577-578, 1999.

27. Teitelbaum DH, Cilley RE, Sherman NJ, et al: A decade of experience with the primary pull-through for Hirschsprung disease in the newborn period: A multicenter analysis of outcomes. Ann Surg 232:372-380, 2000.

28. Georgeson KE, Cohen RD, Hebra A, et al: Primary laparoscopic-assisted endorectal colon pull-through for Hirschsprung's disease: A new gold standard. Ann Surg 229:678-683, 1999.

29. Peña A, Hong A: Advances in the management of anorectal malformations. Am J Surg 180:370-376, 2000.

30. Georgeson KE, Inge TH, Albanese CT: Laparoscopically assisted anorectal pull-through for high imperforate anus—a new technique. J Pediatr Surg 35:927-931, 2000.

31. Langer JC: Gastroschisis and omphalocele. Semin Pediatr Surg 5:124-128, 1996.

32. Wiener ES, Touloukian RJ, Rodgers BM, et al: Hernia survey of the Section on Surgery of the American Academy of Pediatrics. J Pediatr Surg 31:1166-1169, 1996.

33. Miltenburg DM, Nuchtern JG, Jaksic T, et al: Laparoscopic evaluation of the pediatric inguinal hernia—a meta-analysis. J Pediatr Surg 33:874-879, 1998.

34. Grosfeld JL: Current concepts in inguinal hernia in infants and children. World J Surg 13:506-515, 1989.

35. Lotan G, Klin B, Efrati Y, et al: Laparoscopic evaluation and management of nonpalpable testis in children. World J Surg 25:1542-1545, 2001.

36. Tackett LD, Wacksman J, Billmire D, et al: The high intra-abdominal testis: Technique and long-term success of laparoscopic testicular autotransplantation. J Endourol 16:359-361, 2002.

37. Reickert CA, Hirschl RB, Atkinson JB, et al: Congenital diaphragmatic hernia survival and use of extracorporeal life support at selected level III nurseries with multimodality support. Surgery 123:305-310, 1998.

38. Harrison MR, Adzick NS, Bullard KM, et al: Correction of congenital diaphragmatic hernia in utero VII: A prospective trial. J Pediatr Surg 32:1637-1642, 1997.

39. Flake AW, Crombleholme TM, Johnson MP, et al: Treatment of severe congenital diaphragmatic hernia by fetal tracheal occlusion: Clinical experience with fifteen cases. Am J Obstet Gynecol 183:1059-1066, 2000.

40. Boloker J, Bateman DA, Wung JT, et al: Congenital diaphragmatic hernia in 120 infants treated consecutively with permissive hypercapnea/spontaneous respiration/elective repair. J Pediatr Surg 37:357-366, 2002.

41. Stolar CJ: What do survivors of congenital diaphragmatic hernia look like when they grow up? Semin Pediatr Surg 5:275-279, 1996.

42. Nuss D, Kelly RE Jr, Croitoru DP, et al: A 10-year review of a minimally invasive technique for the correction of pectus excavatum. J Pediatr Surg 33:545-552, 1998.

43. Adzick NS, Harrison MR, Crombleholme TM, et al: Fetal lung lesions: Management and outcome. Am J Obstet Gynecol 179:884-889, 1998.

44. Balistreri WF, Grand R, Hoofnagle JH, et al: Biliary atresia: Current concepts and research directions—summary of a symposium. Hepatology 23:1682-1692, 1996.

45. Zerbini MC, Gallucci SD, Maezono R, et al: Liver biopsy in neonatal cholestasis: A review on statistical grounds. Mod Pathol 10:793-799, 1997.

46. Balistreri WF: Bile acid therapy in pediatric hepatobiliary disease: The role of ursodeoxycholic acid. J Pediatr Gastroenterol Nutr 24:573-589, 1997.

47. Ryckman FC, Alonso MH, Bucuvalas JC, et al: Biliary atresia: Surgical management and treatment options as they relate to outcome. Liver Transpl Surg 4:S24-S33, 1998.

48. Alonso-Lej F, Rever WB, Pessagno DJ: Congenital choledochal cyst, with a report of 2, and an analysis of 94 cases. Int Abst Surg 108:1-30, 1959.

49. Yamataka A, Ohshiro K, Okada Y, et al: Complications after cyst excision with hepaticoenterostomy for choledochal cysts and their surgical management in children versus adults. J Pediatr Surg 32:1097-1102, 1997.

50. Bown N, Cotterill S, Lastowska M, et al: Gain of chromosome arm 17q and adverse outcome in patients with neuroblastoma. N Engl J Med 340:1954-1961, 1999.

51. Shimada H, Chatten J, Newton WA Jr, et al: Histopathologic prognostic factors in neuroblastic tumors: Definition of subtypes of ganglioneuroblastoma and an age-linked classification of neuroblastomas. J Natl Cancer Inst 73:405-416, 1984.

52. Haase GM, Perez C, Atkinson JB: Current aspects of biology, risk assessment, and treatment of neuroblastoma. Semin Surg Oncol 16:91-104, 1999.

53. Huff V: Wilms' tumor genetics. Am J Med Genet 79:260-267, 1998.

54. Shamberger RC: Pediatric renal tumors. Semin Surg Oncol 16:105-120, 1999.

55. Raney RB, Anderson JR, Barr FG, et al: Rhabdomyosarcoma and undifferentiated sarcoma in the first two decades of

life: A selective review of Intergroup Rhabdomyosarcoma Study group experience and rationale for Intergroup Rhabdomyosarcoma Study V. J Pediatr Hematol Oncol 23:215-220, 2001.

56. Neville HL, Andrassy RJ, Lobe TE, et al: Preoperative staging, prognostic factors, and outcome for extremity rhabdomyosarcoma: A preliminary report from the Intergroup Rhabdomyosarcoma Study IV (1991–1997). J Pediatr Surg 35:317-321, 2000.

57. Schnater JM, Aronson DC, Plaschkes J, et al: Surgical view of the treatment of patients with hepatoblastoma: Results from the first prospective trial of the International Society of Pediatric Oncology Liver Tumor Study Group. Cancer 94:1111-1120, 2002.

58. Reyes JD, Carr B, Dvorchik I, et al: Liver transplantation and chemotherapy for hepatoblastoma and hepatocellular cancer in childhood and adolescence. J Pediatr 136:795-804, 2000.

59. Kitano Y, Flake AW, Crombleholme TM, et al: Open fetal surgery for life-threatening fetal malformations. Semin Perinatol 23:448-461, 1999.

CHAPTER 71

NEUROSURGERY

Lawrence S. Chin, M.D.,   E. Francois Aldrich, M.D.,
Arthur J. DiPatri, M.D.,   and   Howard M. Eisenberg, M.D.

Cerebrovascular Disorders	**Functional Neurosurgery**
Central Nervous System Tumors	**Surgery for Congenital Abnormalities**
Traumatic Head Injury	**Central Nervous System Infections**
Degenerative Disorders of the Spine	

In this chapter, we consider diseases or conditions of the central nervous system and spine that are commonly managed by neurosurgeons. In some cases, these conditions can be considered solely "neurosurgical"; in others, depending on the style of individual practices, there is an overlap with specialty areas of neurointensivists, neuroradiologists, radiation and medical oncologists, neuro-otologists, plastic surgeons, and orthopedic surgeons. The chapter is divided into subsections: *cerebrovascular disorders,* which includes subarachnoid hemorrhage, intracerebral hemorrhage, aneurysm, and arteriovenous malformation (AVM); *central nervous system tumors,* which includes neoplasms of the brain, cranial nerves, spinal cord and their coverings, and lesions of the skull base; *traumatic head injury; degenerative diseases of the spine; functional neurosurgery,* which includes stereotaxis, epilepsy surgery, surgery for the management of pain and movement disorder, and stereotactic radiosurgery; *surgery for congenital abnormalities* of the brain, skull, facial bones, spinal cord, and spine; and neurosurgical management of *central nervous system infections.*

CEREBROVASCULAR DISORDERS

The term *brain attack* has been coined to increase the awareness of stroke among not only physicians but also the general public. As a public health concern, this disease is the third leading cause of death in the United States. A brain attack is defined as the sudden onset of neurologic worsening, including a loss of consciousness and focal neurologic deficits. The etiology can be classified as either ischemic or hemorrhagic depending on whether or not

blood is seen on a computed tomography (CT) scan of the brain. Among the ischemic causes for brain attack is thromboembolism, which leads to cerebral infarction, but this is a disease traditionally treated by neurologists and is beyond the scope of this chapter. Instead, the focus here is on the management of hemorrhagic stroke, of which there are two types: subarachnoid hemorrhage and intracerebral hemorrhage.

Spontaneous Subarachnoid Hemorrhage

Spontaneous subarachnoid hemorrhage (SAH) is defined as bleeding into the subarachnoid space, particularly the basal cisterns of the brain, which is not caused by trauma. It can range from a small, focal amount of blood to a large, diffuse clot throughout the basal cisterns. Extensive SAH can be associated with intracerebral hematomas and/or intraventricular hemorrhage (IVH). The most common cause of SAH is the rupture of an intracranial aneurysm; other causes include hypertension and AVMs (Table 71-1). Subarachnoid hemorrhage accounts for approximately 10% of all strokes, with an annual incidence of 10 per 100,000 population, resulting in an estimated 30,000 cases in the United States per year. It affects adults of all ages but peaks in the 4th to 5th decades of life; 60% of patients are women.

Signs and Symptoms

Subarachnoid hemorrhage is characterized by the sudden onset of very severe headaches that patients often describe as the worse headache of their life. Other symptoms may include nausea and vomiting, loss of consciousness, and seizures.[1] Depending on the severity of the bleed, the patient's neurologic condition may vary from awake and oriented to moribund with severe neurologic deficits. In the first few hours following SAH, the subarachnoid blood causes an aseptic meningitis characterized by nuchal rigidity, low-grade fever, and photophobia. Warning symptoms preceding SAH from aneurysmal rupture have been reported in up to 40% of patients and are usually attributed to aneurysm enlargement or a minor bleed (sentinel hemorrhage). These symptoms are usually headaches or dizziness, and unfortunately many go unrecognized. Various activities, including heavy lifting and bending (12%), emotional strain (4%), defecation (4%), and coitus (4%), have been blamed for initiating SAH, but approximately 30% of cases occur during sleep. It is estimated that smoking increases the chances of a subarachnoid hemorrhage by a factor of four.[2] Cardiac abnormalities are common after SAH: most patients are hypertensive, and frequent electrocardiographic (ECG) changes such as prolonged QT intervals, elevated or depressed ST segments, and ventricular arrhythmias are present. It is believed that these ECG findings are caused by increased serum levels of catecholamines after SAH, thus resulting in subendocardial ischemia.

Diagnosis and Management of Subarachnoid Hemorrhage

If the clinical history suggests that a patient may have suffered an SAH, the diagnosis should be confirmed by CT scan, or lumbar puncture (LP) if the CT scan is negative. A high index of suspicion by the primary care physician or emergency physician is necessary because misdiagnosis on presentation is the most common preventable factor leading to a poor outcome after a ruptured aneurysm. A delay in diagnosis of subarachnoid hemorrhage occurs in up to 25% of patients and is most likely in alert patients who have only a headache or in patients with no mental status changes or focal neurologic signs.

An unenhanced CT scan is the preferred procedure for detection of subarachnoid hemorrhage and is positive in more than 90% of patients in the first 24 hours and more than 50% in the first week.[3] The sensitivity of CT scan for SAH drops off dramatically after the first week. Subarachnoid hemorrhage appears as areas of increased density in the subarachnoid spaces along the base of the skull and within the sylvian fissure (Fig. 71-1A). The location of the subarachnoid hemorrhage may frequently suggest the site of the aneurysm, and, rarely, the aneurysm itself might be

TABLE 71-1.	Causes of Spontaneous Subarachnoid Hemorrhage	
Cause	**Percentage**
Aneurysm	51
Hypertension	15
Arteriovenous malformation	6
Other (blood diseases, coagulopathies, tumors, angiopathy, etc.)	6
No cause found	22

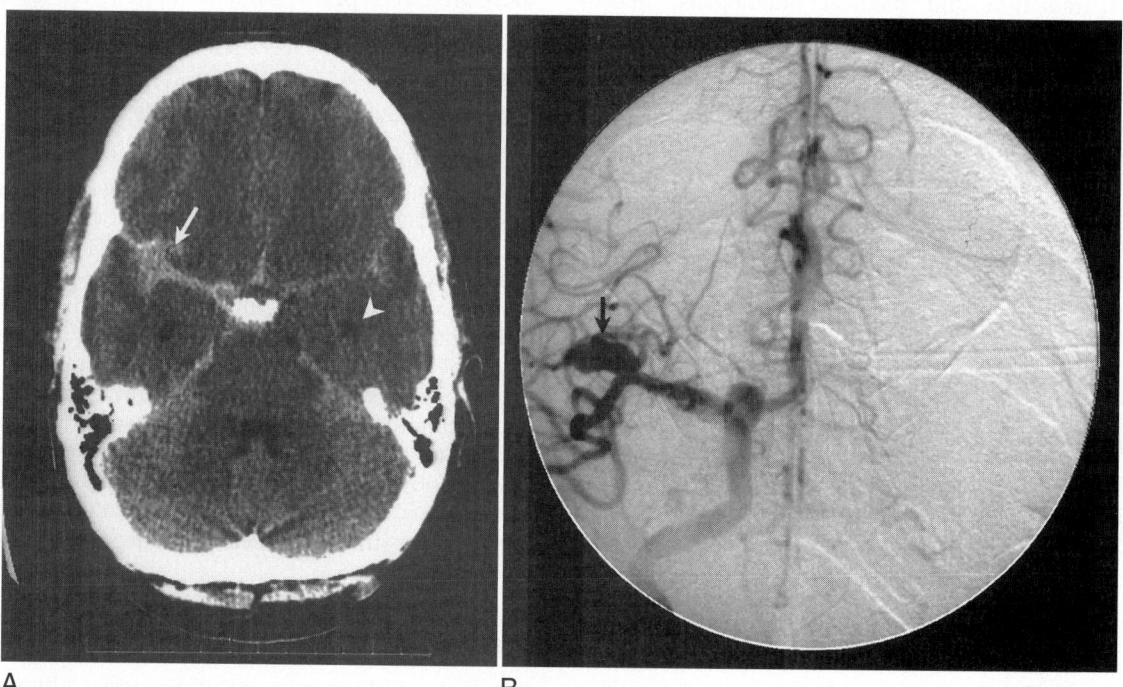

FIGURE 71-1. **A,** CT scan of brain showing subarachnoid blood in the basal cisterns. A focal deposition of blood in the distal sylvian fissure *(arrow)* suggests a middle cerebral artery aneurysm. Dilated temporal horns *(arrowhead)* indicate the presence of hydrocephalus. **B,** Cerebral angiogram shows a right middle cerebral artery aneurysm *(arrow)*.

visible (Fig. 71-1B). Other abnormalities, such as intracerebral hematomas, IVH, and hydrocephalus, can also be diagnosed by CT scans. CT angiography is rapidly becoming an important screening tool in the diagnosis of cerebral aneurysms.[4] Its advantages are the avoidance of arterial puncture, high sensitivity, and three-dimensional reconstruction and visualization. Unlike catheter angiography, however, hemodynamic information on aneurysm filling is not available.

Magnetic resonance imaging (MRI) is not recommended in the acute management of patients with subarachnoid hemorrhage because it is difficult to manage acutely sick patients within the environment of an MRI suite, and SAH is poorly seen on MRI. For patients with unruptured aneurysms, however, MRI and magnetic resonance angiography are excellent screening procedures to detect and follow intracranial aneurysms, and aneurysms as small as 3 mm have been identified in high-quality MRI studies.[5]

If SAH is suspected but the CT scan is negative, an LP should be performed, provided the patient does not have an intracerebral hematoma or other lesion causing mass effect. When an LP is performed, a few milliliters of cerebrospinal fluid (CSF) should be saved for centrifugation, and the appearance of the supernatant fluid should be noted. Oxyhemoglobin appears in the CSF a few hours after the hemorrhage, followed by the appearance of bilirubin, which persists for 2 to 3 weeks and causes the centrifuged CSF to appear yellow. These blood breakdown products result in CSF xanthochromia, which indicate that bleeding has occurred, and that bloody CSF is not the result of a traumatic LP. Similarly, when CSF is obtained more than 1 to 3 weeks after hemorrhage, red blood cells are not usually present, and xanthochromia may be the only proof that bleeding occurred. Further indications of SAH are an elevated CSF pressure and a low glucose content.

Once the diagnosis of a subarachnoid hemorrhage has been established, it is best for the patient to be transferred to a neurosurgical center where surgical treatment can be offered. An angiogram is optional before transfer because it is preferable for the angiogram to be performed at the institution where the surgical management will be provided to ensure good-quality studies and adequate views of the aneurysm. To minimize the risk of missing an aneurysm, a complete four-vessel cerebral angiogram should be performed, including the origin of both posterior inferior cerebellar arteries. If an aneurysm is found, special views are necessary to identify the anatomy of the aneurysm neck and the surrounding blood vessels (Fig. 71-2A). With modern techniques, more than 85% of aneurysms are identified on the first study, but if the study is negative, a second angiogram is usually performed within 7 to 10 days after the initial study, yielding an additional 10%. If both angiograms are negative, other causes of SAH need to be excluded. Additional studies to order may include a contrast-enhanced brain MRI to exclude an intracranial tumor, as well as a thorough medical work-up to exclude a bleeding disorder or vasculitis. After the diagnosis of aneurysmal SAH, the patient should receive strict bed rest, calcium-channel blockers (nimodipine) to combat vasospasm, anticonvulsants, blood pressure control, and pain relief, but oversedation should be avoided.

Cerebral Aneurysms

The normal cerebral artery consists of three layers: (1) an outer adventitia consisting of loosely woven collagen; (2) a smooth muscle layer called the *media;* and (3) an inner layer called the *intima,* which includes the internal elastic lamina, a thin collagen layer, and the endothelium. Cerebral artery aneurysms (also known as *berry* or *saccular aneurysms*) typically develop at vessel bifurcations,

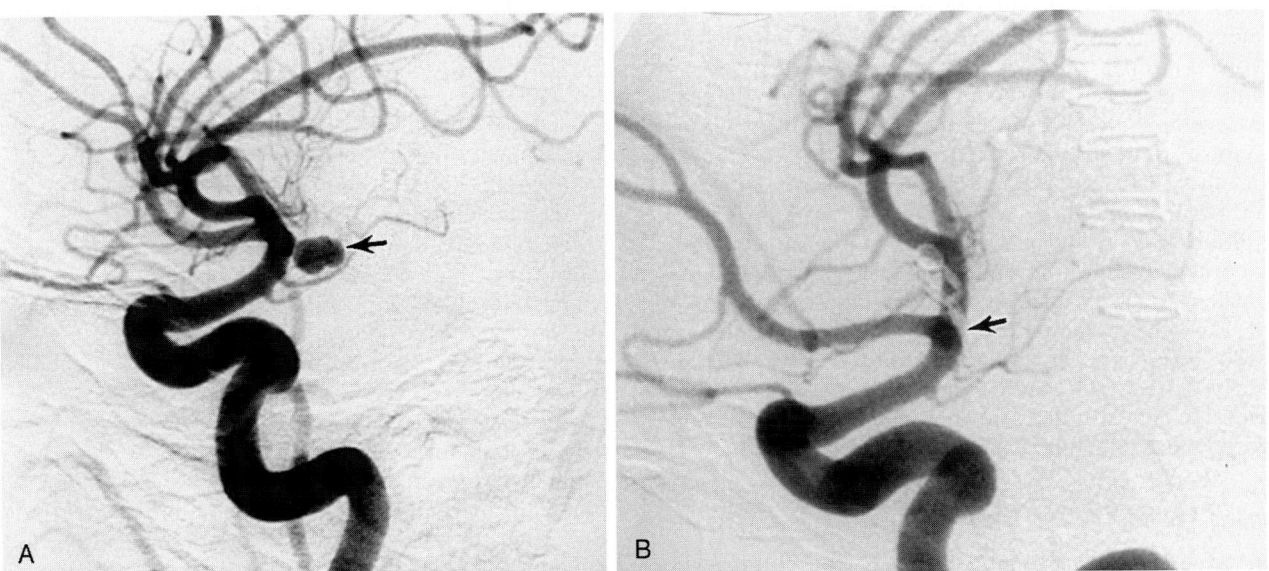

■ **FIGURE 71-2.** **A,** Subtracted carotid angiogram shows a 4 × 6-mm berry aneurysm *(arrow)* originating from the distal internal carotid artery. **B,** Postoperative carotid angiogram shows clip placement *(arrow)* with total obliteration of the aneurysm.

where defects in the media are common, and have been postulated to arise from degenerative changes in the wall of the vessel. As an aneurysm enlarges, the internal elastic lamina becomes fragmented and defects in the media enlarge, resulting in an aneurysm dome that consists primarily of the residual intima and the adventitia. Turbulent blood flow entering the aneurysm through its relatively narrow neck contributes to its enlargement and to the laminations of thrombus that are frequently deposited within its sac. Berry aneurysms can occur anywhere along the arterial circle of Willis, but they are most common in the anterior circulation: at the junction of the posterior communicating artery and the internal carotid artery, at the junction of the anterior communicating artery and anterior cerebral artery, or at the first major branch of the middle cerebral artery. In the posterior circulation, the most common location is at the terminal bifurcation of the basilar artery. Multiple aneurysms are found in approximately 20% of patients with aneurysms.

The natural history of intracranial aneurysms has been the focus of numerous studies. Approximately 10% to 15% of patients die from aneurysmal SAH before reaching the hospital. If the patient survives the initial hemorrhage, rebleeding is the most likely cause of death, with a peak incidence in the first 24 hours after the initial event. If the aneurysm is left unsecured, the rebleed rate is 20% in the first 2 weeks, 50% in the first 6 months, and thereafter 3% to 4% per year.[6] Compared to ruptured aneurysms, incidentally found or unruptured aneurysms have a lower risk of bleeding that depends on aneurysm size. The yearly risk is approximately 0.05% to 0.5% for aneurysms smaller than 1 cm in diameter and 1% to 2% for aneurysms larger than 1 cm.[6]

Besides rebleeding, cerebral vasospasm is the main cause of complications and death in patients with aneurysmal SAH. The peak incidence for vasospasm is between the 3rd and 10th day following SAH. Once it develops, it can persist for weeks. Vasospasm is caused by a cascade of events initiated by blood breakdown products in the subarachnoid space leading to narrowing of the arterial lumen. This results in decreased blood flow through the involved arteries, and depending on the severity, it may manifest as cerebral ischemia or infarction. The risk for developing vasospasm is proportional to the amount of clot in the subarachnoid space and can be estimated from the thickness of blood in the basal cisterns as seen on the CT scan.[7]

Blood and proteinaceous debris in the subarachnoid space can occlude the arachnoid villi and other arachnoidal channels that facilitate the normal absorption of CSF. This causes a communicating hydrocephalus that can last for days to weeks until the blood has been absorbed. The blood can also cause scarring in the subarachnoid space, which can lead to permanent communicating hydrocephalus in approximately 20% of cases.

Surgical Treatment of Aneurysms

After an aneurysm has been identified, a surgical decision must be made regarding the technique and timing of obliteration. In the past, surgery was often delayed until the 2nd or 3rd week after the initial hemorrhage to avoid the complications of operating on a swollen brain. With delayed surgery the surgical morbidity and mortality rates were acceptable, but the overall results were not always good because of a high incidence of rebleeding and difficulty in managing vasospasm.[8] Currently, most experts advocate early surgical intervention preferably within the first 48 hours after hemorrhage.[9] The standard approach for an anterior circulation aneurysm is a pterional craniotomy, which exposes the frontal and temporal lobes and allows access to the sylvian fissure. The operating microscope provides illumination and magnification for the neurosurgeon to dissect the aneurysm free from its parent vessels and to allow a definitive clip to be placed across the neck, thus obliterating blood flow into the aneurysm. Aneurysm clips are manufactured in a variety of shapes, sizes, and lengths and are MRI compatible. Temporary aneurysm clips have less closing force than permanent clips, and when placed on the surrounding blood vessels provide safety during dissection and are indispensable during an intraoperative aneurysm rupture. Intraoperative evoked potential monitoring and advanced neuroanesthesia techniques are critical to avoid ischemic complications from temporary clipping. Ideally, the end result is an aneurysm that is excluded from the normal circulation without compromise of the adjacent vessels or the small perforating vessels, which provide blood for critical deep brain structures such as the internal capsule (Fig. 71-2B). With experienced surgeons, the operative mortality rate is less than 5%. After surgery, a postoperative angiogram can confirm good clip placement with total obliteration of the aneurysm and patent surrounding vessels. Alternatively, though technically challenging, an intraoperative angiogram can be performed, which allows the neurosurgeon to reposition the aneurysm clip without requiring reoperation.

During the past decade, endovascular methods have been refined to treat intracranial aneurysms. Initially, only endovascular balloon occlusion of a feeding artery was feasible. Now, the direct obliteration of an aneurysm lumen using either balloons or microcoils is possible. The most popular technique, initially described by Guglielmi and colleagues, uses a platinum microcoil that is soft and can be detached from the stainless-steel guide by passing a very small direct current that causes electrolysis at the solder junction.[10,11] This technique is most successful in aneurysms with a small neck (Fig. 71-3A and B). In current practice, endovascular techniques are best suited for posterior fossa aneurysms because of the higher surgical risks associated with these aneurysms. No direct comparisons are now available between surgical and endovascular therapy and long-term follow-up with aneurysm coiling is still lacking.

Despite successful obliteration of the aneurysm, patients remain at significant risk for vasospasm, hydrocephalus, and medical complications and should be treated in an intensive care setting for at least 7 to 10 days. Operative complications represent only a small portion of the morbidity and mortality rates associated with ruptured intracranial aneurysms.[12] Vasospasm most commonly presents as a deterioration in mental status or the develop-

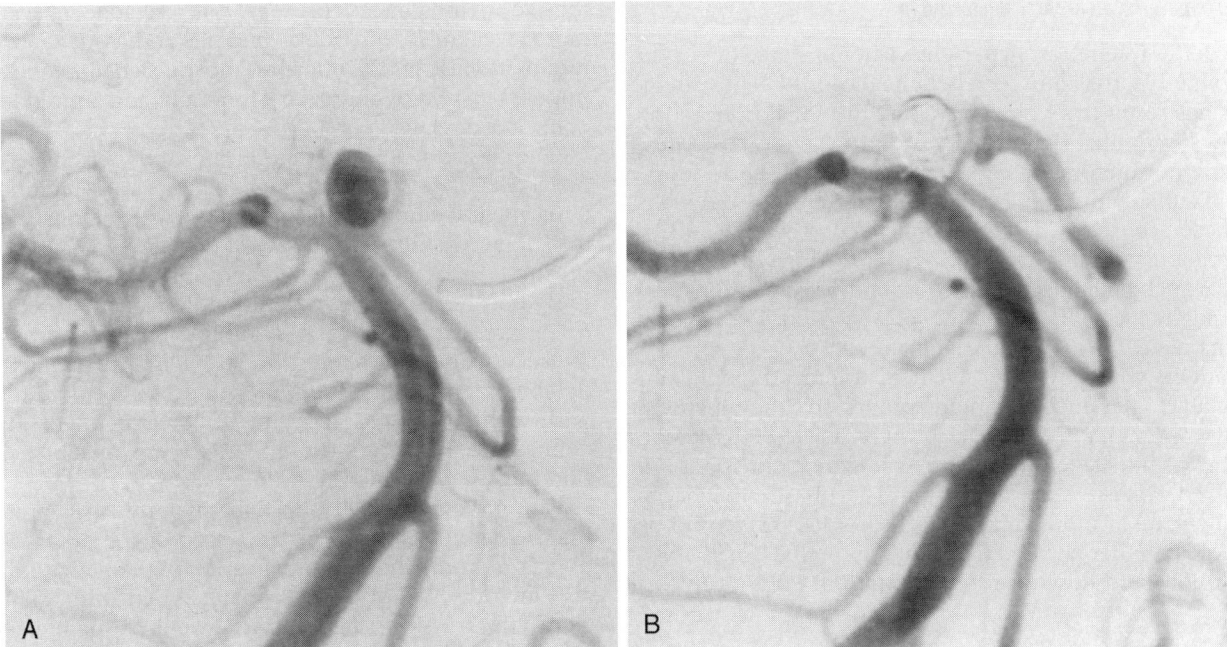

FIGURE 71-3. **A,** Subtracted vertebral angiogram shows a basilar tip aneurysm. **B,** Subtracted vertebral angiogram after the placement of coils demonstrates excellent obliteration of the aneurysm and preservation of adjacent vessels.

ment of focal neurologic deficits, most commonly hemiparesis or dysphasia. A CT scan should be performed to exclude hydrocephalus, rebleed, stroke, or cerebral edema, but it is unable to provide proof of vasospasm. The transcranial Doppler is a frequently used noninvasive diagnostic tool that is sensitive to caliber changes in the larger vessels of the circle of Willis, and in vasospasm it can detect an increase in cerebral blood flow velocity. When in doubt, a cerebral angiogram can confirm the diagnosis. Vasospasm must be aggressively managed and avoided if possible because it causes ischemia and can lead to infarction resulting in permanent disability or death. On admission, all patients are placed on the calcium-channel blocker nimodipine for 21 days to prevent and treat vasospasm. Once the aneurysm is secured, all patients are treated aggressively with hypertension, hypervolemia, and hemodilution (also known as HHH) therapy, which counteracts vasospasm by maintaining cerebral blood flow. In refractory cases, endovascular treatments using transluminal balloon angioplasty or intra-arterial papaverine injection may be beneficial (Box 71-1).

Acute hydrocephalus, which raises the intracranial pressure (ICP) and causes neurologic deterioration, should be treated by insertion of an intraventricular catheter (IVC) to provide CSF drainage. Permanent communicating hydrocephalus can develop in approximately 20% of patients and requires a shunting procedure, usually a ventriculoperitoneal or lumboperitoneal shunt.

Spontaneous Intracerebral Hemorrhage

A spontaneous intracerebral hematoma (SICH) is a blood clot in brain parenchyma that arises in the absence of

---

Box 71-1. Management of Vasospasm

Prevention of arterial narrowing
  Subarachnoid blood removal
  Prevention of dehydration and hypotension
  Calcium-channel blockers (nimodipine)
Reversal of arterial narrowing
  Intra-arterial papaverine
  Transluminal balloon angioplasty
Prevention and reversal of ischemic neurologic deficit
  Hypertension, hypervolemia, and hemodilution

---

trauma and has a variety of causes, the most important being hypertension (Box 71-2). SICH accounts for 10% of all strokes, and there are approximately 40,000 cases of SICH annually in the United States.[1] Age is an important predisposing factor, as illustrated by the fact that at age 45, there is a 2 per 100,000 population per year incidence, whereas at age 80 or older, there is a 350 per 100,000 population per year incidence. In young adults, SICH is most likely due to AVM, aneurysm, or drug abuse, whereas in the elderly, hypertension, tumor, or amyloid angiopathy is most common. Diagnosis of the underlying lesion causing the intracerebral hematoma is critical, particularly if the hematoma causes significant mass effect and the patient needs surgery. The surgical approach, instrumentation, and postoperative follow-up need to be tailored to the specific etiology. The remainder of this section covers the management of hypertensive SICH.

Hypertensive Intracerebral Hemorrhage

In order of frequency, hypertensive hemorrhage occurs in the putamen, thalamus, cerebellum, or pons.[13] These hemorrhages result from bleeding along the small perforating arteries of the brain such as the lenticulostriates, thalamoperforators, or midline basilar artery perforators. When subjected to long-standing hypertension, the walls of these arteries undergo fibrinoid necrosis, and miliary microaneurysms known as *Charcot-Bouchard aneurysms* appear. Rebleeding seldom occurs, although patients may deteriorate several days after presentation as cerebral edema develops around the hematoma.

Patients with a hypertensive hematoma in the putamen typically experience a rapidly progressive hemiparesis, hemisensory loss, and hemianopsia contralateral to the side of the hemorrhage. When the dominant hemisphere is involved, aphasia is usually present. Thalamic hemorrhages usually cause a greater hemisensory loss than motor weakness. Other characteristic findings include small reactive pupils and downward eye deviation. Pontine hyper-tensive hemorrhages present with headache, vertigo, motor weakness, and ocular findings and carry a mortality rate of at least 75%.[14] Poor prognostic signs include small pupils, bilateral pyramidal dysfunction, and a rapid loss of consciousness.

The classic symptoms of a cerebellar hypertensive hemorrhage are headache, dizziness, nausea, and vomiting. On neurologic examination, patients may demonstrate an ipsilateral dysmetria and gait imbalance. Focal motor, sensory, visual field deficits, and aphasias are conspicuously absent. Neurologic deterioration occurs secondary to progressive brain stem compression and obstructive hydrocephalus and should be suspected in patients that demonstrate obtundation, motor weakness, and difficulty with conjugate eye movement. Treatment of hydrocephalus by ventriculostomy and emergent clot evacuation must be considered in these cases.[15]

The radiographic diagnosis of hypertensive intracerebral hematoma is made by a CT scan of the brain, which reveals not only the size and location of the hematoma but also the presence of hydrocephalus, brain shift, and brain stem compression (Fig. 71-4A). In elderly patients with a well-known history of hypertension and a classic CT appearance of a hematoma in the putamen, thalamus, cerebellum, or pons, further diagnostic studies are usually not indicated, and treatment plans can be based on the CT scan. However, in patients younger than 40 years; those without hypertension; those with a history of neoplasm, blood dyscrasias, or bacterial endocarditis; and specifically those with blood in the subarachnoid space or an atypical location or appearance of the blood clot, further diagnostic studies are indicated. An MRI with contrast medium is preferred because it can reveal tumors, AVMs, and aneurysms larger than 3 mm. If a vascular cause for the intracerebral hematoma is suspected, a four-vessel cerebral angiogram should be performed, which may be positive in more than 50% of younger patients. In cases with negative imaging results, a thorough medical work-up for coagulopathy and vasculitis should be performed.

Box 71-2. Causes of Spontaneous Intracerebral Hemorrhage

Hypertension
Vascular anomaly
   Cerebral aneurysm
   Arteriovenous malformation
   Cavernous malformation
Cerebral infarction (stroke) transformation
Cerebral amyloid angiopathy
Coagulopathy
Tumors
Drug abuse
Other

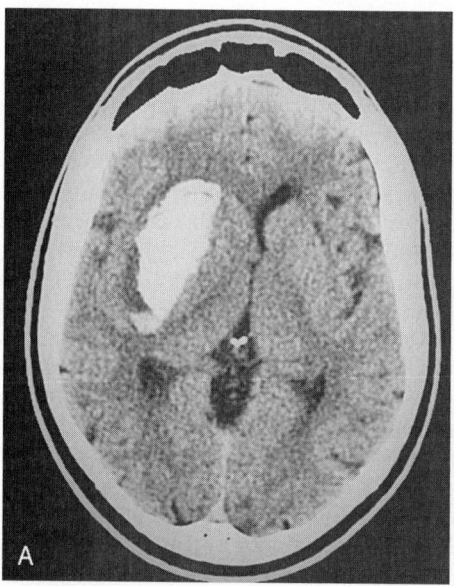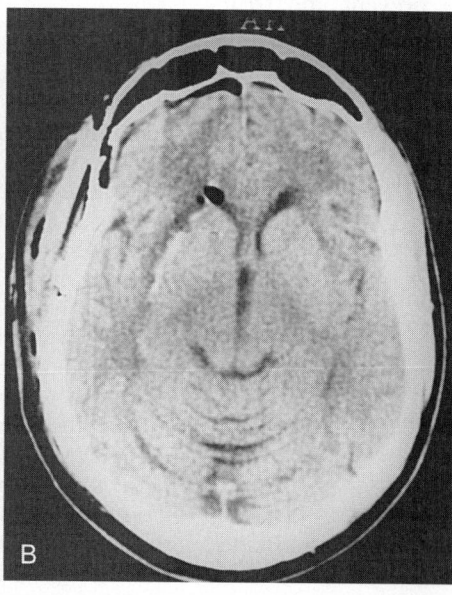

FIGURE 71-4. Nonenhanced CT scan of the head. **A,** Spontaneous hypertensive intracerebral hematoma in the nondominant hemisphere. **B,** Immediate postoperative CT scan shows near-total removal of intracerebral hematoma.

Treatment

Neurologic deficit caused by damaged brain tissue cannot be reversed; however, treatment can be directed at preventing and reversing secondary brain damage caused by edema, intracranial hypertension, brain shift, and direct pressure on the surrounding brain parenchyma. Most patients need to be managed in an intensive care unit where close neurologic examinations can be performed and cardiopulmonary complications minimized. ICP may need monitoring via an intraparenchymal fiberoptic probe or an IVC, which has the advantage of both providing pressure readings as well as being able to drain CSF to lower ICP. Arterial hypertension should be controlled, but care should be taken to preserve cerebral perfusion pressure to at least 70 to 80 mm Hg.

The role and timing of surgical intervention for a hypertensive intracerebral hemorrhage remain controversial. The patient's age, medical condition, level of consciousness, and neurologic examination must be considered while making a decision for surgery. Furthermore, the CT scan appearance—namely, the size, location, midline shift, signs of raised ICP, and whether the blood clot is on the dominant or nondominant side of the brain—is important in the decision-making process. In elderly, moribund patients with a large dominant hemisphere hematoma, surgery is not indicated. Similarly, in an alert patient with minimal neurologic deficit and a small hematoma, surgery will not be beneficial. Brain stem and deep basal ganglia hemorrhages, especially in the dominant hemisphere, are usually not treated surgically, whereas peripherally located hematomas as a group are much better surgical candidates. Patients with an initial good neurologic examination who then deteriorate, especially if the clot is on the nondominant side, should undergo immediate surgery (Fig. 71-4B). In general, cerebellar hematomas carry a much better prognosis than most hypertensive bleeds, and they should be removed in most patients regardless of how poor their neurologic examination may be (Fig. 71-5). Most neurosurgeons have had the experience of a moribund patient that made an excellent recovery following removal of a cerebellar hemorrhage.

There are two basic surgical methods for removing intracerebral hematomas. The first is to perform a stereotactic needle aspiration of the blood clot using fibrinolytic agents or mechanical assistance to break up the clot. Clot removal is incomplete, but enough can be removed to lower the ICP and to diminish local brain compression. Achieving hemostasis can be a problem, and tumors, AVMs, and other vascular pathology can be missed. Although this technique is used in certain centers, it is not widely accepted as the method of choice to treat intracerebral hematomas. The second and more commonly used method is by craniotomy for evacuation of the hematoma. The craniotomy is centered over the area of the brain where the hematoma comes closest to the surface, and once the brain has been exposed, ultrasonography can confirm the location of the blood clot under the cortex. Intraoperative techniques include the use of the operating microscope for magnification and illumination, gentle brain retraction, and bipolar

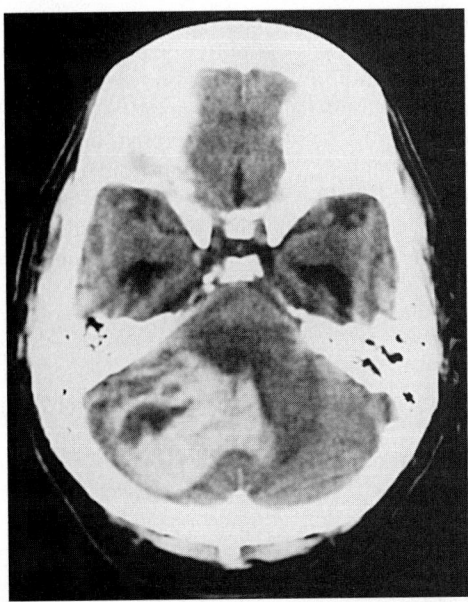

FIGURE 71-5. Nonenhanced CT scan of brain shows a large hypertensive intracerebellar hematoma with obstruction of the fourth ventricle and enlargement of the temporal horns indicating obstructive hydrocephalus.

coagulation to control intraoperative bleeding. After the hematoma has been removed, the walls of the cavity should be carefully inspected for abnormalities that should undergo biopsy.

IVH may be an isolated problem caused by hypertension, or it can occur in combination with intracerebral hematomas or subarachnoid hemorrhage. By obstructing the normal CSF flow out of the lateral ventricles, IVH leads to hydrocephalus and raised ICP. Placement of an IVC relieves this blockade, lowers the ICP, and allows drainage of the hematoma. Instilling fibrinolytics such as tissue plasminogen activator through the IVC dissolves the clots quicker and reduces the time patients need to have an IVC in place. Additionally, this therapy may also prevent development of hydrocephalus.[16]

Vascular Malformations

Pathologists differentiate vascular malformations into four categories: capillary telangiectasias, venous angiomas, cavernous angiomas, and AVMs. Capillary telangiectasias are benign lesions that are often found in the brain stem. Venous angiomas typically have a "caput medusa" appearance of a single large vein fed by smaller draining veins. There is intervening normal parenchyma between the vessels, and the malformation often provides essential venous drainage to an area of brain. Venous angiomas have an extremely low potential for bleeding and should not be removed. Cavernous angiomas are developmental malformations within the brain substance that are best demonstrated by MRI, which detects the presence of recurrent small hemorrhages (mixed signal intensity) surrounded by a hemosiderin ring (low signal intensity). Cavernous angiomas are usually angiographically occult because they lack feeding arteries and draining veins. Patients typically present with seizures or a neurologic deficit from a hemorrhage. Not uncommonly they are found as incidental lesions on an MRI obtained for an unrelated reason. A cavernous angioma that has had more than one clinically significant bleed should be removed by craniotomy, if it is in a surgically accessible location. The natural history of incidentally found cavernous angiomas is not dangerous enough to warrant their routine removal. The benefit of stereotactic radiosurgery has not yet been established in these lesions.

AVMs are abnormal collections of blood vessels where arterial blood flows directly into draining veins without an intervening capillary bed. Classically, they are congenital lesions that consist of a feeding artery or arteries, a nidus or center, and draining veins that carry arterialized blood and appear red. The dysplastic vessels found in the nidus do not have intervening normal brain parenchyma, although in some pediatric patients, AVMs may appear as large, diffuse lesions that contain normal brain tissue. The superficial portion of an AVM may cover part of the cerebral surface, but the lesion tapers down like a cone to the ventricular surface. AVMs usually present with an intracranial bleed, seizure, or focal ischemia caused by arteriovenous shunting of blood from adjacent brain ("steal" phenomenon). When large, AVMs can be diagnosed by CT and MRI, but four-vessel cerebral angiography is needed to demonstrate the anatomy and hemodynamic characteristics (Fig. 71-6).

AVMs tend to bleed earlier in life than aneurysms, with a peak incidence in teenagers and young adults and an annual risk between 3% and 4%.[17] The rate of rebleed after an initial hemorrhage is higher than 3% to 4% for the initial few years but then returns to baseline. Compared to aneurysms, AVMs do not have a tendency to rebleed in the first 24 hours, and, consequently, they do not require urgent surgery unless a hemorrhage with significant mass effect needs to be removed.

The management of AVMs falls into three categories: microsurgical excision, glue embolization, and stereotactic radiosurgery. Depending on the characteristics of the AVM (size, location, arterial supply, and venous drainage) and the clinical condition of the patient, a decision is made regarding which of these three modalities should be used. Stereotactic radiosurgery is indicated for surgically inaccessible or unruptured AVMs that are smaller than 3 cm in diameter. Also, AVMs found in eloquent cortex are suitable for radiosurgery. After irradiation, the patient is not protected from hemorrhage until complete obliteration of the AVM occurs, which can take 2 or 3 years. The rate of obliteration depends directly on the dose of radiation delivered to the nidus. A small AVM that is given a dose of 25 Gy has a 98% chance of being obliterated. Larger AVMs cannot be given as high a dose of radiation because of radiation-induced side effects and therefore have a lower rate of obliteration. Large, inoperable AVMs are candidates for stereotactic radiosurgery in combination with pretreatment embolization to diminish the lesion size. Alternatively, the AVM is divided into smaller sections that are individually radiated over a period of months to years, or the entire AVM is treated to a low dose that reduces the size of the nidus for a second treatment years later, which is also performed at a low dose to reduce the risk of complications.

Endovascular embolization is a proven method to reduce the size and blood flow through AVMs, but they are rarely obliterated by this technique alone. Microsurgical resection with or without embolization is still the most commonly used modality to treat AVMs, particularly in patients who have suffered a hemorrhage. Using the angiogram to guide the resection, the neurosurgeon dissects out the feeding arteries and then divides them. Next, the nidus is separated from the surrounding brain, and the draining veins are transected. It is important that the entire nidus be removed as documented by postoperative angiography because even a small residual malformation can lead to future hemorrhage.

CENTRAL NERVOUS SYSTEM TUMORS

Intracranial Tumors

Intracranial tumors are commonly described as *primary* or *secondary,* depending on their site of origin. Primary intracranial tumors arise from cells found in the brain, the pituitary gland, or the coverings of the brain. The incidence of primary brain tumors in the United States is 11.5 in 100,000, or approximately 35,000 per year.[18] Secondary intracranial tumors are derived from tumors that arise from outside the brain. They may represent local extension of regional tumors such as chordoma or glomus tumors, or more commonly, they are blood-borne metastases from primary malignancies outside the brain. It is estimated that there are 150,000 to 250,000 patients with secondary brain tumors per year.

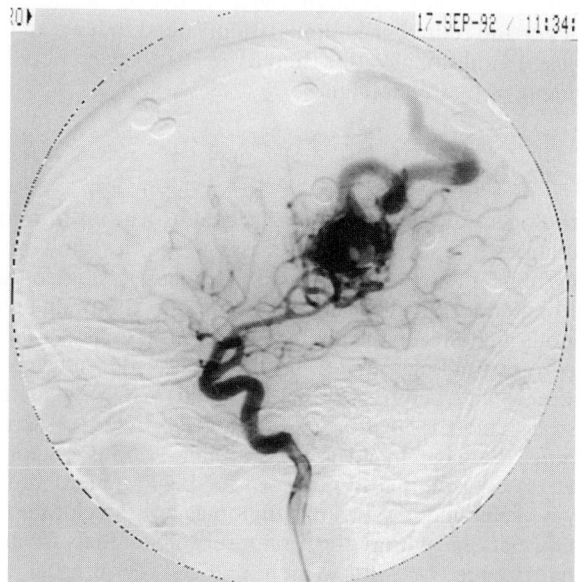

FIGURE 71-6. Subtracted carotid angiogram shows an arteriovenous malformation fed by the middle cerebral artery and drained by a superficial vein into the superior sagittal sinus.

Clinical Presentation

Intracranial tumors primarily present in two ways: One is by a generalized increase in ICP, and the other is from focal compression or irritation of the brain. An increase in ICP may be produced by direct mass effect from tumor bulk or hemorrhage, or it may occur indirectly through hydrocephalus. A tumor may obstruct the ventricular system at the foramen of Monro, aqueduct of Sylvius, or the fourth ventricle, thus producing noncommunicating hydrocephalus. Alternatively, tumor debris or hemorrhage can obstruct the arachnoid villi, causing the symmetrical enlargement of the entire ventricular system (communicating hydrocephalus). The most common symptoms of increased ICP are headache, nausea, vomiting, and reduction in the level of consciousness. The headaches are usually worse in the morning, which are caused by an exacerbation of ICP during sleep because of the recumbent position and a rise in Pco_2 during deep sleep. Vomiting is due to pressure exerted by high ICP or direct compression on the area postrema in the floor of the fourth ventricle. These symptoms may be mild or unnoticed until the tumor has become very large, if the tumor growth rate is slow, or if the tumor is peripherally located. On the other hand, a small, strategically located tumor (e.g., foramen of Monro) may cause early symptoms due to hydrocephalus. Patients experiencing long-standing elevations of ICP usually exhibit papilledema, which is found during the funduscopic examination. Rarely, patients have a unilateral or bilateral abducens nerve palsy. Herniation of the medial aspect of the temporal lobe over the edge of the tentorium can cause brain stem compression and abnormalities of the ipsilateral third nerve (dilated pupil). Vital sign changes include an elevation of the systolic blood pressure, bradycardia, and abnormal ventilatory patterns (Cushing's response).

The second presentation pattern relates to focal compression (neurologic deficit) or irritation of the brain (seizure). Tumor growth in a brain region typically results in the loss of neurologic function and may be detected by a careful neurologic examination. The development of an aphasia and right-sided weakness might suggest a tumor that is compressing the left hemisphere in a right-handed individual. A bitemporal hemianopsia with galactorrhea and amenorrhea in a young woman is indicative of a prolactin-secreting, pituitary macroadenoma. Tinnitus and a progressive, unilateral hearing loss are a common presentation for a cerebellopontine angle meningioma or a vestibular nerve schwannoma.

Radiology

Clinical presentation alone is not sufficiently sensitive or specific to establish the diagnosis of a brain tumor. Furthermore, the presence of specific neurologic findings may help localize the tumor in the brain but does not establish the histology. Radiologic studies are therefore critical to confirm the clinical diagnosis.

The modern era of tumor diagnosis began with the widespread use of CT scans in the 1970s and then MRI in the 1980s. Previously, diagnostic studies were indirect and relied on the interpretation of blood vessel shifts as seen in cerebral angiography or ventricular changes in air ventriculography. Both CT and MRI provided a direct view of the mass and the brain surrounding it. In addition, the digital acquisition of the information allowed reconstruction of the images in axial, coronal, and sagittal planes, thus permitting evaluation of the tumor in three-dimensional space, which is critical for preoperative planning. With current advances in computer and optical technology, it is now practical to use these imaging studies for intraoperative stereotactic localization. The development of small, portable MRI magnets now allows the surgeon to obtain an MRI scan without leaving the operating room. Consequently, a small area of residual brain tumor can be detected and removed without requiring a reoperation.

The recommendation for the initial screening of a patient suspected to have a brain tumor is a gadolinium-enhanced MRI. MRI is more sensitive than CT for detecting abnormalities in the brain and offers superior anatomic localization. MRI is superior to CT in the posterior fossa because there is no interference from bony artifact. The use of enhancement is critical because many brain tumors are not seen unless contrast medium is used.

Although MRI is the preferred imaging method, it may not be indicated for all patients. MRI does not expose patients to x-rays, but the strong magnetic field can interfere with the function of pacemakers and other implanted devices. Further, patients who are claustrophobic may not tolerate the traditional "closed" MRI scanner. "Open" MRIs are not as confining but sacrifice magnet strength and therefore have poorer spatial resolution.

For detecting bony abnormalities, CT scans are more sensitive and are less costly and time consuming to perform. They are useful in the postoperative period when patients may need multiple follow-up studies, or if patients are critically ill and the speed and ease of imaging become important.

Cerebral angiography is indicated when highly vascular or skull base tumors are suspected. In these cases, preoperative localization of feeding arteries and nearby venous structures may influence the surgical approach. Preoperative embolization can reduce intraoperative blood loss and make surgery safer.

Surgery

A number of technical advances have made tumor surgery safer and more effective. Bipolar electrocautery allows the neurosurgeon to precisely cauterize tissues and vessels between two points. Because the current spread is minimized, the bipolar can be used near critical structures such as the brain stem, optic nerve, and carotid artery. The ultrasonic aspirator simultaneously breaks up tough tumors and sucks away the debris. This device is frequently used to internally debulk large tumors, which then allows the tumor capsule to be collapsed inward and removed. Intraoperative ultrasonography provides real-time images of tumors and cysts beneath the brain surface and is useful for locating and then following the removal of a subcortical tumor or hematoma. The operating microscope provides superior illumination and magnification through small cranial openings. This allows the neurosurgeon to resect tumors from critical areas in the brain and along the skull base. Image-guided (CT or MRI) stereotactic techniques allow highly accurate biopsies to be performed through a small burr hole. The evolution of frameless stereotactic systems allows instant and precise localization of a probe during craniotomy by displaying the point on a preoperative MRI or CT. The fusion of stereotactic imaging with the operating microscope via a "heads-up" display translates three-dimensional images into the vision of the neurosurgeon while he or she is operating.

There are two main principles in the surgical management of intracranial tumors: histologic diagnosis and reduction of tumor mass effect. Diagnosis may be accomplished by image-directed stereotactic needle biopsy or from specimens obtained at craniotomy. The decision between biopsy and craniotomy is influenced by the location and size of the tumor and the clinical presentation of the patient. In general, a tumor causing mass effect or neurologic symptoms in a relatively noneloquent area of the brain should be removed, provided the patient can undergo general anesthesia. Exceptions are made for tumors that are unusually sensitive to radiation or chemotherapy, such as lymphoma or germinoma. Tumors found in deep brain structures should undergo stereotactic biopsy.

Primary Brain Tumors

Primary tumors of the brain are commonly divided into those that arise from either within the brain parenchyma (intra-axial) or outside the parenchyma (extra-axial). This distinction is important because the tumor types as well as surgical approaches and expectations are quite different.

Intra-axial Brain Tumors

Of the cells within the brain that are at risk for becoming neoplastic, most are derived from the glia (astrocytes, oligodendrocytes, and ependymal cells) and are called *gliomas*. Neurons are almost exclusively postmitotic and therefore at very low risk for becoming a tumor. Despite having low metastatic potential (a consequence of the blood-brain barrier and the lack of brain lymphatics), the prognosis of malignant gliomas is poor because of their ability to infiltrate widely. Even low-grade gliomas infiltrate into normal brain and have a propensity to transform into a higher-grade glioma. Glioma cells spread preferentially along white matter tracts and may cross the corpus callosum into the contralateral hemisphere. Glioma cells also tend to be resistant to both radiation and chemotherapy.

Astrocytoma. These tumors are the most common type of glioma and account for 50% of all primary brain tumors. Under the World Health Organization classification system, astrocytomas are divided into four groups (grades 1 to 4) based on light-microscopy characteristics.[19] Four attributes are evaluated by pathologists: degree of cellularity, mitotic figures, endothelial proliferation, and necro-

sis. Grade 1 astrocytomas are a special category reserved for well-circumscribed tumors with essentially no ability to transform into higher grades. Low-grade, or grade 2, astrocytomas contain only one attribute, usually increased cellularity, and have a lower growth rate than higher-grade tumors. Unlike grade 1 tumors, these astrocytomas are infiltrative and lack distinct boundaries. Grade 3, or anaplastic, astrocytomas have two attributes: usually increased cellularity and either endothelial proliferation or mitotic figures. Grade 4 tumors, or *glioblastoma multiforme* (GBM), have three or more attributes and characteristically have necrosis. GBMs are the most aggressive and most common of all gliomas. Although many exceptions exist, low-grade gliomas are generally seen in younger patients (<50 years), whereas high-grade gliomas are seen in older patients (>50 years). Recent investigations into the genetic abnormalities of astrocytomas have shown frequent mutations in the *p53* gene, abnormalities in chromosome 10, and overexpression of the epidermal growth factor receptor.[20]

The most common grade 1 astrocytoma is the *pilocytic astrocytoma.* This tumor is most frequently seen in the cerebellar hemisphere and hypothalamus of children and young adults. On MRI, they appear as peripherally enhancing lesions, often with a mural nodule. Despite favorable biologic characteristics, hypothalamic tumors may carry a poor prognosis because the hypothalamus and optic nerve make surgical resection impossible without high morbidity rates. Pilocytic astrocytomas in the cerebrum and cerebellum are well circumscribed, surgically accessible, and therefore curable by complete resection.[21] Chemotherapy and radiation do not normally play a role in their treatment.

Low-grade astrocytomas often have subtle characteristics on MRI and may be completely missed on CT scans. They appear as a hypodense area on T1 sequences and a bright signal on T2, and they lack contrast enhancement (Fig. 71-7A and B). Because they are infiltrative, complete surgical resection is impossible, but most studies find that a more complete surgical resection improves prognosis. There is some evidence supporting the use of radiation therapy, but no evidence suggests that chemotherapy plays a role in treatment.[22] Underscoring the fact that these are not benign tumors, the median survival time is 5 to 7 years.

High-grade astrocytomas appear as irregularly enhancing areas on MRI. There are mass effect and extensive areas of edema that contain infiltrating tumor cells (Fig. 71-8A). The best treatment involves surgical resection followed by fractionated external-beam radiation to a dose of 60 Gy (6000 rads) (Fig. 71-8B to D). Chemotherapy may improve survival slightly in selected patients. Bis-chloroethyl-nitrosourea (BCNU)-impregnated biodegradable wafers (Gliadel) also offer a small survival advantage and may replace intravenous chemotherapy in some patients.[23] Favorable prognostic variables for survival include younger age, more complete surgical resection, radiation therapy, and good performance status. The median survival is 2 years for anaplastic astrocytomas and 1 year for GBMs.

Oligodendroglioma. This tumor is typically found in the frontal, temporal, or parietal lobes. On CT scans, calcifi-

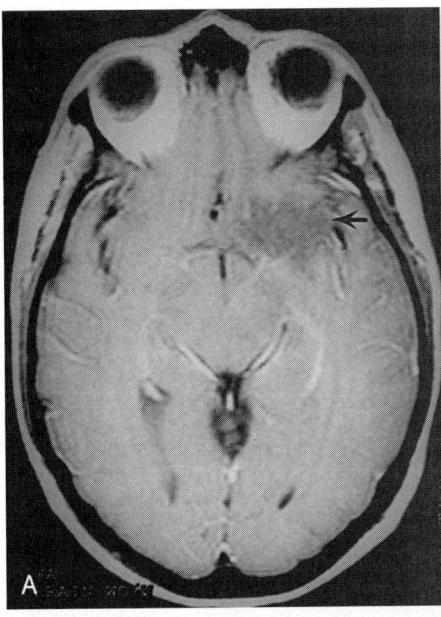 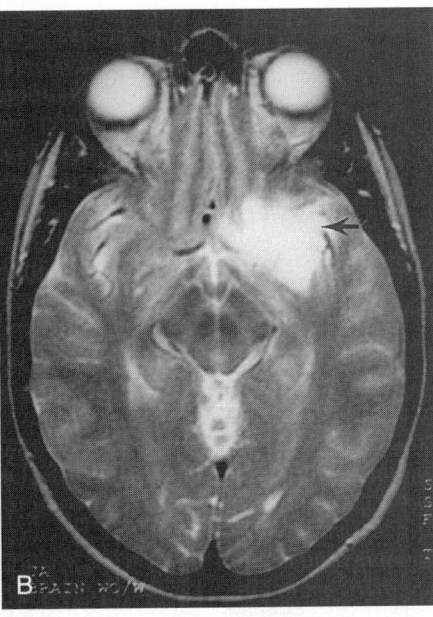

FIGURE 71-7. Low-grade astrocytoma. **A,** A nonenhancing, low-density region *(arrow)* in the left inferior frontal lobe is seen on the T1-weighted MRI study. There is no significant mass effect, but the edges of the lesion are not well circumscribed, thus indicating infiltration. **B,** The same region appears hyperdense on the T2-weighted MRI study.

cation and hemorrhage are more often seen in oligodendrogliomas than in the other primary brain tumors. Its MRI characteristics are similar to those of the astrocytomas. The treatment for oligodendrogliomas is similar to the astrocytomas, with the exception that chemotherapy may be more effective in oligodendroglioma.[24] Frequent losses of chromosomes 1p and 19q are found in these tumors and signal a better prognosis. The median survival time is 7 to 10 years.

Ependymoma. Ependymomas are most frequently diagnosed in younger patients. The peak incidence is in childhood, when they typically present as a mass in the fourth ventricle and cause hydrocephalus. Typical symptoms include headache, nausea and vomiting, papilledema, gait ataxia, vertigo, and diplopia. Ependymomas appear as inhomogenously enhancing masses arising from the floor of the fourth ventricle and often conforming to the shape of the ventricle. The primary treatment consists of surgical resection and postoperative radiation therapy. Anaplastic ependymomas may spread through the CSF pathways, signaling a poor prognosis. Craniospinal axis radiation is indicated when this occurs. The median survival time is 7 to 10 years, with younger children faring worse than older ones. A complete surgical resection is associated with a good prognosis and should be attempted when feasible.

Medulloblastoma. Accounting for 20% to 25% of all pediatric brain tumors, this is the most common primary brain tumor in children. Derived from an undifferentiated precursor to both astrocytes and neurons, medulloblastomas are most often found in the cerebellar vermis. Like ependymomas in this location, they present with symptoms of hydrocephalus and midline cerebellar signs. In adults, these tumors have a propensity for the lateral cerebellar hemisphere and present with dysmetria. Outside the posterior fossa, these tumors are called *primitive neuroectodermal tumors.* Histologically, they are highly cellular with the potential for both astrocytic and neuronal differentiation. Treatment consists of maximal sur-

gical resection followed by radiation therapy. Because these tumors can spread through the CSF system, craniospinal axis radiation is advocated. Since the deleterious effects of radiation on the developing spine and brain are well known, chemotherapy is used in younger children in an attempt to delay or avoid craniospinal radiation.[25] The once dismal prognosis associated with this tumor has improved with advances in surgery and radiation delivery. The median survival time is 7 to 10 years, with complete surgical resection and lack of CSF spread being the most favorable prognostic factors.

Hemangioblastoma. After metastases, hemangioblastomas are the most common posterior fossa tumor in adults and are rarely seen in the pediatric population. They are histologically benign tumors composed of capillaries, dilated vessels, and foamy stromal cells. Most hemangioblastomas occur spontaneously, but this tumor can occur as part of von Hippel-Lindau (VHL) disease, which is an autosomal dominant disorder. The gene associated with VHL disease has been mapped to chromosome 3p25 and functions as a tumor suppressor gene.[26] Other tumors found in VHL disease include retinal angiomas, renal and pancreatic cysts, pheochromocytoma, and renal cell carcinoma. Patients typically present with cerebellar findings: headaches, ataxia, vertigo, and dysmetria. Although most commonly found in the cerebellum, they also occur in the brain stem and spinal cord. Radiographically, these tumors present as a solid enhancing mass or as a cystic tumor with an enhancing mural nodule. The recommended treatment is complete surgical removal of the solid component or nodule; cyst removal is not required for a cure. The prognosis with a gross total resection is favorable.

Primary Central Nervous System Lymphoma. This once rare intracranial tumor has been rising disproportionately in incidence during the past 20 years. Two distinct populations develop primary central nervous system lymphomas. The first is elderly patients and the second is immunocompromised patients, especially those with end-stage

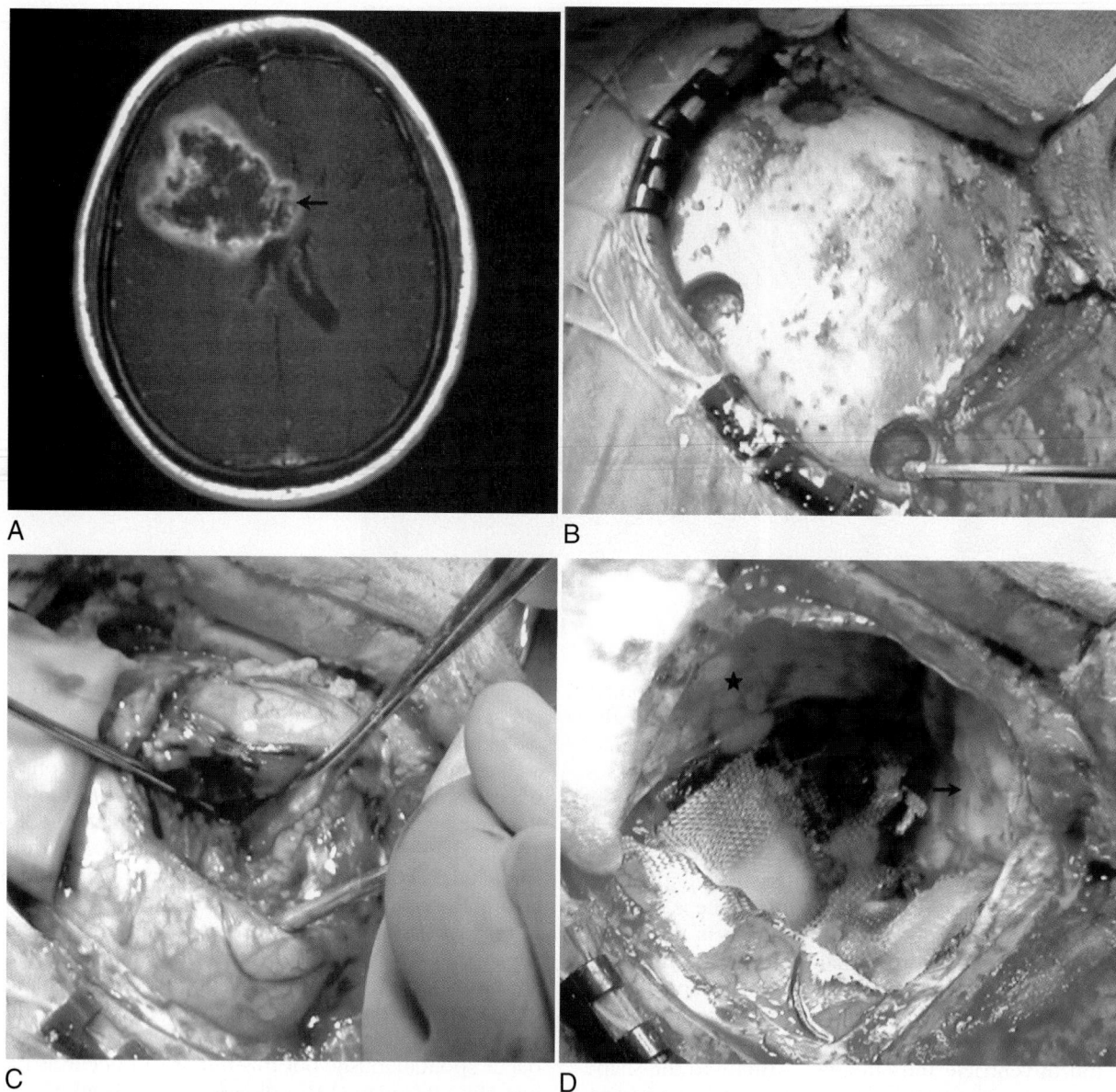

FIGURE 71-8.   MRI and intraoperative pictures of a patient with a right frontal glioblastoma multiforme (GBM). **A,** A right frontal GBM is seen on axial T1-weighted MRI. The enhancing lesion demonstrates central necrosis and is causing mass effect. Infiltration along the corpus callosum is also shown *(arrow)*. **B,** A frontal craniotomy is being performed. Burr holes have been placed and will be connected for bony removal. **C,** The brain has been incised and the tumor is being removed using a combination of suction and blunt dissection. **D,** The tumor and frontal lobe have been resected. The cut edge of the brain is seen at the lower left. The falx is seen along the midline *(star)* and the orbital roof is exposed *(arrow)*. The resection cavity has been lined with Gliadel wafers and covered with a layer of Surgicel for hemostasis.

acquired immunodeficiency syndrome (AIDS). This tumor is highly sensitive to radiation, and surgical resection is not indicated. Suspected patients should undergo a stereotactic biopsy followed by radiation therapy. The addition of chemotherapy may reduce the time to recurrence. Despite being a radiosensitive tumor, the prognosis is still poor. The median survival time is 4 years in persons without AIDS and 3 to 6 months in persons with AIDS.[27]

Germ Cell and Pineal Region Tumors. Germ cell tumors are a broad category that includes germinoma, embryonal carcinoma, choriocarcinoma, and endodermal sinus tumor. These tumors are characteristically found in the pineal or

hypothalamic region of children and young adults. Germ cell tumors often release tumor markers into the CSF, which can be detected by LP. α-Fetoprotein is characteristic of endodermal sinus tumors, and β-human chorionic gonadotropin is secreted by choriocarcinoma and any tumor with trophoblastic elements. Placental alkaline phosphatase can be found in the CSF of patients with germinoma. The finding of these tumor markers in the CSF is pathognomonic for a germ cell tumor and can preclude the need for biopsy. The presence of large veins in the pineal region makes stereotactic needle biopsy hazardous because of the risk of hemorrhage. Many surgeons opt for craniotomy to obtain sufficient tissue for an accurate diagnosis. Germinoma is a radiosensitive tumor and may be curable. The other germ cell tumors carry a poor prognosis and frequently require both radiation and chemotherapy.

Pineal gland tumors originate in the posterior aspect of the third ventricle, and, when large, may cause hydrocephalus from occlusion of the aqueduct of Sylvius (Fig. 71-9). These relatively rare tumors are found in adults as pineocytomas and in children as pineoblastoma. Other tumors found in this location include meningiomas and astrocytomas. Parinaud's syndrome describes the classic symptoms associated with a pineal region tumor: paralysis of upward gaze, pupils that constrict on accommodation but fail to react to light, and nystagmus retractorius. Two approaches are commonly used to access the pineal region: the infratentorial supracerebellar, which requires the patient to be placed in the sitting position; and the occipital transtentorial. The vein of Galen complex must be dealt with carefully: if damaged, these veins can lead to hemorrhage and venous infarcts in the thalamus. Tumors in this area should be resected totally if possible. When residual tumor is left, stereotactic radiosurgery or fractionated radiation therapy is indicated.

Extra-axial Brain Tumors

Meningioma. Meningiomas are the second most common primary brain tumor, accounting for 20% of the total. Arising from arachnoidal cap cells, they are benign tumors that originate in the dura and displace the brain as they grow. Meningiomas do not invade the brain unless they are malignant, but they can invade and erode the skull, or they can cause a hyperostotic reaction. The most common

locations are the parasagittal region, cerebral convexities, subfrontal region, and cerebellopontine angle. These tumors are usually found in adults and are more common in women. Meningiomas appear isointense to brain on T1 and T2 MRI sequences but enhance strongly and homogeneously (Fig. 71-10A and B). The primary treatment should be surgery because the patient may be cured by a complete resection. This requires complete removal of the tumor, dural origin, and involved skull. However, even with a gross total resection, 10% of patients have a recurrence within 10 years.[28]

Certain locations make a complete resection difficult or impossible to accomplish because of the surrounding structures. For example, meningiomas in the medial sphenoid wing or petroclival region are entwined with the carotid artery and cranial nerves entering the cavernous sinus. Leaving some tumor behind is often better than risking the loss of neurologic function for the sake of obtaining a complete removal. The development of stereotactic radiosurgery using the gamma knife or linear accelerator offers a new tool for the control of residual tumor growth.[29] These devices allow a high dose of radiation (12 to 20 Gy) to be given in a single fraction with millimeter accuracy to the tumor while sparing the surrounding brain from a significant radiation exposure. Large (>3 cm) residual or recurrent meningiomas may require treatment with conventional fractionated radiation therapy. Chemotherapy does not play a significant role in the treatment of this tumor.

Schwannoma. These benign tumors arise from Schwann cells that form the myelin sheath around cranial nerves after their emergence from the brain stem. The most common type—vestibular schwannoma or acoustic neuroma—originates from the vestibulocochlear nerve (cranial nerve VIII) and presents with unilateral hearing loss, tinnitus, dizziness, and, when the tumor is large, facial numbness. Facial motor weakness is a rare presenting symptom, and it indicates the presence of a facial nerve (cranial nerve VII) schwannoma or a malignant tumor. Other commonly affected nerves are the trigeminal (cranial nerve V), followed by the glossopharyngeal and vagus (cranial nerves IX and X, respectively). Schwannomas appear isointense to brain on T1 MRI and usually enhance well. MRI scans show an enhancing mass in the cerebellopontine angle that enters the internal auditory canal—a distinguishing feature of acoustic tumors compared to cerebellopontine angle meningiomas (Fig. 71-11).

Bilateral vestibular schwannomas are associated with the neurocutaneous disorder, neurofibromatosis 2. Individuals with this disorder present with multiple schwannomas, meningiomas, and ependymomas. The inheritance is autosomal dominant, and the gene has been mapped to 22q12.2.[30] The most common neurocutaneous disorder, neurofibromatosis 1 (*NF-1*), is caused by an inherited defect (autosomal dominant) in the neurofibromin gene, which codes for a tumor suppressor and is found on 17q11.2.[31] This gene is quite large, and there is a high spontaneous mutation rate that explains why as many as 50% of patients with *NF-1* represent new cases without a previous family history. The list of associated conditions and tumors with *NF-1* is extensive and only partially listed

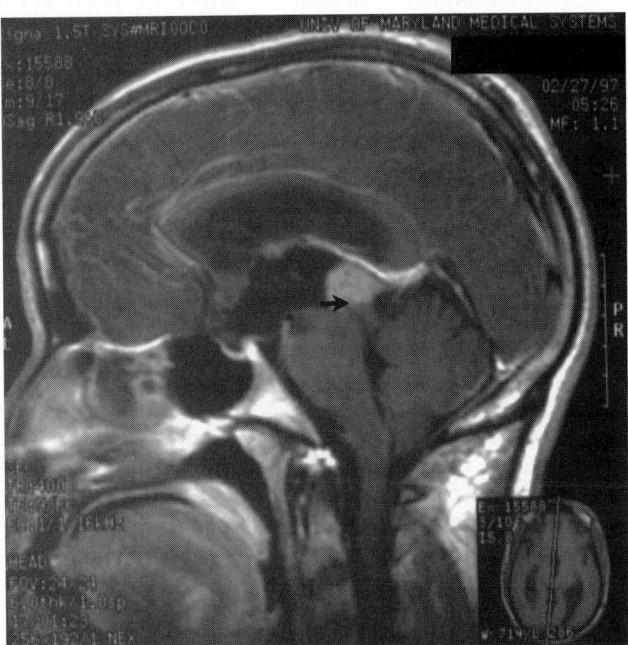

FIGURE 71-9. A pineocytoma is seen on T1-weighted MRI. The patient has hydrocephalus caused by obstruction of the top of the aqueduct of Sylvius by the tumor (*arrow*).

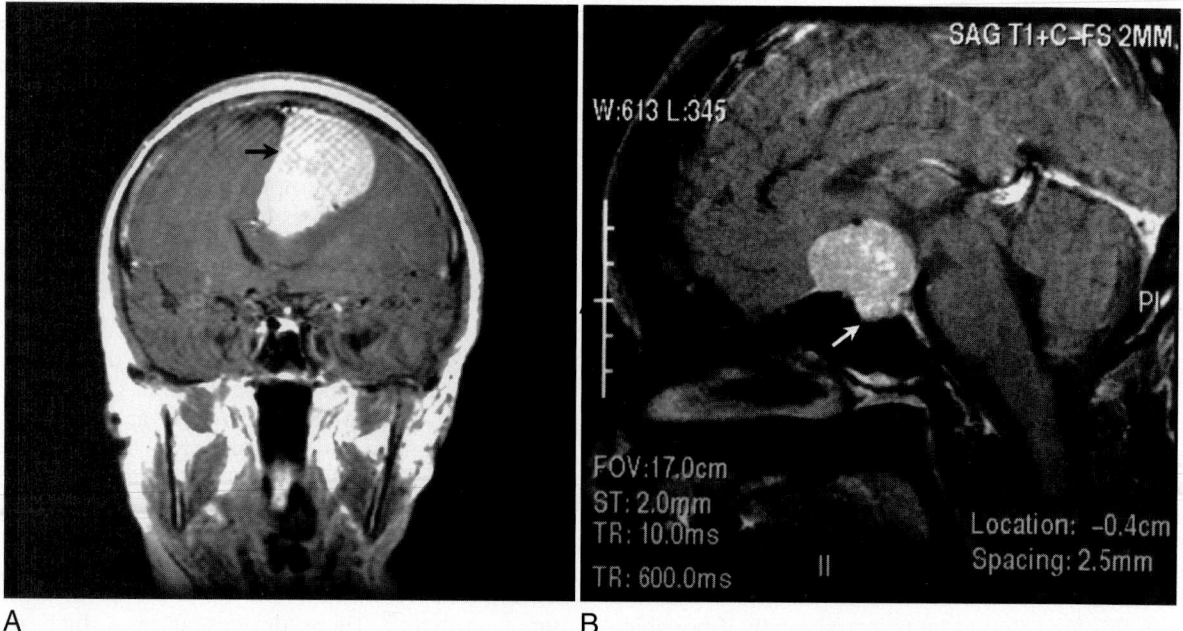

A   B

FIGURE 71-10.   Two examples of meningioma are seen on T1-weighted MRI. **A,** Coronal image shows a meningioma based on the falx *(arrow)* causing compression of the left frontal lobe. **B,** Sagittal MRI demonstrates a tuberculum sella meningioma causing compression of the optic chiasm. Although this tumor appears similar to a pituitary macroadenoma, the presence of a normal sella turcica *(arrow)* indicates a suprasellar origin and makes meningioma a more likely diagnosis.

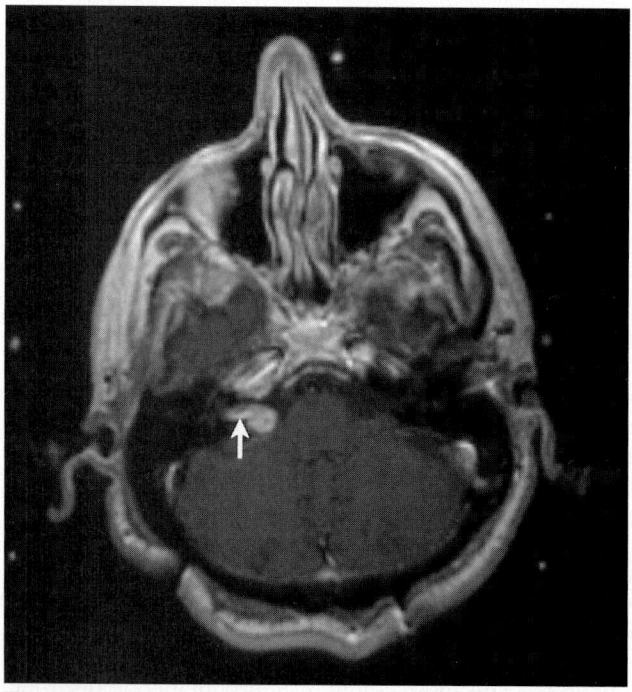

FIGURE 71-11.   Patient with a right vestibular schwannoma seen on T1-weighted MRI. It is characteristic for these tumors to extend into and, frequently, enlarge the internal auditory canal *(arrow).*

here: café au lait spots, neurofibromas, axillary freckling, optic and hemispheric gliomas, Lisch nodules in the iris, bone abnormalities, scoliosis, and macrocephaly.

Like meningiomas, a complete surgical resection may result in a cure. The primary risks of surgery are related to cranial nerve injury from tumor dissection and removal. Most schwannomas in the posterior fossa are removed via a retromastoid craniectomy: an incision is made behind the ear, followed by removal of the lateral suboccipital bone. After the dura is opened, the cerebellum is retracted to expose the tumor. In addition to the operating microscope, intraoperative brain stem auditory evoked potentials and facial nerve electromyographic monitoring are crucial for identifying the facial nerve and monitoring hearing and facial function during tumor removal. Small vestibular schwannomas can be resected through a retromastoid approach with little risk of facial nerve weakness, but still only a few patients have hearing preservation. Large acoustic tumors are primarily resected through a retromastoid craniectomy, but the risk of facial weakness is higher, and there is no chance for hearing to be preserved. For small tumors found principally in the internal auditory canal, the middle fossa approach, which provides exposure to the tumor by elevating the temporal lobe, can be used to remove the tumor while attempting hearing preservation. The last commonly used surgical technique, the translabyrinthine approach, destroys hearing because the labyrinth is removed during the temporal bone drilling, but it provides the surgeon a direct view of the tumor with minimal brain retraction and is useful in patients with medium to small tumors and no serviceable hearing. Although surgery is still considered the standard treatment, small to medium schwannomas can also be effectively treated with stereotactic radiosurgery, which provides tumor control with very low morbidity and no mortality.[32] This modality is also useful for patients with residual or recurrent schwannomas.

Pituitary Adenoma. Cells in the anterior pituitary gland give rise to benign pituitary adenomas. These tumors are described as functional or nonfunctional depending on whether excessive hormone secretion by the tumor can be detected. Functional tumors cause an endocrinopathy from excessive hormone production. These endocrine abnormalities may be evident even in microadenomas (<1 cm) that are otherwise too small to cause neurologic deficit. The most common functional tumor is the *prolactinoma*, which causes amenorrhea and galactorrhea in women. Men are relatively insensitive to excessive prolactin secretion, and, often, they are not diagnosed until their tumor becomes large and headaches or visual symptoms occur. A mildly elevated prolactin level is not necessarily indicative of a prolactinoma but may be caused by compression of the pituitary stalk by a large adenoma. This phenomenon led to the identification of dopamine inhibition by the hypothalamus on prolactin-secreting cells. Oral administration of a dopamine agonist such as bromocriptine can shrink prolactinomas in 80% of cases. Overproduction of adrenocorticotrophic hormone by a pituitary adenoma causes Cushing's disease, which is characterized by centripetal obesity, moon facies, buffalo hump, purple striae, glucose intolerance, and psychiatric disturbance. A growth hormone–secreting adenoma causes acromegaly, which results in growth of the hands, feet, lower jaw, and supraorbital ridge. Because most of the changes occur in soft tissue, they may be reversible with proper treatment. More serious effects of acromegaly are hypertension, cardiomegaly, and hyperglycemia. Although it does not supplant surgery, the subcutaneous injection of a somatostatin analogue (octreotide) can reduce the effects of excessive growth hormone production. Tumors that secrete thyroid-stimulating hormone, luteinizing hormone, or follicle-stimulating hormone are rare and not encountered in a general neurosurgery practice.

Nonfunctional pituitary adenomas typically present with mass effect on adjacent structures, notably the optic chiasm. Because the optic pathways from the medial half of each retina cross in the chiasm, compression in this area affects both temporal visual fields. The patient experiences a loss of peripheral vision and describes a bitemporal field cut on formal visual field testing. Although cavernous sinus invasion is common with pituitary macroadenomas (>1 cm), it is unusual to see deficits in cranial nerves III to VI. Some anterior pituitary hypofunction may result from compression of normal pituitary gland by large macroadenomas, but it is highly unusual to have posterior pituitary dysfunction such as diabetes insipidus. The presence of diabetes insipidus suggests the possible diagnosis of a hypothalamic tumor, germ cell tumor, craniopharyngioma, pituitary carcinoma, or metastasis.

On MRI, the anterior pituitary enhances strongly and rapidly because it lacks a blood-brain barrier. As a result, pituitary microadenomas appear as a nonenhancing area within the pituitary gland that is seen best on coronal images (Fig. 71-12A). Macroadenomas erode and enlarge the sella turcica in addition to elevating the optic chiasm (Fig. 71-12B). The MRI shows a variable degree of enhancement and cannot usually distinguish between tumor and normal pituitary. A full endocrine work-up is essential in all patients, and formal visual field testing should be performed in all patients with a macroadenoma.

The unique anatomy of the pituitary sella allows tumors in this region to be approached through the nose via a trans-sphenoidal craniotomy. A sublabial or intranasal incision is used to gain access to the septal cartilage and perpendicular plate of the ethmoid. These structures are followed posteriorly to the rostrum of the sphenoid sinus, which is opened widely. The surgeon then has a direct

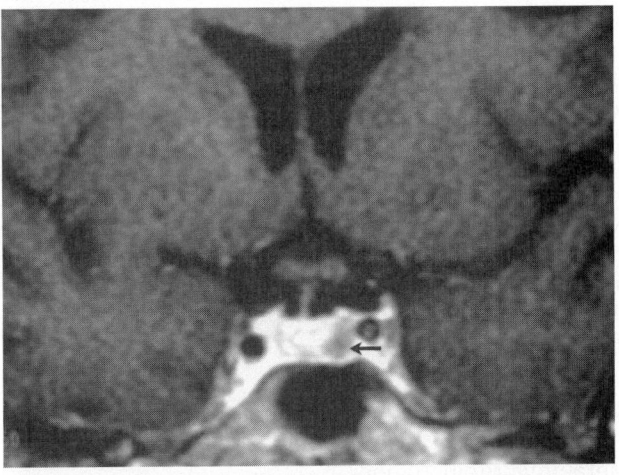

A

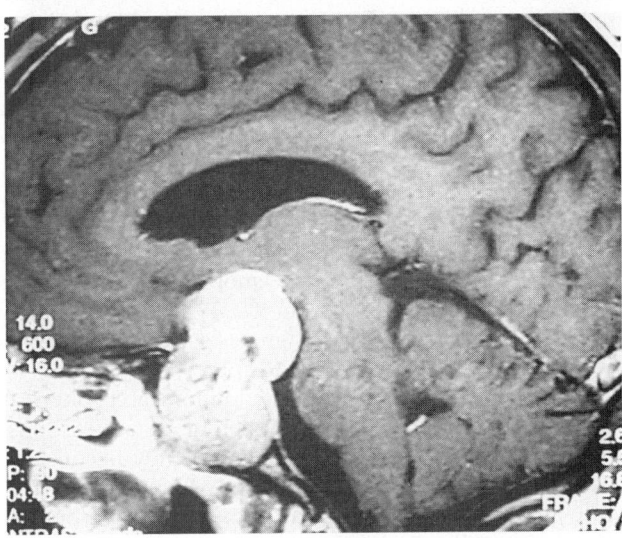

B

■ FIGURE 71-12. Pituitary adenomas seen on MRI. **A,** The left side of the pituitary gland contains a microadenoma that appears hypodense on coronal MRI *(arrow)*. Slight deviation to the pituitary stalk to the right is seen. **B,** Sagittal T1-weighted MRI shows a pituitary macroadenoma characteristically expanding the sella and elevating the optic chiasm.

view of the sella floor, which is usually quite thin with macroadenomas. Once the sella is removed, the tumor is removed using pituitary ring curettes. Care must be taken with tumors invading the cavernous sinus to avoid lacerating the carotid artery. Since it is not uncommon to see a flattened layer of normal pituitary gland on the sella floor, care must also be taken in preserving the remaining gland to prevent postoperative hypopituitarism. After the tumor has been removed, the suprasellar arachnoid must be inspected for CSF leak. If a leak is suspected, an abdominal fat graft can be harvested and used to seal the sella. Even large macroadenomas can be removed safely by this technique, but complete removal may be impossible when there is extensive cavernous sinus invasion or if the consistency of the tumor does not allow the suprasellar component of the tumor to descend into the field. Conventional intracranial surgery is chosen when the tumor is primarily suprasellar tumor or when there is residual suprasellar tumor that causes a persistent visual defect. For some neurosurgeons, a primary endoscopic approach is used, but the limitations related to the lack of stereoscopic vision, and reduced surgical maneuverability may keep this technique from becoming standard. Patients with complete tumor removal should be evaluated with yearly MRI scans for recurrence. A good option for patients with a small residual tumor is radiosurgery, which can prevent further tumor growth with few side effects. If the residual tumor contacts the optic nerve, fractionated radiation therapy is indicated because the large single fraction used in radiosurgery will cause optic nerve injury.

Secondary Brain Tumors

Metastatic Brain Tumors

By virtue of its disproportionately high blood flow, the brain is a common site for metastases. The incidence depends on whether only symptomatic or autopsy studies are cited, and it varies from 15% to 30% of all patients with cancer.[33] The distribution of metastases in the brain is directly related to the amount of blood flow to each part of the brain; therefore, more metastases are found in the frontal lobe, given its larger size compared with other brain regions. The most common primary sites are lung (35%), breast (20%), skin (melanoma) (10%), kidney (10%), and gastrointestinal tract (5%). For reasons that are unclear, prostate cancer rarely metastasizes to the brain but frequently metastasizes to the spine.

On imaging studies, metastatic tumors are spherical and homogeneously enhancing. When metastases are suspected, MRI is the preferred screening study because of its sensitivity. They are most frequently found at the gray-white junction where the end-arteries narrow and branch into arterioles (Fig. 71-13). Because the tumors are distinct from the surrounding brain tissue, they do not appear infiltrative or diffuse. Mass effect and edema are also commonly seen on MRI. The treatment is dependent on the number of lesions, their size, and the physical condition of the patient. A large (>3 cm) metastasis causing neurologic compromise should be resected, if surgically acces-

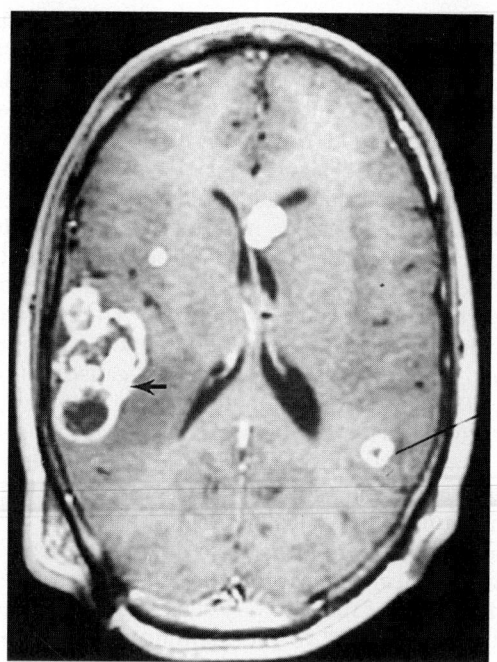

FIGURE 71-13. Multiple brain metastases on axial T1-weighted MRI study. Four metastatic lesions are seen in this image. Although metastases usually appear round and regular, they can also be irregular and exhibit central necrosis (arrow).

sible, and then the patient should be treated with whole-brain radiation therapy (WBRT). A small, single metastasis causing neurologic deficit may be removed or treated with radiosurgery followed by WBRT.[34] Multiple metastases are also usually treated with radiosurgery and WBRT or with WBRT alone. The average survival time with optimal treatment ranges from 7 to 12 months. Prognosis is improved when the primary tumor is controlled and the extent of metastatic disease is limited. Chemotherapy is not useful in most brain metastases, with the exception of small cell lung cancer and seminomas.

Regional Bone Tumors

The regional skull-base tumors most frequently encountered by neurosurgeons are the clivus chordoma and chondrosarcoma. Chordomas are locally invasive tumors derived from remnants of the primitive notochord. Headaches, diplopia, and other cranial nerve deficits are the most common presenting symptoms. Local bone destruction is noted on CT and MRI. There may be mass effect on the brain stem with large tumors. The primary treatment for these tumors is surgery, usually via a specialized skull base approach, followed by radiosurgery if there is residual or recurrent tumor.

Intraspinal Tumors

Intraspinal tumors are commonly divided into three groups: extradural, intradural extramedullary, and intradural intramedullary. Each group has a characteristic presentation and radiographic appearance.

Extradural Tumors

These tumors originate in the vertebral body, or less commonly, the epidural space. Most are malignant and represent metastatic tumors, particularly from lung, breast, and prostate. Other common extradural tumors are lymphoma and multiple myeloma. As these tumors grow, they destroy the vertebrae, causing pathologic fractures and spinal cord compression. On plain film radiograph, the vertebral bodies and pedicles may appear destroyed or collapsed. Although metastases are usually lytic, prostate metastases may be blastic and appear hyperdense on plain film. MRI is the preferred radiographic study because of its superior resolution of the spinal cord and its ability to show axial, sagittal, and coronal views (Fig. 71-14). Contrast agent administration is critical for differentiating tumor from the surrounding soft tissues. CT scanning is useful for determining the extent of bony involvement.

Metastatic tumors most commonly involve the thoracic spine, and the earliest symptom is usually pain both along the spine and around the trunk in a radicular pattern. As the tumor enlarges, it causes progressive spinal cord injury. Myelopathic symptoms such as motor weakness, spasticity, and hyperreflexia are common findings. A sensory level appropriate to the spinal level of involvement may also be found.

If a patient presents with an extradural tumor and no primary cancer is known, a diagnosis must be obtained. A CT-guided needle biopsy may be sufficient to make this diagnosis. Treatment consists of a combination of surgery and radiation therapy. Surgery is required if the biopsy is inadequate or if there is a progressive neurologic deficit. Tumor found in the posterior epidural space or bony elements is best treated by laminectomy. Provided that the anterior spine is not affected, laminectomy should not destabilize the spine, and the patient can proceed with postoperative radiation therapy. When there is significant destruction of the vertebral bodies or anterior compression of the spinal cord, an anterior surgical approach must be used. A transthoracic or a lateral extracavitary approach may be used to perform a vertebrectomy along with stabilization by a bone graft with metal plate internal fixation or a methyl methacrylate construct. External-beam radiation is indicated if multilevel extradural disease exists or if there is minimal neurologic compromise. Corticosteroid therapy is frequently used to reduce tumor edema and can improve or stabilize a neurologic deficit.

Intradural, Extramedullary Tumors

Intradural, extramedullary tumors are found within the dura but outside the substance of the spinal cord. Most intradural, extramedullary tumors are benign and arise from the meninges (meningioma) or nerve roots (schwannoma and neurofibroma). Less commonly seen are malignant tumors, which usually spread through the spinal subarachnoid space from a primary brain tumor such as ependymoma or medulloblastoma. Primary tumors from outside the brain (e.g., lymphoma) can also seed the spinal subarachnoid space, thus resulting in meningeal carcinomatosis.

Spinal meningiomas are most frequently found in the thoracic region, and they are much more commonly found in women rather than men. They tend to originate from the anterior spinal dura and compress the spinal cord. Schwannomas and neurofibromas originate from nerve roots and can be found at any spinal level. Schwannomas are more commonly seen coming off the sensory nerve roots (dorsal) than the motor nerve roots (ventral). These nerve sheath tumors may occasionally grow extradurally out the intervertebral foramen. Benign intradural, extramedullary tumors typically present with myelopathy and radiculopathy.

Plain spine films may show an enlarged intervertebral foramen, but they are otherwise of little diagnostic value. Intradural, extramedullary tumors have a characteristic CT-myelogram appearance consisting of a displaced spinal cord and a meniscus corresponding to the outline of the tumor. The relationship of the tumor to the spinal cord and its enhancement characteristics are best seen on MRI. Involvement over multiple levels is also best assessed by the sagittal MRI. When meningeal carcinomatosis is suspected, an LP for cytology should be performed.

Meningiomas, schwannomas, and neurofibromas should be surgically resected. A laminectomy is usually adequate to gain access to the tumor, although certain tumors may require a lateral or even an anterior approach to facilitate complete removal. The removal of nerve sheath tumors may require sacrifice of the affected nerve root, but ordinarily this is of minor consequence because the ventral motor roots are not involved. A cure is possible when the entire schwannoma or neurofibroma tumor can be grossly removed. Malignant tumors are too diffuse and widespread to be completely removed by surgery, and

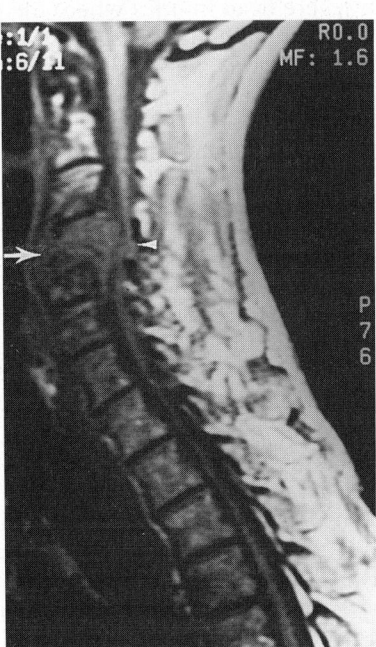

■ **FIGURE 71-14.** Spinal metastasis on sagittal T1-weighted MRI study. The C4 vertebral body has been extensively infiltrated with metastatic tumor *(arrow)*. There is severe compression of the cervical spinal cord at this level *(arrowhead)*.

external-beam radiation therapy is the best treatment for these patients.

Intramedullary Tumors

Intramedullary tumors originate in the substance of the spinal cord. The two most common tumors are astrocytoma and ependymoma. Patients usually experience myelopathy and sensory disturbance below the spinal level of involvement. Tumors at the level of the conus medullaris and below cause a cauda equina syndrome, which classically presents with perineal anesthesia, bowel and bladder incontinence, and lower extremity pain and weakness.

Plain films are not sensitive enough to detect the presence of an intramedullary tumor. A CT-myelogram may demonstrate a block of contrast flow with expansion of the spinal cord; however, an MRI with contrast is the preferred imaging study (Fig. 71-15). An enlarged spinal cord that shows contrast enhancement from within is suggestive of an intramedullary tumor. Tumor cysts or an associated syrinx can also be detected by MRI.

The primary treatment for an intramedullary tumor is laminectomy followed by tumor resection or biopsy. Intraoperative ultrasound is useful for determining the extent of tumor and syrinx location. The ultrasonic aspirator and operating microscope are indispensable tools in the surgical treatment of intramedullary tumors. The histology of the tumor often determines whether it can be grossly

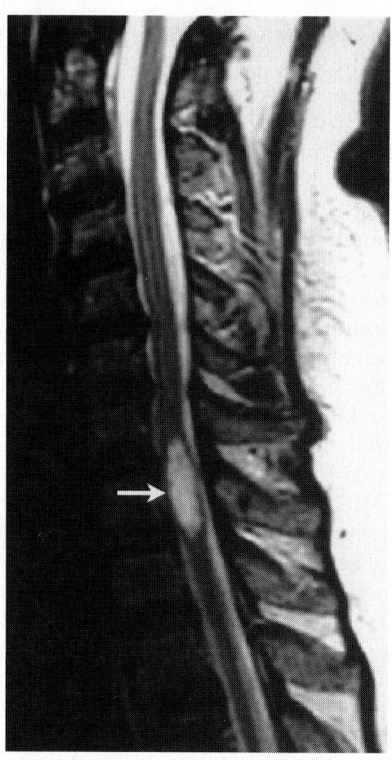

FIGURE 71-15. A spinal cord ependymoma is seen on T2-weighted MRI. The cord at the T1 level is dilated by the intramedullary tumor *(arrow)*, which appears distinct from the surrounding spinal cord.

removed. Ependymomas typically have a cleavage plane between tumor and spinal cord, which makes gross total resection feasible. The prognosis is good when this is accomplished. Any residual tumor should be treated with fractionated, external-beam radiation therapy. Spinal cord astrocytomas, like their intracranial counterparts, are infiltrative and impossible to remove completely. An attempt to do so may cause unacceptable injury to the spinal cord. Postoperative radiation therapy should be given for most astrocytomas. Other less common intramedullary tumors that should be treated surgically include hemangioblastoma and dermoid and epidermoid tumors.

TRAUMATIC HEAD INJURY

Virtually everyone who takes the trouble to open a surgical textbook already knows that traumatic injury is a social and health problem of enormous proportion. For example, statistics available from the mid 1990s indicate that trauma caused approximately 150,000 deaths in the United States annually, and about half were the result of head injury. In addition, there were 10,000 new spinal cord injuries annually, and approximately 200,000 people in the United States are living with disabilities caused by these injuries. The financial cost is high not only for acute care but also for the costs of chronic long-term care and lost wages because those injured are frequently young (mean age in the 30s).

This section considers traumatic injury of the central nervous system but focuses mainly on severe head injury. Although severe head injury is only a relatively small part of the overall head injury picture, mild and moderate injuries combined are probably at least five times as common, and surgeons are more involved in the care of patients with severe head injuries where the care is obviously more complicated and the risk of dying and severe disability is much greater.

Initial Evaluation of the Patient with Severe Head Injury

Severe head injury is generally defined as a coma-producing injury where coma is not related to extracranial conditions (e.g., severe intoxication) and is sustained at least beyond the period of acute resuscitation. Using the well-established Glasgow Coma Scale (GCS), the most common method for the diagnosis of traumatic coma, patients who do not open their eyes even to a painful stimulus, utter words, or follow even the simplest commands are considered to be in a coma.

The neurologic evaluation of a patient with traumatic coma includes, at a minimum, an assessment according to the GCS and an evaluation of the pupils. The GCS evaluates and scores three elements of the physical examination: intensity of stimulation that will or will not cause eye opening, vocal responses, and motor responses (Table 71-2). The score is weighted by the motor evaluation, which can establish whether there is cortical control of the motor system or only brain stem responses, thus indicating a functional disconnection between the cortex and brain stem. These brain stem responses are arranged in

TABLE 71-2. **Scoring with the Glasgow Coma Scale**

Eye-Opening Response		Verbal Response		Motor Response	
Score	Response	Score	Response	Score	Response
4	Spontaneous	5	Oriented	6	Obeys commands
3	To speech	4	Confused	5	Localizes to painful stimulus
2	To pain	3	Inappropriate responses	4	Withdraws to painful stimulus
1	No response	2	Incomprehensible responses	2	Extension to painful stimulus
		1	No response	1	No response

hierarchical order and indicate severity and perhaps the anatomic level of the brain stem injury. Scoring is frequently confounded; examples include the eye-opening response confounded by traumatic facial swelling, the vocal response confounded by intubation, and the motor response confounded by the presence of paralytic agents. However, a score of 8 or less is frequently used to designate coma, provided the motor system can be evaluated and the patient is not following commands; missing eye and vocal responses are by convention scored 1 (see Table 71-2).

The presence of an unresponsive pupil, particularly a dilated pupil, is significantly correlated with a poor outcome and therefore an important part of the examination. A dilated pupil, particularly in cases where traumatic injury of the globe can be excluded, often indicates the side of a mass lesion, such as a hematoma where the clot has displaced the mesial-temporal lobe structures causing compression the ocular motor nerve.

In addition to this abbreviated physical examination, imaging of the brain is an important method for evaluation of these patients. For acute evaluation, a CT scan has much greater efficacy than either the least complicated method of evaluation, plain skull films, or the more complicated MRI. The CT scan can be used to assess the presence and location of hematomas, contusions, brain swelling, and the presence of herniation either across the midline or across the tentorium where there is actual or incipient compression of the upper brain stem. Transtentorial herniation is best diagnosed by evaluating the CSF spaces around the midbrain (the mesencephalic cisterns) (Fig. 71-16). The absence or occlusion of the mesencephalic cisterns usually indicates dislocation of supratentorial structures below the tentorial notch.

Primary and Secondary Injuries

Before proceeding to the specifics of management, it is useful to consider that although the brain is injured immediately at impact (primary injury), these injuries are frequently followed by later events that cause secondary injuries. Primary injury includes diffuse axonal injury, contusion, hematoma, and traumatic subarachnoid hemorrhage. Diffuse axonal injury, which is an injury to the white matter, can occur in minor as well as severe brain injury and is due to anatomic or functional disrup-

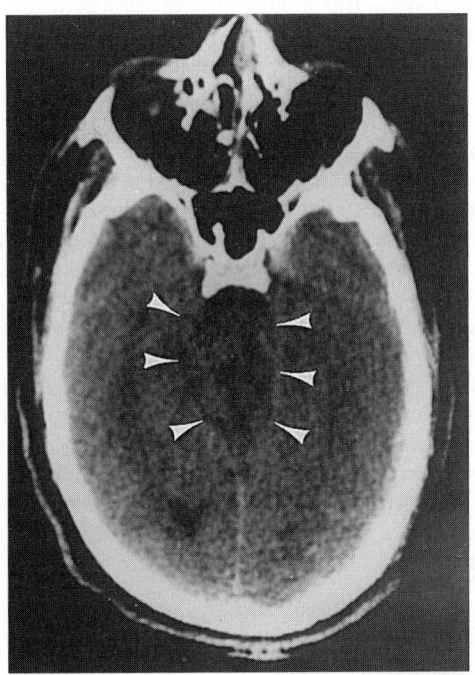

FIGURE 71-16. CT scan of the head in a patient with a closed head injury. Severe compression of mesencephalic cisterns is seen, indicating midbrain compression *(arrowheads)*. Compare with Figure 71-17*A*.

tion of axons. The CT scan "footprint" of diffuse axonal injury consists of small petechial hemorrhages in the white matter, most frequently seen in the corpus callosum and the dorsal rostral brain stem. Extensive diffuse axonal injury in the brain stem can cause coma and is in fact the most likely cause of coma in patients without evidence of mass effect and herniation.

Although contusions and hematomas usually are evident immediately after an impact, they can increase in size, particularly during the first 12 to 24 hours, and a very early CT scan may not be sufficient to evaluate their full effect; in most centers a second delayed CT scan is the routine. Hematomas include intracerebral clots, where there is a spectrum from contusion to pure clot. Extra-axial clots include acute subdural hematoma and epidural hematoma (discussed in detail later). Like contusions, these clots can increase in size or first appear after a few hours, or even days, after injury.

Secondary injuries are potentially preventable and treatable. These include the effects of hypotension, hypoxia, and herniation with elevated ICP due to mass effect. Hypoxia or shock has been found to be associated, independent of injury severity, with poor outcome. Both are frequent occurrences, not only in the prehospital phase but later as well, and have been regularly found even when patients are treated in sophisticated intensive care settings. The correction of shock and hypoxia is the first level of management of head-injured patients, and any head-injured patient who is suspected of having poor ventilation should be intubated urgently (if possible, at the scene).

Secondary brain stem injury frequently occurs from mass effect, which is almost always supratentorial; herniation then occurs across the tentorium with secondary brain stem compression. If progress of this herniation is unabated, there ultimately is loss of vital functions as specific centers in the brain stem are injured. In addition, herniation can cause destruction of the brain stem as the downward movement of the stem exceeds the dislocation of its nutrient arteries, resulting in hemorrhagic infarctions, frequently but not always a terminal event that can be documented by CT scan. These lesions (Duret's hemorrhages) usually occur in the central portion of the brain stem and are usually larger than those associated with diffuse axonal injury.

Mass effect leading to herniation is almost always associated with increased ICP, and the monitoring of ICP can be used to assess the risk of secondary brain injury. In addition, increased ICP can reduce vascular profusion to the point of ischemia. The cerebral profusion pressure (CPP), an index of perfusion, is the difference between mean arterial blood pressure and ICP.

Intracranial Pressure

Evaluation of the patient with severe head injury during the acute period relies on rigorous and frequent monitoring of the patient's neurologic examination, GCS score, pupils, arterial blood gases, and, in many cases, ICP. ICP monitoring is usually started after the initial CT scan in patients not taken to the operating room for evacuation of a mass lesion. Even patients taken to the operating room frequently have ICP monitors placed at the end of the operation because later brain swelling may still be a problem, even after the successful evacuation of a mass. In some centers, young comatose patients with high GCS scores (e.g., 7 or 8) and completely normal CT scans are not immediately monitored, whereas in other centers, virtually all comatose patients, regardless of the CT scan findings, are monitored. The risk of increased ICP in a comatose patient with a completely normal CT scan is considerably lower than that with scans showing any abnormality, a risk estimated at 10% to 15%, but it is still higher than the risk of inserting an ICP monitor.

ICP monitoring devices can be considered of two types: IVCs and devices that measure pressure from sites other than the ventricles, including the brain parenchyma, or extra-axial spaces, including the subarachnoid space or the subdural or epidural space. The ventricular catheter is generally preferred because it is assumed to be the most accurate, and CSF can be drained as a method to reduce mass effect. Of the other methods, the intraparenchymal device is most commonly used. Ventricular catheters are sometimes avoided when the chance of accessing the ventricle is reduced—specifically, when the ventricles are occluded or significantly shifted by brain swelling. The complications of ICP monitoring are inaccuracy of the information due to occlusion of the catheter by blood or necrotic brain or other causes of dampening and baseline drift. Infection, which occurs in approximately 5% of insertions, can be mitigated by watertight closure around the device tunneling catheters and can possibly be reduced by use of prophylactic antibiotics (either peri-insertion or chronic) and periodic changing of the device (after 5 to 7 days). Hematomas around the catheter occur in 1% to 2% of cases, and, sometimes unfortunately, become large enough to cause mass effect that requires operative removal.

Other methods of invasive monitoring, while in limited use, are potentially important and should be considered at this time experimental without proved efficacy. These methods include the measurement of jugular venous gases and glucose and lactate to evaluate oxygenation and nutrition of the brain, brain temperature and oxygen probes, and brain microdialysis.

Nonoperative Management

The initial management, as noted earlier, is assessment and treatment of shock and hypoxia, as well as the search for other injuries and an evaluation of the patient's clotting ability with rapid correction if necessary, because coagulopathy will delay urgently required operations, increase the risk of expansion of hematomas and contusions, and delay the placement of invasive monitoring devices, particularly for the measurement of ICP. Although plain skull films are no longer considered mandatory, a lateral cervical spine film that visualizes the cervical spine from the cranial cervical junction to the C7, T1 interspace is extremely important, and a concerted effort must be made to evaluate the entire cervical spine for fractures and dislocations.

A team approach to the initial evaluation and later management has been shown to be important, but the neurosurgeon must be an involved member of that team. Once stabilization has been successfully started, a CT scan of the head is made. A patient with a significant clot or contusion should be taken to the operating room for evacuation, provided there is no severe coagulopathy. Patients requiring other operations to achieve cardiovascular stability or to correct other emergent conditions can undergo cranial and extra-axial operations simultaneously. When no operative lesion is found by CT, which occurs in approximately 70% of cases, the patient is treated by medical management primarily directed at normalization of ICP. However, a repeat CT scan should be made routinely during the first 12 to 24 hours, as mentioned earlier, and again if ICP becomes elevated, particularly when refractory to medical management.

The following steps should be considered in patients without significant mass effect as well as in patients after evacuation of the mass. The head of the bed is elevated to 30 degrees, and the head is placed in a neutral position. A firm collar should be used until stability of the cervical spine can be shown at a later time by flexion/extension views of the neck. ICP should be maintained below 20 mm Hg, and CPP should be maintained above 70 mm Hg. Hypotension, particularly a mean arterial blood pressure of less than 90 mm Hg, should be prevented or treated, and dehydration should be avoided. In elderly patients or patients suspected of having cardiac dysfunction, cardiac indices and hydration should be carefully evaluated by appropriate methods. ICP elevations of more than 20 mm Hg should be actively treated. The first line of management is the drainage of ventricular fluid when possible, that is, the placement of a ventricular catheter and the use of short-acting sedatives and muscle relaxants, even though the accuracy of neurologic examination is hindered and greater reliance is placed on ICP monitoring and CT scanning. However, these drugs can be intermittently discontinued so that the patient may be evaluated periodically.

If ICP elevations still occur, mannitol or other diuretics are used. Mannitol is given in boluses of 0.25 to 1 g/kg and repeated every 4 to 6 hours. Serum osmolarity is followed to monitor dosage; in addition, an osmolarity of greater than 320 is associated with the risk of renal failure. The mechanism of action of mannitol was once thought to be due only to a reduction in brain water but is now considered to be due to improvement in cerebral blood flow via plasma expansion and reduced blood viscosity. Other diuretics and hypertonic saline are used in some centers in addition to mannitol or in its place.

The role of hyperventilation has become controversial. The mechanism of action is reduction in brain blood volume and thereby mass effect via a change in cerebrovascular tone (vasoconstriction). However, although brain blood volume is reduced, so is cerebral blood flow, and ischemia has been shown to be a common event in patients with severe head injury. A decrease in cerebral blood flow is then potentially harmful, and the period of greatest risk of ischemia is considered to be the first 3 days after injury. Therefore, normal ventilation or only mild hyperventilation to a Paco$_2$ of no less than 35 is generally recommended initially. Nonetheless, Paco$_2$ must be carefully monitored because high Paco$_2$ causes vasodilation and unwanted increase in brain blood volume. In patients with traumatic subarachnoid hemorrhage, calcium-channel blockers have been shown to improve outcome and are used by some centers (see later).

Optimum therapy maintains ICP below 20 and CPP above 70 mm Hg. A controversy, however, has developed among neurosurgeons and neurointensivists as to which is most important—ICP or CPP. In some cases, a CPP higher than 70 mm Hg can be maintained only with elevation of blood pressure. However, the loss of vasomotor tone, which is known to occur in patients with severe head injury, and an increase in blood pressure can combine to cause high elevations of ICP. Contradictory evidence is used to support both sides, and the controversy is unsettled. Some neurosurgeons who believe in the ultimate importance of CPP also disagree with the idea of elevating the patient's head.

When ICP becomes refractory to these strategies, a CT scan is mandatory, particularly if the mannitol dosage has been optimized, to look for newly formed or expanded mass lesions. In cases without new mass lesions, barbiturate therapy to lower ICP has been advocated. The major risk is hypotension. Another option for lowering ICP is decompressive craniectomy (see later).

Although all of the strategies outlined earlier should be considered crude with regard to mechanism of action, there has been in fact a considerable effort to study the role of subcellular mechanisms in traumatic brain injury. A number of candidate mechanisms have been advanced, including free radical formation; the release of excitatory amino acids, particularly glutamate; and the release of lactic acid. Many drugs, particularly those targeting free radicals and excitatory amino acids, have been highly successful in animal models of head injury, but despite multiple rigorously designed randomized clinical trials, none of these drugs has shown efficacy, with exception of one study of a calcium-channel blocker in patients with traumatic subarachnoid hemorrhage.

Prospective but nonrandomized studies have shown that head-injured patients lose significant amounts of nitrogen and that the replacement of 100% to 140% of resting metabolic expenditure with 15% to 20% nitrogen calories improves outcome.

Operative Management

Clots or contusions larger than 25 to 30 cm^3 are generally considered to cause significant mass effect capable of causing neurologic deterioration and progressive brain injury. The diagnosis, size, and location of these lesions are virtually always made by CT. It is sometimes difficult to distinguish between an epidural and an acute subdural hematoma. The epidural hematoma is frequently but not always located in the middle fossa and has a more lenticular appearance than the acute subdural hematoma (Fig. 71-17). Clots on the lateral surface of the brain are most often removed by creating a large "trauma flap" that extends down to the zygoma to expose the middle fossa and a large portion of the lateral surface of the brain. A bleeding source is not always found in the case of acute subdural hematoma and is frequently from the middle meningeal artery or one of its branches in the case of an epidural hematoma.

In the past, for patients with intractable ICP, a large decompression has been advocated. There has been a recent renewal of interest in this option, and a National Institutes of Health–supported study of its efficacy is about to begin. The decompression should include the dura, and expansion of the dura using a graft is generally recommended; however, the opening should be large enough so that the brain does not herniate through the created

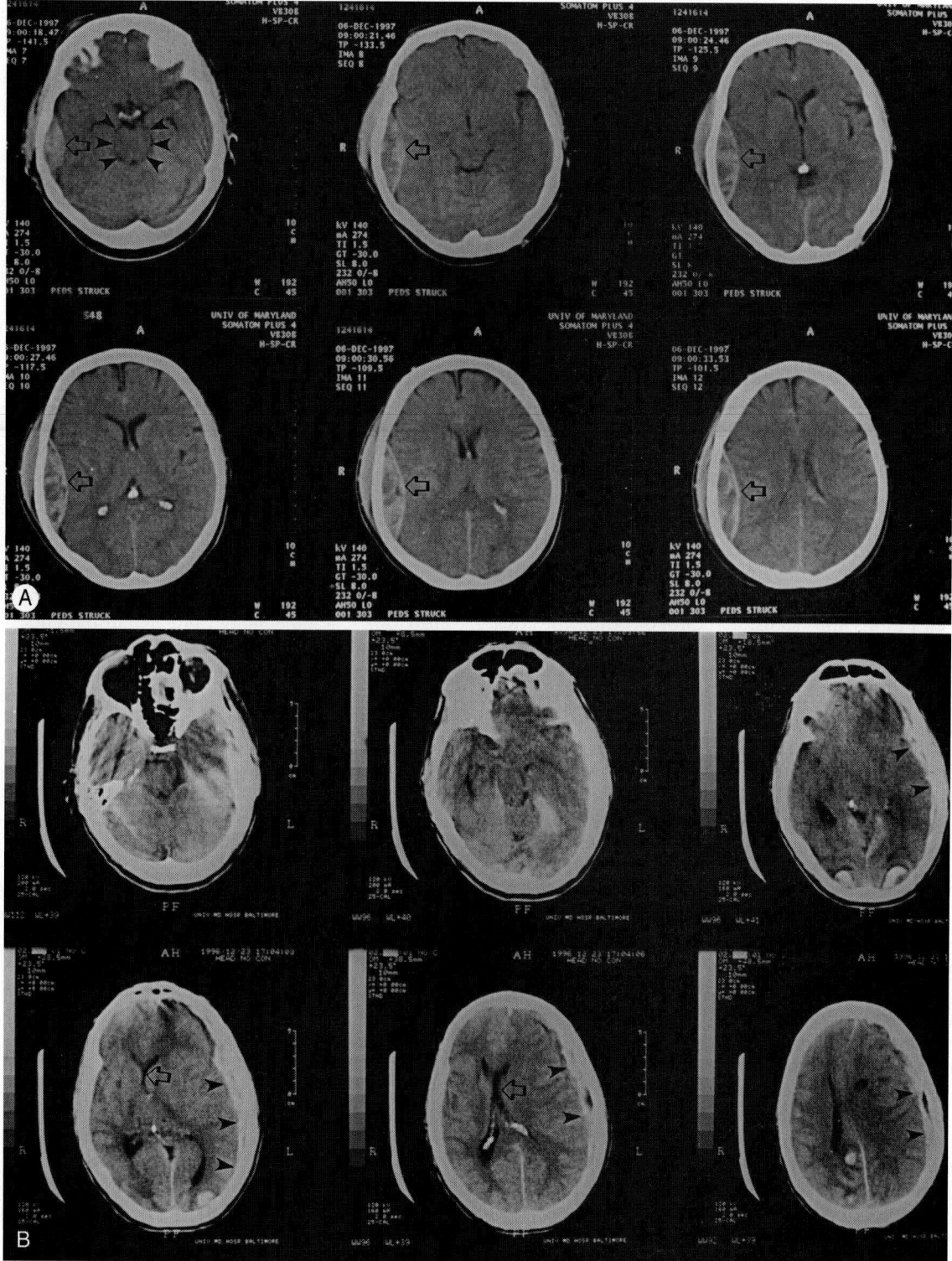

■ FIGURE 71-17.   CT scans of two patients with closed head injury. **A,** This patient has a right temporal epidural hematoma *(arrows)*. The mesencephalic cisterns are patent in the top left, indicating a lack of brain stem compression despite mass *(arrowheads)*. Compare with Figure 71-16. **B,** This patient has suffered an acute left subdural hematoma *(arrowheads)* with midline shift *(arrows)*.

hole and strangulate its blood supply, as seen with strangulated bowel.

Outcome

With a comparison of studies that were conducted at different times and potentially flawed by bias due to differences in cohorts, it appears that outcome has improved since the mid 1970s, when information on severity was first available with the GCS score. Both morbidity and mortality rates seem to have decreased; mortality rates have decreased from approximately 50% to less than 30%.

Penetrating Injuries

The outcome for nonpenetrating injury has improved, but the high mortality rate for patients rendered comatose after missile injury appears to have not changed. Noncomatose patients almost always survive, although with deficits depending on the path of the bullet; the risk of death in the comatose patient in most studies is approximately 90%. However, despite this high mortality rate, many centers use the same medical management as for comatose patients with nonpenetrating injury. Most patients with gunshot wounds do not have large hematomas or contusion, but operative therapy of the missile tract is debated. The current standard in most centers is débridement of the first few centimeters of the tract followed by a watertight dural closure. However, reports from Middle East conflicts in which patients were treated without any débridement but with only simple skin closure of the bullet hole did not indicate a worse outcome.

Other Conditions and Complications of Head Injury

Epilepsy. The overall incidence of epilepsy (delayed seizures) after head injury is approximately 5%. The risk is greater in patients with penetrating injuries or clots. However, randomized studies of the use of prophylactic antiepileptic drugs in the acute period have shown efficacy only in the first week.

Hydrocephalus. Hydrocephalus is a known complication of head injury and can be associated with poor recovery. However, severe head injury is also associated with ventricular dilation due to brain atrophy. The diagnosis of hydrocephalus can then be problematic but is most easily made when there is ventricular dilation and abnormal CSF pressure, yet little in the way of sulcal (cortical surface) dilation.

Cerebrospinal Fluid. CSF leak, otorrhea, and rhinorrhea are well-known complications of head injury, particularly when there is a basal skull fracture, which can be identified by CT scan, particularly using bone windows with coronal views. Otorrhea may be also associated with facial nerve (cranial nerve VII) injury, but the leak frequently regresses spontaneously, whereas rhinorrhea is more likely to persist. The risk of a persistent leak is meningitis. The leak may initially be treated by lumbar drainage in the chronic phase when there is no risk of herniation. If the leak persists, operative intervention either through the sinuses, possibly with endoscopy, or transcranially with dura repair is mandatory.

Traumatic Aneurysms. Traumatic aneurysms can occur when vessels are injured and are a cause of delayed subarachnoid hemorrhage and delayed death and complications after head injury. When a patient has a penetrating injury or fracture at the skull base near major arteries, an arteriogram is indicated.

Carotid Dissection. Carotid dissection rarely occurs with head injury but can be the cause of delayed deterioration, particularly when there is an injury to the neck; the diagnosis is made by angiography.

Chronic Subdural Hematoma. Chronic subdural hematomas most frequently occur after minor injury and present with headaches, confusion, altered consciousness, and occasionally focal deficit. The diagnosis is made by CT scan, and treatment is generally done either by twist drill drainage or by burr holes.

DEGENERATIVE DISORDERS OF THE SPINE

Degenerative Disease of the Lumbar Spine

Between 50% and 90% of the population experience back pain at some point in life. Fortunately, most of these symptoms last for no longer than a few weeks, but when one considers the direct medical costs, decreased productivity, and lost wages, the expense to society is staggering. Low back pain and other disorders of the lumbar spine are some of the more common reasons adults seek attention from their primary care providers. Certainly, these disorders as a whole represent one of the most frequent reasons for referral to neurosurgeons.

The lumbar spine in a normal individual is composed of five lumbar vertebrae and five lumbar discs. Because the lumbar spine must support the weight of the entire spinal column and is subject to the greatest loads within the spine, the individual vertebrae are relatively large structures. Each vertebra is made up of a vertebral body and a dorsal neural arch. Each neural arch is in turn composed of laminae, pedicles, facet joints, and a spinous process. Several ligaments connect the lumbar vertebrae to each other. The anterior longitudinal ligament is a continuous structure that spans the length of the spinal column and is more closely adherent to the concave ventral surface of the vertebral bodies than to the intervertebral discs. The posterior longitudinal ligament also runs the entire length of the spinal column. This structure spreads out at each disc level and tends to thin out laterally over the intervertebral disc. The paired ligamentum flava are thick elastic structures that connect the undersurfaces of adjacent laminae. These ligaments are discontinuous at each midvertebral level and in the midline and function to limit flexion of the spine. The interspinous and intertransverse ligaments connect adjacent spinous and transverse processes, respectively.

Between each lumbar vertebra lies an intervertebral disc. Each disc is made up of three components: the *annulus fibrosus,* a circular structure made up of concentric circles of fibrous tissue; the *nucleus pulposus,* the soft, semigelatinous central portion of the disc; and the *cartilaginous endplate,* an unossified portion of the vertebral body. The disc functions as a physiologic shock absorber and allows for limited motion of each intervertebral segment. The lumbar region normally has a lordotic curvature that is convex ventrally.

At each spinal level, a nerve root containing both motor and sensory components exits on each side of the spine. These nerve roots leave the thecal sac, cross the intervertebral disc space, and then travel a short distance within the lateral recesses of the spinal canal. After passing around the pedicle, the nerve root enters the neural foramen, where it leaves the spine. The spinal cord usually terminates at the caudal aspect of the L1 vertebral body. The cauda equina continues distally and is composed of the lumbar and sacral nerve roots that have not yet exited through their respective neural foramina.

Lumbar Radiculopathy

Lumbar discs are particularly prone to desiccation and herniation, in part due to the heavy loads they must bear and the significant motion they must endure. Under these stresses, the nucleus pulposus may herniate either through the cartilaginous endplate or through the annulus fibrosis. As individuals age, the annulus normally desiccates, and because of this process, it becomes more susceptible to tearing or rupture. Disc herniations can occur in any direction, but the most clinically significant are those that occur posterolaterally. Disc material extruded in this location may compress a nerve root or the cauda equina, causing radicular symptoms and signs in the anatomic distribution of the affected nerve root. Large, central herniations may compress the cauda equina or result in bilateral radicular symptoms. In many cases, symptoms related to disc herniations are self-limited due to reparative processes that can occur. Desiccation of the herniated disc material can lead to shrinkage of the herniated fragment with resolution of the patient's signs and symptoms.

In the lumbar spine, at least 90% of disc herniations occur at the L5-S1 or L4-5 levels. L3-4 herniations make up only 5% of cases, with the remainder occurring at L2-3 and L1-2. The typical posterolateral disc herniation compresses a nerve root as it exits from the dural sac. Clinically, a herniated disc at one level usually affects the nerve root that exits at the level below. For instance, a left L4-5

disc herniation usually compresses the left L5 nerve root. Patients typically present with signs and symptoms that are attributable to compression of a particular nerve root. Initial complaints are backache, and in most of those affected, there is no history of antecedent trauma. Prior similar complaints of back pain or sciatica are common complaints. The patient's back pain is usually followed by severe pain that radiates into the lower extremities. Numbness or paresthesias may occur in the same distribution as the pain, and weakness of selected muscle groups can occur. With a large centrally herniated fragment, compression of the cauda equina may result in bilateral radicular signs and even sphincter disturbances. Table 71-3 summarizes the most common clinical presentations.

On physical examination, the patient with a herniated lumbar disc and an active radiculopathy appears uncomfortable. The spine may appear normal, but mild flexion or even scoliosis can be observed. Paraspinal muscle spasm is frequently present, and bending of the spine is limited. Radicular pain on flexion of the straight leg at the hip (Lasègue's sign) is one of the most important tests in the diagnosis of a herniated disc. The neurologic examination is important in localizing the level of disc herniation and should include complete motor, sensory, and reflex testing. Although many of the physical examination findings are stereotypical for a particular disc herniation syndrome, variability does occur and may be due to subtle neuroanatomic differences in patients or to specific characteristics of the actual disc herniation (i.e., fragment size or location).

Initially, unless the patient's signs are associated with sphincter disturbance or significant weakness in a radicular distribution, most patients are treated medically for at least 2 weeks. A large number of nonoperative therapies are available and include rest, analgesics, muscle relaxants, and the application of heat. After the acute period of pain has resolved, physical therapy with attention to lumbosacral exercises may prevent recurrences. If conservative measures fail to relieve the patient's symptoms or if sphincter disturbances or weakness occurs, imaging of the spine is indicated. Plain radiographs are obtained to exclude other conditions such as fractures or neoplasm. MRI is the preferred method for imaging the spine, but in selected patients postmyelography CT may be helpful.

Indications for surgery include radicular pain that does not improve with conservative measures, recurrent episodes of incapacitating pain, disc herniations associated with significant weakness in the appropriate muscle

TABLE 71-3.	Clinical Findings of Common Lumbar Disc Herniations				
Disc	**Nerve Root**	**Pain**	**Sensory Change**	**Motor Deficits**	**Reflex Loss**
L3–4	L4	Anterior thigh, anterior leg, and medial ankle	Anterior leg	Quadriceps	Knee jerk
L4–5	L5	Posterior hip and posterolateral thigh and leg	Medial dorsum of foot and occasionally medial ankle	Foot and toe extension	None
L5–S1	S1	Hip, buttock, and posterior thigh and leg	Lateral foot and ankle	Plantar flexion	Ankle jerk

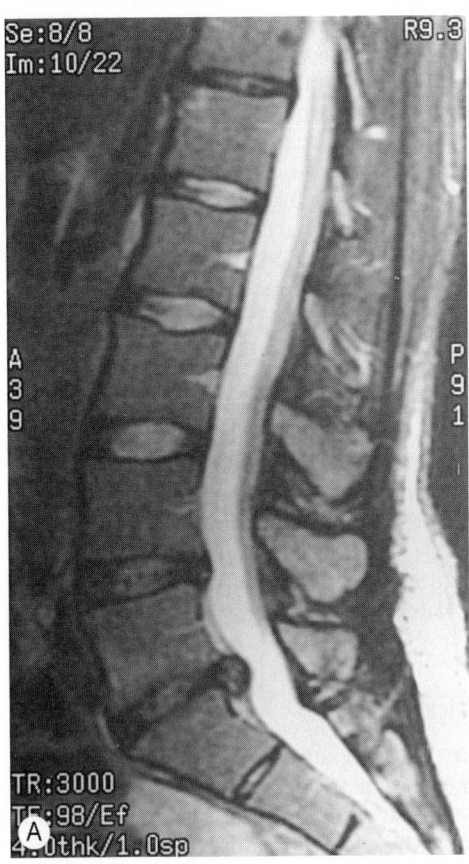

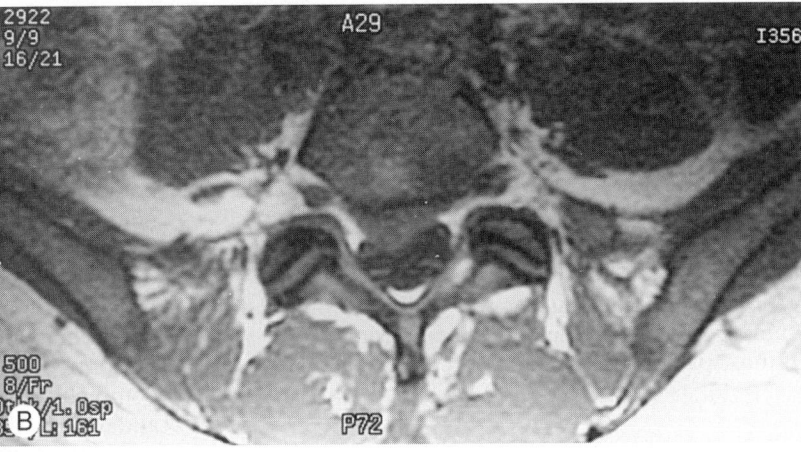

FIGURE 71-18.   Lumbar spine MRI in a patient with a right S1 radiculopathy. **A,** Sagittal T2-weighted image shows disc desiccation (disc space is darker), loss of disc height, and protrusion at the L5–S1 level. **B,** Axial T1-weighted MRI illustrates a right paramedian disc herniation causing compression of the right S1 nerve root.

groups, and massive midline herniations with signs of cauda equina compression (Fig. 71-18A and B).

The standard treatment of these disorders uses a midline incision over the affected interspace followed by a hemilaminectomy to expose the dural sac and nerve root. Gentle medial retraction of these structures exposes the herniated disc fragments, which are removed along with any loose disc material identified within the disc space. The nerve root is then explored thoroughly along its course to ensure that it is adequately decompressed. In cases of large disc herniations or in those cases with a free, extruded disc fragment, a complete laminectomy at the appropriate level may be necessary. Most patients recover sufficiently to be discharged within 1 or 2 days of surgery. Nearly 90% of patients treated surgically have good results. Five percent of patients experience a recurrence of their pain and require reoperation.

Lumbar Spinal Stenosis

Lumbar radiculopathy can occur in patients without disc herniation when significant lumbar spinal canal narrowing is present. Secondary or acquired spinal stenosis is a condition that occurs when degenerative changes narrow the spinal canal to such a degree that constriction of the neural elements occurs and causes neurologic deficits. The symptoms and signs of central canal stenosis can mimic the cauda equina syndrome, whereas lateral recess stenosis may cause a radiculopathy that is indistinguishable from that seen with a herniated lumbar disc.

With progressive degeneration of the lumbar spine, lumbar disc degeneration, ligamentous hypertrophy, and articular spondylosis occur, which leads to direct mechanical compression of the cauda equina. Patients classically demonstrate signs of neurogenic claudication: pain, numbness, paresthesias, and weakness in the legs that occurs with standing or walking, which increases the lumbar lordosis and causes an infolding of the ligamentum flavum. Flexion of the spine or simply leaning forward typically relieves these symptoms by stretching the ligamentum flavum, thus leading to an increased spinal canal diameter. The pathogenesis of radiculopathy associated with neurogenic claudication has not been fully defined, but it is thought to occur as a result of nerve root ischemia. When activity-related increases in the metabolic rate of nerve roots cannot be met, the resulting microvascular deficiency leads to an ischemic radiculopathy. Neurogenic claudication is distinguished from vascular claudication by the presence of good pulses in the lower extremities and the requirement for sitting or leaning forward to relieve the pain rather than just stopping.

The physical examination may be normal in many of these patients unless they are examined immediately after activity. Therefore, the clinical history becomes important if lumbar spinal stenosis is suspected. In general, these histories tend to be less acute than those encountered in patients with disc herniations. Lumbar spine MRI has become the imaging modality of choice in these cases and is capable of defining the relationships between the spinal and neural elements. Medical therapy including bed rest, analgesics, and either steroidal or nonsteroidal anti-inflammatory agents may reduce inflammation and relieve symptoms, but the relief is brief because symptoms usually recur with the resumption of activity. Surgery is indicated in patients with recurrent and disabling pain that limits their usual activity or in the rare patient with signs of nerve root or cauda equina compression. The standard procedure involves performing a wide laminectomy at those levels determined to be stenotic on preoperative imaging studies. Care must be exercised to avoid postsurgical instability. Success rates after decompression for lumbar stenosis are high and range from 80% to 90%, with most patients returning to premorbid activity levels (Fig. 71-19).

Lumbar Instrumentation and Fusion

Once rarely performed by neurosurgeons, lumbar instrumentation and fusion have become procedures that are now part of the general neurosurgical repertoire.[35] In general, lumbar instrumentation and fusion are performed simultaneously: The instrumentation provides immediate rigid fixation while the spine completes the process of forming a bony fusion that ensures long-term stabilization. Lumbar fusion is effective in reducing mechanical and discogenic back pain, which must be distinguished from lumbar radiculopathy, neurogenic claudication, lumbar facet arthropathy, and myofascial lumbar strain. The most common indications for fusion and instrumentation are spondylolisthesis (slippage of a vertebral body on an adjacent level) and intractable pain associated with disc degeneration.[36] The preoperative evaluation includes plain films to evaluate bony anatomy, a CT scan to determine the size and shape of the pedicles and vertebral bodies, and an MRI scan to evaluate disc degeneration and neural compression. The lumbar spine exposure is more generous than usually performed for a simple laminectomy or discectomy: the entire facet joint and transverse process complex is identified. A generous laminectomy, which may include a partial or complete facetectomy, is performed to relieve neural compression followed by a complete discectomy. The interspace is then distracted and filled with bone or a biomechanical spacer. Under fluoroscopic guidance, and using the position of the transverse process as a landmark, screws are inserted through the pedicles into the vertebral body and attached to rods (Fig. 71-20A and B). Finally, autologous bone is placed along the lateral gutters between the transverse processes to form a posterolateral fusion mass.

Degenerative Cervical Lesions

Neck pain and radiculopathy are among the most common symptoms seen by primary care practitioners. Lesions of the cervical intervertebral discs are in many ways analogous to those affecting the lumbar area, but important anatomic differences introduce variations in symptoms, signs, and treatment.

Anatomy

The cervical disc, like the lumbar disc, is composed of a tough outer annulus fibrosis and a softer inner nucleus pulposus. It is separated from the vertebral bodies above and below it by cartilaginous endplates. An important distinction from the lumbar spine is that the spinal canal in the cervical area contains the spinal cord rather than the lumbar nerve roots, so a reduction in the size of the spinal canal by spondylosis or a midline disc herniation causes compression of the spinal cord, which results in significantly more dangerous complications. The cervical spine contains the joints of Luschka, which are not present elsewhere in the spine. These joints, one on each side of the disc, can give rise to bony spurs or ridges (osteophytes), as can the main facet joints (apophyseal joints) and the edges of the vertebral bodies adjacent to the intervertebral disc. The exiting nerve root on each side travels between these joints and can be compressed by osteophytes extending into the intervertebral foramen from any or all of these three sources or from a posterolateral soft disc herniation.

In the cervical area, the nerves exit transversely. There are seven cervical vertebrae but eight pairs of cervical nerves. The nerve roots exit on each side at the level of the intervertebral disc, and the number of the nerve root corresponds to the vertebral body below the foramen (e.g., at the C5–6 foramen, the C6 nerve root exits), except for C7–T1, where the C8 nerve root exits.

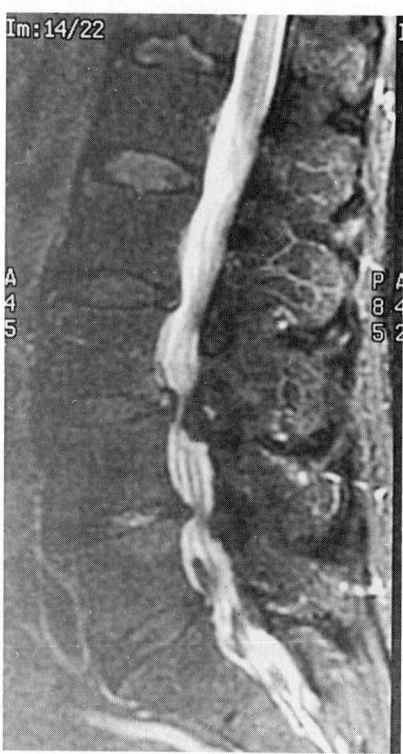

FIGURE 71-19.   Sagittal T2-weighted MRI study in a patient with neurogenic claudication. Degenerative changes are noted at multiple levels with severe spinal stenosis at the L3–4 and L4–5 levels.

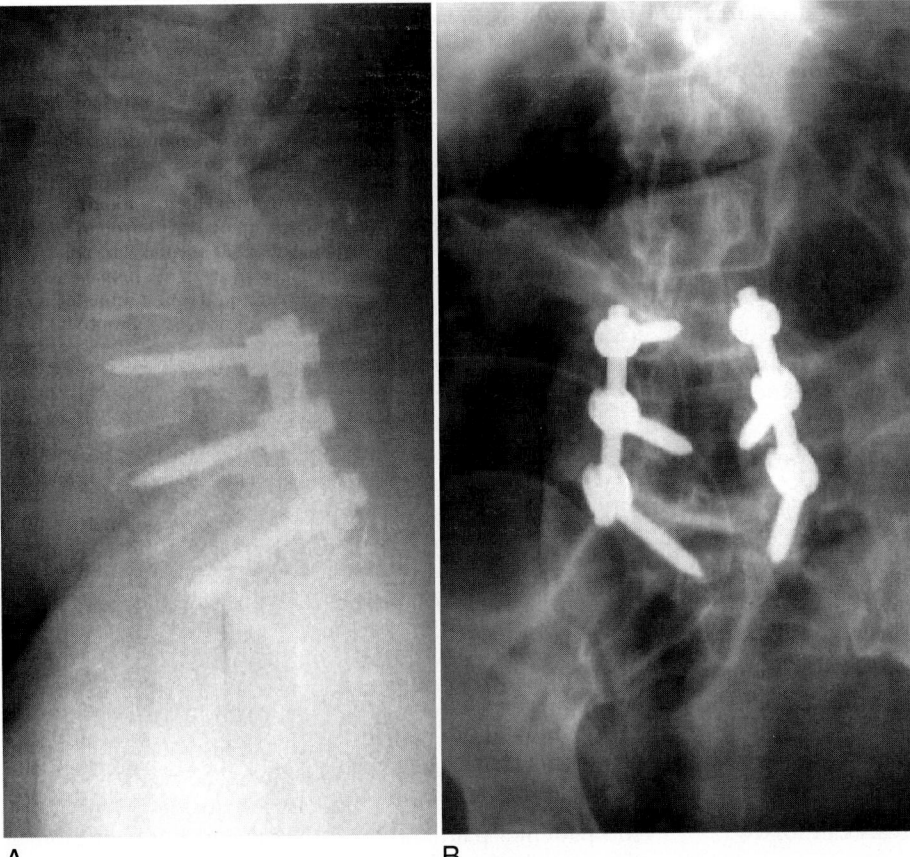

A   B

■ **FIGURE 71-20.** Plain lumbar films of a patient who underwent L4–5, L5–S1 laminectomy with pedicle screw instrumentation and posterolateral bony fusion. **A,** Lateral film showing pedicle screws in the L4, L5, and S1 vertebral bodies. **B,** Anteroposterior view of the pedicle screw and rod construct.

Pathology

Disc degeneration is a dynamic process that begins early in life and progresses at a variable rate. Degenerative changes in the cervical intervertebral disc can take two main forms: (1) the nucleus pulposus can herniate out of its normal confined space (soft disc) or (2) the entire disc can slowly lose substance, with loss of disc height resulting in osteoarthritis of the facet joints and the joints of Luschka. The combination of degenerative disc disease and osteophyte formation is called *cervical spondylosis.*

Three pathologic entities are recognized in the cervical area: (1) mechanical neck pain, (2) cervical radiculopathy, and (3) cervical myelopathy. Any of these can occur in isolation or in combination with each other. Compression of a nerve root in the intervertebral foramina by either a soft disc herniation or osteophyte can lead to cervical radiculopathy. Motor root dysfunction leads to weakness and atrophy, whereas sensory root compression causes pain, sensory loss, and paresthesias in the nerve root distribution. Anterior compression of the spinal cord can be caused by acute or chronic central disc herniation, osteophytic ridges, or posterior compression by thickening of the ligamentum flavum and hypertrophic facet joints. This stenosis leads to spinal cord compression manifesting as cervical myelopathy. A congenitally narrow spinal canal predisposes patients to developing cervical myelopathy.

Cervical Radiculopathy

A patient's history is of great importance in the evaluation of neck and arm pain. Symptoms usually develop acutely with the usual posterolateral disc rupture but more gradually and chronically in spondylosis. The usual history is that of a proximal radiating arm pain with numbness and paresthesias distally in the nerve root distribution. The pain and paresthesias may be intensified by neck movement, especially by extension or by lateral flexion of the side of the compression and by coughing or straining. In severe cases, patients notice a motor weakness in the same nerve root distribution.

On examination, the patients usually exhibit restriction of neck movement, especially in extension. Downward head compression by the examiner, as well as flexing the neck to the side of the involvement, usually aggravates the pain. Nerve root compression in the upper cervical spine is unusual. Compression of C2 causes occipital neuralgia, but if C3 and C4 are compressed, it usually causes non-specific neck and shoulder pain without any muscle weakness. Compression of the C5 root leads to shoulder and deltoid pain with weakness in the deltoid muscle (abduction of the arm). The most common root compression syndromes are those involving the sixth and seventh cervical roots. With C6 root compression, the pain is in a radicular distribution down the arm, distal to the elbow, with paresthesias or sensory loss over the thumb and index finger. Biceps weakness (flexion of the elbow), as well as weakness in extension of the wrist, is present, and diminution of the biceps and brachioradialis reflex may be present. With C7 root compression, the pain radiates down the back of the arm distal to the elbow. Paresthesias in the middle finger that also involve the index finger or ring finger or both may be present. Because of overlapping of the C6 and C8 roots, the sensory loss may be minimal or absent. Triceps muscle weakness (extension of the elbow), as well as weakness in flexion of the wrist, is a hallmark of this nerve root compression. The triceps reflex may be diminished or absent. Eighth nerve root compression causes pain down the arm as well as sensory changes that involve the ulnar side of the hand, but they usually present with intrinsic hand muscle weakness.

Myelopathy

Compression of the spinal cord can lead to cervical myelopathy, which is manifested by motor neuron dysfunction at the level of compression and upper motor neuron dysfunction (spasticity, clonus, increased deep tendon reflexes, Babinski's sign, and Hoffmann's sign) below that level. In cases of acute central disc herniation, these symptoms may occur acutely, but in cases caused by cervical spondylitic stenosis, the onset is much more gradual and insidious. These patients usually complain of poor muscle coordination, especially in their hands and when walking. In chronic and severe cases, symptoms of spasticity become clear and quadriparesis can follow.[37]

Diagnostic Studies

Plain radiographs of the cervical spine are obtained to assess the presence and degree of spondylosis but especially to identify a cause of neck and arm pain other than disc disease such as neoplasm or infection. If conservative treatment fails, other diagnostic studies are indicated to make a diagnosis of the cause of the patient's symptoms.

MRI is the procedure of choice as an initial diagnostic tool to evaluate cervical radiculopathy and myelopathy. In some cases where the diagnosis is not immediately apparent, a cervical myelogram followed by CT scanning could yield definitive information. In cases where the clinical diagnosis is in doubt and other causes, such as plexopathies or peripheral nerve compressions must be excluded, electromyography and nerve conduction studies are helpful.

Treatment

The initial treatment of a patient with acute radiculopathy is conservative and consists of restriction of activity, soft cervical collar, and medication for pain and muscle spasm. After the acute phase, physical therapy with intermittent cervical halter traction may be beneficial. Anti-inflammatory and antispasmodic medication may be of value over a prolonged period to reduce the discomfort of cervical spondylosis. Most of the patient's symptoms improve with conservative treatment.

There are two indications to perform surgery in patients with cervical radiculopathy: (1) failed medical management with intolerable arm pain and (2) progressive and significant motor loss. The aim of surgery is to provide nerve root decompression, and this can be accomplished by either a posterior approach through a foraminotomy or by an anterior approach through the intervertebral disc. Both approaches lead to excellent results, and the choice of which to use is tailored by the patient's specific pathology.[38]

With anterior pathology (paracentral disc herniation or large uncovertebral osteophytes), an anterior cervical discectomy, nerve root decompression, and fusion are indicated. This approach is performed through the plane between the carotid sheath laterally and the esophagus and trachea medially. The procedure is performed with the aid of the operating microscope, and after the disc is removed, the foramen is widely opened from the anterior. A fusion is then performed with a bone plug obtained either from the patient's iliac crest or fibular allograft. Most neurosurgeons place an anterior locking plate, especially if two or more levels are performed (Fig. 71-21A to C).[39,40] The rationale of a locking plate is that it offers immediate rigid fixation, diminishes the patient's neck pain, avoids complication with the bone plug, and causes a solid fusion in virtually all cases. If an anterior locking plate is not placed, the patient should be kept in a cervical collar for 6 weeks, and regular follow-up radiographs are necessary to monitor the fusion. The results obtained from this procedure are excellent, causing resolution of the patient's pain and paresthesias and normalization of the neurologic deficit.[41]

A posterior approach is indicated in patients with unilateral radicular symptoms without significant neck pain where the pathology can be resected from the posterior. This includes foraminal disc herniations or foraminal stenosis caused by thickening of the ligamentum flavum and from hypertrophic facet joints. An approach similar to a lumbar microdiscectomy is used with a small unilateral approach. With the aid of the operating microscope, a small foraminotomy is performed with a high-speed drill, thereby decompressing the affected nerve root and allowing the removal of small foraminal discs. This procedure does not require any fusions, and equally excellent results can be obtained.[42,43]

In contrast to cervical radiculopathy, cervical myelopathy poses a far greater surgical challenge. Conservative therapy plays only a minor role in these patients, and surgery is indicated far more urgently than radiculopathy because compression of the spinal cord poses a significant risk to the patient's spinal cord function. Acute central disc herniations are always treated through an anterior approach as described, and if the patient can be operated on before permanent damage occurs, the prognosis is usually good.

In patients with chronic spondylosis in whom there is compression from anterior as well as posterior, complex surgery might be necessary. A significant number of these patients have already sustained some permanent spinal cord damage, and the results of surgical decompression can be less optimal. The decompression can be performed either from anterior or posterior, or in some cases, from a combination of both (Fig. 71-22A to C). Anterior verte-

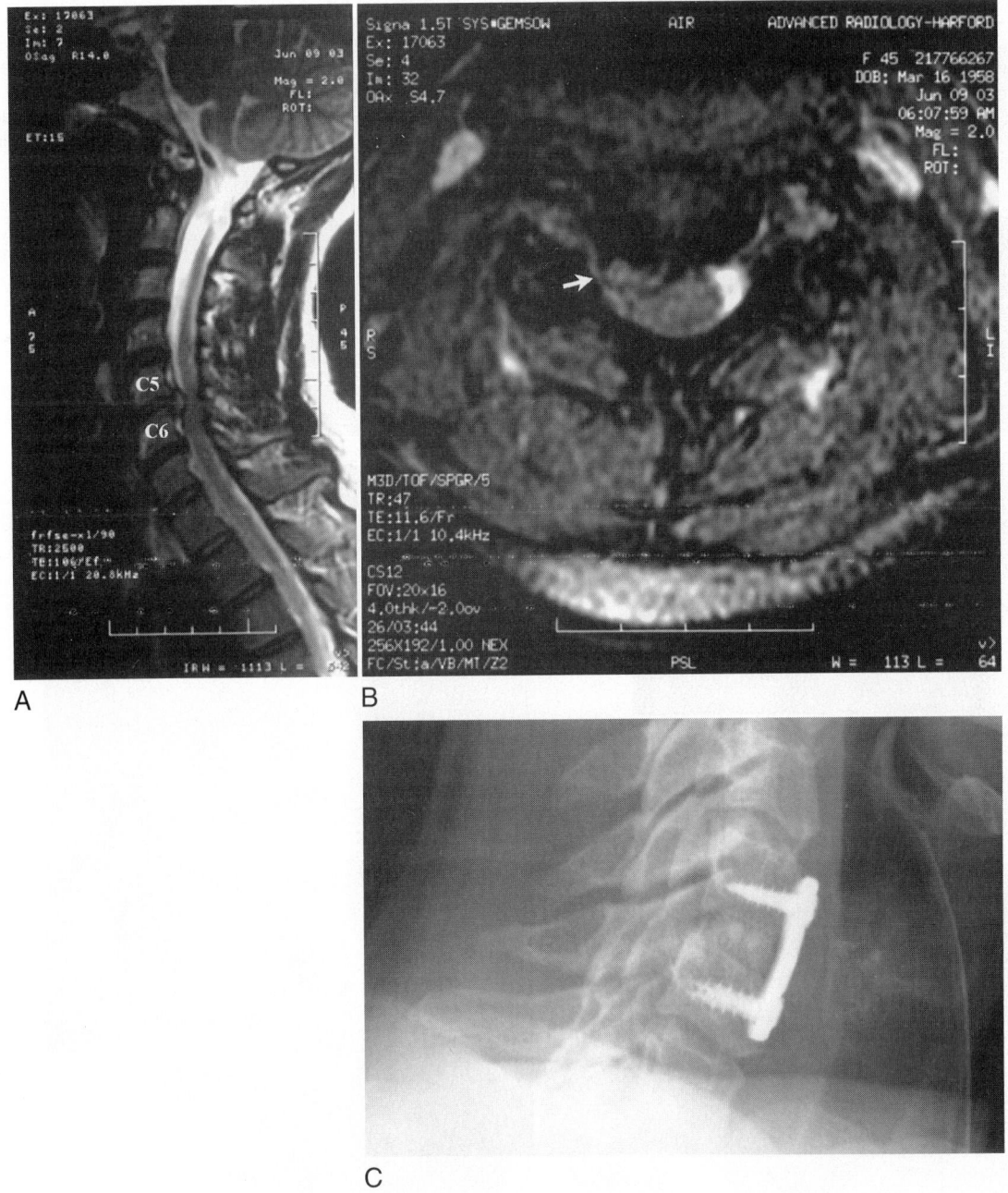

FIGURE 71-21. A patient with a right C5-6 disc herniation and C6 radiculopathy. **A,** Sagittal T2-weighted MRI study shows a disc herniation with compression of the spinal subarachnoid space. **B,** A large paramedian disc herniation is shown compressing the right C6 nerve root and spinal cord *(arrow).* **C,** A postoperative lateral plain film shows a fibular allograft in the C5-6 disc space and an anterior plate with screws in the C5 and C6 bodies.

bral osteophytic ridges or chronic disc herniations must be decompressed anteriorly, and because multiple levels might be involved, multilevel discectomies or even corpectomies (removal of the central 18 mm of vertebral body) to achieve decompression might be necessary. After spinal cord decompression, a fibula or an iliac crest bone graft is positioned, followed by an anterior locking plate.[44]

If the patient has a congenitally narrow canal and most of the compression is from posterior, cervical laminectomies can be performed to decompress the spinal canal. This can be accomplished with or without lateral mass plate fusion for stability. Because of the intrinsic spinal cord damage, the multilevel involvement, and the chronic nature of the disease, the results are sometimes less satisfactory than those for cervical radiculopathy. However, with modern microsurgical techniques, the prognosis has improved, and in most patients, improvement in the neurologic function can be accomplished.

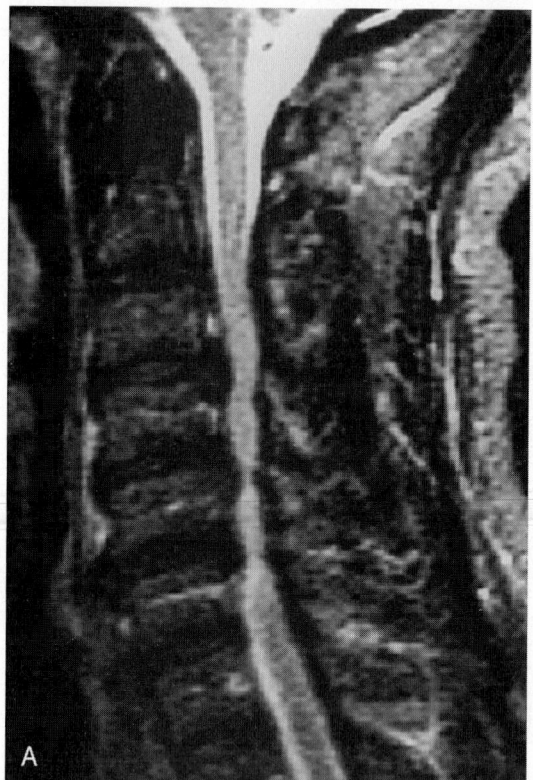

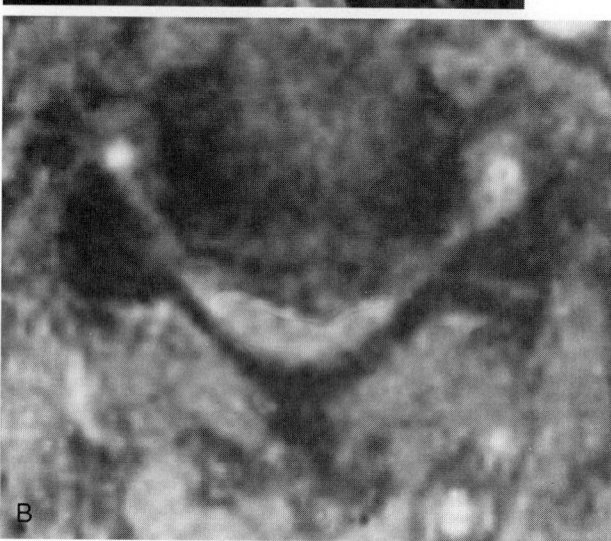

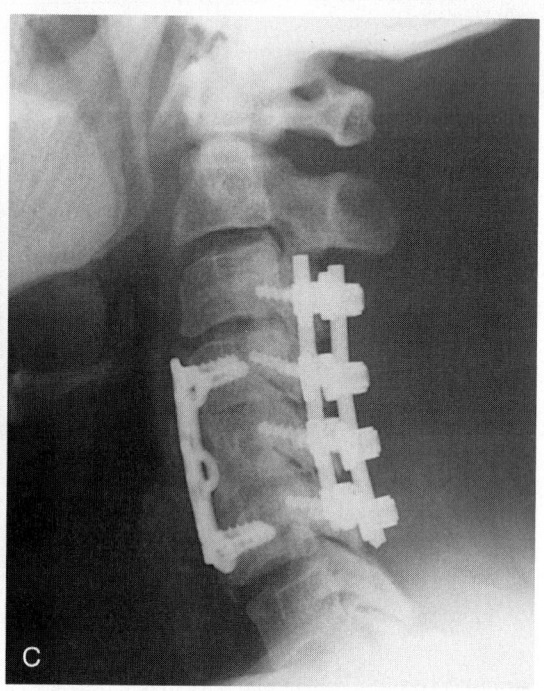

FIGURE 71-22. A patient with multilevel cervical stenosis who presented with myelopathy. **A,** T2-weighted sagittal MRI study shows severe cervical spinal stenosis at the C3–4, C4–5, and C5–6 levels. **B,** T2-weighted axial image shows chronic disc and osteophyte protrusion causing anterior compression. **C,** Postoperative lateral radiograph. A two-staged procedure was performed: a C5 corpectomy with an iliac bone graft and anterior locking plating, followed by a cervical laminectomy of C3–C7 with additional stabilization by lateral mass instrumentation.

FUNCTIONAL NEUROSURGERY

This section includes a discussion of the principles of stereotactic surgery and its application to brain biopsy, radiosurgical ablation of lesions, lesion generation and electrode implantation for movement disorder, and the surgical management of epilepsy and pain.

Stereotactic Neurosurgery

Stereotactic neurosurgery is defined as the use of a coordinate system to provide accurate navigation to a point or region in space. The coordinates for any point in the brain are determined by a fixed stereotactic frame that is rigidly attached to the skull, or they may be based on a frameless system that uses fiducial markers placed on the scalp that are then correlated with MRI or CT results. The most commonly used frame-based systems are the Leksell Model G and the Cosman-Roberts-Wells frames (Fig. 71-23). Both frames are rigidly attached to the skull, usually under local anesthesia, by four threaded pins that penetrate only the outer table of the skull. A box containing fiducial markers that appear on MRI or CT is then attached to the frame, which allows precise determination of X, Y, and Z coordinates of any point within the frame. Finally, a stereotactic arc is mounted on the frame, and the proper coordinates are positioned before the procedure is performed.

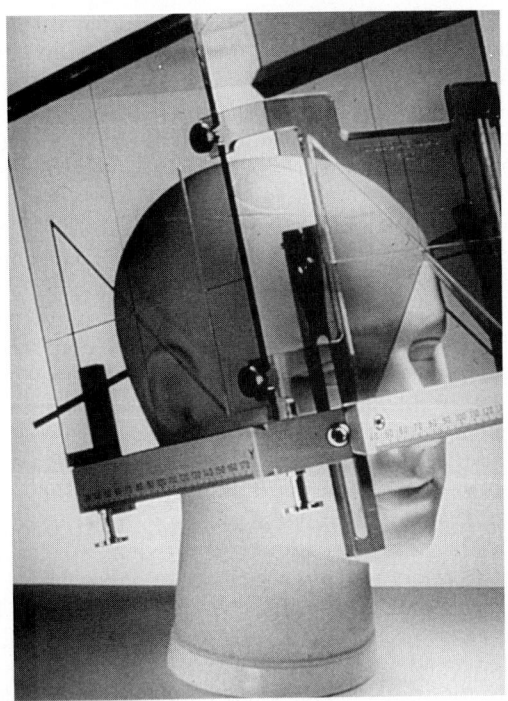

FIGURE 71-23. The Leksell stereotactic coordinate frame is rigidly attached to the head by four threaded pins. The fiducial box is mounted on the frame during the imaging (MRI or CT) study. *X, Y,* and *Z* coordinates are determined directly from the imaging study. The center of the frame is arbitrarily given the coordinates 100, 100, 100.

Frame-Based Stereotactic Procedures

Frame-based stereotactic surgery provides the most accurate and stable method for accessing deep targets within the brain. This is most commonly used to perform biopsies, implant electrodes or make lesions, and as guidance for radiation delivery. By attaching a guide mounted on an arc to the stereotactic frame, any point within the brain may be approached from a wide variety of entry points and angles. Drill and biopsy guides are rigidly attached to the arc and allow accurate positioning. Suspected tumors or infections deep to the surface make ideal targets for stereotactic biopsies. Complications after biopsy are unusual, but care must be taken to avoid biopsy of a vascular lesion. A small hematoma at the biopsy site is not unusual and is rarely clinically significant.[45] The morbidity rate for a stereotactic biopsy is less than 5%, and the mortality rate is less than 1%.[46] The diagnostic yield is approximately 90%.[47]

Deep Brain Lesion and Stimulation. The original rationale for stereotactic surgery was to create deep brain lesions in patients with movement disorders.[48] Early stereotactic localization was based on the use of ventriculography to outline the anterior and posterior boundaries of the third ventricle (AC-PC line); this line was then used as the reference for determining the location of surrounding deep brain structures such as the ventro-intermediate nucleus (VIM) of the thalamus and the medial globus pallidus (GPi). Because anatomic and physiologic target confirmation and lesioning techniques remained crude, the results

were inconsistent, and when pharmacologic therapy with L-dopa was found to be effective, stereotactic surgery quickly fell out of favor.[49] Long-term follow-up of patients treated with dopamine agonists has revealed limitations with these drugs, and modern stereotactic surgery, due largely to refinements in intracranial imaging and microelectrode recording, once again plays a prominent role in the treatment of patients with tremors, rigidity, and dyskinesias.[50] In the early 1990s, a resurgence of interest by neurosurgeons in Parkinson's disease was led by the rediscovery of Leksell's technique of making radiofrequency lesions in the posteroventral GPi for dyskinesias and rigidity.[51] The accuracy and safety of creating these lesions have been improved with the development of reliable microelectrode recording that provides instant feedback on the position of the electrode tip by detecting characteristic neuronal bursting patterns in different brain structures. Deep brain lesion procedures are limited by their inherent irreversibility and prohibitive complications with bilateral lesions (e.g., severe psychomotor retardation in GPi). The evolution of surgical treatment for Parkinson's disease has led to the development of deep brain stimulation (DBS) to replace lesion making and the subthalamic nucleus (STN) as a target.[52] Despite its central role in modulating the GPi, the STN was avoided as a potential target because hemiballismus was observed in patients with STN damage. By using DBS, which induces a reversible inhibition of neuronal activity, instead of ablation, the STN became a viable target and is now substantiated as the preferred target for Parkinson's disease. In addition, bilateral DBS can used in a patient allowing treatment of bilateral symptoms without risk of the deficits seen in bilateral GPi lesions.[53,54] When tremor alone is the primary symptom, DBS of the VIM thalamus is the most effective treatment.[55]

Stereotactic Radiosurgery. Stereotactic radiosurgery, first proposed by Leksell in 1951, uses the stereotactic frame to determine the coordinates of a lesion and then delivers a concentrated dose of radiation to that point.[56] Gamma knife and modified linear accelerator systems are the most widely used radiosurgery devices, and they use photons to deliver their effect. Indications for stereotactic radiosurgery include metastatic tumors, malignant gliomas, benign brain tumors, AVMs, and trigeminal neuralgia. More than 90% of metastatic tumors are initially controlled with stereotactic radiosurgery, and 80% are controlled long term.[34] Stereotactic radiosurgery has the greatest impact on survival in patients with single brain metastases, but it is also suitable for patients with multiple lesions and controlled primary disease and also for patients with recurrence in the brain at distant sites. According to preliminary results from a recent Radiation Therapy Oncology Group study, stereotactic radiosurgery as part of the initial treatment does not prolong survival in patients with GBM; however, it may play a role in patients with recurrent gliomas. Approximately 95% of benign tumors are controlled with stereotactic radiosurgery, and it is useful in the treatment of postsurgical residual disease. Patients with trigeminal neuralgia are frequently elderly and are often not fit for conventional surgery. Of the different stereotactic radiosurgery techniques, only Gamma knife has the documented accuracy and clinical results to support its use in treating trigeminal neuralgia. Eighty percent to 85% of patients have significant improvement in their pain following Gamma knife, but as many as 40% recur within 5 years.[57] The primary risk of radiosurgery is radiation necrosis, which occurs 6 to 24 months after treatment and is related to the dose delivered and the volume treated.[58] There is essentially no mortality associated with stereotactic radiosurgery.

Frameless Stereotactic Procedures

The new generation of frameless stereotactic devices allows the neurosurgeon to correlate MRI and CT images with pointing devices that may be a simple probe, a robotic arm, or an actual surgical instrument such as an endoscope or biopsy probe.[59] Furthermore, these images may be fused with the display in a surgical microscope.[60] These devices allow the surgeon to efficiently plan skin incisions, bone openings, and location within the brain during a procedure. Without a rigidly attached frame, the surgeon no longer has to deal with the physical obstruction from the frame, but there may be a sacrifice in accuracy.

Epilepsy Surgery

Because *epilepsy* is a complex condition not associated with a single cause, the definition must to some extent be arbitrary. A useful definition, however, is recurrent seizures not due to an active provoked cause. With this definition, recurrent seizures during acute head injury are not considered epilepsy, but chronic recurrent seizures as a sequela of head injury are considered epilepsy. Regardless of the definition used, the condition is pervasive; the prevalence in North America of chronic use of an antiepileptic drug is 70 per 100,000 population. The prevalence is higher in childhood and in elderly persons, when cerebrovascular disease becomes an important cause. The risk of developing epilepsy is 3% over a lifetime; in the United States, there are more than 100,000 new cases a year. Of these, 60,000 are temporal lobe epilepsy, characterized most frequently by partial complex seizures, and of these, 25% are medically intractable—either not controlled by antiepileptic drugs or controlled with unacceptable side effects. Of this intractable group, one third are probably candidates for seizure surgery, in this particular case a partial anterior temporal lobectomy. This equates to 5000 new cases per year. Other types of epilepsy can be managed by other types of operations, such as partial excision at sites other than the temporal lobe, hemispherectomy, and section of the corpus callosum (corpus callosotomy). These other cases add to the cohort of surgical candidates but in much smaller numbers.

The implantation of vagal nerve stimulators was approved by the U.S. Food and Drug Administration for the control of seizures. Although this device (discussed later) virtually never results in complete cessation of all seizures, it is gaining acceptance and the indications are

expanding, so a large percentage of patients with intractable seizures without, or even some with, anatomically defined single foci may be candidates. It is conceivable then, that although this methodology does not replace ablative surgery, which is potentially curative, it may become the most frequent operation for intractable seizures.

The consequences of epilepsy that lead a patient and physician to consider seizure surgery when medical therapy is not efficacious include injuries due to falls and other accidents occurring during the seizures, seizures as a cause of sudden death, limitations of employability, restrictions against driving, limitation of social interactions, and problems related to learning and education due either to the seizures themselves or the side effects of drugs. In addition, novel drugs appear with regular frequency and obviously should be tried on patients intractable to conventional therapy, but none have resulted in a therapeutic breakthrough, so for many patients, surgery remains the ultimate hope.

The symptoms of seizures and the side effects of drugs vary greatly in severity, and there are no nationally accepted guidelines for direct referral of intractable patients for surgery. For some patients, the inability to legally drive is incentive enough. Also, there is a growing tendency to refer young patients for surgery rather than wait for the condition to "burn out." The rationale is that seizures frequently persist after adolescence; "mirror" foci can become established as independent foci, making ablative surgery impossible. Perhaps more important, epilepsy establishes psychological problems and dependency during childhood that might not be significantly mitigated even if later surgery results in a major decrease in seizures or even a seizure-free life. Furthermore, drug side effects that are tolerable to adults may interfere with learning, education, and socialization in children.

The Work-Up

The initial work-up is the search for remediable or treatable causes for chronic, recurrent seizures. To surgeons, most important is the diagnosis of structural lesions, particularly brain tumors and cerebrovascular abnormalities such as AVMs or cavernous malformations. When seizures are associated with structural lesions, removal of the lesion itself, or "lesionectomy" (early in the course of the seizures), is frequently sufficient to result in a seizure-free life. However, later, once seizures become more established, the removal of adjacent brain may be required.

As part of the initial work-up, the neurologist must establish that the events are associated with paroxysmal electrical events in the brain—that they are not pseudoseizures. Although many of these pseudoseizures can be diagnosed by the medical history or by witnessing an event, other cases mimic real seizures so well that diagnosis can be made only by video monitoring the patient with simultaneous electroencephalographic recording. (Phase I monitoring is considered in more detail later.)

Imaging

CT or, in most cases, MRI is an important part of the initial work-up. As structure, lesions can be identified, as can areas of atrophy related to past trauma or infection. In temporal lobe epilepsy, particularly with partial, complex seizures, special attention is paid to the mesial temporal structures to locate gliosis and atrophy of the hippocampus. Unilateral atrophy or gliosis is frequently indicative of the side of the focus and is a predictor of a good outcome after surgery. Examination of these structures requires special MR slices and imaging techniques. T2-weighted images are most sensitive to focal gliosis (Fig. 71-24), as are low-grade tumors and small hamartomas. Thin sections of even 5 to 7 mm also increase the sensitivity. Enhancement with a paramagnetic contrast agent (gadolinium) using T1-weighted images helps in the detection of structural lesions. Finally, MR volume measurements showing a reduction in hippocampal volume on the side of resection strongly predict outcome.

Positron-emission tomographic (PET) imaging has aided the work-up of patients with focal seizures. Interictal studies show hypometabolism and reduced cerebral blood flow in the area of the focus, whereas ictal studies show a relative increase in metabolism and flow. Single-photon emission CT is less expensive and more widely available than PET. Commercially available stable isotopes are used. Most important, ictal single-photon emission CT scans can be obtained much more easily than ictal PET because markers with much longer half-lives can be held at the bedside and given during an event and then imaged after the seizure is over.

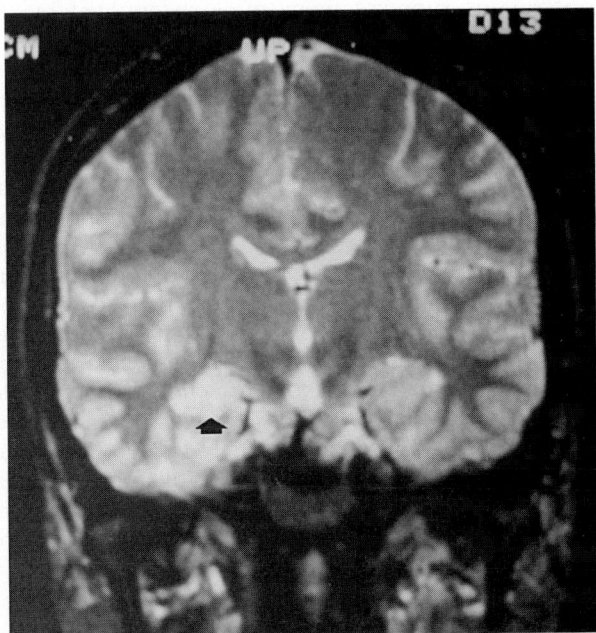

FIGURE 71-24. T2-weighted coronal MRI study shows gliosis of mesial temporal structures (*arrow*).

Correlation of Electroencephalography and Clinical Seizures: Phase 1 Monitoring

Phase I monitoring is used as an initial part of the work-up of patients suspected as having a single focus, most frequently in the temporal lobe. Chronic electroencephalographic recording performed while patients are actively surveyed by television monitors allows simultaneous comparison of clinical events and electroencephalograms. This establishes that the patient's clinical seizures are related to paroxysmal electrical discharges from the brain. In most cases, laterality (i.e., the side of the brain), and in some cases, further localization (e.g., temporal versus frontal lobe) can be established. Multiple seizures are recorded in the hospital after the patient's antiepileptic drugs are reduced or discontinued. The correlation is simplest when the patient's seizures are stereotyped. Patients with more than one type of clinical seizure are more difficult to evaluate, but in these cases, this type of monitoring is particularly important. As mentioned earlier, this method can be used to distinguish real seizures from pseudoseizures.

Establishment of Hemispheric Dominance of Language and Memory. The intracarotid amobarbital test (Wada test) is the most widely used and best established method for determining the dominant hemisphere for language and memory. The test is used most frequently for patients under consideration for a temporal lobectomy. Each carotid artery is injected in turn using a catheter passed from the femoral artery as is done for standard carotid arteriograms. Language and memory are individually assessed while each hemisphere is exposed to small injections of amobarbital. The patient is carefully monitored during testing to make certain that recirculation has not affected both sides simultaneously during testing. Many centers insist on Wada tests even when a clearly right-handed patient is diagnosed with a right temporal focus.

Other methods that are less invasive have shown promise with regard to the localization of cortical function, even language. Magnetoencephalography records electrical events as dipoles and therefore can be used to localize function, even to the extent of mapping language. However, these methods should be considered experimental, and the availability is severely limited. It seems possible that language mapping would also be feasible with functional MRI.

Intracranial Electrical Recording. The most common of these methods involve stereotactically implanted depth electrodes (Fig. 71-25), implanted strip electrodes, and implanted grids (Fig. 71-26). All are used to further localize the focus. Electrode grids can also be used to map language (Fig. 71-27). The indications for use of these arrays varies from center to center, particularly depending on whether the surgeon is willing to operate on awake patients; language mapping and resection can then take place during the same craniotomy.

Stereotactic-implanted depth electrodes are frequently placed in each frontal and temporal lobe to provide information about side and sometimes site, frontal versus temporal lobe, in cases in which site and side have not been

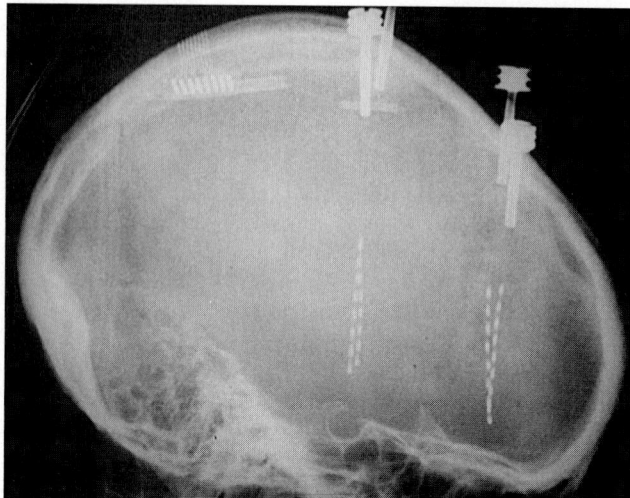

FIGURE 71-25.   Skull radiograph shows implanted depth electrodes.

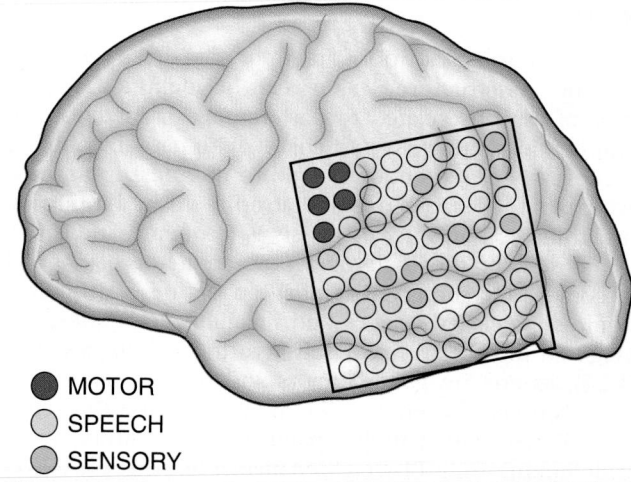

- ● MOTOR
- ○ SPEECH
- ○ SENSORY

FIGURE 71-27.   Language and sensory motor map.

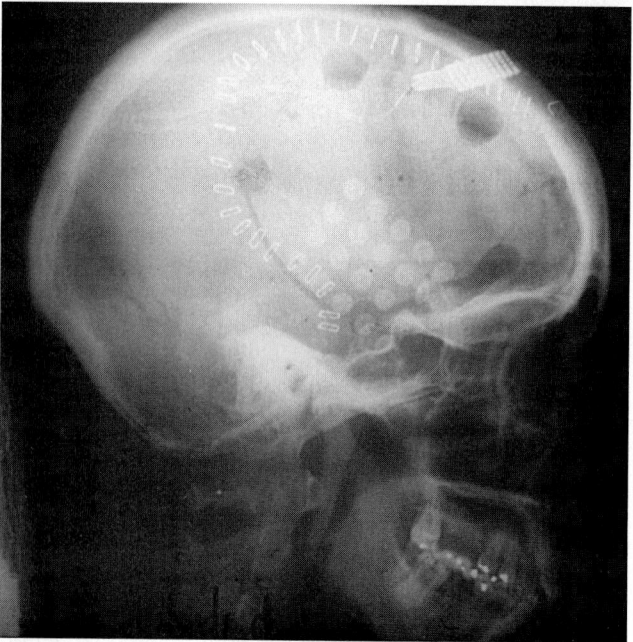

FIGURE 71-26.   Skull radiograph shows an implanted grid.

resolved by phase I monitoring (see earlier). Language mapping using grids or a movable dipole electrode on the exposed cortex of awake patients establishes cortical sites involved in language. The grids require a separate craniotomy for implantation. The method, however, is essentially the same: A current passes between two electrodes. If the current blocks language, the underlying cortex is considered eloquent for language and spared at the time of resection. Negative results are obviously harder to interpret than are positive results that cause language arrest, and when language is not blocked, the current strength is progressively increased to, if possible, the threshold for after-discharges. The risk of implanted electrodes is a hematoma, particularly with depth electrodes, for which the risk is

approximately 1%. In addition, there is a low risk of infection as the electrode wires are let out through the skin.

Resection of a Focus

The most frequent operation of this kind is *temporal lobectomy*. Usually, the lateral and inferior cortices are removed after a temporal craniotomy exposes the anterior temporal lobe. The mesiotemporal structures, including the amygdala and hippocampus, are excised. The extent of the resection is guided by the location of the focus and language mapping in the dominant lobe. At some centers, surgeons do not map language in the dominant temporal lobe and then perform a more lateral limited resection. The extent of the hippocampal resection can be influenced by a depth electrode implanted at the time the hippocampus is exposed and by the extent to which the hippocampus supports memory as determined by the Wada test (see earlier). However, a hippocampal resection of at least 2.0 to 2.5 cm from the anterior tip appears to be correlated with better outcomes than are smaller resections. The medial temporal structures can also be resected without removal of lateral temporal cortex by developing a plane for exposure through opening of the sylvian fissure and resection of the amygdala and hippocampus from that vantage point.

Cortical resections can also be made to remove a focus in other parts of the hemisphere. The second most common site after a temporal lobectomy is the frontal cortex. The results here, however, are in general less predictable than with temporal lobe resections. Although eloquent cortex is spared, a focus that includes motor or sensory cortex still can be surgically treated. Instead of resection, multiple gyral cortical incisions perpendicular to the axis of the involved gyrus are made, interrupting the local association fibers but sparing the deeper projecting fibers.

Other Cranial Operations for Generalized Seizures

Section of the corpus callosum is used to interrupt the spread of severe seizures and mitigate generalization.

Indications are otherwise not specific, but the operation is usually reserved for severe cases, frequently where there are drop attacks (atonic seizures) and thereby a significant risk of injury. However, the presence of atonic attacks does not ensure a good outcome from this operation.

The corpus callosum is approached through the interhemispheric fissure. Usually, the operation is staged so that the anterior two thirds of the corpus callosum are divided at the first operation. The section is completed at a second craniotomy only if the initial section does not provide a satisfactory result. Complications include hydrocephalus and, in some cases, a serious disconnection syndrome with language and behavioral impairment.

Hemispherectomy is an operation usually restricted to children with extensive unilateral epileptiform activity. Many or most of these children have developmental abnormalities of the brain, including abnormal cellular migration and hemiplegia. Although initially the entire cortex of the hemisphere was removed, sparing the basal ganglion, the operative technique has been modified so that portions of the hemisphere are left with their vascular connections intact but disconnected from the remainder of the brain by sectioning of adjacent white matter.

The results of this operation can be rewarding with regard not only to seizures but also to function, because the seizures may have caused functional impairment. However, the operation is associated with a high morbidity rate, including hydrocephalus, aseptic meningitis, and superficial cerebral hemosiderosis, which is thought to significantly contribute to mortality and morbidity rates, although the cause remains obscure. Partial hemispherectomy or functional hemispherectomy as described earlier is thought to mitigate this problem.

Vagal Nerve Stimulator

As mentioned at the beginning of this section, vagal nerve stimulators are novel and are a newly approved method to manage intractable seizures. The mechanism of action is not entirely clear, but it is well known that most vagal nerve fibers are afferent. These fibers project to many structures in the brain, including the hippocampus, amygdala, and thalamus. The efficacy in vagal nerve stimulation has been shown in animal models of epilepsy. Although stimulation of either vagus nerve is effective in animal models, the left nerve is always chosen because stimulation is less likely to cause cardiac effects than is stimulation of the right nerve. Like a cardiac pacemaker, the stimulator can be programmed after insertion. The predominant side effect is hoarseness during stimulation. Reduction in seizure frequency is usually 50%, which is similar to the result of many drugs but without drug side effects. Long-term stimulation, for 6 months or longer, seems to be associated with a greater rather than a lesser effect. However, unlike ablative operations, such as temporal lobectomy, only 1% of patients with vagal nerve stimulators become seizure free.

Neurosurgical Treatments for Pain

Pain is the most common symptom that prompts patients to see a physician. Unfortunately, it is still poorly understood, and many patients are inadequately treated as a result. Further complicating treatment is the lack of an objective measure of pain. There are two broad categories of pain: nociceptive and neuropathic. *Nociceptive pain* is caused by the activation of peripheral sensory receptors from an unusually strong stimulus. Examples include low back pain or cancer infiltration in bone. *Neuropathic pain* is poorly understood and is characterized by a lack of peripheral sensory stimulation, such as central pain that occurs after a stroke or phantom limb pain after amputation. It frequently contains elements of burning, tingling, or electric shocks and is poorly responsive to narcotic medications. Neurosurgical treatments may be either neuroablative or neuroaugmentative. Ablation involves making a lesion, whereas augmentation usually takes the form of electrical stimulation or infusion of opioids. Both types of treatment may be performed at any point along the pain pathway.

Sensation occurs with the activation of peripheral receptors by external stimuli. Nociceptors consist primarily of free nerve endings that transmit signals through small unmyelinated A delta and C nerve fibers. The cell bodies of these first-order neurons are found in the dorsal root ganglia and send their axons into the dorsal gray of the spinal cord to synapse with second-order neurons. These neurons comprise the spinothalamic tract, which decussates at the spinal cord level and ascends to the thalamus. The parallel paleospinothalamic tract includes connections with multiple interneurons in the periaqueductal gray of the brain stem and is involved in the perception of poorly localized, longer-lasting pain.

Trigeminal Neuralgia

Trigeminal neuralgia is characterized by brief attacks of a severe, lancinating pain experienced in one or a combination of the three branches of the trigeminal nerve. Also known as *tic douloureux*, it causes a patient's face to wince and spasm in pain. Typically unilateral and without sensory deficits, it is more prevalent in older patients except for patients who have multiple sclerosis, in whom it may present earlier and bilaterally. The pathogenesis is believed to be arterial compression of the trigeminal nerve, which causes demyelination and axonal crosstalk, along its root entry zone near the pons (Fig. 71-28). The initial treatment is medical; carbamazepine (Tegretol) and gabapentin (Neurontin) are effective in most patients, although a significant percentage develop resistance to their medication or have intolerable side effects. Three forms of surgical therapy are effective: microvascular decompression, percutaneous nerve ablation, and Gamma knife surgery. Microvascular decompression is performed through a retromastoid craniectomy that exposes the transverse and sigmoid sinus junction. Arterial compression on the trigeminal nerve is relieved, and the nerve is protected from further indentation by interposed, shredded Teflon pledgets.[61] Immediate pain relief is seen in

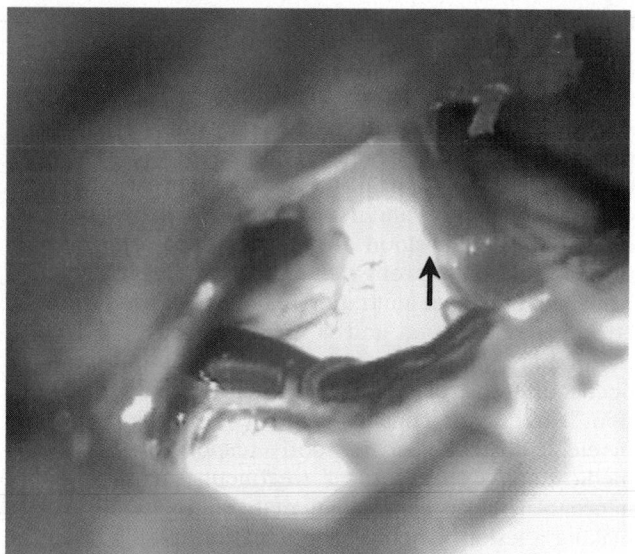

FIGURE 71-28. An intraoperative photograph through the operative microscope in a patient with typical trigeminal neuralgia. The left trigeminal nerve is compressed superiorly by an arterial branch of the superior cerebellar artery *(arrow)*.

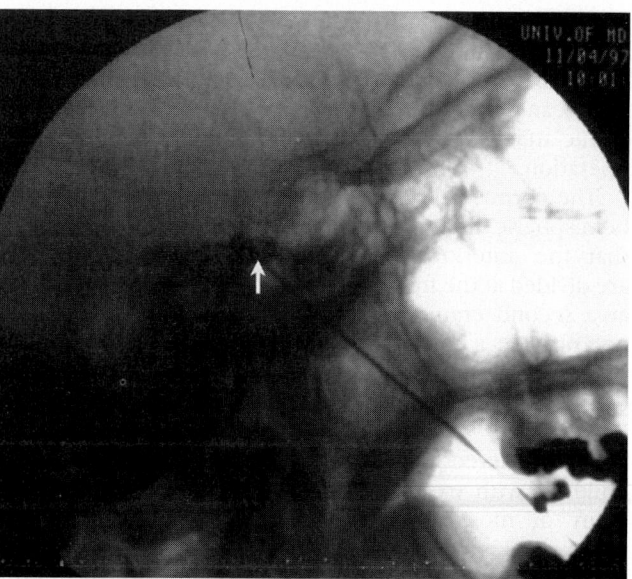

FIGURE 71-29. A lateral skull film in a patient undergoing glycerol rhizotomy for typical trigeminal neuralgia. A 20-gauge spinal needle is directed to the foramen ovale and nonionic contrast agent is injected to outline the trigeminal ganglion *(arrow)*.

nearly all patients, but pain recurrence is seen in 10% to 30% by 10 years. The percutaneous approaches avoid anesthesia and craniotomy risks associated with microvascular decompression but have slightly lower success rates. A spinal needle is directed to the foramen ovale under fluoroscopic guidance, and a radiofrequency lesion, glycerol injection, or balloon compression is performed on the trigeminal ganglion (Fig. 71-29).[62] In conjunction with pain relief, most patients experience facial numbness. Gamma knife surgery uses 201 beams of cobalt 60–derived photons focused on the trigeminal nerve to interrupt pain impulses.[57] This procedure is effective in 80% of patients.

Neuroablation Procedures

Neurectomy. Transection of a peripheral nerve results in numbness and may temporarily relieve pain, but it is not a viable long-term therapy. The pain may recur and become neuropathic in nature. Because most peripheral nerves are mixed sensorimotor, neurectomy will result in motor loss as well.

Rhizotomy. Open ablation of the sensory root can be performed via an intradural or extradural approach or percutaneously using radiofrequency coagulation or phenol injection.[63] The lesion should be made proximal to the dorsal root ganglion, and multiple roots need to be resected because of sensory overlap between adjacent dermatomes. Rhizotomy may be useful for pain with distribution in a limited number of dermatomes.

Dorsal Root Entry Zone Lesion. Using a specially designed radiofrequency electrode, multiple lesions are made along the dorsal roots that ablate the dorsal horn gray matter, including the second-order neurons. This treatment is most successful for nerve root or brachial plexus avulsion and spinal cord injury.[64] It has also been used for postherpetic neuralgia and post-thoracotomy pain. The most

common complication is ipsilateral motor weakness caused by injury to the adjacent corticospinal tract. Extension of this concept to the trigeminal nucleus caudalis, where second-order neurons from cranial nerves V, VII, IX, and X carry pain and temperature information, has been used to treat anesthesia dolorosa, atypical facial pain, and postherpetic neuralgia.[65] Lesions are made from the C2 dorsal roots moving rostrally along the medial edge of cranial nerve XI rootlets to the level of the obex. The most significant risk is ataxia caused by injury to the spinocerebellar tract, which overlies the nucleus caudalis. Good to excellent pain relief has been reported in 74% of patients, with a 39% risk of ataxia.

Cordotomy. This procedure is performed percutaneously with radiofrequency lesioning of the spinothalamic tract in the anterior portion of the cervical spinal cord. Localization is performed with radiographic guidance, myelography, and an impedance change when the cord is penetrated.[66] Stimulation of a properly placed electrode results in paresthesias on the contralateral side with no ipsilateral motor responses. Cordotomy is primarily indicated for cancer patients who have unilateral pain. Bilateral cordotomy is not advised because of the risk of Ondine's curse (loss of involuntary respiratory drive).

Myelotomy. Splitting the spinal cord at and above the level of pain divides the spinothalamic tract as it crosses in the anterior spinal cord. This procedure is most often used for bilateral, nociceptive pain due to cancer.

Midbrain Tractotomy. This procedure ablates the spinothalamic tract in the brain stem with the use of stereotactic guidance. The periaqueductal gray is often included in the lesion to also affect the paleospinothalamic pathway. The most common indication is for face and shoulder pain from head and neck cancer.

Thalamotomy. This type of lesion is now rarely used. Thalamic stimulation has proved to be more effective.

Cingulotomy. Using stereotactic guidance, bilateral radiofrequency lesions are made in the white matter deep to the cingulate gyrus, resulting in interference to Papez's limbic circuit. This procedure is most useful when depression is the dominant feature of the pain syndrome.

Sympathectomy. Sympathectomy is indicated for the treatment of causalgia, reflex sympathetic dystrophy, or Raynaud's phenomenon, but the specific mechanism of pain relief is not clear. To avoid a Horner's syndrome (ptosis, miosis, anhidrosis, and apparent enophthalmos), the T1 sympathetic ganglion should not be resected. The endoscopic approach is preferred to supraclavicular, transaxillary, and posterior costotransversectomy.[67]

Neuroaugmentation Procedures

Spinal Cord Stimulation. Spinal cord or dorsal column stimulation as a treatment for pain is based on the gate control theory, which postulates that nonpainful stimuli carried through large, myelinated nerves in the dorsal columns of the spinal cord modulate perception of painful stimuli through unmyelinated fibers.[68] In general, spinal cord stimulation is indicated for neuropathic pain syndromes, including peripheral nerve injury, reflex sympathetic dystrophy, deafferentation pain, and postherpetic neuralgia. Patients should be screened by temporary test electrode stimulation that produces a paresthesia over the painful area. Lower extremity pain is best treated with a low thoracic placement. Short-term success is seen in 80% of patients, with 50% having long-term pain relief.[69]

Deep Brain Stimulation. Two primary deep brain sites have been used for the relief of pain: periaqueductal gray and the sensory thalamus. Periaqueductal gray has been used primarily for nociceptive pain and likely activates endogenous opioids.[70] Thalamic stimulation is based on the gate control theory and is used for neuropathic pain.

Intrathecal Narcotic Infusion. The direct application of narcotics provides a more potent activation of opioid receptors in the substantia gelatinosa of the spinal cord. The onset of action is rapid (5 to 10 minutes), and serum levels are negligible. Continuous delivery of intrathecal morphine is made possible by an implantable, programmable pump.[71] Most patients are able to decrease or eliminate oral narcotics, and the quality of life improvement is frequently significant. This treatment modality is usually used for nociceptive cancer pain. Drug tolerance can develop with use.

SURGERY FOR CONGENITAL ABNORMALITIES

Embryology

Neural tube defects are common congenital disorders that can affect any portion of the neuraxis. A basic understanding of the development of the nervous system is helpful when trying to understand the structural characteristics of a particular malformation and its associated neurologic findings. During the 2nd week of gestation, ectodermal cells proliferate near the midline of the embryo, forming the neural plate. At approximately day 17 of gestation, the neural plate invaginates and the lateral portions thicken, forming the neural folds. As the neural folds move closer together in the midline, adhesion occurs and the neural tube closes. At the cephalic end, the cranial neuropore closes on approximately day 24 of gestation. The caudal neuropore is thought to close a short time later. Immediately after neural tube closure, the superficial ectoderm joins in the midline and then separates from the underlying neural tube. Mesenchymal tissue will migrate between these two layers and will later form the skull, vertebral column, meninges, and paraspinal musculature. This process has been termed *primary neurulation* and is usually complete by day 25.

Formation of the neural tube below the caudal neuropore occurs via a process termed *canalization* or *secondary neurulation*. In this process, an undifferentiated aggregate of pluripotential cells termed the *caudal cell mass* forms in close proximity to the developing hindgut and genitourinary structures. Within this cell mass, vacuoles form, enlarge, coalesce, and eventually make contact with the central canal of the neural tube formed during primary neurulation. A process of *retrogressive differentiation* then continues for approximately 7 weeks and is responsible for the formation of the most caudal portions of the spinal cord—the conus medullaris and the filum terminale.

Disordered primary neurulation results in defects in the axial skeleton, meninges, and overlying dermal structures. Examples include craniorachischisis totalis, the total failure of neural tube closure, as well as anencephaly, encephalocele, and myelomeningocele. Disorders of caudal neural tube formation result in occult dysraphic states. These abnormalities of the sacral and coccygeal segments form beneath intact dermal elements and have no exposed neural tissue. Examples include lipomyelomeningocele, diastematomyelia, and congenital dermal sinus. These caudal spinal anomalies may be associated with other abnormalities, such as imperforate anus, malformed genitalia, and renal dysplasias as part of a broader *caudal regression syndrome*.

Myelomeningoceles

Myelomeningoceles represent the most important clinical examples of disordered neurulation because most affected infants survive. The essential defect is a failure of closure of the caudal neuropore. The resulting lesion by definition involves the spinal cord, a deficient axial skeleton, and an incomplete meningeal and dermal covering. Instead of forming into a tube, the neural folds persist as a flat plate of tissue referred to as the *neural placode*. This structure has the appearance of a filleted spinal cord with an often visibly open central canal (Fig. 71-30). The ventral half of the spinal cord is usually less affected than the dorsal half that incompletely neurulated, and the dorsal roots exit from the anterior surface of the spinal cord just lateral to the ventral roots. Spinal defects include a lack of fusion of

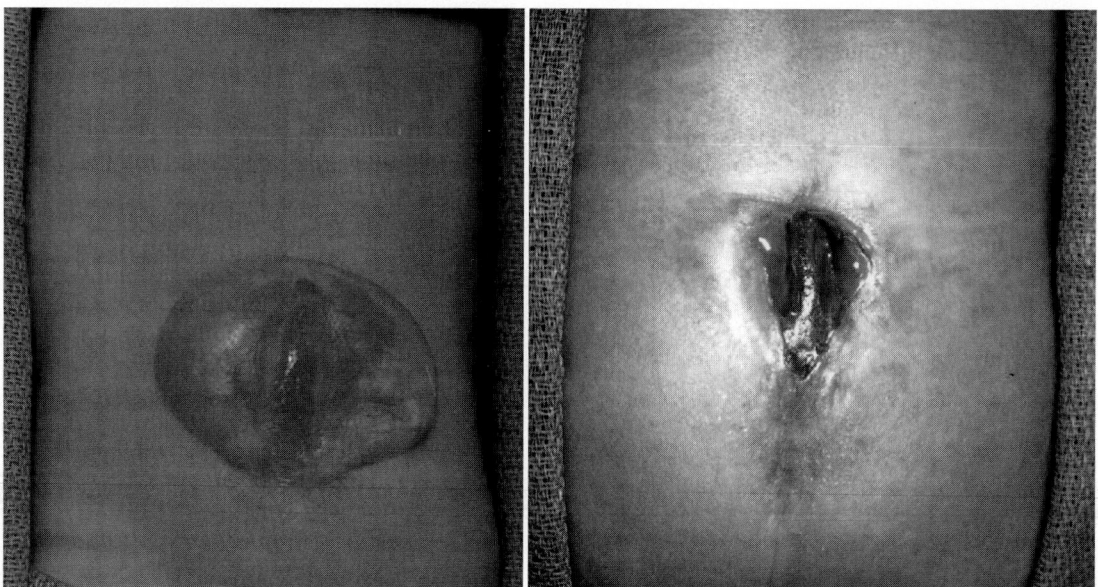

FIGURE 71-30.   Two examples of myelomeningoceles. The neural placode, a flat plate of dysraphic neural elements, is exposed.

the vertebral arches, laterally displaced pedicles, and a widened spinal canal. Nondisjunction of the superficial ectoderm from the neural tube results in the neural placode and meninges being continuous laterally with the dermal elements. An enlarged subarachnoid space ventral to the placode usually results in a dorsally protruding sac on which the neural placode is visible. The thoracolumbar junction is the most common level affected (45%), followed by lumbar (20%), lumbosacral (20%), and sacral (10%). More rostral locations are involved in only 5% of cases. The cause of myelomeningocele has not been determined precisely, but both environmental and genetic factors have been implicated. Improvements in prenatal screening for neural tube defects and folic acid supplementation around the time of conception have contributed to a worldwide decline in the birth prevalence of myelomeningocele. In the United States, the incidence is approximately 1 per 1000 live births.

Virtually all children born with a myelomeningocele also have a constellation of associated anomalies of the skull, brain, spine, and spinal cord that have been collectively described as the *Chiari II malformation*. The exact cause of this anomaly is unknown, but the failure of neural tube closure with drainage of CSF through the open neural tube into the amniotic fluid has been implicated. According to this hypothesis, collapse of the primitive ventricular system results in a decrease in the inductive influences on the overlying axial mesenchyme, a defect that ultimately affects development of the skull. Major features of this complex include a small posterior fossa with inferior displacement of the medulla, fourth ventricle, and cerebellar vermis through the foramen magnum; formation of a medullary kink within the cervical spinal canal; and various midbrain anomalies such as a beaked tectum and abnormalities of the ventricular system. Between 80% and 90% of children born with myelomeningocele develop hydrocephalus and require shunting. Fourth ven-

tricular outlet obstruction and obliteration of the posterior fossa subarachnoid cisterns are the likely causes of hydrocephalus in these children, although abnormalities of the cerebral aqueduct are also known to occur.

The first step in the management of a newborn with myelomeningocele is a careful clinical assessment with particular emphasis on motor, sensory, reflex, and sphincter function. A complete system review should also be completed to determine the presence of associated anomalies, and orthopedic and urologic consultations are requested. Daily occipital-frontal circumference measurements should be recorded, and a baseline ultrasound examination of the brain is obtained. Open defects should be covered with a saline-moistened nonadherent dressing to prevent injury to and desiccation of the neural placode. Neurotoxic substances are avoided, and the child should be kept prone or in a lateral recumbent position until surgery. If the initial assessment has excluded other systemic disorders, and the child is not critically ill, the myelomeningocele is repaired shortly after birth, usually within the first 48 hours. Surgical goals include elimination of CSF leakage, preservation of neurologic function, and prevention of infection. The general procedure for closure includes separation of the neural placode from the surrounding epithelial tissue followed by identification and mobilization of the dura mater. Some surgeons advocate reconstruction of the neural placode to prevent retethering when the dura is closed. Fascial closure followed by multilayer skin closure completes the procedure.

In most cases, hydrocephalus develops rapidly after myelomeningocele closure, with many children becoming symptomatic within the first few weeks after closure. Although most children with myelomeningocele are ambulatory, many require braces or crutches. Children with S1 motor levels can usually walk unaided, whereas children with lesions at or above L2 are usually wheelchair dependent. Approximately 75% of children with the myelomeningocele/Chiari II complex have normal intelligence. This figure decreases to near 60% in children requiring shunts. Owing to the complexity of the problems presented by the management of these children, their care is best addressed through a multidisciplinary team approach that involves pediatricians, neurosurgeons, orthopedic surgeons, and urologists.

Encephaloceles

Disordered closure of the cranial neuropore can also result in various defects that are known to cause substantial neurologic dysfunction. One of the more extreme forms, *anencephaly*, results from failure of cranial neuropore closure. This affects both the forebrain and brain stem and is not compatible with survival. Encephaloceles are also thought to occur due to a defect in cranial neuropore closure, but the precise cause is not known. One widely held hypothesis attributes their formation to a failure of the development of the overlying mesenchymal tissue with local cerebral herniation occurring at approximately 8 to 12 weeks of gestation. The worldwide incidence is nearly 1 in 5000 live births. Encephaloceles are usually classified by their location over the skull and can occur either over the convexities or through the skull base. In Western populations, 85% of these lesions occur in the occipital region, whereas in Southeast Asian populations, frontal lesions are relatively more common. Occipital encephaloceles are often large and have variable contents (Fig. 71-31A and B). The brain contained within these defects is usually dysplastic, and encephaloceles that contain a large amount of neural tissue have a poor prognosis. Frontal encephaloceles are frequently located near the nasion, and the prognosis is usually better in these

more anteriorly located lesions. Regardless of the location, encephaloceles are frequently associated with other intracranial abnormalities, such as partial or complete agenesis of the corpus callosum, Dandy-Walker malformations, hydrocephalus, or holoprosencephaly. Neurosurgical intervention is indicated in most situations, with the exception of patients with large defects and associated microcephaly. At surgery, the contents of the encephalocoele are relocated into the cranium or they are resected. A watertight dural closure is then performed, and the skull and skin is reconstructed for an acceptable cosmetic result.

Occult Spinal Dysraphism

The term *occult spinal dysraphism* refers to those embryologic defects that occur due to disordered retrogressive differentiation. Owing to an increasing clinical awareness of these conditions as well as improvements in imaging techniques, the occurrence of these abnormalities is becoming increasingly important in clinical practice. Most of these disorders occur in the lumbar region and are frequently associated with abnormal cutaneous markings such as hemangiomas, focal hirsutism, soft tissue masses, or a sinus tract. Although most cases of *spina bifida occulta* have no clinical significance, the presence of these markings often signal an underlying dysraphic state in an infant. In an older child, the finding of various orthopedic, urologic, or neurologic signs may suggest the presence of one of these states. Children with highly arched feet, leg-length discrepancies, and scoliosis require a more detailed investigation. Persistent urinary tract infections in a child, or the new onset of incontinence in a child who was previously toilet trained, as well as lower extremity weakness, sensory abnormalities, or radicular pain, is also

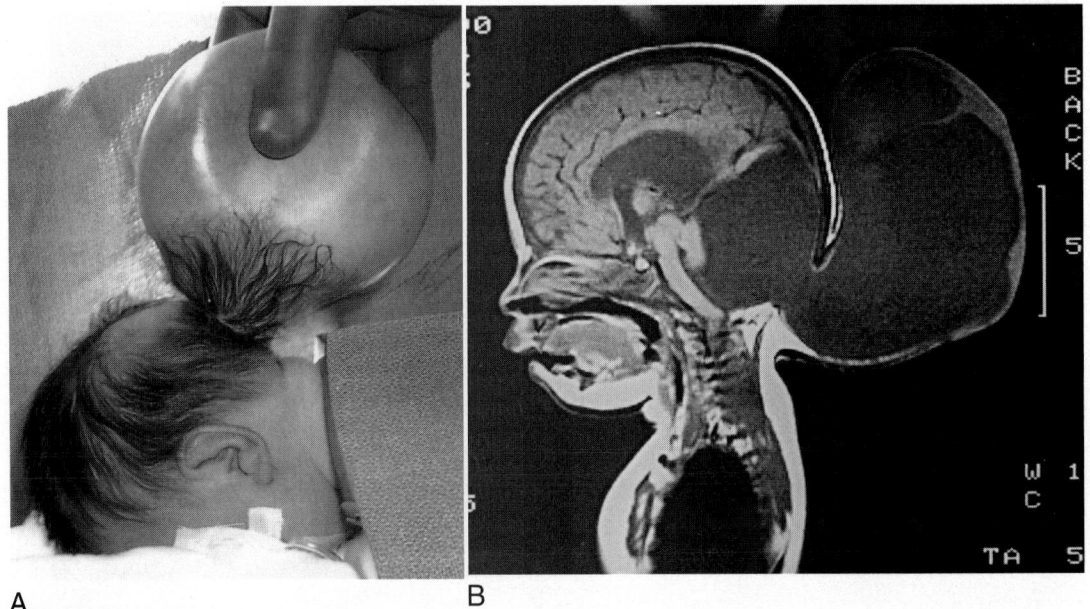

A   B

■ **FIGURE 71-31.**   An infant with a large occipital encephalocoele. **A,** The large skin-covered encephalocoele is visible. **B,** A sagittal MRI study in a newborn with a large occipital encephalocele. At surgery, the sac contained herniated dysplastic cerebellar tissue as well as cerebrospinal fluid.

associated with an occult dysraphic disorder. In a child suspected of having a dysraphic lesion, MRI has become the imaging modality of choice. Although the radiologic findings vary depending on the particular abnormality, tethering of the spinal cord can lead to worsened neurologic function due to repeated trauma with flexion and extension of the spine. Surgery is usually indicated in patients with occult spinal dysraphism to prevent later neurologic deterioration.

Lipomyelomeningoceles

Lipomyelomeningoceles are skin-covered malformations in which a subcutaneous lipoma is connected through a fibroadipose stalk to an intramedullary, intradural lipoma. These defects are thought to occur when the superficial ectoderm separates prematurely from the underlying neural ectoderm, allowing the migration of mesenchymal tissue into the neural tube. This intramedullary adipose tissue remains continuous with the subcutaneous tissue and results in one of the more common clinical causes of spinal cord tethering. Most children present with a midline soft tissue mass that may or may not distort the gluteal crease. Dimples and hemangiomas are frequently present. Scoliosis, foot deformities, motor or sensory deficits, and neurogenic bladder are common presentations. Neurologic deterioration is thought to be secondary to either direct injury by stretching of the spinal cord or vascular compromise. Most surgeons advocate releasing the tethered cord before the development of neurologic symptoms. The goals of treatment include the release of the tethering elements, preservation of neurologic function, debulking of the intramedullary mass, dural reconstruction, and acceptable cosmesis.

Diastematomyelia

Diastematomyelia is an uncommon dysraphic lesion in which the spinal cord is split longitudinally at one or more continuous levels and separated by a bony, cartilaginous, or fibrous spur. These abnormalities are frequently associated with an overlying cutaneous marker such as a hairy patch. The precise embryogenesis is not well understood. Presenting complaints are similar to those seen in children with other forms of occult spinal dysraphism such as abnormal cutaneous markings, orthopedic deformities, or neurologic dysfunction. Surgical goals include untethering the spinal cord by removing the bony or fibrous median septum and reconstructing the dural sac.

Dermal Sinus Tracts

Congenital dermal sinus tracts are often inconspicuous-appearing lesions that can occur in either the lumbosacral or occipital regions and may be associated with significant neurologic complications. These defects typically appear as a small ostium or dimple near the midline and represent the superficial extent of an epithelium-lined tract that can extend intradurally (Fig. 71-32). They can be associated with intracranial or intraspinal dermoid or epidermoid tumors and may also allow passage of bacteria into the subarachnoid space with resulting meningitis. When indicated, the entire tract is removed by following the cutaneous ostium to its termination, which may extend into the intradural space. Shallow pits at the tip of the coccyx are normal variants detected in some infants and have no clinical significance.

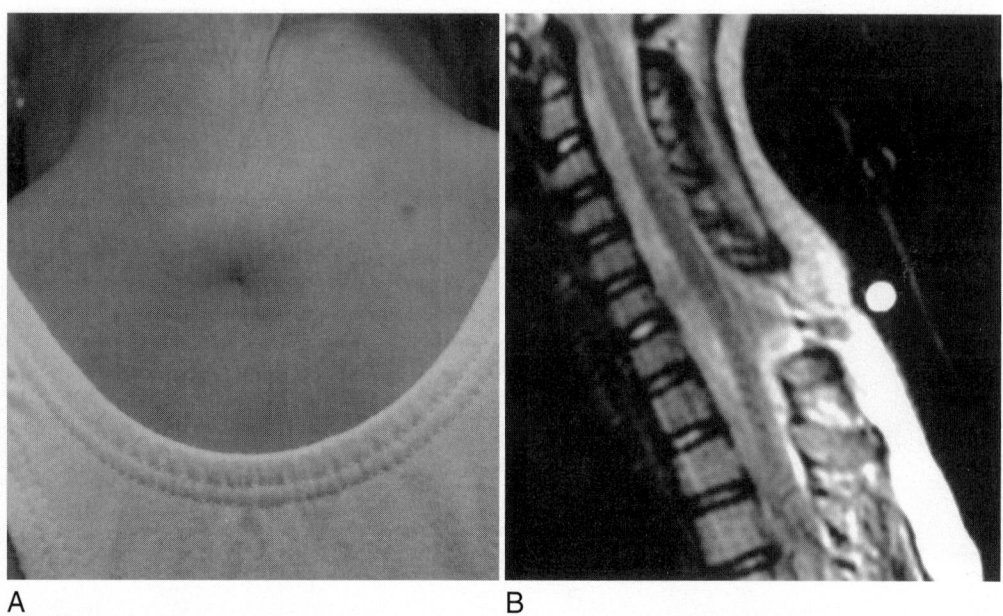

A   B

FIGURE 71-32. **A,** Dermal sinus tract in a 10-year-old girl who presented with purulent drainage. **B,** Sagittal T2-weighted MRI study shows a connection of the sinus tract with the thecal sac.

Hydrocephalus

Hydrocephalus is a condition that results from an imbalance between the production and absorption of CSF. This mismatch leads to the accumulation of CSF within the intracranial compartment, and, ultimately, ventricular enlargement and intracranial hypertension. Historically, hydrocephalus has been classified into broad categories. In the most clinically useful classification, communicating hydrocephalus is present when an obstruction to the flow of CSF occurs outside of the ventricular system, usually at the level of the basal subarachnoid cisterns or at the arachnoid granulations. Noncommunicating hydrocephalus results from lesions that create an obstruction to CSF flow within the ventricular system. This most commonly occurs at the level of the aqueduct of Sylvius but is also seen at the foramina of Monro or at the foramina of Luschka and Magendie in the fourth ventricle. In nearly all cases, hydrocephalus results from the decreased absorption of CSF. Only in the rare case of a choroid plexus papilloma has increased CSF production been implicated.

Hydrocephalus can occur in either congenital or acquired forms. Although the true incidence of hydrocephalus in children is difficult to determine, as an isolated *congenital* form, it is estimated to occur in approximately 1 per 1000 live births. When one considers all types of hydrocephalus that present in infancy, the incidence is nearly 3 or 4 per 1000. Aqueductal stenosis is a major cause of hydrocephalus in the newborn and is responsible for nearly one third of congenital cases. True narrowing of the aqueduct lumen, subependymal gliosis secondary to in utero infection or hemorrhage, or a malformed aqueduct may be responsible. Children born with myelomeningocele have a high incidence of hydrocephalus due to the associated Chiari II malformation, a complex malformation that involves the hindbrain, spine, and supratentorial structures. Nearly 80% to 90% of these children develop hydrocephalus due to fourth ventricular outlet obstruction and compromise of the posterior fossa subarachnoid cisterns. The Dandy-Walker malformation is another cause of congenital hydrocephalus and is characterized by the absence of the cerebellar vermis, cystic expansion of the fourth ventricle, and hydrocephalus. Viral and parasitic exposure in utero is a well-known cause of congenital hydrocephalus, with cytomegalovirus and toxoplasmosis having been implicated in many cases. Intracranial tumors, arachnoid cysts, and other abnormalities such as vein of Galen malformations can also lead to congenital hydrocephalus.

Acquired forms of hydrocephalus usually occur after IVH or after an episode of meningitis. Posthemorrhagic hydrocephalus is most commonly seen in the premature infant after a germinal matrix/IVH. Meningitis in the newborn period may induce leptomeningeal fibrosis and, ultimately, hydrocephalus. Tumors or other mass lesions can also cause hydrocephalus in older children (Fig. 71-33A and B).

The clinical features of hydrocephalus are related to the development of elevated ICP. In the newborn, excessive head enlargement with an enlarged, tense anterior fontanelle and open cranial sutures are common presentations. Irritability, vomiting, and lethargy may also be present. The presentation in an older child is more acute because the moderating effects of open cranial sutures are not present. Severe headache, vomiting, and lethargy are the usual presenting signs in these children.

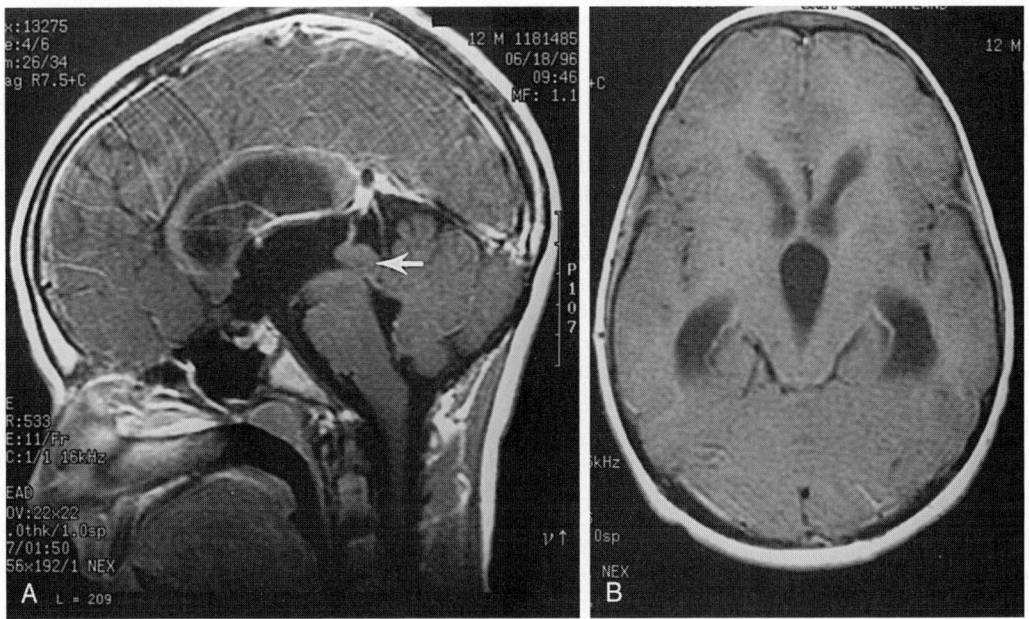

■ FIGURE 71-33. MRI studies in a 12-year-old boy with hydrocephalus. **A,** Sagittal T1-weighted MRI study demonstrates a small tectal glioma *(arrow)* causing aqueductal stenosis and the typical pattern of triventricular hydrocephalus. **B,** Axial MRI study demonstrating a dilated third ventricle and enlarged temporal horns.

In the newborn period, ultrasonography can easily determine the presence of ventriculomegaly. CT scanning remains the most commonly used imaging technique for screening or emergent indications and is preferred when a more detailed assessment of intracranial morphology is required. MRI frequently provides a much clearer depiction of the intracranial structures and is becoming the imaging modality of choice in many clinical situations.

The goal of any treatment for hydrocephalus is to prevent or possibly reverse the neurologic injury that may occur from distortion of the normal intracranial structures or from elevated ICP. Most cases are treated by diversion of CSF from the cerebral ventricles to the peritoneal cavity via a ventriculoperitoneal shunt. Other less favored sites for diversion include the pleural cavity and the superior vena cava. Although shunts are responsible for improving the quality of life for many patients with hydrocephalus, they are also associated with significant complication rates. Approximately 5% to 10% of shunt operations are complicated by infection. Most are caused by skin flora, which infect the device at the time of implantation. Other complications include obstruction of the shunt, disconnection or fracture of the hardware, intracerebral hematomas, and peritonitis.

Endoscopic third ventriculostomy is another technique used in the treatment of hydrocephalus that has come into much wider use due to advances in endoscopic equipment and techniques. In this procedure, a small fenestration is created in the floor of the anterior third ventricle under endoscopic guidance, thus allowing CSF to directly enter the subarachnoid space. This technique is indicated only in certain forms of noncommunicating hydrocephalus and has the added benefit of avoiding a lifetime of shunt dependency if successful.

The prognosis in a child diagnosed with hydrocephalus varies and is more likely to depend on the etiologic mechanism that led to the hydrocephalus than on the hydrocephalus itself. Cognitive abilities appear to be best in those children with communicating forms and the myelomeningocele/Chiari II complex. In children with congenital aqueductal stenosis or Dandy-Walker malformations, the high degree of cerebral dysgenesis in these conditions is associated with significant cognitive impairment in most cases. Most children with hydrocephalus due to a congenital central nervous system infection have a grim developmental prognosis due to the significant degree of parenchymal destruction. The outcome in hydrocephalus associated with meningitis in the newborn period varies and depends on the organism and the degree of injury to the cerebrum.

Craniosynostosis

The term *craniosynostosis* refers to the premature closure or fusion of a cranial suture. Usually, the cranial sutures serve as a site of bone deposition in the growing calvarium. This separation of the calvarial bones allows for progressive enlargement of the skull with growth of the brain. When one or more of these sutures close prematurely, cranial deformity can occur. Primary nonsyndromic forms of craniosynostosis are the most common and affect nearly 1 in 2500 children. Craniosynostosis can also occur as part of a recognized syndrome or secondary to a systemic disorder. The diagnosis of nonsyndromic craniosynostosis is based on recognition of the characteristic abnormal skull shape. The demonstration of a prematurely fused suture on plain skull radiography or CT scanning with bone windows is helpful in confirming the diagnosis. Not all abnormalities of skull shape are caused by craniosynostosis. Asymmetry of the calvarium can also occur when deformational forces are applied to the growing calvarium over a prolonged period. These children with "positional molding" must be distinguished from those with true craniosynostosis because they will improve with time and will not require surgery.

Isolated sagittal synostosis is the most common form of craniosynostosis and accounts for approximately 40% to 60% of craniosynostoses. Closure of the sagittal suture typically results in *scaphocephaly,* with a long, narrow skull and varying degrees of compensatory frontal and occipital bossing. Premature closure of the coronal suture accounts for approximately 20% to 30% of all cases and is characterized by asymmetry of the forehead, flattening of the ipsilateral frontal and parietal bones, bulging of the contralateral frontal region, and bulging of the ipsilateral temporal bone. The orbits are asymmetrical, and the nasal root is deviated toward the fused suture. Unilateral cases outnumber bilateral forms by 2:1. Metopic synostosis accounts for fewer than 10% of all cases of craniosynostosis. Premature fusion of the metopic suture results in a skull with a characteristic triangular shape, or *trigonocephaly,* with a prominent midline frontal ridge, recessed orbital rims, and hypotelorism. True lambdoid synostosis is rare and must be distinguished from posterior positional molding.

Parents of children with single-suture synostosis should understand that aesthetics or cosmesis is the only consideration. There is little evidence to support claims of an increased incidence of seizures, mental retardation, or other neurologic deficits in children with simple forms of craniosynostosis. Affected children who do not undergo corrective surgery invariably face social stigmatization due to their abnormal appearance. For this reason, many parents are willing to accept the low risks of craniofacial surgery to prevent socialization or psychological problems in the future. Although the specific surgical technique varies depending on the affected suture, most craniofacial surgeons agree that early surgery is preferable for the simple reason that one can capitalize on the period of rapid brain growth to ameliorate any minor postoperative asymmetries in skull shape. The timing of surgery varies from center to center, but surgery is recommended as soon as the child can safely tolerate the physiologic stress of surgery, usually between 3 and 9 months of age.

CENTRAL NERVOUS SYSTEM INFECTIONS

Acute bacterial meningitis is an infection of the subarachnoid spaces and meninges. The bacteria responsible may spread to the subarachnoid space from an infection of a contiguous structure such as the paranasal sinuses or through the bloodstream. The causative organism varies depending on the patient's age. Newborns tend to be infected by gram-negative enteric organisms such as *Escherichia coli* and *Klebsiella.* In children, *Haemophilus influenzae, Pneumococcus,* and *Meningococcus* are the predominant organisms. Meningitis in adults is usually caused by either pneumococcal or meningococcal infection. Symptoms are due to leptomeningeal irritation and elevated ICP, and they usually include fever, neck stiffness, and headache. An impaired level of consciousness and seizures are other common findings. Once meningitis is suspected, antibiotic treatment should begin immediately, sometimes even before obtaining a CSF specimen if the clinical suspicion is high. If hydrocephalus develops, a ventriculoperitoneal shunt may be required once the CSF is sterilized. In a child with recurrent episodes of meningitis, a dermal sinus tract must be considered; if it is found, exploration and complete excision are necessary.

Brain Abscess

The brain may be infected by a multitude of organisms, including bacterial, viral, fungal, and parasitic forms. The mode of infection varies depending on the particular organism and can include direct spread from adjacent structures, hematogenous seeding, or direct inoculation as would occur after surgery or trauma. Brain abscesses may be solitary or multiple, and the pathogenesis of these two presentations varies slightly. Multiple abscesses usually occur with systemic infections that spread hematoge-

nously. Solitary lesions are more likely to occur after direct spread from an infected parameningeal structure such as the middle ear or paranasal sinus. The responsible agents vary and depend on the immune status of the host. In a normal host, anaerobic *Streptococcus, Staphylococcus, Enterobacteriaceae, H. influenzae,* or anaerobes may spread from dental, pulmonary, cutaneous, cardiac, or other sources. In immunocompromised hosts, the responsible organisms usually include *Nocardia asteroides, Listeria monocytogenes, Candida* species, *Cryptococcus neoformans, Mucor* species, and *Aspergillus.*

Most patients present with altered mental status, focal neurologic signs, seizures, and signs of elevated ICP. Unless the patient has a systemic infection, a fever and an elevated white blood cell count are often absent. Contrast CT or MRI shows a ring-enhancing lesion within the brain parenchyma, usually at the gray-white junction. Differentiating between an abscess and brain tumor can often be difficult because their contrast enhancement patterns are similar; however, recent studies indicate that diffusion-weighted (DW) MRI can improve the diagnostic accuracy.[72] DW MRI characterizes brownian motion in tissues and allows measurement of the apparent diffusion coefficient. Diffusion is unrestricted in CSF, which appears dark on DW MRI; infarcts create restricted diffusion in brain and can be detected by DW MRI earlier than by conventional MRI or CT. Purulent brain abscesses also have decreased molecular motion because of high viscosity and inflammatory cells, thus resulting in a bright signal on DW MRI (Fig. 71-34A and B). By contrast,

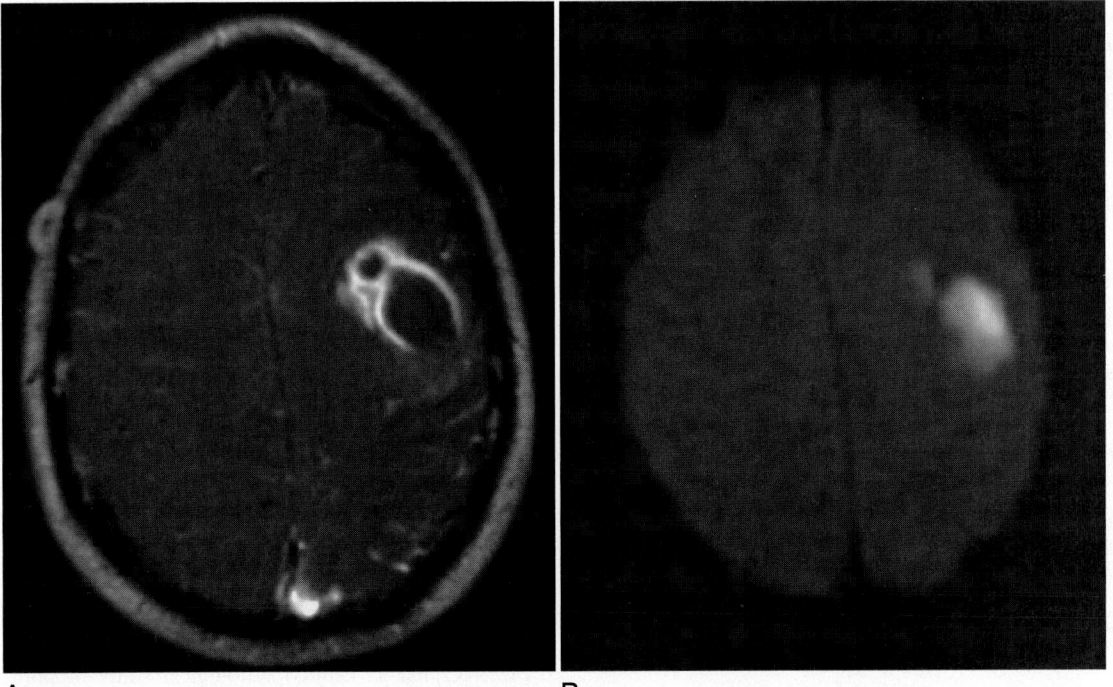

A   B

■ FIGURE 71-34. This patient presented with a right hemiparesis of several days' duration. **A,** Axial T1-weighted MRI study with contrast agent shows a peripherally enhancing lesion with surrounding edema. This lesion is compatible with either malignant tumor or abscess. **B,** The lesion appears bright on diffusion-weighted MRI, indicating a high likelihood of abscess. The patient underwent a craniotomy, where the abscess was drained.

malignant brain tumors (glioma and metastatic) appear hypointense.

Despite improved diagnostic techniques and the availability of effective broad-spectrum antibiotics, the surgical treatment of brain abscesses remains important. Surgery is indicated when the diagnosis is unclear, when mass effect or neurologic deficit exists, when the organism cannot be obtained, and when abscesses fail to resolve with antibiotic treatment. Open, stereotactic, or ultrasound-guided procedures can be used for resection or drainage of abscesses.

Spinal Abscess

Bacterial infections can also affect the spinal column. Spinal epidural abscess is a rare condition in which pyogenic organisms proliferate within the confines of the spinal epidural space. Infection usually occurs via hematogenous spread or from direct extension of discitis or osteomyelitis. Predisposing factors include diabetes mellitus, an immunocompromised state, renal disorders, intravenous drug abuse, and recent spinal surgery. Fever and back pain are the most common initial symptoms. Because this is a rare condition, there is often a delay in diagnosis. It is noteworthy that these patients can progress from normal to complete paralysis within hours, and because the effects of spinal cord compression can be devastating, this condition should be considered a neurosurgical emergency. If evidence of spinal cord compression exists, a contrast MRI is done to confirm the site of the extradural lesion. Urgent decompressive surgery with abscess drainage is then indicated. In milder infections with little or no spinal cord compression, management is usually medical, with close neurologic evaluation and imaging studies.

Selected References

Albright AL, Pollack IF, Adelson PD: Principles and Practice of Pediatric Neurosurgery. New York, Thieme, 1999.

> **A multiauthored reference extensively covers the subject of pediatric neurosurgery. The editors emphasize "clinical pearls" following each chapter, and extensive bibliographies are provided for more detailed reference.**

Apuzzo MLJ (ed): Malignant Cerebral Glioma. Park Ridge, IL, American Association of Neurological Surgeons, 1990.

> **This single volume provides an excellent review of malignant gliomas, including pathology, surgical results, radiation therapy, and chemotherapy.**

Benzel EC: Spine Surgery: Techniques, Complication Avoidance, and Management. Philadelphia, Churchill Livingstone, 1999.

> **A multiauthored text that emphasizes the fundamentals of spine surgery and practical considerations in the management of spinal disorders. A large number of expert authors provide an excellent discussion of the subjects as well as extensive references for further study.**

Eisenberg HM, Aldrich EF (eds): Management of Head Injury. Neurosurg Clin North Am 2:[entire issue], 1991.

> **A review of the management of head injury.**

Engel J Jr, Pedley TA (eds): Epilepsy: A Comprehensive Textbook, Vols 1-3. Philadelphia, Lippincott-Raven, 1998.

> **A three-volume comprehensive epilepsy text.**

Germano IM (ed): Neurosurgical Treatment of Movement Disorders. Park Ridge, IL, American Association of Neurological Surgeons, 1998.

> **An excellent review of all aspects of movement disorder surgery. Detailed chapters describe a variety of surgical approaches, including implantation of neurostimulators.**

References

1. Broderick JP, Brott T, Tomsick T, et al: Intracerebral hemorrhage more than twice as common as subarachnoid hemorrhage. J Neurosurg 78:188-191, 1993.
2. Bell BA, Symon L: Smoking and subarachnoid haemorrhage. BMJ 1:577-578, 1979.
3. Inoue Y, Saiwai S, Miyamoto T, et al: Postcontrast computed tomography in subarachnoid hemorrhage from ruptured aneurysms. J Comput Assist Tomogr 5:341-344, 1981.
4. Matsumoto M, Sato M, Nakano M, et al: Three-dimensional computerized tomography angiography-guided surgery of acutely ruptured cerebral aneurysms. J Neurosurg 94:718-727, 2001.
5. Ross JS, Masaryk TJ, Modic MT, et al: Intracranial aneurysms: Evaluation by MR angiography. AJR Am J Roentgenol 155:159-165, 1990.
6. Unruptured intracranial aneurysms—risk of rupture and risks of surgical intervention. International Study of Unruptured Intracranial Aneurysms Investigators. N Engl J Med 339:1725-1733, 1998.
7. Fisher CM, Kistler JP, Davis JM: Relation of cerebral vasospasm to subarachnoid hemorrhage visualized by computerized tomographic scanning. Neurosurgery 6:1-9, 1980.
8. Kassell NF, Torner JC, Haley EC Jr, et al: The International Cooperative Study on the Timing of Aneurysm Surgery: I. Overall management results. J Neurosurg 73:18-36, 1990.
9. Kassell NF, Torner JC, Jane JA, et al: The International Cooperative Study on the Timing of Aneurysm Surgery: II. Surgical results. J Neurosurg 73:37-47, 1990.
10. Guglielmi G, Vinuela F, Sepetka I, et al: Electrothrombosis of saccular aneurysms via endovascular approach: I. Electrochemical basis, technique, and experimental results. J Neurosurg 75:1-7, 1991.
11. Guglielmi G, Vinuela F, Dion J, et al: Electrothrombosis of saccular aneurysms via endovascular approach: II. Preliminary clinical experience. J Neurosurg 75:8-14, 1991.
12. Juvela S, Porras M, Heiskanen O: Natural history of unruptured intracranial aneurysms: A long-term follow-up study. J Neurosurg 79:174-182, 1993.
13. Ojemann RG, Heros RC: Spontaneous brain hemorrhage. Stroke 14:468-475, 1983.
14. Nakajima K: Clinicopathological study of pontine hemorrhage. Stroke 14:485-493, 1983.
15. Ott KH, Kase CS, Ojemann RG, et al: Cerebellar hemorrhage: Diagnosis and treatment—a review of 56 cases. Arch Neurol 31:160-167, 1974.
16. Mayfrank L, Lippitz B, Groth M, et al: Effect of recombinant tissue plasminogen activator on clot lysis and ventricular

dilatation in the treatment of severe intraventricular haemorrhage. Acta Neurochir (Wien) 122:32-38, 1993.

17. Ondra SL, Troupp H, George ED, et al: The natural history of symptomatic arteriovenous malformations of the brain: A 24-year follow-up assessment. J Neurosurg 73:387-391, 1990.

18. Central Brain Tumor Registry of the United States: 1997 Annual Report (*www.cbtrus.org*). 1998.

19. Kleihues P, Louis DN, Scheithauer BW, et al: The WHO classification of tumors of the nervous system. J Neuropathol Exp Neurol 61:215-225, 2002.

20. Kleihues P, Ohgaki H: Primary and secondary glioblastomas: From concept to clinical diagnosis. Neuro-oncol 1:44-51, 1999.

21. Palma L, Guidetti B: Cystic pilocytic astrocytomas of the cerebral hemispheres: Surgical experience with 51 cases and long-term results. J Neurosurg 62:811-815, 1985.

22. Shaw EG, Daumas-Duport C, Scheithauer BW, et al: Radiation therapy in the management of low-grade supratentorial astrocytomas. J Neurosurg 70:853-861, 1989.

23. Brem H, Piantadosi S, Burger PC, et al: Placebo-controlled trial of safety and efficacy of intraoperative controlled delivery by biodegradable polymers of chemotherapy for recurrent gliomas. The Polymer-Brain Tumor Treatment Group. Lancet 345:1008-1012, 1995.

24. Paleologos NA, Cairncross JG: Treatment of oligodendroglioma: An update. Neuro-oncol 1:61-68, 1999.

25. Packer RJ, Sutton LN, Elterman R, et al: Outcome for children with medulloblastoma treated with radiation and cisplatin, CCNU, and vincristine chemotherapy. J Neurosurg 81:690-698, 1994.

26. Seizinger BR, Rouleau GA, Ozelius LJ, et al: Von Hippel-Lindau disease maps to the region of chromosome 3 associated with renal cell carcinoma. Nature 332:268-269, 1988.

27. Kaufmann T, Nisce LZ, Coleman M: A comparison of survival of patients treated for AIDS-related central nervous system lymphoma with and without tissue diagnosis. Int J Radiat Oncol Biol Phys 36:429-432, 1996.

28. Simpson D: The recurrence of intracranial meningiomas after surgical treatment. J Neurol Neurosurg Psychiatry 20:22-39, 1957.

29. Lee JY, Niranjan A, McInerney J, et al: Stereotactic radiosurgery providing long-term tumor control of cavernous sinus meningiomas. J Neurosurg 97:65-72, 2002.

30. Lutchman M, Rouleau GA: Neurofibromatosis type 2: A new mechanism of tumor suppression. Trends Neurosci 19:373-377, 1996.

31. Marchuk DA, Saulino AM, Tavakkol R, et al: cDNA cloning of the type 1 neurofibromatosis gene: Complete sequence of the *NF1* gene product. Genomics 11:931-940, 1991.

32. Petit JH, Hudes RS, Chen TT, et al: Reduced-dose radiosurgery for vestibular schwannomas. Neurosurgery 49:1299-1306, 2001.

33. Posner JB, Chernik NL: Intracranial metastases from systemic cancer. Adv Neurol 19:579-592, 1978.

34. Sansur CA, Chin LS, Ames JW, et al: Gamma knife radiosurgery for the treatment of brain metastases. Stereotact Funct Neurosurg 74:37-51, 2000.

35. Cloward RB: The treatment of ruptured lumbar intervertebral discs by vertebral body fusion: I. Indications, operative technique, after care. J Neurosurg 10:154-168, 1953.

36. Booth KC, Bridwell KH, Eisenberg BA, et al: Minimum five-year results of degenerative spondylolisthesis treated with decompression and instrumented posterior fusion. Spine 24:1721-1727, 1999.

37. Montgomery DM, Brower RS: Cervical spondylotic myelopathy: Clinical syndrome and natural history. Orthop Clin North Am 23:487-493, 1992.

38. Raynor RB: Anterior or posterior approach to the cervical spine: An anatomical and radiographic evaluation and comparison. Neurosurgery 12:7-13, 1983.

39. Wang JC, McDonough PW, Endow K, et al: The effect of cervical plating on single-level anterior cervical discectomy and fusion. J Spinal Disord 12:467-471, 1999.

40. Wang JC, McDonough PW, Endow KK, et al: Increased fusion rates with cervical plating for two-level anterior cervical discectomy and fusion. Spine 25:41-45, 2000.

41. Bohlman HH, Emery SE, Goodfellow DB, et al: Robinson anterior cervical discectomy and arthrodesis for cervical radiculopathy: Long-term follow-up of one hundred and twenty-two patients. J Bone Joint Surg Am 75-A:1298-1307, 1993.

42. Aldrich F: Posterolateral microdisectomy for cervical monoradiculopathy caused by posterolateral soft cervical disc sequestration. J Neurosurg 72:370-377, 1990.

43. Henderson CM, Hennessy RG, Shuey HM Jr, et al: Posterior-lateral foraminotomy as an exclusive operative technique for cervical radiculopathy: A review of 846 consecutively operated cases. Neurosurgery 13:504-512, 1983.

44. Saunders RL, Bernini PM, Shirreffs TG Jr, et al: Central corpectomy for cervical spondylotic myelopathy: A consecutive series with long-term follow-up evaluation. J Neurosurg 74:163-170, 1991.

45. Kulkarni AV, Guha A, Lozano A, et al: Incidence of silent hemorrhage and delayed deterioration after stereotactic brain biopsy. J Neurosurg 89:31-35, 1998.

46. Hall WA: The safety and efficacy of stereotactic biopsy for intracranial lesions. Cancer 82:1749-1755, 1998.

47. Chandrasoma PT, Smith MM, Apuzzo ML: Stereotactic biopsy in the diagnosis of brain masses: Comparison of results of biopsy and resected surgical specimen. Neurosurgery 24:160-165, 1989.

48. Gildenberg PL: Spiegel and Wycis—the early years. Stereotact Funct Neurosurg 77:11-16, 2001.

49. Hughes RC, Polgar JG, Weightman D, et al: L-Dopa in parkinsonism and the influence of previous thalamotomy. BMJ 1:7-13, 1971.

50. Kelly PJ, Gillingham FJ: The long-term results of stereotaxic surgery and L-dopa therapy in patients with Parkinson's disease: A 10-year follow-up study. J Neurosurg 53:332-337, 1980.

51. Laitinen LV, Bergenheim AT, Hariz MI: Leksell's posteroventral pallidotomy in the treatment of Parkinson's disease. J Neurosurg 76:53-61, 1992.

52. Limousin P, Krack P, Pollak P, et al: Electrical stimulation of the subthalamic nucleus in advanced Parkinson's disease. N Engl J Med 339:1105-1111, 1998.

53. Gross C, Rougier A, Guehl D, et al: High-frequency stimulation of the globus pallidus internalis in Parkinson's disease: A study of seven cases. J Neurosurg 87:491-498, 1997.

54. Limousin P, Pollak P, Benazzouz A, et al: Effect of parkinsonian signs and symptoms of bilateral subthalamic nucleus stimulation. Lancet 345:91-95, 1995.

55. Benabid AL, Pollak P, Gervason C, et al: Long-term suppression of tremor by chronic stimulation of the ventral intermediate thalamic nucleus. Lancet 337:403-406, 1991.

56. Leksell L: The stereotaxic method and radiosurgery of the brain. Acta Chir Scand 102:316-319, 1951.

57. Petit JH, Herman JM, Nagda S, et al: Radiosurgical treatment of trigeminal neuralgia: Evaluating quality of life and treatment outcomes. Int J Radiat Oncol Biol Phys 56:1147-1153, 2003.

58. Chin LS, Ma L, DiBiase S: Radiation necrosis following Gamma knife surgery: A case-controlled comparison of treatment parameters and long-term clinical follow up. J Neurosurg 94:899-904, 2001.

59. Barnett GH, Kormos DW, Steiner CP, et al: Use of a frameless, armless stereotactic wand for brain tumor localization with two-dimensional and three-dimensional neuroimaging. Neurosurgery 33:674-678, 1993.

60. Roberts DW, Nakajima T, Brodwater B, et al: Further development and clinical application of the stereotactic operating microscope. Stereotact Funct Neurosurg 58:114-117, 1992.

61. McLaughlin MR, Jannetta PJ, Clyde BL, et al: Microvascular decompression of cranial nerves: Lessons learned after 4400 operations. J Neurosurg 90:1-8, 1999.

62. Lunsford LD: Treatment of tic douloureux by percutaneous retrogasserian glycerol injection. JAMA 248:449-453, 1982.

63. van Kleef M, Spaans F, Dingemans W, et al: Effects and side effects of a percutaneous thermal lesion of the dorsal root ganglion in patients with cervical pain syndrome. Pain 52:49-53, 1993.

64. Nashold BS Jr, Ostdahl RH: Dorsal root entry zone lesions for pain relief. J Neurosurg 51:59-69, 1979.

65. Bernard EJ Jr, Nashold BS Jr, Caputi F, et al: Nucleus caudalis DREZ lesions for facial pain. Br J Neurosurg 1:81-91, 1987.

66. Lahuerta J, Bowsher D, Lipton S, et al: Percutaneous cervical cordotomy: A review of 181 operations on 146 patients with a study on the location of "pain fibers" in the C2 spinal cord segment of 29 cases. J Neurosurg 80:975-985, 1994.

67. Kux M: Thoracic endoscopic sympathectomy for treatment of upper-limb hyperhidrosis. Lancet 1:1320, 1977.

68. Melzack R, Wall PD: Pain mechanisms: A new theory. Science 150:971-979, 1965.

69. North RB, Kidd DH, Zahurak M, et al: Spinal cord stimulation for chronic, intractable pain: Experience over two decades. Neurosurgery 32:384-394, 1993.

70. Young RF, Chambi VI: Pain relief by electrical stimulation of the periaqueductal and periventricular gray matter: Evidence for a non-opioid mechanism. J Neurosurg 66:364-371, 1987.

71. Hassenbusch SJ, Pillay PK, Magdinec M, et al: Constant infusion of morphine for intractable cancer pain using an implanted pump. J Neurosurg 73:405-409, 1990.

72. Guzman R, Barth A, Lovblad KO, et al: Use of diffusion-weighted magnetic resonance imaging in differentiating purulent brain processes from cystic brain tumors. J Neurosurg 97:1101-1107, 2002.

CHAPTER 72

PLASTIC SURGERY

John L. Burns, M. D. and **Steven J. Blackwell, M. D.**

General Plastic Surgical Principles and Techniques	**Lower Extremity**
	Breast and Aesthetic Surgery
Head and Neck	**Conclusion**
Trunk and External Genitalia	

Plastic surgery takes its name from the Greek term "plastikos," which means to mold and reshape. Plastic surgery is an extremely diverse surgical specialty whose chief purpose is to restore form and function. The American Board of Plastic Surgery states,

> The specialty of plastic surgery deals with the repair, replacement, and reconstruction of physical defects of form or function involving the skin, musculoskeletal system, craniomaxillofacial structures, hand, extremities, breast and trunk, and external genitalia. It uses aesthetic surgical principles not only to improve undesirable qualities of normal structures, but in all reconstructive procedures as well.

The diverse nature of this discipline lends itself to many areas of further specialization. These include, but are not limited to, hand and microvascular surgery, craniomaxillofacial surgery, acute and reconstructive burn surgery, and aesthetic surgery. Several of these areas, including hand surgery, burns, wound care, and cutaneous malignancies, are covered in separate chapters. Herein we offer medical students, residents, and general surgeons only an overview of plastic surgery with an emphasis on reconstruction.

GENERAL PLASTIC SURGICAL PRINCIPLES AND TECHNIQUES

Skin Incisions and Excisions

Because plastic surgery is a specialty dealing with difficult wounds and wound problems, meticulous attention is focused on wound closure and avoidance of unsightly scars. Skin incisions are carefully planned so as to avoid an obvious scar. Skin creases and hair-bearing areas are useful places to camouflage incisions. For example, facial incisions can be hidden in the pretragal crease, subciliary crease, or nasolabial fold.[1] Breast incisions can be hidden in the periareolar skin, the inframammary crease, or the axilla.

Tension should be avoided across skin incisions because it will result in wide and unsightly scars. In 1861, Carl Langer noted that tension is unevenly distributed in skin and that human skin is less distensible in the direction of tension lines than across them. "Langer's lines" can be used to design skin incisions and diminish tension across the incision. When possible, incisions should be placed perpendicular to the long axis of the underlying muscle. Relaxed skin tension lines (RSTLs) are lines of minimal tension, which often appear as wrinkle lines or natural skin lines.[2] RSTLs lie perpendicular to the underlying muscle and are accentuated by contraction of the muscle (Fig. 72-1). An example of this principle is transverse wrinkling of the forehead, which is perpendicular to the underlying vertically oriented frontalis muscle. Anatomic areas where tension is excessive should be avoided if possible. The shoulders, back, and anterior chest are high tension and mobile areas where wide scarring is difficult to avoid. Patients should also be questioned as to propensity for development of hypertrophic scars or keloid formation. Ears, anterior chest, and shoulders are areas prone to these problematic scars.[3,4]

When possible, incisions should not be placed over weight-bearing or high-use surfaces. Incisions placed on the palm of the hand, sole of the foot, or fingertips occasionally result in painful and functionally impairing scars. Linear scars contract up to 20% in the longitudinal direction. For this reason, cutaneous scars that cross the flexor

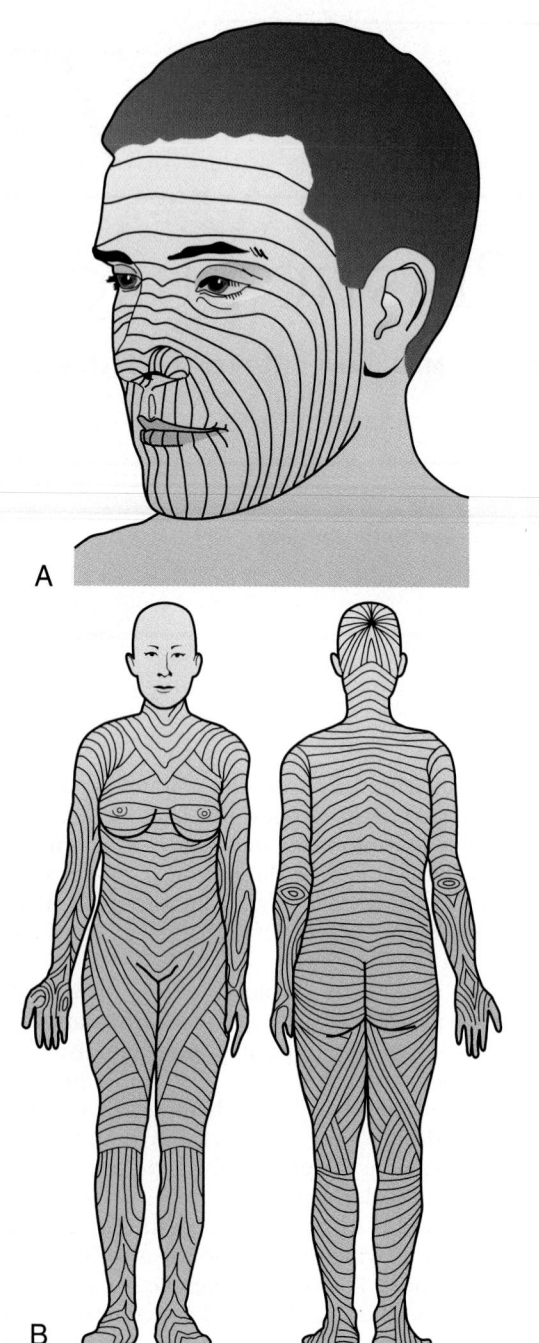

FIGURE 72-1.   A, Facial relaxed skin tension lines (RSLTs). **B,** RSLTs of the entire body. (**A** and **B,** From Trott A: Wounds and Lacerations: Emergency Care and Closure, 2nd ed. St. Louis, Mosby, 1997, p 51.)

surface of joints can restrict the ability of the joint to extend. This problem is obviated by designing elective incisions across flexor creases in a zigzag pattern.

The most favorable excision design is the double-lenticular or elliptical design with a 4:1 length-to-width ratio.[5] This results in an ability to close the wound without a mound of skin at the extremes of the incision ("dog-ear

deformity). A circular excision deforms spontaneously to an ovoid defect according to Langer's principle, allowing an elliptical pattern to be easily implemented for a more aesthetic closure.

Open Wounds

Wound closure by primary healing or first intention involves closure of the wound by direct skin approximation, flap, or skin graft. The result is transformation of an open to a closed wound in a single operative session. Spontaneous healing, or secondary intention, involves wound healing without surgical manipulation. Tertiary healing, healing by third intention, or delayed primary closure combines tenants of both primary healing and spontaneous healing. In this case, a contaminated wound is left open for several days to allow the normal host defenses to débride the wound. The wound is then closed primarily and tensile strength develops normally.

An open wound that is undergoing spontaneous healing can be induced to heal if etiologic factors are recognized and treatments optimized. Wound healing is negatively affected by systemic, regional, or local factors (Fig. 72-2). Systemic factors include active history of tobacco use, diabetes, malnutrition, anemia, hypoxemia, congestive heart failure or coronary artery disease, immunosuppression, cancer, and genetic factors. Regional factors include peripheral atherosclerosis, venous hypertension, and peripheral neuropathy. Local causes include trauma, burns, pressure, infection, radiation, and infiltration. These issues must be recognized when evaluating an open wound, and treatment must address both the open wound and any factors that threaten to impair healing.

Two common problems encountered in chronic open wounds are malnutrition and bacterial inoculation. Larger chronic open wounds can serve as a source of protein loss. A serum albumin level less than 2.5 g/dL reflects inadequate nutritional reserve and impaired ability to heal a wound.[6] Careful attention to diet and protein replacement is critical for normal wound healing to occur.

Because of the fear of bacterial invasion, primary wound closure beyond 6 to 8 hours after injury was historically proscribed. However, several scientific studies have since shown that when blood supply to a wound is adequate and bacterial invasion is absent, wounds can be safely closed at any time following proper débridement and irrigation.[7] Routine swab cultures of wound surfaces offer both inadequate and inaccurate reflections of the risk for wound infection. Quantitative bacteriology is a highly effective test whereby a biopsy of viable wound tissue can accurately assess the risk for unfavorable outcome for contemplated wound closure ($>10^3$ bacteria per gram of tissue for β-hemolytic *Streptococcus* and $>10^5$ bacteria per gram of tissue for all other bacterial species). Wounds with counts lower than those stated can be expected to heal.

Wound Closure

In general, expeditious closure of wounds is one of the goals of plastic surgery and should follow a reconstructive

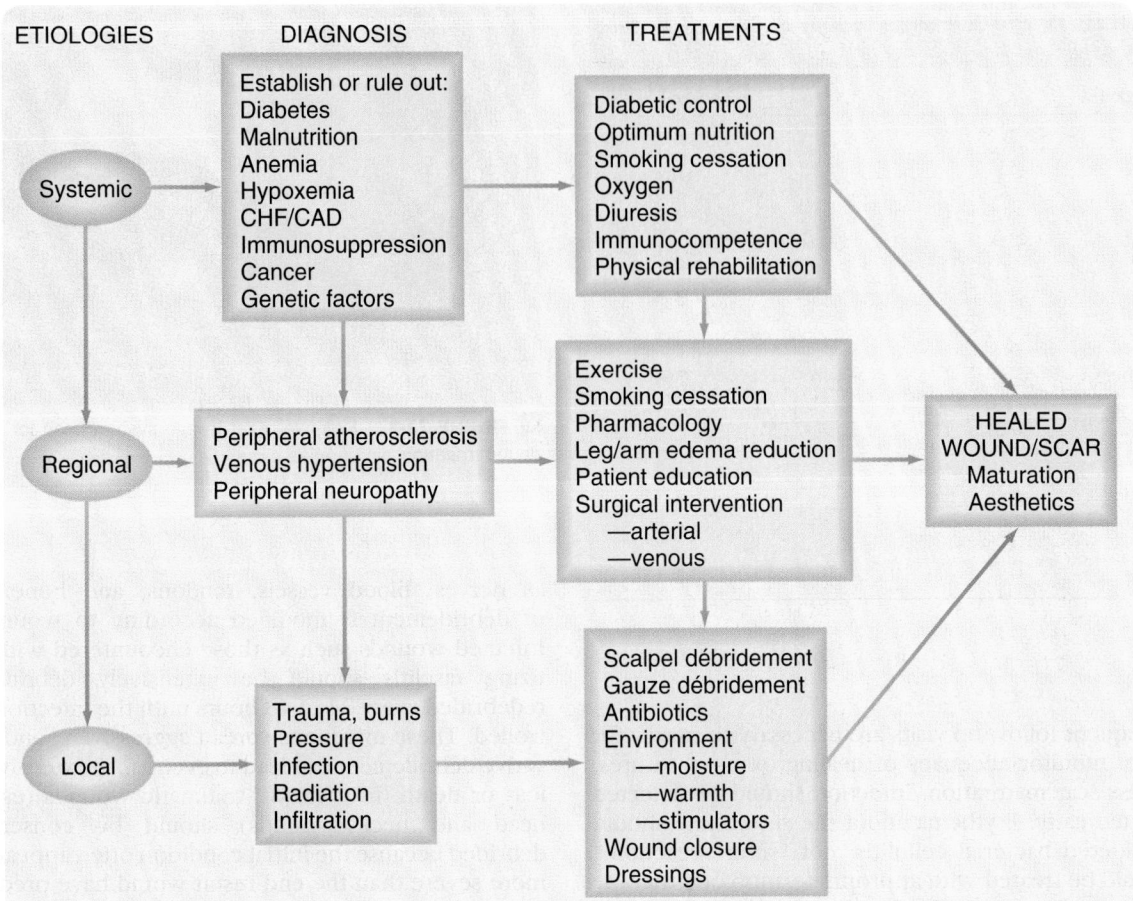

FIGURE 72-2.   Impediments to wound healing. CHF, congestive heart failure; CAD, coronary artery disease. (From Russel R [ed]: Plastic Surgery Educational Foundation: Instructional Courses, Vol 4. St. Louis, Mosby, 1991, p 252.)

Box 72-1. Reconstructive Ladder

Linear closure	Myocutaneous flaps
Skin grafts	Free flaps
Skin flaps	

---

ladder beginning with the simple and advancing to the complex as the wound dictates (Box 72-1). An optimal linear closure is seen when the skin edges are coapted under minimal tension without redundant skin mounds (dog ears) at the incisional poles. Undermining adjacent skin, either just deep to the dermis or just superficial to the fascia is commonly used to alleviate tension. Layered closure of wounds describes the technique whereby the separate anatomic planes of the wound are reapproximated, like with like. Dermal approximation is of paramount importance, because it should bear most of the tension dispersed across the skin interface. Dermal sutures are placed with the knot buried. Dermal sutures can be placed vertically, obliquely, or horizontally to approximate the dermis. On completion of a correct dermal closure, the skin edges should be perfectly aligned, even slightly everted, along the length of the wound.

Epidermal skin sutures function for fine alignment of skin edges. Interrupted sutures are less constrictive than running sutures. The needle should enter and exit the skin at 90 degrees to evert the skin edges. These skin sutures should be removed as soon as adequate intrinsic bonding strength is sufficient. Skin sutures left in place too long result in an unsightly track pattern. On the other hand, removing sutures prematurely risks wound dehiscence. Nonabsorbable sutures on the face are typically removed after 5 days. Sutures in the hand, foot, or across areas that are acted on by motion should be left for 14 days or longer (Table 72-1). Alternatively, by employing the running intradermal suturing technique, the time constraints of suture removal may be disregarded, and these sutures may be left in place longer without risking a track pattern scar. Finally, epidermal approximation can be achieved without suture using a medical-grade cyanoacrylate adhesive such as Dermabond. Such adhesives are applied across the coapted skin edges only and contribute no tensile strength. Tape closure strips such as Steri-Strips can be applied at the completion of wound closure to help splint the coapted skin edges.

TABLE 72-1.	Guidelines for Day of Suture Removal by Area
Body Region	**Removal (days)**
Scalp	6–8
Ear	10–14
Eyelid	3–4
Eyebrow	3–5
Nose	3–5
Lip	3–4
Face (other)	3–4
Chest/abdomen	8–10
Back	12–14
Extremities	12–14
Hand	10–14
Foot/sole	12–14

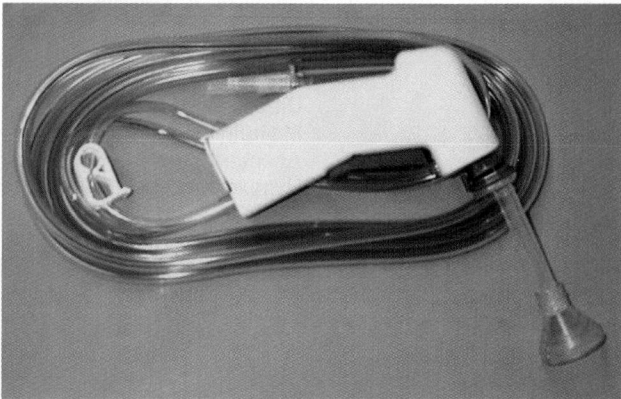

FIGURE 72-3. Example of jet lavage system used for wound irrigation.

Subsequent follow-up visits are necessary to survey for infection, monitor adequacy of healing, remove sutures, and assess scar maturation. Infection should be detected and treated early. Erythema about the suture line should be considered bacterial cellulitis, not "suture reaction," and should be treated with appropriate antibiotic therapy and topical antimicrobials. Undiagnosed infection can lead to dehiscence of the wound and problematic scars. Patients should be instructed to avoid ultraviolet radiation exposure to immature scars because it risks local hyperpigmentation changes. Although barrier protection is best, sunscreens can also be used. For patients with firm and tender scars, scar massage using moisturizing lotion can soften the scar and lessen the discomfort.

Certain patients may demonstrate a propensity for hypertrophic or keloid scar formation.[3] Preoperative discussion must review the increased risk of untoward scar consequences in these susceptible patients. When wounds demonstrate these tendencies, several treatment options are available. Antipruritic medication is often necessary to manage complaints of itching of the scar. Scar massage with lotion can be used to soften and soothe these scars. Although the mechanism is still in question, topical application of silicone gel strips or sheets have shown value for improving such problematic scars.[8] Intralesional injection of steroids into a keloid scar can inactivate and shrink the scar; such therapy is not indicated for hypertrophic scars. Interval follow-up assessments are necessary to gauge therapeutic response.

Débridement and Irrigation

While technically easy, proper wound débridement requires astute surgical judgment and careful inspection. Débridement implies the removal of devitalized and contaminated tissues while preserving critical structures such as nerves, blood vessels, tendons, and bone. Extent of débridement is modified according to wound type. Infected wounds such as those encountered with necrotizing fasciitis should be extensively débrided and redébrided every 24 to 48 hours until the infection is controlled. These infections spread aggressively, and conservative débridement can lead to even more extensive tissue loss or death. In contrast, traumatic wounds (especially head and neck wounds) should be conservatively débrided because the initial condition often appears much more severe than the end result would have predicted.

After débridement, open wounds should be kept moist. Allowing these wounds to desiccate results in loss of proteinaceous fluid and necrosis of the superficial wound layers. The popular technique of wet-to-dry dressing changes should be viewed as a surface débridement technique and not a substitute for an appropriate wound dressing. The wet-to-dry dressing technique, when used on a clean and viable wound bed, may cause injury to granulation tissue and delay wound healing.

In addition to débridement, wound irrigation, with or without antibiotics, should be a mainstay of infection control. Wounds suspected of harboring bacteria should be evaluated using quantitative bacteriology as discussed earlier. Numerous jet lavage systems exist (Fig. 72-3) that forcefully apply irrigant to the wound surface and act to decrease the bacterial load.[9] Generally, jet lavage irrigation decreases the bacterial load on the wound surface by 10^2. The amount of irrigant used averages 1.5 L, with larger wounds requiring a greater volume of irrigant.

Grafts and Flaps

As a rule, the surgeon should apply the concept of a reconstructive ladder when assessing possibilities for wound closure (see Box 72-1). The reconstructive ladder should be followed so that simple options are used before complex solutions are considered. A secondary plan should be available in case the primary plan fails. This ensures that the surgeon does not compromise a future option while performing an initial closure.

Grafts

Ascending the reconstructive ladder, skin grafts follow only linear closure in complexity. Skin grafts can be divided, based on thickness, into full-thickness and split-thickness grafts (Fig. 72-4). Full-thickness grafts include epidermis with the entirety of the dermis; the donor site must be closed separately. Split-thickness grafts vary in the amount of dermis included in the graft. The modern power-driven dermatome allows precise selection of graft thickness. Typically a split-thickness graft is harvested at 10/1000 of an inch. For split-thickness grafts, the donor site is most often closed with an occlusive or medication-impregnated meshed gauze. The donor site re-epithelizes spontaneously. Because of this healing ability of the donor site, split-thickness grafts are especially valuable to close larger wounds. Because split-thickness donor sites can be reharvested after re-epithelization, this method of wound closure is the workhorse for burn injuries. Thin split-thickness grafts contract to a greater extent than thick split-thickness or full-thickness grafts. Full-thickness grafts resist deformation more than thinner split-thickness grafts and are therefore more suitable for reconstruction where late contracture is expected to compromise the functional or aesthetic outcome.

The skin graft must be applied to a well-vascularized recipient wound bed. It will not adhere to exposed bone, cartilage, or tendon devoid of periosteum, perichondrium, or peritenon, respectively, or devoid of its vascularized, perimembranous envelope. There are three steps in the "take" of a skin graft: imbibition, inosculation, and revascularization.[10,11] Imbibition occurs up to 48 hours after graft placement and involves the free absorption of nutrients into the graft. Inosculation designates the period in which donor and recipient capillaries become aligned. There remains a debate as to whether new channels are formed or if preexisting channels reconnect. Finally, after approximately 5 days, revascularization occurs and the graft demonstrates both arterial inflow and venous outflow.

Reasons for skin graft failure are well understood. The most common causes of skin graft failure are hematoma (or seroma), infection, and movement (shear).[12,13] Hematoma is most often the consequence of inadequate intraoperative hemostasis, and can be identified before irreversible damage has occurred. By examining the skin graft before the 4th postoperative day, a hematoma or seroma can be evacuated, and the mechanical obstruction to revascularization of the graft is thus removed. Some surgeons make stab incisions in the graft preemptively to create small outlets for fluid to drain from beneath the graft, a technique know as "pie crusting." Others might use a mesh expander device that creates a chain-link fence pattern in the graft. Although these methods may provide egress portals for serous fluid or blood, an unsightly meshed pattern results, making this technique unsuitable for aesthetic reconstruction. Bacterial contamination of a wound results in graft loss. Topical or systemic antimicrobials or both can be used to control bacterial proliferation. Finally, movement of the graft results in shearing of delicate capillary alignments and graft loss. Graft immobilization is critical to graft take and can be accomplished with a variety of methods including a bolster dressing, light compression wraps, or a vacuum-assisted closure (VAC) device, just to name a few.

Special considerations in choosing a skin graft donor site include skin quality and color from the donor region that best matches the recipient site. For example, skin harvested from the blush zone above the clavicles is best suited for facial grafting. Skin grafts harvested from areas caudal to the waist result in tallow discoloration and pos-

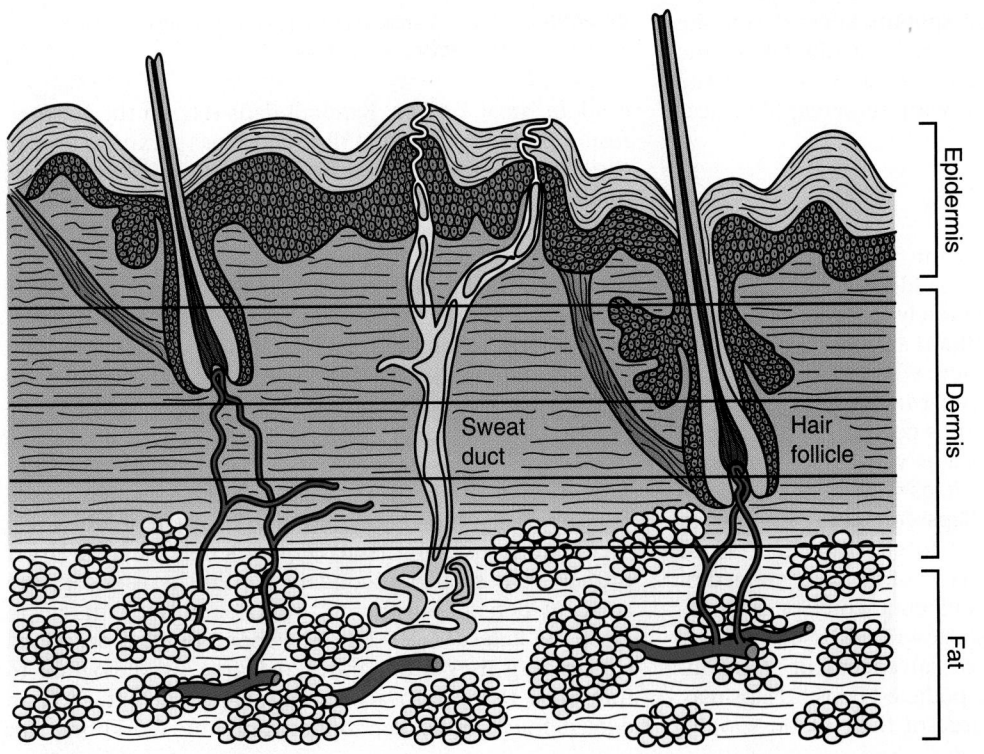

FIGURE 72-4. Cross section of skin depicting levels contained in split-thickness and full-thickness skin grafts.

Epidermis

Dermis

Fat

Sweat duct

Hair follicle

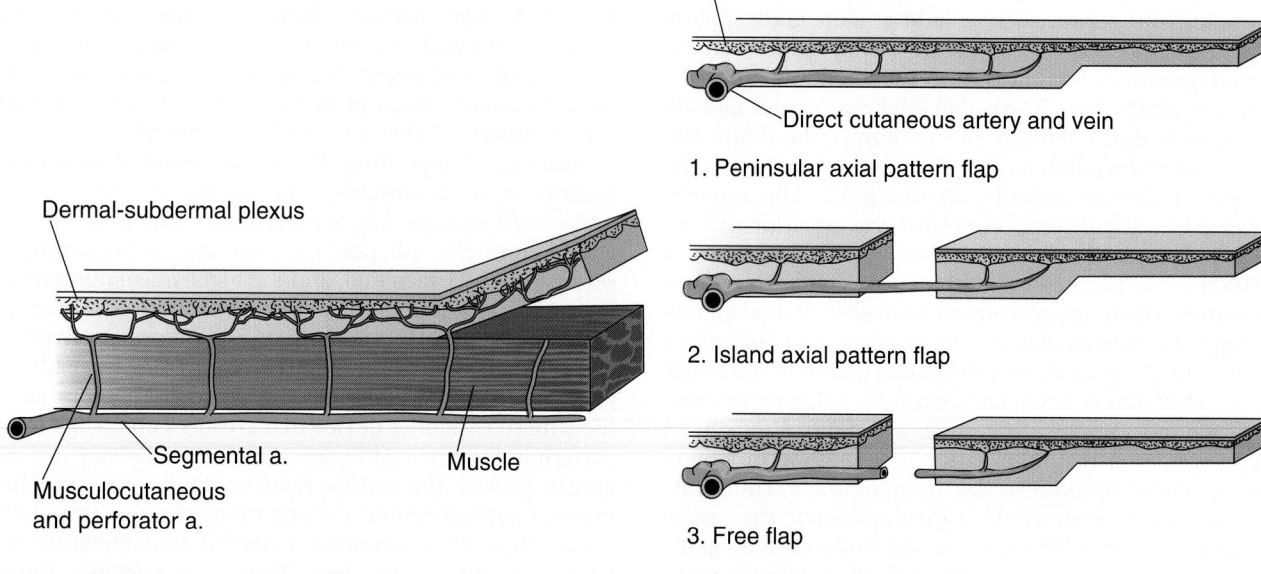

A Random pattern skin flap

B Axial pattern skin flaps

FIGURE 72-5. **A** and **B,** Vascular patterns of random pattern and axial skin flaps. (**A** and **B,** From Place MJ, Herber SC, Hardesty RA: Basic techniques and principles in plastic surgery. *In* Aston SJ, Beasley RW, Thorne CHM [eds]: Grabb and Smith's Plastic Surgery, 5th ed. Philadelphia, Lippincott-Raven, 1997, p 21.)

sible unwanted hair growth. Because split-thickness donor sites permanently scar, it is wise to choose a donor site that can be concealed. When a large amount of graft is needed, the thighs and buttocks are areas that can be hidden with everyday clothes. The inner arm or groin crease are each fine sources for full-thickness grafts because both areas offer relatively glabrous skin sources, the donor sites of which can be easily hidden with clothes. One often overlooked split-thickness donor site is the scalp; taking extreme care to avoid taking the graft below the level of the hair follicle, this donor site heals quickly, painlessly, and with imperceptible scar consequences.

Flaps

Flap reconstruction represents the next order of complexity along the reconstructive ladder (Fig. 72-5). A *flap* is defined as a partially or completely isolated segment of tissue perfused with its own blood supply. Flaps are the reconstructive option of choice where a padded and durable cover is needed to reconstruct an integumentary defect over vital structures, tissues devoid of perivascular membrane, or over implants. Flaps vary greatly in terms of complexity from simple skin flaps with a random blood supply to microvascular free flaps containing composite tissue. Numerous schemes exist to classify flaps.[14] Flaps may be classified based on the type of tissue contained in the flap: fasciocutaneous, musculocutaneous, or osteocutaneous flaps.[15,16] Flaps are also described based on their design and method of transfer: advancement, rotation, transposition, interpolation, or pedicled flaps.[17] Flaps may be further defined by the source of their blood supply:

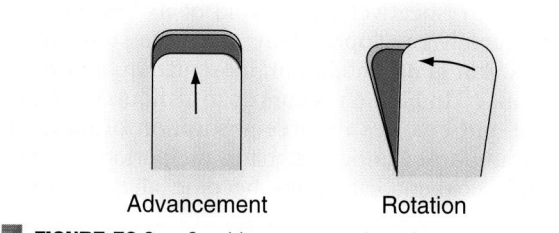

Advancement   Rotation

FIGURE 72-6.   Graphic representation of commonly used local flaps: advancement and rotation flaps.

random, axial, or free. Random flaps rely on the low-perfusion pressures found in the subdermal plexus to sustain the flap and not a named blood vessel.[18,19] Nevertheless, random flaps are used widely in reconstruction of cutaneous defects. These local flaps recruit adjacent tissue based on geometric design patterns.

Advancement and rotation flaps represent commonly used random-patten skin flaps (Fig. 72-6). The Z-plasty, bilobed flap, rhomboid, and V-Y (or Y-V) advancement flaps are commonly used random flaps. Z-plasty involves transposing two adjacent triangular-shaped flaps to redirect and lengthen an existing scar (the central limb) (Fig. 72-7). The angles of the Z-plasty can be increased to provide greater length. Typically a 60-degree angle is used that lengthens the central limb by 75%. The bilobed flap is commonly used for nasal reconstruction[20]; here, a larger primary and smaller secondary flap are transposed into adjacent defects borrowing the loose adjacent tissue to close the defect (Fig. 72-8). The rhomboid flap described by Limberg uses a 60- and 120-degree parallelogram to transpose tissue into a diamond-shaped defect. It is an extremely versatile flap option and the workhorse for

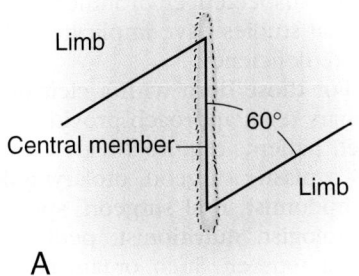

A

FIGURE 72-7.   **A** to **C,** Graphic representation of the Z-plasty transposition flap commonly used for scar contracture release. (**A** to **C,** From Aston SJ, Beasley RW, Thorne CHM [eds]: Grabb and Smith's Plastic Surgery, 5th ed. Philadelphia, Lippincott-Raven, 1997, p 20.)

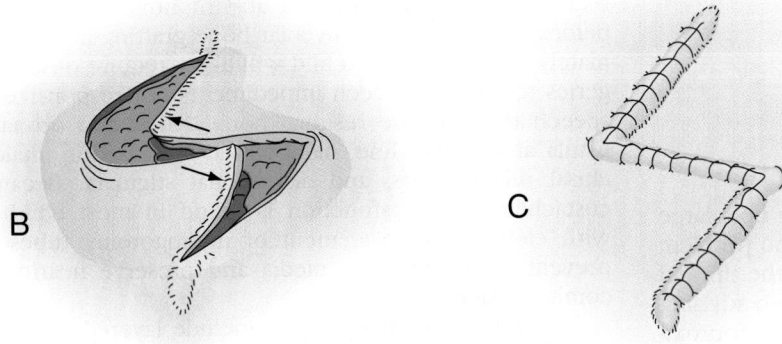

B   C

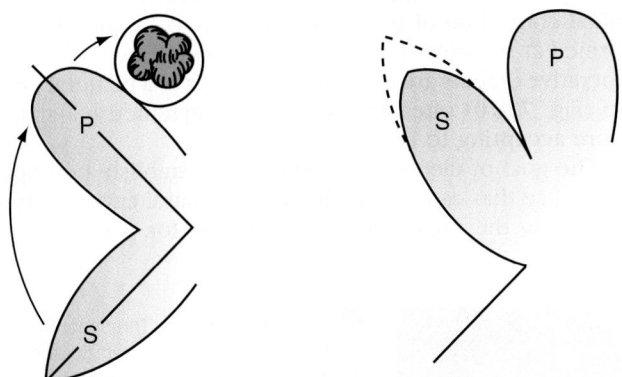

FIGURE 72-8.   Graphic representation of the bilobed flap commonly used for nasal reconstruction. P, primary flap; S, secondary flap. (From Aston SJ, Beasley RW, Thorne CHM [eds]: Grabb and Smith's Plastic Surgery, 5th ed. Philadelphia, Lippincott-Raven, 1997, p 23.)

most plastic surgeons.[20] Finally, the V-Y (or Y-V) advancement flaps are commonly used to lengthen scars around the nose and mouth. A backcut at the base of a flap may decrease tension at a flap's tip, creating a greater arc of rotation; overzealous backcut or tension at flap inset can each cause ischemia to the flap and threaten its survival.

An axial flap is based on a named blood vessel and can provide a reproducible and stable skin or skin/muscle (myocutaneous) flap. Flaps can also be raised with the underlying fascia (fasciocutaneous), which recruits the fascial blood supply and thereby increases the predictable vascularity to the flap. Because of its reliable blood supply, the axial flap can be used to provide much-needed length and bulk that the random flap cannot. An axial flap that remains attached to its proximal blood supply and is transposed to a defect is known as a *pedicled flap*. Alternately, the vascular pedicle can be completely transected, the paddle of tissue transferred and reanastomosed to recipient vessels in a remote location. This technique requires the use of an operating microscope and is known as *microsurgery*.

The relatively recent advent of microsurgery has dramatically altered the practice of plastic surgery and allows the surgeon a plethora of reconstructive options that were not previously available.[21] The human eye is capable of visualizing objects as small as 100 μm. Operating microscope can magnify an object up to 40 ×, allowing the surgeon precise control. Microsutures vary in size from 8-0 to 11-0, which allows the surgeon to suture vessels less than 1.0 mm in diameter. The principles and techniques of microsurgery are similar to vascular surgery. However, laboratory training with an operating microscope using small animals is essential before progressing into clinical surgery. In addition, experience in recognizing the causes and solutions of flap failure is mandatory. Despite numerous techniques such as Doppler probing and temperature monitoring, clinical assessment remains the gold standard for free flap monitoring.[22,23] The most common cause of flap failure is venous congestion. If a problem is suspected, the first response must include removal of enough sutures at the bedside that will relieve pressure on the flap. The standard of care dictates a rapid return to the operating room to release tension, evacuate any fluid collections, eliminate sources of vascular pedicle kinking, and examine and possibly revise the arterial and/or venous anastomosis. Numerous pharmacologic agents have been used to manipulate vascular tone and the clotting cascade and to reduce the ill effects of the inflammatory mediators liberated through the arachidonic acid pathway. Leech therapy may occasionally salvage flaps that suffer from significant venous congestion. Despite these many therapies, nothing can replace meticulous operative technique and diligent postoperative clinical assessment.

HEAD AND NECK

Congenital and Craniomaxillofacial

Cleft Lip and Palate

Congenital defects of the head and neck make up a large percentage of pediatric plastic surgery. Here, no problem is more common than congenital clefting of the lip and palate. Epidemiologic analysis is important when advising expectant parents. Cleft lip and palate occurs in approximately 1 in 1000 live births. Racial differences are noted, with greatest prevalence found in Mexican Americans and Asians, then whites, and least common in African Americans. An isolated cleft palate occurs in approximately 1 in 2000 live births. Cleft lip and/or palate occurs as an isolated event in 86% of cases but is combined with other malformations in 14% of cases. When one sibling has a cleft lip or palate, the probability of the next child being affected is 4%. When both a parent and child are affected, the likelihood of the next child having a cleft lip or palate increases to 17%.[24] The etiology of clefting of the lip and palate remains unknown, but a multifactorial combination

of heredity with environmental factors seems most plausible. Suspected environmental agents based purely on animal studies have implicated phenytoin,[25] ethanol, and folate deficiency.

For those born with a cleft lip or palate, a multidisciplinary team approach provides the highest level of care. Cleft patients require a wide variety of specialists, including a plastic surgeon, otolaryngologist, pediatric dentist, orthodontist, oral surgeon, speech-language pathologist, audiologist, nutritionist, pediatrician, psychologist, and social worker. Such organized teams generally employ more experienced surgeons who perform a large number of these procedures and are more familiar with variant cases. The timing of cleft repair is important and a general recommendation is lip repair at 3 months, palate repair before 12 months, and alveolar bone grafting at approximately 9 years.[26-28] The child will likely require other surgeries to address speech impediments not responsive to speech therapy, the residual bony deficit and oronasal fistula at the gum line, nasal airway obstruction, malocclusal relationships, and distortional stigmata. Because eustachian tube dysfunction is found in most children with cleft palate, placement of myringotomy tubes to prevent recurrent otitis media and preserve hearing is commonplace.

Principles of cleft lip repair include layered repair of the skin, muscle, and mucous membrane to restore symmetrical length and function. The Millard rotation-advancement unilateral cleft lip repair (Fig. 72-9) has become a widely applied and reproducible model.[29] An initial correction of the nasal deformity is frequently performed at the time of the lip repair. Even though the preoperative defects are more severe, repair of a bilateral cleft lip (Fig. 72-10) often results in better symmetry, a status more accepting to the casual eye.

The goal of cleft palate repair is to establish a competent valve that can isolate the oral and nasal cavities, thus recreating the muscular sling necessary for palatal eleva-

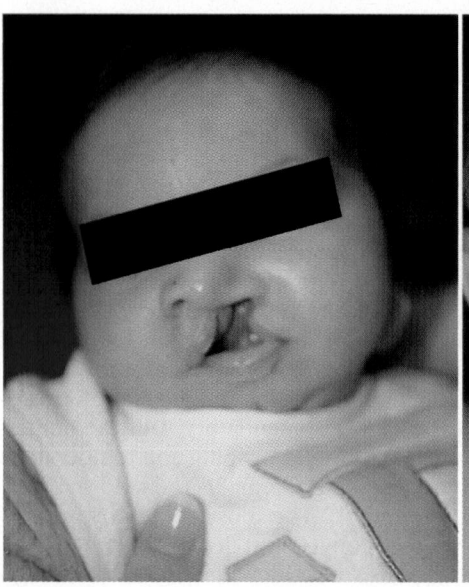
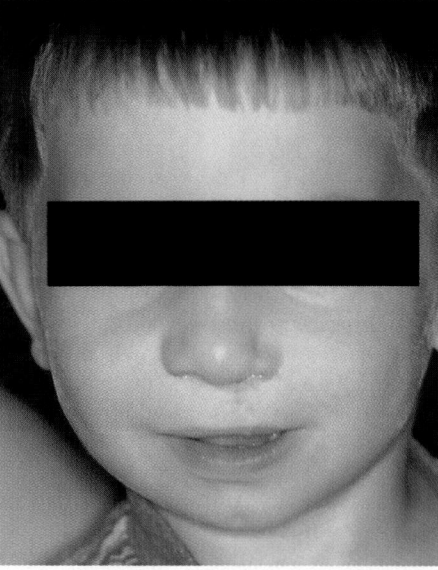

A   B

■ **FIGURE 72-9.** **A,** Three-month-old boy with a unilateral cleft lip and palate. **B,** Postoperative photograph, age 5 years, after Millard rotation-advancement cleft lip repair.

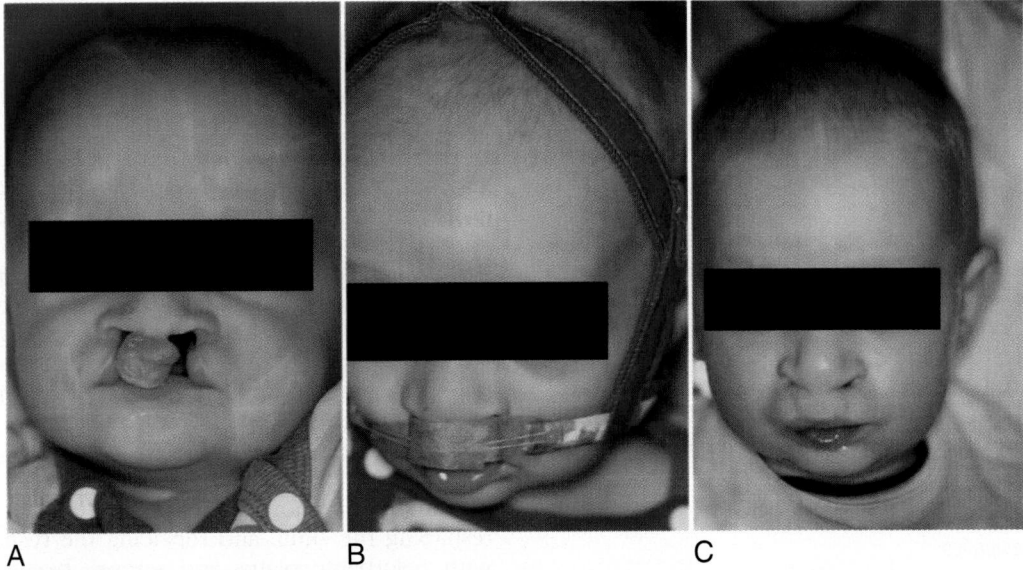

FIGURE 72-10. **A,** Preoperative photographs of a 3-month-old boy with a bilateral cleft lip and palate. **B,** Wearing orthodontic appliance to push back prominent premaxilla. **C,** Postoperative view 6 months after lip repair.

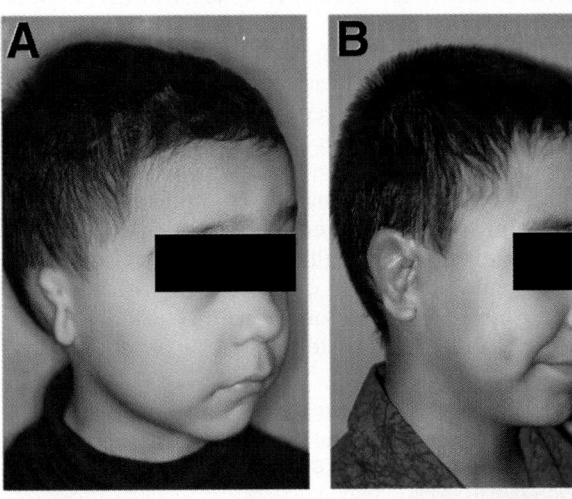

FIGURE 72-11. **A,** Preoperative photograph of 3-year-old boy with microtia. **B,** Postoperative photography, age 7 years, one year after ear reconstruction with autologous rib graft and subsequent ear lobule rotation.

tion. Just before school age, both speech assessment and speech diagnostic studies determine if there is residual hypernasal speech; additional surgery of pharyngeal flap or pharyngoplasty might be necessary to remedy the problem.

Other Congenital Anomalies

Embryologic development of the head and neck begins at the 4th week with the formation of the branchial apparatus. Branchial cleft cyst, sinus, or fistula represents remnants from epithelial-lined tracts in the lateral neck along the anterior border of the sternocleidomastoid muscle. Clinically, the sinus or fistula may connect with the skin and/or oropharynx, and later in life, if surgical excision is

not carried out, malignant transformation or infection may occur.

The thyroid develops embryologically at the base of the tongue and descends along a midline tract to its final pretracheal position in the neck. Thyroglossal duct cysts arise from remnant tissue left during the embryonic descent of the thyroid tissue. Usually, the thyroglossal duct disappears with development. However, duct remnants may be present as sinuses or cysts along the migration pathway. These are most commonly present in the midline at the level of the hyoid bone and are treated with excision.

Ear deformities are commonly encountered in newborn infants and vary widely in severity. Anotia (complete absence) and microtia (vestigial remnants or absence of part of the ear) require extensive surgery and can be associated with other craniofacial deformities. Minor abnormalities in ear shape can sometimes be overcome with early splinting or taping of the newborn's ear; this is possible because the effect of maternal estrogen makes the ear cartilage extremely pliable and amenable to reshaping in the neonate. For anotia or microtia, surgical repair is recommended at 7 years of age. By this age, the contralateral ear has developed to near adult size and the child will begin to experience the expectations of schoolmates. Although numerous synthetic implants exist for reconstruction of an absent ear, the gold standard remains autologous rib cartilage graft taken from the contralateral cartilaginous portion of the ribs (Fig. 72-11).[30] The graft is shaped and placed into a subcutaneous pocket over a suction drain. Autologous rib grafts have been shown to be superior to synthetic implants because of their resistance to extrusion and infection.

Prominent ears provide a frequent source of peer teasing in school-age children. When ears protrude excessively from the temporal scalp, otoplasty provides the surgical correction. Ear prominence must be carefully analyzed because it can occur due to conchal constriction or hypertrophy, a poorly defined or absent antihelical fold, or a conchoscaphal angle greater than 90 degrees. Knowledge of normal ear position is critical to attaining an acceptable postoperative result. A normal ear's anatomic bounds extend from the eyebrow superiorly to the base of the nasal columella inferiorly; it inclines posteriorly approximately 20 degrees off vertical and protrudes at its midpoint 16 to 18 mm from the scalp. For conchal excess, an ellipse of conchal cartilage can be excised adjacent to the mastoid and the reduced concha can be recessed additionally by suture fixation to the mastoid fascia.[31] The antihelical fold is recreated using both scoring anteriorly to weaken the cartilage and mattress suturing posteriorly to attain the desired natural appearing convexity (Fig. 72-12). Ideally, it is better to overcorrect a bit, because most patients are sensitive to even minor residual prominence.

Less Common Anomalies

Craniofacial surgery is a reconstructive discipline that addresses the skull, the facial skeleton, and soft tissues of the face. Using this approach both neurosurgeon and plastic surgeon are able to address pathology due to congenital anomalies, post-traumatic deformities, and defects after tumor ablation. Access to the craniofacial skeleton is accomplished through inconspicuous incisions such as the bicoronal, lower eyelid, and upper buccal sulcus incisions. Following craniotomy, the dura and brain are retracted to provide safe exposure that will allow selective osteotomies of the craniofacial skeleton that are repositioned and then rigidly fixed using plates and screws.

Congenital anomalies involving the skull and facial skeleton are rare but severely deforming. Premature fusion of the cranial sutures is known as *craniosynostosis* and occurs once in 2000 live births.[32] Craniosynostosis can limit the skull's volume and increase intracranial pressure.[33] Skull deformities may also arise from extrinsic causes such as torticollis or as a result of intrauterine head molding during pregnancy. These skull deformities are responsive to nonsurgical measures. Where synostosis also affects the cranial base, the conditions are called *craniofacial syndromes*. Here, restricted skull and facial growth result in a constricted and deformed cranial vault, shallow orbits with exorbitism, and midface retrusion that is manifest as nasopharyngeal airway narrowing and severe dental malocclusion. Examples of such syndromes include Apert's (craniosynostosis, exorbitism, midface hypoplasia, and complex syndactylies) and Crouzon's (similar to Apert's syndrome but without syndactyly). When premature skull fusion is documented, surgical correction is performed in conjunction with a neurosurgeon. This involves removing the involved portion of the skull, reshaping the skull, and replacing the reshaped portion with resorbable plates and screws; best outcomes are obtained when this surgery is carried out before 1 year of age.[34] Other conditions that may require craniofacial surgery include facial clefts that extend beyond the lip and palate, hemifacial microsomia, and various rare craniofacial syndromes.

Maxillofacial surgery addresses dental occlusion with selective osteotomies of facial bones. Preoperative management usually involves cephalometric analysis of the facial skeleton as it relates to dentition. Preoperative orthodontic alignment of the teeth with dental models is also necessary. When the maxilla is implicated, a maxillary osteotomy (Le Fort I osteotomy) can be performed to advance or impact the maxilla with its dentition.[35] Likewise, the mandible can be osteotomized with its intact dentition to restore centric or normal occlusion.[36] Similar procedures can be used to address facial asymmetry.

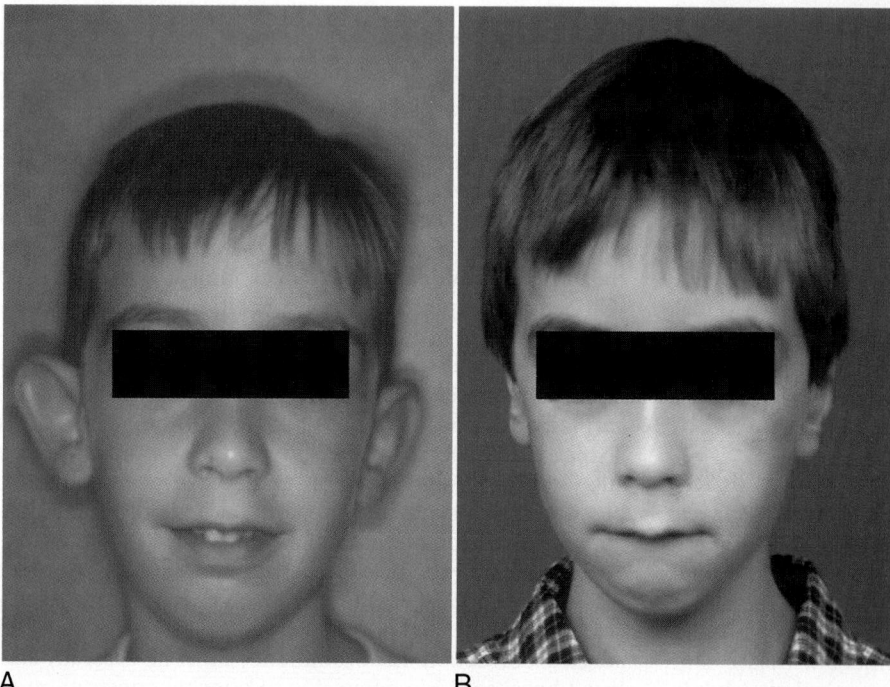

FIGURE 72-12. **A,** Preoperative view of 7-year-old boy with prominent ears. **B,** Postoperative view 3 months after otoplasty.

A   B

Trauma

Facial soft tissue injuries are frequently encountered in the emergency department. Common etiologies include abrasions, lacerations, blast injuries, and human or animal bites. For more severe injuries, a trauma evaluation is mandatory with establishment of a secure airway and cervical spine clearance prior to management of the facial injury.[37] Patients with extensive facial bony fractures deserve special attention because traumatic edema and intraoral bleeding can quickly compromise the airway as occurs with bilateral subcondylar mandible fractures. Radiologic evaluation is mandatory to rule out bony fractures. Physical examination should include careful attention to facial nerve (cranial nerve VII) function and parotid duct integrity. Foreign bodies should be removed and the wound irrigated, but radical débridement of damaged tissue is never indicated because facial soft tissues have an exceptional blood supply. Meticulous reapproximation of the anatomy should be undertaken as soon as the patient's general medical condition allows. This includes careful realignment of the eyebrows, eyelids, and vermilion border of the lips. When possible, facial wounds should be irrigated and closed within 8 hours of the injury. Primary closure may be delayed up to 24 hours if the wounds are irrigated, sterile dressings are applied, and antibiotics are instituted. Tetanus prophylaxis should be administered. Treatment of dog and cat bites usually includes a single antibiotic (e.g., amoxicillin or doxycycline), but for human bites, a second antibiotic aimed at anaerobic coverage should be prescribed.

Common fractures of the facial skeleton include nasal fractures, mandible fractures, zygomatic complex, maxilla (Le Fort I to III), naso-orbital-ethmoid complex (NOE), and frontal sinus fractures. Nasal fractures are the most common facial fractures. The diagnosis is most frequently made clinically and radiographic study offers little added value. On physical examination, it is mandatory to assess the nasal septum for a possible septal hematoma; an undrained septal hematoma can result in necrosis and erosion of the nasal septum. Most nasal fractures can be treated with closed reduction and splinting including intranasal packing.[38] Postoperatively, these patients should be covered with appropriate antibiotics because toxic shock syndrome has been reported with intranasal packing. NOE fractures are the result of a high-energy impact. These patients classically present with a complex nasal fracture including a saddle-nose deformity, a wide nasal root with loss of anterior projection, and telecanthus (wide interpupillary distance resulting from a fracture of the medial orbital wall and ethmoids with displacement of the medial canthal tendons laterally).[39] NOE fractures can involve damage to the nasolacrimal duct that can be repaired over a stent. In addition, care must be taken to accurately reposition the medial canthal tendons and restore nasal projection.

Fractures of the frontal sinus are most frequently seen in association with NOE fractures. In such injuries, damage to the nasofrontal duct and posterior wall of the frontal sinus must be identified.[40,41] Where nasofrontal duct injury is missed, duct obstruction and future muco-cele may occur. When recognized, obliteration of the sinus remains the mainstay of treatment. Cerebrospinal fluid rhinorrhea indicates fracture involvement of the posterior wall of the frontal sinus; in this case, neurosurgical comanagement is essential. Selection of a proper surgical plan takes into account the forehead deformity, potential for nasofrontal duct obstruction, and evidence of breached bony confines of the anterior cranial fossa.

Midface fractures involving the zygoma and maxilla often result in loss of facial height and symmetry. Facial height and projection depend on a complex bony buttressing system.[42] These buttresses represent the thickest bony supports for the facial skeleton. In the vertical dimension, the nasomaxillary, zygomaticomaxillary, and pterygomaxillary buttresses maintain facial height. Anterior projection of the face is maintained by the horizontal buttresses: the mandible, palate, orbital rims, and frontal bar. The primary goals of repairing midface fractures are restoration of facial height, projection, and symmetry. Once the fractures are anatomically reduced, plates and screws placed across the buttresses allow for rigid union.[43]

Fractures of the zygoma, or malar bone, are known as *zygomatic complex fractures*. Because of the zygoma's anatomic contribution to the bony orbit, these patients present with eye findings such as periorbital ecchymosis, subconjunctival hemorrhage, paresthesia of the infraorbital nerve, tenderness at the infraorbital rim, and enophthalmos.[44] Axial and coronal view computed tomographic (CT) imaging is the most valuable study for assessing the damage. Classically, these fractures involve the lateral orbital wall (zygomaticofrontal region), infraorbital rim, zygomaticomaxillary buttress, and zygomatic arch. Surgical reduction and plate fixation is challenging—the three-dimensional spatial relationships must be anatomically perfect since volumetric changes within the orbit may cause permanent double vision, and enophthalmos may result.[45,46] Isolated zygomatic arch fractures can be approached by incising below the deep temporal fascia and placing a lever below the fractured arch to lift the depressed segment (i.e., the Gillies approach). For fractures involving the orbital floor, indications for surgical exploration include diplopia, extraocular muscle entrapment, and enophthalmos.[47] Orbital injury that affects the superior orbital fissure is a surgical emergency. The set of nerve palsies resulting is called *superior orbital fissure syndrome*: eyelid ptosis, globe proptosis, motionless globe (cranial nerve III, IV, and VI paralyses), and ophthalmic division (cranial nerve V_1) anesthesia.[48] If blindness is seen in addition to these findings, the term *orbital apex syndrome* is used.[49]

Midface fractures involving the maxilla can be classified by fracture patterns know as Le Fort I, II, and III (Fig. 72-13).[50] These patterns also represent progressive gradation of severity and reflect increasing causal impact energies. Le Fort I fractures traverse the maxilla horizontally at the level of the piriform rim. Le Fort II fractures involve the nasofrontal junction, the nasal process of the maxilla, medial portion of the inferior orbital rim, and across the anterior maxilla. Le Fort III fractures refer to complete disjunction of the facial skeleton from the skull base.

Le Fort I level

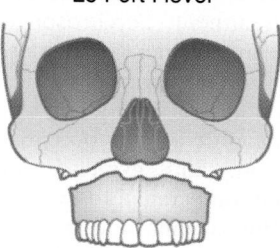

Le Fort III level

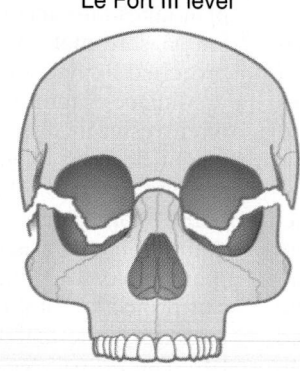

Le Fort II level

■ **FIGURE 72-13.**   Representation of facial fractures at the Le Fort I, II, and III levels. (From manson PN: Facial injuries. *In* McCarthy JG [ed]: Plastic Surgery, Vol. 2, The Face. Philadelphia, Saunders, 1990, pp 867-1141.)

Operative reduction of maxillary fractures begins with placement of arch bars to the maxillary and mandibular dentition. The dentition is then brought into normal occlusion before the fractures are plated. This procedure, known as interdental or intermaxillary (IMF) fixation, is necessary to re-establish the proper dentoskeletal relationships, immobilize the fractured bones, and ensure normal postoperative occlusion. Facial buttresses are then plated to restore normal facial height and projection.[51]

Mandible fractures are second only to nasal fractures in frequency. Because the mandible is the largest and strongest of the facial bones, the force required to fracture the mandible can also damage the cervical spine. Cervical spine clearance is recommended as up to a 10% coincident of cervical spine trauma is reported in association with mandible fractures.[37,52] In addition, the airway can be compromised in patients with bilateral subcondylar mandible fractures because support for the posterior oropharynx is lost. Recommended radiographic evaluation of a mandible fracture includes a panoramic radiograph (Panorex) and Towne's view radiograph. As in midface fractures, restoration of dental occlusion forms the foundation for fracture management. IMF prior to fracture exposure and plating is necessary. Most mandibular fractures can be plated using intraoral incisions.[53] If necessary, a small stab incision can be made for a percutaneous approach to the fracture. This technique, which requires intraoral exposure and an externally placed trocar, eliminates the need for a larger external incision. If an external incision is necessary, care must be taken to avoid trauma to the marginal mandibular branch of the facial nerve. Many patients with mandibular fractures experience trauma to the inferior alveolar nerve (a branch of the trigeminal nerve), which runs through a canal within the body of the mandible and terminates in the lower lip as the mental nerve. These patients may experience permanent numbness of the lower lip and teeth on the affected side. Fractures of the coronoid process of the mandible can result in trismus (inability to open the mouth) as the coronoid process normally passes beneath the zygomatic arch with mouth opening. Condylar and subcondylar mandible fractures are most often treated by IMF alone.[54] Surgical exposure of the temporomandibular joint places the facial nerve at risk and exposes the joint to possible injury and dysfunction. Medical management of mandibular fractures involves a puree-type diet, interdental fixation for several weeks, 1% chlorhexidine mouth rinses, and antibiotics.

Facial Nerve Palsy

The facial nerve, cranial nerve VII, is responsible for innervating muscles of facial expression (mimetic muscles). Facial expression is a unique trait of each individual and loss of facial nerve function is psychologically and functionally problematic. Facial nerve anatomy is complex and oftentimes variable.[55] Detailed knowledge of facial nerve anatomy is paramount in facial surgery to avoid iatrogenic injury. There are five distinct branches of the facial nerve: frontal (temporal), zygomatic, buccal, marginal mandibular, and cervical. After the facial nerve exits the stylomastoid foramen, it can branch in a variety of patterns (Fig. 72-14). Despite differing arborization patterns, the branches are always found in precise anatomic planes.[56] Therefore, a three-dimensional understanding of facial nerve anatomy is essential to identify or protect a nerve branch. For example, the frontal branch of the facial nerve travels in the superficial temporal fascia.[57] Dissecting in planes superficial or deep to this layer protects the frontal branch. The buccal, zygomatic, and marginal mandibular branches travel just deep to the superficial musculoaponeurotic system (SMAS) after traversing the substance of the parotid gland and emerging from its anterior

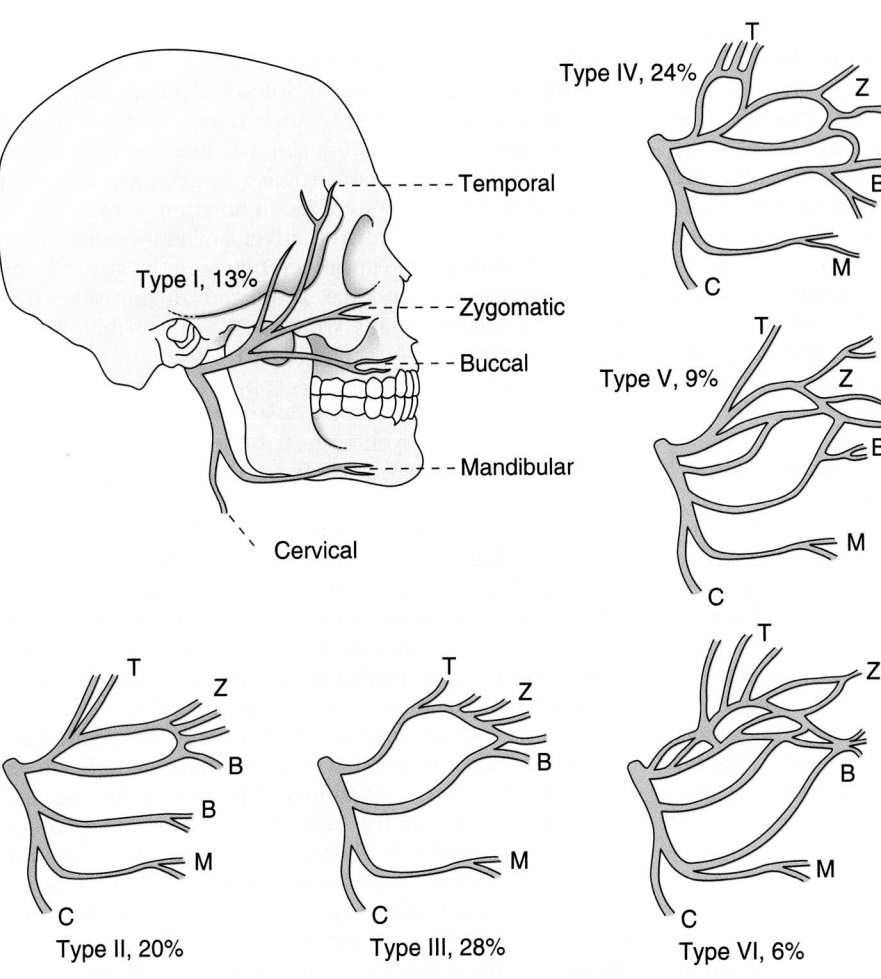

FIGURE 72-14. Facial nerve anatomy and common branching patterns. (From May M: The Facial Nerve. New York, Thieme, 1986, p 55.)

Type IV, 24%

Type I, 13%

- - - - Temporal

- - - - Zygomatic

- - Buccal

- - - Mandibular

Cervical

Type V, 9%

Type II, 20%

Type III, 28%

Type VI, 6%

border. Dissecting superficial to this layer protects these facial nerve branches.

The most common cause of facial paralysis is Bell's palsy. In most cases it is idiopathic and occurs in 1 in 5000 individuals per year in the United States.[58] Bell's palsy is commonly associated with pregnancy and diabetes mellitus. Most patients with Bell's palsy have a complete remission, but the chance for remission decreases with age. Bell's palsy is commonly treated with corticosteroids in an effort to reduce nerve edema and restore normal circulation.[59] Surgical decompression of the nerve within the bony facial canal is reserved for cases refractory to conservative measures.[60]

Trauma in the form of temporal bone fractures or deep facial lacerations is the second most frequent cause of facial palsy. When possible, immediate exploration and primary repair of the facial nerve affords the best chance to regain nerve function.[61] When this is not possible because of a nerve gap, then nerve grafting should be attempted.[62] When this is not possible, cross-face nerve grafting may be indicated[63]; here, a minor branch of the nerve on the normal side is sectioned, and the proximal end of this branch is then anastomosed to the distal nerve end on the paralyzed side with the use of nerve grafts. Other alternatives include muscles transfers, such as the temporalis or masseter muscles, to provide motion to the

corner of the mouth. Free innervated tissue transfer has been successful using the gracilis muscle.[64] For elderly and very ill patients, static procedures can be implemented. These include gold implants in the upper eyelid with tightening of the lower lid to allow eyelid closure. Tensor fascia lata and dermis grafts offer autogenous donor sources that can be used to statically suspend the corner of the mouth. Although techniques to re-establish facial balance in repose are largely successful, obtaining facial symmetry with animation has remained an elusive outcome.

TRUNK AND EXTERNAL GENITALIA

Chest Wall Reconstruction

Chest wall defects most frequently occur as a consequence of ablative tumor resection or from extensive trauma. The resulting defects range from soft tissue only to complex defects involving skin, muscle, and bone. Simple defects involving only soft tissue can be skin grafted. However, more complex defects usually require flap reconstruction. For example, advanced cases of breast cancer mandate extensive resection of skin and muscle;

in such cases then, simple solutions such as primary closure or skin grafting may not be possible. In addition, where postoperative radiation is planned, skin graft coverage is a poor choice because radiation changes and breakdown are predictable. In these patients, choice of a myocutaneous flap brings vascularized tissue into the defect to cover exposed ribs and provides healthy tissue that can sustain postoperative radiation. Larger defects, larger than 10 cm with loss of more than three adjacent ribs, can risk flail chest with attendant compromised respiratory function.[65] To prevent this outcome, skeletal integrity can be restored using autogenous split rib grafts or alloplastic material such as polypropylene mesh.[66] Once again, muscle or myocutaneous flaps are called on to provide final coverage over this defect.

Wound infection and dehiscence occur in approximately 2% of median sternotomies and increase morbidity for cardiothoracic patients. These wounds can be successfully managed with removal of sternal wires, generous débridement of necrotic bone and cartilage, culture-based antimicrobial therapy, and flap closure.[67] In addition to providing soft tissue coverage, a muscle flap also recruits much-needed blood supply to the area to assist in healing and controlling infection. Muscle flaps most frequently used for closure of sternal wounds include the pectoralis major or rectus abdominis. Release of sternal wire fixation has not been shown to result in chest wall instability and is generally well tolerated.

Breast Reconstruction

Breast cancer is the most common malignant neoplasm in women, affecting approximately 1 in 8 women in the United States.[68] Although the loss of a breast can be a psychologically devastating reality, the opportunity to reconstruct the breast is rewarding for both the plastic surgeon and the patient. Since it has been conclusively shown that postmastectomy reconstruction does not adversely influence survival outcomes or recurrence rates, preoperative consultation should be offered to all women desiring breast reconstruction, and the option of not reconstructing the breast should also be discussed.[69]

With rare exception, the nipple-areolar complex (NAC) is excised with the breast. After removal of the breast, there is usually only enough skin to close the defect over a flat chest wall. The reconstructive surgeon must account for this deficient skin envelope in an attempt to re-create the breast mound. With the advent of immediate breast reconstruction, a team approach between the ablative and reconstructive surgeon has produced an improved aesthetic outcome for many women. When possible, a skin-sparing mastectomy is performed so as to provide a sufficient skin envelope to support a reconstructed breast.[70] Immediate breast reconstruction has been shown be safe, and the psychological benefit of waking from anesthesia with a reconstructed breast mound cannot be underestimated.

The simplest form of breast reconstruction is tissue expansion followed by placement of permanent breast implants (Fig. 72-15).[71] A tissue expander is an inflatable silicone bag that contains an integrated or remote port for access during expansion using injectable saline. This implant is placed beneath a muscular pocket created using the pectoralis major muscle superiorly and medially and the serratus muscle inferiorly and laterally. These muscles are raised from the chest wall and sutured together over the uninflated tissue expander. The skin is closed and allowed to heal over the next 2 to 3 weeks. Inflation of the tissue expander is performed weekly until a volume slightly larger than desired is reached. The skin is allowed to remodel for several weeks. In a separate procedure, the expander is exchanged for a permanent breast implant. Tissue expansion has the benefit of a relatively short procedure, limiting other body scars, and no sacrifice of muscle to support a flap. Drawbacks include difficulty creating natural breast ptosis, capsular contracture, weekly office visits for expansion, and the need for a second procedure. This is the most popular mode of breast reconstruction.

The breast mound can be created using myocutaneous flaps such as the transverse rectus abdominis myocuta-

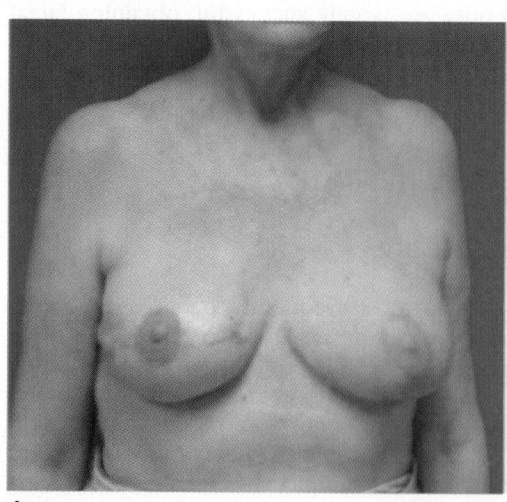
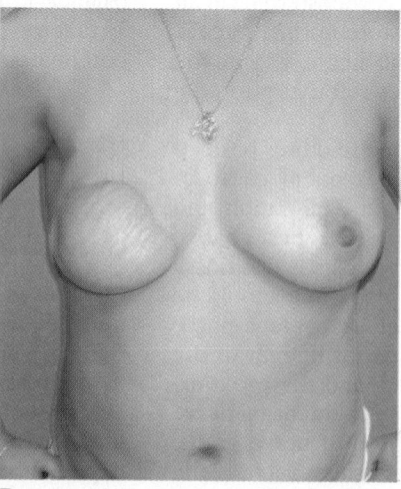

FIGURE 72-15. **A,** A 63-year-old woman after right mastectomy with tissue expander followed by implant reconstruction, right nipple reconstruction with tattooing of the nipple-areolar complex, and contralateral full-scar mastopexy. **B,** A 43-year-old woman after right mastectomy with autologous tissue reconstruction with a transverse rectus abdominis myocutaneous flap.

A   B

neous (TRAM) flap (see Fig. 72-15) or the latissimus dorsi myocutaneous flap. The TRAM flap uses the infraumbilical and suprapubic fat that derives its blood supply from the underlying rectus abdominis muscle. This flap may be executed in a pedicled fashion based on the superior epigastric vessels.[72] This technique can leave the patient with a bothersome epigastric bulge. Using microvascular technique, the TRAM flap can be transferred as a free flap based on the deep inferior epigastric vessels that are anastomosed to branches of the thoracodorsal in the axilla or the internal mammaries at the sternocostal junction.[73] Free TRAM flaps have been shown to have a more robust blood supply than pedicled TRAM flaps and can be used in patients who smoke. Advantages of the TRAM flap include ability to create a natural breast appearance that contains a generous volume of autogenous fat, virtually identical to the resected breast. In addition, many women like the flattened appearance of their abdomen, which is similar to that achieved with abdominoplasty. Drawbacks to the TRAM flap include a longer operative time, a visible scar on the lower abdomen, and a slight weakening of the abdominal wall. Recently, free TRAM flaps have been performed using perforating vessels from the rectus muscle. These flaps, known as *perforator flaps*, spare the rectus muscle, thereby eliminating weakness in the abdominal wall.

The latissimus dorsi muscle can be used with a skin paddle to make up for the deficient skin envelope after mastectomy. Based on the thoracodorsal vessels, this method of reconstruction commonly requires placement of a small breast implant beneath the flap to achieve adequate size.[74] Natural breast appearance and ptosis can be achieved in a single procedure using the latissimus dorsi flap. Implants covered by the latissimus dorsi muscle undergo less capsular contracture following postoperative radiation treatment as compared with primary expander/implant reconstructions as mentioned earlier. Disadvantages include sacrifice of the latissimus dorsi muscle, a wide scar on the back, and difficult operative positioning. In addition to breast reconstruction, the latissimus dorsi is commonly relied on for other chest wall reconstructive needs.

The contralateral breast should always be considered as part of the total reconstructive procedure. When needed, reduction mammaplasty or mastopexy should be performed to match the reconstructed breast. At times, breast augmentation may be necessary if the reconstructed breast is larger. Nipple reconstruction using local flaps and tattooing of the NAC are performed after the breast mound reconstruction has been completed. Using these techniques, a natural-appearing breast mound can be created and symmetry can be restored.

Abdominal Wall Reconstruction

The abdominal wall is a complex structure strengthened by a precise arrangement of abdominal wall musculature and fascia. Abdominal wall defects are frequently encountered and may or may not include a hernia component. Prosthetic fabrics such as polytetrafluoroethylene and polypropylene are widely used to span preperitoneal defects.[75] Exposure of such alloplastic material results in the harboring of bacteria in the interstices of the mesh fabric.[76] In the case of infection, the mesh must be removed and the infection cleared before closure is attempted. Temporary (interim) closure is often achieved using autogenous skin graft placed directly on the well-vascularized bowel serosa.[77] Final and permanent closure requires fascial, muscular, and skin reconstruction. Lower abdominal defects can be closed using a tensor fascia lata or rectus femoris flap. Large abdominal hernias, which have failed mesh repair, may be amenable to closure by component separation.[78,79] In this procedure, muscular layers of the abdominal wall are meticulously separated and allowed to slide, making mobilization possible to cover large defects. Postoperative issues of increased intra-abdominal pressure and respiratory insufficiency can be expected and appropriate ventilator support might be required for a while. To foster uneventful healing and maintenance of the repair integrity, use of an abdominal binder or compression garment and avoidance of strenuous activity are necessary.

Pressure Sores

One of the most costly problems in modern medicine is pressure sores that are derived from prolonged immobility. Spinal cord injuries with paralysis, elderly nursing home patients, and severely ill intensive care patients represent patient groups most commonly at risk for pressure sores. Prevention of pressure sore formation requires a high level of patient compliance and support from ancillary staff. Given today's economic environment and nursing shortage, this level of care is frequently not available for these high-demand patients. Prevention of pressure sores requires pressure relief in the form of specialized mattresses and wheelchair cushions combined with manually moving the patient. Skin should be kept clean and dry.

Pressure sores commonly occur over pressure-bearing surfaces such as the occipital scalp, elbows, heels, iliac crests, greater trochanters, ischial tuberosities, and sacrum.[80] Pressure sores result from tissue ischemia occurring from prolonged pressure exceeding capillary arterial pressure of 32 mm Hg. In the supine position, pressure of 40 to 60 mm Hg occurs over the occiput, sacrum, and heel. In the sitting position, pressures of 100 mm Hg occur over the ischial tuberosities.[81] Constant pressure applied for 2 hours can result in muscle necrosis.

Numerous grading schemes have been devised to classify pressure sores (Box 72-2). The simplest involves four grades: grade I (skin erythema), grade II (skin ulceration with necrosis into subcutaneous tissue), grade III (necrosis involving the underlying muscle), and grade IV (exposed bone/joint).[80] On inspection, a pressure sore usually appears much smaller than it actually is. This occurs because deeper tissues adjacent to bone are exposed to higher pressure than the cutaneous tissue. The deep (muscle) layer is more susceptible to ischemic insult than the overlying fat or skin.[82] Surgical débridement discloses the true extent of pressure-induced injury.

Box 72-2. Classification System for Pressure Ulcers

Stage I: Nonblanchable erythema of intact skin; impending skin ulceration

Stage II: Partial-thickness skin loss involving epidermis and/or dermis; ulcer is superficial and presents clinically as an abrasion, blister, or shallow crater

Stage III: Full-thickness skin loss involving damage or necrosis of subcutaneous tissue that may extend down to, but not through, underlying fascia; ulcer presents clinically as a deep crater with or without undermining of adjacent tissue

Stage IV: Full-thickness skin loss with extensive destruction, tissue necrosis, or damage to muscle, bone, or supporting structures

---

Treatment of these wounds requires a multidisciplinary approach with focus on prevention of reoccurrence. Initially, a pressure sore should be débrided of nonviable tissue to include quantitative microbiologic testing. Antibiotic therapy should be culture based with the knowledge that wounds with more than 10^5 organisms per gram of living tissue are infected and will not heal. Wound care should be initiated with appropriate topical antimicrobials. The patient should be given a pressure-relieving mattress and seat cushion, and the caregiver should be instructed to turn the patient a minimum of every 2 hours. The nutritional status of the patient must be assessed, including nutrition consultation and serum protein and albumin levels. Nutritionally depleted patients cannot heal their wounds regardless of the quality of care.

Surgical closure of these wounds involves flap closure to pad bony prominences, and myocutaneous flaps may be chosen to recruit blood supply to the wound.[83] Unfortunately, numerous studies have demonstrated that most surgically closed wounds eventually reoccur.[84] For those who are ambulatory, surgical closure should never compromise the patient's ability to mobilize. Most ambulatory patients heal with good local wound care, nutritional support, and avoidance of pressure.

The recent advent of VAC devices has dramatically improved the outcomes for many of these difficult wounds.[85] Using a specialized suction apparatus applied over a sponge and occlusive dressing, VAC therapy can shrink these wounds and stimulate the formation of granulation tissue and healing by secondary intention without the need for flap surgery closure. This form of therapy is notably proprietary and requires the use of a specialized device and additionally trained health care personnel. However, many third-party payers have come to accept VAC therapy as a cost-effective means of managing these wounds.

External Genitalia

Deformities of the external genitalia can be congenital or secondary to trauma, neoplastic defects, and infections.

For those infants with ambiguous external genitalia, gender reassignment (usually female) should be done by 18 months of age. Causes of ambiguous genitalia include hormonal imbalance (congenital adrenal hyperplasia), maternal drug use, and hermaphroditism. Of primary importance in gender reassignment is functional anatomic potential with lesser consideration given to potential fertility and karyotype.

Following cutaneous avulsion injury to the male genitalia, a temporizing measure of burying the penis and testes in adjacent soft tissues of the upper thigh allows salvage until permanent reconstruction is possible. Both the penile shaft and testes are amenable to split-thickness skin graft coverage. If the injury is sharp in nature, the penis can be replanted using microvascular technique. Total penile reconstruction is complex because of the need to re-establish both external and internal (urethral) function. Urethral reconstruction can be accomplished with free grafts of buccal mucosa or glabrous skin. The standard for penile shaft reconstruction is the free radial forearm flap microvascular transfer. Penile rigidity can be obtained using either an external device or an implanted prosthesis. Vaginal reconstruction performed by plastic surgeons is most often accomplished using pudendal groin flaps or skin grafts.[86]

Infections in the groin region can be problematic. Hidradenitis suppurativa results from chronic infection of apocrine sweat glands. Incision and drainage or wide excision are often necessary in addition to culture directed antibiotic therapy to reduce the bacterial load in these wounds. Skin graft success to cover these wounds can be compromised if infection is incompletely controlled and if the skin grafts are in adequately immobilized areas. Fournier's gangrene is a mixed aerobic and anaerobic infection that spreads rapidly along fascial planes. Diabetic patients are particularly susceptible. Radical surgical débridement and jet lavage irrigation are mandatory in addition to antibiotic therapy. Patients so affected frequently require serial operating room sessions for débridement before the wound bed is deemed ready for definitive wound coverage. Once the infection is controlled, closure is achieved with skin grafts or local flaps.

LOWER EXTREMITY

Trauma

Trauma to the lower extremity is frequently complex and can require a team of specialists to include orthopedic, plastic, and vascular surgery disciplines to deliver all the care needs. Re-establishment of normal or near-normal ambulation in a sensate extremity is the goal in lower extremity trauma. Patients presenting with traumatic injuries to the lower extremity frequently have other life-threatening injuries mandating strict adherence to Advanced Trauma Life Support protocol. Of foremost concern should be ensuring good vascular supply to the affected extremity. Fasciotomy is often required to prevent ischemic changes in muscle and nerve tissues following high-energy or crush injuries. When necessary, revascularization by primary repair or bypass grafting can salvage a compromised extremity.[87] Degloved tissue should be conservatively débrided and its viability carefully assessed clinically or with the aid of intravenous fluorescein testing whereby cutaneous survival can be predicted. Copious jet lavage irrigation should always accompany initial débridement. Thigh injuries can generally be managed with delayed primary closure or skin grafting alone. Extensive soft tissue loss may require local flap reconstruction to cover exposed bone, blood vessels, or nerves; several local muscle flaps or myocutaneous flaps are typically available to address such exposures.

Lower leg trauma is more complex due the paucity of tissue surrounding the anterior tibia. Fractures of the lower leg are most often classified according to the Gustilo system (Table 72-2).[87] The proximal third of the lower leg including the knee joint is amenable to closure using the medial or lateral head of the gastrocnemius muscle.[88] Defects involving the middle third of the lower leg can be closed using a pedicled soleus muscle flap with or without addition of the flexor digitorum longus muscle as well.[87] Distal third defects, those defects above the ankle, are problematic and not infrequently necessitate free tissue transfer to provide adequate soft tissue coverage with a reliable blood supply.[89] Foot wounds can often be closed with local flaps such as the sural artery island flap for heel defects.[90]

Venous Stasis, Ischemic, and Diabetic Ulcers

Lower extremity ulcers may have a similar appearance but often have differing etiologies and treatment needs. Treatment success and healing depend on proper identification of the underlying problem, good wound hygiene, and surgical intervention that addresses all the pathologic issues.

Venous stasis ulcers result from venous hypertension that is usually caused by valvular incompetence. These ulcers are characteristically present over the medial malleolus and are usually nontender but may be associated with pruritus. Other typical findings include increased lower extremity edema and hyperpigmentation in the adjacent skin resulting from increased hemosiderin deposition. Treatment regimens focus on increasing venous return

and decreasing edema. Compression stockings or wraps combined with frequent elevation of the extremity and avoidance of prolonged standing are commonly prescribed.[91] The wound should be kept clean by washing, and judicious use of topical antimicrobials should be instituted. Either surgical or enzymatic débridement of nonviable tissue acts to facilitate wound healing. It is important that arterial inflow be checked using noninvasive Doppler studies that record the ankle/brachial index (ABI). Compression techniques should be avoided for those patients with an ABI less than 0.8 because vascular compromise may ensue.

Ischemic lower extremity ulcers are due to arterial insufficiency from proximal arterial occlusion. These are typically painful, punched out in appearance, demonstrate minimal edema, and have no change in surrounding pigmentation. They are typically located in a more distal location than venous ulcers, such as the lateral aspects of the great and fifth toes, as well as the dorsum of the foot. These ulcers indicate advanced peripheral vascular disease and are associated with very low ABI readings (between 0.1 and 0.3). Typically, these ulcers do not heal without surgical revascularization of the extremity.[92] Once revascularized, these wounds can be expected to heal with either simple wound care or skin grafting.

Diabetic ulcers commonly result from decreased protective sensation. Diabetic peripheral neuropathy is common in the hands and feet (stocking-and-glove distribution).[93] Diabetic ulcers are usually found on the plantar surface of the foot over the metatarsal heads or heel. Edema is usually mild with no change in surrounding pigmentation. Treatment is focused on preventing further damage to the area with devices such as custom-fitted orthopedic shoes to eliminate pressure over the metatarsal heads. Necrotic tissue must be judiciously débrided, and topical antimicrobials are needed to control local infection. In some cases, resection of the underlying bony prominence may improve wound healing. Diabetic patients must be educated to examine their feet routinely. This is paramount to prevent recurrence of these problematic wounds.

Lymphedema

Lymphedema is an accumulation of protein and fluid in the subcutaneous tissue. Functional disability and gross disfigurement can occur. Congenital lymphedema is seen in 10% of cases. When the condition presents first in early puberty, it is called *lymphedema praecox*. Lymphedema tarda is congenital lymphedema that becomes manifest only in middle age. The most common cause of secondary lymphedema in developed nations is resection of regional nodal basins for cancer. In subtropical and tropical underdeveloped nations, filariasis accounts for the primary etiology of secondary lymphedema. Treatment of lymphedema is difficult and often frustrating for both patient and surgeon alike. Nonoperative management includes compression garments or intermittent compression machines, elevation of the affected extremity, antiparasitic medications where appropriate, and systemic

Type	Description
TABLE 72-2.	**Gustilo Classification of Open Fractures of the Tibia**
I	Open fracture with a wound < 1 cm
II	Open fracture with a wound > 1 cm without extensive soft tissue damage
III	Open fracture with extensive soft tissue damage
IIIA	III with adequate soft tissue coverage
IIIB	III with soft tissue loss with periosteal stripping and bone exposure
IIIC	III with arterial injury requiring repair

antibiotics to treat recurrent bouts of cellulitis.[94] Surgical techniques offer only symptomatic relief, and there is no procedure that reliably produces a cure. The most common procedures include circumferential excision and skin grafting,[95] serial excision of subcutaneous tissues, or serial liposuction reduction[96] of the subcutaneous tissues. Microlymphatic bypass has been attempted but has met with only marginal success. The postoperative leg deformities can be nearly as grotesque as the presenting swelling; however, functional improvement with both decreased weight of the affected extremity and reduced cutaneous infection incidence offers net gains in quality of life.

BREAST AND AESTHETIC SURGERY

Because plastic surgery is a specialty that deals with outwardly visible concerns, the psychological state of a patient must be considered. In this specialty, where outward appearance remains a benchmark for success, it is necessary to maintain an objective but compassionate perspective. It is difficult to put an accurate value on a patient's self esteem. As humans, our psyche is intimately related to our perception of the way we appear to those around us. Although cosmetic or aesthetic surgery is medically unnecessary, its importance to the overall well-being of patients cannot be underestimated. Patient selection is paramount, and realistic postoperative outcomes should be carefully explained.

Elective breast surgery addresses both functional and aesthetic concerns. Breasts can be reduced, enlarged, or lifted to produce a more normal appearance. Macromastia (abnormally large breasts) is a functionally difficult and psychologically devastating problem for some women (Fig. 72-16). From a functional standpoint, macromastia can result in neck and back pain, painful bra-strap shoulder grooving, inframammary intertrigo, and difficulty finding appropriate clothing. Breast reduction surgery (reduction mammaplasty) involves moving the nipple and areola to a position on the chest wall opposite the infra-

mammary fold. The NAC may remain attached to the native underlying breast or in gigantomastia (extremely large breasts) may be transferred as a full-thickness graft. The keyhole pattern represents the most popular incisional design to achieve the desired recontouring. Alterations in nipple sensation and compromised ability to breast-feed infants may be experienced. Despite these potential risks, most patients are happily relieved from both the discomfort and psychological concerns associated with abnormally large breasts.[97]

For men, the problem of large breasts (gynecomastia) also can be psychologically devastating. Most adolescents experience some degree of breast tissue enlargement. However, if this does not resolve by the late teens or early 20s, surgery may be indicated. Breast cancer can occur in men, and suspicious masses (hard, unilateral, or nodular) should undergo biopsy. Gynecomastia can be due to abnormal hormone levels, so endocrine system assessment is advisable. Most cases of gynecomastia are amenable to simple liposuction with minimal glandular resection through a periareolar incision as necessary. Redundant skin will usually redrape over the chest in a cosmetically acceptable manner, thereby limiting the need for skin resection to extreme cases only.[98]

On the opposite extreme, many women suffer from concern surrounding abnormally small breasts (micromastia) (Fig. 72-17). For appropriate candidates, breast augmentation can restore a feminine ideal of sexual attractiveness. Breast augmentation is usually accomplished through discrete incisions placed around the areola, at the inframammary fold, or in the axilla. Breast implant volume is determined by a woman's breast diameter. Most breast implants are constructed of a silicone envelope that is filled with sterile saline. Silicone-filled breast implants are now used only by select centers and physicians to reconstruct mastectomy defects and for exchange of previous silicone-filled implants. Breast implants can be inserted above or below the pectoralis major muscle. The decision of which approach to use factors in any need to better camouflage the implant, associated breast ptosis, and both physician and patient preference.[99]

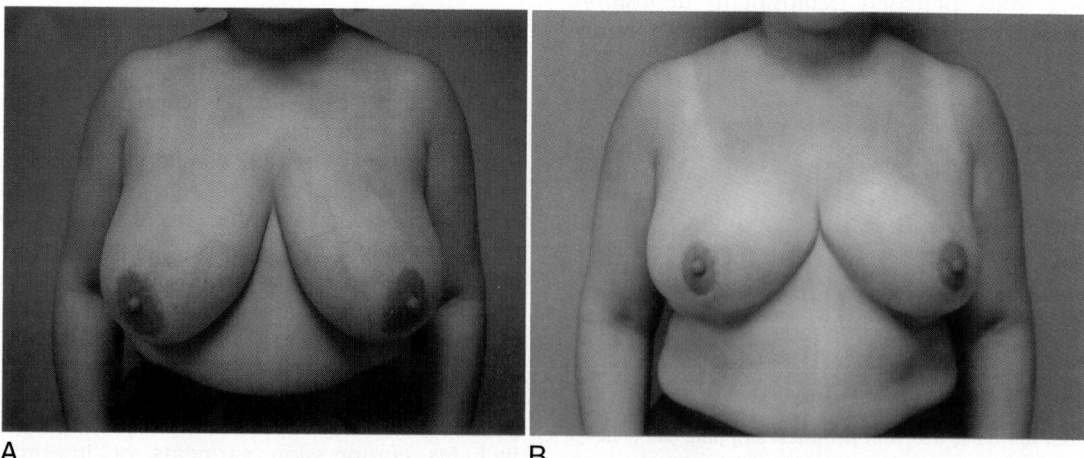

A   B

■ **FIGURE 72-16.** A 35-year-old woman with macromastia (**A**) and after reduction mammaplasty (**B**) using an inferior pedicle with Wise (keyhole) pattern.

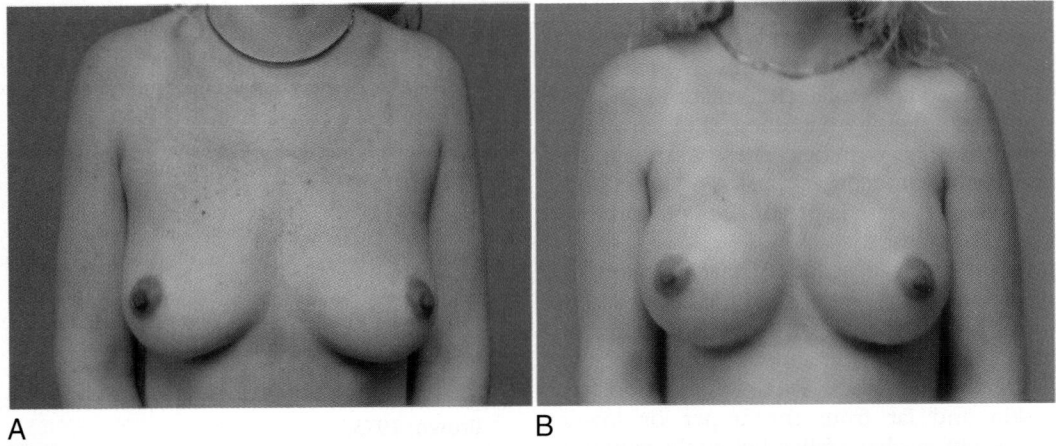

FIGURE 72-17. **A,** Preoperative view of a 28-year-old G0P0 woman. **B,** Postoperative view 6 months after a bilateral submuscular augmentation mammaplasty through an inflammatory approach.

With age and childbearing, breasts sag below the level of the inframammary crease, resulting in breast ptosis. Breast ptosis is graded based on the position of the NAC in relation to the inframammary crease. In addition, breasts may involute with childbearing and age, resulting in worsening ptosis. Breast ptosis is classified as grade I (NAC position at the level of the inframammary fold), grade II (NAC position below the inframammary fold), and grade III (NAC position well below the inframammary fold and pointing down).[100] The goal of breast lifting or mastopexy is to restore a normal position of the NAC in relation to the inframammary fold. For grade I ptosis, simple breast augmentation may restore upper-pole breast volume and also correct NAC position. For grades II and III ptosis, skin recontouring and NAC repositioning are necessary. Mastopexy incisions can involve a superior NAC incision (crescent mastopexy), circumareolar incision (donut mastopexy), or a keyhole incision that involves skin excision in the vertical and horizontal dimensions similar to the pattern used for breast reduction surgery. Some women may require a combination of both incisional recontouring (mastopexy) and implant placement (augmentation) to achieve the desired result.

Lipodystrophy, excess fatty deposits in distinct anatomic areas, and redundant skin can be addressed through suction-assisted lipectomy or excisional techniques, respectively. Body contouring involves creating a more ideal body shape given a patient's preoperative anatomy and goals. Many patients present complaining of an inability to lose fatty deposits in problem areas such as the infraumbilical region, hips, flanks, buttocks, thighs, and knees. Patients who are candidates for suction-assisted lipectomy have good skin turgor without abundant laxity or striae. Liposuction does not remedy cellulite. Following infiltration of a tumescent solution containing a dilute solution of local anesthetic with epinephrine, specialized hollow cannulas attached to tubing that connects to a vacuum aspirator device are used to extract the targeted areas of excess subcutaneous fat. Up to 30 mg/kg of lidocaine is typically injected first into the targeted areas to be liposuctioned. This is well tolerated because the solution contains epinephrine, which slows absorption and is injected directly into fat, which has a minimal blood supply. Although large-volume liposuction has been reported in the literature, the surgeon must be cautious because large intravascular fluid shifts may occur when volumes in excess of 5000 mL are aspirated.[101] Severe infections that spread along fascial planes can occur when sterile technique is compromised.

Excision techniques are necessary in cases where redundant skin, abundant striae, or ptotic changes are present. When this procedure is performed to address the upper inner arm, it is called *brachioplasty*, whereas for the upper inner thigh it is commonly referred to as a *thigh lift*. In the abdomen, when a patient presents with a hanging abdominal panniculus or if following weight loss or multiple pregnancies there is the problem of loose, hanging skin or lower abdominal stretch marks, the excisional procedure that addresses these issues is called *abdominoplasty*. Skin and fat are excised as a modified transverse ellipse from the lower abdomen, and an abdominal flap is raised to the costal margin laterally and the xiphoid centrally. The underlying fascia may be plicated to correct any diastasis between the paired rectus muscles. The umbilicus is left attached to its underlying vascular stalk and then relocated through a midline stab incision as the abdominal flap is closed devoid of the wrinkled infraumbilical and suprapubic skin and fat.

Facial rejuvenation is a complex area of plastic surgery requiring a detailed understanding of facial anatomy. Facial aging, although unavoidable, can be drastically hastened with sun exposure, smoking, and poor skin care. Facial aging is associated with increased facial wrinkles (rhytids), descent and loss of facial fat, as well as splotchy pigmentation. Skin care products that stimulate collagen, decrease sun (ultraviolet light) exposure, and smooth irregular pigmentation can be instituted early in the treatment process. Numerous nonsurgical methods exist to smooth facial rhytids and involve removing the epidermis and superficial dermis. These include nonablative laser treatments, chemical peels, and microdermabrasion. Recently, botulinum toxin (Botox) has been used to correct mild upper facial rhytids by temporarily paralyzing underlying hyperactive facial muscles, thereby decreasing fine skin wrinkles.[102] Ablative lasers (carbon dioxide laser) and deeper chemical peels (phenol) remove a layer of epidermis and superficial dermis, which heals by re-epithelialization and neocollagen formation. The net effect is a smoother, slightly tightened skin envelope with reduction in fine-line wrinkles. These more aggressive facial resurfacing procedures heal like a second-degree burn, so recovery time is prolonged compared to the nonablative techniques.

Problematic brow ptosis, descent of facial fat involving the nasolabial fold and jowls, and loss of the cervicomental angle requires a combination of browlift, facelift, or necklift. Isolated excesses of skin and fat in the upper or lower eyelids can be addressed with a blepharoplasty (excision of skin and fat from the upper or lower eyelids).[103] If the eyebrows have fallen below the superior orbital rim, a browlift is needed to bring the brow back to its normal position and rejuvenate the forehead region as well.[104] When facial or neck resuspension cannot be accomplished with nonsurgical means, a rhytidectomy or facelift should be considered. Using a combination temporal, preauricular, and postauricular incision, the facial skin with or without the underlying SMAS fascia is undermined, advanced, and finally secured to rid facial rhytids and sagging neck and resuspend facial fat. Sometimes, to maximize the refinement sought for recontouring the neck, additional liposuction and tightening by plication of the platysma muscle is necessary. These procedures alone or in combination are successful toward achieving a well-rested and more youthful facial appearance.[105]

Finally, nasal deformities can be corrected with rhinoplasty.[106] An open technique using a transcolumellar incision is preferred where moderate sculpting of the nasal alar cartilage is necessary and where septal surgery is needed at the same time. Alternatively, a closed approach using intranasal incisions can be used for more minor corrections. Careful preoperative assessment of the deformity and nasal airway is essential. Different techniques exist to shape the nose, including suture plication, cartilage resection, cartilage grafting, controlled fracturing of the nasal bones, and rasping of cartilage or bone. Nasal obstruction can be corrected by removing the offending buckle of a deviated septum and internally splinting the dorsal septum with a septal cartilage graft. Postoperative nasal packing is instilled to prevent hematomas, and antibiotics are given to prevent *Staphylococcus* infection. Postoperative nasal edema takes months to completely resolve, and revisional surgery should not be considered before a 12-month period has elapsed, because the distortion from postsurgical induration and swelling is not cleared before then.

CONCLUSION

Plastic surgery is an extremely diverse surgical specialty whose primary goal is to restore both form and function. Important areas of plastic surgery such as thermal injury, hand and upper extremity surgery, and wound care are covered in other chapters within this text. Herein, we have offered only a superficial overview of the realm of plastic surgery.

Selected References

Achauer B, Eriksson E, Vander Kolk C, et al (eds): Plastic Surgery: Indications, Operations, and Outcomes. St. Louis, Mosby, 2000.

A five-volume comprehensive text of plastic and reconstructive surgery.

Aston SJ, Beasley RW, Thorne CH (eds): Grabb and Smith's Plastic Surgery, 5th ed. Philadelphia, Lippincott-Raven, 1997.

A concise single-volume text of plastic and reconstructive surgery.

Borges A: Elective Incisions and Scar Revision. Boston, Little, Brown, 1973.

A concise review of designing elective incision and scar treatment, with particular attention to local flaps such as the Z-plasty.

Bostwick J: Plastic and Reconstructive Breast Surgery. St. Louis, Quality Medical, 2000.

An excellent single-authored text dedicated to aesthetic and reconstructive breast surgery.

Jackson IT: Local Flaps in Head and Neck Reconstruction. St. Louis, Mosby, 1985.

An excellent and concise overview of local flaps for head and neck reconstruction with clear visual explanations.

Mathes S, Nahai F: Reconstructive Surgery: Principles, Anatomy, and Technique. New York, Churchill Livingstone, 1997.

A clear and clinically relevant text dedicated to flap-based reconstructive surgery.

Millard D: Cleft Craft—The Evolution of Its Surgery. Boston, Little, Brown, 1976.

A comprehensive review of the history and techniques of cleft lip and palate surgery.

References

1. Ferraro J (ed): Fundamentals of Maxillofacial Surgery. New York, Springer-Verlag, 1997, p 207.
2. Borges AF: Relaxed skin tension lines (RSTL) versus other skin lines. Plast Reconstr Surg 73:144, 1984.
3. Rahban SR, Garner WL: Fibroproliferative scars. Clin Plast Surg 30:1, 2003.
4. Rockwell WB, Cohen IK, Ehrlich HP: Keloids and hypertrophic scars: A comprehensive review. Plast Reconstr Surg 84:827, 1989.
5. Grabb WC: Basic techniques of plastic surgery. In Grabb WC, Smith JW (eds): Plastic Surgery, 3rd ed. Boston, Little, Brown, 1979, p 3.
6. Ruberg RL: Role of nutrition in wound healing. Surg Clin North Am 64:705, 1984.
7. Robson MC, Krizek TJ, Southwick WO: Quantitative bacterial analysis of comparative wound irrigations. Ann Surg 181:819, 1975.
8. Mustoe TA, Cooter RD, Gold MH, et al: International clinical recommendations on scar management. Plast Reconstr Surg 110:560, 2002.

9. Gross A, Cutrigut DE, Bhaskar SN: Effectiveness of pulsating water jet lavage in treatment of contaminated crushed wounds. Am J Surg 124:373, 1972.

10. Converse JM, Uhlschmid GK, Ballantyne DL: "Plasmatic circulation" in skin grafts. Plast Reconstr Surg 28:274, 1975.

11. Converse JM, Smahel J, Ballantyne DL, et al: Inosculation of vessels of skin graft and host bed: A fortuitous encounter. Br J Plast Surg 28:274, 1975.

12. Teh BT: Why do skin grafts fail? Plast Reconstr Surg 63:323, 1979.

13. Robson MC, Krizek TJ: Predicting skin graft survival. J Trauma 13:213, 1973.

14. Lamberty BGH, Healy C: Flaps: Physiology, principles of design, and pitfalls. In Cohen M (ed): Mastery of Plastic and Reconstructive Surgery. Boston, Little, Brown, 1995, p 56.

15. Cormach GC, Lamberty GGH: A classification of fasciocutaneous flaps according to their patterns of vascularization. Br J Plast Surg 37:80, 1984.

16. McCraw JB, Vasconez LO: Musculocutaneous flaps: Principles. Clin Plast Surg 7:9, 1980.

17. Kunert P: Structure and construction: The system of skin flaps. Ann Plast Surg 27:509, 1991.

18. Yousif NJ, Ye Z, Grunert BK, et al: Analysis of the distribution of cutaneous perforators in cutaneous flaps. Plast Reconstr Surg 101:72, 1998.

19. Timmons MJ: Landmarks in the anatomical study of the blood supply of the skin. Br J Plast Surg 38:197, 1985.

20. Jackson IT: Local Flaps in Head and Neck Reconstruction. St. Louis, Mosby, 1985.

21. Armstrong MB, Masri N, Venugopal R: Reconstructive microsurgery: Reviewing the past, anticipating the future. Clin Plast Surg 28:671, 2001.

22. Cho BC, Shin DP, Byun JS, et al: Monitoring flap for buried free tissue transfer: Its importance and reliability. Plast Reconstr Surg 110:1249, 2002.

23. Furnas H, Rosen JM: Monitoring in microvascular surgery. Ann Plast Surg 26:265, 1991.

24. Murray JC: Gene/environment causes of cleft lip and/or palate. Clin Genet 61:248, 2002.

25. Carstens MH: Development of the facial midline. J Craniofac Surg 13:129, 2002.

26. Stal S, Klebuc M, Taylor TD, et al: Algorithms for the treatment of cleft lip and palate. Clin Plast Surg 25:493, 1998.

27. Rohrich RJ, Byrd HS: Optimal timing of cleft palate closure: Speech, facial growth, and hearing considerations. Clin Plast Surg 17:27, 1990.

28. Rosenstein SW, Grasseschi M, Dado DV: A long-term retrospective outcome assessment of facial growth, secondary surgical need, and maxillary lateral incisor status in a surgical-orthodontic protocol for complete clefts. Plast Reconstr Surg 111:1, 2003.

29. Schendel SA: Unilateral cleft lip repair—state of the art. Cleft Palate Craniofac J 37:335, 2000.

30. Brent B: Technical advances in ear reconstruction with autogenous rib cartilage grafts: Personal experience with 1200 cases. Plast Reconstr Surg 104:319, 1999.

31. Yugueros P, Friedland JA: Otoplasty: The experience of 100 consecutive patients. Plast Reconstr Surg 108:1045, 2001.

32. Robin NH: Molecular genetic advances in understanding craniosynostosis. Plast Reconstr Surg 103:1060, 1999.

33. Panchal J, Uttchin V: Management of craniosynostosis. Plast Reconstr Surg 111:2032, 2003.

34. Marchac D, Renier D: Craniofacial Surgery for Craniosynostosis. Boston, Little, Brown, 1982.

35. Kawamoto HJ: Simplification of the Le Fort I osteotomy. Clin Plast Surg 16:777, 1989.

36. Emshoff R, Scheiderbauer A, Gerhard S: Stability after rigid fixation of simultaneous maxillary impaction and mandibular advancement osteotomies. Int J Oral Maxillofac Surg 32:137, 2003.

37. Manson P: Management of facial fractures. Perspect Plast Surg 2:1, 1988.

38. Staffel JG: Optimizing treatment of nasal fractures. Laryngoscope 112:1709, 2002.

39. Ellis E III: Sequencing treatment for naso-orbito-ethmoid fractures. J Oral Maxillofac Surg 51:543, 1993.

40. Gerbino G, Roccia F, Benech A, et al: Analysis of 158 frontal sinus fractures: Current surgical management and complications. J Craniomaxillofac Surg 28:133, 2000.

41. Xie C, Mehendale N, Barrett D, et al: Thirty-year retrospective review of frontal sinus fractures: The Charity Hospital experience. J Craniomaxillofac Trauma 6:7, 2000.

42. Manson PN, Clark N, Robertson B, et al: Subunit principles in midface fractures: The importance of sagittal buttresses, soft tissue reductions, and sequencing treatment of segmental fractures. Plast Reconstr Surg 103:1287, 1999.

43. Gruss JS, Mackinnon SE: Complex maxillary fractures: Role of buttress reconstruction and immediate bone grafts. Plast Reconstr Surg 78:9, 1986.

44. Grossman MD, Roberts DM, Barr CC: Ophthalmic aspects of orbital injury: A comprehensive diagnostic and management approach. Clin Plast Surg 19:17, 1992.

45. Zingg M, Laedrach K, Chen J, et al: Classification and treatment of zygomatic fractures: A review of 1,025 cases. J Oral Maxillofac Surg 50:778, 1992.

46. Rohrich RJ, Hollier LH, Watumell D: Optimizing the management of orbitozygomatic fractures. Clin Plast Surg 19:149, 1992.

47. Burnstine MA: Clinical recommendations for repair of isolated orbital floor fractures: An evidence-based analysis. Ophthalmology 109:1207, 2002.

48. Rohrich RJ, Hackney FL, Parikh RS: Superior orbital fissure syndrome: Current management concepts. J Craniomaxillofac Trauma 1:44, 1995.

49. Rohrich RJ: The orbital apex syndrome: Compromised vision associated with high-velocity orbitozygomatic fractures. Perspect Plast Surg 6:149, 1992.

50. Luce EA: Developing concepts and treatment of complex maxillary fractures. Clin Plast Surg 19:125, 1992.

51. Markowitz BL, Manson PN: Panfacial fractures: Organization of treatment. Clin Plast Surg 16:105, 1989.

52. Andrew CT, Gallucci JG, Brown AS, et al: Is routine cervical spine radiographic evaluation indicated in patients with mandibular fractures? Am Surg 58:369, 1992.

53. Nishioka GS, Van Sickels JE: Transoral plating of mandibular angle fractures: A technique. Oral Surg 66:531, 1988.

54. Bos RR, Ward Booth RP, de Bont LG: Mandibular condyle fractures: A consensus. Br J Oral Maxillofac Surg 37:87, 1999.

55. Freilinger G, Gruber H, Happak W, et al: Surgical anatomy of the mimetic muscle system and the facial nerve: Importance for reconstructive and aesthetic surgery. Plast Reconstr Surg 80:686, 1987.

56. Rudolph R: Depth of the facial nerve in face lift dissections. Plast Reconstr Surg 85:537, 1990.

57. Stuzin JM, Wagstrom L, Kawamoto HK, et al: Anatomy of the frontal branch of the facial nerve: The significance of the temporal fat pad. Plast Reconstr Surg 85:29, 1990.

58. Merren MD: Nonepidemic incidence of Bell's palsy. Am J Otol 9:159, 1988.

59. Austin SR, Peskind SP, Austin SG, et al: Idiopathic facial nerve paralysis: A randomized double-blind controlled study of placebo versus prednisone. Laryngoscope 103:1326, 1993.

60. Myckatyn TM, Mackinnon SE: The surgical management of facial nerve injury. Clin Plast Surg 30:307, 2003.

61. Falcioni M, Taibah A, Russo A: Facial nerve grafting. Otol Neurotol 24:486, 2003.

62. Spector JG, Lee P, Peterein J, et al: Facial nerve regeneration through autologous nerve grafts: A clinical and experimental study. Laryngoscope 101:537, 1991.

63. Inigo F, Ysunza A, Rojo P: Recovery of facial palsy after crossed facial nerve grafts. Br J Plast Surg 47:312, 1994.

64. Buncke HJ, Buncke GM, Kind GM, et al: Cross-facial and functional microvascular muscle transplantation for longstanding facial paralysis. Clin Plast Surg 29:551, 2002.

65. Mansour KA, Thourani VH, Losken A: Chest wall resections and reconstruction: A 25-year experience. Ann Thorac Surg 73:1720, 2002.

66. Arnold PG, Pairolaro PC: Chest wall reconstruction: An account of 500 consecutive patients. Plast Reconstr Surg 98:804, 1996.

67. Jones G, Jurkiewicz MJ, Bostwick J: Management of the infected median sternotomy wound with muscle flaps: The Emory 20-year experience. Ann Surg 225:766, 1997.

68. Jemal A, Thomas A, Murray T, et al: Cancer statistics 2002. CA 52:23, 2002.

69. Shons AR, Cox CE: Breast cancer: Advances in surgical management. Plast Reconstr Surg 107:541, 2001.

70. Kroll SS, Khoo A, Singletary SE, et al: Local recurrence risk after skin-sparing and conventional mastectomy: A 6-year follow-up. Plast Reconstr Surg 104:421, 1999.

71. Spear SL, Spittler CJ: Breast reconstruction with implants and expanders. Plast Reconstr Surg 107:177, 2001.

72. Shestak KC: Breast reconstruction with a pedicled TRAM flap. Clin Plast Surg 25:167, 1998.

73. Schusterman MA, Kroll SS, Miller MJ, et al: The free transverse rectus abdominis musculocutaneous flap for breast reconstruction: One center's experience with 211 consecutive cases. Ann Plast Surg 32:234, 1994.

74. Papp C, McCraw JB: Autogenous latissimus breast reconstruction. Clin Plast Surg 25:261, 1998.

75. Deligiannidis N, Papavasiliou I, Sapalidis K, et al: The use of three different mesh materials in the treatment of abdominal wall defects. Hernia 6:51, 2002.

76. Szczerba SR, Dumanian GA: Definitive surgical treatment of infected or exposed ventral hernia mesh. Ann Surg 237:437, 2003.

77. Girotto JA, Chiaramonte M, Menon NG: Recalcitrant abdominal wall hernias: Long-term superiority of autologous tissue repair. Plast Reconstr Surg 112:106, 2003.

78. Ramirez OM, Ruas E, Dellon AL: "Components separation" method for closure of abdominal wall defects: An anatomic and clinical study. Plast Reconstr Surg 86:519, 1990.

79. Shestak KC, Edington HJD, Johnson RR: The separation of anatomic components technique for the reconstruction of massive midline abdominal wall defects: Anatomy, surgical technique, applications, and limitations revisited. Plast Reconstr Surg 105:731, 2000.

80. Barczak C, Barnett R, Childs E, et al: Fourth National Pressure Ulcer Prevalence Survey. Adv Wound Care 10:18, 1997.

81. Lindan O, Greenway RM, Piazza JM: Pressure distribution of the surface of the human body: Evaluation of lying and sitting positions using a bed of springs and nails. Arch Phys Med Rehabil 6:378, 1965.

82. Nola GT, Vistnes LM: Differential response of skin and muscle in the experimental production of pressure sores. Plast Reconstr Surg 66:728, 1980.

83. Schryvers OI, Stranc MF, Nance PW: Surgical treatment of pressure ulcers: 20-year experience. Arch Phys Med Rehabil 81:1556, 2000.

84. Disa JJ, Carlton JM, Goldberg NH: Efficacy of operative cure in pressure sore patients. Plast Reconstr Surg 89:272, 1992.

85. Wanner MB, Schwarzl F, Strub B, et al: Vacuum-assisted wound closure for cheaper and more comfortable healing of pressure sores: A prospective study. Scand J Plast Reconstr Surg Hand Surg 37:28, 2003.

86. McGraw JB, Horton CE, Horton CE Jr: Basic techniques in genital reconstructive surgery. *In* McCarthy JG (ed): Plastic Surgery, Vol 6 (The Trunk and Lower Extremity). Philadelphia, WB Saunders, 1990, p 4121.

87. Byrd HS, Spicer TE, Cierny G III: Management of open tibial fractures. Plast Reconstr Surg 76:719, 1985.

88. Chung YJ, Kim G, Sohn BK: Reconstruction of a lower extremity soft tissue defect using the gastrocnemius musculoadipofascial flap. Ann Plast Surg 49:91, 2002.

89. Heller L, Levin LS: Lower extremity microsurgical reconstruction. Plast Reconstr Surg 108:1029, 2001.

90. Erdmann MW, Court-Brown CM, Quaba AA: A five-year review of islanded distally based fasciocutaneous flaps on the lower limb. Br J Plast Surg 50:421, 1997.

91. Mayberry JC, Moneta GL, Taylor LM Jr, et al: Fifteen-year results of ambulatory compression therapy for chronic venous ulcers. Surgery 109:575, 1991.

92. Treiman GS, Oderich GS, Ashrafi A, et al: Management of ischemic heel ulceration and gangrene: An evaluation of factors associated with successful healing. J Vasc Surg 31:1110, 2000.

93. Stevens MJ, Feldman EL, Greene DA: The aetiology of diabetic neuropathy: The combined roles of metabolic and vascular defects. Diabet Med 12:566, 1995.

94. Cohen SR, Payne DK, Tunkel RS: Lymphedema: Strategies for management. Cancer 92(4 Suppl):980, 2001.

95. Miller TA, Wyatt LE, Rudkin GH: Staged skin and subcutaneous excision for lymphedema: A favorable report of long-term results. Plast Reconstr Surg 102:1486, 1999.

96. Brorson H, Svensson H: Liposuction combined with controlled compression therapy reduces arm lymphedema more effectively than controlled compression therapy alone. Plast Reconstr Surg 102:1058, 1998.

97. Collins ED, Kerrigan CL, Kim M, et al: The effectiveness of surgical and nonsurgical interventions in relieving the symptoms of macromastia. Plast Reconstr Surg 109:1556, 2002.

98. Fruhstorfer BH, Malata CM: A systematic approach to the surgical treatment of gynaecomastia. Br J Plast Surg 56:237, 2003.

99. Hidalgo DA: Breast augmentation: Choosing the optimal incision, implant, and pocket plane. Plast Reconstr Surg 105:2202, 2000.

100. Regnault P: Breast ptosis: Definition and treatment. Clin Plast Surg 3:193, 1976.

101. Commons GW, Halperin B, Chang CC: Large-volume liposuction: A review of 631 consecutive cases over 12 years. Plast Reconstr Surg 108:1753, 2001.

102. Fagien S: Botox for the treatment of dynamic and hyperkinetic facial lines and furrows: Adjunctive use in facial aesthetic surgery. Plast Reconstr Surg 103:701, 1999.

103. Jelks GW, Jelks EB: Preoperative evaluation of the blepharoplasty patient: Bypassing the pitfalls. Clin Plast Surg 20:213, 1993.

104. Chiu ES, Baker DC: Endoscopic brow lift: A retrospective review of 628 consecutive cases over 5 years. Plast Reconstr Surg 112:628, 2003.

105. Pitanguy I: Facial cosmetic surgery: A 30-year perspective. Plast Reconstr Surg 105:1517, 2000.

106. Sheen JH: Rhinoplasty: Personal evolution and milestones. Plast Reconstr Surg 102:2148, 1998.

CHAPTER 73

HAND SURGERY

T. M. Sunil, M.S. Orth., D.N.B. Orth.,   Harold E. Kleinert, M.D.,

John H. Miller, M.D.,   and   Sandeep S. Jejurikar, M.D.

Clinical Anatomy	**Nerve Compression Syndromes**
Clinical Evaluation of the Injured Hand	**Tumors**
Diagnostic Aids	**Infection**
Anesthesia	**Congenital Anomalies**
Tourniquet	**Tenosynovitis**
Soft Tissue Injuries	**Arthritis**
Fractures and Dislocations	**Contractures**
Amputation and Replantation	**Conclusion**

The human hand represents the evolutionary pinnacle of appendages in all living organisms. Whereas it is no surprise that the hand is far more intricate than the shapeless pseudopodia of a humble ameba, it is amazing to note the enormous gap that separates the human hand from our immediate living predecessor, the ape. Functions such as writing, playing musical instruments and handling of tools that we take for granted are well nigh impossible even for the most well trained of apes. The functions of the human hand range from the tangible to the intangible. They may broadly be divided into motor, sensory, stereognostic, and expressive. The motor component enables one to manipulate the external environment while the sensory component permits recognition of the same. Stereognosis is a higher mental function that involves the amalgamation of both motor and sensory skills, permitting recognition of objects without visual assistance. Indeed, this latter function is honed to an exquisite degree in blind people whose hands are their windows to the external world. The use of hands as organs of expression is uniquely human and is a component that is yet to be fully understood.

The field of hand surgery may have evolved as a separate specialty only recently, but its birth is lost somewhere in the dim past of medicine. The first writings on tendon repair come from Avicenna, an Arabian surgeon of the 10th century who advocated suturing of ruptured tendons. However, this was rarely followed in Europe because of the strong influence of Galen, who taught that tendons and nerves had the same characteristics and repair of either would result in gangrene and convulsions. These misconceptions stemmed from a poor and often fanciful understanding of anatomy. The exhaustive and amazingly accurate treatises on anatomy by Leonardo da Vinci (1452-1519) and Andreas Vesalius (1514-1564) paved the way for modern scientific surgery. Interest in the hand as a separate entity can be traced to the pioneering works of Allen Kanavel in the early part of the 20th century, who wrote extensively on the anatomy of the hand, highlighting its intricacy and beauty. He established the world's first dedicated hand care unit at the Northwestern University Medical School, which, with the efforts of his disciples, Sumner Koch, Michael Mason, and Harvey Allen, would soon go on to become famous as the Chicago School of Hand Surgery. The creation of hand surgery as a separate specialty can be credited to Sterling Bunnel. His monumental experience and excellent organizational skills led to the organization of specialized hand care centers in various military hospitals throughout the United States. He was also responsible for the birth of the world's first hand surgical society, the American Society for Surgery of the Hand, in 1946. The next few decades saw the birth of hand societies all over the world, and the International Federation of Societies for Surgery of the Hand (IFSSH) was established in 1966. Currently, the IFSSH has more than 40 member hand societies, representing in excess of 5000 physicians worldwide. The birth of hand surgery as a specialty was followed by the need for a specialized training in the field; and, soon, fellowship programs arose all over the world. In 1973, the American Board for Medical Specialties recognized a certification in hand surgery as an added qualification to basic training in general, orthopedic, or plastic surgery. Currently, Sweden, Singapore, and India have recognized hand surgery as an entirely independent specialty.

CLINICAL ANATOMY

Internationally, the nomenclature of digits has been standardized. The hand has five digits, namely, the thumb and four fingers (note that the thumb is not called a finger). The four fingers are called the index, long, ring, and small fingers. The use of numbers to designate digits is no longer acceptable.

The anatomic structures of the hand can be broadly classified into six groups depending on the principal function they perform. These are covering structures, supporting structures, restraining structures, feeding structures, controlling structures, and moving structures. The skin and nails are covering structures that serve the principal function of protecting the hand from external elements. The bones, joints, as well as capsuloligamentous elements provide support, while aponeuroses, retinacula, and tendon sheaths act as restraints, retaining structures within their anatomic confines. Vascular structures primarily nourish the hand, while the neural elements including nerves and their specialized end organs permit the brain to exercise exquisite control on the functioning of the hand. Lastly, the muscular elements are the organs that move the hand in all its intricate and complex activities.

Covering Structures

The skin of the hand is highly specialized. It is thin and pigmented on the dorsum but is thick, glabrous, and extremely sensitive on the palmar surface. The palmar skin, especially at the fingertips, is endowed with a profusion of sensory end organs, such as pacinian bodies, Merkel discs, and Meissner corpuscles. Furthermore, the palmar skin is fixed to the underlying aponeurosis by retinacula cutis at the skin creases. These represent skin joints and enable efficient gripping of objects. The nail is a hardened keratinous outgrowth from skin and protects the dorsal aspect of the sensitive fingertip.

Supporting Structures

The skeletal elements of the hand comprise the distal radius and ulna, eight carpal bones, five metacarpals, and 14 phalanges. The thumb has only two phalanges whereas the other four digits have three each. The bones of the hands form a number of joints that are connected in series. The significance of this arrangement is described later in the section dealing with muscles.

The wrist joint is the foundation on which the hand rests. It is a complex articulation of the distal radius and ulna with the carpal bones. The carpal bones are arranged in two transverse rows. These rows are concave volar-

ward and form the floor of the carpal tunnel. The proximal carpal row comprising the scaphoid, lunate, and triquetrum (with the exception of the outlying pisiform) is devoid of any muscular insertion. It hence forms an intercalated segment between the distal forearm and distal carpal row, which is formed by the trapezium, trapezoid, capitate, and hamate. Recognition of this arrangement is of significance in understanding the various patterns of wrist instability. Flexion and extension of the wrist principally occur at the midcarpal joint whereas radial and ulnar deviations occur mainly at the radiocarpal articulation.

The carpometacarpal joint (CMCJ) of the thumb is the most mobile of all joints in the hand. It takes the form of a double saddle joint between the trapezium and first metacarpal and permits a wide range of movements in all three dimensions, making the human thumb unique in the living world. The index and long finger metacarpals are essentially devoid of independent mobility. The metacarpals of the ring and small fingers are capable of rotating axially at their respective carpometacarpal joints (CMCJ). This enables cupping of the hand, thus increasing efficiency of grip. The metacarpophalangeal joints (MCPJ) are condyloid joints and can move in three planes. Flexion-extension occur on a transverse axis in the sagittal plane, abduction-adduction take place on an anteroposterior axis in the coronal plane, and a small amount of rotation occurs on the longitudinal axis of each metacarpal in the transverse plane. This enables the hand to grasp objects of all shapes and sizes. This is best illustrated by grasping a spherical object and looking at the fingers end on (Fig. 73-1). The interphalangeal joints (IPJ) are essentially hinge joints and principally permit flexion and extension. The capsules of the metacarpophalangeal and interphalangeal joints are reinforced on either side by collateral ligaments. In addition, the volar capsules of these joints display a specialized fibrocartilaginous thickening termed the *volar plate*. These plates are firmly attached to the base of the distal bone of each joint and loosely attached proximally. This arrangement permits them to freely glide over the head of the proximal bone during flexion-extension, effectively increasing the area of articulation between the adjacent bones.

Restraining Structures

The palmar aponeurosis consists mainly of three components: a central triangular portion with thenar and hypothenar slips on either side. The thenar slip overlies the ball of the thumb, providing support as well as attachment to the thenar intrinsic muscles. Similarly, the hypothenar slip covers as well as provides attachment to the hypothenar muscles. The central triangular part of the palmar aponeurosis accounts for the hollow of the palm and from its distal end sends out four fibrous slips. These individually enter each finger, blending on their deep aspect with the corresponding fibrous flexor sheath.

The fibrous flexor sheath is a specialized osteofibrous tunnel through which the long flexor tendons of the digits pass. The flexor sheath of each finger displays localized

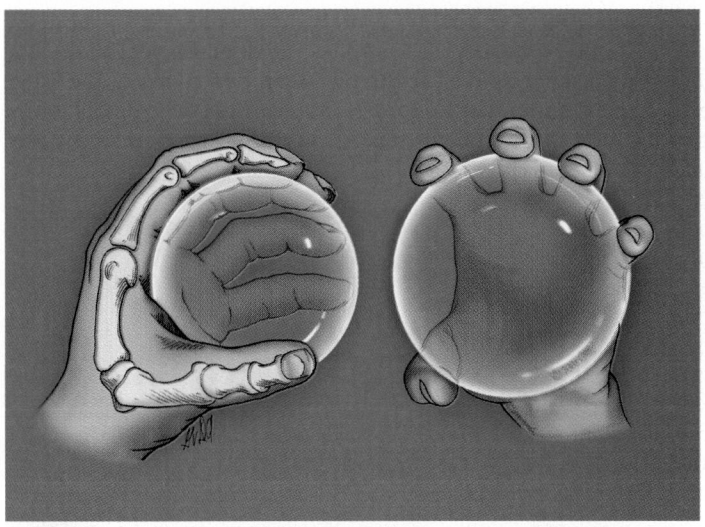

FIGURE 73-1. The ability of the fingers to abduct and rotate at the MCP joint permits grasping of spherical objects. Rotation of the digits is appreciated by looking at the plane of the nails.

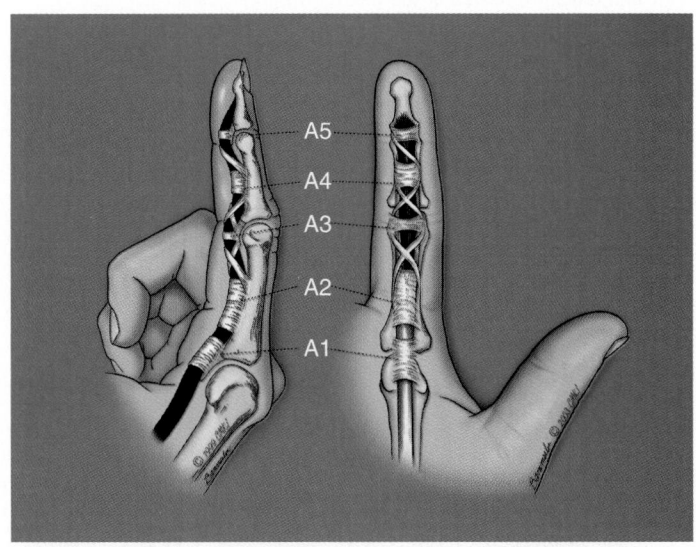

FIGURE 73-2. Cruciate and annular pulleys of the fibrous flexor sheath.

A5
A4
A3
A2
A1

thickenings known as pulleys that are particularly important in preventing bowstringing of the tendons. These pulleys may be annular or cruciate. The annular pulleys are formed by transversely running collagen fibers and are five in number. The odd-numbered annular pulleys—A1, A3, and A5—overlie the volar plates of the metacarpophalangeal (MCP), proximal interphalangeal (PIP), and distal interphalangeal (DIP) joints, respectively. The A2 and A4 pulleys overlie the shafts of the proximal and middle phalanges. There are three cruciate pulleys, C1, C2, and C3, which lie between A2-A3, A3-A4, and A4-A5, respectively. These are formed by collagen fibers that are oriented in a criss-cross pattern and permit longitudinal foreshortening of the fibrous flexor sheath during flexion of the fingers (Fig. 73-2).

The flexor retinaculum spans the transverse arch of the carpus and forms the roof of the carpal tunnel. It prevents bowstringing of the long flexor tendons during flexion of the wrist. On the dorsal side, this function is taken over by the extensor retinaculum, which restrains the long extensors of the wrist and digits. The extensor retinaculum in addition sends down septa between the extensor tendons, dividing them into six distinct compartments. This is discussed in detail in the section on extensor muscles.

Feeding Structures

The blood supply to the hand is principally from the radial and ulnar arteries (Fig. 73-3). In about 0.5% of the population, a persistent median artery may be seen. The radial and ulnar arteries each divide in the proximal part of the wrist into superficial and deep branches. The corresponding branches then unite to form the superficial and deep palmar arches. The superficial palmar arch is usually dominated by the ulnar artery. From it arise common metacarpal arteries that go on to divide into digital arteries, supplying adjacent digits of the second, third, and fourth web spaces. The ulnar digital artery of the small finger also arises from the superficial palmar arch. In contrast, the deep palmar arch is usually dominated by the radial artery. It gives rise to the principal arteries of the thumb and radial border of the index finger. The digital arteries of the thumb are located entirely on the volar aspect of the thumb. On the other hand, the digital arteries of the fingers are located on either side of the flexor sheath. In this location, they lie deeper and more central to their respective digital nerves.

Controlling Structures

The median, ulnar, and radial nerves are the principal nerves of the hand (Fig. 73-4). The median and ulnar nerves supply the long flexors of the wrist and fingers in the forearm while the radial nerve supplies all the exten-

sors (Fig. 73-5). Within the hand proper, the radial nerve is purely sensory and supplies the dorsal aspect of the first web space as well as the proximal two thirds of the radial three and a half digits. The median nerve supplies motor fibers to the thenar muscles and the first two lumbricals.

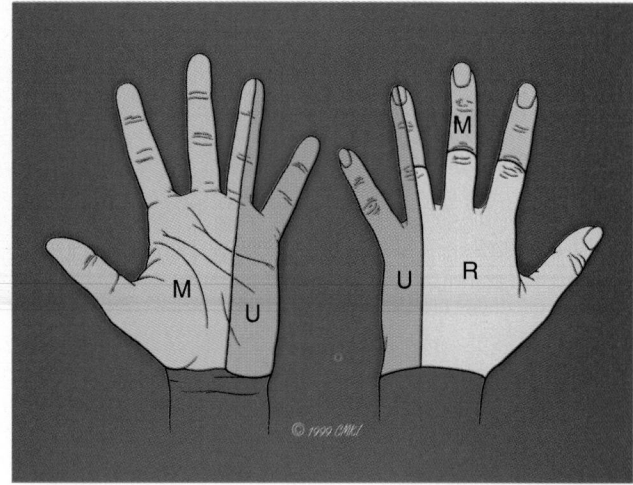

■ **FIGURE 73-4.**   Sensory areas of the median (M), ulnar (U), and radial (R) nerves of the hand.

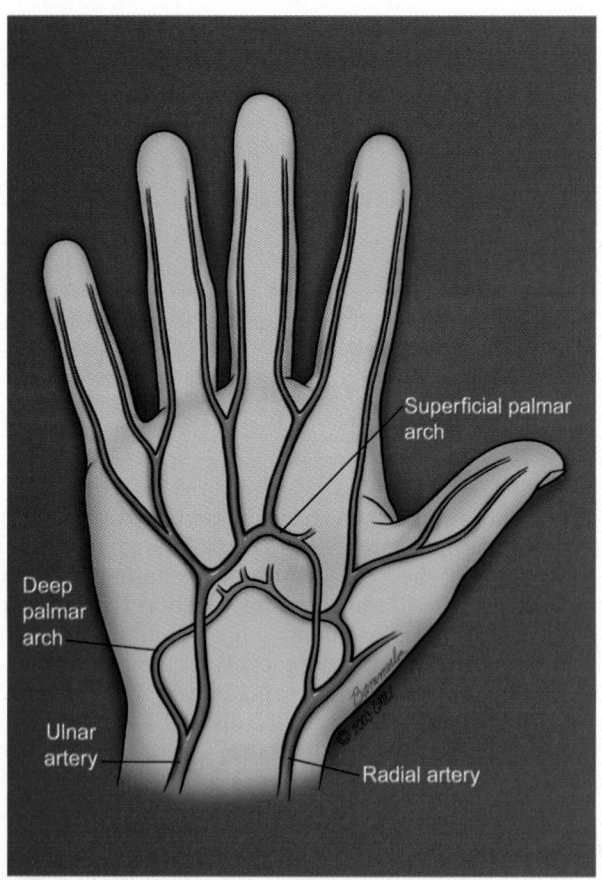

■ **FIGURE 73-3.**   The major arterial arcades of the hand.

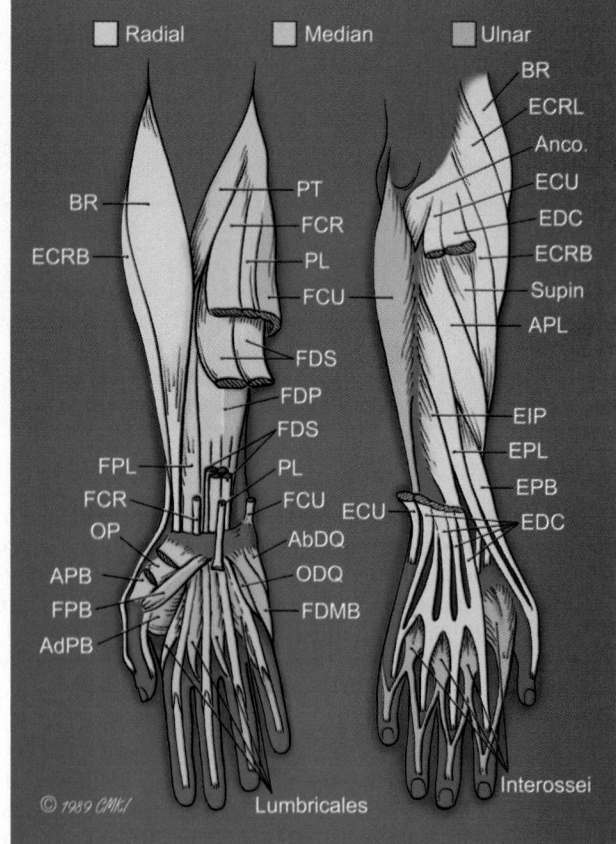

■ **FIGURE 73-5.**   Muscles of the forearm and hand, colored according to their innervation.

It also carries sensory fibers from the entire volar aspect as well as the distal thirds of the dorsal aspects of the radial three and a half digits. The ulnar nerve supplies motor fibers to the hypothenar muscles, all the interossei, the third and fourth lumbricals, the adductor pollicis, and the deep belly of the flexor pollicis brevis. It also carries all the sensory fibers from the ulnar one and a half digits and ulnar border of the hand.

Moving Structures

The musculotendinous units of the hand are classified into extrinsic and intrinsic groups. Precise knowledge of their anatomy allows the surgeon to formulate an accurate clinical assessment.

Extrinsic Muscles

The extrinsic muscles originate proximal to the wrist and comprise the long flexors and extensors of the wrist and digits (see Fig. 73-5). As they pass distally toward their respective insertions, these musculotendinous units may cross one or more proximally located joints. It may be recollected at this stage that the joints of the hand are arrayed proximodistally in series. Consequent to this arrangement, any muscle that moves a distally located joint will also have a corresponding effect on the more proximally located joints that they have crossed.

The extensors are located dorsally and can be divided into three subgroups. The lateral subgroup is termed the *mobile wad* and consists of the brachioradialis (BR), extensor carpi radialis longus (ECRL), and extensor carpi radialis brevis (ECRB). The ECRL and ECRB extend and deviate the wrist radially. The second subgroup forms a superficial layer and comprises three muscles: the extensor carpi ulnaris (ECU), the extensor digiti quinti (EDQ), and the extensor digitorum communis (EDC). The ECU extends and deviates the wrist toward the ulna, while the EDQ and EDC act primarily to extend the MCP joints of the small and remaining fingers, respectively. The third subgroup is deep and consists of four muscles, all of which act on the thumb and index finger. The abductor pollicis longus (APL), extensor pollicis longus (EPL), and extensor pollicis brevis (EPB) act on the thumb, whereas the extensor indicis proprius (EIP) extends the MCP joint of the index finger. The supinator is the last of the deep muscles and is located proximally in the forearm. All of these muscles are supplied either directly by the radial nerve or by its principal motor division, the posterior interosseous nerve.

The extensor tendons pass through six compartments under the extensor retinaculum. From radial to ulnar, they are as follows: The first compartment contains the APL and EPB, which form the radial boundary of the *anatomic snuff box.* The second compartment contains the radial wrist extensors, the ECRL and ECRB. The third compartment contains the EPL, which forms the ulnar boundary of the anatomic snuff box. The EIP and EDC pass through the fourth compartment whereas the EDQ passes through the fifth compartment, overlying the distal radioulnar joint. The final and sixth compartment contains the ECU.

The long finger extensor tendons broaden out to form a hood over the MCP joints. At this level, the proximal part of the hood, termed the *sagittal band,* loops around the MCP joint and blends into its volar plate. It thus forms a "lasso" around the base of the proximal phalanx through which it extends the MCP joint. Distal and dorsal to the axis of the MCP joint, the extensor hood receives the insertions of the interossei and lumbricals. Then, through a complex arrangement of fibers on the dorsal aspect of the fingers, the extensor hood drops an insertion to the base of the middle phalanx. This is termed the *central slip* and extends the PIP joint. Finally, the extensor hood inserts through its *terminal slip* into the base of the distal phalanx, thus extending the DIP joint.

The flexor muscles are located volarly and are arranged in three layers (see Fig. 73-5). The superficial layer consists of four muscles: pronator teres (PT), flexor carpi radialis (FCR), flexor carpi ulnaris (FCU), and palmaris longus (PL). The intermediate layer consists of the flexor digitorum superficialis (FDS), which provides independent flexion at the PIP joints of each finger. The deep group contains three muscles: flexor pollicis longus (FPL), which flexes the IP joint of the thumb; flexor digitorum profundus (FDP), which flexes the DIP joints of the fingers; and pronator quadratus, which lies in the distal part of the forearm and supports pronation of the forearm. The FCU and ulnar half of the FDP (moving the ring and small fingers) are supplied by the ulnar nerve whereas all the other muscles on the volar side of the forearm are supplied by the median nerve.

Intrinsic Muscles

The intrinsic muscles originate within the hand at or distal to the wrist. The thenar eminence consists of the abductor pollicis brevis (APB), flexor pollicis brevis (FPB), and opponens pollicis (OP). There are four dorsal interossei that arise from adjacent sides of each metacarpal and provide abduction of the MCP joints of the index, middle, and ring fingers. There are three palmar interossei that adduct the index, ring, and small fingers toward the middle finger. Four lumbricals originate on the FDP tendons in the palm and insert on the radial sides of the extensor hoods. They, along with the interossei, bring about flexion at the MCP and extension at the IP joints of the fingers. A small muscle termed the *palmaris brevis* is located transversely in the skin at the base of the hypothenar eminence. It is innervated by the ulnar nerve and helps in cupping the skin of the palm during grip.

CLINICAL EVALUATION OF THE INJURED HAND

The first rule of evaluating an injured hand is to remember that there is a human being attached to it. It is very easy for one to be distracted by the dramatic appearance of a mangled extremity and miss other more serious injuries elsewhere in the body. Once this possibility has been ruled out, examination proceeds in a systematic manner.

An accurate history is imperative to fully understand the extent of injury sustained. The importance of this is best illustrated by taking the example of machinery injuries, which are usually the most common cause of major hand injuries. They can, however, cause a wide spectrum of damage depending on how sharp or blunt the working tool is, whether it rotates or presses, and whether it is hot or not while in use. The mere fact that a machine tool is hot while in use adds the element of thermal damage to the injury spectrum. The presence of toxic chemicals in the machine further complicates issues. The type of work that a machine is used for determines the amount of contamination, as for instance, a piece of farmyard equipment is obviously more contaminated than one used to cut metal.

The first step of examination is visual inspection of the entire upper extremity. The color of the hand can provide valuable information about its vascular status whereas deformities suggest underlying skeletal injuries. The fingers are normally held in slight flexion while at rest, and the amount of flexion progressively increases from the index to the small fingers. Loss of this normal cascade of flexion can indicate flexor tendon injury. Exposure of vital structures needs to be carefully assessed and loss of any soft tissue cover noted. Prolonged exposure of vital structures such as nerves, arteries, tendons, and joints to the exterior can lead to their desiccation and death.

First, assess for vascularity of the hand because its very survival depends on this. Pressure on the tip of the nail causes blanching of the nail bed, and release of the pressure should result in a prompt return of color. Inadequate or sluggish return of color suggests arterial injury whereas a very rapid return of color or a persistent dusky coloration suggests venous obstruction. Obstruction of major arterial trunks usually leads to diminished or absent pulses distally. On occasion, however, collateral flow may result in the preservation of peripheral pulses. Active bleeding should be controlled with pressure and elevation. Partial transaction of vessels results in prolonged active bleeding because the protective spasm of the vessel walls ends up opening the rent. Ligation or clamping of vessels in the emergency department should be avoided. The radial and ulnar arteries can be assessed for patency by the Allen test, in which they are occluded by the examiner and the patient is asked to open and close the hand a few times. Pressure on one of the arteries is then released and perfusion is assessed. Capillary refill should occur throughout the entire hand within 5 seconds. The test is then repeated for the other artery.

It is imperative to rule out compartment syndrome of the forearm or hand. The interstitial pressure of the tissues in the body is usually below 30 mm Hg. Any rise in this pressure can potentially block capillary blood flow, leading to ischemia. The forearm and intrinsic compartments of the hands are unyielding osteofascial chambers, bounded deeply by bone and interosseous membranes and superficially by investing fascial layers. Any increase in volume of the contents of these compartments—as can occur after muscle swelling, mass lesions, or bleeding into

the compartment—can cause the intracompartmental pressure to rise with consequent capillary shutdown. This is termed *compartment syndrome* and is a surgical emergency. The most reliable test for this condition is the "stretch" test. Passive flexion or extension of the digits stretches the antagonistic group of muscles. Pain indicates an increased pressure in the compartment housing that group of muscles. Similarly, placing the fingers in the intrinsic minus position of hyperextension at the MCP and flexion at the IP joints stretches the intrinsic muscles, indicating a corresponding rise in compartmental pressure of the hand. These conditions require emergency fasciotomy to relieve the pressure or else serious vascular compromise may ensue.

Bones and joints should be evaluated carefully. Deformities are noted, and each joint is assessed for its passive and active range of motion. The opposite hand, if uninjured, is the best guide to assess this. All fingers when flexed at the MCP and PIP joints point toward the scaphoid tubercle. Gross deviation or crossing of fingers, also known as scissoring, signifies a rotational deformity of the metacarpal or phalanges of that ray. Abnormal or excessive mobility of joints may be the result of injury to the collateral ligaments or capsule.

Nerves are assessed for both sensory and motor function. Sensibility is assessed separately on both the ulnar and radial halves of the pulp by the two-point discrimination test. A bent paper clip can be used to perform this test, and the minimum distance between the two points of the clip that the patient can distinguish as separate is recorded. A two-point sensibility greater than 8 mm suggests nerve injury.[1-3] Knowledge of the sensory distribution of the various nerves of the hand helps localize the lesion. Regeneration of sensory nerves can be clinically assessed by eliciting Tinel's sign. The injured nerve is percussed along its course from distal to proximal. At the site of regeneration, the patient feels paresthesia along the distal distribution of the nerve. Because nerves regenerate at the rate of a millimeter a day (or about an inch a month), the site at which Tinel's sign is elicited also progresses distally. Such a distal progression of Tinel's sign is taken as clinical evidence of nerve regeneration.

Assessing the muscles of the hand helps detect injuries of musculotendinous units as well as nerves. The integrity of the FDP is assessed by asking the patient to flex the DIP joint while passively stabilizing the PIP joint in extension. The FTP tendons to the long, ring, and small fingers arise from intimately interconnected muscle bellies and hence cannot function independent of one another. This is useful when assessing the action of the FDS to these digits. Asking the patient to flex any one of these three fingers while passively stabilizing the PIP and DIP joints of the other two in extension immobilizes the FDP. The patient can now only use the FDS and thus flexes the tested finger only at the PIP joint. Inability to flex the finger indicates loss of FDS activity. Examination of the EDC is usually straightforward and can be assessed by asking the patient to extend the MCP joints of the fingers. The tendons of the EDC are interconnected over the dorsum of the hand by juncturae tendinae and hence cannot move entirely independent of one another. This property is used to test for the integrity of the EIP and EDM muscles, which are additional extensors of the index and small fingers, respectively. The integrity of these tendons is assessed by having the patient flex the middle and ring fingers while maintaining the index and small fingers in extension at their MCP joints. The integrity of the flexor and extensor tendons can also be tested objectively by squeezing the corresponding muscle bellies more proximally in the forearm. This should cause the digits to passively flex or extend, respectively. Along the same lines, passive flexion or extension of the wrist tightens the extensor or flexor muscles, respectively, causing the fingers to either extend or flex. The thenar muscles are tested by abducting or opposing the thumb against resistance while feeling for contraction of the muscle belly. The intrinsics, if functioning, can hold the fingers in the "intrinsic plus" position of flexion at the MCP and of extension at the IP joints.

DIAGNOSTIC AIDS

Radiography

The standard views for hand imaging are the posteroanterior and lateral views. Viewing the radiograph begins with a systematic assessment of soft tissue shadows. The presence of foreign bodies or air is looked for. Metal and glass are radiopaque whereas wood and similar vegetable matter may be radiolucent. Subtle fractures result in small hematomas that lift the periosteum and adjacent soft tissues off the surface of the injured bone. This is evident in some areas like the distal radius as an indirect indicator of a fracture and is termed the *fat pad sign*. Attention is next turned to the structural integrity of individual bones. Fractures are usually obvious, and the direction of deformity is noted. Angulations are named after the direction in which the apex lies. Rotatory deformities show up as a mismatch of the diameters of bones at the fracture line. Undisplaced crack fractures can be detected either by looking for indirect soft tissue signs, as described earlier, or by looking for breaks in individual trabeculae under a magnifying glass. Attention is finally turned to assessing the alignment of bones with respect to one another. Loss of joint congruity suggests a luxation. Widening of spaces between bones is an indicator of ligamentous disruption or laxity. This is of particular significance with respect to the carpal bones and is often the only indicator of instability. Comparison with radiograms of the opposite uninvolved hand helps distinguish injury-induced instability from congenital laxity. Additional special views can be obtained depending on the pathologic process that is suspected. Sometimes, dynamic or stress views are taken to unmask ligamentous injuries.

Angiography

This modality is now limited in its application to the detection of subtle vascular anomalies or injuries. It is being increasingly replaced by MR angiography, which is proving to be a valuable noninvasive alternative.

CT and MRI

Injuries of carpal bones can be missed in conventional radiographs because the carpal bones are quite twisted and small in their structure. CT helps pick up most of these fractures. In addition, intraosseous lesions are best delineated by CT. Sometimes, three-dimensional CT is used to help assess the exact extent of deformity of a bone before reconstruction.

Soft tissue lesions, subtle ligamentous disruptions, and early avascular necrosis of bones and tumors can often be detected only by MRI. MR angiography is now increasingly being relied on to detect vascular malformations. Gadolinium-enhanced MRI helps pick up inflammatory lesions.

Ultrasound and Doppler Scans

On occasion, ultrasound scans can help detect soft tissue lesions. Their use in picking up occult ganglia and intramuscular masses is well known but suffers from being very observer specific.

A hand-held Doppler unit is an invaluable tool in the armamentarium of the hand surgeon. It can be used to detect obstructions to blood flow in vessels as well as to help look for potential feeding vessels while planning flaps for reconstruction.

ANESTHESIA

Most upper extremity anesthesia is performed under local or regional anesthesia. Lidocaine (1%) often combined with a long-acting agent such as bupivacaine (0.25%) is used for digital nerve blocks.[4] It is important to ensure that vasoconstrictive agents such as norepinephrine are not used with local anesthetics, lest they cause shutdown of distal circulation with disastrous consequences. Digital anesthesia distal to the PIP joint can be obtained by injection of the anesthetic agent into the tendon sheath at the A1 pulley. The entire hand can be anesthetized by a wrist block whereas the entire upper extremity can be anesthetized by interscalene, supraclavicular, or axillary blocks.[5,6]

Prolonged surgery requires the patient to remain immobile for extended periods of time, and this can get very uncomfortable. In such circumstances, it may be wise to appropriately sedate patients as well as catheterize their bladders before draping.

Tourniquet

Virtually all hand and upper extremity surgery is performed under tourniquet control. This not only minimizes blood loss but also provides for a clear visualization of the operative field. A rubber ring rolled down from distal to proximal can be used to exsanguinate a digit and then be left on at the base as a digital tourniquet. Tourniquets around the wrist and forearm are not very popular because they increase flexion of the digits and make surgery difficult. Upper extremity tourniquets can remain inflated for no longer than 2 hours. If required for longer periods, they can be deflated for a period of 20 minutes and reinflated again. The interval between deflation and reinflation should be at least 5 minutes for every 30 minutes of tourniquet ischemia. This minimizes the ischemic effects of tourniquet pressure on muscle and nerve.[7] Tourniquet pressures should be maintained at 80 to 100 mm Hg above the patient's systolic blood pressure. Never fail to remove a tourniquet at the conclusion of surgery. The consequences of not doing so can be catastrophic.

SOFT TISSUE INJURIES

Fingertip Injuries

Fingertip injuries are the most common of all hand injuries. They often appear innocuous but, owing to the fact that they involve the most sensitive part of the digit, can lead to significant disability.[8] A thorough knowledge of anatomy of the fingertip is necessary for appropriate treatment.[9-11] The fingertip is covered by a richly innervated glabrous skin, which contains many sensory end organs. The pulp skin is firmly anchored to the underlying distal phalanx by fibrous septa, which enables efficient grasp. The dorsum of the fingertip is protected by the nail plate, which lies on a bed of nail matrix. The proximal third of the nail matrix contributes to nail growth and is called the *germinal matrix.* The distal two thirds of the matrix is largely supportive and is called the *sterile matrix.* Injury to the nail matrix is often accompanied by an associated avulsion of the nail plate. Sometimes, however, the nail plate may remain intact and the nail matrix injury presents as a subungual hematoma. If this hematoma occupies more than 50% of the surface of the nail plate, it is better to surgically remove the nail and repair the matrix tear.[12] Nail bed injuries are repaired with 7-0 absorbable sutures under loupe magnification. Adequate bone support must be present under the nail matrix, or else it leads to the development of a hook-nail deformity.[13]

Any surgical technique used to restore soft tissue coverage of a fingertip must take into account the nature of injury and the patient's age. Goals of treatment include maintaining length, sensibility, motion, and contour. Primary closure of open wounds can be performed if adequate soft tissue is present.[14] Most fingertip defects smaller than 1 cm² heal by secondary intention, provided no bone is exposed. Sometimes, amputated fingertips can be defatted and replaced as composite tissue grafts. These tend to do well in children, but their survival is often a matter of chance in adults. Defects larger than 1 cm² can be covered with full-thickness skin grafts. Good color matching can be achieved by harvesting such grafts from the hypothenar eminence or from the radial aspect of the thumb MCP joint. On occasion, the distal phalanx can be shortened to achieve a tension-free closure. Local flaps, such as the V-Y advancement flap, are frequently used to cover exposed bone of the fingertip (Fig. 73-6).[15] This flap is created by

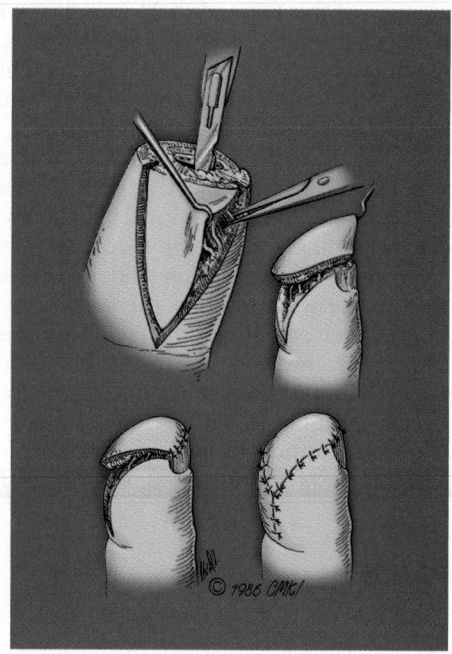

■ FIGURE 73-6.   V-Y advancement flap for coverage of the fingertip.

making a V- shaped incision over the remaining pulp. It is then raised by freeing the fibrous septa from the underlying phalanx, taking care to preserve the neurovascular bundles on either side of the digit. The flap is then advanced distally to cover the exposed tip. Other options for fingertip coverage include lateral V-Y flaps, cross-finger flaps, thenar flaps, and hypothenar flaps.[16,17] Specialized flap coverage for thumb-tip amputation includes the Moberg advancement flap.[18] Loss of the entire pulp skin requires replacement by a sensate glabrous tissue. This is achieved by harvesting a part of the pulp of the great toe along with its neurovascular pedicle and transferring it to the injured digit as a microvascular free flap. A significant complication of fingertip injury is residual hypersensitivity. This may be due to the formation of end-neuromas or as a result of entrapment of injured nerve endings in scar tissue. Restoration of adequate soft tissue coverage and institution of early sensory re-education programs can minimize this problem.

Flexor Tendon Injuries

Flexor tendon injuries are most commonly caused by lacerations or puncture wounds on the palmar surface of the hand.[19] On occasion, flexor tendons can be avulsed from their bony insertions by sudden violent contractions. Flexor tendon injuries should ideally be treated by a surgeon experienced in the management of these injuries.[20] It is important to look for associated injuries to adjacent neurovascular and skeletal structures. Severed flexor tendons generally retract proximally because of reflex muscle contraction. Consequently, the cut ends of the tendon do not lie at the site of skin injury. In such circumstances, it may be necessary to extend the skin wound by making incisions either proximally or distally to retrieve the tendon ends. This will have to be informed to the patient before surgery lest the surgeon be accused of making the wound bigger than it was! If the tendon ends have withdrawn into the flexor sheath, additional exposure is obtained by incising cruciate pulleys, taking care to avoid injury to the critical A2 and A4 pulleys. During repair, the tendon should be grasped only in the central portion of the cut end to avoid traumatizing the smooth external gliding surface of the tendon.

At the wrist, the four FDS tendons lie superficial to the four FDP tendons. As it passes through the flexor sheath, each FDS tendon divides into two slips. The FDP tendon passes through this "decussation" of the FDS tendon and continues into the finger toward its final insertion at the base of the distal phalanx. The slips of the FDS tendon then wrap around the FDP tendon and reunite deep to it at the chiasma before finally inserting on either side of the shaft of the middle phalanx. Thus, in the finger the FDS tendon actually lies deep to the FDP tendon, which is hence more vulnerable to injury at this location.

The basic technique of tendon repair involves the placement of a "core suture" within the substance of the tendon. Although there are many techniques for placing the core suture, our preferred method is the six-stranded loop suture (Fig. 73-7).[21] A core suture primarily bridges the injury gap and provides most of the strength of the repair. Nonabsorbable 4-0 Prolene or Ti-Cron sutures are the preferred material. After placing a core suture, the approximated ends of the tendon can be smoothed out by placing running epitendinous sutures of 6-0 nylon or Prolene. This suture also contributes to the strength of the repair. Depending on when a flexor tendon is sutured,

the repair is termed *primary, delayed primary, early secondary,* or *late secondary.* Primary repair is usually carried out within 24 hours of injury. This is the best time for repair because the wound is free of scar tissue and there is less risk of infection. Delayed primary repairs are those that are performed after 24 hours but before 10 days of injury whereas early secondary repairs are performed between 10 days and 6 weeks after injury. By 6 weeks, the muscle-tendon unit has shortened, making direct repair difficult. In such circumstances a staged tendon repair with the use of interposition tendon grafts may be required.

Flexor tendon injuries are divided into five zones (Fig. 73-8).[22] Treatment and prognosis are influenced by the zone of injury. Zone I lies distal to the insertion of the FDS tendon and affects only the FDP tendon. If adequate tendon length is available distally, a conventional repair as described earlier can be performed. Sometimes, the tendon ruptures very near to its insertion into the distal phalanx, leaving no or insufficient distal tendon for a conventional repair. In such situations, a core suture is placed in the proximal cut end of the tendon and pulled through drill holes in the distal phalanx onto the dorsal surface of the digit. The suture is secured here by tying it over a button on the dorsal surface of the nail plate.

Zone II is the zone of the pulleys and extends from the beginning of the fibrous flexor sheath at the distal palmar crease to the insertion of the FDS. It contains the FDS and FDP tendons enclosed in a narrow fibrous canal. Zone II was in the past referred to as "no-man's land" because it was thought that primary repairs should not be performed here and most surgeons favored secondary repair with tendon grafting. This is no longer the case today, and conventional tendon repair techniques are recommended. Favorable results can be consistently obtained in zone II injuries by meticulous primary repair and early controlled motion.[20,23-25]

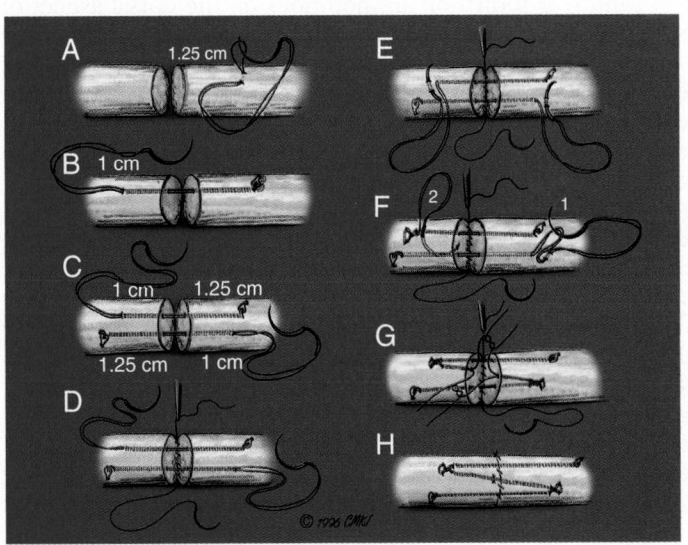

■ **FIGURE 73-7.** The six-stranded Tsai suture technique. **A,** Placement of superficial locking suture at medial palmar quadrant of proximal tendon. **B,** Placement of core suture in medial palmar quadrant with needle inserted close to the locking suture and parallel to the tendon fibers. **C,** Placement of superficial locking suture at lateral palmar quadrant of distal tendon. **D,** Placement of running epitenon sutures in posterior wall of tendon. **E,** Placement of locking sutures at ends of first set of core sutures. **F,** Locking the suture in E by placing the needle through the loop suture. **G,** Intratendinous knotting of the loop sutures. **H,** Running epitenon sutures (anterior wall).

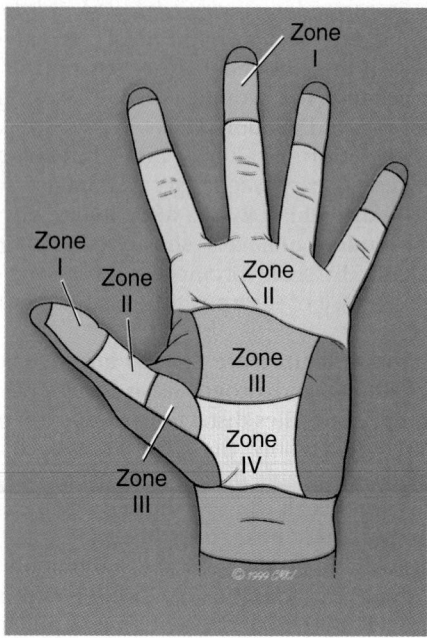

FIGURE 73-8. Zones of flexor tendon injury.

The Louisville method incorporates active extension and passive flexion of the fingers with protection from hyperextension. The injured limb is placed in a dorsal below-elbow splint with the wrist in slight flexion and the MCP joint in 60 degrees of flexion. This allows for full extension of the IP joints. Hooks are then glued to the nail plates and rubber bands of predetermined tension are attached to them. These rubber bands then pass under a transverse bar in the palm and are attached to a tension device. The patient is encouraged to actively extend his or her fingers to the limits of the splint while the rubber bands passively flex the tendons. This permits a continuous motion of the tendons and prevents the development of contracture of the flexor muscle fibers. The passive force exerted by the rubber bands protects the repair from forceful active flexion. Clinical and laboratory studies have demonstrated that dynamic splinting aids in flexor tendon healing by improving tensile strength, remodeling scar tissue, and minimizing adhesion, thus improving range of motion.[26,27]

Zone III is located between the distal carpal ligament and the distal palmar crease. This is the area of the lumbrical muscles, which take origin from the tendons of the FDP. These injuries heal favorably because of good blood supply and the absence of a tight osteofibrous tunnel.

Zone IV is the area of the carpal tunnel and lies deep to the transverse carpal ligament. These injuries can be problematic because of the passage of many structures through a confined space. It may be necessary to repair the transverse carpal ligament and maintain the wrist in flexion until healing occurs to prevent bowstringing of the flexor tendons.

Zone V is located in the forearm. Tendon repairs in this zone almost universally have a favorable prognosis. Technical difficulties may be experienced in suturing injuries at the musculotendinous junction.

It is imperative to institute an intensive postoperative physiotherapy regimen after a flexor tendon repair. The principal goal is to keep the tendons moving. This prevents adhesions from developing between the repaired tendons and surrounding structures. Currently, there are three basic regimens in practice. Our preferred method in Louisville is one of passive flexion followed by active extension. The other two methods are the passive flexion/passive extension regimen of Duran and Houser and the active extension/active extension method also known as the Belfast method. These different methods with many subtle variations of the same theme are all in current use throughout the world. No one method has been shown to be better or worse than the other.

Extensor Tendon Injuries

The subcutaneous location of extensor tendons makes them susceptible to crush, laceration, and avulsion injuries. The presence of juncturae tendinae prevents proximal retraction of severed EDC tendons.[28] Extensor tendons have been divided into nine zones that ascend numerically from the nail bed to the forearm. The odd-numbered zones begin at the DIP joint and are located over the joints, whereas the even-numbered zones are located between the joints.[25]

Extensor tendons are anatomically thinner than flexor tendons and over the digits are spread out in the form of a hood. Although it may be possible to use conventional tendon repair techniques in the proximal parts of the tendons, this may not be the case in the extensor hood. Here, horizontal mattress sutures, figure-of-eight mattress sutures, or a weaving Kirchmayr suture may be needed.

Rehabilitation after repair of extensor tendons follows similar principles as for repair of the flexors. Adhesions and scar formation are notorious on the dorsal aspect of the metacarpals that responds to zone VI of extensor tendons. Injuries located in this zone require particular care to avoid tethering of the tendons, which can lead to loss of active extension and restriction of flexion. Distal injuries of the extensor tendons over the DIP and PIP joints can be protected in small finger-based splints. Injuries of the terminal slip of the extensor tendon affect only movement of the DIP joint. Repairs at this level can be immobilized in a dorsal splint that holds the DIP joint in extension. Injuries of the central slip affect primarily PIP motion and these repairs are immobilized in a Capener splint. This is a finger-based dynamic splint that permits active flexion of the PIP while passively extending it. More proximal extensor tendon injuries are protected by dynamic extensor outrigger splints that permit active flexion while passively extending the digits at the MCP joints. Immediately after repair there is a transient loss of tensile strength and gliding of the tendon. Early protected motion can increase tensile strength through collagen remodeling and improve tendon glide by preventing adhesions.[29-31]

Nerve Injuries

Nerve injuries have been variously classified depending on the extent of injury.[32,33] The time-honored method is the Seddon classification of injuries into three types: neurapraxia, axonotmesis, and neurotmesis. Neurapraxia is a physiological block of impulse conduction without anatomic disruption of the nerve fiber. A certain amount of demyelination may however be present. Neurapraxia is seen after prolonged pressure on a nerve, as may occur after prolonged use of a tourniquet or compression in confined places such as the carpal tunnel. Once the offending cause has been removed, spontaneous recovery is the rule but may take up to 6 weeks or more. Axonotmesis refers to injuries in which the axonal fibers are completely divided but the covering neural tubes are intact. Such injuries usually accompany traction injuries of nerves that rupture the weaker axons, leaving the stronger nerve sheaths intact. Unless precluded by unfavorable surroundings, these divided axons regenerate in a reliable and predictable fashion through the retained neural tubes, and a distal march of Tinel's sign can always be elicited. Neurotmesis is the highest degree of nerve injury and refers to a complete transection of the nerve. This is usually the result of direct sharp trauma or a very violent traction injury. Accurate approximation of the cut nerve ends and a meticulous repair is mandatory for good recovery. A distally progressing Tinel sign is indicative of a successful repair.

An important factor for functional recovery after nerve injury is the state of the nerve end organs. This is of particular significance in motor nerves where the muscle end plates start to undergo atrophy after loss of neural stimulation. Unless reinnervated, their number progressively dwindles with time and by 12 to 18 months may be insufficient to restore adequate function of a muscle. This factor combined with the expected time it takes a nerve to grow from the site of injury to the affected muscle determines the expected functional outcome after nerve repair.

A good nerve repair can only be accomplished under magnification. Use of an operating microscope makes it possible to approximate individual nerve fascicles and suture them together with extremely fine sutures. Repairs should be tension free and are accomplished by epineurial or perineurial repair, or both.[34] If direct repair of the cut ends cannot be accomplished without tension, an interposition nerve graft is used. The sural nerve and terminal branch of the posterior interosseous nerve are good sources of donor nerves.[35] In small nerves like the digital nerves, gaps of less than 2 cm can be bridged with vein grafts.[36]

The mechanism of nerve injury can influence the results of repair. Sharp transactions tend to do better than crushing or avulsion nerve injuries. Age of the patient also plays a role, and children do much better than adults. It has also been noted that pure motor nerves tend to regenerate better than mixed nerves and these do better than pure sensory nerves.

Vascular Injuries

Vascular injuries of the extremities can occur as a result of direct or indirect trauma. Direct trauma can be mechanical, thermal, or chemical. Mechanical trauma, in turn, can take the form of penetrations, lacerations, crushing injuries, or contusions of the vessel. This may be caused by external objects or by internal structures, such as the sharp spike of a fractured bone. Penetrating injuries can give rise to two additional injury patterns. If only the adventitia and outer part of the media are injured, the vessel wall is considerably weakened and with time the vessel may balloon out to form a pseudoaneurysm. Penetrating injuries can also on occasion lead to the development of arteriovenous fistulas. These can cause significant shunting of blood, resulting in a steal syndrome with chronic ischemic effects on the extremity. Indirect vascular trauma is caused either by traction injuries, which can avulse vessels, or repetitive microtrauma from vibratory tools, which can lead to thrombosis. The latter usually affects the ulnar artery in Guyon's canal at the wrist and is called the *ulnar hammer syndrome.* Irrespective of their cause, vascular injuries may lead to a critical compromise of circulation in the extremity and hence need to be treated on an emergent basis.

Arterial repair is indicated to prevent ischemic complications and is best accomplished under magnification. The transected vessels are examined under the operating microscope and sequentially resected until normal-looking intima is obtained. This often results in fairly large gaps between the cut ends of the vessels. As in nerves, the primary goal is a tension-free repair. To achieve this in the presence of a gap defect, interposition reversed-vein grafts are used. The saphenous vein is the preferred donor for larger vessels like the brachial, radial, or ulnar arteries. Veins on the volar surface of the forearm or dorsum of the foot are harvested to bridge gaps in digital vessels.

Major injuries that cause damage to both the radial and ulnar arteries can lead to dangerous vascular compromise. Restoration of circulation in such situations is a surgical emergency and is termed *revascularization.* This is in contrast to the term *replantation,* which is used to describe reattachment of a completely amputated part. The classic surgical sequence is to first restore stability of the limb by fixing skeletal injuries and only then repair soft tissues, including vessels. Sometimes, however, the duration may be beyond the 2 to 3 hours of warm ischemia that muscles can tolerate. In such circumstances, an immediate vascular conduit is established with the help of a vein graft to restore temporary circulation. Surgery then proceeds in the routine sequence of fixing bones followed by repair of tendons. At this stage, the temporary conduit can be resected and a definitive vascular repair performed.

Muscles often swell after prolonged periods of ischemia. This can lead to an increase of pressures within the closed compartments of the forearm, resulting in a compartment syndrome. It is hence the practice of most surgeons to perform a routine fasciotomy to decompress the forearm compartments after revascularization. Under ischemic conditions, muscle tissue switches over to anaerobic respiration, and this can result in a build-up of dangerous levels of toxic substances such as lactic acid. Furthermore, myonecrosis might occur, leading to the release of myoglobin from within the muscle cells. Restoration of circulation to such a limb can cause a sudden flooding of the circulation by these toxic substances. This is termed *reperfusion syndrome* and can lead to multiorgan failure, especially affecting the renal and cardiac systems.

Emboli may lodge in arteries at points where the vessel branches and obstruct blood flow. Such emboli usually originate from the heart or proximal arterial aneurysms. This requires embolectomy followed by anticoagulant therapy to prevent propagation of the clot. Embolectomy in larger vessels can be achieved through endovascular balloon catheters, but smaller vessels require an arteriotomy. Thrombolytic enzymes such as urokinase can also be used to dissolve emboli or thrombi but require careful monitoring in the presence of open wounds.

Digital arterial injury may accompany frostbite.[37] This is caused by both a direct injury to the endothelial cells as well as hemoconcentration with consequent hypercoagulability. Division of the sympathetic innervation of these vessels, termed *digital sympathectomy,* may improve blood flow in these conditions.

Venous injuries in the hand or upper extremity often result from intravenous cannulations with subsequent thrombophlebitis. Treatment consists of elevation, antibiotics, and warm compresses. Injuries of large veins with severe bleeding require ligation or repair of the offending vessel. Chronic compression syndromes can produce venous thrombosis in the subclavian or axillary veins, causing venous edema in the extremity. This can usually be treated by elevation, anticoagulation, and even thrombolytic therapy. Severe cases of compression of the subclavian vein at the thoracic outlet require excision of the first rib with resection of the scalene muscles.

FRACTURES AND DISLOCATIONS

Fractures are categorized according to their anatomic location within each bone.[38] Accordingly, they may occur in the head, neck, shaft, or base of a bone and may be intra-articular or extra-articular. They may be open or closed depending on whether they communicate with the exterior. Fractures can be further classified by the shape of the fracture line as transverse, oblique, spiral, or comminuted. Bending forces produce transverse or oblique fractures whereas torsional forces produce spiral fractures. Axial forces tend to cause fractures at the ends of bones, and these are often comminuted.

Distal Phalanx Fractures

Fractures of the distal phalanx are the most commonly encountered fractures in the hand.[39] They may involve the tuft, shaft, or base and are most often associated with nail bed injuries. If undisplaced or minimally displaced, they can be treated with a "gutter" or "thimble" splint for a period of 3 to 4 weeks. Unstable transverse shaft fractures require fixation with 0.035-inch diameter Kirschner wires.

Mallet Finger

A mallet finger can result from an avulsion fracture of the attachment terminal slip of the extensor mechanism at the base of the distal phalanx. The distal phalanx adopts a dropped attitude and cannot be actively extended (Fig. 73-9). Most closed mallet injuries are managed by splinting the DIP joint in extension, provided the fracture involves less than 30% of the joint surface and is displaced by less than 2 mm.[40] Grossly displaced or large intra-articular fragments may require internal fixation with a Kirschner wire.[41]

Jersey Finger

This is an avulsion fracture of the insertion of the FDP tendon into the distal phalanx. It occurs after a violent pull of the FDP against resistance, as can occur when a footballer catches onto the jersey of an opponent and forcefully pulls. The avulsed fragment may lie rarely as far proximally as in the palm. This fracture generally requires open reduction and internal fixation with a mini-screw or Kirschner wires.

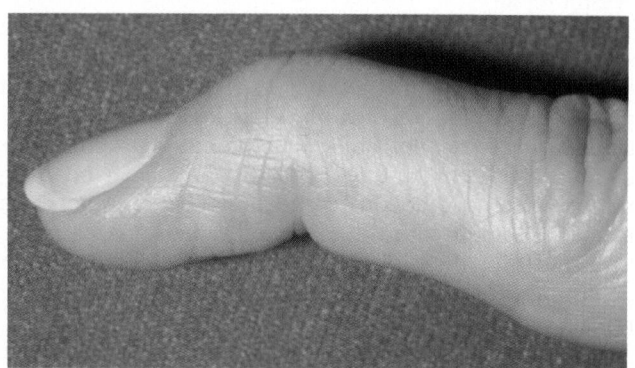

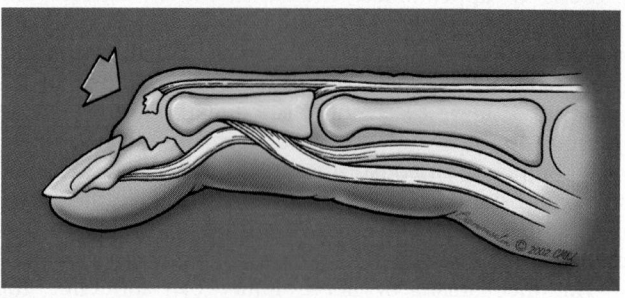

FIGURE 73-9. **A** and **B,** Mallet finger deformity.

Middle Phalanx, Proximal Phalanx, and Metacarpal Fractures

These fractures may involve the head, neck, shaft, or base of the bone. Head and base fractures are usually intra-articular. Fractures of the head are usually due to axial compression forces. If undisplaced, they can be treated by splinting. Phalangeal fractures can be immobilized in finger splints whereas metacarpal fractures are treated in a splint with the wrist in 20 to 30 degrees of dorsiflexion, the MCP joints in 70 degrees of flexion, and the IP joints fully extended. This is termed the *universal position of immobilization* of the hand. Gross displacement requires accurate restoration of the articular surface by surgery. Reduction can then be maintained by traction through an external device or by fixing the fragments with mini-screws or Kirschner wires.

Neck fractures are generally due to a combination of axial compression and bending. They are also called "booby-trap" fractures in the middle phalanx and "boxer's fracture" if involving the metacarpal of the little finger. If undisplaced, these fractures can be splinted, but if displaced or angulated more than 10 degrees, they require open reduction and internal fixation with crossed Kirschner wires or plates and screws. Dorsal angulation at the fracture with associated palmar prominence of the metacarpal head may lead to pain in the palm when gripping.[42] Angular deformities also lead to extensor lag deformity. The index and long finger metacarpals are less mobile than the ring and small finger metacarpals. Therefore, a maximum of 15 degrees of angular deformities can be tolerated in the index and long metacarpals while up to 20 to 40 degrees may be acceptable in the ring and small fingers.

Shaft fractures are caused by bending, torsional, or crushing forces. In the middle phalanx, displacement occurs as a result of forces exerted by the insertions of the FDS and the central slip (Fig. 73-10). If the fracture lies distal to the FDS insertion, the proximal fragment is flexed by this muscle, resulting in a volar angulation. In contrast, if the fracture occurs proximal to the FDS insertion, the proximal fragment is extended by the central slip of the extensor mechanism while the distal part is flexed by the FDS. This results in a dorsal angulation. Most shaft fractures of the proximal phalanx fractures tend to angulate volarward (Fig. 73-11). This is caused by the interossei, which flex the proximal fragment, and the central slip, which, via the PIP joint, extends the distal fragment. Shaft fractures that are undisplaced or those that are stable after reduction can be treated by splints. Sometimes, "buddy taping" the finger to the adjacent uninjured one suffices. This protects the interphalangeal joints and allows collateral ligaments to heal. It also permits early motion, thus preventing tendon adhesions.[43] Metacarpal fractures, however, require immobilization in the "universal position." Displaced and unstable fractures require open reduction followed by fixation with Kirschner wires or plates and screws.

Base fractures are caused by axial forces with or without an associated bending component and may be intra-articular. An abducted fracture of the base of the proximal phalanx of the little finger is called the "extra octave" injury. A special fracture in this category is an

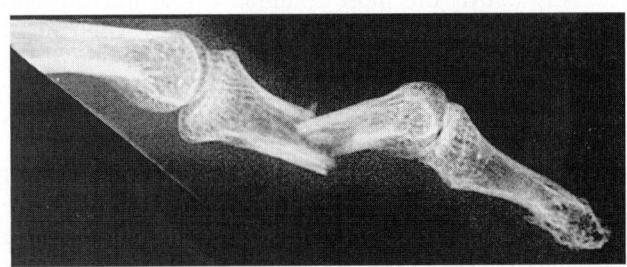

■ **FIGURE 73-10.** Middle phalanx fracture.

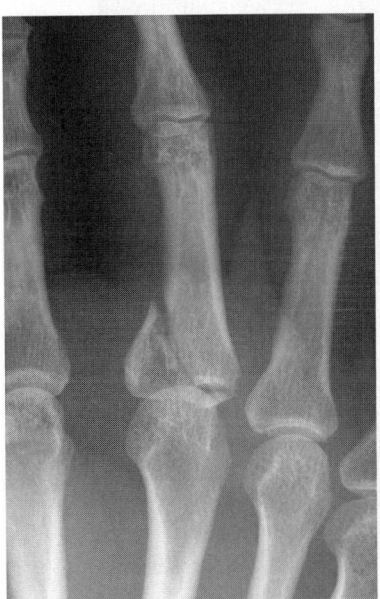 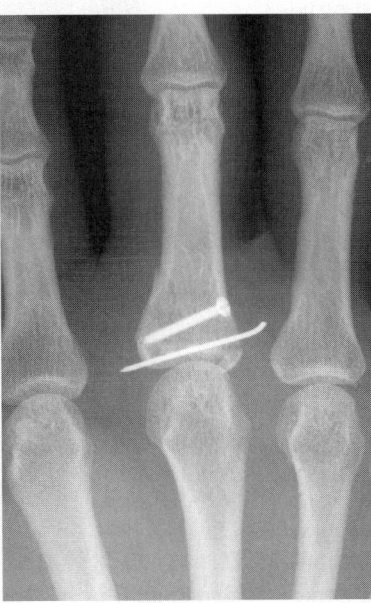

■ **FIGURE 73-11.** Intra-articular fracture of proximal phalanx.

A B

intra-articular fracture of the base of the thumb metacarpal, called Bennett's injury. Here, the large distal fragment is pulled proximally and into adduction by the abductor pollicis longus and adductor pollicis acting in tandem. The small proximal fragment is held in its anatomic location by the ulnar collateral ligament.[44] An intra-articular comminuted fracture of the base of the thumb metacarpal is known as Rolando's fracture. If undisplaced, most of the just-mentioned fractures can be treated by percutaneous pinning with Kirschner wires followed by appropriate splinting. Displaced intra-articular fractures require accurate open reduction followed by fixation with mini-screws and Kirschner wires (see Fig. 73-11). Often, isolated fractures of the bases of middle and ring finger metacarpals do not require splinting because they are immobilized quite adequately by the other intact metacarpals.

Complications that may occur after phalangeal or metacarpal fractures include malrotation, malunion, nonunion, and stiffness of the digit owing to tendon adhesions and joint contractures.

Carpal Fractures

Scaphoid Fracture

The scaphoid is the most common carpal fracture and accounts for nearly 60% of all carpal injuries. The patient may present with a diffuse pain over the radial side of the wrist. Examination reveals tenderness over the anatomic snuff box and also over the scaphoid tubercle. If a scaphoid fracture is suspected, initial radiographic examination must include posteroanterior, lateral, and a special scaphoid view, which is a posteroanterior view with the wrist in full ulnar deviation. Quite often, immediate postinjury radiographs may not reveal a fracture. CT may help in such situations, or one may opt to apply an empirical splint and repeat radiographs after 2 weeks. Blood vessels enter the scaphoid mainly through its distal half, and fractures through the "waist" may deprive the proximal half of its blood supply, leading to avascular necrosis in as many as 30% of cases.[45] Treatment of nondisplaced fractures is with a long-arm cast including the base of the thumb. This is called a thumb spica and is maintained for 6 weeks, followed by a short-arm cast for an additional 6 weeks. Displaced fractures require open reduction with screw fixation. Nonunion is a notorious problem in the scaphoid and is seen in a third of cases. These can be treated with cancellous bone grafts or pedicled vascularized bone grafts. Electrical stimulation has also been shown to be effective in tackling this problem.[46]

Hook of Hamate Fracture

An often overlooked carpal fracture is the hook of the hamate fracture, which produces hypothenar pain and tenderness. This injury has to be suspected in patients with persistent ulnar-sided wrist pain after a blow to the palm. The fracture can be demonstrated by special radiographic views or CT scans. Long-standing hook of the hamate fractures are usually treated with resection of the hook.

Fractures in Children

Fractures in children differ from adults in many ways. The growth plates are still open and injuries affecting the physis can alter bone growth. The fact that the pediatric bones are still growing also permits greater remodeling. Hence, moderate angular or translational displacements at fractures tend to correct with age. Rotational deformities never correct and are hence totally unacceptable. The pediatric skeleton is more elastic, and fractures are generally less common and less likely to be displaced. The epiphyses are located proximally in the phalanges and distally in the metacarpals, with the exception of the thumb metacarpal, where it is located proximally. The Salter-Harris classification describes five types of epiphyseal injuries (Fig. 73-12).[47] Accurate reduction and stabilization either in splints or by internal fixation is required for treatment. It is important to remember that implants that cross the physeal must cause minimal damage; hence, smooth Kirschner wires are usually preferred to threaded devices such as screws.

Dislocations

A dislocation is described according to the direction of displacement of the distal bone in the involved joint. They are more frequently seen in the PIP joint than any other joint in the hand. An important dislocation is a dorsal dislocation of the MCP joint. Here, the proximal phalanx displaces dorsally and the metacarpal head volarward. Often the metacarpal head buttonholes through and gets trapped in a fibrous space bounded by the longitudinally oriented fibers of the palmar fascia and flexor tendons on either side, the superficial transverse metacarpal ligament proximally, and the natatory ligament distally. This is

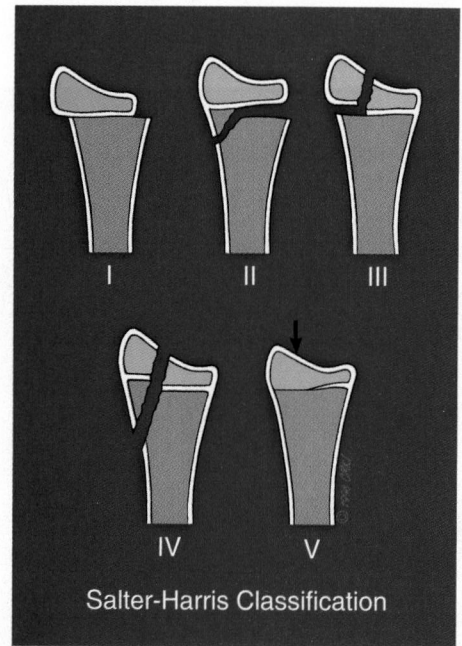

FIGURE 73-12.   Salter-Harris classification of epiphyseal injuries.

called Kaplan's lesion and is most common in the index finger. The condition invariably requires open reduction by surgical release of the offending structures. Dislocations of the carpal bones are relatively uncommon but, owing to the fact that the carpal bones are so deeply located, do not cause visible deformities. They are hence easily missed in the clinic. This problem is further compounded by the fact that the carpal bones are so twisted in their normal shapes that malalignments are not very obvious on radiographs. Dislocations need to be reduced at the earliest and immobilized in appropriate splints. Delayed recognition and inadequate treatment of these injuries can have long-term repercussions in the form of secondary degenerative arthropathy.

Traumatic Joint Instabilities

Disruption or laxity of the capsuloligamentous supports of joints can lead to various instability patterns. These can occur in the PIP and DIP joints as a result of collateral ligament and volar plate tears. Most injuries are incomplete and can be treated in a protective splint for 3 weeks, followed by buddy splinting to an adjacent normal finger for an additional 3 weeks. Infrequently, complete collateral ligament tears are seen and may require open repair.

Gamekeeper's Thumb

This injury results from rupture of the ulnar collateral ligament of the thumb MCP joint. The collateral ligament lies immediately deep to the insertion of the adductor pollicis aponeurosis at this location. Often, the avulsed collateral ligament folds back on itself and at that moment the adductor aponeurosis gets interposed between it and the bone. This is called the Stener lesion and invariably requires surgery because healing is impossible without open reduction and reattachment of the ligament.[48]

AMPUTATION AND REPLANTATION

Increasing industrialization and mechanization has led to a proportional increase in the number of severe hand injuries seen. Total amputation of parts or whole of the upper extremity at various levels is seen quite often and requires reattachment. Such a procedure is termed *replantation,* and its feasibility depends on various factors, including the level and type of amputation; the patient's age, occupation, and medical history; and associated risk factors. Another obvious factor is the surgical expertise of the treating surgeon. Clean-cut or sharp amputations are easier to replant, whereas crushing or avulsion injuries are less amenable to salvage. Nerve regeneration is better in children and accordingly better functional recovery can be expected. It has also been noted that replantations at more distant levels like the wrist or at the level of the digits tend to recover better because nerves can reinnervate their end organs faster, before atrophy sets in. At the digital levels, replantation should always be attempted if the thumb is involved in view of its importance in hand function. Multiple digital amputations also require serious attempt at replantation. Single digital amputations and ring avulsion amputations are relative indications because functional recovery is often suboptimal even if the replanted part survives.

Contraindications to replantation include medical conditions that are not compatible with a long duration of anesthesia. Relative contraindications include vascular disorders, diabetes, hypertension, multiple injury levels, gross contamination, ring avulsion injuries, prolonged ischemia, and advanced age. Before embarking on replantation, the patient must be made aware of the many months of postoperative care and rehabilitation that are mandatory to recover useful function.

Transportation of the amputated part to the replantation center is of paramount importance and significantly affects the success of surgery. The severed part is cleaned with a sterile isotonic solution, wrapped in moist sterile gauze, and then sealed in a waterproof bag. This bag is placed in a container of ice and sent to the replantation center. Muscle is very poorly tolerant of ischemia and hence the more proximal the amputation, the lesser the permissible ischemia time before replantation. With proper preservation and cooling, the permissible ischemia time can be extended to 8 hours for proximal amputations, whereas in digits it can be as long as 12 hours or more.

The sequence of replantation has been standardized and but for minor variations is the same all over the world (Fig. 73-13). The first step is to meticulously dissect and débride the amputated part under magnification and identify all structures. It is essential to find at least one good artery and two good veins for a problem-free replantation. Next, the proximal stump is débrided, explored, and corresponding structures identified. Restoration of skeletal stability is then restored by stable fixation. Often, it is essential to shorten the skeleton to achieve a tension-free vascular repair. This is then followed by repair of the flexor tendons, arteries, nerves, veins, and, finally, skin. In more proximal replantations, a forearm fasciotomy is usually performed to preclude a compartment syndrome from developing. Sometimes, ischemia is very prolonged and it becomes imperative to restore perfusion before all else. In such circumstances, a "table-top" arterial conduit can be established with an interposition vein graft. Surgery then proceeds in the usual fashion. It is also helpful in such circumstances to flush out the amputated part with isotonic intravenous solutions to get rid of potential toxic metabolites, as described earlier in the section on vascular trauma.

After a replantation, a bulky dressing is applied to the limb, which is then placed in a well-padded splint. The limb is kept warm, and anticoagulant therapy in the form of a mixture of 5000 units of heparin in 500 mL of low-molecular-weight dextran is administered over 24 hours. The replanted part is then scrupulously monitored for adequacy of circulation by regularly checking its turgor, color, and capillary refill. Thermocouples can be used to monitor the temperature while plethysmography helps in monitoring the circulatory status of the replant.

Excessive turgor, dusky purple discoloration, and a very rapid capillary refill indicate venous obstruction. Treatment

FIGURE 73-13.   Replantation. **A,** Radiograph of hand with multiple-digit amputation. **B,** Radiograph of severed digits. **C,** Severed digits with fairly sharp amputation edges. **D,** Immediately after replantation (palmar view). **E,** Immediately after replantation (dorsal view). **F,** Three-year follow-up showing extension. **G,** Three-year follow-up showing flexion. (**A** to **G,** Courtesy of Tsu-Min Tsai, M.D.)

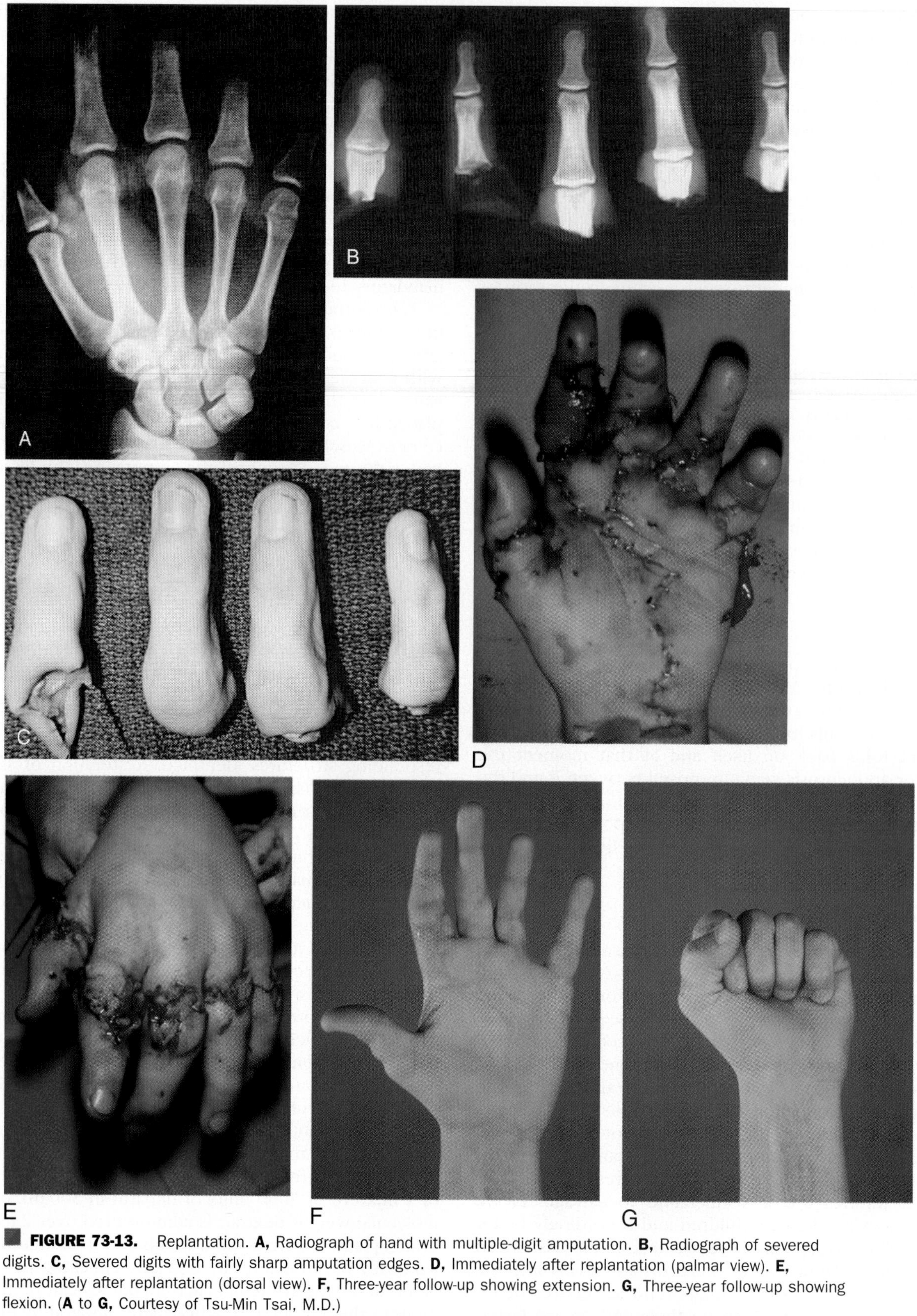

includes releasing tight dressings and sutures, removing the nail plate, and applying heparin-soaked pledgets to the nail bed. Sometimes, medicinal leeches are used to aid in decongestion. Blood loss should be monitored when using any of these methods. Medicinal leeches, although usually safe, can harbor *Aeromonas hydrophila*, requiring prophylactic antimicrobial treatment. A cold, flaccid, pale part with poor or no capillary refill suggests arterial occlusion. This usually requires immediate reexploration under magnification. It has been our experience that 50% of replantations with subsequent vascular compromise can be salvaged by prompt and appropriate intervention.

NERVE COMPRESSION SYNDROMES

Nerves pass through several anatomic bottlenecks along their course in the upper extremity (Fig. 73-14). These are potential sites of nerve compression syndromes and lead to sensory and motor deficits distal to the site of entrapment.

Median Nerve Compression

The median nerve can potentially be compressed at five sites in the upper extremity. From distal to proximal these are the carpal tunnel at the wrist, the fibrous arch between the two heads of FDS in the proximal forearm, the two heads of the pronator teres just distal to the elbow, the lacertus fibrosus at the elbow, and the ligament of Struthers in the lower arm. Compression under the carpal tunnel produces carpal tunnel syndrome whereas compression at any of the other four sites is loosely grouped under pronator syndrome.

Carpal Tunnel Syndrome

The carpal tunnel is a tight osseofibrous tunnel at the wrist traversed by the median nerve and all nine long digital flexor tendons. Its floor is formed by the carpal bones and

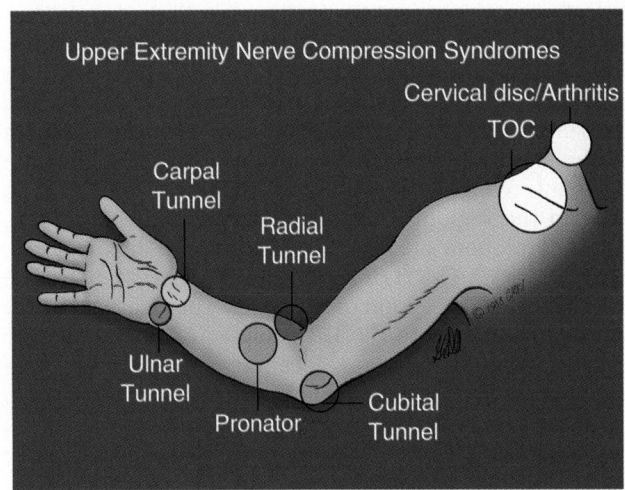

FIGURE 73-14. Potential sites of nerve compression. TOC, thoracic outlet compression.

its roof by the flexor retinaculum. Normal pressures in this tunnel are 20 to 30 mm Hg. Any rise in pressure above this causes progressive conduction blocks in the nerve with subsequent sensory and motor dysfunction. Pain and paresthesia are the earliest symptoms and are characteristically more at night or after prolonged activity. The patient may also complaint of clumsiness of his or her hands with a proclivity for dropping objects.

Flexor synovitis is the most common cause of carpal tunnel syndrome, but it may also follow traumatic derangement of the carpal alignment. Other less common causes include space-occupying lesions in the carpal tunnel or a persistent median artery.

Sensory evaluation may reveal a widened two-point discrimination and a positive Tinel sign over the wrist. Holding the wrist in acute flexion may elicit paresthesia along the median nerve distribution. This is called the Phalen test and is considered positive if symptoms develop in less than a minute.[49] Thenar weakness or wasting is usually a late finding and suggests a severe degree of compression. Nerve conduction studies and electromyography can be useful adjuncts to clinical examination.

Initial treatment of carpal tunnel syndrome is nonoperative and includes the use of wrist splints or local corticosteroid injections. Modifications in work patterns help, such as avoiding vibratory machinery and repetitive motion. Persistence of symptoms is an indication for surgical decompression. This is achieved by longitudinally dividing the flexor retinaculum by open or endoscopic means. Synovectomy and removal of any mass lesion is also necessary if that is the cause for the problem.

Pronator Syndrome

Compression of the median nerve at any of the four sites proximal to the wrist produces symptoms that are largely similar to those of carpal tunnel syndrome. However, nocturnal symptoms are relatively uncommon although the palm may feel more numb because the palmar cutaneous branch is also involved. Symptoms are reproduced or worsened by attempting pronation against resistance, the so-called pronator stress test. Resisted flexion of the long finger may also worsen symptoms, indicating compression under the FDS arch. Nevertheless, it is difficult to be categorical of the exact site that is causing the pronator syndrome and, hence, surgical decompression may involve release of all the four potential sites of compression.

Ulnar Nerve Compression

The ulnar nerve has three potential sites of compression. Starting distally, these are Guyon's canal at the wrist, the cubital tunnel at the elbow, or the medial intermuscular septum in the distal arm.

Guyon's Canal

Guyon's canal is bounded by the hook of the hamate, pisiform, pisohamate ligament, and palmar carpal ligament.[50]

Compression of the ulnar nerve known to occur at this site is most often idiopathic.[51] Trauma, mass lesions, and synovitis are some of the other causes. Motor and sensory deficits of the ulnar nerve develop. A positive Tinel sign and worsening of symptoms by direct compression are clinical means of detecting Guyon's canal syndrome. Treatment is surgical and consists of dividing the palmar carpal ligament as well as removing any offending mass in the region.

Cubital Tunnel Syndrome

As it passes into the forearm, the ulnar nerve curves tightly around the grooved posterior and inferior surfaces of the medial humeral epicondyle. This groove is bridged by Osborne's ligament proximally and the two heads of the FCU distally. Compression of the ulnar nerve in this osteofibrous tunnel is termed the *cubital tunnel syndrome.* Motor and sensory symptoms develop along the distribution of the ulnar nerve and are worsened by adopting a flexed attitude at the elbow. Examination reveals a positive Tinel sign over the tunnel and aggravation of symptoms by sustained hyperflexion of the elbow.

Initial treatment is nonoperative and consists of splinting of the elbow in extension at night followed during the day by soft extension pads to prevent elbow flexion or direct pressure on the nerve. Failure of nonoperative means is an indication for surgical decompression. The fascia overlying the cubital tunnel is divided either by open or endoscopic means. If this also fails, the ulnar nerve is freed of all fibrous restraints around the elbow and transposed anterior to the medial epicondyle into a subcutaneous or submuscular position.

Radial Nerve Compression

Sites of radial nerve compression starting proximally include the triangular space in the axilla, the spiral groove in the arm, and the lateral intermuscular septum proximal to the elbow. More distally, the posterior interosseous nerve, which is the principal motor division of the radial nerve, can get compressed near the annular ligament of the radial head or within the substance of the supinator muscle. This may result in variable degrees of paresis of muscles innervated by the radial nerve.[52] Initial treatment is splinting the arm; and, if this fails, the nerve is surgically decompressed.

Thoracic Outlet Syndrome

All the neurovascular structures that enter the upper extremity do so through the thoracic outlet. This is a narrow space at the base of the neck bounded by the first rib medially, the scalenus anticus muscle and clavicle anteriorly, and the scalenus medius muscle posteriorly.[53] All the elements of the brachial plexus as well as the subclavian artery and vein can be potentially compressed at this site. Thoracic outlet syndrome usually occurs in women between the ages of 18 and 35 years. It can be idiopathic or triggered by injuries and repetitive strains. Symptoms include easy fatigability as well as diffuse pains radiating down the entire upper extremity.

Clinical examination may be unremarkable or reveal a confusing mass of findings. A positive Tinel sign can often be elicited at both the supraclavicular and infraclavicular regions. Roos' test is performed by asking the patient to hold both the arms overhead in a "surrender" position while opening and closing the fist. This reproduces symptoms within 1 minute. Adson's test involves palpating the radial pulse while the patient turns the chin toward the same side, inhales deeply, and holds his or her breath. The test is termed positive if the radial pulse disappears or diminishes in volume and if the maneuver reproduces symptoms. The costoclavicular compression test involves sustained downward pressure on the clavicle and is positive if symptoms are reproduced. An anteroposterior radiogram of the lower cervical spine may reveal a cervical rib. Nerve conduction studies are often normal but may reveal slowing of nerve conduction velocities at more peripheral sites of compression, a condition termed *double-crush syndrome.*

Treatment of the thoracic outlet syndrome is primarily nonoperative. Neck and thoracic muscle exercises are instituted, and activities that precipitate the symptoms are modified or curtailed. Injection of a local anesthetic agent with corticosteroid into the anterior scalene muscles may relieve symptoms in some cases. Persistent symptoms particularly if supported by electrophysiologic and radiologic evidence of potential compression require surgical decompression. This is accomplished by a transcervical or transaxillary resection of the first rib, often with release of the scalene muscles.

TUMORS

Tumors are uncommon in the hand, and nearly 95% are benign.

Ganglion Cyst

Ganglions account for 70% of all tumors in the hand. They are formed by an outpouching of the synovial membrane from a joint or tendon sheath and contain a thick jelly-like mucinous substance, similar in composition to synovial fluid. Sixty percent of ganglions occur on the dorsal aspect of the wrist and arise in the region of the scapholunate ligament. Volar wrist ganglions are fewer and tend to arise in the region of the scaphotrapeziotrapezoid joint. Another frequent site for these tumors is the flexor sheath, especially at the level of the A1 pulley where they can be felt to move with flexion of the finger. They can also occur after osteoarthritis of the DIP joints and are erroneously called mucus cysts. In this location, a ganglion cyst can exert pressure on the germinal matrix of the nail bed, resulting in a deformed or grooved nail.

Ganglions are more common in women and occur usually around the third decade of life. By themselves, these tumors are innocuous and can be left alone.

Treatment is required only for cosmetic purposes or to relieve pressure effects on adjacent structures. Aspiration of the mucinous substance with a large-bore needle followed by instillation of a corticosteroid into the sac may suffice. If this fails, the ganglion is surgically excised. Particular care is taken to trace and resect the root or pedicle of the tumor right down from the joint or sheath from which it arises. The volar wrist ganglion is often very closely related to the radial artery. The Allen test is performed before surgery to determine the adequacy of ulnar arterial flow, lest accidental injury to the radial artery during excision lead to ischemia of the hand. Sometimes it may be necessary to leave behind a cuff of ganglion wall attached to the radial artery to avoid injuring it. At the level of the DIP joint, optimal treatment includes meticulous excision followed by removal of osteophytes from the joint.[54]

Giant Cell Tumor

Giant cell tumor, also known as pigmented villonodular synovitis (PVNS), is the second most common hand tumor and arises from the synovial membrane of joints or tendon sheaths. It is yellow-brown on gross appearance and contains multinucleated giant cells on microscopy. The tumor is almost invariably benign in the hand and generally asymptomatic, although it may produce notching of adjacent bones by pressure. Giant cell tumors can also envelop digital neurovascular bundles or extend along the tendon sheaths. Treatment is surgical and consists of excision of the tumor along with any involved synovium.

Epidermal Inclusion Cyst

Epidermal inclusion cysts are also known as implantation dermoids and occur after trauma. Epidermal cells become accidentally lodged in the subcutaneous tissue and continue to grow there. They occur more often in men and are usually found fixed to the palmar skin. Symptoms are related to the size and location of the cyst. Treatment is surgical excision, and recurrence is rare.

Lipoma

Lipomas make up 3% of hand tumors and can be located anywhere, although the thenar eminence is the most frequent site. They are usually painless but may become symptomatic by compressing on adjacent nerves. Recurrence is rare, but resection can be tedious if the tumor is large.

Pyogenic Granuloma

Pyogenic granuloma is a misnomer for an exuberant outgrowth of granulation tissue at sites of previous trauma. The lesions are highly vascular with a thin epithelial cover and are friable, bleed easily, and can grow rapidly. They occur most commonly on the fingertips and respond to either curettage or simple excision.

Verruca Vulgaris

Verruca vulgaris are viral warts and occur usually on the digits especially in the nail bed region. They are treated most effectively by coagulation, curettage, or excision. Recurrence is not uncommon, especially in the region of the nail bed.

Vascular Malformations

These may be hemangiomas or arteriovenous malformations and may present at any time before or after birth. They are frequently associated with massive hypertrophy of the involved area and can invade and envelop virtually all tissue planes of the hand. Compression garments can be tried but give unpredictable results. Injury can result in uncontrolled bleeding, and involved digits can be so massive as to hamper hand function. Selective embolization has been tried in cases in which a definite feeder vessel could be identified. More often than not, amputation of the involved ray may be required.

INFECTION

Infection of the hand is fairly common and assumes significance because of the severe functional compromise that may result from improper or inadequate treatment.

Paronychia

Paronychia refers to infection of the lateral nail folds and usually results from a penetrating injury. The most common causative organism is *Staphylococcus aureus*. Treatment for early cases is with antibiotics, preferably a penicillin in combination with a β-lactamase inhibitor such as sulbactam or clavulanic acid. Once an abscess develops, surgical drainage is required. Traditionally, this has been achieved by making a longitudinal incision just lateral and parallel to the nail fold; however, recent recommendations are to merely remove the nail and let the pus drain out from under the nail fold.

Felon

A felon is an abscess of the pulp space and usually accompanies paronychia. Because the pulp space contains rigid fibrous septa fixing the skin to the periosteum of the distal phalanx, collections in this region can lead to a build-up of high pressures that can be severely painful. Appropriate treatment is surgical incision and drainage of the abscess followed by appropriate antibiotics. Complications include septic tenosynovitis, skin necrosis, and osteomyelitis of the distal phalanx.

Suppurative Tenosynovitis (Acute and Chronic)

Acute suppurative tenosynovitis most commonly affects the flexor tendon sheaths. They usually arise after penetrating trauma and are caused by *Staphylococcus aureus*. Kanavel described four cardinal signs in the digit: a fusiform swelling, a flexed attitude, tenderness over the tendon sheath, and pain on passive extension.[55] Early cases may respond to nonoperative treatment, including elevation, warm soaks, and intravenous antibiotics. Unresponsive or late cases require surgical drainage. The flexor sheath is opened through two separate incisions proximally at the level of the A1 pulley and distally at the level of the A5 pulley. A small catheter or infant feeding tube is passed down the flexor sheath through these incisions and continuously irrigated with isotonic saline or lactated Ringer's solution for 36 to 48 hours. Antibiotics are required for at least 1 or 2 weeks. More severe infections or a delay in treatment may lead to necrosis of the tendon sheath, osteomyelitis, and abscesses. These are best treated by thorough débridement through an extensive exposure.

Chronic tenosynovitis is usually of a granulomatous type and is caused by *Mycobacterium tuberculosis*, atypical mycobacteria, or fungi. Treatment includes administration of appropriate antimicrobial agents combined with surgical excision of the involved synovium. Chronic infective synovitis needs to be differentiated from other causes of chronic granulomatous synovitis, such as sarcoidosis and amyloidosis.

Deep Space Infections

Kanavel described fascial spaces in the hand where infections tend to localize.[55] There are three palmar spaces lying deep to the palmar aponeurosis, namely, the midpalmar, thenar, and hypothenar spaces. A fourth space, termed *Parona's space,* is in the distal forearm and overlies the pronator quadratus muscle. On the dorsal aspect of the hand, the subaponeurotic space lies deep to the extensor tendons over the dorsal interosseous muscles.

Deep infections can lead to the collection of pus in any of these areas and require surgical drainage followed by appropriate antibiotic therapy.

Web space fissures, cuts, or blisters can become infected. This may progress dorsally, involving the space between the superficial and deep transverse metacarpal ligaments. The web space assumes an hourglass shape, which is referred to as a "collar-stud" abscess. The abscess is best drained by both dorsal and palmar incisions. Transverse incisions should be avoided because they may lead to contracture and narrowing of the web space.

Herpes Infection

Herpetic infection or "whitlow" of a digit is caused by the herpes simplex virus and is frequently seen in health care personnel in which the source is usually orotracheal secretions of patients. The organism incubates for 2 to 14 days before forming fluid-filled vesicles on the fingertip. These lesions can sometimes mimic paronychia or felons. The diagnosis is made from a potassium hydroxide prep and Tzanck smear. Viral cultures and immunofluorescence with radioisotope-tagged antibodies can be helpful. Clinically, herpetic infections must be differentiated from bacterial infections. Herpetic infections are self-limiting, and treatment is nonoperative. Surgical incision and drainage can lead to systemic involvement and possible viral encephalitis.

Bites

Animal and human bites are quite common on the hand. Of them, human bites carry the worst prognosis. Human bites are contaminated by mixed oral flora and if untreated can lead to severe infection with rapid destruction of local tissue. Common organisms infecting human bites are *Staphylococcus, Streptococcus, Bacteroides,* and *Eikenella corrodens.*[56] Most human bite injuries on the hand occur when an individual strikes another person in the mouth with a clenched fist. A tooth produces a puncture wound that may even penetrate into the MCP joint. Clinical examination should focus on the possibility of extensor tendon injury and joint penetration. Surgical exploration, débridement, and lavage are mandatory in the treatment of these injuries. Human bite wounds should not be closed primarily and are treated with penicillins or cephalosporins after surgery.

CONGENITAL ANOMALIES

Congenital hand anomalies are sporadic in their incidence. Their causes may be genetic, teratogenic, or idiopathic and may have syndromic association with anomalies elsewhere in the body. The most common hand anomalies are syndactyly and polydactyly.

Syndactyly

Syndactyly is most prevalent in the Western Hemisphere and is classified as failure of differentiation of parts or structures. It is characterized as fusion of adjacent digits and can involve part or whole of the length of involved digits (Fig. 73-15). If fusion is limited to skin and soft tissues only, the syndactyly is termed "simple" and if skeletal fusion occurs, it is called "complex." Apert's syndrome is a severe form of syndactyly. Treatment is a surgical separation of the digits within the first year of life. Local flaps and full-thickness skin grafts are necessary to achieve full coverage of the separated digits.

Polydactyly

Polydactyly is more prevalent in the African continent and is classified as a duplication of digits. It is very variable in its clinical presentation and ranges from simple skin tags to a complete supernumerary digit, most often the thumb (Fig. 73-16). Treatment is removal of the extra appendage. Tissue parts from the excised appendage can be used to reconstruct the resected region.

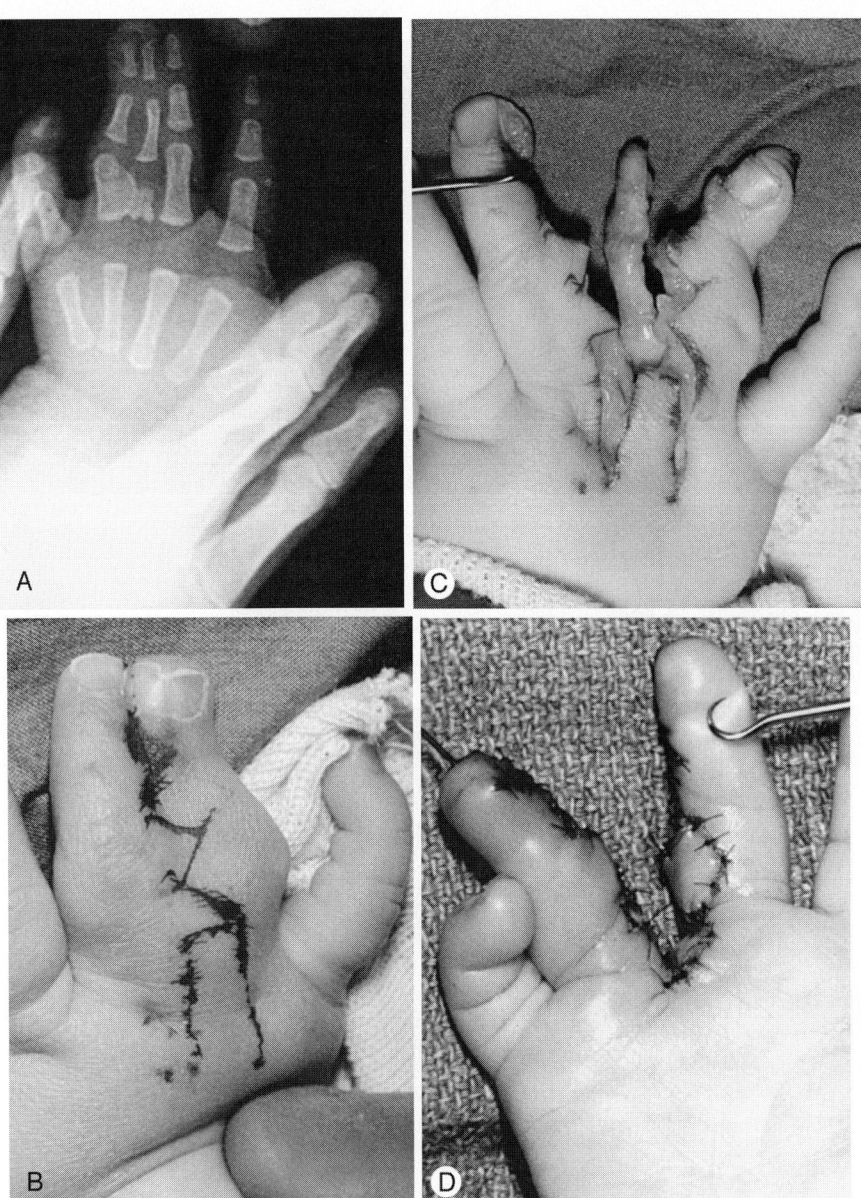

■ FIGURE 73-15.   Syndactyly.
A, Radiograph showing hidden polydactyly between third and fourth digits.
B, Marking the planned incisions to prevent scar contractures.
C, Intraoperative photography showing excision of hidden extra digit.
D, Immediate postoperative photograph.

Growth Arrests

Growth arrests can affect parts or whole of the upper extremity. Brachydactyly is failure of longitudinal growth of digits. Partial or complete longitudinal growth deficits affecting the radius or ulna produce radial and ulnar "club hands," respectively. Radial club hand, or manus valgus, is the more common of the two and can be associated with other anomalies, such as thrombocytopenia, Fanconi's anemia, or the VACTERL complex (*V*ertebral defects, *A*norectal malformation, *C*ardiac anomalies, *T*racheoesophageal fistula, *E*sophageal atresia, *R*enal dysplasia, and *L*imb anomalies). Poland's syndrome is a condition characterized by ipsilateral chest wall and limb hypoplasia. Treatment of any of these problems involves lengthening and realignment of existing structures.

Constriction Band Syndrome

Constriction band syndrome is secondary to intrauterine amniotic bands. These can act like tourniquets and threaten the viability of digits, limbs, and other parts. This condition often results in congenital amputation. It is important to differentiate congenital amniotic bands from acquired bands that may occur in infants because of neglected external ligatures, termed the *hair-thread-tourniquet syndrome.*

Clinodactyly

Clinodactyly is a deviation of digits toward the radial or ulnar direction. This usually involves the distal phalanx

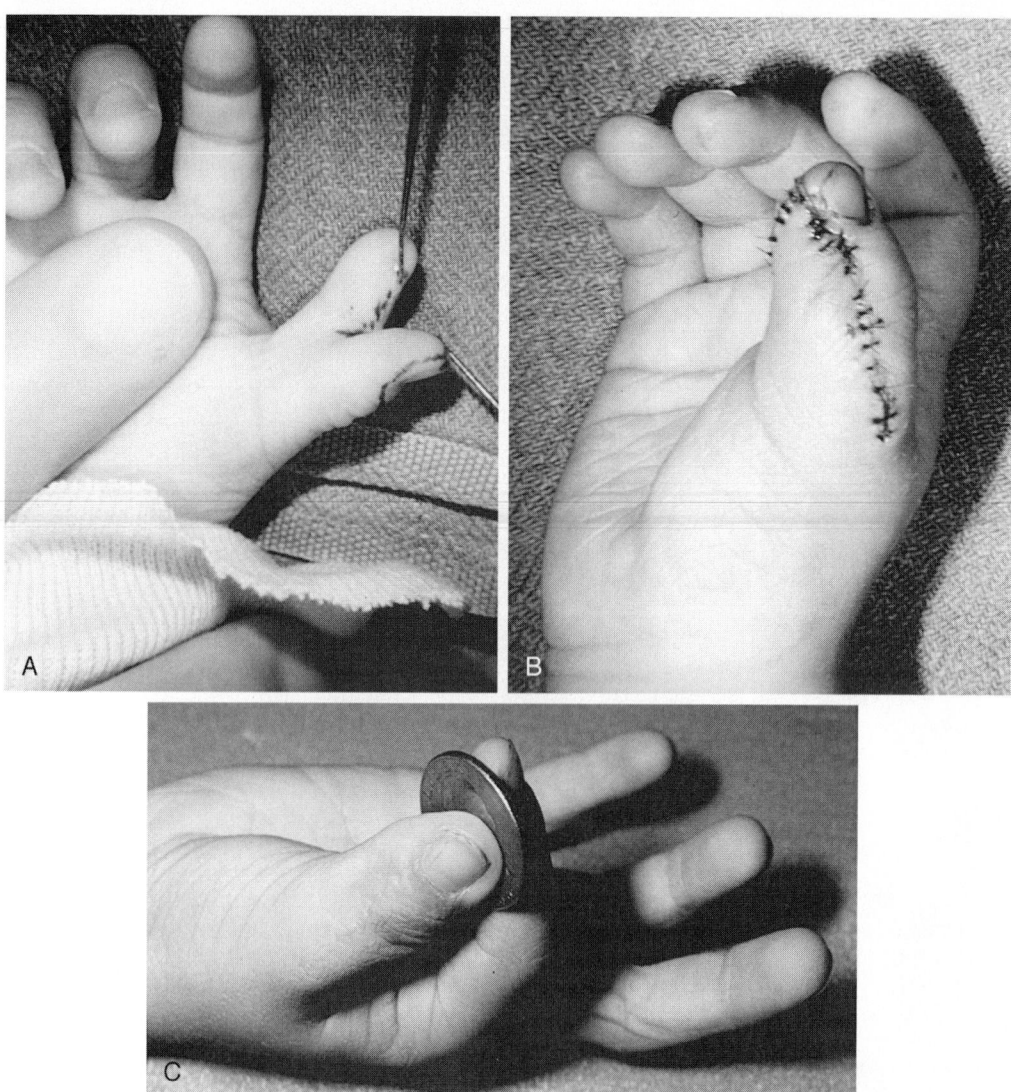

FIGURE 73-16.   Thumb duplication. **A,** Preoperative view. **B,** Immediate postoperative view. **C,** At 5-year follow-up, normal thumb function.

and is commonly seen with the presence of a triangular middle phalanx termed the *delta phalanx*. Treatment is required if the problem is affecting function and involves corrective osteotomy.

Camptodactyly

Camptodactyly is a congenital flexion deformity of digits occurring in the sagittal plane. It is most common and severe in the small finger at the PIP joint. Initial treatment is by serial splinting or distraction histogenesis with an external fixator. If this does not correct the deformity, surgical correction by Z-plasties of the skin is performed. It is important to remember that camptodactyly is usually accompanied by deficient skin, and surgical correction may require the additional use of skin grafts.

TENOSYNOVITIS

De Quervain's Disease

De Quervain's disease is a constricting tenosynovitis affecting the tendons of EPB and APL in the first extensor compartment. The main symptom is pain worsened by activity. There may be a fusiform swelling of the tendon sheath, and the region is tender to palpate. Finkelstein described a test in which ulnar deviation of the wrist with the thumb grasped in a fist causes pain.[57] The opposite hand should also be tested to unmask subclinical affectations.

De Quervain's disease is initially treated nonoperatively by local corticosteroid injection and rest in a thumb spica splint. If these measures fail, surgical decompression of the first dorsal compartment is performed. Care is taken to protect the radial sensory nerve branches, which course just under the skin in this area because trauma or transection leads to painfully disabling neuromas.

Trigger Finger

Trigger finger is a constricting tenosynovitis of the flexor tendons at the level of the A1 pulley. The condition is divided into four grades of increasing severity. Grade I is characterized by pain and tenderness at the A1 pulley. Grade II is associated with the development of a palpable nodule in the flexor tendon, but the tendon still glides in and out of the flexor sheath. Grade III is when the characteristic "triggering" occurs. The patient can flex the digit, but the nodule catches at the proximal edge of the A1 pulley, locking the PIP joint in this flexed position. Attempts at extending the digit cause it to suddenly snap back, much like the trigger of a gun. Often, the patient needs to use the opposite hand to unlock and extend the digit. Grade IV is when the constriction is so tight that the patient either cannot flex the digit or it gets fixed in the flexed position and can no longer be fully extended.

Nonoperative treatment includes local injection of a corticosteroid preparation. Ultrasound massage of the A1 pulley has also been tried to help increase its viscoelasticity and thus expand it to some extent. If this regimen fails, the A1 pulley is longitudinally divided under direct vision. Triggering can also occur in the thumb and is treated similarly. The annular pulley is divided longitudinally on its radial side to avoid accidental division of the oblique pulley that lies immediately distal to the ulnar border of the annular pulley.

Extensor Carpi Ulnaris Tenosynovitis

The ECU tendon and its subsheath are important dorsal supports of the distal radioulnar joint (DRUJ) and triangular fibrocartilage complex (TFCC). Inflammation of this tendon may occur after repetitive strain and forms an important cause of the enigmatic ulnar-sided wrist pain syndrome (USWP). Differential diagnosis includes TFCC tears as well as arthropathy and sprains of the DRUJ and pisotriquetral and lunotriquetral joints. Diagnosis is made by eliciting tenderness along the ECU tendon as well as pain on resisted ulnar extension of the wrist. Treatment includes splinting and local corticosteroid injection.

Intersection Syndrome

This is an ill-understood condition characterized by pain and crepitus at the point where the APL and EPB tendons intersect the tendons of ECRL and ECRB. Initial treatment is by splinting, local corticosteroid injection, and anti-inflammatory medication. Refractory cases require surgical excision of involved tenosynovial membranes and local fascial thickening, which is frequently seen.

Other sites of tenosynovitis include the FCR and FCU tendons. These can be treated by splinting and local corticosteroid injection.

ARTHRITIS

Osteoarthritis (Primary and Secondary)

Primary osteoarthritis is a degenerative joint disease that generally occurs later in life and is seen in 90% of women and 80% of men by the eighth decade of life. An injury to a joint that leaves the articular surfaces incongruous can precipitate a secondary osteoarthritis within 5 to 6 years after injury. The condition is relentlessly progressive and usually affects the hands and large weight-bearing joints.

Osteoarthritis begins with a biochemical alteration of the water content of articular cartilage. Soon the cartilage weakens and develops small cracks, a condition termed *fibrillation.* Progressive erosion and thinning of the cartilage leads to increased stress on the subchondral bone, which becomes highly sclerotic and polished like ivory. This is termed *eburnation.* The overloaded joint tries to compensate by forming new bone around the edges of the articular cartilage. These bony outcroppings are called *osteophytes.*

Osteoarthritis most commonly affects the DIP and PIP joints in the fingers and the carpometacarpal joint of the thumb. Osteophytes at the DIP joints are called Heberden's nodes, and those at the PIP joint are called Bouchard's nodes. The involved joints are painful and stiff. They may be deformed or may subluxate. Compression with a rotatory movement along the long axis of the digit is called the "grinding test" and produces pain. Radiography reveals narrowing of the joint space, sclerosis of subchondral bone, and the presence of osteophytes.

Initial treatment consists of local corticosteroid injection and splinting. Chondroprotective agents such as glucosamine and chondroitin sulfate have demonstrated ability to reduce symptoms if started early. If this does not provide relief, surgical intervention is required. Synovectomy and joint débridement are often all that may be required. In very advanced cases, the DIP joints respond best to resection of osteophytes, followed by arthrodesis (surgical fusion) of the joint. PIP joints require replacement by silicone prosthesis, although arthrodesis can also be selectively used. The thumb CMC joint is treated by arthrodesis in the young because it provides greater stability and can tolerate loads better. In the elderly, excision of the trapezium followed by a suspension-interposition arthroplasty is preferred. The arthroplasty consists of interposing a length of tendon, rolled into a ball, in the space created by excising the trapezium. In addition, the first metacarpal is suspended from the second with the help of a surgically constructed tendinous sling. This provides greater stability but is less tolerant of heavy activity, a factor that should not be of great concern in the elderly.

Rheumatoid Arthritis

Rheumatoid arthritis is a chronic, systemic, autoimmune disorder of uncertain origin.[58] The condition can affect all connective tissue elements and leads to damage of joints, tendons, and ligaments. About 2 million people are affected by this disorder in the United States. Women are two to three times more susceptible to rheumatoid arthritis, and the disease usually begins in the fourth decade of life. Management of this disorder requires a team effort and is primarily at two levels. The rheumatoid disease process needs medical management by a rheumatologist whereas the mechanical deformities are managed by orthopedic and hand surgeons. Psychiatrists, physiotherapists, orthotists, and prosthetists form the remaining members of the team. In the hand, surgical intervention is required for basically two purposes: reduction of pain and restoration of normal mechanics.

Synovial hypertrophy can be severely painful, and the patient presents with swollen, inflamed joints. Local corticosteroid injections may help, but, sometimes, synovectomy is indicated. Excising unhealthy synovium also can protect the joint from destruction by reducing pannus formation. Treatment of the disease process continues at the same time with nonsteroidal anti-inflammatory drugs (NSAIDs) as well as disease-modifying antirheumatoid drugs (DMARDs).

Mechanical derangements occur at all joints and usually follow characteristic patterns. At the wrist this usually takes the form of radial deviation, whereas in the digits more complex deformity patterns occur.

Boutonnière Deformity

This deformity of digits is characterized by a flexion at the PIP and hyperextension at the DIP joints (Fig. 73-17). It is usually caused by attenuation and eventual rupture of the central slip of the extensor mechanism. The head of the proximal phalanx then luxates dorsally and "buttonholes" between the lateral bands of the extensor mechanism. This causes an over-pull on the terminal slip, leading to hyperextension of the DIP joint. If seen early, the condition can be treated by dynamic splinting. Late cases require surgical correction.

Swan-Neck Deformity

Swan-neck deformity is the mechanical opposite of a boutonniere deformity and is characterized by hyperextension at the PIP joint and flexion at the DIP joint (Fig. 73-18). The deformity can be caused by a variety of factors, including synovitis and volar plate inadequacy at the PIP joint, tightness of the intrinsic muscles, and adhesions of the FDS tendon in the flexor sheath with subsequent loss of volar support of the PIP joint. Attenuation or rupture of the terminal slip of the extensor mechanism can cause a mallet deformity with secondary over-pull of the central slip producing the deformity. As in boutonnière deformity, swan neck deformity may respond to splinting if seen early. Late cases require surgical correction.

Ulnar Drift

This deformity occurs typically at the MCP joints and is accompanied by an ulnar subluxation of the long extensor tendons. In combination with a radial deviation of the wrist, ulnar drift of the fingers produces a characteristic "Z" deformity of the hand (Fig. 73-19). The radial collateral ligaments of the MCP joints are grossly attenuated whereas the ulnar collateral ligaments shorten, maintaining the deformity. Often, the joints are volarly luxated as well. If seen early, dynamic splinting helps correct the deformity and also decreases synovial inflammation. Late cases require surgery. If the MCP joints are not eroded or grossly volar luxated, soft tissue realignment suffices. Eroded and grossly luxated MCP joints require additional prosthetic replacement.

CONTRACTURES

Mobility is the most important prerequisite for normal hand function. Various conditions cause stiffness and contractures of hand joints and include post-traumatic contractures, Dupuytren's disease, and Volkmann's ischemic contracture. Post-traumatic contractures are by far the

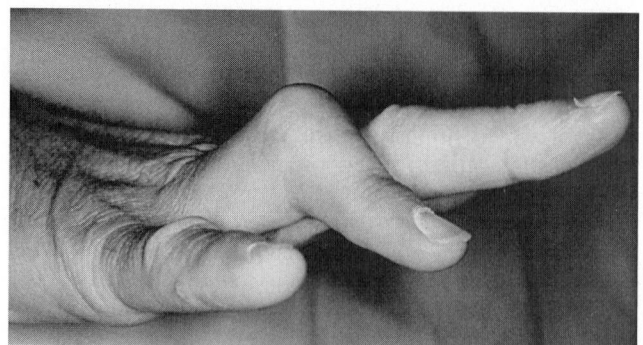

■ FIGURE 73-17. Boutonnière deformity.

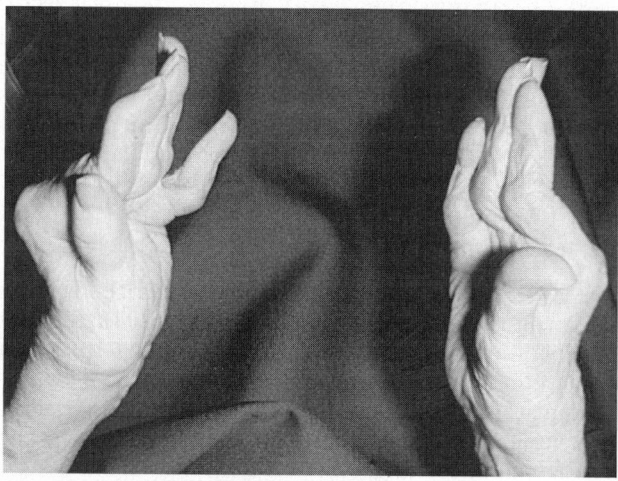

■ FIGURE 73-18. Swan neck deformity.

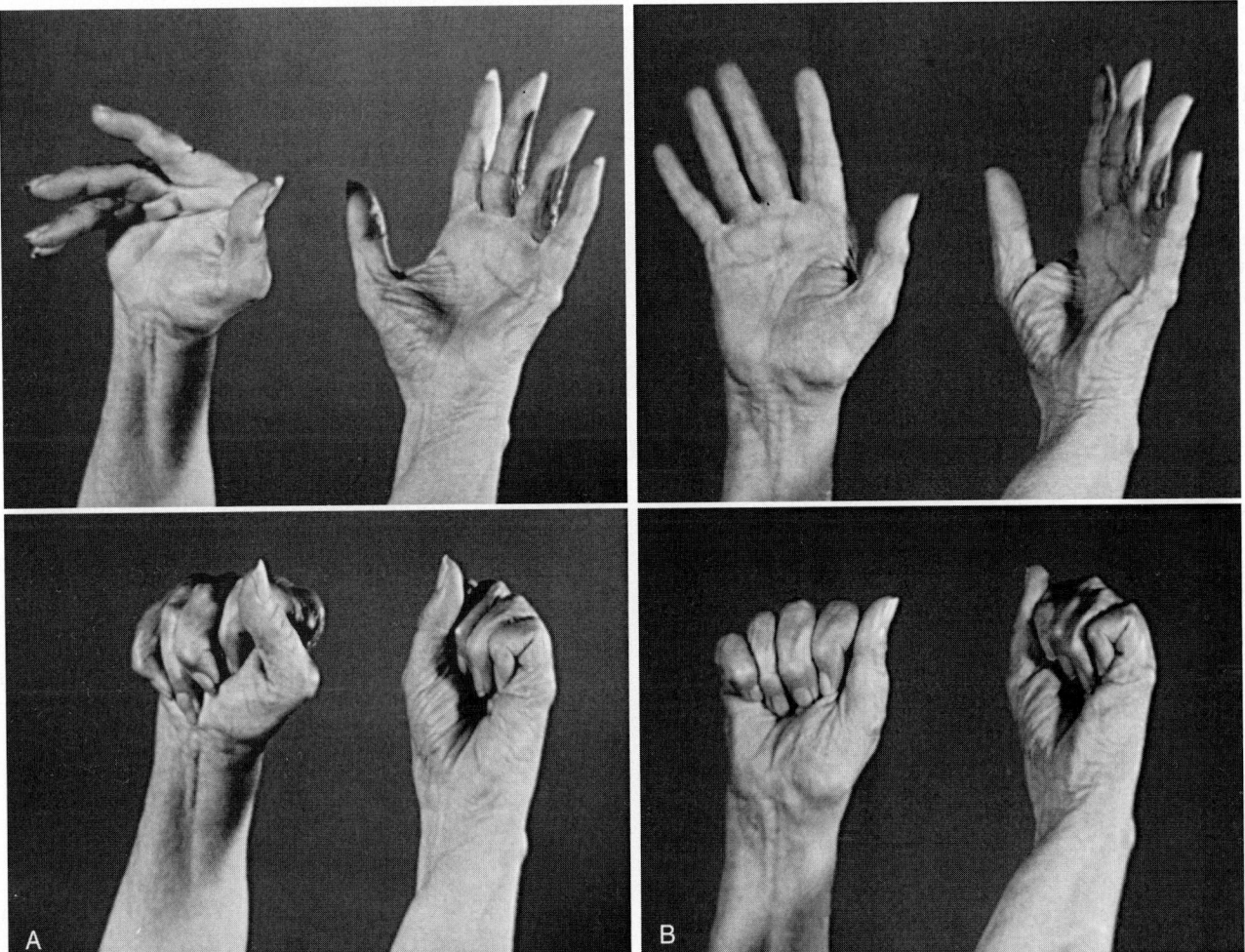

FIGURE 73-19. Z deformity with radial deviation of wrist and ulnar drift of fingers. **A,** Rheumatoid arthritis of uncorrected right hand. The left hand, which was more severely deformed, is shown after surgical correction. **B,** After bilateral surgical correction, both hands functioned normally.

most common and need to be prevented by appropriate treatment of the primary injury, followed by an intensive course of physiotherapy to minimize scarring as well as maintain the suppleness of soft tissues and joints. Once they develop, contractures, if mild, can be stretched out by rigorous physiotherapy, including exercises, ultrasound massage, and splinting at night. If severe, surgical release of the contracture is indicated.

Dupuytren's Disease

Dupuytren's disease is a contracture of the palmar aponeurosis, extending into the digits. It is more common in men and is largely of familial origin typically affecting those with Scandinavian ancestry. It is usually seen after 50 years of age and is autosomal dominant with variable penetrance. There is some evidence to suggest that it may be more common in patients with a history of epilepsy, alcoholism, diabetes, and myocardial infarction.[59] The disease usually begins in the ring and small fingers, with the index being the least involved of all digits.

McFarlane, in a landmark article, analyzed in great detail the patterns of fascial involvement in Dupuytren's disease.[60] Accordingly, the disease mainly involves the longitudinally oriented fibers of the palmar aponeurosis, sparing the superficial transverse metacarpal ligament. Contracture of the natatory ligaments leads to adduction contractures of the web spaces. In the fingers, the spiral band of Gosset, the lateral digital sheath, and varying parts of Cleland's and Grayson's ligaments get involved in a common contracted mass termed the *spiral cord.* This produces flexion contractures at the MCP and PIP joints as well as displaces the digital neurovascular bundles into a more superficial and midline position. The latter fact has to be borne in mind during surgical correction and extreme caution exercised to avoid injuring the neurovascular bundles.

Mere thickening of the palmar fascia into cords or nodules does not require treatment. There is anecdotal evidence that stretching exercises and high doses of vitamin E (800 mg/day) may help slow down the progression of deformity. Fasciectomy is the surgery of choice and is reserved for patients with greater than 30 degrees of MCP joint flexion contracture or any degree of PIP joint flexion contracture. In the palm, this is best carried out through a transverse incision, whereas in the digits vertical incisions are used. After removal of the offending cords, the transverse palmar incisions can be left open or partly closed while the longitudinal digital incisions are converted into Z-plasties and closed in a tension-free manner. Frequently, local flaps or skin grafts may be required. Postoperative management includes static night splinting with joint mobilization and stretching exercises. Complications include hematoma, reflex sympathetic dystrophy, and recurrence of contracture.

Volkmann's Ischemic Contracture

Volkmann's ischemic contracture develops as a result of myofascial contractures in response to prolonged ischemia. The most common cause for this is an unattended compartment syndrome of the forearm or hand, which has been discussed earlier in the chapter. The involved muscles become necrotic and are replaced by fibrous tissue, which produces contractures that are refractory to passive stretch.

The FDP and FPL muscles are the most commonly and severely affected ones in the forearm. The digits are characteristically flexed, and passive extension of the wrist worsens the flexion deformity. This is termed *Volkmann's sign.* In the hand, intrinsic contractures are assessed by Bunnel's test, in which passive extension of the MCP joints produces flexion of the PIP and DIP joints.

If the contracture is mild, passive stretching exercises and serial splinting may solve the problem. If it is severe, the contracture can be released by "Z" lengthening of tendons or by performing a muscle slide operation. This latter procedure involves subperiosteal elevation of the common flexor origin from the humerus and allowing it to slide distally until the contracture is corrected. Rarely, a relative lengthening of the flexor muscles can be achieved by shortening the skeleton. This is done by performing a carpectomy or by resecting a segment of forearm bones and fixing them in the shortened position with plates and screws. In its most severe form, Volkmann's ischemic contracture may involve all muscles of a group, leaving no functioning muscle units behind. In such cases, tendon transfers from adjacent uninvolved groups can provide some return of function.

CONCLUSION

The hand is a human being's most effective mechanical tool, and any compromise in its function can have serious repercussions on day-to-day activities. Increasing mechanization of the world has led to a dramatic increase in the incidence of hand injuries, accounting for almost 25% of all emergency department visits. Seventy percent of major hand injuries occur as a result of machinery injuries and are most often preventable. It has been reported that in as many as 81% of industrial injuries, appropriate safety precautions were either not available or were ignored.[61] This raises serious questions because such injuries occur in the controlled environment of an industrial workshop, which should make them eminently preventable. In the United States, about 18 million new hand injuries are reported annually, accounting for one fourth of all work-related disabilities. The financial burden of these injuries is obvious and is caused both by money spent for treatment as well as in lost days of work.

The future of hand surgery is exciting. The absolute explosion of scientific development in the last century has blurred the lines between scientific fact and fiction. Allograft hand transplantation has been successful and, with continued improvement in immunosuppressive therapy, may become a routine procedure. Genetic engineering has led to the synthesis of various tissue substitutes, increasing the limits of reconstructive possibilities. Arthroscopic-guided laser surgery has already shown its advantages as a minimally invasive method for large joint synovectomy and may soon play a role in the smaller joints of the hand. Telecommunications and computerization have caused national borders to disappear overnight and have made accurate and instant recall of information possible. Specialized centers are springing up all over the world to perpetuate spread of knowledge. It is up to the future generations of surgeons to dedicate themselves to this growing field of hand surgery and help keep its torch burning brightly in the world of medicine.

Selected References

Ashbell TS, Kleinert HE, Putcha SM, Kutz JE: The deformed finger nail, a frequent result of failure to repair nail bed injuries. J Trauma 7:177-190, 1967.

Excellent article on the consequences of neglecting the common fingertip injury.

Kleinert HE, Kutz JE, Ashbell TS, Martinez E: Primary repair of lacerated flexor tendon in no man's land [Abstract]. J Bone Joint Surg Am 49:577, 1967.

Excellent abstract on flexor tendon injuries and early mobilization.

Kleinert HE, Verdan C: Report of the Committee on Tendon. J Hand Surg 8:794-798, 1983.

Excellent article on classification of flexor and extensor tendon injuries by zones.

McFarlane RM: Patterns of diseased fascia in the fingers in Dupuytren's contracture: Displacement of the neurovascular bundle. Plast Reconstr Surg 54:31-44, 1974.

A citation classic for patterns of fascial contracture in Dupuytren's disease.

Millesi H: Nerve grafting. Clin Plast Surg 11:105-113, 1984.

This article describes the anatomic compression sites and clinical classifications of radical nerve compression.

Seddon HJ: Three types of nerve injury. Brain 66:237, 1943.

Landmark article and information on nerve injury types and classification.

Wilgis EF: Observations on the effects of tourniquet ischemia. J Bone Joint Surg Am 53:1343-1346, 1971.

> **Thorough review of the principles of tourniquet use, risks, and potential complications.**

References

1. Dellon AL: The moving two-point discrimination test: Clinical evaluation of the quickly adapting fiber/receptor system. J Hand Surg [Am] 3:474-481, 1978.
2. Gellis M, Pool R: Two-point discrimination distances in the normal hand and forearm: Application to various methods of fingertip reconstruction. Plast Reconstr Surg 59:57-63, 1977.
3. Mackinnon SE, Dellon AL: Two-point discrimination tester. J Hand Surg [Am] 10:906-907, 1985.
4. Wilhelmi BJ, Blackwell SJ, Miller J, et al: Epinephrine in digital blocks: Revisited. Ann Plast Surg 41:410-414, 1998.
5. Kasdan ML, Kleinert HE, Kasdan AP, et al: Axillary block anesthesia for surgery of the hand. Plast Reconstr Surg 46:256-261, 1970.
6. Kleinert HE, Desimone K, Gaspar HE, et al: Regional anesthesia for upper extremity surgery. J Trauma 3:3-12, 1963.
7. Wilgis EF: Observations on the effects of tourniquet ischemia. J Bone Joint Surg Am 53:1343-1346, 1971.
8. Kleinert HE: Finger tip injuries and their management. Am Surg 25:41-51, 1959.
9. Van Beek AL, Kassan MA, Adson MH, et al: Management of acute fingernail injuries. Hand Clin 6:23-35; discussion 37-28, 1990.
10. Verdan CE, Egloff DV: Fingertip injuries. Surg Clin North Am 61:237-266, 1981.
11. Zook EG, Van Beek AL, Russell RC, et al: Anatomy and physiology of the perionychium: A review of the literature and anatomic study. J Hand Surg [Am] 5:528-536, 1980.
12. Brown RE: Acute nail bed injuries. Hand Clin 18:561-575, 2002.
13. Ashbell TS, Kleinert HE, Putcha SM, et al: The deformed finger nail, a frequent result of failure to repair nail bed injuries. J Trauma 7:177-190, 1967.
14. Rosenthal EA: Treatment of fingertip and nail bed injuries. Orthop Clin North Am 14:675-697, 1983.
15. Atasoy E, Ioakimidis E, Kasdan ML, et al: Reconstruction of the amputated finger tip with a triangular volar flap: A new surgical procedure. J Bone Joint Surg Am 52:921-926, 1970.
16. Cronin TD: The cross finger flap: A new method of repair. Am Surg 17:419-425, 1951.
17. Kutler W: A new method for fingertip amputation. JAMA 133:29, 1947.
18. Moberg E: Aspects of sensation in reconstructive surgery of the upper extremity. J Bone Joint Surg Am 46:817-825, 1964.
19. Pennington G, et al: Flexor tendon injuries. In First Hand News: Topics in Upper Extremity Care. Louisville, KY, Christine M. Kleinert Institute for Hand and Micro Surgery, 1993, vol 5(2), pp 1-4.
20. Kleinert HE, Kutz JE, Atasoy E, et al: Primary repair of flexor tendons. Orthop Clin North Am 4:865-876, 1973.
21. Lim BH, Tsai TM: The six-strand technique for flexor tendon repair. Atlas Hand Clin 1:65-77, 1996.
22. Verdan CE: Primary repair of flexor tendons. Am J Orthop 42A:647-657, 1960.
23. Kleinert HE, Kutz JE, Ashbell TS, et al: Primary repair of lacerated flexor tendon in no man's land [Abstract]. J Bone Joint Surg 49A:577, 1967.
24. Kleinert HE, Spokevicius S, Papas NH: History of flexor tendon repair. J Hand Surg [Am] 20:S46-S52, 1995.
25. Kleinert HE, Verdan C: Report of the Committee on Tendon Injuries (International Federation of Societies for Surgery of the Hand). J Hand Surg [Am] 8:794-798, 1983.
26. Duran RJ: Controlled passive motion following flexor tendon repair in zones 2 & 3. In AAOS Symposium on Tendon Surgery in the Hand. St. Louis, CV Mosby, 1974, p 105.
27. Werntz JR, Chesher SP, Breidenbach WC, et al: A new dynamic splint for postoperative treatment of flexor tendon injury. J Hand Surg [Am] 14:559-566, 1989.
28. Wehbe MA: Junctura anatomy. J Hand Surg [Am] 17:1124-1129, 1992.
29. Chow JA, Dovelle S, Thomes LJ, et al: A comparison of results of extensor tendon repair followed by early controlled mobilisation versus static immobilisation. J Hand Surg [Br] 14:18-20, 1989.
30. Evans RB: Immediate active short arc motion following extensor tendon repair. Hand Clin 11:483-512, 1995.
31. Evans RB, Burkhalter WE: A study of the dynamic anatomy of extensor tendons and implications for treatment. J Hand Surg [Am] 11:774-779, 1986.
32. Seddon HJ: Three types of nerve injury. Brain 66:237, 1943.
33. Sunderland S: Nerves and Nerve Injuries, 2nd ed. Edinburgh, Churchill Livingstone, 1978, pp 69-141.
34. Kleinert HE, Griffin JM: Technique of nerve anastomosis. Orthop Clin North Am 4:907-915, 1973.
35. Millesi H: Nerve grafting. Clin Plast Surg 11:105-113, 1984.
36. Chiu DT, Strauch B: A prospective clinical evaluation of autogenous vein grafts used as a nerve conduit for distal sensory nerve defects of 3 cm or less. Plast Reconstr Surg 86:928-934, 1990.
37. House JH, Fidler MO: Frostbite of the hand. In Green DP (ed): Operative Hand Surgery, 3rd ed. New York, Churchill Livingstone, 1993, pp 2033-2041.
38. Stern PJ: Fractures of the metacarpals and phalanges. In Green DP (ed): Operative Hand Surgery, 3rd ed. New York, Churchill Livingstone, 1993, p 695.
39. Schneider LH: Fractures of the distal phalanx. Hand Clin 4:537-547, 1988.
40. McFarlane RM, Hampole MK: Treatment of extensor tendon injuries of the hand. Can J Surg 16:366-375, 1973.
41. Hamas RS, Horrell ED, Pierret GP: Treatment of mallet finger due to intra-articular fracture of the distal phalanx. J Hand Surg [Am] 3:361-363, 1978.
42. McNealy RW, Lichtenstein ME: Fractures of the metacarpals and phalanges. West J Surg Obstet Gynecol 43:156-161, 1935.
43. Strickland JW, Steichen JB, Kleinman WB, et al: Phalangeal fractures: Factors influencing digital performance. Orthop Rev 11:39-50, 1982.
44. Bennett EH: Fractures of the metacarpal bones. Dublin J Med Sci 73:72-75, 1882.
45. Taleisnik J, Kelly PJ: The extraosseous and intraosseous blood supply of the scaphoid bone. J Bone Joint Surg Am 48:1125-1137, 1966.
46. Frykman GK, Taleisnik J, Peters G, et al: Treatment of nonunited scaphoid fractures by pulsed electromagnetic field and cast. J Hand Surg [Am] 11:344-349, 1986.
47. Salter RB, Harris WR: Injuries involving the epiphyseal plate. J Bone Joint Surg 45A:587-622, 1963.
48. Stener B: Displacement of the ruptured ulnar collateral ligament of the metacarpophalangeal joint of the thumb: A clinical and anatomical study. J Bone Joint Surg Br 44:869-879, 1962.

49. Phalen GS: The carpal-tunnel syndrome: Clinical evaluation of 598 hands. Clin Orthop 83:29-40, 1972.

50. Guyon F: Note sur une disposition anatomique proper à la face anterieure de la region du poignet et non encores décrité par la docteur. Bull Soc Anat Paris (2nd series) 36:184-186, 1861.

51. Murata K, Shih JT, Tsai TM: Causes of ulnar tunnel syndrome: A retrospective study of 31 subjects. J Hand Surg [Am] 28:647-651, 2003.

52. Lister GD, Belsole RB, Kleinert HE: The radial tunnel syndrome. J Hand Surg [Am] 4:52-59, 1979.

53. Atasoy E: Thoracic outlet compression syndrome. Orthop Clin North Am 27:265-303, 1996.

54. Kleinert HE, Kutz JE, Fishman JH, et al: Etiology and treatment of the so-called mucous cyst of the finger. J Bone Joint Surg Am 54:1455-1458, 1972.

55. Kanavel AB: A Guide to the Surgical Treatment of Acute and Chronic Suppurative Processes in the Fingers, Hand, and Forearm, 7th ed. Philadelphia, Lea & Febiger, 1943.

56. Goldstein EJ, Barones MF, Miller TA: *Eikenella corrodens* in hand infections. J Hand Surg [Am] 8:563-567, 1983.

57. Finkelstein H: Stenosing tendovaginitis at the radial styloid process. J Bone Joint Surg 12:509-540, 1930.

58. Kleinert HE, Frykman G: The wrist and thumb in rheumatoid arthritis. Orthop Clin North Am 4:1085-1096, 1973.

59. Rayan GM: Palmar fascial complex anatomy and pathology in Dupuytren's disease. Hand Clin 15:73-86, vi-vii, 1999.

60. McFarlane RM: Patterns of the diseased fascia in the fingers in Dupuytren's contracture: Displacement of the neurovascular bundle. Plast Reconstr Surg 54:31-44, 1974.

61. al Zahrani S, Ikram MA, al-Qattan MM: Predisposing factors to industrial hand injuries in Saudi Arabia. J Hand Surg [Br] 22:131-132, 1997.

CHAPTER 74

GYNECOLOGIC SURGERY

Stephen S. Entman, M.D.,   Cornelia R. Graves, M.D.,   Barry K. Jarnagin, M.D.,   and   Lynn P. Parker, M.D.

Pelvic Embryology and Anatomy

Reproductive Physiology

Clinical Evaluation

Management of Preinvasive and Invasive Disease of the Female Genital Tract

Alternatives to Surgical Intervention

Technical Aspects of Surgical Options

Surgery During Pregnancy

Gynecology, along with the co-specialty of obstetrics, represents the art and science of the female reproductive tract. The global knowledge base for the specialty demands an understanding of embryology and anatomy of female pelvic organs, the hypothalamic-pituitary-ovarian hormonal axis, ovulation, the endometrial response to the hormonal milieu, oocyte fertilization and implantation, embryogenesis, fetal health and development, maternal adaptation to pregnancy, and labor and delivery. Additionally, obstetric and gynecologic care requires knowledge of functional and pathologic variations and abnormalities in these processes, including dysfunctional hormonal and endometrial cycling, ovarian accidents, pelvic infection, benign and malignant neoplasms, abnormal pregnancy implantation, teratogenesis, fetal and maternal complications of pregnancy, and abnormal labor. The full range of this knowledge is beyond the scope of one chapter. Instead, the focus here is to provide the surgeon with sufficient understanding of the basic information for effective care of the female patient in need of surgical evaluation and care. The potential settings for this care include the following:

- Evaluation of women with abdominopelvic complaints in the emergency setting
- Request for intraoperative assistance or consultation by a gynecologic surgeon
- Unanticipated pelvic pathologic processes in the operative setting
- Emergency surgical care in the absence of an obstetrician-gynecologist
- Surgical care of the pregnant patient

To these ends, the chapter is structured to provide the following information:

1. Anatomy, with attention to surgical anatomic relationships
2. Reproductive physiology
3. Clinical evaluation of the female patient, including important elements of history, physical examination and ancillary tests
4. Special considerations related to gynecologic malignancies
5. Medical alternatives to surgical management of common gynecologic conditions
6. Surgical technique for common gynecologic procedures, vulnerabilities for surgical injury, and specific issues related to surgical judgment
7. Physiologic changes in pregnancy and perioperative and intraoperative care of the pregnant patient
8. Surgical technique for obstetrical procedures

PELVIC EMBRYOLOGY AND ANATOMY

Embryology

The female external genitalia are derived embryologically from the genital tubercle, which in the absence of testosterone fails to undergo fusion and devolves to the vulvar structures. The labial structures are of ectodermal origin. The urethra, the vaginal introitus, and the vulvar vestibule are derived from uroepithelial entoderm. The lower third of the vagina develops from the invagination of the urogenital sinus.

The internal genitalia are derived from the genital ridge. The ovaries develop from the incorporation of primordial germ cells into coelomic epithelium of the mesonephric (wolffian) duct, and the tubes, uterus, cervix, and upper two thirds of the vagina develop from the paramesonephric (müllerian) duct. The embryologic ovaries migrate caudad to the true pelvis. Primordial ovarian follicles develop but remain dormant until stimulation in adolescence by gonadotropins. The paired müllerian ducts migrate caudad and medially to form the fallopian tubes and fuse in the midline to form the uterus, cervix, and upper vagina. The wolffian ducts regress. Failure or partial failure of these processes can result in distortions of anatomy and potential diagnostic dilemmas (Table 74-1).

Anatomy

External Genitalia

The external genitalia consist of the mons veneris, labia majora, labia minora, clitoris, vulvar vestibule, urethral meatus, and the ostia of the accessory glandular structures (Fig. 74-1). These structures overlie the fascial and muscle layers of the perineum. The perineum is the most caudal region of the trunk and includes the pelvic floor and those structures occupying the pelvic outlet. It is bounded superiorly by the funnel-shaped pelvic diaphragm and inferiorly by the skin covering the external genitalia, the anus, and adjacent structures. Laterally, the perineum is bounded by the medial surface of the inferior pubic rami, the obturator internus muscle below the origin of the levator ani muscle, the coccygeus muscle, the medial surface of the sacrotuberous ligaments, and the overlapping margins of the gluteus maximus muscles (Fig. 74-2).

The pelvic outlet can be divided into two triangles separated by a line drawn between the ischial tuberosities. The anterior or urogenital triangle has its apex anteriorly at the symphysis pubis, and the posterior or anal triangle has its apex at the coccyx.

The urogenital triangle contains the urogenital diaphragm, a muscular shelf extending between the pubic

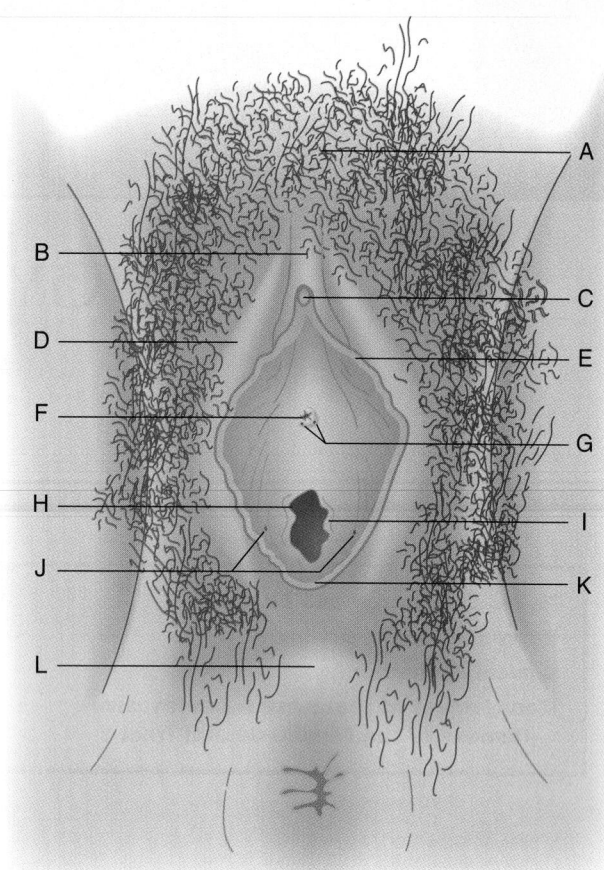

FIGURE 74-1.   The external genitalia. A, mons pubis; B, prepuce; C, clitoris; D, labia majora; E, labia minora; F, urethral meatus; G, Skene ducts; H, vagina; I, hymen; J, Bartholin glands; K, posterior fourchette; L, perineal body.

rami and penetrated by the urethra and vagina and the external genitalia, consisting of the mons pubis, the labia majora and minora, the clitoris, and the vestibule. The mons pubis is a suprapubic fat pad covered by dense skin appendages. The labia majora extend posteriorly from the mons, forming the lateral borders of the vulva. They have a keratinized stratified squamous epithelium with all of the normal skin appendages and extend posteriorly to the lateral perineum. Within the confines of the labium are fat and the insertion of the round ligament. Medial to the labia majora are interlabial grooves and the labia minora, which are of similar cutaneous origin but devoid of hair follicles. The labia minora are richly vascularized, with an erectile venous plexus. The bilateral roots of the clitoris fuse in the midline to form the glans at the lower edge of the pubic symphysis. The labia minora fuse over the clitoris to form the hood and, to a variable degree, below to create the clitoral frenulum.

Contiguous to the medial aspect of the labia minora, demarcated by Hart's line, is the vulvar vestibule extending to the hymeneal sulcus. The vestibular surface is a stratified, squamous mucous membrane that shares embryology and has similar characteristics to the distal urethra and urethral meatus. The Bartholin glands at 5 and

TABLE 74-1. Selected Anatomic Abnormalities as a Result of Disrupted Embryogenesis	
Organ	**Abnormality**
Ovary	Duplication of ovary; secondary ovarian rests; paraovarian cysts (wolffian remnants)
Tube	Congenital absence; paratubal cyst (hydatid of Morgagni)
Uterus	Agenesis; complete or partial duplication of the uterine fundus
Cervix	Agenesis; complete or partial duplication of the cervix
Vagina	Agenesis; transverse or longitudinal septum; paravaginal (Gartner's duct) cyst
Vulva	Fusion; hermaphroditism; cyst of the canal of Nuck (round ligament cyst)

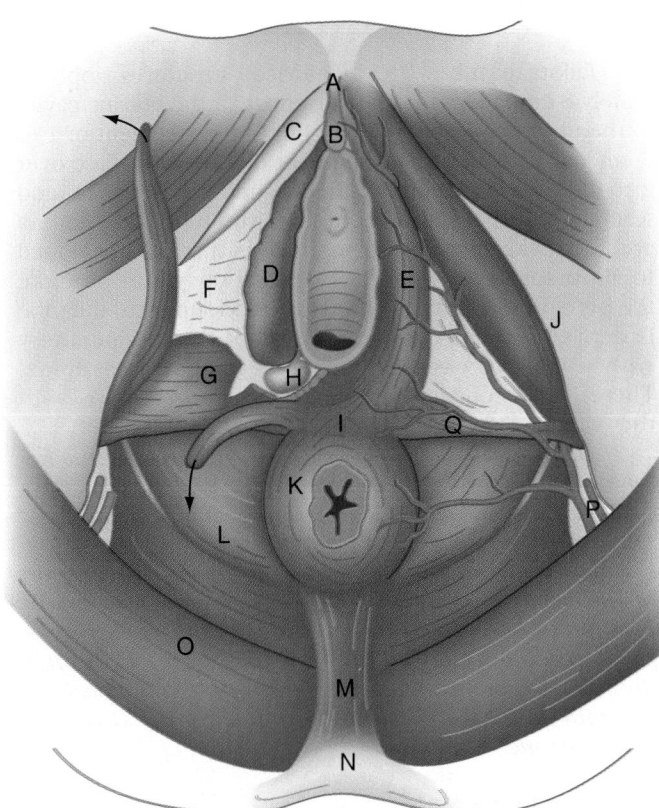

■ FIGURE 74-2.   The muscles and fascia of the perineum.
A, suspensory ligament of clitoris; B, clitoris; C, crus of clitoris;
D, vestibular bulb; E, bulbocavernosus muscle; F, inferior fascia of
urogenital diaphragm; G, deep transverse perineal muscle;
H, Bartholin gland; I, perineal body; J, ischiocavernosus muscle;
K, external anal sphincter; L, levator ani muscle; M, anococcygeal
body; N, coccyx; O, gluteus maximus muscle; P, pudendal artery
and vein; Q, superficial transverse perineal muscle.

7 o'clock, the paraurethral Skene glands, and minor
vestibular glands positioned around the lateral vestibule
are all under the vestibular bulb, subjacent to the bulbocavernosus muscle. The ostia of these glands pass through
the vestibular mucosa, directly adjacent to the hymeneal
ring.

The muscles of the external genitalia consist of the
deep and superficial transverse perineal muscles, the
paired ischiocavernosus muscles that cover the crura of
the clitoris, and the bulbocavernosus muscles lying on
either side of the vagina covering the vestibular bulbs.

The anal triangle contains the anal canal with surrounding internal and external sphincters, the ischiorectal fossa, filled with fatty tissue, the median raphe, and the
overlying skin.

Blood supply to the perineum is predominantly from a
posterior direction from the internal pudendal artery,
which, after arising from the internal iliac artery, passes
through Alcock's canal, a fascial tunnel along the obturator internus muscle below the origin of the levator ani
muscle. On emerging from Alcock's canal, the internal
pudendal artery sends branches to the urogenital triangle
anteriorly and to the anal triangle posteriorly. Anteriorly,
there is blood supply to the mons pubis from the inferior

epigastric, a branch of the femoral artery. Laterally, the
external pudendal artery arises from the femoral artery
and supplies the lateral aspect of the vulva. Venous return
from the perineum accompanies the arterial supply and,
therefore, drains into the internal iliac and femoral veins.

*It is important for the surgeon dissecting the external
genitalia to be cognizant of the variability of direction
from which the blood supply of the operative field is
derived.*

The major nerve supply to the perineum comes from
the internal pudendal nerve, which originates from S2 to
S4 anterior rami of the sacral plexus and travels through
Alcock's canal in company with the internal pudendal
artery and vein. Anterior branches supply the urogenital
diaphragm and the external genitalia while the posterior
branch, the inferior rectal nerve, supplies the anus, the
anal canal, the ischiorectal fossa and the adjacent skin.
Branches of the posterior femoral cutaneous nerve from
the sacral plexus innervate the lateral aspects of the
ischiorectal fossa and adjacent structures. The mons pubis
and anterior labia are supplied by the ilioinguinal and genitofemoral nerves from the lumbar plexus; they travel
through the inguinal canal and exit through the superficial inguinal ring. All of these paired nerves routinely cross
the midline for partial innervation of the contralateral side.
The visceral efferent nerves responsible for clitoral erection are derived from the pelvic splanchnic nerves and
reach the external genitalia in company of the urethra and
vagina as they pass through the urogenital diaphragm.

*Surgical injury to the pelvic nerve plexus can result
in neuropathic pain and diminished sexual, voiding,
and excretory function.*

The lymphatic drainage of the perineum including both
the urogenital triangle and anogenital triangle travels for
the most part with the external pudendal vessels to the
superficial inguinal nodes. The deep parts of the perineum
including the urethra, the vagina, and the anal canal drain,
in part, through the lymphatics that accompany the internal pudendal vessels and into the internal iliac lymph
nodes.

The fascia and fascial spaces of the perineum are important regarding spread of extravasated fluids and both
superficial and deep infections. Fascia covers each of
the muscles bounding the perineum, including the deep
surface of the levator ani, the obturator internus, the
coccygeus, as well as other perineal muscles such as the
urogenital diaphragm. The fascia of the levator ani
muscles fuses with the obturator internus fascia and the
pubic rami, creating well-defined fascial spaces, the
ischiorectal fossae. Beneath the skin of the external genitalia is a layer of fat, and deep to this is Colles' fascia,
which is attached to the ischiopubic rami laterally and the
posterior edge of the urogenital diaphragm. Anteriorly,
Colles' fascia of the vulva is continuous with Colles' fascia
of the anterior abdominal wall.

Infections or collections of extravasated urine deep to
the urogenital diaphragm are usually confined to the
ischiorectal fossa, including the anterior recess, which is
superior to the urogenital diaphragm. Collections of fluid
or infections superficial to the urogenital diaphragm may
pass to the abdominal wall deep to Colles' fascia. Because

of various fascial fusions, infections spreading from the vulva to the anterior abdominal wall do not spread into the inguinal regions or the thigh.

Internal Genitalia

The internal genitalia consist of the ovaries, fallopian tubes, uterus, cervix, and vagina with associated blood supply and lymphatic drainage (Figs. 74-3 to 74-5).

Ovary

The oblong ovaries, which are glistening white, vary in size, a factor that is dependent on age and status of the ovulatory cycle. In the prepubescent girl, the ovary will appear as a white sliver of tissue less than a centimeter in any dimension. The ovary of a woman during her reproductive years will vary in size and shape. The size of the nonovulating ovary will typically be in the range of $3 \times 2 \times 1$ cm. When a follicular or corpus luteum cyst is present, the size may extend up to 5 to 6 cm. A follicular cyst is an asymmetrical, translucent clear structure. A corpus luteum cyst will generally be characterized by areas of golden yellow and, occasionally, a hematoma. The ovaries are suspended from the lateral sidewall of the pelvis below the pelvic brim by the infundibulopelvic ligament and attach to the superolateral aspect of the uterine fundus with the utero-ovarian ligament.

The primary blood supply to the ovary is the ovarian artery. It arises directly from the aorta and courses with the vein through the infundibulopelvic ligament into the medulla on the lateral aspect of the ovary. The right ovarian vein generally drains to the inferior vena cava and the left drains to the common iliac vein; however, variations commonly occur. There is a rich, anastomotic arterial complex arising from the uterine artery that spreads across the broad ligament and the mesosalpinx. The venous return accompanies that arterial supply. There is no somatic innervation to the ovary, but the autonomic fibers arise from the lumbar sympathetic and the sacral parasympathetic plexuses. Lymphatic drainage parallels the iliac and aortic arteries.

There are three important relationships to be considered in surgical dissection. The infundibulopelvic ligament, with the ovarian blood supply, crosses over the ureter as it descends into the pelvis. As the surgeon divides and ligates the ovarian vessels, it is critical that this relationship be identified to avoid transecting, ligating, or kinking the ureter. The risk of ureteral injury is greater with a more proximal dissection of the ligament. Additionally, in its natural position, the suspended ovary drops along the pelvic sidewall along the course of the midureter. If there are adhesions between the ovary and the peritoneum of the pelvic sidewall, careful dissection is necessary to avoid tenting the peritoneum with the attached ureter and creating injury. The third surgical relationship is the complex of external iliac vessels and the femoral nerve that courses along the iliopsoas muscle, directly below the course of the ovarian vessels; with anterior adhesions of an ovary, these structures may be subjacent to the malpositioned ovary.

Fallopian Tubes

The fallopian tubes are cylindrical structures approximately 8 cm in length. They originate at the uterine cavity in the uterine cornua, with an intramural segment of 1 to 2 cm and narrow isthmic segment of 4 to 5 cm, flare over 2 to 3 cm to the funnel of the infundibular segment, and terminate in the fimbriated end of the tube. The fimbria are fine, delicate mucosal projections that are positioned to allow for capture of the extruded oocyte to promote the potential for fertilization. The blood supply to the tube is derived primarily from branches of the uterine artery with a delicate cascade of vessels in the mesosalpinx. There is a secondary supply from the anastomosis with the ovarian vessels.

The surgeon must be aware of the fragility of the fallopian tube and handle this structure delicately, especially in women wishing to preserve their fertility. The mucosa lining the tubal lumen, especially at the fimbriated end, is highly specialized to facilitate transport of the oocyte and the fertilized zygote. Traumatic manipulation of the tube can induce tubal infertility or predispose to later tubal pregnancy, either through damage to the mucosa or by distortion of tubal position by adhesions, thereby interfering with the access or transport mechanisms.

Uterus and Cervix

The uterus with the cervix is a midline, pear-shaped organ suspended in the midplane of the pelvis by the cardinal and uterosacral ligaments. The cardinal ligaments are dense fibrous condensations arising from the fascial covering of the levator ani muscles of the pelvic floor and inserting into the lateral portions of the uterocervical junction. The uterosacral ligaments arise posterolaterally from the uterocervical junction and course obliquely in a posterolateral direction to insert into the parietal fascia of the pelvic floor at the sacroiliac joint. The round ligaments of the uterus arise from the anterolateral superior aspect of the uterine fundus, course anterolaterally to the internal inguinal ring, and insert into the labia majora. The round ligaments are highly stretchable and serve no function in pelvic organ support. The broad ligaments are composed of a visceral peritoneal surface containing loose adventitious tissue. These ligaments also provide no pelvic organ support but do allow access to an avascular plane of the pelvis through which the retroperitoneal vasculature and ureter can be exposed.

The size of the uterus is influenced by age, hormonal status, prior pregnancy, and common benign neoplasms. The normal uterus during the reproductive years is approximately $8 \times 6 \times 4$ cm and weighs about 100 g. The prepubertal and postmenopausal uterus is substantially smaller. The mass of the uterus is almost exclusively made up of myometrium, a complex of interlacing bundles of smooth muscle. The uterine cavity is 4 to 6 cm from the internal cervical os to the uterine fundus, shaped as an inverted triangle, 2 to 3 mm wide at the cervix, and 3 to 4 cm across the fundus, extending from cornua to cornua. It is only a few millimeters of depth between anterior and posterior walls, with no defined lateral walls in the non-

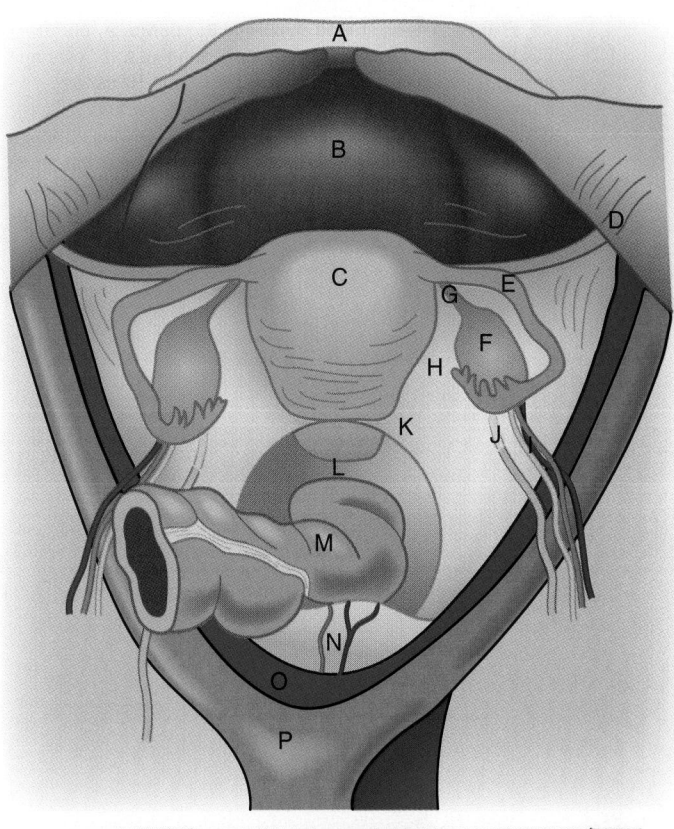

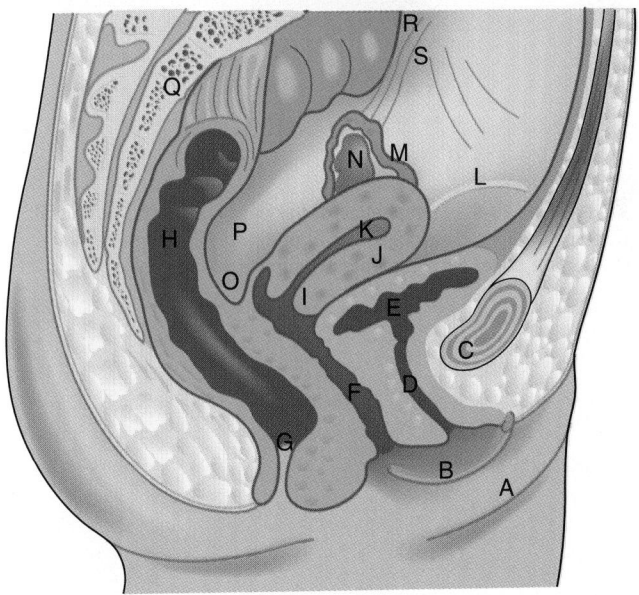

FIGURE 74-3. The internal genitalia. **Front view:** A, symphysis pubis; B, bladder; C, corpus uteri; D, round ligament; E, fallopian tube; F, ovary; G, utero-ovarian ligament; H, broad ligament; I, ovarian artery and vein; J, ureter; K, uterosacral ligament; L, cul-de-sac; M, rectum; N, middle sacral artery and vein; O, vena cava; P, aorta. **Side view:** A, labium majus; B, labium minus; C, symphysis pubis, D, urethra; E, bladder; F, vagina; G, anus; H, rectum; I, cervix uteri; J, corpus uteri; K, endometrial cavity; L, round ligament; M, fallopian tube; N, ovary; O, cul-de-sac; P, uterosacral ligament; Q, sacrum; R, ureter; S, ovarian artery and vein.

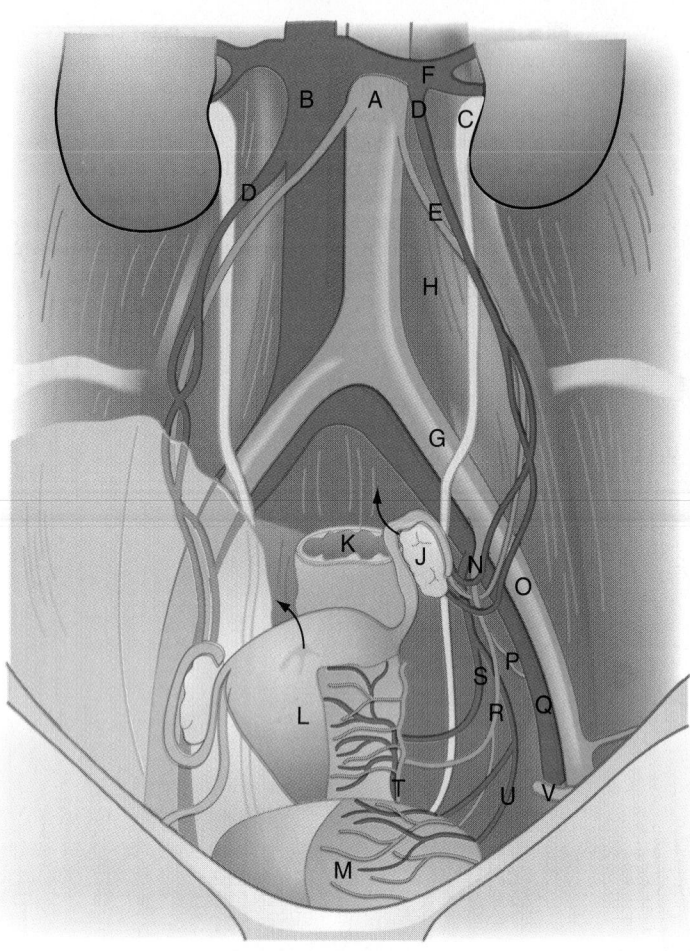

■ FIGURE 74-4.   Blood supply of the pelvis. A, aorta; B, inferior vena cava; C, ureter; D, ovarian vein; E, ovarian artery; F, renal vein; G, common iliac artery; H, psoas muscle; I, middle sacral artery; J, ovary; K, rectum; L, corpus uteri; M, bladder; N, internal iliac (hypogastric) artery, anterior branch; O, external iliac artery; P, obturator artery; Q, external iliac vein; R, uterine artery; S, uterine vein; T, vaginal artery; U, superior vesicle artery; V, inferior epigastric artery.

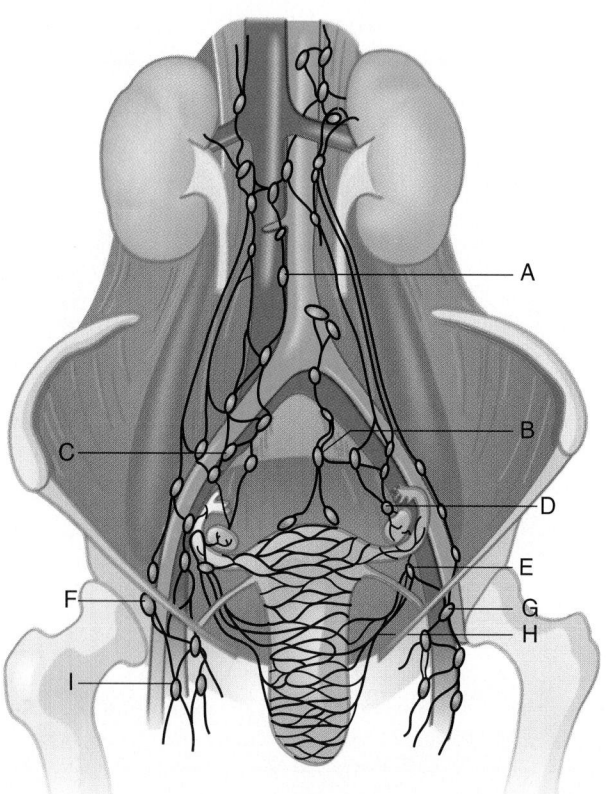

■ FIGURE 74-5.   Lymphatics of the pelvis. A, aortic; B, sacral; C, common iliac; D, hypogastric; E, obturator; F, deep inguinal; G, Cloquet node; H, parametrial; I, superficial inguinal.

pregnant state. The most common reason for variation in size is current pregnancy, followed by uterine fibroids.

If, during a surgical procedure, the surgeon encounters an enlarged uterus, undiagnosed pregnancy must be considered. The morphologic differences between a uterus enlarged by a pregnancy and one enlarged by fibroid include symmetrical enlargement in pregnancy with generally asymmetrical enlargement with fibroids. If symmetrical, consider the origin of the round ligaments. With pregnancy, the round ligaments stretch as the uterus grows and continue to originate from the normal site; even with an apparently symmetrical fibroid uterus, the origin of the round ligaments is frequently displaced from the top of the uterine fundus or asymmetrical course through the pelvis. Finally, the pregnant uterus is usually dusky and soft, whereas fibroids are generally firm and nodular masses can be palpated in the myometrial wall.

The uterine cavity is lined by the endometrium, a complex epithelial-stromal-vascular secretory tissue. The arterial supply to the endometrium is derived from branches of the uterine artery that perforate the myometrium to the inactive basalis layer. There they form the arcuate vessels, which produce radial branches extending through the functional layer toward the compacted surface layer. The menstrual cycle is further described later in the chapter, but during the postovulatory phase these vessels differentiate into spiral arteries, uniquely suited to allow menstruation and subsequent hemostasis.

The uterine cervix is histologically dynamic, with changes in cervical mucus production during the ovarian cycle. In the follicular phase, under estrogen stimulation, copious clear mucus is produced that facilitates the transport of sperm through the cervical canal to ascend through the uterine cavity to the fallopian tubes. During progesterone-dominant states, either luteal phase or with exogenous hormones, the mucus becomes viscous and plugs the cervix. The secretory epithelium of the endocervical canal has a dynamic metaplastic interaction with the stratified squamous epithelium of the portio vaginalis of the ectocervix under hormonal stimulation.

Because the cervical canal is continuous with the vagina, surgical procedures involving the uterus and tubes are considered to be clean-contaminated cases.

The major sources of blood supply for the uterus and cervix are the uterine arteries, which are branches of the anterior division of the internal iliac (hypogastric) arteries. Although the origin of the uterine artery is usually a single, identifiable vessel, it divides into multiple ascending and descending branches as it courses medially to the lateral margins of the cervicouterine junction. The distance from the uterus at which this division occurs is highly variable. Venous return from the uterus flows into the companion internal iliac vein. Lymphatics from the cervix and upper vagina drain primarily through the internal iliac nodes, but from the uterine fundus, drainage occurs primarily along a presacral path directly to the para-aortic nodes.

The primary surgical consideration for managing the uterine vessels is the close proximity of the ureter, which courses approximately 1 cm below the artery and 1 cm lateral to the cervix. If the surgeon loses control of one of the branches of the vessel, it is important to use techniques that avoid clamping or kinking the ureter. Often, the most prudent way to secure the uterine artery is to expose its origin and place hemostatic clips on the vessel.

Innervation of the uterus and cervix is derived from the autonomic plexus. Autonomic pain fibers are activated with dysmenorrhea, in labor, and with instrumentation of the cervix and uterus.

In the retroperitoneal space lateral to the uterus is the obturator nerve, which arises from the lumbosacral plexus and passes through the pelvic floor via the obturator canal to innervate the medial thigh. With relatively normal pelvic anatomy it is unlikely to be subjected to injury, but under circumstances in which the surgeon must dissect the retroperitoneal or paravaginal spaces, this relatively subtle structure can be injured with significant neuropathic residual.

Vagina

The vagina originates at the cervix and terminates at the hymeneal ring. The anatomic axis of the upper vagina is posterior to anterior in a caudal direction. The anterior and posterior walls of the upper two thirds of the vagina are normally apposed to each other to create a transverse potential space, distensible through pliability of the lateral sulci. The lower third of the vagina has a relatively vertically oriented caudal lumen. The mucosa of the vagina is nonkeratinized, stratified, squamous epithelium that responds to estrogen stimulation.

The blood supply to the vagina is provided by descending branches of the uterine artery and vein and ascending branches of the internal pudendal artery and its companion vein. These vessels course along the lateral walls of the vagina. Innervation is derived from the autonomic plexus and the pudendal nerve, which track with the vessels.

Traumatic lacerations of the vagina are most commonly located along the lateral sidewalls. The degree to which there is major injury to the vessels can be associated not only with significant evident hemorrhage but also concealed hemorrhage. Spaces in which a hematoma can be concealed are the retroperitoneum of the broad ligaments, the paravesicular and pararectal spaces, and the ischiorectal fossa. Because of the proximity of the pudendal nerve, attempts to ligate the vessels require maintaining orientation to the location of Alcock's canal to avoid creating neuropathic injury. In the absence of an accumulating hematoma, often the best approach to management is a bulk vaginal pack to achieve tamponade. To accomplish this requires significant sedation or anesthesia and an indwelling urinary catheter.

The uterus, cervix, and vagina with their fascial investments comprise the middle compartment of the pelvis. The structures of the anterior compartment, the bladder and urethra, and the posterior compartment, the rectum, are each invested with a fascial layer. Avascular planes of loose areola tissue separate the posterior fascia of the bladder and the anterior fascia of the vagina and also the anterior fascia of the rectum and the posterior fascia of the vagina. Anteriorly, the bladder is attached to the lower uterine segment by the continuous visceral peritoneum. This vesicouterine fold can be incised transversely with minimal difficulty to expose the plane and allow dissection of the bladder from the cervix and vagina. Posteriorly, the proximity of the rectum to the posterior vagina is significant only below the peritoneum of the cul-de-sac of Douglas, unless the cul-de-sac anatomy is distorted by dense adhesions.

Operative technique for gynecologic procedures is optimized by careful identification of these planes to separate and protect the adjacent organs from operative injury. The surgeon can create an incidental cystotomy, which may or may not be recognized, or devitalize the bladder wall with a crush or stitch, with delayed development of a vesicovaginal fistula.

In the lower pelvis, the ureter courses anteromedially after it passes under the uterine vessels and progresses toward the trigone of the bladder through a fascial tunnel on the anterior vaginal wall. The fixation of the ureter by the tunnel precludes effective displacement from the operative site by retracting. While the location of the fascial tunnel is generally 1 to 2 cm safely below the usual site for vaginotomy during hysterectomy, in cases with a large cervix, a distorting uterine myoma, a prior cesarean section, or bleeding from the bladder base or vaginal wall, the ureter can be transected, crushed, or kinked with a stitch.

The rectovaginal septum is surgically relevant during repair of episiotomy or obstetric laceration, repair of rectovaginal fistula, or pelvic support procedures. Identification of the fascial layers investing the subjacent structures and utilizing the tissue strength is critical to an optimal repair.

REPRODUCTIVE PHYSIOLOGY

The development of a differential diagnosis of gynecologic complaints is facilitated by an understanding of the reproductive cycle and eliciting a careful menstrual history. Many conditions are a direct consequence of aberrations in the hypothalamic-pituitary-ovarian (HPO) cycle and of the effects of the hormonal milieu on the endometrium. Others tend to be mere variation in the presentation of different phases of the cycle. A detailed description of the cycle is beyond the scope of this text, but the surgeon needs to have a basic understanding of the relationships in this complex process to elicit an adequate history, interpret the findings on physical examination, use ancillary tests appropriately, and formulate the differential diagnosis (Fig. 74-6).

Ovarian Cycle

Under the stimulus of hypothalamic secretion of gonadotropin-releasing hormone (GnRH) to the pituitary gland, follicle-stimulating hormone (FSH) is released into the systemic circulation. During this secretory phase of

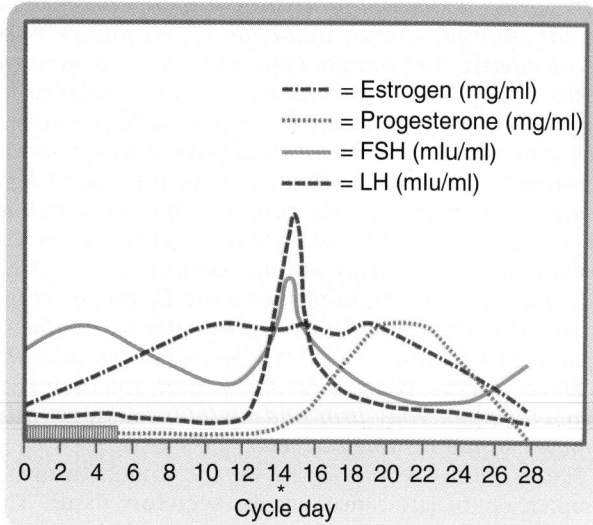

HORMONAL CHANGES DURING THE MENSTRUAL CYCLE

—·—·— = Estrogen (mg/ml)
·········· = Progesterone (mg/ml)
———— = FSH (mIu/ml)
– – – – = LH (mIu/ml)

Cycle day

■ **FIGURE 74-6.**   Hormonal changes during the menstrual cycle. Menses, days 0-5; ovulation, day 14. FSH, follicle-stimulating hormone; LH, luteinizing hormone.

the ovarian cycle, the primordial follicles of the ovary are targeted and stimulated toward growth and maturity. Multiple follicles are recruited in each cycle, but generally only one follicle becomes dominant, destined to reach maturity and extrusion at ovulation. The effects of the maturation process include not only the completion of the meiotic germ cell development but also the stimulation of the granulosa cells that surround the follicle to secrete estradiol and other estrogenic compounds and inhibin. As the estradiol level increases in the circulation it has a positive regulatory effect on GnRH, which in turn stimulates the pituitary gland to release a surge of luteinizing hormone (LH). The LH surge stimulates the release of the oocyte from the follicle. After the release, the follicle site converts to the corpus luteum; and the dominant hormone secreted during this luteal phase is progesterone. This sequence of hormonal events prepares the cervix, uterus, and tubes for sperm transport into the upper genital tract, fertilization, implantation, and support of the early gestation. In the absence of conception, through mechanisms not yet known, the corpus luteum undergoes atresia and the next ovarian cycle begins.

Endometrial Cycle

The hormonal sequence of the ovarian cycle controls the physiologic changes in the endometrium. By convention, each endometrial cycle begins on day 1, defined as the onset of menses. In an idealized cycle, the LH surge and ovulation occur on day 14. Atresia of the corpus luteum occurs on day 28, and menses begin the next day, cycle day 1 of the new cycle.

During the follicular phase of the ovarian cycle, estrogen exerts a stimulatory effect on the endometrium, producing the proliferative phase of the endometrial cycle. The endometrial tissues that are affected include the surface and glandular epithelium, the stromal matrix, and the vascular bed. The stromal layer thickens, the glandular elements elongate, and the terminal arterioles of the endometrial circulation extend from the basalis toward the endometrial surface. The mucous secretions of the glands of the endometrium (and the endocervix) become profuse and watery, facilitating ascent of spermatozoa for potential fertilization.

During the luteal phase of the ovarian cycle, corresponding to the secretory phase of the endometrial cycle, progesterone domination converts the endometrium toward receptivity for implantation of the fertilized oocyte. Several endometrial changes occur under progesterone stimulation. The growth of the endometrial stroma is terminated, the surface layer of the endometrium becomes compacted, the glandular secretions become more viscous, and the terminal arterioles become coiled, creating the spiral arterioles. Cervical mucus similarly becomes more viscous and tenacious, creating a relative barrier between the vagina and the uterine cavity.

In the absence of fertilization, and with the withdrawal of progesterone due to atresia of the corpus luteum, there is a complex sequence of arteriolar spasm, leading to ischemic necrosis of the endometrial surface and endometrial shedding, or menses. Normal menses, in the absence of structural pathology, is an orderly process because these arteriolar changes occur in the entire mucosa simultaneously and universally, with vasospasm and coagulation occluding the terminal vessels. Bleeding associated with normal menses is notable for the absence of clotting because of fibrinolysis within the uterine cavity before flow. With fertilization and implantation, menses are absent (amenorrhea). Alternatively, a disordered ovarian cycle leads to a disordered endometrial cycle and abnormal uterine bleeding patterns.

Early Pregnancy

A brief description of the events leading to pregnancy is useful for understanding the possible complications of early pregnancy. Coitus during the 48 hours before ovulation or within the periovulatory period establishes the conditions for fertilization. As just noted, sperm transport is facilitated by the estrogenic environment and the spermatozoa ascend through the cervix and uterine cavity and to the fallopian tube. When a mature oocyte and spermatozoa come into contact in the distal fallopian tube, fertilization can occur. This usually occurs 3 to 5 days after ovulation. During tubal transport, the zygote undergoes multiple divisions to reach the stage of the morula by the time it reaches the cavity. Implantation generally occurs 5 to 7 days after fertilization.

There are two significant clinical implications to delay in the fertilization-transport sequence. If the zygote has not matured adequately before reaching the endometrial cavity, implantation will not occur and a preclinical, unrecognized pregnancy will be lost. If there is delay in the fertilization-transport sequence, whether because of the randomness of coital timing or because of altered tubal structure or function, the zygote can reach the stage at which it is programmed to adhere to genital mucosa while still in the fallopian tube, resulting in an ectopic pregnancy.

Amenorrhea and Abnormal Menses

A disrupted sequence of the hypothalamic-pituitary-ovarian interaction has a profound effect on the endometrium and menses. There are two broad classes of amenorrheic disorders: hypogonadotropic and anovulatory. Although the details of the pathology and evaluation are beyond the scope of this text, hypogonadotropic conditions result from central disruption of hypothalamic-pituitary axis. Common causes for this condition include stress, hyperprolactinemia, and low body mass (anorexia nervosa; athletes such as distance runners, gymnasts, ballerinas). Because of the hypogonadotropic state, follicles are not stimulated, estrogen is not secreted, and endometrial proliferation does not occur. The result is an atrophic endometrium.

Atrophic endometrium can be identified with ultrasound by measuring the endometrial bilayer. Although local equipment and operator experience will vary, an endometrial bilayer of less than 5 mm in a young amenorrheic woman is highly supportive of the diagnosis. This must then be followed by a thorough investigation of the entire axis.

Anovulation results from a disrupted sequence of the axis from failure of the feedback loop to trigger the LH surge. The patient may have normal or elevated FSH levels, but FSH continues to stimulate continuous production of estrogen from the granulosa cells. The chronic unopposed estrogen promotes continuous proliferation of the endometrium, without the maturing sequence induced by progesterone. The proliferation of the endometrium results in excessive thickness. This becomes clinically manifest by prolonged amenorrhea, often followed by prolonged and profuse uterine bleeding (hypermenorrhea, menorrhagia). The most common cause for this presentation is polycystic ovarian disease (PCOD), but physiologic or social stress can produce a similar clinical scenario.

Ultrasound measurement of the endometrial bilayer can exceed 20 mm. Patients with chronic anovulation with chronic unopposed estrogen are at risk for endometrial hyperplasia and even endometrial cancer. The evaluation of the patient must address both the etiology for the chronic anovulation and the endometrial consequences. Histologic diagnosis requires an endometrial biopsy or curettage.

After prolonged amenorrhea with excessive proliferation of the endometrial lining, hypermenorrhea and menorrhagia may occur because of four parallel mechanisms. The growth of tissue from basalis to surface extends beyond the terminal branches of the arterioles, resulting in surface ischemia and necrosis. The volume of endometrial tissue is obviously increased. The normal hemostatic mechanisms of the spiral arterioles in the menstrual cycle are absent. Finally, the shedding of the endometrial surface is not a universal event but rather is random and leads to multiple foci of bleeding that are dyssynchronous and occurring over a prolonged time. Frequently, the rate of bleeding exceeds the capacity of normal intracavitary fibrinolytic processes and blood clots are common in the flow.

CLINICAL EVALUATION

In the urgent or acute setting, the gynecologic history focuses on the variation from normal ovarian and menstrual physiology as it relates to the reproductive life cycle. Patients will typically present with aberrant bleeding patterns, pelvic-abdominal pain or ill-defined discomfort, or a combination of these symptoms. With a focused history, the differential diagnosis can be constructed with further refinement from physical findings and ancillary tests. The key elements to be elicited are age, pregnancy history, recent and past menstrual history, sexual history, contraception, prior gynecologic disease and procedures, and the evolution of the current complaints.

History

Age

Patient age is primarily relevant because of the phases of the reproductive life cycle: menarche at adolescence, perimenopause in middle age, and menopause.

At time of menarche, the synchrony of the hypothalamic-pituitary-ovarian axis is immature and the sequence of hypergonadotropic anovulatory amenorrhea-hypermenorrhea is common. Similarly, this is the age group in which emotional stress, anorexia nervosa, and excessive athleticism commonly occur, and the amenorrheic patient may have hypogonadotropic amenorrhea. Finally, however, the young patient may be fertile and sexually active, so pregnancy with complications must always be considered.

In the perimenopausal years, the ovary is less responsive to the gonadotropic stimulus and anovulation with the amenorrhea-hypermenorrhea sequence is common. In this age group, however, anatomic abnormalities such as uterine leiomyomas or endometrial polyps may confound the presentation.

Menopause is defined as cessation of menses for 1 year or more. Any postmenopausal woman who presents with uterine bleeding must be presumed to have uterine pathology and have an appropriate evaluation for possible hyperplastic or neoplastic endometrial pathology.

Pregnancy History

The commonly used notation for describing pregnancy history is GTPAL, for gravidity (number of pregnancies), term births, preterm births, abortions (spontaneous, induced, or ectopic), and living children. Additional comment is made if there have been recurring spontaneous abortions, ectopic pregnancies, or multiple gestation.

Although any pregnancy can develop complications, the patient with a history of poor outcomes in prior pregnancies will be at higher risk for another adverse outcome. In the acute setting, with pain and/or bleeding, pregnancy complications must be considered.

Menstrual History

The date of the last menstrual period (LMP) and the prior menstrual period (PMP) must be determined as accurately as possible. It is often necessary to elicit menstrual events over several prior months to establish a pattern. Additionally, it is important to obtain a description of any variation from the patient's normal pattern of quantity and duration of menstrual flow. Within the context of this menstrual history, one can place the current complaints of bleeding and/or pain in perspective.

The amenorrhea-hypermenorrhea sequence was described earlier. The patient who describes "two periods this month" may merely be describing a normal 28-day cycle beginning early and then late in the same calendar month. Alternating episodes of light bleeding with normal flow may suggest breakthrough bleeding at time of ovulation or on oral contraceptives. Excessive flow (menorrhagia) associated with regular cycles at normal intervals suggests structural abnormalities of the endometrial cavity, most commonly submucous leiomyomas or endometrial polyps. Random or intermittent bleeding episodes during the cycle should prompt consideration of a lesion of the cervix, endometrial hyperplasia, or, occasionally, adenocarcinoma of the endometrium.

Dysmenorrhea (menstrual cramps) is generally considered to occur only with ovulatory cycles. The patient who typically has dysmenorrhea but who currently denies cramps, even with a current episode of heavy flow, may be having an anovulatory bleeding episode, regardless of the interval between periods. Patients with high-volume flow, with insufficient intracavitary fibrinolysis, may experience cramps as the uterus contracts to expel the clot.

Bleeding associated with threatened pregnancy loss or from an extrauterine pregnancy must be considered, whether heavy or light flow, continuous or episodic, or anteceded by reported normal cycles or after amenorrhea.

Bleeding after menopause demands consideration of endometrial pathology and appropriate work-up to rule out hyperplasia or carcinoma.

Postcoital bleeding suggests cervical lesions, including cervicitis, polyps, or neoplasia.

Sexual History

As a sensitive and personal subject that is often difficult to elicit reliably in the acute setting, sexual activity may significantly influence the formulation of the differential diagnosis. Beyond the possibility of pregnancy, the patient who will acknowledge unprotected coitus with casual sexual partners should be considered to be at high risk for sexually transmitted diseases. Reliable reports of the use of barrier contraception reduce, but do not eliminate, the possibility of a sexually transmitted disease.

Pregnancy must be ruled out in any circumstance in which there is a clinical presentation that is not inconsistent with complications of pregnancy.

Contraception

Reliable use of contraception does not totally preclude the possibility of pregnancy but should raise other possible diagnoses to a higher level in the differential diagnosis.

Breakthrough bleeding on hormonal contraception is typically low volume and is rarely associated with cramps or pain. In the presence of other symptoms, pregnancy complications and genital tract infections should be considered. Patients with an intrauterine contraceptive device (IUD) may have spotting and cramping, but because the IUD increases the risk of endometrial infection and because a disproportionate percentage of pregnancies that are conceived with an IUD are extrauterine, these patients need careful evaluation.

Patients with previous tubal sterilization have a 1% to 3% lifetime risk of pregnancy, with a disproportionate number of extrauterine pregnancies. Irregular bleeding associated with pain mandates careful evaluation.

Prior Gynecologic Diseases and Procedures

Past gynecologic history may give direction to recurring conditions suggesting lifestyle issues that create risk of recurrence or raise consideration of complications of previous interventions.

Tubal ligation, prior tubal injury from an ectopic pregnancy, endometriosis, or pelvic inflammatory disease all increase the risk of extrauterine pregnancy. Endometriosis with intraperitoneal inflammatory response may cause significant pain. Patients with a history of functional ovarian cysts with or without intraparenchymal hemorrhage have a higher risk for recurrence. Previous pelvic surgery with periovarian adhesions can cause significant pain even with benign, self-limited ovarian cyst accidents but also may predispose to ovarian torsion.

The ovarian remnant syndrome is an interesting and confusing entity. It can cause pelvic pain in ill-defined patterns. The etiology of the syndrome is a retained fragment of ovarian capsule after previous ovarian surgery. The fragment is adherent to the peritoneum and remains viable through a parasitic blood supply. Active follicles can be recruited through gonadotropin stimulation, and the dynamics of peritoneal inflammation can be severely symptomatic. These remnants are most commonly found after resection of a densely adherent ovary with endometriosis or purulent infection of the pelvis. They are frequently located along the course of the ureter and may present with flank pain from urinary obstruction.

History of Present Illness

The surgeon elicits the historical elements described earlier to construct the evolution of the presenting complaint and formulate a plan for further evaluation and treatment. In this section the focus is on the most common emergency presentations: bleeding and pain.

Bleeding

- When did bleeding begin?
- How does the current flow compare with normal? Are there clots in the menstrual flow normally? Currently?
- How did the timing of onset relate to previous menses? Was there any prolongation of the interval between the last period and the onset of the current bleeding event?
- Were recent menses normal? Expected timing, flow, duration?
- Are menstrual periods normally associated with menstrual cramps? Is the current episode associated with similar cramps? No cramps? More intense discomfort?

Pain

- When did the pain begin? Relationship to last menses? Ovulatory?
- What is the character of the pain? Cramping? Sharp? Pressure? Stabbing? Colicky?
- What is the pattern of the pain? Constant? Intermittent? Episodic?
- Where is the pain located? Generalized? Midline suprapubic? Lateralized?
- Does the pain radiate? Vagina? Rectum? Legs? Back? Upper abdomen? Shoulder?
- Were there changes in the character, pattern, or location of the pain over time; for example, did cramping midline pain become acute sharp lateralized pain, followed by relief, evolving to generalized abdominal pain radiating to the shoulder? Did lateralized constant intense pressure evolve to acute sharp pain or intermittent colicky pain?
- Is there exacerbation of the pain with movement? Intercourse? Coughing?
- Are there any urinary tract symptoms? Dysuria?
- Are there any intestinal symptoms? Constipation? Obstipation? Diarrhea?

Physical Examination

The approach to the physical examination of the gynecologic patient must account for the threat to dignity and modesty that genital examination poses. In the emergency setting, against a background of fear and/or pain, and especially among the young and elderly patients, the patient must be afforded maximum comfort. This includes an adequate sense of physical privacy, the continuous presence of a chaperone, a comfortable examination table on which to assume the lithotomy position, and patience by the examiner.

Although the chief complaint might suggest that only a focused pelvic examination is necessary, the examiner will enhance comfort and trust by a more general examination before the pelvic one. The examiner must remember that the patient cannot see and cannot anticipate what she will experience next; the examiner or the assistant should inform the patient at every step in the process what the next sensation will be.

At the beginning of the pelvic examination, the examiner should encourage relaxation and exposure by having the patient relax her medial thighs to allow the knees to drop out toward laterally placed hands. The knees should never be pushed apart by the examiner. Before contacting the genitalia, gentle touch of the gloved hand on the medial thigh with gentle pressure and movement toward the vulva will orient the patient to the progress of the examination. The external genitalia are inspected for lesions and evidence of trauma. This is followed by the insertion of a properly sized, lubricated vaginal speculum. The patient should be prepared for the speculum by placing a finger on the perineum and exerting gentle pressure with encouragement to relax the introital muscles. The speculum is placed at the hymeneal ring at a 30-degree angle from the vertical to minimize lateral or urethral pressure. After the leading edge is through the introitus, the speculum is rotated to the horizontal plane as it is advanced toward the apex of the vagina. The blades are gently separated as the midvagina is approached so that the cervix can be visualized, and the blades are spread to surround the cervix. During the advancement and subsequent withdrawal, the walls of the vagina are visualized for lesions or trauma. The cervix is inspected for lesions, lacerations, dilation, products of conception, or purulent discharge. Support of the pelvic structures in the anterior, posterior, and superior compartments is evaluated. Vaginal swabs for microscopic wet mount examination of the vaginal environment, for gonorrhea and *Chlamydia*, and a Papanicolaou smear should be obtained as indicated.

After the speculum examination, the index and middle fingers of the dominant hand are inserted into the vagina. Before placing the abdominal hand, the examining fingers gently palpate the vaginal walls to elicit tenderness or to detect fullness or mass. The cervix is palpated for size and consistency. The examining fingers are placed sequentially along the side in all four quadrants of the cervix, and gentle pressure is exerted to move the cervix in the opposite direction to elicit cervical motion tenderness.

Because the major supporting structures for the uterus are the cardinal and uterosacral ligaments that insert at the cervicouterine junction, the junction serves as the fulcrum for leverage. As the cervix is moved in one direction, it is likely that the uterine fundus is being displaced in the opposite direction. Tenderness with cervical motion may be related to traction on the ligamentous attachments, collision of the cervix against a structure in the direction to which the cervix is being displaced, or collision of the fundus against a structure on the opposite side.

The bimanual examination is performed with gentle pressure from the nondominant hand systematically mobilizing pelvic contents against the vaginal fingers. Except with large masses that are palpable on abdominal examination, the primary information gathered is detected by the vaginal fingers. Specifically note lateralized tenderness and masses. The rectovaginal examination provides additional perspective, especially for the cul-de-sac and adnexal structures.

Very young women and some elderly women will not tolerate insertion of two fingers or occasionally even one. Under these circumstances, a rectal finger along with the abdominal placement of the other hand can simulate a bimanual examination.

Diagnostic Considerations

Although there are always atypical crossover presentations for any of the possible diagnoses, the most common considerations for the differential diagnosis of symptom complexes are as follows:

Bleeding Without Pain

- Anovulatory cycle
- Threatened or spontaneous abortion (miscarriage of intrauterine pregnancy)
- Vaginal laceration
- Vaginal or cervical neoplasm

Bleeding Associated With Midline Suprapubic Pain

- Dysmenorrhea
- Threatened or spontaneous abortion (miscarriage of intrauterine pregnancy)
- Endometritis associated with pelvic infection
- Uterine fibroids
- Early presentation of a complication of extrauterine pregnancy
- Vaginal laceration

Bleeding Associated With Lateralized Pelvic Pain

- Extrauterine pregnancy, prerupture
- Functional ovarian cyst
- Ruptured functional ovarian cyst
- Ruptured corpus luteum with or without an intrauterine pregnancy
- Vaginal trauma

Bleeding Associated With Generalized Pelvic Pain

- Ruptured extrauterine pregnancy
- Ruptured corpus luteum with or without an intrauterine pregnancy
- Septic spontaneous or induced abortion
- Vaginal trauma

Midline Pelvic Pain Without Bleeding

- Endometritis/pelvic inflammatory disease
- Endometriosis
- Pelvic neoplasm
- Urinary tract infection
- Constipation

Lateralized Pelvic Pain Without Bleeding

- Extrauterine pregnancy
- Functional ovarian cyst, with or without intraparenchymal hemorrhage
- Functional ovarian cyst with rupture
- Functional or neoplastic ovarian cyst with intermittent torsion
- Pedunculated paratubal or paraovarian cyst with intermittent torsion
- Endometriosis
- Ovarian remnant syndrome
- Ureteritis
- Constipation

Generalized Abdominal Pain Without Bleeding

- Ruptured extrauterine pregnancy
- Ruptured ovarian cyst
- Pelvic inflammatory disease with pelvic peritonitis
- Endometriosis

Obstipation

- Cul-de-sac hematoma
- Cul-de-sac adnexal mass
- Posterior uterine fibroid
- Pelvic abscess
- Endometriosis

Flank Pain

- Pyelonephritis
- Ureteral obstruction
- Ovarian remnant syndrome with or without ureteral obstruction

Other Acute Clinical Presentations

Acute vulvovaginitis is a common presenting emergency complaint. Presenting symptoms are intense pruritus or cutaneous pain with discharge. The most frequent pathogens are mycotic or herpes simplex. Mycotic infections are generally characterized by a thick, white, cottage cheese discharge. Primary herpetic infections will often present as profuse watery discharge, inguinal adenopathy, and signs of a viremia. In contrast, other common vaginal infections, such as bacterial vaginosis and trichomoniasis, may cause irritative symptoms and malodorous discharge but rarely cause pain.

Common acute vulvar complaints include infection of skin appendages: folliculitis, furunculosis, and cellulitis. The ostium of Bartholin's gland may become occluded, with or without infection. Sterile cysts are only minimally uncomfortable, but a Bartholin abscess is exquisitely painful.

Necrotizing fasciitis is a life-threatening infection that can occur in the vulva. It can begin as a cellulitis, from infected skin appendages, or after biopsy or episiotomy. Once established, it can quickly extend through the fascial planes. Women at risk are patients with obesity, diabetes, and corticosteroid or other immunosuppressive drug use. Management is immediate surgical débridement. Patients may require several débridements to determine the extent of the fascial involvement. Skin grafts are often needed to repair large defects. It is very important that women with risk factors for necrotizing fasciitis who present with a vulvar cellulitis be admitted for intravenous therapy with antibiotics and possible surgical treatment.

Pelvic Masses

Masses identified in the pelvis can be functional, congenital, neoplastic, hemorrhagic, or inflammatory and can arise from the ovary or the uterus. Additionally, the anatomy of the cul-de-sac of Douglas in its dependent position in the pelvis facilitates restriction of pelvic infection as collections or abscesses to that location.

Common ovarian masses include functional cysts, hemorrhagic cysts, paraovarian or paratubal wolffian remnants, endometrioma, and benign or malignant tumors (epithelial, germ cell, stromal).

The most common neoplastic mass in young women is the benign cystic teratoma. Because of the sebaceous content of these lesions, they frequently "float" to the anterior cul-de-sac between the uterus and the bladder.

Diagnostic considerations for differentiating among ovarian masses of the various causes are discussed in detail in the later section on ovarian cancer.

Common uterine masses include leiomyoma, adenomyoma, and bicornuate uterus. Common inflammatory masses include tubo-ovarian abscess, pelvic collection, and appendiceal or diverticular abscess.

Inflammatory masses in the anterior cul-de-sac most commonly originate from sigmoid diverticular disease.

Ancillary Tests

Imaging

The single most effective and efficient modality for assessing pelvic anatomy and pathology is real-time ultrasound, especially with a transvaginal transducer. This technique allows not only assessment of the size and relationship of the pelvic structures but also, by clear delineation of echogenicity, can provide strong suspicion of the nature of a pathologic process. With real-time Doppler flow assessment, blood flow to an organ or mass and fetal heart motion are readily apparent.

Axial tomography and magnetic resonance imaging (MRI) rarely provide additional information for benign pelvic pathology but are valuable techniques for assessing malignancies.

Intravenous pyelography may be useful if ultrasound assessment of the urinary tract is inadequate to delineate obstruction or anatomic distortion.

Pregnancy Tests

There are two endocrine tests that are useful for determining the presence and health of a pregnancy: human chorionic gonadotropin (HCG) and progesterone.

Modern pregnancy tests measure the β subunit of HCG, and the sensitivity of the qualitative urine assay can be as low as 20 mIU/mL. This is sufficiently low as to virtually exclude all but the earliest of gestations. Unless a viable fetus can be detected clinically or by ultrasound, a positive urine test, in the clinical setting that could suggest an ectopic pregnancy, must be followed with a quantitative serum radioimmunoassay. A result less than 5 mIU/mL is a negative test. In most laboratories, and depending on the quality of the ultrasound equipment and the experience of the sonographer, a healthy intrauterine pregnancy that has produced 2000 mIU/mL of β-HCG should be visualized. In the absence of that threshold, serial β-HCG tests should be scheduled at 2-day intervals.[1]

In the "typical" healthy intrauterine pregnancy, serum β-HCG levels double every 48 hours. However, this description is based on pooled, aggregated data; within the datasets there are many patients with successful pregnancies who will have intervals with a lower slope of rise followed by an interval with steep rise. A decline in value over a 2-day period is always ominous and, therefore, demands a clinical decision about intrauterine versus extrauterine failed pregnancy. The greater challenge occurs when the rate of increase is less than 60% over 48 hours. This is ambiguous, and if the β-HCG level is below the discriminatory value of 2000 mIU, clinical presentation and clinical judgment are vital to determine whether continued observation or intervention is the appropriate course.[2]

Caveat: There are three commonly used reference standards for β-HCG, and significant interlaboratory variation in test results. It is critical to understand the standard used and to be certain that the sequential tests are performed in the same laboratory. If a change in laboratories is necessary, repeat parallel testing in the new laboratory, using the residual serum from the original sample, will resolve the question.

Significantly elevated β-HCG levels should suggest a hydatidiform mole or a germ cell tumor.

Determining serum progesterone levels can be a useful adjunct in assessing the viability of a pregnancy. The quantitative relationship with pregnancy status is not as discrete. Progesterone levels less than 5 ng/mL are rarely associated with successful pregnancies. Among women whose levels exceed 25 ng/mL, only a small fraction will have failed or ectopic pregnancies.[3]

Serum Hormone Assays

Other than the assessment of pregnancy, there is relatively little value to ordering reproductive hormone levels in the acute setting. These tests are relatively expensive and the sequence of ordering them should be determined by the clinical findings. The laboratory turnaround time is rarely less than a day.

Cervicovaginal Cultures, Gram Stain, and Wet Prep

Because the healthy vagina is a polymicrobial environment, there are only four organisms for which cervicovaginal cultures are clinically useful: gonococcus, *Chlamydia trachomatis,* herpes simplex, and, in pregnancy, group B β-hemolytic *Streptococcus.* Current technology links the tests for gonococcus and *Chlamydia* in a single swab/medium kit for molecular analysis of the organisms.

Gram stain of purulent cervical discharge is useful in the emergency setting for identification of the gram-negative intracellular diplococci, which is diagnostic of gonococcus. The test may also be useful in helping identify *Trichomonas vaginalis.*

Culture and Gram stain of purulent material from an abscess of Bartholin's gland may allow the physician to select a narrow-spectrum antibiotic as an adjunct to drainage.

The vaginal wet mount is useful in diagnosis of the offending organism in acute vaginitis. A sample of discharge is taken, both from the vaginal pool and by rubbing the vaginal walls with a cotton swab. The swab is placed in 1 to 2 mm of saline in a tube to create a slurry. A drop of the slurry is placed on a slide with a coverslip and viewed under low- and high-power light microscopy. The specimen is examined for polymorphonuclear leukocytes, clue cells, trichomonads, hyphae, and budding yeast forms. If hyphae and budding yeast forms are not identified, a second slide is prepared by mixing a drop of the slurry with a drop of potassium hydroxide, which will lyse the epithelial cells and highlight the fungal organisms.

The clue cell is an epithelial cell with densely adherent bacteria, creating a stippled effect. To make this diagnosis, the density of bacteria must obscure cell margins in a substantial percentage of the cells. These, along with a strong amine odor, are diagnostic of bacterial vaginosis. There is rarely a significant white cell response to this condition because it is not an infection per se but rather a shift in the normal vaginal ecosystem.

Trichomonads are often obvious as flagellated, motile organisms similar in size to white blood cells. The organism is fragile, however, and motility can be inhibited by severe infection or cooling of the specimen during a delay before inspecting.

Lower Genital Cytology

The Papanicolaou cytologic technique has had significant public health impact and reduced the incidence of invasive cervical cancer. While the processing time for the smear limits usefulness in the acute setting, there are two important reasons to consider obtaining the sample. The first is to take the opportunity of the visit to test a previously noncompliant patient. The second is to satisfy any significant concern about a high-grade cervical lesion before surgical manipulation of the cervix. (See the later section on cervical cancer.)

There are two fundamental approaches to obtaining and preparing the specimen. In the older technique, a cervical spatula is placed in the cervical os and rotated circumferentially against the cervical epithelium. This is followed by a cotton swab placed in the cervical canal and rotated on its long axis. As each step is completed, the instrument is wiped across a glass slide and spray fixative is applied. In the more recent technique, the specimen from the instrument is swirled in a fluid-based preservative that is processed to provide a more homogeneous slide for Papanicolaou staining. Although the cost of the fluid-based technique is greater, the improved accuracy and the reduction of both false-positives and false-negatives make this more cost effective.

MANAGEMENT OF PREINVASIVE AND INVASIVE DISEASE OF THE FEMALE GENITAL TRACT

Staging guidelines for various types of neoplasia may be found at the website for the Federation of International Gynecologic Oncology (www.figo.org) or see the selected references at the end of this chapter.[4]

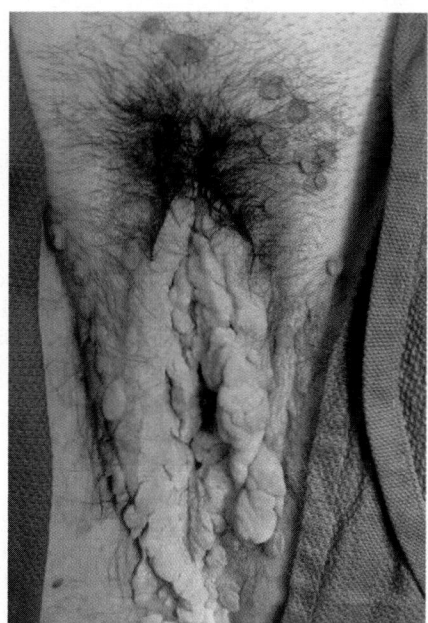

FIGURE 74-7. Condylomata. (Courtesy of Lynn Parker, M.D., Vanderbilt University Medical Center.)

Preinvasive Vulvar Squamous Lesions

Dysplasia of the vulva usually presents as persistent symptoms of vulvar pruritus, occasionally because the patient has seen a visible lesion, and, rarely, because of bleeding. Vulvar dysplasia and condylomata tend to be multifocal and can involve any area on the vulva (Fig. 74-7). On physical examination, the dysplasia can appear as white thickened epithelium, pigmented, erythematous, exophytic, or a combination of these findings. Because appearance can be variable, a 4- or 5-mm punch biopsy should be performed to differentiate dysplasia from an invasive lesion. Vulvar dysplasia is related to exposure to the human papillomavirus, but unlike cervical cancer there is not a direct relationship between preinvasive disease and cancer.

Evaluation of the patient with vulvar dysplasia should include colposcopy of the vulva, vagina, and cervix because 15% to 20% of patients will have dysplasia in more than one of these sites. Colposcopy is the use of a microscope to better visualize the area of concern. A 4% acetic acid solution is applied to the skin to make more apparent any areas of preinvasive disease. Changes can appear as thickened white epithelium, vascular changes, or any of the possible appearances described previously. A biopsy specimen should be taken of any suspicious lesion and sent for pathologic study. Pathologic classification is based on the extent of epithelial involvement: up to one third of the epithelium is called vulvar intraepithelial neoplasia (VIN I); up to two thirds, VIN II; and greater than two thirds, VIN III.

Treatment of dysplasia of the vulva includes wide local excision with a 5-mm margin around the lesion and little, if any, removal of the underlying subcutaneous tissue. This approach is best used in patients with a focal lesion. Patients who have multifocal disease will benefit from laser ablation with a CO_2 laser. Depth of ablation depends on whether the area is hair bearing or not. Hair-bearing areas require ablation to a depth of 2 to 2.5 mm. Non–hair-bearing areas are ablated to a depth of 1 to 2 mm. Postoperative care of the treatment area includes application of Silvadene cream three times a day.

An alternative treatment is imiquimod (Aldara) cream. The mechanism of action is thought to be stimulation of the patient's immune system to reverse the effect of the human papillomavirus. The most common side effect of the cream is an area of irritation involving the treatment area.

Invasive Vulvar Squamous Lesions

The most common vulvar cancer is squamous cell carcinoma (90%). It tends to present in women older than the age of 65. Other risk factors include immunocompromised state, cigarette smoking, obesity, and lichen sclerosus. Patients may present with a visible lesion, bleeding, pain, or dysuria. The lesion may be exophytic, ulcerative, or nodular. Any suspicious lesion on the vulva should be sampled with a 3- or 4-mm punch biopsy to rule out malignancy. Any lesion with greater than 1 mm depth of invasion requires treatment not only of the primary lesion but also evaluation of the inguinal lymph nodes.

Treatment of vulvar cancer is primarily surgical. For early-stage disease, primary therapy is wide radical excision, which is removal of a 1.5- to 2-cm margin around the primary tumor and removal of the subcutaneous tissue down to the level of the endopelvic fascia. If the lesion is lateralized, the ipsilateral inguinal lymph nodes only need to be removed. If the lesion is midline, bilateral inguinal lymph nodes should be removed. If more than two lymph nodes are positive, the patient should receive postoperative radiation therapy. If one node is positive and only ipsilateral nodes were done, the other groin should be dissected. For advanced stage disease (stage III or IV), chemotherapy and irradiation are the treatments of choice. If there are large inguinal lymph nodes, however, surgical debulking may have value before chemotherapy and irradiation (Table 74-2).

Vulvar cancer may recur locally or distally. With local recurrence, wide radical excision can be used with removal of ipsilateral nodes if they have not previously been removed. Distal sites can include nodal areas, liver, lung, and subcutaneous nodules in the skin. Unless there is an isolated lesion that can be excised, distal disease is best treated with chemotherapy.

Verrucous carcinoma is a specific variant of vulvar carcinoma that presents as a fungating mass. It has a papillary architecture with pushing borders. Microscopically, there is little or mild nuclear atypia, which distinguish it from warty squamous cell carcinomas. In general, this type of vulvar cancer is best treated with surgery. As opposed to other vulvar malignancies, it may get larger if treated with radiation therapy.

TABLE 74-2.   Treatment of Vulvar Cancer

Diagnosis	Treatment
Invasion < 1 mm	Wide local excision
Stage I or II lesion lateral location	Wide radical excision + unilateral inguinofemoral lymphadenectomy
Stage I or II midline lesion	Wide radical + bilateral inguinofemoral lymphadenectomy
Lesion with extension into vagina, anus, or distal urethra	Wide radical excision with bilateral inguinofemoral lymphadenectomy or chemoradiation followed by excision of residual tumor
Any size lesion with groin nodes	Excision of groin followed by chemoradiation therapy
Distant metastases	Palliative chemotherapy

Melanoma of the Vulva

Melanoma is the second most common type of malignancy involving the vulva, primarily occurring in older women. Clinical presentation and appearance is similar to melanoma at other sites, and lesions are staged by the same criteria. Standard treatment is wide local excision with a 2-cm margin around the lesion. Melanomas of the vulva follow lymphatic pathways just as they do in other locations in the body, but the role of lymphadenectomy in the treatment of vulvar melanoma is controversial. Lymphadenectomy in this disease appears to be prognostic instead of therapeutic and helps identify patients who would benefit from adjuvant therapy.

Bartholin's Gland Carcinoma

Bartholin's gland carcinomas can be adenocarcinomas arising from the gland itself or squamous cell carcinomas that arise from the duct or adenoid cystic carcinomas. Histologically, there must be a transition between normal gland or duct and cancer to make the diagnosis. Unlike squamous cells cancers, lymph node involvement is common and can be bilateral. Treatment is wide radical excision with bilateral lymph node dissection.

Basal Cell Carcinoma

Just like basal cell carcinomas in other locations, vulvar basal cell carcinoma is a local tumor with little risk of lymph node metastasis. Therefore, treatment includes wide local excision only.

Paget's Disease of the Vulva

Paget's disease of the vulva occurs in postmenopausal women. It presents as a red, velvety lesion with pruritus and, occasionally, bleeding. It can occur anywhere on the vulva. Microscopically, the disease extends far beyond the visible lesion. Paget's disease may be intraepithelial, invasive beyond the basement membrane, or associated with an underlying adenocarcinoma (Paget's cells involving the epithelium plus an adenocarcinoma in the subcutaneous tissue). Paget's disease of the vulva is also associated with coexisting malignancies, such as those at breast, colon, or genitourinary locations. Work-up of patients with this diagnosis should include screening for other malignancies. Treatment is wide local excision for patients with intraepithelial Paget's disease, but wide radical excision and lymph node dissections should be considered in patients with invasive Paget's or intraepithelial Paget's disease with an underlying adenocarcinoma.

Vulvar Sarcomas

Vulvar sarcomas can occur with many histologic subtypes. In general, the treatment is wide radical excision followed by radiation therapy and, in some cases, postoperative chemotherapy.

Preinvasive Vaginal Lesions

Dysplasia of the vagina, with or without overt condylomata, can occur, typically presenting as an abnormal Papanicolaou smear result. On colposcopic examination, lesions appear as thickened white epithelium or areas of vascular change. In patients with an intact uterus, vaginal dysplasia is typically seen in conjunction with cervical dysplasia. Therefore, colposcopy of the cervix should also include evaluation of the vagina. Any abnormal area on colposcopy should be sampled to confirm the diagnosis and rule out invasion.

Treatment of vaginal dysplasia includes laser ablation or wide excision of the vaginal mucosa. An alternative treatment for women who are poor surgical candidates is intravaginal 5-fluorouracil.

Invasive Vaginal Lesions

Although far less common than squamous cell carcinomas of the cervix or vulva, this lesion is the most common type of cancer in the vagina. Tumors may be identified through an abnormal Papanicolaou smear or by a visible lesion. They can occur at any location in the vagina but are most likely to occur at the vaginal apex. These tumors can present as a second primary site in patients with previous cervical carcinoma. Diagnosis is made with biopsy or wide local excision. It is important to exclude a cervical cancer with vaginal involvement or recurrent cervical or endometrial carcinoma. If a vaginal primary lesion is confirmed, staging is based on examination and evaluation of the paravaginal areas and sidewall. If the disease is apical, pelvic nodal disease should be the most likely site of spread. If the disease is in the lower vagina, inguinal node involvement must be ruled out. Computed tomography (CT) of the abdomen and pelvis should be done to rule out nodal involvement. A chest radiograph must be done to rule out pulmonary metastasis.

Treatment options for vaginal cancer include surgical resection or chemotherapy and irradiation for stage I tumors and for more advanced disease. Recurrence can be local or remote. If recurrence is local after irradiation, pelvic exenteration can be considered. For remote recurrence, chemotherapy is used.

Vaginal adenocarcinomas occur rarely. Most well known is the correlation of clear cell carcinoma of the vagina in patients who were exposed in utero to diethylstilbestrol (DES). Because DES has not been used for many years, this problem, and diagnosis, has decreased in occurrence. Other epithelial types can include endometrioid or papillary serous carcinomas. Treatment of adenocarcinomas is the same as that outlined for squamous malignancies. Neuroendocrine carcinomas can occur in the vagina. Evaluation for metastasis should include not only evaluation of the chest, abdomen, and pelvis but also that of the head and bones. As opposed to squamous malignancies, chemotherapy and irradiation is most appropriate.

Melanomas can occur in the vagina, with the same variations of presentation as other body sites. Treatment options include anterior or posterior exenteration depending on the location of the lesion in the vagina. Pelvic radiation can also be considered. Prognosis is poor for these patients even if surgical margins are negative.

Rhabdomyosarcoma can occur in the vagina and mainly occurs in young girls. Combined modality therapy with surgery, chemotherapy, and irradiation has been the most effective in this tumor.

Preinvasive Disease of the Cervix

Human papillomavirus (HPV) is a DNA virus that has an affinity for cells in the junction of squamous and glandular cells in the cervix (transformation zone). High-risk HPV types, most notably types 16 and 18, enter the cell and use the cell's system to produce viral products like E6 and E7. These viral products interfere with the cell's natural apoptotic mechanism that makes the cell immortal. This is the mechanism for the transition to malignancy for HPV-related cancers. Dysplasia or precancer can occur in the cervix and typically arises in the transformation zone.

Papanicolaou smears are a screening test for dysplasia and malignancy. Over the years there have been several classifications of Papanicolaou smears, of which the most recent is the revised Bethesda Classification. In that classification, patients who require further evaluation with colposcopy include those with glandular lesions and atypical cells in whom a high-grade lesion cannot be ruled out as well as those with low-grade and high-grade squamous intraepithelial lesions. Biopsy at the time of colposcopy can confirm the histologic diagnosis of mild, moderate, or severe dysplasia. At the time of colposcopy, comment should be made as to whether the entire lesion and transformation zone can be seen. If the patient has an adequate colposcopic examination, has a low-grade lesion (mild dysplasia), and is compliant, she can be expectantly managed because regression may occur in up to 70% of patients over 2 years. If the patient is noncompliant or has other factors of concern, treatment could include

cryotherapy, large-loop excision of the transformation zone (LEEP), or laser ablation. For high-grade lesions such as moderate or severe dysplasia, LEEP or laser is a consideration.

Cone biopsy is recommended for patients who have glandular lesions, a Papanicolaou smear of concern for invasion or microinvasion, a positive result of endocervical curetting, an inadequate colposcopy, or a two-step discrepancy between Papanicolaou smear and biopsy specimens. The technique for cone biopsy is discussed later.

Invasive Disease of the Cervix

Ninety percent of invasive cancers of the cervix are squamous cell carcinomas. Other histologic types include adenocarcinoma, adenosquamous carcinoma, neuroendocrine carcinoma, basal cell carcinoma, and, rarely, signet ring cell carcinoma. Patients may present with postcoital bleeding, irregular bleeding, malodorous discharge, an abnormal Papanicolaou smear, or a visible lesion. Advanced lesions may present with symptoms of sidewall involvement, which include back pain that radiates down the leg, unilateral edema of the leg, or flank pain. Whether there is a grossly visible lesion or abnormal cytology and abnormal colposcopy, diagnosis requires tissue biopsy. Cervical cancer is staged clinically. These lesions invade into the stroma of the cervix and then expand into the lymphatics accompanying the ligamentous supporting tissues of the cervix and upper vagina. As they extend, pelvic sidewall involvement may cause ureteral obstruction and hydronephrosis. The bladder or rectum may become involved. Although lymphatic spread is common, staging criteria do not include node involvement. That being said, however, metastasis to lymph nodes significantly impacts prognosis.

When the diagnosis of cervical cancer is made from a LEEP or a cone biopsy, it is important to determine as accurately as possible the depth of invasion involved. The type of treatment recommended varies significantly based on depth of invasion.

Once the diagnosis is confirmed histologically, bimanual and rectovaginal examination should be done to determine if there is any vaginal, parametrial, or pelvic sidewall extension. This completes clinical staging. Other evaluation should include chest radiography, either CT or intravenous pyelography to rule out hydronephrosis, and either CT or lymphangiography to rule out lymph node involvement. Treatment varies with stage of disease (Table 74-3).

For example, a tumor with 1 to 3 mm of invasion is a microinvasive cancer of the cervix that can be treated with simple hysterectomy or, in selected cases, can be managed with a cone biopsy in patients who strongly desire fertility. However, a tumor with greater than 5 mm depth of invasion or 7 mm on horizontal extent is a stage IB1 tumor with 10% risk of pelvic lymph node metastasis and requires a radical hysterectomy for treatment. Therefore, if depth of invasion cannot be accurately determined or if the invasive component involves the endocervical margin, a repeat cone biopsy should be done.

TABLE 74-3.   Treatment of Cervical Cancer

Diagnosis	Treatment
Stage IA1	Simple hysterectomy
Stage IA2	Modified radical hysterectomy and pelvic lymphadenectomy
Stage IB1	Radical hysterectomy and pelvic lymphadenectomy; or pelvic radiation therapy followed by brachytherapy
Stage IB2	Chemotherapy and irradiation
Stage IIA-IVA	Chemotherapy and irradiation
Stage IVB	Palliative radiation with chemotherapy

Treatment of Stage IA1 Disease

Stage IA1 disease is typically a total abdominal hysterectomy. However, some European studies have described treating this disease with cold knife conizaton in patients who strongly desire fertility and will be compliant with follow-up.

Treatment of Stage IA2 Disease

Stage IA2 disease is treated with modified radical hysterectomy. Modified radical hysterectomy differs from radical hysterectomy in that the uterine artery is ligated at the level of the ureter instead of at the origin.

Treatment of Stage IB1 Disease

Patients with stage IB1 disease have equal cure rates with radiation therapy or radical hysterectomy with pelvic lymphadenectomy. Radiation therapy includes 45 to 50 Gy of whole-pelvic radiation followed by brachytherapy. The goal dose is 85 to 90 Gy to point A, which is a point measured 2 cm above and 2 cm lateral to the cervix. Radical hysterectomy involves removal of the uterus, parametrial tissue, and 1 cm of the upper vagina. It does not necessarily include oophorectomy. Cure rates are between 85% and 90%. Risks and benefits of both treatment options should be discussed with the patient and a treatment plan agreed on.

Pelvic lymphadenectomy involves removal of all visible lymph tissue from the level of the bifurcation of the iliac arteries down to the transverse circumflex iliac vein. Laterally, the tissue is separated from the genitofemoral nerve and the external iliac artery and vein. The bundle is then separated medially from the hypogastric and superior vesical artery. Inferiorly, the bundle is separated from the obturator nerve.

In patients who have more than one positive pelvic lymph node, deep invasion of the cervix, or a positive margin, pelvic irradiation is recommended postoperatively.

Treatment of Stage IB2 Disease

Stage IB2 or bulky IB2 disease can be treated in a variety of ways. Some would favor radical hysterectomy with a high likelihood of postoperative radiation therapy. Others would favor chemotherapy and irradiation as primary treatment. Finally, some patients respond to pelvic radiation and one brachytherapy followed by extrafascial hysterectomy.

Treatment of Stages IIA to IVA

Stage IIA disease can be treated with radical hysterectomy, but most gynecologic oncologists would currently treat these patients with chemotherapy and irradiation. For stage IIB to IVA tumors, treatment is a combination of radiation therapy with cisplatin-based chemotherapy. In 1999, Morris and colleagues compared extended-field radiation therapy versus chemotherapy and irradiation for patients with stage IB2 to IVA tumors. There was a survival advantage seen for patients receiving both chemotherapy and irradiation. Current regimens include cisplatin possibly in combination with 5-fluorouracil.

Treatment of Stage IVB Disease

Stage IVB disease involves distant metastasis. Most commonly affected are the lung and liver. In this instance, radiation therapy is changed to palliative and chemotherapy is the focus of treatment. First-line agents typically include cisplatin or 5-fluorouracil.

Treatment of Patients With Enlarged Lymph Nodes

When enlarged lymph nodes are seen on initial CT evaluation, patients may benefit from retroperitoneal lymph node dissection to remove the bulky disease. Radiation therapy alone cannot sterilize bulky adenopathy. Retroperitoneal node dissection allows the nodes to be debulked and to determine if para-aortic lymph nodes are involved. Para-aortic lymph node involvement is a poor prognostic factor. Nodal dissection is undertaken with a retroperitoneal approach through a paramedian or midline incision. A retroperitoneal approach has a much lower risk of fistula formation or bowel obstruction than an intraperitoneal approach.

Treatment of Neuroendocrine Tumors

Neuroendocrine carcinomas of the cervix are among the most rare and aggressive types. Five-year survivals have been reported in the 5% to 10% range. As with other neuroendocrine tumors, the disease can metastasize to bone, brain, lung, or liver. Assessment should include evaluation of these areas before treatment. As opposed to other cervical cancers, chemotherapy and irradiation regimens can include other agents in addition to cisplatin, such as etoposide.

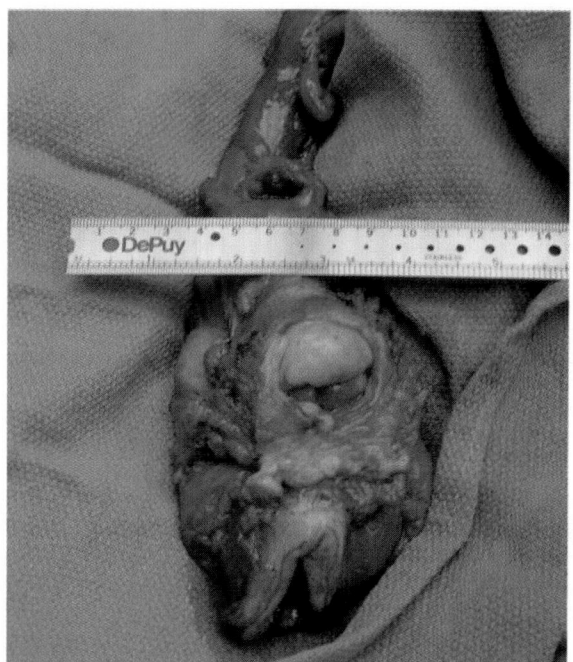

FIGURE 74-8. Pelvic exenteration. (Courtesy of Lynn Parker, M.D., Vanderbilt University Medical Center.)

Treatment of Recurrent Disease

If the patient has evidence of local recurrence on pelvic examination, distant disease must be ruled out by imaging studies. Once this has been completed, sidewall involvement must be ruled out. Patients with central recurrence of cervical cancer who have received previous radiation therapy can be cured with pelvic exenteration (Fig. 74-8). Survival rates are between 30% and 40%.

Postoperative morbidity and mortality for the procedure can be as high as 10%. Isolated distant metastasis, such as a single lung lesion or an incisional recurrence, may be treated with surgical resection followed by radiation therapy. In patients with multiple, distant metastases or sidewall involvement, chemotherapy is palliative and an average life expectancy is 9 to 12 months.

Special Considerations in Management of Cervical Cancer and Treatment Complications

Inappropriate Surgical Management

One of the most frequent and deleterious errors in surgical management of cervical cancer is failure to recognize the importance of block dissection of the tumor. The so-called cut-through procedure in which the surgeon transects active cancer extending beyond the cervix results in a reduction of 5-year survival from the 50% to 85% range to the 20% to 30% range. This error may occur because of inadequate preoperative evaluation of the diagnosed cancer or be encountered at the time of hysterectomy for presumed (and perhaps, coexistent) benign disease.

Treatment of the Pregnant Patient

Cervical cancer diagnosed early in pregnancy is a difficult situation. By continuing the pregnancy, the mother may be risking her own life. Recommendations in the first trimester are to consider radical hysterectomy in stage IB1 lesions and chemotherapy and irradiation in higher-stage lesions. If the radiation is given, spontaneous abortion will occur in 4 to 6 weeks. In the second trimester and later, the patient may be expectantly managed until maturity of the fetus with plans for treatment after delivery. Typically, delivery is expedited at 34 weeks once lung maturity is confirmed.

Management of the Cervical Cancer Patient with Acute Hemorrhage

Some patients with cervical cancer present with acute hemorrhage. When this occurs, do not attempt a surgical resection. The vagina should be packed with Monsel's solution applied to the gauze and a Foley catheter placed. The patient should be transfused and then transferred to a center where evaluation and treatment can begin.

Management of Radiation Complications

Typical complications after radiation therapy can include hemorrhagic cystitis, hemorrhagic proctitis, small bowel obstruction, and fistula formation.

Hemorrhagic cystitis can be managed with placement of a large three-way Foley catheter with continuous bladder irrigation. Hydrocortisone can be added as well. Cystoscopy and focal cauterization can also stop focal bleeding sites. Transfusion is commonly required.

Hemorrhagic proctitis can be managed with cortisone enemas and transfusion. Colonoscopy with focal cautery can also be used. However, biopsies should be avoided because of the risk of fistula formation. In some cases, colostomy with resection of the affected bowel may be indicated. Small bowel obstruction tends to occur in the ileum in patients who had previous surgery before irradiation. When conservative management fails, laparotomy with small bowel resection and reanastomosis may be required. Sharp dissection is important to use to avoid injury to surrounding structures.

Fistula formation occurs in 3% to 5% of patients treated with radiation therapy. Patients at higher risk include diabetics, patients with peripheral vascular disease, or those with collagen vascular disease. Rectovaginal fistula in a radiated field typically is not treatable with more conservative surgeries, and colostomy is required. In vesicovaginal fistulas, a urinary conduit is usually required.

Endometrium

The patient who presents with postmenopausal bleeding or abnormal bleeding after chronic anovulatory amenorrhea must be evaluated for endometrial hyperplasia or endometrial carcinoma. Although suspicion may be heightened by an abnormal endometrial ultrasound, diagnosis of these lesions requires tissue confirmation. Ultrasound measurement of the thickness of endometrial stripe can assist in avoiding unnecessary biopsies. The postmenopausal woman who has an endometrial bilayer stripe less than 5 mm without an irregularity in the cavity is very unlikely to have a carcinoma. If patient comfort or cervical stenosis precludes office endometrial biopsy, dilatation and curettage may be necessary to make the diagnosis.

Hyperplasia

Endometrial hyperplasia is an overgrowth of the lining of the uterus. There are several different histologic types, including simple hyperplasia, simple hyperplasia with atypia, complex hyperplasia, and complex hyperplasia with atypia. These are listed in an order of increasing risk of development into endometrial adenocarcinoma. Patients with complex hyperplasia with atypia have a 20% to 30% chance of developing or having a coexisting adenocarcinoma. Risk factors for hyperplasia include obesity, hypertension, diabetes, anovulation, and unopposed estrogen use. Simple hyperplasia can be managed with progestin therapy, followed by a repeat endometrial biopsy after 3 months. In patients with complex atypical hyperplasia who have completed childbearing, hysterectomy is recommended.

Endometrial Adenocarcinoma

There are many histologic types of endometrial cancer. The most common type is endometrioid, but other types include papillary, papillary serous, squamous, clear cell, and neuroendocrine. Papillary serous, clear cell, and neuroendocrine tumors behave aggressively with a high risk of recurrence of disease.

Because bleeding is an early sign, most patients present with early-stage disease; and potential for survival is high. Staging of endometrial adenocarcinoma is surgical. The procedure involves obtaining pelvic washings on entering the abdomen, total abdominal hysterectomy with bilateral salpingo-oophorectomy, and possible bilateral pelvic and para-aortic lymphadenectomy. Table 74-4 outlines the criteria for patients who require lymphadenectomy as well as those who require postoperative radiation therapy. However, management or patients with advanced-stage disease is variable, with chemotherapy, radiotherapy, and even adjunctive surgical debulking of tumor.

Risk factors for recurrence include grade of tumor, depth of invasion, lymphovascular space invasion, cervical involvement, stage of disease, and histologic subtype. Table 74-4 outlines treatment recommendations for postoperative vaginal brachytherapy or pelvic irradiation.

Papillary serous adenocarcinoma of the endometrium behaves more like an ovarian carcinoma than an endometrial cancer. Most patients experience recurrence with intra-abdominal disease and carcinomatosis. This is a rare histologic type so numbers reported in the literature are small. Postoperative chemotherapy is indicated.

Treatment options for local recurrence of endometrial cancer in the pelvis include radiation therapy if the patient has not been previously irradiated or pelvic exenteration in the irradiated patient. Remote disease must be ruled out

TABLE 74-4.	Treatment of Endometrial Cancer
Diagnosis	Treatment
Grade 1 or 2, stage IA or IB, < 30% myometrial invasion, no lymph or vascular invasion	No further therapy
Grade 1 or 2 with one third to two thirds of myometrial invasion; or grade 1 or 2 with cervical involvement; no lymph or vascular invasion	Vaginal brachytherapy
Grade 1 or 2 with more than two thirds of myometrial invasion; grade 3 with myometrial invasion and lymph and vascular invasion	Whole pelvic radiation therapy
Stage IIIC disease	Extended-field radiation therapy
Stage IVB disease	Postoperative chemotherapy

before these therapies. Fifty percent of patients who did not receive postoperative radiation can be salvaged in this situation. Isolated metastases involving the abdominal wall, lung, or bone can be treated with surgical resection or focused radiation therapy. Multifocal remote or nodal disease is treated with hormonal therapy or chemotherapy.

Endometrial Cancer in Young Women

If a young woman still desires children, she may be treated with high doses of progestins and followed with hysteroscopy and dilatation and curettage. These patients must have no evidence of myometrial invasion on MRI. They also must actively pursue pregnancy, at times with the help of a reproductive endocrinologist, once the cancer has been cleared because of their risk factors for recurrence.

Endometrial Sarcomas

Endometrial sarcomas can present as vaginal bleeding or a rapidly growing uterus. The sarcoma can be homologous (arising from tissue normally found in the uterus such as smooth muscle) or heterologous (arising from tissue normally not found in the uterus such as cartilage). Sarcomas are classified based on tissue type, necrosis, and degree of atypia. Leiomyosarcoma is the most common type. Diagnosis is made on hypercellularity, moderate nuclear atypia, high mitotic rate (10 mitotic figures/10 high-power fields), and tumor necrosis. Two of the last three criteria are required for diagnosis.

Endometrial stromal sarcomas tend to occur in younger women and are low grade with typically fewer than 3 mitotic figures per high-power field. High-grade endometrial sarcomas are rare and tend to be aggressive.

Management of these patients is surgical, with staging performed as noted for endometrial adenocarcinomas.

These tumors are vascular, and patients often require intraoperative transfusion. Unlike endometrial adenocarcinomas, these tumors spread hematogenously so recurrences can occur in the pelvis, lung, or liver. Postoperative radiation therapy decreases risk of pelvic recurrence but does not improve overall survival.

Mixed Müllerian Tumors of the Uterus

Malignant mixed müllerian tumors of the uterus (MMMT) are a combination of epithelial adenocarcinoma and sarcoma that coexist in the uterus. The most common epithelial component is papillary serous carcinoma. It is the epithelial component that metastasizes, typically to the abdomen with carcinomatosis or to the lung or liver. Staging is performed as in other endometrial cancers with the addition of omental biopsy because abdominal metastases are common. In patients with stage I and II disease, Molpus and colleagues[5] reported an increased survival in patients who received postoperative radiation therapy. For comparison, 5-year survival with endometrioid adenocarcinoma stage I is around 90% but in MMMT 5-year survival is 50%. In patients with advanced disease, multiagent chemotherapy is indicated.

Management of a Pelvic Mass

When a pelvic mass is discovered on examination, ultrasound can be helpful in determining characteristics that are worrisome for malignancy. In general, a simple cyst in a premenopausal patient will not be cancerous. However, a mass with complex features such as septations, papillations, and solid components is more worrisome. Several benign lesions such as endometriomas, hemorrhagic corpus luteum, and dermoid cysts can have these features and must be in the differential diagnosis (Table 74-5).

Tubo-ovarian abscess can also appear worrisome on ultrasound, so the clinical scenario is important in determining the treatment plan.

In a premenopausal patient with a simple cyst, an ultrasound examination should be repeated in 6 to 8 weeks to see if it is hemorrhagic corpus luteum. However, in a postmenopausal patient with a complex adnexal mass, evaluation should include CT to rule out omental disease or other site of primary tumor and barium enema to rule out colonic involvement or primary tumor.

CA-125 is a glycoprotein that is produced by certain tumors. It, unfortunately, is not specific for ovarian cancer and may be elevated in lung, appendiceal, and signet ring cell carcinomas and other malignancies. In the premenopausal patient, benign findings such as leiomyomas, endometriosis, menstruation, pregnancy, and pelvic inflammatory disease may elevate CA-125. Other diseases such as cirrhosis of the liver may also elevate the value. CA-125, therefore, should not be checked in the premenopausal patient with a pelvic mass because the false-positive rate is too high. However, in the postmenopausal patient with a pelvic mass and an elevated CA-125, ovarian cancer is diagnosed in 80% of these patients. This is the population in which the test is helpful.

Definitive diagnosis of a pelvic mass requires visual inspection and histologic diagnosis. Laparoscopy or laparotomy can be done depending on the clinical suspicion of malignancy. In patients with potential for carcinomatosis, laparoscopy should not be done because of port site metastasis that occurs quickly and can make debulking difficult. At the time of surgery, pelvic washings should be done. The mass should be visually inspected to augment prior information from ultrasound. If all indications are that the lesion is benign, ovarian cystectomy or drainage (see section on Technical Aspects of Surgical Options) is indicated, with evaluation of cyst cytology or gross or microscopic evaluation of the tissue to confirm a benign lesion. If there is a higher level of suspicion or the patient is menopausal, oophorectomy is performed and frozen section histologic diagnosis is provided.

Serous and mucinous cystadenomas are very common benign tumors of the ovary that can occur in any age group. Treatment can be cystectomy or oophorectomy, depending on the amount of ovary involved. Brenner tumors are benign transitional cell tumors of the ovary that can also be managed in a similar fashion

If the lesion is an invasive, epithelial ovarian cancer, treatment should include a hysterectomy, bilateral salpingo-oophorectomy, omentectomy, peritoneal biopsies of the diaphragms, bilateral paracolic gutters, bilateral pelvis, and cul-de-sac and lymph node sampling. If the cell type is mucinous, an appendectomy should also be performed to rule out a metastasis from the appendix.

Extensive disease mandates tumor debulking to remove all possible tumor. Patients who undergo optimal tumor reductive surgery (< 2 cm of visible disease) have a survival advantage over patients who cannot be or are not optimally debulked. Complete staging is very important because patients who have a grade 1 or 2 stage IA ovarian cancer do not require chemotherapy. With other stages, surgery is followed by chemotherapy.

TABLE 74-5.	Differential Diagnosis of Ovarian Masses
Mass	**Differential Diagnosis**
Benign disease	Hemorrhagic corpus luteum; endometrioma; tubo-ovarian abscess; ectopic pregnancy; serous or mucinous cystadenoma; cystadenofibroma; fibroma; Brenner tumor; dermoid
Malignant	
Epithelial	Serous borderline tumor; mucinous borderline tumor; invasive cancer (papillary serous; endometrioid; transitional cell; clear cell; neuroendocrine or small cell; malignant mixed müllerian tumor)
Germ cell	Dysgerminoma; endodermal sinus tumor; choriocarcinoma; immature teratoma; embryonal carcinoma; polyembryoma
Stromal	Sertoli-Leydig cell tumor; granulosa cell tumor
Metastasis	Colon cancer, stomach cancer, breast cancer, lymphoma

Borderline tumors do not behave like invasive ovarian cancers. Typically, they are treated with surgery alone and do not require chemotherapy. They tend to occur in younger women. If found at frozen section and the patient is finished with childbearing, pelvic washings, hysterectomy, bilateral salpingo-oophorectomy, omentectomy, peritoneal biopsies, and lymph node biopsies should be performed. If the patient desires future fertility, a unilateral oophorectomy, omentectomy, peritoneal biopsies, and lymph node biopsies on the side of the tumor can be performed. The other ovary can then be monitored with ultrasound. Staging should be done in the event an invasive ovarian cancer is found at the time of final pathologic diagnosis. Mucinous borderline tumors have also been associated with abnormalities in the appendix. Therefore, an appendectomy should be performed in conjunction with other staging.

Other types of ovarian tumors include sex cord stromal tumors such as granulosa cell tumors or Sertoli-Leydig cell tumors. These typically appear solid but, occasionally, can have a cystic appearance. Hysterectomy, bilateral salpingo-oophorectomy, and staging should be performed. For stage I tumors of adult type, no further therapy is needed. For patients with higher stages, postoperative chemotherapy or radiation therapy should be added.

Among girls and young women, germ cell tumors must be considered. The most common cell type is a dysgerminoma. Ninety percent of dysgerminomas are diagnosed at stage I. Conservative surgery with unilateral oophorectomy and staging can be performed, leaving the uterus and other tube and ovary in place. No further therapy is needed.

Other germ cell tumors include endodermal sinus tumor, choriocarcinoma, immature teratoma, and embryonal carcinoma. A mixture of these cancers can be present. Tumor markers such as β-HCG, α-fetoprotein (AFP), and lactate dehydrogenase (LDH) may be detected in certain germ cell tumors. Patients who have a gonadoblastoma must be evaluated with chromosomes. If XY chromosomes are discovered, the gonads should be removed to prevent development of dysgerminoma. This may occur in 20% of patients with gonadoblastoma.

Because these are potentially very aggressive tumors, postoperative chemotherapy should be implemented with the diagnoses of teratoma (stage IA, grade 2 or 3 immature teratoma or any higher stage), dysgerminomas (stage II and higher), any endodermal sinus tumor, or choriocarcinoma.

ALTERNATIVES TO SURGICAL INTERVENTION

There are valid indications for medical or observational management of many acute gynecologic conditions, even if there is also a surgical option available. Because acute pelvic pathologic processes are often accompanied by severe pain or bleeding to a degree that the general surgeon would consider it a surgical emergency in the upper abdomen, we provide some guidance to the clinical judgment to allow the surgeon to avoid, or defer, surgery. We also provide an overview approach to the medical management and the points to observe during follow-up observation.

Dysfunctional Uterine Bleeding

As described earlier, this condition is a manifestation of dyssynchronous endometrial physiology. In the acute setting, medical management does not require a tissue or even an ultrasound diagnosis. Emergency implementation of dilatation and curettage is not necessary. The episode can be truncated by inducing acute proliferation and regeneration of the endometrium with high doses of estrogens, followed by induction of a secretory endometrium with a progestin.

An oral or intravenous bolus of estrogens (e.g., conjugated estrogens, 5 mg PO every 6 hours for four to six doses or 25 mg IV for two doses 6 hours apart) with simultaneous administration of an active progestin (micronized progesterone, 100 mg PO bid, or medroxyprogesterone, 10 mg four times a day) will stabilize the endometrium. The progestin must be continued for at least 7 days and then withdrawn to simulate atresia of the corpus luteum. This will mimic the orderly menses of an ovulatory cycle, although perhaps with heavy bleeding. The patient should receive oral contraceptives for several months to stabilize iron stores, allow for orderly evaluation of structural pathology, and initiate a plan to assess underlying HPO pathology.

Spontaneous Abortion

First-trimester pregnancies fail 10% to 15% of the time, often with minimal symptoms. For the patient who does present with pain or bleeding, it must be confirmed that this is an early gestation. On inspection of the cervix, one can observe whether there is placental tissue in a dilated cervical os; if so, it can often be removed with a sponge forceps and resolve the event. The need for acute surgical intervention with curettage is wholly dependent on the amount of blood loss and intensity of pain. The patient who is hemodynamically stable and has pain control may spontaneously complete her miscarriage without a procedure.

Ectopic Pregnancy

Ruptured ectopic pregnancy is a surgical emergency, but there are two other tubal pregnancy scenarios that are amenable to less aggressive management in the patient who is hemodynamically stable and has limited intraperitoneal blood loss: the tubal abortion and the unruptured ectopic pregnancy. The tubal abortion results when the pregnancy is extruded from the fimbriated end of the tube. Pain is often described as lateralized cramping, and the volume of blood identified in the cul-de-sac is only about 100 mL. These events may be self-limited; and if pain and hemodynamic status are under control during observation, surgery may be avoided.

A patient may present with pain and vaginal bleeding, and an intact tubal pregnancy is identified by ultrasound. There are varying sets of criteria for medical management of the unruptured tubal pregnancy, based on gestational size (<3 cm or < 5 cm) and the presence of fetal cardiac activity, but the physician should actively consider medical rather than surgical management.

Surgical procedures for managing an ectopic pregnancy include salpingectomy, salpingostomy, or segmental resection. For the patient desiring to maintain maximal future fertility, preservation of the tube is preferable.

Medical management of tubal pregnancy relies on the cytotoxic effect of methotrexate. Several protocols for dosage (e.g., 1 mg/kg) and follow-up are available. Consultation with an experienced gynecologist before initiation is advisable.

Pelvic Infection

The diagnosis of pelvic inflammatory disease (PID) can be challenging. Most commonly, the differential diagnosis includes appendicitis, urinary tract infection, ruptured ovarian cyst, or ectopic pregnancy, all of which share some of the signs and symptoms of PID. The diagnosis of PID should be made only when the patient has fever, leukocytosis, purulent discharge from the cervix, bilateral adnexal tenderness on gentle palpation, and peritoneal signs limited to the pelvis. Appendicitis is differentiated by anteceding gastrointestinal symptoms, the evolving pain pattern, absence of cervical discharge, and generalized peritonitis. Lower urinary tract infection is distinguished by dysuria and obvious pyuria. Rarely do ovarian cysts or ectopic pregnancy present as significant fever or leukocytosis. In a classic study, Wolner-Hanssen and colleagues concluded that the sensitivity and specificity of clinical assessment for PID was so poor that laparoscopic inspection of the pelvis is necessary to make a firm diagnosis.[6] Although that may be unduly aggressive in many cases, this diagnosis must be applied cautiously, because it is stigmatizing and labels the patient, disproportionately among women of color, from lower socioeconomic status or with counterculture lifestyles.

Acute PID, as a polymicrobial infection, is a medical not a surgical disease. The major acute complication of this disease is a tubo-ovarian abscess (TOA). In contrast to abscesses related to the intestine, however, initial management of a TOA is administration of broad-spectrum intravenous antibiotics. Indications for surgical intervention are ruptured TOA with generalized peritonitis or failure to respond to medical therapy.

A pelvic inflammatory collection is a clinical variant of a TOA. Whereas an abscess is an infectious process bounded by inflammatory response across natural tissue planes, the collection, which may be indistinguishable on ultrasound or CT scan, is bounded by anatomic surfaces of the posterior cul-de-sac, rectum, uterus, and intestine. Pelvic collections are more common than true abscesses and much more likely to respond to medical therapy than abscesses.

Functional Ovarian Cysts

Rupture of a follicle or corpus luteum cyst or intraparenchymal hemorrhage in the corpus luteum can result in extreme pain, with signs of localized peritoneal irrita-

tion. If ultrasound evaluation reveals a simple cyst and does not demonstrate significant intraperitoneal bleeding, and if Doppler flow study rules out an ovarian torsion, this acute condition will resolve in 12 to 24 hours. Fluids and analgesic support are all that is necessary.

If the event is on the right ovary, the acuity clearly will force consideration of appendicitis, but prior gastrointestinal symptoms, fever, and leukocytosis are rarely present.

Ovarian torsion is a surgical emergency and sometimes mandates oophorectomy. However, unless the ovary is obviously necrotic at the time of laparoscopic inspection, the surgeon should untwist the ovarian pedicle and directly observe for return of blood flow before considering removal.

Uterine Leiomyomas

These benign myometrial tumors are present in up to 40% of women and more prevalent among women of African descent. With clinical or ultrasound confirmation of the diagnosis, observation for stability over time is indicated. Surgical intervention is warranted if the patient has unresponsive menorrhagia, intolerable pressure symptoms, rapid growth, or change in consistency of palpable masses. Leiomyosarcoma is a sufficiently rare event that hysterectomy or myomectomy to rule out malignancy carries greater statistical risk than the lesion itself.

Observational management is especially valid in women who are approaching menopause, because leiomyomas are estrogen dependent and with the decline in estrogen production, typically the lesions will decrease in size. Continued observation is important after menopause because progressive growth in this time period may reflect malignant transformation.

Endometriosis and Endometriomas

This is a complex disease created by the presence of ectopic endometrial tissue in the peritoneal cavity or adnexa. This endometrial tissue transforms and bleeds with the ovarian cycle. This process induces a sterile inflammatory response, resulting in pain, pelvic adhesions, and, when located within the ovary, a complex hemorrhagic mass known as an endometrioma. First-line therapy for this disease is medical induction of temporary menopause and suppression of ovarian estrogen. Surgical management for younger women is conservative, with local destruction of lesions and maximum conservation of reproductive organs. Women who have completed their reproductive plans will benefit from hysterectomy and oophorectomy.

TECHNICAL ASPECTS OF SURGICAL OPTIONS

Surgery for Menorrhagia and Abnormal Uterine Bleeding

Dilation and curettage (D&C) is the classic gynecologic procedure for the evaluation and possible therapeutic treatment of menorrhagia, menometrorrhagia, and abnormal uterine bleeding. It is now understood that its therapeutic success is 25% or less and usually temporary. Because it is a blind procedure, it is difficult to ensure that the entire endometrium is curetted uniformly, much like attempting to scoop cake batter out of a bowl with a spoon. Therefore, more commonly now, hysteroscopy is used in conjunction with D&C so that the cavity can be visualized and any pathologic process seen can be directly sampled or removed. The combination of the two adds both to the evaluation and the therapeutic success.

In addition, ablative techniques now are being used for improved therapy for nonstructural bleeding abnormalities.[7,8] These ablative techniques (rollerball, thermal balloon, hydrotherapy, cryotherapy, microwave) are advanced techniques best reserved for a surgeon with extensive experience in hysteroscopy and the evaluation and manipulation of the endometrial cavity.

Technique: Fractional Dilation and Curettage

A weighted speculum and anterior retracting blade or a bivalve Graves speculum are used in the vagina to visualize the cervix. The cervix is grasped transversely on the anterior lip with a single-toothed tenaculum. A Kevorkian curette is used to curette the endocervix for a specimen. A sound is placed through the cervix and into the uterus and gently tapped on the fundus of the uterus to measure the depth of the cavity. This step is important to help prevent and/or recognize uterine perforation for the remainder of the procedure. The cervix is dilated with graduated dilators of increasing diameter. At this time, if hysteroscopy is going to be performed, the hysteroscope is introduced through the cervix and into the uterus for visualization of the endometrial cavity, with glycine or saline commonly used as a distention medium. The curettage phase is performed. A sharp curette (the largest diameter that will easily fit through the cervix) is introduced gently into the cervix and endometrial cavity. This should be done without excessive pressure or undue force. The fundus should be found, and a firm withdrawal stroke should be applied until the curette reaches the cervicouterine junction. This should be repeated while moving circumferentially around the uterine cavity, attempting to curette as much of the endometrial cavity as possible. The procedure is terminated; the instruments are removed with careful attention to the cervix, which may bleed when the tenaculum is removed. The bleeding usually stops with pressure and/or silver nitrate or Monsel's solution.

Potential Complications

As with any surgical procedure, infection from instrumenting the cavity or bleeding from the denuded endometrial lining can occur. In addition, perforation of the uterine cavity is possible and can occur in any of the phases of the procedure. However, it occurs most commonly during the sounding of the uterus, and bleeding from the perforated area can occur. The perforation is usually midline and self-limiting. Usually, observation for 24 hours is all that is required. If there is continued bleeding, as evidenced by decreasing hemoglobin or increased abdominal pain, or if other symptoms present, exploration by laparoscopy or laparotomy may be required. Injury to the bowel is possible, although rare, with perforation.

Treatment of Bartholin Gland Cyst or Abscess

Large, symptomatic Bartholin gland cysts or painful abscesses may not respond to conservative treatment. The surgical treatment options for this include (1) incision and drainage with Word catheter placement, (2) marsupialization, or (3) excision of the gland itself. Excision of the gland is rarely indicated. Typically, incision and drainage with appropriate follow-up and/or marsupialization is all that is needed to treat this condition.

Incision and drainage generally is made on the vestibular side at the hymeneal ring in a lower dependent portion of the cyst or abscess using a sharp knife. The cyst is stabilized, and an incision is made into the cyst itself. A small Word catheter is placed into the cyst for drainage and the lesion is reevaluated on a weekly basis. Patients with abscesses should be pretreated with antibiotics.

To perform a marsupialization, an elliptical incision is made in the vestibular mucosa down to the wall of the gland. The wall of the gland is incised the entire length of the ellipse. The contents are evacuated, and the wall of the cyst is sutured to the vestibular mucosa with 3-0 synthetic absorbable suture, either in an interrupted fashion or by using a baseball stitch (Fig. 74-9). The patient is placed on a regimen of hot sitz baths. If the lesion is an abscess, the patient is given adequate antibiotic coverage. Whether marsupialization or incision and drainage has been performed, sexual intercourse should be avoided until the area has completely healed.

Cone Procedure

Conization can be performed with a cold knife or a LEEP. A LEEP conization entails removal of the transformation zone with an ectocervical loop followed by a removal of an endocervical specimen with an endocervical loop. This is called a top-hat procedure and allows for sampling of the canal. If a cold knife conization is done in the operating room, a single-tooth tenaculum is placed on the anterior lip of the cervix. Vicryl 0 figure-eight retention sutures are placed at the 3 and 9 o'clock positions. A circumferential incision is made around the transformation zone and the lesion. The specimen is grasped with Allis clamps to maintain orientation, and a deeper circumferential incision is made in the cervix. The specimen is removed with a scalpel or Mayo scissors. A marking stitch is placed at the 12 o'clock position on the specimen, and an endocervical curetting is performed above the cone biopsy. Risk of recurrence of dysplasia is dependent on the status of the endocervical and ectocervical margins as well as if the endocervical curetting is positive for dysplasia.

Surgery for Ovarian Cysts

Ovarian cysts are common, especially functional cysts. Benign ovarian cysts have been discussed previously.

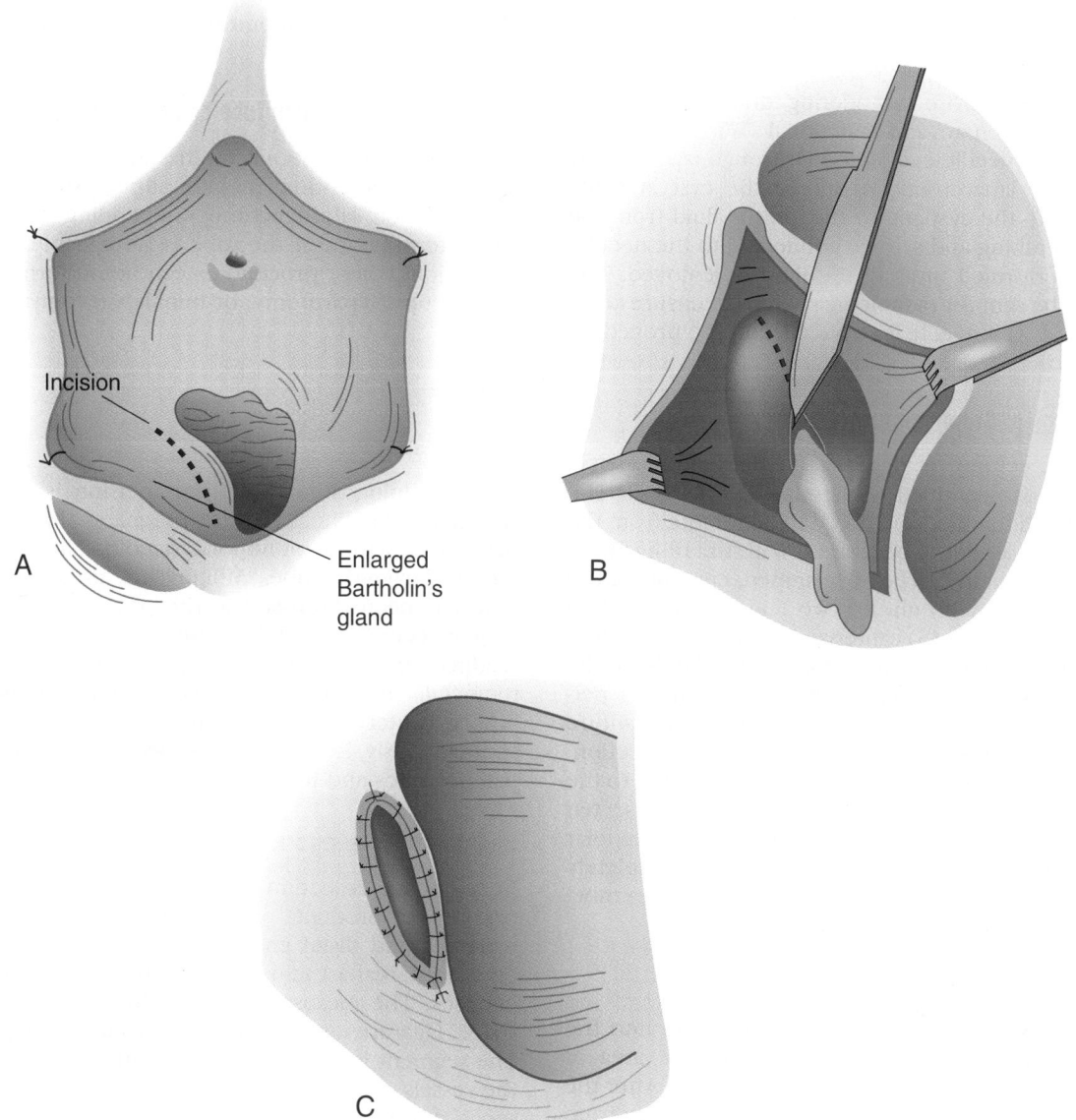

FIGURE 74-9. Bartholin's gland marsupialization. **A,** Retraction of the labia and incision over the mucosa of the vagina. **B,** Wall of the gland is excised. **C,** Completed marsupialization. (Modified from Mitchell CW, Wheeless CR: Atlas of Pelvic Surgery, 3rd ed. Baltimore, Lippincott Williams & Wilkins, 1997.)

When found, the decision is, "What management is most appropriate?" Treatment is individualized to each patient, depending on the clinical scenario. When an ovarian cyst is an incidental finding at the time of other surgery, it is important to know what, if any, the patient's symptoms are, where the patient is in her menstrual cycle, and what size of follicle is normal for that part of the cycle.

It is critical to remember that any time surgery is performed on the adnexal structures there is a risk of adhesion formation that might inhibit fertility. If the patient has been asymptomatic with a small functional cyst, observation, especially in the younger patient, is most appropriate. If the functional ovarian cyst is large (>5.0 to 6.0 cm) and/or symptomatic, aspiration may be considered. If the cyst is larger or is not consistent with functional lesion, oophorectomy may be considered if the patient is closer to menopause. As an alternative, ovarian cystectomy may be considered. This option removes the cyst but preserves the function of the ovary. It also reduces the risk of recurrence as compared with ovarian cyst drainage.

Technique

Ovarian Cyst Drainage

It is imperative, before considering drainage, that the ovarian cyst is benign and functional. With this being noted, a hollow needle can be used, through laparoscopy or exploratory laparotomy, to pierce the cyst at a 90-degree angle to the cyst and to suction the fluid from the cyst through tubing and syringe connected to the needle. Suction is performed until all the fluid is removed. The fluid should be sent for pathologic analysis to ensure accurate diagnosis. The needle is removed, and the procedure is terminated.

Oophorectomy ± Salpingectomy

When oophorectomy is desired, the infundibulopelvic (IP) ligament is identified and isolated. The ipsilateral ureter must be identified and noted to be remote from the area of the IP ligament to be ligated. With the IP ligament isolated, the ligament can be (1) clamped, cut, and suture ligated; (2) ligated with one or two Endoloops and then surgically dissected; or (3) cauterized with bipolar cautery and sharply dissected. If the ipsilateral tube is to be removed, the dissection across the mesosalpinx is performed, either with clamp, sharp dissection, and suture ligation or with bipolar coagulation and sharp dissection. If the uterus is present, attention should be directed to the utero-ovarian ligament. This ligament should be dissected in a similar fashion, as described previously, with bipolar cautery or the clamping technique. The ovary, completely dissected, possibly in conjunction with the fallopian tube, can be removed.

Ovarian Cystectomy

To begin an ovarian cystectomy, a surgical line into the ovarian capsule is developed sharply over the area of the cyst, on the antimesovarian side of the ovary. After the incision into the capsule, the cyst is dissected away from the capsule with sharp and/or blunt dissection. Scissors, knife, Kittner dissector, hydrodissection, or a combination of these may be used for this dissection, being careful to avoid rupture of the cyst. Once the cyst is removed in toto, the base of the ovarian capsule will usually have some bleeding. Hemostasis can be obtained at the base, either with electrocautery or by suturing. Once hemostasis is obtained, most surgeons do not suture the capsule but rather approximate the edges loosely together to heal spontaneously on its own. It is believed that this reduces the risk of adhesion formation. Interceed or other adhesion barriers can be used at this time to reduce adhesion formation.

Potential Complications

Bleeding from the large vascular pedicles is the most dangerous potential risk. If hemostasis is not completely obtained, the large vessels can bleed profusely very quickly. The more chronic complication from adnexal surgery is adhesion formation with infertility or subfertility. Injury to

the ureter is always a concern during this surgery if the ureteral course is not monitored appropriately.

Surgery for the Fallopian Tube or Ectopic Pregnancy

There are many options for treatment of ectopic pregnancy. Surgical options include salpingostomy, segmental resection, or salpingectomy, depending on desire for future fertility and if the tube is salvageable. As in prior discussions, these procedures can be performed through laparoscopy, laparotomy, or mini-laparotomy.

Technique

Salpingostomy

With a salpingostomy, a linear incision is made in the antisalpingetic line over the pregnancy. This is usually performed with a monopolar needle. The pregnancy is removed from the tube. "Milking" the pregnancy from the tube has been discussed in the past. However, it is no longer recommended because of an increased risk of retained tissue. Once the pregnancy is completely removed, hemostasis is achieved with monopolar or bipolar cautery. The tube is not sutured but left open to spontaneously heal. This has been shown to improve patency rates and fertility (Fig. 74-10).

Segmental Resection

In segmental resection, the portion of the tube encompassing the products of conception is resected and the proximal and distal ends are left in situ. This gives the option of reanastomosis at a later date if the patient chooses. The mesosalpinx is perforated in an avascular space. Ligatures are placed on each side of the pregnancy. The segment is sharply resected within the ligatures, and the vessels of the mesosalpinx are inspected for injury and secured if necessary.

Salpingectomy

In salpingectomy, the tube is grasped and the mesosalpinx is secured using bipolar cautery, an Endoloop, or clamps with a suture ligation. The tube is sharply excised. The area is examined closely for hemostasis (Fig. 74-11).

In rare cases, the ectopic pregnancy is in the abdomen and not in the fallopian tube. In these cases, the fetus is removed with ligation of the umbilical cord near its insertion into the placenta. Because of the vascularity of the placenta, the placenta is left in situ, with subsequent medical therapy with methotrexate.

Potential Complications

The vascular supply of the tube in pregnancy is markedly increased and, therefore, bleeding is a risk both during and after the surgery is completed. If the tube is preserved, there is a risk of subsequent recurrent ectopic pregnancy. Also, there is a risk of retained placental tissue

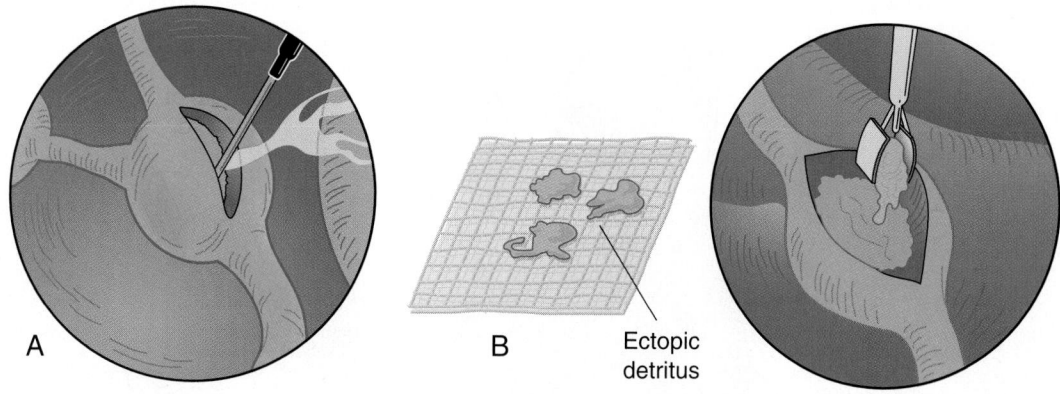

A

B
Ectopic
detritus

FIGURE 74-10. Salpingostomy. **A,** Fallopian tube is opened in a longitudinal manner. **B,** Trophoblastic tissue removed in pieces. (Modified from Mitchell CW, Wheeless CR: Atlas of Pelvic Surgery, 3rd ed. Baltimore, Lippincott Williams & Wilkins, 1997.)

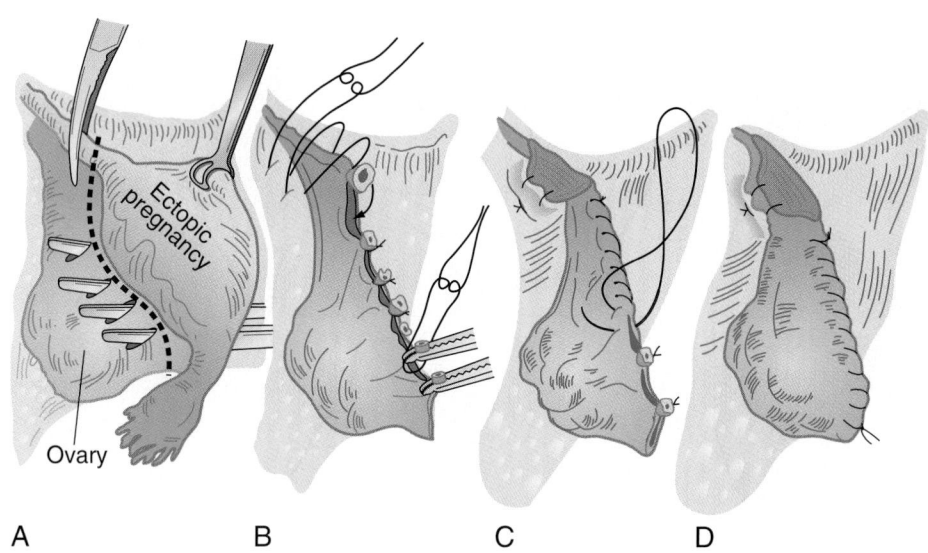

Ectopic
pregnancy

Ovary

A   B   C   D

FIGURE 74-11. Salpingectomy. **A,** Tube is excised from the cornual portion across the mesosalpinx to the fimbria. **B,** Pedicles tied, peritoneal lining is re-established, and cornual portion of the tube is buried into the posterior segment of the uterine cornu. **C,** Mesosalpinx is reperitonealized. **D,** Mesosalpinx is closed and the procedure completed. (Modified from Mitchell CW, Wheeless CR: Atlas of Pelvic Surgery, 3rd ed. Baltimore, Lippincott Williams & Wilkins, 1997.)

in the tube and persistent ectopic pregnancy. Adhesions of the affected adnexa are also a significant risk, whether the tube is preserved or removed.

Hysterectomy

Hysterectomy is one of the most common procedures performed. The route of hysterectomy depends on the indication for surgery, the size of the uterus, the descent of the cervix and uterus, the shape of the vagina, the size of the patient, and the skill and preference of the surgeon.

Because of the significant impact of the transvaginal approach on appreciating anatomic relationships, vaginal hysterectomy and laparoscopically assisted hysterectomy should only be performed by an experienced vaginal surgeon.

Technique

Any lower abdominal incision (vertical, Pfannenstiel, Maylard, Cherney) can be used. The bowel is packed from the pelvis and the patient placed in Trendelenburg position. The ureters are identified, and the following steps are performed bilaterally (Fig. 74-12).

The round ligament is identified, incised between clamps, and ligated with 0 absorbable suture. The leaves of the broad ligament are sharply opened anteriorly and posteriorly, with the anterior leaf open to the vesicouterine fold. If the ovary is to be preserved, the proximal tube and utero-ovarian ligament are clamped, incised, and ligated. If the tube and ovary are to be removed, the infundibulopelvic ligament is doubly clamped, incised, and doubly ligated with a 0 absorbable tie and a 0 synthetic absorbable suture. After this has been performed

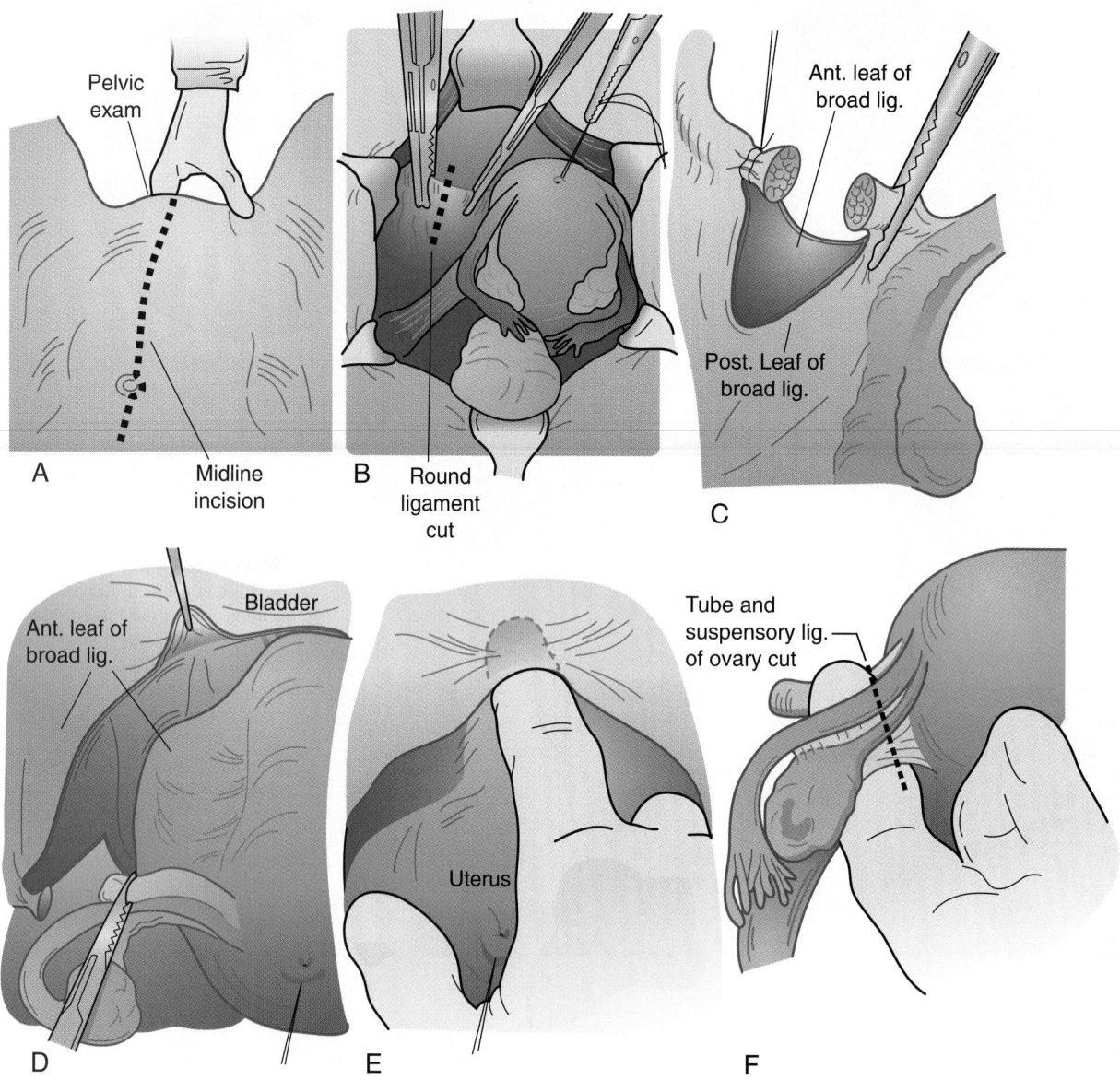

FIGURE 74-12. **A** to **N**, Hysterectomy. (Modified from Mitchell CW, Wheeless CR: Atlas of Pelvic Surgery, 3rd ed. Baltimore, Lippincott Williams & Wilkins, 1997.)

Continued

bilaterally, the vesicoperitoneal fold is elevated and incised. The filmy attachments of the bladder to the pubovesical fascia are sharply dissected, mobilizing the bladder off the cervix. The filmy adventitious tissue surrounding the uterine vessels is skeletonized sharply, dissecting the tissue to expose the uterine vessels. The uterine vessels are clamped, incised, and ligated at the level of the lower uterine segment. This is accomplished by placing the tip of the clamp on the uterus at right angle to the axis of the cervix and sliding or stepping off the uterus. The pedicle is incised and a simple absorbable 0 suture ligature is placed. The cardinal and uterosacral ligaments are sequentially clamped, incised, and suture ligated with a Haney double transfixion suture. Each clamp is placed medial to the previous pedicle to allow for the ureter to passively retract laterally. The anterior vagina can be entered by a stab incision and cut across with either a scalpel or scissors. Alternatively, right angle clamps can be used to clamp the angle of the vagina, below the distal cervix. The tissue above this angle clamp is then incised and ligated with a Haney stitch. With the lumen of the vagina now exposed, sharp dissection is used to complete the vaginal transection. The vaginal wall, incorporating perivaginal fascia, muscularis, and mucosal edge is closed with a series of figure-of-eight 0 absorbable sutures with the angle stitches incorporating the ipsilateral uterosacral ligament. Ligatures should be snug but not strangulate the vaginal edges. The pelvic peritoneum does

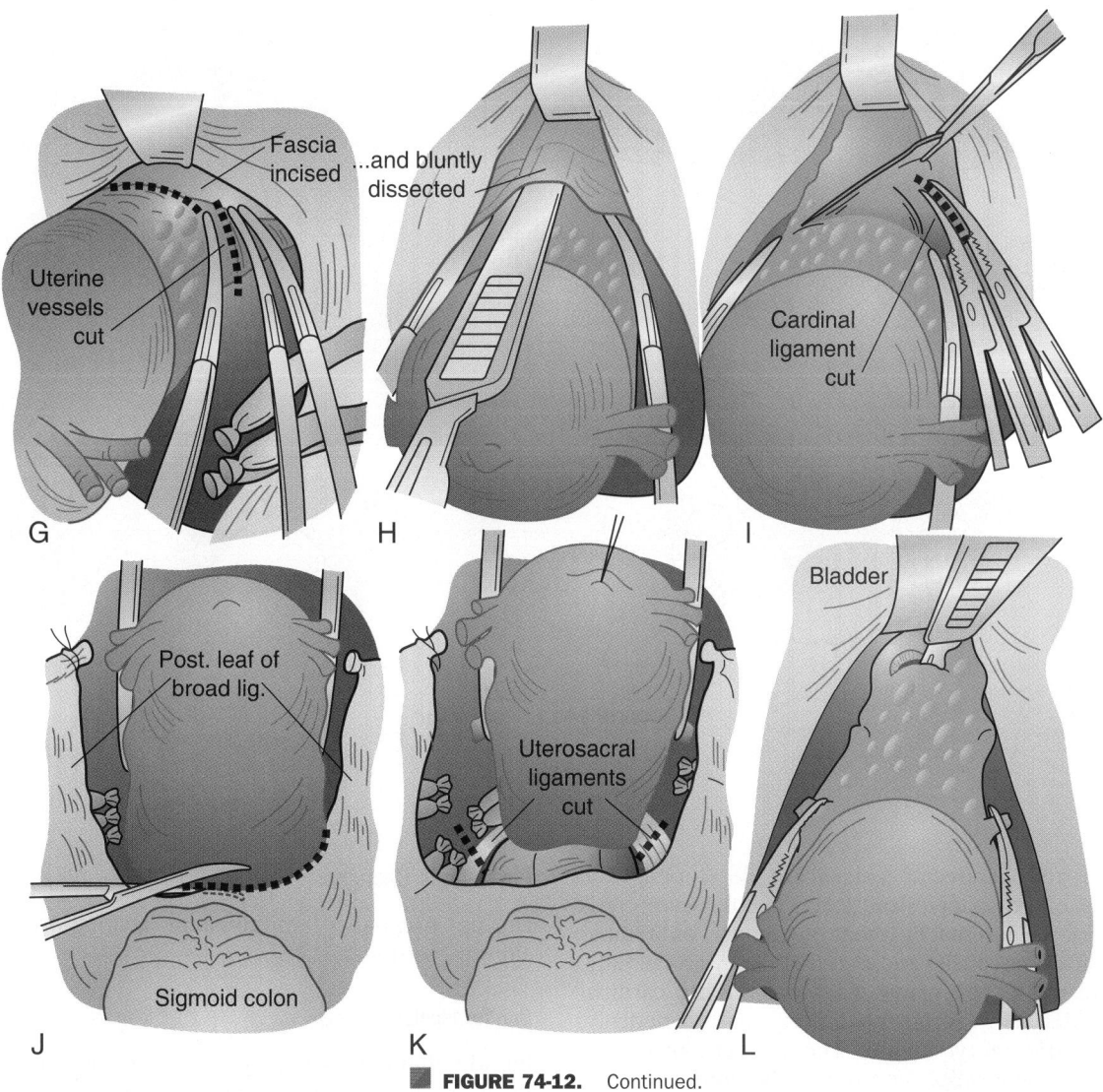

G — Fascia incised — Uterine vessels cut — ...and bluntly dissected

H

I — Cardinal ligament cut

J — Post. leaf of broad lig. — Sigmoid colon

K — Uterosacral ligaments cut

L — Bladder

FIGURE 74-12.   Continued.

not need to be closed. The pelvis is irrigated, hemostasis is ensured, and the abdominal incision closed routinely.

Potential Complications

Because of the proximity of the ureter to the cervix, uterine vessels, and infundibulopelvic ligament, the ureter can be injured during the hysterectomy and, with the dissection necessary between the bladder and cervix, injury to the bladder is likewise a common complication. It is imperative that these injuries be recognized and repaired intraoperatively, if possible. Fistulas, such as vesicovaginal or ureterovaginal, likewise can form postoperatively secondary to ischemic injury caused by denudation of the bladder muscularis or partial entrapment with a vaginal closure stitch.

The vascular supply to the uterus and ovaries is rich. Intraoperative and postoperative bleeding is a concern. A previously secure pedicle can begin to bleed acutely in the postoperative period. A vaginal stump vessel, missed

because of operative vasospasm, can cause a pelvic cuff hematoma. Thromboembolism originating from the pelvic vasculature is also a potential postoperative problem. Hysterectomy is considered a clean-contaminated procedure because of entering the vagina. Pelvic cuff infection is common, despite the routine use of prophylactic antibiotics.

There has been increased discussion recently regarding the effect of hysterectomy on the pelvic floor. Failure to reapproximate the endopelvic fascia or failure to heal results in a large, apical endopelvic fascial defect. This results in an apical enterocele that progresses in size over time. It is estimated that 60% of women by 60 years of age have significant pelvic support defects.

Radical Hysterectomy

Radical hysterectomy can be performed through a vertical, Cherney, or Maylard incision. Once the pelvis is entered, the retroperitoneal space is opened and the

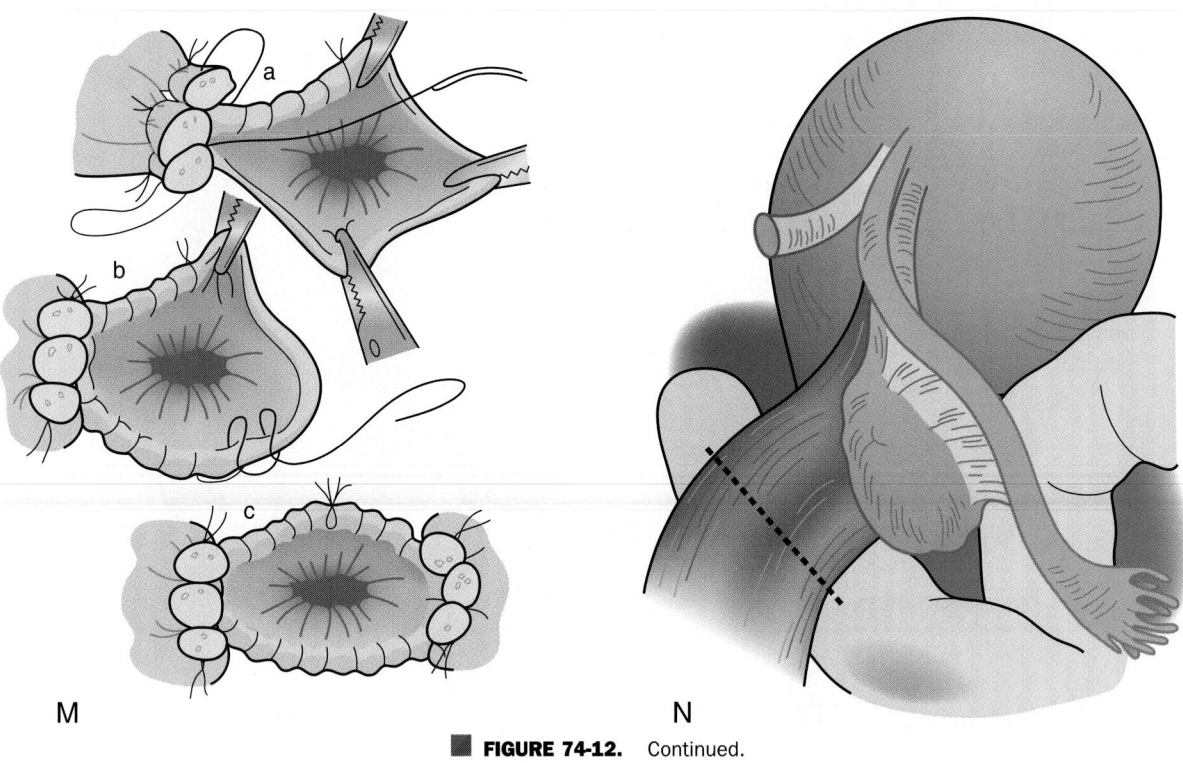

FIGURE 74-12. Continued.

paravesical and pararectal spaces are developed. The boundaries of the paravesical space are the symphysis pubis anteriorly, cardinal ligament posteriorly, obliterated umbilical artery medially, and external iliac vein laterally. The boundaries of the pararectal space are the cardinal ligament anteriorly, sacrum posteriorly, ureter medially, and hypogastric artery laterally. The bladder flap is then developed to the level of the vagina. The uterine arteries are isolated back to the origin and are ligated. The ureter is then separated from the medial leaf of the broad ligament, and the parametrial tunnel is developed. The ureter is separated from the parametrial tissue and is rolled laterally. The rectovaginal space is then entered, and the uterosacral ligaments are transected two thirds of the way to the sacrum. The amount of postoperative urinary retention is related to how close to the sacrum the uterosacral ligament is ligated. The parametrium is then taken at the sidewall. The specimen is removed when the vagina is entered 1 cm below the cervix. The angle sutures are secured with 0 Vicryl Heaney sutures, and the cuff is closed with 0 Vicryl figure-eight sutures.

SURGERY DURING PREGNANCY

Surgery is required in 0.1% to 2.2% of pregnant women. Changes in maternal-fetal physiology, the enlarging gestation, and changes in maternal organ placement can make diagnosis and treatment challenging. In this section, important issues for the surgeon to consider before proceeding to the operating room are considered.

Physiologic Changes

During pregnancy, multisystem adaptations result in altered physiology.

Cardiovascular System

Blood volume increases by 45% to 50% at term. Placental hormone production stimulates maternal erythropoiesis, which increases red cell mass by approximately 20%. This results in a functional hemodilution, manifested by a physiologic anemia. Therefore, pregnancy should be considered a hypervolemic state.

Maternal heart rate increases as early as 7 weeks. In late pregnancy, maternal heart rate is increased by approximately 20% over antepartum values.

Systemic vascular resistance decreases by 20% but gradually increases near term. This results in a decrease in systolic and diastolic blood pressure during pregnancy, with a gradual recovery to nonpregnant values by term. Because there is increased pressure in the venous system, there is decreased return from the lower extremities, resulting in dependent edema.

Respiratory System

In pregnancy, minute volume is increased while functional residual volume is decreased (Table 74-6). Although it seems intuitive that lung volume would be decreased during pregnancy, an increase in minute volume in association with an expansion of the anterior and posterior

TABLE 74-6. Physiologic Changes of Pregnancy

System	Changes	Result
Cardiovascular/hemodynamic	Blood volume increased by 50%; red cell mass increased by 20%; cardiac output increased by 50%; heart rate increased by 20%; systemic vascular resistance decreased by 20%	High output cardiac state with a hemodilutional anemia
Respiratory	Minute volume increased by 20%; functional residual capacity decreased by 15%; tidal volume increased by 20% to 30%; oxygen consumption increased by 20%	Compensated respiratory alkalosis
Gastrointestinal	Smooth muscle relaxation; delayed gastrointestinal emptying	Full stomach; constipation
Coagulation	Fibrinogen increased by 30%; protein S level decreased by 30% to 40%	Hypercoagulable state regardless of risk factors
Renal	Glomerular filtration rate increased by 50%; serum creatinine concentration decreased 40%; physiologic hydronephrosis	Increased urination; increased risk of upper urinary tract infection

diameter of the chest results in increased tidal volume, thereby also increasing minute ventilation. These changes result in a compensated respiratory alkalosis. Normal PCO_2 in pregnancy ranges from 28 to 35 mm Hg. PO_2 is usually greater than or equal to 100 mm Hg. Oxygen consumption and basal metabolic rate are also increased during pregnancy by approximately 20%.

These physiologic changes result in less pulmonary reserve for the acutely ill pregnant patient, reducing time needed for deterioration of respiratory distress to respiratory failure. Early intervention is mandatory.

Gastrointestinal Tract

During pregnancy there is a decrease in gastrointestinal motility. This is caused by mechanical changes in the abdomen with the enlarging uterus and the smooth muscle relaxation induced by high production of progesterone in pregnancy. Gastric emptying may be delayed for up to 8 hours. Pregnant women should be considered to have a functionally full stomach at all times. In addition, a decrease in large intestine motility may result in constipation severe enough to cause significant abdominal pain.

Coagulation Changes

Pregnancy is a hypercoagulable state. Fibrinogen is increased approximately 30% over baseline values. The hypercoagulable state of pregnancy is associated with increased risk of deep venous thrombosis and pulmonary embolus. This is particularly compounded when bed rest or immobilization occurs during the gestational period.

Renal Changes

Pregnancy increases blood flow to the renal pelvis approximately 50%. This results in an increased glomerular filtration rate. Frequent urination is common. Serum creatinine concentration is approximately 40% less than in a nonpregnant state. Therefore, a creatinine value of 1 mg/dL during gestation should be considered abnormal.

Ureteral diameter increases in pregnancy secondary to compression and smooth muscle relaxation. Peristalsis is delayed, and reflux occurs freely from the bladder into the lower ureteral segment. This results in an increased incidence of pyelonephritis during pregnancy. Therefore, asymptomatic bacteriuria should be aggressively treated.

Imaging Techniques

The most common imaging technique used during pregnancy is ultrasound. Ultrasound is considered the safest modality and is used for fetal assessment. In patients with abdominal pain, an ultrasound study should be considered the first-line diagnostic test. During ultrasonography, the presence of an intrauterine pregnancy should be documented if possible. In addition, evaluation of the cul-de-sac for fluid, the ureter for dilatation or stones, the gallbladder for the presence of gallstones, and the placenta for abnormalities can be obtained.

MRI can be also used during pregnancy. There are no data to suggest any increased risk from this modality; in fact, MRI is now used to diagnose fetal abnormalities, especially abnormalities of the central nervous system.

Although there are theoretical risks associated with ionizing radiation, fortunately, most diagnostic radiographic procedures are associated with minimal or no risk to the fetus. Existing evidence suggests that there is no increased risk to the fetus with regard to congenital malformations, growth restriction, or abortion from radiographic procedures that expose the fetus to doses of 5 rads or less. In 1995, the American College of Obstetrics and Gynecology published guidelines regarding diagnostic imaging during pregnancy. These published outlines reflect the opinions of the authors. Women should be reassured that concern about radiation exposure should not prevent medically indicated diagnostic procedures. It cannot be stressed enough that maternal well-being is of the utmost importance, and appropriate diagnostic procedures should be obtained to facilitate a rapid diagnosis.

Clinical Evaluation During Pregnancy

Abdominal pain during pregnancy can be confusing to the clinician. It is natural for the clinician to attribute most abdominal pain to the pregnancy; however, other organ systems during pregnancy are affected at the rate of the general population. In addition to these diagnoses, diagnosis specific to pregnancy should also be considered.

Appendicitis

Appendicitis is one of the most common surgical complications of pregnancy, with an incidence of approximately 2 per 1000. This incidence is not increased over the general population; however, appendiceal location during pregnancy changes with the upward displacement of the appendix with advancing gestation (Fig. 74-13). Nevertheless, the most common presenting symptom is pain in the right lower quadrant. This presents regardless of gestational age. The diagnosis of appendicitis in pregnancy may be difficult, because many of the symptoms of appendicitis are seen during pregnancy. Pain in the right lower quadrant may be mistaken for round ligament pain, and nausea, vomiting, and abdominal discomfort may be mistaken for hyperemesis gravidarum. Because mild leukocytosis is commonly seen in pregnancy, it may confound the diagnosis. However, other symptoms such as fever and anorexia can help the clinician establish the diagnosis. Ultrasonography may be used, but it is of limited value if bowel loops are distended. CT without contrast medium enhancement can be used, if needed, to assist in the diagnosis.

Rupture of the appendix during pregnancy increases perinatal morbidity and mortality. This is particularly true when rupture occurs after 20 weeks' gestation. Peritonitis increases the risk of preterm labor and preterm delivery. Therefore, it is prudent that the clinician make an early diagnosis and proceed immediately with surgical intervention.

Cholelithiasis

After appendicitis, biliary tract disease is the second most common general surgical condition encountered during pregnancy. Cholelithiasis of pregnancy usually develops from obstruction of the cystic duct. Clinical presentation ranges from intermittent attacks of biliary colic to persistent pain radiating into the subcapsular area in cases where the common bile duct is obstructed by a stone. Ultrasound is helpful in detecting the presence of stones. The differential diagnosis of acute cholelithiasis includes acute pain in the liver of pregnancy, HELLP (hemolysis, elevated liver enzymes, low platelets) syndrome, and severe preeclampsia. Initial attacks may be treated conservatively with intravenous fluids, antibiotics, and antispasmodics; however, without prompt resolution of symptoms, surgery should be considered. Delay of surgery in a patient with cholecystitis may increase perinatal morbidity. Despite the potential difficulty of operating on a pregnant woman, lower morbidity has been shown in those patients managed surgically, particularly in the case involving obstruction. In early gestations, laparoscopic cholecystectomy can be considered.

Although rare, pancreatitis may present during pregnancy. The most common cause of pancreatitis in pregnant women is cholelithiasis. However, pancreatitis can be a complication of severe preeclampsia or HELLP syndrome. Pancreatitis caused by milk-alkali toxicity may be seen in patients with excessive intake of antacids.[9]

Intestinal Obstruction

The incidence of intestinal obstruction is similar to that of the general population. Patients present with classic symptoms of abdominal colicky pain associated with hyperactive peristalsis. Nausea and vomiting is present in approximately 80% of the cases. Bowel distention is marked. Laparotomy should be performed before bowel necrosis and perforation occur. If perforation occurs during pregnancy, there is a significant increase in maternal and perinatal morbidity and mortality.

Ovarian Masses

With frequent use of ultrasound in early pregnancy, the corpus luteum cyst of pregnancy is frequently identified. This is physiologic and, in the absence of symptoms of torsion, requires only follow-up to ensure the diagnosis. The progesterone produced in the first 14 weeks of gestation is necessary to support the pregnancy until placental production of progesterone replaces it. Therefore, if surgery is required for symptoms of torsion or bleeding, every effort should be made to preserve the corpus luteum in the first trimester.

Obstetric Complications Resulting in Abdominal Pain

Abruption

Placental abruption usually occurs in the third trimester. It may be associated with excruciating abdominal pain. Contrary to popular belief, overt vaginal bleeding does not need to be present for the diagnosis to be made. Ultrasonography is of little use, because only 5% to 10% of abruptions can be seen. Therefore, the diagnosis of abrup-

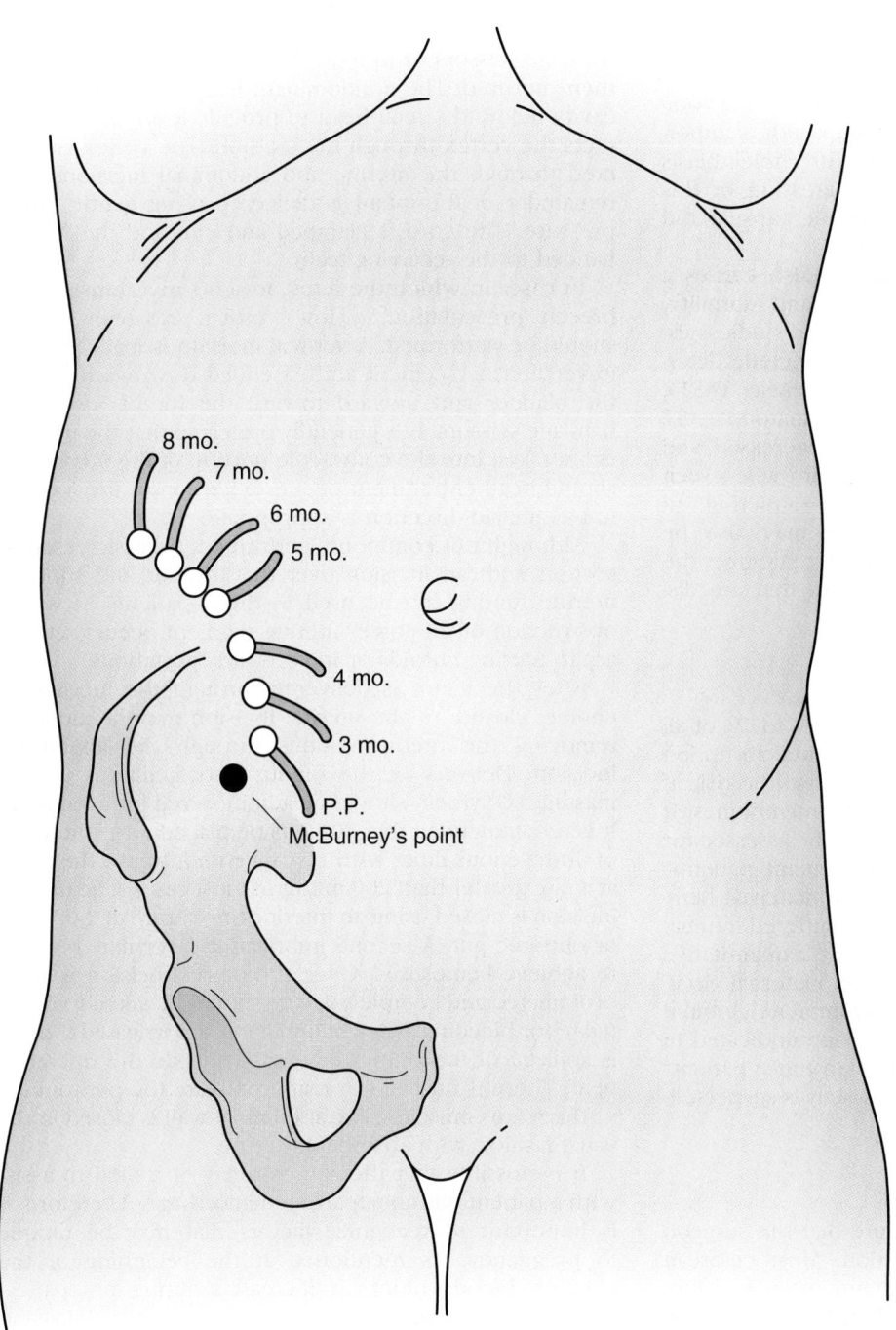

FIGURE 74-13. Location of the appendix in pregnancy. As modified from Bauer and colleagues (JAMA, 1932), the approximate location of the appendix during succeeding months of pregnancy is diagrammed. In planning an operation, it is better to make the abdominal incision over the point of maximum tenderness unless there is a great disparity between that point and the theoretical location of the appendix. (From Ludmir J, Stubblefield PG: Surgical procedures in pregnancy. *In* Gabbe S, Nubyl JR, Simpson JL [eds]: Obstetrics: Normal and Problem Pregnancies, 4th ed. Philadelphia, Churchill Livingstone, 2002, p 617.)

tion is clinical. Abruptions are usually associated with uterine hypertonicity, resulting in fetal heart rate abnormalities. It is important for the clinician to make a rapid diagnosis of abruption.

Trauma may increase the risk of abruption. There are three distinct mechanisms for post-traumatic placental abruption. First, blunt trauma to the uterus (e.g., assault or seat belt placement) can cause a direct injury to the placental implantation site. Second, the sudden acceleration-deceleration cycle that occurs in motor vehicle accidents can cause a contrecoup shearing injury. Finally, even in the absence of any overt physical injury, the acute adrenergic reaction to stress can result in sufficient uterine vasospasm to create ischemic necrosis at the implantation site; with reperfusion, a subplacental hematoma can dissect the plane of the implantation site.

The pregnant patient and her fetus who experience trauma should be monitored for at least 4 hours, with the possibility of prolonged monitoring for 24 hours. Abruption may quickly become a surgical emergency, requiring immediate delivery of the fetus. Laboratory studies that may be helpful in the diagnosis of abruption include a platelet count and fibrinogen. As the retroplacental hematoma expands, clotting factors, especially fibrinogen and platelets, are consumed. This may assist the clinician in the diagnosis in occult cases.

Pregnancy-Related Hepatic Complications

HELLP syndrome and acute fatty liver of pregnancy can present as right upper quadrant pain and nausea and vomiting. HELLP is a form of severe preeclampsia. It is important that the clinician not mistake this for cholelithiasis or other gastrointestinal pathology. Progression of this disease can result in rupture of the hepatic capsule and maternal death if the diagnosis is missed.

Acute fatty liver of pregnancy, which also carries a serious risk of maternal and fetal morbidity and mortality, can present in similar fashion. Laboratory studies are useful in the diagnosis of these entities to include determination of LDH, aspartate aminotransferase (AST), platelet count, creatinine, uric acid, and hematocrit. AST and LDH will be elevated, platelets will be decreased, and the hematocrit may be increased, especially when seen in association with intravascular volume depletion. In patients with acute fatty liver, glucose may also be decreased. It is important that the clinician remember the physiologic changes in interpreting values that are discussed at the beginning of this chapter.

Trauma

Trauma from accidental injuries occurs in 6% to 7% of all pregnancies. In addition to the risk of placental abruption noted earlier, blunt trauma may also increase the risk of preterm labor and preterm rupture of the membranes. It is important that pregnant trauma patients be assessed for the same spectrum of injuries as nonpregnant patients. Multiple studies have established that fetomaternal hemorrhage is increased in women who have suffered trauma. Women who are RhD negative should have a quantitative assessment of the volume of fetal cells in maternal circulation and an appropriate dose of anti-D immune globulin administered. Peritoneal lavage is not contraindicated in pregnancy and can be performed safely in those patients in whom the possibility of a ruptured viscus is suspected.

Common Obstetric Surgical Procedures

The most common obstetric procedure that the surgeon will encounter is the cesarean section. Most cesarean sections are performed through a Pfannenstiel incision; however, a vertical subumbilical midline incision can be used, especially in obese patients and in those patients in which rapid entry into the abdominal cavity is indicated. After the placement of a bladder catheter, entry into the peritoneal cavity can be undertaken. In most cases, the peritoneum of the vesicouterine fold is transected transversely and the bladder is gently dissected from the lower uterine segment. The lower uterine segment is palpated to check for malrotation to ensure that a transverse uterine incision centers on the midline. The underlying fetal part should be palpated. If the presenting part is the fetal head, the incision is marked 1 to 2 cm above the original margin of the bladder. A small transverse incision is made with a scalpel across the midline of the lower uterine segment down to the fetal membranes. The incision may be extended in a transverse fashion using bandage scissors or in blunt fashion. The membranes are then ruptured. The nondominant hand is placed into the cavity below the fetal head to provide leverage that redirects the vertex through the incision. The vertex is delivered through the uterine and abdominal incisions. The remainder of the infant is delivered using gentle fundal pressure. The cord is clamped and cut, and the fetus is handed to the receiving team.

In cases in which the fetus presents in a transverse or breech presentation, a low vertical cesarean section should be performed. A vertical incision is made into the lower uterine segment and extended downward toward the bladder and upward toward the fundus using the bandage scissors. It is generally preferred that the incision is not taken into the contractile portion of the uterus; but should head entrapment occur, extension of the incision in a cephalad direction is appropriate.

Although not commonly performed, a classic cesarean section with an incision over the anterior and superior uterine fundus can be used in those patients in which obstruction of the lower uterine segment occurs secondary to uterine fibroids or in very early gestations.

After the infant is delivered through the incision of choice, closure of the uterine incision may be aided by removing the uterine fundus through the abdominal incision. Delivery of the fundus also facilitates uterine massage. Oxytocin should be administered intravenously. It is recommended that 20 units be placed into a liter bag of intravenous fluid, with care taken not to run the fluids at a rate greater than 200 mL/hr in most cases. The uterine incision is closed using an interlocking suture of 1-0 Vicryl or chromic gut. A second imbricating layer may be used to achieve hemostasis. Once the uterus incision is reapproximated and completed, care should be taken to investigate for bleeding. The abdomen may be irrigated if there is spillage of meconium or vernix outside the operative field. There is no need to reapproximate the peritoneum or the rectus muscles. The abdominal wall is closed in the usual fashion with absorbable suture.

It is possible that the surgeon may be called to assist with a patient with postpartum hemorrhage. Therefore, it is important to recognize factors that may be unique to pregnancy. As mentioned at the beginning of the chapter, blood volume is increased during pregnancy. Hemorrhage in pregnancy is defined as blood loss in excess of 1000 mL. It should be noted, however, that because of the increase in blood volume by term, the patient may lose 1500 to 2000 mL before symptoms. The most common cause of postpartum hemorrhage is uterine atony. Risk factors for uterine atony include prolonged labor, uterine infection, cesarean section, and overdistention of the uterus. Hemorrhage can also be seen in abruption of the placenta and in those patients with placenta previa, either before or after delivery. It is recommended that therapy be initiated after the loss of 600 mL.

The first step is to assess for vaginal, cervical, or uterine lacerations. If negative and uterine atony is the mechanism, manual exploration of the uterus should be initiated to ensure complete removal of the placenta and aggressive fundal massage should be begun. If this is unsuccessful, the administration of a solution of oxytocin (20 units in a liter of physiologic saline solution at a rate of 200 mL/hr) may assist with uterine contractility. A rate of as high as 500 mL in 10 minutes can be administered without significant cardiovascular complications; however, maternal hypotension may occur with an intravenous bolus injection of as low as 5 units.

When oxytocin fails to provide adequate response, a synthetic 15-methyl-$F_{2\alpha}$ prostaglandin (carboprost) should be administered intramuscularly or in the uterine wall. In addition, methergine, 0.2 mg, may be administered intramuscularly. Methergine is contraindicated in those patients with hypertension. Prostaglandin $F_{2\alpha}$ is contraindicated in patients with asthma. Misoprostol (Cytotec) also has uterotonic properties and can be used at a dose of 1000 µg per rectum.

When pharmacologic measures fail to control hemorrhage, then surgical measures should be undertaken. If the hemorrhage is secondary to uterine atony, ligation of the uterine vessels may be successful. The first step in ligating the uterine arteries is at the anastomosis of the uterine and the ovarian artery high on the fundus just below the utero-ovarian ligament. A large suture on the atraumatic needle can be passed from the uterus around the vessel and tied. If bilateral utero-ovarian vessel ligation does not stop bleeding, temporary atraumatic occlusion of the ovarian arteries in the infundibulopelvic ligaments may be attempted. By decreasing perfusion pressure, thrombosis in the vascular bed may produce hemostasis.

If conservative measures are unsuccessful, cesarean hysterectomy may need to be performed before sequelae of coagulopathy and hemorrhagic shock occur. In the case of postpartum hemorrhage, supracervical hysterectomy is often the procedure of choice. As in the gynecologic hysterectomy described earlier, the superior attachments of the uterus are separated, but, after the ligation of the uterine arteries the fundus of the uterus is amputated from the cervix, which is closed with figure-eight sutures. This procedure also maintains the integrity of the uterosacral ligaments.

It is difficult to remove the cervix, especially after a vaginal delivery secondary to dilatation of the lower uterine segment. Only surgeons who are skilled in this procedure should proceed without consultation.

Other Procedures

On rare occasions, the surgeon may be consulted to assist with repair of an episiotomy and extension. Episiotomy is an incision into the perineal body made to help facilitate delivery. Most episiotomies are cut in the midline from posterior fourchette toward the rectum. While more comfortable for the patient, these incisions may extend through the anal sphincter (third degree) or through the rectal wall (fourth degree). An inappropriate repair may result in a rectovaginal fistula. These fistulas present with the same symptoms as seen in other rectal fistulas associated with Crohn's disease but are much easier to repair and have a lower rate of recurrence.

Repair of an episiotomy requires reapproximation of the vaginal tissue and the perineal body. Repair of the anal sphincter requires that the fascial capsule that usually retracts posteriorly be identified and reapproximated. If the rectal wall has been compromised, a multilayer closure, using 2-0 or 3-0 absorbable suture of mucosa, muscularis, rectovaginal fascia, anal sphincter, vaginal muscularis, and vaginal mucosa will provide the best opportunity to avoid a fistula. Because of the increased vascularity associated with pregnancy, with an adequate closure without stitch-induced tissue necrosis healing is not usually a problem.

Selected References

Baggish MS, Karram M (eds): Atlas of Pelvic Anatomy and Gynecologic Surgery. Philadelphia, WB Saunders, 2001.

Detailed pelvic anatomy and comprehensive coverage is presented of gynecologic procedures.

Clarke S, Phelan JP, Cotton DB (eds): Critical Care Obstetrics, 3rd ed. Boston, Blackwell Scientific, 1997.

This book provides a comprehensive pathophysiology of pregnancy.

Fleming ID, Cooper JS, Henson DE, et al: AJCC Cancer Staging Manual, 5th ed. Philadelphia, Lippincott-Raven, 1998.

Comprehensive cancer staging is described.

Rock J, Jones HWJ III (eds): TeLinde's Operative Gynecology, 9th ed. Philadelphia, Lippincott Williams and Wilkins, 2003.

Encyclopedic coverage addresses all areas of gynecologic surgery with an expanded oncology section.

Speroff L, Glass RH, Kase NG (eds): Clinical Gynecologic Endocrinology and Infertility, 6th ed. Philadelphia, Lippincott Williams & Wilkins, 1999.

A comprehensive description of reproductive physiology is presented.

References

1. Kadar N, Friedman M, Zacher M: Further observations on the doubling time of human chorionic gonadotropin in early asymptomatic pregnancies. Fertil Steril 54:783-787, 1990.
2. Keith SC, London SN, Weitzmen GA, et al: Serial transvaginal ultrasound scans and β-human chorionic gonadotropin levels in early singleton and multiple pregnancies. Fertil Steril 59:1007-1010, 1993.
3. Gelder MS, Boots LR, Younger JB: Use of a single random serum progesterone value as a diagnostic aid for ectopic pregnancy. Fertil Steril 55:497-500, 1991.
4. Federation of International Gynecology and Obstetrics. 1998. FIGO Staging of Gynecologic Cancer: http://www.figo.org/default.asp?id=32
5. Molpus KL, Redlin-Frazier S, Reed G, et al: Postoperative pelvic irradiation in early stage mixed müllerian tumors. Eur J Gynaecol Oncol 19:541-546, 1998.

6. Wolner-Hanssen P, Mardh P-A, Svensson L, et al: Laparoscopy in women with chlamydial infection and pelvic pain: A comparison of patients with and without salpingitis. Obstet Gynecol 61:299-303, 1983.

7. Loffer FD: Three-year comparison of thermal balloon and rollerball ablation in treatment of menorrhagia. J Am Assoc Gynecol Laparosc 8:48-54, 2001.

8. Loffer FD, Grainger D: Five-year follow-up of patients participating in a randomized trial of uterine balloon therapy versus rollerball ablation for treatment of menorrhagia. J Am Assoc Gynecol Laparosc 9:429-435, 2002.

9. Marcovici I, Marzano D: Pregnancy-induced hypertension complicated by postpartum renal failure and pancreatitis: A case report. Am J Perinatol 19:177-179, 2002.

10. Mitchell CW, Wheeless CR Jr (eds): Atlas of Pelvic Surgery, 3rd ed. Baltimore, Williams & Wilkins, 1997.

11. Ludmir J, Stubblefield PG: Surgical Procedures in Pregnancy. *In* Gabbe S, Nubyl JR, Simpson JL (eds): Obstetrics: Normal and Problem Pregnancies, 4th ed. Philadelphia, Churchill Livingstone, 2002, p 368.

CHAPTER 75

SURGERY IN THE PREGNANT PATIENT

Paul R. Beery II, M.D., and **E. Christopher Ellison**, M.D.

Physiologic Changes of Pregnancy
Radiology Safety Concerns in Pregnancy
Anesthesia Safety Concerns in Pregnancy
Prevention of Preterm Labor
Abdominal Pain and the Acute Abdomen in
 Pregnancy
Minimally Invasive Surgery in Pregnancy
Breast Masses in Pregnancy

Hepatobiliary Disease in Pregnancy
Endocrine Disease in Pregnancy
Small Bowel Disease in Pregnancy
Colon and Rectum in Pregnancy
Vascular Disease in Pregnancy
Trauma in Pregnancy
Summary

Pregnant women are subject to the same surgical diseases as their nonpregnant counterparts. An estimated 1% to 2% of pregnant women require surgical procedures, with nonobstetric surgery necessary in up to 1% of pregnancies in the United States each year. Most indications for surgical intervention are those that are common for the patient's age group and unrelated to pregnancy, such as acute appendicitis, symptomatic cholelithiasis, breast masses, or trauma. The pregnant patient offers unique challenges to the surgeon. Changes in maternal anatomy and physiology and safety of the fetus are among the issues of which the surgeon must be cognizant. The presentation of surgical diseases in the pregnant patient may be atypical or may mimic signs and symptoms associated with a normal pregnancy, and a standard evaluation may be unreliable due to pregnancy-associated changes in diagnostic tests or laboratory values. Finally, many physicians may be more conservative in diagnostic evaluation and treatment. Any of these factors may result in a delay in diagnosis and treatment, adversely affecting maternal and fetal outcome. Although consultation with an obstetrician is ideal when caring for a pregnant patient, the surgeon needs to be aware of certain fundamental principles when such a resource is unavailable. This chapter discusses the key points in caring for the pregnant patient who presents with nonobstetric surgical disease.

PHYSIOLOGIC CHANGES OF PREGNANCY

Progesterone and estrogen, two of the principal hormones of pregnancy, mediate many of the maternal physiologic changes in pregnancy. These changes may mimic pathophysiology that occurs in nonpregnant individuals, most notably cardiac or liver disease. Elevated progesterone levels as well as decreased serum motilin result in smooth muscle relaxation, producing multiple effects in several organ systems. In the stomach, this decreased smooth muscle tone results in diminished gastric tone and motility. The lower esophageal sphincter tone is also lower and, when combined with increased intra-abdominal pressure, results in an increase in the incidence of gastroesophageal reflux. Small bowel motility is reduced, increasing small bowel transit time. Absorption of nutrients, however, remains unchanged, with the exception of iron absorption, which is increased due to increased iron requirements. In the colon, pregnancy-related changes usually manifest as constipation. This is due to a combination of increased colonic sodium and water absorption, decreased motility, and mechanical obstruction by the gravid uterus. An increase in portal venous pressure and therefore an increase in the pressure in the collateral venous circulation results in dilation of the veins at the gastroesophageal junction. This is of importance only if the patient had esophageal varices prior to becoming pregnant. The most common result of the increased portal venous pressure is the dilation of the hemorrhoidal veins leading to the well-known complaint of hemorrhoids by the patient.

In addition to alterations in smooth muscle tone and motility, other notable changes occur in the gastrointestinal tract. The function of the gallbladder is altered, as is the chemical composition of bile. During the second and third trimester, the volume of the gallbladder may be twice that found in the nonpregnant state, and gallbladder emptying is markedly slower. In a pregnant baboon model, an increased biliary cholesterol saturation and a decreased proportion of chenodeoxycholic acid were noted, although there are limited data in human subjects.[1] It is unknown if the increased biliary stasis, changes in bile composition, or a combination of the two factors results in an increased risk of gallstone formation, but the risk of developing gallstones increases with multiparity. However, the incidence of symptomatic cholelithiasis during pregnancy is similar to the incidence in age-related nonpregnant patients.[2]

Some of the changes of pregnancy closely resemble liver disease. These include spider angiomata and palmar erythema from elevated serum estrogen levels, hypoalbuminemia, and elevated serum cholesterol, alkaline phosphatase, and fibrinogen levels. Serum bilirubin and hepatic transaminase levels remain unchanged during pregnancy.

In the cardiovascular system, peripheral vascular resistance is decreased as a consequence of diminished vascular smooth muscle tone. Cardiac output increases by as much as 50% during the first trimester of pregnancy. Initially, this is due to an increased stroke volume resulting from an increase in plasma volume and red blood cell mass, but a gradual increase in maternal heart rate also contributes. Cardiac output falls back to nearly normal late in pregnancy, usually during the 36th to 40th weeks' gestation. During the third trimester, cardiac output is dramatically decreased when the mother is lying supine. This is due to compromised venous return from the lower extremity from compression of the inferior vena cava by the gravid uterus. In the supine position, the inferior vena cava may be completely occluded; venous drainage of the lower extremities is through collateral channels. With this drop in preload, an increase in sympathetic tone usually maintains peripheral vascular resistance and blood pressure. However, up to 10% of patients may experience supine hypotensive syndrome in which the sympathetic response is not adequate to maintain blood pressure. During anesthesia induction in the operating room, anesthetic agents may inhibit the compensatory sympathetic response, causing a more precipitous fall in blood pressure. From a surgeon's perspective, it may be necessary to place the patient in left lateral decubitus position during procedures performed during the third trimester, relieving caval compression by the enlarged uterus.

Oxygen consumption increases during pregnancy. Minute ventilation increases by 30% to 40% due to an increase in tidal volume, which appears to be a result of elevated serum progesterone level. Progesterone not only increases the sensitivity of the respiratory centers to CO_2

but also acts as a direct stimulant to the respiratory centers.[1] As a consequence of the increased minute ventilation, maternal PaO_2 levels during late pregnancy range from 104 to 108 mm Hg and maternal $PaCO_2$ ranges from 27 to 32 mm Hg. Renal compensation maintains normal maternal pH. The decreased $PaCO_2$ increases the CO_2 gradient from the fetus to the mother, facilitating CO_2 transfer from the fetus to the mother. The oxygen-hemoglobin dissociation curve of maternal blood is shifted to the right; this, coupled with the increased affinity for oxygen of fetal hemoglobin, results in increased oxygen transfer to the fetus. Elevation of the diaphragm by as much as 4 cm results in a decrease in total lung volume by 5%. Diminished expiratory reserve volume and residual volume result in a functional residual capacity that is 20% lower than that in the nonpregnant woman. Vital capacity and inspiratory reserve volume remain stable.

In the kidney, there is an increase in the glomerular filtration rate by 50% that accompanies a 75% increase in renal plasma flow. Urinary glucose excretion increases as a direct consequence of the increased glomerular filtration rate. Blood urea nitrogen decreases by 25% during the first trimester and maintains at that level for the remainder of pregnancy. Serum creatinine also decreases by the end of the first trimester from a nonpregnant value of 0.8 mg/dL to 0.7 mg/dL and may be as low as 0.5 mg/dL by term. A fivefold to tenfold increase in serum renin occurs with a subsequent fourfold to fivefold increase in angiotensin. Although the pregnant patient is apparently less sensitive to the hypertensive effects of the increased angiotensin, elevated aldosterone levels result in an increase in sodium reabsorption, overcoming the natriuresis produced by elevated progesterone. Serum sodium levels are decreased, however, as the increase in sodium reabsorption is less than the increase in plasma volume. Serum osmolality is decreased to 270 to 280 mOsm/kg.[1]

The increase in plasma volume and red blood cell mass is accompanied by a progressive rise in the leukocyte count during pregnancy. During the first trimester, the white blood cell count ranges from 3000 to 15,000 cells/mm^3, increasing to a range of 6000 to 16,000 cells/mm^3 during the second and third trimesters.[1] Platelet count progressively declines throughout pregnancy, while the mean platelet volume tends to increase after 28 weeks' gestation. As previously stated, fibrinogen levels are elevated to a range of 400 to 500 mg/dL. Plasma levels of factors VII, VIII, IX, and X also rise progressively, whereas levels of factors XI and XIII decline and levels of factors II, V, and XII remain unchanged. In spite of these alterations in the coagulation cascade and platelet count, bleeding time and clotting time are unchanged.

RADIOLOGY SAFETY CONCERNS IN PREGNANCY

Radiographic studies remain useful diagnostic tools in the pregnant patient. Of greatest concern with radiation exposure is the risk to the fetus from the exposure. The accepted maximum dose of ionizing radiation during the entire pregnancy is 5 rads (0.05 Gy). The fetus is at the highest risk from radiation exposure from the preimplantation period to approximately 15 weeks' gestation. Primary organogenesis occurs during this time, and the teratogenic effects of radiation, particularly to the developing central nervous system, are at their highest. Perinatal radiation exposure has also been associated with childhood leukemia and certain childhood malignancies. The radiation dose that has been associated with congenital malformation is higher than 10 rads (0.1 Gy).[3] As demonstrated in Table 75-1, radiation exposure to the fetus with the doses from the more common radiology procedures is well below that threshold. Nonetheless, prudence on the part of the clinician is required to avoid unnecessary fetal exposure to ionizing radiation, especially during the first trimester and early second trimester when the risk from exposure is greatest.

Magnetic resonance imaging (MRI) avoids exposure to ionizing radiation but poses an unknown risk to the fetus. Animal studies have shown no teratogenic effect or increased incidence of fetal death or congenital malformations from the electromagnetic radiation, static magnetic field, radiofrequency magnetic fields, or intravenous contrast agents used during MRI. Theoretically, the gradient magnetic fields may produce electric currents within the patient, and the high-frequency currents induced by radiofrequency fields may cause local generation of heat. The long-term effect of exposure is not known.[4] Currently, the National Radiological Protection Board advises against the use of MRI during the first trimester of pregnancy.

Ultrasonography is routinely used by obstetricians during pregnancy. Although tissue heating and cavitation are theoretical effects of ultrasound exposure, such effects have never been reported. Ultrasound may be a helpful alternative diagnostic tool when trying to avoid exposure to ionizing radiation, but it does have some limitations. Deeper structures are difficult to visualize and may be obscured by superficial structures that are more echodense. Ultrasound imaging has a limited field of view and is highly operator dependent. Despite these limitations, certain disease processes, such as a palpable breast mass, may be evaluated effectively and safely.

ANESTHESIA SAFETY CONCERNS IN PREGNANCY

Anesthesia concerns during pregnancy include the safety of both the mother and the fetus. The fetus may be affected by exposure to teratogenic effects of anesthetic agents, risk of preterm labor, and the risk from changes in maternal physiology as a consequence of anesthesia. Changes in uterine blood flow and maternal acid-base status may result in hypoxemia or asphyxia for the fetus. These can be a result of maternal hypotension or hypoxia, maternal hyperventilation, or the placental passage of anesthetic agents that affect the fetal central nervous or cardiovascular systems.

The effects of anesthesia during pregnancy can be divided into direct, or active, and indirect, or passive, effects. The direct effects are those effects that relate to the possible teratogenic or embryotoxic properties of the drugs used for anesthesia, some of which do cross the placenta. The indirect effects are those mechanisms by which an anesthetic agent or surgical procedure may interfere with maternal or fetal physiology and in doing so harm the fetus. For the most part, the fetus experiences indirect effects as a consequence of anesthetic agents administered to the mother and hemodynamic changes of the mother from blood loss or anesthetic agents. The most profound effects on the fetus are related to decreased uterine blood flow or decreased oxygen content of uterine blood. Unlike circulation to other vital organs, most notably the brain, the uterine circulation is not autoregulated. During the third trimester, uterine circulation represents nearly 10% of cardiac output. When treating maternal hypotension, vasopressors such as dopamine and epinephrine, while increasing the maternal systemic pressure, have little or no effect on uterine circulation.[5] Other maneuvers, such as fluid bolus, Trendelenburg position, compression stockings, or leg elevation, have a larger impact on increasing uterine blood flow.

In addition to the risks related to maternal hypoxia or hypotension, the risk of spontaneous abortion and teratogenesis related to anesthetic agents is of major concern. Many nonhuman studies have demonstrated different teratogenic effects with similar agents but have not led to definitive conclusions regarding teratogenic potential in humans. For a congenital defect to result, exposure to the teratogen must occur during the vulnerable differentiation stage of the affected organ system. As previously noted, differentiation of the major organ systems occurs during the first trimester of human embryonic development. Therefore, delaying semielective surgical procedures until after the first trimester may reduce the risk of teratogenicity. However, large survey studies have demonstrated an increased risk of spontaneous abortions, intrauterine growth retardation, and low-birth-weight neonates in women who require surgery during pregnancy. These studies lacked information on the indications for the nonobstetric surgical procedures. It is therefore difficult to separate the effects of anesthesia on the fetus from the effects of the underlying disease process on the mother and fetus.[6]

Elective surgical procedures should be delayed until at least 6 weeks after delivery, when maternal physiology has

TABLE 75-1. Fetal Radiation Exposure with Radiographic Imaging	
Examination Type	Estimated Fetal Radiation Exposure (rads)
Two-view chest radiograph	0.00007
Cervical spine radiograph	0.002
Pelvis radiograph	0.04
Head CT	<0.050
Abdomen CT	2.60
Upper GI series	0.056
Barium enema	3.986
Hepatobiliary (HIDA) scan	0.150

CT, computed tomography; GI, gastrointestinal.

returned to the nonpregnant state and when the impact on the fetus is no longer a concern. When emergent procedures are required, obviously, the life of the mother takes priority, although an experienced anesthesiologist will be able to modify the anesthesia used according to maternal physiology and fetal well-being. For semielective surgical procedures, attempts should be made to delay surgery until after the first trimester whenever possible. This needs to be determined on an individual case basis, because continued exposure to the underlying disease process may be more harmful than the operative risk to both the mother and the fetus. During the second trimester, after organ system differentiation has occurred, there is almost no risk of anesthetic-induced malformation or spontaneous abortion. Later in pregnancy, during the third trimester, the risk of preterm delivery is at its highest.

When the pregnant patient requires surgical intervention, consultation with the obstetrician and possibly a perinatologist is essential. The specialist is helpful in determining the optimum technique to monitor fetal status and is able to assist with perioperative management and diagnose and manage preterm labor. Typically, when emergent surgery occurs during the first trimester or early second trimester, fetal heart tones should be obtained before and after anesthesia exposure. During the late second trimester and third trimester, when the fetus is of viable age, continuous intraoperative monitoring should be performed when possible. Transvaginal ultrasound can be used when the surgical field involves the abdomen. Continuous monitoring should be used if a significant blood loss is possible or anticipated to assess fetal well-being.

Fetal heart rate for fetal status and tocometer monitoring for uterine activity should be obtained before and after the procedure even if intraoperative monitoring is not believed necessary or is not available.

PREVENTION OF PRETERM LABOR

The incidence of preterm labor associated with nonobstetric surgery is related to both gestational age and the indication for surgery. Gestational age at treatment and severity of the underlying disease are the most predictive indicators of patients at risk for preterm labor. The later in gestation the patient is, the higher the risk of preterm contractions or preterm labor. Intraperitoneal surgeries and disease processes with intraperitoneal inflammation are the most likely to have postoperative courses complicated by preterm contractions and preterm labor. In multiple studies, a significant difference was found in the number of patients with preterm contractions based on the average time from onset of symptoms to operative intervention. A delay in treatment does appear to increase the chance of preterm labor, likely related to the primary disease process. Laparoscopic and open techniques have an equal incidence of preterm labor.

There is no general consensus on the use of prophylactic tocolytics after nonobstetric surgery during pregnancy. Tocolytic use varies widely between centers and among physicians. Most studies suggest that tocolytics be used only if contractions are noted during postoperative monitoring or are appreciated by the patient. Tocolytics used as needed are generally successful at preventing preterm labor and preterm delivery when postoperative contractions are detected. Terbutaline, magnesium, and indomethacin (Indocin) all have been used in different studies with equivalent results. Nearly 100% of patients with postoperative contractions were successfully tocolyzed and delivered at term. In general, for patients with postoperative contractions before 32 weeks, indomethacin would be a reasonable treatment, whereas terbutaline could be used first line for patients at greater than 32 weeks' gestation. The use of prophylactic tocolysis should be individualized, depending on the patient's gestational age and the underlying disease process.

ABDOMINAL PAIN AND THE ACUTE ABDOMEN IN PREGNANCY

When the pregnant patient presents with abdominal pain, it may be difficult to distinguish a pathophysiologic cause from normal pregnancy-associated symptoms. Changes in the position and orientation of abdominal viscera from the enlarging uterus as well as alterations in physiology already described may modify the perception or manifestation of an intra-abdominal process. If early in the pregnancy, the woman may not know that she is pregnant. Additionally, some intra-abdominal processes are exclusive to pregnancy, such as ectopic pregnancy, HELLP (hemolysis, elevated liver enzymes, low platelets) syndrome, or acute fatty liver of pregnancy. Thirdly, both patient and physician may attribute the patient's complaints to normal pregnancy, resulting in a delay in evaluation and treatment. These delays in diagnosis and definitive intervention are the most serious adverse event affecting maternal and fetal outcome. It is usually not the treatment but the delay in diagnosis and severity of the primary disease process that poorly impact outcomes.[7] Box 75-1 lists the more common causes of abdominal pain in the pregnant patient, classified according to location.

MINIMALLY INVASIVE SURGERY IN PREGNANCY

When laparoscopic techniques were initially described, pregnancy was considered a contraindication to laparoscopy. Effects of CO_2 pneumoperitoneum on venous return and cardiac output, uterine perfusion, and fetal acid-base status were unknown. Laparoscopy was safely used in several series where the technique was used to evaluate pregnant patients for ectopic pregnancy. Those patients with an intrauterine pregnancy had no increase in fetal loss or observed negative effect on long-term outcome.[8,9] When comparing laparoscopic and open techniques in nonpregnant patients, those patients who underwent laparoscopic procedures had decreased pain, shorter hospital stays, and a quicker return to normal activity.

Major concerns of laparoscopy during pregnancy include injury to the uterus, decreased uterine blood flow,

Box 75-1. Common Causes of Abdominal Pain in the Pregnant Patient

Right Upper Quadrant

Gastroesophageal reflux
Peptic ulcer disease
Acute cholecystitis
Biliary colic
Acute pancreatitis
Hepatitis
Acute fatty liver of pregnancy
HELLP syndrome
Preeclampsia
Pneumothorax
Pneumonia
Acute appendicitis
Hepatic adenoma
Hemangioma

Right Lower Quadrant

Acute appendicitis
Ectopic pregnancy
Renal or ureteral colic
Pelvic inflammatory disease
Tubo-ovarian abscess
Endometriosis
Adnexal torsion
Ruptured ovarian cyst
Ruptured corpus luteum

Lower Abdomen

Threatened, incomplete, or complete abortion
Abruptio placentae
Preterm labor
Pelvic inflammatory disease
Tubo-ovarian abscess
Inflammatory bowel disease
Irritable bowel syndrome
Pyelonephritis

Flank

Pyelonephritis
Hydronephrosis of pregnancy
Acute appendicitis (retrocecal appendix)

Diffuse Abdominal Pain

Early acute appendicitis
Small bowel obstruction
Acute intermittent porphyria
Sickle cell crisis

HELLP, *hemolysis, elevated liver enzymes, low platelets.*

Box 75-2. Advantages and Disadvantages of Laparoscopy over Laparotomy in Pregnancy

Advantages

Decreased fetal depression secondary to decreased narcotic requirement
Decreased risk of wound complications
Diminished postoperative maternal hypoventilation
Decreased manipulation of the uterus

Disadvantages

Possible uterine injury during trocar placement
Decreased uterine blood flow
Preterm labor risk secondary to the increased intra-abdominal pressure
Increased risk of fetal acidosis and unknown effects of CO_2 pneumoperitoneum

abdominal pressure occur normally during pregnancy during maternal Valsalva maneuvers. The risk of pneumoperitoneum may also be less than the risk of direct uterine manipulation that occurs with laparotomy. Fetal respiratory acidosis with subsequent fetal hypertension and tachycardia were observed in a pregnant ewe model but were reversed by maintaining maternal respiratory alkalosis.[10] Additionally, in the small series comparing laparoscopy and open techniques, no significant difference in preterm labor or delivery-related side effects was observed.[11] Box 75-2 illustrates the general comparison between laparoscopic and open technique.

The Society of American Gastrointestinal Endoscopic Surgeons recommends the following guidelines for laparoscopic surgery during pregnancy:

1. Obstetric consultation should be obtained preoperatively.
2. When possible, operative intervention should be deferred until the second trimester, when fetal risk is lowest.
3. Pneumoperitoneum enhances lower extremity venous stasis already present in the gravid patient, and pregnancy induces a hypercoagulable state. Therefore, pneumatic compression devices should be used whenever possible.
4. Fetal and uterine status, as well as maternal end-tidal CO_2 and/or arterial blood gases, should be monitored.
5. The uterus should be protected with a lead shield if intraoperative cholangiography is a possibility. Fluoroscopy should be used selectively.
6. Given the enlarged gravid uterus, abdominal access should be attained using an open technique.
7. Dependent positioning should be used to shift the uterus off the inferior vena cava.
8. Pneumoperitoneum pressures should be minimized to 8 to 12 mm Hg and not allowed to exceed 15 mm Hg.[12]

Trocar placement in the pregnant patient should not differ radically from placement in the nonpregnant patient early in pregnancy. Later in pregnancy, as the gravid

fetal acidosis, and preterm labor from increased intra-abdominal pressure. During the second trimester the uterus is no longer contained within the pelvis. The open technique for abdominal access reduces the risk of injury. Decreased uterine blood flow from pneumoperitoneum remains theoretical, because significant changes in intra-uterus enlarges superiorly, adjustments in trocar placement must be made to avoid uterine injury and to improve visualization. The camera port must be placed in a supraumbilical location, and the remaining ports are placed under direct camera visualization. An angled scope may aid in viewing over or around the uterus. The uterus should be manipulated as little as possible.

Alternatively, a gasless laparoscopic technique has been described. Called the abdominal wall lift technique, it avoids the need for pneumoperitoneum. Early results have shown a decrease in respiratory acidosis and improvement in intraoperative ventilatory function, although operative times are significantly higher.[13] Further evaluation is needed before this technique can be recommended in the pregnant patient.

BREAST MASSES IN PREGNANCY

Pregnancy-associated breast cancer is defined as breast cancer that is diagnosed during pregnancy or within 1 year following pregnancy. It has become increasingly more prominent as more women delay childbearing until they are in their 30s and 40s; the incidence of breast cancer is higher in women of those age groups. Overall, pregnancy-associated breast cancer has been reported to occur in 1 in 10,000 to 1 in 3000 pregnancies.[14,15] It is the most common nongynecologic malignancy associated with pregnancy. It usually presents as a painless palpable mass with or without nipple discharge. Recent studies have demonstrated that pregnancy-associated breast cancer may be more common in women with a genetic predisposition to breast cancer. In a group of 292 women diagnosed with breast cancer prior to age 40 years, those patients with a known *BRCA1* or *BRCA2* mutation were more likely to develop cancer during pregnancy.[16] In a group of 383 women in Japan, a family history of breast cancer was three times more common in patients who were diagnosed with breast cancer while pregnant or lactating when compared to nonpregnant patients with breast cancer.[17] As is true in nonpregnant patients, ductal carcinoma is the most common pathologic type of tumor, accounting for 75% to 90% of breast cancers in pregnant patients.[18]

Delays in diagnosis and treatment are common, although this has recently improved. Previous studies demonstrated delays in diagnosis of nearly 6 months, but more recent data show a mean delay of 1 to 2 months. Given a tumor doubling size of 130 days, a delay in diagnosis and treatment of 1 month increases the risk of nodal metastasis by 0.9%, whereas a delay of 6 months increases the risk by 5.1%.[18] Although the initial reports of pregnancy-associated breast cancer more than 100 years ago proposed a dismal prognosis, more recent literature has suggested that this is due to a more advanced stage at the time of diagnosis.[15,19] When compared with age-matched nonpregnant controls, women with pregnancy-associated breast cancer present with a larger primary tumor and a higher risk of positive axillary lymph nodes.[19] However, women with pregnancy-associated breast cancer have a similar stage-related prognosis compared to nonpregnant controls. Overall, these women bear a worse prognosis because of the more advanced disease at presentation. Pregnancy is a hyperestrogenic state and may correlate with rapid tumor proliferation and axillary lymph node metastases,[20] although pregnant women and nonpregnant young women have a higher percentage of estrogen receptor–negative cancers than older women.[21] In a series comparing 75 patients with pregnancy-associated breast cancer and 182 nonpregnant patients with breast cancer, 42% of cancers were estrogen receptor negative in the pregnant group and 21% were estrogen receptor negative in the nonpregnant control group.[22] This higher incidence of estrogen receptor–negative cancer is likely due to a down-regulation of estrogen receptors during pregnancy. Physiologic changes of breast engorgement, rapid cellular proliferation, and increased vascularity make a reliable physical examination difficult; masses of similar size that would be easily palpable in the nonpregnant state may be obscured, or palpable masses may be attributed to normal pregnancy-related changes. Benign breast lesions such as galactoceles, mastitis, abscesses, lipomas, fibroadenomas, lobular hyperplasia, and lactational adenomas account for 80% of breast masses that occur during pregnancy or during lactation. However, any palpable mass that persists for 4 weeks or longer should be evaluated.

Because of the changes in the breast tissue with pregnancy, imaging modalities may be difficult to interpret. If used with appropriate shielding, mammography carries a limited risk to the fetus. Mammography has a high false-negative rate due to the increased density of the fibroglandular breast tissue, however, so it has limited usefulness in the evaluation of the pregnant patient. Ultrasonography can safely be performed as an initial evaluation or in conjunction with mammography. Ultrasound is able to distinguish solid from cystic lesions in 97% of patients and is helpful in guiding fine-needle aspiration or biopsy. MRI of the breast is highly sensitive but only moderately specific and is being used more frequently in the nonpregnant patient. Its usefulness in the pregnant patient is yet to be determined. Although MRI does not use ionizing radiation, the two main risks to the fetus from the magnetic field and electromagnetic radiation are heating and cavitation. The gadolinium contrast is listed as a pregnancy category C drug, to be used only if the potential benefit outweighs the potential risk. Gadolinium crosses the placenta and has been associated with fetal abnormalities in rats. With other reliable imaging modalities available, MRI is not currently recommended for breast imaging in the pregnant patient.

Tissue diagnosis is essential. Core-needle biopsy with or without ultrasound guidance is a safe and reliable method for obtaining tissue. The major risks are hematoma formation and milk fistula development. A pressure dressing should be applied following the biopsy to minimize the risk of hematoma from the hypervascularity of the breasts. The risk of milk fistula may be reduced by stopping lactation for several days prior to biopsy and by emptying the breast of milk just prior to the procedure. If the biopsy is done postpartum, a 1-week course of bromocriptine may also be given prior to biopsy. Fine-needle aspiration may be a reliable alternative to core-needle or open biopsy. It can be performed safely with ultrasound guidance under local anesthesia without exposing the patient and fetus to the risks involved with general anesthesia, but its accuracy is dependent on the pathologist's experience in distinguishing the proliferative changes of pregnancy from cancer. In a series of 214 patients, none of the patients with negative fine-needle aspiration cytology developed cancer during the 18- to 24-month follow-up period.[21]

The mainstay of therapy for pregnancy-associated breast cancer is surgical resection. Modified radical mastectomy has long been considered the appropriate choice for local control. It eliminates the need for adjuvant radiation and its risk to the fetus. More recent data have suggested that the combination of local control and adjuvant therapy may be tailored to the patient according to the stage of pregnancy as well as the stage of the cancer.[18] In stages I and II cancers, mastectomy with axillary dissection is preferred. Axillary dissection is necessary because of the aggressive nature of pregnancy-associated breast cancer and the higher incidence of nodal metastasis. Sentinel node biopsy poses an unknown risk to the fetus and should be avoided until the safety of the radioisotope is determined.

In patients diagnosed during the late second trimester or later, immediate breast-conserving lumpectomy and axillary dissection followed with radiation postpartum is a treatment option. If the diagnosis of breast cancer is made in the first or early second trimester of pregnancy, lumpectomy and axillary dissection can be followed by chemotherapy after the first trimester and radiation after delivery. Chemotherapy is indicated for node-positive cancers or node-negative tumors greater than 1 cm. Current chemotherapeutic regimens are relatively safe after the first trimester, when the teratogenic risk is greatest. The increased plasma volume, the hypoalbuminemia, and the fact that almost all chemotherapeutic agents cross the placenta change the pharmacokinetics of the drugs and make accurate dosing difficult. Antimetabolites such as methotrexate should be avoided due to the high risk of spontaneous abortion even after the first trimester. Other agents have been associated with congenital malformations and complications such as preterm delivery, low birth weight, hyaline membrane disease, transient leukopenia, transient tachypnea of the newborn, and intrauterine growth retardation, but most of these effects occurred when the chemotherapeutic agent was administered during the first trimester. Twenty-four patients with pregnancy-associated breast cancer were given a chemotherapeutic regimen during the second and third trimester that included fluorouracil, cyclophosphamide, and doxorubicin. None of the infants had congenital malformations, and the median age at delivery was 38 weeks.[23] Long-term effects of the chemotherapeutic agents used for pregnancy-associated breast cancer on growth and development of children are not known. Cyclophosphamide and doxorubicin can enter breast milk; breast-feeding is contraindicated during chemotherapy.

Radiation is typically not offered during pregnancy because of its teratogenic risk and its risk of induction of childhood malignancies. The risk is directly related to both dose and developmental stage. During the preimplantation stage and continuing to 15 weeks after conception, during organogenesis, the rapidly proliferating cells of the fetus are most sensitive to radiation, and exposure greater than 1 Gy during this period has a high likelihood of causing fetal death. The standard therapeutic course of 5000 rads (50 Gy) results in a varying exposure to the fetus, depending on the gestational age and proximity of the gravid uterus to the radiation bed. Even with abdominal shielding, the greatest fetal exposure is due to scatter. Although there are several case reports of healthy infants born after maternal radiation exposure, radiation is not recommended during pregnancy due to the risks to the fetus.

Elective termination of the pregnancy to receive appropriate therapy without the risk of fetal malformation is no longer routinely recommended because no improvement in survival has been demonstrated.[18] With the treatment options available to the pregnant patient with breast cancer, a combined approach among the patient, surgeon, oncologist, and maternal-fetal medicine specialist should ensure optimal treatment of the disease while minimizing risk to the patient and the fetus. A suggested algorithm for the management of breast masses in pregnancy is shown in Figure 75-1.

HEPATOBILIARY DISEASE IN PREGNANCY

Liver abnormalities during pregnancy can be classified as occurring exclusively during pregnancy as a direct result of conditions during pregnancy, occurring simultaneously but not exclusively during pregnancy, or developing prior to the pregnancy. Examples of liver disorders unique to pregnancy include acute fatty liver of pregnancy, intrahepatic cholestasis of pregnancy, and liver disease related to preeclampsia or eclampsia, specifically HELLP syndrome and spontaneous hepatic hemorrhage or rupture. Preexisting liver disorders that may manifest with complications during pregnancy include hepatic adenoma and hepatocellular carcinoma.

The etiology of acute fatty liver of pregnancy is unknown, although it is more common in first pregnancies, in twin pregnancies, and in women who are pregnant with a male fetus. Although it has been diagnosed as early as the 26th week of gestation, it usually occurs during the third trimester, typically around the 35th week of gestation. Acute fatty liver of pregnancy carries a 20% maternal and fetal mortality rate. Initial nonspecific symptoms such as malaise, nausea, vomiting, and right upper quadrant pain are followed by signs of significant liver dysfunction within 2 weeks of onset of symptoms. Progression to fulminant hepatic failure quickly leads to preterm labor and an increased risk of fetal mortality. Although there is no specific treatment for acute fatty liver of pregnancy, prompt delivery after diagnosis may prevent progression to fulminant hepatic failure and reduce the risk of fetal death. Liver function typically returns to normal after delivery.

Approximately 10% of women with preeclampsia or eclampsia have associated liver involvement,[24] ranging

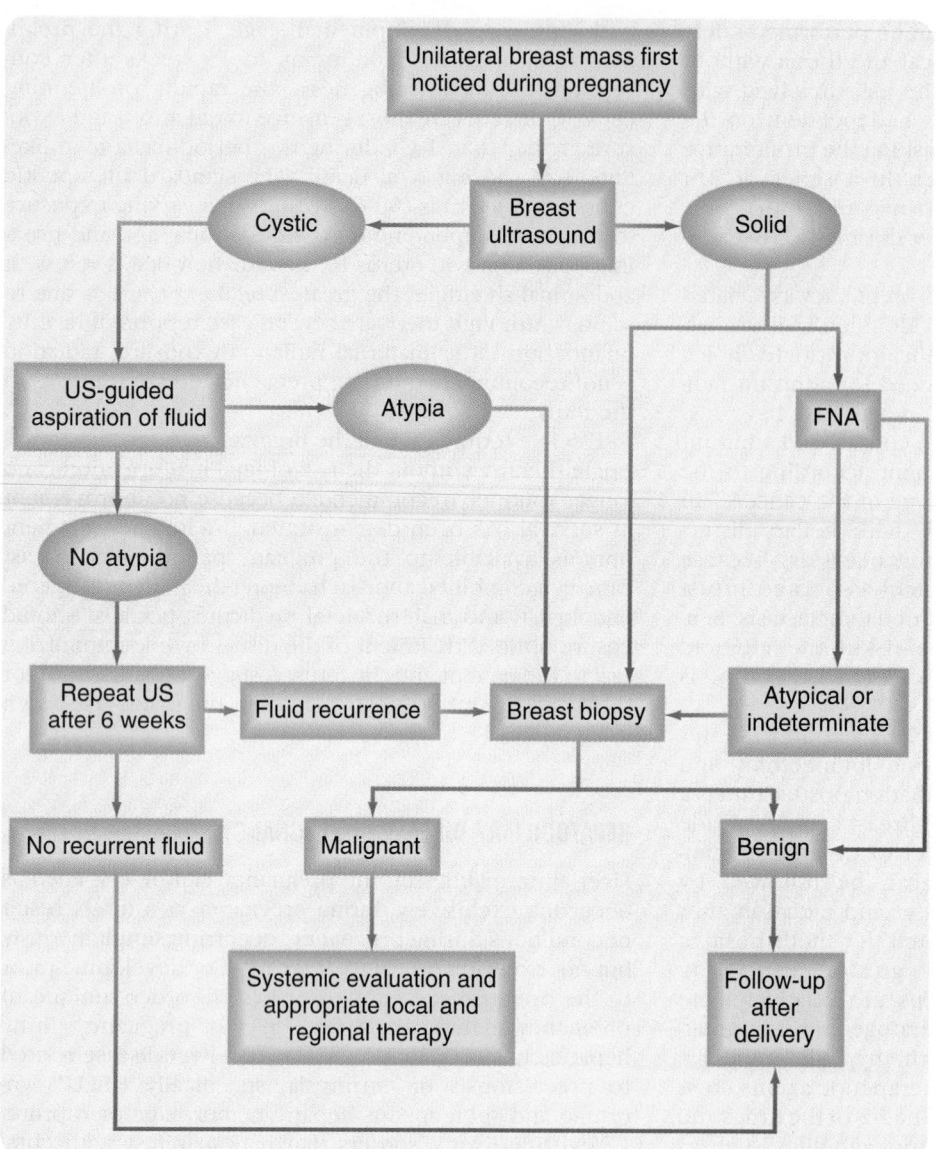

■ **FIGURE 75-1.**   Algorithm for the management of a breast mass during pregnancy. US, ultrasound; FNA, fine-needle aspiration.

from severe elevation of hepatic enzymes to HELLP syndrome to hepatic rupture. Hepatic hemorrhage or rupture occurs primarily during the third trimester or can develop up to 48 hours after delivery. Right upper quadrant pain is the initial manifestation, followed by hepatic tenderness, peritonitis, chest and right shoulder pain, or the development of hemodynamic instability within a few hours. The diagnosis should be suspected in a pregnant patient with preeclampsia who develops right upper quadrant pain. A computed tomographic (CT) scan of the abdomen is highly sensitive and specific in diagnosis; ultrasonography findings are usually nonspecific and have a higher incidence of false-negative studies. The diagnosis may also be made during cesarean section.[25] Management depends on suspicion of ongoing intraperitoneal hemorrhage or vascular instability. Hepatic hematomas without evidence of ongoing bleeding in hemodynamically stable patients may be managed nonoperatively with serial imaging and close monitoring, and these lesions typically heal without intervention. If there is evidence or suspi-

cion of rupture, immediate intervention is required because maternal and fetal mortality from hepatic hemorrhage is 49% and 59%, respectively.[24] Immediate laparotomy with either abdominal packing or hepatic artery ligation reduces maternal and fetal mortality. Coagulopathy should be corrected aggressively. If the patient is relatively stable or abdominal packing has been unsuccessful in controlling hemorrhage, angiography with selective embolization may be performed. Angiography is most useful when the diagnosis is made postpartum.[25]

Hepatic adenomas are uncommon, benign lesions that are usually associated with oral contraceptive use in young women.[26] Hepatic adenomas are also associated with glycogen storage disease, diabetes, exogenous steroids, and pregnancy. They are usually solitary lesions but may be multifocal, and they have a low potential for malignant transformation. Although the specific etiology is unknown, it has been hypothesized that a change in hormone levels, specifically the sex steroids, leads to hepatotoxicity or exposes a hereditary defect in carbohydrate metabolism that results in hepatocyte hyperplasia and adenoma formation. The observation that adenomas may resolve after cessation of exogenous steroid or oral contraceptive use supports this hypothesis. The association of hepatic adenomas with pregnancy supports the hypothesis that elevated levels of endogenous hormones may contribute to adenoma formation, although no data exist showing regression of a hepatic adenoma after pregnancy. Similarly, the true incidence of hepatic adenomas during pregnancy is not known.

The major risk of a hepatic adenoma during pregnancy is spontaneous rupture, which carries a mortality rate of approximately 60% for both mother and fetus[27] even with operative intervention.[28] When spontaneous rupture does occur, the presentation may be similar to that described previously for hepatic hemorrhage associated with preeclampsia: right upper quadrant pain with referred right shoulder pain with progression to shock. Immediate laparotomy should be performed with cesarean section, control of hemorrhage, and resection of the adenoma if possible.

Because of the high mortality associated with rupture of a hepatic adenoma, elective resection may be performed. Resection during the second trimester minimizes operative risk to the mother and fetus and does not interfere with the remainder of the pregnancy or subsequent pregnancies.[26] Because of the unknown recurrence risk, however, subsequent pregnancy and oral contraceptive use may be discouraged in these patients.

Cholecystectomy for symptomatic cholelithiasis is second to appendectomy as the most common nonobstetric surgical procedure performed during pregnancy. As stated earlier, pregnancy is associated with an increased incidence of cholelithiasis. Most pregnant women are asymptomatic. Although an estimated 2% to 4% of pregnant women may be found to have gallstones by ultrasound, only 0.05% to 0.1% of those women will be symptomatic. The symptoms of biliary colic are the same in pregnant and nonpregnant patients. In patients with symptoms consistent with cholelithiasis, ultrasound is the diagnostic examination of choice. In pregnant patients, ultrasound is as accurate in identifying gallstones and signs of inflammation as it is in nonpregnant patients.

Historically, pregnant patients with a clear operative indication, such as obstructive jaundice, gallstone pancreatitis, and choledocholithiasis underwent cholecystectomy regardless of gestational age. Patients with recurrent biliary colic or acute cholecystitis that responded to medical management were treated expectantly until after delivery, at which time they underwent cholecystectomy. As it has become understood that adverse maternal and fetal outcomes are related more to the disease process and not the surgical intervention, management patterns have changed. Additionally, complications from nonoperative management of gallstone disease result in an increase in maternal and fetal mortality. With gallstone pancreatitis during pregnancy, maternal mortality of 15% and fetal mortality of 60% has been reported.[29] Of those patients managed nonoperatively, 35% to 58% developed biliary colic refractory to medical management, requiring multiple hospitalizations.[30] Therefore, surgical intervention should be considered as primary management of gallstones in pregnancy.

The timing of cholecystectomy for biliary colic depends on the gestational age and the severity of symptoms. A spontaneous abortion rate of 12% with open cholecystectomy during the first trimester falls to 5.6% and 0% during the second and third trimesters, respectively. The risk of preterm labor is nearly zero during the second trimester and 40% during the third trimester.[2] The optimum time for cholecystectomy is the second trimester, when the risk of spontaneous abortion and preterm labor are the least, unless the patient develops a complication of cholelithiasis.

Laparoscopic cholecystectomy is relatively safe during the second trimester. The gravid uterus is not usually large enough at this gestational age to interfere with visualization; the uterus also is less likely to be inadvertently instrumented at this size. The open technique using the Hasson trocar is recommended for obtaining access to the abdomen. If intraoperative cholangiography or endoscopic retrograde cholangiopancreatography is indicated for choledocholithiasis, the uterus should be protected with appropriate shielding. If the severity of symptoms prevents delaying surgical intervention until after delivery, laparoscopic cholecystectomy can be safely performed during the third trimester, although the risk of preterm labor is substantially increased. In several small series of patients, preterm labor was successfully managed with tocolytics, and the patients delivered healthy term infants.[30,31]

ENDOCRINE DISEASE IN PREGNANCY

Pheochromocytomas originate from chromaffin cells in the adrenal medulla or from extramedullary paraganglion cells. They are hormonally active tumors, secreting the catecholamines norepinephrine, epinephrine, and, less commonly, dopamine. Pheochromocytomas are usually described by the "rule of 10," which states that 10% of pheochromocytomas are extra-adrenal, 10% are bilateral, 10% are malignant, and 10% are familial. These tumors can occur sporadically or as part of a syndrome, such as multiple endocrine neoplasia (MEN) type 2a, MEN 2b, or von Hippel-Lindau disease.

Although pheochromocytomas are uncommon in pregnancy, they have devastating effects for both mother and fetus. Pheochromocytomas that remain undiagnosed during pregnancy have a postpartum maternal mortality as high as 55%, with fetal mortality also exceeding 50%. The greatest risk occurs from the onset of labor to 48 hours following delivery. The index of suspicion should be high in any patient with preeclampsia, paroxysmal hypertension, or unexplained fever following delivery. With diagnosis and appropriate treatment, maternal mortality is reduced to nearly 0%, and fetal mortality is decreased to 15%.[32] Diagnosis is made by elevated urine catecholamines; urinary catecholamines in the pregnant patient without a pheochromocytoma are the same as in the nonpregnant patient. Lack of proteinuria also helps eliminate preeclampsia as a cause of hypertension.

Metaiodobenzylguanidine (MIBG) imaging is not recommended during pregnancy, because the small molecule may cross the placenta; use of MIBG imaging has not been evaluated in pregnancy.

Surgical resection should be performed prior to 20 weeks' gestation, when spontaneous abortion is less likely and the size of the gravid uterus does not interfere with the procedure. If the diagnosis is made late in the second trimester or during the third trimester, medical management followed by combined cesarean section and resection of the pheochromocytoma may be an option. It is unknown if the standard preoperative management with α blockade or calcium-channel blockade followed by perioperative β blockade in nonpregnant patients is safe during pregnancy. The long-term effects of the α blocker phenoxybenzamine on the fetus have not been determined, although calcium-channel blockers are safe to use during pregnancy. β Blockers are frequently used during pregnancy with close monitoring for intrauterine growth retardation. Consultation with a maternal-fetal medicine specialist is essential to determine the preoperative management that will ensure the optimal postoperative result for the patient and fetus. In nonpregnant patients, the method of approach depends on suspected malignancy, unilateral versus bilateral tumors, extra-adrenal location, size of the tumor, and surgeon's preference and experience. In all series comparing the different approaches, including open versus laparoscopic technique, pregnant patients were not included. In a small series, two pregnant patients who underwent transperitoneal laparoscopic adrenalectomy delivered healthy infants at term.[33]

SMALL BOWEL DISEASE IN PREGNANCY

Intestinal obstruction is the third most common nonobstetric surgical issue in pregnancy behind acute appendicitis and acute cholecystitis. The incidence of small bowel obstruction during pregnancy is similar to that in the general population (1/3000). Adhesions resulting from prior abdominal and pelvic surgeries are the most frequent causes for intestinal obstruction in pregnancy, accounting for 53% to 59% of cases.[34] Other causes of small bowel obstruction in the pregnant patient include volvulus, intussusception, malignancy, or hernia, although the displacement of the small bowel out of the pelvis by the enlarging uterus makes this a rare cause. There has been one reported case of spontaneous bowel obstruction in a patient pregnant with triplets with none of the risk factors for small bowel obstruction.[34]

The symptoms of an obstruction are identical to those in the nonpregnant patient and consist of the triad of abdominal pain, vomiting, and obstipation. Pain, present in 85% to 98% of cases, is usually colicky in nature and located in the mid-abdomen, although the character and duration are highly variable. Nausea and vomiting are seen in 80% of pregnant patients with small bowel obstruction; however, nausea and vomiting are not uncommon during the first trimester of normal pregnancy. Nausea and vomiting that persist or begin later in pregnancy should arouse suspicion and be evaluated. Bowel distention may be marked but difficult to assess due to the gravid uterus. Diagnosis is made by serial examination and plain abdominal radiograph.

Treatment for small bowel obstruction in pregnancy is identical to that in the nonpregnant patient. Therapy consists of nasogastric decompression and intravenous fluids. However, a lower threshold for operative management is necessary. If after 6 to 8 hours of nonoperative treatment there is no satisfactory patient response, a laparotomy should be performed before perforation or bowel necrosis occurs. Maternal mortality ranges from 6% to 20% due to sepsis and multisystem organ failure, and fetal loss is as high as 26% to 50%.[34] To avoid the risk to the mother and fetus, a more aggressive approach should be used.

COLON AND RECTUM IN PREGNANCY

Acute appendicitis is the most common nonobstetric surgical problem in the pregnant patient, occurring in 1 in 1500 pregnancies. The incidence of acute appendicitis is fairly evenly distributed among the trimesters of pregnancy, with a slight predominance during the second trimester. Timely and accurate diagnosis is challenging because the typical clinical findings of nausea, vomiting, abdominal pain, and mild leukocytosis may be findings in a normal pregnancy. Delay in diagnosis results in an increased perforation rate of 10%. This has significant consequences for the patient and fetus. Fetal mortality increases from 5% in acute appendicitis to 30% in perforated appendicitis.[35-38] Preterm labor and premature delivery rates are as high as 40% in perforated appendicitis[36-38] compared to a 13% rate of preterm labor and 4% rate of premature delivery in acute appendicitis.[39] As early as 1908, Babler indicated the significance of this problem when he wrote, "The mortality of appendicitis complicating pregnancy is the mortality of delay."[40]

In 1932, Baer studied 78 normal pregnant women with radiographic studies at regular intervals from the second month of pregnancy to 10 days postpartum. Patients were given barium meals 18 hours before examinations. Upright and dorsal films were taken. The films showed that the enlarging uterus pushes the appendix upward with a counterclockwise rotation of the appendiceal tip. From this progressive displacement of the appendix toward the right upper quadrant, Baer deduced that early in pregnancy pain from appendicitis is low and that as the gestation progresses (and appendiceal displacement occurs), the pain is located higher in the abdomen.[41] He postulated that the nearer the pregnancy to term, the higher the point of maximum tenderness. Some controversy exists, however. A review of 45 pregnant patients with acute appendicitis demonstrated that pain in the right lower quadrant is the most common symptom regardless of gestational age (first trimester, 86%; second trimester, 83%; third trimester, 85%).[39] Despite the inconsistency, acute appendicitis should be included in the differential diagnosis of every pregnant woman who presents with right-sided abdominal pain.

The treatment for suspected acute appendicitis in the pregnant patient is emergent appendectomy. Although helical CT scans have demonstrated higher than 90% sensitivity and specificity in the diagnosis of acute appendicitis, little data are available in pregnant patients. In nonpregnant patients, a 10% to 15% negative laparotomy rate is considered to be acceptable. Because of the increased risk to both mother and fetus with appendiceal perforation, a negative rate of 30% to 33% is acceptable. The debate is then for open or laparoscopic technique. The argument for open appendectomy is that the laparoscopic approach exposes the fetus to the risks of pneumoperitoneum and trocar placement without the benefit of a significantly smaller incision. The laparoscopic technique enables examination of a larger portion of the abdomen with less uterine manipulation and allows location of the appendix as the appendix is pushed into the right upper quadrant by the enlarging uterus.

Colonic pseudo-obstruction, or Ogilvie's syndrome, is a functional obstruction, or adynamic ileus, without a mechanical etiology. Ten percent of all cases of Ogilvie's syndrome occur in postpartum patients. It is characterized by massive abdominal distention with cecal dilation. Although neostigmine is an effective first-line therapy in nonpregnant patients, its safety in pregnancy is unknown. It can be used safely in the postpartum period. Colonoscopic decompression has been described in postpartum patients, with laparotomy indicated only in suspected perforation.

VASCULAR DISEASE IN PREGNANCY

Of more than 400 cases of ruptured splenic artery aneurysms in the literature, about 100 cases of ruptured splenic artery aneurysm during pregnancy have been reported, with only 12 cases of maternal and fetal survival.[42] Rupture occurred during the third trimester in two thirds of the cases and was typically misdiagnosed as splenic rupture or uterine rupture. Maternal mortality was 75% with a fetal mortality of 95%. Increased portal pressures, high splenic artery flow due to distal aortic compression, and progressive arterial wall weakening are contributing factors. Multiparity may increase the risk; 78% of patients with ruptured splenic artery aneurysms have been in their third pregnancy. Survival is most likely related to a "two-stage rupture," in which the lesser sac temporarily tamponades the bleeding aneurysm.

When treated electively in nonpregnant patients, mortality is only 0.5% to 1.3%. When the diagnosis is made in a woman of childbearing age or in a pregnant patient, a splenic artery aneurysm of 2 cm or larger should be treated electively due to the increased risk of rupture during pregnancy.[42]

Acute iliofemoral venous thrombosis is six times more frequent among pregnant than nonpregnant patients. Pregnancy may increase the risk of thrombosis through a number of factors, including mechanical obstruction of venous drainage by the enlarging uterus, decreased activity in late pregnancy and at time of delivery, intimal injury from vascular distention or surgical manipulation during cesarean section, and abnormal levels of coagulation factors already described.[43] Additionally, a wide spectrum

of pathologic abnormalities such as the presence of lupus anticoagulant antibodies and deficiencies of proteins C and S may further increase the risk of thrombotic disease. Protein S serves as a cofactor for activated protein C, which has anticoagulant activity. Therefore, a deficiency of protein S leads to spontaneous, recurrent thromboembolic complications in nonpregnant adults. Even in normal individuals, protein S levels are substantially reduced during pregnancy.

The management of acute iliofemoral venous thrombosis during pregnancy is controversial because thrombolytic therapy poses hazards to the fetus. The risk of pulmonary thromboembolism with manipulation of the clot during thrombectomy would have catastrophic effects on both the patient and the fetus. Techniques that have been described include interruption of the inferior vena cava via a right retroperitoneal approach or interruption of the inferior vena cava passage of a Fogarty catheter through the unaffected contralateral femoral vein. The disadvantage of the retroperitoneal approach is that an extensive dissection is required. The disadvantages of the Fogarty catheter are that the catheter may still dislodge clots that have extended into the vena cava and that once the catheter is removed, an inferior vena cava filter must still be placed. However, the most effective technique is filter placement in the inferior vena cava via the internal jugular vein using ultrasound guidance, followed by thrombectomy.

TRAUMA IN PREGNANCY

Trauma is the leading nonobstetric cause of maternal mortality and occurs in as many as 7% of pregnancies.[44] The most common mechanisms of injury are from falls or from motor vehicle crashes.[45] When compared to age-matched pregnant controls, pregnant women who sustained trauma had a higher incidence of spontaneous abortion, preterm labor, fetomaternal hemorrhage, abruptio placentae, and uterine rupture.[46] Multiple studies have attempted to identify risk factors that predict morbidity and mortality in the pregnant trauma patient. The maternal Injury Severity Score, mechanism of injury, and physical findings are unable to adequately predict adverse outcomes such as abruptio placentae and fetal loss.[47] Early involvement of an available obstetrician is important to evaluate both maternal and fetal well-being.

In the management of the pregnant trauma patient, the critical point is that resuscitation of the fetus is accomplished by resuscitation of the mother. Therefore, the initial evaluation and treatment of the pregnant injured patient is identical to that of the nonpregnant injured patient. Rapid assessment of the maternal airway, breathing, and circulation and ensuring an adequate airway avoids maternal and fetal hypoxia. In the later stages of pregnancy, as already described, uterine compression of the vena cava may result in hypotension from diminished venous return, so the pregnant trauma patient should be placed in left lateral decubitus position. If spinal cord injury is suspected, the patient may be secured to a backboard and then tilted to the left.

The increased blood volume associated with pregnancy has important implications in the trauma patient. Signs of blood loss such as tachycardia and hypotension may be delayed until the patient loses nearly 30% of her blood volume. As a result, the fetus may be experiencing hypoperfusion long before the mother manifests any signs. Early and rapid fluid resuscitation should be administered even in the pregnant patient who is normotensive.

As with the primary survey, the secondary survey should proceed in a similar fashion as in the nonpregnant patient. Special attention should be given to the abdominal examination. The uterus remains protected by the pelvis until approximately 12 weeks' gestation and is relatively well sheltered from the abdominal injury until that time. As the uterus grows, it becomes more prominent and more vulnerable to injury. Measurement of fundal height provides a rapid approximation of gestational age. At 20 weeks' gestation, it should be at the level of the umbilicus and should be approximately 1 cm per week of gestation. Intrauterine hemorrhage or uterine rupture may result in a discrepancy in measurement. A pelvic examination should be performed, by an obstetrician if possible, to evaluate for vaginal bleeding, ruptured membranes, or a bulging perineum. Vaginal bleeding may indicate abruptio placentae, placenta previa, or preterm labor. Rupture of the amniotic fluid may result in umbilical cord prolapse, which compresses the umbilical vessels and compromises fetal blood flow. This requires immediate cesarean section. If cloudy white or greenish fluid is seen from the cervical os or perineum, the presence of amniotic fluid is confirmed by Nitrazine paper, which changes from green to blue.

The Kleihauer-Betke (K-B) test for the assessment of fetomaternal transfusion is useful after maternal trauma and should be ordered with the initial laboratory studies that include a type and crossmatch. Because of the sensitivity of the K-B test, a small amount of fetomaternal transfusion may be undetected. Therefore, all Rh-negative pregnant trauma patients should be considered for Rh immunoglobulin (RhoGAM) therapy.

The most common cause of fetal death after blunt injury is abruptio placentae. Deceleration of the fetal heart rate may be the earliest sign of abruption. The uterus should be evaluated for contractions, rupture, or abruptio placentae. Early initiation of cardiotocographic fetal monitoring adequately warns of deterioration in the condition of the fetus.

SUMMARY

Pregnant patients are susceptible to the same surgical diseases as nonpregnant patients of similar age. Maternal physiologic changes as well as the enlarging uterus may result in atypical presentation of surgical disease, or symptoms may be attributed to normal pregnancy. A delay in diagnosis and treatment of surgical illnesses in pregnancy poses a greater risk to maternal and fetal well-being than the risks of anesthesia or of surgical intervention. Early consultation with an obstetrician, maternal-fetal medicine specialist, and perinatologist can ensure optimal out-

comes and avoid pitfalls. Laparoscopy is becoming increasingly accepted in the pregnant patient, and future advances will hopefully make it even safer for obstetric patients. Preterm labor prevention should be individualized given the patient's gestational age and underlying disease process.

Selected References

Babler EA: Perforative appendicitis complicating pregnancy. JAMA 51:1310, 1908.

> **Landmark article first describing appendicitis in pregnancy.**

Baer JL: Appendicitis in pregnancy. JAMA 98:1359, 1932.

> **Landmark article illustrating the change in appendiceal location during pregnancy.**

Brodsky JB, Cohen EN, Brown BW Jr, et al: Surgery during pregnancy and fetal outcome. Am J Obstet Gynecol 138:1165, 1980.

> **Large series that first looked at fetal outcomes in nonobstetric surgery.**

Mourad J, Elliott JP, Erickson L, et al: Appendicitis in pregnancy: New information that contradicts longheld clinical beliefs. Am J Obstet Gynecol 182:1027, 2000.

> **This paper, which retrospectively reviewed more than 66,000 deliveries and found 45 pregnant patients with appendicitis, challenged the original landmark paper by Baer regarding the presentation of acute appendicitis in pregnant patients.**

Society of American Gastrointestinal Endoscopic Surgeons: Guidelines for laparoscopic surgery during pregnancy. Surg Endosc 12:189, 1998.

> **Current guidelines for laparoscopy in pregnancy.**

Tarraza HM, Moore RD: Gynecologic causes of the acute abdomen and the acute abdomen in pregnancy. Surg Clin North Am 77:1371, 1997.

> **Current review that accurately describes the increased risk to the mother and fetus due to the underlying pathology as opposed to the risk imposed by surgical intervention.**

Woo JC, Yu T, Hurd TC: Breast cancer in pregnancy. Arch Surg 138:91, 2003.

> **The most current comprehensive review of breast cancer in pregnancy, including the ongoing trends in treatment.**

References

1. Cruikshank DP, Wigton TR, Hays PM: Maternal physiology in pregnancy. *In* Gabbe SG (ed): Obstetrics: Normal and Problem Pregnancies. New York, Churchill Livingstone, 1996, pp 91-109.
2. Ghumman E, Barry M, Grace PA: Management of gallstones in pregnancy. Br J Surg 84:1646, 1997.
3. Mayr NA, Wen BC, Saw CB: Radiation therapy during pregnancy. Obstet Gynecol Clin North Am 25:301, 1998.
4. Pelsang R: Diagnostic imaging modalities during pregnancy. Obstet Gynecol Clin North Am 25:287, 1998.

5. Rosen MA: Management of anesthesia for the pregnant surgical patient. Anesthesiology 91:1159, 1999.

6. Brodsky JB, Cohen EN, Brown BW Jr, et al: Surgery during pregnancy and fetal outcome. Am J Obstet Gynecol 138:1165, 1980.

7. Tarraza HM, Moore RD: Gynecologic causes of the acute abdomen and the acute abdomen in pregnancy. Surg Clin North Am 77:1371, 1997.

8. Lemaire BMD, van Erp WFM: Laparoscopic surgery during pregnancy. Surg Endosc 11:15, 1997.

9. Thomas SJ, Brisson P: Laparoscopic appendectomy and cholecystectomy during pregnancy: Six case reports. J Soc Laparoendosc Surg 2:41, 1998.

10. Hunter JG, Swanstrom L, Thornburg K: Carbon dioxide pneumoperitoneum induces fetal acidosis in a pregnant ewe model. Surg Endosc 9:272, 1995.

11. Curet MJ: Special problems in laparoscopic surgery: Previous abdominal surgery, obesity, and pregnancy: Surg Clin North Am 80:1093, 2000.

12. Society of American Gastrointestinal Endoscopic Surgeons: Guidelines for laparoscopic surgery during pregnancy. Surg Endosc 12:189, 1998.

13. Uen Y, Liang A, Lee H : Randomized comparison of conventional carbon dioxide insufflation and abdominal wall lifting for laparoscopic cholecystectomy. J Laparoendosc Surg 12:7, 2002.

14. Anderson B, Petrek J, Bryon D, et al: Pregnancy influences breast cancer stage at diagnosis in women 30 years and younger. Ann Surg Oncol 3:204, 1996.

15. Falkenberry SS: Breast cancer in pregnancy. Obstet Gynecol Clin North Am 29:225, 2002.

16. Johannsson O, Loman N, Borg A, Olsson H.: Pregnancy-associated breast cancer in *BRCA1* and *BRCA2* germ-line mutation carriers. Lancet 352:1359, 1998.

17. Ishida T, Yokoe T, Kasumi F, et al: Clinicopathological characteristics and prognosis of breast cancer patients associated with pregnancy and lactation: Analysis of case-control study in Japan. Jpn J Cancer Res 83:1143, 1992.

18. Woo JC, Yu T, Hurd TC: Breast cancer in pregnancy. Arch Surg 138:91, 2003.

19. Gemignani ML, Petrek JA, Borgen PI, et al: Breast cancer and pregnancy. Surg Clin North Am 79:1157, 1999.

20. Petrek J, Dukoff R, Rogatko A: Prognosis of pregnancy associated with breast cancer. Cancer 67:869, 1991.

21. Gupta R, McHutchinson A, Dowle C, et al: Fine-needle aspiration cytodiagnosis of breast masses in pregnant and lactating women and its impact on management. Diagn Cytopathol 9:156, 1993.

22. Bonnier P, Romain S, Dilhuydy J, et al: Influence of pregnancy on the outcome of breast cancer: A case-control study. Int J Cancer 72:720, 1997.

23. Berry D, Theriault R, Holmes F, et al: Management of breast cancer during pregnancy using a standardized protocol. J Clin Oncol 17:855, 1999.

24. Borum ML: Hepatobiliary diseases in women. Med Clin North Am 82:51, 1998.

25. Stain SC, Woodburn DA, Stephens AL: Spontaneous hepatic hemorrhage associated with pregnancy. Ann Surg 224:72, 1996.

26. Hill MA, Albert T, Zieske A, et al: Successful resection of multifocal hepatic adenoma during pregnancy. South Med J 90:357, 1997.

27. Monks PL, Fryar BG, Biggs WW: Spontaneous rupture of an hepatic adenoma in pregnancy with survival of mother and fetus. Aust N Z J Obstet Gynaecol 26:155, 1986.

28. Rosel HD, Baier A, Mesewinkel F: Exsanguination caused by liver cell adenoma and rupture of the hepatic capsule as cause of maternal death. Zentralbl Gynakol 112:1363, 1990.

29. Printen KJ, Ott RA: Cholecystectomy during pregnancy. Am Surg 44:432, 1978.

30. Gouldman JW, Sticca RP, Rippon MB: Laparoscopic cholecystectomy in pregnancy. Am Surg 64:93, 1998.

31. Eichenberg BJ, Vanderlinden J, Miguel C, et al: Laparoscopic cholecystectomy in the third trimester of pregnancy. Am Surg 62:874, 1996.

32. Janetschek G, Finkenstedt G, Gasser R, et al: Laparoscopic surgery for pheochromocytoma: Adrenalectomy, partial resection, excision of paragangliomas. J Urol 160:330, 1998.

33. Janetschek G, Neumann HPH: Laparoscopic surgery for pheochromocytoma. Urol Clin North Am 28:1, 2001.

34. Meyerson S, Holtz T, Ehrinpreis M, et al: Small bowel obstruction in pregnancy. Am J Gastroenterol 90:299, 1995.

35. Gurbuz AT, Peetz ME: The acute abdomen in the pregnant patient: Is there a role for laparoscopy? Surg Endosc 11:98, 1997.

36. Kammerer WS: Nonobstetric surgery during pregnancy. Med Clin North Am 63:1157, 1979.

37. Kort B, Katz VI, Watson WJ: The effect of nonobstetric operation during pregnancy. Surg Gynecol Obstet 177:371, 1993.

38. Schreiber JH: Laparoscopic appendectomy in pregnancy. Surg Endosc 4:100, 1990.

39. Mourad J, Elliott JP, Erickson L, et al: Appendicitis in pregnancy: New information that contradicts long-held clinical beliefs. Am J Obstet Gynecol 182:1027, 2000.

40. Babler EA: Perforative appendicitis complicating pregnancy. JAMA 51:1310, 1908.

41. Baer JL: Appendicitis in pregnancy. JAMA 98:1359, 1932.

42. Herbeck M, Horbach T, Putzenlechner C, et al: Ruptured splenic artery aneurysm during pregnancy: A rare case with both maternal and fetal survival. Am J Obstet Gynecol 181:763, 1999.

43. Neri E, Civeli L, Benvenuti A, et al: Protected iliofemoral venous thrombectomy in a pregnant woman with pulmonary embolism and ischemic venous thrombosis. Tex Heart Inst J 29:130, 2002.

44. Esposito TJ, Gens DR, Smith LG, et al: Trauma during pregnancy: A review of 79 cases. Arch Surg 126:1073, 1991.

45. Schiff MA, Holt VL, Daling JR: Maternal and infant outcomes after injury during pregnancy in Washington State from 1989 to 1997. J Trauma 53:939, 2002.

46. Pak LL, Reece EA, Chan L: Is adverse pregnancy outcome predictable after blunt abdominal trauma? Am J Obstet Gynecol 179:1140, 1998.

47. Pearlman MD, Tintinalli JE, Lorenz RP: A prospective controlled study of outcome after trauma during pregnancy. Am J Obstet Gynecol 162:1502, 1990.

UROLOGIC SURGERY

Aria F. Olumi, M.D. and **Jerome P. Richie, M.D.**

Anatomy	Neurogenic Bladder
Urologic Trauma	Benign Prostatic Hyperplasia
Emergent Urologic Conditions	Scrotal Masses
Nephrolithiasis	Urologic Malignancies

The field of urology has undergone unprecedented advances over the past decade. Advances in treatment of erectile dysfunction, laparoscopic and minimally invasive surgery, and reconstructive urology are some of the highlights. The focus in this chapter is on general urologic issues with special emphasis on issues pertinent to the general surgeon. We review anatomy of the genitourinary system, urologic trauma, emergent urologic conditions, nephrolithiasis, neurogenic bladder, benign prostatic hyperplasia, scrotal masses, and urologic malignancies.

ANATOMY

Retroperitoneum

The retroperitoneum is bounded anteriorly by the peritoneal sac and its contents (Fig. 76-1), is separated from the thorax superiorly by the muscular diaphragm, and is contiguous with the extraperitoneal portions of the pelvis inferiorly. The body wall creates the posterior and lateral limits of the retroperitoneum, and incisions through the posterolateral abdominal wall, or flank, provide the most direct routes to the structures of the retroperitoneum.

Adrenal Glands

The adrenal, or suprarenal glands are paired, yellow-orange, solid endocrine organs that lie within the perirenal (Gerota's) fascia superomedial to either kidney, buried within the perinephric fat. Although closely applied to the upper poles of the kidneys, the adrenals are embryologically and functionally distinct and are physically separated

from the kidneys by connective tissue septa in continuity with Gerota's fascia as well as by varying amounts of perinephric adipose tissue. Thus, in cases of renal ectopia, the adrenal gland is usually found in approximately its normal anatomic position and does not follow the kidney. Similarly, in cases of renal agenesis, the adrenal on the involved side is typically present (in greater than 90% of such cases).

The normal adult adrenal gland weighs approximately 5 g and measures 3 to 5 cm in greatest transverse dimension. In the neonate, the adrenals are relatively much larger in size compared with total body mass and may be one third of the size of the kidney at birth (Fig. 76-2). Both adrenals are somewhat flattened in the anteroposterior axis, the left more so than the right. The right gland assumes a more pyramidal shape and rests more superior to the upper pole of the right kidney. The left gland is more crescentic and rests more medial to the upper pole of the left kidney; in fact, it may lie directly atop the renal vessels at the left renal hilum. The right adrenal thus tends to lie more superiorly in the retroperitoneum than does the left adrenal. This is in contradistinction to the fact that the right kidney lies, in general, slightly more inferiorly than the left, and this fact must be taken into account in the planning of incisions for adrenal surgery.

Each adrenal is a composite of two separate and functionally distinct glandular elements: cortex and medulla. The medulla, which forms the central core of each adrenal, consists of chromaffin cells derived from the neural crest and intimately related to the sympathetic nervous system. The cells of the medulla produce neuroactive catecholamines, primarily epinephrine and norepinephrine, which are released directly into the bloodstream through an extensive venous drainage system. The adrenal cortex is mesodermally derived, com-

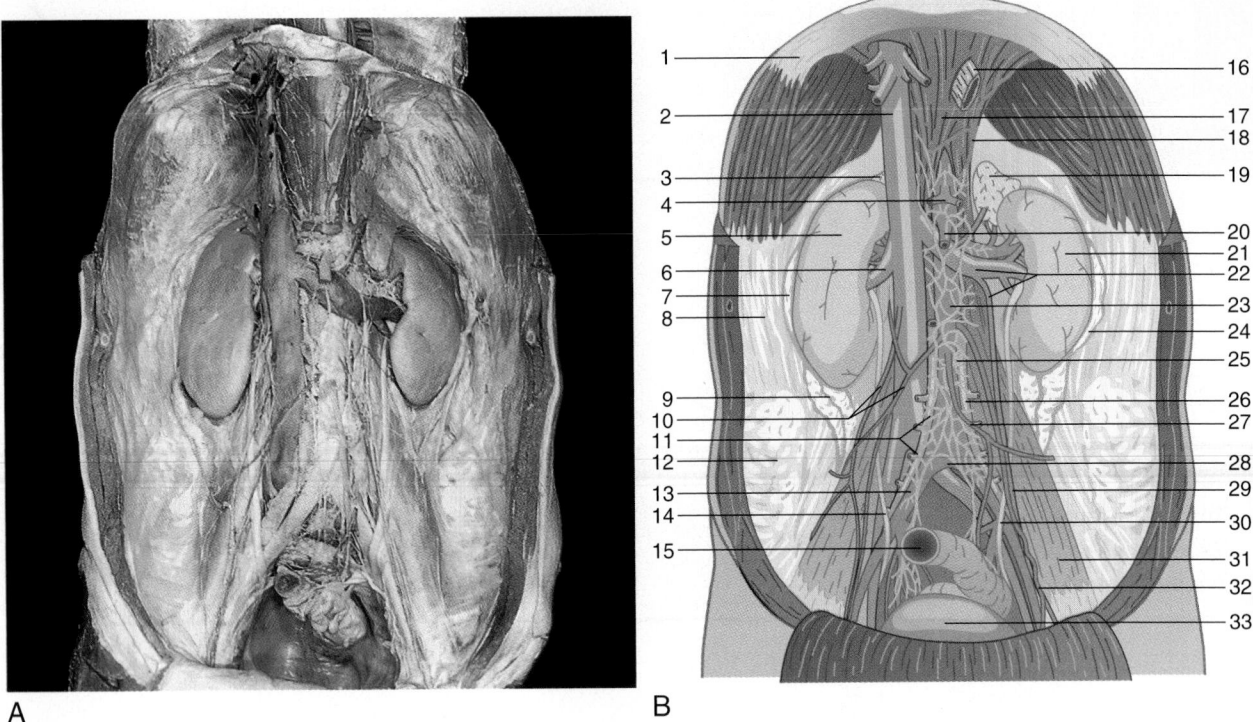

FIGURE 76-1. **A** and **B,** The retroperitoneum dissected. The anterior perirenal fascia (Gerota's fascia) has been dissected. 1, diaphragm; 2, inferior vena cava; 3, right adrenal gland; 4, upper pointer at celiac artery, lower pointer at celiac autonomic nervous plexus; 5, right kidney; 6, right renal vein; 7, Gerota's fascia; 8, pararenal retroperitoneal fat; 9, perinephric fat; 10, upper pointer at right gonadal vein, lower pointer at right gonadal artery; 11, lumbar lymph node; 12, retroperitoneal fat; 13, right common iliac artery; 14, right ureter; 15, sigmoid colon (cut); 16, esophagus (cut); 17, right crus of diaphragm; 18, left inferior phrenic artery; 19, upper pointer at left adrenal gland, lower pointer at left adrenal vein; 20, upper pointer at superior mesenteric artery, lower pointer at left renal artery; 21, left kidney; 22, upper pointer at left renal vein, lower pointer at left gonadal vein; 23, aorta; 24, perinephric fat; 25, aortic autonomic nervous plexus; 26, upper pointer at Gerota's fascia, lower pointer at inferior mesenteric ganglion; 27, inferior mesenteric artery; 28, aortic bifurcation into common iliac arteries; 29, left gonadal artery and vein; 30, left ureter; 31, psoas major muscle covered by psoas sheath; 32, cut edge of peritoneum; 33, pelvic cavity.

pletely surrounds and encases the medulla, and forms the bulk of the adrenal gland, which is 80% to 90% by weight. Three cell layers can be identified in the cortex. The outermost layer is the zona glomerulosa, which produces aldosterone in response to stimulation by the renin-angiotensin system. Centripetally located are the zona fasciculata and zona reticularis, which produce glucocorticoids and sex steroids, respectively. Unlike the zona glomerulosa, these latter functions are regulated by pituitary release of adrenocorticotropic hormone (ACTH). The substance of the adrenal gland is inherently quite friable but is enclosed by a thick, collagenous capsule; yet it still can be readily torn with aggressive handling at the time of operation.

The adrenals, concordant with their key role in the body's hormonal milieu, are highly vascularized. The arterial supply is relatively symmetrical bilaterally. Multiple small arteries supply each adrenal gland. These are branch vessels, which can be traced to three major arterial sources for each gland: (1) superior branches from the

inferior phrenic artery, (2) middle branches directly from the aorta, and (3) inferior branches from the ipsilateral renal artery. In contrast to the multiple arteries, usually a single large adrenal vein exits each gland from its hilum anteromedially. On the right side, this vein is very short and enters directly into the inferior vena cava on its posterolateral aspect. The adrenal vein on the left is more elongated and is typically joined by the left inferior phrenic vein before entering the superior aspect of the left renal vein. The adrenal lymphatics in general exit the glands along the course of the venous drainage and eventually empty into para-aortic lymph nodes.

The adrenal medulla receives greater autonomic innervation than any other organ in the body. Multiple preganglionic sympathetic fibers enter each adrenal along the course of the adrenal vein and synapse with chromaffin cells in the medulla. This rich sympathetic innervation of the medulla reaches the adrenal via the splanchnic nerves and celiac ganglion. In contrast, the adrenal cortex is believed to receive no innervation.

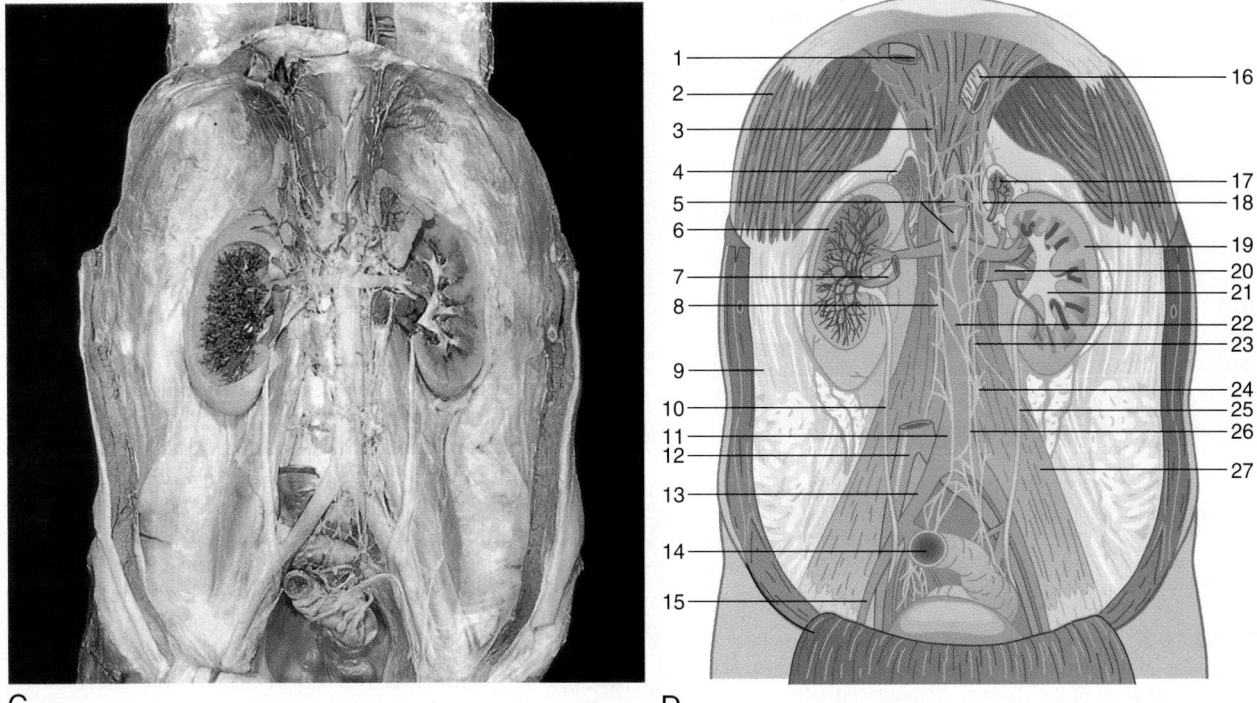

FIGURE 76-1—Continued   C and **D,** The retroperitoneum dissected. Kidneys and adrenal glands have been sectioned and the inferior vena cava has been excised over most of its intra-abdominal course. 1, inferior vena cava (cut); 2, diaphragm; 3, right inferior phrenic artery; 4, right adrenal gland; 5, upper pointer at celiac artery, lower pointer at superior mesenteric artery; 6, right kidney; 7, upper pointer at right renal artery, lower pointer at right renal vein (cut); 8, lumbar lymph node; 9, transversus abdominis muscle covered with transversalis fascia; 10, right ureter; 11, anterior spinous ligament; 12, inferior vena cava (cut); 15, right external iliac artery; 16, esophagus (cut); 17, left adrenal gland; 18, celiac ganglion; 19, left kidney; 20, upper pointer at left renal artery, lower pointer at left renal vein (cut); 21, left renal pelvis; 22, aorta; 23, aortic autonomic nervous plexus; 24, inferior mesenteric ganglion; 25, left ureter; 26, inferior mesenteric artery; 27, psoas major muscle covered by psoas sheath. (Reproduced with permission from Kabalin J: Surgical anatomy of the retroperitoneum, kidneys, and ureters. In Walsh PC, Retik AB, Vaughan ED Jr, et al [eds]: Campbell's Urology, 8th ed. Philadelphia, Elsevier, 2002, pp 4-7).

Kidneys and Ureters

The kidneys are paired solid organs that lie in the retroperitoneum along the borders of the psoas muscle (see Fig. 76-1). The kidneys and associated adrenal glands are surrounded by perirenal fat, which is enclosed in perinephric fascia, known as Gerota's fascia. Gerota's fascia forms an important anatomic barrier around the kidney and tends to contain pathologic processes originating from the kidney. Superiorly, Gerota's fascia fuses and tapers to disappear over the inferior diaphragmatic surface. Medially, Gerota's fascia extends across the midline and is contiguous with Gerota's fascia on the contralateral side, although the anterior and posterior leaves are generally fused and inseparable as they cross the great vessels. Inferiorly, Gerota's fascia remains an open potential space, containing the ureter and gonadal vessels on either side.

Each kidney is positioned obliquely, and awareness of the anatomic relationship of the kidneys to the surrounding organs is paramount. The posterior relations of the kidneys to the abdominal wall musculature are relatively symmetrical (Fig. 76-3). The 12th rib crosses the upper third of each kidney. Because the left kidney lies more cephalad than the right kidney, the 11th rib lies directly posterior to the upper aspect of the left kidney and not the right kidney (see Fig. 76-3). As a result of the contour of the psoas muscle, both kidneys lie obliquely with the upper pole more medially located than the lower pole. In addition, each kidney does not lie in a simple coronal plane and the lower pole is pushed more anteriorly than the upper pole of each kidney.

In contrast to the similarities of posterior anatomic relations in each kidney, the anterior relation of each kidney is significantly different. The right kidney lies behind the liver, and it is separated from the liver by reflection of the peritoneum, except for a small area of its upper pole, which comes into direct contact with the liver's retroperitoneal bare spot. The extension of parietal peritoneum

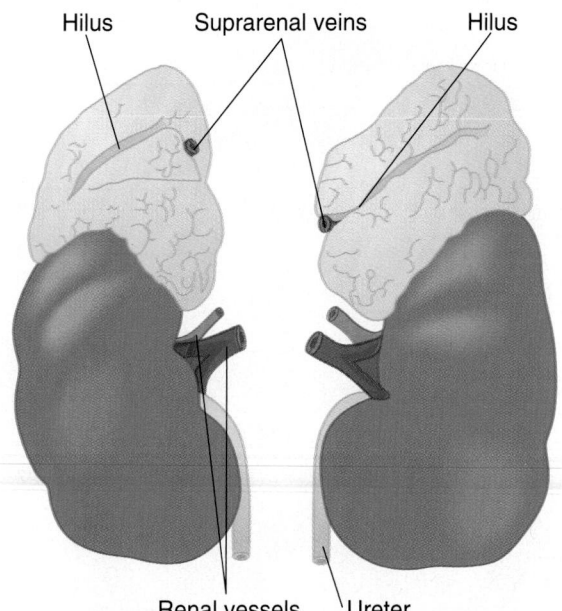

■ FIGURE 76-2. Kidneys and adrenal glands from neonate. Note large size of the adrenal glands relative to the kidneys, and note the fetal lobation of the kidneys. (Reproduced with permission from Kabalin J: Surgical anatomy of the retroperitoneum, kidneys, and ureters. In Walsh PC, Retik AB, Vaughan ED, et al [eds]: Campbell's Urology, 8th ed. Philadelphia, Elsevier, 2002, p 21.)

that bridges between the perirenal fascia covering the upper pole of the right kidney and the posterior aspect of the liver is called the *hepatorenal ligament.* Excessive traction on this attachment or the hepatocolic ligament during right renal surgery may produce hepatic parenchymal tears. The duodenum is applied directly to the medial aspect and hilar structures of the right kidney (see Figs. 76-1 and 76-3). The hepatic flexure of the colon, which also is extraperitoneal, crosses the lower pole of the right kidney. The adrenal gland covers the superomedial aspect of the upper poles of both right and left kidneys, as already discussed.

On the left, the retroperitoneal tail of the pancreas and the related splenic vessels are applied directly to the upper to middle portion and hilum of the kidney. Superior to the pancreatic tail, the left kidney is covered by peritoneum of the lesser sac and here is related to the posterior gastric wall. Below the pancreatic tail, the medial aspect of the kidney is covered by peritoneum of the greater sac and is related to the jejunum. The lower pole of the left kidney is crossed by the splenic flexure of the colon, generally in an extraperitoneal position. The spleen is separated from the upper lateral portion of the left kidney by peritoneal reflection. However, there is typically a peritoneal extension between the perirenal fascia covering the upper pole of the left kidney and the inferior splenic capsule, called the *splenorenal,* or *lienorenal,* ligament. Just as with the adjacent and often contiguous

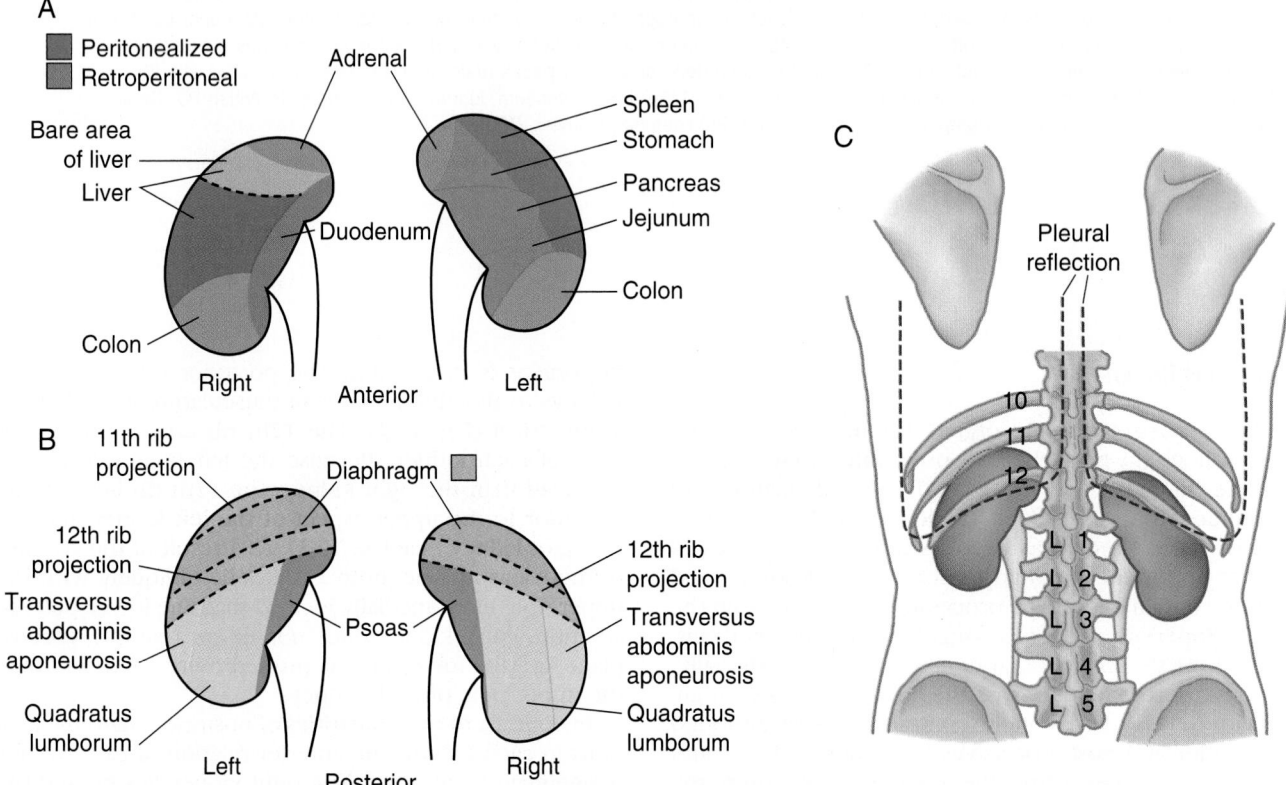

■ FIGURE 76-3. Anatomic relations of the kidneys. **A,** Anterior relations to the abdominal organs. **B,** Posterior relations to the muscles of the posterior body wall and ribs. **C,** Relations to the pleural reflections and skeleton posteriorly. (Reproduced with permission from Kabalin J: Surgical anatomy of the retroperitoneum, kidneys, and ureters. In Walsh PC, Retik AB, Vaughan ED Jr, et al [eds]: Campbell's Urology, 8th ed. Philadelphia, Elsevier, 2002, pp 49-87.)

splenocolic ligamentous attachment, care must be taken not to exert undue tension on the splenorenal ligament during operative procedures on the left kidney, to avoid inadvertent tearing of the spleen. Such tearing may necessitate splenectomy during left nephrectomy. Both splenocolic and splenorenal ligaments, and the contralateral hepatocolic and hepatorenal ligaments, are typically avascular and can be divided sharply with safety.

The renal artery and vein typically branch from the aorta and inferior vena cava, respectively, to supply each kidney (see Fig. 76-1). The renal vein is more anterior than the renal artery, whereas the urinary collecting system (i.e., the renal pelvis) is the most posteriorly located structure of the renal hilum. The renal arteries and veins typically branch from the aorta and inferior vena cava at the level of the second lumbar vertebral body, below the level of the anterior takeoff of the superior mesenteric artery. The right renal artery passes behind the inferior vena cava in its course and is considerably longer than the left renal artery. The main renal artery typically divides into four or more segmental vessels, with five branches most commonly described. The first and most constant segmental division is a posterior branch, which usually exits the main renal artery before it enters the renal hilum and proceeds posteriorly to the renal pelvis to supply a large posterior segment of the kidney. The remaining anterior division of the main renal artery typically branches as it enters the renal hilum (Fig. 76-4). The renal arteries are end branch vessels and do not communicate with each other. This is in contrast to the renal venous system, which contains many intrarenal anastomoses.

The right renal vein is short (2 to 4 cm) and enters the right lateral aspect of the inferior vena cava directly, usually without receiving other venous branches. The left renal vein is generally three times the length of the right (6 to 10 cm) and must cross anterior to the aorta to reach the left lateral aspect of the inferior vena cava (see Fig. 76-1). Lateral to the aorta, the left renal vein typically receives the left adrenal vein superiorly, a lumbar vein posteriorly, and the left gonadal vein inferiorly.

The renal collecting system includes the calyces, the renal pelvis, and the ureter (Fig. 76-5). There are usually

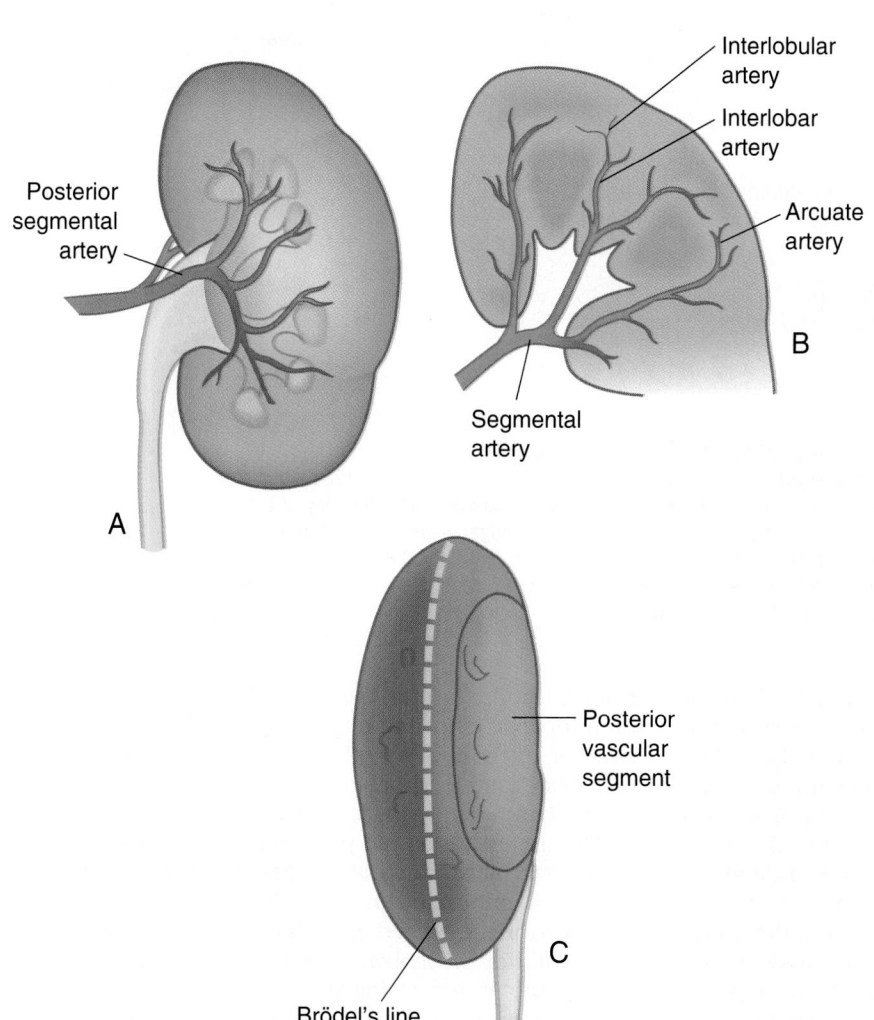

Posterior segmental artery

Segmental artery

Interlobular artery

Interlobar artery

Arcuate artery

A

B

Posterior vascular segment

Brödel's line

C

FIGURE 76-4. **A,** The posterior branch of the renal artery and its distribution to the central segment of the posterior surface of the kidney. **B,** Branches of the anterior division of the renal artery supplying the entire anterior surface of the kidney as well as the upper and lower poles at both surfaces. The segmental branches lead to interlobar, arcuate, and interlobular arteries. **C,** The lateral convex margin of the kidney. Brödel's line, which is 1 cm from the convex margin, is the bloodless plane demarcated by the distribution of the posterior branch of the renal artery. (A and C, From Tanagho E: Anatomy of the genitourinary tract. In Smith's General Urology, 14th ed. Norwalk, CT, Appleton & Lange, 1995, pp 1-16. With permission of the McGraw-Hill Company.)

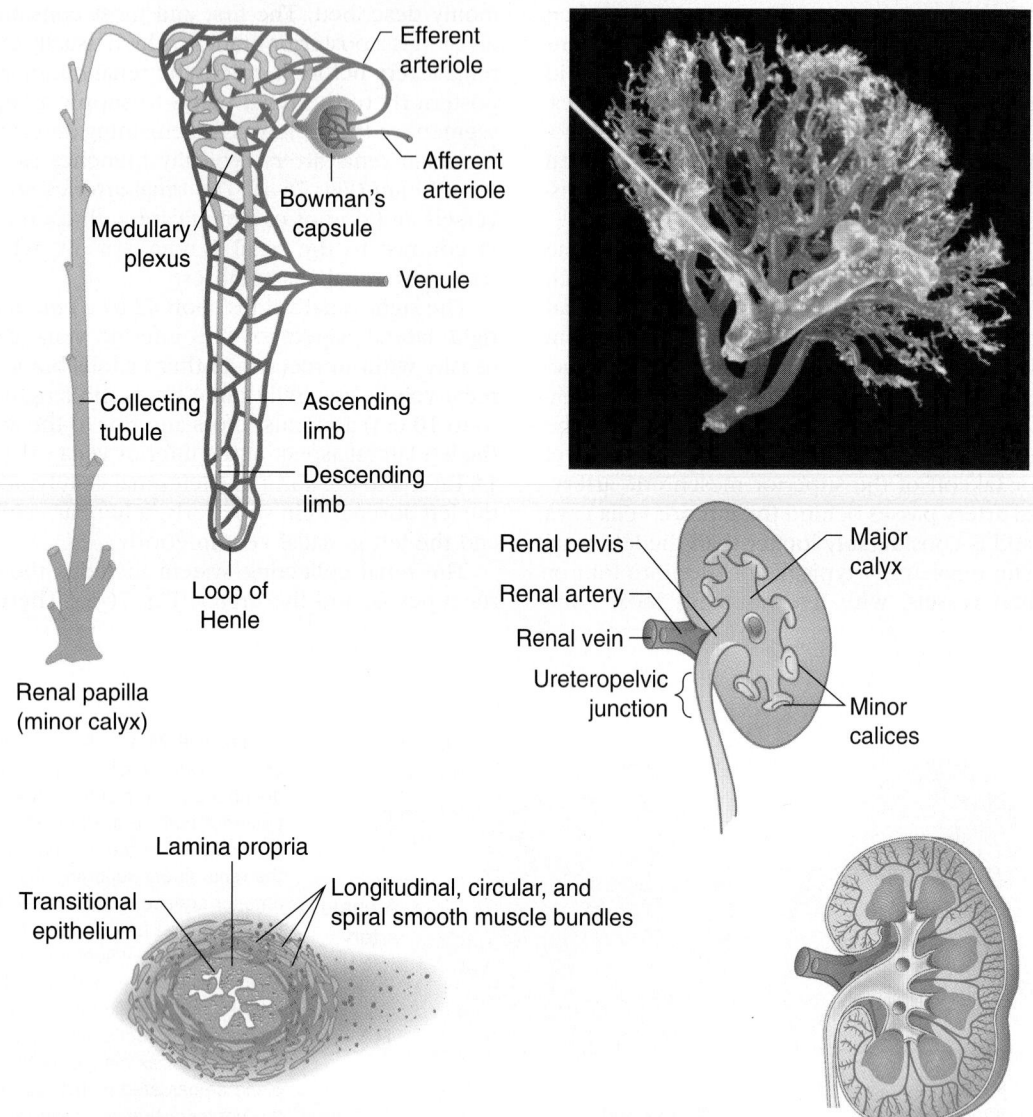

FIGURE 76-5. Anatomy and histology of the kidney and ureter. **Upper left,** Diagram of the nephron and its blood supply. **Upper right,** Cast of the pelvic calyceal system and the arterial supply of the kidney. **Middle,** Renal calyces, pelvis, and ureter (posterior aspect). **Lower left,** Histology of the ureter. The smooth muscle bundles are arranged in both a spiral and a longitudinal manner. **Lower right,** Longitudinal section of kidney showing calyces, pelvis, ureter, and renal blood supply (posterior aspect). (From Tanagho E, McAninch JW [eds]: Smith's General Urology, 15th ed. New York, McGraw-Hill, 2000. Reproduced with permission of the McGraw-Hill Company.)

8 to 12 minor calyces that unite to form 2 to 3 major calyces, which in turn join to form the renal pelvis. The renal pelvis tapers to form the ureter inferomedially. The adult ureter is usually 25 to 30 cm long. The ureter is arbitrarily divided into segments for the purposes of surgical or radiographic demonstration. The "abdominal" ureter extends from the renal pelvis to the iliac vessels, and the "pelvic" ureter extends from the iliac vessels to the bladder (Fig. 76-6). For radiographic purposes, the ureter is divided into three segments. The upper, middle, and lower ureter is commonly described from the renal pelvis to the upper border of sacrum, upper border to lower border of sacrum, and lower border of sacrum to the bladder, respectively. There are three areas of relative nar-rowing in the ureter that are of clinical importance: ureteropelvic junction, the point where the ureter crosses anterior to the iliac vessels, and the ureterovesical junc-tion. For example, spontaneous passage of ureteral stones can be hampered at these relative areas of narrowing.

The ureters lie on the psoas muscle and pass medially to the sacroiliac joints and cross the iliac vessels ante-riorly. An important anatomic landmark for easy iden-tification of the ureters is at the site where the ureters cross anterior to the iliac vessels. After crossing the iliac vessels, the ureters swing laterally near the ischial spines before passing medially to penetrate the base of the bladder. In the male, the vasa deferentia pass anterior to the ureters as they exit the internal inguinal ring. In the

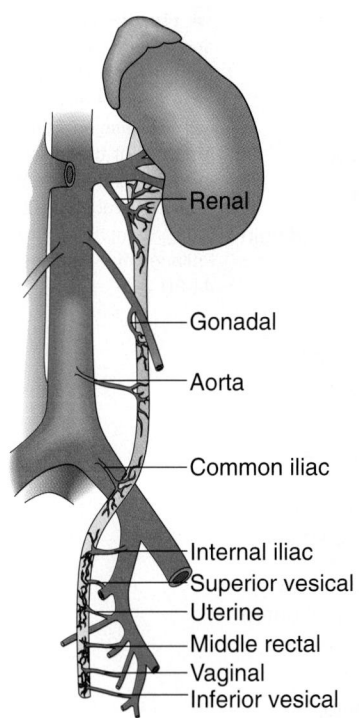

FIGURE 76-6. Sources of arterial blood supply to the ureter. (Reproduced with permission from Kabalin J: Surgical anatomy of the retroperitoneum, kidneys, and ureters. In Walsh PC, Retik AB, Vaughan ED Jr, et al [eds]: Campbell's Urology, 8th ed. Philadelphia, Elsevier, 2002, pp 49-87.)

female, the uterine arteries are closely related to the lower ureters.

The blood supply to the calyces, pelvis, and upper ureter are derived from the renal arteries (see Fig. 76-6). The lower ureter obtains its blood supply from the common and internal iliac arteries and the internal spermatic and vesical arteries.

Bladder

The bladder is a hollow muscular organ that functions to store and evacuate urine. In adulthood, it has a capacity of approximately 500 mL. The cephalad portion of the bladder is attached to the anterior abdominal wall by the urachus, a fibrous remnant of the cloaca that attaches the bladder to the anterior abdominal wall. The obliterated umbilical artery in the medial umbilical fold serves as an important landmark for the surgeon (Fig. 76-7). It may be traced to its origin from the internal iliac artery to locate the ureter, which lies on its medial side. The superior aspect of the bladder is covered by peritoneal reflection. Inferiorly, the bladder is attached to the pubic bone by dense condensations to the posterior aspect of the pubic bone, known as the puboprostatic ligaments in males and pubovesical ligaments in females.

The superior, middle, and inferior vesical arteries, which are branches of the hypogastric artery are the major source of blood supply to the bladder. In females, additional branches from the vaginal and uterine arteries

supply the bladder. The veins of the bladder coalesce into the vesicle plexus and drain into the internal iliac vein. Lymphatics from the lamina propria and muscularis drain to channels on the bladder surface, which run with the superficial vessels within the thin visceral fascia. Small paravesical lymph nodes can be found along the superficial channels. The bulk of the lymphatic drainage passes to the external iliac lymph nodes. Some anterior and lateral drainage may go through the obturator and internal iliac nodes, whereas portions of the bladder base and trigone may drain into the internal and common iliac groups.

A transitional epithelial layer lines the bladder mucosa. Lamina propria, a thin elastic connective tissue, lies between the transitional epithelial cell layer and the muscularis propria. The muscularis propria, also known as the detrusor muscle, is composed of interlacing smooth muscle bundles with no distinct layers.

Prostate and Seminal Vesicles

The prostate is a fibromuscular organ that lies just inferior to the bladder. The normal prostate weighs approximately 20 g and contains the prostatic urethra. The prostate is supported anteriorly by the puboprostatic ligament and inferiorly by the urogenital diaphragm (Fig. 76-8). The ejaculatory ducts exit in the posterior portion of the prostate across the verumontanum, a mound within the prostate gland (see Fig. 76-8). The prostate has a peripheral zone, a central zone, and a transitional zone; an anterior segment; and a preprostatic sphincteric zone (Fig. 76-9). Benign prostatic hyperplasia develops from the periurethral glands at the site of the median or lateral lobes, whereas the posterior lobe is prone to cancerous formation. The prostate is separated from the rectum by the two layers of Denonvilliers' fascia, serosal rudiments of the pouch of Douglas, which once extended to the urogenital diaphragm (Fig. 76-10).

The arterial supply to the prostate is derived from the inferior vesical, internal pudendal, and middle rectal (hemorrhoidal) arteries. The veins from the prostate drain into the periprostatic plexus, which has connections with the deep dorsal vein of the penis and the internal iliac (hypogastric) veins.

The neurovascular bundles responsible for erection are located near the posterolateral surface of the urethra and prostate gland (see Fig. 76-30). Special care in preserving these nerves is crucial to maintaining potency after radical prostatectomy.[1]

The seminal vesicles lie just cephalad to the prostate under the base of the bladder. They are about 6 cm long and quite soft. Each vesicle joins its corresponding vas deferens to form the ejaculatory duct. The ureters lie medial to each, and the rectum is contiguous with their posterior surfaces.

Penis and Urethra

The penis is composed of two corpora cavernosal bodies (responsible for erectile function of the penis) and one corpora spongiosum where the urethra courses through.

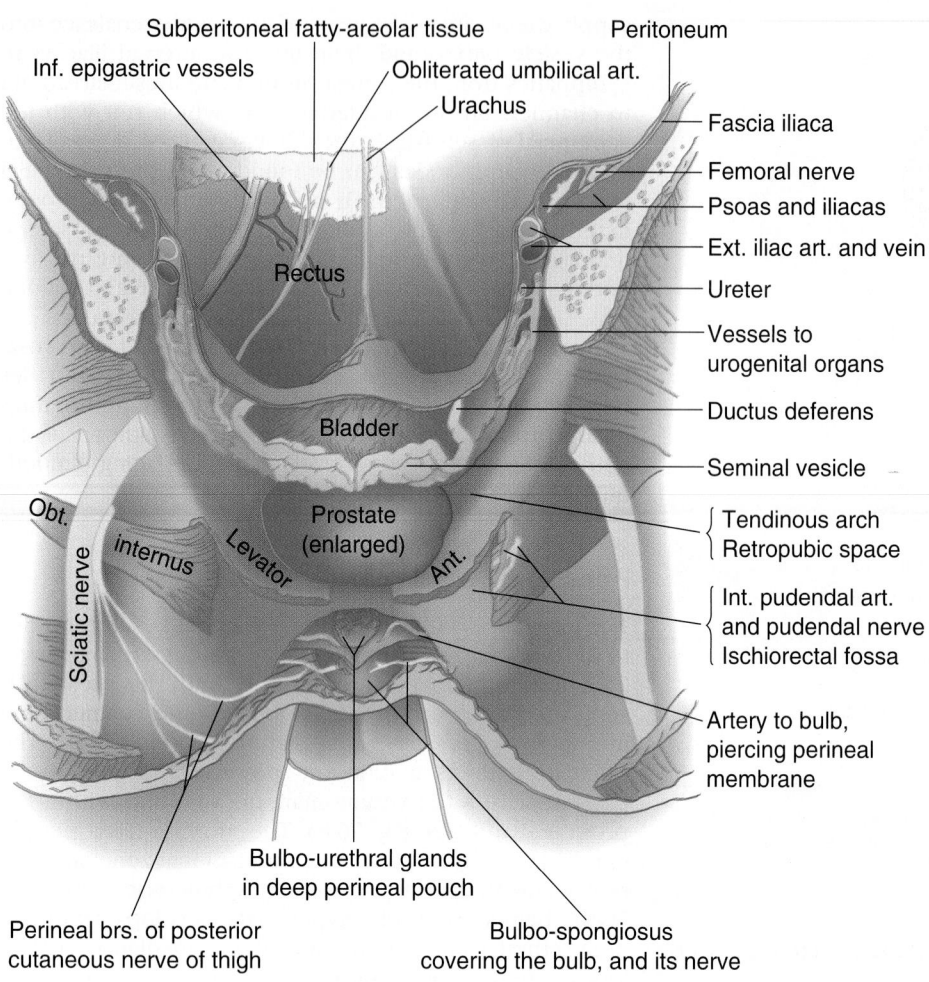

Subperitoneal fatty-areolar tissue

Inf. epigastric vessels

Obliterated umbilical art.

Urachus

Peritoneum

Fascia iliaca

Femoral nerve

Psoas and iliacas

Ext. iliac art. and vein

Ureter

Vessels to urogenital organs

Ductus deferens

Seminal vesicle

Tendinous arch
Retropubic space

Int. pudendal art. and pudendal nerve
Ischiorectal fossa

Artery to bulb, piercing perineal membrane

Rectus

Bladder

Prostate (enlarged)

Obt.

internus

Levator

Ant.

Sciatic nerve

Bulbo-urethral glands in deep perineal pouch

Perineal brs. of posterior cutaneous nerve of thigh

Bulbo-spongiosus covering the bulb, and its nerve

FIGURE 76-7. Male pelvis and anterior abdominal wall viewed from behind. The sacrum and ilia have been removed. (Reproduced with permission from Brooks JD: Anatomy of the lower urinary tract in male genitalia. In Walsh PC, Retik AB, Vaughan ED Jr, et al [eds]: Campbell's Urology, 8th ed. Philadelphia, Elsevier, 2002, pp 41-80.)

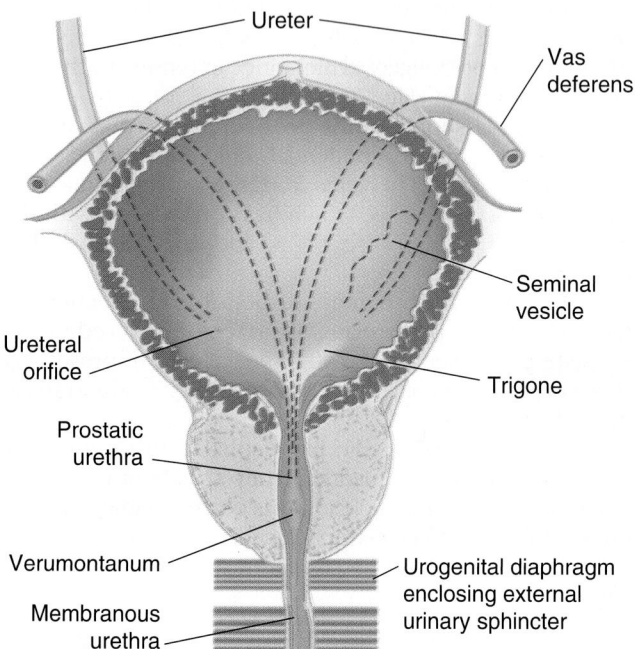

Ureter

Vas deferens

Seminal vesicle

Ureteral orifice

Trigone

Prostatic urethra

Verumontanum

Membranous urethra

Urogenital diaphragm enclosing external urinary sphincter

FIGURE 76-8. Anatomy and relations of the ureters, bladder, prostate, seminal vesicles, and vasa deferentia (anterior view). (Reproduced with permission from Tanagho EA, McAninch JW [eds]: Smith's General Urology, 15th ed. New York, McGraw-Hill, 2000)

Each corporal body is covered by tunica albuginea (Fig. 76-11), and collectively all corporal bodies are covered by a thick layer of Buck's fascia. All corporal bodies are capped by the glans of the penis (see Fig. 76-10).

The male urethra, which is approximately 20 cm long, is divided into four anatomic sections: prostatic, membranous, bulbous, and penile. The voluntary external urinary sphincter lies within the urogenital diaphragm and is an important anatomic landmark to preserve the function of the urinary sphincter after prostatic or urethral surgery. The female urethra is approximately 4 cm and lies below the pubic symphysis and anterior to the vagina.

Spermatic Cord, Epididymis, and Testes

The two spermatic cords extend from the internal rings through the internal canals to the testes. Each cord contains the vas deferens, internal and external spermatic arteries, artery of the vas, spermatic vein, lymphatics, and nerves.

The epididymis is connected to the testis by efferent ducts from the testis. It consists of a markedly coiled duct. At its lower pole the epididymis becomes continuous with the vas deferens (Fig. 76-12).

The average testis is $4 \times 3 \times 2.5$ cm. Tunica albuginea, which is a dense fascial covering, overlies the testis. The

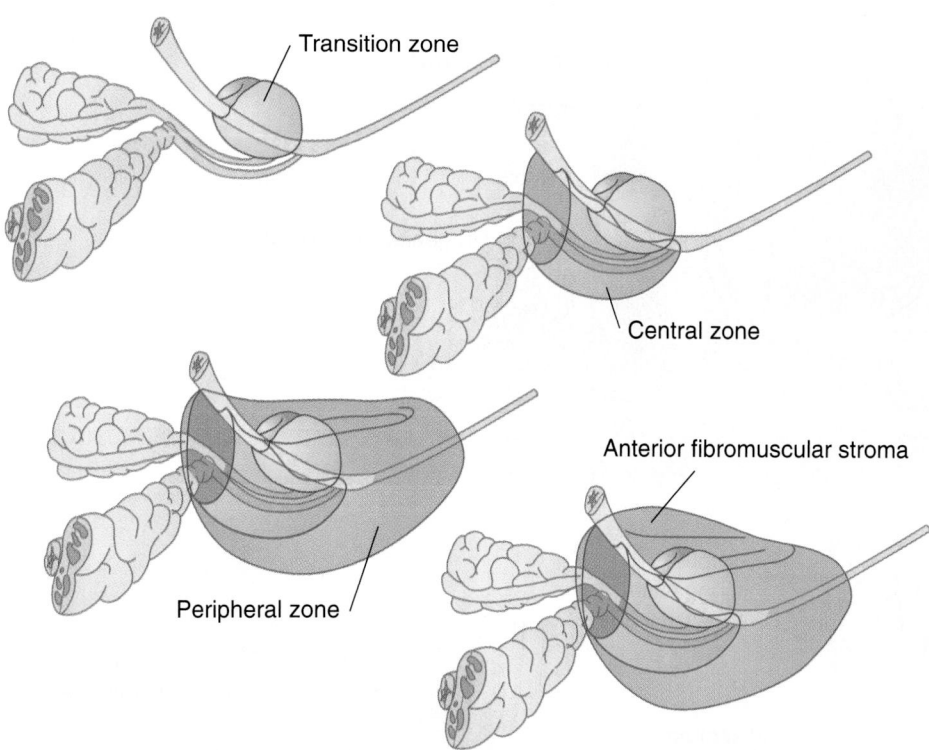

Transition zone

Central zone

Anterior fibromuscular stroma

Peripheral zone

FIGURE 76-9. Zonal anatomy of the prostate as described by J. E. McNeal (Am J Surg Pathol 12:619-633, 1988). The transition zone surrounds the urethra proximal to the ejaculatory ducts. The central zone surrounds the ejaculatory ducts and projects under the bladder base. The peripheral zone constitutes the bulk of the apical, posterior, and lateral aspects of the prostate. The anterior fibromuscular stroma extends from the bladder neck to the striated urethral sphincter. (Reproduced with permission from Brooks J: Anatomy of the lower urinary tract and male genitalia. In Walsh PC, Retik AB, Vaughan ED Jr, et al [eds]: Campbell's Urology, 8th ed. Philadelphia, Elsevier, 2002, p 112.)

tunica albuginea forms a dense fibrous mediastinum that connects with the lobules within the testis (see Fig. 76-12). The testis is covered anteriorly and laterally by the visceral layer of the serous tunica vaginalis.

UROLOGIC TRAUMA

Approximately 10% of all injuries seen in the emergency department involve the genitourinary system to some extent. Many of the injuries are subtle and difficult to define and require great diagnostic expertise. Initial assessment in order of importance includes the following: A, airway with cervical spine protection; B, breathing; C, circulation and control of external bleeding; D, disability or neurologic status; E, exposure (undress) and environment (temperature control).[2]

Resuscitation may require intravenous lines and urethral catheterization in seriously injured patients. In men, before the Foley catheter is inserted the urethra should be carefully inspected for presence of any blood.

A detailed history and description of the accident is obtained. In cases of gunshot wounds, the type and caliber of the weapon should be determined, because high-velocity projectiles cause much more extensive damage.

Renal Trauma

The urologic examination should focus on the abdomen and genitalia. Fractures of the lower ribs are often associated with renal injuries to the retroperitoneum (see Fig. 76-3), whereas pelvic fractures can be accompanied by bladder and urethral injuries.

The assessment of the extent of injury should be done in an orderly fashion for proper staging. The algorithm in Figure 76-13 outlines the staging for blunt trauma in adults as it pertains to the urologic evaluation and is further discussed in the following section.

Hematuria is the best indicator of traumatic injury to the urinary system. Microscopic hematuria (> 5 red blood cells per high-power field), heme-positive urine dipstick, and gross hematuria are the strongest indicators of genitourinary injury. However, the degree of hematuria does not necessarily correlate with degree of injury. The combination of systemic shock (systolic blood pressure > 90 mm Hg) and microscopic hematuria is strongly associated with severe renal injuries.[3,4] The best urine sample for assessment of hematuria in the trauma patient is the first aliquot of voided or catheterized specimen, because a later sample can often be diluted by diuresis.

A classification and grading system for renal injuries (Figs. 76-13 and 76-14) has helped in proper identification and better communication of the extent of injury between different members of the trauma team. Use of appropriate imaging studies enables the trauma team to appropriately stage the extent of the renal injury. All victims of blunt trauma with gross hematuria and those patients with microscopic hematuria and shock (systolic blood pressure of less than 90 mm Hg any time during evaluation and resuscitation) should undergo renal imaging, usually CT with intravenous contrast medium enhancement. Adult patients with microscopic hematuria and without shock can be observed without imaging studies, because an extremely low percentage of these patients (less than 0.0016%) have any significant renal injuries.[5] In contrast, pediatric patients with blunt trauma and microscopic

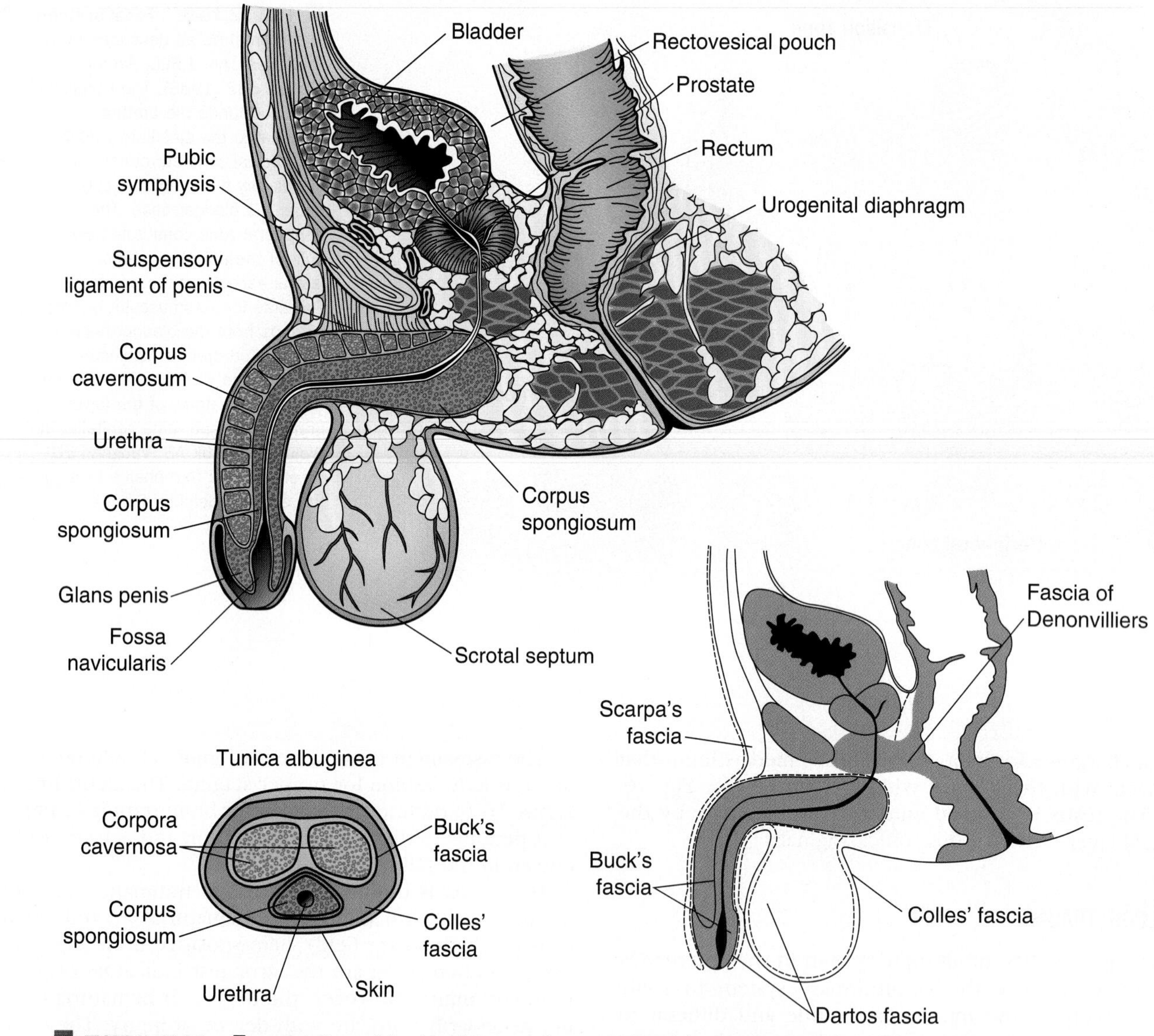

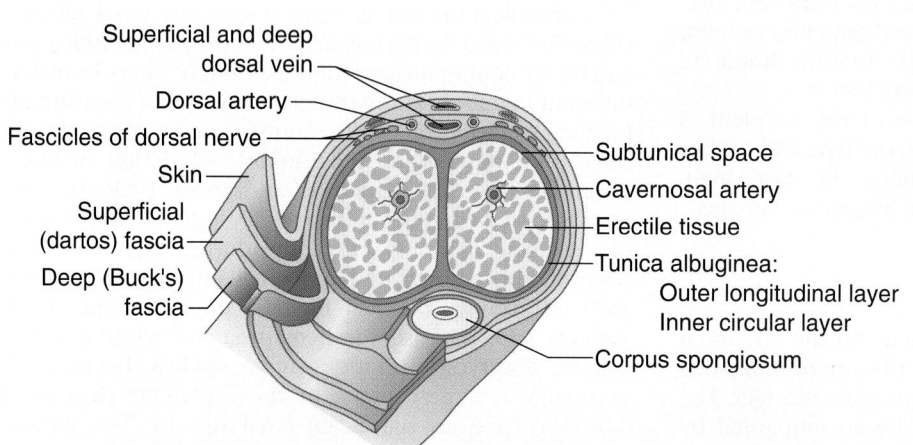

FIGURE 76-10.   Top, Relations of the bladder, prostate, seminal vesicles, penis, urethra, and scrotal contents.
Lower left, Transverse section through the penis. The paired upper structures are the corpora cavernosa. The single lower body surrounding the urethra is the corpus spongiosum. **Lower right,** Fascial planes of the lower genitourinary tract. (Reproduced with permission from Tanagho EA, McAninch JW [eds]: Smith's General Urology, 15th ed. New York, McGraw-Hill, 2000.)

FIGURE 76-11.   Cross section of the penis, demonstrating the relationship between the corporeal bodies, penile fascia, vessels, and nerves. (Reproduced with permission from Devine CJ, Angermeier KW: AUA Update Series 13(2):10, 1994.)

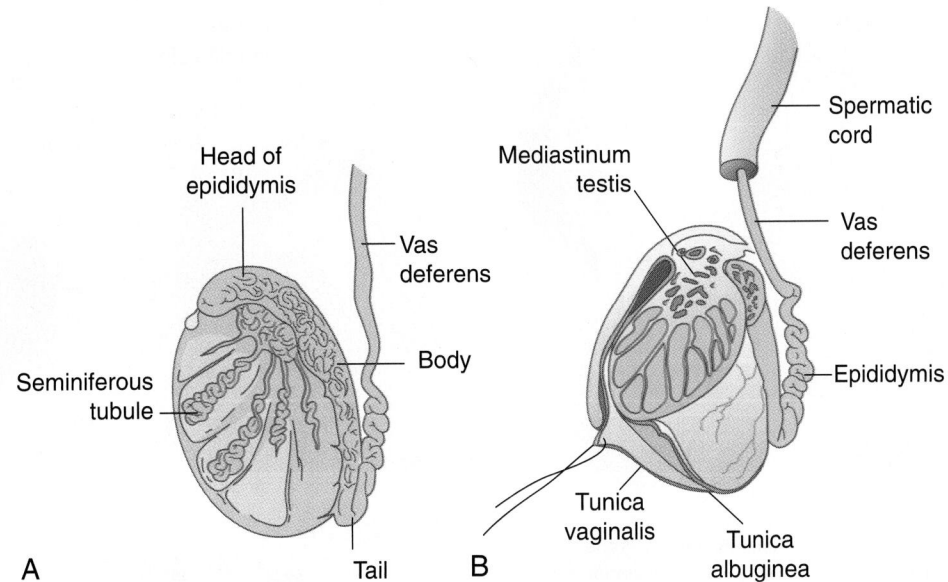

FIGURE 76-12.   Testis and epididymis. **A,** One to three seminiferous tubules fill each compartment and drain into the rete testis in the mediastinum. Twelve to 20 efferent ductules become convoluted in the head of the epididymis and drain into a single coiled duct of the epididymis. The vas is convoluted in its first portion. **B,** Cross section of the tunica vaginalis, showing the mediastinum and septations continuous with the tunica albuginea. The parietal and visceral tunica vaginalis are confluent where the vessels and nerves enter the posterior aspect of the testis. (Reproduced with permission from Brooks J: Anatomy of the lower urinary tract and male genitalia. In Walsh PC, Retik AB, Vaughan ED Jr, et al [eds]: Campbell's Urology, 8th ed. Philadelphia, Elsevier, 2002, pp 89-128.)

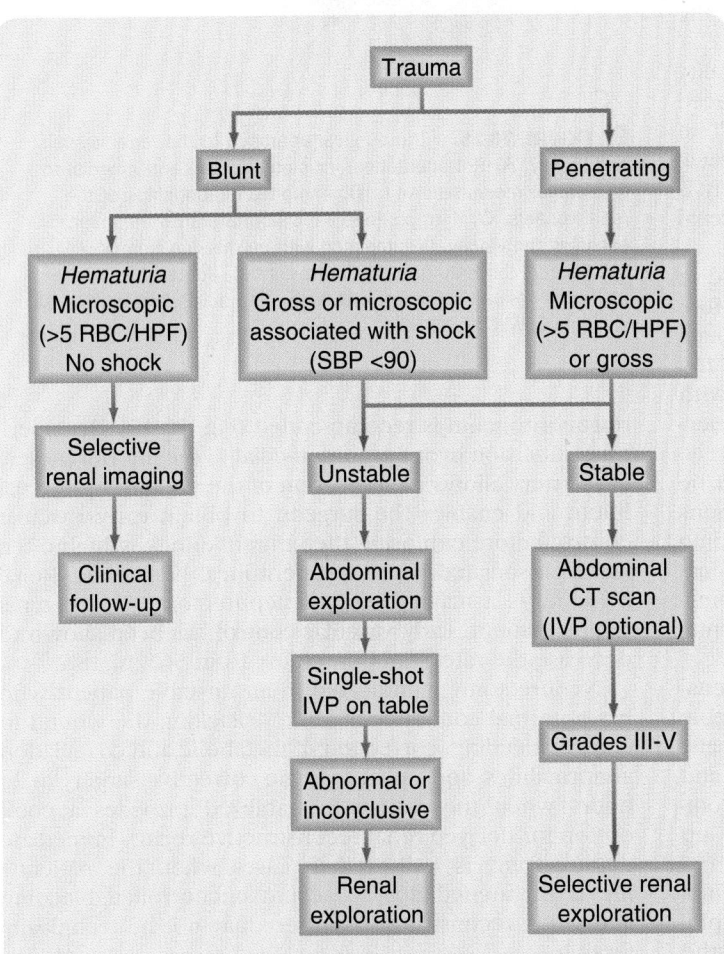

FIGURE 76-13.   Flow chart for adult renal injuries to serve as a guide for decision making. (Reproduced with permission from McAninch JW, Santucci RA: Genitourinary trauma. In Walsh PC, Retik AB, Vaughan ED Jr, et al [eds]: Campbell's Urology, 8th ed. Philadelphia, Elsevier, 2002, p 3711.)

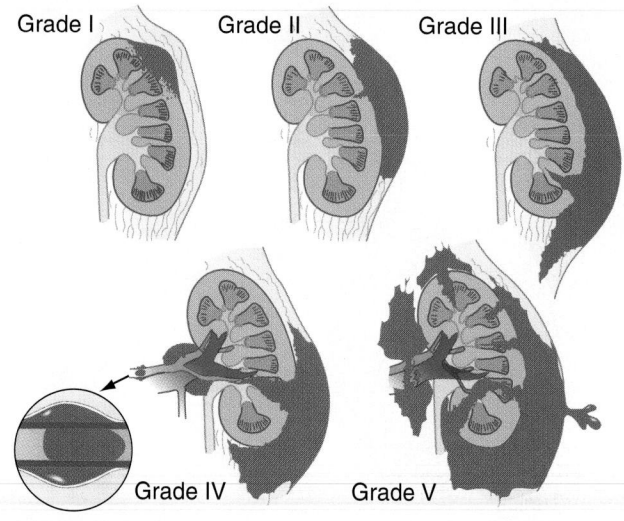

FIGURE 76-14. Classification of renal injuries by grade (based on the organ injury scale of the American Association for the Surgery of Trauma). (Reproduced with permission from McAninch JW, Santucci RA: Genitourinary trauma. In Walsh PC, Retik AB, Vaughan ED Jr, et al [eds]: Campbell's Urology, 8th ed. Philadelphia, Elsevier, 2002, p 3709.)

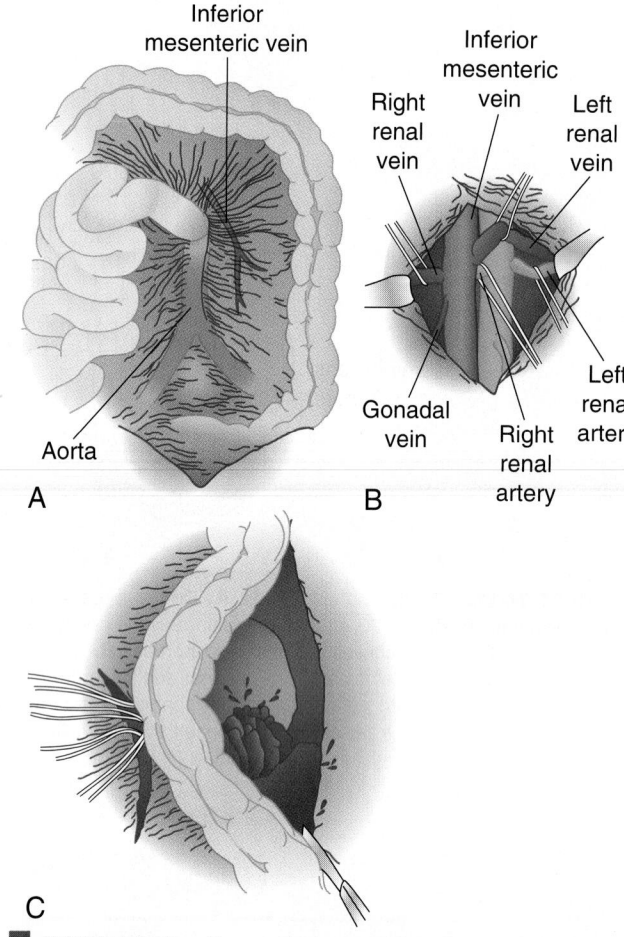

FIGURE 76-15. The surgical approach to the renal vessels and kidney. **A,** Retroperitoneal incision over the aorta medial to the inferior mesenteric vein. **B,** Anatomic relationships of the renal vessels. **C,** Retroperitoneal incision lateral to the colon, exposing the kidney. (Reproduced with permission from McAninch JW: Surgery for renal trauma. In Novick AC, Pontes ES, Streem SB [eds]: Stewart's Operative Urology, 2nd ed. Baltimore, Williams & Wilkins, 1989.)

hematuria require an imaging modality (CT scan or ultrasound). Pediatric patients have a high catecholamine output; therefore, shock is not a good predictor of the degree of renal injury.

Excretory urography used to be the imaging modality for assessment of renal trauma, but it has been replaced for the most part by contrast medium–enhanced CT in most emergency departments for evaluation of renal injuries.[6] Occasionally, single-shot excretory urography is used for immediate intraoperative assessment of renal trauma.[7]

Significant injuries (grades II through V) are found in only 5.4% of renal trauma cases (see Fig. 76-14).[7] More than 98% of all renal injuries can be managed nonoperatively. More often high-grade renal injuries (grades IV and V) would require surgical management; however, with proper staging of the renal injury and careful patient selection, even these injuries can be managed nonoperatively.

Indications for renal exploration after trauma can be separated into absolute and relative.[8] Absolute indications include evidence of persistent renal bleeding, expanding perirenal hematoma, and pulsatile perirenal hematoma. Relative indications include urinary extravasation, nonviable tissue, delayed diagnosis of arterial injury, segmental arterial injury, and incomplete staging.

Segmental renal artery injury with an associated renal laceration results in a substantial amount of nonviable tissue (usually more than 20%), and such injuries usually resolve more quickly with surgical reconstruction and tissue removal. This approach often avoids the high complication rate noted when this group is followed up without renal exploration.[9]

When surgical exploration for renal trauma is indicated, using a transabdominal approach and early exploration of the renal hilum and vasculature before the

retroperitoneum is recommended (Fig. 76-15). Retroperitoneal incision over the aorta medial to the inferior mesenteric artery allows identification of the left and right renal hilum and enables the surgeon to obtain early vascular control before exploring the injured kidney, which often has an associated large retroperitoneal hematoma. Renal bleeding is a major cause of nephrectomy in the renal trauma patient. Early vascular control has been shown to decrease the rate of nephrectomy from 56% to 18%.[10]

Nephrectomy is indicated in an unstable patient who has a normal contralateral kidney. Packing the wound to control bleeding, correction of metabolic and coagulation abnormalities, and a plan to begin corrective surgery in 24 hours when the patient is stabilized provides a good option for delayed renal reconstructive repair. Immediate nephrectomy is indicated in cases when the patient's life is threatened due to severe uncontrolled bleeding and when reconstructive surgery may not be technically feasible.

Ureteral Injuries

Ureteral injuries occur in less than 4% and 1% of all penetrating and blunt traumas, respectively. Ureteropelvic junction (UPJ) disruption after blunt trauma is rare and can be missed because patients often do not exhibit hematuria. Diagnosis of UPJ disruption is made by a high index of suspicion in cases of high deceleration injury. Delayed CT contrast images, which visualize the renal collecting system and proximal ureter with excreted contrast material, are the best way to assess the UPJ's integrity. When delayed contrast images are not possible because of a patient's hemodynamic instability, an intraoperative "one-shot" intravenous pyelogram (2 mg/kg intravenous contrast material given 10 minutes before flat plate abdominal radiography) is performed in patients with hypotension or a history of significant deceleration, despite absence of gross hematuria. Intraoperative palpation of the UPJ is usually not sensitive enough to assess any UPJ disruption.

Iatrogenic Ureteral Injury

Management of iatrogenic ureteral injuries is dependent on timing of the injury and the location of the ureteral injury. Frequency of ureteral injuries is rare. Iatrogenic ureteral injuries are often associated with large pelvic masses (benign or malignant) that may displace the ureter from its normal anatomic position. Inflammatory pelvic disorders such as endometriosis may encase the ureter in a similar way and account for inadvertent ureteral injury during pelvic surgery. Extensive carcinoma of the colon may invade areas outside the colon wall and directly involve the ureter; thus, resection of the ureter may be required along with resection of the tumor mass. Devascularization may occur with extensive pelvic lymph node dissections or after radiation therapy to the pelvis for pelvic cancer. In these situations, ureteral fibrosis and subsequent stricture formation may develop along with ureteral fistulas.

Injuries to the *lower third of the ureter* allow several options in management. The procedure of choice is reimplantation into the bladder combined with a psoas-hitch procedure to minimize tension on the ureteral anastomosis.[11] The bladder is dissected after catheter instillation of saline. The urachus and contralateral obliterated umbilical artery are divided (Fig. 76-16A). Peritoneum is mobilized off the anterior and posterior aspect of the bladder. These maneuvers allow more extensive mobilization of the bladder. The bladder is incised in midline or obliquely to allow mobilization of bladder to the ipsilateral psoas muscle (see Fig. 76-16B). It is sutured to the psoas muscle, but care is taken to avoid the genitofemoral nerve on the surface of the muscle or the femoral nerve deep in the psoas muscle (see Fig. 76-16C). An antireflux ureteral anastomosis should be done when possible to minimize potential damage to upper urinary tract from long-standing urinary reflux (see Fig. 76-16D).

Primary ureteroureterostomy can be used in lower-third injuries when the ureter has been ligated without transection. The ureter is usually long enough for this type of anastomosis. A bladder tube flap (Boari flap) can be used when the ureter is shorter.

Transureteroureterostomy may be used in lower-third injuries if extensive urinoma and pelvic infection have developed. This procedure allows anastomosis and reconstruction in an area away from the pathologic processes. Caution must be utilized to prevent tension on the normal recipient ureter.

Midureteral injuries can be managed with primary ureteroureterostomy if there is not a significant loss of viable ureter between the proximal and distal sites of injury; otherwise, transureteroureterostomy is a good option.

Upper ureteral injuries are best managed by primary ureteroureterostomy. If there is extensive loss of the ureter, autotransplantation of the kidney and transposition of bowel to replace the ureter are potential surgical options.

Bladder Injuries

Bladder injury after blunt trauma is relatively rare, owing to the protected intrapelvic position of the bladder. Bladder injuries are associated with 6% to 10% of all pelvic fractures. Conversely, in the presence of a bladder injury, the majority of patients (83% to 100%) suffer from other pelvic fractures. Bladder injuries can be classified into two types: *extraperitoneal* and *intraperitoneal*. Extraperitoneal ruptures are thought to result from direct laceration, usually by bone spicules from the fractured pelvis. Extraperitoneal bladder rupture can most commonly be managed conservatively with catheter drainage, resulting in spontaneous healing of the bladder injury.[12] However, some authors have listed several contraindications to such conservative management: bone fragment projecting into the bladder (which is unlikely to heal), open pelvic fracture, and rectal perforation.[13] Another relative indication for surgical repair of extraperitoneal bladder injury is concomitant other abdominal and/or pelvic injuries requiring surgical management. In this setting, surgical repair of the bladder injury can potentially decrease the risk of vesicocutaneous fistula.[14]

Intraperitoneal bladder rupture accounts for 25% of all bladder injuries. The postulated mechanism of intraperitoneal bladder injury is thought to be caused by rapid rise of intra-abdominal pressure during blunt trauma.[15] In contrast to extraperitoneal bladder injuries, intraperitoneal bladder rupture requires operative repair with two-layer closure of the bladder injury and placement of a perivesical drain.

Retrograde cystography is the traditional imaging modality to diagnosis bladder rupture. It is critical to obtain filling and drainage cystography films, because 13% of bladder injuries are diagnosed by the drainage cystography plain films.[16] CT can also be used for diagnosis of bladder injury (Fig. 76-17). The preferred method of assessing for bladder injury is retrograde filling of the bladder with 300 to 400 mL of contrast material (or until the patient experiences discomfort) through the Foley catheter and obtaining images both during the filled and drained phases of the study.

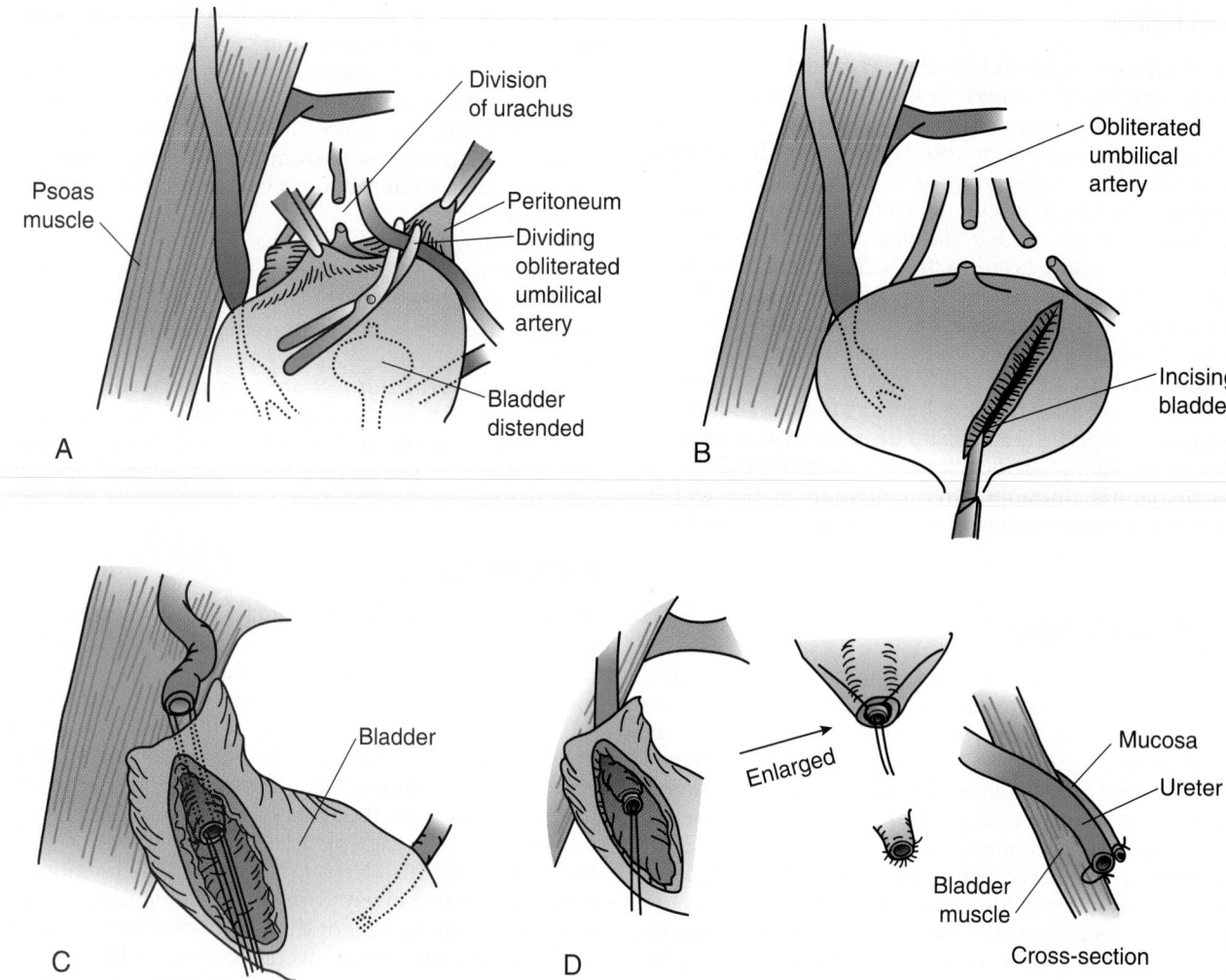

FIGURE 76-16.   **A,** After the midline incision is made, a retroperitoneal approach delineates the bladder. The bladder is dissected after catheter instillation of saline. The urachus and contralateral obliterated umbilical artery are divided. The peritoneum is mobilized off the posterior aspect of the bladder. These maneuvers allow more extensive mobilization of bladder. **B,** The bladder is incised in midline or obliquely to allow mobilization of bladder to right psoas muscle. **C,** The bladder is sutured to psoas muscle, but care is taken to avoid genitofemoral nerve on surface of muscle. It is important not to place the sutures too deeply in psoas muscle because femoral nerve branches can be injured. **D,** Antireflux submucosal ureteral reimplantation is then constructed. The ureter is advanced in a submucosal tunnel. Anchoring absorbable sutures are placed in mucosa and muscle. (Modified from Mathews R, Marshall F: Versatility of the adult psoas hitch ureteral reimplantation. J Urol 158:2078-2082, 1997.)

Urethral Injuries

Urethral injuries are associated with 4% to 14% of all pelvic fractures[17,18] and are more common in cases of bilateral pelvic injuries.[19,20] Diagnosis of urethral injuries is made by a high index of suspicion in the presence of blood at the urethral meatus, inability to urinate, and/or a palpable full bladder on abdominal examination. When blood is present at the meatus, retrograde urethrography aids in diagnosis of any urethral injury. In the presence of minor urethral injury, a catheter can be placed by an experienced urologist with or without the aid of a cystoscope.[21]

Urethral injuries are classified as those confined to the posterior urethra (above the urogenital diaphragm) and to the anterior urethra (below the urogenital diaphragm).

Posterior urethral injuries are further subclassified as type I (urethral stretch), type II (urethral disruption proximal to the urogenital diaphragm), and type III (proximal and distal disruption of the urogenital diaphragm).

For treatment of posterior urethral injuries, early endoscopic realignment has become more accepted as an excellent initial treatment option.[22] Realignment of the damaged urethra with a stented Foley catheter can lead to complete healing of the urethral injury or need for future endoscopic treatment of developed urethral strictures. If realignment of the damaged urethra cannot be achieved, then suprapubic catheterization, followed by delayed combined antegrade and retrograde endoscopic repair or open surgical repair are the potential treatment options.

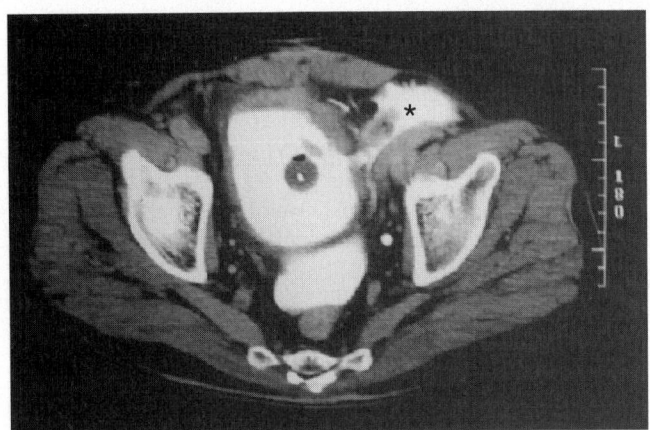

FIGURE 76-17. Extraperitoneal bladder injury. Contrast agent is extravasated to the space of Retzius *(asterisk)* after retrograde filling of the bladder through the indwelling Foley catheter.

In contrast to posterior urethral injuries that are often associated with many other pelvic injuries, anterior urethral injuries are often isolated and often associated with straddle injuries. The bulbar urethra is often the site of injury. The best initial treatment modality for anterior urethral injuries is not well defined; however, most would agree that primary realignment with Foley catheter, if possible, is the best initial treatment. In cases of severe anterior urethral injury, a suprapubic catheter may be required, followed by delayed open surgical repair.[23]

External Genitalia Injuries

The most common cause of penile amputation is genital self-mutilation.[24] If the amputated penis is available, reattachment of the penis is recommended by most authors; however, the clinician is often challenged by the overriding psychiatric issues that led to the act of penile amputation. Psychiatric consultation should always be sought to assess the risk of further self-mutilation.[25]

Penile "fracture" or rupture of the corpus cavernosum (see Figs. 76-10 and 76-11) from trauma to the erect penis most commonly occurs by striking the symphysis pubis or the perineum during sexual intercourse. Presentation of penile fracture includes trauma to the erect penis, followed by a "popping" sound, pain, and immediate detumescence. Penile fracture is associated with urethral injuries in 38% of cases.[26,27] Therefore, urethrography should be performed in suspected cases when the patient has blood at the meatus, gross hematuria, or inability to void. Immediate repair of the penile injury is recommended because there is a lower risk of penile deformity, faster recover, and less morbidity.[28,29]

Risk of testicular rupture after blunt trauma to the scrotum is greater than 50%. The most common causes are assaults and sports injuries and motor vehicle accidents.[30-32] Surgical exploration and repair of significant hematocele, intratesticular hematoma, or rupture of tunica albuginea is recommended.[33,34]

EMERGENT UROLOGIC CONDITIONS

Fournier's Gangrene

Fournier's gangrene is a necrotizing fasciitis of the male genitalia and perineum that involves mainly subcutaneous tissues. Mortality is dependent on severity of disease but can exceed 50% in some series.[35] The disease can rapidly progress. The most common cause is from infections of the colon, rectum, or lower genitourinary tract or cutaneous infection of the genitalia, perineum, or anus. Most common risk factors are diabetes mellitus, alcohol use, and immunocompromised states. Infections can spread along the dartos and Colles' and Scarpa's fascia because these fascial planes are continuous. The spread of the infection rarely involves the deep fascial planes and musculature.

Both aerobic and anaerobic organisms can cause the infection. The most common isolated organism is *Escherichia coli,* and other commonly cultured organisms include *Enterococcus, Staphylococcus, Streptococcus, Bacteroides fragilis,* and *Pseudomonas aeruginosa.*

The presenting sign is usually a painful swelling and induration of the penis, scrotum, or perineum. Cellulitis, eschar, necrosis, crepitus, foul odor, and/or fever may be some other accompanying signs.

Aggressive surgical débridement of all necrotic, ischemic, and infected tissue along with copious irrigation is critical. Infected tissue should be cultured and initial broad-spectrum intravenous antibiotic coverage (e.g., ampicillin, gentamicin, and clindamycin) instituted. Suprapubic catheter placement can help divert the urine and decrease the risk of further bacterial seeding of the wound.

If a colonic source is suspected, proctoscopy under general anesthesia can be performed, and, if necessary, diverting colostomy may be indicated. Additional débridement in 24 hours after the initial débridement may be necessary. Wet to dry dressing changes along with strict control of diabetes, metabolites, and adequate nutritional support are critical to proper wound healing.

Testicular Torsion

Testicular torsion is a urologic emergency that requires rapid diagnosis and intervention to maintain viability to the testis. There are two types of testicular torsion: extravaginal and intravaginal. Extravaginal torsion is diagnosed in the newborn, and the cause is due to nonadherence of the tunica vaginalis to the dartos layer. As a result, the spermatic cord and tunica vaginalis are rotated as a unit. Intravaginal torsion is usually diagnosed in males 12 to 18 years of age, but it can occur at any age. The etiology of intravaginal torsion is malrotation of the spermatic cord with the tunica vaginalis. Both extravaginal (newborn) and intravaginal (adolescent) types of testicular torsion lead to strangulation of blood supply to the testis.

Presentation of testicular torsion is acute onset of testicular pain and/or swelling, and some may have episodic symptoms of pain suggestive of intermittent torsion. Physical examination may reveal a tender firm testis, high-riding testis, horizontal lie of testis, absent cremasteric reflex, and no pain relief with elevation of the testis. The spermatic cord may appear thickened. The posteriorly positioned epididymis may be positioned differently.

Diagnosis of testicular torsion is made mainly by clinical suspicion. When one is uncertain, color Doppler ultrasound evaluation or a nuclear testicular scan may help with the diagnosis. In case of epididymo-orchitis, a Doppler ultrasound study may demonstrate increased blood flow and increased radionuclide activity by radionuclide scan; testicular torsion would show no blood flow or poor radionuclide tracer uptake on each respective study.

Immediate surgical exploration is indicated if testicular torsion is suspected. If treated within the first 4 to 6 hours of onset of symptoms, the chance of testicular salvage is high. During surgical exploration the testis is rotated to its normal position to restore blood flow. If the testis is viable, orchiopexy of the affected and the contralateral testis is completed. If the affected testis is nonviable, orchiectomy of the affected testis and orchiopexy of the contralateral side are performed.

If an operating facility is not immediately available, manual detorsion by external rotation of the testis toward the thigh for intravaginal (adolescent) torsion can be attempted.

Priapism

Priapism is a pathologic condition of a penile erection that persists beyond or is unrelated to sexual stimulation. Except in cases of the nonischemic type, priapism is often accompanied by pain and tenderness. It can occur in all age groups, including the newborn, but the peak incidence is seen from ages 5 to 10 and 20 to 50 years. In the younger group, priapism is most often associated with sickle cell disease or neoplasm; in the older group, priapism is often caused by pharmacologic agents. Low-flow (veno-occlusive [type I]) priapism accounts for the majority of instances of priapism (Box 76-1). Because of decreased venous outflow and increase in intracavernosal pressure, low-flow priapism is associated with a painful, fully erect penis causing local hypoxia and acidosis. In addition, the penile glans is engorged as well.

In contrast to low-flow priapism, high-flow (type II) priapism is associated with increased arterial inflow without increased venous outflow resistance, thus resulting in high inflow and high outflow (see Box 76-1). As a result, the penis is erect but nontender in high-flow priapism states. The penile glans is usually soft and nontender.

Low-flow priapism can be distinguished from high-flow priapism by obtaining a corporeal blood gas value. Findings of PO_2 less than 30 mm Hg, PCO_2 greater than 60 mm Hg, and pH less than 7.25 are consistent with low-flow priapism. If the patient has a history of sickle cell disease or trait, then intravenous hydration, alkalinization with bicarbonate in intravenous fluid, analgesia, and supplemental oxygen can help reduce the veno-occlusive state

---

Box 76-1. Causes of Low-Flow and High-Flow Priapism

Low-Flow Priapism

Sickle cell trait and disease
Leukemia (especially chronic myelogenous leukemia)
Total parenteral nutrition (especially with 20% lipid infusion)
Medications (e.g., sildenafil, trazodone, chlorpromazine, topical and systemic cocaine)
Intracavernosal injections
Malignant penile infiltration
Hyperosmolar IV contrast
Spinal cord injury (usually self-limiting and no treatment required)
Spinal or general anesthesia (usually self-limiting and no treatment required)

High-Flow Priapism

Perineal or penile trauma

TABLE 76-1. Intracavernous Vasoconstrictor Therapy for Low-Flow Priapism*

Drug	Recommended Dosage
Epinephrine	10-20 μg
Phenylephrine	250-500 μg
Ephedrine	50-100 mg

*Intracavernous injection every 5 minutes until detumescence after aspiration of 10 to 20 mL of blood.

---

in the corporeal bodies. If the low-flow priapism persists in the patient with sickle cell disease, red blood cell transfusion to increase the hemoglobin value above 10 mg/dL and reduce the hemoglobin S value below 30% of total hemoglobin can help reduce the severity of priapism.

Low-flow priapism may require corporal irrigation with normal saline. The midshaft of the penis can be injected with a small-gauge butterfly needle and irrigated with 10 to 20 mL of normal saline. After irrigation with normal saline, an α-adrenergic intracorporeal injection every 5 minutes until detumescence can be used to correct low-flow priapism (Table 76-1). A patient's blood pressure and pulse should be monitored during intracorporeal α-adrenergic treatments. In severe cases when intracorporeal α-adrenergic treatment fails to treat low-flow priapism, surgical procedure with shunts (corporoglandular, corporospongiosal, or corporosaphenous) may be necessary to divert the occluded corporal blood.

High-flow priapism can be confirmed by a perineal Doppler ultrasound or arteriography to identify an arterial-lacunar fistula responsible for the priapism. High-flow priapism can be treated expectantly, and, if not resolved, arterial embolization or open surgical arterial ligation may be required.

NEPHROLITHIASIS

The prevalence of renal calculi varies with the population studied, and rates of nephrolithiasis vary regionally. Three to 12 percent of the population will develop symptomatic nephrolithiasis during their lifetime.[36] Eighty percent of patients with nephrolithiasis form calcium stones, most of which are composed primarily of calcium oxalate or, less often, calcium phosphate.[37] The other main types include uric acid, struvite (magnesium ammonium phosphate), and cystine stones. A combination of different stone types may exist within a single stone.

Stone formation occurs when normally soluble material (e.g., calcium) supersaturates the urine and begins the process of crystal formation. It is not clear how crystals formed in the tubules become a stone rather than being washed away by the high rate of urine flow. It is presumed that crystal aggregates become large enough to be anchored (usually at the end of the collecting ducts) and then slowly increase in size over time. This anchoring is thought to occur at sites of epithelial cell injury, perhaps induced by the crystals themselves.

Major risk factors associated with idiopathic nephrolithiasis, which accounts for the majority of symptomatic stones include the following:

- Low urine volume
- Hypercalciuria
- Hyperoxaluria
- Hyperuricosuria
- Dietary factors
  - Low fluid intake
  - Types of fluid intake: sodas, apple juice, grapefruit juice
  - High sodium chloride intake
  - High protein intake
  - Low calcium intake
- History of prior nephrolithiasis
- Hyperoxaluria (enteric hyperoxaluria, short bowel syndrome)
- Type I renal tubular acidosis

Patients may occasionally be diagnosed with asymptomatic nephrolithiasis when a radiologic imaging study of the abdomen is performed for other purposes. Symptoms are usually produced when stones pass from the renal pelvis into the ureter. Pain is the most common symptom and varies from a mild and barely noticeable ache to severe pain requiring parenteral analgesics. Pain typically waxes and wanes in severity and develops in waves or paroxysms that are related to movement of the stone in the ureter and associated ureteral spasm. The site of obstruction from the stone generally determines the location of pain. The referred pain associated with the renal colic usually originates from the flank and radiates to the front upper abdomen for kidney-related pain or radiates to the front toward the groin (Fig. 76-18). Often, microscopic hematuria and, less commonly, gross hematuria are associated with the patient with acute nephrolithiasis; however, lack of hematuria does not rule out nephrolithiasis.

The diagnosis of nephrolithiasis is initially suspected by the clinical presentation. Confirmatory radiologic tests include abdominal plain film (KUB), intravenous pyelography (IVP), ultrasonography, and nonenhanced CT. At our institution, nonenhanced CT is the test of choice for accurate and rapid diagnosis of symptomatic nephrolithiasis (Fig. 76-19).

Many patients with acute renal colic can be managed conservatively with pain medication and hydration until the stone passes spontaneously. Based on axial dimension of the stone determined by CT, the spontaneous rate of stone passage is dependent on the stone size and location of the stone (Table 76-2).[38]

Treatment of urinary lithiasis is dependent on the size and location of the stone in addition to the severity of symptoms associated with the stone. Patients who are suspected of having uric acid stones (those with urine pH < 6.5 or radiolucent calculi on plain films) can be treated with oral bicarbonate or potassium citrate supplementation to alkalinize the urine. If urine pH is alkalinized above 7.0, the chance of spontaneous dissolution of the stone by 3 months is great. Open surgery for nephrolithiasis is seldom performed in the United States, because of advances in minimally invasive techniques using extracorporeal shock wave lithotripsy (mainly for renal and proximal ureteral stones less than 2 cm), percutaneous lithotripsy (mainly for renal stones larger than 2 cm), and ureteroscopy (for renal and ureteral stones).

NEUROGENIC BLADDER

Micturition is a complex process, involving the central nervous system, autonomic nervous system, and the detrusor and sphincter muscle systems. The storage phase of micturition requires a bladder that can accommodate large urine volumes with low bladder pressure, which is accomplished by reflex inhibition of detrusor muscle. The relationship between change in bladder volume and bladder pressure is referred to as *compliance* of the bladder. Normal micturition begins with relaxation of the external sphincter, followed by relaxation and opening of the bladder neck and contraction of the detrusor. Complex interactions in the central nervous system are coordinated between cerebral motor cortex, basal ganglia, cerebellum, pontine nuclei, and sacral cord nuclei. Disruption in any of the central nervous system, autonomic nervous system, or the detrusor/sphincter mechanisms can lead to a neurogenic bladder.

To determine the mechanism responsible for a neurogenic bladder, a detailed history and physical examination and evaluation of the voiding pattern using a voiding diary are essential. Detailed questioning about the sensation of filling and urgency assesses sensory function. Urodynamics evaluations, which include a cystometrogram, help to analyze the strength and timing of detrusor contraction and bladder compliance. Cystometrography can assess the presence of any uninhibited or hyperreflexic bladder contractions. The urinary sphincter is assessed by urethral pressure profiles and electromyography. Postvoid residual volume can help determine the efficiency of voiding. Fluoroscopic voiding studies help determine the anatomic position of the bladder and the urethra during the storage

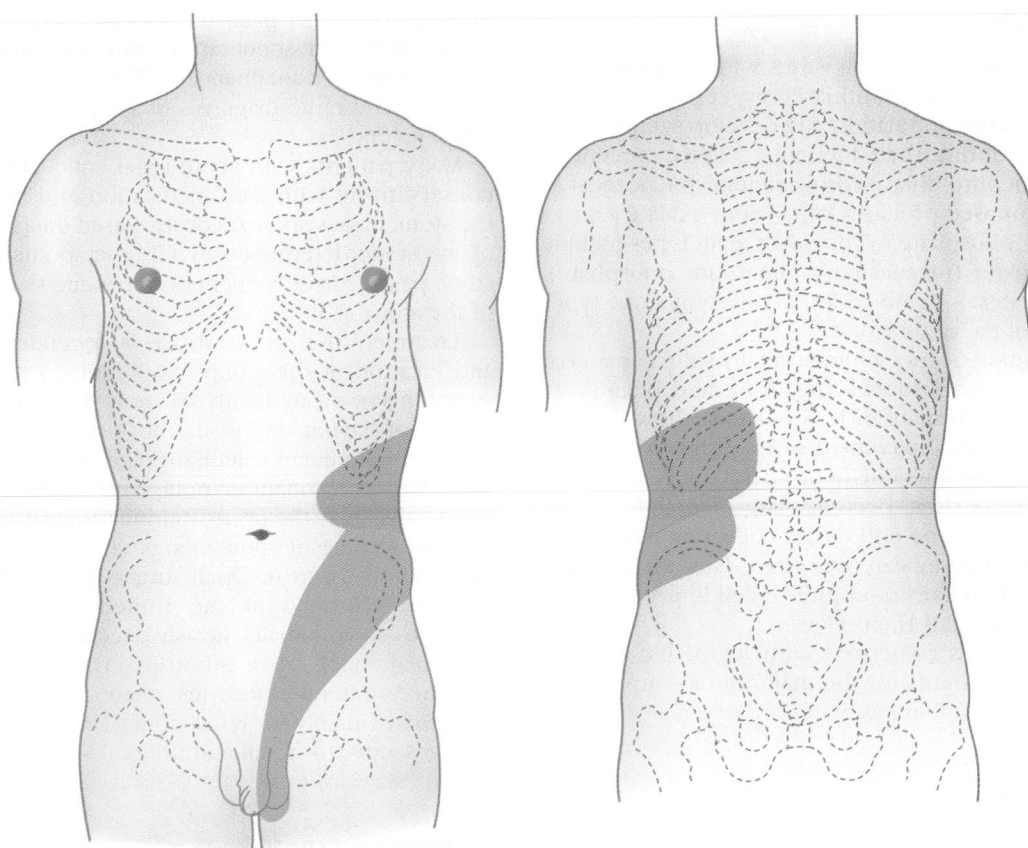

FIGURE 76-18. Referred pain from kidney *(dotted areas)* and ureter *(shaded areas)*. (Reproduced with permission from Tanagho E, McAninch JW [eds]: Smith's General Urology, 15th ed. New York, McGraw-Hil, 2000.)

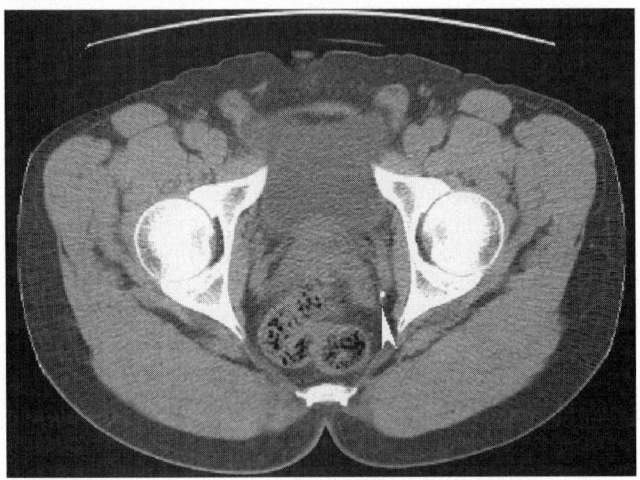

FIGURE 76-19. CT scan of the pelvis demonstrating ureterolithiasis in the distal left ureter *(arrowhead)*.

TABLE 76-2. Spontaneous Rate of Renal Stone Passage Based on Size and Location of Stone	
	Rate of Stone Passage (%)
STONE SIZE (mm)	
1	87
2-4	76
5-7	60
7-9	48
>9	25
STONE LOCATION	
Proximal ureter	48
Mid ureter	60
Distal ureter	75
Ureterovesical junction	79

From Coll DM, Varanelli MJ, Smith RC: Relationship of spontaneous passage of ureteral calculi to stone size and location as revealed by unenhanced helical CT. AJR Am J Roentgenol 178:101-103, 2002.

and the micturition phases. Renal ultrasound assesses for any potential hydronephrosis associated with high bladder pressures.

The primary therapeutic goal of treating patients with neurogenic bladder is preservation of renal function and restoring normal urinary patterns. Anticholinergic therapy can help in decreasing the frequency and severity of any uninhibited bladder contractions and improving bladder compliance. α-Adrenergic compounds can be used to increase sphincteric resistance when necessary. Clean intermittent catheterization is an efficient, relatively easy and safe method of ensuring bladder emptying with a wide range of applications. Because of a lower rate of urinary tract infection, clean intermittent catheterization is the preferred method of ensuring efficient bladder emptying than chronic indwelling urethral catheterization. Many patients may require a combination of medicines and manipulations to minimize urinary incontinence, improve bladder emptying, prevent urinary infections, and preserve renal function.

BENIGN PROSTATIC HYPERPLASIA

Benign prostatic hyperplasia (BPH) is a common entity among elderly men and is responsible for significant disability, but it is an infrequent cause of death. In men 20 to 30 years of age the prostate weighs approximately 20 g; however, the mean prostatic weight increases after the age of 50.[39] The prevalence of histologically diagnosed prostatic hyperplasia increases from 8% in men aged 31 to 40, to 40% to 50% in men aged 51 to 60, to over 80% in men older than age 80. The Baltimore Longitudinal Study of Aging compared the age-specific prevalence of pathologically defined BPH at autopsy with the clinical prevalence based on history and the results of digital rectal examination.[40] There was good agreement between the clinical prevalence and autopsy incidence in men of all ages.

The natural history of BPH as studied by a population-based study in Olmstead County, Minnesota, demonstrated that lower urinary tract symptoms associated with BPH increase with age.[41] In most men, symptoms are progressive and will eventually require medical or surgical treatment. Men with symptomatic BPH who are not treated have a 2.5% risk per year to develop urinary retention. Predictive risk factors associated with a chance of developing urinary retention include age, symptoms, urinary flow rate, and prostate size.[41]

Race has some influence on the risk for BPH severe enough to require surgery. Although the age-adjusted relative risk of BPH necessitating surgery is similar in black and white men, black men younger than 65 years old may need treatment more often than white men.[42] In the American Male Health Professional Study, men of Asian ancestry were less likely (relative risk 0.4, 95% confidence interval 0.2 to 0.8) to undergo surgery for BPH as compared with white men, and black men had a similar risk to white men.[43]

Androgens are necessary for both normal and abnormal development of prostate. Testosterone is converted to a more potent androgen, dihydrotestosterone, by the enzyme 5α-reductase type 2. The type 1 form of the enzyme is present in liver and skin.

Men who congenitally lack 5α-reductase type 2 have normal serum testosterone levels but lack dihydrotestosterone.[44] Men with this disorder have a rudimentary prostate throughout life but rarely experience bladder outlet obstruction secondary to BPH. These findings suggest that the active androgen, dihydrotestosterone, is important in promoting growth of prostate that would eventually lead to symptomatic BPH.

The majority of the prostatic nodules responsible for the bladder outlet obstructive symptoms associated with BPH arise in the periurethral tissue (see Fig. 76-9). The hyperplastic nodules comprise primarily stromal components and, to a lesser degree, epithelial cells; stereologic measurements have revealed a fourfold increase in stroma and a twofold increase in glandular components.[45] It has been suggested that the stromal-epithelial component of prostatic tissue significantly increases in men with symptomatic BPH.[46] Because BPH is primarily a disease of the stroma, the stroma might have intrinsic properties that enable it to proliferate and also to induce hyperplasia of the epithelium. In the presence of androgen, mesenchymal tissue derived from the urogenital sinus can induce differentiation of prostate epithelium.[47] In contrast, stroma lacking functional androgen receptors cannot induce differentiation of normal epithelium. These observations emphasize the importance of the stroma in development of the prostate.

The common symptoms of BPH are increased frequency of urination, nocturia, hesitancy, urgency, and weak urinary stream. These symptoms typically appear slowly and progress gradually over a period of years. However, they are not specific for BPH. Furthermore, the correlation between symptoms and the presence of prostatic enlargement on rectal examination is poor.[48] This discrepancy probably results from changes in bladder function that occurs with aging and from enlargement of the transitional zone of the prostate that is not always evident on rectal examination (see Fig. 76-9).

It is critical to exclude other causes of lower urinary tract symptoms other than BPH before institution of any medical or surgical treatment. The differential diagnosis of lower urinary tract symptoms in addition to BPH includes the following:

- Urethral stricture
- Bladder neck contracture
- Carcinoma of the prostate
- Carcinoma of the bladder
- Bladder calculi
- Urinary tract infection and prostatitis
- Neurogenic bladder

Physical examination should include a detailed examination of the abdomen, genitalia and prostate size, consistency, nodularity, and symmetry. Urinalysis and determination of serum prostate-specific antigen (PSA) and serum creatinine levels are routine laboratory evaluations for men with lower urinary tract symptoms.

Clinical testing with uroflowmetry and assessment of postvoid residual can help the clinician in determining the severity of bladder outlet obstruction. In some cases, detailed urodynamics evaluations that include pressure flow studies, cystometrogram, and cystourethroscopy may be helpful in the diagnosis of other causes responsible for lower urinary tract symptoms other than BPH. The American Urological Association (AUA) symptom score was developed to better assess the severity of patients' lower urinary tract symptoms secondary to BPH (Fig. 76-20).[49] The AUA symptom score can be a useful tool to compare a patient's urinary symptoms before and after initiating therapy.

Medical treatment for BPH has played a major role in improving the symptomatology associated with bladder

1. Incomplete emptying: Over the past month, how often have you had a sensation of not emptying your bladder completely after you finished urinating?

Not at all	Less than 1 time in 5	Less than half the time	About half the time	More than half the time	Almost always	Your score
0	1	2	3	4	5	

2. Frequency: Over the past month, how often have you had to urinate again less than 2 hours after you finished urinating?

Not at all	Less than 1 time in 5	Less than half the time	About half the time	More than half the time	Almost always	Your score
0	1	2	3	4	5	

3. Intermittency: Over the past month, how often have you found that you stopped and started again several times when you urinated?

Not at all	Less than 1 time in 5	Less than half the time	About half the time	More than half the time	Almost always	Your score
0	1	2	3	4	5	

4. Urgency: Over the past month, how often have you found it difficult to postpone urination?

Not at all	Less than 1 time in 5	Less than half the time	About half the time	More than half the time	Almost always	Your score
0	1	2	3	4	5	

5. Weak stream: Over the past month, how often have you had a weak stream?

Not at all	Less than 1 time in 5	Less than half the time	About half the time	More than half the time	Almost always	Your score
0	1	2	3	4	5	

6. Straining: Over the past month, how often have you had to push or strain to begin urination?

Not at all	Less than 1 time in 5	Less than half the time	About half the time	More than half the time	Almost always	Your score
0	1	2	3	4	5	

7. Nocturia: Over the past month or so, how many times did you get up to urinate from the time you went to bed until the time you got up in the morning?

None	1 time	2 times	3 times	4 times	5 or more times	Your score
0	1	2	3	4	5	

Add up your scores for total AUA score = _____

Quality of life due to urinary symptoms: If you were to spend the rest of your life with your urinary condition just the way it is now, how would you feel about that? (Bold, highlight or underline)

Delighted   Pleased   Mostly satisfied   Mixed   Mostly dissatisfied   Unhappy   Terrible

FIGURE 76-20. American Urological Association Urinary System Score. (From Barry MJ, et al: J Urol 148:1549-1557, 1992.)

outlet obstruction. Although one decade ago surgical treatment may have been at the forefront of therapy for BPH, medical treatment is now the first-line therapy for BPH. Medical therapy focuses on two aspects of the pathophysiology of BPH:

- A dynamic (physiologic, reversible) component related to the tension of prostatic smooth muscle in the prostate, prostate capsule, and bladder neck

- A fixed (structural) component related to the bulk of the enlarged prostate impinging on the urethra

The two classes of drugs, α-adrenergic antagonists (release smooth muscle tension) and 5α-reductase inhibitors (reduce the enlarged prostate size) act on each of the components mentioned earlier.

The three most common α-adrenergic antagonists used in the United States are terazosin, doxazosin, and tamsulosin. α_1-Adrenergic antagonists act against the dynamic component of bladder outlet obstruction. Prostatic tissue contains two types of α-adrenergic receptors: α_1- and α_2.[50] The α_1 receptors are abundant in the prostate and base of the bladder and sparse in the body of the bladder.[50,51] The density of these receptors is increased in hyperplastic prostatic tissue.[52] In one report there was a direct relationship between the smooth muscle content of prostatic tissue and the increase in maximal urinary flow rate in men with BPH treated with terazosin.[53]

The most common 5α-reductase inhibitor used in the United States is finasteride. It acts by blocking the conversion of testosterone to the more potent androgen dihydrotestosterone. The decreased serum and prostatic levels of dihydrotestosterone lead to reduction in prostatic size over time.

α-Adrenergic blockers have been shown to be more efficacious than 5α-reductase inhibitors by improving the lower urinary tract symptoms associated with BPH. In a Veterans Administration Cooperative trial, 1229 men with BPH were randomly assigned to receive placebo, terazosin (10 mg/day), finasteride (5 mg/day), or a combination of terazosin and finasteride.[54] The study concluded the following:

- Terazosin lowered the symptom score by 6.1 points (from 16.2 to 10.1) versus 2.6 points with placebo.
- Terazosin increased the peak urinary flow rate by 2.7 mL/sec versus 1.4 mL/sec with placebo.
- Finasteride alone was no better than placebo.
- The combination of finasteride and terazosin was no better than terazosin alone.

Although the Veterans Administration Cooperative trial did not find a benefit for the combination of finasteride and terazosin after only 1 year of therapy,[54] the Medical Therapy of Prostatic Symptoms (MTOPS) was designed as a multicenter randomized, placebo-controlled, double-masked clinical trial with a 4-year follow-up to assess whether a combination of finasteride and terazosin was beneficial in reducing the risk of progression of BPH.[55] The MTOPS trial demonstrated that finasteride and the combination of finasteride and doxazosin (another α blocker equivalent to terazosin) significantly reduced the risk of progression from BPH requiring invasive therapy (Fig. 76-21).

Surgical Treatments for Benign Prostatic Hyperplasia

Transurethral Resection of Prostate

Transurethral resection of prostate (TURP) is a proven surgical technique that significantly improves lower urinary tract symptoms associated with BPH.[56] The most common reasons that intervention is recommended in a patient with symptoms of bladder outlet obstruction and irritability are that the symptoms are moderate to severe, are bothersome, and interfere with the patient's quality of life. Although symptoms constitute the primary reason for recommending intervention, in patients with an obstructing prostate there are some absolute indications. These are acute urinary retention, recurrent infection, recurrent hematuria, and azotemia.

CUMULATIVE INCIDENCE OF BPH-RELATED INVASIVE THERAPY (%)

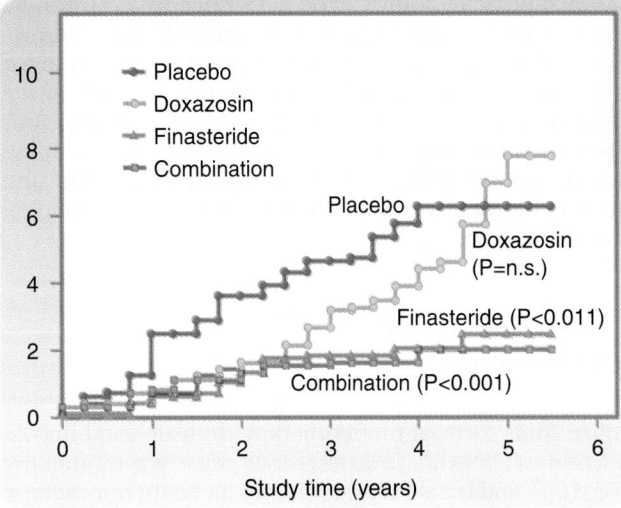

FIGURE 76-21. Medical Therapy of Prostatic Symptoms (MTOPS) trial demonstrating that finasteride when used alone or in combination with doxazosin (an α-adrenergic blocking agent) can reduce the cumulative incidence of invasive therapy related to benign prostatic hypertrophy. (Courtesy of Dr. Claus Roehrborn, University of Texas, Southwestern Medical Center.)

TUR syndrome is an immediate postoperative complication that happens in 2% of all TURPs. Glycine is the solution used during TURP. Excessive systemic absorption of glycine can lead to dilutional hyponatremia. The symptoms associated with TUR syndrome include mental confusion, nausea, vomiting, hypertension, bradycardia, and visual disturbance. Usually, the patients do not become symptomatic until the serum sodium concentration reaches 125 mEq/dL. The risk is increased if the gland is larger than 45 g, the resection time is longer than 90 minutes, or the irrigant fluid is greater than 70 cm H_2O above the patient. All of these factors lead to greater fluid absorption and increase the risk of TUR syndrome. Other potential causes of TUR syndrome could be due to conversion of glycine to glycolic acid and ammonium. Ammonium intoxication has been suggested as a possible cause of the TUR syndrome or direct toxic effect of the glycine.

Furosemide (Lasix) can be used to treat the hyponatremia associated with the TUR syndrome. Combination of diuretic and decreasing fluid overload gradually treats the hyponatremia over 8 to 12 hours. In severe cases, slow infusion of 3% saline can be utilized to slowly correct the hyponatremia.

Open Prostatectomy

Indications for open prostatectomy are the same as for TURP. Open prostatectomy instead of TURP is the preferred technique for treatment of bladder outlet obstruction from BPH when the prostate is estimated to weight more than 100 g. Open prostatectomy should also be considered when a man presents with ankylosis of the hip or other orthopedic conditions, preventing proper positioning in dorsal lithotomy for TURP.

Open prostatectomy can be performed by a retropubic or a suprapubic approach. With either technique the prostatic adenoma (periurethral central zone) is removed while the prostatic capsule or the peripheral zone of the prostate remains behind (see Fig. 76-9). Patients after open prostatectomy still remain at risk of developing prostate cancer in the peripheral zone of the prostate and should continue to be monitored for risk of developing prostate cancer.

Minimally Invasive Therapy for Benign Prostatic Hyperplasia

Over the past few years minimally invasive therapies that utilize some form of thermotherapy (transurethral needle ablation [TUNA],[57] transurethral microwave therapy [TUMT],[58] and transurethral water-induced thermotherapy [WIT][59]) for ablation of the enlarged prostate gland have been developed (for a recent review see Tunuguntal and Evans[60]). The advantage of these procedures is that they have less morbidity than TURP and open prostatectomy. Most notably, prostate thermotherapy for treatment of BPH has fewer sexual side effects such as retrograde ejaculation than TURP and open prostatectomy. However, findings on long-term efficacy, safety, and re-treatment are lacking at this time. Minimally invasive therapies are particularly useful in patients on anticoagulants, patients who are poor surgical candidates, and younger men who are sexually active and would like to avoid the risk of retrograde ejaculation commonly encountered with surgical therapies for BPH.

SCROTAL MASSES

For the clinician to differentiate between the emergent and urgent scrotal conditions such as testicular torsion and testis cancer, knowledge of the anatomy of the scrotum and potential scrotal masses is essential. Scrotal and paratesticular masses are mostly benign conditions.

Hydrocele

A *hydrocele* consists of a collection of fluid within the tunica or processus vaginalis. Although it may occur within the spermatic cord, it is most often seen surrounding the testis (Fig. 76-22). Surgical correction is only required if a patient is symptomatic secondary to the size and/or discomfort associated with the hydrocele. *Communicating hydrocele* of infancy and childhood is secondary to a patent processus vaginalis, which is continuous with the peritoneal cavity. It is also a form of indirect inguinal hernia. Most communicating hydroceles spontaneously close by 1 year of age. However, persistent communicating hydroceles and presence of bowel content within the hydrocele sac may require surgical correction.

Spermatocele

A *spermatocele* is a painless fluid-filled sac with sperm that is often located above and posterior to the testis. Although most spermatoceles are less than 1 cm, some may become large and hard, mimicking a solid neoplasm. Spermatocele is differentiated from hydrocele of the tunica vaginalis in that the latter covers the entire anterior surface of the testis. Spermatoceles do not require any intervention unless the patient experiences discomfort.

Torsion of Testicular Appendix and Epididymis

At the upper pole of the testis and epididymis there are small vestigial appendices that can spontaneously undergo torsion. A very reactive inflammatory reaction leading to testicular and scrotal swelling can follow ischemic necrosis of the appendix testis. It may be difficult to differenti-

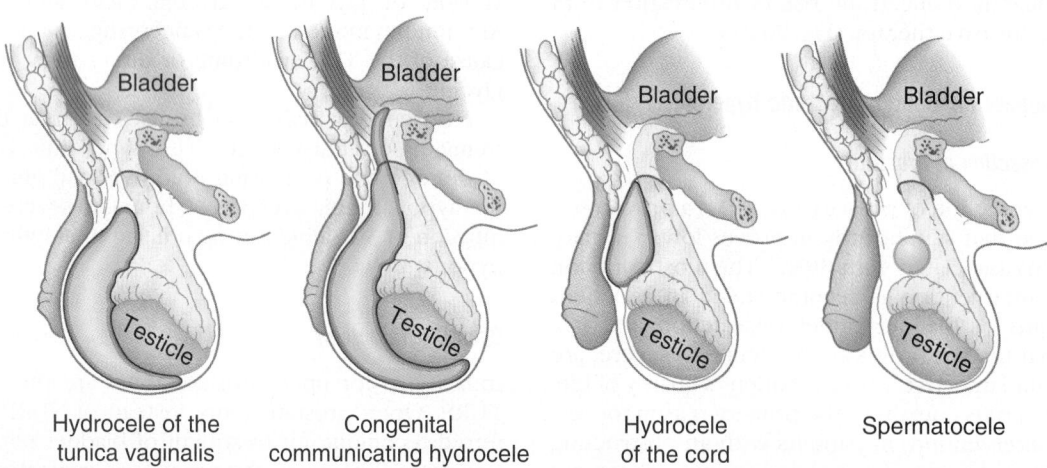

Hydrocele of the tunica vaginalis   Congenital communicating hydrocele   Hydrocele of the cord   Spermatocele

FIGURE 76-22.   Hydrocele of the tunica vaginalis and cord; spermatocele. (Reproduced with permission from Tanagho E, McAninch JW [eds]: Smith's General Urology, 15th ed. New York, McGraw-Hill, 2000.)

ate between torsion of the testicular appendix and torsion of the spermatic cord. If clinical diagnosis is uncertain, immediate surgical exploration is necessary, because in the case of spermatic cord torsion, time is of the essence to restore blood supply to a viable testis.

Varicocele

Varicocele is a result of dilatation of veins that drain into the internal spermatic veins. Approximately 10% of young men have varicoceles, with the left side most commonly affected. Most commonly, varicoceles arise secondary to incompetent internal spermatic vein valves. However, presence of unilateral right-sided varicocele should raise the suspicion of poor drainage at the junction of right testicular vein and right renal vein, which could be secondary to a large right-sided renal mass. In addition, the sudden onset of varicocele in an older man should raise the suspicion of a retroperitoneal mass, leading to inadequate drainage of the testicular veins.

Examination of a man with varicocele when he is upright reveals a mass of dilated, tortuous veins lying posterior to and above the testis. It may extend up to the external inguinal ring, and the Valsalva maneuver can increase the degree of dilatation.

Sperm concentration and motility can be significantly decreased in 65% to 75% of subjects. Infertility is observed in a higher percentage of individuals with varicoceles than the rest of the population. Surgical ligation for the dilated internal spermatic veins may restore fertility; however, in the absence of infertility, poor testicular growth in the adolescent, or patient discomfort, surgical intervention is not indicated.

UROLOGIC MALIGNANCIES

Renal Cell Carcinoma

Renal cell carcinomas, which originate within the renal cortex, are responsible for 80% to 85% of all primary renal neoplasms. Transitional cell carcinomas of the renal pelvis are the next most common (approximately 8%). Other parenchymal epithelial tumors, such as oncocytomas, collecting duct tumors, and renal sarcomas, occur infrequently. Nephroblastoma or Wilms' tumor is common in children (5% to 6% of all primary renal tumors).

Patients with renal cell carcinoma present with a range of symptoms, but many are asymptomatic until the disease is advanced. At presentation, approximately 25% of individuals either have distant metastases or significant local disease. Other patients, despite having only localized disease, present with a wide array of symptoms and/or laboratory abnormalities. Fever, cachexia, amyloidosis, anemia, hepatic dysfunction, and hormonal abnormalities are some manifestations of the paraneoplastic syndrome complex associated with renal cell carcinoma. Renal cell carcinomas may produce a host of hormones, including erythropoietin, parathyroid hormone–related protein (PTHrP), gonadotropins, human chorionic gonadotropin,

an ACTH-like substance, renin, glucagon, and insulin.[61] Because of this unusual paraneoplastic characteristic, renal cell carcinoma has been labeled the "internist's tumor." The classic triad of renal cell carcinoma, which is defined as flank pain, hematuria, and a palpable abdominal renal mass, is uncommon (9% of patients); when present, it strongly suggests metastatic disease.[62]

With increasing use of radiologic modalities there has been a significant rise in the incidence of renal cancer in the United States. Over the past decade CT has replaced intravenous pyelography and ultrasound to become the radiologic modality of choice to evaluate renal masses. Characteristic features of renal cell carcinoma on CT include enhancement of lesion after injection of intravenous contrast medium (Fig. 76-23), thickened irregular walls, thickened or enhanced septa within the mass, or multilocular mass. Magnetic resonance imaging (MRI) can be used for defining poorly characterized renal masses on CT or when CT is contraindicated in cases of allergy to intravenously administered contrast agent or poor renal function. In addition, MRI is very helpful in defining the extent of tumor extension into the renal vein or inferior vena cava.

Clinical staging (Table 76-3) using the best available radiologic modality is crucial before therapy. Surgical therapy is principally offered to patients with early renal cell carcinoma, in whom it may be curative. This includes patients in whom preoperative staging suggests that the tumor is either stage I or stage II, representing small (<7 cm) or large (>7 cm) growths limited to the kidney without evidence of lymph node or metastatic disease.[63]

Slightly different surgical considerations involve patients in whom preoperative evaluation suggests that the renal cell carcinoma is stage III. Patients with this stage of disease include those with tumor invasion into the adrenal gland or perinephric tissues (but not extending beyond Gerota's fascia), those with enlarged abdominal

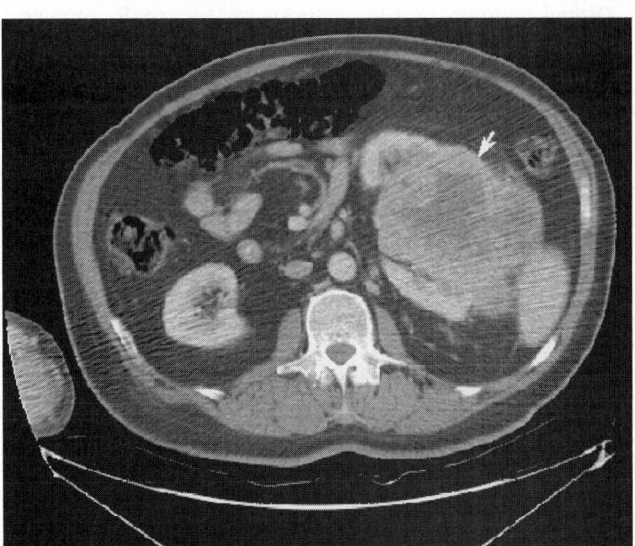

■ FIGURE 76-23. CT scan of abdomen demonstrates a large enhancing left renal mass consistent with renal cell carcinoma *(arrow)*.

TABLE 76-3.   Staging of Renal Cell Carcinoma

PRIMARY TUMOR (T)

TX	Primary tumor cannot be assessed
T0	No evidence of primary tumor
T1	Tumor 7 cm or less in greatest dimension, limited to the kidney
T1a	Tumor 4 cm or less in greatest dimension, limited to the kidney
T1b	Tumor more than 4 cm but not more than 7 cm in greatest dimension, limited to the kidney
T2	Tumor more than 7 cm in greatest dimension, limited to the kidney
T3	Tumor extends into major veins or invades adrenal gland or perinephric tissues but not beyond Gerota's fascia
T3a	Tumor directly invades adrenal gland or perirenal and/or renal sinus fat but not beyond Gerota's fascia
T3b	Tumor grossly extends into the renal vein or its segmental (muscle-containing) branches or the vena cava below the diaphragm
T3c	Tumor grossly extends into the vena cava above diaphragm or invades the wall of the vena cava
T4	Tumor invades beyond Gerota's fascia

REGIONAL LYMPH NODES (N)

NX	Regional lymph nodes cannot be assessed
N0	No regional lymph node metastases
N1	Metastases in a single regional lymph node
N2	Metastases in more than one regional lymph node

DISTANT METASTASIS (M)

MX	Distant metastasis cannot be assessed
M0	No distant metastasis
M1	Distant metastasis

From American Joint Committee on Cancer, 2003.

lymph nodes, and those with invasion of the major veins (renal vein or inferior vena cava).

Among those with radiologic evidence of abdominal lymph node involvement, a standard radical nephrectomy should also be offered as a possible curative procedure, because many nodes initially suspected of harboring tumor radiologically are enlarged only because of reactive inflammation.[63] Patients with stage IV disease are defined as those with large tumors extending beyond Gerota's fascia, obvious evidence of extensive disease in regional lymph nodes, and frank metastases. Nephrectomy may be indicated for palliative reasons or as a component of clinical trials.

Renal cancer is not responsive to irradiation and chemotherapy; therefore, radical nephrectomy remains the cornerstone of treatment of localized renal cancer. Radical nephrectomy consists of early ligation of the renal artery and vein and excision of the kidney and Gerota's fascia. Routine removal of the ipsilateral adrenal gland is uncommon, unless the tumor involves a large portion of the upper pole of the kidney or there is suggestion of adrenal gland involvement on preoperative radiologic examinations.[64]

Immunotherapy has demonstrated a modest response in patients with advanced renal cancer, and its utility is under intense investigation.[65] The combination of cytoreductive nephrectomy followed by immunotherapy may be beneficial for patients with metastatic renal cell carcinoma.[66,67]

Urothelial Carcinoma

The epithelial lining composing the renal pelvis, ureter, bladder, and proximal urethra is from transitional cell epithelium. Transitional cell carcinomas (TCCs) comprise more than 90% of all urothelial cancers in the United States. Adenocarcinoma (2%), squamous cell carcinoma (5% to 10%), undifferentiated carcinomas (2%), and mixed carcinomas (4% to 6%) are other types of urothelial malignancies. TCCs commonly appear as papillary and exophytic lesions.

TCCs of the renal pelvis or ureter account for less than 5% of all renal tumors and less than 1% of genitourinary neoplasms. The ratio of tumors of the bladder, renal pelvis, and ureter is 51 to 3 to 1.[68] However, in the Balkan countries (Bulgaria, Greece, Romania, Yugoslavia), an endemic familial nephropathy predisposes to renal pelvic neoplasms, which account for almost 50% of all renal tumors.[69] The incidence of upper tract urothelial neoplasms has modestly increased over the past 20 years in the United States. The age-adjusted annual incidence in the National Cancer Institute Surveillance, Epidemiology and End Results (SEER) database increased from 0.69 to 0.73/100,000 person-years over the time period 1973 to 1996.[70]

Cancer of the bladder is the fourth most common cancer in men and the tenth in women. More than 56,000 people (41,500 males and 15,000 females) develop bladder cancer each year in the United States, and 12,600 individuals (8,600 males and 4,000 females) are expected to die of the disease.[71]

The surface epithelium (urothelium) that lines the mucosal surfaces of the entire urinary tract is exposed to potential carcinogens that may be excreted in the urine or activated in the urine by hydrolyzing enzymes. Environmental exposures are thought to account for most cases of urothelial cancer. For example, a link between environmental factors and TCC of the urothelium was first suggested by the increased incidence of TCC in industrialized societies and urban dwellers. Second, increased incidence of renal pelvis and bladder carcinoma has been reported in aniline dye workers.[72] Exposure to chemicals used in the aluminum, dye, paint, petroleum, rubber, and textile industries has been estimated to account for up to 20% of all bladder cancer cases.[73] Hairdressers and barbers have an excess risk of bladder cancer that is thought to be related to long-term exposure to permanent hair dyes.[74] In most cases, the suspect carcinogens are arylamines or their derivatives that take several years to accumulate, thus accounting for the long latency period before the development of bladder cancer.

Clinical manifestations of urothelial carcinoma include gross or microscopic hematuria, which is the most common symptom at the time of presentation, occurring in 70% to 95% of patients. In patients with renal pelvis and ureteral malignancies, flank pain occurs in 8% to 40% and may be precipitated by obstruction of the ureter or ureteropelvic junction due to the tumor mass. Bladder irritation, or constitutional symptoms, occurs in less than 10% of urothelial malignancies.

Diagnosis of renal pelvis and ureteral malignancies is commonly made by radiologic modalities, which may include CT, IVP, or retrograde pyelography (Fig. 76-24). Ureteroscopy has been used for confirming any upper urinary tract malignancies when radiologic modalities are not confirmatory.[75] Cystoscopy is the main procedure used for diagnosing bladder carcinoma (Fig. 76-25).

Staging of urothelial malignancy is dependent on the depth of invasion of the tumor through the submucosal musculature or adjacent organs. Figure 76-26 demonstrates the staging system most commonly used for bladder carcinoma. More than 70% of all newly diagnosed bladder cancers are superficial, 50% to 70% are stage Ta, 20% to 30% are stage T1, and 10% are carcinoma in situ.

The standard treatment of renal pelvis and upper ureteral urothelial carcinomas includes complete nephroureterectomy with excision of the distal ureteral cuff from the bladder. Distal ureteral tumors can be treated with segmental resection followed by reimplantation of the remainder of the ureter into the bladder. The initial treatment options for bladder carcinoma are dictated by the tumor stage, grade, size, and number of tumors detected. In general, low-grade superficial tumors are treated by transurethral resection (TUR) of bladder tumor with or without intravesical treatment, whereas muscle-invasive tumors (stage T2 or higher) are treated with radical cystectomy with or without systemic chemotherapy (see Figure 76-26 for staging of bladder carcinoma). Bacille Calmette-Guérin (BCG) is an attenuated strain of *Mycobacterium bovis* rendered completely avirulent by long-term cultivation on bile-glycero-potato medium and used in BCG vaccine for immunization against tuberculosis. BCG introduced intravesically has been shown to induce a major histocompatibility complex–mediated immune response against bladder cancer. Intravesical treatment with BCG has been shown to decrease the rate of bladder cancer recurrence and risk of tumor progression. Table 76-4 summarizes the general guidelines for treatment of bladder carcinoma.

After radical cystectomy a portion of small and/or large bowel is often used for diversion of urine. Knowledge of the anatomy and of potential metabolic complications associated with various urinary diversions is important for proper management of patients after urinary diversion. Ureteroileal urinary diversion is the most common method of urinary diversion in the United States. The conduit is constructed from a segment of the ileum 15 to 20 cm proximal to the ileocecal valve (Fig. 76-27). In contrast to the ileal loop urinary diversion that requires constant drainage of urine into a drainage bag, continent

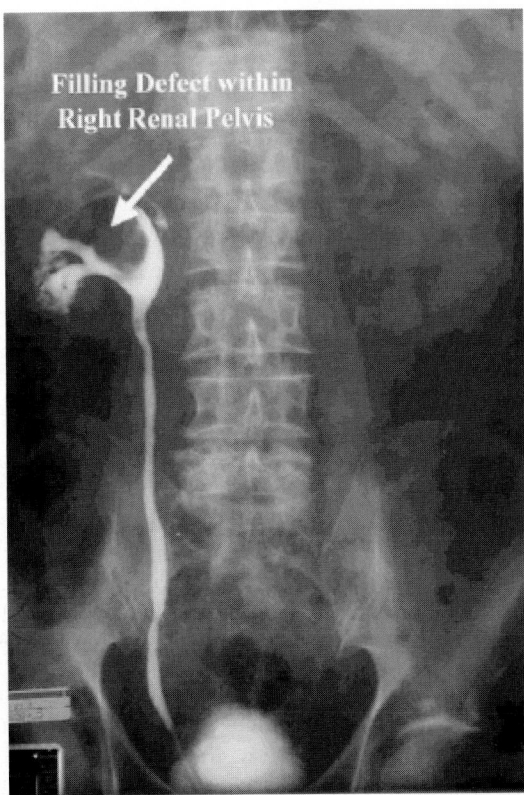

FIGURE 76-24. Retrograde pyelography demonstrating a filling defect in the right renal pelvis consistent with transitional cell carcinoma of renal pelvis.

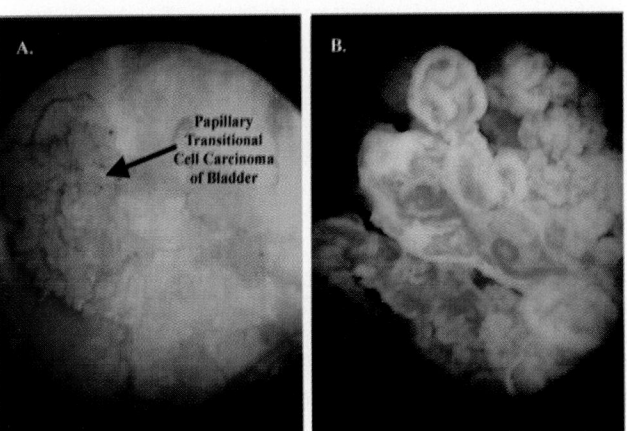

FIGURE 76-25. Cystoscopic views of papillary transitional cell carcinoma of the bladder with low (**A**) and high (**B**) magnifications.

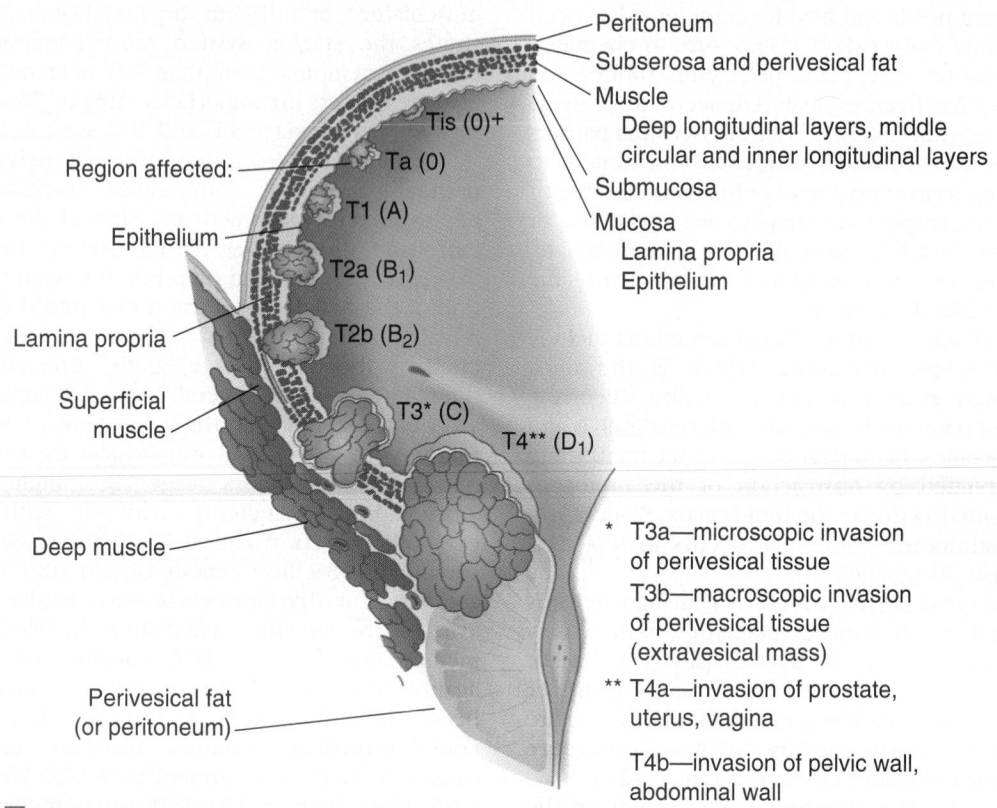

Peritoneum
Subserosa and perivesical fat
Muscle
   Deep longitudinal layers, middle
   circular and inner longitudinal layers
Submucosa
Mucosa
   Lamina propria
   Epithelium

Tis (0)+
Ta (0)
T1 (A)
T2a (B₁)
T2b (B₂)
T3* (C)
T4** (D₁)

Region affected:
Epithelium
Lamina propria
Superficial muscle
Deep muscle
Perivesical fat (or peritoneum)

* T3a—microscopic invasion
  of perivesical tissue
  T3b—macroscopic invasion
  of perivesical tissue
  (extravesical mass)

** T4a—invasion of prostate,
   uterus, vagina

   T4b—invasion of pelvic wall,
   abdominal wall

FIGURE 76-26. Staging of bladder cancer. (Reproduced with permission from Tanagho E, McAninch JW [eds]: Smith's General Urology, 15th ed. New York, McGraw-Hill, 2000.)

TABLE 76-4.   Guidelines for Treatment of Transitional Cell Bladder Carcinoma

Cancer Stage	Initial Treatment Option
Tis	TUR + intravesical immunotherapy (BCG)
Ta (single, small focus)	TUR
Ta (large, multifocal)	TUR + BCG or intravesical chemotherapy
T1 (low grade)	TUR + BCG or intravesical chemotherapy
T1 (high grade)	TUR + (BCG or intravesical chemotherapy) or radical cystectomy
T2-T4	Radical cystectomy Neoadjuvant chemotherapy + radical cystectomy Radical cystectomy + adjuvant chemotherapy Neoadjuvant chemotherapy + cystectomy + irradiation
Any T, N+, M+	Systemic chemotherapy followed by selective surgery or irradiation

TUR, transurethral resection; BCG, bacille Calmette-Guérin.

urinary reservoirs (Fig. 76-28) are catheterized four to six times per day to drain the urine and do not require appliance of an abdominal urinary stoma. The biggest advance in urinary diversion over the past two decades has been the ability to perform continent orthotopic urinary diversion (Fig. 76-29) in both male and female patients.[76-78]

Early complications after urinary diversion include excessive bleeding, intestinal obstruction, urinary extravasation, and/or rupture and infection. Late complications include metabolic disorders, stomal stenosis, pyelonephritis, and formation of calculi. Metabolic abnormalities associated with colonic urinary diversions are dependent on the length and segment of bowel used in the urinary diversion. In general, when ileum and/or large bowel are used for urinary diversion then hyperchloremic metabolic acidosis may manifest. A potential complication of chronic long-term metabolic acidosis may be decreased bone calcium content and osteomalacia.

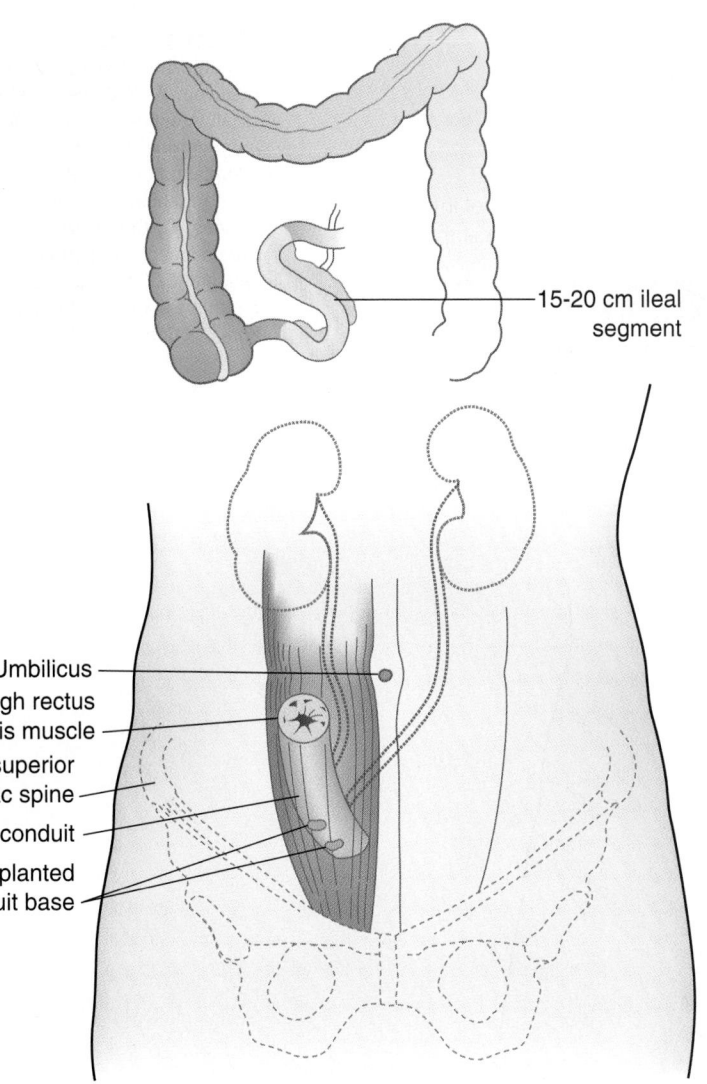

FIGURE 76-27. Ileal conduit urinary reservoir. (Reproduced with permission from Tanagho E, McAninch JW [eds]: Smith's General Urology, 15th ed. New York, McGraw-Hill, 2000.)

15-20 cm ileal segment

Umbilicus

Stoma through rectus abdominis muscle

Anterior superior iliac spine

Ileal conduit

Ureters reimplanted in conduit base

Prostate Carcinoma

Prostate cancer is the most common cancer in men in the United States except for nonmelanoma skin cancer. It is estimated that 189,000 men will be diagnosed with prostate cancer in 2002 and that 30,200 deaths will occur.[71] Prostate cancer has been detected with increasing frequency. The increase in detection is due in part to the widespread availability of tests for serum prostate-specific antigen (PSA) and to increased public awareness and increased screening for the disease.

The clinical presentation of prostate cancer has significantly changed ever since the introduction and wide use of PSA. Fifteen years ago, before common use of PSA, prostate cancer was first detected by digital rectal examination or because the patient had urinary symptoms. Urinary symptoms could include urgency, nocturia, frequency, and hesitancy, which are similar clinical symptoms as those of BPH. Ever since the 1990s prostate cancer is often diagnosed after a man has been found to have a high serum PSA concentration with a normal prostate

examination. Only 20% of newly detected prostate cancers are associated with an abnormal digital rectal examination as the first clinical sign of prostate cancer.

Serum PSA elevation is often the first sign of prostatic pathology. Both BPH and prostate cancer can lead to an elevation of serum PSA; however, the rate of rise of PSA associated with prostate cancer is usually higher than compared with BPH.[79] Other causes of elevated PSA include prostate inflammation and perineal trauma.

A total serum PSA concentration greater than 4.0 ng/mL is considered abnormal in most assays and is suggestive of prostate cancer. To improve the accuracy of PSA as a cancer screening tool, age-related[80] and race-related[81] PSA values have been recommended and are widely used by clinicians for early diagnosis of prostate cancer.

The normal range for age-related PSA levels is as follows[80]:

- 40 to 49 years old: 0 to 2.5 ng/mL
- 50 to 59 years old: 0 to 3.5 ng/mL
- 60 to 69 years old: 0 to 4.5 ng/mL
- 70 to 79 years old: 0 to 6.5 ng/mL

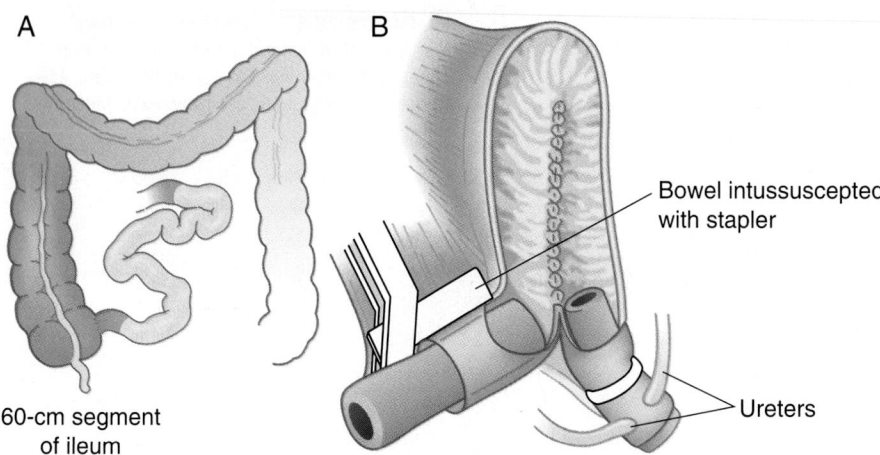

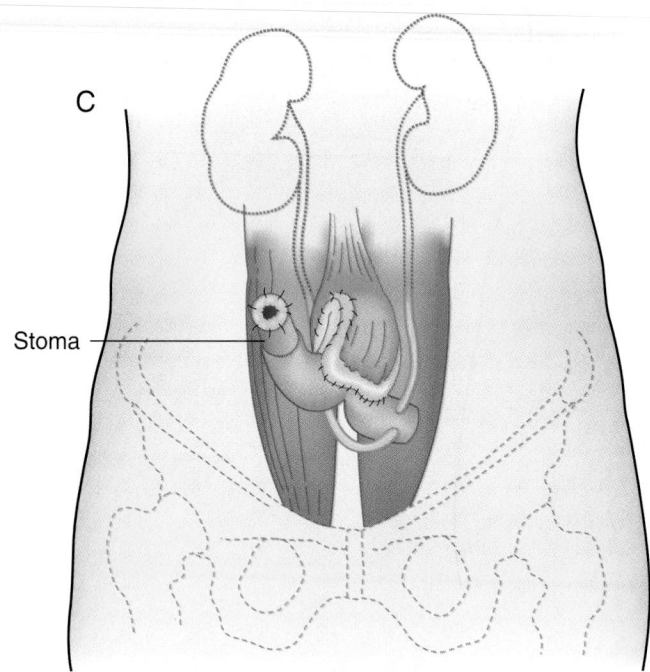

A
60-cm segment
of ileum

B
Bowel intussuscepted
with stapler

Ureters

C
Stoma

FIGURE 76-28. Continent catheterizable Kock pouch urinary reservoir. **A,** Sixty centimeters of small intestine selected. **B,** Afferent (nonrefluxing) limb for ureteral reimplantation and efferent limb for stoma fashioned using stapling devices. **C,** Completed reservoir. (Reproduced with permission from Tanagho E, McAninch JW [eds]: Smith's General Urology, 15th ed. New York, McGraw-Hill, 2000.)

The normal range for age-related and race-related PSA levels includes[81]:

- 40 to 49 years old: 0 to 2.0 ng/mL (blacks); 0 to 2.5 (whites)
- 50 to 59 years old: 0 to 4.0 ng/mL (blacks); 0 to 3.5 (whites)
- 60 to 69 years old: 0 to 4.5 ng/mL (blacks); 0 to 3.5 (whites)
- 70 to 79 years old: 0 to 5.5 ng/mL (blacks); 0 to 3.5 (whites)

Prostate biopsy is the gold standard for prostate cancer diagnosis. Transrectal biopsy is a relatively simple office technique that can be performed without sedation or analgesia. If a prostate biopsy specimen is interpreted as containing carcinoma, additional evaluation or clinical staging may be required to determine the extent of spread. Clinical and pathologic staging of prostate cancer is listed in Table 76-5.

The most effective therapy for an individual man with early stage prostate cancer is not clear. Management options include surgery, radiation therapy (external beam or brachytherapy, with or without hormone therapy), or observation, also termed *watchful waiting.* Issues to be considered in making the choice between treatments include the following:

- The man's general medical condition, age, and comorbidity
- The histologic grade (Gleason score) of the tumor on prostate biopsy
- Pretreatment serum PSA value
- Extent of tumor involving the prostate biopsy needle cores
- The clinical stage of the disease and the likelihood of the cancer being confined to the prostate gland, and, therefore, potentially amenable to cure
- An estimation of the outcome associated with the alternative treatments for prostate cancer

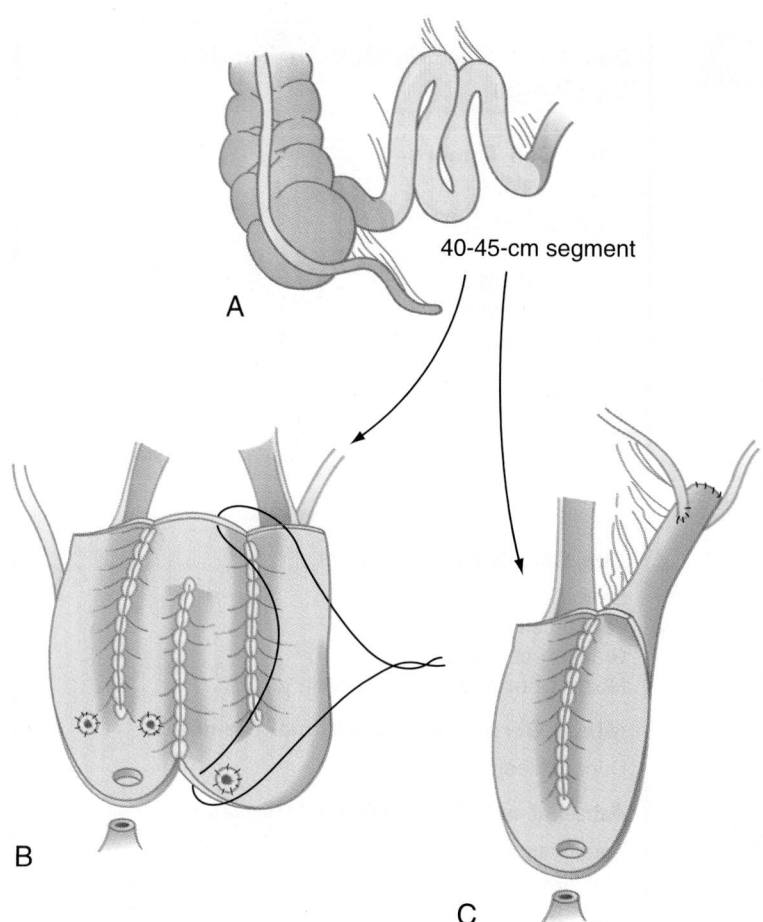

■ **FIGURE 76-29.** Orthotopic neobladder. Bladder substitutes constructed entirely of small intestine. **A,** Forty to 45 cm of small intestine is selected. **B,** Small intestine is opened and fashioned into a "W". The ureters are reimplanted into the second and third limbs of the reservoir, and the reservoir is attached to the urethra. **C,** Small intestine is folded into a "J" with the most proximal portion of the segment not opened. The ureters are reimplanted into the intact ileal segment of the reservoir, and the reservoir is attached to the urethra. (Reproduced with permission from Tanagho EA, McAninch JW [eds]: Smith's General Urology, 15th ed. New York, McGraw-Hill, 2000.)

40-45-cm segment

■ The potential side effects associated with the different forms of treatment for early-stage disease

For purposes of this chapter, only an overview of the surgical treatment (radical retropubic prostatectomy) is explained. After gaining access to the retropubic space of Retzius, the endopelvic fascia is incised (Fig. 76-30A), the puboprostatic ligament is divided, the dorsal venous complex is followed by obtaining hemostasis, and the urethra is incised (see Fig. 76-30B). After incising the urethra and releasing the rectourethralis fascia, care is taken not to harm the neurovascular bundle, which is responsible for maintaining potency. Excision of lateral pelvic fascia is followed by division of the bladder neck and excision of the seminal vesicles (see Fig. 76-30D). Reconstruction of the bladder neck and anastomosis to the remnant urethra (see Fig. 76-30E) completes the procedures.

Because prostate cancer has a high prevalence in elderly men, prostate cancer prevention is an attractive treatment strategy. In a recent large randomized trial that included 18,000 men, the effect of finasteride as a chemopreventive agent on development of prostate cancer was examined.[82] It has long been appreciated that prostate cancer is an androgen-dependent cancer and that removal of androgens reduces the progression of prostate cancer. Finasteride blocks the conversion of testosterone to the more potent androgen dihydrotestosterone by blocking the enzyme 5α-reductase type 2. The hypothesis of this study was to determine whether elimination of dihydrotestosterone would reduce the risk of developing prostate cancer. The study determined that finasteride may prevent or delay the appearance of prostate cancer but that men using finasteride are at increased risk of developing more advanced high-grade prostate cancers. The study concludes that the potential benefits of finasteride are reducing/delaying prostate cancer and improving the men's lower urinary tract symptoms. However, the potential benefits need to be weighed against the sexual side effects and the increased risk of developing high-grade prostate cancer.[82]

Testicular Carcinoma

Testicular cancer, although relatively rare, is the most common malignancy in men in the 15- to 35-year age group and evokes widespread interest for several reasons. Testicular cancer has become one of the most curable solid neoplasms and serves as a paradigm for the multimodal treatment of malignancies. The dramatic improvement in survival resulting from the combination of effective diagnostic techniques, improved tumor markers, effective multidrug chemotherapeutic regimens, and mod-

TABLE 76-5.   Staging of Prostate Carcinoma: TNM Classification for Prostate Carcinoma

PATHOLOGIC: PRIMARY TUMOR (T)

pT2	Organ confined
pT2a	Unilateral, one half of one lobe or less
pT2b	Unilateral, involving more than one half of lobe but not both lobes
pT2c	Bilateral disease
pT3	Extraprostatic extension
pT3a	Extraprostatic extension
pT3b	Seminal vesicle invasion
pT4	Invasion of bladder, rectum

CLINICAL: PRIMARY TUMOR (T)

TX	Primary tumor cannot be assessed
T0	No evidence of primary tumor
T1	Clinically inapparent tumor neither palpable nor visible by imaging
T1a	Tumor incidental histologic finding in 5% or less of tissue resected
T1b	Tumor incidental histologic finding in more than 5% of tissue resected
T1c	Tumor identified by needle biopsy (e.g., because of elevated prostate-specific antigen)
T2	Tumor confined within prostate
T2a	Tumor involves one half of one lobe or less
T2b	Tumor involves more than one half of one lobe but not both lobes
T2c	Tumor involves both lobes
T3	Tumor extends through the prostate capsule
T3a	Extracapsular extension (unilateral or bilateral)
T3b	Tumor invades seminal vesicle(s)
T4	Tumor is fixed or invades adjacent structures other than seminal vesicles: bladder neck, external sphincter, rectum, levator muscles, and/or pelvic wall

PATHOLOGIC: REGIONAL LYMPH NODES (N)

pNX	Regional nodes not sampled
pN0	No positive regional nodes
pN1	Metastases in regional node(s)

CLINICAL: REGIONAL LYMPH NODES (N)

NX	Regional lymph nodes were not assessed
N0	No regional lymph node metastasis
N1	Metastasis in regional lymph node(s)

CLINICAL AND PATHOLOGIC: DISTANT METASTASIS (M)

MX	Distant metastasis cannot be assessed (not evaluated by any modality)
M0	No distant metastasis
M1	Distant metastasis
M1a	Nonregional lymph node(s)
M1b	Bone(s)
M1c	Other site(s) with or without bone disease

From American Joint Committee on Cancer, 2003.

Box 76-2.   Classification of Testicular Carcinoma

Germ Cell Tumors

Seminoma
  Classic (typical)
  Atypical
  Spermatocytic
Nonseminomatous
  Embryonal carcinoma
  Teratoma
    Mature
    Immature
    Mature or immature with malignant transformation
  Choriocarcinoma
  Yolk sac tumor (endodermal sinus tumor)

Sex Cord-Stromal Tumors

Sertoli cell tumor
Leydig cell tumor
Granular cell tumor
Mixed types (e.g., Sertoli-Leydig tumor)

Mixed Germ Cell and Stromal Elements

Gonadoblastoma

Adnexal and Paratesticular Tumors

Adenocarcinoma of rete testis
Mesothelioma

Miscellaneous Tumors

Carcinoid
Lymphoma
Testicular metastasis

Testicular cancer has become one of the most curable cancers in the United States because of advances in medical and surgical therapy since the 1970s.[84] Cisplatin-based chemotherapy regimens have improved the response rates for testicular cancer.[85] In addition, detailed identification of the retroperitoneal lymph nodes and metastatic landing sites has been a major advance in surgical treatment of patients at high risk for advanced cancers.[84,86]

Testicular tumors usually present as a nodule or painless swelling of one testis, which may be noted incidentally by the patient or by his sexual partner.[83] Occasionally, a man with a previously small atrophic testis will note enlargement. Thirty to 40 percent of patients complain of a dull ache or heavy sensation in the lower abdomen, perianal area, or scrotum, whereas acute pain is the presenting symptom in 10%. Gynecomastia, which occurs in about 5% of men with testicular germ cell tumors, is a systemic endocrine manifestation of these neoplasms.

Examination should include a detailed evaluation of the neck, chest, and abdominal contents. Patients with testicular tumors often have a palpable parenchymal testis

---

ifications of surgical technique has led to a decrease in patient mortality from more than 50% before 1970 to less than 5% in 1997.[83] Germ cell tumors account for 95% of testicular cancers (Box 76-2). They may consist of one predominant histologic pattern or represent a mix of multiple histologic types. For treatment purposes, two broad categories of testis tumors are recognized: pure seminoma (no nonseminomatous elements present) and all others, which together are termed *nonseminomatous germ cell tumors* (see Box 76-2).

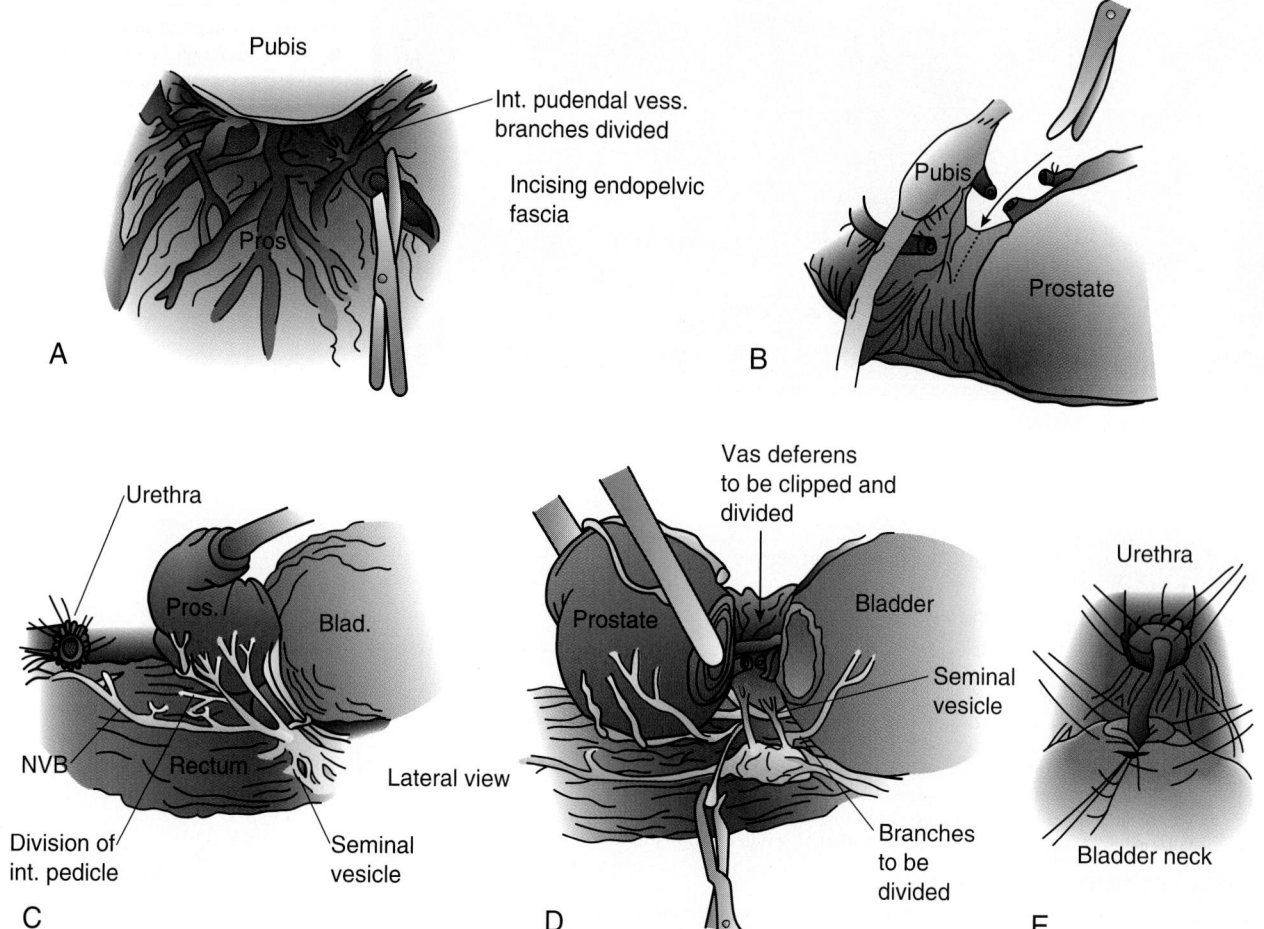

Pubis

Int. pudendal vess.
branches divided

Incising endopelvic
fascia

Pros.

A

Pubis

Prostate

B

Urethra

Pros.

Blad.

NVB   Rectum

Division of
int. pedicle

Seminal
vesicle

Lateral view

C

Vas deferens
to be clipped and
divided

Prostate   Bladder

Seminal
vesicle

Branches
to be
divided

D

Urethra

Bladder neck

E

■ **FIGURE 76-30.** Anatomic radical retropubic prostatectomy. **A,** The incision in the endopelvic fascia is made at the junction with the pelvic sidewall well away from the prostate and bladder. Anteriorly, near the puboprostatic ligaments, small arterial and venous branches from the internal pudendal vessels are often encountered. These are clipped and divided. **B,** Transection of the puboprostatic ligaments and exposure of the anterior urethra. **C,** Posterior dissection of the prostate gland (side view) by reflecting the prostate off of the rectum. Special care is taken to preserve the neurovascular bundle. **D,** Transection of the prostate from the bladder neck and transection of the vas deferens. **E,** Anastomosis between the bladder neck and the urethra after removal of the prostate and seminal vesicles. (Reproduced with permission from Walsh PC, Retik AB, Vaughan ED Jr, et al (eds): Campbell's Urology, 8th ed. Philadelphia, Elsevier, 2002, pp 3113-3126.)

mass, which can be better appreciated if compared with the contralateral normal testis. The examiner needs to differentiate between intraparenchymal testicular masses, which are often malignant, and extraparenchymal testicular masses, which are often benign (see section on benign testicular masses). Scrotal ultrasound can distinguish intrinsic from extrinsic testicular lesions with a high degree of accuracy and can detect intratesticular lesions as small as 1 to 2 mm in diameter (Fig. 76-31).

Further radiologic work-up will include high-resolution CT of the abdomen and pelvis and chest radiography. Regional metastases first appear in the retroperitoneal lymph nodes. Although CT is the imaging modality of choice to evaluate the retroperitoneum, false-negative rates as high as 44% have been described.[87] Occult micrometastases are responsible for most of these false negatives, as evidenced by a retroperitoneal relapse rate of 20% to 25% in men with clinical stage I disease who

do not undergo retroperitoneal lymph node dissection (RPLND).[88,89]

In men suspected of having testicular tumor serum markers of α-fetoprotein (AFP), the β subunit of human chorionic gonadotropin (β-HCG) and lactate dehydrogenase (LDH) should be obtained. Serum levels of AFP and/or β-HCG are elevated in 80% to 85% of men with nonseminomatous germ cell tumors (see Box 76-2), even when nonmetastatic. In contrast, serum β-HCG is elevated in fewer than 20% of testicular seminomas and AFP is not elevated in pure seminomas. Neither serum β-HCG nor AFP alone or in combination is sufficiently sensitive or specific to establish the diagnosis of testicular cancer in the absence of histologic confirmation. Serum LDH concentrations are elevated in 30% to 80% of men with pure seminoma and in 60% of those with nonseminomatous tumors.[90,91] LDH is a less sensitive and less specific tumor marker than β-HCG or AFP for men

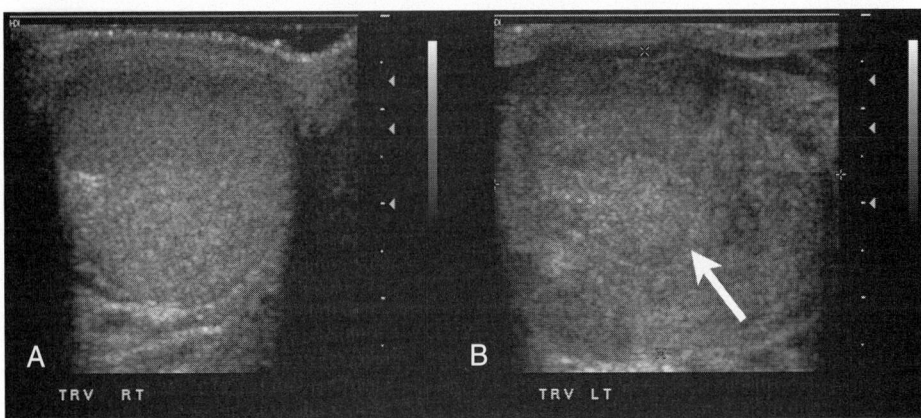

Normal right testis   Heterogeneous mass in left testis

FIGURE 76-31.   **A,** Normal ultrasound image of testis. **B,** Heterogeneous mass in left testicle (arrow) that is very irregular. Pathology was consistent with embryonal cell carcinoma with extensive lymphovascular invasion.

TABLE 76-6.   Staging of Testicular Carcinoma

PATHOLOGIC: PRIMARY TUMOR (T)

pTX	Primary tumor cannot be assessed (if no radical orchiectomy has been performed, TX is used)
pT0	No evidence of primary tumor (e.g., histologic scar in testis)
pTis	Intratubular germ cell neoplasia (carcinoma in situ)
pT1	Tumor limited to the testis and epididymis without vascular/lymphatic invasion; tumor may invade into the tunica albuginea but not the tunica vaginalis
pT2	Tumor limited to the testis and epididymis with vascular/lymphatic invasion, or tumor extending through the tunica albuginea with involvement of the tunica vaginalis
pT3	Tumor invades the spermatic cord with or without vascular/lymphatic invasion
pT4	Tumor invades the scrotum with or without vascular/lymphatic invasion

CLINICAL: PRIMARY TUMOR (T)

Tumor stage is generally determined after orchiectomy, at which time a pathologic stage is assigned.

PATHOLOGIC: REGIONAL LYMPH NODES (N)

pNX	Regional lymph nodes cannot be assessed
pN0	No regional lymph node metastasis
pN1	Metastasis with a lymph node mass 2 cm or less in greatest dimension and less than or equal to 5 nodes positive, none more than 2 cm in greatest dimension
pN2	Metastasis with a lymph node mass more than 2 cm but not more than 5 cm in greatest dimension; or more than 5 nodes positive, none more than 5 cm; or evidence of extranodal extension of tumor
pN3	Metastasis with a lymph node mass more than 5 cm in greatest dimension

CLINICAL: REGIONAL LYMPH NODES (N)

NX	Regional lymph nodes cannot be assessed
N0	No regional lymph node metastasis
N1	Metastasis with a lymph node mass 2 cm or less in greatest dimension; or multiple lymph nodes, none more than 2 cm in greatest dimension
N2	Metastasis with a lymph node mass more than 2 cm but not more than 5 cm in greatest dimension; or multiple lymph nodes, any one mass greater than 2 cm but not more than 5 cm in greatest dimension
N3	Metastasis with a lymph node mass more than 5 cm in greatest dimension

DISTANT METASTASIS (M)

MX	Distant metastasis cannot be assessed
M0	No distant metastasis
M1	Distant metastasis
M1a	Nonregional nodal or pulmonary metastasis
M1b	Distant metastasis other than to nonregional lymph nodes and lungs

SERUM TUMOR MARKERS (S)

SX	Marker studies not available or not performed
S0	Marker study levels within normal limits
S1	LDH < 1.5 × N *and* HCG (mIu/mL) > 5,000 *and* AFP (ng/mL) < 1,000
S2	LDH 1.5-10 × N *or* HCG (mIu/mL) 5,000-50,000 *or* AFP (ng/mL) 1,000-10,000
S3	LDH > 10 × N *or* HCG (mIu/mL) > 50,000 *or* AFP (ng/mL) > 10,000

LDH, lactate dehydrogenase; N, indicates upper limit of normal for LDH assay.
From American Joint Committee on Cancer, 2003.

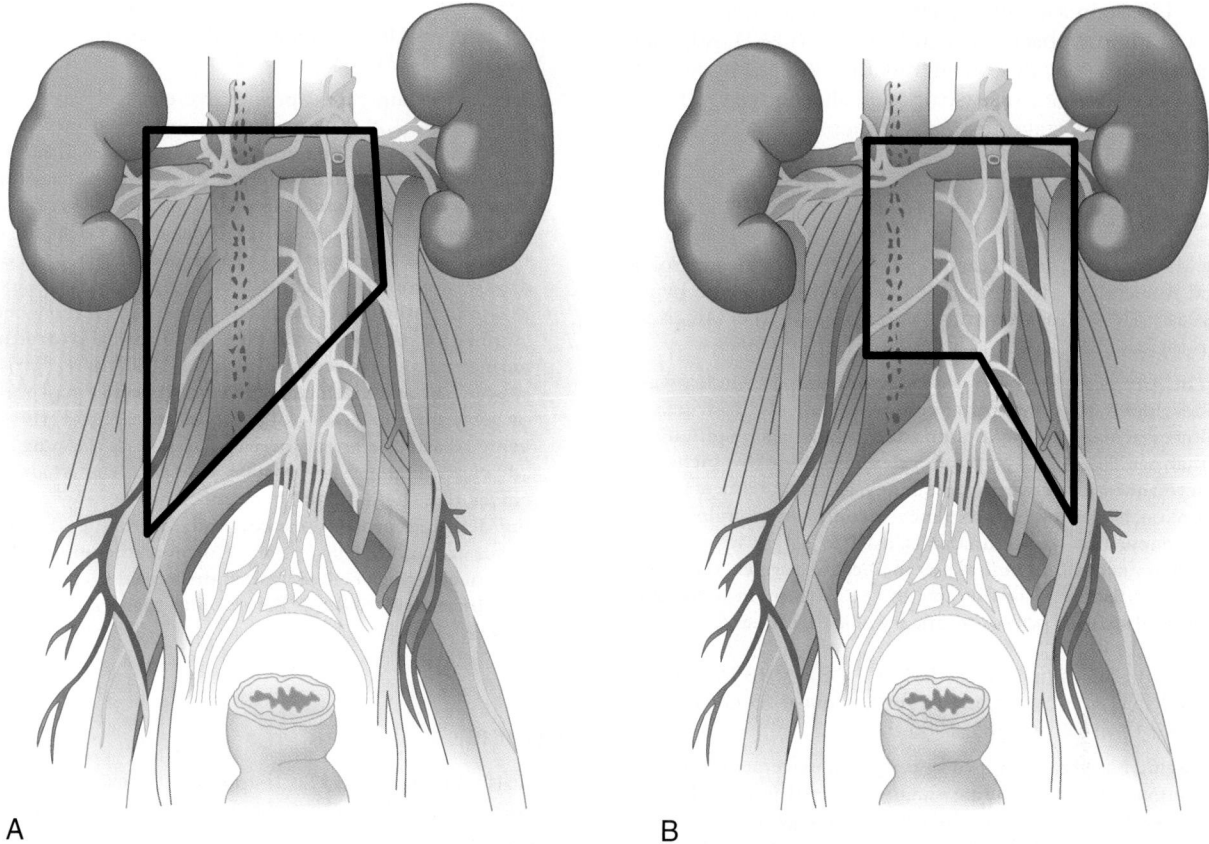

FIGURE 76-32.   Surgical template for modified, left-sided (**A**) and right-sided (**B**) retroperitoneal lymph node dissection. (Reproduced with permission from Sheinfeld J, McKierman J, Bosl GJ: Surgery of testicular tumors. In Walsh PC, Retik AB, Vaughan ED Jr, et al [eds]: Campbell's Urology, 8th ed. Philadelphia, Elsevier, 2002, pp 2926-2927.)

A   B

with nonseminomatous germ cell tumors, but it may be the only marker that is elevated in seminomas. In addition, a significantly elevated serum LDH has independent prognostic value in men with advanced seminoma.

A radical *inguinal* orchiectomy with high ligation of the spermatic cord near the internal inguinal ring should be performed to permit histologic evaluation of the primary tumor and to provide local tumor control. Scrotal violation through a scrotal incision or an attempt to "biopsy" the testis should be avoided because of concern for changing the lymphatic channels available to the testis tumor and potential for a poorer outcome.[92]

The serum half-lifes of HCG and AFP are 18 to 36 hours and 5 to 7 days, respectively. If testicular cancer produces any of these serum markers, following their progressive change after radical orchiectomy is an important consideration in determining the adequacy of therapy. As an example, rapid normalization after orchiectomy for stage 1 disease suggests elimination of the tumor, whereas persistence of tumor markers after the period during which normalization is expected to occur may be the only evidence of persistent occult disease.[93]

After determination of the histologic subtype of the testis cancer, several parameters may identify patients at

high risk of metastasis to the retroperitoneum despite absence of lymphadenopathy on staging CT. For nonseminomatous germ cell tumors those factors include (1) vascular or lymphatic invasion, (2) primary tumor (T) stage T2 to T3 (Table 76-6), and (3) embryonal carcinoma component greater than 40% of total tumor volume. Patients with these risk factors who have no bulky retroperitoneal lymphadenopathy and have normal tumor markers after radical orchiectomy may be candidates for retroperitoneal lymph node dissection (RPLND).

The principles underlying the modern surgical treatment of testicular germ cell tumors are based on the stepwise predictable metastatic pattern of these tumors,[94] with the notable exception of choriocarcinoma. RPLND is the only reliable method to identify nodal micrometastases and is the gold standard for providing accurate pathologic staging of the retroperitoneum. Both the number and size of involved retroperitoneal lymph nodes have prognostic importance (see Table 76-6).[95] As surgical therapy for metastatic testicular cancer has evolved, the full bilateral RPLND used in the past evolved first to a *template-type* (Fig. 76-32) dissection and then to a *nerve-sparing* modification with a unilateral template.[96,97] The evolution of the modified nerve-sparing RPLND has resulted in decreased morbidity with ejaculatory dysfunctions commonly observed with bilateral RPLND. Adjuvant chemotherapy may be considered after RPLND in patients with resected stage 2 disease or as an alternative to RPLND in men with low-stage testicular cancer.

Selected References

Barry MJ, Fowler FJ Jr, O'Leary MP, et al: The American Urological Association symptom index for benign prostatic hyperplasia. The Measurement Committee of the American Urological Association. J Urol 148:1549-1557, 1992.

> The American Urological Association symptom index was developed to standardize and assess men's obstructive lower urinary tract symptoms due to BPH in a quantitative manner. The AUA symptom index questionnaire includes seven questions covering frequency, nocturia, weak urinary stream, hesitancy, intermittency, incomplete emptying, and urgency. The questionnaire is used to assess a patient's urinary symptoms before any medical or surgical therapy. After initiation of the therapy, the AUA symptom score can be used again to assess the efficacy of the treatment.

Bretan PN Jr, McAninch JW, Federle MP, Jeffrey RB Jr: Computerized tomographic staging of renal trauma: 85 consecutive cases. J Urol 136:561-565, 1986.

> Staging has greatly helped in proper management of renal trauma patients. Accurate staging of renal injuries by CT has significantly helped in proper management of renal trauma patients. This article is one of the first articles that described staging of renal injuries using CT.

Carter HB, Pearson JD, Metter EJ, et al: Longitudinal evaluation of prostate-specific antigen levels in men with and without prostate disease. JAMA 267:2215-2220, 1992.

> This was a case-control prospective longitudinal study that assessed the rate of prostate-specific antigen change in men with and without prostate diseases. This study was one of the first studies to demonstrate that the rate of prostate-specific antigen change can be an early determinant of differentiating between benign prostatic hyperplasia and prostate cancer.

Coll DM, Varanelli MJ, Smith RC: Relationship of spontaneous passage of ureteral calculi to stone size and location as revealed by unenhanced helical CT. AJR Am J Roentgenol 178:101-103, 2002.

> Noncontrast CT has become an important imaging modality in diagnosis and management of acute renal colic. This study nicely demonstrates the likelihood of spontaneous passage of renal/ureteral stones in relation to the size and location of the stone.

Einhorn LH, Donohue JP: Improved chemotherapy in disseminated testicular cancer. J Urol 117:65-69, 1977.

> Testicular cancer has become one of the most curable cancers in the United States because of advances in medical and surgical therapy since the 1970s. Addition of cisplatin to chemotherapy regimens significantly improved the long-term survival and curability of metastatic testicular cancer. This reference is a classic landmark article demonstrating the efficacy of platinum-based chemotherapy for testicular cancer patients.

Thompson IM, Goodman PJ, Tangen CM, et al: The influence of finasteride on the development of prostate cancer. N Engl J Med 349:215-224, 2003.

> This large randomized prospective clinical trial included 18,000 men, and the investigators examined the effect of finasteride in development of prostate cancer. It has been long appreciated that prostate cancer is an androgen-dependent cancer, and removal of androgens reduces the progression of prostate cancer. Finasteride blocks the conversion of testosterone to the more potent androgen dihydrotestosterone by blocking the enzyme 5α-reductase type 2. The hypothesis of this study was to determine whether elimination of the more potent androgen dihydrotestosterone would reduce the risk of developing prostate cancer. The study determined that finasteride may prevent or delay the appearance of prostate cancer; however, men using finasteride are at increased risk of developing more advanced high-grade prostate cancers. The study concludes that the potential benefits of finasteride are reducing/delaying prostate cancer and improving the men's lower urinary tract symptoms. However, the potential benefits need to be weighed against the sexual side effects and the increased risk of developing high-grade prostate cancer.

References

1. Walsh PC, Lepor H, Eggleston JC: Radical prostatectomy with preservation of sexual function: Anatomical and pathological considerations. Prostate 4:473-485, 1983.
2. American College of Surgeons Committee on Trauma: Advanced Trauma Life Support for Doctors. Chicago, American College of Surgeons, 1997.
3. Nicolaisen GS, McAninch JW, Marshall GA, et al: Renal trauma: Re-evaluation of the indications for radiographic assessment. J Urol 133:183-187, 1985.
4. Mee SL, McAninch JW, Robinson AL, et al: Radiographic assessment of renal trauma: A 10-year prospective study of patient selection. J Urol 141:1095-1098, 1989.
5. Miller KS, McAninch JW: Radiographic assessment of renal trauma: Our 15-year experience. J Urol 154:352-355, 1995.
6. Bretan PN Jr, McAninch JW, Federle MP, Jeffrey RB Jr: Computerized tomographic staging of renal trauma: 85 consecutive cases. J Urol 136:561-565, 1986.
7. Morey AF, McAninch JW, Tiller BK, et al: Single shot intraoperative excretory urography for the immediate evaluation of renal trauma. J Urol 161:1088-1092, 1999.
8. McAninch JW, Carroll PR, Klosterman PW, et al: Renal reconstruction after injury. J Urol 145:932-937, 1991.
9. Husmann DA, Gilling PJ, Perry MO, et al: Major renal lacerations with a devitalized fragment following blunt abdominal trauma: A comparison between nonoperative (expectant) versus surgical management. J Urol 150:1774-1777, 1993.
10. McAninch JW, Carroll PR: Renal trauma: Kidney preservation through improved vascular control—a refined approach. J Trauma 22:285-290, 1982.
11. Mathews R, Marshall FF: Versatility of the adult psoas hitch ureteral reimplantation. J Urol 158:2078-2082, 1997.
12. Hayes EE, Sandler CM, Corriere JN Jr: Management of the ruptured bladder secondary to blunt abdominal trauma. J Urol 129:946-948, 1983.
13. Corriere JN Jr, Sandler CM: Mechanisms of injury, patterns of extravasation and management of extraperitoneal bladder rupture due to blunt trauma. J Urol 139:43-44, 1988.

14. Kotkin L, Koch MO: Morbidity associated with nonoperative management of extraperitoneal bladder injuries. J Trauma 38:895-898, 1995.

15. Peters PC: Intraperitoneal rupture of the bladder. Urol Clin North Am 16:279-282, 1989.

16. Carroll PA: Urothelial tumors. *In* Tanagho EA, McAninch JW (eds): Smith's General Urology, vol 14. Norwalk, CT, Appleton & Lange, 1995, pp 353-371.

17. Colapinto V, McCallum RW: Injury to the male posterior urethra in fractured pelvis: A new classification. J Urol 118:575-580, 1977.

18. Mitchell JP: Injuries to the urethra. Br J Urol 40:649-670, 1968.

19. Lowe MA, Mason JT, Luna GK, et al: Risk factors for urethral injuries in men with traumatic pelvic fractures. J Urol 140:506-507, 1988.

20. Koraitim MM, Marzouk ME, Atta MA, Orabi SS: Risk factors and mechanism of urethral injury in pelvic fractures. Br J Urol 77:876-880, 1996.

21. Guille F, Cippola B, el Khader K, Lobel B: Early endoscopic realignment for complete traumatic rupture of the posterior urethra—21 patients. Acta Urol Belg 66:55-58, 1998.

22. Asci R, Sarikaya S, Buyukalpelli R, et al: Voiding and sexual dysfunctions after pelvic fracture urethral injuries treated with either initial cystostomy and delayed urethroplasty or immediate primary urethral realignment. Scand J Urol Nephrol 33:228-233, 1999.

23. Iverson AJ, Morey AF: Radiographic evaluation of suspected bladder rupture following blunt trauma: Critical review. World J Surg 25:1588-1591, 2001.

24. Aboseif S, Gomez R, McAninch JW: Genital self-mutilation. J Urol 150:1143-1146, 1993.

25. Romilly CS, Isaac MT: Male genital self-mutilation. Br J Hosp Med 55:427-431, 1996.

26. Zargooshi J: Penile fracture in Kermanshah, Iran: Report of 172 cases. J Urol 164:364-366, 2000.

27. Fergany AF, Angermeier KW, Montague DK: Review of Cleveland Clinic experience with penile fracture. Urology 54:352-355, 1999.

28. Kalash SS, Young JD Jr: Fracture of penis: Controversy of surgical versus conservative treatment. Urology 24:21-24, 1984.

29. Mellinger BC, Douenias R: New surgical approach for operative management of penile fracture and penetrating trauma. Urology 39:429-432, 1992.

30. Schuster G: Traumatic rupture of the testicle and a review of the literature. J Urol 127:1194-1196, 1982.

31. Vaccaro JA, Davis R, Belville WD, Kiesling VJ: Traumatic hematocele: Association with rupture of the testicle. J Urol 136:1217-1218, 1986.

32. MacDermott JP, Gray BK, Stewart PA: Traumatic rupture of the testis. Br J Urol 62:179-181, 1988.

33. Altarac S: Management of 53 cases of testicular trauma. Eur Urol 25:119-123, 1994.

34. McAninch JW, Kahn RI, Jeffrey RB, et al: Major traumatic and septic genital injuries. J Trauma 24:291-298, 1984.

35. Morpurgo E, Galandiuk S: Fournier's gangrene. Surg Clin North Am 82:1213-1224, 2002.

36. Johnson CM, Wilson DM, O'Fallon WM, et al: Renal stone epidemiology: A 25-year study in Rochester, Minnesota. Kidney Int 16:624-631, 1979.

37. Coe FL, Parks JH, Asplin JR: The pathogenesis and treatment of kidney stones. N Engl J Med 327:1141-1152, 1992.

38. Coll DM, Varanelli MJ, Smith RC: Relationship of spontaneous passage of ureteral calculi to stone size and location as revealed by unenhanced helical CT. AJR Am J Roentgenol 178:101-103, 2002.

39. Berry SJ, Coffey DS, Walsh PC, Ewing LL: The development of human benign prostatic hyperplasia with age. J Urol 132:474-479, 1984.

40. Guess HA, Arrighi HM, Metter EJ, Fozard JL: Cumulative prevalence of prostatism matches the autopsy prevalence of benign prostatic hyperplasia. Prostate 17:241-246, 1990.

41. Girman CJ, Jacobsen SJ, Guess HA, et al: Natural history of prostatism: Relationship among symptoms, prostate volume and peak urinary flow rate. J Urol 153:1510-1515, 1995.

42. Sidney S, Quesenberry CP Jr, Sadler MC, et al: Incidence of surgically treated benign prostatic hypertrophy and of prostate cancer among blacks and whites in a prepaid health care plan. Am J Epidemiol 134:825-829, 1991.

43. Platz EA, Kawachi I, Rimm EB, et al: Race, ethnicity and benign prostatic hyperplasia in the health professionals follow-up study. J Urol 163:490-495, 2000.

44. Imperato-McGinley J, Gautier T, Zirinsky K, et al: Prostate visualization studies in males homozygous and heterozygous for 5 alpha-reductase deficiency. J Clin Endocrinol Metab 75:1022-1026, 1992.

45. Rohr HP, Bartsch G: Human benign prostatic hyperplasia: A stromal disease? New perspectives by quantitative morphology. Urology 16:625-633, 1980.

46. Shapiro E, Becich MJ, Hartanto V, Lepor H: The relative proportion of stromal and epithelial hyperplasia is related to the development of symptomatic benign prostate hyperplasia. J Urol 147:1293-1297, 1992.

47. Cunha GR, Donjacour AA, Cooke PS, et al: The endocrinology and developmental biology of the prostate. Endocr Rev 8:338-363, 1987.

48. Barry MJ, Cockett AT, Holtgrewe HL, et al: Relationship of symptoms of prostatism to commonly used physiological and anatomical measures of the severity of benign prostatic hyperplasia. J Urol 150:351-358, 1993.

49. Barry MJ, Fowler FJ Jr, O'Leary MP, et al: The American Urological Association symptom index for benign prostatic hyperplasia. The Measurement Committee of the American Urological Association. J Urol 148:1549-1557; discussion 1564, 1992.

50. Andersson KE: Alpha 1 adrenergic receptor blockade in the male lower urinary tract and other body systems. Scand J Urol Nephrol Suppl 168:13-19, 1995.

51. Lepor H: Alpha blockade for the treatment of benign prostatic hyperplasia. Urol Clin North Am 22:375-386, 1995.

52. Price DT, Schwinn DA, Lomasney JW, et al: Identification, quantification, and localization of mRNA for three distinct alpha 1 adrenergic receptor subtypes in human prostate. J Urol 150:546-551, 1993.

53. Shapiro E, Hartanto V, Lepor H: The response to alpha blockade in benign prostatic hyperplasia is related to the percent area density of prostate smooth muscle. Prostate 21:297-307, 1992.

54. Gormley GJ, Stoner E, Bruskewitz RC, et al: The effect of finasteride in men with benign prostatic hyperplasia. The Finasteride Study Group. N Engl J Med 327:1185-1191, 1992.

55. Bautista OM, Kusek JW, Nyberg LM, et al: Study design of the Medical Therapy of Prostatic Symptoms (MTOPS) trial. Control Clin Trials 24:224-243, 2003.

56. Wasson JH, Reda DJ, Bruskewitz RC, et al: A comparison of transurethral surgery with watchful waiting for moderate symptoms of benign prostatic hyperplasia. The Veterans Affairs Cooperative Study Group on Transurethral Resection of the Prostate. N Engl J Med 332:75-79, 1995.

57. Cimentepe E, Unsal A, Saglam R: Randomized clinical trial comparing transurethral needle ablation with transurethral resection of the prostate for the treatment of benign prostatic hyperplasia: Results at 18 months. J Endourol 17:103-

107, 2003.

58. Osman Y, Wadie B, El-Diasty T, Larson T: High-energy transurethral microwave thermotherapy: Symptomatic vs urodynamic success. BJU Int 91:365-370, 2003.

59. Muschter R, Schorsch I, Danielli L, et al: Transurethral water-induced thermotherapy for the treatment of benign prostatic hyperplasia: A prospective multicenter clinical trial. J Urol 164:1565-1569, 2000.

60. Tunuguntla HS, Evans CP: Minimally invasive therapies for benign prostatic hyperplasia. World J Urol 20:197-206, 2002.

61. Gold PJ, Fefer A, Thompson JA: Paraneoplastic manifestations of renal cell carcinoma. Semin Urol Oncol 14:216-222, 1996.

62. Skinner DG, Colvin RB, Vermillion CD, et al: Diagnosis and management of renal cell carcinoma: A clinical and pathologic study of 309 cases. Cancer 28:1165-1177, 1971.

63. Vogelzang NJ, Stadler WM: Kidney cancer. Lancet 352:1691-1696, 1998.

64. Tsui KH, Shvarts O, Barbaric Z, et al: Is adrenalectomy a necessary component of radical nephrectomy? UCLA experience with 511 radical nephrectomies. J Urol 163:437-441, 2000.

65. Atkins MB: Interleukin-2: Clinical applications. Semin Oncol 29:12-17, 2002.

66. Flanigan RC, Salmon SE, Blumenstein BA, et al: Nephrectomy followed by interferon alfa-2b compared with interferon alfa-2b alone for metastatic renal-cell cancer. N Engl J Med 345:1655-1659, 2001.

67. Mickisch GH, Garin A, van Poppel H, et al: Radical nephrectomy plus interferon-alfa–based immunotherapy compared with interferon alfa alone in metastatic renal-cell carcinoma: A randomised trial. Lancet 358:966-970, 2001.

68. Williams CB, Mitchell JP: Carcinoma of the renal pelvis: A review of 43 cases. Br J Urol 45:370-376, 1973.

69. Petronic VJ, Bukurov NS, Djokic MR, et al: Balkan endemic nephropathy and papillary transitional cell tumors of the renal pelvis and ureters. Kidney Int Suppl 34:S77-S79, 1991.

70. Munoz JJ, Ellison LM: Upper tract urothelial neoplasms: Incidence and survival during the last 2 decades. J Urol 164:1523-1525, 2000.

71. Jemal A, Thomas A, Murray T, Thun M: Cancer statistics, 2002. CA Cancer J Clin 52:23-47, 2002.

72. Oyasu R, Hopp ML: The etiology of cancer of the bladder. Surg Gynecol Obstet 138:97-108, 1974.

73. Jung I, Messing E: Molecular mechanisms and pathways in bladder cancer development and progression. Cancer Control 7:325-334, 2000.

74. Gago-Dominguez M, Castelao JE, Yuan JM, et al: Use of permanent hair dyes and bladder-cancer risk. Int J Cancer 91:575-579, 2001.

75. Blute ML, Segura JW, Patterson DE, et al: Impact of endourology on diagnosis and management of upper urinary tract urothelial cancer. J Urol 141:1298-1301, 1989.

76. Hautmann RE, Miller K, Steiner U, Wenderoth U: The ileal neobladder: 6 years of experience with more than 200 patients. J Urol 150:40-45, 1993.

77. Stein JP, Stenzl A, Esrig D, et al: Lower urinary tract reconstruction following cystectomy in women using the Kock ileal reservoir with bilateral ureteroileal urethrostomy: Initial clinical experience. J Urol 152:1404-1408, 1994.

78. Stein JP, Cote RJ, Freeman JA, et al: Indications for lower urinary tract reconstruction in women after cystectomy for bladder cancer: A pathological review of female cystectomy specimens. J Urol 154:1329-1333, 1995.

79. Carter HB, Pearson JD, Metter EJ, et al: Longitudinal evaluation of prostate-specific antigen levels in men with and without prostate disease. JAMA 267:2215-2220, 1992.

80. Oesterling JE, Jacobsen SJ, Chute CG, et al: Serum prostate-specific antigen in a community-based population of healthy men: Establishment of age-specific reference ranges [see comments]. JAMA 270:860-864, 1993.

81. Morgan TO, Jacobsen SJ, McCarthy WF, et al: Age-specific reference ranges for prostate-specific antigen in black men. N Engl J Med 335:304-310, 1996.

82. Thompson IM, Goodman PJ, Tangen CM, et al: The influence of finasteride on the development of prostate cancer. N Engl J Med 349:215-224, 2003.

83. Bosl GJ, Motzer RJ: Testicular germ-cell cancer. N Engl J Med 337:242-253, 1997.

84. Einhorn LH: Treatment of testicular cancer: A new and improved model. J Clin Oncol 8:1777-1781, 1990.

85. Einhorn LH, Donohue JP: Improved chemotherapy in disseminated testicular cancer. J Urol 117:65-69, 1977.

86. Richie JP: Clinical stage 1 testicular cancer: The role of modified retroperitoneal lymphadenectomy. J Urol 144:1160-1163, 1990.

87. Richie JP, Garnick MB, Finberg H: Computerized tomography: How accurate for abdominal staging of testis tumors? J Urol 127:715-717, 1982.

88. Read G, Stenning SP, Cullen MH, et al: Medical Research Council prospective study of surveillance for stage I testicular teratoma. Medical Research Council Testicular Tumors Working Party. J Clin Oncol 10:1762-1768, 1992.

89. Gels ME, Hoekstra HJ, Sleijfer DT, et al: Detection of recurrence in patients with clinical stage I nonseminomatous testicular germ cell tumors and consequences for further follow-up: A single-center 10-year experience. J Clin Oncol 13:1188-1194, 1995.

90. Weissbach L, Bussar-Maatz R, Mann K: The value of tumor markers in testicular seminomas: Results of a prospective multicenter study. Eur Urol 32:16-22, 1997.

91. Fossa A, Fossa SD: Serum lactate dehydrogenase and human choriogonadotropin in seminoma. Br J Urol 63:408-415, 1989.

92. Leibovitch I, Baniel J, Foster RS, Donohue JP: The clinical implications of procedural deviations during orchiectomy for nonseminomatous testis cancer. J Urol 154:935-939, 1995.

93. Saxman SB, Nichols CR, Foster RS, et al: The management of patients with clinical stage I nonseminomatous testicular tumors and persistently elevated serologic markers. J Urol 155:587-589, 1996.

94. Donohue JP, Zachary JM, Maynard BR: Distribution of nodal metastases in nonseminomatous testis cancer. J Urol 128:315-320, 1982.

95. Richie JP, Kantoff PW: Is adjuvant chemotherapy necessary for patients with stage B1 testicular cancer? J Clin Oncol 9:1393-1396, 1991.

96. Pizzocaro G: Retroperitoneal lymphadenectomy in clinical stage I nonseminomatous germinal testis cancer. Eur J Surg Oncol 12:25-28, 1986.

97. Donohue JP, Foster RS, Rowland RG, et al: Nerve-sparing retroperitoneal lymphadenectomy with preservation of ejaculation. J Urol 144:287-291; discussion 291-292, 1990.

Index

Note: Page numbers followed by an f indicate illustrations; page numbers followed by a t refer to tables; page numbers followed by a b signal boxes.